Normal tomographic ^{201}Tl study obtained using a rotating gamma scintillation camera. Plates A-1, B-1, and C-1 show selected tomographic slices at stress and redistribution in the short axis, horizontal long axis, and vertical long axis. Note the uniform homogeneous uptake of ^{201}Tl in the myocardium. Functional quantitative images ("bull's-eye displays") are shown in Plates A-2, B-2, and C-2. Each short-axis tomographic slice from apex to base is subjected to maximal count circumferential profile analysis. These profiles then are displayed as a series of concentric circles with the apex at the center and with the base at the periphery. These are positioned in the same way as are the short-axis tomographic slices shown in Plate A-1. The bull's-eye displays in Plates A-2 and B-2 were obtained from stress and delayed images. Plate C-2 shows the bull's-eye for ^{201}Tl washout. Note that there is uniform uptake of ^{201}Tl at stress and redistribution and that the washout bull's-eye also is uniform with no abnormal zones depicted. (See Chapter 109, "Techniques of Nuclear Cardiology," by Zaret and Berger.)

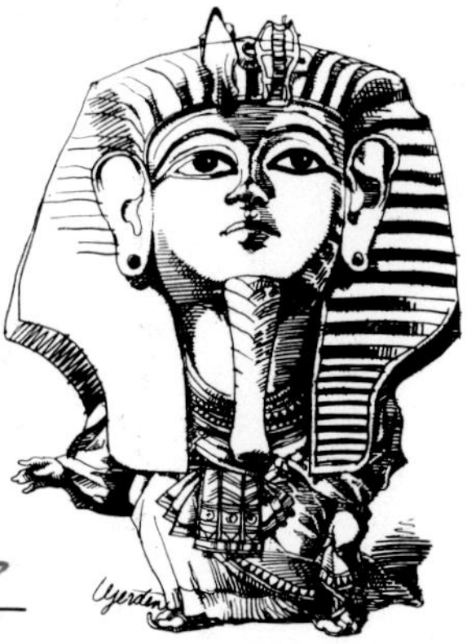

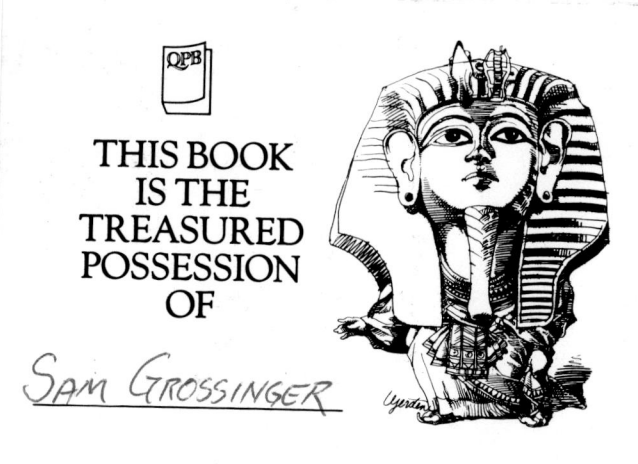

THE HEART

Arteries and Veins

THE HEART

Sixth Edition

Arteries and Veins

Editor-in-Chief
J. Willis Hurst, M.D.
Candler Professor of Medicine (Cardiology)
Chairman, Department of Medicine
Emory University School of Medicine
Chief, Medical Service and Cardiology
Emory University Hospital
Chief, Medical Service
Grady Memorial Hospital
Head, Medical Section and Cardiology
Emory University Clinic
Atlanta, Georgia

Editors
R. Bruce Logue, M.D.
Professor Emeritus of Medicine (Cardiology)
Emory University School of Medicine
Director, Carlyle Fraser Heart Center
Crawford W. Long Memorial Hospital
Atlanta, Georgia

Charles E. Rackley, M.D.
Anton and Margaret Fuisz Professor of Medicine
Chairman, Department of Medicine
Georgetown University Medical Center
Washington, D.C.

Robert C. Schlant, M.D.
Professor of Medicine (Cardiology)
Director, Division of Cardiology
Emory University School of Medicine
Chief of Cardiology, Grady Memorial Hospital
Atlanta, Georgia

Edmund H. Sonnenblick, M.D.
Olson Professor of Medicine
Chief, Division of Cardiology
Department of Medicine
Albert Einstein College of Medicine
Bronx, New York

Andrew G. Wallace, M.D.
Kempner Professor of Medicine and
Vice Chancellor for Health Affairs
Duke University Medical Center
Durham, North Carolina

Nanette Kass Wenger, M.D.
Professor of Medicine (Cardiology)
Department of Medicine
Emory University School of Medicine
Director, Cardiac Clinics, Grady Memorial Hospital
Atlanta, Georgia

MCGRAW-HILL BOOK COMPANY
New York St. Louis San Francisco Auckland
Bogotá Guatemala Hamburg Johannesburg
Lisbon London Madrid Mexico Montreal
New Delhi Panama Paris San Juan São Paulo
Singapore Sydney Tokyo Toronto

NOTICE
Medicine is an ever-changing science. As new research and clinical experience broaden our knowledge, changes in treatment and drug therapy are required. The editors and the publisher of this work have made every effort to ensure that the drug dosage schedules herein are accurate and in accord with the standards accepted at the time of publication. Readers are advised, however, to check the product information sheet included in the package of each drug they plan to administer to be certain that changes have not been made in the recommended dose or in the contraindications for administration. This recommendation is of particular importance in regard to new or infrequently used drugs.

THE HEART
Arteries and Veins

3 4 5 6 7 8 9 0 DOCDOC 8 9 8 7

ISBN 0-07-031485-3
ISBN 0-07-031486-1
ISBN 0-07-031487-X
ISBN 0-07-079440-5

This book was set in Baskerville by Waldman Graphics, Inc. The editors were Beth Kaufman Barry, Donna McIvor, and T. Fiore Lavery; the production supervisor was Avé McCracken; the cover was designed by Edward R. Schultheis; the index was prepared by Philip James.

R. R. Donnelley & Sons Company was printer and binder.

Library of Congress Cataloging in Publication Data
Main entry under title:

The Heart, arteries and veins.

Issued also in 2v.
Includes bibliographies and index.
1. Cardiovascular system—Diseases. I. Hurst, J. Willis (John Willis), date. [DNLM:
1. Cardiovascular Diseases. WG 100 H435]
RC667.H42 1986 616.1 85-13254
ISBN 0-07-079440-5 (set)

RC667.H42 1986b 616.1 85-14876
ISBN 0-07-031485-3 (combined)
ISBN 0-07-031486-1 (vol 1)
ISBN 0-07-031487-X (vol 2)

DEDICATION

To Paul Dudley White (1886–1986) on his 100th birthday* with appreciation for leading the way.

*Dr. Paul Dudley White was born in Roxbury, Massachusetts, on June 6, 1886.

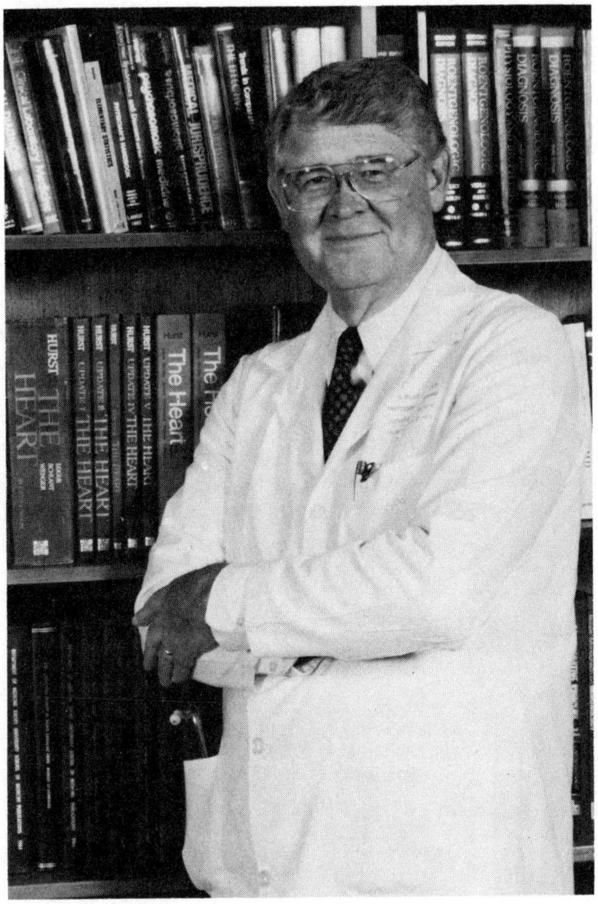

J. Willis Hurst received his M.D. degree in 1944 and served his medical residency at the Medical College of Georgia before going to Massachusetts General Hospital where he was cardiology fellow to Paul Dudley White, M.D. Between 1946 and 1947 he served in the Army at Fitzsimons General Hospital in Denver. In 1954 and 1955 he served in the Navy at the United States Naval Hospital in Bethesda, Maryland, and, in 1955, became Chief of Cardiology there. In 1957 he was appointed to his present position as Professor of Medicine and Chairman of the Department of Medicine at Emory University School of Medicine.

Dr. Hurst has served on the organizing bodies of several government and professional groups, including the National Heart, Lung and Blood Council, the Subspecialty Board of Cardiology of which he served as Chairman from 1967 to 1970, the Paul Dudley White Society, and the American Heart Association, of which he was President from 1971 to 1972. He is a member of the College of Cardiology. He served as President of the Association of Professors of Medicine in 1984–1985. For 18 years, Dr. Hurst was President Lyndon Johnson's cardiologist.

An outstanding educator, Dr. Hurst has received numerous honors in recognition of his teaching abilities. In 1974 he was given the Gifted Teacher Award by the American College of Cardiology. The same organization also conferred on him the Master Teacher Award in 1970 and 1974. The American Heart Association presented him with both the Gold Heart and Herrick Awards; the American College of Physicians designated him as a Master in the College and recently selected him for the Distinguished Teacher Award.

A skilled and disciplined writer and editor, he has piloted the internationally appreciated text, *The Heart,* through six editions. His daily work, which begins at 4 A.M., consists of writing, running a large department of medicine at a dynamic medical school, teaching, clinical research, and consultative cardiology practice at Emory University Hospital.

Contents

List of Contributors xix

Preface xxvii

Prologue: The Growth of Knowledge xxix
Howard B. Burchell, M.D., Ph.D.

PART I The Normal Heart and Blood Vessels 1

1 Embryology of the Heart 3
L. H. S. Van Mierop, M.D., and Lynn M. Kutsche, M.D.

2 Anatomy of the Heart 16
Robert C. Schlant, M.D., and Mark E. Silverman, M.D.

3 Normal Physiology of the Cardiovascular System 37
Robert C. Schlant, M.D., and Edmund H. Sonnenblick, M.D.

4 Electrical Activity of the Heart 73
Andrew G. Wallace, M.D.

5 Metabolic Regulation and Myocardial Function 85
Howard E. Morgan, M.D., and James R. Neely, Ph.D.

PART II Methods Used to Collect Data on Every Patient (The "Routine" Examination) 101

6 The Approach to the Patient: Goals and Cardiac Appraisal 103
J. Willis Hurst, M.D.

7 The History: Past Events and Symptoms Related to Cardiovascular Disease 109
J. Willis Hurst, M.D., Douglas C. Morris, M.D., I. Sylvia Crawley, M.D., and Edward R. Dorney, M.D.

8 Inspection of the Patient 122
Mark E. Silverman, M.D., and J. Willis Hurst, M.D.

9 Physical Examination of the Arteries and Veins (Including Blood Pressure Determination) 138
Robert A. O'Rourke, M.D.

10 Inspection and Palpation of the Precordium 152
Ernest Craige, M.D.

11 Auscultation of the Heart 157
Aubrey Leatham, F.R.C.P., Graham J. Leech, M.A., W. Proctor Harvey, M.D., and Antonio C. de Leon, Jr., M.D.

12 Examination of the Retina 198
W. Banks Anderson, Jr., M.D.

13 Physical Examination of the Chest, Abdomen, and Extremities 204
J. Willis Hurst, M.D., and Paul H. Robinson, M.D.

14 The Resting Electrocardiogram 206
Agustin Castellanos, M.D., and Robert J. Myerburg, M.D.

15 The Chest Roentgenogram 230
James T. T. Chen, M.D.

PART III Methods and Strategy Used to Collect Data on Selected Patients (The Assessment of Specific Problems) 245

16 Assessment of Structural Abnormalities and Blood Flow 247
Joseph K. Perloff, M.D.

17 Assessment of Cardiac Function and Myocardial Contractility 265
John Ross, Jr., M.D.

18 Assessment of Electrical Abnormalities 281
Douglas P. Zipes, M.D., and R. Joe Noble, M.D.

19 Assessment of Myocardial Ischemia 299
Richard M. Steingart, M.D., and James Scheuer, M.D.

PART IV Disorders of the Cardiovascular System 317

20 Pathophysiology of Heart Failure 319
Robert C. Schlant, M.D., and Edmund H. Sonnenblick, M.D.

21 The Recognition and Management of Heart Failure 345
James F. Spann, Jr., M.D., and J. Willis Hurst, M.D.

22 Pathophysiology of Hypotension and Shock 370
Francois M. Abboud, M.D.

23 The Recognition and Management of Shock 383
David W. Ferguson, M.D., and Francois M. Abboud, M.D.

24 High-Cardiac-Output States 395
Noble O. Fowler, M.D.

25 Mechanisms of Arrhythmias and Conduction Abnormalities 406
Warren M. Smith, M.B., and John J. Gallagher, M.D.

26 Recognition of Arrhythmias and Conduction Abnormalities 431
Henry J. L. Marriott, M.D., and Robert J. Myerburg, M.D.

27 Management of Arrhythmias and Conduction Abnormalities 475
Warren M. Smith, M.B., and Andrew G. Wallace, M.D.

28 Artificial Cardiac Pacemakers 486
Harry G. Mond, M.D., and J. Graeme Sloman, E.D.

29 Syncope: Pathophysiology and Differential Diagnosis 507
Arnold M. Weissler, M.D., and James V. Warren, M.D.

30 Cardiac Syncope: Diagnosis, Mechanism, and Management 521
Harisios Boudoulas, M.D., and Richard P. Lewis, M.D.

31 Pathology and Mechanisms of Sudden Death 529
Giorgio Baroldi, M.D.

32 Predictors and Prevention of Sudden Cardiac Death 538
Leonard A. Cobb, M.D., and Jeffrey A. Werner, M.D.

33 Cardiopulmonary Resuscitation and the Subsequent Management of the Patient 546
Myron L. Weisfeldt, M.D., and Nisha Chibber Chandra, M.D.

PART V Diseases of the Heart and Blood Vessels 555

34 Incidence, Prevalence, and Mortality of Cardiovascular Diseases 557
William B. Kannel, M.D., and Thomas J. Thom, B.A.

35 Genetics and the Cardiovascular System 566
W. Jape Taylor, M.D.

Section A Congenital Heart Disease 580

36 The Pathology, Abnormal Physiology, Clinical Recognition, and Medical and Surgical Treatment of Congenital Heart Disease 580
Elizabeth W. Nugent, M.D., William H. Plauth, Jr., M.D., Jesse E. Edwards, M.D., Robert C. Schlant, M.D., and Willis H. Williams, M.D.

Section B Valvular Heart Disease 729

37 Aortic Valve Disease 729
Charles E. Rackley, M.D., Jesse E. Edwards, M.D., Robert B. Wallace, M.D., and Nevin M. Katz, M.D.

38 Mitral Valve Disease 754
Charles E. Rackley, M.D., Jesse E. Edwards, M.D., and Robert B. Karp, M.D.

39 Combined Aortic and Mitral Valve Disease 785
Charles E. Rackley, M.D., Jesse E. Edwards, M.D., and Robert B. Karp, M.D.

40 Tricuspid and Pulmonary Valve Disease 792
Charles E. Rackley, M.D., Jesse E. Edwards, M.D., Robert B. Wallace, M.D., and Nevin M. Katz, M.D.

Section C Coronary Heart Disease 801

41 Factors Influencing Atherogenesis 801
Russell Ross, Ph.D.

42 Prevention of Coronary Atherosclerosis 817
Nanette Kass Wenger, M.D., and Robert C. Schlant, M.D.

43 Pathology of Coronary Atherosclerotic Heart Disease 839
Bernadine Healy Bulkley, M.D.

44 Pathophysiology of Myocardial Ischemia 856
Stephen M. Factor, M.D., and Edward S. Kirk, Ph.D.

45 Atherosclerotic Coronary Heart Disease: Recognition, Prognosis, and Treatment 882
J. Willis Hurst, M.D., Spencer B. King III, M.D., Gottlieb C. Friesinger, M.D., Paul F. Walter, M.D., and Douglas C. Morris, M.D.

46 Coronary Artery Spasm 1009
D. Gregg Hopkins, M.D., and Donald C. Harrison, M.D.

47 Nonatherosclerotic Coronary Heart Disease 1016
Donald S. Baim, M.D., and Donald C. Harrison, M.D.

48 Rehabilitation of the Patient with Atherosclerotic Coronary Heart Disease 1025
Nanette Kass Wenger, M.D., and Gerald F. Fletcher, M.D.

Section D Systemic Arterial Hypertension 1038

49 Pathophysiology of Hypertension 1038
Harriet P. Dustan, M.D.

50 Diagnostic Evaluation of the Patient with Hypertension 1048
W. Dallas Hall, M.D., Gary L. Wollam, M.D., and Elbert P. Tuttle, Jr., M.D.

51 Treatment of Systemic Hypertension 1071
Gary L. Wollam, M.D., and W. Dallas Hall, M.D.

Section E Pulmonary Hypertension and Pulmonary Heart Disease 1091

52 Pulmonary Hypertension: Mechanism and Recognition 1091
Hiroshi Kuida, M.D.

53 Primary Pulmonary Hypertension 1099
Hiroshi Kuida, M.D.

54 Pulmonary Embolism 1105
James E. Dalen, M.D., and Joseph S. Alpert, M.D.

55 Chronic Cor Pulmonale 1120
Joseph C. Ross, M.D., and John H. Newman, M.D.

Section F Endocarditis 1130

56 Infective and Noninfective Endocarditis 1130
David T. Durack, M.B., D.Phil.

Section G Myocardial Disease 1158

57 Myocarditis 1158
Nanette Kass Wenger, M.D., Walter H. Abelmann, M.D., and William C. Roberts, M.D.

58 Cardiomyopathy and Myocardial Involvement in Systemic Disease 1181
Nanette Kass Wenger, M.D., John F. Goodwin, M.D., and William C. Roberts, M.D.

Section H The Pericardium and Its Diseases 1249

59 Diseases of the Pericardium 1249
Ralph Shabetai, M.D.

Section I Traumatic Heart Disease 1276

60 Traumatic Heart Disease 1276
Panagiotis N. Symbas, M.D., and Daniel Arensberg, M.D.

Section J Neoplastic Disease of the Heart 1284

61 Neoplastic Heart Disease 1284
Robert J. Hall, M.D., and Denton A. Cooley, M.D.

Section K Rheumatic Fever 1306

62 Acute Rheumatic Fever and Its Management 1306
Gene H. Stollerman, M.D.

Section L Syphilis and the Cardiovascular System 1314

63 Syphilis and the Cardiovascular System 1314
J. O'Neal Humphries, M.D., and Bernadine Healy Bulkley, M.D.

Section M Diseases of the Blood Vessels 1321

64 Diseases of the Aorta 1321
Joseph Lindsay, Jr., M.D., Michael E. DeBakey, M.D., and Arthur C. Beall, Jr., M.D.

65 Diseases of the Peripheral Arteries 1339
Jess R. Young, M.D.

66 Cerebrovascular Disease and Neurological Manifestations of Heart Disease 1354
Gary R. Kilgo, M.D., James F. Toole, M.D., and Terence B. McGhee, M.D.

67 Vascular Disease of the Digestive System 1364
W. Scott Brooks, Jr., M.D.

68 Diseases of the Peripheral Veins and the Venae Cavae 1372
Garland D. Perdue, Jr., M.D., and Robert B. Smith III, M.D.

PART VI The Heart and Other Medical Problems 1381

Section A The Heart and Certain Physiological Conditions 1383

69 Heart Disease and Pregnancy 1383
John H. McAnulty, M.D., James Metcalfe, M.D., and Kent Ueland, M.D.

70 The Heart in Athletes 1398
Andrew G. Wallace, M.D.

71 Cardiovascular Aging and Adaptation to Disease 1403
Myron L. Weisfeldt, M.D., and Gary Gerstenblith, M.D.

Section B Cardiac Involvement in Systemic Disease 1412

72 The Heart and Endocrine Diseases 1412
John R. K. Preedy, M.D., Stephen D. Clements, Jr., M.D., and Harry K. Delcher, M.D.

73 The Heart and Collagen Vascular Disease 1435
Bernadine Healy Bulkley, M.D., and J. O'Neal Humphries, M.D.

74 The Heart, Alcoholism, and Nutritional Disease 1446
Timothy J. Regan, M.D.

75 The Heart and Obesity 1452
James K. Alexander, M.D.

76 The Heart and Chronic Renal Failure 1458
Susan K. Fellner, M.D.

77 Electrolytes and the Heart 1466
Charles Fisch, M.D.

78 Effect of Noncardiac Drugs, Radiation, Electricity, and Poisons on the Heart 1479
I. Sylvia Crawley, M.D.

Section C The Heart and Anesthesia 1494

79 Anesthesia and the Patient with Cardiovascular Disease 1494
Carl C. Hug, Jr., M.D., Ph.D.

80 Evaluation and Management of Patients with Heart Disease Who Undergo Noncardiac Surgery 1511
R. Bruce Logue, M.D.

Section D Emotional Stress, Psychiatric Conditions, and the Heart 1520

81 The Heart and Emotional Stress 1520
James C. Buell, M.D., and Robert S. Eliot, M.D.

82 Psychiatric Disorders in Cardiac Patients 1530
Arthur M. Freeman III, M.D., and David G. Folks, M.D.

83 Iatrogenic "Heart Disease" 1536
Peter C. Gazes, M.D., and J. Willis Hurst, M.D.

Section E The Heart and Environmental Factors 1543

84 The Influence of Environmental Factors on the Cardiovascular System 1543
Robert F. Grover, M.D., Ph.D., John T. Reeves, M.D., Loring B. Rowell, Ph.D., Claude A. Piantadosi, M.D., and Herbert A. Saltzman, M.D.

Section F Insurance, Legal, and Occupational Problems 1556

85 Insurance Problems of Patients with Heart Disease 1556
Joseph A. Wilber, M.D.

86 Cardiac Examinations for Legal Purposes 1563
Elliot L. Sagall, M.D.

87 Occupation and Cardiovascular Disease 1577
Nanette Kass Wenger, M.D.

PART VII The Pharmacology of Cardiac Drugs and the Techniques of Special Procedures 1581

Section A The Pharmacology of Cardiac Drugs 1583

88 Drugs Used to Control Vascular Resistance and Capacitance 1583
Jay N. Cohn, M.D.

89 Drugs Used to Treat Cardiac Arrhythmias 1593
Warren M. Smith, M.B., and Andrew G. Wallace, M.D.

90 Beta-Adrenergic Blocking Drugs 1606
William H. Frishman, M.D., and Edmund H. Sonnenblick, M.D.

91 Calcium Channel Blockers 1624
William H. Frishman, M.D., and Edmund H. Sonnenblick, M.D.

92 Digitalis 1639
Frank I. Marcus, M.D., and Shoei K. Huang, M.D.

93 Nondigitalis Cardiac Inotropic Agents 1652
Thierry H. LeJemtel, M.D., and Edmund H. Sonnenblick, M.D.

94 Diuretics 1657
Vera Delaney, M.D., and Edmund Bourke, M.D.

95 Anticoagulants, Platelet-Controlling Drugs, and Thrombolytic Agents 1667
Sol Sherry, M.D., and Arthur Belber, M.D.

Sections B through H Techniques of Special Procedures 1687

Section B Techniques of Vectorcardiography, Specialized Electrocardiography, Electrophysiology, and Electrical Treatment of Arrhythmias 1687

96 Technique of Vectorcardiography 1687
A. Calhoun Witham, M.D.

97 Technique of Esophageal Electrocardiography 1690
Ross D. Fletcher, M.D., and Robert C. Saunders, M.D.

98 Techniques of Exercise Testing 1704
Robert F. DeBusk, M.D.

99 Technique of QRS Signal Averaging 1716
Paul F. Walter, M.D., and Scott J. Pollak, M.D.

100 Techniques of Long-Term Continuous Electrocardiographic Recording 1720
R. Joe Noble, M.D., and Douglas P. Zipes, M.D.

101 Techniques of His Bundle Recordings: Clinical Value and Indications 1727
Douglas L. Packer, M.D., John J. Gallagher, M.D., and Andrew G. Wallace, M.D.

102 Techniques of Programmed Stimulation, Atrial Pacing, and Electrical Assessment of Drug Therapy 1734
Harold C. Strauss, M.D., Lawrence D. German, M.D., and Andrew G. Wallace, M.D.

103 Cardioversion and Defibrillation 1741
Bernard Lown, M.D., and Regis A. de Silva, M.D.

104 Artificial Cardiac Pacemakers: Transvenous Implantation Techniques 1747
Harry G. Mond, M.D.

105 Artificial Cardiac Pacemakers: Testing Methods 1755
Harry G. Mond, M.D.

106 The Implantable Cardioverter-Defibrillator 1761
M. Mirowski, M.D.

Section C Techniques of Diagnostic Radiography, Nuclear Cardiology, Radiographic Guided Intervention, and Nuclear Magnetic Resonance 1764

107 Technique of Cardiac Fluoroscopy 1764
James T. T. Chen, M.D.

108 Techniques of Cardiac Catheterization Including Coronary Arteriography 1768
Robert H. Franch, M.D., Spencer B. King III, M.D., and John S. Douglas, Jr., M.D.

109 Techniques of Nuclear Cardiology 1809
Barry L. Zaret, M.D., and Harvey J. Berger, M.D.

110 The Use of Digital Subtraction Imaging in Cardiac Disease 1858
William J. Casarella, M.D.

111 Computed Tomography of the Heart 1864
Murray G. Baron, M.D.

112 Studies of the Carotid Artery and Its Branches 1874
Ira F. Braun, M.D., J. Timothy Fulenwider, M.D., and Robert B. Smith III, M.D.

113 Radionuclide Lung Imaging and Pulmonary Angiography 1881
Peter J. Sones, M.D., and William A. Fajman, M.D.

114 Phlebography 1885
Renate L. Soulen, M.D.

115 Magnetic Resonance Imaging of the Heart and Great Vessels 1889
William J. Casarella, M.D., and Harvey J. Berger, M.D.

116 Radiologically Guided Intervention in the Heart and Great Vessels 1897
William J. Casarella, M.D.

117 Technique of Percutaneous Transluminal Angioplasty of the Coronary, Renal, Mesenteric, and Peripheral Arteries 1901
David Petrie Hall, M.D., and Andreas R. Gruentzig, M.D.

118 Techniques of Achieving Pulmonary, Peripheral, and Coronary Thrombolysis 1916
James F. Spann, Jr., M.D., Sol Sherry, M.D., and Ronald N. Rubin, M.D.

119 The Use of the Laser in the Treatment of Coronary Artery Obstruction 1922
George S. Abela, M.D., and C. Richard Conti, M.D.

Section D Echocardiography and Doppler Techniques 1926

120 Echocardiography 1926
Joel M. Felner, M.D.

121 Doppler Methods for Analysis of Arterial and Venous Disorders 1974
D. E. Strandness, Jr., M.D.

122 The Use of Doppler in the Evaluation of Cardiac Disorders and Function 1978
Alan S. Pearlman, M.D.

Section E Phonocardiography and Pulse Wave Tracing 1990

123 Technique of Phonocardiography and Pulse Wave Tracings 1990
Ernest Craige, M.D.

Section F Techniques of Monitoring Seriously Ill Patients with Heart Disease and Computer-Based Monitoring after Cardiac Surgery 1998

124 Techniques of Monitoring the Seriously Ill Patient with Heart Disease (Including Use of Swan-Ganz Catheter) 1998
H. J. C. Swan, M.D., Ph.D.

125 Techniques of Computer-Based Monitoring after Cardiac Surgery 2004
Louis C. Sheppard, Ph.D.

Section G Cardiovascular Surgical Techniques 2008

126 Surgical Management of Pericardial Disease 2008
Joseph I. Miller, Jr., M.D.

127 Treatment of Tachycardia by Cardiac Surgery 2013
Edward L. C. Pritchett, M.D., and Andrew G. Wallace, M.D.

128 Techniques for Insertion of Epicardial Pacemakers 2016
Kamal A. Mansour, M.D.

129 Techniques of Using the Intraaortic Balloon Pump 2021
Joseph M. Craver, M.D., and Charles R. Hatcher, Jr., M.D.

130 Techniques of Cardiopulmonary Bypass 2025
Robert A. Guyton, M.D., Willis H. Williams, M.D., and Charles R. Hatcher, Jr., M.D.

131 Techniques of Valvular Surgery 2030
Robert A. Guyton, M.D., and Charles R. Hatcher, Jr., M.D.

132 Techniques for the Surgical Treatment of Atherosclerotic Coronary Artery Disease and Its Complications 2036
Ellis L. Jones, M.D., and Charles R. Hatcher, Jr., M.D.

133 Techniques of Surgical Treatment of Diseases of the Aorta 2043
Panagiotis N. Symbas, M.D., and Charles R. Hatcher, Jr., M.D.

134 Technique of Carotid Artery Surgery 2052
Robert B. Smith III, M.D.

135 Technique of Surgical Treatment of Peripheral Vascular Disease 2057
Robert B. Smith III, M.D.

136 Technique of Cardiac Transplantation 2062
John C. Baldwin, M.D., Edward B. Stinson, M.D., Philip E. Oyer, M.D., Ph.D., Stuart W. Jamieson, M.D., and Norman E. Shumway, M.D., Ph.D.

137 Technique of Using the Mechanical Heart 2069
William C. DeVries, M.D.

Section H Opening the Heart at Necropsy 2077

138 Examining the Heart at Necropsy 2077
William C. Roberts, M.D.

Epilogue: The Future of Cardiology 2081
J. Willis Hurst, M.D.

Index I-1

Contributors

Francois M. Abboud, M.D.
Professor and Chairman, Department of Internal Medicine; Professor of Physiology, Department of Physiology and Biophysics; University of Iowa College of Medicine, Iowa City, Iowa

George S. Abela, M.D.
Assistant Professor of Medicine, University of Florida College of Medicine, Gainesville, Florida

Walter H. Abelmann, M.D.
Professor of Medicine, Harvard Medical School; Physician, Beth Israel Hospital, Boston, Massachusetts

James K. Alexander, M.D.
Professor of Medicine, Baylor College of Medicine; Chief of Cardiology, Veterans Administration Hospital, Houston, Texas

Joseph S. Alpert, M.D.
Professor of Medicine; Director, Division of Cardiovascular Medicine, University of Massachusetts Medical School, Worcester, Massachusetts

W. Banks Anderson, Jr., M.D.
Professor of Ophthalmology, Duke University Eye Center, Durham, North Carolina

Daniel Arensberg, M.D.
Associate Professor of Medicine (Cardiology), Department of Medicine, Emory University School of Medicine, Atlanta, Georgia

Donald S. Baim, M.D.
Assistant Professor of Medicine, Harvard Medical School; Cardiovascular Division, Beth Israel Hospital, Boston, Massachusetts

John C. Baldwin, M.D.
Clinical Assistant Professor of Cardiovascular Surgery, Stanford University School of Medicine, Stanford, California

Giorgio Baroldi, M.D.
Professor of Pathology and Chairman Cardiovascular Pathology, Institute of Biomedical Sciences, Department of Pathological Anatomy, Medical School, University of Milan; Director, Department of Pathology, Institute of Clinical Physiology CNR, University of Pisa; Director of Milan Section, Institute of Clinical Physiology, Niguarda Hospital, Milan, Italy

Murray G. Baron, M.D.
Professor and Associate Chairman, Department of Radiology, Emory University School of Medicine, Atlanta, Georgia

Arthur C. Beall, Jr., M.D.
Professor of Surgery, Baylor College of Medicine, Houston, Texas

Arthur Belber, M.D.
Clinical Instructor of Medicine, Temple University School of Medicine, Philadelphia, Pennsylvania

George A. Beller, M.D.
Professor of Medicine, Head, Division of Cardiology, University of Virginia School of Medicine, Charlottesville, Virginia

Harvey J. Berger, M.D.
Professor of Radiology and Medicine (Cardiology), Emory University School of Medicine; Director, Division of Nuclear Medicine, Emory University Hospital, Atlanta, Georgia

Harisios Boudoulas, M.D.
Professor of Medicine and Pharmacy, The Ohio State University College of Medicine, Columbus, Ohio

Edmund Bourke, M.D.
Professor of Medicine (Nephrology and Inorganic Metabolism), Director, Division of Nephrology and Inorganic Metabolism, Emory University School of Medicine, Atlanta, Georgia

Ira F. Braun, M.D.
Assistant Professor of Radiology, Emory University School of Medicine, Atlanta, Georgia

W. Scott Brooks, Jr., M.D.
Associate Professor of Medicine (Digestive Diseases), Department of Medicine, Emory University School of Medicine, Atlanta, Georgia

James C. Buell, M.D.
Associate Director and Director of Research of the National Center of Preventive and Stress Medicine, Phoenix, Arizona; Assistant Professor of Medicine, University of Nebraska Medical School, Omaha, Nebraska

Bernadine Healy Bulkley, M.D.
Professor of Medicine and Associate Professor of Pathology, The Johns Hopkins Hospital, Baltimore, Maryland

Howard B. Burchell, M.D., Ph.D.
Emeritus Professor of Medicine, University of Minnesota Medical School, Minneapolis, Minnesota

William J. Casarella, M.D.
Professor and Chairman, Department of Radiology, Emory University School of Medicine, Atlanta, Georgia

Agustin Castellanos, M.D.
Professor of Medicine, Director, Clinical Electrophysiology, University of Miami School of Medicine, Miami, Florida

Nisha Chibber Chandra, M.D.
Assistant Professor of Medicine, The Johns Hopkins University School of Medicine, Baltimore, Maryland

James T. T. Chen, M.D.
Professor of Radiology, Director of Cardiopulmonary Radiology, Duke University Medical Center, Durham, North Carolina

Stephen D. Clements, Jr., M.D.
Professor of Medicine (Cardiology), Department of Medicine, Emory University School of Medicine, Atlanta, Georgia

Leonard A. Cobb, M.D.
Professor of Medicine, University of Washington; Director, Division of Cardiology at Harborview Medical Center, Seattle, Washington

Jay N. Cohn, M.D.
Professor of Medicine and Head, Cardiovascular Division, University of Minnesota Medical School, Minneapolis, Minnesota

C. Richard Conti, M.D.
Professor of Medicine, Director, Division of Cardiology, University of Florida College of Medicine, Gainesville, Florida

Denton A. Cooley, M.D.
Surgeon-in-Chief, Texas Heart Institute, Houston, Texas; Clinical Professor of Surgery, University of Texas Medical School, Houston, Texas

Ernest Craige, M.D
Professor of Medicine, Henry A. Foscue Distinguished Professor of Cardiology, University of North Carolina School of Medicine, Chapel Hill, North Carolina

Joseph M. Craver, M.D.
Associate Professor of Surgery (Cardio-Thoracic), Emory University School of Medicine, Atlanta, Georgia

I. Sylvia Crawley, M.D.
Professor of Medicine (Cardiology), Department of Medicine, Emory University School of Medicine; Chief, Cardiology Section, Atlanta Veterans Administration Medical Center, Atlanta, Georgia

James E. Dalen, M.D.
Professor and Chairman, Department of Medicine, University of Massachusetts Medical School; Physician-in-Chief, University of Massachusetts Hospital, Worcester, Massachusetts

Michael E. DeBakey, M.D.
Chancellor, Chairman of the Department of Surgery, Olga Keith Wiess Professor of Surgery; Director, Cardiovascular Research and Training Center and The DeBakey Heart Center, Baylor College of Medicine, Houston, Texas

Robert F. DeBusk, M.D.
Associate Professor of Medicine, Stanford University School of Medicine; Director, Stanford Cardiac Rehabilitation Program, Stanford, California

Vera Delaney, M.D.
Assistant Professor of Medicine (Nephrology and Inorganic Metabolism), Department of Medicine, Emory University School of Medicine, Atlanta, Georgia

Harry K. Delcher, M.D.
Clinical Associate Professor of Medicine (Endocrinology), Emory University School of Medicine; Associate Medical Director, Atlanta Regional Diabetes Center, Atlanta, Georgia

Antonio C. de Leon, Jr., M.D.
Medical Director, St. John Cardiovascular Institute; Clinical Professor of Medicine and Chief of Cardiology, University of Oklahoma Tulsa Medical College, Tulsa, Oklahoma

Regis A. de Silva, M.D.
Assistant Clinical Professor of Medicine, Harvard Medical School, Boston, Massachusetts

William C. DeVries, M.D.
Director of the Total Artificial Heart Implant Project, Humana Heart Institute, International, Louisville, Kentucky

Edward R. Dorney, M.D.
Professor of Medicine (Cardiology), Department of Medicine, Emory University School of Medicine, Atlanta, Georgia

John S. Douglas, Jr., M.D.
Associate Professor of Medicine (Cardiology) and Assistant Professor of Radiology (Cardiac Radiology), Emory University School of Medicine, Atlanta, Georgia

David T. Durack, M.B., D.Phil.
Professor of Medicine, Microbiology and Immunology; Chief, Division of Infectious Diseases, Duke University Medical Center, Durham, North Carolina

Harriet P. Dustan, M.D.
Professor of Medicine and Director, Cardiovascular Research and Training Center, University of Alabama in Birmingham, School of Medicine, Birmingham, Alabama

Jesse E. Edwards, M.D.
Professor of Pathology, University of Minnesota, Minneapolis, Minnesota; Senior Consultant Anatomic Pathology, United Hospitals, St. Paul, Minnesota

Robert S. Eliot, M.D., F.A.C.C.
Director, The National Center of Preventive and Stress Medicine, Phoenix, Arizona

Stephen M. Factor, M.D.
Professor of Pathology and Associate Professor of Medicine (Cardiology); Director, Anatomic Pathology of the Bronx Municipal Hospital Center, Albert Einstein College of Medicine, Bronx, New York

William A. Fajman, M.D.
Associate Professor of Radiology; Emory University School of Medicine, Atlanta, Georgia

Susan K. Fellner, M.D.
Associate Professor of Medicine, Pritzker School of Medicine, University of Chicago, Chicago, Illinois

Joel M. Felner, M.D.
Professor of Medicine (Cardiology), Emory University School of Medicine, Atlanta, Georgia

David W. Ferguson, M.D.
Former Assistant Professor, Division of Cardiovascular Diseases, Department of Internal Medicine, University of Iowa College of Medicine, Iowa City, Iowa; currently Director, Cardiac Intensive Care Unit, Medical Center Hospital of Vermont, University of Vermont College of Medicine, Burlington, Vermont

Charles Fisch, M.D.
Distinguished Professor of Medicine and Director, Cardiovascular Division and Krannert Institute of Cardiology, Indiana University School of Medicine, Indianapolis, Indiana

Gerald F. Fletcher, M.D.
Professor of Medicine (Cardiology), Medical Director, Emory Health Enhancement Program, Emory University School of Medicine, Atlanta, Georgia

Ross D. Fletcher, M.D.
Chief, Cardiology Section, Veterans Administration Medical Center; Associate Professor of Medicine, Georgetown University School of Medicine, Washington, D.C.

David G. Folks, M.D.
Assistant Professor of Psychiatry, University of Alabama School of Medicine, Birmingham, Alabama

Noble O. Fowler, M.D.
Professor of Medicine, Director, Division of Cardiology, University of Cincinnati College of Medicine, Cincinnati, Ohio

Robert H. Franch, M.D.
Professor of Medicine (Cardiology), Emory University School of Medicine, Atlanta, Georgia

Arthur M. Freeman III, M.D.
Professor and Vice Chairman, Department of Psychiatry, University of Alabama School of Medicine, Birmingham, Alabama

Gottlieb C. Friesinger, M.D.
Professor of Medicine, Director, Division of Cardiology, Vanderbilt University School of Medicine, Nashville, Tennessee

William H. Frishman, M.D.
Professor of Medicine, Albert Einstein College of Medicine; Director of Medical Service, Hospital of The Albert Einstein College of Medicine, Bronx, New York

J. Timothy Fulenwider, M.D.
Assistant Professor of Surgery, Emory University School of Medicine, Atlanta, Georgia

John J. Gallagher, M.D.
Sanger Clinic and Heineman Medical Research Center, Charlotte, North Carolina

Peter C. Gazes, M.D.
Professor of Medicine, Director, Cardiovascular Division, Medical University of South Carolina, Charleston, South Carolina

Lawrence D. German, M.D.
Assistant Professor of Medicine, Director, Clinical Electrophysiology Laboratory, Duke University Medical Center, Durham, North Carolina

Gary Gerstenblith, M.D.
Associate Professor of Medicine, Johns Hopkins University School of Medicine, Baltimore, Maryland

John F. Goodwin, M.D.
Emeritus Professor of Clinical Cardiology; Honorary Consulting Physician, Royal Postgraduate Medical School, Hammersmith Hospital, London, England

Robert F. Grover, M.D., Ph.D.
Professor Emeritus of Medicine, University of Colorado School of Medicine, Denver, Colorado

Andreas R. Gruentzig, M.D.
Professor of Medicine (Cardiology) and Radiology, Emory University School of Medicine; Director of Interventional Cardiovascular Medicine, Emory University Hospital, Atlanta, Georgia

Robert A. Guyton, M.D.
Associate Professor of Surgery (Cardio-Thoracic), Director, Cardio-Thoracic Research Laboratory, Crawford W. Long Memorial Hospital, Atlanta, Georgia

David Petrie Hall, M.D.
Former Fellow in Medicine (Cardiology), Emory University School of Medicine, Atlanta, Georgia; Clinical Staff, St. Thomas Hospital; Private Practice, Cardiology Consultants, P.C., Nashville, Tennessee

Robert J. Hall, M.D.
Clinical Professor of Medicine, Baylor College of Medicine and the University of Texas Medical School at Houston; Medical Director, Texas Heart Institute; Director, Division of Cardiology, St. Luke's Episcopal Hospital, Houston, Texas

W. Dallas Hall, M.D.
Professor of Medicine (Hypertension); Director, Division of Hypertension, Emory University School of Medicine, Atlanta, Georgia

Donald C. Harrison, M.D.
Professor of Medicine; William G. Irwin Professor of Cardiology; Chief, Division of Cardiology, Stanford University School of Medicine, Stanford, California

W. Proctor Harvey, M.D.
Professor of Medicine, Department of Medicine, Division of Cardiology, Georgetown University Medical Center, Washington, D.C.

Charles R. Hatcher, Jr., M.D.
Professor of Surgery (Cardio-Thoracic); Chief of Cardiovascular Surgery, Division of Cardio-Thoracic Surgery, Emory University School of Medicine; Vice President for Health Affairs and Director of The Woodruff Health Sciences Center, Emory University, Atlanta, Georgia

Theodore Hersh, M.D.
Professor of Medicine (Digestive Diseases), Emory University School of Medicine, Atlanta, Georgia

D. Gregg Hopkins, M.D.
Former Fellow in Cardiology, Stanford University School of Medicine, Stanford, California

Shoei K. Huang, M.D.
Assistant Professor of Medicine, Arizona Health Sciences Center, University of Arizona, Tucson, Arizona

Carl C. Hug, Jr., M.D., Ph.D.
Professor of Anesthesiology and Pharmacology, Director, Cardiothoracic Anesthesia, Emory University School of Medicine, Atlanta, Georgia

J. O'Neal Humphries, M.D.
O.B. Mayer Sr. and Jr. Professor of Medicine; Chairman, Department of Medicine; Dean, School of Medicine, University of South Carolina, Columbia, South Carolina

J. Willis Hurst, M.D.
Candler Professor of Medicine (Cardiology); Chairman, Department of Medicine, Emory University School of Medicine, Chief, Medical Service and Cardiology, Emory University Hospital; Chief, Medical Service, Grady Memorial Hospital; Head, Medical Section and Cardiology, Emory University Clinic, Atlanta, Georgia

Stuart W. Jamieson, M.D.
Associate Professor of Cardiovascular Surgery, Stanford University School of Medicine, Stanford, California

Ellis L. Jones, M.D.
Professor, Thoracic and Cardiovascular Surgery, Emory University School of Medicine, Atlanta, Georgia

William B. Kannel, M.D., M.P.H.
Professor of Medicine; Chief of Section, Preventive Medicine and Epidemiology; Department of Medicine; Adjunct Professor of Public Health (Epidemiology and Biostatistics); Boston University Medical Center, Boston, Massachusetts; Evans Research Foundation, Boston, Massachusetts

Robert B. Karp, M.D.
Professor of Surgery; Chief, Cardiac Surgery Section, University of Chicago Medical Center, Chicago, Illinois

Nevin M. Katz, M.D.
Assistant Professor of Surgery, Georgetown University Medical Center, Washington, D.C.

Gary R. Kilgo, M.D.
Chief Resident, Department of Neurology, Bowman Gray School of Medicine, Winston-Salem, North Carolina

Spencer B. King III, M.D.
Professor of Medicine (Cardiology); Professor of Radiology; Director of Cardiac Catheterization Laboratory, Emory University Hospital, Atlanta, Georgia

Edward S. Kirk, Ph.D.
Professor of Medicine, Departments of Medicine and Physiology and Biophysics, Albert Einstein College of Medicine, Bronx, New York

Hiroshi Kuida, M.D.
Professor of Internal Medicine; Professor of Physiology; University of Utah School of Medicine, Salt Lake City, Utah

Lynn M. Kutsche, M.D.
Assistant Professor of Pediatrics (Cardiology and Research), Department of Pediatrics, University of Florida College of Medicine, Gainesville, Florida

Aubrey Leatham, F.R.C.P.
Physician to St. George's Hospital and the National Heart Hospital, London, England

Graham J. Leech, M.A.
Senior Lecturer in Biomedical Engineering, St. George's Hospital Medical School, London, England

Thierry H. LeJemtel, M.D.
Associate Professor of Medicine, Division of Cardiology, Department of Medicine, Albert Einstein College of Medicine, Bronx, New York

Richard P. Lewis, M.D.
Professor of Medicine; Director, Division of Cardiology, Ohio State University College of Medicine, Columbus, Ohio

Joseph Lindsay, Jr., M.D.
Professor of Medicine, The George Washington University; Chairman, Section of Cardiology, The Washington Hospital Center, Washington, D.C.

R. Bruce Logue, M.D.
Professor Emeritus of Medicine (Cardiology), Emory University School of Medicine; Director, Carlyle Fraser Heart Center, Crawford W. Long Memorial Hospital, Atlanta, Georgia

Bernard Lown, M.D.
Professor of Cardiology, Harvard School of Public Health; Physician, Brigham and Women's Hospital, Boston, Massachusetts

John H. McAnulty, M.D.
Professor of Medicine, Oregon Health Sciences University, Portland, Oregon

Terence B. McGhee, M.D.
Mountain Neurological Center, Asheville, North Carolina

Kamal A. Mansour, M.D.
Associate Professor of Surgery (Cardio-Thoracic), Emory University School of Medicine, Atlanta, Georgia

Frank I. Marcus, M.D.
Professor of Medicine, Cardiology Section, University of Arizona College of Medicine, Tucson, Arizona

Henry J. L. Marriott, M.D.
Clinical Professor of Medicine (Cardiology), Emory University School of Medicine, Atlanta, Georgia; Clinical Professor of Pediatrics (Cardiology), University of Florida, Gainesville, Florida; Director, Clinical Research, Rogers Heart Foundation, St. Petersburg, Florida

James Metcalfe, M.D.
Professor of Medicine, Oregon Heart Associate Chair of Cardiovascular Research, Oregon Health Sciences University, Portland, Oregon

Joseph I. Miller, Jr., M.D.
Associate Professor of Thoracic and Cardiovascular Surgery, Emory University School of Medicine, Atlanta, Georgia

M. Mirowski, M.D.
Director, Coronary Care Unit; Professor of Medicine, The Johns Hopkins University School of Medicine, Baltimore, Maryland

Harry G. Mond, M.D. (Australia), F.R.A.C.P., F.A.C.C.
Physician to Pacemaker Clinic, Department of Cardiology, The Royal Melbourne Hospital, Victoria, Australia

Howard E. Morgan, M.D.
Evan Pugh Professor and Chairman of Physiology, The Milton S. Hershey Medical Center, The Pennsylvania State University, Hershey, Pennsylvania

Douglas C. Morris, M.D.
Associate Professor of Medicine (Cardiology), Emory University School of Medicine; Director of the Cardiac Catheterization Laboratory, Chief of Cardiology, Crawford W. Long Memorial Hospital, Atlanta, Georgia

Robert J. Myerburg, M.D.
Professor of Medicine and Physiology, Director of the Division of Cardiology, University of Miami Medical School, Miami, Florida

James R. Neely, Ph.D.
Professor of Physiology, The Pennsylvania State University College of Medicine, Hershey, Pennsylvania

John H. Newman, M.D.
Associate Professor of Medicine; Elsa S. Hanigan Chair in Pulmonary Medicine, Vanderbilt University School of Medicine and St. Thomas Hospital, Nashville, Tennessee

R. Joe Noble, M.D.
Consulting Cardiologist, St. Vincent Hospital and Health Care Center, Indianapolis, Indiana; Clinical Professor of Medicine, Indiana University School of Medicine, Indianapolis, Indiana

Elizabeth W. Nugent, M.D.
Associate Professor of Pediatrics, Cardiology Division, Emory University School of Medicine, Atlanta, Georgia

Robert A. O'Rourke, M.D.
Charles Conrad and Anna Sahm Brown Professor of Medicine; Chief, Cardiology Division, University of Texas Health Science Center, San Antonio, Texas

Philip E. Oyer, M.D., Ph.D.
Associate Professor of Cardiovascular Surgery, Stanford University Medical Center, Stanford, California

Douglas L. Packer, M.D.
Fellow in Cardiology and Electrophysiology, Duke University Medical Center, Durham, North Carolina

Alan S. Pearlman, M.D.
Associate Professor of Medicine and Bioengineering, University of Washington School of Medicine, Seattle, Washington

Garland D. Perdue, Jr., M.D.
Associate Dean for Clinical Affairs, Emory University School of Medicine, Professor of Surgery; Clinic Director, The Emory Clinic; Medical Director, Emory University Hospital, Atlanta, Georgia

Joseph K. Perloff, M.D.
Steisand/American Heart Association Professor of Medicine and Pediatrics, University of California at Los Angeles School of Medicine, Los Angeles, California

Claude A. Piantadosi, M.D.
Assistant Professor of Medicine, Duke University Medical Center, Durham, North Carolina

William H. Plauth, Jr., M.D.
Professor of Pediatrics, Emory University School of Medicine, Atlanta, Georgia

Scott J. Pollak, M.D.
Fellow in Medicine (Cardiology), Emory University School of Medicine, Atlanta, Georgia

John R. K. Preedy, M.D.
Professor of Medicine (Endocrinology), Emory University School of Medicine; Associate Chief of Staff for Research and Development, Veterans Administration Medical Center, Atlanta, Georgia

Edward L. C. Pritchett, M.D.
Associate Professor of Medicine, Division of Cardiology, Duke University Medical Center, Durham, North Carolina

Charles E. Rackley, M.D.
Anton and Margaret Fuisz Professor of Medicine, Chairman, Department of Medicine, Georgetown University Medical Center, Washington, D.C.

John T. Reeves, M.D.
Professor of Medicine; Associate Director, Cardiovascular-Pulmonary Research Laboratory, University of Colorado Health Sciences Center, Denver, Colorado

Timothy J. Regan, M.D.
Professor of Medicine; Director, Division of Cardiovascular Diseases; University of Medicine and Dentistry of New Jersey, New Jersey Medical School, Newark, New Jersey

William C. Roberts, M.D.
Chief, Pathology Branch, National Heart, Lung and Blood Institute, Bethesda, Maryland; Clinical Professor of Pathology and Medicine (Cardiology), Georgetown University, Washington, D.C.

Paul H. Robinson, M.D.
Associate Professor of Medicine (Cardiology), Emory University School of Medicine, Atlanta, Georgia

John Ross, Jr., M.D.
Professor of Medicine, Head, Division of Cardiology, Department of Medicine, University of California, San Diego; Attending Physician, UCSD Medical Center, La Jolla, California

Joseph C. Ross, M.D.
Professor of Medicine; Associate Vice Chancellor for Health Affairs, Vanderbilt University, Nashville, Tennessee

Russell Ross, Ph.D.
Professor and Chairman of Pathology; Adjunct Professor of Biochemistry, University of Washington, Seattle, Washington

Loring B. Rowell, Ph.D.
Professor, Physiology and Biophysics, Professor of Medicine (Cardiology), University of Washington School of Medicine, Seattle, Washington

Ronald N. Rubin, M.D.
Associate Professor of Medicine and Thrombosis, Department in Internal Medicine and the Specialized Center for Thrombosis Research, Temple University Hospital and School of Medicine, Philadelphia, Pennsylvania

Elliot L. Sagall, M.D.
Assistant Clinical Professor of Medicine, Harvard Medical School, Boston, Massachusetts

Herbert A. Saltzman, M.D.
Professor of Medicine, Duke University, Durham, North Carolina

Robert C. Saunders, M.D.
Chief, Medical Intensive Care and Coronary Care Unit, Veterans Administration Medical Center, Washington, D.C.; Assistant Professor of Medicine, George Washington University School of Medicine, Washington, D.C.

James Scheuer, M.D.
Professor of Medicine and Physiology, Albert Einstein College of Medicine; Chief of Cardiology, Montefiore Hospital and Medical Center, Bronx, New York

Robert C. Schlant, M.D.
Professor of Medicine (Cardiology); Director, Division of Cardiology, Emory University School of Medicine; Chief of Cardiology, Grady Memorial Hospital, Atlanta, Georgia

Ralph Shabetai, M.D.
Professor of Medicine, University of California San Diego; Chief of Cardiology, San Diego Veterans Administration Medical Center, San Diego, California

Louis C. Sheppard, Ph.D.
Professor and Chairman, Department of Biomedical Engineering, School of Engineering, The University of Alabama at Birmingham, Birmingham, Alabama

Sol Sherry, M.D., D.Sc. (Hon.)
Distinguished Professor and Dean, Temple University School of Medicine, Philadelphia, Pennsylvania

Norman E. Shumway, M.D., Ph.D.
Professor and Chairman, Department of Cardiovascular Surgery, Stanford University School of Medicine, Stanford, California

Mark E. Silverman, M.D.
Professor of Medicine (Cardiology), Emory University School of Medicine and Piedmont Hospital, Atlanta, Georgia

J. Graeme Sloman, E.D., B.Sc., F.R.C.P. (LOND.), F.R.C.P. (EDIN.), F.R.A.C.P., F.A.C.C.
Director of Cardiology and Chairman, Cardiovascular Unit, Epworth Medical Centre, Richmond, Victoria, Australia

Robert B. Smith III, M.D.
Professor of Surgery and Head of General Vascular Surgery, Emory University School of Medicine; Chief, Surgical Service, Veterans Administration Medical Center, Atlanta, Georgia

Warren M. Smith, M.B.
Cardiologist, Department of Cardiology, Green Lane Hospital, Epsom, Auckland, New Zealand

Burton E. Sobel, M.D.
Professor of Medicine, Director of Cardiovascular Division, Department of Medicine, Washington University School of Medicine; Cardiologist-in-Chief at Barnes Hospital, St. Louis, Missouri

Peter J. Sones, M.D.
Clinical Professor of Radiology, Emory University School of Medicine, Atlanta, Georgia

Edmund H. Sonnenblick, M.D.
Olson Professor of Medicine, Chief, Division of Cardiology, Albert Einstein College of Medicine, Bronx, New York

Renate L. Soulen, M.D.
Professor of Radiology; Chief, Section of Cardiovascular Radiology; Vice Chairman, Department of Diagnostic Imaging, Temple University Health Sciences Center, Philadelphia, Pennsylvania

James F. Spann, Jr., M.D.
Professor of Medicine, Director, Cardiology Division, Director, Gazes Cardiac Research Institution, Medical University of South Carolina, Charleston, South Carolina

Richard M. Steingart, M.D.
Assistant Professor of Medicine (Cardiology and Nuclear Cardiology), Montefiore Medical Center, Bronx, New York

Edward B. Stinson, M.D.
Professor of Cardiovascular Surgery, Stanford University School of Medicine, Stanford, California

Gene H. Stollerman, M.D.
Professor of Medicine, Boston University School of Medicine, Boston, Massachusetts

D. E. Strandness, Jr., M.D.
Professor of Surgery; Head, Section of Vascular Surgery, University of Washington School of Medicine, Seattle, Washington

Harold C. Strauss, M.D., C.M.
Professor of Medicine and Associate Professor of Pharmacology, Duke University Medical Center, Durham, North Carolina

H. J. C. Swan, M.D., Ph.D.
Director, Division of Cardiology, Cedars-Sinai Medical Center; Professor of Medicine, University of California at Los Angeles School of Medicine, Los Angeles, California

Panagiotis N. Symbas, M.D.
Professor of Surgery, Thoracic and Cardiovascular Surgery Division, Emory University School of Medicine, Atlanta, Georgia

W. Jape Taylor, M.D.
Distinguished Service Professor of Medicine, University of Florida College of Medicine, Gainesville, Florida

Thomas J. Thom, B.A.
Epidemiology and Biometry Program, National Heart, Lung and Blood Institute, Bethesda, Maryland

James F. Toole, M.D.
Teagle Professor of Neurology, Bowman Gray School of Medicine, Winston Salem, North Carolina

Elbert P. Tuttle, Jr., M.D.
Professor of Medicine (Nephrology and Inorganic Metabolism), Emory University School of Medicine, Atlanta, Georgia

Kent Ueland, M.D.
Professor of Gynecology and Obstetrics; Chief, Section of Maternal-Fetal Medicine, Stanford University School of Medicine, Stanford, California

L. H. S. Van Mierop, M.D.
Professor of Pediatrics (Cardiology and Research) and Pathology; Graduate Research Professor, Department of Pediatrics, University of Florida College of Medicine, Gainesville, Florida

Andrew G. Wallace, M.D.
Kempner Professor of Medicine and Vice Chancellor for Health Affairs, Duke University Medical Center, Durham, North Carolina

Robert B. Wallace, M.D.
Professor and Chairman, Department of Surgery, Georgetown University Medical Center, Washington, D.C.

Paul F. Walter, M.D.
Professor of Cardiology, Emory University School of Medicine, Atlanta, Georgia

James V. Warren, M.D.
Professor of Medicine, The Ohio State University College of Medicine, Columbus, Ohio

Nanette Kass Wenger, M.D.
Professor of Medicine (Cardiology), Department of Medicine, Emory University School of Medicine; Director, Cardiac Clinics, Grady Memorial Hospital, Atlanta, Georgia

Myron L. Weisfeldt, M.D.
Professor of Medicine; Director, Cardiology Division, The Johns Hopkins Hospital, Baltimore, Maryland

Arnold M. Weissler, M.D.
Professor and Chairman, Department of Medicine, Rose Medical Center, Denver, Colorado

Jeffrey A. Werner, M.D.
Consulting Cardiologist, Redmond Medical Center, Redmond, Washington; Clinical Associate Professor of Medicine, University of Washington School of Medicine, Seattle, Washington

Joseph A. Wilber, M.D.
Clinical Associate Professor of Medicine, Emory Univer-

sity School of Medicine; Vice President and Medical Director, Georgia International Life Insurance Company; Medical Consultant, Adult Health, Georgia Department of Human Resources, Atlanta, Georgia

Willis H. Williams, M.D.
Chief of Surgery, Henrietta Egleston Hospital for Children; Associate Professor of Surgery (Cardiothoracic); Assistant Professor of Pediatrics, Emory University School of Medicine, Atlanta, Georgia

A. Calhoun Witham, M.D.
Professor of Medicine, Medical College of Georgia, Augusta, Georgia

Gary L. Wollam, M.D.
Associate Professor of Medicine (Hypertension), Emory University School of Medicine, Atlanta, Georgia

Jess R. Young, M.D.
Head, Department of Peripheral Vascular Disease, Cleveland Clinic Foundation, Cleveland, Ohio

Barry L. Zaret, M.D.
Robert W. Berliner Professor of Medicine, Professor of Diagnostic Radiology, Chief, Section of Cardiology, Yale University School of Medicine, New Haven, Connecticut

Douglas P. Zipes, M.D.
Professor of Medicine, Indiana University School of Medicine; Senior Research Associate, Krannert Institute of Cardiology, Indianapolis, Indiana

Preface

Our goal in the sixth edition of *The Heart* is, as it was in previous editions, to create a book which will assist the physician who takes care of patients. Accordingly, we have designed and written an easy-to-use, complete treatise on disease of the heart and blood vessels. We believe the book is well-suited to specialists and nonspecialists, and residents and students. Since our treatment is extensive, we urge the reader to use the introductions placed at the beginning of each part to gain a clear view of the purposes of the book and our methods for achieving them.

An effective planning session for the sixth edition of *The Heart* was held in 1983. The editors discussed feedback from readers and agreed on the necessary changes. We added 29 new chapters to the 109 found in the fifth edition. All other chapters were brought up to date and many were extensively revised. Some of the chapters were shortened to make room for "the new." It was not feasible to include all new ideas, procedures, and techniques, but we believe we have been reasonable in selecting those new developments which are important and will become part of standard practice in the future. Whenever possible unnecessary duplication of information was avoided. The duplication that does exist was planned in order to make the material easier for the reader to comprehend. All chapters were compiled with care and checked several times for accuracy and clarity. Painstaking efforts were made to attribute the sources of all borrowed material.

An important new concept, first introduced in the fifth edition, receives continued and expanded attention in the sixth. In the last edition we recognized the increasing impact of modern technology and developed ground rules for governing its use. In this edition our discussion is grouped in three portions. First, in Part II, we emphasize that most cardiovascular problems can be solved by carefully performing the "routine" examination. Second, in Part III, we highlight the value of special technology in the detection and treatment of heart disease; but we also stress the importance, before choosing a procedure, of asking the proper questions—those which lead to the selection of specific methods for accurate diagnosis. Third, in Part VII, we describe and detail the use of the procedures themselves.

In our efforts to make the contents of *The Heart* as accessible as possible to readers, we have organized the text clearly and logically into seven parts. Part I, "The Normal Heart and Blood Vessels," contains discussions of the embryology, anatomy, and biochemistry the practicing physician should know in order to understand the heart and its diseases. The fundamental information given here serves as a reference to the cardiovascular problems examined in subsequent parts.

Part II, "The Methods Used to Collect Data on Every Patient (The 'Routine' Examination)," discusses history-taking, performing a physical examination, analyzing the electrocardiogram, and studying the chest x-ray. These conventional methods for collecting data on the patient are fully described and evaluated. These methods, if they do not lead to a diagnostic conclusion, also aid in determining which further tests are needed.

Accordingly, Part III, "Methods and Strategy Used to Collect Data on Selected Patients (The Assessment of Specific Problems)," presents strategies and techniques used to answer specific questions not answered by the routine examination. Four important manifestations of cardiovascular problems are addressed: structural abnormalities and blood flow, cardiac function and myocardial contractility, electrical abnormalities, and myocardial ischemia. The details of the techniques themselves are discussed in Part VII (B through H).

Part IV, "Disorders of the Cardiovascular System," focuses on those cardiovascular problems which are consequences of a disease process. Included here are chapters on the treatment and management of heart failure, hypotension and shock, hyperdynamic circulation, arrhythmias, pacemakers, syncope, sudden cardiac death, and cardiopulmonary resuscitation. The discussions of hypotension and shock, arrhythmias, and syncope have been expanded in this edition.

Part V, "Diseases of the Heart and Blood Vessels" concentrates on the fundamental abnormalities of the cardiovascular system. There are complete sections on the incidence, prevalence, and mortality of cardiovascular disease, congenital heart disease, valvular heart disease, coronary heart disease, arterial hypertension, pulmonary hypertension, endocarditis, myocardial disease, pericardial disease, traumatic heart disease, neoplastic heart disease, rheumatic fever, and syphilitic heart disease, and diseases of the blood vessels are examined in terms of recognition, management, treatment, and prevention. The discussions of atherosclerosis have been thoroughly revised and expanded, and all chapters have been updated.

Part VI, "The Heart and Other Medical Problems," presents more general physiological and psychological conditions, as well as certain relevant socioeconomic subjects, which involve the heart and blood vessels. Among the topics discussed are pregnancy, athletics, aging, endocrine disease, collagen disease, alcohol and nutrition, obesity, renal disease, electrolytes, noncardiac drugs, anesthesia, and emotional stress.

Part VII, "The Pharmacology of Cardiac Drugs and the Techniques of Special Procedures," represents one of the most revised and expanded portions of the sixth edition.

Section A deals with the pharmacology of commonly used cardiac drugs. Throughout the book readers can find discussions of the drugs used to treat diseases and disorders without being mentally side-tracked with the details of pharmacology; here, complete coverage of the pharmacology of cardiac drugs is found. New to this edition are chapters on drugs used to control vascular resistance and capacitance; drugs used to treat cardiac arrhythmias; beta blockers; calcium blockers; digitalis; nondigitalis cardiac inotropic agents; diuretics; and anticoagulants and platelet-controlling drugs.

Sections B through H deal with the techniques involved in performing certain diagnostic and therapeutic procedures. The discussion highlights the types of high-technological procedures available and describes the indications and limitations of their use while stressing the information a physician needs to understand surgical procedures. Of the 43 chapters here, 18 are completely new. They include internal defibrillation; digital subtraction imaging; CT; pulmonary angiography; NMR; thrombolysis; lasers; Doppler; valvular and carotid surgery; and the use of the artificial heart and other timely topics.

The careful reader will detect a slight difference in the opinions expressed by different authors writing on the same subject—differences which were not as obvious in earlier editions of the book. Such differences have increased as new techniques and procedures have been added to the diagnostic and therapeutic strategies related to patient care. Appropriately, the editor-in-chief has not attempted to obtain a consensus of ideas. If such could be done, it would not accurately depict the current state of the art. Readers should collate the information that is presented here. They can then use their own judgment in applying a strategy of work-up and treatment for their patients. It is important to remember that the strategy is often determined by the quality of the results of the components of a diagnostic and therapeutic system. For example, if nuclear cardiology at an institution is not reliable, the physician may rely more often on coronary arteriography to solve the problems of coronary disease. If an institution excels at coronary angioplasty, the procedure will be used more often than it will at an institution where the technique is being used with less success.

I wish to thank Dr. Richard Krause, Dean of Emory University School of Medicine, for his leadership, friendship, and encouragement. His wisdom and scholarship are awesome and inspirational. Dr. Charles Hatcher, Vice-President for Health Affairs of Emory University, has, in addition to his administrative duties as Director of the Woodruff Medical Center, developed an outstanding cardiac surgical team at Emory University. Cardiology cannot flourish without excellent cardiac surgery and its support systems of cardiac anesthesiology and cardiac nursing. He and his staff have contributed significantly to the creation of this book.

I wish to thank Carol Miller for her tireless efforts to achieve perfection. She is a genius at work. She is able to decipher my scribbles and place them with lightning speed into the word processor. The thousands of pieces that make up the whole of this book must be filed for quick retrieval. She can do that too with a misfile record approaching zero and, with it all, she is happy!

I thank the authors and five editors of this volume for answering my numerous letters and telephone calls and for writing and rewriting the manuscripts. They are busy experts who took the time to teach us all through their writing. Their secretaries are indispensable to their efforts and we appreciate their help.

I thank Robert McGraw, Donna McIvor, Joseph Brehm, Beth Kaufman Barry, Terry Fiore Lavery, and Camille Truchel of McGraw-Hill. Phil James has tackled the important job of indexing and, once again, he has done a superb job.

To Nelie, my wife, I thank with love. She has made our house a home and has made far more of me than I would have been. No Nelie, no book.

J. Willis Hurst, M.D.

PROLOGUE

The Growth of Knowledge

Howard B. Burchell, M.D., Ph.D.

As credulity is the cause of error, so incredulity oftentimes of not enjoying truth.

Sir Thomas Browne, 1646[1]

This sixth edition of *The Heart* appears 20 years after the first edition. If one accepts estimates that in this century the sum of information more than doubles every 10 years, then in 20 years, new data on the circulation would have quadrupled. With regard to technology, I suspect this may well be so, but in terms of caring for the patient, i.e., properly applying the new information and understanding the uniqueness of a patient's problem and reactions, the extent of growth in the information load has not been so gross.

In the second and third editions, Paul White wrote the prologue, highlighting the cardiac discoveries over the centuries, continuing a climactic emphasis on preventive cardiology. His exhortation to the profession and public was "heart disease before 80 is our fault, not God's or Nature's will." He also directed attention to the importance of preventive efforts against heart disease in early life, "a children's crusade." Paul White's own textbook[2] appeared just over a half century ago, became popular, and was kept up-to-date for over two decades. It is still a text to be perused in any study of a cardiac problem if one is interested in gaining a historical perspective. He added a provocative list of unanswered questions about heart disease in the appendix of the first edition (1931). Using these as a base for a catechism, one may appreciate the growth of clinical knowledge during the following 50 years (1930 to 1980).

I have been privileged to write the prologue for the last three editions of this text; in these editions I have outlined the growth of cardiological knowledge, the explosive increase in technological developments, and the emergence of a large community of accredited heart specialists. *The Heart* has always had an undercurrent stress on the history of cardiac disease; one could cite, for example, the photographs of Osler at the bedside in the second and third editions, and the reproductions of the mural of Diego Rivera in the Cardiologic Institute of Mexico, enshrining the cardiological "greats" in the fourth edition. In addition, the fourth edition was dedicated to the memory of William Harvey on the 400th anniversary of his birth (1578).

The nature of the growth of knowledge has fascinated both the scientist and the philosopher. Progress in understanding has always seemed to plateau following momentous contributions, and it may take years, or centuries, for discoveries of exceptions and flaws in a system of thought to become so numerous that new paradigms are needed. Such shifts in belief are revolutionary; sometimes they are recognized as such by the creator, e.g., Harvey, but often not. Kuhn's explorations of the mechanisms of scientific revolutions are enlightening.[3] He discusses the complex background from which discoveries have evolved and how the new paradigms have replaced the old and become accepted as the new truth.

William Harvey is properly acclaimed as the father of cardiology, but he belongs to no specialist sect. It is of less importance to debate whether conceptually or experimentally Harvey was the first to *discover* the circulation than to recognize the all-persuasive evidence that the quality and quantity of his theoretical calculations, his logic, and his experimental work *proved* the existence of the circulation. Others had undoubtedly glimpsed the truth; Harvey's demonstrations established it, though some of his contemporaries were slow to accept it. The story of his work has been told and retold. Of the voluminous literature available for study, two appraisals that I have particularly enjoyed reading are Osler's Harverian Lecture, "The Growth of Truth as Illustrated in the Discovery of Circulation,"[4] and Bylebyl's "The Growth of Harvey's 'De Motu Cordis.' "[5] A newly edited translation of Harvey's classic by Whitteridge is now available and is a great asset to any scholar; particularly helpful are her extensive footnotes.[6]

As beginnings of a historical reference shelf for cardiology, my suggestions are *Cardiac Classics,* edited by Willius and Keys[7] (a third companion volume has recently been published by Callahan, Keys, and Key[7a]); *Circulation of the Blood, Men and Ideas,* by Fishman and Richards;[8] *A Short History of Cardiology,* by Herrick;[9] a *History of Electrocardiography,* by Burch and Pasquale;[10] *The History of Coronary Heart Disease,* by Leibowitz;[11] the *History of Cardiac Surgery,* by Johnson;[12] and *The Surgeon's Heart,* by Richardson.[13] To reacquaint myself with the development of cardiac catheterization and angiography, I turn to the reports of Cournand[14] and Doby,[15] respectively. For reminiscent portrayals of developments in cardiology in this century, I suggest "History and Perspectives in Cardiology," a small monograph edited by Snellen and associates.[16]

Physicians have been interested in the symptoms caused by heart disease since ancient times, and the early insights into the nature of pulmonary congestion from heart failure are outlined in the scholarly work of Saul Jarcho, *The Concept of Heart Failure from Avicenna to Albertini.*[17]

My favorite early textbook at the beginning of my specialty orientation was that of James Hope;[18] with the development of more narrowed interests, my more modern treasured volume is *The Graphic Registration of the Heart Beat* by Thomas Lewis.[19] Among modern collectors of books on heart disease was Evan Bedford, and his library has been retained largely intact and is now housed in the Royal College of Physicians Library in London.[20] One of our famed American physicians, James Herrick,[21] known best, along with Osler and Dock, for the clarification of the dynamic nature of coronary obstructive disease, was history-minded; this being exemplified by his learned address on "Textbooks of the Early Nineteenth Century."

It is not long ago that the opportunities for advanced study were minimal in the United States for a young, eager American medical graduate. Many scientific treks by Americans occurred in the eighteenth century, particularly to Edinburgh, London, and sometimes Leyden. The role of Benjamin Franklin in sponsoring such trips is noteworthy.[22] Later, in the first half of the nineteenth century, there were frequent travelers to Paris, where, in particular, the clinics of Louis and of Laennec were the attractions. Among these young American medical graduate visitors to Paris was Oliver Wendell Holmes. Holmes is well known to cardiologists for his lighter side through "Stethoscope Verses," which facetiously outlines in rhyme the perils to the young man back from France after giving an overinterpretation of sounds heard over the heart.[23] In the mid-nineteenth century, Dublin was attracting students of heart disease, and in the latter part of the century, the German clinics (so well described in Osler's letters to his students in 1872 to 1874) gained a dominant position. It was from Carl Ludwig's laboratory that Henry Bowditch returned to America to establish at Harvard the first modern American physiology laboratory.[24] The experimental approach began thus to supersede the didactic curriculum; the latter was exemplified by the teaching of erudite young Robley Dunglison, brought from England by Thomas Jefferson at the formation of the University of Virginia. Dunglison's *Human Physiology* appeared in 1832.

At the beginning of this (twentieth) century, the revolutionary clinical insights of James Mackenzie,[25] initially a general practitioner, with his rather crude apparatus to record the pulse, created a new dimension in cardiology. His work gave the impetus for Thomas Lewis[26] to develop as one of the first true "clinical investigators." Lewis established London as an outstanding cardiological center. He edited the English specialty journal *Heart,* which was launched in 1909. It was in London that a large number of Americans later to become leaders in cardiology made their entrance on the heart stage, a fact in part determined by World War I (1914 to 1918). In the two decades following this war, the Vienna cardiology clinics also attracted many graduate students.

In consequence of the racial madness in central Europe, before the midcentury, the American cardiological community benefited from the arrival of émigrés, both students and established physicians, from many countries. These illustrious persons have made a lasting imprint on American cardiology.

To mention an often reiterated point, as physicians we should remember that our debts to basic science investigators and to industrial laboratories are tremendous ones. Not infrequently, it has been a basic scientist or a clinical investigator not specifically categorized as "heart-oriented" who has had a new insight into, or has made observations which have clarified, a puzzling cardiovascular phenomenon. Generally, progress has occurred in the basic science field without there having been much prior thought about the practical applications. Logically, it would follow that one could not predict when a scientific discovery would have therapeutic implications. However, when a real "breakthrough" relating to treatment has become evident, basic scientists have accelerated their effort to explain and assess that treatment, this activity being the natural outgrowth of basic scientists' interest in helping their fellow human beings and perhaps sometimes an expectation of liberal financial support. The development of open heart surgery exemplifies how a therapeutic triumph depended on many years of work in the basic science laboratory with success dependent on technological breakthroughs.[27]

The growth of knowledge widely viewed includes the dissemination of newly discovered facts as well as the accumulation of data and a recording of the discoveries. One visualizes in the last part of this century a revolution occurring relative to computer storage and management of knowledge equivalent to that of 500 years ago when the printed book replaced the manuscript. Boorstin points out that while in earlier centuries "physicians and lawyers locked their knowledge in a learned language," the printing press made it increasingly difficult to keep a secret, and that it greatly altered the meaning of owning an idea.[28] Priority became a prize, a situation which has continued, both as a help and occasionally as a plague to us.

There is an ancient admonition to the physician to be neither the first to try the new, nor the last to lay the old aside. I have not liked its seemingly condescending tone, but truly it contains a valid message concerning how we should utilize technological advances. These must not take precedence over the well-known total needs of a patient during an illness because of their novelty alone.

References

1. Wilkin, S. (ed.): "Sir Thomas Browne's Works," William Pickering, London, 1836, Vol. II, p. 210.
2. White, P. D.: "Heart Disease," Macmillan Publishing Company, New York, 1931.
3. Kuhn, T. S.: "The Essential Tension: Second Thoughts on Paradigms," The University of Chicago Press, Chicago, 1977.
4. Osler, W.: "The Growth of Truth as Illustrated by the Discovery of the Circulation of the Blood, Being the Harverian Oration Delivered at the Royal College of Physicians, London, October 18, 1906," H. Frowde, London, 1906.
5. Bylebyl, H. J.: The Growth of Harvey's "De Motu Cordis," *Bull. Hist. Med.,* 47:427, 1973.
6. Harvey, W.: "An Anatomical Disputation Concerning the Movement of the Heart and Blood in Living Creatures," G. Whitteridge (trans.), Blackwell Scientific Publications, Ltd., Oxford, 1976 (Lippincott, distributors, United States).
7. Willius, F. A., and Keys, T. E. (eds.): "Cardiac Classics," The C. V. Mosby Company, St. Louis, 1941.

7a. Callahan, J. C., Keys, T. E., and Key, J. D. (eds.): "Classics of Cardiology," vol. 3, Robert E. Krieger Publishing Co., Malabar, Florida, 1983.

8. Fishman, A. P., and Richards, D. W. (eds.): "Circulation of the Blood, Men and Ideas," Oxford University Press, Fair Lawn, N.J., 1964.
9. Herrick, J.: "A Short History of Cardiology," Charles C Thomas, Publisher, Springfield, Ill., 1942.
10. Burch, G. E., and Pasquale, N. P.: "A History of Electrocardiography," The Year Book Publishers, Inc., Chicago, 1964.
11. Leibowtiz, J. O.: "The History of Coronary Heart Disease," Wellcome Institute of the History of Medicine, University of California Press, Berkeley, Calif., 1970.
12. Johnson, S. L.: "The History of Cardiac Surgery, 1896–1955," The Johns Hopkins Press, Baltimore, 1970.
13. Richardson, R. G.: "The Surgeon's Heart: A History of Cardiac Surgery," Heinemann Medical Books, Ltd., London, 1969.
14. Cournand, A.: Cardiac Catheterization, *Acta Med. Scand. (Suppl.)*, 579:7, 1975.
15. Doby T.: "Development of Angiography and Cardiovascular Catheterization," Publishing Sciences Group, Littleton, Mass., 1976.
16. Snellen, H. A., Dunning, A. J., and Arntzenius, A. C.: "History and Perspectives of Cardiology," Leiden University Press, Boston, 1981.
17. Jarcho, S.: "The Concept of Heart Failure from Avicenna to Albertini," Harvard University Press, Cambridge, 1980.
18. Hope, J.: "A Treatise on the Diseases of the Heart and on the Affections That May Be Mistaken for Them," Lea & Blanchard, Philadelphia, 1842 (first available American edition based on third London edition published by C. W. Pennock).
19. Lewis, T.: "The Graphic Registration of the Heart," Hoeber, New York, 1920.
20. Bedford, D. E.: Introduction, in C. Newman, "The Evan Bedford Library of Cardiology Catalog of Books, Pamphlets and Journals," London, Royal College of Physicians, 1977.
21. Herrick, J. B.: Certain Textbooks on Heart Disease of the Early Nineteenth Century, *Bull. Hist. Med.,* 10:136, 1941.
22. Larabee, L. W. (ed.): "The Papers of Benjamin Franklin," Yale University Press, New Haven, Conn., 1966, vol. 9, pp. 219, 377.
23. Holmes, O. W.: "Stethoscope Verses," in F. A. Willius and T. E. Keys (eds.), "Cardiac Classics," The C. V. Mosby Company, St. Louis, 1941.
24. "Dictionary of American Biography," Charles Scribner's Sons, New York, 1927–1957, vol. I, pp. 494–496 [H. P. Bowditch (1840–1911)].
25. Mair, A.: "Sir James Mackenzie, M. D.: General Practitioner, 1853–1925," Churchill Livingstone, Edinburgh, 1973.
26. Clegg, H.: "Dictionary of National Biography, 1941–1950," Oxford University Press, New York, 1959, pp. 501–502 [Sir T. Lewis (1881–1945)].
27. Comroe, J. H., and Dripps, R. D.: Ben Franklin and Open Heart Surgery, *Circ. Res.,* 35:661, 1974.
28. Boorstin, D. J.: "The Discoverers—A History of Man's Search to Know His World and Himself," Random House, New York, 1983, p. 409.

Volume I

PART I

The Normal Heart and Blood Vessels

The purpose of Part I is to describe the normal heart. An entire book could be written on this subject, but the discussion included here has been refined to emphasize the knowledge that will interest the practicing physician.

The science that is basic to the understanding of the heart and blood vessels may be approached in two different ways. Some physicians may recognize their need to know more about the science that is basic to the entire field of cardiology. They may have no specific patient in mind as they read. They read simply to understand how the heart works. Other physicians may recognize they cannot understand a specific patient's disease process or its management without understanding the scientific basis for it. Part I has been designed to meet both these objectives.

1

Embryology of the Heart

L. H. S. Van Mierop, M.D.   Lynn M. Kutsche, M.D.

Interest in cardiovascular embryology, not only among embryologists and anatomists but also among clinicians, has been stimulated by the spectacular advances made in the diagnosis and surgical treatment of congenital heart disease since the 1940s. There are many different cardiac anomalies, some of great complexity, and embryology of the heart, rather than being a difficult subject having little relevance to clinical medicine, has proved to be of enormous value in the understanding of the pathology and pathogenesis of these anomalies.

Development of the Heart

The Heart Prior to Septation

Early Vasculogenesis
The vascular system first appears in embryos of about 3 weeks' ovulation age as scattered masses of angiogenic cell clusters, or "blood islands," which rapidly increase in size and number, acquire a lumen, and become confluent to form a vascular plexus.[1] Part of the plexus differentiates into main channels, resulting in a bilaterally symmetrical vascular system. At the cephalic end of the embryo (on each side of the midsagittal plane) a section of main channel specializes further. Each acquires contractile elements within its wall, producing a pair of heart tubes which come to lie parallel and close to each other within the cephalic part of the developing body cavity (intraembryonic coelom), ventral to the foregut.

Fusion of the heart tubes results in the formation of a single tube (Fig. 1-1), the wall of which consists of an external myocardial mantle 1 to 2 cell layers thick and a single layer of endothelial cells internally, separated from each other by a relatively thick, acellular, and almost structureless third layer called *cardiac jelly*.[2,3] From this tube will develop initially the embryonic ventricle and bulbus cordis (hence the term *bulboventricular tube*) and later the ventricles and their outflow tracts. A more detailed account of the foregoing has been given elsewhere.[4,5]

Formation of the Heart Loop
At the beginning of the next phase of development, the embryo is about 2 mm long and 23 days old. The dilated cephalic, extrapericardial portion of the bulboventricular tube is called the *aortic sac*. From it originates the first pair of aortic arches and later also the second, third, fourth, and sixth arches (the fifth pair of aortic arches does not normally develop in mammals or is very rudimentary). The caudal half of the bulboventricular tube expands and represents the early embryonic ventricle. The atria are paired and lie extrapericardially, caudal to the embryonic ventricles, embedded in mesenchyme.

The growing bulboventricular tube bends to the right and anteriorly, initially in the shape of the letter *C*, and later into a compound sigmoid structure: the bulboventricular loop. The deepening concavity on the left side of the bulboventricular loop is referred to as the bulboventricular or conoventricular groove or sulcus. Since the bending of the heart tube involves the entire cardiac wall, the bulboventricular sulcus corresponds internally to a fold, the bulboventricular, or conoventricular, fold. At this stage the descending limb of the loop is called the embryonic ventricle, the ascending limb the bulbus cordis.

Cardiac looping appears to be due to a fundamental property of the myocardium[6–9] rather than being a passive phenomenon brought about by the necessity for the rapidly lengthening bulboventricular loop to accommodate itself to the smaller available space in the coelomic (pericardial) cavity as was thought previously.[10,11]

Since the arterial and venous poles of the heart tube are fixed, bending of the tube imparts upon it a certain amount of torsion which is at least in part responsible for the spiral disposition of the later developing truncoconal septum. The atrioventricular junction, which at first lies in the midline, is crowded laterally to the left. The embryonic ventricle moves to the left side of the pericardial cavity and the right side of this cavity is now occupied by the rapidly enlarging bulbus cordis.

Initial changes within the endocardial tube are concerned mainly with the development of local expansions throughout its length (Figs. 1-2, 1-3). The atrial portion of the heart dilates to form a large common atrium. The atrioventricular junction, the atrioventricular canal, remains relatively narrow and shifts cephalad and mesiad. The ventricle and the proximal one-third of the bulbus cordis expand, while the junction between them, the primary interventricular foramen, remains narrow and comes to lie approximately in the midsagittal plane (Figs. 1-2, 1-3).[11]

Anomalies *Ventricular Inversion with Transposition of the Great Arteries.* If the cardiac loop is formed to the left and anterior rather than to the right and anterior, then all structures derived from the bulboventricular loop, i.e., the atrioventricular valves, the ventricles, and the arterial roots, will develop in

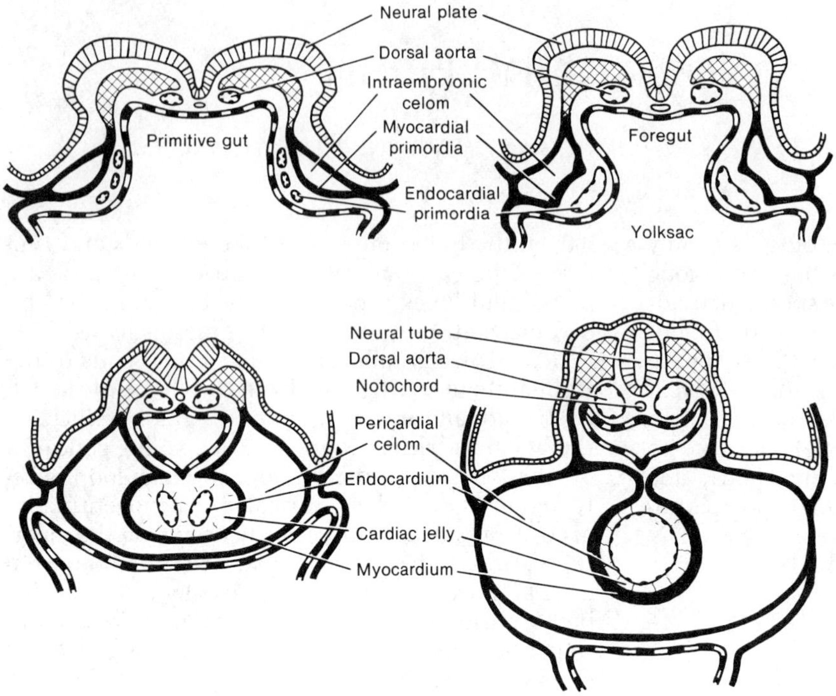

FIGURE 1-1 Schematic transverse sections through embryos of different ages, showing formation of the single heart tube. (*Adapted from several sources.*)

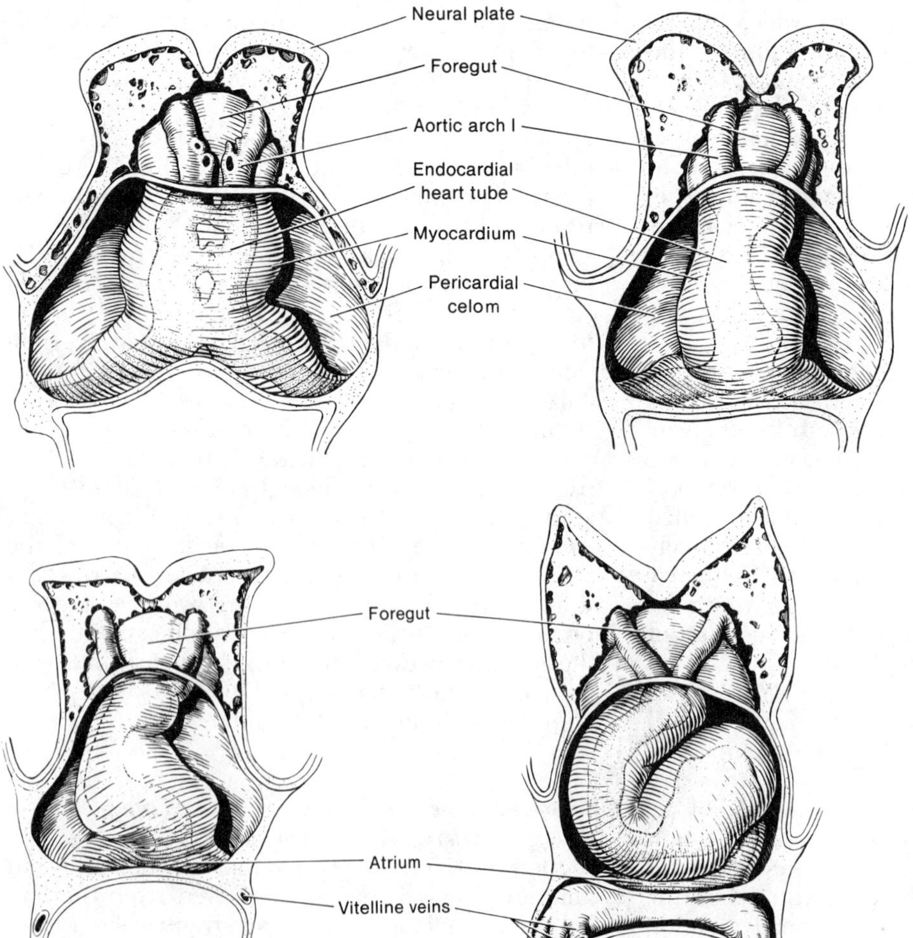

FIGURE 1-2 Schematic ventral dissections of human embryos of different ages, showing formation of the heart loop. (*From C. L. Davis, Development of the Human Heart from Its First Appearance to the Stage Found in Embryos of Twenty Paired Somites, Contrib. Embryol., 19:245, 1927. Adapted from and reproduced with permission from Carnegie Institution of Washington.*)

an inverted position. Since the truncoaortic sac, the atria, and the sinus venosus all lie extrapericardially, these parts of the heart will be normally located. The aorticopulmonary septum also develops in a normal fashion, but since partitioning of the inverted truncus arteriosus takes place in mirror-image fashion, the end result is transposition of the great arteries with the aorta arising anteriorly from a left-sided, morphologically right ventricle and the pulmonary trunk posteriorly from a right-sided left ventricle, hence the term *corrected transposition* commonly used for this anomaly.

The Primitive Ventricles, the Conus Cordis, and the Truncus Arteriosus

At the close of this phase of development, diverticula appear in two sharply defined areas along the right and left ventrolateral borders of the endocardial tube just proximal to, and distal from, the primary interventricular foramen[12] (i.e., in the early embryonic ventricle and in the proximal one-third of the bulbus cordis; Fig. 1-3). These diverticula develop initially at the expense of the cardiac jelly, and later also penetrate the myocardium as the latter increases in thickness, producing a spongy mass of trabeculae. Thus, the capacity of the heart is increased.

Although externally the appearance of the heart has changed considerably, functionally it still consists essentially of a single tube. The trabeculated, embryonic ventricle may now be called the primitive left ventricle, since it will contribute the major portion of the definitive left ventricle (Fig. 1-3). Similarly, the proximal one-third of the bulbus cordis, also trabeculated, may be called the *primitive right ventricle.*[13]

At this stage of development the embryo is approximately 3 mm long, and has an ovulation age of about 25 days.[2] The heart completely occupies the pericardial cavity, with the primitive left ventricle located on the left side and the bulbus cordis on the right. Because of future developments, it now becomes helpful to distinguish three sections in the bulbus cordis, of which the proximal trabeculated one-third is the primitive right ventricle. From the adjacent middle one-third of the bulbus, the conus cordis, the outflow portions of both ventricles will be derived. The terminal one-third of the bulbus, after partitioning, develops into the aortic and pulmonary roots and may, therefore, be appropriately called the *truncus arteriosus.* The distalmost portion of the truncus arteriosus, together with the adjoining aortic sac from which the aortic arches arise, is called the *truncoaortic sac.*

The rapid growth and expansion of the primitive atria causes the truncoconal section of the bulbus cordis to shift from its initial far lateral position to a more medial location. The result is that the truncus arteriosus comes to lie in a midsagittal position, in a depression of the atrial roof between the primitive right and left atria; the conus cordis assumes an oblique position and lies between the roof of the primitive left ventricle and the anteromedial wall of the right atrium. In an embryo of approximately 4 to 5 mm crown-rump (C-R) length (ovulation age of approximately 27 days), the external shape of the heart already suggests its future four-chambered condition. The stage is now set for septation of the heart, and no major changes in the external ap-

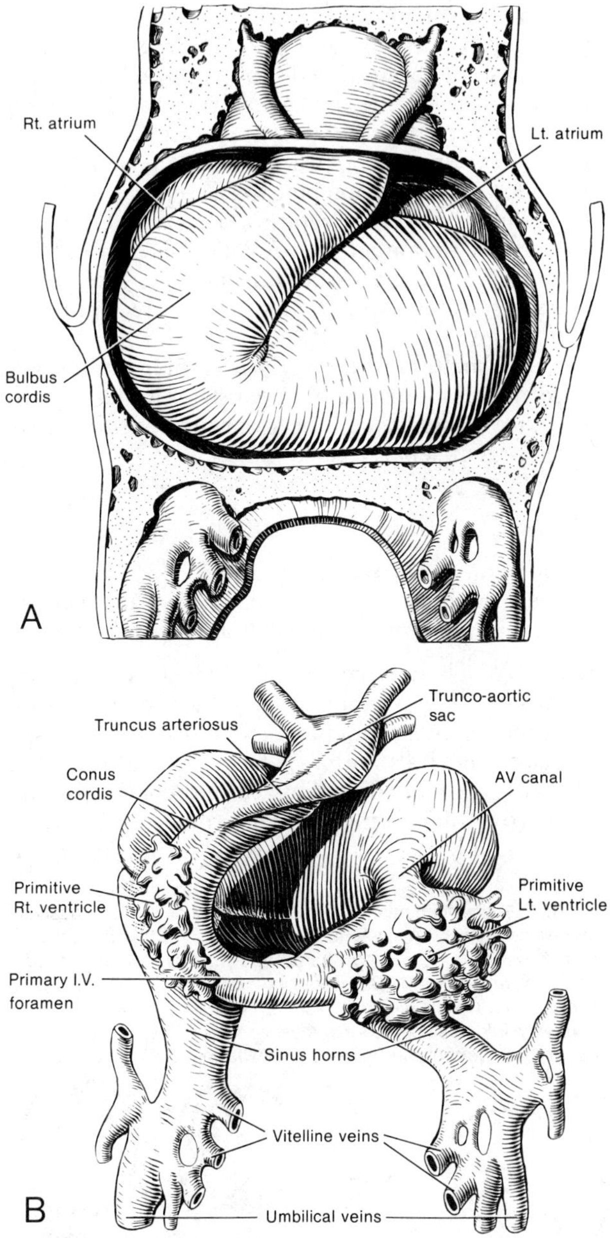

FIGURE 1-3 Twenty human somite embryos, ovulation age about 25 days. *A.* Ventral dissection. *B.* Reconstruction of cardiac lumen. [*Adapted from an original painting by Frank H. Netter, M.D., that appeared in L.H.S. Van Mierop, Embryology of the Heart, in F. H. Netter (ed.), "The CIBA Collection of Medical Illustrations," CIBA Pharmaceutical Company, Summit, N.J., 1969, vol. 5, pt. I, p. 112. Copyright by CIBA Pharmaceutical Company, Division of CIBA-GEIGY Corporation. Reproduced with permission from the publisher, editor, and author.*]

pearance of the heart other than size will take place while that process goes on over the next 10 days.

Because of rapid growth and continually changing curvature of the embryo during the following period of growth and development, it becomes difficult to continue to appreciate spatial relations. In the following discussion on cardiac septation, therefore, the diaphragm (septum transversum) is assumed to maintain an approximately horizontal position as in the adult, standing person. The terms *anterior, posterior, superior,* and *inferior* are employed accordingly.

The formation of the various cardiac septa takes place more or less simultaneously; for descriptive purposes, however, it is necessary to consider their development separately.

Septation of the Heart

Mechanisms of Cardiac Septation

There are three ways in which a septum can be formed in a hollow organ such as the heart:[5]

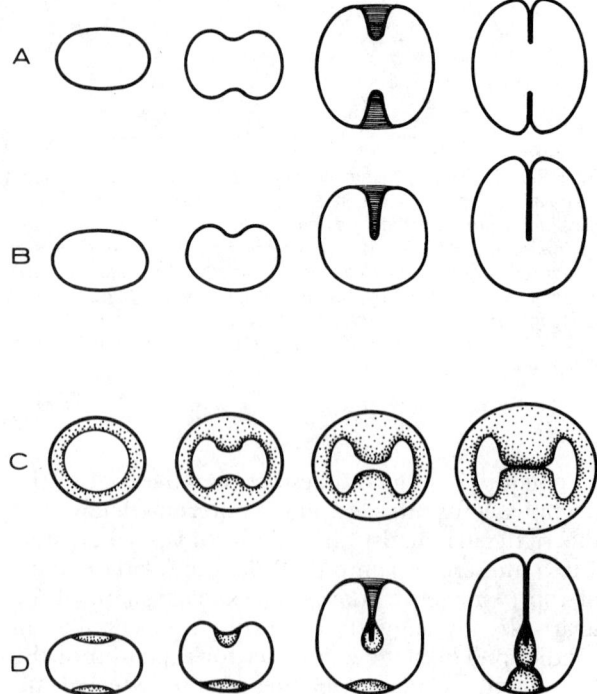

1. A relatively narrow segment increases in diameter only slowly or not at all, while on either side of the segment, rapid and expansive growth takes place (Fig. 1-4*A* and *B*). The portion of the walls of the expanded regions on either side of the narrow intervening segment come to face each other, appose, and fuse. If growth takes place more or less equally everywhere, the particular portion of the heart, after fusion of the opposing walls, is transformed into a structure containing a diaphragm with a central opening. Usually, however, expansive growth takes place mainly in one direction, resulting in the formation of a septum with an eccentrically placed communication between the two adjoining chambers. A septum formed in this fashion is simply a duplication of the wall of the organ and can never be complete: there is always an opening in it somewhere. If fusion of the apposing walls occurs very early and keeps pace with the expansive growth of the cardiac section involved, the fact that the septum is a duplication may never be very obvious, and it may look more like a ridge or a membrane.
2. An entirely different mechanism of septum formation may be observed in portions of the heart which possess a well-developed layer of cardiac mesenchyme ("endocardial cushion tissue") between the myocardium and the endocardium (e.g., the atrioventricular canal, the conus cordis, and the truncus arteriosus). This cardiac mesenchymal tissue is derived from, or at any rate replaces, the earlier cardiac jelly. Local elaborations of such cardiac mesenchyme form two opposing masses of tissue, grow toward each other, and fuse. These masses of mesenchymal tissue have a characteristic appearance in microscopic sections, stain lightly, and contain relatively fewer nuclei than the surrounding tissue. They are large and bulky and are called "cushions." When fully formed, septa developed in this manner are complete, and their thickness characteristically equals or exceeds their height in the early phases of their development (Fig. 1-4*C*).
3. Occasionally a septum in its initial phases of development is formed passively, but is completed by actively growing cushion tissue present along its free edge (Fig. 1-4*D*).

FIGURE 1-4 Mechanisms of cardiac septation. *A, B.* Passively formed septum. *C.* Actively formed septum. *D.* Combination of *B* and *C.* [*From L. H. S. Van Mierop, Morphological Development of the Heart, in R. M. Berne (ed.), "Handbook of Physiology," sec. 2: "The Cardiovascular System," vol. 1: "The Heart," American Physiological Society, Bethesda, Md., 1979, p. 11. Reproduced with permission from the publisher, editor, and author.*]

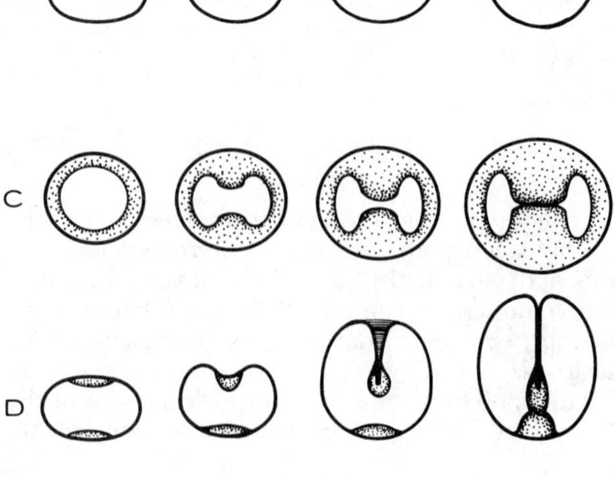

Partitioning of the embryonic heart is accomplished by the formation of seven septa. Of these, three are formed passively (septum secundum of the atrium, the muscular portion of the ventricular septum, and the aorticopulmonary septum), three are formed actively (the septum of the atrioventricular canal, the conal septum, and the truncal septum). One, the atrial septum primum, starts out as a passively formed septum, but it is completed by actively growing tissue along its border, probably derived from the atrioventricular endocardial cushions.

The Ventricles

In the 3-mm embryo, the primitive right and left ventricles are little more than local expansions of the original cardiac tube.[2] They are connected to each other by the smooth-walled, relatively narrow primary interventricular foramen, and trabeculae

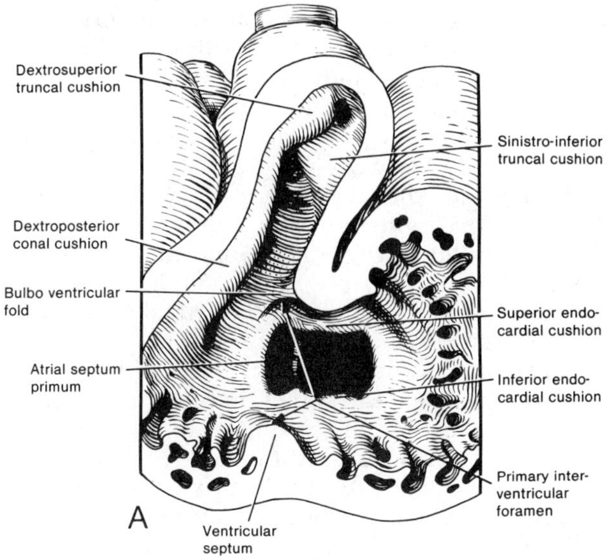

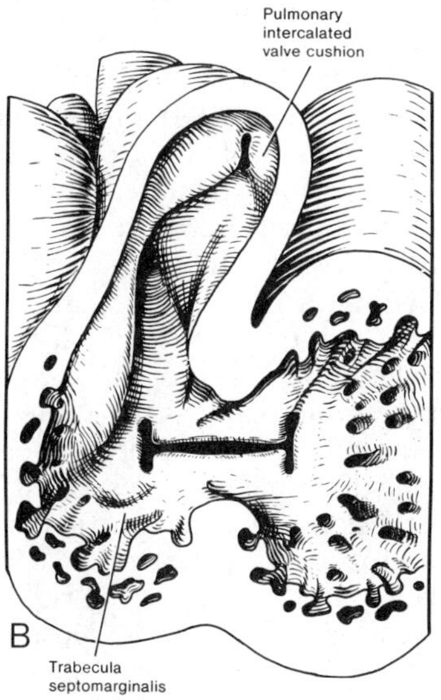

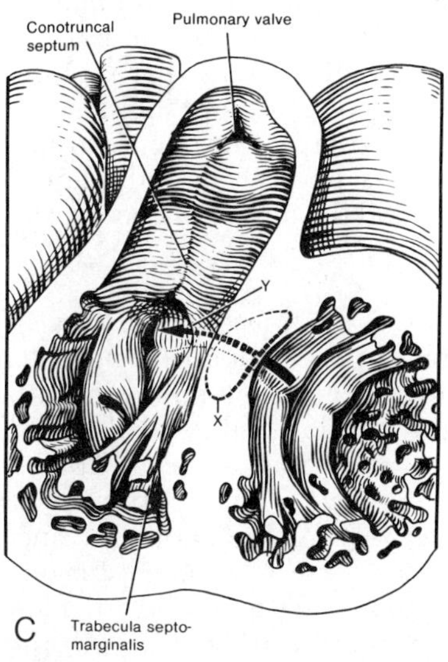

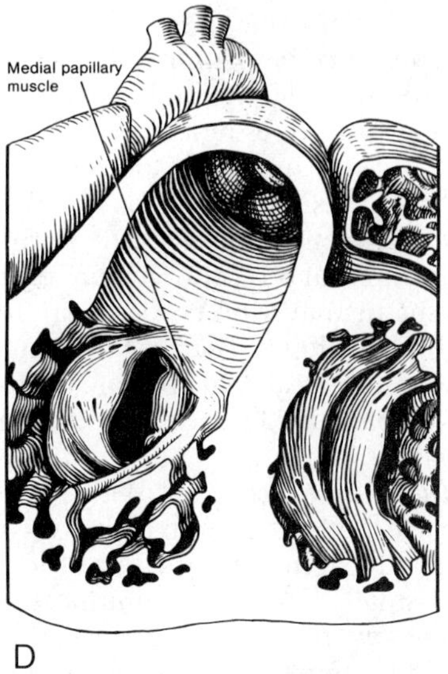

FIGURE 1-5 Schematic frontal section through the heart of embryos of *A.* 6.5 mm, *B.* 9 mm, *C.* 16 mm, *D.* 40 mm C-R length. X = primary interventricular foramen; Y = secondary interventricular foramen. (*From L. H. S. Van Mierop, R. D. Alley, H. W. Kausel, and A. Stranahan, The Anatomy and Embryology of Endocardial Cushion Defects, J. Thorac. Cardiovasc. Surg., 43:71, 1962. Redrawn with permission from the publisher and author.*)

have just begun to make their appearance in each (Fig. 1-3).

In an embryo of about 5 mm C-R length, the atrioventricular (AV) canal leads exclusively into the primitive left ventricle and blood can reach the primitive right ventricle only by way of the primary interventricular foramen, the borders of which are formed by the developing muscular interventricular septum inferiorly and anteriorly, and by the bulboventricular fold superiorly and posteriorly (Fig. 1-5*A*). The interventricular septum and the bulboventricular fold are continuous with each other anterosuperiorly.

The ventricles enlarge by centrifugal growth of the myocardium, closely followed by increasing diverticulation and formation of trabeculae internally to prevent the compact outer layer of the myocardium from becoming too thick.

The medial walls of the growing and expanding ventricles appose and fuse, forming the major portion of the muscular ventricular septum.[11,14–16] On the right side, a large trabecula, the trabecula septomarginalis,[17] appears early (in embryos of about 9 mm C-R length) and runs from the anteroinferior border of the primary interventricular foramen toward the apex (Fig. 1-5*B*).

The primary interventricular foramen never closes but actually enlarges, and in the fully developed heart gives access to the aortic infundibulum, or vestibule.[11,16,18]

Anomalies *Single Ventricle, Left Ventricular Type with Rudimentary Outflow Chamber.* If the early embryonic atrioventricular canal fails to shift medially, retains its far leftward position, and divides into right and left atrioventricular ostia, then both these ostia continue to empty into the primitive left ventricle. The proximal one-third of the bulbus (primitive right ventricle) therefore does not receive the right atrioventricular ostium, its inflow portion will not develop, and as a result it remains small. The communication between the large ventricular chamber and the rudimentary outflow chamber represents the persistent primary interventricular foramen of the young embryo heart. Because the main chamber has the morphological features of a left ventricle, this anomaly has also been referred to as a *double inlet left ventricle.*

Double Inlet Right Ventricle. With a double inlet right ventricle both atrioventricular valves enter a morphologically right ventricle, and the left ventricle is a very small chamber communicating with the right ventricle by means of a basilar ventricular septal defect. This anomaly can be thought of as being due to excessive rightward shift of the atrioventricular canal. Generally, both great arteries arise from the right ventricle as well; i.e., a double outlet right ventricle is associated.

Double Outlet Right Ventricle. A double outlet right ventricle appears to be due to a lack of medial shift of the conus cordis, which retains its original embryological relation with the right ventricle only. The bulboventricular fold is retained and separates the two arterial ostia from the atrioventricular ostia (aortic-mitral valve discontinuity).

The Atrioventricular Canal

Division of the atrioventricular canal into a right and left atrioventricular orifice is executed by a pair of opposing masses of mesenchymal tissue, the superior and inferior atrioventricular endocardial cushions, which make their appearance at the superior and inferior borders of the canal in embryos of about 6 mm C-R length (Fig. 1-5). At this time, the atrioventricular canal and the truncoconal region of the heart have begun to realign themselves, and both have shifted medially from the far lateral position seen in younger specimens. At 6 mm, this shift has not been completed as yet: the atrioventricular canal gives access to the primitive left ventricle only and is separated from the conus cordis by the bulboventricular fold. With further development, the central portion of this fold recedes, and blood can now enter the primitive right ventricle directly from the atrium (Fig. 1-5). In embryos of about 9 mm C-R length, the left-sided portion of the fold is seen to terminate almost midway along the base of the superior endocardial cushion and is much less prominent (Fig. 1-5*B*); the right-sided portion becomes part of the parietal band. In older embryos, both the shift to the left and the effacement of the central part continue until this portion eventually becomes unrecognizable as such. As a result, the plane of the primary interventricular foramen (the posterosuperior border of which is formed, as we have seen, by the bulboventricular fold) inclines more and more to the left from an originally vertical position. As a further result, direct access is gained from the primitive left ventricle to the posteromedial portion of the conus cordis (by way of the primary interventricular foramen) and therefore to the aorta.

Meanwhile, the atrioventricular canal has enlarged to the right while the growing endocardial cushions project progressively into the lumen and approach each other (Fig. 1-5*B*). Similar but much smaller cushions appear on the lateral borders of the atrioventricular canal.

In embryos of about 10 mm C-R length, the major cushions reach each other and fuse, resulting in a complete division of the canal into right and left atrioventricular orifices. At the same time the cushions also bend, and after fusion they eventually form an arch which has its concavity directed anteriorly and toward the left ventricle[11,19] and its convexity directed posteriorly toward the atria (Figs. 1-5*C*, 1-8). The free margin of the atrial septum primum meets the convex atrial side of the fused endocardial cushions about midway between their extremities and fuses with them (Fig. 1-7*C*). That portion of the endocardial cushions to the left of the septum primum, i.e., the left limb of the arch, eventually becomes incorporated into the anterior or aortic cusp of the mitral valve, and therefore does not participate in the formation of the cardiac septum.

With deepening of the endocardial cushion arch or bay, the right half of the fused endocardial cushions comes to lie more and more in a sagittal plane, i.e., in about the same plane as but somewhat to the right of the muscular interventricular septum. The communication still remaining between right and left ventricles, the secondary interventricular foramen, is bordered at this point by the muscular ventricular septum inferiorly and anteriorly, the right extremity of the fused endocardial cushions posteriorly, and the conal septum superiorly (Fig. 1-5*C*). The plane of the secondary interventricular foramen, therefore, inclines somewhat to the right, while that of the primary interventricular foramen, as we have seen, has come to deviate to the left. They share, however, the top of the muscular septum as part of their inferior borders. Before the closure of the secondary interventricular foramen can be discussed, it is necessary first to direct our attention to the truncus arteriosus and the developments which have taken place there.

Anomalies *Persistent Atrioventricular Canal.* There are several forms of persistent atrioventricular canal, all due to various degrees of failure of fusion of the superior and inferior endocardial cushions of the embryonic atrioventricular canal. Total lack of fusion results in a single atrioventricular ostium, i.e., the complete form of the anomaly. Since the arch or bay normally formed after the fusion of the endocardial cushions fails to develop, the lower border of the atrial septum cannot fuse with the endocardial cushions. The result is a low-lying, large interatrial communication, and the atrioventricular part of the cardiac septum is absent. The upper part of the ventricular septum remains deficient to a greater or lesser degree, and there is an interventricular communication.

In the partial forms of the anomaly the endocardial cushions fuse centrally only and the arch is generally not formed. The result is an interatrial communication or so-called ostium primum–type atrial septal defect. The upper part of the muscular ventricular septum remains deficient, but this area of the ventricular septum is closed by fibrous tissue. Because the left side of the endocardial cushions does not fuse, the anterior or aortic cusp of the mitral valve is cleft. Occasionally the arch is formed well enough so that the atrial septum does fuse with the partially fused endocardial cushions, producing a form of partial persistent atrioventricular canal with an intact atrial septum but with an interventricular communication and a cleft anterior mitral valve cusp. The aortic valve in all forms of persistent atrioventricular canal cannot descend to assume its proper position and therefore is located somewhat higher and farther to the right than in a normal heart. This, in addition to the deficiency of the basilar part of the muscular ventricular septum, accounts for the elongated left ventricular outflow tract ("gooseneck" deformity) characteristic of this group of anomalies.

Ventricular Septal Defect. Some forms of perimembranous ventricular septal defect may be due to failure of fusion of the right extremity of the fused endocardial cushions and the upper border of the muscular ventricular septum and also the conal septum. Since the endocardial cushions fuse normally, there is no cleft in the anterior mitral valve cusp, nor is there an interatrial communication.

The Truncus Arteriosus

Septation of the truncoconal area of the bulbus cordis begins in embryos of about 6 mm C-R length with the appearance of two opposing truncal cushions (Fig. 1-5). One of these is located on the dextrosuperior wall of the truncus (dextrosuperior truncal cushion), the other on the sinistroinferior wall (sinistroinferior truncal cushion).

The cushions rapidly enlarge and fuse to form the truncal septum, thus dividing the truncus into aortic and pulmonary channels. The truncus is the first part of the heart to become partitioned (embryos of about 7 mm C-R length). The truncal cushions (and therefore the truncal septum) are large and bulky, and to accommodate them the initially slender truncal area of the heart expands.

Meanwhile, the truncal cushions proximally meet the distal extremities of a similar pair of mesenchymal masses developing in the conus cordis: the conal cushions. With further growth, the distal surface of the fused truncal cushions presents a front which faces the origin of the sixth aortic arches (Fig. 1-5). The distal, still undivided portion of the truncus, together with the adjacent aortic sac, dilates to form the truncoaortic sac. At the same time, the sixth arches move closer together and to the left, their most proximal portions probably fusing for a short distance. The origins of the fourth aortic arches (from the roof of the truncoaortic sac) shift somewhat to the right. As a result, the sixth arches become aligned with the pulmonary channel and the fourth arches with the aortic channel. At the same time, the dorsal wall of the truncoaortic sac between the origins of the fourth and sixth arches invaginates to form a vertical septum, the aorticopulmonary septum, the leading edge of which approaches the distal face of the truncal septum with which it fuses.[11,13,20,21]

Partitioning of the truncoaortic area is complete in embryos of about 9 mm C-R length.

Anomalies *Persistent Truncus Arteriosus.* If the truncal cushions remain hypoplastic and fail to fuse, partitioning of the truncus arteriosus does not take place. If, in addition to the hypoplastic truncal cushions, both intercalated valve cushions are present, these structures may each form a valve cusp, and the result is a quadricuspid truncal valve. Fusion between adjacent valve anlagen may produce a tricuspid truncal valve in which one of the cusps is larger than the other two and contains a raphe indicating its dual origin. This is the most commonly seen condition. In the great majority of cases, the aorticopulmonary septum does develop and a short common pulmonary trunk arises from the persistent trunk. In the few cases where it does not, the two pulmonary arteries arise independently from the major trunk. Usually the conal cushions also fail to fuse and the infundibular septum therefore is absent as well. The ductus arteriosus is almost always absent, except when interruption of the aortic arch is associated.

Aorticopulmonary Septal Defect. Aorticopulmonary septal defect appears to be due to failure of fusion between the distal extremity of the truncal septum and the aorticopulmonary septum. Both arterial valves are present, but there is a communication of varying size between the ascending aorta and the pulmonary trunk.

The Conus Cordis

The conal cushions make their appearance at about the same time as do the truncal cushions (Fig. 1-5). One is located on the dextrodorsal wall, the other on the sinistroventral wall of the conus cordis. The dextrodorsal conal cushion becomes continuous with the dextrosuperior truncal cushion, and the sinistroventral conal cushion with the sinistroinferior truncal cushion. Fusion of the conal cushions begins proximally, progressing rapidly in a distal direction to complete the partition of the truncoconal part of the heart in embryos of about 14 to 15 mm C-R length.

With completion of the conal septum, the originally large interventricular communication becomes much reduced in size, and in a 15- to 16-mm embryo the remaining small secondary interventricular foramen is bordered by the conal septum, by the top of the muscular ventricular septum, and by the right extremities of the fused endocardial cushions, all of which contribute to its closure. This region is initially quite thick, and only much later (fetus of about 3 months), and with the formation of the anterior portion of the septal (medial) cusp of the tricuspid valve, does an area of variable extent become thin and fibrous: the interventricular part of the membranous septum. That part of the endocardial cushion arch or bay between the junction with the septum primum and the ventricular septum also becomes the atrioventricular portion of the membranous septum (Fig. 1-6).

Anomalies *Ventricular Septal Defect, Eisenmenger Type.* Hypoplasia or absence of the conal cushions results in a large basilar septal defect, dextroposition of the aortic valve, and a hypoplastic or absent infundibular septum.

Ventricular Septal Defect, Supracristal Type. This type of interventricular communication is due either to simple failure of fusion of truncal and conal septa or to malalignment between these septa which makes fusion impossible.

Tetralogy of Fallot. The basic anomaly in tetralogy of Fallot appears to be an anterior displacement of varying degree of the conal septum which leads to unequal partitioning of the conus at the expense of the right ventricular infundibulum, hence the infundibular stenosis. The displaced conal septum cannot participate in the closure of the interventricular foramen. There is therefore a very large basilar ventricular septal defect and dextroposition of the aortic valve. Pulmonary valvar anomalies, while commonly associated, are not an essential feature of tetralogy of Fallot.

The Sinus Venosus

In a 4-mm embryo, the sinus venosus consists of a central unpaired part, the transverse portion of the sinus venosus, and the right and left sinus horns (Figs. 1-3, 1-7). It receives three pairs of veins: the omphalomesenteric (vitelline) veins, the umbilical (allantoic) veins, and the common cardinal veins. At

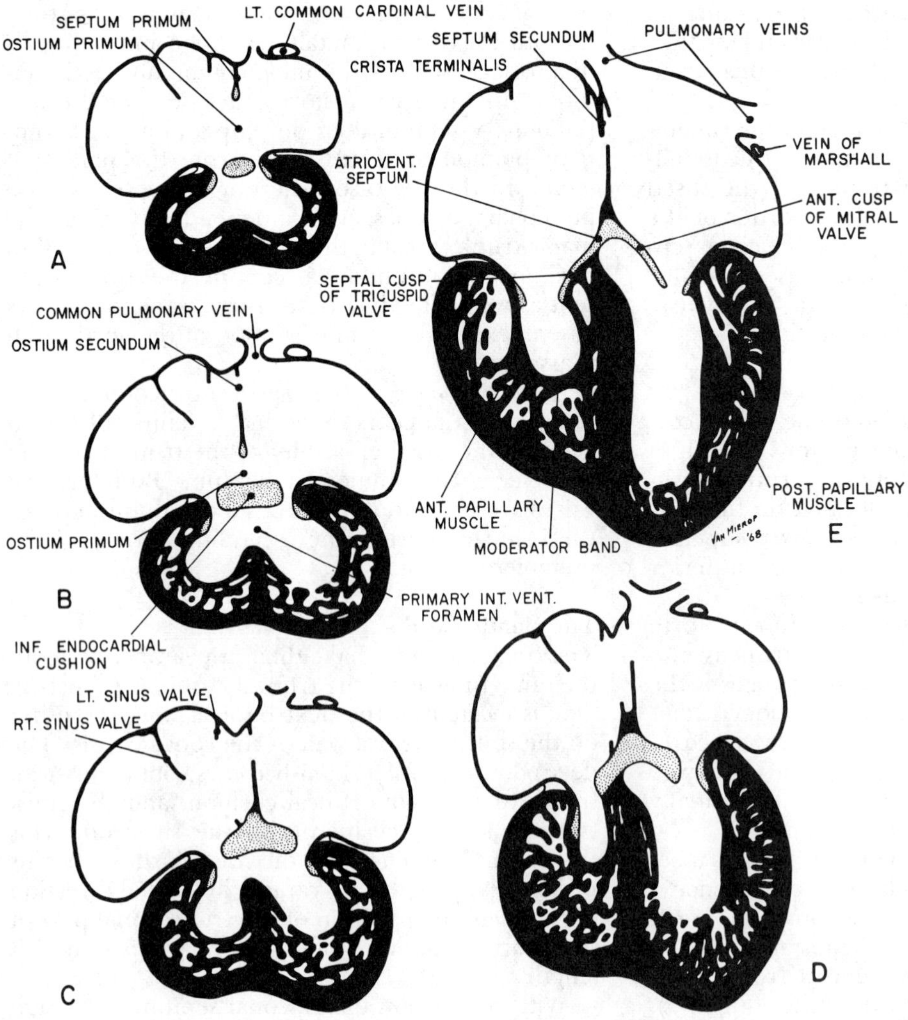

FIGURE 1-6 Sections through heart of embryos of different ages. Diagrammatic. *A.* 6 mm. *B.* 9 mm. *C.* 12 mm. *D.* 17 mm. *E.* 40 mm. [*From L. H. S. Van Mierop, Embryology of the Atrioventricular Canal Region, in R. H. Feldt (ed.), "Atrioventricular Canal Defects," W. B. Saunders Company, Philadelphia, 1976, p. 6. Reproduced with permission from the publisher, editor, and author.*]

first, the sinus venosus is not well demarcated from the atrium. Later, the left horn and the transverse portion of the sinus venosus become more and more separated from the left side of the atrium by the development of a deep fold which, in the fully developed heart, represents the wall between the coronary sinus and the left atrium (Fig. 1-7*B* to *D*). The proximal portions of the umbilical veins soon disappear. Owing to the development of anastomotic channels between right and left systemic veins and preferential flow of blood to the right side, the right sinus horn and proximal cardinal and vitelline veins gain in size and importance, while their left counterparts become greatly attenuated. The right sinus horn attains a vertical position, becomes incorporated into the right atrium to form the smooth-walled, intercaval part of the atrium, and the communication between the sinus venosus and the atrium is now limited to this horn. The transverse portion and the proximal left sinus horn become the coronary sinus; the distal left sinus horn and left common cardinal vein normally obliterate (ligament of Marshall).

On the right side, the cardiac wall at the sinoatrial junction also folds in, as on the left, and forms the right sinus valve (Figs. 1-3, 1-6). Another, smaller fold, the left sinus valve, appears somewhat later on the left side of the sinoatrial junction, so that in a 4- to 6-mm embryo the vertical sinoatrial orifice is flanked on either side by a valvelike structure (Fig. 1-6). Superiorly, the sinus valves join to form a single fold, the septum spurium. The sinus valves, particularly the right sinus valve, are relatively very large in a 16-mm embryo, but later they usually disappear almost completely. The left sinus valve fuses with the atrial septum. The inferior part of the right sinus valve is divided into a larger inferior vena caval (eustachian) valve and a smaller coronary sinus (thebesian) valve; the remainder usually disappears.

Anomalies *Cor Triatriatum Dexter.* Total persistence of the right sinus valve of the embryonic heart produces a septum in the right atrium separating the intercaval part of the right atrium from the atrial body. The remaining opening may be quite small and restrictive.

Persistent Left Superior Vena Cava. Persistence of the left sinus horn and left common cardinal vein results in a left superior vena cava entering the coronary sinus.

The Atria, Atrial Septum, and Pulmonary Veins

In a 3-mm embryo expansion of the atrial portion of the heart is well underway (Fig. 1-3). Owing to the presence of the truncus arteriosus, a depression is formed in the roof of the common atrium. As expansion proceeds, the depression deepens, corresponding internally to a sickle-shaped crest. This is the first indication of the septum primum. Its free edge is directed toward the atrioventricular canal, and the foramen between the left and right primitive atria which it borders is the ostium primum (Fig. 1-6). Extensions from the superior and inferior endocardial cushions grow along the edge of the septum primum. Proliferation of this tissue with the concomitant fusion of the endocardial cushions brings about closure of the ostium primum, a process which is completed in embryos of about 10 to 11 mm C-R length. Meanwhile, perforations have appeared in the septum primum posterosuperiorly. These rapidly coalesce to form the ostium secundum, thus ensuring continued free communication between the right and left primitive atria. Expansive growth of the atria and infolding of the atrial wall between the

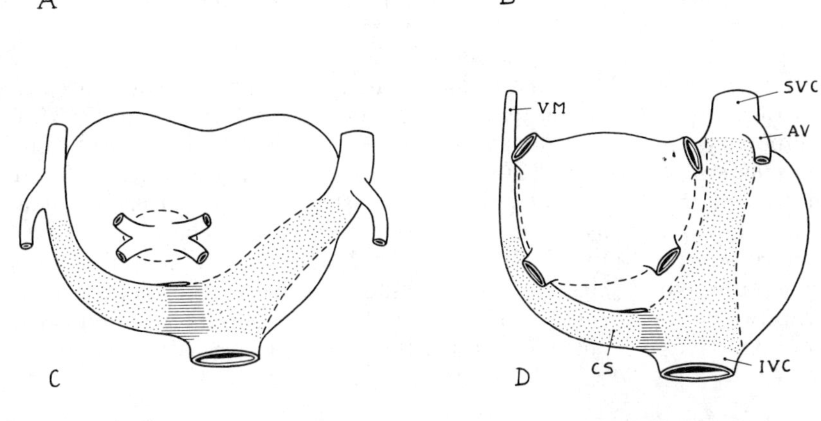

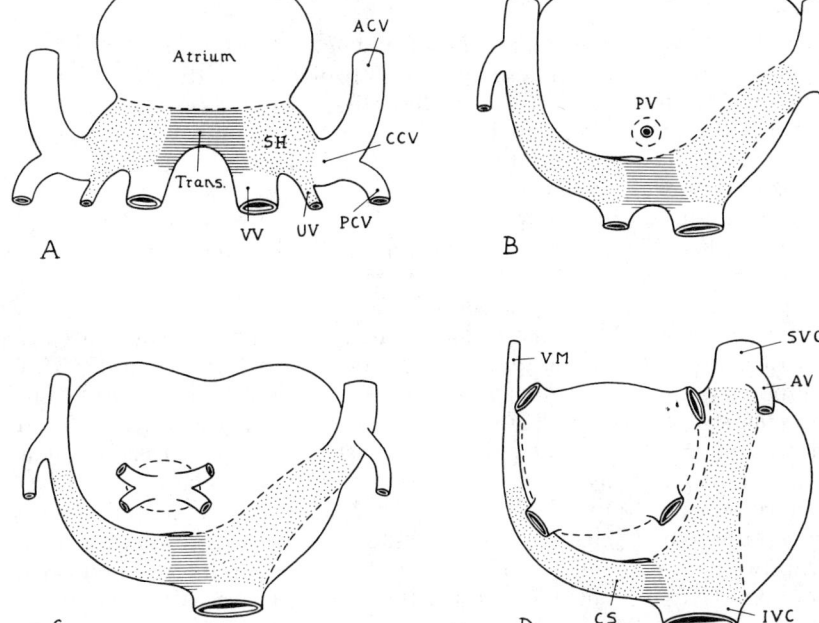

FIGURE 1-7 Posterior view of the atria and sinus venosus in embryos of *A.* 3 mm, *B.* 5 mm, *C.* 12 mm, C-R length. *D.* Postnatal. Diagrammatic. A(C)CV = anterior (common) cardinal vein; AV = azygos vein; CS = coronary sinus; IVC = inferior vena cava; PCV = posterior cardinal vein; PV = pulmonary vein; SH = sinus horn; UV = umbilical vein; VM = vein of Marshall; VV = vitelline vein; SVC = superior vena cava. (*From L. H. S. Van Mierop and F. W. Wiglesworth, Isomerism of the Cardiac Atria in the Aplenia Syndrome, Lab. Invest., 11:1303, 1962. Reproduced with permission from the publisher and author.*)

left sinus valve and septum primum produces the posterosuperior part of the septum secundum. The anteroinferior part of the septum secundum is believed to have a different origin.[22–24] The opening bordered by the free edge of the septum secundum is the foramen ovale. Postnatally, after fusion of the septum primum and the septum secundum, the foramen ovale becomes the fossa ovalis, and the free edge of the septum secundum is then called the *limbus fossae ovalis.*

The single embryonic pulmonary vein, already well developed in a 5- to 6-mm embryo (Figs. 1-6, 1-7), develops as an outgrowth of the posterior left atrial wall near the atrial floor just to the left of the septum primum, and gains connections with the splanchnic plexus of veins in the region of the developing lung buds.[25–27] Later in development, the vein itself and parts of its first four branches expand tremendously and become incorporated into the embryonic left atrium to form the larger smooth part of the adult left atrium. In the fully developed heart, the original embryonic left atrium is represented by little more than the trabeculated atrial appendage. The intrapulmonary part of the splanchnic venous plexus ultimately loses its connections with the systemic veins and drains exclusively by way of the pulmonary veins.

Anomalies *Atrial Septal Defect at the Fossa Ovalis.* This anomaly, also referred to as a *secundum-type atrial septal defect,* is due to overresorption of the septum primum, producing a very large ostium secundum which cannot be guarded adequately by the septum secundum. Frequently, the septum secundum is also hypoplastic, further enlarging the atrial septal defect. In some cases the ostium secundum is normal but the septum secundum is absent. Total absence of both septum primum and septum secundum (common atrium) is rare and almost always associated with a form of persistent atrioventricular canal.

Anomalous Pulmonary Venous Connection. The total form of anomalous pulmonary venous connection presumably is due either to lack of development of the embryonic common pulmonary vein or to early involution and disappearance of this vein. One or more of the early embryonic channels connecting the pulmonary venous bed to the systemic venous circulation is retained. Depending upon which of these channels drains the pulmonary vascular bed, a number of types of total anomalous pulmonary venous connections are recognized. Partial anomalous pulmonary venous return is due to retention of a connection between part of the pulmonary venous system with the systemic venous circulation.

Cor Triatriatum Sinister. If incorporation of the common pulmonary vein into the left atrium does not take place and the common pulmonary venous ostium remains narrow, the result is a septum-like structure that divides the left atrium into two components, one of which receives the pulmonary veins and the other gives access to the mitral valve and left atrial appendage.

Development of the Heart Valves

The Atrioventricular Valves

In an embryo of about 10 to 12 mm C-R length, both atrioventricular orifices are surrounded by mesenchymal endocardial cushion-type tissue which has a provisional valve function.

The definitive atrioventricular valves, however, are derived only in very small part from this tissue. Nearly all the material contributing to the atrioventricular valve cusps is elaborated from the (muscular) ventricular wall, the internal layer of which is liberated by a process of diverticulation and undermining described earlier (Fig. 1-6). A "skirt" of ventricular muscle is formed at each atrioventricular orifice, originating from the atrioventricular junction and attached lower down to the ventricular walls or septum by trabeculae retained for this purpose.[5] All atrioventricular valve cusps are therefore thick and fleshy at first, and only later in development are they transformed into thin and fibrous cusps.[13]

As with the cusps themselves, the chordae tendineae are initially thick, muscular, and few in number; only later are they transformed into delicate fibrous strands. The papillary muscles remain muscular.

The atrioventricular valve cusps are not all formed at the same time. The anterior cusp of the mitral valve is the first to develop (12- to 14-mm embryo), followed shortly by the anterior cusp of the tricuspid valve and by the posterior cusp of the mitral valve (14- to 16-mm embryo). The posterior and septal cusps of the tricuspid valve are "liberated" much more slowly, and even in a 10- to 12-week-old fetus (50-mm C-R length) the anteriormost part of the septal cusp has not been formed.[11]

Anomalies *Tricuspid Valve Atresia, Mitral Valve Atresia.* These anomalies probably are due to fusion of endocardial cushion tissue which borders the atrioventricular canal in very young embryos, during or shortly after partitioning of the atrioventricular canal.

Ebstein's Anomaly of the Tricuspid Valve. Ebstein's anomaly is very likely due to an abnormality of the process of undermining of the myocardium.

The Arterial Valves

The primordia of the semilunar valves are already visible as small tubercles in a 9-mm embryo, just after partitioning of the truncus has been completed. Each truncal cushion carries a tubercle on the extremity of its distal face. One of each pair is assigned to pulmonary and aortic channels, respectively. On the walls of both aortic and pulmonary channels, opposite the fused truncus cushions, a third small cushion appears. These two intercalated valve cushions[20] form the third member of each arterial valve primordium (Figs. 1-5, 1-8). Beginning at the tubercles, the semilunar valve cusps and sinuses of Valsalva are probably formed by a process of excavation of the truncal and intercalated valve cushions in a proximal direction. This process appears well advanced in a 16-mm embryo, and is virtually completed in a 40-mm embryo. This could explain the "migration" of the arterial valves, which at first lie far distal to the more proximal position found in the fully developed heart.[18,28] Both the aortic and pulmonary roots, therefore, consisting of the sinuses of Valsalva and the semilunar valves, are derived from the truncus arteriosus and the truncal and intercalated valve cushions.

Anomalies *Bicuspid Arterial Valves.* A bicuspid aortic or pulmonary valve is due either to failure of development of an intercalated valve cushion, resulting in a valve with two approximately equal-sized cusps, neither containing a raphe, or, more commonly, to fusion of adjacent valve anlagen, in which case the cusps are generally unequal in size, with the larger containing a raphe of varying height.

Arterial Valve Stenosis or Atresia. Fusion of two or all three of the arterial valve anlagen produces stenosis or atresia of the valve.

Absent Arterial Valves. Absence of the pulmonary or aortic valve, particularly the latter, is a rare anomaly, and presumably is due to failure of development of arterial valve anlagen.

FIGURE 1-8 Development of the arterial valves. Diagrammatic.

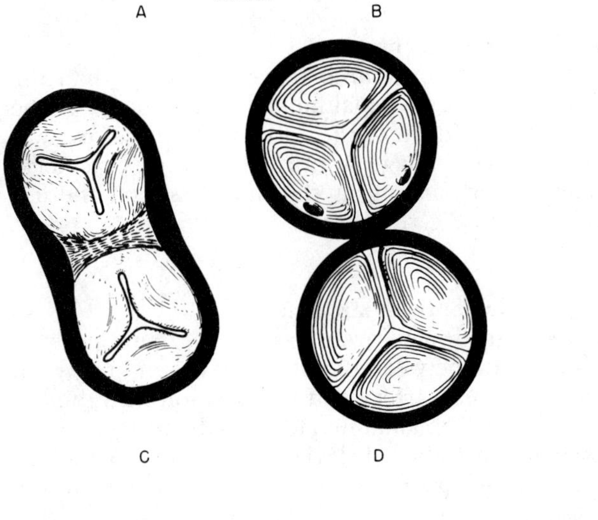

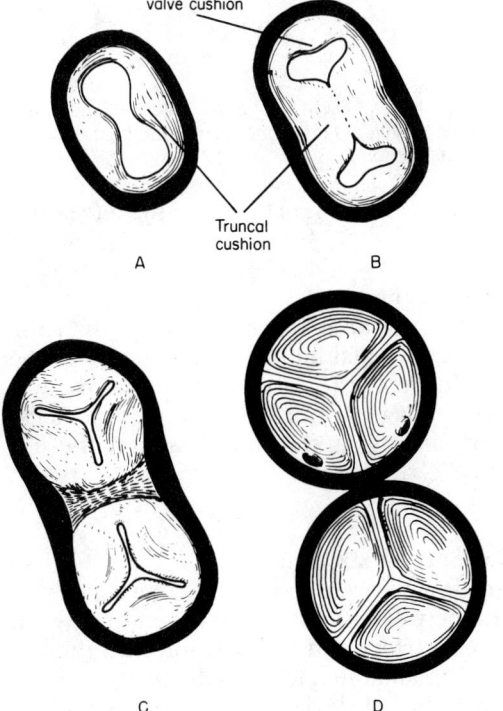

Development of the Aortic Arch System

In an embryo of about 3 mm the first pair of aortic arches is large and the second pair is just forming (Figs. 1-3, 1-9*A*). The dilated junction of the truncus arteriosus and the first pair of aortic arches is the aortic sac, from which subsequent aortic arches will originate, new arches being added caudally. A true ventral aorta is not present in mammalian embryos. Caudally the dorsal aortas fuse to form a single vessel; this fusion progresses craniad.

In a 4-mm embryo the first arch has largely disappeared with only a part of it persisting as a portion of the maxillary artery (Fig. 1-9*B*). The second aortic arch has also retrogressed; eventually all that remains is the tiny stapedial artery. The third aortic arch is well developed and the fourth and sixth arches are being formed as ventral and dorsal sprouts of the aortic sac and dorsal aorta, respectively. The ventral portion of the sixth arch already has as its major branch the primitive pulmonary artery even though the arch itself has not yet been completed. The fifth aortic arch in mammals is rudimentary and present only for a very brief time.

In a 10-mm embryo the first two aortic arches are no longer present as such and the third, fourth, and sixth are large (Fig. 1-9*C*). The truncoaortic sac has been divided by the formation of the aorticopulmonary septum so that the sixth arches are now continuous with the pulmonary trunk. Of the cervical intersegmental arteries the seventh pair will play an important role in the formation of the subclavian arteries. They are located at about the level where the dorsal aortas join each other.

In a 14-mm embryo the aortic arch system has largely lost its original symmetrical pattern (Fig. 1-9*D*). The segments of the dorsal aortas between the third and fourth arches, the carotid ducts, have disappeared, and the third arches begin to elongate as the heart descends farther into the thorax. This descent has also caused a relative shortening of the paired portion of the dorsal aorta. The dorsal portion of the right sixth arch has disappeared; its counterpart on the left persists until birth as the ductus arteriosus. The seventh intersegmental arteries have migrated craniad. The aortic sac has been "pulled out" on both sides: on the right it forms the brachiocephalic (innominate) trunk; on the left it becomes part of the definitive arch of the aorta up to the origin of the left third arch (common carotid artery).

In a 17-mm embryo the right dorsal aorta between its junction with the left dorsal aorta and the origin of the right seventh intersegmental artery has become attenuated and later disappears (Fig. 1-9*E*). The remainder of the right dorsal aorta persists and, with the right fourth aortic arch, forms the proximal subclavian artery.

After birth the distal part of the left sixth aortic arch, the ductus arteriosus, normally also obliterates

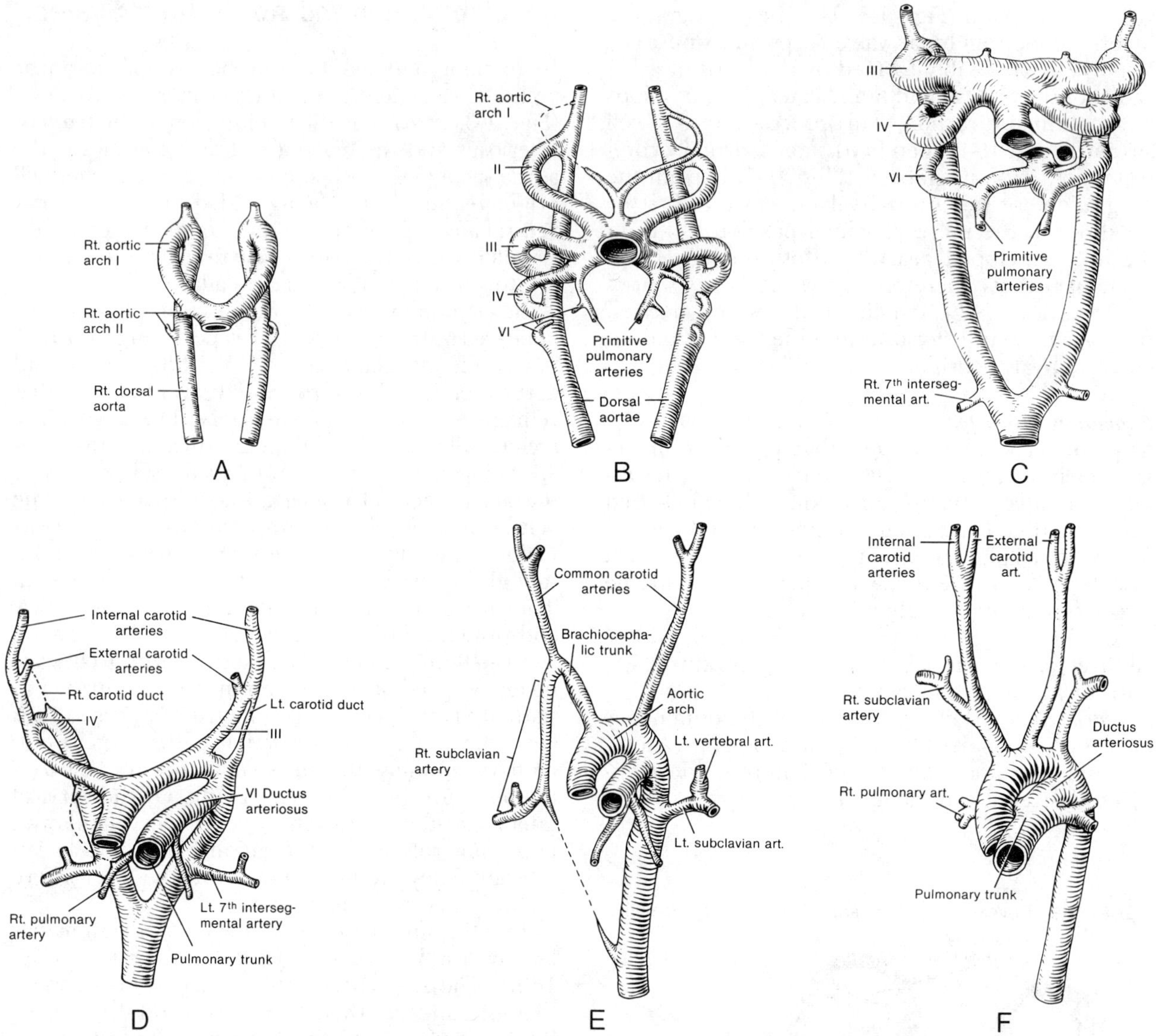

FIGURE 1-9 Development of the aortic arch system. Embryos of *A.* 3 mm, *B.* 4 mm, *C.* 10 mm, *D.* 14 mm, *E.* 17 mm C-R length, and *F.* neonate. (*From E. D. Congdon, Transformation of the Aortic Arch System during the Development of the Human Embryo, Contrib. Embryol., 14:47, 1922. Reproduced with permission from the Carnegie Institution of Washington.*)

and is converted to the ligamentum arteriosum. Thus the adult aortic arch system is established. See Table 1-1 for the ultimate fate of the various components of the embryonic aortic arch system.

Anomalies

Most aortic arch anomalies can be explained as being due to abnormal retention or disappearance of various segments.

Patent Ductus Arteriosus

A ductus arteriosus is anomalous only if it remains patent after birth.

Double Aortic Arch

A double aortic arch is the result of persistence and continued patency of the segment of the right dorsal aorta between the origin of the right seventh intersegmental artery and its junction with the left dorsal aorta.

Right Aortic Arch

With a right aortic arch the right rather than the left dorsal aorta is maintained in its entirety. The branching pattern of the aortic arch, therefore, will be the mirror image of normal with the brachiocephalic artery arising as the first vessel on the left rather than the right side.

Anomalous Subclavian Artery

If the right fourth arch disappears, then the right dorsal aorta between the origin of the right seventh intersegmental artery and the junction with the left dorsal aorta is maintained to form the proximal portion of the right subclavian artery. Because of its genesis, such a subclavian artery will arise from the

TABLE 1-1 Components of the Heart and Their Embryonic Origins

Embryonic Origin	Component of the Heart
1. Truncus arteriosus	Aortic and pulmonary roots
2. Aortic sac	Ascending aorta, brachiocephalic (innominate) artery, and aortic arch up to origin of left common carotid artery
3. First arches	Parts persist as components of the maxillary arteries
4. Second arches	Parts persist as the stapedial arteries
5. Third arches	Common carotid arteries and proximal segment of internal carotid arteries
6. Fourth arches	
a. Right	Most proximal segment of the right subclavian artery
b. Left	Aortic arch segment between the left common carotid and left subclavian arteries
7. Fifth arches	No known derivations; transient and never well developed
8. Sixth arches	
a. Right	Proximal part becomes proximal segment of the right pulmonary artery; distal part disappears early
b. Left	Proximal part becomes proximal segment of the left pulmonary artery; distal part persists, until birth, as ductus arteriosus
9. Right dorsal aorta	Cranial portion becomes part of the right subclavian artery; remainder disappears
10. Left dorsal aorta	Distal aortic arch
11. Right seventh intersegmental artery	Part of right subclavian artery
12. Left seventh intersegmental artery	Left subclavian artery

aortic arch distal to the left subclavian artery and course behind the esophagus to enter the right arm.

Interrupted Aortic Arch

In this anomaly the left fourth arch disappears. The ascending aorta has no connection with the descending aorta, which receives its blood from the pulmonary trunk by way of a patent ductus arteriosus. If both fourth arches disappear, then the right subclavian artery will arise anomalously, usually from the descending aorta, and the ascending aorta terminates into the two carotid arteries.[29]

Absent Left Pulmonary Artery

The left pulmonary artery almost always is absent only in the sense that it arises from a left-sided ductus arteriosus (or ligamentum arteriosum). The anomaly is the result of disappearance of the proximal left sixth arch. If, in this anomaly, the aortic arch is on the left side, then the ductus arteriosus which feeds the intrapulmonary part of the left pulmonary artery arises from the usual position on the underside of the arch. If the aortic arch is on the right, then the ductus arteriosus will arise from the brachiocephalic trunk with the left common carotid and left subclavian arteries as a trifurcation.

References

1. Davis, C. L.: Development of the Human Heart from Its First Appearance to the State Found in Embryos of 20 Paired Somites, *Contrib. Embryol.,* 19:245, 1927.
2. Davis, C. L.: Description of a Human Embryo Having 20 Paired Somites, *Contrib. Embryol.,* 15:1, 1923.
3. Davis, C. L.: The Cardiac Jelly of the Chick Embryo, *Anat. Rec.,* 27:201, 1924.
4. Van Mierop, L. H. S.: Embryology of the Heart, in F. H. Netter (ed.), "The CIBA Collection of Medical Illustrations," CIBA Pharmaceutical Co., Summit, N.J., 1969, vol. 5, pt. I, p. 112.
5. Van Mierop, L. H. S.: Morphological Development of the Heart, in R. M. Berne (ed.), "Handbook of Physiology," sec. 2: "The Cardiovascular System," vol. 1: "The Heart," American Physiological Society, Bethesda, Md., 1979, p. 1.
6. Castro-Quezada, A., Nadal-Ginard, B., and de la Cruz, M. V.: Experimental Study of the Formation of the Bulboventricular Loop in the Chick, *J. Embryol. Exp. Morphol.,* 27:623, 1972.
7. Manasek, F. J., Burnside, M. B., and Waterman, R. E.: Myocardial Cell Shape Change as a Mechanism of Embryonic Heart Looping, *Dev. Biol.,* 29:9, 1972.
8. Stalsberg, H.: Origin of Heart Asymmetry: Right and Left Contributions to the Early Chick Embryo Heart, *Dev. Biol.,* 19:109, 1969.
9. Stalsberg, H.: Mechanism of Dextral Looping of the Embryonic Heart, *Am. J. Cardiol.,* 25:265, 1970.
10. Patten, B. M.: The Formation of the Cardiac Loop in the Chick, *Am. J. Anat.,* 30:273, 1922.
11. Van Mierop, L. H. S., Alley, R. D., Kausel, H. W., and Stranahan, A.: Pathogenesis of Transposition Complexes: I. Embryology of the Ventricles and Great Arteries, *Am. J. Cardiol.,* 12:216, 1963.
12. Streeter, G. L.: Developmental Horizons in Human Embryos: Description of Age Groups XI, 13–20 Somites, and Age Group XII, 21–29 Somites, *Contrib. Embryol.,* 30:211, 1942.
13. Van Mierop, L. H. S., Alley, R. D., Kausel, H. W., and Stranahan, A.: The Anatomy and Embryology of Endocardial Cushion Defects, *J. Thorac. Cardiovasc. Surg.,* 43:71, 1962.
14. Streeter, G. L.: Developmental Horizons in Human Embryos: Description of Age Groups XV, XVI, XVII, XVIII, Being the Third Issue of a Survey of the Carnegie Collection, *Contrib. Embryol.,* 32:113, 1948.
15. Mall, F. P.: On the Development of the Human Heart, *Am. J. Anat.,* 13:249, 1912.
16. Keith, A.: The Hunterian Lectures on Malformation of the Heart, *Lancet,* 2:359, 433, 519, 1909.
17. Tandler, J.: Anatomie des Herzens, in "Bardeleben's Handbuch der Anatomie des Menschen," Gustav Fischer Verlag, Jena, 1913, p. 1.
18. Grant, R. P.: Embryology of Ventricular Flow Pathways in Man, *Circulation,* 25:756, 1962.
19. Los, J. A.: Embryology, in H. Watson (ed.), "Paediatric Cardiology," The C. V. Mosby Company, St. Louis, 1968, p. 1.
20. Kramer, T. C.: The Partitioning of the Truncus and Conus and the Formation of the Membranous Portion of the Interventricular Septum in the Human Heart, *Am. J. Anat.,* 71:343, 1942.
21. Shaner, R. F.: Anomalies of the Heart Bulbus, *J. Pediatr.,* 61:233, 1962.

22. Asami, I.: Beitrag zur Entwicklungsgeschichte des Vorhofseptums im menschlichen Herzen, eine lupenpraparatorisch-photographische Darstellung, *Z. Anat. Entwicklungsgesch.*, 139:55, 1972.
23. Christie, G. A.: Development of the Limbus Fossae Ovalis in the Human Heart—A New Septum, *J. Anat.*, 97:45, 1963.
24. Odgers, R. N. B.: The Formation of the Venous Valves, the Foramen Secundum and the Septum Secundum in the Human Heart, *J. Anat.*, 69:412, 1935.
25. Auer, J.: The Development of the Human Pulmonary Veins and Its Major Variations, *Anat. Rec.*, 101:581, 1948.
26. Los, J. A.: The Development of the Human Pulmonary Veins and the Coronary Sinus in the Human Embryo, Thesis, University of Leiden, 1958.
27. Neill, C. A.: Development of the Pulmonary Veins, *Pediatrics*, 18:880, 1956.
28. Waterston, D.: The Development of the Heart in Man, *Trans. R. Soc. Edinburgh*, 52:257, 1918.
29. Kutsche, L. M., and Van Mierop, L. H. S.: Cervical Origin of the Right Subclavian Artery in Aortic Arch Interruption: Pathogenesis and Significance, *Am. J. Cardiol.*, 53:892, 1984.

2

Anatomy of the Heart

Robert C. Schlant, M.D.   Mark E. Silverman, M.D.

In nature a difference in form always hints at a difference in function.

B. Kisch, 1956[1]

Gross Anatomy of the Heart and Blood Vessels

An appreciation of cardiac anatomy provides an essential framework for understanding cardiac physiology and pathophysiology, examining the patient, and interpreting noninvasive and invasive tests of the heart.[2–7]

The heart is situated in the middle mediastinum, where it is partially overlapped by the neighboring lungs (Fig. 2-1). The sternum and costal cartilages of the third, fourth, and fifth ribs overlie the heart anteriorly. About two-thirds of the heart is left of the midline. The heart rests upon the diaphragm and is tilted forward and to the left so that the apex is anterior to the rest of the heart. The normal apex impulse can be palpated in the fourth or fifth intercostal space near the midclavicular line. The weight and size of the heart vary considerably depending on age, sex, body length, epicardial fat, and general nutrition.

The borders of the normal cardiac silhouette in a frontal view are formed by the following structures (Fig. 2-1).[3] The top of the cardiac silhouette is formed by the transverse and ascending aorta. The upper right margin is contributed by the superior vena cava. The right atrium provides the remaining right lateral cardiac border. Most of the inferior border is composed of right ventricle. The apex and the lower left lateral cardiac border consist of left ventricle. The left atrial appendage perches atop the left ventricle and to the side of the pulmonary artery, interjecting on the cardiac border between the left ventricle and pulmonary outflow tract. The pulmonary outflow area produces the rest of the upper left border.

External Features

The atria are separated from the ventricles externally by the *coronary sulcus (atrioventricular sulcus),* which circles the heart between the atria and ventricles (Fig. 2-1). The right coronary artery, after leaving the aorta, travels in this sulcus between the right atrium and right ventricle until it descends on the posterior surface of the heart. Similarly, the left circumflex artery is found in the coronary sulcus between the left atrium and left ventricle until the artery ramifies posteriorly.

Externally the two ventricles are delineated by *interventricular sulci,* which descend from the coronary sulcus toward the apex. Epicardial fat often obscures these landmarks. The anterior interventricular sulcus contains the *left anterior descending coronary artery* and courses over the muscular ventricular septum between the right and left ventricles to the apex. It then turns the apex and is continued as the posterior interventricular sulcus on the diaphragmatic surface of the heart (Fig. 2-1).

The posterior interventricular sulcus is the pathway for the *posterior descending coronary artery,* which is usually the terminal branch of the right coronary artery or, less frequently, of the left circumflex artery. The two atria may be delineated externally by a groove on the posterior surface between the right pulmonary veins and the venae cavae.

The *crux* of the heart refers to the area on the

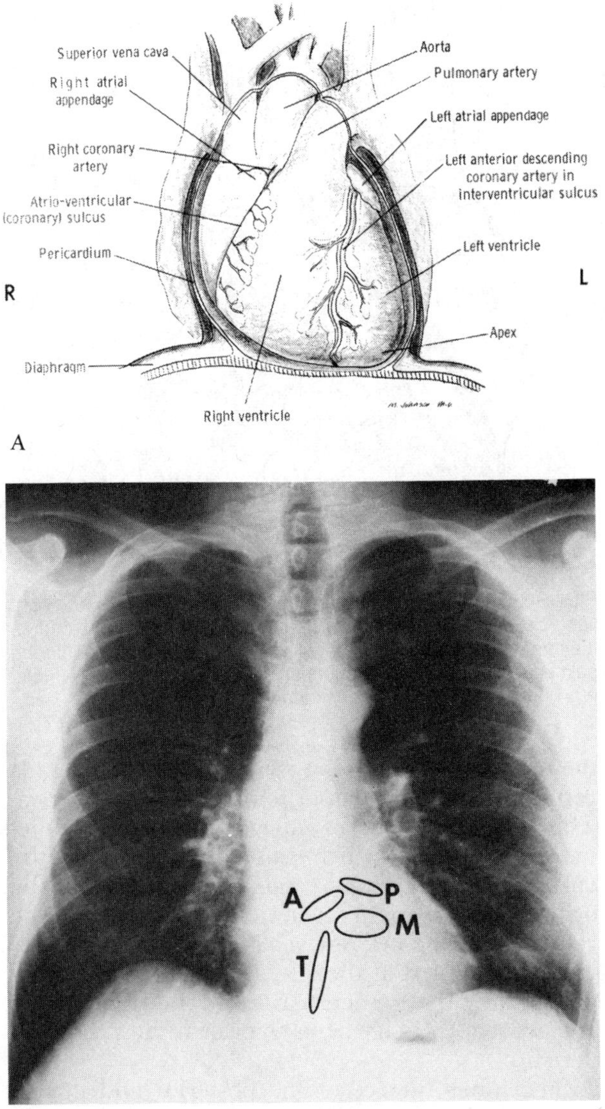

FIGURE 2-1 *A.* Diagram showing the normal relations of the pericardium, great vessels, ventricles, and atria as viewed in the frontal position. R = right; L = left. *B.* Frontal (AP) roentgenogram of the heart. The components which form the cardiac silhouette can be readily identified from *A.* A = aortic valve ring; P = pulmonary valve ring; M = mitral valve ring; T = tricuspid valve ring. (*Diagram by McClaren Johnson, Jr., M.D.*)

posterior-basal surface where the coronary sulcus meets the posterior interventricular sulcus. Internally at this junction, the atrial septum joins the ventricular septum. The coronary artery that crosses this area makes a sharp inward turn at the crux and provides a small artery to the nearby atrioventricular node. The area of the heart below the crux is referred to as the diaphragmatic, or inferior, surface of the heart. A transverse section through the heart is extremely helpful in demonstrating the relations of the cardiac chambers (Fig. 2-2). The ventricular and atrial septa are aligned obliquely 45° to the left of the midline with the planes of the septa directed approximately from right scapula to left nipple.[6] The entire right side of the heart is to the right of this plane, placing most of the right atrium anterior to the left atrium and most of the right ventricle anterior to the left ventricle.

Fibrous Skeleton

A fibrous tissue framework affords a firm anchorage for the attachments of the atrial and ventricular musculature as well as the valvular tissue (Fig. 2-3).[8] At the center of the heart the *central fibrous body* (right fibrous trigone) fuses together the medial aspect of the mitral and tricuspid valves and the aortic roots. The left fibrous trigone is formed by compact bundles of connective tissue that course from the central fibrous body to the left, posteroinferiorly and anteriorly. Continuations of fibroelastic tissue from the central fibrous body (right fibrous trigone) and left fibrous trigone partially encircle the mitral and tricuspid valves. These rings of tissue are the *mitral* and *tricuspid annuli,* which serve as attachments for the mitral and tricuspid valves as well as for the atrial and ventricular muscle. A triple scalloped line of heavy collagenous tissue extends anteriorly from the left and right fibrous trigones to provide a three-pointed, crownlike skeletal support for the aortic root and cusps. A substantial ligament of tissue, the conus ligament, passes from the right side of the aortic root to a similar arrangement of scalloped tissue that surrounds the pulmonic root.

An important extension of the fibrous skeleton, the *membranous ventricular septum,* extends inferiorly and anteriorly from the central fibrous body (right fibrous trigone).[6,7,9] This membranous septum is lo-

FIGURE 2-2 Diagram of a transverse section through the heart at approximately the level of the eighth thoracic vertebra. The plane of the atrial and ventricular septa slants approximately 45° to the left of the midline. RA = right atrium; LA = left atrium; R = right; L = left.

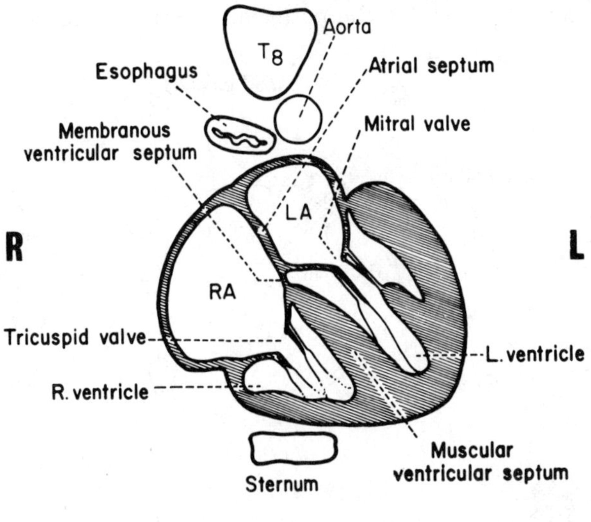

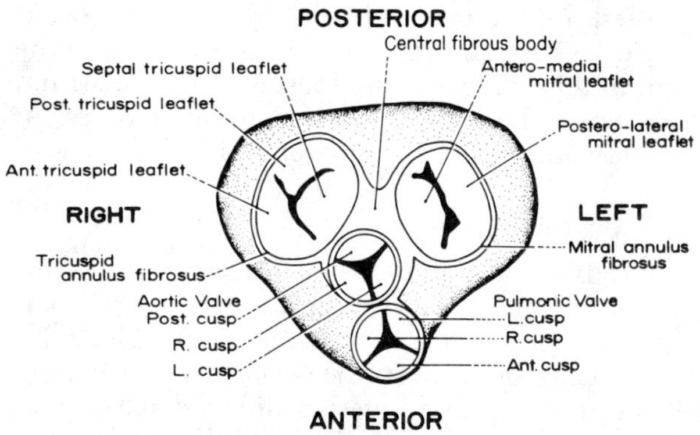

FIGURE 2-3 Schematic anterosuperior view of the heart with the atria removed. The components of the fibrous skeleton and the orientation of the leaflets of each valve are demonstrated.

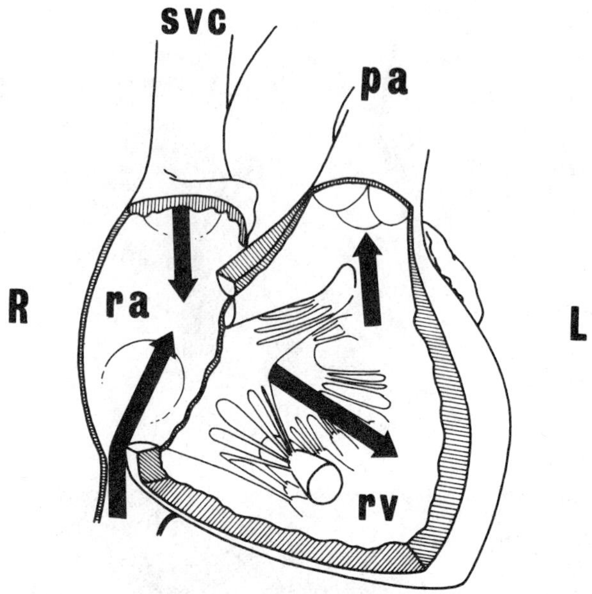

FIGURE 2-4 Schematic frontal view of the right atrium and right ventricle. The arrows indicate the general orientation of blood as it enters the right atrium and right ventricle and is ejected into the pulmonary artery. SVC = superior vena cava; ra = right atrium; rv = right ventricle; pa = pulmonary artery; R = right; L = left.

cated at the summit of the muscular ventricular septum, where it provides support for the right coronary and noncoronary aortic cusps. A portion of the membranous ventricular septum extends slightly above the tricuspid valve, forming a small portion of the medial wall of the right atrium (Fig. 2-2).[9] The *bundle of His* penetrates the central fibrous body and travels along the inferior margin of the membranous portion of the ventricular septum.[10] At the crest of the muscular septum, about the level of the junction of the right coronary and posterior (noncoronary) aortic cusps, the His bundle separates into a *left bundle branch* and a *right bundle branch.*

Right Atrium

Venous blood returns to the heart via the superior and inferior venae cavae into the right atrium, where it is stored during right ventricular systole. During ventricular diastole, blood flows from the right atrium into the right ventricle (Fig. 2-4). The right atrium forms the right lateral cardiac border and is above, behind, and to the right of the right ventricle (Figs. 2-2 and 2-4). Most of the right atrium is anterior to the left atrium as well as to the right of it (Fig. 2-5). Anteromedially, the right atrial appendage protrudes from the right atrium and overlaps the aortic root (Fig. 2-1). On the posterior external surface of the right atrium a ridge, the *sulcus terminalis,* extends vertically from the superior to the inferior vena cava. This corresponds to an internal muscular bundle, the *crista terminalis,* which runs along the edge of the entrance to the atrial appendage to the front of the orifice of the superior vena cava and then to the right side of the inferior vena cava.[6] The *sinus node* is usually located at the lateral margin of the junction of the superior vena cava with the right atrium and atrial appendage beneath or near the sulcus terminalis.

The inner surface of the posterior and medial (septal) walls of the right atrium is smooth, while the surfaces of the lateral wall and of the right atrial appendage are composed of parallel muscle bundles, the *pectinate* muscles.[6] The right atrial wall measures almost 2 mm in thickness. The superior and inferior venae cavae enter the right atrium pos-

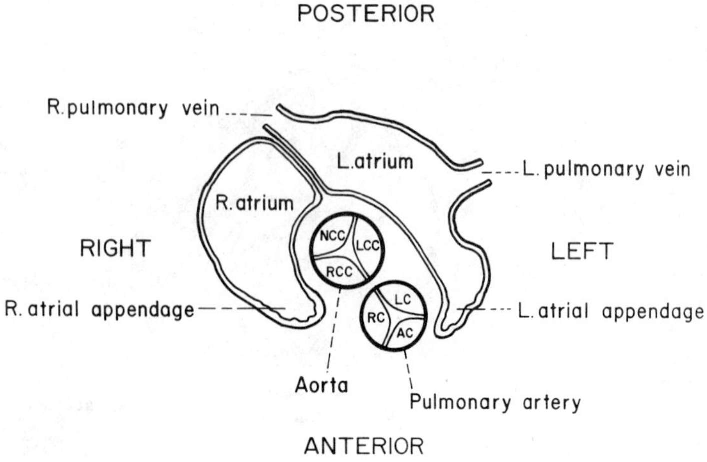

FIGURE 2-5 Schematic transverse section through the heart at approximately the level of the second intercostal space. The relation between the left and right atria and the interatrial septum is illustrated. The relative positions of the aortic and pulmonary valves and their cusps are shown. AC = anterior cusp; RC = right cusp; LC = left cusp of the pulmonary valve; LCC = left coronary cusp; RCC = right coronary cusp; NCC = noncoronary cusp of the aortic valve.

teriorly and medially at its superior and inferior aspects. The orifice of the superior vena cava usually has no valve; the orifice of the inferior vena cava is flanked anteriorly by an inconstant, rudimentary valve, the *eustachian valve,* formed by a crescentic fold. The caval orifices may vary in shape and diameter depending upon the phase of respiration, the cardiac cycle, and the contraction or relaxation of surrounding muscular bands. The variation in the orifice may play some role in promoting venous return or preventing atrial reflux.

The medial wall of the right atrium includes the atrial septum and is also important because of its proximity to several structures.[6] Anteriorly, the posterior (noncoronary) cusp and the right coronary cusp of the aortic root lean against the medial right atrium, forming a normal slight bulge known as the *torus aorticus,* which is a useful landmark during transseptal catheterization of the left side of the heart. The proximal right coronary artery is in the immediate vicinity as it enters the coronary sulcus. The proximity of the aortic root to the right atrium permits an aneurysm of the sinus of Valsalva to rupture into the right atrium.

The *atrial septum* is found in the posteroinferior portion of the medial wall of the right atrium and extends obliquely forward from right to left (Fig. 2-5).[11] Near the center of the atrial septum there is a shallow depression, the *fossa ovalis,* which often has a prominent fold, or limbus, anteriorly. The ostium of the *coronary sinus* is located between the inferior vena cava and the tricuspid valve. The orifice of the coronary sinus is guarded by a rudimentary flap of tissue, the *Thebesian valve.* The *atrioventricular (AV) node* is anterior and medial to the coronary sinus, just above the septal leaflet of the tricuspid valve. The sinus and atrioventricular nodes, as well as the entire conducting pathways, are not grossly visible.

Right Ventricle

The right ventricle receives venous blood from the right atrium during ventricular diastole and propels blood into the pulmonary circulation during ventricular systole (Fig. 2-4).

The right ventricle is normally the most anterior cardiac chamber, lying directly beneath the sternum (Fig. 2-2). Enlargement or hyperactivity of the right ventricle may often be detected by palpation of the sternum or the lower left sternal border. The right ventricle is partially below, in front of, and medial to the right atrium, but anterior and to the right of the left ventricle. Most of the entire inferior border of the frontal roentgenogram view of the heart consists of the right ventricle (Fig. 2-1).

The striking difference in configuration between the two ventricles is illustrated by a transverse section (Fig. 2-6). The left ventricular chamber is an ellipsoidal sphere surrounded by relatively thick musculature (8 to 15 mm at autopsy), well suited to ejecting against the high resistance of the systemic vessels. The right ventricle, which normally contracts against very low resistance, has a crescent-shaped chamber and a thin outer wall measuring 4 to 5 mm in thickness.[12] The anterior right ventricular wall curves over the ventricular septum, which bulges into the right ventricular cavity. Although the ventricular septum forms the medial wall of both ventricles, it seems to contribute predominantly to left ventricle function in normal subjects. The anterior and inferior walls of the right ventricular cavity are lined by muscle bundles, the *trabeculae carneae,* which often form ridges along the inner surface of the wall or cross from one wall to the other. A rather constant muscle, the *moderator band,* crosses from the lower ventricular septum to the anterior wall, where it joins the anterior papillary muscle (Fig. 2-7). The right bundle branch, after traveling through the muscular ventricular septum, courses through the moderator muscle to the endocardium of the right ventricle.

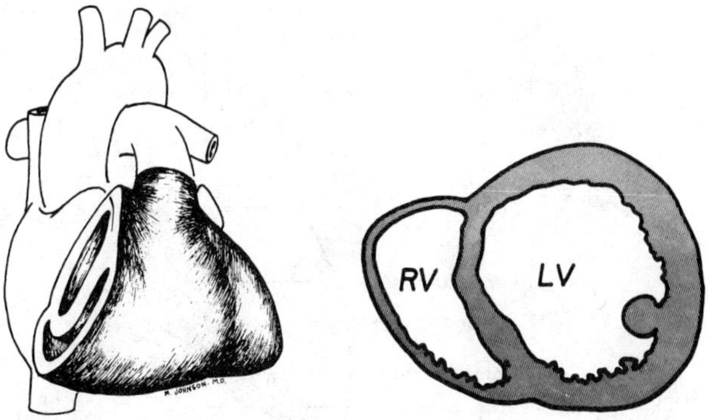

A B

FIGURE 2-6 Diagrams of the heart to illustrate the differences in shape of the right and left ventricles. *A.* Ventricles in approximate anatomic position. *B.* Cross section, illustrating the more nearly circular dimensions of the left ventricle. (*Diagrams by McClaren Johnson, Jr., M.D.*)

Functionally, the right ventricle can be partitioned into an inflow and an outflow tract. The inflow tract, consisting of the tricuspid valve and the trabecular muscles of the anterior and inferior walls, directs entering blood anteriorly, inferiorly, and to the left at an angle of 60° to the outflow tract[13] (Fig. 2-4). The smooth-walled outflow tract, also referred to as the *infundibulum,* forms the superior portion of the right ventricle. It is separated from the inflow tract by a thick muscle, the *crista supraventricularis,* which arches from the anterolateral wall over the anterior leaflet of the tricuspid valve to the septal (medial) wall, where it joins other constrictor bands of muscle that encircle the outflow tract (Fig. 2-7). Blood entering the infundibulum is ejected superiorly and posteriorly into the pulmonary artery.

Left Atrium

The left atrium receives blood from the pulmonary veins and serves as the reservoir during left ventricular systole and as a conduit during left ventricular

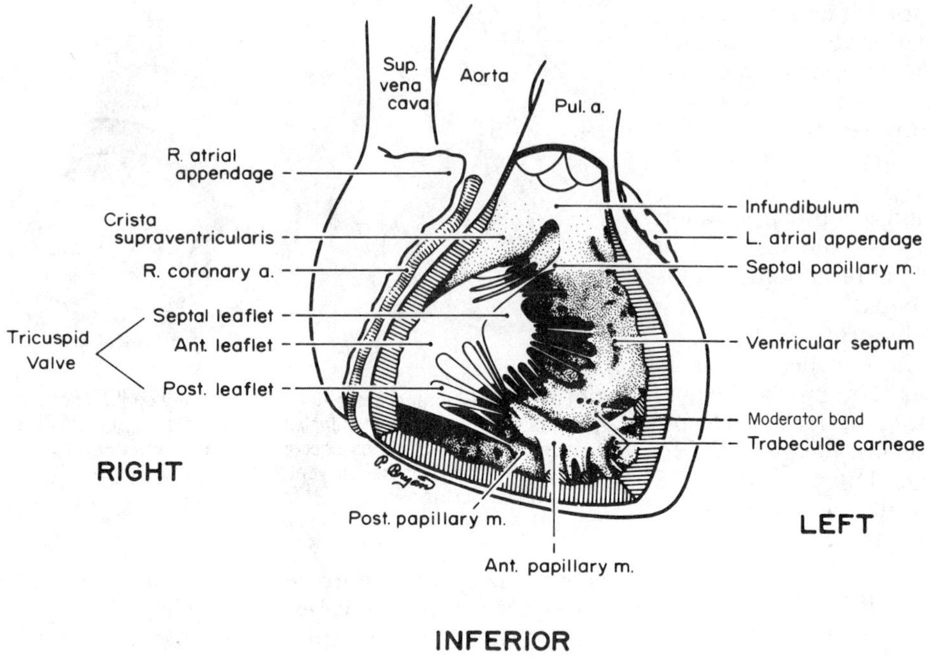

FIGURE 2-7 Schematic representation of a frontal view of the heart. The anterior right ventricular wall has been removed to demonstrate the orientation of the tricuspid leaflets and the papillary muscles. The anterior papillary muscle is sectioned. The trabeculated inflow portion of the right ventricle is contrasted with the smooth infundibular (outflow) area.

filling. In addition, left atrial contraction provides a significant increment of blood to the left ventricle, stretching the ventricle and priming it for ventricular ejection. This is sometimes referred to as the "atrial kick."

The left atrium is located superiorly, in the midline, and posterior to the other cardiac chambers (Figs. 2-2, 2-5, and 2-8). As a consequence of this posterior position, the left atrium is not normally seen in the frontal roentgenogram. The esophagus abuts directly upon its posterior surface, while the aortic root impinges upon its anterior wall. The right atrium is to the right and anterior (Fig. 2-5). The left ventricle is to the left, anterior, and inferior. The posterior position of the left atrium makes it impossible to palpate externally unless it is massively dilated. With severe mitral regurgitation, however, expansion of the left atrium from the regurgitation and the ejection recoil of the anteriorly located ventricles may force the heart anteriorly, producing a late systolic sternal lift. The left atrium usually enlarges posteriorly and laterally in mitral stenosis or regurgitation, occasionally even reaching the right or left lateral chest wall.

The wall of the left atrium is 3 mm thick, slightly thicker than that of the right atrium. Two pulmonary veins enter posterolaterally on each side, conveying oxygenated blood from the lungs. Though there are no true valves at the junction of the pulmonary veins and the left atrium, sleeves of atrial muscle extend from the left atrial wall around the pulmonary veins for 1 or 2 cm and may exert a partial sphincter-like influence, tending to lessen reflux during atrial systole or mitral regurgitation.

The endocardium of the left atrium is smooth and slightly opaque. Pectinate muscles are present only in the *left atrial appendage*, which projects from the anterolateral left atrium, alongside the pulmonary artery (Fig. 2-1). The atrial septum is smooth but may contain a central shallow area corresponding to the fossa ovalis.

Left Ventricle

The left ventricle receives blood from the left atrium during ventricular diastole and ejects blood into the systemic arterial circulation during ventricular systole (Figs. 2-8 and 2-9). The left ventricle is roughly bullet-shaped with the blunt tip directed anteriorly, inferiorly, and to the left, where it contributes, with the lower ventricular septum, to the apex of the heart (Fig. 2-2).[14] Although the left ventricle forms the lower left lateral cardiac border in the frontal roentgenogram, the major portion of its external surface is posterolateral (Fig. 2-2). The left ventricle is posterior and to the left of the right ventricle and inferior, anterior, and to the left of the left atrium. The left ventricular chamber is approximately an ellipsoidal sphere, surrounded by thick muscular walls measuring 8 to 15 mm, or approximately two to three times the thickness of the right ventricular wall. The tip of the left ventricular apex is often thin, sometimes measuring 2 mm or less. The medial wall of the left ventricle is the *ventricular septum*, which is shared with the right ventricle (Fig. 2-6). The septum, which is roughly triangular in shape with the base of the triangle at the level of the aortic cusps, is entirely muscular except for the small membranous septum, located superiorly just below the right coronary and the posterior coronary cusps (Fig. 2-2).[9] The upper third of the septum is smooth endocardium. The remaining two-thirds of the septum and the remaining ventricular walls are ridged

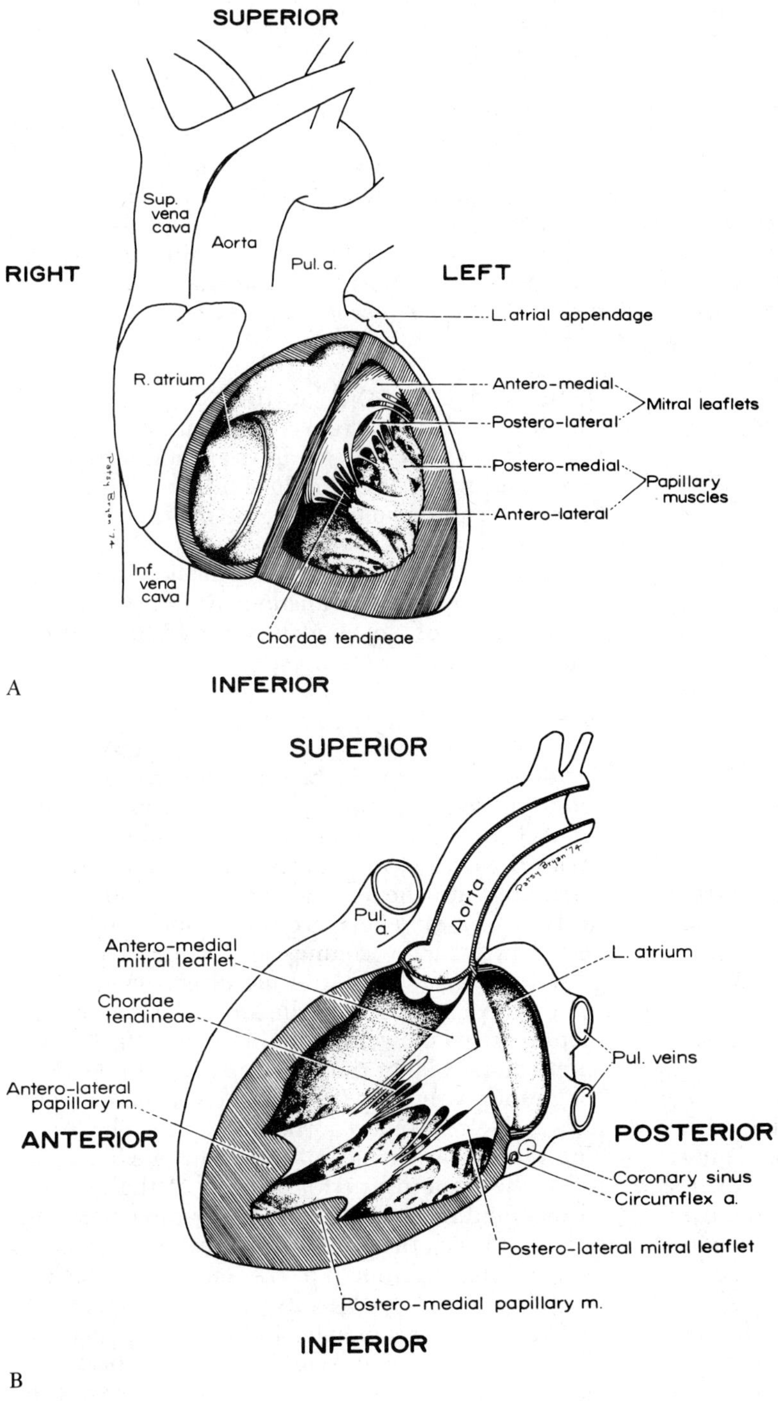

FIGURE 2-8 Schematic drawings illustrating the components of the mitral complex (mitral annulus, mitral leaflets, chordae tendineae, and papillary muscles). *A.* Frontal view; right ventricle and ventricular septum removed. *B.* Left lateral view; lateral wall of left atrium and left ventricle partially removed.

by interlacing muscles, the trabeculae carneae. The ventricular wall exclusive of the septum is often referred to as the free wall of the left ventricle.

The *anteromedial leaflet* of the mitral valve, which is the larger and more mobile of the two mitral leaflets, extends from the top of the posteromedial septum across the ventricular cavity to the anterolateral ventricular wall and separates the left ventricular cavity into an inflow and an outflow tract. The funnel-shaped inflow tract, which is formed by the *mitral annulus* and by both mitral leaflets and their *chordae tendineae,* directs the entering atrial blood inferiorly, anteriorly, and to the left (Fig. 2-9). The outflow tract, surrounded by the inferior surface of the anteromedial mitral leaflet, the ventricular septum, and the left ventricular free wall, orients the blood flow from the left ventricular apex to the right and superiorly at an angle of 90° to the inflow tract.[6] With the onset of ventricular systole, both mitral leaflets are propelled together and upward, converting the entire left ventricle into an expulsion chamber.

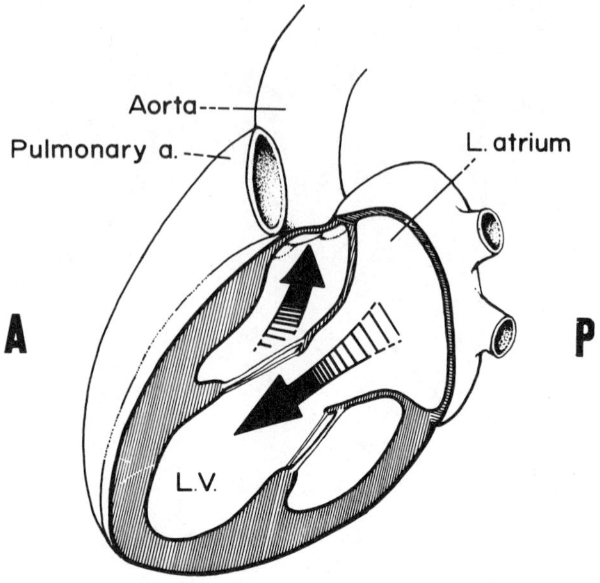

FIGURE 2-9 Schematic left lateral view of the left side of the heart. The arrows indicate the general orientation of blood flow from left atrium to left ventricle to aorta. A = anterior; P = posterior.

Semilunar Valves[15–17]

The semilunar aortic and pulmonary valves are similar in configuration, except the aortic cusps are slightly thicker. They are situated at the summit of the outflow tract of their corresponding ventricle, the pulmonary valve being anterior, superior, and slightly to the left of the aortic valve (Figs. 2-3, 2-5). Each valve is composed of three fibrous cusps. The U-shaped convex lower edges of each cusp are attached to and suspended from the root of the aorta or pulmonary artery, with the upper free valve edges projecting into the lumen. The cusps, which are often slightly unequal in width, circle the inside of the vessel root.[18] Behind each cusp the vessel wall bulges outward, forming a pouchlike dilatation known as the *sinus of Valsalva.* The free edge of each cusp is concave, with a nodular interruption at the center of the leaflet, the *nodulus Arantii.* The portion of the cusp adjacent to the rim is not as thick and may normally contain small perforations. During ventricular systole, the cusps are passively thrust upward away from the center of the aortic lumen. During ventricular diastole, the cusps fall passively into the lumen of the vessel as they support the column of blood above. The noduli Arantii meet in the center and contribute to the support of the leaflets. The geometry of the cusps and the strong fibrous tissue support provide excellent approximations of the leaflets and prevent regurgitation of blood.

The pulmonary cusps are called *anterior, right,* and *left* (Figs. 2-3 and 2-5). The designation of the aortic cusps is best related to the coronary arteries (Fig. 2-5). The two anterior cusps are referred to as the right and left coronary cusps. The remaining cusp is the noncoronary, or posterior, cusp. Since the plane of the aortic valve is oblique, with the right posterior side lower than the left anterior side, the origin of the left coronary artery is slightly superior to that of the right coronary artery.[19] The ostia of the coronary arteries are located in the upper third of their respective sinus of Valsalva. The right coronary artery passes anteriorly and to the right, while the left coronary artery courses anteriorly and to the left. In some hearts there is a separate ostium in the right coronary sinus of Valsalva for the *conus artery,* sometimes called the *third coronary artery.*

Mitral and Tricuspid Complex[6,20–22]

The flow of blood across the mitral and tricuspid orifice is regulated by an intricate interaction between the atrium, the annulus fibrosus, the valvular tissue, the chordae tendineae, the papillary muscles, and the ventricular wall. These six components, constituting the mitral and tricuspid "complex," should be considered functionally as a unit, since derangement of any one part may allow serious hemodynamic consequences.[22]

Mitral Valve

The orifice of the mitral valve faces anterolaterally and directs the left atrial blood inferiorly, anteriorly, and to the left. The fibroelastic valvular tissue, which is attached to the annulus fibrosus, completely encircles the orifice, providing a cone-shaped funnel extending into the recesses of the left ventricular cavity (Fig. 2-8). There are two major leaflets connected by bridging commissural tissue. The triangular *anteromedial leaflet* stretches diagonally from the posteromedial aspect of the muscular ventricular septum across the ventricular cavity to attach to the anterolateral wall of the left ventricle. This leaflet is continuous with supporting tissues of the noncoronary and left coronary aortic cusps, which lie above. The ventricular surface of the anteromedial leaflet forms the posterosuperior portion of the left ventricular outflow tract. There are pathological conditions in which the outflow tract may be obstructed by abnormal attachment of the anteromedial leaflet or by an eccentric pull by its papillary muscles.

The longer, less mobile, and quandrangular *posterolateral leaflet* encircles about two-thirds of the circumference of the mitral valve orifice. It is attached superiorly to the annulus fibrosus and circles from anterolateral to posteromedial ventricle (Fig. 2-3). This leaflet is more restricted in its movements than the anteromedial leaflet. Although the two mitral leaflets differ greatly in height and mobility, both contribute importantly to effective valve closure.

Tricuspid Valve[23]

The right atrioventricular (tricuspid) orifice, which is larger than the mitral orifice, is oriented with its plane in a semivertical axis, and directs the right atrial blood anteriorly, inferiorly, and to the left (Fig. 2-4). Its relatively superficial position below the lower left sternal border allows tricuspid murmurs to be heard best in this area. The tricuspid leaflets differ from the mitral leaflets in being thinner, more translucent, and less easily separated into well-defined leaflets. There are usually three major leaflets of unequal size (Fig. 2-6). The largest leaflet is the *anterior leaflet,* which stretches from the infundibular area downward to the inferolateral wall of the ventricle. The *septal (medial) leaflet* attaches to both the membranous and muscular portions of the ventricular septum. At times this leaflet may partially or completely occlude small ventricular septal defects of the outflow tract. The *posterior leaflet,* which is usually the smallest, is attached to the tricuspid ring along its posteroinferior border.

The rapid opening and closing of the mitral and tricuspid leaflets is possible because of their remarkable mobility that is facilitated by attachments at only the basilar and apical aspects, a specific gravity approximating that of blood, a smooth surface minimizing friction, and a large area of coaptation between the leaflets.

Papillary Muscles[20,22–24]

The papillary muscles of both ventricles are located below the commissures of the atrioventricular valves. These muscles project from the trabeculae carneae and may be single, bifid, or occasionally a row of muscles arising from the ventricular wall. In the left ventricle the two groups of papillary muscles, located below the anterolateral and posteromedial commissures, arise from the junction of the apical and middle third of the ventricular wall (Fig. 2-10). In the right ventricle there are usually three papillary muscles (Fig. 2-7). The largest is the *anterior papillary muscle,* which is found below the commissure between the anterior and posterior leaflets, originating from the moderator band as well as from the anterolateral ventricular wall. The *posterior papillary muscle* lies beneath the junction of the posterior and septal leaflets. A small *septal papillary muscle,* originating from the wall of the infundibulum, tethers the anterior and septal leaflets high against the infundibular wall. At times this muscle is virtually absent, and the chordae tendineae arise from a small tendinous connection to the infundibulum.

The papillary muscles, because of their relatively parallel alignment to the ventricular wall and their chordal attachments to two adjacent valve leaflets, pull the leaflets of the mitral and tricuspid valves together and downward at the onset of isovolumic ventricular contraction (Fig. 2-11).

FIGURE 2-10 Papillary muscle of the left ventricle, demonstrating its origin from the trabeculae carneae. The chordae tendineae are shown reaching from the papillary muscle to both mitral valve leaflets. A= anteromedial mitral leaflet; P = posterolateral mitral leaflet; PM = papillary muscle.

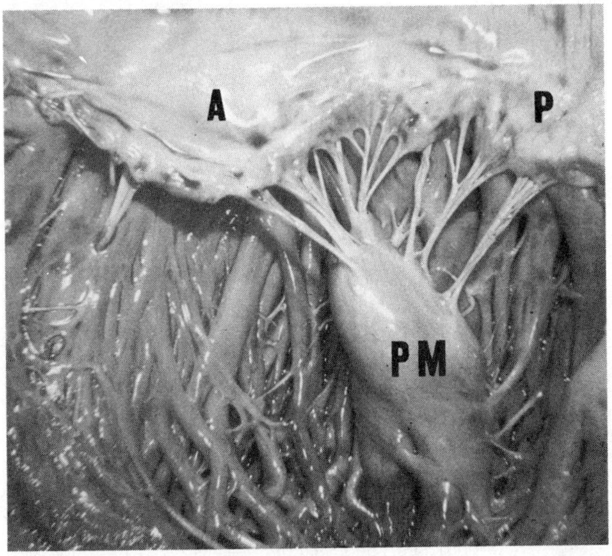

Chordae Tendineae[25]

Strong cords of fibrous tissue, the chordae tendineae, spring from the tip of each papillary muscle (Figs. 2-6, 2-10, and 2-11). They often subdivide and interconnect before they attach to the two leaflets directly above. The chordae may attach directly into a fibrous band running along the free edge of the valves, or they may become incorporated into the ventricular surface of the leaflet a few millimeters back from the edge. Additional chordae run directly from the ventricular wall into the undersurface of the posterolateral leaflet of the left ventricle and the septal and posterior leaflets of the right ventricle.

The chordae tendineae, by their attachments to most of the free valvular border and by their numerous cross connections, allow the valve leaflets to balloon upward and against each other and evenly distribute the forces of ventricular systole. Dysfunction or rupture of a papillary muscle or rupture of a chorda tendinea may undermine the support of one or more valve leaflets, producing regurgitation.

Pericardium[26]

The heart is enclosed by the pericardium, the two surfaces of which can be visualized by considering

FIGURE 2-11 The left ventricular wall and papillary muscle are shown to have a parallel orientation. PM = papillary muscle; LV = left ventricle.

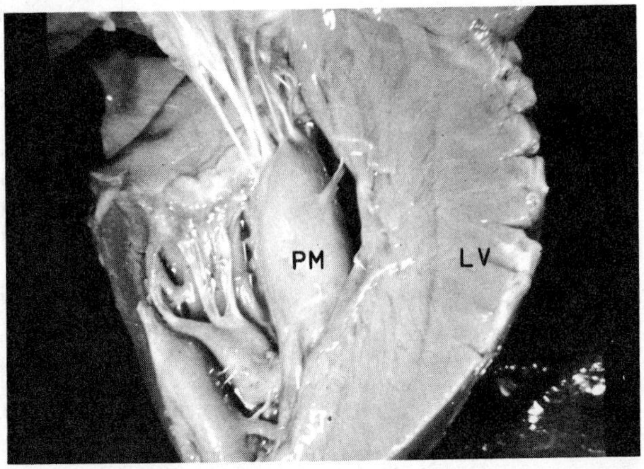

the heart as a fist that is plunged into a large balloon (Fig. 2-1). The surface of the balloon in intimate contact with the fist is analogous to the *visceral pericardium,* or *epicardium.* This surface encases the heart, extending several centimeters onto each of the great vessels. It is then reflected back, as is the outer surface of the balloon, to form the *parietal pericardium.* The two pericardial surfaces are lined by smooth, glistening serous tissue and are separated by a thin layer of lubricating fluid which allows the heart to move freely within the parietal pericardium. The parietal pericardium is attached by ligaments to the manubrium, the xiphoid process, the vertebral column, and the diaphragm. There is normally about 10 to 20 ml of thin, clear pericardial fluid, which moistens the contracting surfaces of the visceral and parietal pericardium.

Innervation of the Heart[27–29]

Although the sinus or sinoatrial (SA) node, the AV node, and specialized conduction system of the heart possess the inherent ability for spontaneous, rhythmic initiation of the cardiac excitation impulse, the autonomic nervous system has an important role in the regulation of the rate of impulse formation. The autonomic nervous system also influences the rate of spread of the excitation impulse, the depolarization and repolarization of the myocardium, and the contractility of both the atria and the ventricles.

The parasympathetic innervation of the heart originates in the medulla and passes through the right and left vagus nerve (Fig. 2-12). Two sets of cardiac nerves arise from each vagus nerve: the superior (superior and inferior cervical) cardiac nerves, which arise from the vagi in the neck, and the inferior (thoracic) cardiac nerves, which arise from either the vagus nerves or the recurrent branches of the vagi. The sympathetic innervation of the heart passes from the spinal cord to the upper four or five thoracic ganglia. Some fibers from the upper thoracic ganglia pass up the cervical sympathetic to the superior, middle, or inferior cervical ganglia. The

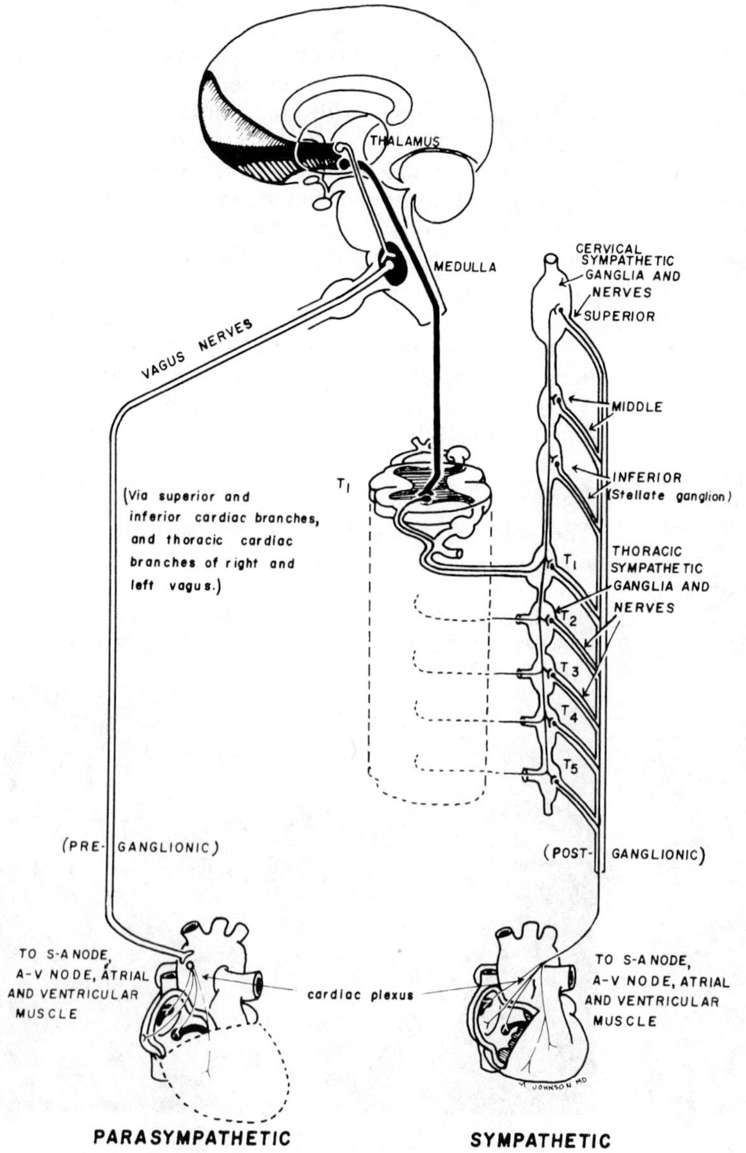

FIGURE 2-12 A simplified, diagrammatic representation of the efferent autonomic innervation of the heart. The parasympathetic and sympathetic nerves to the heart, many of which closely accompany each other in and through the various cardiac and coronary plexuses, have been separated for illustrative purposes. See text for details. (*Diagram by McClaren Johnson, Jr., M.D.*)

superior (cervical), middle (cervical), and inferior (cervical) cardiac nerves originate from their respective ganglia and pass downward through the deep and superficial parts of the cardiac plexus to the heart. When the inferior cervical and first thoracic ganglia are fused together, the resulting ganglion is known as the *stellate ganglion.* Additional cardiac branches arise from the upper four or five thoracic ganglia and pass to the *cardiac plexus,* which surround the root and arch of the aorta near the tracheal bifurcation. The cardiac and coronary plexuses are formed by cardiac branches from both the sympathetic and parasympathetic systems. Both sympathetic and parasympathetic fibers influence the SA node, the AV node, and both the atrial and ventricular myocardium although vagal fibers to the ventricles are rather sparse. Sympathetic fibers are dense to the epicardial coronary arteries and veins and are moderate to intramural vessels. Sympathetic stimulation to the heart is mediated by the release of the neurohormone norepinephrine. Cardiac parasympathetic impulses are transmitted by acetylcholine.

Afferent impulses from chemoreceptors and mechanoreceptors in the pericardium, connective tissue, adventitia, and walls of the heart pass by peripheral sensory axons through sympathetic plexuses and through the lower two cervical and upper four thoracic sympathetic ganglia to thoracic dorsal ganglia, where the cell bodies of the neurons are located. The impulses are carried by the central axon of this neuron through the dorsal roots to the posterior gray column of the spinal cord, where the fibers synapse with the second-order neuron. From this neuron, fibers cross the median plane, ascend in the ventral spinothalamic tract, and terminate in the posteroventral nucleus of the thalamus. Some afferent vagal ganglia have been found in the left coronary artery system. Impulses passing through these neurons and ganglia are thought to be important in the Bezold-Jarisch reflex.

The Lymphatic System of the Heart[30,31]

The lymphatic drainage of the heart flows from subendocardial vessels to an extensive capillary plexus lying throughout the subepicardium. These capillaries converge into collecting lymphatic channels that run alongside the coronary vessels: a *posterior interventricular trunk* paralleling the posterior descending coronary artery up to the crux of the heart and then circling around to the right from posterior to anterior in the right coronary sulcus; an *anterior interventricular trunk* ascending from the apex to the base next to the left anterior descending coronary artery; and an *obtuse marginal trunk* running alongside the left circumflex artery (Fig. 2-13).

The two major left ventricular lymphatic channels—the anterior interventricular trunk and the obtuse marginal trunk—join near the base of the pulmonary artery to form the left coronary channel. More often, the right coronary channel unites with the left coronary channel to become a main supracardiac channel, the *principal cardiac lymphatic,* which passes upward beneath the left atrial appendage, behind the pulmonary artery, to enter a pretracheal node between the arch of the aorta and the pulmonary artery. One or two lymphatic channels then connect this pretracheal node to the *cardiac lymph node* located between the superior vena cava and the right brachiocephalic artery. From there the *right lymphatic duct* runs cephalad in the mediastinum to drain into the junction of the internal jugular and right subclavian veins.

Aorta and Great Vessels

The origins of the aorta and pulmonary artery[30,31] are similar in that they are both derived from the division of the embryonic truncus arteriosus. Although at birth the walls of these vessels are of approximately equal thickness, in adult life the wall of the

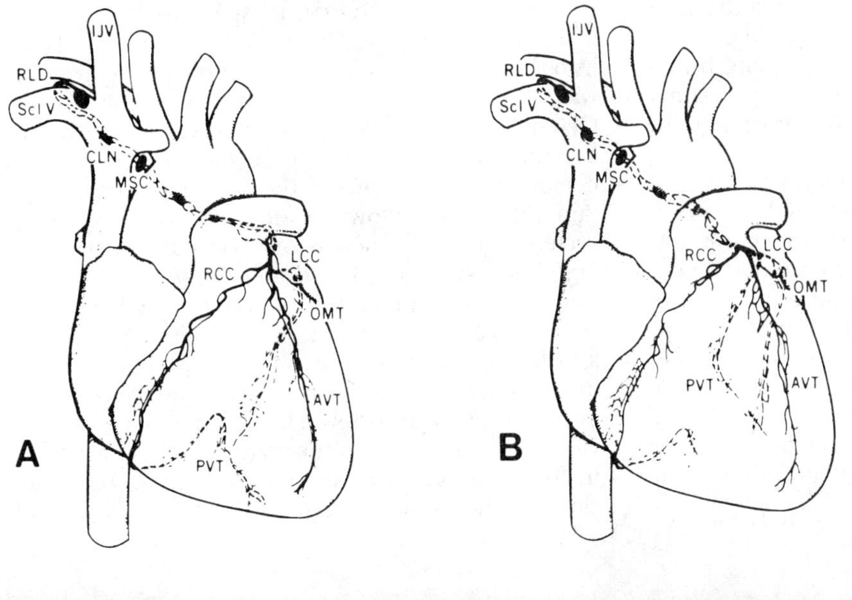

FIGURE 2-13 Diagrams of two different anatomical patterns (*A* and *B*) of lymphatic drainage channels of the heart. PVT = posterior interventricular trunk; RCC = right coronary channel; LCC = left coronary channel; AVT = anterior interventricular trunk; OMT = obtuse marginal trunk; MSC = main supracardiac channel; CLN = cardiac lymph node; RLD = right lymphatic duct; SclV = right subclavian vein; IJV = internal jugular vein. (*From M. Feola, R. Merklin, S. Cho, and S. K. Brockman, The Terminal Pathway of the Lymphatic System of the Human Heart, Ann. Thorac. Surg., 24:531, 1977. Reproduced with permission from the publisher and authors.*)

aorta is considerably thicker than that of the pulmonary artery. This is presumably a result of the decreased pulmonary artery pressure after birth. The aorta has many elastic fibers, which allow it to function as a compression chamber or reservoir for blood during the rapid ejection from the left ventricle. The term *windkessel* (from the German word for the air compression chamber in water pumps that converts pulsatile flow to nearly continuous flow) is customary in the literature for this function. Aging changes in the aorta may reduce the windkessel effect and result in a higher pulse pressure.

Arteries

The systemic arteries originate from the aorta and its branches, and they branch successively to become individually smaller. As the total cross-sectional area of the arteries, arterioles, and capillaries increases, the average velocity of blood flow decreases. The arteries eventually branch into small arterioles, which are the major areas of resistance in the systemic circulation. At the junction of the arterioles and the capillaries, there are often vascular sphincters. These precapillary sphincters have a basal myogenic tone that is continuously modified by local and systemic physical, chemical, and neural influences that profoundly affect the perfusion of the capillaries in the region. In addition, there may be small vascular shunts between small arterioles and venules that are capable of shunting blood past the capillary bed.

Capillaries

The capillaries are small vessels, usually consisting of single endothelial cells. At times the capillaries seem capable of holding several red blood cells transversely; at other times the red blood cells appear to pass singly through the capillaries. In a given capillary bed, there is frequently a stasis of flow in some capillaries and at the same time there is an active flow in other capillaries. This periodic flow through different capillary beds is thought to have a normal physiological function of increasing nutrition in these areas. Under conditions of maximal flow, the entire capillary bed may be maximally dilated. Under normal flow conditions, there may be some gravitational layering of red blood cells, white blood cells, and plasma in the capillaries. Under certain conditions, such as acute stress, shock, or toxemia, or uncontrolled diabetes, there may be a sludging or congregation of red blood cells in the capillaries. The normal capillary pressure in the systemic circulation is estimated to be approximately 25 to 35 mmHg. In contrast, the normal pulmonary capillary pressure is 7 to 10 mmHg. It is estimated that the systemic capillary bed, under basal resting conditions, has a volume of approximately 5 percent of the total blood volume.

Veins

The veins of the body collect the blood from the capillaries and successively join one another to form progressively larger vessels that return the blood to the heart by way of the superior and inferior venae cavae. There is normally a slight pressure gradient between the systemic veins and the right atrium. In addition, the flow of blood returning to the heart is aided by the presence of valves in many of the larger veins, particularly those of the legs. This allows the muscular contraction of the arms and legs (the "muscular pump") and the normal pressure changes in the thoracic (the "respiratory pump") and abdominal cavities to contribute to the return of blood to the heart. Since they are normally subjected to less pressure than arteries, veins are considerably thinner walled. Their pressure-volume characteristics are also significantly different from those of arteries. As a result, veins are capable of accommodating much larger volumes of blood with very slight changes in pressure. For this reason the veins are often referred to as *capacitance vessels.* The veins, as well as the arteries, are capable of changing their pressure-volume characteristics in response to hormonal or neural stimulation. At times this change in venomotor "tone" enables the veins to increase the return of blood to the heart and to make available blood needed in other areas. In a sense, such shifts in the distribution of blood volume are a type of internal blood transfusion. At rest, about 50 to 65 percent of the blood volume is located in the venous portions of the circulation.

Systemic Lymphatic Vessels[32,33]

Although the cardiovascular system is sometimes considered to be a closed fluid system, there is a large volume of fluid with small amounts of protein filtered in the renal glomeruli and a considerable quantity of similar filtration through the systemic capillaries into the interstitial spaces.

Fluid and protein filtered from blood capillaries into the interstitial fluid must return to the heart by way of either the veins or the lymphatic circulation. Generally, the smallest lymphatic vessels in the tissues are closed, permeable vessels similar to blood capillaries. Like the veins, the lymphatic vessels contain valves that allow the flow of lymph to be directed centrally. The major terminal vessel of the lymphatic system is the *thoracic duct.* The thoracic duct usually terminates by joining the left brachiocephalic vein at the junction of the internal jugular and left subclavian veins. Occasionally, it may end in branches of the left brachiocephalic vein or may even subdivide into branches ending separately in various great veins. On the right side there are three major lymphatic vessels: the right jugular, right subclavian, and right mediastinal lymphatic ducts. Although they usually enter the right internal jugular, subclavian, and brachiocephalic veins, respectively, occasionally the right jugular and right subclavian ducts unite to form a *right lymphatic duct,* which usually enters the right brachiocephalic vein. The right mediastinal lymphatic vessel almost always enters the right brachiocephalic vein separately. The significance of other lymphaticovenous connections, such as those present in the abdomen, is uncertain at present.

Some of the importance of the lymphatic system becomes apparent when one realizes that in 24 h the thoracic duct alone returns to the circulation a volume of fluid about equal to the total plasma volume and containing 50 to 100 percent of the total circulating plasma protein.

The importance of the myocardial lymphatic vessels in the maintenance of normal myocardial nutrition and in the response to injury of the heart, particularly the endocardium and heart valves, has been emphasized. Undoubtedly, a more significant role will be shown for the lymphatic system in many other conditions, particularly pulmonary edema and valvular disease.

Pulmonary Circulation[34]

The basic function of the pulmonary circulation is the uptake of oxygen and the liberation of carbon dioxide by the blood. This function is efficiently accomplished by the pulmonary circuit, which normally carries all the cardiac output through the lungs at a pressure in the adult approximately one-sixth that of the systemic circulation. It is obvious, therefore, that its resistance to blood flow (the ratio of pressure difference across the pulmonary circuit to flow through the pulmonary circulation) is one-sixth that of the systemic circulation.

The pulmonary circulation differs from the systemic circulation in several important ways. The pulmonary arterial vessels have thinner walls and less medial muscle than their counterparts in the systemic circulation with the same luminal cross-sectional area. The main pulmonary artery, which in the fetus is histologically similar to the aorta, becomes much thinner walled than the aorta after birth. There is normally a conspicuous fragmentation of the elastic fibers in the pulmonary artery following birth, unless there is a congenital heart defect that allows pulmonary hypertension to persist. In general, the pulmonary circulation may be said to be relatively passive. In comparison with systemic vessels, its blood vessels in most instances react relatively less to neural, humoral, or pharmacologic agents. In some cases the reactions are the opposite of those produced in systemic vessels; e.g., arterial hypoxia and hypercapnia may both produce vasoconstriction in the pulmonary circulation, whereas in the systemic circulation their effect is generally vasodilatation. Although pulmonary vasoconstriction has been demonstrated experimentally to occur under autonomic nervous system stimulation and as a result of carotid sinus and carotid body reflexes, the importance of these mechanisms in the normal control of the pulmonary circulation is uncertain. Two mechanisms that help to maintain the normal relation between pulmonary ventilation and blood flow in different areas of the lung (normal ventilation perfusion ratio) are local regional vasoconstriction produced by alveolar hypoxia and local bronchoconstriction in underperfused areas, possibly produced by a lack of normal carbon dioxide concentration.

In the normal person at rest in the upright position, there is relatively little perfusion of the upper segments of the lung, and consequently there is little exchange of oxygen and carbon dioxide in these areas. This pattern of blood flow is the result of the relatively low pulmonary artery pressure, which is barely adequate to perfuse the upper areas of the lungs. When an individual lies on one side, there is correspondingly a greater flow of blood to the dependent parts of the lung.

In contrast to systemic capillaries, which have a pressure of 25 to 35 mmHg, the pulmonary capillaries at rest have a pressure of only 7 to 10 mmHg. This is of distinct advantage, since pulmonary capillary pressure must be elevated to 25 to 30 mmHg before pulmonary edema occurs if the serum proteins, capillary walls, and lymphatic drainage are normal (referred to as *pulmonary capillary reserve*). Actually, the net effect on the low pressure in the pulmonary capillaries combined with a normal oncotic pressure of blood causes the pulmonary circulation to keep the interstitial tissues of the lung in a relatively "dehydrated" state.

The total pulmonary blood volume in normal adults is probably about 500 ml. As in the systemic circulation, about 50 to 65 percent of this volume is on the venous side. Normal pulmonary capillary blood volume at rest is about 100 ml. The total surface area of the pulmonary capillaries is estimated to be 50 to 100 m^2.

The flow through the lungs of a normal person can increase about threefold before there is a significant increase in the required driving pressure, or pressure difference between the main pulmonary artery and the left atrium. This is usually attributed to the utilization of vascular channels not used at rest and to dilatation of other vessels. In the presence of pulmonary vascular disease or lung disease, this reserve may be markedly diminished.

The Coronary Arteries[6,7,19,35–38]

The ostia of the two coronary arteries are located behind the aortic cusps near the top of the sinuses of Valsalva. These cusps are designated the *right or left coronary cusp,* depending on the coronary artery originating from it. The remaining coronary cusp is

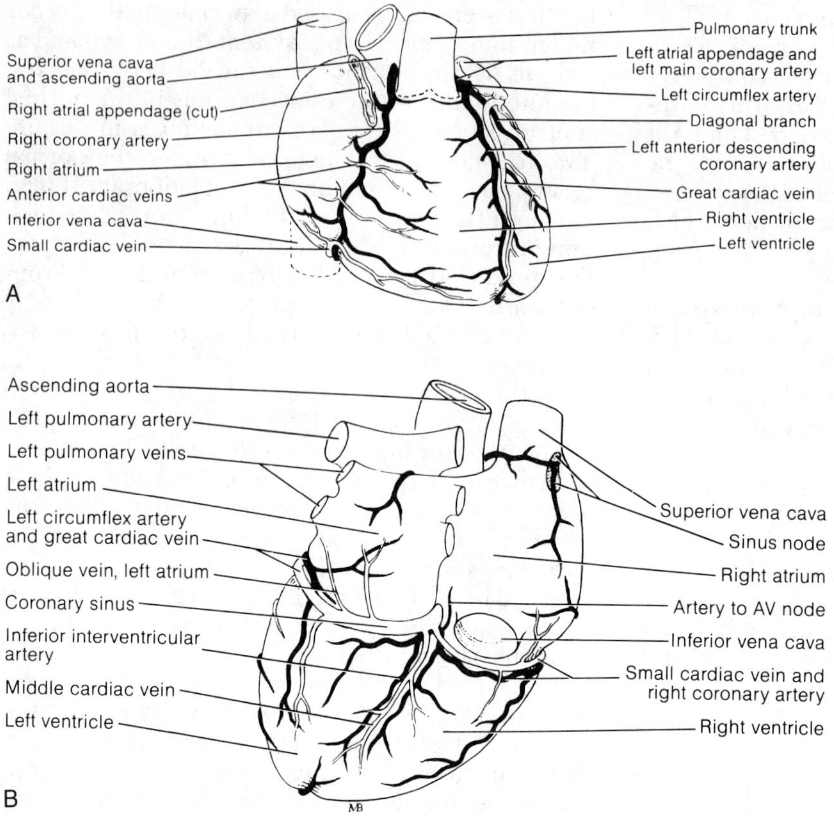

FIGURE 2-14 Diagram illustrating the principal arteries and veins (*A*) on the anterior surface of the heart and (*B*) on the posterior and inferior surfaces of the heart. Part of the right atrial appendage has been resected to show the proximal right coronary artery. In *B* the heart is shown more vertically oriented to expose the inferior surface. (*From R. Walmsley and H. Watson, "Clinical Anatomy of the Heart," Churchill Livingstone, New York, 1978. Reproduced with permission from the publisher and authors.*)

the *noncoronary (or posterior) cusp*. The plane of the aortic root is rotated and tilted slightly so that the ostium of the left coronary artery is superior and posterior to the right coronary ostium. (See also Chap. 107.)

Left Main Coronary Artery

The *left main coronary artery* (LMCA) travels anteriorly, slightly inferiorly, and leftward from the left aortic sinus to emerge from behind the pulmonary trunk. Within a short distance, usually 2 to 10 mm, the left main stem divides into two or more major arteries of nearly equal diameter—the *left anterior descending coronary artery,* the *left circumflex coronary artery,* and sometimes a *diagonal* (*or "intermediate"*) *coronary artery* (Fig. 2-14*A* and *B*).

Left Anterior Descending Coronary Artery

The left anterior descending (LAD) coronary artery is a direct continuation from the left main stem coursing anteriorly and caudally over the ventricular septum within the anterior interventricular sulcus. It usually circles around the apex and terminates in the inferior aspect of the cardiac apex. The branches of this artery, in their usual order of origin, are the first diagonal, the first septal perforator, right ventricular branches (not always seen in normal hearts), other septal perforators, and other diagonal branches. There may be two to six diagonal arteries, including the first diagonal, which may originate separately from the left main trunk. These diagonal branches course laterally over the free wall of the left ventricle in the angle between the left anterior descending and the left circumflex arteries. There are also three to five septal branches, which leave the LAD at a right angle and plunge deeply into the ventricular septum (Fig. 2-15). The LAD and its branches nourish most of the ventricular septum; the anterior, lateral, and apical wall of the left ventricle; most of the right and left bundle branches; and the anterolateral papillary muscle of the left ventricle. When the posterior descending artery is provided by the circumflex artery, the entire septum is vascularized by the left coronary system.[39] The LAD can also provide collateral circulation to the anterior right ventricle via the circle of Vieussens, to the posterior ventricular septum by the septal perforators, and to the posterior descending artery from the distal LAD or a diagonal branch.

Left Circumflex Coronary Artery

The left circumflex artery arises from the left main trunk at an obtuse angle and turns posteriorly as it courses around the left side of the heart within the left atrioventricular sulcus. In about 85 to 90 percent of patients it will terminate near the obtuse margin of the left ventricle; in the remaining patients it continues around to the crux of the heart, where it provides the posterior descending artery. The branches of the left circumflex are variable but

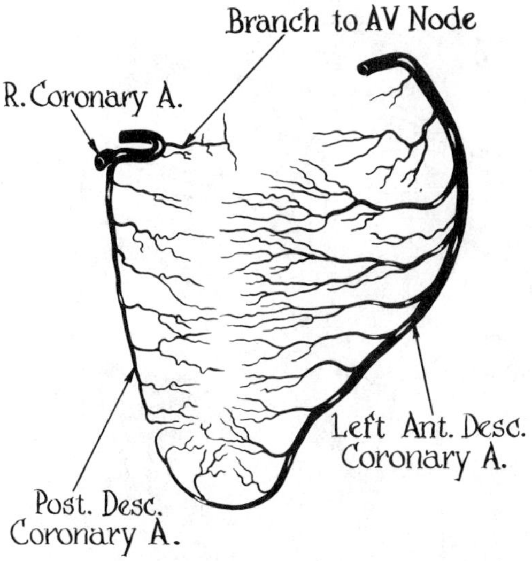

FIGURE 2-15 Drawing demonstrating the normal blood supply of the human ventricular septum. (*From T. N. James and G. E. Burch, Blood Supply of the Human Interventricular Septum, Circulation, 17:391, 1958. Reproduced with permission from the American Heart Association, Inc. and the authors.*)

may include the sinus node artery (40 to 50 percent), the left atrial circumflex branch, the anterolateral marginal, the distal circumflex, one or more posterolateral marginals, and the posterior descending artery (10 to 15 percent). The anterolateral marginal, which is usually the largest branch, is directed along the anterolateral wall toward the apex.

The left circumflex artery normally supplies blood to the left atrial wall, the posterior and lateral left ventricle, the anterolateral papillary muscle, and, in 40 to 45 percent of hearts, the sinus node. When it provides the posterior descending artery, it also supplies the AV node, the proximal bundle branches, the remainder of the inferoposterior left ventricular wall, a small portion of the posterior-basalar ventricular septum, and the posteromedial papillary muscle of the left ventricle.

Right Coronary Artery

The right coronary artery leaves the right aortic sinus and descends in the right atrioventricular groove curving posteriorly at the acute margin of the right ventricle. In 85 to 90 percent of hearts, it makes a 90° turn at the crux of the heart and continues downward in the posterior AV groove, finally terminating as a left ventricular branch. The branches of the right coronary artery include the conus artery (which may originate from a separate ostia in the right aortic sinus in 40 to 50 percent of hearts) to the right ventricular outflow area, the artery to the sinus node (50 to 60 percent), several anterior right ventricular branches, right atrial branches, the acute marginal branch, the artery to the AV node and proximal bundle branches, the posterior descending artery, and terminal branches to the left ventricle and left atrium. When the sinus node artery originates from the right coronary artery, it runs along the anterior right atrium to the superior vena cava, which it encircles in a clockwise or counterclockwise direction before it penetrates the sinus node.[40] In 40 to 50 percent of hearts, the sinus node artery originates from the proximal left circumflex artery and crosses behind the aorta and in front of the left atrium to reach the superior vena cava. Along its course, the sinus node artery supplies the atrial myocardium, the crista terminalis, and the atrial septum. The artery to the AV node arises at or near the inward U-shaped turn of the posterior descending coronary at the level of the crux of the heart (Fig. 2-15).[41] Usually the posterior descending artery begins proximal to the crux and courses toward the apex within the posterior interventricular sulcus. The right coronary artery provides blood flow to the sinus node (50 to 60 percent), the right ventricular wall, the crista supraventricularis, and the right atrium. In 85 to 90 percent of hearts the posterior descending branch supplies the basal one-half to two-thirds of the posterior ventricular septum, the AV node, the proximal His bundle, half the diaphragmatic surface, and the posteromedial papillary muscle of the left ventricle. The right coronary artery is an important collateral to the anterior descending coronary artery via the conus coronary artery and through communicating vessels in the ventricular septum (Fig. 2-14). *Kugel's artery,* which may originate from either the proximal right or left coronary artery, runs from anterior to posterior along the base of the atrial septum and is an important collateral to the AV node and the posterior circulation.[42]

The Coronary Veins[6,19,37]

An extensive intercommunicating network of veins provides venous drainage for the coronary circulation. Three venous drainage systems can be considered: the *coronary sinus* and its tributaries, the *anterior right ventricular veins,* and the *Thebesian veins* (Fig. 2-14).

The coronary sinus, located in the posterior atrioventricular groove near the crux of the heart, receives venous blood from the great, middle, and small cardiac veins, the posterior veins of the left ventricle, and the left atrial oblique vein (of Marshall). The coronary sinus drains blood predominantly from the left ventricle. The anterior interventricular vein lies in the anterior interventricular sulcus, parallel to the left anterior descending coronary artery. It ascends to near the bifurcation of the left main coronary artery and then turns leftward to circle posteriorly under the left atrium in the left atrioventricular sulcus, where it is referred to as the *great cardiac vein.* Along its posterior course, the great cardiac vein receives venous blood from large marginal and posterior left ventricular branches and then becomes the coronary sinus near the posterior margin of the left atrium. The *posterior interventricular vein* (*middle cardiac vein*) arises near the posterior aspect of the cardiac apex and ascends in the posterior interventricular sulcus next to the posterior descending coronary artery and drains either into the right atrium directly or into the coronary sinus just before it empties into the right atrium. The *oblique vein of Marshall* runs along the posterior left atrium and joins the great cardiac vein at the point where the latter becomes the coronary sinus. The coronary sinus extends 2 to 3 cm within the posterior atrioventricular groove before it opens into the inferior-posterior-medial aspect of the right atrium, between the orifice of the inferior vena cava and the septal tricuspid leaflet. A crescent-shaped, rudimentary valve, the Thebesian valve, can be seen at its entrance. The total distance from the bifurcation of the left coronary artery to the Thebesian valve is about 9 cm. About 85 percent of the coronary venous blood, including the drainage from the ventricular septum, the left ventricle, both atria, and some of the right ventricle, is carried by this elaborate system of veins. It is important to note that studies involving catheterization of the coronary sinus often require placing the tip of a catheter in the coronary sinus beyond the entrance of the posterior interventricular vein or other major veins draining the posterior left ventricle.

There are two to four *anterior cardiac veins* that originate in and drain the anterior right ventricular wall, travel superiorly to cross the right atrioventricular sulcus, and enter either directly into the right atrium anteriorly or into a collecting vein at the base of the right atrium. The *small cardiac vein,* which receives some branches from the right ventricle and the right atrium, winds around the right side of the heart in the atrioventricular sulcus and terminates in either the coronary sinus or the right atrium. The Thebesian veins are tiny venous outlets draining directly into the cardiac chambers, primarily into the right atrium and right ventricle.

The Conduction System of the Heart[6,7,43–45]

The Sinus Node

The sinus node, described by Keith and Flack in 1907,[45a] is located within the sulcus terminalis at the confluence of the superior vena cava, right atrial appendage, and lateral wall of the right atrium. The node is spindle-shaped and measures 10 to 20 mm in length and about 3 mm at its widest point. The sinus node artery, which originates from the right coronary artery in 50 to 60 percent of hearts and the left circumflex in the remainder, passes through the center of the sinus node.

Internodal Pathways

Three conducting pathways that facilitate conduction of the electrical impulse between the sinus and the AV nodes have been described by James.[46–48] These three pathways are designated the *anterior, middle, and posterior internodal tracts* (Figs. 2-16 and 2-17). The anterior internodal tract, or *Bachman's bundle,* courses anteriorly around the superior vena cava and down the atrial septum to the AV node. Fibers from this tract also branch off to the left atrium. The middle internodal tract leaves the sinus node and courses posteriorly around the superior vena cava and then descends within the atrial septum to the AV node. The posterior internodal tract runs posteriorly through the crista terminalis and then through the posterior atrial septum to reach the AV node.

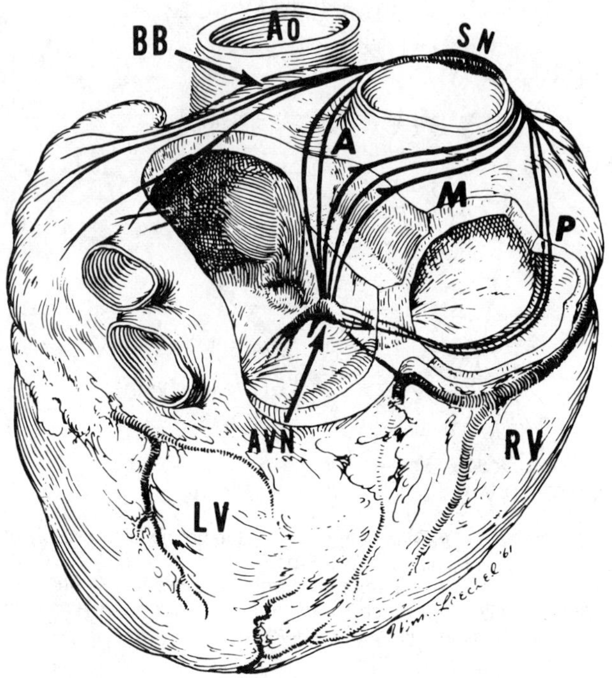

FIGURE 2-16 Drawing depicting the three internodal pathways: anterior (A), middle (M), and posterior (P). Bachman's bundle (BB) contains the major interatrial pathway as well as the initial portion of the anterior internodal pathway. Ao = aorta; LV = left ventricle; RV = right ventricle; SN = sinus node; AVN = AV node. *[From T. N. James and L. Sherf, P Waves, Atrial Depolarization, and Pacemaking Site, in R. C. Schlant and J. W. Hurst (eds.), "Advances in Electrocardiography," Grune & Stratton, New York, 1972, p. 37. Reproduced with permission from the publisher and author. Modified from T. N. James, The Connecting Pathways between the Sinus Node and the A-V Node and between the Right and the Left Atrium in the Human Heart, Am. Heart J., 66:489, 1963.]*

The AV Node and Bundle of His

Described by Tarawa in 1906,[48a] the *AV node* is located in the medial floor of the right atrium at the base of the atrial septum and between the coronary sinus ostium and the insertion of the septal leaflet of the tricuspid valve. The *bundle of His* begins imperceptibly at the anterior extension of the AV node and then penetrates through the central fibrous body at the crest of the muscular ventricular septum, just below the inferior margin of the membranous ventricular septum and between the right and noncoronary aortic cusps (Fig. 2-18). Over a distance of 5

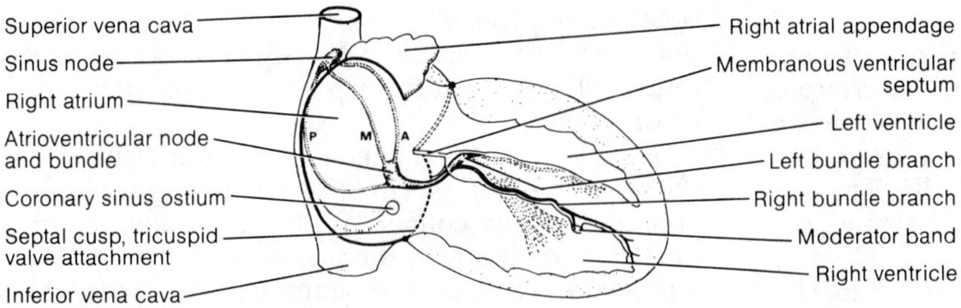

FIGURE 2-17 Diagram of the heart illustrating the principal features of the human conduction system in a lateral view. The drawing is not intended to represent a true anatomic section. A, M, and P refer to the anterior, middle, and posterior internodal pathways. (*From R. Walmsley and H. Watson, "Clinical Anatomy of the Heart," Churchill Livingstone, New York, 1978. Reproduced with permission from the publisher and authors.*)

to 15 mm, fibers of the left bundle depart from the common bundle and then fan out widely within the subendocardium of the left side of the ventricular septum. About midway to the apex the left bundle separates into two major divisions, the anterior-superior and posterior-inferior fascicles, which continue to the base of the two papillary muscles and the adjacent myocardium. A third, or middle, division has also been described. The right bundle branch originates from the distal end of the common bundle as a relatively slender bundle about 1 mm wide. From the right side of the ventricular septum, near the inferior edge of the membranous septum, it courses toward the right ventricular apex with some branches passing through the moderator band to the anterior papillary muscle of the right ventricle while other branches innervate nearby areas of the apex of the right ventricle.

FIGURE 2-18 Diagram of the human AV node and His bundle, showing their relation to the two AV valves and the atrial and ventricular septa, including the membranous portion of the latter. As the bundle courses medially and inferiorly along the lower margin of the membranous interventricular septum, it gives rise early to a single right branch but continues providing multiple left branches, which form virtually a sheet of fibers down the left septal endocardium. Only a few fibers from the internodal pathways are shown in order to avoid obscuring details of the AV node, but these may be seen entering the superior and posterior margins of the node (its crest) as well as the lower portion of the convex right atrial surface of the node. A few internodal fibers terminate in the base of the tricuspid valve, and rarely (almost exclusively in infants) a few may penetrate directly to the ventricular septum. (*From T. N. James, Morphology of the Human Atrioventricular Node with Remarks Pertinent to Its Electrophysiology, Am. Heart J., 62:756, 1961. Reproduced with permission from the publisher and author.*)

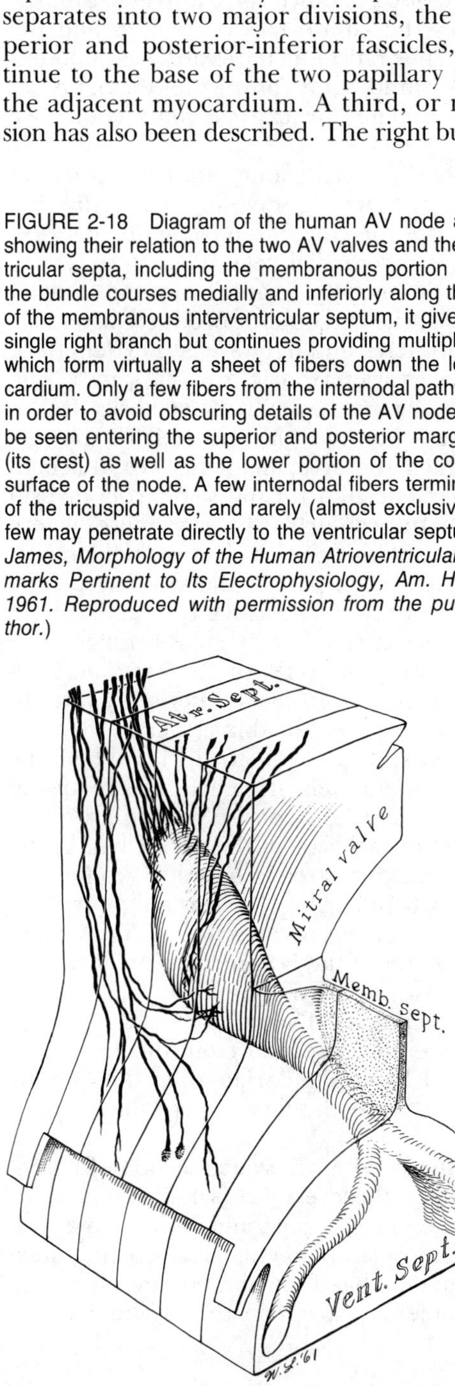

Ultrastructure of the Myocardium

The functions of the heart may be classified into three types: electrical, mechanical, and endocrine. Many myocardial cells are specialized for one of these functions. The myocardial cells concerned primarily with mechanical shortening are similar, although there are some differences between atrial and ventricular myocardium.[49] Several different types of cells have electrical or endocrine activity as a major function, and the structure of such cells is significantly different from that of contractile, or "working," myocardial cells.[43,46,47,50–53]

Some special cells of the heart are particularly developed for the generation and very rapid conduction of an electrical impulse to the working cells.[46] There are four types of cells generally recognized in this system of impulse formation and rapid conduction. These are the *P cells, transitional cells, ameboid cells,* and *Purkinje cells.* P cells are numerous in the sinus node, and are also present in the AV node and internodal pathways.[54] Transitional cells are found predominantly in the sinus node, the AV node, and internodal pathways, and for considerable distances in the atrial tissue adjacent to both nodes. Ameboid cells are found primarily in the eustachian ridge area. Purkinje cells are found at the margins of the sinus node; in the internodal pathways, which also contain intermingled transitional cells and ordinary working myocardial cells; adjacent to the AV node; and in the His bundle and its branches. The His bundle consists primarily of Purkinje cells, while the bundle branches consist of Purkinje cells intermingled with ordinary working cells.

P cells are so named[51,52] because of their pale appearance on microscopy and their resemblance to primitive myocardial cells, and because they are thought to be the site of origin of the pacemaker impulse. They are usually ovoid or rounded in contrast to the usual elongated shape of other myocardial cells. They measure 5 to 10 μm in greatest diameter and are the smallest type of myocardial cell.

Transitional cells are a heterogeneous group of cells that include all cells with a microscopic appearance intermediate between the P cells and the more complex working myocardial cells. They are more elongated than P cells but shorter and narrower than working myocardial cells.

Ameboid cells have been described[55,56] in electron micrographs from the eustachian ridge. They may be elongated, triangular, oval, or nongeometric in shape. They have multilobular nuclei and pseudopodic prolongations that fill the spaces between neighboring cells and are often filled with a heavy concentration of electron-opaque granules, which tends to give the cells a dark appearance. They have many mitochondria and myofibrils. Although the exact function of the ameboid cells is unknown, they may act as an auxiliary pacemaker or may be a source of atrial natriuretic factor (see Chap. 3).

Purkinje cells are identified primarily on the basis of their ultrastructure. Purkinje cells tend to be both broader and shorter than working myocardial cells and measure from 10 to 30 μm in cross section and 20 to 50 μm in length.

Contractile, or working, myocardial cells are similar, whether they are from atrial or ventricular myocardium. They are characterized by hundreds of myofibrils in a special arrangement. Working myocardial cells are arranged longitudinally in series, with multiple cells forming a "fiber." Multiple fibers are generally arranged in parallel. Although cardiac muscle fibers have many lateral and end-to-side connections, the contractile cells are not a true anatomic syncytium. Intercalated disks at the terminal margins and junctions of contractile cells form a specialized, transversely oriented cell boundary.[57] The myofibrils of working myocardial cells insert in the region of the intercalated disk. Contractile cells have many mitochondria and a nucleus which tends to be centrally located and slightly elongated. These myocardial cells are about 10 to 20 μm in diameter and 50 to 100 μm in length.

Contractile cells contain an intricate *sarcotubular system* of tubules, vesicles, and cisternae.[58,59] One component of this system consists of the periodic invagination of the sarcolemma by *transversely oriented tubules* known as the *T system.* Focal dilatations of the T-system tubules are seen in the area of the *Z band,* forming a cisternlike structure, the *intermediary vesicle.*[60] A second component of the sarcotubular system is the series of interconnecting longitudinal tubules that tend to be oriented parallel to the myofibrils, which they surround. Near the Z band, these tubules have local dilatations—*lateral sacs,* or *terminal cisternae*—which, together with the intermediary vesicle, form a *triad.* A triad consists of an intermediary vesicle from the T system and two lateral sacs from the longitudinal system. Although the three components of the triad are very close to each other, they probably are not in direct communication. The term *subsarcolemma cisternae* describes both central (T system) and peripheral (sarcolemma) sites of proximity.

Transverse tubules are arranged perpendicularly to the long axis of the cell, but branch longitudinally, and can directly connect with other transverse tubules.[61,62] In contrast, the internal longitudinal system (or sarcoplasmic reticulum) is a plexiform labyrinth of vesicles and tubules, some of which may also be transversely oriented.[63]

The sarcotubular system plays an important role in both electrical impulse conduction[64] and electromechanical coupling.[60] The impulse spreads rapidly on the surface of cells, down the transverse tubules, and stimulates the lateral sacs or vesicles and the entire sarcoplasmic reticulum to release large amounts of calcium around the contractile elements of the cell and initiate myocardial contraction (see Chap. 3).[65]

The myofibrils form longitudinally oriented strands of interdigitating myosin and actin filaments, which are the contractile elements of working, contractile myocardial cells (Figs. 2-19, 2-20). The repeating morphologic and functional unit of contractile cells, the sarcomere, produces a regular band pattern of dark and light areas. The length of each sarcomere varies from 1.5 to 2.2 μm.[66] The dark Z bands, where the intercalated disks are located, provide a boundary at the ends of the sarcomere to which the actin filaments are attached. These thin filaments of actin and some tropomyosin B project into the center of the sarcomere, where they interdigitate with the thick myosin filaments which lie in the central part of the sarcomere. The thick filaments of myosin measure 1.5 μm and have small excrescences produced by cross-bridges.[67]

The dark and light zones of the sarcomere on microscopy are produced by the periodic, interdigitating relations between the thin actin and the thick myosin filaments (Figs. 2-19 to 2-21). When the myofibrils are moderately stretched, the following pattern is seen: the *I band* consists of thin actin filaments attached to each side of the dark Z band. The *A band* is the wide dark area in between two peripherally located I bands. The *H zone* is a lighter band of thick myosin filaments in the center of the A band. Crossing the center of the H zone is a thin dark line, the *M line,* consisting of the knoblike excrescences of the myosin filaments. The portions of the A band that extend in either direction from the H zone to each adjacent I band are darker than the H zone because they contain both thin actin and thick myosin filaments.

The appearance of a transverse section of myofibril depends upon the level of the sarcomere at which the cut is made. The H-zone and M-line area contain only thick myosin filaments arranged in a hexagonal pattern; the I band contains only evenly spaced thin actin filaments, except in the H zone; the A

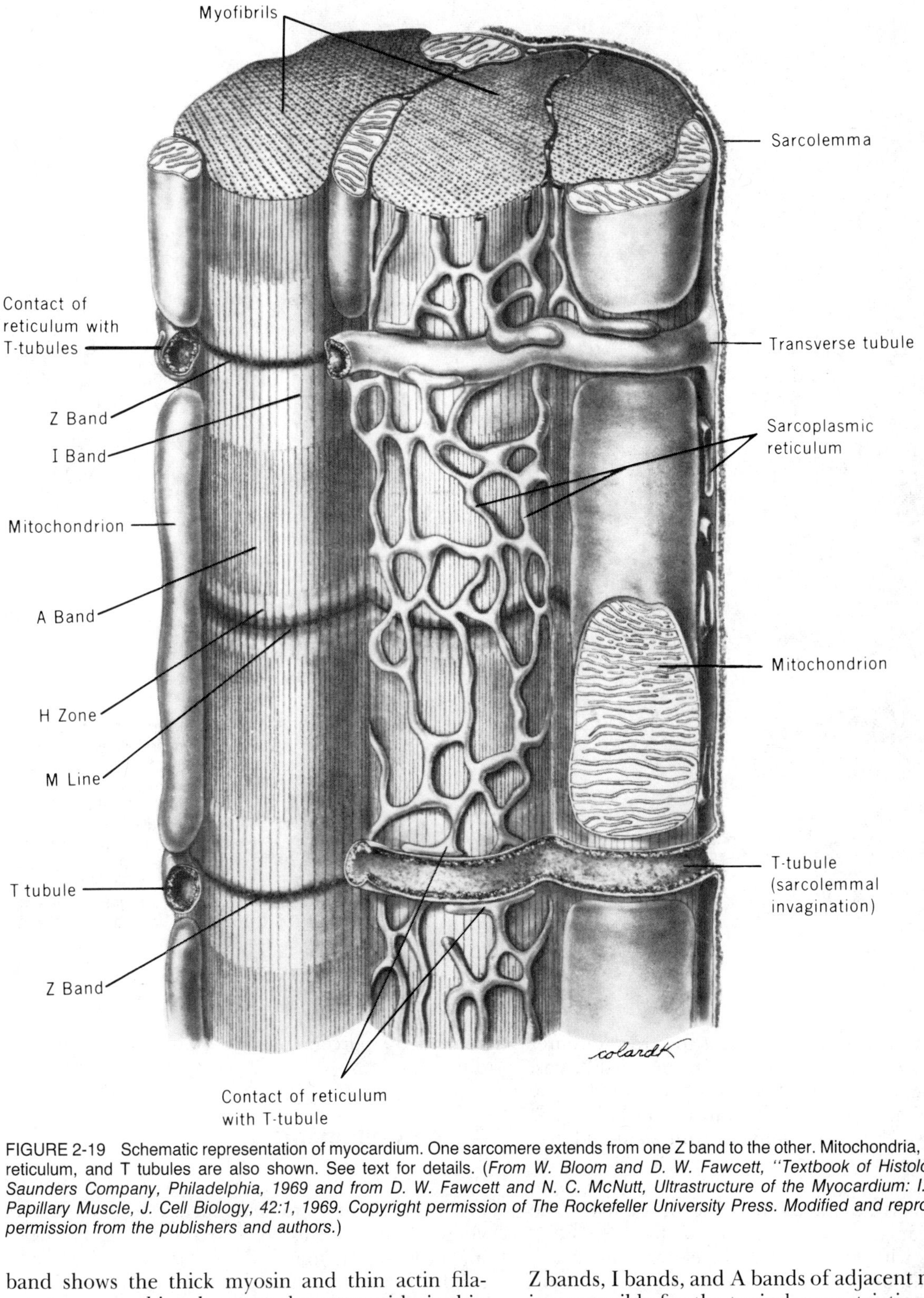

FIGURE 2-19 Schematic representation of myocardium. One sarcomere extends from one Z band to the other. Mitochondria, sarcoplastic reticulum, and T tubules are also shown. See text for details. (*From W. Bloom and D. W. Fawcett, "Textbook of Histology," W. B. Saunders Company, Philadelphia, 1969 and from D. W. Fawcett and N. C. McNutt, Ultrastructure of the Myocardium: I. Ventricular Papillary Muscle, J. Cell Biology, 42:1, 1969. Copyright permission of The Rockefeller University Press. Modified and reproduced with permission from the publishers and authors.*)

band shows the thick myosin and thin actin filaments arranged in a hexagonal pattern with six thin actin filaments surrounding each thick myosin filament (Fig. 2-22).

Each working myocardial cell contains hundreds of parallel myofibrils with rows of mitochondria between them (Figs. 2-19 to 2-21). The alignment of Z bands, I bands, and A bands of adjacent myofibrils is responsible for the typical cross striations seen on light microscopy.

Many studies have supported the application of Huxley and Hanson's "sliding filament hypothesis"[68–70] to both skeletal and myocardial muscle. In their theory, linkages between the actin and myosin

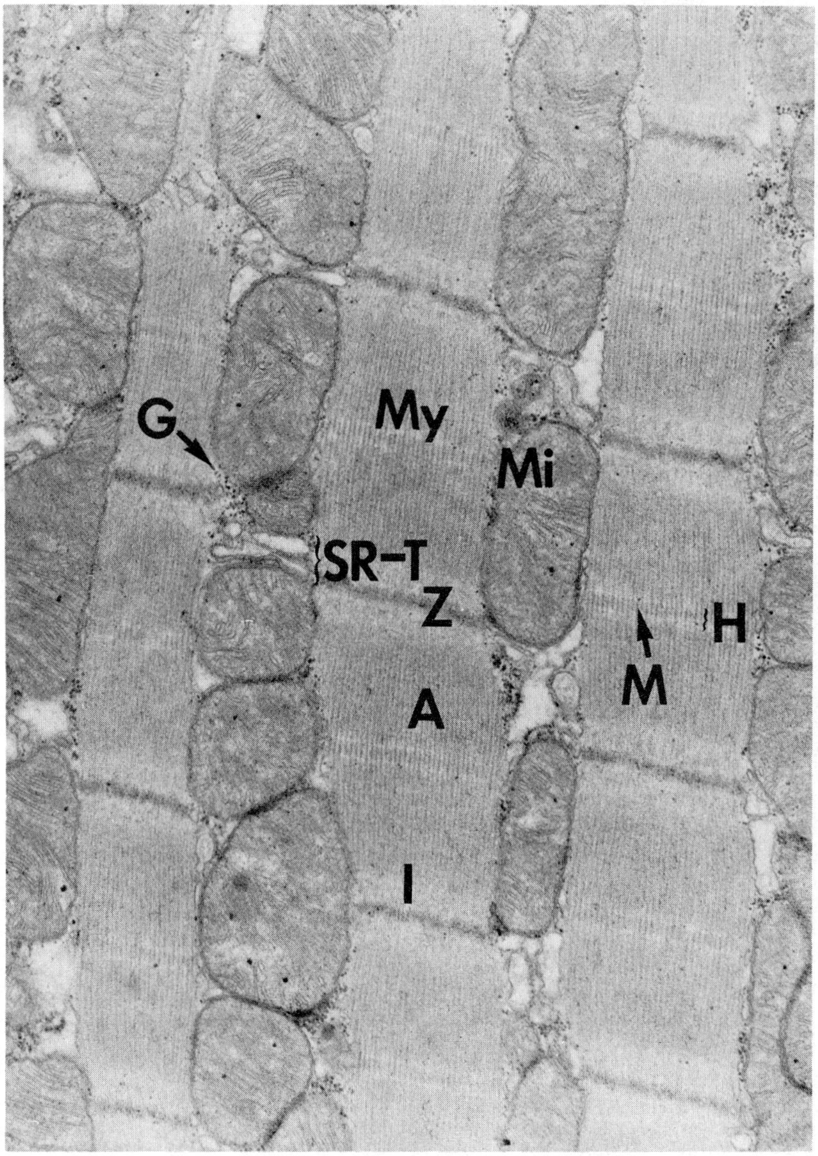

FIGURE 2-20 Electron micrograph of hamster myocardium, longitudinal section. Thick myosin and thin actin filaments are arranged into myofibrils (My) which exhibit the characteristic banding pattern. Mi = mitochondrion; G = glycogen particles; SR-T = elements of sarcoplasmic reticulum and T-tubule system; A = A band; Z = Z band; I = I band; M = M line; H = H zone. (*Courtesy of Claudia R. Adkison, Ph.D., Department of Anatomy, Emory University, Atlanta, Ga.*)

pull or propel the actin filaments toward the center of the sarcomere. The two sets of filaments slide past each other causing the muscle fiber to shorten. The myosin component for the linkage is heavy (H) meromyosin,[69] which combines with actin and also contains the ATPase necessary to split the ATP to provide the energy for contraction. When a myocardial cell is activated, the concentration of free intracellular Ca^{2+} increases markedly. The Ca^{2+} combines with troponin and releases the actin-myosin inhibition, thereby permitting the actin and myosin fibers to slide and the muscle fiber to shorten. (See Chap. 3.)

The *mitochondria* of working myocardial cells (Figs. 2-19 to 2-21) are cylindrically shaped and measure 2 by 0.5 μm. They have many infoldings, or *cristae,* which project inward from the membrane. Mitochondria are very numerous and comprise between 25 and 50 percent of the total mass of myocardium.[66]

Acknowledgments

We would like to thank Dr. Thomas James for his many contributions to chapters and sections in previous editions of this book, particularly those dealing with the anatomy of the coronary artery and conducting system, the ultrastructure of the heart, and the pathophysiological correlations in disease of the conduction system. Dr. Libi Sherf contributed significantly to chapters and sections on myocardial ultrastructure. We are indebted to both Dr. James and Dr. Sherf for all they have taught us. We are responsible for any possible misinterpretation in this chapter of their research studies and teachings.

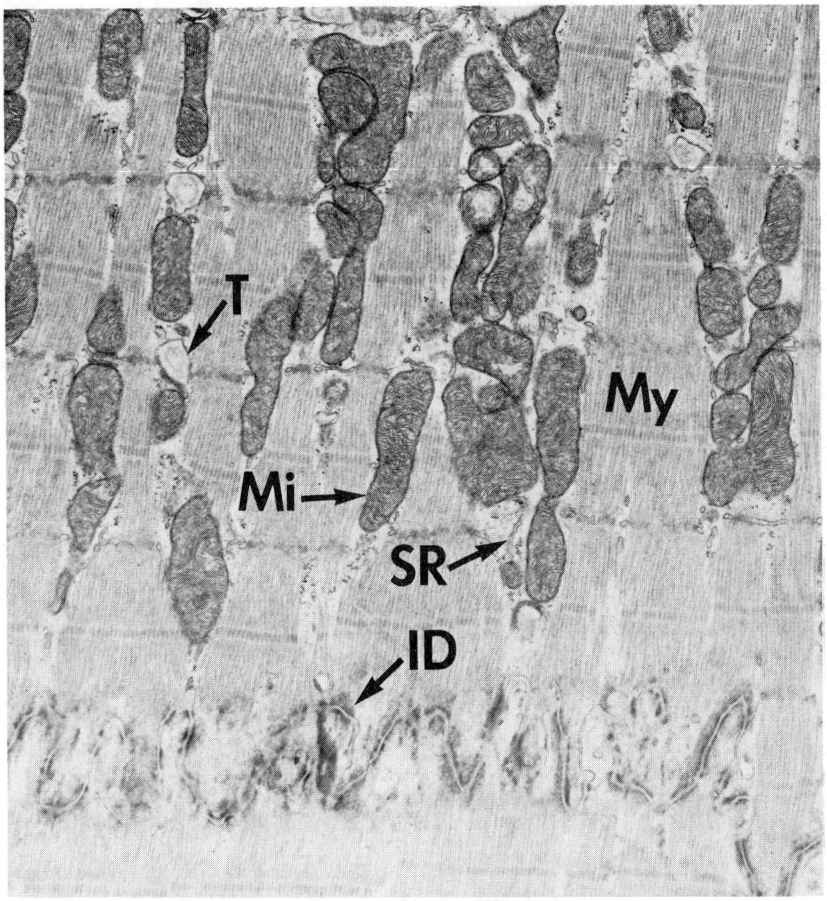

FIGURE 2-21 Electron micrograph of human myocardium, longitudinal section. Cytoplasm is packed with a regular array of myofibrils (My), showing the distinct banding pattern. Mitochondria (Mi) and elements of the sarcoplasmic reticulum (SR) and the T-tubule system (T) are arranged around the myofibrils. Portions of two cells are shown joined end to end at the intercalated disk (ID). (*Courtesy of Claudia R. Adkison, Ph.D., Department of Anatomy, Emory University, Atlanta, Ga.*)

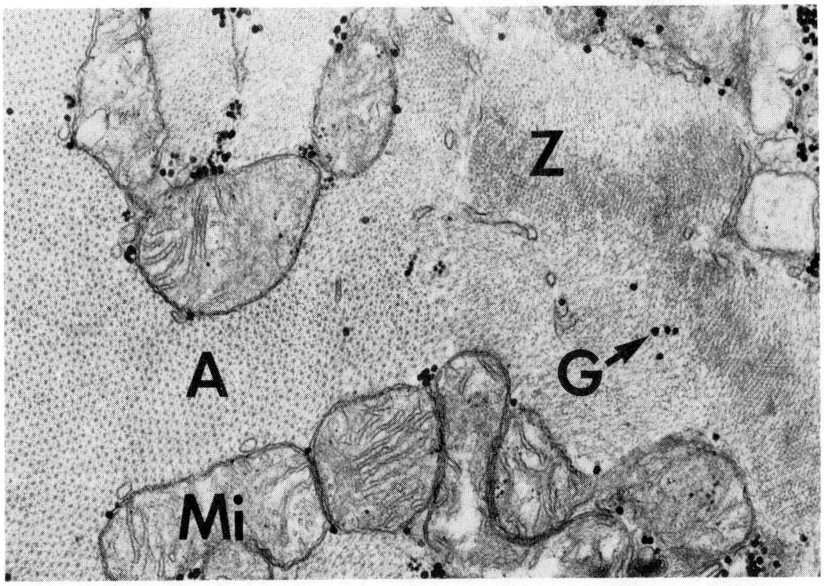

FIGURE 2-22 Electron micrograph of dog myocardium, cross section. Thin actin and thick myosin filaments form a hexagonal array in the A band (A) of a myofibril. Z = Z band; G = glycogen particles; Mi = mitochondrion. (*Courtesy of Claudia R. Adkison, Ph.D., Department of Anatomy, Emory University, Atlanta, Ga.*)

References

1. Kisch, B.: Electron Microscopy of the Atrium of the Heart: I, *Guinea Pig Exp. Med. Surg.*, 14:99, 1956.
2. Burton, A. C.: The Importance of the Shape and Size of the Heart, *Am. Heart J.*, 54:801, 1957.
3. Zimmerman, J.: The Functional and Surgical Anatomy of the Heart, *Ann. R. Coll. Surg. Engl.*, 39:348, 1966.
4. Davies, M. J., Pomerance, A., and Lamb, D.: Techniques in Examination and Anatomy of the Heart, in A. Pomerance and M. J. Davies (eds.), "The Pathology of the Heart," Blackwell Scientific Publications, Ltd., Oxford, 1975, p. 1.
5. McAlpine, W. A.: "Heart and Coronary Arteries," Springer-Verlag New York Inc., New York, 1975.
6. Walmsley, R., and Watson, H.: "Clinical Anatomy of the Heart," Churchill Livingstone, New York, 1978.
7. Anderson, R. H., and Becker, A. E.: "Cardiac Anatomy," Churchill Livingstone, London, 1980.
8. Lev, M., and Bharati, S.: The Fibrous Skeleton of the Heart, in J. W. Hurst (ed.), "Update IV: The Heart," McGraw-Hill Book Company, New York, 1982, p. 7.
9. Rosenquist, G. C., and Sweeney, L. J.: The Membranous Ventricular Septum in the Normal Heart, *Johns Hopkins Med. J.*, 135:9, 1974.
10. Titus, J. L.: Normal Anatomy of the Human Cardiac Conduction System, *Mayo Clin. Proc.*, 48:24, 1973.
11. Sweeney, L. J., and Rosenquist, G. C.: The Normal Anatomy of the Atrial Septum: In the Human Heart, *Amer. Heart J.*, 98:194, 1979.
12. Prakash, R.: Determination of Right Ventricular Wall Thickness in Systole and Diastole: Echocardiographic and Necropsy Correlation in 32 Patients, *Br. Heart J.*, 40:1257, 1978.
13. Grant, R. P., Downey, F. M., and MacMahon, H.: The Architecture of the Right Ventricular Outflow Tract in the Normal Heart and in the Presence of Ventricular Septal Defects, *Circulation*, 24:223, 1961.
14. Kennedy, J. W., Baxley, W. A., Figley, M. M., Dodge, H. T., and Blackmon, J. R.: Quantitative Angiocardiography: I. The Normal Left Ventricle in Man, *Circulation*, 34:272, 1966.
15. Zimmerman, J.: The Functional and Surgical Anatomy of the Aortic Valve, *Isr. Med. J.*, 5:862, 1969.
16. Merklin, R. J.: Position and Orientation of the Heart Valves, *Am. J. Anat.*, 125:375, 1969.
17. Davies, M. J.: "Pathology of Cardiac Valves," Butterworth Scientific Publications, London, 1980.
18. Vollebergh, F. E. M. G., and Becker, A. E.: Minor Congenital Variations of Cusp Size in Tricuspid Aortic Valves: Possible Link with Isolated Aortic Stenosis, *Br. Heart J.*, 39:1006, 1977.
19. Gensini, G. F.: "Coronary Arteriography," Futura Publishing, New York, 1975.
20. Silverman, M. E., and Hurst, J. W.: The Mitral Complex, *Am. Heart J.*, 76:399, 1968.
21. Ranganathan, N., Lam, J. H. C., Wigle, E. D., and Silver, M. D.: Morphology of the Human Mitral Valve: II. The Valve Leaflets, *Circulation*, 41:459, 1970.
22. Perloff, J. K., and Roberts, W. C.: The Mitral Apparatus: Functional Anatomy of Mitral Regurgitation, *Circulation*, 46:227, 1972.
23. Silver, M. D., Lam, J. H. C., Ranganathan, N., and Wigle, E. D.: Morphology of the Human Tricuspid Valve, *Circulation*, 43:333, 1971.
24. Estes, E. H., Jr., Dalton, F. M., Entman, M. L., Dixon, H. D. II, and Hackel, D. B.: The Anatomy and Blood Supply of the Papillary Muscles of the Left Ventricle, *Am. Heart J.*, 71:356, 1966.
25. Lam, J. H. C., Ranganathan, N., Wigle, E. D., and Silver, M. D.: Morphology of the Human Mitral Valve: I. Chordae Tendineae, *Circulation*, 41:449, 1970.
26. Holt, J. P.: The Normal Pericardium, *Am. J. Cardiol.*, 26:455, 1970.
27. Mitchell, G. A. G: "Cardiovascular Innervation," The Williams & Wilkins Company, Baltimore, 1956.
28. Ellison, J. P., and Williams, T. H.: Sympathetic Nerve Pathways to the Human Heart and Their Variations, *Am. J. Anat.*, 124:149, 1969.
29. Randall, W. C. (ed.): "Nervous Control of Cardiovascular Function," Oxford University Press, New York, 1984.
30. Feola, M., Merklin, R., Cho, S., and Brockman, S. K.: The Terminal Pathway of the Lymphatic System of the Human Heart, *Ann. Thorac. Surg.*, 24:531, 1977.
31. Miller, A. J.: "Lymphatics of the Heart," Raven Press, New York, 1982.
32. Rusznyak, I.: "Lymphatics and Lymph Circulation: Physiology and Pathology," L. Youlten (ed.), 2d English ed., Oxford, Pergamon Press, New York, 1967.
33. Yoffey, J. M., and Courtice, F. C.: "Lymphatics, Lymph and Lymphomyeloid Complex," Academic Press, New York, 1970.
34. Fishman, A. P., and Hecht, H. H. (eds.): "The Pulmonary Circulation and Intestinal Space," The University of Chicago Press, Chicago, 1969.
35. Laurie, W., and Woods, J. D.: Anastomoses of the Coronary Circulation, *Lancet*, 2:812, 1958.
36. Pepler, W. J., and Meyer, B. J.: Interarterial Coronary Anastomoses and Coronary Arterial Pattern, *Circulation*, 22:14, 1960.
37. James, T. N.: "Anatomy of the Coronary Arteries," Hoeber Medical Division, Harper & Row Publishers, Inc., New York, 1961.
38. James, T. N.: The Delivery and Distribution of Coronary Collateral Circulation, *Chest*, 58:183, 1970.
39. James, T. N., and Burch, G. E.: Blood Supply of the Human Interventricular Septum, *Circulation*, 17:391, 1958.
40. Anderson, K. R., Ho, S. Y., and Anderson, R. H.: Location and Vascular Supply of Sinus Node in Human Heart. *Br. Heart J.*, 41:28, 1979.
41. James, T. N.: A Useful Landmark for Interpreting Angiocardiograms, *Radiology*, 75:804, 1963.
42. Kugel, M. A.: Anatomical Studies on the Coronary Arteries and Their Branches: I. Arteria Anastomotica Auricularis Magna, *Am. Heart J.*, 3:260, 1927.
43. James, T. N.: Anatomy of the Human Sinus Node, *Anat. Rec.*, 141:109, 1961.
44. Anderson, R. H., Becker, A. E., Tranum-Jensen, J., and Janse, M. J.: Anatomico-Electrophysiological Correlations in the Conduction System—A Review, *Br. Heart J.*, 45:67, 1981.
45. Massing, G. K., and James, T. N.: Anatomic Configuration of the His Bundle and Bundle Branches in the Human Heart, *Circulation*, 53:609, 1976.

45a. Keith, A., and Flack, M.: The Form and Nature of the Muscular Connections between the Primary Divisions of the Vertebrate Heart, *J. Anat. Physiol.*, 41:172, 1907.

46. James, T. N.: The Connecting Pathways between the Sinus Node and the A-V Node and between the Right and the Left Atrium in the Human Heart, *Am. Heart J.*, 66:498, 1963.
47. James, T. N., and Sherf, L.: Specialized Tissues and Preferential Conduction in the Atria of the Heart, *Am., J. Cardiol.*, 28:414, 1971.
48. James, T. N., and Sherf, L.: P Waves, Atrial Depolarization, and Pacemaking Site, in R. C. Schlant and J. W. Hurst (eds.), "Advances in Electrocardiography," Grune & Stratton, Inc., New York, 1972, p. 37.

48a. Tawara, S.: "Das Reizleitungssystem des Saugetierherzens," G. Fischer, Jena, 1906.

49. McNutt, N. S., and Fawcett, D. W.: The Ultrastructure of the Cat Myocardium: II. Atrial Muscle, *J. Cell Biol.*, 42:46, 1969.
50. James, T. N.: Morphology of the Human Atrioventricular Node, with Remarks Pertinent to Its Electrophysiology, *Am. Heart J.*, 62:756, 1961.
51. James, T. N., Sherf, L., Fine, G., and Morales, A. R.: Com-

parative Ultrastructure of the Sinus Node in Man and Dog, *Circulation,* 34:139, 1966.
52. James, T. N., and Sherf, L.: Ultrastructure of the Human Atrioventricular Node, *Circulation,* 37:1049, 1968.
53. James, T. N., Sherf, L., and Urthaler, F.: Fine Structure of the Bundle Branches, *Br. Heart J.,* 36:1, 1974.
54. James, T. N., and Sherf, L.: Specialized Tissues and Preferential Conduction in the Atria of the Heart, *Am. J. Cardiol.,* 28:414, 1971.
55. Sherf, L., and James, T. N.: Fine Structure of Cells and Their Histological Organization within Internodal Pathways of the Heart: Clinical and Electrocardiographic Implications, *Am. J. Cardiol.,* 44:345, 1979.
56. Sherf, L., and James, T. N.: Functional Anatomy and Ultrastructure of the Internodal Pathways, in R. C. Little (ed.), "Physiology of Atrial Pacemakers and Conductive Tissues," Futura Publishing Co., Inc., Mount Kisco, N.Y., 1980, p. 67.
57. Sjostrand, F. S., and Andersson-Cedergren, E.: Intercalated Discs of Heart Muscle, in G. H. Bourne (ed.), "The Structure and Function of Muscle," Academic Press, Inc., New York, 1960, p. 421.
58. Porter, K. R., and Palade, G. E.: Studies on the Endoplastic Reticulum: III. Its Form and Distribution in Striated Muscle Cells, *J. Biophys. Biochem. Cytol.,* 3:269, 1957.
59. Hoffman, B. F.: Physiology of Atrioventricular Transmission, *Circulation,* 24:506, 1961.
60. Essner, E., Novikoff, A. B., and Quintana, N.: Nucleoside Phosphatase Activities in Rat Cardiac Muscle, *J. Cell Biol.,* 25:201, 1965.
61. Fawcett, D. W., and McNutt, N. S.: The Ultrastructure of the Cat Myocardium: I. Ventricular Papillary Muscle, *J. Cell Biol.,* 42:1, 1969.
62. Forssmann, W. G., and Giardier, L.: A Study of the T System in Rat Heart, *J. Cell Biol.,* 44:1, 1970.
63. Sommer, J. R., and Johnson, E. A.: A Comparative Study of Purkinje Fibers and Ventricular Fibers, *J. Cell Biol.,* 36:497, 1968.
64. Huxley, A. F., and Taylor, R. E.: Local Activation of Striated Muscle Fibres, *J. Physiol.,* 144:426, 1958.
65. Huxley, A. F.: The Links between Excitation and Contraction, *Proc. R. Soc. London Ser. B,* 160:486, 1964.
66. Braunwald, E., Ross, J., Jr., and Sonnenblick, E. H.: Mechanisms of Contraction of the Normal and Failing Heart, *N. Engl. J. Med.,* 277:794, 1967.
67. Hasselbach, W.: ATP Driven Active Transport of Ca in the Membranes of the Sarcoplasmic Reticulum, *Proc. R. Soc. London Ser. B,* 160:501, 1964.
68. Huxley, H. E., and Hanson, J.: Changes in the Cross-Striations of Muscle during Contraction and Stretch and Their Structural Interpretation, *Nature,* 173:973, 1954.
69. Huxley, H. E.: Structural Arrangement and the Contraction Mechanism in Striated Muscle, *Proc. R. Soc. London Ser. B,* 160:442, 1964.
70. Huxley, H. E.: Structural Evidence Concerning Mechanism of Contraction in Striated Muscle, in W. M. Paul, C. M. Kay, and G. Monckton (eds.), "Muscle," Pergamon Press, Toronto, 1965, p. 3.

3

Normal Physiology of the Cardiovascular System

Robert C. Schlant, M.D.
Edmund H. Sonnenblick, M.D.

The cardiovascular system has these three basic functions: to transport oxygen and other nutrients to the cells of the body, to remove metabolic waste products from the cells, and to carry substances such as hormones from one part of the body to another. In addition, the heart and blood vessels have important neurohumoral functions. With every beat, the performance of the heart may be considered the net result of the following three major determinants: preload, afterload, and contractility (the inotropic state). The heart rate then determines the performance of the heart relative to time. Cardiac performance is further influenced by atrial function, neural control, hormones and metabolic products, the synchrony of ventricular contraction, anesthesia, and drugs. This chapter will review myocardial excitation-contraction coupling, fundamentals of muscle mechanics, the major factors influencing cardiac performance, the cardiac cycle, the major mechanisms of cardiac reserve, the response to exercise, and the coronary circulation. Detailed discussions are found in the general reference sources.[1–14] The evaluation of cardiac and myocardial function is discussed further in Chap. 17.

Myocardial Excitation-Contraction Coupling[11,15–33]

In recent years there has been a great increase in our understanding of the mechanisms by which the action potential stimulus initiates the contractile process in heart muscle. All these studies have emphasized the central role in excitation-contraction coupling of the calcium ion (Ca^{2+}), which has been known to be essential for myocardial contraction since the classic studies of S. Ringer.[15a] The Ca^{2+} ion is now known to have two major roles in excitation-contraction, i.e., the initiation of contraction (trigger substance) and the regulation of myocardial contraction (regulating factor).

With the initiation of the action potential in ventricular myocardium (Fig. 3-1), there is a very rapid influx of Na^+ (or change in Na^+ *conductance*) which produces the rapid electrical spike and overshoot during phase zero (see Chap. 4). During the plateau of the action potential (phase 2), there is a slow inward flux of Ca^{2+} across the myocardial cell membrane, or sarcolemma, into the intracellular fluid (sarcoplasm or cytosol). One view maintains that the extracellular Ca^{2+} ions are temporarily bound on special sites on the membrane for one or more beats prior to being transported into the sarcoplasm by subsequent action potentials.[23,31] As indicated schematically in Fig. 3-2, the action potential also spreads from the myocardial cell membrane down the extensive *transverse (T) tubular system,* which consists of sarcolemma invaginations especially near the Z bands that are in direct continuity with the extracellular or interstitial space (see Chap. 2 for anatomic details). Although not definitely established, it appears probable that during the passage of the action potential the T system contributes qualitatively to intracellular Ca^{2+} in the same manner as does the regular sarcolemma. The action potential descends the T system near the Z bands into *triadic junctions,* in which a single T-system tubule is in extremely close proximity to, but not open communication with, two terminal *cisternae,* or extensions (*lateral sacs*) of the *sarcoplasmic reticulum* (SR). The SR is an extensive system of intracellular tubules more or less floating in the sarcoplasm, with many branches near the transverse tubules and the surface membranes (sarcolemma) and investing every myofibril in the cell. While the SR is present in all mammalian cardiac cells, the T system is present where the cells are relatively large and serves to take the surface membrane deep into the fiber. In small atrial fibers and the conduction system, the T system is generally absent. The exact mechanism by which the action potential "signal" is transferred from the sarcolemma and the T system to the intracellular sarcoplasmic reticulum is unknown, though it has been suggested with substantial evidence that the relatively small transsarcolemmal flux of calcium mediates this role.[33] Once the sarcoplasmic reticulum is depolarized, however, the excitation spreads rapidly throughout the SR, resulting in the release into the sarcoplasma of relatively large amounts of free Ca^{2+}, which then activates the fibril to contract. It appears probable that the Ca^{2+} is released particularly from the terminal cisternae (vesicles, lateral sacs) of the SR. Mitochondria can also release Ca^{2+} into the intracellular fluid, but it is doubtful that this mechanism contributes significantly to intracellular Ca^{2+} in human myocardium.[34,35] It is likely that the relatively small amount of inward Ca^{2+} movement actually produced by the action potential is the initiating stimulus for this calcium-triggered or "regenerative" release of Ca^{2+} from SR and mitochondria.[33]

FIGURE 3-1 Schematic action potential of human ventricular myocardium together with probable electrolyte movements. The initial phase 0 spike and overshoot is related to a sudden influx of Na^+. This is followed by a slower, maintained influx of Ca^{2+} during the plateau phase 2. The phase of Ca^{2+} efflux is not well defined for human ventricular myocardium, but presumably it occurs during phase 4.

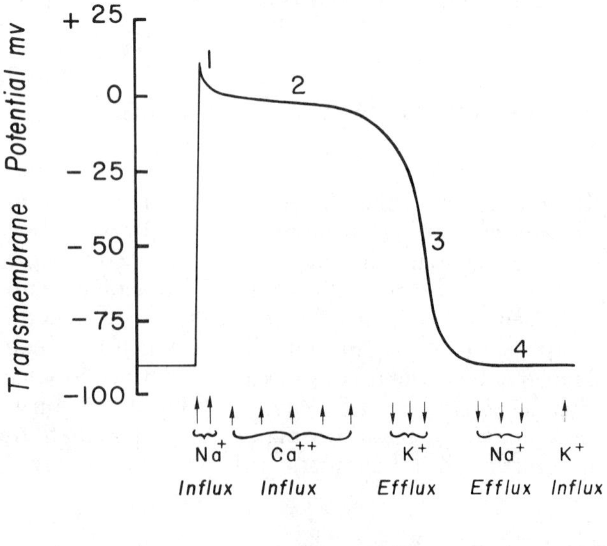

The increased sarcoplasmic "free," or "activating," Ca^{2+} diffuses to the myofibrils, where it binds to subunits of troponin, troponin C, which are located periodically along the thin actin filaments. In the absence of Ca^{2+}, troponin works through tropomyosin, which courses along the actin filament, to prevent actin from acting with myosin. Once Ca^{2+} attaches to troponin C, however, the inhibitory effect of troponin and tropomyosin upon the interaction of actin and myosin is released.[36–39] This loss of inhibition, or "derepression," allows enzyme sites on myosin bridges to interact with actin so that the resultant actomyosin ATPase, in the presence of bound adenosine triphosphate (ATP) and magnesium, can produce bridge motion and thus myocardial contraction by the sliding filament mechanism. An increase in the free Ca^{2+} concentration from 5×10^{-7} to 6×10^{-6} M results in the production of approximately 90 percent of the maximum force. The exact fraction of myofibrillar Ca^{2+} bound by troponin C and necessary for activation is unknown, though about 22 μmol is needed by the myofibril for 50 percent activation and 90 μmol for maximal activation. The increased sarcoplasmic Ca^{2+} also influences myocardial metabolism by activating glycogen phosphorylase, which results in increased glycogenolysis. The energy for myocardial contraction is obtained from molecules of magnesium ATP that are split by an ATPase site on the myosin filament heads during each interaction with actin (see Chap. 5).

Relaxation is initiated by an unknown stimulus (or loss of inhibition) that produces an increased binding, uptake, or sequestration of sarcoplasmic Ca^{2+}. It is not certain exactly where or how this decrease in intracellular Ca^{2+} occurs in human myocardium. It has been suggested that Ca^{2+} up-

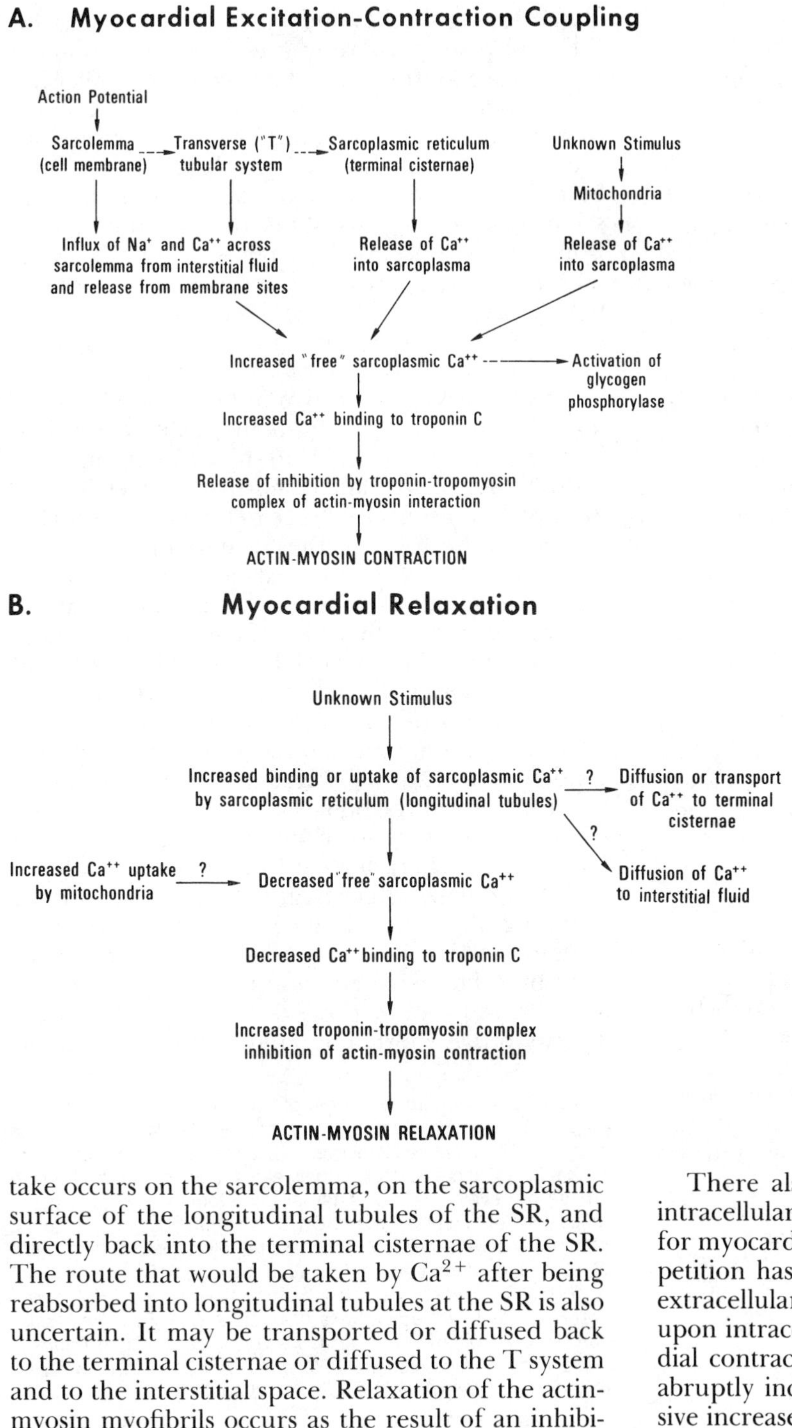

FIGURE 3-2 Schematic diagram of the events producing (*A*) excitation-contraction coupling and (*B*) relaxation in myocardium. The relative contribution of the sarcolemma, the T system, and the mitochondria to the increase in free sarcoplasmic Ca^{2+}, which is responsible for the initiation of contraction, is uncertain in human myocardium. The mechanisms and the pathways by which sarcoplasmic Ca^{2+} is taken up or sequestrated during relaxation are not well defined for human myocardium.

take occurs on the sarcolemma, on the sarcoplasmic surface of the longitudinal tubules of the SR, and directly back into the terminal cisternae of the SR. The route that would be taken by Ca^{2+} after being reabsorbed into longitudinal tubules at the SR is also uncertain. It may be transported or diffused back to the terminal cisternae or diffused to the T system and to the interstitial space. Relaxation of the actin-myosin myofibrils occurs as the result of an inhibition produced by the troponin-tropomyosin complex in the presence of low intracellular Ca^{2+}.

The amount of Ca^{2+} available to inhibit troponin and induce contraction of the actin-myosin myofilaments is directly related to the rate and to the amount of tension developed. It is likely that many drugs (such as digitalis,[23,31,40–42] sympathomimetic amines,[43–45] xanthines[46]) or conditions (acidosis, an increase in heart rate,[47–48] postextrasystolic potentiation[49]) have their influence upon myocardial contractility through their effect upon available intracellular Ca^{2+}.[50,51]

There also appears to be competition between intracellular sodium (Na^+) and calcium (Ca^{2+}) ions for myocardial sarcolemma binding sites. Such competition has been used to explain the influence of extracellular and intracellular Na^+ concentration upon intracellular Ca^{2+} concentration and myocardial contractility.[10,17,19,21,23] When the heart rate is abruptly increased, there is an associated progressive increase in contractile force, known as the *Bowditch staircase phenomenon,* or *treppe.* Langer has suggested that the increased heart rate results in a temporary increase in intracellular Ca^{2+} secondary to the internal shift of Na^+.[23,31] Drugs such as digitalis which inhibit membrane sodium-potassium-activated ATPase also might produce some of their effects by influencing intracellular Na^+, which, in turn, influences intracellular Ca^{2+} and contractile force.[17,23,31,40–42,52] Studies have also suggested that defects in the kinetics of intracellular calcium may be present in the myocardium of patients with heart failure[6,16,18,21,23,26,53] (see Chap. 20).

Muscle Mechanics

The basic mechanics of contraction of the heart is regulated by four distinct, although interrelated factors: (1) the *preload* (Starling's law of the heart), which is the passive load that establishes the initial muscle length of the cardiac fibers prior to contraction; (2) the *afterload,* which is the sum of all the loads against which the myocardial fibers must shorten during systole, which are created by the end-diastolic volume of the ventricle, the aortic impedance, the arterial resistance, the peripheral vascular resistance, the mass of blood in the aorta and great arteries, and the viscosity of the blood; (3) the *contractility,* or *inotropic state,* of the heart, which reflects the speed and shortening capacity of the myocardium for a given set of loading conditions; and (4) the *heart rate,* or frequency of contraction. As will be described, the fiber length appears to influence quantitatively the number of active force-generating sites in the myocardium, whereas a change in the contractile state (or contractility) is related to a qualitative change in the force generated by the sites, i.e., their activations, with or without a change in their number. Before one reviews these mechanisms, however, a brief review of fundamental myocardial mechanics as described by force-velocity-length relations is appropriate. More detailed discussions are presented in specialized reviews.[6,54–59]

Fundamentals of Muscle Mechanics[4,54–78]

A. V. Hill[79,80] suggested a model for muscular contraction which has been exceedingly useful for understanding myocardial mechanics and predicting their changes under a number of different circumstances. In this model (Fig. 3-3) muscle contraction behaves as if there were a *contractile element* (CE) which is capable of developing force and of shortening, a *series elastic component* (SE) which is passively stretched by shortening the CE, and a *parallel elastic component* (PE) which supports resting tension but plays little role during contraction. The precise anatomic sites of the components or, indeed, their exact arrangement is uncertain. These factors may be in the contractile filaments, in the cell membranes, or in both. Several other models have been proposed using the same basic components. While the "working" model is useful for conceptual purposes, one must recognize that anatomic reality is not implied. In isolated muscle preparations, this SE is created by damaged elastic ends of the muscle; in the intact heart, the SE includes valves and elastic structures.

After activation of a strip of heart muscle that is not allowed to shorten (isometric contraction, Fig. 3-4), the CE rapidly begins to shorten at its maximal velocity (V_{max}). As the CE shortens, it stretches the SE, which transmits the force to the external attachments. As the force in the SE develops, however, the velocity of shortening declines in accord with a basic inverse relation between force and velocity of muscle contraction. Because of the time required to stretch the SE, the external developed force lags behind the theoretical maximal force of the CE that it could develop (P_0) if no SE were present. Three hypothetical isometric contractions under different conditions are shown in Fig. 3-5. Curve *A* represents the control contraction; curve *B* represents the changes produced by an increase in initial muscle length and is characterized by a greater peak force P_0, which occurs after about the same time interval following stimulation; and curve *C* represents an increased frequency of contraction from curve *B*, illustrating the increased contractility manifested by an increased rate of force development (increased velocity of CE shortening) and shortened duration

FIGURE 3-3 A. V. Hill's three-component model for muscle. See text. [*From E. H. Sonnenblick, The Mechanics of Myocardial Contraction, in S. A. Briller and H. L. Conn, Jr. (eds.), "The Myocardial Cell: Structure, Function, and Modification by Cardiac Drugs," University of Pennsylvania Press, Philadelphia, 1966, p. 173. Reproduced with permission from the publisher, editor, and author.*]

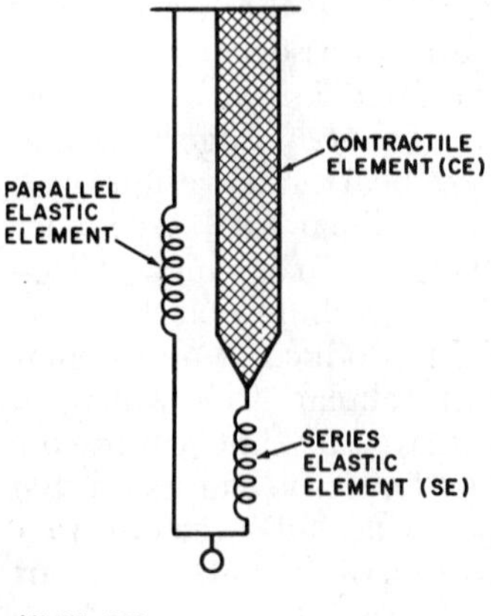

FIGURE 3-4 Schematic model of an isometric contraction of a strip of heart muscle. *Left:* The muscle model with a contractile element (CE) and a series elastic component (SE). The initial length of the SE (l_0) increases by Δl between *A* and *B*. *Right:* The time course of development of external force together with the hypothetical instantaneous force of CE which it might develop if no SE attachments were present. Point *A*, the initial resting state; point *B*, some time during active activation. See text. [*From E. H. Sonnenblick, The Mechanics of Myocardial Contraction, in S. A. Briller and H. L. Conn, Jr. (eds.), "The Myocardial Cell: Structure, Function, and Modification by Cardiac Drugs," University of Pennsylvania Press, Philadelphia, 1966, p. 173. Reproduced with permission from the publisher, editor, and author.*]

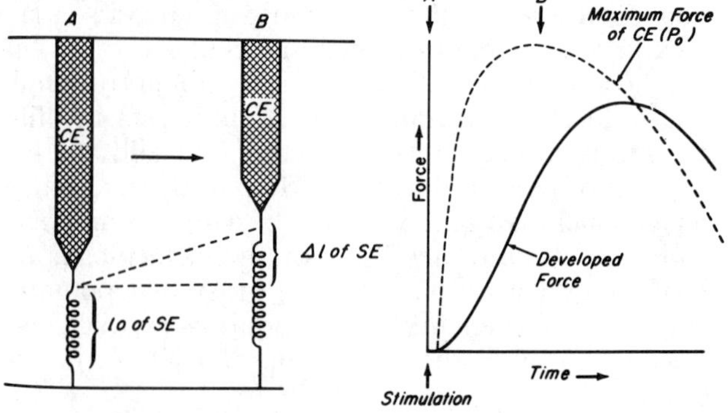

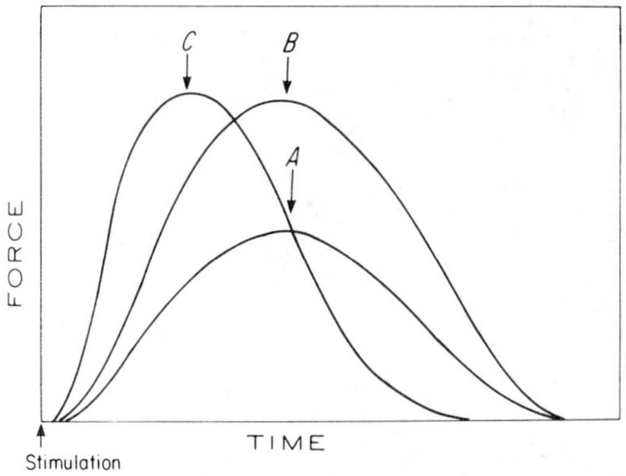

FIGURE 3-5 Hypothetical isometric force developed by three hypothetical contractions. *A.* Control. *B.* Increased initial muscle length. *C.* The muscle in curve *B* contracting more frequently. See text. [*From E. H. Sonnenblick, The Mechanics of Myocardial Contraction, in S. A. Briller and H. L. Conn, Jr. (eds.), "The Myocardial Cell: Structure, Function, and Modification by Cardiac Drugs," University of Pennsylvania Press, Philadelphia, 1966, p. 173. Reproduced with permission from the publisher, editor, and author.*]

of the active state, rather than by an increase in peak force.

The *preload* is the load that stretches the muscle to its initial length *prior* to contraction as related to the resting length-tension (load) curve of the muscle. The *afterload* is the load the muscle must move after it starts to contract.

When myocardium contracts against a constant afterload and is allowed to shorten (an *isotonic contraction,* Fig. 3-6), the CE initially shortens and stretches the SE while developing enough external force to overcome the afterload. The initial slope of the shortening curve relative to time on the right is used to calculate the initial velocity of shortening for the particular load *P*. With progressively increasing afterloads, the time interval from stimulus to the onset of shortening is prolonged, but the time to maximal shortening is unchanged (Fig. 3-7). In addition, the initial velocity of isotonic shortening for each load, which is obtained by drawing a tangent to the initial shortening slope, decreases markedly with increasing loads. This basic relation is further illustrated in Figs. 3-8 and 3-9, in which the force-velocity relations of isolated papillary muscles are plotted to illustrate the basic principle of a decrease in the initial velocity of shortening with increasing loads. As shown in Fig. 3-8, extrapolation of the curve to zero yields the theoretic maximal velocity (V_{max}) of shortening of the contractile elements in the unloaded muscle. V_{max} in turn is altered by factors that modify the activation of the muscle but not by a change in initial muscle length within physiological resting lengths. Thus, it has been a useful

FIGURE 3-6 An afterloaded isotonic contraction of myocardium. On the left is the muscle model attached to a load *P* which is supported when the muscle is at rest (*A*). This type of load *P* that is encountered by the CE only when the CE attempts to shorten is the afterload, whereas the small load used to stretch the system to its initial length is the preload. With stimulation of the system, the CE begins to shorten at maximum speed V_{max}. During the isometric portion of the contraction, between *A* and *B*, the CE shortens and the SE matches the load *P*, and the load starts to move. Once the load begins to move to point *B*, the SE remains constant in length, and shortening of the system reflects shortening of the CE alone. The curves on the right reflect force and shortening as functions of time after stimulation. The tangent to the slope of the curve of initial shortening is used to obtain the *initial velocity* of *isotonic shortening* for a given load. After plotting the initial velocity of shortening for different loads, one may extrapolate the curve to zero load to obtain the theoretic intrinsic or maximal velocity V_{max}. See Fig. 3-8. [*From E. H. Sonnenblick, The Mechanics of Myocardial Contraction, in S. A. Briller and H. L. Conn, Jr. (eds.), "The Myocardial Cell: Structure, Function, and Modification by Cardiac Drugs," University of Pennsylvania Press, Philadelphia, 1966, p. 173. Reproduced with permission from the publisher, editor, and author.*]

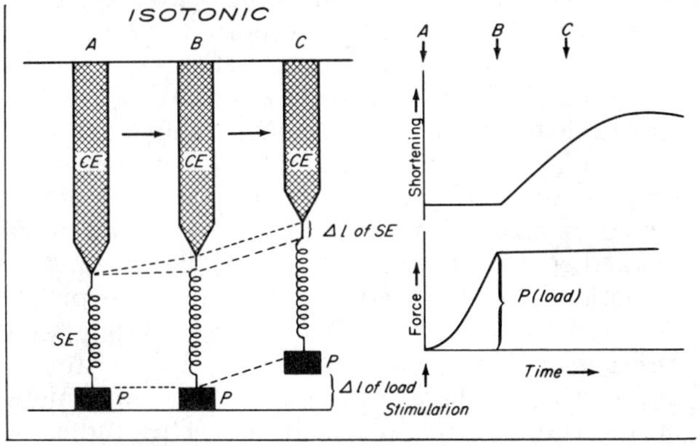

FIGURE 3-7 A series of superimposed tracings made from isolated papillary muscle which was arranged in such a manner that both initial isometric contraction and subsequent isotonic shortening are possible. *Below:* Serial isometric contraction at increasing afterloads (horizontal lines). *Above:* Successive isotonic shortening corresponding to the increasing afterloads in the lower tracing (dashed lines). The dashed lines on the upper tracing represent the initial velocity of shortening. As the afterload increases, the initial velocity of shortening decreases and the extent of shortening decreases, but the isometric relaxation phase increases. [*From E. H. Sonnenblick, The Mechanics of Myocardial Contraction, in S. A. Briller and H. L. Conn, Jr. (eds.), "The Myocardial Cell: Structure, Function, and Modification by Cardiac Drugs," University of Pennsylvania Press, Philadelphia, 1966, p. 173. Reproduced with permission from the publisher, editor, and author.*]

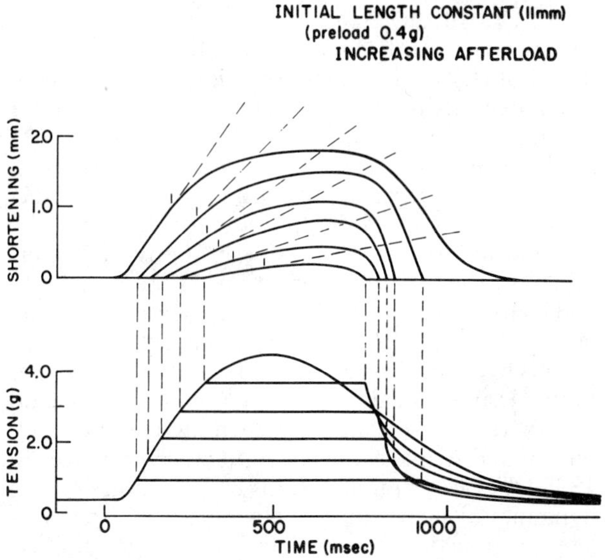

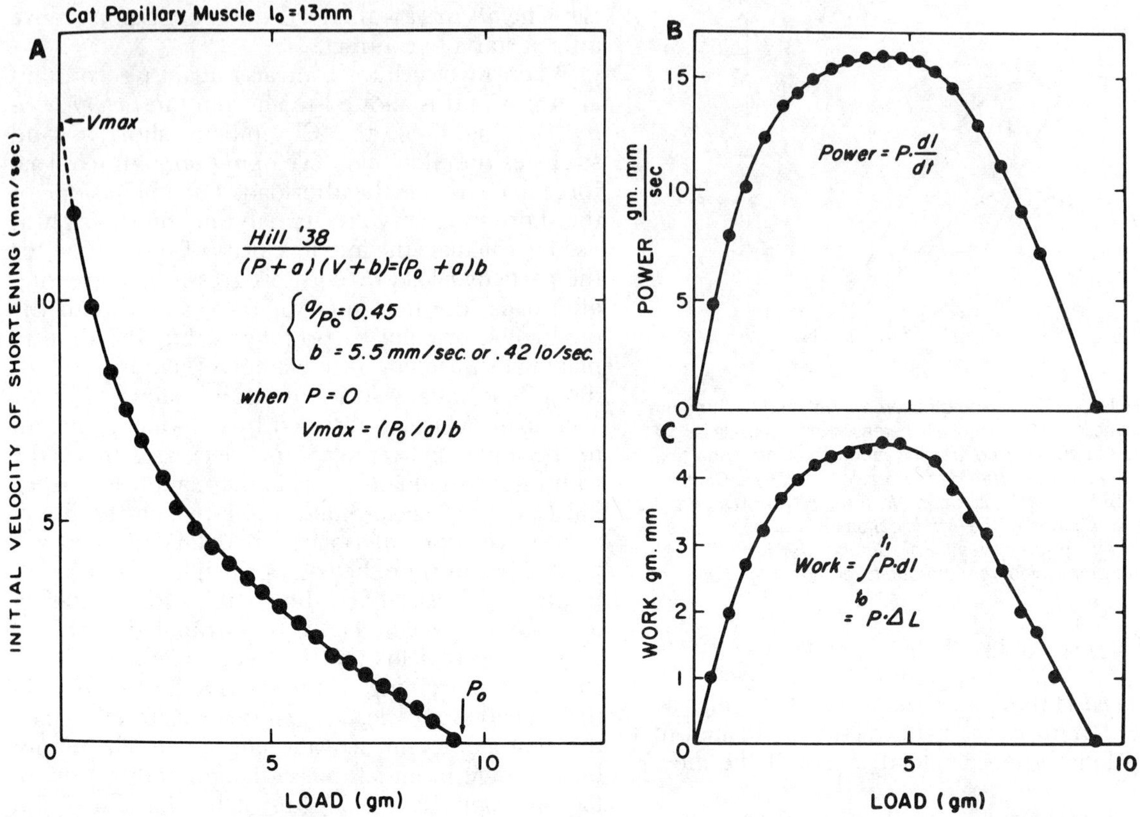

FIGURE 3-8 *A.* Force-velocity relations of a papillary muscle, illustrating the decreasing initial velocity of shortening with increasing loads. The insert gives Hill's equation for muscular contraction with the derived constants. When the curve is extrapolated to zero load, one obtains the V_{max}, or the intrinsic velocity of shortening. When the load is increased to the point at which no shortening can occur (an isometric contraction), the maximum force is manifest (P_0 or intrinsic force). *B.* The load versus the power (force versus velocity of shortening). *C.* The load versus work (force or load versus displacement). Note that peak power and work are obtained at loads approximately 50 percent of the maximal force of contraction P_0 obtained during isometric conditions. Instantaneous force-velocity curves similar to those in *A* are also obtained when the velocity of shortening is measured at a constant time after stimulation by quick-release techniques. [*From E. H. Sonnenblick, The Mechanics of Myocardial Contraction, in S. A. Briller and H. L. Conn, Jr. (eds.), "The Myocardial Cell: Structure, Function, and Modification by Cardiac Drugs," University of Pennsylvania Press, Philadelphia, 1966, p. 173. Reproduced with permission from the publisher, editor, and author.*]

index of the contractility of the myocardial fibers being examined.

Preload: The Frank-Straub-Wiggers-Starling Principle

In 1871 H. P. Bowditch[81] showed that if the condition of the heart muscle remains unaltered, contractions remain equal in strength regardless of the strength of stimuli applied. This principle, which has become known as the *all-or-nothing law of the heart,* implied that cardiac muscle either does not contract at all or responds to the fullest extent, but that the magnitude of the all-or-none response is determined by the inherent "condition" of the muscle. In 1884 Howell and Donaldson[82] presented unequivocal evidence that the heart itself has intrinsic mechanisms by which its output is adjusted to the venous input. Using a heart-lung preparation, they found that increasing the venous return increased cardiac output and stroke as well as right atrial pressure. In 1895 O. Frank[83] published his classic studies on the dynamics of heart muscle. His object was to correlate the reactions of cardiac muscle with the responses of skeletal muscle, the force of contraction of which had been previously shown by A. Fick,[84] J. von Kries,[85] and M. Blix[86] to be related to the initial length and resting tension. Frank studied the frog atria and ventricles and showed that, within limits, stepwise increases in diastolic volume and pressure just before contraction—the *presystolic* or *end-diastolic* volume and pressure—determine the magnitude of the all-or-none response. His studies emphasized the dependence of the cardiac response on hemodynamic events immediately preceding excitation. In 1914 Wiggers[87] reported experiments that were the first to demonstrate that the reactions established by Frank for the frog's ventricle are also applicable to the naturally beating right ventricle of dogs. He concluded that the rate of isometric pressure rise and the peak systolic pressure are determined by changes in the initial tension, as long as marked changes in inherent contractility are not simultaneously produced by experimental procedures. Also in 1914, Straub[88] and Starling and associates[89,90] independently reported their studies of the effect of changes in initial tension and length on the response of isolated hearts. The studies of

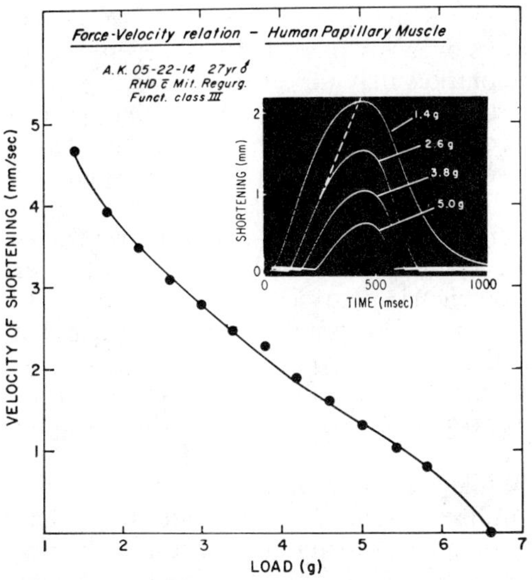

FIGURE 3-9 Relation between the initial velocity of isotonic shortening and afterload of a human papillary muscle stimulated at a rate of 12 stimuli per minute. Preload was 1.4 g with a muscle length of 15 mm. Note the significant decrease in initial velocity as the load increases. The insert shows four recordings with different afterloads; the decrease in rate of shortening with increasing afterload is apparent from the altered slopes of the length-time curves. *(From E. H. Sonnenblick, E. Braunwald, and A. G. Morrow, The Contractile Properties of Human Heart Muscle: Studies on Myocardial Mechanics of Surgically Excised Papillary Muscles, J. Clin. Invest., 44:966, 1965. Reproduced with permission from The American Society for Clinical Investigation and author.)*

Starling and associates have received the greatest amount of attention in the English-speaking areas of the world, and, in deference to Otto Frank, the general principle is often referred to as the *Frank-Starling law of the heart.*[91] Starling and associates, on the basis of highly suggestive, but not quite conclusive, studies on the heart-lung preparation, concluded, "The mechanical energy set free on passage from the resting to the constricted state depends on the area of 'chemically active surfaces,' i.e., on the length of the muscle fibers."[90] Wiggers[92] has pointed out that although there is a general impression that the often-reproduced representation of the law by Starling and associates was based on data from their own experiments, the careful reader will discover that the published curves were acknowledged to be reproductions of graphs previously published by Blix and by Frank. From the earlier studies of Frank, Straub, and Wiggers, it was not certain whether the responsiveness of the heart was fundamentally related to changes in presystolic pressure (initial tension) or to changes in volume (initial length). The conclusion by Starling that cardiac responsiveness was primarily related to presystolic *fiber length* has been validated by nearly all investigators, but it is clear that fiber length and resting tension are interrelated. Wiggers has emphasized the importance of other factors affecting the responsiveness of the myocardium and has stressed that the statement of the law of the heart, in which the energy of contraction is a function of the length of the muscle fiber, should be modified by the phrase, "under equivalent states of responsiveness."[92] Sarnoff and Berglund[93,94] demonstrated this principle by showing that a "family of curves" relating stroke work to left atrial pressure exists for each ventricle and that many other factors, such as humoral agents, neural influences, and metabolic condition of the myocardium, determine which particular "curve" the ventricle is operating on at a given moment. The studies of Braunwald and associates[6,95,96] have shown the applicability of the law of the heart in both the normal and the diseased human heart.

The fact that initial fiber length rather than intraventricular pressure is important in influencing the strength of contraction is of great significance. Although these two factors are usually related to each other, the relation may vary considerably because of changes in ventricular *distensibility* or *compliance,* i.e., the ratio of change in ventricular volume to change in ventricular diastolic pressure ($\Delta V/\Delta P$), while ventricular *stiffness* is the reciprocal, or the change in pressure for a given change in volume ($\Delta P/\Delta V$).[97–106] Most of the recognized changes in ventricular compliance occur chronically owing to ventricular distension or hypertrophy. Except in response to ischemia, significant acute changes in the pressure-volume relation or in distensibility of ventricles probably do not occur, nor are there significant, acute changes due to inotropic agents.[97,107] On the other hand, ventricular distensibility is often significantly influenced by filling of the opposite ventricle, especially when filling pressures are elevated and within the constraints of the pericardium.[107,108] Thus, the pressure-volume relationships of one ventricle can be immediately influenced by acute changes in the filling of the contralateral ventricle. At cardiac catheterization it is possible to obtain reasonable estimations of ventricular end-diastolic and end-systolic volumes and very accurate measurements of end-diastolic pressure. As discussed in Chap. 17, the ventricular end-diastolic pressure may be elevated either by an altered compliance due to myocardial ischemia or failure or by ventricular hypertrophy itself.[6,97–110] The term *lasitrophy* has been used to refer to the diastolic properties of myocardium and cardiac chambers.

The Frank-Starling law of the heart is the major mechanism by which the normal right and left ventricles maintain equal minute outputs even though their stroke outputs may vary considerably during normal respiration. Thus, if the right ventricle temporarily pumps more blood into the pulmonary circulation than the left ventricle pumps into the systemic circulation, the proper balance between the two pumps is soon achieved, since the venous return to the left atrium and ventricle causes the left ventricular end-diastolic fiber length to be greater, increasing left ventricular stroke output. In addition, a decreased left ventricular stroke output would eventually lead to decreased return of blood to the right atrium and ventricle, producing a decrease in right ventricular stroke output. By this mechanism the two ventricles, which function as two pumps in series, are able to balance their outputs and prevent pulmonary edema despite marked variations in stroke volumes.

A left ventricular "function curve" is shown in Fig. 3-10, in which left ventricular stroke volume is plotted as a function of left ventricular end-diastolic pressure. Although similar curves may be obtained by plotting ventricular stroke volume against left atrial mean pressure or left ventricular volume (which is more difficult to measure), the basic determinant is probably fiber length. Because end-diastolic fiber length and intraventricular pressure are normally related to each other, it is common in clinical situations to measure left ventricular end-diastolic pressure, since fiber length is difficult to determine in patients. In Fig. 3-10, curve *A* represents a hypothetical normal left ventricular function curve. Curve *B* represents a "shift to the left" of the function curve of the same ventricle under the influence of sympathetic stimulation or the infusion of epinephrine, norepinephrine, or other catecholamines. Curve *C* represents a "shift to the right" of curve *A*, such as might occur with myocardial depression from hypoxia, cardiodepressant drugs, or myocardial "failure." Note that under normal conditions (curve *A*) very slight changes in fiber length, which can be produced by small changes in filling pressure, are associated with significant increases in stroke volume. As mentioned above, this is one of the major mechanisms by which the two ventricles have balanced outputs over any period of time, even though their stroke outputs may vary considerably from beat to beat, particularly during the respiratory cycle. It should be emphasized that sympathetic stimulation may increase cardiac output, not only by producing an increase in heart rate but also by increasing the contractile force of both the atria and the ventricles, with a resultant increase in stroke volume. The increase in ventricular contractile force produced by sympathetic stimulation may be depicted graphically as a shift to the left of the ventricular function curve. Thus, sympathetic impulses can produce an increase in ventricular stroke volume without the necessity of a change in end-diastolic fiber length or pressure. While there is good evidence that the normal heart utilizes alterations in preload (or the Starling law of the heart) during normal resting circumstances or during exercise, the failing, dilated heart may have little such reserve remaining. Thus, the hearts of patients with heart failure and cardiac dilatation have most of their fibers chronically extended to the top (L_{max}) of their force-length curve where sarcomere lengths are about 2.2 μm after fixation (see Fig. 3-12). Accordingly, many such hearts appear to be operating chronically at their ideal maximal length and are therefore unable to respond significantly to increased filling or stretch with a greater force of contraction.

FIGURE 3-10 Relation between left ventricular end-diastolic pressure and left ventricular stroke volume. Curve *A*, the normal function. Curve *B*, the shift to the left of the original curve associated with increased contractility, such as might result from sympathetic stimulation of the ventricle or the infusion of epinephrine or norepinephrine. Curve *C*, a shift to the right of the original curve associated with decreased contractility, such as might result from ventricular failure from ischemia or myocardial depressant drugs. A ventricle functioning on a curve *C* might be restored to a curve *A* by the action of digitalis or inotropic drugs, such as norepinephrine or epinephrine. Similar but not identical curves are obtained when left ventricular stroke volume or cardiac output is plotted against left ventricular end-diastolic pressure or left atrial mean pressure. Function curves such as these may be obtained from both ventricles and both atria.

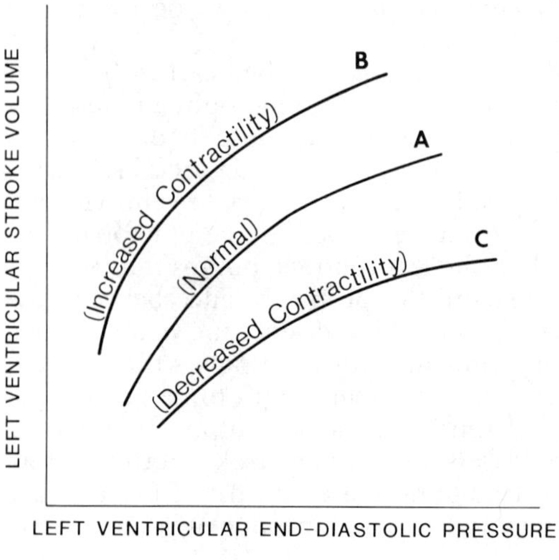

Figure 3-11 illustrates the interrelation between ventricular end-diastolic volume, end-diastolic pressure, and stroke work. As indicated in Fig. 3-11*A*, the relation between stroke volume and end-diastolic volume is nearly linear. On the other hand, the relation between end-diastolic pressure and volume (Fig. 3-11*B*) is curvilinear, with a definite volume at zero pressure and with a rather sharp increase in pressure above a certain volume. Figure 3-11*C* illustrates the familiar curvilinear relation between ventricular end-diastolic pressure and stroke volume.

Ultrastructural Basis of Starling's Law[6,66,109–122]

The length-tension relation of a papillary muscle is shown in Fig. 3-12. The length of a myocardial sarcomere at which maximal force develops is approximately 2.2 μm after fixation, at which length the thin actin and thick myosin myofilaments are optimally overlapped to provide the greatest number of force-generating sites. When the sarcomere is stretched beyond about 2.2 μm, the developed force decreases as the myofilaments become partially disengaged and fewer contractile sites are brought into play. At a length of 3.65 μm, the actin and myosin myofilaments are completely disengaged, and developed tension drops to zero. These long sarcomeres are seen only in skeletal fibers since cardiac sarcomeres are too stiff to be that overstretched. While consistent with a "sliding-filament" mechanism, such longer sarcomere lengths at which force falls are not seen physiologically. At sarcomere lengths

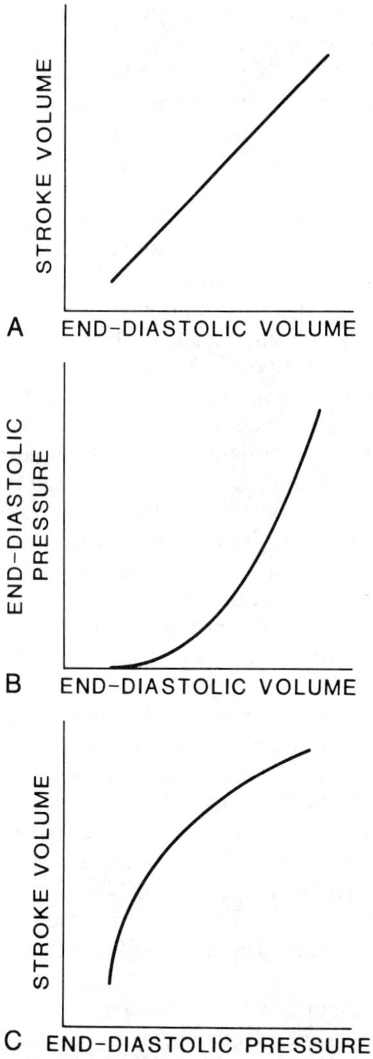

FIGURE 3-11 Illustration of the interrelations between stroke work, ventricular end-diastolic volume, and end-diastolic pressure. As indicated in *A*, the relation between stroke volume and end-diastolic volume is actually nearly linear. On the other hand, the relation between end-diastolic pressure and end-diastolic volume (*B*), is curvilinear, with a definite volume at zero pressure and with a rather sharp increase in pressure above a certain volume. *C* illustrates the familiar curvilinear relation between stroke volume and ventricular end-diastolic pressure, similar to Fig. 3-10.

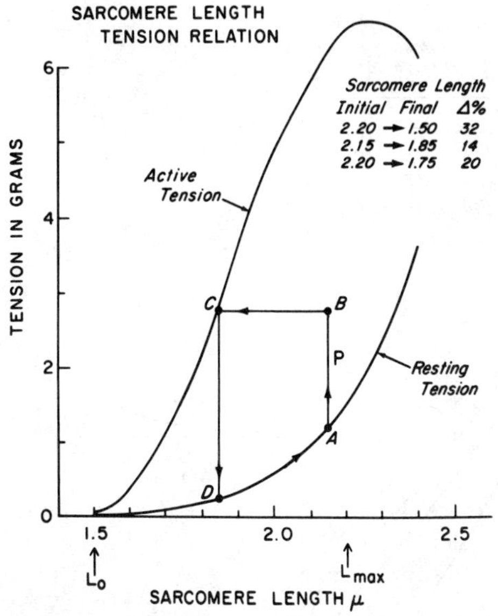

FIGURE 3-12 The relation between papillary sarcomere length, resting tension, and developed or active tension. Note that active tension increases up to a sarcomere length of 2.2 μm (L_{max}) and then decreases. The resting tension increases markedly above a sarcomere length of 2.0 to 2.2 μm, which corresponds to an end-diastolic pressure of about 10 to 12 mmHg. The course of a normal contraction is shown in *ABCD.* Contraction starts at point *A* and develops a force equal to an imposed load *P*, reaching point *B.* The fiber then shortens until the active tension curve is reached at *C,* when relaxation occurs and returns the course to *D* at the end of systole. Normally, the ventricle functions on the ascending limb of the active tension curve at length below L_{max}, where greatest active tension develops, with sarcomere lengths between 1.8 and 2.2 μm. The descending limb of the length-active tension curve occurs at sarcomere lengths greater than L_{max}. There is normally a modern heterogeneity of sarcomere lengths in the heart, sarcomeres in the subendocardial layers tending to be longer and to shorten more than sarcomeres from the midwall or epicardium. In patients with marked ventricular dilatation, most of the dilatation is due to rearrangement and plastic "slippage" of the muscle fibers and myofibrils together with an increase in length of fibers due to synthesis of sarcomeres in series rather than to stretching of individual sarcomeres. [*From E. H. Sonnenblick, H. M. Spotnitz, and D. Spiro, Role of the Sarcomere in Ventricular Function and the Mechanism of Heart Failure, Circ. Res., 15(suppl. 2):70, 1964. Reproduced with permission from the American Heart Association, Inc., and the author.*]

of less than 2.2 μm, the actin myofilaments first pass into the center of the sarcomere, and at 2.0 μm, they bypass one another and developed tension decreases. The reason for the fall in force with shortening sarcomere length in this physiological portion of the curve is not clear. Among explanations have been interference of the thin filaments, restoring forces, and a decrease in Ca^{2+} sensitivity of the sarcomere at short lengths. The latter explanation has received recent support.[123] As the papillary muscle in Fig. 3-12 is increasingly stretched, the resting tension increases, at first slowly and then more markedly. The *stiffness* of myocardial muscle can be defined as the slope of the curve relating the change in resting tension (ΔT) to the change in length (ΔL).

It is also significant that a sarcomere length of 2.2 μm, which produces peak active tension (L_{max}), occurs in normal dogs at about the upper limit of normal ventricular filling pressure, 10 to 12 mmHg. Theoretically, the normal ventricle may have an ejection fraction of 55 percent with a shortening of individual sarcomere length of only 13 percent.[6,112,113] One study has suggested that perhaps 50 percent of the normal stroke volume can theoretically be accounted for by a pistonlike effect produced by ventricular thickening;[124] however, the physiological significance of this phenomenon is uncertain.

Influences of Fiber Length and Heart Rate upon Force-Velocity Relations

The influence of increased initial fiber length on the force-velocity relation of a papillary muscle is shown in Fig. 3-13. With increasing fiber length there is an

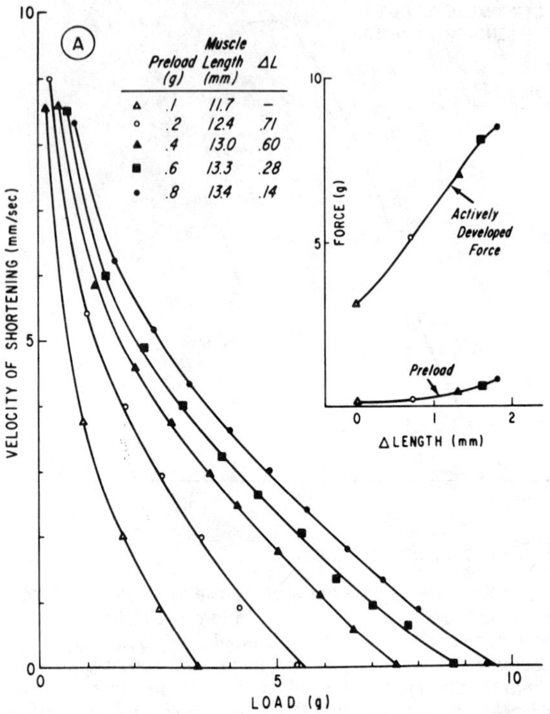

FIGURE 3-13 The effects of increasing initial muscle length on the force-velocity relation. The initial velocity of shortening is plotted against preload, increases in which increase the initial length. In the insert, the maximal force developed is plotted against the change in muscle length. It is apparent that an increased muscle length produces little or no increase in V_{max}, the velocity of shortening at zero load obtained by extrapolation, but increases the actively developed maximal force P_0, which is produced under isometric conditions when the load is increased so much that no shortening can occur. *(From E. H. Sonnenblick, Series Elastic and Contractile Elements in Heart Muscle: Changes in Muscle Length, Am. J. Physiol., 207:1330, 1964. Reproduced with permission from the publisher and author.)*

increase in the maximal actively developed force which the fiber can develop (P_0) at zero velocity of shortening or isometric contraction for each fiber length. In contrast, there is little or no change in the maximal velocity of shortening (V_{max}).[125] The increase in intrinsic force P_0 with unchanged V_{max} produced by increased initial muscle length is probably related to an increased number of active contractile sites rather than to an increase in their contractility per se. The increase in contractility associated with an increase in heart rate occurs in both atrial and ventricular muscle and is termed the *Bowditch effect,* or *treppe.*[47,48,64,66,69,126–130]

Contractility and the Inotropic State[6,10,54–78,131–161]

The second major mechanism by which myocardial function is altered is by a change in the inotropic state (contractility) of the muscle independent of a change in fiber length. The actual biochemical events at or near the ultrastructural contractile sites that are responsible for increases in contractility, or inotropism, remain the subject of very active investigation and appear related to an enhanced degree of activation of cardiac muscle for a given contraction.[27–33] Abbott and Mommaerts[162] and Sonnenblick and his associates[6,54,60,63–71,125,131,163] have noted that an increase in the contractile state of a muscle is characterized by an increase in V_{max}, with or without a change in P_0, the maximal force under isometric conditions at zero velocity.

An increase in heart rate increases the contractile state, as shown by an increase in the velocity of shortening at any level of tension and by changes in location of V_{max}, obtained by extrapolating to zero load, without a change in P_0. Strophanthidin and norepinephrine both produce a significant shift to the right in the force-velocity curves, and an increase in both V_{max} and P_0 in association with a decrease in the time from stimulation to peak shortening.[65] Increased contractility can also be illustrated by ventricular function curves (Fig. 3-10); however, a function curve tends to be a less sensitive indicator of changes in the contractile state of isolated myocardium than a force-velocity curve. Thus, function curves, which relate end-diastolic pressure to stroke volume and stroke work, may show only small changes at a time when significant changes are apparent in the force-velocity curves.[69] The increased contractility produced by an increase in heart rate (the *force-frequency relation* or the *Bowditch phenomenon*[47,48,68,126–130]) affects primarily the speed of contraction and is thus more readily shown by force-velocity curves than by ventricular function curves. The increased contractility produced by large amounts of norepinephrine or by large increases in heart rate may, however, be apparent in both types of curves.

The complex interrelations between *force, velocity,* and *length* of both isolated myocardium and intact ventricles can best be represented by a three-dimensional graph.[6,67] Figure 3-14 is a diagram of such a graph for a ventricle with the superimposed course of a single contraction; Fig. 3-15 illustrates the effect of increasing preload or initial muscle length; Fig. 3-16 illustrates the effects of an increased contractile state. This indicates that when contractility is augmented, the myocardium shortens faster at any given muscle length, for any given load, and also shortens further or generates more force. It should be noted that myocardial contractility at any one moment is best defined by the *surface* of the curved surface relating force, velocity, and length.

When sympathetic stimulation causes the heart to beat with increased contractility and at a faster rate, not only is the contraction more forceful and faster, but the relaxation and elastic recoil of the ventricular musculature ("diastolic suction") are also more rapid. Both the more forceful contraction and the more vigorous relaxation tend to increase stroke volume of the next beat, since the diastolic filling period is longer than it would otherwise be and since, with the more rapid elastic recoil, the ventricular pressure will be lower earlier and more rapidly, and possibly lower absolutely, than it otherwise would

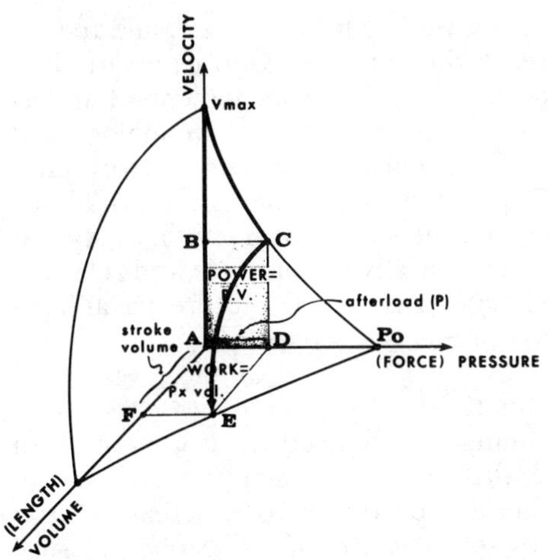

FIGURE 3-14 Force-velocity-length (force-velocity-volume) diagram of the intact ventricle. The force is the equivalent of load, which is the sum of preload (end-diastolic pressure) and afterload (aortic pressure). The length axis is derived from intraventricular volume. The superimposed dark line portrays the course of a single contraction. Starting at *A,* with activation, the CE velocity rises toward V_{max}. With CE shortening, force is built up and velocity of shortening decreases to *C.* This represents the isometric (isovolumic) phase of contraction. At *C,* the force equals the load, and shortening begins from *C* to *E.* During muscle shortening between *C* and *E,* velocity of shortening changes as a function of the decrease in muscle length which ensues. Shaded area on the force-velocity (vertical) plane represents calculated power (*ABCD*); shaded area on the base represents work for a load *P* (*ADEF*). [*From E. H. Sonnenblick, The Mechanics of Myocardial Contraction, in S. A. Briller and H. L. Conn, Jr. (eds.), "The Myocardial Cell: Structure, Function, and Modification by Cardiac Drugs," University of Pennsylvania Press, Philadelphia, 1966, p. 173. Reproduced with permission from the publisher, editor, and author.*]

be. The increased emptying produced by increased contractility also means that the fiber length will be less at the beginning of the next diastole. This tends to increase distensibility of the ventricle and to allow greater filling at a lower filling pressure.

Afterload: Aortic Impedance

It has been known since O. Frank's experiments[83] that ventricular ejection and performance are importantly influenced by the resistance against which the ventricles contract.[6,54,57–65,76,87,89,92,144,145,164–171] For the left ventricle the major peripheral factors are the aortic impedance, the peripheral vascular resistance, the arterial wall (or stiffness) resistance, the mass of the column of blood in the aorta, and the viscosity of blood; the corresponding factors for the right ventricle are the main pulmonary artery impedance, the pulmonary vascular resistance, the mass of blood in the pulmonary circulation, and the viscosity of blood. In addition to these peripheral factors, the preload, or end-diastolic volume of each ventricle, is a major determinant of ventricular afterload. Thus, the amount of blood in the ventricle at end diastole directly determines the radius of the ventricle at the onset of systole and thereby (by the Laplace relationship) the amount of myocardial wall tension necessary during the next ventricular ejection.

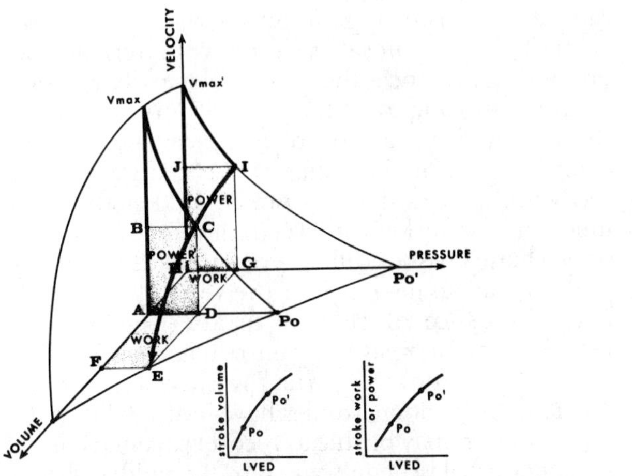

FIGURE 3-15 The effect of increasing preload (left ventricular end-diastolic pressure) on the force-velocity-volume relation. Blood pressure remains the same. Maximum isometric force increases from P_0 to P_0'; work increases from *ADEF* to *HGEF,* while power increases from *ABCD* to *HGIJ.* This increase in the end-diastolic volume of the ventricle does not represent a change in the contractile state of the myocardium, since V_{max} is not changed. The insert in the lower right shows the predicted relations of stroke volume, stroke work, and stroke power to *LVED* (left ventricular end-diastolic pressure), reflecting changes in work and power areas from the three-dimensional diagram. [*From E. H. Sonnenblick: The Mechanics of Myocardial Contraction, in S. A. Briller and H. L. Conn, Jr. (eds.), "The Myocardial Cell: Structure, Function, and Modification by Cardiac Drugs," University of Pennsylvania Press, Philadelphia, 1966, p. 173. Reproduced with permission from the publisher, editor, and author.*]

In conditions in which the volume of blood in the left ventricle decreases rapidly after the onset of systole (such as mitral regurgitation or ventricular septal defect), the total impedance to left ventricular emptying rapidly decreases during systole, thereby

FIGURE 3-16 The effect of increasing the contractile state on the force-velocity-volume relation of the ventricle. Both V_{max} and P_0 are augmented, while the load (pressure) has been kept constant. Work and power are augmented. [*From E. H. Sonnenblick, The Mechanics of Myocardial Contraction, in S. A. Briller and H. L. Conn, Jr. (eds.), "The Myocardial Cell: Structure, Function, and Modification by Cardiac Drugs," University of Pennsylvania Press, Philadelphia, 1966, p. 173. Reproduced with permission from the publisher, editor, and author.*]

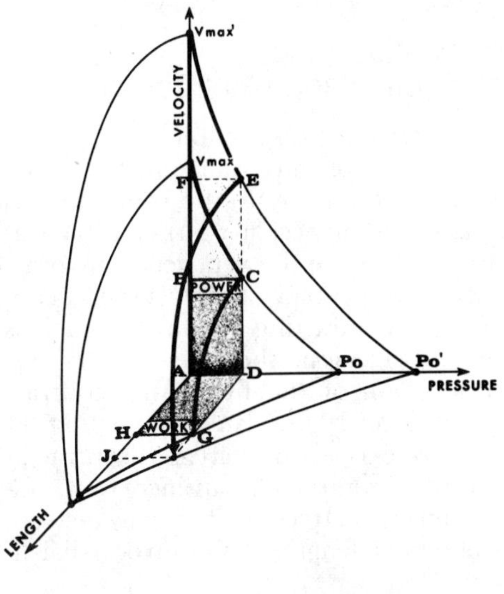

rapidly decreasing significantly the load upon the ventricle.[169] In general, the effects of afterload continuously influence the force-velocity-length-time relations throughout the course of myocardial shortening. Since afterload influences the rate and extent of systolic emptying of the ventricles, it directly influences the ventricular end-systolic volume; thus, afterload indirectly influences the diastolic characteristics (filling pressure and volume or preload) of the next beat of the ventricle. An additional influence of changes in afterload is manifested by an increase in ventricular performance several beats after the aortic pressure is raised (the *Anrep effect*).[172] Some studies have indicated that this phenomenon may be due to recovery from transient subendocardial ischemia caused by the sudden change in arterial pressure.[6,173]

Heart Rate

The fourth major determinant of cardiac function is the heart rate, or the frequency of cardiac contraction. This is probably the major mechanism by which most individuals increase their cardiac output during periods of modest increased demand or exercise. An increase in pulse rate may also increase myocardial contractility; this force-interval relation is known as *treppe,* the *staircase phenomenon,* or the *Bowditch effect.*[6,47,48,68,69,81,126–130,174] This effect is much more apparent in the anesthetized animal or depressed heart than in the intact, conscious individual.[6,128,175] Even in the intact individual, however, the duration of each systole decreases as the heart rate increases, within limits. Nevertheless, since there are more systoles per minute, the total time per minute spent in systole increases.[176] Presumably, the increase in heart rate results in more Ca^{2+} being released from the stores within the myocardial cell, thus enhancing myofibrillar contraction. The "recuperative effect of a long pause" upon the strength of contraction is known as the *Woodworth phenomenon,* or as the negative, or reverse, staircase phenomenon.[177,178]

Other Factors Influencing Ventricular Function and Contractility

Sequence of Ventricular Contraction

An additional concept of importance in the application of the law of the heart to the ventricle as a whole concerns the sequence of ventricular activation and contraction. Since the ventricular myocardial fibers contract sequentially, the strength of contraction of the later-contracting myocardial fibers is influenced by the strength, the rate, and the sequence of contraction of the fibers that contract earlier and that stretch the later-contracting fibers.[179–182] Since one aspect of increased contractility is a faster rate of contraction, an increased contractility of the initially contracting fibers may increase the end-diastolic fiber length of the myocardial fibers that have not yet begun to contract, and thereby directly increase the force of contraction of those fibers that contract later. This phenomenon has been referred to as *idioventricular kick,*[182] in analogy with the increased ventricular filling and performance, the *atrial kick,* produced by atrial systole. An abnormal sequence of ventricular contraction, or dyssynergia, is also mechanically less efficient and relatively wasteful of energy, particularly if there are areas of akinesis or dyskinesis (see Chap. 44).

Ventricular Suction

Ventricular filling is enhanced by any increases in the pressure difference between the atrium and ventricle, whether produced by increased atrial pressure or by lower ventricular diastolic pressure. The latter phenomenon, which can be produced by increased elastic recoil, is referred to as *diastolic suction.* One form is present normally during early diastole, immediately following opening of the atrioventricular (AV) valve, and its extent is inversely related to ventricular volume. During this earliest phase of rapid ventricular filling, the pressure in the ventricle *decreases* despite a rapid *increase* in ventricular volume. Other forms of diastolic suction have been reviewed by Brecher,[183] although the physiological significance of the phenomena is still uncertain. This phenomenon enhances filling of the ventricle in early diastole, especially when the end-systolic volume is small.[184] Such a mechanism would be of especial value during exercise, where tachycardia may limit the time for filling. Interestingly, increases in contractility not only increase the rate of pressure change during systole (dP/dt) but also increase the rate of relaxation, reflected as negative dP/dt.[185] In the failing ventricle, where ventricular volume is large, diastolic suction is much less and higher mean atrial pressures are needed to fill the ventricle.

Atrial Function[2,6,186–193]

There are two main functions of the atria: a transport, or pump, function and a reservoir function to contain blood available for rapid ventricular filling. Like the ventricles, the atria respond to an increase in fiber length by an increased force of contraction. Increased atrial contractility characterized by a shift to the left of atrial function curves (or a shift to the right of their force-velocity curves) may be produced by increased sympathetic stimulation, by inotropic agents such as digitalis or catecholamines, or by decreased vagal stimulation. Each of these causes the atrium to pump a greater amount of blood forward into the ventricle, with a resultant increase in ventricular end-diastolic fiber length and pressure (the atrial kick), thereby causing the ventricle to increase its force of contraction. When the atrial transport function is lost (i.e., by atrial fibrillation) in a person with an otherwise normal heart, the normal circulatory reserve mechanisms are able to maintain the cardiac output at rest within normal limits, although the response of the cardiac output to strenuous exercise is usually diminished. In a patient with ventricular disease, however, even the resting cardiac output may be diminished significantly by this form of *atrial failure* (see Chap. 20).

The atria have also been shown to produce atriopeptigen, which undergoes selective proteolytic cleavage to form atriopeptin I and atriopeptin II. Both have natriuretic and diuretic actions, and both relax intestinal smooth muscle. Atriopeptin II also relaxes vascular muscle.[194–202] It is possible that an elevation in blood volume produces atrial distension and triggers the release of atriopeptigen leading to diuresis and natriuresis and restoring normal blood volume. Atrial natriuretic factor has also been found to inhibit the production of aldosterone.[203] The importance of atrial peptides such as atrial natriuretic factor in normal homeostasis, congestive heart failure, or essential hypertension are under active investigation.

Nervous Control[1–10,204–212]

The nerve endings of sympathetic fibers, which lie between the myocardial fibers, synthesize norepinephrine and store it in granules. Upon stimulation, these sympathetic fibers cause the local release of norepinephrine, which acts locally upon beta receptors which are present on the fiber surface locally to enhance the activity of adenyl cyclase, which in turn catalyzes the conversion of ATP to cyclic AMP (adenosine 3′, 5′-monophosphate, or "second messenger").[213–215] Once nerve stimulation stops, the same nerve endings take up and store norepinephrine for reutilization. A small amount of the norepinephrine is also metabolized locally. Sympathetic nerve fibers reach the entire atria and ventricles, as well as the sinus or sinoatrial (SA) and AV nodes, while vagal fibers, which cause the local release of acetylcholine, influence predominantly the atrial musculature and SA and AV nodes. Some vagal innervation, however, has also been shown to reach the ventricles, and vagal stimulation can decrease ventricular contractility.[216] In general, sympathetic stimulation increases atrial and ventricular contractility, increases heart rate, and speeds the spread of excitation through the AV node and, very slightly, through the ventricles.[217] Recent studies have also suggested that the coronary vessels and heart muscle may produce neuropeptides that can influence coronary vascular resistance and myocardial contractility.

Vagal stimulation generally has opposite effects to sympathetic stimulation. At any given instant, the effect of the nervous system on the heart is the net balance of these two opposing controls, which usually vary reciprocally. It is probable that the vagal parasympathetic stimulation, which is generally inhibitory, normally predominates in the conscious state and maintains the usual resting heart rate of about 65 to 75 beats per minute.[6,218] The resting bradycardia of exercise training is due predominantly to a slowing of the intrinsic rate of the sinus node pacemaker due to enhanced vagal activity in association with a decrease in the adrenergic influence.[219] Neural reflexes, particularly from stretch receptors in the carotid sinus and aorta, form a major extrinsic control mechanism that influences myocardial performance directly and indirectly.[210] When carotid sinus stretch decreases, as with arterial hypotension, a reflex venoconstriction is produced by the sympathetic nervous system that increases venous return and thereby increases ventricular end-diastolic fiber length. Simultaneously, carotid sinus hypotension produces reflex arterial vasoconstriction, increasing peripheral vascular resistance and aortic impedance. In addition, carotid sinus hypotension elicits reflexes that increase atrial and ventricular contractility. Stimulation of the carotid sinus nerve, such as might occur with carotid sinus hypertension, produces opposite effects.

Drugs and Hormones

Myocardial contractility is increased by increased activation of the myocardium, which is mediated in one form or another by an enhanced availability of Ca^{2+} ions inside the cell.[32,33] Increased Ca^{2+} bathing the heart produces this action. Catecholamines including norepinephrine, epinephrine, and isoproterenol act through beta receptors on the myocardial cell, which activate the adenyl cyclase system, which ultimately affects membrane systems within the cells that deliver Ca^{2+} to the contractile proteins. Phosphorylation of these membranes also enhances relaxation.[10] Digitalis glycosides enhance contractility but act by inhibiting the $Na\text{-}K^{+}$-stimulated ATPase in the cell surface membrane, thereby leaving larger amounts of Ca^{2+} within the fiber.[23,31,40–42] Contractility is also increased to some degree by corticosteroids, aldactone, angiotensin, serotonin,[220] and glucagon.[221–223] The physiologic role of other substances such as prostaglandins[224–226] and polypeptide systems such as kinekard,[227] neuropeptide Y, and cardioglobulin[228] in the regulation of myocardial contractility is unclear. The actions of thyroxine on myocardial contractile functions are complex,[229–232] but in general its effects are to increase contraction and relaxation rate. Myocardial contractility is decreased by hypoxia and by many drugs, including barbiturates, quinidine, procainamide, disopyramide, lidocaine, most beta blockers, and calcium antagonists. Acidosis also depresses myocardial contractility, particularly if the sympathoadrenal system function is impaired.[233] Morphine produces a negative inotropic effect upon isolated myocardial strips, but in the conscious dog it produces a beta-adrenergic-mediated increase in myocardial contractility and alpha-adrenergic-mediated coronary vasoconstriction.[234]

In recent years, a number of neuropeptides have been shown to have significant effects upon myocardial contractility and coronary vascular resistance. Some of these occur in significant amounts in the heart and may play important roles in the normal regulation of myocardial contractility and coronary blood flow.

Anesthesia

General anesthesia from halothane or pentobarbital may depress myocardial contractility significantly.[174] In addition, the reflex control mechanisms influencing heart rate may be significantly altered by anesthesia. For example, under anesthesia, the reflex bradycardia of acute hypertension is caused mainly by withdrawal of sympathetic stimulation, while in the conscious state, it is caused almost entirely by parasympathetic restraint.[175,194,205] In the intact conscious animal, the force-frequency relation, or the Bowditch phenomenon, appears to influence myocardial contractility relatively little, whereas an increase in heart rate causes a much larger increase in contractility if the level of contractility is first depressed by generalized anesthesia.[175] Similarly, in anesthetized animals, the increase in heart rate produced by acute volume loading and presumed stimulation of low-pressure receptors in the atria (the *Bainbridge reflex*) is erratic; on the other hand, the reflex is consistently found in conscious animals and can be blocked by the combination of atropine and propranolol.[235] In contrast, the *Anrep effect,* or the positive inotropic effect of an acute increase in afterload, has been demonstrated in the anesthetized animal but is difficult to demonstrate in the conscious subject with low spontaneous heart rates.[175]

Anesthesia also influences the response to many drugs. The relative increase in myocardial contractility produced by digitalis is much less apparent in the conscious state than if the myocardium is depressed by general anesthesia or propranolol. In addition, intravenous ouabain given to the conscious subject produces substantial coronary vasoconstriction and mesenteric vasodilatation, in contrast to effects that are produced during anesthesia.[175] The coronary vasoconstriction produced by norepinephrine or morphine sulfate, which is due to alpha-adrenergic stimulation, and the coronary vasoconstriction produced by dopamine are much more apparent with the subject in the conscious state than under general anesthesia.[175,236]

Postextrasystolic Potentiation

When an extraventricular depolarization is imposed or occurs spontaneously between normal beats, the subsequent normal beat is potentiated. The extent of *postextrasystolic potentiation* is generally related to the closeness of the extra beat to the prior normal beat. Advantage has even been taken clinically of this phenomenon by placing an electrically induced extra beat close to the spontaneous beat and continuing this.[237–239] This "paired electrical stimulation" markedly increases myocardial contractility and stroke output, although the cardiac output per minute is not increased unless it was previously decreased. The mechanism of this type of postextrasystolic potentiation is probably related to increased availability of the calcium ions near the contractile sites of the actin and myosin myofilaments. Unfortunately, current methods for the use of this mechanism for the treatment of the failing heart have the danger of inducing ventricular fibrillation.

Mechanisms of Cardiac Reserve

The normal homeostatic mechanisms regulate cardiac output to meet the demands of the body and can enable the heart to increase its output five- to sixfold during exercise. It is not possible to separate sharply those mechanisms by which the cardiovascular system is normally controlled and those mechanisms of *cardiac reserve* (Table 3-1) that the heart may utilize to meet increased demands on the normal heart and/or to maintain cardiac function in the presence of disease of the heart or circulatory system. Many of these homeostatic and regulatory mechanisms act synergistically in the intact organism; others, such as the sympathetic and parasympathetic nervous control of the heart, are in a state of constantly varying balance. Although it is often possible to separate and even quantify the relative contributions of each mechanism in the experimental animal, it is at present difficult, if not impossible, to separate the possible mechanisms functioning at one instant in a human being. Indeed, the demonstration of mechanisms during physiological experiments indicates only *potential* mechanisms of reserve or control, not what actually happens in the intact organism. Furthermore, most of the mechanisms are interrelated and affect one another, so that the contribution of one mechanism depends upon, and changes with, the contribution of the other mechanisms. In the following discussion, we shall consider some of these mechanisms from the standpoint of their use as forms of *cardiac reserve,* although many of these same mechanisms are utilized in the *normal circulatory regulation.*[6,145,150,240–243] (See also Chaps. 17 and 20.)

The two basic mechanisms of cardiac reserve by which the heart or any other pulsatile pump can increase its minute output in the face of increased demands (or attempt to maintain output in the pres-

TABLE 3-1 Mechanisms of Cardiac Reserve

Increased heart rate
Increased stroke volume
Increased oxygen extraction
Redistribution of blood flow
Anaerobic metabolism
Cardiac dilatation
Cardiac hypertrophy

ence of myocardial disease) are (1) change in rate and (2) change in stroke volume.

Heart Rate

A change in pulse rate is one of the simplest and most effective ways of increasing cardiac output. It is probably the most important and most commonly employed mechanism for effecting rapid changes in cardiac output, particularly in untrained individuals under conditions of moderately increased demands. An increase in heart rate by itself may increase cardiac output about four- to fivefold in highly trained athletes. Above certain limits, however, cardiac output may actually begin to fall as heart rate rises. This rate is about 170 to 180 beats per minute for most normal young individuals, but may be 200 to 220 in trained athletes or only 120 to 140 in older, untrained persons or in patients with heart disease. The decrease in cardiac output above a certain rate is due largely to the shortening of the time of diastole, limiting both the time for adequate filling of the ventricles and for coronary blood flow, which occurs predominantly during diastole in the left ventricle. Although an increase in heart rate does produce a rather slight increase in myocardial contractility and a shortening in the absolute duration of systole,[6,47,66–68,126–130,174] negative inotropic effects of tachycardia can become apparent above a certain rate.[174] Most changes in pulse rate are effected by decrease in vagal inhibition and/or by sympathetic stimulation of the sinus node of the heart.[204–212]

Stroke Volume

In a normal individual in the recumbent position, the ratio of left ventricular stroke volume (SV) to end-diastolic volume (EDV), termed the *ejection fraction,* is about 60 to 75 percent as estimated angiographically. Increased contractility may increase the ejection fraction and the stroke volume with a decreased end-systolic volume (ESV), with the EDV either decreasing or remaining the same. An increased stroke volume can also be produced either by a primary increase in venous return, which increases the end-diastolic fiber length of the atria and ventricles, or by a decrease in afterload, which permits enhanced emptying of the ventricle. In the early stages of heart failure, there is often an increase in end-diastolic volume and fiber length, which tends to maintain the stroke volume, although the ejection fraction is decreased. A decrease in ejection fraction is a hallmark of ventricular failure (see Chaps. 17 and 20).

Increased Oxygen Extraction

When the tissue requirements for oxygen increase, or the supply of blood decreases, the tissues may, up to a point, extract more oxygen from each volume of blood passing through the tissue. The entry of oxygen into myocardial cells is facilitated by myoglobin, which has oxygen dissociation characteristics favorable to the diffusion of oxygen into the cells.[244] Increased oxygen extraction is a major reserve mechanism utilized by the tissues of the body acutely during extreme exertion or chronically when the cardiac output is diminished. This reserve mechanism is of less value to the myocardium, which even normally extracts about 75 percent of its arterial oxygen content (see below and Chap. 19).

Redistribution of Blood Flow[1–14,207,245–253]

The redistribution of cardiac output is a major mechanism of reserve for the body under conditions of increased demand, as during exercise or under conditions of diminished cardiac output. The general result is to maintain blood flow to the brain and the heart and to the tissues acutely requiring blood flow, while sacrificing blood flow to tissues and organs not being utilized or less essential to the immediate survival of the person. The mechanisms by which this redistribution occurs are complex. Although the following explanation is oversimplified, the redistribution may be considered to be the integrated response of two mechanisms: (1) a local autoregulation of the metabolically active tissue or organ, by which local changes in P_{O_2}, P_{CO_2}, pH, potassium ion (K^+) concentration, and other metabolic products affect the local blood vessels to reduce small vessel resistance and increase blood flow (see below); and (2) an integrated response of the central nervous system, mediated by the sympathetic and parasympathetic nervous systems, to produce vasodilatation of the active or exercising organ and vasoconstriction of many other tissues and organs. In addition, there often appears to be a venoconstriction mediated by the sympathetic nervous system which increases venous return to the heart and performs a type of internal transfusion or shifting blood from the large venous reservoirs to the heart, arterial system, and active organs.

Anaerobic Metabolism

Many tissues, particularly skeletal muscle, may also utilize anaerobic metabolism as a reserve mechanism, although the value of this mechanism for the myocardium is also quite limited (see Chaps. 5 and 19). In a normal individual during moderate exercise, anaerobic metabolism may account for about 5 percent of the energy utilized; patients with heart failure may obtain 30 percent of their immediate total energy requirements by anaerobic metabolism during exercise.

Dilatation and Hypertrophy

Dilatation and hypertrophy are forms of compensatory reserve, although they are also swords of Damocles for the heart. Their effects in heart failure are discussed in Chaps. 17 and 20, and their significance in athletes is discussed in Chap. 70.

Sequential Phases of the Cardiac Cycle[11,243–247]

The successive mechanical events of the cardiac cycle may be described by a modification (Plate 1) of Wiggers' classic diagram, which divided the cardiac cycle into two *periods,* systole and diastole, and subdivided these periods into *phases* of cardiac activity.[254–258] In the following discussion, the cardiac cycle is divided according to events on the left side of the heart. Corresponding periods and phases may also be described for events on the right side of the heart, with some differences (see below).

The first phase of ventricular systole is *isovolumic* (*isovolumetric* or *isochoric*) *contraction.* This phase begins with the first detectable rise in left ventricular pressure after the *z point;* it is associated with the initial, mitral component (MC) of the first heart sound and the beginning of the isovolumic contraction (IC) wave of the apexcardiogram. The end of the isovolumic contraction phase and the beginning of the succeeding *rapid ventricular ejection* phase are indicated by the opening of the aortic valve (AO), a rise in aortic pressure, a decrease in ventricular volume, and the peak of the ejection E wave of the apexcardiogram. The onset and termination of the next phase of *reduced ventricular ejection* are less well defined; however, this phase may be said to begin when the shape of the ventricular volume curve indicates a significant decrease in the rate of ejection. This normally occurs prior to the peak systolic pressure in the left ventricle and aorta. The phase of reduced ejection lasts until the end of actual ventricular ejection and the beginning of diastole, which occurs just prior to the recording of the *incisura,* or the sharp downward deflection on the aortic pressure tracing. The brief initial phase of diastole preceding the incisura is referred to as *protodiastole* and represents the time required for the reversal of flow in the aorta and for closure of the aortic valve, which is responsible for the incisura of the aortic pressure tracing.

The beginning of the next phase of isovolumic relaxation of the left ventricle is signified by the closure of the aortic valve as indicated by the aortic component (AC) of the second heart sound and by an inward isovolumic relaxation (IR) wave of the apexcardiogram. Isovolumic relaxation lasts until the left ventricular pressure falls below the left atrial pressure and blood begins to flow from the atrium into the ventricle. Usually, the left ventricular pressure falls below the left atrial pressure tracing slightly *after* the peak of the left atrial *v* wave, since there is a slight fall in left atrial pressure caused by a decrease in the upward bulging of the AV valve structures during ventricular isovolumic relaxation. In a sense, this is the opposite of the mechanism thought to produce the *c* wave in the atria during early ventricular systole.

The end of the isovolumic relaxation phase and the beginning of the *rapid ventricular filling phase* are indicated by an increase in the ventricular volume curve, and by the 0 point of the apexcardiogram, which coincides with the opening of the mitral valve (MO). If the mitral valve is diseased, the opening of the valve may be audible as an "opening snap" (OS). This rapid ventricular filling phase is associated with a continuation of the decrease in atrial pressure (the *y descent*) begun during isovolumic relaxation, a rapid increase in ventricular volume, and an outward rapid-filling wave (RFW) in the apexcardiogram.

The end of the rapid ventricular filling phase and the beginning of the *slow ventricular filling phase* are evidenced by a change in the slope of the ventricular volume curve, which indicates a change in the rate of ventricular filling. At times, the end of rapid ventricular filling is associated with low-frequency vibrations or a sound, termed the S_3 or *ventricular gallop,* which occurs very shortly before the nadir of the *y* descent of the atrial pressure tracing. On the apexcardiogram the end of the rapid ventricular filling phase (and the identification of S_3) is indicated at the moment when an abrupt change in slope occurs at the transition from the RFW to the slow-filling wave (SFW). This may be associated with a brief outward pulsation which is referred to as an *F wave,* or *peak,* on the apexcardiogram; frequently it is both visible and palpable.

During the phase of slow ventricular filling, or diastasis, the pressures in the left atrium and left ventricle slowly increase until the next atrial systole produces the *a wave* in the left atrial pressure tracing. At times, an *h wave* is present in late diastasis prior to the *a* wave. Atrial contraction and the increased ventricular filling produced by atrial contraction are reflected in an increase in ventricular pressure, an increase in ventricular volume, and an outward *a* wave of the apexcardiogram. Toward the peak or the second half of the atrial *a* wave there may be a sound (S_4), particularly if there is a vigorous atrial contraction and relaxation. After the *a* wave of atrial contraction and relaxation, there is a very brief period or point (*z point*) when atrial and ventricular pressures are essentially equal in normal individuals. The next cardiac cycle begins when the next ventricular contraction causes a definite sharp rise in pressure from the *z* point.

As one would expect from the location of the sinus node, contraction of the right atrium and opening of the tricuspid valve occur slightly before the corresponding events on the left side of the heart (Plates 1 and 2). On the other hand, excitation and contraction of the left ventricle begins prior to contraction of the right ventricle, although the beginning of ejection of blood into the pulmonary artery slightly precedes ejection into the aorta, since the pressure in the right ventricle does not have to increase to such a high level before ejection begins

(Plate 2). Interestingly, right ventricular ejection lasts beyond left ventricular ejection, producing the normal interval between the aortic component of the second heart sound (A_2) and the pulmonic component of the second heart sound (P_2). The shorter duration of the left ventricle ejection is related to the greater contractile force of the left ventricle and to differences in the aorta and the pulmonary artery impedance and compression-chamber (windkessel) characteristics.

During the brief phase of left ventricular isovolumic systole, the central aortic pressure pulse may show a slight positive wave that is produced by slight bulging of the aortic valve due to the rapidly increasing left ventricular pressure. There is evidence that during left ventricular ejection, the left ventricular pressure exceeds aortic pressure only during the early part of ejection, and actually is slightly less than aortic pressure during most of systole.[259] It should also be noted that though several components of the first and second heart sounds are referred to by the name of the valve commonly associated with the production of that sound, the sounds are not produced by the actual closure or striking together of the valve leaflets. *The sounds are more properly considered to be produced by the sudden acceleration and deceleration of blood with tensing of the entire valve structures and by vibrations of all cardiac structures.* Actually, there is evidence that the atrioventricular valves and the aortic valve may be closed physiologically at a different time than when these sounds occur.[260–266] In most clinical situations, the two components of the first heart sound, the mitral (M) and the tricuspid (T) component, are produced by sudden acceleration-deceleration of blood, the valves, and cardiac structures in association with abrupt closure of the mitral and tricuspid valves, respectively.

The shape of an apexcardiogram tracing varies significantly depending on the particular instrumentation used to record it. The tracing shown in Plate 1 was obtained with a piezo crystal, which is widely used for timing despite some inherent distortion (see Chaps. 10 and 122).

The Arterial Pulse

The arterial pressure pulse is produced by the ejection of blood from the left ventricle into the aorta and great vessels at a rate faster than its runoff into the peripheral circulation. In humans, an average left ventricular stroke volume of 60 to 100 ml is ejected in about 0.25 s, and of this volume, approximately two-thirds is ejected during the rapid-ejection phase. Although the peak rate of ejection of blood occurs prior to the peak pressure in the left ventricle or aorta, the pressure continues to rise in the aorta as long as blood is ejected into the aorta faster than it runs off into the peripheral arteries. Sometimes there is a slight notch in the central arterial pulse wave during or toward the end of the rapid-ejection phase. This is referred to as the *anacrotic notch,* or *shoulder;* it is accentuated in valvular aortic stenosis. At the end of ventricular ejection (and after the brief phase of protodiastole), the aortic valve closes. In central aortic pressure tracings, this event is reflected by a sharp downward deflection, or *incisura,* on the descending limb of the pressure tracing and a gradual fall during diastole. At times left ventricular isovolumic contraction causes a slight positive deflection in central arterial tracings just prior to the onset of the main arterial pulse wave.

As the arterial pressure pulse wave passes to the periphery, there are significant changes in its form (Fig. 3-17).[267] As the pulse moves away from the heart, the initial upstroke of the pulse becomes steeper, there is normally no anacrotic pause on the ascending limb, and the systolic maximum becomes peaked and increased in magnitude. The *dicrotic notch,* or *halt,* which corresponds to the incisura recorded more centrally, tends to occur later and lower and to be smoother in contour than the incisura. The positive wave that follows the dicrotic notch is referred to as the *dicrotic wave;* in many peripheral arteries this is normally more prominent than the slight upward deflection recorded centrally following the incisura. Although the systolic pressure may increase as the wave moves to the periphery, the diastolic and mean arterial pressures decrease slightly. The major factors responsible for these changes in the arterial pulse contour are (1) distortion of the components of the pulse waves as they travel peripherally, (2) different rates of transmission of various components of the pulse wave, (3) amplification or distortion of different components of the pulse by *standing* or *reflected waves,* (4) differences in elastic behavior and in caliber of the arteries, and (5) conversion of some kinetic energy to hydrostatic energy. Further details of the arterial pulse are discussed in Chap. 9.

The Venous Pulse[186,268]

The form of the venous pressure pulse is determined by the rate of return of the blood from the peripheral tissues into the venous segment, the pressure-volume characteristics of the segment of the vein, the nature of the resistance to flow or distensibility offered by the right atrium and ventricle during the different phases of the cardiac cycle, and, to a slight degree, the tissues overlying the veins at the point of observation. Although the venous pressure pulse wave travels peripherally away from the heart, there is at the same time a venous flow of blood in the opposite direction toward the heart.

The *a* wave of the venous pressure pulse is related to contraction of the right atrium and is followed by the *z* point immediately preceding ventric-

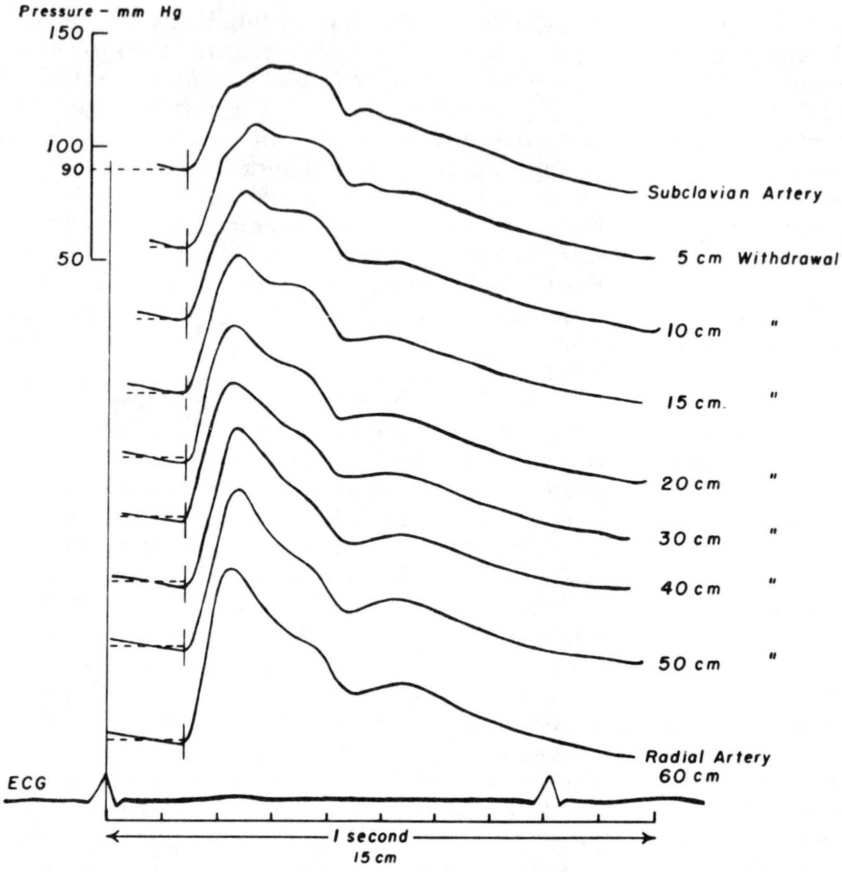

FIGURE 3-17 Pulse contours in a healthy 30-year-old man, showing transformation of pressure pulse in subclavian-radial system. Pressure pulses were recorded consecutively during withdrawal of tip of arterial catheter from subclavian artery near aorta to radial artery in left arm. Onsets of pressure pulses are aligned for purposes of comparison. As the pulse wave moves peripherally, initial wave steepens and increases in magnitude, dome-shaped systolic maximum becomes peaked, and dicrotic halt moves down and to the right and becomes slurred. Low-amplitude, central postdicrotic wave is not seen after catheter has been withdrawn 10 cm or more. Prominence of radial dicrotic wave is due, in part, to change in position of dicrotic halt. Horizontal broken line intersecting onset of each pulse contour is calibration reference point (90 mmHg). Interval of time from peak of R wave of electrocardiogram to onset of systolic upswing of each pulse wave is indicated by duration of each tracing to left side of short vertical lines, which mark onset of systole from each pulse. [*From H. W. Marshall, H. F. Helmholz, and E. H. Wood, Physiologic Consequences of Congenital Heart Disease, in W. F. Hamilton and P. Dow (eds.), "Handbook of Physiology," sec. 2; "Circulation," American Physiological Society, Washington, D.C., 1962, vol. 1, p. 417. Reproduced with permission of the publisher and authors.*]

ular systole. In the jugular venous pulse, the *c wave* as usually recorded is produced predominantly by the systolic impulse in the adjacent carotid artery, with some contribution by right ventricular contraction and upward bulging of the tricuspid valve. In the early part of ventricular systole and following the brief *c* wave, there is a rapid inflow of blood to the right atrium produced in part by descent of the tricuspid valve ring, which produces the normal negative venous wave during ventricular systole, the negative *x* wave, or *x descent* (systolic collapse). The latter is also produced by the ejection of blood from both ventricles, which decreases the intrapericardial pressure and therefore the pressure in both atria. As the venous inflow continues into the atria after the *x* descent, the pressure in the atria and in the veins builds up, producing the *v wave* during approximately the second half of ventricular systole. The *v* wave continues to build up until the right ventricle passes through the phase of isovolumic relaxation and begins its phase of rapid ventricular filling. The peak of the right atrial *v* wave occurs shortly before or simultaneously with opening of the tricuspid valve and the beginning of the phase of rapid right ventricular filling. During early ventricular diastole, the rapid flow of blood from the great veins and right atrium into the right ventricle produces the negative *y descent* (or diastolic collapse) of the peripheral venous pulse wave. The venous pulse wave is somewhat damped when recorded externally, and even when recorded directly, the waves are usually less steep in rise and descent than the corresponding waves of the atria. In part this is due to the damping effect of the large veins, which can accommodate markedly different volumes of blood without a marked change in pressure. Clinically, venous pulse waves are particularly difficult to evaluate in the presence of tachycardia, obesity, or shock, or during the administration of drugs that produce venoconstriction. Further details of the venous pulse are discussed in Chap. 9.

Normal Pressures and Flow Rates in the Cardiovascular System[269–272]

In general, the pressure in the systemic arteries is about five or six times greater than in the pulmonary arteries, though the amount of blood flowing in each unit is essentially the same. The left ventricular output may be very slightly greater than the right ventricular output because of the small amount of bronchial artery flow that returns in the pulmonary veins and the drainage of a few Thebesian veins into the left atrium and ventricle. In order to compare measurements between individuals of different sizes, measurements of flow and resistance are often expressed in terms of square meters of body surface area; i.e., instead of comparing cardiac output in absolute number of liters per minute, the output of the heart is expressed as the *cardiac index,* or liters per minute per square meter of body surface area. There is still a need for additional data to establish the limits of "normal" for vascular pressures, flow, and resistance for normal individuals of all ages under conditions of rest, exercise, or emotional stress. Furthermore, some of the slight differences in normal values reported from different laboratories are related to the use of different methods of measurement or different baselines for measurement of pressure. Table 3-2 lists the mean and range of hemodynamic measurements for normal resting adults, and Table 3-3 gives the distribution of systemic blood flow and oxygen consumption in a hypothetical 70-kg normal resting male.

TABLE 3-2 Hemodynamic Values of Normal Recumbent Adults

	Mean	Range
Caridan index, liters/min/m²	3.4	2.8–4.2
Stroke index, ml/beat	47	30–65
Arteriovenous oxygen difference, ml per liter of blood	38	30–48
Arterial saturation, %	98	94–100
Pressure,* mmHg		
Brachial artery		
Systolic	130	90–140
Diastolic	70	60–90
Mean	85	70–105
Left ventricle		
Systolic	130	90–140
End-diastolic	7	4–12
Left atrium		
Maximum	13	6–20
Minimum	3	−2–+9
Mean	7	4–12
Pulmonary artery wedge ("PC")		
Maximum	16	9–23
Minimum	6	1–12
Mean	9	6–15
Pulmonary artery		
Systolic	24	15–28
Diastolic	10	5–16
Mean	16	10–22
Right ventricle		
Systolic	24	15–28
End-diastolic	4	0–8
Right atrium		
Maximum	7	2–14
Minimum	2	−2–+6
Mean	4	−1–+8
Venae cavae		
Maximum	7	2–14
Minimum	5	0–8
Mean	6	1–10
End-diastolic volume		
Left ventricular, ml/m²	70	50–90
Resistance, dyn·s/cm⁵		
Total systemic	1150	900–1400
Systemic arteriolar	850	600–900
Total pulmonary	200	150–250
Pulmonary arteriolar	70	45–120

*Baseline for pressure measurements one-half of anteroposterior chest diameter: 1 mmHg = 133.332 Pascal (Pa) = 0.133 kPa.

Response to Exercise[6,14,66,273–305]

The mechanisms utilized to increase the cardiac output during dynamic exercise vary, depending on the age, condition, posture, and athletic training of the person. In particular, the relative contribution of heart rate and stroke volume has been of considerable interest. It would appear that most "normal" but untrained individuals in the supine position increase their cardiac output during mild to moderate dynamic exercise predominantly by an increase in pulse rate rather than by an increase in stroke volume. With more extreme exercise, even this type of individual will increase stroke volume about 10 to 15 percent in the supine position and by 30 to 100 percent in the upright position, despite a considerably shortened systolic ejection period. In normal persons who are more accustomed to physical exertion, there is an earlier and more marked increase in stroke volume in both positions, and stroke volume often doubles during extreme upright exercise. In general, pulse rate may increase threefold (or even fivefold in some highly trained athletes), whereas stroke volume increases considerably less. With extreme increases in rate, stroke volume may even decline slightly.

Dynamic exercise results in increased sympathetic adrenergic nervous activity to the resistance vessels of the kidney and splanchnic area and to the uninvolved muscles, while increasing blood flow to the exercising muscles by sympathetic vasodilatation and, probably, by local autoregulation. The increase in sympathetic nervous system activity is roughly proportional to the intensity of exercise. The arterial systolic blood pressure often increases 40 to 60 mmHg during moderate or severe exercise, although the mean arterial blood pressure increases much less. The diastolic pressure may increase slightly, decrease slightly, or stay the same. Calculated total arterial resistance normally decreases considerably during exercise. An increase in cardiac output is further aided by an increase in venous return produced by the combination of vasodilatation of the exercising muscles and the increased mechanical activity of the skeletal muscles, which rhythmically compress the peripheral veins, and by the rhythmic increase and decrease of the pressure in the peritoneal and thoracic cavities. The latter is sometimes referred to as the *abdominothoracic pump.* Exercise also produces a decrease in the volume of blood in venous reservoirs, especially the splanchnic blood volume. The result of these shifts is to make more blood available to the heart, arterial vessels, and exercising muscles. On the other hand, during prolonged exercise, plasma volume may decrease significantly, with a resultant increase in hematocrit.[306,307] An increase in venous return to the atria may also produce an increase in heart rate by the Bainbridge reflex; this is more apparent in patients with a low resting heart rate or with hypervolemia in association with hemodilution. Isometric exercises of relatively mild degree may produce

TABLE 3-3 Distribution of Systemic Blood Flow and Oxygen Consumption in a Normal Subject* at Rest in a Comfortable Environment

Circulation	Blood Flow, ml/min	Percentage of Total Flow	AV† O_2 Difference, ml/dl	O_2 Consumption, ml/min	Percentage of Total Consumption
Splanchnic	1400	24	4.1	58	25
Renal	1100	19	1.3	16	7
Cerebral	750	13	6.3	46	20
Coronary	250	4	11.4	27	11
Skeletal muscle	1200	21	8.0	70	30
Skin	500	9	1.0	5	2
Other organs	600	10	3.0	12	5
Total body	5800	100	4.0	234	100

*Weight, 70 kg; surface area, 1.7 m^2.
†AV = arteriovenous.
Source: Wade, O. L., and Bishop, J. M.: "Cardiac Output and Regional Blood Flow," Blackwell Scientific Publications, Ltd., Oxford, 1962. Reproduced with permission from the publisher and authors.

significant increases in blood pressure and pulse rate,[308–317] factors of considerable importance in patients with coronary artery disease (see Chaps. 19, 44, and 45).

During exercise, there is a significant redistribution of the elevated cardiac output. During mild to moderate dynamic exercise, coronary blood flow and blood flow to the active skeletal muscles increases, and cerebral flow is maintained whereas renal and splanchnic flows diminish. During more severe exercise, these changes are exaggerated, and flow to the resting skeletal muscles may decrease. During maximal exercise, cerebral flow may also decrease, in association with hyperventilation and respiratory alkalosis. Skin blood flow may decrease initially during exercise, but it increases with continued exercise and contributes to the elimination of body heat.

In general, there is evidence of a generalized sympathetic discharge during exercise that in certain organs is overridden by local vasodilator metabolites and changes in P_{O_2}, P_{CO_2}, pH, and K^+. The plasma levels of both norepinephrine and epinephrine increase during dynamic exercise, but the level of norepinephrine is increased much less during isometric exercise. In exercising skeletal muscles, there may be increased activity of sympathetic vasodilator fibers in addition to decreased vasoconstrictor activity. Venoconstriction during exercise tends to shift blood toward the central circulation and to the active skeletal muscles. Similar venoconstriction may occur in response to cold, emotion, hyperventilation, or norepinephrine.

Myocardial Oxygen Consumption

The hemodynamic determinant of myocardial oxygen consumption ($M\dot{V}_{O_2}$) was related in 1907 by Barcroft and Dixon to external work, or the product of aortic pressure and flow.[318] In 1912, Rohde concluded that ventricular pressure and heart rate together determined myocardial oxygen consumption,[319] and in 1915 Evans and Matsuoka reported "a relation between the tension set up on contraction and the metabolism of the contractile tissue."[320] They noted that volume work was performed more economically (i.e., with less oxygen consumed) than was an equal amount of calculated pressure work, and they also called attention to the fact that the tension change in the wall of the heart "varies roughly as the endocardiac pressure and as the square of the radius of the heart cavities," the now-familiar Laplace relation. Since their paper was published, many studies have confirmed the importance of active intramyocardial tension, or wall stress, developed by the ventricle, or a related variable, as major determinants of myocardial oxygen consumption.[321–324,379] Some of the related variables that have been correlated with $M\dot{V}_{O_2}$ include the product of pressure and heart rate, the product of integrated ventricular pressure and heart rate (the tension-time index),[325] developed wall tension, and contractile element work.

The inotropic state or contractility, or the velocity of contraction, is the second major determinant of myocardial oxygen consumption. It can account for the variations in $M\dot{V}_{O_2}$ when various calculations of developed tension or work, under various positive or negative inotropic interventions, either do not change or change in the opposite direction.[321–327] The results of several earlier studies relating $M\dot{V}_{O_2}$ to ventricular end-diastolic fiber length or diastolic volume were probably related to changes in developed tension or velocity of contraction. Similarly, the net effect on myocardial oxygen consumption of various positive inotropic interventions, such as sympathetic nerve stimulation or excitement, paired electrical stimulation, or the infusion of digitalis glycosides, catecholamines, or calcium, depends to a large degree upon the relative effects upon the tension developed and on the contractile state, as reflected in V_{max}, the maximum velocity of shortening of the unloaded muscle.[321–324] Most of the increase in myocardial oxygen uptake produced by catecholamines is related to the hemodynamic alterations that they induce, although large doses can increase oxygen uptake in the nonbeating heart by a small amount. The effect of digitalis on $M\dot{V}_{O_2}$ depends upon its relative effects upon the contractile state of the heart, which it increases, causing $M\dot{V}_{O_2}$ to increase, and upon ventricular wall tension, which can decrease $M\dot{V}_{O_2}$ significantly if the heart radius decreases sufficiently.[324,327,328]

As shown in Table 3-4, the seven determinants of myocardial oxygen consumption can be classified as four major determinants and three minor determinants. The oxygen cost of electrical activation is probably less than 1 percent of the total $M\dot{V}_{O_2}$, and the costs for contractile-state activation and deactivation and for the maintenance of the active state are also small.[322–325] Clinically, it is sometimes useful to calculate an estimate of relative myocardial oxygen requirements by determining the product of systolic blood pressure and heart rate, the *tension-time index,*[325] or pressure time per minute.[329] One may also factor the product of pressure and heart rate by the total duration of systole per minute.

Coronary flow and pressure affect oxygen consumption in the nonworking heart but have variable effects in the beating heart.[330] Alcohol stimulates the myocardial uptake of oxygen, whereas hypothermia markedly decreases oxygen consumption.

Regulation of Regional Blood Flow[1–10,12,13,205,207,245,249,331,332]

The amount of blood flowing to an individual organ of the body is determined by the difference between the arterial and venous pressures in the vessels supplying the organ and by the vascular resistance of the organ. Although the arterial and venous pressures change in situations such as exercise, eating, or emotional stress, most of the alterations in the distribution of blood flow are the consequence of changes in vascular resistance of the organ.

The major mechanisms by which decreases in organ vascular resistance are effected are an increase in caliber of the vessels and an opening of new vascular channels. Since most of the vascular resistance appears to be located at the level of the small arteries and arterioles, it is probable that most of the regulation occurs by changes in caliber of these vessels, although changes in the capillaries and veins may at times play an important role.

TABLE 3-4 Determinants of Myocardial Oxygen Consumption

Major determinants
Myocardial mass
Intramyocardial tension or wall stress (pressure × volume)
Inotropic state (contractility)
Heart rate
Minor determinants
External work (load × shortening)
Basal oxygen requirements
Activation energy

In a consideration of the local control of blood flow, several fundamental relations and definitions should first be introduced.

The *resistance* to blood flow through a given portion of the circulation is usually expressed by the ratio of mean pressure difference between two points in the vascular system to the mean amount of blood passing from one point to the other. It is usually calculated using mean pressures and flows, although most vascular flow is pulsatile. If it were possible to measure accurately instantaneous pressure differences and flows, it would be theoretically more proper to calculate vascular *impedance,* which is the ratio of pulsatile pressure to pulsatile flow and which varies with the frequency of the pulse. Vascular resistance may be expressed in various units, i.e., *peripheral resistance units* (PRU), pressure gradient (mmHg) per unit blood flow (ml/s); by Aperia's formula to give results in absolute or metric (cgs, or centimeter-gram-second) units by multiplying PRU units by a conversion factor of 1332 to express resistance in terms of $dyn \cdot s/cm^5$; or by the ratio of pressure gradient (mmHg) to blood flow expressed in liters per minute to give *R units.* R units may be converted approximately to $dyn \cdot s/cm^5$ by multiplying by 80. Minor changes in calculated resistance are usually of no significance, not only because of possible errors in pressure or flow measurements, but also because changes in apparent resistance may result from the distending effect of inflow or exit pressure. Conversely, alteration in the distending force may mask changes in the vascular bed. Because of such considerations and the nonlinear relation between pressure and flow of most vascular beds, changes in calculated resistance cannot be equated simply with vasoconstriction or vasodilatation. This is particularly true if there are changes in both pressure and flow.

The relation of the various factors affecting the resistance to fluid flow in rigid tubing is expressed by Poiseuille's equation:

$$\text{Fluid flow} = \frac{\pi(\text{pressure difference})(\text{radius})^4}{8(\text{vessel length})(\text{fluid viscosity})}$$

Since the experiments from which the equation was derived were performed in straight rigid tubes with steady streamlined flow of an ideal, viscous fluid, it is not possible to apply this relation directly to the vascular system, in which the vessels are neither straight nor rigid, the blood is not a simple viscous fluid, and the flow is not always streamlined. Nevertheless, the predominant influence on flow of the radius of the vessel, which is raised to the *fourth* power in the above equation, is apparent. Of the other factors, changes in vessel length are thought to be ordinarily relatively unimportant; however, changes in viscosity related to changes in hematocrit, temperature, and serum proteins are often of marked significance, particularly in small blood vessels. It should also be noted that in most vascular beds, most of the blood vessels are connected in parallel rather than in series. The total resistance of vessels connected in parallel is calculated by adding the *conductance* of each individual vessel ($1/R$, the reciprocal of the individual resistance) to obtain the total conductance of all the vessels (Fig. 3-18). Because of these relations for vessels in parallel and in accordance with Poiseuille's laws, the resistance of four small tubes in parallel is four times as great as that of a single large tube of equal total cross-sectional area. Actually, it requires 16 small tubes with four times the total cross-sectional area to have a resistance as low as a single wide tube or vessel.

Since all normal blood vessels are distensible at least to some extent, it follows that increasing the *intraluminal pressure* will increase the *transmural pressure* on the vessel wall and increase the diameter and radius of the vessel. This effect is seen in Fig. 3-19, which illustrates the pressure-flow and pressure-resistance curves of an isolated peripheral vascular bed. Note that as the distending pressure is increased from 20 to 40 mmHg, there is a marked decrease in calculated resistance associated with an increase in flow. The pressure at about 20 mmHg, at which flow ceases entirely, has been sometimes referred to as the *critical closure pressure;* however, it is perhaps better referred to as the *critical flow pressure,* since it is unlikely that there is often complete anatomic closure of the vessels.

The amount of distension present in an individual blood vessel is dependent on the stiffness, or *tone,* of the vessel and on the *distending* or *transmural pressure,* i.e., the difference between the intraluminal pressure, which tends to expand the vessel, and the external pressure, which tends to compress the vessel. The tone, or stiffness, of a blood vessel is determined by the geometry of the vessel and by the mechanical properties of the vessel wall. Important relations between the distending pressure and the tension in the wall of a blood vessel are expressed in the following form of the *law of Laplace:*

$$\text{Wall tension} = \text{distending pressure} \times \frac{\text{vessel radius}}{2 \times \text{wall thickness}}$$

From this equation it is apparent that the tension in the wall of a blood vessel tending to expand it is greater if the radius of the vessel is greater or if the blood vessel wall is thinner. Thus, veins with greater radii and thinner walls than their arterial counterparts have a greater wall tension than their arterial counterparts *at the same pressure.* The degree of stretching of the vessel wall produced by wall tension depends on the elastic stiffness of the vessel wall. The term *distensibility* is usually defined by the pressure-volume characteristics of a given vessel and is dependent on the above and other factors.

The regulation of vascular stiffness achieved by alterations in the physicochemical-mechanical properties of vascular smooth muscle is referred to as *vasomotion.* The major factors by which changes in vasomotion and changes in vessel caliber are accomplished are (1) metabolic, chemical, and hormonal substances carried in the blood and/or locally produced, and (2) the activity of fibers from autonomic nervous system innervating the blood vessels and locally releasing norepinephrine or acetylcholine. The relative importance of these two mechanisms varies markedly from one vascular bed to another. Although it was formerly thought that the release of

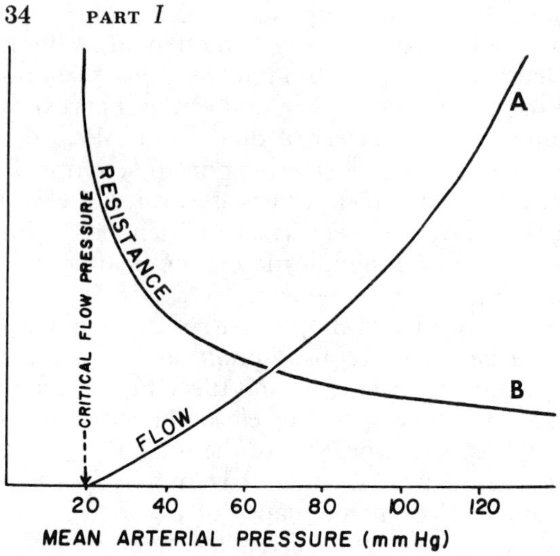

FIGURE 3-19 Relations among pressure, flow, and resistance of a peripheral vascular bed. In *A,* no flow is apparent below about 20 mmHg, the critical flow pressure, or critical closure pressure. At pressure above this value, the flow increases progressively more for each unit of pressure rise as the resistance of the vascular bed is decreased by the pressure within the vessels. *B.* Marked decrease in calculated resistance. (*From A. C. Guyton, "Textbook of Medical Physiology," 6th ed., W. B. Saunders Company, Philadelphia, 1981. Adapted and reproduced with permission of the publisher and author.*)

FIGURE 3-18 Comparison of the calculation of vascular resistance of vessels in series and in parallel. In most vascular beds most of the blood vessels of the same size are connected in parallel.

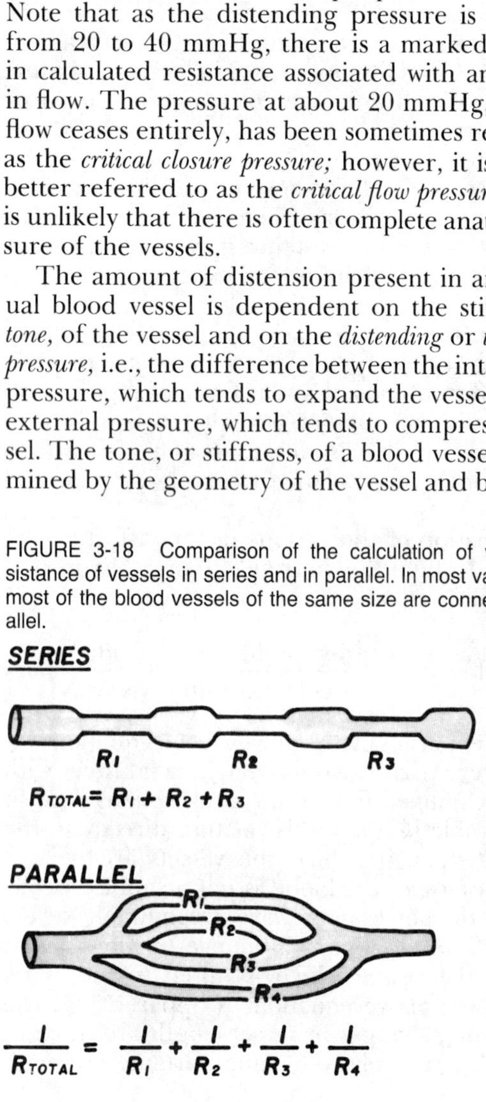

epinephrine and norepinephrine from the adrenal medulla played an important role in the normal physiologic control of vascular tone, this mechanism is not currently thought to be important except under conditions of extreme stress when the adrenal medulla releases significant quantities of these substances.

Most systemic arteries, and probably veins, respond to hypoxia and/or an increase in P_{CO_2} with vasodilatation.[245–247,249,252,253] The vasodilatation produced by hypoxia in many vascular beds is significantly augmented by an increase in K^+ concentration. Other substances that may be important in the local control of vasomotion include prostaglandins,[227,250,251,333] lactic acid, histamine, neuropeptides and other vasoactive peptides, and unknown "metabolic products." The cerebral vessels are particularly sensitive to P_{CO_2},[248,249] whereas the coronary vessels respond strikingly to changes in P_{O_2},[334,335] although qualitatively similar changes are found in most other systemic vessels. It is probable that the myocardial vasodilatation produced by hypoxia is ordinarily mediated by the metabolite adenosine rather than by a direct effect of lowered P_{O_2}, unless the hypoxia is extreme.[334–336] Local prostaglandins and neuropeptides released in the heart may also be important.[225,226,250,333] In most organs, the effects of P_{O_2}, P_{CO_2}, K^+, prostaglandins, and metabolic products work synergistically with the autonomic nervous system to regulate regional blood flow. In contrast to systemic vessels, the pulmonary vessels seem to respond in the opposite manner to changes in P_{CO_2}, pH, and P_{O_2}. In addition to their regional effects, P_{O_2} and P_{CO_2} in the mixed venous blood returned to the heart appear to be involved in the control of the total output of the heart through poorly understood mechanisms.

Neural Control of Blood Vessels[2,6,12,205,207,208,253,331,332]

Three main types of nerve fibers are important in the control of blood vessels: (1) sympathetic vasoconstrictor fibers, (2) sympathetic vasodilator fibers, and (3) parasympathetic vasodilator fibers.

Sympathetic vasoconstrictor fibers are found in both arteries and veins throughout the body, but not in capillaries. These fibers appear to effect vasoconstriction by the release of norepinephrine at the nerve fiber endings. Vasodilatation may be produced by inhibition of the discharge rate of these nerve fibers. These fibers are important in responding to local or regional stimuli of many types. In addition, they are the major pathways for reflex changes in peripheral resistance secondary to changes in carotid sinus and aortic stretch receptors, as well as reflex changes from the carotid body chemoreceptors and from stretch receptors in the low-pressure areas of the intrathoracic vascular bed. They are thought to be the principal mechanism by which impulses from the cortical and subcortical areas of the brain influence total and regional peripheral resistance. The effect of these nerve fibers on the coronary and cerebral blood vessels is ordinarily very slight, being overshadowed by the influence of P_{O_2} and P_{CO_2}.[248–253] The influence of sympathetic stimulation and coronary reflexes is considered in Chap. 44.

Sympathetic vasodilator fibers appear to be of importance in skeletal muscles, although it is possible that some cutaneous blood vessels and coronary vessels also receive this type of fiber. It is probable that these fibers are not normally active tonically and that they are not significantly influenced by the carotid sinus or aortic arch stretch receptors. They are thought to be important in increasing blood flow to muscles during exercise. The effector agent at the nerve fiber ending is thought to be acetylcholine.

Parasympathetic vasodilator fibers are restricted to the tongue and salivary glands and to the sacral area, particularly the erectile vessels of the genital organs. In the sacral area these nerves take part in the local regulation of blood flow according to the needs of local activity, but they are not thought to play an important role in the reflex control of major cardiovascular functions. The transmitted substance at their nerve root endings is acetylcholine.

Parasympathetic stimulation of the salivary glands causes the release of a *kallikrein,* which acts on kininogen, a plasma α_2 globulin synthesized in the liver, to form lysyl bradykinin, which is converted by a plasma aminopeptidase to *bradykinin,* a substance with powerful vasodilator properties. The sweat glands of the skin, innervated by sympathetic cholinergic fibers, may also liberate a kallikrein, and there is evidence that a kallikrein precursor in plasma may be activated by certain physical and chemical factors. In addition, the release of kallikrein and the formation of kinins have been suggested as contributing factors in the hypotension associated with endotoxin and anaphylactic shock, the dumping syndrome, and carcinoid syndrome.[337,338]

In general, vasoconstriction occurs as the result of increased activity of the sympathetic nervous system, which causes the local release of norepinephrine at the nerve fiber endings in blood vessels, whereas vasodilatation is produced by the inhibition of sympathetic vasoconstrictor impulses and/or by metabolic products and local environmental conditions (P_{O_2}, P_{CO_2}, pH, K^+, etc). Localized vasodilatation may also be produced in exercising muscle by sympathetic vasodilator fibers, and in the sacral area and salivary glands by parasympathetic fibers. In some areas vasodilatation may be produced by the formation of neuropeptides and other polypeptides under autonomic nervous system influence.[339] Prostaglandins are also very important in local circulatory control.[39,224–226,250]

It is not possible to present a succinct but accurate description of the anatomic pathways by which the central nervous system helps to control cardiovascular function. Nor is it possible to describe simply the mechanisms by which the nervous system is able to integrate impulses from all levels—the cortex and limbic system, reticular system, diencephalon, mesencephalon, medulla oblongata, spinal cord, etc.—and to synthesize these impulses in order to provide the organism with responses varying from the massive sympathetic discharge associated with shock to very discrete vasomotor changes. There appear to be three major pools of spontaneously active neurons important to the control of both the heart and the peripheral blood vessels: the cardiovascular-excitatory center (pressor area), which is located in the rostrolateral portion of the medulla; the cardiovascular inhibitory center (depressor area), which is located in the mediocaudal portion of the medulla; and the dorsal motor nucleus of the vagus nerve, which exerts a cardiac-inhibitory influence.[2] It is also apparent that impulses from high levels at times bypass lower integrative areas. There is unfortunately little information regarding the nature of the processes by which conditioning involving the autonomic nervous system occurs.

Coronary Circulation[334–336,340–343]

The normal coronary circulation is able to provide oxygen to the heart under a wide range of conditions and is able to increase its flow five or six times the value at rest.[341–345] The *coronary vascular reserve* refers to the capacity of the coronary circulation to provide additional oxygenated blood to the myocardium. At rest, however, the coronary blood flow (CBF) is approximately 70 to 90 ml per 100 g per minute and the oxygen consumption of the heart approximately 8 to 10 ml per 100 g per minute.[334–336,342–347] Even at rest, however, the heart, which is normally aerobic (Chap. 5), utilizes most of the oxygen contained in its blood supply. Consequently, the oxygen content of the blood in the coronary sinus is about 5 ml per 100 ml blood, which corresponds to about 30 percent saturation and a P_{O_2} of 18 to 20 mmHg.[340,346,347] As a result, relatively little additional oxygen can be made available to the heart by greater oxygen extraction, and any increase in demand for oxygen by the heart must be met by an increase in coronary blood flow.[346,348] Thus, any increase in the myocardial oxygen requirement (Table 3-4) will normally result in proportional increase in coronary blood flow.

Determinants of Coronary Blood Flow

Physical Factors
Aortic diastolic pressure is a direct, major determinant of coronary blood flow; however, excessively elevated diastolic pressure does not result in unneeded perfusion because of autoregulation.[331] On the other hand, when the perfusion pressure is very low, the coronary circulation is maximally dilated and coronary blood flow is linearly related to the perfusion pressure. Arterial or inflow pressure can influence coronary vascular resistance by distending the coronary vessels.[349] Coronary blood flow may be decreased by factors decreasing effective coronary perfusion pressure, such as congenital anomalies of the coronary arteries or obstruction of a coronary artery by atherosclerosis, thrombosis, or vasoconstriction. In general, it is necessary to decrease the lumen or cross-sectional area of an epicardial coronary vessel by two-thirds or more to cause a significant decrease in coronary flow, although this varies with the length and character of the obstruction; lesser degrees of obstruction can cause a significant decrease in flow, especially under conditions that increase the need for coronary blood flow.

Extravascular Compressive Forces During ventricular systole, the left ventricular intramyocardial pressure exceeds left ventricular cavitary pressure or aortic systolic pressure. As a consequence, the penetrating coronary vessels in the wall of the left ventricle are markedly compressed, or "throttled," markedly decreasing any forward flood flow and often producing retrograde flow.[346,350] In addition to the physical systolic compression of the vessels, coronary flow is impeded by increased shear caused by twisting of the coronary vessels during systole.[351] The effect of these forces upon coronary blood flow during systole are much greater for the high-pressured left ventricle, which therefore receives the majority of its coronary blood flow during diastole, than for the right ventricle, where coronary blood flow is more nearly equal during systole and diastole (Fig. 3-20). In patients with coronary artery disease or even with marked left ventricular hypertrophy, tachycardia can predispose to myocardial ischemia not only by the direct increase in oxygen consumption, but by significantly limiting the amount of time occupied by diastole, when the left ventricle receives most of its blood supply.

Tissue pressure and especially ventricular diastolic pressure also influence and can decrease coronary blood flow, especially to the subendocardium of a "failing" left ventricle and particularly if arterial hypotension is also present. The outlet pressure in the coronary sinus or right atrium can offer some impediment to coronary perfusion, although this is seldom a significant factor in the absence of severe coronary artery disease. Blood viscosity is an additional factor that may contribute to a limitation of coronary blood flow, particularly in the presence of coronary artery disease. Whether or not a myogenic mechanism contributes to the autoregulation of coronary blood flow is uncertain. Additional physical factors affecting the adequacy of coronary blood flow include the total myocardial mass and the diffusion distance of oxygen from coronary capillaries to the center of hypertrophied myocardial cells.

Metabolic Factors
Coronary blood flow normally increases linearly with increased myocardial oxygen requirements, and most

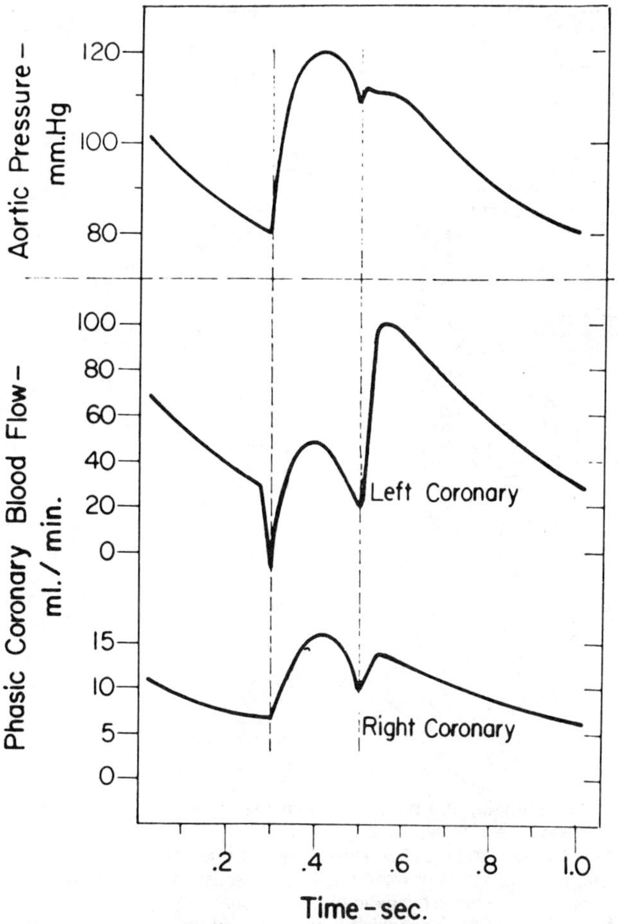

FIGURE 3-20 Comparison of phasic coronary blood flow in the left and right coronary arteries. Note the marked decrease in flow in the left coronary artery during systole. (*From R. M. Berne and M. N. Levy, "Cardiovascular Physiology," 4th ed., C. V. Mosby Company, St. Louis, 1981. Reproduced with permission from the publisher and authors.*)

of the increase in coronary blood flow is by coronary vasodilatation secondary to metabolic autoregulation. In general, any influence that increases myocardial oxygen requirements (Table 3-4) will result in a proportional increase in coronary blood flow. It is likely that several mediators or metabolic vasodilators are responsible for the metabolic autoregulation of the coronary circulation. Adenosine, which is formed by dephosphorylation of AMP and which has strong coronary vasodilator properties, appears to fulfill most of the criteria for the physiological regulation of coronary blood flow and to play a major role in the metabolic control of coronary resistance (Fig. 3-21).[334–336,341–343,351–353] Other substances that are potential mediators include other nucleotides,[352] prostaglandins, carbon dioxide, and pH concentration. On the other hand, it is unlikely that K^+, Ca^{2+}, or osmolality function as mediators in the normal control of coronary circulation.[343,351,354] The oxygen tension appears to influence coronary resistance secondarily by influencing the release of other mediators rather than by a direct influence upon the coronary vessels. Changes in pH and P_{CO_2} also have a slight effect upon myocardial oxygenation by producing changes in the oxygen-hemoglobin dissociation curve.

Although many prostaglandins can produce coronary vasodilatation, at present they are not thought to play a major role in the normal control of coronary resistance. Some studies, however, have suggested that thromboxane A_2, an extremely strong coronary vasoconstrictor, may be important in producing coronary spasm.[355–359] Local atherosclerosis may also potentiate the vasoconstrictor effects of alpha agonists,[360] norepinephrine, serotonin,[361–363] or histamine.[364] Such potentiation could cause coronary spasm (see Chap. 46).

Neural Factors

Sympathetic Nerves As described in Chap. 2, sympathetic nerves to the heart and coronary vessels arise from the three sympathetic ganglia and the first four thoracic sympathetic ganglia. Sympathetic adrenergic fibers extensively innervate both the epicardial and the intramural arteries and veins. Large coronary vessels appear to have both alpha_2 and beta_2 receptors, while small vessels have predominantly beta_2 receptors. The coronary vessels do not appear to have beta_1-adrenergic receptors, which appear to be limited to the myocardium, or sympathetic cholinergic fibers.[365–368]

Stimulation of cardiac sympathetic nerves produces a direct vasoconstriction of the coronary arteries. This vasoconstriction, however, is normally overwhelmed by vasodilatation secondary to the increase in myocardial metabolism secondary to the sympathetic stimulation of heart rate and myocardial contractility. Coronary vascular beta receptors are not thought to contribute to the response to nerve stimulation.[354]

Parasympathetic Nerves Experimentally, stimulation of the vagus nerves produces some direct coronary vasodilatation that is mediated by the release of acetylcholine and can be blocked by atropine.[369] In the intact organism, however, vagal stimulation produces bradycardia and may decrease myocardial contractility, both of which decrease myocardial oxygen requirements and which result in secondary coronary vasoconstriction.

Coronary Reflexes Although coronary vascular resistance is primarily determined by metabolic autoregulation, it is also modulated by the sympathetic nervous system in response to changes in arterial pressure that are sensed by baroreceptors in the carotid sinus. Carotid chemoreceptors, which may be initiated by acidosis, hypoxemia, or hypercapnia, can also influence coronary resistance by a predominant vasodilator effect mediated by the vagi and, perhaps, by a lesser vasoconstrictor effect mediated by the sympathetic nerves and only apparent if the vagal reflex is blocked. There is no convincing evi-

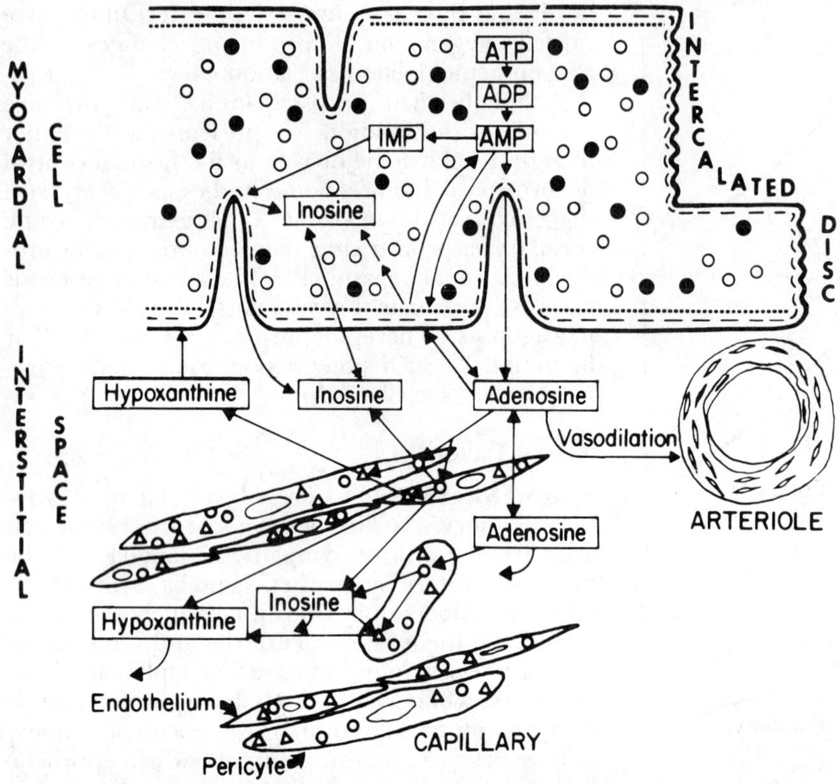

FIGURE 3-21 Diagram depicting a myocardial cell, interstitial space, an arteriole, and a capillary with the localization of enzymes involved in formation and fate of adenosine. Adenosine formed by 5′-nucleotidase from AMP (which in turn arises from ATP) can enter the interstitial space. There it can induce arteriolar dilatation and reenter the myocardial cell, where it is either phosphorylated to AMP by adenosine kinase or deaminated to inosine by adenosine deaminase, or enter the capillaries and leave the tissue. A large fraction of adenosine that crosses the capillary wall is deaminated to inosine, which in turn is split to hypoxanthine and ribose-1-PO_4 by nucleoside phosphorylase located in the endothelial cells, pericytes, and erythrocytes. Most of the adenosine is taken up by the myocardial cells, and that escaping in the circulation is largely in the form of inosine and hypoxanthine. Since adenylic acid deaminase (which deaminates AMP to IMP) is in low concentration in heart muscle, the major degradative pathway from AMP is via dephosphorylation to adenosine. Open circle = Adenosine deaminase; solid circle = adenylic acid deaminase; triangle = nucleoside phosphorylase; dashes = 5′-nucleotidase; dots = adenosine kinase. [*From R. M. Berne and R. Rubio, Coronary Circulation, in R. M. Berne (ed.), "Handbook of Physiology," sec. 2: "The Cardiovascular System," vol. 1: "The Heart," American Physiological Society, Bethesda, Md., 1979, p. 873. Reproduced with permission of the publisher and authors.*]

dence, however, of a coronary-to-coronary reflex except following the intracoronary administration of veratridine, which is known to elicit the Bezold-Jarisch reflex, a coronary-to-periphery reflex producing hypotension and bradycardia.[336] There is evidence of reflex vasodilation of some peripheral vascular beds as well as changes in heart rate and contractility following coronary occlusion.[336] On the other hand, there is little substantial evidence of reflex vasoconstriction of coronary vessels from peripheral phenomena such as gastritis or cholecystitis. There is good evidence for a pulmonary inflation reflex that produces coronary vasodilatation in part mediated by a withdrawal of sympathetic tone.[370]

Coronary Collateral Circulation

The exact stimuli and mechanisms for the development of coronary collaterals are not known. Hypoxia appears to play a major role. It has been postulated that hypoxia releases vasodilator metabolites that dilate preexisting microscopic collateral vessels, increasing their pressure and tangential wall stress and damaging the vessel walls. This initial damage is then followed by reparative processes and the development of large-lumen, thick-walled collateral vessels.[336,371–374] In human beings, the presence of coronary collaterals usually signifies the presence of significant coronary artery disease.[348,361–374]

Humoral Factors

Norepinephrine stimulates alpha receptors in the coronary vessels and produces direct coronary vasoconstriction but indirectly produces coronary vasodilatation and an increase in coronary blood flow due to the marked increase in myocardial contractility.[236,375–377] Epinephrine substantially increases myocardial oxygen demand and coronary blood flow.[375] The effects of dopamine upon the coronary circulation vary markedly with the dose administered, but in general it produces mild coronary vasodilatation. Isoproterenol stimulates beta vasodilator receptors and produces an increase in coronary venous oxygen saturation in normal animals.[378,379]

Angiotensin II produces coronary vasoconstriction although this effect is partially obscured by its effect of increasing myocardial oxygen consumption by increases in systemic pressure and left ventricular wall stress, heart rate, and myocardial contractility. It may also release prostaglandins E_2 and F, which produce coronary vasodilatation.[380,381]

High concentrations of vasopressin produce direct coronary vasoconstriction.[353,382–384] Coronary vascular tone is probably not significantly affected by changes in concentration of Na^+, K^+, Ca^{2+}, or Mg^{2+} although studies have suggested that Ca^{2+} produces mild vasoconstriction; Mg^{2+} produces vasodilatation; Na^+ produces no effect; and K^+ produces a biphasic response, with small doses producing vasodilatation and large doses vasoconstriction.

Thyroid hormone produces coronary vasodilatation secondary to its effects upon heart rate and myocardial contractility.[385–390] Adrenal steroids affect coronary blood flow and resistance secondarily by their tendency to produce systemic hypertension and left ventricular hypertrophy. Glucagon produces coronary vasodilatation that is secondary to an increase in heart rate and contractility. Beriberi is associated with increased coronary blood flow and decreased myocardial oxygen extraction,[391] perhaps as part of generalized arterial vasodilatation.

Adenosine and acetylcholine both produce marked coronary vasodilatation.[336,353] Histamine produces coronary vasodilatation, both directly and indirectly by its positive inotropic and chronotropic effects.[343] Serotonin also produces direct and, to a lesser degree, indirect coronary vasodilatation.

Polypeptides are possibly important in the regulation of coronary blood flow.[336,339,342,351] Bradykinin increases coronary blood flow, possibly by the actions of prostaglandins.[392–394] Substance P produces moderate coronary vasodilatation, but its role in the normal regulation of coronary blood flow is unknown.[395,396] Vasoactive intestinal polypeptide (VIP) appears to produce both direct coronary vasodilatation and indirect vasodilatation owing to its positive inotropic effects.[396,397] Neuropeptide tyrosine Y (NPY), which was recently discovered in the pig brain and gut and which appears to be one of the most widespread neuropeptides, coexists with norepinephrine in the peripheral nervous system including nerves to coronary blood vessels. NPY may play a role in some instances of coronary spasm.[398]

Many prostaglandins produce coronary vasodilatation, especially prostacyclin (PGI_2).[225,399] Thromboxane A_2 is a very strong coronary vasoconstrictor and may be important in producing episodic, vasospastic decreases in coronary blood flow (see Chap. 46).

Distribution of Coronary Blood Flow

Current evidence indicates that the blood flow to the left ventricle is closely related to its oxygen demands. In experimental animals, this is also true within the left ventricle, where the left ventricular subendocardium at rest consumes 10 to 30 percent more oxygen per gram than the subepicardium and has a proportionately higher blood flow.[400–410] During tachycardia or other conditions that increase myocardial oxygen requirements and coronary blood flow in experimental animals, however, coronary blood flow is more nearly equal to that of different layers of the left ventricular myocardium. The few estimates of coronary blood flow distribution in human beings, however, have suggested a fairly homogeneous distribution of coronary flow in the layers of the left ventricle at rest.[411,412] Although still not completely agreed upon, most studies have indicated that the left ventricular subendocardium, which has a very dense vasculature, has a higher systolic intramyocardial pressure, calculated wall stress, and oxygen consumption than the subepicardium.[403,413] Coronary flow to the left ventricular subendocardium is especially likely to be compromised by elevation of left ventricular diastolic pressure. The latter may be seen chronically in patients with hypertension, aortic stenosis, or hypertrophic cardiomyopathy or may occur acutely secondary to myocardial infarction.

References

1. Hamilton, W. F., and Dow, P. (eds): "Handbook of Physiology," sec. 2: "Circulation," American Physiological Society, Washington, D.C., 1962–1965, vols. 1–3.
2. Guyton, A. C., Jones, C. E., and Coleman, T. G.: "Circulatory Physiology: Cardiac Output and Its Regulation," 2d ed., W. B. Saunders Company, Philadelphia, 1973, 556 pp.
3. Guyton, A. C., and Jones, C. E. (eds.): "Cardiovascular Physiology," University Park Press, Baltimore, 1974, vol. I, 349 pp.
4. Guyton, A. C., Taylor, A. E., and Granger, H. J.: "Circulatory Physiology," vol. II: "Dynamics and Control of the Body Fluids," W. B. Saunders Company, Philadelphia, 1975, 397 pp.
5. Guyton, A. C., and Young, D. B.: "Cardiovascular Physiology," vol. III: "Arterial Pressure and Hypertension," University Park Press, Baltimore, 1979, 564 pp.
6. Braunwald, E., Ross, J., Jr., and Sonnenblick, E. H.: "Mechanisms of Contraction of the Normal and Failing Heart," 2d ed., Little, Brown and Company, Boston, 1976, 417 pp.
7. Rushmer, R. F.: "Cardiovascular Dynamics," 4th ed., W. B. Saunders Company, Philadelphia, 1976, 584 pp.
8. Levine, H. J. (ed.): "Clinical Cardiovascular Physiology," Grune & Stratton, Inc., New York, 1976, 945 pp.
9. Vasalle, M. (ed.): "Cardiac Physiology for the Clinician," Academic Press, Inc., New York, 1976, 263 pp.
10. Katz, A. M.: "Physiology of the Heart," Raven Press, New York, 1977, 450 pp.
11. Noble, M. I. M.: "The Cardiac Cycle," Blackwell Scientific Publications, Ltd., Oxford, 1979.
12. Berne, R. M. (ed.): "Handbook of Physiology," sec. 2: "The Cardiovascular System," vol. 1: "The Heart," American Physiological Society, Bethesda, Md., 1979.
13. Shepherd, J. T., and Vanhoutte, P. M.: "The Human Cardiovascular System: Facts and Concepts," Raven Press, New York, 1979.
14. Braunwald, E., and Ross, J., Jr.: Control of Cardiac Performance, in R. M. Berne (ed.), "Handbook of Physiology," sec. 2: "The Cardiovascular System," vol. 1: "The Heart," American Physiological Society, Bethesda, Md., 1979, p. 533.
15. Ebashi, S., and Endo, M.: Calcium Ion and Muscle Contraction, *Prog. Biophys. Mol. Biol.*, 18:123, 1968.
15a. Ringer, S.: A Further Contribution regarding the Influence

of the Different Constituents of the Blood on the Contraction of the Heart, *J. Physiol.* (London), 4:29, 1882.
16. Harris, P., and Opie, L.: "Calcium and the Heart," Academic Press, Inc., New York, 1971, 198 pp.
17. Kones, R. J.: The Molecular and Ionic Basis of Altered Myocardial Contractility, *Res. Commun. Chem. Pathol. Pharmacol.,* 5(suppl. 1):1, January 1973
18. Inesi, G.: Active Transport of Calcium Ion in Sarcoplasmic Membranes, *Annu. Rev. Biophys. Bioenerget.,* 1:191, 1973.
19. Morad, M., and Goldman, Y.: Excitation-Contraction Coupling in Heart Muscle: Membrane Control of Development of Tension, *Prog. Biophys. Mol. Biol.,* 27:257, 1973.
20. Trautwein, W.: Membrane Currents in Cardiac Muscle Fibers, *Physiol. Rev.,* 53:793, 1973.
21. Reuter, H.: Exchange of Calcium Ions in the Mammalian Myocardium: Mechanisms and Physiological Significance, *Circ. Res.,* 34:599, 1974.
22. Levy, M. N., and Martin, P. J.: Cardiac Excitation and Contraction, in A. C. Guyton and C. E. Jones (eds.), "Cardiovascular Physiology," University Park Press, Baltimore, 1974, vol. I, p. 49.
23. Langer, G. A.: Ionic Movements and the Control of Contraction, in G. A. Langer and A. J. Brady (eds.), "The Mammalian Myocardium," John Wiley & Sons, Inc., New York, 1974, p. 193.
24. Schwartz, A.: Active Transport in Mammalian Myocardium, in G. A. Langer and A. J. Brady (eds.), "The Mammalian Myocardium," John Wiley & Sons, Inc., New York, 1974, p. 81.
25. Nayler, W. G., and Seabra-Gomes, R.: Excitation-Contraction Coupling in Cardiac Muscle, *Prog. Cardiovasc. Dis.,* 18:75, 1975.
26. Katz, A. M., Tada, M., and Kirchberger, M. A.: Control of Calcium Transport in the Myocardium by the Cyclic AMP Protein Kinase System, *Adv. Cyclic Nucleotide Res.,* 5:453, 1975.
27. Ebashi, S.: Excitation-Contraction Coupling, *Annu. Rev. Physiol.,* 38:293, 1976.
28. Fozzard, H. A.: Heart: Excitation-Contraction Coupling, *Annu. Rev. Physiol.,* 39:201, 1977.
29. Endo, M.: Calcium Release from the Sarcoplasmic Reticulum, *Physiol. Rev.,* 57:71, 1977.
30. Fabiato, A., and Fabiato, F.: Calcium Release from the Sarcoplasmic Reticulum, *Circ. Res.,* 40:119, 1977.
31. Langer, G. A.: Ionic Basis of Myocardial Contractility, *Annu. Rev. Med.,* 28:13, 1977.
32. Winegrad, S.: Electromechanical Coupling in Heart Muscle, in R. M. Berne (ed.), "Handbook of Physiology," sec. 2: "The Cardiovascular System," vol. 1: "The Heart," American Physiological Society, Washington, D.C., 1979, p. 393.
33. Fabiato, A., and Fabiato, F.: Calcium and Cardiac Excitation-Contraction Coupling. *Annu. Rev. Physiol.,* 41:473, 1979.
34. Lehninger, A. L.: Ca^{2+} Transport by Mitochondria and Its Possible Role in the Cardiac Contraction-Relaxation Cycle, *Circ. Res.,* 35:83, 1974.
35. Carafoli, E., Tiozzo, R., Lugli, G., Crovetti, F., and Kratzing, C.: The Release of Calcium from Heart Mitochondria by Sodium, *J. Mol. Cell. Cardiol.,* 6:361, 1974.
36. Young, M.: The Molecular Basis of Muscle Contraction, *Annu. Rev. Biochem.,* 38:913, 1969.
37. Katz, A. M.: Biochemical Basis for Cardiac Contraction, in I. Mirsky, D. N. Ghista, and H. Sandler (eds.), "Cardiac Mechanics: Physiological, Clinical, and Mathematical Considerations," John Wiley & Sons, Inc., New York, 1974, p. 67.
38. Katz, A. M.: Contractile Proteins, in G. A. Langer and A. J. Brady (eds.), "The Mammalian Myocardium," John Wiley & Sons, Inc., New York, 1974, p. 51.
39. Noble, M. I., and Pollack, G. H.: Molecular Mechanisms of Contraction, *Circ. Res.,* 40:333, 1977.
40. Akera, T.: Membrane Adenosine Triphosphatase: A Digitalis Receptor, *Science,* 198:569, 1977.
41. Akera, T., and Brody, T. M.: The Role of Na^+, K^+-ATPase in the Inotropic Action of Digitalis, *Pharmacol. Rev.,* 29:187, 1977.
42. Langer, G. A.: Relationship between Myocardial Contractility and the Effects of Digitalis on Ionic Exchange, *Fed. Proc.,* 36:223, 1977.
43. Katz, A. M., Bailin, G., Kirchberger, M. A., and Today, M.: Regulation of Myocardial Cell Function by Agents that Increase Cyclic AMP Production in the Heart, in A. P. Fishman (ed.), "Heart Failure," Hemisphere Publishing Corp., Washington, D.C., 1978, pp. 11–28.
44. Keely, S. L., and Corbin, J. D.: Involvement of cAMP-dependent Protein Kinase in the Regulation of Heart Contractile Force, *Am. J. Physiol.,* 233:H269, 1977.
45. Hicks, M. J., Shigekawa, M., and Katz, A. M.: Mechanism by Which Cyclic Adenosine 3′:5′-Monophosphate-Dependent Protein Kinase Stimulates Calcium Transport in Cardiac Sarcoplasmic Reticulum, *Circ. Res.,* 44:384, 1979.
46. Luttgau, H. C.: Caffeine, Calcium, and the Activation of Contraction, in A. W. Cuthbert (ed.), "Calcium and Cellular Function," St. Martin's Press, New York, 1970, p. 241.
47. Arentzen, C. E., Rankin, J. S., Anderson, P. A. W., Feezor, M. D., and Anderson, R. W.: Force-Frequency Characteristics of the Left Ventricle in the Conscious Dog, *Circ. Res.,* 42:64, 1978.
48. Johnson, E. A.: Force-Interval Relationship of Cardiac Muscle, in R. M. Berne (ed.): "Handbook of Physiology," sec. 2: "The Cardiovascular System," vol. 1: "The Heart," American Physiological Society, Bethesda, Md., 1979, p. 475.
49. Hoffman, B. F., Bindler, E., and Suckling, E. E.: Postextrasystolic Potentiation of Contraction in Cardiac Muscle, *Am. J. Physiol.,* 185:95, 1956.
50. Langer, G. A.: Heart: Excitation-Contraction Coupling, *Annu. Rev. Physiol.,* 35:55, 1973.
51. Sperelakis, N., and Schneider, J. A.: A Metabolic Control Mechanism for Calcium Ion Influx That May Protect the Ventricular Myocardial Cell, *Am. J. Cardiol.,* 37:1079, 1976.
52. Akera, T., and Brody, T. M.: The Role of Na^+, K^+-ATPase in the Inotropic Action of Digitalis, *Pharmacol. Rev.,* 29:187, 1978.
53. Schwartz, A., Sordahl, L. A., Entman, M. L., et al.: Abnormal Biochemistry in Myocardial Failure, in D. T. Mason (ed.), "Congestive Heart Failure: Mechanisms, Evaluation and Treatment," Yorke Medical Books, New York, 1976, p. 25.
54. Brutsaert, D. L., and Sonnenblick, E. H.: Cardiac Muscle Mechanics in the Evaluation of Myocardial Contractility and Pump Function: Problems, Concepts and Directions, *Prog. Cardiovasc. Dis.,* 16:337, 1973.
55. Langer, G. E., and Brady, A. J.: "The Mammalian Myocardium," John Wiley & Sons, Inc., New York, 1974, 310 pp.
56. Mirsky, I., Ghista, D. N., and Sandler, H.: "Cardiac Mechanics: Physiological, Clinical, and Mathematical Considerations," John Wiley & Sons, Inc., New York, 1974, 490 pp.
57. Skelton, C. L., and Sonnenblick, E. H.: Physiology of Cardiac Muscle, in H. J. Levine (ed.), "Clinical Cardiovascular Physiology," Grune & Stratton, Inc., New York, 1976, p. 57.
58. Brady, A. J.: Mechanical Properties of Cardiac Fibers, in R. M. Berne (ed.), "Handbook of Physiology," sec. 2: "The Cardiovascular System," vol. 1: "The Heart," American Physiological Society, Washington, D.C., 1979, p. 461.
59. Alpert, N. R., Hamrell, B. B., and Mulieri, L. A.: Heart Muscle Mechanics, *Annu. Rev. Physiol.,* 41:521, 1979.
60. Sonnenblick, E. H.: Implications of Muscle Mechanics in the Heart, *Fed. Proc.,* 21:975, 1962.
61. Fry, D. L., Griggs, D. M., Jr., and Greenfield, J. C., Jr.: Myocardial Mechanics: Tension-Velocity-Length Relationships of Heart Muscle, *Circ. Res.,* 14:73, 1964.
62. Evans, J. R. (guest ed.): Symposium: Structure and Function of Heart Muscle, *Circ. Res.,* 15(suppl. 2):1, 1964.
63. Sonnenblick, E. H.: Instantaneous Force-Velocity-Length Determinants in the Contraction of Heart Muscle, *Circ. Res.,* 16:441, 1965.

64. Sonnenblick, E. H., Braunwald, E., and Morrow, A. G.: The Contractile Properties of Human Heart Muscle: Studies on Myocardial Mechanics of Surgically Excised Papillary Muscles, *J. Clin. Invest.*, 44:966, 1965.
65. Glick, G., Sonnenblick, E. H., and Braunwald, E.: Myocardial Force-Velocity Relations Studied in Intact Unanesthetized Man, *J. Clin. Invest.*, 44:978, 1965.
66. Sonnenblick, E. H., Braunwald, E., Williams, J. F., Jr., and Glick, G.: Effects of Exercise on Myocardial Force-Velocity Relations in Intact Unanesthetized Man: Relative Roles of Changes in Heart Rate, Sympathetic Activity, and Ventricular Dimensions, *J. Clin. Invest.*, 44:2051, 1965.
67. Sonnenblick, E. H.: The Mechanics of Myocardial Contraction, in S. A. Briller and H. L. Conn, Jr. (eds.), "The Myocardial Cell: Structure, Function and Modification by Cardiac Drugs," University of Pennsylvania Press, Philadelphia, 1966, p. 173.
68. Sonnenblick, E. H., Morrow, A. G., and Williams, J. F., Jr.: Effects of Heart Rate on the Dynamics of Force Development in the Intact Human Ventricle, *Circulation*, 33:945, 1966.
69. Covell, J. W., Ross, J., Jr., Sonnenblick, E. H., and Braunwald, E.: Comparison of the Force-Velocity Relation and the Ventricular Function Curve as Measures of the Contractile State of the Intact Heart, *Circ. Res.*, 19:364, 1966.
70. Braunwald, E., Sonnenblick, E. H., Ross, J., Jr., and Gault, J. H.: Insights into Cardiovascular Physiology Derived from Muscle Mechanics, *Am. J. Cardiol.*, 20:705, 1967.
71. Pool, P. E., and Sonnenblick, E. H.: Mechanochemistry of Heart Muscle: I. The Isometric Contraction, *J. Gen. Physiol.*, 50:951, 1967.
72. Gault, J. H., Ross, J., Jr., and Braunwald, E.: Contractile State of the Left Ventricle in Man: Instantaneous Tension-Velocity-Length Relations in Patients with and without Disease of the Left Ventricular Myocardium, *Circ. Res.*, 22:451, 1968.
73. Pool, P. E., Chandler, B. M., Seagren, S. C., and Sonnenblick, E. H.: Mechanochemistry of Cardiac Muscle: II. The Isotonic Contraction, *Circ. Res.*, 22:465, 1968.
74. Barns, J. W., Covell, J. W., and Ross, J., Jr.: The Mechanics of Isotonic Left Ventricular Contractions, *Am. J. Physiol.*, 224:725, 1973.
75. Huxley, A. F.: Muscular Contraction, *J. Physiol. London*, 243:1, 1974.
76. Mahler, F., Ross, J., Jr., O'Rourke, R. A., and Covell, J. S.: Effects of Changes in Preload, Afterload and Inotropic State on Ejection and Isovolumic Phase Measures of Contractility in the Conscious Dog, *Am. J. Cardiol.*, 36:626, 1975.
77. Abbott, B. C., and Gordon, D. G.: A Commentary on Muscle Mechanics, *Circ. Res.*, 36:1, 1975.
78. Jewell, B. R.: A Re-Examination of the Influence of Muscle Length on Myocardial Performance, *Circ. Res.*, 40:221, 1977.
79. Hill, A. V.: The Heat of Shortening and the Dynamic Constants of Muscle, *Proc. R. Soc. London Ser. B*, 126:136, 1938.
80. Hill, A. V.: "First and Last Experiments in Muscle Mechanics," University Press, Cambridge, 1970, p. 141.
81. Bowditch, H. P.: Ueber die Eigenthumlichkeiten der Reizbarkeit, welche die Muskelfasern des Herzens zeigen, *Verh. K. Sachs Ges. Wochenshr, Leipzig Math. Phys. Cl.*, 23:652, 1871.
82. Howell, W. H., and Donaldson, F., Jr.: Experiments upon the Heart of the Dog with Reference to Maximum Volume of Blood Sent Out by Left Ventricle in a Single Beat, *Philos. Trans. R. Soc. London Ser. B*, 175:139, 1884.
83. Frank, O.: Zur Dynamik des Herzmuskels, *Z. Biol.*, 32:370, 1895, C. B. Chapman and E. Wasserman (trans.), *Am. Heart J.*, 58:282,467, 1959.
84. Fick, A.: "Mechanische Arbeit und Warmeentwickelung bei der Muskeltatigheit," F. A. Brockhaus, Leipzig, 1882.
85. Kries, J. von: Untersuchungen zur Mechanik der quergestreiften Muskels, *Arch. Physiol. Leipzig*, 1880, p. 348; 1885, p. 67.
86. Blix, M.: Die Lange und die Spannung des Muskels, *Skand. Arch. Physiol.*, 5:173, 1895.
87. Wiggers, C. J.: Some Factors Controlling the Shape of the Pressure Curve in the Right Ventricle, *Am. J. Physiol.*, 33:382, 1914.
88. Straub, H.: I. Dynamik des Saugetierherzens; II. Mitteilung Dynamik des Rechten Herzens, *Dtsch. Arch. Klin. Med.*, 115:531, 116:409, 1914.
89. Patterson, S. W., and Starling, E. H.: On the Mechanical Factors Which Determine the Output of the Ventricles, *J. Physiol.*, 48:357, 1914.
90. Patterson, S. W., Piper, H., and Starling, E. H.: The Regulation of the Heart Beat, *J. Physiol.*, 48:465, 1914.
91. Starling, E. H.: "The Linacre Lecture on the Law of the Heart," Longmans, Green & Co., Ltd., London, 1918.
92. Wiggers, C. J.: Determinants of Cardiac Performance, *Circulation*, 4:485, 1951.
93. Sarnoff, S. J., and Berglund, E.: Ventricular Function: I. Starling's Law of the Heart Studied by Means of Simultaneous Right and Left Ventricular Function Curves in the Dog, *Circulation*, 9:706, 1954.
94. Sarnoff, S. J.: Myocardial Contractility as Described by Ventricular Function Curves: Observations on Starling's Law of the Heart, *Physiol. Rev.*, 35:107, 1955.
95. Braunwald, E., and Ross, J., Jr.: Applicability of Starling's Law of the Heart to Man, in J. R. Evans (guest ed.), Symposium: Structure and Function of Heart Muscle, *Circ. Res.*, 15(suppl. 2):169, 1964.
96. Braunwald, E.: The Control of Ventricular Function in Man, *Br. Heart J.*, 27:1, 1965.
97. Levine, H. J.: Compliance of the Left Ventricle, *Circulation*, 46:423, 1972.
98. Templeton, G. H., Ecker, R. R., and Mitchell, J. H.: Left Ventricular Stiffness during Diastole and Systole: The Influence of Changes in Volume and Inotropic State, *Cardiovasc. Res.*, 6:95, 1972.
99. Covell, J. S., and Ross, J., Jr.: Nature and Significance of Alterations in Myocardial Compliance, *Am. J. Cardiol.*, 32:449, 1973.
100. Grossman, W., McLaurin, L. P., Moos, S. P., Stefandouros, M. A., and Young, D. T.: Wall Thickness and Diastolic Properties of the Left Ventricle, *Circulation*, 49:129, 1974.
101. Gaasch, W. H., Cole, J. S., Quinones, M. A., and Alexander, J. K.: Dynamic Determinants of Left Ventricular Diastolic Pressure-Volume Relations in Man, *Circulation*, 51:317, 1975.
102. Mirsky, I.: Assessment of Passive Elastic Stiffness of Cardiac Muscle: Mathematical Concepts, Physiologic and Clinical Considerations, Directions for Future Research, *Prog. Cardiovasc. Dis.*, 18:277, 1976.
103. Grossman, W., and McLaurin, L. P.: Diastolic Properties of the Left Ventricle, *Ann. Intern. Med.*, 84:316, 1976.
104. Gaasch, W. H., Levine, H. J., Quinones, M. A., and Alexander, J. K.: Left Ventricular Compliance: Mechanisms and Clinical Implications. *Am. J. Cardiol.*, 38:645, 1976.
105. Wisnecki, J. A., and Bristow, J. D.: Left Ventricular Stiffness, *Annu. Rev. Med.*, 29:475, 1978.
106. Lewis, B. S., and Gotsman, M. S.: Current Concepts of Left Ventricular Relaxation and Compliance, *Am. Heart J.*, 99:101, 1980.
107. Bemis, C. E., Serur, J. R., Borkenhagen, D., Sonnenblick, E. H., and Urshel, C. W.: Influence of Right Ventricular Filling Pressure on Left Ventricular Pressure and Dimension, *Circ. Res.*, 34:498, 1974.
108. Little, W. C., Badke, F. R., and O'Rourke, R. A.: Effect of Right Ventricular Pressure on the End-Diastolic Left Ventricular Pressure-Volume Relationship before and after Chronic Right Ventricular Pressure Overload in Dogs without Pericardia, *Circ. Res.*, 54:719, 1984.
109. Braunwald, E., and Ross, J., Jr.: The Ventricular End-Diastolic Pressure Appraisal of Its Value in the Recognition of Ventricular Failure in Man, *Am. J. Med.*, 34:147, 1963.
110. DiDonna, G., LeWinter, M., Johnson, A., and Peterson, K.: Effects of Left Ventricular Hypertrophy on Diastolic Wall Stiffness, *Circulation*, 50(suppl. 3):45, 1974.
111. Spiro, D., and Sonnenblick, E. H.: The Structural Basis of the Contractile Process in Heart Muscle under Physiological

and Pathological Conditions, *Prog. Cardiovasc. Dis.*, 7:295, 1965.
112. Spiro, D.: The Fine Structure and Contractile Mechanism of Heart Muscle, in S. A. Briller and H. L. Conn, Jr. (eds.), "The Myocardial Cell: Structure, Function, and Modification by Cardiac Drugs," University of Pennsylvania Press, Philadelphia, 1966, p. 13.
113. Ross, J., Jr., Sonnenblick, E. H., Covell, J. W., Kaiser, G. A., and Spiro, D.: Architecture of the Heart in Systole and Diastole: Technique for Rapid Fixation and Analysis of Left Ventricular Geometry, *Circ. Res.*, 21:409, 1967.
114. Sonnenblick, E. H., Ross, J., Jr., Covell, J. W., Spotnitz, H. M., and Spiro, D.: The Ultrastructure of the Heart in Systole and Diastole: Changes in Sarcomere Length, *Circ. Res.*, 21:423, 1967.
115. Sonnenblick, E. H., and Ross, J., Jr.: Some Ultrastructural Considerations in Myocardial Failure: Sarcomere Overextension and Length Dispersion, in R. D. Tanz, F. Kavaler, and J. Roberts (eds.), "Factors Influencing Myocardial Contractility," Academic Press, Inc., New York, 1967, p. 43.
116. Leyton, R. A., and Sonnenblick, E. H.: The Sarcomere as the Basis of Starling's Law of the Heart in the Left and Right Ventricles, in E. Bajusz and G. Jasmin (eds.), "Methods and Achievements in Experimental Pathology," S. Karger A. G., Basel, 1971, vol. 5, p. 22.
117. Spotnitz, H. M., Leyton, R. A., Kelly, D. T., et al.: "Outstretched" Sarcomere in Subacute Volume Pressure Loading of Dog Right Ventricle, *Circulation,* 46(suppl. 2):44, 1972.
118. Sonnenblick, E. H., Skelton, C. L., Spotnitz, W. D. and Feldman, D.: Redefinition of the Ultrastructural Basis of Cardiac Length-Tension Relations, *Circulation,* 48(suppl. 4):65, 1973.
119. Yoran, C., Covell, J. W., and Ross, J., Jr.: Structural Basis for the Ascending Limb of Left Ventricular Function, *Circ. Res.,* 32:197, 1973.
120. Sonnenblick, E. H., and Skelton, C. L.: Reconsideration of the Ultrastructural Basis of Cardiac Length-Tension Relations, *Circ. Res.*, 35:517, 1974.
121. Skelton, C. L., Sponitz, W. W., Feldman, D., Serur, J. R., Mirsky, I., and Sonnenblick, E. H.: Ultrastructural and Functional Correlates of Acute Cardiac Distention, *Clin. Res.*, 22:304a, 1974.
122. Sonnenblick, E. H., Spotnitz, H. M., and Spiro, D.: Role of the Sarcomere in Ventricular Function and the Mechanism of Heart Failure, *Circ. Res.,* 15(suppl. 2):70, 1964.
123. Allen, D. G., and Kurihara, S.: Calcium Transients at Different Muscle Length in Rat Ventricular Muscle, *J. Physiol. London,* 292:68P, 1979.
124. Dodge, H. T., Frimer, M., and Stewart, D. K.: Functional Evaluation of the Hypertrophied Heart in Man, *Circ. Res.,* 35(suppl. 2):122, 1974.
125. Sonnenblick, E. H.: Series Elastic and Contractile Elements in Heart Muscle: Changes in Muscle Length, *Am. J. Physiol.,* 207:1330, 1964.
126. Vatner, W. F., and Braunwald, E.: Cardiac Frequency: Control and Adjustments to Alterations, *Prog. Cardiovasc. Dis.,* 14:431, 1972.
127. Anderson, P. A. W., Manring, A., and Johnson, E. A.: Force-Frequency Relationship: A Basis for a New Index of Cardiac Contractility?, *Circ. Res.,* 33:665, 1973.
128. Higgins, C. B., Vatner, S. F., Franklin, D., and Braunwald, E.: Extent of Regulation of the Heart's Contractile State in the Conscious Dog by Alteration in the Frequency of Contraction, *J. Clin. Invest.,* 52:1187, 1973.
129. Mahler, F., Yoran, C., and Ross, J., Jr.: Inotropic Effect of Tachycardia and Poststimulation Potentiation in the Conscious Dog, *Am. J. Physiol.,* 227:569, 1974.
130. Stone, H. L.: Effect of Heart Rate on Left Atrial Systolic Shortening in the Dog, *J. Appl. Physiol.,* 38:1110, 1975.
131. Tanz, R. D., Kavaler, F., and Roberts, J. (eds.): "Factors Influencing Myocardial Contractility," Academic Press, Inc., New York, 1967.
132. Mason, D. T., Spann, J. F., and Zelis, R.: Quantification of the Contractile State of the Intact Human Heart: Maximal Velocity of Contractile Element Shortening Determined by the Instantaneous Relation between the Rate of Pressure Rise and Pressure in the Left Ventricle during Isovolumic Systole, *Am. J. Cardiol.,* 26:248, 1970.
133. Sonnenblick, E. H., Parmley, W. W., Urschel, C. W., and Brutsaert, D. L.: Ventricular Function: Evaluation of Myocardial Contractility in Health and Disease, *Prog. Cardiovasc. Dis.,* 12:449, 1970.
134. Mason, D. T., Spann, J. F., Jr., Zelis, R., and Amsterdam, E. A.: Alterations of Hemodynamics and Myocardial Mechanics in Patients with Congestive Heart Failure: Pathophysiologic Mechanisms and Assessment of Cardiac Function and Ventricular Contractility, *Prog. Cardiovasc. Dis.,* 12:507, 1970.
135. Mirsky, I., Ellison, R. C., and Hugenholtz, P. G.: Assessment of Myocardial Contractility in Children and Young Adults from Ventricular Pressure Recordings, *Am. J. Cardiol.,* 27:359, 1971.
136. Braunwald, E.: On the Difference between the Heart's Output and Its Contractile State, *Circulation,* 43:171, 1971.
137. Mason, D. T., Braunwald, E., Covell, J. W., Sonnenblick, E. H., and Ross, J., Jr.: Assessment of Cardiac Contractility: The Relation between the Rate of Pressure Rise and Ventricular Pressure during Isovolumic Systole, *Circulation,* 44:47, 1971.
138. Karliner, J. S., Gault, J. H., Eckberg, D., Mullins, C. B., and Ross, J., Jr.: Mean Velocity of Fiber Shortening: A Simplified Measure of Left Ventricular Myocardial Contractility, *Circulation,* 44:323, 1971.
139. Graham, T. P., Jr., Jarmakani, J. M., Canent, R. V., Jr., and Anderson, P. A. W.: Evaluation of Left Ventricular Contractile State in Childhood: Normal Values and Observations with a Pressure Overload, *Circulation,* 44:1043, 1971.
140. Grossman, W., Brooks, H., Meister, S., Sherman, H., and Dexter, L.: New Technique for Determining Instantaneous Myocardial Force-Velocity Relations in the Intact Heart, *Circ. Res.,* 28:290, 1971.
141. Wolk, M. J., Keefe, J. F., Bing, O. H. L., Finkelstein, L. J., and Levine, H. J.: Estimation of V_{max} in Auxotonic Systoles from the Rate of Relative Increase of Isovolumic Pressure: (dp/dt) kP, *J. Clin. Invest.,* 50:1276, 1971.
142. Mirsky, I., Pasternac, A., and Ellison, R. C.: General Index for the Assessment of Cardiac Function, *Am. J. Cardiol.,* 30:483, 1972.
143. Noble, M. I. M.: Problems Concerning the Application of Concepts of Muscle Mechanics to the Determination of the Contractile State of the Heart, *Circulation,* 45:252, 1972.
144. Mitchell, J. H., Hefner, L. L., and Monroe, R. G: Performance of the Left Ventricle, *Am. J. Med.,* 53:481, 1972.
145. Ross, J., Jr., and Sobel, B. E.: Regulation of Cardiac Contraction, *Annu. Rev. Physiol.,* 34:47, 1972.
146. Mason, D. T., Zelis, R., Amsterdam, E. A., and Massumi, R. A.: Clinical Determination of Left Ventricular Contractility by Hemodynamics and Myocardial Mechanics, in P. N. Yu and J. F. Goodwin (eds.), "Progress in Cardiology," Lea & Febiger, Philadelphia, 1972, vol. I, p. 121.
147. Blinks, J. R., and Jewell, B. R.: The Meaning and Measurement of Myocardial Contractility, in D. H. Bergel (ed.), "Cardiovascular Fluid Dynamics," Academic Press, Inc., New York, 1972, p. 225.
148. Ross, J., Jr., and Peterson, K. L.: On the Assessment of Cardiac Inotropic State, *Circulation,* 47:435, 1973.
149. Dodge, H. T., Kennedy, J. W., and Peterson, J. L.: Quantitative Angiocardiographic Methods in the Evaluation of Valvular Heart Disease, *Prog. Cardiovasc. Dis,,* 16:1, 1973.
150. Mason, D. T.: Regulation of Cardiac Performance in Clinical Heart Disease: Interactions between Contractile State Mechanical Abnormalities and Ventricular Compensatory Mechanisms, *Am. J. Cardiol.,* 32:437, 1973.
151. Benzing, G., III, Stockert, J., Nave, E., and Kaplan, S.: Evaluation of Left Ventricular Performance: Circumferential Fiber Shortening and Tension, *Circulation,* 49:925, 1974.
152. Peterson, K. L., Skloven, D., Ludbrook, P., Uther, J. B., and Ross, J., Jr.: Comparison of Isovolumic and Ejection

Phase Indices of Myocardial Performance in Man, *Circulation,* 49:1088, 1974.
153. Morkin, E., and LaRaia, P. J.: Biochemical Studies on the Regulation of Myocardial Contractility, *N. Engl. J. Med.,* 290:445, 1974.
154. Davidson, D. M., Covell, J. W., Malloch, C. I., and Ross, J., Jr.: Factors Influencing Indices of Left Ventricle Contractility in the Conscious Dog, *Cardiovasc. Res.,* 8:299, 1974.
155. Mirsky, I., and Parmley, W. W.: Force-Velocity Studies in Isolated and Intact Heart Muscle, in I. Mirsky, D. N. Ghista, and H. Sandler (eds.), "Cardiac Mechanics: Physiological, Clinical, and Mathematical Considerations," John Wiley & Sons, Inc., New York, 1974, p. 87.
156. Mirsky, I., Pasternac, A., Ellison, R. C., and Hugenholtz, P. G.: Clinical Applications of Force-Velocity Parameters and the Concept of a "Normalized Velocity," in I. Mirsky, D. N. Ghista, and H. Sandler (eds.), "Cardiac Mechanics: Physiological, Clinical, and Mathematical Considerations," John Wiley & Sons, Inc., New York, 1974, p. 293.
157. Mirsky, I.: Review of Various Theories for the Evaluation of Left Ventricular Wall Stresses, in I. Mirsky, D. N. Ghista, and H. Sandler (eds.), "Cardiac Mechanics: Physiological, Clinical, and Mathematical Considerations," John Wiley & Sons, Inc., New York, 1974, p. 381.
158. Brady, A. J.: Mechanics of the Myocardium, in G. A. Langer and A. J. Brady (eds.), "The Mammalian Myocardium," John Wiley & Sons, Inc., New York, 1974, p. 163.
159. Abel, F. L.: Comparative Evaluation of Pressure and Time Factors in Estimating Left Ventricular Performance, *J. Appl. Physiol.,* 40:196, 1975.
160. Naqvi, S. Z., Chisholm, S. Z., Standen, J. R., and Shane, S. J.: Relative Insensitivity of Isovolumic Phase Indices in Assessment of Left Ventricular Function, *Am. Heart J.,* 91:577, 1976.
161. Sonnenblick, E. H., and Strobeck, J. E.: Derived Indices of Ventricular and Myocardial Function, *N. Engl. J. Med.,* 296:978, 1977.
162. Abbott, B. C., and Mommaerts, W. F. H. M.: A Study of Inotropic Mechanisms in the Papillary Muscle Preparation, *J. Gen. Physiol.,* 42:533, 1959.
163. Parmley, W. W., Chuck, L., and Sonnenblick, E. H.: Relation of V_{max} to Different Models of Cardiac Muscle, *Circ. Res.,* 30:34, 1972.
164. Sarnoff, S. J., and Mitchell, J. H.: The Control of the Function of the Heart, in W. F. Hamilton and P. Dow (eds.), "Handbook of Physiology," sec. 2; "Circulation," American Physiological Society, Washington, D.C., 1962, vol. 1, p. 489.
165. Imperial, E. S., Levy, M. N., and Zieske, H. J., Jr.: Outflow Resistance as an Independent Determinant of Cardiac Performance, *Circ. Res.,* 9:1145, 1961.
166. Sonnenblick, E. H., and Downing, S. E.: Afterload as a Primary Determinant of Ventricular Performance, *Am. J. Physiol.,* 204:604, 1963.
167. Levine, H. J., Forwand, S. A., McIntyre, K. M., and Schecter, E.: Effect of Afterload on Force-Velocity Relations and Contractile Element Work in the Intact Dog Heart, *Circ. Res.,* 18:729, 1966.
168. Evans, G. L., Smulyan, H., and Eich, R. H.: Role of Peripheral Resistance in the Control of Cardiac Output, *Am. J. Cardiol.,* 20:216, 1967.
169. Urschel, C. W., Covell, J. W., Sonnenblick, E. H., Ross, J., Jr., and Braunwald, E.: Myocardial Mechanics in Aortic and Mitral Valvular Regurgitation: The Concept of Instantaneous Impedance as a Determinant of the Performance of the Heart, *J. Clin. Invest.,* 47:867, 1968.
170. MacGregor, D. C., Covell, J. W., Mahler, F., Dilley, R. B., and Ross, J., Jr.: Relations between Afterload, Stroke Volume, and the Descending Limb of Starling's Curve, *Am. J. Physiol.,* 227:884, 1974.
171. Milnor, W. R.: Arterial Impedance as Ventricular Afterload, *Circ. Res.,* 36:565, 1975.
172. Von Anrep, G.: On the Part Played by Suprarenals in the Normal Vascular Reactions of the Body, *J. Physiol.,* 45:307, 1912.
173. Vatner, S. F., Monroe, R. G., and McRitchie, R. J.: Effects of Anesthesia Tachycardia and Autonomic Blockade on Anrep Effect in Intact Dogs, *Am. J. Physiol.,* 226:1450, 1974.
174. Koch-Weser, J. and Blinks, J. R.: The Influence of the Interval between Beats on Myocardial Contractility, *Pharmacol. Rev.,* 15:601, 1963.
175. Vatner, S. F., and Braunwald, E.: Cardiovascular Control Mechanisms in the Conscious State, *N. Engl. J. Med.,* 293:970, 1975.
176. Boudoulas, H., Rittgers, S. E., Lewis, R. P., Leier, C. V., and Weissler, A. M.: Changes in Diastolic Time with Various Pharmacologic Agents: Implications for Myocardial Perfusion, *Circulation,* 60:164, 1979.
177. Woodworth, R. S.: Maximal Contraction, "Staircase" Contraction, Refractory Period, and Compensatory Pause of the Heart, *Am. J. Physiol.,* 8:213, 1902.
178. Hajdu, S.: Mechanism of the Woodworth Staircase Phenomenon in Heart and Skeletal Muscle, *Am. J. Physiol.,* 216:206, 1969.
179. Hawthorne, E. W.: Instantaneous Dimensional Changes of the Left Ventricle in Dogs, *Circ. Res.,* 9:110, 1961.
180. Schlant, R. C., Dixon, F., Elson, S. H., Rawls, W. J., and Williamson, F. R., Jr.: Modification of the Law of the Heart: Influence of Early Contracting Areas, *Circulation,* 30(suppl. 3):153, 1964.
181. Schlant, R. C., Rawls, W. J., Dixon, F., and Elson, S.: Intraventricular Kick: An Additional Determinant of Ventricular Performance, *Clin. Res.,* 13:62, 1965.
182. Schlant, R. C.: Idioventricular Kick, *Circulation,* 34(suppl. 3):209, 1966.
183. Brecher, G. A.: Experimental Evidence of Ventricular Diastolic Suction, *Circ. Res.,* 4:513, 1956.
184. Sonnenblick, E. H.: The Structural Basis and Importance of Restoring Forces and Elastic Recoil for the Filling of the Heart, *Eur. Heart J.,* 1(suppl. A):107, 1980.
185. Weisfeldt, M. L., Scully, H. E., Frederiksen, J., et al.: Hemodynamic Determinants of Maximum Negative DP/DT and the Periods of Diastole, *Am. J. Physiol.,* 227:613, 1974.
186. Brecher, G. A., and Galletti, P. M.: Functional Anatomy of Cardiac Pumping, in W. F. Hamilton and P. Dow (eds.), "Handbook of Physiology," sec. 2: "Circulation," American Physiological Society, Washington, D.C., 1963, vol. 2, p. 759.
187. Mitchell, J. H., Gilmore, J. P., and Sarnoff, S. J.: The Transport Function of the Atrium: Factors Influencing the Relation between Mean Left Atrial Pressure and Left Ventricular End Diastolic Pressure, *Am. J. Cardiol.,* 9:237, 1962.
188. Braunwald, E.: Hemodynamic Significance of Atrial Systole, *Am. J. Med.,* 37:665, 1964.
189. Burchell, H. B.: A Clinical Appraisal of Atrial Transport Function, *Lancet,* 1:775, 1964.
190. Williams, J. F., Jr., Sonnenblick, E. H., and Braunwald, E.: Determinants of Atrial Contractile Force in the Intact Heart, *Am. J. Physiol.,* 209:1061, 1965.
191. Mitchell, J. H., Gupta, D. N., and Payne, R. M.: Influence of Atrial Systole on Effective Ventricular Stroke Volume, *Circ. Res.,* 17:11, 1965.
192. Payne, R. M., Stone, H. L., and Engelken, E. L.: Atrial Function during Volume Loading, *J. Appl. Physiol.,* 31:326, 1971.
193. Suga, H.: Importance of Atrial Compliance in Cardiac Performance, *Circ. Res.,* 35:39, 1974.
194. de Bold, A. J., Borenstein, H. B., Veress, A. T., and Sonnenberg, H.: A Rapid and Potent Natriuretic Response to Intravenous Injection of Atrial Myoscardial Extract in Rats, *Life Sci.,* 28:89, 1981.
195. de Bold, A. J.: Tissue Fractionation Studies on the Relationship between an Atrial Natriuretic Factor and Specific Atrial Granules. *Can. J. Physiol. Pharmacol.,* 60:324, 1982.
196. de Bold, A. J.: Atrial Natriuretic Factor of the Rat Heart: Studies on Isolation and Properties, *Proc. Soc. Exper. Biol. Med.,* 170:133, 1982.
197. Keller, R.: Atrial Natriuretic Factor Has a Direct, Prostaglandin-Independent Action on Kidneys, *Can. J. Physiol. Pharmacol.,* 60:1078, 1982.

198. Sonnenberg, H., Milojevic, S., Chong, C. K., and Veress, A. T.: Atrial Natriuretic Factor: Reduced Cardiac Content in Spontaneously Hypertensive Rats, *Hypertension,* 5:672, 1983.
199. Borenstein, H. B., Cupples, W. A., Sonnenberg H., and Veress, A. T.: The Effect of a Natriuretic Atrial Extract on Renal Haemodynamics and Urinary Excretion in Anesthetized Rats, *J. Physiol. London,* 334:133, 1983.
200. Currie, M. G., Geller, D. M., Cole, B. R., et al.: Bioactive Cardiac Substances: Potent Vasorelaxant Activity in Mammalian Atria, *Science,* 221:71, 1983.
201. Thibault, G., Garcia, R., Cantin, M., and Genest, J.: Atrial Natriuretic Factor: Characterization and Partial Purification, *Hypertension,* 5:175, 1983.
202. Currie, M. G., Geller, D. M., Cole, B. R., et al.: Purification and Sequence Analysis of Bioactive Atrial Peptides (Atriopeptins), *Science,* 223:67, 1984.
203. Atarashi, K., Mulrow, P. J., Franco-Saenz, R., Snajdar, R., and Rapp, J.: Inhibition of Aldosterone Production by an Atrial Extract, *Science,* 224:992, 1984.
204. Higgins, C. B., Vatner, S. F., and Braunwald, E.: Parasympathetic Control of the Heart, *Pharmacol. Rev.,* 25:119, 1973.
205. Sagawa, K., Kumada, M., and Schramm, L. P.: Nervous Control of the Circulation, in A. C. Guyton and C. E. Jones (eds.), "Cardiovascular Physiology," Physiology ser. I, University Park Press, Baltimore, 1974, vol. 1, p. 197.
206. Linden, R. J.: Reflexes from the Heart, *Prog. Cardiovasc. Dis.,* 18:201, 1975.
207. Abboud, F. M., Heistad, D. D., Mark, A. L., and Schmid, P. G.: Reflex Control of the Peripheral Circulation, *Prog. Cardiovasc. Dis.,* 18:371, 1976.
208. Kirchheim, H. R.: Systemic Arterial Baroreceptor Reflexes, *Physiol. Rev.,* 56:100, 1976.
209. Levy, M. N., and Martin, P. J.: Neural Control of the Heart, in R. M. Berne (ed.), "Handbook of Physiology," sec. 2: "The Cardiovascular System," vol. 1: "The Heart," American Physiological Society, Bethesda, Md., 1979, p. 581.
210. Brown, A. M.: Cardiac Reflexes, in R. M. Berne (ed.), "Handbook of Physiology," sec. 2: "The Cardiovascular System," vol. 1: "The Heart," American Physiological Society, Bethesda, Md., 1979, p. 677.
211. Korner, P. I.: Central Nervous Control of Autonomic Cardiovascular Function, in R. M. Berne (ed.), "Handbook of Physiology," sec. 2: "The Cardiovascular System," vol. 1: "The Heart," American Physiological Society, Bethesda, Md., 1979, p. 691.
212. Randall, W. C. (ed.): "Nervous Control of Cardiovascular Function," Oxford University Press, New York, 1984.
213. Sutherland, E. W.: On the Biological Role of Cyclic AMP, *JAMA,* 214:1281, 1970.
214. Hardman, J. G., Robison, G. A., and Sutherland, E. W.: Cyclic Nucleotides, *Annu. Rev. Physiol.,* 3:311, 1971.
215. Sobel, B. E., and Mayer, S. E.: Cyclic Adenosine Monophosphate and Cardiac Contractility, *Circ. Res.,* 32:407, 1973.
216. DeGeest, H., Levy, M. N., Zieske, H., and Lipman, R. I.: Depression of Ventricular Contractility by Stimulation of the Vagus Nerves, *Circ. Res.,* 17:222, 1965.
217. Wallace, A. G., and Sarnoff, S. J.: Effects of Cardiac Sympathetic Nerve Stimulation on Conduction in the Heart, *Circ. Res.,* 14:86, 1964.
218. Glick, G., and Braunwald, E.: Relative Roles of the Sympathetic and Parasympathetic Nervous Systems in the Reflex Control of Heart Rate, *Circ. Res.,* 16:363, 1965.
219. Badeer, H. S.: Resting Bradycardia of Exercise Training: A Concept Based on Currently Available Data, in P. E. Roy and G. Rona (eds.), "The Metabolism of Contraction," vol. 10: "Recent Advances in Studies on Cardiac Structure and Metabolism," University Park Press, Baltimore, 1975, p. 553.
220. Buccino, R. A., Covell, J. W., Sonnenblick, E. H., and Braunwald, E.: Effects of Serotonin on the Contractile State of the Myocardium, *Am. J. Physiol.,* 213:483, 1967.
221. Parmley, W. W., Glick, G., and Sonnenblick, E. H.: Cardiovascular Effects of Glucagon in Man, *N. Engl. J. Med.,* 279:12, 1968.
222. Glick, G., Parmley, W. W., Wechsler, A. S., and Sonnenblick, E. H.: Glucagon: Its Enhancement of Cardiac Performance in the Cat and Dog in Persistence of Its Inotropic Action Despite Beta-Receptor Blockade and Propranolol, *Circ. Res.,* 22:789, 1968.
223. Glick, G.: Glucagon: A Perspective, *Circulation,* 45:513, 1972.
224. Higgins, C. B., and Braunwald, E.: The Prostaglandins: Biochemical, Physiologic and Clinical Considerations, *Am. J. Med.,* 53:92, 1972.
225. Dusting, G. J., Moncada, S., and Vane, J. R.: Prostaglandins, Their Intermediates and Precursors: Cardiovascular Actions and Regulatory Roles in Normal and Abnormal Circulatory System, *Prog. Cardiovasc. Dis.,* 21:405, 1979.
226. Bloor, C. M., White, F. C., and Sobel, B. E.: Coronary and Systemic Haemodynamic Effects of Prostaglandins in the Unanaesthetized Dog, *Cardiovasc. Res.,* 7:156, 1973.
227. Lowe, T. E.: The Clinical Significance of Kinekard, *Am. J. Cardiol.,* 20:304, 1967.
228. Leonard, E., and Hajdu, S.: Cardioglobulin: Clinical Correlations, *Circ. Res.,* 9:891, 1961.
229. Gold, H. K., Spann, J. F. J., and Braunwald, E.: Effect of Alterations in the Thyroid State on the Intrinsic Contractile Properties of Isolated Rat Skeletal Muscle, *J. Clin. Invest.,* 49:849, 1970.
230. Gunning, J. F., Harrison, C. E., Jr., and Coleman, H. J. III: Myocardial Contractility and Energetics following Treatment with D-Thyroxine, *Am. J. Physiol.,* 226:1166, 1974.
231. Strauer, B. E., and Scherpe, A.: Experimental Hyperthyroidism: I. Hemodynamics and Contractility in Situ, *Basic Res. Cardiol.,* 70:115, 1975.
232. Skelton, C. L., Su, J. Y., and Pool, P. E.: Influence of Hyperthyroidism on Glycerol-Extracted Cardiac Muscle from Rabbits, *Cardiovasc. Res.,* 10:380, 1976.
233. Rocamora, J. M., and Downing, S. E.: Preservation of Ventricular Function by Adrenergic Influences during Metabolic Acidosis in the Cat, *Circ. Res.,* 24:373, 1969.
234. Vatner, S. F., Marsh, J. D., and Swain, J. D.: Effects of Morphine on Coronary and Left Ventricular Dynamics in Conscious Dogs, *J. Clin. Invest.,* 55:207, 1975.
235. Horwitz, L. D., and Bishop, V. S.: Effect of Acute Volume Loading on Heart Rate in the Conscious Dog, *Circ. Res.,* 30:316, 1972.
236. Vatner, S. F., Higgins, C. B., and Braunwald, E.: Effects of Norepinephrine on Coronary Circulation and Left Ventricular Dynamics in the Conscious Dog, *Circ. Res.,* 34:812, 1974.
237. Frommer, P. L., Robinson, B. F., and Braunwald, E.: Paired Electrical Stimulation: A Comparison of the Effects on Performance of the Failing and Nonfailing Heart, *Am. J. Cardiol.,* 18:738, 1966.
238. Cranefield, P. F., and Hoffman, B. F.: The Physiologic Basis and Clinical Implications of Paired Pulse Stimulation of the Heart, *Dis. Chest,* 49:561, 1966.
239. Braunwald, E., Sonnenblick, E. H., Frommer, P. L., and Ross, J., Jr.: Paired Electrical Stimulation of the Heart: Physiologic Observations and Clinical Implications, *Adv. Intern. Med.,* 13:61, 1967.
240. Braunwald, E.: Regulation of the Circulation, *N. Engl. J. Med.,* 290:1124, 1974.
241. Neill, W. A.: Regulation of Cardiac Output, in H. J. Levine (ed.), "Clinical Cardiovascular Physiology," Grune & Stratton, Inc., New York, 1976, p. 121.
242. Oberg, B.: Overall Cardiovascular Regulation, *Annu. Rev. Physiol.,* 38:537, 1976.
243. Parmley, W. W., and Talbot, L.: Heart as a Pump, in R. M. Berne (ed.), "Handbook of Physiology," sec. 2: "The Cardiovascular System," vol. 1: "The Heart," American Physiological Society, Bethesda, Md., 1979, p. 429.
244. Wittenberg, J. B.: Myoglobulin-Facilitated Oxygen Diffusion: Role of Myoglobin in Oxygen Entry into Muscle, *Physiol. Rev.,* 50:559, 1970.
245. Rodbard, S. (guest ed.): Local Regulation of Blood Flow, *Circ. Res.,* 18–19(suppl. 1):1, 1971 (American Heart Association Monograph 33).
246. Shepherd, A. P., Granger, H. J., Smither, E. E., and Guy-

ton, A. C.: Local Control of Tissue Oxygen Delivery and Its Contribution to the Regulation of Cardiac Output, *Am. J. Physiol.*, 225:747, 1973.
247. Hutchins, P. M., Bond, R. F., and Green, H. D.: Participation of Oxygen in the Local Control of Skeletal Muscle Microvasculature, *Circ. Res.*, 34:85, 1974.
248. Lassen, N. A.: Control of Cerebral Circulation in Health and Disease, *Circ. Res.*, 34:749, 1974.
249. Korner, P. I.: Control of Blood Flow to Special Vascular Areas: Brain, Kidney, Muscle, Skin, Liver, and Intestine, in A. C. Guyton and C. E. Jones (eds.), "Cardiovascular Physiology," Physiology ser. I, University Park Press, Baltimore, 1974, vol. 1, p. 123.
250. Berger, H. J., Zaret, B. L., Speroff, L., Cohen, L. S., and Wolfson, S.: Regional Cardiac Prostaglandin Release during Myocardial Ischemiain Anesthetized Dogs, *Circ. Res.*, 38:566, 1976.
251. Messina, E. J., Weiner, R., and Kaley, G.: Prostaglandins and Local Circulatory Control, *Fed. Proc.*, 35:2367, 1976.
252. Abboud, F. M., Schmid, P. G., Heistad, D. D., and Mark, A. L.: Regulation of Peripheral and Coronary Circulation, in H. J. Levine (ed.), "Clinical Cardiovascular Physiology," Grune & Stratton, Inc., New York, 1976, p. 143.
253. Zelis, R. (ed.): "The Peripheral Circulations," Grune & Stratton, Inc., New York, 1975, p. 417.
254. Wiggers, C. J.: Studies on the Consecutive Phases of the Cardiac Cycle: I. The Duration of the Consecutive Phases of the Cardiac Cycle and the Criteria for Their Precise Determination, *Am. J. Physiol.*, 56:415, 1921.
255. Wiggers, C. J.: Studies on the Consecutive Phases of the Cardiac Cycle: II. The Laws Governing the Relative Durations of Ventricular Systole and Diastole, *Am. J. Physiol.*, 56:439, 1921.
256. Braunwald, E., Fishman, A. P., and Cournand, A.: Time Relationship of Dynamic Events in the Cardiac Chambers, Pulmonary Artery and Aorta in Man, *Circ. Res.*, 4:100, 1956.
257. Wooley, C. F., Levin, H. S., Leighton, R. F., Goodwin, R. S., Ryan, J. M., and Rieser, G. F.: Intracardiac Sound and Pressure Events in Man, *Am. J. Med.*, 42:248, 1967.
258. Schlant, R. C.: Events during Cardiac Cycle, in P. L. Altman and D. S. Dittmer (eds.), "Respiration and Circulation," 2d ed., Federation of American Society for Experimental Biological Proceedings, Bethesda, Md., 1973, p. 304.
259. Spencer, M. P., and Greiss, F. C.: Dynamics of Ventricular Ejection, *Circ. Res.*, 10:274, 1962.
260. Grant, C., Greene, D. G., and Bunnell, I. L.: The Valve-Closing Function of the Right Atrium: A Study of Pressures and Atrial Sounds in Patients with Heart Block, *Am. J. Med.*, 34:325, 1963.
261. MacCanon, D. M., Arevalo, F., and Meyer, E. C.: Direct Detection and Timing of Aortic Valve Closure, *Circ. Res.*, 14:387, 1964.
262. Piemme, T. E., Barnett, G. O., and Dexter, L.: Relationship of Heart Sounds to Acceleration of Blood Flow, *Circ. Res.*, 18:303, 1966.
263. Delman, A. J.: Hemodynamic Correlations of Cardiovascular Sounds, *Annu. Rev. Med.*, 18:139, 1967.
264. Craige, E., and Fortuin, N. J.: Genesis of Heart Sounds and Murmurs as Demonstrated by Echocardiography, in C. R. Joyner (ed.), "Ultrasound in the Diagnosis of Cardiovascular-Pulmonary Disease," Year Book Medical Publishers, Inc., Chicago, 1974, p. 119.
265. Burgraf, G. W., and Craige, E.: First Heart Sound and Ejection Sounds: Echocardiographic and Phonocardiographic Correlation with Valvular Events, *Am. J. Cardiol.*, 35:346, 1975.
266. Chandraratna, P. A. N., Lopez, J. M., and Cohen, L. S.: Echocardiographic Observations on the Mechanism of Production of the Second Heart Sound, *Circulation*, 51:292, 1975.
267. Marshall, H. W., Helmholz, H. F., and Wood, E. H.: Physiologic Consequences of Congenital Heart Disease, in W. F. Hamilton and P. Dow (eds.), "Handbook of Physiology," sec. 2; "Circulation," American Physiological Society, Washington, D.C., 1962, vol. 1, p. 417.
268. Mackay, I. F. S.: The True Venous Pulse Wave, Central and Peripheral, *Am. Heart J.*, 74:48, 1967.
269. Barratt-Boyes, B. G., and Wood, E. H.: Cardiac Output and Related Measurements and Pressure Values in the Right Heart and Associated Vessels, Together with an Analysis of the Hemodynamic Response to the Inhalation of High Oxygen Mixtures in Healthy Subjects, *J. Lab. Clin. Med.*, 51:72, 1958.
270. Braunwald, E., Brockenbrough, E. C., Frahm, C. J., and Ross, J.: Left Atrial and Left Ventricular Pressures in Subjects without Cardiovascular Disease, *Circulation*, 24:267, 1961.
271. Wade, O. L., and Bishop, J. M.: "Cardiac Output and Regional Blood Flow," Blackwell Scientific Publications, Ltd., Oxford, 1962.
272. Grossman, W.: "Cardiac Catheterization and Angiography," 2d ed., Lea & Febiger, Philadelphia, 1980.
273. Dexter, L., Whittenberger, J. L., Haynes, F. W., Goodale, W. T., Gorlin, R., and Sawyer, C. G.: Effect of Exercise on Circulatory Dynamics of Normal Individuals, *J. Appl. Physiol.*, 3:439, 1951.
274. Barratt-Boyes, B. G., and Wood, E. H.: Hemodynamic Response of Healthy Subjects to Exercise in the Supine Position while Breathing Oxygen, *J. Appl. Physiol.*, 11:129, 1957.
275. Wang, Y., Marshall, R. J., and Shepherd, J. T.: The Effect of Changes in Posture and of Graded Exercise on Stroke Volume in Man, *J. Clin. Invest.*, 39:1051, 1960.
276. Braunwald, E., Goldblatt, A., Harrison, D. C., and Mason, D. T.: Studies on Cardiac Dimensions in Intact, Unanesthetized Man: III. Effects of Muscular Exercise, *Circ. Res.*, 13:460, 1963.
277. Ross, J., Jr., Gault, J. H., Mason, D. T., Linhart, J. W., and Braunwald, E.: Left Ventricular Performance during Muscular Exercise in Patients with and without Cardiac Dysfunction, *Circulation*, 34:597, 1966.
278. Epstein, S. E., Beiser, G. D., Stampfer, M., Robinson, B. F., and Braunwald, E.: Characterization of the Circulatory Response to Maximal Upright Exercise in Normal Subjects and Patients with Heart Disease, *Circulation*, 35:1049, 1967.
279. Braunwald, E., Sonnenblick, E. H., Ross, J., Jr., Glick, G., and Epstein, S. E.: An Analysis of the Cardiac Response to Exercise, *Circ. Res.*, 20(suppl. 1):1, 1967.
280. Chapman, C. B. (ed.): Physiology of Muscular Exercise, *Circ. Res.*, 20(suppl. 1):1, 1967.
281. Bevegard, B. S., and Shepherd, J. T.: Regulation of the Circulation during Exercise in Man, *Physiol. Rev.*, 47:178, 1967.
282. Ekelund, L. G.: Circulatory and Respiratory Adaptation during Prolonged Exercise, *Acta Physiol. Scand.*, vol. 70(suppl. 292):1, 1967.
283. Astrand, P. O., and Rodahl, K.: "Textbook of Work Physiology: Physiological Bases of Exercise," 2d ed., McGraw-Hill Book Company, New York, 1977.
284. Luepker, R. V., Holmberg, S., and Varnauskas, E.: Left Atrial Pressure during Exercise in Hemodynamic Normals, *Am. Heart J.*, 81:494, 1971.
285. Shappell, S. D., Murray, J. A., Bellingham, A. J., Woodson, R. C., Detter, J. C., and Lenfant, C.: Adaptation to Exercise: Role of Hemoglobin Affinity for Oxygen and 2,3-Diphosphoglycerate, *J. Appl. Physiol.*, 30:827, 1971.
286. Simonson, E.: Evaluation of Cardiac Performance in Exercise, *Am. J. Cardiol.*, 30:722, 1972.
287. Vatner, S. F., Franklin, D., Higgins, C. B., Patrick, T., and Braunwald, E.: Left Ventricular Response to Severe Exertion in Untethered Dogs, *J. Clin. Invest.*, 51:3052, 1972.
288. Horwitz, L. D., Atkins, J. M., and Leshin, S. J.: Role of the Frank-Starling Mechanism in Exercise, *Circ. Res.*, 31:868, 1972.
289. Guyton, A. C., Jones, C. E., and Coleman, T. G.: Cardiac Output in Muscular Exercise, in A. C. Guyton, C. E. Jones, and T. G. Coleman (eds.), "Circulatory Physiology: Cardiac Output and Its Regulation," 2d ed., W. B. Saunders Company, Philadelphia, 1973, p. 436.
290. Randall, D. C., and Smith, O. A.: Ventricular Contractility

during Controlled Exercise and Emotion in the Primate, *Am. J. Physiol.*, 226:1051, 1974.
291. Scheuer, J., Penpargkul, P., and Bhan, A. K.: Experimental Observations on the Effects of Physical Training upon Intrinsic Cardiac Physiology and Biochemistry, *Am. J. Cardiol.*, 33:744, 1974.
292. Scheuer, J., and Tipton, C. M.: Cardiovascular Adaptations of Physical Training, *Annu. Rev. Physiol.*, 39:221, 1977.
293. Adams, W. C., McHenry, M. M., and Bernauer, E. C.: Long-Term Physiologic Adaptations to Exercise with Special Reference to Performance and Cardiorespiratory Function in Health and Disease, *Am. J. Cardiol.*, 33:765, 1974.
294. Vatner, S. F.: Effects of Exercise on Distribution of Regional Blood Flows and Resistances, in R. Zelis (ed.), "The Peripheral Circulations," Grune & Stratton, Inc., New York, 1975, p. 211.
295. McRitchie, R. J., Vatner, S. F., Boettcher, D., Heyndricks, G. R., Patrick, T. A., and Braunwald, E.: Role of Arterial Baroreceptors in Mediating Cardiovascular Response to Exercise, *Am. J. Physiol.*, 230:85, 1976.
296. Smith, E. E., Guyton, A. C., Manning, R. D., and White, R. J.: Integrated Mechanisms of Cardiovascular Response and Control during Exercise in the Normal Human, *Prog. Cardiovasc. Dis.*, 18:421, 1976.
297. Schlant, R. C.: Physiology of Exercise, in G. F. Fletcher (ed.), "Exercise in the Practice of Medicine," Futura Publishing, Mount Kisco, N.Y., 1982, p. 1.
298. Christensen, N. J., and Galbo, H.: Sympathetic Nervous Activity during Exercise, *Annu. Rev. Physiol.*, 45:139, 1983.
299. Ludbrook, J.: Reflex Control of Blood Pressure during Exercise, *Annu. Rev. Physiol.*, 45:155, 1983.
300. Blomqvist, C. G., and Saltin, B.: Cardiovascular Adaptations to Physical Training, *Annu. Rev. Physiol.*, 45:169, 1983.
301. Brengelmann, G. L.: Circulatory Adjustments to Exercise and Heat Stress, *Annu. Rev. Physiol.*, 45:191, 1983.
302. Stone, H. L.: Control of the Coronary Circulation during Exercise, *Annu. Rev. Physiol.*, 45:213, 1983.
303. Mitchell, J. H., Kaufman, M. P., and Iwamoto, G. A.: The Exercise Pressor Reflex: Its Cardiovascular Effects, Afferent Mechanisms, and Central Pathways, *Annu. Rev. Physiol.*, 45:229, 1983.
304. Vatner, S. F., and Pagani, M.: Cardiovascular Adjustments to Exercise: Hemodynamics and Mechanisms, *Prog. Cardiovasc. Dis.*, 19:91, 1976.
305. Bertrand, M. E., Carre, A. G., Ginestet, A. P., Lefebvre, J. M., Desplanque, L. A., and Lekieffre, J. P.: Maximal Exercise in Normal Subjects, *Eur. J. Cardiol.*, 5/6:481, 1977.
306. Astrand, P. O., and Saltin, B.: Plasma and Red Cell Volume after Prolonged Severe Exercise, *J. Appl. Physiol.*, 19:819, 1964.
307. Lundvall, J., Mellander, S., Westling, H., and White, T.: Fluid Transfer between Blood and Tissues during Exercise, *Acta Physiol. Scand.*, 85:258, 1972.
308. Lind, A. R., Taylor, S. H., Humphreys, P. W., Kennelly, B. M., and Donald, K. W.: The Circulatory Effects of Sustained Voluntary Muscle Contraction, *Clin. Sci.*, 27:299, 1964.
309. Lind, A. R., and McNicol, G. W.: Local and Central Circulatory Responses to Sustained Contractions and the Effect of Free or Restricted Arterial Inflow on Postexercise Hyperaemia, *J. Physiol.*, 192:575, 1967.
310. Lind, A. R., and McNicol, G. W.: Circulatory Responses to Sustained Hand-Grip Contractions Performed during Other Exercise, Both Rhythmic and Static, *J. Physiol.*, 192:595, 1967.
311. Lind, A. R., and McNicol, G. W.: Cardiovascular Responses to Holding and Carrying Weights by Hand and by Shoulder Harness, *J. Appl. Physiol.*, 25:261, 1968.
312. Nutter, D. O., Schlant, R. C., and Hurst, J. W.: Isometric Exercise and the Cardiovascular System, *Mod. Concepts Cardiovasc. Dis.*, 41:11, 1972.
313. Fisher, M. L., Nutter, D. O., Jacobs, W., and Schlant, R. C.: Haemodynamic Responses to Isometric Exercise (Hand-Grip) in Patients with Heart Disease, *Br. Heart J.*, 35:422, 1973.
314. Haissly, J.-C., Messin, R., Degre, S., Vandermoten, P., Demaret, B., and Denolin, H.: Comparative Response to Isometric (Static) and Dynamic Exercise Tests in Coronary Disease, *Am. J. Cardiol.*, 33:791, 1974.
315. Martin, C. E., Shaver, J. A., Leon, D. F., Thompson, M. E., Reddy, P. S., and Leonard, J. J.: Autonomic Mechanism in Hemodynamic Responses to Isometric Exercise, *J. Clin. Invest.*, 54:104, 1974.
316. Stefadouros, M. A., Grossman, W., Shahawy, M. E., and Whitham, A. C.: The Effect of Isometric Exercise on the Left Ventricular Volume in Normal Man, *Circulation*, 49:1185, 1974.
317. McCloskey, D. I., and Streatfield, K. A.: Muscular Reflex Stimuli to the Cardiovascular System during Isometric Contractions of Muscle Groups of Different Mass, *J. Physiol.*, 250:431, 1975.
318. Barcroft, J., and Dixon, W. E.: The Gaseous Metabolism of the Mammalian Heart, *J. Physiol.*, 35:182, 1907.
319. Rohde, E.: Uber den Einfluss der mechanischen Bedingungen auf die Tatigkeit und den Sauerstoffverbrauch des Warmbluterherzens, *Arch. Exp. Pathol. Pharmakol.*, 68:401, 1912.
320. Evans, C. L., and Mutsuoka, Y.: The Effect of Various Mechanical Conditions on the Gaseous Metabolism and Efficiency of the Mammalian Heart, *J. Physiol.*, 49:378, 1915.
321. Graham, T. P., Jr., Covell, J. W., Sonnenblick, E. H., Ross, J., Jr., and Braunwald, E.: Control of Myocardial Oxygen Consumption: Relative Influence of Contractile State and Tension Development, *J. Clin. Invest.*, 47:375, 1968.
322. Sonnenblick, E. H., Ross, J., Jr., and Braunwald, E.: Oxygen Consumption of the Heart: Newer Concepts of Its Multifactoral Determination, *Am. J. Cardiol.*, 22:328, 1968.
323. Braunwald, E.: Control of Myocardial Oxygen Consumption: Physiologic and Clinical Consideration, *Am. J. Cardiol.*, 27:416, 1971.
324. Sonnenblick, E. H., and Skelton, C. L.: Oxygen Consumption of the Heart: Physiological Principles and Clinical Implications, *Mod. Concepts Cardiovasc. Dis.*, 40:9, 1971.
325. Sarnoff, S. J., Braunwald, E., Welch, G. H., Case, R. B., Stainsby, W. N., and Macruz, R.: Hemodynamic Determinants of Oxygen Consumption of the Heart with Special Reference to the Tension-Time Index, Index, *Am. J. Physiol.*, 192:148, 1958.
326. Sonnenblick, E. H., Ross, J., Jr., Covell, J. W., Kaiser, G. A., and Braunwald, E.: Velocity of Contraction as a Determinant of Myocardial Oxygen Consumption, *Am. J. Physiol.*, 209:919, 1965.
327. Covell, J. W., Braunwald, E., Ross, J., Jr., and Sonnenblick, E. H.: Studies on Digitalis: XVI. Effects on Myocardial Oxygen Consumption, *J. Clin. Invest.*, 45:1535, 1966.
328. Coleman, H. N., III: Role of Acetylstrophanthidin in Augmenting Myocardial Oxygen Consumption: Relation of Increased O_2 Consumption to Changes in Velocity of Contraction, *Circ. Res.*, 21:487, 1967.
329. Neill, W. A., Levine, H. J., Wagman, R. J., and Gorlin, R.: Left Ventricular Oxygen Utilization in Intact Dogs: Effect of Systemic Hemodynamic Factors, *Circ. Res.*, 12:163, 1963.
330. Gregg, D. E.: Effect of Coronary Perfusion Pressure or Coronary Flow on Oxygen Usage of the Myocardium, *Circ. Res.*, 13:497, 1963.
331. Shepherd, J. T., and Vanhoutte, P. M.: "Veins and Their Control," W. B. Saunders Company, Philadelphia, 1975, p. 269.
332. Abboud, F. M., Schmid, P. G., Heistad, D. D., Mark, A. L., and Barnes, R.: The Venous System, in H. J. Levine (ed.), "Clinical Cardiovascular Physiology," Grune & Stratton, Inc., New York, 1976, p. 207.
333. Needleman, P.: The Synthesis and Function of Prostaglandins in the Heart, *Fed. Proc.*, 35:2376, 1976.
334. Rubio, R., and Berne, R. M.: Regulation of Coronary Blood Flow, *Prog. Cardiovasc. Dis.*, 18:105, 1975.
335. Klocke, F.: Coronary Blood Flow in Man. *Prog. Cardiovasc. Dis.* 19:117, 1976.
336. Berne, R. M., and Rubio, R.: Coronary Circulation, in R. M. Berne (ed.), "Handbook of Physiology," sec. 2: "The

Cardiovascular System," vol. 1: "The Heart," American Physiological Society, Bethesda, Md., 1979, p. 873.
337. Kellermeyer, R. W., and Graham, R. C., Jr.: Kinins—Possible Physiologic and Pathologic Roles in Man, *N. Engl. J. Med.*, 279:754, 1968.
338. Schachter, M.: Kallikreins and Kinins, *Physiol. Rev.*, 49:509, 1969.
339. Sander, G. E., and Huggins, C. G.: Vasoactive Peptides, *Annu. Rev. Pharmacol.*, 12:227, 1972.
340. Gregg, D. E., and Fisher, L. C.: Blood Supply to the Heart, in W. F. Hamilton and P. Dow (eds.), "Handbook of Physiology," sec. 2: "Circulation," American Physiological Society, Washington, D.C., 1963, vol. 2, p. 1517.
341. Berne, R. M.: Regulation of Coronary Blood Flow, *Physiol. Rev.*, 44:1, 1964.
342. Klocke, F. J., and Ellis, A. K.: Control of Coronary Blood Flow, *Annu. Rev. Med.*, 31:489, 1980.
343. Marcus, M. L.: "The Coronary Circulation in Health and Disease," McGraw-Hill Book Company, New York, 1983.
344. Coffman, J. D., and Gregg, D. E.: Reactive Hyperemia Characteristics of the Myocardium, *Am. J. Physiol.*, 199:1143, 1960.
345. Marcus, M., Wright, C., Doty, D., Eastham, C., Laughlin, D., Krumm, P., Fastenow, C., and Brody, M.: Measurement of Coronary Velocity and Reactive Hyperemia in the Coronary Circulation of Humans, *Circ. Res.*, 49:877, 1981.
346. Gregg, D. E.: "Coronary Circulation in Health and Disease," Lea & Febiger, Philadelphia, 1950.
347. Gorlin, R.: Measurement of Coronary Blood Flow in Health and Disease, in A. Morgan Jones (ed.), "Modern Trends in Cardiology," Paul B. Hoeber, Inc., New York, 1961, p. 191.
348. Messer, J. V., Wagman, R. J., Levine, H. J., Neill, W. A., Krasnow, N., and Gorlin, R.: Patterns of Myocardial Oxygen Extraction during Rest and Exercise, *J. Clin. Invest.*, 41:725, 1962.
349. Hanley, F. L., Messina, L. M., Grattan, M. T., and Hoffman J. I.: The Effect of Coronary Inflow Pressure on Coronary Vascular Resistance in the Isolated Dog Heart, *Circ. Res.*, 54:760, 1984.
350. Wiggers, C. J.: The Interplay of Coronary Vascular Resistance and Myocardial Compression in Regulating Coronary Flow, *Circ. Res.*, 2:271, 1954.
351. Bache, R. J., and Dymek, D. J.: Local and Regional Regulation of Coronary Vascular Tone, *Prog. Cardiovasc. Dis.*, 24:191, 1981.
352. Berne, R. M.: Nucleotide Degradation in the Hypoxic Heart and Its Possible Relation to Regulation of Coronary Blood Flow, *Fed. Proc.*, 20:101, 1961.
353. Berne, R. M.: The Role of Adenosine in the Regulation of Coronary Blood Flow, *Circ. Res.* 47:807, 1980.
354. Mark, A. L., and Abboud, F. M.: Myocardial Blood Flow: Neurohumoral Determinants, R. Zelis (ed.), "Peripheral Circulation," Grune & Stratton, Inc., New York, 1975, p. 95.
355. Folts, J. D., Crowell, E. B., Jr., and Rowe, G. G.: Platelet Aggregation in Partially Obstructed Vessels and Its Elimination with Aspiring, *Circulation*, 54:365, 1976.
356. Uchida, Y., Yoshimoto, N., and Murao, S.: Prostaglandin E_2 and Epinephrine Participate in Cyclical Reduction of Coronary Blood Pressure and Flow, *Jpn. Heart J.*, 19:281, 1978.
357. Kuzuya, T., Tada, M., Inoue, M., et al.: Increased Levels of Thromboxane A_2 in Peripheral and Coronary Circulation in Patients with Angina Pectoris, *Am. J. Cardiol.*, 45:454, 1980.
358. Robertson, R. M., Robertson, D., Roberts, L. J., et al.: Thromboxane A_2 in Vasotonic Angina Pectoris, *N. Engl. J. Med.*, 304:998, 1981.
359. Esumi, K., Tada, M., Kuzuya, T., et al.: Thromboxane A_2 and Prostaglandin I_2 in Canine Circulation during Transient Myocardial Ischemia, *Circulation*, 64(suppl. 4):266, 1981.
360. Yokoyama, M., Goldman, M., and Henry, P. D.: Supersensitivity of Atherosclerotic Arteries to Ergonovine Partially Mediated by a Serotonergic Mechanism, *Circulation*, 60(suppl. 2):100, 1979.
361. Heistad, D. D., Armstrong, M. L., Marcus, M. L., Piegors, D. J., and Mark, A. L.: Augmented Responses to Vasoconstrictor Stimuli in Hypercholesterolemic and Atherosclerotic Monkeys, *Circ. Res.*, 54:711, 1984.
362. Mudge, G. H., Jr., Goldberg, S., Gunther, S., Mann, T., and Grossman, W.: Comparison of Metabolic and Vasoconstrictor Stimuli on Coronary Vascular Resistance in Man. *Circulation*, 59:544, 1979.
363. Johannsen, U. J., Mark, A. L., Marcus, M. L., and Armstrong, M. L.: Effects of Dietary Hyperlipoproteinemia on Coronary Vascular Responsiveness in Vivo, *Circulation*, 64(suppl. 4):267, 1980.
364. Shimokawa, H., Tomoike, H., Nabeyama, S., Yamamoto, H., Araki, H., and Nakamura, M.: Coronary Artery Spasm Induced in Atherosclerotic Miniature Swine, *Science*, 221:560, 1983.
365. Bohr, D. R.: Adrenergic Receptors in Coronary Arteries, *Ann. N. Y. Acad. Sci.*, 139:799, 1967.
366. Gross, G. J., and Feigl, E. O.: Analysis of Coronary Vascular Beta Receptors in Situ, *Am. J. Physiol.*, 228:1909, 1975.
367. Hamilton, F. N., and Feigl, E. O.: Coronary Vascular Sympathetic Beta-Receptor Innervation, *Am. J. Physiol.*, 230:1569, 1976.
368. Stiles, G. L., and Lefkowitz, R. J.: Cardiac Adrenergic Receptors, *Annu. Rev. Med.*, 35:149, 1984.
369. Feigl, E. O.: Parasympathetic Control of Coronary Blood Flow in Dogs, *Circ. Res.*, 25:509, 1969.
370. Vatner, S. F., and McRitchie, R. J.: Interaction of the Chemoreflex and the Pulmonary Inflation Reflex in the Regulation of Coronary Circulation in Conscious Dogs, *Circ. Res.*, 37:644, 1975.
371. Schaper, W.: "The Collateral Circulation of the Heart," North Holland Publishing Company, Amsterdam, 1971.
372. Wechsler, A. S.: Development of Coronary Collateral Circulation. *Annu. Rev. Med.*, 28:341, 1977.
373. Schaper, W.: Collateral Circulation, in W. Schaper (ed.), "The Paraphysiology of Myocardial Perfusion," Elsevier/North Holland Biomedical Press, Amsterdam, 1979.
374. Gregg, D. E., and Patterson, R. D.: Functional Importance of the Coronary Collaterals, *N. Engl. J. Med.*, 303:1404, 1980.
375. Berne, R. M.: Effect of Epinephrine and Norepinephrine on the Coronary Circulation, *Circ. Res.*, 6:664, 1958.
376. Yurchak, P. M., Rolett, E. L., Cohen, L. S., and Gorlin, R.: Effects of Norepinephrine on the Coronary Circulation in Man, *Circulation*, 30:180, 1964.
377. Sullivan, J. M., and Gorlin, R.: Effect of L-Epinephrine on the Coronary Circulation in Human Subjects with and without Coronary Artery Disease, *Circ. Res.*, 21:919, 1967.
378. Krasnow, N., Rolett, E. L., Yurchak, P. M., Hood, W. B., Jr., and Gorlin, R.: Isoproterenol and Cardiovascular Performance, *Am. J. Med.*, 37:514, 1964.
379. Braunwald, E.: Control of Myocardial Oxygen Consumption: Physiologic and Clinical Consideration, *Am. J. Cardiol.*, 27:416, 1971.
380. Dusting, G. J., Moncada, S., and Vane, J. R.: Prostaglandins, Their Intermediates and Precursors: Cardiovascular Actions and Regulatory Roles in Normal and Abnormal Circulatory Systems, *Prog. Cardiovas. Dis.*, 21:405, 1979.
381. Gunther, S., and Cannon, P. J.: Modulation of Angiotensin II Coronary Vasoconstriction by Cardiac Prostaglandin Synthesis, *Am. J. Physiol.*, 238:H895, 1980.
382. Nakano, J.: Cardiovascular Actions of Vasopressin. *Jpn. Circ. J.*, 37:363, 1973.
383. Nakano, J.: Cardiovascular Responses to Neurohypophysial Hormones, in R. O. Greep and E. B. Astwood (eds.), "Handbook of Physiology," sec. 7: Endocrinology," American Physiological Society, Washington, D.C., 1974, vol. 4, chap. 15, p. 395.
384. Hays, R. M.: Agents Affecting the Renal Conservation of Water, in A. G. Gilman, L. S. Goodman, and A. Gilman (eds.), "The Pharmacological Basis of Therapeutics," Macmillan Company, London, 1980, chap. 37, p. 916.

385. Leight, L., Defazio, V., Talmers, F. N., Regan, T. J., and Hellems, H. K.: Coronary Blood Flow, Myocardial Oxygen Consumption and Myocardial Metabolism in Normal and Hyperthyroid Human Subjects, *Circulation,* 14:90, 1956.
386. Buccino, R. A., Spann, J. F., Jr., Pool, P. E., et al.: Influence of Thyroid State on the Intrinsic Contractile Properties and Energy Stores of the Myocardium, *J. Clin. Invest.,* 46:1669, 1967.
387. Corliss, R. J., McKenna, D. H., Sigler, S., O'Brien G. S., and Rowe, G. G.: Systemic and Coronary Hemodynamic Effects of Vasopressin, *Am. J. Med. Sci.,* 5:293, 1968.
388. Amidi, M., Leon, D. F., deGroot, W. J., et al.: Effect of the Thyroid State on Myocardial Contractility and Ventricular Ejection Rate in Man, *Circulation,* 38:229, 1968.
389. Skeleton, C. L., Pool, P. E., Seagren, S. C., and Braunwald, E.: Mechanochemistry of Cardiac Muscle: V. Influence of Thyroid State on Energy Utilization, *J. Clin. Invest.,* 50:463, 1971.
390. Skelton, C. L., and Sonnenblick, E. H.: Cardiovascular System, in S. C. Werner and S. H. Ingbar (eds.), "Hyperthyroidism," Harper & Row Publishers, Inc., New York, 1978, chap. 36, p. 688.
391. Hackel, D. B., and Kleinerman, J.: Effects of Thiamin Deficiency on Myocardial Metabolism in Intact Dogs, *Am. Heart J.,* 46:1, 1953.
392. Hilton, S. M., and Lewis, G. P.: Relationship between Glandular Activity, Bradykinin Formation and Functional Vasodilatation in the Submandibular Salivary Gland, *J. Physiol.,* 134:471, 1956.
393. Needleman, P., Marshall, G. R., and Sobel, B. E.: Hormone Interactions in the Isolated Rabbit Heart: Synthesis and Coronary Vasomotor Effects of Prostaglandins, Angiotensin, and Bradykinin, *Circ. Res.,* 37:802, 1975.
394. Regoli, D., Barabe, J., and Therialult, B.: Does Indomethacin Antagonize the Effects of Peptides and Other Agents on the Coronary Circulation of Rabbit Isolated Hearts? *Can. J. Physiol. Pharmacol.,* 55:307, 1977.
395. Losay, J., Mroz, E. A., Treagear, G. W., Leeman, S. E., and Gamble, W. J.: Action of Substance P on the Coronary Blood Flow in the Isolated Dog Heart, in U. S. von Euler and B. Pernow (eds.), "Substance P," Raven Press, New York, 1976.
396. Said, S. I.: VIP: Overview, in S. R. Bloom (ed.), "Gut Hormones," Churchill Livingstone, Edinburgh, 1978, chap. 73, p. 465.
397. Said, S. I.: Vasoactive Intestinal Polypeptide (VIP) as a Neural Peptide, in A. Miyoshi (ed.), "Gut Peptides, Secretion, Function and Clinical Aspects," Kodansha Ltd., Tokyo, 1979.
398. Gu, J., Adrian, T. E., Tatemoto, K., Polak, J. M., Allen, J. M., and Bloom, S. R.: Neuropeptide Tyrosine (NPY)—A Major Cardiac Neuropeptide, *Lancet,* 1:1008, 1983.
399. Needleman, P., and Kaley, S.: Cardiac and Coronary Prostaglandin Synthesis and Function, *N. Engl. J. Med.,* 298:1122, 1978.
400. Kirk, E. S., Turbow, M. E., Urschel, C. S., and Sonnenblick, E. H.: Non-uniform Contractility across the Heart Wall Caused by Redistribution of Coronary Flow, *J. Clin. Invest.,* 49:51A, 1970.
401. Downey, J. M., and Kirk, E. S.: Distribution of the Coronary Blood Flow Across the Canine Heart Wall During Systole, *Circ. Res.,* 34:251, 1974.
402. Cobb, F. R., Bache, R. J., and Greenfield, J. C., Jr.: Regional Myocardial Blood Flow in Awake Dogs, *J. Clin. Invest.,* 53:H1618, 1974.
403. Hoffman, J. I. E., and Buckberg, G. D.: Transmural Variations in Myocardial Perfusion, in P. N. Yu and J. F. Goodwin (eds.), "Progress in Cardiology," Lea & Febiger, Philadelphia, 1976, chap. 3, p. 37.
404. Hoffman, J. I. E.: Determinants and Prediction of Transmural Myocardial Perfusion, *Circulation,* 58:381, 1978.
405. Fedor, M., McIntosh, D. M., Rembert, J. C., and Greenfield, J. C., Jr.: Coronary and Transmural Myocardial Blood Flow Responses to Transient Ischemia in Awake Domestic Pigs, *Am. J. Physiol.,* 235:H435, 1978.
406. Mueller, T. M., Marcus, M. L., Kerber, R. E., Young, Y. A., Barnes, R. W., and Abboud, F. M.: Effect of Renal Hypertension and Left Ventricular Hypertrophy on the Coronary Circulation in Dogs, *Circ. Res.,* 42:543, 1978.
407. Murray, P. A., Baig, H., Fishbein, M. C., and Vatner, S. F.: Effects of Experimental Right Ventricular Hypertrophy on Myocardial Blood Flow in Conscious Dogs, *J. Clin. Invest.,* 64:421, 1979.
408. Vinten-Johansen, J., and Weiss, H. R.: Oxygen Consumption in Subepicardial and Subendocardial Regions of the Canine Left Ventricle: The Effect of Experimental Acute Valvular Aortic Stenosis, *Circ. Res.,* 46:139, 1980.
409. Manohar, M., Thurmon, J. C., Tranquilli, W. J., Devous, M. D., Sr., Theodarakis, M. C., Shawley, R. V., Feller, D. L., and Benson, J. G.: Regional Myocardial Blood Flow and Coronary Vascular Reserve in Unanesthetized Young Calves with Severe Concentric Right Ventricular Hypertrophy, *Circ. Res.,* 48:785, 1981.
410. Wangler, R. D., Peters, K. G., Marcus, M. L., and Tomanek, R. J.: Effects of Duration and Severity of Arterial Hypertension on Cardiac Hypertrophy and Coronary Vasodilator Reserve, *Circ. Res.,* 51:10, 1982.
411. Schelbert, H. R., Phelps, M. E., Hoffman, E. J., Huang S.-C., Selin, C. E., and Kuhl, D. E.: Regional Myocardial Perfusion Assessed with N-13 Labeled Ammonia and Positron Emission Computerized Axial Tomography, *Am. J. Cardiol.,* 43:209, 1979.
412. Vogel, R. A., Kirch, D. L., LeFree, M. T., Rainwater, J. O., Jensen, D. P., and Steel, P. P.: Thallium-201 Myocardial Perfusion Scintigraphy: Results of Standard and Multi-Pinhole Tomographic Techniques, *Am. J. Cardiol.,* 43:787, 1979.
413. Hoffman, J. I. E.: The Effect of Intramyocardial Forces on the Distribution of Intramyocardial Blood Flow, *J. Biomed. Eng.,* 1:33, 1979.

4

Electrical Activity of the Heart

Andrew G. Wallace, M.D.

If a pair of electrodes (zinc covered by chamois leather and moistened with brine) are strapped to the front and back of the chest, and connected with a Lippmann's capillary electrometer the mercury in the latter will be seen to move slightly but sharply at each beat of the heart. . . . Each beat of the heart is seen to be accompanied by an electrical variation.

A. D. Waller, 1887[1]

Each contraction of the heart is initiated by an electrical event that occurs because cardiac muscle is an excitable tissue. There is a difference in electrical potential between the inside and the outside of nearly all cells of the body. This difference is called the *transmembrane potential.* In the heart, the transmembrane potential is substantial in size and the cells are also excitable; that is, an appropriate stimulus leads to a change in membrane properties as a consequence of which ions flow across the membrane and elicit an *action potential.*

Certain cells in the heart do not require an external stimulus to initiate the membrane changes that lead to an action potential. Such cells undergo slow, spontaneous diastolic depolarization; and when membrane potential has fallen to threshold, an action potential ensues. The property by which excitation is initiated in the absence of an external stimulus is referred to as *automaticity.* Numerous regions throughout the specialized conduction system are capable of automatic behavior under normal physiological conditions. The frequency of automatic impulse formation is greatest in the sinoatrial (SA) node, and for this reason the sinus node normally functions as the pacemaker of the heart.

When current is injected into any single cardiac cell through a microelectrode, membrane potential is displaced not only in that cell, but also in neighboring cells over some distance from the electrode. This phenomenon demonstrates that heart cells are connected through couplings that offer a low resistance to the flow of electric current, and as a consequence an action potential elicited in one cell is capable of being transmitted to another and to another, that is, conducted.

The atrial chambers are thin-walled. Specialized fibers are found in the atria, but they are not organized into specialized tracts or bundles as they are within the ventricles. Rather, in selected regions working atrial musculature becomes more densely packed and longitudinally oriented, creating routes of preferential propagation at a velocity relatively greater than in other thinner, less organized parts of the atrial chambers. (See also Chap. 2.) Activation of the atrial musculature is responsible for the P wave on the surface electrocardiogram. The morphology of the P wave is determined primarily by the site of impulse formation within the SA node. A second factor in determining the morphology of the P wave is the relative mass of the two atria. Finally, the preferential routes of atrial propagation play an important role in intraatrial conduction, influencing the conduction time from sinus node to atrioventricular (AV) node and from sinus node to left atrium.

The AV node is the only normal avenue over which an impulse can be transmitted from atrium to ventricle. It has a number of unique properties, the most important of which is its exceedingly low conduction velocity. The long time required for conduction through the AV node and the resulting delay between atrial and ventricular activation are responsible for the PR interval of the electrocardiogram.

In the ventricles, the bundle branches and their distal ramifications consist of highly specialized *Purkinje fibers.* This system or network is characterized by an extremely rapid conduction velocity and by an anatomic organization that provides nearly simultaneous excitation of the inner shells of both ventricles. Subsequent activation of ventricular muscle is responsible for generating the QRS complex on the electrocardiogram. The form of the QRS complex is determined primarily by the sequence of ventricular activation and by the thickness of the two ventricles. The specialized conduction system plays a key role in initiating and coordinating the activity of a complex and very nonhomogeneous organ (Fig. 4-1). It is remarkable, indeed, that we know as much as we do about disturbances of cardiac rhythm and activation since the activity of the specialized conduction system is silent on the ordinary surface electrocardiogram. Studies in animals, and more recently in human beings, have been able to record the activity of these specialized tissues. These recordings have contributed importantly to clarifying the role of the specialized conduction system in the normal heart and elucidating the mechanisms responsible for many electrocardiographic abnormalities.

Transmembrane Potential

In heart cells, as in all living cells, ions are distributed unequally across the cell membrane. This disequilibrium has two important features. First, for any given ion the concentration is different on the

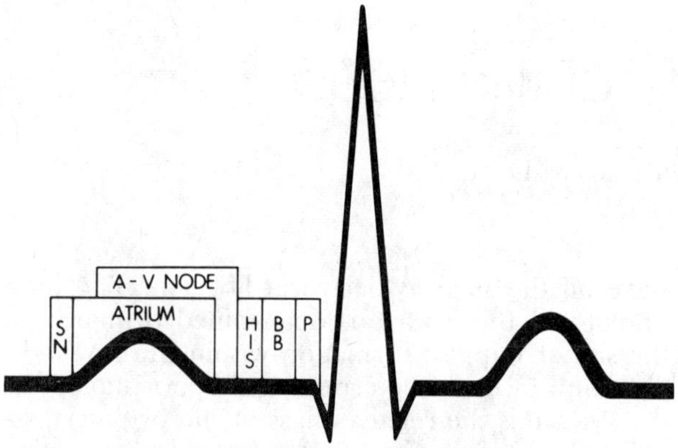

FIGURE 4-1 Normal electrocardiographic complex. Also shown is the sequence of activity in the specialized conducting system. SN = sinus node; HIS = His bundle; BB = bundle branches; P = peripheral Purkinje tissue.

inside and outside of the cell. Second, the electrical potential is different on the inside and outside of the cell.[2] These conditions create two passive forces which tend to promote ionic movement. In the first case, ions in solution tend to move from areas of higher to areas of lower concentration as a result of diffusion forces, and the force promoting diffusion is proportional to the concentration gradient. For ions, movement is also promoted by electrical forces. For example, when the inside of a cell is electrically negative with respect to the outside, positively charged ions will tend to move to the inside and negatively charged ions will tend to move to the outside; this electrical force is proportional to the transmembrane voltage gradient. Each ion, whether on the inside or outside of the cell, has a potential energy which is the net consequence of the diffusion and electrical forces acting on it. When this net potential energy is the same on both sides of the cell membrane, no movement will occur for the ion in question and an equilibrium state exists. The transmembrane electrical potential that exists when electrical and diffusion forces are exactly equal is referred to as the *equilibrium potential* for the ion in question.

The concentration of potassium is approximately 35 times greater on the inside of heart cells than on the outside, and the concentration of sodium is approximately 4.5 times greater on the outside of the cell than on the inside. The diffusion force (P_c) which tends to move potassium out of the cell is directly proportional to its concentration difference across the membrane, and the potential energy of potassium ions attributable to this force is expressed by the following equation:

$$P_c = RT \ln \frac{[\mathrm{K}]_i}{[\mathrm{K}]_o} \tag{4-1}$$

where R = the gas constant
T = the absolute temperature
K_i = intracellular K^+ concentration
K_o = extracellular K^+ concentration
ln = the natural logarithm, or log to the base e (= 2.718)

The inside of a resting heart cell, however, is about 90 mV negative with respect to the outside (Fig. 4-2). This electrical force will tend to move potassium in the opposite direction, that is, from outside to inside the cell. The potential energy of potassium attributable to this electrical force (P_e) is proportional to transmembrane potential and is expressed by the equation:

$$P_e = ZFE_m \tag{4-2}$$

where Z = the valence of the ion
F = 96,500 (the Faraday number)
E_m = the transmembrane potential

In a steady state the potential energy due to electrical and diffusion forces is equal and no net ionic movement occurs. Thus:

$$ZFE_m = RT \ln \frac{[\mathrm{K}]_i}{[\mathrm{K}]_o} \tag{4-3}$$

or at 37.5°C:

$$E_\mathrm{K} = 61.5 \ln \frac{[\mathrm{K}]_i}{[\mathrm{K}]_o} \tag{4-4}$$

Equation (4-4) is the *Nernst equation* and describes the equilibrium potential for potassium that must exist to exactly counteract the diffusion force resulting from the difference in concentration across the cell membrane. When this equation is solved using actual data for the concentration of potassium inside and outside a heart cell, $E_K = -90$ mV, a value almost identical to the measured resting transmembrane potential in cardiac cells.

The above calculation has been developed for potassium; however, when membrane potential is stable, as it is during diastole, the sum of all currents related to ionic movement across the cell membrane must equal zero. Furthermore, in addition to diffusion and electrical forces the actual movement of any particular ion will be influenced by the permeability of the membrane to the ion in question. This has led to a more general equation, the Hodgkin and Katz modification of Goldman's constant field equation, which describes transmembrane potential at any time and accounts for the influence of ions other than potassium. This equation is noted below:

$$V_m = \frac{RT}{F} \ln \frac{P_\mathrm{K}[\mathrm{K}]_i + P_\mathrm{Na}[\mathrm{Na}]_i + P_\mathrm{Cl}[\mathrm{Cl}]_o + \cdots}{P_\mathrm{K}[\mathrm{K}]_o + P_\mathrm{Na}[\mathrm{Na}]_o + P_\mathrm{Cl}[\mathrm{Cl}]_i + \cdots} \tag{4-5}$$

Solution of Eq. (4-5) gives a value for V_m of -90 mV if we assume that during diastole the membrane is permeable to potassium but not to sodium, a fact supported by direct observations. Similarly, if permeability to sodium is increased abruptly (as with the upstroke of the action potential), solution of Eq. (4-5) gives a positive value for V_m consistent with the actual measured transmembrane potential.

The sodium and potassium concentration gradients across the cell membrane are created by the

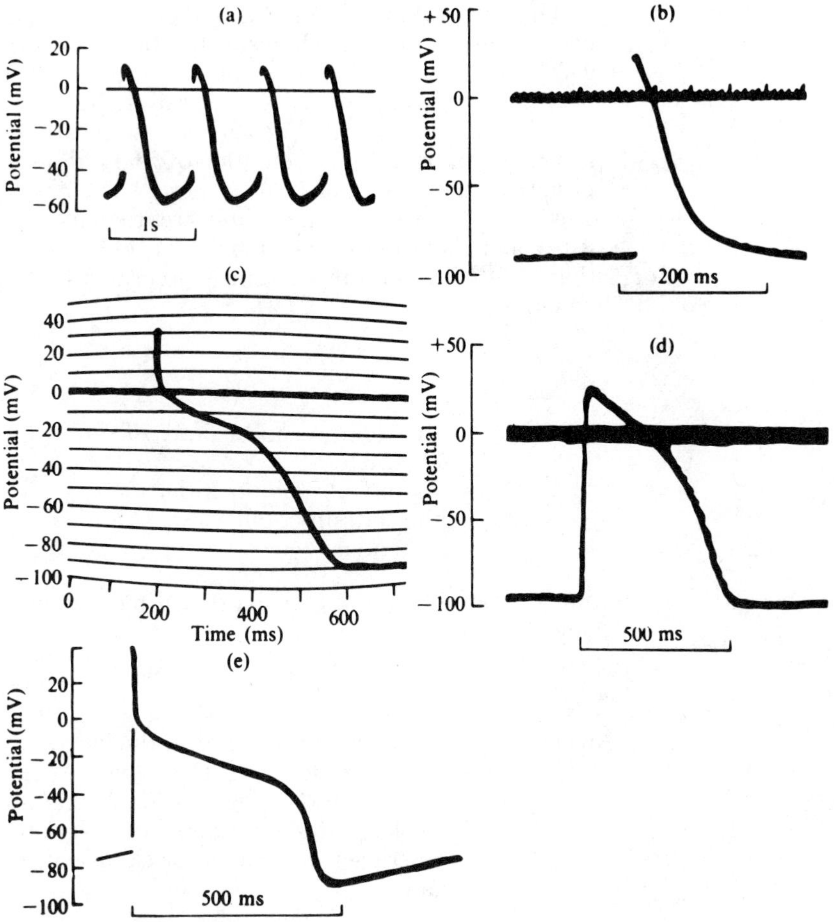

FIGURE 4-2 Action potentials recorded from different parts of the heart. *a*. Sinus node. *b*. Atrium. *c*. Quiescent Purkinje fiber. *d*. Ventricle. *e*. Automatic Purkinje fiber. Transmembrane potential at rest varies from −50 mV in SA node to −95 mV in atrium, Purkinje, and ventricle. (*From D. Noble, "The Initiation of the Heart Beat," Oxford University Press, Clarendon Press, Oxford, 1975. Reproduced with permission from the publisher and author.*)

activity of a Na^+-K^+ exchange pump that accumulates K inside the cell and pumps Na to the outside. The pump includes an enzyme that requires ATP for its activity and is subject to inhibition by uncoupling oxidative phosphorylation or by perfusion with a solution deficient in oxygen.[3] The activity of the enzyme is stimulated by Na and K through two separate loci (an internal site with high affinity for Na and an external site with high affinity for K). The activity of the enzyme is further dependent on pH and is inhibited by high concentrations of ouabain. For many years, Na and K exchange was felt to be tightly coupled and thus electroneutral; however, recent data indicate that more Na is pumped out than K is pumped in and hence there is a net outward current that contributes to the negative intracellular potential. This interpretation implies that the Na^+-K^+ pump is electrogenic, that it contributes to the transmembrane potential, and that transmembrane potential can be changed by agents that affect the activity of the pump.

Excitability and the Action Potential

The term *excitability* is used to describe the fact that when a resting cardiac cell is depolarized to a critical level (called *threshold*), the membrane becomes permeable and a regenerative inward current causes an action potential. It is well known that cells found in different parts of the heart have different transmembrane potentials, different thresholds, and action potentials of different shapes (Fig. 4-3). Recently these action potentials have been grouped into two general types: fast and slow responses (Fig. 4-4). Fast responses are characteristic of ordinary working atrial and ventricular muscle cells and of Purkinje fibers. In these fibers resting membrane potential is −80 to −90 mV, the upstroke velocity of the action potential is 100 to 500 V/s, and conduction velocity is rapid.[4] Slow responses are characteristic of the normal sinus and AV nodal cells. In these fibers, resting potential is −40 to −70 mV, upstroke velocity of the action potential is 1 to 10 V/s, and conduction velocity is very slow.[5] The membrane properties and ionic currents responsible for each type of action potential are different.

Much of what is known about excitable cells was initially derived from studies of squid axon and cardiac Purkinje fibers, both of which have fast responses. Consequently, we know more about the ionic basis for the action potential in fast cells. It is of great interest and importance, however, that when fast-responding cardiac cells become depressed and depolarized, they assume many of the characteristics of slow cells. Thus, mechanisms responsible for the slow response are relevant to both the normal and abnormal function of the heart.

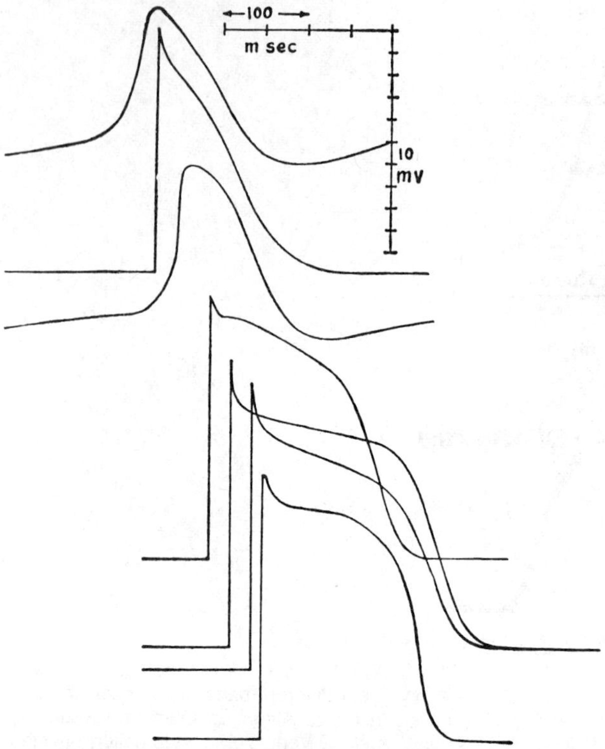

FIGURE 4-3 Transmembrane action potentials recorded from (*top* to *bottom*) SA node, atrium, AV node, His bundle, false tendon, peripheral Purkinje, ventricle. Note differences in shape, amplitude, and duration of action potentials. (*From B. F. Hoffman and P. F. Cranefield, "Electrophysiology of the Heart," McGraw-Hill Book Company, New York, 1960, p. 261. Reproduced with permission from the publisher and author.*)

In Purkinje fibers, threshold potential is approximately −70 mV, and when the cell is depolarized to that level either by a stimulus or by a propagated action potential, membrane sodium conductance (permeability) increases abruptly. As a consequence, positively charged sodium ions enter the cell rapidly, causing further depolarization (phase 0 of the action potential). Membrane potential reaches approximately +20 mV, but never quite equals the value predicted by the sodium equilibrium potential (Fig. 4-5). This is because activation of the fast channel for sodium conductance lasts only a millisecond or two and then becomes inactivated.[6]

The fast sodium channel is currently viewed as being guarded by a mechanism that functions as a gate and that probably represents a charged electric field between components of the phospholipid matrix of the membrane.[1,7] The gate is closed in a resting fiber because of the orientation of charged phospholipids that block the entry of positively charged ions. With depolarization, the lipids reorient and the gates open, allowing sodium to move inside the fiber (Fig. 4-5). The sodium current is described by the equation

$$I_{Na} = g_{Na}(V_m - V_{Na}) \qquad (4\text{-}6)$$

where g_{Na} = the sodium conductance of the channel
V_m = the membrane potential
V_{Na} = the sodium equilibrium potential

g_{Na} is a variable parameter expressed by the equation

$$g_{Na} = \bar{g}_{Na} m^3 h \qquad (4\text{-}7)$$

where $\bar{g}_{Na}$ = the maximal sodium conductance
m = a voltage-dependent variable describing activation (opening) of the gates
h = a voltage- and time-dependent variable describing inactivation or closing of the gates

In this two-component model of the sodium channel, m changes much more rapidly than h in response to a change of membrane potential (V_m). Assume, for example, in a resting cell with transmembrane potential of approximately −90 mV, that $h = 1$ (open) and $m = 0$ (closed): the value for m^3h will be 0 and the gate will be closed. Once the cell is depolarized to threshold, m changes rapidly to 1 and the gate is open for sodium to move into the cell. After depolarization, h changes slowly from 1 to 0, and as it does the value of m^3h decreases toward 0, closing the gate and inactivating the sodium current. In this model the term m^3h describes the kinetics of the sodium channel or gate.

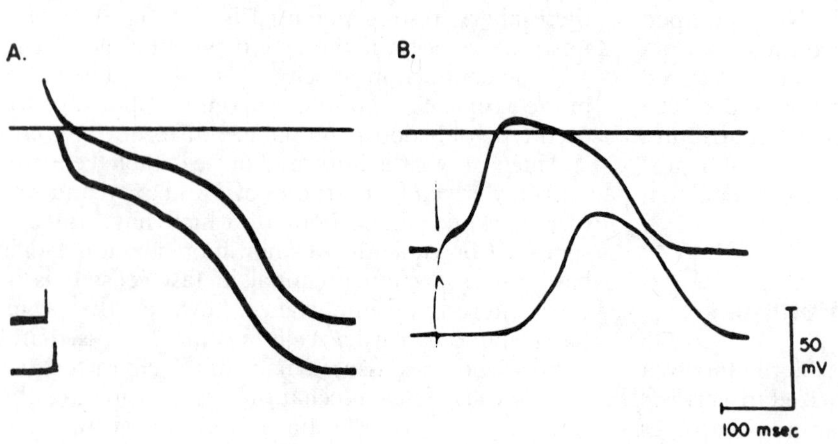

FIGURE 4-4 Action potentials typical of fast (*A*) and slow (*B*) responses.

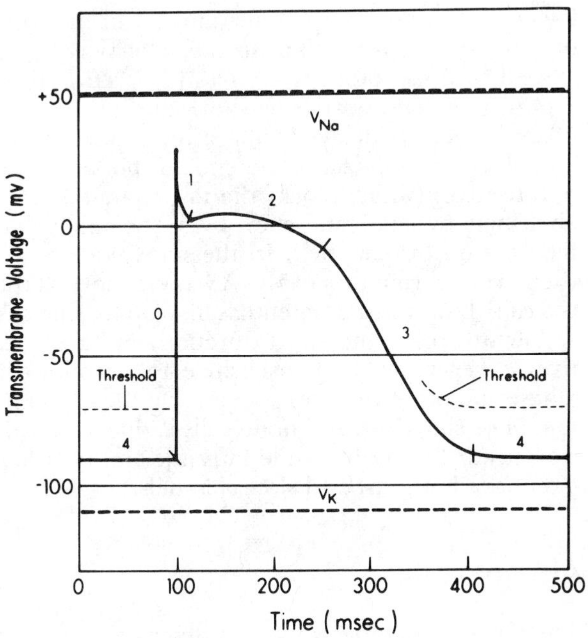

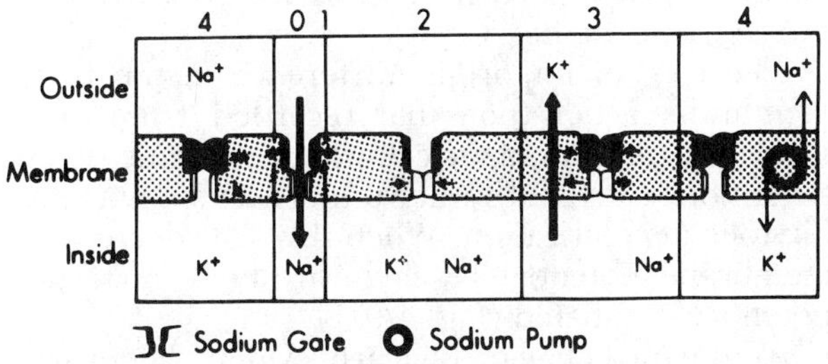

FIGURE 4-5 Schematic representation of the cardiac action potential and the sequence of events that determine the time change in voltage. V_{Na} = sodium equilibrium potential; V_K = potassium equilibrium potential. The four phases of the action potential are noted above. Below are shown the cardiac membrane, the gates which open and close to allow Na and K ions to move across the membrane, causing depolarization and then repolarization. Finally, the activity of the pump which restores Na and K during phase 4 is illustrated. [*From T. Bigger, Jr., Antiarrhythmic Drugs in Ischemic Heart Disease, Hospital Practice, 7(11), 1972, and from E. Braunwald (ed.), "The Myocardium: Failure and Infarction," H. P. Publishing Company, Inc., New York, 1974, p. 296. Drawn by Bunji Tagawa. Redrawn and reproduced with permission from the publisher and author.*]

In addition to this early inward sodium current, there is a second and much more slowly inactivated inward current that appears to contribute to the plateau of the action potential in cardiac fibers. Current evidence suggests that this inward current develops about 10 ms after phase 0 and is most likely attributable to calcium ions[8] or to a separate slow sodium channel.

Following the plateau of the action potential, potassium permeability, which had decreased while the cell was depolarized, returns to its higher level. With this increase in potassium conductance, positively charged potassium ions move from inside to outside the membrane. The potassium current I_K is described by the equation

$$I_K = g_K(V_m - V_K) \qquad (4\text{-}8)$$

where g_K = the potassium conductance
V_m = the membrane potential
V_K = the potassium equilibrium potential

As a consequence of the egress of positively charged potassium, the cell repolarizes (Fig. 4-6). In cardiac fibers the onset and rate of repolarization are influenced primarily by agents that increase or decrease potassium conductance.[1]

In summary, in muscle and Purkinje fibers the action potential is brought about by an initial fast inward movement of sodium (phase 0) that ends abruptly (phase 1). During the plateau of an action potential (phase 2), membrane voltage is influenced by slow inward currents carried by calcium and/or sodium and an outward potassium current (ix_1). This latter current (ix_1) is slow to start but turns on in a time-dependent manner and, when maximal, causes the cell to rapidly repolarize (phase 3).

Under normal circumstances, recovery of the sodium-carrying system is closely coupled to repolarization. However, under the influence of a number of agents, including reduced temperature and drugs, repolarization and recovery of responsiveness can be dissociated in time such that recovery from inactivation occurs only long after repolarization.

It has already been noted that in normal Purkinje fibers there is evidence of a second inward current

FIGURE 4-6 A model of the cardiac action potential based on modifications of the Hodgkin-Huxley theory. The action potential is shown above. Change in sodium conductance (g_{Na+}), solid curve, and potassium conductance (g_{K+}), dashed curve, are shown below. See text for description. (*From D. Noble, "The Initiation of the Heart Beat," Oxford University Press, Clarendon Press, Oxford, 1975. Reproduced with permission from the publisher and author.*)

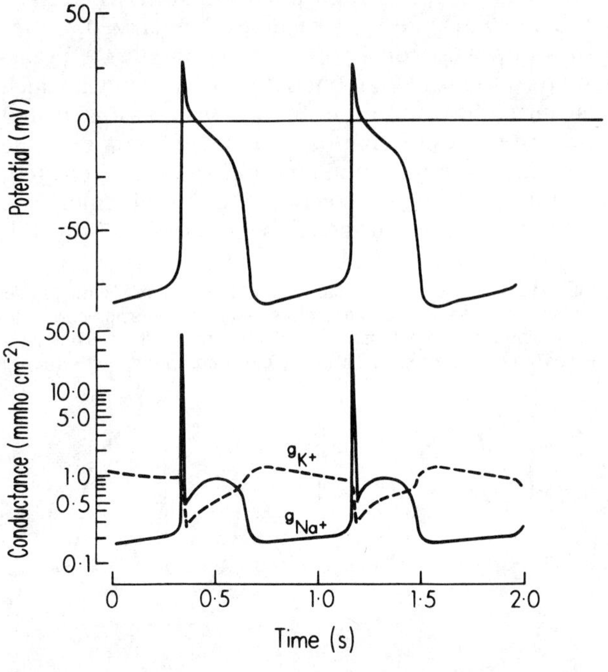

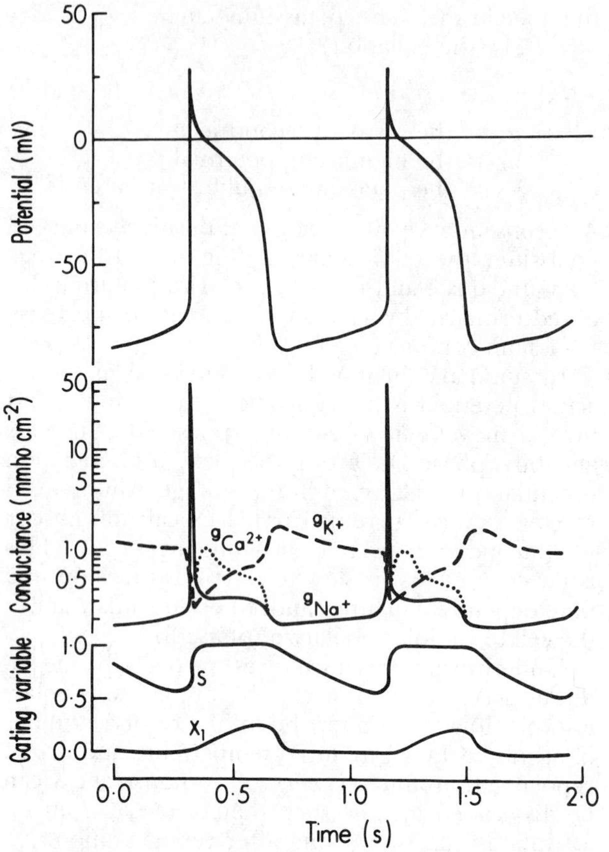

FIGURE 4-7 A model of the cardiac action potential, similar to that shown in Fig. 4-6, except that changes in calcium conductance ($g_{Ca^{2+}}$) have been added to indicate the slow-channel current. *S* and X_1 are variables which control potassium conductances (g_{K+}) and are analogous to *m* and *h*, which control sodium conductance (g_{Na+}). (*From D. Noble, "The Initiation of the Heart Beat," Oxford University Press, Clarendon Press, Oxford, 1975. Reproduced with permission from the publisher and author.*)

that is delayed in onset and is carried by calcium and/or sodium through a slow channel (Fig. 4-7). When a Purkinje fiber becomes depolarized, either by an applied voltage or by a high external potassium concentration, the rapid sodium channel, which is normally responsible for phase 0, is inactivated (i.e., the gates or channels are closed). Under these circumstances an action potential can still be elicited, and it is attributable solely to the slow channel (Fig. 4-8). A slow-response action potential has the following characteristics: (1) threshold is in the range of −50 to −35 mV, (2) upstroke velocity is 1 to 10 V/s, (3) action potential amplitude is reduced, (4) action potential duration is short, and (5) recovery of excitability is delayed long after repolarization. The slow-response action potential is not altered by tetrodotoxin (which blocks the fast channel), but is abolished by manganese or by verapamil (which blocks the slow channel). In the sinus node and in the N region (middle) of the AV node, normal cells typically have resting potentials of −50 to −60 mV, a slow upstroke, and short duration, and are sensitive to verapamil and insensitive to tetrodotoxin. These and other features suggest that the action potential of sinus and AV node cells is due solely to a slow inward current,[9] while Purkinje and muscle fibers have both fast and slow channels.

Automaticity

The term *automaticity* is used to describe a property of some cardiac cells to initiate an action potential spontaneously. Many cells have the capacity of becoming automatic, but only the group of cells that initiate a propagated impulse is referred to as the *pacemaker* of the heart.

There is an important difference in the transmembrane action potential recorded from automatic cells. In automatic cells the membrane potential is not steady, but rather undergoes spontaneous diastolic depolarization. When this slow decrease in membrane potential reaches threshold, an action potential is initiated (Fig. 4-9).

Automatic behavior is clearly evident under normal conditions in the sinus node and in Purkinje fibers. On the other hand, the maximal diastolic potential, the rate of spontaneous depolarization, and other features of the action potential are distinctly different in the sinus node and in Purkinje fibers. It follows that the mechanisms responsible for automaticity in the sinus node and in Purkinje fibers may not be the same.

The mechanisms responsible for automaticity and its control have been reviewed recently.[10] It should be recalled that in all cardiac cells there is an inward (leakage) current, which is presumably carried by

FIGURE 4-8 Action potential recorded from a calf Purkinje fiber in the presence of adrenalin. Panel *a* is control. Panels *b* to *e* show action potentials recorded in the presence of increasing concentrations of tetrodotoxin. Tetrodotoxin blocks the fast sodium channel, and the residual action potential (*e*) is due entirely to the slow channel. (*From D. Noble, "The Initiation of the Heart Beat," Oxford University Press, Clarendon Press, Oxford, 1975. Reproduced with permission from the publisher and author.*)

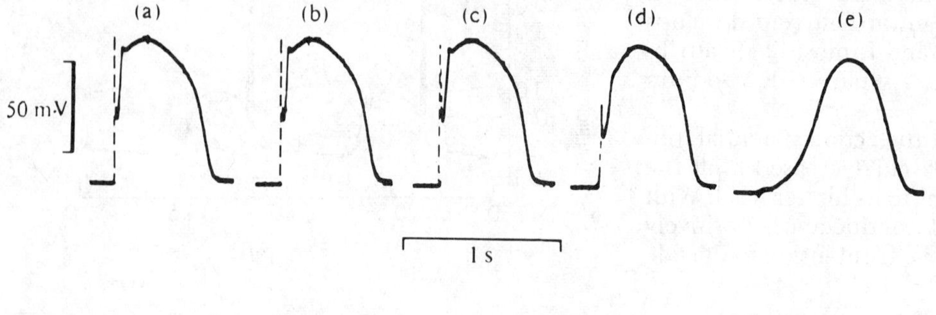

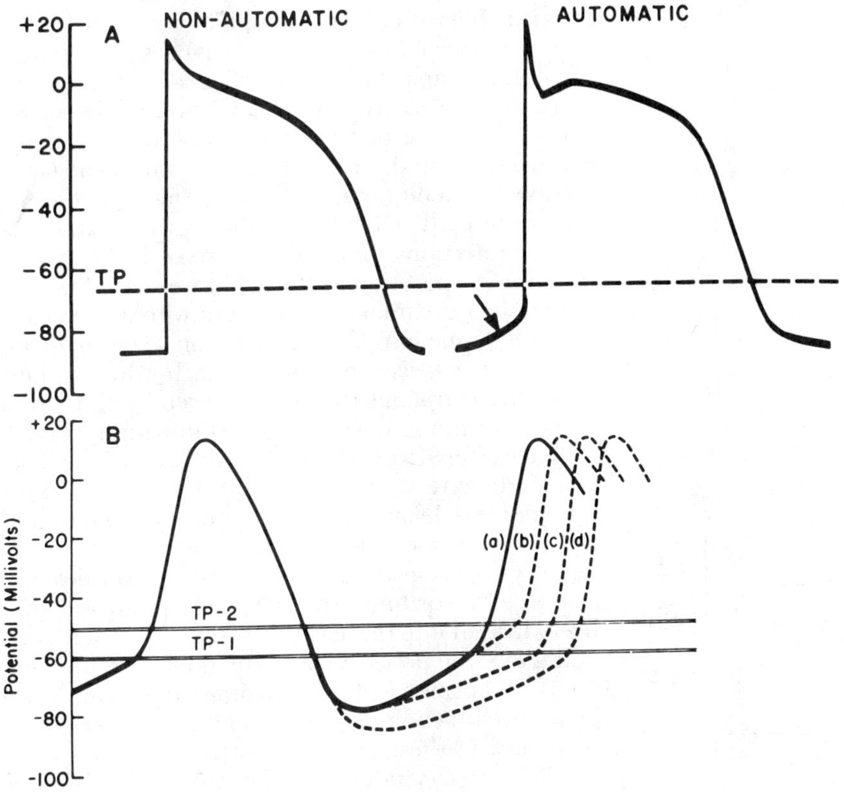

FIGURE 4-9 Schematic representation showing the difference in action potential characteristics of a nonautomatic and automatic cell. (*A*). *B* shows that changes in the rhythmicity of an automatic cell can result from a change in threshold (*b*), a reduced rate of diastolic depolarization (*c*), or hyperpolarization (*d*).

positively charged sodium ions. If this leakage current is not offset in diastole by an electrically equal outward ion flux, then diastolic depolarization will ensue.

In the sinus node the action potential is short. Potassium conductance is activated by depolarization and increases further with time to cause repolarization. The subsequent diastolic decrease of the outward potassium current (ix_1), especially at a low membrane potential, allows the inward sodium leakage current to dominate membrane potential and to cause diastolic depolarization.

In Purkinje fibers the action potential is long. Furthermore, the cells repolarize to a membrane potential of −85 to −95 mV. Voltage clamp studies have shown that when a Purkinje fiber is clamped at −60 mV an outward potassium current i_{K2} is maximally activated. At −90 mV, however, i_{K2} is completely inactivated, although this deactivation is slow and time-dependent. Thus, during repolarization, when membrane potential reaches −60 mV, i_{K2} is maximal. Further repolarization to −90 mV deactivates i_{K2} but only with a time delay (Fig. 4-10). Hence in Purkinje fibers there is a slow fall of potassium conductance in diastole, as in the sinus node, which allows the inward sodium current to cause spontaneous diastolic depolarization. In the sinus node it is delayed inactivation of ix_1, while in Purkinje fibers it is delayed inactivation of i_{K2}, that causes the pacemaker current.

Vagal nerve stimulation slows impulse initiation by the sinus node, while sympathetic nerve stimulation speeds impulse formation. The major consequence of vagal nerve stimulation is hyperpolarization of sinus node cells. This hyperpolarization is induced by acetylcholine, which increases potassium conductance. Both hyperpolarization and a reduced rate of spontaneous diastolic depolarization contribute to a reduced frequency of sinus node firing (Fig. 4-11). The ionic basis for the ability of adrenergic stimuli to enhance firing in the sinus node is not known.

During normal rhythm, impulse formation takes place in the sinus node and this region functions as the pacemaker.

Conduction

Once an action potential has been initiated at any given site in the heart, excitation is propagated away from that site. Because the resistivity of the cytoplasm is low, current flows with ease through the cytoplasm from excited to unexcited regions of the cell. This current is sufficient to discharge the capacitance of the distal membrane and hence to bring the membrane to threshold, where its resistance drops, allowing more inward current as a source to discharge still more distant units of membrane. Propagation from one cell to another occurs at sites of low-resistance coupling between cells, allowing current derived from one cell to discharge an adjacent cell.[11]

In its simplest and theoretical form the cardiac cell in a steady state has been viewed as behaving as though it were a segment of a cable. This cable is

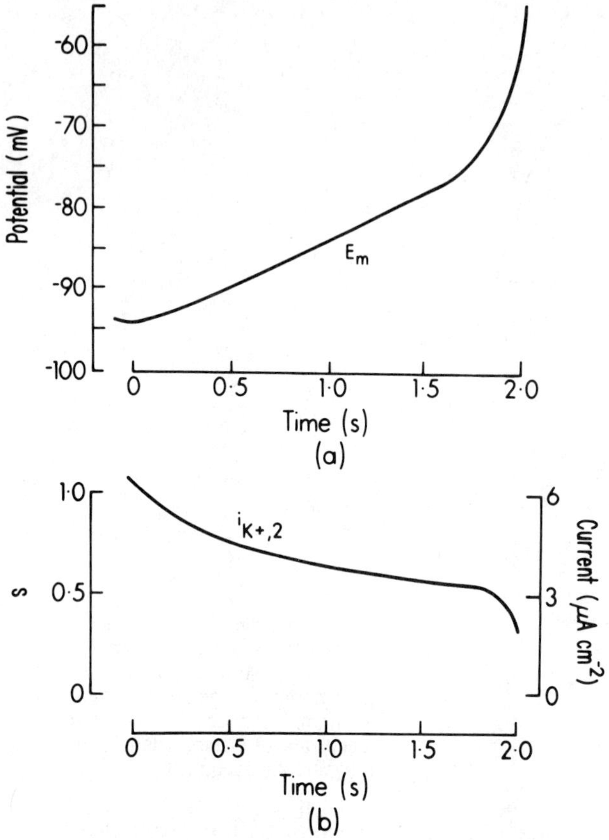

FIGURE 4-10 Mechanism of pacemaker activity in Purkinje fibers. The upper panel shows diastolic depolarization of the transmembrane potential (E_m) characteristic of a pacemaker potential. The lower curve depicts the slow diastolic decrease in outward potassium current ($i_{K+,2}$). The decrease in this outward potassium current allows the inward sodium leakage current to depolarize the cell. See text. *(From D. Noble, "The Initiation of the Heart Beat," Oxford University Press, Clarendon Press, Oxford, 1975. Redrawn and reproduced with permission from the publisher and author.)*

made up of a membrane (the sarcolemma) surrounding the myoplasm. The membrane has a resistance (i.e., the inverse of conductance), and conductance reflects permeability to the ion in question. Membrane conductance is low (i.e., resistance is high) in the resting fiber. The cell membrane also behaves like a capacitor, evident from the fact that when a step function of current is applied across the membrane, transmembrane potential changes more slowly. Membrane capacitance is presumed to reflect primarily the structure and composition of the sarcolemma. The resistivity of the cytoplasm and of the extracellular fluid are considered constant and small relative to membrane resistance. Although the geometry of cardiac tissue and the nature of intercellular connections may seem to make it difficult to treat the preparation as though it were a cable (and in fact such treatments are fraught with interpretive difficulty), one important conclusion seems inescapable: cardiac cells are joined to each other by low-resistance couplings that allow current to flow from one cell to the next with minimal impediment.

FIGURE 4-11 Membrane potential recorded from pacemaker cell of the frog sinus venosus during vagal nerve stimulation. Note that hyperpolarization and a reduced slope of diastolic depolarization both contribute to the slowing of the pacemaker. *(From M. M. Hutter and M. M. Trautwein, Vagal and Sympathetic Effects on Pacemaker Fibers in the Sinus Venosus of the Heart, J. Gen. Physiol., 39:715, 1956. Reproduced with copyright permission from The Rockefeller University Press and author.)*

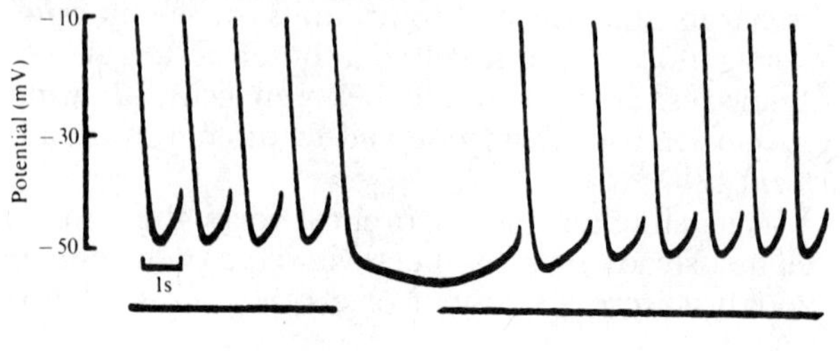

Recordings from the region of the atrioventricular node have revealed that this structure accounts for the long delay between the end of atrial excitation and the emergence of activation in the His-Purkinje system. On the basis of anatomic studies and single cell recordings, the atrioventricular node has been divided into three regions: the atrionodal junction (AN), the node (N), and the nodal-His junction (NH). Transmembrane recordings from the N region reveal action potentials of the slow response type, and in these cells the upstroke velocity is insensitive to tetrodotoxin. Electron micrographic studies show a paucity of intercellular connections and a more or less random array of slender cells. Conduction velocity is exceedingly slow in the N region, and these electrophysiological and anatomic findings seem sufficient to account for the observed slow propagation.

Genesis of the Electrocardiogram

Excitation and repolarization of the heart creates an electric field that is distributed throughout the body. These currents produce potentials on the body surface, and when two electrodes are placed on the body and connected through an appropriate amplifier, an electrocardiogram, or graphic recording of the potential difference between sites, is obtained. Ordinarily, voltage is plotted on the vertical axis and time on the horizontal axis over an interval of time that is equal to at least one complete cardiac cycle. Voltage displacements with respect to time occur during excitation and recovery of the atrium and ventricle.

The form of the electrocardiogram is determined by the sequence of excitation and recovery, by the resulting potential differences on the surface of the heart (i.e., the generator), and by factors that determine current flow within a three-dimensional, bounded, nonhomogeneous conductor such as the torso. These latter factors help to explain the relation between epicardial potentials and their projection onto the body surface.

During normal rhythm, activation of the atrium begins in the sinus node (Fig. 4-12). The excitation

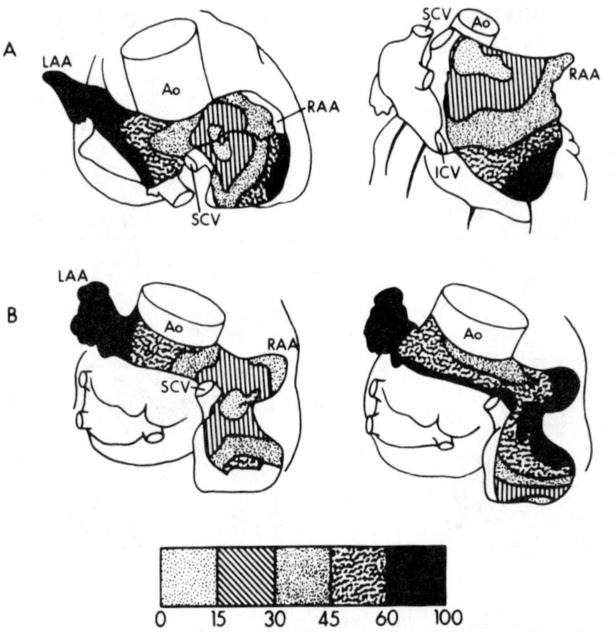

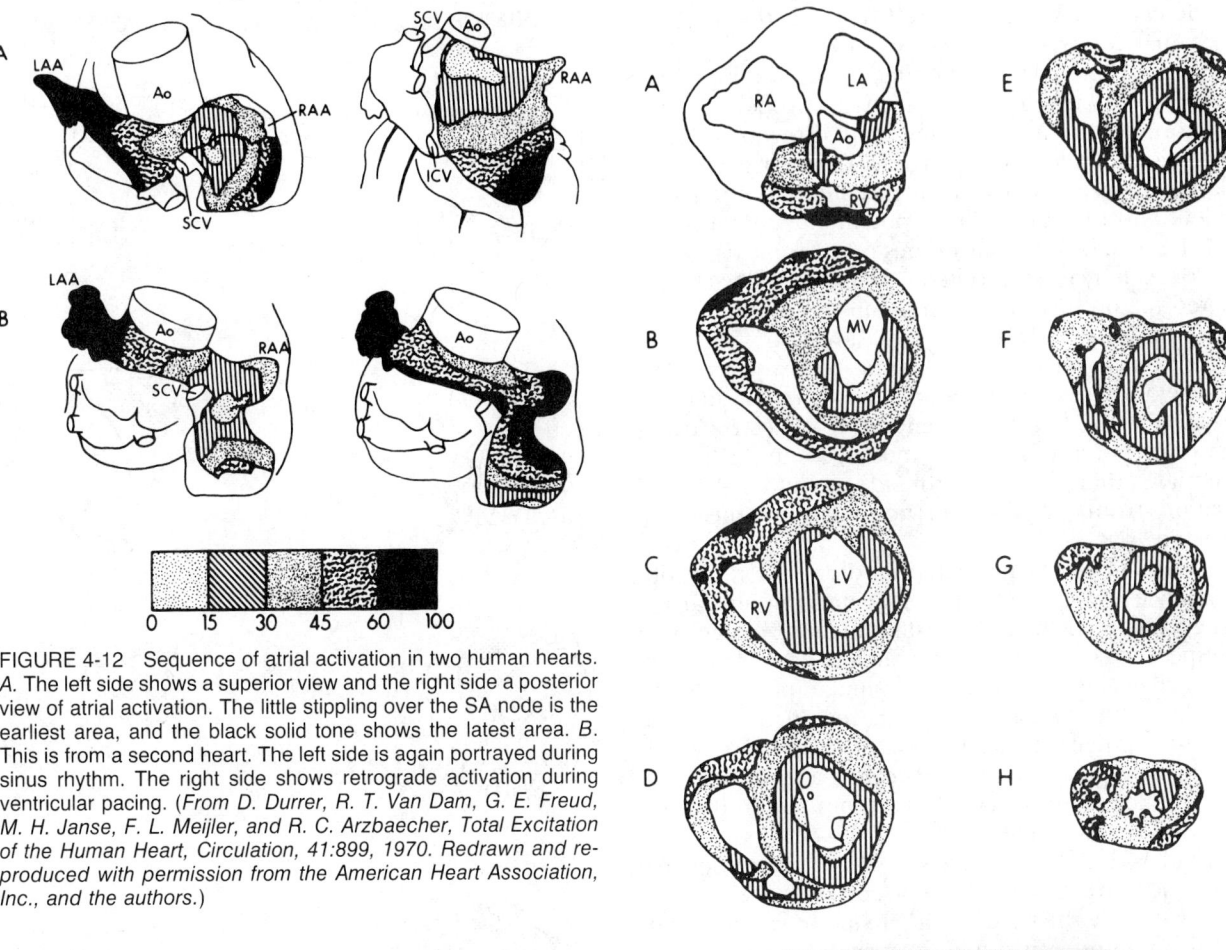

FIGURE 4-12 Sequence of atrial activation in two human hearts. *A*. The left side shows a superior view and the right side a posterior view of atrial activation. The little stippling over the SA node is the earliest area, and the black solid tone shows the latest area. *B*. This is from a second heart. The left side is again portrayed during sinus rhythm. The right side shows retrograde activation during ventricular pacing. (*From D. Durrer, R. T. Van Dam, G. E. Freud, M. H. Janse, F. L. Meijler, and R. C. Arzbaecher, Total Excitation of the Human Heart, Circulation, 41:899, 1970. Redrawn and reproduced with permission from the American Heart Association, Inc., and the authors.*)

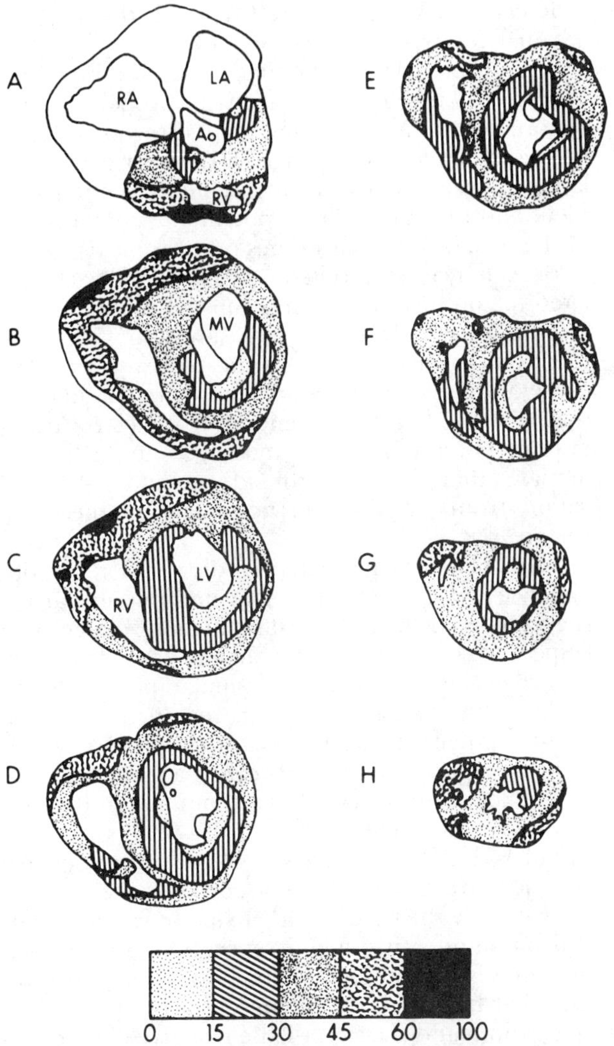

FIGURE 4-13 The normal sequence of activation of the human ventricle. *A* to *H*. Transverse sections from base to apex. In each section regions of similar activation times are enclosed by isochronous lines, and the temporal sequence is depicted in the legend. RA = right atrium; LA = left atrium; Ao = aorta; MV = mitral valve; RV = right ventricle. See text. (*From D. Durrer, R. T. Van Dam, G. E. Freud, M. H. Janse, F. L. Meijler, and R. C. Arzbaecher, Total Excitation of the Human Heart, Circulation, 41:899, 1970. Redrawn and reproduced with permission of the American Heart Association, Inc., and the authors.*)

wave spreads over the right atrium, from the head of the sinus node into the left atrium, and down the interatrial septum.[12] Because all three of these structures have thin walls, endocardial to epicardial spread is an insignificant factor in determining P-wave morphology. Because there are areas of preferential impulse propagation in the atrial walls and septum (see Chap. 2), the advancing wave front is irregular. However, the overall direction of the wave front is downward and from right to left.

As might be expected from the anatomic distribution of the Purkinje system, the general sequence of ventricular activation is from apex to base.[13] Initial excitation begins on the left side of the interventricular septum near the apex (Fig. 4-13). This is followed by activation of the endocardial surface of the right ventricle near the apex. Within a few milliseconds the impulse spreads rapidly over the entire Purkinje network and there are shells of depolarized endocardial muscle that encircle the cavities of both ventricles. Excitation first reaches the epicardial surface of the right ventricle at its margin with the interventricular septum. At the same time, wave fronts in the left ventricle are still confined to the intramural portions of the free wall. Midway through the QRS complex, epicardial breakthrough has been completed around the thinner right ventricle. The terminal portions of the QRS complex result from persisting activity in the basal regions of the left ventricle and upper interventricular septum.

The traditional approach for relating the activation sequence of the heart to the electrocardiogram is to assume (1) that the boundary between excited and still unexcited cells is a smooth, continuous surface, and (2) that any component of this surface is a potential dipole, one side of which is a source and the other a sink for current flow. The dipole theory also assumes that current flow is oriented perpendicular to the direction of propagation and that the strength of the dipole is related to its surface area. The potential at any site remote from the dipole is then proportional to the solid angle subtended by that dipole surface.

Recent work has indicated that this theory is inadequate to explain the electrocardiogram.[14,15] The critical problem is that the theory was developed for isotropic tissues in which electrical properties such as conductivity are the same in all directions. Heart muscle, however, is anisotropic. In the heart the relation between the spatial intracellular potential gradient and the extracellular potential is the opposite of that predicted from studies of isotropic tissue. As a consequence, extracellular potential is directly related to conduction velocity, and the orientation of a dipole is perpendicular to a slowly moving wave front but parallel to a high-velocity wave front. Because of these considerations, most current analyses that view the heart as a generator of electrocardiographic potentials use the measured epicardial potential rather than isochrons demarcating the activation fronts to simulate potentials on the body surface.[16]

Maps of epicardial potential distribution are obtained by placing electrodes at multiple epicardial sites and recording the instantaneous voltage with respect to some remote site such as the left leg. At any given instant, regions of similar potentials are enclosed by *isopotential lines;* a region of maximal positive potential is called a *maximum,* and a region of peak negative potential is called a *minimum.*

The location of maxima and minima on the epicardial surface change during the process of activation as does the relative size of regions of positive and negative potential. As a consequence, on the body surface the potential at any point varies in sign and amplitude throughout excitation. In general, the sign of the potential will be positive at recording sites that face a source of current arising from the epicardium and the sign will be negative if a recording site faces a current sink on the epicardium. The amplitude of a potential is a function of the distance between a recording electrode and the heart, but it is also influenced by the electrical resistivity of tissues between the heart and the electrode.[17]

During atrial activation excitation starts at the sinus node, creating an epicardial zone of negative potential (sink) with positive potentials over the still unactivated left atrium.[18] As a consequence, the right shoulder is in a negative portion of the resulting field and the left chest and back are in a positive portion of the field. For these reasons the P wave is negative in lead aV_R and tends to be positive (upright) in leads II, aV_F, V_5, and V_6.

During ventricular activation initial left-to-right activation of the septum (Fig. 4-13) produces positive epicardial potentials over the right ventricle and negative potentials over the left ventricle (Fig. 4-14). As a consequence the field on the chest is positive anteriorly and negative on the back (Fig. 4-15). Subsequently, with epicardial breakthrough over the right ventricle the right ventricular surface potential becomes negative while the left ventricle is positive (Fig. 4-14), and the consequence is negative potentials over the right shoulder and anterior chest and positive surface potentials over the left chest and back. Finally, as epicardial breakthrough develops over the apical portion of the left ventricle as well as the entire right ventricle (only the posterior base of the left ventricle is positive), the field on the chest is negative everywhere except on the back (Fig. 4-15). This sequence produces a QRS complex that is initially positive anteriorly (V_1), dominantly positive in inferior leads (II, III, aV_F) throughout midexcitation, and finally dominantly positive to the left and posteriorly (V_6) during late activation.

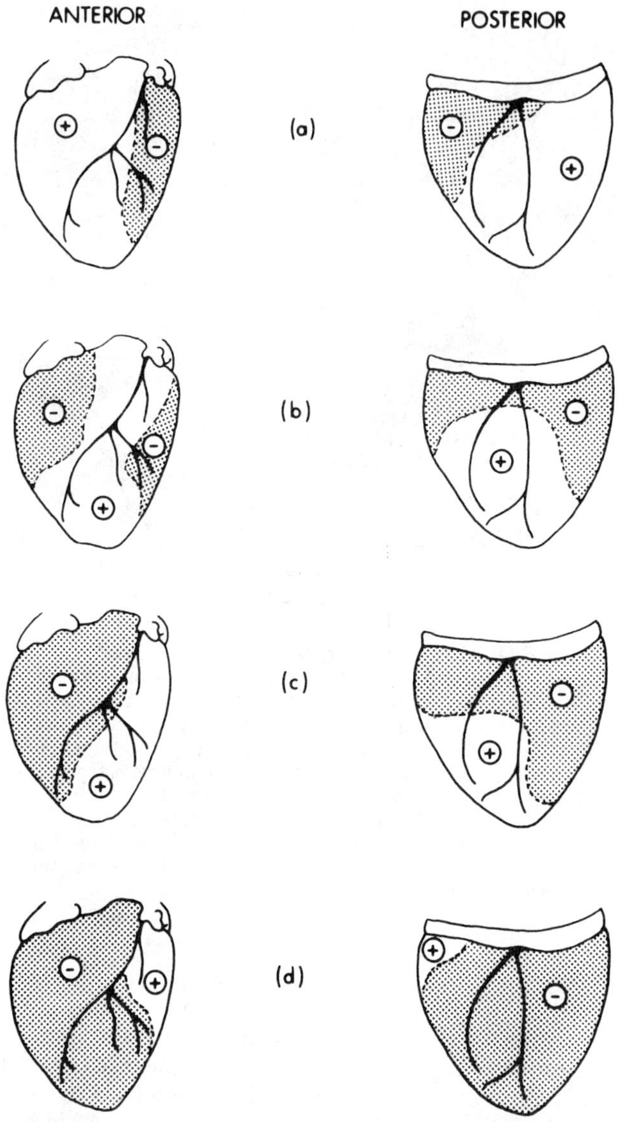

FIGURE 4-14 Epicardial potential distributions throughout the QRS complex. *a.* Very early ventricular activation. *b.* Approximately 20 ms into QRS. *c.* Approximately 50 ms into QRS. *d.* During terminal ventricular activation. Adapted from data regarding detailed isopotential maps of chimpanzee. See text. *(From M. S. Spach, R. C. Barr, C. F. Lanning, and P. C. Tucek, Origin of Body Surface QRS and T Wave Potentials from Epicardial Potential Distributions in the Intact Chimpanzee, Circulation, 55:268, 1977. Reproduced with permission of the American Heart Association, Inc., and the authors.)*

The action potential of ventricular muscle is long lasting (250 to 300 ms) relative to the duration of

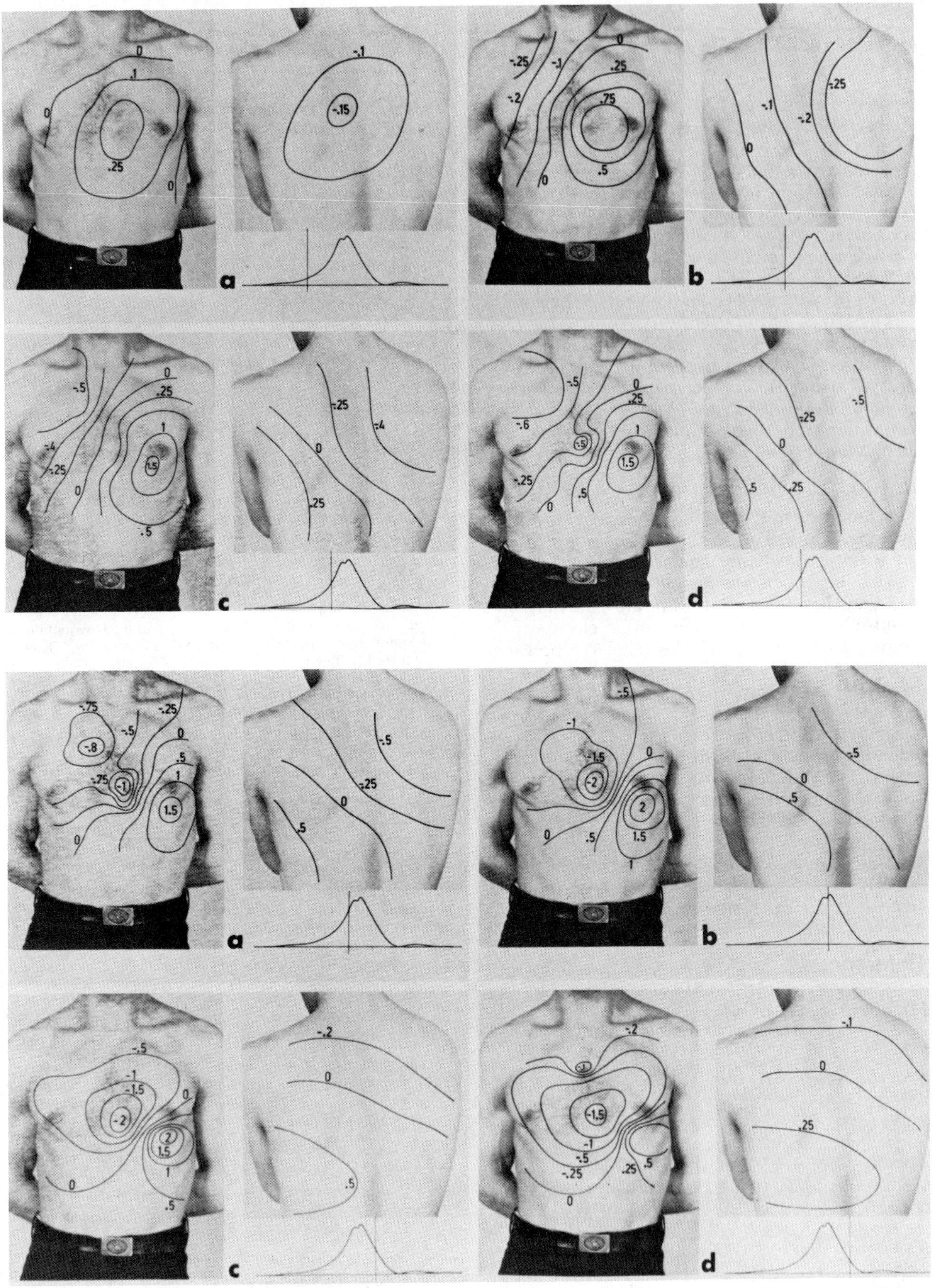

FIGURE 4-15 Isopotential maps of the thoracic surface in normal subject. *Top: a.* Onset of ventricular activation. There is one anterior maximum and one dorsal minimum. *b.* Early activation, dorsal minimum moves to right shoulder. *c.* The anterior maximum moves to the left nipple and negative potentials appear over the right anterior chest. *d.* A new minimum appears on right anterior chest. *Bottom* (continued from same subject): *a.* There are two anterior minima. *b.* The two anterior minima merge. *c.* Late QRS. *d.* Terminal QRS with maximum at lower left anterior axillary line and lower left back. See text. (*From B. Taccardi, Distribution of Heart Potentials on the Thoracic Surface of Normal Human Subjects, Circ. Res., 12:341, 1963. Reproduced with permission of the American Heart Association, Inc., and author.*)

the excitation process and the QRS complex (70 to 80 ms). Much of this long interval is accounted for by the plateau phase of the action potential: all cells are depolarized, the difference in potential between cells is negligible, the potential on the epicardial surface is uniform, and no appreciable electric field is created or recorded on the body surface. On the electrocardiogram this relative isoelectric interval corresponds to the ST segment, separating the end of the QRS and the beginning of the T wave.

The T wave of the electrocardiogram is the manifestation on the body surface of a changing electric field produced by repolarization of ventricular muscle. At a cellular level repolarization corresponds to phase 3 of the cardiac action potential. Because all cells do not repolarize simultaneously, voltage gradients exist leading to a distribution of positive and negative potentials on the epicardial surface. Several studies have demonstrated that repolarization starts later and lasts longer in the endocardium than in the epicardium. Hence, the sequence of repolarization is opposite to the sequence of excitation. This reversal in sequence is thought to account for the fact that the QRS and T wave are generally both positive or negative in any given electrocardiographic lead even though the cellular process underlying the QRS and T are opposite transmembrane electrical events. Generally, the amplitude of the T wave is less than that of the QRS because the magnitude of potential gradients in the heart at any time during repolarization is less than during excitation. The duration of the T wave is longer than the QRS, in part because repolarization takes longer at a cellular level, and in part because repolarization is not propagated. Whereas changes in conduction or ventricular mass dominate in causing changes of the QRS complex, metabolic factors and drugs dominate as causes of change in the T wave.

References

1. Waller, A. D.: Demonstration on Man of Electromotive Changes Accompanying the Heart's Beat, *J. Physiol,* 8:229, 1887.
2. Noble, D.: "The Initiation of the Heart Beat," Clarendon Press, Oxford, 1975.
3. Carmeliet, E.: Cardiac Transmembrane Potentials and Metabolism, *Circ. Res.,* 42:577, 1978.
4. Cranefield, P. F.: "The Conduction of the Cardiac Impulse," Futura Publishing, Mt. Kisco, N.Y., 1975.
5. Zipes, D. P.: Recent Observations Supporting the Role of Slow Currents in Cardiac Electrophysiology, in H. J. J. Wellens, K. I. Lee, and M. J. Janse (eds.), "The Conduction of the Cardiac Impulse," Stanfertdroese, B. V., Leiden, 1976.
6. McAllister, R. E., Nobel, D., and Tsein, R. W.: Reconstruction of the Action Potential of Cardiac Purkinje Fibers, *J. Physiol.,* 251:1, 1975.
7. Cahalan, M.: Molecular Properties of Sodium Channels in Excitable Membranes, in C. W. Cotman, G. Poste, and G. L. Nicolson (eds.), "The Cell Surface and Neuronal Function," Elsevier Publishing Company, Amsterdam, 1980.
8. Beeler, G. W., and Reuter, H.: Reconstruction of the Action Potential of Ventricular Myocardial Fibers, *J. Physiol.,* 268:177, 1977.
9. Wit, A. L., and Cranefield, P. F.: Effect of Verapamil on the Sinoatrial and Atrioventricular Nodes of the Rabbit and the Mechanism by Which It Arrests Reentrant Atrioventricular Nodal Tachycardia, *Circ. Res.,* 35:413, 1974.
10. Vassale, M.: Cardiac Automaticity and Its Control, *Am. J. Physiol.,* 233:H625, 1977.
11. Lieberman, M., Kootsey, J. M., Johnson, E. A., and Sawanobori, T.: Slow Conduction in Cardiac Muscle, *Biophys, J.,* 13:37, 1973.
12. Boineau, J. P., Moone, C. R., Hudson, R. D., Hugh, D. G., Erdin, R. A., Jr., and Wylds, A. C.: Observation in Reentrant Excitation Pathways and Refractory Period Distributions in Spontaneous and Experimental Atrial Flutter, in H. Kulbertus (ed.), "Reentrant Arrhythmias: Mechanisms and Treatment," University Park Press, Baltimore, 1976, chap. 6.
13. Durrer, D., Van Dam, R. T., Freud, G. E., Janse, M. H., Meijler, F. L., and Arzbaecher, R. C.: Total Excitation of the Human Heart, *Circulation,* 41:899, 1970.
14. Corbin, L. A., and Scher, A. M.: The Canine Heart as an Electrocardiographic Generator: Dependence on Cell Orientation, *Circ. Res.,* 41:58, 1977.
15. Spach, M. S., Miller, W. T., Jones, E. M., Warren, R. B., and Barr, R. C.: Extracellular Potentials Related to Intracellular Action Potentials during Impulse Conduction in Anisotropic Cardiac Muscle, *Circ. Res.,* 45:188, 1979.
16. Spach, M. S., Barr, R. C., Lanning, C. F., and Tucek, P. C.: Origin of Body Surface QRS and T Wave Potentials from Epicardial Potential Distributions in the Intact Chimpanzee, *Circulation,* 55:268, 1977.
17. Rudy, Y., Plonsey, R., and Liebman, J.: The Effects of Variations in Conductivity and Geometric Parameters on the Electrocardiogram Using an Electric Sphere Model, *Circ. Res., 44:104, 1979.*
18. Scher, A. M., and Spach, M. S.: Cardiac Depolarization and Repolarization and the Electrocardiogram, in R. M. Berne, N. Sperelakis, and S. R. Geiger (eds.), "The Handbook of Physiology," American Physiological Society, Bethesda, Md., 1979, p. 357.

5

Metabolic Regulation and Myocardial Function

Howard E. Morgan, M.D. James R. Neely, Ph.D.

Cardiac metabolism is a dynamic process that regulates production of high-energy phosphates on a beat-to-beat basis and turnover of heart proteins within periods of a few hours to several days. Energy reserves within the heart are severely limited; for example, as much as 5 percent of the total of ATP and creatine phosphate are consumed per beat, and the glycogen and triglyceride contents are able to support high levels of ventricular pressure development for no more than 6 and 12 min, respectively. As a result, the heart is dependent upon a continuous supply of substrate from the plasma to maintain energy production. Furthermore, both oxygen and substrates must be available because production of ATP by anaerobic glycolysis is limited to no more than 5 to 7 percent of normal energy production. The dynamics of energy production and utilization are best illustrated by measuring changes in high- and low-energy phosphate compounds during the cardiac cycle. Measurements of this type have not been technically feasible in mammalian hearts in the past because of the lack of methods to stop cardiac contraction during various phases of the cycle and the relatively small changes in total high-energy phosphate content that occur with each beat. The ability to make measurements during defined portions of the cycle has been obtained by use of phosphorus nuclear magnetic resonance (^{31}P-NMR) spectroscopy.[1] With this technique, the nuclei of phosphate compounds within the heart are induced to resonate by placement of the heart in a high magnetic field where it is bombarded with bursts of radio waves. Time resolution using this technique is approximately 2 ms, and potentially allows for 100 estimates to be made during each cardiac cycle. In well-oxygenated hearts that are perfused in vitro and supplied with only glucose as substrate, ATP and creatine phosphate levels are maximal during diastole and lowest during systole (Fig. 5-1). Conversely, inorganic orthophosphate (P_i) and the sum of low-energy compounds, P_i, sugar phosphates, and NAD are highest during systole and lowest during diastole. These data emphasize the dynamic nature of cardiac energy production and demonstrate directly the utilization and production of ATP and creatine phosphate during each beat of the heart.

Although turnover of protein and other macromolecular components of the heart occurs on a much longer time base than the high-energy phosphate reserves, the half-time for turnover of heart proteins and RNA varies from 1 h to several days.[2] The significance of the rapid turnover rate is that myofibrillar or enzymatic components of the heart can change in quantity or in type of isozyme over short time periods. For example, if synthesis of a specific cardiac protein with a half-life of 2 h were inhibited in ischemic hearts while normal rates of protein degradation were maintained, more than 95 percent of that protein would disappear after 12 h. If this protein were an essential component in energy production or contractile activity, functional capacity would be severely compromised. Fortunately, both synthesis and degradation of proteins are energy-requiring processes. Consequently, degradation of existing protein is reduced at the same time that synthesis of new protein is inhibited, and turnover rate is slowed greatly.

This chapter will focus on the biochemical mechanisms that sustain energy production and macromolecular synthesis and degradation by the heart. Fine control of the regulatory mechanisms is necessary to sustain the function of this vital organ.

General Features of Metabolic and Functional Alterations

Cardiac metabolism is regulated in a manner that sustains production of high-energy phosphate and contractile and synthetic activity despite large fluctuations in availability of carbohydrates, lipids, amino acids, and hormones. The metabolic versatility of the heart allows a wide range of substrates to be oxidized for energy production. Increased cardiac work stimulates substrate uptake and oxidation as well as biosynthetic processes in proportion to the need of the tissue.[3,4] As a result, metabolic and functional alterations that threaten cell survival occur only when coronary flow is reduced to the point that oxygen delivery and removal of metabolic products are severely compromised. However, lesser degrees of impairment can result from marked hormonal deficiency or during hypertrophy that is associated with overload of the left ventricle.

Modification of Function by Availability of Oxidative Substrates and Hormones

Fatty acids are the major fuel of the heart in normal animals, but glucose and lactate can make a large contribution following a meal that elevates insulin levels. When insulin is lacking, as in the diabetic, fatty acids and ketone bodies account for practically all of the oxidative fuel of cardiac muscle. Glucose utilization in the diabetic heart is impaired both by insulin lack and by indirect inhibitory effects of ox-

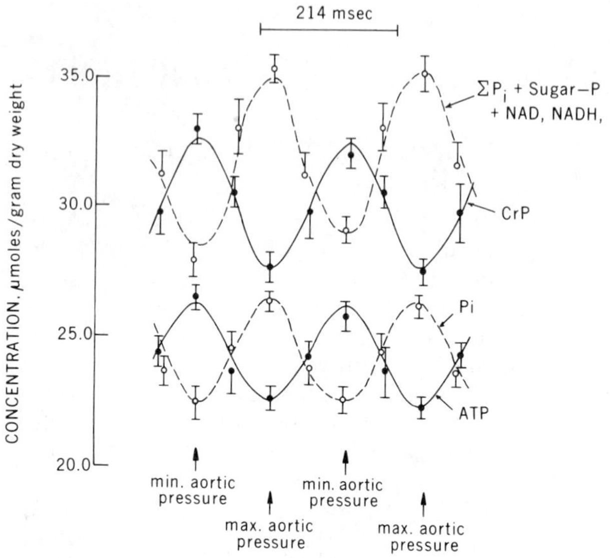

FIGURE 5-1 Concentration of ATP, creatine phosphate, P_i, and the sum of P_i plus sugar phosphates, NAD, and NADH in isolated working rat hearts that were perfused at an aortic pressure of 115/70 mmHg and provided 11 m*M* glucose in Krebs-Henseleit bicarbonate buffer. Maximal and minimal aortic pressures occurred at the times indicated. *(From E. T. Fossell, H. E. Morgan, and J. S. Ingwall, Measurement of Changes in High-Energy Phosphates in the Cardiac Cycle Using Gated P-31 Nuclear Magnetic Resonance, Proc. Natl. Acad. Sci. U.S.A.., 77:3654, 1980. Adapted and reproduced with permission from the publisher and author.)*

idation of fatty acids and ketone bodies on entry of glucose into the cell, on the glycolytic pathway, and on mitochondrial oxidation of pyruvate, the product of glycolysis. As a result, the small amount of glucose that is taken up is diverted to glycogen, and glycogen levels increase. Functional consequences of insulin lack may be observed when energy generation is dependent on glucose uptake and oxidation. An impairment of function has been observed in vitro when hearts from diabetic animals are supplied only glucose as exogenous substrate,[5] and an improvement of function has been observed in human diabetics who had impaired ventricular function following cardiac surgery and were treated with glucose and insulin.[6]

Modification of Function Mediated by Altered Protein Turnover and Gene Expression

Heart proteins have half-lives averaging approximately 5 days.[2] As a result, a complete complement of new protein is synthesized about every 3 weeks; from this point of view, a person has essentially a "new heart" each month. Maintenance of constant cardiac mass depends on equal rates of synthesis and degradation of protein. Similarly, constant levels of a specific enzyme or myofibrillar protein indicate that rates of synthesis and degradation of that particular protein are the same. Insulin, fatty acids, oxygen availability, and cardiac work affect rates of both synthesis and degradation. Synthetic rates can be modified by availability of ribosomes, messenger RNA, and enzymatic components (capacity for synthesis) or by the rate at which the components that are present are used to form protein (efficiency of synthesis). Efficiency of synthesis generally is well maintained, and changes in cardiac mass are accounted for by modifications in the capacity of the pathway. It should be noted that cellular components with short half-lives are particularly susceptible to derangements in protein synthesis or degradation. In hypoxic muscle, for example, degradation of mitochondria is accelerated; restoration of normal oxidative capacity is dependent upon rapid resynthesis of these organelles when normoxia is restored.

Gene expression also is under hormonal and metabolic control in heart muscle. Perhaps the best example of these changes occurs in relation to the isozymes of myosin.[7] The Ca^{2+}- and actin-activated splitting of ATP by one isozyme is faster than with the other. Speed of contraction in muscle correlates closely with myosin ATPase activity. Expression of the gene for the isozyme with high as compared with low ATPase activity is dependent upon the presence of physiological levels of thyroid and adrenocortical hormones and upon development of normal levels of ventricular pressure. For example, Ca^{2+}-activated myosin ATPase and speed of contraction are reduced in hypertrophied or hypothyroid hearts. However, the mechanisms that control expression of myosin genes are not understood.

General Mechanisms of Metabolic Control

Regulation of flux through a metabolic pathway occurs by four major mechanisms: (1) changes in levels of enzymes in the pathway, (2) changes in substrate availability, (3) allosteric control of key enzymes, and (4) covalent modification of enzymes.

Regulation Dependent upon Enzyme Levels

Regulation dependent upon enzyme levels involves changes in the rate of synthesis and/or degradation of the enzyme and generally occurs after exposure for a few hours to several days to altered substrate or hormone availability or work load.[2] As noted above, however, levels of enzymes with short half-lives can change rapidly. For example, the synthesis of ornithine decarboxylase, an enzyme associated with rapid formation of polyamines in hypertrophying hearts, increases within a few hours following imposition of increased afterload or induction of hyperthyroidism. In addition, availability of substrates or other substances that bind to the substrate site of an enzyme can decrease degradation and lead to increased tissue levels. An example of this type of regulation is provided by another enzyme in the synthetic pathway for polyamines, *S*-adenosylmethionine decarboxylase. In this case, a substrate analogue, methylglyoxal-bis(guanylhydrazone) (MGBG) binds to the substrate site, inhibits degradation, and leads to a tenfold increase in tissue levels of the protein after 24 h.

Regulation Dependent upon Substrate Availability

If a substrate is present at concentrations below that required for saturation of the pathway, substrate concentration can influence the rate of its utilization. For example, relative rates of glucose and fatty acid utilization depend to a large extent on the plasma concentrations of fatty acids. Fatty acid oxidation is increased when the plasma concentration is elevated above the usual physiological level and inhibition of glucose utilization occurs. On the other hand, rates of glucose utilization depend more upon availability of insulin and fatty acids and the levels of ventricular pressure development than upon the plasma levels of carbohydrate.

Regulation Dependent upon Allosteric Modification of the Enzyme

Various metabolites may bind to a site on an enzyme other than the substrate site and either increase or decrease the catalytic activity.[3,4] The rate of several glycolytic enzymes, including phosphofructokinase and phosphorylase *b* (Fig. 5-2), is controlled, at least in part, by this mechanism. Tissue levels of metabolites that increase in hypoxic muscle, including inorganic phosphate, 5′-AMP, ADP, and fructose-1,6-diphosphate, enhance catalytic activities of these enzymes, while metabolites that are present in high amount in well-oxygenated muscle inhibit catalytic activity. The rate that is expressed in vivo depends on the relative amounts of activators and inhibitors. This type of regulation is rapid and accounts for much of the fine control of metabolism.

Regulation Dependent upon Covalent Modification

The activities of several glycolytic enzymes, as well as other enzymes that are involved in amino acid metabolism and protein synthesis, are regulated by a phosphorylation-dephosphorylation mechanism.[3,4,8] Several of the enzymes are phosphorylated by the cyclic AMP–dependent protein kinase, but protein kinases that are regulated by Ca^{2+} and metabolic intermediates are involved in many cases (Fig. 5-3). Activation of glycogen phosphorylase is mediated by phosphorylase kinase, but this kinase is, in turn, activated by the cyclic AMP–dependent protein kinase. On the other hand, cyclic AMP has not been demonstrated to influence the activity of pyruvate dehydrogenase, either directly or indirectly. Phosphorylation may either increase the catalytic activity (phosphorylase, phosphorylase kinase, or phosphofructokinase) or inhibit the enzyme (glycogen synthase and pyruvate dehydrogenase). Although covalent modification is involved, the phosphorylation-dephosphorylation reactions are rapid and account for changes in catalytic activity over periods of seconds to minutes.

Regulation of the Glycolytic Pathway

Utilization of glucose and glycogen by heart muscle is regulated at a number of steps in the conversion of these substrates to acetyl CoA or lactate,[3,4] the final products of the pathway (Fig. 5-4). The activities of glucose transport, phosphofructokinase, glyceraldehyde-3-phosphate dehydrogenase, pyruvate dehydrogenase, glycogen synthase, and glycogen phosphorylase have been identified as regulatory sites that are affected by factors such as insulin, epinephrine, cardiac work, ischemia, availability of fatty acids, and diabetes.

Glucose Transport

Glucose movement across the cell membrane of heart muscle involves carrier-mediated transport of sugar

Effector	Change in concentration in hypoxic heart	Effect on catalytic activity	
		Phosphofructokinase	Phosphorylase b
Inorganic phosphate	↑	↑	↑
5′ - AMP	↑	↑	↑
ADP	↑	↑	↔
ATP	↓	↓	↓
Glucose - 6 - P	↓	↔	↓
Fructose - I, 6 - P	↑	↑	↔
Citrate	↓	↓	↔

FIGURE 5-2 Factors accounting for allosteric activation of phosphofructokinase and phosphorylase *b* in hypoxic heart.

Enzyme	Protein kinase	Effect of phosphorylation on catalytic activity
Glycogen phosphorylase	Phosphorylase kinase	↑
Phosphorylase kinase	Cyclic AMP - dependent protein kinase	↑
Glycogen synthase	Cyclic AMP - dependent protein kinase	↓
Phosphofructokinase	Cyclic AMP - dependent protein kinase	↑
Pyruvate dehydrogenase	Pyruvate dehydrogenase kinase	↓

FIGURE 5-3 Effect of covalent modification on the activities of glycolytic enzymes.

down a concentration gradient and, as such, may only equilibrate intracellular and extracellular glucose concentrations (Fig. 5-4). The transport system shows saturation kinetics, stereospecificity, and competition between different sugars, suggesting that binding of sugar to a membrane component involves a limited number of binding sites which behave in a manner similar to substrate binding to an enzyme.[3,4] Binding of insulin or an increase in ventricular pressure development somehow alters the rate of movement of glucose across the membrane. In the absence of insulin, the rate of transport is slow, intracellular glucose concentrations are low, and transport represents the major restriction to glucose utilization. When insulin is present, transport is accelerated and intracellular glucose concentrations approach the extracellular value. In these circumstances, intracellular phosphorylation of sugar

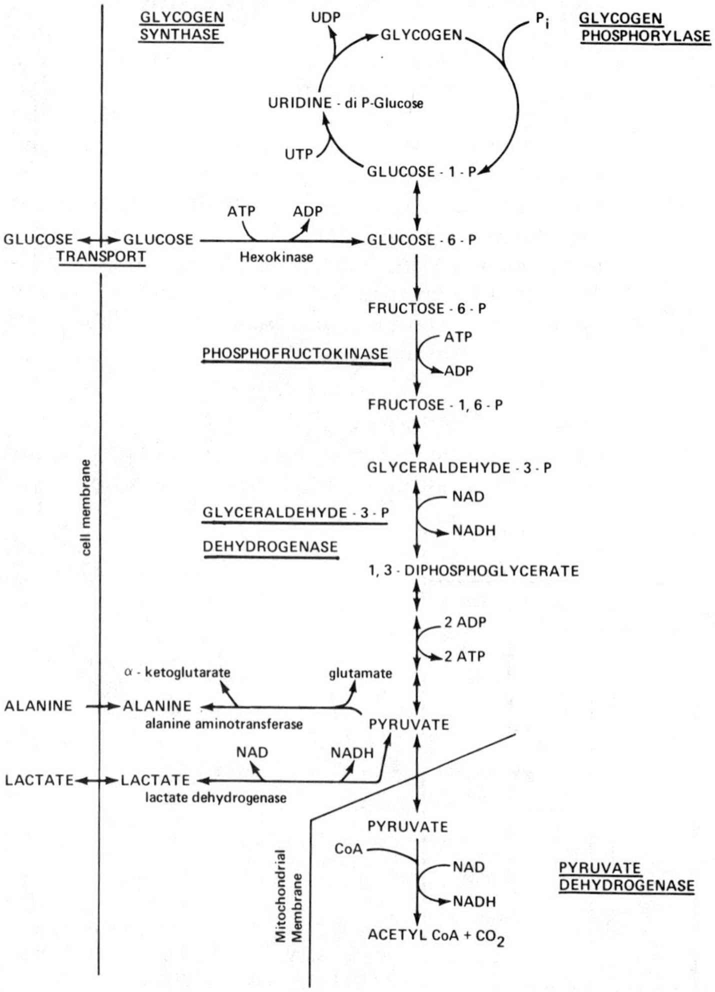

FIGURE 5-4 Simplified pathway of glucose and glycogen metabolism in heart. Sites of metabolic regulation are indicated by underlining the name of the reaction.

restricts the overall rate of utilization. In the diabetic heart, transport is less sensitive to stimulation by insulin; for example, a given concentration of insulin within the physiological range results in less acceleration of transport in diabetic as compared with normal hearts. Transport is inhibited in normal hearts by oxidation of fatty acids, and the decreased sensitivity to insulin in diabetic hearts has been associated with increased plasma and tissue levels of fatty acid. Hypophysectomy of diabetic animals restores insulin sensitivity perhaps because there is less mobilization of fatty acid from adipose tissue. Inhibition of fatty acid oxidation in isolated hearts restores insulin sensitivity toward normal. Increased cardiac work accelerates transport both in the presence and absence of insulin, but not in the presence of high concentrations of fatty acid. The mechanism of this work effect is now known.

In addition to increased cardiac work and insulin, hypoxia accelerates glucose transport in hearts from normal animals. In addition, hypoxia renders the transport system more sensitive to stimulation by insulin. In hearts of diabetic animals, however, there is less acceleration of transport as a result of hypoxia or increased cardiac work. These observations suggest that hypoxia, increased cardiac work, and oxidation of fatty acids exert control on glucose transport principally by altering insulin sensitivity rather than through direct effects on the carrier system.

Glycogen Metabolism

Glycogen synthesis and degradation occur by separate pathways (Fig. 5-4). Synthesis involves transfer of the glucose moiety from uridine diphosphoglucose to glycogen and is catalyzed by glycogen synthase. Glycogen synthase occurs in two forms, *a* and *b*. Conversion of one form to the other depends upon a phosphorylation-dephosphorylation mechanism.[3,4,8] The *a*, or active, form is dephosphorylated (Fig. 5-3). Synthase *a* is converted to the *b* form by phosphorylation that is catalyzed by a cyclic AMP–dependent protein kinase. The activities of both forms are increased by glucose-6-phosphate, but the activity of the *b* form is completely dependent upon this allosteric effector.

Phosphorylase catalyzes the transfer of a glucose residue from glycogen to glucose-1-phosphate. Phosphorylase also occurs in two forms, *a* and *b*. The *a* form is the phosphorylated form of the enzyme and is active in the absence of AMP (Fig. 5-3). Activity of the *b* form is dependent upon AMP for activity, and the activity is inhibited by ATP and glucose-6-phosphate (Fig. 5-2). Conversion of phosphorylase *b* to phosphorylase *a* is catalyzed by phosphorylase kinase, an enzyme whose activity also is controlled by phosphorylation-dephosphorylation (Fig. 5-3).

Turnover of glycogen is regulated both by hormonal and nonhormonal factors. Epinephrine activates adenylate cyclase, increases cyclic AMP levels, and results in conversion of phosphorylase to the *a* form and synthase to the *b* form.[8] Glycogen breakdown ensues. Insulin increases the fraction of synthase in the *a* form and raises glycogen levels. Hypoxia also results in *b*-to-*a* conversion and, in addition, activates the *b* form by a decrease in ATP and an increase in 5′-AMP and P_i concentrations. Glycogenolysis is rapid under these conditions. Myocardial glycogen metabolism differs from that of skeletal muscle in that starvation and diabetes increase the glycogen concentration. These effects appear to depend upon increased plasma levels of free fatty acids and ketone bodies. Oxidation of these substrates increase tissue levels of glucose-6-phosphate, as will be discussed in the next section. Glucose-6-phosphate activates glycogen synthase and inhibits phosphorylase; these changes in enzyme activity appear to account for the glycogen accumulation.

Glucose Phosphorylation

Glucose is phosphorylated by hexokinase using ATP as the energy donor.[3,4] The enzyme occurs both in soluble (30 percent) and particulate (70 percent) forms; both forms are inhibited by the product of the reaction, glucose-6-phosphate. The major factor regulating the rate of glucose phosphorylation is the concentration of glucose-6-phosphate. The principal reaction that controls glycolysis and glycogen metabolism and determines the tissue level of glucose-6-phosphate is phosphofructokinase. The activity of this enzyme is regulated by allosteric effectors and by covalent modification. In general, situations that lead to decreased tissue levels of high-energy phosphates, such as hypoxia and increased cardiac work, increase phosphofructokinase activity, while conditions that increase energy levels and provide alternative oxidative substrates, such as diabetes and elevated plasma levels of fatty acid, decrease activity. These inhibitory effects appear to be mediated both by higher energy levels and accumulation of citrate, a product of fatty acid oxidation. Intracellular pH also appears to have a large effect on phosphofructokinase activity. As pH decreases from 7.3 to 6.9, enzyme activity falls and control by allosteric effectors is much more marked. In contrast to regulation of phosphofructokinase activity by allosteric effectors, the physiological role of covalent modification is not understood at present.

Activation of phosphofructokinase leads to accumulation of fructose-1,6-diphosphate, and a shift in the rate-limiting step of glycolysis to glyceraldehyde-3-phosphate dehydrogenase in hearts that are perfused under anoxic or ischemic conditions and in aerobic hearts at very high levels of cardiac work. Factors that restrict activity of the dehydrogenase include accumulation of NADH, H^+, and lactate. Because high levels of these intermediates accumulate during ischemia, glycolysis may be blocked at the dehydrogenase step. In these cases, increased cytosolic NADH appears to be most important in restricting the rate.

Pyruvate Metabolism

Pyruvate that is formed by glycolysis can be released from the heart as lactate or alanine or can be oxidized within the mitochondria to acetyl CoA and CO_2 (Fig. 5-4). Both lactate dehydrogenase and alanine aminotransferase catalyze near-equilibrium reactions that are dependent upon the levels of NAD, NADH, α-ketoglutarate, and glutamate in the cytosol. When NADH and pyruvate levels are increased, such as in hypoxic muscle, production of lactate and alanine are raised. Oxidation of pyruvate to acetyl CoA is an intramitochondrial reaction that is catalyzed by the pyruvate dehydrogenase complex.[3,4] Because of its localization, the complex is in direct competition with beta oxidation of fatty acids for CoA and NAD.

Pyruvate dehydrogenase is a complex of five enzymes, three of which are involved with pyruvate metabolism (pyruvate dehydrogenase, dihydroxylipoyltransacetylase and dihydroxylipoyl dehydrogenase). The other two enzymes modify the activity of the pyruvate dehydrogenase component by phosphorylation and dephosphorylation of the enzyme (pyruvate dehydrogenase kinase and pyruvate dehydrogenase phosphatase). Phosphorylation decreases the activity, while dephosphorylation by the phosphatase activates. High NADH/NAD and acetyl CoA/CoA ratios decrease the activity of the complex. This effect is due, in part, to product inhibition (NADH and acetyl CoA are both inhibitors) and to inactivation by phosphorylation. Pyruvate dehydrogenase kinase is activated by acetyl CoA and NADH and is inhibited by CoA and NAD; the active kinase inhibits pyruvate dehydrogenase by phosphorylation.

In hearts from normal animals, approximately 20 percent of pyruvate dehydrogenase is in the active form. Activity is decreased in hearts from diabetic animals, in association with higher tissue levels of acetyl CoA and NADH. Furthermore, activation of the enzyme by cardiac work is blocked in diabetic tissue.[9] These effects of diabetes probably are examples of secondary alterations in glucose metabolism of the heart that result from increased fatty acid mobilization in the periphery and oxidation of the fatty acid by the heart. Inhibition and inactivation of pyruvate dehydrogenase can be produced in hearts from normal animals by perfusion with fatty acids or ketone bodies; these conditions result in high mitochondrial levels of acetyl CoA and NADH.

Integrated Control of Carbohydrate Metabolism in Heart

Both in vivo and in isolated hearts, fatty substrates are used in preference to glucose and glycogen. In well-oxygenated hearts that are developing normal levels of ventricular pressure, glucose transport is the major restriction to utilization of exogenous glucose, and glycogen breakdown is restrained at the phosphorylase reaction. The rate of transport depends upon the levels of insulin bound to the tissue and the availability of fatty substrates. Glycogen breakdown is restrained because phosphorylase is almost entirely in the *b* form and the activity of this form is inhibited by high levels of ATP and glucose-6-phosphate and low levels of 5′-AMP and P_i. The activity of phosphofructokinase is very low because of high levels of ATP and citrate. Under these circumstances glucose utilization is markedly reduced and most of the substrate that is taken up is diverted to glycogen. The final site at which fatty acid restrains glycolysis is at the pyruvate dehydrogenase reaction. Increased levels of acetyl CoA and NADH, products of the oxidation of fatty acids, inhibit the enzyme and lead to conversion of a larger fraction of the pyruvate that is formed to lactate.

An increase in ATP and O_2 consumption in heart muscle accompanies increased ventricular pressure development, or heart rate, or the presence of inotropic agents, such as epinephrine. When plasma fatty acid levels are low, an increase in ventricular pressure development accelerates glucose uptake and oxidation. This effect is accounted for by more rapid rates of glucose transport, glucose phosphorylation, and phosphofructokinase. Activation of phosphofructokinase is accounted for by lower tissue levels of ATP and citrate and higher levels of P_i. In these circumstances, pyruvate dehydrogenase is activated as a result of low NADH/NAD and acetyl CoA/CoA ratios in the mitochondria, and glucose oxidation is rapid. When plasma fatty acid levels are high, the heart preferentially utilizes this substrate because of the inhibition of pyruvate dehydrogenase, phosphofructokinase, phosphorylase, and glucose transport. Pyruvate dehydrogenase is inhibited by higher levels of NADH and acetyl CoA, while phosphofructokinase is inhibited by elevated levels of citrate and lower concentrations of P_i. Glucose phosphorylation and glycogen breakdown are restrained by higher tissue levels of glucose-6-phosphate that are secondary to inhibition of phosphofructokinase.

The most common causes of decreased ATP production in heart muscle are restriction of oxygen supply by hypoxia (decreased oxygen tension) or ischemia (decreased coronary flow of well-oxygenated blood).[3] Hypoxia results in a tenfold increase in glucose uptake and a rapid rate of glycogen breakdown. These effects are accounted for by acceleration of glucose transport, hexokinase, phosphorylase, and phosphofructokinase as a result of increased intracellular levels of ADP, AMP, and P_i, and decreased levels of ATP and glucose-6-phosphate. Because of lack of oxygen, conversion of pyruvate to lactate and alanine is rapid. It should be emphasized that the accelerated rate of glycolytic flux in the hypoxic tissue generates only 5 to 7 percent of the ATP that is formed in well-oxygenated hearts. As a result, tissue levels of high-energy phosphates fall. Ventricular failure is rapid in severe hypoxia.

In contrast to the sustained increase in glycolytic flux in hypoxic muscle, ischemia results in only a transient elevation that is followed by inhibition.[3,10] Inhibition occurs despite higher tissue levels of ADP, AMP, and P_i. Inhibition of the glycolytic rate is not overcome by insulin. In this circumstance, the rate-controlling step appears to be glyceraldehyde-3-phosphate dehydrogenase, whose activity is restricted by high levels of NADH, lactate, and H^+. In ischemic muscle, accumulation of lactate and hydrogen ions is more marked than in hypoxic hearts.

Regulation of Fatty Acid Metabolism

The rate of fatty acid uptake and utilization by the heart depends to a large extent on the concentration of fatty acid in the blood, but even more upon the metabolic activity of the myocardium.[11] The fatty acid that is taken up may be used for synthetic purposes, but in the heart it is used primarily for oxidation to produce energy. Cardiac muscle oxidizes fatty acids as the principal fuel for ATP production.

Because the overall rate of fatty acid utilization is determined primarily by the energy demands of the heart, an increased supply in the plasma has a limited ability to accelerate fatty acid uptake. The upper limit is reached when the supply exceeds the capacity of the cells to bind the fatty acids and to convert them to CO_2 and, to a much lesser extent, to form complex lipids and metabolic intermediates.

Fatty Acid Uptake and Activation

Fatty acids are supplied to the heart from the blood, where they are carried either as the free acid, usually bound to albumin, or as triglycerides in chylomicrons and lipoproteins (Fig. 5-5). The free fatty acid (FFA) is the principal form that is utilized by heart. The triglycerides are hydrolyzed to FFA by lipoprotein lipase prior to their utilization. The majority of plasma FFA is bound to albumin. The amount that is free in solution is small and is determined by the FFA/albumin molar ratio; the portion that is free is less than 1 percent of the total. The unbound pool of FFA is in equilibrium with albumin-bound plasma FFA and a tissue pool of FFA (Fig. 5-5). The exact nature of the tissue pool is not known, but probably is composed of FFA in the cytoplasm and FFA bound to intracellular membranes and soluble proteins. The uptake of FFA by cells does not require energy and functions only to maintain an equilibrium between plasma and cellular pools of FFA. When plasma FFA is raised to about 0.5 m*M*, uptake increases in proportion. With further elevations in plasma concentration, uptake is not proportional to concentration and finally reaches a plateau. Because the net rate of FFA uptake depends on the concentration gradient across the cell membrane, the rate of uptake is increased when removal of intracellular FFA is increased by raising the rate of oxidation, as with increased ventricular pressure development. Thus, the predominant control of fatty acid uptake in the heart appears to be related to the plasma content of unbound fatty acid, which is determined by diet and hormonal control of fatty acid mobilization from liver and adipose tissue, and the level of intracellular fatty acid, which is determined by the rates of FFA removal by cellular metabolism.

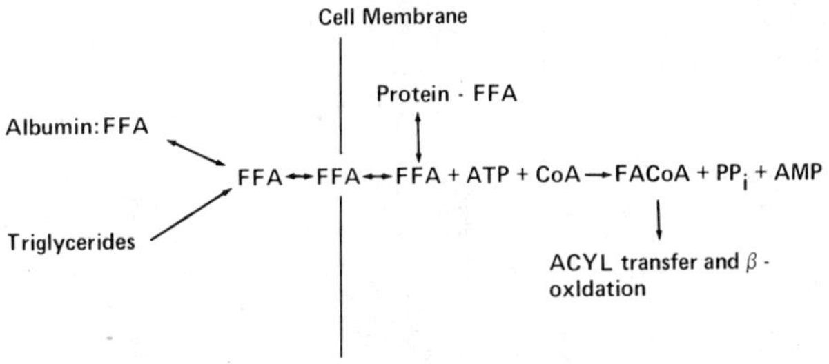

FIGURE 5-5 Fatty acid uptake and activation.

The first step in the cellular metabolism of fatty acids is their conversion to long-chain fatty acyl CoA (FACoA) esters. This process, referred to as *activation,* is catalyzed by long-chain acyl CoA synthases (Fig. 5-5). In heart muscle, these enzymes are located on the outer mitochondrial membrane. Fatty acyl CoA is relatively insoluble in water and is bound to cellular proteins and lipid membranes. The activities of the synthases are inhibited by all three of their products and are restrained by the low concentration of CoA in the cytosol. As a result, fatty acid activation is controlled by the FACoA/CoA and ATP/AMP ratios.

Mitochondrial Transport of Fatty Acyl Residues and Beta Oxidation

After FACoA is formed, it can be used either for synthesis of complex lipids in the cytosol or for oxidation in the mitochondria. Prior to mitochondrial oxidation, the fatty acyl moiety undergoes reactions that function to move the acyl group from the site of activation on the outer mitochondrial membrane to the mitochondrial matrix, where it is oxidized (Fig. 5-6). First, the acyl group is transferred from CoA to carnitine, and second, it is transported across the inner mitochondrial membrane. Transport of acylcarnitine involves an exchange reaction in which acylcarnitine moves across the mitochondrial membrane in exchange for free carnitine and is independent of metabolic energy. The third reaction in this segment is the transfer of the acyl group from carnitine to matrix CoA and forms FACoA in the matrix that is used for beta oxidation. In hearts that are developing low levels of ventricular pressure and are perfused with a range of palmitate concentrations in the buffer, the ratios of FACoA to CoA and fatty acylcarnitine to carnitine vary over a wide range,

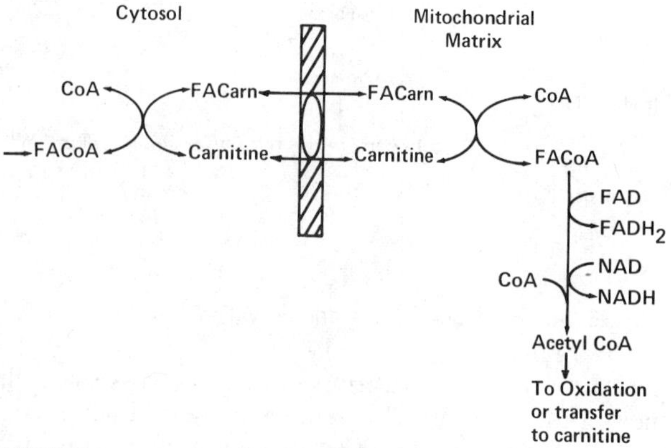

FIGURE 5-6 Acyl transfer, transport, and oxidation.

but a linear relation exists between the fractions of CoA and carnitine in the fatty acyl forms, suggesting that the transfer and transport systems are in equilibrium in the intact cell. With higher levels of pressure development and more rapid oxidation, however, the tissue level of fatty acylcarnitine (FACarn) increases while that of FACoA decreases. This observation suggests that, with rapid rates of oxidation, beta oxidation removes mitochondrial FACoA faster than either acylcarnitine transport or the transferase in the inner mitochondrial membrane can replenish the supply. If beta oxidation is inhibited, as occurs in ischemic hearts, most of the total CoA and carnitine are converted to their long-chain acyl derivatives within 5 min. Under ischemic conditions, the increase in FACoA/CoA is linearly related to the rises in FACarn/carnitine, again indicating that the system of transferases, as a whole, remained in equilibrium. Therefore, changes in the rates of these reactions on a short-term basis are most likely brought about by increased levels of substrates and/or faster rates of product removal. However, the reduction in fatty acid oxidation that occurs in the presence of high serum lactate, as might be found in an exercising person, results from inhibition of the outer carnitine-acyl CoA transferase.[12] This effect of lactate, or another metabolite whose level may be altered by lactate, suggests that this transferase reaction is regulated by factors other than levels of substrates and products. It is known that the isolated enzyme is inhibited by malonyl CoA and that cardiac muscle contains malonyl CoA.[13] However, it is not known if the lactate inhibition is mediated by changes in malonyl-CoA levels. On a longer time scale, the activities of the enzymes that are involved in fatty acid oxidation may be increased by synthesis of more enzyme, as has been demonstrated in exercising skeletal muscle.[14]

After production of FACoA in the matrix, the next major sequence of reactions involved in the oxidation of fatty acids is the beta-oxidation system that leads to production of acetyl CoA (Fig. 5-6). The most likely means of controlling these reactions is through the availability of one or more of the substrates: FACoA, CoA, NAD, or FAD. For example, acceleration of beta oxidation that results from increased work in cardiac muscle is associated with a decrease in the acetyl CoA/FACoA and NADH/NAD ratios. In ischemic hearts, levels of acetyl CoA decrease and levels of FACoA increase, indicating that beta oxidation is inhibited in association with a large increase in the NADH/NAD ratios. These observations indicate that the rate of beta oxidation depends on rates of oxidation of NADH and $FADH_2$ by electron transport and of acetyl CoA by the citric acid cycle.

In heart muscle, acetyl CoA that is produced by beta oxidation is used at appreciable rates only for oxidation by the citric acid cycle. The only alternative route for disposal of mitochondrial acetyl CoA is to transfer the acetyl unit across the mitochondrial membrane to cytosolic carnitine, where it is stored as acetylcarnitine. The acetyl transferase system has a very high activity in cardiac muscle, but the purpose of storing acetylcarnitine is not clear. Because there is about 10 times as much carnitine as CoA in the heart, storage of excess acetyl units as cytosolic acetylcarnitine may provide a buffer against large changes in mitochondrial acetyl CoA and may act as a reservoir of readily available substrate for oxidation.

Control of CoA and Carnitine Availability

Myocardial levels of CoA and carnitine vary with the nutritional and hormonal state of the animal. With fasting, CoA levels increase, and in diabetic animals, myocardial CoA increases by about 50 percent and carnitine levels decrease by about 30 percent. Thus there is a very large change in the carnitine/CoA ratio which may be important in shunting fatty acids to triglyceride synthesis under these conditions. Cardiac muscle does not synthesize carnitine, and regulation of its levels is mediated by changes in serum carnitine concentration and rates of membrane transport of carnitine into the cells. CoA, on the other hand, is synthesized by the heart using pantothenic acid taken up from the blood. Control of this pathway occurs at the level of pantothenate kinase, which is subject to strong regulation by external factors other than substrates and products.[15] Insulin is a powerful inhibitor in the presence of glucose, and a decrease in insulin levels may account for increased myocardial CoA synthesis in diabetes.

Integrated Control of Fatty Acid Metabolism in Heart

The control of uptake by the heart will be discussed for five conditions: (1) increased availability of extracellular fatty acids as a determinant of fatty acid uptake at low levels of cardiac work, (2) increased fatty acid oxidation that results from increased cardiac work, (3) decreased oxidation that results from restriction of oxygen availability in ischemic muscle, (4) decreased oxidation that results from the presence of alternative substrates, and (5) increased oxidation in diabetic hearts. The entire pathway of fatty acid oxidation is geared to replenish acetyl CoA, as this intermediate is oxidized in the citric acid cycle. Flux through the citric acid cycle is coupled to the rate of myocardial oxygen consumption through feedback control of the cycle by changes in levels of high-energy phosphates and NADH.

Increased availability of extracellular fatty acids raises the rate of uptake but uptake is limited when the capacity to oxidize fatty acids is reached. When hearts are perfused with high levels of fatty acids at low levels of cardiac work (Fig. 5-7), flux through the citric acid cycle occurs at a constant rate. Under these conditions, the rate of FFA oxidation is limited by the rate of acetyl CoA oxidation, and, as a result, acetyl CoA accumulates. Excess acetyl units that are produced from beta oxidation are transferred to the cytosol and stored there as acetyl derivatives of CoA and carnitine. Long-chain acyl derivatives of both CoA and carnitine also accumulate, but to a lesser extent than the acetyl derivatives. As a result of increased levels of acetyl and long-chain derivatives of CoA and carnitine, the levels of free CoA and carnitine decrease and limit activation and transfer of acyl units. Higher tissue levels of FFA result.

When cardiac work is accelerated and the rate of substrate oxidation increases, flux through the citric acid cycle is faster and levels of acetyl CoA and acetylcarnitine are diminished rapidly (Fig. 5-8); beta oxidation is stimulated and levels of long-chain acyl CoA decrease. Simultaneously, levels of free CoA and free carnitine increase, the rate of FFA activation accelerates, and FFA uptake increases in association with decreased cellular levels of fatty acids. Under these conditions, the slowest step for fatty acid utilization appears to be the capacity of the cells to transport acyl units across the inner mitochondrial membrane. The rise in FACarn most likely occurs in the cytosol, and this increase probably accounts for faster rates of transport into the mitochondria because of a higher cytosolic-to-matrix gradient.

Under oxygen-deficient conditions, i.e., ischemia and hypoxia, the amount of oxygen that is available to support oxidation by the citric acid cycle is reduced. Levels of $FADH_2$ and NADH increase, and beta oxidation is inhibited. Long-chain acyl derivatives of CoA and carnitine increase to very high levels (Fig. 5-9), and activation and uptake of FFA is reduced. High levels of fatty acyl CoA inhibit enzymes in both a specific and nonspecific manner.[16] Free fatty acids and long-chain acylcarnitine have a detergent effect at high concentrations and inhibit Na-K-ATPase.[17,18] Therefore, in addition to reducing capacity for ATP synthesis, myocardial ischemia also results in accumulation of compounds that potentially are detrimental to myocardial function and metabolism.

The presence of certain alternate substrates in the serum can modify the rates of fatty acid oxidation by the heart. For example, when serum lactate increases to 3 to 5 m*M*, oxidation of fatty acids is reduced and oxidation of lactate is increased. These concentrations of lactate would easily occur in the serum of exercising individuals. The inhibition by lactate occurs at the level of carnitine palmitoyl-CoA transferase I and represents another example of integrated control of the energy-producing pathways. The oxidation of fatty acids inhibits glucose utilization but glucose has little effect on fatty acid oxidation. This is probably because the fatty acid

FIGURE 5-7 Pathway for fatty acid oxidation in heart muscle. Metabolic intermediates that are elevated when hearts are perfused with 1.2 m*M* fatty acid at 60 mmHg ventricular pressure development are shown in boldface. This figure illustrates the two transferase systems for acyl units, each located on the inner and outer surfaces of the inner mitochondrial membrane. It includes compartmentation of CoA in two nonexchangeable pools (cytosolic and mitochondrial matrix); carnitine translocase is shown on the inner mitochondrial membrane between the two transferase systems. At low rates of energy utilization and excess fatty acid supply, most of the CoA and carnitine are converted to their acetyl derivatives. (See text for additional discussion.) [*From J. A. Idell-Wenger and J. R. Neely, Regulation of Uptake and Metabolism of Fatty Acids by Muscle, in J. M. Dietschy, A. M. Gotto, Jr., and J. A. Ontko (eds.), "Disturbances in Lipid and Lipoprotein Metabolism," American Physiological Society, Bethesda, Md., 1978. Reproduced with permission from the publisher, editor, and author.*]

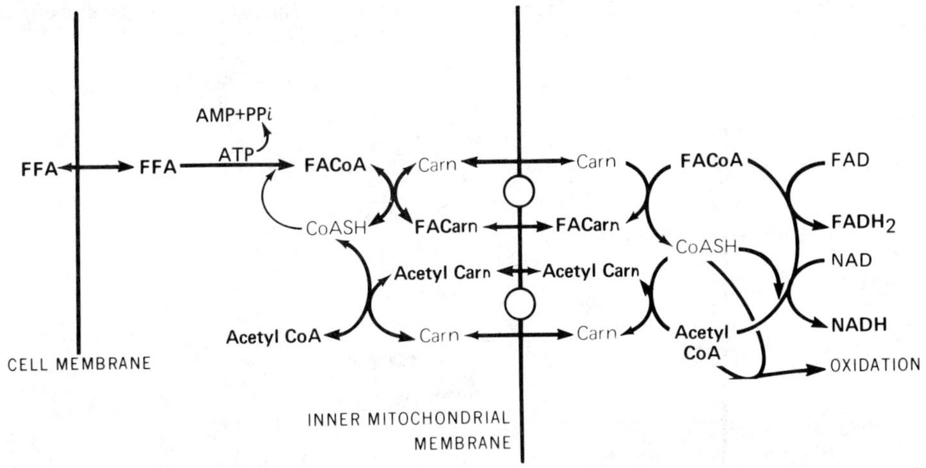

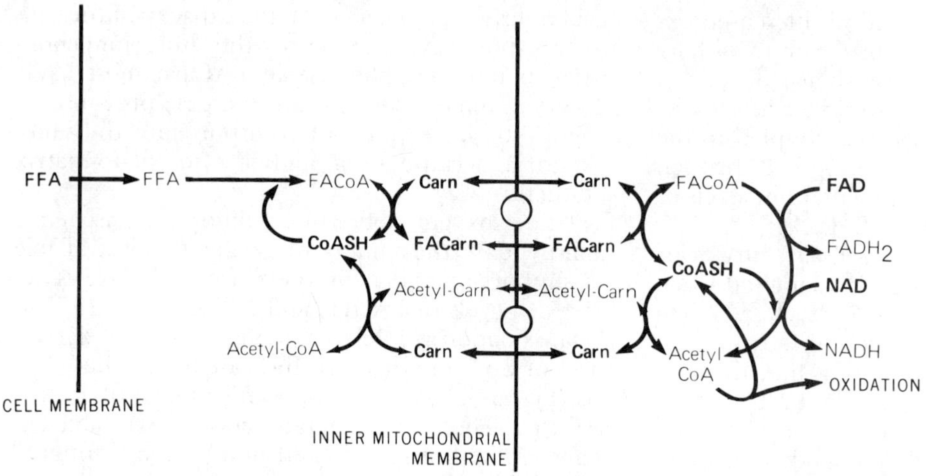

FIGURE 5-8 Pathway for fatty acid oxidation in which metabolic intermediates that are elevated when hearts are perfused with 1.2 m*M* fatty acid at 120 mmHg ventricular pressure are shown in heavier print. Levels of FACarn increased, but it is uncertain if the increase occurs in both cellular compartments. Most, if not all, of the increase was restricted to the cytosolic compartment. (See text for additional discussion.) [*From J. A. Idell-Wenger and J. R. Neely, Regulation of Uptake and Metabolism of Fatty Acids by Muscle, in J. M. Dietschy, A. M. Gotto, Jr., and J. A. Ontko (eds.), "Disturbances in Lipid and Lipoprotein Metabolism," American Physiological Society, Bethesda, Md., 1978. Reproduced with permission from the publisher, editor, and author.*]

inhibition of glucose transport and phosphofructokinase does not allow enough glycolytic flux to increase pyruvate or lactate to levels that are inhibitory for fatty acid oxidation.

As mentioned above, the heart of a diabetic animal oxidizes almost entirely fatty acids and ketone bodies for energy production. Alterations of fatty acid metabolism in the diabetic heart include increased tissue levels of long-chain acyl CoA and acylcarnitine esters, increased rates of esterification to complex lipids, and higher tissue levels of triglycerides. The increased acyl CoA and acylcarnitine esters result, at least in part, from a greater supply of plasma fatty acids and higher tissue content of CoA. This increase in total CoA may also contribute to the higher levels of long-chain acyl CoA and, because of the equilibrium position of the transferase enzymes, to higher acylcarnitine. The high levels of acyl CoA could account for increased triglycerides as a result of a mass action effect on triglyceride synthesis and an inhibition of triglyceride lipase.

Regulation of Protein Turnover

Disorders of ventricular function, high-energy phosphate formation, and substrate oxidation may result from inhibition of synthesis or accelerated degradation of specific heart proteins. Hypertrophy and reduction in cardiac mass depend upon changes in the relative rates of synthesis and degradation of all heart proteins. As mentioned earlier, turnover of heart proteins is a dynamic process that results in rapid replacement of proteins. The $t_{\frac{1}{2}}$ for turnover of cardiac myosin is 5 to 6 days. Protein turnover in the heart is affected by availability of hormones, oxidative substrates, and oxygen. Decreased availabil-

FIGURE 5-9 Pathway for fatty acid oxidation illustrating metabolic intermediates that are elevated during ischemia in hearts perfused with 1.2 m*M* fatty acid. (See text for additional discussion.) [*From J. A. Idell-Wenger and J. R. Neely, Regulation of Uptake and Metabolism of Fatty Acids by Muscle, in J. M. Dietschy, A. M. Gotto, Jr., and J. A. Ontko (eds.), "Disturbances in Lipid and Lipoprotein Metabolism," American Physiological Society, Bethesda, Md., 1978. Reproduced with permission from the publisher, editor, and author.*]

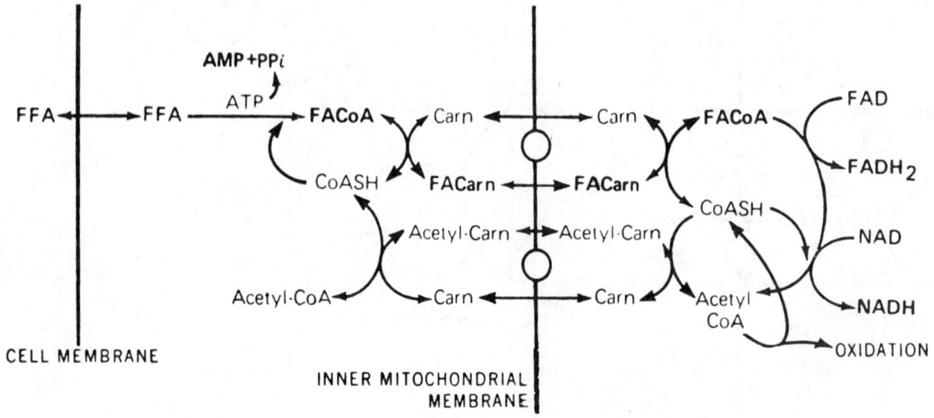

ity of these factors may perturb protein balance of the heart.

Regulation of Protein Synthesis

The pathway of protein synthesis is shown in Fig. 5-10.[2] Transport of amino acids into the intracellular pool is considered to be the first step in protein synthesis. On the other hand, extracellular availability of amino acids does not appear to restrain protein synthesis in the heart when normal plasma levels of amino acids are present. At least six transport systems for various classes of amino acids are present in most cell types:

1. The A system transports alanine, glycine, and other neutral amino acids with short side chains. It is Na^+-dependent and transports amino acids against a concentration gradient.
2. The L system is leucine-preferring, is not Na^+-dependent, and has highest affinity for neutral amino acids with branched-chain or aromatic rings.
3. The ASCP system transports alanine, serine cysteine, and proline and is Na^+-dependent.
4. Basic amino acids, such as lysine, arginine, and ornithine, are transported by the lysine system.
5. Acidic amino acids, such as glutamic and aspartic acids, are transported by the dicarboxylate carrier.
6. The beta system is a low-affinity system that transports beta-alanine and taurine.

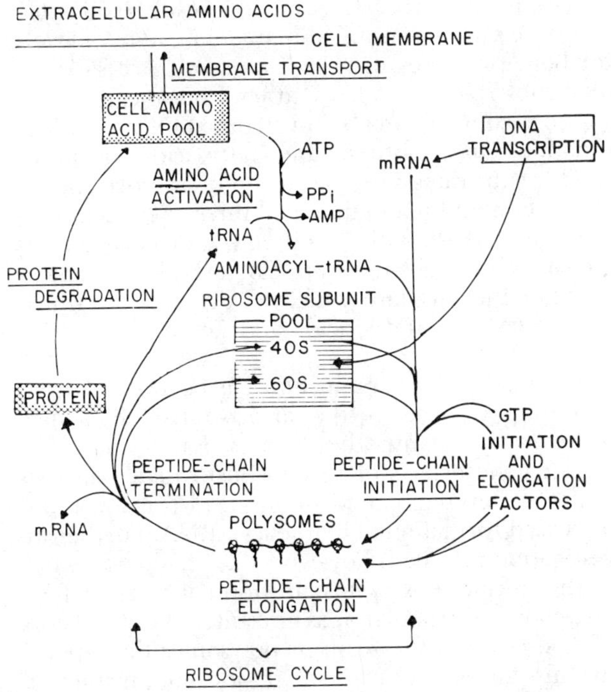

FIGURE 5-10 Pathway of protein turnover. Amino acids are supplied to the intracellular pool by either membrane transport or protein degradation. Intracellular amino acids are activated to form aminoacyl derivatives by combination with transfer RNA (tRNA). Polymerization of activated amino acids into protein is catalyzed by a series of ribosome-catalyzed reactions that make up the ribosome cycle. These reactions include initiation of peptide chains on the ribosomes and elongation and termination of chains. Peptide-chain initiation refers to binding of messenger RNA (mRNA) and initiator tRNA (methionyl tRNA$_f$) to the small ribosomal subunit (40 S), followed by the binding of the large subunit (60 S). Both steps require GTP and initiation factors. Peptide-chain elongation refers to successive addition of activated amino acids as determined by the code contained within mRNA. This process is dependent on elongation factors. When the protein is complete, the peptide chain and ribosomal subunits are released into the cytoplasm. Protein degradation refers to reactions catalyzed by proteases and results in the release of free amino acids into the intracellular pool. (See text for additional discussion.) [*From H. E. Morgan, D. E. Rannels and E. E. McKee, Protein Metabolism of the Heart, in R. M. Berne (ed.), "Handbook of Physiology," sec. 2: "The Cardiovascular System," American Physiological Society, Bethesda, Md., 1979. Reproduced with permission from the publisher, editor, and author.*]

The contents of amino acids within the intracellular pool are determined by (1) the rate of entry from the extracellular space; (2) the rate of exit from the cell; (3) rates of formation or destruction of the compound by transamination, oxidation, or other metabolic processes; and (4) rates of protein synthesis and degradation. As a result, intracellular levels of amino acids may fall even though protein synthesis is accelerated. These findings, in addition to the observation that 90 percent of the tRNA is in the aminoacyl form, indicate that steps that occur later in the protein synthetic pathway, such as peptide-chain initiation and elongation, are rate-limiting for protein synthesis in vivo.

The heart contains a pool of ribosomes that is present as either subunits or polysomes. These particles cycle from the subunit pool into polysomes through the peptide-chain initiation reactions. Initiation consists of the binding of mRNA, an initiator tRNA, and 40- and 60-S subunits, and is followed by translation of the mRNA to form a protein. Initiation of peptide chains in the heart is controlled by insulin, epinephrine, and glucagon; the availability of amino acids, fatty substrates, and oxygen; and the aortic pressure to which the heart is exposed.[19] As a result of the breadth of factors that regulate initiation, these reactions remain sufficiently rapid to keep most of the ribosomal subunits in polysomes and to shift the rate-limiting step to elongation and termination of peptide chains. These reactions are limited by the supply of ribosomes, elongation factors, aminoacyl tRNA, and guanosine triphosphate (GTP). In anoxic or ischemic hearts, high-energy phosphate reserves are depleted, including the GTP levels, and rates of protein synthesis are inhibited at the level of these ribosome-catalyzed reactions.

Regulation of Protein Degradation

The exact pathway by which proteins are degraded to free amino acids is not known, but lysosomes appear to be involved.[2] These organelles contain a number of hydrolytic enzymes, including acid proteases that are capable of degrading protein to free amino acids. Wildenthal and Crie demonstrated that chloroquine, a drug that is sequestered by lysosomes and inhibits their function, lowers the rate of proteolysis in fetal mouse hearts.[20] Similarly, it has been shown that swelling of lysosomes by exposure of isolated perfused hearts to amino acid methyl esters restrains the rate of protein degradation.[21] Lysosomal proteases have pH optima that are in the range of 2 to 4, a value much lower than the overall intracellular pH. One mechanism of the energy requirement of protein degradation appears to involve maintenance of low intralysosomal pH. Lysosomes often appear in the perinuclear region of myocardial cells and in the rows of mitochondria.

Changes in the total activity of lysosomal enzymes and the morphology of cardiac lysosomes are found to accompany a number of physiological and pathological changes in the heart.[22] The total activity of cathepsin D, a lysosomal protease, changes during thyrotoxic cardiac hypertrophy and its regression.[23] These findings suggest that changes in the lysosomal system are linked to physiological events that modify protein turnover.

In addition to acid proteases, proteolytic enzymes that have pH optima in the neutral and alkaline range are present in the heart. These enzymes include a soluble Ca^{2+}-activated protease that removes Z lines from myofibrils and particulate proteases that degrade protein to free amino acids. The physiological role of these particulate proteases is in doubt, however, because much of the activity appears to be localized in a nonmuscle cell, the mast cell. This finding illustrates one of the difficulties in defining the proteolytic pathway, namely, the presence within the heart of a variety of cell types, including fibroblasts, endothelial cells, mast cells, and phagocytic cells. Some of these cells are rich in proteolytic enzymes, but these proteases may play little or no role in normal protein turnover.

The energy requirement for proteolysis may involve not only maintenance of intralysosomal pH, but other steps in the proteolytic pathway. These steps include internalization of cytoplasmic components in lysosomes and an ATP-dependent proteolytic system in the cytosol.[24] The latter system has been investigated, particularly in reticulocytes, where it is active in the hydrolysis of abnormal proteins, for example, those that contain amino acid analogues. The energy requirement appears to involve initial steps in the proteolytic pathway because factors that reduce levels of high-energy phosphates, such as anoxia and ischemia, prevent the loss of activity of a specific enzyme, *S*-adenosylmethionine decarboxylase, and do not lead to the accumulation of the products of proteolysis, peptides and free amino acids, within the heart. In regard to effects of reduced oxygen delivery on protein degradation in the heart, it is important that the initial step in the pathway be blocked. Otherwise, proteolysis would proceed and result in inactivation of enzymes and contractile proteins and would contribute to irreversible damage in ischemic myocardium.

Factors other than activity or availability of proteases affect rates of protein degradation. Susceptibility of individual proteins to proteolytic attack is correlated with molecular weight, isoelectric point, and conformational state. In general, large proteins are degraded more rapidly than smaller ones; more acidic proteins have shorter half-lives; and alteration of conformation by cofactor or substrate binding decreases the degradative rate.

Integrated Control of Protein Metabolism in Heart

A wide range of factors affect either protein synthesis or degradation in heart muscle. These include (1) availability of amino acids, and particularly leucine, (2) supply of oxidative substrates, (3) availability of hormones, (4) adequacy of oxygen delivery, and (5) the level of aortic pressure. Many of these factors have opposite effects on the synthetic as compared with the degradative pathway; for example, insulin accelerates synthesis and inhibits degradation. These combined changes result in a marked reduction in net amino acid release.

Over long periods of time, protein synthesis depends on the availability of free amino acids in the plasma. Over short time intervals, however, the content of amino acids in the heart is usually well beyond what is required to saturate the synthetic pathway. Leucine appears to play a unique role in accelerating synthesis and inhibiting degradation. Plasma concentrations of leucine are increased during fasting and in diabetic animals and contribute to maintenance of cardiac mass in these insulinopenic states. The leucine effect may involve a direct effect of the amino acid on enzymes in the pathway or may result indirectly through its oxidation.

Both protein synthesis and degradation are energy-requiring processes, and, as a result, oxidizable substrate must be supplied to maintain energy levels for both processes. Glucose can serve as a satisfactory substrate for ATP synthesis but is unable to support control rates of protein synthesis or degradation. On the other hand, fatty acids and other similar substrates are able to both support energy generation and maintain equal rates of protein synthesis and degradation and nitrogen balance. Effects of these substrates appear to be important in insulin-deficient states, such as diabetes, in which plasma levels of fatty acids and ketone bodies are elevated.

For nearly 50 years, insulin has been recognized as an important factor that affects nitrogen balance in heart and many other tissues. Early studies attributed the effects of insulin on protein synthesis to an accelerated rate of amino acid transport and increased formation of aminoacyl tRNA. Further investigation revealed, however, that the major effect of the hormone is to sustain optimal rates of peptide-chain initiation and, as a result, to keep the pool of ribosomes in the form of polysomes that are active in synthesizing protein. In addition, insulin inhibits protein degradation and prevents formation of autophagic vacuoles from primary lysosomes.[25] In the presence of physiological levels of the hormone, rates of synthesis and degradation are equal and the heart is in nitrogen balance.[26]

Hypertrophy that results from increased ventricular pressure development involves greater efficiency and capacity of the synthetic pathway. As shown in Table 5-1, working hearts that are developing peak systolic pressures of about 145 mmHg have a rate of protein synthesis that is equal to the rate of protein degradation. High efficiency of synthesis is maintained in these experiments by inclusion of a substrate and hormone mixture that simulates normal plasma and by development of a physiological systolic aortic pressure. The more important factor accounting for growth of the heart is increased concentration of RNA within the heart. RNA levels are elevated within 1 to 3 days after imposition of a high work load, and increased capacity for synthesis is a major factor leading to increased cardiac mass. Whether the increase in RNA concentration is due to faster synthesis and processing of precursor forms of RNA or to reduced RNA degradation is unresolved. After the phase of rapid growth is over, RNA concentrations return to their original value.

Factors accounting for accumulation of more RNA in the early phases of hypertrophy are still unknown, but stretch of the ventricular wall appears to be the mechanical parameter responsible for maintenance of the efficiency of synthesis.[19,29–31] An elevation in aortic pressure from 60 to 120 mmHg increased protein synthesis in Langendorff perfused hearts. When ventricular pressure development was abolished by draining, protein synthesis still increased as aortic pressure was raised. In arrested hearts, protein synthesis was elevated in response to a higher aortic pressure despite the fact that no intraventricular pressure was developed. Stretch of the ventricular wall as a consequence of increased aortic pressure, the so-called garden-hose effect, may be the mechanical parameter most closely related to faster protein synthesis.

As described above, both protein synthesis and degradation are energy-requiring processes and are inhibited in tissues that are depleted of ATP and other high-energy compounds. After 1 h of ischemia (Table 5-1), rates of both synthesis and degradation are inhibited about 80 percent; but these rates are equal, indicating that loss of rapidly turning over proteins will be no greater in ischemic than in well-oxygenated tissue.

In hearts of diabetic animals, rates of protein synthesis are lower than in control aerobic hearts (Table 5-1). This reduction is due to reduced capacity (decreased RNA) for synthesis. The negative nitrogen balance of the diabetic heart is intensified by an increase in the rate of proteolysis. Furthermore, high levels of insulin are unable to normalize rates of protein synthesis in diabetic hearts. These findings indicate the precarious nature of the balance that maintains heart size in severely diabetic animals.

Relation of Metabolic Disorders to Myocardial Function

The ability of the heart to utilize a variety of carbon substrates helps to ensure a constant supply of ATP to support mechanical function even under adverse conditions of substrate supply. In addition, a disorder in one pathway is less likely to limit ATP production because the heart simply uses another substrate. The switch in metabolism of hearts in diabetic animals, as discussed above, is an example of the benefits derived from diverse metabolic capacities. The central role of oxygen and the complete dependence of the heart on oxidative production of ATP, however, makes this tissue particularly susceptible to decreased oxygen supply. Thus, hypoxia or ischemia greatly affects mechanical function. Other examples of metabolic disorders that affect mechanical activity are the alterations of protein metabolism that develop in different thyroid states. These two conditions, i.e., decreased oxygen supply and altered protein metabolism, will be discussed below.

Myocardial Ischemia

Cardiac muscle has the highest rate of oxygen consumption and the largest fractional extraction of ar-

TABLE 5-1 Effects of Cardiac Hypertrophy, Myocardial Ischemia, and Diabetes on Protein Turnover*

Conditions of Perfusion and Animal	Working Heart: Protein Synthesis	Working Heart: Protein Degradation
Aerobic perfusion, control	100 ± 3	107 ± 6
Aerobic perfusion, hypertrophying heart	124 ± 4	103 ± 2
Ischemic perfusion	23 ± 1	22 ± 7
Aerobic perfusion, diabetic	67 ± 2	137 ± 7

*Rat hearts were perfused in vitro as working or ischemic preparations with buffer that simulated the substrate and hormone levels of normal plasma.[27,28] Synthesis was measured by following incorporation of ^{14}C-phenylalanine into protein, and degradation was assessed by measuring release of phenylalanine. Rates are expressed as a percentage of the aerobic control rate of protein synthesis (954 ± 25 nmol phenylalanine incorporated into protein per gram of dry heart per hour).

terial oxygen of any tissue in the body.[3,4] The extraction of oxygen is about 70 percent compared with less than 10 percent for carbon substrates. Therefore, oxygen is the first substrate whose supply becomes limited when coronary flow is reduced. The small fractional extraction of carbon substrates coupled with decreased utilization of these substrates during ischemia (see above) suggests that their supply would never limit ATP production. Although the primary metabolic disorder of ischemic tissue is a subnormal oxygen supply, the metabolism and function of the heart is disrupted at all levels. The reduced oxygen supply results in a cascade of events that eventually affect every metabolic and functional process of the heart. In addition to reduced ATP production, slow flux through electron transport causes an accumulation of NADH in both the mitochondrial and cytosolic compartments. In the mitochondria, increased NADH inhibits the citric acid cycle, pyruvate oxidation, and β oxidation of fatty acids. The slowed rate of β oxidation results in accumulation of FACoA and FACarn (Fig. 5-9), and potential detrimental effects of these naturally occurring detergents are discussed above. In the cytosol, elevated NADH causes increased lactate production and inhibits anaerobic production of ATP by glycolysis. The lower oxidative neutralization of H^+ also results in decreased cellular pH, which affects a number of enzymes and cellular functions.

Perhaps the most significant secondary consequence of reduced oxidative metabolism is the net loss of adenine nucleotides from the total pool of ATP, ADP, and AMP. ATP is hydrolyzed to ADP, which cannot be rephosphorylated by either oxidative phosphorylation or glycolysis. Tissue levels of AMP increase because adenylate kinase converts 2ADP to ATP and AMP. Associated with this increase in AMP, production of its degradation products (adenosine, inosine, and hypoxanthine) is accelerated. In contrast to the phosphorylated nucleotides, these dephosphorylated degradation products can penetrate cell membranes and are lost from the cells. The removal of nucleotide products results in a net loss of the adenine nucleotides. Mechanical function of the heart depends on an adequate supply of ATP, and the loss of nucleotides is associated with onset of irreversible damage to the tissue. Unfortunately, cardiac muscle cannot rapidly restore the nucleotide pool, and tissue levels of ATP remain low with reperfusion of ischemic tissue. Several hours to days are required for restoration of normal ATP levels. Thus, one of the major advances in open heart surgery in recent years has been the use of cardioplegic solutions to preserve ATP levels during exposure of the heart to ischemia.

In addition to the loss of adenine nucleotides, accumulation of metabolic products cause damage to the heart that is independent of low ATP levels. Depletion of myocardial glycogen prior to exposing the heart to experimentally induced ischemia or inhibition of glycolysis prevents the large accumulation of lactate and other products of glycolysis that otherwise would occur during ischemia. Reducing product accumulation by these procedures greatly delays the onset of irreversible damage (Neely, unpublished observations).

Cardioplegic solutions vary considerably, depending on the institution, but the most important common ingredient is high $[K^+]$ to achieve cardiac arrest. Maintenance of contractility in the first few seconds of ischemia consumes large amounts of ATP at a time when production is suppressed. Cardiac arrest prior to induced ischemia prevents this energy wasting, and maintenance of arrest preserves adenine nucleotide levels. Hypothermic conditions also reduce ATP utilization by cellular processes other than mechanical contraction and help to preserve cellular ATP. Many combinations of substrates have been employed in attempts to improve anaerobic production of ATP, but these can be expected to have little beneficial effects on energy levels. Not only are the substrate-utilizing pathways inhibited by ischemia as discussed above, but hypothermic conditions have the same slowing effect on energy-producing as on energy-utilizing pathways. Attempts to preserve the viability of ischemic tissue should, however, include measures to prevent metabolic products from accumulating.

Myosin ATPase Activity and Cardiac Function

Velocity of contraction in skeletal muscle correlates with myosin ATPase activity. In cardiac muscle, myosin ATPase activity is highest in those species that have the fastest heart rate. Increased cardiac contractility is associated with elevated myosin ATPase activity in hyperthyroid animals.[7] In addition, decreased contractility is associated with depressed myosin ATPase in a number of pathological conditions.[32] These alterations in myosin ATPase activity and mechanical function of the heart are due to control of gene expression that results in a change in the content of the various myosin isoenzymes.

The myosin molecule consists of two heavy chains (subunits) that contain a tail region and a globular head region which possesses the actin-binding sites and the ATPase activity. The molecule also contains two light chains which are noncovalently bound to the head region of the heavy chains and may be important in controlling the ATPase activity. Ventricular muscle contains three isoenzymes of myosin that are referred to as V_1, V_2, and V_3. These isoenzymes are structurally distinct because they consist of different combinations of the two heavy-chain subunits. The ATPase activity is greatest for V_1 and least for V_3. The activity that is expressed in the intact muscle depends on the ratio of the different isoenzymes that are present.

Hyperthyroidism is associated with increased contractility of the heart in those species with low ATPase activity and slow heart rate, and hypothyroid states result in depressed myosin ATPase activity and contractility.[7] The ratio of V_1 to V_3 isoenzymes is highest in hyperthyroid animals and lowest in hypothyroid states. Thyroxine increases the synthesis of V_1 and suppresses synthesis of V_3.[33] Recently, these changes in isomyosin synthetic rates were shown to correlate with the levels of their respective mRNA, suggesting that regulation of myosin isoenzyme synthesis occurs at a pretranslational level.[34] Thus, effects of thyroxine on cardiac contractility are mediated through control of gene expression, which, in turn, determines the type of myosin isoenzyme that is present and, therefore, the activity of actin-activated myosin ATPase. This effect of thyroxine on isomyosins may account for the decrease in myosin ATPase activity in hearts of diabetic rats where serum thyroxine levels are greatly reduced.[35]

Concluding Remarks

The obvious question that arises from a more comprehensive understanding of myocardial metabolism is how this information can be used to describe the pathophysiology of heart disease and to plan therapy. In this section, three examples will be considered that represent either practical or potential applications of metabolic principles.

Perhaps the best example of a practical use of an understanding of metabolism is in the intraoperative protection of ischemic myocardium. As outlined above, therapy must be planned to reduce energy utilization rather than to increase high-energy phosphate production via greater substrate availability. This conclusion is based on the facts that substrate availability does not limit ATP synthesis in ischemic hearts and that factors such as hypothermia reduce both ATP utilization and production at the same time. Only increased oxygen delivery or agents that stop mechanical activity of the heart can be expected to prevent irreversible damage.

A second area in which an understanding of metabolic principles is of value is cardiomyopathies that are dependent on endocrine disorders. In the diabetic heart, optimal contractility is dependent upon substantial levels of free fatty acids or ketone bodies in plasma or upon adequate treatment with insulin. This situation results from the inability of the heart of severely diabetic animals to utilize glucose at a sufficient rate to support ATP production. In hypothyroid animals, contractility can be restored as a result of an effect of thyroid hormone on expression of the genes for myosin isoenzymes.

Finally, the potential exists for facilitating hypertrophy of muscle cells in response to an increased afterload or to loss of myocardial mass as a result of infarction. An improved understanding of factors that regulate RNA synthesis and protein turnover should aid in providing optimal conditions for growth of muscle cells and for recovery of ventricular function.

References

1. Fossell, E. T., Morgan, H. E., and Ingwall, J. S.: Measurement of Changes in High-Energy Phosphates in the Cardiac Cycle Using Gated P-31 Nuclear Magnetic Resonance, *Proc. Natl. Acad. Sci. U.S.A.*, 77:3654, 1980.
2. Morgan, H. E., Rannels, D. E., and McKee, E. E.: Protein Metabolism of the Heart, in R. M. Berne (ed.), "Handbook of Physiology," sec. 2: "The Cardiovascular System," American Physiological Society, Bethesda, Md., 1979, p. 845.
3. Neely, J. R., and Morgan, H. E.: Relationship between Carbohydrate and Lipid Metabolism and Energy Balance of Heart Muscle, *Annu. Rev. Physiol.*, 36:413, 1974.
4. Randle, P. J., and Tubbs, P. K.: Carbohydrate and Fatty Acid Metabolism, in R. M. Berne (ed.), "Handbook of Physiology," sec. 2: "The Cardiovascular System," American Physiological Society, Bethesda, Md., 1979, p. 805.
5. Miller, T. B., Jr.: Cardiac Performance of Isolated Perfused Hearts from Alloxan Diabetic Rats, *Am. J. Physiol.*, 236:4808, 1979.
6. Muller, J. E., Mochizuki, S., Koster, J. K., Collins, J. J., Cohn, L. H., and Neely, J. R.: Insulin Therapy for the Syndrome of Low Cardiac Output Following Cardiopulmonary Bypass, *Am J. Cardiol.*, 41:1215, 1978.
7. Morkin, E.: Stimulation of Cardiac Myosin Adenosine Triphosphatase in Thyrotoxicosis, *Circ. Res.*, 44:1, 1979.
8. Stull, J. T., and Mayer, S. E.: Biochemical Mechanisms of Adrenergic and Cholinergic Regulation of Myocardial Contractility, in R. M. Berne (ed.), "Handbook of Physiology," sec. 2: "The Cardiovascular System," American Physiological Society, Bethesda, Md., 1979, p. 741.
9. Kobayashi, K., and Neely, J. R.: Effects of Increased Cardiac Work on Pyruvate Dehydrogenase Activity in Hearts from Diabetic Animals, *J. Mol. Cell. Cardiol.*, 15:347, 1983.
10. Rovetto, M. J., Whitmer, J. T., and Neely, J. R.: Comparison of the Effects of Anoxia and Whole Heart Ischemia on Carbohydrate Utilization in Isolated Working Rat Hearts, *Circ. Res.*, 32:699, 1973.
11. Idell-Wenger, J. A., and Neely, J. R.: Regulation of Uptake and Metabolism of Fatty Acids by Muscle, in J. M. Dietschy, A. M. Gotto, Jr., and J. A. Ontko (eds.), "Disturbances in Lipid and Lipoprotein Metabolism," American Physiological Society, Bethesda, Md., 1978, p. 269.
12. Bielefeld, D. R., Vary, T. C., and Neely, J. R.: Site of Inhibition of Fatty Acid Oxidation by Lactate and Oxfenicine in Cardiac Muscle, *Fed. Proc.*, 42:1258, 1983.
13. McGarry, J. D., Mills, S. E., Long, C. S., and Foster, D. W.: Observations on the Affinity for Carnitine, and Malonyl-CoA Sensitivity, of Carnitine Palmitoyl-Transferase I in Animal and Human Tissues: Demonstration of the Presence of Malonyl-CoA in Non-Hepatic Tissues of the Rat, *Biochem. J.*, 214:21, 1983.
14. Mole, P. A., Oscai, L. B., and Holloszy, J. O.: Adaptations of Muscle to Exercise: Increase in Levels of Palmitoyl-CoA Synthetase, Carnitine Palmityl-Transferase and Palmityl-CoA Dehydrogenase and in the Capacity to Oxidize Fatty Acids, *J. Clin. Invest.*, 50:2323, 1971.
15. Robishaw, J. D., and Neely, J. R.: Pantothenate Kinase and Control of CoA Synthesis in Heart, *Am. J. Physiol.*, 246:H532, 1984.
16. Morel, F., Lanquin, G., Lumardi, J., Duszynski, J., and Vignais, P. V.: An Appraisal of the Functional Significance of the Inhibitory Effect of Long Chain Acyl-CoA's on Mitochondrial Transports, *FEBS Lett.*, 39:133, 1974.
17. Lamers, J. M. J., and Hulsmann, W. C.: Inhibition of (Na^+ + K^+)-Stimulated ATPase of Heart by Fatty Acids, *J. Mol. Cell. Cardiol.*, 9:343, 1977.
18. Wood, J. M., Busch, B., Pitts, B. J. R., and Schwartz, A.: Inhibition of Bovine Hearts Na^+, K^+-ATPase by Palmityl Carnitine and Palmityl-CoA, *Biochem. Biophys. Res. Commun.*, 74:677, 1977.
19. Kira, Y., Kochel, P. J., Gordon, E. E., and Morgan, H. E.: Aortic Perfusion Pressure as a Determinant of Cardiac Protein Synthesis, *Am. J. Physiol.*, 246:C247, 1984.

20. Wildenthal, K., and Crie, J. S.: Lysosomes and Cardiac Protein Catabolism, in K. Wildenthal (ed.), "Degradative Processes in Heart and Skeletal Muscle," North-Holland Biomedical Press, Amsterdam, 1980, p. 113.
21. Long, W. M., Chua, B. H. L., Lautensack, N., and Morgan, H. E.: Effects of Amino Acid Methyl Esters on Cardiac Lysosomes and Protein Degradation, *Am. J. Physiol.*, 245:C101, 1983.
22. Morgan, H. E., Chua, B., and Beinlich, C. J.: Regulation of Protein Degradation in Heart, in K. Wildenthal (ed.), "Degradative Processes in Heart and Skeletal Muscle," North-Holland Biomedical Press, Amsterdam, 1980, p. 87.
23. Wildenthal, K.: Lysosomes and Lysosomal Enzymes in the Heart, in J. T. Dingle and R. T. Dean (eds.), "Lysosomes in Biology and Pathology," North-Holland Publishing Company, Amsterdam, 1975, p. 167.
24. Hershko, A., Ciechanover, A., Heller, H., Haas, A. L., and Rose, I. A.: Proposed Role of ATP in Protein Breakdown: Conjugation of Proteins with Multiple Chains of the Polypeptide of ATP-Dependent Proteolysis, *Proc. Natl. Acad. Sci. U.S.A.*, 77:1783, 1980.
25. Long, W. M., Chua, B. H. L., Munger, B. L., and Morgan, H. E.: Effects of Insulin on Cardiac Lysosomes and Protein Degradation, *Fed. Proc.*, 43:1295, 1984.
26. Flaim, K. E., Kochel, P. J., Kira, Y., Kobayashi, K., Fossel, E. T., Jefferson, L. S., and Morgan, H. E.: Insulin Effects on Protein Synthesis Are Independent of Glucose and Energy Metabolism, *Am. J. Physiol.*, 245:C133, 1983.
27. Williams, I. H., Chua, B. H. L., Sahms, R. H., Siehl, D., and Morgan, H. E.: Effects of Diabetes on Protein Turnover in Cardiac Muscle, *Am. J. Physiol.*, 239:E178, 1980.
28. Chua, B., Kao, R. L., Rannels, D. E., and Morgan, H. E.: Inhibition of Protein Degradation by Anoxia and Ischemia in Perfused Rat Hearts, *J. Biol. Chem.*, 254:6617, 1979.
29. Arnold, G., Kosche, F., Miessner, E., Neitzert, A., and Lochner, W.: The Importance of Perfusion Pressure in the Coronary Arteries for the Contractility and Oxygen Consumption of the Heart, *Pflügers Archiv.*, 299:339, 1968.
30. Takala, T.: Protein Synthesis in the Isolated Perfused Rat Heart: Effects of Mechanical Work, Diastolic Ventricular Pressure, and Coronary Flow on Amino Acid Incorporation and Its Transmural Distribution into Left Ventricular Protein, *Basic Res. Cardiol.*, 76:44, 1981.
31. Vogel, W. M., Apstein, C. S., Briggs, L. L., Gaasch, W. H., and Ahn, J.: Acute Alterations in Left Ventricular Diastolic Chamber Stiffness: Role of the "Erectile" Effects of Coronary Arterial Pressure and Flow in Normal and Damaged Hearts, *Circ. Res.*, 51:465, 1982.
32. Scheuer, J., and Bhan, A. K.: Cardiac Contractile Proteins, Adenosine Triphosphatase Activity and Physiological Function, *Circ. Res.*, 45:1, 1979.
33. Hoh, J. F. Y., and Egerton, L. J.: Action of Triiodothyronine on the Synthesis of Rat Ventricular Myosin Isoenzyme, *FEBS Lett.*, 101:143, 1979.
34. Everett, A. W., Sinha, A. M., Umeda, P. K., Jakovcic, S., Rabinowitz, M., and Zak, R.: Regulation of Myosin Synthesis by Thyroid Hormone: Relative Change in the α and β-Myosin Heavy Chain mRNA Levels in Rabbit Heart, *Biochemistry*, 23:1596, 1984.
35. Garber, D. W., Everett, A. W., and Neely, J. R.: Cardiac Function and Myosin ATPase in Diabetic Rats Treated with Insulin T_3 and T_4, *Am. J. Physiol.*, 244:H592, 1983.

PART II

Methods Used to Collect Data on Every Patient (The "Routine" Examination)

The wise physician always views abnormalities of the cardiovascular system in the context of abnormalities of other organ systems. Good clinical judgment is not possible without such an approach. Accordingly, the physician attempts to identify the abnormalities of *all* organ systems. As part of this effort the physician must determine if cardiovascular abnormalities are present and, if present, what are their causes. This can be achieved by answering the following four questions.

- Is there an abnormality of cardiovascular structure and blood flow?
- Is there an abnormality of cardiac function and myocardial contractility?
- Is there an abnormality of cardiac rhythm or cardiac conduction (electrical abnormality)?
- Is there a metabolic abnormality such as myocardial ischemia?

When the *etiology,* altered *anatomy,* and altered *physiology* have been determined it is essential to identify the effect the disease process has on the present and will have on the future status of the patient. The consequences of the disease process are termed the *cardiac status* and *prognosis.* With this information, and after considering the abnormalities in the other organ systems, it is possible to offer rational medical and surgical treatment to the patient.

The questions listed above can usually be answered by utilizing the history, physical examination, electrocardiogram, and chest roentgenogram from all patients (or potential patients). These procedures are used when performing the *"routine" examination.* The more skilled the physician is in performing the routine examination the fewer additional procedures will be needed to answer the physician's questions about the patients and to solve the patient's problems. When additional procedures are needed, the physician should be able to select the proper procedures with greater precision. *The purpose of Part II is to discuss the clinical skills required to perform the routine examination and to highlight the approach to the patient (goals and cardiac appraisal).* If the routine examination does not solve the patient's problems or answer all of the physician's questions, the physician should consider whether it is necessary to answer these questions, i.e., if the answers to the questions can provide information necessary for the improvement of the patient's condition. If the answer is yes, the physician should then determine what to do next. *The strategy and techniques used to answer carefully thought-out questions that are not answered by the routine examination, but that should be answered, are discussed in Part III and Part VIIB through H.*

6

The Approach to the Patient: Goals and Cardiac Appraisal

J. Willis Hurst, M.D.

The professional man is in essence one who provides service. But the service he renders is something more than that of the laborer, even the skilled laborer. It is a service that wells up from the entire complex of his personality. True, some specialized and highly developed techniques may be included, but their mode of expression is given its deepest meaning by the personality of the practitioner. In a very real sense his professional service cannot be separate from his personal being. He has no goods to sell, no land to till; his only asset is himself. It turns out that there is no right price for service, for what is a share of a man worth? If he does not contain the quality of integrity, he is worthless. If he does, he is priceless. The value is either nothing or it is infinite.

So do not try to set a price on yourselves. Do not measure out your professional services on an apothecary's scale and say, "Only this for so much". Do not debase yourselves by equating your souls to what they will bring in the market. Do not be a miser, hoarding your talents and abilities and knowledge, either among yourselves or in your dealings with your clients, patients, or flock. Rather be reckless and spendthrift, pouring out your talent to all to whom it can be of service. Throw it away, waste it; and in the spending it can be of service. Do not keep a watchful eye lest you slip and give away a little bit of what you might have sold. Do not censor your thoughts to gain a wider audience. Like love, talent is useful only in its expenditure, and it is never exhausted. Certain it is that man must eat, so set what price you must on your service. But never confuse the performance, which is great, with the compensation, be it money, power, or fame, which is trivial.

Judge Elbert P. Tuttle, Sr., 1957[1,*]

From its beginning in 1966, *The Heart* has been written for physicians who take care of patients who have heart disease. Accordingly, it seems appropriate to set down some of the attributes of good physicians that seem to be timeless and to highlight some of the concerns of patients that are also timeless. Heart disease and its treatment should then be viewed in the context of the performance of good physicians and the concerns of the patients.

Attributes of Good Physicians[1]

The practice of medicine should be viewed as a bridge between medical competence and compassion. Compassionate physicians care about their patients and strive to be competent in what they do. In other words, compassion stimulates good physicians to be competent.

- Good physicians are trustworthy. Patients often assume that all physicians upon graduating from medical school are equally competent. This indicates that our predecessors produced a record of excellence by which we are all judged. Whether or not we are competent can only be answered by ourselves and by colleagues, but the trust patients have in physicians must not be violated by any of us.
- Good physicians are intelligent but they must be more than memory experts. The modern definition of intelligence is the ability to learn how to learn. Good physicians appreciate the essence of self-education. They are constantly asking themselves questions and pursuing the answers.
- Good physicians have an interest in scientific matters, especially in how the body works. The latter includes an intense interest in human behavior.

Physicians of today must know more than the physicians of yesterday about experimental design, statistics (e.g., Bayes' theorem), and the sensitivity, specificity, predictive value, and efficiency of test results. Sensitivity indicates the frequency of a positive test result in a population of patients with a certain disease. Specificity indicates the frequency of a negative test result in a population of patients without a certain disease. The predictive value of a positive test result indicates the frequency of diseased patients in a population of patients in which all of the test results are positive. The predictive value of a negative test result indicates the frequency of nondiseased patients in a population of patients in which all the test results are negative. The efficiency of a test indicates the percentage of patients correctly classified by the test. Bayes' theorem states that the predictive value of a test result is predetermined by the prevalence of the disease in the population being studied.

Physicians have learned to apply these descriptive terms to laboratory tests. The same descriptive terms should be applied to the results of the history and physical examination. For example, every story of chest discomfort does not have the same predictive value as a diagnostic marker of coronary atherosclerosis, and rales in the lungs are not perfect markers of heart failure.

- Good physicians must be able to read and understand the medical literature, to use test results

*Reproduced with the permission of the publisher and author.

properly, and to discuss medical matters with their colleagues. Tutors are not always available. Accordingly, physicians must be able to think and learn on their own. The medical literature becomes increasingly important to physicians who are sufficiently compassionate to wish to remain competent. Obviously then, physicians must be able to interpret what they read or hear, and to apply it to their daily work with patients.

- Good physicians are highly motivated people. They stand in awe at the wonders of the human body and how it works. They want to understand it. They care about the welfare of their patients and want to do all they can to help them. Their motivation is stimulated by their innate curiosity about body functions and the compassion they feel for their patients.
- Good physicians aspire to have good common sense. Common sense in medicine implies that physicians have sound pathophysiological or biochemical bases for their ideas and actions. This is very important, for all physicians must deal with variations of illnesses that are not exactly similar to those reported in the latest medical journal. Common sense in medicine can also be defined as a logical and defensible extension of the medical concepts that have been passed on to us by our predecessors. This implies that physicians who have a scholarly view of their profession trace the origin of the great ideas in medicine. They learn about those who had the ideas and how their ideas were challenged by some and accepted by others. They learn that what we currently say and do has come to us over the centuries and after much debate. Therefore, if one knows the origin of an idea, it is possible to extend it a bit, feeling that another step along a path that has stood the test of time is a reasonably safe step compared with a lateral step into the unknown.
- Good physicians have a sense of pertinence. They can separate trivia from meaningful material.
- Good physicians have a highly developed sense of priority. They can receive all the scientific and emotional stimuli that bombard them during a busy day and determine what they should do first, next, or last. This ability is extremely important since many, many lab tests can be ordered and many things can be done. The list of possible diagnoses may be long, and the physicians must determine the order in which each possibility should be explored.
- Good physicians recognize that it is necessary to establish realistic goals for patients. Is the goal to cure; to relieve; to stand by until the end comes; for the patient to return to work; or for the patients to simply feed themselves?
- Good physicians have good clinical judgment. Like common sense, this term is difficult to define. Physicians who display good clinical judgment seem to have considerable common sense (as defined above), a refined sense of pertinence, and a keen sense of priority. In addition, they have a demonstrated track record of making sound decisions in complex situations.

  The physician who is able to make good judgments on patients never views one body system as an isolated system. A physician who makes good judgments views the disorders of one organ system in the context of the disorders of other organ systems.
- Good physicians keep good records. Their records need not be long but they should indicate what they discovered in the patient; the data they used to make decisions; what they did for the patient's problems; and how they followed up on what they did (see later discussion).
- Good physicians have considerable organizational ability. Physicians recognize that it is not possible to render the medical care they wish to deliver unless they can lead nonphysicians to assist them in accomplishing their goals in the care of patients and in medicine generally. This attribute is more important now than it was in the past because medicine is more complex and more people are required to deliver proper care.
- Good physicians make themselves available. There is, of course, a limit to endurance, and good physicians must have appropriate rest. The patients of good physicians know that their physicians want to be available to them and, when they are not available, that appropriate "coverage" has been arranged.
- Good physicians are professionals. Judge Elbert P. Tuttle, Sr., offers us the finest definition of professionalism I know.[1] This definition is recorded at the beginning of this chapter.

I have not listed attributes such as honesty, integrity, and kindness as being attributes of good physicians. Of course, they are. But they are the attributes of all good people. What I have discussed here are the attributes of good *physicians*. I have assumed that good people have chosen medicine and that many fine qualities were learned in the home long before medical school matriculation. Older physicians in medical schools and hospitals should, however, teach by their actions how the kindness one possesses can be translated to the care of the patient. Very often a physician needs to prescribe a bit more of himself or herself for the patient rather than a tranquilizer. That is, the time spent talking to a patient may be better medicine than the latest drug.

Concerns of Patients

Some years ago, I had a serious illness. Therefore, I qualify as a patient and can express my concerns from that point of view.

- As a patient I do not like to be called a *consumer of health care*. This statement is dehumanizing. For the same reason I do not want the physicians who care for me to be called *purveyors of health care*.

- I believe that most patients want a physician they can talk to and who cares about their well-being and sees them as human beings.
- Patients want physicians to be honest but they do not demand that every rare and unusual complication be discussed to the point that they see themselves as exceptions who are doomed to the ravages of every simple illness.
- Patients can identify good physicians by the frequency with which physicians state they do not know. No physician knows everything and it is arrogant to present such a picture. Patients can identify good physicians by the sensitivity they have to the need for another medical opinion. Patients expect their physicians to assist them in their health problems and this includes obtaining proper consultation. Respect for physicians by patients is increased when the physicians express by words and actions that they want the best for their patients.
- Patients want their physicians to be available. They know that every human needs rest. They do not object to that. They do object to a poorly defined system of coverage when their physician is unavailable.
- Patients trust their physicians. This places the weight on medical schools, house staff and fellow programs, licensing agencies, and hospital staffs to determine whether individual physicians can do what they claim they can do.

The Whole Is Greater Than the Part

Mortimer Adler points out that truth is difficult to define but offers "the whole is greater than the part" as an example of a truth that is self-evident.[2] The human body is made up of organs and the whole body is greater than any organ. This is one way of emphasizing that the identification and management of the diseases of an organ (such as the heart) should not be the specific goal of any physician. *The proper perspective should be to view problems related to one organ in the context of the problems of other organs.* Coronary arteries are not admitted to coronary care units—*people* with coronary arteries are admitted to coronary care units. Many decisions regarding the management of heart disease are influenced by the diseases that are present in the other organs as well as by the personality of the patient. This is why physicians who have good clinical judgment manage the same disease differently in different patients. The old cliché is still true—*know* the patient and treat the whole patient.

Data Collection, Problem Formulation, Planning, and Follow-Up[3]

The medical data that physicians collect from their patients should be determined by the goals they set for themselves and their patients. If physicians are to render primary comprehensive care to patients, they must collect medical data from the patient that permits them to do that. If physicians are called upon to give opinions about the heart and blood vessels, they must collect data which will give insight about these structures, but they must also collect data about all other organs in order to make a decision about the heart and circulation.

Weed has pointed out the four steps a physician must take to transfer medical knowledge to the care of the patient.[3,4]

The data to be collected on every patient can be defined in advance and is called a *defined data base.* The cardiovascular data to be collected on every patient is discussed in Part II of this book.

After the facts (data) have been collected, the physician must analyze them and synthesize them into a list of "problems." The problems may be highly resolved (diagnoses), and no additional diagnostic work may be needed. On the other hand, the problems may be poorly resolved and may represent a symptom, a structural abnormality, a physiological derangement, a biochemical abnormality, etc., and additional work may be needed. It is useful to list and number the problems on a single sheet of paper which should be the first item in the office or hospital record. The *problem list* serves as the table of contents to the health of the patient. It makes it possible for a physician to view one problem in the context of all other problems. For example, the cardiovascular problems can be viewed in the context of the cerebral or gastrointestinal disorders.

Once the problem list has been carefully formulated, listed and numbered, it is then essential to develop and record the *initial plans* for each problem or to state why plans should not be developed for the problem. The problem for which plans are to be written is numbered and titled just as it is listed on the problem list. It is useful to develop a differential diagnosis for those problems that are poorly resolved and to develop and record the *diagnostic workup* that is planned for each possibility. The physician's sense of priority determines the sequence in which a workup progresses. The initial plans for each problem must indicate what *therapy* is to be used at that point in time. In many instances the physician should record the *instructions* given the patient (education of the patient). For example, the operative risks for coronary bypass surgery might be recorded as follows: "The patient and the family have been instructed that the operative risk in our hospital is about 1 percent."

Progress notes should be written for appropriate problems. They too should be numbered and titled to match the number and titles on the problem list and initial plans. Such notes should include the subjective and objective data related to the specific problem, the assessment of the new data, and new plans.

This is not the place to discuss the value of organizing data and action in the manner described above. The virtue of having a system in one's work is self-evident.[3,4] The system discussed above is teachable and serves to link data gathering and data analysis to the plans that are designed to improve a patient's well-being.

The Proper Use of Technology

The introductions to each part of this book should be read carefully. The introductions to Parts II and III are germane to the discussion here. The defined data base indicates the information that should be gathered on every patient. The tools used to gather the information are the history, physical examination, chest x-ray, electrocardiogram, and other routine laboratory tests. This data-gathering process can be implemented in almost all offices and hospitals. This technique permits the physician to identify the patient's cardiovascular problem at a high level of resolution most of the time. By performing the routine examination the physician should be able to determine if there is a structural abnormality or an abnormality of blood flow, an abnormality of cardiac function or myocardial contractility, an electrical abnormality (abnormal rhythm or conduction disturbance), or a metabolic abnormality such as myocardial ischemia. *The types of data to be gathered routinely are discussed in Part II.* If the problem is identified at a low level of resolution, the physician should ask whether further refinement of the problem is necessary. Can further clarification of the questions be translated into improved treatment of the patient? If the answer is yes, the physician should state the problems and phrase the questions in such a way that it is clear which test or procedure should be done next. Thus, the tests and procedures are chosen in order to answer specific questions. Accordingly, the tests and procedures that yield results that have predictive values that are sufficiently great to make decisions are utilized. *This important strategy is discussed in the introduction to Part III.* This approach makes technology the physician's servant rather than the reverse. This approach inhibits the approach in which the physician learns certain techniques and then tries to apply them and hopes that the results are useful. This approach is not only one of sound scientific medicine but it is, in my judgment, the only way the cost of medical care will be contained. A discussion of the techniques which are used to answer these questions can be found in Part VIIB through H.

The Cardiac Appraisal

The physician must ask the following questions. Is heart or blood vessel disease present? What other diseases or disorders does the patient have that require treatment or that might modify the treatment ordinarily used for the patient's heart disease? Do I really know all that I need to know about the patient's heart disease? This question leads to the purpose of the discussion in this section.

Dr. Paul White highlighted the elements of a "complete cardiac diagnosis" in 1914.[5] He translated his concept into action when he designed special cards that were to be filled out for every patient. The original cards had four surfaces; later he designed the cards so that a *defined data base* was displayed on six surfaces. The face of the cards showed his concept of a complete cardiac diagnosis. By the early 1920s this concept had been independently introduced and well established in the Massachusetts General Hospital in Boston and the Bellevue Hospital in New York City.[6] A committee of the New York Heart Association wrote the first edition of *Criteria for the Classification and Diagnosis of Heart Disease* in 1928.[7] There have been eight editions of this book and the title has changed a little over the years. The eighth edition was published in 1979 and is titled *Nomenclature and Criteria for Diagnosis of Diseases of the Heart and Great Vessels.*[8]

The series of eight editions of this book has had an enormous impact on the practice of medicine generally and cardiology specifically. The book should be read by all students, house officers, cardiac fellows, and physicians who are interested in the diseases of the heart and blood vessels. The book emphasizes correct nomenclature (which is essential for communication) and throws a spotlight on the elements of a complete cardiac diagnosis. The first six editions required the physician to establish the *etiology* of the heart disease, the altered *anatomy* of the heart disease, the altered *physiology* of the heart disease, and the *functional capacity* of the patient. The latter was determined by assessing the degree of symptoms, angina or dyspnea, expressed by the patient. Class 1 implied the patient had no symptoms. Class 2 implied that the patient had symptoms with more than usual activity. Class 3 implied that the patient had symptoms with usual activity. Class 4 implied the patient had symptoms at rest. The prognosis was then based on the functional classification. While the presence of symptoms is very important, symptoms do not always determine the seriousness of a disease process or enable one to determine whether a patient can work. Therefore the Criteria Committee of the New York Heart Association made a rather marked change in the seventh edition of *Nomenclature and Criteria for the Diagnosis of Diseases of the Heart and Great Vessels.* The following paragraphs are reproduced from the seventh edition and indicate in more detail the method of determining the *cardiac status* and *prognosis* of a patient. (These new categories replaced the *functional* and *therapeutic* classifications that were presented in earlier editions.)

The following excerpts from the 7th edition are reprinted below with permission from the New York Heart Association and its Criteria Committee, and Little, Brown and Company.[9]

From the preface:

The Functional and Therapeutic Classification of previous editions required that the physician classify the patient's cardiac status on the basis of symptoms alone, without regard to the etiologic, anatomic, or physiologic diagnoses. Although a consideration of symptomatology is essential for a correct physiologic diagnosis, it is now recognized that a classification of cardiac status based on symptoms alone may be misleading. Symptoms may be absent in the presence of serious anatomic and physiologic abnormalities, and the necessity for medical or surgical intervention may not be appreciated. In addition, symptoms may appear only after serious changes have taken place in the heart and lungs, which can prevent an effective attack upon the underlying defect. Further, some therapies may alter the symptoms and the course of the disease only briefly, whereas others may fundamentally change the course of the disease. Recommendations for therapy can rarely be based on a single diagnostic category; the implications of the other two categories also must be considered.

With these considerations in mind, a new classification, Cardiac Status and Prognosis, is presented. This classification should reflect an accurate assessment of each patient based on the etiologic, anatomic, and physiologic diagnoses and on an understanding of the benefits of present therapies.

From the introduction:

The *etiologic, anatomic,* and *physiologic* diagnoses of cardiovascular disease depend upon a careful analysis of the patient's history, a thorough physical examination, and, when indicated, a variety of laboratory examinations. Some of the latter are not specific for evaluation of the cardiovascular system, but represent an attempt to delineate the major problem. Others, such as electrocardiography, phonocardiography, echocardiography, cardiac catheterization, and a variety of radiologic techniques, are employed to detect the cause of heart disease or to identify specific anatomic and physiologic abnormalities.

The diagnostic categories are frequently dependent upon one another and, in the final synthesis, their compatibility should be examined.

The *etiology* of heart disease should be determined by considering both structural and functional disturbances. If two or more possible causes of heart disease are present, each should be mentioned. . . .

Anatomic lesions of the heart and great vessels usually can be recognized clinically. In some instances their manifestations are so specific that the anatomic abnormality is easily identified. Frequently, however, the presence of a structural lesion is inferred from a recognition of the cause of the heart disease, the identification of a physiologic disturbance known to result from it, or both. More than one anatomic abnormality may be present in any one patient; each should be included in the anatomic diagnosis.

Different *physiologic* disturbances often have similar clinical manifestations; the identification of the cause of the disturbance may therefore rest upon knowledge of the etiologic or anatomic diagnoses. Frequently, more than one physiologic abnormality is present; all should be included in the physiologic diagnosis. If no disturbance is present, the physiologic diagnosis is simply: Normal Sinus Rhythm.

Each of the diagnostic items has been assigned a code number. The grading of *Cardiac Status* and *Prognosis* is also coded numerically.

A complete cardiac diagnosis should include one or more titles from each of the principal diagnostic categories of this nomenclature: *etiologic, anatomic, physiologic,* and *cardiac status* and *prognosis.*

Certain patients may have symptoms, abnormal physical signs, or both which are referable to the heart, but which after detailed study cannot be ascribed with certainty to structural or functional cardiac disease. In such cases the diagnosis should be *No Heart Disease, Unexplained Manifestation.* Patients who have a disease such as systemic arterial hypertension, which can cause heart disease but which at the time of observation has not done so, are to be designated as having *No Heart Disease, Predisposing Etiologic Factor* (systemic arterial hypertension).

From the discussion regarding the cardiac status and prognosis:

The purpose of this classification, "Cardiac Status and Prognosis," is to assess the present cardiac status of the patient and to make a prognosis of the future status as modified by optimal therapy. *Cardiac status* represents a total assessment of the etiologic, anatomic, and physiologic diagnoses. *Prognosis* is based on an assessment of the potential effects of optimal current medical and surgical therapies. The classification should be reviewed frequently and revised when indicated. This appraisal should communicate to others the physician's opinion of the patient's status and prognosis without consideration of details of management.

Recommendations for further diagnostic procedures, medical and surgical therapies, and limitation of physical activity should be detailed at the end of this classification.

Cardiac Status	**Prognosis**
1 Uncompromised	1 Good
2 Slightly compromised	2 Good with therapy
3 Moderately compromised	3 Fair with therapy
4 Severely compromised	4 Guarded despite therapy

Specific Recommendations: (Further diagnostic procedures; medical or surgical correction of the underlying defect; limitation of physical activity; use of antibiotics, digitalis glycosides, diuretics; dietary restrictions; and so forth.)

The changes made in the seventh edition (1973[9]) and carried on in the eighth edition (1979[8]) of the book are significant. In years to come the change will be viewed as the time in history when physicians began to accept the new information made possible by the technology of the era. It will represent the time when physicians recognized that physiological abnormalities, discovered only in the laboratory, should at times be used to determine the severity and natural history of certain disease processes.

The proper understanding of a cardiovascular problem requires that the physician establish the *etiologic, anatomic, physiologic* diagnosis. After that is completed the physician should review *all* the data (not just the patient's symptoms) and establish the patient's *cardiac status* and *prognosis.*

The following example serves to make the point. A 54-year-old man had mild, recent-onset angina pectoris. The patient continued to work as a machinist and developed angina with moderate exercise.

Prior to 1973, when the seventh edition of *Nomenclature and Criteria for Diagnosis of Diseases of the Heart and Great Vessels* was published, one would have viewed and recorded the complete diagnosis of a patient as follows.

Etiology: Coronary atherosclerosis.
Anatomy: Obstruction of coronary arteries (location and extent of disease unknown).
Physiology: Unstable angina pectoris (recent onset).
Function: Class 1.
Therapeutic: Good with drug therapy and avoidance of moderate activity. (This assumption was based on the fact the angina was mild and could be prevented by avoiding moderate exercise.)

Now, one would view the same patient differently. A coronary arteriogram would be ordered even though the recent onset of angina was mild. Let us suppose the arteriogram showed 95 percent cross-sectional obstruction of the left main coronary artery (as it is likely to do in more than 10 percent of such patients). The new record would be as follows.

Etiology: Coronary atherosclerosis.
Anatomy: 95 percent cross-sectional obstruction of the left main coronary artery.
Physiology: Unstable angina pectoris (recent onset). Good contractility.
Cardiac status: Class 4. Severely compromised. (Even though the symptoms are mild and controllable, it has been clearly established that left main coronary artery obstruction is a potentially lethal lesion.)
Prognosis: Class 2. Good with surgical therapy. (Five-year survival rate is about 90 percent in patients who have successful bypass surgery.)

TABLE 6-1 Grading of Angina Effort by the Canadian Cardiovascular Society

1. Ordinary physical activity does not cause . . . angina, such as walking and climbing stairs. Angina with strenuous or rapid or prolonged exertion at work or recreation.
2. Slight limitations of ordinary activity. Walking or climbing stairs rapidly, walking uphill, walking or stair climbing after meals, or in cold, or in wind, or under emotional stress, or only during the few hours after awakening. Walking more than two blocks on the level and climbing more than one flight of ordinary stairs at a normal pace and in normal conditions.
3. Marked limitation of ordinary physical activity. Walking one to two blocks on the level and climbing one flight of stairs in normal conditions and at normal pace.
4. Inability to carry on any physical activity without discomfort—anginal syndrome *may* be present at rest.

Source: L Campeau, Letter to the Editor, *Circulation,* 54:522, 1976. Reproduced with permission from the American Heart Association, Inc., and author.

Specific recommendations: Coronary bypass surgery plus medical management.

A functional classification is still needed, especially in patients with angina pectoris, to determine the indications for certain forms of therapy, to assess the response to therapy, in order to judge the degree of disability, and for the investigation of patients who enter important clinical trials. A classification determined by symptoms must not be used alone, however, to predict survival chances for a patient. The Canadian Cardiovascular Society classification of *functional* is currently being used for the purposes mentioned above, and the New York Heart Association designation of *cardiac status* is used to describe the prognosis (including survival) of a patient with cardiac disease. The Canadian Cardiovascular Society functional classification is shown in Table 6-1.[10]

Summary

This chapter is merely one physician's approach to patients with heart disease. There are many other equally good approaches to the problem. The approach detailed here, however, attempts to be all-encompassing since it describes some of the attributes of a good physician; some concerns of patients; the heart and its diseases viewed in the context of all organs and their diseases; data collection, problem formulation, planning, and follow-up of the patients' problems; and an approach to patients based on the concepts emphasized in the seventh and eighth editions of *Nomenclature and Criteria for Diagnosis of Diseases of the Heart and Great Vessels.*[8,9] The cardiac status and the prognosis are determined by the New York Heart Association criteria, and the functional capacity of a patient is designated according to the Canadian Cardiovascular Society criteria.

This approach can serve as a goal for all of us. It links the good physician to a concerned patient. It guides one's thinking in establishing a complete diagnosis and improves communication. It translates medical knowledge to medical care.

References

1. Tuttle, E. P., Sr.: An excerpt from "Heroism in War and Peace," an address given at the commencement exercises of the professional and graduate schools of Emory University, June 7, 1957, *The Emory University Quarterly,* 13(3):129–139, October 1957.
2. Adler, M. J.: "Great Ideas from the Great Books," Washington Square Press, Inc., New York, 1963.
3. Weed, L. L.: "Medical Records, Medical Education, and Patient Care," The Press of Case Western Reserve, Cleveland, 1969, p. 273.
4. Hurst, J. W., and Walker, H. K.: "The Problem-Oriented System," MEDCOM, New York, 1972.
5. White, P. D.: "Heart Disease," 1st ed., The Macmillan Company, New York, 1931.

6. White, P. D.: "Heart Disease," 4th ed., The Macmillan Company, New York, 1951, p. 9.
7. The Criteria Committee for the New York Heart Association: "Criteria for the Classification and Diagnosis of Heart Disease," 1st ed., New York Heart Association, Inc., New York, 1928.
8. The Criteria Committee of the New York Heart Association: "Nomenclature and Criteria for Diagnosis of Diseases of the Heart and Great Vessels," 8th ed., New York Heart Association, Inc., New York, 1979.
9. The Criteria Committee of the New York Heart Association: "Nomenclature and Criteria for Diagnosis of Diseases of the Heart and Great Vessels," 7th ed., New York Heart Association, Inc., New York, 1973.
10. Campeau, L.: Letter to the Editor, *Circulation,* 54:522, 1976.

7

The History: Past Events and Symptoms Related to Cardiovascular Disease

J. Willis Hurst, M.D.
Douglas C. Morris, M.D.
I. Sylvia Crawley, M.D.
Edward R. Dorney, M.D.

The due appreciation of the patient's sensations is essential to a knowledge of the condition of the heart.

Sir James Mackenzie, M.D., 1916[1]

The purpose of this chapter is to discuss the important technique of history taking and to present a panoramic view of the symptoms due to cardiovascular disease. The symptoms produced by cardiovascular disease are discussed in greater detail in the chapters dealing with the conditions that cause them.

History Taking

The Purpose of History Taking

The objective of history taking is to collect medical information from the patient and to establish a doctor-patient relationship.

Eliciting the History

The art and science of obtaining an accurate medical history, including the symptoms of a patient, is the hallmark of an excellent physician.

Dr. Paul White, a master clinician, made the following points regarding history taking. (From P. D. White, "Heart Disease," Macmillan Publishing Co., Inc., New York, 1931. Copyright 1931 by Macmillan Publishing, Co., Inc. Reprinted with permission from the publisher.)

> First and most important of all is the story of the patient together with a careful consideration of his personality and reactions as he himself tells the story. If told by someone else, especially in the absence of the patient, the story has a certain amount of value dependent on the narrator's intelligence and the closeness of his acquaintanceship with the patient, but this procedure prevents insight into the case that may come only by listening to the patient's own discussion of his history and symptoms.
>
> If the confidence of the patient is secured at the start and he is put at once at his ease, the results for both patient and doctor may mean the difference between success and failure in the proper handling of the case, which is more than simply the establishment of the correct diagnosis and the outline of the special cardiovascular treatment. Sometimes trivial remarks, actions, or occurrences may destroy the confidence or ease of the patient and so prevent the successful evolution of the case. It is at the very outset that the physician must use the greatest care.[2]

Dr. Paul Wood, a brilliant cardiologist, expressed his view of history taking as follows. (Reprinted with permission from the publisher.[3])

> To take an accurate and relevant history is one of the most difficult and important arts in medicine. Sometimes, a complete diagnosis can be made from the history alone, and not infrequently the possibilities can be whittled down to two or three. A good history should at least indicate the system involved, or it should point unerringly to some group or groups of diseases. A common mistake is the failure to analyze any given symptoms sufficiently; in cardiovascular work this applies especially to pain, breathlessness, palpitations, and syncope. The student is usually taught to encourage the patient to tell his story in his own words, and to record them more or less verbatim. Yet such an account may be verbose, irrelevant, inaccurate, and misleading. It is an axiom that the leading questions must be avoided at all cost; yet again, an experienced physician must know that the ability to put the appropriate leading question at the right moment, and the intelligent interpretation of its reply, are invaluable. It is not pretended that leading questions may not lead to false

> information, if the power of their suggestion is not appreciated by the questioner; and it is agreed that much may be lost by failure to allow the patient freedom and time to express his complaints in his own way; but the average patient will not mention half the available information until he is pressed, and the data freely given must be checked as at the bar. For example, in the differential diagnosis between a neural and non-neural somatic lesion, an accurate description of the quality of the pain may determine the issue immediately; yet the majority of patients will volunteer no information concerning the quality of pain, and if asked to describe it will do so inadequately. They may say it is aching or sharp, but fail to enlarge on this, even when urged to do so. In answer to the leading question, "Does it tingle?" however, they may reply at once in the affirmative. It is essential to realize that the matter does not end there: that such a positive reply to a leading question is satisfied that the pain really does tingle, and that the patient is not merely saying so because it seems the easier answer. It is scarcely too much to say that the best history taker is the one who can best interpret the answer to a leading question. Appropriate leading questions can only be asked, however, when the proffered history has provided sufficient data upon which to work, and if the physician has sufficient knowledge of the possibilities then entailed. It is this latter factor which makes it easier for the expert than for the student.[3]

Dimsdale (quoted with the permission of the author and publisher) has recently emphasized that "learning how to take a history requires effort, patience, and tact as well as an organized, coherent framework for processing the information."[4] Feinstein[5] and Engle[6] have also written eloquently on the subject.

Errors Made in History Taking

The Inhumane Interview

As stated above, one of the objectives of history taking is to establish a doctor-patient relationship. When the history-taking period is over patients should realize that the physician knows a lot about them and cares a lot about their well-being. When patients perceive that physicians give of themselves they will, in return, give their trust to the physician.

Unfortunately, history taking does not always accomplish the goal of creating a good and proper doctor-patient relationship. In fact, the interview may establish adversary roles for the physician and the patient. The interview will fail if the interviewer is too hurried; demands precise answers and displays irritation when such are not given; shows disdain when the answers to questions are not known; insists on probing deeper in certain areas that are too emotionally painful to the patient to be discussed; fails to look up from the desk during the interview; receives multiple telephone calls during the interview; seems to treat dreaded diseases casually; gives nonverbal signals of personal unhappiness; and seems to be automated rather than understanding. In this case, the interview will be perceived by the patient as the most inhumane and cruel portion of the entire medical workup. Today we hear a great deal about the inhumanness of medicine. The inhumanness usually is blamed on machines and technology. However, machines are either used or misused by physicians and their helpers, and machines do not talk—people do. In fact, considerable inhumanness can be displayed during the "old-fashioned" interview. When the medical interview fails, the physician will be unable to establish a workable relationship with the patient and the medical "facts" will often be wrong because the patient wishes to avoid the cold process of interrogation.

The "Flaw" in Dealing with the Chief Complaint

Physicians are taught to ask patients to state their "chief complaint." Sometimes the physician forgets that a patient's chief complaint may not help to identify the patient's most serious problem. The physician, however, must always deal with the patient's chief complaint. Make no mistake about that. Not to do so will lead to instant patient dissatisfaction since the patient perceives the chief complaint as the most serious one and feels that the physician is caloused when it is ignored. The physician, however, must not fail to find and pursue other symptoms that may be more serious.

The "Flaw" in Dealing with the Present Illness

Physicians have been taught to elicit the details related to the chief complaint. The details indicate the sequence of events related to the chief complaint and all aspects of the complaint itself. The details related to the chief complaint are labeled "the present illness." Should the interviewer's mind be dominated by this lock-step sequence, he or she may not pursue all the patient's complaints. It is far better to ask patients to enumerate *all* their symptoms and to establish "present illnesses" for all the symptoms the physician judges to be of significance.

The Use and Abuse of Medical Questionnaires

A medical questionnaire can be helpful or harmful depending upon the manner in which the physician uses it.

The questionnaire is helpful when it is given to (or sent to) the patient well in advance of the interview. Then the patient can record certain data more accurately because they will have time to think about the question, ask others about the question, and look up in personal papers details about the question. When there is insufficient time to send the patient the questionnaire, it can be handed out in the physician's office. The abnormalities perceived by the patient should be probed, and related areas should be pursued by the physician. This approach, when properly implemented, should ensure that nothing important has been overlooked and will permit more time for the physician to personalize the interview.

The medical questionnaire may be harmful if the physician allows it to act as a substitute for interaction with the patient or fails to show the patient that it is a very important part of the medical record.

Failure to Properly Interpret the Past History
Physicians may make an error when they accept a past event as fact. We seem willing to accept a past history of rheumatic fever as fact but demand strict criteria for the current diagnosis of the disease. We seem willing to accept the past diagnosis of myocardial infarction when the basis of the belief may be hearsay evidence. The "past history" is very important but, at times, it can mislead the physician (see later discussion).

Failure to Talk with the Family
Every experienced physician knows that successful care of the patient is frequently determined by the physician's relationship with members of the patient's family. An essential part of doctoring is to establish a physician-family relationship as well as a doctor-patient relationship. It is also important to obtain information from family members about the patient's symptoms and the patient's reaction to the illness.

Failure to Assess the Patient's Feelings
The history can be obtained and the physician may or may not really know the patient. Good historians will know their patient's reaction to illness, feelings about disability, feelings about surgical intervention, and emotional reactions. Good physicians know their patients as human beings. The physician should remember that, when the interview is over, the patient will have a perception of the physician. Obviously, physicians want to be perceived as knowledgeable and caring people. Remember that the patient's perception of the physician begins with the interview; the patient "examines" the physician while the physician is examining the patient.

Failure to "Live through a Day" with the Patient
It is important for the physician to live through a day with the patient. This is accomplished by simply asking the patient to enumerate the activities of the day, beginning with getting up in the morning and ending with getting up 24 h later. When this is done, many new insights about the patients and their lives will be discovered.

Symptoms as Diagnostic Markers

The Predictive Value of Symptoms

The value of a patient's medical history (including symptoms) has been emphasized in the past. It was thought that, of the useful medical information for a given patient, 70 percent was contained in the medical history, 20 percent was contained in the physical examination, and 10 percent was found in the results of the laboratory procedures. This concept did not survive because laboratory technology, including electrocardiography, roentgenography, and cardiac catheterization, became highly developed and the value of laboratory tests became apparent. The emphasis was misleading even before new laboratory procedures became available. In fact, the diagnostic value of the medical history (including symptoms) is predetermined by the type of disease that the patient has. For example, faint aortic regurgitation is usually identified by hearing the heart murmur with the stethoscope. The history in such a patient might reveal no information regarding the patient's heart disease. The Wolff-Parkinson-White syndrome might be suspected in a patient with a history of paroxysmal atrial tachycardia, but the electrocardiographic evidence of a short PR interval and a wide QRS duration can only be identified by inspecting the electrocardiogram. Angina pectoris due to myocardial ischemia secondary to coronary atherosclerosis can only be recognized by eliciting the appropriate symptom.

The proper way to view the various methods of data collection (history, physical examination, and laboratory tests) is to recognize that all three methods are needed to detect the presence and severity of cardiovascular disease. Which method or methods yield the proper diagnosis is largely predetermined by the nature and severity of the disease process. The challenge of today is to determine the proper content of the history, physical examination, and laboratory examination.

Physicians have an enormous respect for the diagnostic value of the patient's symptoms. However, it must be remembered that symptoms do not always reveal the presence of or indicate the seriousness of disease. Modern medicine requires that physicians understand the sensitivity, specificity, and predictive value of test results. Physicians, as a rule, apply these standards to laboratory test results but have not applied them to symptoms and physical signs. It is, in fact, as important to know the sensitivity, specificity, and predictive value of the response to a question or the presence or absence of a physical sign as it is to know the sensitivity, specificity, and predictive value of laboratory test results.

The physician must learn the predictive value of symptoms and determine whether the history obtained is sufficiently adequate to be used in the decision-making process about the patient. The physician then adds this information to the results (with their predictive value) obtained from the physical examination, electrocardiogram, and chest x-ray and determines whether a definite decision can be made. If definitive decisions cannot be made, the physician then asks whether or not more information is needed. If the answer is yes, the physician determines what should be done next.

The Presence and Magnitude of Symptoms in Relation to Heart Disease

If the absence of certain symptoms always signified the absence of heart disease and the presence of certain symptoms always signified the presence and severity of heart disease, a physician would only have to ask, "How do you feel?" If the patient answered "Fine," the physician could pronounce the patient well. The inadequacy of this approach is highlighted by the fact that many patients who undergo sudden death due to atherosclerotic coronary heart disease have had *no* warning symptom before the tragic event occurred. Patients with treacherous ventricular rhythm disturbances may not know that the abnormal rhythm is occurring. Patients with evidence of pulmonary congestion on the chest x-ray may not have dyspnea. Patients with high-grade obstruction of the left main coronary artery due to coronary atherosclerosis (a dangerous lesion) may have *mild* symptoms of angina pectoris.

Patients may, however, have many symptoms as the result of minor disorders. For example, a patient with occasional premature ventricular contractions may feel each abnormal beat and be petrified with the fear of death. The patient with severe and terrifying angina pectoris due to coronary atherosclerosis may have only a high-grade obstruction of the right coronary artery. Such a lesion is accompanied by a fairly good long-term prognosis compared with the very poor long-term prognosis of a patient with high-grade obstruction of the left main coronary artery.

Some patients deny the presence of symptoms, often at a deep psychological level, since they cannot face the reality of the problem, while others may willfully withhold information from the physician because they might, for example, lose their job if the truth were known.

Some patients whose symptoms are dependent on effort will have no symptoms because they do not do enough to produce them. Elderly patients, sedentary patients, and patients whose physical activity is limited by another illness fall into this category. Some patients with angina pectoris due to coronary atherosclerosis or shortness of breath due to mitral stenosis may consciously or unconsciously walk more slowly in order to avoid symptoms. In fact, physicians frequently advise such patients to do less walking in order to avoid symptoms. The patient follows the physician's advice and then returns for follow-up examination, and sometimes the physician erroneously concludes that the patient is "better" because he or she describes fewer symptoms.

Elderly patients with cerebral atrophy may not be able to recall symptoms and may become frustrated when the details of symptoms are pursued. Patients who are psychiatrically disturbed may be unable to perceive symptoms or to give a meaningful account of their distress.

One must conclude that symptoms are extremely important in the recognition of heart disease and its complications. One must also conclude that the absence of symptoms does not guarantee the absence of heart disease and that the presence and magnitude of symptoms do not always parallel the seriousness of the heart disease.

The Interpretation of Symptoms

The interpretation of symptoms is not always easy. Symptoms considered to be due to heart disease may in reality be arising from another organ. For example, dyspnea may be due to pulmonary disease, not heart disease.

Symptoms attributed to noncardiovascular disease may in reality be due to heart disease. For example, pain in the jaw may be considered to be due to a toothache when it is actually due to angina pectoris secondary to coronary atherosclerosis.

The Determinants and Value of Symptoms

The determinants and value of symptoms depend upon the following factors: the presence of cardiovascular disease that has reached a level of severity that can produce symptoms; the ability of the patients to perceive, observe, and relate their symptoms; and the ability of physicians to elicit the symptoms from their patients without misleading the patients, to interpret the meaning of patients' symptoms, to determine the predictive value of various types of symptoms, and to correlate the symptoms with the results of the physical examination and laboratory data.

The Past History

Although the past history is at times misleading, it may offer an important clue to disease. There may be a history of congenital heart disease in the family. The patient's mother may give a history of rubella during the first 2 months of pregnancy, making more likely patent ductus, pulmonary valve stenosis, coarctation of the pulmonary arteries, and aortic septal defect. Viral disease during the last trimester may involve the fetal heart. A definite history of rheumatic fever may be helpful in the effort to establish the cause of a heart murmur, whereas a negative history of rheumatic fever does not eliminate it as a cause of a heart murmur. The history of hypertension in the family increases the chances that a patient's high blood pressure is essential hypertension. Death from coronary disease in family members under the age of 40 to 50 increases a patient's chances of having the disease. Trauma may cause pericarditis, myocardial infarction, acute severance of the aorta, septal rupture, and aortic and mitral valve disease. Old trauma may be responsible for a thoracic aortic aneurysm. Drugs may directly or indirectly cause heart disease. Accordingly, a detailed history of the use of medication is essential.

Symptoms Associated with Cardiovascular Disease

Pain

The ability to evaluate pain and discomfort, especially that related to cardiovascular disease, is a direct index of the expertise of the physician. In order for the physician to evaluate pain it is necessary to determine its location, its radiation, its quality, how long it has been present, how long each episode lasts, the factors that produce it, and the factors that relieve it.

Chest Pain

Pain Due to Myocardial Ischemia The most common cause of myocardial ischemia is atherosclerotic coronary heart disease (see Chap. 45). Other causes of myocardial ischemia include aortic stenosis and regurgitation (Chap. 37), cardiomyopathy (Chap. 58), and rare forms of coronary artery disease including coronary artery spasm (Chaps. 46 and 47).

Chest pain or discomfort occurs when coronary atherosclerosis reaches a critical degree of severity and the lumen of the coronary arteries becomes sufficiently narrow to cause ischemia of the cardiac muscle. Myocardial ischemia may develop when the coronary flow, which is adequate at rest, is not adequate when the demands of the heart are increased or when spasm or thrombosis impedes coronary flow when the patient is at rest. The altered physiology responsible for myocardial ischemia due to coronary atherosclerosis is discussed in Chap. 44. Myocardial ischemia due to valve disease or cardiomyopathy also signifies the severity of the conditions. (See Chaps. 37 and 58.)

Brief "Pain" of Myocardial Ischemia (Angina Pectoris). One manifestation of myocardial ischemia is angina pectoris. This serious disorder is discussed in Chap. 45. The diagnosis of angina pectoris may be missed if the physician inquires only about pain.

Many patients with angina pectoris deny the sensation of pain but complain of an aching, heavy, or squeezing sensation in the chest; chest pressure; chest tightness and dyspnea; or indigestion located in the chest.

Angina pectoris occurs during effort but may occur at rest. It is precipitated by emotions, especially anger, and exposure to cold, and may follow meals.

The unpleasant sensation is usually located in the retrosternal region of the chest or across the anterior portion of the upper part of the chest. The discomfort usually affects an area about the size of a clenched fist. As a matter of fact, the patient frequently clenches his or her fist and places it on the region of the chest where the discomfort is located.

It is always useful to have the patient circumscribe the extent of the pain by indicating its location, using a single finger. The pain may radiate to the neck, jaw, hard palate, tongue, left arm, right arm, shoulder, elbow, wrist, back, or upper part of the abdomen. On rare occasions the discomfort may be more pronounced in these areas or may be felt only in one or more of the areas mentioned.

The pain usually lasts from 1 to 3 min if the provoking cause is discontinued. Patients soon learn to stop walking or to slow their pace when they feel this discomfort. The duration of the angina pectoris provoked by anger may last longer than it does when it is caused by effort but rarely lasts longer than 10 min.

Angina pectoris is usually relieved promptly after nitroglycerin is placed under the tongue.

The electrocardiogram may be normal at rest and show ST-segment displacement only during effort.

Angina pectoris may be aggravated by many other medical conditions, including all types of emotional stress, obesity, anemia, and thyrotoxicosis.

The subsets of angina pectoris include *stable angina pectoris, unstable angina pectoris, Prinzmetal's angina* (variant angina), and *postinfarction angina.* These subsets are described in detail in Chap. 45. Prinzmetal's angina does not follow the pattern described above in one major respect. This type of angina usually occurs at rest and is accompanied by ST-segment elevation in the electrocardiogram. The syndrome is thought to be due to coronary artery spasm alone or with coexistent fixed obstructive coronary disease. (See Chaps. 45 and 46.)

It is important to identify the subset to which the patient belongs because treatment is usually linked to a particular subset (see Chap. 45).

Angina Equivalents. Some patients with myocardial ischemia note abrupt exhaustion, faintness, and dyspnea rather than chest discomfort, and such symptoms may lead the physician away from the correct diagnosis. (See Chap. 45.)

Prolonged "Pain" Due to Myocardial Ischemia. Prolonged pain due to myocardial ischemia is said to be present when the chest discomfort lasts longer than 10 to 20 min. The difference in duration occurs because the pathophysiology of angina pectoris, which is brief, is often different from the pathophysiology of more prolonged myocardial ischemia (see Chap. 44). The discomfort may develop when the patient is doing very little. In fact, it may awaken the patient from sleep. The patient may become restless and occasionally walk the floor in search of comfort. The discomfort is commonly, but not always, more severe than the discomfort of angina.

The pain of prolonged myocardial ischemia is rarely aggravated by deep breathing or turning. Many patients with prolonged pain due to myocardial ischemia may have *no* abnormalities demonstrated in the electrocardiogram, and the blood level of cardiac enzymes may not become elevated. Some patients may exhibit only ST-T wave changes in the electrocardiogram; others may have ST-T wave changes with elevation of blood cardiac enzymes; and some patients may exhibit QRS changes with elevation of cardiac enzymes.

Infarction of the myocardium is said to be present when two of the following three conditions exist: a history of prolonged chest discomfort characteristic of myocardial ischemia; abnormal ST-T or Q waves in the electrocardiogram; and elevation of blood cardiac enzymes.

Patients with prolonged chest discomfort due to

myocardial ischemia may fall into one of several subsets (see Chap. 45). *It is mandatory to identify the subset of chest pain due to myocardial ischemia to which the patient belongs because treatment is usually linked to a particular subset* (see Chap. 45).

Pain Due to Dissecting Aneurysm of the Aorta Acute dissection of the aorta is usually associated with excruciating pain. (See Chaps. 45 and 64.) The pain is usually located in the anterior portion of the chest, lasts for hours, and is frequently of maximal intensity at the onset. More than the usual amount of opiates may be needed for relief. This pain tends to radiate into the thoracic portion of the back more often than the pain of myocardial infarction, and it may be felt predominantly in the back. It is not aggravated by deep breathing or turning. It may be located in the abdomen if the arteries of the abdominal viscera are involved. Occasionally, the pain seems to shift from one area in the chest to a lower portion as the dissection progresses.

Pain Due to Aortic Aneurysm A thoracic aortic aneurysm (see Chap. 64) may erode a vertebral body and produce constant severe pain.

Pain Due to Acute Pericarditis The pain of acute pericarditis (see Chap. 59) is not related to effort but is usually aggravated by deep breathing. It is often described as feeling "sharp." It is usually located in the precordial area and may radiate to the upper portion of the shoulders or sides of the neck. The patient tends to avoid deep breaths or even normal respiration because of the intense aggravation of the discomfort associated with this activity. Turning the body from side to side may aggravate the pain, as may swallowing. Leaning forward may occasionally relieve the discomfort. The absence of a pericardial friction rub does not exclude pericarditis.

Pain Due to Pulmonary Emboli The majority of small pulmonary emboli (see Chap. 54) produces no chest pain. In fact, the patient may not identify any symptoms that are directly due to pulmonary emboli, which is why the majority of emboli are not diagnosed. The pain of pulmonary embolism may, at times, be similar to that of myocardial ischemia. Acute distressing dyspnea may be the only clue to pulmonary embolism. The diagnosis is frequently based on circumstantial evidence. When pulmonary infarction develops, pleuritis may be identified. The pain in such cases is located in the lateral portion of the chest and is aggravated by breathing.

Pain Related to Pulmonary Hypertension The chest pain associated with pulmonary hypertension (see Chaps. 52 and 53) may simulate angina pectoris and occurs, most often, in patients with mitral stenosis or Eisenmenger's syndrome. The pain has been thought to be due to dilatation of the pulmonary artery, but we believe it is due to right ventricular myocardial ischemia.

Discomfort Due to Noncardiovascular Causes There are many noncardiovascular causes of chest pain and many of them can simulate the pain of myocardial ischemia (see Chap. 45). Only one of the common causes of noncardiovascular discomfort will be discussed here.

The most common cause of chest pain is not related to cardiovascular disease but is associated with *anxiety.* The discomfort is usually located in the left inframammary region and rarely radiates to other locations. The pain does not occur during effort but may occur after effort. It is not aggravated by breathing but is associated with other signs of anxiety such as periodic deep-sighing respiration, hyperventilation, sinus tachycardia, fatigue, and a fear of "closed-in" places. The discomfort may be characterized as a series of short sticks and stabs lasting no longer than it takes to snap one's fingers, or it may be a dull ache lasting for hours to days at a time. This type of discomfort may be disabling to patients and may consume their every thought. The discomfort may also be located in the substernal area and anterior chest region (Chap. 45). The discomfort may be so similar to myocardial ischemia that it is not possible to separate the two conditions without a coronary arteriogram.

Since angina pectoris and the discomfort associated with anxiety (or other causes) may—and frequently do—coexist, great skill is needed to clarify such problems. The medical history may offer the major diagnostic clue in such a situation because the patient's major complaint may be due to anxiety even if obstructive coronary disease is found on coronary arteriography.

The chest pain associated with the *shoulder-hand syndrome; esophageal rupture; esophageal spasm; esophageal reflux; diseases of the spine, shoulder girdle, pleura, lung,* and *mediastinum (including mediastinal emphysema); stomach* and *duodenal disorders; gallbladder disease; thrombophlebitis of the chest wall; herpes zoster;* and *other chest wall syndromes* must be considered in the differential diagnosis. (See Chap. 45.)

Pain in the Extremities

Intermittent claudication of the lower extremities due to peripheral atherosclerosis (see Chaps. 65 and 68) is frequently overlooked because the physician thinks that the discomfort ought to be localized in the calf of the leg. Whenever discomfort develops in the arch of the foot, calf of the leg, thighs, hips, or gluteal region during effort, then peripheral arterial vascular disease must be considered.

The symptoms associated with acute arterial occlusion of the lower extremities may at the onset be no more than the effects of hypesthesia (interpreted by the patient as "the leg going to sleep").

Intermittent claudication of the upper extremities and masseter muscle may occur. This symptom is usually due to a nonatherosclerotic cause of arterial disease such as arteritis.

The pain of Raynaud's disease may be noted in the fingers after exposure to cold. The patient may note pallor of the fingers prior to feeling pain. This symptom should lead the physician to inquire about dysphagia and look for the skin changes of scleroderma.

Head Pain

The pain of myocardial ischemia may be felt in the jaw, hard palate, cheek, and rarely even deep in the ear canal.

The pain of temporal arteritis may be localized to the temporal region and be associated with visual difficulty and polymyalgia rheumatica.

Migraine headache is vascular in origin and may be quite severe. Other clues include nausea, scotoma, and intolerance to light.

Hypertension does not usually produce headache but severe headache may occur in patients with severe hypertension.

Pain in the Abdomen

The pain due to an expanding or rupturing atherosclerotic abdominal aneurysm is discussed in Chap. 64.

Abdominal angina due to vascular disease of the mesenteric arteries is discussed in Chap. 67.

The pain of myocardial ischemia or pericarditis may be located in the upper portion of the abdomen.

The liver may become painful and tender as a result of heart failure. Liver discomfort may be aggravated by effort in such patients.

Joint Pain

Almost all forms of arthritis may be associated with heart disease. Rheumatic fever, rheumatoid arthritis, psoriatic arthritis, ankylosing spondylitis, gonococcal arthritis, Reiter's disease, and Lyme arthritis are all associated with heart or pericardial disease.

Dyspnea (Difficult Breathing)

Dyspnea is a very distressing symptom. The patient complains of "shortness of breath" or that he or she "can't get enough breath."

There are many causes of dyspnea. The investigation of dyspnea must include a search for the factors that precipitate and relieve dyspnea and must identify the body position associated with the complaint.

Obviously, an infant or small child does not complain of shortness of breath. Therefore, other clues to respiratory distress are required (Chap. 36). The rate of breathing is greatly increased in this age group when there is heart failure or acute lung disease. The respiratory rate of adults with heart failure is not as greatly increased as would be expected from the degree of dyspnea noted by the patient.

Dyspnea is always abnormal when it occurs at rest or when it occurs with slight activity. Dyspnea at rest, but not with effort, in apparently healthy persons suggests an emotional cause of the shortness of breath.

Chronic dyspnea can be caused by heart failure, pulmonary disease, obesity, poor physical fitness, pleural effusions, and effort asthma.

Acute dyspnea may occur with acute pulmonary edema, hyperventilation, pneumothorax, pulmonary embolus, pneumonia, and airway obstruction.

Dyspnea on Effort

Dyspnea on effort (see Chaps. 21 and 55) is a common complaint. It is usually due to congestive heart failure or chronic pulmonary disease. It is necessary to establish the degree of activity required to produce dyspnea. This may be done by inquiring about the daily activity of each patient. It is useless to ask, "Do you get short of breath climbing stairs?" if the patient never climbs stairs. The patient may, however, climb a hill near home every day. It is also valuable to determine when the patient began to notice increasing dyspnea. For example, if the patient only recently has had difficulty in climbing, the dyspnea is more likely to be due to heart failure than to lung disease. The dyspnea could be related to chronic lung disease, but it would then be wise to look for recent complications such as pneumothorax, atelectasis, and asymptomatic pulmonary infection in order to explain the recent increase in symptoms.

Dyspnea related to effort may be the equivalent of angina pectoris in some patients with coronary atherosclerosis who develop transient global myocardial ischemia during effort. (See Chap. 45.)

Wheezing

When a patient complains of wheezing associated with dyspnea, he or she may have lung disease or heart disease. (See Chaps. 21 and 55.) If the patient is an adult, especially over the age of 40, heart failure should be foremost in the mind of the physician, and this should prompt a search for other clues indicating heart disease. When the wheezing is due to heart disease, the patient is said to have cardiac asthma. If there is a history of periodic wheezing and dyspnea since childhood, then, of course, bronchial asthma and lung disease are more likely to be the cause. One must remember, however, that patients who have had bronchial asthma for many years may also develop heart disease and heart failure. When this occurs the heart failure may precipitate more bronchial asthma, but the physician may be misled into assuming the patient's problem remains that of uncomplicated bronchial asthma. The point is that the patient who wheezes from bronchial asthma may wheeze more when he or she develops left ventricular failure.

Wheezing on effort may be due to either heart failure or chronic lung disease. Wheezing due to chronic lung disease becomes apparent because the effort evokes deeper respiratory excursions and, in some patients, precipitates "effort asthma."

Orthopnea

Orthopnea is a special type of dyspnea (see Chaps. 20 and 21). It implies that patients have less difficulty breathing in the sitting position than in the recumbent position. The patient relates that he or she places two or three pillows under the head in order to have a restful night. This symptom is often associated with congestive heart failure but may also be associated with severe chronic lung disease.

The fatigue associated with the effort of breathing seems to be less when the dyspnea is due to chronic pulmonary disease than when it is due to heart failure.

Paroxysmal Nocturnal Dyspnea

Paroxysmal nocturnal dyspnea is a very important variety of shortness of breath (see Chaps. 20 and 21). The predictive value of this symptom as a sign of heart failure is excellent but not perfect. Characteristically, patients have little difficulty falling asleep in the recumbent position. One or two hours later they are awakened from sleep with acute shortness of breath. They seek relief by sitting upright on the side of the bed or even in a chair. They occasionally go to the open window searching for air. After a time, they become comfortable and return to bed. They may then sleep comfortably the remainder of the night.

The only other causes for this unusual sequence of events are hyperventilation syndrome due to anxiety and pulmonary emboli. It would be most unusual for pulmonary emboli to occur for many nights at the same hour. The hyperventilation syndrome due to anxiety is not so clearly relieved by sitting up and is associated with other signs and symptoms of anxiety. Heart failure and anxiety may coexist since both are common.

Acute Pulmonary Edema

Acute pulmonary edema is usually due to disease of the left ventricle or to mitral valve disease (see Chaps. 20 and 21). The patient experiences the sudden development of dyspnea and cough, and may produce frothy, blood-tinged sputum. The symptoms may occur without previous warning as in myocardial infarction, or may be preceded by dyspnea on effort or cardiac asthma.

Pulmonary edema may be due to noncardiac causes.

Cheyne-Stokes Breathing

Cheyne-Stokes breathing is characterized by periods of hyperpnea which alternate with periods of apnea (see Chaps. 20 and 21). This type of breathing usually occurs in older patients with heart failure. Patients with Cheyne-Stokes respiration usually have cerebral vascular disease and heart disease of the left side of the heart.

Patients with Cheyne-Stokes respiration rarely complain of dyspnea, perhaps because they are so sick. They are occasionally aware of acute shortness of breath during the hyperpneic phase of the cycle.

The type of breathing associated with the hypoventilation syndrome of obesity, or the Pickwickian syndrome, may be periodic in nature but is not identical with Cheyne-Stokes breathing. Cheyne-Stokes respiration rarely occurs in older children or in patients with cor pulmonale. Normal newborn babies, however, may exhibit a breathing pattern that is somewhat similar to Cheyne-Stokes respiration.

Dyspnea Due to Pulmonary Embolism

The sudden dyspnea of acute pulmonary embolism (see Chap. 54) may be profound and is often the only symptom associated with this often sudden, catastrophic event. This condition should be suspected when sudden dyspnea occurs during the postsurgical or postpartum period or in a patient who has chronic heart failure.

Dyspnea Due to Anxiety

Dyspnea due to anxiety, a common cause of breathing difficulty, has no relation to heart disease but is often mistaken by patient and physician as being due to heart disease. (See Chaps. 45 and 81.)

The shortness of breath associated with anxiety assumes two forms, both of which may be terrifying to patients. They may simply feel as though the air "does no good," or "does not go down far enough"; or say that they "can't get a good, satisfying breath." Normal breathing is interrupted by deep sighs. Some patients experience claustrophobia. Fatigue, palpitation, and precordial "aching" or "sticks" may also be present. The patient may develop prolonged periods of hyperventilation which are frequently associated with numbness of the arms, hands, and lips, tetany, and unreal sensation.

This type of dyspnea can occur in patients who also have pulmonary or heart disease, thereby testing the diagnostic acumen of the physician.

Dyspnea Due to Hypoxia

The dyspnea associated with congenital heart disease (see Chap. 36) with right-to-left shunt is related to hypoxia. The dyspnea is usually related to effort, but the young child may have episodes of breathlessness and increased cyanosis. The child may become unconscious during the terrifying episodes (Chap. 36).

Severe anemia may be the sole cause of dyspnea on effort and is a frequent contributing factor (Chap. 36).

Methemoglobinemia may also be responsible for dyspnea on effort and, like anemia, may be a contributing factor.

Dyspnea Due to Thyrotoxicosis

The dyspnea of thyrotoxicosis (see Chap. 72) is due to associated myopathy and an increase in the body's need for oxygen.

The "Dyspnea" of Pregnancy and Acidosis
The full-term pregnant female may "huff and puff" with effort but has a curious reaction to the audible respiratory effort (see Chap. 69). She seems quite conscious of her labored breathing but is rarely, if ever, alarmed by it. Accordingly, she is not truly dyspneic.

Patients with compensatory hyperpnea associated with metabolic acidosis due to diabetes mellitus or uremia rarely complain of true dyspnea.

Cough

A dry, nonproductive cough may be related to the pulmonary congestion associated with heart failure. It may develop with effort but may also occur at rest. Although dyspnea is usually present, cough may dominate the clinical picture.

The cough which accompanies pulmonary edema is often associated with frothy, pink-tinged sputum, whereas the sputum associated with chronic bronchitis is usually white and mucoid. The sputum accompanying pneumonia is often thick and yellow. The sputum associated with pulmonary infarct may be bloody as may be the sputum associated with cancer of the lung or bronchiectasis.

Palpitation

The term *palpitation* is used by patients to describe a disagreeable awareness of the heartbeat. (See Chaps. 18, 26, and 100 to 102.) The patient may use some other term and report a "pounding," "stopping," "jumping," or "racing" in the chest. A parent may observe an abnormal heart rhythm when looking at or feeling a child's precordium.

The sensitivity of the nervous system determines whether the patient complains of palpitation. The complaint is not directly related to the seriousness of the heart disease or to the exact type of arrhythmia. For example, one patient may feel every premature contraction when there is no evidence of heart disease, while another patient may not detect ventricular tachycardia associated with serious heart disease.

When a patient feels a premature cardiac contraction, he or she rarely feels the early beat which has occurred out of cadence and usually feels the subsequent beat which is associated with a large stroke volume. On rare occasions a patient may be aware of his or her heartbeat after digitalis medication has been given because of the increased force of contraction induced by the drug. When this occurs, ectopic beats due to digitalis intoxication may also be noted by the patient. Patients may be aware of a cardiac arrhythmia by detecting an uncomfortable sensation in their necks. This is probably due to distension of the neck veins when the right atrium contracts against a closed tricuspid valve.

Patients may complain when the heartbeat is slow or fast and when the heartbeat is regular or irregular. The patient may detect if the onset and offset of the rapid beat is abrupt or gradual. The patient may complain of forceful, regular heartbeats. Conditions associated with an increased stroke output may produce a feeling of forceful contraction of the heart. The best example of this is perhaps found in patients with aortic regurgitation. Ectopic beats, atrial fibrillation, and other arrhythmias may be more troublesome to patients with aortic regurgitation because in such cases the variations of the stroke output are so radically different from normal.

Patients may complain of palpitation of the heart when the rhythm and rate are entirely normal or when the regular cadence of rhythm is interrupted by ectopic contractions, paroxysmal rapid heartbeat, or extreme bradycardia, including complete heart block. The rhythm responsible for the palpitation may not be present when the patient is seen and other means of detection may be needed (Chap. 18).

It is useful to ask if anyone counted the patient's pulse during an episode of tachycardia. The heart rate of 150 beats per minute suggests atrial flutter or sinus tachycardia. A heart rate of 180 beats per minute suggests atrial tachycardia. The patient may know if the Valsalva maneuver aborted an attack of regular tachycardia. The patient may give a history of increased urine output during atrial tachycardia, atrial fibrillation, and flutter.

Syncope

Syncope (see Chaps. 29 and 30) is defined as the transient loss of consciousness due to an inadequate cerebral blood flow. Near syncope may be applied to the clinical situation in which the patient feels dizzy and weak, and tends to lose postural tone but does not lose consciousness. Although epilepsy may produce similar symptoms, cerebral vascular disease is a more common problem in differential diagnosis.

Although some patients seek medical advice because of frequent episodes of syncope, many others do not give such a history spontaneously. In such cases the patient either has forgotten the episodes or has been unaware of their occurrence. Also it is not uncommon for the physician to forget to inquire about the occurrence of syncope while interviewing the patient and the family. When a patient gives a definite history of one episode of syncope, it is wise to assume that more than one episode has occurred.

Syncope may occur in many types of heart disease and circulatory disorders, including atherosclerotic coronary heart disease, aortic stenosis, aortic regurgitation, mitral stenosis, idiopathic hypertrophic cardiomyopathy, left atrial tumor, primary pulmonary hypertension, pulmonary arteriolar disease secondary to left-to-right shunts, pulmonary stenosis, tetralogy of Fallot, paroxysmal rapid heartbeat, sinus arrest (sick sinus syndrome), ventricular standstill or fibrillation related to atrioventricular block, Adams-Stokes attacks due to coronary atherosclerosis or perhaps more commonly to Lev's disease or Lenègre's disease, acute blood loss, pulmonary embolism, etc. Syncope may also take various forms, such as carotid sinus syncope, cough syncope, micturition syncope, vagovagal syncope, and vasodepressor syncope.

Other Symptoms That Worry Patients

Patients may hear or feel several worrisome cardiovascular events other than palpitation (see later discussion). Patients with severe tricuspid regurgitation may feel the expanding venous pulse in the neck. Some feel the pulse wave hit the ear, and others note that their collar is "too tight" when the heart beats. Patients may complain of recurring single or double sounds in the head that are synchronous with the heartbeat. These sounds are usually heard at night. Patients with aortic regurgitation may feel a throbbing sensation in the neck. Benign venous hums may cause a distracting noise in the ear, and patients may hear their own intracerebral arteriovenous malformation or fistula.

History of "Swelling of the Legs," Weight Gain, or Enlarging Girth

Edema may be found on physical examination although the patient may be unaware of its existence. On the other hand, there may be a history of "swelling," and edema may not be found at the time of examination. (See Chaps. 20 and 21.)

In the past generalized edema was required before a diagnosis of heart failure could be made. Although this extreme degree of edema is not required to establish the diagnosis of heart failure today, it is unfortunate that many physicians still demand the presence of at least some edema before seriously considering the diagnosis of congestive heart failure. Of course, patients are seen today with considerable peripheral edema due to heart failure, but it must be stated emphatically that edema is a late sign of congestive heart failure. Many other subtle signs of heart failure are usually present before the appearance of edema.

Considerable weight gain due to retention of extracellular fluid may occur without associated edema. This may, at times, be as much as 10 to 15 lb. On the other hand, there are numerous causes of edema other than congestive heart failure, and its presence is not diagnostic of congestive heart failure. When the diagnosis of heart failure is delayed until edema develops or when heart failure is diagnosed simply because edema is present, the approach to the diagnostic problem is clearly superficial.

Local factors play a major role in determining the distribution of fluid in the body. Pulmonary edema due to mitral stenosis provides a good illustration of the importance of local factors. When ventricular diastole is shortened to a critical point, pulmonary edema develops because the right ventricle continues to pump more blood into the lungs than can pass the stenosed mitral valve. Under these circumstances there will be no weight gain or peripheral edema. The body fluid has simply been redistributed and it accumulates in the lungs. The patient with chronic congestive heart failure who has gained weight because of retention of sodium and water secondary to altered renal function may detect edema of the ankles and lower legs during the day and note that it diminishes during the night. The edema occurs in the legs because of local hydrostatic factors which are related to the upright position.

It is important to ascertain whether edema of the extremities preceded or followed dyspnea on effort. Although there are many exceptions, the edema due to poor function of the left ventricle, mitral stenosis, or cor pulmonale is usually preceded by dyspnea.

Edema may be due to hypoproteinemia such as occurs in nephrosis and starvation. As with heart failure, the edema may occur in the dependent portion of the body. Such edema usually occurs when the total blood protein is below 5 g/dl.

Edema of one leg is usually due to local factors such as varicose veins, thrombophlebitis, or lymphedema. When there is bilateral leg edema due to heart failure, there may be more on one side than the other if a local factor is also present. Edema may shift from the extremities to the sacral region when a patient is confined to bed.

Periorbital edema is more common in children than in adults. Although this finding on history of physical examination may be due to renal disease, it also occurs in heart failure. It simply indicates that salt and water have been retained and that the tissue pressure around the eyes of the child is low. Rare causes of periorbital edema include trichinosis and superior vena caval obstruction.

Ascites may be recognized by the patient as an increase in girth or swelling of the abdomen. Ascites due to congestive heart failure is not common today and invariably follows peripheral edema. A local factor, such as cirrhosis, is also suggested when ascites, associated with heart failure, seems to be out of proportion to peripheral edema. Constrictive pericarditis and restrictive cardiomyopathy should also be thought of in this setting (Chaps. 58 and 59). The distribution of extracellular fluid is somewhat different in the child with heart failure compared with the adult. The child with heart failure forms ascites more readily than does the adult.

Hemoptysis (Coughing Up Blood)

When a patient gives a history of "coughing blood," it is necessary to ascertain the exact nature of the sputum. The sputum must be examined both grossly and microscopically.

It is useful to determine whether the material that is coughed up contains large volumes of liquid blood (hemoptysis), which indicates brisk bleeding, or whether it contains smaller quantities of dark or clotted blood, which would indicate slow bleeding from low-pressure vessels or subsiding bleeding. Brisk bleeding, for example, is commonly associated with specific focal ulceration of the bronchus, such as bronchogenic carcinoma, a foreign body, bronchiectasis, or a bleeding aortic aneurysm. Slow bleeding strongly suggests venous bleeding which is more likely to be the result of increased pulmonary vascular resistance with secondary increase in flow through the bronchial venous system such as may occur as a result of mitral stenosis or bronchiectasis.

It is also helpful to notice whether the expectorated blood is intimately mixed with sputum (blood-streaked sputum) or pus, because this is a valuable clue to the possible site of the origin of the bleeding. Intimate mixtures of blood and pus are excellent signs of a deep-seated site of pulmonary suppuration.

At times, posterior epistaxis associated with systemic hypertension may cause blood-streaked sputum. On rare occasions localized disease of the nose may give a similar clinical picture. As a rule, however, epistaxis is obvious and is not usually confused with bloody sputum.

Pink, frothy sputum is frequently associated with acute pulmonary edema. Blood-streaked sputum may occur with acute pulmonary congestion when the classic findings of acute pulmonary edema are not fully developed. The blood comes from pulmonary capillaries which have ruptured under high intravascular pressure.

Hemoptysis may be due to pulmonary tuberculosis, pneumonia, bronchiectasis, bronchogenic carcinoma, primary pulmonary hemosiderosis, Osler-Rendu-Weber disease with a pulmonary arteriovenous aneurysm, and necrotic pulmonary arterial lesions due to periarteritis nodosa or lupus erythematosus. Four cardiovascular conditions must never be overlooked as causes of hemoptysis: mitral stenosis, pulmonary infarction, Eisenmenger physiology, and aortic aneurysm.

Mitral Stenosis

Hemoptysis due to mitral stenosis (see Chap. 38) is frequently induced by physical exercise, sexual intercourse, or marked excitement. It may be the first symptom of mitral stenosis and may occur during pregnancy. The blood comes from a break in the pulmonary veins which have ruptured under very high pressure. The bleeding is due to rupture of endobronchial vessels that form collateral channels between the bronchial veins and pulmonary venous system. Episodes of pulmonary hemorrhage of this type tend to subside as the veins adapt to the high pressure and as pulmonary arteriolar disease develops.

Pulmonary Infarction

Many pulmonary emboli do not lead to pulmonary infarction, but when they do, frank hemoptysis occurs in the minority of instances (see Chap. 54). Despite this, when hemoptysis occurs in a patient with heart failure, pulmonary infarction is likely. The bloody sputum usually appears from a few hours to a day after the embolus and is due to necrosis and hemorrhage into the alveoli.

Eisenmenger Physiology

Patients with severe pulmonary hypertension associated with an interventricular septal defect, patent ductus arteriosus, or atrial septal defect may have hemoptysis, presumably secondary to rupture of pulmonary capillaries (see Chap. 36).

Aortic Aneurysms

An aortic aneurysm (see Chap. 64) may rupture into the tracheobronchial tree and produce lethal hemoptysis. Aneurysms due to syphilis, atherosclerosis, and dissection may cause this catastropic event.

Fatigue and Weakness

There are many causes of fatigue and weakness (see Chaps. 20, 21, and 45), and therefore these symptoms are not specific for heart disease. The most common cause of these symptoms is anxiety, increased emotional tension, and depression. Anemia and other chronic disease states may be associated with fatigue and weakness. The least common cause is Addison's disease.

When a patient with heart disease is waterlogged or when there is pulmonary congestion due to heart disease, the patient is likely to complain of dyspnea. Now, with modern therapy, these complaints may be supplanted by the feelings of fatigue and weakness. The actual physiological mechanism of the fatigue associated with heart failure is not known, but it is probably related to an inadequate cardiac output. The heart fails in its prime objective of nourishing all the tissues and organs of the body, including the skeletal muscles. Potassium depletion due to the use of diuretics without adequate potassium replacement may be the cause of weakness.

A patient may experience exhaustion related to effort as a manifestation of transient global myocardial ischemia due to atherosclerotic coronary heart disease (Chap. 45). Dyspnea and hypotension may also occur at the time such a patient detects the exhaustion. The complaint of exhaustion may occur before, during, or following myocardial infarction (Chap. 45).

A patient may feel weak after massive diuresis. In this case the symptom relates to potassium depletion, altered blood volume, and postural hypotension. Patients on antihypertensive drug therapy may complain of weakness because of postural hypotension.

Fatigue and weakness may be due to anxiety rather than to heart disease. As a rule, the fatigue due to heart disease is related to effort, whereas the fatigue of anxiety occurs continuously.

Cyanosis and Other Skin Color

Finally, many drugs, such as beta blockers, may produce fatigue and weakness. (See Chaps. 21, 36, 54, and 55.) Patients or their family members may detect cyanosis of the lips and relate their observation to the physician. Four grams per deciliter of reduced hemoglobin are needed for cyanosis to occur. Arterial oxygen saturation must be about 85 percent or less for cyanosis to develop. Cyanosis cannot occur when the hemoglobin is less than 33 percent of normal since reduced hemoglobin cannot be produced in an amount sufficient to cause the bluish color. When the hemoglobin is normal, about one-third of it must be in the reduced form for the bluish color to appear.

Accordingly, family members cannot detect minor degrees of cyanosis. Physicians have the same problem. This explains why errors are made when congenital heart disease is divided into cyanotic and noncyanotic groups. Such a division may be useful when cyanosis is definitely present, but lesser degrees of arterial oxygen unsaturation are not recognized with regularity.

A bluish tint to the skin may not be due to congenital heart disease with a right-to-left shunt or pulmonary disease since it may be due to argyria or methemoglobinemia.

Cyanosis in the patient with chronic congestive heart failure should suggest the possibility of associated pulmonary embolism.

The patient or a family member may detect that the cyanosis is more intense in the feet than the hands (Chap. 36). This suggests a right-to-left shunt through the patent ductus arteriosus. Cyanosis may be associated with clubbing of the fingers (Chap. 36).

A history of flushing sometimes precipitated by alcohol should lead one to search for the other signs and symptoms of carcinoid heart disease (Chap. 61).

A history of a change in normal skin color to bronze plus a history of diabetes suggests hemochromatosis.

Squatting

Young children with tetralogy of Fallot learn that their dyspnea is relieved when they squat. (See Chap. 36.) Squatting increases peripheral arterial resistance, which decreases the right-to-left shunt and increases pulmonary blood flow. This compensatory mechanism does not occur when such a patient is submerged in water.

Recurrent Bronchitis and Pulmonary Infection

Recurrent coughing due to heart failure is often thought to be due to bronchitis. Patients with chronic bronchitis may cough more when heart failure ensues. Patients with increased blood flow to the lungs due to left-to-right shunts are subject to severe attacks of pulmonary infection. Patients with high pulmonary venous pressure are more prone to the development of pulmonary edema when they have viral pneumonitis than are patients with normal pulmonary venous pressure. This is especially true in patients with mitral stenosis. The high pulmonary venous pressure plus injury to the alveolar wall by the virus increases the transudation of fluid into the alveoli.

Insomnia

There are many causes of insomnia. The most common causes are mental conflict, emotional disturbances, and depression. Heart failure, however, may be the cause of insomnia. The patient with Cheyne-Stokes respiration may sleep during the apneic phase and wake during the hyperpneic phase of the condition. Patients with pulmonary congestion due to heart failure as a result of disease of the left side of the heart may have insomnia before they detect nocturnal dyspnea.

Cerebral Symptoms

Patients may have dizziness, near syncope, and syncope, as discussed under "Syncope" earlier in this chapter.

Patients with decreased cardiac output secondary to heart failure may become mentally confused and disoriented. This may be due to hypoxia, drugs that are invariably prescribed for such patients, or renal or hepatic failure.

Cerebral symptoms may be associated with a transient ischemic attack of the brain, a cerebral vascular accident due to lacunar infarcts, cerebral hemorrhage, a cerebral embolus from an atheromatous ulcer in the carotid system, infective endocarditis, recent myocardial infarction or atrial fibrillation with or without mitral stenosis, or clots on a prosthetic valve.

Convulsions rarely occur as a result of heart disease. Convulsions may be related to cardiac standstill when unilateral intracranial disease or unilateral carotid disease make localizing signs possible.

Coma rarely occurs as a result of heart disease. The patient in shock or the patient with violent tachycardia who also has considerable intracranial or extracranial vascular disease may have such severe cerebral hypoxia that coma occurs. Hypoxic coma may follow cardiac resuscitation.

Hoarseness

Hoarseness is usually unrelated to cardiovascular disease. It can occur in patients with an aortic aneurysm that involves the left recurrent laryngeal nerve. Mitral stenosis may occasionally produce hoarseness, but this is rarely seen today since mitral stenosis is usually corrected surgically before it produces such a symptom. The hoarseness in such patients is due to the pressure of a large pulmonary artery or left atrium on the recurrent laryngeal nerve.

Pericardial effusion may be related to myxedema, which may be associated with a coarse, low-pitched voice. A woman with myxedema may be disturbed when her voice is mistaken for a man's voice. This often occurs when the patient talks on the telephone.

Hoarseness and loss of voice may occur following the use of an endotracheal tube during cardiac surgery.

Epistaxis

Severe nosebleed may occur in patients with hypertension. This disturbs the patient a great deal. This can, on rare occasions, be so severe as to place the life of a patient in danger because of exsanguination. Epistaxis was once said to occur in acute rheumatic fever, but this is rarely seen in the United States today. Trauma is the most common cause of nosebleed.

Anorexia, Nausea, and Vomiting

Nausea and vomiting are often due to digitalis in patients with heart disease. Patients with myocardial infarction may complain of nausea and exhibit vomiting, but opiates may, and often do, cause the symptoms in such patients. Patients with heart failure may have anorexia and nausea without any other apparent cause.

Indigestion

Many patients with angina pectoris due to coronary atherosclerosis erroneously attribute their symptoms to "indigestion" or "heartburn," while patients with heartburn, esophageal reflux, and esophageal spasm may believe they have angina pectoris.

Hiccups

Hiccups may occur in patients with myocardial infarction and are common during the postoperative period after cardiac surgery.

Jaundice

Jaundice may be detected by the patient or a member of the family. As a rule, hepatic congestion due to heart failure will not produce jaundice. When jaundice does occur in a patient with heart failure, it is appropriate to consider pulmonary infarction in addition to the hepatic congestion or cirrhosis of the liver. The hemolysis of red blood cells may occur in patients with prosthetic valves and this may produce jaundice. On rare occasion hemolytic anemia and jaundice may be caused by severe aortic valve stenosis.

Patients with cyanosis and jaundice may have a faint green appearance. This color is sometimes noted in patients with tricuspid stenosis and in patients with long-standing heart failure and tricuspid regurgitation.

Dysphagia

Dysphagia may occur in patients with scleroderma which may be associated with heart disease. Aortic arch anomalies may produce dysphagia. An extremely large left atrium may also, on rare occasion, produce dysphagia.

Weight Loss, Malnutrition, and Cachexia

Patients with long-standing heart failure may give a history of eating poorly and weight loss. Therefore, calorie, protein, and vitamin malnutrition may occur.

Urinary Symptoms

Patients with chronic heart failure may note oliguria during the day and polyuria at night. Men with borderline urinary tract obstruction due to enlargement of the prostate may have more difficulty voiding when heart failure ensues, and this in turn may make the heart failure worse. Polyuria may occur during atrial tachycardia, atrial fibrillation, or flutter. Massive infarction of the prostate may occur following cardiac surgery in patients with hyperplasia when hypotension develops and pressor agents are used.[7]

Fever and Chills

Patients with rheumatic fever do not have chills unless aspirin has been used for treatment. Chills are common in patients with bacterial endocarditis. Fever may also be due to pericarditis. Myalgia, chills, and fever may, on very rare occasions, be related to myocardial infarction, presumably because of some form of autoimmune response to necrotic myocardial tissue.

It is important to inquire whether there has been any recent dental work (including cleaning) in patients with heart murmurs and fever, since this may be a clue to the diagnosis of endocarditis.

Noises Heard by the Patient

A loud heart murmur may be heard by a patient or a member of the family. For example, the murmur of interventricular septal defect is often heard by the patient. A patient may hear the murmur associated with retroversion of an aortic valve cusp, rupture of the chordae tendineae of the mitral valve, and retroversion of a porcine mitral valve. Some noises from the chest can even be heard at a considerable distance. It is not uncommon for individuals to become aware of their heartbeat by hearing arterial bruits or heart sounds when the side of their head is placed on a pillow. The murmur of an arteriovenous fistula located near the ear or a cervical venous hum may be heard by the patient.

Abnormal Movements

Patients may complain that their neck veins are distended or move vigorously, and patients with aortic regurgitation may complain that their head "bobs." Patients and their family members may be disturbed by the uncontrollable movements of chorea.

Patients Who Say They Have Had a Heart Attack

Many patients state that they have had a heart attack because, to them, any abrupt incident thought to be related to the heart is considered to be a heart attack. This includes prolonged myocardial ischemia without infarction, a cardiac arrhythmia, pulmonary edema, or hyperventilation. Accordingly, one should not automatically conclude that a patient has had a myocardial infarction when the patient says he or she has had a heart attack.

References

1. Mackenzie, J.: "Principles of Diagnosis and Treatment in Heart Affections," Oxford Medical Publications, London, 1916, p. 48.
2. White, P. D.: "Heart Disease," The Macmillan Company, New York, 1931, pp. 4, 9.
3. Wood, P. D.: "Diseases of the Heart and Circulation," 2d ed., J. B. Lippincott Company, Philadelphia, 1957, p. 1.
4. Dimsdale, J. E.: Delays and Slips in Medical Diagnosis, *Perspect. Biol. Med.*, 27(2):213, 1984.
5. Feinstein, A. R.: "Clinical Judgment," Kreiger, Melbourne, Fla., 1967.
6. Engle, G., and Morgan, W.: "Interviewing the Patient," W. B. Saunders Company, Philadelphia, 1973.
7. Taussig, A. S., Hurst, J. W., Ambrose, S. S., and Sewell, C. W.: Massive Prostatic Infarction Following Aortocoronary Bypass Surgery: A Report of Two Cases, *Clin. Cardiol.*, 7(2):113, 1984.

8

Inspection of the Patient

Mark E. Silverman, M.D.   J. Willis Hurst, M.D.

You can observe a lot just by watching.

Yogi Berra[1,*]

The purpose of this chapter is to discuss the clues to the presence of heart disease that an astute clinician can discover by inspection of the patient.

Body Configuration

In Marfan's syndrome the findings include an arm span greater than the body height, an upper segment/lower segment ratio of less than 0.85, kyphoscoliosis, pectus excavatum, and pectus carinatum.[2–4] Patients with homocystinuria may also have long extremities, pectus carinatum, and kyphoscoliosis.[4] The cardiac involvement differs. Homocystinuria is associated with thrombosis of intermediate-sized arteries; while patients with Marfan's syndrome may suffer aortic, mitral, or tricuspid regurgitation, aortic dilatation or dissection, coronary artery involvement, pulmonary artery dilatation, redundant chordae tendineae, calcified mitral annulus, or aneurysms of the sinus of Valsalva or descending aorta.

With extreme obesity biventricular cardiac hypertrophy, arrhythmias, particularly during sleep, and increased cardiac output may be present.[5] The Pickwickian syndrome may occur, with somnolence, respiratory acidosis, and cor pulmonale.

The Ellis–van Creveld syndrome is characterized by dwarfism due to short extremities. A large atrial septal defect or atrioventricular (AV) canal defect is frequent.[6] In osteogenesis imperfecta the legs are short with marked bowing, saber shins, and pseudoarthroses. Calcification of the arteries, aortic root dilatation, and aortic and mitral regurgitation may occur.[4,7]

Congenital heart disease has been noted in Klinefelter's syndrome.[8] This syndrome may be recognized because of gynecomastia, tall stature, long extremities, and eunuchoid configuration of the body.

Skin

The cream-colored plaques of xanthelasma around the eyes or xanthomatous lumps over the Achilles tendons, knuckles, and tendons may warn of hyperlipidemia as a cause of atheroma lining or occluding coronary arteries. Aortic stenosis may also

*Reproduced with permission of the publisher.

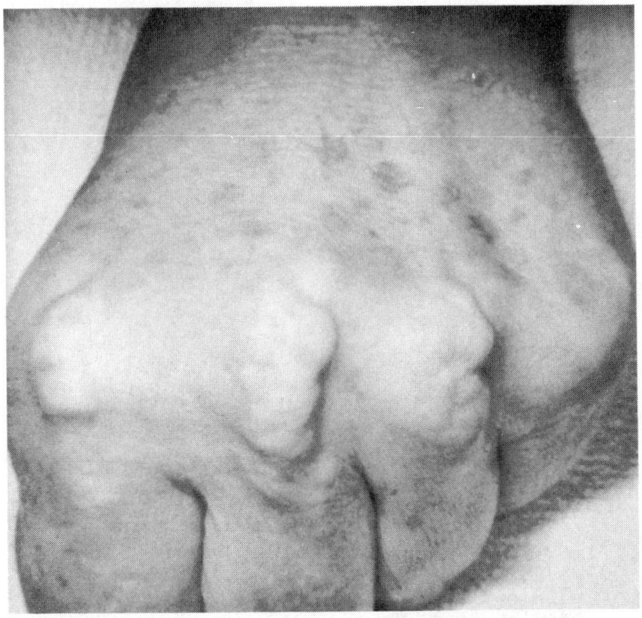

FIGURE 8-1 Xanthomatosis. Xanthoma around the knuckles associated with coronary atherosclerosis.

occur[9] (Fig. 8-1). Xanthoma and a yellow hue to the skin are physical findings in Cori's disease (type III glycogenosis). This disease may involve the myocardium.[9] Infarctions of the skin, nodules, petechiae, livedo reticularis, cyanosis, and gangrenous changes in the extremities may be due to polyarteritis, which may produce myocardial infarction, hypertension, arrhythmias, congestive heart failure, and pericarditis (Fig. 8-2).[10]

The contracted shiny skin of scleroderma gives the face a tight, bony appearance and contracts the fingers. Cor pulmonale secondary to pulmonary fibrosis or pulmonary artery involvement is the most common cardiac difficulty; however, myocardial fibrosis, valvular thickening, conduction defects, arrhythmias, and pericarditis may occur (Fig. 8-3).[11]

FIGURE 8-2 Polyarteritis. Distal gangrene of the fingers may be associated with coronary arteritis. (*From M. E. Silverman and J. W. Hurst, The Hand and the Heart, Am. J. Cardiol., 22:718, 1968. Reproduced with permission from the publisher.*)

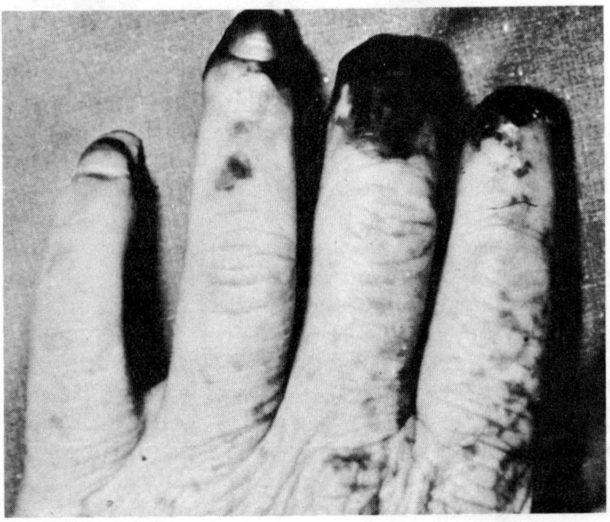

In Werner's syndrome the skin is tightly stretched over the bones. There is marked loss of subcutaneous tissue, and ulcerations occur over the legs. Severe coronary atherosclerosis often causes myocardial infarction at an early age.[12]

The presenting sign of systemic lupus erythematosus may be the typical butterfly-shaped inflammation, malar depigmentation, a vascular blush over the phalanges, a brownish-red palmar rash, discoid plaques or papules, Raynaud's phenomenon, urticaria, vitiligo, or hyperpigmentation (Fig. 8-4). Pericarditis, myocarditis, verrucous endocarditis, coronary artery disease, valvular disease, and conduction defects are the cardiovascular abnormalities.[13] Congenital complete heart block is a complication in the newborn of mothers with lupus erythematosus.[14] The affected baby may have a butterfly facial rash.

Hyperelastic skin, "cigarette paper" scars, and hyperextensible joints are found in the Ehlers-Danlos

FIGURE 8-3 Scleroderma. Indurated, depigmented skin with flexion contractures of the fingers associated with severe systemic hypertension.

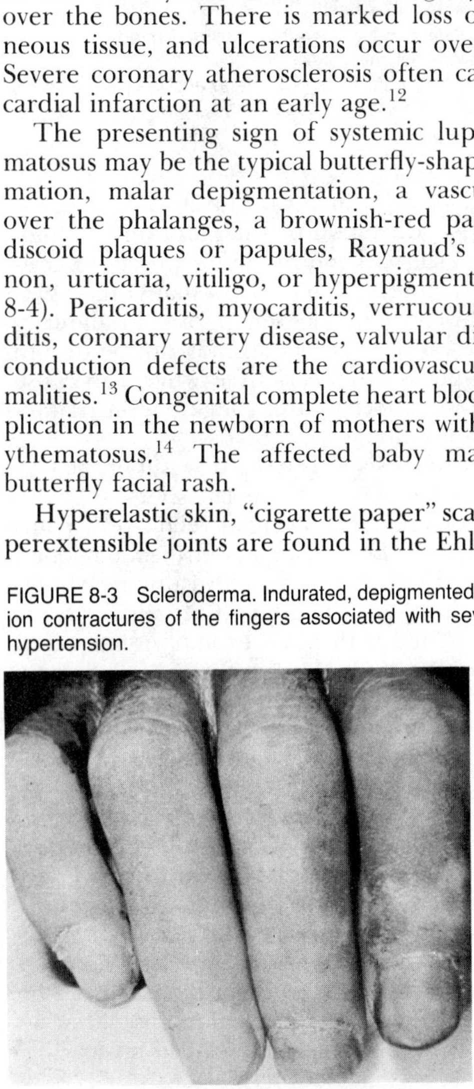

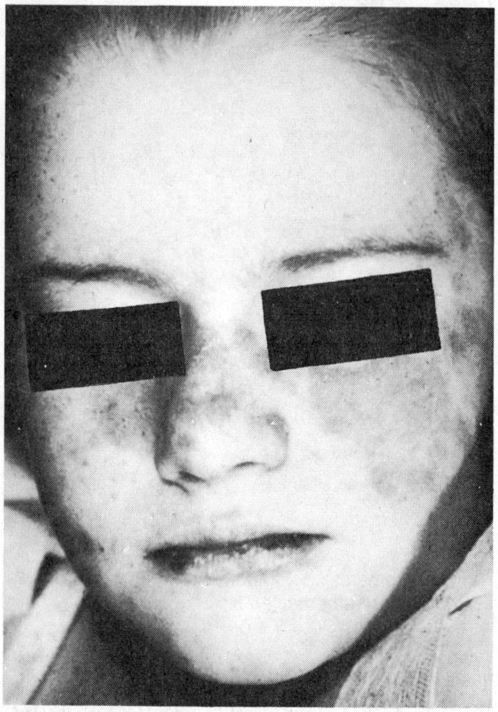

FIGURE 8-4 Systemic lupus erythematosus. Butterfly rash. Associated with pericardial, myocardial, and endocardial disease. (*From M. E. Silverman and J. W. Hurst, The Hand and the Heart, Am. J. Cardiol., 22:718, 1968. Reproduced with permission from the publisher and authors.*)

syndrome (Fig. 8-5*A* and *B*). Mitral and tricuspid valve prolapse, dilatation of the aorta and pulmonary artery, arterial rupture, and a variety of congenital heart diseases may accompany this syndrome.[15] A progressive looseness of skin allowing pendulous folds and droopy eyelids can be due to cutis laxa, a generalized elastolysis which can cause aortic dilatation and rupture, congestive heart failure, and cor pulmonale.[16]

Tuberous sclerosis is revealed by subungual fibromas of the fingers, café au lait spots, subcutaneous nodules, and a scattering of yellow-brown angiofibromas on the face (Plate 3*A*).[17] Rhabdomyomas may be found in the heart and may cause heart failure, obstruction, or arrhythmia. Café au lait spots are also associated with pheochromocytoma, renal artery stenosis, multiple lentigenes syndrome, Turner's syndrome, and pulmonic valve stenosis. Sweating is an important sign of congestive heart failure in an infant, as well as a clue to a pheochromocytoma in an adult.

In hemochromatosis the skin may develop a speckled, bronze, or slate-gray coloration. Myocardial or pericardial infiltration with iron deposits may cause arrhythmias, dilated or rarely restrictive cardiomyopathy, congestive heart failure, or pericarditis.[9,18]

The rash of dermatomyositis is scaly and red, and is often localized over the joints of the fingers. The eyelids may be decorated by a lavender discoloration (Plate 3*B*). Pericarditis, heart block, and myocardial disease are the cardiac findings.[19]

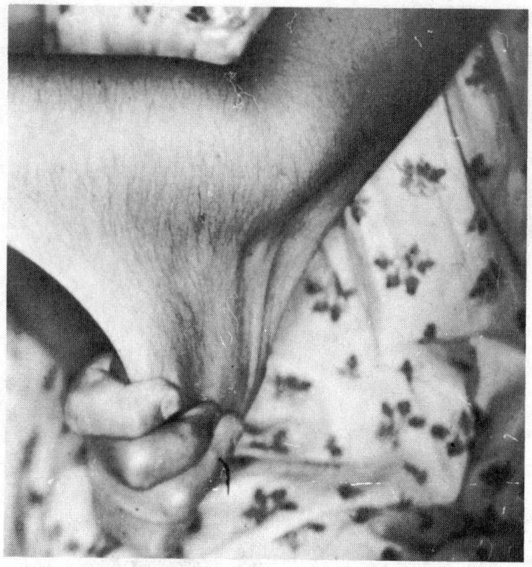

A

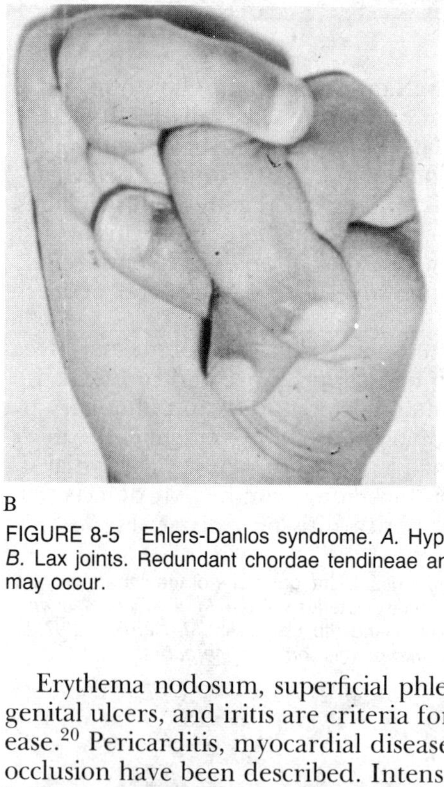

B

FIGURE 8-5 Ehlers-Danlos syndrome. *A.* Hyperextensible skin. *B.* Lax joints. Redundant chordae tendineae and arterial rupture may occur.

Erythema nodosum, superficial phlebitis, oral and genital ulcers, and iritis are criteria for Behçet's disease.[20] Pericarditis, myocardial disease, and arterial occlusion have been described. Intense flushing episodes, a chronic reddish cyanotic hue, and telangiectasia of the face are part of the dramatic presentation of the carcinoid syndrome. The usual cardiac lesions are a combination of stenosis and regurgitation of the tricuspid and pulmonary valves; however, with a patent ductus arteriosus, lung metastases, or a patent foramen ovale, lesions can also occur on the left side of the heart.[21]

The skin of pseudoxanthoma elasticum is thickened, lax, and yellowish, particularly over the axillary folds, antecubital area, and neck (Fig. 8-6). The skin around the mouth may sag. The arteries may be calcified, and the aortic and mitral valves thickened. Angina pectoris and claudication are frequent

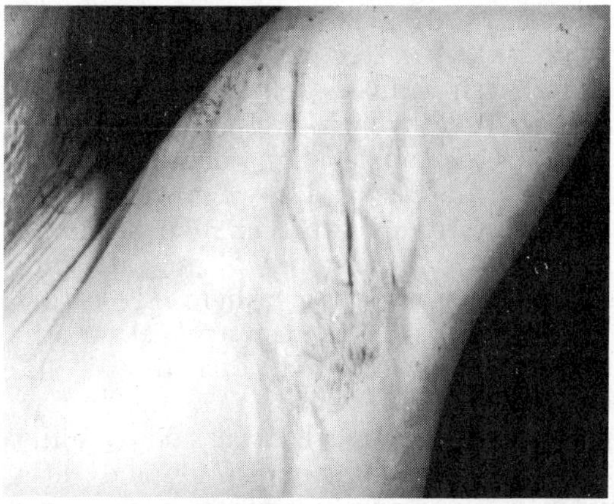

FIGURE 8-6 Pseudoxanthoma elasticum. Grooved, lax skin in a typical location. Arterial calcification may occur.

symptoms.[4,22] Aortic regurgitation and mitral valve prolapse may occur.

Elevated, waxy nodules of the skin and eyelids that may become hemorrhagic when stroked ("pinch purpura") may be associated with conduction abnormalities or myocardial disease due to amyloidosis.[23]

Degos' disease (malignant atrophic papulosis) is announced by a crop of asymptomatic, oval cutaneous lesions which have a white center and surrounding erythema. Occlusive fibrosis of small- and medium-sized arteries causing pleuritis and pericarditis is part of this rapidly fatal problem.[24]

Vitiligo, typically on the palms and soles, is a sign of Graves' disease.

Extensive skin lesions, particularly Kaposi's sarcoma or exfoliative dermatitis due to psoriasis, may divert the vascular supply through shunts in the skin to produce high-output cardiac failure.[25] Hemangiomas of the skin may also signify multinodular hemangiomatosis of the liver, a cause of high-output congestive heart failure in infancy. An underlying arteriovenous fistula with high-output failure may be evidenced by a barely discernible scar or surgical incision. Port wine stains, hemangioma of the skin, and varicose veins may be accompanied by asymmetric lengthening and overgrowth of an extremity or digit or hemihypertrophy as a result of congenital peripheral arteriovenous fistulas (Fig. 8-7).[26]

Telangiectasia of the fingertips, lips, and tongue and pulmonary and hepatic arteriovenous fistulas are associated with hereditary hemorrhagic telangiectasia (HHT).[27] (See Plate 3*C* and *D*.)

The skin involvement in sarcoidosis includes lupus pernio, erythema nodosum, plaques, pigmentary changes, subcutaneous nodules, and alopecia. Arrhythmias, altered conduction, congestive heart failure, and sudden death can occur.[24]

Erythema marginatum, a migratory, annular eruption, and subcutaneous nodules may herald the appearance of acute rheumatic fever. Pericarditis, myocarditis, and valvular inflammation are the well-known cardiac possibilities. An expanding erythema

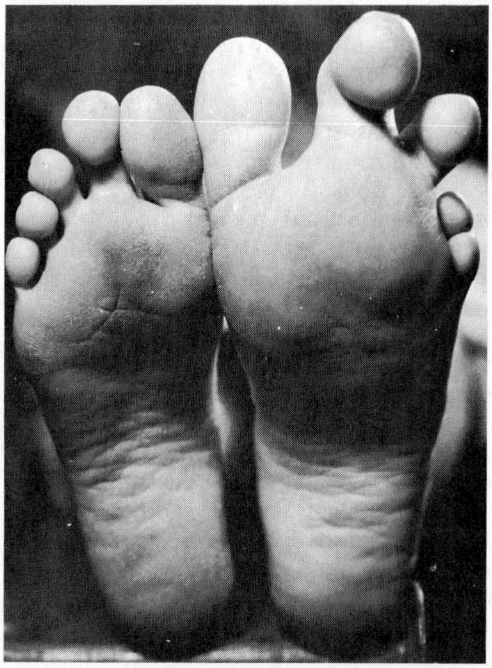

FIGURE 8-7 Congenital peripheral arteriovenous fistulas. Asymmetric enlargement of an extremity or digit associated with unusual varicose veins may occur in patients with congenital peripheral arteriovenous fistulas. Grotesque enlargement of the toes and foot on the right.

with a bright red border which may be followed by central clearup, vesiculation, or necrosis (erythema chronicum migrans) precedes the joint involvement and possible AV block, bundle branch block, or myopericarditis that is seen in Lyme arthritis.[25]

The multiple lentigines syndrome, consisting of small, dark brown macular lesions on the neck and trunk, has been associated with abnormal electrocardiographic conduction, T-wave changes, pulmonic stenosis, hypertrophic subaortic stenosis, and a leftward or superior mean QRS axis (Fig. 8-8).[26]

The purplish, pinpoint angiokeratomata of Fabry's disease present on the lip, penis, and trunk.

FIGURE 8-8 Multiple lentigines syndrome. Dark brown macular lesions on the abdomen associated with hypertrophic subaortic stenosis.

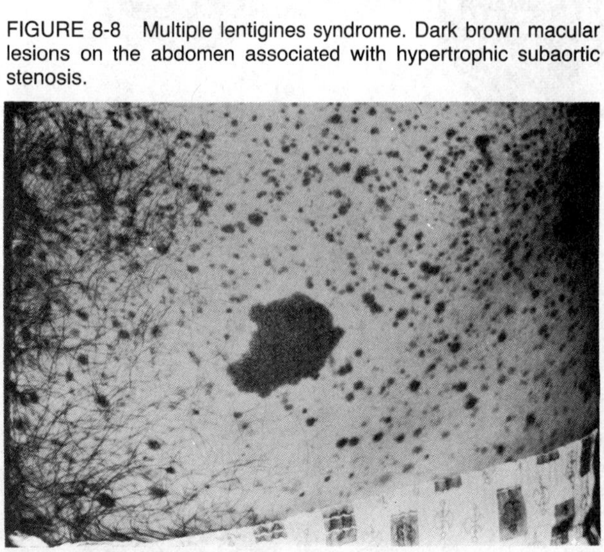

Involvement of the myocardium and blood vessels with ceramide trihexoside may result in angina pectoris, myocardial infarction, mitral regurgitation, hypertrophic cardiomyopathy, congestive heart failure, and arrhythmias.[9]

The skin lesion known as *keratosis blennorrhagica* is almost pathognomonic for Reiter's syndrome. This rash begins as erythematous macules progressing to hyperkeratotic papules which coalesce and crust over the palms and soles. Arthritis, conjunctivitis, iritis, and urethritis complete the clinical presentation. Pericarditis, myocarditis, aortic regurgitation, and conduction defects may be sequelae.[28]

Urochrome pigmentation of the skin and uremic frost are cutaneous findings of far-advanced renal disease. Patients on chronic dialysis may develop severe atherosclerosis and metastatic calcification of the myocardium, resulting in heart failure, conduction disturbances, pericarditis, severe coronary artery disease, and sudden death.[29]

Cyanosis of the skin often suggests congenital heart disease with right-to-left shunting of blood.

Gait

An unusual gait can suggest a neuromuscular disorder that may also involve the heart.[30] An ataxic, wide-based gait associated with kyphoscoliosis, hammertoe, equinovarus, nystagmus, and oscillation of the head and trunk is seen in Friedreich's ataxia (Fig. 8-9). Heart disease is virtually always present and includes myocardial disease, angina pectoris, hypertrophic subaortic stenosis, sinus node artery occlusion, and arrhythmias.[30,31] Refsum's disease, a lipidosis characterized by high levels of phytanic acid, associates cerebellar ataxia, night blindness, deafness, ichthyosis, cataracts, and polyneuropathy with myocardial disease and conduction abnormalities.[32] Patients with muscular dystrophy of the Duchenne type walk in a slow, waddling fashion. Myocardial disease, often diagnosable by distinctive electrocardiographic changes, tachycardia, arrhythmias, and mitral valve prolapse, are relatively common.[30,33] The patient with ankylosing spondylitis walks slowly, stiffly, and bent over because of a rigid, painful spine. Heart block and aortic and, rarely, mitral regurgitation are part of this illness.[34]

Squatting is a classic sign of tetralogy of Fallot.

FIGURE 8-9 Friedreich's ataxia with secondary kyphoscoliosis. Severe cardiomegaly occurred before the kyphoscoliosis developed.

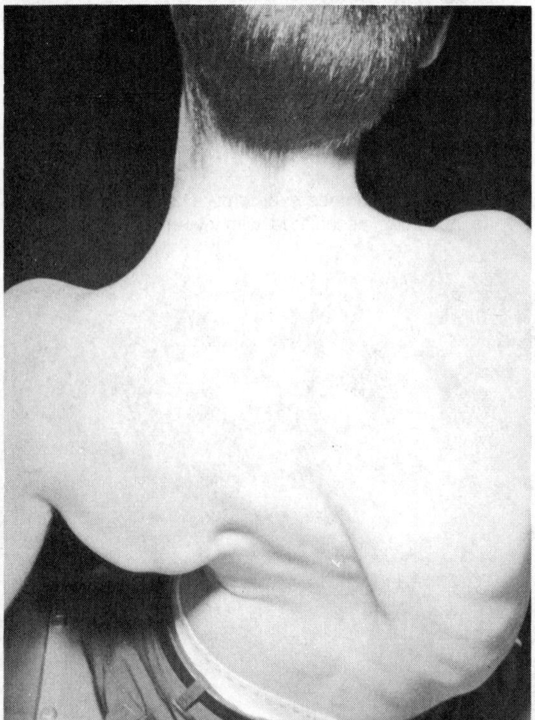

Face[35]

In the mucopolysaccharidoses, the head is large and boat-shaped. The nose is broad and the nostrils flare. Large lips, small and widely spaced teeth, and a large protuberant tongue are oral findings.[3,9] Hurler's syndrome has a high incidence of heart disease because of mucopolysaccharide deposition in the coronary arteries, endocardial fibroelastosis, and thickening of the valves (Fig. 8-10).[36] Primary myocardial disease and aortic regurgitation are the cardiovascular abnormalities in Morquio's syndrome. Aortic regurgitation also occurs in Scheie's syndrome.

The head in Marfan's syndrome and homocystinuria is long and narrow (Fig. 8-11*A*). The palate is often arched. Ectopia lentis may be obvious or may be detected by finding a tremulous iris when the head is shaken from side to side (Fig. 8-11*A* to *D*).

Cornelia de Lange syndrome is a rare disorder characterized by mental retardation; bushy, confluent eyebrows; hirsutism; long eyelashes; a small

FIGURE 8-10 Hurler's syndrome. Coarse features and bushy eyebrows. Mucopolysaccharides may be abnormally deposited in the valves, coronary arteries, and aorta.

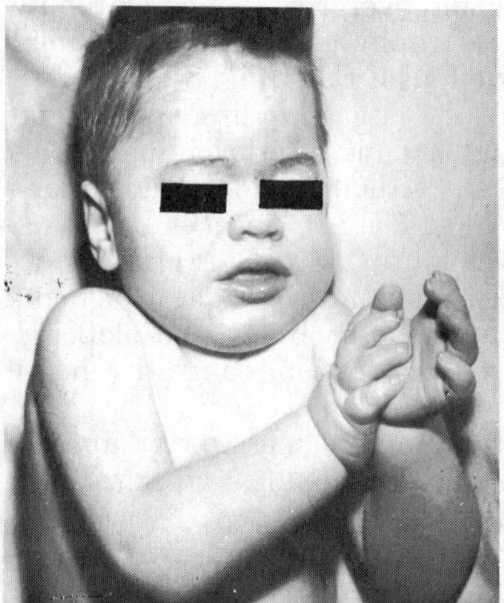

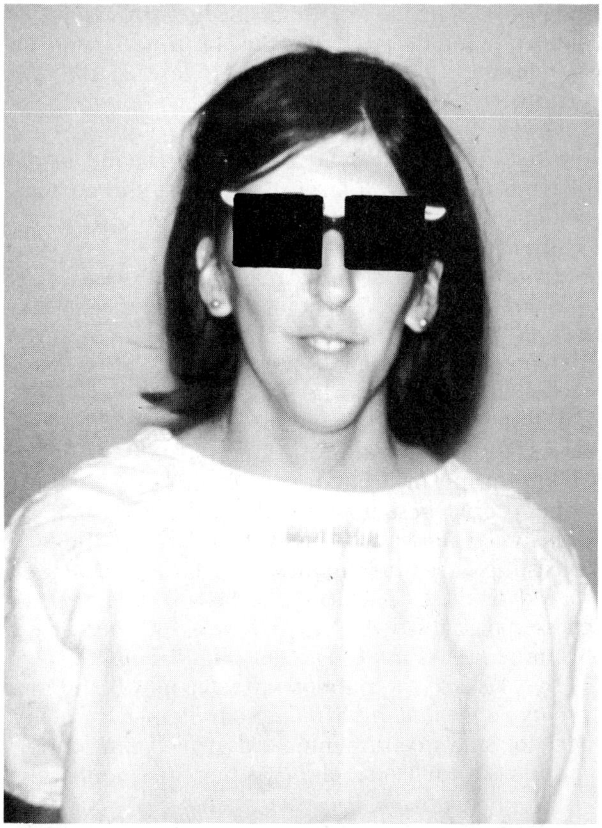

A

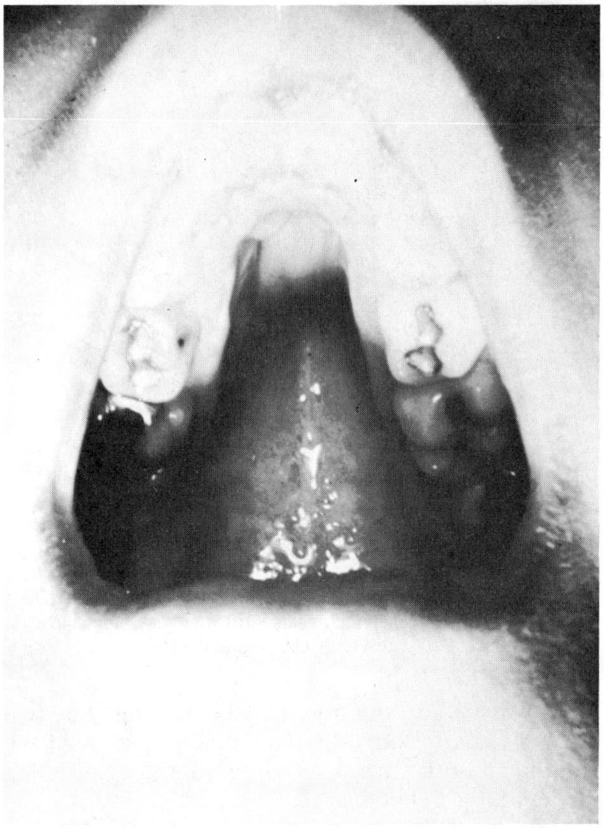

C

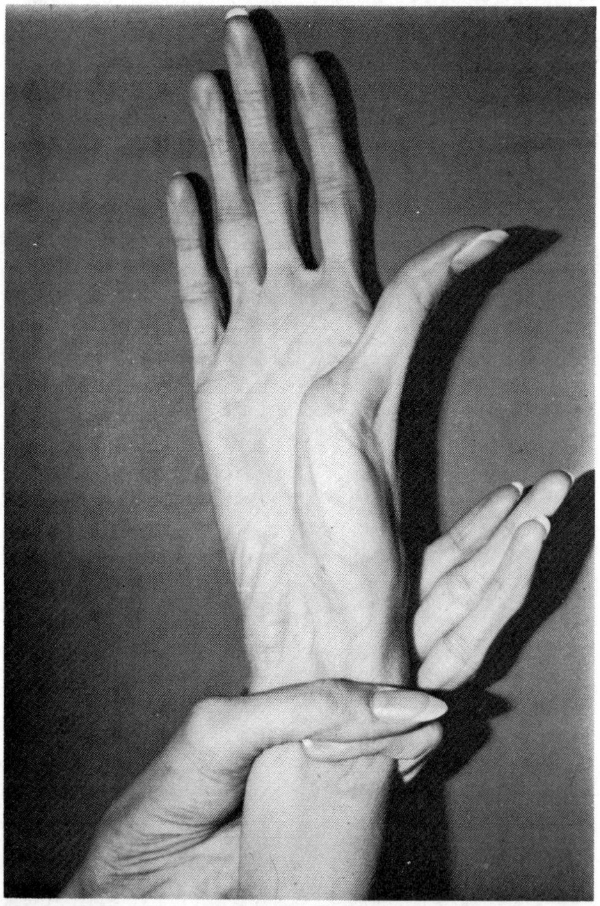

B

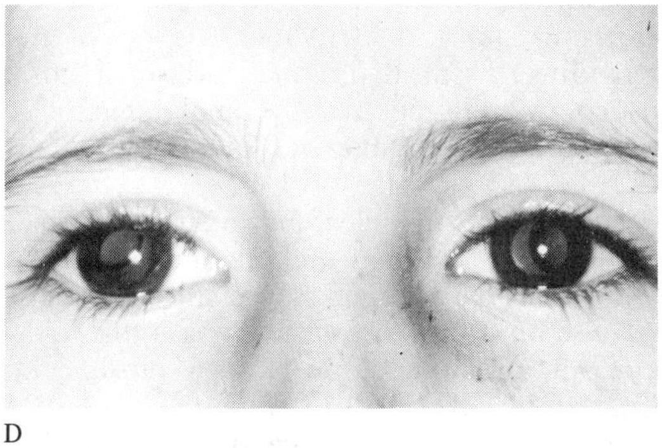

D

FIGURE 8-11 Marfan's syndrome. *A.* Long, narrow face. *B.* Arachnodactyly and positive wrist sign. *C.* High arched palate. *D.* Ectopia lentis associated with aortic aneurysm and severe aortic regurgitation in a teenage girl.

mandible; a broad, flat upturned nose; and an antimongoloid slant to the eyes in conjunction with a variety of congenital heart defects (Fig. 8-12).

In Werner's syndrome the patients have a beaked nose and premature graying and balding.

The alterations in the Rubinstein-Taybi syndrome include a prominent forehead; a thin, beaked nose or a broad nasal bridge; large, low-set ears; and an antimongoloid slant of the eyes. A variety of congenital heart defects occur.[37]

The trisomy syndromes offer almost pathognomonic facial clues, and all have a high association with cardiovascular anomalies.[38] In trisomy 13–15 syndrome the infants have a cleft palate and lip. The

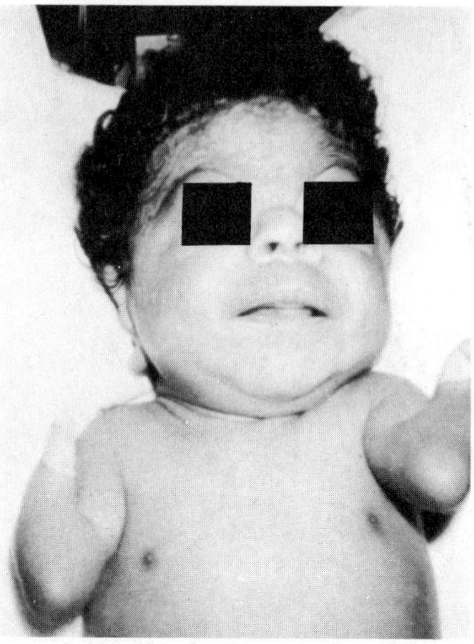

FIGURE 8-12 Cornelia de Lange syndrome. Low hairline, hirsutism, bushy eyebrows, phocomelia, and a single thumblike digit. May be associated with ventricular septal defect.

ocular tissue and the nose may be missing. The features of the trisomy 18 syndrome are a small triangular mouth with a receding chin, a small mandible, and a webbed neck.

The familiar face of Down's syndrome (trisomy 21) is recognized because of the small head; shallow orbits; epicanthal folds; slanted palpebral fissures; hypertelorism; cataracts; Brushfield's spots of the iris; protruding, fissured tongue; and small nose. The most common lesions are AV canal defect, ventricular septal defect, tetralogy of Fallot, and patent ductus.[39]

A low hairline, a small jaw, and a short, webbed neck are physical findings in both Turner's syndrome and the Klippel-Feil syndrome. Turner's syndrome also includes short stature, epicanthal folds, hypertelorism, pigmented moles, and ptosis (Fig. 8-13). Coarctation of the aorta, aortic stenosis, and hypertrophic cardiomyopathy are the usual cardiovascular considerations.[40] The Klippel-Feil syndrome may cause facial asymmetry, cleft palate, torticollis, deafness, strabismus, and hydrocephaly (Fig. 8-14). Ventricular septal defect is the usual cardiac problem.[41]

Patients with Noonan's syndrome are sometimes confused with those having Turner's syndrome because they share in common short stature, webbed neck, and hypogonadism. They differ, however, in that they are often mentally retarded and have dental malocclusion, antimongoloid slanting of the eyes, and normal chromosomes. Valvular pulmonic stenosis is the defect most likely to be present. Obstructive and nonobstructive cardiomyopathy and other congenital defects have been recognized (Fig. 8-15).[40,42]

The term *mulibrey nanism* has been coined to describe a syndrome which involves muscle, liver, brain, and eyes. These patients have a triangular face, bulging forehead, low nasal bridge, growth retardation, pigmentary changes in the fundus, and hemangiomas. The cardiac lesion is constrictive pericarditis.[43]

A variety of congenital heart defects are seen in the velocardiofacial syndrome. The face in this disorder is long with a large fleshy nose, broad nasal bridge, flattened malar region, narrow, palpebral fissures, and deep overbite.[44]

In myotonia dystrophica the patient may have a masklike expression, drooping eyelids, sunken cheeks, a receding hairline, and cataracts. Conduction disturbances, arrhythmias, mitral valve prolapse, or myocardial disease may be present.[45] Permanent atrial paralysis has been documented in patients who have facioscapulohumeral muscular dystrophy.

The origin of a harsh systolic murmur over the upper right chest may be resolved in favor of supravalvular aortic stenosis if the characteristic face, consisting of a wide mouth with large lips, widely spaced teeth, elfin features, a broad forehead, depressed nasal bridge, long philtrum, full cheeks, and prominent ears, is recognized (Fig. 8-16).[46]

Dysplasia of the pulmonary valve may be familial and is suggested by a triangular-shaped face, hypertelorism, ptosis, mental and growth retardation, and low-set ears. A similar dysplastic pulmonic valve

FIGURE 8-13 Turner's syndrome. Epicanthal folds, pigmented moles, hypertelorism, and scars on the neck where webs have been removed may be associated with coarctation of the aorta.

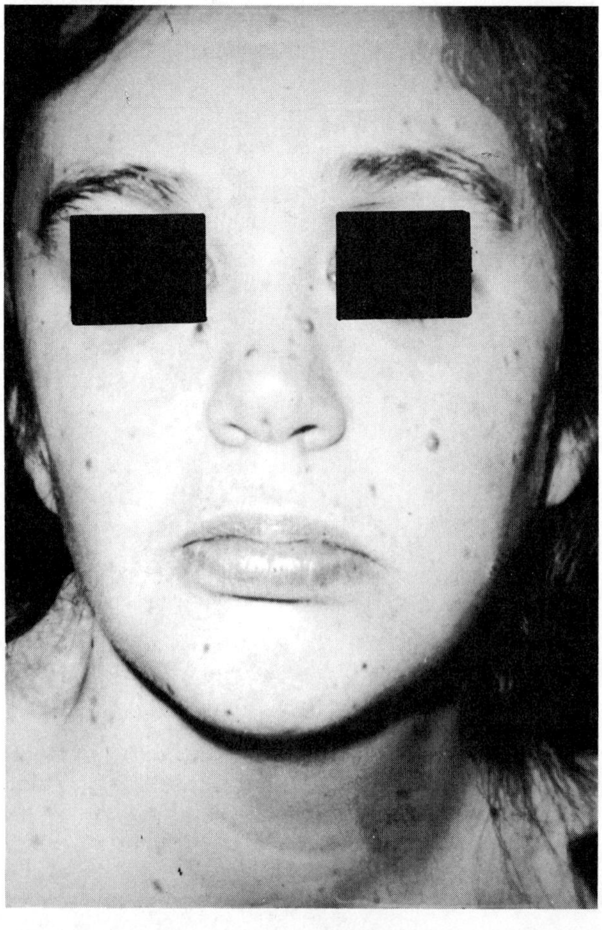

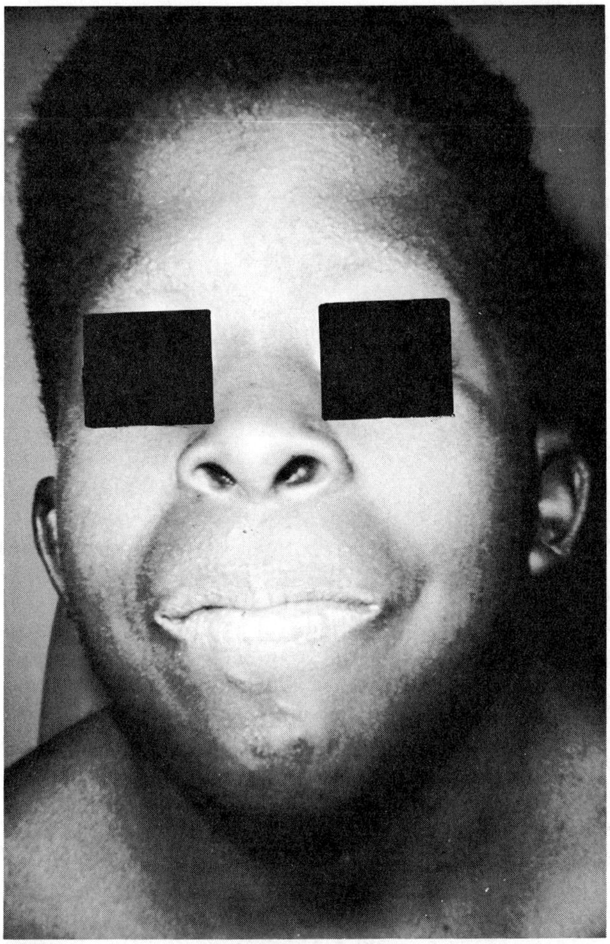

FIGURE 8-14 Klippel-Feil syndrome. Marked webbing of the neck and low-set ears associated with a ventricular septal defect.

is described in Noonan's, Watson's, and the multiple lentigines syndromes.[47]

A variety of congenital heart defects are associated with the Smith-Lemli-Opitz syndrome. The clinical findings are mental and growth retardation, hypertonia, anteverted nares, micrognathia, broad maxillary ridge, ptosis, epicanthal folds, cleft palate, and cataracts.[48]

Inflammatory destruction of the cartilage of the

FIGURE 8-15 Noonan's syndrome. Ptosis, hypertelorism, and low-set ears were associated with valvular pulmonic stenosis.

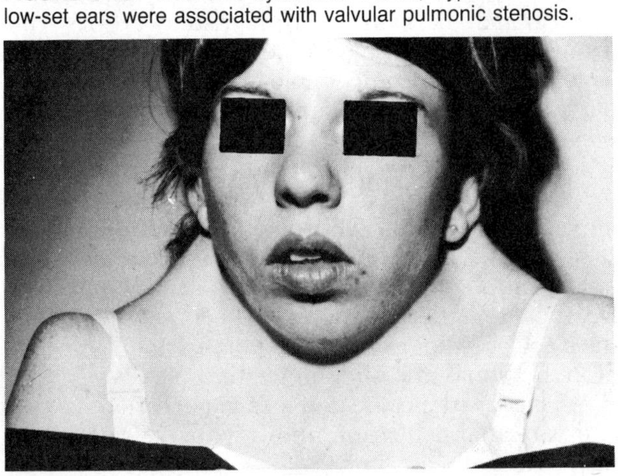

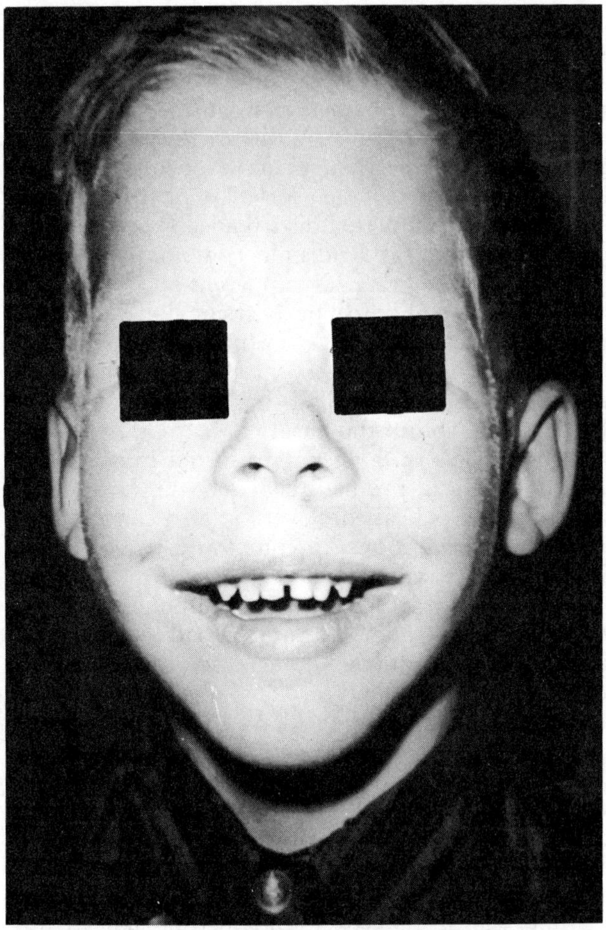

FIGURE 8-16 Supravalvular aortic stenosis. Turned-up nose, broad cheeks, large mouth with peg-shaped teeth, and large ears.

face resulting in a saddle-shaped collapse of the nose or a cauliflower ear may occur together with inflammation of the aortic ring, pericarditis, and aneurysm or dissection of the aorta when polychondritis is the culprit (Fig. 8-17*A* and *B*).[49]

The calamitous onset of cyanosis of the head and neck, sweating of the forehead, prominent jugular venous *a* waves, and dyspnea is virtually diagnostic of a pulmonary embolus.

The mucocutaneous lymph node syndrome (Ka-

FIGURE 8-17 Polychondritis. *A.* Destruction of cartilage of nose, producing a "saddle nose" (*B*), in association with aortic regurgitation. (*Courtesy of Dr. Warren Sarrell, Anniston, Ala.*)

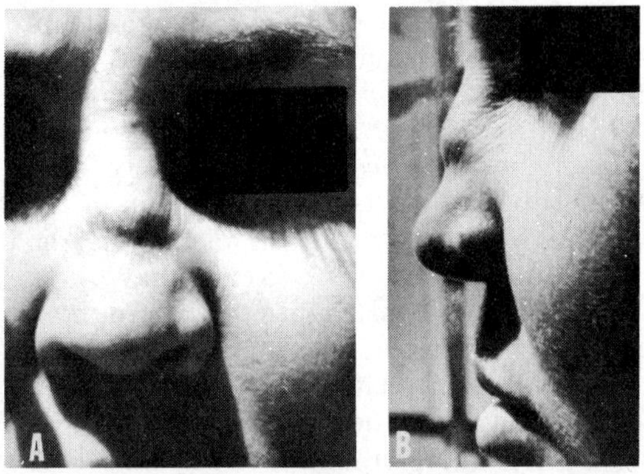

wasaki's disease) presents with conjunctivitis; erythema of the oral mucosa, palms, and fingertips; fissuring of the lips; cervical adenopathy; and a polymorphous desquamative rash in young children and occasionally adults. A diffuse perivasculitis is responsible for the frequent occurrence of coronary artery obstruction or aneurysm, pericarditis, myocarditis, and conduction disturbance.[50]

The cardiofacial syndrome combines unilateral partial lower-face weakness, apparent on crying, with ventricular septal defect or, occasionally, other congenital heart defects.[51] A seventh nerve palsy has been noted in children with diastolic blood pressure exceeding 120 mmHg. This has been attributed to hemorrhage within the facial nerve.[52]

Progeria is a rare, peculiar disorder in which the face is small and prematurely aged, the eyes bulge, and the nose is beaked. Severe atherosclerosis with myocardial infarction is a common cause of death in the early years.[53]

An excessive growth of the facial bones provides the protruding mandible and broad forehead in acromegaly. Conduction defects, myocardial hypertrophy and fibrosis, and coronary atherosclerosis may be the cardiac consequences.[54]

In hypothyroidism, the face is distorted by thickened skin, dry hair, puffy eyelids, and an enlarged tongue. Pericardial effusion, hypercholesterolemia, asymmetric septal thickening, and possibly premature myocardial infarction are the cardiac possibilities.[55]

Blue sclerae may be found in osteogenesis imperfecta. The patients may have aortic regurgitation, mitral regurgitation, deafness, and a history of numerous fractures.[7]

Patients under age 40 who have arcus senilis should be evaluated for hyperlipidemia.

The differential diagnosis of cataracts includes myotonia dystrophica, Marfan's syndrome, homocystinuria, Down's syndrome, Laurence-Moon-Biedl-Bardet syndrome, Friedreich's ataxia, Werner's syndrome, polychondritis, Refsum's disease, Hallermann-Streiff syndrome, rubella syndrome, and diabetes. The Laurence-Moon-Biedl-Bardet syndrome and the Hallermann-Streiff syndrome display a variety of congenital heart defects.[56] Diabetes is a strong risk factor for coronary atherosclerosis. The association of cataracts, deafness, nystagmus, and patent ductus or pulmonary artery stenosis constitutes the rubella syndrome (Fig. 8-18). A fibrous stenosis of cerebral, renal, and aortic vessels is a late aftermath.[57]

A coloboma (fissure) of the iris and choroid is a major sign of the cat's-eye syndrome and is found with various cardiac defects.[58]

External ophthalmoplegia, ptosis, myocardial disease, and complete heart block (Kearns-Sayre syndrome) may be due to ocular muscular dystrophy.[59]

In severe right-sided congestive heart failure or massive tricuspid regurgitation the venous pressure may be so elevated that the eyes protrude or even pulsate. Exophthalmos may also be secondary to hyperthyroidism and lead to the etiologic diagnosis of unexplained tachycardia, tricuspid regurgitation, atrial arrhythmias, or high-output congestive heart failure. In the elderly patient with apathetic thyrotoxicosis the expected physical findings may not be present. Instead these patients have a small thyroid, marked temporal muscle wasting, altered mentation, sunken eyes, and atrial fibrillation.

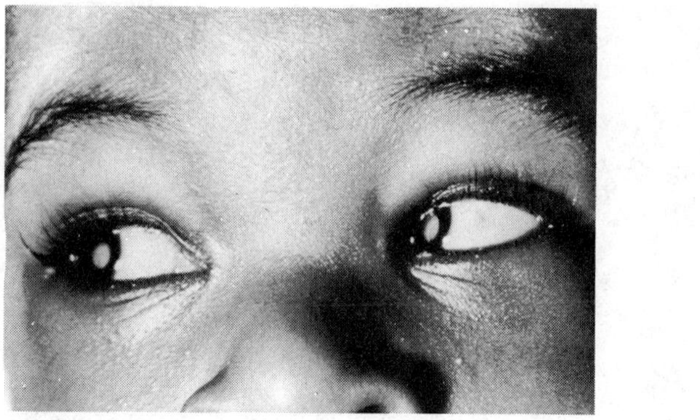

FIGURE 8-18 Rubella syndrome. Cataracts associated with peripheral pulmonic stenosis.

Facial swelling may be an early sign of carcinoma involving the pericardium or superior vena cava. Patients with bacterial endocarditis may present with severe ophthalmitis as the initial sign. Persistent searching of the upper and lower eyelids for subconjunctival hemorrhage or petechiae may lead to the diagnosis of bacterial endocarditis. Conjunctivitis may be associated with Reiter's syndrome and the mucocutaneous lymph node syndrome.

Ears

Low-set ears are a nonspecific congenital abnormality and are common to syndromes which have a high cranial vault, a short mandibular ramus, a short neck, or a hyperextended head. This is a finding in Down's, Noonan's, Cornelia de Lange, Turner's, and the Rubinstein-Taybi syndromes, trisomy 8 mosaicism, and trisomy 13–15, trisomy 18, and the Smith-Lemli-Opitz, Klippel-Feil, and Pierre Robin syndromes.[60] The ear may be malformed in trisomy 13–15 syndrome, Klippel-Feil syndrome, Turner's syndrome, Goldenhar's syndrome (oculoauriculovertebral dysplasia),[61] chromosome 9 and 22 abnormalities, and polychondritis.

Deafness is common to Hurler's syndrome, Klippel-Feil syndrome, Turner's syndrome, osteogenesis imperfecta, rubella syndrome, familial pulmonic stenosis, the multiple lentigines syndrome, and familial mitral regurgitation with skeletal anomalies. Deafness together with a prolonged QT interval on the electrocardiogram may be familial and forewarn of arrhythmias and sudden death.

An increased incidence of a diagonal earlobe crease and ear-canal hair are found in patients with coronary artery disease.[62, 62a]

Mouth

An enlarged tongue may be an important clue that amyloidosis or glycogen storage disease is the cause of an unexplained cardiomyopathy.[9,23] The amyloid deposits may also depress the submaxillary glands, giving a misleading impression of lymphadenopathy. The tongue is also enlarged in Hurler's syndrome, Down's syndrome, and in hypothyroidism.

Orange, large lobulated tonsils are a feature of Tangier disease, a type of hyperlipidemia in which there is a deficiency of high-density lipoprotein and an incidence of coronary artery disease.[9]

The upper lip may be tied down to the alveolar ridge in the Ellis–van Creveld syndrome (Fig. 8-19). The teeth may be absent, dysplastic, or peg-shaped.

Enlarged tonsils and adenoids may block the airways enough to result in respiratory acidosis. Infants with this problem often have flaring nostrils and an adenoidal expression. Cor pulmonale secondary to pulmonary hypertension, which is reversible following extirpation of the tonsils and adenoids, is the cardiac manifestation.[63] Upper airway obstruction may produce increased vagal tone, sinus bradycardia, or sinus arrhythmia, and first degree AV block in the massively obese.[64]

A high arched palate can be observed in Marfan's syndrome (Fig. 8-11*C*), Cornelia de Lange syndrome, trisomy 18 syndrome, Rubinstein-Taybi syndrome, Turner's syndrome, and the Pierre Robin syndrome.

There appears to be an increased incidence of congenital heart disease with cleft palate or lip. The exact type is variable.[65] In the familial third and fourth pharyngeal pouch syndrome, a cleft palate, micrognathia, and low-set ears are seen and truncus arteriosus may be present.

A cleft palate is also a common occurrence in the Pierre Robin syndrome. The invariable feature of this syndrome is a hypoplastic mandible with a "shrewlike" face (Fig. 8-20). The posteriorly displaced tongue produces severe respiratory problems and may cause cor pulmonale.[66] Cardiovascular disease is frequent.

FIGURE 8-19 Ellis–van Creveld syndrome. *A.* Typical "lip tie" due to multiple frenulum. *B.* Polydactyly. This patient had a large atrial septal defect.

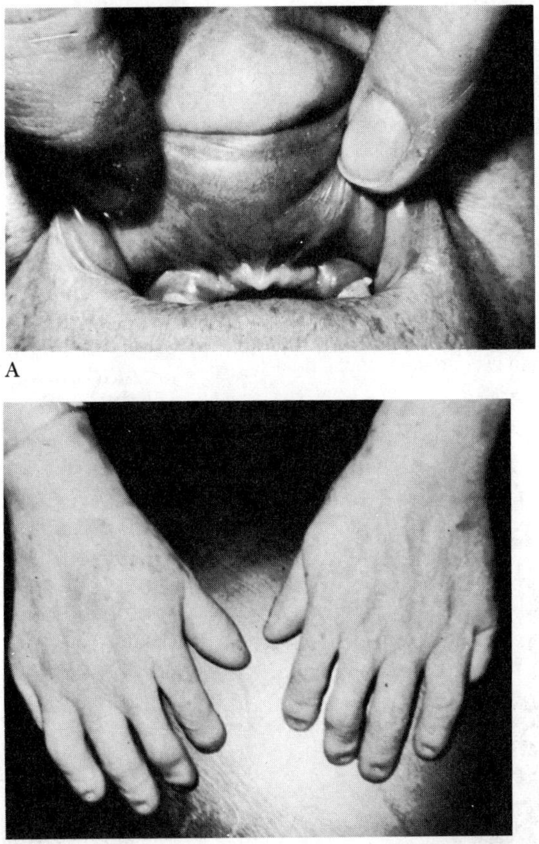

A

B

Extremities[67]

The upper extremities may have a greater muscular development than the legs in coarctation of the aorta. Underdevelopment of musculature is seen in large left-to-right intracardiac shunts. Pseudohypertrophy of the calves is a manifestation of muscular dystrophy.

Warm, moist hands with a fine tremor and occasionally with clubbing of the fingers suggest hy-

FIGURE 8-20 Pierre Robin syndrome. Hypoplastic mandible associated with a ventricular septal defect.

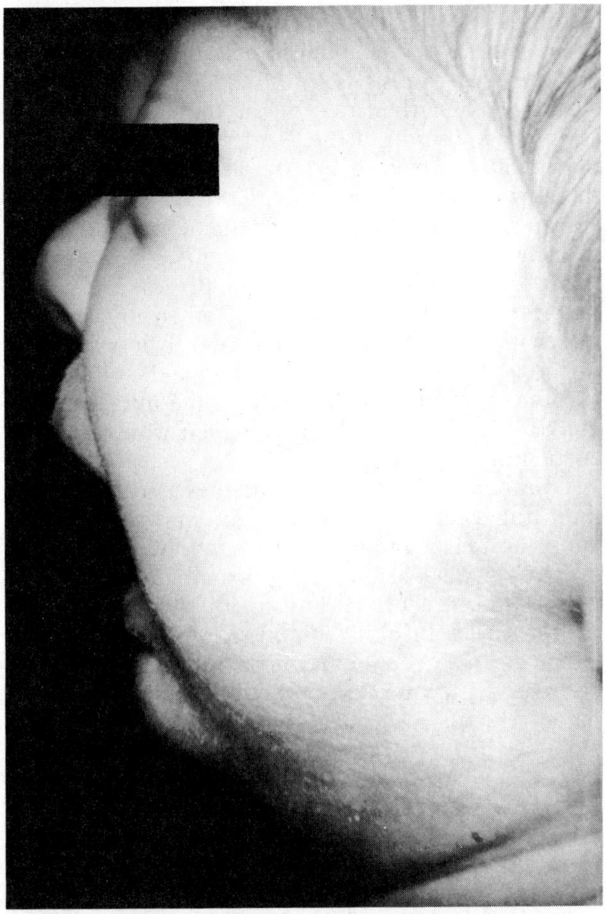

perthyroidism. A cold hand with coarse, puffy skin may be due to hypothyroidism.

A spadelike hand with "sausage" fingers is one of the many flagrant external changes in acromegaly.

A myocardial infarction or arterial occlusion may be followed by the development of the shoulder-hand syndrome, which displays a hand that is swollen, shiny, discolored, and stiff. Painful swelling of the dorsal surface of the hands and feet is an early clinical sign of sickle cell disease. High-output cardiac failure with cardiomegaly, systolic and occasionally diastolic murmurs, and pulmonary vascular thromboses are the cardiovascular complications.

Hypoplastic fingernails, lymphedema, clinodactyly, and a shortened fifth finger are found in Turner's syndrome.

Clubbing of the fingers and cyanosis are typical of congenital heart disease or pulmonary arteriovenous fistulas with a right-to-left shunt (Plate 4*A*). Red fingertips, or "tuft erythema," may signify small or intermittent right-to-left shunts with only slight reduction in arterial oxygen saturation (Plate 4*B*).

Cyanosis and clubbing with a high cardiac output, presumably related to small arteriovenous shunts in the lung, are infrequent physical signs of cirrhosis of the liver. Diseases of the lungs, such as emphysema, scleroderma, and sarcoidosis, may produce clubbing and may also lead to cor pulmonale. Acute painful clubbing or hypertrophic osteoarthropathy is a manifestation of bronchogenic carcinoma, which may invade or metastasize to the heart or pericardium.

Specific anatomic implications can be made when differential cyanosis is found.[68,69] Cyanosis of the fingers greater than that of the toes suggests complete transposition of the great vessels with either a preductal coarctation or complete interruption of the aortic arch, pulmonary hypertension, and a reversed shunt through a patent ductus arteriosus delivering oxygenated blood to the lower extremities (Plate 4*C*). In this abnormality the presence of coarctation of the aorta can be separated from complete interruption of the aortic arch. Slightly less cyanosis of the left arm when compared with the right arm favors coarctation of the aorta, while intense, symmetric cyanosis of both arms is seen with complete aortic interruption.

Cyanosis and clubbing of the toes associated with pink fingernails of the right hand and minimal cyanosis and clubbing in the left hand are due to pulmonary hypertension with normally related great vessels and a reversed shunt through a patent ductus arteriosus bringing unoxygenated blood to the left arm and lower extremities (Plate 4*D*). This is also true with interruption of the aortic arch and a patent ductus arteriosus delivering unoxygenated blood to the legs. If the right subclavian artery arises proximal to the aortic obstruction, then the right hand may be pink and the left hand cyanotic. When the right subclavian artery originates anomalously from the descending aorta, then both hands are cyanotic.

Pallor of the nail bed suggests anemia and possible high-output cardiac failure or a superimposed burden on an ischemic myocardium.

Splinter hemorrhages of the nails may lead to the diagnosis of bacterial endocarditis but may also occur in a wide variety of unrelated diseases, in embolism from other sources, and in healthy people. Other clues to bacterial endocarditis include Osler's nodes, Janeway lesions, petechiae, and clubbing of the fingers (Plate 3*E* and *F*).[70] Osler's nodes are typically reddish-purple, tender nodules in the distal pad of the finger or toe. There may be a white center. Janeway lesions appear in the palms or soles and are nontender, hemorrhagic, and slightly raised. Petechiae may be found in the mouth, around the clavicle, or on the legs.

A variation in the size or number of fingers is an excellent indication of congenital or inherited heart disease. In the Ellis–van Creveld syndrome polydactyly and dystrophic nails are found (Fig. 8-19).[6] Polydactyly is part of the Laurence-Moon-Biedl-Bardet syndrome. Polydactyly in combination with retroflexible thumbs, transverse creases, hyperconvex narrow nails, and flexion of the fingers and hands is classic for trisomy 13–15 syndrome.[38]

Hypoplasia or absence of the radial aspect of the hand has a very striking connection with septal defects. In the Holt-Oram syndrome, an autosomal dominant disorder, the thumbs may resemble a finger, being hypoplastic and in the same plane as the rest of the fingers, or they may be triphalangeal, absent, or longer than normal (Fig. 8-21). The forearms are short, and supination and pronation are limited. The usual cardial defect is a secundum atrial septal defect.[71] An identical thumb, or absence of the thumb or radius, occurs with a ventricular septal defect in ventriculoradial dysplasia; this is not felt to be a heritable disorder (Fig. 8-22).[72]

Arachnodactyly and lax joints are salient features of both Marfan's syndrome and homocystinuria.[4] When patients with Marfan's syndrome clench their hand around the flexed thumb, the thumb pro-

FIGURE 8-21 Holt-Oram syndrome. Fingerized thumb (arrow) associated with an atrial septal defect.

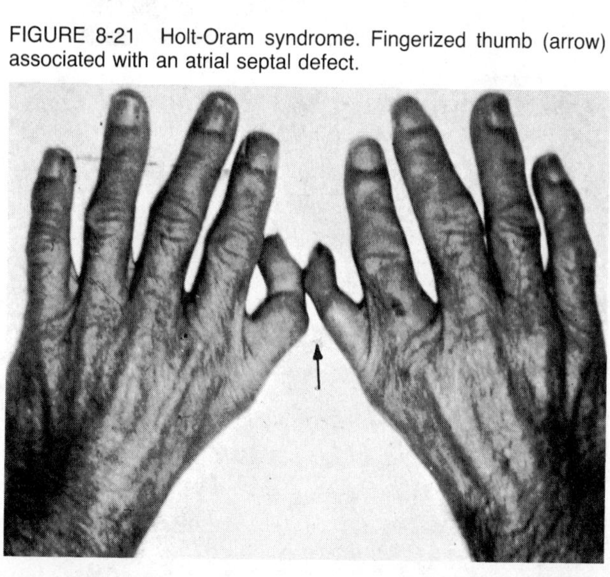

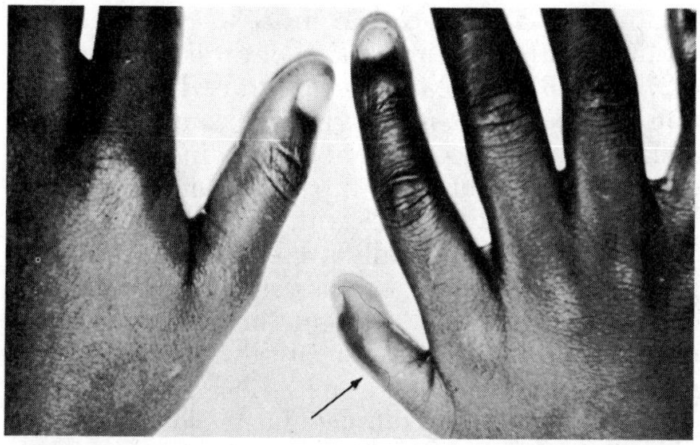

FIGURE 8-22 Ventriculoradial dysplasia. Hypoplastic thumb (arrow) associated with a ventricular septal defect. (*From M. E. Silverman and J. W. Hurst, The Hand and the Heart, Am. J. Cardiol., 22:718, 1968. Reproduced with permission from the publisher and authors.*)

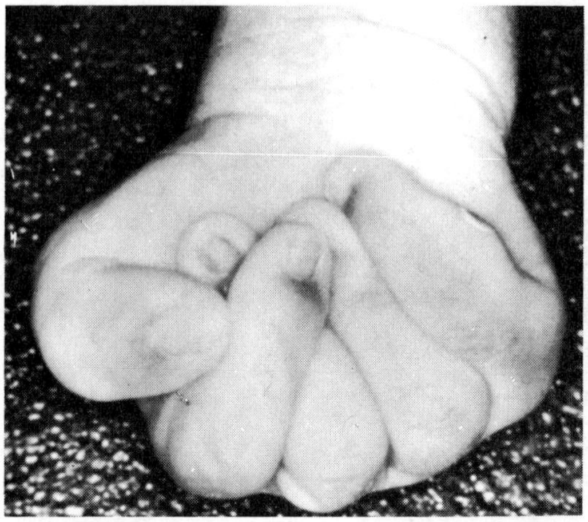

FIGURE 8-24 Trisomy 18 syndrome. Tightly clenched fist with overlapping index and fifth fingers. A ventricular septal defect was present.

trudes past the ulnar side of the hand. They can also easily encircle their wrist by grasping it with the fifth finger and thumb of the other hand (Fig. 8-11*B*). The fingers may be contracted in homocystinuria.

Broad thumbs and great toes are the hallmark of the Rubinstein-Taybi syndrome (Fig. 8-23*A* and *B*).[37]

The hand in trisomy 18 syndrome is characteristic, consisting of a tightly clenched fist, an index finger overlapping the third finger, a fifth finger overlapping the fourth finger, and stubby fingers (Fig. 8-24).[38]

Transverse creases of the palms are not diagnostic but are common in Down's syndrome (Fig. 8-25).

Cornelia de Lange syndrome is a rare disorder featuring a "chicken wing" appendage, or a proximal thumb, or short, tapering digits (Fig. 8-12).

Ulnar deviation of the fingers, thickening of the middle interphalangeal joints, boxing of the wrists, and subcutaneous nodules typify rheumatoid arthritis, which has a high incidence of cardiac disease including pericarditis, coronary arteritis, or granulomatous inflammation involving the myocardium or the base or cusps of the aortic and mitral valves.[73,74] Jaccoud's arthritis is usually due to repeated attacks of rheumatic fever and may cause marked ulnar deviation at the metacarpophalangeal joints, resembling rheumatoid arthritis (Fig. 8-26).[75] The fingers, however, can be moved freely into a correct alignment. Acute rheumatic fever may express itself by inflammation of the joints.

FIGURE 8-23 Rubinstein-Taybi syndrome. *A*. Broad thumb. *B*. Broad great toe. May be associated with a variety of congenital heart defects. (*A, from M. E. Silverman and J. W. Hurst, The Hand and the Heart, Am. J. Cardiol., 22:718, 1968. Reproduced with permission from the publisher and authors.*)

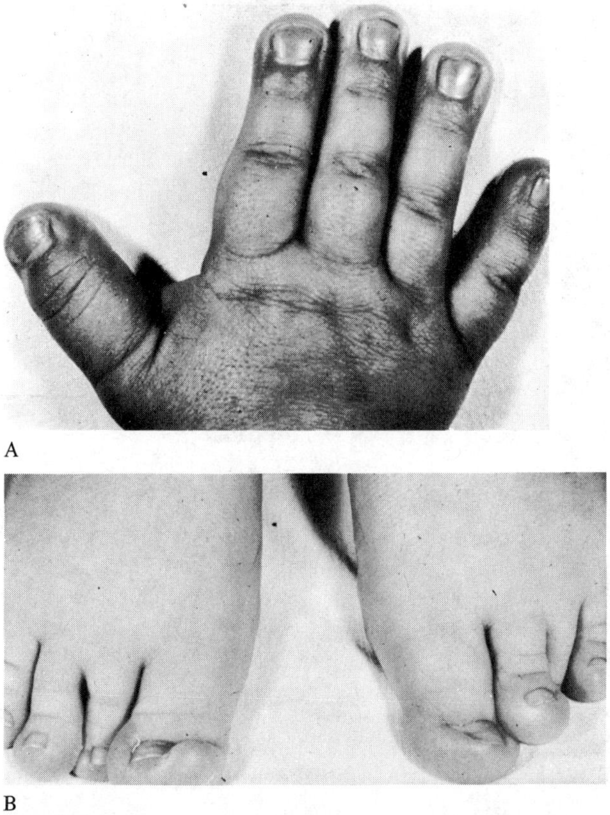

A

B

FIGURE 8-25 Down's syndrome. Simian crease associated with an atrioventricular defect. (*From M. E. Silverman and J. W. Hurst, The Hand and the Heart, Am. J. Cardiol., 22:718, 1968. Reproduced with permission from the publisher and authors.*)

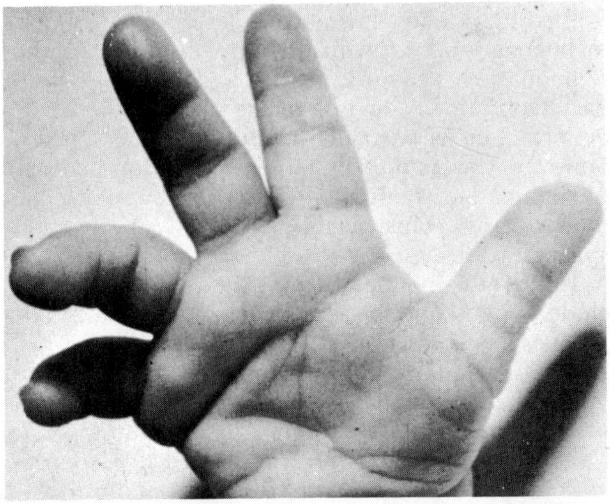

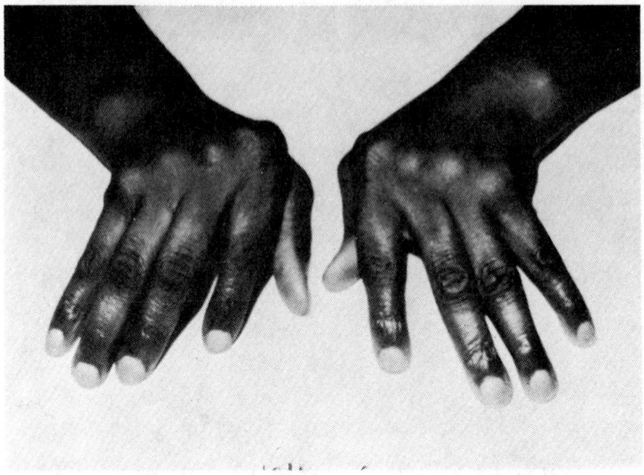

FIGURE 8-26 Jaccoud's arthritis. Ulnar deviation of the fingers suggesting rheumatoid arthritis; however, the fingers could be freely moved back into a normal alignment. (*Courtesy of Dr. Albert Raizner, Baylor University, Houston, Tex.*)

The diagnosis of Whipple's disease may be neglected unless the polyarthritis is connected to the abdominal pain and diarrhea. Pericarditis, endocarditis, coronary artery disease, aortic regurgitation, and arrhythmias may be present and may antedate the malabsorption.[76]

Uric acid crystals, causing gouty arthritis, may also occur in the heart, resulting in nodules in the myocardium, valves, or conducting system.[77]

Blue-black pigmentation of atheroma, mitral and aortic valvulitis, myocardial infarction, and arthritis can be due to an accumulation of homogentisic acid in alkaptonuria.[9]

Arthritis is also common to lupus erythematosus, polychondritis, polymyositis, sickle cell disease, and Lyme arthritis and Behçet's disease.

Elbow contractures, humeroperoneal weakness, and sinus node dysfunction are the manifestations of Emery-Dreifuss muscular dystrophy.[78]

Thorax and Neck

Structural deformity and neuromuscular disorders of the thorax may alter normal respiration, leading to hypoxia and vasoconstriction, distortion of the pulmonary vasculature, and impedance to pulmonary blood flow. Cor pulmonale may be the consequence. This is particularly true in kyphoscoliosis; however, cor pulmonale may also develop because of rheumatoid spondylitis, osteogenesis imperfecta, thoracoplasty, poliomyelitis, muscular dystrophy, and spinal cord disease.

In the mucopolysaccharidoses the deformities include kyphoscoliosis, pectus carinatum, and a barrel-shaped chest with a short neck. The Klippel-Feil syndrome is identified by a short neck due to congenital fusion of the cervical vertebrae and scoliosis, in addition to many other bony deformities.[42]

The straight-back syndrome, as well as pectus excavatum, may displace the heart to the left, producing a misleading impression of cardiomegaly (Fig. 8-27*A* and *B*). Systolic and even a rare diastolic murmur may be heard, although significant cardiac impairment rarely occurs. There is an increased incidence of a straight back in patients with congenital heart disease, particularly with atrial septal defects. Scoliosis is also commonly present in cyanotic congenital heart disease. There is a significant incidence of pectus excavatum, straight thoracic spine, and scoliosis in patients with mitral valve prolapse.[79]

Ankylosing spondylitis may be associated with aortic regurgitation, complete heart block, and cardiomyopathy.[79a]

Other important clues may be gained from a close scrutiny of the thorax. Bilateral prominence of the anterior part of the chest, with bulging of the upper two-thirds of the sternum and indrawing of the lower one-third, is an effect of ventricular septal defect in children. A unilateral bulge at the fourth and fifth intercostal spaces at the lower left sternal border is found in adults with ventricular septal defects. A bulge in the area of the second and third intercostal spaces at the left sternal border may be due to an underlying atrial septal defect.[80]

An underlying aneurysm of the ascending aorta may be suggested by a pulsating sternoclavicular joint

FIGURE 8-27 Chest deformities that may produce murmurs. *A.* Straight-back syndrome. *B.* Pectus excavatum. (*A, from A. C. De Leon, Jr., J. K. Perloff, H. Twigg, and M. Majd, The Straight Back Syndrome: Clinical Cardiovascular Manifestations, Circulation, 32:193, 1965. Reproduced with permission from the American Heart Association, Inc., and authors.*)

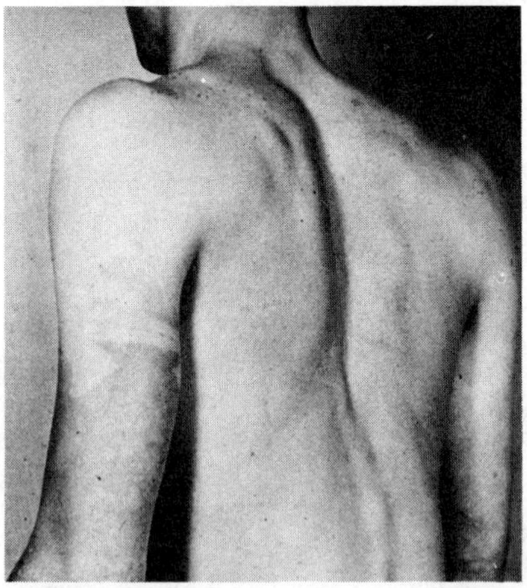

A

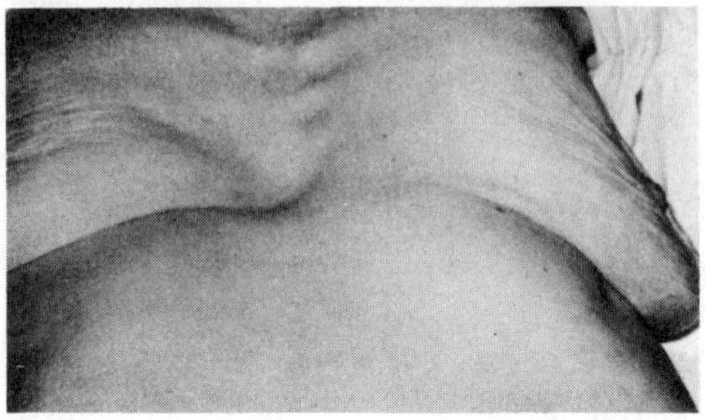

B

or by an abnormal bulge over the upper right sternal border.

In Turner's syndrome the chest is broad, with widely spaced nipples (shield chest), hypoplastic breast tissue, and a webbed neck.

Tortuous vessels along the lateral chest wall or surrounding the scapula result from coarctation of the aorta. Buckling of the right common carotid artery is often mistaken for an aneurysm. Distension of the left external jugular vein may develop when the aorta becomes enlarged and sclerotic or dissected, compressing the left brachiocephalic vein against the sternum. Unilateral distension of the neck veins may lead to a diagnosis of mediastinal tumor. Bilateral distension of the neck veins, plus evidence of collateral venous circulation over the upper part of the chest, suggests superior vena cava obstruction.

Tachypnea may be an early sign of congestive heart failure, particularly in infants. Sighing respirations or tachypnea may heighten the suspicion that an atypical chest pain or dizzy spells are related to hyperventilation. The respirations in patients with pericarditis and pulmonary infarction are shallow, because the patient is afraid of increasing the pleuritic pain. In pulmonary edema, the respirations are desperately deep and labored. Wheezing may be audible in patients suffering from a pulmonary embolus or pulmonary edema.

Miscellaneous

An imperforate anus may be associated with a cardiovascular malformation.[81] This may occur as an isolated finding or as a component of the Vater association, the asplenia syndrome, the CHARGE syndrome (*c*oloboma, *h*eart disease, *a*tresia choanae, *r*etarded growth, *g*enital hypoplasia, *e*ar anomalies),[82] or the cat's-eye syndrome. The Vater association also includes vertebral defects, tracheoesophageal fistulas, and radial and renal dysplasia.[83] The asplenia syndrome has a striking incidence of complex congenital heart disease.[84] Cardiovascular malformations are found in 15 to 25 percent of newborns with omphalocele.[85]

Abnormalities involving chromosomes 1, 9, 11, and 22 have been described with congenital heart disease.[86] The findings in chromosome 1 include a peaked nose, micrognathia, and long, tapering fingers. Children with chromosome 9 abnormalities have a prominent forehead, hypertension, anteverted nostrils, long upper lip, short neck, mental retardation, and external ear malformations. A chromosome 11 abnormality shares similar features, and, in addition, there is retraction of the lower lip. Psychomotor retardation, coloboma, hypertelorism, antimongoloid slanting of the eyes, and preauricular tags or fistulas are clues to a chromosome 22 defect.

Congenital heart disease, primarily patent ductus arteriosus, has now been linked to the 49,XXXXY syndrome. This rare syndrome should be suspected when the infant has psychomotor retardation, hypoplastic genitals, prognathism, clinodactyly (inward curving of the fifth finger), and radioulnar synostoses.

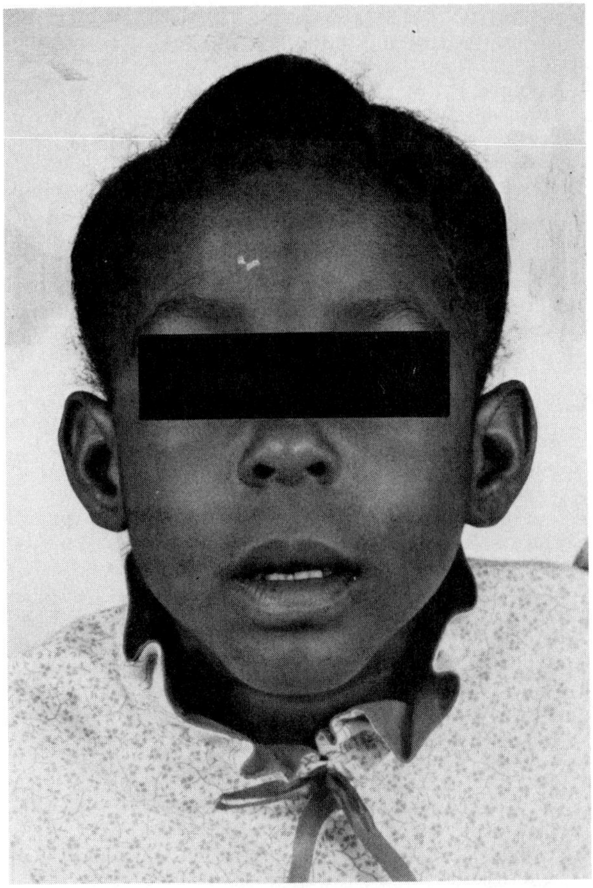

FIGURE 8-28 Fetal alcohol syndrome. Midface hypoplasia, absent philtrum, and microcephaly associated with a ventricular septal defect.

Offspring of chronic alcoholic mothers have been observed to share similar characteristics. These include microcephaly, short palpebral fissures, hypoplastic face with thinned vermilion border and diminished to absent philtrum, epicanthal folds, growth deficiency, joint anomalies, and septal defects (Fig. 8-28).[87]

The presence of any congenital somatic abnormality should always stimulate a search for heart disease. In a recent study extracardiac abnormalities were found in 25 percent of infants seen during the first year for significant cardiac disease. The defects were commonly found in the musculoskeletal system or associated with a specific syndrome.[88]

References

1. Hollander, P., and Hollander, Z. (eds.): "The Masked Marvels," Random House, Inc., New York, 1982, p. 81.
2. Pyeritz, R. E., and McKusick, V. A.: The Marfan Syndrome, *N. Engl. J. Med.*, 300:772, 1979.

3. Roberts, W. C., and Honig, H. S.: The Spectrum of Cardiovascular Disease in the Marfan Syndrome, *Am. Heart J.*, 104:115, 1982.
4. Beighton, P.: The Inherited Disorders of Connective Tissue: I. Pseudoxanthoma Elasticum, Ehlers-Danlos, Marfan's Syndrome, Homocystinuria, Osteogenesis Imperfecta, *Bull. Rheum. Dis.*, 23:696, 1972–1973 ser.
5. Messerli, F. H., Sundgaard-Riise, K., Reisin, E., Dreslinski, G., Dunn, F. G., and Frohlich, E.: Disparate Cardiovascular Effects of Obesity and Arterial Hypertension, *Am. J. Med.*, 74:808, 1983.
6. da Silva, E. O., Janovitz, D., and de Albuquerque, S. C.: Ellis–van Creveld Syndrome, *J. Med. Genet.*, 17:349, 1980.
7. White, N. J., Winerals, G. C., and Smith, R.: Cardiovascular Abnormalities in Osteogenesis Imperfecta. *Am. Heart J.*, 106:1416, 1983.
8. Rosenthal, A.: Cardiovascular Malformations in Klinefelter's Syndrome: Report of Three Cases, *J. Pediatr.*, 80:471, 1972.
9. Blieden, L. C., and Miller, J. H.: Cardiac Involvement in Inherited Disorders of Metabolism, *Prog. Cardiovasc. Dis.*, 16:1615, 1974.
10. Przybojewski, J. Z.: Polyarteritis Nodosa in the Adult: Report of a Case with Repeated Myocardial Infarction and a Review of Cardiac Involvement, *S. Afr. Med. J.*, 60:512, 1982.
11. Botstein, G. R., and LeRoy, E. C.: Primary Heart Disease in Systemic Sclerosis (Scleroderma): Advances in Clinical and Pathologic Features, Pathogenesis, and New Therapeutic Approaches, *Am. Heart J.*, 102:913, 1981.
12. Nakao, Y., Kishikara, M., Yoshimi, H., Inoue, Y., Tanaka, K., Sakamota, N., et al.: Werner's Syndrome: In Vivo and In Vitro Characteristics As a Model of Aging, *Am. J. Med.*, 65:919, 1978.
13. Borenstein, D. G., Fye, W. B., Arnett, F. C., and Stevens, M. B.: The Myocarditis of Systemic Lupus Erythematosus, *Ann. Intern. Med.*, 89:619, 1978.
14. Esscher, E., and Scott, J. S.: Congenital Heart Block and Maternal Systemic Lupus Erythematosus, *Br. Med. J.*, 1:1235, 1979.
15. Leier, C. V., Call, T. D., Fulkerson, P. K., and Wooley, C. F.: The Spectrum of Cardiac Defects in the Ehlers-Danlos Syndrome, Types I and III, *Ann. Intern. Med.*, 92:171, 1980.
16. Harris, R. B., Heaphy, M. R., and Perry, H. O.: Generalized Elastolysis (Cutis Laxa), *Am. J. Med.*, 65:815, 1978.
17. Fenoglio, J. J., Jr., McAllister, H. A., Jr., and Ferrans, V. J.: Cardiac Rhabdomyoma: A Clinicopathologic and Electron Microscopic Study, *Am. J. Cardiol.*, 38:241, 1976.
18. Candell-Riera, J., Lu, L., Seres, L., et al.: Cardiac Hemochromatosis: Beneficial Effects of Iron Removal Therapy, *Am. J. Cardiol.*, 52:824, 1983.
19. Haupt, H. M., and Hutchins, G. M.: The Heart and Cardiac Conduction System in Polymysitis-Dermatomyositis: A Clinicopathologic Study of 16 Autopsied Patients, *Am. J. Cardiol.*, 50:998, 1982.
20. James, D. G., and Thompson, A.: Recognition of the Diverse Cardiovascular Manifestations in Behçet's Disease, *Am. Heart J.*, 103:457, 1982.
21. Callahan, J. A., Wrolewski, E. M., Reeder, G. S., Edwards, W. D., Seward, J. B., and Tajik, A. J.: Echocardiographic Features of Carcinoid Heart Disease, *Am. J. Cardiol.*, 50:762, 1982.
22. Strole, W. E., Jr., and Margolis, R. J.: Gastrointestinal Bleeding with Ocular and Cutaneous Abnormalities, *N. Engl. J. Med.*, 308:579, 1983.
23. Roberts, W. C., and Waller, B. F.: Cardiac Amyloidosis Causing Cardiac Dysfunction: Analysis of 54 Necropsy Patients, *Am. J. Cardiol.*, 52:137, 1983.
24. Virmani, R., Bures, J. C., and Roberts, W. C.: Cardiac Sarcoidosis; a Major Cause of Sudden Death in Young Individuals, *Chest*, 77:423, 1980.
25. Steere, A. C., Bartenhagen, N. H., Craft, J. E., et al.: The Early Clinical Manifestations of Lyme Disease, *Ann. Intern. Med.*, 99:76, 1983.
26. St. John Sutton, M. G., Tajik, A. J., Giuliana, E. R., Gordon, H., and Daniel Su, W. P.: Hypertrophic Obstructive Cardiomyopathy and Lentiginosis: A Little Known Neural Ectodermal Syndrome, *Am. J. Cardiol.*, 47:214, 1981.
27. Hodgson, C. H., Burchell, H. B., Good, C. A., and Clagett, O. T.: Hereditary Hemorrhagic Telangiectasia and Pulmonary Arteriovenous Fistula: Survey of a Large Family, *N. Engl. J. Med.*, 261:625, 1959.
28. Ruppert, G. B., Lindsay, J., and Barth, W. F.: Cardiac Conduction Abnormalities in Reiter's Syndrome, *Am. J. Med.*, 73:335, 1982.
29. Scharf, S., Wexler, J., Longnecker, R. E., and Blanfox, M. D.: Cardiovascular Disease in Patients on Chronic Hemodialytic Therapy, *Prog. Cardiovasc. Dis.*, 22:343, 1980.
30. Perloff, J. K.: Cardiomyopathy Associated with Heredofamilial Neuromyopathic Diseases, *Mod. Concepts Cardiovasc. Dis.*, 40:23, 1971.
31. Gottdiener, J. S., Hawley, R. J., Maron, B. J., Bertorini, T. F., and Engle, W. K.: Characteristics of the Cardiac Hypertrophy in Friedreich's Ataxia, *Am. Heart J.*, 103:525, 1982.
32. Lewis, H. D., Jr., White, H. H., and Dunn, M.: Refsum's Syndrome: A Neurological Disease with Interesting Cardiovascular Manifestations, *Circulation*, 34(suppl. 3):157, 1966.
33. Sanyal, S. K., and Johnson, W. N.: Cardiac Conduction Abnormalities in Children with Duchenne's Progressive Muscular Dystrophy, *Circulation*, 66:863, 1982.
34. Bergfeldt, L., Edhag, O., Vedin, L., and Vallin, H.: Ankylosing Spondylitis: An Important Cause of Severe Disturbances of the Cardiac Conduction System, *Am. J. Med.*, 73:187, 1982.
35. Goodman, R. M., and Gorlin, R. J.: "Atlas of the Face in Genetic Disorders," 2d ed., The C. V. Mosby Company, St. Louis, 1977.
36. Brosius, F. C., and Roberts, W. C.: Coronary Artery Disease in the Hurler Syndrome, *Am. J. Cardiol.*, 47:649, 1981.
37. Gellis, S. S., and Feingold, M.: Rubinstein-Taybi Syndrome, *Am. J. Dis. Child.*, 121:327, 1971.
38. Scarbrough, P. R., Finley, W. H., and Finley, S. C.: A Review of Trisomies 21, 18, and 13, *Ala. J. Med. Sci.*, 19:174, 1982.
39. Greenwood, R. D., and Nadas, A. S.: The Clinical Course of Cardiac Disease in Down's Syndrome, *Pediatrics*, 58:893, 1976.
40. Van der Hauwaert, L. G., Fryns, J. P., Dumoulin, M., and Logghe, N.: Cardiovascular Malformations in Turner's and Noonan's Syndrome, *Br. Heart J.*, 40:500, 1978.
41. Helmi, C., and Pruzansky, S.: Craniofacial and Extracranial Malformations in the Klippel-Feil Syndrome, *Cleft Palate J.*, 17:65, 1980.
42. Pearl, W.: Cardiovascular Anomalies in Noonan's Syndrome, *Chest*, 71:677, 1977.
43. Turiteri, L., Perheentupa, J., and Rapola J.: The Cardiopathy of Mulibrey Nanism: A New Inherited Syndrome, *Chest*, 65:628, 1974.
44. Young, D., Shprintzen, R. J., and Goldbery, R. B.: Cardiac Malformations in the Velocardiofacial Syndrome, *Am. J. Cardiol.*, 46:643, 1980.
45. Motta, J., Guilleminult, C., Billingham, M., Barry, W., and Mason, J.: Cardiac Abnormalities in Myotonic Dystrophy: Electrophysiologic and Histopathologic Studies, *Am. J. Med.*, 67:467, 1979.
46. Jones, K. L., and Smith, D. W.: The Williams Elfin Facies Syndrome, *J. Pediatr.*, 86:718, 1975.
47. Yurchak, P. M.: A Nine-Year-Old Girl with Congenital Heart Disease and Dysmorphic Facies, *N. Engl. J. Med.*, 295:92, 1976.
48. Robinson, C. D., Perry, L. W., Barlee, A., and Mella, G. W.: Smith-Lemli-Opitz Syndrome with Cardiovascular Abnormality, *Pediatrics*, 47:844, 1971.
49. McAdam, L. P., O'Hanlan, M. A., Bluestone, R., and Pearson, C. M.: Relapsing Polychondritis: Prospective Study of 23 Patients and a Review of the Literature, *Medicine*, 55:193, 1976.
50. Hiraishi, S., Yashiro, K., Oguchi, K., Kausana, K., Ishii, K., and Nakazawa, K.: Clinical Course of Cardiovascular Involvement in the Mucocutaneous Lymph Node Syndrome: Relation between Clinical Signs of Carditis and Development of Coronary Arterial Aneurysm, *Am. J. Cardiol.*, 47:323, 1981.

51. Cayler, G. G., Blumenfeld, C. M., and Anderson, R. L.: Further Studies of Patients with the Cardiofacial Syndrome, *Chest,* 60:161, 1971.
52. Moore, P., and Fiddler, G. I.: Facial Palsy in an Infant with Coarctation of the Aorta and Hypertension, *Arch. Dis. Child.,* 55:315, 1980.
53. DeBush, F. L.: The Hutchinson-Gilford Progeria Syndrome: Report of Four Cases and Review of the Literature, *J. Pediatr.,* 80:697, 1972.
54. Lie, J. T., and Grossman, S. J.: Pathology of the Heart in Acromegaly: Anatomic Findings in 27 Autopsied Patients, *Am. Heart J.,* 100:41, 1980.
55. Santos, A. D., Miller, R. P., Mathew, P. K., Wallace, W. A., Cave, W. T., Jr., and Hinojosa, L.: Echocardiographic Characterization of the Reversible Cardiomyopathy of Hypothyroidism, *Am. J. Med.,* 68:675, 1980.
56. Nadjmi, B., Flanagan, M. J., and Christian, J. R.: Laurence-Moon-Biedl Syndrome, *Am. J. Dis. Child.,* 117:352, 1969.
57. Fortuin, N. J., Morrow, A. G., and Roberts, W. C.: Late Vascular Manifestations of the Rubella Syndrome: A Roentgenographic-Pathologic Study, *Am. J. Med.,* 51:134, 1971.
58. Ho, C. K., Kaufman, R. L., and Podos, S. M.: Ocular Colobomata, Cardiac Defect, and Other Anomalies, *J. Med. Genet.,* 11:289, 1975.
59. Roberts, N. K., Perloff, J. K., and Kark, R. A. P.: Cardiac Conduction in the Kearns-Sayre Syndrome (A Neuromuscular Disorder Associated with Progressive External Ophthalmoplegia and Pigmentary Retinopathy), *Am. J. Cardiol.,* 44:1396, 1979.
60. Robinow, M., and Roche, A. F.: Low-Set Ears, *Am. J. Dis. Child.,* 125:482, 1973.
61. Friedman, S., and Saraclar, M.: The High Frequency of Congenital Heart Disease in Oculo-auriculo-vertebral Dysplasia (Goldenhar's Syndrome), *J. Pediatr.,* 85, 873, 1974.
62. Elliott, W. J.: Ear Lobe Crease and Coronary Artery Disease, *Am. J. Med.,* 75:1024, 1983.
62a. Wagner, R. F., Jr., Weinfeld, H. B., Wagner, K. D., et al.: Ear-Canal Hair in the Ear-Lobe Crease as Predictors for Coronary-Artery Disease, *N. Engl. J. Med.,* 311:1317, 1984.
63. Levin, D. L., Muster, A. J., Pachman, L. M., Wessel, H. V., Paul, M. W., and Koshaba, J.: Cor Pulmonale Secondary to Upper Airway Obstruction, *Chest,* 68:167, 1975.
64. Tilkian, A. G., Guilleminault, C., Schroeder, J. S., Lehrman, K. L., Simmons, F. B., and Dement, W. C.: Sleep-Induced Apnea Syndrome: Prevalence of Cardiac Arrhythmias and Their Reversal after Tracheostomy, *Am. J. Med.,* 63:348, 1977.
65. Shah, C. V., Pruyansky, S., and Harris, W. S.: Cardiac Malformations with Facial Clefts, *Am. J. Dis. Child.,* 119:238, 1970.
66. Johnson, G. M., and Todd, D. W.: Cor Pulmonale in Severe Pierre Robin Syndrome, *Pediatrics,* 65:152, 1980.
67. Silverman, M. E., and Hurst, J. W.: The Hand and the Heart, *Am. J. Cardiol.,* 22:718, 1968.
68. Aziz, K., Sanyal, S. K., and Goldblatt, E.: Reversed Differential Cyanosis, *Br. Heart J.,* 30:288, 1968.
69. Chesler, E., Moller, J. H., and Edwards, J. E.: Anatomic Basis for Delivery of Right Ventricular Blood into Localized Segments of the Systemic Arterial System, *Am. J. Cardiol.,* 21:72, 1968.
70. Proudfit, W. L.: Skin Signs of Infective Endocarditis, *Am. Heart J.,* 106:1451, 1983.
71. Smith, A. T., Sack, G. H., Jr., and Taylor, G. J.: Holt-Oram Syndrome, *J. Pediatr.,* 95:538, 1979.
72. Harris, L. C., and Osborne, W. P.: Congenital Absence or Hypoplasia of the Radius with Ventricular Septal Defect, *J. Pediatr.,* 68:265, 1966.
73. Nomeir, A. M., Turner, R. A., and Watts, L. E.: Cardiac Involvement in Rheumatoid Arthritis, *Arthritis Rheum.,* 22:561, 1979.
74. Sibbitt, W. L., Jr., and Williams, R. C., Jr.: Cutaneous Manifestations of Rheumatoid Arthritis, *Int. J. Dermatol.,* 21:563, 1982.
75. Bittle, J. A., and Perloff, J. K.: Chronic Post-Rheumatic Fever Arthropathy of Jaccoud, *Am. Heart J.,* 105:515, 1983.
76. James, T. N., and Bulkley, B. H.: Abnormalities of the Coronary Arteries in Whipple's Disease, *Am. Heart J.,* 105:481, 1983.
77. Curtiss, E. I., Miller, T. R., and Shapiro, L. S.: Pulmonic Regurgitation Due to Valvular Tophi, *Circulation,* 67:699, 1983.
78. Hopkins, L. C., Jackson, J. A., and Elsas, L. J.: Emery-Dreifuss Humeroperoneal Muscular Dystrophy: An X-Linked Myopathy with Unusual Contractures and Bradycardia, *Ann. Neurol.,* 10:230, 1981.
79. Udoshi, M. B., Shah, A., Fisher, V. J., and Dolgin, M.: Incidence of Mitral Valve Prolapse in Subjects with Thoracic Skeletal Abnormalities—A Prospective Study, *Am. Heart J.,* 97:303, 1979.
79a. Roberts, W. C., Hollingsworth, J. F., Bulkley, B. H., Jaffe, R. B., Epstein, S. E., and Stinson, E. B.: Combined Mitral and Aortic Regurgitation in Ankylosing Spondylitis: Angiographic and Anatomic Features, *Am. J. Med.,* 56:237, 1974.
80. Arosemena, E., Elliot, L. P., and Eliot, R. S.: Chest Deformity in Adults with Congenital Heart Disease, *Am. J. Cardiol.,* 20:309, 1967.
81. Greenwood, R. D., Rosenthal, A., and Nadas, A. S.: Cardiovascular Malformations Associated with Imperforate Anus, *J. Pediatr.,* 86:576, 1975.
82. Pagon, R. A., Graham, J. M., Jr., Zonana, J., and Yong, S. L.: Coloboma, Congenital Heart Disease, and Choanal Atresia with Multiple Anomalies: CHARGE Association, *J. Pediatr.,* 99:223, 1981.
83. Quan, L., and Smith, D. W.: The Vater Association, *J. Pediatr.,* 82:104, 1973.
84. Freedom, R. M.: The Asplenia Syndrome: A Review of Significant Extracardiac Structural Abnormalities in 29 Necropsied Patients, *J. Pediatr.,* 81:1130, 1972.
85. Greenwood, R. D., Rosenthal, A., and Nadas, A. S.: Cardiovascular Malformations Associated with Omphalocele, *J. Pediatr.,* 85:818, 1974.
86. Lewandowski, R. C., Jr., and Yunis, J.: New Chromosomal Syndromes, *Am. J. Dis. Child.,* 129:515, 1975.
87. Steeg, C. N., and Woolf, P.: Cardiovascular Malformations in the Fetal Alcohol Syndrome, *Am. Heart J.,* 98:635, 1979.
88. Jaigesimi, P., and Antia, A. V.: Extra Cardiac Defects in Children with Congenital Heart Disease, *Br. Heart J.,* 42:475, 1979.

9

Physical Examination of the Arteries and Veins (Including Blood Pressure Determination)

Robert A. O'Rourke, M.D.

Most of the derangements in the circulation, occasioned by the diseases of the heart, are exhibited externally by phenomena sensible to the sight or touch.

The state of the pulse, in the first periods of the disease of the heart, presents some peculiar characters either by themselves or by comparison of their relation with the nature of the strokes of the heart.

From the state alone of the pulse, the various characters just mentioned, especially from its continued irregularity, can the diagnosis of an organic affection of the heart be established? I answer in the affirmative, in case the disease has advanced; I think I can go farther, and say that the action of the heart is so essentially established in the beginning even of its affections, that by studying cautiously, at this period, the state of the pulse, which must afford signs of the disease, that is, if I may be allowed the expression, yet merely sketched; once confirmed, the pulse only must announce its existence to the enlightened and observing physician.

It is surprising that physicians have not attended to this singularity, when by feeling the pulse in both arms of the patient, they found it strong or weak on one side, while on the other its character was quite different; that the pulse on the right side, for example, had often a certain force, when it was impossible to find or feel it on the left side.

J. N. Covisart, 1806[1]

The Measurement of Systemic Blood Pressure*

The indirect measurement of the arterial blood pressure using cuff sphygmomanometry is one of the most commonly applied techniques for assessing the status of the circulation and the interaction between the heart and arterial system. Alterations from normal frequently provide important diagnostic information in patients with a variety of cardiac and noncardiac diseases.

Physical Determinants of the Blood Pressure

The arterial blood pressure, a measure of the lateral force per unit area of vascular wall, is expressed as millimeters of mercury or dynes per square centimeter. The peak systolic pressure is determined by the volume and velocity of left ventricular ejection, the peripheral arteriolar resistance, the distensibility of the arterial wall, the viscosity of the blood, and the end-diastolic volume in the arterial system. The subsequent reduction in pressure during diastole is in turn influenced by blood viscosity, arterial distensibility, peripheral resistance to flow, and the length of the cardiac cycle.[1a] Important physical factors affecting arterial distensibility include (1) the elastic modulus of the arterial wall, the ratio of stress (force acting to deform the wall) to strain (the proportional deformation produced); and (2) the geometry of the arterial wall, i.e., the internal radius (r) and wall thickness (h), which govern wall tension (T) according to the modified Laplace equation, $T = Pr/h$, where P = intravascular pressure. A decrease in elasticity or an increase in radius results in diminished distensibility and a greater rise in pressure per unit volume of blood.[1a]

Techniques for Measuring the Blood Pressure

Direct Methods

In 1733 Stephen Hales recorded the arterial pressures in animals by cannulation and a blood-filled glass column.[2] Current techniques for the direct and continuous measurement of arterial pressure utilize the electromanometer, a transducer which converts mechanical energy into an electric signal suitable for amplification, display, and recording. The artery is cannulated with a saline-filled catheter or needle which mechanically couples the circulation to the arterial manometer. Pressures are recorded using atmospheric pressure as the "zero" reference level, and intravascular pressures are further referenced to the level of the heart by addition or subtraction of a gravitation factor. The gravitation factor is expressed by the formal pgh, where p is the density of blood (g/ml), g is the acceleration due to gravity (980 cm/s), and h is the transducer height (cm) above or below the horizontal plane of the heart.

The strain gauge manometer commonly is used for the precise and accurate measurement of blood pressure. However, error may originate in the catheter or coupling system, in which the properties of inertia, friction, and elasticity interact to produce damping of the frequency response. Systems may be overdamped or underdamped, both resulting in signal distortion. Nevertheless, the appropriate combination of an inelastic cardiac catheter and con-

*The portion of this chapter entitled The Measurement of Systemic Blood Pressure appeared in the fifth edition of *The Heart*. It was written by Dr. Donald Nutter and is reproduced here, with slight modification, with the permission of Dr. Nutter.

necting tube filled with bubble-free fluid produces "critical" damping in which the system response is constant to some desirable frequency level and adequate for the clinical recording of intravascular pressures.[1a]

Measurement errors also occur when an end-hole catheter is positioned axial to flow in a vessel, and may become important during high arterial flow when kinetic energy may exceed 10 percent of the total fluid energy. The use of a side-hole catheter positioned in a large, patent artery allows measurement of the true blood pressure. Also, pressure transients due to catheter whip can falsely elevate the measured arterial pressure.[1a]

Miniature, self-flushing strain gauge manometers attached directly to an intravascular catheter or needle eliminate many of the problems related to transducer mounting and flushing, and overdamping by connective tubing. However, the most satisfactory method for reducing measurement errors is the use of intravascular electromanometers mounted on cardiac catheters or surgically implanted in the vascular wall.

Indirect Methods

The development of the indirect measurement of blood pressure is due primarily to the invention of the inflatable cuff manometer (Riva-Rocci, 1896) and the discovery and use of the arterial sounds (Korotkov, 1905). Current technique is based on the auscultatory detection of low-pitched Korotkov sounds over a peripheral artery at a point distal to cuff compression of the artery. McCutcheon and Rushmer[3] described two major components of these sounds: the initial transient (k_i) and the compression murmur (k_c), which coincide with the opening tap and rumble sounds of Rodbard.[4] The initial sound k_i occurs when cuff pressure reaches arterial pressure and likely results from abrupt arterial opening and vascular distension. The intensity of this initial sound depends on the slope of the pressure pulse and the level of the distal arterial pressure at the time of arterial opening, the sound being louder with vasodilatation and high-velocity flow and softer with arterial constriction or circulatory collapse. The initial transient probably is caused by oscillation of the arterial wall as the occluded segment is suddenly opened by systolic pressure and the compression murmur by a turbulent jet of flow distal to the partially compressed segment.

The Korotkov sounds have been divided into five phases occurring in sequence as the occluding pressure declines. Phase I consists of clear tapping sounds (k_i) which occur when the cuff pressure has fallen to the arterial peak systolic level. These sounds are initially soft, and gradually become louder as cuff pressure falls. Phase II consists of k_i sounds followed by swishing sounds or murmurs (k_c). Phase III is an augmentation of phase II sounds as an increased volume of blood passes through the partially compressed artery. Phase IV is signaled by the abrupt, distinct muffling of the sounds, resulting in a blowing quality that slowly diminishes in intensity. It is due to diminution and loss of component k_i as cuff pressure approaches arterial diastolic levels, and reduction in component k_c as the flow period lengthens and velocity decreases. Phase V, complete cessation of sound, occurs when the artery is no longer compressed to an extent which produces turbulent flow. The cuff pressure at which sound disappears may be extremely low or nonexistent when high-flow velocities (e.g., from exercise, anemia, fever) already exist in the circulation.

Proper technique is important for obtaining accurate measurements of blood pressure by the indirect method. The inflatable rubber bag within the compression cuff should have a width that is 20 percent greater than the limb diameter and a length adequate to encompass at least half the limb. The cuff should be applied snugly, with the inflatable bag positioned over the artery, at the level of the heart. Before auscultation the peak systolic pressure should be estimated as the cuff pressure which obliterates the distal arterial pulse.[1a] The stethoscope is then applied lightly but firmly over the artery and auscultatory pressure is determined by inflating the cuff to a level approximately 30 mmHg above the peak systolic pressure and noting the onset and behavior of the Korotkov sounds as the cuff is deflated at a rate of 2 to 3 mmHg/s. When the sounds disappear, the bag should be rapidly decompressed and 1 or 2 min allowed to pass before repeat determinations are made. A 1980 American Heart Association report[5] recommends that the systolic pressure be recorded as the point at which the first tapping sound occurs for two consecutive beats (phase I), and that the diastolic pressure be recorded in adults as the point at which sounds become inaudible. In children and in adults with a hyperkinetic circulation, the diastolic pressure should be recorded as the point at which muffling of the sounds occurs (onset of phase IV). The arterial pressures at both the onset of muffling and the disappearance of sound should be recorded. The mean blood pressure can be estimated by the addition of one-third the pulse pressure (systolic pressure minus diastolic pressure) to the diastolic pressure.

The method of sphygmomanometry contains several sources of error related to inadequate apparatus, inaccurate detection of the Korotkov sounds, and observer techniques.[1a] For example, a cuff of less than the recommended width may inadequately transmit pressure to the artery and falsely elevate the recorded blood pressure. The standard blood pressure cuff may often be unsatisfactory for pressure measurement in the arms or in the legs of very obese subjects; higher blood pressures in obese subjects have been attributed to the use of a cuff too narrow for the increased arm girth. When the bag fails to enclose the arm, the pressure is falsely elevated and varies with arm circumference, cuff width, and the level of blood pressure. When the cuff is deflated too slowly or is immediately reinflated for multiple pressure determinations, the resultant venous congestion may artificially elevate the diastolic pressure and may falsely decrease the systolic pressure by decreasing the intensity of phase I or phase II sounds to an inaudible level. Rapid deflation of the cuff may also cause the first (systolic) sounds to be missed. An erroneously low systolic pressure may also result from the failure to detect the presence of an auscultatory gap, a silent interval occasionally present just below the systolic pressure level.[1a]

Studies correlating direct and indirect blood pressure measurements have been characterized by considerable variability between individual subjects but in general have shown a good correlation between indirect and direct measurements of blood pressure in the arm.[6] The observed trend has been for the indirect method to underestimate systolic pressure by several millimeters of mercury, to overestimate diastolic pressure by several millimeters of mercury when phase IV is used as an end point, and to slightly underestimate diastolic pressure in normal individuals when phase V is taken as the end point.

Normal Blood Pressure

The normal range usually has been obtained by performing a frequency distribution on a population sample and defining arbitrary percentages of subjects above and below the mean as normal, borderline, or abnormal. The normal blood pressure range varies with age, sex, and socioracial grouping. In the United States, the pressure increases rapidly during the first few days of life and then increases gradually, with a slightly greater increment in systolic than in diastolic values, throughout life. The pressure tends to be higher in western, industrialized societies than in Asian and African and technically underdeveloped societies.[1a]

The normal blood pressure limits for adults (younger than 40 and of mixed sex and race) living in the United States are approximately 100 to 140 mmHg systolic and 60 to 90 mmHg diastolic. However, in an individual subject, baseline pressures above or below these levels do not define a pathological state, since the physiological range of normal for an individual may overlap with the statistical range of abnormality.[1a]

It has been demonstrated in mildly to moderately hypertensive persons that the blood pressure "casually" recorded by a physician is significantly higher than the average value of a series of intermittent indirect determinations or continuous direct recordings made during normal activity. To estimate basal blood pressure, measurements have been obtained during sleep, when the subject first awakens in the morning while still recumbent, or after several hours of reclining.

Many factors contribute to variations in an individual's blood pressure during daily activities. These include (1) body posture; (2) state of muscular, cerebral, or gastrointestinal activity; (3) emotional or painful stimuli; (4) environmental factors such as temperature and noise level; and (5) the use of tobacco, coffee, and other drugs with direct or neutrally mediated vasomotor properties.[1a] Twenty-four-hour pressures, obtained from normal and hypertensive subjects with an automatic recorder, have shown considerable variability with activity and emotional stimuli.[7,8] The average diurnal pattern of blood pressure consists of an increase throughout the day and early evening and a significant, rapid decline to a low point during the early, deep stage of sleep.

With normal respiration the peak systolic blood pressure is greater during expiration by as much as 10 mmHg than during inspiration. An augmentation of this difference occurs in patients with pericardial tamponade (pulsus paradoxicus; see Chap. 59) and during hyperventilation.

Dynamic exercise in both the supine and upright positions produces a moderate increase in blood pressure (systolic pressure greater than mean greater than diastolic pressure). Sustained isometric muscular contractions produce an abrupt increase is systolic, mean, and diastolic blood pressure that is dependent on the strength of the contraction.[9]

Abnormal Blood Pressure

Increased Pulse Pressure

An increase in arterial pulse pressure is commonly observed during routine sphygmomanometric recordings. This usually results from an increase in stroke volume and ejection velocity, often associated with a decrease in peripheral resistance. Fever, anemia, hot weather, exercise, hyperthyroidism, or arteriovenous fistulas may produce this change. Several cardiac diseases, such as aortic regurgitation, patent ductus arteriosus, or truncus arteriosus, often result in a widened pulse pressure. An increased pulse pressure due to a large stroke volume may occur with complete heart block or marked sinus bradycardia.[1a]

Atherosclerosis of the large arteries often reduces arterial compliance, a normal or even decreased stroke volume resulting in an elevated systolic pressure. The so-called systolic hypertension of the elderly does not necessarily represent a change in arteriolar resistance; efforts to lower this type of systolic pressure elevation can significantly reduce peripheral perfusion. Less common is the increased pulse pressure associated with systemic arteriovenous fistulas, where a relative tachycardia and wide pulse pressure may be the only clinical clues.

Reduced Pulse Pressure

A narrow pulse pressure is uncommon in normal subjects but may result from an increased peripheral resistance (increased circulating catecholamines in heart failure), decreased stroke volume (severe aortic stenosis), and/or markedly decreased intravascular volume (diabetic ketoacidosis).[1a]

Unequal Pulse Pressures

The diagnostic importance of blood pressure differences between right and left arms has been enhanced in recent years by the recognition of supravalvular aortic stenosis[10] in children and the subclavian steal syndrome in adults. Most patients with the former have greater than 20 mmHg higher blood pressure in the right arm. The subclavian steal syndrome, often accompanied by symptoms of cerebrovascular insufficiency, usually results in a pronounced lowering or absence of brachial artery pressure in the ipsilateral extremity.[1a]

A progressive rise in systolic pressure normally occurs as the point of measurement is moved peripherally from the central aorta. However, the increment in systolic pressure is equivalent in the large arteries of the upper arm and the thigh. Direct recordings of femoral and brachial arterial pressures (systolic, diastolic, and mean) in adults[11] and children[12] and indirect measurement of popliteal and brachial pressures using appropriate pressure cuffs[13] have demonstrated that pressures are equal in these sites. A difference in arm and leg pressures may occur because of coarctation of the aorta or acquired problems such as aortic dissection, aortic arch syndrome, and the subclavian steal syndrome.[1a]

Pulsus Alternans

The sphygmomanometer can be used to identify the beat-to-beat variation in pressure that accompanies pulsus alternans. (See Chap. 20.) The heart rhythm must be normal when the "test" is performed.

Pulsus alternans is discussed later in this chapter. It occurs in patients with severe heart disease who exhibit poor left ventricular contraction. It can occur for a few beats following atrial tachycardia in normal persons. It can also occur when the respiratory rate is half the pulse rate. This may be apparent when pulsus paradoxus is present in patients with cardiac tamponade.

Pulsus Paradoxus

A normal person may exhibit a 10- to 12-mmHg drop in systolic pressure during inspiration. A fall in pressure greater than this amount may be identified in patients with acute cardiac tamponade, constrictive pericarditis, severe obstructive lung disease, and restrictive cardiomyopathy.

The "test" is performed by inflating the blood pressure cuff above systolic pressure and then slowly releasing it. As the cuff pressure is gradually reduced, the blood pressure sounds become audible during expiration. The difference in pressure between the first audible sound heard on expiration and the pressure level at which the sounds are heard during all phases of respiration gives a measurement of magnitude of pulsus paradoxus.

The mechanism of pulsus paradoxus is discussed in Chap. 59.

The Arterial Pulse

Palpation of the arterial pulse was one of the earliest forms of physical diagnosis, and there is still no physical sign more basic or important in clinical medicine. Any discussion of the arterial pulse must include recent advances in measurement of arterial hemodynamics, assessment of the arterial wave contour, and frequency analysis of the pressure pulse.[14–18]

Physical Determinants of the Arterial Pulse

Origin of the Arterial Pulse

Pressure and blood flow measurements in the ascending aorta result from the interaction between the heart and arterial system. The rise in left ventricular pressure, upon exceeding the aortic pressure, becomes the driving force for the movement of blood into the ascending aorta.[19,20] This driving force is dependent upon the intrinsic contractility of ventricle muscle, the size and shape of the left ventricle, and the heart rate. It is opposed by several forces which impede the development of flow and are interrelated in a complex manner. Three major factors contributing to arterial impedance include (1) resistance, (2) inertia, and (3) compliance. Resistance is related to blood viscosity and the geometry of the vasculature, opposes flow, and is unaffected by changes in heart rate. Inertia is related to the mass of the blood, opposes the rate of change of arterial blood flow (i.e., acceleration), and is heart rate–dependent. Compliance is related to the distensibility of the vascular walls, opposes changes in arterial blood volume, and is also heart rate–dependent. The heart rate dependency of inertia and compliance introduces phase shifts between instantaneous pressure and flow in a pulsatile system.[19] Inertia and compliance are important determinants of the character of ventricular ejection, especially in early systole when flows and pressures are changing rapidly.

The arterial pulse wave begins with aortic valve opening and the onset of left ventricular ejection. Aortic pressure rises rapidly in early systole since the left ventricular stroke volume enters the aorta faster than it flows to distal sites. The rapid-rising portion of the arterial pressure curve is often termed the *anacrotic limb* (from a Greek word meaning "upbeat").[21] Recent studies in experimental animals and in patients indicate that peak proximal aortic flow velocity occurs slightly earlier than peak pressure.[15] After its peak, aortic pressure declines as ventricular ejection slows and peripheral blood flow continues. During isovolumic relaxation, there is a transient reversal of flow from the central arteries toward the ventricle just prior to aortic valve closure which is associated with an incisura on the descending limb of the aortic pressure pulse. The subsequent smaller, secondary positive wave has been attributed to the elastic recoil of the aorta and aortic valve but is partially due to reflected waves from more distal arteries. Beyond this, aortic pressure decreases again as further "runoff" in the peripheral circulation occurs in diastole.

The proximal aortic pulse pressure is directly proportional to the ratio of stroke volume to arterial distensibility, but multiple factors influence this complex relationship.[21] Arterial distensibility diminishes as the distending arterial pressure increases. Accordingly, the pulse pressure for a constant stroke volume will be larger if the mean blood pressure is elevated. In addition, arterial distensibility varies inversely with the rate of rise of intraluminal pressure. When the systolic ejection rate increases, the stiffer arterial wall results in a greater pulse pressure. Finally, the arterial pulse pressure may be modified by reflected pressure waves and by the rate of blood flow from arterioles to veins.

Arterial Pulse Contour

Pulsatile changes in arterial diameter are virtually identical to the pressure pulse, with minor differences explained in terms of nonlinear elasticity and viscosity of the arterial wall. In 1939, Hamilton and Dow explained the pressure wave contour in different arteries in terms of wave reflection between the aortic valve and peripheral sites.[22] In their hypothesis, the arterial pulse bounded back and forth between the aortic valve and peripheral reflecting sites, setting up a system of "standing waves" in the aorta. However, the standing wave hypothesis is not completely accurate since some attenuation to the wave in travel occurs and there is incomplete reflection of the wave.[23]

More precise information about the arterial pulse has been obtained from quantitative studies in which a regularly repeated pressure or flow wave is considered as a series of harmonics.[14,24] Each harmonic component has a definite modulus (amplitude) and a definite phase (delay) from a set point of reference. Given modulus and phase of the different harmonics of the pulse, the original wave can be resynthesized, and corresponding components of waves recorded simultaneously can be compared. By measuring and correlating mean values of the waves, vascular resistance can be calculated and the resistance properties of vessels downstream can be interpreted. The corresponding frequency components of pressure and flow can be compared in order to determine vascular impedance, the relation of pressure to flow at frequencies which are multiples of the heart rate.[14]

Usually, there is a linear relation between pressure and flow at the same point in an artery and between pressure and pressure at different points in the arterial system. From impedance curves, it is possible to identify the factors responsible for the relation between pulsatile pressure and flow.[15,16,20,25] Furthermore, the coefficient of reflection in peripheral vessels can be calculated from the relation of resistance to the minimal and subsequent values of impedance modulus. The peripheral arterial pressure wave recorded is the summation of the incident (initial) and reflected waves. The systemic circulation may be represented by a simple asymmetric T-tube model which emphasizes the importance of wave reflection at two arteriolar reflecting sites in the upper and lower parts of the body.[14,17]

Peripheral Transmission of the Arterial Pulse

As the normal aortic pulse wave is transmitted peripherally, significant changes in its contour occur due to (1) distortion and damping of pulse wave components; (2) different rates of transmission of various components; (3) distortion or exaggeration by reflected, resonant, or standing waves; (4) conversion of kinetic energy into hydrostatic or potential energy; (5) differences in distensibility and caliber of the arteries; and (6) changes in the vessel wall due to age and/or disease.[26]

The arterial pressure pulse enters the proximal aorta and travels distally at a velocity many times faster than maximum blood flow. The pressure wave is accompanied by a traveling wave distending the arterial wall, the pulse wave velocity increasing as arterial wall distensibility diminishes.[21] This normally occurs distally, as the arteries branch into smaller channels and their walls become stiffer. However, with increasing age and with systemic hypertension, arterial wall distensibility diminishes and pulse wave velocity is correspondingly greater.[14,27,28]

The pulse wave arrives progressively later at more peripheral sites when timed from the QRS complex on the ECG. Representative time delays are as follows: carotid, 30 ms; brachial, 60 ms; radial, 80 ms; and femoral, 75 ms.

The arterial pulse wave undergoes a progressive change in shape during its transmission distally (Fig. 9-1). The pulse pressure and systolic amplitude increase, and the ascending limb of the pulse wave becomes steeper. The incisura of the central aortic pulse is gradually replaced by a smoother, somewhat later, dicrotic notch which occurs at lower pressure levels. The dicrotic notch and the following positive secondary or dicrotic wave probably result from the summation of the forward pulse wave and reflected waves from the peripheral vessels.

Examination of the Arterial Pulse

All major arterial pulses should be examined bilaterally both for patency and for waveform characteristics (Chap. 65). The thickness and hardness of the arterial walls often can be assessed by "rolling" the vessel against underlying tissue. A pulse in the

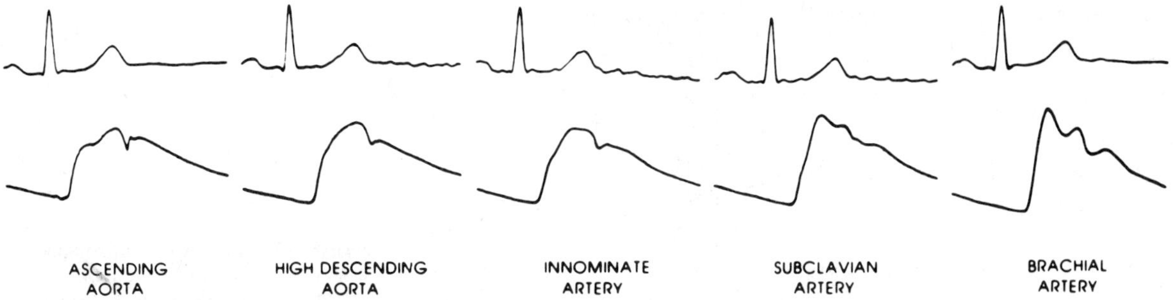

FIGURE 9-1 Changes in the contour of the arterial pressure pulse during a pullback of a micromanometer catheter from the central aorta to the brachial artery.

foot should not be considered absent unless examined with the foot in the dependent position. Otherwise, the arterial pulses usually are examined with the patient supine and with the trunk of the body slightly elevated.

The examiner uses tactile receptors in the tips of the fingers to sense movement of the arterial wall associated with the pressure pulse as it passes the site of palpation. Measurements in the proximal aorta show cyclic movement in both diameter and length proportional to the pulse pressure.[29] However, in more peripheral arteries with connective tissue attachments, the detectable movement is small and variable, with radial expansion by only about 2 percent of the end-diastolic cross-sectional area.[30]

The usual technique for palpating the arterial pulse is to press with the examining fingers until the maximum pulse is sensed. The pulse is felt as changing displacement superimposed on the "baseline" displacement produced by compressing the artery. The examiner should apply varying degrees of pressure while concentrating on the separate phases of the pulse wave. This method, referred to as *trisection,* is useful for assessing the upstroke, systolic peak, and diastolic slope of the arterial pulse.[26] Controversy exists as to how many fingers should be used to palpate the pulse, and the examiner should use whichever method he or she prefers, being careful not to perceive the examining fingertip pulse as well.

Palpation of the carotid artery is preferred for assessing cardiac performance, since the carotid pulse corresponds more closely to the central aortic pressure. However, in certain cardiac diseases (e.g., aortic regurgitation), the abnormalities detected in the carotid pulse are accentuated in the peripheral pulses. For determining the cardiac rate and rhythm, the radial pulse most often is used, but if it is irregular, cardiac auscultation often provides more reliable information. To evaluate the integrity of the peripheral arterial blood supply and to localize any lesions that exist, the arterial pulses in all four extremities should be examined and compared (Chap. 65).

Inspection of the carotid arterial and jugular venous pulsations should be performed at the same time. The carotid pulse usually is best examined with the sternocleidomastoid muscles relaxed and with the head rotated slightly toward the examiner. The carotid pulse may be timed from the first heart sound, which is heard slightly before the pulsation. The carotid pulse should be palpated in the lower half of the patient's neck in order to avoid carotid sinus compression. Occasionally, it is useful to palpate two arteries simultaneously (e.g., radial and femoral) to detect an apparent pulse wave delay such as occurs in patients with coarctation of the aorta.

The examination of arterial pulses in the abdomen and upper and lower extremities should be performed carefully in all patients and compared using a scale such as 0 = complete absence of pulsation; 1+ = small or reduced pulsation; 2+ = normal or average pulsation; and 3+ = large or bounding pulsation. Furthermore, auscultation over the major arteries should be performed since an audible bruit may be a clue to partial occlusion or may (e.g., carotid) indicate transmission of a cardiac murmur.

Normal Arterial Pulse

The normal carotid pulse has a smooth, rapid upstroke or ascending limb to a smooth, dome-shaped summit (Fig. 9-2). Then a downstroke occurs which is somewhat less rapid than the upstroke. The dicrotic notch and secondary diastolic wave usually are not felt, but may be palpable in some normal individuals or during fever, exercise, or excitement. The dicrotic notch usually occurs about 300 ms after the onset of the pulse wave when corrected for heart rate.

In arteries distal to the carotid, the pulse wave arrives later and has a steep initial wave that rises to a high peak pressure, whereas the diastolic pressure and the mean pressure are slightly lower. The systolic upstroke time (onset of pulse wave to its peak) tends to be shorter and the left ventricular ejection time (onset of pulse wave to incisura) longer in more peripheral arterial pulses. In the brachial artery, the heart rate–corrected systolic upstroke time averages 120 ms (range, 90 to 160 ms) and the systolic ejection time about 320 ms (range, 280 to 360 ms).

Graphic recordings of the arterial pulses frequently show two positive deflections during systole, the first shoulder being referred to as the *percussion wave* and the second as the *tidal wave.* In the normal

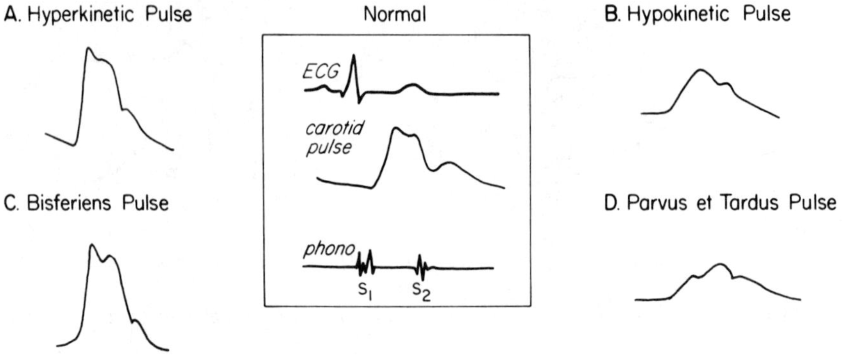

FIGURE 9-2 Schematic representation of the normal carotid pulse and four types of abnormal pulses. ECG = electrocardiogram; phono = phonocardiogram, S_1 and S_2 = first and second heart sounds.

proximal aortic pulse, the percussion wave is due to arrival of the impulse generated by left ventricular ejection, the tidal wave is its echo from the upper part of the body, and the dicrotic or diastolic wave is its reflection from the lower part of the body.[1] The contour of the distal pulses can be explained in similar terms with altered time relations between incident and reflected waves at different distances from peripheral reflecting sites.

With aging, there is a relative increase in the second (tidal) systolic wave and the height of the incisura relative to the first systolic wave.[18,27,31] The systolic upstroke time is longer, and the amplitude and duration of the diastolic wave tends to be less prominent.

Abnormal Arterial Pulses

In hypertension and arteriosclerosis, the pressure pulse amplitude is increased, the tidal wave is prominent, and the diastolic wave is absent. All features of the pulse can be explained by increased wave velocity.[14,27] The reflected wave from the lower body returns to the proximal aorta during late systole, merging with the echo from the upper body sites to augment the tidal wave and increase systolic pressure.[14] With systemic hypotension, the pulse wave velocity is decreased and the tidal and diastolic waves are further displaced from the percussion wave.

Impairment of one or both carotid arteries usually is produced by atherosclerosis, but multiple other causes include thrombosis, embolus, arteritis, and diseases of the aortic arch. Kinking of the carotid or brachiocephalic artery is relatively frequent, particularly in hypertensive patients, and may simulate aneurysmal dilatation. Femoral pulses may be diminished in the child and young adult as a result of coarctation of the aorta. However, in most adults it is caused by atherosclerosis of the abdominal aorta, aortic bifurcation, or the ileofemoral arteries (Chap. 65).

Hyperkinetic Arterial Pulse

Large, bounding arterial pulses usually indicate the rapid ejection of an increased volume of blood from the left ventricle (Fig. 9-2). Commonly, the arterial pulse pressure is increased and the peripheral arterial resistance is diminished. The hyperdynamic arterial pulse is sometimes referred to in terms which describe a particular component of the pulse wave. Thus, the water-hammer pulse, named after a Victorian toy, refers to an extremely rapid, forceful ascending limb of the arterial pulse wave.[32] By contrast, "collapsing pulse" refers to a quick, marked decrease in the arterial pulse wave following its peak. Hyperkinetic pulses often are more prominent in the brachial, radial, or femoral arteries than in the carotid artery. The term *Quincke pulse* refers to visible small pulsations in the nail bed of patients with hyperdynamic arterial pulses from any cause including aortic regurgitation.

Hyperkinetic arterial pulses occur in normal subjects with a hyperkinetic circulation (e.g., exercise, fever), patients with cardiovascular diseases associated with increased stroke volume, and patients with marked bradycardia and an extremely large stroke volume. A hyperdynamic arterial pulse also occurs in patients with an abnormally rapid runoff of blood from the arterial system (e.g., patent ductus arteriosus, peripheral arteriovenous fistulas). Patients on chronic hemodialysis often have hyperdynamic pulses produced by the combination of a surgical arteriovenous fistula, anemia, and hypertension.

In aortic regurgitation, the rapid-rising, bounding arterial pulse results from an increase in stroke volume and the rate of left ventricular ejection. The early systolic flow often produces palpable vibrations manifested as a thrill on the steep ascending limb. Later in systole, the rate of ventricular ejection and the arterial pulse wave decrease sharply, often resulting in systolic collapse.[21]

Bisferiens Arterial Pulse

The bisferiens (from Latin, "twice beating") pulse has a waveform characterized by two positive waves during systole (Fig. 9-2). The pulse wave upstroke rises rapidly and forcefully, producing the first systolic peak. A brief decline in pressure is followed by a smaller and somewhat slower-rising positive pulse wave (tidal wave). Abnormalities of left ventricular ejection and reflected waves from peripheral arteries both contribute to the prominence of the second systolic wave in the bisferiens pulse. The bisferiens pulse, usually felt in the carotid artery, is sometimes more readily palpable in a brachial or radial artery. A bisferiens pulse often occurs in patients with aortic regurgitation and in patients with combined aortic stenosis and severe aortic regurgitation.[33–36]

However, it also occurs commonly in other conditions associated with the rapid ejection of an increased stroke volume from the left ventricle (e.g., exercise, fever, patent ductus arteriosus).

The bisferiens pulse often is present in patients with hypertrophic cardiomyopathy, many of whom have dynamic left ventricular outflow obstruction.[37] In this syndrome, the midsystolic negative wave usually coincides with a marked decrease in the rate of left ventricular ejection. The second systolic wave, or tidal wave, most likely is produced by reflected waves from the periphery. The bisferiens pulse may be elicited by maneuvers that decrease the left ventricular size or increase its contractility. However, the most characteristic aspect of the arterial pulse in hypertrophic obstructive cardiomyopathy is its rapid rate of rise. A physical finding nearly specific for hypertrophic cardiomyopathy is a much smaller arterial pressure pulse in the cardiac cycle following a premature ventricular contraction.

Hypokinetic Arterial Pulse

A small, weak arterial pulse frequently is present in patients with a diminished stroke volume (Fig. 9-2). In most instances, the decreased stroke output is associated with both a decreased rate and duration of left ventricular ejection, and there is a narrow arterial pulse pressure despite an increased arterial resistance. Common causes include hypovolemia, left ventricular failure, and mitral or aortic valve stenosis. It is frequent in patients with valvular aortic stenosis.

Parvus et Tardus Pulse

Patients with moderate or severe valvular aortic stenosis often have an arterial pulse that is small and has a delayed systolic peak.[38,39] Occasionally, there may be a detectable shoulder on the upstroke of the carotid pulse, referred to as anacrotic (Fig. 9-2).[40] Palpable coarse vibrations are often present as a systolic thrill over the slowly rising carotid pulse. The parvus et tardus pulse is much easier to detect in the carotid arteries than in more distal arteries.

Most middle-aged patients with uncomplicated severe aortic stenosis have a parvus et tardus pulse, but this pulse may also occur in relatively mild stenosis. Furthermore, an apparently normal arterial pulse is not unusual in elderly patients with severe aortic stenosis due to the decreased distensibility of the large arteries, which also alters the character of the arterial pulse. Severe left ventricular failure often results in a small, weak pulse which may be difficult to distinguish from that in aortic stenosis.

Dicrotic Arterial Pulse

The dicrotic (from a Greek word meaning "double beating") pulse is a twice-peaked pulse with one peak in systole and the second in diastole, the latter due to an accentuated and palpable dicrotic wave that follows the second heart sound (Figs. 9-2 and 9-3).[41] It is usually felt best in the carotids, although it may also be palpated over more peripheral arteries. Major abnormalities include a short systolic ejection phase, a low dicrotic notch, a large diastolic valve, a narrow pulse pressure, a diminished rate of rise of the pulse, and the lack of distinct percussion and tidal waves. The dicrotic pulse is most common in young or middle-aged patients with poor left ventricular performance. It is usually associated with a low cardiac output, markedly diminished stroke volume, elevated left ventricular end-diastolic pressure, and high systemic arterial resistance. In general, the dicrotic wave becomes less prominent with age, hypertension, generalized atherosclerosis, and diabetes. Rarely, the dicrotic wave can be palpated in young febrile patients in whom none of the other abnormal features of the dicrotic pulse are present.

Pulsus Alternans

Pulsus alternans is a characteristic pulse pattern in which the beats occur at regular intervals but in which there is a regular attenuation of the height of the pressure pulses (Fig. 9-3).[42,43] Rarely, pulsus alternans is so marked that the weaker pulses are not felt at all. When pulsus alternans is noticed first after a premature contraction, the extent of the difference in systolic pressure in alternating beats declines for several cycles until the pulse amplitude is again constant. The initiation of post-premature ventricular contraction pulsus alternans is probably related to the increased duration of left ventricular filling after the extrasystole, resulting in a greater end-diastolic volume and hence increased contractile force due to the Frank-Starling mechanism.[44]

Severe depression of left ventricular performance often results in sustained pulsus alternans. There is an alteration in aortic flow, systolic left ventricular pressure, aortic systolic pressure, left ventricular *dP*/

FIGURE 9-3 Intraarterial pressure curve showing both pulsus alternans and a dicrotic waveform in a patient with congestive cardiomyopathy. ECG = electrocardiogram; S = systole; D = diastole.

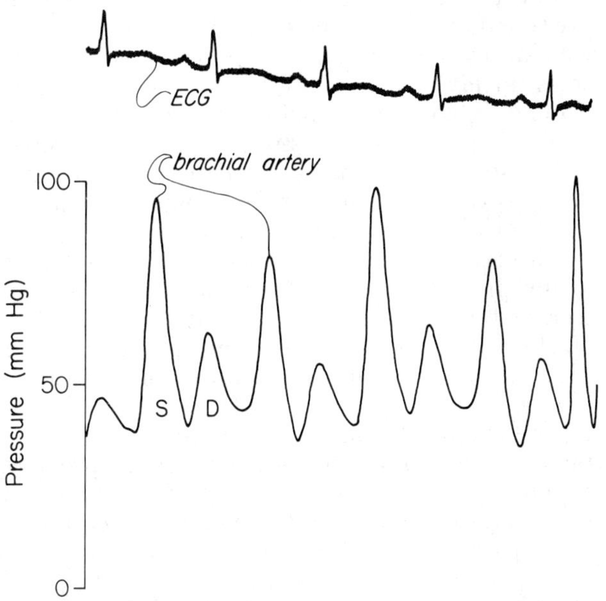

dt, and left ventricular end-diastolic pressure. Sustained pulsus alternans likely is due to alteration of the contractile state of at least part of the myocardium, which may be caused by the failure of electromechanical coupling in some cells during the weaker contraction.[45] A subsequent stronger contraction would then represent contraction of all cells, some of which were potentiated.

Pulsus alternans may be better appreciated when palpating a distal artery that has a slightly wider pulse pressure than the carotid artery. It is often brought out or accentuated when the patient assumes the upright position, thus decreasing venous return. The patient's respiration should be held since the small changes in arterial pressure caused by normal respiration may obscure the recognition of pulsus alternans. Pulsus alternans can be confirmed by using a sphygmomanometer and is usually associated with a left ventricular third heart sound.

Pulsus Parodoxus

A paradoxical pulse (see Chap. 59) is defined as a marked decrease in the pulse amplitude during normal quiet inspiration or a decrease in the systolic arterial pressure by more than 10 mmHg. The normal small decline in systolic blood pressure probably is produced predominantly by relative pooling of blood in the pulmonary vessels during inspiration, and may also reflect the delayed transmission through the lungs of the preceding expiratory fall in venous pressure and right ventricular cardiac output.[26]

In patients with cardiac tamponade, fluid accumulation in the pericardium increases intrapericardial pressure, and the heart's filling capacity is reduced. During inspiration, the expected augmentation of venous return to the right side of the heart occurs despite the elevated intrapericardial pressure.[46] The diminished thoracic pressure also causes a pooling of blood in the pulmonary capillary bed and diminishes pulmonary venous return to the left atrium. Since the high intrapericardial pressure limits flow to the heart and the total cardiac filling capacity is limited, the increase in right-sided heart volume with inspiration causes an obligatory decrease in left-sided heart filling. This, along with the pooling of blood in the pulmonary bed, produces a decline in left ventricular stroke volume and systolic blood pressure during inspiration.[47] Pulsus paradoxus is common with cardiac tamponade but infrequent with constrictive pericarditis.

Different hemodynamic mechanisms contribute to the production of paradoxical pulse in certain patients with superior vena cava obstruction, asthma, or obstructive airway disease, and in some patients with pulmonary embolism, shock, or postthoracotomy.[26]

The extent of pulsus paradoxicus can be quantitated by cuff sphygmomanometry as the pressure difference between the first discernible Korotkov sound on expiration and the pressure level during which Korotkov sounds are audible during all phases of respiration.

Effects of Arrhythmias on the Arterial Pulse

Premature Ventricular Depolarizations

A premature ventricular depolarization may be associated with no pulse, a small-amplitude pulse, or a normal arterial pulse, depending upon timing and whether the left ventricular pressure generated is able to open the aortic valve. The arterial pulse following a premature depolarization usually is greatly enhanced because of decreased aortic impedance, increased left ventricular filling, and augmented left ventricular contractility. At times, premature ventricular depolarizations are so common as to produce an irregularly irregular pulse. Then, the presence of cannon *a* waves in the jugular venous pulse should alert one to the correct diagnosis.

Tachyarrhythmias

The ECG usually is needed for the definitive diagnosis of any abnormality of heart rate or rhythm. However, careful observation of the arterial and jugular venous pulses frequently leads to the correct diagnosis.

Most tachycardias associated with a regular pulse are of supraventricular origin. In sinus tachycardia, the arterial pulse will gradually slow with carotid sinus pressure and then again gradually increase. Paroxysmal atrial tachycardia has an "all-or-none" response. Carotid sinus pressure will increase the block at the atrioventricular (AV) junction in patients with atrial flutter, the pulse rate slowing and subsequently returning to its original rate in a "jerky" fashion.

In patients with ventricular tachycardia and AV dissociation, the variation in the atrial-ventricular sequence of contraction and resulting pulse amplitude may often be detected by palpation.

An irregularly irregular pulse with a varying pulse pressure is usually the result of atrial fibrillation. However, multifocal atrial tachycardia is also a common cause of this finding in patients with severe chronic obstructive lung disease.

Bradyarrhythmias

An unusually slow heart rate frequently is associated with a decrease in the rate of rise and amplitude of the arterial pressure pulse. Complete heart block is readily diagnosed by the variability in the arterial pulse amplitude, the changing intensity of the first heart sound, and intermittent cannon *a* waves in the jugular venous pulse.

Venous Pulse

The evaluation of the venous pulse is an integral part of the physical examination, the venous pulse reflecting both the mean right atrial pressure and the hemodynamic events in the right atrium. Factors influencing the right atrial and central venous pressure (CVP) include the total blood volume, the distribution of blood volume, and right atrial contraction.

Venous blood returning from the systemic capillaries has a nonpulsatile flow. Changes in volume flow created by skeletal muscles and respiratory pump are nonsynchronous with the pulsatile activity of the heart. However the changes in flow and pressure, caused by right atrial and ventricular filling, give rise to pulsations in the central veins that are transmitted toward the peripheral veins, opposite to the direction of blood flow. With the possible exception of the *c* wave, which is the combined result of carotid arterial impact and an upward movement of the tricuspid valve, the pulsations observed in the neck are produced by right atrial and ventricular activity.[48]

Examination of the Jugular Venous Pulse

The two main objectives of the bedside examination of the neck veins are the estimation of the CVP and the inspection of the waveform. In most cases, the right internal jugular vein is superior for both purposes. In most normal subjects, the maximum pulsation of the internal jugular vein is observed when the trunk is inclined by less than 30°. In patients with an elevated venous pressure, it may be necessary to elevate the trunk farther, sometimes to as much as 90°.[49] When the neck muscles are relaxed, shining a beam of light gently across the skin overlying the internal jugular vein exposes its pulsations. Simultaneous palpation of the left carotid artery aids the examiner in deciding which pulsations are venous.

Measurements of Venous Pressure

The difference between venous distension and venous pressure elevation must be considered. Veins may be markedly dilated with minimal increase in pressure, or may not be visibly distended despite a very high venous pressure. Venous pressure may be estimated by examing the veins in the dorsum of the hand. With the patient sitting or lying at a 30° elevation or greater, the arm is slowly and passively raised from a dependent position. When the venous pressure is normal, the veins collapse when the dorsum of the hand reaches the level of the sternal angle of Louis. Unfortunately, local venous obstruction or augmented peripheral venous constriction may affect adversely the accuracy of estimating CVP by this method.

The external or internal jugular veins may also be used to estimate venous pressure. The more direct route to the right atrium makes the internal jugular vein superior for the estimation of venous pressure and assessment of the venous waveform.[50] The patient is examined at the optimum degree of trunk elevation for visualization of venous pulsations (Fig. 9-4). In the average patient, the center of the right atrium lies approximately 5 cm below the sternal angle regardless of body position. The vertical distance from the top of the oscillating venous column to the level of the sternal angle is generally found to be less than 3 cm (3 cm + 5 cm = 8 cm). Severely elevated venous pressure may be missed by failing to elevate adequately the patient's head. It may be necessary to actually have the patient sit upright. If the "pulsating meniscus" is very high, pulsations may be inapparent in the lower neck. When venous engorgement is marked, the patient's earlobe may pulsate and even the veins on the top of the heart may be distended.

In patients suspected of right ventricular failure, but who have normal resting venous pressures, the hepatojugular reflux test is useful. With the patient breathing normally, firm pressure is applied with the palm of the hand to the upper quadrant of the abdomen for 30 to 60 s. The patient should be instructed to continue to breathe normally during the test. Normally, the jugular venous pressure is not altered significantly. However, the abnormal right ventricle is unable to accept the increase in blood volume due to enhanced venous return without a marked increase in its filling pressure, which is transmitted to the neck veins. Normally, the height of the neck vein distension does not increase more than 3 cm during abdominal compression. Ducas et

FIGURE 9-4 Method of measuring the mean jugular venous pressure as the vertical distance above the sternal angle of Louis, the latter being 5 cm above the mid-right atrium regardless of trunk elevation.

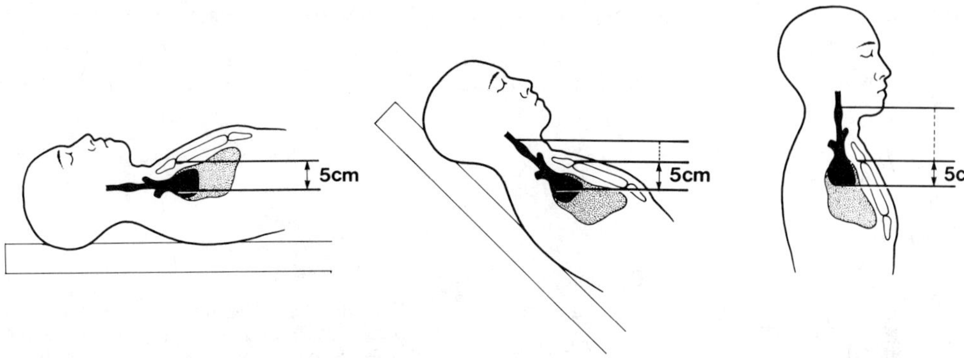

al. have studied this test and have attested to the accuracy of the test results.[51]

Analysis of Venous Waveforms

Again the patient's trunk should be inclined to whatever elevation is necessary to reveal the top of the oscillating venous column.[52] Having the patient take a slow, deep inspiration will increase the amplitude of the presystolic *a* wave while decreasing the mean right atrial pressure. This is also a useful technique for identifying the site at which the pulsations will be best visualized. Simultaneous palpation of the left carotid artery aids the examiner in relating the venous pulsations to the timing of the cardiac cycle.

Normal Venous Pulse

The normal jugular venous pulse (JVP) reflects phasic pressure changes in the right atrium and consists of three positive waves and two negative troughs (Fig. 9-5). In considering this pulse, it is useful to refer to the events of the cardiac cycle. The positive presystolic *a* wave is produced by right atrial contraction and is the dominant wave in the JVP, particularly during inspiration.

During atrial relaxation, the venous pulse descends from the summit of the *a* wave. Depending on the PR interval, this descent may continue until a plateau (z point) is reached just prior to right ventricular systole. More often, the descent is interrupted by a second positive venous wave, the *c* wave, which is produced by bulging of the tricuspid valve into the right atrium during right ventricular isovolumetric systole and by the impact of the carotid artery adjacent to the jugular vein.[53] Following the summit of the *c* wave, the JVP contour declines, forming the normal negative systolic wave, the *x* wave. The *x* descent is due to a combination of atrial relaxation and the downward displacement of the tricuspid valve during right ventricular systole.

The positive late systolic *v* wave in the JVP results from the increase in blood volume in the venae cavae and right atrium during ventricular systole when the tricuspid valve is closed. After the peak of the *v* wave is reached, the right atrial pressure decreases because of the diminished bulging of the tricuspid valve into the right atrium and the decline in right ventricular pressure which follow tricuspid valve opening. The latter occurs at the peak of the *v* wave in the JVP. Following the summit of the *v* wave, there is a negative descending limb, referred to as the *y* descent or diastolic collapse, which is due to the tricuspid valve opening and the rapid inflow of blood into the right ventricle. The initial *y* descent corresponds to the right ventricular rapid-filling phase. The trough of the *y* wave occurs in early diastole and is followed by the ascending limb of the *y* wave, which is produced by continued diastolic inflow of blood into the right side of the heart. The velocity of this ascending pressure curve depends on the rate of venous return and the distensibility of the right heart chambers. When diastole is long, the ascending limb of the *y* wave is often followed by a small, brief, positive wave, the *h* wave, which occurs just prior to the next *a* wave. At times, there is a plateau phase rather than a distinct *h* wave. With increasing heart rate, the *y* trough and *y* ascent are followed immediately by the next *a* wave.

Usually, there are three visible major positive waves (*a, c, v*) and two negative waves (*x, y*) when the pulse rate is below 90 beats per minute and the PR interval is normal. With faster heart rates, there is often fusion of some of the pulse waves, and an accurate analysis of the waveform is more difficult.

Abnormal Venous Pulse

Elevated Venous Pressure

The most common cause of an elevated jugular venous pressure is an elevated right ventricular pressure such as occurs in patients with pulmonic stenosis, pulmonary hypertension, or right ventricular failure secondary to right ventricular infarction. The venous pressure also is elevated when obstruction to right ventricular inflow occurs, such as with tricuspid stenosis or right atrial myxoma, or when constrictive pericardial disease impedes right ventricular inflow. It may also result from vena cava obstruction and, at times, an increased blood volume. Patients with obstructive pulmonary disease may have an elevated venous pressure only during expiration.

Kussmaul's Sign

Normally there is an increase in the *a* wave of the JVP but a decrease in the mean jugular venous pressure during inspiration as a result of the increased filling of the right side of the heart associated with

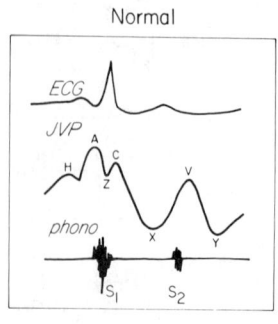

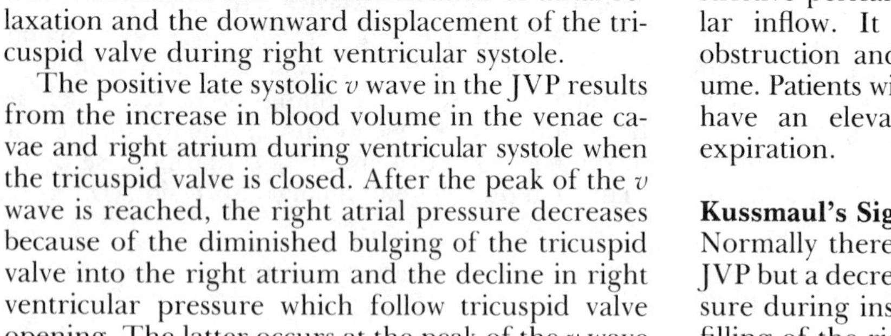

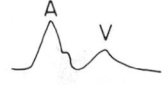

FIGURE 9-5 The normal jugular venous pulse (JVP) and four types of abnormal JVPs. See text for definitions of A, X, V, Y, and H.

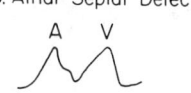

the decline in intrathoracic pressure. However, an inspiratory increase in the venous pressure occurs in patients with severe constrictive pericarditis when the heart is unable to accept the increase in right ventricular volume without a marked increase in the filling pressure.[54] However, while Kussmaul's sign was first described in patients with constrictive pericarditis, its most common cause is severe right-sided heart failure, regardless of etiology. The presence of Kussmaul's sign is useful in the diagnosis of right ventricular infarction.[55]

Abnormalities of the *a* Wave

The *a* wave in the JVP is absent when there is no effective atrial contraction, such as in atrial fibrillation (Fig. 9-6*A*). In certain other conditions, the *a* wave may not be apparent. In sinus tachycardia the *a* wave may fuse with the preceding *v* wave, particularly if the PR interval is prolonged. In some patients with sinus tachycardia, the *a* wave may occur during the *v* or *y* descent and may be small or absent. In the presence of first degree AV block, a discrete *a* wave with ascending and descending limbs is often completed prior to the first heart sound and the *ac* interval is prolonged (Fig. 9-6*B*).

Large *a* waves are of considerable diagnostic value (Fig. 9-5). When giant *a* waves are present with each beat, the right atrium is contracting against an increased resistance. This may result from obstruction at the tricuspid value (tricuspid stenosis or atresia, right atrial myxoma) or increased resistance to right ventricular filling. A giant *a* wave is more likely to occur in patients with pulmonic stenosis or pulmonary hypertension in whom both the atrial and ventricular septums are intact.

Cannon *a* waves occur when the right atrium contracts while the tricuspid valve is closed during right ventricular systole. Cannon waves may occur either regularly or irregularly and are most common in the presence of arrhythmias (Fig. 9-6*C*).

Abnormalities of the *x* Wave

The most important alteration of the normally negative systolic collapse (*x* wave) of the JVP is its obliteration or even replacement by a positive wave. This is usually due to tricuspid regurgitation.[56,57] Although atrial relaxation may contribute to the normal *x* descent, the development of atrial fibrillation does not obliterate the *x* wave except in the presence of tricuspid regurgitation. Accordingly, the occurrence of a positive wave in the JVP during ventricular systole is strong evidence of tricuspid regurgitation (Figs. 9-5 and 9-7). Mild tricuspid regurgitation lessens and shortens the downward *x* wave as the regurgitation of blood into the right atrium produces a positive wave which diminishes the usual systolic fall in venous pressure. In some patients with moderate tricuspid regurgitation, there is a fairly distinct positive wave during ventricular systole between the *c* and *v* waves.

In patients with constrictive pericarditis, the *x* descent wave during systole is often more prominent than the early diastolic *y* wave (Fig. 9-5).

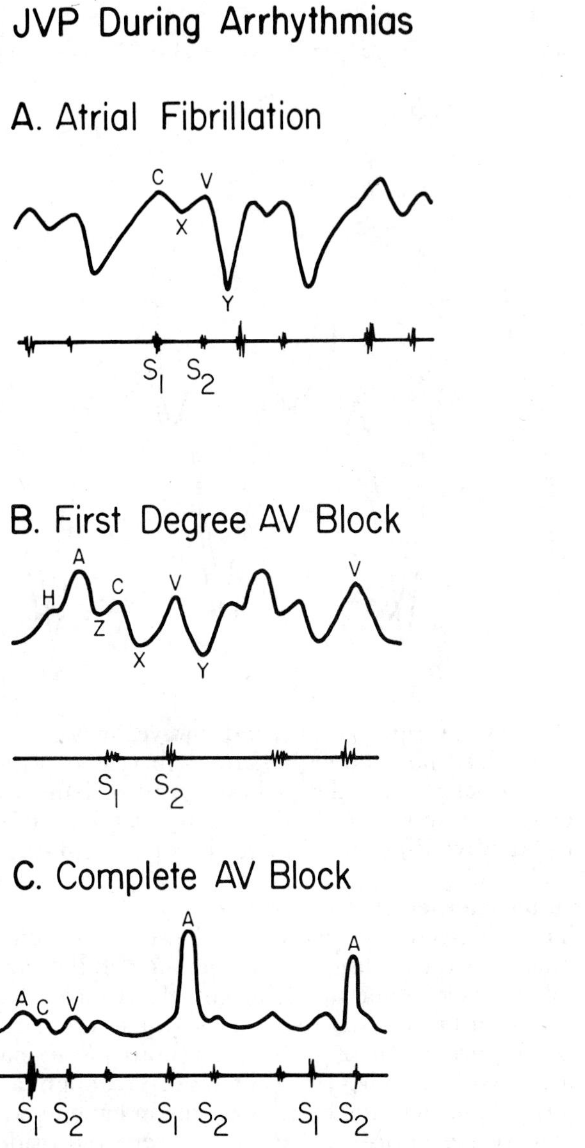

FIGURE 9-6 Abnormal jugular venous pulse in three common arrhythmias (see text).

Abnormalities of the *v* Wave

The positive, late systolic *v* wave results from the increasing right atrial blood volume during ventricular systole when the tricuspid valve normally is closed. With mild tricuspid regurgitation, the *v* wave becomes more prominent, and when tricuspid regurgitation becomes severe, the prominent *v* wave and the obliteration of the *x* descent result in a single, large positive systolic wave (ventricularization) (Figs. 9-5 and 9-7).

Normally the *v* wave is lower in amplitude than the *a* wave in the JVP. However, in patients with an atrial septal defect, the higher left atrial pressure is transmitted to the right atrium and the *a* and *v* waves are often equal in the right atrium and the JVP.[58] In patients with constrictive pericarditis and sinus

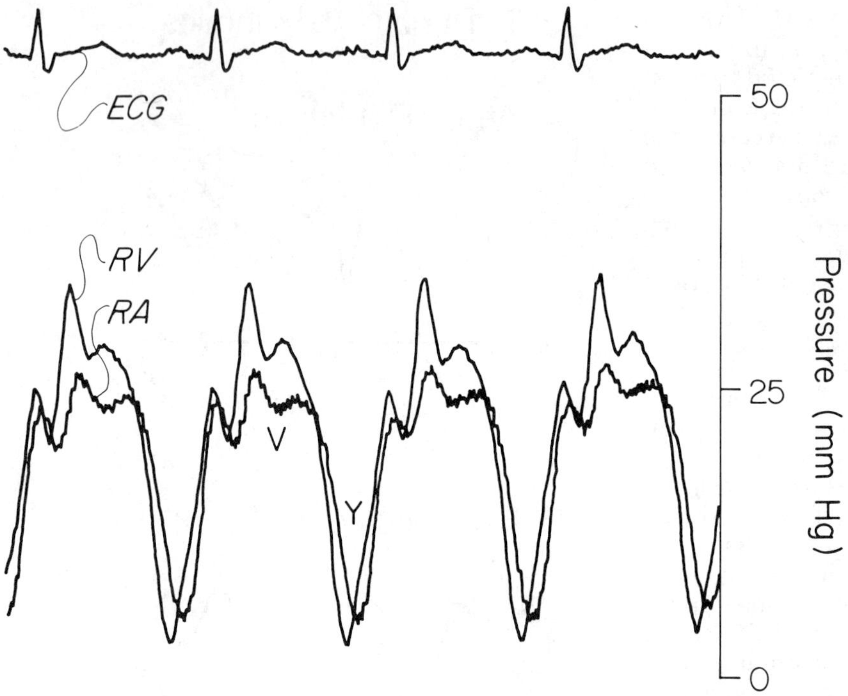

FIGURE 9-7 Right atrial (RA) and right ventricular (RV) pressure curves in a patient with severe tricuspid regurgitation. Note ventricularization of RA pressure curve. ECG = electrocardiogram.

rhythm, the right atrial *a* and *v* waves may also be equal, but the venous pressure is increased, which is unusual with atrial septal defect. In patients with constrictive pericarditis who are in atrial fibrillation, the *cv* wave is prominent and the *y* descent rapid.

Abnormalities of the *y* Trough
The *y* descent, or diastolic collapse, is produced mainly by the tricuspid valve opening and the rapid inflow of blood into the right ventricle. A rapid, deep *y* descent in early diastole occurs with severe tricuspid regurgitation (Fig. 9-5). A venous pulse characterized by a sharp *y* descent, a deep *y* trough, and a rapid ascent to the baseline is seen in patients with constrictive pericarditis or with severe right-sided heart failure. A slow *y* descent in the JVP suggests an obstruction to right ventricular filling and may be the only abnormal finding in patients with tricuspid stenosis or right atrial myxoma (Fig. 9-5).[59] In both constrictive pericarditis and severe right-sided heart failure, the venous pressure is elevated with a sharp *y* dip in the JVP. The presence of a large positive systolic venous wave favors the diagnosis of severe heart failure.

Effects of Arrhythmias of the Venous Pulse

Large *a* waves in the JVP during arrhythmias equate with the P wave (atrial contraction) occurring between the onset of the QRS complex and the termination of the T wave (Fig. 9-6). Such cannon *a* waves may occur regularly in junctional rhythm. More commonly, they occur irregularly when AV dissociation accompanies premature ventricular depolarizations, ventricular tachycardia, or complete heart block. The *a* wave is absent in patients with atrial fibrillation, and flutter *a* waves at a regular rate of 250 to 300 per minute frequently are observed in patients with atrial flutter and varying degrees of AV block. Patients with multifocal atrial tachycardia often have prominent and somewhat variable *a* waves in the JVP. In these patients, many of whom have pulmonary hypertension secondary to lung disease, the *a* waves are often very large.

References

1. Covisart, J. N.: "An Essay of the Organic Diseases and Lesions of the Heart and Great Vessels," C. E., Horeau, Paris, 1806.
1a. Nutter, D. O.: Measurement of the Systolic Blood Pressure, in J. W. Hurst (ed.), "The Heart," McGraw-Hill Book Company, New York, 1982.
2. Hales, S.: "Statistical Essays: Containing Haema-staticks; or, an Account of Some Hydraulick and Hydrostatical Experiments Made on the Blood and Blood-Vessels of Animals," W. Innys and R. Manby, London, 1733.
3. McCutcheon, E. P., and Rushmer, R. F.: Korotkov Sounds: An Experimental Critique, *Circ. Res.,* 20:149, 1967.
4. Rodbard, S.: The Components of the Korotkov Sounds, *Am. Heart J.,* 74:278, 1967.
5. Kirkendall, W. M., Feinleib, M., Freis, E. D., and Mark, A. L.: AHA Committee Report: Recommendations of Human Blood Pressure Determination by Sphygmomanometers, *Circulation,* 62:1146A, 1980.
6. Neilsen, P. E., and Janniche, H.: The Accuracy of Auscultatory Measurement of Arm Blood Pressure in Very Obese Subjects, *Acta. Med. Scand.,* 195:403, 1974.
7. Littler, W. A., Honour, A. J., Pugsley, D. J., and Sleight, P.: Continuous Recording of Direct Arterial Pressure in Unrestricted Patients, *Circulation,* 51:1101, 1975.
8. Richardson, D. W., Honour, A. T., Fenton, D. W., Stott, F. H., and Pickering, G. W.: Variation in Arterial Pressure throughout the Day and Night, *Clin. Sci.,* 26:445, 1964.
9. Donald, K. W., Lind, A. R., McNicol, G. W., Humphreys, P. W., and Staunton, H. P.: Cardiovascular Responses to Sustained Contractions, *Circ. Res.,* 20(suppl. 1):15, 1967.
10. Wooley, C. F., Hosier, D. M., Booth, R. W., Molnar, W.,

Sirak, H. D., and Ryan, J. M.: Supravalvular Aortic Stenosis, *Am. J. Med.*, 31:717, 1961.
11. Pascarelli, E. F., and Betrand, C. A.: Comparison of Blood Pressure in the Arms and Legs, *N. Engl. J. Med.*, 270:693, 1964.
12. Park, M. K., and Guntheroth, W. G.: Direct Blood Pressure Measurements in Brachial and Femoral Arteries in Children, *Circulation*, 41:231, 1970.
13. Felix, W. R., Hochbert, H. M., George, M. E. D., Schmalzbach, E. L., and Vaserberg, R.: Ultrasound Measurement of Arm and Leg Blood Pressures, *JAMA*, 226:1096, 1973.
14. O'Rourke, M. F.: The Arterial Pulse in Health and Disease, *Am. Heart J.*, 82(5):687, 1971.
15. Murgo, J. P., Westerhof, N., Giolma, J. P., and Altobelli, S. A.: Aortic Input Impedance in Normal Man: Relationship to Pressure Wave Shapes, *Circulation*, 62:106, 1980.
16. O'Rourke, M. F.: Pressure and Flow Waves in Systemic and the Anatomical Design of the Arterial System, *J. Appl. Physiol.*, 23:139, 1967.
17. O'Rourke, M. F., and Auido, A. P.: Pulsatile Flow and Pressures in Human Systemic Arteries: Studies in Man and in a Multibranched Model of the Human Systemic Arterial Tree, *Circ. Res.*, 46:363, 1980.
18. Murgo, J. P., Westerhof, N., Giolma, J. O., and Altobelli, S. A.: Effects of Exercise on Aortic Impedance and Pressure Wave Shapes in Normal Man, *Circ. Res.*, 48:334, 1981.
19. Murgo, J. P., Altobelli, S. A., Dorethy, J. F., Logsdon, J. R., and McGranaham, G. M.: Normal Ventricular Ejection Dynamics in Man during Rest and Exercise, *Circulation*, 46:92, 1975.
20. Westerhof, N., Murgo, J. P., Sipkema, P., Giolma, J. P., and Elzingor, G.: Arterial Impedance, in N. H. C. Hwang, D. R. Gross, and D. J. Patel (eds.), "Quantitative Cardiovascular Studies," University Park Press, Baltimore, 1979, pp. 111–150.
21. Marx, H. J., and Yu, P. N.: Clinical Examination of the Arterial Pulse, *Prog. Cardiovasc. Dis.*, 10:207, 1967.
22. Hamilton, W. F., and Dow, P.: An Experimental Study of the Standing Waves in the Pulse Propagated through the Aorta, *Am. J. Physiol.*, 125:48, 1939.
23. McDonald, D. A., and Taylor, M. G.: The Hydrodynamics of the Arterial Circulation, *Prog. Biophys.*, 9:105, 1959.
24. McDonald, D. A.: The Relation of Pulsatile Pressure to Flow in Arteries, *J. Physiol.*, 127:533, 1955.
25. O'Rourke, M. F., and Taylor, M. G.: Input Impedance of the Systemic Circulation, *Circ. Res.*, 20:365, 1967.
26. Schlant, R. C., and Felner, J. M.: The Arterial Pulse—Clinical Manifestations, *Curr. Prob. Cardiol.*, 2(5):1, 1977.
27. O'Rourke, M. F., Blazek, J. V., Morreels, C. L., Jr., and Krovetz, L. J.: Pressure Wave Transmission along the Human Aorta: Changes with Age and Hypertension, *Circ. Res.*, 23:567, 1968.
28. Freis, E. D., Heath, W. C., Luchsinger, P. C., and Snell, R. E.: Changes in the Carotid Pulse Which Occur with Age and Hypertension, *Am. Heart J.*, 71:757, 1966.
29. Patel, D. J., Greenfield, J. C., and Dry, D. L.: In Vivo Pressure Length-Radius Relationships of Certain Blood Vessels in Man and Dog, in E. O. Attinger (ed.), "Pulsatile Blood Flow," McGraw-Hill Book Company, New York, 1964, chap. 17, p. 293.
30. Stead, E. A., and Greenfield, J. C.: Pressures and Pulses, *Physiol. Phys.*, 2:1, 1964.
31. Freis, E. D., and Kyle, M. C.: Computer Analysis of Carotid and Brachial Pulse Waves: Effects on Age in Normal Subjects, *Am. J. Cardiol.*, 22:691, 1968.
32. Corrigan, D. J.: On Permanent Patency of the Mouth of the Aorta, or Inadequacy of the Aortic Valves, *Edinburgh Med. Surg.*, 37:225, 1832.
33. Clarke, J. M.: On the Pulsus Bisferiens of Aortic Regurgitation, *Lancet*, 2:1529, 1894.
34. Broadbent, W.: Pulsus Bisferiens, *Br. Med. J.*, 1:75, 1899.
35. Fleming, P. R.: The Mechanism of the Pulsus Bisferiens, *Br. Heart J.*, 19:519, 1951.
36. Ikram, H., Nixon, P. G. F., and Fox, J. A.: The Hemodynamic Implications of the Bisferiens Pulse, *Br. Heart J.*, 26:452, 1964.
37. Wigle, E. D.: The Arterial Pressure Pulse in Muscular Subaortic Stenosis, *Br. Heart J.*, 25:97, 1963.
38. Steell, G.: The Pulse in Aortic Stenosis, *Lancet*, 2:1206, 1894.
39. Feil, H. S., and Katz, L. N.: The Transformation of the Central into the Peripheral Pulse in Patients with Aortic Stenosis, *Am. Heart J.*, 2:12, 1926.
40. Dow, P.: The Development of the Anacrotic and Tardus Pulse of Aortic Stenosis, *Am. J. Physiol.*, 131:432, 1940.
41. Ewy, G. A., Rios, J. C., and Marcus, F. I.: The Dicrotic Arterial Pulse, *Circulation*, 39:655, 1969.
42. White, P. D.: Alternation of the Pulse: A Common Clinical Condition, *Am. J. Med. Sci.*, 150:82, 1915.
43. Cohn, K. E., Sandler, H., and Hancock, E. W.: Mechanisms of Pulsus Alternans, *Circulation*, 36:372, 1967.
44. Mitchell, J. H., Sarnoff, S. J., and Sonnenblick, E. H.: Alternating End-Diastolic Fiber Length as a Causative Factor, *J. Clin. Invest.*, 42:55, 1963.
45. Pace, J. B., Priola, D. V., and Randall, W. C.: Alterations in Cardiac Synchrony and Contractility during Induced Pulsus Alternans, *Physiologist*, 9:259. 1966.
46. Shabetai, R., Fowler, N. O., Fenton, J. C., and Masagkay, M.: Pulsus Parodoxus, *J. Clin. Invest.*, 44:1882, 1965.
47. Shabetai, R., Fowler, N. O., and Guntheroth, W. G.: The Hemodynamics of Cardiac Tamponade and Constrictive Pericarditis, *Am. J. Cardiol.*, 20:480, 1970.
48. Hurst, J. W., and Schlant, R. C.: Examination of the Veins, in "The Heart," 4th ed., McGraw-Hill Book Company, New York, 1978, chap. 15, p. 193.
49. Fowler, N. O., and Marshall, W. J.: Cardiac Diagnosis from Examination of Arteries and Veins, *Circulation*, 30:272, 1964.
50. Ewy, G. A., and Marcus, F. I.: Bedside Estimation of the Venous Pressure, *Heart Bull.*, 17:41, 1968.
51. Ducas, J., Magder, S., and McGregor, M.: Validity of the Hepatojugular Reflux as a Clinical Test for Congestive Heart Failure, *Am. J. Cardiol.*, 52(10):1299, 1983.
52. Fowler, N. O.: Inspection and Palpation of Venous and Arterial Pulses, in "Examination of the Heart," American Heart Association, New York, 1972, pp. 1–41.
53. Wood, P.: "Diseases of the Heart and Circulation," 2d ed., J. B. Lippincott Company, Philadelphia, 1957, p. 47.
54. Kussmaul, A.: Uber Schwielige Mediastino-pericarditis und Den Parodoxen Pulse, *Berl. Klin. Wochenschr.*, 10:433, 1873.
55. Dell'Italia, L., Starling, M. R., and O'Rourke, R. A.: Physical Examination for Exclusion of Hemodynamically Important Right Ventricular Infarction, *Ann. Intern. Med.*, in press.
56. Messer, A. L., Hurst, J. W., Rappaport, M. B., and Sprague, H. B.: A Study of the Venous Pulse in Tricuspid Valve Disease, *Circulation*, 1:388, 1950.
57. Mueller, O., and Shillingford, J.: Tricuspid Incompetence, *Br. Heart J.*, 16:195, 1954.
58. Dexter, L.: Atrial Septal Defect, *Br. Heart J.*, 18:209, 1956.
59. Perloff, J. K., and Harvey, W. P.: Clinical Recognition of Tricuspid Stenosis, *Circulation*, 22:346, 1960.

10

Inspection and Palpation of the Precordium

Ernest Craige, M.D.

Quod erigitur cor, et inmucronem se sursum elevat, sic ut illo tempore ferire pectus, et foris sentiri pulsatio possit.

[*The heart erects, and raises itself into a point, so that at this moment it strikes the chest wall, and externally a pulsation can be felt.*]

William Harvey, M.D., 1628[1]

In these days of increasing dependence on expensive technological methods in cardiac diagnosis, there is a tendency to give only passing attention to the physical examination. Even among the traditional features of the physical examination, inspection and palpation are often passed over as the physician limits the examination of the heart to laying on the stethoscope. This trend is unfortunate since a great deal of information of diagnostic value can be obtained by simple bedside methods which are rapid, inexpensive, and nontraumatic. Inspection, palpation, and auscultation can often lead one toward an accurate diagnosis, or, even when further technological studies are required, the questions to be asked and the protocol to be followed can be worked out with greater precision and economy.

Inspection of the Precordium

Many valuable clues in cardiac diagnosis are provided by inspection of the neck and thorax. This has been described in Chap. 8. Attention to the precordium in particular can be rewarding. Pulsations in this area can best be appreciated with the help of a light beam directed tangentially across the surface. Another simple method utilizes a wand—a cotton-tipped swab impaled in the hole of a pediatric suction electrode used in precordial electrocardiography. The suction electrode is attached to the moving chest wall, and the exaggerated movements imparted to the cotton-tipped end of the swab may provide vivid clarification of an otherwise confusing undulation. Asymmetry of the thorax can often be detected by inspecting the patient from the foot of the bed. A convex bulging of the precordium suggests the presence of heart disease beginning early in life when the thorax is still capable of being molded to accommodate a dilated right ventricle, as in atrial septal defect. Generalized cardiac enlargement due to rheumatic heart disease in early childhood can result in a similar configuration.

Pulsations Due to the Heartbeat

Precordial pulsations occur principally in five areas:

1. The cardiac apex, which is normally occupied by the left ventricle
2. The left sternal border at third and fourth interspaces, where a visible heave in systole may represent right ventricular enlargement
3. Higher along the left border in the second intercostal space, where pulsation of the pulmonary artery may be seen when that vessel is dilated
4. Upper right sternal border, occasionally the site of pulsations due to dilatation or aneurysm of the aortic root
5. The midprecordium, third or fourth intercostal spaces at the midclavicular line, where bulging of the ischemic or aneurysmal anterior surface of the left ventricle may be perceptible

The precordium may less commonly be drawn inward during systole, as with constrictive pericarditis or isolated tricuspid regurgitation.

All these visible signs are also palpable and will therefore be considered in greater detail below.

Palpation of the Precordium[2] (See Fig. 10-1)

Physiology of Tactile Perception

Physiologists have demonstrated that the human hand is endowed with certain neurons which are primarily sensitive to *positional change* and others that are sensitive to the time rate of positional change, or *velocity*.[3] Information has, however, been limited with respect to the frequency response of the human hand, especially in the spectrum of frequencies encountered in precordial motion. This problem has been investigated by Smith and Craige using an in vitro palpating device in which amplitude and frequency of a sinusoidal waveform can be independently manipulated.[4] Their results show that the fingers are insensitive to movements of relatively large *amplitude* when frequency is very low (< 5 Hz). Sensitivity improves with increasing frequency, where presumably neurons activated by changes in *velocity* assume a larger role in tactile perception. These observations are supported by clinical observations: for instance, the stethoscope can be *seen* to ride up and down with movements of the precordium, but, with the eyes averted, these same movements of the precordium may be imperceptible by *palpation*. On the other hand, higher-frequency phenomena such as thrills and the "shocks" associated with aortic or pulmonary components of the second sound of exaggerated intensity are easily palpable although the amplitude of their movement is insufficient to be visible. In palpating the impulse at the cardiac apex, ordinarily only the initial brisk outward component is perceptible. This portion of the apical motion is characterized by a major contribution of higher-frequency vibrations. The low-frequency diastolic phenomena—filling wave and *a* wave—are usually imperceptible except when greatly exaggerated in amplitude or composed of higher-frequency elements as in some pathologic states.[5]

It is apparent therefore that the fingers represent a very imperfect transducer for transferring the information contained in precordial movement to our centers of perception in the brain. In addition, in the design of graphic methods to represent precordial movement it is probably futile to try for a system that simulates on paper exactly what one perceives by palpation. Tactile perception by even the most experienced bedside clinician is still a very primitive form of examination. Thus, the analogy from auscultation-phonocardiography that the most useful phonocardiograms for clinical purposes are those which most nearly reproduce what one hears is not transferable to palpation and its graphic counterpart. Despite these limitations in the information which one can hope to obtain from palpation, the method provides definite advantages which continue to warrant its inclusion in the physical examination.

The Apex Beat

Source of the Apex Beat

The apex beat results from the impact of the left ventricle against the chest wall in early systole. It is affected by the pressure pulse in the left ventricle, the stroke volume, and a kaleidoscopic complex effect of ballistic recoil and torsion of the heart during systole further modified by chest wall thickness, fluid, emphysema, etc. Palpable phenomena in diastole are principally the result of ventricular filling. From the location of the apex beat one can make an estimate of heart size, and from its character one can sometimes obtain clues regarding physiologic or morphologic abnormalities.

Technique of Palpation

For the most accurate appraisal of heart size it is best to feel for the apex impulse with the patient sitting up, leaning forward in expiration. The center (not the outermost border) of the point of maximal impulse will be found to correlate within approximately 1 cm with the outer border of the heart as measured in a standard chest roentgenogram. The position of the apex impulse should be described in terms of its distance from the midsternal line and the intercostal space in which it is located. Normally the impulse of the cardiac apex lies at or medial to the midclavicular line.

The apex impulse is often palpated, for convenience, with the patient supine. In this position its pulsations are feeble because of the heart's having fallen away from contact with the chest wall and the location of the apex may be displaced upward and laterally by the higher position of the diaphragm. For optimal appreciation of the waveforms constituting the apex impulse, and particularly for its diastolic constituents, it is best to palpate with the patient in the left lateral decubitus position.[6] The observer should stand at the right side of the bed. It is often very helpful to magnify the apical movements by holding the base of a wand—a Bic pencil is ideal—in the interspace where the impulse has been located, with the impulse itself acting as a fulcrum and the point thus providing a moving indicator of pulsatile systolic and diastolic phenomena. If there is any doubt about the timing of palpable movements, one should *listen* with the stethoscope while feeling the precordium. If S_1 and S_2 are clearly identified, the timing of palpable events should not be difficult.

Character of the Impulse

The normal apex beat usually consists merely of a thrust at the beginning of systole during the period of isovolumic contraction. (See Fig. 10-1.) The impulse is small in amplitude and brief in duration. It is exaggerated in thin, youthful subjects and with the patient in the left lateral decubitus position. Therefore, as with other physical signs, one must make observations in a large number of individuals in order to appreciate the wide range of normalcy and the alterations that may be expected with age, body build, pregnancy, etc. Diastolic waves are usually imperceptible in normal individuals.

A hyperkinetic cardiac impulse is characterized by an increase in amplitude but retention of the brief duration that is found in the normal beat. The hyperdynamic impulse occurs in a variety of circumstances where the stroke volume is augmented, as with mitral regurgitation, thyrotoxicosis, severe anemia, and left-to-right shunts such as ventricular septal defect or patent ductus arteriosus.[7,8] The same type of exaggerated impulse may be found in young, thin normal individuals, especially with exercise and excitement. Not infrequently, where the stroke volume is increased, a filling wave may be palpable in early diastole, with the patient lying in the left lateral decubitus position. This corresponds to the audible third heartbeat sound.

A hypokinetic or imperceptible apical impulse may be encountered with obesity, emphysema, pericardial effusion, or constriction. In shock also the apical impulse may be feeble or absent.

A sustained apex beat is a heave that has greater duration than the impulses previously described. It is swift in upstroke and exaggerated in amplitude. This type of powerful thrust of the left ventricle is

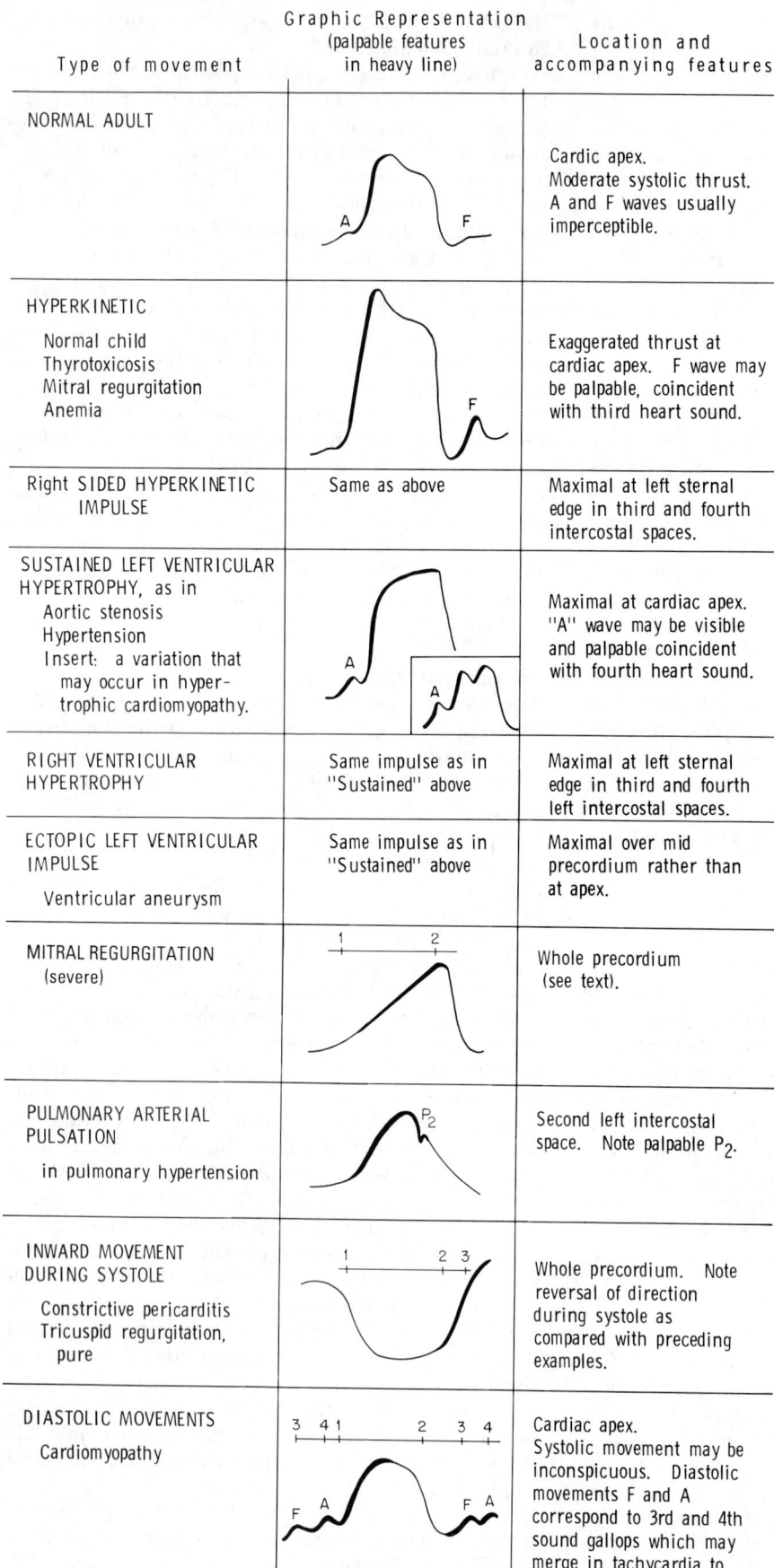

Type of movement	Graphic Representation (palpable features in heavy line)	Location and accompanying features
NORMAL ADULT	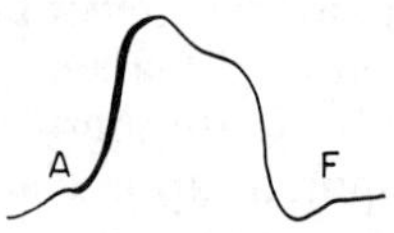	Cardic apex. Moderate systolic thrust. A and F waves usually imperceptible.
HYPERKINETIC Normal child Thyrotoxicosis Mitral regurgitation Anemia	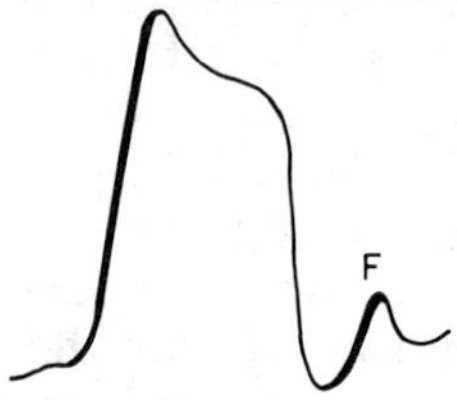	Exaggerated thrust at cardiac apex. F wave may be palpable, coincident with third heart sound.
Right SIDED HYPERKINETIC IMPULSE	Same as above	Maximal at left sternal edge in third and fourth intercostal spaces.
SUSTAINED LEFT VENTRICULAR HYPERTROPHY, as in Aortic stenosis Hypertension Insert: a variation that may occur in hyper-trophic cardiomyopathy.	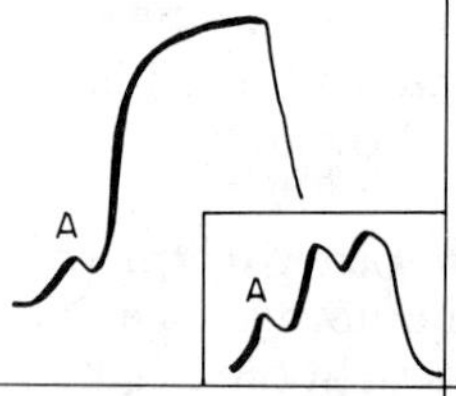	Maximal at cardiac apex. "A" wave may be visible and palpable coincident with fourth heart sound.
RIGHT VENTRICULAR HYPERTROPHY	Same impulse as in "Sustained" above	Maximal at left sternal edge in third and fourth left intercostal spaces.
ECTOPIC LEFT VENTRICULAR IMPULSE Ventricular aneurysm	Same impulse as in "Sustained" above	Maximal over mid precordium rather than at apex.
MITRAL REGURGITATION (severe)	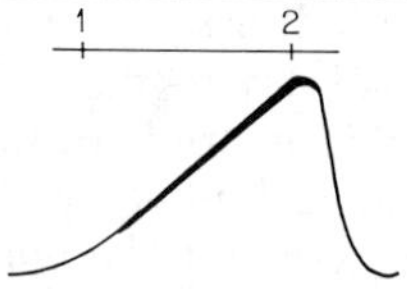	Whole precordium (see text).
PULMONARY ARTERIAL PULSATION in pulmonary hypertension	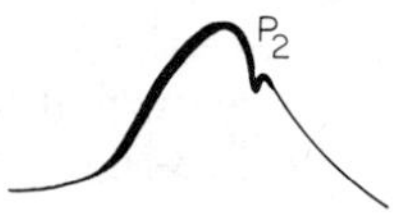	Second left intercostal space. Note palpable P_2.
INWARD MOVEMENT DURING SYSTOLE Constrictive pericarditis Tricuspid regurgitation, pure	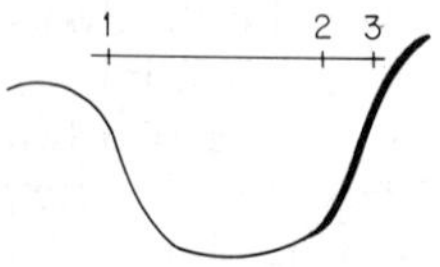	Whole precordium. Note reversal of direction during systole as compared with preceding examples.
DIASTOLIC MOVEMENTS Cardiomyopathy	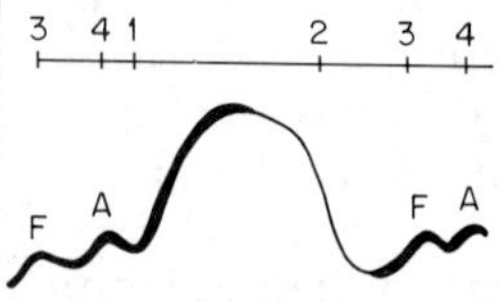	Cardiac apex. Systolic movement may be inconspicuous. Diastolic movements F and A correspond to 3rd and 4th sound gallops which may merge in tachycardia to form a summation sound.

FIGURE 10-1 Graphic representation of apical movements in health and disease. Palpable features are indicated by a heavy line.

seen in association with aortic stenosis, systemic hypertension, and idiopathic hypertrophic subaortic stenosis—all conditions characterized by left ventricular hypertrophy.[8,9] Usually a palpable *a* wave is perceptible in presystole with the patient lying on the left side.[5,6,10] A sustained thrust can also be felt with cardiomyopathy, but its amplitude is less and the velocity of its upstroke is lower, giving the impression of a weaker impulse. Prominent waves in diastole corresponding to third and fourth sounds are a frequent accompaniment in cardiomyopathy.

Right Ventricular Impulse

In the presence of right ventricular hypertrophy (RVH) there may be a sustained thrust at the left sternal edge. This is usually best appreciated as a systolic heave in the third and fourth left intercostal spaces.[11,12] This type of impulse occurs in association with high systolic pressures in the right ventricle, as in pulmonary hypertension or pulmonary stenosis. A hyperkinetic impulse characterized by increased amplitude but brief duration may be appreciated in the same location in conditions where there is an increased stroke volume but without excess pressure as in atrial septal defect[13] or pulmonary regurgitation. It should be noted that in tetralogy of Fallot, despite the presence of systemic pressures in the right ventricle, one does not encounter a right ventricular heave. There may be brief palpable vibrations at the time of S_1 and S_2, but the precordium is motionless during systole.[14] Absence of a sustained right ventricular thrust in the tetralogy is apparently due to the escape route for blood from right ventricle to aorta in this condition in contrast to the obstructive situation in pulmonary stenosis with intact ventricular septum. Another congenital cardiac condition affecting the right ventricle, but characterized by absence of a precordial heave or thrust, is Ebstein's anomaly of the tricuspid valve.[15]

Ectopic Impulses

Precordial Bulges in Ischemic Heart Disease

Precordial bulges in the third or fourth interspaces several centimeters from the sternum may occur in ischemia of the left ventricle.[16] They may be noted occasionally during an attack of angina pectoris, presumably as a result of transitory dyskinesis of the ventricular wall. With aneurysm of the anterior surface of the left ventricle a systolic bulge may persist in this location. A prominent presystolic *a* wave is an almost invariable accompaniment.

Mitral Regurgitation

In severe mitral regurgitation, in addition to the hyperkinetic impulse at the cardiac apex described above, there may be a generalized heave in systole over the whole precordium.[17] This movement is distributed over a wider area of the chest wall than the localized thrust of RVH, and it peaks later in systole. This delayed systolic wave mimics in timing the *v* wave in the left atrium and, like the *v* wave, is thought to be due to expansion of the left atrium by the regurgitant mass of blood and consequent lifting of the whole heart forward during systole.

Pulmonary Arterial Pulsation

Where the pulmonary artery is greatly swollen due to increased flow or pressure or poststenotic dilatation, there may be a palpable systolic bulge in the second left intercostal space.[18] However, a pulsation in this area is occasionally encountered in a young normal subject with a thin chest wall and hyperactive circulation.

Pulsation at Second Right Intercostal Space

In the presence of a dilated or aneurysmal aortic root there may be a systolic pulsation at the upper right sternal edge or sternoclavicular junction.

Exaggerated Movements in Diastole

Diastolic waves may be encountered in a variety of circumstances where their audible counterparts (third and fourth heart sounds or gallops) occur. These diastolic movements may be of large amplitude, as for instance in cardiomyopathy, but owing to their low velocity, they may not be readily perceived in a casual examination. The method described above of using a wand as a lever or visible marker at the apex beat provides a vividly exaggerated manifestation of these diastolic movements that may be edifying to the observer and is a readily available way to demonstrate bedside diagnostic phenomena to others.

Inward Retraction of the Precordium in Systole

An inward movement of the precordium during systole occurs principally in two situations: (1) constrictive pericarditis[19,20] and (2) pure tricuspid regurgitation, i.e., imcompetence of the valve as a primary abnormality rather than secondary to pulmonary hypertension and right ventricular failure. When the precordium moves *inward* during systole, it moves *outward,* of course, in early diastole at the time of ventricular filling. A careless observer utilizing palpation by itself can easily fall into the trap of reversing systole and diastole. If, however, one *listens* while palpating, the thrust of the diastolic heartbeat should be obvious.[21]

Palpable Heart Sounds

Heart sounds are frequently palpable in normal, young, thin individuals, as when exaggerated in disease states. For example, S_1 becomes snapping and accentuated in mitral stenosis and is responsible for the "tapping" apical impulse which is characteristic of that condition. A similarly accentuated and palpable S_1 is encountered in left atrial myxoma.

S_2 is increased and palpable in conditions associated with elevated pressures in the great vessels. Thus, A_2 may be palpable at the second right intercostal space in systemic hypertension or coarctation of the aorta. P_2 may be palpable at the second left intercostal space in pulmonary hypertension. An exaggerated single second sound palpable in this location but of aortic origin occurs in the uncommonly encountered corrected transposition of the great vessels where the source of the vibration lies close to the chest wall. The high-frequency vibrations associated with closure of the semilunar valves are sometimes called *shocks* because of their percussion quality and brief duration. They must be differentiated from the more sustained movements described above that are due to ventricular contractions.

Thrills

A *thrill* by definition is a palpable sensation resulting from the intense vibration of a loud murmur. It provides no specific diagnostic information beyond that yielded by the murmur itself. Thrills are often most readily perceived by applying the sensitive area of the hand at the base of the fingers, whereas all the other palpable phenomena described above are best appreciated by the fingertips.

References

1. Harvey, W.: "Exercitatio Anatomica de Motu Cordis et Sanguinis in Animalibus," Frankfort, 1628.
2. Abrams, J.: Precordial Motion in Health and Disease, *Mod. Concepts Cardiovasc. Dis.,* 49:55, 1980.
3. Kneibestol, M., and Vallbo, A. B.: Single Unit Analysis of Mechanoreceptor Activity from the Human Glabrous Skin, *Acta Physiol., Scand.,* 80:178, 1970.
4. Smith, D., and Craige, E.: Enhancement of Tactile Perception as Employed in Palpation, *Circulation,* 62:1114, 1980.
5. Denef, B., DeGeest, H., and Kesteloot, H.: The Clinical Value of the Calibrated Apical A Wave and its Relationship to the Fourth Heart Sound, *Circulation,* 60:1412, 1979.
6. Bethell, H. J. N., and Nixon, P. G. F.: Examination of the Heart in Supine and Left Lateral Positions, *Br. Heart J.,* 35:902, 1973.
7. Craige, E., and Sutton, G. C.: Quantitation of Precordial Movement: II. Mitral Regurgitation, *Circulation,* 35:483, 1967.
8. Sutton, G. C., Prewitt, T. A., and Craige, E.: Relationship between Quantitated Precordial Movement and Left Ventricular Function, *Circulation,* 41:179, 1970.
9. Benchimol, A., Legler, J. F., and Dimond, E. G.: The Carotid Tracing and Apex Cardiogram in Subaortic Stenosis and Idiopathic Myocardial Hypertrophy, *Am. J. Cardiol.,* 11:427, 1963.
10. Gibson, T. C., Madry, R., Grossman, W., McLaurin, L. P., and Craige, E.: The A Wave of the Apex Cardiogram and Left Ventricular Diastolic Stiffness, *Circulation,* 49:441, 1974.
11. Schmidt, R. E., and Craige, E.: Precordial Movements over the Right Ventricle in Children with Pulmonary Stenosis, *Circulation,* 32:241, 1965.
12. Kesteloot, H., and Willems, J.: Relationship between the Right Apexcardiogram and Right Ventricular Dynamics, *Acta Cardiol.,* 22:64, 1967.
13. Eddleman, E. E., Holt, J. H., and Bancroft, W. H., Jr.: Computer Analysis of the Kinetocardiogram from Patients with Atrial Septal Defects, *Am. Heart J.,* 71:435, 1966.
14. Craige, E.: Apexcardiography, in A. M. Weissler (ed.), "Noninvasive Cardiology," Grune & Stratton, Inc., New York, 1974, p. 30.
15. Genton, E., and Blount, S. G., Jr.: The Spectrum of Ebstein's Anomaly, *Am. Heart J.,* 73:395, 1967.
16. Eddleman, E. E., Jr., and Harrison, T. R.: The Kinetocardiogram in Patients with Ischemic Heart Disease, *Prog. Cardiovasc. Dis.,* 6:189, 1963.
17. Basta, L. L., Wolfson, P., Eckberg, D. L., and Abboud, F. M.: The Value of Left Parasternal Impulse Recordings in Assessment of Mitral Regurgitation, *Circulation,* 48:1055, 1973.
18. Sakamoto, T., Matuhisa, M., Inoue, K., Hayashi, T., and Ito, U.: Clinical and Hemodynamic Observation of Indirect Pulmonary Artery Pulse Tracing, *Cardiovasc. Sound Bull.,* 3:127, 1973.
19. Boicourt, O. W., Nagle, R. E., and Mounsey, J. P. D.: The Clinical Significance of Systolic Retraction of the Apical Impulse, *Br. Heart J.,* 27:379, 1965.
20. El-Sherif, A., and El-Said, G.: Jugular, Hepatic and Precordial Pulsations in Constrictive Pericarditis, *Br. Heart J.,* 33:305, 1971.
21. Mounsey, J. P. D.: Inspection and Palpation of the Cardiac Impulse, *Prog. Cardiovasc. Dis.,* 10:187, 1967.

11

Auscultation of the Heart

I was consulted in 1816 by a girl who presented the general symptoms of heart disease and in whom palpation and percussion gave little information on account of the patient's obesity. Her age and sex forbade an examination [by direct auscultation]. Then I remembered a well-known acoustic fact, that if the ear be applied to one end of a plank it is easy to hear a pin's scratching at the other end. I conceived the possibility of employing this property of matter in the present case. I took a quire of paper, rolled it very tight, and applied one end of the roll to the precordium; then inclining my ear to the other end, I was surprised and pleased to hear the beating of the heart much more clearly than if I had applied my ear directly to the chest.

Rene Theophile Hyacinthe Laennec, 1826[1]

The Principles of Auscultation

Aubrey Leatham, F.R.C.P.
Graham J. Leech, M.A.

The Evolution of Cardiac Auscultation

An account of the history of auscultation is given in the fourth edition of this textbook, and greater detail is given in McKusick's scholarly monograph *Cardiovascular Sound in Health and Disease.*[2]

In the last 30 years, the origin of the high-frequency components of heart sounds has been attributed by most practicing physicians to the final halt of closing valves; this theory is compatible with the effects of asynchronous left and right ventricular contractions as with bundle branch block, ventricular ectopics, and pacing. This view was challenged by Luisada[13] (see "The First and Second Heart Sounds," below), but in the last decade echocardiography, with its ability to time valve movements exactly, has confirmed the valve theory.

Basic Physics of Sound Waves

The word *sound* describes a sensation produced when pressure waves having certain characteristics strike the eardrum. Pressure waves are generated by a vibrating object that disturbs the particles of the medium surrounding it. The particles pass the vibrations on to their neighbors, and the disturbance is propagated through the medium like ripples spreading out across a pond. The particles do not travel through the medium but simply vibrate to and fro. The disturbance or wave travels in a direction parallel to that of the particle vibrations and is transmitted by the elastic coupling between them.

If waves are generated continuously in a regular pattern by a vibrating piston, the resulting alternating compressions and rarefactions can be described as follows. The *wavelength* is the distance between two successive peaks or troughs; the *amplitude* is the difference between maximum and minimum pressures. A complete segment comprising one peak and one trough is called a *cycle.* The number of cycles passing a particular point in one second is the *frequency.* Frequency, wavelength, and propagation velocity are related as follows:

$$\text{Frequency} \times \text{wavelength} = \text{propagation velocity}$$

For a given medium, propagation velocity is fixed, and so frequency and wavelength are inversely related. In air, pressure waves travel 300 m/s; in soft tissue, about 1550 m/s; and in bone, 4000 m/s. Thus, at a frequency of 256 Hz, or cycles per second, which is the pitch of middle C on a piano, the wavelength sound in air is about 1.3 m.

Waves from a small source surrounded by a uniform medium radiate outward in all directions, the intensity diminishing as the square of the distance. Intensity is further diminished by imperfect transfer of energy within the medium; water, for example, is a very good transmission medium, but air is some five times less efficient.

Pressure waves exhibit the same properties as other wave phenomena (e.g., light), the apparent differences being due to the relative sizes of the wavelength (100 cm for sound, compared with 0.00005 cm for light). Thus, when waves encounter an extensive boundary between two different transmission media, some of the energy is reflected and some transmitted, the path of the latter being deviated by refraction. Small obstacles scatter some of the incident energy in all directions. Diffraction allows waves to "bend" around a large obstacle; waves can also interact to produce interference effects and generate *standing waves,* i.e., zones of maximum and minimum amplitude.

If pressure waves encounter an object that is free to move in the direction of wave propagation, the object is caused to oscillate at the wave frequency. If an object that is constrained by some elastic force is disturbed, it vibrates at a frequency determined by its mass, the spring characteristics, and the degree of frictional damping present. This effect is called *resonance.* If such an object is disturbed by a wave train with a frequency that is identical to the resonant frequency, the resulting oscillations will have a very large amplitude. Thus, if, for example, a bank of tuning forks is placed in the path of sound waves, all the forks will vibrate a little, but the one with a resonant frequency that is closest to the wave frequency will "sing."

The Human Ear

The human hearing apparatus is very complex. It comprises the ear, which can be divided into the external, middle, and inner ears; the cochlear nerve; and those portions of the brain concerned with hearing perception.

Incoming pressure waves are collected by the pinna and led into the external auditory canal, which slopes forward and downward and is terminated by the eardrum. The waves cause the eardrum to vibrate, and the vibrations are transmitted to the oval window of the cochlea across the middle ear cavity by the three ossicles. The relatively small area of the oval window coupled with the large area of the eardrum improves energy transfer across the impedance mismatch between the air and the fluid within the cochlea.

The cochlea is a spiral canal rather like a snail shell and is separated along its length by two membranes into three compartments, the outer two of which join at its apex. The oval window connects to one of the outer compartments, which are filled with perilymph. The channel winds up the spiral, then down the other side, terminating in the round window which connects to the middle ear again. Between the two outer sections is the cochlear duct, filled with endolymph. Within the cochlear duct is the organ of Corti containing some 25,000 fine, hairlike fibers which form the terminal elements of the cochlear nerve. Pressure waves are transmitted from the perilymph, across the separating membrane, into the endolymph. The nerve fibers act rather like the array of tuning forks described earlier. Those near the bottom of the spiral are stimulated by high-frequency vibrations; those near the apex, by lower frequencies.

The fibers of the cochlear nerve lead, via several synaptic junctions, to the primary auditory reception center in the anterior transverse temporal gyrus; the neurons of this center fire at rates corresponding to the amplitude and frequency of the pressure waves. Through complex and little-understood interaction between these cells and those of the associated cerebral cortex, the sensation of sound is generated.

Sound perception is a complex subject, but some aspects relevant to cardiac auscultation must be mentioned. The most striking feature of human hearing is its almost incredible sensitivity; at its best it can detect pressure levels of 0.0002 dyn/cm^2 (equivalent to 10^{-16} W/cm^2). Although relatively crude by the standards of the animal kingdom, this is far superior to any manufactured microphone and amplifier. The sensitivity of the ear is, however, greatly influenced by wave frequency. It performs best between 2 and 4 kHz; outside this range, sensitivity falls progressively, and below 30 Hz or above 18 kHz is effectively zero. The manner in which sensitivity varies with frequency depends on the amplitude of the waves. For very high amplitudes, sensitivity varies little within the overall frequency range, but for lower amplitudes, the variation is greater. Heart sounds and murmurs generally have very low intensity, close to the threshold of hearing; furthermore, most lie in the frequency range of 1 to 500 Hz, well below the optimal range of the ear. In this region, the response characteristically approximates a straight line with a slope of 15 dB per octave. This means that if one tone has half the frequency of another, it must have 5.6 times the amplitude in order to appear to be equally loud. The substantial proportion of the heart's vibrational energy that lies below 30 Hz cannot be heard at all (though high-amplitude components may be detected by palpation).

Another psychoacoustic perception peculiarity of the ear is that it takes up to 1 s after the onset of a sound for its full intensity to be perceived, and this serves to lower the effective sensitivity for brief noises. Similarly, once the ear is accustomed to a relatively loud sound, a softer sound is not well heard. Thus, in a patient with a ventricular septal defect, it may be difficult to hear a faint P_2 component immediately after the loud systolic murmur. The smallest time interval that the ear can resolve is about 20 ms (0.02 s), so splitting of the first heart sound will only be apparent if the interval between the two components exceeds this amount. Finally, the ear has a remarkable ability to separate "wanted" from "unwanted" sounds. Thus, although a quiet environment is undoubtedly best for auscultation, the skilled practitioner can to a large extent ignore interference from extraneous sources and from respiratory noise and borborygmi which would render a phonocardiographic recording useless.

The Origin of Cardiac Sounds and Murmurs

The vibratory phenomena associated with the action of the heart can broadly be divided into *heart sounds,* brief noises which generally mark the beginning or end phases of the cardiac cycle, and *murmurs,* which last longer and are associated with blood flow.

Although heart sounds have been studied for over 150 years, there is no universally accepted theory for their origin. In 1830, Rouanet[3] pumped water through an animal heart while holding it to his ear to listen to the sounds generated. He observed that there were two major noises from each side of the heart, one at the beginning and one at the end of systole. He attributed these to "tensioning" of the leaflets of the atrioventricular (AV) and semilunar valves, respectively. Similar experiments by Dock[4] and others supported this view. Thus the *valvular* theory holds that the first heart sound has two major components, associated with mitral and tricuspid closure, and similarly the second sound has aortic and pulmonary components.

Although satisfactory for clinical purposes, the valvular theory came under attack in the 1960s as a result of studies of intracardiac pressures using high-

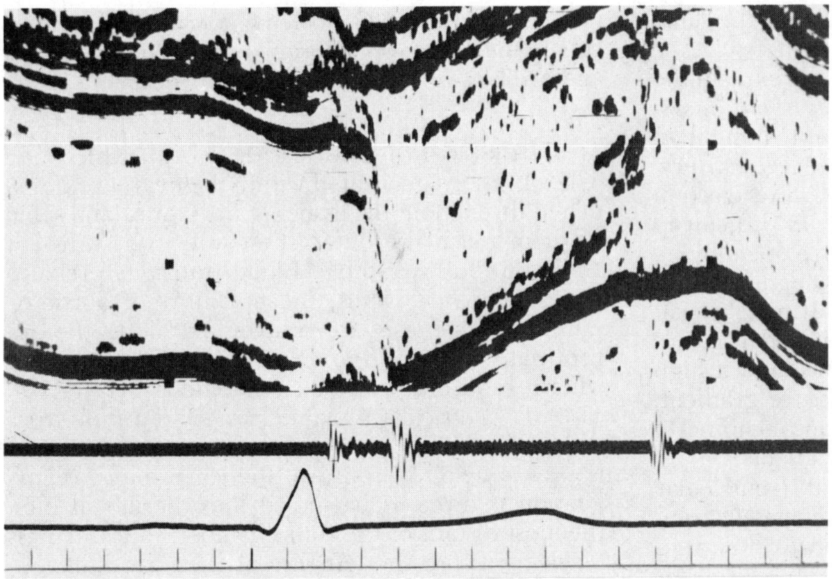

FIGURE 11-1 High-speed echophonocardiogram from a patient with a nonstenotic bicuspid aortic valve showing the relation of heart sounds to valve movements. The onset of the vibrations of the ejection sound occurs precisely at the moment when the motion of the diseased valve is suddenly halted. (See also Fig. 11-2.)

fidelity micromanometers. These showed that the timing of reversal of the pressure gradient across valves did not coincide with the associated sound components, and, since the valves are passive structures, it was assumed that they opened and closed at the moment of gradient reversal. Thus, it appeared that valve closure was not synchronous with the sound events, and so alternative mechanisms involving the tensioning of the ventricles and great vessels were proposed.[5] There is fallacy in this argument, however, since blood flowing through an open valve has momentum and the reversed pressure gradient takes a finite time to halt flow before the valve can close. Gradient crossover thus precedes valve closure by a variable interval influenced by the flow rate and the impedance characteristics of the downstream vessels.

More recently, echocardiography has provided a method for timing the motions of valves directly against sound phenomena and has vindicated the valvular theory by demonstrating invariable coincidence between the sound components and the abrupt halting of the valve leaflets as they tense under the influence of moving masses of blood (Figs. 11-1 and 11-2). Thus, the components of the first and second heart sounds, opening snaps, early systolic

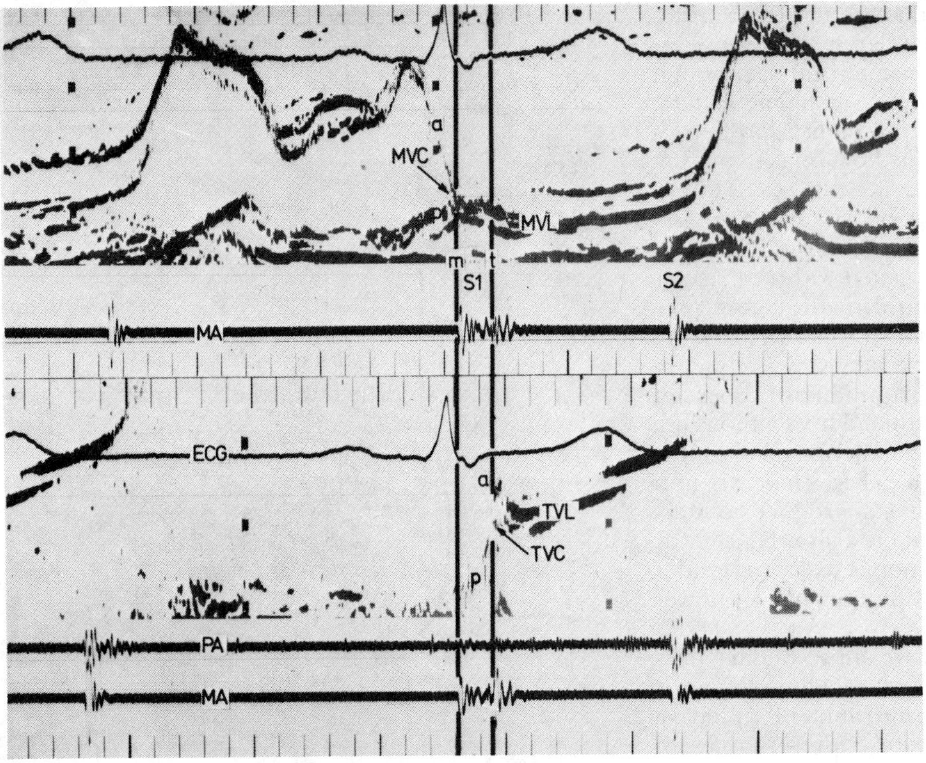

FIGURE 11-2 Echophonocardiogram from a normal subject with physiological splitting of the first heart sound. The tracings from the mitral and tricuspid valves were not recorded simultaneously, but the subject was in regular rhythm, and the tracings were aligned using the ECG. It will be seen that the first component of the first sound coincides with the terminal halt of the closing mitral valve (MCV) and the second component with that of the tricuspid valve (TVC).

ejection clicks, and prolapse clicks all have the same underlying mechanism.[6,7]

This concept does not, however, fully explain the early systolic "root" sounds sometimes heard in systemic or pulmonary hypertension and thought to arise from sudden distension of an enlarged artery. Their timing is identical to that of valve ejection sounds, and this makes the root theory difficult to accept, since at the moment when valve opening becomes maximal, ejection has already begun but has not yet achieved maximum velocity. It may be that some fibrous thickening of the semilunar cusps, known to occur in hypertensive states, and a high rate of increase of accelerating pressure gradient, which is due to late onset of ejection, combine to generate an audible sound in these patients.

There are also the third and fourth (ventricular filling) sounds. The former is approximately coincident with the transition from rapid to slow ventricular filling, and the latter occurs about 150 ms after the ECG P wave. Their precise origin is not certain, although they appear to arise as a result of a "shudder" of the left ventricular muscle in reaction to a sudden change in filling rate. In support of this concept is the fact that a sharp deflection of the interventricular septum coincident with a third sound can sometimes be seen on echocardiographic recordings.

When fluid flows through a pipe, if the flow velocity exceeds a certain value, flow becomes turbulent and some energy is dissipated in vortices which generate audible vibrations. Unstable flow can also arise when fluid passes through a small hole in a plate which partly occludes a pipe, when the pipe diameter changes abruptly, when a jet impinges on a surface, or when two streams having different directions of flow interact. Similar mechanisms underlie the generation of cardiac murmurs, although the complex geometry of the cardiohemic system, together with the nonlinear mechanical properties of blood vessels and pulsatile flow, makes mathematical analysis very difficult.

The audible characteristics of a murmur are determined mainly by the size and velocity of the jet. Thus, a high-velocity jet associated with ventricular septal defect or aortic or mitral regurgitation produces a high-frequency murmur, whereas a low-velocity jet in mitral stenosis generates a low-frequency murmur. Unfortunately, murmur intensity does not necessarily indicate flow volume. Thus, although a very small jet does not usually generate a loud murmur, torrential flow through a large hole, as in a large ventricular septal defect, can produce no murmur at all. It must be remembered also that the ear perceives higher-frequency noises as being louder than those of the same amplitude but of lower frequency.

Finally, murmurs can arise from secondary phenomena such as vibrations of chordae tendineae or torn semilunar cusps. These murmurs often have a characteristic "musical" quality. Other sources of noises within the heart, such as pericardial friction rubs, generally have different audible characteristics and are best not considered as murmurs at all.

Transmission of Sounds and Murmurs

The vibrations generated within the heart are transmitted throughout the tissues of the thorax, and some of them reach the outer chest wall with sufficient amplitude to be audible. Blood transmits pressure waves very well. Thus, the murmurs of aortic or pulmonary stenosis are transmitted along the appropriate artery and are best detected at the point where they come closest to the chest surface (Fig. 11-3). In ventricular septal defect, the murmur arises within the right ventricle, close to the chest wall, and is easy to hear. In contrast, the jet in mitral regurgitation is directed backward into the left atrium, the most distant of the four chambers, but the mass of blood within the left side of the heart still conducts the sounds fairly well to the apex, where they are best heard.

Transmission is aided by bringing the heart into contact with the chest wall without intervening lung tissue, which strongly attenuates sound waves. Thus, it helps to lean the patient forward and listen during held expiration to hear the murmur of aortic regurgitation, and to turn the patient to the left so that the apical beat can be palpated, indicating that the heart is in contact with the chest wall, when listening to the diastolic murmur of mitral stenosis.

FIGURE 11-3 Sites for auscultation and nomenclature. PA = pulmonary area. Pulmonary sounds or murmurs are usually maximal in the second or third left spaces but may extend inferiorly; LSE = lower left sternal edge or tricuspid area; AA = aortic area; MA = mitral area. (*From A. Leatham, "Examination of the Cardiovascular System," 2d ed., Oxford Medical Publications, Oxford, 1979. Reproduced with permission from the publisher, editor, and author.*)

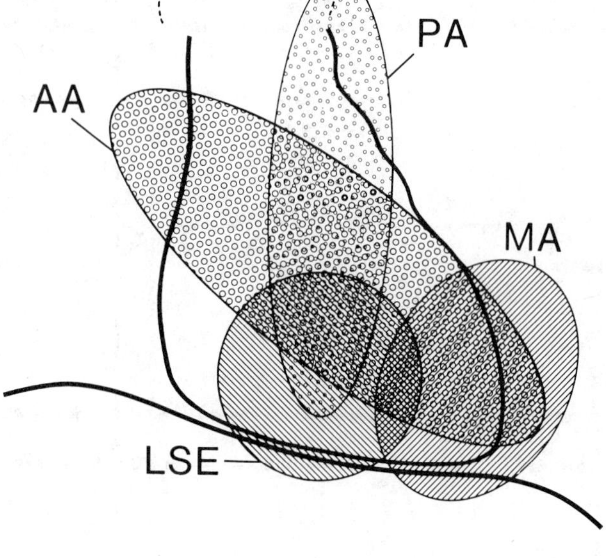

The chest wall itself has relatively high attenuation and is far from homogeneous, with the result that significant losses occur at interfaces between bones and muscle. The structure of the chest wall is such that most transmission is probably not via compression waves but via longitudinal shear waves, which transfer energy less effectively. Finally, the characteristics of the chest wall are somewhat frequency-dependent, with optimal transmission occurring between 100 and 200 Hz.[8]

For practical purposes, modification of heart sounds during transmission to the precordium is uncontrollable and largely unknown, so auscultatory findings are based on the characteristics of the vibrations as they appear on the chest surface. However, the build of the patient should be borne in mind when assessing their significance. Thus, a soft ejection murmur in a thin adolescent in whom the main pulmonary artery lies directly beneath the chest wall is less likely to be pathological than a murmur of the same intensity heard in an obese patient.

Vibrations reaching the chest wall, from whatever origin, combine to produce a compound wave. This can be considered on the basis of Fourier analysis to be comprised of a series of pure tones. The lowest frequency present, called the *fundamental,* is the frequency of the heart rate, typically 1 Hz (60 beats per minute). Added to it are numerous harmonics, with frequencies that are exact multiples of the fundamental and amplitudes that generally decrease with increasing frequency. The higher-frequency harmonics are most evident at the time of transient events such as halting of blood masses associated with valve closures. Because of their high frequency, these components do not excite resonant vibrations within the large masses of the heart and chest structures, and they die away very rapidly. Thus, if one wants to identify precisely the timing of transient events, it is best to remove all the low-frequency components. This is particularly necessary when two or more events occur in rapid succession, such as the closure of the AV or semilunar valves. The low-frequency vibrations merge together; but if they are eliminated and only the high-frequency components are detected, the vibrations from the first event end before those from the second begin, and the two can be distinguished (Fig. 11-4).

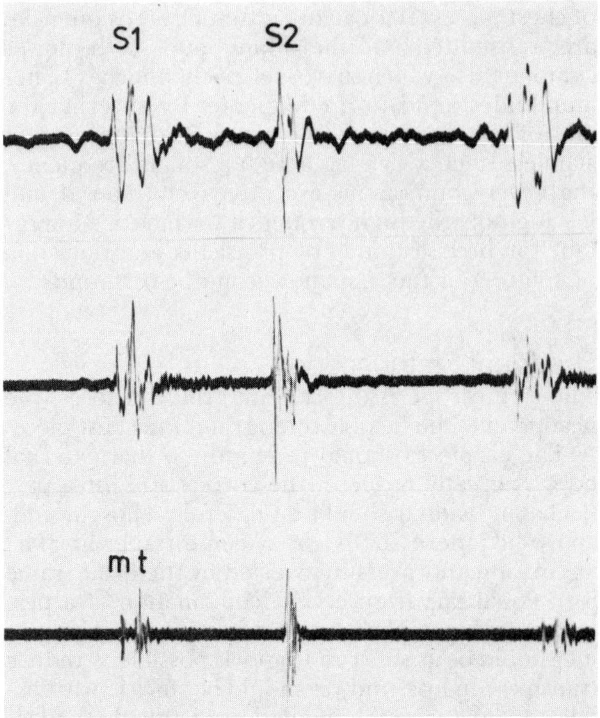

FIGURE 11-4 Phonocardiograms recorded from a normal subject to illustrate the effect of electronic filtering. At the top, there is very little filtering, so low-frequency sound components dominate the tracing. The center and bottom tracings have progressively greater attenuation of low frequencies and correspond approximately to the stethoscope bell and diaphragm, respectively. Physiological splitting of the first heart sound is revealed only when the low-frequency aftervibrations are totally eliminated.

The Physical Principles of Auscultation

Most sound energy reaching our ears is transmitted under so-called free field conditions in which the intensity diminishes as the square of the distance from the source. Waves arising from very low amplitude vibrations, such as those of the precordium, would thus be audible only if the ear were placed very close to the chest. As Laennec found, however, this is not always practical, so he rolled some paper to form a tube, one end of which he held on the patient's chest and the other he applied to his ear.

The stethoscope channels almost all the vibrational energy from the area of the precordium underneath the chest piece directly to the observer's eardrum. It is analogous to the catheter manometer system used to measure intravascular pressures, in which pressure signals are conducted along a fluid-filled tube to a remote sensing gauge. The following general principles govern the operation of the stethoscope. It should contact as large an area of the chest wall as possible, since by this means a given amplitude of precordial vibration will generate the greatest air volume displacement within the stethoscope. The internal volume of the tubing should be small, and its walls as rigid as possible, consistent with maneuverability, so that the volume displacement is converted into the maximum pressure fluctuation. It must make a perfect air seal against the chest wall, and the earpieces must fit perfectly into the external auditory canal; otherwise the pressure fluctuations will "leak out" and not be transmitted to the eardrum at maximal amplitude.

The frequency characteristics of the sounds are somewhat modified by the stethoscope tubing, which behaves rather like an organ pipe and resonates at certain frequencies determined primarily by its length.[9] However, the relatively low compliance of even thick-walled rubber tubing damps the resonant peaks considerably. Greater control of frequency response can be achieved by the use of different types of chest pieces. With an open funnel, all frequencies are transmitted into the tubing, and so the lower components, which have relatively much greater amplitudes, tend to predominate. By covering the end of the funnel with a thin rigid diaphragm of stainless steel, which has a high resonant frequency, the lower components are effectively filtered out, leaving only the high frequencies, which are important for precise timing of transients and detection of splitting of the first and second heart sounds.

The Ideal Stethoscope

The stethoscope is divisible into the earpieces, the head frame, the flexible tubing, and the chest piece.

The earpieces should fit exactly so that external noise is greatly reduced; the correct size for a particular individual should be carefully chosen, and, above all, there should be a comfortable fit. The angulation and pressure exerted by the head frame is of equal importance. The combination of a perfect fit with complete comfort is essential. The tubing should be as short and rigid as possible to reduce transmission loss, and yet should be sufficiently flexible to allow varying angulation of the chest piece without movement of the earpieces in the external meatus; this movement not only interferes with a close fit but may also cause meatitis. It is seldom practical to reduce the length of the tubing to less than 12 in, and double tubing is apparently more efficient than single tubing for transmitting high frequencies.[10]

The greatest variations occur in the stethoscope chest piece. The essential principle is that a rigid diaphragm transmits the high frequencies preferentially by resonating with them, thus acting as a filter. On the other hand, a bell transmits all frequencies with minimal loss, provided that it is not applied so firmly to the chest wall that the skin acts as a diaphragm. The larger the bell, the greater the intensity of sound collected, but the limiting factor with a large bell is the difficulty of obtaining a good fit over the rib cage of thin individuals; thus, ideally both a large and a small bell are required, and it is possible for the two to be combined.

The small bell has an additional advantage for localization of sounds and murmurs, particularly in pediatric cardiology. The diaphragm chest piece can cover a large area, since a perfect fit on the chest wall is not needed, and should be rigid (0.003-in stainless steel is as good as anything so far known). It should now be clear that the minimum requirement for an efficient stethoscope for cardiac auscultation is the combination of a bell chest piece and a diaphragm chest piece in a single instrument with a good changeover switch. Unfortunately, most popular stethoscopes have small and inefficient bells and large floppy diaphragms passing a high volume of sound, but with no filtration. It is strongly emphasized that a diaphragm with great rigidity is required for listening to high-frequency sounds, splitting of sounds, and high-frequency murmurs, and that a bell, which should be as large as possible, should be used for listening to low-frequency sounds and murmurs. Since auscultation of the heart is normally conducted near the lower threshold of the human hearing mechanism, an efficient stethoscope carries a great advantage in the practice of clinical cardiology. It might be thought that electronic amplification would be useful for bedside auscultation, but unfortunately no portable apparatus is yet as efficient as a good stethoscope. The greatest problem is the enormous variation in amplitude of vibrations useful for diagnosis in a typical heart cycle. Thus, high gain is required for low-intensity vibrations, and loud vibrations then produce distortion.

The Technique of Auscultation

Auscultation is the most difficult part of examination of the cardiovascular system but is greatly simplified if the physician knows what to listen for. It should therefore be preceded by the history and physical examination. For example, a history of paroxysmal nocturnal dyspnea should direct attention to listening for an opening snap or mitral diastolic murmur as evidence of mitral stenosis, or for a third heart sound as evidence of left ventricular failure. The finding of a slow-rising carotid pulse helps immensely in the interpretation of an apical systolic murmur when it is impossible to determine whether it is a pansystolic regurgitant murmur or a midsystolic aortic ejection murmur because of inaudibility of the second heart sound.

A quiet room is essential for accurate auscultation, and it is equally important that the patient be relaxed and comfortable. Often a background noise from contraction of chest wall muscles can be reduced by asking the patient to relax. Poor transmission of sound occurs with obesity and with hyperinflation. Particularly with the latter, aortic systolic murmurs are distant in the aortic and pulmonary areas.

At the start of auscultation, the patient is usually reclining comfortably at an elevation of 30 to 40°, as for the preceding examination of the venous and arterial pulses, and it is convenient to start auscultation in the pulmonary area, i.e., second and third left spaces. Figure 11-3 shows the usual auscultatory areas—note the considerable overlap between the aortic and mitral areas. The first and second heart sounds should be identified easily enough in most cases since systole is shorter than diastole. With tachycardia, systole and diastole may be of the same duration; accordingly, the carotid pulse should be palpated since its upstroke occurs very soon after the first heart sound. Auscultation in the pulmonary area using the diaphragm of the stethoscope usually reveals splitting of the second heart sound during the inspiratory phase of phasic respiration. The first and greater component is due to closure of the aortic valve (A_2), and the second and smaller component is due to closure of the pulmonary valve (P_2). The sounds should fuse in the expiratory phase of continuous respiration when the patient is reclining at 30 to 40°. If splitting remains obvious in expiration, the patient should be requested to breathe a little slower and deeper; fusion should then occur. Persistence of splitting suggests that there is a prolongation of right ventricular systole or shortening of left. Appreciation of normal and abnormal splitting of the second sound is the single most important step in the examination of children, since physiological right ventricular outflow ejection systolic murmurs are frequently present and cause difficulty in diagnosis.

If the order of valve closure is reversed (P_2 before A_2), the splitting is maximal in expiration and disappears on inspiration as P_2 delays, and this indicates prolongation of left ventricular systole. The pulmonary component of the second sound in a normal subject may be transmitted to the lower left sternal edge, but seldom to the apex.

The diaphragm of the stethoscope should then be moved to the lower left sternal edge, where in normal subjects the first heart sound is usually split into mitral and tricuspid components. These are both high-pitched sounds, and the interval between them is very small. The first component is usually louder and is due to closure of the mitral valve; the second component is usually much softer, sometimes inaudible, and is due to closure of the tricuspid valve. The splitting is particularly obvious in patients with sternal depression, owing to the juxtaposition of the heart to the stethoscope.

The diaphragm is then moved to the apex or mitral area, where the dominant component of the first heart sound is mitral closure and tricuspid closure is difficult to hear. In fact, obvious "splitting of the first heart sound" at the apex, particularly when separation of the two components is a little more than usual, should suggest audibility of an early systolic ejection sound from the aortic valve. The second heart sound at the apex should be single and is solely due to the closure of the aortic valve. In diastole in a normal subject, careful auscultation of the apex with the bell gently but accurately applied to the skin should reveal a low-pitched sound, which is the third heart sound and is due to rapid ventricular filling. This sound is obvious in thin children, tends to become progressively softer with increasing age, and disappears to auscultation (but not to a phonocardiogram) after the age of 40 to 45 years. The rapid ventricular filling sound is heard more easily if the patient leans to the left in the reclining position.

Many physicians prefer to reverse the order for auscultation, starting with the bell and then diaphragm at the apex and continuing with the diaphragm at the lower left sternal edge and pulmonary areas.

Auscultation should now be directed toward hearing abnormal sounds. Preceding the first sound, there may be a low-pitched sound due to ventricular filling following atrial contraction. This is easily confused with splitting of the first heart sound but is maximal at the apex (when left ventricular in origin) with the patient lying on the left side, and it is best heard with the bell rather than with the diaphragm. The aortic ejection sound, best recognized at the apex, has already been mentioned. In the pulmonary area, an early systolic sound will suggest the presence of a pulmonary ejection sound. Soon after the second heart sound, there may be an opening snap of the mitral valve. This is of high frequency, best heard with the diaphragm, and resembles P_2 in quality but is heard over a wider area, including the apex; during inspiration it should be possible to hear A_2, P_2, and the snap all close together. Attention is then paid to the possibility of a systolic murmur: its site of maximum intensity is noted and its intensity is graded. Even more important is the decision as to whether the murmur is a midsystolic ejection murmur or a pansystolic regurgitant murmur which extends to the relevant component of the second heart sound, since the site of maximum intensity may be misleading (Fig. 11-3) and aortic murmurs are often maximal at the mitral area, particularly in elderly subjects.

In diastole, there may be a high-pitched early diastolic murmur from aortic or pulmonary regurgitation, starting with the relevant component of the second heart sound. It should be remembered that the aortic valve underlies the third or fourth left intercostal space, and an aortic diastolic murmur is usually heard in this area with the diaphragm; often it is best heard in the patient upright and in held expiration since respiration mimics the quality of the murmur. An aortic diastolic murmur may also be transmitted to the apex. Maximal intensity in the aortic area to the right of the sternum suggests that the aorta is dilated. A pulmonary diastolic murmur secondary to pulmonary hypertension (the usual cause) is indistinguishable in site, timing, and quality from an aortic diastolic murmur, and should only be diagnosed if there is clinical and electrocardiographic evidence of right ventricular hypertrophy, a loud P_2 on auscultation, and a large pulmonary artery on x-ray.

Ventricular filling murmurs due to flow through the mitral or tricuspid valves occur a little later in diastole. They are low-pitched because of the much lower velocity of flow and therefore are best heard with the bell gently but accurately applied to the apex with the patient inclined to the left in the case of a mitral murmur or applied at the lower end of the sternum particularly during inspiration in the case of a tricuspid murmur. It is important to grade the intensity of the murmur and particularly its duration, since this is an approximate measure of the degree of obstruction. Next, it is important to listen in other areas, particularly at the aortic area to the right of the upper sternum where aortic systolic murmurs may be maximal, and also below the left clavicle where the murmur of patent ductus arteriosus is maximal and may be confined to that area; an identical continuous murmur may, however, be due to normal return of venous blood from the head and neck (venous hum), but this disappears when the patient is in the horizontal position. When congenital heart disease is suspected, it is necessary to listen to the whole chest since, for example, the continuous murmur found in pulmonary atresia may be maximal posteriorly; in coarctation of the aorta, the systolic murmur is usually as loud over the spine as it is over the front of the chest. Most murmurs are heard best when the patient is horizontal, since this causes increased venous return, or after exercise with the patient in this position. The patient should also be examined in the upright position for systolic sounds or murmurs secondary to a floppy mitral valve, since diminished stroke volume with the patient in the upright position may allow greater prolapse of floppy cusps. Left ventricular outflow obstruction and the resulting systolic murmur in obstructive cardiomyopathy also increase with diminished stroke volume when the patient assumes the upright position.

The First and Second Heart Sounds

Aubrey Leatham, F.R.C.P.
Graham J. Leech, M.A.

Heart sounds are of two varieties: those due to halting of closing or opening valves, and those due to halting of the ventricular walls at their limit of filling. Not surprisingly, the quality and timing of each group are completely different.

Valve closing and opening sounds result from the sudden halt of valve cusps which were moving at high velocity, and for this reason they are composed of high-frequency vibrations which sound high-pitched and are relatively loud because of the ear's great sensitivity to high frequencies.

The valve origin of the high-frequency heart sounds was described by Dock[4] nearly 50 years ago and has been accepted by many clinicians for the last 30 years mainly for indirect reasons[11] and particularly because of the findings with asynchronous ventricular contraction in bundle branch block, ventricular ectopic beats, and pacing.[12] This concept was challenged by Luisada,[13] but the development of cineangiography and later of echocardiography permitted for the first time an exact relation to be established between valve motion and heart sounds. Echoes taken synchronously with phonocardiograms at fast paper speeds have now established that the final halting of closing and opening valves is exactly coincident with the major high-frequency heart sounds.[14–16]

The First Heart Sound

Physiological Splitting of the First Heart Sound
Contraction of the left ventricle closely precedes that of the right.[17] Thus, the first valve to halt after closure as a result of the rise of ventricular pressure in early systole is the mitral, and this is responsible for the initial major components of the first heart sound. The first heart sound is maximal at the apex or mitral area where the apex of the left ventricle strikes the chest wall as it rotates in early systole. Fractionally later, the tricuspid valve closes, and this coincides with a rather smaller high-frequency vibration that is maximal at the lower left sternal edge over the tricuspid valve. This asynchrony of mitral and tricuspid valve closure accounts for the normal splitting of the first heart sound (Fig. 11-5), which can usually be heard at the lower end of the sternum, particularly in thin patients and children. The origin of the second component of the first heart sound had been controversial for many years; it was stated that closure of the tricuspid valve was noiseless and that the second component of the first sound arose on the left side of the heart, but echophonocardiography has now firmly established the tricuspid origin of this sound (Fig. 11-2).[14,16,18] Splitting of the first heart sound in normal subjects measures 20 to 50 ms and is wider than would be expected from the slight asynchrony of onset of left and right ven-

FIGURE 11-5 Physiological splitting of the first sound by 20 ms, best heard over the tricuspid valve at the lower left sternal edge where the second component (tricuspid closure) is maximal. The first component is much the louder sound in all other areas, particularly the mitral area. Echophonocardiography (Fig. 11-2) has confirmed the strong clinical suspicion that the first component is due to closure of the mitral valve, the second to the tricuspid valve. (*From A. Leatham, Splitting of the First and Second Heart Sounds, Lancet, 2:607, 1954. Reproduced with permission from the publisher and author.*)

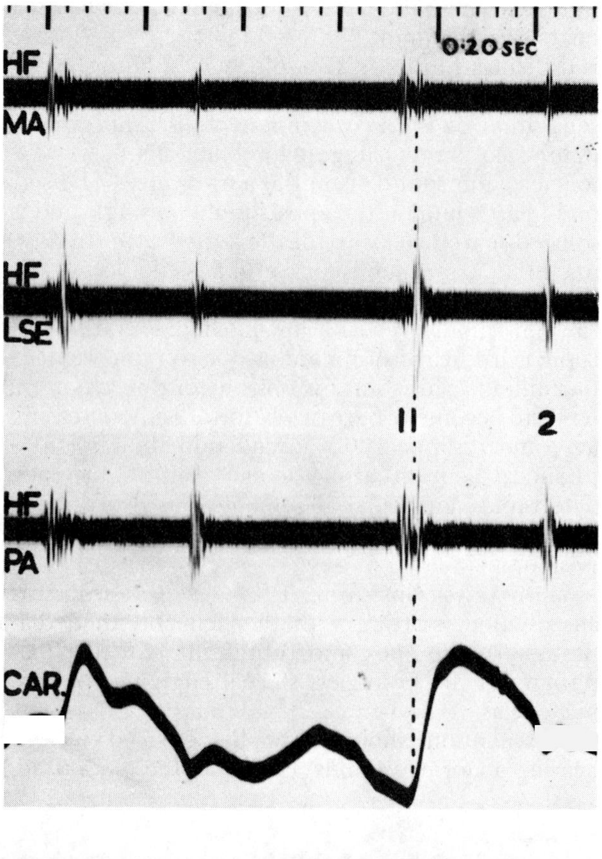

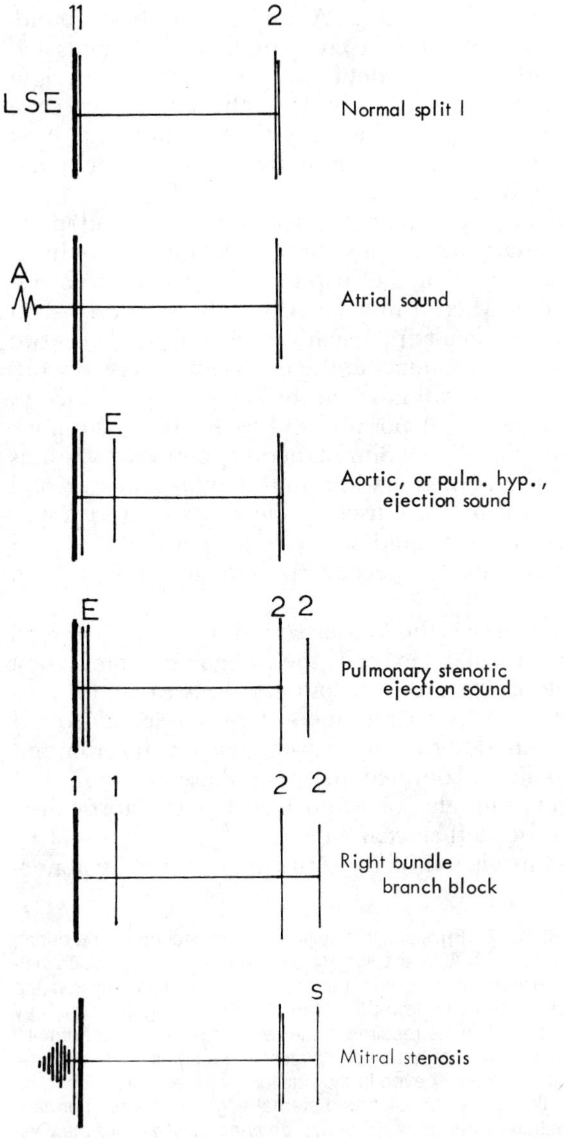

FIGURE 11-6 Differential diagnosis of physiological splitting of first sound. *(From A. Leatham, "Auscultation of the Heart and Phonocardiography," Churchill Livingstone, Edinburgh, 1970, p. 19. Reproduced with permission from the publisher and author.)*

tricular contraction. It appears that at normal PR intervals, the preceding atrial contraction has not only reopened the mitral valve but in addition has nearly closed it so that the slightest rise of the first part of the left ventricular (LV) pressure pulse is sufficient to complete closure. The tricuspid valve, however, starts from a wide-open position (right atrial contraction is less efficient than left in exerting closure forces) and thus takes longer to reach its final closed position.[19]

The differential diagnosis of splitting of the first heart sound is shown in Fig. 11-6.

Abnormally Wide Splitting of the First Heart Sound

Delay in onset of right ventricular contraction, causing delay in onset of tricuspid closure, is the usual cause of abnormally wide splitting of the first heart sound. It is found in most cases of complete right bundle branch block, particularly when this is an isolated finding, and also when ventricular contraction is initiated by an ectopic or pacemaker impulse arising in the left ventricle.[12] Late tricuspid closure cannot always be heard, however, in complete right bundle branch block, and the echo shows that in these cases tricuspid closure is not delayed and produces only minor vibrations; presumably this indicates that the block is peripheral with slowing of the right ventricular upstroke rather than delay in onset.[20] Peripheral block seems more likely to be associated with advanced myocardial or conducting tissue disease. In keeping with the division of right bundle branch block into proximal and peripheral block, depending on the timing of tricuspid closure, a loud late tricuspid closure sound is the almost invariable finding in Ebstein's anomaly,[18] in which the right bundle is stunted and the peripheral branches fail to develop. In partial right bundle branch block, there may be slight delay of tricuspid closure; but when an ECG of similar pattern denotes hypertrophy, as in atrial septal defect, there is no delay of tricuspid closure and no abnormally wide splitting of the first heart sound.[21]

In left bundle branch block, abnormal splitting of the first heart sound is rare because there is usually no delay in onset of mitral closure and the block seems to be at arborization level in most cases.[12] High left atrial pressure, as in mitral stenosis or myxoma, may cause reversed splitting of the first sound, with tricuspid closure preceding the greatly delayed mitral closure, which is also extremely loud (see below).

In patients with pacemakers, we were puzzled by the frequent finding of a high-frequency sound preceding not only the first sound but also the ventricular pressure pulse. On investigation it was found to be due to contraction of chest wall skeletal muscle, which has a shorter electromechanical interval than cardiac muscle.[22]

Intensity of the First Heart Sound

The intensity of the mitral and tricuspid valve closure sound depends on several factors:

- Adequacy of AV cusps to halt ventricular flow
- Mobility of cusps
- Position of cusps and rate of ventricular contraction

Regurgitation has to be very severe for deficiency of cusp tissue to fail to cause an abrupt halt of closing cusps with ventricular contraction. Fibrosis or calcification of the mitral valve cusps is a much more common cause of a faint first heart sound (and absent opening snap) and may produce difficulty in the diagnosis of mitral stenosis, which is invariably present under these conditions and would be expected to cause a loud first sound.

The position of the AV cusps, whether wide open or semiclosed, has long been known to be the most important factor responsible for the intensity of the first heart sound.[23–26] The distance of travel of flimsy cusps with little mass did not seem to be an adequate explanation, but it has recently been shown that the variable delay in closure, depending on the distance of travel, is the basic underlying factor.[27] A valve which is semiclosed at the end of diastole will come to its final halt at the very beginning of the left ventricular pressure pulse when the rate of rise is slow; the resulting sound is soft. A valve that is wide open at the end of diastole takes longer to come to its final halt, which occurs on a later and steeper part of the left ventricular pressure pulse; the resulting sound is loud.

The loudest first heart sounds are found with mitral stenosis (and mobile left atrial myxoma). Delay of mitral valve closure has been known since the beginnings of phonocardiography to be due to the longer time required for the rising left ventricular pressure pulse to exceed the elevated left atrial pressure.[28] It is only recently, with the advent of high-speed echophonocardiography, that it has been shown that the same principle of the relation between the halt and the ventricular pressure pulse accounts for nearly all variations in intensity of the first heart sound.[27] Echocardiography has shown that when left atrial contraction precedes ventricular contraction by a moderate or long interval (PR interval > 0.16 s), not only has the mitral valve been reopened at the end of diastole but eddies from ventricular filling have almost completely closed the valve so that its final halt occurs at the very beginning of the left ventricular pressure pulse at a low rate of pressure change and generates a soft sound. With shorter PR intervals, the valve is still wide open from the closely preceding atrial contraction; it therefore takes longer to reach its final halt position, which then occurs later at a more steeply rising part of the left ventricular pressure pulse, so the greater rate of pressure change generates a loud sound. Other causes of a wide-open valve at the end of diastole and consequently a loud first sound are high-output states, left-to-right shunts, and tachycardia, which shortens ventricular filling time.

With shunts, either the mitral or the tricuspid valve may be selectively affected; so, for example, a loud tricuspid component of the first heart sound is the rule in atrial septal defect.[21] It is also possible that the condition of the ventricular wall plays a part in the intensity of the first sound. In aortic stenosis, the first sound tends to be faint for a given PR interval; perhaps atrial contraction is unusually effective in closing the mitral valve because of its increased force of contraction in the face of inelastic ventricle.

The Second Heart Sound

The physiological asynchrony of the left and right ventricles becomes even more important with the second heart sound. Separation of its aortic (A_2) and pulmonary (P_2) components is the key to auscultation of the heart. Once A_2 and P_2 have been found, their intensities can be compared, nearby sounds and murmurs can be identified, the duration of right and left ventricular systole in the same heart cycle can be compared, and an estimate can be made of the effect of respiration on the loading of right and left ventricles.

Normal splitting of the second heart sound in the pulmonary area, well known to Potain,[29] is confined to the height of the inspiratory phase of free respiration, when it may be very wide (e.g., 0.10 s). It is more difficult and usually impossible to detect two distinct components in the expiratory phase of continuous respiration when the subject is examined in the semiupright position (30 to 40° from the horizontal, Fig. 11-7). Simultaneous phonocardiograms from the pulmonary and mitral areas and a carotid pulse tracing were used to identify the two components of the second sound, and it was found that aortic normally precedes pulmonary closure (Fig. 11-7).

A_2 is much the louder sound, being heard in all areas; it usually exceeds the pulmonary component in intensity even in the pulmonary area, and is normally the only component of the second sound transmitted to the mitral area. P_2 is much softer and normally is confined to the pulmonary area and nearby, though it is often heard at the aortic area and lower left sternal edge.

Transmission of P_2 to the apex is usually abnor-

FIGURE 11-7 Physiological splitting of the second sound during inspiration, with A_2 preceding P_2, as shown by simultaneous indirect carotid tracing and high-frequency phonocardiograms from the pulmonary area and lower left sternal edge. During the expiratory phase of continuous respiration the two components are normally fused completely or nearly completely in the semiupright posture. A_2 is louder than P_2 even in the pulmonary area. P_2 is seen to be fainter than A_2 at the lower left sternal edge, and is not normally transmitted to the apex. (*From A. Leatham, Splitting of the First and Second Heart Sounds, Lancet, 2:607, 1954. Reproduced with permission from the publisher and author.*)

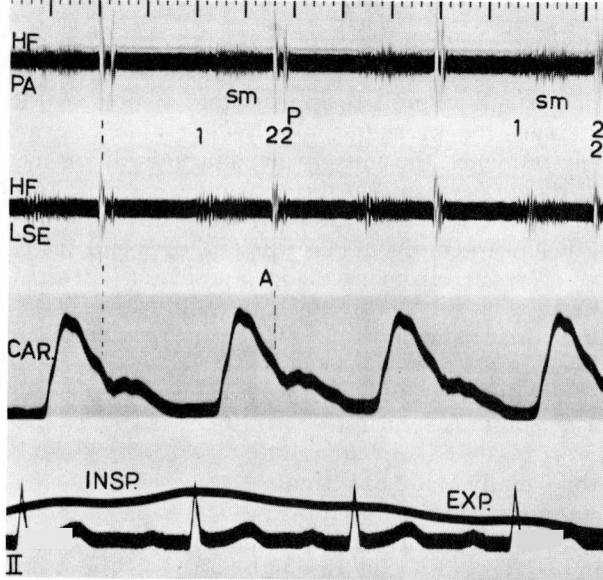

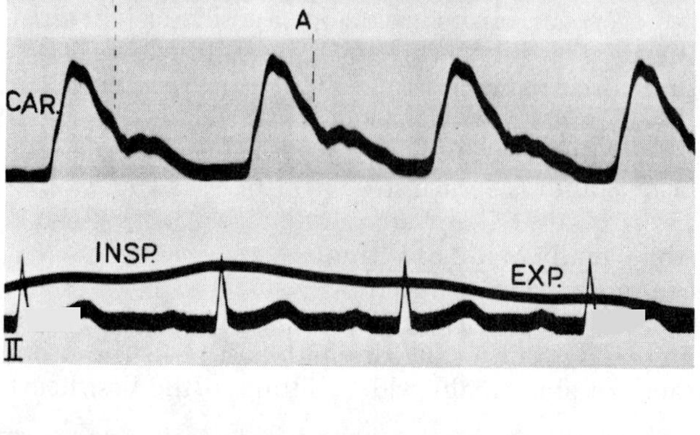

mal in adults. Fusion or close splitting of the second sound in the expiratory phase of continued respiration *almost* excludes right-sided lesions, such as atrial septal defect and pulmonic stenosis, and thus has great practical importance in the examination of children referred because of a systolic murmur. If there is doubt about too-obvious splitting of the second sound in expiration, the splitting will disappear in almost all normal subjects in the semiupright position (about 40° from the horizontal), especially when respiration becomes a little slower and deeper; splitting may persist, however, in normal subjects during expiration in the recumbent position, because of increased venous return, or during held expiration. There are a few normal subjects, however, with obvious expiratory splitting of the second sound (normal inspiratory increase) and unusually wide splitting of the first sound, suggesting delay in contraction of the right ventricle, yet with a normal ECG. When catheterization was performed in two patients to exclude atrial septal defect, a delayed onset of the right ventricular pressure pulse was found. In a few other normal subjects, unusually wide splitting of the first and second sounds appeared to be associated with a depressed sternum, but this was probably simply due to increased audibility of sounds from proximity.

The variations in splitting of the second sound are probably caused by ventricular increase in stroke volume causing delay in valve closure. During inspiration, blood is drawn by the negative pressure in the chest into the right side of the heart from the extrathoracic venous reservoir, but not immediately into the left side where the venous reservoir is intrathoracic. The splitting during inspiration has been thought to be caused mainly by the inspiratory increase in stroke volume of the right ventricle with consequent delay in pulmonary closure.[11,16,30] However, aortic closure also moves with respiration,[31] though only slightly (35 percent of total movement).[32] It must be appreciated that the immediate inspiratory increase in stroke volume of the right ventricle is followed after 1 to 3 s by a similar increase in stroke volume of the left ventricle, and that it is necessary to study the effect of inspiration after a period of apnea to prevent superimposition of one respiratory cycle on another.[33] This concept was applied by Shafter[34] to the second heart sound in adult subjects, and similar results have been produced in children.[35] Following halted respiration, inspiration has no effect on A_2, but causes an immediate delay in P_2 because of increased stroke volume of the right ventricle as blood is drawn from the extrathoracic venous reservoir; 1 to 3 s later, there is a delay in A_2 as the inspiratory increase in stroke volume reaches the left ventricle (Fig. 11-8). At normal respiratory rates, diminished stroke volume of the left ventricle with earlier A_2 coincides with the inspiratory increase in stroke volume of the right ventricle and later P_2 (wide split). Increased stroke volume of the left ventricle and later A_2 coincides with the ex-

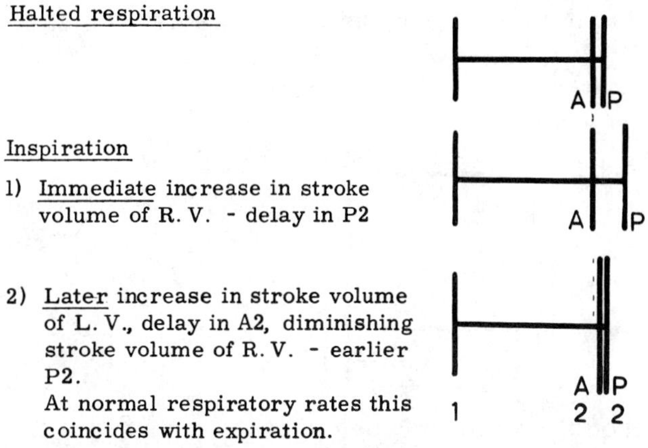

Halted respiration
A P
Inspiration
1) Immediate increase in stroke volume of R. V. - delay in P2
A P
2) Later increase in stroke volume of L. V., delay in A2, diminishing stroke volume of R. V. - earlier P2.
At normal respiratory rates this coincides with expiration.
1
A P
2 2

FIGURE 11-8 Mechanism of normal splitting of the second sound.

piratory diminution in stroke volume of the right ventricle and earlier P_2 (narrow split or fusion). It should be mentioned, however, that changes in capacitance of the pulmonary vascular tree with respiration have also been suggested as the cause of variations in splitting of the second heart sound with respiration.

Thus, we are testing first the ability of the right ventricle to increase its stroke volume; provided that the right ventricle achieves this, we are then testing the function of the left ventricle in the same way. To enable the individual variations in stroke volume of the two ventricles to take place, the interatrial septum must be intact.

It follows that fixed splitting of the second heart sound may be due either to inability of the right ventricle to vary its stroke volume, causing a constant duration of systole, or to approximately equal inspiratory delay of A_2 and P_2, indicating that the two ventricles share a common venous reservoir (Fig. 11-9). Right ventricular failure or disease may produce true fixed splitting of the second sound. Inability of the right ventricle to vary its stroke volume means that a constant flow reaches the left ventricle, which will not therefore vary its stroke volume either, even if it has normal function. In right ventricular failure, fixed splitting of the second sound is often obvious, particularly as P_2 may be a little late. It was puzzling that in constrictive pericarditis, with its fixed ventricular capacity, inspiratory splitting of the second sound appeared to be retained, but it has now been shown[36] that although P_2 is fixed, A_2 becomes earlier on inspiration, fitting in with the known inspiratory diminution in left ventricular stroke volume with pericardial constriction.

In atrial septal defect, either with normal or with high pulmonary vascular resistance (including an Eisenmenger's reaction), the fixed or nearly fixed splitting of the second sound is a highly valuable physical sign (Figs. 11-9 to 11-11). The key point is that aortic closure usually delays *immediately* with inspiration,[34] simultaneously with the normal delay of pulmonary closure; this indicates that the stroke volume of the left ventricle is increasing at the same

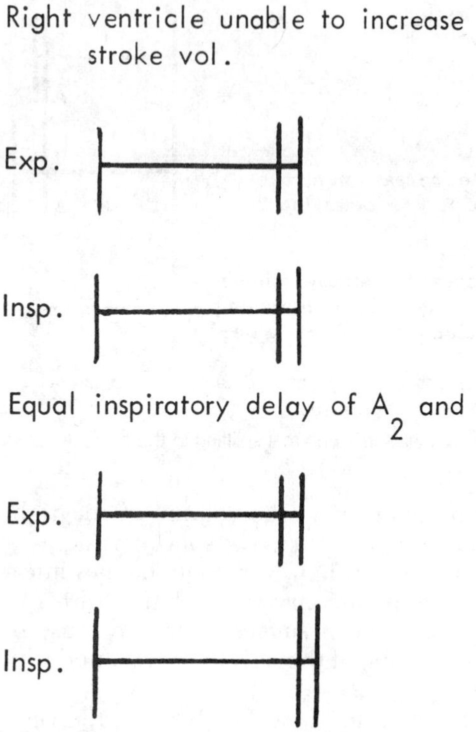

FIGURE 11-9 Fixed splitting of second sound. (*From A. Leatham, "Auscultation of the Heart and Phonocardiography," Churchill Livingstone, Edinburgh, 1970, p. 66. Reproduced with permission from the publisher and author.*)

time as the right, either because of a transient right-to-left shunt or because of lessening of the left-to-right shunt at that moment. With anomalous pulmonary venous return and an intact interatrial septum, one would not expect fixed splitting from simultaneous inspiratory delay of A_2 and P_2; in the rare patients who have been studied, no such fixed

FIGURE 11-10 Atrial septal defect (normal low pulmonary vascular resistance). Wide splitting of the second sound due to delay of P_2 with little variation ("fixed split") throughout the respiratory cycle, shown by measurement from the onset of systole to be due to nearly equal delay of both A_2 and P_2 on inspiration. (*From A. Leatham and I. Gray, Auscultatory and Phonocardiographic Signs of Atrial Septal Defect, Br. Heart J., 43:138, 1956. Reproduced with permission from the publisher and author.*)

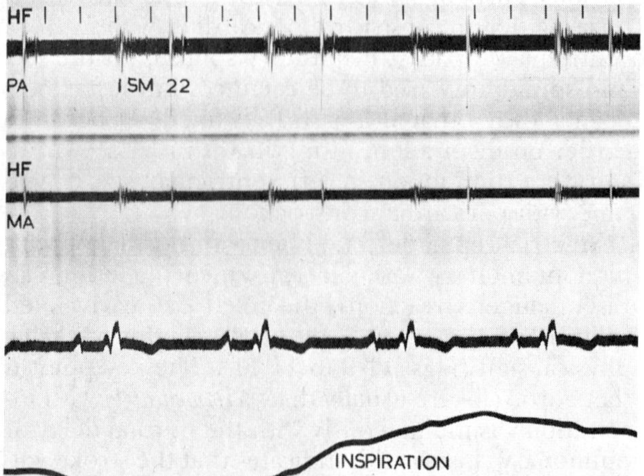

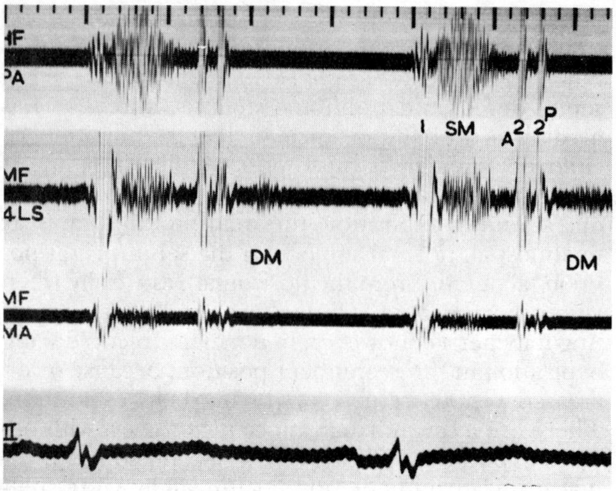

FIGURE 11-11 Atrial septal defect with left-to-right shunt (pulmonary artery pressure, 22.6 mmHg). Despite the low PVR, P_2 is as loud as A_2 in the pulmonary area and is transmitted to the mitral area. (*From A. Leatham and I. Gray, Aucultatory and Phonocardiographic Signs of Atrial Septal Defect, Br. Heart J., 43:138, 1956. Reproduced with permission from the publisher and author.*)

splitting has been found. Thus, with the relatively common sinus venosus type of defect, in which the interatrial communication is small, there is usually some respiratory variation in splitting of the second sound.[34] With interventricular communications it is only with very large defects or a single ventricle, always with extreme pulmonary hypertension (Eisenmenger's syndrome), that both A_2 and P_2 delay immediately on inspiration,[37] thus accounting for the single second sound (Fig. 11-12). A complicating factor is that extreme increase in stroke volume may not allow further inspiratory delay.

Wide Splitting of Second Heart Sound

Splitting of the second sound, which is too wide in the expiratory phase of phasic respiration to be physiological, is usually due to delay in pulmonary closure from right-sided lesions or disease (Fig. 11-13). Identification of the two components is usually easy, especially when respiratory variations are retained (i.e., when there is no right ventricular failure or atrial septal defect), for P_2 will be later on inspiration, increasing the splitting; in addition, P_2 is usually the fainter component and is usually not transmitted to the mitral area. In complete right bundle branch block, the electrical delay in activation of the right ventricle usually results in a late rise of the right ventricular pressure pulse, and the whole of right ventricular systole is late, resulting in late pulmonary closure. The normal respiratory variations can usually be detected, though sometimes with great difficulty, and a further clue to the diagnosis is usually given by the abnormally wide splitting of the first sound due to delayed tricuspid closure. Occasionally, in a subject who is normal or who has a small ventricular septal defect, abnormally wide splitting is a sign of right-sided electromechanical

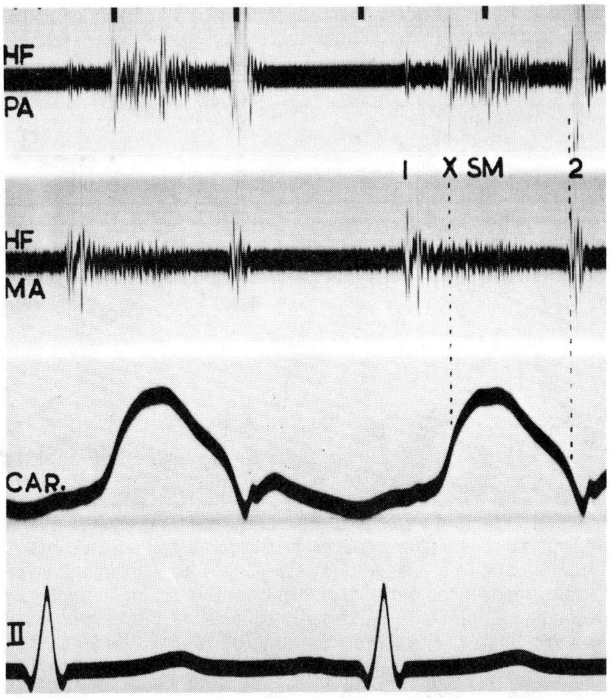

FIGURE 11-12 Pulmonary hypertension. Eisenmenger's ventricular septal defect. Complete fusion of A_2 and P_2 in expiration and inspiration (when A_2 and P_2 delay equally) is found only where there is a large ventricular septal defect or single ventricle *and* equal pulmonary and systemic vascular resistances. (*From A. Leatham, "Auscultation of the Heart and Phonocardiography," Churchill Livingstone, Edinburgh, 1970, p. 81. Reproduced with permission from the publisher and author.*)

FIGURE 11-13 Right-sided heart abnormalities causing delay of P_2 and thus abnormally wide splitting of second sound. (*From A. Leatham, "Auscultation of the Heart and Phonocardiography," Churchill Livingstone, Edinburgh, 1970, p. 55. Slightly modified and reproduced with permission from the publisher and author.*)

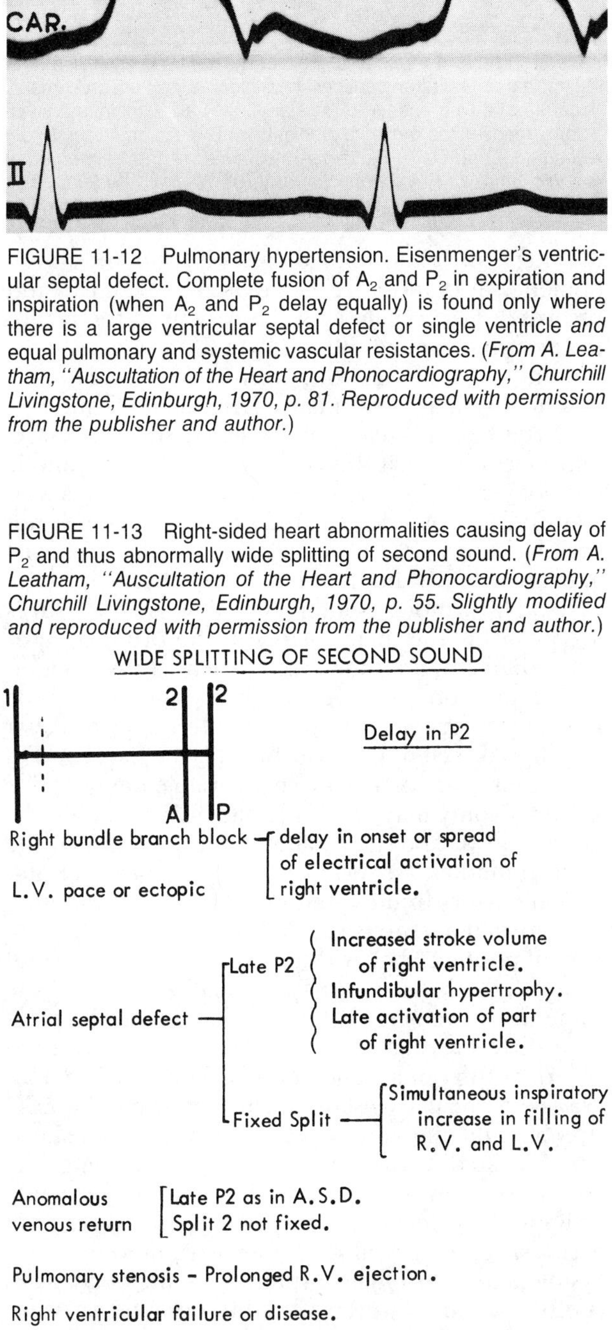

delay (prolonged Q-RV upstroke) without an electrocardiographic abnormality. In incomplete right bundle branch block accompanying right ventricular hypertrophy, there is usually no abnormality of the second (or the first) heart sound, and the Q-RV time is normal.

In atrial septal defect (Fig. 11-10), the abnormal behavior of the second sound with respiration has already been considered, but a second abnormality is delay in pulmonary closure. This is probably due in most cases to the large stroke volume of the right ventricle compared with the left, and there is a similar delay in P_2 with anomalous venous return. Following repair of an interatrial defect, respiratory variations in splitting appear at once; but in some cases delay in pulmonary closure persists for a time (without complete right bundle branch block), and there must be less easily reversible changes in the right ventricle to account for this.

In pulmonary valve stenosis with intact ventricular septum, the right ventricular pressure can rise above systemic level and achieve almost normal resting pulmonary flow and pressure. A faint and greatly delayed pulmonary closure sound can usually be heard and recorded at the pulmonary area, except in some extremely severe cases. The earlier aortic closure sound is frequently drowned in the pulmonary systolic murmur but can be identified at the apex (Fig. 11-14). These findings are similar in pure infundibular stenosis (Fig. 11-15). In the presence of an associated right-to-left shunt through a ventricular septal defect (cyanotic tetralogy of Fallot), pulmonary flow and pressure are so greatly reduced

FIGURE 11-14 Isolated pulmonary valve stenosis (RVP., 100 mmHg—A_2 to P_2, 0.09 s). Because of prolongation of right ventricular ejection compared with left, the pulmonary systolic murmur may drown A_2 in the pulmonary area, but stops before the greatly delayed P_2, which is usually audible or at least recordable. A_2 may be heard and recorded at the mitral area so that A_2 to P_2 interval can be measured and gives a surprisingly accurate assessment of the severity of the stenosis. (*From A. Leatham, "Auscultation of the Heart and Phonocardiography," Churchill Livingstone, Edinburgh, 1970, p. 56. Reproduced with permission from the publisher and author.*)

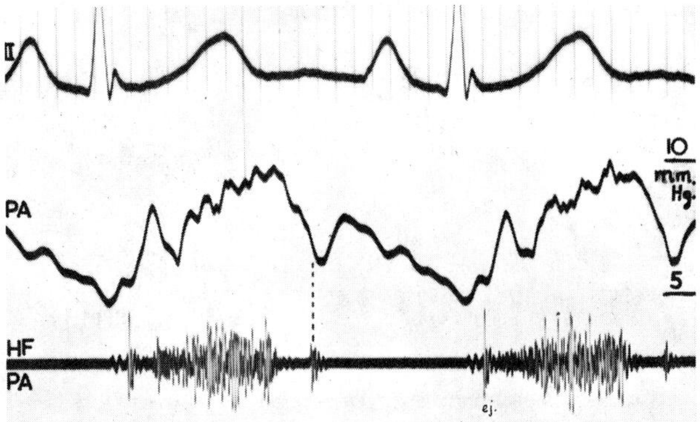

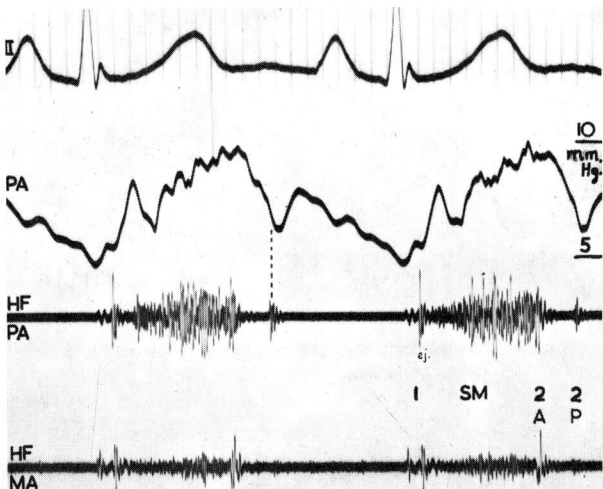

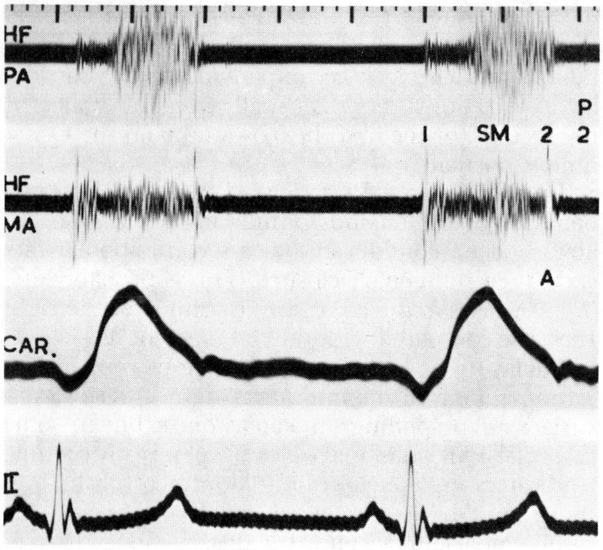

FIGURE 11-15 Isolated pulmonary infundibular stenosis. Prolongation of right ventricular systole and delay of P_2 (0.09 s after A_2), as with valve stenosis (but no ejection sound). (*From A. Leatham, "Auscultation of the Heart and Phonocardiography," Churchill Livingstone, Edinburgh, 1970, p. 57. Reproduced with permission from the publisher and author.*)

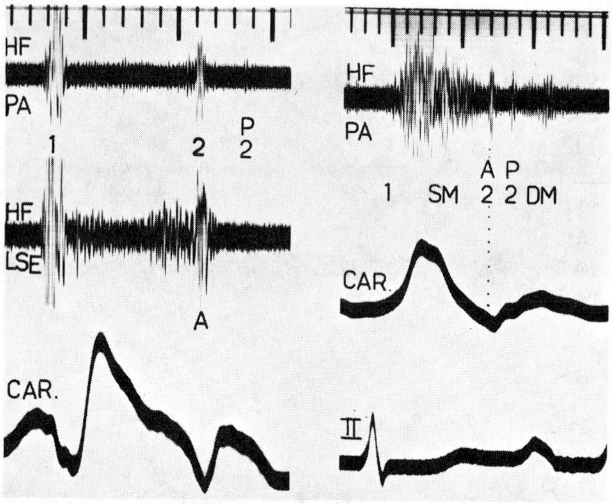

FIGURE 11-17 Tetralogy of Fallot. The delayed P_2 (0.1 s after A_2) appeared first after a successful Blalock operation, presumably because of an increase in pulmonary flow. Later a pulmonary valvotomy reduced the pressure gradient and P_2 became earlier. (*From A. Leatham and D. W. Weitzman, Auscultatory and Phonocardiographic Signs of Pulmonary Stenosis, Br. Heart J., 19:303, 1957. Reproduced with permission from the publisher and author.*)

that it is rare to hear or record pulmonary closure (Fig. 11-16;[38] a useful point in identifying pure pulmonic stenosis with cyanosis due to a reversed interatrial shunt), though it may first appear in tetralogy of Fallot as a late sound following a Blalock operation or valvotomy (Fig. 11-17). In infants with

FIGURE 11-16 Severe pulmonic stenosis with ventricular septal defect and right-to-left shunt (tetralogy of Fallot); P_2 cannot be heard or recorded even with extra gain in channel 2 (+ voltage limitation distorting murmur). (*From A. Leatham, "Auscultation of the Heart and Phonocardiography," Churchill Livingstone, Edinburgh, 1970, p. 58. Reproduced with permission from the publisher and author.*)

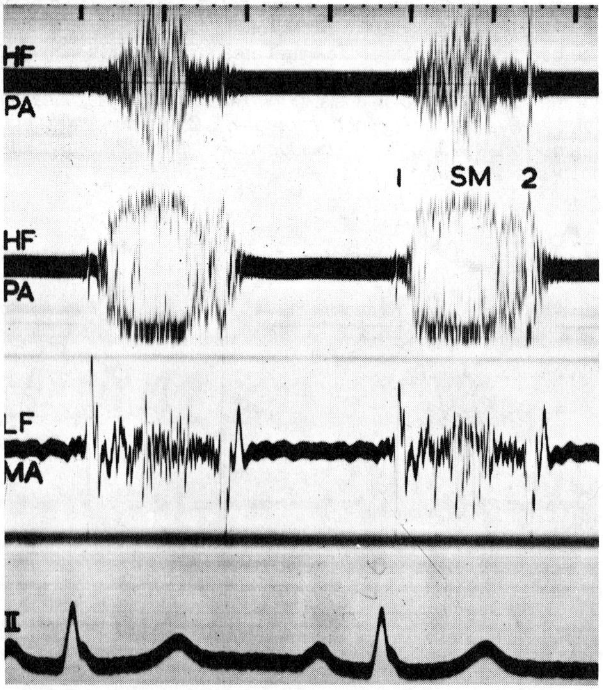

tetralogy of Fallot, before or soon after the development of cyanosis, P_2 can often be heard and recorded,[39] especially with the patient in the reclining position. Indeed the late P_2 at the acyanotic stage in infancy may be the only way to differentiate this potentially fatal abnormality from a small and unimportant ventricular septal defect, since the ECG may be equivocal at this stage. In so-called acyanotic tetralogy of Fallot (moderate pulmonic stenosis with ventricular septal defect), the pulmonary flow is not greatly reduced, and late P_2 can usually be heard and recorded, though it is notably absent in some cases. Thus, though pulmonary flow and pressures are probably the main factors in the production of an audible P_2, another factor, such as the relation of the pulmonary valve to the chest wall, may be important, for the outflow tract in tetralogy of Fallot is often directed posteriorly and the large aorta overlies it anteriorly, both to a variable degree. The valve anatomy may be a third factor. P_2 may also be audible in tetralogy of Fallot if the pressure in the main pulmonary artery is elevated by bilateral pulmonary artery branch stenosis, and it can sometimes be recorded if venous return is increased in the horizontal position. The width of splitting of the second sound (i.e., the delay of P_2 in relation to A_2 in the same heart cycle) is closely associated with the pressure difference across the valve and thus with the severity of the pulmonic stenosis (Fig. 11-18).[38] This may be particularly useful in children when the ECG may be difficult to interpret; it also obviates the need for repeated catheterization when following the course of stenosis too mild for surgery or when judging the effect of surgery which should result in a return to a normal duration of right ventricular systole and physiological splitting. Some delay of P_2 is often found, however, with the very mild pressure

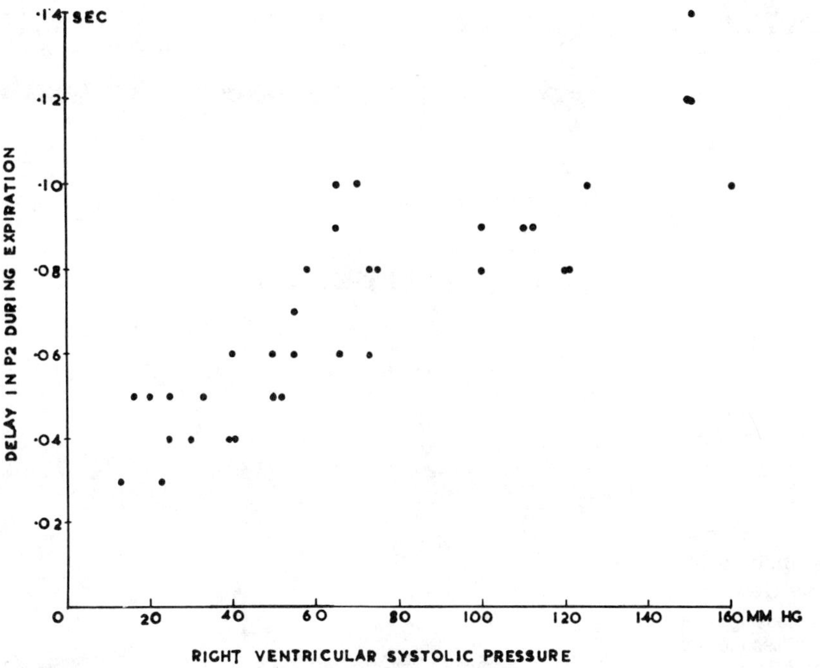

FIGURE 11-18 In pulmonic stenosis there is an approximate but useful correlation between the delay of P_2 (width of splitting) and the right ventricular systolic pressure. (*From A. Leatham and D. W. Weitzman, Auscultatory and Phonocardiographic Signs of Pulmonary Stenosis, Br. Heart J., 19:303, 1957. Reproduced with permission from the publisher and author.*)

differences associated with idiopathic dilatation of the pulmonary artery or minimal pulmonic stenosis, so that an elasticity factor has been invoked as another cause of delay.[40] In only one or two cases over the last 15 years has there been expiratory fusion of A_2 and P_2 with pulmonic stenosis, and the right ventricular pressure has always been less than 50 mmHg.

Though delay of P_2 compared with A_2 is frequent when there is right-sided heart failure with raised venous pressure and may be transient (e.g., with pulmonary embolism), it may occur with right ventricular disease without failure. A late P_2 may persist after successful pulmonary valvotomy (even with abolition of the gradient and no right bundle branch block, Fig. 11-19) and also after complete closure of an atrial septal defect, particularly when the shunt has been large and the patient is relatively old; presumably, persistence of a late P_2 in these cases is due to irreversible, or only slowly reversible, changes in the right ventricle or pulmonary vasculature.

FIGURE 11-19 Postpulmonary valvotomy. Two years after abolition of the pressure gradient, P_2 remains 0.08 s after A_2, presumably because of irreversible changes in the right ventricle. Preoperatively the patient had a greatly raised venous pressure. (*From A. Leatham, "Auscultation of the Heart and Phonocardiography," Churchill Livingstone, Edinburgh, 1970, p. 62. Reproduced with permission from the publisher and author.*)

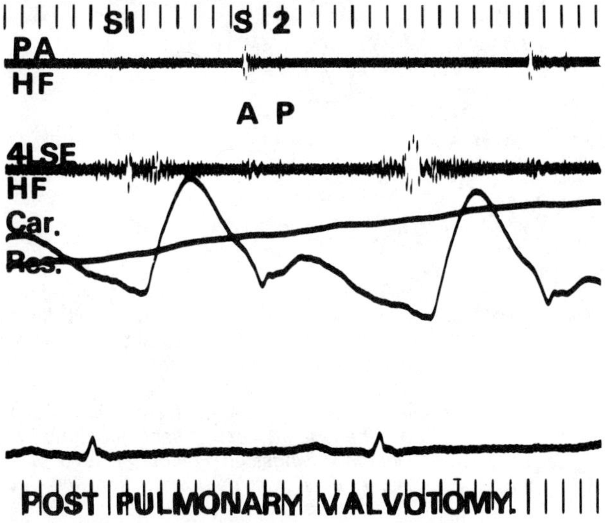

Abnormally wide splitting of the second sound with the normal order of valve closure, A_2 before P_2, is sometimes due to left-sided abnormalities (Fig. 11-20). In left-to-right shunting ventricular septal defect, even when small, pulmonary closure is often abnormally late, though with normal respiratory variation; this appears to be mainly because of delayed activation of the right ventricle, even without delay on the ECG, and also because of shortening of the isovolumic time of the left ventricle from diastolic overloading. The loud pansystolic murmur may make it difficult to hear aortic closure, and an apparently single second sound (thought to be A_2) then raises the possibility of pulmonic stenosis; but a search around the pulmonary area and above it, using a rigid stethoscope diaphragm, is usually successful in picking up two components of the second sound in ventricular septal defect, even in very young infants, with insufficient splitting for the loud murmur to be due to pulmonic stenosis (Fig. 11-21). As mentioned earlier, a P_2 with only slight or moderate delay may be the only characteristic differentiating a harmless ventricular septal defect from early tetralogy of Fallot in an infant whose only obvious physical sign is a loud systolic murmur. In mitral regurgitation, there is frequently wide splitting of the second sound (Fig. 11-22); this can be attributed to shortening of left ventricular ejection time resulting

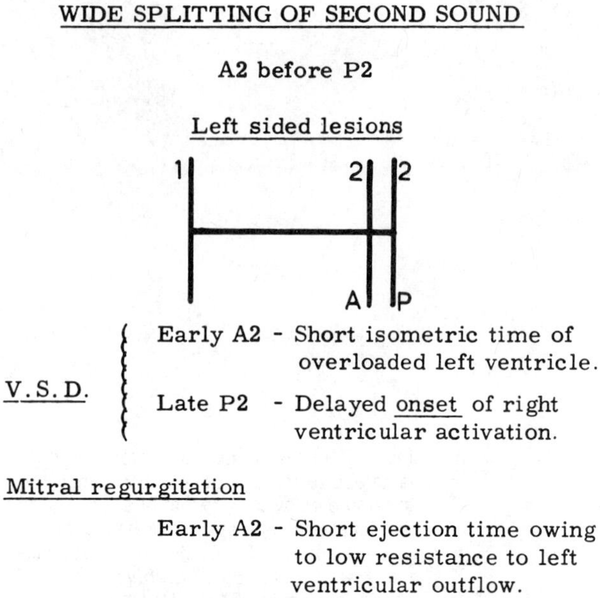

WIDE SPLITTING OF SECOND SOUND
A2 before P2
Left sided lesions
1
2
2
A
P
V.S.D.
Early A2 - Short isometric time of overloaded left ventricle.
Late P2 - Delayed onset of right ventricular activation.
Mitral regurgitation
Early A2 - Short ejection time owing to low resistance to left ventricular outflow.

FIGURE 11-20 Left-sided heart abnormalities, causing early A_2 or late P_2 and thus abnormally wide splitting of second sound. (*From A. Leatham, "Auscultation of the Heart and Phonocardiography," Churchill Livingstone, Edinburgh, 1970, p. 63. Reproduced with permission from the publisher and author.*)

from the diminished resistance to left ventricular outflow,[41] a physical sign which may disappear when the left ventricle is more severely affected.

Reversed Splitting of Second Heart Sound

Delay in aortic closure sufficient to allow P_2 to precede A_2 results in reversed splitting of the second heart sound. The splitting will then be maximal on expiration and disappear or lessen on inspiration, with delay of pulmonary closure (Fig. 11-23).[11,42]

The most common cause of obvious reversed splitting of the second sound is left-sided electrical

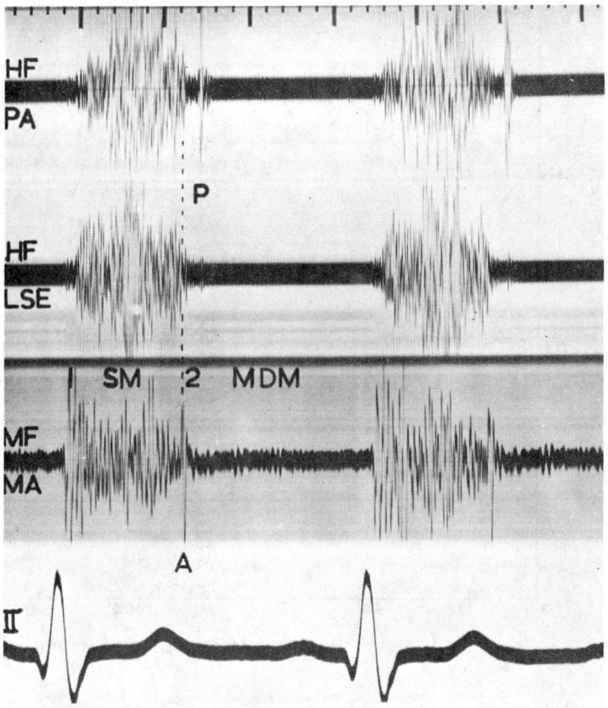

FIGURE 11-21 Ventricular septal defect with large left-to-right shunt. The loud pansystolic murmur tends to drown A_2 except at the mitral area, but the very wide splitting can usually be detected. P_2 is much louder than A_2 in the pulmonary area, and this was a useful indication of pulmonary hypertension, mainly hyperkinetic in this case (pulmonary artery systolic pressure 50, PVR 5 units). (*From A. Leatham, Auscultation of the Heart, Lancet, 2:793, 1958. Reproduced with permission from the publisher and author.*)

delay from left bundle branch block; the width of splitting is in keeping with the width of the QRS complex and may be very great. Identification of the reversed order of valve closure may be possible by judging intensity and distribution of each compo-

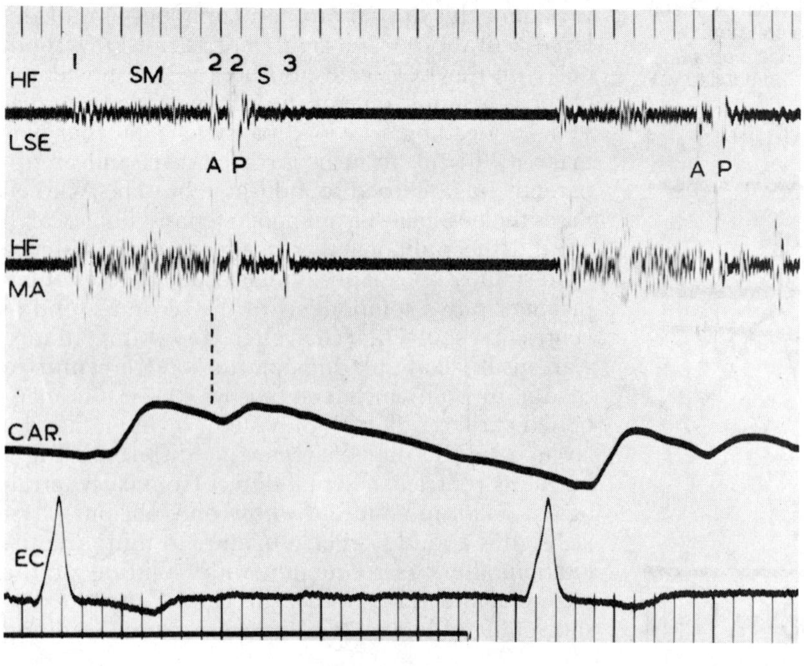

FIGURE 11-22 Mitral regurgitation. Abnormally wide splitting of second sound due to shortening of left ventricular ejection time from diminished resistance to left ventricular outflow, which is both into the aorta and into the left atrium. (*From A. Leatham, "Auscultation of the Heart and Phonocardiography," Churchill Livingstone, Edinburgh, 1970, p. 64. Reproduced with permission from the publisher and author.*)

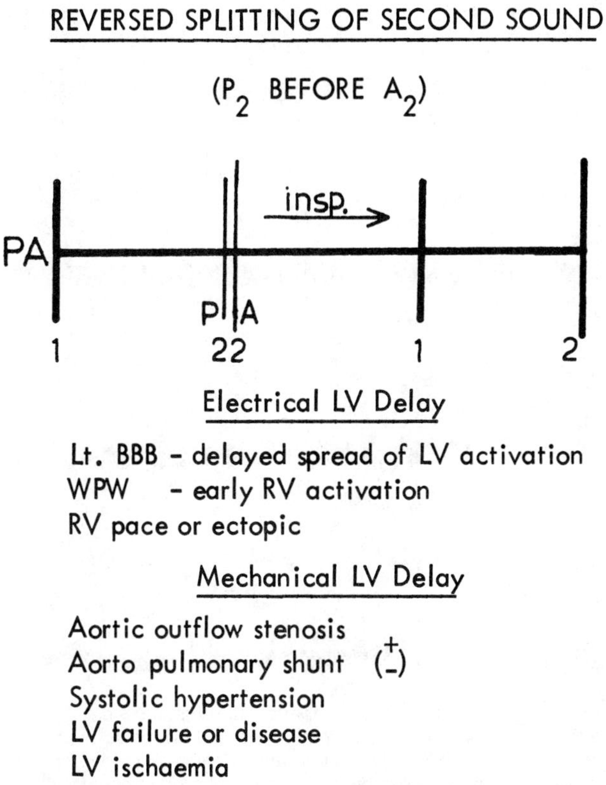

FIGURE 11-23 Prolongation of left ventricular systole (or delay in onset of left ventricular systole) causes reversed splitting of the second sound, P_2 before A_2 in expiration. The inspiratory delay of P_2 will cause lessening of the split or fusion of A_2 and P_2 paradoxically, on inspiration. (*From A. Leatham, "Auscultation of the Heart and Phonocardiography," Churchill Livingstone, Edinburgh, 1970, p. 69. Reproduced with permission from the publisher and author.*)

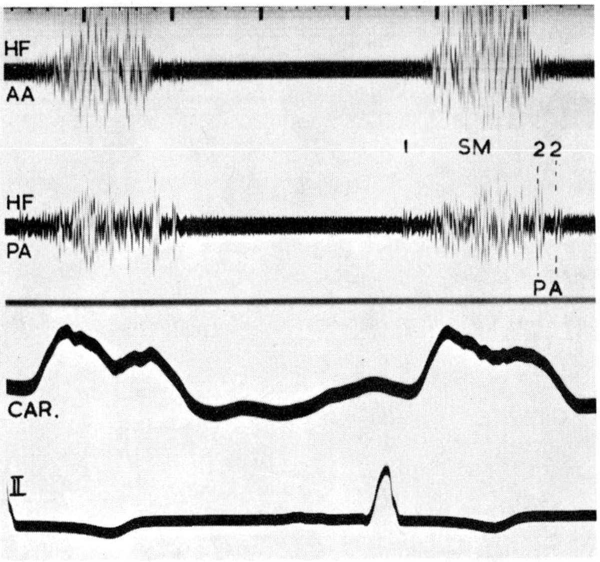

FIGURE 11-24 Aortic stenosis. Prolongation of left ventricular systole with delay in A_2, causing reversal of the normal order of valve closure. P_2, however, may be drowned in the murmur and difficult to hear unless accentuated from pulmonary hypertension secondary to left ventricular failure. (*From A. Leatham, "Auscultation of the Heart and Phonocardiography," Churchill Livingstone, Edinburgh, 1970, p. 71. Reproduced with permission from the publisher and author.*)

nent, but often P_2 is as loud as A_2 because of pulmonary hypertension from left ventricular failure. The narrowing or disappearance of the split on inspiration is of much greater help in diagnosing reversed splitting by auscultation, but disappearance of a soft P_2 may be due to inspiratory insulation rather than to fusion with A_2. Lesser degrees of left-sided delay or preexcitation of the right ventricle (Wolff-Parkinson-White syndrome) may result in only slight precedence of P_2 in expiration (reversed split) but normal splitting (P_2 last) on inspiration.

Delayed electrical activation of the left ventricle from a right ventricular ectopic beat or pacing usually causes reversed splitting of both first and second sounds as expected; but with right ventricular endocardial pacing, splitting is sometimes physiological, suggesting prior stimulation of left bundle fibers in the septum.

Mechanical prolongation of left ventricular systole, resulting in reversed splitting of the second sound, may be caused by obstruction to left ventricular outflow (Fig. 11-24). It may be difficult to distinguish the earlier pulmonary component because it may be drowned in the prolonged aortic ejection murmur, unless it is accentuated by pulmonary hypertension secondary to left ventricular failure. Furthermore, in calcific aortic stenosis, the aortic component may be inaudible. In the absence of bundle branch block and aortic stenosis, reversed splitting may be a sign of prolongation of left ventricular systole because of cardiac ischemia, nicely documented by Yurchak and Gorlin,[43] or because of myocardial disease. Unfortunately, reversed splitting also occurs not infrequently with unimportant systolic hypertension. Often in such cases the delay is slight and the splitting is reversed only on expiration, becoming physiological on inspiration, when P_2 is delayed.

Relative Intensity of A_2 and P_2 and Pulmonary Hypertension

Comparison of the intensity of the undivided second sound in various areas has little significance, since even in the pulmonary area aortic closure usually contributes more than pulmonary closure, except in neonates.[44] Separation of the two components during respiration, however, allows a comparison to be made of their relative intensities. In the pulmonary area (second left space) of normal subjects, A_2 was never exceeded by P_2 in size on a high-frequency sound recording (resembling auscultation with a diaphragm stethoscope); and A_2 equaled P_2 in only 3 of 162 normal subjects, and these 3 subjects were all less than 20 years old.[45] P_2 is so much the lesser component that transmission to the mitral area was found in only 9 of the 162 normal subjects, and these 9 subjects were all less than 20 years old also. Thus, splitting of the second sound at the mitral area should immediately suggest that P_2 is abnormally loud.

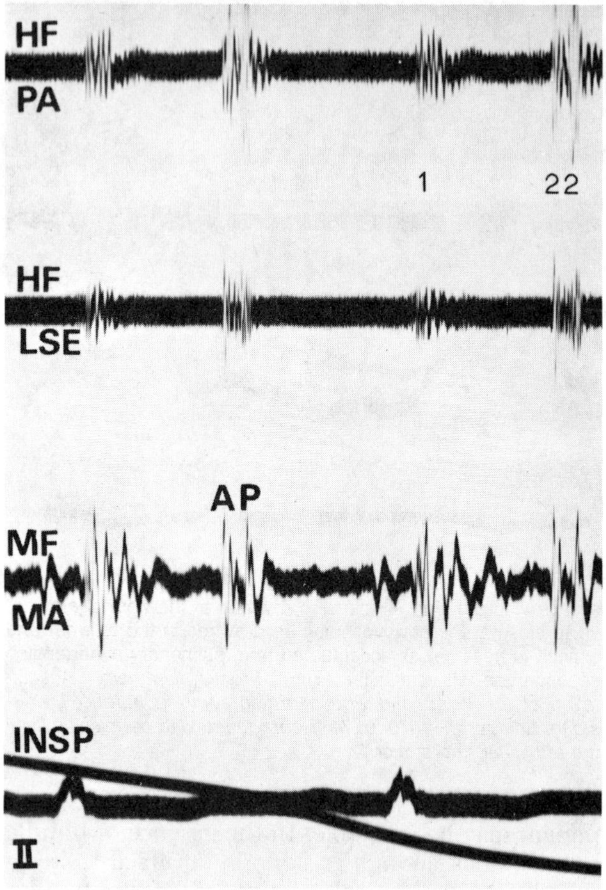

FIGURE 11-25 Pulmonary hypertension. Eisenmenger's atrial septal defect with bidirectional shunt. P_2 is abnormally loud at the pulmonary area. The transmission of P_2 to the mitral area is abnormal, and furthermore the split can be detected more easily at the mitral area, where the two components are similar in size. (*From A. Leatham, "Auscultation of the Heart and Phonocardiography," Churchill Livingstone, Edinburgh, 1970, p. 77. Reproduced with permission from the publisher and author.*)

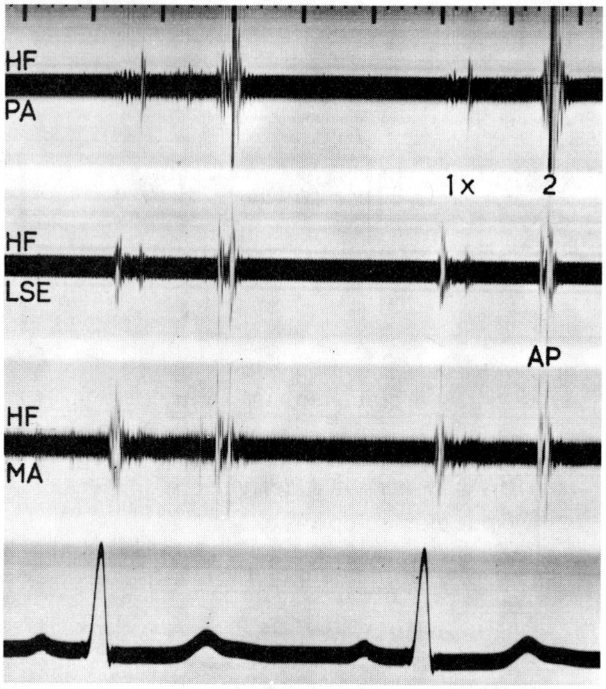

FIGURE 11-26 Pulmonary hypertension. Eisenmenger's patent ductus arteriosus. P_2 is abnormally loud and dwarfs A_2 at the pulmonary area, causing difficulty in auscultation of the two components. The transmission of P_2 to the mitral area is abnormal; furthermore, the split can be detected more easily at the mitral area, where the two components are similar in size. (*From A. Leatham, "Auscultation of the Heart and Phonocardiography," Churchill Livingstone, Edinburgh, 1970, p. 83. Reproduced with permission from the publisher and author.*)

In atrial septal defect with normal pulmonary arterial pressure, P_2 is abnormally loud; it equals or exceeds A_2 in the pulmonary area in most patients and is transmitted to the mitral area in about half of them (Fig. 11-11).[37] In normotensive atrial septal defect, the increased intensity and wide transmission of P_2—easily heard because of the wide "fixed" splitting—may be a function of the sharp pulmonary arterial pulse, because of the abnormally low pulmonary vascular resistance; an additional factor is probably the dilated right ventricle reaching to the apex.

Concerning pulmonary hypertension, lip service is still being paid to "accentuation of the second sound in the pulmonary area" by those who do not understand the large contribution of A_2 to this sound. Occasionally, however, when splitting cannot be detected, one has to fall back on this sign, which may be cautiously interpreted as suggesting pulmonary hypertension if the second sound is sufficiently intense to be palpated selectively in the pulmonary area. The widespread idea that splitting of the second sound disappears in pulmonary hypertension is incorrect; this splitting disappears only in patients with a large ventricular septal defect or a single ventricle who have equal pulmonary and systemic vascular resistance and bidirectional shunt and in whom the left and right ventricles have been undertaking the same work for years and function as a single chamber. It was found that A_2 and P_2 fused together delayed equally on inspiration.[37] Otherwise, in pulmonary hypertension, the second sound splits normally on inspiration. In the pulmonary area, however, it may be difficult to detect a relatively soft A_2 preceding a very loud P_2, but in the mitral area the two components are often similar in size (Fig. 11-25) and can be heard more easily, which also indicates that P_2 is abnormally loud (as in atrial septal defect or pulmonary hypertension). However, wide splitting of the second sound, as in some normal subjects during deep inspiration, is rare with pulmonary hypertension, unless there is right ventricular failure. In contrast to the single second sound of Eisenmenger's ventricular septal defect, there is physiological splitting with Eisenmenger's patent ductus (Fig. 11-26), and wide fixed splitting with Eisenmenger's atrial septal defect (Fig. 11-25); these differences are often the only way of diagnosing the underlying defect in Eisenmenger's syndrome, as pointed out by Paul Wood in 1958 without the aid of phonocardiography.[46]

P_2 greater than A_2 in the pulmonary area, or transmitted to the mitral area, is a useful physical sign of pulmonary hypertension from mitral valve disease or from left-to-right shunting ventricular septal defect (Fig. 11-21), and of primary, embolic, or respiratory pulmonary hypertension. It is not a sign of pulmonary hypertension in atrial septal defect, in which pulmonary hypertension may be difficult to diagnose unless a delayed ejection sound is present. An abnormal A_2/P_2 ratio ($A_2 \leq P_2$) in the pulmonary area is more useful in the detection of pulmonary hypertension in mitral stenosis and ventricular septal defect than transmission of P_2 to the mitral area, which is surprisingly rare in these two situations.[37] In mitral regurgitation, P_2 may exceed A_2 in the pulmonary area without pulmonary hypertension, possibly because A_2 is reduced in intensity.

Single Second Heart Sound

A single second heart sound (Table 11-1) throughout the respiratory cycle is usually a result of the relatively faint pulmonary component being inaudible. Such inaudibility is rare in healthy children and young adults, and is uncommon even in older persons, under good auscultatory conditions, if a rigid stethoscope diaphragm is used. Respiration must be slow and adequate in depth, and the patient must remain relaxed while the search is made at and around the pulmonary area and lower left sternal edge. Hyperinflation, making the heart sounds distant, is perhaps the most common cause of inability to hear pulmonary closure, and a misdiagnosis of reversed splitting must be avoided when inspiratory insulation causes a soft P_2 to disappear. Separation of the components without the inspiratory loss of intensity may sometimes be achieved with increased venous return in the reclining position. Pulmonary closure is completely fused with aortic closure throughout the respiratory cycle only in Eisenmenger's syndrome, with a large ventricular septal defect or single ventricle. Otherwise, in pulmonary hypertension splitting is retained (even with a single ventricle if pulmonary vascular resistance is less than systemic), though it may be difficult to detect in the pulmonary area. With chronic right ventricular failure, the right ventricle is usually unable to increase its stroke volume with inspiration, and fusion of P_2 is abnormally late and easily detectable throughout the respiratory cycle. With constrictive pericarditis and fixed stroke volume of the right ventricle, inspiratory splitting can be detected because A_2 comes earlier. Drowning of the relatively early P_2 by a prolonged left-sided ejection murmur in patients with aortic stenosis has already been stressed (Fig. 11-24). Inaudibility of P_2 because of true diminution in intensity is relatively rare and suggests tetralogy of Fallot or pulmonary atresia. Even in neonates and infants, physiological splitting of the second sound can usually be detected by an experienced observer, and a single second sound should arouse suspicion if other signs suggest congenital heart disease.

Failure to detect aortic closure in any area is much less common. In pulmonary hypertension, the fainter earlier sound (A_2) may be dwarfed and rendered inaudible by a greatly accentuated P_2 at the pulmonary area, and the splitting may then be easier to detect at the mitral area. Aortic closure may be drowned by a loud systolic murmur, but only at the site of maximum intensity of the murmur. Thus, in the pulmonary area, the loud prolonged ejection systolic murmur of pulmonary stenosis may drown an earlier A_2 which, however, is audible in the mitral area. In the mitral area, a loud regurgitant pansystolic murmur may drown A_2, but not at the base, where both A_2 and P_2 are clear and often widely separated. Finally, it is only with severe aortic stenosis (usually calcific) that A_2 may become truly inaudible.

TABLE 11-1 Single Second Heart Sound

1. P_2 *not detected* despite rigid stethoscope diaphragm, relaxation of subject, adequate respiration, search in many areas, reclining position of patient
   a. Because its intensity is diminished
      (1) Poor transmission (hyperinflation + inspiration)
      (2) Tetralogy of Fallot (severe) or pulmonary atresia, etc. (rarely pure pulmonic stenosis)
   b. Because it is synchronous with A_2: Eisenmenger's ventricular septal defect or single ventricle
   c. Because it is concealed by systolic murmur: aortic stenosis
2. A_2 *not detected*
   a. Because its intensity is diminished; calcific aortic stenosis
   b. Because it is synchronous with P_2: Eisenmenger's ventricular septal defect or single ventricle
   c. Because it is concealed by
      (1) Loud P_2 (in pulmonary area only) in pulmonary hypertension
      (2) Loud pansystolic murmur (mitral regurgitation and ventricular septal defect)
      (3) Loud prolonged ejection systolic murmur (pulmonic stenosis)

Source: A. Leatham, "Auscultation of the Heart and Phonocardiography," Churchill Livingstone, Edinburgh, 1970, pp. 86–87. Reproduced with permission from the publisher and author.

Mistaken Diagnosis of Abnormal Splitting of Second Heart Sound

Very wide inspiratory separation of the two components can of course be found in many normal subjects at certain respiratory rates, but obvious splitting of the second sound (> 0.02 s) in the expiratory phase of *continued* respiration in the semi-upright position is most unusual in healthy patients, particularly when respiration is slow and deep. It is more common to make a misdiagnosis of abnormal *fixed* splitting of the second sound (Table 11-2). This is particularly likely in infants when a rapid respiratory rate causes less variation in right ventricular

TABLE 11-2 Conditions Misdiagnosed as Fixed Split of Second Heart Sound

1. Rapid respiration in children, e.g., inspiration coinciding with alternate beats
2. Many ectopic beats
3. Wide split, e.g., right bundle branch block, especially if stroke volume is varying (atrial fibrillation)
4. Close opening snap or late systolic click

Source: A. Leatham, "Auscultation of the Heart and Phonocardiography," Churchill Livingstone, Edinburgh, 1970, p. 88. Reproduced with permission from the publisher and author.

stroke volume. The addition of many ventricular ectopic beats may cause difficulty, particularly when irregularities from atrial fibrillation is added. Though the ear can easily detect the respiratory variations between a narrow and a wide split, a wide split increasing still further on inspiration (e.g., in isolated complete right bundle branch block) may be thought to be fixed. Finally, a late systolic click preceding A_2 and an opening snap following A_2 may be misdiagnosed as fixed splitting of the second sound, if inspiratory splitting (or at least slurring) of the second sound has been missed.

Auscultation of the heart should start with identification of aortic and pulmonary closure and their separation in relation to respiration. It is then possible to identify other sounds and relate murmurs to sounds, and make a comparison of the duration of systole of the right and left ventricles as a test of ventricular function and of an intact interatrial septum.

The Normal Third Heart Sound and Gallops

W. Proctor Harvey, M.D.
Antonio C. de Leon, Jr., M.D.

Ventricular Filling Sounds

The ventricular filling sounds may occur in either or both ventricles. They include the atrial (S_4) gallop sound, the ventricular (S_3) gallop sound, the summation gallop sound, and the normal physiological third heart sound. Most commonly these sounds originate in the left ventricle, but when the total evaluation of the patient is considered, right-sided filling sounds (gallops) may be properly identified. A helpful clue is the fact that the right-sided filling sounds of the right ventricle may selectively increase with inspiration.

The mechanism of production of these filling sounds is probably related to the cessation of filling of blood from the atria to the ventricles, probably resulting in distension and vibrations of the ventricular wall, papillary muscles, and chordae. The valves apparently are not implicated in production of these low-frequency sounds since the ECG does not show specific valvular movement at this time. As a rule, these are low-frequency vibrations producing the sounds that we detect with our stethoscope. One should use the bell of the stethoscope (barely making an air seal with the skin) and listen over a very localized spot in order to hear these important sounds. The filling sounds of the left ventricle (atrial S_4) and ventricular (S_3) gallops (physiological third heart sounds) can best be heard by placing the bell of the stethoscope on the apical impulse and with the patient turned to the left lateral position.

The physician can usually palpate these filling sounds with the examining fingers. It is often said that these sounds (vibrations) can be felt (and sometimes seen) better than they can be heard. If one listens carefully and specifically for the filling sounds, however, they will generally be heard.

The ventricular filling sounds are sometimes picked up by the phonocardiogram, since the low-frequency vibrations can be accentuated to such an extent that the phonocardiogram records what the human ear cannot hear. It is important to remember, however, that the audible and palpable sounds have more clinical relevance than do inaudible sounds recorded on the phonocardiogram.

Gallop Rhythm

The term *gallop rhythm* describes an auscultatory phenomenon in which a tripling or quadrupling of heart sounds resembles the canter of a horse. Almost a century ago, Potain presented to the Medical Society of the Hospital of Paris a paper entitled "Du rhythme cardiaque appelé bruit de galop."[47] In this paper he acknowledged that his professor Bouillaud was the one who gave this rhythm the name by which it is still known today.

Although gallop rhythm was described 100 years ago, the great majority of gallops go unrecognized, are misinterpreted, or are considered unimportant. This is unfortunate because a gallop sound, depending on the type, is often one of the earliest clinical clues to heart disease and affords valuable bedside information concerning diagnosis, prognosis, and treatment.[48,49] Gallops are diastolic events and appear to be related to two periods of filling of the ventricles: the rapid-filling phase (the ventricular diastolic gallop) and the presystolic filling phase related to atrial systole (atrial gallop). Since gallops are diastolic sounds, extra sounds occurring in the heart cycle must therefore be separated into being systolic or diastolic events. In the past a sound occurring in systole was often referred to as a *systolic gallop*. It is wise to abandon this label in favor of more descriptive terminology, such as systolic sound, ejection sound, or systolic click. Thus, the application of the term *gallop rhythm* is restricted to diastolic events. Whether extra sounds are systolic or diastolic is readily determined by a simple technique known as *inching* (Fig. 11-27).[48,49] The second sound over the aortic area is almost always louder than the first sound. The stethoscope is moved, or "inched," from the aortic area of the heart to the apex, and

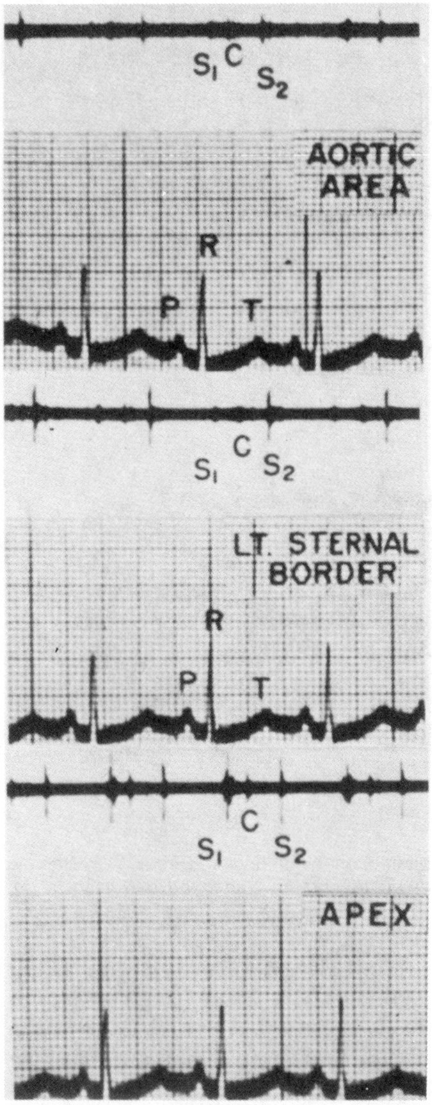

FIGURE 11-27 The stethoscope is "inched" from the aortic area to the apex. The extra sound (C) is systolic and is louder at the apex. (*From S. A. Levine and W. P. Harvey, "Clinical Auscultation of the Heart," 2d ed., W. B. Saunders Company, Philadelphia, 1959, p. 71. Reproduced with permission from the publisher and author.*)

at the same time attention is focused on the second heart sound. If the extra sound is noted to occur in systole before the second heart sound, it is obviously a systolic sound. On the other hand, if the extra sound comes after the second sound or before the first heart sound, then it is in diastole and represents a diastolic event. Even with a heart rate more rapid than normal, the inching technique permits easy and accurate timing of this sound. Sounds occurring in diastole, then, are identified as to their timing and possible etiology.

Although both gallops are sounds resulting from filling of the ventricles, the atrial gallop, generally in presystole, is related to atrial contraction and can be identified on the phonocardiogram following the P wave of the ECG (Fig. 11-28). The atrial gallop is not present with atrial fibrillation since there is no

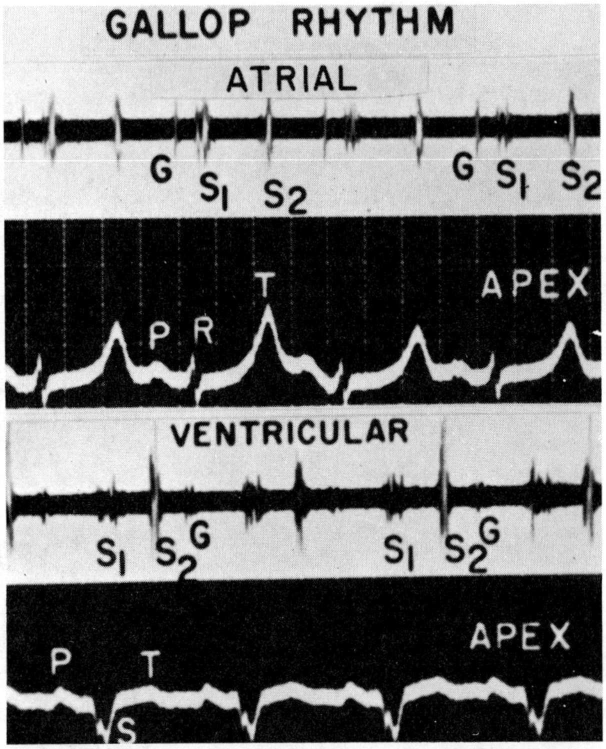

FIGURE 11-28 Gallops are diastolic sounds. The atrial gallop (G, upper tracing) is related to atrial systole. The ventricular gallop (G, lower tracing) occurs in early diastole at the end of rapid ventricular filling. (*From S. A. Levine and W. P. Harvey, "Clinical Auscultation of the Heart," 2d ed., W. B. Saunders Company, Philadelphia, 1959, p. 68. Reproduced with permission from the publisher and author.*)

atrial contraction. A ventricular diastolic gallop, on the other hand, occurs 0.14 to 0.16 s after the second heart sound (Fig. 11-28). Both atrial and ventricular diastolic gallops frequently occur in the same patient. When the two gallops occur in close proximity, low-frequency vibrations with duration may result in a diastolic rumble. Rarely both gallop sounds occur at the exact same time, producing what is known as a *summation gallop*. This summation gallop can be prominent, even at times louder than either the first or second sounds.

Atrial (S_4) Gallop[50]

An atrial (S_4) gallop sound (Fig. 11-29) is related to atrial contraction and may occur with or without any clinical evidence of cardiac decompensation. Both left and right atrial gallops are usually best heard along the lower left sternal border at apex. At times, the S_4 originating from the right side is louder during inspiration. An atrial gallop sound is a frequent finding in patients with cardiomyopathy, coronary artery disease, hypertension (systemic and pulmonary), and with the more severe degrees of aortic and pulmonic stenosis. It can also occur when there is a delay in AV conduction (prolongation of the PR interval on the ECG) and, in addition, may be heard in some normal hearts. If one searches carefully for an atrial sound or gallop, it is most commonly heard

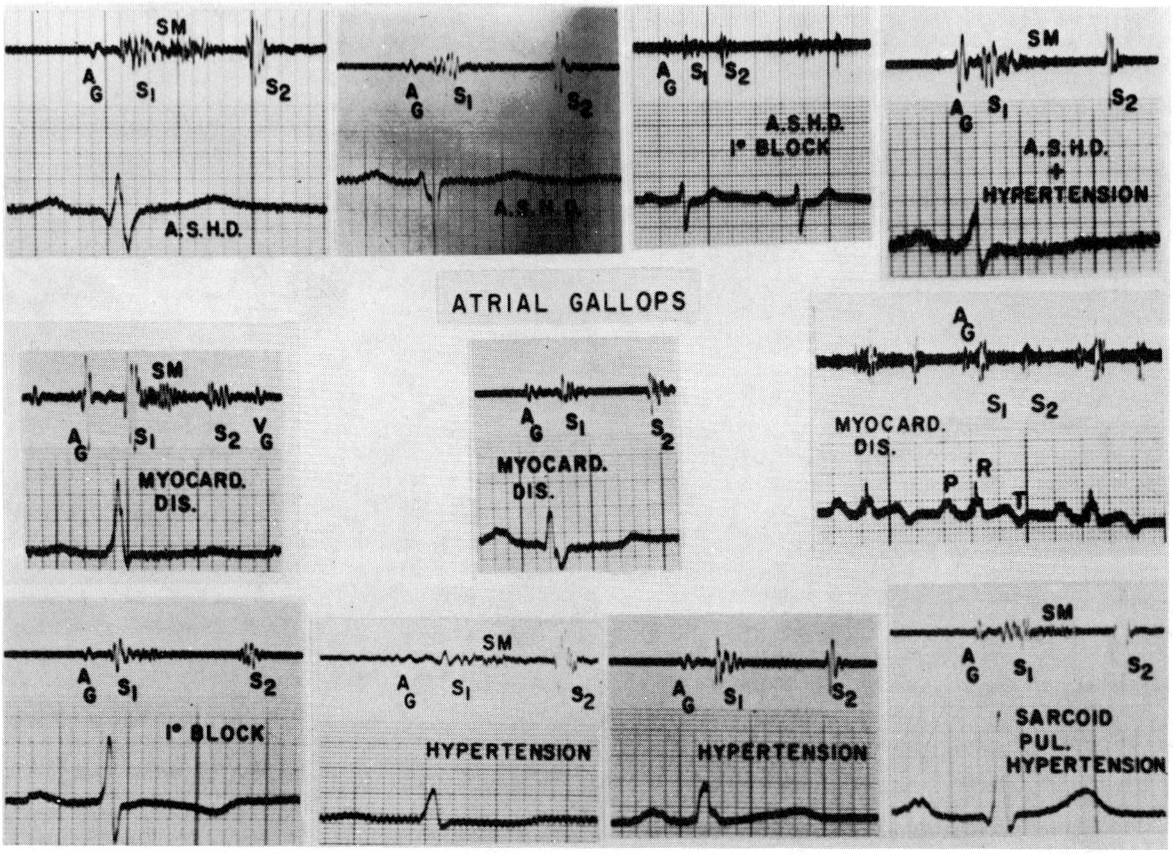

FIGURE 11-29 Composite of various atrial gallops which represent a common, although often overlooked, finding. (*From W. P. Harvey, Heart Sounds and Murmurs, Circulation, 30:269, 1964. Reproduced with permission from the author and the American Heart Association, Inc.*)

in patients with coronary artery disease, and at times this may be one of the first clues from the physical examination as to the presence of underlying heart disease. It would be unusual not to hear a faint atrial gallop sound in a patient who has had a previous myocardial infarction. In a study of 107 patients with recently documented myocardial infarction, an atrial gallop was detected in 105 on clinical auscultation as well as on the phonocardiogram.[51] Of the two patients who did not have an atrial gallop, one had mitral stenosis in addition to myocardial infarction. The other patient had atrial infarction with extensive fibrosis of the left atrium documented at postmortem examination. In the same series of cases of acute myocardial infarction, an atrial gallop was present (i.e., noted clinically with the stethoscope and also documented on the phonocardiogram) in all of the 20 patients examined within an hour of admission to the hospital.

The atrial gallop sound associated with myocardial infarction may be easily heard, or it may be faint—more commonly, it is faint. The sound is often louder during an episode of acute myocardial ischemia and pain, or during the initial phases of myocardial infarction. Subsequently, usually with improvement of the patient, the gallop sound becomes fainter but, if carefully searched for, can generally be heard. It is worthy of emphasis, however, that special techniques are often necessary to "bring out" or detect a faint gallop. Listening at the point of maximum impulse of the left ventricle, with the patient turned to the left lateral position, is often necessary to adequately detect the gallop. The gallop sound equivalent can also be palpated by the physician's examining fingers placed over the point of maximum impulse, again with the patient in the left lateral position. Careful inspection of the precordium with the naked eye, or observing the movements of a lightweight pencil, wooden stick, or broom straw held or taped over the point of maximum impulse, will also demonstrate the precordial movements which correlate with gallop sounds heard with the stethoscope.

An atrial gallop sound is heard in the majority of patients with cardiomyopathy who have normal sinus rhythm.[52] (Ventricular gallops are also frequent.) As a rule, the atrial gallop persists in patients with cardiomyopathy, although in some, with clinical improvement, the gallop may become faint and occasionally disappear. With the exacerbation of symptoms it generally becomes louder.

Atrial gallop sounds are common in patients with systemic arterial hypertension and are more likely to be a constant finding in a patient who has persistent blood pressure elevation. With sustained significant hypertension, an atrial gallop sound may be present for years even though there may be no evidence of heart failure.

Aortic stenosis, particularly in those patients having higher degrees of aortic valve obstruction, is associated with an atrial gallop sound. The results of the study indicated that an atrial gallop sound with aortic stenosis appeared to correlate with a systolic gradient of 70 mmHg or more with a left ventricular end-diastolic pressure of 15 mmHg or more.[53] Personal observations, particularly in the older age group, indicate that an atrial sound may be misleading when one attempts to relate it to severity of aortic stenosis. Older patients may have an atrial gallop sound when there is a minimal or moderate aortic valve gradient, indicating that an additional myocardial disease factor, such as coronary artery disease, is obviously playing a significant role in the production of the atrial gallop. In a patient under 40 years of age, however, there seems to be a better clinical correlation of an atrial gallop sound with the severity of stenosis.[54]

A right ventricular atrial gallop sound may occur in patients with pulmonary valve obstruction.[8,9] The more severe the obstruction is, the more likely it is to be associated with an atrial gallop sound. Also, the atrial gallop sound is not unusual in patients with pulmonary hypertension from various causes, such as atrial septal defect, ventricular septal defect, patent ductus arteriosus, recurrent pulmonary emboli, and primary pulmonary hypertension. The atrial gallop sound appears, therefore, to be related to changes in the myocardium—either the left or the right ventricle, or both—in which there is a change in ventricular compliance and increased resistance to filling.

In addition, an atrial gallop sound may be heard when cardiac output and stroke volume are increased, as in some patients with thyrotoxicosis, anemia, and large arteriovenous fistulas. It is also a common finding in patients with first, second, or third degree heart block.[2] Usually, an atrial gallop sound is not normally detected, since in patients with a normal PQ (PR) interval on the ECG (normal AV conduction), the atrial gallop sound occurs at an interval after atrial contraction (approximately 0.16 s after the beginning of the P wave of the ECG). Although a faint sound may normally be present, it is often not specifically identified or is merged with the first heart sound. When the PR interval is prolonged, i.e., 0.22 to 0.26 s, an atrial gallop sound is usually heard in addition to a faint first heart sound. (These two simple auscultatory findings provide the physician with an immediate bedside clue to first degree heart block.) With second degree block, the atrial gallop sound is easily heard. In patients with a constant 2:1 AV block, the atrial sound often occurs at the approximate timing of the normal third heart sound of ventricular diastole, resulting in a prominent sound in the early part of diastole. In complete heart block, in which there is AV dissociation, atrial gallop sounds are frequently heard. Careful auscultation in a quiet room is usually necessary to detect these sounds, which resemble faint footsteps on a carpet.

The importance of the atrial gallop sound is not sufficiently appreciated, and only in recent years has its value in assessing the various types of heart disease been realized.

Ventricular (S_3) Diastolic Gallop

The ventricular (S_3) diastolic gallop (Fig. 11-28) has clinical connotations different from those of the atrial (S_4) gallop.[48,49] It is frequently one of the first signs that one can detect indicating serious heart disease and/or cardiac decompensation. This gallop appears in the early part of diastole, later than the opening snap of mitral stenosis but at the same time as the normal physiological third heart sound heard in the young. If searched for, the ventricular diastolic gallop is a common finding and can appear in a great variety of diseased states of the heart, including those due to coronary disease; hypertensive, rheumatic, and congenital heart disease; cardiomyopathy; and others. A ventricular diastolic gallop is usually present in patients with cardiac decompensation. *In fact, it may be one of the earliest clinical findings of cardiac dysfunction.* The majority of these gallop sounds are faint, and because of this they are frequently overlooked.

Since most gallop sounds are faint, a special technique must be employed to detect them. The patient should be recumbent and examined in a quiet room. Closing the door that leads to the corridor of the hospital, closing windows, or turning off fans or the air conditioner may make the difference as to whether or not a gallop is heard. If one exerts normal pressure with the flat diaphragm of the stethoscope, the gallop, though present, may not be heard, or may be greatly diminished. Very light pressure with the bell of the stethoscope is necessary to hear the low-frequency vibrations. Gallop sounds from the left ventricle are often best heard by having the patient turn to the left lateral position; the physician then listens at the point of maximum impulse in the apical area (this is similar to the maneuver that one uses when listening for the localized rumble of mitral stenosis). It is of great importance to use palpation first to detect this point of maximum impulse of the left ventricle after the patient has turned to the left lateral position. The stethoscope is then placed over this localized area, and the gallop sound is either heard for the first time or is accentuated in intensity. A ventricular gallop sound is frequently well heard along the lower left sternal border and apex and with the patient recumbent. Right ventricular (S_3) gallop sounds may become louder with inspiration. Both atrial and ventricular gallops generally become fainter when the patient sits or stands. At times the gallop sounds are better heard after slight physical effort, and when the blood flow and heart rate are somewhat accelerated. Having the patient cough five or six times may bring out the faint gallop. Occasionally, a gallop sound is detected when one listens after the patient has had brief exertion, such as walking, climbing a flight of stairs, or performing a number of sit-ups on the examining table. The quality of sounds simulating a horse galloping is more likely to be noticed when the heart rate is increased. It should be emphasized, however, that a gallop occurring at a slow rate still has the same significance that it would have when heard at a faster rate.

Gallops are usually faint sounds. They frequently wax and wane with normal phases of respiration; this is particularly true of ventricular gallops. At times, instead of being detected with every heartbeat, they are heard with every third or fourth beat. If the patient has any degree of emphysema or increase in anteroposterior diameter of the chest, the gallop sound is damped. In such instances auscultation over the xiphoid process or just under the rib cage at the attachment of the diaphragm may be advantageous. The same gallop which is easily heard during sinus tachycardia (e.g., 100 to 120 beats per minute) may be poorly heard at a rate of 70 beats per minute, unless one mentally "tunes in" to this low-frequency sound and uses the above-described techniques.

When atrial and ventricular diastolic gallops occur in close proximity to each other, although not exactly simultaneously, a diastolic rumble can thereby be produced; this is not an uncommon finding in a patient with dilated cardiomyopathy, or in others in whom myocardial dysfunction presents a problem. It is more common in patients with a sinus tachycardia, and the two gallop sounds merge closer together and may produce a diastolic rumble. This combination of low-pitched sounds may simulate the murmur of mitral stenosis. The authors have personally observed several patients referred for surgery of mitral stenosis who, instead, had dilated cardiomyopathy with atrial and ventricular diastolic gallops producing a rumble.

Prognosis of Ventricular Diastolic Gallops To date, there has been no satisfactory study of life expectancy once a gallop sound is detected. Modern therapy has prolonged the life of cardiac patients, and in many earlier studies only the louder type of gallop was observed. As has been previously emphasized, the prognosis depends on the type of gallop present. It is obvious that the atrial diastolic gallop which occurs in the absence of cardiac decompensation does not carry as grave a prognosis as that associated with the ventricular diastolic gallop. In general, it appears that the average life expectancy after a persistent, easily heard ventricular gallop has been found is approximately 4 to 5 years. There are, of course, individual variations, with some patients dying weeks or months later and still others living 10 years or longer. Some clinical points concerning gallops are worthy of discussion. The louder the gallop, the poorer the prognosis. The prognosis is worse if gallop rhythm persists despite adequate medical management. For example, it is relatively common to hear a ventricular diastolic gallop following acute myocardial infarction during the earlier stages. In the usual case, the gallop disappears in time (several days to several weeks). When it is particularly loud and persists months after the acute episode, however, it generally is associated with significant permanent heart damage and chronic cardiac decompensation, thus indicating a poorer prognosis. Another patient with an acute myocardial infarction may have a ventricular diastolic gallop during the acute phase, but subsequently no ventricular gallop or other signs of heart failure may be evident. This represents a temporary sign of heart failure with subsequent recovery, and indicates a better myocardial reserve. The prognosis in such an individual would then be related to other aspects of the underlying heart disease rather than to congestive heart failure. It also appears that loud persistent gallops, together with slight sinus tachycardia, are additional evidence of serious heart failure, the elevation of heart rate being a further sign of compensatory mechanism for the cardiac dysfunction.

The faint ventricular gallop that has the better prognosis is the one which is detected as an early sign of congestive heart failure and which disappears after treatment for the failure. As a rule such treatment needs to be continued. A ventricular diastolic gallop is frequently associated with a slight pulsus alternans. On the other hand, the finding of a pulsus alternans that is readily detected on palpation is almost always associated with a ventricular diastolic gallop. Both these findings indicate a failing myocardium, and too little attention has been paid to them in the past. In addition, alternation of the intensity of heart sounds and/or murmurs is frequent when a ventricular diastolic gallop and pulsus alternans are present. Nearly all these findings are clues indicating some degree of cardiac decompensation. The patient may have a gallop rhythm and concomitant extrasystoles. For a few beats following the extrasystoles, the intensity of the gallop sound is often accentuated. This is known as *postextrasystolic accentuation* of the gallop. On the other hand, after extrasystoles, an occasional patient with a normal heart will have a few transient beats with an early diastolic third sound which is of no prognostic significance. In addition, coincident with and sometimes persistent for a period after cessation of the tachycardia, such as in atrial tachycardia, a gallop rhythm may be heard temporarily. This is likewise usually benign.

Normal Physiological Third Heart Sound

A ventricular diastolic gallop occurs with the same timing as the normal physiological third sound, approximately 0.14 to 0.16 s after the second heart sound (Fig. 11-30). The technique employed to discover the normal third sound is the same as the technique used to find a ventricular gallop sound. The third sound is a normal finding in young adults.

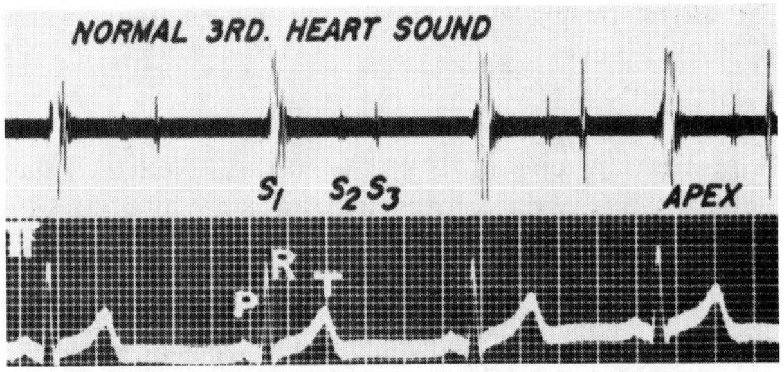

FIGURE 11-30 Note variation in intensity of normal third sound (S_3). *(From S. A. Levine and W. P. Harvey, "Clinical Auscultation of the Heart," 2d ed., W. B. Saunders Company, Philadelphia, 1959. Similar to Fig. 59 on p. 63. Reproduced with permission from the publisher and author.)*

Members of our division of cardiology examined approximately 1200 schoolchildren, ages about 8 to 12. Approximately 100 were personally examined by one of the authors (W. P. Harvey). All the subjects had a normal third heart sound and a venous hum; an innocent systolic precordial murmur was heard in approximately 80 percent of the subjects. Short innocent bruits were heard in the neck of one-fourth to one-third of the subjects.

The normal third sound waxes and wanes in intensity with respiration. It is therefore preferable to listen while the patient continued to breathe in a normal fashion, since this aids the left ventricular blood flow and production of the third sound. It is not heard as well when the patient is sitting or standing.

At times, the low-frequency vibrations that constitute a normal physiological third sound may be of sufficient length to produce a short rumble; this can be misinterpreted as the rumble of mitral stenosis. The third heart sound becomes less frequent in the years 20 to 30 and less frequent still after 30. Most men have lost their normal third heart sound by the age of 30; occasionally women at this age retain this normal sound. As a rule, a low-pitched sound with this timing in a person in the forties, fifties, or over represents a ventricular diastolic gallop. It is ironic that a sound which in youth represents a normal, healthy condition should in later years be an unhealthy sign denoting a failing heart. Since this diastolic sound occurs at the time of the normal physiological third sound, it is frequently asked how one can tell the difference between a normal physiological third sound and a ventricular diastolic gallop. Practically, this differentiation is not difficult: after putting together all aspects of the cardiovascular evaluation, and considering the patient's age, one can generally make a correct identification. For example, a patient at the age of 23 having a third heart sound occurring 0.15 s after the aortic component of the second heart sound, no history or symptoms of heart disease, a normal ECG and roentgenogram, and no other laboratory evidence indicating a heart problem, is assumed to have a normal physiological third heart sound. On the other hand, a faint heart sound occurring with the identical timing in a man aged 55 would immediately alert the physician to the presence of underlying heart disease. A total cardiovascular evaluation of such a patient will generally afford confirmatory evidence of heart disease in the history, ECG, x-ray, etc.

Timing of Atrial and Ventricular Diastolic Gallops

When the heart rate is slow or normal, the timing of gallops is not difficult. The atrial gallop sound follows the atrial contraction in presystole and therefore precedes the first heart sound. The ventricular gallop sound occurs at the time of the physiological third sound in early diastole and is easily identified when the rate is normal. With a more rapid heart rate, however, differentiation of the atrial gallop sound from the ventricular gallop sound may be difficult, if not impossible, until the heart rate becomes slower. For this differentiation, stimulation of the carotid sinus has been valuable. When slowing is produced with carotid sinus pressure, the atrial gallop will be heard in relation to the first heart sound in presystole, whereas the ventricular gallop remains in conjunction with the second heart sound, occurring shortly after it. Frequently when carotid sinus pressure causes a sudden slowing of the heart rate, there may be a temporary period of several beats when neither the atrial nor the ventricular gallop is detected; but with the gradual resumption of the faster rate, the extra sound can be identified without difficulty in its proper place. This test should not be used unless it is deemed important to obtain the information and the information cannot be obtained by other safer means.

Combination of Gallops

Not uncommonly one hears two sounds in diastole producing not a triple rhythm but a quadruple rhythm. An atrial gallop can be heard for a number of years in a person who has hypertension but no signs or symptoms of cardiac decompensation. Once failure ensues, however, a ventricular gallop may also become evident—thus making two gallop sounds in addition to the two normal sounds. Or an individual who has coronary artery disease may have an atrial gallop in the absence of other evidence of cardiac disease, and may keep the atrial gallop for a number of years before a ventricular diastolic gallop appears. Both atrial and ventricular diastolic gallop sounds occurring in the same person can be identified by first focusing one's attention on a sound in presystole and then concentrating on a sound occurring in the early part of diastole. As previously discussed, when both atrial and ventricular diastolic gallops occur in close proximity, although not simultaneously, a rumble may be heard which simulates the rumble of mitral stenosis, or a flow rumble such as may occur with left-to-right shunts.

Summation Gallops

Uncommonly, the atrial and ventricular diastolic gallop sounds occur simultaneously. This often results in a very loud diastolic gallop sound, which may be louder than either of the two normal heart sounds. When this situation is analyzed on the phonocardiogram, it may be seen that the two gallop sounds occur at exactly the same time; for this reason, the condition is designated as a *summation gallop*. When the heart rate slows (normally or with carotid sinus pressure), it may be possible to separate the atrial from the ventricular gallop sounds, neither of which is as loud as the summation gallop.

Classification of Gallop Rhythm

Some physicians have suggested abandoning the term *gallop rhythm* in favor of *filling sounds*. However, it is doubtful this will take place, since gallop rhythm is firmly ingrained in our medical terminology and it is "catchy" and descriptive.

Use of terms such as *protodiastolic, mesodiastolic,* and *presystolic* has been purposely avoided in this discussion because it appears that this terminology has contributed to the present and past confusion about gallop rhythm. For example, in a patient with atrial fibrillation three observers listening to the same gallop sound in diastole may each call it a different type of gallop. Depending on the length of the diastolic pause when the first observer listens, the diastolic sound may be termed *protodiastolic* by this observer. The next observer may concentrate on the same sound, feel that it is middiastolic, and thus term it mesodiastolic. If the third observer decides that the diastolic sound is closer to the first sound, he or she will designate it a presystolic gallop. Actually, the same gallop is heard by each person. If the diastolic gallops were classified as atrial or ventricular, such confusion would not exist since there is no atrial contraction. If atrial fibrillation is present, the gallop is necessarily ventricular in type. If the rhythm is regular and the rate somewhat rapid, slowing the rate makes it possible to identify the sound as either atrial or ventricular, or both.

Another approach used today, and obviously gaining in popularity, is that of labeling the sounds as third and fourth heart sounds (S_3 and S_4 gallops). At times, however, one may hear five or six sounds in the heart. The terminology of atrial and ventricular gallop is a personal preference, as it appears to have a more physiological basis.

Ejection Sounds: Systolic Clicks, Systolic "Whoops," Opening Snaps, and Other Sounds

W. Proctor Harvey, M.D.
Antonio C. de Leon, Jr., M.D.

Ejection Sounds[38,55]

An ejection sound is produced in early systole at the time of ejection of blood from the left ventricle into the aorta, or from the right ventricle into the pulmonary artery.[56]

Pulmonary Ejection Sound

A pulmonary ejection sound is usually heard in patients with valvular pulmonic stenosis.[57] It occurs in early systole when forward motion of the stenotic valve abruptly halts. The pulmonary ejection sound is best heard over the pulmonary area or third left intercostal space near the sternal border and is often misinterpreted as the first heart sound. To avoid this confusion one should always keep this possibility in mind and remember that the first heart sound is not well heard in this area. The pulmonary ejection sound, however, is usually poorly heard or absent at the apex. It is characteristic for the pulmonary ejection sound to diminish in intensity (Fig. 11-31) or disappear with inspiration and become louder with expiration. During inspiration, the right ventricular end-diastolic pressure exceeds the pressure in the main pulmonary artery, and no ejection sound can be heard or recorded.[11] With expiration, the right ventricular end-diastolic pressure is lower and an ejection sound can be heard. These findings support a previous suggestion[58] that during inspiration the inflow of blood to the right ventricle may move the stenotic pulmonary valve leaflets to the forward, more "open," position, thereby resulting in less movement with systole. During expiration, the valve leaflets are in a "closed" position, and with systole the stenosed valve is forced forward until it abruptly stops, producing the systolic ejection sound. An ejection sound is a common finding in pulmonary valve stenosis, particularly of mild to moderate degree. It may not be detected in the more severe forms of stenosis, or it may occur close to the first heart sound, thereby making specific identification difficult. An ejection sound is not heard with isolated infundibular stenosis.

The pulmonary ejection sound is useful in differentiating between atrial septal defect and mild pulmonic stenosis. At times this differential may be difficult, since both conditions may have a grade 2 to 3 systolic murmur over the pulmonary area in addition to a wide "fixed" splitting of the second heart sound. It is useful to recall that an ejection sound occurs frequently in patients with mild to moderate pulmonic stenosis but is uncommon in patients with atrial septal defect. When it is heard in a patient with an atrial septal defect, it is more likely to be associated with a variable degree of pulmonary hypertension. As a rule, a pulmonary ejection sound is not heard in the uncomplicated ostium secundum atrial defect, although exceptions have been observed. Since atrial septal defect and mild pulmonic stenosis may occur together, a pulmonary ejection sound in a patient displaying the typical clinical features of atrial septal defect should suggest the possibility of an associated pulmonic stenosis. A pulmonary ejection sound may be heard in patients with pulmonary hypertension associated with various conditions (Fig. 11-31), including ventricular septal

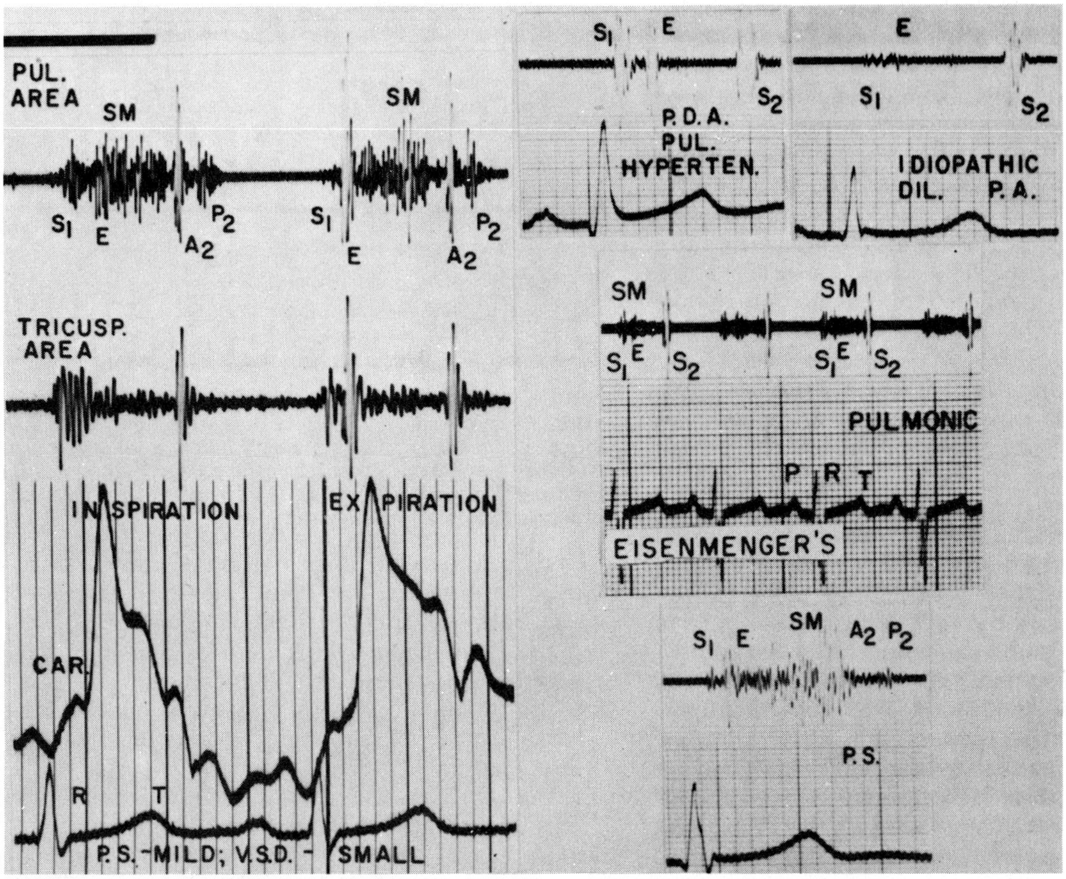

FIGURE 11-31 Composite of various pulmonary ejection sounds (E). *Left.* Pulmonic stenosis (PS), mild with small ventricular septal defect (VSD). Note striking decrease in ejection sound (E) with normal inspiration. *Upper middle.* Patent ductus arteriosus with pulmonary hypertension. *Upper right.* Idiopathic dilatation of the pulmonary artery. *Right middle.* Eisenmenger's syndrome. *Right lower.* Pulmonic stenosis (PS). [*From W. P. Harvey, Heart Sounds and Murmurs, Circulation, 30:265, 1964 (except right middle portion). Reproduced with permission from the author and the American Heart Association, Inc.*]

defect, primary pulmonary hypertension, and recurrent pulmonary emboli. With pulmonary hypertension, the second sound is usually closely split and the pulmonic component of the sound is accentuated.

A pulmonary ejection sound may also be heard in patients who do not have pulmonary hypertension or valvular stenosis. It may occur in patients with hyperthyroidism, idiopathic dilatation of the pulmonary artery, or other conditions, including aneurysmal dilatation, that cause enlargement of the pulmonary artery.[59] In these instances, the cause of the ejection sound cannot be related to the abrupt stopping of a stenotic valve, as in congenital valvular pulmonic stenosis.

Aortic Ejection Sound

The aortic ejection sound (Fig. 11-32)[48,56,60] is heard in patients with valvular aortic stenosis. Such a sound is heard in patients with congenital bicuspid aortic valve stenosis. Uncommonly, it may also be heard in some patients with rheumatic aortic stenosis of a milder or moderate degree in which the valve is still mobile. The ejection sound may not be heard in patients with severely calcified valve leaflets.

The congenital bicuspid aortic valve is one of the most common congenital heart lesions. It presents with a spectrum of findings. An ejection sound may be heard in a patient with a bicuspid valve when no murmur is audible. The ejection sound may be heard at the apex as well as at the base. More commonly, a short midsystolic murmur of grade 2 or 3 intensity

FIGURE 11-32 Examples of aortic ejection sounds (E). Note that the ejection sound is well heard at the apex, as well as over the aortic area. (*From W. P. Harvey, Heart Sounds and Murmurs, Circulation, 30:264, 1964. Reproduced with permission from the author and the American Heart Association, Inc.*)

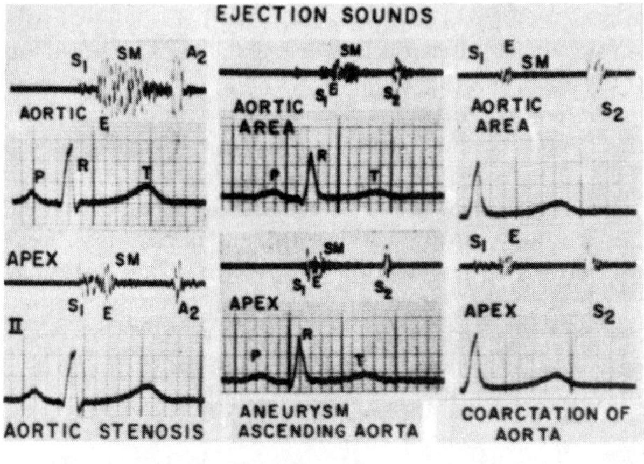

is heard, together with the ejection sound and a prominent aortic valve closure sound. An early blowing aortic diastolic murmur plus an ejection sound and easily heard aortic valve closure may be present. Bicuspid aortic valve stenosis may progress over the years. The valve may become heavily calcified in the fifth to seventh decades of life, producing symptoms of congestive failure, syncope, dizziness, and myocardial ischemia, and aortic valve replacement may then be necessary. A bicuspid aortic valve may have regurgitation as its only abnormality; the regurgitation may vary from mild to severe.

An ejection sound can also be heard with aortic regurgitation, coarctation of the aorta, aneurysm of the ascending aorta, and occasionally tetralogy of Fallot. If a systolic ejection sound is heard at the apex and/or over the aortic area in a patient who has coarctation of the aorta, an associated bicuspid aortic valve is likely to be present. The ejection sound is usually produced by the bicuspid valve and not by the coarctation; however, an ejection sound can occur with coarctation and appears related to dilatation of the descending aorta. An aortic ejection sound with aortic stenosis provides clinical support of the likelihood that the stenosis is of valvular type rather than infundibular, supravalvular, or idiopathic hypertrophic subaortic stenosis. Aortic ejection sounds, in contrast to the pulmonary ejection sounds, are usually well heard at the apex and have no respiratory variation. The aortic ejection sound occurs at the time of the abrupt stopping of the forward motion of the valve in early systole. With a stenotic bicuspid valve, it coincides with the "doming" of the valve in systole as seen on cineangiograms. The aortic ejection sound is composed of higher frequencies than the ventricular filling sounds (gallops), from which it can usually be differentiated by simple techniques (to be discussed later). The aortic ejection sound is often better heard at the apex than at the base of the heart. A harsh midsystolic ejection murmur of aortic stenosis over the aortic area may compete with detection of the ejection sound, or even mask it in some patients.

Systolic Clicks

The systolic click is an extra sound occurring in systole[48] (Fig. 11-33, upper tracing). Usually only a single click is heard; however, at times, several or even multiple, rapidly occurring clicking sounds can be detected. Although the position of the click in the cardiac cycle is usually constant, occasionally it may vary slightly.

Change in position can alter the click-murmur auscultatory findings. For example, clicks may move toward the latter part of systole when the patient is in the squatting position and return to early or midsystole on standing. Systolic clicks may be heard at early, mid-, or late systole, although most commonly they occur at midsystole. Though they are often found in otherwise normal patients, they are frequently overlooked and sometimes misinterpreted as murmurs or friction rubs. They are very common, particularly in young females. It is now well established that these auscultatory findings are related to systolic prolapse of the mitral valve leaflets (generally posterior, although the anterior leaflet can also prolapse).[61–68] Prolapse of the tricuspid valve also occurs. A systolic click is usually decreased in intensity or is absent at the base of the heart; it is seldom heard over the aortic area. Having the patient recumbent and in the left lateral position often helps in finding clicks; also some clicks are better heard when the patient is sitting, standing, or squatting. Systolic clicks were formerly considered to be benign or even extracardiac in origin. A possible relation to pericardial disease had also been postulated. Various descriptive terms have been used, such as *systolic click-murmur syndrome, prolapsing mitral leaflet syndrome, Barlow's syndrome, "billowing" mitral valve, posterior leaflet deformity,* or *"floppy" valve.* The term *mitral valve prolapse,* however, is the one most commonly used today. Of great importance and still not fully appreciated, however, is the fact that bacterial endocarditis may occur on the mitral valve in such cases.[61,67]

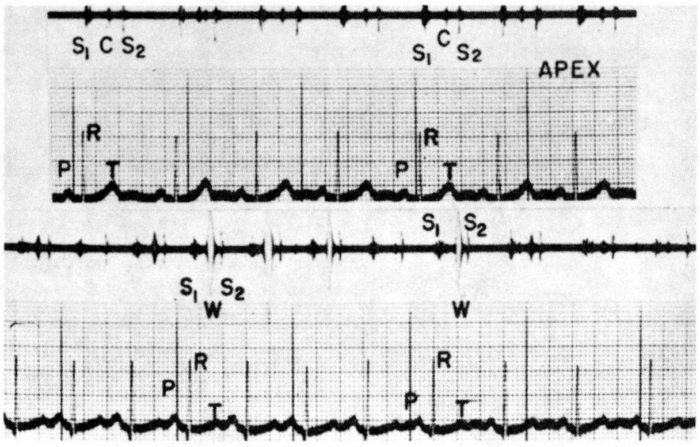

FIGURE 11-33 Asymptomatic patient with a systolic click (C) and musical systolic "whoop" (W) sound. Note in the lower tracing that whoop occurred in latter part of systole. (*From S. A. Levine and W. P. Harvey, "Clinical Auscultation of the Heart," 2d ed., W. B. Saunders Company, Philadelphia, 1959, p. 553. Reproduced with permission from the publisher and author.*)

Sudden death has occurred, although it is rare, and too much emphasis has been placed on the possibility of this dire event; as a result many patients have been unnecessarily frightened and made unduly anxious. Rupture of chordae tendineae spontaneously or with infective endocarditis has evolved as the most serious complication, but this too is uncommon. Patients with Marfan's syndrome, or variants of this syndrome and osteogenesis imperfecta, may have varying degrees of mitral valve involvement. A systolic click or clicks may be the only indication of a minimal involvement, or the click sounds may be associated with the late apical systolic murmur; other patients have severe mitral insufficiency with a pansystolic murmur, a result of rupture of chordae tendineae.

For a number of years it has been known that the great majority of patients having auscultatory findings of mitral valve prolapse (systolic clicks and/or a late apical systolic murmur) usually have a good prognosis and have been able to live essentially normal lives.

Systolic Whoops

Systolic whoops[48,66] are characterized by a loud, sometimes inconstant, short musical murmur heard at the apex and occurring in the latter part of systole, often without other evidence of significant heart disease (Fig. 11-33). Preceding the whoop there is often a systolic sound or click, which also, like the whoop, is sometimes transient. As with the late apical systolic murmur and systolic click, the whoop was for years considered benign, the postulation being that it was related either to a vibrating portion of the valve structure or to an extracardiac phenomenon. However, during follow-up periods of a decade or more, the whoop in some patients has been observed to develop the usual characteristics of a systolic murmur, although it is more prominent in the latter part of systole. The whoop, therefore, is usually due to pathological change in the mitral valve. Uncommonly, it originates from the tricuspid valve. Another term given this peculiar murmur is *precordial honk*,[69,70] since the sound is reminiscent of that made by a goose. There is evidence that the descriptive terms *whoop* and *honk* refer to similar pathological change, most frequently in the mitral valve. Evidence for this probability was a report on eight patients with precordial honks or whoops who were studied with complete catheterizations of the right and left side of the heart and left ventricular cineangiography.[70] Five patients had no other evidence of heart disease. Ballooning of the mitral valve into the left atrium during ventricular systole was seen on the cineangiogram and was associated with late systolic mitral regurgitation in four of the five patients. It is likely that what would be described as a whoop by some would be designated as a honk by others, and that the difference in terms probably has been a matter of semantics. These patients are also subject to bacterial endocarditis.

Opening Snaps

Opening Snap of the Mitral Valve

The opening of a normal mitral valve is acoustically silent. However, in the presence of disease caused by the pathological changes of rheumatic mitral stenosis, a clear sound is definitely audible in early diastole, occurring 0.04 to 0.12 s after the aortic valve closure of the second heart sound. It is best heard at the apex but is usually widely transmitted. It can be heard in the aortic area (second right intercostal space near the sternum) and the pulmonary area (second and third left intercostal space near the sternum), where it is misinterpreted as a split second sound. This is the *opening snap of mitral stenosis;* the term is now well ingrained in the literature and is in common use today. The opening snap occurs in early diastole when there is a sudden halt of a downward movement of the mitral valve structure. This occurs when the left ventricular pressure is falling. The higher the atrial pressure, the more rapid the downward descent of the mitral valve structure, and in turn, the earlier the opening snap. This sound occurs later than the usual splitting of the second heart sound but earlier than the physiological third heart sound. The opening snap often affords the first clue to the diagnosis of mitral stenosis; further supporting evidence is a loud first heart sound and an accentuated pulmonary valve closure of the second heart sound. Listening at a localized area at the point of maximum impulse of the left ventricle, with the patient turned to the left lateral position, one may hear the characteristic and diagnostic rumble of mitral stenosis. Remember, the rumble of mitral stenosis may be localized to the apex, but the opening snap is widely transmitted.

The opening snap is present in normal sinus rhythm as well as in atrial fibrillation. It persists after mitral commissurotomy (although there may be a decrease in its intensity) and usually occurs later after the second heart sound compared with before the operation. The opening snap is present in well over 90 percent of patients with mitral stenosis; rarely, when absent, it is likely to be associated with heavily calcified, thickened immobile stenotic valves. The second heart sound associated with mitral stenosis is often loud and closely split, with the degree of splitting increasing slightly coincident with inspiration. The opening snap heard over the pulmonary area is sometimes misinterpreted as a split second sound. By focusing attention carefully on the components of the second heart sound, however, one may note that three components are heard coincident with inspiration; this "trill" effect of three sounds is the result of slightly wider splitting of the second heart sound coincident with inspiration, plus the opening snap. This simple auscultatory point is often of important diagnostic application in the differential diagnosis of atrial septal defect versus mitral stenosis. In some cases of atrial septal defect, a diagnostic flow rumble may be heard, the second heart sound is accentuated, and the wide splitting of the second heart sound is misinterpreted as a second sound and an opening snap. In fact, a number of cases of congenital atrial septal defect have for many years been labeled as rheumatic heart disease. By paying strict attention to the splitting of the second heart sound, an important clue to the correct diagnosis can be appreciated. If only two components of the second heart sound persist, then the diagnosis of atrial septal defect should be entertained. On the other hand, the presence of the three components, i.e., the split second sound plus the opening snap, would be confirmatory evidence of rheumatic heart disease.

Opening Snap of the Tricuspid Valve

The characteristics of the opening snap of tricuspid stenosis are similar to those of the opening snap of mitral stenosis. The opening snap of the tricuspid valve is best heard along the lower left sternal border. Occasionally it is better heard along the lower right sternal border. Since practically all patients with rheumatic tricuspid stenosis have concomitant mitral stenosis, the possibility of confusing the two snaps always exists. In addition, the tricuspid opening snap is more likely to occur later after the second sound than the mitral opening snap; because of this, the mitral diastolic rumble may "drown out" the tricuspid opening snap, making identification difficult. An occasional rare case of tricuspid stenosis occurs unassociated with mitral stenosis, however, and the opening snap can then be easily identified as tricuspid. The clinical diagnosis of tricuspid stenosis is obviously better made by the combination of all the clinical findings. These include the observation of a large *a* wave in the jugular venous pulse; a slow *y* descent, suggesting obstruction at the tricuspid valve. Of importance is an increase in intensity of the diastolic rumble coincident with inspiration. Although with normal sinus rhythm there is a presystolic accentuation of the rumble, it may frequently taper off and not crescendo to the first sound, which is more typically present with mitral stenosis.

Occasionally, an opening snap of the tricuspid valve is heard in a patient with atrial septal defect.

Other Sounds

Pericardial Knock

The pericardial knock[48,71] occurs early in diastole, generally 0.10 to 0.12 s after the second heart sound, and is common in patients with constrictive pericarditis (Fig. 11-34). It has also been termed the *early diastolic sound* or the *third heart sound of constrictive pericarditis*. In a study of 26 patients with constrictive pericarditis, the pericardial knock was the most common clinical finding, being heard in 24 of 26 patients.[72] The knock, which may be present with or without calcification of the pericardium, is produced in the rapid-filling phase of ventricular diastole. The extra sound is a filling sound, with the pericardium acting as a constricting shell, preventing the usual relaxation of the ventricles in diastole. The pericardial knock occurs in the early part of diastole, usually slightly later than the opening snap of mitral stenosis but earlier than the normal physiological third sound or the ventricular diastolic gallop sound. Occasionally, the pericardial knock comes earlier, thereby simulating the opening snap of mitral stenosis. The typical rumble of mitral stenosis, however, is generally absent. Detection of this early diastolic sound in a patient who does not have the customary signs of coronary, hypertensive, or rheumatic valvular disease should always make one suspect the presence of pericardial disease. The pericardial knock sound may be single and sharp, or

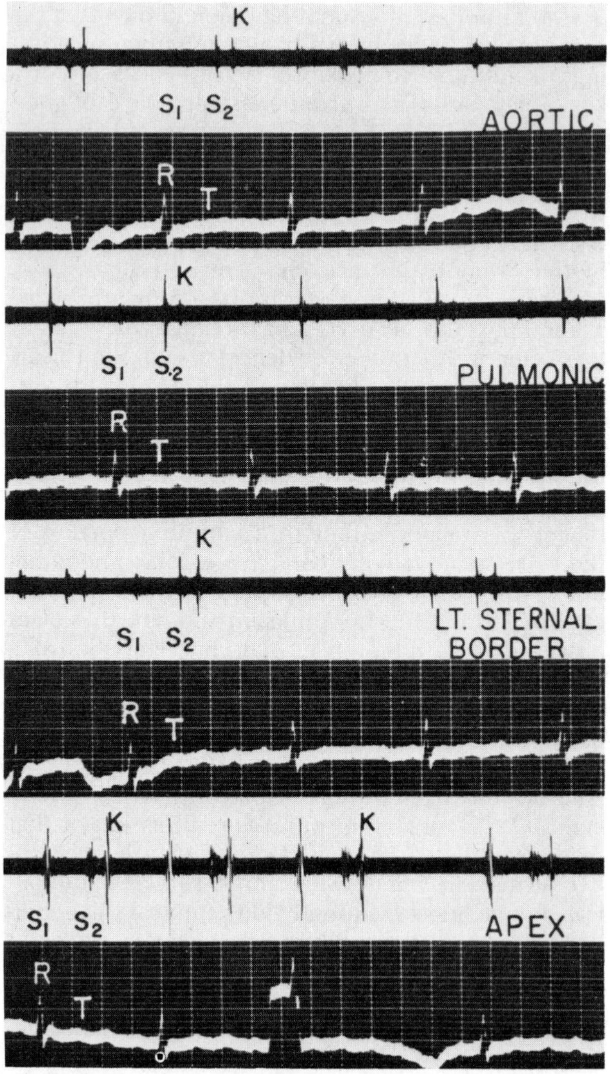

FIGURE 11-34 Pericardial knock: constrictive pericarditis. (*From S. A. Levine and W. P. Harvey, "Clinical Auscultation of the Heart," 2d ed., W. B. Saunders Company, Philadelphia, 1959, p. 535. Reproduced with permission from the publisher and author.*)

occasionally it may show considerable variation in intensity as well as in the number of components. It may also vary with normal respiration. The sound or sounds may persist after surgery on the pericardium, although to a lesser degree, or they may be absent. In other patients, a diastolic sound occurs later after the second sound, simulating the timing of the ventricular diastolic gallop or a normal physiological third sound. It is likely that the pericardial knock and ventricular diastolic gallops are related to similar mechanisms concerned with the filling of the ventricles in early diastole; when the constriction is removed and the myocardium is still in a state of decompensation, the filling sound comes later, consistent with the timing of a ventricular diastolic gallop.

Artificial Valve Sounds and Murmurs[48,73]

Since the beginning of the use of prosthetic valves in human beings in 1951 by Hufnagel, whose artificial ball valve was placed in the first portion of the descending aorta, there has been a succession of various types of prosthetic and other valves, including artificial leaflets, caged-ball valves of the Starr-Edwards type, disk valves, homografts, heterografts, and many variants and modifications of these (Fig. 11-35). Artificial valves have usually been inserted in the aortic and mitral valve areas, but occasionally and less commonly, the tricuspid valve has also been replaced. In some cases, three artificial valves have been used to replace the tricuspid valve.

Sounds vary considerably with the different types of prosthetic valves. The caged-ball or disk valve has an opening sound and a closing sound. Some, such as the caged-ball type, produce sounds that are louder than the normal heart sounds and have a different quality; others, like the porcine valve, produce sounds more like those of a normal heart. With a double valve replacement, each valve may have an opening sound and a closing sound. At times, more than one sound of a normally functioning valve is made at the time of opening and/or closing.

The physician should become familiar with the characteristics of the sounds made by the various artificial valves. Complications following surgery include infection and dislodgment of the valve. Clot formation and emboli have unfortunately been frequent. *Ball variance,* a term used to describe physical changes in a caged ball, occurred in the past but does not appear to be a problem with the newer balls currently used. Ball variance includes changes in the ball's contour and size. Disintegration of the ball has also taken place, particularly in the past. Various unusual sounds may occur when the valve is not functioning properly. Therefore, a series of rattles or clicks, which may simulate the rolling of dice or a ball traversing a roulette wheel, may be heard. Rarely, sounds are multiple rather than single, occurring in systole and/or diastole. When such sounds are present, the possibility of clot formation or some other complication of the artificial valve must be suspected. Multiple sounds are more common when the ball is enclosed in a cage. More than one sound coincident with opening and closing might be expected with any changes in contour of the ball, or when the ball seats itself in the cage that contains it. It should be emphasized, however, that multiple sounds can occur in a normally functioning prosthetic valve. This is particularly more likely to occur with an aortic caged-ball prosthesis during systole.

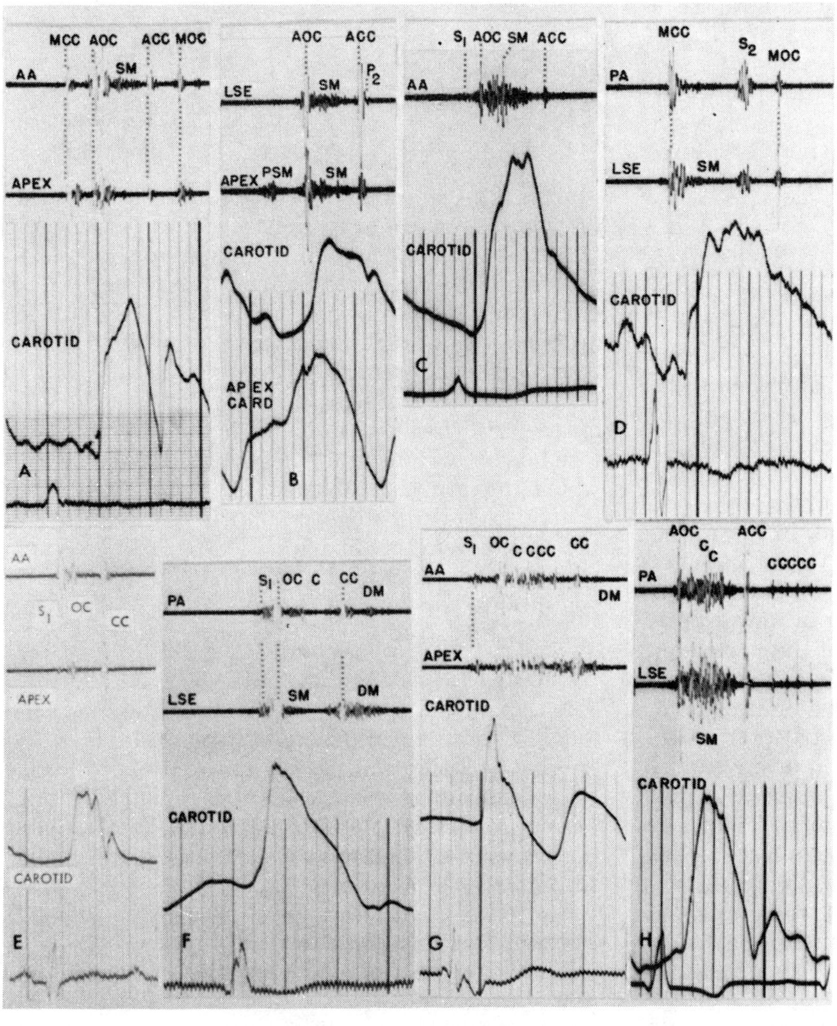

FIGURE 11-35 Composite of patients with various artificial prosthetic valves. AA, aortic area; MCC, mitral closing click; AOC, aortic opening click; ACC, aortic closing click; MOC, mitral opening click; SM, systolic murmur; DM, diastolic murmur. *A.* Aortic and mitral valves replaced with Starr-Edwards prostheses. *B.* Original Hufnagel ball valve (inserted in first portion of descending aorta). *C.* Aortic leaflets (three). *D.* Mitral discoid valve. Note interval from second sound (S_2) to mitral opening click. *E.* Trileaflet "unitized" aortic valve. Opening click (OC) resembles ejection sound. *F.* Hufnagel aortic discoid valve. Note systolic click (C) in addition to opening (OC) and closing (CC) clicks. *G.* Ball valve. Multiple extra sounds (CCCC) occur in systole. *H.* Aortic discoid valve. Extra prosthetic valve sounds (CCCCC) are heard in diastole.

Cineangiograms in such instances may show the ball "bobbing" against the top of the cage during systole. A change in the time of occurrence or intensity of the normally functioning prosthetic valve sounds may be the first sign of malfunction. This was illustrated by a patient who had an opening click sound (of her mitral prosthetic valve) that was so close to the second heart sound it gave the initial impression of being the aortic component of a widely split second sound. However, this short interval between this opening sound and the second sound indicated restricted movement of her caged-ball mitral prosthesis. This was confirmed at surgery, when ball variance was noted. A new mitral valve replaced the old one, with prompt relief of her severe congestive heart failure. On the other hand, if there is a delayed opening sound of a Starr-Edwards mitral prosthetic valve, this may also be an indication of valve malfunction. The late opening sound after the second sound can be caused by a clot or by ball variance; it also may result from obstruction to movement of the prosthetic ball (or disk) by the ventricular wall or septum, when the left ventricular cavity is too small for the size of the prosthetic valve. Disruption of sutures of a prosthetic valve can occur, resulting in disappearance of the valve sounds. When this complication follows insertion of a mitral valve prosthesis, with resulting deterioration of the patient's condition, the opening click sound and a systolic murmur may be absent.[74] At times, a prosthetic valve, such as a discoid type of mitral valve, may get stuck in its open position; the murmur of mitral regurgitation may again be regularly heard, or heard intermittently if the valve only occasionally sticks in its open position.

The bioprosthetic valves usually do not produce an audible opening sound in the aortic position but a distinct, well-defined closing sound is expected. A grade 2 to grade 6 early systolic murmur (see below) is often present, but a diastolic murmur should be considered an abnormal finding. In the mitral position, an opening sound can be heard in half the cases, and a short, soft, middiastolic murmur can be a normal finding.[75] Degenerative changes of the bioprosthetic (porcine) valve occurs and, in the mitral position, results in the alteration of peak frequency characteristic of its closing sound.[76,77]

The occurrence of a new murmur or new sounds should be a clue to a complication of the prosthetic valve. An aortic diastolic murmur indicates regurgitation, and it may occur with both a bioprosthetic or a mechanical prosthetic valve. Obstruction occurring in a porcine valve in the aortic position may produce a significant louder systolic murmur, often in association with a diastolic murmur of regurgitation. The appearance of a diastolic mitral rumble in a porcine valve in the mitral position indicates malfunction causing stenosis of the valve. This is especially true in children where there is a likelihood of rapid early calcification and obstruction taking place. A pansystolic murmur of mitral regurgitation is a complication of all artificial valves.

The degenerated porcine valve can cause a musical murmur; this probably results from flutter of an insufficient leaflet.[78] In addition, a succession of systolic clicks of a porcine valve can indicate degeneration of the valve.

Extracardiac Sounds Produced by Cardiac Pacemakers

It is now well established that the pacemaker can produce a sound in presystole that is related to skeletal muscle contraction rather than being of cardiac origin.[79] At times one can see precordial muscle contraction coincident with the sound, and the patient may be aware of it, occasionally feeling some discomfort. Also, uncommonly, the pacemaker can produce unusual auscultatory findings. This may result in peculiar musical murmurs such as a whoop or honk. These are often loud and occur in late systole. In one patient personally observed, a murmur having a musical quality resembling a "grunt" or "groan" (also described as sounding like "the croaking of a frog") was heard in systole, and at times in diastole. Apparently this was related to the position of the pacing catheter across the tricuspid valve, since repositioning it resulted in disappearance of the murmurs.

Murmurs

W. Proctor Harvey, M.D.
Antonio C. de Leon, Jr., M.D.

Murmurs are audible successive sounds with distinct duration, as opposed to "heart" sounds such as the first or second heart sounds, which are short, transient auditory events. The currently accepted pathogenetic mechanism of cardiac murmurs is that they are the result of turbulence created by blood flow.[80] A critical level of turbulence must be achieved to produce a sound that is clinically appreciated. The characteristics of the murmur depend upon the velocity of blood flow and the surrounding structures which are caused to vibrate.

It is useful to categorize murmurs according to their location in the cardiac cycle. Accordingly, murmurs are identified as being systolic, diastolic, or continuous.

Systolic Murmurs

The classification of systolic murmurs[81] into (1) systolic ejection murmurs and (2) pansystolic, or regurgitant systolic, murmurs has proved to be of great clinical usefulness. These two broad categories are usually readily recognized and immediately enable the clinician to limit diagnostic considerations (Fig. 11-36).

Systolic Ejection Murmurs

A systolic ejection murmur implies turbulent blood flow at the time of right and/or left ventricular ejection into its corresponding great vessel. Its origin is

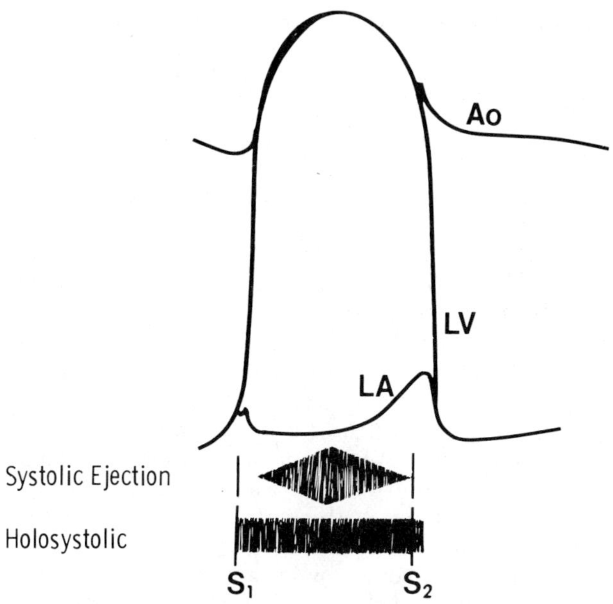

FIGURE 11-36 Characteristics of a systolic ejection murmur and a holosystolic (pansystolic) regurgitant systolic murmur.

therefore likely to be along the ventricular outflow, at the semilunar valve level, or at the immediate great vessel. Since actual blood flow is an essential ingredient to the genesis of turbulence responsible for the murmur, the murmur starts after semilunar valve opening (i.e., after isometric period of ventricular contraction) and ends upon cessation of flow with closure of the same semilunar valve. The characteristics of the left ventricular pressure curve (Fig. 11-36) causes the murmur to be typically crescendo-decrescendo or diamond-shaped. Peak intensity of the murmur could be in early, mid-, or late systole, depending upon the factors influencing turbulent blood flow, i.e., large volume and/or rapid velocity of ventricular ejection or turbulence created by varying degrees of obstruction to ventricular outflow.

The Innocent Systolic Ejection Murmur Data from intracardiac phonocardiography suggest that turbulent flow (and hence murmur) is invariably present in the great vessels at the time of ventricular ejection.[82] The intensity of the murmur, as influenced by stroke volume and/or velocity of ejection, and proximity of the great vessels to the chest wall (influenced by body build) determine whether the murmur is audible with the stethoscope. These factors are most often met in children and young adults; i.e., they tend to have a brisk circulation and a smaller chest cage with a narrow anteroposterior (AP) diameter. Hence, systolic murmurs are most commonly encountered as normal findings. The murmur tends to be of medium frequency, peaks in early to midsystole, usually ends well before the second heart sound, and is best heard along the left sternal border or at the left or right second interspace. It may be the result of turbulent flow into the pulmonary artery,[83] the aorta,[84] or both. On occasion, a musical, vibratory "twanging" or "groaning" murmur is noted along the left sternal border—the Still's murmur; the second is distinctive and, once heard, is easily recognized as a variation of the innocent systolic murmur. The exact genesis of the Still's murmur has not been conclusively established. It has been proposed to originate from the right heart and result from vibrations of the right ventricular moderator band or pulmonary valve,[62] and more recently, the aortic or subaortic region has been proposed as its source.[85]

Although the innocent systolic murmur is usually best heard over an area such as the pulmonary or left sternal border, it is also commonly heard over the lower left sternal border, apex, and aortic areas.

The innocent murmur is generally grade 1 to 3 intensity (grade scale of 1 to 6; see below).

There are also several forms of extracardiac innocent systolic murmurs. One form is the systolic murmur which originates from branches of the aortic arch and presents as a cervical systolic murmur[86] from the increased vascularity which occurs in lactating breast or thyrotoxicosis.[48]

Systolic Murmurs Due to Obstruction of Right Ventricular Outflow (Pulmonic Stenosis) A useful clinical correlation has been demonstrated between the length and peak of the systolic murmur and the severity of obstruction in isolated pulmonic stenosis.[87,88] In mild stenosis, the murmur is short and peaks in early systole. With severe obstruction, the duration of right ventricular ejection is prolonged, thus resulting in delay of the pulmonic closure sound (P_2), which is also diminished in intensity. The murmur is long, and while it does end with the pulmonic closure sound (P_2), it can extend beyond the aortic closure sound (A_2). The peak of the murmur's intensity occurs in late systole (Fig. 11-37). A valvular location of the obstruction is usually indicated by the presence of a pulmonic ejection sound immediately preceding the onset of the ejection systolic murmur. A pulmonic ejection sound is not heard when the obstruction is at the infundibular portion of the right ventricle. The site of maximal murmur intensity in valvular pulmonic stenosis is the left second interspace, with radiation to the left side of the neck and clavicular area. With infundibular obstruction, the murmur may be maximal in intensity at the third left interspace.

Significant pulmonic stenosis occurring in association with a large ventricular septal defect (tetralogy of Fallot) results in a systolic ejection murmur across the obstruction which must be interpreted in a manner directly opposed to isolated pulmonic stenosis.[89] In this instance, more severe pulmonic stenosis results in more right-to-left shunting across the ventricular septal defect and hence a smaller volume of flow across the obstruction. The converse occurs with a lesser degree of obstruction. Thus, in tetralogy of Fallot, the systolic murmur tends to get shorter with more severe degrees of cyanosis and is longest in the patient with minimal or no detectable cyanosis.

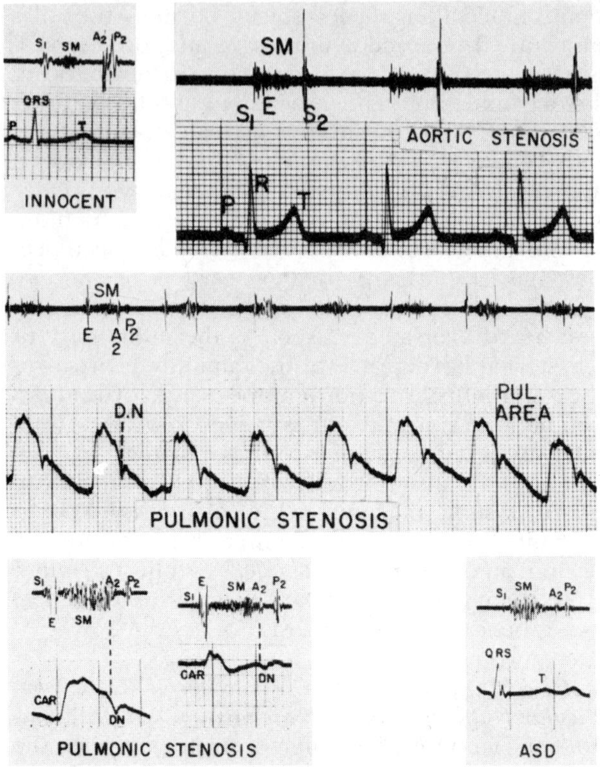

FIGURE 11-37 Comparison with innocent systolic murmur. Composite of several systolic ejection murmurs. Note the ejection sound preceding the murmur (AS and PS) and the fixed split second sound (ASD). (*Most segments are from S. A. Levine and W. P. Harvey, "Clinical Auscultation of the Heart," 2d ed., W. B. Saunders Company, Philadelphia, 1959, p. 200. Reproduced with permission from the publisher and author.*)

Several recognized pathological entities are associated with a systolic ejection murmur across the right ventricular outflow tract. As a rule, the murmur is short and limited to early or midsystole, heard best at the second left intercostal space. Among the conditions are atrial septal defect,[90] idiopathic dilatation of the pulmonary artery,[91] and congenital low-pressure pulmonary valve regurgitation.[92] Their specific recognition is determined not by the systolic murmur but by other auscultatory events: "fixed splitting" of the second heart sound, a pulmonic ejection sound with a physiological S_2 and radiologic evidence of a dilated pulmonary artery, or a medium- or low-frequency early to middiastolic murmur, respectively.

Pulmonary artery branch stenosis is also often associated with a systolic ejection murmur (rarely, a continuous murmur). Its length varies according to the degree of pulmonary artery constriction. The diagnostic hallmark at the bedside is the wide distribution of the murmur throughout the thoracic cage—such that it is equally well heard posteriorly, in both midaxillary regions, as well as anteriorly.[93] Occasionally, patients with a large shunt due to an atrial septal defect will have a similar, widely distributed peripheral pulmonary arterial systolic murmur as a result of increased pulmonary blood flow.[94]

Systolic Murmur Due to Obstruction of Left Ventricular Outflow (Aortic Stenosis) There is a general correlation between the length of the murmur across a fixed obstruction to left ventricular outflow and the severity of obstruction (Fig. 11-38). The murmur tends to be harsh, has a crescendo-decrescendo configuration, and ends at or before aortic valve closure. With *supravalvular* obstruction, the murmur tends to be louder and best heard higher, i.e., at the suprasternal notch and carotid arteries. In fixed *subvalvular* obstruction, it may be loudest along the third left sternal border and is frequently associated with aortic regurgitation. With *dynamic obstruction* such as occurs with idiopathic hypertrophic subaortic stenosis (IHSS), the murmur is loudest at the apex and left sternal border, with poor radiation to the second interspace. Responses to bedside maneuvers, which are discussed later in this chapter, also aid in recognition. *Valvular* aortic stenosis on a congenital basis is usually preceded by an aortic ejection sound, unless the aortic valve is calcified to the extent of

FIGURE 11-38 *Top.* Mild congenital aortic valvular stenosis—aortic ejection sound followed by a very short ejection murmur. *Middle.* Moderate aortic stenosis—longer systolic murmur occupying one-half to two-thirds of systole. *Bottom.* Severe aortic stenosis with long ejection systolic murmur occupying almost all of systole. (*Bottom from S. A. Levine and W. P. Harvey, "Clinical Auscultation of the Heart," 2d ed., W. B. Saunders Company, Philadelphia, 1959, p. 330. Reproduced with permission from the publisher and author.*)

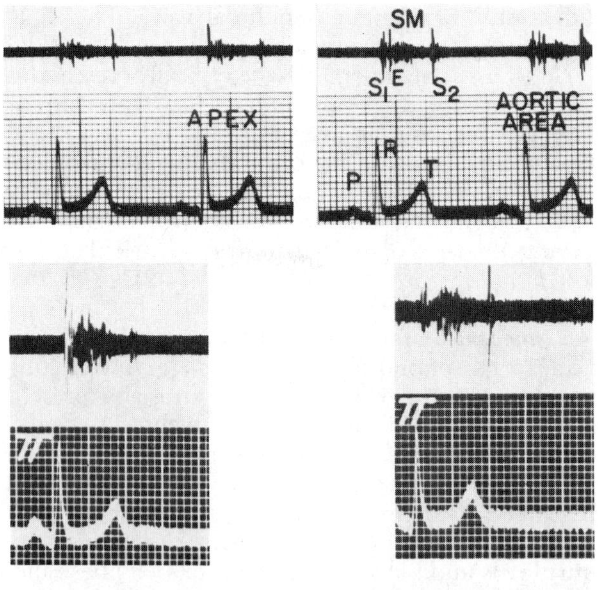

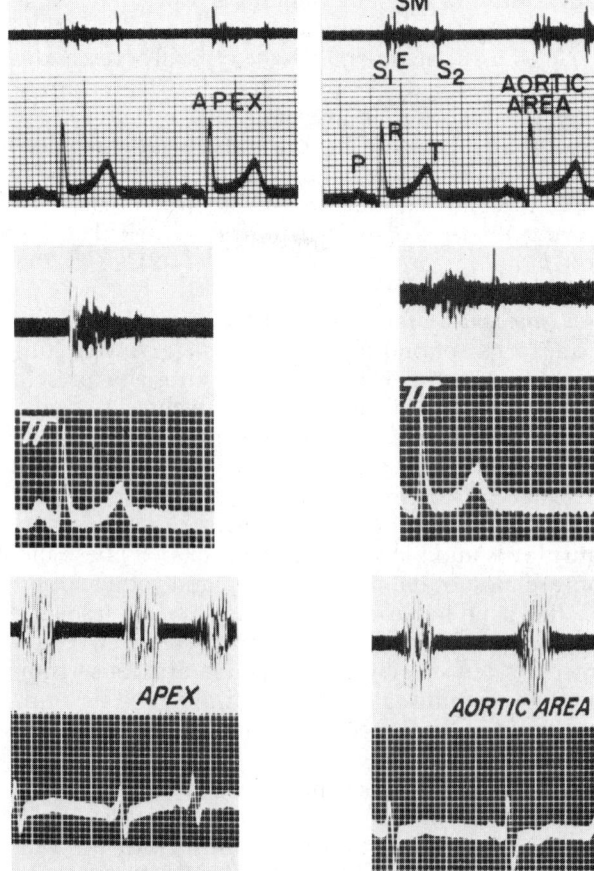

rendering it immobile. The murmur may be loudest at the cardiac apex, although it is also heard at the second right interspace, suprasternal notch, and carotid arteries. A long murmur, especially associated with a paradoxical second heart sound (no left bundle branch block), implies severe obstruction. A short, early-peaking systolic murmur is expected with mild obstruction. It should be remembered, however, that in severe stenosis with left ventricular failure and diminished cardiac output, the murmur may be short and, in a few instances, even absent.

Holosystolic (Pansystolic) Murmurs

These murmurs represent *regurgitant murmurs,* i.e., mitral regurgitation, tricuspid regurgitation, and ventricular septal defect (Fig. 11-39). The murmur begins as soon as the AV valve closes and continues beyond semilunar valve closure. Because the pressure difference (gradient) between ventricle and recipient chamber (atrium or right ventricle) is considerable throughout systole, the murmur tends to have an even or plateau configuration.

Variants Mitral valve regurgitation may be present with a variety of murmur configurations. In acute, severe mitral regurgitation, the giant left atrial v wave results in a smaller late systolic left ventricular to left atrial gradient. Hence, the murmur tends to decrease in intensity or be absent in late systole.[96] Mitral valve prolapse frequently presents with a late systolic murmur that is crescendo-decrescendo or crescendo to the second heart sound.[97] When the murmur is holosystolic, a late systolic accentuation may be present. A systolic click (or clicks) may be associated with a systolic murmur, or may occur without a murmur. Papillary muscle dysfunction may present as a holosystolic, midsystolic, late systolic, or early systolic murmur.[98]

The murmur of tricuspid regurgitation may also be altered from its typical holosystolic configuration. It may decrease in late systole, and in wide-open tricuspid regurgitation the murmur may be absent or confined to early systole. Selective inspiratory increase in intensity of the murmur is typical of this lesion.

FIGURE 11-39 *Top.* Holosystolic murmur of chronic mitral regurgitation. *Middle.* Holosystolic murmur of ventricular septal defect. *Bottom.* Holosystolic murmur of tricuspid regurgitation with inspiratory augmentation of murmur. [*Top and bottom from S. A. Levine and W. P. Harvey, "Clinical Auscultation of the Heart," 2d ed., W. B. Saunders Company, Philadelphia, 1959, pp. 335, 341. Reproduced with permission from the publisher and author.*]

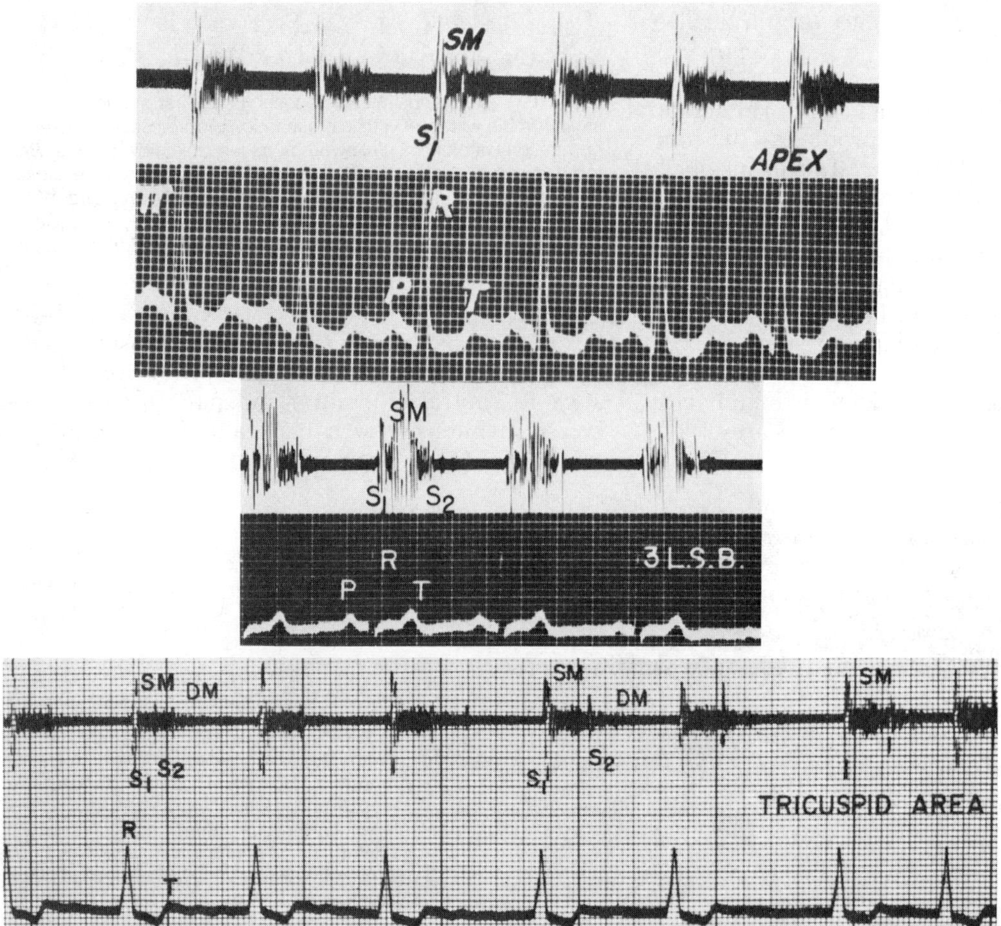

The typical holosystolic murmur of ventricular septal defect usually peaks in midsystole. It may also be modified by the onset of pulmonary hypertension. This results in the progressive shortening of the systolic murmur as the degree of pulmonary hypertension increases.[99] Commonly, the murmur of ventricular septal defect heard in infants and young children may subsequently disappear because of spontaneous closure of the defect. In small muscular ventricular septal defects, physiological closure of the defect toward the latter part of systole accounts for the less than holosystolic murmur in some cases.[100]

Diastolic Murmurs

Murmurs in diastole can occur across two locations: (1) across the AV valves (mitral or tricuspid) or (2) across the semilunar valves (aortic and pulmonic).

Diastolic Murmurs across the AV Valves

Mitral Diastolic Murmurs Mitral diastolic murmurs begin after mitral valve opening and hence do not start immediately after the second heart sound. The onset is more in middiastole and is the result of turbulent blood flow across the valve; the murmur is usually of low frequency or rumbling in character. Certain lesions of hemodynamic severity result in increased diastolic mitral blood flow which result in a middiastolic rumble in the absence of mitral valve obstruction. Included in these lesions are *ventricular septal defect, patent ductus arteriosus,* and *mitral regurgitation* (Fig. 11-40). On the other hand, rheumatic or congenital *mitral valve stenosis* produces a diastolic rumbling murmur (Fig. 11-40).[101] In this instance, the turbulent blood flow results from the pressure gradient between left atrium and left ventricle, and hence the length of the rumble can reflect the severity of obstruction. In normal sinus rhythm, the diastolic murmur increases in intensity at the time of atrial contraction (presystolic crescendo).

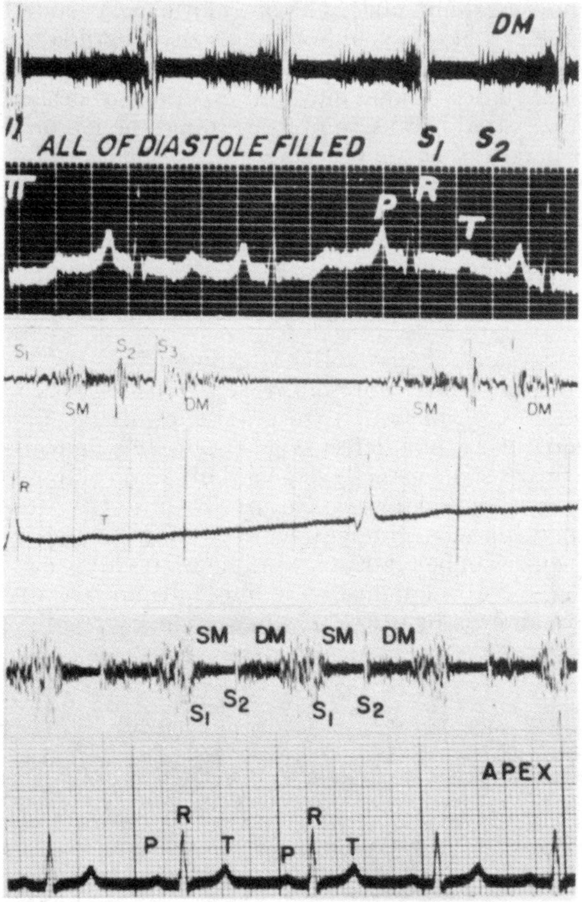

FIGURE 11-40 *Top.* Mitral stenosis. Loud first sound (S_1); diastolic rumble with presystolic crescendo. *Middle.* Severe mitral regurgitation with loud S_3 followed by middiastolic flow rumble. *Bottom.* Severe aortic insufficiency with apical diastolic rumble (Austin Flint) mimicking mitral stenosis. (*From S. A. Levine and W. P. Harvey, "Clinical Auscultation of the Heart," 2d ed., W. B. Saunders Company, Philadelphia, 1959, p. 252, 241, 295. Reproduced with permission from the publisher and author.*)

Tricuspid Diastolic Murmurs Like their mitral valve counterpart, tricuspid diastolic murmurs are of low frequency but differ in that they are usually best heard at the lower left sternal border (versus the apex for mitral murmurs) and may selectively increase in intensity with respiration.[102] A murmur

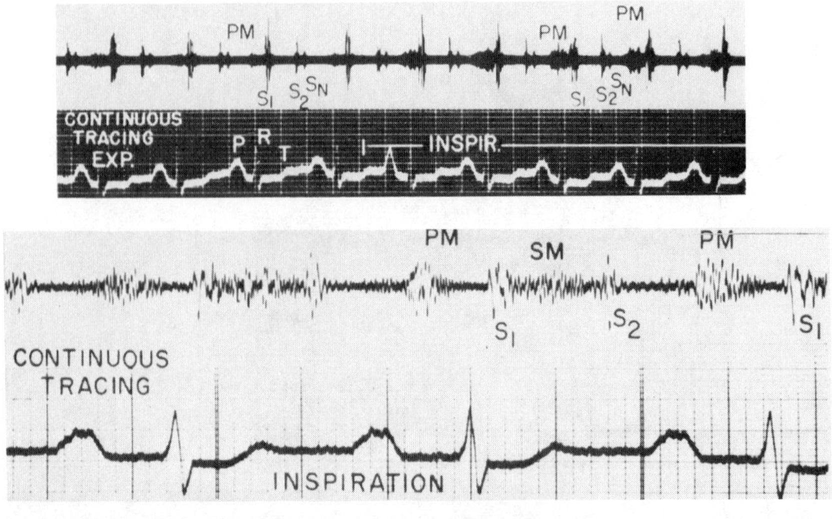

FIGURE 11-41 *Top.* Tricuspid stenosis with inspiratory increase of presystolic murmur. *Bottom.* Tricuspid stenosis and insufficiency with 1° AV block showing presystolic murmur during atrial systole well before S_1. (*From S. A. Levine and W. P. Harvey, "Clinical Auscultation of the Heart," 2d ed., W. B. Saunders Company, Philadelphia, 1959, pp. 344, 345. Reproduced with permission from the publisher and author.*)

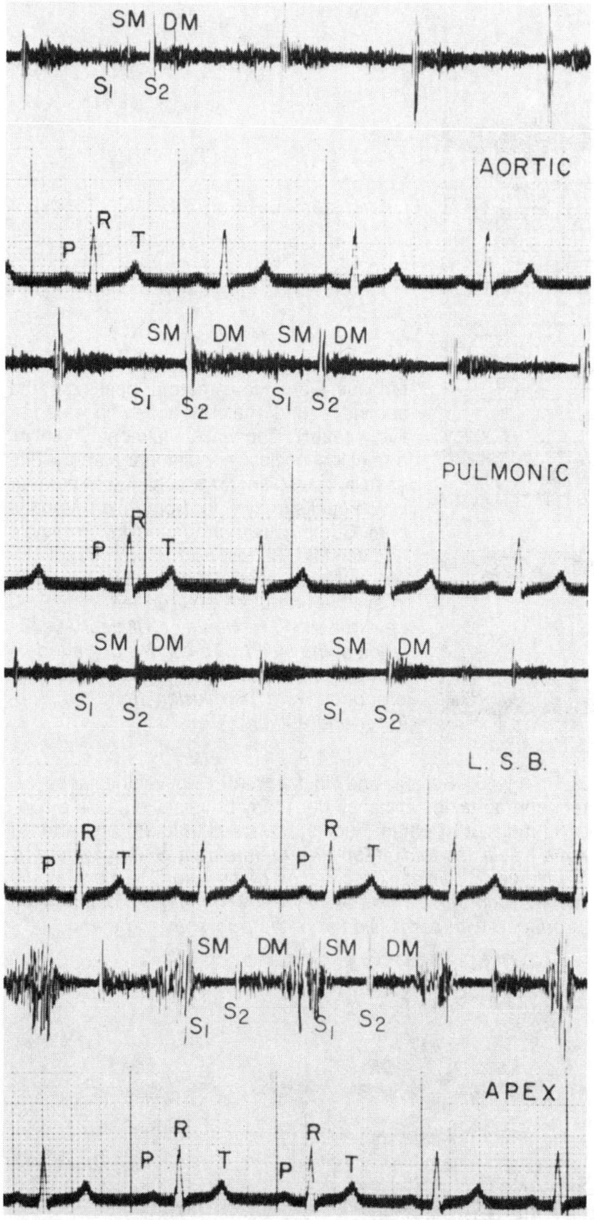

FIGURE 11-42 Phonocardiogram of a patient with severe aortic insufficiency showing a diastolic rumble (Austin Flint) at apex. (*From S. A. Levine and W. P. Harvey, "Clinical Auscultation of the Heart," 2d ed., W. B. Saunders Company, Philadelphia, 1959, p. 295. Reproduced with permission from the publisher and author.*)

caused by an increased volume of blood flow without valve obstruction occurs with a large left-to-right shunt in *atrial septal defect* and *tricuspid valve regurgitation*. Tricuspid stenosis also results in a diastolic rumbing murmur which can have a late diastolic (presystolic) crescendo-decrescendo component as a result of right atrial systole (Fig. 11-41).

Diastolic Murmurs across the Semilunar Valves

Aortic Valve Regurgitation The murmur of aortic regurgitation begins immediatly after the aortic valve closure sound (A_2) and typically is of high frequency with a decrescendo configuration. It is usually best heard along the left sternal border but may also be noted at the second right interspace and cardiac apex. In cases due to dilatation or aneurysm of the ascending aorta, the diastolic murmur may be louder at the right second, third, and fourth interspaces compared with the left.[103] These are called "right-sided" aortic diastolic murmurs and usually are associated with dilatation and rightward displacement of the aortic root.

With significant aortic regurgitation, a medium- to low-frequency, blubbery type of diastolic murmur with or without presystolic crescendo may be noted at the cardiac apex (Austin Flint murmur) (Fig. 11-42).

Pulmonary Valve Regurgitation The murmur of *pulmonary valve regurgitation* in the presence of *pulmonary hypertension* results in a high-frequency, decrescendo diastolic murmur starting from the pulmonic valve closure sound (P_2) and best heard along the second and third left sternal border (Graham Steell murmur) (Fig. 11-43). It may also show a selective inspiratory increase in intensity. The pulmonic component of the second sound (P_2) is accentuated and is palpable over the pulmonic area of the precordium.

Low-pressure pulmonary valve regurgitation results in a low- or medium-pitched murmur. Often, the onset is at some interval after the pulmonic valve closure (P_2), resulting in the middiastolic rather than early diastolic murmur. In some cases, the murmur starts just after the pulmonic valve closure (P_2), but the rumbling low-frequency characteristic of the murmur makes it distinctive.[92]

FIGURE 11-43 Graham Steell murmur, mitral stenosis. (*From S. A. Levine and W. P. Harvey, "Clinical Auscultation of the Heart," 2d ed., W. B. Saunders Company, Philadelphia, 1959, p. 271. Reproduced with permission from the publisher and author.*)

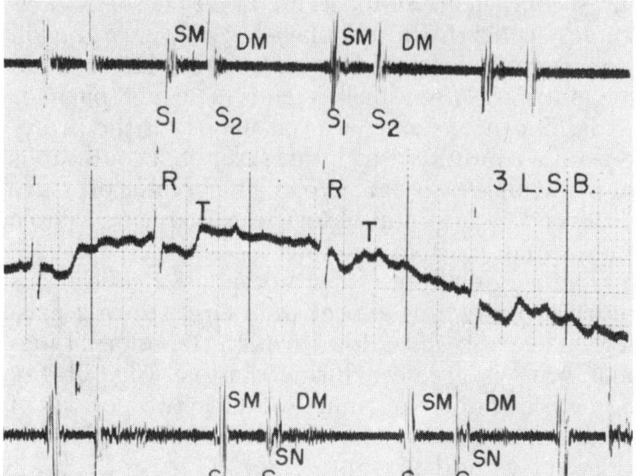

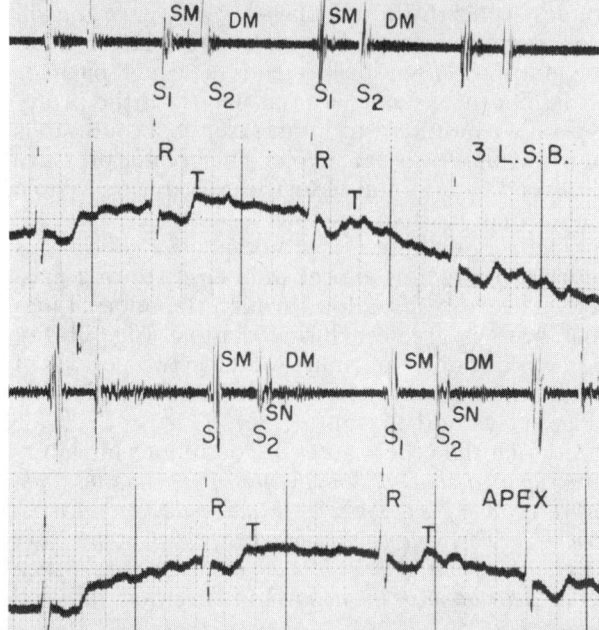

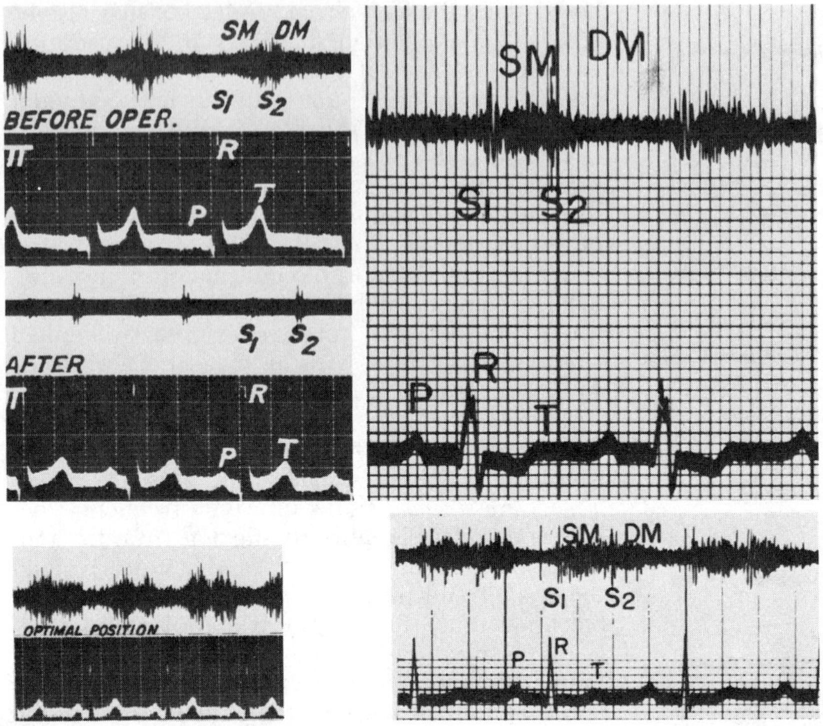

FIGURE 11-44 *Top left.* Patent ductus arteriosus. Continuous murmur peaking at the second sound (before) absent postoperatively (after). *Top right.* Pulmonary emboli producing occlusive pulmonary artery disease and resulting in a continuous murmur which peaks in systole. *Bottom left.* Venous hum. Continuous murmur peaking in systole and diastole. *Bottom right.* Coronary arteriovenous fistula; continuous murmur peaks both in systole and diastole. (*Top left from S. A. Levine and W. P. Harvey, "Clinical Auscultation of the Heart," 2d ed., W. B. Saunders Company, Philadelphia, 1959, p. 368. Reproduced with permission from the publisher and author.*)

Continuous Murmurs

Murmurs which extend from systole into diastole, thus going beyond the second heart sound, are called *continuous murmurs.* For such a murmur to occur, blood flow must be able to continue from a high pressure to a lower pressure area despite semilunar valve closure. Thus, the location or source of the murmur determines to a large extent whether the murmur itself peaks in intensity in systole, at the second heart sound, or in diastole.

Patent ductus arteriosus is the prototype of an entity causing a continuous murmur that peaks at the second heart sound (Fig. 11-44). Usually, it is loudest beneath the left clavicle, and, if large, will have sharp sounds (eddy sounds) interspersed within the murmur. When small, it tends to be high-pitched.

Significant systemic arterial stenosis is the prototype of a condition which can result in a continuous murmur that peaks in systole. The greater pressure difference across the obstruction is during systole rather than diastole.

The venous hum is a prototype of a continuous murmur that tends to peak in intensity during diastole. This is so since flow through the internal jugular veins is greatest during diastole (Fig. 11-44). Some continuous murmurs will have two periods of peak intensity, one in systole and another in diastole (Figs. 11-44 and 11-45).

Among the other causes of continuous murmurs are *ruptured sinus of Valsalva aneurysm into the right heart, coronary arteriovenous fistula, pulmonary arteriovenous fistulas, systemic arteriovenous fistulas,* some cases of *branch stenosis of the pulmonary artery, collaterals* (such as in *coarctation of the aorta*) and surgically induced

FIGURE 11-45 Systolic and diastolic murmur of ventricular septal defect and aortic insufficiency (*top*) may be mistaken for the continuous murmur of patent ductus arteriosus (*middle*) and arteriovenous fistula (*bottom*). (*Top and middle from S. A. Levine and W. P. Harvey, "Clinical Auscultation of the Heart," 2d ed., W. B. Saunders Company, Philadelphia, 1959, p. 442, bottom, p. 488. Reproduced with permission from the publisher and author.*)

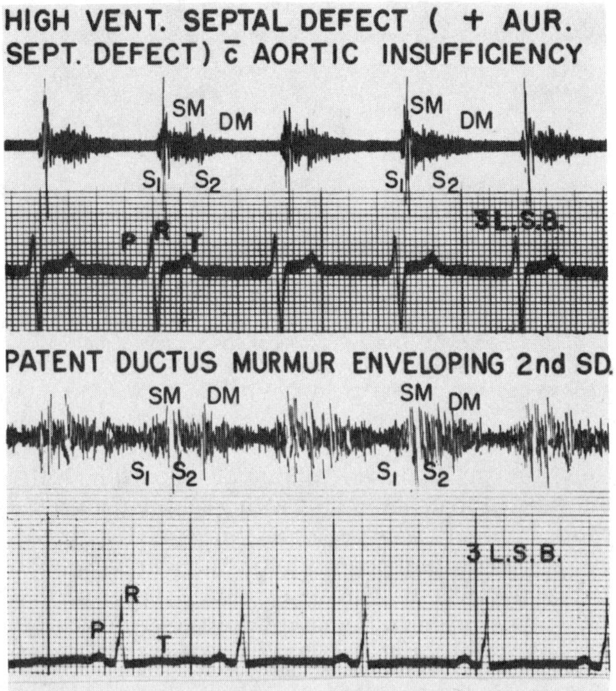

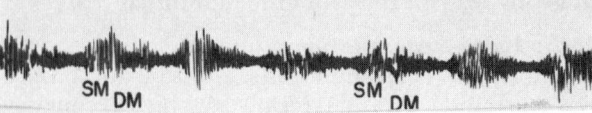

shunts such as the *Blalock-Taussig anastomosis, Waterston shunt,* and the *arteriovenous shunt for renal hemodialysis.*

Murmurs Related to Artificial Valves

For murmurs related to artificial valves, see "Artificial Valve Sounds and Murmurs," above.

The Grading of Murmurs

The most commonly utilized method of grading the intensity of murmurs is based upon the recommendation of Levine.[48] Murmur intensity is divided into six grades:

Grade 1 is a faint murmur heard only after a period of concentration or "tuning in."
Grade 2 is a faint murmur heard immediately on auscultation.
Grade 3 is a moderate-intensity murmur.
Grade 4 is a loud murmur usually associated with a thrill.
Grade 5 is a loud murmur, but it cannot be heard unless the stethoscope is touching the chest wall.
Grade 6 is a loud murmur which can be heard with the entire stethoscope chest piece held off the chest wall.

Aids to Auscultation

Cycle Length

The ejection systolic murmur caused by obstruction to the right or left ventricular outflow tract (with intact interventricular septum) increases in intensity after a long diastolic filling period. Thus, in the beat following a premature beat with a compensatory pause, the murmur increases in intensity. This can be useful in distinguishing a long ejection systolic murmur (especially when loudest at the cardiac apex) from a holosystolic or regurgitant murmur, such as mitral regurgitation which does not appreciably change in intensity following a premature beat.

Valsalva Maneuver[104]

A sustained Valsalva maneuver causes a decrease in venous return, a fall in systemic arterial pressure, and a small ventricular volume (phase 2 of the maneuver). Hence, such a maneuver results in intensification of the murmur of hypertrophic cardiomyopathy (idiopathic subaortic stenosis), and can also bring out a late systolic murmur or convert one into a holosystolic murmur in mitral valve prolapse.

Isometric Handgrip

The isometric handgrip maneuver results in the elevation of systemic resistance and blood pressure. Thus, in hypertrophic cardiomyopathy, the murmur may diminish in intensity. The diastolic murmur of aortic regurgitation increases, and the click in mitral valve prolapse may occur later in systole.

Prompt Squatting

Prompt squatting results in an initial increase in venous return and elevation of systemic arterial pressure. Accordingly, the murmur of hypertrophic cardiomyopathy tends to decrease or may be abolished. In some cases of mitral valve prolapse, it also may result in the decrease or abolition of the late systolic murmur. In tetralogy of Fallot, the maneuver results in less right-to-left shunting and thus an increase in the length and intensity of the murmur across the stenotic right ventricular infundibular and/or pulmonary valve.

Pharmacologic Agents[104,105]

Two agents are commonly employed: one is a vasodilator, amyl nitrite; the other is a vasopressor, usually methoxamine or phenylephrine.

Amyl nitrite causes systemic vasodilatation and hence a fall in systemic blood pressure. This is promptly followed by a reflex tachycardia and increased venous return to the right side of the heart. Thus, administration of the drug results in a decrease in intensity of the murmurs of *mitral regurgitation, ventricular septal defect, aortic regurgitation,* and the *Austin Flint rumble.* Conversely, it results in an increase in intensity of the murmurs of *obstruction to right (intact septum)* and *left ventricular outflow (hypertrophic cardiomyopathy* and *aortic stenosis), tricuspid stenosis,* and *regurgitation,* and *mitral stenosis.*

Drugs such as methoxamine and phenylephrine, have an effect that is opposite to that caused by amyl nitrite inhalation and is similar to that obtained by a properly peformed isometric handgrip or prompt squatting.

Note: Unless otherwise stated, most of the illustrations used by Drs. Harvey and de Leon are from S. A. Levine and W. P. Harvey, "Clinical Auscultation of the Heart," 2d ed., W. B. Saunders Company, Philadelphia, 1959. We wish to thank W. B. Saunders for permitting us to reproduce the illustrations. Whenever possible, the exact source (page numbers) is listed. The exact page number for some of the segments of the collages are not listed.

References

1. Laennec, R. T. H.: "Traité de l'auscultation médiate," 2d ed., Brosson et Chaude, Paris, 1826, vol. 1, p. 5.
2. McKusick, V. A.: "Cardiovascular Sound in Health and Disease," The Williams & Wilkins Company, Baltimore, 1958.
3. Rouanet, J.: Analyse des bruits de coeur. Thesis 252, Paris, 1832.
4. Dock, W.: Mode of Production of First Heart Sound, *Arch. Intern. Med.,* 50:737, 1933.
5. Luisada, A., MacCanon, D. M., Kumar, S., et al.: Changing Views on the Mechanism of the First and Second Heart Sounds, *Am. Heart J.,* 88:503, 1974.
6. Mills, P. G., Chamusco, R., Moos, S., et al.: Echophonocardiographic Studies of the Contribution of the Atrioventricular Valves to the First Heart Sound, *Circulation,* 54:944, 1976.
7. Leech, G., and Leatham, A.: Correlation of Heart Sounds

and Valve Motion, in P. Hanrath and D. Mathey (eds.), "Evaluation of Cardiac Dynamics by Ultrasound," Springer-Verlag, Berlin, 1980.

8. Zalter, R., Hardy, H. C., and Luisada, A.: Acoustic Transmission Characteristics of the Thorax, *J. Appl. Physiol.*, 18:428, 1963.
9. Ertel, P. Y., Lawrence, M., Brown, R. K., et al.: Stethoscope Acoustics: I. The Doctor and His Stethoscope, *Circulation*, 34:889, 1966.
10. Ertel, P. Y., Lawrence, M., Brown, R. K., and Stern, A. M.: Stethoscope Acoustics: II. Transmission and Filtration Patterns, *Circulation*, 34:899, 1966.
11. Leatham, A.: Splitting of the First and Second Heart Sounds, *Lancet*, 2:607, 1954.
12. Haber, E., and Leatham, A.: Splitting of Heart Sounds from Ventricular Asynchrony in Bundle Branch Block, Ventricular Ectopic Beats, and Artificial Pacing, *Br. Heart J.*, 27:691, 1965.
13. Luisada, A. A.: Tricuspid Component of the First Heart Sound, in D. F. Leon and J. A. Shaver (eds.), "Physiologic Principles of Heart Sounds and Murmurs," American Heart Association, New York, 1975, p. 19.
14. Leatham, A., and Leech, G.: Observations on the Relationship between Heart Sounds and Valve Movements by Simultaneous Echo and Phonocardiography, *Br. Heart J.*, 37:557, 1975. (Abstract.)
15. Waider, W., and Craige, E.: First Heart Sound and Ejection Sounds: Echocardiographic and Phonocardiographic Correlation with Valvular Events, *Am. J. Cardiol.*, 35:3, 1975.
16. Leatham, A.: "Auscultation of the Heart and Phonocardiography," 2d ed., J. & A. Churchill, Ltd., London, 1975.
17. Braunwald, E., Fishman, A., and Cournand, A.: Time Relationship of Dynamic Events in the Cardiac Chambers, Pulmonary Artery and Aorta in Man, *Circ. Res.*, 4:100, 1956.
18. Crews, T., Pridie, R., Benham, R., and Leatham, A.: Auscultatory and Phonocardiographic Findings in Ebstein's Anomaly: Correlation of First Heart Sound with Ultrasonic Recordings of Tricuspid Valve Movement, *Br. Heart J.*, 34:681, 1972.
19. Brooks, N., Leech, G., and Leatham, A.: Factors Responsible for Normal Splitting of First Heart Sound: High Speed Echophonocardiographic Study of Valve Movement, *Br. Heart J.*, 42:695, 1979.
20. Brooks, N., Leech, G., and Leatham, A.: Complete Right Bundle Branch Block. Echophonocardiographic Study of First Heart Sound and Right Ventricular Contraction Times, *Br. Heart J.*, 41:637, 1979.
21. Leatham, A., and Gray, I.: Auscultatory and Phonocardiographic Signs of Atrial Septal Defect, *Br. Heart J.*, 18:193, 1956.
22. Harris, A.: Pacemaker "Heart Sound," *Br. Heart J.*, 29:608, 1967.
23. Wolferth, C., and Margolies, A.: Certain Effects of Auricular Systole and the Prematurity of Beat on the Intensity of the First Heart Sound, *Trans. Assoc. Am. Physicians*, 45:44, 1930.
24. Levine, S., and Harvey, W.: Clinical Auscultation of the Heart, W. B. Saunders Company, Philadelphia, 1949.
25. Shah, P., Kramer, D., and Gramiak, R.: Influence of the Timing of Atrial Systole on Mitral Valve Closure and on the First Heart Sound in Man, *Am. J. Cardiol.*, 26:231, 1970.
26. Burgraaf, G. W., and Craige, E.: The First Heart Sound in Complete Heart Block: Phonoechocardiographic Correlations, *Circulation*, 50:17, 1974.
27. Leech, G., Brooks, N., Green-Wilkinson, A., and Leatham, A.: Mechanism of Influence of PR Interval on Loudness of First Heart Sound, *Br. Heart J.*, 43:138, 1980.
28. Weiss, O., and Joachim, G.: Registrierung von Herztonen und Herzgeraischen mittles des Phonoskops und ihre Beziehungen zum Elektrokardiogramm, *Arch. klin Med.*, 73:240, 1911.
29. Potain, C.: Note sur les dédoublements normales des bruits du coeur, *Bull. Soc. Méd. Hôp. Paris*, ser. 2, 3:138, 1866.
30. Leatham, A., and Towers, M.: Splitting of the Second Heart Sound in Health, *Br. Heart J.*, 13:575, 1951.
31. Boyer, S. H., and Chisholm, A. W.: Physiologic Splitting of the Second Heart Sound, *Circulation*, 18:1010, 1958.
32. Castle, F. R., and Jones, K. L.: The Mechanism of Respiratory Variations in Splitting of the Second Heart Sound, *Circulation*, 24:180, 1961.
33. Dornhorst, A. C., Howard, P., and Leathart, G. L.: Respiratory Variations in Blood Pressure, *Circulation*, 6:553, 1952.
34. Shafter, H. A.: Splitting of the Second Heart Sound, *Am. J. Cardiol.*, 6:1013, 1960.
35. Leatham, A., Segal, B., and Shafter, H.: Auscultatory and Phonocardiographic Findings in Healthy Children with Systolic Murmurs, *Br. Heart J.*, 4:451, 1963.
36. Beck, W., Schrire, V., and Vogelpoel, L.: Splitting of the Second Heart Sound in Constrictive Pericarditis, with Observations on the Mechanism of Pulsus Paradoxus, *Am. Heart J.*, 64:765, 1962.
37. Sutton, G., Harris, A., and Leatham, A.: Second Heart Sound in Pulmonary Hypertension, *Br. Heart J.*, 30:743, 1968.
38. Leatham, A., and Weitzman, D. W.: Auscultatory and Phonocardiographic Signs of Pulmonary Stenosis, *Br. Heart J.*, 19:303, 1957.
39. Tofler, O. B.: The Pulmonary Component of the Second Heart Sound in Fallot's Tetralogy, *Br. Heart J.*, 25:509, 1963.
40. Schrire, V., and Vogelpoel, L.: The Role of the Dilated Pulmonary Artery in Abnormal Splitting of the Second Heart Sound, *Am. Heart J.*, 63:501, 1962.
41. Brigden, W., and Leatham, A.: Mitral Incompetence, *Br. Heart J.*, 15:55, 1953.
42. Gray, I.: Paradoxical Splitting of the Second Heart Sound, *Br. Heart J.*, 18:21, 1956.
43. Yurchak, P. M., and Gorlin, R.: Paradoxical Splitting of the Second Heart Sound in Coronary Heart Disease, *N. Engl. J. Med.*, 269:741, 1963.
44. Craige, E., and Harned, H. S.: Phonocardiographic and Electrocardiographic Studies in Normal Newborn Infants, *Am. Heart J.*, 65:180, 1963.
45. Harris, A., and Sutton, G.: Second Heart Sound in Normal Subjects, *Br. Heart J.*, 30:739, 1968.
46. Wood, P.: The Eisenmenger Syndrome or Pulmonary Hypertension with Reversed Central Shunt, *Br. Med. J.*, 2:701, 1958.
47. Potain, Pierre C.: Du rhythme cardiaque appelé bruit de gallop, in A. Ruskin (ed.), "Classics in Arterial Hypertension," Charles C Thomas, Publisher, Springfield, Ill., 1956. (Reference, courtesy of Dr. Robert C. Tarazi)
48. Levine, S. A., and Harvey, W. P.: "Clinical Auscultation of the Heart," 2d ed., W. B. Saunders Company, Philadelphia, 1959.
49. Harvey, W. P., and Stapleton, J.: Clinical Aspects of Gallop Rhythm with Particular Reference to Diastolic Gallops, *Circulation*, 18:5, 1017, 1958.
50. Leonard, J. J., Weissler, D. M., and Warren, J. V.: Observations on the Mechanism of Atrial Gallop Rhythm, *Circulation*, 17:1007, 1958.
51. Hill, J. L., O'Rourke, R. A., Lewis, R. P., and McGranahan, G. M.: The Diagnostic Value of the Atrial Gallop in Acute Myocardial Infarction, *Am. Heart J.*, 78:194, 1969.
52. Harvey, W. P., Segal, J. P., and Gurel, T.: The Clinical Spectrum of Primary Myocardial Disease, *Prog. Cardiovasc. Dis.*, 7:17, 1964.
53. Goldblatt, A., Aygen, M. M., and Braunwald, E.: Hemodynamic-Phonocardiographic Correlations of the Fourth Heart Sound in Aortic Stenosis, *Circulation*, 26:92, 1962.
54. Caulfield, W. H., de Leon, A. C., Perloff, J. K., and Steelman, R. B.: The Clinical Significance of the Fourth Heart Sound in Aortic Stenosis, *Am. J. Cardiol.*, 28:179, 1971.
55. Perloff, J. K.: Recognition and Differential Diagnosis of Pulmonary Stenosis, in B. L. Segal (ed.), "The Theory and Practice of Auscultation," F. A. Davis Company, Philadelphia, 1959.
56. Leatham, A.: Auscultation of the Heart, *Lancet*, 2:793, 1958.
57. Hultgren, H. N., Reeve, R., Cohn, K., and McLeod, R.: The Ejection Click of Valvular Pulmonic Stenosis, *Circulation*, 40:631, 1969.

58. Reeve, R.: Variations of the Ejection Click in Valvular Pulmonic Stenosis, *Clin. Res.*, 14:129, 1966. (Abstract.)
59. Leatham, A., and Vogelpoel, L.: The Early Systolic Sound in Dilatation of the Pulmonary Artery, *Br. Heart J.*, 16:21, 1954.
60. Hancock, E. W.: Origin of the Ejection Sound in Aortic Stenosis, *Clin. Res.*, 13:209, 1965.
61. LeBauer, E. J., Perloff, J. K., and Keliher, T. F.: Isolated Systolic Click with Bacterial Endocarditis, *Am. Heart J.*, 73:534, 1967.
62. Humphries, J. O., and McKusick, V. A.: Differentiation of Organic and "Innocent" Systolic Murmurs, *Prog. Cardiovasc. Dis.*, 5:152, 1962.
63. Leon, D. F., Leonard, J. J., Kroetz, F. W., Page, W. L., Shaver, J. A., and Lancaster, J. F.: Late Systolic Murmurs, Clicks, and Whoops Arising from the Mitral Valve: Transseptal Intracardiac Phonocardiographic Analysis, *Am. Heart J.*, 72:325, 1966.
64. Ronan, J. A., Perloff, J. K., and Harvey, W. P.: Systolic Clicks and the Late Systolic Murmur: Intracardiac Phonocardiographic Evidence of Their Mitral Valve Origin, *Am. Heart J.*, 70:319, 1965.
65. Barlow, J. B., and Bosman, C. K.: Aneurysmal Protrusion of the Posterior Leaflet of the Mitral Valve: An Auscultatory-Electrocardiographic Syndrome, *Am. Heart J.*, 71:166, 1966.
66. Harvey, W. P.: Some Newer or Poorly Recognized Findings on Clinical Auscultation, *Mod. Concepts Cardiovasc. Dis.*, 37:85, 1968.
67. Lachman, A. S., Bramwell-Jones, D. M., Lakier, J. B., Pocock, W. A., and Barlow, J. B.: Infective Endocarditis in the Billowing Mitral Leaflet Syndrome. *Br. Heart J.*, 37:326, 1975.
68. Harvey, W. P., and Capone, M. A.: Bacterial Endocarditis Related to Cleaning and Filling of Teeth: With Particular Reference to the Inadequacy of Present-Day Knowledge and Practice of Antibiotic Prophylaxis for All Dental Procedures, *Am. J. Cardiol.*, 8:793, 1961.
69. Rackley, C. E., Whalen, R. E., Floyd, W. L., Orgain, E. S., and McIntosh, H. D.: Precordial Honk, *Am. J. Cardiol.*, 17:609, 1966.
70. Behar, V. S., Whalen, R. E., and McIntosh, H. D.: Ballooning Mitral Valve in Patients with the "Precordial Honk" or "Whoop," *Am. J. Cardiol.*, 20:789, 1967.
71. Mounsey, P.: The Early Diastolic Sound of Constrictive Pericarditis, *Br. Heart J.*, 17:143, 1955.
72. Dayem, M. K. A., Wasfi, R. M., Bentall, H. H., Goodwin, J. F., and Cleland, W. P.: Investigation and Treatment of Constrictive Pericarditis, *Thorax*, 22:242, 1967.
73. Dayem, M. K. A., and Raftery, E. B.: Phonocardiogram of the Ball-and-Cage Aortic Valve Prosthesis, *Br. Heart J.*, 29:446, 1967.
74. Leachman, R. D., and Cokkinos, D. V. P.: Absence of Opening Click in Dehiscence of Mitral Valve Prosthesis, *N. Engl. J. Med.*, 281:461, 1969.
75. Smith, N. D., Raisada, V., and Abrams, J.: Auscultation of the Normally Functioning Prosthetic Valve, *Ann. Intern. Med.*, 95:593, 1981.
76. Magilligan, D. J., Jr., Lewis, J. W., Jr., Jara, F. M., et al.: Spontaneous Degeneration of Porcine Bioprosthetic Valves, *Ann. Thorac. Surg.*, 30:259, 1980.
77. Stein, P. D., Sabbah, H. N., Lakien, J. B., Magilligan, D. J., and Goldstein, S.: Frequency of the First Heart Sound in the Assessment of Stiffening of Mitral Bioprosthetic Valves, *Circulation*, 63:200, 1981.
78. Stein, P. D., Sabbah, H. N., Magilligan, D. J., Jr., and Lakier, J. B.: Mechanism of a Musical Systolic Murmur Caused by a Degenerative Porcine Bioprosthetic Valve, *Am. J. Cardiol.*, 49:1874, 1982.
79. Kramer, D. H., Moss, A. J., and Shah, P. M.: Mechanisms and Significance of Pacemaker-Induced Extracardiac Sound, *Am. J. Cardiol.*, 25:367, 1970.
80. Sabbah, H. N., and Stein, P. D.: Turbulent Flow in Humans: Its Primary Role in the Production of Ejection Murmurs, *Circ. Res.*, 38:513, 1976.
81. Leatham, A.: A Classification of Systolic Murmurs, *Br. Heart J.*, 17:574, 1955.
82. Lewis, D. H.: Phonocardiography, in "Handbook of Physiology," sec. 2: "Circulation," American Physiological Society, Bethesda, Md., 1962, vol. 1, chap. 22.
83. de Leon, A. C., Perloff, J. K., Twigg, H., and Majd, M.: The Straight Back Syndrome, *Circulation*, 32:193, 1965.
84. Stein, P. D., and Sabbah, H. N.: Aortic Origin of Innocent Murmurs, *Am. J. Cardiol.*, 39:665, 1977.
85. Wennevold, A.: The Origin of the Innocent "Vibratory" Murmur Studied with Intracardiac Phonocardiography, *Acta Med. Scand.*, 181:1, 1967.
86. Fowler, N. O., and Marshall, W. S.: The Supraclavicular Arterial Bruit, *Am. Heart J.*, 69:410, 1965.
87. Vogelpoel, L., and Schrire, V.: Auscultatory and Phonocardiographic Assessment of Pulmonary Stenosis with Intact Ventricular Septum, *Circulation*, 22:55, 1960.
88. Gamboa, R., Hugenholtz, P. E., and Nados, A. S.: Accuracy of the Phonocardiogram in Assessing Severity of Aortic and Pulmonic Stenosis, *Circulation*, 30:35, 1964.
89. Vogelpoel, L., and Schrire, V.: Auscultatory and Phonocardiographic Assessment of Fallot's Tetralogy, *Circulation*, 22:73, 1960.
90. Barber, J. M., Magidson, O., and Wood, P.: Atrial Septal Defect with Special Reference to Electrocardiogram, Pulmonary Artery Pressure, and Second Heart Sound, *Br. Heart J.*, 12:277, 1950.
91. Deshomukh, M., Guvenc, S., Bartivoglio, L., and Goldberg, H.: Idiopathic Dilation of the Pulmonary Artery, *Circulation*, 27:710, 1960.
92. Criscitiello, M. G., and Harvey, W. P.: Clinical Recognition of Congenital Pulmonary Valve Insufficiency, *Am. J. Cardiol.*, 20:765, 1967.
93. D'Cruz, I. A., Agustsson, M. H., Bicoff, J. P., Weinberg, M, Jr., and Arcilla, R. A.: Stenotic Lesions of the Pulmonary Arteries, *Am. J. Cardiol.*, 13:441, 1964.
94. Perloff, J. K., Caulfield, W. H., and de Leon, A. C.: Peripheral Pulmonary Artery Murmur of Atrial Septal Defect, *Br. Heart J.*, 29:411, 1967.
95. Oakley, C. M., and Hallidic-Smith, K. A.: Assessment of Site and Severity in Congenital Aortic Stenosis, *Br. Heart J.*, 29:367, 1967.
96. Ronan, J. A., Jr., Steelman, R. B., de Leon, A. C., Jr., Waters, T. J., Perloff, J. K., and Harvey, W. P.: The Clinical Diagnosis of Acute Severe Mitral Insufficiency, *Am. J. Cardiol.*, 27:284, 1971.
97. Barlow, J. B., Bosman, C. K., Pocock, W. A., and Marchand, P.: Late Systolic Murmurs and Nonejection (Mid-Late) Systolic Clicks, *Br. Heart J.*, 30:203, 1968.
98. Burch, G. E., DePasquale, N. P., and Phillips, J. H.: The Syndrome of Papillary Muscle Dysfunction, *Am. Heart J.*, 75:399, 1968.
99. Perloff, J. K.: Auscultatory and Phonocardiographic Manifestations of Pulmonary Hypertension, *Prog. Cardiovasc. Dis.*, 9:303, 1967.
100. Nadas, A. S., Scott, L. P., Hauck, A. J., and Rudolph, A. M.: Spontaneous Functional Closure of Ventricular Septal Defects, *N. Engl. J. Med.*, 264:309, 1961.
101. Wood, P.: An Appreciation of Mitral Stenosis, *Br. Heart J.*, 1:1051, 1954.
102. Perloff, J. K., and Harvey W. P.: Clinical Recognition of Tricuspid Stenosis, *Circulation*, 22:346, 1960.
103. Harvey, W. P., Corrado, M. A., and Perloff, J. K.: "Right-Sided" Murmurs of Aortic Insufficiency, *Am. J. Med. Sci.*, 245:533, 1963.
104. Dohan, M. C., and Criscitiello, M. G.: Physiological and Pharmacological Manipulations of Heart Sounds and Murmurs, *Mod. Concepts Cardiovasc. Dis.*, 39:121, 1970.
105. de Leon, A. C., Jr., and Harvey, W. P.: Pharmacologic Agents and Auscultation, *Mod. Concepts Cardiovasc. Dis.*, 44:23, 1975.

12

Examination of the Retina

W. Banks Anderson, Jr., M.D.

The study of retinal changes associated with vascular disease is of unusual importance, interest and difficulty. Of importance, because of the unique opportunities offered in the eye of observing . . . the intimate changes in the vascular tree. Of interest, because many of the most fascinating and complicated problems in medicine are bound up in the derangements of the cardiovascular system. . . . Of difficulty, because today, after more than a century of research and study, we are still far from possessing the plan of the maze into which the search for ultimate causes of these extremely common problems had led us.

Sir Stewart Duke-Elder, 1967[1,*]

Inspection of the smaller vessels of the body is possible in only three areas: the retina, the conjunctiva, and the nail beds. Helmholtz's gift of the ophthalmoscope has made the retina by far the easiest and most rewarding of these observation sites. Viewing this two-dimensional vascular display is generally much easier, especially in the aged, if the pupils are dilated. One drop of tropicamide 1% ophthalmic solution (Mydriacyl) will dilate the pupils in 15 or 20 min. Care should be taken to make pulse and blood pressure determinations prior to instillation of such rapidly acting mydriatics as both the pulse and the blood pressure may increase after absorption of the drops. Although complications of mydriasis are rare, patients in whom the iris seems closely apposed to the cornea or those with a history of closed-angle glaucoma are best left undilated.

Examination of the retina should proceed methodically. Best pupillary dilatation is maintained if the optic disk is observed first. Look for evidence of edema and blurred margins and for cupping with sharp contours. Rule out neovascularization or the pallor of optic atrophy. Next scan along the superior temporal arcade, inspecting the arteries carefully for embolic plaques at each bifurcation. Note the arteriovenous crossings for evidence of obscuration of the vein and for pronounced nicking and banking of the vessels. The lower arcade and the nasal vessels may be inspected next. Avoid the macular area until all else has been viewed, as the pupil constricts most intensely when this area is illuminated. To find diabetic microaneurysms early, look just temporal to the fovea along the horizontal raphe. To discover cotton-wool infarcts, look circularly around the disk two disk diameters out. With such a plan in mind the retina can be efficiently searched for evidence of cardiovascular disease. (See Table 12-1.)

An appreciation of the pathophysiological variations in retinal architecture is essential for recognizing its disease processes. The following sections describe morphologic changes helpful in assessing the cardiac patient.

TABLE 12-1 Retinal Topography

Finding	Most Common Location
Arteriovenous crossings	Upper temporal quadrant
Cotton-wool spots	Around optic disk
Hard exudates	Between disk and fovea
Microaneurysms	Temporal to fovea
Emboli	Arterial bifurcations
Diabetic new vessels	Nerve head and arcades

Retinal Vessel Caliber Changes

Caliber changes along the course of a single artery or vein are of much greater significance than are estimates of arteriovenous ratios or absolute vascular diameter. Estimates of the degree of tortuosity or straightening are also generally valueless, except in the situation where the veins are large, dark, and tortuous. This constellation of findings implies outflow obstruction, arterial inflow obstruction, hypoxia, or all three.[2] Such dark and dilated veins may occur in patients with large left-to-right shunts and in the leukemias and hyperviscosity syndromes.

Autonomic innervation of the retinal vessels does not exist.[3] Nevertheless the retinal vessels may change in caliber both acutely and chronically. Autoregulation of the retinal vessels does occur, and oxygen is the most active vasomotor substance. With hyperoxia there is rapid constriction of both the arteries and veins, while in hypoxia vasodilatation occurs.[4] Elevated carbon dioxide tension is also a retinal vasodilator.[5] A striking clinical example of these combined effects is the vasodilatation, darkening of the blood column, and retinal and disk edema seen in patients with marked pulmonary insufficiency and right-sided cardiac failure.[6] At the opposite extreme the marked vasoconstrictor effect of oxygen may produce retinal vasoobliteration in immature infants with resulting retrolental fibroplasia.

Estimates of arteriovenous ratios are of little clinical utility.[7] Of much greater significance are variations in the caliber of a single vessel. These changes may take the form of focal narrowing, sometimes called *beading* or *spasm*. Beading is produced by an abnormal constriction which may be contiguous with an abnormally dilated segment. Usually seen in the venous system where there is venous outflow ob-

*Reproduced with permission from the publisher.

struction, such beading is particularly common in diabetic retinopathy. Beading of the arteries is *not* generally associated with systemic disease but is seen in congenital conditions such as von Hippel's angiomatosis, Coats's disease, and Leber's miliary aneurysms.

Segmental narrowing or spasm of the retinal vessels has been much described in the older literature. Most descriptions of rapid waves of "spasm" were probably observations of patients with moving fibrin or platelet emboli. Narrowing of the retinal vessels has been observed in response to injections of norepinephrine and angiotensin.[8] Autoregulatory narrowing of the retinal vessels is a response to hypertension, and upon occasion may be focal. This narrowing is chronic, and spasm is not an apt description.

Vascular Wall Thickening

Normally only the blood column is visible when the retinal vessels are viewed. When changes in the walls do occur, they are most visible along the sides of the vessels since in this location the tangential line of sight presents a greater thickness to the viewer. Vessels at the disk often appear sheathed. This normal variant may be associated with a veil of tissue in front of the disk (Bergmeister's papilla). More peripheral retinal vessels become sheathed or cuffed in response to intraocular inflammation, vasculitis, or multiple sclerosis. Fatty exudate (hard exudate) may collect along venous walls (never arteries), particularly in diabetic exudative retinopathy. These deposits are not intrinsic to the wall itself. After venous obstructive disease of some duration, a white uniform line may develop along either side of the retinal veins in the involved area. Ballantyne terms this *halo sheathing*,[9] and Kennedy and Wise have found it to consist of increased collagen deposition in the vessel wall.[10]

Arteriosclerosis

Should the retinal arterial circulation be considered arterial or arteriolar? If one accepts the criteria of Bloom and Fawcett[11] that blood vessels less than 0.3 mm in diameter are arterioles, then all the retinal arterial circulation may be considered arteriolar. Nevertheless Hogan and Feeney have demonstrated smooth-muscle cells several layers thick in the media of the retinal arterial vessels both posteriorly and in the periphery.[12] These physicians suggest that the term *arteriole* be applied only to the smallest precapillary vessels. We will use the term *arteriosclerosis* rather than *arteriolosclerosis* and *artery* rather than *arteriole* without respect to the size of the vessel.

In arteriosclerosis the medial smooth muscle (which may hypertrophy in chronic hypertension) becomes hyalinized with the deposition of collagen. As the wall thickens, the light reflex broadens and the vessel takes on a burnished coppery luster which, with further thickening, may transmute to silver. Obscuration of the venous blood column at arterial crossings is early evidence of this process. Even when the artery walls have become so thick as to look like "silver wires," flow can ordinarily still be demonstrated by fluorescein angiography.

Arteriovenous Compression

Arteriovenous compression or "nicking" has as its histologic basis the sharing by the artery and vein of a common adventitial sheath at their crossings. Arteriosclerotic thickening impedes venous outflow at these locations with venous tortuosity, engorgement, and darkening of the blood column distal to the compression. Where the vein dives beneath the thick artery wall, sometimes "banking" to intersect at right angles, its blood column is obscured and it appears nicked.

Atherosclerosis

Atherosclerosis, or fatty infiltration of the intima, was once thought not to occur in the retina. Clinicopathologic confirmation of retinal atherosclerosis has been obtained.[13] Retinal atheromata have a predilection for the bifurcations and bends within the first two branches of the central retinal artery, appearing as segments of irregular yellowish sheathing and having the crystalline knobbiness of a salted pretzel stick. On occasion the thickening may progress to the point where no blood column is visible, although total obstruction is rare.

Cotton-Wool Spots

Cotton-wool spots are generally a sign of serious systemic disease. They may be seen in patients with severe hypertension, blood dyscrasias, collagen diseases, or hemorrhagic shock. Cotton-wool spots are also frequently seen in patients with acquired immunodeficiency syndrome (AIDS) and are a poor prognostic sign.[14] They are almost invariably found within three disk diameters of the optic disk and have a feathery, woolly character because of their anterior involvement of the nerve fiber layer. (See Plate 5*B* and *C*.) Cotton-wool spots may at times be confused with persistent myelinization of the nerve fiber layer. Cotton-wool "exudates" are *not* exudates but consist of a cluster of cell-like swollen ends of fragmented axones (cytoid bodies) in an area of edematous retina. They are evanescent and will often disappear in a few weeks, leaving behind no observable trace of their presence. Ischemia is almost certainly the cause of these spots, which may occur secondary to occlusion of peripapillary capillaries or occlusion of a small artery, or secondary to hypoxia. The presence of these cotton-wool spots is usually indicative of serious systemic disease.

Hard Exudates

Hard exudates are most probably edema residues. They occur in situations where the vessels become leaky, and as the more watery component of the extravasation is resorbed, the lipid residue forms hard, yellow, waxy deposits. They may surround the leaking vessel in a circinate ring or may accumulate in the macula, radiating from the fovea in the spokes of a macular "star." Histologically found deep in the retina, these exudates will disappear in some months if the source of the leakage is eliminated. These exudates indicate a loss of vascular wall integrity and are associated with hypertension, diabetes, venous outflow obstruction, and retinal angiomas. They are not ischemic in origin but indicate chronic fluid extravasation and retinal edema.

Microaneurysms

Microaneurysms are not unique to diabetes but occur in many disease states, including retinal venous obstructive disease, sickle cell disease, the dysproteinemias, Behçet's disease, sarcoidosis, and other forms of uveitis. A common factor in all these conditions seems to be the presence of both retinal hypoxia and viable capillary endothelial cells. Microaneurysms are outpouchings in capillary walls that range in size from 20 to 100 μm. Commonly found adjacent to zones of capillary obliteration or "dropout," it has been suggested that they represent abortive attempts at revascularization of a compromised capillary bed. Their etiology is, however, still unknown.

Neovascularization

Neovascularization also occurs in conditions where microaneurysms are found. The new vessels generally originate from capillaries or from the venous side of the circulation and are associated with greater or lesser degrees of fibrosis. In all cases, however, the new vessels are incorporated in an associated fibrous membrane. Some of the channels appear to function as shunts, and in cases of venous outflow obstruction may serve to bypass the obstructed site. Other neovascular channels branch in a fanlike fashion toward an avascular zone or forward into the vitreous cavity, proliferating along a posterior hyaloid membrane. Such a rete mirabile does not appear to have any shunting function and is more suggestive of an attempt at revascularization of an unperfused tissue. Clinically the likelihood of blinding vitreous hemorrhage is greatly increased in the presence of such neovascularization.[15]

Retinal Vessel Leakage

Normally the retinal vessels are permeable only to quite small molecules. This *blood-retina barrier* is analogous to the blood-brain barrier and is facilitated by the overlapping of the endothelial cells and the tight endothelial cell junctions in retinal vessels. Enclosed within the basement membrane of the capillary is an intramural pericyte whose investment may contribute to the relative impermeability of these vessels.

The sodium fluorescein molecule normally does not traverse this vascular barrier, and by fluorescein angiography abnormal sites of leakage can be conveniently defined. With this technique, neovascular channels are found to leak profusely, as do microaneurysms. In severe hypertension small areas of leakage may be seen along tiny arteries in the vicinity of cotton-wool spots.[16] Vessels damaged by emboli may leak, as do obstructed veins or inflamed vessels. Retinal edema and hard exudates are the consequences of this leakage.

Retinal Hemorrhage

Hemorrhage into the retina indicates further breakdown in the integrity of the vascular wall. When the hemorrhage occurs in the inner retina, as in hypertension, it assumes a feathery flame shape as it is molded and dispersed by the nerve fibers coursing toward the disk. Deeper hemorrhages, such as those in diabetics, take on a more rounded dot or blot shape. Diabetic neovascularization may result in large hemorrhages beneath the retinal internal limiting membrane or into the vitreous, which obscures the underlying retina. In obstructions of the central retinal vein, the fundus may be splattered with blood as if a tomato had ruptured on the disk. (See Plate 6*A*.) Small hemorrhages are difficult to differentiate from microaneurysms, but hemorrhages usually fade within several weeks while microaneurysms may persist for months to years.

Hemorrhage may occur *beneath* the retina and usually originates not from the retinal vessels but from proliferation of a choroidal neovascular membrane growing through Bruch's membrane. These hemorrhages commonly occur beneath the macula and may destroy central vision. They have the appearance of a gray-black mass with a red fringe and have been mistaken for malignant melanomas of the choroid.

Vascular Occlusion

When the central artery or one of its branches is occluded, the nonperfused retinal area becomes cloudy in a matter of minutes. At the fovea where the retina is one cell layer thick and nourished by the choroid, the normal color and transparency persist. By contrast with the surrounding pallor, the fovea then has a cherry-red appearance. Occlusion at the capillary level is identified by the surrounding microaneurysms or adjacent cotton-wool spots. With fluorescein angiography such areas can be directly identified by their lack of perfusion.

Occlusion of the central retinal vein results in retinal edema and the "squashed tomato" hemorrhages as noted above (Plate 6*A*). Occlusions of branches of the central vein produce edema and hemorrhage in the drained area. These branch vein occlusions always occur at arteriovenous crossings. Examination of the retina of the opposite eye of such patients will generally reveal significant arteriovenous compression. As collateral drainage channels develop, the edema and hemorrhagic retinopathy subside, leaving white-walled veins, neovascularization, and microaneurysms in the affected area. Hemorrhage into the vitreous may occur as a late complication from the neovascularization. There is a very high incidence of hypertension in patients with venous obstructive disease,[17] and retinal and systemic arteriosclerosis is usually present.

Optic Disk Edema

Increased intracranial pressure, retinal venous outflow obstruction, inflammation, and ischemia are the four major causes of optic disk edema. The term *papilledema* is reserved by ophthalmologists and neurologists for that form of disk edema which is the result of increased intracranial pressure. It therefore has an etiologic connotation and is not used generally to mean optic disk edema. Patients with papilledema see well, while other forms of disk edema are associated with poor vision. *Papillitis* is the term applied to inflammatory disk edema. Patients with ischemic optic neuritis commonly have a pale edematous disk with an altitudinal field defect. When associated with elevations of the sedimentation rate, such patients should be suspected of having giant cell arteritis (temporal arteritis). If this diagnosis can be established, steroid therapy is indicated to prevent visual loss in the opposite eye.

Optic Atrophy

With the resolution of disk edema in papillitis or ischemic optic neuritis, the disk will become flat and pale. Both pallor and impaired visual function are necessary for the diagnosis of optic atrophy since both the color and vascularity of the disk are highly variable. If the disk is atrophic and cupped with a shift of the vessels to the nasal side, glaucoma should be suspected. Optic atrophy without cupping may indicate intracranial tumor and should be investigated. It is unlikely that tumor has caused the atrophy if vision was once poor and has returned to near-normal levels. This is the situation often observed in patients with demyelinating disease.

Embolism

Embolism from the heart and great vessels occurs more commonly than is generally appreciated. A sudden increase in tinnitus in one ear, a fleeting woozy sensation, a scintillating scotoma, a transient monocular visual loss all may be symptoms of embolic ischemia. This clinical suspicion may be confirmed by ophthalmoscopy. In Table 12-2 we have listed characteristics of retinal emboli of cardiovascular significance. Of these, platelet emboli are at once the most common and the most evanescent. Within minutes after vision has returned, platelet emboli have usually broken into fragments too small to identify ophthalmoscopically. Most other emboli persist for days or years and are more lasting evidence of an embolic episode. Hollenhorst cholesterol plaques may be identified at the same bifurcations for months to years after the embolic shower.

Platelet emboli, Hollenhorst plaques (Fig. 12-1), and calcium emboli are usually seen along the course of a retinal artery. Roth spots (see Plate 6*C*) and fat emboli may not appear to be intravascular and may not be associated with a vessel which is ophthalmoscopically visible.

TABLE 12-2 Emboli of Cardiovascular Significance

Type	Appearance	Significance
Platelet	Dull pink to gray often with associated fibrin	Downstream vegetations, mural thrombi
Hollenhorst plaque	Glistening yellow-orange plaques at bifurcations	Downstream atheroma (containing cholesterol)
Calcium plaque	Glistening white plaques	Calcific aortic stenosis
Roth spot	Hemorrhage with gray-white center (Plate 6*C*)	Blood dyscrasia or septic embolus as in SBE
Fat embolus	Fuzzy-bordered gray-white spot without hemorrhage	Severe trauma with long bone fractures; prognosis grave
Myxoma	Disk edema, retinal edema in arterial supply zone	Life-threatening atrial myxoma

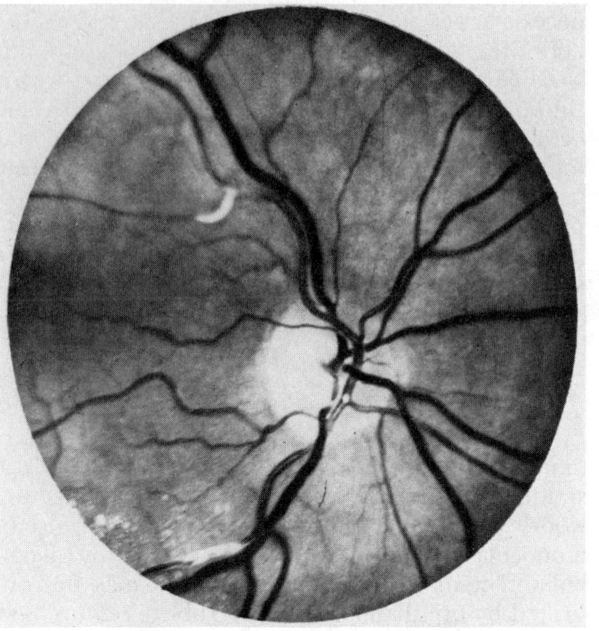

FIGURE 12-1 Retinal emboli often lodge at bifurcations, as in this patient with carotid atherosclerosis. Note that the embolic material often seems larger than the containing vessel, as in the embolus at the lower left edge of the photograph. Emboli may damage the vessel wall and cause leakage, as can be seen by the exudate deposited about the inferior embolus. Hollenhorst cholesterol plaques rarely completely obstruct arterial flow, and this patient maintained vision.

Diseases

The eye is a major target for two extremely common diseases of cardiovascular significance: diabetes and hypertension. Blindness from the former now ranks as the second leading cause of acquired adult blindness in the United States, and these diabetic changes are commonly paralleled by severe renal and cardiac vasculopathy.

Diabetes

The average diabetic develops ophthalmoscopically visible retinal changes after 16 years of the disease. Focal loss of a portion of the capillary bed is followed by microaneurysm formation and vascular dilatation around the borders of the area of capillary dropout. Vascular leakage occurs with dot and blot hemorrhages and deposits of hard exudate (Fig. 12-2). New blood vessels develop along the vascular arcades and at the optic nerve head (Fig. 12-3). The proliferation of new blood vessels with their associated membranes often results in blinding hemorrhage into the vitreous cavity and tractional detachment of the retina.

The clinician must recognize early proliferative diabetic retinopathy, for not only are these changes associated with renal and cardiac disease but im-

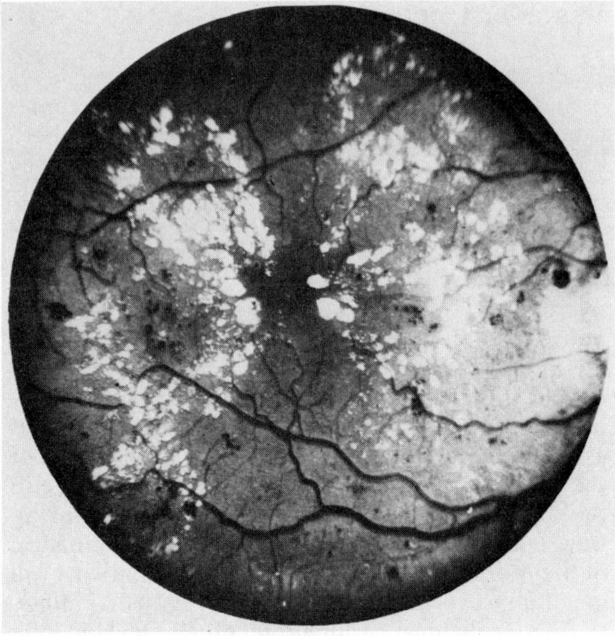

FIGURE 12-2 Exudative diabetic retinopathy, right eye, illustrating microaneurysms, dot and blot hemorrhages, and venous engorgement with extensive deposits of hard, yellow exudate.

mediate laser photocoagulation of the retina may be sight-saving.[18] Control of the hypertension which is commonly associated is also of great importance, as elevations of systemic blood pressure compound the difficulty in controlling retinal vascular leakage.

FIGURE 12-3 Proliferative diabetic retinopathy, left eye. There is extensive neovascularization of the disk with an associated small intravitreal hemorrhage which obscures the upper temporal vessels. Along the inferior temporal arcade is another area of neovascularization. These new vessels are incorporated in fibrous membranes which may tent up the vessels and cause traction detachments of the retina, as at the lower right edge of the photograph.

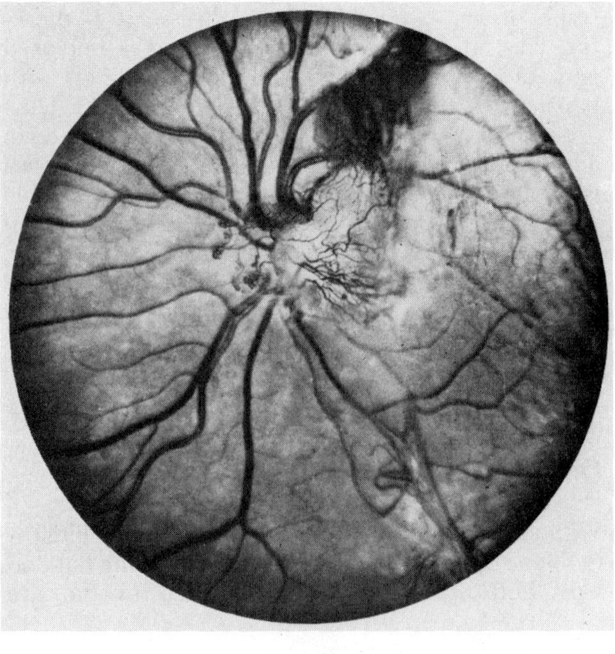

Hypertension

When the systemic blood pressure rises, the retinal circulation becomes especially vulnerable since its capillary pressure floor is determined by the intraocular pressure (about 16 mmHg) and not by the jugular or cavernous sinus pressure. The intraocular pressure does not increase in hypertension, and increases in systemic blood pressure would be directly reflected in increased retinal capillary perfusion pressure were it not for the homeostatic responses of the retinal vasculature. Vasoconstriction of the arterial tree and thickening of the arterial vessel walls with consequent reduction in lumen diameter are homeostatic responses to hypertension. (See Plates 5*A* to *D* and 6*B* and *D*.) Arteriosclerotic narrowing of the vessels acts to insulate the capillary bed from the elevated arterial supply pressure. These arteriosclerotic changes are visible as narrowing, increases in central light reflexes, and copper and silver wiring of the arteries. (See Plate 5*C*.) If, however, increases in the systemic blood pressure are either very marked or very rapid, these homeostatic mechanisms are overwhelmed. The resulting decompensation of the capillary bed results in accumulations of fluid in the retina and optic nerve head. The aqueous portion of the fluid is more rapidly cleared than the lipid component, which accumulates as hard exudate. Hemorrhage may occur in the inner retinal layers in a characteristic flame pattern, and focal ischemia in the nerve fiber layer may result in cotton-wool microinfarcts. In severe hypertensive decompensation the optic nerve head becomes swollen and edematous. In the Scheie[19] and Keith-Wagener[20] classifications, patients with disk edema would be assigned to the grade IV category. (See Plate 5*C*.) Patients with eclampsia or pheochromocytoma may have such marked and rapid elevations of capillary pressure that edema fluid floats the retina off the choroid, producing an exudative (nonrhegmatogenous) detachment of the retina.

Such retinal signs of capillary bed decompensation are usually paralleled by severe renal vasculopathy, and aggressive therapeutic efforts are indicated immediately. The likelihood that the patient suffers from a nonessential variety of hypertension is also markedly increased, especially if the patient is Caucasian.[21] It is clinically useful therefore to categorize hypertensive patients as to whether or not their retinal circulation is compensated, or has decompensated with observable edema, cotton-wool spots, flame hemorrhages, or swelling of the optic disk.

References

1. Duke-Elder, S., (ed.): "System of Ophthalmology, vol. X." Diseases of the Retina, (by Duke-Elder, S., and Dobree, J. H.), The C. V. Mosby Company, St. Louis, 1967, p. 277.
2. Wise, G. N., Dollery, C. T., and Henkind, P.: "The Retinal Circulation," Harper & Row Publishers, Inc., New York, 1971, p. 220.
3. Laties, A. M.: Central Retinal Artery Innervation: Absence of Adrenergic Innervation to the Intraocular Branches, *Arch. Ophthalmol.*, 77:405, 1967.
4. Cusick, P. L., Benson, O. O., and Boothby, W. M.: Effect of Anoxia and of High Concentrations of Oxygen on the Retinal Vessels, *Proc. Mayo Clin.*, 15:500, 1940.
5. Frayser, R., and Hickam, J. B.: Retinal Vascular Response to Breathing Increased Carbon Dioxide and Oxygen Concentrations, *Invest. Ophthalmol.*, 3:427, 1964.
6. Stevens, P. M., Austen, F., and Knowles, J. H.: Prognostic Significance of Papilledema in Course of Respiratory Insufficiency, *JAMA*, 183:161, 1963.
7. Stokoe, W. L., and Turner, R. W.: Normal Retinal Vascular Pattern: Arteriovenous Ratio as a Measure of Arterial Caliber, *Br. J. Ophthalmol.*, 50:21, 1966.
8. Dollery, C. T., Hodge, J. V., and Hill, D. W.: The Response of Normal Retinal Blood Vessels to Angiotensin and Noradrenaline, *J. Physiol.*, 165:500, 1963.
9. Ballantyne, A. J.: The State of the Retina in Diabetes Mellitus, *Trans. Ophthalmol. Soc. U.K.*, 66:503, 1966.
10. Kennedy, J. E., and Wise, G. N.: Clinicopathologic Correlation of Retinal Lesions: 2. Retinochoroidal Vascular Anastomosis in Uveitis, *Am. J. Ophthalmol.*, 71:1221, 1971.
11. Bloom, W., and Fawcett, D. W.: "A Textbook of Histology," 10th ed., W. B. Saunders Company, Philadelphia, 1975, p. 397.
12. Hogan, M. J., and Feeney, L.: The Ultrastructure of the Retinal Blood Vessels, *J. Ultrastruct. Res.*, 9:10, 1963.
13. Brownstein, S., Font, R. L., and Alper, M. G.: Atheromatous Plaques of the Retinal Blood Vessels: Histologic Confirmation of Ophthalmoscopically Visible Lesions, *Arch. Ophthalmol.*, 90:49, 1973.
14. Rosenberg, P. R., Uliss, A. E., Friedland, G. H., Harris, C. A., Small, C. B., and Klein, R. S.: Acquired Immunodeficiency Syndrome—Ophthalmic Manifestations in Ambulatory Patients, *Ophthalmology*, 90:874, 1983.
15. The Diabetic Retinopathy Study Research Group: Four Risk Factors for Severe Visual Loss in Diabetic Retinopathy. The Third Report, *Arch. Ophthalmol.*, 97:654, 1979.
16. Hodge, V. J., and Dollery, C. T.: Retinal Soft Exudates: A Clinical Study by Color and Fluorescence Photography. *Q. J. Med.*, 33:117, 1964.
17. Klien, B. A., and Olwin, J. H.: A Survey on the Pathogenesis of Retinal Venous Occlusion, *Arch. Ophthalmol.*, 56:207, 1956.
18. The Diabetic Retinopathy Study Research Group: Photocoagulation Treatment in Proliferative Diabetic Retinopathy. The Second Report of Diabetic Retinopathy Study Findings, *Ophthalmology*, 85:82, 1978.
19. Scheie, H. G.: Evaluation of Ophthalmoscopic Changes of Hypertension and Arteriolar Sclerosis, *Arch. Ophthalmol.*, 49:117, 1953.
20. Keith, N. M., Wagener, H. P., and Barker, N. W.: Some Different Types of Essential Hypertension: Their Course and Prognosis, *Am. J. Med. Sci.*, 197:332, 1939.
21. Davis, B. A., Crook, J. E., Vestal, R. E., and Oates, J. A.: Prevalence of Renovascular Hypertension in Patients with Grade III or IV Hypertensive Retinopathy, *N. Engl. J. Med.*, 301:1273, 1979.

13

Physical Examination of the Chest, Abdomen, and Extremities

J. Willis Hurst, M.D. Paul H. Robinson, M.D.

This is not the proper place to discuss the details of the physical examination of the chest, abdomen, and extremities. This important subject is discussed in other books.[1] It *is* the place to emphasize that portion of the examination that relates to the cardiovascular system and to clarify a few common misconceptions that are related to it.

The Physical Examination of the Chest

The shape of the thorax is important. It may be "barrel-shaped," suggesting severe emphysema. There may be a skeletal abnormality, such as kyphoscoliosis or a depressed sternum, that may distort the ECG, produce heart murmurs, or cause cardiac dysfunction.

The physical examination of the lungs is a crude method for detecting disease, but it must be learned and utilized for two reasons: (1) It is painless and noninvasive; it is easy to percuss the chest and listen to the lungs because no special equipment other than a stethoscope is needed. Since a chest x-ray cannot be made hourly or even daily, the abnormalities found on physical examination often determine *when* an x-ray of the chest should be made. (2) Although the chest x-ray is superior to the physical examination in detecting the presence of congestive heart failure, pleural fluid, pulmonary infiltrates, and pneumothorax, the chest x-ray will *not* detect wheezing or a pleural rub. The latter two conditions are detected only by auscultation of the lungs.

The patient with pulmonary infarction may have a pleural friction rub. Pleural fluid may be produced by pulmonary infarction or heart failure. Pleural fluid due to heart failure is usually located in the right pleural space. When pleural fluid is located on the left side or is predominant on the left, it is wise to consider a cause other than (or in addition to) heart failure. For example, pulmonary infarction may be responsible for such a clinical finding. A pneumothorax may develop as part of spontaneous mediastinal emphysema or may be secondary to a procedure. Increased resonance and decreased breath sounds may be due to pulmonary emphysema. Signs of pulmonary consolidation may be due to pneumonia or pulmonary infarction. Wheezing and rales may be due to bronchial disease. Heart failure may be associated with rales in the lung bases, wheezing, and pleural fluid. On the other hand, heart failure is frequently not associated with rales. In fact, interstitial pulmonary edema does not produce rales. Experienced and skilled clinicians rarely use the presence of rales to diagnose heart failure. They use other clues that have a higher predictive value to determine the presence or absence of heart failure.

The Physical Examination of the Abdomen

The size of the abdominal aorta must be determined in every patient. The technique of doing this is discussed in Chap. 64. An abdominal aortic aneurysm may be overlooked because the physician may ignore the area above the umbilicus and concentrate on the area below the umbilicus.

Patients with heart disease may develop certain abnormalities of the abdomen. The liver may become large and tender in patients with heart failure or constrictive pericarditis. The liver edge may move in patients with tricuspid regurgitation. Such movement is due to downward displacement of the liver by a column of regurgitant blood and to engorgement of the liver during systole.

The spleen may become palpable in patients with severe heart failure and in patients with infective endocarditis. Splenomegaly is a poor sign of heart failure or endocarditis since heart failure must be severe and endocarditis must be present a long time before the spleen enlarges. An x-ray of the abdomen may detect splenomegaly that is not detected on physical examination.

When ascites occurs, one should consider cirrhosis of the liver since this is the most common cause of the condition. Patients with heart failure alone may have ascites, but this is less common today than it was prior to the modern era of diuretic therapy. Patients with destruction of the tricuspid valve by infective endocarditis may develop grotesque systolic pulsation of the internal jugular veins in the neck; a large, moving, and pulsating liver; and ascites. When there is evidence of minimal heart failure and considerable ascites, it is wise to consider the presence of both heart failure and separate cirrhosis of the liver. Constrictive pericarditis is still common, but it is discovered earlier now than it was formerly, and therefore ascites is not commonly due to this condition. The "old-fashioned" variety of constrictive pericarditis still occurs, however, and it is wise to consider the possibility of its presence when ascites is out of proportion to the peripheral edema.

The heart is of normal size or only slightly enlarged, a pericardial "knock" is heard, and there are strutted external neck veins with a rapid *x* or *y* descent in the internal jugular vein pulsation. Restrictive cardiomyopathy can mimic constrictive pericarditis in that there may be ascites, strutted neck veins, and little or no leg edema. The heart is usually large in patients with restrictive cardiomyopathy.

A peripheral arteriovenous fistula produces a continuous murmur. When the fistula is in the abdomen, the murmur may be heard over the abdomen. Fistulas due to trauma and surgery may occur. For example, a fistula between the renal artery and renal vein may produce a continuous murmur which is heard in the region of the kidney. The best example of a continuous murmur heard in a region which is adjacent to the abdomen is the one heard over the lumbar area following lumbar disk surgery.

A systolic bruit may be heard over the kidney areas and may signify obstructive lesions in the renal arteries. A systolic bruit may be heard over the abdominal aorta, but its presence is not sufficient to make a diagnostic decision regarding disease of the aorta.

The Physical Examination of the Extremities

Many diagnostic clues can be identified in the hands and feet. (See Chap. 8.)

The physical examination of the aorta and the arteries and veins of the upper and lower extremities is discussed in Chaps. 64, 65, and 68. The identification of arterial disease and thrombophlebitis is important. Atherosclerosis of the peripheral arteries may produce intermittent claudication of the arch of the foot, calf, thigh, or buttock and, in extreme form, may result in tissue damage of the toes. Peripheral atherosclerosis is a risk factor for ischemic heart disease—its presence increases the likelihood of coronary atherosclerosis (Chap. 45). Thrombophlebitis may produce pain in the calf or thigh, or edema, and thus should act as a warning that pulmonary emboli may occur.

Edema of the lower extremities has been the time-honored sign of heart failure. Edema is a late sign of heart failure, however, and its predictive value as a diagnostic sign is poor. Considerable heart failure may be present and edema may be absent. Edema of the lower extremities may be due to local factors such as varicose veins or thrombophlebitis. Under such circumstances, the edema may occur only in one leg.

Edema may be the result of tight garters and venous stasis secondary to a long trip in an airplane. Edema may be due to primary kidney disease with its associated salt and water retention. When edema is found, the physician should think first in terms of local factors and, if local factors can be excluded, then think in terms of salt and water retention. It is then necessary to determine the cause of the salt and water retention by finding evidence of heart disease and other signs of heart failure or evidence of primary renal disease. The salt and water retention of heart failure is due to renal dysfunction related to a poor cardiac output and the alteration of certain levels of hormones. (See Chap. 20.) The salt and water retention due to primary renal disease is due to disease within the kidney itself.

Reference

1. Walker, H. K., Hall, W. D., and Hurst, J. W.: "Clinical Methods: The History, Physical, and Laboratory Examinations," 2d ed., Butterworths, Boston, 1980, pp. 200, 628–640, 726, 740–775.

14

The Resting Electrocardiogram

Agustin Castellanos, M.D. Robert J. Myerburg, M.D.

The interpretation of the electrocardiogram is not a matter of memorizing a few characteristic patterns; there are many unusual variations and combinations of electrocardiographic phenomena which must be studied, analyzed and correlated one with another and with other available data before any meaningful conclusion is possible. These situations demand some acquaintance with the electrical and physiological principles by which they are determined.

Frank N. Wilson, 1952*

In the early thirties, Frank N. Wilson undertook the arduous task of translating electrocardiographic theory into clinical medicine. The contributions made by Wilson and those whom he inspired have been so great that, despite the extensive amount of work done on this subject, most of what is known about the resting electrocardiogram (ECG) can be directly or indirectly attributed to them.[1–4] A thorough knowledge of conventional theory is fundamental in the eighties to avoid serious conceptual misunderstandings when attempting to correlate electrocardiographic information with that provided by the various presently available and soon to be introduced noninvasive methods, such as nuclear magnetic resonance, used to study the electromechanical and metabolic activity of the heart.

Classically, there are two major subdivisions of nonexercise, nonambulatory electrocardiography:[1] (1) the study of the resting 12-lead ECG, which deals with the electric forces produced by the atria and ventricles during the cardiac cycle as recorded at the body surface, and (2) the analysis of arrhythmias. The former will be discussed in this chapter and the latter is dealt with in Chap. 26. Likewise, the source of cardiac electrical activity, which resides at the cellular level, is described in Chap. 25.

Normal Activation of the Heart

After emerging from the sinus node, the cardiac impulse propagates throughout the atria in its journey toward the atrioventricular (AV) node. The *normal* P wave (resulting from activation of both atria) is a consequence of, but does not directly represent, sinus node activity. During sinus rhythm the right atrium is activated before the left atrium.[3] This explains why high-fidelity recordings of the P waves of some normal persons show a small notch at the top. The latter simply reflects the normal asynchrony existing between both atria. Because of the anatomic position of the node, atrial depolarization can be represented by a vector pointing inferiorly, to the left, and somewhat posteriorly.[4] The normal P waves are always positive in leads I, II, aV_F, and V_3 to V_6 and always negative in lead aV_R. According to the anatomic position of the heart, the P wave may be diphasic in leads V_1, III, and aV_L or negative in the latter lead. Atrial repolarization, also called T_a, is directly opposite in polarity to the P wave. It is usually not seen because it coincides with PR segment and QRS complex. Since the cardiac impulse reaches the AV node before the end of atrial depolarization, arrival of excitation at the AV node occurs at an undetermined moment (which can be roughly estimated by catheter recordings) within, but before the end of, the P wave. The latter is further described in *Update V: The Heart*.[4a]

Activation of the ordinary ventricular muscle (onset of the QRS complex) starts as soon as the impulse emerging from the most distal ramifications of the bundle branches depolarizes a sufficiently large number of cells.[3,4] Therefore, the PR interval (used to estimate AV conduction time) includes conduction through the "true" AV structures (AV node, His bundle, bundle branches, and main divisions of the left bundle branch) as well as through those parts of the atria located between the sinus and AV nodes.[5]

Conventional ECG theory holds that the onset of ventricular depolarization (given by the beginning of the normal q wave) reflects activation of the left side of the interventricular septum.[1,3–13] This has been attributed to the fact that the left bundle system is shorter than the right bundle branch. In addition, the large, fanlike distribution of the terminal ramifications of the fascicles of the left bundle branch on the left septal surface produces activation of a greater number of ordinary muscle cells per unit of time. For this reason, the normal initial vectors (0.01 to 0.02 s) point from left to right, therefore explaining the small q wave in lead V_6 and the small r wave in lead V_1. After the cardiac impulse descending through the right bundle branch reaches the right septal surface, the interventricular septum is activated in both directions. Septal activation is thereafter encompassed within, or neutralized by, free wall activation. The most distal ramifications of both bundle branches (Purkinje fibers) form networks within the subendocardial regions of both ventricular walls. The latter are activated as soon as the multiple ramifications emerge from the Purkinje fibers. The greater number of ordinary muscle fibers on the thicker left ventricular free wall explains why events of the left ventricular free wall overpower those of the interventricular septum and right ventricular free wall.

*Reproduced with the permission of the publisher.

Ventricular Depolarization and Repolarization

In the human heart, for example, in the free left ventricular wall, the *sequence* of ventricular depolarization is from endocardium to epicardium. Depolarization has been described as a moving wave with the *positive charges in front* of the negative charges.[2,6–9] An electrode, such as V_6, overlying the epicardium of the left ventricle will record a positivity because it consistently faces positive charges throughout the entire depolarization sequence.[2,6–9]

On the other hand, the *sequence* of ventricular repolarization is from epicardium to endocardium. However, the *negative charges travel in front* since repolarization tends to reestablish the resting, polarized state of the previously depolarized cells. As a consequence, V_6 will record a positive deflection (T wave) because it constantly faces positive charges throughout the entire repolarization sequence[2,6–9] The earlier epicardial onset of repolarization has been attributed to the shorter duration of repolarization that epicardial cells have in comparison with endocardial cells.[4,7,9] Thus, repolarization finishes at the epicardium while it still has not been completed at the endocardium. Hence, the sequence of repolarization is, as previously stated, from epicardium to endocardium.

Einthoven Triangle Hypothesis and Bipolar Standard Leads

In 1913, Einthoven, Fahr, and de Waart developed a method of studying the electrical activity of the heart by representing it graphically in a two-dimensional geometric figure, namely, an equilateral triangle.[14] While this representation is not strictly mathematically true, it has provided the clinician with a practical point with which to work. In spite of the many objections to the theory, it still stands.[6,12] There are several simplifying assumptions upon which Einthoven's hypothesis is founded:[12,14]

- The body is a homogeneous volume conductor. Although the conductivity of the various tissues is not the same, the differences are not great enough to invalidate this assumption.
- The sum of all the electric forces, or the mean of all the forces generated during the cardiac cycle, can be considered as originating in a dipole located in the electrical center of the heart.
- Electrodes placed on the right arm, left arm, and left leg are used to pick up the potential variations on these extremities. Standard (bipolar) leads I, II, and III are obtained by recording, respectively, the potential differences between left arm and right arm, left leg and right arm, and left leg and left arm. These leads record potential variations in the frontal plane only.
- Attachment between the limb electrodes form the apices of an equilateral triangle with reference to a dipole located in its center. Anatomically, of course, these extremities in no sense form an equilateral triangle. But if the cardiac field does originate in a central dipole, then the distances from it to the extremities are great enough to be assumed to approach infinity.
- The position of the electrodes on the forearms and limbs corresponds to a position in the root of the corresponding limb. For example, an electrode in the right forearm records the electrical activity which reaches the right shoulder. It should be pointed out that when the electrodes are placed proximally to the roots of the extremities they lose their relatively "far" distance from the heart. Hence, Einthoven's equilateral triangle theory does not hold. This explains why leads placed proximally to the roots of the extremities, such as those used for coronary care unit and Holter monitoring, by being only "equivalent" to the corresponding bipolar leads, are in some cases markedly different than the "true" standard bipolar leads.

Wilson Central Terminal

The sum of the potentials from right arm, left arm, and left leg is equal to zero throughout the cardiac cycle with respect to any point at the body surface.[2,3,6,12] If leads are connected to electrodes in these points, their potential is zero with respect to any other electrode on the body surface. When this common point—Wilson's central terminal—is attached to the negative pole of the electrocardiographic machine through 5000-Ω resistors and an "exploring" electrode is connected to the positive pole, the potential variations recorded will be those of the positive pole only. A lead taken by this method is called a *unipolar lead.* Actually, the potential of the central terminal is not zero because the right arm, left arm, and left leg are not equidistant from each other and from the heart; the body tissues vary in resistance; and the heart and the extremities do not lie in exactly the same plane in the body. The potential of the central terminal has been said to average around 0.3 mV.[6]

Unipolar Extremity Leads

Unipolar extremity leads were initially recorded by a system in which the central terminal of Wilson constituted the indifferent electrode and the exploring electrode was one of the three limb electrodes. These leads were known as VR, VL, and VF. At present, unipolar extremity leads are obtained by disconnecting the input to the central terminal of Wilson from the extremity being explored. This results in $1\frac{1}{2}$-fold increase in the observed morphological pattern. These augmented (a) extremity leads are the ones usually used for clinical electrocardiography and are labeled aV_R, aV_L, and aV_F.[6,12]

Electrical Axis

The *electrical axis* may be defined as a vector originating in the center of Einthoven's equilateral triangle.[12] A vector is a mathematical value expressed as an arrow which has direction, sense, and magnitude. The direction of the electrical axis is also the direction of the activation process as projected in the plane of the limb leads. Its length represents the manifest potential of the dipole in the center of the triangle.

These general considerations apply either to the instantaneous electrical axis (vector indicating the direction of the impulse at the instant at which it is determined) or to the mean electrical axis (which is the resultant of all instantaneous electrical axes). Although the mean electrical axis can be calculated from any of the deflections of the ECG (P, T, or QRS) it is generally used in reference to the QRS.

There are many methods for determining the mean electrical axis. The one recommended by electrocardiographers of the classical school consists of calculating the net areas enclosed by the QRS complexes in leads I, II, and III.[3,6,10,12] The net area is the absolute sum of the positive and negative areas of the QRS complex in the corresponding lead. One of the drawbacks of this method is that the absolute values of the net area cannot be determined *accurately* by inspection. Since the absolute magnitude of the electrical axis is not of fundamental clinical importance, it has been recommended that arbitrary units be used.

When this is done the results can be counterchecked by using Einthoven's law. For example, if in a given case lead I is +4 units, lead II is +2 units, and lead III is −2 units, the calculation is accurate since the sum of leads I and III [+4 + (−2)] = lead II (+2). After having determined the net area, the results are plotted on the sides of the triangle and perpendiculars dropped from two or from all three leads. The perpendiculars will meet at a point away from the center of the triangle. A line drawn from the latter to the former defines the mean electrical axis.

A simpler, though less precise, method of calculating the quadrant (or parts of a quadrant) in which the electrical axis is located consists of using the maximal QRS deflections in leads I and aV_F and, when necessary, in lead II (Fig. 14-1). This method is inexact from the mathematical viewpoint, but has the value of simplicity.[13]

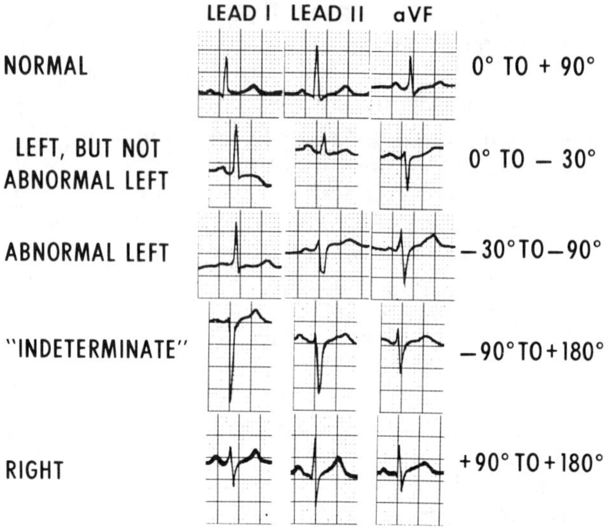

FIGURE 14-1 Determination of the quadrant, or parts of the left superior quadrant, in which the electrical axis can be located according to maximal ventricular deflections. The "indeterminate" quadrant is also called the *right superior* or *northwest* quadrant.

Unipolar Precordial (Chest) Leads

Since the dipolar theory was from the early days of electrocardiography applied to the standard and unipolar extremity leads, it appeared logical to extend that concept to the chest leads as well. Thus arose the vectorial approach to the chest leads, which, when applied to the 12-lead ECG, can be properly called *vectorial electrocardiography*.[15–17] This method is no doubt the most widely used in ECG teaching and interpretation throughout the world. Instantaneous or mean (maximal) vectors are constructed with the standard and unipolar extremity leads being utilized for frontal plane projections and the chest leads being used for projections in the horizontal plane. All vectors are considered to originate in the previously mentioned electrical center of the heart. Although "spatial" vectorcardiography is not discussed in this chapter, an important difference between it and vectorial electrocardiography must be understood to appreciate the morphology resulting from improperly placed, or mispositioned, chest leads. Both *frontal plane spatial vectorcardiographic* projections and *frontal plane vector electrocardiographic* projections (construed from the standard leads) only record forces moving either superiorly or inferiorly and to the left or to the right. On the contrary, whereas the *horizontal plane spatial vectorcardiographic projections* are said to exclusively record electric forces moving anteriorly or posteriorly and to the left or to the right, the *horizontal plane vector electrocardiographic* projections may also record forces moving inferiorly or superiorly. The latter occurs because normal chest leads are not, even in theory, located at the same horizontal level at which the electrical center of the heart is located.[17] What is important is that any unipolar chest lead facing positive electric charges will yield positive (QRS, ST, or T) deflections, while those facing negative charges will result in negative deflections (below the baseline).

Electrocardiographic "Injury"

In orthodox electrocardiographic language *injury* implies *abnormal* ST-segment changes; *necrosis, ab-*

normal Q waves; and *ischemia, symmetrical* T-wave inversion (or elevation).[2–8,10–12,13] Following the work of Wilson et al.,[18] several authors consider that electrocardiographic injury occurs because the affected cells are unable to maintain their normal polarization during diastole.[2–8,10,11,19] Various hypotheses have been postulated to explain how this diastolic hypopolarization, or generalized diastolic depolarization, is manifested as abnormal ST-segment shifts in the surface ECG.

One hypothesis is based on the existence of a diastolic current of injury. During the control (diastolic) period, both membrane resting potential and the surface ECG baseline are at their normal levels. At the onset of injury the resting intracellular potential decreases (for example, from −90 to −70 mV) and the ECG baseline shifts below its preinjury level. Because the injured cells leak negative ions, their *exterior* becomes relatively negative (or less positive) than that of the normal cells. Thus, a current of injury flows between the negative ("injured") zone and the positive (normal) region. This produces a negative displacement of the surface electrocardiographic *baseline* in the leads facing the injured region.

In the surface ECG, depolarization (by virtue of the electrical negativization of the nonaffected area) practically reduces the potential difference between noninjured and injured regions. Therefore, the ST segment remains at the preinjury level, which is relatively *elevated* in reference to the injury baseline. In consequence, the ST segment appears to be abnormally displaced above the latter. Note that the apparent presence of a systolic current of injury actually reflects disappearance of the diastolic current of injury. Finally, after the end of repolarization, the current of injury between injured and noninjured regions is reestablished and the ECG baseline is again depressed (as it was immediately before depolarization). Since the precise moment at which injury starts is not recorded in the surface ECG, the baseline that is almost invariably recorded is the postinjury baseline, which has been placed at an apparently adequate position by the recording instrument or by the ECG technician.

It also has been shown that the abnormal ST-segment elevation in leads facing the affected zone does not merely represent the (passive) return of the baseline to its preinjury level, but that it reflects a true, active, positive displacement. Thus, when depolarization of both normal and injured regions has occurred, the surface of the normal cells, on account of their greater initial polarization, will be able to accumulate more negative ions. Hence, the normal regions become more negative than the injured regions, which are relatively more positive. In consequence, the ST segment becomes actively elevated above and beyond the preinjured baseline because of the relative potential difference existing at the end of depolarization. Most likely injury reflects both disappearance of diastolic baseline shifts plus active ST elevation.[20,21]

The mechanism of abnormal ST-segment elevation in anatomically defined ventricular aneurysms has not been fully established. Some authors consider that it results from the earlier repolarization of a ring of persistently viable (but nevertheless affected) tissue surrounding the aneurysm.[7] Other investigators consider that chronic ST-segment elevation reflects functional (echocardiographic) dyskinesia, thus not necessarily being due to a pathological ventricular aneurysm.[22]

It is important to remember that, according to the concept of vectorial electrocardiography, injury can be represented by an ST-segment vector pointing *toward* the injured zone.

Abnormal Q Waves

Abnormal Q waves appearing several hours after total occlusion of a coronary artery result from the necrosis secondary to the decreased blood supply. The number of affected cells has to be large enough so as to produce changes reflected at the body surface. In general, the depth of the Q wave is proportional to wall thickness involvement.[4] Thus, in leads I and V_4 to V_6, a QS complex reflects transmural necrosis. The duration of the Q wave is proportional to the extent of the area of necrosis parallel to the epicardial surface.[4] If the latter starts in the subendocardium and extends toward, but does not quite reach, the epicardium, the corresponding leads will record QR or Qr complexes depending upon the amount of living tissue located between dead tissue and recording electrode. Therefore, abnormal Q waves may occur in infarctions which are not completely transmural.[4] In this chapter, however, abnormal Q waves will be considered as reflecting transmural involvement.

Abnormal Q waves seen very early in the course of the clinical entity known as acute myocardial infarction or in Prinzmetal's variant angina may not be due to anatomic necrosis. For instance, when the degree of cellular affectation (injury) is severe enough to produce a significant degree of hypopolarization (to, let us say, around −60 mV), the cells become electrically inexcitable even though they are not anatomically (irreversibly) necrotic.[4,5,13] Hence, abnormal Q waves occur. Because the cells are only severely affected (significantly hypopolarized) but not necrotic, interventions (pharmacologic or mechanical) improving cellular metabolism and oxygenation can restore the normal polarization. If these cells again become excitable, then the abnormal Q waves disappear or vanish. On the other hand, Q waves appearing several hours after the onset of an episode of chest pain leading to the clinical diagnosis of myocardial infarction reflect anatomic necrosis resulting from persistent lack of blood flow. More recently, it has been observed that Q waves due to anatomic necrosis can appear earlier in time, almost immediately after reperfusion. These Q waves, which represent cellular death due to sudden reperfusion, can be distinguished pathologically from necrosis due to sustained deprivation of blood supply. In any case, as time goes on, the necrotic cells eventually are replaced by fibrous tissue. Then the abnormal Q waves reflect fibrosis, not necrosis. It should be stressed that chronic, fibrotic Q waves, although most frequently due to coronary artery disease, may also result from any process, such as severe myocarditis, capable of producing death of a sufficiently large number of myocardial cells.

Electrocardiographic "Ischemia"

Symmetrical T waves (inverted or upright) characteristic of electrocardiographic ischemia have been considered to reflect a type, or degree, of cellular affectation resulting only in action potentials of increased duration.[4,8] Because the QT interval recorded at the body surface can be considered as the sum of all action potentials (that is, of the QT intervals of individual cells), any process (such as electrocardiographic ischemia) which increases action potential duration will cause prolongation of ventricular repolarization and the QT interval.

The previously mentioned, normal, shorter repolarization of epicardial cells (due to their shorter action potentials in comparison with that of the endocardial cells) and the concomitant epicardial-to-endocardial spread of repolarization with the negative charge in front and the positive charges facing the epicardium explain why V_5 and V_6 normally show positive T waves.

Thus, in subendocardial ischemia the increased duration of the action potentials occurs in a group of cells where it was already longer than in the epicardium. Because this is an exaggeration of normal, repolarization, though taking a longer time than usual, still spreads from epicardium to endocardium. In consequence, the QT interval is prolonged and the T wave appears symmetrically positive. On the other hand, the increase in action potential duration that occurs in epicardial ischemia results not only in delayed repolarization (QT prolongation) but also in a change in the sequence of repolarization, which now starts at the earlier repolarized endocardium, thereafter spreading toward the epicardium with the negative charges in front. The latter produces the characteristic symmetrical T-wave inversion.

Transmural Myocardial Infarction

The most frequently detected initial ECG manifestation of transmural myocardial infarction is abnormal ST-segment elevation in the leads reflecting the electrical activity of the affected zone. In addition, the T waves become taller and appear as an upward extension of the rising ST segments.[4,10] These T waves have been called "hyperacute" when appearing before the ST-segment elevation.[10] The abnormal Q waves first seen coexist several hours later with ST-segment elevation. Subsequently, if the ECG evolution is "typical," there is a gradual return of the ST segment to the baseline with the T wave becoming progressively deeper. The model sequence described above is by no means invariable since time relations cannot be predicted with absolute accuracy because of the differences which exist among patients. However, there is always some evolution along similar lines.[10] Schamroth considers that when ST elevation persists for 6 months or more, an anatomic ventricular aneurysm is most probably present.[7] Yet an anatomic aneurysm or its functional, echocardiographic equivalent may exist if only chronic abnormal Q waves are recorded.[13]

Location of the Site of Transmural Myocardial Infarctions

Table 14-1 shows the location of the infarction according to the leads in which abnormal Q waves appear.[23] In addition, it depicts other processes, which by also producing abnormal Q waves of different etiologies, result in false patterns of myocardial infarction. It has to be understood that in the classification of the location of an infarction by the leads where abnormal Q waves occur, the "affected" zone produced by the occlusion or spasm of a given vessel may (and in fact does) extend beyond the area of necrosis. For example, a single lesion of the posterior descending coronary artery may be located so

TABLE 14-1 Electrocardiographic Location of Infarction Sites according to the Leads Showing Abnormal Q Waves

Site	Leads	False Patterns
Inferior (diaphragmatic)	II, III, aV_F	WPW type B; IHSS*
"True" posterior (posterobasal)	V_1†	WPW type A; right ventricular hypertrophy; "atypical" incomplete right bundle branch block
Inferoposterior	II, III, aV_F, V_1†	WPW type A; IHSS
Anteroseptal	V_1–V_2	Left ventricular hypertrophy; chronic lung disease; left bundle branch block
Anterolateral	I, aV_L, V_4–V_6	IHSS; ventricular septal defect
Extensive anterior	I, aV_L, V_1–V_6	
High anterolateral	I, aV_L	
Apical (apicoanterior)	V_2–V_4	
Posterolateral	V_1, V_4–V_6	IHSS; WPW type A; Duchenne's muscular dystrophy

*Idiopathic hypertrophic subaortic stenosis.
†Tall R wave, reciprocal to changes in "indicative" back lead.

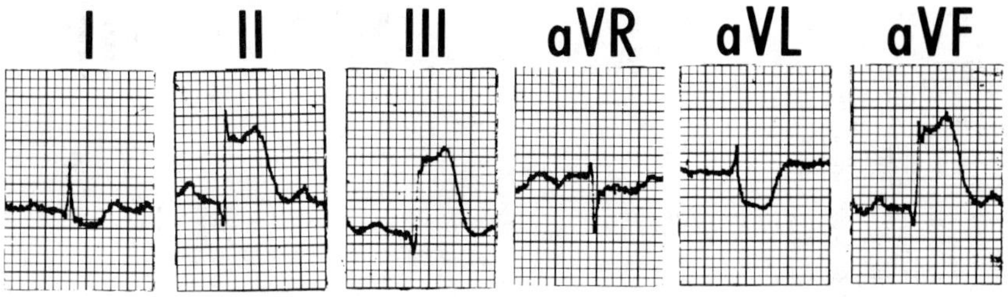

FIGURE 14-2 Acute inferior (diaphragmatic) myocardial infarction showing "indicative" ST-segment elevation in leads whose positive poles face the inferior wall (II, III, and aV_F). Reciprocal changes are seen in the diametrically opposed leads (I and aV_L) located in the same (frontal) plane.

as to produce necrosis and injury in the inferior (diaphragmatic) wall but only injury in the posterobasal (true posterior) wall, both being a consequence of the same occlusion. Thus, the affected zone involves (though in different ways) the inferior as well as the posterobasal (true posterior) walls. In other words, the region where *normal* Q waves and abnormal ST-segment elevation are present is not one to which the infarction (defined by presence of abnormal Q waves) extended but is part of the originally affected zone. If we classify the infarction as inferior (the site of abnormal Q waves), it is incorrect to state either that an extension to the posterobasal wall occurred or that the affected zone was exclusively inferior. For, as previously stated, the affected zone included both inferior and posterobasal (true posterior) walls, in such a way that the former was necrotic and injured and the latter only injured.

Reciprocal ST-Segment Changes

According to the theory of vectorial electrocardiography, in a posteroinferior infarction with abnormal Q waves and ST-segment elevation limited to this wall (that is, *without* the "affectation" of the posterobasal, true posterior wall), the reciprocal ST-segment changes will occur in diametrically opposed leads located in the *same* plane. For example, "indicative" ST elevation in leads III and aV_F, which record the electrical activity of the inferior (posteroinferior or diaphragmatic) wall, yield "reciprocal" ST-segment depression in leads I and aV_L because they face the superior (anterolateral) wall (Fig. 14-2).[10] For this reason, an inferior wall injury not affecting the posterobasal wall cannot produce reciprocal changes in a lead, such as V_2, which is located in a plane perpendicular to the frontal plane. The perpendicularity between vertical lead aV_F and horizontal lead V_2 can also be seen in a left sagittal plane where lead aV_F faces the inferior (diaphragmatic wall) and lead V_2 the anteroseptal and posterobasal walls (Fig. 14-3, left).

In addition, as previously stated, the ST-segment vector of injury points toward the injured zone. As a consequence of this postulate ST-segment depression in lead V_2 may reflect injury in the anterior subendocardial wall as well as injury in the posterobasal or (true posterior) wall (Fig. 14-3, right). It should be emphasized that the ECG by itself cannot distinguish between these two possibilities. The differential diagnosis can perhaps best be done by myocardial imaging with ionic tracers with the patient in the left lateral position.

Subendocardial Myocardial Infarction

Although, as previously mentioned, abnormal Q waves can occur in subendocardial infarction, the "typical" pattern has been said to consist of abnormal ST-segment depression in all leads save aV_R, which shows ST-segment elevation (Fig. 14-4). Clas-

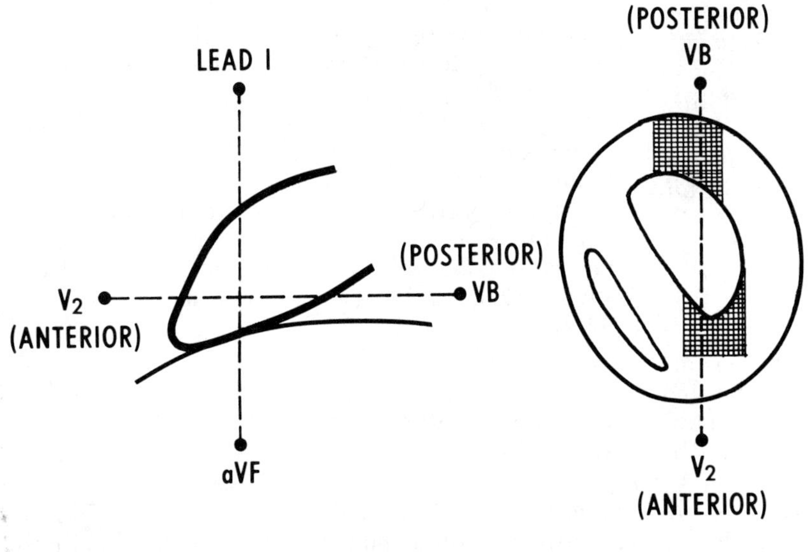

FIGURE 14-3 Diagrammatic representation explaining why, in a left lateral plane (left lateral x-ray view), anterior chest lead V_2 cannot be reciprocal to inferior lead aV_F (left). The right-hand schematic shows that ST-segment depression in anterior chest lead V_2 may reflect either anteroseptal wall subendocardial injury or posterobasal (true posterior) injury (transverse view from above corresponding to the electrovectorcardiographic horizontal plane). VB = unipolar chest lead (V) placed on the back of the thorax.

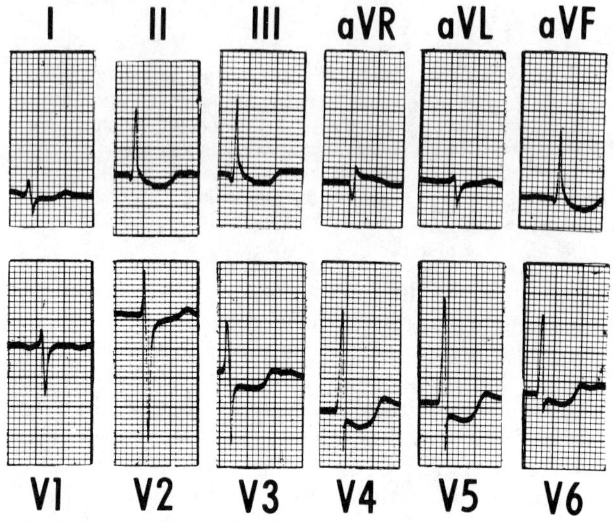

FIGURE 14-4 Classic subendocardial infarction manifested by abnormal ST-segment depression in all leads except aV_R, which shows ST-segment elevation. (*From L. Lemberg and A. Castellanos, Jr., "Vectorcardiography," 2d ed., Appleton-Century-Crofts, Inc., New York, 1975. Reproduced with permission from the publisher and authors.*)

sically, the abnormal repolarization changes persist for several days, rather than disappearing in minutes or hours as is the case with the transitory ST changes of the syndromes of coronary insufficiency.[23] Yet most cardiologists make the diagnosis of subendocardial infarction when clinical, enzymatic, and, at times, radionuclide findings are associated with not only the previously mentioned repolarization changes but also with nonspecific ST-segment and T-wave changes and, even, with a normal ECG.

Right Ventricular Infarction

According to Braat et al. an ST-segment elevation of 1 mm or more in lead V_4R in patients *with acute inferior myocardial infarction* (MI) has a sensitivity of 100 percent, a specificity of 87 percent, and a predictive accuracy of 92 percent for the diagnosis of right ventricular infarction (Fig. 14-5). These changes disappeared within 10 to 18 h after the onset of chest pain in 50 percent of their patients and after 72 h in the remaining patients.[24] Most authors agree that the ECG diagnosis of right ventricular infarction by the changes in V_4R has to be made within the initial 24 h.

Pericarditis

The electrocardiographic pattern of acute pericarditis not due to MI is produced by the associated epicardial myocarditis, which, in turn, results in diffuse epicardial "injury." The ST segments can be elevated in all leads except aV_R and, rarely, in V_1 (Fig. 14-6). Symmetrical T-wave inversion (due to epicardial "ischemia") usually develops after the ST

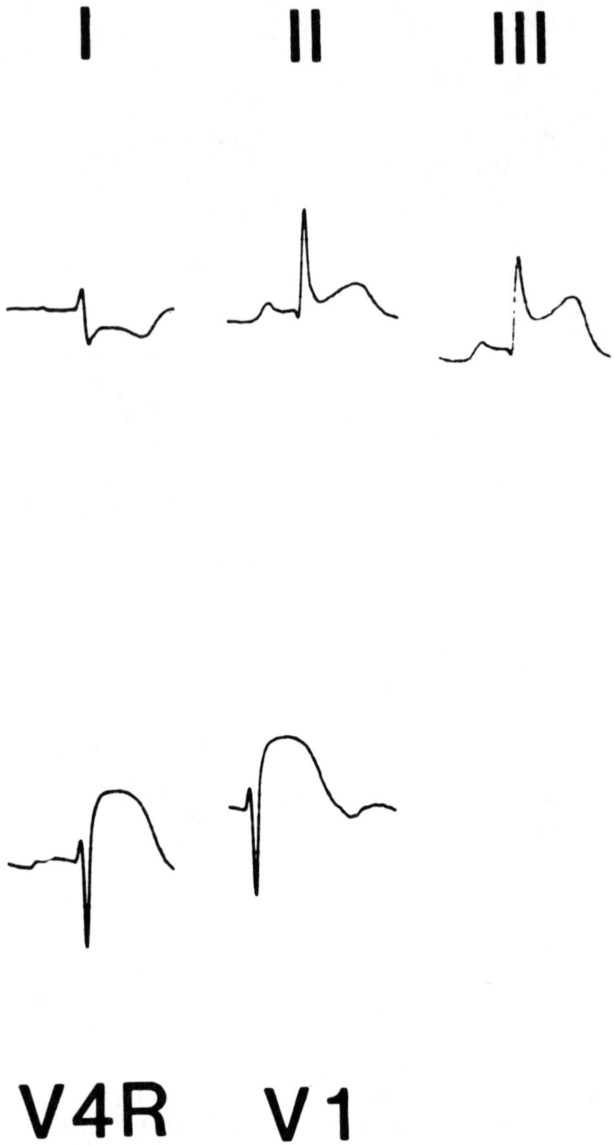

FIGURE 14-5 Acute inferior (diaphragmatic) myocardial infarction with coexisting right ventricular infarction. Note ST-segment elevation in lead V_4R (and also in V_1). The ECG was taken 4 h after the onset of chest pain.

segments have returned to the baseline (but can appear during the injury stage). Neither reciprocal ST-segment changes nor abnormal Q waves are seen. The ECG pattern of acute pericarditis has to be differentiated from that occurring in some normal young persons which is often referred to, incorrectly, as "early repolarization." The pattern consists, in the left chest leads, of normal ST-segment elevation associated with large R waves which have small r′ deflections starting *above* the baseline (Fig. 14-7).

Intraventricular Conduction Disturbances

The nomenclature of the different types of intraventricular conduction disturbances has produced

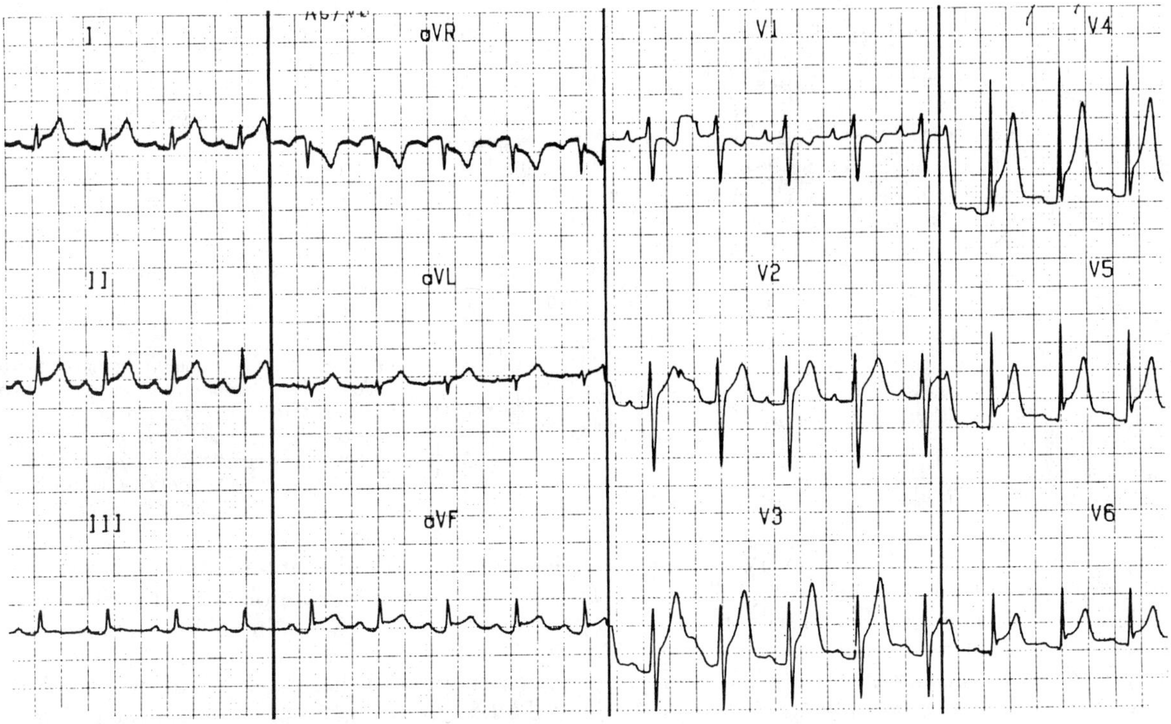

FIGURE 14-6 Acute nonspecific pericarditis showing ST-segment elevation in all leads except V_1 and aV_R.

almost insurmountable difficulties in the understanding of concepts.[5,13] In view of the multiple terms currently in use, it seems as if attempts to establish a consistently accepted nomenclature are practically utopian. Still, a working classification is necessary, primarily for didactic reasons, in order to make the proper concepts understandable.

Left Anterior Hemiblock

In left anterior hemiblock the posteroinferior regions of the left ventricular endocardium are activated abnormally before the anterosuperior left ventricular area.[5] After emerging from the posteroinferior division of the left bundle branch, the impulse first propagates in an inferior, rightward, and usually anterior direction for a short period of time. This orientation is responsible for the small q waves in leads I and aV_L and for the r waves in leads II, III, and aV_F (Fig. 14-8).

FIGURE 14-7 Normal variant. ST elevation (not due to pericarditis) in a healthy 21-year-old male. Note large R wave with a notch (arrows) in its terminal part appearing as a small r′ wave starting a few millimeters above the baseline.

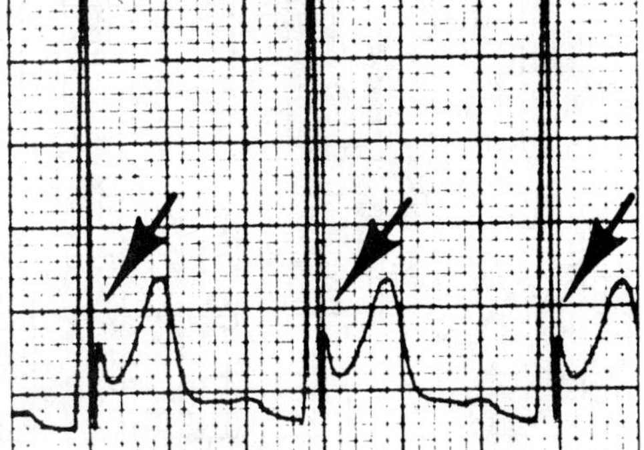

Although the posteroinferior division is "posterior" (dorsal) in reference to the anterosuperior division of the left bundle branch and the anterolateral wall of the left ventricle, it is "anterior" (ventral) in reference to the most posteriorly located part of the left ventricle.[13] This spatial location of the posteroinferior division explains why in left anterior hemiblock the right chest leads show (as in patients without left anterior hemiblock) a predominantly negative deflection, indicating that the activation front is moving in a posterior direction (away from V_1).[13]

If the posteroinferior division were to end at the posteriormost part of the left ventricle, the right chest leads would show predominantly positive deflections, since the activation front would be moving toward V_1 and V_2. From the electrocardiographic viewpoint, the divisions of the left branch behave more as if they were "superior" and "inferior" rather than anterior and posterior. For this reason, the most significant abnormalities produced by left anterior and left posterior hemiblock (in absence of "complete" right bundle branch block) occur in the standard and unipolar extremity leads rather than in the precordial leads.[13] "Pure" left anterior hemiblock usually produces abnormal left axis deviation, that is, an electrical axis pointing superiorly and to the left, between -30 and $-90°$ (Fig. 14-8). However, other processes can also produce abnormal left axis deviation (Table 14-2).[13] But in left anterior hemiblock the peak of the r wave in lead III occurs before the peak of the r wave in lead II.[25,26] Both aV_L and aV_R show predominantly positive deflec-

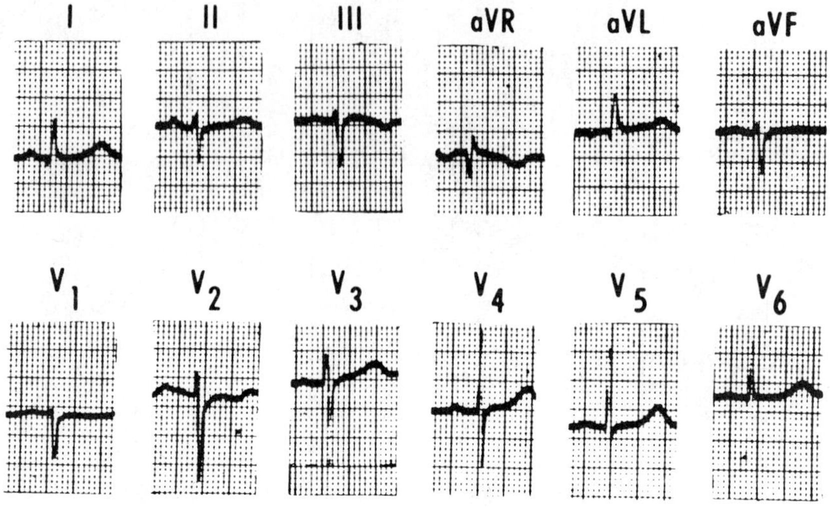

FIGURE 14-8 Left anterior hemiblock in a patient with "primary" conduction system disease. (*From A. Castellanos and R. J. Myerburg, "The Hemiblocks in Myocardial Infarction," Appleton-Century-Crofts, Inc., New York, 1976. Reproduced with permission from the publisher and authors.*)

tions, with the peak of the R wave in aV_L being inscribed before that of the R wave in aV_R.[25,26]

When left anterior hemiblock coexists with certain types of congenital right ventricular enlargements and extensive anterolateral MI, the electrical axis can be located in the "indeterminate" (right superior) quadrant. Evidently, the most constant feature of the axis deviation produced by left anterior hemiblock is its *superior* orientation, not necessarily its *superior and leftward* orientation (abnormal left axis deviation). The differentiation between the indeterminate electrical axis produced by complicated left anterior hemiblock and that resulting exclusively from some "atypical" types of right ventricular enlargement can best be made by lead aV_L (Fig. 14-9). Other causes of a right superior axis location are shown in Table 14-3.

Because of the multiple interconnections between the divisions of the left bundle branch system, the appearance of left anterior hemiblock does not increase QRS duration by more than 0.025 s. Therefore, a left anterior hemiblock pattern with prolonged QRS duration generally indicates the presence of additional conduction disturbances such as right bundle branch block, myocardial infarction, "focal" block, or combinations of the above (Figs. 14-10 and 14-11).[27]

The diagnosis of left anterior hemiblock in presence of MIs of different locations is shown in Fig. 14-12.

Left Posterior Hemiblock

In "pure" left posterior hemiblock, the impulse, after emerging from the unblocked anterosuperior divi-

TABLE 14-2 Causes of Abnormal (−30 to −90°) Left Axis Deviation

Cause	Characteristic Features
1. Left anterior hemiblock	rS complexes in lead II with positive T waves
2. Extensive inferior wall myocardial infarction	Qr complexes in lead II with ST-segment elevation and/or T-wave inversion
3. Extensive inferior wall myocardial infarction with possible left anterior hemiblock	QS pattern in leads II, III, and aV_F with ST-segment elevation and/or T-wave inversion
4. WPW syndrome, usually type B	Short PR interval; delta wave
5. Hyperkalemia	Wide QRS complexes; peaked T waves
6. Pulmonary emphysema	Low voltage; peaked P waves
7. Right ventricular apical pacing	Pacemaker spikes; predominantly negative ventricular deflection in V_1
8. Middle cardiac vein pacing	Pacemaker spikes; predominantly positive QRS deflection in V_1
9. Left coronary arteriography	Knowledge that dye was injected in left coronary artery

FIGURE 14-9 Indeterminate, right superior, or northwest electrical axis produced by right ventricular hypertrophy as seen in some patients with congenital heart disease (*top*) and in left anterior hemiblock (*bottom*). Lead aV_L is the most important lead to establish the differential diagnosis since in right ventricular hypertrophy this lead shows a predominantly negative deflection, whereas in left anterior hemiblock it shows a predominantly positive deflection.

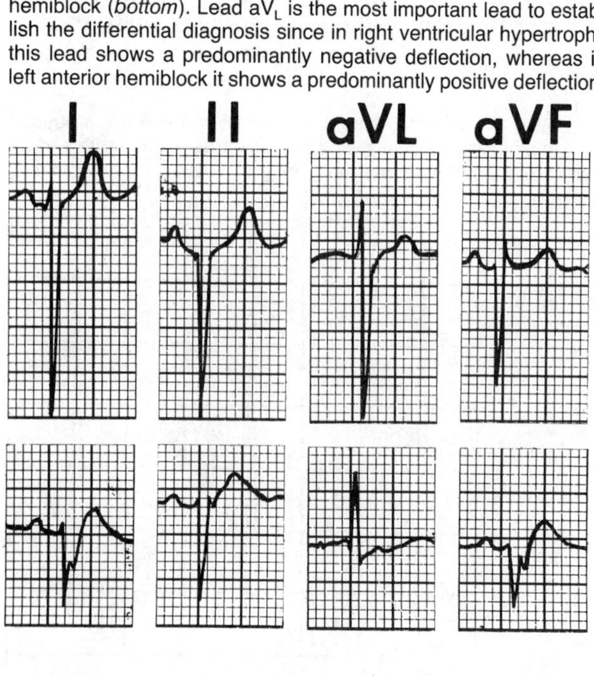

TABLE 14-3 Causes of Right Superior (Indeterminate or Northwest) Axis Deviation

Cause	Characteristic
1. Left anterior hemiblock with right ventricular hypertrophy	Radiological and echocardiographic evidence of right ventricular hypertrophy; predominantly positive deflection in lead aV_L
2. Left anterior hemiblock with extensive lateral myocardial infarction	Qr complexes in I
3. Right ventricular hypertrophy	rS complexes in aV_L; large, narrow R waves in V_1
4. Pulmonary emphysema	Low voltage, peaked P waves
5. S_1–S_2–S_3 pattern	Abnormal anatomic position of heart or thoracic chest wall abnormalities

sion, first moves in a superior, leftward, and somewhat anterior direction.[5] This produces the small q waves in leads II, III and aV_F, and the deep S waves in leads I and aV_L (Figs. 14-13 and 14-14, top row).

Radiological studies of the human heart in situ have shown that the paraseptal regions of the posteroinferior (diaphragmatic) surface of the anatomic *left* ventricle are located, spatially, more to the *right* than certain anterior portions of the anatomic right ventricle. Since the portions of the left ventricle that are spatially located to the right are less significant than those located superiorly, the degree of right axis deviation produced by pure left posterior hemiblock is of lesser magnitude than that of left axis deviation produced by left anterior hemiblock. The hallmark of left posterior hemiblock is, therefore, an "inferior" axis shift as much as "right" axis deviation (Fig. 14-14).

Because a similar sequence of ventricular activation can also occur in right ventricular hypertrophy, pleuropulmonary disease (acute or chronic), and extremely vertical anatomic heart positions due to a slender body build or chest wall deformities, it is evident that the diagnosis of pure left posterior hemiblock cannot be made from the ECG alone. Additional clinical, radiological, or pathological information is required for this purpose.[27] Other processes producing right axis deviation are given in Table 14-4.

The diagnosis of left posterior hemiblock in presence of MI is shown in Fig. 14-14 (middle and bottom rows).

FIGURE 14-10 Left anterior hemiblock with wide QRS complexes. Whereas *A* shows left anterior hemiblock with right bundle branch block, in *B* these conduction disturbances coexist with diffuse septal and inferoposterior fibrosis. Consequently, the expected small q wave and the wide S wave in lead I are not present. This pattern has been called "masquerading" bundle branch block since the standard leads suggest left bundle branch block while the chest leads are diagnostic of right bundle branch block.

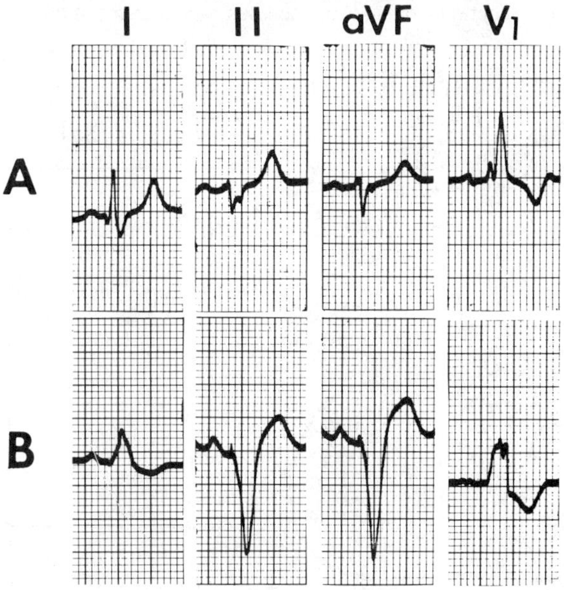

"Complete" Right Bundle Branch Block

It is now known that a complete right bundle branch block pattern (with QRS duration greater than 0.11 s) does not necessarily reflect the existence of a complete conduction block in the right branch. This pattern only indicates that the totality, or majority, of both ventricles are activated by the impulse emerging from the left branch.[13,28–31] Thus, a significant degree of conduction delay ("high-grade" or "incomplete" right bundle branch block) can produce a similar pattern. This is best seen when the QRS changes are intermittent, or when spontaneous (or induced) premature atrial beats produce different degrees of functional right bundle branch block. Whereas in Fig. 14-15 the next-to-last QRS complex has a duration compatible with the diagnosis of complete right bundle branch block, the last ventricular complex is even wider (0.15 s), therefore suggesting that the former was not due to a total conduction block in the right branch.

"Incomplete" Right Bundle Branch Block

For many years it has been recognized what has recently been proved with endocardial (catheter) and epicardial mapping, namely, that incomplete right bundle branch block patterns can be produced by the following:[27–41] (1) different degrees of conduction delays through the main trunk of the right bundle branch; (2) an increased conduction time through an elongated right bundle branch, stretched because of a concomitant enlargement of the right septal surface (as in congenital volume overloading of the right ventricle); (3) a diffuse Purkinje-myocardial delay due to right ventricular stretch or dilatation; (4) ventriculotomy- or disease-related interruption of the major ramifications of the right branch ("distal" right bundle branch block or "right hemiblocks"); (5) congenital variations of the distribution of the major distal ramifications resulting in a slight delay in activation of the crista supraventricularis.

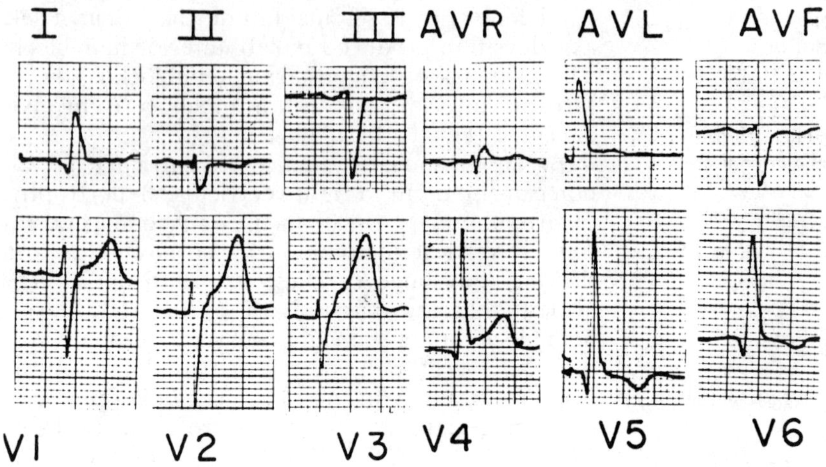

FIGURE 14-11 Left anterior hemiblock with wide QRS complexes due to coexisting left ventricular focal (anterolateral periinfarction) block. Note that there is an exclusively terminal delay (best seen in leads I and V_5) located to the left and posteriorly.

Concealed Right Bundle Branch Block

A conduction delay in the main trunk of the right bundle branch or in its major ramifications may not be manifested in the surface ECG when there are coexisting conduction disturbances (and of greater degree) in the main left bundle branch, the anterosuperior division of the left bundle branch, and/or in the free left ventricular wall.[5,13] A right bundle branch block can also be concealed in some patients with Wolff-Parkinson-White syndrome, type B, provided that the ventricular insertion of the accessory pathway (Kent bundle) causes preexcitation of the right ventricular regions that would be activated late because of the right bundle branch block.[41,42]

FIGURE 14-12 Diagnosis of left anterior hemiblock associated with myocardial infarction. *A.* Left anterior hemiblock and anteroseptal myocardial infarction. *B.* Left anterior hemiblock and anterolateral myocardial infarction. *C.* Left anterior hemiblock and anterolateral myocardial infarction with electrical axis in right superior (indeterminate) quadrant. *D.* Left anterior hemiblock and inferior wall myocardial infarction.

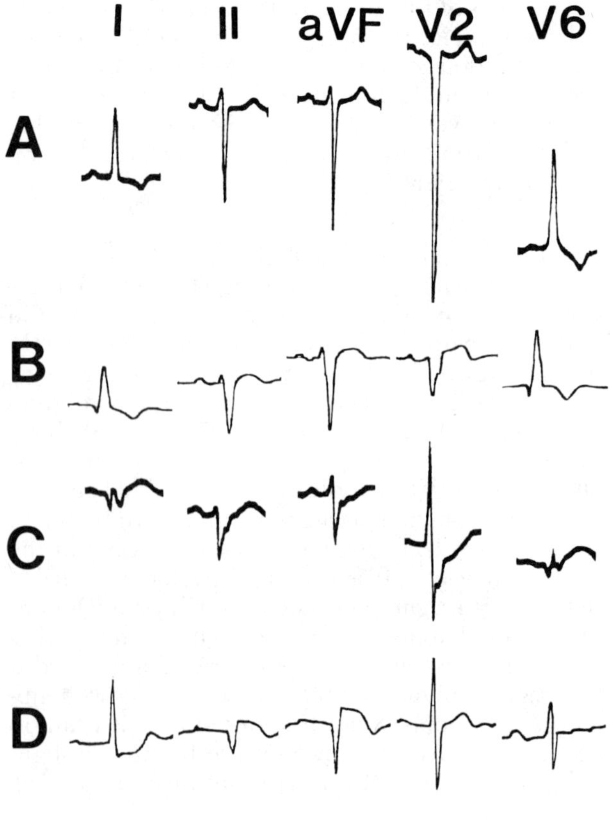

"Focal" Block

Several names have been applied to the conduction disturbances occurring in the left-sided Purkinje-myocardial junctions, left septal surface, or free wall of the left ventricle: arborization block, diffuse (nonspecific) intraventricular block, periinfarction block, parietal block, etc.[5,43–48] Although readers might disagree with what we are hereby considering (in keeping with Rosenbaum's concepts) as focal block,

FIGURE 14-13 Electrogenesis of right axis deviation due to left posterior hemiblock (*top*) and right ventricular hypertrophy (*bottom*). In the former, right axis deviation is due to the hemiblock-related reorientation of electric forces within the anatomically predominant left ventricle. In right ventricular hypertrophy right axis deviation is due to the increase in size of the now anatomically predominant right ventricle. It should be emphasized that the differentiation between these two processes cannot be made on the basis of the ECG alone.

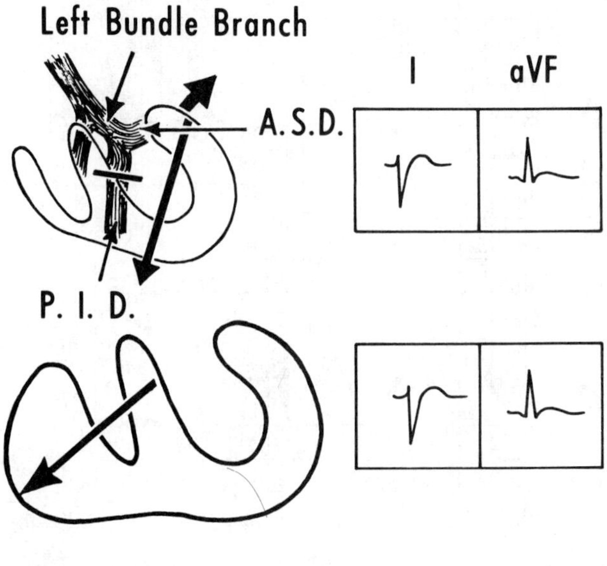

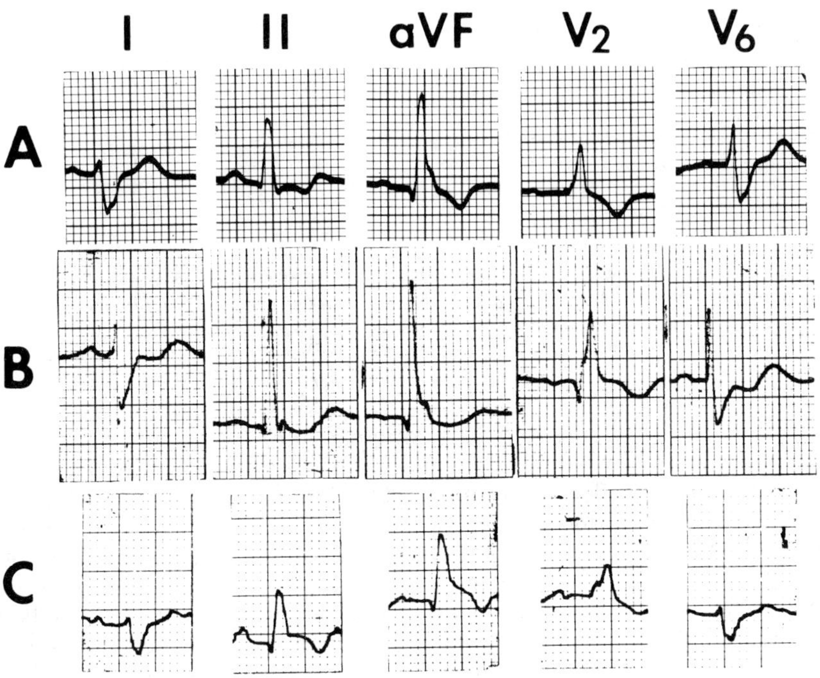

FIGURE 14-14 *A.* Left posterior hemiblock without myocardial infarction. *B.* Left posterior hemiblock coexisting with anteroseptal myocardial infarction. *C.* Left posterior hemiblock with inferior myocardial infarction diagnosed only by evolutionary ST-T changes.

they must nevertheless have a clear understanding of the concept that it implies.[5]

These conduction disturbances have different electrogenetic mechanisms.[5,43] Thus, the cellular "affectation" due to acute injury resulting from coronary artery disease, hyperkalemia, drugs (Fig. 14-16), and intracoronary injections of contrast material occurs within (inside) the affected regions. Focal blocks occurring in subacute or chronic MI after the appearance of abnormal Q waves (periinfarction block), as well as those occurring in the presence of diffuse myocardial fibrosis (of noncoronary etiology), are due to the circuitous and irregular activation of living cells surrounded by (or surrounding) areas of fibrotic tissue.

TABLE 14-4 Causes of Right Axis Deviation (> +90°)

Cause	Characteristic Feature
1. No apparent cause; occurs in some normal individuals	Anatomic vertical heart position
2. Pulmonary emphysema (without right ventricular hypertrophy)	Anatomic vertical heart position
3. Right ventricular hypertrophy	Increase in right ventricular mass
4. Left posterior hemiblock	Absence of radiological and echocardiographic right ventricular hypertrophy
5. Extensive anterolateral myocardial infarction	Qr complexes in lead I with abnormal ST segment and T waves
6. WPW syndrome, type A	Short PR interval; delta waves
7. Left ventricular pacing	Pacemaker spikes; predominantly positive deflection in V_1
8. Reversed right arm and left arm electrodes	Negative P wave in lead I; aV_L in aV_R position and vice versa
9. Dextrocardia without concomitant heart disease	Position of heart in right hemithorax

"Complete" Left Bundle Branch Block

The conduction disturbance of complete left bundle branch block is characterized by wide (greater than 0.11 s) QRS complexes. The diagnostic criteria consist of prolongation of the QRS complexes (over 0.11 s) with neither a q nor an S wave in leads I and in the *properly placed* V_6. A wide R wave with a notch on its top ("plateau") is seen in these leads. In hearts with an electrical (and anatomic) vertical position a small q wave may be seen in aV_L in the absence of MI. Right chest leads V_1 may or may not show an initial r wave, but the latter should be present in lead V_2. Unfortunately, as mentioned in reference to complete right bundle branch block, these morphological patterns can be recorded in patients with high-degree (not necessarily complete) left bundle branch block.

The direction of the electrical axis in patients showing QRS changes typical of complete left bundle branch has been a widely discussed subject. In the majority of the human hearts the site of exit from the right bundle branch does not seem to be at the lowermost right ventricular region (in pacemaker nomenclature called the *right ventricular apex*). If this were the case, all complete left bundle branch blocks would show (as when the right ventricular apex is paced) abnormal left axis deviation. The electrical axis in uncomplicated complete left bundle branch block usually is not located beyond −30°.

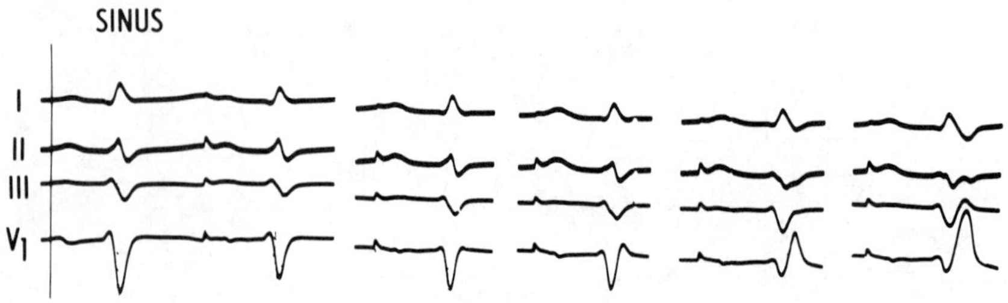

FIGURE 14-15 Right bundle branch block induced by premature right atrial stimulation. Whereas the first beat is of sinus origin, the others show increasing (from left to right) grades of right bundle branch block aberration. Note that the slightest degree of right bundle branch block only produces a decrease in the size of the S wave in V_1 (second ventricular complex). (*From A. Castellanos and R. J. Myerburg, "The Hemiblocks in Myocardial Infarction," Appleton-Century-Crofts, Inc., New York, 1976. Reproduced with permission from the publisher and authors.*)

Complete Left Bundle Branch Block with Myocardial Infarction

When a complete left bundle branch block is present, the impulse emerges from the right bundle branch and propagates inferiorly, to the left, and slightly anteriorly. This orientation of the initial forces tends to abolish previously present inferiorly and laterally located abnormal Q waves characteristic of inferior, and lateral, wall myocardial infarctions.[13] However, if the infarction is anteroseptal the impulse cannot propagate toward the left. Instead, the initial vectors point toward the free wall of the right ventricle because now the right ventricular free wall forces are not neutralized by the normally preponderant initial left ventricular free wall forces. Thus, a small q wave will be recorded in leads I, V_5, and V_6, where it is not normally recorded *in complete left bundle branch block* (Fig. 14-17).

FIGURE 14-16 Left ventricular focal (inferior periinfarction) block. Arrows point toward the terminal delay located to the left and posteriorly (notch in the descending position of the R wave in V_6) and inferiorly (r wave of 0.04 s in lead aV_F).

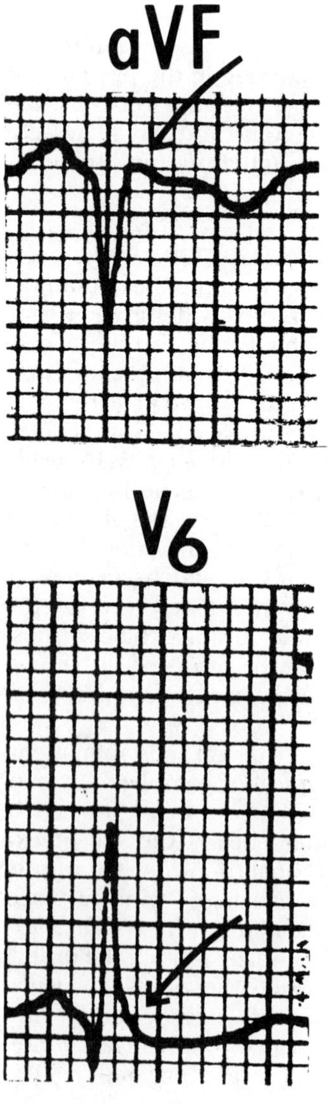

Complete Left Bundle Branch Block with Abnormal Left Axis Deviation

The surface electrocardiographic pattern of complete left bundle branch block with abnormal (-30 to $-60°$) left axis deviation, one of the most difficult to categorize, has been attributed to the following:[13] (1) the coexistence of a high degree conduction delay in the trunk of the left bundle branch ("incomplete" left bundle branch block) with a left anterior hemiblock; (2) the association of a high-degree conduction delay in the posterior division of the left bundle branch ("incomplete" left posterior hemiblock) with a left anterior hemiblock; (3) the coexistence of complete left bundle branch block with diffuse left ventricular focal block; (4) complete left bundle branch block combined with an extensive MI of the low anterolateral wall (Fig. 14-18); (5) the

FIGURE 14-17 Complete left bundle branch block with anteroseptal infarction. There is a small q wave in front of the otherwise typical wide ventricular complexes in leads I and V_6. A small r wave is present in V_1.

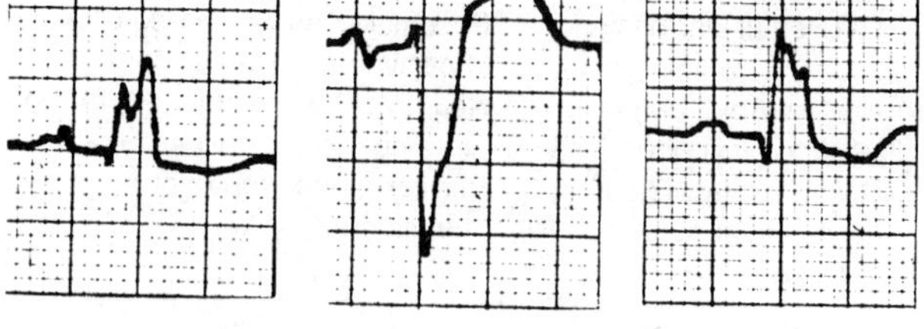

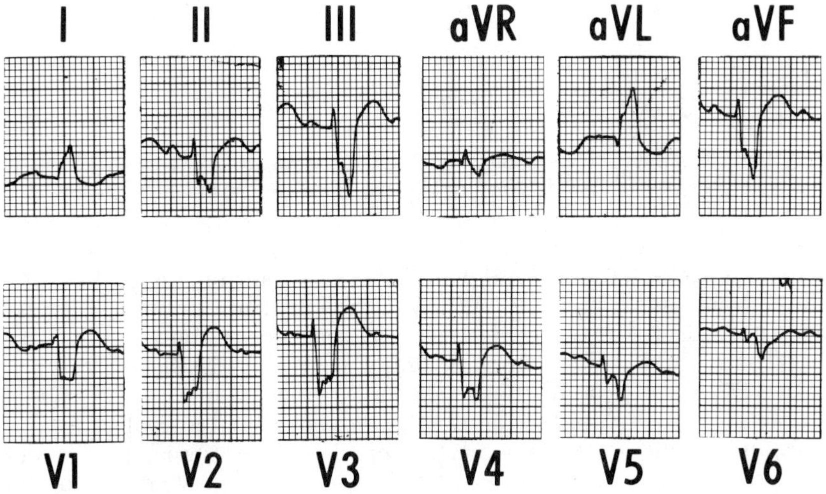

FIGURE 14-18 Complete left bundle branch block with *abnormal* left axis deviation. Necropsy showed an old myocardial infarction not involving the septum but affecting the entire low anterolateral wall.

association of complete left bundle branch block with a block in the superior subdivision of the right bundle branch (right superior hemiblock); and (6) complete left bundle branch block occurring in a patient with abnormal anatomic rotation of the heart due to thoracic chest wall deformities or pleuropericardial disease. However, in some cases of complete left bundle branch block with abnormal left axis deviation, no cause for the latter can be found (applying presently available knowledge).

"Incomplete" Left Bundle Branch Block Pattern

An incomplete left bundle branch block pattern can be diagnosed in a heart with an electrically horizontal (or semihorizontal) heart position when leads I and V_6 show an R wave with a slurring in its upstroke (not on its top as in complete left bundle branch block). Leads V_1 shows rS or QS complexes and lead V_2 rS complexes. Although QRS duration usually ranges between 0.08 and 0.11 s, this pattern can be observed with QRS durations of 0.12 and 0.13 s. Not surprisingly, an incomplete left bundle branch block pattern can be produced by various processes, namely: (1) conduction delays in the main trunk of the left bundle branch; (2) conduction delays (of more or less equal degree) in the divisions of the left bundle branch; (3) diffuse septal fibrosis; (4) small septal infarctions; (5) left ventricular enlargements (generally pressure overloading) in patients with congenital heart disease; and (6) combinations of all the above.

Wide QRS Complexes Occurring in Patients with Bypass Tracts

Wolff-Parkinson-White Syndrome

The characteristic pattern of Wolff-Parkinson-White (WPW) syndrome consists of a short PR interval (reflecting faster-than-normal conduction through an accessory pathway of the Kent bundle type) preceding a wide QRS complex.[49] The latter shows an initial slurring (delta wave) followed by a terminal, slender part. The usual ventricular complex is a fusion beat resulting from ventricular activation by two wave fronts. One, traversing the accessory pathway, produces the delta wave. The other, emerging from the normal AV pathway, is responsible for the terminal, more normal parts of the QRS complex. The degree of preexcitation (amount of muscle activated through the Kent bundle) depends on many factors. Foremost among these are the distance between the sinus node and atrial insertion of accessory pathway and, more important, the differences in conduction time through the normal pathway and accessory pathway. Other things being equal, a patient with rapid, or enhanced, AV nodal conduction will have a smaller delta wave than a patient with slow conduction through the AV node. Moreover, if there is total block at the AV node or His-Purkinje system, the impulse will be conducted exclusively via the Kent bundle.[50] When this occurs, the QRS complexes are no longer fusion beats since the ventricles are then activated exclusively from the preexcited site. Consequently, the delta wave disappears and the QRS complexes are as wide as (really simulating) those produced by artificial or spontaneous beats arising in the vicinity of the ventricular end of the accessory pathway.[50]

The most used (and frequently misinterpreted) ECG classification of the WPW syndrome is the one proposed by Rosenbaum et al. in 1945, which is based on the polarity of the *major QRS deflection* (not of the delta wave) in leads V_1 and V_2.[51] In type A of this classification the R wave is the largest deflection in these leads, and, in type B, "the S or QS is the chief deflection in at least one of them."[51] However, invasive (catheter) electrophysiological studies have shown that this classification is not always exact to predict the location of the accessory AV pathway (Kent bundle), especially when the degree of preexcitation is not maximal.[50,52–57] According to the results obtained from intracardiac studies, information from the standard and unipolar extremity leads

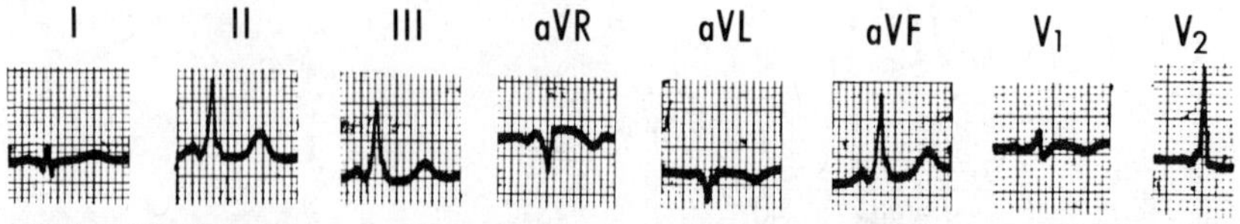

FIGURE 14-19 WPW syndrome, type A, according to the classification of Rosenbaum et al. There were predominantly positive deflections in V_1 and V_2. The delta wave pointed anteriorly and to the right (thus being negative in leads I and aV_L), as well as inferiorly. The electrical axis was vertical. The patient had a left lateral accessory pathway.

may also be of importance. For example, (1) predominantly positive deflections (R or Rs complexes) in V_1 and V_2 with negative delta waves in leads I and aV_L with positive delta waves in III and aV_F suggest a left lateral accessory pathway (WPW syndrome, type A) (as in Fig. 14-19); (2) predominantly negative deflections (QS or rS complexes) in V_1 and V_2 with superior electrical axis and positive delta waves in I and aV_L suggest a right lateral accessory pathway (WPW syndrome, type B) (as in Fig. 14-20); and (3) some cases, classified as type B according to the criteria of Rosenbaum et al. because of predominantly negative (rS) complexes in V_1 and V_2, may have left lateral accessory pathways if the delta wave is negative in leads I and aV_L and positive in the inferior leads (Fig. 14-21).

Posteroseptal pathways are most difficult to diagnose during sinus rhythm. In general, their presence can be suspected when, with a superior electrical axis, V_1 shows a predominantly negative deflection and V_2 a predominantly positive deflection, or if there are R waves in both leads (Fig. 14-21 to 14-23). Anteroseptal pathways show a vertical axis with negative deflections in V_1 and V_2.

Nodoventricular (Mahaim) Fibers

The surface ECG in patients having, exclusively, nodoventricular (Mahaim) fibers usually shows a normal PR interval without a distinct delta wave.[58] We have observed that a q wave is usually absent in leads I, V_5, and V_6. These tracts terminate in the right ventricle but the supraventricular impulse traversing the Mahaim tract reaches the ventricles (during sinus rhythm) only 0.01 to 0.015 s before the impulse traversing the normal pathway. This causes only a slight, earlier-than-normal arrival of excitation at the right septal surface, similar to that occurring in a small degree of incomplete left bundle branch block (Fig. 14-24).

FIGURE 14-20 WPW syndrome, type B, according to the classification of Rosenbaum et al. Note predominantly negative deflections in leads V_1 and V_2. The delta wave pointed posteriorly, to the left, and superiorly. There was abnormal (left superior) axis deviation. Invasive electrophysiological studies revealed the existence of a right lateral accessory pathway (Kent bundle). *(From L. Lemberg and A. Castellanos, Jr., "Vectorcardiography," 1st ed., Appleton-Century-Crofts, Inc., New York, 1969. Reproduced with permission from the publisher and authors.)*

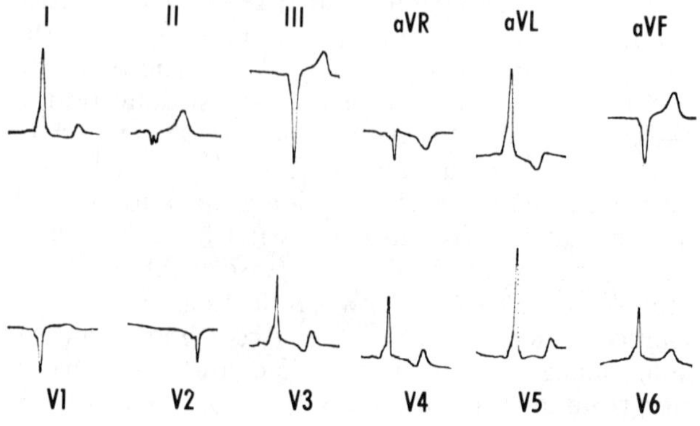

Wide QRS Complexes Produced by Ventricular Pacing from Different Sites

In determining the location of the stimulating electrodes, special care should be taken so as not to consider that the distortion produced by large unipolar spikes constitutes parts of the pacing-induced QRS complexes. It is best not to describe the electrically produced ventricular beats as having a right or left bundle branch morphology since what is relevant is the polarity of the properly positioned V_1 and V_2

FIGURE 14-21 WPW syndrome, type B, according to the terminology of Rosenbaum et al., due to predominantly negative deflections (rS complexes) in lead V_1. However, the patient did not have a right lateral, or posteroseptal, accessory pathway, but a *left* lateral accessory pathway since the delta wave was oriented to the right (because it was negative in lead I and aV_L), anteriorly, and inferiorly. The electrical axis pointed to the left and inferiorly.

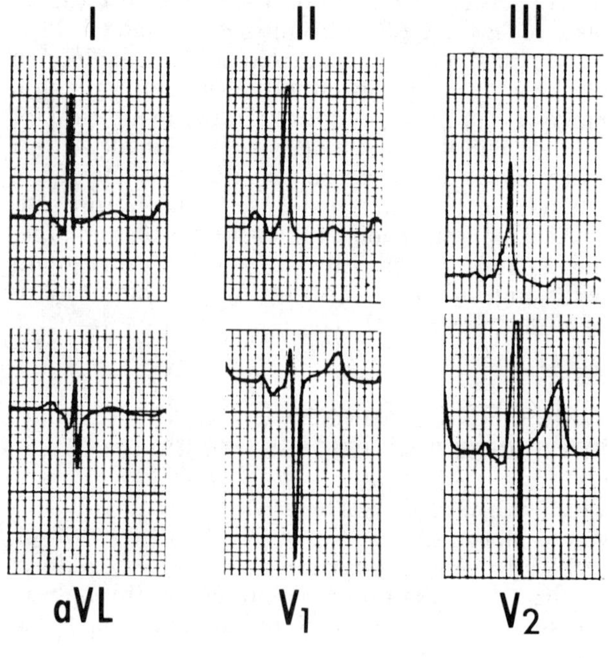

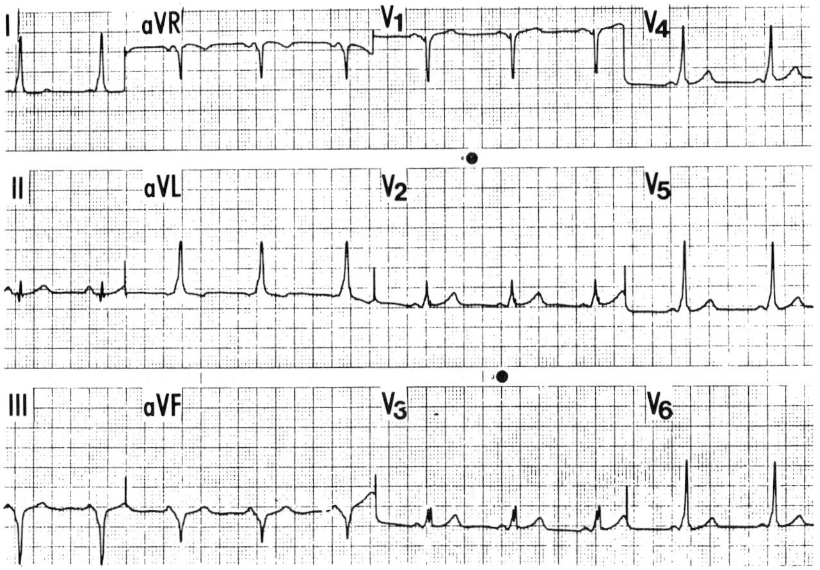

FIGURE 14-22 WPW syndrome, type B, according to the classification of Rosenbaum et al. However, in contrast, to Fig. 14-20, the predominantly negative deflection in V_1 was associated with an R wave in V_2. The delta wave was oriented anteriorly, to the left, and superiorly. The electrical axis pointed superiorly and to the left. The patient had a posteroseptal (or left paraseptal) accessory pathway.

electrodes and the direction of the electrical axis (Fig. 14-25).[59,60] For example, endocardial or epicardial stimulation of the *anteriorly* located right ventricle at any site, apical (inferior), middle, or outflow tract (superior), yields predominantly negative deflections in the right chest leads owing to the *posterior* spread of activation. The reverse (positive deflections in V_1 and V_2) occurs when the epicardial stimulation of the superior and lateral portions of the posterior left ventricle by catheter electrodes in the distal coronary sinus or great and middle cardiac veins (or by implanted electrodes in the nearby muscle) result in *anteriorly* oriented forces. On the other hand, *superior* deviation of the electrical axis only indicates that an *inferior* ventricular site has been stimulated, regardless of whether this site is the apical portion of the right ventricle or the inferior part of the left ventricle (paced through the middle cardiac vein). Conversely, an *inferior* vertical axis is simply a consequence of pacing from a *superior* site, which can be the endocardium of the right ventricular outflow tract or the epicardium of the posterosuperior and lateral portions of the left ventricle.

Left Ventricular Hypertrophy

The sensitivity and specificity of the various ECG criteria used to diagnose left (and right) ventricular hypertrophy are discussed in *Update I: The Heart*.[61] Hence, only certain points will be elaborated. For example, all ECG criteria of left ventricular hypertrophy include "high" voltage. Yet, the latter may not be present because of extracardiac factors such as lung and mediastinal diseases, pleural and pericardial effusion, anasarca, and obesity. Moreover,

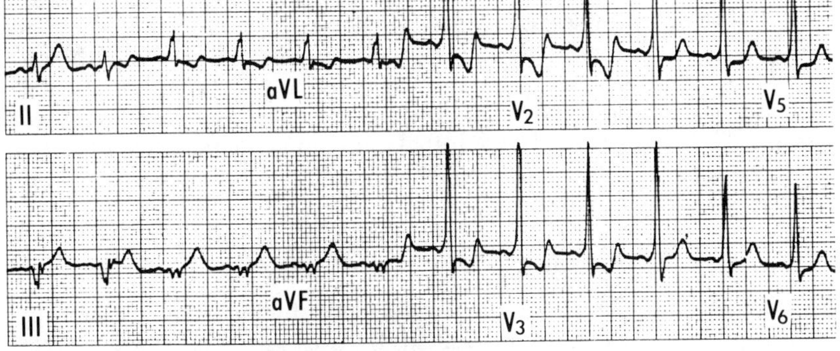

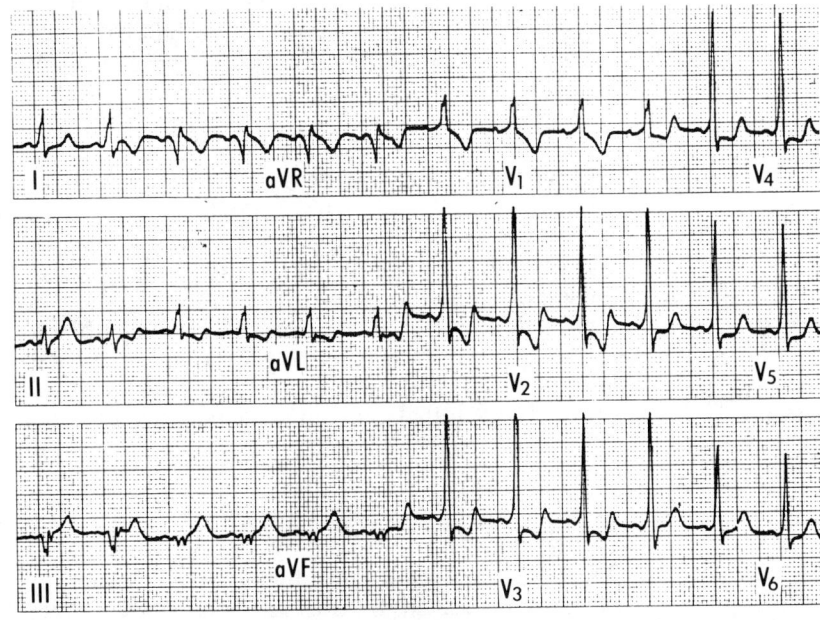

FIGURE 14-23 WPW syndrome, type A, according to the classification of Rosenbaum et al. There were all-positive complexes (R waves) in V_1 and V_2. The delta wave was oriented anteriorly, to the left, and inferiorly. The electrical axis pointed superiorly and to the left. The patient had a posteroseptal (left paraseptal) accessory pathway.

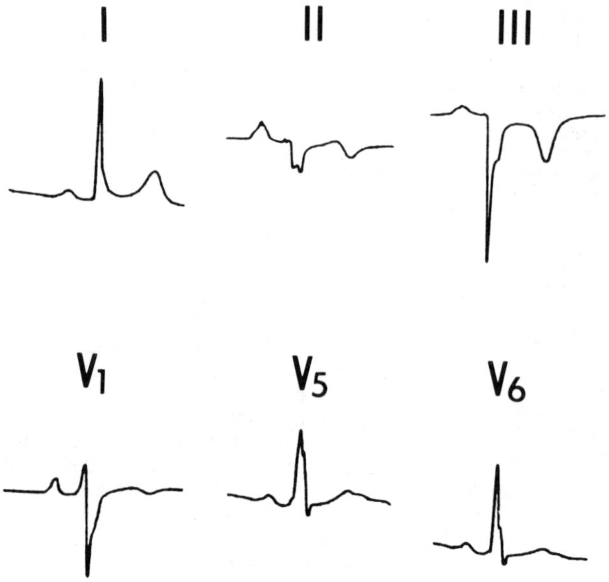

FIGURE 14-24 ECG from a normal 17-year-old male who had recurrent, sustained supraventricular tachycardia with a complete left bundle branch block and abnormal left axis deviation morphology. During sinus rhythm the PR intervals and QRS complexes (without a delta wave) had a normal duration. Small q waves were also absent in leads I, aV_L (not shown), V_5, and V_6. Note left superior axis deviation and posttachycardia T-wave inversion in leads II and III. The patient had a nodoventricular (Mahaim) fiber.

voltage (reflecting the electrical activity of living muscle) can also be decreased by intracardiac factors such as diffuse myocardial processes or infarction, as well as by the type of, or varieties of stimuli leading to, hypertrophy. On the other hand, high voltage may occur without left ventricular hypertrophy in some normal young individuals and in patients with left bundle branch block, left anterior hemiblock, and WPW syndrome.

FIGURE 14-25 QRS changes (location of the electrical axis and polarity of lead V_1) produced by pacing from right ventricular apex (RVA), right ventricular outflow tract (RVOT), great cardiac vein (GCV), and middle cardiac vein (MCV).

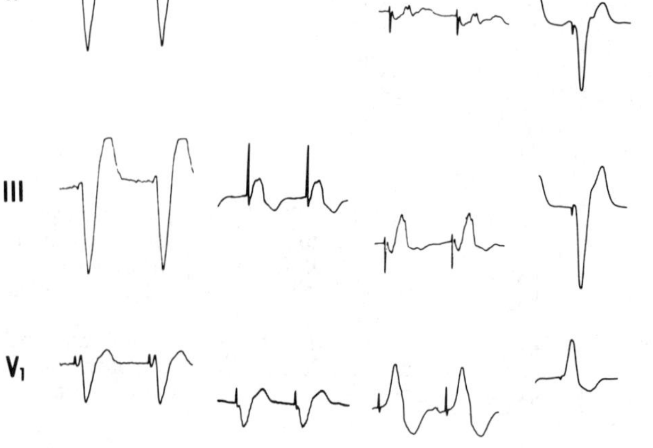

In regard to the correlation of the ECG and other methods used to diagnose left ventricular hypertrophy the following should be kept in mind:[62–64] (1) conventional x-rays and necropsy criteria, which measure radiological left ventricular size and pathological left ventricular weight, respectively, include living *and* fibrotic tissue; (2) angiographic and M-mode echocardiographic criteria have a higher sensitivity, specificity, and predictive value than electrocardiographic criteria; and (3) in the future, it is very likely that nuclear magnetic resonance will become the "golden" standard.

Processes Producing, or Leading to, Right Ventricular Hypertrophy and Enlargement

Right ventricular hypertrophy will be manifested in the ECG only when the right ventricular forces predominate over those of the left ventricle. Since the latter has, roughly, three times more mass than the former, the right ventricle may double in size (when the left ventricle is normal) or triple its weight (when there is significant left ventricular hypertrophy) and still not result in the necessary requirements to pull the electric forces anteriorly and to the right. For these reasons, right ventricular hypertrophy cannot be recognized easily in adult patients.

In spite of these limitations, the ECG is helpful in the diagnosis of pulmonary emphysema (Fig. 14-26), "pure" mitral stenosis (Fig. 14-27), and some congenital malformations such as atrial septal defect (Fig. 14-28) and pulmonic stenosis (Fig. 14-29).[11] False positive diagnosis of right ventricular hypertrophy may occur in patients with true posterior (basal) myocardial infarction, complete right bundle branch block, left posterior hemiblock and type A WPW syndrome.

Electrolyte Imbalances

Because multiple factors can affect ventricular repolarization in diseased hearts, the finding characteristic of a specific electrolyte abnormality may be modified, and even mimicked, by various pathological processes and certain drugs. In practice, the major problem with the electrocardiographic diagnosis of electrolyte imbalance is not the negative ECG but the production of similar changes by other conditions.[65]

Hyperkalemia

The initial effect of acute hyperkalemia is the appearance of peaked T waves with a narrow base (Fig.

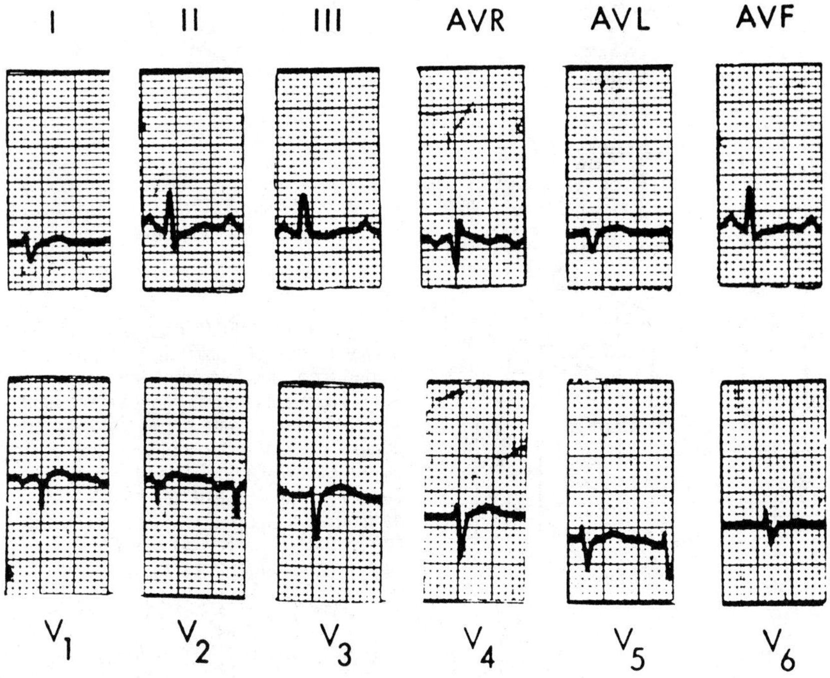

FIGURE 14-26 ECG taken on a patient with pulmonary emphysema, showing slight right axis deviation with small rS complexes in lead I, a vertical heart position, overall tendency to low voltage, and rS complexes in all chest leads. (*From L. Lemberg and A. Castellanos, Jr., "Vectorcardiography," 2d ed., Appleton-Century-Crofts, Inc., New York, 1975. Reproduced with permission from the publisher and authors.*)

14-30, left). The diagnosis of hyperkalemia is almost certain when the duration of the base is 0.20 s or less (with rates between 60 and 110 beats per minute). As the degree of hyperkalemia increases, the QRS complex widens, with the electrical axis usually being deviated abnormally to the left and only rarely to the right (Fig. 14-30, right). In addition, the PR interval is prolonged, and the P wave flattens until it disappears. If the patient remains untreated, death ensues due either to a coarse slow ventricular fibrillation or to ventricular standstill. Quinidine, procainamide, and disopyramide toxicity (not idiosyncrasy) and large doses of tricyclic depressants (especially when ingested for suicidal purposes) can also produce death through progressive QRS widening (Fig. 14-31, right). These processes, however, are associated with prolonged QT (or QU) intervals. On the other hand, wide QRS complexes with narrow-based T waves are almost pathognomonic of hyperkalemia. (Compare Fig. 14-30, right, with Fig. 14-31, right.)

Hypokalemia

The abnormal and delayed repolarization that occurs in hypokalemia is best expressed as QU, rather than QT, prolongation, since at times it can be difficult to differentiate between notching of the T wave

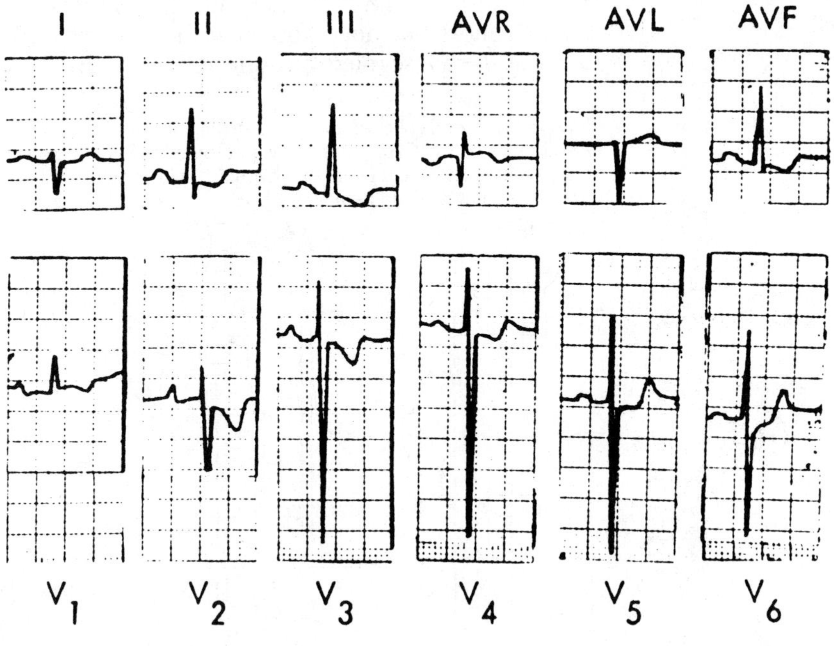

FIGURE 14-27 ECG from a patient with right ventricular hypertrophy due to pure mitral stenosis showing P "mitrale," right axis deviation, an all-positive deflection (R wave of only around 5 mm) in V_1, and rS complexes from V_2 to V_6. (*From L. Lemberg and A. Castellanos, Jr., "Vectorcardiography," 2d ed., Appleton-Century-Crofts, Inc., New York, 1975. Reproduced with permission from the publisher and authors.*)

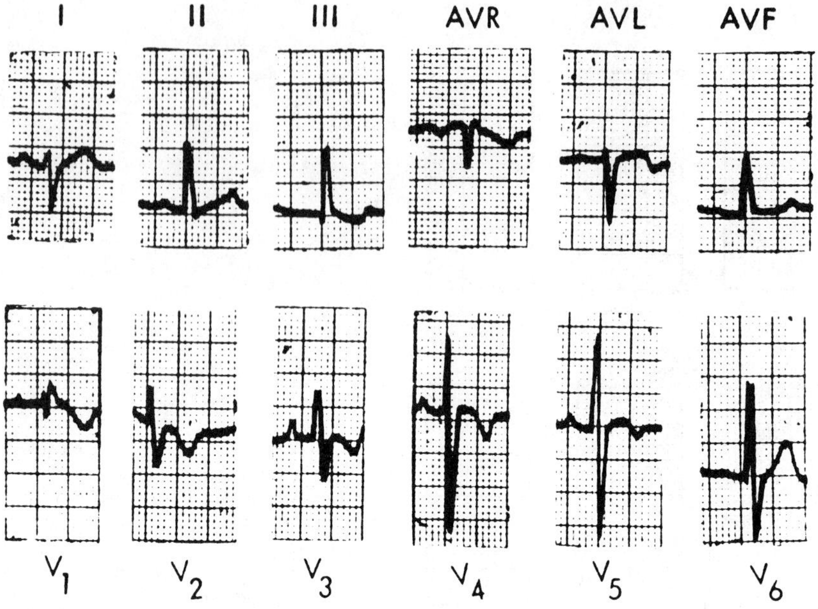

FIGURE 14-28 ECG from a patient with right ventricular enlargement (volume overload in type) due to a small atrial septal defect (ostium secundum). Right axis deviation was associated with an incomplete right bundle branch block pattern (rsR′ complexes of low voltage in lead V_1). (*From L. Lemberg and A. Castellanos, Jr., "Vectorcardiography," 2d ed., Appleton-Century-Crofts, Inc., New York, 1975. Reproduced with permission from the publisher and authors.*)

and T- and U-wave fusion. The earliest change consists of the U wave being taller than the T wave. As the serum potassium falls, the ST segment becomes more depressed and there is a gradual blending of T waves into what appears to be a tall U wave (Fig. 14-32).

An ECG pattern similar to that of hypokalemia can be produced by some antiarrhythmic drugs, especially quinidine (Fig. 14-31, left). These quinidine-induced repolarization changes need not indicate quinidine "toxicity" but may only reflect that the patient is taking this drug. However, when repolarization is greatly prolonged, they can lead to characteristic ventricular arrhythmias. Classic quinidine toxicity is characterized by QRS widening (greater than 25 percent of control values) not due to bundle branch block, generally coexisting with a prolonged repolarization (Fig. 14-31, right).

FIGURE 14-29 ECG from a 17-year-old patient who had right ventricular enlargement (pressure overloading in type) due to severe pulmonic stenosis. Note extreme right axis deviation, overall high voltage, and qR complexes in lead V_1 *without* an incomplete right bundle branch block pattern. (*From L. Lemberg and A. Castellanos, Jr., "Vectorcardiography," 2d ed., Appleton-Century-Crofts, Inc., New York, 1975. Reproduced with permission from the publisher and authors.*)

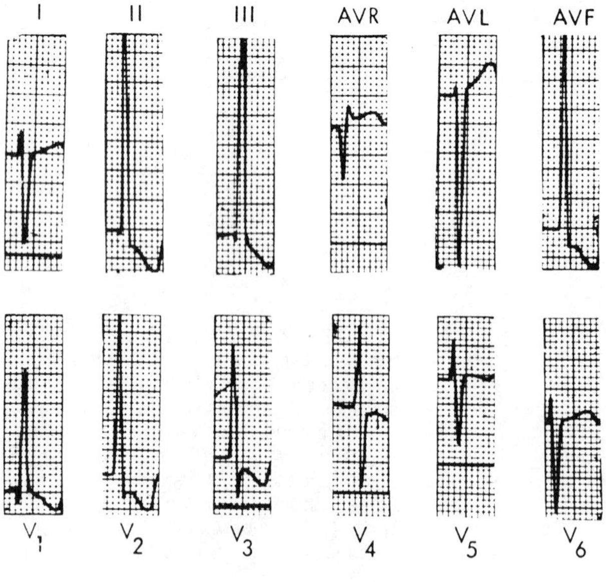

Hypomagnesemia

Hypomagnesemia does not produce QU prolongation unless the coexisting hypokalemia (with which it is almost invariably associated) is severe.[65] Although long-standing, or severe, magnesium deficiency lowers the amplitude of the T wave and depresses the ST segment, it does not prolong the QT interval.

Hypercalcemia

During sinus rhythm with normal rates the QT interval is short but does not show the upward concavity of the ST segment produced by digitalis. This

FIGURE 14-30 Electrocardiographic manifestations of early hyperkalemia (narrow QRS complex, with a peaked T wave having a very narrow base) and advanced hyperkalemia (absent P wave, wide QRS complex, and peaked T wave).

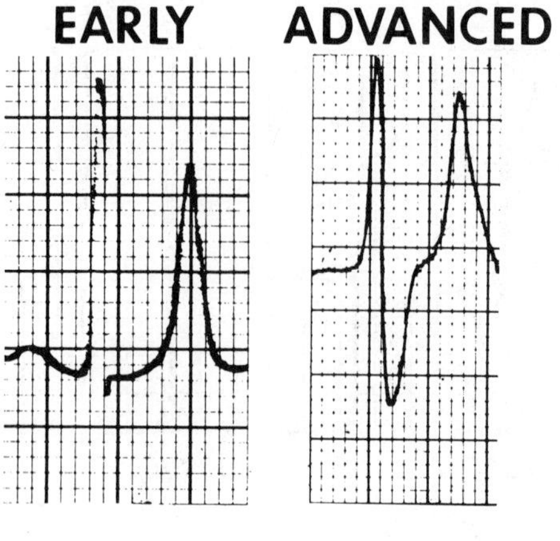

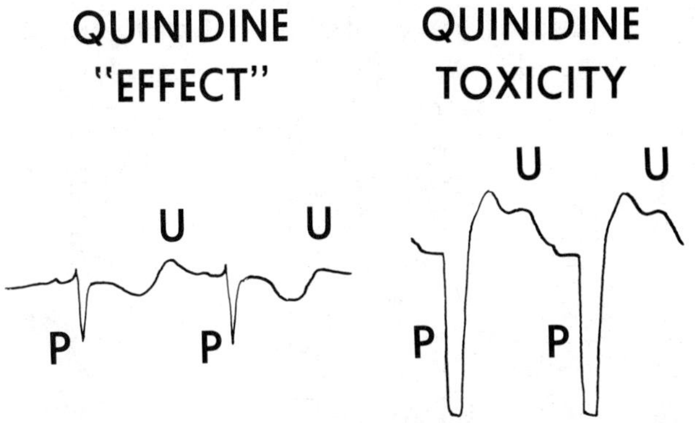

FIGURE 14-31 The left panel shows the delayed repolarization pattern (due to quinidine effect) which may be a precursor of, or coexist with, quinidine-induced *torsades de pointes*. Note that the QRS complexes were narrow. The right panel shows delayed repolarization syndrome (associated with drug-induced QRS widening) which is seen in classic quinidine toxicity.

drug, which also shortens the QT interval, produces its characteristic effects in leads where the R waves predominate. The classic upward concavity of the ST segment is seen in the left chest leads in patients with left ventricular hypertrophy, and in V_1 and V_2 when there is right ventricular hypertrophy with predominantly positive deflections in these leads.

Hypocalcemia

The typical electrocardiographic pattern of hypocalcemia consists of QT prolongation at the expense of the ST segment. The T wave is usually of normal width, but can be narrow-based if there is coexistent (moderate) hyperkalemia (Fig. 14-33). A very marked subendocardial ischemia (with the so-called hyper-acute ST-T changes) can produce a similar pattern, but in those cases the T wave, though peaked, is not as narrow-based as in Fig. 14-33. It has been said that hypocalcemia per se does not produce T-wave inversion. When present, T-wave inversion is usually a reflection of coexisting processes such as left ventricular hypertrophy and incomplete left bundle branch block. An ECG pattern similar to that of hypocalcemia can be produced by some organic abnormalities of the central nervous system, and by congenitally prolonged QT intervals such as are found in Jervell-Lange-Nielsen's syndrome and the Romano-Ward syndrome.

FIGURE 14-32 Electrocardiographic manifestations of hypokalemia (intermediate precordial lead). The top recording is the control showing a small, but normal, U wave. The remaining recordings are arranged to show increasing degrees of hypokalemia.

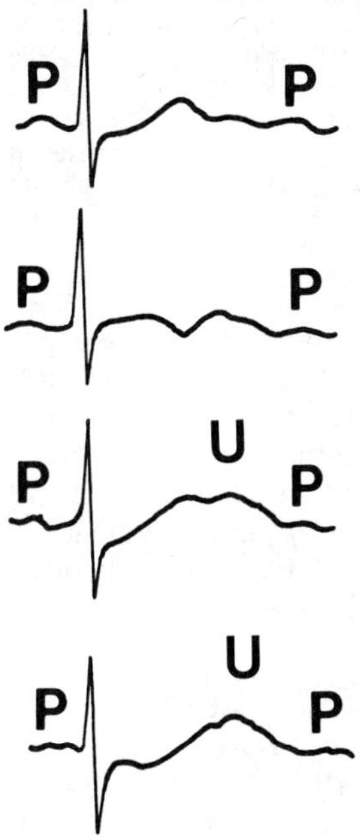

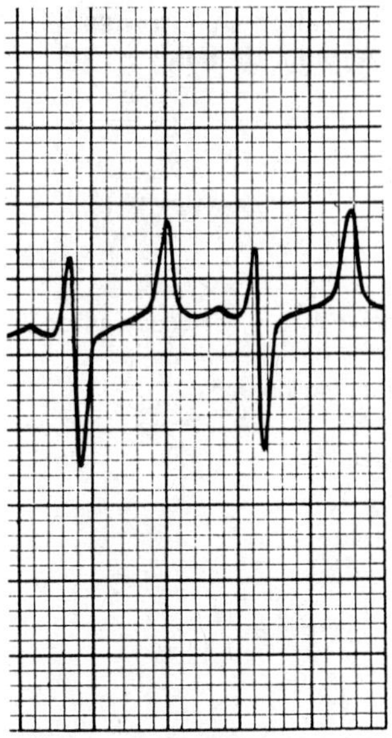

FIGURE 14-33 The most frequently diagnosed (by the ECG) hypocalcemic pattern is that occurring with hyperkalemia (due to renal disease). Although in this tracing the QT interval was not prolonged, the narrow-based (0.08 s), peaked T wave (diagnostic of hyperkalemia) was associated with an ST segment of 0.16 s duration. The latter finding indicates the coexistence of hypocalcemia, in spite of the normal QT interval.

Delayed Repolarization Syndromes

Although it is not always easy to differentiate between prolonged QT and QU intervals, determining the existence of prolonged repolarization is not difficult especially if intermediate (V_3 and V_4) chest leads are analyzed. For these reasons, it has been recommended that the single more comprehensive delayed depolarization syndrome be used (Table 14-5).[65–70] In these cases, long strips should be obtained since the duration of depolarization, though greater at slower rates (or longer cycle lengths) than under normal conditions, differs from normal in the magnitude of bradycardia dependency.

Artifacts

During the last few years the number and types of instruments used for noninvasive and invasive (elec-

TABLE 14-5 Delayed Depolarization Syndromes (Prolonged QT and/or QU Intervals, Usually Bradycardia-Dependent)

1. Electrolyte disturbances
   a. Hypokalemia
   b. Hypocalcemia
   c. Hypomagnesemia
2. Drugs
   a. Class 1B antiarrhythmic agents (quinidine, disopyramide, procainamide)
   b. Class 3 antiarrhythmic agents (amiodarone)
   c. Psychotropic drugs
3. Central nervous system diseases
   a. Subarachnoid hemorrhage
   b. Ruptured berry aneurysm
   c. Cryptococcal meningitis
4. Congenital syndromes
   a. Jervell and Lange-Nielsen's syndrome
   b. Romano-Ward syndrome
5. Electrocardiographic "ischemia"
6. Arrhythmias
   a. Posttachycardia syndrome
   b. Cardiac arrest of any etiology
   c. Chronic idioventricular rhythms

trical or nonelectrical) study of cardiac functions have multiplied exponentially. Naturally, physicians and hospital administrators have concentrated their attention on them. Technicians have been more interested in being in charge of more lucrative services. These factors have downgraded the importance of the 12-lead ECG, relegating it to a tertiary role. Not surprisingly, the technical quality of ECGs has deteriorated in many centers. Optimal quality can only be achieved if the parties involved understand what is happening. The following are some of the artifacts commonly seen in 1984 in routine ECG tracings.

Muscle Tremor and Alternating Current Interference

Muscle tremor and alternating current interference are the most frequently encountered artifacts because some patients will continue to have disease processes producing tremor and because the number of electronic devices causing interference used in a hospital environment has increased.

Improper Limb Lead Positioning

Improper limb lead positioning has become fairly common because of relaxation of quality control. It is more frequent in those institutions with inadequate standards for hiring technicians and with poor on-site training. Since mixing up the cables from the electrocardiographic machine has gone beyond switching the right arm and cables, the various types of electrodal confusion are illustrated in Fig. 14-34. The method depicted in this illustration, based on the use of unipolar extremity leads only, is simpler than those methods based on the analysis of bipolar standard leads.[10,12] Not recognized in any textbook of electrocardiography is the incontrovertible fact

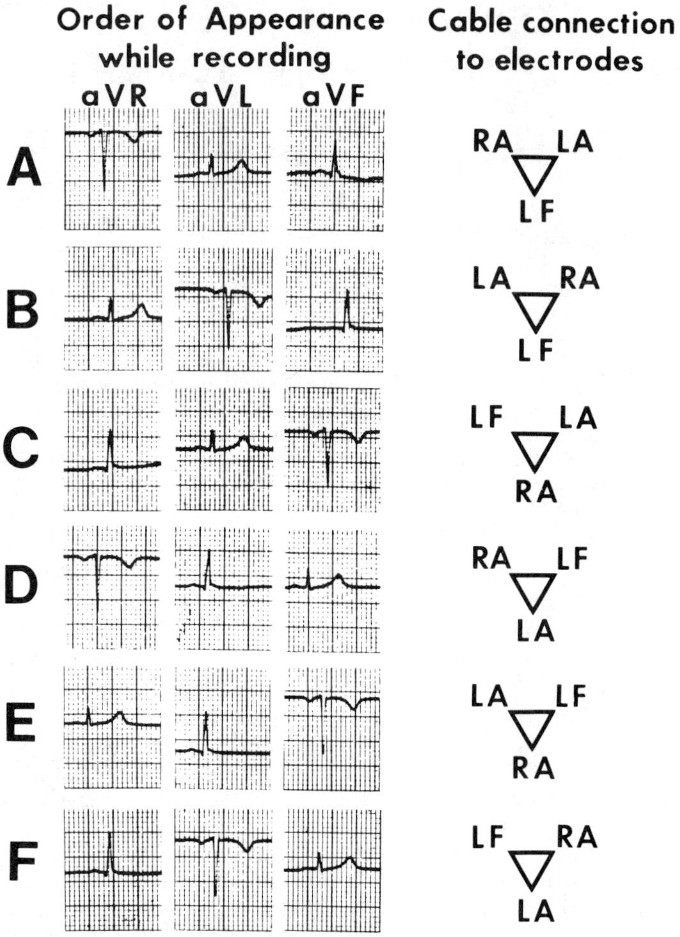

FIGURE 14-34 Identification of improper connections of the *cables* from the electrocardiographic machine to the electrodes placed on the patient's limbs. Note that aV_R, aV_L, and aV_F invariably refer to *whatever morphological pattern* is recorded when, while the ECG is being obtained, the corresponding knobs are turned in this order (regardless of whether the cables are properly or improperly attached). On the other hand, right arm, left arm, and left leg correspond to the *normal morphological pattern* obtained when the cables are properly attached. This method of identification, based solely on the analysis of the unipolar extremity leads, is simpler than the method based on the study of the bipolar standard leads. *A.* Normal. *B.* Left arm in aV_R; right arm in aV_L; left leg in aV_F. *C.* Left leg in aV_R; left arm in aV_L; right arm in aV_F. *D.* Right arm in aV_R; left leg in aV_L; left arm in aV_F. *E.* Left arm in aV_R; left leg in aV_L; right arm in aV_F. *F.* Left leg in aV_R; right arm in aV_L; left arm in aV_F.

that in some centers even the "sanctity" of the attachment of the right leg (ground) cable to the right leg electrode has been violated. In our experience, this results in recordings which may be recognized as artifactual in some instruments but not in others. Most frequently (depending on which limb the right leg electrode was placed), this problem may be identified because one of the bipolar leads records practically no electrical activity whatsoever.

Variation in Chest Lead Placement

Variation in chest lead placement is a problem more common now than when, in 1961, Simonson noted the "considerable variation in chest lead placement in the same patients by different technicians and even by the same technician in several ECG's in the same patient."[17] This author stated that, in a controlled study, placement of the V_2 electrode varied 10 cm vertically and 8 cm horizontally in 103 healthy subjects.[17] Moreover, Kerwin, McLean, and Tegelaar found a rather large error in placement of chest electrodes (2 to 3 cm in both horizontal and vertical directions) in repeated trials in the same patients by the same technicians.[71]

Overshoot, Overdamping, and Running Down of the Standardization Battery

Overshoot, overdamping, and running down of the standardization battery, by causing significant changes in QRS voltage and ST segments, may be of enough importance to cause errors in the diagnosis of ventricular hypertrophy and coronary artery disease.

Wandering Baseline

Wandering baseline is usually due to unclear electrodes.

Inconstant, Irregular, and Bizarre Deflections

Inconstant, irregular, and bizarre deflections are produced by small bits of metal in the electrode parts, loose connections, or broken wires.

Computer Applications

It has been more than 20 years since the first attempts were made to apply computer technology to the interpretation of ECGs.[72] During this time the field has progressed from initial attempts at the recognition of normal tracings to some of today's more sophisticated programs.[73] In general, computer systems for true analysis of ECGs have as their main component a program usually having four basic functions:[74,75] (1) the measuring of ECG parameters, which includes an automatic wave front recognition section and a measurement section that extracts the wave fronts, a set of values, and contour; (2) the interpretation of previously acquired information, responsible for the final statements generated by the program; (3) the identification of various rhythms, both normal and abnormal; and (4) the comparison with previous ECGs by means of which significant changes between tracings are recognized.

A problem not sufficiently emphasized in the literature is one faced by physicians and hospital administrators who decide to computerize their ECG operation: the process of selecting from the multiple available programs. Substantial differences exist between available programs with regard to measurement definitions and classification criteria and terminology. As every electrocardiographer knows there is a lack of standardized, universally agreed upon diagnostic terms and criteria. However, this problem is not solely related to computers but concerns also all ECG interpretations, whether performed by individuals or machines. It has to be remembered that the program used depends on criteria imposed on it by human programmers. General guidelines relating to the selection of a program are not easy to give at this time. Physicians making the selection should be familiar with the diagnostic criteria employed (supplied by the manufacturers) and with the program's practical performance. In some cases, the latter information can be obtained by communicating directly with other users. Of particular importance is knowledge of the manufacturer's service performance.

Finally, the program selected has to be, at present, "tuned in" to the operational environment (community hospital or teaching institution; urban center or rural area, etc.) in which it has to perform.

Once a program has been selected and is in use it requires initial and periodic evaluation. The most practical method consists of accepting as a standard constrained human observers who are given a set of measurements or criteria agreed upon before the evaluation. In academic centers attempts to determine sensitivity and specificities should be made, applying as standards electrocardiographic-independent evidence obtained using *more than one* of the currently available in vivo, noninvasive methods, as well as (when possible) postmortem information.

Proper computerization has definite advantages:

- Speed in providing reports with the resulting improved turnaround time
- Optimal utilization of emergency electrocardiographic services
- Reproducibility of measurements
- Improvements in quality control
- Possible decrease in physician's reading time and more consistency in interpretations
- Enhancement of the capacity to handle large volumes of ECGs
- Substantial improvement in record storage and retrieval with better comparison with previous tracings

Because presently digital recording ECGs are being viewed as sources of change in the socioeconomic sphere of medicine, computerized ECG programs have to be evaluated using standard methods of measuring cost-effective methods as they apply to the corresponding operational environment. That is, the economic factors involved—initial investment, operational costs, payroll, overhead, professional fees—have to be compared with those of the preexisting system in the same hospital. As computer technology advances, institutions will have to evaluate these considerations according to the specific requirements of each installation.

References

1. Wilson, F. N.: Foreword, in J. M. Barker, "The Unipolar Electrogram: A Clinical Interpretation," Appleton-Century-Crofts, Inc., New York, 1952, p. xii.

2. Johnston, F. D., and Lepeschkin, E. (eds.): "Selected Papers of Dr. Frank N. Wilson," Edwards Brothers, Inc., Ann Arbor, Mich., 1955.
3. Sodi-Pallares, D., and Calder, R. M.: "New Bases of Electrocardiography," The C. V. Mosby Company, St. Louis, 1956, pp. 169, 373.
4. Sodi-Pallares, D., Medrano, G. A., Bisteni, A., and Ponce de Leon Jurado, J.: "Deductive and Polyparametric Electrocardiography," Instituto Nacional de Cardiologia de Mexico, Mexico D. F., 1970, pp. 36, 136.
4a. Hurst, J. W. (ed.): "Update V: The Heart," McGraw-Hill Book Company, New York, 1981.
5. Rosenbaum, M. B., Elizari, M. V., and Lazzari, J. O.: "The Hemiblocks," Tampa Tracings, Oldsmar, Fla., 1970.
6. Lipman, B. S., Massie, E., and Kleiger, R. E.: "Clinical Scalar Electrocardiography," 6th ed., Year Book Medical Publishers, Inc., Chicago, 1972, pp. 210–215.
7. Schamroth, L.: "The Electrocardiology of Coronary Artery Disease," Blackwell Scientific Publications, London, 1975.
8. Castellanos, A., and Lemberg, L.: "A Programmed Introduction to Electrical Axis and Action Potential," Tampa Tracings, Oldsmar, Fla., 1974, pp. 34, 114–153.
9. Lewis, T., and Rothschild, M. A.: The Excitatory Process in the Dog's Heart: II. The Ventricles, *Try. R. Soc.*, 206:181, 1915.
10. Marriott, H. J. L.: "Practical Electrocardiography," 7th ed., The Williams & Wilkins Company, Baltimore, 1983.
11. Cabrera, E., and Gaxiola, A.: Teoria y Practica de la Electrocardiografia," 2d ed., La Prensa Medica Mexicana, Mexico D. F., 1966.
12. Barker, J. M.: "The Unipolar Electrocardiogram: A Clinical Interpretation," Appleton-Century-Crofts, Inc., New York, 1952.
13. Castellanos, A., and Myerburg, R. J.: "The Hemiblocks in Myocardial Infarction," Appleton-Century-Crofts, Inc., New York, 1976.
14. Einthoven, W., Fahr, G., and de Waart, A.: Über die Richtung und die manifeste grosse der Potentialschwankungen im menshlichen Herzen und über den Einfluss der Herzlage auf die Form des Elektrokardiogramms, *Arch. f. d. g. Physiol.*, 150:275, 1913.
15. Grant, R. P.: Spatial Vector Electrocardiography: A Method for Calculating the Spatial Electrical Vectors of the Heart from Conventional Leads, *Circulation*, 2:676, 1950.
16. Grant, R. P., and Estes, E. H., Jr.: "Spatial Vector Electrocardiography," Blakiston Co., New York, 1951.
17. Simonson, E.: "Differentiation between Normal and Abnormal in Electrocardiography," The C. V. Mosby Company, St. Louis, 1961, p. 262.
18. Wilson, F. N., Hill, I. G. W., and Johnston, F. D.: The Form of the Electrocardiogram in Experimental Myocardial Infarction: I. Septal Infarcts and the Origin of the Preliminary Deflections of the Canine Electrocardiogram, in F. D. Johnston and E. Lepeschkin (eds.), "Selected Papers of Dr. Frank N. Wilson," Edwards Brothers, Inc., Ann Arbor, Mich., 1955, pp. 572–590.
19. Bayley, R. H.: An Interpretation of Injury and the Ischemic Effects of Myocardial Infarction in Accordance with the Laws Which Determine the Flow of Electric Current in Homogeneous Volume Conductors, and in Accordance with Relevant Pathologic Changes, *Am. Heart J.*, 24:514, 1942.
20. Bruyneel, K. J. J.: Use of Moving Epicardial Electrodes in Defining ST-Segment Changes after Acute Coronary Occlusion in the Baboon: Relation to Primary Ventricular Fibrillation, *Am. Heart J.*, 89:731, 1975.
21. Holland, R. P., and Brooks, H.: TQ-ST Segment Mapping: Critical Review and Analysis of Current Concepts, *Am. J. Cardiol.*, 40:110, 1977.
22. Arvan, S., and Varat, M. A.: Persistent ST-Segment Elevation and Left Ventricular Wall Abnormalities: A 2-Dimensional Echocardiographic Study, *Am. J. Cardiol.*, 53:1542, 1984.
23. The Criteria Committee of the New York Heart Association: "Nomenclature and Criteria for Diagnosis of Diseases of the Heart and Great Vessels," 8th ed., Little, Brown and Company, Boston, 1979, p. 94.
24. Braat, S. H., Brugrada, P., den Dulk, K., van Ommen, V., and Wellens, H. J. J.: Value of Lead V4R for Recognition of the Infarct Coronary Artery in Acute Inferior Myocardial Infarction, *Am. J. Cardiol.*, 53:1538, 1984.
25. Warner, R. A., Hill, N. E., Mookherjee, S., and Smucyan, H.: Improved electrocardiographic criteria for the diagnosis of left anterior hemiblock, *Am. J. Cardiol.*, 51:723, 1983.
26. Milliken, J. A.: Isolated and Complicated Left Anterior Fascicular Block: A Review of Suggested Electrocardiographic Criteria, *J. Electrocardiol.*, 16:199, 1983.
27. Rosenbaum, M. B., Elizari, M. V., and Lazzari, J. O.: The Differential Electrocardiographic Manifestations of Hemiblocks, Bilateral Bundle Branch Blocks and Trifascicular Blocks, in R. C. Schlant and J. W. Hurst (eds.), "Advances of Electrocardiography," Grune & Stratton, New York, 1972.
28. Wilson, F. N., Johnston, F. D., Rosenbaum, F. F., et al.: The Precordial Electrocardiogram, in F. D. Johnston and E. Lepeschkin (eds.), "Selected Papers of Dr. Frank N. Wilson," Edwards Brothers, Inc., Ann Arbor, Mich., 1954, p. 364.
29. Wilson, F. N., and Herrman, G. R.: An Experimental Study of Incomplete Bundle Branch Block and of the Refractory Period of the Heart of the Dog, in F. D. Johnston and E. Lepeschkin (eds.), "Selected Papers of Dr. Frank N. Wilson," Edwards Brothers, Inc., Ann Arbor, Mich., 1954, p. 749.
30. Rothberger, C. J., and Winterberg, H.: Experimentelle Beitrage zur Kenntnis der Reizleitungstorungen in den Kammern des Saugetierherzens, *Ges. Exp. Med.*, 5:264, 1917.
31. Barker, J. M., and Valencia, F.: The Precordial Electrocardiogram in Incomplete Right Bundle Branch Block, in F. D. Johnston and E. Lepeschkin (eds.), "Selected Papers of Dr. Frank N. Wilson," Edwards Brothers, Inc., Ann Arbor, Mich., 1954, p. 884.
32. Grishman, A., and Scherlis, L.: "Spatial Vectorcardiography," W. B. Saunders Company, Philadelphia, 1952, p. 107.
33. Kossmann, C. E., Berger, A. R., Rader, B., Brumlik, J., Briller, S. A., and Donnelly, J. H.: Intracardiac and Intravascular Potentials Resulting from Electrical Activity of the Normal Human Heart, *Circulation*, 2:10, 1950.
34. Blount, S. G., Mumyan, E. A., Jr., and Hoffman, M. S.: Hypertrophy of the Right Ventricular Outflow Tract: A Concept of the Electrocardiographic Findings in Atrial Septal Defect, *Am. J. Med.*, 22:784, 1957.
35. Cabrera, E., and Gaxiola, A.: A Critical Re-evaluation of Systolic and Diastolic Overloading Patterns, *Prog. Cardiovasc. Dis.*, 2:219, 1959.
36. Moore, E. N., Hoffman, B. F., Patterson, D. F., and Stuckey, J. H.: Electrocardiographic Changes Due to Delayed Activation of the Wall of the Right Ventricle, *Am. Heart J.*, 68:347, 1964.
37. Fahr, G.: Some Fundamental Principles of Electrocardiography, *Arch. Intern. Med.*, 27:126, 1921.
38. Punja, M. M., Schneebaum, R., and Cohen, J.: Bifascicular Block Induced by Hyperkalemia, *J. Electrocardiol.*, 6:71, 1973.
39. Sung, R. J., Tamer, D. M., Agha, A. S., Castellanos, A., Myerburg, R. J., and Gelband, H.: Etiology of the Electrocardiographic Pattern of "Incomplete Right Bundle Branch Block" in Atrial Septal Defect: An Electrophysiologic Study, *J. Pediatr.*, 87:1182, 1975.
40. Castellanos, A., Ramirez, A. V., Mayorga-Cortes, A., et al.: Left Fascicular Blocks during Right-Heart Catheterization Using the Swan-Ganz Catheter, *Circulation*, 64:1271, 1981.
41. Pickoff, A. S., Wolff, G. S., Tamer, D., and Gelband, H.: Arrhythmias and Conduction System Disturbances in Infants and Children—Recent Advances and Contributions of Intracardiac Electrophysiology, in A. Castellanos and A. N. Brest (eds.), "Cardiac Arrhythmias—Mechanisms and Management," *Cardiovasc. Clin.*, 11:203, 1980.
42. Garcia, O. L., Castellanos, A., Sung, R. J., and Gelband, H.: Exposure of Concealed Right Bundle Branch Block in Wolff-Parkinson-White Type B by Pacing from the Vicinity of the A-V Node, *Am. Heart J.*, 96:662, 1978.
43. Grant, R. P.: Peri-Infarction Block, *Prog. Cardiovasc. Dis.*, 27:237, 1959.
44. Oppenheimer, B. S., and Rothschild, M. A.: Electrocardio-

graphic Changes Associated with Myocardial Involvement: With Special Reference to Prognosis, *JAMA*, 69:429, 1917.
45. Castle, C. H., and Keane, W. M.: Electrocardiographic "Peri-Infarction Block": A Clinical and Pathologic Correlation, *Circulation*, 31:403, 1965.
46. Corne, R. A., Parkin, T. W., Brandenburg, R. O., and Brown, A. L., Jr.: Peri-Infarction Block: Postmyocardial Infarction Intraventricular Conduction Disturbance, *Am. Heart J.*, 69:150, 1965.
47. First, S. R., Bayley, R. H., and Bedford, D. R.: Peri-Infarction Block, *Circulation*, 2:31, 1950.
48. Watt, T. B., Jr., and Pruitt, R. B.: Electrocardiographic Findings Associated with Experimental Arborization Block in Dogs, *Am. Heart J.*, 69:642, 1965.
49. Wolff, L., Parkinson, J., and White, P. D.: Bundle-Branch Block with Short P-R Interval in Healthy Young People Prone to Paroxysmal Tachycardia, *Am. Heart J.*, 5:685, 1930.
50. Castillo, C. A., and Castellanos, A.: His Bundle Recordings in Patients with Reciprocating Tachycardias and Wolff-Parkinson-White Syndrome, *Circulation*, 42:271, 1970.
51. Rosenbaum, F. F., Hecht, H. H., Wilson, F. N., and Johnston, F. D.: The Potential Variations of the Thorax and the Esophagus in Anomalous Atrioventricular Excitation (Wolff-Parkinson-White Syndrome), *Am. Heart J.*, 29:281, 1945.
52. Wallace, A. G., Sealy, W. C., Gallagher, J. J., and Kasell, J.: Ventricular Excitation in Wolff-Parkinson-White Syndrome, in H. J. J. Wellens, K. I. Lie, and M. J. Janse (eds.), "The Conduction System of the Heart: Structure, Function and Clinical Implications," H. E. Stenfert Kroese BV, Leiden, 1976, pp. 613.
53. Befeler, B., Castellanos, A., Castillo, C. A., Agha, A. S., Vagueiro, M. C., and Myerburg, R. J.: Arrival of Excitation at the Right Ventricular Apical Endocardium in Wolff-Parkinson-White Syndrome Type B, *Circulation*, 48:655, 1973.
54. Castillo, C. A., Castellanos, A., Jr., Befeler, B., Myerburg, R. J., Agha, A. S., and Vagueiro, M. C.: Arrival of Excitation at Right Ventricular Apical Endocardium in Wolff-Parkinson-White Syndrome Type A, with and without Right Bundle Branch Block, *Br. Heart J.*, 35:594, 1973.
55. Castellanos, A., Agha, A. S., Portillo, B., and Myerburg, R. J.: Usefulness of Vectorcardiography Combined with His Bundle Recordings and Cardiac Pacing in Evaluation of the Pre-excitation (Wolff-Parkinson-White) Syndrome, *Am. J. Cardiol.*, 30:623, 1972.
56. Wellens, H. J. J.: Contribution of Cardiac Pacing to our Understanding of the Wolff-Parkinson-White Syndrome, *Br. Heart J.*, 37:231, 1975.
57. Gallagher, J. J., Sealy, W. C., Kasell, J., and Wallace, A. G.: Multiple Accessory Pathways in Patients with the Pre-excitation Syndrome, *Circulation*, 54:571, 1976.
58. Gallagher, J. J., Smith, W. M., Kasell, J. H., Benson, D. W., Jr., Sterba, R., and Grant, A. O.: Role of Mahaim Fibers in Cardiac Arrhythmias in Man, *Circulation*, 64:176, 1981.
59. Castellanos, A., Jr., Ortiz, J. M., Pastis, N., and Castillo, C. A.: The Electrocardiogram in Patients with Pacemakers, *Prog. Cardiovasc. Dis.*, 13:190, 1970.
60. Castellanos, A., Jr., Lemberg, L., Salhanick, L., and Berkovits, B. V.: Pacemaker Vectorcardiography, *Am. Heart J.*, 75:6, 1968.
61. Hurst, J. W. (ed.): "Update I: The Heart," McGraw-Hill Book Company, New York, 1979.
62. Ter Keurs, H. E. D. J., and Schipperheyn, J. J.: "Cardiac Left Ventricular Hypertrophy," Martinus Nijhoff Publishers, Boston, 1983.
63. Murphy, M. L., Thenabadu, P. N., De Soyza, N., et al.: Reevaluation of Electrocardiographic Criteria for Left, Right and Combined Cardiac Ventricular Hypertrophy, *Am. J. Cardiol.*, 53:1140, 1984.
64. Woythaler, J. N., Singer, S. L., Kwan, O. L., et al.: Accuracy of Echocardiography versus Electrocardiography in Detecting Left Ventricular Hypertrophy: Comparison with Postmortem Mass Measurements, *J. Am. Coll. Cardiol.*, 2:305, 1983.
65. WanderArk, C. R., Ballantyne, F. III, and Reynolds, E. W.: Electrolytes and the Electrocardiogram, *Cardiovasc. Clin.*, 5:268, 1973.
66. Schwartz, P. J., and Wolf, S.: QT Interval Prolongation as Predictor of Sudden Death in Patients with Myocardial Infarction, *Circulation*, 57:1074, 1978.
67. Burch, G. E.: The EKG, the Heart, the CNS, and Autonomic Nervous System, in P. J. Schwartz, A. M. Brown, A. Malliani, and A. Zanchetti (eds.), "Neural Mechanisms in Cardiac Arrhythmias," Raven Press, New York, 1978, pp. 43–53.
68. James, T. N., Froggatt, P., Atkinson, W. J., Jr., et al.: De Subitaneis Mortibus: Observations on the Pathophysiology of the Long QT Syndromes with Special Reference to the Neuropathology of the Heart, *Circulation*, 57:1221, 1978.
69. Schwartz, P. J., and Stone, H. L.: Unilateral Stellectomy and Sudden Death, in P. J. Schwartz, A. M. Brown, A. Malliani, and A. Zanchetti (eds.), "Neural Mechanisms in Cardiac Arrhythmias," Raven Press, New York, 1978, pp. 107–122.
70. Myerburg, R. J., and Castellanos, A.: The Diagnosis and Management of Patients with Prolonged Q-T Intervals, *Cardiology* (weekly update), 1:2, 1979.
71. Kerwin, A. J., McLean, R., and Tegelaar, H.: A Method for the Accurate Placement of Chest Electrodes in the Taking of Serial Electrocardiographic Tracings, *Can. Med. Assoc. J.*, 82:258, 1960.
72. Taback, L., Marden, E., Mason, H. L., and Pipberger, H. V.: Digital Recording of Electrocardiographic Data for Analysis by a Digital Computer. *I.R.E. Trans. Med. Elect.*, 6:167, 1959.
73. Pipberger, H. V., and Cornfeld, J.: What ECG Computer Program to Choose for Clinical Application: The Need for Consumer Protection, *Circulation*, 47:918, 1973.
74. Tenth Bethesda Conference Report: Optimal Electrocardiography, *Am. J. Cardiol.*, 41:111, 1978.
75. Laks, M. M., and Ginzton, L.: Computerized Electrocardiographic Interpretation—A Practical Adjunct to the Electrocardiographer, *Pract. Cardiol.*, 5:127, 1979.

15

The Chest Roentgenogram

James T. T. Chen, M.D.

They were the footprints of a gigantic hound!
Sir Arthur Conan Doyle, 1902[1]

A systematic approach to cardiac roentgenology is simple and effective.[2] First of all, to prevent the observer from being biased by an opinion which may occasionally be oversimplified or even mistaken, an objective observation of all roentgen signs is made *without* the clinical information. For example, a patient was referred to our pulmonary division because the patient had "bronchial asthma" refractory to therapy for 20 years. The routine chest roentgenograms, however, showed typical signs of severe mitral stenosis. As soon as the appropriate treatment was instituted, the patient's cardiac asthma disappeared for the first time in two decades. Likewise, an ostium secundum atrial septal defect may be misinterpreted as mitral stenosis because of similar physical signs. The split second sound may be misinterpreted as the opening snap. The diastolic rumble through the tricuspid valve which is the result of increased flow may mimic the diastolic murmur of mitral stenosis. The x-ray signs, however, are quite different between the two entities (Figs. 15-4*B* and 15-5*A*).

The *final* radiological conclusion, however, should be drawn only after correlating the x-ray findings with both the clinical information and the laboratory data.

Major Steps of Roentgenologic Examination

Objective Analysis

Roentgenographic Examination of Anatomy

An Overview The first step is to survey the roentgenograms and look at the entire situation, searching particularly for noncardiac conditions that may reflect heart disease. For instance, a right-sided stomach with an absent inferior vena cava may direct our attention to the possibility of congenital interruption of inferior vena cava with azygos continuation[3,4] (Fig. 15-1). A narrowed anteroposterior diameter of the thorax may be the cause of an innocent murmur.[5] Rib notching (Fig. 15-10*A*) is an important clue to the diagnosis of coarctation of the aorta.[6,7]

Pulmonary Vasculature The lung may be likened to a mirror which faithfully reflects the underlying pathophysiology of the heart.[2,8–11] By careful evaluation of the pulmonary vasculature one may narrow down the diagnostic possibility to a manageable level. For example, if uniform dilatation of all pulmonary vessels is present, the diagnosis of a left-to-right shunt (Fig. 15-4*B*) is preferred to a left-sided obstructive lesion. The latter typically shows a cephalad pulmonary blood flow pattern (Fig. 15-5*A*). More detailed analysis of the pulmonary vascularity will be given separately below.

Lung Parenchyma[9] The lung is a reflector of the heart. When the right side of the heart fails, the lung becomes unusually radiolucent because of decreased pulmonary blood flow. On the other hand, significant left-sided heart failure is characterized by the presence of pulmonary edema and a cephalad blood flow pattern (see page 235).

Cardiac Size[10,12,13] A significantly enlarged heart is always abnormal, while mild cardiomegaly may reflect a higher than average cardiac output from a normal heart, as seen in athletes in active training. The cardiothoracic ratio remains the simplest and the most practical yardstick for the assessment of cardiac size. The mean value for adults in deep inspiration is 44 percent. More accurate roentgen measurements of the cardiac size have been well documented[14,15] and are out of the scope of the present discussion. The nature of cardiomegaly can usually be determined by the specific roentgen appearance. As a rule, when the pulmonary blood flow pattern remains normal, cardiac lesions with volume overload tend to present a greater degree of cardiomegaly than lesions with pressure overload alone. For example, patients with aortic stenosis typically show an increase in convexity of the left ventricle but very little cardiac enlargement. In such a condition, there is only hypertrophy of the myocardium without dilatation of the cardiac lumen. On the other hand, the left ventricle both dilates and hypertrophies in the case of aortic insufficiency, producing a much larger heart even before congestive heart failure takes place. Both right-sided and left-sided heart failure can cause gross cardiac enlargement. The associated vascular abnormality in each case is, however, drastically different (see below under "Pulmonary Vascularity"). A heart smaller than average is encountered in patients with chronic obstructive pulmonary disease (Fig. 15-7*A*), Addison's disease, anorexia nervosa, and starvation. However, an abnormally small heart is difficult to define except in a retrospective fashion when the heart has returned to its normal capacity following successful

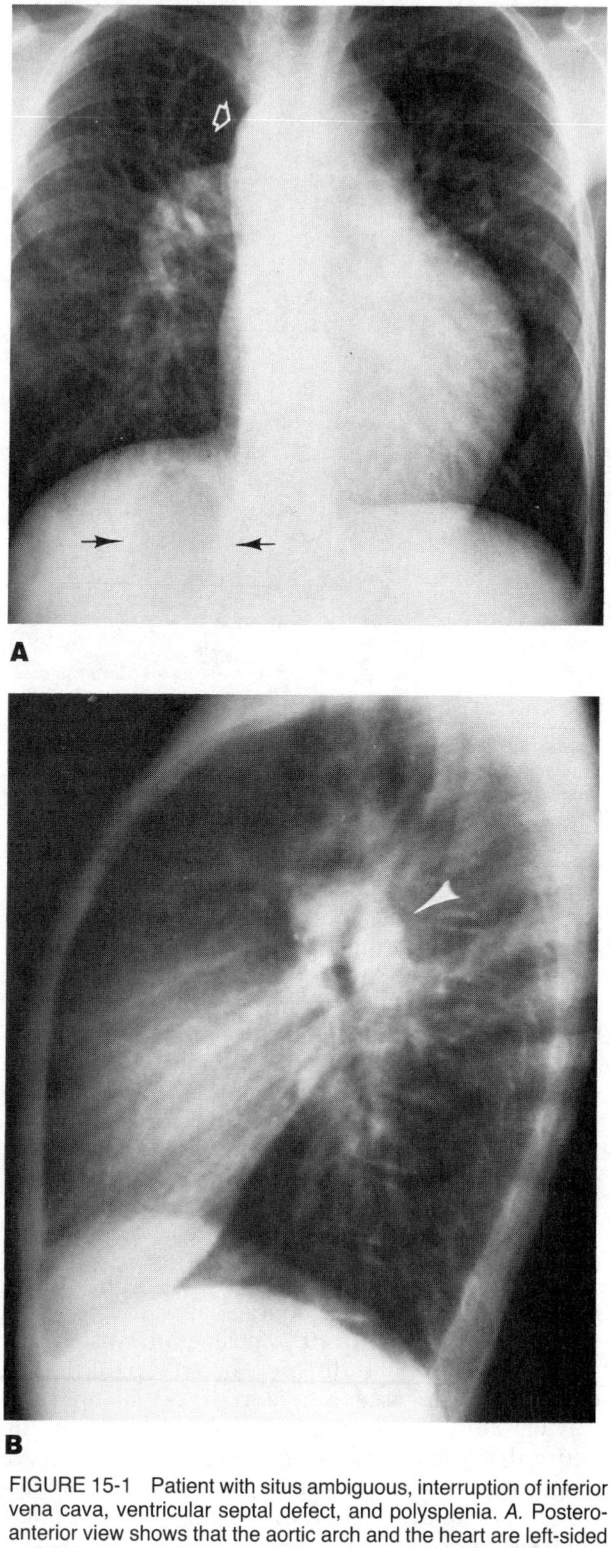

FIGURE 15-1 Patient with situs ambiguous, interruption of inferior vena cava, ventricular septal defect, and polysplenia. *A.* Posteroanterior view shows that the aortic arch and the heart are left-sided and the stomach (lower arrows) is right-sided. The azygos vein (upper arrow) is markedly enlarged. The heart is mildly enlarged, and there is moderate increase in pulmonary vascularity. *B.* Lateral view shows an absent image of the inferior vena cava. The azygos arch (arrow) is markedly dilated.

therapy. For example, in patients with Addison's disease, the heart, in response to steroid therapy, may become significantly larger.

Cardiac Contour Any significant deviations from the normal cardiovascular contour may serve as a clue to the correct diagnosis. For instance, coeur en sabot, or a "boot-shaped" heart (Fig. 15-4*C*), is characteristic of tetralogy of Fallot. A bulge along the left cardiac border with a retrosternal double density is virtually diagnostic of left ventricular aneurysm (Fig. 15-2). A markedly widened right cardiac contour in association with a straightened left cardiac border is frequently seen in patients with severe mitral stenosis leading to tricuspid insufficiency (Fig. 15-7*D*).

Abnormal Densities Besides the familiar double density cast by an enlarged left atrium, other increased densities may be found within the confines of the heart by a variety of dilated vascular structures, e.g., tortuous descending aorta, aortic aneurysm, coronary artery aneurysm, pulmonary varix, etc.[2] Furthermore, large cardiac calcifications are easily seen, particularly in the lateral and oblique views. If smaller calcific deposits are suspected, they should be promptly verified or ruled out by cardiac fluoroscopy. Any radiologically detectable calcification in the heart is of clinical importance. The heavier the calcification, the more significant it becomes (Fig. 15-10*E*). As a rule, the extent of valvular calcification is proportionate to the severity of the valve stenosis regardless of the other roentgen signs of the disease.[2] Calcification of the coronary artery is almost always of atherosclerotic nature. Mönckeberg's medial calcification of the coronary system is extremely rare. A radiologically detectable coronary calcification is correlated with major-vessel occlusion in 94 percent of patients with chest pain.[16]

Abnormal Lucencies The abnormal lucencies in and about the heart include (1) the displaced subepicardial fat lines caused by effusion or thickening of the pericardium (see Chap 107), (2) pneumopericardium, and (3) pneumomediastinum. Pneumomediastinum is differentiated from pneumopericardium by the fact that the former shows a more superior extension of the air strip beyond the confines of the pericardium.

Cardiac Malpositions[3,4]

Dextrocardia By definition dextrocardia is a mirror image of the heart and the abdominal viscera (situs inversus). A ninefold increase in the incidence of congenital cardiac defects is found in patients with dextrocardia (5 percent) as compared with the general population (0.6 to 0.8 percent). Also known is the tendency for these patients to develop noncardiac lesions known as Kartagener's triad: dextrocardia, sinusitis, and bronchiectasis.

Dextroversion Dextroversion represents an anomaly with situs solitus and a right-sided heart (the apex of the ventricles points to the right side and inferi-

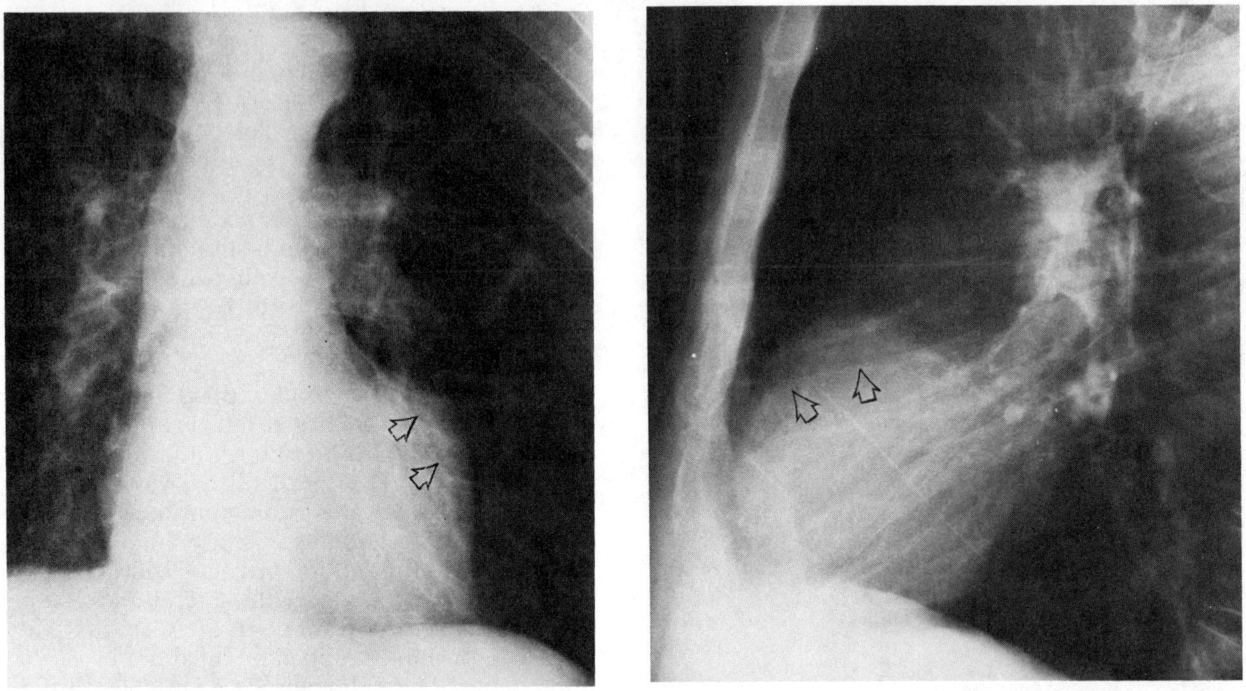

A B

FIGURE 15-2 Left ventricular aneurysm. *A.* Posteroanterior view showing the typical bulge (arrows) along the left cardiac border representing the anterolateral wall left ventricular aneurysm. *B.* Lateral view showing a double density with sharp borders anteriorly and superiorly (arrows). This is the left ventricular aneurysm that casts a shadow on the normal right ventricle. Fluoroscopically it is easy to confirm its origin and to separate it from the right ventricle by rotating the patient under direct vision.

orly). Roentgenographically situs solitus is a certainty when both the aortic knob and the gastric air bubble are on the left side. Situs solitus also means that both the abdominal viscera and the atria are normal. Under these circumstances, if the ventricles fail to swing from their primitive right-sided position to their normal left-sided position, abnormal relations between the ventricles and the rest of the cardiovascular structures are bound to occur.

The incidence of congenital cardiac defects was estimated at 98 percent in patients with dextroversion. Of these patients over 80 percent had congenitally corrected transposition (or *l*-loop transposition) of the great arteries. The next commonly associated lesions were a combination of ventricular septal defect and pulmonary stenosis, a tetralogy-like pathophysiology (Fig. 15-3*D*). Therefore, from the statistical point of view it is important to be able to differentiate dextroversion from dextrocardia, and this is readily accomplished on grounds of the roentgenogram alone.

Levoversion Levoversion is a mirror image of dextroversion, consisting of a combination of situs inversus and a left-sided heart. The extremely high incidence of cyanotic congenital cardiac defects in patients with levoversion is comparable to that with dextroversion.

Cardiac Malpositions with Indeterminate Situs In this group of malpositions the patient's heart may be either left-sided or right-sided. The situs is ambiguous, with the roentgenogram showing aortico-gastric bubble discordance. In other words, the aortic knob and the stomach are not on the same side, and therefore, the situs is unpredictable, though the left atrium tends to be on the side of the aorta. Under these circumstances, interruption of inferior vena cava with azygos continuation is almost always present (Fig. 15-1). The next most commonly associated lesions are polysplenia and a left-to-right shunt, most frequently a ventricular septal defect. The only exception to the rule of indeterminate situs is an isolated right-sided arch.

Other Abnormalities

Great Vessels[9,12,13] The roentgen appearance of the great vessels often provides valuable information for the diagnosis of heart disease. For example, selective dilatation of the ascending aorta is the hallmark of valvular aortic stenosis; generalized dilatation of the entire thoracic aorta, on the other hand, favors the diagnosis of aortic insufficiency or systemic hypertension, or both, depending on the size of the left ventricle. A larger left ventricle is associated with aortic insufficiency because of volume overload (see Chap. 107). In atrial septal defect and mitral stenosis the pulmonary trunk is quite large and the aortic knob is usually small (Figs. 15-4*B* and 15-5*A*). This is explained on the basis of a leftward cardiac rotation which occurs when an enlarged right ventricle coexists with a normal-sized left ventricle. When the heart rotates to the left, the aorta folds on itself

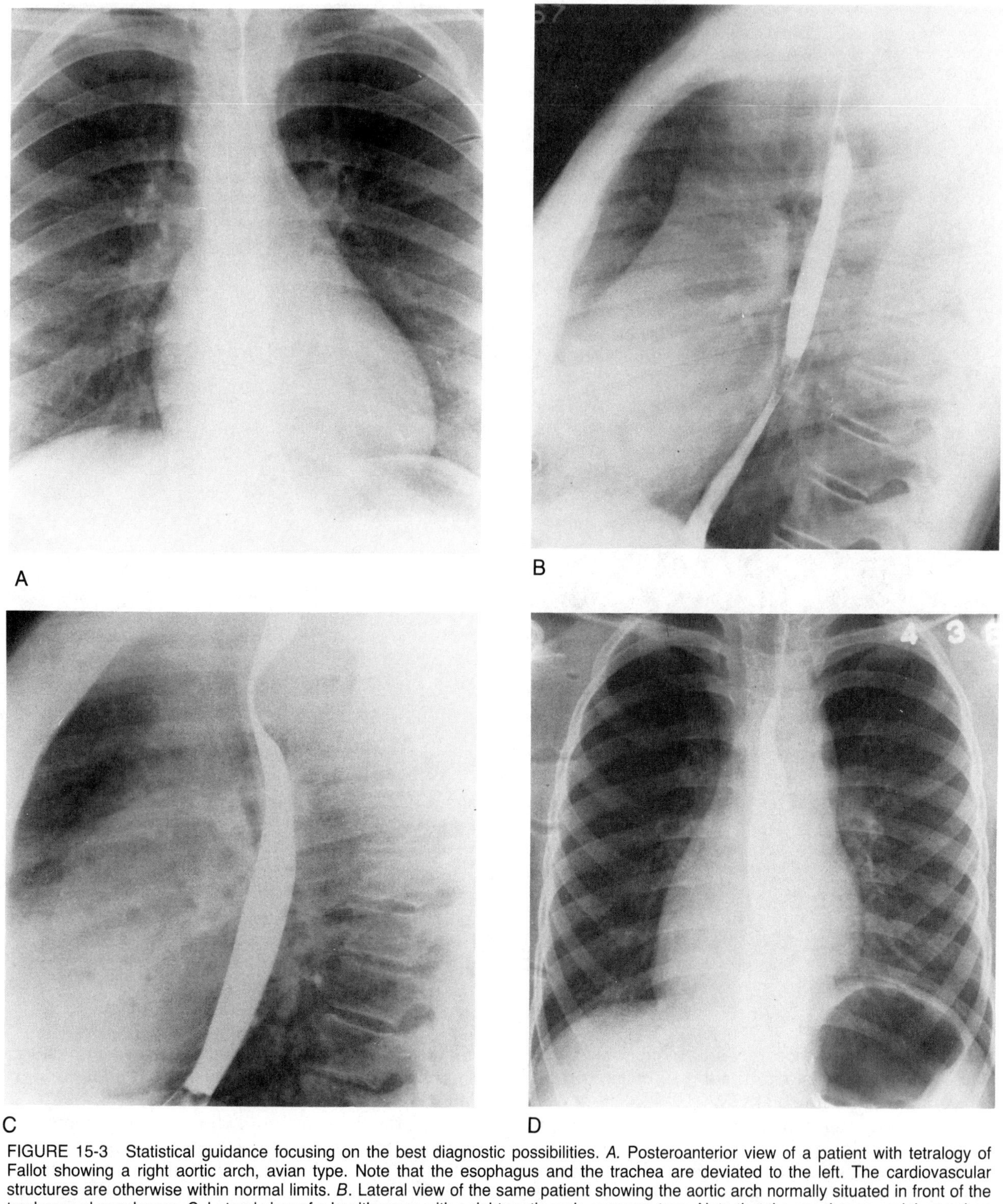

FIGURE 15-3 Statistical guidance focusing on the best diagnostic possibilities. *A.* Posteroanterior view of a patient with tetralogy of Fallot showing a right aortic arch, avian type. Note that the esophagus and the trachea are deviated to the left. The cardiovascular structures are otherwise within normal limits. *B.* Lateral view of the same patient showing the aortic arch normally situated in front of the trachea and esophagus. *C.* Lateral view of a healthy man with a right aortic arch, common type. Note that the esophagus and the trachea are markedly displaced anteriorly by a huge aortic diverticulum from which arises the aberrant left subclavian artery. The posteroanterior view of his chest (not shown) is very similar to that of the patient shown in *A. D.* Posteroanterior view of a patient with dextroversion. Note that the aortic arch and the stomach air bubble are both on the left (situs solitus), and the apex of the ventricles is pointing to the right inferiorly. As was predictable from statistics and proved by cardiac catheterization, this patient had the typical combination of corrected transposition of great arteries, ventricular septal defect, and pulmonary stenosis. He was cyanotic. The pulmonary vascularity appears decreased.

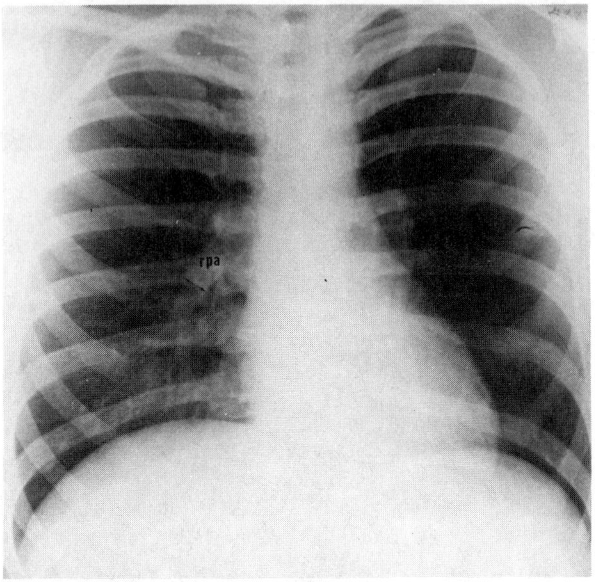

A

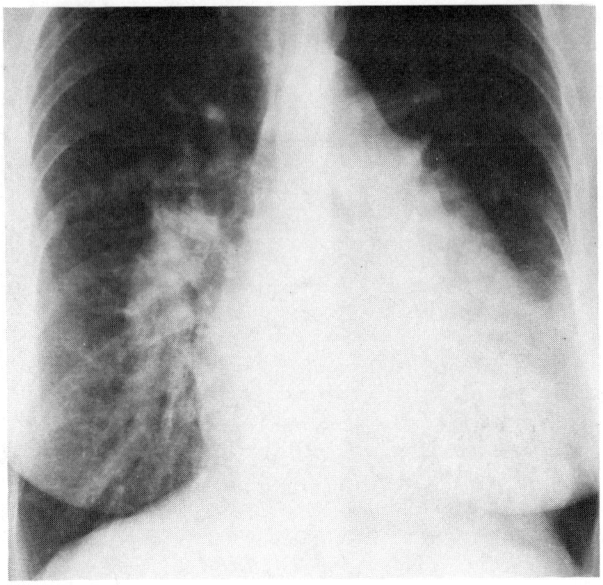

B

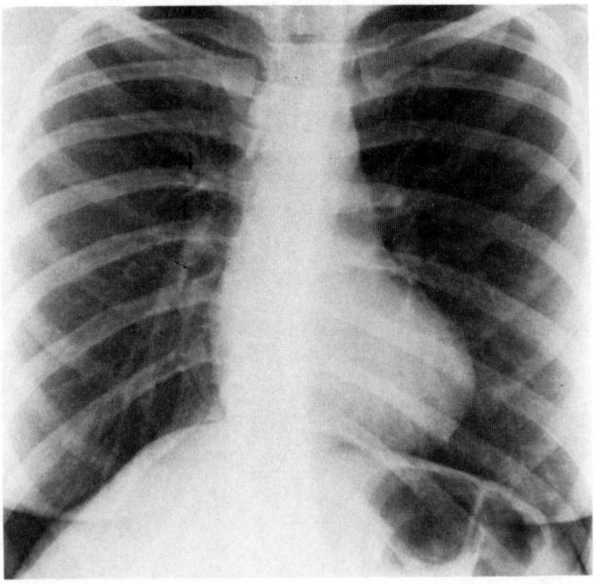

C

FIGURE 15-4 Roentgenographic assessment of the volume of pulmonary blood flow. *A.* Normal: There is caudalization of the pulmonary vascularity due to gravity. The right descending pulmonary artery (rpa) measures (arrows) 13 mm in diameter in this young adult male patient. *B.* Increased: Patient with secundum atrial septal defect showing uniform increase in pulmonary vascularity bilaterally. The right descending pulmonary artery is markedly enlarged, measuring 27 mm. *C.* Decreased: Patient with tetralogy of Fallot showing a boot-shaped heart and uniform decrease in pulmonary vascularity. The right descending pulmonary artery is markedly decreased, measuring 6 mm.

in the midline and becomes inconspicuous. Meanwhile the pulmonary trunk is brought laterad and looks larger than it actually is.

As already mentioned, prominence of the pulmonary trunk is a reliable secondary sign of a right ventricular enlargement, with the following exceptions: (1) tetralogy of Fallot with hypoplasia of the pulmonary trunk, (2) idiopathic dilatation of the pulmonary artery, (3) patent ductus arteriosus prior to the development of Eisenmenger physiology, and (4) straight-back syndrome, pectus excavatum, and scoliosis with narrowed anteroposterior diameter of the chest. In the latter circumstances the heart is compressed, displaced, and rotated to the left, giving rise to a falsely enlarged pulmonary artery.

In coarctation of aorta, the engorged aortic knob and the poststenotic dilatation of the descending aorta cause an E sign on the barium-filled esophagus, outlining the site of coarctation[6] (Fig. 15-10*B*).

The abnormal size and distribution of both the pulmonary and the systemic veins are important clues to the presence of certain heart disease, e.g., anomalous pulmonary venous connections and interruption of inferior vena cava with azygos continuation.

The significance of aortic arch anomalies will be discussed in the section on statistical guidance.

Mediastinal Structures[10,12,13,17,18] The mediastinal organs are frequently affected by the cardiovascular structures because of their close spatial interrelationships. An enlarged left atrium not only displaces the esophagus and the descending aorta but

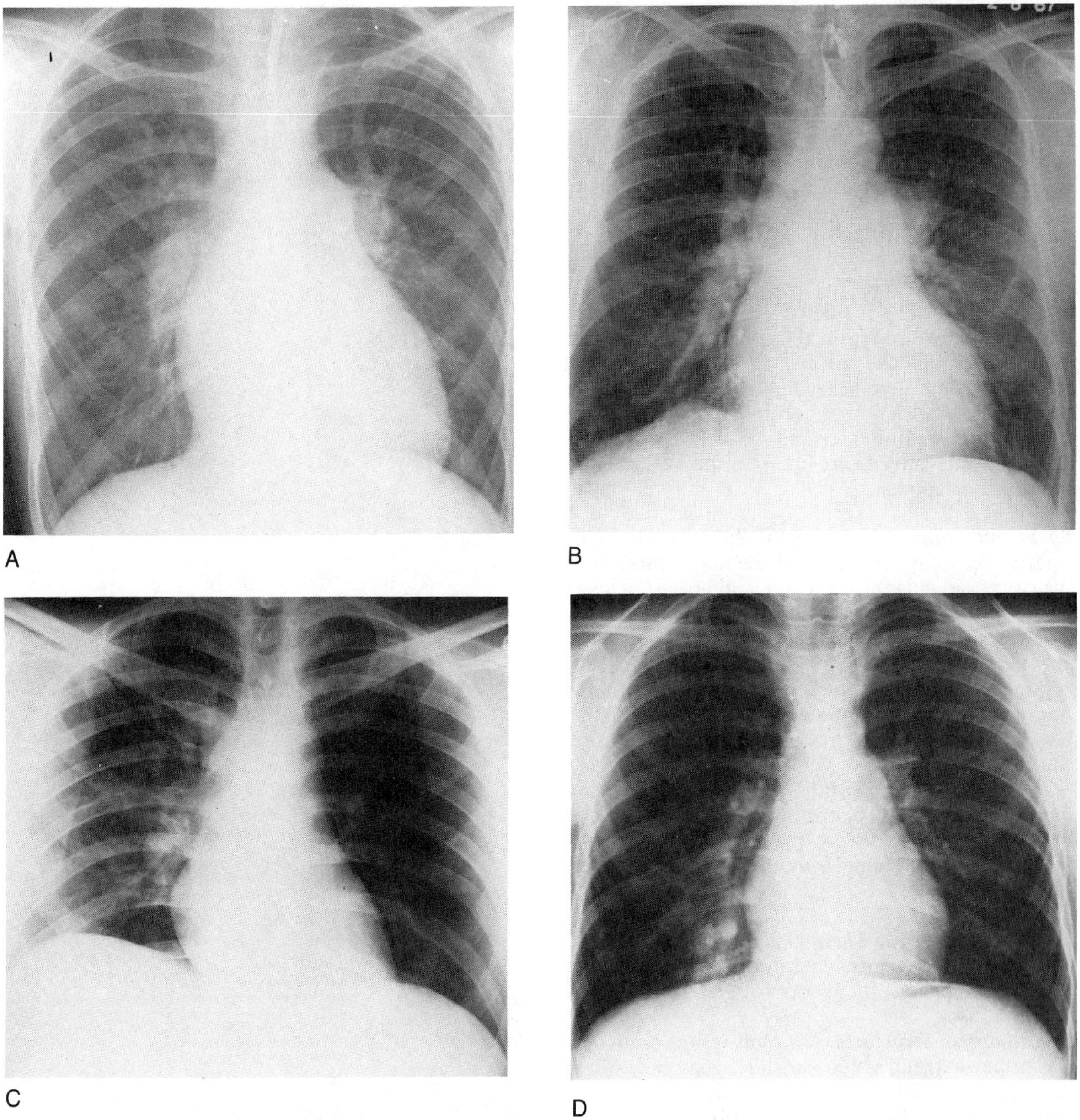

FIGURE 15-5 Abnormal pulmonary blood flow patterns. *A.* Cephalization: Patient with severe mitral stenosis showing dilatation of the upper vessels with constriction of the lower vessels. *B.* Centralization: Patient with Eisenmenger's atrial septal defect and ventricular septal defect showing marked dilatation of the pulmonary trunk and the central segments of both pulmonary arteries with pruning of the peripheral branches. *C.* Lateralization: Patient with massive pulmonary embolism obstructing the left main pulmonary artery. Note the uneven distribution of blood flow between the two lungs in favor of the right. *D.* Localization: A cyanotic child showing localized vascular changes representing a large pulmonary arteriovenous fistula in the right lower lobe (*Parts A and B from J. T. T. Chen et al., Roentgen Appearance of Pulmonary Vascularity in the Diagnosis of Heart Disease, Am. J. Roentgenol., 112:559, 1971. Reproduced with permission from the publisher and author.*)

also elevates and compresses the left stem bronchus. A double aortic arch may compress both the trachea and the esophagus. Patients with an anomalous origin of the left pulmonary artery from the right pulmonary artery (the pulmonary artery sling) usually present compression symptoms of the right stem bronchus. On the other hand, malignant processes may invade the heart and great vessels, causing cardiac tamponade or superior vena cava syndrome, for example. More frequently than not, these mediastinal changes are evident on the chest roentgenogram and should be recognized promptly.

Lung Parenchyma[9] When the right side of the heart fails, the lung becomes unusually radiolucent on account of decreased pulmonary blood flow. On the other hand, significant left-sided heart failure is easily recognized on the chest roentgenogram by the presence of pulmonary edema and cephalad blood flow pattern (Fig. 15-6*A*). Longstanding severe pulmonary venous hypertension may lead to hemosiderosis and/or ossification of the lung. When right-sided heart failure occurs as a result of severe left-sided heart failure, the preexisting pulmonary congestion will improve because of the decreased pulmonary blood flow (Fig. 15-6*B*).

Pleura A right-sided pleural effusion is typically present when the left side of the heart is failing. A bilateral hydrothorax, on the other hand, suggests bilateral heart failure or a noncardiac etiology of the effusion. Congestive heart failure is also known to be associated with a pseudotumor, or "vanishing," tumor, representing interlobar collection of pleural fluid. As congestive heart failure improves, the "tumor" will disappear.

Bones and Joints Notching of the ribs has many origins. Basically any of the three major intercostal structures can enlarge, compress, and erode the lower borders of the ribs, producing areas of notching. These structures are the intercostal arteries, veins, and nerves. Coarctation of the aorta[6] (Fig. 15-10*A*) represents the most common cause of rib notching due to dynamic dilatation and tortuosity of the arteries. Superior vena cava syndrome may cause a similar phenomenon of venous origin. Neurofibromatosis is known to produce rib notching by numerous intercostal neurofibromas. Patients with rheumatoid heart disease may show typical rheumatoid arthritic changes in the acromioclavicular joints.

Soft Tissues over the Chest Patients with renal failure may show severe edema in the soft tissues over the chest as part of the picture of general anasarca.

Extrathoracic Structures In Holt-Oram syndrome the upper-extremity abnormalities may be evident in a chest roentgenogram or on other films in the patient's x-ray folder. A large arteriovenous malformation with curvilinear calcifications may be seen in the neck, thereby providing a clue as to the etiology of the patient's congestive heart failure. Radiographic evaluation of the patient's abdominal viscera is an integral part of the workup for cardiac malpositions.[3,4]

Fluoroscopic Observation for Dynamics

Cardiac fluoroscopy is a valuable adjunct to the chest roentgenogram. Its many advantages and limitations are detailed in Chap. 107.

Comparison

In order to appreciate the acuteness or chronicity of the disease or its response to therapy, one must carefully compare the serial roentgenograms. As

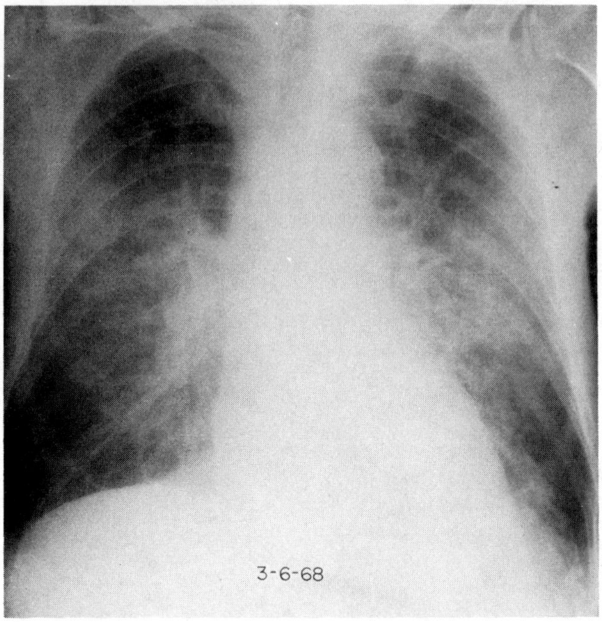

A

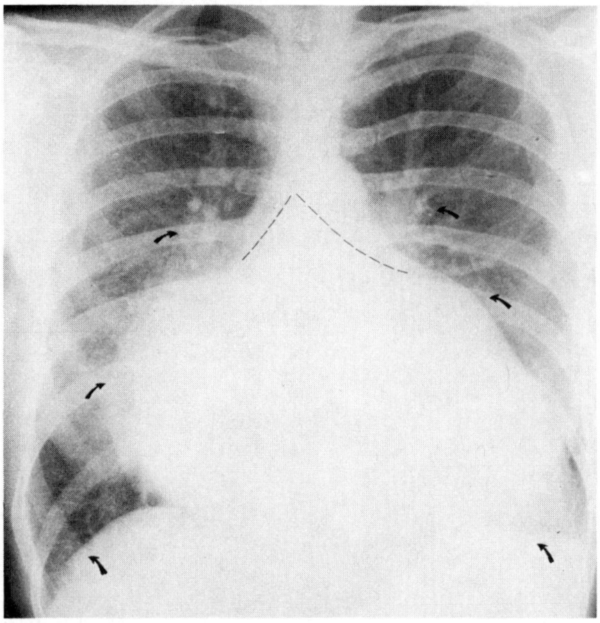

B

FIGURE 15-6 Roentgen appearance of left-sided heart failure. *A.* Acute: Patient with acute myocardial infarction showing "bat wings" appearance of severe alveolar type of pulmonary edema and a normal-sized heart. *B.* Chronic: Patient with severe rheumatic heart disease (severe mitral and tricuspid insufficiency and mild aortic insufficiency). This is a predominantly left-sided failure pattern. Note the giant left atrium forming the border of the right side of the heart (middle right arrow) and a bulging left atrial appendage along the border of the left side of the heart (left middle arrow). The peribronchial cuff of edema fluid is indicated by the upper left arrow. The Kerley B lines are marked by the lower right arrow. The upper right arrow points to the markedly dilated right superior pulmonary vein. The lower vessels were constricted. The left ventricle was enlarged with its apex marked by the lower left arrow. The markedly widened subcarinal angle is outlined by the retouched lower margin of both main stem bronchi. (*Part A from J. T. T. Chen et al., Roentgen Appearance of Pulmonary Vascularity in the Diagnosis of Heart Disease, Am. J. Roentgenol., 112:559, 1971. Reproduced with permission from the publisher and author.*)

demonstrated in Fig. 15-7*B*, the heart could neither be considered enlarged nor failing if the baseline study made 3 years before (Fig. 15-7*A*) were not available for comparison (see below under "Heart Failure"). Similarly, a rapidly enlarging heart with a normal pulmonary vascularity is highly suggestive of pericardial effusion.

Statistical Guidance

Certain roentgenologic findings are by themselves diagnostic of a disease; other signs are indirectly suggestive of the diagnosis on the basis of statistics. Nevertheless, the latter can be quite useful by virtue of their high predictive value of a certain disease or a group of similar diseases. Therefore, one should

FIGURE 15-7 Roentgen appearance of right-sided heart failure. *A.* Patient with severe obstructive emphysema showing overaeration of the lungs, centralized flow pattern, and a small heart size. *B.* Three years later the patient was in frank right-sided heart failure. Note that the heart got bigger as his emphysema got worse. The centralized flow pattern became more severe. *C.* Patient with Ebstein anomaly showing gross cardiomegaly with severe decrease in pulmonary vascularity. The right cardiac border represents the huge right atrium, and the left cardiac border represents the giant right ventricle. *D.* Patient with rheumatic mitral stenosis showing a giant right atrium (arrow) representing severe functional tricuspid insufficiency secondary to unrelenting left-sided failure. The pulmonary venous congestion had improved following the onset of right-sided heart failure.

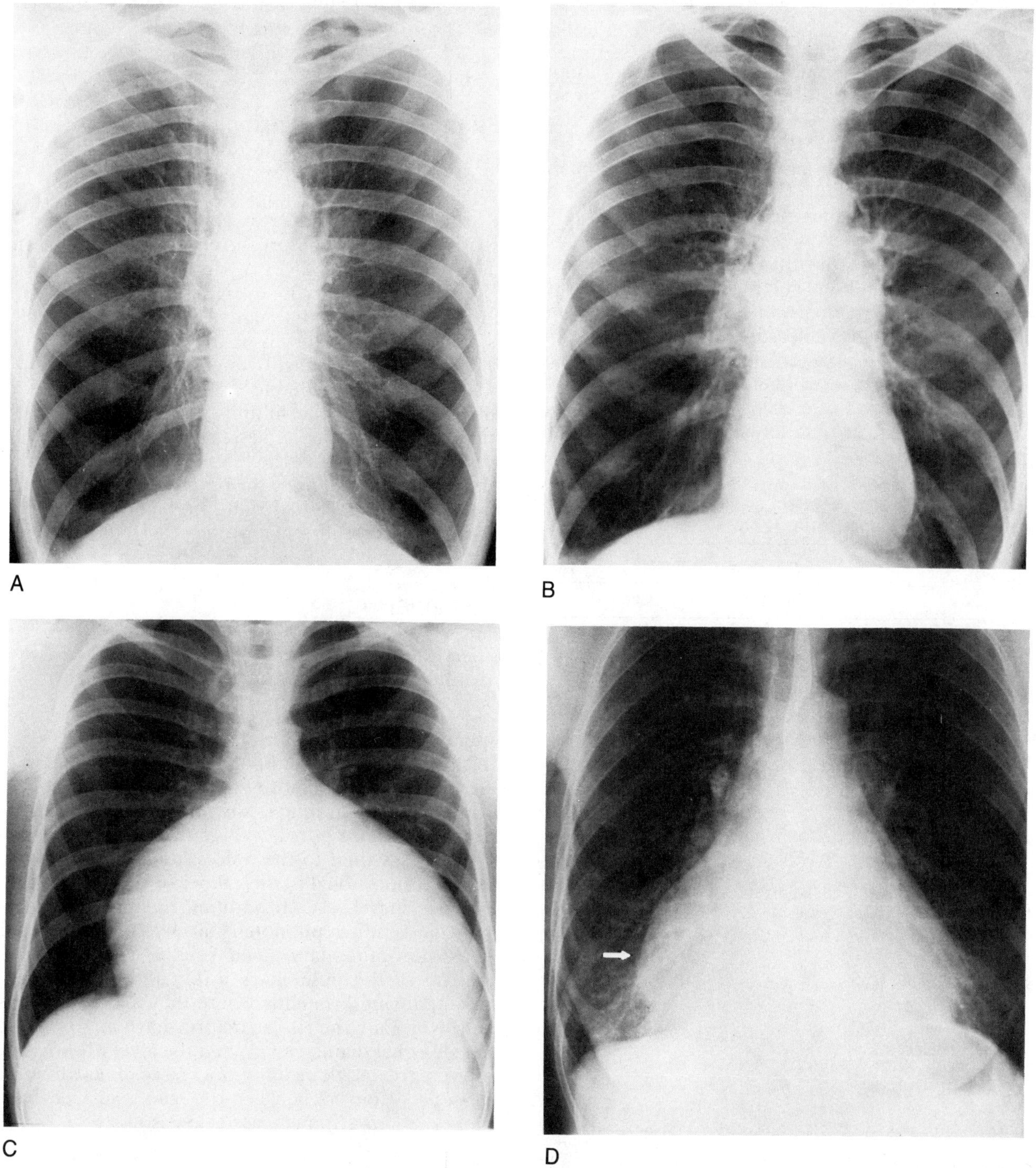

A B C D

always keep the statistical information in mind in the practice of cardiac roentgenology.

In addition to what has been mentioned in the section on cardiac malpositions, other anatomic settings may also provide useful statistical guidance for making a more precise radiographic diagnosis. Different types of aortic arch anomalies are good examples.

When a right-sided aortic arch is present, the incidence of congenital heart disease increases from 10- to 100-fold, depending on the anatomic details of the anomaly.[17,18] Of practical importance, there are only two types of right-sided aortic arch. The first has been called the *avian type*, implying a normal status for the birds but a seriously wrong one for human beings. The overwhelming majority of humans with this type would be born with cyanotic congenital heart disease. The second category may be called the *common type* because of a higher incidence of occurrence. Most patients with this type are physiologically normal, and their arch anomaly is usually discovered incidentally on routine chest x-rays or during a barium-meal study. The x-ray findings of the two types are similar in the posteroanterior view but are quite different in the lateral view (Fig. 15-3*A*, *B*, and *C*). The incidence of congenital heart disease in patients with a right-sided aortic arch[18] is shown in Table 15-1. In the presence of the avian type of right aortic arch the patient has only a 2 percent chance of being physiologically normal. The diagnosis of tetralogy of Fallot should be seriously considered under such conditions until proven otherwise.

TABLE 15-1 Cardiac Defects Associated with Each Type of Right-Sided Aortic Arch

	Type of Anomaly	
	Avian	**Common**
Anatomic details	With mirror-image branching; the arch is anterior to the trachea	With aberrant left subclavian artery arising from a large aortic diverticulum which is posterior to the esophagus
Patients with cardiac defects, %	98	12
Type of defects, %:		
Tetralogy of Fallot	90	71
Truncus arteriosus	2.5	
Transposition of great arteries	1.5	
Atrial septal defect and/or ventricular septal defect	0.5	21
Coarctation of aorta		7
Others	5.5	1

Patients with a double aortic arch, on the other hand, rarely have congenital heart disease, though they tend to be symptomatic in infancy because of a compressing vascular ring.[17]

Clinical Correlation

The next step in the examination is to correlate the roentgenologic findings with the clinical information and other laboratory parameters for the final conclusion. It may become necessary at this point to reexamine the radiograph, or to review the fluoroscopic observation, or both. After detailed analysis of some finer points, a wrong impression may be corrected or a correct diagnosis reinforced.

Pulmonary Vascularity

Normal

The normal roentgen appearance of the pulmonary vascularity is typified by a caudad flow pattern because of gravity. The pressure differential between the apex and the base of the lung is approximately 22 mmHg in adults in upright position.[19] Therefore, more flow under higher distending pressure is expected in the vessels of the lower lobe than of the upper lobe. Normally one sees little vascularity above the hilum, whereas more and larger vessels are found below the hilum. Since the pulmonary resistance is normal, all vessels taper gradually in a treelike manner from the hilum toward the periphery of the lung. The right descending pulmonary artery measures 10 to 15 mm in diameter in males and 9 to 14 mm in females (Fig. 15-4).[20]

Abnormal

The abnormal pulmonary vasculature can be classified into two categories, either in terms of volume or in terms of distribution.[9,11]

Abnormalities in Volume

In the evaluation of pulmonary vasculature the caliber of the vessels is more important than the length or the number. As long as the pulmonary blood flow pattern remains normal, with greater amount of flow to the bases than to the apices, the volume of the flow is proportional to the caliber of the pulmonary arteries (Fig. 15-4). In addition to measuring the right descending pulmonary artery, one may also assess the pulmonary blood volume by comparing the size of the pulmonary artery with that of the accompanying bronchus where they are viewed on end. Normally the two structures have an approximately equal diameter.[21] When the artery/bronchus ratio is greater than unity, increased blood flow is suggested. Conversely, when the ratio is smaller than unity (Fig. 15-4*C*), decreased flow is likely.

Increased Pulmonary Blood Flow

In the case of mild to moderate left-to-right shunts, for example, the vessels dilate in proportion to the increased flow with no significant change in pressure, resistance, or flow pattern. This phenomenon is also called *shunt vascularity* or *equalization*. The last expression is based on the fact that the distribution of blood flow tends to be equalized between the upper and lower lung zones; however, this change is not marked, and the lower lobes still receive a great deal more blood than the upper. Mild increase in pulmonary vascularity with slight cardiomegaly is commonly found in pregnant women and trained athletes with greater cardiac output and supranormal performance of the heart.

Decreased Pulmonary Blood Flow

Patients with tetralogy of Fallot frequently show decreased pulmonary vascularity with smaller and shorter pulmonary arteries and more radiolucent lungs (Fig. 15-3*A*). Marked reduction in pulmonary blood flow is also encountered in patients with right-sided heart failure without a right-to-left shunt (Fig. 15-7). This is attributed to the significant decrease in cardiac output from both ventricles.

Abnormalities in Distribution

An abnormal distribution of flow (or an abnormal flow pattern) always reflects a changed pulmonary vascular resistance, either locally or diffusely.

Cephalization In the presence of postcapillary pulmonary hypertension the physiological disturbances may begin when the total intravascular pressure exceeds the oncotic pressure of the blood. As a result fluid leaks out of the vessels and collects in the interstitium before pouring into the alveoli.

Pulmonary edema interferes with gas exchange, resulting in a state of hypoxia. Hypoxia has a profound influence to contract on the pulmonary vessels. Since there is a greater pressure increase in the lung bases than in the apices, the basilar vessels begin to constrict, forcing the blood to flow upward. This phenomenon actually represents a reversal of the normal blood flow pattern, redistribution or *cephalization* of the pulmonary vascularity. Cephalization occurs in one of these three conditions: (1) left-sided obstructive lesions, e.g., mitral stenosis (Fig. 15-5*A*)[20] and aortic stenosis; (2) left ventricular failure, e.g., coronary heart disease and cardiomyopathies; or (3) severe mitral insufficiency even before pump failure of the left ventricle occurs. It should be emphasized that unless there is obvious constriction of the lower-lobe vessels, the diagnosis of cephalization should not be made. Dilatation of the upper-lobe vessels is of secondary importance and can be found without narrowing of the basilar vessels in a number of entities, most noticeably, left-to-right shunts.

Centralization In the presence of a large left-to-right shunt, reactive pulmonary arteriolar spasms may cause significant elevation of pulmonary vascular resistance, which in turn produces a centralized pulmonary flow pattern (Eisenmenger syndrome) (Fig. 15-5*B*). The pulmonary trunk and central pulmonary arteries now dilate in response to increased pressure in addition to increased volume. The distal pulmonary arteries constrict in a concentric fashion from the hilum toward the periphery of the lung. A similar flow distribution is seen in patients with severe obstructive emphysema, representing severe precapillary pulmonary hypertension (Fig. 15-7*A* and *B*).

Lateralization Massive unilateral pulmonary embolism may cause a lateralized flow pattern. Since one major pulmonary artery is obstructed, the blood is forced to flow through the healthy lung only. The paucity of pulmonary vascularity in the diseased lung is termed *Westermark sign* (Fig. 15-5*C*).

Localization A localized abnormal flow pattern is exemplified by the arteriovenous fistula in a cyanotic child (Fig. 15-5*D*).

Combined Abnormalities

In reality an abnormal pulmonary vascularity is more frequently than not of the mixed type. There is a great variety of possible combinations, e.g., cephalization plus decreased flow in severe mitral stenosis (Fig. 15-5*A*), centralization with increased flow in Eisenmenger's atrial septal defect and ventricular septal defect (Fig. 15-5*B*).

Summary

Roentgen analysis of the pulmonary vasculature is accomplished in two steps. First, the volume of the pulmonary flow can be estimated by the degree of pulmonary arterial enlargement as long as the flow pattern remains normal. Second, the distribution of the pulmonary flow is compared with the normal caudad flow pattern. Any deviation from that indicates an altered pulmonary vascular resistance. The volume and the distribution of pulmonary blood flow may change singly or in combination depending on the nature and the severity of the underlying heart disease.

In Heart Failure

In addition to specific chamber enlargement, the pulmonary vasculature uniquely portrays the underlying pathophysiology of heart failure. In the chronic setting, decreased flow with increased pulmonary lucency is the hallmark of right-sided failure (Fig. 15-7); striking cephalization of the pulmonary vasculature is typical for left-sided decompensation (Figs. 15-5*A* and 15-6*B*).

Left-Sided

Acute Left-Sided Heart Failure The pulmonary vascular changes associated with acute left ventricular failure are usually not discernible for two reasons: (1) The resultant severe pulmonary edema obscures the pulmonary vasculature. (2) The redistribution of pulmonary blood flow secondary to acute left-sided heart failure is usually relatively mild. The combination of alveolar pulmonary edema and a normal-sized heart is the hallmark of acute left-sided heart failure,[9] most commonly seen in acute myocardial infarction (Fig. 15-6*A*). The edema fluid in this circumstance tends to distribute in a butterfly pattern.[22] The reason for that is poorly understood.

Chronic Left-Sided Heart Failure Chronic left-sided heart failure is characterized by striking cephalization of the pulmonary vasculature and interstitial pulmonary edema or fibrosis with multiple distinct Kerley B lines (Fig. 15-6*B*). Pulmonary hemosiderosis, ossification, or both, may result from long-standing severe postcapillary pulmonary hypertension.

Right-Sided

Acute Right-Sided Heart Failure Acute right-sided heart failure most commonly results from massive pulmonary embolism. The typical roentgen signs are rapidly developing centralization of the pulmonary vasculature and dilatation of the right-sided cardiac chambers and the venae cavae. In addition the lungs may show localized or lateralized oligemia, the Westermark sign. Eventually opacities in either or both lungs may develop as a result of pulmonary infarction.

Chronic Right-Sided Heart Failure Chronic right-sided heart failure has a number of causes. The common ones include congenital pulmonary stenosis, Ebstein's anomaly, severe chronic obstructive pulmonary disease, and recurrent pulmonary thromboembolic disease. Diffusely decreased pulmonary vascularity with unusually lucent lungs is seen in patients with right-sided heart failure without pulmonary hypertension (Fig. 15-7*C*). Centralized pulmonary flow pattern is encountered when the right-sided heart failure is secondary to precapillary pulmonary hypertension (Fig. 15-7*A* and *B*). Cephalized flow pattern with unusually lucent lungs is found in patients with right-sided heart failure secondary to severe left-sided heart failure (Fig. 17-7*D*). The degree of right-sided chamber enlargement is proportional to the severity of tricuspid insufficiency.

Combined

It is generally believed that the most common right-sided heart failure is caused by severe left-sided heart failure. This is exemplified by patients with severe mitral stenosis leading to severe tricuspid insufficiency (Fig. 15-7*D*). Other examples of bilateral heart failure are cardiac tamponade and constrictive pericarditis when both sides of the heart are affected (Fig. 15-8).

FIGURE 15-8 Patient with calcific constrictive pericarditis. Typically there is only mild postcapillary pulmonary hypertension due to left-sided constriction. Severe pulmonary venous congestion is prevented by the concurrent right-sided constriction. *A.* Posteroanterior view shows moderate cardiomegaly and mildly cephalad pulmonary blood flow pattern. *B.* Lateral view shows heavy calcification of the pericardium (arrows) and left atrial enlargement deviating the barium-filled esophagus.

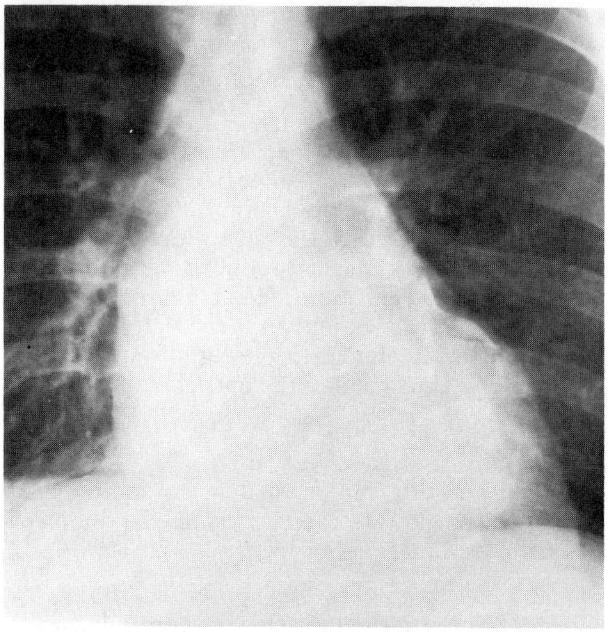

A

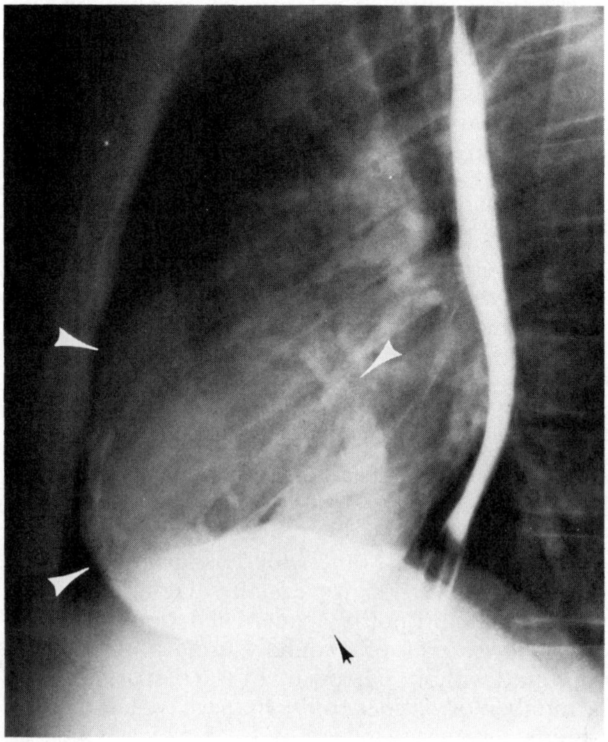

B

Four-View Cardiac Series[4,12,13]

To examine all aspects of the heart, a four-view cardiac series is recommended. It should be obtained in the workup of each new patient. For follow-up studies, posteroanterior and lateral views are sufficient. The normal interrelationships of cardiac chambers and great vessels in each view are illustrated in Fig. 15-9. For many years after the discovery of x-rays, fluoroscopy played a greater role than

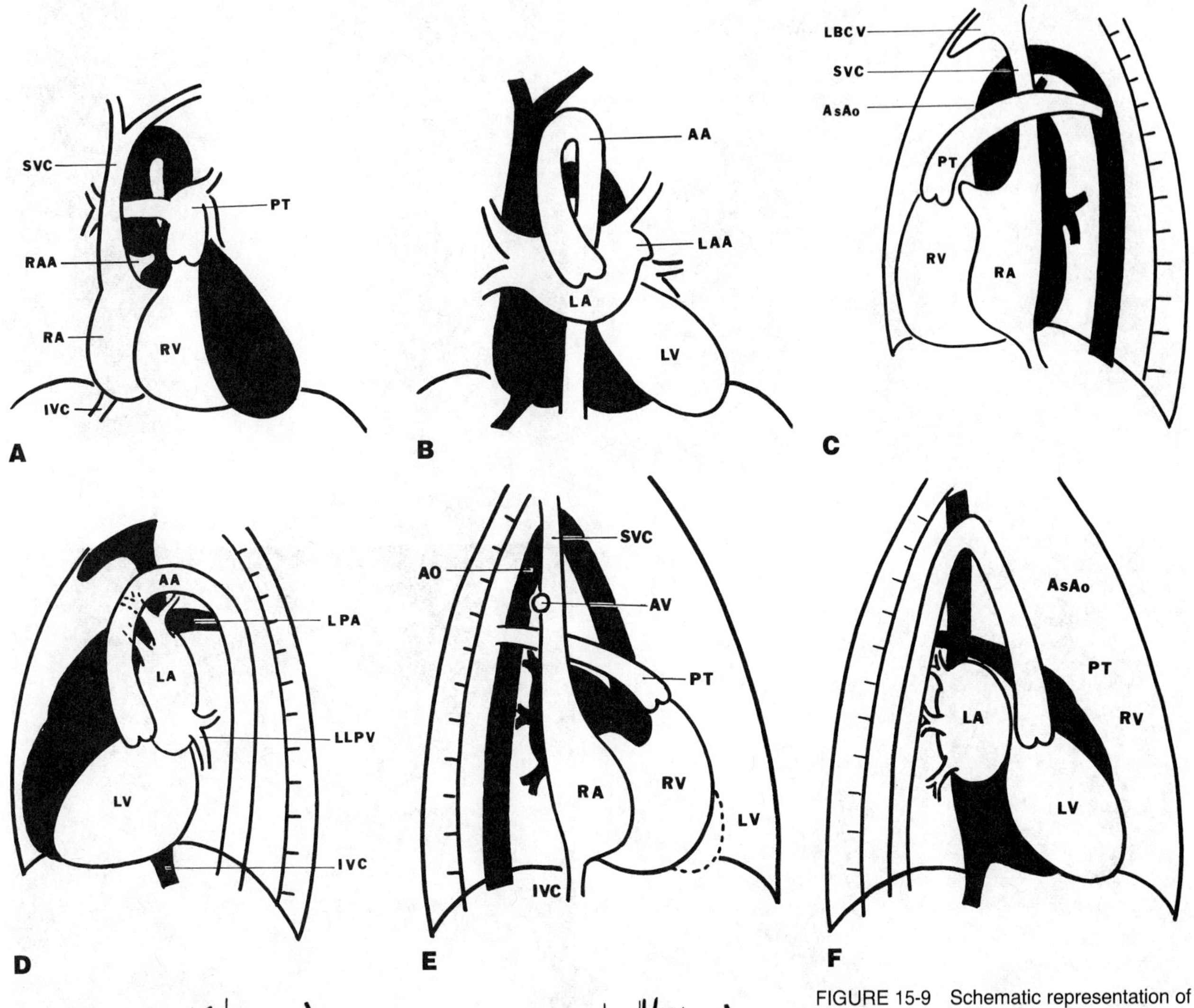

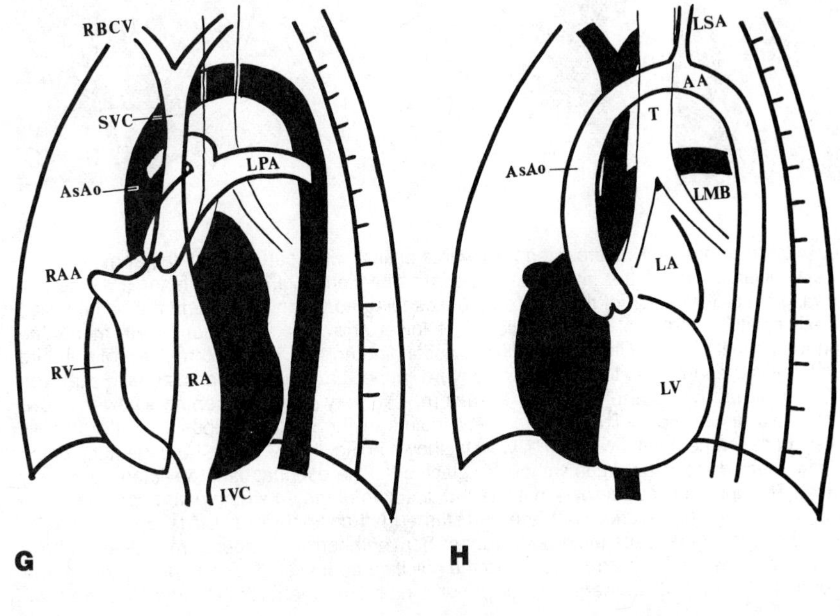

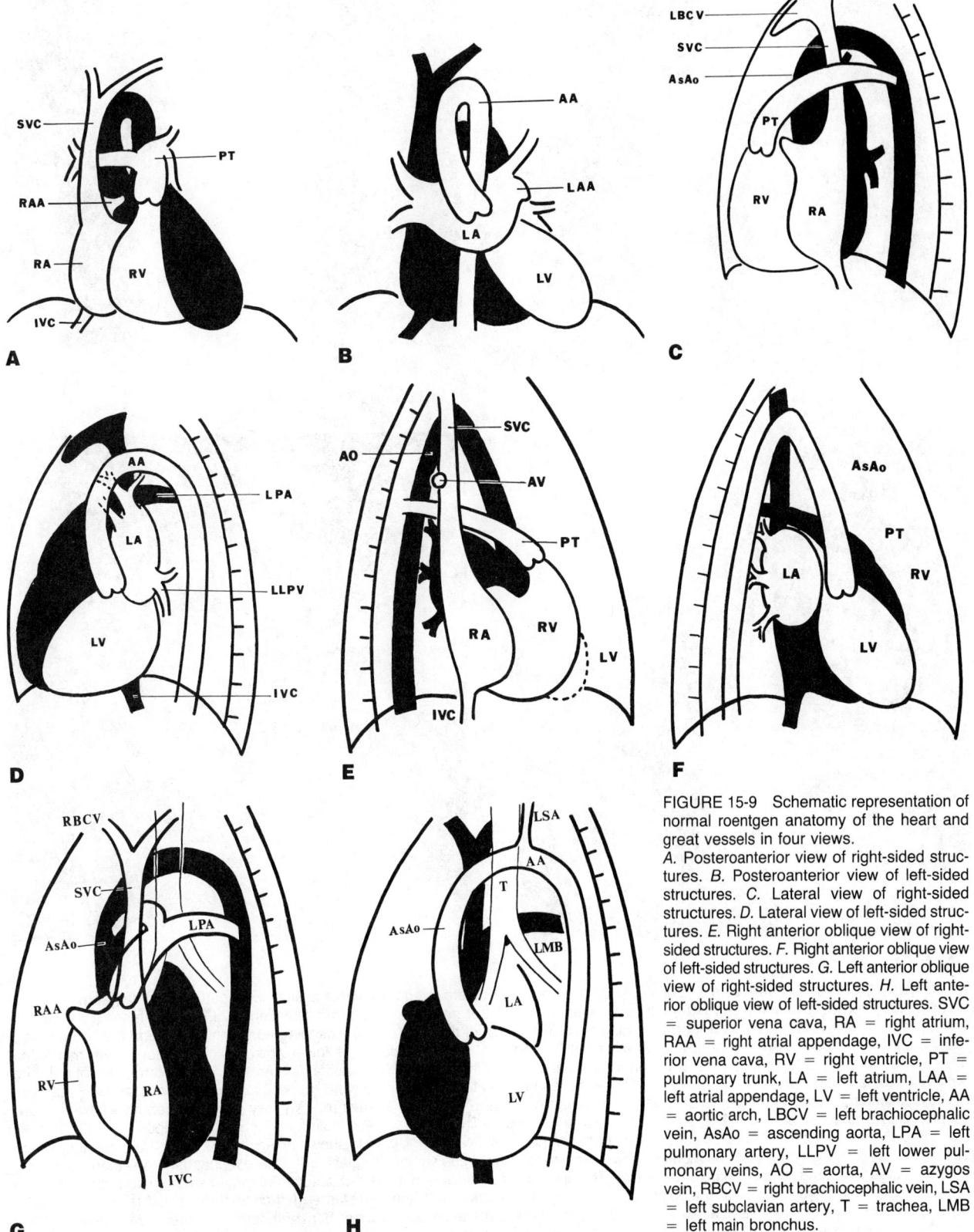

FIGURE 15-9 Schematic representation of normal roentgen anatomy of the heart and great vessels in four views. *A.* Posteroanterior view of right-sided structures. *B.* Posteroanterior view of left-sided structures. *C.* Lateral view of right-sided structures. *D.* Lateral view of left-sided structures. *E.* Right anterior oblique view of right-sided structures. *F.* Right anterior oblique view of left-sided structures. *G.* Left anterior oblique view of right-sided structures. *H.* Left anterior oblique view of left-sided structures. SVC = superior vena cava, RA = right atrium, RAA = right atrial appendage, IVC = inferior vena cava, RV = right ventricle, PT = pulmonary trunk, LA = left atrium, LAA = left atrial appendage, LV = left ventricle, AA = aortic arch, LBCV = left brachiocephalic vein, AsAo = ascending aorta, LPA = left pulmonary artery, LLPV = left lower pulmonary veins, AO = aorta, AV = azygos vein, RBCV = right brachiocephalic vein, LSA = left subclavian artery, T = trachea, LMB = left main bronchus.

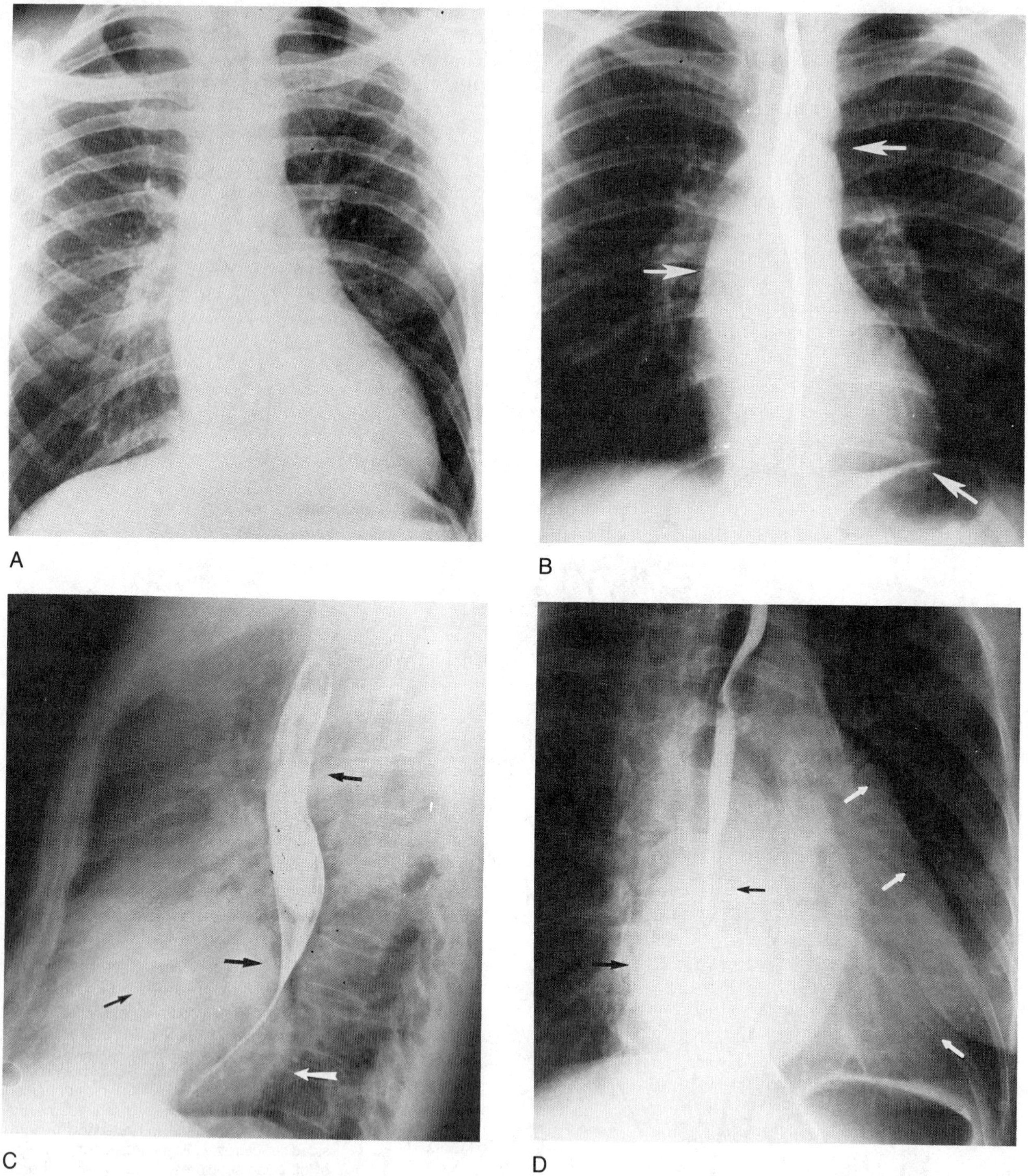

FIGURE 15-10 Practical application of four-view cardiac series. *A.* Posteroanterior view in a patient with coarctation of the aorta showing areas of rib notching bilaterally and left ventricular enlargement in the inferior and leftward direction. *B.* Posteroanterior (PA) view of another patient with coarctation of the aorta showing figure-three sign of the deformed descending aorta, and E sign on the barium-filled esophagus. The upper arrow (on the patient's left) points to the level of coarctation. The lower arrow (on the patient's left) marks the apex fo the enlarged left ventricle. The arrow on the patient's right indicates the dilated ascending aorta. *C.* Left lateral view of the third patient with coarctation of the aorta showing barium-filled esophagus to be pushed forward (upper arrow) by the poststenotic dilatation of the descending aorta, and pushed backward (middle arrow) by the enlarged left atrium. The very large left ventricle (lower arrow) simply casts a shadow behind the esophagus without displacing it. The oblique arrow points to the calcium deposits in the stenotic bicuspid aortic valve. *D.* Right anterior oblique view of the same patient whose PA view is shown in Fig. 15-7*D*. Note the huge right atrium casting a triangular density (lower horizontal arrow) behind the esophagus without displacing it. The esophagus is deviated posteriorly by the enlarged left atrium (upper horizontal arrow). The upper oblique arrows indicate the direction of the enlarging pulmonary trunk and right ventricle. The lower oblique arrow points to the normal left ventricle with the undisturbed left costophrenic sulcus. *E.* Left anterior oblique view of a patient with valvular aortic stenosis. The dilated ascending aorta (upper horizontal arrow) is found immediately above the flat anterior border of the normal right ventricle. The lower oblique arrow points to the calcified aortic valve. The upper oblique arrow marks the elevated left stem bronchus, which is due to left atrial enlargement. The lower horizontal arrow marks the enlarged left ventricle.

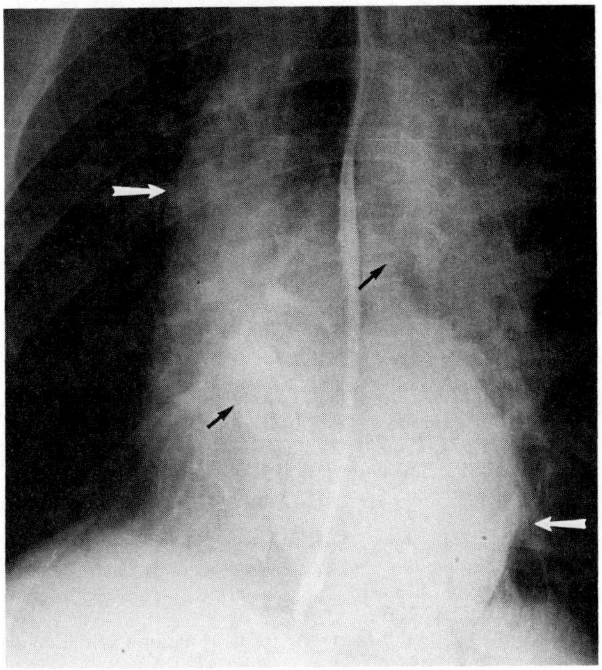

E

radiography in diagnostic roentgenology. Therefore, traditionally the roentgenogram is viewed on the illuminator in such a fashion that it is as if the viewer were examining the patient under the fluoroscope. The examiner is facing the patient and the oncoming x-rays in the posteroanterior view. The left lateral aspect of the patient's chest is closest to the examiner (or the fluoroscopic screen) when a left lateral view is taken. Likewise, the right or left anterior aspect is facing the examiner when the right or left anterior oblique view, respectively, is taken.

Posteroanterior View

The posteroanterior view is the most familiar of all views (Fig. 15-9*A* and *B*). It is particularly useful in the evaluation of pulmonary vasculature and in the assessment of the overall cardiac size. The barium-filled esophagus helps outline the aorta (Figs. 15-3*A* and *D* and 15-10*B*) and the left atrium.

Left Lateral View

The left lateral view (Fig. 15-9*C* and *D*) is indispensable in the evaluation of pericardial disease (see Fig. 107-4) and cardiac calcification (see Fig. 107-2). The barium-filled esophagus helps diagnose aortic arch anomalies (Figs. 15-3*B* and *C* and 15-10*C*), left atrial enlargement (Figs. 15-8*B* and 15-10*C*), and right coronary artery calcification (see Figs. 107-2 and 107-3*B*).

Right Anterior Oblique View at 45°

The right anterior oblique view (Fig. 15-9*E* and *F*) effectively separates the four cardiac chambers. Each chamber enlarges in a different direction: the right ventricle expands anteriorly, superiorly, and leftward; the left ventricle expands inferiorly and leftward; the left atrium expands posteriorly, rightward, and superiorly; the right atrium expands rightward, posteriorly, and inferiorly. The esophagus in the right anterior oblique view is a very sensitive indicator of left atrial enlargement, second only to that in the lateral view (Fig. 15-10*D*).

Left Anterior Oblique View at 60°

In the left anterior oblique view at 60° (Fig. 15-9*G* and *H*) the thoracic aorta is seen in its entirety (Fig. 15-10*E*). This view is also useful in the assessment of ventricular enlargement (Fig. 15-10*E*) and in the detection of left coronary artery calcification (see Fig. 107-3*D*). The barium study is usually omitted in this view in order to make it possible to see the tracheal bifurcation clearly and to evaluate the effect of an enlarged left atrium on the left stem bronchus.

Cardiac Chamber Enlargement[2]

Critical assessment of individual cardiac chamber requires a complete cardiac series in four views with fluoroscopy. Left atrial enlargement is the easiest to detect. Basically a barium swallow will show the typical rightward and posterior displacement of the esophagus in all views except the left anterior oblique. A double density, a bulging left atrial appendage, and an elevated left stem bronchus are the other manifestations of left atrial enlargement (Figs. 15-6*B* and 15-10*C* and *D*). Left ventricular enlargements are manifested by a leftward inferior and posterior extension of the left lower cardiac border (Fig. 15-10*A*, *C*, and *E*). Right ventricular enlargement is best appreciated in the lateral and left anterior oblique views as an anterior bulge of the heart. In addition, the anterior cardiac border also gets longer and taller from the level of the diaphragm upward. A large pulmonary trunk is a secondary sign of right ventricular enlargement (Figs. 15-4*B*, 15-5*A* and *B*, and 15-7*B*). Lastly, when the right ventricle enlarges, the left side of the heart is displaced in the superolateral direction, forming a gentle convexity along the left upper cardiac border (Fig. 15-4*B*). Right atrial enlargement is best tested in posteroanterior and right anterior oblique views. In the adult population greater than 5.5-cm extension of the border of the right side of the heart from the midline is considered a definite evidence of right atrial enlargement (Fig. 15-7*C* and *D*). In the right anterior view, the enlarged right atrial chamber casts a triangular shadow behind the barium-filled esophagus without displacing it (Fig. 15-10*D*). Occasionally the enlarged right atrial appendage may form a shelflike projection over the upper anterior border of the heart immediately below the ascending aorta in the left anterior oblique view. However, this is a rare sign. When the right atrium is huge, it may cast a double density in the lateral view continuous with the dilated inferior vena cava.[2]

References

1. Doyle, A. C.: "The Hound of the Baskervilles," Grosset & Dunlop, New York, 1902.
2. Chen, J. T. T.: The Plain Radiograph in the Diagnosis of Cardiovascular Disease, in C. Putman (ed.), "Symposium on Cardiopulmonary Imaging," *Radiol. Clin. North Am.*, 21:609, 1983.
3. Elliott, L. P., Jue, K. L., and Amplatz, K.: A Roentgen Classification of Cardiac Malpositions, *Invest. Radiol.*, 1:17, 1966.
4. Elliott, L. P., and Schiebler, G. L.: "X-Ray Diagnosis of Congenital Cardiac Disease," 2d ed., Charles C Thomas, Publisher, Springfield, Ill., 1979.
5. de Leon, A. C., Perloff, J. K., and Twigg, H. L.: The Straight Back Syndrome: Clinical and Cardiovascular Manifestations, *Circulation*, 32:193, 1965.
6. Figley, M.: Accessory Roentgen Signs of Coarctation of the Aorta, *Radiology*, 62:671, 1954.
7. Juhl, J. H.: "Essentials of Roentgen Interpretation," 4th ed., Harper & Row, Publishers, Philadelphia, 1981.
8. Edwards, J. E., Carey, L. S., Neufeld, H. N., and Lester, R. G.: "Congenital Heart Disease," W. B. Saunders Company, Philadelphia, 1965.
9. Chen, J. T. T., Capp, M. P., Johnsrude, I. S., Goodrich, J. K., and Lester, R. G.: Roentgen Appearance of Pulmonary Vascularity in the Diagnosis of Heart Disease, *Am. J. Roentgenol.*, 112:559, 1971.
10. Swischuck, L. E.: "Plain Film Interpretation in Congenital Heart Disease," 2d ed., The Williams & Wilkins Company, Baltimore, 1979.
11. Milne, E. N. C.: Some New Concepts of Pulmonary Blood Flow and Volume, *Radiol. Clin. North Am.*, 16:515, 1978.
12. Meszaros, W. T.: "Cardiac Roentgenology," Charles C Thomas, Publisher, Springfield, Ill., 1969.
13. Cooley, R. N., "Radiology of the Heart and Great Vessels," 3d ed., The Williams & Wilkins Company, Baltimore, 1978.
14. Lusted, L. B., and Keats, T. E.: "Atlas of Roentgenographic Measurement," 4th ed., Year Book Medical Publishers, Chicago, 1978.
15. Chickos, P. M., Figley, M. M., and Fisher, L.: Correlation between Chest Film and Angiographic Assessment of Left Ventricular Size, *Am. J. Roentgenol.*, 128:367, 1977.
16. Margolis, J. R., Chen, J. T. T., Kong, Y., et al.: The Diagnostic and Prognostic Significance of Coronary Artery Calcification: A Report of 800 Cases, *Radiology*, 137:609, 1980.
17. Shuford, W. H., and Sybers, R. G.: "The Aortic Arch and Its Malformations," Charles C Thomas, Publisher, Springfield, Ill., 1974.
18. Stewart, J. R., Kincaid, O. W., and Titus, J. L.: Right Aortic Arch: Plain Film Diagnosis and Significance, *Am. J. Roentgenol.*, 97:377, 1966.
19. Fraser, R. G., and Pare, J. A. P.: "Diagnosis of the Diseases of the Chest," 2nd ed., W. B. Saunders Company, Philadelphia, 1979, p. 97.
20. Chen, J. T. T., Behar, V. S., Morris, J. J., McIntosh, H. D., and Lester, R. G.: Correlation of Roentgen Findings with Hemodynamic Data in Pure Mitral Stenosis, *Am. J. Roentgenol.*, 102:280, 1968.
21. Wojtowicz, J.: Some Tomographic Criteria for an Evaluation of the Pulmonary Circulation, *Acta Radiol. (Diag.)*, 2:215, 1964.
22. Fleischner, F. G.: The Butterfly Pattern of Acute Pulmonary Edema, *Am. J. Cardiol.*, 20:39, 1967.

PART III

Methods and Strategy Used to Collect Data on Selected Patients (The Assessment of Specific Problems)

Most of the investigation about the heart and circulation can be brought into focus by answering four questions.

- Is there an abnormality of cardiovascular structure and blood flow?
- Is there an abnormality of cardiac function and myocardial contractility?
- Is there an abnormality of cardiac rhythm or cardiac conduction (electrical abnormality)?
- Is there a metabolic abnormality such as myocardial ischemia?

The "routine" examination (discussed in Part II) does not always answer these questions. When this occurs the physician must consider whether it is absolutely necessary to pursue the answers because, unfortunately, there are times when the answers will not enable the physician to manage the patients' conditions in a new and different manner. Should the decision be made that obtaining the answers to the questions could be beneficial to the patient, then carefully selected tests may be ordered. Accordingly, the purpose of Part III is to discuss the four questions and to describe the strategy and nonroutine tests used to answer these questions. The discussion of equipment itself and the technique of using it is presented in Part VII B through H.

The organization of Parts II, III, and VII B through H was created in an effort to inhibit a trend of modern cardiology to become technique-oriented and technique-dominated. *This unique organization is utilized to emphasize that specialized tests and procedures must be used to answer the specific questions of a perceptive physician and should not be used before the questions have been brought into proper focus.* Tests must not be ordered because the results of the tests might be interesting or because specialized equipment is available for use.

Finally, as emphasized in the introduction to Part II, the physician must view the disorder of the cardiovascular system in the context of the problems found in other organ systems. Good judgment regarding the management of a patient's cardiovascular disease cannot be rendered without understanding all the health problems, including psychological problems, of the patient.

16

Assessment of Structural Abnormalities and Blood Flow

Joseph K. Perloff, M.D.

One does not then make just any experiment but does what must be done.

John Cage, 1976[1]

The chief objectives of the clinical cardiovascular examination are to determine whether or not disease is present and to characterize the disease so identified. The history, physical examination, electrocardiogram, and chest roentgenograms may provide a sufficient basis for judgment so that additional information is not required, at least at that time. Conversely, there may be important unanswered questions that are appropriately answered in clinical diagnostic laboratories. Access to such facilities permits resolution of most, if not all, diagnostic problems confronting the cardiac clinician. In fact, the laboratory armamentarium is presently so vast and its capabilities so great that the physician is faced not only with a virtual tyranny of options but also with the potential for detecting clinically unimportant disease or variations of normal incorrectly interpreted as disease. The physician responsible for patient care remains the ultimate arbiter, and must decide whether and which laboratory studies are required and in what sequence. Nothing replaces the judgment of that physician. If certain questions do not require immediate answer, laboratory study can be deferred, but if those questions can be resolved by safe, painless, and inexpensive investigation, there is often a legitimate inclination to proceed. The physician has an unassignable obligation to select the safest, most painless, least inconvenient, and least costly study or studies that can answer a given question. The purpose of this chapter is to improve the practitioner's strategy in making these decisions. Laboratory investigation is a logical extension of clinical thinking, not a substitute for it. There should be a constant interplay between clinical and laboratory diagnoses and between pragmatic considerations and intellectual curiosity. Important insights gained apart from cardiac diagnostic laboratories must be continually cultivated by polishing bedside talents, but the complete cardiac physician must be as comfortable and as well versed in dealing with laboratory information as in dealing with information personally secured at the bedside.

In this chapter, I shall discuss acquired and congenital valvular heart disease, nonvalvular congenital heart disease with expected adult survival, the cardiomyopathies, and pericardial disease. Abnormalities of myocardial contractility, electrical activity, and myocardial ischemia will be considered in Chaps. 17, 18, and 19. Since the scalar electrocardiogram and chest x-ray are routine, my focus will be on other laboratory modalities.

Valvular Heart Disease—Acquired and Congenital

The Aortic Valve

This section concerns the functionally normal bicuspid aortic valve, valvular aortic stenosis (congenital aortic stenosis and acquired nonrheumatic stenosis in the aged), and aortic regurgitation (mild, severe, chronic, acute).

Bicuspid Aortic Valve

A soft, grade I-II/VI midsystolic murmur most prominent in the second right intercostal space in a child or young adult arouses suspicion of a functionally normal bicuspid aortic valve. Auscultation is virtually confirmatory when it detects an aortic ejection sound (typically loudest at the apex) and a soft, high-frequency, mid-left sternal edge murmur of aortic regurgitation. It is important to confirm the presence of a functionally normal bicuspid aortic valve because of the high susceptibility to infective endocarditis[2] and because the long-term course may culminate in calcific aortic stenosis on the one hand,[2,3] or aortic regurgitation on the other.[4] The problem is most taxing when suspicion depends on the right basal midsystolic murmur alone, with the ejection sound in doubt and the murmur of aortic regurgitation undetected.

The first laboratory procedure is the echocardiogram, both M-mode and two-dimensional imaging. The laboratory request should give precise instructions to the technologist to concentrate on the aortic valve, particularly in the two-dimensional short axis, although the eccentric diastolic closure line on the M-mode remains useful (Fig. 16-1).[5–7] The technologist should also be instructed to record meticulously images of the anterior mitral leaflet on the M-mode tracing, since the fine flutter of aortic regurgitation serves to return the clinician to the bedside in search of the faint, high-frequency, early diastolic murmur.[8,9]

If the M-mode and two-dimensional echocardiograms are nondiagnostic, and if high-quality echocardiograms were recorded by a skilled technologist and read by an experienced echocardiographer, the

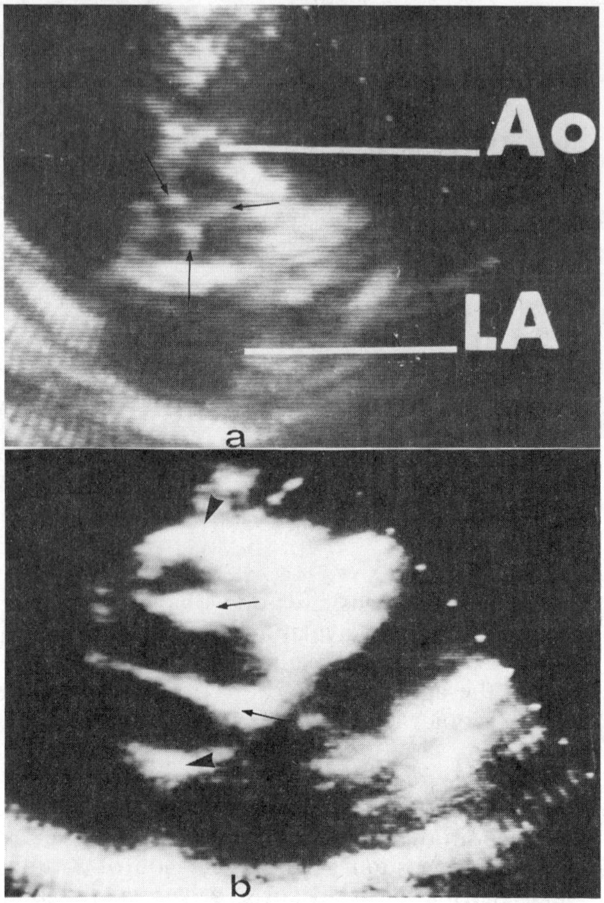

FIGURE 16-1 *a.* Two-dimensional echocardiogram in the short axis showing a normal trileaflet (arrows) aortic valve in diastole. Ao = aorta, LA = left atrium. *b.* Two-dimensional echocardiogram in the short axis showing an open bicuspid aortic valve in systole (arrows) with horizontal commissures. Arrowheads point to the anterior and posterior aortic walls.

issue need not be pursued further. Thoracic aortography, another sensitive means of identifying a bicuspid aortic valve, is not justified, given the above constraints. If suspicion of a bicuspid aortic valve lingers because the echocardiogram is not technically satisfactory, reassessment after an interval of a year or so is appropriate.

Aortic Stenosis

For the purpose of this discussion, let us deal with two forms of congenital valvular aortic stenosis: intrinsic stenosis from birth and fibrocalcific thickening of a bicuspid aortic valve that was functionally normal at birth (see above). Clinical assessment of severity poses comparatively little difficulty at the far ends of the spectrum—very mild or very severe—but when the degree of obstruction is less certain, the clinician is confronted with the taxing problem of the timing, type, and sequence of laboratory investigations. The preadolescent child or teenager with a mobile, intrinsically stenotic congenital aortic valve is typically an asymptomatic, healthy, active male in whom a resting 12-lead ECG is normal or may exhibit only an ambiguous increase in QRS voltage, and in whom the chest x-ray is normal except for poststenotic dilatation of the aortic root.[2]

The first step in laboratory evaluation is the echocardiogram. In assessing severity, the importance of the echocardiogram lies in imaging below the aortic valve.[10–12] Imaging of the valve per se does not provide reliable insight into severity. If septal–left ventricular free wall thicknesses are greater than normal, it can be assumed that there has been an adaptive increase in left ventricular mass in response to afterload imposed by the obstruction. The M-mode echocardiogram is reliable in estimating left ventricular peak systolic pressure employing a simple wall thickness/cavity dimension ratio (Bennett's formula).[10–13] Given the estimated peak systolic pressure derived from this formulation, the gradient is the difference between that pressure and the cuff manometric systolic pressure. The echocardiogram, especially two-dimensional imaging, nicely defines the mobile stenotic valve and dilated aortic root.[8] Doppler echocardiography for aortic stenotic gradients is valuable in infants and children, less so in adults.[14]

Exercise electrocardiography is next selected as a simple, safe, and inexpensive diagnostic tool, shedding light on the capacity of the afterloaded left ventricle to withstand additional physical stress.[15] Significant depression of the ST segments in an exercising young person with a stenotic aortic valve selects that patient out as one who is at risk. In young patients with M-mode echocardiographic evidence of an increase in left ventricular mass, an accurately calculated elevation in left ventricular peak systolic pressure (see above) and two-dimensional echocardiographic evidence of the mobile, dome aortic valve, cardiac catheterization, and angiocardiography are likely to be confirmatory, but are not presently applied. However, when the M-mode echocardiogram does not clearly indicate an increase in septal–left ventricular free wall thicknesses or a significant calculated elevation in left ventricular peak systolic pressure, and the exercise electrocardiogram exhibits an ischemic response, the logical step in resolving the clinical problem is cardiac catheterization.

Planning of diagnostic interventions is especially sensitive when dealing with a bicuspid aortic valve that is undergoing progressive obstruction (gradual fibrocalcific thickening). The valve may, for a time, remain mobile enough to generate an aortic ejection sound. Fluoroscopy (image intensification) can be used to identify incipient calcification, but valve mobility and thickening can also be examined safely and simply by echocardiography. Abundant aortic valve calcium at fluoroscopy predicts severe stenosis, but an analogous conclusion cannot be securely drawn from dense aortic valve images on echocardiography. Conclusions regarding the degree of obstruction are difficult if not impossible when echocardiography focuses on the valve alone.[6] Meticulous use of sequential echocardiographic observations (especially M-mode determinations of septal–free wall thicknesses) and exercise electrocardiography is important in determining when cardiac catheterization is best performed in anticipation of surgery. It is not uncommon for progression to be represented first by ST-segment depressions in the exercise electrocardiogram rather than by echocardiographic evidence of a significant increase in ventricular septal–free wall thicknesses. However, the M-mode echocardiogram can be used to apply Bennett's formula, provided the patient is still a relatively young adult without aortic regurgitation. Evidence of progression in the exercise electrocardiogram and echocardiogram set the stage for cardiac catheterization.

A relatively common concomitant of aging is the insidious development of ridgelike, fibrous or fibrocalcific thickenings at the bases of previously normal trileaflet aortic cusps as they insert into the sinuses of Valsalva.[2,16] Early morphological changes are confined to the base of the cusps, and occur without commissural fusion, without impairment of cusp mobility, and, accordingly, without obstruction.[2] It is appropriate to designate the accompanying murmur as *aortic sclerotic.* What begins as an innocent aortic systolic murmur, however, represents one end of a continuum that culminates at the other end in severe calcific aortic stenosis as calcium is progressively deposited on the aortic surfaces of previously normal trileaflet valves that stiffen and obstruct even though commissural fusion remains absent.[2,17] The distinction between aortic *sclerosis* and *stenosis* as herein defined and a clinical estimate of the magnitude of obstruction can be difficult. Clinical signs that might shed light on the severity of this form of aortic stenosis are commonly unreliable.[16] Echocardiography of the aortic valve per se is useful in excluding significant stenosis if mobile leaflets are recorded, but is otherwise of relatively little help, since dense echoes can be reflected from sclerotic but nonstenotic valves.[12] A simple but important diagnostic intervention is cardiac fluoroscopy. It is a good rule of thumb that absence of fluoroscopic calcification is presumptive evidence of a sclerotic but nonstenotic valve, while the presence of dense calcification is a sign of significant stenosis. Cardiac catheterization remains the means of determining not only the degree of obstruction (gradient and orifice size) but also the presence and degree of atherosclerotic coronary disease which usually coexists. The patients in question should be selected for catheterization and angiography only when valve replacement is a viable therapeutic option. This form of aortic stenosis typically occurs above age 65 years, and often in the seventies or eighties.

Since coronary artery disease is common in this age group, a trying question is the relative effect on left ventricular function of coronary arterial obstruction versus aortic valvular obstruction. Thallium 201 imaging may not determine the relative contributions of coronary arterial and aortic valvular obstruction. However, ^{99m}Tc ventriculography together with coronary angiocardiography and left ventriculography usually—but by no means invariably—permits reasoned conclusions.

Aortic Regurgitation

In patients with *chronic severe aortic regurgitation,* the selection of diagnostic studies and the timing of surgical intervention are disputed clinical problems. The normal left ventricle adapts to gradual, progressive volume loads by increasing its internal dimensions with proportionate increases in septal–free wall thickness.[17] The purpose of diagnostic investigations in chronic severe aortic regurgitation is to identify the transition beyond a normal adaptive response, that is, to determine when the left ventricle has begun to exceed its capacity to handle excess volume as a normal pump. Cardiac catheterization and angiocardiography (thoracic aortography, left ventriculography) are not required to establish that the chronic aortic regurgitation is *severe,* a point that should be clinically evident. Determinations of left ventricular function can be assessed—and serially reassessed with individual patients as their own controls—at rest and during exercise by safe, relatively inexpensive, noninvasive techniques (see below).[18–21]

A fundamental question requiring resolution in *symptomatic* patients with chronic severe aortic regurgitation is whether left ventricular performance has deteriorated to a point that precludes an acceptable response to valve replacement at a reasonable operative risk. In answering this pivotal question, several important indexes of left ventricular function—end-systolic dimension, ejection fraction, and percent fractional shortening—are amenable to noninvasive assessment. The echocardiogram is the simplest, safest, and least expensive first step.[18,19] A second and more refined technique is radionuclide angiography using ^{99m}Tc (see above).[20] Gated cardiac scintigraphy is more expensive than echocardiography, but it is safe, provides two-dimensional information on septal and free wall motion, is an accurate means of determining ejection fraction, and permits observations at rest and during graded exercise.[20] As a rule, all necessary information except the anatomy of the coronary arteries can be established by echocardiography and radionuclide angiography. Accordingly, in *young* patients (30 to 40 years of age), cardiac catheterization and angiocardiography are not required preoperative procedures. In patients above age 40 years, especially males (who constitute most subjects with chronic severe valvular aortic regurgitation), and especially if left ventricular function is depressed, catheterization is employed chiefly to study the coronary arteries, even though in the majority of instances the coronary arteries are large and dilated.

An equally important and perhaps more taxing problem is the *asymptomatic* patient with chronic severe aortic regurgitation. When should such patients undergo aortic valve replacement? Which diagnostic procedures are important in answering this question? Clinical assessment serves to establish the presence of chronic severe aortic regurgitation, but laboratory investigation is required to determine the insidious transition from the normal adaptive response of the volume-loaded left ventricle to incipient, asymptomatic deterioration of function. Let us again focus on left ventricular end-systolic dimension, fractional shortening, and ejection fraction. The echocardiogram permits quantification of these indexes,[22] and also provides a baseline for safe, simple, convenient reassessment at appropriate intervals.[18,19] A progressive increase in left ventricular end-systolic volume with a reciprocal decrease in fractional shortening selects out even asymptomatic patients with chronic severe aortic regurgitation. A single assessment with no basis for comparison makes interpretation difficult, but an appreciable increase in end-systolic dimension (in excess of 55 mm) with a reduced ejection fraction warrants careful scrutiny. Two-dimensional echocardiography sheds considerable light on chamber size and wall motion, while technetium radionuclide angiography (see above) provides data on wall motion and ejection fraction both at rest and in response to exercise.[20] In the relatively young (30- to 40-year-old) asymptomatic patient, cardiac catheterization and angiocardiography offer little or no important information beyond that provided by the echocardiogram and radionuclide angiography as described above.

A common cause of *acute severe aortic regurgitation* is infective endocarditis on a previously unrecognized, functionally normal bicuspid aortic valve.[4] The clinical manifestations are in contrast to those of *chronic* severe aortic regurgitation.[4] Sudden imposition of a large volume load finds the left ventricle unprepared, since there is no adaptive response. Time is of the essence since acute severe aortic regurgitation is, by and large, life-threatening, requiring prompt identification and surgical relief.[4] Given the clinical suspicion, the diagnosis must be confirmed without delay and the etiology established beyond reasonable doubt. The simplest, most important initial study is the echocardiogram.[4] In the presence of acute severe aortic regurgitation, the steep rise in left ventricular diastolic pressure exceeds left atrial pressure in latter diastole, prematurely closing the mitral valve, sometimes before the inscription of the P wave of the electrocardiogram.[4,23] The M-mode echocardiogram recorded with the electrocardiogram as a reference tracing permits relatively precise identification of the important sign of premature mitral valve closure. The M-mode and two-dimensional images shed light on etiology by detecting vegetations on the aortic valve (infective endocarditis) or the double aortic wall of a dissecting aneurysm.[4] Swift decisions are in order; the next diagnostic procedure is thoracic aortography to confirm that the acute aortic regurgitation is *severe* and to clarify further the etiology, especially if dissecting aneurysm is suspected. Given the suspicion of acute severe aortic regurgitation due to infective endocarditis, multiple blood cultures should be secured and antimicrobial therapy begun, but it should be underscored that surgical intervention is generally obligatory before a bacteriologic cure can be effected.[4]

The Mitral Valve

In this section, three mitral valve disorders will be dealt with: prolapse, severe regurgitation (chronic or acute), and obstruction at the mitral orifice.

Mitral Valve Prolapse

The first necessity is to recognize a long-suspected matter of fact—that superior systolic movement of the mitral leaflets is not necessarily abnormal.[24,25] The high sensitivity of the two-dimensional echocardiogram permits detection of mild to moderate superior displacement within the Gaussian distribution of normal. The clinical diagnosis of *pathological* mitral valve prolapse rests more securely on a number of major critera (Table 16-1). One or more of these criteria reliably establishes the diagnosis. Intermediate criteria (listed in Table 16-2) are not necessarily abnormal and are therefore insufficient in themselves to establish a secure diagnosis of *pathological* mitral valve prolapse. Follow-up is therefore appropriate. Minor criteria are listed in Table 16-3. Since these criteria occur in other disease states or in normal persons, they should not be used alone as evidence for pathological mitral prolapse. When minor criteria coexist with intermediate or major criteria, the security of the diagnosis rests on the higher-order criteria.

Patients with major criteria require prophylaxis for infective endocarditis, and those with intermediate criteria probably do. However, persons with only minor criteria not only require no prophylaxis, but should not have their potential fears reinforced by such advice.

Twenty-four-hour ambulatory electrocardiograms (more useful than exercise stress testing for

TABLE 16-1 Mitral Valve Prolapse: Major Criteria

Mid to late systolic clicks(s) and a late systolic murmur at the cardiac apex
Multiple mid to late systolic clicks at the cardiac apex
Apical late systolic murmur in the young
Apical late systolic "whoop"
Marked superior systolic motion of mitral leaflet(s) on two-dimensional echocardiography
Moderate to marked superior systolic motion of mitral leaflet(s) on two-dimensional echocardiography with chordal rupture
Moderate superior systolic motion of mitral leaflet(s) with late systolic mitral regurgitation on Doppler echocardiography
Superior systolic motion of mitral leaflet(s) with moderate to marked annular dilation on two-dimensional echocardiography
Apical holosystolic murmur with moderate to marked angiographic or two-dimensional echocardiographic superior systolic motion of mitral leaflet(s)

TABLE 16-2 Mitral Valve Prolapse: Intermediate Criteria

Moderate superior systolic motion of mitral leaflet(s) on two-dimensional echocardiography
Moderate superior systolic motion of mitral *and* tricuspid leaflets on two-dimensional echocardiography
Single mid to late systolic click at the cardiac apex
Moderate superior systolic motion of mitral leaflets on two-dimensional echocardiography in a patient whose first-degree relative(s) have major criteria
Focal neurological attacks or amaurosis fugax in the young

detection of arrhythmia in this setting) are best reserved for patients whose palpations have not been properly characterized and whose symptoms are sufficient to warrant pharmacological suppression.[26] Intracardiac electrophysiological studies are generally unnecessary, and apply to those rare patients believed to be at risk of unsuppressed, sustained ventricular tachycardia.

Chronic Severe Mitral Regurgitation

Insidious progression of mitral regurgitation allows the left ventricle time to adapt to the augmented volume. In addition, left atrial size usually increases appreciably, sometimes reaching giant proportions, especially in chronic severe rheumatic mitral regurgitation. The larger the left atrium, the more likely that the chamber will handle regurgitant flow with little or no elevation of its pressure.[27]

Diagnostic investigation should address left ventricular size and function, left atrial size, and mitral valve structure. The echocardiogram is the first step, both for accurate confirmation of left atrial size (which can also be inferred with relative accuracy from a cardiac series with barium esophogram) and more importantly, for left ventricular function and mitral valve structure. Left ventricular internal dimensions can be determined, and both the excursions and the thickness of septum–free wall can be quantified. The echocardiogram sheds light on when the adaptive response of the volume-loaded left ventricle is exceeded, i.e., identification of a progressive increase in end-systolic dimensions and a progressive fall in left ventricular ejection fraction (increased E point–septal separation)[28] and fractional shortening. Echocardiographic assessment of the mitral valve may also clarify etiology, especially pathological mitral prolapse with ruptured chordae tendineae. The two-dimensional echocardiogram is the simplest and most definitive diagnostic study when "mitral regurgitation" occurs with congenitally corrected transposition of the great arteries (see below) (Fig. 16-2).[2] The degree of mitral regurgitation is usefully studied with Doppler echocardiography.[9,29] Estimates of regurgitant flow with Doppler echocardiography correlate well with selective left ventriculography.[29] Left ventricular function can be determined by the safe, noninvasive technique of radionuclide angiography employing ^{99m}Tc (see above).[20–22] The method not only provides accurate quantification of ejection fraction at rest but also can

TABLE 16-3 Mitral Valve Prolapse: Minor Criteria

"Atypical" chest pain, dyspnea, fatigue
Giddiness, dizziness, syncope
Psychological disturbances
PVCs singly or repetitive at rest, with exercise, or on ambulatory ECG in the young
Supraventricular tachycardia
T-wave inversions in inferior leads or lateral precordial leads in the young
Mild to moderate thoracic bony abnormalities
Hypomastia
Mild superior systolic motion of the mitral valve
Mild superior systolic motion of mitral and tricuspid leaflets

FIGURE 16-2 *a.* Two-dimensional echocardiogram (apical four-chamber view) from a patient with congenitally corrected transposition of the great arteries and systemic AV valve regurgitation. The tricuspid valve (TV) is in the left side of the heart and is dramatically recessed into the cavity of an anatomic systemic right ventricle (RV). This is left-sided Ebstein's anomaly. The left atrium (LA) is enlarged. The mitral valve (MV) and left ventricle (LV) are in the right side of the heart (inverted position). *b.* Similar image in a patient with Ebstein's anomaly of a right-sided (noninverted) tricuspid valve (TV) which is dramatically recessed into the cavity of the right ventricle (RV). The right atrium (RA) is enlarged.

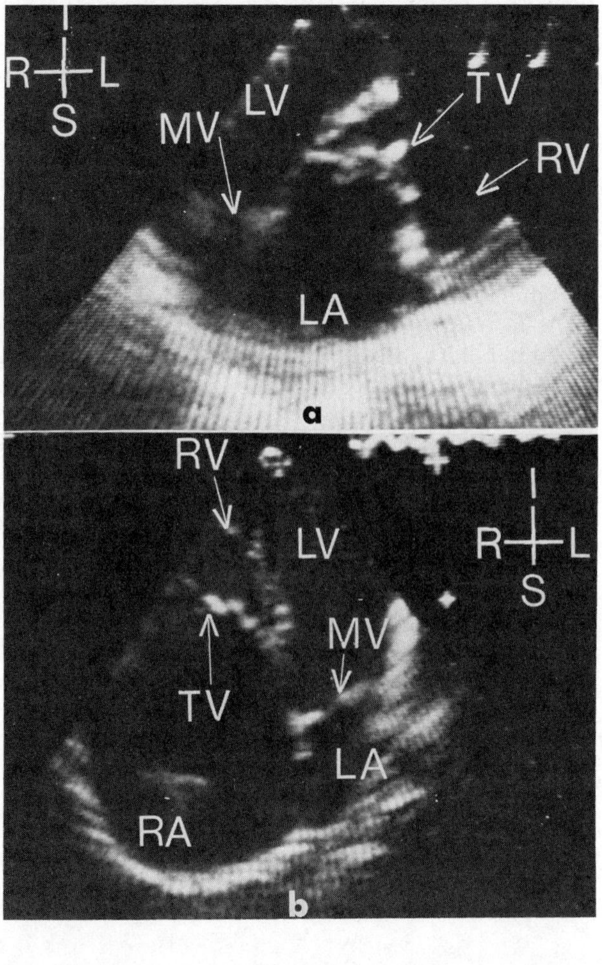

give important information in response to exercise. Furthermore, preoperative data can be used as a basis for comparison with postoperative ventricular function. Careful assessment using the above modalities reduces the need for cardiac catheterization and angiocardiography, which are best applied when the presence and magnitude of coexisting aortic valve disease are unsettled, and when older subjects are suspected of having coronary artery disease.

Acute Severe Mitral Regurgitation
Severe mitral regurgitation of acute onset due to rupture of primary chordae tendineae or papillary muscle is a fundamentally different clinical problem from that just discussed.[30] Acute severe mitral regurgitation due to rupture of primary chordae tendineae is a case in point. A previously normal but physiologically unprepared left ventricle and left atrium are suddenly called upon to handle a dramatic augmentation in volume. Ventricular filling pressure increases sharply while cardiac output falls. As the normal-sized left atrium suddenly receives marked regurgitant flow, its steeply rising diastolic pressure is transmitted via the pulmonary veins to the pulmonary artery so that pulmonary hypertension ensues.[30] The diagnostic study that has the virtues of low cost, safety, and high yield is the echocardiogram, which accurately examines left ventricular internal dimensions and percent fractional shortening, mitral valve structure, and left atrial size. The echocardiogram is sensitive in detecting ruptured chordae tendineae and is moderately sensitive in identifying elevated pulmonary arterial pressure.[6] Doppler interrogation of the left atrium adds useful semiquantitative information.[29] Cardiac catheterization and left ventriculography are desirable but not obligatory before operation to measure the left atrial (or wedge) and pulmonary arterial pressures, to confirm the degree of regurgitant flow, and in older subjects, to study the coronary arteries.

Acute severe mitral regurgitation due to ruptured papillary muscle is more ominous and urgent, since the tear typically occurs in the setting of recent cardiac infarction, so that sudden severe volume load is imposed upon a left ventricle that is suffering from fresh necrosis.[31,32] To distinguish between ruptured papillary muscle and perforated ventricular septum is obligatory. The echocardiogram, which can be done at the bedside in the intensive care unit, points the way by identifying a flail mitral valve. A flotation catheter is then placed in the pulmonary artery[33] to measure left atrial pressure (wedge) which is appreciably elevated (see above), and to determine the oxygen saturations in the right side of the heart, confirming the absence of a shunt and hence the absence of a perforated ventricular septum. Salvage is possible if the rupture is due to discontinuity of a head of a papillary muscle rather than of the entire papillary muscle trunk. Coronary arteriography is necessary to plan bypass at the time of mitral valve replacement. During cardiac catheterization in these critically ill patients, safety is increased by using contrast echocardiography with agitated indicator dye injected into the left ventricle to confirm the degree of mitral regurgitation.

Mitral Stenosis
Careful clinical assessment generally provides most if not all the important anatomic and physiological information in young subjects with pure, isolated rheumatic mitral stenosis. Echocardiography is, however, a major extension, giving information on mitral valve thickness and mobility, orifice size, left atrial size, right ventricular internal dimensions, and ventricular septal motion (normal or paradoxical), while Doppler echocardiography is accurate in estimating orifice size[33] (Fig. 16-3). The pulmonary valve echo sheds light on pulmonary hypertension.

The average young (30- to 40-year-old) patient with pure severe rheumatic mitral stenosis does not require cardiac catheterization before operation. Catheterization with angiography is best reserved to establish the coronary arterial anatomy in older subjects, especially males, and to quantify the degree of pulmonary hypertension.

FIGURE 16-3 Mitral pressure half-time ($t_{½}$) calculated from the Doppler velocity profile. The $t_{½}$ is the time necessary for the initial pressure to fall to half its peak value. An estimate of the mitral valve area is obtained by dividing 220 by the $t_{½}$ in milliseconds. Here, 220/240 = 0.9 cm^2.

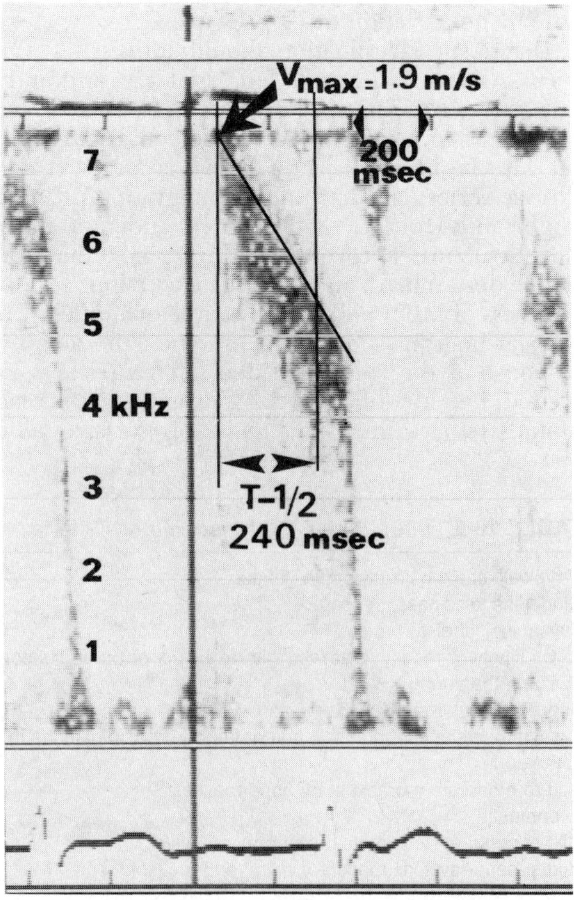

Left Atrial Tumors
An additional form of obstruction at the mitral orifice deserves comment, namely, myxoma of the left atrium.[35] Use of the echocardiogram, especially the two-dimensional image, is a major step forward in identifying myxoma, both within the left atrium proper and as the mobile tumor seats in diastole within the mitral orifice.[6] Cardiac catheterization and left ventriculography are important in determining the degree of mitral regurgitation, underscoring the question of integrity of the mitral leaflets ("wrecking ball" effect of traumatic impact) that may require valve replacement. Clinical suspicion and echocardiographic confirmation of a mobile left atrial mass warn the catheterizer that myxoma is present, so that transseptal catheterization of the left side of the heart is avoided.

The Tricuspid Valve

Tricuspid Regurgitation with Elevated Right Ventricular Pressure
The commonest form of tricuspid regurgitation occurs in patients with morphologically normal tricuspid valves that are rendered incompetent by elevated right ventricular pressure (pulmonary hypertension) and right ventricular failure.[35] Pulmonary hypertensive rheumatic mitral stenosis serves as a useful point of departure. It is necessary to underscore the importance of identifying the presence and degree of tricuspid regurgitation, which, when severe, requires tricuspid reconstruction (seldom replacement) during operation for mitral stenosis. Registration of the pulmonary valve echo partially addresses the problem of pulmonary hypertension, although atrial fibrillation, by eliminating the *a* wave, compromises the value of the observation. The echocardiogram can measure the internal dimensions of the right ventricle and right atrium and can record ventricular septal motion, which in the presence of tricuspid regurgitation (right ventricular volume overload) exhibits abnormal (paradoxical) movement during systole. Doppler echocardiography serves to identify and semiquantify tricuspid regurgitation; contrast echocardiography (intravenous injection) is even more accurate (Fig. 16-4). Cardiac catheterization and angiography are useful but not obligatory in confirming the degree of tricuspid regurgitation.

Tricuspid Regurgitation with Normal Right Ventricular Pressure
"Low-pressure" tricuspid regurgitation (normal right ventricular and pulmonary arterial systolic pressures) differs from the tricuspid regurgitation described above. Consider two varieties of low-pressure tricuspid regurgitation: (1) congenital (Ebstein's anomaly),[2] and (2) acquired (tricuspid infective endocarditis). In Ebstein's anomaly, two-dimensional echocardiography provides definitive images of the anatomy of the deformed tricuspid valve recessed into the right ventricular cavity (Fig. 16-2).[6] Cardiac catheterization is unnecessary in identifying the portion of right side of the heart that is mechanically atrial but electrically ventricular,[2] and the degree of tricuspid regurgitation can be estimated by Doppler or contrast echocardiography. Surgical intervention in Ebstein's anomaly addresses the morphological and hemodynamic faults as well as bypass tracts (Wolff-Parkinson-White syndrome).[38] Preoperative electrophysiological studies are seldom necessary, however, since bypass tracts are consistently right-sided[2] and can be interrupted at open operation.

An acquired form of tricuspid regurgitation without right ventricular–pulmonary hypertension occurs with tricuspid infective endocarditis, generally in intravenous drug abusers. The clinical signs, especially auscultatory, may be subtle, since the murmur is often localized at the left or right lower sternal edge and is soft, medium-frequency, early systolic decrescendo, augmenting or appearing only on inspiration (Fig. 16-5).[37] The first diagnostic steps include a series of blood cultures and serial chest x-rays (septic pulmonary emboli). The echocardiogram provides important information on both structure and function; the tricuspid valve is often visu-

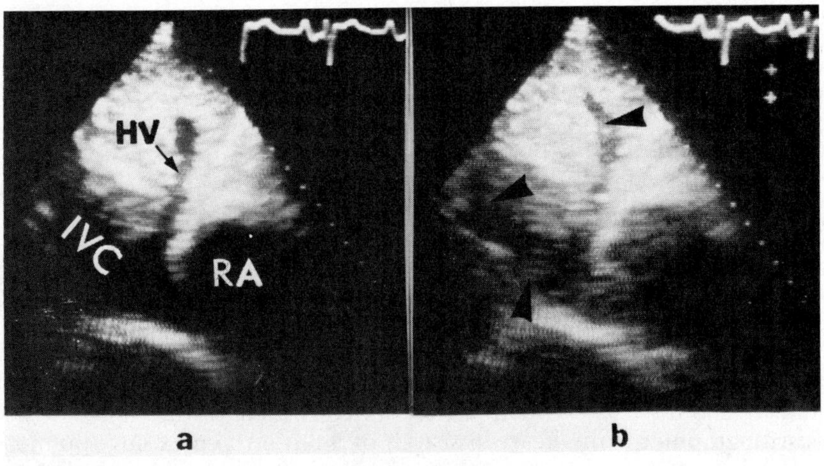

FIGURE 16-4 *a.* Two-dimensional echocardiogram of right atrium (RA), inferior vena cava (IVC), and hepatic vein (HV) in the control state. *b.* After injection of saline into the right antecubital vein, a cloud of echoes appears not only in the RA, but also in IVC and HV (tricuspid regurgitation).

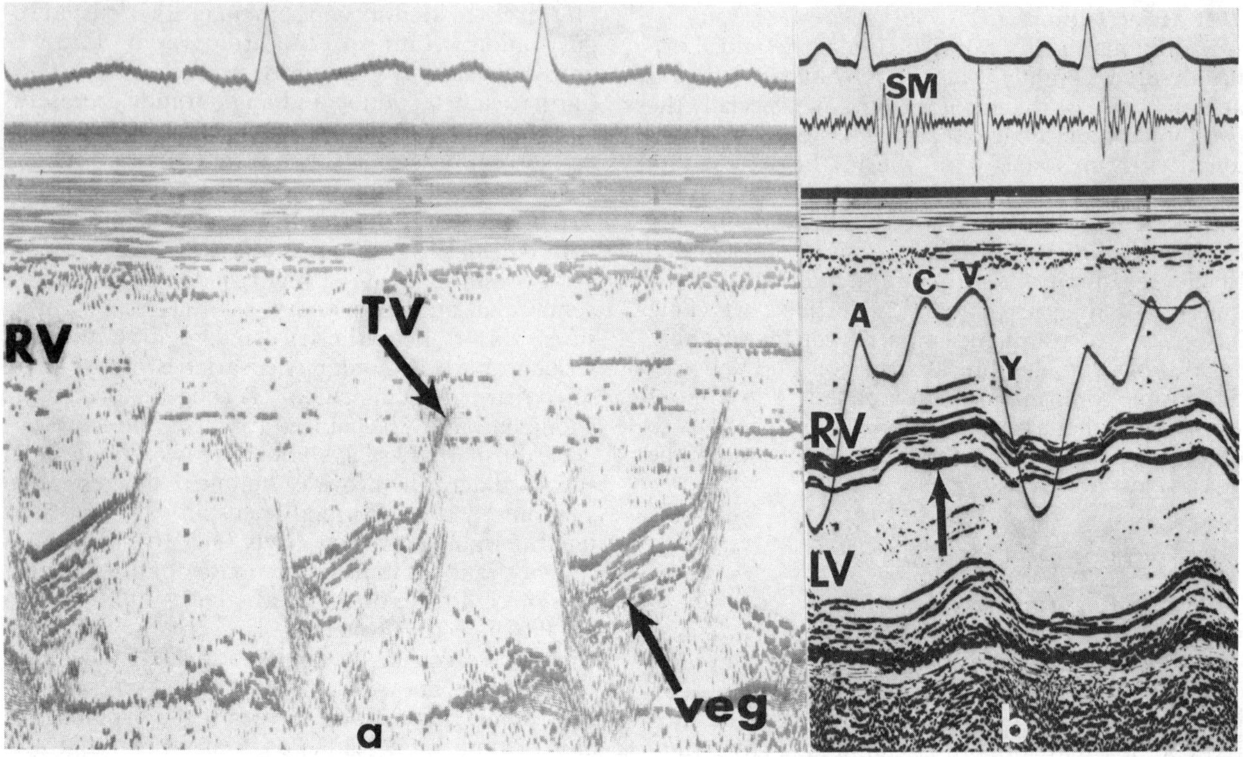

FIGURE 16-5 Tracings from a 28-year-old woman with tricuspid infective endocarditis (heroin abuse). *a.* The transducer beam traverses the right ventricle (RV), imaging the tricuspid valve (TV) (upper arrow), which is thickened by vegetations (veg) (lower arrow). *b.* Simultaneous ECG, phonocardiogram, and echocardiogram with superimposed jugular venous pulse. The phonocardiogram shows the typical early systolic murmur (SM) of low-pressure tricuspid regurgitation. The right ventricular (RV) internal dimensions are increased, and there is paradoxical motion of the ventricular septum (arrow) reflecting right ventricular volume overload. The jugular venous pulse shows an *a* wave with obliterated *x* descent, a dominant *v* wave with brisk *y* descent, and the carotid pulse (C).

alized and vegetations identified (Fig. 16-5), while right atrial and right ventricular internal dimensions are measured and ventricular septal motion (paradoxical) is recorded because of the presence of volume overload (Fig. 16-5). Doppler echocardiography is an important step forward in confirming tricuspid regurgitation, which is generally mild to moderate. Eradication of infection sometimes requires surgical removal of the tricuspid valve followed by further antibiotic therapy. The dramatic clinical picture of acute, severe, low-pressure tricuspid regurgitation emerges postoperatively. The echocardiogram allows sequential comparison of right ventricular internal dimensions during the course of therapy. Cardiac catheterization and angiography are not indicated in simple tricuspid infective endocarditis with mild to moderate regurgitation, and are unnecessary, as a rule, after surgical excision.

Tricuspid Stenosis

The finding of rheumatic tricuspid stenosis implies with virtual certainty the presence of rheumatic mitral stenosis.[39] Despite long-established clinical diagnostic criteria,[39] tricuspid stenosis is still often overlooked. Yet, clinical suspicion is necessary if diagnostic methods for confirmation are to be properly executed. Given the suspicion, we should deliberately seek high-quality echocardiographic recordings of the tricuspid valve, which can usually be identified as stenotic. Fortuitous identification sometimes occurs when echocardiograms are recorded in patients with rheumatic mitral stenosis. Two-dimensional imaging confirms right atrial enlargement. Doppler interrogation provides a good estimate of the severity of obstruction, but cardiac catheterization is the most reliable standard. Simultaneous high-sensitivity pressures should be recorded on both sides of the tricuspid valve in the control state, during active respiration, and, if nondiagnostic, during exercise.

Right Atrial Tumor

Evidence of tricuspid obstruction in the *absence* of mitral stenosis arouses suspicion of right atrial myxoma.[35] The tumor commonly causes not only obstruction but incompetence of the tricuspid valve (traumatic impact). The two-dimensional echocardiogram is dramatic and diagnostic, identifying the mobile mass within the right atrium in systole and within the tricuspid orifice in diastole. Angiocardiography is not necessary to confirm these observations. Myxoma of either right or left atrium is often associated with *biatrial* tumors. Accordingly, two-dimensional echocardiograms should routinely study both atria. Catheterization of the right side of the heart in search of a left atrial myxoma (pulmonary arteriography with levo phase) may be compromised by the presence of an unsuspected right atrial myxoma.

The Pulmonary Valve

Pulmonary Regurgitation Due to Pulmonary Hypertension

The causes of pulmonary hypertension are legion,[36,40] but I shall deal only with its presence, not its etiology. The M-mode echocardiogram is useful in identifying the flat EF slope and absent *a* wave in the pulmonary valve tracing, an increase in right ventricular wall thickness and internal dimensions (regurgitant flow in addition to afterload), abnormal ventricular septal motion (volume overload of the right ventricle), and the fine flutter which is sometimes present on the tricuspid valve.[41] It should be borne in mind that an increase in right ventricular internal dimensions and abnormal septal motion may be due to coexisting tricuspid regurgitation (see above). The two-dimensional image in the short-axis view records the right ventricular outflow tract and pulmonary trunk, which are likely to be enlarged, in addition to the right ventricular cavity, free wall, and septum. Cardiac catheterization remains the best method for quantifying the degree of pulmonary hypertension and for determining pulmonary vascular resistance. Doppler interrogation of the right ventricular outflow tract is useful in confirming the high-frequency diastolic Graham Steell murmur rather than aortic regurgitation, a distinction not reliably made by auscultation.

Low-Pressure Pulmonary Regurgitation

Low-pressure pulmonary regurgitation, congenital or acquired, is in contrast to the hypertensive pulmonary regurgitation described above.[2] In congenital pulmonary valve regurgitation, the morphological abnormalities of the leaflets range from mild derangement to virtual or complete absence of valve tissue; the degree of pulmonary incompetence varies accordingly. The accompanying murmur is a soft, medium-frequency, middiastolic murmur as opposed to the typical Graham Steell murmur. The abnormalities of flow and structure are reflections of a range of pure right ventricular volume overload. Accordingly, the echocardiogram is useful in establishing the internal dimensions of the right ventricle and paradoxical motion of the ventricular septum, and Doppler echocardiography can identify pulmonary valve incompetence. With heightened clinical suspicion and the above echocardiographic confirmation, cardiac catheterization is not required, and is less useful in confirming the diagnosis than in establishing the degree of regurgitant flow.

Acquired low-pressure pulmonary regurgitation is a feature of infective endocarditis on a previously normal pulmonary valve (intravenous drug abuse) or of postoperative repair of valvular pulmonary stenosis or the tetralogy of Fallot.[42] In the presence of infective endocarditis, the first diagnostic steps are multiple blood cultures and plain film roentgenography to identify septic pulmonary emboli from the infected valve. The echocardiogram can image the pulmonary valve and its vegetations, sometimes dramatically.

Obstruction to Right Ventricular Outflow

Obstruction to right ventricular outflow can be acquired or congenital, supravalvular, valvular, or subvalvular, but for the purpose of this discussion, let us focus on congenital valvular pulmonary stenosis. The clinical diagnosis can be established with high probability, and the degree of obstruction relatively accurately estimated.[2] The chief role of the laboratory is the more refined appraisal of severity and, when the ejection sound is equivocal, identification of a thickened or dysplastic valve. The echocardiogram is a useful first step. There is a relation between the degree of pulmonary stenosis, the force of right atrial contraction, and the depth of the *a* wave in the pulmonary valve M-mode image.[43] There is also a relation between severity and right ventricular free wall and ventricular septal thicknesses. Occasionally the septum is thicker than the posterior left ventricle (disproportionate septal thickness). The two-dimensional echocardiogram records in the short axis the dilated pulmonary trunk and the mobile domed pulmonary valve, whereas Doppler interrogation is relatively accurate in predicting the gradient[44] (Fig. 16-6).

In patients with a secure diagnosis of mild valvular pulmonary stenosis, cardiac catheterization is unnecessary, since surgical intervention is not a consideration. When severity appears sufficient to warrant surgical intervention, catheterization and angiography are employed to confirm the gradient, to identify secondary hypertrophic subpulmonary stenosis (which may require resection), and to clarify valve thickness and mobility.

Nonvalvular Congenital Heart Disease with Expected Adult Survival

Ostium Secundum Atrial Septal Defect

Ostium secundum atrial septal defect, in its uncomplicated form, is readily amenable to clinical diagnosis, especially in children and young adults.[2] The first confirmatory laboratory procedure is the echocardiogram that provides evidence of right ventricular volume overload—increased right ventricular internal dimensions and paradoxical motion of the ventricular septum.[6] The tricuspid valve is easily imaged and shows increased mobility and occasionally fine diastolic vibrations. The incidence of superior systolic movement of the mitral leaflets (prolapse) is

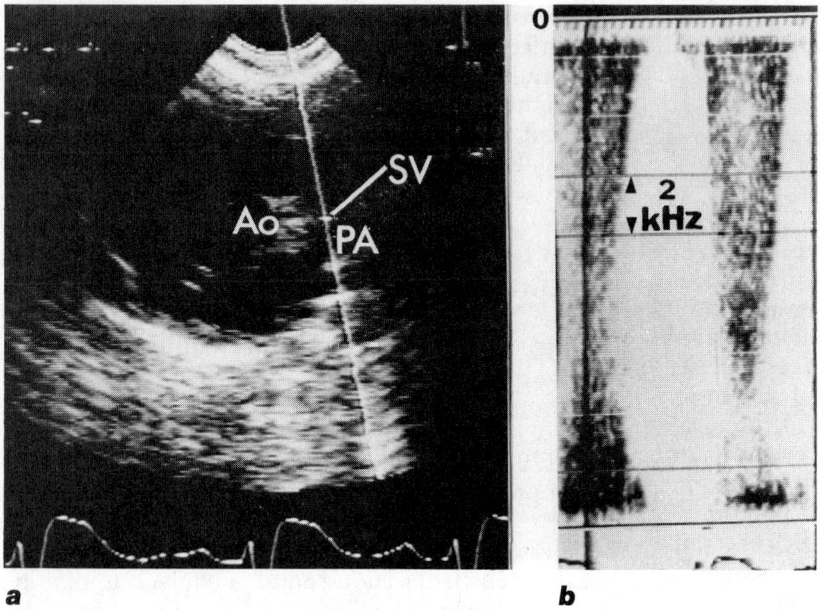

FIGURE 16-6 *a.* Cursor showing sample volume (SV) in the pulmonary artery (PA) distal to a stenotic pulmonic valve. Ao = aorta, PA = pulmonary artery. *b.* The Doppler records a 13 kHz frequency shift away from the sample volume, a peak velocity of 3.25 m/s, and a calculated gradient of 42 mmHg ($4 \times V_m^2$). The catheterization gradient was 40 mmHg.

more often than not due to alterations in shape and a decrease in size of the left ventricular cavity rather than pathological prolapse caused by a connective tissue abnormality.[45] The two-dimensional echocardiogram is capable of identifying the presence, location, and size of the defect in the atrial septum, and often identifies one or more normally draining pulmonary veins in addition to the large right atrium. Is there need for cardiac catheterization and angiography? Given secure clinical and echocardiographic evidence of an uncomplicated, non-pulmonary hypertensive, low-resistance, high-flow ostium secundum atrial septal defect in the young, what further data *can* the catheterization laboratory provide? If the right superior pulmonary vein connects anomalously to the superior vena cava, an experienced surgeon readily identifies this variation as soon as the chest is opened; it makes little difference during surgical repair if right pulmonary veins connect within the atria on the right atrial side of the septal rim.

Although uncomplicated ostium secundum atrial septal defects in the young are easily diagnosed, similar defects can be surprisingly difficult to recognize in adults.[2,46] Cardiac catheterization and angiography are then necessary in anticipation of surgery. Older subjects with ostium secundum atrial septal defects and pulmonary hypertension can be safely and beneficially operated on if the left-to-right shunt is in excess of 2:1. In such patients, catheterization is required not only to establish the anatomic diagnosis, but to determine pulmonary vascular resistance, the magnitude of the left-to-right shunt, and the anatomy of the coronary arteries.

Coarctation of the Aorta

The diagnosis of coarctation of the aorta in adults is almost always made based on physical signs and chest x-rays, even though the latter occasionally display surprisingly little or no rib notching despite auscultatory evidence of murmurs of collateral circulation.[2,46] However, information from the diagnostic laboratories remains desirable. The presence of a coexisting bicuspid aortic valve should be sought, especially in the male, and is usually established with echocardiography (see above). Cardiac catheterization is important chiefly for the morphological details on aortography, but the same information can be obtained less invasively with digital vascular imaging (Fig. 16-7). The coarctation, as well as the proximal and distal aorta and collaterals, are well visualized by this technique. In subjects with mild coarctation, exercise stress testing is an important adjunct, provoking disproportionate systolic hypertension and an augmented gradient (arm-leg blood pressure) in response to stress.

FIGURE 16-7 Digital vascular image (DVI) in an 18-year-old patient with coarctation of the aorta (arrowhead) just distal to the left subclavian artery (LSA). The contrast material was injected into the superior vena cava. A Ao = ascending aorta, D Ao = descending aorta.

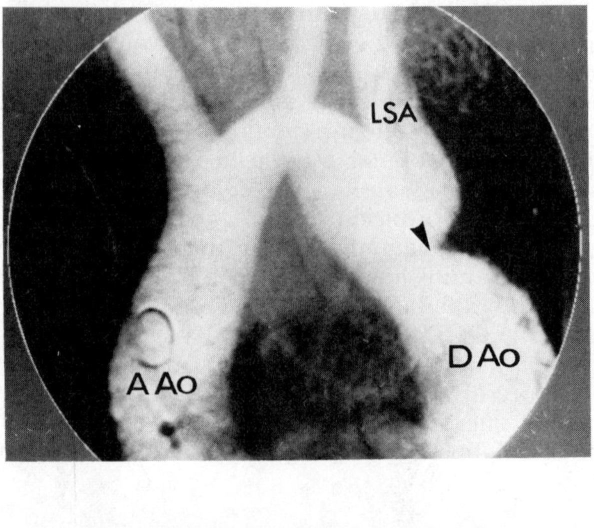

Patent Ductus Arteriosus

Surprisingly, a patent ductus arteriosus is sometimes overlooked until adulthood.[2,46] In the small, nonpulmonary hypertensive ductus, diagnosis depends upon detection of the characteristic continuous murmur. Two-dimensional echocardiography in the short axis sometimes identifies the ductus as it joins the pulmonary trunk.[5] Catheterization is seldom required unless categoric exclusion of coronary arteriovenous fistula to the pulmonary trunk is considered desirable. Even patients with large patent ductus and left-to-right shunts sometimes await diagnosis until adulthood, and their disease must be separated from aorticopulmonary septal defects, a distinction that two-dimensional echocardiography generally achieves. Calcification of the ductus complicates repair in adults, so chest x-rays and fluoroscopy should be applied meticulously in search of ductal calcium. The adult with patent ductus arteriosus, pulmonary hypertension, and suprasystemic pulmonary vascular resistance is recognized by differential cyanosis (cyanotic feet, acyanotic hands).[2] This simple physical sign not only establishes the anatomic and physiological diagnoses, but indicates inoperability since suprasystemic pulmonary vascular resistance channels unoxygenated blood from the pulmonary trunk through the ductus into the aorta distal to the left subclavian artery.

Coronary Arteriovenous Fistula

In coronary arteriovenous fistula both coronary arteries arise from the aorta, but a fistulous branch of one or more than one of these vessels communicates directly with a cardiac chamber or with the pulmonary trunk, coronary sinus, or vena cava.[2] A continuous murmur is the hallmark of a coronary arterial fistula, and differs from the murmur of patent ductus by its configuration and site of maximal intensity. It is a good rule of thumb to consider the diagnosis whenever an asymptomatic acyanotic patient exhibits a precordial continuous murmur that does not peak around the second heart sound and that is maximal at an atypical site. Definitive diagnosis depends upon selective coronary arteriography which accurately identifies not only the vessel or vessels of origin but also the drainage site.

Tetralogy of Fallot

In patients with nonrestrictive, malalignment ventricular septal defects, the presence of obstruction to right ventricular outflow does not increase the afterload on the right ventricle and may serve the useful purpose of regulating pulmonary blood flow so that volume overload of the left heart is avoided while adequate oxygenation occurs. Tetralogy of Fallot remains the commonest cyanotic congenital cardiac anomaly in adults,[2] and the clinical diagnosis can, as a rule, be made with a high degree of accuracy. Echocardiography establishes the posterior aortic wall–to–mitral valve continuity and the biventricular aorta (Fig. 16-8) and identifies the ventricular septal defect.[6,47] Cardiac catheterization with right ventriculography is obligatory before surgical intervention to define the morphology of the right ventricular outflow tract from the infundibulum through the pulmonary valve to the pulmonary trunk and its branches. In addition, it is important to know whether the left anterior descending coronary artery arises anomalously from the right coronary and crosses the infundibulum.

Situs Inversus

Complete situs inversus of both thoracic and abdominal viscera implies mirror-image dextrocardia, so that all that is required is simple recognition of the cardiac malposition, which is securely accomplished by the physical signs, electrocardiogram, and chest x-ray. No further diagnostic investigations are required, provided the heart is otherwise normal, which is usually the case.

Situs Solitus with Right Thoracic Heart

When the thoracic and abdominal viscera are in their normal or situs solitus positions but the cardiac apex is on the right, congenital anomalies almost always coexist, and the types are generally predictable. The commonest anomalies are congenitally corrected transposition of the great arteries, pulmonary stenosis, and ventricular or atrial septal defects.[2] These lesions occur singly or in combination. Although additional diagnostic investigation is seldom necessary to establish the cardiac malposition per se, assuming that the spleen is present and single, laboratory investigation is required to clarify the presence and degree of complicating anomalies. Situs solitus of the lungs and atria and the presence of a single spleen rest relatively securely upon radiographic identification of an anatomic right bronchus and an anatomic left bronchus. A frontal chest x-ray, perhaps deliberately overpenetrated, may be all that is required to visualize the right bronchus (wide and straight) and the morphological left bronchus (narrower, "sway-backed," and running in a more horizontal course). The right atrium and the trilobed (right) lung are concordant with the anatomic right bronchus, while the left atrium and bilobed (anatomic left) lung are concordant with the anatomic left bronchus.[2] Visualization of morphological right *and* left bronchi and a liver that is *not* transverse on chest x-ray minimizes concern that asplenia or polysplenia complicates the cardiac malposition.

If doubt remains, three safe, inexpensive, and accurate diagnostic tests resolve the problem. The first and simplest is a smear of peripheral blood to search for the Howell-Jolly bodies and Heinz bodies of asplenia. The second is two-dimensional echocardiography of the abdomen for identification of a transverse liver. The third is scanning with an isotope taken up by the spleen and therefore capable of

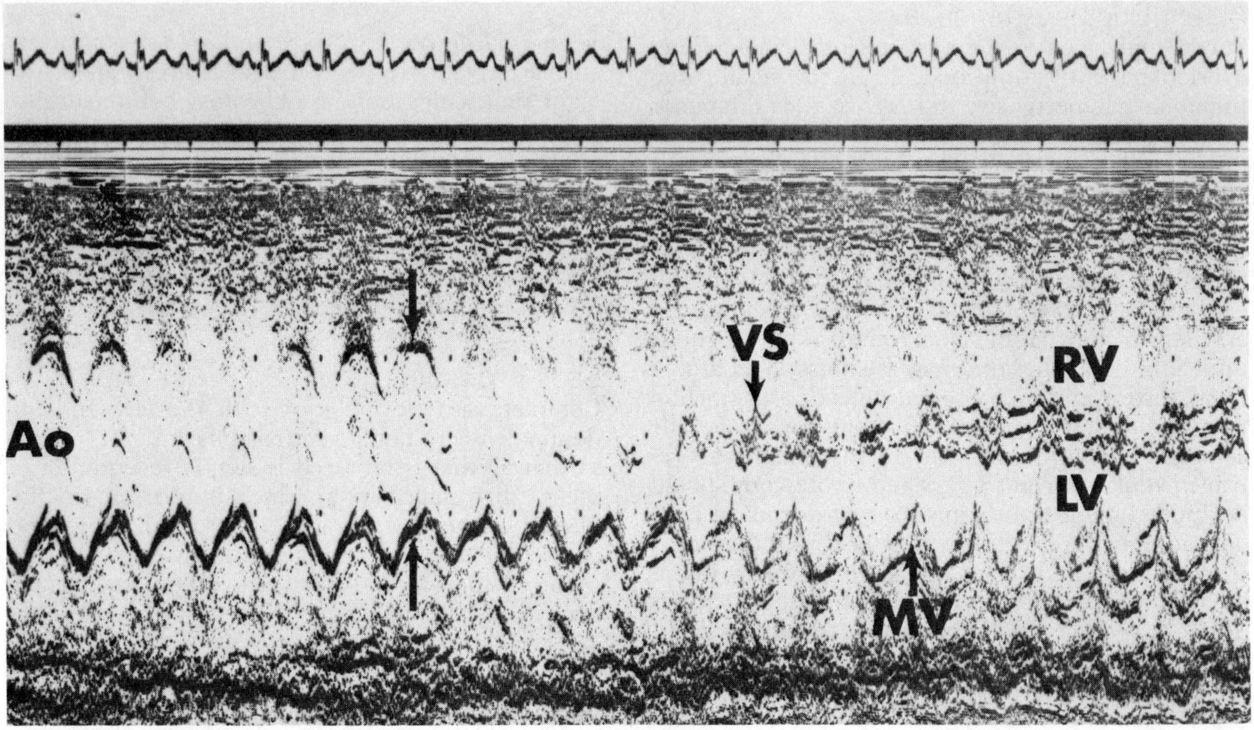

FIGURE 16-8 Typical tetralogy of Fallot with M-mode sweep from dilated aorta (Ao) through mitral valve (MV) and ventricular septum (VS). The anterior aortic wall (left upper arrow) is anterior to the plane of the ventricular septum (right upper arrow); the posterior aortic wall (left lower arrow) is in continuity with the anterior mitral leaflet (right lower arrow). Thus, the dilated aorta takes origin from both left (LV) and right (RV) ventricles.

revealing the absence, presence, and type (single, multiple) of splenic tissue.

Congenitally Corrected Transposition of the Great Arteries

Congenitally corrected transposition of the great arteries is characterized by the presence of a tricuspid valve and morphological right ventricle in the left side of the heart, and a mitral valve and morphological left ventricle in the right side of the heart.[2] Despite right-to-left interchange (inversion) of the ventricles and their atrioventricular (AV) valves, right atrial blood flows into the pulmonary trunk, albeit across a mitral valve and through an anatomic left ventricle, while left atrial blood flows into the aorta, albeit across a tricuspid valve and through an anatomic right ventricle.[6] There is ventricular–great artery discordance, i.e., "transposition," but the transposition is "corrected" as the above flow patterns attest. Two-dimensional echocardiography can identify the relative positions of the great arteries as well as the shape and internal architecture of the ventricles. There is a common association with ventricular septal defect, abnormalities of the systemic AV (tricuspid) valve, obstruction to outflow of the venous (morphological left) ventricle, and prolonged AV conduction.[2]

In adults, congenitally corrected transposition is often associated with incompetence of the left AV valve misdiagnosed as "mitral" regurgitation (see above). Attention to the chest x-ray and electrocardiogram arouses suspicion. Two-dimensional echocardiograms can be conclusive, since the anatomic derangement that gives rise to left AV valve regurgitation is an Ebstein-like anomaly identified as tricuspid leaflet tissue recessed into the systemic ventricle (Fig. 16-2). Doppler echocardiography semiquantifies left AV valve regurgitation which, if still in doubt, can be resolved by systemic ventriculography.

The increased PR interval or prolonged AV conduction in patients with congenitally corrected transposition sometimes culminates in late complete heart block. Occasionally such patients with no other coexisting congenital cardiac anomaly present in adulthood with complete AV block misdiagnosed as "acquired."

Perforated Sinus of Valsalva Aneurysm

The common form of congenital aortic sinus aneurysm originates from either the right or noncoronary sinus and perforates into the right ventricle or right atrium.[2] The physiological consequences attending the ruptures of these aneurysms depend upon the amount of blood flowing through the abnormal communication, the rapidity with which the perforation develops, and the chamber that receives the shunt. Ruptured sinus of Valsalva aneurysms occur predominantly in males, with a ratio of 4:1. The substantial majority of ruptures develop well after puberty, but before age 30 years. The clinical disorder therefore typically expresses itself in young adult males. Two-dimensional echocardiography sheds light on the morphological defect, identifying the aneurysm as well as the chamber that receives it; diagnosis of the latter is materially improved by Doppler echocardiography. Cardiac catheterization and selective aortography quantify the shunt and confirm the morphology of the defect and the chamber into which it perforates.

The Cardiomyopathies

Three categories of cardiomyopathy will be considered: hypertrophic, dilated, and restrictive.[48,49] Hypertrophic cardiomyopathy, obstructive or nonobstructive, is a genetic disorder characterized by two anatomic hallmarks, namely, disproportionate ventricular septal thickness and septal cellular disarray.[50] Dilated cardiomyopathy is a pathophysiological, not an etiologic, classification, indicating that the primary target of disease is left ventricular myocardium which responds by dilatation without an increase in septal–free wall thicknesses.[51] Restrictive cardiomyopathy is also a pathophysiological rather than an etiologic classification,[52] implying that left and right ventricular diastolic distensibility and systolic fiber shortening are restricted because of disease of ventricular myocardium.

Hypertrophic Cardiomyopathy

The clinical diagnosis of *hypertrophic cardiomyopathy* can be firmly established by noninvasive diagnostic means. The presence or absence—though not necessarily the degree—of obstruction to left ventricular outflow can also be estimated.[50] The echocardiogram is well suited to provide information on key features of the diagnosis, namely, the increase in ventricular septal thickness with a septal/posterior wall ratio equal to or greater than 1.5:1, a relatively hypokinetic septum, systolic anterior motion of the anterior mitral leaflet, increased velocity of posterior wall systolic movement, and abnormal aortic valve motion (midsystolic notch followed by flutter) (Fig. 16-9).[53,54] Doppler echocardiography is useful in identifying mitral regurgitation. Technetium 99m gated blood pool scans dramatically show in real time the dynamic contraction of the left ventricular free wall with cavity obliteration, and the diastolic frames nicely outline the thickened ventricular septum (Fig. 16-10). Thus, virtually all necessary information can be secured safely, simply, accurately, and relatively inexpensively by noninvasive means. In patients who are potential candidates for operation, catheterization of the right and the left sides of the heart is done together with left ventriculography to confirm the presence and degree of right and left ventricular outflow obstruction and the degree of mitral regurgitation.

Dilated Cardiomyopathy

Dilated cardiomyopathy can be acute, subacute, or chronic, inflammatory or noninflammatory.[51] Let us take as a point of departure acute, inflammatory cardiomyopathy (myocarditis) that is believed to be infectious. Virtually all categories of infectious agents have been implicated, but for practical clinical purposes in western Europe and the United States, the prevailing causes by far are the enteroviruses (Coxsackie, echo, and polio viruses).[55–57] Vaccine has dramatically decreased the incidence of polio, and echovirus myocarditis is now relatively uncommon. The high-order associations for acute infectious (inflammatory) cardiomyopathies in the human host are the Coxsackie A virus types 4 and 16, and

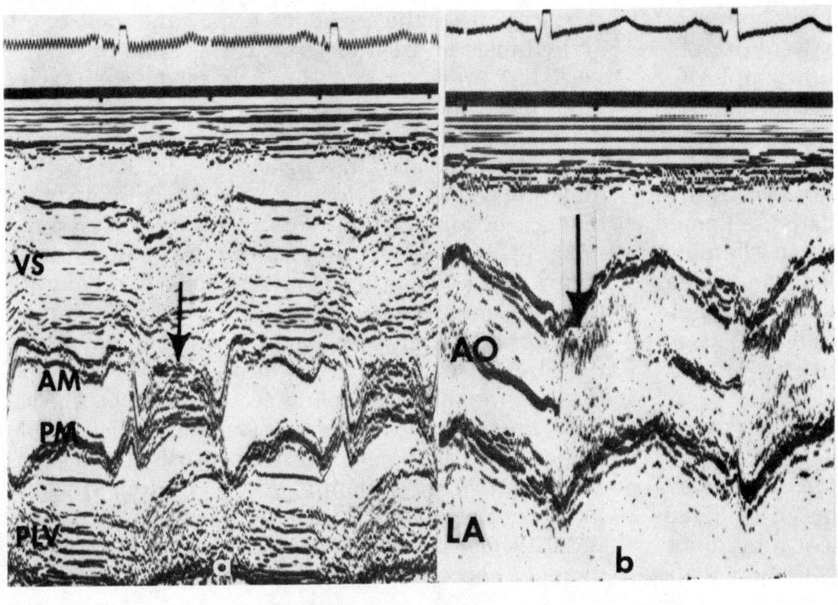

FIGURE 16-9 M-mode echocardiogram from a 9-year-old boy with genetic hypertrophic obstructive cardiomyopathy. *a.* The ultrasonic beam is directed through the ventricular septum (VS), which is hypokinetic and much thicker than the posterior left ventricular wall (PLV). The arrow points to systolic anterior motion of the anterior mitral leaflet, which touches the septum during most of systole. AM = anterior mitral leaflet in diastole, PM = posterior mitral leaflet in diastole. *b.* Arrow points to typical aortic valve preclosure followed by abnormal vibrations of the aortic leaflets. AO = aorta, LA = left atrium.

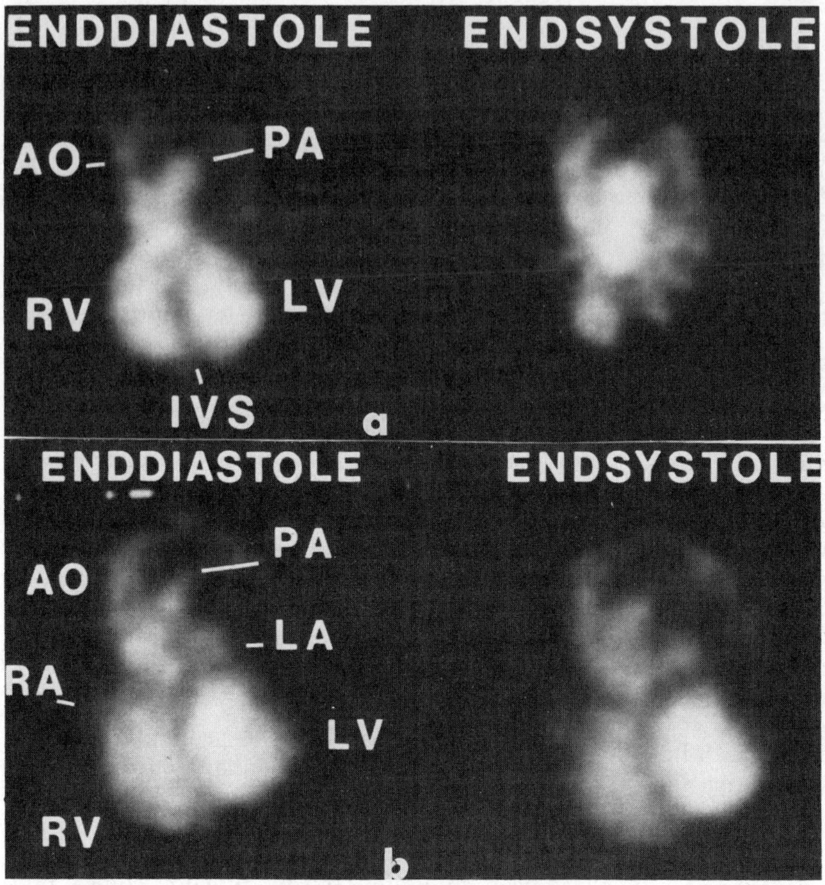

FIGURE 16-10 ^{99m}Tc multiple gated acquisition scan from a patient with hypertrophic obstructive cardiomyopathy (left anterior oblique position). The end-systolic frame shows virtual obliteration of the left ventricular (LV) cavity. RV = right ventricle, IVS = interventricular septum, AO = aorta, PA = main pulmonary artery. *b.* Similar study from a patient with chronic dilated cardiomyopathy. From end diastole to end systole, there is virtually no change in the dimensions of the dilated hypokinetic left ventricle (LV), and little change in the right ventricle (RV). RA = right atrium, LA = left atrium.

Coxsackie B virus types 1 through 5.[57] Thus, despite a wide range of potential infectious etiologies, the practical clinical concerns center on Coxsackie groups A and B.

The group B Coxsackie virus is myonecrotic and therefore exposes the patient to high risk.[57,58] The group A is largely interstitial, causing little or no myofiber injury.[57] If acute inflammatory cardiomyopathy is believed to be due to a Coxsackie B virus, and the patient comes under care during the earliest phases of the illness, throat and stool cultures for virus should be accompanied by serum samples for type-specific antibodies.[57] The initial serum can then be used for comparison with subsequent antibody titers. Acute infectious inflammatory cardiomyopathy puts the patient at risk on several counts, namely, mechanical failure of the dilated, inflamed left ventricle, electrical instability of that chamber, and systemic emboli from diseased left ventricular endocardium (endocardial clot). Patients are generally ill enough to require hospitalization in an intensive care unit, and surveillance with electrocardiographic monitoring may prove critical.

After an initial tissue-invasive phase of acute infectious cardiomyopathy, virus quits the heart, and the disease, especially with Coxsackie B, enters a subacute phase of inflammation believed to be autoimmunologic.[56,57] Ventricular electrical instability continues as a threat, together with further dilatation and failure of the diseased left ventricle; the risk of systemic emboli persists. If the patient comes under observation at this stage of the natural history, throat and stool cultures are negative. Type-specific antibody titers may still be used but less so, especially if there is no basis for comparison with acute phase serum. Two important diagnostic steps are desirable, namely, characterization of ventricular structure and function by echocardiography, and clarification of the presence, type, and degree of arrhythmias by 24-h electrocardiographic monitoring. The first step is the echocardiogram (Fig. 16-11). An increase in internal dimensions at end diastole can be measured precisely. Septal–free wall thickness (normal or diminished) can be determined and ventricular function assessed (fractional shortening, ejection fraction, etc.).[22,28] Two-dimensional imaging also provides important information on left ventricular endocardial clot. The occasional salutary therapeutic response to steroids is predicated on the assumption that myocardial inflammation persists in the absence of virus in the myocardium, and that the inflammation is amenable to immunosuppression. There is evidence that ^{67}Ga imaging is capable of detecting active myocardial necrosis that accompanies subacute inflammation.[60] Endomyocardial biopsy can be obtained with the Konno or the Olympus catheter via the right ventricle with relative safety in experienced hands.[61] Once virus leaves the heart,

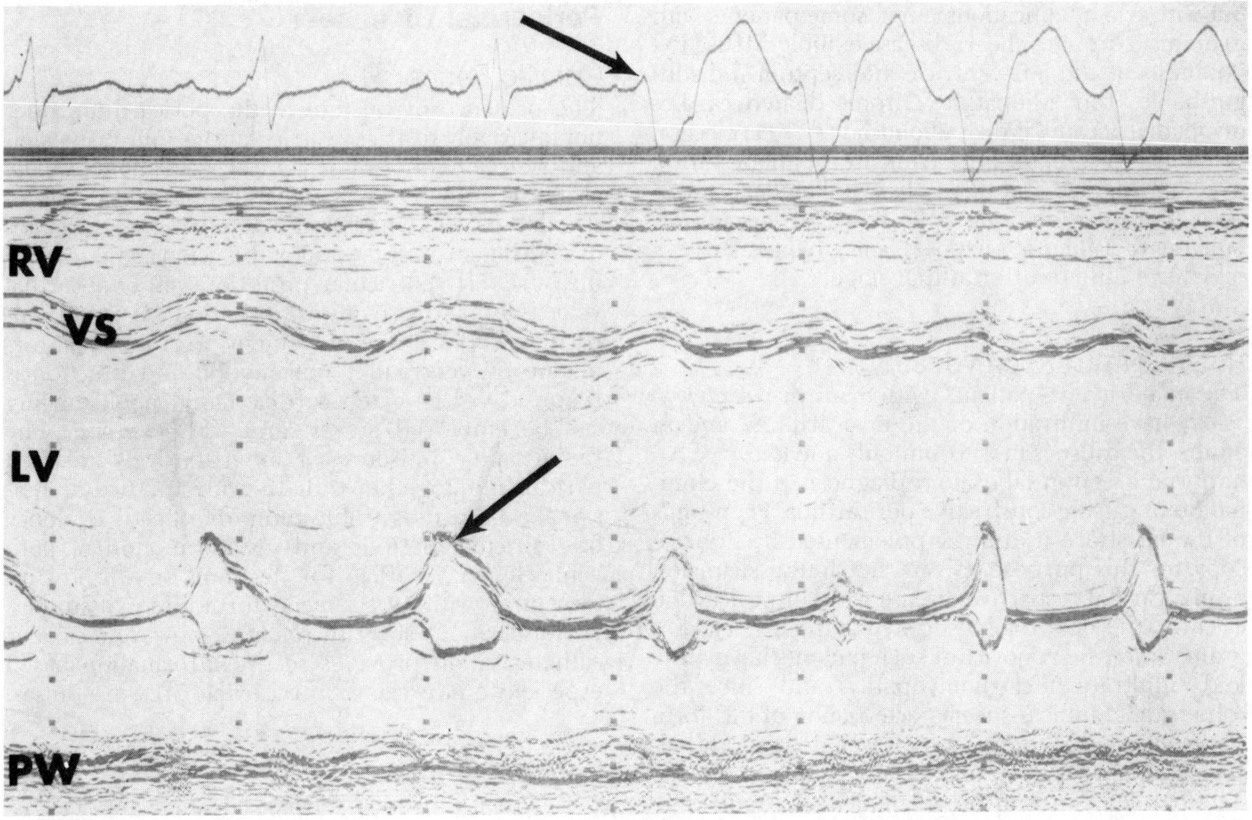

FIGURE 16-11 M-mode echocardiogram from a 20-year-old woman with chronic dilated cardiomyopathy. The ultrasonic beam traversed the right ventricle (RV), ventricular septum (VS), and left ventricle (LV). The mitral valve (lower arrow) is conspicuously separated from both ventricular septum and posterior wall (PW), which is virtually akinetic. The increase in distance from anterior mitral leaflet (E point) to ventricular septum reflects a marked depression in left ventricular ejection fraction. The upper arrow identifies the beginning of ventricular tachycardia, a common complication of dilated cardiomyopathy, especially in the chronic, subacute phase.

fresh tissue offers a paucity of *etiologic* information, but biopsy together with ^{67}Ga can provide useful information on persistent inflammation potentially amenable to immunosuppression.[61]

Chronic dilated cardiomyopathy is thought to represent the fibrotic end stage of preexisting acute and subacute infectious myocarditis (see above). Diagnostic information during this phase of the natural history centers on appraisal of ventricular function, potential left ventricular endocardial clot, and the persistent though perhaps diminished risk of electrical ventricular instability. The initial step, especially if the patient comes under observation for the first time at this stage, is the echocardiogram. The increase in left ventricular internal dimensions can be astonishing; septal–posterior wall motion and increased E point–septal separation (reduced ejection fraction) are dramatically abnormal (Fig. 16-11).[28,62] Endocardial clot may be found at the left ventricular apex. The echocardiogram permits accurate pathophysiological characterization of the cardiomyopathy, but the proper etiologic designation becomes *idiopathic dilated cardiomyopathy*.

In young subjects, the distinction between this stage of idiopathic dilated cardiomyopathy and *dilated ischemic cardiomyopathy* is not important because of the high improbability of the latter. It should be pointed out, however, that chest pain from myocardial necrosis is common, especially during the acute myonecrotic phase and often during the subacute phase of infectious inflammatory cardiomyopathy. In males beyond age 40 years and in most post-menopausal females, the distinction from cardiac dilatation due to ischemia (coronary heart disease) becomes important.[62] It is chiefly in this setting that coronary arteriography sometimes provides useful diagnostic information.

Apart from establishing the presence of obstructive coronary artery disease in older subjects whose ventricular pathophysiology resembles chronic dilated cardiomyopathy, cardiac catheterization and left ventriculography offer little additional information. In subjects with chronic dilated cardiomyopathy, the echocardiogram can be supplemented by ^{99m}Tc radionuclide imaging, which not only refines the observations on left ventricular function but also gives information on segmental ventricular wall motion (Fig. 16-10).[22] The young patient with a dilated, diffusely hypokinetic left ventricle and no segmental wall abnormalities on two-dimensional imaging and radionuclide-gated blood pool scans does not require invasive studies. The older individual with two-dimensional or radionuclide evidence of segmental wall disease is selected out as noted above, but with two qualifications. First, some patients with ischemic (coronary) heart disease exhibit diffuse hypokinesis of the left ventricle and septum indistinguishable from idiopathic, chronic dilated cardiomyopathy. Second, if the radionuclide (^{99m}Tc) ejection fraction is less than 25 percent in a patient with a markedly dilated and diffusely hypokinetic left ventricle, coronary arteriography becomes less important for therapeutic purposes, since bypass surgery may have little to offer at that stage.

Restrictive Cardiomyopathy

The majority of patients with *restrictive cardiomyopathy* have infiltration of the myocardium, and in adults, the cause is most commonly amyloid.[63,64] An important step in laboratory diagnosis is the elimination of calcific constrictive pericarditis. Plain films of the chest are usefully supplemented by fluoroscopy for this purpose. Given the clinical suspicion of myocardial restrictive disease without pericardial calcium, the next diagnostic step is the echocardiogram. Since the majority of such patients have amyloid (infiltrative) cardiomyopathy, and since the echocardiographic tissue characterization of this form of restrictive cardiomyopathy is well defined, the information is sensitive and relatively characteristic. The parallel bands in the M mode and the distinctive myocardial "sparkling" in two-dimensional real time, together with a symmetrical increase in septal, left ventricular, and right ventricular wall thicknesses, diffuse hypokinesis, and small left ventricular internal dimensions at end diastole, weigh strongly in favor of amyloid restrictive cardiomyopathy.[63,64] The reliability of these echocardiographic criteria generally makes endomyocardial biopsy confirmation unnecessary. In addition, careful search for systematized amyloid often sets the stage for an extracardiac tissue diagnosis (biopsy) which adds weight to the echocardiographic findings.

It is difficult to make the distinction between noncalcific constrictive pericarditis, endocardial restriction, and restrictive cardiomyopathy. The difference is important since surgical intervention is indicated in the former but not in the latter two disorders. If the clinical setting makes the distinction obligatory, then cardiac catheterization is required with simultaneous, high-sensitivity recordings of biventricular diastolic pressures. Since restrictive cardiomyopathy and endocardial restriction seldom cause identical changes in right and left ventricular distensibility characteristics, right and left ventricular filling pressures will differ or can be made to differ with physical interventions such as induced premature ventricular beats, exercise (isotonic or isometric), and Valsalva maneuver. Conversely, since constrictive pericarditis almost invariably results in the *same* degree of restriction of both ventricles, the elevated filling pressures will be identical despite physical interventions.

Pericardial Diseases

Calcific Pericarditis

The presence of calcium in the pericardium does not invariably restrict ventricular diastolic distension and systolic motion, but clinical assessment usually establishes whether or not significant myocardial restriction exists. A first step in confirming restriction of ventricular wall motion is the echocardiogram to measure left ventricular posterior wall endocardial velocity and to provide information on right ventricular endocardial movement. If further information on ventricular wall motion and function is required, ^{99m}Tc gated cardiac blood pool imaging can be employed at rest and with exercise. The radiographic presence of an extensively calcified pericardium together with M-mode and two-dimensional echocardiographic and radionuclide evidence of restricted diastolic and systolic motion of both ventricles may suffice for deciding on surgical intervention without the need for additional studies. If doubt about severity remains, however, cardiac catheterization provides secure information based especially on the classic intracardiac pressure pulses.

Pericardial Effusion

Let us deal with mild to marked *chronic* pericardial effusion on the one hand,[65] and sudden pericardial effusion with tamponade on the other.[66,67] Echocardiography is a major step forward in the safe, painless, accurate diagnosis of mild to marked pericardial effusion (Fig. 16-12). Attention should focus on both posterior and anterior pericardium, as well as on distortions of motion of intracardiac structures that occur with large effusions. Two echocardiographic features indicate the presence of pericardial effusion, namely, the separation of visceral and parietal pericardium, i.e., a posterior or posterior and anterior echo-free space, and failure of the parietal pericardium to move with the ventricular wall, seen most clearly in the posterior wall echoes. A posterior pericardial effusion is, as a rule, visualized behind the left ventricle, but disappears behind the left atrium. Identification of pericardial fluid from echocardiographic data permits quantitative conclusions. The echocardiogram is sensitive in detecting small amounts of fluid; the transition from normal to abnormal is well defined and clinically seldom important. When the left ventricular posterior wall (epicardium) is never in contact with the parietal pericardium, the effusion is at least moderate. If this feature coexists with an obvious anterior effusion, the probability of 500 to 1000 ml of fluid is substantial. A large effusion permits the heart to "swing" within it, so that conclusions drawn from motion of septum, mitral leaflets, etc., must be deferred.

The principal value of the echocardiogram in patients clinically suspected of cardiac tamponade is

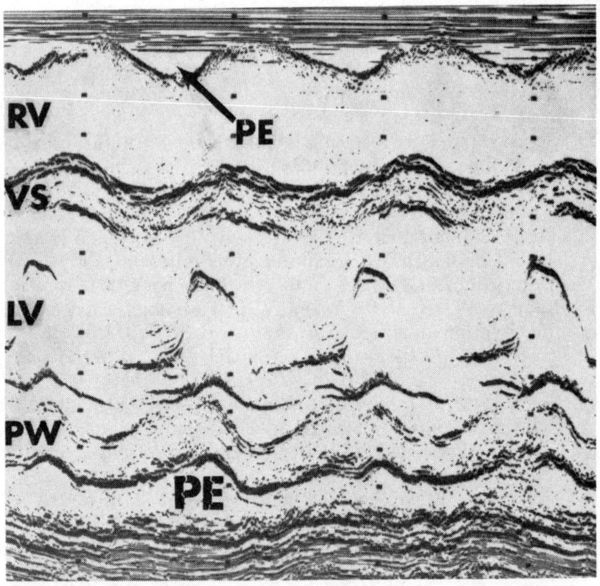

FIGURE 16-12 M-mode echocardiogram in a patient with a large pericardial effusion. The ultrasonic beam traverses the right ventricle (RV), ventricular septum (VS), left ventricle (LV), and posterior wall (PW). The posterior pericardial effusion (PE) is represented by an echo-free space behind the posterior wall in both systole and diastole. In addition, there is an anterior pericardial effusion (arrow) represented by an anterior echo-free space.

the identification of pericardial fluid, as noted above. Tamponade per se is generally not a secure echocardiographic diagnosis.[68,69] In pericardial tamponade, the echocardiogram sometimes identifies a selective inspiratory increase in right ventricular internal dimensions with reciprocal decrease in left ventricular internal dimensions. A more important sign is a characteristic indentation of the right atrial wall generally best seen on the apical four-chamber view.[68] Nevertheless, the diagnosis of pericardial tamponade is secure when significant echocardiographic pericardial effusion occurs in the presence of dyspnea, orthopnea, tachycardia, elevated systemic venous pressure, hepatomegaly, decreased systolic arterial pressure, narrow pulse pressure, pulsus paradoxus, normal to diminished heart sounds, etc. In this setting, further diagnostic information is not required before proceeding with pericardiocentesis. When large pericardial effusion or tamponade of unknown cause are treated by pericardial tap, it is wise after removal of the fluid to inject air and then to secure an upright chest x-ray. This simple technique sometimes permits identification of pericardial tumor seen on profile in the air-filled pericardial space. Such a procedure can be accomplished with no risk and little additional cost.

References

1. Cage, J.: "Silence—Lectures and Writings," Wesleyan University Press, Middletown, Connecticut, 1976.
2. Perloff, J. K.: "The Clinical Recognition of Congenital Heart Disease," 2d ed., W. B. Saunders Company, Philadelphia, 1978.
3. Roberts, W. C.: The Congenitally Bicuspid Aortic Valve: A Study of 85 Autopsy Patients, *Am. J. Cardiol.*, 26:72, 1970.
4. Morganroth, J., Perloff, J. K., Zeldis, S., et al.: Acute Severe Aortic Regurgitation: Pathophysiology, Clinical Recognition and Management, *Ann. Intern. Med.*, 87:223, 1977.
5. Nanda, N. C., Gramiak, R., Manning, J., et al.: Echocardiographic Recognition of the Congenital Bicuspid Aortic Valve, *Circulation*, 49:870, 1974.
6. Hagen, A. D., DiSessa, T. G., Bloor, C. M., and Calleja, H. B.: "Two-Dimensional Echocardiography," Little, Brown and Company, Boston, 1983, p. 484.
7. Tajik, A. J., Seward, J. B., Hagler, D. J., et al.: Two-Dimensional Real-Time Ultrasonic Imaging of the Heart and Great Vessels, *Mayo Clin. Proc.*, 53:271, 1978.
8. Skorton, D., Child, J. S., and Perloff, J. K.: Accuracy of the Echocardiographic Diagnosis of Aortic Regurgitation, *Am. J. Med.*, 69:377, 1980.
9. Quinones, M. D., Young, J. B., Waggoner, A. D., et al.: Assessment of Pulsed Doppler Echocardiography in Detection and Quantification of Aortic and Mitral Regurgitation, *Br. Heart J.*, 44:612, 1980.
10. Bennett, D. H., Evans, D. W., and Raj, M. V. J.: Echocardiographic Left Ventricular Dimensions in Pressure and Volume Overload: Their Use in Assessing Aortic Stenosis, *Br. Heart J.*, 37:971, 1975.
11. Blackwood, R. A., Bloom, K. R., and Williams, C. M.: Aortic Stenosis in Children: Experience with Echocardiographic Prediction of Severity, *Circulation*, 57:263, 1978.
12. Abbasi, A. S.: "Echocardiographic Interpretation," Charles C Thomas, Publisher, Springfield, Ill., 1981, pp. 101, 103.
13. Hagen, A. D., DiSessa, T. G., Samtoy, L., et al.: Reliability of Echocardiography in Diagnosing and Quantifying Valvular Aortic Stenosis, *Cardiovasc. Med.*, 4:391, 1980.
14. Stamm, R. B., and Randolph, P. M.: Quantification of Pressure Gradients across Stenotic Values by Doppler Ultrasound, *J. Am. Coll. Cardiol.*, 2:707, 1983.
15. Borer, J. S., Bacharach, S. L., Green, M. V., et al.: Left Ventricular Function in Aortic Stenosis: Response to Exercise and Effects of Operation, *Am. J. Cardiol.*, 41:382, 1978.
16. Roberts, W. C., Perloff, J. K., and Costantino, T.: Severe Valvular Aortic Stenosis in Patients over 65 Years of Age, *Am. J. Cardiol.*, 27:497, 1971.
17. Perloff, J. K.: Development and Regression of Increased Ventricular Mass, *Am. J. Cardiol.*, 50:605, 1982.
18. Henry, W. C., Bonow, R. B., Rosing, D. R., et al: Observations on the Optimum Time for Operative Intervention for Aortic Regurgitation: II. Serial Echocardiographic Evaluation of Asymptomatic Patients, *Circulation*, 61:484, 1980.
19. Henry, W. L., Bonow, R. O., Borer, J. S., et al.: Observations on the Optimum Time for Operative Intervention for Aortic Regurgitation: I. Evaluation of the Results of Aortic Valve Replacement in Symptomatic Patients, *Circulation*, 61:471, 1980.
20. Borer, J. S., Bacharach, S. L., Green, M. V., et al.: Exercise-Induced Left Ventricular Dysfunction in Symptomatic and Asymptomatic Patients with Aortic Regurgitation: Assessment with Radionuclide Cineangiography, *Am. J. Cardiol.*, 42:351, 1978.
21. Burow, R. D., Strauss, H. W., Singleton, R., et al.: Analysis of Left Ventricular Function from Multiple Gated Acquisition Cardiac Blood Pool Imaging, *Circulation*, 56:1024, 1977.
22. Shine, K. I., Perloff, J. K., Child, J. S., et al.: Non-invasive Assessment of Myocardial Function, *Ann. Intern. Med.*, 92:78, 1980.
23. Welch, G. H., Braunwald, E., and Sarnoff, S. J.: Hemodynamic Effects of Quantitatively Varied Experimental Aortic Regurgitation, *Circ. Res.*, 5:546, 1975.
24. Perloff, J. K.: Mitral Valve Prolapse: Evolving Concepts, *N. Engl. J. Med.*, 307:369, 1982.
25. Shrivastava, S., Guthrie, R. B., and Edwards, J. E.: Mitral Valve Prolapse, *Mod. Concepts Cardiovasc. Dis.*, 46:57, 1977.

26. Winkle, R. A., Lopez, M. G., and Fitzgerald, J. W.: Arrhythmias in Patients with Mitral Valve Prolapse, *Circulation,* 52:73, 1975.
27. Ross, J., Braunwald, E., and Morrow, A. G.: Clinical and Hemodynamic Observations in Pure Mitral Insufficiency, *Am. J. Cardiol.,* 2:11, 1958.
28. Child, J. S., Perloff, J. K., and Krivokapich, J.: Effect of Left Ventricular Size on Echocardiographic E Point to Ventricular Septal Separation, *Am. Heart J.,* 101:797, 1981.
29. Abassi, A. S., Allen, M. W., DeCristofaro, D., et al.: Detection and Estimation of Degree of Mitral Regurgitation by Range-Gated Pulsed Doppler Echocardiography, *Circulation,* 61:143, 1980.
30. Ronan, J. A., Steelman, R. B., DeLeon, A. C., et al.: The Clinical Diagnosis of Acute Severe Mitral Regurgitation, *Am. J. Cardiol.,* 27:284, 1971.
31. Perloff, J. K., and Roberts, W. C.: The Mitral Apparatus: Functional Anatomy of Mitral Regurgitation, *Circulation,* 46:227, 1972.
32. Roberts, W. C., and Perloff, J. K.: Mitral Valvular Disease: A Clinicopathologic Survey of the Conditions Causing the Mitral Valve to Function Abnormally, *Ann. Intern. Med.,* 77:939, 1972.
33. Thuiilez, C., Theroux, P., Bourassa, M. G., et al.: Pulsed Doppler Echocardiographic Study of Mitral Stenosis, *Circulation,* 61:381, 1982.
34. Swan, H. J. C., Ganz, W., Forrester, J. S., et al.: Catheterization of the Heart in Man with Use of a Flow-Directed Balloon Tipped Catheter, *N. Engl. J. Med.,* 283:447, 1970.
35. Nasser, W. K., Davis, R. H., Dillon, J. C., et al.: Atrial Myxoma: I. Clinical and Pathologic Features in Nine Cases; II. Phonocardiographic, Echocardiographic, Hemodynamic and Angiographic Features in Nine Cases, *Am. Heart J.,* 83:694, 810, 1972.
36. Perloff, J. K.: Auscultatory and Phonocardiographic Manifestations of Pulmonary Hypertension, *Prog. Cardiovasc. Dis.,* 9:303, 1967.
37. Rios, J. C., Massumi, R. A., Breesman, W. T., et al.: Auscultatory Features of Acute Tricuspid Regurgitation, *Am. J. Cardiol.,* 23:4, 1969.
38. Gallagher, J. J., Pritchett, E. L. C., Sealy, W. C., et al.: The Pre-excitation Syndromes, *Prog. Cardiovasc. Dis.,* 20:285, 1978.
39. Perloff, J. K., and Harvey, W. P.: The Clinical Recognition of Tricuspid Stenosis, *Circulation,* 22:346, 1960.
40. Perloff, J. K., and Szidon, J. P.: Pulmonary Hypertension: Etiologies, Recognition, Consequences, in J. T. Willerson and C. A. Sanders (eds.), "Clinical Cardiology," Grune & Stratton, New York, 1977.
41. Weyman, A. E., Dillon, J. C., Feigenbaum, H., et al.: Echocardiographic Patterns of Pulmonary Valve Motion with Pulmonary Hypertension, *Circulation,* 50:905, 1974.
42. Engle, M. A., and Perloff, J. K.: "Congenital Heart Disease after Surgery," Yorke Medical Books, New York, 1983, p. 255.
43. Weyman, A. E., Dillon, J. C., Feigenbaum, H., and Chang, S.: Echocardiographic Patterns of Pulmonic Valve Motion in Pulmonic Stenosis, *Am. J. Cardiol.,* 34:644, 1974.
44. Lima, C. O., Sahn, D. J., Valdez-Cruz, L. M., et al.: Noninvasive Prediction of Transvalvular Pressure Gradient in Patients with Pulmonary Stenosis by Quantitative Two-Dimensional Echocardiographic Doppler Studies, *Circulation* 67:866, 1983.
45. Schreiber, T. L., Feigenbaum, H., Weyman, A. E.: Effect of Atrial Septal Defect Repair on Left Ventricular Geometry and Degree of Mitral Valve Prolapse, *Circulation,* 61:888, 1980.
46. Perloff, J. K.: Overlooked Congenital Heart Disease in the Adult, *Cardiovasc. Med.,* 5:535, 548, 1980.
47. Morris, D. C., Felner, J. M., Schlant, R. C., et al.: Echocardiographic Diagnosis of Tetralogy of Fallot, *Am. J. Cardiol.,* 36:908, 1975.
48. Goodwin, J. F., and Oakley, C. M.: The Cardiomyopathies, *Br. Heart J.,* 34:545, 1972.
49. Goodwin, J. F.: Prospects and Predictions for the Cardiomyopathies, *Circulation,* 50:210, 1974.
50. Maron, B. J., and Epstein, S. E.: Hypertrophic Cardiomyopathy. Recent Observations Regarding the Specificity of Three Hallmarks of the Disease: Asymmetric Septal Hypertrophy, Septal Disorganization and Systolic Anterior Motion of the Anterior Mitral Leaflet, *Am. J. Cardiol.,* 45:141, 1980.
51. Roberts, W. C., and Ferrans, V. J.: Pathologic Anatomy of the Cardiomyopathies, *Hum. Pathol.,* 6:287, 1975.
52. Ziady, G. M., Oakley, C. M., Raphael, M. J., et al.: Primary Restrictive Cardiomyopathy, *Br. Heart J.,* 37:556, 1975.
53. Shah, P. M., Gramiak, R., Adelman, A. G., et al.: Role of Echocardiography in Diagnosis and Hemodynamic Assessment of Hypertrophic Subaortic Stenosis, *Circulation,* 44:891, 1971.
54. Falicov, R., Resnekov, L., Bharati, S., et al.: Mid-zone Ventricular Obstruction: A Variant of Obstructive Cardiomyopathy, *Am. J. Cardiol.,* 37:432, 1976.
55. Abelmann, W. H.: Virus and the Heart, *Circulation,* 44:950, 1971.
56. Lerner, A. M., Wilson, F. M., and Reyes, M. P.: Enteroviruses and the Heart: I. Epidemiological and Experimental Studies, *Mod. Concepts Cardiovasc. Dis.,* 44:7, 1975.
57. Lerner, A. M., Wilson, F. M., and Reyes, M. P.: Enteroviruses and the Heart: II. Observations in Humans, *Mod. Concepts Cardiovasc. Dis.,* 44:11, 1975.
58. Reyes, M. P., Ho, K.-L., Smith, F., and Lerner, A. M.: A Mouse Model of Dilated-type Cardiomyopathy Due to Coxsackievirus B3, *J. Infect. Dis.,* 144:232, 1981.
59. El-Khatib, M. R., Chason, J. L., and Lerner, A. M.: Ventricular Aneurysms Complicating Coxsackievirus Group B, Types 1 and 4 Murine Myocarditis, *Circulation* 59:412, 1979.
60. Robinson, J. A., O'Connell, J., Henkin, R. E., et al.: Gallium-67 Imaging in Cardiomyopathy, *Ann. Intern. Med.,* 90:198, 1979.
61. Mason, J. W., Billingham, M. E., and Ricci, D. R.: Treatment of Acute Inflammatory Myocarditis Assisted by Endomyocardial Biopsy, *Am. J. Cardiol.,* 45:1037, 1980.
62. Corya, B. C., Feignebaum, H., Rasmussen, S., et al.: Echocardiographic Features of Congestive Cardiomyopathy Compared with Normal Subjects and Patients with Coronary Artery Disease, *Circulation,* 49:1153, 1974.
63. Child, J. S., Levisman, J. A., Abbasi, A. S., and MacAlpin, R. N.: Echocardiographic Manifestations of Infiltrative Cardiomyopathy: A Report of Seven Cases Due to Amyloid, *Chest,* 70:726, 1976.
64. Child, J. S., Krivokapich, J., and Abbasi, A. S.: Increased Right Ventricular Wall Thickness on Echocardiography in Amyloid Infiltrative Cardiomyopathy, *Am. J. Cardiol.,* 44:1391, 1979.
65. Brown, A. K.: Chronic Idiopathic Pericardial Effusion, *Br. Heart J.,* 28:609, 1966.
66. Reddy, P. S. Curtiss, E. I., O'Toole, J. D., et al.: Cardiac Tamponade: Hemodynamic Observations in Man, *Circulation,* 58:265, 1978.
67. Shabetai, R., Fowler, N. O., and Guntheroth, W. G.: The Hemodynamics of Cardiac Tamponade and Constrictive Pericarditis, *Am. J. Cardiol.,* 26:480, 1970.
68. Gillman, L. D., Guyer, D. E., Gibson, T. C., et al.: Hydrodynamic Compression of the Right Atrium: A New Echocardiographic Sign of Cardiac Tamponade, *Circulation,* 68:294, 1983.

17

Assessment of Cardiac Function and Myocardial Contractility

John Ross, Jr., M.D.

Dilatation causes weakness of the cardiac walls, diminishes the vigor of their contraction, and is therefore the reverse of hypertrophy. So long as compensation is maintained, the enlargement of a cavity may be considerable. The limit is reached when the hypertrophied walls in the systole can no longer expel all the contents, part of which remain, so that at each diastole the chamber is abnormally full.

W. Osler, 1892[1]

In evaluating the patient with cardiac dysfunction, a high index of suspicion about the underlying pathophysiological process after careful clinical examination and routine tests will aid greatly in the selection of additional procedures (if any) that may be needed to establish a diagnosis or to direct therapy. Before discussing the use of special tests and their application to selected clinical problems, it will be useful to consider first some general concepts about overall failure of the heart, myocardial failure, and the effects of altered loading conditions on cardiac function. The end result of these processes is often the sequence described above by Osler,[1] an early conceptualization of reduced ejection fraction.

Is Heart Failure Present or Not?

Failure of the heart as a *pump* (*overall heart failure*) is not synonymous with *myocardial failure.*

Overall Heart Failure

Ideally, we would like to have two measures that determine the effects of heart failure on the tissues of the body: (1) the amount of blood pumped per minute relative to body surface area (the cardiac index) and (2) the pressures behind the pumping chambers (ventricular "filling pressures," reflected either by the mean atrial or the ventricular end-diastolic pressures) both at rest and during stress.

In clinical terms, failure of the right side of the heart at rest is evidenced by the presence of an elevated right-sided heart filling pressure (mean venous pressure 8 cm H_2O or greater) in the resting state, which may be associated with signs of congestion (peripheral edema, hepatomegaly, ascites). Left-sided heart failure at rest is evidenced by the presence of an abnormally elevated filling pressure of the left side of the heart sufficient to cause pulmonary venous congestion on the chest roentgenogram, and may be associated with pulmonary rales or pleural effusion. A low cardiac index (less than 2.4 liters min/m^2) would provide supportive evidence of overall heart failure at rest.

Further identification of overall heart failure is provided by inability of the left side of the heart to produce a normal increase in cardiac output with exercise (less than 600-ml increase in cardiac output per deciliter increase in V_{O_2}),[2] often with an abnormal increase in the right- or left-sided filling pressures or both during exercise.[3] The finding of impaired functional capacity, reflected by a reduced maximal oxygen consumption (V_{O_2}) during exercise, also signifies overall heart failure since this measure correlates with the cardiac output and indicates that *cardiac reserve* is impaired.[4] However, it has been shown that some patients with poor left ventricular function at rest (ejection fraction below 30 percent) can exhibit good exercise capacity and oxygen uptake during a graded treadmill exercise test.[5] Therefore, the presence of *abnormal ventricular function at rest does not necessarily indicate that overall heart failure is present, nor does the absence of overall cardiac failure necessarily mean that ventricular function is normal.*

The above descriptions of overall heart failure say nothing about the *cause* of the failure, and with such a broad description heart failure may be due to such diverse etiologies as generalized myocardial disease, mitral stenosis, chronic pulmonary disease, or constrictive pericarditis. Nevertheless, such descriptions provide a starting point for the identification of right- and left-sided heart failure, or both, from which one may proceed to determine whether or not signs of overall heart failure are due to myocardial disease, mechanical factors, or both. Regardless of cause, the manifestations of heart failure may be aggravated by other conditions such as fever, anemia, dysrhythmia, fluid overload, or metabolic disorders.

Myocardial Failure

Depression of myocardial function (reduced myocardial contractility or inotropic state) constitutes one cause of overall heart failure. Myocardial failure can be defined as the inability of each unit of muscle in the ventricle to shorten a normal distance at a normal velocity against a normal level of systolic load (afterload); it can also be described as the inability of the left ventricle to develop pressure or tension at a normal rate during isovolumetric contraction.[6] The direct causes of most forms of myocardial failure remain unknown, but a few can be identified, such as acute depression of contractility produced by myocarditis, certain drugs, acidosis, or ischemia; chronic depression of contractility can be caused by scarring or patchy myofibrillar loss, or damage to muscle cells caused by inflammation and other processes.

Most commonly, the clinical problem is to determine whether or not *basal myocardial contractility is depressed* in hearts of greatly differing size, or in the same heart at different points in time under different loading conditions (for example, in serial studies after cardiac valve replacement).[7–10] To compare one heart with another, it is necessary to "normalize," or to correct for a given initial heart size. Therefore, when used to detect depressed contractility, systolic function is usually expressed as percentage change of the diastolic volume produced by systole (the ejection fraction), as discussed subsequently.

Ideally, systolic loading on the ventricles (afterload) should also be known and expressed in normalized terms, since afterload affects wall shortening. Systolic pressure in the aorta or the left ventricle is often used to provide an index of afterload, but a variation of the Laplace equation should be applied if possible to define force per unit of cross-sectional area of the ventricular wall (wall stress).[6] Thus, it is generally recognized that a large, thin-walled ventricle maintaining a normal systolic pressure in the resting state is carrying a higher than normal systolic wall stress, whereas a ventricle that is concentrically hypertrophied may be creating a very high systolic pressure, but carrying a normal level of systolic wall stress.

Under some circumstances, excessive cardiac loading conditions can produce failure of the heart as a pump, even though myocardial contractility is not depressed. Under other circumstances, favorable loading conditions and/or compensatory events may mask the presence of depressed myocardial contractility. In addition, impaired cardiac filling due to a variety of causes can produce changes in overall cardiac performance without impaired myocardial systolic function. Finally, severe segmental contraction disorders can coexist with areas of supranormal regional contraction, to yield normal overall cardiac function. These general categories of dissociation between cardiac pump function and myocardial contractility are summarized in Table 17-1.

TABLE 17-1 Dissociations between Pump Function and Myocardial Function

OVERALL HEART FAILURE WITHOUT MYOCARDIAL FAILURE
Acute mechanical overload
Acute cor pulmonale
Malignant hypertension
Acute volume overload (valvular regurgitation)
Chronic severe overload
High cardiac output states (Paget's disease, beriberi)
Valvular and congenital heart disease
Impaired cardiac filling
Pericardial restriction
Restrictive myocardial disease
Mechanical obstruction (mitral and tricuspid stenosis, tumor)
Tachycardias
Low cardiac output due to heart block or bradycardia
MYOCARDIAL FAILURE WITHOUT OVERALL HEART FAILURE
Systolic unloading of the ventricle
Mitral regurgitation
Vasodilator drugs
Compensated myocardial failure
Segmental contraction disorders
Transient myocardial ischemia
Myocardial infarction

Heart Failure without Myocardial Failure

Mechanical Overload and Afterload Mismatch

The level of contractility or inotropic state of the myocardium significantly affects the behavior of the heart. However, *cardiac performance* must be distinguished from *myocardial contractility* per se, since performance is also importantly influenced by the interplay between the preload and the afterload. For example, severe acute hypertension or sudden aortic regurgitation can quickly lead to left ventricular pump failure without myocardial depression; this situation can be described within a framework termed *afterload mismatch with limited preload reserve.*[11] Afterload mismatch can be simply defined as *inability of the ventricle operating at any stable level of inotropic state to maintain a normal forward stroke volume against the prevailing systolic load.*

Afterload mismatch tends to occur when preload reserve is unavailable and the ventricle is therefore unable to compensate for altered afterload (Table 17-2).[8,11] Thus, when the normal heart is pushed to the limit of its preload reserve, a further increase in afterload (as by acute hypertension which leads to augmentation of systolic wall stress) can produce a reduction in wall shortening and in the forward stroke volume of the left ventricle (Fig. 17-1).[12] This situation resembles that in the normal heart under experimental circumstances where the preload is controlled and held constant and only the afterload is varied; there is an *inverse* relation between the systolic pressure and the stroke volume.[12,13] Similarly, in the failing heart, when preload reserve is fully utilized, if aortic pressure is increased, the ventricle

TABLE 17-2 Factors Causing Limited Preload Reserve Which Predispose to Afterload Mismatch

Peripheral	Cardiac
Venous return held constant experimentally	Acute volume loading to limit of ventricular filling
Venous return limited by peripheral factors	Chronic cardiac dilation
	Increased impedance to cardiac filling

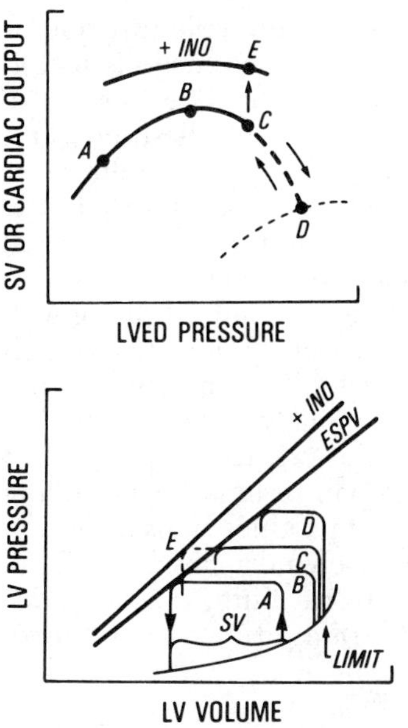

FIGURE 17-1 Two different frameworks for describing ventricular function, and the effects of afterload mismatch and alterations in contractility. *Upper panel:* Relation between left ventricular end-diastolic (LVED) pressure and stroke volume (SV) or cardiac output in the presence of mild depression of ventricular function but with considerable preload reserve. Points A to B show the effects of a volume load: the stroke volume and cardiac output increase. Points B to C show the response to a small dose of a vasopressor, such as angiotensin II or phenylephrine, and points C to D show the effect of a high dose of vasopressor: a marked increase in left ventricular systolic pressure and an apparent descending limb of cardiac function [increased LVED pressure with decreased stroke volume, as the LV reaches the limit of preload reserve (heavy dashed line to point D)]. Reduction of the aortic pressure (correction of afterload mismatch) would move the ventricle back to point C. Point D may also be seen as operation of the ventricle on a downwardly displaced "cardiac output curve," the curve being displaced by the effects of increased resistance to ventricular ejection as defined by Guyton.[114] Also seen are the effects of a positive inotropic drug (+INO), administered at point C, which shifts the function curve upward allowing the delivery of a larger stroke volume or cardiac output from the same LVED pressure (point E). *Lower panel:* Diagram of the same responses in another framework: left ventricular (LV) pressure-volume loops and the linear end-systolic pressure-volume relation (ESPV).[115] The curved lower line represents the diastolic pressure-volume relation. Beat A is a control contraction (corresponding to point A in upper diagram), showing the counterclockwise loop during LV isovolumetric contraction, ejection, and isovolumetric relaxation, and the stroke volume (SV) is indicated. With volume loading there is a mild pressure increase as the ventricle moves to beat B. With infusion of a vasopressor in low dose, the ventricle moves to point C and continues to reach the linear ESPV relation at end ejection; the stroke volume drops slightly (point C). With a marked pressor stress (beat D), the ventricle reaches the limit of its preload reserve; it cannot compensate for the increased systolic pressure and the stroke volume drops markedly (beat D, corresponding to point D in panel above). This response is due to afterload mismatch, and *not* to change in myocardial contractility. The effect of a positive inotropic agent (+INO) to shift the linear end-systolic pressure volume relation upward and to the left as described by Sagawa[114] is shown, and the stroke volume increases (beat E compared to beat C).

cannot compensate and stroke volume falls,[14] yielding an apparent descending limb of function due to afterload mismatch (Fig. 17-1). That is, the failing ventricle behaves *as if* its preload were fixed, and any increase in systolic pressure induces afterload mismatch. Afterload mismatch can also occur in the normal heart when a vasopressor drug is administered and the venous return is inadequate to allow the ventricle to maintain stroke volume;[11] reflex venodilation or other peripheral regulatory factors may be responsible for such responses. Finally, afterload mismatch can occur even without intervention when the filling ventricle is unable to deliver a normal stroke volume at the existing level of normal aortic pressure.[8,11] Under all of these conditions in which the reserve provided by increasing preload is limited or unavailable, the *stroke volume becomes inversely related to the afterload.* An apparent "descending limb" of ventricular function under these conditions is undoubtedly due primarily to excess afterload (afterload mismatch) rather than to sarcomere overstretch.[8,11]

These principles are illustrated in Fig. 17-1 using two different schemes for describing cardiac function (ventricular function curves, and pressure-volume loops with end-systolic pressure-volume relations). Of course, all of these responses, which reflect alterations in ventricular performance due to induced changes in loading, can be altered by changes in the inotropic state. In *acute* overall heart failure due to *afterload mismatch* (apparent descending limb, point D, Fig. 17-1), reduction of the overload by vasodilator therapy or by replacement of a defective valve with a prosthesis should promptly reverse the pump failure since myocardial contractility is basically intact.[11] Augmentation of the inotropic state with a positive inotropic drug will further improve ventricular performance (Fig. 17-1, point E).

In *chronic* mechanical overload, such as that due to valvular heart disease or a large left-to-right shunt, adaptations occur primarily through the development of concentric or eccentric hypertrophy, which compensates for the overload and prevents overall cardiac failure.[15–17] In most of these conditions, heart failure does not occur until myocardial damage supervenes due to long-standing hypertrophy. However, as discussed subsequently, critical aortic stenosis can produce afterload mismatch and heart failure *without* irreversible depression of myocardial contractility (Fig. 17-2). Less is known about heart failure due to the overload of high-output states, such as Paget's disease or beriberi, although it is likely that in these conditions altered sodium balance with fluid retention can lead to a congested state in the absence of myocardial failure.

Impaired Cardiac Filling

There is evidence that impaired cardiac filling can lead to heart failure (Table 17-1). It has been well documented that decreased forward cardiac output and elevation of cardiac filling pressures are often associated with normal systolic function in chronic constrictive pericarditis and in acute cardiac tamponade.[18] There is also experimental evidence that acute volume overload, as by overtransfusion, can cause elevated cardiac filling pressures and im-

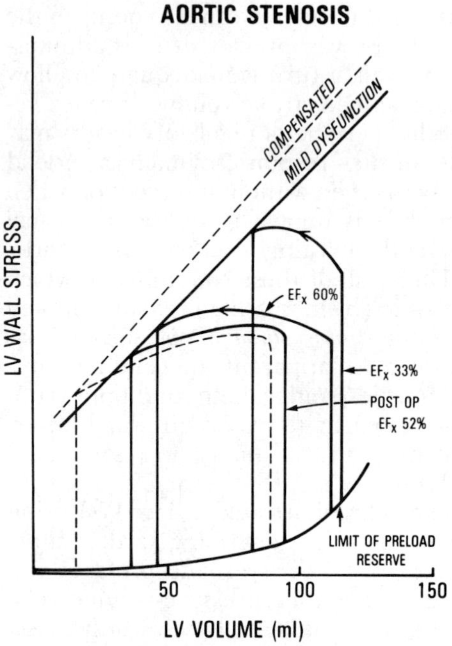

FIGURE 17-2 Diagrammatic examples of left ventricular (LV) function in valvular aortic stenosis. Loops of LV volume versus wall stress are shown during single contractions. The curved relation between diastolic left ventricular volume and wall stress is also shown, along with the linear end-systolic wall stress–volume relation. In compensated aortic stenosis (dashed lines), the LV volume and the left ventricular wall stress–volume loop are normal, with a fall of wall stress during ejection and a normal level of systolic wall stress despite elevated systolic pressure, due to concentric LV hypertrophy (see text). With development of mild depression of myocardial contractility, the linear end-systolic relation is shifted somewhat to the right, the left ventricle enlarges to encroach on its preload reserve, and the wall stress rises somewhat during ejection, although the ejection fraction (EF_X) is well maintained at 60 percent. With further progression of critical stenosis, the ventricle reaches the limit of its preload reserve, the wall stress rises markedly during ejection as the ventricle is unable to unload itself, and the stroke volume drops sharply (EF_X = 33 percent). This response is due to afterload mismatch, not to further depression of myocardial contractility. Following aortic valve replacement, there is persistence of mild depression of myocardial contractility, but the afterload mismatch is corrected and the ejection fraction returns to near normal postoperatively (EF_X = 52 percent).

paired filling of the left side of the heart due to limitation of pericardial expansion as the right side of the heart overfills.[19–21] This response is associated with elevation of the *intrapericardial pressures,* with *apparent* depression of the ventricular function curve. It also leads to a shift upward of the entire diastolic pressure-volume relation of the left and right ventricles, due to changes of intrapericardial pressure, and the shift can be corrected by bleeding or by the use of a vasodilator such as nitroprusside.[19,20] Such responses may explain acute shifts downward of the left ventricular diastolic pressure-volume relation observed clinically with vasodilators,[22,23] and elevated intrapericardial pressures could play a role in producing the high filling pressures in severe acute heart failure.

Restrictive disease of the ventricular chambers also leads to elevated diastolic ventricular and atrial pressures despite normal systolic contractile function of the myocardium.[24] Mechanical obstructions to filling of the ventricles include mitral and tricuspid valve stenosis, cor triatriatum, fibrosing mediastinitis, and intraatrial clots or tumors which lead to pulmonary or systemic venous hypertension. Very rapid ventricular and atrial tachyarrhythmias, including atrial fibrillation, can cause marked reduction of the diastolic ventricular filling time per minute, along with inappropriate timing or loss of atrial systole, which can lead to elevated cardiac filling pressures and a fall in cardiac output. Finally, marked bradyarrhythmias can impair the cardiac output. All of these conditions which impair or limit cardiac filling in diastole (Table 17-1) can produce signs of overall heart failure despite relatively normal systolic function of the ventricular myocardium, that is, a dissociation between cardiac pump function and myocardial contractility.

Myocardial Failure without Heart Failure

As might be anticipated, the converse of afterload mismatch can occur when the preload is adequate but the afterload or wall stress on the myocardial fibers is abnormally low. The best example is mitral regurgitation, in which the low impedance leak into the left atrium may result in maintenance of a normal ejection fraction until late in the clinical course, when depression of myocardial contractility has already occurred.[25] Thus, favorable loading conditions can mask depressed contractility which, under normal loading conditions, would produce a low ejection fraction (Fig. 17-3).

Favorable loading conditions can be produced by treatment of the failing heart with a vasodilator drug which lowers the afterload during ejection.[26–28] Experimental studies indicate that in acute heart failure, favorable effects of a vasodilator such as nitroprusside on the cardiac output result from both decreased afterload and peripheral circulatory effects.[29,30] In this setting, left ventricular unloading by nitroprusside produces a large shift of blood volume from the distended central circulation to the peripheral bed, which is sufficient to counterbalance the peripheral pooling of blood due to the drug's dilating action on the veins; this shift of blood volume, when coupled with reduced resistance to ventricular ejection, allows the venous return to increase and hence leads to an increase in the output of the failing heart by the vasodilator.[30] Overall heart failure may thereby be relieved despite severe persistent depression of myocardial contractility.

Which Special Procedure Should Be Selected?

Special diagnostic procedures to identify and quantify cardiac dysfunction or myocardial failure must be selected with careful regard to the question being

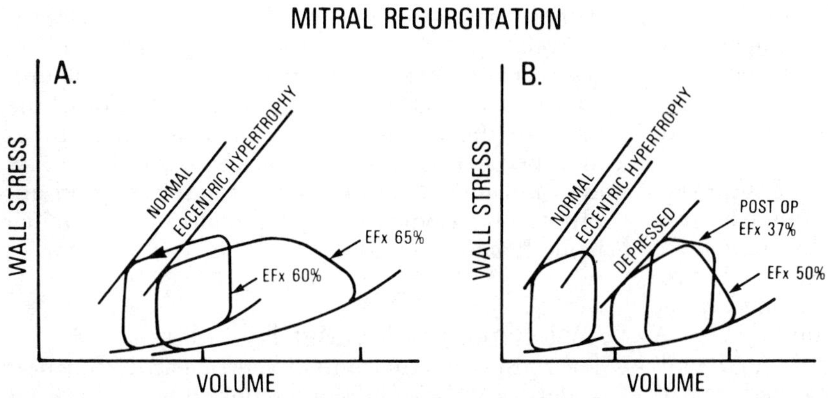

FIGURE 17-3 Diagrammatic examples of left ventricular (LV) function in mitral regurgitation. *A.* Volume overload hypertrophy (eccentric hypertrophy) causes displacement to the right of the curved diastolic pressure-volume relation and the linear end-systolic volume–wall stress relation, and the loop of a single LV contraction (volume versus wall stress) shows delivery of a very large total stroke volume. Because of the low-impedance leak into the left atrium, the ejection fraction is maintained at high-normal level (EF_X = 65 percent). *B.* The development of markedly depressed myocardial contractility shifts the linear end-systolic volume–wall stress relation downward and to the right. In this setting, prior to mitral valve replacement, the ventricle can still maintain a relatively low mean systolic wall stress, wall stress being reduced in particular early and late during ejection because of the regurgitant leak; therefore the total stroke volume remains high and ejection fraction is only mildly reduced (EF_X = 50 percent). Following mitral valve replacement, despite some reduction in end-diastolic volume in this example, the LV must now eject entirely into the aorta with its high impedance of the aorta, the wall stress early and late during ejection rises, and the ejection fraction falls (postoperative EF_X = 37 percent). This postoperative response, the opposite of that in the patient with aortic stenosis (Fig. 17-2), is again due to altered systolic loading conditions rather than a change in myocardial contractility produced by the operation. *(From J. Ross, Jr.: Left Ventricular Function and the Timing of Surgical Treatment of Valvular Heart Disease, Ann. Intern Med., 94:498, 1981. Modified and reproduced with permission from the publisher and author.)*

asked, as well as the overall safety, usefulness, and cost of each procedure (Table 17-3). For example, if the question can be answered by an extremely safe, noninvasive procedure such as M-mode and two-dimensional echocardiography or treadmill exercise testing, there is little reason to use a more expensive procedure which requires intravenous injection of a radioisotope. If the problem is to evaluate symptoms and the degree of functional impairment in a patient with heart disease of known etiology, then an exercise test for functional capacity or for ischemic changes on the ECG may be all that is needed to guide therapy. If the problem is to confirm a suspected diagnosis of depressed left ventricular function due to primary myocardial disease, an echocardiogram may provide an adequate answer, as well as information about whether valvular heart disease, hypertrophic cardiomyopathy, pericardial disease, or restrictive myocardial disease can be implicated. If, for technical reasons, the echocardiogram is not conclusive for evaluating the degree of left ventricular dysfunction, a radionuclide angiographic determination of the ejection fraction provides an appropriate next step. The systolic time intervals, particularly the preejection period/left ventricular ejection time (PEP/LVET) ratio, sometimes are useful, particularly in comparing groups of patients.[31,32] However, if such noninvasive tests do not provide a diagnosis that is sufficiently accurate to allow effective medical or surgical therapy, then cardiac catheterization may be indicated. In the presence of acute, severe heart failure with or without hypotension, and sometimes in severe chronic heart failure, right-sided heart catheterization in the intensive care unit setting may be highly useful, both in the diagnosis of causative factors and in the guiding of the responses to acute therapy.

Assessment of Overall Heart Failure

In evaluating symptoms of severe dyspnea, orthopnea, or edema, special procedures are usually not required for identifying the presence of right- or left-sided heart failure at rest. Knowledge of the cardiac output is generally not required, and filling pressures can be estimated. However, it is likely that in the future, Doppler echocardiographic determination of resting cardiac output will find increasing clinical application.[33] Also, a noninvasive method for measuring the cardiac output in patients with heart failure, the carbon dioxide rebreathing technique, has been validated.[34]

TABLE 17-3 Potential Steps in Assessing Ventricular Dysfunction

Exercise capacity
Echocardiography
Two-dimensional, M mode for ventricular size; ejection phase indexes; Doppler studies
Radionuclide angiography for ejection fraction, if echocardiography inadequate
Fluoroscopy for calcium
Balloon catheterization of right side of the heart
Cardiac output, filling pressures, systemic vascular resistance
Formal cardiac catheterization
Hemodynamic variables; quantitative ventriculography; ejection fraction (isovolumic phase indexes); coronary arteriography

Exercise Capacity
By the use of a treadmill or bicycle ergometer, exercise capacity can be determined from the maximum workload that the patient is able to carry out. The $\dot{V}_{O_2}$ when the patient performs a truly maximum effort is the best indicator of overall cardiac function, since it equals the product of the maximum cardiac output and the maximum arteriovenous O_2 difference. Noninvasive measurement of respiratory gas exchange during exercise has provided a useful approach for characterizing cardiac functional class based on the maximum $\dot{V}_{O_2}$: class A (normal) > 20 ml/min/kg; class B = 16 to 20 ml/min/kg; class C = 10 to 15 ml/min/kg; and class D < 10 ml/min/kg.[35] In class D patients, for example, there is an inability to increase the stroke volume during exercise, although the resting cardiac output is reduced to the same degree as in class C patients.[35] Maximum $\dot{V}_{O_2}$ in METS (multiple of resting $\dot{V}_{O_2}$) can also be estimated from the workload performed, and this can provide a useful clinical estimate of functional capacity.

Determination of the exercise capacity can be highly useful for objectively evaluating the significance of symptoms in patients with chronic cardiomyopathy or chronic valvular heart disease, even though it is not possible in the latter instance to determine the relative contributions of myocardial dysfunction and hemodynamic abnormalities due to the valve disease. (In severe aortic stenosis exercise testing is usually contraindicated.) Exercise testing can also be valuable for following responses to various forms of treatment, such as vasodilator therapy in chronic heart failure.[27]

The response to exercise is determined primarily by the exercise cardiac output, but many other factors, including adaptations in the skeletal muscles and the peripheral vascular bed, cardiovascular reflexes, motivation, and drug therapy, are also operative. It is therefore not surprising that good functional capacity has been reported in some individuals who have markedly impaired left ventricular function at rest, and vice versa.[5,36,37] For example, Franciosa et al. reported some patients with ejection fractions of only 25 percent who were able to exercise for 17 min, and others with normal ejection fractions who had exercise times of less than 5 min.[36]

Right Heart Catheterization
Catheterization of the pulmonary artery by the Swan-Ganz technique (Chap. 99) may be useful for evaluation and management of severe overall heart failure in certain clinical settings. This approach is frequently employed for evaluating severe heart failure in acute myocardial infarction,[38] particularly when complicated by hypotension (Chap. 124). For example, a test of left ventricular function can be performed by using a small volume load (200- to 200-ml dextrose infusion), and by measuring the response of the cardiac output, stroke volume, or stroke work index relative to the accompanying rise in pulmonary artery wedge pressure.[39] A flat or descending relation indicates that left ventricular function is severely depressed with maximum use of the preload reserve. Catheterization of the right side of the heart in the intensive care unit is also sometimes indicated to quantitate chronic refractory heart failure, and it may be invaluable for selecting an appropriate vasodilator and monitoring its initial hemodynamic effects.[38]

Assessment of Myocardial Failure

The most common cause of ventricular dysfunction is depressed systolic contraction due to reduced myocardial fiber shortening. The first step is the *detection* of such an abnormality; then, further steps may be needed to define its cause (e.g., overload due to valvular disease, or primary myocardial failure). In chronic disease, such an abnormality is almost always accompanied by diastolic enlargement of the ventricle. Less commonly, systolic function is preserved and diastolic dysfunction (increased myocardial stiffness, pericardial disease) is responsible for high filling pressures. Often, the basic problem is to distinguish reduced ventricular performance due to mechanical abnormalities from that due to myocardial failure. Several measures of ventricular function, obtained by a variety of methods, can be used for this purpose.

Contractility Indexes
For evaluating *basal contractility* in many types of heart disease it is *not* necessary to rely on hemodynamic indexes of contractility that are independent of preload and afterload. In effect, when preload reserve has been fully utilized, depressed myocardial contractility will result in an "afterload mismatch" in the resting state, which will be expressed by inability of the ventricle to maintain normal performance *per unit* of its circumference or volume. In this setting, the afterload (wall stress) may be somewhat increased (and further contribute to impaired performance), but this increase occurs *because* depressed myocardial function has produced chamber enlargement. Therefore, measurement of normalized ejecting performance will effectively detect depressed myocardial contractility.

In the resting state, the so-called ejection phase indexes based on measurements of the left ventricular chamber size are perhaps the *most useful and practical* means of detecting depressed myocardial function. Such indexes include the percentage of the end-diastolic volume that is ejected (the *ejection fraction,* for which 55 percent is the lower limit of normal), the percentage shortening of the ventricular end-diastolic diameter (the *fractional shortening,* for which the lower limit of normal is 28 percent), and the mean velocity of internal diameter or circumferential fiber (CF) shortening, the *mean* V_{CF} (lower limit of normal is 1.2 circumference/second). The ejection fraction is most commonly employed, and a reduced value measured in the resting state usually can detect depressed basal ventricular contractility. Like all of the "ejection-phase" measures it is highly sensitive to *changes in afterload* and under some conditions may not reflect depressed basal myocardial contractility when the level of afterload is *low* or *high.* The ejection phase indexes effectively separate normal patients from patients with clear-cut left ventricular myocardial disease.[40,42] The ejection phase measures have the advantage that they can be determined noninvasively by echocardiography or radionuclide angiography, and good agreement with measurements made from angiograms has generally been found.

Analyses of right ventricular function have been limited, primarily because of the complex shape of this chamber and the difficulty of computing right ventricular volumes angiographically. However, radionuclide techniques (nongeometric) have permitted assessment of the left and right ventricular ejection fractions at rest and during stress.[42,43] At rest, the lower limit of normal of the right ventricular ejection fraction is approximately 40 to 43 percent.[43] Two-dimensional echo techniques allow qualitative assessment of right ventricular size and function.

In chronic, compensated valvular heart disease or chronic hypertension, the left ventricular wall undergoes hypertrophy of the volume or pressure overload type, so that the mean systolic wall stress is often maintained at relatively normal or only mildly elevated levels.[44] In sudden aortic or mitral regurgitation, in acute hypertension or with long-standing severe hypertension, the ejection phase measures may become unreliable for evaluating myocardial contractility, since a reduced ejection fraction can be due to afterload mismatch (Table 17-1). Alternatively, the systolic unloading of the left ventricle in chronic mitral regurgitation may yield a normal ejection fraction even when myocardial contractility is depressed.[25] Under such circumstances, *limitations* of the ejection phase measures for identifying impaired myocardial contractility *must be recognized.* If measurement of the degree of depression of myocardial contractility or lack thereof is desired, normalized ventricular performance can be examined at the operating level of systolic *wall stress* and compared with the performance of the normal ventricle at a comparable level of wall stress.

Calculation of wall stress remains largely a research technique although it can be done noninvasively using echocardiography.[45] However, it is rarely necessary to determine wall stress for effective clinical management if one keeps in mind the above caveats about loading conditions. Several techniques have been described for assessing myocardial contractility under abnormal loading conditions using analysis of wall stress. Each involves determining the inverse relation between afterload and some normalized measure of systolic function (velocity, wall shortening, or stroke volume) over a range of loading conditions in the normal heart (produced by a graded pressor infusion), and then comparing the function of the heart in question with this normal range. These approaches have included the relation between wall stress and fractional shortening (e.g., see Fig. 17-4)[46] and between force (wall stress) and velocity, and the relation between end-systolic vol-

FIGURE 17-4 Example of one approach, employed by Borow et al.,[46] for defining basal myocardial contractility when systolic loading conditions are abnormal. Shown are the relations between left ventricular (LV) fractional shortening [percent change of left ventricular (LV) internal diameter, D, determined by echocardiography] over a range of LV end-systolic wall stress values. The LV systolic pressure and wall stress were varied in these normal patients by graded infusions of phenylephrine to produce the linear regression shown (standard deviations indicated). Using such a plot, a patient with normal end-systolic wall stress (70 g/cm², for example) in the resting state could be characterized as having myocardial failure if the fractional shortening were below approximately 30 percent. Alternatively, in a patient with aortic stenosis in whom the end-systolic wall stress is elevated (120 g/cm²), fractional shortening might be below 25 percent, but this reduction is due to afterload mismatch rather than to depressed myocardial contractility (see also Fig. 17-2). (*From R. M. Borow, L. H. Greene, W. Grossman, and E. Braunwald: Left Ventricular End-Systolic Stress-Shortening and Stress-Length Relations in Humans, Am. J. Cardiol. 50:1301, 1982. Reproduced with permission from the publisher and author.*)

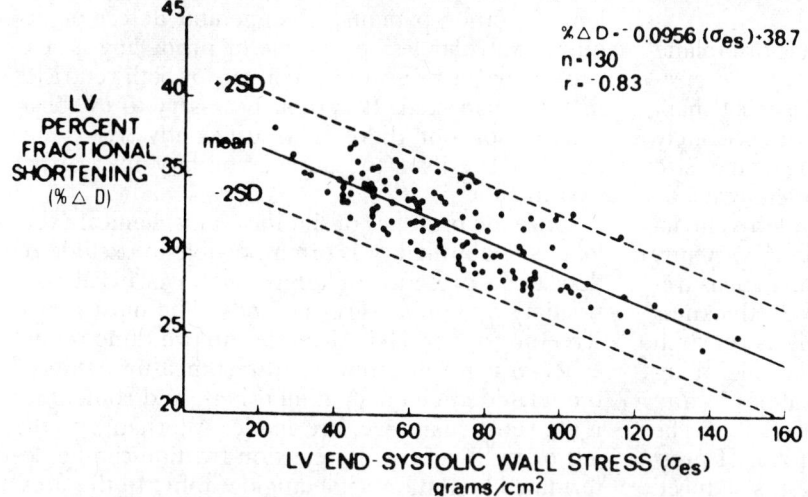

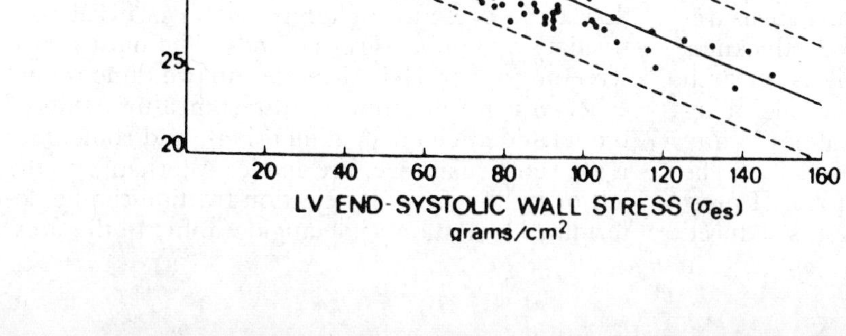

ume and wall stress.[45,46,49] The ejection fraction can also be compared at similar levels of systolic wall stress.

Noninvasive Methods

Echocardiography (Chap. 120) is the current method of choice for assessing myocardial function; it also allows identification of mechanical cardiac disorders and provides clues to impaired filling, which are signaled by reduced EF slope of the mitral valve and by left atrial enlargement. Chamber enlargement can be confirmed (left ventricular end-diastolic size is increased if the dimension is over 5.2 cm or 3.8 cm/m^2 body surface area). All of the above-mentioned ejection phase indexes of contractility can be calculated, together with chamber wall thickness, and using two-dimensional echocardiography left ventricular end-diastolic volume and myocardial mass can be determined.[49–51]

Radionuclide angiography (Chap. 109) is particularly suitable for determining the ejection fraction of the ventricles, and it correlates well with angiography.[52] Measurements of absolute ventricular volumes and diastolic filling rates have also been reported.[54–56] This approach is valuable when technically adequate echo studies cannot be obtained as, for example, in chronic obstructive pulmonary disease, or when assessment of global function independent of ventricular geometry and regional wall motion is needed in the presence of coronary heart disease. An abnormal response (less than 5 percent increase) in the left or right ventricular ejection fraction during exercise occurs during regional myocardial ischemia in patients with coronary heart disease, but it is not specific for ischemia.[55]

Cardiac Catheterization and Angiography

In the evaluation of cardiac and myocardial dysfunction, because of expense and some risk to the patient (Chap. 108), formal cardiac catheterization and coronary arteriography are undertaken only when a precise diagnosis is critical to the selection of appropriate medical or surgical therapy and when that diagnosis cannot be achieved by noninvasive techniques.

Selective ventriculography using single or biplane left ventriculographic studies to calculate the ejection fraction or other ejection phase measures (Chap. 108) has long provided the standard for accurately quantifying the basal level of left ventricular size and function.[58,59] Chamber enlargement can be identified, the upper limit of normal of left ventricular end-diastolic volume being 110 ml/m^2 body surface area (2 SD).[60] High-fidelity pressure measurements together with volume and wall thickness calculations have also been used, largely as research tools, to study systolic wall stress,[61] diastolic filling rates,[62] diastolic stress-strain abnormalities,[63] and "isovolumic-phase indexes" of contractility.[7,64,65] The simplest such index is the peak rate of rise of pressure (dP/dt) of the left ventricle: when it is reduced below about 1400 mmHg/s, myocardial contractility is usually depressed. This measure is affected by a number of factors, however. In the author's view, various contractile indexes derived from isovolumic systole are generally less reliable than ejection phase indexes in the individual patient.[7,40,41,66]

Myocardial Biopsy

When cardiac catheterization studies fail to reveal a specific cause for unexplained severe cardiac failure, myocardial biopsy (Chap. 108) can sometimes reveal evidence of an unsuspected infiltrative cardiomyopathy, microvascular disease, or evidence of inflammation. In the past, the diagnostic yield of such myocardial biopsies has been relatively low;[64] more recently, using electron and fluorescence microscopy, over 60 percent of one group of patients with unexplained congestive heart failure showed evidence of inflammation, and some responded to immunosuppressive therapy.[65]

How Should Special Procedures Be Used to Solve Specific Clinical Problems?

Recognition of Mechanical Factors Sufficient to Cause Heart Failure

In assessing the patient who has clinical signs of acute or chronic overall heart failure, it is important at the outset to consider the possibility that mechanical factors rather than myocardial depression are primarily responsible (Table 17-1). Impaired cardiac filling due to pericardial disease or other cause should be carefully excluded, as discussed subsequently in the section on myocardial disease. In some patients, a mechanical cause for secondary heart failure may be relatively obvious, as in severe systemic hypertension, coarctation of the aorta, or arteriovenous fistula due to trauma or other cause. In those settings, extensive evaluation of the associated cardiac dysfunction may not be necessary, since treatment of the primary disorder will correct the cardiac problem. In other patients, a congenital defect or acquired valvular lesion capable of producing an excessive flow or pressure load on one or both ventricles may be suspected. It is then necessary to establish whether or not there is a sufficiently *severe* mechanical overload to cause secondary myocardial dysfunction.

Once the presence of significant mechanical overload is established, it is often possible to exclude or detect the presence of depressed myocardial contractility by noninvasive methods. The most useful screening approach is M-mode and two-dimensional echocardiography, in which direct measurements of the left-sided chamber dimensions, and sometimes right ventricular size, are made. Alternatively, the left or right ventricular ejection fraction can be determined by radionuclide angiography. In the presence of chronic volume overload, the finding of normal systolic contractile function by echocardiography or a normal radionuclide ejection fraction, despite the presence of a moderately increased ventricular end-diastolic dimension, usually indicates the absence of significant depression of myocardial contractility. An important exception occurs in chronic mitral regurgitation, as discussed further in the section on myocardial function in valvular heart disease which follows below. If coronary artery disease and regional wall motion abnormalities coexist with valvular heart disease, the M-mode echocardiogram is often unreliable. Calculation of left ventricular volume by the two-dimensional echo technique may be feasible, or the ejection fraction may be determined by the radionuclide technique.

In heart failure due to sudden, severe volume overload (consequent to infective endocarditis of the aortic or mitral valves, ruptured chordae tendineae infarction of a papillary muscle, or ruptured interventricular septum) noninvasive studies should be performed and may provide clues to the diagnosis as well as to the presence of severe ventricular dysfunction. M-mode echocardiographic studies when associated with two-dimensional studies may allow the identification of a flail mitral valve leaflet, ventricular septal defect, or vegetations on the aortic, mitral, or tricuspid valves. Diastolic fluttering of the anterior mitral valve leaflet may be noted in aortic valve regurgitation, and with acute severe aortic regurgitation preclosure of the mitral valve in mid-diastole may be identified on the M-mode echocardiogram (Chap. 120). The echocardiogram will also allow identification of the reduction in fractional shortening and ejection fraction of the left ventricle that usually accompanies severe acute overload; this may be due to full utilization of the preload reserve with acute afterload mismatch rather than significant depression of myocardial contractility.[11] In the further diagnosis and treatment of heart failure due to sudden cardiac overload in the intensive care setting, insertion of a balloon catheter usually is advisable to measure the wedge pressure, to search for a left-to-right shunt, and to guide vasodilator and other therapy. Before considering surgical treatment, full cardiac catheterization should usually be performed to ascertain the severity of the mechanical lesion and the state of the left ventricle, and to examine the coronary arteries.

Recognition of Myocardial Failure in Chronic Valvular Heart Disease

Valvular lesions that overload the left ventricle (aortic stenosis, aortic regurgitation, and mitral regurgitation) can, over time, produce severe left ventricular hypertrophy, which eventually is associated with myocardial fibrosis or other subcellular changes[69] and left ventricular dysfunction.[69,70] Such dysfunction may persist even after surgical correction of the valve defect; patients with chronic valvular heart disease must therefore be carefully managed to avoid irreversible left ventricular dysfunction.[71] The types of special studies on the left ventricle and the frequency with which they should be performed vary somewhat among the three valvular lesions.

Valvular Aortic Stenosis

In the young patient suspected of having severe aortic stenosis, cardiac catheterization studies are generally carried out early. Operation is undertaken if the suspicion of severe stenosis is confirmed, since the risk of surgery appears to be less than the risk of sudden death in such individuals.[70] In these patients, the question of myocardial dysfunction does not usually pose a significant problem. The adult with clinical features of significant aortic stenosis who develops symptoms of left ventricular dysfunction, syncope, or angina pectoris must be catheterized promptly. Sometimes, particulary in older individuals with heart failure, the aortic systolic murmur may not be loud, and sometimes the pulse pressure may be normal, even in the presence of severe stenosis (Chap. 37). In such individuals, echocardiography, phonocardiography, and fluoroscopy for aortic calcification may contribute useful information, but if there is unexplained left ventricular dysfunction with signs of aortic stenosis, hemodynamic studies should usually be done. Cardiac catheterization should document whether or not the aortic valve narrowing is signficant (valve orifice area less than 0.75 cm^2 or 0.6 cm/m^2 body surface area are approximate guidelines),[71] whether associated coronary atherosclerosis is contributing to the patient's symptoms, and whether or not there is depressed contractile function. Generally, if the stenosis is severe and symptoms are present, operation is undertaken, since the outlook with medical therapy is poor.[70,72]

In the adult patient who does not have significant symptoms but has physical findings of aortic stenosis, the chest roentgenogram will typically reveal a normal heart size, and the electrocardiogram may be nonspecific. A baseline M-mode echocardiogram should be obtained to document thickening of the aortic valve, to determine the degree of thickening of the left ventricular walls, and to ensure that the left ventricular end-diastolic dimension, fractional shortening, and ejection fraction are all within the normal range. Such patients can be followed by clinical examination, and watched closely for onset of symptoms.

Serial echocardiographic or catheterization studies carried out after aortic valve replacement for aortic stenosis indicate that hypertrophy regresses and left ventricular function remains normal in most patients, and even if it is moderately depressed preoperatively, ventricular function tends to return toward normal during the first 6 months postoperatively.[73–75] Even in patients with severely depressed ventricular function preoperatively, the average ejection fraction returns to near normal or normal, although in a few patients it remains somewhat depressed.[76] These findings suggest that mechanical overload per se (afterload mismatch), rather than irreversibly depressed myocardial contractility, is usually responsible for the reduced left ventricular function preoperatively.[71] The development of some dilation of the left ventricular chamber at end diastole, with relative thinning of the ventricular wall and reduced fractional shortening, may be due to increasing severity of critical aortic stenosis, as well as to early left ventricular decompensation. Most likely, when mild to moderate depression of left ventricular function develops,[77] the preload reserve becomes fully utilized, and then any further progression of the critical aortic stenosis will result in afterload mismatch with a fall in the ejection fraction (Figure 17-2).[8,71] In some patients, marked hypertrophy may result in impaired ventricular filling because of reduced ventricular compliance, so that the preload reserve is not fully utilized.[8,11] It has also been suggested that sometimes an inadequate degree of hypertrophy may develop relative to the level of afterload.[78] In any case, aortic valve replacement allows the ventricle to eject normally, with marked improvement of the ejection fraction in most instances (correction of afterload mismatch) (Fig. 17-2), and irreversible myocardial changes postoperatively have now become relatively uncommon.

Serial echocardiographic studies of left ventricular function may not be as important in patients with aortic stenosis as in patients with chronic volume overload (see below) for reaching a decision concerning operation. The current criteria for surgical treatment, which are based largely on the development of significant symptoms, remain appropriate. Thus, aortic stenosis operation need not be considered *solely* to protect the left ventricle from irreversible myocardial damage. In addition, the data suggest that even in the patient with severe left ventricular dysfunction and an ejection fraction as low as 18 to 20 percent, operation should *not be denied,* since ventricular function frequently will improve postoperatively.[71]

Aortic Regurgitation

In following the asymptomatic patient with chronic mild to moderate aortic regurgitation (Chap. 37) and a heart that appears minimally enlarged by physical examination and chest roentgenogram, serial clinical examinations can be done relatively infrequently. On the other hand, when the patient has clinically severe aortic regurgitation with symptoms of left ventricular dysfunction or angina pectoris, it is generally advisable to proceed directly with cardiac catheterization and consideration of surgical treatment.[79] Such studies will characterize the severity of the regurgitation, the status of left ventricular function, and the presence or absence of associated coronary artery disease. Initial echocardiographic or radionuclide studies in such individuals may help to confirm the need for catheterization studies (see below).

In the patient without symptoms who has severe aortic regurgitation and whose heart size is increased on the chest roentgenogram and by physical examination, a baseline echocardiogram should be obtained for measurement of the left ventricular dimensions. If moderate enlargement of the left ventricle, with normal fractional shortening and calculated ejection fraction is found, and the patient remains asymptomatic, serial echocardiographic studies about every 1½ to 2 years can be recommended to ensure that progressive cardiac enlargement and deterioration of left ventricular function do not occur. If the left ventricular enlargement is marked (end-diastolic diameter of the ventricle 70 mm or more), annual follow-up should be advised. Studies have shown that in the great majority of such patients the development of symptoms and the onset of depression of the fractional shortening occur nearly simultaneously, and that operative results in this setting are good.[80]

When angiographic or echocardiographic analyses have been made before and after aortic valve replacement for severe aortic regurgitation in patients with marked cardiomegaly and very severely depressed function, irreversible left ventricular dysfunction is sometimes seen to persist postoperatively.[81] When there is only moderate cardiomegaly and normal or mild depression of left ventricular function, by 6 months to 1 year after aortic valve replacement the heart size has diminished, hypertrophy has regressed,[74,82,83] and left ventricular function has returned toward normal.[82,83] This sequence most likely reflects correction by operation of afterload mismatch,[71] since the high systolic aortic pressure and volume overload preoperatively in aortic regurgitation make the systolic wall stress elevated (and higher than in mitral regurgitation).[84] However, when there is more marked cardiomegaly and left ventricular function is moderately impaired (ejection fraction 25 to 40 percent), in a few patients left ventricular size and function remain abnormal in the postoperative period, and postoperative mortality appears increased.[81,85–87] It would clearly be desirable to avoid such an occurrence, and there is a growing tendency to consider operation even in patients with relatively mild symptoms if there is evidence of considerable left ventricular dysfunction as reflected by echocardiography.[71,83,86,88]

These general criteria may be summarized as follows: if the left ventricular end-diastolic diameter approaches 75 mm or 3.8 cm/m^2 body surface area,[87] the end-systolic diameter is 55 mm or greater,[86] the fractional shortening falls below 25 percent, the calculated ejection fraction is below 40 percent, the ratio of ventricular radius to wall thickness exceeds 3.8,[87,88] or the peak systolic pressure multiplied by the ratio of ventricular end-diastolic radius to end-diastolic wall thickness exceeds 600,[87] confirmation of these findings by cardiac catheterization[24] and consideration of operation are advisable.[71] Because of shape changes, there is a relatively wide margin of error when left ventricular dimensions measured by echocardiography are compared with those measured by angiography.[89]

During cardiac catheterization of patients with aortic regurgitation, the possibility of detecting myocardial dysfunction by infusion of a vasopressor agent has been explored.[90] A fall in forward stroke volume during this stress in the face of a rise in end-diastolic pressure has been considered to indicate depression of myocardial contractility. However, the role of increased aortic regurgitation in the face of enhanced systemic arterial pressure and the possibility of limited preload reserve with acute afterload mismatch occurring during this stress prohibits direct determination by this approach of whether or not myocardial contractility is chronically depressed. Moreover, the status of left ventricular function after valve replacement in patients with an abnormal response to pressor stress has not yet been reported. The significance of a fall in the radionuclide ejection fraction during exercise in some patients[91] also deserves further study.

Mitral Regurgitation

Relatively infrequent examinations are required for asymptomatic patients with clinical evidence of only moderate chronic mitral regurgitation (Chap. 38) and in whom the left ventricle is only mildly enlarged on physical examination and chest roentgenogram. If the patient has limiting symptoms of left ventricular failure that are refractory to medical treatment, echocardiography should be carried out, followed by cardiac catheterization to confirm the severity of the regurgitation, assess its etiology, evaluate the degree of left ventricular dysfunction, and examine whether or not associated disease of other valves or the coronary arteries is contributory. In such patients, provided left ventricular function is not severely depressed, replacement or surgical repair of the mitral valve is usually undertaken.

In the relatively asymptomatic patient with severe mitral regurgitation, the possibility of developing "silent" irreversible myocardial dysfunction poses an important problem.[71] As discussed earlier, mitral regurgitation places relatively favorable systolic loading conditions on the left ventricle, and eccentric hypertrophy coupled with low wall stress due to the low-impedance leak early and late in systole allows maintenance of a high normal ejection fraction when contractility is normal (Fig. 17-3*A*).[92] Even when myocardial contractility becomes depressed, a relatively normal ejection fraction can be maintained (Fig. 17-3*B*), although mean V_{CF} is sometimes reduced.[92] Thus, if significant cardiomegaly is seen on the chest roentgenogram or found on physical examination in such patients, a baseline echocardiographic study should be obtained to assess left ventricular performance.

In contrast to aortic regurgitation, studies before and after mitral valve replacement indicate that left ventricular function tends to fall to some degree following operation in most patients, even though it may remain within the normal range postoperatively.[25] Moreover, when cardiomegaly remains only moderate, there is a progressive reduction in ventricular size and mass after valve replacement.[25,93] However, when there is a marked increase in left ventricular end-diastolic and particularly end-systolic dimensions preoperatively, with the fractional shortening and ejection fraction at low-normal or mildly depressed levels, ventricular function usually deteriorates further at 6 months to 1 year following mitral valve repair or replacement, and ventricular hypertrophy and dilation fail to regress.[25,93] The marked fall in the ejection fraction following mitral valve replacement in these patients suggests that the ejection fraction was maintained at an artificially high value preoperatively, masking depression of myocardial function (Fig. 17-3*B*).[71] Following correction of the low-impedance leak, the depression of ventricular function becomes manifest, since all of the ventricular ejection is now into the aorta with its high impedance and the ejection fraction falls, reflecting afterload mismatch induced by relief of the regurgitant leak (Fig. 17-3*B*).

In the follow-up of the patient with severe mitral regurgitation who has relatively few symptoms but who has cardiomegaly, serial echocardiographic studies should be performed annually. If on initial or serial studies the left ventricular end-diastolic diameter approaches 8.0 cm and the end-systolic diameter exceeds 5.0 cm (2.6 cm/m^2 body surface area), and, in addition, the fractional shortening falls below 30 percent[25,93] or the calculated ejection fraction falls below 55 percent, cardiac catheterization should be undertaken to confirm the degree of mitral regurgitation and the status of left ventricular function.[81] Angiography may also provide information as to the etiology of the mitral regurgitation (prolapse, rheumatic or coronary disease), and in patients over 50 years of age the coronary arteries should be studied. If the echocardiographic findings are confirmed, operative intervention to prevent further deterioration of myocardial function should then be considered.[81] However, in contrast to aortic valve disease, since severe further deterioration of ventricular function appears to occur postoperatively in patients with significantly depressed left ventricular function, it may not be advisable to recommend operation if the ejection fraction is reduced below 40 to 45 percent, although additional confirmation of initial studies[25,93] would be desirable.

Recognition of Myocardial Failure following Heart Surgery

Signs of left or right ventricular failure in the early or late postoperative period after aortic or mitral valve replacement can be due to irreversible myocardial disease existing preoperatively. Occasionally, the failure is due to intraoperative myocardial infarction, or damage due to inadequate myocardial preservation of the hypertrophied heart, although the advent of hypothermic cardioplegia has made this occurrence less common. Heart failure in this setting can also be due to a paravalvular leak causing severe valvular regurgitation,[94] or to prosthetic valve dysfunction due to clotting or fibrosis[95] producing obstruction or regurgitation.

It is very important to identify a mechanical cause of the heart failure so that reoperation can be considered. However, in the postoperative setting physical findings are often not definitive; for example, a severe paravalvular leak around a prosthetic mitral valve can occur with little or no systolic murmur.[94] Echocardiography may be useful for detecting severe left ventricular dysfunction, and a radionuclide study may also reveal a depressed ejection fraction, but these approaches are not always satisfactory for excluding a mechanical abnormality of the prosthetic valve; in the future Doppler flow studies may be useful for this purpose. To definitively establish the cause of postoperative heart failure, it is usually advisable to proceed promptly with diagnostic cardiac catheterization and ventriculography, together with coronary arteriography.

Recognition and Evaluation of Primary Myocardial Disease

In suspected myocardial disease, the initial goal should be to establish by the simplest possible methods whether or not myocardial dysfunction is present. The physiological pattern of the disease and its cause should then be sought, although complete information may not be necessary to decide upon appropriate treatment.

Is Myocardial Disease Present?

The most useful and inexpensive initial screening test is the M-mode echocardiogram, supplemented if necessary by a two-dimensional study. If these are technically unsatisfactory or inconclusive, a radionuclide angiogram can be performed to detect a depressed ejection fraction of either the left or right ventricle.

If the left ventricular end-diastolic chamber diameter is increased on the echocardiogram without a significant increase in wall thickness, and the fractional shortening or calculated ejection fraction is reduced, it is likely that a cardiomyopathy (or myocarditis) of the dilated type is present (Chaps. 57 and 58); the right ventricular internal diameter may also be increased in this condition. This diagnosis is particularly likely in the absence of a heart murmur, hypertension, prior myocardial infarction, or other cause for secondary ventricular enlargement and dysfunction.

In some endurance-trained athletes, the internal chamber diameter of the right or left ventricle, or both, may be abnormally large and associated with electrocardiographic evidence of ventricular hypertrophy. However, measures of systolic contractile function by echocardiography (fractional shortening, calculated ejection fraction, and V_{CF}) are normal in such individuals.[96–98]

If the echocardiogram shows an abnormally thickened left ventricular wall, but the end-diastolic chamber diameter and systolic function are normal, hypertrophic cardiomyopathy is likely, provided hypertension or aortic stenosis are absent (Chap. 120). The echocardiogram will usually allow further differentiation into the symmetrical or asymmetrical type of hypertrophy, and if systolic anterior motion of the mitral valve is associated with a heart murmur, hypertrophic obstruction to left ventricular outflow should be considered.

If there is a significantly reduced EF slope of an otherwise normal mitral valve, together with significant left atrial enlargement, a restrictive pathophysiology is suggested, and a granular sparkling appearance with other features may suggest amyloidosis.[99] Echocardiography may detect a thickened pericardium or pericardial effusion, valvular abnormalities, or unexpected wall motion disorders. In some patients with cardiomyopathy, radionuclide angiography during exercise can demonstrate an abnormal decrease or a failure to increase of the ejection fraction, even when coronary heart disease is absent.[42,57] Thus, for simply establishing the presence or absence of significant myocardial disease, cardiac catheterization is rarely necessary.

When Should Cardiac Catheterization Be Done?

Whenever the patient with myocardial disease is refractory to therapy, or there is a deteriorating clinical course, as complete a pathophysiological diagnosis as possible should be reached by cardiac catheterization. When diagnostic cardiac catheterization is undertaken, right- and left-sided heart catheterization, left ventriculography, and coronary arteriography should generally be done since even if a specific etiology is not identified, such studies often assist in management. In some patients, endomyocardial biopsy of either the right or the left ventricle may be performed to search for a tissue diagnosis, as discussed earlier.

One major goal of the cardiac catheterization study is to exclude the presence of surgically treatable disease, such as unsuspected congenital heart disease with a left-to-right shunt (atrial septal defect is often missed clinically), unexpectedly severe valvular aortic stenosis or mitral regurgitation, a severe obstructive component of hypertrophic cardiomyopathy, constrictive pericarditis, or a significant contribution from unsuspected coronary atherosclerosis (see next section).

Another major goal is to establish the pathophysiological pattern of the myocardial disease in order to allow more rational selection of therapy. Basically, there are three patterns: congestive, restrictive, and obstructive (or several of these patterns may coexist) (Chap. 108). The congestive type is most common, and the pure restrictive type is quite rare. A restrictive pattern can be mimicked by constrictive pericarditis, and that condition should be carefully excluded (Chap. 108).[18] Selective ventriculography and analysis of pressure tracings from the right and left ventricles and atria will generally establish whether the disorder is primarily due to congestive cardiomyopathy with dilation of the chambers, wall thinning, and reduced systolic function, or to restrictive disease. In restrictive disease, the chamber size and systolic function may be normal, although this is not always the case;[24,100] there may be a thickened left ventricular wall; and there is evidence of reduced ventricular diastolic compliance with impaired filling of the left ventricle.[62] Characteristically, there is an early diastolic dip followed by a rapid rise and then a plateau of pressure during diastasis, a prominent *a* wave with an elevated end-diastolic pressure, and a delayed *y* descent on the pulmonary artery wedge pressure or left atrial tracing indicating impaired atrial emptying into the diseased ventricle.[24,62,100] The right ventricle may also exhibit these phenomena. These features resemble constrictive pericarditis (Chap. 108), although typically in restrictive disease the right- and left-sided diastolic pressures do not equilibrate. In congestive cardiomyopathy, these features generally are absent, although the ventricular end-diastolic pressure is usually elevated, and the early diastolic pressure is also high. Thus, the dominant physiological pattern, congestive or restrictive, can usually be identified.[18] Which pattern is present carries important implications for therapy since vigorous use of diuretics and positive inotropic stimuli are appropriate for the congestive pattern, whereas such therapy in the patient with restrictive pathophysiology can lead to decreased ventricular filling pressures and volumes with further impairment of the filling of the stiffened ventricle, and a reduction of cardiac output.[24] Likewise, afterload reduction therapy by vasodilators is more appropriate in the congestive setting, since in restrictive cardiomyopathy ventricular systolic emptying may already be near maximum, and dilating properties of these agents on the veins may also lead to reduced diastolic filling.

The restrictive type of pathophysiology may blend with that due to outflow tract obstruction in hypertrophic cardiomyopathy, and surgical relief of a severe resting outflow gradient identified at cardiac catheterization may become necessary in occasional patients who are refractory to medical therapy.[101] Also, there is now evidence that pharmacological agents that block the calcium slow channel (such as verapamil) may be effective in relieving symptoms in hypertrophic obstructive cardiomyopathy, and they may alter the diastolic properties of the hypertrophied ventricle as well.[102]

Coronary arteriography should accompany diagnostic studies to exclude the possibility of silent ischemia in the patient with cardiomyopathy. Ischemic cardiomyopathy sometimes cannot be distinguished from other types of cardiomyopathy without such studies.

There are some settings in which limited cardiac catheterization should be considered. In the patient with established myocardial disease associated with heart failure that is refractory to treatment, if vasodilator therapy is being considered, it may be advisable to undertake balloon catheterization of the right side of the heart in order to characterize the hemodynamic setting.[38] Moreover, serial measurements following single oral doses of the proposed therapeutic regimen (e.g., a balanced arteriolar and venodilator such as prazosin or captopril, a venodilator such as isosorbide dinitrate, or combination therapy with isosorbide dinitrate and the arteriolar dilator hydralazine) can allow selection of the most appropriate drugs.[27] Alternatively, the finding of an unexpectedly low cardiac filling pressure with a normal cardiac output, together with lack of response to a therapeutic test of vasodilators, may contraindicate the use of chronic vasodilator therapy.

Recognition and Evaluation of Ischemic Myocardial Dysfunction

Ischemic Cardiomyopathy

In the patient with cardiomyopathy, the clinical symptoms and the electrocardiogram may not suggest prior myocardial infarction or recurrent ischemia, yet coronary heart disease may be the underlying process.[103–105] In some patients, attacks of dyspnea without pain or atypical pain may reflect recurrent myocardial ischemia or subendocardial infarction, and "silent" or painless myocardial ischemia is being recognized with increasing frequency[106] even in the absence of diabetes mellitus, which is known to be associated with silent ischemia and infarction.[107] The finding of coronary artery calcification on image intensification fluoroscopy may be very helpful in suggesting the diagnosis, and among a group of younger patients with cardiomyopathy those shown on coronary arteriography to have an ischemic type invariably showed calcification of either two or three coronary arteries.[103] Thallium perfusion imaging during and after exercise may also indicate the presence of myocardial scar at rest, or show transient exercise-induced perfusion defects, and a fall in the radionuclide ejection fraction with exercise has been reported to be more indicative of ischemia than idiopathic cardiomyopathy. Generally, however, if this diagnosis is suspected, cardiac catheterization with coronary arteriography will be required to fully characterize the degree of coronary atherosclerosis. In the more typical patient with "ischemic cardiomyopathy" a clear history of several previous myocardial infarctions and angina pectoris will be obtained. Such patients should usually undergo cardiac catheterization as well, even if heart failure without angina pectoris is the presenting picture, since myocardial revascularization has resulted in improvement of dyspnea and heart failure, or transient attacks of myocardial ischemia, in a few patients with ischemic cardiomyopathy.[108] Generally, however, the surgical results have not been satisfactory.[109]

In the patient with established coronary heart disease who has angina pectoris and cardiomegaly, noninvasive studies of left ventricular size and function may be important in selecting medical therapy. For example, if there is left ventricular enlargement, the combination of digitalis with propranolol may reduce heart size and diminish the severity of anginal attacks.[110]

Ventricular Aneurysm

Sometimes heart failure or low cardiac output due to a left ventricular aneurysm is suggested by the ECG or the chest roentgenogram. The M-mode echocardiogram may exhibit relatively normal septal and posterior wall systolic shortening in the presence of an apical aneurysm, but the use of two-dimensional echocardiography has proved much more reliable in detecting the presence of an aneurysm.[111] The radionuclide angiogram is also useful for this purpose,[112] and recently nuclear magnetic resonance has allowed imaging of areas of wall thinning and left ventricular aneurysm in patients with coronary heart disease.[113] If a ventricular aneurysm is seriously suspected in a patient who has significant symptoms due to heart failure, cardiac catheterization should be carried out to define the extent of the aneurysm and to assess the degree of coronary artery disease prior to considering corrective operation (Chap. 108).

References

1. Osler, William: "The Principles and Practice of Medicine," D. Appleton & Company, New York, 1892, p. 637.
2. Harvey, R. M., Ferrer, M. I., Samet, P., Bader, R. A., Bader, M. E., Cournand, A., and Richards, D. W.: Mechanical and Myocardial Factors in Rheumatic Heart Disease with Mitral Stenosis, *Circulation,* 11:531, 1955.
3. Ross, J., Jr., Gault, J. H., Mason, D. T., Linhart, J. W., and Braunwald, W.: Left Ventricular Performance during Muscular Exercise in Patients with and without Cardiac Dysfunction, *Circulation,* 34:597, 1966.
4. Bruce, R. A.: Exercise Testing for Evaluation of Ventricular Function, *N. Engl. J. Med.,* 296:671, 1977.
5. Benge, W., Litchfield, R. L., and Marcus, M. L.: Exercise Capacity in Patients with Severe Left Ventricular Dysfunction, *Circulation,* 61:955, 1980.
6. Braunwald, E., Ross, J., Jr., and Sonnenblick, E. H.: "Mechanisms of Contraction of the Normal and Failing Heart," 2d ed., Little, Brown and Company, Boston, 1976.
7. Ross, J., Jr., and Peterson, K. L.: On the Assessment of Cardiac Inotropic State, *Circulation,* 47:435, 1973. (Editorial.)
8. Ross, J.: Cardiac Function and Myocardial Contractility: A Perspective, *J. Am. Coll. Cardiol.,* 1:52, 1983.
9. Ross, J., Jr.: The Assessment of Myocardial Performance in Man by Hemodynamic and Cineangiographic Techniques, *Am. J. Cardiol.,* 23:511, 1969.
10. Braunwald, E., and Ross, J., Jr.: Control of Cardiac Performance, in R. M. Berne, N. Sperelakis, and S. R. Geiger (eds.) "Handbook of Physiology," Waverly Press, Baltimore, 1979, p. 533.
11. Ross, J., Jr.: Afterload Mismatch and Preload Reserve: A Conceptual Framework for the Analysis of Ventricular Function, *Prog. Cardiovasc. Dis.,* 18:255, 1976.
12. MacGregor, D. C., Covell, J. W., Mahler, G., Dilley, R. B., and Ross, J., Jr.: Relations between Afterload, Stroke Volume, and Descending Limb of Starling's Curve, *Am. J. Physiol.,* 227:884, 1974.
13. Ross, J., Jr., Covell, J. W., Sonnenblick, E. H., and Braunwald, E.: Contractile State of the Heart Characterized by Force-Velocity Relations in Variably Afterloaded and Isovolumic Beats, *Circ. Res.,* 18:14.149, 1966.
14. Ross, J., Jr., and Braunwald, E.: The Study of Left Ventricular Function in Man by Increasing Resistance to Ventricular Ejection with Angiotensin, *Circulation,* 29:739, 1964.
15. Ross, J., Jr.: Adaptation of the Left Ventricle to Chronic Volume Overload, *Circ. Res.,* 35(suppl. 2):64, 1974.
16. Sasayama, S., Ross, J., Jr., Franklin, D., Bloor, C. M., Bishop, S., and Dilley, R. B.: Adaptations of the Left Ventricle to Chronic Pressure Overload, *Circ. Res.,* 38:172, 1976.
17. Ross, J., Jr.: Pathophysiology of the Human Heart: Function of the Heart under Abnormal Loading Conditions, in H. P. Krayenbuehl and W. Kubler (eds.), "Kardiologie in Klinik und Praxis," Georg Thieme Verlag, Stuttgart, 1981, Vol. I, Chap. 31, pp. 9–28.
18. Shabetai, R., Mangiardi, L., Bhargava, V., Ross, J., Jr., and Higgins, C. B.: The Pericardium and Cardiac Function, *Prog. Cardiovasc. Dis.,* 22:107, 1979.
19. Shirato, K., Shabetai, R., Bhargava, V., Franklin D., and Ross, J., Jr.: Alteration of the Left Ventricular Diastolic Pressure-Segment Relation Produced by the Pericardium: Effects of Cardiac Distension and Afterload Reduction in Conscious Dogs, *Circulation,* 57:1191, 1978.
20. Glantz, S. A., Misbach, G. A., Moores, W. Y., Mathey, D. G., Lekven, J., Stowe, D. F., Parmley, W. W., and Tyberg, J. V.: The Pericardium Substantially Affects the Left Ventricular Diastolic Pressure-Volume Relationship in the Dog, *Circ. Res.,* 42:443, 1978.
21. Stokland, O., Miller, M. M., Lekven, J., and Hebekk, A.: The Significance of the Intact Pericardium for Cardiac Performance in the Dog, *Circ. Res.,* 47:27, 1980.
22. Alderman, E. L., and Glantz, S. A.: Acute Hemodynamic Interventions Shift the Diastolic Pressure-Volume Curve in Man, *Circulation,* 54:662, 1976.
23. Brodie, B. R., Gross, W., Mann, T., and McLaurin, L. P.: Effects of Sodium Nitroprusside on Left Ventricular Diastolic Pressure-Volume Relations, *J. Clin. Invest.,* 59:59, 1977.
24. Meaney, E., Shabetai, R., Bhargava, V., Shearer, M., Weidner, C., Mangiardi, L., Smalling, R., and Peterson, K.: Cardiac Amyloidosis, Constrictive Pericarditis, and Restrictive Cardiomyopathy, *Am. J. Cardiol.,* 38:547, 1976.
25. Schuler, G., Peterson, K., Johnson, A., Francis, G., Dennish, G., Utley, J., Daily, P., Ashburn, W., and Ross, J., Jr.: Temporal Response of Left Ventricular Performance to Mitral Valve Surgery, *Circulation,* 59:1218, 1979.
26. Franciosa, J. A., and Cohn, J. N.: Hemodynamic Responsiveness to Short- and Long-acting Vasodilators in Left Ventricular Failure, *Am. J. Med.,* 65:126, 1978.
27. Chatterjee, K., and Parmley, W. W.: Vasodilator Therapy for Acute Myocardial Infarction and Chronic Congestive Heart Failure, *J. Am. Coll. Cardiol.,* 1:33, 1983.
28. Ross, J., Jr.: Role of Vasodilator Therapy, in J. Karliner and G. Gregoratos (eds.), "Coronary Care," Churchill Livingstone, New York, 1980, pp. 497–509.
29. Pouleur, H., Covell, J. W., and Ross, J., Jr.: Effects of Alterations in Aortic Input Impedance on the Force-Velocity-Length Relationship in the Intact Canine Heart, *Circ. Res.,* 45:126, 1979.
30. Pouleur, H., Covell, J. W., and Ross, J., Jr.: Effects of Nitroprusside on Venous Return and Central Blood Volume in the Absence and Presence of Acute Heart Failure, *Circulation,* 61:328, 1980.
31. Gillian, R. E., Parnes, W. P., Khan, M. A., Bouchard, R. J., and Warbasse, J. R.: The Prognostic Value of Systolic Time Intervals in Angina Pectoris Patients, *Circulation,* 60:268, 1979.
32. Garrard, C. L., Jr., Weissler, A. M., and Dodge, H. T.: Relationship of Alterations in Systolic Time Intervals to Ejection Fraction in Patients with Cardiac Disease, *Circulation,* 42:455, 1970.
33. Fisher, D. C., Sahn, D. J., Friedman, M. J., Larson, D.,

Valdes-Cruz, L. M., Horowitz, S., Goldberg, S. J., and Allen, H. D.: The Mitral Valve Orifice Method for Noninvasive Two-dimensional Echo Doppler Determinations of Cardiac Output, *Circulation,* 67:872, 1983.
34. Franciosa, J. A.: Evaluation of the CO_2 Rebreathing Cardiac Output Method in Seriously Ill Patients, *Circulation,* 55:449, 1977.
35. Weber, K. T., Kinasewitz, G. T., Janicki, J. S., and Fishman, A. P.: Oxygen Utilization and Ventilation during Exercise in Patients with Chronic Cardiac Failure, *Circulation,* 65:1213, 1982.
36. Franciosa, J. A., Park, M., and Levine, T. B.: Lack of Correlation between Exercise Capacity and Indexes of Resting Left Ventricular Performance in Heart Failure, *Am. J. Cardiol.,* 47:33, 1981.
37. Engler, R. L., Ray, R., Higgens, C. B., McNally, C., Buxton, W., Bhargava, V., and Shabetai, R.: The Clinical Assessment of Follow-up of Functional Capacity in Patients with Chronic Congestive Cardiomyopathy, *Am. J. Cardiol.,* 49:1832, 1982.
38. Swan, H. J. C., and Ganz, W.: Hemodynamic Measurements in Clinical Practice: A Decade in Review, *J. Am. Coll. Cardiol.,* 1:103, 1983.
39. Raphael, L. D., Mantle, J. A., Moraski, R. E., Rogers, W. J., Russell, R. O., and Rackley, C. E.: Quantitative Assessment of Ventricular Performance in Unstable Ischemic Heart Disease by Dextran Function Curves, *Circulation,* 55:858, 1977.
40. Peterson, K. L., Sklovan, D., Ludbrook, P., Uther, J. B., and Ross, J., Jr.: Comparison of Isovolumetric and Ejection Phase Indices of Myocardial Performance in Man, *Circulation,* 49:1088, 1974.
41. Kreulen, T., Bove, A. A., McDonough, M. T., Sands, M. J., and Spann, J. F.: The Evaluation of Left Ventricular Function in Man: A Comparison of Methods, *Circulation,* 51:677, 1975.
42. Schoolmeester, W. L., Simpson, A. G., Sauerbrunn, B. J., and Fletcher, R. D.: Radionuclide Angiographic Assessment of Left Ventricular Function during Exercise in Patients with a Severely Reduced Ejection Fraction, *Am. J. Cardiol.,* 47:804, 1981.
43. Berger, H. J., Johnstone, D. E., Sands, J. M., Gottschalk, A., and Zaret, B. L.: Response of Right Ventricular Ejection Fraction to Upright Bicycle Exercise in Coronary Artery Disease, *Circulation,* 60:1292, 1979.
44. Grossman, W., Jones, D., and McLaurin, L. P.: Wall Stress and Patterns of Hypertrophy in the Human Left Ventricle, *J. Clin. Invest.,* 56:56, 1975.
45. Takahashi, M., Sasayama, S., Kawai, C., and Kotoura, H.: Contractile Performance of the Hypertrophied Ventricle in Patients with Systemic Hypertension, *Circulation,* 62:116, 1980.
46. Borow, K. M., Green, L. H., Grossman, W., and Braunwald, E.: Left Ventricular End-Systolic Stress-Shortening and Stress-Length Relations in Humans, *Am. J. Cardiol.,* 50:1301, 1982.
47. Gault, J. H., Ross, J., Jr., and Braunwald, E.: Contractile State of the Left Ventricle in Man: Instantaneous Tension-Velocity-Length Relations in Patients with and without Disease of the Left Ventricular Myocardium, *Circ. Res.,* 22:451, 1968.
48. Peterson, K. L., Uther, J. B., Shabetai, R., and Braunwald, E.: Assessment of Left Ventricular Performance in Man: Instantaneous Tension-Velocity-Length Relations Obtained with the Aid of an Electromagnetic Velocity Catheter in the Ascending Aorta, *Circulation,* 47:924, 1973.
49. Sasayama, S., Franklin, D., and Ross, J., Jr.: Hyperfunction with Normal Inotropic State of the Hypertrophied Left Ventricle, *Am. J. Physiol.,* 232:H418, 1977.
50. Cooper, R. H., O'Rourke, R. A., Karliner, J. S., Peterson, K. L., and Leopold, G. R.: Comparison of Ultrasound and Cineangiographic Measurements of the Mean Rate of Circumferential Fiber Shortening in Man, *Circulation,* 46:914, 1972.
51. Mason, S. J., and Fortuin, N. J.: The Use of Echocardiography for Quantitative Evaluation of Left Ventricular Function, *Prog. Cardiovasc. Dis.,* 21:119, 1978.
52. Schiller, N. B., Acquatella, H., Ports, T. A., Drew, D., Goerke, J., Ringertz, H., Silverman, N. H., Brundage, B., Botvinick, E. H., Boswell, R., Carlsson, E., and Parmley, W. W.: Left Ventricular Volume from Paired Biplane Two-Dimensional Echocardiography, *Circulation,* 60:547, 1979.
53. Ashburn, W. L., Schelbert, H. R., and Verba, J. W.: Left Ventricular Ejection Fraction—A Review of Several Radionuclide Angiographic Approaches Using the Scintillation Camera, *Prog. Cardiovasc. Dis.,* 20:267, 1978.
54. Slutsky, R., Karliner, J., Ricci, D., Kaiser, R., Pfisterer, M., Gordon, D., Peterson, K., and Ashburn, W.: Left Ventricular Volumes by Gated Equilibrium Radionuclide Angiography: A New Method, *Circulation,* 61:556, 1980.
55. Pitt, B., Kalff, V., Rabinovitch, M. A., Buda, A. J., Colfer, H. T., Vogel, R. A., and Thrall, J. A.: Impact of Radionuclide Techniques on Evaluation of Patients with Ischemic Heart Disease, *J. Am. Coll. Cardiol.,* 1:63, 1983.
56. Starling, M. R., Dell'Italia, L. J., Walsh, R. A., Little, W. C., Benedetto, A. R., and Nusynowitz, M. L.: Accurate Estimates of Absolute Left Ventricular Volumes from Equilibrium Radionuclide Angiographic Count Data Using a Simple Geometric Attenuation Correction, *J. Am. Coll. Cardiol.,* 3:789, 1984.
57. Bodenheimer, M. M., Banka, V. S., and Helfant, R. H.: Nuclear Cardiology. I. Radionuclide Angiographic Assessment of Left Ventricular Contraction: Uses, Limitations and Future Directions, *Am. J. Cardiol.,* 45:661, 1980.
58. Dodge, H. T., and Sheehan, F. H.: Quantitative Contrast Angiography for Assessment of Ventricular Performance in Heart Disease, *J. Am. Coll. Cardiol.,* 1:73, 1983.
59. Dodge, H. T., and Baxley, W. A.: Left Ventricular Volume and Mass and Their Significance in Heart Disease, *Am. J. Cardiol.,* 23:528, 1969.
60. Kennedy, J. W., Baxley, W. A., Figley, M. M., Dodge, H. T., and Blackmon, J. R.: Quantitative Angiocardiography: I. The Normal Left Ventricle in Man, *Circulation,* 34:272, 1966.
61. Mirsky, I., and Parmley, W. W.: Force-Velocity Studies in Isolated and Intact Heart Muscle, in I. Mirsky, D. N. Ghista, and H. Sandler (eds.), "Cardiac Mechanics: Physiological, Clinical, and Mathematical Considerations," John Wiley & Sons, New York, 1974, p. 87.
62. Tyberg, T. I., Goodyear, A. V. N., Hurst, V. W., III, Alexander, J., and Langou, R. A.: Left Ventricular Filling in Differentiating Restrictive Amyloid Cardiomyopathy and Constrictive Pericarditis, *Am. J. Cardiol.,* 47:791, 1981.
63. Peterson, K. L., Tsuji, J., Johnson, A., DiDonna, J., and LeWinter, M. M.: Diastolic Left Ventricular Pressure-Volume and Stress-Strain Relations in Patients with Valvular Aortic Stenosis and Left Ventricular Hypertrophy, *Circulation,* 58:77, 1978.
64. Nejad, N. S., Klein, M. D., Mirsky, E., and Lown, B.: Assessment of Myocardial Contractility from Ventricular Pressure Recordings, *Cardiovasc. Res.,* 5:15, 1971.
65. Mahler, F., Covell, J. W., O'Rourke, R. A., and Ross, J., Jr.: Effects of Acute Changes in Loading and Inotropic State on Left Ventricular Performance and Contractility Measures in the Conscious Dog, *Am. J. Cardiol.,* 35:626, 1975.
66. Ross, J., Jr., and Sobel, B. E.: Regulation of Cardiac Contraction, *Ann. Rev. Physiol.,* 34:47, 1972.
67. Olsen, E. G. J.: Endomyocardial Biopsy, *Br. Heart J.,* 40:95, 1978.
68. Chi-sung, Z., Cheng, C. T., Palmer, D. C., Codd, J. E., Pennington, G., and Williams, G. A.: High Incidence of Myocarditis by Endomyocardial Biopsy in Patients with Idiopathic Congestive Cardiomyopathy, *J. Am. Coll. Cardiol.,* 3:63, 1984.
69. Schwarz, F., Schaper, J., Kittstein, D., Flameng, W., Walter, P., and Schaper, W.: Reduced Volume Fraction of Myofibrils in Myocardium of Patients with Decompensated Pressure Overload, *Circulation,* 63:1299, 1981.
70. Ross, J., Jr., and Braunwald, E.: Aortic Stenosis, *Circulation,* 37 (suppl. 5):61, 1968.

71. Ross, J., Jr.: Left Ventricular Function and the Timing of Surgical Treatment in Valvular Heart Disease, *Ann. Intern. Med.*, 94:498, 1981.
72. Frank, S., Johnson, A., and Ross, J., Jr.: Natural History of Valvular Aortic Stenosis, *Br. Heart J.*, 35:41, 1973.
73. Kennedy, J. W., Doces, J., and Stewart, D. K.: Left Ventricular Function before and following Aortic Valve Replacement, *Circulation*, 56:944, 1977.
74. Pantely, G., Morton, M., and Rahimtoola, S. H.: Effects of Successful, Uncomplicated Valve Replacement on Ventricular Hypertrophy, Volume, and Performance in Aortic Stenosis and in Aortic Incompetence, *J. Thorac. Cardiovasc. Surg.*, 75:383, 1978.
75. Henry, W. L., Bonow, R. O., Borer, J. S., Kent, K. M., Ware, J. H., Redwood, D. R., Itscoitz, S. B., McIntosh, C. L., Morrow, A. G., and Epstein, S. E.: Evaluation of Aortic Valve Replacement in Patients with Valvular Aortic Stenosis, *Circulation*, 61:814, 1980.
76. Smith, N., McAnulty, J. H., and Rahimtoola, S. H.: Severe Aortic Stenosis with Impaired Left Ventricular Function and Clinical Heart Failure, Results of Valve Replacement, *Circulation*, 58:255, 1978.
77. Peterson, K. L.: Instantaneous Force-Velocity-Length Relations of the Left Ventricle: Methods, Limitations, and Applications in Humans, in A. P. Fishman (ed.), "Heart Failure," Hemisphere Publishing, Washington, 1978.
78. Gunther, S., and Grossman, W.: Determinants of Ventricular Function in Pressure-Overload Hypertrophy in Man, *Circulation*, 59:679, 1979.
79. Slutsky, R., Karliner, J., Battler, A., Pfisterer, M., Swanson, S., and Ashburn, W.: Reproducibility of Ejection Fraction and Ventricular Volume by Gated Radionuclide Angiography after Myocardial Infarction, *Radiology*, 132:155, 1979.
80. Bonow, R. O., Rosing, D. R., McIntosh, C. L., Jones, M., Marm, B. J., Gordon Lan, K. K., Lakatos, E., Bacharach, S. L., Green, M. V., and Epstein, S. E.: The Natural History of Asymptomatic Patients with Aortic Regurgitation and Normal Left Ventricular Function, *Circulation*, 68:509, 1983.
81. Gault, J. H., Covell, J. W., Braunwald, E., and Ross, J., Jr.: Left Ventricular Performance following Correction of Free Aortic Regurgitation, *Circulation*, 42:773, 1970.
82. Schwarz, F., Flameng, W., Thormann, J., Sesto, M., Langebartels, F., Hehrlein, F., and Schlepper, M.: Recovery from Myocardial Failure after Aortic Valve Replacement, *J. Thorac. Cardiovasc. Surg.*, 75:854, 1978.
83. Schuler, G., Peterson, K. L., Johnson, A. D., Francis, G., Ashburn, W., Dennish, G., Daily, P. O., and Ross, J., Jr.: Serial Non-invasive Assessment of Left Ventricular Hypertrophy and Function after Surgical Correction of Aortic Regurgitation, *Am. J. Cardiol.*, 44:585, 1979.
84. Wisenbaugh, T., Spann, J. F., and Carabello, B. A.: Differences in Myocardial Performance and Load Between Patients with Similar Amounts of Chronic Aortic Versus Chronic Mitral Regurgitation, *J. Am. Coll. Cardiol.*, 3:916, 1984.
85. Clark, D. G., McAnulty, J. H., and Rahimtoola, S. H.: Valve Replacement in Aortic Insufficiency with Left Ventricular Dysfunction, *Circulation*, 61:411, 1980.
86. Henry, W. L., Bonow, R. O., Borer, J. S., Ware, J. H., Kent, K. M., Redwood, D. R., McIntosh, C. L., Morrow, A. G., and Epstein, S. E.: Observations on the Optimum Time for Operative Intervention for Aortic Regurgitation: I. Evaluation of the Results of Aortic Valve Replacement in Symptomatic Patients, *Circulation*, 61:471, 1980.
87. Gaasch, W. H., Carroll, J. D., Levine, H. J., and Criscitiello, M. G.: Chronic Aortic Regurgitation: Prognostic Value of Left Ventricular End-Systolic Dimension and End-Diastolic Radius/Thickness Ratio, *J. Am. Coll. Cardiol.*, 1(3):775, 1983.
88. Gaasch, W. H., Andrias, C. W., and Levine, H. J.: The Effect of Aortic Valve Replacement on Left Ventricular Volume, Mass and Function, *Circulation*, 58:825, 1978.
89. Abdulla, A. M., Frank, M. J., Canedo, M. I., and Statadourus, M. A.: Limitations of Echocardiography in the Assessment of Left Ventricular Size and Function in Aortic Regurgitation, *Circulation*, 61:148, 1980.
90. Bolen, J. L., Holloway, E. L., Zener, J. C., Harrison, D. C., and Alderman, E. L.: Evaluation of Left Ventricular Function in Patients with Aortic Regurgitation Using Afterload Stress, *Circulation*, 53:132, 1976.
91. Borer, J. S., Bachrach, S. L., Green, M. V., Kent, K. M., Henry, W. L., Rosing, D. R., Seides, S. F., Johnston, G. S., and Epstein, S. E.: Exercise-Induced Left Ventricular Dysfunction in Symptomatic and Asymptomatic Patients with Aortic Regurgitation: Assessment with Radionuclide Cineangiography, *Am. J. Cardiol.*, 42:351, 1978.
92. Eckberg, D. L., Gault, J. H., Bouchard, R. L., Karliner, J. S., and Ross, J., Jr.: Mechanics of Left Ventricular Contraction in Chronic Severe Mitral Regurgitation, *Circulation*, 47:1252, 1973.
93. Zile, M. R., Gaasch, W. H., Carroll, J. D., and Levine, H. J.: Chronic Mitral Regurgitation: Predictive Value of Preoperative Echocardiographic Indexes of Left Ventricular Function and Wall Stress, *J. Am. Coll. Cardiol.*, 3:235, 1984.
94. Rockoff, S. D., Ross, J., Jr., Oldham, N. H., Mason, D. T., Morrow, A. G., and Braunwald, E.: Left Ventricular Performance during Muscular Exercise in Patients with and without Cardiac Dysfunction, *Circulation*, 34:597, 1966.
95. Copans, H., Lakier, J. B., Kinsley, R. H., Colsen, P. R., Fritz, V. U., and Barlow, J. B.: Thrombosed Bjork-Shiley Mitral Prostheses, *Circulation*, 61:169, 1980.
96. Morganroth, J., Maron, B. J., Henry, W. L., and Epstein, S. E.: Comparative Left Ventricular Dimensions in Trained Athletes, *Ann. Intern. Med.*, 82:521, 1975.
97. Roeske, W. R., O'Rourke, R. A., Klein, A., Leopold, G., and Karliner, J. S.: Noninvasive Evaluation of Ventricular Hypertrophy in Professional Athletes, *Circulation*, 53:286, 1976.
98. Gilbert, C. A., Nutter, D. O., Felner, J. M., Perkins, J. B., Heymsfield, S. B., and Schlant, R. C.: Echocardiographic Study of Cardiac Dimensions and Function in the Endurance-Trained Athlete, *Am. J. Cardiol.*, 40:528, 1977.
99. Siquera-Filho, A. G., Cunha, C. L. P., Tajik, A. J., Seward, J. B., Schattenberg, T. T., and Giuliani, E. R.: M-Mode and Two-Dimensional Echocardiographic Features in Cardiac Amyloidosis, *Circulation*, 63:188, 1980.
100. Benotti, J. R., Grossman, W., and Cohn, P. F.: Clinical Profile of Restrictive Cardiomyopathy, *Circulation*, 61:1206, 1980.
101. Maron, B. J., Merrill, W. H., Freier, P. A., Kent, K. M., Epstein, S. E., and Morrow, A. G.: Long-Term Clinical Course and Symptomatic Status of Patients after Operation for Hypertrophic Subaortic Stenosis, *Circulation*, 57:1205, 1978.
102. Rosing, D. R., Kent, K. M., Borer, J. S., Seides, S. F., Maron, B. J., and Epstein, S. E.: Verapamil Therapy: A New Approach to the Pharmacologic Treatment of Hypertrophic Cardiomyopathy: I. Hemodynamic Effects, *Circulation*, 60:1201, 1979.
103. Johnson, A. D., Laiken, S. L., and Shabetai, R.: Noninvasive Diagnosis of Ischemic Cardiomyopathy by Fluoroscopic Detection of Coronary Artery Calcification, *Am. Heart J.*, 96:521, 1978.
104. Burch, G. E., Giles, T. D., and Colclough, H. L.: Ischemic Cardiomyopathy, *Am. Heart J.*, 79:291, 1970.
105. Dash, H., Johnson, R. A., Dinsmore, R. E., and Hawthorne, J. W.: Cardiomyopathic Syndrome Due to Coronary Artery Disease: I. Relation to Angiographic Extent of Coronary Disease and to Remote Myocardial Infarction, *Br. Heart J.*, 39:733, 1977.
106. Chierchia, S., Lazzari, M., Freedman, B., Brunelli, C., and Maseri, A.: Impairment of Myocardial Perfusion and Function during Painless Myocardial Ischemia, *J. Am. Coll. Cardiol.*, 1:924, 1983.
107. Lloyd-Mostyn, R. H., and Watkins, P. J.: Defective Innervation of Heart in Diabetic Autonomic Neuropathy, *Br. Med. J.*, 3:15, 1975.

108. Mundth, E. D., Hawthorne, J. W., and Buckley, M. J.: Direct Coronary Arterial Revascularization: Treatment of Cardiac Failure Associated with Coronary Artery Disease, *Arch. Surg.*, 103:529, 1971.
109. Yatteau, R. F., Peter, R. H., Behar, V. S., Bartel, A. G., Rosati, R. A., and Kong, Y.: Ischemic Cardiomyopathy: The Myopathy of Coronary Artery Disease, Natural History and Results of Medical Versus Surgical Treatment, *Am. J. Cardiol.*, 34:520, 1974.
110. Crawford, M. H., LeWinter, M. M., O'Rourke, R. A., Karliner, J. S., and Ross, J., Jr.: Combined Propranolol and Digoxin Therapy in Angina Pectoris, *Ann. Intern. Med.*, 83:449, 1975.
111. Kotler, M. N., Mintz, G. S., Segal, B. L., and Parry, W. R.: Clinical Uses of Two-dimensional Echocardiography, *Am. J. Cardiol.*, 45:1061, 1980.
112. Froehlich, R. T., Falsetti, H. L., Doty, D. B., and Marcus, M. L.: Prospective Study of Surgery for Left Ventricular Aneurysm, *Am. J. Cardiol.*, 45:923, 1980.
113. Higgins, C. B., Lanzer, P., Stark, D., Botvinick, E., Schiller, N. B., Crooks, L., Kaufman, L., and Lipton, M. J.: Imaging by Nuclear Magnetic Resonance in Patients with Chronic Ischemic Heart Disease, *Circulation*, 69:523, 1984.
114. Guyton, A. C., Jones, C. E., and Coleman, T. G.: "Circulatory Physiology: Cardiac Output and Its Regulation," 2d ed., W. B. Saunders Company, Philadelphia, 1973.
115. Sagawa, K.: The Ventricular Pressure-Volume Diagram Revisited, *Circ. Res.*, 43:677, 1978.

18

Assessment of Electrical Abnormalities

Douglas P. Zipes, M.D. R. Joe Noble, M.D.

The hierarchy of steps taken to evaluate and treat a patient suspected of having an arrhythmia generally proceeds from simple, noninvasive, and inexpensive outpatient tests to more complex, expensive, and invasive studies performed in the hospital. The nature of the rhythm disturbance and its effects on the patient determine the order of the tests chosen. Some rhythm disturbances such as sustained ventricular tachycardia or ventricular fibrillation are hazardous in and of themselves while others, such as a sustained supraventricular tachycardia (SVT), must be evaluated according to the context in which they occur. Supraventricular tachycardia at a rate of 180 beats per minute in a young patient who complains only of palpitations or mild anxiety is approached quite differently than supraventricular tachycardia that precipitates angina in a patient with coronary artery disease, or syncope in a patient with aortic stenosis, or ischemic symptoms in a patient with peripheral vascular disease. Thus, the physician evaluates a *patient* who has a rhythm disturbance rather than an isolated rhythm disturbance. Before obtaining a test, it is important to question whether the information provided by the test is sufficiently important to justify its risk and expense. Whenever possible, tests with maximal sensitivity, specificity, and predictive accuracy are chosen.

The initial evaluation always begins with a history and physical examination followed by routine tests such as the 12-lead electrocardiogram and chest x-ray, and often an echocardiogram and stress test. For patients who have electrical abnormalities, we consider long-term (24-h) electrocardiographic recording (or a modification of this approach; see Chap. 100) a routine test. All of these tests are not obtained in all patients, but selected ones are useful in many patients suspected of having electrical abnormalities.

Other techniques including cardiac catheterization, esophageal electrocardiography, vectorcardiography, mapping from the body surface or from the heart itself, and a variety of methods to condition the cardiac electrical signal are useful in selected circumstances. In certain patients neurological assessment including electroencephalography is important.

Information Provided by the History

A great deal of overlap between the features of various rhythm disturbances exists at this stage of the initial evaluation of the patient; nevertheless, the history provides some direction and diagnostic clues as the first step in the assessment. While some patients may be referred for assessment of electrical abnormalities noted incidentally during evaluation of another problem, the symptomatic patient generally complains of palpitations described as a thumping, irregularity in the chest, or a pause in heart action, at times producing anxiety or fatigue. Many patients are acutely aware of any cardiac irregularity while others are oblivious even to short runs of rapid ventricular tachycardia. Premature atrial or ventricular complexes are probably the most common cause of palpitations and are often perceived by the patient as skipped or dropped beats.

Tachycardia may produce syncope or presyncope, angina, or shortness of breath.

Useful information regarding possible precipitating factors includes the use of potentially cardioactive drugs found in some decongestants, bronchial dilators, or other over-the-counter drugs, or the ingestion of alcohol[1] or excessive caffeine-containing foods. Symptoms may be precipitated by a certain activity, or may occur at a certain time of day or month (e.g., associated with menses). Knowledge of the typical onset and termination of the arrhythmia is helpful: abrupt and paroxysmal onset is consistent with such tachycardias as an atrioventricular (AV) nodal reentrant tachycardia, while a gradual speeding and slowing is more in keeping with a sinus tachycardia. Termination by Valsalva maneuver or carotid massage suggests a supraventricular rather than a ventricular tachycardia.

The rate of the arrhythmia often narrows diagnostic possibilities. Ventricular rates at 150 beats per minute should always raise the potential diagnosis of atrial flutter with 2:1 AV block, while most supraventricular tachycardias, such as those caused by AV nodal reentry or associated with an overt or concealed accessory pathway, occur at rates in excess of 150 beats per minute. Ventricular tachycardia commonly occurs at rates similar to supraventricular tachycardias but also faster and slower.

Information Provided by the Physical Examination

Physical examination offers the opportunity to gain two important pieces of information: the nature of the arrhythmia, if it is present, assessed by determining heart rate and rhythm, jugular venous pulse, heart sounds, and blood pressure, and the nature of associated structural heart disease, if any. Although it is well known that patients without structural heart disease may have supraventricular tachyarrhythmias, it is less commonly appreciated that they may have ventricular tachyarrhythmias that are on occasion even life-threatening,[2,3] Thus, a normal physical examination, even in a young person, does not preclude the diagnosis of ventricular tachycardia; some of these patients may have structural heart disease that goes unrecognized.[4]

Physical findings can provide certain clues to an arrhythmia if the patient has structural heart disease. The presence of a left ventricular aneurysm in a patient with a history of myocardial infarction who complains of palpitations raises the question of ventricular tachyarrhythmia and also provides some information about prognosis.[5] The patient with hypertrophic[6] or dilated cardiomyopathy commonly has ventricular arrhythmias, while the patient with mitral stenosis or thyrotoxicosis might have an atrial tachyarrhythmia.

Information Provided by Laboratory Tests

Usually the chest x-ray and echocardiogram provide adjunctive information about the diagnosis derived after a careful history and physical examination, and help establish the presence or absence of structural heart disease, its extent, and its type. Echocardiography[7] and phase imaging[8] may be useful to identify the origin of ventricular ectopy.

The presence of wall motion abnormalities determined by echocardiography or left ventriculography has been shown, using a stepwise discriminant analysis, to be useful prognostically. Septal akinesia or dyskinesia is a major predictor of ventricular tachycardia.[9] Left ventricular ejection fraction can be useful in predicting the development of ventricular tachycardia following myocardial infarction. Those patients with a radionuclide left ventricular ejection fraction less than 40 percent have been found to have a greater risk of developing ventricular tachycardia within a few weeks after a myocardial infarction.[10] A stress test gives information on the functional cardiovascular capabilities of the patient but also may be useful in precipitating certain cardiac arrhythmias (see below). Ventricular arrhythmias recorded during stress testing may add independent prognostic information to the noninvasive evaluation.[11] Serial exercise testing may be an appropriate means of assessing efficacy of therapy in patients with exercise-induced ventricular tachycardia if reproducibility is established in two control tests before therapy is begun.[12]

Long-term ECG recording provides the most direct laboratory test to evaluate electrical abnormalities, and it, or a similar procedure, is often the first definitive noninvasive approach taken to understand the nature of the electrical disturbance (see below). Prolonged recording of the ECG in patients engaged in normal daily activity (Holter monitoring, ambulatory monitoring) has dramatically expanded the physician's capability to detect disturbances in cardiac rhythm, particularly transient ones, to quantitate the frequency and complexity of the rhythm disturbance, to correlate these alterations with symptoms, and to evaluate the effect of antiarrhythmic therapy on the arrhythmia.[13–16] In addition, such recordings can document alterations in QRS, ST, and T contour. Long-term ECG recording is the most sensitive noninvasive test to demonstrate transient arrhythmias and is usually the first test to be obtained.

For the test to be specific, the patient must have both the arrhythmia and symptoms at the same time. If symptoms occur without an arrhythmia, the latter can be excluded as a cause. Also, recording important arrhythmias without symptoms precludes a definitive causal relation between symptoms and arrhythmia, and reduces the specificity of the test. The likelihood of recording the causal arrhythmia varies greatly from patient to patient, at different times in the same patient, and in different disease states. Thus, the sensitivity of the test is quite variable. Events that occur frequently can be detected during short recording periods, but the minimum time recommended is 24 h. The various techniques by which the electrocardiogram can be reported over a prolonged period are discussed in Chap. 100.

Electrocardiographic recordings can be accomplished out of the hospital, either using tape recorders or transmitting the electrocardiographic signal transtelephonically[17–19] to a receiver in the physician's office or clinic. In patients with more serious rhythm disturbances, the recording is done in the hospital, using bedside monitors, telemetry, or an ambulatory portable recorder. The therapeutic and prognostic implications of many of the rhythm disturbances noted by continuous, long-term ECG recording are unknown, and therefore the physician must integrate data obtained from long-term ECG recording with the patient's clinical problem. Telephone transmission of the ECG may be useful in some patients with symptoms suggestive of a cardiac arrhythmia. However, in one study of 41 patients, half were unable to transmit their episodes of palpitations because they were too brief or did not recur. In the other half nine of those who did transmit had abnormal ECGs.[19]

In the future, signal conditioning techniques such as signal averaging,[20] fast Fourier transform analysis of signal averaged ECGs,[21] and line beat-by-beat recording of microvolt potentials[22] may be used noninvasively to detect patients at risk of developing sustained ventricular tachycardia.

Invasive electrophysiological studies provide important information when a particular abnormality can be demonstrated, but absence of proof is not the same as proof of absence. Failure to demonstrate an abnormality does not exclude the possibility that it may be present on another occasion and still be responsible for the patient's symptoms. Thus, the sensitivity of an electrophysiological study may be low depending on the nature of the rhythm disturbance. Its specificity depends on the abnormality induced as well as the stimulation protocol used to induce it. Ideally, the methodology of the electrophysiological study would permit induction of only clinically and prognostically important cardiac arrhythmias in all patients who are at risk of spontaneous life-threatening arrhythmia and in no patient without such risk. This is difficult to achieve. For example, to induce ventricular tachyarrhythmias, at least two ventricular extrastimuli are required in a majority of patients known to have ventricular tachycardia. In some instances, two ventricular extrastimuli fail to induce arrhythmias in patients who are susceptible, yet using three or more ventricular extrastimuli increases the likelihood of producing nonspecific or nonclinical arrhythmias. Two extrastimuli appear to represent a reasonable compromise.[23,24]

Stimulating more than one right ventricular site and using multiple cycle lengths increases the sensitivity without apparently decreasing the specificity significantly.[25] Left ventricular stimulation, altering the characteristics of the stimuli, or infusing drugs such as isoproterenol each may increase the percent of ventricular arrhythmias induced at the expense of sacrificing specificity. Ideally, we seek to induce the patient's clinical arrhythmia along with replication of the symptoms, but this is not always achieved.

Electrophysiological studies also can be used to assess response to antiarrhythmic drugs. The most reliable criterion from such studies is conversion of inducible sustained ventricular tachyarrhythmia to one that is either nonsustained or not inducible at all.[26] Other endpoints are less reliable.

Approach to the Patient with Palpitations

History

Evaluation of the patient with palpitations begins with an assessment of the severity of the arrhythmia by the symptoms it produces. Does the patient complain simply of isolated "thumps" or pauses suggesting single premature beats or do the palpitations occur in flurries or long runs, perhaps associated with syncope or presyncope? The next important fact to establish is whether the patient has a history of structural heart disease and, if so, the diagnosis and extent of disease. This finding significantly affects the importance of the palpitations (see below). Patients who have frequent ventricular ectopic beats (greater than 100 per day) and no evidence of underlying cardiac disease may have a high prevalence of complex ventricular ectopy. The ectopy tends to persist over short-term intervals, but most patients remain asymptomatic and have little risk of progression to serious, sustained tachyarrhythmias. Additional studies are necessary to determine long-term natural history for these patients.[27] Ventricular ectopy can be found in healthy individuals, even teenage boys,[28] and does not necessarily forbode a serious clinical prognosis. Finding the same degree of ectopy in patients with coronary artery disease may distinguish groups at increased risk for syncope or sudden cardiac death, however. For example, ventricular arrhythmias and left ventricular dysfunction are independently related to risk of mortality after myocardial infarction.[29]

Physical Examination

Physical examination confirms the presence or absence of structural heart disease, but generally does not provide much information regarding the nature of the palpitations.

Laboratory Tests

Chest x-ray and echocardiography help establish the presence or absence of structural heart disease.

In patients with palpitations the cardiac rhythm is recorded to document the suspected disturbance, which is essential to rational management. After obtaining the 12-lead ECG, long-term ECG recording would be the next noninvasive test chosen. In one study long-term ECG recording had a sensitivity of 69 percent and a specificity of 90 percent in 85 patients complaining of palpitations.[30] The first step in evaluation is to determine if the rhythm disturbance is an isolated premature beat or pause, if it is of supraventricular or ventricular origin, and if it is accompanied by tachycardia or bradycardia. Of equal importance is the determination that symptoms that potentially owe their origin to cardiac arrhythmias are correlated temporally with the recorded rhythm disturbance. Palpitations may be quite bothersome to some patients, and the responsible rhythm disturbance can range from sinus arrhythmia to a complex ventricular tachyarrhythmia. In each instance, the documentation of a rhythm disturbance and resultant symptoms establishes the need for therapy as well as the clinical therapeutic approach. It is important to stress that patients without heart disease may have complex arrhythmias, the significance of which is often unclear (Fig. 18-1).[31–34]

Once therapy is deemed essential and an agent is administered, the efficacy of the agent should be established. Prolonged ECG recording is the best method available to accurately and quantitatively document the efficacy and lack of toxicity of a drug.[15] The cardiac rhythm also can be correlated with serum concentrations and time of administration of an antiarrhythmic agent. For example, if ventricular ectopy increases markedly just prior to the next due dose of an antiarrhythmic agent, and the serum concentration falls to a subtherapeutic level at the same time, perhaps the drug should be given more frequently.

When pacemaker surveillance clinics fail to document pacemaker dysfunction or other arrhythmias that are suspected to be intermittent, long-term ECG recording is the preferable diagnostic technique, both to evaluate pacemaker function and to detect pacemaker-induced arrhythmias. Care must be taken to place leads to optimally visualize the pacemaker artifact.

Often patients with ischemic heart disease complain of palpitations, and these patients may need a 24-h ECG recording. Whereas it is clear that recording frequent and complex ventricular ectopy in patients with ischemic heart disease implies a worse prognosis, it is unclear precisely which frequency or degree of complexity requires therapy; the optimal duration of recording required to detect these abnormalities and the optimal times for recording (immediately prior to discharge from the hospital after a myocardial infarction, for example, or at some interval post hospitalization) are unknown. Finally the efficacy of antiarrhythmic therapy in altering the ultimate prognosis has not yet been established.

Although it may seem likely that the ventricular ectopy of these patients is etiologically related to the pathogenesis of ventricular fibrillation, it has not been demonstrated that suppressing the ventricular ectopy reduces the likelihood of sudden death. Consequently, though prolonged ECG recording provides a means of detecting arrhythmias in patients with coronary heart disease, this detection has not yet been equated with specific therapeutic recommendations. Hence, routine recording, though informative, cannot be advised for all such patients. The combination of serious impairment in left ventricular function and complex ventricular ectopy clearly implies a worse prognosis, which probably justifies aggressive therapy. Thus, it would seem reasonable to record an ambulatory ECG in postinfarction patients with significant left ventricular dysfunction.[35–37]

Most patients with ischemic heart disease, particularly those recovering from recent infarction, exhibit premature ventricular complexes (PVCs) when monitored for extended periods. The simple demonstration of PVCs is of little therapeutic or prognostic significance. However, the following characteristics of ventricular ectopy have been associated with a worse prognosis in patients with ischemic heart disease: (1) frequent PVCs; (2) multiform PVCs; (3) early coupling intervals (R-on-T phenomenon); (4) pairs of PVCs; (5) bigeminy; and (6) ventricular tachycardia. There is no universal agreement as to the significance of each of these characteristics. Even if it is conceded that more complex forms of ventricular ectopy imply an increased risk of sudden cardiac death, it is not known whether ectopy is causally related to death or is only a marker identifying the patient at increased risk.

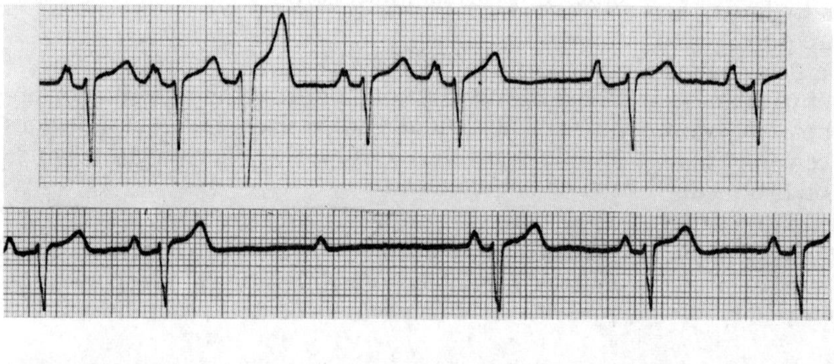

FIGURE 18-1 Twenty-four-hour recording in a young adult without heart disease complaining of palpitations. A premature ventricular complex (third complex), nonconducted premature atrial complex (in T wave of fourth sinus-conducted complex), and first degree AV block are present during sleep. In the lower tracing, lengthening of the P-P interval and a nonconducted sinus P wave are probably due to a transient increase in vagal tone, not type II AV block. Monitor lead.

Palpitations in patients with hypertrophic[6,38,39] and dilated[40] cardiomyopathy may be important. Since sudden death in patients with hypertrophic cardiomyopathy does not correlate with the degree of outflow obstruction, arrhythmias such as ventricular tachycardia seem the likely cause. Long-term ECG recording frequently has demonstrated potentially serious tachyarrhythmias or frequent and complex ventricular ectopy in these patients.

Patients with mitral valve prolapse often complain of palpitations,[41,42] and when studied with 24-h ECG recording, most of them with symptoms demonstrate arrhythmias. Nearly every known rhythm may occur in such patients; sinus bradycardia, sinus arrest, wandering atrial pacemaker, premature atrial complexes (PACs), brief runs of supraventricular tachycardia, and frequent PVCs occur in about one-third to one-half of them, including some with complex ventricular ectopy. The patient's clinical characteristics and symptoms bear little relation to the frequency or severity of the rhythm disturbance recorded. Furthermore, the prognostic significance of these rhythm disturbances is totally unknown. Ventricular tachycardia or fibrillation does not necessarily occur in patients who have complex ventricular rhythm disturbances; and sudden cardiac death has occurred in patients with no documented arrhythmia on prolonged monitoring.[43]

A stress test would be indicated next, particularly if the patient complained of palpitations with exertion. In response to exercise testing, about one-third of normal subjects develop ventricular ectopy, usually in the form of occasional, uniform PVCs. The PVCs are more likely to occur at higher heart rates and are not reproducible from one test to the next. Multiform PVCs, pairs of PVCs, and ventricular tachycardia infrequently develop in response to exercise in normal patients; however, since they may be recorded in normal patients, their presence does not establish the existence of ischemia or heart disease. Exercise-induced supraventricular premature complexes are of no known prognostic significance.[44,45]

Many patients with documented coronary artery disease develop PVCs in response to exercise, and the frequency and complexity of ventricular ectopy correlates generally with the presence of more severe coronary artery involvement. Ventricular ectopy appears at lower heart rates (less than 130 beats per minute) than in a normal population, and often occurs in the early recovery period as well (Fig. 18-2). The ectopy is more reproducible from one test to the next in patients with coronary disease. More frequent PVCs (greater than 10 per minute), multiform PVCs, and ventricular tachycardia are more likely to occur in patients with coronary disease than in normal patients. PVCs at rest may be suppressed by exercise in patients with documented coronary disease, so that this observation does not necessarily imply a benign prognosis nor absence of underlying structural heart disease. The incidence of sudden cardiac death is increased in patients with coronary disease who develop ventricular ectopy at heart rates less than 130 beats per minute with exercise, and in whom the ectopy is associated with ST-segment changes, presumably as a manifestation of the relation between ventricular ectopy and ischemia. Those patients with more extensive coronary disease and more significant impairment in left ventricular function have the greatest prevalence of frequent and complex forms of ventricular ectopy. Ventricular arrhythmias induced by exercise in the postinfarction patient correlate with the severity of coronary disease and left ventricular impairment.[46,47] Whereas exercise-induced ventricular arrhythmias are of interest in population studies, they are of little or no help in determining the presence or severity of organic heart disease in an individual patient.

Previously undetected arrhythmias also may be elicited by exercise in patients with heart disease such as hypertrophic cardiomyopathies, but in studies reported thus far, long-term ECG recording detects all of the serious arrhythmias recorded during exercise.[38,39] Exercise may induce arrhythmias in as much as 75 percent of patients with mitral valve prolapse, and complex types of previously unsuspected arrhythmias may be found. For instance, atrial fibrillation or ventricular tachycardia not previously

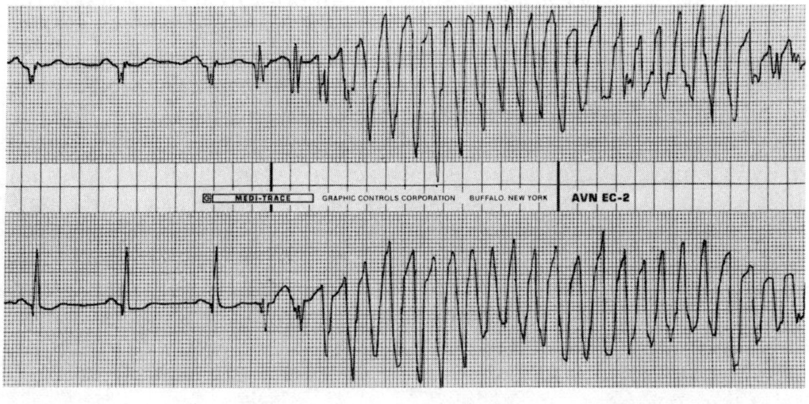

FIGURE 18-2 Onset of sustained ventricular tachycardia during the cooldown period after a treadmill stress test in a patient with coronary artery disease. Lead II, *top*; modified V_5, *bottom*.

recorded on resting ECG may be elicited by exercise.[48] Most of these arrhythmias would be detected by long-term ECG recording.

Stress testing is indicated in most patients recovering from myocardial infarction.[47–50] Ventricular arrhythmias correlate with the presence and extent of coronary disease and the degree of left ventricular dysfunction and may constitute a separate risk factor.[50] The exact frequency and complexity of ventricular ectopy that might benefit from antiarrhythmic therapy is unknown; however, sustained ventricular tachycardia in response to stress would clearly indicate further diagnostic and therapeutic considerations.

Whenever any complex ventricular arrhythmia is detected by any other means, stress testing may be indicated to detect more complex grades of ectopy;[51] to determine the relation of the arrhythmia to activity; and to aid in choosing antiarrhythmic therapy. For instance, ventricular tachycardia detected only at a certain, critical heart rate and a given degree of activity may suggest that therapy include beta-blocking drugs or activity limitations. If serious arrhythmias are detected by prolonged recording or resting ECG, stress testing may be helpful in directing therapy and establishing the limits of patient activity. In selected patients in whom an arrhythmia is suspected on the basis of symptoms but has not been detected by long-term ECG recording, stress testing is also indicated.

For the same reasons, whenever ventricular ectopy is judged sufficient to warrant therapy, stress testing may be indicated. However, the test must be interpreted with caution. Intuitively, one would expect a decrease in ventricular ectopy between a pre- and posttherapy test to indicate efficacy of antiarrhythmic agents. However, as mentioned earlier, in normal patients results from consecutive tests are not reproducible.[51] In patients with coronary disease, the test results are more reproducible, but not dependably so.[44] When two tests are performed 45-min apart, less ectopy is consistently recorded on the second test.[52] Hence, a decrease in the frequency of PVCs on the posttherapy test cannot necessarily be taken as evidence of drug efficacy. Conversely, sustained ventricular tachycardia on a second test at least indicates that the current antiarrhythmic therapy is inadequate.

Prolonged electrocardiographic recording may be compared with exercise testing to detect arrhythmias.[53] Some investigators have recorded more frequent and potentially more serious ventricular arrhythmias during an exercise test than during a 24-h recording period with normal activity,[54] while others have reported the opposite—that is, prolonged recording appears more sensitive than exercise testing in detecting ventricular arrhythmias.[55] Clearly, the choice of the best method for detecting arrhythmias must be individualized. If symptoms of a rhythm disturbance develop during exertion, or are related to ischemia, then exercise testing probably would be preferable; conversely, if the arrhythmia develops at rest, unprovoked by exertion, then long-term ECG recording would be the logical first choice.

The etiology of the heart disease is another determinant of the comparative sensitivity of the two techniques. For instance, long-term ECG recording is more sensitive than exercise testing in detecting rhythm disturbances and particularly in detecting complex ventricular arrhythmias in patients with hypertrophic cardiomyopathy[39] or mitral valve prolapse.[42] However, one technique may detect important rhythm disturbances the other technique may not detect, regardless of the specific sensitivity, in all varieties of heart disease and in all types of rhythm disturbances. Furthermore, each technique provides different sorts of information, such as the frequency of the rhythm disturbance (continuous recording), the relationship of the rhythm disturbance to activity, and the hemodynamic manifestations of the rhythm disturbance (stress testing). The techniques are complementary, and occasionally both are necessary to identify fully a rhythm disturbance.

Arrhythmias detected by either stress testing or long-term recording are not specific for any disease process, nor do most arrhythmias necessarily imply disease at all. Consequently, even though stress testing and ambulatory recording are extremely helpful in defining arrhythmias and on occasion in guiding antiarrhythmic therapy, neither technique is highly sensitive or specific for a particular cardiac abnormality.

Electrophysiological studies employing programmed stimulation of the heart, though extremely informative and useful in selected patients, are invasive procedures that provide data during a circumscribed and somewhat artificial time period. Detection of a spontaneously occurring rhythm disturbance by long-term ECG recording which elicits simultaneous symptoms is of considerable help to the clinician in selecting therapy and has a certain "real life" value attached to it. As with exercise testing, electrophysiological studies and prolonged ECG recording also supplement each other and the choice for a specific patient must be individualized. Examples of patients in whom invasive electrophysiological study would be superior to long-term recording include those whose rhythm disturbance occurs so infrequently that prolonged recording would be impractical and patients in whom knowledge of the electrophysiological mechanism responsible for the arrhythmia would be helpful therapeutically. In still other patients with serious ventricular arrhythmias it may be essential to establish the efficacy of antiarrhythmic management expeditiously; in such patients, electrophysiological studies may provide this information quickly; waiting for an arrhythmic event to occur spontaneously may involve unknown periods of time. With these exceptions, long-term recording may prove more sensitive and cost-effective in the detection of rhythm disturbances.

Approach to the Patient with Syncope (see Chap. 30)

Syncope caused by a cardiac arrhythmia results from a decrease in cerebral blood flow due to heart rates that are too fast or too slow to maintain normal cardiac output. Presyncope may also occur, and it is often related by the patient as a feeling of graying out, an awareness of one's surroundings but an inability to interact, lightheadedness, faintness, or weakness, in contrast to complete loss of consciousness. Some patients may report palpitations prior to the syncopal or presyncopal spell. Generally, vertigo is not a feature of cardiogenic syncope. While determining the cause of syncope often is exceedingly simple—an ECG recording during the syncopal spell is usually sufficient—the difficulty of achieving an ECG recording at the precise time that syncope occurred creates significant diagnostic and therapeutic problems.

History

A careful history can elicit the potential causes of syncope, as discussed in Chaps. 29 and 30. Cardiac syncope refers to fainting related primarily to a sudden and marked decrease in cardiac output. Cardiac arrhythmia may be an independent cause of syncope or can contribute in the setting of organic heart disease or cerebrovascular disease. The hemodynamic response to a cardiac arrhythmia may differ depending on whether the patient is standing or lying when the arrhythmia occurs. Syncope from a cardiac rhythm disturbance generally begins without an aura, is sudden and brief (if the patient recovers), may be associated with bodily injury if the patient falls, generally is without epileptiform movements or involuntary bladder or bowel movements unless the loss of consciousness is protracted, and is usually not followed by postictal depression. Common arrhythmic causes include bradyarrhythmias due to sinus nodal dysfunction or AV block or tachycardias, most often ventricular but also supraventricular on occasion. Bradycardia may follow tachycardia, and treatment of both may be necessary (Fig. 18-3). Neurological causes for syncope must be considered, particularly in older age groups, and a thorough neurological evaluation is mandatory.

Physical Examination

Physical examination in general confirms the findings obtained in the history and helps establish the presence of organic heart disease. Physical examination also may reveal the presence of bradycardia or tachycardia. Simple tests such as carotid sinus pressure or rise from a recumbent position are included.

Laboratory Tests

In the absence of structural heart disease, chest x-ray and echocardiogram are not likely to be revealing. Blood chemistry for hypoglycemia or other metabolic causes of syncope may be useful. In general, a stress test is nonrevealing. Most commonly, prolonged 24-h ECG recording is indicated first, but its yield is often low. Potentially remediable rhythm disturbances may be recorded;[56] however, a symptom-related arrhythmia is recorded infrequently.[57] High-grade AV block, ventricular tachycardia, or tachycardia-bradycardia syndrome infrequently manifest themselves during the recording period. In one study of elderly patients with episodic cerebral symptoms and unexpected falls, the authors concluded that ambulatory electrocardiography was of no more value than standard electrocardiography to detect arrhythmias causing cerebral symptoms.[58] A retrospective analysis of 121 patients admitted for syncope revealed that electrocardiographic monitoring for more than 24 h was helpful in only 7 of 67 patients. In this study the average hospital stay was approximately 9 days with a cost of \$2500 (range \$240 to \$12,000).[59] In a prospective study by the same authors, prolonged electrocardiographic monitoring was diagnostic in 29 of 190 patients (15 percent). After 1 year, almost one-quarter of those patients in whom a cardiac cause of syncope was diagnosed had experienced sudden death compared with only 4 percent if a noncardiac cause of syncope was found. Thus, cardiac causes of syncope appear important to identify.[60]

The yield of electrophysiological testing to determine the cause of syncope is influenced by whether patients have structural heart disease.[61–64] In almost

FIGURE 18-3 AV block follows spontaneous termination of ventricular tachycardia. Several seconds elapse before return of 1:1 conduction. Symptoms could be generated by the ventricular tachycardia or the AV block. Monitor lead.

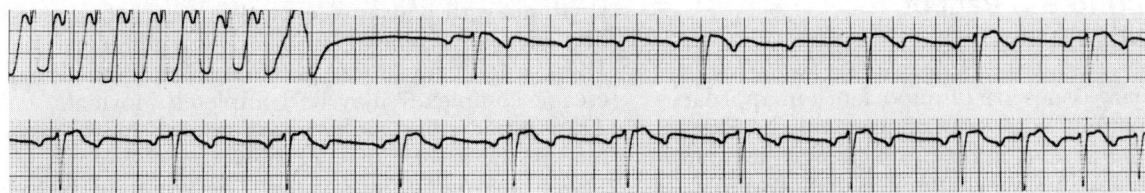

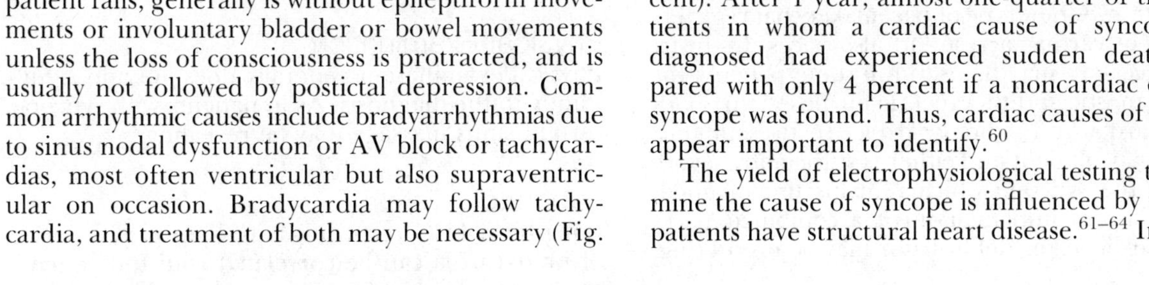

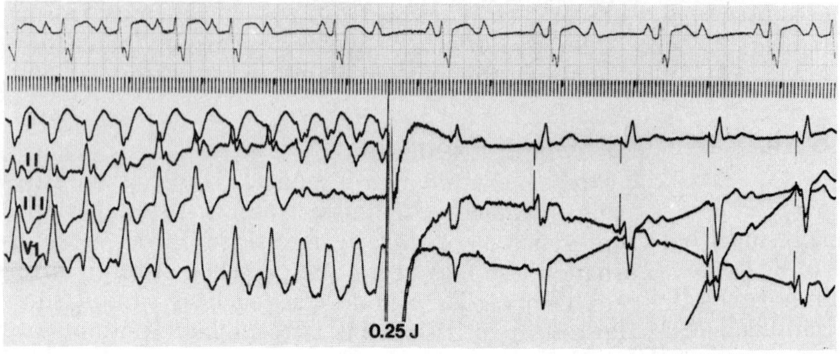

FIGURE 18-4 Ventricular tachycardia and AV block. The patient has intermittent 2:1 AV block (monitor lead, *top*). In addition he has spontaneous and electrically inducible ventricular tachycardia (*bottom* recording, leads I, II, III, and V_1) treated with an implantable pacemaker-cardioverter. At the dark vertical line, a shock of 0.25 J terminates the ventricular tachycardia, which is then followed by AV block. The implanted unit now functions as a pacemaker to maintain an adequate ventricular rate.

three-quarters of patients who have syncope and structural heart disease, an electrophysiological study yields diagnostically useful data. This percentage decreases to 20 percent in those without heart disease. Thus, electrophysiological testing is recommended for patients who have near syncope or syncope that remains unexplained after a thorough evaluation including a complete neurological evaluation and a 24-h electrocardiographic recording. Since both bradycardia and tachycardia can be responsible for syncope, one cannot assume the cause based on anything less than a recording of the ECG during the syncopal event or replication during an electrophysiological study of a cardiac rhythm disturbance that produces the same or similar symptoms in the patient.

In some patients, even after a thorough evaluation including an electrophysiological study, a cause of the syncope still cannot be found. Repeated 24-h electrocardiographic recordings may be indicated in these patients. If the patient still experiences recurrent syncope and there is some indication of bradyarrhythmia (such as the presence of an intraventricular conduction disturbance, prolongation of the His-Purkinje conduction time, or abnormal sinus nodal function), at times pacemaker implantation may be necessary without further definitive information. A new type of pacemaker that registers episodes of cardiac arrest and also paces the heart when necessary may be useful in some patients for both diagnostic and therapeutic purposes.[65] If both a tachycardia and a bradycardia are present in a symptomatic patient and either is sufficiently severe to cause the syncope which remains unexplained, evaluation and implantation of a combined pacemaker-cardioverter-defibrillator may be useful (Fig. 18-4).[66]

Approach to the Patient with Bradycardia

Two primary issues are of importance in approaching the patient with a bradyarrhythmia. First is whether the patient is symptomatic and has symptoms while the bradyarrhythmia is demonstrated. If that is determined, for example, by a 24-h ECG recording, further diagnostic studies may not be indicated. Second, patients may be minimally symptomatic but have arrhythmias that permit definitive decisions. For example, in patients who have type II second degree AV block, the demonstration of His-Purkinje block, even in the minimally symptomatic or possibly asymptomatic individual, may be sufficient evidence to conclude that pacemaker therapy is indicated, based on the natural history of this disorder. We will consider sinus node dysfunction and AV conduction disturbances separately.

Approach to Patients Who Have Sinus Node Dysfunction

History

The history in patients with sinus node dysfunction may be one of palpitations, presyncope or syncope, or symptoms consistent with low cardiac output due to persistent bradycardia, such as fatigue or even the symptoms of congestive heart failure. Some patients may have associated tachycardia (bradycardia-tachycardia syndrome), which also may produce symptoms. The important feature is to establish causality between symptoms and bradycardia.

Physical Examination

Physical examination generally does not add significantly to the diagnosis. As in patients with syncope, carotid sinus massage may be revealing.[67]

Laboratory Tests

Long-term ECG recordings are helpful if a period of bradycardia can be correlated with the patient's symptoms (Fig. 18-5). However, it is important to remember that asymptomatic sinus bradycardia with heart rates of 35 to 40 beats per minute, sinus arrhythmia with pauses of even 2-s, Wenckebach second degree AV block, particularly during sleep (Fig. 18-1), wandering atrial pacemaker and junctional escape complexes may be completely normal.[32–34] Transient cardiac arrhythmias appear more common in the elderly than in the young.[58]

Modulating autonomic tone, for example, by carotid sinus massage,[67] to expose the patient with the

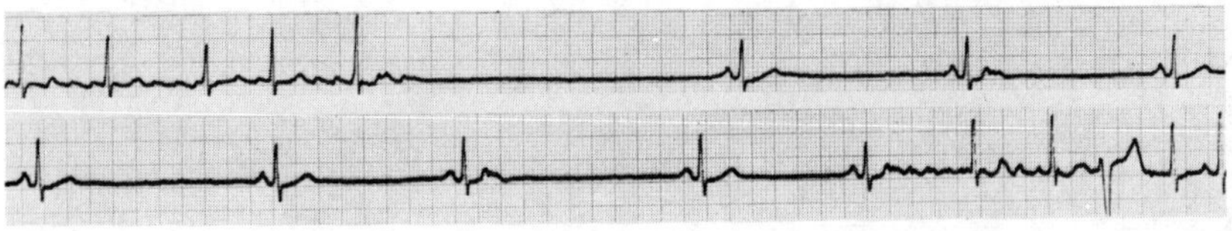

FIGURE 18-5 Long-term ECG recording in a patient with sick sinus syndrome associated with bradycardia-tachycardia. Following termination of atrial fibrillation, a 3.2-s pause occurs. The patient had written in her diary, "lightheaded feeling," thus suggesting a causal relation between the ECG recording and symptoms.

hypersensitive carotid sinus reflex, stress testing,[68] or the administration of atropine,[69,70] isoproterenol,[71] propranolol,[72] or combined atropine and propranolol[71] to produce pharmacological denervation may uncover abnormal sinus nodal responses and identify the patient with sinus node dysfunction. Still, however, correlating bradycardia with the patient's symptoms is of utmost importance. Such autonomic studies may be particularly useful in the patient who has symptoms suggestive of being caused by sinus bradycardia, and who has intermittent sinus bradycardia demonstrated by ECG recordings. If the bradycardia does not attain the slow rates that produce symptoms, and if a clear causal relation between sinus nodal dysfunction and symptoms has not been established, manipulation of autonomic tone may be revealing. Invasive electrophysiological studies to evaluate sinus nodal function include assessment of sinus nodal automaticity and sinoatrial conduction time.[73–77] Such studies are indicated when a causal relationship between the presence of sinus bradycardia, sinus pauses, or sinus nodal exit block and the patient's symptoms has not been established despite repeated 24-h ECG recordings and stress tests.[78,79] Additional candidates considered for electrophysiological studies are patients with known sinus nodal dysfunction who need a pacemaker to assess anterograde and retrograde AV conduction in order to determine the appropriate site and method of pacing.

Patients who are possible candidates for electrophysiological studies include those who have had a complex surgical procedure involving the atria, such as a Mustard procedure, or those in whom it is desirable to establish mechanisms responsible for sinus nodal dysfunction, for example, excessive or inappropriate vagal tone, so that adequate therapy can be achieved with drugs such as aminophylline rather than with pacing. Patients who are not considered candidates are those who have asymptomatic bradycardia or in whom symptoms have clearly been related causally to sinus nodal dysfunction. Electrophysiological testing combined with long-term ECG recording may be more useful than either test alone in revealing sinus nodal dysfunction in patients with sinus bradycardia.[80]

At the time of electrophysiological study, overdrive suppression appears to be one of the most useful and sensitive tests to evaluate sinus nodal dysfunction. Prolonged sinus nodal recovery time has been found in 35 to 93 percent of patients suspected of having sinus nodal dysfunction.[79] Many patients who have ECG evidence only of sinus bradycardia have normal corrected sinus node recovery times, and this probably accounts for the wide range of responses in this group. Generally, measurement of the sinoatrial conduction time is not a sensitive indicator of sinus nodal dysfunction and is prolonged in less than half of the patients with clinical findings of sinus node disease. A new technique to record sinus nodal activity with extracellular electrodes may permit more accurate characterization of sinus nodal automaticity and sinoatrial conduction with more reliable identification of patients who have sinus nodal dysfunction.[81] In patients with sinus nodal dysfunction, directly measured sinoatrial conduction time appears longer than that measured in people with normal sinus function and may not correlate with the sinoatrial conduction time measured indirectly.[82]

It is necessary to evaluate AV nodal and His-Purkinje function in patients with sinus nodal dysfunction since they may also exhibit impaired AV nodal conduction.[83]

Approach to the Patient with AV Block

History

The history is similar to that found in patients with symptomatic sinus bradycardia.

Physical Examination

Physical examination may be helpful if second or third degree AV block is present. Prior to the "dropped" (blocked) beat, due to progressive PR prolongation of type I (Wenckebach) second degree AV block, the patient may have progressive increase in the AC venous pulse interval, progressive quickening of the ventricular rate, and progressive decrease in the intensity of S_1. Usually, however, these findings are too subtle to recognize. In type II second degree AV block, the PR interval remains fixed prior to the block and so does the AC interval and intensity of S_1. Intermittent "gallop" sounds due to atrial systole "marching through" the cardiac cycle, variable peak systolic blood pressure, and intermittent cannon *a* waves in the jugular venous pulse may be present during complete AV block because of the accompanying complete AV dissociation.

Laboratory Tests

The ECG is the most important laboratory test since the site of block usually dictates the clinical course

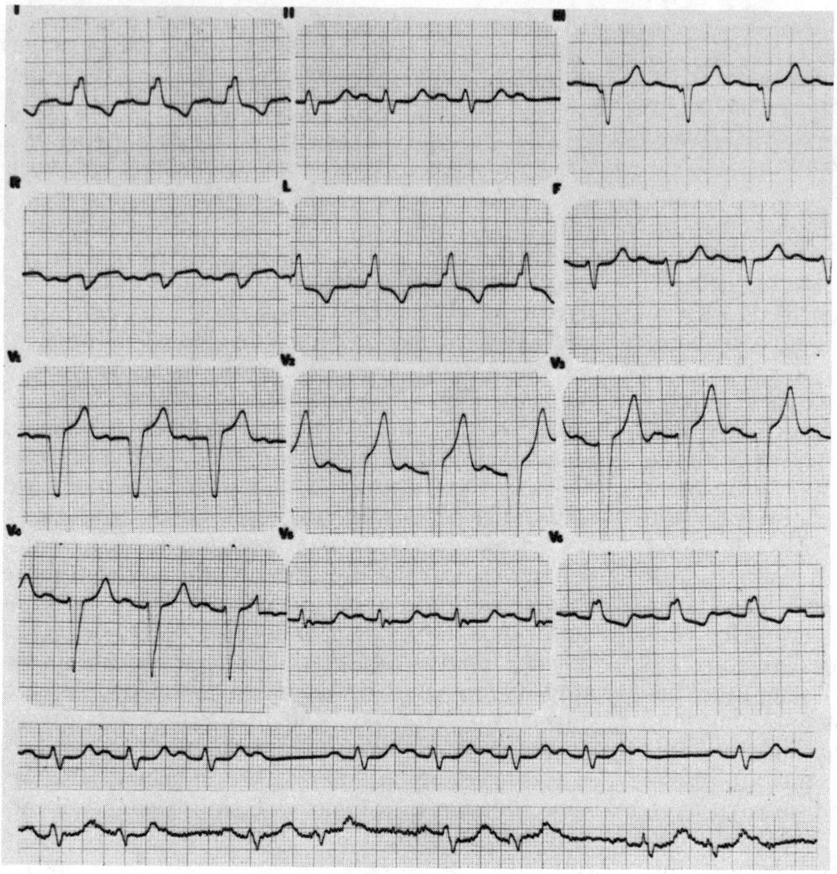

FIGURE 18-6 Type II second degree AV block. The 12-lead ECG demonstrates a left bundle branch block. The rhythm strip below illustrates the onset of type II second degree AV block. Note fixed PR interval prior to the block. In the second rhythm strip (note movement artifacts), the patient sat up, increasing the sinus rate as well as the ratio of blocked P waves.

of the patient and whether or not a pacemaker is needed.[84,85] Generally, the site of AV block can be determined from an analysis of the scalar ECG (Fig. 18-6).[84-88] However, if the block is intermittent, a considerable number of 24-h ECG recordings may be necessary to record it.

When the site of block cannot be determined from such an analysis and when it is imperative to know the site of block in order to make a clinical decision, an invasive electrophysiological study is indicated.[87,88] Patients with block in the His-Purkinje system more commonly become symptomatic and require pacemaker implantation because of periods of bradycardia or asystole than do patients who have AV nodal block. Thus, candidates for electrophysiological study include those in whom His-Purkinje block is suspected and cannot be diagnosed by the scalar ECG, such as patients with (1) type I Wenckebach second degree AV block with bundle branch block; (2) fixed 2:1 AV block, particularly when associated with bundle branch block; (3) possible intra-His AV block in patients who have AV block that appears to be located in the AV node; and (4) apparent type II AV block with a normal QRS complex.

Patients who *might* be considered for electrophysiological evaluation include those with (1) concealed junctional extrasystoles suspected as the cause of AV block; (2) asymptomatic complete AV block to test the automaticity of the escape focus; (3) first degree AV block with symptoms (presyncope, syncope); (4) postoperative development of AV block; (5) the need to determine mechanisms of block that may influence therapy such as heightened vagal tone treated by aminophylline or other drugs rather than pacemaker implantation.

Patients *not* considered for study include (1) those in whom symptoms in the presence of AV block have been correlated by scalar ECG; (2) the asymptomatic patient with AV nodal (Wenckebach) block; (3) the asymptomatic patient with periodic AV block of short duration often associated with sinus node slowing (Fig. 18-1), such as AV nodal block during sleep or atrial fibrillation and intermittent slow ventricular rate; and finally (4) the symptomatic (presyncope, syncope) patient with type II second degree or third degree AV block. Sometimes patients in this category can be considered for an electrophysiological study if, for example, ventricular tachycardia is also suspected.

Autonomic manipulation may be used to help establish the site of block. Atropine or isoproterenol shorten AV nodal conduction time while vagal maneuvers prolong the AV nodal conduction time (AH interval). Little change occurs in His-Purkinje time (HV interval). Exercise or atropine may shorten the PR interval or increase the ratio of conducted P waves during type I (Wenckebach) AV nodal block, while exercise may increase the number of blocked P waves in type II second degree AV block (Fig. 18-6).

Patients who have complete AV block and a normal QRS complex at a rate exceeding 40 to 60 beats per minute and are asymptomatic do not require study. Neither do symptomatic patients who have complete AV block and a prolonged QRS complex at a rate generally less than 40 beats per minute. The former patients usually have AV nodal block and do not require therapy, while pacemaker implantation is indicated for the latter patients since they usually have His-Purkinje block. Prophylactic permanent pacemaker implantation may be indicated for the asymptomatic patient who has acquired complete AV block, and therefore that patient may not require an electrophysiological study.

Approach to the Patient with an Intraventricular Conduction Defect

History

Most patients with an intraventricular conduction defect (IVCD) are asymptomatic and remain so. Those who complain of palpitations, syncope, or presyncope may be experiencing intermittent AV block or episodes of a tachyarrhythmia, usually ventricular (see below). Commonly these patients have structural heart disease and may relate a history appropriate for diseases such as calcific aortic stenosis or ischemic heart disease.

Physical Examination

Unless the patient has structural heart disease, the physical examination generally is noncontributory.

Laboratory Tests

The asymptomatic patient who has an IVCD does not require evaluation. The patient with palpitations, syncope, or presyncope requires investigation to determine the cause of the symptoms; many patients with IVCD and syncope have a ventricular tachyarrhythmia responsible for the syncope. In the symptomatic patient, a long-term ECG recording is ordered first. If symptoms occur infrequently, a negative study is most likely; in these patients various event recorders or telephonic transmitters may be useful. A stress test is not particularly useful, but it may reveal the presence of ischemic heart disease or precipitate the causal arrhythmia in some patients.

For patients with an intraventricular conduction defect, an electrophysiological study provides information on the duration of the HV interval, a measure of His-Purkinje conduction time, which can be prolonged with a normal PR interval or normal with a prolonged PR interval. A prolonged HV interval is associated with a greater likelihood of developing AV block, of having organic heart disease, and of experiencing death.[89] Finding very long HV intervals, exceeding 100 ms, may identify patients at significant risk of developing AV block.

There is some controversy regarding the importance of a prolonged HV interval.[89,90] The development of heart block in asymptomatic patients with chronic bifascicular block occurs at a rate of approximately 2 percent per year. This small incidence of progression to bifascicular block and the relatively high prevalence rate of prolonged HV interval in patients with bifascicular block may preclude the usefulness of the HV interval in predicting the occurrence of heart block. The difference between the usefulness of recording an HV interval in asymptomatic and symptomatic patients may relate to the Bayesian theorem, which states that the predictive value of a given test relates to the given prevalence of the disease being tested for in a given population.

In a recent publication[91] patients with bundle branch block and an HV interval > 70 ms progressed more often to spontaneous second and third degree AV block than did those whose HV interval was less than 70 ms. AV block occurred in 25 percent of those with HV intervals > 100 ms. The incidence of all deaths and cardiac deaths was higher for those who had HV intervals > 70 ms. However, there was no difference in the incidence of relief from symptoms or incidence of cardiac or sudden death between those who received pacemakers and those who did not. Thus, a markedly prolonged HV interval may predict the subsequent development of spontaneous AV block, but prophylactic pacing has been shown to be of no value to relieve symptoms or prolong life.

In patients with IVCD, electrophysiological study should be considered (1) to explain symptoms of syncope or presyncope in patients in whom no other cause can be found, and (2) to differentiate aberrancy due to IVCD from ventricular tachycardia. Occasionally, patients considered for study might be those who postoperatively develop an IVCD. Atrial pacing can be used to uncover abnormal His-Purkinje conduction. In addition to stressing the His-Purkinje system by pacing the atria at fast rates and short premature intervals, drug infusions such as with procainamide or ajmaline sometimes expose abnormal His-Purkinje conduction. It should be remembered that patients with an IVCD may have symptoms due to sinus node dysfunction or a tachyarrhythmia and not just AV block. Patients who are totally asymptomatic and have IVCD should not be studied electrophysiologically.

Approach to the Patient with Tachycardia

History

Patients with tachycardia may complain of sustained palpitations and be able to indicate both the rate and rhythm (see "Information Provided by the History" at beginning of this chapter). Alternatively, they may relate a history of syncope or presyncope, congestive heart failure, or angina.

Physical Examination

Physical examination may provide some clues if the patient has structural heart disease. For example, findings consistent with ventricular disorders such as hypertrophic[38] or dilated[40] cardiomyopathy or coronary artery disease[36] suggest that the tachycardia may be ventricular in origin. A supraventricular tachycardia may be suspected in an otherwise healthy, young individual with a normal physical examination who complains of sustained palpitations. This diagnosis is supported even more if a patient relates a history of tachycardia beginning at a very young age. However, it is important to remember that even very young patients with no apparent structural heart disease may have recurrent ventricular tachycardia.[4,92] If the tachycardia is present during the examination, its rate, rhythm, and response to carotid sinus massage (Fig. 18-7) are determined, and signs indicating the presence of AV dissociation are noted.

Laboratory Tests

Following the initial evaluation, the first approach should be to document the presence of tachycardia electrocardiographically. Ideally, a 12-lead ECG should be obtained during the tachycardia. For infrequently occurring episodes, a 24-h ECG recording or similar test is chosen. If the QRS complex is normal and identical to that present during sinus rhythm, the tachycardia must be supraventricular, and the differential diagnosis now relates to its mechanism. The 12-lead ECG provides many diagnostic clues in this regard (Fig. 18-8). In the absence of evidence suggesting the presence of anterograde conduction over an accessory pathway, such as the lack of a delta wave during sinus rhythm and atrial fibrillation, and in the absence of significant symptoms such as angina, syncope, or congestive heart failure, the initial diagnostic and therapeutic approaches for supraventricular tachycardias can be performed on an outpatient basis. For patients with sustained ventricular tachycardia and most forms of nonsustained ventricular tachycardia and for patients resuscitated from ventricular fibrillation, hospitalization is necessary with monitored evaluation.

If the tachycardia is present at the time of evaluation, its nature can be assessed, and appropriate

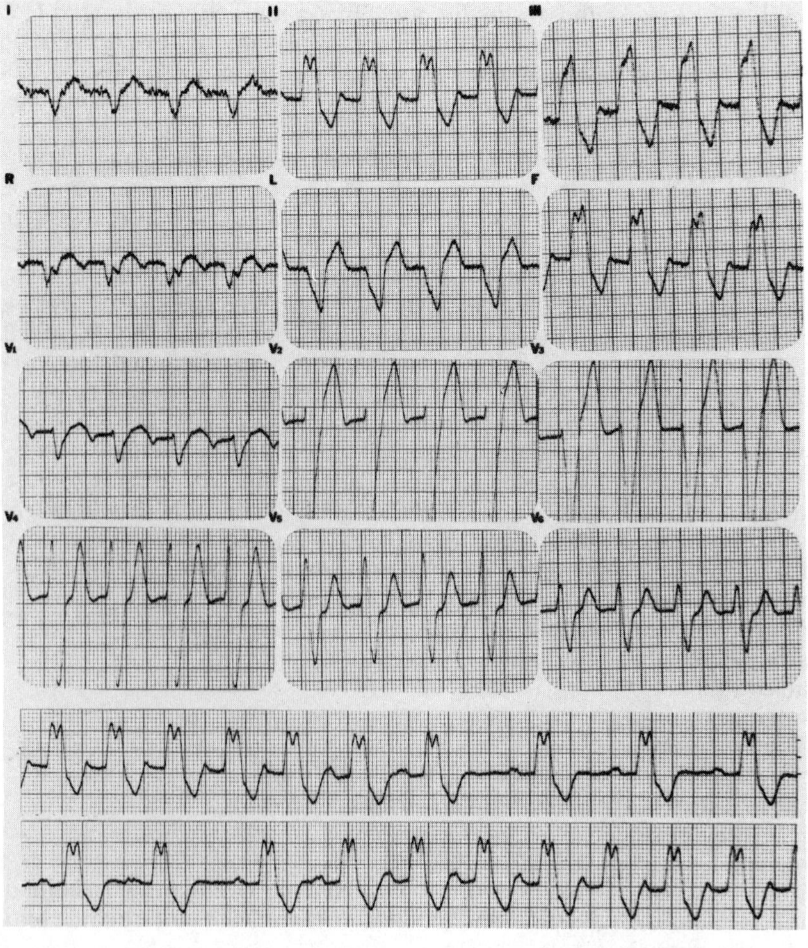

FIGURE 18-7 Sinus tachycardia with an IVCD. The 12-lead ECG illustrates an IVCD of a left bundle branch block type with right axis deviation. In the continuous recording of lead II (*bottom*), carotid sinus massage produces slowing of the sinus rate and documents that the rhythm is a sinus tachycardia.

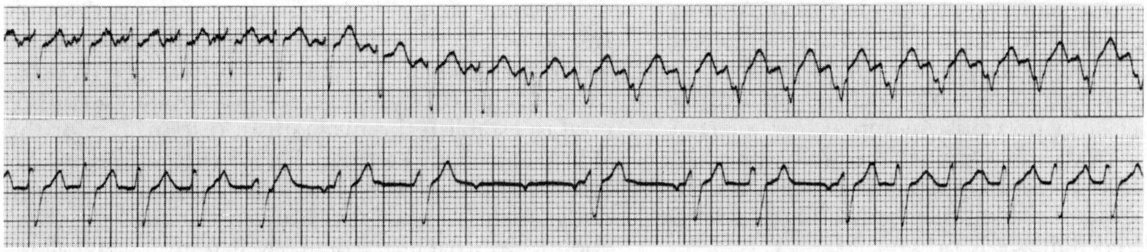

FIGURE 18-8 Supraventricular tachycardia (160 beats per minute). In the middle of the top strip, the QRS changes configuration without a rate change due to development of a delta wave and conduction over a right-sided accessory pathway (documented by electrophysiological study). A reentrant circuit utilizing the accessory pathway first retrogradely and then anterogradely is possible. In the lower strip, transient AV block results, uncovering the atrial tachycardia without its termination. Such a finding excludes participation of an AV circuit in the maintenance of the tachycardia.

therapy can be begun. Esophageal recording (Fig. 18-9) and stimulation may be very useful in diagnosing and sometimes treating the tachycardia and should be performed when atrial activity cannot be discerned from the scalar ECG.[93] If an accessory pathway is present or if the diagnosis of the tachycardia is in doubt, it is often preferable to admit the patient to the hospital for evaluation.

Echocardiography and chest x-ray are useful to establish the presence and extent of structural heart disease. Often, in patients with ventricular tachyarrhythmias being considered as surgical candidates for therapy, phase imaging or echocardiography can be used to help establish the origin of the tachycardia. Cardiac catheterization and coronary arteriography may be necessary, particularly in patients with ischemic heart disease.

In patients who have exercise-induced ventricular tachycardia or fibrillation (Fig. 18-2), coronary artery bypass surgery is an effective therapeutic ap-

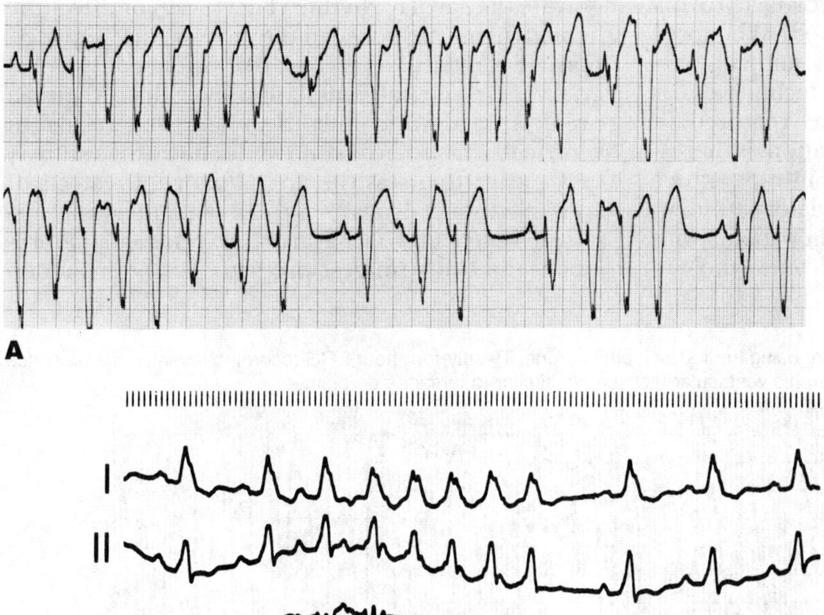

A

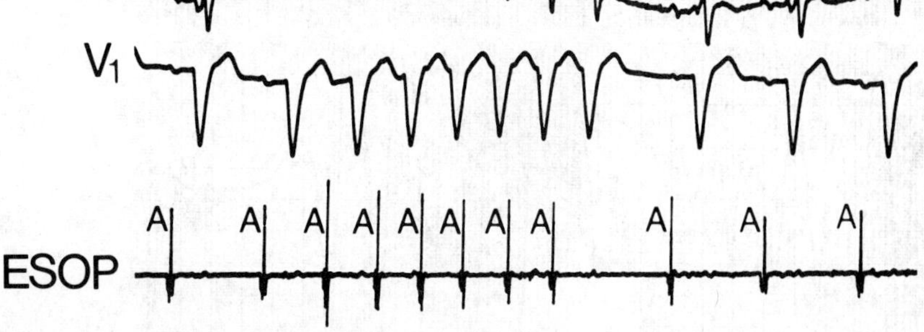

B

FIGURE 18-9 *A.* A wide QRS tachycardia somewhat resembles the sinus-initiated QRS complexes, but with more aberrancy. Distinct atrial activity during tachycardia is not seen in this monitor lead. *B.* Esophageal recording illustrates short runs of atrial flutter responsible for the tachycardia. Left bundle branch block is present.

proach. In these patients, electrophysiological studies may not induce the arrhythmia. In patients with left ventricular wall motion abnormalities following myocardial infarction or with localized myocardial damage such as a previous operative scar, electrophysiological studies may induce the arrhythmia (see below) while exercise may not; operative mapping and endocardial resection may be useful techniques when localized damage is present.[94]

Following these routine evaluations, an electrophysiological study is often indicated. We would consider as candidates for an electrophysiological study those who have recurrent drug-resistant supraventricular or ventricular tachycardia or have a tachycardia that produces life-threatening or potentially life-threatening symptoms. Additional candidates are those in whom it is necessary to differentiate a supraventricular tachycardia with aberrant ventricular conduction of any type from a ventricular tachycardia. Often atrial pacing at rates faster than the rate of the tachycardia can be accomplished with esophageal pacing or right atrial pacing to demonstrate a ventricular origin of the wide QRS tachycardia by producing fusion and capture beats and normalization of the HV interval if the latter is recorded. Patients who have had a serious arrhythmia only while receiving drug therapy (Fig. 18-10) can be tested electrophysiologically for tachycardia when the drug has been discontinued. Whenever nonpharmacological therapy such as antitachycardia pacing devices, catheter ablation techniques, or preoperative surgical evaluation are required, a thorough electrophysiological evaluation is necessary. For example, preoperative and intraoperative electrophysiological mapping is mandatory to identify the site of the accessory pathway in patients with Wolff-Parkinson-White (WPW) syndrome who are undergoing surgical interruption of the pathway.[95] In addition to these indications, in patients who have a supraventricular tachycardia (including WPW syndrome), electrophysiological study should be considered to establish the mechanism responsible for the supraventricular tachycardia,[96] for example, to differentiate a concealed accessory pathway from AV nodal reentry, since this often crystallizes the therapeutic approach, particularly if nonpharmacological forms of therapy are indicated. Electrophysiological mechanisms responsible for most ventricular tachycardias are less clearly defined and less helpful in determining therapy.

Electrophysiological studies permit evaluation of drug efficacy by testing the effect of drugs on initiation and maintenance of tachycardia. Serial drug testing is a major reason for performing electrophysiological studies in patients[97–99] and is very useful when the tachycardia is sporadic and paroxysmal since induction in the laboratory and serial electrophysiological testing appears to be cost-effective.[100] Electrophysiological studies permit an objective assessment of drug efficacy or response to other therapy such as electrical devices[101] or surgery[102] in patients with inducible tachycardias. They also allow the safety of such therapy to be measured, which is particularly important when drugs potentially aggravate the cardiac rhythm (Fig. 18-10) or affect the hemodynamic response to the tachycardia. Suppression of ventricular tachycardia induced by programmed electrical stimulation by a drug regimen predicts freedom from both spontaneous recurrent ventricular tachycardia and sudden death, and may be a means to assess the arrhythmogenic effects of antiarrhythmic drugs.[26,97–99] In patients with sustained ventricular tachycardia or ventricular fibrillation, the two strongest predictors of both sudden

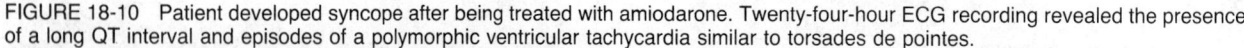

FIGURE 18-10 Patient developed syncope after being treated with amiodarone. Twenty-four-hour ECG recording revealed the presence of a long QT interval and episodes of a polymorphic ventricular tachycardia similar to torsades de pointes.

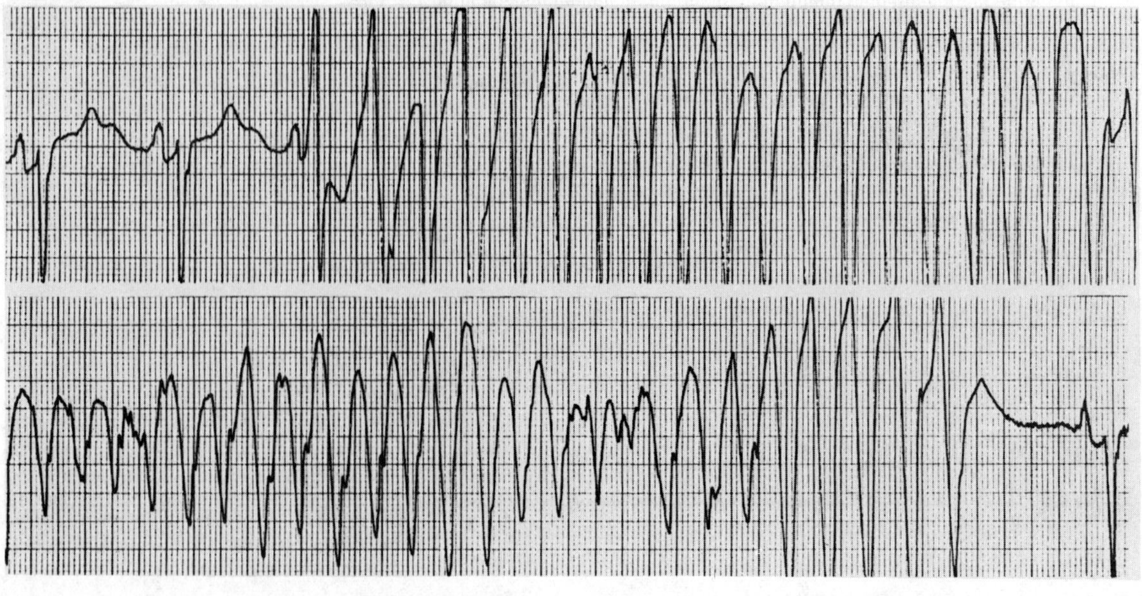

death and cardiac death were a higher New York Heart Association functional classification and the failure of any therapy to be identified as potentially effective on the basis of electrophysiological study.[97] Discriminant analysis of multiple clinical factors may allow development of a predictor function that can be used to estimate the probability of benefit from drug therapy.

Potential candidates for electrophysiological studies are those who are asymptomatic with well-tolerated or infrequent episodes of nonsustained ventricular tachycardia. Patients who have asymptomatic nonsustained ventricular tachycardia or only complex premature ventricular beats in the absence of structural heart disease are probably not candidates for electrophysiological studies at the present time.

It has been suggested that electrophysiological testing may be used to identify patients at risk for the subsequent development of ventricular tachycardia or sudden death following myocardial infarction.[103,104] However, this approach at present must be considered experimental and cannot be recommended as a clinical tool or as a routine part of the evaluation of patients after myocardial infarction. If a sufficient number of premature ventricular stimuli are used, many nonclinical cardiac arrhythmias may be produced.[23,24] Nonsustained polymorphic ventricular tachycardia and ventricular fibrillation are nonspecific responses to aggressive stimulation protocols and can be produced by using three or four extrastimuli in patients without a history of ventricular tachycardia. These facts reduce the prognostic specificity of electrophysiological testing.

Approach to the Patient with Cardiac Arrest

History

Patients who have survived an episode of out-of-hospital cardiac arrest not associated with acute myocardial infarction make up a diverse group in whom a variety of factors may combine to cause ventricular tachycardia or ventricular fibrillation.[105] Seventy-five percent have significant coronary artery disease while the remaining 25 percent have a variety of cardiac disturbances.[106,107] The recurrence rate of ventricular tachyarrhythmias, particularly ventricular fibrillation, and sudden cardiac death in patients who are resuscitated from out-of-hospital ventricular fibrillation and do not evolve a myocardial infarction is 25 percent to 30 percent at 1 year.[106]

Physical Examination

Physical examination may show signs consistent with a cardiac arrhythmia and the underlying heart disease for that particular patient. They are not unique for the patient with cardiac arrest.

Laboratory Tests

Sudden cardiac death during ambulatory recording may be characterized by a bradycardia in 25 percent of patients. Some patients may have an increase in sinus rate and in the frequency of premature ventricular complexes and ventricular tachycardia in the hours prior to ventricular fibrillation. The latter in almost all instances is initiated by ventricular tachycardia. A ventricular tachyarrhythmia is usually found on long-term ECG recording during sudden cardiac death in hospitalized patients.[108–110] Because patients may have many months without another episode of cardiac arrest, long-term ECG recording to document the event and provide therapeutic assessment generally has not proved sensitive enough. Stress testing uncommonly provokes the arrhythmia that triggers the cardiac arrest.

Each patient should be considered individually; each should undergo a comprehensive cardiac evaluation directed at the optimal evaluation and management of such factors such as ischemia, heart failure, valvular heart disease, and sensitivity to antiarrhythmic drugs. Because the treatment of these factors alone, without addition of specific antiarrhythmic therapy, is frequently insufficient to prevent a recurrence, we feel the present data most convincingly support invasive electrophysiological evaluation.[106,111,112] In approximately 75 percent of these patients, programmed electrical stimulation of the heart initiates a ventricular tachyarrhythmia. Conventional or investigational antiarrhythmic drugs and surgery suppress inducible ventricular arrhythmias in 60 to 70 percent of these patients. Suppression predicts freedom from a recurrence of ventricular tachyarrhythmias or sudden cardiac death in 85 to 95 percent of patients followed for a mean of 2 years. In contrast, recurrence rates among patients with ventricular arrhythmias still inducible after therapy range between 25 and 40 percent.[106] Thus, an electrophysiological study should be considered early in the management of patients with cardiac arrest without myocardial infarction.

References

1. Engle, T. R., and Luck, J. C.: Effect of Whiskey on Atrial Vulnerability and "Holiday Heart," *J. Am. Coll. Cardiol.*, 1:816, 1983.
2. Pedersen, D. H., Zipes, D. P., Foster, P. R., and Troup, P. J.: Ventricular Tachycardia and Ventricular Fibrillation in a Young Population, *Circulation*, 60:988, 1979.
3. Rahilly, G. T., Jr., Prystowsky, E. N., Zipes, D. P., Naccarelli, G. V., Jackman, W. M., and Heger, J. J.: Clinical and Electrophysiologic Findings in Patients with Repetitive Monomorphic Ventricular Tachycardia and Otherwise Normal Electrocardiograms, *Am. J. Cardiol.*, 50:459, 1982.
4. Garson, A., Jr., Gillette, P. C., and Titus, J. L., et al.: Surgical Treatment of Ventricular Tachycardia in Infants, *N. Engl. J. Med.*, 310:1443, 1984.
5. Cohen, M., Weiner, I., Pichard, A., Holt, J., Smith, H. Jr., and Gorlin, R.: Determinants of Ventricular Tachycardia in Patients with Coronary Artery Disease and Ventricular Aneurysm, *Am. J. Cardiol.*, 51:61, 1983.

6. Kowey, P. R., Eisenberg, R., and Engel, T. R.: Sustained Arrhythmias in Hypertropic Obstructive Cardiomyopathy, *N. Engl. J. Med.*, 310:1566, 1984.
7. Torres, M. A., Corday, E., Meerbaum, S., Sakamaki, T., Peter, T., and Uchiyama, T.: Characterization of Left Ventricular Mechanical Function during Arrhythmias by Two-dimensional Echocardiography, *J. Am. Colt. Cardiol.*, 1:819, 1983.
8. Botvinick, E., Frais, M., and O'Connell, W., et al.: Phase Image Evaluation of Patients with Ventricular Preexcitation Syndromes, *J. Am. Coll. Cardiol.*, 3:799, 1984.
9. Cohen, M., Weiner, I., Pichard, A., Holt, J., Smith, H. Jr., and Gorlin, R.: Determinants of Ventricular Tachycardia in Patients with Coronary Artery Disease and Ventricular Aneurysm, *Am. J. Cardiol.*, 51:61, 1983.
10. Braat, S. H., DeZwaan, C., Brugada, P., and Wellens, H. J. J.: Value of Left Ventricular Ejection Fraction in Extensive Anterior Infarction to Predict Development of Ventricular Tachycardia, *Am. J. Cardiol.*, 52:686, 1983.
11. Califf, R. M., McKinnis, R. A., and McNeer, J. F., et al.: Prognostic Value of Ventricular Arrhythmias Associated with Treadmill Exercise Testing in Patients Studied with Cardiac Catheterization for Suspected Ischemic Heart Disease, *J. Am. Coll. Cardiol.*, 2:1060, 1983.
12. Woelfel, A., Foster, J. R., Simpson, J. R., Jr., and Gettes, L. S.: Reproducibility and Treatment of Exercise-Induced Ventricular Tachycardia, *Am. J. Cardiol.*, 53:751, 1984.
13. Holter, N. J.: "New Method for Heart Studies: Continuous Electrocardiography of Active Subjects over Long Periods Is Now Practical," *Science*, 134:1214, 1961.
14. Winkle, R. A.: Curriculum in Cardiology, Current Status of Ambulatory Electrocardiography, *Am. Heart J.*, 102:757, 1981.
15. Sami, M., Kraemer, H., and Harrison, D. C., et al.: A New Method for Evaluating Antiarrhythmic Drug Efficacy, *Circulation*, 62:1172, 1980.
16. Morris, S. N., and McHenry, P. L.: Cardiac Arrhythmias during Exercise Testing and Exercise Conditioning, *Cardiovasc. Clin.*, 9:57, 1978.
17. Grodman, R. S., Capone, R. J., and Most, A. S.: Arrhythmia Surveillance by Transtelephonic Monitoring: Comparison with Holter Monitoring in Symptomatic Ambulatory Patients, *Am. Heart J.*, 98:459, 1979.
18. Judson, P., Holmes, D. R., and Baker, W.: Evaluation of Outpatient Arrhythmias Utilizing Transtelephonic Monitoring, *Am. Heart J.*, 97:759, 1979.
19. Fyfe, D. A., Holmes, D. R., Jr., Newbauer, S. A., and Feldt, R. H.: Transtelephonic Monitoring in Pediatric Patients with Clinically Suspected Arrhythmias, *Clin. Ped.*, 23:139, 1984.
20. Simson, M. B.: Clinical Application of Signal Averaging, *Cardiol. Clin.*, 1:109, 1983.
21. Cain, M. E., Ambos, H. D., Witkowski, F. X., and Sobel, B. E.: Fast Fourier Transform Analysis of Signal Averaged Electrocardiograms for Identification of Patients Prone to Sustained Ventricular Tachycardia, *Circulation*, 69:711, 1984.
22. Flowers, N. C., Shvartsman, F., Horan, L. G., Palakurthy, P., Sohi, G. S., and Sridharan, M. R.: Analysis of PR Subintervals in Normal Subjects and Early Studies in Patients with Abnormalities of the Conduction System using Surface His Bundle Recordings, *J. Am. Coll. Cardiol.*, 2:939, 1983.
23. Brugada, P., Green, M., Abdollah, H., and Wellens, H. J. J.: Significance of Ventricular Arrhythmias Initiated by Programmed Ventricular Stimulation: The Importance of the Type of Ventricular Arrhythmia Induced and the Number the Premature Stimuli Required, *Circulation*, 69:87, 1984.
24. Buxton, A. E., Waxman, H. L., Marchlinsiki, F. E., Untereker, W. J., Waspy, L. E., and Josephson, M. E.: Role of Triple Extrastimuli during Electrophysiologic Study of Patients with Documented Sustained Ventricular Tachyarrhythmias, *Circulation*, 69:532, 1984.
25. Prystowsky, E. N., Heger, J. J., Lloyd, E. A., and Zipes, D. P.: Clinical Electrophysiology of Ventricular Tachycardia, in D. P. Zipes (ed.), "Cardiology Clinics," W. B. Saunders Company, Philadelphia, 1983, p. 253.
26. Ruskin, J. N., Schoenfeld, M. H., and Graran, H.: Role of Electrophysiologic Techniques in the Selection of Antiarrhythmic Drug Regimens for Ventricular Arrhythmias, *Am. J. Cardiol.*, 52:41C, 1983.
27. Montague, T. J., McPherson, D. D., MacKenzie, B. R., Spencer, C. A., Manton, M. A., and Horacek, B. M.: Frequent Ventricular Ectopic Activity without Underlying Cardiac Disease: Analysis of 45 Subjects, *Am. J. Cardiol.*, 52:980, 1983.
28. Dickinson, D. F., and Scott, O.: Ambulatory Electrocardiographic Monitoring in 100 Healthy Teenage Boys, *Br. Heart J.*, 51:179, 1984.
29. Bigger, J. T., Fleiss, J. L., Krieger, R., Miller, J. P., and Rolnitzky, L. M.: Multicenter Post-Infarction Research Group: The Relationships among Ventricular Arrhythmias, Left Ventricular Dysfunction, and Mortality in the Two Years after Myocardial Infarction, *Circulation*, 69:250, 1984.
30. Diamond, T. H., Smith, R., and Myerburgh, D. T.: Holter Monitor—A Necessity for the Evaluation of Palpitations, *S. Afr. Med. J.*, 63:5, 1983.
31. Pilcher, G. F., Cook, A. J., Johnston, B. L., and Gletcher, G. F.: 24-Hour Continuous Electrocardiography during Exercise and Free Activity in 80 Apparently Healthy Runners, *Am. J. Cardiol.*, 52:859, 1983.
32. Kostis, J. B., McCrone, K., and Moreyra, A. E., et al.: Premature Ventricular Complexes in the Absence of Identifiable Heart Disease, *Circulation*, 63:1351, 1981.
33. Brodsky, M., Wu, D., Dennis, P., Kanakis, C., and Rosen, K. M.: Arrhythmias Documented by 24-Hour Continuous Electrocardiographic Monitoring in 50 Male Medical Students without Apparent Heart Disease, *Am. J. Cardiol.*, 39:390, 1977.
34. Sobotka, P. A., Mayer, J. H., Bauernfeind, R. A., Kanakis, C., annd Rosen, K. M.: Arrhythmias Documented by 24-Hour Continuous Ambulatory Electrocardiographic Monitoring in Young Women without Apparent Heart Disease, *Am. Heart J.*, 101:753, 1981.
35. Winkle, R. A., Peters, F., and Hall, R.: Characterization of Ventricular Tachyarrhythmias on Ambulatory ECG Recordings in Post-Myocardial Infarction Patients: Arrhythmia Detection and Duration of Recording, Relationship between Arrhythmia Frequency and Complexity, and Day-to-Day Reproducibility, *Am. Heart J.*, 102:162, 1981.
36. Marchlinski, F., Buxton, A. E., Waxman, H. L., and Josephson, M. E.: Identifying Patients at Risk of Sudden Death after Myocardial Infarction: Value of the Response to Programmed Stimulation, Degree of Ventricular Ectopic Activity and Severity of Left Ventricular Dysfunction, *Am. J. Cardiol.*, 52:1190, 1983.
37. Bigger, J. T., Jr., Fleiss, J. L., Kleiger, R., Miller, J. P., Rolnitzky, L. M., and the Multicenter Post-Infarction Research Group: The Relationships among Ventricular Arrhythmias, Left Ventricular Dysfunction, and Mortality in the Two Years after Myocardial Infarction, *Circulation*, 69:250, 1984.
38. McKenna, W. J.: Arrhythmia and prognosis in hypertrophic cardiomyopathy, *Eur. Heart J.*, 4(suppl. f):225, 1983.
39. Savage, D. D., Seides, S. F., Maron, B. J., Myers, D. H., and Epstein, S. E.: Prevalence of Arrhythmias during 24-Hour Electrocardiographic Monitoring and Exercise Testing in Patients with Obstructive and Nonobstructive Hypertrophic Cardiomyopathy, *Circulation*, 59:866, 1979.
40. Meinhertz, T., Hoffman, T., and Kasper, W.: Significance of Ventricular Arrhythmias in Idiopathic Dilated Cardiomyopathy, *Am. J. Cardiol.*, 53:902, 1984.
41. Winkle, R. A., Lopez, M. G., Popp, R. L., and Hancock, E. W.: Life-threatening Arrhythmias in the Mitral Valve Prolapse Syndrome, *Am. J. Med.*, 60:961, 1976.
42. DeMaria, A. N., Amsterdam, E. A., Vismara, L. A., Neumann, A., and Mason, D. T.: Arrhythmias in the Mitral Valve Prolapse Syndrome, *Ann. Intern. Med.*, 84:656, 1976.
43. Shappell, S. D., Marshall, C. E., Brown, R. E., and Bruce, T. A.: Sudden Death and the Familial Occurrence of Mid-

systolic Click, Late Systolic Murmur Syndrome, *Circulation,* 48:1128, 1984.
44. McHenry, P. L., Morris, S. N., Kavalier, M., and Jordan, J. W.: Comparative Study of Exercise-Induced Ventricular Arrhythmias in Normal Subjects and Patients with Documented Coronary Artery Disease, *Am. J. Cardiol.,* 37:609, 1976.
45. Morris, S. N., and McHenry, P. L.: Cardiac Arrhythmias during Exercise Testing and Exercise Conditioning, *Cardiovasc. Clin.,* 9:57, 1978.
46. Miller, D. H., and Borer, J. S.: Exercise Testing Early after Myocardial Infarction, *Am. J. Med.,* 72:427, 1982.
47. Theroux, P., Marpole, D., Derek, G. F., and Bourassa, M. G.: Exercise Stress Testing in the Post-Myocardial Infarction Patient, *Am. J. Cardiol.,* 52:664, 1983.
48. Gooch, A. F., Vicencio, F., Maranhao, V., and Goldberg, H.: Arrhythmias and Left Ventricular Asynergy in the Prolapsing Mitral Leaflet Syndrome, *Am. J. Cardiol.,* 29:611, 1972.
49. Goldschlager, N.: Exercise-Testing in Patients with Recent Myocardial Infarction, *Council Clin. Cardiol. Newsletter,* 5:1, 1980.
50. Weld, F. M., Chu, K., Bigger, J. T., Jr., and Rolnitzky, L. M.: Risk Stratification with Low-Level Exercise Testing Two Weeks after Acute Myocardial Infarction, *Circulation,* 64:306, 1981.
51. Faris, J. V., McHenry, P. L., Jordan, J. W., and Morris, S. N.: Prevalence and Reproducibility of Exercise-Induced Ventricular Arrhythmias during Maximal Exercise Testing in Normal Men, *Am. J. Cardiol.,* 38:617, 1976.
52. Sheps, D. S., Ernst, J. C., and Briese, F. R.: Decreased Frequency of Exercise-Induced Ventricular Ectopic Activity in the Second of Two Consecutive Treadmill Tests, *Circulation,* 55:891, 1977.
53. Kennedy, H. L.: Comparison of Ambulatory Electrocardiography and Exercise Testing, *Am. J. Cardiol.,* 47:1359, 1981.
54. Kosowsky, B. D., Lown, B., Whiting, R., and Gufney, T.: Occurrence of Ventricular Arrhythmias with Exercise as Compared to Monitoring, *Circulation,* 44:826, 1971.
55. Crawford, M., O'Rourke, R. A., Ramakrishna, N., Henning, H., and Ross, J. Jr.: Comparative Effectiveness of Exercise Testing and Continuous Monitoring for Detecting Arrhythmias in Patients with Previous Myocardial Infarction, *Circulation,* 50:301, 1974.
56. Lipski, J., Cohen, L., Espinoza, J., Motro, M., Dack, S., and Donoso, E.: Value of Holter Monitoring in Assessing Cardiac Arrhythmias in Symptomatic Patients, *Am. J. Cardiol.,* 37:102, 1976.
57. Gibson, T., and Heitzman, M. R.: Diagnostic Efficacy of 24-Hour Electrocardiographic Monitoring for Syncope, *Am. J. Cardiol.,* 53:1013, 1984.
58. Taylor, I. C., and Stout, R. W.: Is Ambulatory Electrocardiography A Useful Investigation in Elderly People with "Funny Turns"? *Age Aging,* 12:211, 1983.
59. Kapoor, W. N., Karpf, M., Maher, Y., Miller, R. A., and Levey, G. S.: Syncope of Unknown Origin: The Need for a More Cost-Effective Approach to Its Diagnostic Evaluation, *JAMA,* 247:2687, 1982.
60. Kapoor, W. N., Karpf, M., Wieand, S., Peterson, J. R., and Levey, G. S.: A Prospective Evaluation and Follow-up of Patients with Syncope, *N. Engl. J. Med.,* 309:197, 1983.
61. DiMarco, J. P., Garan, H., Hawthorne, J. W., and Ruskin, J. N.: Intracardiac Electrophysiologic Techniques and Recurrent Syncope of Unknown Cause, *Ann. Intern. Med.,* 95:542, 1981.
62. Gulamhusein, S., Naccarelli, G. V., Ko, P. T., et al.: Value and Limitations of Clinical Electrophysiologic Study and Assessment of Patients with Unexplained Syncope, *Am. J. Med.,* 73:700, 1982.
63. Morady, F., Shen, E., and Schwartz, A.: Long-term Follow-up of Patients with Recurrent Unexplained Syncope Evaluated by Electrophysiologic Testing, *J. Am. Coll. Cardiol.,* 2:1053, 1983.
64. Akhtar, M., Shenasa, M., Denker, S., Gilbert, C. J., and Rizwi, N.: Role of Cardiac Electrophysiologic Studies in Patients with Unexplained Recurrent Syncope, *PACE,* 6:192, 1983.
65. Shaw, D. B., Kekwick, C. A., Veale, D., and Whistance, T. W.: Unexplained Syncope—A Diagnostic Pacemaker? *PACE,* 6:720, 1983.
66. Zipes, D. P., Heger, J. J., Miles, W. M., et al.: Early Experience with the Implantable Cardioverter, *N. Engl. J. Med.,* 311:485, 1984.
67. Probst, P., Muhlberger, V., Lederbauer, M., Pachinger, O., Kaliman, J., and Steinbach, K.: Electrophysiologic Findings and Carotid Sinus Massage, *PACE,* 6:689, 1983.
68. Holden, W., McAnnulty, J. H., and Rahimtoola, S. H.: Characterization of Heart Rate Response to Exercise in the Sick Sinus Syndrome, *Br. Heart J.,* 40:923, 1978.
69. Jose, A. D.: Effect of Combined Sympathetic and Parasympathetic Blockage on Heart Rate and Cardiac Function in Man, *Am. J. Cardiol.,* 18:476, 1966.
70. Jordan, J. A., Yamaguchi, I., and Mandel, W. J.: Studies on the Mechanisms of Sinus Node Dysfunction in a Sick Sinus Syndrome, *Circulation,* 57:217, 1978.
71. Cleaveland, C. R., Rangno, R. E., and Shand, D. G.: A Standardized Isoproterenol Sensitivity Test: The Effects of Sinus Arrhythmia, Atropine and Propranolol, *Arch. Intern. Med.,* 130:147, 1972.
72. Stern, S., and Eisenberg, S.: The Effects of Propranolol (Inderal) on the Electrocardiogram of Normal Subjects, *Am. Heart J.,* 77:192, 1969.
73. Mandel, W. J., Hayakawa, H., Danzig, R., and Marcus, H. S.: Evaluation of Sinoatrial Node Function in Man by Overdrive Suppression, *Circulation,* 44:59, 1971.
74. Narula, O. S., Samet, P., and Javier, R. P.: Significance of the Sinus Node Recovery Time, *Circulation,* 45:140, 1972.
75. Breithardt, G., Seipel, L., and Loogen, F.: Sinus Node Recovery Time and Calculated Sinoatrial Conduction Time in Normal Subjects and Patients with Sinus Node Dysfunction, *Circulation,* 56:43, 1977.
76. Benditt, D. G., Strauss, H. C., Scheinmann, M. M., Behar, V. S., and Wallace, A. G.: Analysis of Secondary Pauses following Termination of Rapid Atrial Pacing in Man, *Circulation,* 54:436, 1976.
77. Kerr, C. R., Grant, A. O., Wenger, T. L., and Strauss, H. T.: Sinus Node Dysfunction, *Cardiol. Clin.,* 1:187, 1983.
78. Gann, D., Tolentino, A., and Samet, P.: Electrophysiologic Evaluation of Elderly Patients with Sinus Bradycardia, *Ann. Intern. Med.,* 90:24, 1979.
79. Prystowsky, E. N.: The Sick Sinus Syndrome—Diagnosis and Treatment, in E. Donoso (ed.), "Advances and Controversies in Cardiology," Grune & Stratton, New York, 1981, p. 93.
80. Reiffel, J. A., Bigger, J. T., Jr., Krammer, M., and Reid, D. S.: Ability of Holter Electrocardiographic Recording and Atrial Stimulation to Detect Sinus Node Dysfunction in Symptomatic and Asymptomatic Patients with Sinus Bradycardia, *Am. J. Cardiol.,* 40:189, 1977.
81. Hariman, R. J., Krongrad, E., Boxer, R. A., Weiss, M. B., Steeg, C. N., and Hoffman, B. N.: Method for Recording Electrical Activity of the Sinoatrial Node and Automatic Atrial Foci during Cardiac Catheterization in Human Subjects, *Am. J. Cardiol.,* 45:775, 1980.
82. Julliard, A., Guillerm, F., Chuong, H. V., Barrillon, A., and Gerbaux, A.: Sinus Nodal Electrogram Recordings in 59 Patients, *Br. Heart J.,* 50:75, 1983.
83. Narula, O. S.: Atrioventricular Conduction Disturbances in Patients with Sinus Bradycardia, *Circulation,* 44:1096, 1971.
84. Langendorf, R., and Pick, A.: Atrioventricular Block, type II (Mobitz): Its Nature and Clinical Significance, *Circulation,* 38:819, 1968.
85. Dhingra, R., Denes, P., Wu, D., Chuquimia, R., and Rosen, K. M.: The Significance of Second-Degree Atrioventricular Block and Bundle Branch Block: Observations Regarding Site and Type of Block, *Circulation,* 49:638, 1978.
86. Dhingra, R. C., Wyndham, C., and Bauernfeind, R.: Significance of Block distal to the His Bundle Induced by Atrial

Pacing in Patients with Chronic Bifascicular Block, *Circulation,* 60:1455, 1979.
87. Zipes, D. P.: Second Degree Atrioventricular Block, *Circulation,* 60:465, 1979.
88. Puech, P., and Wainwright, R. J.: Clinical Electrophysiology of Atrioventricular Block, *Cardiol. Clin.,* 1:209, 1983.
89. Dhingra, R. C., Palileo, E., and Strasberg, B., et al.: Significance of the HV Interval in 517 Patients with Chronic Bifascicular Block, *Circulation,* 64:265, 1981.
90. McAnnulty, J. H., Rahimtoola, S. H., and Murphy, E.: Natural History of "High Risk" Bundle Branch Block: Final Report of a Prospective Study, *N. Engl. J. Med.,* 307:137, 1982.
91. Scheinman, M. M., Peters, S. W., Suave, M., et al.: Value of the HQ Interval in Patients with Bundle Branch Block and Role of Prophylactic Permanent Pacing, *Am. J. Cardiol.,* 50:1316, 1982.
92. Pedersen, D. H., Zipes, D. P., Foster, P. R., and Troup, P. J.: Ventricular Tachycardia and Ventricular Fibrillation in a Young Population, *Circulation,* 60:988, 1979.
93. Benson, D. W., Jr., Sanford, M., Dunnigan, A., and Benditt, D. G.: Transesophageal Atrial Pacing Threshold, Role of Intraelectrode Spacing, Pulse Width and Catheter Insertion Depth, *Am. J. Cardiol.,* 53:63, 1984.
94. Moran, J. M., Kehoer, F., Loeb, J. M., Sanders, J. H., Jr., Tommaso, C. L., and Michaelis, L. L.: Operative Therapy of Malignant Ventricle Rhythm Disturbances, *Ann. Surg.,* 198:479, 1983.
95. Klein, G. J., and Guiraudon, G. M.: Surgical Therapy of Cardiac Arrhythmias, *Cardiol. Clin.,* 1:323, 1983.
96. Sung, R. J., Chang, M. S., and Chiang, B. N.: Clinical Electrophysiology of Supraventricular Tachycardia, *Cardiol. Clin.,* 1:225, 1983.
97. Swerdlow, C. D., Winkle, R. A., and Mason, J. W.: Determinants of Survival in Patients with Ventricular Tachyarrhythmias, *N. Engl. J. Med.,* 308:1436, 1983.
98. Spielman, S. R., Schwartz, J. S., and McCarthy, D. M., et al.: Predictors of the Success or Failure of Medical Therapy in Patients with Chronic Recurrent Sustained Ventricular Tachycardia: A Discriminant Analysis, *J. Am. Coll. Cardiol.,* 1:408, 1983.
99. Heger, J. J., Prystowsky, E. N., and Zipes, D. P.: Drug Therapy of Cardiac Arrhythmias, *Cardiol. Clin.,* 1:305, 1983.
100. Ferguson, D., Saksena, S., Greenberg, E., and Craelius, W.. Management of Recurrent Ventricular Tachycardia: Economic Impact of the Therapeutic Alternatives, *Am. J. Cardiol.,* 53:531, 1984.
101. Zipes, D. P., Heger, J. J., and Prystowsky, E. N.: Pacing and Tranvenous Cardioversion to Control Tachyarrhythmias, *Cardiol. Clin.,* 1:341, 1983.
102. Page, P. L., Arcinighas, J. G., and Plumb, V. J.: Value of Early Postoperative Epicardial Programmed Ventricular Stimulation Studies after Surgery for Ventricular Tachyarrhythmias, *J. Am. Coll. Cardiol.,* 2:1046, 1983.
103. Hamer, A., Vohra, J., Hund, D., and Sloman, G.: Prediction of Sudden Death by Electrophysiologic Studies in High Risk Patients Surviving Acute Myocardial Infarction, *Am. J. Cardiol.,* 50:223, 1982.
104. Richards, D. A., Cody, D. V., Deniss, A. R., Russell, P. A., Young, A. A., and Uther, J. B.: Ventricular Electrical Instability: A Predictor of Death after Myocardial Infarction, *Am. J. Cardiol.,* 51:75, 1983.
105. Marchlinski, F. E., Buxton, A. E., Waxman, H. L., and Josephson, M. E.: Identifying Patients at Risk of Sudden Death after Myocardial Infarction, *Am. J. Cardiol.,* 52:1190, 1983.
106. Ruskin, J. N., and Garan, J.: Electrophysiologic Observations in Survivors of Out-of-Hospital Cardiac Arrest Related to Ischemic Heart Disease, *Cardiol. Clin.,* 1:287, 1983.
107. Southworth, W. F., and Ruffy, R.: Evaluation and Treatment of Survivors of Sudden Cardiac Death or Nonbradycardic Syncope Unrelated to Coronary Artery Disease, *Cardiol. Clin.,* 1:275, 1983.
108. Clark, M. B., Dwyer, E. M., Jr., and Greenburg, H.: Sudden Death during Ambulatory Monitoring, Analysis of Six Cases, *Am. J. Med.,* 75:801, 1983.
109. Pratt, C. M., Francis, M. J., Luck, J. C., Wundam, C. R., Miller, R. R., and Quinones, M. A.: Analysis of Ambulatory Electrocardiograms in Fifteen Patients during Spontaneous Ventricular Fibrillation with Special Reference to Preceding Arrhythmic Events, *J. Am. Coll. Cardiol.,* 2:789, 1983.
110. Panidis, I. P., and Morganroth, J.: Sudden Death in Hospitalized Patients: Cardiac Rhythm Disturbances Detected by Ambulatory Electrocardiographic Monitoring, *J. Am. Coll. Cardiol.,* 2:798, 1983.
111. Dennis, R., Waxman, H. L., Kienzle, M. G., Buxton, A. E., Marchlinski, F. E., and Josephson, M. E.: Clinical Characteristics of Long-term Follow-up in 119 Survivors of Cardiac Arrest: Relation to Inducibility at Electrophysiologic Study, *Am. J. Cardiol.,* 52:969, 1983.
112. Garan, H., Ruskin, J. N., DiMarco, J. P., et al.: Electrophysiologic Studies before and after Myocardial Revascularization in Patients with Life-threatening Ventricular Arrhythmias, *Am. J. Cardiol.,* 51:519, 1983.

19

Assessment of Myocardial Ischemia

Richard M. Steingart, M.D. James Scheuer, M.D.

Definition of Ischemic Heart Disease

Ischemic heart disease is defined by the World Health Organization as "myocardial impairment due to imbalance between coronary blood flow and myocardial requirements caused by changes in the coronary circulation."[1] According to this definition, atherosclerotic coronary artery disease is the major, but not the only, pathophysiological cause of ischemia. This chapter focuses on ischemia as a manifestation of pathological changes in the epicardial coronary arteries (see Chap. 45).

Scope of the Problem

Despite a decrease in age-adjusted mortality during the last decade,[2] coronary artery disease still caused 566,000 deaths in 1980.[3] An estimated 5.4 million individuals have coronary artery disease manifested by either chronic angina or healed myocardial infarction. At the other end of the spectrum, however, there are many more individuals between the ages of 40 and 70 years without symptoms of ischemic heart disease. Of these, between 3 to 12 percent have occult coronary artery disease.[4,5]

The clinical manifestations of myocardial ischemia caused by coronary artery disease include chronic stable angina, unstable angina, prolonged myocardial ischemia without evidence of infarction, acute myocardial infarction, congestive heart failure, ventricular arrhythmias, and sudden death. Any one of these clinical syndromes may be the first overt manifestation of the disease (see Chap. 45).

General Approach to Problem Solving in Patients with Suspected or Proven Ischemic Heart Disease

The clinician managing patients with suspected ischemic heart disease should pose five somewhat related questions: (1) Is coronary artery disease present? (2) If it is present, what is the patient's prognosis? (3) Are symptoms related to the underlying disease? (4) Is therapy available that is effective in relieving symptoms? (5) Is therapy available that can improve the prognosis?

Modern medical therapy can ameliorate symptoms in most patients with typical angina pectoris (Chap. 45). If intensive drug therapy does not allow the patient an acceptable life-style, however, coronary bypass surgery and angioplasty are highly effective in producing symptomatic relief and can be accomplished with low morbidity and mortality in competent hands (Chap. 45).[6,7] Several carefully conducted prospective trials have demonstrated that in selected subgroups of patients with angina pectoris, coronary bypass grafting can prolong life when compared with medical therapy alone. To date, the strongest evidence that coronary bypass grafting confers an advantage to survival is in patients with $\geq$ 50 percent diameter stenoses of the left main coronary artery.[8,9] There is also convincing evidence that in patients with three-vessel coronary artery disease ($\geq$ 70 percent stenoses) and impaired resting ventricular function (ejection fractions ranging from 30 to 50 percent), coronary bypass grafting can prolong life. The value of bypass grafting in improving survival rates in symptomatic patients with three-vessel disease and normal ejection fractions is less definite but the European coronary artery surgery group[9] as well as others[10] report favorably in this regard. (See Chap. 45 for further discussion of the indications for coronary bypass surgery and angioplasty.)

At present, cardiac catheterization with coronary arteriography is the most accurate test for determining the presence and severity of coronary artery disease. However, the presence of coronary artery disease defined only angiographically does not ensure that the patient's symptoms result from ischemia, nor does it define a population that is homogeneous with respect to either myocardial function or prognosis.

By using the history, physical examination, electrocardiogram, and chest x-ray along with other noninvasive tests, the physician often can make a reasonable judgment of whether significant coronary disease is present or absent. Such noninvasive methods can also be used to measure ventricular function and provide information that permits probability estimates to be made about the extent of coronary involvement. Although some forms of clinical and noninvasive test data, such as ventricular premature beats or ST depression in the electrocardiogram during exercise testing, do not correlate well with resting ejection fraction or the extent of coronary artery disease, they can be used to predict prognosis[11–13] and identify higher-risk patients for further investigation or definitive therapy. Since these noninvasive methods can only provide probability estimates of the severity of coronary disease, *the threshold for proceeding to cardiac catheterization has been set at considerably less than 100 percent certainty for suspected left main or three-vessel coronary disease, particularly when there is evidence of ventricular dysfunction.* Such an approach is effective in discovering appropriate surgical candidates, while at the same time reducing the number of patients unnecessarily subjected to the risk and cost of arteriography.

Data To Be Gathered on All Patients: Initial Estimation of Likelihood of Coronary Disease

At one end of the coronary artery disease spectrum are those individuals who usually require no testing beyond the initial evaluation. These are the asymptomatic individuals who may harbor occult coronary disease; the prevalence of atherosclerotic coronary artery disease in this population averages approximately 5 percent.[5] The likelihood of coronary disease rises with age, male sex, and the presence of multiple risk factors such as cigarette smoking, hypertension, hypercholesterolemia, or diabetes.[14] In general, asymptomatic individuals without significant risk factors who have normal resting electrocardiograms and chest x-rays can be assured of a low probability of coronary disease and even lower likelihood of having a significant coronary event.[5,15] Under special circumstances, such as prior to initiating a vigorous exercise program, electrocardiographic exercise testing may be indicated.[16] There are certain occupations, for instance, airline pilot and bus driver, in which one person is responsible for the safety of many others for which exercise electrocardiographic testing might be useful. Routine exercise testing for the general population is not advisable because of the low yield of true positive results in asymptomatic patients.[15]

In some instances, the initial evaluation leads directly to coronary arteriography to evaluate the patient for angioplasty or bypass grafting. Such an approach is indicated in patients with (1) typical angina pectoris which interferes with life-style despite intensive medical therapy; (2) continuing ischemia soon after myocardial infarction despite medical therapy; and (3) accelerating or unstable angina and in patients with prolonged myocardial ischemia without evidence of infarction who are not easily controlled with medical therapy.

Clinical Circumstances in Which More Noninvasive Testing Is Often Required

Figures 19-1, 19-2, and 19-3 are decision trees that indicate the sequential use of noninvasive tests in patients in whom the initial evaluation does not lead directly to either cardiac catheterization or the conclusion that the patient does not have clinically important coronary disease. The patient's history provides a starting point for use of the decision tree, and the probability of ventricular dysfunction is employed in each part of the tree to guide the physician to the appropriate test.

Patients with Chronic, Stable Chest Pain Syndromes*

The predictive value of chest "pain" for myocardial ischemia is determined by the characteristics of the chest "pain" (Chap. 45). The predictive value of different types of chest "pain" which suggest myocardial ischemia are shown in Table 19-1. The definitions for chest pain were adapted from the Coronary Artery Surgery Study,[17] and have proved to be useful in estimating the likely presence of coronary disease. The likelihood that coronary disease is present increases as the symptoms of chest pain become more "typical" of classic angina pectoris.[5] For a given chest pain syndrome, however, age, sex, and risk factors significantly influence the likelihood of disease.[18] These estimates have been used to categorize patients as having low, moderate or high likelihoods of coronary artery disease (Figs. 19-1, 19-2, and 19-3).

After the baseline characteristics are determined, the duration of the chest pain, its response to medical therapy, and the functional impairment that it has produced should be evaluated. *Obstructive coronary disease is very likely in men and older women with typical angina pectoris* (Table 19-1 and Chap. 45). Such patients with controlled pain syndromes are candidates for further noninvasive testing to define more clearly the risk of a future coronary event and to help determine optimal therapy (Fig. 19-3.) *Patients with chronic "atypical" angina and patients with nonanginal chest pain* are also candidates for further testing to help establish or exclude the diagnosis of coronary disease and at the same time assess prognosis (Figs. 19-1 and 19-2). *Asymptomatic individuals* with multiple risk factors have likelihoods of coronary disease similar to those with very atypical symptoms, and they too may require further evaluation to help establish or exclude the diagnosis of coronary disease (Figs. 19-1 and 19-2).

Patients with a Prior Myocardial Infarction

Early Phase

The patient seen early in the course of an acute myocardial infarction who has continuing ischemia which is not readily responsive to medical therapy *should undergo coronary arteriography and possible angioplasty or bypass grafting* (Chap. 45). On the other hand, if the patient is stable, the approach should concentrate on risk stratification.

*See Table 19-1 for definitions of typical angina, atypical angina, nonanginal chest pain, and asymptomatic patients with myocardial ischemia.

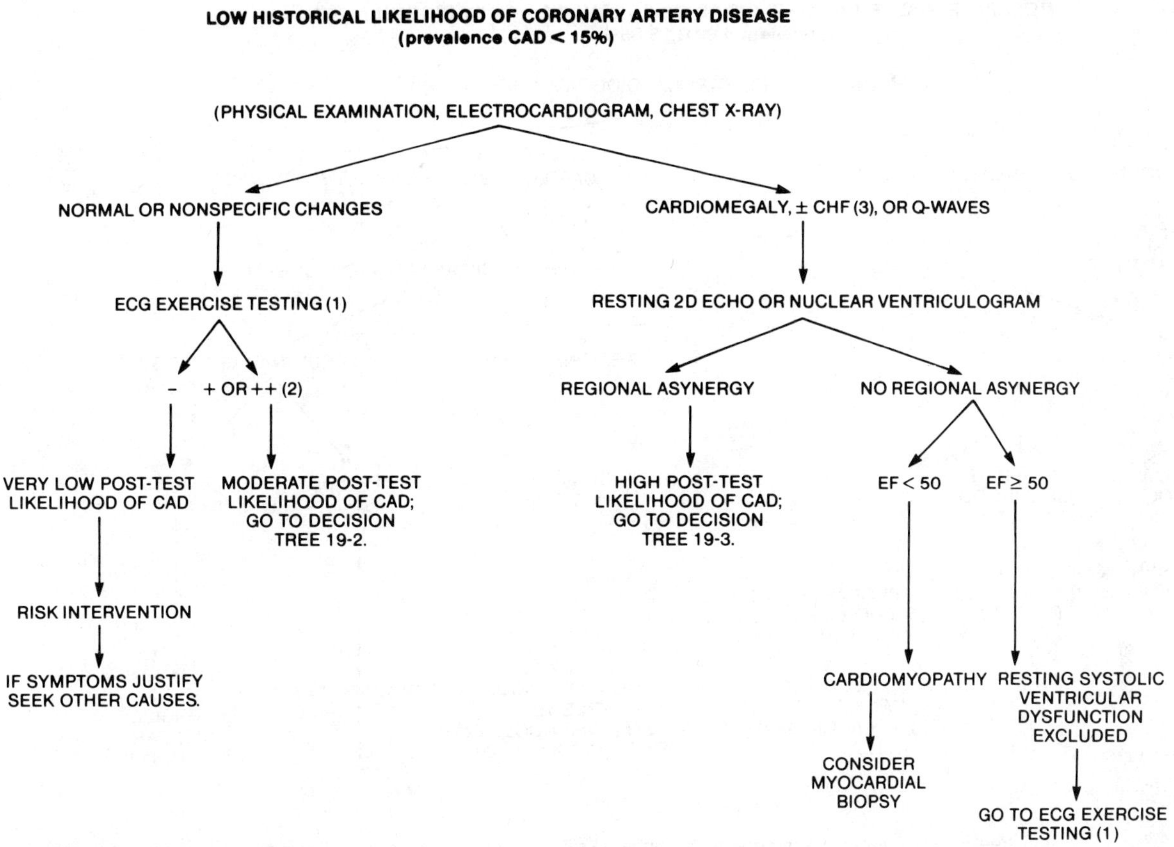

FIGURE 19-1 Decision tree for patients with a low historical likelihood (< 15 percent) of coronary artery disease. (1) Nuclear exercise testing if left bundle branch block, left ventricular hypertrophy, drug therapy, etc., would result in uninterpretable or inconclusive ECG exercise test. (2) Markedly positive tests, although unusual, are reasonably predictive of coronary disease presence and may indicate a high risk for a future coronary event. Consideration should be given to proceeding to cardiac catheterization, particularly in symptomatic patients. (3) Findings of ventricular dysfunction (variable predictive value); e.g., S_3, rales, vascular redistribution on chest x-ray. (*Note by Editor-in-Chief:* Decision-making is always influenced by the physician's judgment regarding the reliability of the test results and the safety of the procedures used to gather the data. Accordingly, each physician must decide if the test results obtained at his or her own facility are indeed reliable and that the procedures can be safely performed. Decision-making is also influenced by the feelings of the physician and patient. For example, the predictive value of a test result that is in the range of 90 percent may be satisfactory for some physicians and patients but not for others. All of this forces one to conclude that there is no rigid way to assess myocardial ischemia and that common sense and practical considerations will continue to prevail. The reader is also referred to Chap. 45 for further discussion.)

In patients under the age of 40 who have had an acute infarction, the delineation of coronary anatomy by *coronary arteriography* is important because the coronary arteries are occasionally normal.[19] However, when obstructive coronary disease is present, *the results of angiography sometimes combined with exercise testing* are needed to determine prognosis and decide on the best course of therapy.[20] In patients over the age of 40 who have had an acute infarction, coronary disease is almost invariably present.[19,21] These patients have a higher cardiac mortality than the general population, but the risk for a given patient is relatively low and seems to be declining, probably due to improved pharmacological therapy. The rate of 1-year mortality for medically treated survivors of acute infarction ranges between 3.5 and 7.5 percent.[22,23] Therefore, risk stratification is important and should be done early because the greatest incidence of recurrent infarction or death in these patients occurs during the first 3 months following an acute infarction.[24]

Information about the patient during the stay in the coronary care unit can be used to predict high risk. The presence of rales above the bases, frequent ventricular premature beats, and a history of limited exercise capacity prior to infarction all have prognostic importance in postinfarction patients.[11] The risk of future coronary events can be more precisely defined by resting ventricular performance and the severity and extent of obstructive coronary disease.[20] However, cardiac catheterization is not indicated in all stable patients recovering from an acute infarction because newer, noninvasive methods appear to be very effective in identifying the relatively small high-risk group.

Chronic Phase

In the patient who is seen at least 3 months after an acute myocardial infarction, the first step is to confirm the diagnosis (Fig. 19-3). The patient's historical recollection should be corroborated by pathological Q waves on the resting electrocardiogram, as

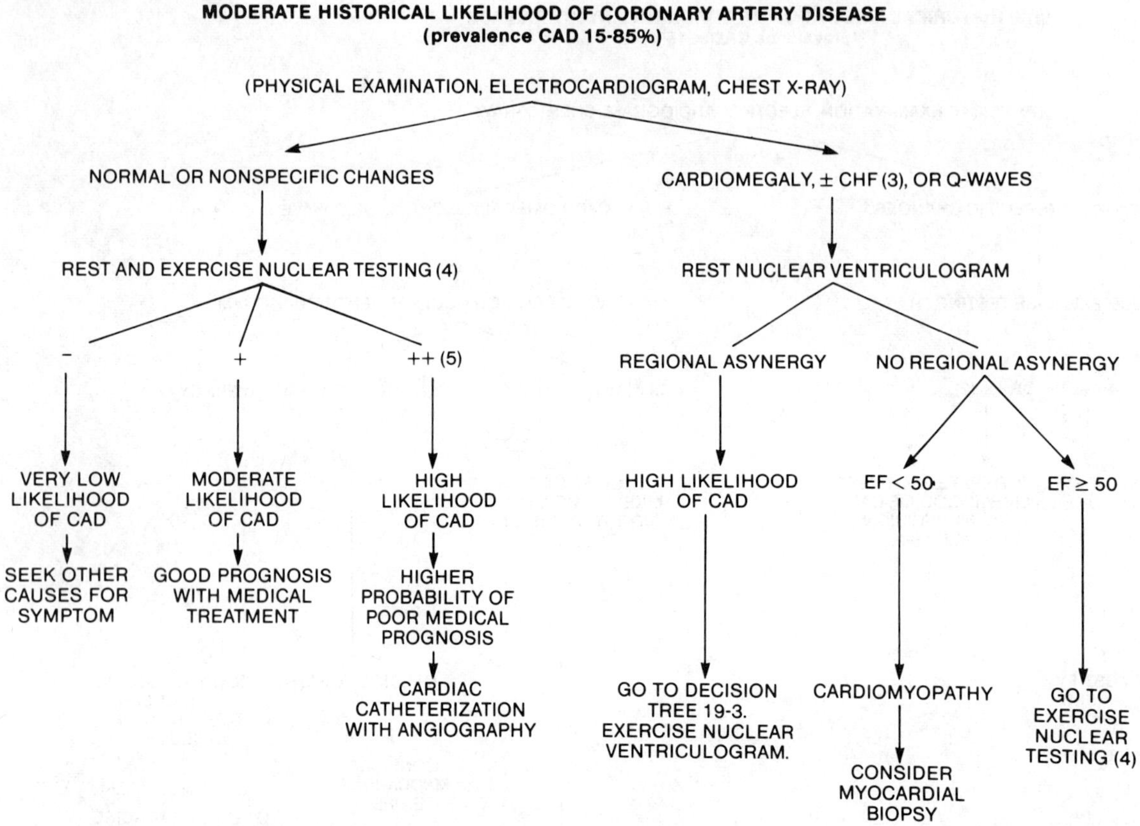

FIGURE 19-2 Decision tree for patients with a moderate historical likelihood of coronary artery disease. (3) Findings of ventricular dysfunction (variable predictive value); e.g., S_3, rales, vascular redistribution on chest x-ray. (4) Assumes sensitivity of ≥ 75 percent, specificity ≥ 85 percent for either thallium scintigraphy or radionuclide ventriculography. (5) Thallium scan: Multiple defects or increased lung uptake. Radionuclide ventriculogram: Resting ejection fraction < 50 percent and positive (+) result or ≥ 10 ejection fraction unit fall with exercise regardless of resting function. Markedly positive ECG result (downsloping ST depression at early workload, fall in systolic blood pressure) may accompany these changes. (See note in Fig. 19-1, as well as Chap. 45.)

these are highly predictive of prior infarction and obstructive coronary disease.[25] Since not all infarcts are accompanied by pathological Q waves, and Q waves can disappear with time, the patient's prior records should be searched for electrocardiographic and muscle-brain creatine kinase (MB-CK) isoenzyme documentation of infarction.[26] Chronic ST-segment and T-wave abnormalities, as well as conduction disturbances, are not specific for ischemia or infarction and thus should not be considered in isolation as evidence of ischemic heart disease.[27]

The patient's symptomatic state should then be assessed. Most data on prognosis and treatment of patients after a myocardial infarction are derived from symptomatic populations. Further, as in patients without prior infarction, these patients can experience noncardiac chest pain. Since coronary disease is almost invariably present, the clinician must decide if the pain is related to ischemia. If the pain is "typical" of angina pectoris, one can safely assume that it is caused by the underlying coronary disease. If the pain is not typical, noninvasive testing is helpful.

If the patient is limited by "typical" angina despite medical therapy, cardiac catheterization is the procedure of choice. If the pain can be managed medically, the clinician should then ask whether medical therapy also minimizes the patient's risk of future infarction and/or premature death. These questions are best answered with information about the function of the patient's ventricle and the extent of coronary disease. Data from the initial clinical evaluation can provide some useful information regarding ventricular function. Absence of pathological Q waves on the resting electrocardiogram in patients with isolated ischemic heart disease is usually associated with a normal left ventricular ejection fraction, although regional dysfunction may be present.[28] Similarly, QRS scores can be used to estimate ventricular performance.[29,30] If the scores are low, the extent of ventricular scarring can be expected to be small. Low scores on electrocardiograms recorded during the first week after an infarction are strongly associated with a normal ejection fraction. A cardiothoracic ratio of > 0.5 on a technically adequate posteroanterior chest x-ray is often associated with marked depression of the ejection fraction. However, the presence of pathological Q waves, moderate or high QRS scores, or a cardiothoracic ratio of < 0.5 may each be associated with either a normal or a depressed ejection fraction.[31] Evidence of congestive heart failure on the chest x-ray, such as pulmonary venous redistribution or pulmonary edema, usually

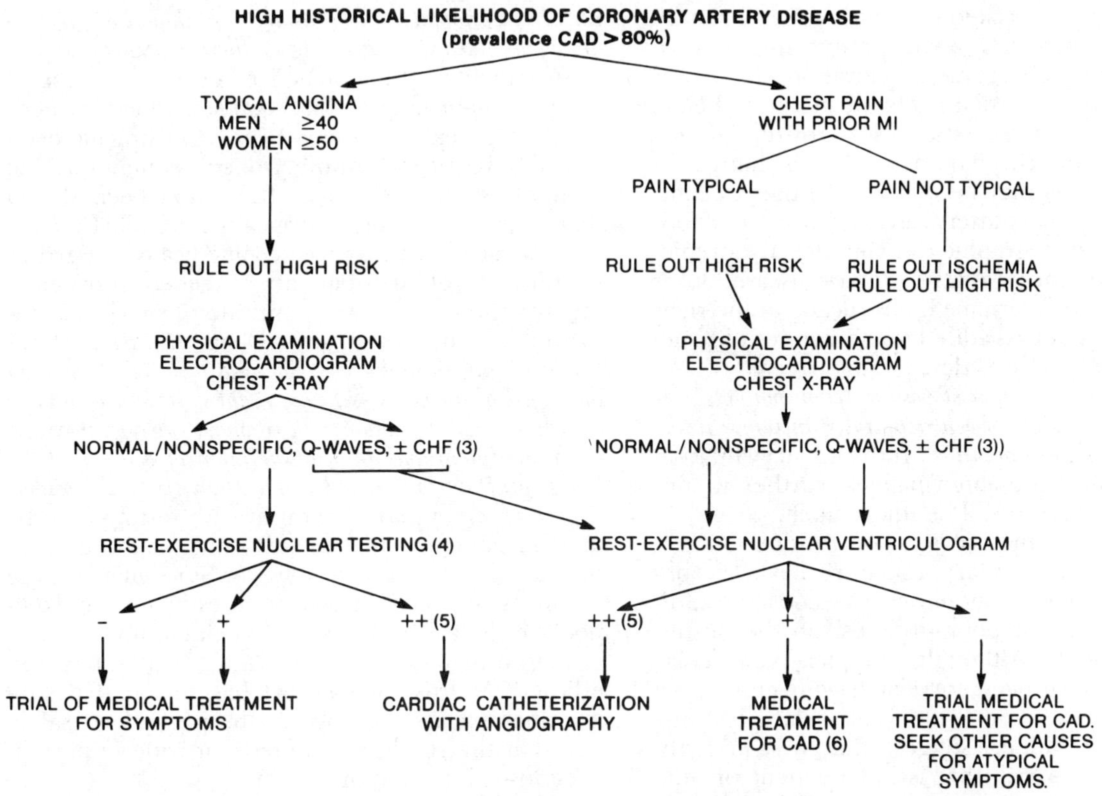

FIGURE 19-3 Decision tree for patients with a high historical likelihood (> 80 percent) of coronary artery disease. (3) Findings of ventricular dysfunction (variable predictive value); e.g., S_3, rales, vascular redistribution on chest x-ray. (4) Assumes sensitivity of > 75 percent, specificity > 85 percent for either thallium scintigraphy or radionuclide ventriculography. (5) Thallium scan: Multiple defects or increased lung uptake. Radionuclide ventriculogram: Resting ejection fraction < 50 percent and positive (+) result or > 10 ejection fraction unit fall with exercise regardless of resting function. Markedly positive ECG result (downsloping ST depression at early workload, fall in systolic blood pressure) may accompany these changes. (6) If resting ejection fraction is depressed, any firm evidence of ischemia during exercise should prompt consideration of cardiac catheterization with angiography. (See note in Fig. 19-1, as well as Chap. 45.)

indicates ventricular dysfunction and a poorer prognosis, but the degree of dysfunction (and the ejection fraction) is difficult to quantify. Similarly, dyspnea, a displaced point of maximal cardiac impulse, or an S_3 gallop are also indicative of ventricular dysfunction and perhaps higher risk[11] but are not precise predictors of the left ventricular ejection fraction. Since the benefit of surgical therapy is greatest within a relatively narrow range of ejection fractions,[6,32] accurate determinations using either radionuclide ventriculography or two-dimensional echocardiography are needed.

The initial evaluation can in some cases provide data on the extent and location of coronary artery disease. A history of disabling angina or evidence on physical examination of ventricular dysfunction

TABLE 19-1 Pretest Likelihood of Coronary Artery Disease according to Age, Sex, and Symptoms*†

	Asymptomatic		Nonanginal Chest Pain		Atypical Angina		Typical Angina	
Age, years	Men	Women	Men	Women	Men	Women	Men	Women
30–39	1.9 ± 0.3	0.3 ± 0.1	5.2 ± 0.8	0.8 ± 0.3	21.8 ± 2.4	4.2 ± 1.3	69.7 ± 3.2	25.8 ± 6.6
40–49	5.5 ± 0.3	1.0 ± 0.2	14.1 ± 1.3	2.8 ± 0.7	46.1 ± 1.8	13.3 ± 2.9	87.3 ± 1.0	55.2 ± 6.5
50–59	9.7 ± 0.4	3.2 ± 0.4	21.5 ± 1.7	8.4 ± 1.2	58.9 ± 1.5	32.4 ± 3.0	92.0 ± 0.6	79.4 ± 2.4
60–69	12.3 ± 0.5	7.5 ± 0.6	28.1 ± 1.9	18.6 ± 1.9	67.1 ± 2.4	54.4 ± 2.4	94.3 ± 0.4	90.6 ± 1.0

*Each value represents the percent ± 1 standard error of the percent.

†Assessment of anginal symptoms: (1) Is chest pain substernal? (2) Is it precipitated by exertion? (3) Is it relieved within 10 min by rest or nitroglycerin? Answers to three of three questions "yes" = typical angina. Answers to two of three questions "yes" = atypical angina. Answers to one of three questions "yes" = nonanginal chest pain. No complaints of discomfort above the diaphragm = asymptomatic.

Source: Adapted from G. A. Diamond and J. S. Forrester, Analysis of Probability as an Aid in the Clinical Diagnosis of Coronary Artery Disease, *N. Engl. J. Med.*, 300:1350, 1979. Reprinted with permission from the publisher and authors.

are only slightly associated with multivessel coronary disease.[33] Abnormal Q waves or dynamic T-wave inversion and ST-segment elevation (but not depression) in precordial leads during an ischemic episode have been related to disease of the left anterior descending coronary artery. Such changes in the inferior leads may be related to either circumflex or right coronary artery disease. Changes in both these electrocardiographic distributions are predictors of two- or three-vessel coronary disease, but it is not possible to determine if obstruction in the right or circumflex artery is added to the signs of obstruction of the left anterior descending artery.[34]

If *the initial evaluation of postinfarction patients suggests multivessel disease or ventricular dysfunction, cardiac catheterization may be indicated.* If the initial evaluation fails to demonstrate abnormalities, further noninvasive testing should still be undertaken.

Ventricular premature beats on routine ECGs,[35] and complex ventricular premature beats[36,37] observed during longer monitoring periods are additional harbingers of poor prognosis in the postinfarction patient. Although complex ventricular arrhythmias have been correlated with multivessel coronary disease and with ventricular dysfunction,[38,39] some evidence suggests that these arrhythmias constitute a risk that is independent of anatomic factors.[37] The practical importance of ventricular arrhythmias is that their presence on routine ECGs or Holter monitors indicates that the postinfarction patient is in a higher-risk category and frequently requires more thorough investigation. The optimal therapeutic approach for patients with asymptomatic arrhythmias is not known at this time.

Patients with Unstable Angina Pectoris or Prolonged Myocardial Ischemia without Infarction

Typical but unstable angina pectoris (defined as angina of new onset or of increasing severity) forms a distinct diagnostic category. The risk of a major cardiac event is greater in patients in this group than in patients with stable angina but less than it is in patients with acute infarction.[40] Patients with prolonged chest pain which is characteristic of myocardial ischemia in whom there are no objective signs of myocardial infarction are also likely to have a major cardiac event such as infarction. *However, normal coronary arteries without provokable spasm may sometimes be seen at coronary arteriography.*

Patients are more likely to have an acute ischemic event if they have any of the following: an unstable syndrome including prolonged chest discomfort; advanced age; prior myocardial infarction; prior symptoms compatible with typical angina pectoris; diaphoresis; new electrocardiographic findings suggestive of infarction or ischemia. Conversely, the absence of these findings suggests a low probability.[41,42] *If symptoms persist despite intensive medical therapy, catheterization with coronary arteriography should be performed promptly, and consideration should be given to angioplasty or bypass grafting to alleviate symptoms.*

In patients with obstructive coronary disease in whom unstable angina has been controlled by medical therapy, early coronary bypass grafting has been shown to reduce the number of subsequent hospital admissions for chest pain. It has not been shown that *all* patients treated surgically have a better rate of survival than those treated medically.[40] Further stratification of such patients is needed in order to identify the patients in whom rate of survival is improved with bypass surgery (Chap. 45). *But, any patient with an unstable syndrome and a moderate or high likelihood of an acute ischemic event may be a candidate for cardiac catheterization with coronary arteriography and left ventriculography for consideration of angioplasty or bypass grafting to reduce future debility from the underlying coronary disease.* If noninvasive testing is to be used in patients with recently controlled pain syndromes, *it should be done promptly.* Since many of the noninvasive procedures used to estimate the likelihood of disease and to stratify risk employ exercise testing, it is important to consider their safety and efficacy. At least one report has shown that submaximal exercise testing can be performed safely and that the results of the tests provide important prognostic information.[43]

Refining the Estimated Likelihood of Coronary Artery Disease Presence or Absence

Probability Analysis Employing Bayes' Theorem as an Aid in Clinical Decision Making

Fundamental to any discussion of decision making is an understanding of the ability of a test to establish the presence or absence of a disease. This is commonly defined as the test's sensitivity, specificity, and predictive value.[44] Table 19-2 gives the definitions for sensitivity, specificity, and predictive value, along with the equations for Bayes' theorem. With a perfectly accurate test both sensitivity and specificity are 1, and the predictive value is always 100 percent for presence of disease if the result is positive and 0 percent for presence of the disease if the result is negative, regardless of pretest disease likelihood. However, since most of the diagnostic tests discussed in this chapter are less than perfectly sensitive and specific, results should be viewed as probability statements about the presence or absence of disease, derived from the interaction of the test result with the patient's pretest likelihood of disease. By employing Bayes' theorem, which incorporates values for pretest disease likelihood in addition to test sensitivity and test specificity, the clinician can calculate the predictive value of a test result.

Once a test has been performed, the question of its predictive value is most relevant. For example, if

TABLE 19-2 Glossary

True positive (TP):	Positive result in patient with disease.
True negative (TN):	Negative result in patient without disease.
False positive (FP):	Positive result in patient without disease.
False negative (FN):	Negative result in patient with disease.
Sensitivity:	$\frac{TP}{TP + FN}$
Specificity:	$\frac{TN}{TN + FP}$
Predictive value of a positive test for disease presence:	$\frac{TP}{TP + FP}$
Predictive value of a negative test for disease absence:	$\frac{TN}{TN + FN}$
Bayes' theorem:	The probability of disease presence with a positive test =

$$\frac{\text{Sensitivity} \times \text{prevalence}}{(\text{Sensitivity} \times \text{prevalence}) + [(1 - \text{specificity}) \times (1 - \text{prevalence})]}$$

The probability of disease presence with a negative test =

$$\frac{(1 - \text{sensitivity}) \times \text{prevalence}}{(1 - \text{sensitivity} \times \text{prevalence}) + [\text{specificity} \times (1 - \text{prevalence})]}$$

a patient gives a history of "typical angina" pectoris, what are the chances that coronary disease is present? Noninvasive testing can be most efficiently utilized if (1) an estimate of the likelihood of disease is made during the initial evaluation, (2) test sensitivity and specificity are known for the population being tested, and (3) the predictive value of the possible test result(s) is calculated using the foregoing data in Bayes' theorem. *To best assess the merits of a given test and decide among alternative procedures, it is important to calculate the predictive values before any testing is pursued.*

As discussed in the introductory section of this chapter, the patient's age, sex, pain syndrome, and risk factors can be translated into the pretest likelihood of disease.[5] Algorithms are now being developed that also utilize data from the patient's resting ECG.[18] Other equations estimate the probability that a patient will survive to a given time.[13] *Since these equations do not encompass all the data available to the physician, they are best used in concert with excellent, experienced clinical judgment.*

Further testing is indicated only when the initial evaluation leaves at least moderate uncertainty as to the presence or absence of disease or the risk of future cardiac events. Uncertainty in this context is taken to mean an intermediate rather than an undefined likelihood. *The clinician should then choose a test that has been validated in a large and representative patient population*[45] *and learn the properties and validity of the proposed test in the local laboratory.*

Perhaps the most difficult step in medical decision making is the integration of a wide variety of clinical and laboratory data into the thought process that leads to the final diagnosis. Several formalized mathematical systems have been developed to aid the clinician in this process. Multiple regression is one such system. In multiple regression, clinical and laboratory parameters are entered alone and in combination into an equation that is designed to predict the presence or absence of a given characteristic (e.g., coronary artery disease). If a parameter (e.g., ECG exercise test result) makes an independent, statistically significant contribution to the prediction of the characteristic in question, it becomes part of the final equation. The magnitude of its contribution to the final prediction is given by its regression coefficient, and this can be compared with the coefficient of other predictors. A particularly powerful aspect of this approach is its ability to examine the added impact of a test result on prediction in the setting of an already extensive data base. For example, one can ask whether an ECG exercise test result improves the prediction of disease presence or absence once the patient's history, physical examination, etc., have been entered into the regression equation.[46]

Bayes' theorem is an alternative, more intuitive, approach to the integration of a large body of data. When using this approach, the posttest likelihood from one test becomes the pretest likelihood for the next test. Tests applied sequentially must meet the criterion of conditional independence; that is, the test should provide insight into differing aspects of the pathophysiological process. For example, ECG exercise testing hinges on electrochemical alterations that result from ischemia, while exercise thallium scintigraphy provides a measure of relative coronary blood flow. In the multiple regression approach, correlations among test results are detected during the analysis, and only the strongest independent predictors are entered into the final equation. When using Bayes' theorem, such exclusions must be made prospectively based on empiric observations and knowledge of pathophysiology. *It is encouraging that when Bayes' theorem and the multiple regression method were compared for their ability to predict the presence or absence of coronary disease, the estimates of disease likelihood were remarkably similar.*[47]

Because of its relative simplicity, we will emphasize the use of Bayes' theorem in integrating the significance of multiple test results. In Fig. 19-4, posttest disease likelihood is shown on the y axis as a function of pretest likelihood on the x axis. Bayes' theorem was used to generate these curves for the ECG, thallium, and radionuclide ventriculogram (MUGA) exercise tests. To illustrate the use of Bayes' theorem, consider a 45-year-old man with "atypical" chest pain. His pretest likelihood for coronary disease is 0.46. Should he have a positive ECG exercise test result, his posttest likelihood of disease would be approximately 0.86. This value becomes his pretest likelihood for an exercise thallium scan. Should the thallium scan be positive, the likelihood of disease would increase to 0.98, but should it be negative, the likelihood of disease would decrease to 0.63. Additional tests can be applied as needed to more

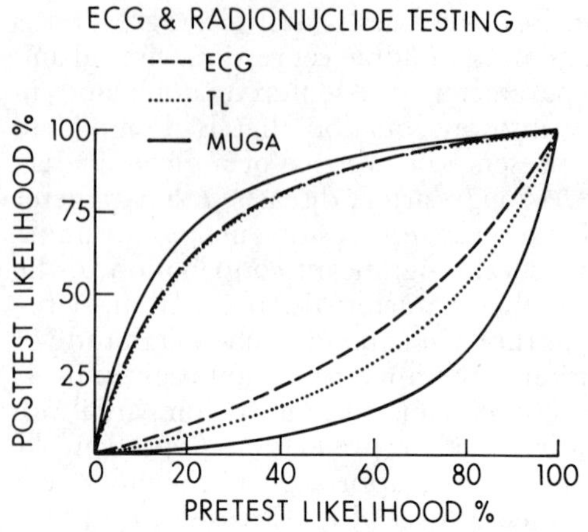

FIGURE 19-4 The use of Bayes' theorem in the diagnosis of coronary artery disease. The impact of exercise ECG, thallium (Tl), and ventriculographic (MUGA) test results as a function of pretest disease likelihood is shown. The curves above the line of identity represent positive test results, while those below the line of identity represent negative test results. See text for additional discussion. (*Adapted from S. E. Epstein, Implications of Probability Analysis on the Strategy Used for Noninvasive Detection of Coronary Artery Disease. Am. J. Cardiol., 46:491, 1980. Reproduced with permission from the publisher and author.*)

firmly establish a final diagnosis, as long as they meet the criterion of conditional independence.

Interaction of Evaluation Techniques with Initial Likelihood Groupings

Rationale for Exercise Testing

In the face of severe stenoses, the diseased coronary artery can still deliver adequate nutrient flow to meet the metabolic needs of the myocardium at rest.[48] The utility of exercise testing rests on the fact that during dynamic exertion in normal subjects, increasing oxygen demand is satisfied by increasing coronary flow.[49] In patients with coronary disease, however, coronary blood flow during exercise cannot increase sufficiently to meet myocardial energy demand, and a supply-demand imbalance results. This imbalance produces myocardial ischemia, manifested by chest pain,[50] electrochemical alterations,[51] regional wall motion abnormalities,[52] and release of nonprotein metabolic products such as potassium, lactate, and adenosine,[53] all of which can be measured by invasive or noninvasive methods.

Electrocardiographic Exercise Testing

Electrocardiographic exercise testing (Chap. 98) capitalizes on the reversible electrochemical alterations that are associated with ischemia. With proper precautions maximal treadmill or bicycle exercise testing can be performed with minimal danger.[54]

Numerous variables influence the diagnostic accuracy of the electrocardiographic exercise test. Left ventricular hypertrophy, hypokalemia, hyperventilation, digitalis therapy, left bundle branch block, and Wolff-Parkinson-White syndrome can produce ST-segment displacement in the absence of obstructive coronary disease.[55] Abnormal ST-segment displacement in patients with these conditions should be considered uninterpretable. ECG exercise testing for most diagnostic purposes also requires that patients be exercised to symptomatic endpoints and achieve at least 85 percent of their age-predicted heart rate in order that the absence of ST-segment displacement be considered a negative result; otherwise, the result is inconclusive.[55] Patients who are likely to have inconclusive or uninterpretable ECG results should be prospectively identified and referred for nuclear exercise tests since uninterpretable results are relatively rare, and though somewhat dependent on maximal exercise, nuclear tests are not so markedly impaired by suboptimal patient performance.

Traditionally the electrocardiographic result has been dichotomized as positive if there is ≥ 1-mm ST depression, and negative if there is < 1-mm ST depression during exercise, as the former increases and the latter decreases the likelihood of disease presence. The sensitivity and specificity of these criteria in coronary disease diagnosis are 0.66 and 0.89, respectively.[55] As more ST-segment depression during exercise is required for a positive test, the specificity rises at the expense of sensitivity. Therefore, each degree of ST-segment depression during exercise has a unique sensitivity and specificity that can be employed to define more precisely the predictive value of the test result.[56]

Nuclear Exercise Testing

An exercise thallium scan (Chap. 109) is considered positive if there is a relative diminution in thallium activity in a significant portion of the heart immediately after exercise, implying a relative diminution in blood flow. If activity becomes more uniform with time, the implication is ischemia. If it does not, the deficiency of activity is considered to be due to myocardial infarction.[57] Since the treadmill protocols used for exercise thallium testing are identical to those used for ECG testing, both the ECG and thallium results are often useful.[58] An exercise radionuclide ventriculogram is considered positive for coronary disease if there is a subnormal ejection fraction increase with exercise in conjunction with regional wall motion abnormalities.[59] The nature of the bicycle protocols used for wall motion tests make the ECG portion of the test less valuable.

Several factors other than myocardial ischemia can also produce "positive" nuclear exercise tests. For example, x-ray attenuation due to an overlying breast can appear to produce a thallium defect. Abnormal ejection fraction responses to exercise may be seen in patients with valvular heart disease[60] and cardiomyopathy.[61] A blunted ejection fraction response may be the result of the normal aging process.[62] For these reasons, regional wall motion abnormalities during exercise should be sought as evidence of ischemia.

In Fig. 19-4, ECG results are dichotomized as positive or negative to illustrate the impact (posttest likelihood or predictive value) of test results over the entire range of possible pretest likelihoods. For comparison, the impact of positive and negative exercise radionuclide studies is shown assuming that the exercise thallium scintigram has a sensitivity of 0.76 and specificity of 0.88 and that the sensitivity and specificity of the exercise radionuclide ventriculogram are both 0.90.

Use of Exercise Tests to Establish the Presence or Absence of Disease

Patients with Low Likelihoods of Disease

In subjects who have low pretest likelihoods of disease (< 15 percent), manipulation of the equations for test accuracy indicates that regardless of which test is chosen, a negative result can be expected in well over 80 percent of the tests performed. An even greater proportion of these negative results will be truly negative. In other words, the posttest likelihood will be extremely low and radionuclide procedures alone or in combination will add little over the ECG exercise test alone. Most positive results are not helpful since for all three tests, positive results are usually falsely positive.

On theoretical grounds, exercise testing in subjects with low likelihoods of disease (including asymptomatic individuals) is best suited to confirming the clinical impression of absence of disease. Only if the ECG exercise test is likely to produce an inconclusive or uninterpretable result should a radionuclide test be substituted. Otherwise, it is most cost-effective to use the ECG exercise test in this low-prevalence population. Testing should not be done routinely, however, since in asymptomatic individuals the diagnostic yield is extremely low.[15]

Even though symptoms remotely suggestive of angina pectoris (nonanginal or atypical chest pain) increase the likelihood of coronary disease, the prevalence of disease is still quite low in younger individuals (particularly women). There are several reasons why ECG exercise testing is clinically useful in this symptomatic but low-prevalence population. While measuring the ST-segment response, the physician can observe and question the patient to clarify uncertainties in the history.[63] If the ST-segment response is negative and the patient has no chest pain during exercise, it is unlikely that coronary disease is responsible for the patient's complaints, and other causes for chest pain should be sought. In those few cases where the patient has a positive ST-segment response, further noninvasive testing is usually necessary since most positive results are mildly positive and not highly predictive. But when symptoms of typical angina occur in conjunction with a slightly positive ST-segment response, medical therapy should be instituted and followed up with testing to confirm its efficacy. In those instances in which the ECG is markedly positive, especially in combination with chest pain and exertional hypotension or markedly diminished exercise capacity, coronary arteriography is indicated and angioplasty or bypass grafting should be considered. Further noninvasive testing in such patients is not productive since such markedly positive ECG results in subjects with more than a trivial pretest likelihood of coronary disease are reasonably predictive of the presence of coronary disease. Under these circumstances, a negative radionuclide result would not lower disease likelihood below that obtained from the initial evaluation alone.[58]

Patients with Intermediate Likelihoods of Disease

Asymptomatic individuals with multiple cardiac risk factors, and most individuals with "atypical" or nonanginal chest pain have intermediate pretest likelihoods (0.16 to 0.84) of having coronary disease (Table 19-1). From Fig. 19-4, it can be seen that for these individuals, the posttest likelihood of coronary disease remains relatively high after a negative ECG result. Further, the predictive value of a positive result will often be less than 0.85. Because of their superior sensitivity, nuclear exercise tests are more suited to excluding disease in these patients. In some patients, positive test results may have to be reinforced with further testing before the diagnosis of ischemic heart disease is finalized. In a study that incorporated both ECG and nuclear exercise test results into the calculation of posttest likelihoods of disease, a firm diagnosis could be made in 74 percent of patients in contrast to 37 percent if ECG exercise testing alone was used.[58] Clearly, the best clinical use of thallium or ventriculographic exercise testing is among subjects with intermediate pretest likelihoods of disease.[64,65]

Patients with High Pretest Likelihoods of Disease

If the clinician's goal is to establish or exclude the diagnosis of coronary disease in the population of patients with high pretest likelihood of disease, only marginal advantage can be gained by further testing (Fig. 19-4). This is particularly true of patients with "typical" angina.

Decision making is more complex when there are atypical complaints and moderate or high likelihoods of disease by virtue of advanced age or multiple risk factors. Observation of the patient during a nuclear exercise test can be useful in clarifying the nature of the pain syndrome. If during a maximal nuclear exercise test, the patient has no chest pain, and the nuclear result is normal, it is very unlikely that obstructive coronary artery disease is responsible for the patient's chest pain syndrome. Atypical chest pain during exercise coupled with a negative nuclear test result should lead to a search for noncardiac causes for the chest pain. The combination of typical symptoms and a negative test result is rarely seen, but when it does occur, a trial of antianginal therapy may be warranted. If drug therapy is unsuccessful, the demonstration of normal coronary arteries without provokable spasm at *cardiac catheterization* is sometimes necessary to reassure the patient of the very low likelihood of a major cardiac event.

When there is "typical" chest pain during the nuclear exercise test accompanied by a positive scan result, myocardial ischemia is almost certainly responsible. The specifics of the scan result can then be used to assign the patient to the best available therapeutic regimen. An ECG exercise test, with or without nuclear scanning, can be helpful in documenting therapeutic efficacy. Atypical pain or no pain during exercise and a positive scan may rarely be seen in these patients. Since the relative merits of surgical and medical therapy are largely unexplored in this group with "silent" ischemia, a medical trial of an "anti-ischemia" regimen is a reasonable approach. If this trial fails to produce symptomatic relief or ameliorate test evidence of ischemia, cardiac catheterization may be indicated, particulary if the noninvasive test results suggest a high risk of a future cardiac event. The demonstration of normal coronary arteries at catheterization is very useful, but the presence of obstructive coronary artery disease in this patient population presents a true dilemma (Chap. 45). Invasive metabolic studies to unearth findings of ischemia along with the chest pain may be useful.

Coronary Arteriography and Ventriculography

Coronary arteriography (Chaps. 45 and 98) is the only current method by which both the presence and the topography of structural coronary disease can be established with certainty. Ventricular function can also be evaluated with the addition of contrast left ventriculography and pressure measurements. The cardiologist should have clear reasons for performing these tests since they are invasive and carry certain risks to the patient, and since the procedures are costly to the medical care system. In general, cardiac catheterization and angiography should be considered in patients who are in the coronary age group and being evaluated for any type of heart surgery; who have unexplained chest pain, when noninvasive evaluations continue to leave serious uncertainty about a diagnosis of coronary disease; or who are asymptomatic but exhibit exercise responses compatible with severe coronary disease.

Coronary Arteriography: Diagnosing the Presence or Absence of Coronary Lesions

When coronary arteriograms are analyzed (Chap. 108), the narrowing is frequently expressed as percent decrease in the diameter of the vessels. The corresponding reduction in cross-sectional area of the lumen is proportional to the square of the decrease in diameter. In humans, 72 percent luminal diameter-narrowing stenosis (92 percent cross-sectional decrease) has been estimated to result in myocardial ischemia at rest, but lesser lesions may produce ischemia during exercise.[66] Long segments of stenosis or multiple lesions appear to reduce coronary flow more markedly than do discrete single, short lesions.[67]

The interpretation of coronary arteriograms is largely subjective, and there is significant intraobserver and interobserver variability in assessing the severity of lesions and in defining the number of coronary vessels involved in any one patient. One finds both inconsistency of readings of the same lesion and substantial disagreement among readers in identifying the number of vessels narrowed by 70 percent or more.[68] Comparison of arteriographically estimated stenoses with measurements made at postmortem examination indicates that angiographers generally underestimate the severity of the obstruction.[69] Technically, contrast arteriograms are two-dimensional representations of a three-dimensional structure. It should be remembered, also, that the coronary lumen may be compromised temporarily or permanently by platelet and/or fibrin thrombi.[21] Finally, the vascular tone may vary, either in the area of the plaque or in the adjacent reference segment, either spontaneously or in response to therapy with vasoactive drugs; thus, the appearance of a lesion may be altered at the time of angiography.[70]

The complexity of the anatomic variations, dynamic changes in coronary stenoses, and subjective interpretations make it difficult to predict the precise physiological effect of many lesions observed in coronary arteriograms. In one study, when direct measurements of reactive hyperemic responses of diseased human coronary vessels were compared with qualitative angiographic readings, no significant correlation was found.[71] Despite the limitations, subjective angiographic readings have provided important prognostic information related to survival from single-, double-, and triple-vessel and left main coronary involvement[6] and are required if coronary bypass grafting or angioplasty is to be done. Arteriographically defined stenoses must, however, be interpreted in the context of complete clinical data.

Not all ischemic syndromes are due to arteriographically demonstrable lesions. Patients with Prinzmetal's angina may have coronary arteries that appear normal at the time of angiography, but can be stimulated to spasm following the intravenous administration of ergonovine (Chap. 98).[72] Spasm, however, more often coexists with structural coronary disease.[73] Ergonovine may be most useful in patients with a characteristic pain pattern but in whom electrocardiograms have not been recorded during pain. Although ergonovine tests are generally safe, there is a risk of producing nitrate-resistant spasm and subsequent infarction. Vasodilating agents should be immediately available to reverse the spasm by intracoronary injection if sublingual nitroglycerin initially fails. Ergonovine should not be given outside the catheterization laboratory.[74]

Coronary Sinus Studies: The Presence or Absence of Ischemia

The observation of coronary lesions by coronary arteriography does not establish the presence of myocardial ischemia. When preangiographic investigation has left doubt as to whether myocardial ischemia is present, invasive techniques may prove helpful. One method for doing this is by coronary sinus studies (Chap. 108). The cardiac metabolic abnormalities reported during myocardial ischemia have been outlined in Chaps. 5 and 44. The technique involves placing a catheter in the coronary sinus to measure coronary blood flow and metabolites, including oxygen, lactate, pyruvate, and free fatty acids.[75]

Coronary blood flow is measured by the washout from the myocardium of foreign materials that are delivered to the heart by intravenous injection, by direct intracoronary injection, or after inhalation of a reference gas.[66] In recent years thermal dilution measurements of cold solution infused into the coronary sinus have frequently been employed.[76] Although consistent abnormalities in coronary blood flow are not present at rest in patients with ischemic heart disease, diminished flow in areas distal to an obstructed vessel can be demonstrated when energy demands are increased or when reactive hyperemia is induced by injection of angiographic contrast medium.[77]

The most frequently employed measure of myocardial ischemia in humans has been the determination of lactate extraction or production across the myocardium. Lactate is normally extracted by the heart. Lactate production by the myocardium is probably abnormal, but low (< 10 percent) or diminishing levels of lactate extraction during stress are not necessarily diagnostic of ischemia in humans.[78] Factors other than ischemia such as fatty acid metabolism, the nutritional state, or levels of circulating catecholamines may alter myocardial lactate metabolism in any individual.[79]

Other metabolites released from the myocardium during ischemia include potassium, phosphate, adenosine, and inosine. These have not proved to be more sensitive than lactate alone.

One problem with coronary sinus studies in ischemic heart disease is that coronary disease is a regional condition whereas myocardial metabolism is heterogeneous. If there is disease of the right coronary artery alone, ischemia might not be detected in coronary sinus studies because much of the sampled blood emanates from the normal left coronary bed and dilutes the abnormal venous drainage from the right coronary bed. Detection of ischemia in the area perfused by the left anterior descending coronary artery is more accurate. Attempts have been made to circumvent this problem by sampling the effluent from different areas of the coronary venous system.[80]

Although metabolic and flow studies are not generally used clinically, they may be helpful in some patients with chest pain and angiographically normal coronary arteries. Some of these patients may have myocardial lactate production induced by atrial pacing.[81] Also, patients with Prinzmetal's angina have been shown to decrease coronary blood flow and produce lactate during ergonovine-induced spasm.[82]

Testing to Assess the Severity of Coronary Disease

Patients with Low Likelihoods of Disease

Limitations of Additional Diagnostic Tests

Patients with a low likelihood of coronary disease have an even lower likelihood of having a future coronary event[15] or high-risk coronary anatomy.[83] Many of the positive tests in this group will be falsely positive. Because of this, investigators have designated only markedly abnormal (highly specific) test results as indicators of multivessel coronary disease or a poor prognosis. If, for instance, during ECG exercise testing, early ST-segment depression, hypotension, and angina are combined into a single criterion for a positive result, the specificity is very high and the predictive value for multivessel coronary disease is reasonably good. However, such amalgamated results severely restrict the sensitivity of the test.[84] Similar problems will exist when nuclear exercise test criteria are altered to enhance the predictive value of a positive result.[85] These considerations make testing to define coronary anatomy or risk impractical if the initial evaluation indicates a low likelihood of disease.

Patients with Intermediate or High Likelihoods of Disease

Rationale of Testing

Patients may fall into the category of high likelihood of disease on the basis of either the initial evaluation alone or the combination of the initial evaluation and positive noninvasive test results. An abnormal test result that increases the likelihood of disease can be examined for its prognostic implications. However, the predictive value for multivessel coronary disease or future coronary events must be interpreted in the context of the lower pretest likelihood of disease.

Using our present knowledge, a left main coronary artery obstruction compromising ≥ 50 percent of the vessel diameter is universally acknowledged as an indication for coronary bypass grafting to prolong life.[8,9] This is found in less than 10 percent of patients studied angiographically. The prevalence of left main disease increases with age, chest pain typical of angina, and unstable angina.[19,83] About one-third of symptomatic patients undergoing arteriography will have three-vessel, and another one-third will have two-vessel, coronary disease. Surgery also appears to prolong life in symptomatic patients with three-vessel disease and depressed ejection fractions.[10] The European Coronary Surgery Study indicates the same is true with patients who have stable angina, three-vessel disease, and good ejection fractions.[9] Although there is some evidence to support the advantage to survival of surgical therapy for most symptomatic patients with multivessel disease, this conclusion is contrary to the findings of the Coronary Artery Surgery Study (Chap. 45).[6] It should be pointed out, however, that 7 percent of the patients (who had no angina or class 1 or 2 stable angina) in the study who had three-vessel disease crossed over to bypass surgery annually because of unacceptable angina.

The survival advantage offered by surgery in substantial segment(s) of the patient population with a high prevalence of coronary artery disease is a compelling reason to proceed with risk stratification beyond the initial evaluation. The initial clinical evaluation is frequently not helpful in distinguishing single-vessel from three-vessel or left main disease in these patients.[83] It is desirable for the clinician to proceed further to "rule out" high-risk lesions.

Exercise Testing to Assess the Severity of Coronary Disease

The sensitivity of both ECG and nuclear exercise testing increases in proportion to the number of coronary arteries with obstructions.[55,86,87] The superior sensitivity of nuclear exercise testing makes it the preferred test (Chap 98). It is very unlikely that a patient with typical angina and three-vessel or left main disease would have a negative nuclear exercise test. Depending on the test type (ECG or nuclear), as much as 50 to 80 percent of patients with single-vessel disease will have positive responses. For this reason, requirements have been stiffened for the diagnosis of multivessel or left main coronary disease. During ECG exercise testing the presence of several manifestations of an extensive ischemic threat are necessary.[84] During thallium scintigraphy, multiple defects corresponding to differing coronary distributions or hang-up of thallium in the lungs will indicate severe ventricular dysfunction during exercise, and this in turn suggests multivessel coronary disease.[85,88] During radionuclide ventriculography, a frank fall in the ejection fraction or regional abnormalities in the distribution of more than one coronary artery is suggestive of multivessel disease.[87] These requirements increase the likelihood that positive test responders are those who may benefit from coronary bypass grafting. Conversely, an entirely normal result is quite predictive of low-risk anatomy. It must be emphasized, however, that failure to demonstrate a *marked* abnormality does not exclude severe coronary disease.

Testing to Assess the Prognosis of Patients with Coronary Disease

Exercise Testing to Assess Prognosis

Exercise testing (Chap. 98) can also be used to stratify risk independent of coronary anatomy. In 1170 medically treated patients with a 49 percent prevalence of significant coronary disease, the 1-year mortality was only 1 percent in 75 percent of the patients who were able to achieve a heart rate of 160 beats per minute, and/or had negative ST-segment responses. Eleven percent of the total population had limited exercise tolerance and a positive test at a low heart rate. Mortality in these patients was 12 percent at 1 year.[89] Data from the Coronary Artery Surgery Study registry indicated that in a population with a 67 percent prevalence of coronary disease, 32 percent of patients had negative ST-segment responses and could exercise to at least stage 3 of a Bruce protocol.[90] Their annual mortality was less than 1 percent. Twelve percent of the population had ≥ 1-mm ST depression and could only exercise into stage 1. Their annual mortality was 5 percent. Evidence of left ventricular dysfunction, either on clinical (reduced exercise tolerance) or ventriculographic grounds (regional wall motion score), added significantly to the future risk, regardless of ST-segment response.

Thus, ECG exercise testing can be used to identify a population of patients with a low risk of death from coronary disease who can safely be managed medically *and higher-risk populations who should have cardiac catheterization.* When the results of catheterization and exercise test data are analyzed in a multivariate fashion, exercise duration and the ST-segment response are shown to be significant predictors of subsequent prognosis, but ventricular function and extent of coronary disease, respectively, are the most powerful predictors. Therefore, patients with less severe anatomic coronary disease and a high-risk exercise test may not have a benign prognosis, especially when ventricular function is abnormal. Some patients with three-vessel disease and preserved ventricular function can exercise beyond stage 4 of a Bruce protocol and have an excellent prognosis.[90]

The few studies on prognosis after nuclear exercise testing are promising but must be interpreted cautiously. In 100 medically treated patients without prior infarction (angiographically proven coronary disease in 42), the number of transient thallium defects was the best predictor of future cardiac events.[91]

In 386 medically treated patients with symptomatic coronary disease followed up to 4 years after exercise radionuclide angiography, multivariate analysis which excluded catheterization data indicated that only the exercise ejection fraction contributed independent information about the likelihood of a future cardiac event.[13] The 19 percent of patients with exercise ejection fractions below 35 percent had a 2-year mortality rate estimated at 40 percent. When the severity of coronary disease was added to the predictive model, this provided independent information, but its additional contribution to the exercise ejection fraction was relatively small.

Cardiac Catheterization and Angiography in the Assessment of Prognosis and Need for Intervention

A number of prognostic indexes using coronary angiographic information have been employed. These include the number of diseased vessels, the number of proximally involved vessels, and several indexes that empirically score the severity of disease.[92] All of these indexes are predictive of survival, but the predictive values are markedly improved by adding ventricular function into the equation. In general, the worse the ventricular function, the more vessels critically stenosed, and the more proximal the stenoses, the poorer the prognosis will be. These features are also useful in predicting which patient will derive the most benefit in terms of improving survival from surgical therapy.

The Resting Ventriculogram

The resting contrast ventriculogram (Chap. 108), or nuclear ventriculogram or two-dimensional echocardiographic ventriculogram, all provide important prognostic information that helps in making a decision for or against surgery. It also helps the surgeon plan the optimal procedure. By measuring the ejection fraction it provides useful information on prognosis and also assists in determining the choice of therapy.[93] The ventriculogram is also useful in assessing regional wall motion. The wall motion may be normal or may show decreased inward movement (hypokinesis), absent movement (akinesis), or paradoxical movement (dyskinesis). Patient mortality with medical therapy varies inversely with the resting ejection fraction and directly with the extent of wall motion abnormalities.[32] The ventriculogram may also demonstrate the presence of a discrete left ventricular aneurysm which may be clinically manifest as congestive heart failure, arrhythmias, or systemic emboli.[94] This is important because it may be necessary to surgically remove the aneurysm and the ectopic electrical foci (guided by electrophysiological studies).[95]

Intervention Ventriculography

The presence of a hypokinetic or akinetic segment on the resting ventriculogram does not ensure the presence of myocardial scar tissue. Regional wall motion may show improvement after the preload is acutely reduced by administration of sublingual nitroglycerin or during the positive inotropic state of postextrasystolic potentiation.[96] This postintervention improvement has been taken as evidence that the affected myocardium is viable but in a depressed functional state because of inadequate myocardial blood flow. An akinetic but viable area may be functionally improved by coronary artery bypass grafting.[96] Recently, noninvasive nuclear methods have been employed to identify dysfunctioning but viable myocardium in the territory supplied by stenotic coronary vessels.[97]

Digital subtraction is a recent advance in radiologically defining left ventricular anatomy and function. This technique permits angiographic evaluation of the left ventricle using small quantities of contrast medium injected selectively into the left ventricle (Chap. 108). Multiple injections can safely be made during interventions. Furthermore, with improving equipment, excellent ventricular angiograms may be obtained with intravenous injections, permitting virtually noninvasive contrast ventriculography to be performed both at rest and with interventions such as exercise and pacing.[98]

The Role of Hemodynamic Evaluation

Groups of patients with coronary artery disease and impaired hemodynamics have poorer medical prognoses than groups of patients with normal hemodynamics. Also, patients with depressed cardiac output tend to have lower rates of survival after surgical therapy than after medical treatment.[99] However, these hemodynamic abnormalities can be correlated with ventriculographic abnormalities that are of prognostic value, and do not appear to add independently to the predictive power of the ventriculogram except in patients with mitral regurgitation, ventricular aneurysm, or ventricular septal defect. In these patients, hemodynamic and angiographic evaluation is important to provide baseline information against which the relative value of medical versus surgical therapy can be measured.

Risks of Catheterization and Coronary Angiography

Numerous complications may arise from coronary arteriography, and the risk of these must be weighed against the risk of not knowing the extent of the patient's disease (Chaps. 45 and 108). A collaborative study demonstrated a 0.2 percent mortality rate within 24 h of catheterization among patients with coronary artery disease and a 0.25 percent nonfatal myocardial infarction rate within 48 h.[100] In patients with greater than 50 percent narrowing of the left main coronary artery, the mortality plus infarction rate was almost seven times as great as in other cases.

Patients with congestive heart failure, hypotension, ejection fractions less than 30 percent, and arrhythmias prior to catheterization also had an increased risk. Thus, patients with the greatest risk from the natural history of their disease have the highest risk from cardiac catheterization and angiography. The risks of angiography vary among different laboratories and the clinician must decide whether the risk of the procedure is outweighed by the potential benefit to be gained from the information (see Chaps. 45 and 108).

Patients Recovering from an Acute Myocardial Infarction

Data gathered from the initial evaluation in the coronary care unit can be used to plot a definitive therapeutic strategy in patients recovering from an acute myocardial infarction. Evidence of ongoing ischemia despite aggressive medical therapy should prompt strong consideration of a surgical approach. Congestive heart failure and ventricular arrhythmias, which may or may not be related to ongoing ischemia, also portend a poor prognosis despite medical therapy.[11] Although patients with these problems are at higher risk of death, there is little firm evidence that in the absence of further ischemia, coronary bypass grafting will reduce this risk. Holter monitoring to assess both the severity of ventricular arrhythmias and the efficacy of any subsequent antiarrhythmic therapy may be indicated in these patients. Once these patients can be stabilized, evidence of a residual ischemic threat should be actively sought. This process should be undertaken early since the greatest risk of dying is in the first 3 months following infarction.

Low-level exercise testing 10 to 14 days after a myocardial infarction is a safe, relatively effective means of stratifying risk.[12] The largest experience to date is with ECG exercise testing. Theroux et al. used 1 mm of ST-segment depression as a criterion to separate a group with a 27 percent 1-year mortality from a group with only 2.1 percent risk.[12] Subsequent studies reported a relative lack of sensitivity for low-level ECG exercise testing.[101]

In a group of 140 stable postinfarction patients, low-level ECG exercise testing, low-level thallium exercise testing, and coronary arteriography were equally effective in identifying patients who died in the follow-up period.[102] However, thallium testing was a superior predictor of recurrent nonfatal infarction and severe angina. Thallium scintigraphy following the intravenous injection of dipyridamole also appears to be an excellent prognosticator[103] and has the advantage of not requiring exercise.

In 61 patients an average of 19 days after infarction, low-level supine exercise radionuclide ventriculography demonstrated that failure of the ejection fraction to increase during exercise was highly sensitive and specific (> 95 percent) and superior to electrocardiographic testing for predicting future cardiac events (including heart failure and coronary surgery) during a 6-month follow-up.[104] Multivariate analyses revealed that only the peak submaximal exercise ejection fraction and a history of previous infarction were predictive of subsequent death, recurrent infarction, or refractory angina.

Thus, ECG, thallium scintigraphy, and radionuclide ventriculography with exercise have all been shown to be useful in identifying patients at high risk for early death. Preliminary data indicate that nuclear exercise testing may be superior to ECG testing for detecting future nonfatal infarctions or refractory angina. Regardless of the test type employed, a positive result requires some manifestation of ischemia to be present. It is logical to assume that procedures aimed at ameliorating the ischemic threat will also ameliorate the higher risk.

Most patients tested to date have been on medical therapy. *Since these tests predict high risk despite medical therapy, it is reasonable to pursue cardiac catheterization in patients with positive tests.* The decision to proceed with bypass grafting or angioplasty, as in patients with chronic angina, must then take into consideration the adequacy of medical therapy, the severity of coronary disease, and ventricular function. At present, however, there are no large-scale randomized clinical trials that have specifically addressed the issue of medical versus surgical therapy in postinfarction patients with high-risk noninvasive test results.

References

1. Report of the Joint International Society and Federation of Cardiology, World Health Organization Task Force on Standardization of Clinical Nomenclature and Criteria for Diagnosis of Ischemic Heart Disease, *Circulation,* 59:607, 1979.
2. Gillum, R. F., Folsom, A., Luepker, R. V., Jacobs, D. R. Jr., Kottke, T. E., Gomez-Marin, O., Prineas, R. J., Taylor, Henry L., and Blackburn, J.: Sudden Death and Acute Myocardial Infarction in a Metropolitan Area, 1970–1980, *N. Engl. J. Med.,* 309:1353, 1983.
3. "Heart Facts, 1980," American Heart Association, Inc., New York, 1979.
4. Epstein, S. E.: Value and Limitations of the Electrocardiographic Response to Exercise in the Assessment of Patients with Coronary Artery Disease, *Am. J. Cardiol.,* 42:667, 1978.
5. Diamond, G. A., and Forrester, J. S.: Analysis of Probability as an Aid in the Clinical Diagnosis of Coronary Artery Disease, *N. Engl. J. Med.,* 300:1350, 1979.
6. CASS Principal Investigators and their Associates: Coronary Artery Surgery Study (CASS): A Randomized Trial of Coronary Artery Bypass Surgery: Survival Data, *Circulation,* 68:939, 1983.
7. CASS Principal Investigators and their Associates: Coronary Artery Surgery Study (CASS): A Randomized Trial of Coronary Artery Bypass Surgery Quality of Life in Patients Randomly Assigned to Treatment Groups, *Circulation,* 68:951, 1983.
8. Takaro, T., Hultgren, H. N., Lipton, M. J., Detre, K. M., and Participants in the Study Group: The VA Cooperative Randomized Study of Surgery for Coronary Occlusive Disease: II. Subgroup with Significant Left Main Lesions, *Circulation,* 54:III–107, 1976.
9. European Coronary Surgery Study Group: Long-term Re-

sults of Prospective Randomized Study of Coronary Artery Bypass Surgery in Stable Angina Pectoris, *Lancet,* 27:1173, 1982.
10. Hammermeister, K. E.: The Effect of Coronary Bypass Surgery on Survival, *Prog. Cardiovasc. Dis.,* 25:297, 1983.
11. The Multicenter Postinfarction Research Group: Risk Stratification and Survival after Myocardial Infarction, *N. Engl. J. Med.,* 309:331, 1983.
12. Theroux, P., Waters, D. D., Halphen, C., Debaisieux, J. C., and Mizgala, H. F.: Prognostic Value of Exercise Testing Soon after Myocardial Infarction, *N. Engl. J. Med.,* 301:341, 1979.
13. Pryor, D. B., Harrell, F. E., Jr., Lee, K. L., Rosati, R. A., Coleman, R. E., Cobb, F. R., Califf, R. M., and Jones, R. H.: Prognostic Indicators from Radionuclide Angiography in Medically Treated Patients with Coronary Artery Disease, *Am. J. Cardiol.,* 53:18, 1984.
14. "Coronary Risk Handbook," American Heart Association, Inc., New York, 1973.
15. Giagnoni, E., Secchi, M. B., Wu, S. C., Morabito, A., Oltrana, L., Mancarella, S., Volpin, N., Fossa, L., Bettazzi, L., Arangio, G., Sachero, A., and Folli, G.: Prognostic Value of Exercise EKG Testing in Asymptomatic Normotensive Subjects, *N. Engl. J. Med.,* 309:1085, 1983.
16. Morris, S. N., and McHenry, P. L.: Role of Exercise Stress Testing in Healthy Subjects and Patients with Coronary Heart Disease, *Am. J. Cardiol.,* 42:659, 1978.
17. Principal Investigators of CASS and their Associates: National Heart, Lung and Blood Institute Coronary Artery Surgery Study, *Circulation,* 63:I–1, 1981.
18. Pryor, D. B., Harrell, F. E., Jr., Lee, K. L., Califf, R. M., and Rosati, R. A.: Estimating the Likelihood of Significant Coronary Artery Disease, *Am. J. Med.,* 75:771, 1983.
19. Betriu, A., Castaner, A., Sanz, G. A., Pare, J. C., Roig, E., Coll, S., Magrina, J., and Navarro-Lopez, F.: Angiographic Findings 1 Month after Myocardial Infarction: A Prospective Study of 259 Survivors, *Circulation,* 65:1099, 1982.
20. Sanz, G., Castaner, A., Betriu, A., Magrina, J., Roig, E., Coll, S., Pare, J. C., and Navarro-Lopez, F.: Determinants of Prognosis in Survivors of Myocardial Infarction: A Prospective Clinical Angiographic Study, *N. Engl. J. Med.,* 306:1065, 1982.
21. DeWood, M. A., Spores, J., Notske, R., Mouser, L. T., Burroughs, R., Golden, M. S., and Lang, H. T.: Prevalence of Total Coronary Occlusion during the Early Hours of Transmural Myocardial Infarction, *N. Engl J. Med.,* 303:897, 1980.
22. Norwegian Multicenter Study Group: Timolol-Induced Reduction in Mortality and Reinfarction in Patients Surviving Acute Myocardial Infarction, *N. Engl. J. Med.,* 304:801, 1981.
23. Beta-Blocker Heart Attack Research Group: A Randomized Trial of Propranolol in Patients with Acute Myocardial Infarction: I. Mortality Results, *JAMA,* 247:1707, 1982.
24. Epstein, S. E., Palmeri, S. T., and Patterson, R. E.: Evaluation of Patients after Acute Myocardial Infarction: Indications for Cardiac Catheterization and Surgical Intervention, *N. Engl. J. Med.,* 307:1487. 1982.
25. Miller, R. R., Amsterdam, E. A., Bogren, J. G., Massumi, R. A., Zelis, R., and Mason, D. T.: Electrocardiographic and Cineangiographic Correlations in Assessment of the Location, Nature and Extent of Abnormal Left Ventricular Segmental Contraction in Coronary Artery Disease, *Circulation,* 49:447, 1974.
26. Grande, P., Christiansen, C., Pedersen, A., and Christensen, M. S.: Optimal Diagnosis in Acute Myocardial Infarction: A Cost-Effectiveness Study, *Circulation,* 61:723, 1980.
27. Friedman, S. E.: "Diagnostic Electrocardiography and Vectorcardiography," 2d ed., McGraw-Hill Book Company, New York, 1977.
28. Helfant, R. H., Bodenheimer, M. M., and Banka, V. S.: Asynergy in Coronary Heart Disease: Evolving Clinical and Pathophysiologic Concepts, *Ann. Intern. Med.,* 87:475, 1977.
29. Ideker, R. E., Wagner, G. S., Ruth, W. K., Alonso, D. R., Bishop, S. P., Bloor, C. M., Fallon, J. T., Gottlieb, G. J., Hackel, D. B., Phillips, H. R., Reimer, K. A., Roark, S. F., Rogers, W. J., Savage, R. M., White, R. D., and Selvester, R. H.: Evaluation of a QRS Scoring System for Estimating Myocardial Infarct Size: II. Correlation with Quantitative Anatomic Findings for Anterior Infarcts, *Am. J. Cardiol.,* 49:1604, 1982.
30. Roark, S. F., Ideker, R. E., Wagner, G. S., Alonso, D. R., Bishop, S. P., Bloor, C. M., Fallon, J. T., Gottlieb, G. J., Hackel, D. B., Phillips, H. R., Reimer, K. A., Rogers, W. J., Ruth, W. K., Savage, R. M., White, R. D., and Selvester, R. H.: Evaluation of a QRS Scoring System for Estimating Myocardial Infarct Size: III. Correlation with Quantative Anatomic Findings for Inferior Infarcts, *Am. J. Cardiol.,* 51:382, 1983.
31. Feild, B. J., Russell, R. O., Jr., Moraski, R. E., Soto, B., Hood, W. P., Jr., Burdeshaw, J. A., Smith, M., Maurer, B. J., and Rackley, C. E.: Left Ventricular Size and Function and Heart Size in the Year following Myocardial Infarction, *Circulation,* 50:331, 1974.
32. Alderman, E. L., Fisher, L. D., Litwin, P., Kaiser, G. C., Myers, W. O., Maynard, C., Levine, F., and Schloss, M.: Results of Coronary Artery Surgery in Patients with Poor Left Ventricular Function (CASS), *Ther. Prevention,* 68:785, 1983.
33. Fisher, L. D., Kennedy, J. W., Chaitman, B. R., Ryan, T. J., McCabe, C., Weiner, D., Tristani, F., Schloss, M., and Warner, H. R.: Diagnostic Quantification of CASS (Coronary Artery Surgery Study) Clinical Exercise Test Results in Determining Presence and Extent of Coronary Artery Disease, *Circulation,* 63:987, 1981.
34. Fuchs, R. M., Achuff, S. C., Grunwald, L., Yin, F. C. P., and Griffith, S. C.: Electrocardiographic Localization of Coronary Artery Narrowings: Studies during Myocardial Ischemia and Infarction in Patients with One-Vessel Disease, *Circulation,* 66:1168, 1982.
35. The Coronary Drug Project Research Group: Prognostic Importance of Premature Beats Following Myocardial Infarction: Experience in the Coronary Drug Project, *JAMA,* 223:116, 1973.
36. Ruberman, W., Weinblatt, E., Goldberg, J. D., Frank, C. W., and Shapiro, S.: Ventricular Premature Beats and Mortality after Myocardial Infarction, *N. Engl. J. Med.,* 297:750. 1977.
37. Bigger, J. T., Jr., Fleiss, J. L., Kleiger, R., Miller, J. P., Rolnitzky, L. M., and the Multicenter Post-Infarction Research Group: The Relationships among Ventricular Arrhythmias, Left Ventricular Dysfunction, and Mortality in the 2 Years after Myocardial Infarction, *Circulation,* 69:250, 1984.
38. Calvert, R. A., Lown, B., and Gorlin, R.: Ventricular Premature Beats and Anatomically Defined Coronary Disease, *Am. J. Cardiol.,* 39:627,1977.
39. Schultz, R. A., Strauss, H. W., and Pitt, B.: Sudden Death in the Year following Myocardial Infarction, *Am. J. Med.,* 62:192, 1977.
40. Cooperative Unstable Angina Study Group: National Cooperative Study Group to Compare Surgical and Medical Therapy: II. In-Hospital Experiences and Initial Follow-up Visits in Patients with One, Two, and Three Vessel Disease, *Am. J. Cardiol.,* 42:839, 1978.
41. Pozen, M. W., D'Agostino, R. B., Mitchell, J. B., Rosenfeld, D. M., Guglielmino, J. T., Schwartz, M. L., Teebagy, N., Valentine, J. M., and Hood, W. B., Jr.: The Usefulness of a Predictive Instrument to Reduce Inappropriate Admissions to the Coronary Care Unit, *Ann. Intern. Med.,* 92(part 1):238, 1980.
42. Goldman, L., Weinberg, M., Weisberg, M., Olshen, R., Cook, E. F., Sargent, R. K., Lamas, G. A., Dennis, C., Wilson, C., Deckelbaum, L., Fineberg, H., Stiratelli, R., and the medical house staffs at Yale–New Haven Hospital and Brigham and Women's Hospital: A Computer-Derived Protocol to Aid in the Diagnosis of Emergency Room Patients with Acute Chest Pain, *N. Engl. J. Med.,* 307:588, 1982.
43. Nixon, J. V., Hillert, M. C., Shapiro, W., and Smitherman,

T. C.: Submaximal Exercise Testing after Unstable Angina, *Am. Heart J.*, 99:772, 1980.
44. Patton, D. D.: Introduction to Clinical Decision Making, *Semin. Nucl. Med.*, 8:273, 1978.
45. Ransohoff, D. F., and Feinstein, A. R.: Problems of Spectrum and Bias in Evaluating the Efficacy of Diagnostic Tests, *N. Engl. J. Med.*, 299:926, 1978.
46. Harrell, F. E., Jr., Califf, R. M., Pryor, D. B., Lee, K. L., and Rosati, R. A.: Evaluating the Yield of Medical Tests, *JAMA*, 247:2543, 1982.
47. Diamond, G. A., and Pollock, B. H.: Computer-Assisted Diagnosis in Noninvasive Evaluation of Coronary Artery Disease, *J. Am. Coll. Cardiol.*, 3:465, 1984.
48. Gould, K. L.: Noninvasive Assessment of Coronary Stenoses by Myocardial Imaging during Pharmacologic Coronary Vasodilation: I. Physiologic Basis and Experimental Validation, *Am. J. Cardiol.*, 41:267, 1978.
49. Brunwald, E., Ross, J., and Sonnenblick, E. H.: "Mechanisms of Contraction of the Normal and Failing Heart," 2nd ed., Little, Brown and Company, Boston, 1976.
50. Gorlin, R.: Pathophysiology of Cardiac Pain, *Circulation*, 32:138, 1965.
51. Scheuer, J., and Brachfeld, N.: Coronary Insufficiency: Relations between Hemodynamic, Electrical, and Biochemical Parameters, *Circ. Res.*, 18:178, 1966.
52. Tennant, R., and Wiggers, C. J.: The Effect of Coronary Occlusion on Myocardial Contraction, *Am. J. Physiol.*, 112:351, 1935.
53. Shell, W. E., and Sobel, B. E.: Biochemical Markers of Ischemic Injury, *Circulation*, 53/54:I–98, 1976.
54. Rochmis, P., and Blackburn, J.: Exercise Tests: A Survey of Procedures, Safety and Litigation Experience in Approximately 170,000 Tests, *JAMA*, 217:1061, 1971.
55. Fortuin, N. J., and Weiss, J. L.: Exercise Stress Testing, *Circulation*, 56:699, 1977.
56. Rifkin, R. D., and Hood, W. B.: Bayesian Analysis of Electrocardiographic Exercise Stress Testing, *N. Engl. J. Med.*, 297:681, 1977.
57. Ritchie, J. L., Zaret, B. L., Strauss, W. B., Pitt, B., Berman, D. S., Schelbert, H. R., Ashburn, W. L., Berger, J. H., and Hamilton, G. W.: Myocardial Imaging with Thallium 201: A Multicenter Study in Patients with Angina Pectoris or Acute Myocardial Infarction, *Am. J. Cardiol.*, 42:345, 1978.
58. Gitler, B., Fishbach, M., and Steingart, R. M.: Use of Electrocardiographic-Thallium Exercise Testing in Clinical Practice, *J. Am. Coll. Cardiol.*, 3:262, 1984.
59. Borer, J. S., Bacharach, S. L., Green, M. V., Kent, K. M., Apstein, S. E., and Johnston, G. S.: Real Time Radionuclide Cineangiography in the Noninvasive Evaluation of Global and Regional Left Ventricular Function at Rest and during Exercise in Patients with Coronary Artery Disease, *N. Engl. J. Med.*, 296:839, 1977.
60. Borer, J. S., Bacharach, S. L., Green, M. V., Kent, K. M., Henry, W. L., Rosing, D. R., Seides, S. F., Johnston, G. S., Epstein, S. E., and Mack, B.: Exercise-Induced Left Ventricular Dysfunction in Symptomatic and Asymptomatic Patients with Aortic Regurgitation: Assessment with Radionuclide Cineangiography, *Am. J. Cardiol.*, 42:351, 1978.
61. Forfar, J. C., Muir, A. L., Sawers, S. A., and Toft, A. D.: Abnormal Left Ventricular Function in Hyperthyroidism: Evidence for a Possible Reversible Cardiomyopathy, *N. Engl. J. Med.*, 307:1165, 1982.
62. Port, S., Cobb, F. R., Coleman, R. E., and Jones, R. H.: Effect of Age on the Response of the Left Ventricular Ejection Fraction to Exercise, *N. Engl. J. Med.*, 303:1133, 1980.
63. Weiner, D. A., McCabe, C., Hueter, D. C., Ryan, T. J., and Hood, W. B., Jr.: The Predictive Value of Anginal Chest Pain as an Indicator of Coronary Disease during Exercise Testing, *Am. Heart J.*, 96:458, 1978.
64. Hamilton, G. W., Trobaugh, G. B., Ritchie, J. L., Gould, K. L., DeRouēn, T. A., and Williams, D. L.: Myocardial Imaging with ^{201}Thallium: An Analysis of Clinical Usefulness Based on Bayes' Theorem, *Semin. Nucl. Med.*, 8:358, 1978.
65. Epstein, S. E.: Implications of Probability Analysis on the Strategy Used for Noninvasive Detection of Coronary Artery Disease, *Am. J. Cardiol.*, 46:491, 1980.
66. Klocke, F. M.: Coronary Blood Flow in Man, *Prog. Cardiovasc. Dis.*, 19:117, 1976.
67. Gould, K. L., and Lipscomb, K.: Effect of Coronary Stenoses on Coronary Flow Reverse and Resistance, *Am. J. Cardiol.*, 34:48, 1974.
68. Detre, K. M., Wright, E., Murphy, J. L., and Takaro, T.: Observer Agreement in Evaluating Coronary Angiograms, *Circulation*, 52:979, 1975.
69. Arnett, E. N., Isner, J. M., Redwood, D. R., Kemt, K. M., Baker, W. P., Ackerstein, J., and Roberts, W. C.: Coronary Artery Narrowing in Coronary Heart Disease: Comparison of Cineangiographic and Necropsy Findings, *Ann. Intern. Med.*, 91:350, 1979.
70. Dhew, C. Y. C., Brown, G. B., Wong, M., Shah, P. M., and Singh, B. M.: The Effects of Verapamil on Coronary Hemodynamics and Vasomobility in Patients with Coronary Artery Disease, *Am. J. Cardiol.*, 45:389, 1980. (Abstract.)
71. White, C. W., Wright, C. B., Doty, D. B., Hiratza, L. F., Eastham, C. L., Harrison, D. G., and Marcus, M. L.: Does Visual Interpretation of the Coronary Arteriogram Predict the Physiologic Importance of a Coronary Stenosis? *N. Engl. J. Med.*, 310:819, 1984.
72. Schroeder, J. S., Bolen, J. L., Quint, R. A., Clark, D. A., Hayden, W. G., Higgins, C. R., and Wexler, L.: Provocation of Coronary Spasm with Ergonovine Maleate: New Test with Results in 57 Patients Undergoing Coronary Arteriography, *Am. J. Cardiol.*, 40:487, 1977.
73. Curry, R. C., Jr., Pepine, C. J., Sabom, M. B., Feldman, R. L., Christie, L. G., and Conti, C. R.: Effects of Ergonovine in Patients with and without Coronary Artery Disease, *Circulation*, 56:803, 1977.
74. Buxton, A., Goldberg, S., Hirshfeld, J. W., Wilson, J., Mann, T., Williams, D. O., Oliva, P., and Kastor, J. A.: Refractory Ergonovine-Induced Coronary Vasospasm: Importance of Intracoronary Nitroglycerin, *Am. J. Cardiol.*, 45:390, 1980. (Abstract.)
75. Mueller, H. S., and Ayres, S. M.: Metabolic Responses of the Heart and Acute Myocardial Infarction, *Am. J. Cardiol.*, 42:363, 1978.
76. Ganz, W., Tamura, K., Marcus, H. S., Donose, R., Yoshid, S., and Swan, H. J. C.: Measurement of Coronary Sinus Blood Flow by Continuous Thermodilution in Man, *Circulation*, 44:181, 1971.
77. Holman, B. L., Cohn, P. F., Adams, D. F., See, J. R., Roberts, B. H., Idoline, J., and Gorlin, R.: Regional Myocardial Blood Flow during Hyperemia Induced by Contrast Agents in Patients with Coronary Artery Disease, *Am. J. Cardiol.*, 38:416, 1976.
78. Gertz, E. W., Wisneski, J. A., Neese, R., Houser, A., Korte, R., and Bristow, J. D.: Myocardial Lactate Extraction: Multi-determined Metabolic Function, *Circulation*, 61:256, 1980.
79. Olson, R. E.: "Excess Lactate" and Anaerobiosis, *Ann. Intern. Med.*, 59:960, 1963.
80. Pepine, C. J., Mehta, J., Webster, W. W., and Nichols, W. W.: In Vivo Validation of a Thermodilution Method to Determine Regional Left Ventricular Blood Flow in Patients with Coronary Disease, *Circulation*, 58:795, 1978.
81. Kemp, H. G., Elliott, W. C., and Gorlin, R.: The Anginal Syndrome with Normal Coronary Arteriography, *Trans. Assoc. Am. Physicians*, 80:59, 1967.
82. Goldberg, S., Lam, W., Mudge, G., Green, L. H., Kushner, F., Hirshfeld, J. W., and Kastor, J. A.: Refractory Ergonovine-Induced Coronary Vasospasm: Importance of Intracoronary Nitroglycerin, *Am. J. Cardiol.*, 45:390, 1980. (Abstract.)
83. Chaitman, B. R., Bourassa, M. G., Davis, K., Rogers, W. J., Tyras, D. H., Berger, R., Kennedy, J. W., Fisher, L., Judkins, M. P., Mock, M. B., and Killip, T.: Angiographic Prevalence of High-Risk Coronary Artery Disease in Patient Subsets (CASS), *Circulation*, 64:360, 1981.
84. San Marco, M. E., Pontius, S., and Silvester, R. H.: Abnor-

mal Blood Pressure Response and Marked Ischemic ST-Segment Depression as Predictors of Severe Coronary Artery Disease, *Circulation,* 61:572, 1980.
85. Dash, J., Massie, B. M., Botvinick, E. H., and Brundage, B. H.: The Noninvasive Identification of Left Main and Three Vessel Coronary Artery Disease by Myocardial Stress Perfusion Scintigraphy and Treadmill Exercise Electrocardiography, *Circulation,* 60:276, 1979.
86. Leppo, J., Yipintsoi, T., Blankstein, R., Bontemps, R., Freeman, L. M., Zohman, L., and Scheuer, J.: Thallium-201 Myocardial Scintigraphy in Patients with Triple Vessel Disease and Ischemic Exercise Stress Tests, *Circulation,* 59:714, 1979.
87. Jones, R. H., McEwan, P., Newman, G. E., Port, S., Rerych, S. K., Scholz, P. M., Upton, M. T., Peter, C. A., Austin, E. H., Leong, K.-H., Gibbons, R. J., Cobb, F. R., Coleman, R. E., and Sabiston, D. C., Jr.: Accuracy of Diagnosis of Coronary Artery Disease by Radionuclide Measurement of Left Ventricular Function during Rest and Exercise, *Circulation,* 64:586, 1981.
88. Kushner, F. G., Okada, R. D., Kirshenbaum, H. D., Boucher, C. A., Strauss, H. W., and Pohost, G. M.: Lung Thallium-201 Uptake after Stress Testing in Patients with Coronary Artery Disease, *Circulation,* 63:341, 1981.
89. McNeer, J. F., Margolis, J. R., Lee, K. L., Kisslo, J. A., Peter, R. H., Kong, Y., Behar, V. S., Wallace, A. G., McCants, C. B., and Rosati, R. A.: The Role of the Exercise Test in the Evaluation of Patients for Ischemic Heart Disease, *Circulation,* 57:64, 1978.
90. Weiner, D. A., Ryan, T. J., McCabe, C. H., Chaitman, B. R., Sheffield, L. T., Ferguson, J. C., Fisher, L. D., and Tristani, F.: Prognostic Importance of a Clinical Profile and Exercise Test in Medically Treated Patients with Coronary Artery Disease, *J. Am. Coll. Cardiol.,* 3:722, 1984.
91. Brown, K. A., Boucher, C. A., Okada, R. D., Guiney, T. E., Newell, J. B., Strauss, H. W., and Pohost, G. M.: Prognostic Value of Exercise Thallium-201 Imaging in Patients Presenting for Evaluation of Chest Pain, *J. Am. Coll. Cardiol.,* 1:994, 1983.
92. Ringqvist, I., Fisher, L. D., Mock, M., Davis, K. B., Wedel, H., Chaitman, B. R., Passamani, E., Russell, R. O., Jr., Alderman, E. L., Kouchoukas, N. T., Kaiser, G. C., Ryan, T. J., Killip, T., and Fray, D.: Prognostic Value of Angiographic Indices of Coronary Artery Disease from the Coronary Artery Surgery Study (CASS), *J. Clin Invest.,* 71:1854, 1983.
93. Nelson, G. R., Cohn, P. F., and Gorlin, R.: Prognosis in Medically Treated Coronary Artery Disease: Influence of Ejection Fraction Compared to Other Parameters, *Circulation,* 52:408, 1975.
94. Cohen, M., Packer, M., and Gorlin, R.: Indications for Left Ventricular Aneurysmectomy, *Circulation,* 67:717, 1983.
95. Horowitz, L. N., Harken, A. H., Kastor, J. A., and Josephson, M. E.: Ventricular Resection Guided by Epicardial and Endocardial Mapping for Treatment of Recurrent Ventricular Tachycardia, *N. Engl. J. Med.,* 302:589, 1980.
96. Steingart, R. M., Wexler, J. P., and Blaufox, M. D.: Pharmacologic Distribution in Cardiovascular Nuclear Medicine Procedures, *Semin. Nucl. Med.,* 1:80, 1981.
97. Rozanski, A., Berman, D., Gray, R., Diamond, G., Raymond, M., Prause, J., Maddahi, J., Swan, H. J. C., and Matloff, J.: Preoperative Prediction of Reversible Myocardial Asynergy by Postexercise Radionuclide Ventriculography, *N. Engl. J. Med.,* 307:212, 1982.
98. Tobis, J., Nalcioglu, O., Johnston, W. D., Seibert, A., Iseri, L. T., Roeck, W., and Henry, W. L.: Digital Angiography in Assessment on Ventricular Function and Wall Motion during Pacing in Patients with Coronary Artery Disease, *Am. J. Cardiol.,* 51:668, 1983.
99. McNeer, J. F., Starmer, C. F., Bartel, A. G., Behar, V. S., Kong, Y., Peter, R. H., and Rosati, R. A.: The Nature of Treatment Selection in Coronary Artery Disease: Experience with Medical and Surgical Treatment of a Chronic Disease, *Circulation,* 49:606, 1974.
100. Davis, K., Kennedy, J. W., Kemp, H. G., Jr., Judkins, M. P., Gosselin, A. J., and Killip, T.: Complications of Coronary Arteriography from the Collaborative Study of Coronary Artery Surgery (CASS), *Circulation,* 59:1105, 1979.
101. Weld, F. M., Chu, K.-L., Bigger, J. T., Jr., and Rolnitzky, L. M.: Risk Stratification with Low-Level Exercise Testing 2 Weeks after Acute Myocardial Infarction, *Circulation,* 64:306, 1981.
102. Gibson, R. S., Watson, D. D., Craddock, G. B., Crampton, R. S., Kaiser, D. L., Denny, M. J., and Beller, G. A.: Prediction of Cardiac Events after Uncomplicated Myocardial Infarction: A Prospective Study Comparing Predischarge Exercise Thallium-201 Scintigraphy and Coronary Angiography, *Circulation,* 68:321, 1983.
103. Leppo, J. A., O'Brien, J., Rothendler, J. A., Getchell, J. D., and Lee, V. W.: Dipyridamole–Thallium-201 Scintigraphy in the Prediction of Future Cardiac Events after Acute Myocardial Infarction, *N. Engl. J. Med.,* 310:1014, 1984.
104. Corbett, J. R., Dehmer, G. J., Lewis, S. E., Woodward, W., Henderson, E., Parkey, R. W., Blomqvist, C. G., and Willerson, J. T.: The Prognostic Value of Submaximal Exercise Testing with Radionuclide Ventriculography before Hospital Discharge in Patients with Recent Myocardial Infarction, *Circulation,* 64:535, 1981.

PART IV

Disorders of the Cardiovascular System

The purpose of Part IV, "Disorders of the Cardiovascular System," is to present a group of conditions that represent, for the most part, the consequences of heart disease.

Many hours were spent trying to identify a word or words that would indicate the difference between a disease process and the consequences of the disease. There are no words that will satisfy the purist because it is not possible to create pigeonholes into which one can force all conditions. The following discussion points out how we view the difference between the words *disease* and *disorder.*

The word *disease* implies the presence of a fundamental abnormality of the heart or blood vessels. The pathologist can usually identify the process when he or she examines the heart and blood vessels. Heart disease may be present without the patient knowing it. The disease process must progress to a certain point before cardiovascular mechanisms become deranged sufficiently to make the patient ill. The disease may be due to a congenital defect or inflammatory disease, or it may be the result of atheroma or a myriad of other causes. On the other hand, the exact cause of the cardiovascular abnormality may be unknown (as it is in many arrhythmias). The basic abnormality of the tissue is designated as heart disease or vascular disease. *Accordingly, whenever a physician identifies a disease process, he or she must ask the following question: Is a disorder present that has resulted from the disease process?*

The word *disorder* implies that the duties assigned to the heart are not being implemented properly. The heart and circulation have the following duties: The heart should function without pain; pump blood properly (not too much and not too little); maintain a proper arterial blood pressure; maintain normal rhythm; prevent transient unconsciousness; and continue beating. A disorder is the result of a derangement of function. A derangement of function may be the consequence of one or several different disease processes. A patient becomes ill because of the derangement of cardiovascular mechanisms that has resulted from the disease process. The pathologist cannot determine whether the patient had chest pain, ventricular dysfunction, shock, a hyperdynamic circulation, arrhythmia, or syncope by examining the heart and blood vessels at autopsy. There may be, of course, indirect evidence of these disorders found in other organs. *Accordingly, whenever a physician identifies a disorder of the cardiovascular system, he or she must ask the following question: What cardiovascular disease or diseases caused the disorder?* This question must be asked because the management of the disease process itself may be quite different from the management of the derangement of function that the disease produced.

Note: Chest pain secondary to cardiovascular disease is a disorder and not a disease. It should, therefore, be discussed in Part IV of this book. In order to prevent unnecessary duplication the reader is referred to the discussions in the individual chapters of Part V where chest pain is discussed in relation to the diseases that produce it.

PLATE 1 Diagram of the cardiac cycle and related cardiovascular events.

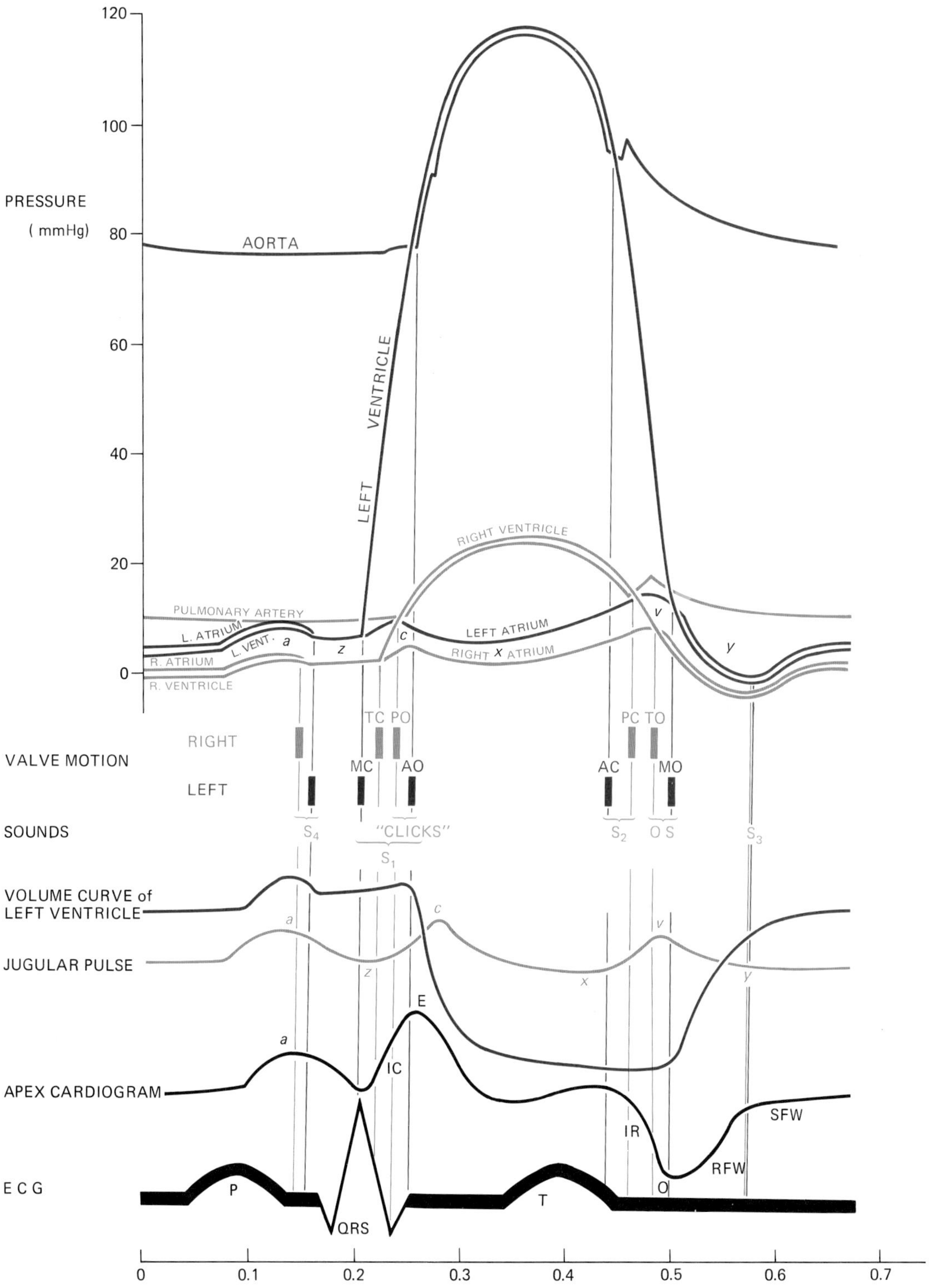

Diagram of the cardiac cycle, showing the pressure curves of the great vessels and cardiac chambers, valvular events and heart sounds, left ventricular volume curve, jugular pulse wave, apex cardiogram (Sanborn piezo crystal), and the electrocardiogram. For illustrative purposes, the time intervals between the valvular events have been modified and the *z* point has been prolonged. Valve motion: MC = mitral component of the first heart sound; MO = mitral valve opening; TC = tricuspid component of the first heart sound; TO = tricuspid valve opening; AC = aortic component of the second heart sound; AO = aortic valve opening; PC = pulmonic valve component of the second heart sound; PO = pulmonic valve opening; OS = opening snap of atrioventricular valves. Apex cardiogram: IC = isovolumic or isovolumetric (isochoric) contraction wave; IR = isovolumic or isovolumetric (isochoric) relaxation wave; O = opening of mitral valve; RFW = rapid-filling wave; SFW = slow-filling wave. (See text in Chap. 3.)

PLATE 2 Relationship between electric and mechanical events and heart sounds.

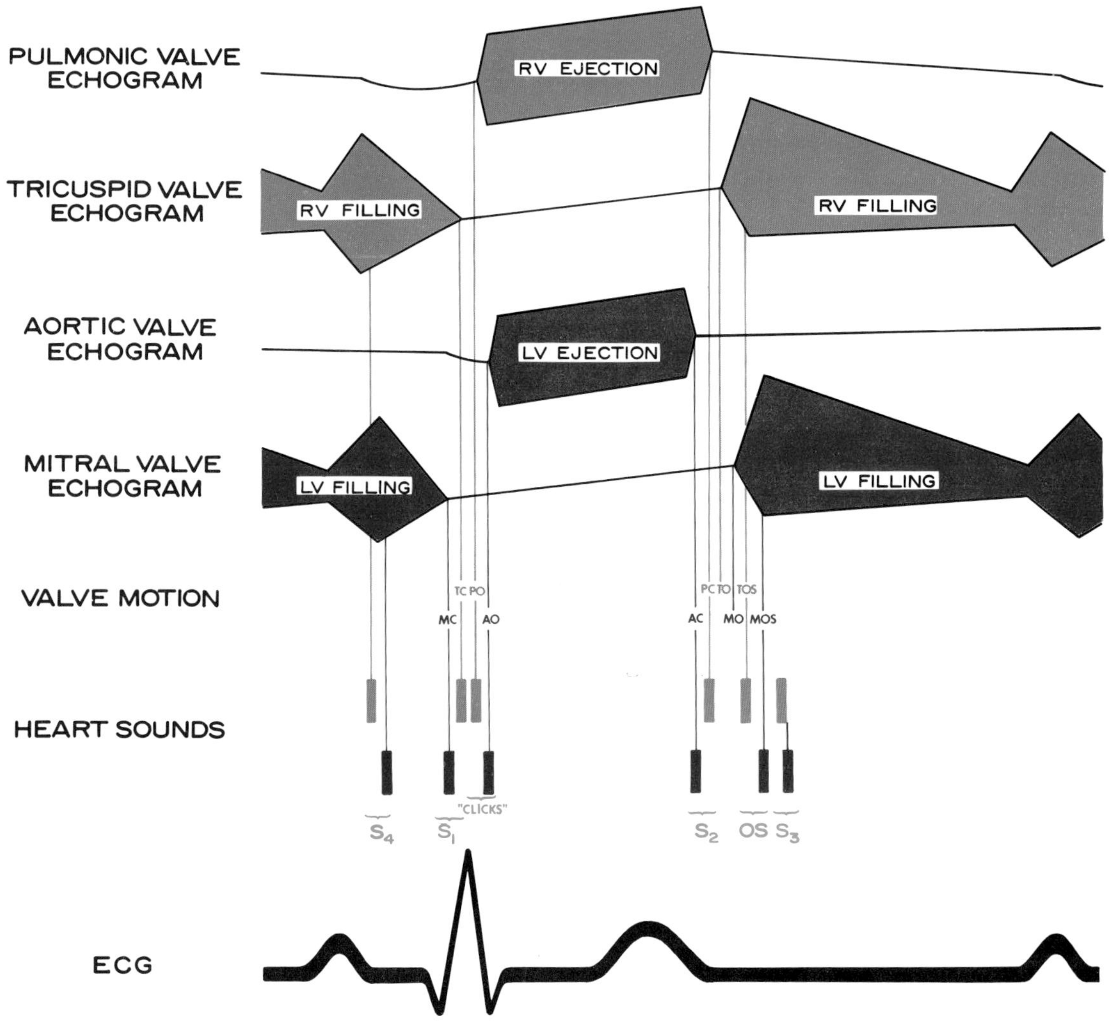

Schematic presentation of the relationships between electrical and mechanical events and heart sounds during the cardiac cycle. The sequence of ejection from, and of filling of, the right ventricle is indicated by the schematic echograms of the pulmonic valve and the tricuspid valve. The corresponding phases of the left ventricle are indicated by the schematic echograms of the aortic valve and the mitral valve. The isovolumic contraction phase for each ventricle occurs in the short phase between the end of filling and the onset of ejection, whereas isovolumic filling occurs in the brief phase between the end of ejection and the onset of filling.

The right atrium starts contracting before the left atrium; on the other hand, the left ventricle starts contracting prior to the contraction of the right ventricle. Because of the relatively higher pressure in the aorta than in the pulmonary artery, the phases of isovolumic contraction and isovolumic relaxation of the left ventricle are much longer than for the right ventricle. As a result, although left ventricular contraction begins first, right ventricular ejection begins prior to left ventricular ejection and also ends after that of left ventricular ejection. Thus, the phase of active ejection for the right ventricle is longer than that of the left ventricle. On the other hand, the total duration of systole, including isovolumic contraction and relaxation, is normally longer for the left ventricle.

The normal sequence of heart sounds and valve motion is schematically depicted: MC = the mitral component of the first heart sound (S_1); TC = the tricuspid component of the first heart sound (S_1); PO = pulmonic valve opening; AO = aortic valve opening; AC = aortic component of the second heart sound (S_2); PC = pulmonic component of the second heart sound (S_2); TO = tricuspid valve opening; TOS = tricuspid opening snap; and MOS = mitral valve opening snap. Normally, the sound produced by the opening of the cardiac valves is not audible; however, in disease states the opening of the mitral or tricuspid valve may produce an "opening snap" which usually occurs about the moment when the respective valve leaflets just reach maximal opening. Similarly, very vigorous tensing and opening of the aortic and pulmonic valves can produce ejection or opening "clicks" or sounds analogous to the opening snaps of the AV valves. An aortic and pulmonic valve opening click or sound may occur anywhere between the onset of valve opening, as illustrated, and the point of maximal opening of the respective valve, where it more commonly occurs. The sound occurring at the end of the rapid-filling phase of the ventricle is referred to as a *third heart sound (S_3), ventricular filling sound, or ventricular gallop.* The sound that occurs during or shortly after the P wave on the electrocardiogram and that is associated with an atrial contribution to ventricular filling is referred to as the *fourth heart sound (S_4).* Both third (S_3) and fourth (S_4) heart sounds may originate from either ventricle. The motion of the valve leaflets is depicted schematically in the valve echograms; for illustrative purposes, not all time intervals are depicted proportionately. (See text in chap. 3)

PLATE 3 Tuberous sclerosis; dermatomyositis; hemorrhagic telangiectasia under fingernails; hemorrhagic telangiectasia on tongue and lips; clubbing of the fingers; Osler's node.

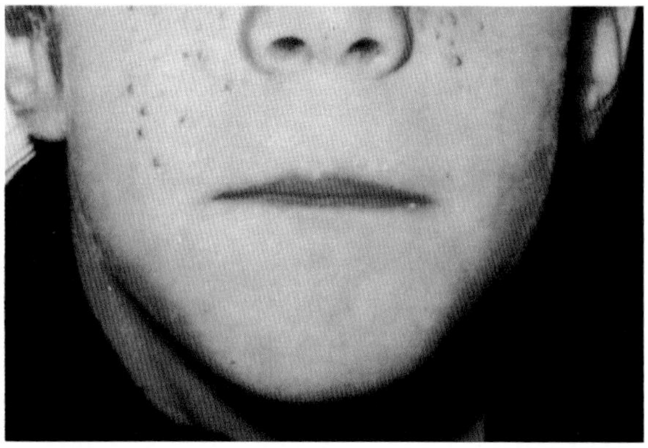

A Tuberous sclerosis. Adenoma sebaceum, may be associated with rhabdomyomas of the myocardium.

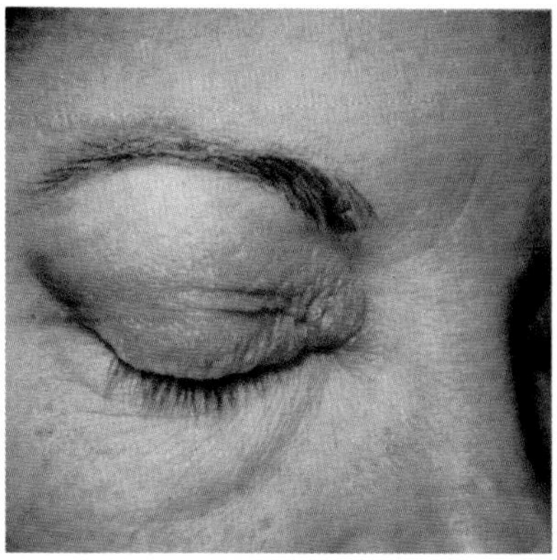

B Dermatomyositis. A violaceous hue and edema of upper eyelid, may be associated with myocardial disease.

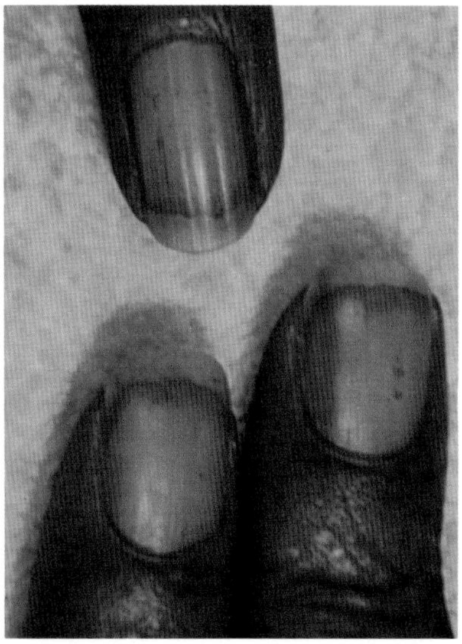

C Hereditary hemorrhagic telangiectasia. Telangiectasia under nails. *(With permission of publisher, from Silverman and Hurst, The Hand and the Heart, Am. J. Cardiol., 22:609, 1968.)*

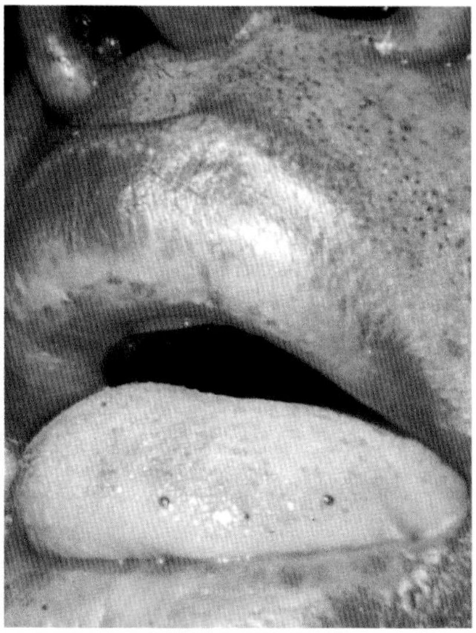

D Hereditary hemorrhagic telangiectasia. Telangiectasia on tongue and lips, may be associated with a pulmonary arteriovenous fistula.

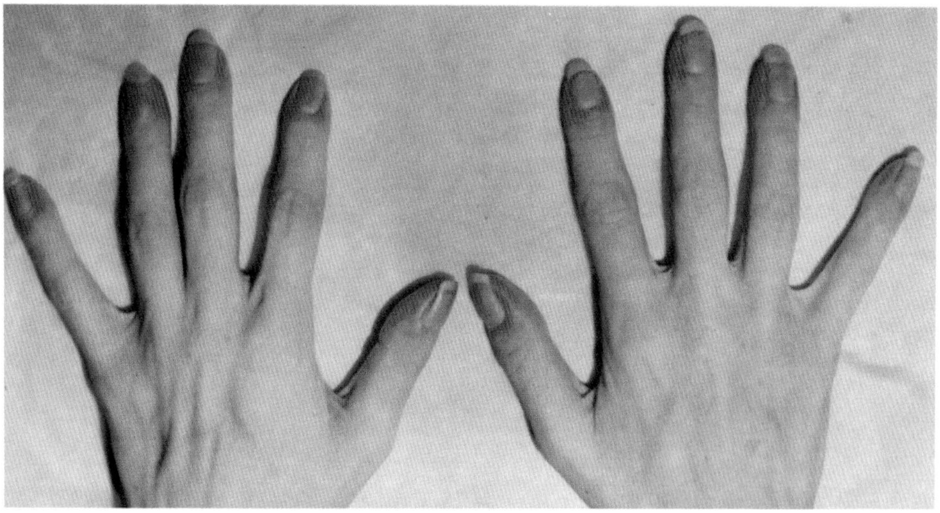

E Clubbing due to bacterial endocarditis.

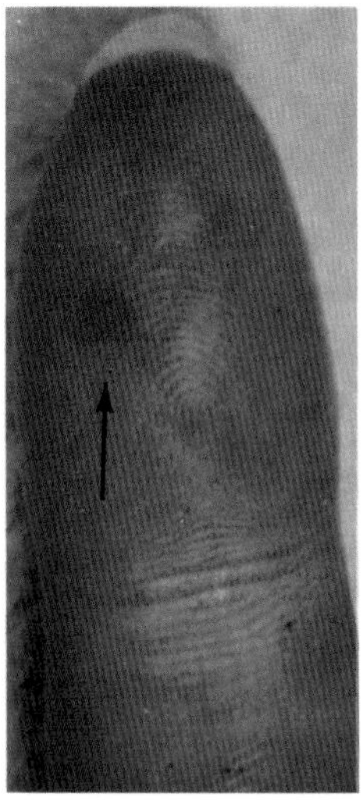

F Osler's node (arrow).

PLATE 4 Symmetric cyanosis; cyanosis of fingers greater than that of toes; cyanosis of left hand and all toes; and tuft erythema.

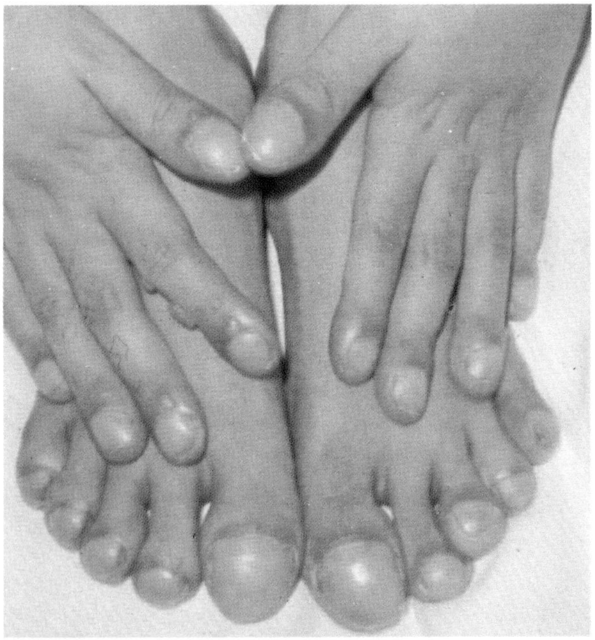

A Symmetric cyanosis. Equal cyanosis and clubbing of hands and feet, due to transposition of great vessels and a ventricular septal defect *without* patent ductus arteriosus.

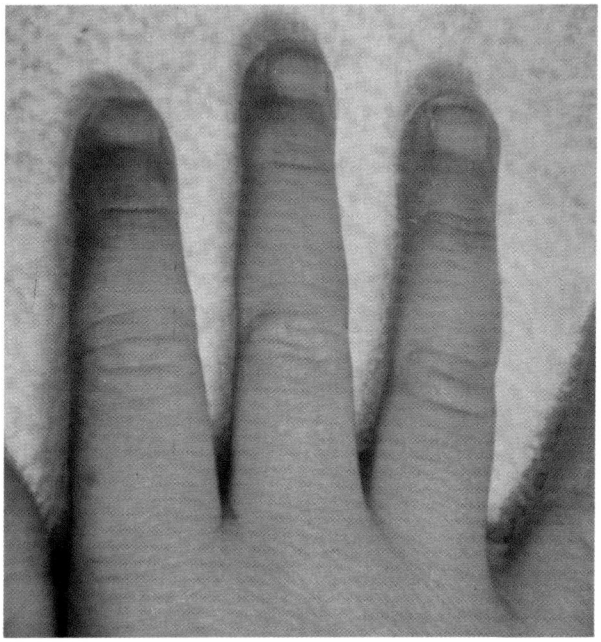

B Tuft erythema. Erythema of fingertips, due to small right-to-left shunt from an AV canal defect.

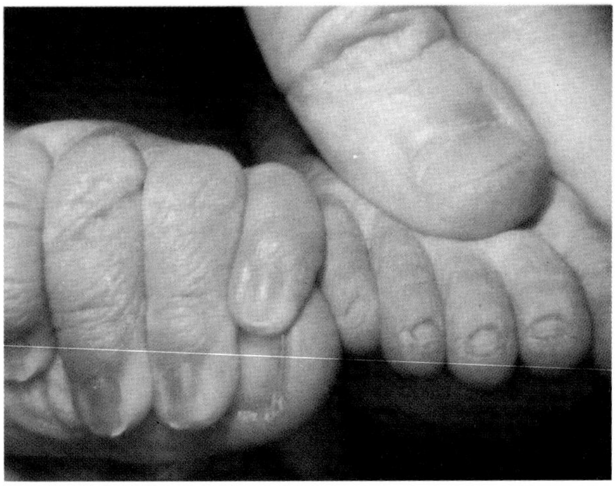

C Differential cyanosis. Cyanosis of fingers (left) greater than that of toes, due to transposition of great vessels *with* patent ductus arteriosus.

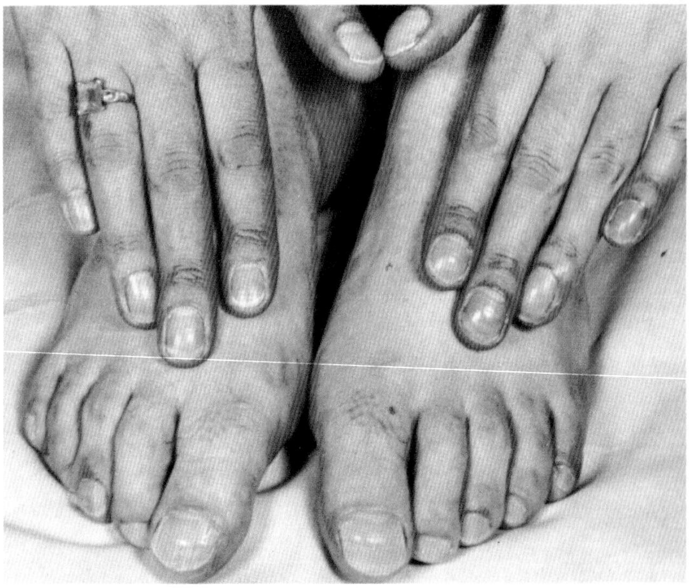

D Differential cyanosis. Clubbing of left hand (compare thumbs) and cyanosis of left hand and all toes, due to patent ductus arteriosus with pulmonary hypertension and normally related great vessels. *(Courtesy of Dr. Joseph K. Perloff, University of California, Los Angeles.)*

PLATE 5 Retinal changes associated with systemic hypertension.

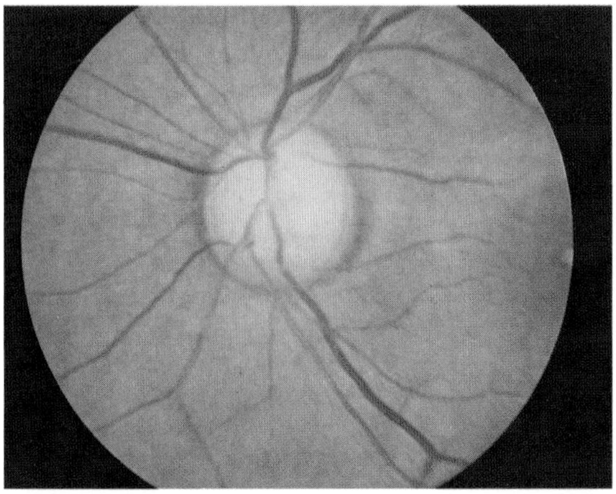

A The retina of a 49-year-old black woman with asymptomatic "essential hypertension" of at least 10 years' duration, showing arteriolar narrowing and straightening, increased light reflex, irregular caliber, loss of small arteriolar branches, and early AV crossing changes. *(Courtesy of Dr. Joseph A. Wilbur.)*

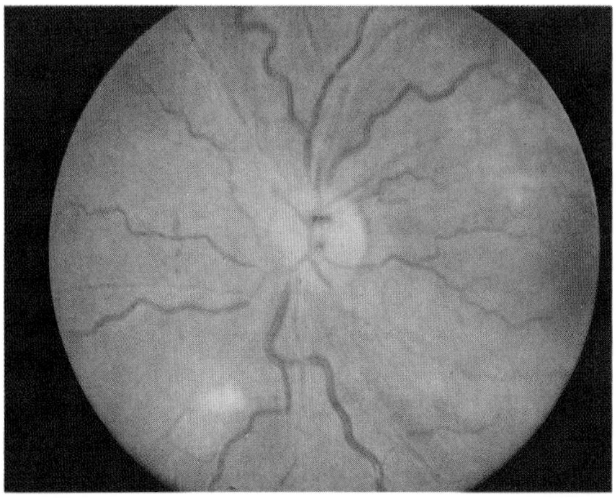

B The retina of a 42-year-old black woman with essential hypertension and blood pressure levels averaging 260/130. She was asymptomatic except for headaches. Note the severe vascular sclerosis seen as marked irregularity of arteriolar caliber, "sheathing," and nearly complete loss of transparency of the arterioles. A "cotton wool" exudate is seen at 7 o'clock. The nasal disk margin is blurred, which may occur normally. *(Courtesy of Dr. Joseph A. Wilbur.)*

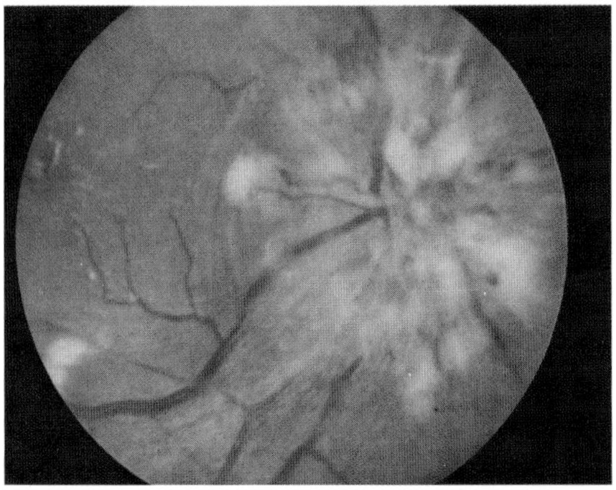

C The retina of a 38-year-old black man with malignant hypertension and with bilateral papilledema and azotemia. There was no visual disturbance. Note the massive edema, hemorrhages, and exudates, completely obscuring the disk and burying the blood vessels. The veins are congested and the arterioles show diffuse thickening ("cooper wire"). There are hard exudates (edema residues) forming in the nerve bundle grooves in the macular region at 10 o'clock. *(Courtesy of Dr. Joseph A. Wilbur.)*

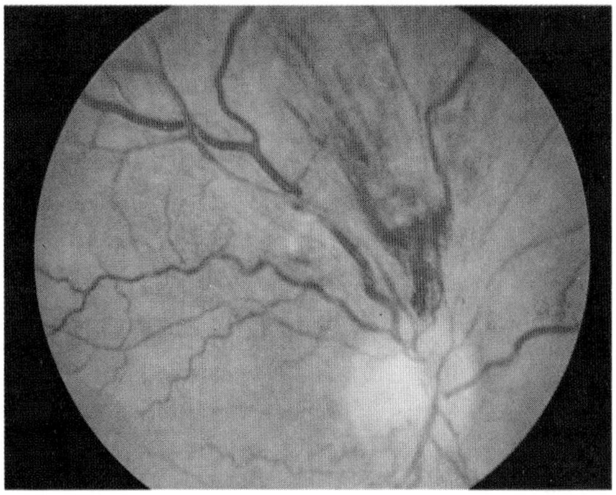

D The retina of a 50-year-old black woman with severe hypertension of 25 years' duration. Arteriosclerosis is shown by the marked narrowing, irregular caliber, increased light reflex, and AV crossing changes. Atherosclerosis is suggested by the large fan-shaped superficial hemorrhage, due to occlusion of a branch of the superior temporal vein as it enters the disk region. *(Courtesy of Dr. Joseph A. Wilbur.)*

PLATE 6 Retinal changes associated with the various diseases: central retinal vein occlusion; diabetes mellitus; acute myeloblastic leukemia and severe anemia; pseudoxanthoma elasticum.

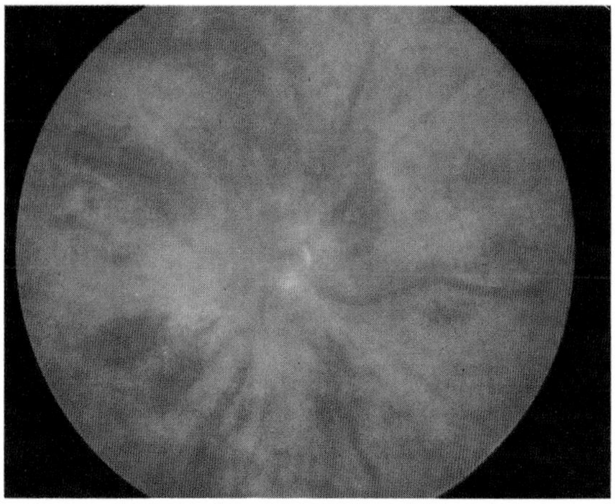

A The retina of a 74-year-old white man with normal blood pressure who complained of sudden loss of vision in one eye. This shows the typical picture of central retinal vein occlusion, probably due to atherosclerosis of its adjacent artery behind the disk. Diffuse edema (loss of retinal detail), massive hemorrhages, and papilledema are present. *(Courtesy of Dr. Joseph A. Wilbur.)*

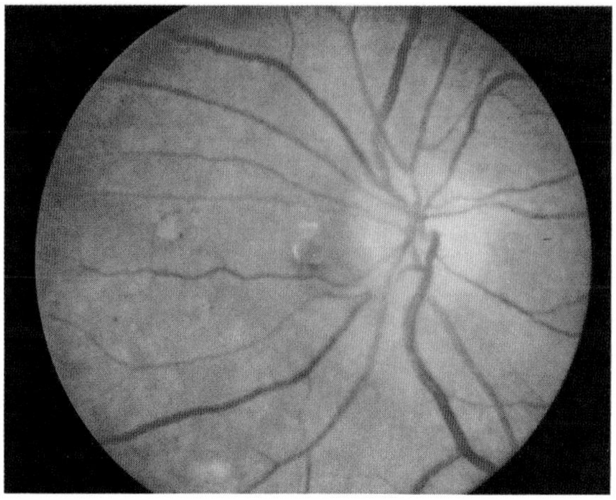

B The retina of a 68-year-old white man with hypertension and mild diabetes mellitus. Note the very small red dots, or capillary aneurysms, scattered between the disk and the macular region. There is also a faint "cotton wool" exudate at 7 o'clock. *(Courtesy of Dr. Joseph A. Wilbur.)*

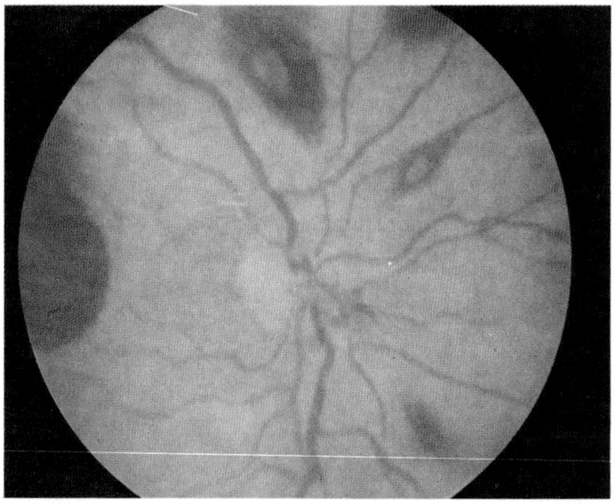

C The retina of a 24-year-old white woman with acute myeloblastic leukemia and severe anemia; the blood pressure was normal. Note the scattered hemorrhages, some with whitish centers (Roth spots), and the portion of the large preretinal hemorrhage at 9 o'clock. The blood vessels are pale but otherwise normal. *(Courtesy of Dr. Joseph A. Wilbur.)*

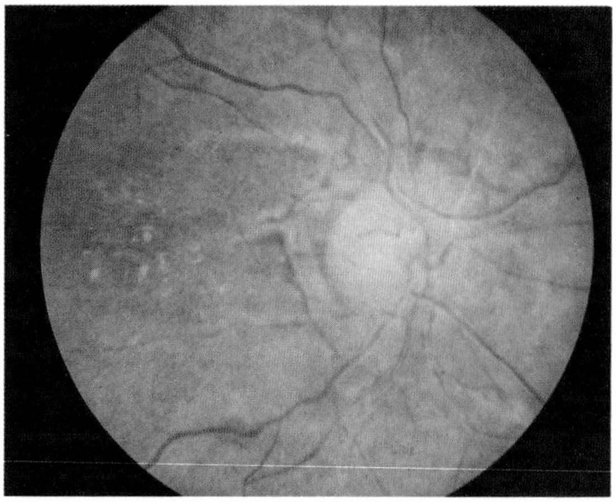

D The retina of a 36-year-old white woman with pseudoxanthoma elasticum. Severe hypertension, marked visual disturbance, and renal insufficiency were present. Note the characteristic brownish angioid streaks around the disk and extending toward the macula. Also seen are marked retinal arteriosclerotic changes, sheathing, irregular caliber, occluded vessels, and hard exudates with a "smudge" hemorrhage at 7 o'clock. *(Courtesy of Dr. Joseph A. Wilbur.)*

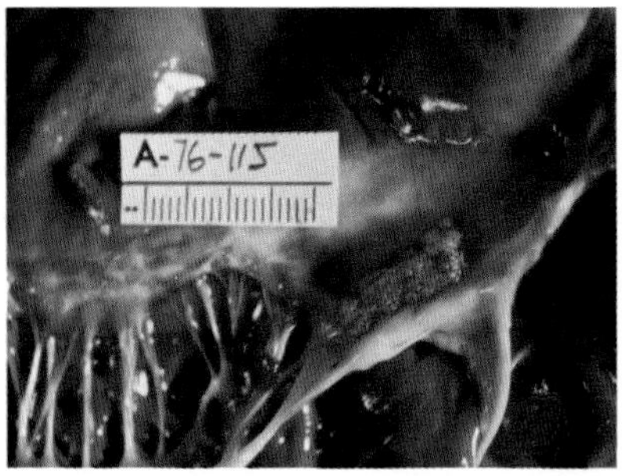

A Typical vegetation of nonbacterial thrombotic endocarditis, found at necropsy in a cachectic patient who died with disseminated lung cancer.

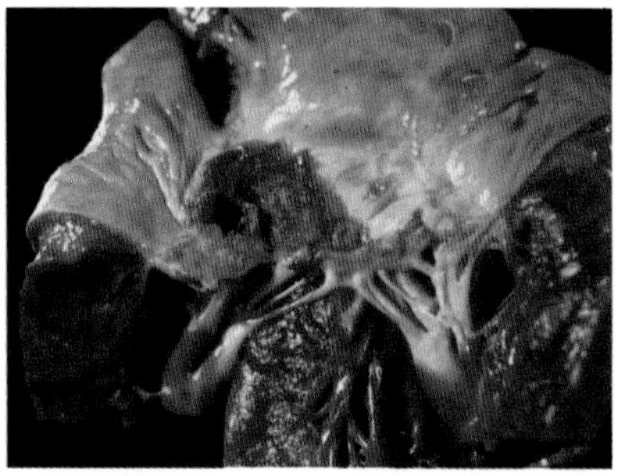

B Typical vegetation of bacteria endocarditis, complicated by perforation of the anterior mitral valve leaflet. Note that the valve shows preexisting chronic rheumatic disease, with thickening, deformity, and fusion of chordae tendineae.

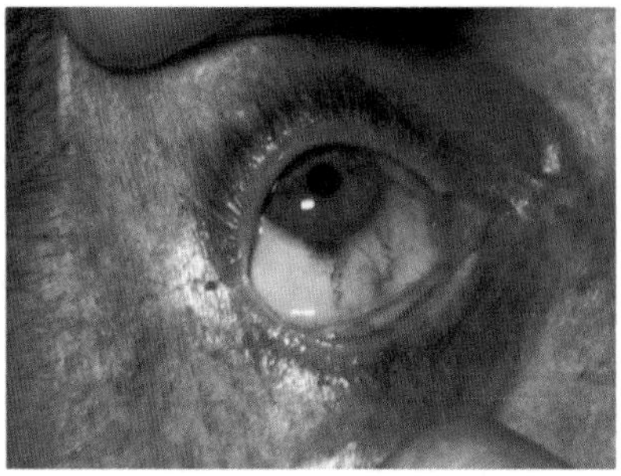

C Typical conjunctival petechia in a patient with SBE due to *Streptococcus sanguis.*

The consequences of embolization from the vegetation shown in a patient with subacute bacterial endocarditis (SBE).

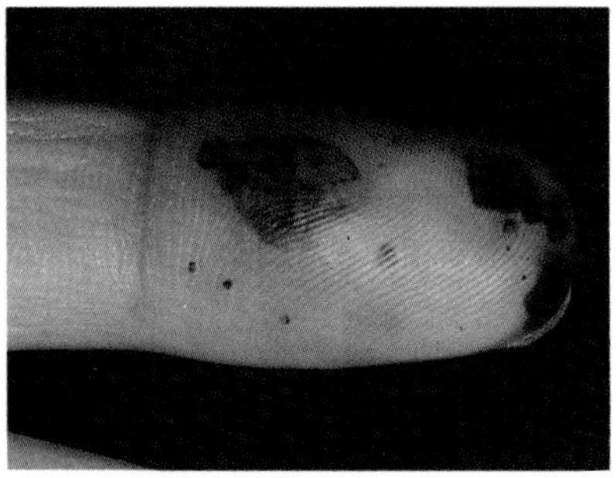

D Ischemic, hemorrhagic, and pustular lesions on the extremities in acute *Staphylococcus aureus* endocarditis.

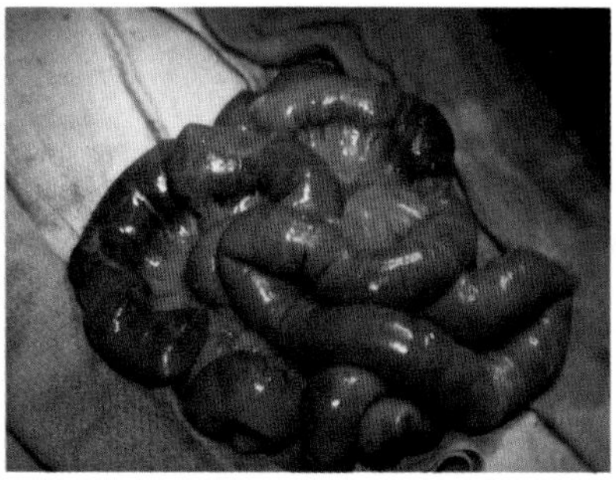

E Segmental ischemia and necrosis in the gut, presenting as acute abdomen.

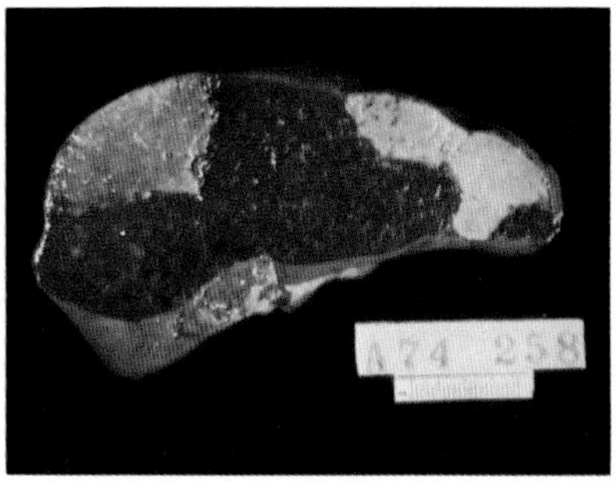

F Infarctions in the spleen.

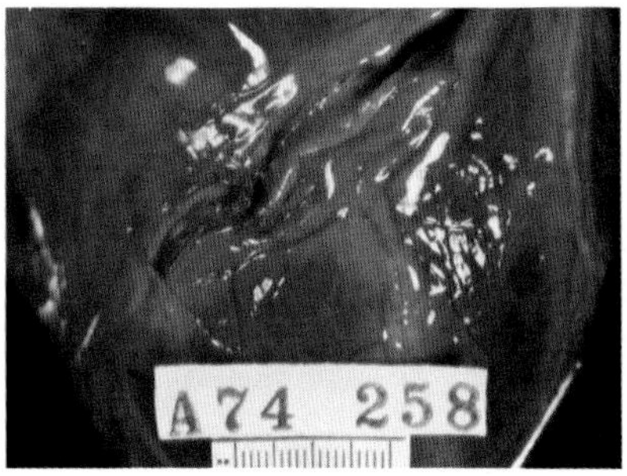

G An infected embolus in a coronary artery.

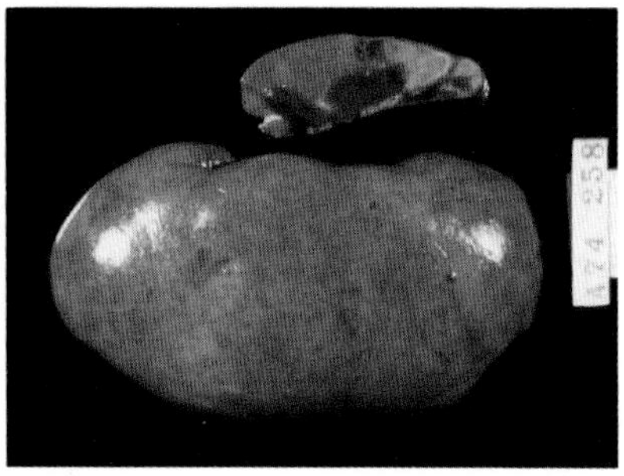

H Kidney from a case of subacute bacterial endocarditis, showing two abnormalities: (1) typical ischemic infarctions due to emboli, and (2) swelling and petechiae ("flea-bitten kidney") due to immune-complex glomerulonephritis.

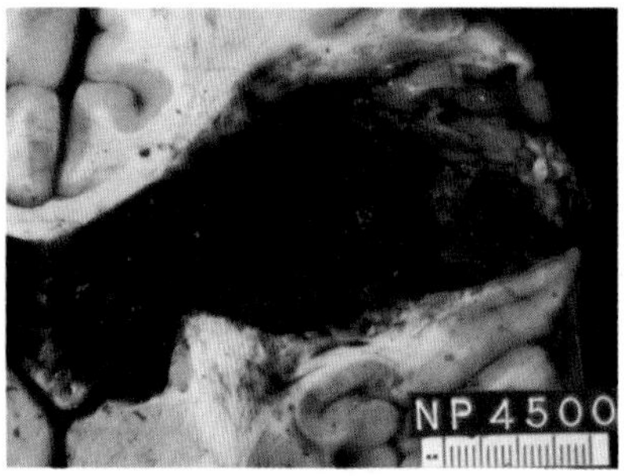

I Massive cerebral hemorrhage with intraventricular extension due to rupture of a small, peripheral mycotic aneurysm (arrowed). The patient had been *bacteriologically* cured of *Staphylococcus epidermidis* endocarditis several weeks previously. Cultures of the blood, valve, and aneurysm taken at necropsy were negative.

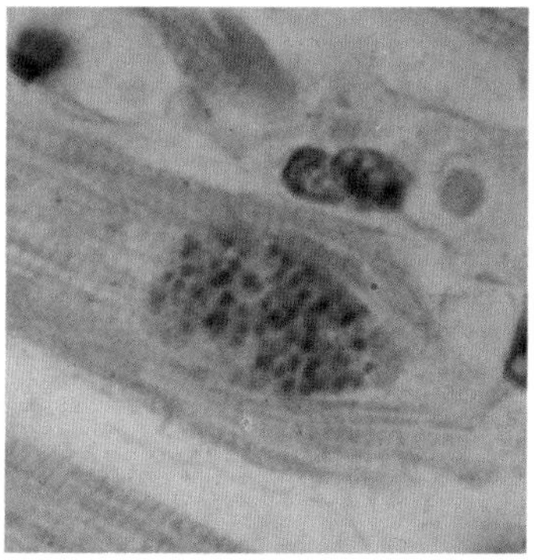

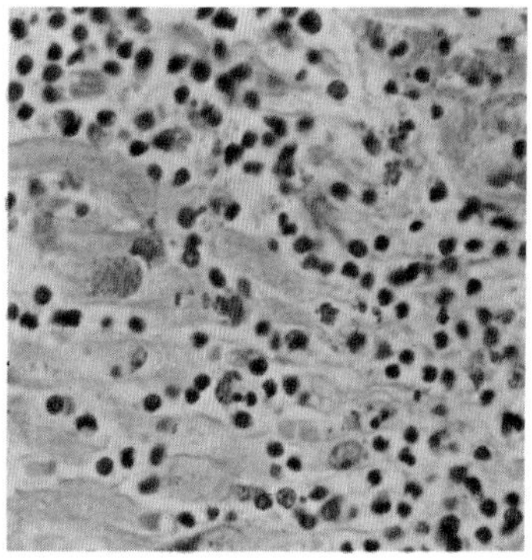

A Toxoplasmosis of the heart in a 27-year-old man with acute lymphocytic leukemia. His illness was characterized by paroxysmal arrhythmias (atrial fibrillation, artrial tachycardia). He died with ventricular fibrillation; *Toxoplasma gondii* organisms were found in myocardial cells. *Right:* Area of focal myocarditis associated with *T. gondii* organisms. *Left:* Close-up view of the encysted organisms. Hematoxylin and eosin stains: ×275 *(right)*, ×915 *(left)*. *(From W. C. Roberts, G. P. Bodey, and P. T. Wertlake, The Heart in Acute Leukemia. A Study of 420 Autopsy Cases, Am. J. Cardiol., 21:388, 1968. Reproduced with permission from the publisher and author.)*

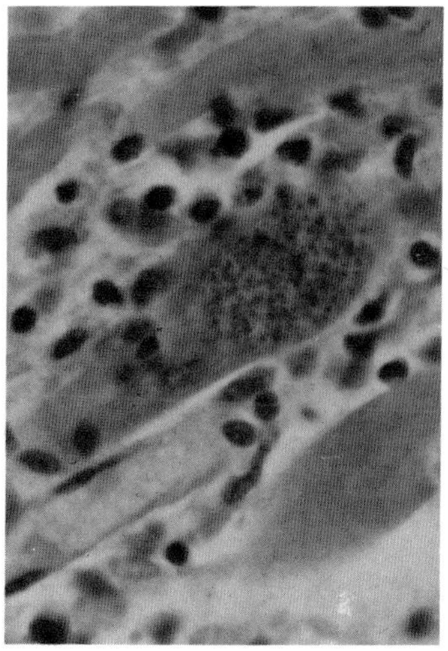

D *Trypanosoma cruzi* in its leishmanial state parasitizing the sarcoplasm of the myocardial cell. The surrounding fiber edema and acute inflammatory reaction are indicative of rupture of the myocardial cell. Hematoxylin and eosin stains: ×125. *(Courtesy of Dr. M. Gravanis, Professor of Pathology, Emory University School of Medicine.)*

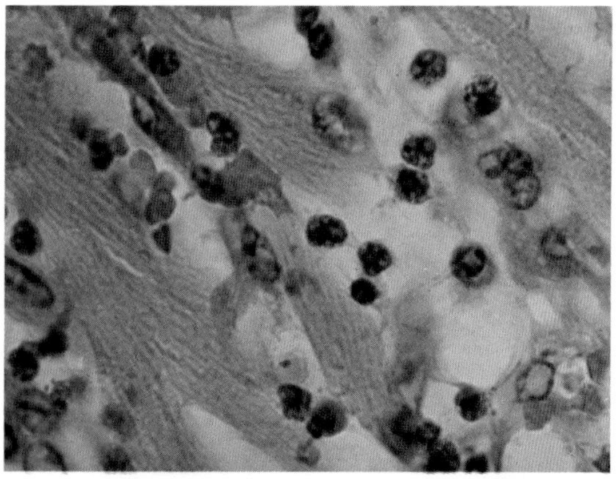

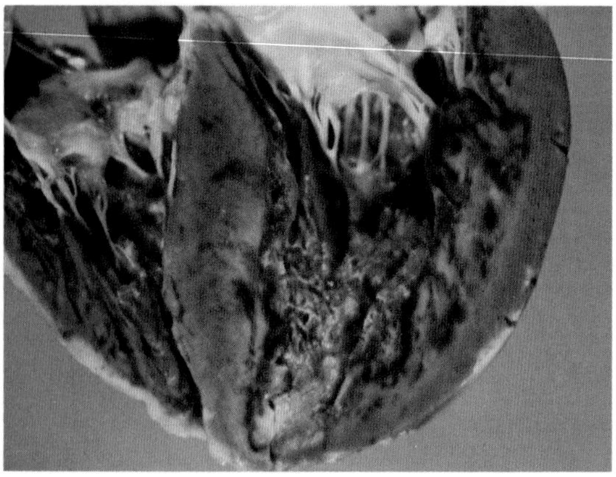

B Trichinosis. Photomicrograph of eosinophilic myocarditis *(upper)* and gross specimen showing left ventricular extensive mural thrombosis *(lower)* in a 46-year-old woman who was well until 13 days before death when she noted fever, headache, neck stiffness, myalgias, dizziness, and pleuritic chest pain. These symptoms worsened, and 3 days before death she was hospitalized. She appeared acutely ill, febrile, and had tachycardia (120 beats per minute). The neck was rigid and the proximal limb muscles very tender. The leukocyte count was 11,000 per cubic millimeter, and the blood smear disclosed 38 percent eosinophils. The ECG was normal except for sinus tachycardia; chest roentgenogram disclosed no abnormalities. She was found dead in bed. After death, it was learned that she often ate raw meat. At necropsy, the heart weighed 260 g; its myocardial walls were filled with extravasated inflammatory cells, mainly eosinophils. Hematoxylin and eosin stain: ×860 *(upper)*. *(From J. J. Andy, J. P. O'Connell, R. C. Daddario, and R. C. Roberts, Trichinosis Causing Extensive Ventricular Mural Endocarditis with Superimposed Thrombosis. Evidence that Severe Eosinophilia Damages Endocardium, Am. J. Med., 63:824, 1977. Reproduced with permission from the publisher and author.)*

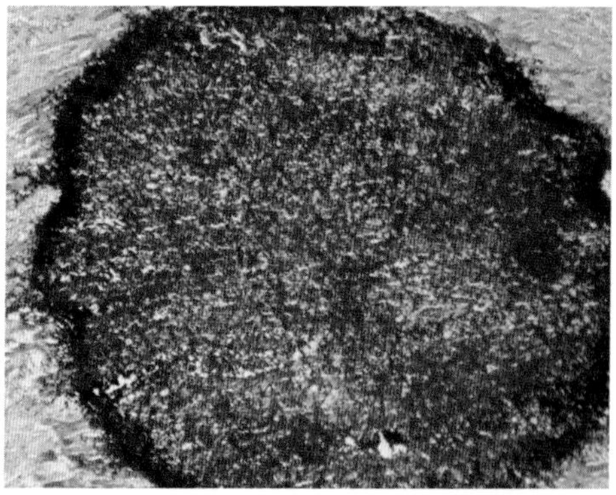

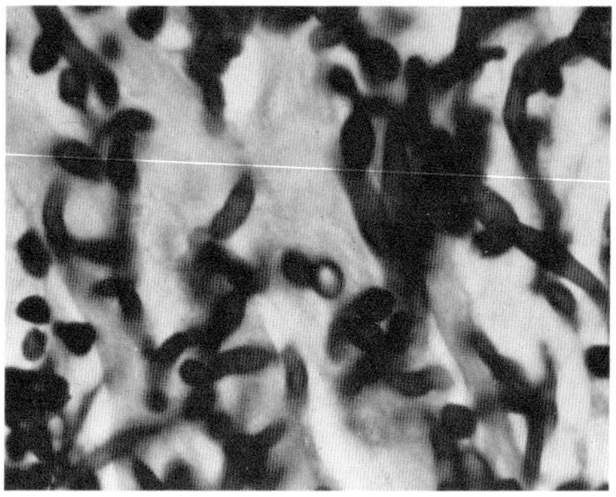

C Cardiac candidiasis in a 20-year-old man with acute myeloblastic leukemia. Gross myocardial abscesses were present in the left and right ventricular free walls, ventricular septum, and papillary muscles. Large myocardial abscess containing massive numbers of *Candida* organisms *(upper)*. Close-up of the *Candida* organisms *(lower)*. Periodic acid Schiff stains: ×12 *(upper)*, ×320 *(lower)*. *(From D. C. Ihde, W. C. Roberts, K. C. Marr, H. D. Brereton, W. P. McGuire, A. S. Levine, and R. C. Young, Cardiac Candidiasis in Cancer Patients, Cancer, 41:2364, 1978. Reproduced with permission from the publisher and author.)*

20

Pathophysiology of Heart Failure

Robert C. Schlant, M.D. Edmund H. Sonnenblick, M.D.

Definitions

In clinical medicine there is an increasing appreciation of the need for precise physiological definitions; nevertheless, at times there is still a considerable difference between the physiological and clinical use of similar terms. This situation is particularly common in considerations of patients with heart failure. The following definitions and classification (Table 20-1) are presented with the realization that future research will allow a much more precise analysis and classification of different types of heart failure based upon differences in their biochemistry and biophysics.[1–7]

Circulatory failure is a general term that refers to an inadequacy of the cardiovascular system in performing its basic functions of providing nutrition to the cells of the body and removing metabolic products from the cells. It may be caused primarily by either cardiac or peripheral (noncardiac) conditions.

TABLE 20-1 Classification of Circulatory Failure and Circulatory Overload

1. Circulatory failure
   a. Heart (cardiac) failure
   b. Noncardiac (peripheral) circulatory failure
      (1) Decreased return of blood to heart, inadequate blood volume
      (2) Increased capacity of vascular bed
      (3) Peripheral vascular abnormalities or disease
      (4) Inadequate oxyhemoglobin
2. Circulatory congestion
   a. Cardiac circulatory overload
      (1) Heart (cardiac) failure
   b. Noncardiac circulatory overload
      (1) Increase in blood volume
      (2) Increase in venous return and/or decrease in peripheral vascular resistance

Noncardiac conditions that can cause circulatory failure include inadequate blood volume, decreased venous return, increased capacity of the vascular system, peripheral vascular abnormalities or disease, and inadequate levels of oxyhemoglobin.

Circulatory overload or congestion is a general term referring to excess blood volume from either cardiac or noncardiac causes.[1] *Noncardiac circulatory overload* may be divided into two categories: (1) those conditions in which the primary defect appears to be an increase in blood volume (the accumulation of excess salt and water due to salt-retaining steroids, excess blood or fluid administration, acute glomerulonephritis, oliguria, or anuria); and (2) those conditions in which the primary defect appears to be an increased venous return and/or decreased peripheral resistance (arteriovenous fistulas, beriberi, cirrhosis, or severe anemia, etc.). Many patients with noncardiac circulatory overload eventually develop secondary "high-output" heart failure (see Chap. 24).

Clinically, the term *congestive heart failure* is used to describe a complicated and variable symptom-sign complex or syndrome that usually, but not necessarily, includes dyspnea and increased fatigability, tachypnea and tachycardia, pulmonary rales, cardiomegaly, ventricular gallop sound(s), and peripheral edema. More precisely, however, congestive heart failure is that state in which abnormal circulatory congestion occurs as the combined result of heart failure and of the peripheral circulatory and sympathetic-renal compensatory mechanisms that are brought into play. When intravascular circulatory congestion is present for any length of time, there is usually increased transudation of fluid from the capillaries into the interstitial spaces. In the pulmonary circulation, if the rate of transudation exceeds the rate of lymphatic drainage, pulmonary edema develops. Initially, this may be detected by x-ray examination, and only later may audible rales be detected on physical examination. In the systemic venous system, venous congestion may be visible and may result in the development of peripheral edema or hepatomegaly. In the majority of patients, congestive heart failure develops chronically and is associated with the retention of sodium and water by the kidneys. In most patients with clinical congestive heart failure due to mechanical or myocardial abnormalities, the heart (pump) failure is preceded by periods of *myocardial* dysfunction and of *myocardial* failure, during which overall cardiac pump function and cardiac output (at least while at rest) may be maintained by compensatory mechanisms.

Acute congestive heart failure can develop following a myocardial infarction of the left ventricle or following the rupture of a cardiac valve or structure. In this situation an acute shift of blood from the systemic circulation to the pulmonary circulation may occur before the retention of significant sodium or water. It should be emphasized that the term *congestive heart failure* should not be used unless the congestion is of cardiac origin. When the cause of the pulmonary or peripheral congestion is not clear, however, it is usually preferable to describe the symptoms or signs, which are nonspecific, and to avoid improperly diagnosing heart failure.

Myocardial dysfunction and *myocardial failure* are terms used to refer to mild ("dysfunction") and to more marked decreased performance ("failure") of the myocardium. In some patients with moderate or more marked myocardial dysfunction or myocardial failure, the decreased myocardial function can be detected by studies of overall cardiac pump function, whereas milder dysfunction in other patients may be detected only by more specific indexes of myocardial contractility (see Chap. 17). In many patients with myocardial "dysfunction," and even more advanced myocardial "failure," the overall cardiac pump function (and cardiac output at rest) may be maintained reasonably well by compensatory mechanisms such as increased ventricular filling or preload (dilatation) and/or cardiac hypertrophy. Myocardial failure may occur due to a loss of cells, i.e., in acute myocardial infarction with segmental loss, in myocarditis with diffuse loss, in toxic cardiomyopathy, or secondary to chronic hypertrophy with scarring or hypertrophy dysfunction (Table 20-2). As compensatory hypertrophy becomes more marked, the unit contractility of the myocardium often declines. Ultimately, the myocardial failure (plus mechanical abnormalities that may be present) often leads to a decrease in systolic pump function that is sufficient to produce overall "pump" or heart failure (see Fig. 20-5). In most patients, significant dysfunction and failure of the myocardium occur before the clinical stages of heart ("pump") dysfunction or failure, and before the clinical syndrome of congestive heart failure (see Chap. 17).

Although myocardial and ventricular dysfunction or failure usually involves both systolic and diastolic dysfunction, it is also frequently useful to consider separately the *systolic* and the *diastolic* properties of the myocardium and of the ventricle.[8,9] Thus, some patients may have marked *systolic ventricular dysfunction* or *failure* at a time when they do not have significant, if any, elevation of diastolic pressures. On the other hand, some patients can have marked elevation of left ventricular diastolic pressure and pulmonary congestion (*diastolic failure of the ventricle*) at a time when the systolic or pumping function of the ventricle is well maintained or even greater than normal. The latter situation may especially occur in some patients with hypertrophic cardiomyopathy or aortic stenosis, in whom the elevated diastolic pressure may be present due to a combination of the effects of ventricular hypertrophy and myocardial diastolic dysfunction at a time when the systolic function or cardiac output may be normal or even slightly elevated. Similarly, some patients with high-output states, primary noncardiac circulatory overload, hypertrophic cardiomyopathy, or aortic stenosis may develop pulmonary congestion and edema secondary to an abnormal elevation of ventricular diastolic pressure at a time when the total cardiac output (systolic or "pump" function) and ejection fraction of the left ventricle is normal or even increased. The latter syndrome can also occur in con-

TABLE 20-2 Causes of Overall Heart "Pump" Failure

1. Mechanical Abnormalities
   a. Increased pressure load
      (1) Central (aortic stenosis, etc.)
      (2) Peripheral (systemic hypertension, etc.)
   b. Increased volume load (valvular regurgitation, shunts, increased preload, etc.)
   c. Obstruction to ventricular filling (mitral or tricuspid stenosis)
   d. Pericardial constriction, tamponade
   e. Endocardial or myocardial restriction
   f. Ventricular aneurysm
   g. Ventricular dyssynergy
2. Myocardial (muscular) abnormalities
   a. Primary
      (1) Cardiomyopathy
      (2) Neuromuscular disorders
      (3) Myocarditis
      (4) Metabolic (diabetes mellitus, etc.)
      (5) Toxic (alcohol, cobalt, etc.)
      (6) Presbycardia
   b. Secondary
      (1) Dysdynamic (secondary to mechanical abnormalities) disorders
      (2) Ischemia (coronary heart disease)
      (3) Metabolic disorders
      (4) Inflammation
      (5) Infiltrative diseases
      (6) Systemic disease
      (7) Chronic obstructive lung disease
      (8) Depression due to drugs
3. Altered cardiac rhythm or conduction sequence
   a. Standstill
   b. Fibrillation
   c. Extreme tachycardia or bradycardia
   d. Electrical asynchrony, conduction disturbances

ditions associated with an increase in blood volume from the accumulation of excess salt and water due to salt-retaining steroids, administration of excess blood or fluid, acute glomerulonephritis, oliguria, or anuria. It may also be found in patients with an abnormally increased venous return and/or decreased peripheral resistance, as might occur with arteriovenous fistulas, beriberi, cirrhosis, severe anemia, etc. In these conditions the chronic volume and/or pressure load upon the ventricle may eventually produce myocardial and ventricular systolic ("pump") dysfunction or failure. Ultimately, this can result in the cardiac output falling to abnormally low levels. When symptoms of pulmonary congestion or pulmonary edema occur while the cardiac output is still normal or elevated, the syndrome is sometimes referred to as *high-output failure* (see also Chap. 24).

Physiologically, heart failure or cardiac failure may be defined as *that condition in which the heart is no longer able to pump an adequate supply of blood for the metabolic needs of the body, provided there is adequate venous return to the heart.* In addition to this primary systolic or "pump" failure, there is often (but not always) an abnormally high diastolic pressure within the ventricle. In patients with mild heart failure, the ventricular end-diastolic pressure and the cardiac output may be normal at rest, but the ventricular end-diastolic pressure often becomes elevated to abnormal levels during stress such as exercise or an increase in afterload, and the increase in cardiac output per deciliter increase in oxygen consumption is decreased. In patients with more severe ventricular failure, both the early and end-diastolic pressures may be elevated even at rest. The elevated left ventricular diastolic pressure is reflected in an elevation of pulmonary venous and capillary pressures and in dyspnea that results from changes in pulmonary compliance due to pulmonary congestion and edema.

Since the basic fundamental of heart failure is an inability of the heart as a pump to supply adequately the demands of the body, it is apparent that the term *heart failure* could be applicable in a very general sense whenever the demands for increased cardiac output are not met as a result of cardiac limitations. This implies that any heart would eventually "fail" if the demands were increased sufficiently. In fact, this might occur in persons with apparently normal hearts during extreme exertion. In most individuals, however, exertion is stopped prior to heart failure by fatigue or breathlessness. In most patients with the clinical syndrome of heart failure, the cardiac output is decreased somewhat at rest and becomes progressively decreased during exercise. It is also apparent that before one reaches the stage of heart failure, as defined above, the body has utilized many compensatory mechanisms after the onset of the initial abnormality or stress and that these compensatory mechanisms eventually have failed to maintain the needs for cardiac output.

As noted in Table 20-2, the causes of overall heart pump failure may be classified into three main categories: (1) failure primarily related to work overloads or mechanical abnormalities, (2) failure primarily related to myocardial abnormalities, and (3) failure related to abnormal cardiac rhythm or conduction sequence. Although heart failure is usually considered as being due to ventricular failure, atrial failure (see below) can contribute significantly.

As indicated in Table 20-2, there are several causes of both "primary" and "secondary" myocardial failure. Myocardial failure is said to be primary when it is caused by (1) idiopathic cardiomyopathy (Chap. 58), (2) cardiomyopathy due to a primary neuromuscular disease (Chap. 58), (3) myocarditis (Chap. 57), (4) metabolic deficiencies of the myocardium, such as beriberi and possibly hyper- or hypothyroidism (Chaps. 24 and 72), (5) toxic effects of chemicals such as alcohol or cobalt, or (6) myocardial changes due to aging (Chap. 71). Myocardial failure is said to be "secondary" (see Table 20-2) when it is produced by (1) "dysdynamic" myocardial failure (see below), (2) myocardial ischemia (which may be either acute, "dynamic" myocardial failure or chronic, static failure due to a loss of myocytes and myocardial fibrosis), (3) metabolic disorders or toxins (Chaps. 5, 58, 72 to 77), (4) myocardial inflammation (Chap. 57), (5) myocardial infiltrative disorders (Chap. 58), (6) systemic diseases (Chaps. 57, 72 to 77), (7) chronic obstructive lung disease, or (8) depression due to drugs. The cause of left ventricular systolic dysfunction in patients with chronic obstructive lung disease is unknown, although the combination of hypoxia and hypercapnia may be important. Left ventricular diastolic dysfunction in such patients is, in part, secondary to the pronounced right ventricular hypertrophy and dilatation and secondary elevation of left ventricular diastolic pressure.

Dysdynamic myocardial failure is a general term used to refer to the common forms of secondary myocardial failure that commonly develop after a period of increased ventricular preload or afterload. The term *dysdynamic* (i.e., "with impaired force or power") *myocardial failure* implies that the systolic mechanical performance or myocardial contractility per unit mass is significantly decreased, often secondary to a chronic mechanical abnormality; initially, however, the overall cardiac (pump) function may be maintained by compensatory mechanisms, and the cardiac output at rest may not be abnormally decreased.

Forward failure and *backward failure* are expressions that have been used at times with somewhat different meanings. In oversimplified terms, "forward failure" has been used to imply that most of the patient's symptoms resulted from a low cardiac output with resultant symptoms of easy fatigability, weakness, or even shock, whereas "backward failure" has implied that most of the patient's symptoms resulted from elevation of venous pressure behind the failing ventricle(s). This elevation of venous pressure *was usually thought* to be caused by the inability of the ventricle to empty itself properly or by obstruction to ventricular filling (mitral or tricuspid stenosis).

The two expressions have also been used in reference to concepts of the pathogenesis of the retention of salt and water. Thus, some early investigators postulated that in backward failure most of the patient's symptoms and signs of pulmonary or peripheral congestion and edema resulted from an elevation of venous pressure behind, or upstream from, the failing ventricle. The cardiac output might be increased or might even be returned to normal by the increased venous pressure behind the ventricle and the resultant increase in diastolic filling or stretch of the ventricle. When right ventricular failure developed, systemic venous and capillary pressures became elevated and peripheral edema developed, producing a decrease in effective circulating blood volume. An increase in tubular reabsorption of salt and water was thought to occur as a result of renal vasoconstriction secondary to the change in "effective" blood volume or secondary to an elevation of renal venous pressure. In forward failure, the decreased cardiac output was postulated to produce tissue edema by an increase in capillary permeability secondary to tissue hypoxia. Later, when this theory became untenable, it was postulated that the decreased cardiac output altered renal plasma flow and glomerular filtration, thereby contributing to the retention of salt and water and producing a secondary increase in blood volume, elevation of venous pressure, and formation of edema. Subsequent studies have demonstrated that while there is still some validity to parts of both the forward-failure and the backward-failure theories, they are oversimplifications of the pathogenesis of salt and water retention and edema formation in heart failure. Accordingly, even though the expressions are oversimplifications in this regard, they may still have some limited usefulness as a form of shorthand to describe a clinical symptom-sign complex. Thus, when the symptoms and signs are predominantly related to pulmonary or systemic venous congestion, backward failure may be said to exist. Conversely, if the symptoms are due to a marked decrease in cardiac output, forward cardiac failure, which is often acute, may be said to exist.

"Left heart" (left-sided) failure and *"right heart" (right-sided) failure* are clinical terms used to refer to conditions in which the primary impairment is of the left side of the heart or of the right side of the heart, respectively. Since both sides of the heart are in a circuit, it is apparent that one side cannot pump significantly more blood than the other side for any length of time in the absence of abnormal shunts, communications, or regurgitation. Furthermore, there is evidence that experimentally produced pure failure of one ventricle may produce significant hemodynamic and biochemical abnormalities of the other ventricle, even without the usual hemodynamic manifestations of ventricular failure. Accordingly, even though the pumping ability of one side may be the primary impairment, the output of the other side is secondarily decreased, and the biochemistry and hemodynamics of the contralateral ventricle can be abnormal even in "pure" one-sided failure.

The most common cause of clinical right-sided heart failure is, of course, left-sided heart failure. Though this right-sided failure is usually said to be secondary to elevation of the pulmonary artery pressure, it is possible that the biochemical changes that may occur in the opposite ventricle in experimental pure unilateral failure may play a significant role. In most situations, the expression *left-sided heart failure* is clinically used in reference to symptoms and signs of elevated pressure and congestion in the pulmonary veins and capillaries, whereas *right-sided heart failure* is used in reference to symptoms and signs of elevated pressures and congestion in the systemic veins and capillaries. Actually, significant amounts of sodium and water retention, with subsequent formation of peripheral edema, may occur with pure left-sided heart failure without hemodynamic evidence of right-sided heart failure.

Latent heart failure is that state in which heart failure is not present at rest but is apparent during periods of increased stress such as exercise, emotion, fever, surgical operations, or after an acute increase in blood volume.

Compensated heart failure is that condition in which heart failure was previously present, but in which cardiac output has been returned to (or maintained at) a normal level by compensatory mechanisms or by therapy. The usual "compensatory" mechanisms include increased sympathetic adrenergic stimulation of the heart, fluid retention by the kidney with increased venous return and increased ventricular preload, and cardiac dilatation and hypertrophy. Clinically, myocardial compensation may be produced by an increase in myocardial contractility by digitalis glycosides or by the use of vasodilator drugs. The term *compensated heart failure* is also used, often less appropriately, in reference to patients with congestive heart failure whose symptoms and signs of pulmonary or peripheral congestion are relieved by diuretic therapy. In such patients, the myocardial function and cardiac output are usually not truly compensated (and cardiac output may actually be further decreased by diuretic therapy), even though the diuretic therapy may produce relief from the clinical symptoms due to congestion.

Atrial failure is that condition in which the atrium fails to provide adequate filling of the ventricle in relation to the venous return to the atrium. Although isolated atrial failure rarely, if ever, produces failure of the entire heart, the development of atrial fibrillation or flutter can precipitate heart failure in patients with compensated heart failure, particularly when marked ventricular hypertrophy or diastolic dysfunction is present and when an "atrial kick" is important to maintaining cardiac output.

TABLE 20-3 Compensatory Mechanisms in Heart Failure

1. Autonomic nervous system
   - *a.* Heart
     - (1) Increased heart rate
     - (2) Increased myocardial contractility
     - (3) Increased rate of relaxation
   - *b.* Peripheral circulation
     - (1) Arterial vasoconstriction (increased afterload)
     - (2) Venous vasoconstriction (increased preload)
2. Kidney: renin-angiotensin-aldosterone
   - *a.* Arterial vasoconstriction (increased afterload)
   - *b.* Sodium and water retention (increased preload and afterload)
   - *c.* Increased myocardial contractility
3. Frank-Starling law of the heart: Increased end-diastolic fiber length, volume, and pressure (increased preload)
4. Hypertrophy
5. Peripheral oxygen delivery
   - *a.* Redistribution of cardiac output
   - *b.* Altered oxygen-hemoglobin dissociation curve
   - *c.* Increased oxygen extraction by tissues
6. Anaerobic metabolism

Compensatory Mechanisms in Heart Failure

Many of the adjustments to heart failure are similar to the homeostatic mechanisms utilized by the body in response to circulatory failure from any cause, such as acute blood loss and acute myocardial infarction. Many of these cardiac reserve mechanisms (Table 20-3) are also utilized by normal subjects during exercise or during periods of increased stress. In human beings with heart failure, it is often impossible to separate the many different, complex mechanisms of adjustment, many of which affect and modify each other. It should also be emphasized that with mild heart failure these compensatory mechanisms are often able to restore to normal or near normal the arterial blood pressure, the organ perfusion, and the cardiac output at rest and perhaps even during moderate exercise. When the failure is mild, there may be few if any symptoms or organ dysfunctions resulting from these "compensatory" mechanisms. Eventually, however, many of the symptoms and organ dysfunctions (even death) that occur in patients with heart failure are the result of "overcompensation" by these same mechanisms (see also Chaps. 17 and 21).

Autonomic Nervous System

One of the more important acute adjustments to heart failure is a reflex increase in autonomic sympathetic excitation to the heart and to most of the arteries and veins.[10–12] In general, the increased sympathetic activity, in combination with increased plasma concentrations of norepinephrine and angiotensin II, produces generalized arterial vasoconstriction and an increase in venous tone. The increased sympathetic adrenergic stimulation of the heart is associated with an inhibition of cardiac parasympathetic activity.[11] An acute increase in sympathetic impulses to the heart normally stimulates the local release of norepinephrine and thereby produces beta stimulation with an increase in heart rate and an increase in myocardial contractility. Norepinephrine also increases the rate of ventricular relaxation, which further contributes to increased ventricular filling. In addition, the generalized increased sympathetic activity and the release of norepinephrine from the adrenal medulla and the peripheral blood vessels contribute toward increasing myocardial contractility.

Patients with chronic congestive heart failure have a significant decrease in the myocardial concentration of norepinephrine.[3,4,13–17] This is associated with decreased activity of myocardial tyrosine hydroxylase, which is the rate-limiting enzyme in the synthesis of norepinephrine.[18] Of interest, when right ventricular hypertrophy and failure is experimentally produced, the myocardial norepinephrine concentration is decreased in both the right and left ventricles.[19] In experimental chronic heart failure, there also is a decrease in the amount of myocardial norepinephrine released per nerve impulse as well as defects in the uptake and the binding of norepinephrine.[17,20] In contrast, the arterial concentration of norepinephrine in patients with moderate to severe congestive heart failure is elevated at rest, and it increases to more than normal during exercise; both of these findings are presumably due to an increased synthesis in the peripheral vasculature and the adrenal medulla.[21] Although the myocardial synthesis of norepinephrine is impaired in congestive heart failure, the myocardium has been said to be normally responsive to exogenous norepinephrine and may even be supersensitive.[19] On the other hand, recent studies have found a decreased catecholamine sensitivity and beta-adrenergic receptor density in failing human hearts.[22] In general, however, most evidence supports the thesis that the failing heart appears to become progressively dependent upon extracardiac, circulating norepinephrine. As a result, congestive heart failure is occasionally made worse by drugs such as beta blockers, guanethidine, or reserpine, all of which may interfere with the myocardial sympathetic-adrenergic system. Overall, however, the defective synthesis and the depletion of myocardial norepinephrine does not appear to be a major, primary cause of myocardial failure, although it may be an important contributing mechanism. Some patients with chronic congestive heart failure also have a significant depression of the normal parasympathetic nervous control of the heart.[14]

In patients with heart failure, the complex reflex actions of the autonomic nervous system and local autoregulatory mechanisms tend to preserve circulation to the brain and heart while decreasing blood flow to the skin, skeletal muscles, spanchnic organs, and kidneys.[3,6,23–29] The increased sympathetic adrenergic stimulation of the peripheral arteries and the increased concentrations of circulating norepinephrine and angiotensin II contribute to the arteriolar vasoconstriction and to the maintenance of arterial pressure, while the sympathetic stimulation of the veins contributes to an increase in venous tone, which helps to maintain venous return and ventricular filling and to support cardiac performance by Starling's law of the heart. The arterial and arteriolar resistance of patients with congestive heart failure is also increased by their increased sodium and water content.[30] The generalized increase in sympathetic nervous system activity also appears to play a facilitative role in sodium and water retention in heart failure.[29]

The increased systemic arteriolar vasoconstriction associated with heart failure is an example of a compensatory mechanism that may have evolved in response to an inadequate cardiac output from other causes, such as hemorrhage or an inadequate blood volume. In such an acute situation, the reflex has obvious acute advantages in maintaining arterial pressure to perfuse the brain and heart, whereas in the patient with chronic heart failure, the compensatory increase in arteriolar resistance may actually make it more difficult for the failing heart to eject blood. One of the cornerstones of the modern therapy of heart failure is the reduction of peripheral vascular resistance by vasodilator drugs (see below and Chaps. 21 and 88).

Kidney: Renin, Angiotensin, and Aldosterone

The compensatory, homeostatic adjustments that occur when the heart fails tend to restore normal ventricular systolic pump function, although often at the price of increased diastolic pressures within the involved ventricle and in the venous system filling the ventricle. One important compensatory mechanism is the increase in ventricular filling pressures produced by an increase in plasma volume as the result of salt and water retention by the kidneys. As indicated in Fig. 20-1, the mechanisms leading to an increase in plasma volume and capillary pressure may ultimately contribute to the formation of interstitial edema.[31] The precise mechanism or stimuli for the initial changes in the kidneys that produce salt and water retention in heart failure are still not clear.[29,32–34] Possible mechanisms include a decrease in the "effective" arterial blood volume, which is sensed by arterial volume receptors and by decreased distending pressure in the carotid sinus and other cardiothoracic receptors in the great arteries and veins, and by sensors in the thorax, kidneys, and atria, and possibly in the ventricles, liver, and central nervous system.[29,35] If there is an increase in renal venous pressure, this may also contribute to sodium retention by the kidneys. The importance of atrial natriuretic factor and other peptides in the pathogenesis of the syndrome of congestive

FIGURE 20-1 Schema of the major events in heart failure that lead to the release of renin by the kidney, the increased secretion of aldosterone, the increased tubular reabsorption of sodium and water, and the production of edema. *(From P. Cannon and M. Martinez-Maldonado, The Pathogenesis of Cardiac Edema, Semin. Nephrol., 3:211, 1983. Reproduced by permission from the publisher and the author.)*

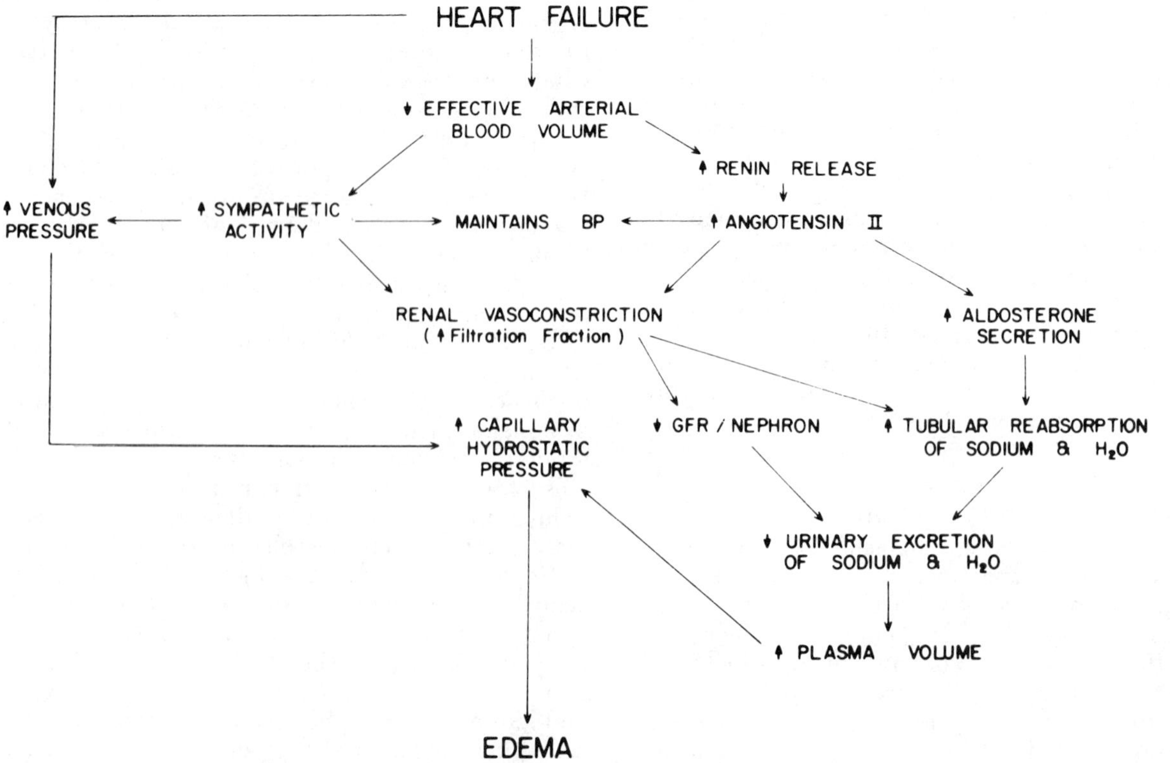

heart failure is unclear.[36–46] There is some evidence that atrial natriuretic factor may inhibit the production of aldosterone.[47]

During the phase of edema formation, patients with heart failure have a significantly reduced ability to excrete a load of either sodium chloride or water. If normal renal perfusion is restored by the expansion of blood volume in patients with mild heart failure, the handling of additional small amounts of sodium may return toward normal; however, patients with severe failure remain unable to excrete solute and water normally despite a marked expansion of blood volume and interstial fluid volume.

The renal vasoconstriction of patients with congestive heart failure is thought to result primarily from increased activity of both the sympathetic nervous system and the renin-angiotensin system.[34] Prostaglandins and vasoactive peptides, especially neuropeptides, may also be involved. In addition to a reduction in total renal blood flow, there is a redistribution of flow that produces a greater reduction of flow in the outer renal cortex with a relative maintenance of perfusion in the juxtamedullary areas.[29,32,48–51]

Patients with mild heart failure may have a normal glomerular filtration rate despite a reduced renal blood flow. This is a result of an increased filtration fraction due to marked efferent renal arteriolar vasoconstriction and decreased hydrostatic pressure in the peritubular capillaries.[52,53] In patients with more severe heart failure, total renal blood flow is even more decreased, and the glomerular filtration rate may be significantly decreased even though the filtration fraction may increase further. In this situation, "prerenal azotemia" is often present, with an increase in the blood urea concentration.

The sympathetic nervous system, which can be activated by lowering of the arterial blood pressure or by direct stimulation of the renal nerves, plays a facilitative role in the renal retention of sodium and water in heart failure. The increased tubular reabsorption of sodium and water in heart failure is aided by the marked redistribution of renal blood flow described above.[29,32,50,51] In addition, the uptake of fluid from the interstitium into the peritubular capillaries is enhanced by the efferent renal arteriolar vasoconstriction, which increases colloid osmotic pressure in the peritubular capillaries. These hemodynamic mechanisms work synergistically to increase sodium and water reabsorption.[29,49,54–59]

Patients with heart failure have significantly decreased excretion rates of sodium chloride due to increased tubular reabsorption, even when the glomerular filtration rate is normal. Most (about 60 to 70 percent) of the glomerular filtrate is normally reabsorbed in the proximal convoluted tubules. Sodium appears to diffuse into proximal tubular cells, from which it is pumped into the lateral and basal intercellular spaces, with chloride and water following passively.[29,32,60,61] At present, it is uncertain whether or not proximal tubular reabsorption is increased in heart failure.[32,62]

About 25 percent of sodium reabsorption normally occurs in the ascending limb in the loop of Henle. In the thick ascending limb, the absorption of chloride is active with sodium following passively.[32] Although it is probable, it is not yet certain that there is increased reabsorption of sodium and water in the thick ascending limb in heart failure.[51,54,62–64]

Most of the remaining 10 percent of filtered sodium is normally reabsorbed in the distal convoluted tubules and collecting ducts by active sodium transport,[51,65,66] and this is linked to the action of aldosterone, which also enhances the excretion of potassium and hydrogen ions. There is strong evidence that experimental heart failure very significantly increases the reabsorption of sodium in the collecting ducts.[32,51,61] It has been suggested that the sensitivity of the cells of the distal tubules and collecting ducts to aldosterone may be increased by an unidentified factor.[29] On the other hand, atrial natriuretic factor appears to decrease the production of aldosterone.[47]

Within hours after the production of heart failure, the kidneys secrete increased amounts of *renin*.[33,67–71] The secretion of renin is controlled by at least the following four mechanisms and agents: (1) changes in wall tension in renal afferent arterioles, (2) a macula densa receptor that detects changes in the rate sodium and/or chloride reach the distal tubule, (3) a negative feedback effect of circulating angiotensin, and (4) the central nervous system, which influences renin secretion by the renal nerves, adrenal medulla, and the posterior pituitary.[70] Carotid sinus or atrial distension may also influence renin secretion.[32,33,72]

Renin acts upon angiotensinogen, which is produced mainly in the liver, to produce angiotensin I, which is converted in the lungs and to a lesser extent in the kidney and blood vessels to angiotensin II.[68–72] Angiotensin II has strong arterial vasoconstrictor properties and contributes to the increase in peripheral vascular resistance and the maintenance of blood pressure in heart failure when "effective" filling of the arterial circulation decreases.[29,67,69,73] Angiotensin II further constricts renal efferent arterioles; in the brain, it stimulates thirst, while in the adrenal gland, it stimulates secretion of *aldosterone*, which very strongly promotes the reabsorption of sodium and chloride in the distal tubules and collecting ducts of the kidney and which is metabolized in the liver. Angiotensin II also has some direct inotropic properties and may augment the release of norepinephrine from nerve endings. Angiotensin II is converted to angiotensin III, which also has vasoconstrictive properties. Glomerular mesangial cells appear to have angiotensin II receptors which may influence mesangial cell contraction and thereby the glomerular surface area available for filtration.[74] There is evidence that in mild experimental heart failure, the secretion of renin and the plasma concentrations of angiotensin II and aldosterone may return to or toward normal after the retention of sodium and water has produced expansion of the blood volume and interstitial fluid volume.[29,75]

There is also evidence in severe heart failure of increased secretion of pituitary antidiuretic hormone, or vasopressin (AVP). Although this may contribute to the decreased ability of some patients to secrete a water load, it is not felt to play a major role in edema formation.[29,76] There is also evidence that a deficiency of "natriuretic factor" might contribute to edema formation; however, its role in heart failure is not clear.[32,71,77–79]

There is good evidence for the presence of bioactive peptides that are made and stored in atrial cells. It has been suggested that increases in extracellular fluid volume and sodium are sensed by atrial receptors, which cause atriopeptigen to be released from storage granules. The atriopeptigen is cleaved to form atriopeptin I and atriopeptin II, both of which have a natriuretic and diuretic effect. Both relax intestinal smooth muscle, and atriopeptin II also relaxes vascular smooth muscle.[36–45] There is also evidence that atrial natriuretic factor may inhibit aldosterone production.[47] The importance of a number of peptides, including atrial peptides and the "atrial natriuretic factor" in normal fluid balance, heart failure, or essential hypertension is the subject of much current research.[44] The neuropeptide tyrosine (PGY), a 36-amino acid peptide, may be important in the control of myocardial contractility and the regulation of myocardial perfusion.[80]

The kidneys synthesize prostaglandins PGE_2 and $PGF_{2\alpha}$ in the interstitial and collecting duct cells of the medulla. These are released into the renal interstitial fluid and renal venous blood, and are metabolized in both the renal cortex and the lungs. PGI_2 (prostacyclin) and PGE_2 can by synthesized by renal vascular and smooth muscle cells.[81,82] Their precise role in the maintenance of normal sodium balance or in heart failure is still unclear.[29,71,83] They may help maintain glomerular filtration in the presence of marked efferent arteriolar vasoconstriction.[84,85] PGI_2 (prostacyclin) and PGE_2 may stimulate the release of renin.[81,82]

There is also suggestive evidence that the vasodilator peptides bradykinin and kallidin, which are formed by the kallikrein-kinin system, may be involved in the intrarenal distribution of blood flow and the excretion of sodium,[40,71,86] but their importance in heart failure is also unknown.

Frank-Starling Law of the Heart

The Frank-Starling law of the heart is immediately brought into play following acute failure of the heart. When the normally filled ventricle fails to eject a normal quantity of blood during one beat, its end-systolic volume increases. Consequently, this increased volume remains and is added to the blood entering the ventricle during the next diastole. The net result is an increased end-diastolic volume for the next beat. This increased "preload" produces an increased amount of stroke work and a larger stroke volume during the next contraction by the Frank-Starling law of the heart (see Chap. 3). Over a period of time, the ventricle may become compensated and may be able to maintain normal or nearly normal stroke volume and work at an increased end-diastolic fiber length and volume (see Fig. 3-10). In many patients with a chronic increase in preload due to aortic or mitral regurgitation, the ventricle dilates markedly and increases its end-diastolic volume strikingly without an increase in pressure. Later, with the onset of diastolic failure of the ventricle, the diastolic pressure becomes progressively elevated. Theoretically, an increase in cardiac output with increased preload would not occur if the heart were operating on a flat or "descending limb" of its function curve. It appears, however, that the heart can function on a "descending limb" for only brief periods.[87–89] Recent studies suggest that the chronically dilatated left ventricle subjected to additional volume load does not utilize the Frank-Starling mechanism to a significant degree at the ultrastructural level.[90–95]

In patients with congestive heart failure the retention of salt and water by the kidneys increases effective blood volume, which tends to increase ven-

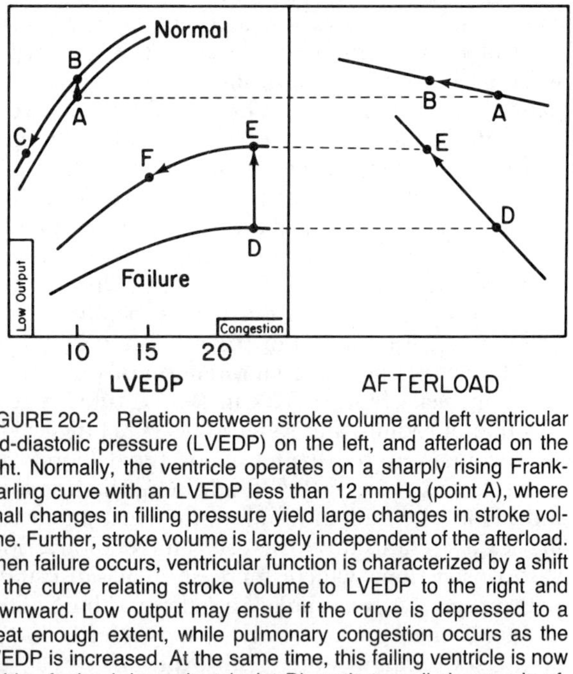

FIGURE 20-2 Relation between stroke volume and left ventricular end-diastolic pressure (LVEDP) on the left, and afterload on the right. Normally, the ventricle operates on a sharply rising Frank-Starling curve with an LVEDP less than 12 mmHg (point A), where small changes in filling pressure yield large changes in stroke volume. Further, stroke volume is largely independent of the afterload. When failure occurs, ventricular function is characterized by a shift of the curve relating stroke volume to LVEDP to the right and downward. Low output may ensue if the curve is depressed to a great enough extent, while pulmonary congestion occurs as the LVEDP is increased. At the same time, this failing ventricle is now highly afterload-dependent (point D) so that small changes in afterload produce large changes in stroke volume.

When afterload is reduced in the normal circulation (i.e., point A to point B) on the right, stroke volume rises very slightly. If venodilatation occurs at the same time, stroke volume falls to point C on the left. The net result is a decrease in stroke volume. On the contrary, when afterload is reduced in the presence of severe ventricular failure, stroke volume is increased (point D to point E) on the right. Since the Frank-Starling curve is relatively flattened, a simultaneous decrease in venous tone leads to a decrease in LVEDP with only a small decrease in stroke volume (point E to point F) on the left. The net result of these opposing consequences may be an increase in stroke volume. These results are observed clinically when nitroprusside is administered as an "unloading" agent for treating the failing ventricle.

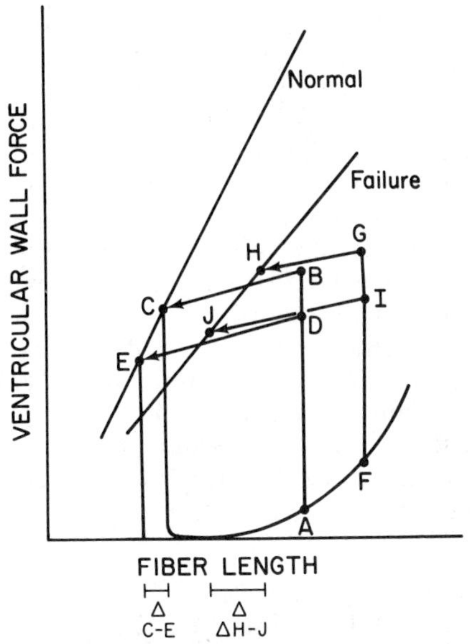

FIGURE 20-3 Relation between ventricular wall force and fiber length. Hypothetical contractile cycles have been portrayed for the normal and failing ventricle. In the normal heart, contraction starts at point A; wall force rises until the aortic valve is opened (point B); the ventricle empties (point B to point C), and relaxation ensues. When arterial pressure (afterload) is reduced, e.g., to point D, ejection starts at point D and procedes to point E.

In the presence of ventricular failure, the fiber length in diastole is increased and ventricular contraction starts at point F. With systolic contraction, ventricular wall force rises to point G, and with ventricular emptying, fiber length decreases to point H. When the afterload is decreased, wall force only needs to reach point I when ventricular wall force begins until emptying to point J.

Of note, for the same relative change in afterload, the increase in shortening is greater in the failing ventricle (ΔH to J) than in the normal heart (ΔC to E) due to the relative flattening of the systolic curve in the former case.

tricular filling volume and to return stroke output toward normal. This basic compensatory mechanism may return stroke output to normal or near normal, but at the expense of increased venous pressure in the pulmonary venous or the systemic venous systems. In some patients this increased filling pressure appears to be chronically necessary for a reasonable cardiac output. Such patients may develop symptoms of decreased cardiac output if the ventricular filling pressure is excessively decreased by diuretics. This need for a high filling pressure is particularly likely to occur in patients with pericardial constriction, aortic stenosis, restrictive cardiomyopathy, or hypertrophic cardiomyopathy (see Chap. 17).

Another characteristic of the failing heart is that it becomes less influenced by preload but more afterload dependent (Figs. 20-2 and 20-3). The normal heart can sustain large changes in systolic loading or afterload with little change in cardiac output and with only minor changes in diastolic volume. When myocardial failure is present and diastolic volume is augmented, however, any further increase in afterload leads to substantial falls in cardiac output. Alternatively, a decrease in afterload in this circumstance may substantially increase the cardiac output.

Hypertrophy of the Heart

Hypertrophy is one of the major adjustments of the heart to chronically increased stress. Experimentally, there is metabolic evidence of hypertrophy within a few hours after an increase in cardiac work.[7,96–103] Hyperplasia, or an actual increase in the total number of myocardial cells, is thought to occur in human beings only if the increased stress occurs within a few months of age. On the other hand, cardiac hypertrophy is associated with a significant increase in the number or size of sarcomeres within each myocardial cell.

Two classic types of left ventricular hypertrophy are recognized: concentric and eccentric. In pure *concentric hypertrophy* of the left ventricle, there is an increase in the thickness of the ventricular wall, but the ventricular chamber does not increase in diameter. In some instances, the ventricular chamber may actually decrease in size. This type of hypertrophy is classically present in patients with isolated valvular aortic stenosis. In pure *eccentric hypertrophy,* the thickness of the left ventricular wall and the internal diameter of the ventricle increase proportionately. This may be seen in normal growth, in endurance athletes, or in patients with volume overload of the left ventricle, as in isolated mitral regurgitation.[104–108] Although the exact myocardial stimulus for hypertrophy is unknown,[7,96–102,109] it has been suggested that an increase in systolic wall tension of the ventricle in conditions associated with increased afterload stimulates the synthesis of sarcomeres in parallel to existing sarcomeres and thereby produces concentric hypertrophy.[104–107] Conversely, it has been suggested that an increase in diastolic wall tension in conditions with increased preload primarily stimulates the synthesis of sarcomeres in series with preexisting sarcomeres and produces eccentric hypertrophy. In compensated hypertrophy, the increase in wall thickness is such that the tension in the wall is maintained in a normal range. There is evidence that there may be differences in the myosin that is synthesized in response to a stimulus to hypertrophy; these differences are more marked in atrial myosin.[110]

It is significant that the increase in individual myocardial cell length in patients with chronically dilated hearts is not adequate to explain the increase in heart size frequently encountered. In such patients, there is also significant myocardial "slippage" or rearrangement, at the level of myofibrils, myocardial fibers, and muscle bundles.[4,104,111–113]

In general, most studies have indicated that the compensatory hypertrophy in many patients with chronic pressure or volume overload can be adequate to return the calculated systolic wall tension to normal although diastolic wall stress may remain abnormal in patients with volume overload.[3,4,6,95,104–107,114–118] Uncompensated failure is commonly characterized by an increase in systolic wall tension despite the compensatory hypertrophy. On the other hand, uncompensated ventricular failure is frequently characterized by a failure to normalize systolic wall tension. Growth hormone, thyroid hormone, hydrocortisone, and increased sympathetic stimulation of the heart appear to be necessary for cardiac hypertrophy to develop in response to stress.[119]

Effect of Cardiac Hypertrophy on Diastolic Compliance

The diastolic compliance or distensibility of ventricles with concentric hypertrophy due to pressure overload is typically much less than that of patients with eccentric hypertrophy due to volume overload in the absence of severe myocardial failure. Thus, the extremely thick hypertrophied ventricle of a patient with concentric hypertrophy from aortic stenosis may require a high left ventricular end-diastolic pressure for normal filling due to the hypertrophy itself. In such patients, an elevation of ventricular diastolic pressure is not necessarily due to myocardial failure. In contrast, many patients with eccentric hypertrophy from mitral or aortic regurgitation may have markedly increased end-diastolic volumes with relatively normal diastolic pressures, often in the presence of significant myocardial and ventricular systolic dysfunction. These findings limit the value of ventricular end-diastolic pressure as an index of left ventricular performance, especially if the diastolic pressure is not correlated with other data (see Chap. 17).[120–128] In addition, left ventricular diastolic pressure-volume relations may be significantly influenced by right ventricular pressure and volume.[129] The term *lusitrophy* has been used to refer to the diastolic relaxation and compliance properties of the ventricles.[130]

Effects of Experimental Cardiac Hypertrophy on Indexes of Myocardial Contractility

When the heart is experimentally caused to become hypertrophied by increasing ventricular preload (volume overload), it is generally agreed that the myocardial contractility per unit mass is not decreased until shortly before the onset of failure.[4,6,91,93–95,131,132] In contrast, there is lack of agreement as to whether or not myocardial contractility per unit mass is decreased soon after the development of hypertrophy that is experimentally produced by increased ventricular afterload (pressure overload), i.e., the experimental equivalent of aortic or pulmonary stenosis. A number of studies of this type of hypertrophy have found that myocardial contractility per unit mass is decreased prior to the development of failure and have suggested that ventricular compensation is maintained by an increase in total myocardial mass.[3,4,19,133–136] It has also been found that this decreased contractility may be reversible if the experimental hypertrophy is reversed by unbanding before the onset of failure.[137] Other studies of pressure-induced hypertrophy have found that myocardial contractility per unit mass may also return to normal if the elevated pressure load is maintained for 24 weeks,[138] whereas other investigators have found normal ventricular function at rest in animals with stable hypertrophy from either volume or pressure overload.[139] Thus, it appears that alterations in myocardial contractility with associated experimental cardiac hypertrophy are variable and depend upon the inciting stimulus and when the ventricle is studied.[132–140] For example, left ventricular hypertrophy induced by high-altitude hypoxia is not associated with a decrease in the indexes of contractility whereas there is a decrease in the indexes with experimental chronic experimental coarctation of the aorta.[94] Part of the discrepancies in different experimental studies may also depend on the acuteness and severity of the overload or preload, the extent of resultant hypertrophy, and the age of the individual when the hypertrophy occurs (see Chap. 17).

Peripheral Oxygen Delivery

Patients with heart failure redistribute the diminished cardiac output. In general, perfusion of the brain and heart are maintained at the expense of circulation to the kidney, splanchnic area, and skin.

The usual decrease in blood flow to the peripheral tissues in heart failure is associated with a progressive decline in the affinity of hemoglobin for oxygen, which is caused by an increase in 2,3-diphosphoglycerate (DPG).[141] This change in affinity, which is reflected in a rightward shift in the oxygen-hemoglobin dissociation curve, facilitates the release of oxygen in the peripheral capillaries of underperfused tissues.

The peripheral tissues in heart failure extract more oxygen per unit of blood flow, with a resultant increase in the body's arteriovenous oxygen difference. This "venous oxygen reserve" is potentially less useful to the myocardium, which even normally extracts about 65 to 75 percent of the oxygen coming to it (see Chaps. 3 and 5), or to the brain.

Some tissues also utilize anaerobic metabolism during transient periods of increased stress such as exercise. Unfortunately, this reserve mechanism is also of only very limited value to the myocardium (see Chap. 5) or the brain.

The Law of Laplace

The law of Laplace and the effects of ventricular dilatation upon the mechanics and energetics of myocardial contraction are important factors in heart failure. On first thought, it might seem that ventricular dilatation is advantageous. With an increased end-diastolic ventricular volume and sarcomere length, each sarcomere would have to shorten less to eject a given volume of blood, and each myocardial fiber would be able to perform more work by virtue of greater preload and the *law of the heart.* In many situations, however, these seeming advantages are negated by several important hymodynamic consequences of dilatation. The more important of these is the need for the myocardial fibers in the

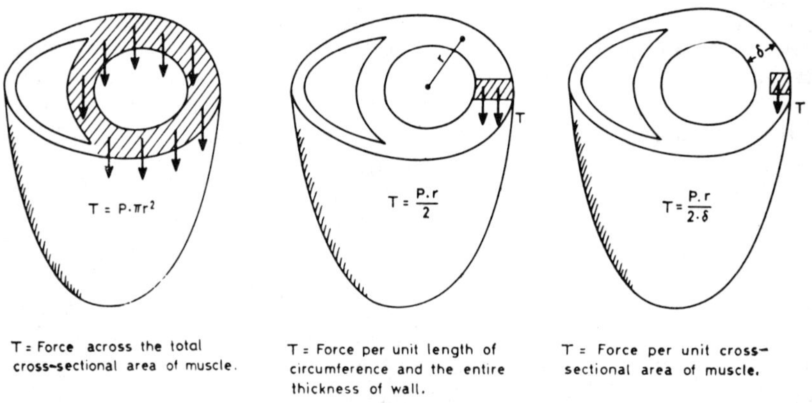

T = P·πr²
T = Force across the total cross-sectional area of muscle.
T = P.r/2
T = Force per unit length of circumference and the entire thickness of wall.
T = P.r/2·δ
T = Force per unit cross-sectional area of muscle.
T
T
δ
r

FIGURE 20-4 Three definitions of contractile force in the myocardium and the formulas based on the law of Laplace used to calculate each. T = contractile tangential tension or force in the wall of the ventricle; P = transmural pressure across the wall of the ventricle; r = average radius of the ventricle, assuming it to be spherical; and δ = ventricular wall thickness. *(From H. S. Badeer, Contractile Tension in the Myocardium, Am. Heart J., 66:432, 1963. Reproduced with permission from the publisher and the author.)*

wall of a dilatated ventricle to develop greater tension in order to produce a given pressure within the ventricle.

In general, ventricular myocardial wall tension is calculated by employing the law of Laplace, which actually applies to a distensible membrane with a spherical or cylindrical shape, and assuming that the ventricle has a spherical cavity. Figure 20-4 illustrates three definitions of contractile tension in the ventricular myocardium, as used by different authors. Badeer[114] has recommended that calculations of myocardial tension be expressed in terms of force per unit of cross-sectional area (formula shown on the right in Fig. 20-4). By all three formulas, it is apparent that as the radius acutely increases, more tension must be developed by each fiber to produce or maintain a given intraventricular pressure. In formula 3, an increased thickness of the ventricular wall tends to decrease the required systolic tension per cross-sectional area.

The law of Laplace expresses an additional disadvantage of the dilated ventricle. In a normal ventricle during ejection, the decrease in average radius of the ventricle is relatively large; consequently, the effect of this decrease in diameter upon instantaneous wall tension is normally greater than the opposite effect of the increasing pressure in the ventricle. As a result, the myocardial fiber tension, or force, may actually *decrease* soon after the beginning of ejection from a normal-sized ventricle, and the tension is usually less at the moment of peak systolic pressure in the ventricle than at the beginning of ejection. On the other hand, if the ventricle is markedly dilated, both the relative and the absolute decrease in average radius is much less during the ejection of an equal volume. In a markedly dilatated ventricle, therefore, the average tension in the myocardial fibers may continue to increase from the beginning of ejection up to the peak systolic pressure.[114,142–144] In a sense, this is an additional type of "afterload" encountered during ejection by ventricles that are significantly dilatated by increased "preload."

A further disadvantage of dilatation is that the increased force, or tension, in the myocardial fibers required to develop a given pressure inside a dilatated ventricle results in a decrease in the *rate* of myocardial fiber shortening (see Chap. 3), further limiting the ability of the ventricle to eject blood.[4,90,92,114,145–147] In mitral regurgitation, the early reduction in afterload (impedance) produced by the relatively rapid emptying of the left ventricle, first into the low-pressure left atrium and then into the aorta, helps to maintain left ventricular function for many years.[2,148]

Basic Mechanisms of Myocardial Failure

The basic biochemical-biophysical mechanisms of myocardial failure remain a very active area of investigation. It is likely that no single mechanism is present in all cases, but rather that different mechanisms (Table 20-4) may exist and contribute under different circumstances.

Energy Production and Utilization

Myocardial Oxygen Consumption in Heart Failure

Most patients with heart failure have a normal coronary blood flow at rest and a normal or elevated

TABLE 20-4 Possible Mechanisms of Myocardial Failure

1. Loss of myocytes
2. Energy production and utilization
   a. Energy supply
   b. Substrate utilization and energy storage
   c. Inadequate mitochondrial mass and function
3. Contractile proteins
   a. Sarcomere "overstretch"
   b. Abnormal myocardial proteins
   c. Defective protein synthesis
   d. Abnormal myosin ATPase
4. Activation of contractile elements
   a. Sarcolemma ATPase
   b. Sarcoplasmic reticulum (SR)
      (1) Ca^{2+} sequestration rate
      (2) Concentration of SR
5. Autonomic nervous system
   a. Depletion of myocardial norepinephrine
   b. Abnormal myocardial receptors
6. Presbycardia

myocardial oxygen consumption per 100 g of tissue.[149] Because of the increased total mass and the increase in myocardial systolic wall tension due to the Laplace relation in patients with heart failure, the total amount of oxygen consumed by the heart may be significantly increased. This may result in a greater amount of oxygen being extracted from each unit of coronary blood flow and a widening of the coronary arteriovenous oxygen difference. Many patients with heart failure are able to increase coronary blood flow during exercise; however, some patients with a dilatated ventricle that increases in diameter during exercise may have a further widening of the coronary arteriovenous oxygen difference during exercise (see Chap. 3). In one study of a group of patients with left ventricular failure, the left ventricular oxygen consumption averaged 16 percent of the total oxygen consumed by the body compared to 5 percent in normal subjects.[150] In one patient with severe aortic valve disease, the left ventricle accounted for 27 percent of the total amount of oxygen consumed by the body.

Substrate Utilization and Energy Storage

Although the myocardial uptake of fatty acids and glucose per 100 g of myocardium is normal in heart failure,[149] there is conflicting evidence on whether or not there is a primary decrease in energy liberation by mitochondrial oxidative phosphorylation.[3,4,6,132,149–160] Although reductions in stores of myocardial high-energy phosphate, creatine phosphate (CP) and/or adenosine triphosphate (ATP) have often been found in heart failure, these changes are usually thought to be secondary and not the primary cause of the failure (see Chap. 5).[3,4,6,158,161,162]

Inadequate Mitochondrial Mass and Function

Several investigators have found a significant decrease in the mass of mitochondria relative to the mass of myofibrils in experimental cardiac hypertrophy.[163,164] As noted elsewhere, there may also be defects in mitochondrial oxidative phosphorylation and in mitochondrial calcium metabolism associated with myocardial failure.

Contractile Proteins

Sarcomere "Overstretch"

As noted in Chap. 3, when myocardial sarcomeres function at lengths up to the L_{max} at about 2.2 μm, they operate on the *ascending limb* of the length-tension curve and develop more active tension with increasing length. When the sarcomeres are stretched beyond the length at which maximal active tension is developed (L_{max}), however, the amount of active tension decreases and the sarcomeres are said to be operating on the *descending limb* of the length-tension curve.[3,4,90–92,111–113,165,166] The existence of a "descending limb" of cardiac function for the entire ventricle is uncertain, however, and much of the apparent decrease in function in some studies was probably due to increased afterload.[87–89] At one time it was thought that sarcomere "overstretch" might be responsible for the decreased myocardial contractility characteristic of many patients with ventricular dilatation and heart failure. Subsequent studies have shown, however, that acute volume loading is associated with an increase in left ventricular midwall mean sarcomere length to about L_{max} (2.2 to 2.4 μm after fixation) and that with chronic volume loading there is additional recruitment of subendocardial and subepicardial sarcomere length to L_{max} but no sarcomere overstretch.[90–95] Other changes that contribute to the marked ventricular dilatation that is frequently present with volume overload include the synthesis of sarcomeres in series with preexisting sarcomeres, slippage of myofibrils and myocardial fibers, and rearrangement of myocardial fibers along cleavage planes of the left ventricle.[3,4,90–93,95,100,111–113,167] Thus, although overstretch of sarcomeres may occasionally be present transiently, it does not appear to be an important primary mechanism of chronic heart failure. The effects of ventricular dilatation upon the law of Laplace have been noted above.

Myosin ATPase

There is substantial evidence of significantly decreased activity of myofibrillar and myosin adenosine triphosphatase (ATPase) in both patients and experimental animals with heart failure.[158,168–176] These changes could significantly interfere with the liberation of energy for myocardial contraction. It has been suggested that the changes in activity of myosin ATPase may be related to associated changes in the number of light chains of myosin.[158,174–176] There are also changes in the characteristics of myosin after the heart is hypertrophied secondary to an increase in afterload. These changes appear to be more marked in atrial myosin than in ventricular myosin.[110]

Defective Protein Synthesis

In most patients with heart failure, there are phases of increased protein synthesis and of stable hyperfunction and hypertrophy which are thought to be initiated by a chronic increase in myocardial stress.[96–102,109,115,177] Meerson has concluded that the subsequent onset of myocardial failure is causally related to a decrease in the synthesis of normal protein due to "wear and tear."[102,109,177] As noted above, experimental hypertrophy may be associated with changes in the characteristics of myosin.[3,110,174–177]

Activation of Contractile Elements

Sarcolemma ATPase

Heart failure may also be associated with defects in the activity of the membrane transport enzyme Na^+,K^+-ATPase,[4,178–180] although the role of this enzyme in the pathogenesis of myocardial failure is less definite.[158]

Sarcoplasmic Reticulum

Calcium Sequestration Rate There is substantial evidence of varying defects in calcium (Ca^{2+}) binding by either sarcoplasmic reticulum or mitochondria in many types of clinical or experimental heart failure.[6,158,181–193] These abnormalities of calcium metabolism appear to be of primary importance in some types of failure, whereas they may be secondary changes in other types. Intracellular acidosis decreases the affinity of troponin-C for Ca^{2+} and may contribute to some forms of heart failure, especially those associated with ischemia.[194] The amount of activator Ca^{2+} available for contraction can also be reduced either by elevation of intracellular Na^+ or by depression of intracellular K^+.[2,186,191–198]

Autonomic Nervous System

As noted above, there is good evidence of defects both in the cardiac sympathetic neurotransmitter and in the cardiac parasympathetic control system in congestive heart failure.[13–22] These changes are not thought to be primary causes of the myocardial failure, although they may contribute significantly.

Senile Cardiomyopathy (Presbycardia or Senile Heart Disease)

In some elderly individuals there may be involutional changes of the myocardium associated with decreased elasticity of the skeleton of the heart and with mild fibrotic changes of the valves. The chemical basis of these aging changes and of the associated brown pigmentation of the heart is not known. This condition, known as *presbycardia, senile heart disease,* or senile cardiomyopathy, probably only rarely produces heart failure by itself; however, it does decrease the contractility and the adaptive reserve capacity of the heart.[199–201] Accordingly, patients with this condition more readily develop heart failure in the presence of other forms of heart disease or, occasionally, even from the increased demands of fever, moderate anemia, mild hyperthyroidism, excess fluid administration, etc. Aged myocardium has also been shown to have a diminished inotropic response to catecholamines and digitalis (see Chap. 71).[202]

Heart Failure Due to Pressure Overload and Volume Overload

Most types of congenital and acquired heart disease result in a mechanical stress upon the heart and myocardium. The two most common general types of mechanical cardiac stress are that resulting from an increased resistance to ventricular emptying of increased afterload (i.e., aortic stenosis, systemic hypertension, etc.) and that resulting from an increased preload or increased ventricular filling (i.e., aortic or mitral regurgitation, ventricular septal defect, etc.). The hemodynamics of several other specific types of mechanical abnormalities are described elsewhere: mitral stenosis (Chap. 38), pericardial tamponade or constriction (Chap. 59), endocardial restriction (Chap. 58), and the several varieties of ventricular dysynergy and aneurysm (Chap. 45).

In some patients with acute mechanical abnormalities, such as the acute rupture of one of the mitral chordae tendineae or of an aortic valve leaflet, the overall function of the heart may fail even though the contractility of the myocardium may initially be relatively normal. Some chronic mechanical abnormalities by themselves can prevent the heart from pumping an adequate amount of blood even without the development of myocardial failure. In the majority of patients with a chronic pressure load (afterload) or a chronic volume load on the left ventricle, however, the development of clinical congestive heart failure or pump failure is preceded by the development of myocardial dysfunction and eventually myocardial failure.

Compensatory Mechanisms in Heart Failure Due to Increased Afterload (Pressure Overload)

Isolated increased afterload ("pressure overload") of the left ventricle is classically seen in patients with systemic hypertension, coarctation of the aorta, or aortic stenosis. The basic reaction of isolated myocardium to an increased afterload is to contract more forcefully but more slowly. In addition, when the heart of experimental animals is acutely subjected to increased afterload, there is metabolic evidence of hypertrophy within a few hours.[96–102] The precise biochemical signal is unknown, but may be related to a chronic increase in systolic wall tension.[102–107] As noted above, the classic type of cardiac hypertrophy associated with aortic stenosis is *concentric hypertrophy,* in which there is marked thickening of the left ventricular walls (including the ventricular septum), but there is no increase in the size of the left ventricular cavity, which may even get smaller.[107] It has been suggested that the increased afterload stimulates myocardial thickening by replication of sarcomeres in parallel.[107] Although the contractility of the myocardium subjected to pressure overload may be decreased per unit mass (see above), overall ventricular compensation is maintained by the increase in myocardial mass. Systolic wall tension may be returned to normal by the concentric hypertrophy and the spherical shape, although diastolic wall stress may remain abnormal.[3,4,7,102–107,114–118,157,162,166] During this phase of adaptive hyperfunction, there may be compensated function of the left ventricle, although at the expense of the adaptive reserve. Eventually, however, both systolic and diastolic myocardial dysfunction and myocardial failure develop, followed by cardiac pump dysfunction and failure or "hyperadaptation" of Meerson.[94,98,102,109] Some of the possible structural and biochemical mechanisms responsible for myocardial failure are discussed above. Figure 20-5 shows the hypothetical changes in myocardial contractility and pump function following the onset of an abnormality such as increased cardiac stress or injury. Note that overall cardiac (pump) function

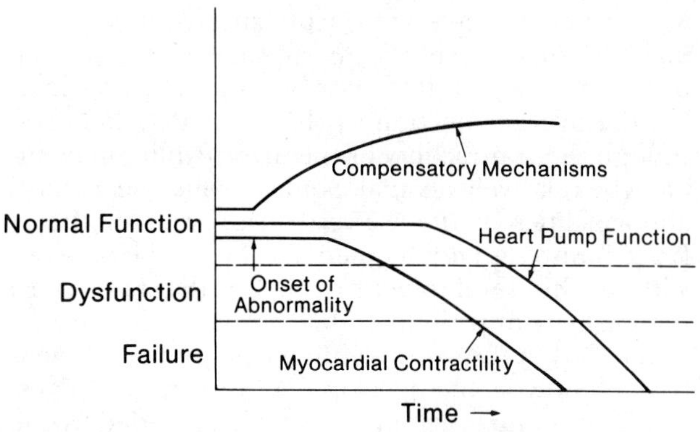

FIGURE 20-5 Hypothetical curves of compensatory mechanisms, overall cardiac or ventricular "pump" performance, and myocardial contractility following the onset of a significant stress such as an increase in ventricular preload or ventricular afterload. Three levels of overall cardiac pump function and myocardial function (contractility) are shown: normal; "dysfunction," or slightly to moderately decreased; and "failure," or markedly decreased function. In general, myocardial function or "contractility" decreases significantly prior to a decrease in overall cardiac "pump" function due to the compensatory mechanisms. Some studies have suggested that myocardial contractility may be decreased very early when hypertrophy occurs due to an increase in afterload. See text for discussion.

may be reasonably maintained by the many compensatory mechanisms until the myocardial failure is moderately severe.

In aortic stenosis there may be special difficulties with the delivery of adequate amounts of oxygen to the myocardial cells, particularly to those in the endocardium. Some of the particular factors responsible for this in aortic stenosis include the elevated myocardial oxygen requirements and the very high intramyocardial pressure, which throttles systolic coronary blood flow even more than usual, especially with tachycardia.[203–205] An elevated ventricular diastolic pressure, which may be necessary to fill the hypertrophied ventricle, will further impede diastolic coronary blood flow to the endocardium (see Chap. 3).[206] In addition, the diffusion distance from myocardial capillaries to the center of the hypertrophied myocardial cells may be significantly increased.[207] Patients with marked concentric hypertrophy from aortic stenosis or other causes frequently have an elevation of left ventricular diastolic filling pressure (and decreased left ventricular compliance or distensibility) due to the hypertrophy itself, rather than to cardiac failure (see "Hemodynamic Characteristics of Heart Failure" below).[117,118,120–128]

Compensatory Mechanisms with Increased Left Ventricular Preload (Volume Overload)

The classic type of ventricular hypertrophy in patients with increased left ventricular preload (volume overload) is the development of *eccentric hypertrophy*, in which the ventricular chamber and the left ventricular wall increase in size proportionately.[96–106] It has been suggested that this type of hypertrophy is produced by a chronic increase in diastolic wall stress and is associated with the synthesis of additional sarcomeres, predominantly in series.[107] Since increased preload also increases systolic wall stress and afterload by the law of Laplace, some replication in parallel also occurs and helps to normalize systolic stress.

When the ventricle is acutely subjected to an increased preload, the ventricle acutely dilates and functions on the "ascending limb" of its length-tension function curve with an increase in the sarcomere length to about 2.2 μm in the midwall of the left ventricle. This length approximates L_{max}, the sarcomere length at which the maximal performance is achieved on the sarcomere length-tension function curve.[112,113] In experimental animals subjected to chronic left ventricular volume loading, the left ventricle may continue to appear to work on a slightly ascending limb of a function curve. In this situation, however, there does not appear to be any additional increase in sarcomere length in the midwall of the left ventricle beyond about 2.2 μm when the ventricle is subjected to increased preload, although there is some additional recruitment in sarcomere length up to about 2.2 μm in the left ventricular endocardial and epicardial area.[90,92,95,112,113,166] Normally, the functioning sarcomere lengths are somewhat less in the endocardium and the epicardium than in the midwall of the left ventricle.[90] The marked ventricular dilatation of chronic volume loading is produced by several mechanisms, including the increase in individual sarcomere length, the synthesis of new sarcomeres in series and parallel with previous sarcomeres, "slippage" between and within myofibrils and fibers, and the rearrangement of myocardial fibers along the normal cleavage planes of the ventricle.[4,90–94,104,111–113,166]

The performance of the ventricle with mitral regurgitation is somewhat aided by the fact that during systole the left ventricle is emptied relatively rapidly by regurgitation into the left atrium and by aortic ejection. This rapid decrease in the mean left ventricular diameter has the effect of rapidly decreasing the systolic wall tension and afterload (impedance) and thus increasing the velocity of contraction.[93,95,146,208] The diastolic capacity of the ventricle with chronically increased volume loads is often markedly increased so that it may accommodate a large volume without excess elevation of diastolic pressure,[95,98] although additional volume loading may produce a precipitous elevation of diastolic pressure indicative of reduced compliance.[91] When the myocardial contractility eventually becomes markedly decreased in patients with chronic volume overload, the many compensatory mechanisms, including ventricular dilatation and hypertrophy, are no longer able to maintain normal compensation, and overall heart "pump" function decreases and may eventually fail (Figs. 20-3 and 20-5).

Atrial Failure and Heart Failure

The two major functions of the atria are pumping and its role as a reservoir. In addition, the atria are the source of atrial natriuretic factor.[36–44] Normally, the atria contribute approximately 15 to 20 percent of ventricular filling, but the relative contribution increases markedly with tachycardia. In normal individuals or patients with mild heart disease, loss of the atrial pumping function may result in no change in cardiac output at rest, although the response to exercise may be diminished. On the other hand, in patients with heart disease and limited cardiac reserve, atrial fibrillation or atrial flutter can produce *atrial failure* with severe detrimental effects on ventricular filling and on the overall pump function of the heart.[209–212]

The more common forms of atrial failure are due to arrhythmia (e.g., atrial fibrillation), mechanical abnormalities (e.g., mitral or tricuspid stenosis), or dysdynamic failure of the atrial myocardium. In some patients with compensated heart disease, congestive heart failure may be precipitated by the onset of atrial fibrillation at times even when the ventricular response rate is controlled by digitalis. In these patients the restoration of normal sinus rhythm may result in a marked improvement in their hemodynamics, presumably by restoration of the normal "booster pump" function of the atria. Interestingly, in some patients following cardioversion and the restoration of normal sinus rhythm, atrial contraction may not occur for several days.[213] Very rarely, atrial fibrillation may produce heart failure in patients with otherwise apparently normal hearts.[214]

Left Atrial Compliance and Heart Failure

The compliance of the left atrium is of great importance in determining the level of left atrial pressure produced by disease of the left side of the heart and especially by mitral regurgitation. Thus, a given volume of mitral regurgitation in a patient with a lax, capacious left atrium may produce only slight elevation of left atrial pressure, whereas the same volume regurgitated into a smaller left atrium with less distensibility may produce marked elevation of left atrial pressure and severe pulmonary congestion (see Chap. 39).[95,212]

Hemodynamic Characteristics of Heart Failure

The major hemodynamic alterations and several of the major compensatory mechanisms that are produced by myocardial and subsequent pump failure are shown in Fig. 20-6. Also indicated are the sites of action of three major therapeutic interventions.

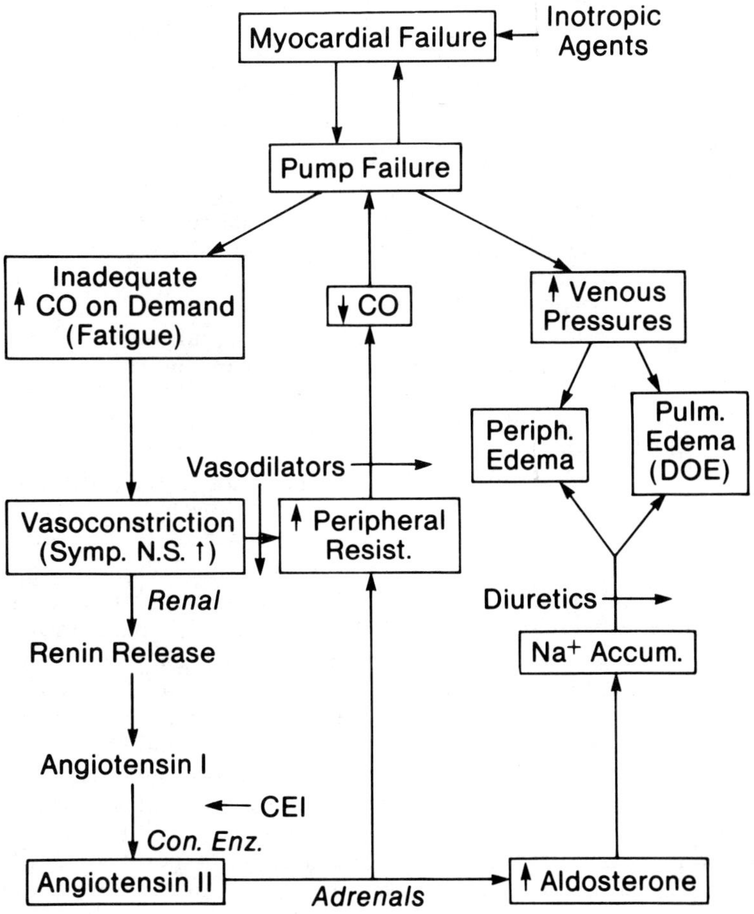

FIGURE 20-6 Schematic diagram of the major hemodynamic alterations and several of the major compensatory mechanisms that result from the development of myocardial failure and pump (heart) failure. Also shown are the sites of action of three major therapeutic inotropic agents, diuretics, and vasodilators.

As described in Chaps. 3 and 17, the performance of the intact heart should generally be assessed at two levels. The first type of analysis is an evaluation of the overall *cardiac pump function* as indicated by the relation between stroke work (or cardiac output) and ventricular end-diastolic volume (or pressure). Ideally, these or other systolic indexes of pump performance are measured at rest and again during exercise or after induced changes in preload or afterload in order to construct a "function curve," although this is seldom done clinically. The second type of assessment is of *myocardial function* (*myocardial contractility* or *inotropic state*). Although decreases in myocardial contractility can sometimes be inferred from studies of overall cardiac function (i.e., when the cardiac output and stroke volume are significantly decreased despite a markedly increased end-diastolic ventricular volume greater than 110 ml/m^2 and the presence of normal afterload and heart rate), more specific and more sensitive quantitative evidence of changes in myocardial contractility in patients is obtained from other special types of analyses. These include the following: (1) *isovolumic phase indexes* utilizing the rate of rise of ventricular pressure (*dP/dt*) or a derivative, (2) *ejection phase indexes* of contractility utilizing circumferential fiber shortening rate (V_{CF}), and (3) *end-systolic indexes,* including analysis of ventricular end-systolic pressure or wall stress–volume relations.[215] The techniques used clinically for evaluation of cardiac function and of myocardial contractility are reviewed in Chap. 17.

Changes in the Contralateral Ventricle

In evaluating left ventricular performance, it is important to keep in mind that experimental right ventricular hypertrophy may be associated with changes in left ventricular end-diastolic pressure or compliance that are probably due in part to a "reversed" Bernheim effect.[129,216–218] In addition, the contralateral left ventricle may have decreased norepinephrine concentration,[19,219] decreased myofibrillar adenosine triphosphatase activity,[169] and increased amounts of collagen.[220] In general, any time there is moderate or marked ventricular hypertrophy, the diastolic pressure-volume relations of the opposite ventricle may be altered.

Secondary Mitral or Tricuspid Regurgitation

"Functional" mitral valve regurgitation may develop secondary to left ventricular myocardial failure, and a similar form of tricuspid regurgitation occurs secondary to right ventricular failure. In both instances the regurgitation is principally the result of failure of the papillary muscles and chordae tendineae of the dilatated ventricle to anchor or constrain the atrioventricular valve leaflets. A secondary mechanism, which is presented in chronic lesions, is dilatation and failure of the valve annulus to constrict properly during systole. If the regurgitation is moderate or severe, the atrial pressure tracings may have a large regurgitant *r* wave ("giant *v* wave").

Pulsus Alternans

Pulsus alternans may occur in patients with heart failure, particularly from aortic stenosis. It may be associated with an alteration of end-diastolic volume or fiber length, with or without an alteration of end-diastolic pressure. In other patients, pulsus alternans may occur in the absence of alteration of either end-diastolic volume or pressure.[221–223] The latter case appears to be associated with an isolated alteration of myocardial contractility. Pulsus alternans is probably related to a defect in the Ca^{2+} release-binding systems involved in excitation-contraction coupling. It may occur briefly in some apparently normal hearts during or following marked tachycardia.

Pulmonary Circulation in Heart Failure

In moderate or severe left ventricular failure, elevated left ventricular diastolic pressure is reflected in an elevation of left atrial, pulmonary capillary, and pulmonary artery diastolic pressures. Initially, the pulmonary artery pressure and right ventricular systolic pressure are abnormally elevated only during exercise, although later they may be chronically elevated to systemic levels at rest, particularly in patients with mitral valve disease (see Chap. 38). In the absence of significant pulmonary vascular disease or tachycardia, the pulmonary artery diastolic pressure can be used as a reasonably good reflection of mean left atrial pressure.

Right Ventricle in Heart Failure

Right ventricular dilatation and failure, with a decreased ejection fraction and rate of ejection, may occur secondary to the chronic pressure load produced by left ventricular failure and, perhaps, secondary to biochemical changes in the contralateral right ventricular myocardium.[3,4,6,19,161,169,219,220] Right ventricular failure may be reflected in a decreased right ventricular stroke volume and ejection fraction, despite an abnormal elevation of the right ventricular end-diastolic volume and pressure, the mean right atrial pressure, and the mean systemic venous pressure. If the failure is mild, these abnormalities may be absent at rest, but may be apparent during exercise. Failure of the right ventricle may also be associated with development of right ventricular pulsus alternans, auscultatory alternans, and a right ventricular diastolic gallop sound. The sequence of severe right ventricular failure secondary to left ventricular failure is frequently associated with the development of tricuspid regurgitation and occasionally associated with the development of functional pulmonary regurgitation due to dilatation of the pulmonary valve ring. Severe pulmonary regurgitation can produce an equalization of the pulmonary artery and right ventricular pressures during mid- or late diastole, although this rarely occurs with functional pulmonary regurgitation. Secondary, or so-called functional, tricuspid regurgitation is caused by the inability of the papillary muscles and chordae tendineae of the dilatated right ventricle to anchor and to maintain adequate closure of the tricuspid valve. Dilatation, or overstretch, of the tricuspid valve ring also contributes to the regurgitation when right ventricular dilatation is severe and chronic. Tricuspid regurgitation may produce large regurgitant *r* waves during systole in the right atrium and systemic veins (see Chap. 40). Clinically, the development of marked right ventricular failure in association with tricuspid regurgitation in a patient with severe left-sided heart failure may occasionally be associated with a significant decrease in the clinical symptoms of pulmonary congestion.

Effects of Exercise in Patients with Myocardial Failure

During exercise in the supine position, the normal ventricle increases its cardiac output predominantly by an increase in rate, although the stroke volume may increase 10 to 20 percent.[224] The increased stroke volume occurs from an unchanged or slightly smaller end-diastolic volume;[225,226] consequently the ejection fraction may increase and the end-systolic volume decrease. The ventricular end-diastolic pressure normally stays the same or slightly decreases, whereas the systolic ejection period shortens and the mean systolic ejection rate increase.[4,6,224–245] In contrast, during exercise in the upright position, the stroke volume may double,[246,247] and during maximal exercise the end-diastolic volume may increase.[4] The calculated efficiency (ratio of external work to oxygen consumed by the heart) increases during exercise in normal individuals, perhaps in part as the result of the decreased average ventricular radius throughout systole.

Conversely, in patients with heart failure due to dysdynamic myocardial failure, exercise may result in the following changes: an elevation of the end-diastolic pressure above 12 mmHg; only a slight increase or an actual decrease in stroke volume despite an increased end-diastolic volume; a decreased ejection fraction;[248] an increased end-systolic volume; and a prolonged preejection phase.[4,144,145,224,227,228,231–233,248] The calculated ventricular efficiency decreases as the result of no increase (or an actual decrease) in stroke volume despite an increased ventricular end-diastolic volume. The latter increases the mean radius of the ventricle and, by the Laplace relation, increases the sarcomere tension necessary to produce a given intraventricular pressure. Not only does the increased tension required by the dilated ventricle increase the myocardial oxygen consumption (MV_{O_2}) but it also decreases the velocity of shortening, further limiting the performance of the ventricle.[4,104,114–116,142–145,249] Exercise may also increase functional atrioventricular valvular regurgitation (see Chap. 17).

In patients with heart failure during dynamic exercise, the cardiac output either does not increase or does not increase adequately relative to the increased oxygen requirements of the body. Usually, the increase in blood flow to the exercising limb(s) is less than normal in clinical heart failure, while there are marked decreases in the already diminished flow to skin, kidneys, and splanchnic organs. Coronary flow usually increases, whereas cerebral flow remains unchanged. The excessive increase in venous tone and central venous pressure during exercise in heart failure may be partially related to a reflex with the afferent limb in the exercising muscle and the efferent limb in the sympathetic nervous system.[1] In addition, the plasma concentration of norepinephrine, which is already increased in moderate or severe congestive heart failure, is further increased. High plasma concentrations of angiotensin II may also contribute to the increase in venous tone.

The fact that the peripheral blood vessels of patients with heart failure have increased sodium and water content and are relatively stiff and relatively unresponsive to local metabolic vasodilator influences during exercise may have a protective influence. For example, if the cardiac output did not increase or even decreased during extensive exercise, the vasodilatation of large skeletal muscle groups could produce an excess fall in the mean arterial pressure.

Effects of Heart Failure on the Peripheral Circulation

In heart failure, there is evidence of a generalized state of arteriolar constriction and venoconstriction, resulting in an elevation of total peripheral vascular resistance and an increase in venous tone (i.e., the venous bed is less distensible than normal).[24–26,28] These changes tend to maintain arterial blood pressure in the face of a decrease in cardiac output at rest or a decrease in the normal increase in organ blood flow during exercise. They are mediated in part by sympathetic vasoconstrictor impulses, related to the generalized increase in sympathetic activity of the body and, perhaps, by mechanical alterations in the distensibility of the resistance (arteriolar) vessels with increased "stiffness" due to increased sodium and water content.[24–26,28,30] In addition, the concentrations of both norepinephrine and angiotensin II are elevated and contribute to both arterial vasoconstriction and the increase in venous tone.[21,73] Increased extravascular fluid or edema can also increase tissue pressure and external pressure on the systemic veins. An increased plasma concentration of vasopressin, or antidiuretic hormone, or of vasoconstrictor peptides or prostaglandins may also contribute to an increase in vascular tone. In some active organs with high oxygen requirements, these vasoconstrictor tendencies may be partially overridden by local metabolic vasodilators or local changes in P_{O_2}, P_{CO_2}, pH, or K^+. In general, however, the usual markedly increased blood flow to exercising muscles is significantly attenuated.

In heart failure associated with a diminished cardiac output, there is a significant redistribution of blood flow which, in part, resembles the normal redistribution occurring during exercise (see Chap. 3). Thus, in heart failure, the renal and skin blood flows are disproportionately reduced early, whereas the decreases in blood flow to the cerebral, splanchnic, and skeletal muscle areas are approximately proportional to the decrease in total cardiac output until the failure is severe. Coronary blood flow per 100 g of tissue tends to remain normal or nearly normal in most patients in heart failure (see Chap. 3). The decreased skin circulation contributes to the heat intolerance and even mild temperature elevations in heart failure, while the decreased flow to the brain and kidneys contributes significantly to the deranged functions of these organs.

As noted above, the increased sympathetic impulses to the kidney and the high blood levels of norepinephrine and angiotensin II produce a redistribution of intrarenal blood flow and lead to further retention of sodium and water.

In addition to a redistribution of blood flow in heart failure, the tissues extract more oxygen per unit of blood flow and utilize anaerobic metabolism to a greater extent than normal, particularly during acute exertion. The increased oxygen extraction results in a widening of the arteriovenous oxygen differences for most organs and for the body as a whole. The pulmonary arteriovenous oxygen difference, which indicates the average of the whole body, is one of the better parameters for judging the adequacy of the heart as a pump to provide oxygen to the tissues.

Physiological Basis of the Therapy of Heart Failure

Heart failure and the resulting compensatory mechanisms described above result in abnormalities in each of the major determinants of myocardial performance: preload, afterload, and contractility. It is useful in selecting the therapy of a patient with heart failure to consider each of these determinants separately (Table 20-5). In general, an excessive increase in preload is treated with either diuretics or venous vasodilators. The relative increase in afterload after associated with heart failure is treated with arterial vasodilators, compounds that inhibit the conversion of angiotensin I to angiotensin II, or compounds that block angiotensin II receptors, while the excess sodium retention with peripheral or pulmonary edema or circulatory congestion is treated with diuretics (see Chap. 21). Figure 20-6 schematically shows the progression from myocardial failure to pump failure and illustrates the major pathophysiological changes in heart failure and the main

TABLE 20-5 Therapy of Heart Failure

Abnormality	Therapy
Preload	Diuretics
	Venous vasodilators
Afterload	Arterial vasodilators
	Angiotensin-converting enzyme inhibitors
	Angiotensin II receptor blockers
Contractility	Inotropic agents

TABLE 20-6 Inotropic Agents

Agent	Action
Digitalis glycosides	Na^+-K^+-ATPase inhibition
Catecholamines:	Stimulate adenylate cyclase; increase cyclic AMP (cAMP); increase slow calcium inward current
Beta$_1$-adrenergic drugs:	
Norepinephrine (NE, IV)	
Epinephrine (IV)	
Isoproterenol (IV,SL)	
Dopamine (IV)	
Dobutamine (IV)	
Prenalterol (IV,PO)	
Levodopa (PO)	Conversion to dopamine, activation of beta-adrenergic receptors, release of NE from sympathetic nerve endings
Propylbutyldopamine (PBDA, IV)	Activates peripheral DA_2 presynaptic and DA_1 postsynaptic dopamine receptors
Beta$_2$ adrenergic drugs:	
Pirbuterol (PO)	
Salbutamol (PO,IV)	
Fenoterol (PO)	
Ibopamine (PO)	
Butopamine (PO)	
Terbutaline (PO)	
Ephedrine (PO)	
Methylxanthines:	
Caffeine	Phosphodiesterase inhibitors; increases cAMP
Aminophylline	
Calcium	
Glucagon	Increases cAMP
Other	
Amrinone (IV)	Phosphodiesterase inhibitor; increases cAMP
Milrinone (IV, PO)	Phosphodiesterase inhibitor; increases cAMP
AY 28,768	
MDL 17,043	
MDL 19,205	
AR 115-BS (Sulmazol)	Phosphodiesterase inhibitor
CI 914	

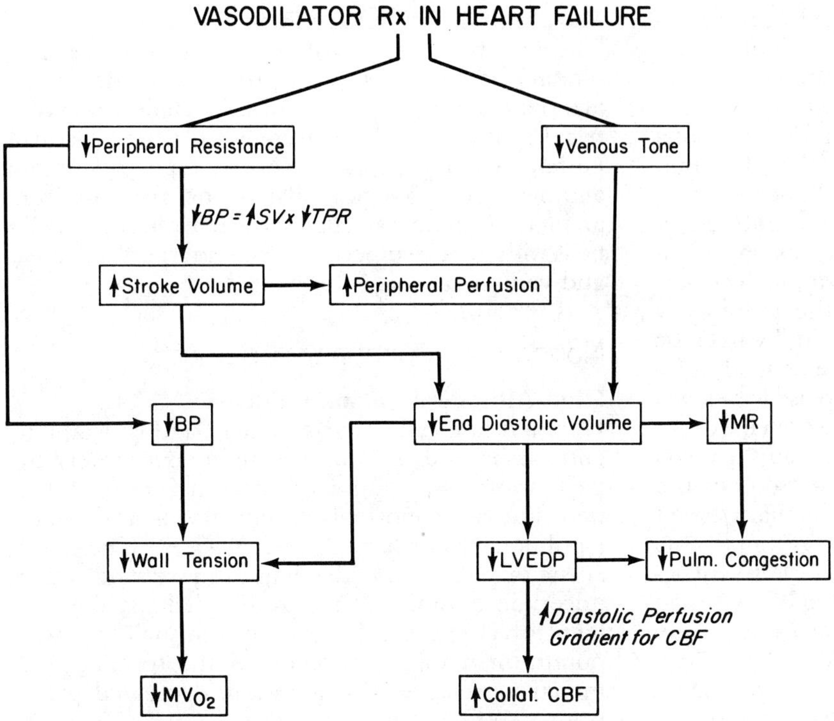

FIGURE 20-7 Schematic diagram of the major actions of vasodilator therapy in heart failure. The decrease in arterial resistance (decreased "afterload") leads to an increase in stroke volume and improved peripheral perfusion. The decrease in arterial pressure combined with a decrease in end-diastolic volume (resulting from the decrease in venous tone) decreases systolic wall tension and myocardial oxygen requirements. The left ventricular end-diastolic volume is decreased as a result of both the improved stroke volume and the decreased venous return. It produces a decrease in left ventricular end-diastolic pressure. The latter reduction may significantly improve coronary blood flow and collateral blood flow to the left ventricle, particularly the subendocardium.

areas of therapeutic attack. Figure 20-7 illustrates schematically the major mechanisms of action of vasodilator therapy in heart failure. Myocardial failure is present in most patients with systolic pump (heart) failure, either as a primary or as a secondary event. Therapy for a decrease in myocardial contractility includes the administration of inotropic (Table 20-6) (see Chaps. 92 and 93). Theoretically, inotropic agents used to treat mild myocardial failure may hasten the progression of the disease, although this potential hazard has not been documented (see Chap. 21 for further details of the treatment of heart failure).[250]

Pulmonary Function and Pulmonary Edema in Congestive Heart Failure

Pulmonary Function

The ventilatory functions of the lungs are frequently impaired due to pulmonary congestion from left ventricular failure or mechanical obstruction at the mitral valve.[251–254] The amount of intrathoracic space available for ventilation may be decreased by fluid in the interstitial, perivascular, and alveolar spaces; by hydrothorax; or in some patients, by an increase in pulmonary blood volume.[255,256] The increased amount of fluid and congestion in the lungs decreases the compliance (increases the stiffness) of the lungs and increases the work and oxygen cost of breathing. Alveolar fluid decreases pulmonary compliance by altering the normal surface tension characteristics, while pericapillary thickening and interstitial edema interfere with alveolar-capillary diffusion of oxygen. The respiratory muscles, which have an increased workload because of the decreased pulmonary compliance, may suffer from relative ischemia and, rarely, may produce pain difficult to distinguish from pain of myocardial origin.

Many patients with moderate pulmonary congestion have compensatory hyperventilation with respiratory alkalosis, although some patients with severe pulmonary edema may have metabolic and respiratory acidosis.[257,258] Pulmonary congestion alters many pulmonary function tests, and it is often difficult to distinguish by such tests between dyspnea due to cardiac causes and dyspnea due to pulmonary causes. In clear-cut instances, however, such a separation is often possible (see Chaps. 21 and 55).[253,254]

Pulmonary Edema

The hydrostatic pressure in the pulmonary capillaries is normally 7 to 12 mmHg at rest in the supine position. When this pressure exceeds plasma oncotic pressure, which is normally 25 to 30 mmHg, net transudation of fluid from the pulmonary capillaries occurs. Pulmonary edema occurs when this rate of transudation exceeds the rate of lymphatic drainage from the tissues.[259–266] If the plasma oncotic pressure is low due to a decreased serum protein concentration, transudation of fluid across the pulmonary capillaries occurs at even lower pressure.[267] There is little evidence that altered capillary permeability due to central nervous system influences or hypoxia is ordinarily an important factor in the production of pulmonary edema in most patients, although changes in capillary permeability can be important in some specialized forms of pulmonary edema due to the "capillary leak syndrome"[268] or in some patients with virus infections of the respiratory tract. The major factor in cardiac pulmonary edema is the pulmonary capillary pressure.[254,259] The pulmonary capillaries have a significant "reserve" compared to systemic capillaries, since the pulmonary capillary pressure can ordinarily increase by 10 to 20 mmHg before significant transudation occurs.

An important consideration in the pulmonary circulation is the normal increase in hydrostatic pressure in both the arteries and veins in the dependent areas of the lungs. This increased pressure accounts, in part, for the initial appearance of pulmonary edema in the lower lobes in many patients with congestive failure. In normal persons in the upright position, relatively little pulmonary blood flow goes to the upper areas of the lungs. In patients with severe mitral stenosis or in severe left ventricular failure, however, the relative blood flow to the upper lobes may equal or even exceed that to the lower lobes. It is as yet uncertain whether this change in distribution of pulmonary blood flow is caused by local vasoconstriction produced by alveolar hypoxia, by a reactive hypertrophy and increased vascular tone of small arteries in the lower lobes secondary to the elevation of pulmonary arterial pressure, or by reflexes from the left atrium or pulmonary veins.

Patients with marked elevation of left atrial pressure for long periods of time may often withstand elevations of pulmonary capillary pressure reasonably well, whereas the same level of pulmonary capillary pressure can produce severe, fulminating pulmonary edema in 5 to 10 min in a patient whose pulmonary circulation is not accustomed to the high-pressure levels. The explanation for this difference may be that patients with chronic transudation of fluid pulmonary capillaries often develop capacious lymphatic channels which are capable of removing large quantities of fluid from the pulmonary interstitial spaces.[269] In addition, the pericapillary thickening and the perivascular edema associated with chronic pulmonary capillary hypertension tend to decrease the rate of fluid transudation. Since pulmonary lymphatic drainage empties into systemic veins, any elevation of central systemic venous pressure tends to decrease pulmonary lymphatic drainage and to worsen pulmonary edema.

It is probable that the occurrence of localized pulmonary edema in areas of acute infection or of previous infection is partially related to permanent alterations in local lymphatic drainage. It is also possible that the relative rareness of pulmonary rales in infants with left ventricular failure is, in part, related to the presence of a pulmonary lymphatic system unscarred by respiratory tract infection. Patients with severe pulmonary disease may have such marked destruction of their pulmonary lymphatics that they develop interstitial pulmonary edema much more readily than normal.

Morphine in Pulmonary Edema

The beneficial effects of morphine in acute pulmonary edema are in part produced by decreased arterial resistance and pressure, which decrease ventricular afterload; by a decrease in venous return, perhaps aided by depression of the respiratory pump; and by "pharmacological phlebotomy" resulting from an increase in the capacity of the peripheral vascular beds with increased perfusion of underperfused areas and venous pooling.[270–273]

Noncardiac Pulmonary Edema[274]

High-Altitude Pulmonary Edema

High-altitude pulmonary edema (HAPE) is apparently associated with marked pulmonary artery hypertension and pulmonary arteriolar vasoconstriction but with normal pulmonary artery wedge ("pulmonary capillary") pressure.[275–280] The mechanism of pulmonary edema in this rare syndrome is uncertain although it is possible that the development of HAPE is related to an unusually marked, nonuniform vasoconstriction of the terminal pulmonary arterioles in response to decreased partial pressure of oxygen in the alveoli. As a consequence, there is excessive blood flow in the other areas of the lung, and the capillary bed may be relatively "unprotected" from the high pulmonary arterial pressure. An additional factor that may be important is the presence of preterminal arterioles, which are short, nonmuscular vessels that arise at right angles from small and medium-sized pulmonary arteries, bypass the pulmonary arterioles, and empty directly into the venous side of the pulmonary capillary bed.[281] These may be important in transmitting the strikingly elevated pulmonary artery pressure directly to the capillary bed in subjects with HAPE. Acute pulmonary hypertension may also damage the arterial walls and lead to direct transarterial leakage of plasma or even blood and allow the formation of microthrombi that may shower the distal capillary bed.[274] Postmortem studies have also suggested that pulmonary vascular obstruction by thrombi may occur in some cases (see Chaps. 54 and 55).

Miscellaneous Forms of Pulmonary Edema

The occasional occurrence of pulmonary edema secondary to pulmonary emboli may be related to "overperfusion edema" similar to that described for high-altitude pulmonary edema; acute left ventricular failure; or to an acute "reversed Bernheim's" effect.[282] The mechanism of pulmonary edema in patients with opiate-induced pulmonary edema (OPE) or heroin intoxication is uncertain, though it may be due to acute apnea with hypoxic pulmonary edema from high-pressure damage to the pulmonary vascular endothelium.[274,283] It may also be due to changes in capillary permeability. Acute cardiomyopathy may also occur.[284] Changes in pulmonary capillary permeability appear to occur in some forms of pulmonary edema associated with infection, inhalation of toxic gases, or with chemicals such as ethchlorvynol or ingested paraquat.[257,274] Changes in capillary permeability also occur in the *a*cute *r*espiratory *d*istress *s*yndrome (ARDS). Vasoconstriction of the pulmonary veins may be an important factor in the pulmonary edema produced by certain endotoxins.[285] Multiple small pulmonary venous thrombi may also produce acute pulmonary edema. Neurogenic pulmonary edema appears to be associated with intensive elevations in systemic arterial and venous pressures and pulmonary arterial, capillary, and venous pressures. The abrupt elevation of pulmonary vascular pressure and volume may damage the vascular endothelium, altering permeability and allowing pulmonary edema to develop.[274,286]

References

1. Eichna, L.: Circulatory Congestion and Heart Failure, *Circulation,* 22:864, 1960.
2. Schlant, R. C., and Nutter, D. O.: Heart Failure in Valvular Heart Disease, *Medicine,* 50:421, 1971.
3. Mason, D. T. (ed.): "Congestive Heart Failure: Mechanisms, Evaluation and Treatment," Yorke Medical Books, New York, 1976, pp. 448.
4. Braunwald, E., Ross, J., Jr., and Sonnenblick, E. H.: "Mechanisms of Contraction of the Normal and Failing Heart," 2d ed., Little, Brown and Company, Boston, 1976, pp. 417.
5. Levine, H. J.: Congestive Heart Failure, in H. J. Levine (ed.), "Clinical Cardiovascular Physiology," Grune & Stratton, New York, 1976, p. 367.
6. Braunwald, E., Mock, M. B., and Watson, J. (eds.): "Congestive Heart Failure: Current Research and Clinical Applications," Grune & Stratton, New York, 1982.
7. Alpert, N. R. (ed.): "Myocardial Hypertrophy and Failure: Perspectives in Cardiovascular Research," vol. 7, Raven Press, New York, 1983.
8. Weber, K. T., and Janicki, J. S.: The Heart As A Muscle-Pump System and The Concept of Heart Failure, *Am. Heart J.* 98:371, 1979.
9. Mirsky, I., Pfeffer, J. M., and Pfeffer, M. A.: Mechanical Properties of Normal and Hypertrophied Myocardium: Is There a Relationship between Diastolic and Systolic Function? in N. R. Alpert (ed.), "Perspectives in Cardiovascular Research," vol. 7, Raven Press, New York, 1983, p. 39.
10. Korner, P. L.: Integrative Neural Cardiovascular Control, *Physiol. Rev.,* 51:312, 1971.
11. Higgins, C. B., Vatner, S. F., and Braunwald, E.: Parasympathetic Control of the Heart, *Pharmacol. Rev.,* 25:119, 1973.
12. Braunwald, E.: Regulation of the Circulation, *N. Engl. J. Med.,* 290:1124, 1420, 1974.
13. Chidsey, C. A., and Braunwald, E.: Sympathetic Activity and Neurotransmitter Depletion in Congestive Heart Failure, *Pharmacol. Rev.,* 18:685, 1966.
14. Eckberg, D. L., Drabinsky, M., and Braunwald, E.: Defective Cardiac Parasympathetic Control in Patients with Heart Disease, *N. Engl. J. Med.,* 285:877, 1971.
15. Rutenberg, H. L., and Spann, J. F., Jr.: Alterations of Cardiac Sympathetic Neurotransmitter Activity in Congestive Heart Failure, *Am. J. Cardiol.,* 32:427, 1973.
16. Goldstein, R. E., Beiser, G. D., Stampfer, M., and Epstein, S. E.: Impairment of Autonomically Mediated Heart Rate Control in Patients with Cardiac Dysfunction, *Circ. Res.,* 36:571, 1975.
17. Rutenberg, H. L., and Spann, J. F., Jr.: Alterations of Cardiac Sympathetic Neurotransmitter Activity in Congestive Heart Failure, in D. T. Mason (ed.), "Congestive Heart Failure: Mechanisms, Evaluation and Treatment," Yorke Medical Books, New York, 1976, p. 85.
18. Pool, P. E., Covell, J. W., Levitt, M., Gibb, J., and Braunwald, E.: Reduction of Cardiac Tyrosine Hydroxylase Activity in Experimental Congestive Heart Failure: Its Role in the Depletion of Cardiac Norepinephrine Stores, *Circ. Res.,* 20:349, 1967.
19. Spann, J. F., Jr., Buccino, R. A., Sonnenblick, E. H., and Braunwald, E.: Contractile State of Cardiac Muscle Obtained from Cats with Experimentally Produced Ventricular Hypertrophy and Heart Failure, *Circ. Res.,* 21:341, 1967.
20. Covell, J. W., Chidsey, C. A., and Braunwald, E.: Reduction of the Cardiac Response to Postganglionic Sympathetic Nerve Stimulation in Experimental Heart Failure, *Circ. Res.,* 19:51, 1966.
21. Thomas, J. A., and Marks, B. H.: Plasma Norepinephrine in Congestive Heart Failure, *Am. J. Cardiol.,* 41:233, 1978.
22. Bristow, M. R., Ginsburg, R., Minobe, W., et al.: Decreased Catecholamine Sensitivity and β-Adrenergic-Receptor Density in Failing Human Hearts, *N. Engl. J. Med.,* 307:205, 1982.
23. Korner, P. I.: Control of Blood Flow to Special Vascular Areas: Brain, Kidney, Muscle, Skin, Liver, and Intestine, in A. C. Guyton and C. E. Jones (eds.), "Cardiovascular Physiology," Physiology Series I, vol. I, University Park Press, Baltimore, 1974, p. 123.
24. Zelis, R., Nellis, S. H., Longhurst, J., Lee, G., and Mason, D. T.: Abnormalities in the Regional Circulations Accompanying Congestive Heart Failure, *Prog. Cardiovasc. Dis.,* 18:181, 1975.
25. Abboud, F. M., Heistad, D. D., Mark, A. L., and Schmid, P. G.: Reflex Control of the Peripheral Circulation, *Prog. Cardiovasc. Dis.,* 18:371, 1976.
26. Zelis, R., Longhurst, J., Capone, R. J., Lee, G., and Mason, D. T.: Peripheral Circulatory Control Mechanisms in Congestive Heart Failure, in D. T. Mason (ed.), "Congestive Heart Failure: Mechanisms, Evaluation and Treatment," Yorke Medical Books, New York, 1976, p. 129.
27. Abboud, F. M., and Thames, M. D.: Interaction of Cardiovascular Reflexes in Circulatory Control, in J. T. Shepherd and F. M. Abboud (eds.), "Handbook of Physiology," American Physiological Society, Bethesda, 1983, pp. 675–754.
28. Vanhoutte, P. M.: Adjustments in the Peripheral Circulation in Chronic Heart Failure, *Eur. Heart J.,* 4(suppl A):67, 1983.
29. Cannon, P., and Martinez-Maldonado, M.: The Pathogenesis of Cardiac Edema, *Semin. Nephrol.,* 3:211, 1983.
30. Zelis, R., Delea C. S., Coleman, H. N., and Mason, D. T.: Arterial Sodium Content in Experimental Congestive Heart Failure, *Circulation,* 41:213, 1970.
31. Casley-Smith, J. R.: Mechanisms in the Formation of Lymph, in A. C. Guyton and J. E. Halls (eds.), "Cardiovascular Physiology IV, International Review of Physiology," vol. 26, University Park Press, Baltimore, 1982, p. 147.
32. deWardener, H.: The Control of Sodium Excretion, in J. Orloff and R. W. Berliner (eds.), "Handbook of Physiology," American Physiological Society, Bethesda, 1973, p. 677.
33. Laragh, J. H., and Sealey, J. E.: The Renin-Angiotensin-Aldosterone Hormonal System and Regulation of Sodium, Potassium, and Blood Pressure Homeostasis, in J. Orloff and R. W. Berliner (eds.), "Handbook of Physiology," American Physiological Society, Bethesda, 1973, p. 831.
34. Hall, J. E.: Regulation of Renal Hemodynamics, in A. C. Guyton and J. E. Halls (eds.), "Cardiovascular Physiology IV, International Review of Physiology," vol. 26, University Park Press, Baltimore, 1982, p. 243.
35. Bishop, V. S., Malliani, A., and Thoren, P.: Cardiac Mechanoreceptors, in J. T. Shepherd and F. M. Abboud (eds.), "Handbook of Physiology," American Physiological Society, Bethesda, 1983, pp. 497–556.

36. de Bold, A. J., Borenstein, H. B., Veress, A. T., and Sonnenberg, H.: A Rapid and Potent Natriuretic Response to Intravenous Injection of Atrial Myocardial Extract in Rats, *Life Sci.,* 28:89, 1981.
37. de Bold, A. J.: Tissue Fractionation Studies on the Relationship between an Atrial Natriuretic Factor and Specific Atrial Granules, *Can. J. Physiol. Pharmacol.,* 60:324, 1982.
38. de Bold, A. J.: Atrial Natriuretic Factor of the Rat Heart: Studies on Isolation and Properties, *Proc. Soc. Exp. Biol. Med.,* 170:133, 1982.
39. Keller, R.: Atrial Natriuretic Factor Has a Direct, Prostaglandin-Independent Action on Kidneys. *Can. J. Physiol. Pharmacol.,* 60:1078, 1982.
40. Sonnenberg, H., Milojevic, S., Chong, C. K., and Veress, A. T.: Atrial Natriuretic Factor: Reduced Cardiac Content in Spontaneously Hypertensive Rats, *Hypertension,* 5:672, 1983.
41. Borenstein, H. B., Cupples, W. A., Sonnenberg, H., and Veress, A. T.: The Effect of a Natriuretic Atrial Extract on Renal Haemodynamics and Urinary Excretion in Anesthetized Rats, *J. Physiol. (Lond.),* 334:133, 1983.
42. Currie, M. G., Geller, D. M., Cole, B. R., et al.: Bioactive Cardiac Substances: Potent Vasorelaxant Activity in Mammalian Atria, *Science,* 221:71, 1983.
43. Thibault, G., Garcia, R., Cantin, M., and Genest, J.: Atrial Natriuretic Factor: Characterization and Partial Purification, *Hypertension,* 5:175, 1983.
44. Schmid, P. G., Sharabi, F. M., and Phillips, M. I.: Peptides and Blood Vessels, in J. T. Shepherd and F. M. Abboud (eds.), "Handbook of Physiology," American Physiological Society, Bethesda, 1983, pp. 815–836.
45. Currie, M. G., Geller, D. M., Cole, B. R., et al.: Purification and Sequence Analysis of Bioactive Atrial Peptides (Atriopeptins), *Science,* 223:67, 1984.
46. Oshima, T., Currie, M. G., Geller, D. M., and Needleman, P.: An Atrial Peptide Is a Potent Renal Vasodilator Substance, *Circ. Res.,* 54:612, 1984.
47. Atarashi, K., Mulrow, P. J., Franco-Saenz, R., Snajdar, R., and Rapp, J.: Inhibition of Aldosterone Production by an Atrial Extract, *Science,* 224:992, 1984.
48. Sparks, H. V., Kopald, H. H., Carriere, S., Chimoskey, J. E., Kinoshita, M., and Barger, A. C.: Intrarenal Distribution of Blood Flow with Chronic Congestive Heart Failure, *Am. J. Physiol.,* 223:840, 1972.
49. Barger, A. C.: Renal Hemodynamics in Congestive Heart Failure, *Ann. N.Y. Acad. Sci.,* 139:786, 1973.
50. Kilcoyne, M. M., Schmidt, D. H., and Cannon, P. J.: Intrarenal Blood Flow in Congestive Heart Failure, *Circulation,* 47:786, 1973.
51. Stein, J. H., Boinjarern, S., Wilson, C. B., and Ferris, T. F.: Alterations in Intrarenal Blood Flow Distribution, *Circ. Res.,* 32-33:61, 1973.
52. Warren, J. V., and Stead, E. A., Jr.: Fluid Dynamics in Chronic Congestive Heart Failure, *Arch. Intern. Med.,* 73:138, 1944.
53. Merrill, A. J.: Edema and Decreased Renal Blood Flow in Patients with Chronic Congestive Heart Failure: Evidence of "Forward Failure" as the Primary Cause of Edema, *J. Clin. Invest.,* 25:389, 1946.
54. Lewy, J. E., and Windhager, E. E.: Peritubular Control of Proximal Tubular Fluid Reabsorption in the Rat Kidney, *Am. J. Physiol.,* 214:943, 1968.
55. Deen, W. M., Robertson, C. R., and Brenner, B. M.: Transcapillary Fluid Exchange in the Renal Cortex, *Circ. Res.,* 33:1–8, 1973.
56. Brenner, B. M., Troy, J. L., and Daugharty, T. M.: Quantitative Importance of Changes in Post-glomerular Colloid Osmotic Pressure in Mediating Glomerular Tubular Balance in the Rat, *J. Clin. Invest.,* 52:190, 1973.
57. Meyers, B. D., Deen, W. M., and Brenner, B. M.: Effects of Norepinephrine and Angiotensin II on the Determinants of Glomerular Ultrafiltration and Proximal Tubule Fluid Reabsorption in the Rat, *Circ. Res.,* 37:101, 1975.
58. Ichikawa, I., and Brenner, B. M.: Importance of Efferent Arteriolar Vascular Tone in Regulation of Proximal Tubule Fluid Reabsorption and Glomerulotubular Balance in the Rat, *J. Clin. Invest.,* 65:1192, 1980.
59. Ichikawa, I., and Brenner, B. M.: Glomerular Response to Severe Congestive Heart Failure in the Rat, *Annual Meeting of the American Society of Nephrology,* Chicago, 1982, p. 152.
60. Windhager, E. E., and Giebisch, G.: Proximal Sodium and Fluid Transport, *Kidney Int.,* 9:121, 1976.
61. deWardener, H. E.: Mechanisms Influencing Urinary Sodium Excretion, in C. J. Dickinson and J. Marks (eds.), "Developments in Cardiovascular Medicine," Baltimore, University Park Press, 1978, p. 179.
62. Levy, M.: Effects of Acute Volume Expansion and Altered Hemodynamics on Renal Tubular Function in Chronic Caval Dogs, *J. Clin. Invest.,* 51:922, 1972.
63. Stumpe, K. O., Solle, H., Klein, H., and Kruch, F.: Mechanism of Sodium and Water Retention in Rats with Experimental Heart Failure, *Kidney Int.,* 4:309, 1973.
64. Mandin, H.: Cardiac Edema in Dogs: I. Proximal Tubular and Renal Function, *Kidney Int.,* 10:591, 1976.
65. Frega, N. S., Davalos, M., and Leaf, A.: Effect of Endogenous Angiotensin on the Efferent Glomerular Arteriole of the Rat Kidney, *Kidney Int.,* 18:323, 1980.
66. Skorecki, K. L., and Brenner, B. M.: Body Fluid Homeostasis in Man, *Am. J. Med.,* 70:77, 1981.
67. Vandongen, R., and Gordon, R. D.: Plasma Renin in Congestive Heart Failure in Man, *Med. J. Austral.* 1:215, 1970.
68. Haber, E.: The Role of Renin in Normal and Pathological Cardiovascular Homeostasis, *Circulation,* 54:849, 1976.
69. Watkins, L., Jr., Burton, J. A., Haber, E., Cart, J. R., Smith, F. W., and Barger, A. C.: The Renin-Angiotensin-Aldosterone System in Congestive Failure in Conscious Dogs, *J. Clin. Invest.,* 57:1606, 1976.
70. Reid, I. A., Morris, B. J., and Ganong, W. F.: The Renin-Angiotensin System, *Ann. Rev. Physiol.,* 40:377, 1978.
71. Baer, P. G., and McGiff, J. C.: Hormonal Systems and Renal Hemodynamics, *Ann. Rev. Physiol.,* 42:589, 1980.
72. Linden, R. J.: Neurocirculatory Control of Sodium and Water Excretion, in C. J. Dickinson and J. Marks (eds.), "Developments in Cardiovascular Medicine," Baltimore, University Park Press, 1978, p. 191.
73. Curtiss, C., Cohn, J. N., Vrobel, T., and Franciosa, J. A.: Role of the Renin-Angiotensin System in the Systemic Vasoconstriction of Chronic Congestive Heart Failure, *Circulation,* 58:763, 1978.
74. Ausiello, D. A., Kreisberg, J. I., Roy, C., and Karnovsky, M. J.: Contraction of Cultured Rat Glomerular Cells of Apparent Mesangial Origin after Stimulation with Angiotensin II and Arginine Vasopressin, *J. Clin. Invest.,* 65:754, 1980.
75. Chonko, A. M., Bay, W. H., Stein, J. H., and Ferris, T. F.: The Role of Renin and Aldosterone in the Salt Retention of Edema, *Am. J. Med.,* 63:881, 1977.
76. Cowley, A. W., Jr.: Vasopressin and Cardiovascular Regulation, in A. C. Guyton and J. E. Halls (eds.), "Cardiovascular Physiology IV, International Review of Physiology," vol. 26, University Park Press, Baltimore, 1982, p. 189.
77. Bahlmann, J., McDonald, S. J., Ventom, M. G., and de Wardener, H. E.: The Effect on Urinary Sodium Excretion of Blood Volume Expansion without Changing the Composition of Blood in the Dog, *Clin. Sci.,* 32:403, 1967.
78. Buckalew, V. M., and Nelson, D. B.: Natriuretic and Sodium Transport Inhibitory Activity in Plasma of Volume Expanded Dogs, *Kidney Int.,* 5:12, 1974.
79. deWardener, H. E.: Natriuretic Hormone, *Clin. Sci. Mol. Med.,* 53:1, 1977.
80. Gu, J., Adrian, T. E., Tatemoto, K., Polak, J. M., Allen, J. M., and Bloom, S. R.: Neuropeptide Tyrosine (NPY)—A Major Cardiac Neuropeptide, *Lancet,* 1:1008, 1983.
81. Berl, T., Henrich, W. L., Erickson, A. L., and Schrier, R. W.: Prostaglandins in the Beta-Adrenergic and Baroreceptor-Mediated Secretion of Renin, *Am. J. Physiol.,* 236:F472, 1979.
82. Levenson, D. J., Simmons, C. E., Jr., and Brenner, B. M.:

Arachidonic Acid Metabolism Prostaglandins and the Kidney, *Am. J. Med.*, 72:354, 1982.
83. McGiff, J., and Itskovitz, H. D.: Prostaglandins and the Kidney, *Circ. Res.*, 33:479, 1973.
84. Lewy, J. E., and Windhager, E. E.: Peritubular Control of Proximal Tubular Fluid Reabsorption in the Rat Kidney, *Am. J. Physiol.*, 214:943, 1968.
85. Schor, N., Ichikawa, I., and Brenner, B. M.: Glomerular Adaptations to Chronic Dietary Salt Restriction or Excess, *Am. J. Physiol.*, 238:F426, 1980.
86. Margolius, H. S., Horwitz, D., Pisano, J. J., and Keiser, H. R.: Relationships among Urinary Kallikrein, Mineralocorticoids and Human Hypertensive Disease, *Fed. Proc.*, 35:203, 1976.
87. Rader, B., Smith, W. W., Berger, A. R., and Eichna, L. W.: Comparison of the Hemodynamic Effects of Mercurial Diuretics and Digitalis in Congestive Heart Failure, *Circulation*, 29:328, 1964.
88. Katz, A. M.: The Descending Limb of the Starling Curve and the Failing Heart, *Circulation*, 32:871, 1965.
89. MacGregor, D. C., Covell, J. W., Mahler, F., Dilley, R. B., and Ross, J., Jr.: Relations between Afterload, Stroke Volume, and the Descending Limb of Starling's Curves, *Am. J. Physiol.*, 227:884, 1974.
90. Ross, J., Jr., Sonnenblick, E. H., Taylor, R. R., Spotnitz, H. M., and Covell, J. W.: Diastolic Geometry and Sarcomere Lengths in the Chronically Dilated Left Ventricle, *Circ. Res.*, 28:49, 1971.
91. McCullagh, W. H., Covell, J. W., and Ross, J., Jr.: Left Ventricular Dilatation and Diastolic Compliance Changes during Chronic Volume Overload, *Circulation*, 45:943, 1972.
92. Spotnitz, H. M., Leyton, R. A., Kelly, D. T., et al.: "Outstretched" Sarcomere in Subacute Volume-Pressure Loading of Dog Right Ventricle, *Circulation*, 46(suppl. 2):44, 1972.
93. Ross, J., Jr., and McCullagh, W. H.: The Nature of Enhanced Performance of Dilated Left Ventricle during Chronic Volume Overloading, *Circ. Res.*, 30:549, 1972.
94. Meerson, F. Z., and Kapelko, V. I.: The Contractile Function of the Myocardium in Two Types of Cardiac Adaptation to a Chronic Load, *Cardiology*, 57:183, 1972.
95. Ross, J., Jr.: Adaptations of the Left Ventricle to Chronic Volume Overload, *Circ. Res.*, 35(suppl. 2):64, 1974.
96. Alpert, N. R. (ed.): "Cardiac Hypertrophy," Academic Press, New York, 1971.
97. Rabinowitz, M., and Zak, R.: Biochemical and Cellular Changes in Cardiac Hypertrophy, *Ann. Rev. Med.*, 23:245, 1972.
98. Meerson, F. Z., Javitz, M. P., Breger, A. M., and Lerman, M. I.: The Mechanism of the Heart's Adaptation to Prolonged Load and Dynamics of RNA Synthesis in the Myocardium, *Basic Res. Cardiol.*, 69:484, 1974.
99. Cohen, J., and Shah, P. M. (eds.): Cardiac Hypertrophy and Cardiomyopathy, *Circ. Res.*, 35(suppl. 2):1, 1974.
100. Rabinowitz, M.: Overview on Pathogenesis of Cardiac Hypertrophy, *Circ. Res.*, 35(suppl. 2):3, 1974.
101. Morkin, E.: Activation of Synthetic Processes in Cardiac Hypertrophy, *Circ. Res.*, 35(suppl. 2):37, 1974.
102. Meerson, F. Z.: Development of Modern Components of the Mechanism of Cardiac Hypertrophy, *Circ. Res.*, 35(suppl. 2): 58, 1974.
103. Grossman, W., Carabello, B. A., Gunther, S., and Fifer, M. A.: Ventricular Wall Stress and the Development of Cardiac Hypertrophy and Failure, in N. R. Alpert (ed.), "Perspectives in Cardiovascular Research," vol. 7, Raven Press, New York, 1983, p. 1.
104. Linzbach, A. J.: Heart Failure from the Point of View of Quantitative Anatomy, *Am. J. Cardiol.*, 5:370, 1960.
105. Badeer, H. S.: Biological Significance of Cardiac Hypertrophy, *Am. J. Cardiol.*, 14:133, 1964.
106. Grant, C. D., Greene, G., and Bunnell, I. L.: Left Ventricular Enlargement and Hypertrophy: A Clinical Angiographic Study, *Am. J. Med.*, 39:895, 1965.
107. Grossman, W., Jones, D., and McLaurin, L. P.: Wall Stress and Patterns of Hypertrophy in the Human Left Ventricle, *J. Clin. Invest.*, 56:56, 1975.
108. Schaper, J.: Hypertrophy in the Human Heart: Evaluation by Qualitative and Quantitative Light and Electron Microscopy, in N. R. Alpert (ed.), "Perspectives in Cardiovascular Research," vol. 7, Raven Press, New York, 1983, p. 177.
109. Meerson, F. Z.: (ed.), "The Failing Heart: Adaptation and Deadaptation," Raven Press, New York, 1983.
110. Gorza, L., Mercadier, J. J., Schwartz, K., Thornell, L. E., Sartore, S., and Schiaffino, S.: Myosin Types in the Human Heart: An Immunofluorescence Study of Normal and Hypertrophied Atrial and Ventricular Myocardium, *Circ. Res.*, 54:694, 1984.
111. Rackley, C. E., Dalldorf, F. G., Hodd, W. P., Jr., and Wilcox, B. R.: Sarcomere Length and Left Ventricular Function in Chronic Heart Disease, *Am. J. Med. Sci.*, 259:90, 1970.
112. Spotnitz, H. M., and Sonnenblick, E. H.: Structural Conditions in the Hypertrophied and Failing Heart, *Am. J. Cardiol.*, 32:398, 1973.
113. Sonnenblick, E. H., and Skelton, C. L.: Reconsideration of the Ultrastructural Basis of Cardiac Length-Tension Relations, *Circ. Res.*, 35:517, 1974.
114. Badeer, H. S.: Contractile Tension in the Myocardium, *Am. Heart J.*, 66:432, 1963.
115. Sandler, H., and Dodge, H. T.: Left Ventricular Tension and Stress in Man, *Circ. Res.*, 13:91, 1963.
116. Hood, W. P., Jr., Rackley, C. E., and Rolett, E. L.: Wall Stress in the Normal and Hypertrophied Human Left Ventricle, *Am. J. Cardiol.*, 22:550, 1968.
117. Grossman, W., McLaurin, L. P., Moos, S. P., Stefandouros, M. A., and Young, D. T.: Wall Thickness and Diastolic Properties of the Left Ventricle, *Circulation*, 49:129, 1974.
118. Sasayama, S., Ross, J., Jr., Franklin, D., Bloor, C. M., Bishop, S., and Dilley, R. B.: Adaptations of the Left Ventricle to Chronic Pressure Overload, *Circ. Res.*, 38:172, 1976.
119. Cohen, J.: Role of Endocrine Factors in the Pathogenesis of Cardiac Hypertrophy, *Circ. Res.*, 35(suppl. 2):49, 1974.
120. Braunwald, E., and Ross, J., Jr.: The Ventricular End-Diastolic Pressure: Appraisal of Its Value in the Recognition of Ventricular Failure in Man, *Am. J. Med.*, 34:147, 1963.
121. Rackley, C. E., Hood, W. P., Jr., Rolett, E. L., and Young, D. T.: Left Ventricular End-Diastolic Pressure in Chronic Heart Disease, *Am. J. Med.*, 48:310, 1970.
122. Levine, H. J.: Compliance of the Left Ventricle, *Circulation*, 46:423, 1972.
123. Covell, J. W., and Ross, J., Jr.: Nature and Significance of Alterations in Myocardial Compliance, *Am. J. Cardiol.*, 32:449, 1973.
124. Grossman, W., and McLaurin, L. P.: Diastolic Properties of the Left Ventricle, *Ann. Intern. Med.*, 84:316, 1976.
125. Gaasch, W. H., Levine, H. J., Quinones, M. A., and Alexander, J. K.: Left Ventricular Compliance: Mechanisms and Clinical Implications, *Am. J. Cardiol.*, 38:645, 1976.
126. Wisneski, J. A., and Bristow, J. D.: Left Ventricular Stiffness, *Ann. Rev. Med.*, 29:475, 1978.
127. Grossman, W., and Barry, W. H.: Diastolic Pressure-Volume Relations in the Diseased Heart, *Fed. Proc.*, 39:148, 1980.
128. Lewis, B. S., and Gotsman, M. S.: Current Concepts of Ventricular Relaxation and Compliance, *Am. Heart J.*, 99:101, 1980.
129. Little, W. C., Badke, F. R., and O'Rourke, R. A.: Effect of Right Ventricular Pressure on the End-Diastolic Left Ventricular Pressure-Volume Relationship before and after Chronic Right Ventricular Pressure Overload in Dogs without Pericardia, *Circ. Res.*, 54:719, 1984.
130. Smith, V. E., and Katz, A. M.: Inotropic and Lusitropic Abnormalities in the Genesis of Heart Failure, *Eur. Heart J.*, 4(suppl. A):7, 1983.
131. Taylor, R. R., and Hopkins, B. E.: Left Ventricular Response to Experimentally Induced Chronic Aortic Regurgitation, *Cardiovasc. Res.*, 6:404, 1972.
132. Cooper, G., IV, Puga, F. J., Zujko, K. J., Harrison, C. E., and Coleman, H. N., III: Normal Myocardial Function and Energetics in Volume-Overload Hypertrophy in the Cat, *Circ. Res.*, 32:140, 1973.

133. Spann, J. F., Jr.: Heart Failure and Ventricular Hypertrophy: Altered Cardiac Contractility and Compensatory Mechanisms, *Am. J. Cardiol.,* 23:504, 1969.
134. Pool, P. E., Chandler, B. M., Spann, J. F., Jr., Sonnenblick, E. H., and Braunwald, E.: Mechanochemistry of Cardiac Muscle: IV. Utilization of High-Energy Phosphates in Experimental Heart Failure in Cats, *Circ. Res.,* 24:313, 1969.
135. Spann, J. F., Jr., Covell, J. W., Eckberg, D. L., Sonnenblick, E. H., Ross, J., Jr., and Braunwald, E.: Contractile Performance of the Hypertrophied and Chronically Failing Cat Ventricle, *Am. J. Physiol.,* 223:1150, 1972.
136. Spann, J. F.: Contractile and Pump Function of the Pressure-Overloaded Heart, in N. R. Alpert (ed.), "Perspectives in Cardiovascular Research," vol. 7, Raven Press, New York, 1983, p. 19.
137. Cooper, G., IV, Satava, R. M., Harrison, C. E., and Coleman, H. N., III: Normal Myocardial Function and Energetics after Reversing Pressure-Overload Hypertrophy, *Am. J. Physiol.,* 226:1158, 1974.
138. Williams, J. F., Jr., and Potter, R. D.: Normal Contractile State of Hypertrophied Myocardium following Pulmonary Artery Constriction in the Cat, *J. Clin. Invest.,* 54:1266, 1974.
139. Malik, A. B., Abe, T., O'Kane, H. O., and Geha, A. S.: Cardiac Performance in Ventricular Hypertrophy Induced by Pressure and Volume Overloading, *J. Appl. Physiol.,* 37:867, 1974.
140. Skelton, C. L., and Sonnenblick, E. H.: Heterogeneity of Contractile Function in Cardiac Hypertrophy, *Circ. Res.,* 35(suppl. 2):83, 1974.
141. Valeri, C. R., and Fortier, N. L.: Red-cell 2,3-Diphosphoglycerate and Creatine Levels in Patients with Red-Cell Mass Deficiency or with Cardiopulmonary Insufficiency, *N. Engl. J. Med.,* 281:1452, 1969.
142. Burch, G. E., Ray, C T., and Cronvich, J. A.: Certain Mechanical Peculiarities of the Human Cardiac Pump in Normal and Diseased States, *Circulation,* 5:504, 1952.
143. Burch, G. E.: Theoretic Considerations of the Time Course of Pressure Developed and Volume Ejected by the Normal and Dilated Left Ventricle during Systole, *Am. Heart J.,* 50:352, 1955.
144. Burch, G. E., DePasquale, N. P., and Cronvich, J. A.: Influence of Ventricular Size on the Relationship between Contractile and Manifest Tension, *Am. Heart J.,* 69:624, 1965.
145. Mason, D. T., Spann, J. F., Jr., Zelis, R., and Amsterdam, E. A.: Alterations of Hemodynamics and Myocardial Mechanics in Patients with Congestive Heart Failure: Pathophysiologic Mechanisms and Assessment of Cardiac Function and Ventricular Contractility, *Prog. Cardiovasc. Dis.,* 12:507, 1970.
146. Brutsaert, D. L., and Sonnenblick, E. H.: Cardiac Muscle Mechanics in the Evaluation of Myocardial Contractility and Pump Function: Problems, Concepts and Directions, *Prog. Cardiovasc. Dis.,* 16:337, 1973.
147. Winegrad, S.: Mechanism of Contraction in Cardiac Muscle, in A. C. Guyton and J. E. Halls (eds.), "Cardiovascular Physiology IV, International Review of Physiology," vol. 26, University Park Press, Baltimore, 1982, p. 87.
148. Urschel, C. W., Covell, J. W., Sonnenblick, E. H., Ross, J., Jr., and Braunwald, E.: Myocardial Mechanics in Aortic and Mitral Valvular Regurgitation: The Concept of Instantaneous Impedance as a Determinant of the Performance of the Intact Heart, *J. Clin. Invest.,* 47:867, 1968.
149. Scheuer, J.: Metabolism of the Heart in Heart Failure, *Prog. Cardiovasc. Dis.,* 13:24, 1970.
150. Levine, H. J., and Wagman, R. J.: Energetics of the Human Heart, *Am. J. Cardiol.,* 9:372, 1962.
151. Sobel, B. E., Spann, J. F., Jr., Pool, P. E., Sonnenblick, E. H., and Braunwald, E.: Normal Oxidative Phosphorylation in Mitochondria from the Failing Heart, *Circ. Res.,* 21:355, 1967.
152. Walker, J. G., and Bishop, S. P.: Mitochondrial Function and Structure in Experimental Canine Congestive Heart Failure, *Cardiovasc. Res.,* 5:444, 1971.
153. Sordahl, L. A., McCollum, W. B., Wood, W. B., and Schwartz, A.: Mitochondria and Sarcoplasmic Reticulum Function in Cardiac Hypertrophy and Failure, *Am. J. Physiol.,* 224, 497, 1973.
154. Henry, P. D., Eckberg, D., Gault, J. H., and Ross, J., Jr.: Depressed Inotropic State and Reduced Myocardial Oxygen Consumption in the Human Heart, *Am. J. Cardiol.,* 31:300, 1973.
155. Gunning, J. F., and Coleman, H. N., III: Myocardial Oxygen Consumption during Experimental Hypertrophy and Congestive Heart Failure, *J. Mol. Cell. Cardiol.,* 5:25, 1973.
156. Cooper, G., Satava, R. M., Harrison, C. E., and Coleman, H. N., III: Mechanism for the Abnormal Energetics of Pressure-Induced Hypertrophy of Cat Myocardium, *Circ. Res.,* 33:213, 1973.
157. Alpert, N. R., Hamrell, B. B., and Halpern, W.: Mechanical and Biochemical Correlates of Cardiac Hypertrophy, *Circ. Res.,* 35(suppl. 2):71, 1974.
158. Schwartz, A., Sordahl, L. A., Entman, M. L., et al.: Abnormal Biochemistry in Myocardial Failure, in D. T. Mason (ed.), "Congestive Heart Failure: Mechanisms, Evaluation and Treatment," Yorke Medical Books, New York, 1976, p. 25.
159. Katz, A. M.: "Physiology of the Heart," Raven Press, New York, 1977.
160. Badeer, H. S.: "Cardiovascular Physiology," Karger, Basel, 1984.
161. Pool, P. E., Spann, J. F., Buccino, R. A., Sonnenblick, E. H., and Braunwald, E.: Myocardial High-Energy Phosphate Stores in Cardiac Hypertrophy and Heart Failure, *Circ. Res.,* 21:365, 1967.
162. Alpert, N. R., and Hamrell, B. B.: Cardiac Hypertrophy: A Compensatory and Anticompensatory Response to Stress, in M. Vassalle (ed.), "Cardiac Physiology for the Clinician," Academic Press, New York, 1976.
163. Goldstein, M. A., Sordahl, L. A., and Schwartz, A.: Ultrastructural Analysis of Left Ventricular Hypertrophy in Rabbits, *J. Mol. Cell. Cardiol.,* 6:265, 1974.
164. Rabinowitz, M., and Zak, R.: Mitochondria and Cardiac Hypertrophy, *Circ. Res.,* 36:367, 1975.
165. Yoran, C., Covell, J. W., and Ross, J., Jr.: Structural Basis for the Ascending Limb of Left Ventricular Function, *Circ. Res.,* 32:297, 1973.
166. Spotnitz, H. M., and Sonnenblick, E. H.: Structural Conditions in the Hypertrophied and Failing Heart, in D. T. Mason (ed.), "Congestive Heart Failure: Mechanisms, Evaluation and Treatment," Yorke Medical Books, New York, 1976, p. 13.
167. Spotnitz, H. M., Spotnitz, W. D., Cottrell, T. S., Spiro, D., and Sonnenblick, E. H.: Cellular Basis for Volume Related Wall Thickness Changes in the Rat Left Ventricle, *J. Mol. Cell Cardiol.,* 6:317, 1974.
168. Alpert, N. R., and Gordon, M. S.: Myofibrillar Adenosine Triphosphate Activity in Congestive Heart Failure, *Am. J. Physiol.,* 202:940, 1962.
169. Chandler, B. M., Sonnenblick, E. H., Spann, J. F., Jr., and Pool, P. E.: Association of Depressed Myofibrillar Adenosine Triphosphatase and Reduced Contractility in Experimental Heart Failure, *Circ. Res.,* 21:717, 1967.
170. Luchi, R. J., Kritcher, E. M., and Thyrum, P. T.: Reduced Cardiac Myosin Adenosine-Triphosphatase Activity in Dogs with Spontaneously Occurring Heart Failure, *Circ. Res.,* 24:513, 1969.
171. Henry, P. D., Ahumada, G. G., Friedman, W. F., and Sobel, B. E.: Simultaneously Measured Isometric Tension and ATP Hydrolysis in Glycerinated Fibers from Normal and Hypertrophied Rabbit Heart, *Circ. Res.,* 31:740, 1972.
172. Conway, G., Heazlitt, R. A., Montag, J., and Mattingley, S. F.: The ATPase Activity of Cardiac Myosin from Failing and Hypertrophied Hearts, *J. Mol. Cell. Cardiol.,* 7:827, 1975.
173. Wikman-Coffelt, J., McPherson, J., Salel, A. F., Kamiyama, T., and Mason, D. T.: Mechanism of Impaired Contractile Protein Function in Aortic Stenosis: Alterations in Myosin ATPase Activity in the Chronically Pressure Overload Canine Left Ventricle, *Am. J. Cardiol.,* 35:177, 1975.

174. Wikman-Coffelt, J., Walsh, R., Fenner, C., Kamiyama, T., Salel, A., and Mason, D. T.: Effects of Severe Hemodynamic Pressure Overload on the Properties of Canine Left Ventricular Myosin: Mechanisms by which Myosin ATPase Activity is Lowered during Chronic Increased Hemodynamic Stress, *J. Mol. Cell. Cardiol.,* 8:263, 1976.
175. Wikman-Coffelt, J., Fenner, C., Salel, A. F., Kamiyama, T., and Mason, D. T.: Myofibrillar Proteins and the Contractile Mechanism in the Normal and Failing Heart, in D. T. Mason (ed.), "Congestive Heart Failure: Mechanisms, Evaluation and Treatment," Yorke Medical Books, New York, 1976, p. 53.
176. Wikman-Coffelt, J., and Mason, D. T.: Mechanism of Decreased Contractility in Chronic Hemodynamic Overload, in D. T. Mason (ed.), "Advances in Heart Diseases," vol. 1, Grune & Stratton, New York, 1977, p. 491.
177. Meerson, F. Z.: The Myocardium in Hyperfunction, Hypertrophy and Heart Failure, *Circ. Res.,* 15(suppl. 2): 11, 1969.
178. Mead, R. J., Peterson, M. D., and Welty, J. D.: Sarcolemmal and Sarcoplasmic Reticular ATPase Activities in the Failing Canine Heart, *Circ. Res.,* 29:14, 1971.
179. Dhalla, N. S., Singh, J. N., Fedelesova, M., Balasubramanian, V., and McNamara, D. B.: Biochemical Basis of Heart Function: XII. Sodium-Potassium Stimulated Adenosine Triphosphatase Activity in the Perfused Rat Heart Made to Fail by Substrate-Lack, *Cardiovasc. Res.,* 8:227, 1974.
180. Beller, G. A., Conroy, J., and Smith, T. W.: Ischemia-Induced Alterations in Myocardial (Na^+ and K^+) ATPase and Cardiac Glycoside Binding, *J. Clin. Invest.,* 57:341, 1976.
181. Harigaya, S., and Schwartz, A.: Fate of Calcium Binding and Uptake in Normal Animals and Failing Human Cardiac Muscle: Membrane Vesicles (Relaxing System) and Mitochondria, *Circ. Res.,* 25:781, 1969.
182. Gertz, E. W., Stam, A. C., Jr., and Sonnenblick, E. H.: A Quantitative and Qualitative Defect in the Sarcoplasmic Reticulum in the Hereditary Cardiomyopathy of the Syrian Hamster, *Biochem. Biophys. Res. Commun.,* 40:746, 1970.
183. McCollum, W. B., Crow, C., Harigaya, S., Bajusz, E., and Schwartz, A.: Calcium Binding by Cardiac Relaxing System Isolated from Myopathic Syrian Hamsters, *J. Mol. Cell Cardiol.,* 1:445, 1970.
184. Suko, J., Vogel, J. H. K., and Chidsey, C. A.: Intracellular Calcium and Myocardial Contractility: III. Reduced Calcium Intake and ATPase of the Sarcoplasmic Reticular Fraction Prepared from Chronically Failing Calf Hearts, *Circ. Res.,* 27:235, 1970.
185. Ueba, Y., Ito, Y., and Chidsey, C. A.: Intracellular Calcium and Myocardial Contractility, *Am. J. Physiol.,* 220:1553, 1971.
186. Harris, P., and Opie, L. (eds.): "Calcium and the Heart," Academic Press, New York, 1971, p. 198.
187. Kaufmann, R. L., Homburger, H., and Wirth, H.: Disorder in Excitation-Contraction Coupling of Cardiac Muscle from Cats with Experimentally Produced Right Ventricular Hypertrophy, *Circ. Res.,* 28:346, 1971.
188. Sulakhe, P. V., and Dhalla, N. S.: Excitation-Contraction Coupling in Heart: VII. Calcium Accumulation in Subcellular Particles in Congestive Heart Failure. *J. Clin. Invest.,* 50:1019, 1971.
189. Katz, A. M., and Repke, D. I.: Calcium-Membrane Interactions in the Myocardium: Effects of Ouabain, Epinephrine and 3′,5′-Cyclic Adenosine Monophosphate, *Am. J. Cardiol.,* 31:193, 1973.
190. Ito, Y., Suko, J., and Chidsey, C. A.: Intracellular Calcium and Myocardial Contractility: V. Calcium Uptake of Sarcoplasmic Reticulum Fraction in Hypertrophied and Failing Rabbit Hearts, *J. Mol. Cell. Cardiol.,* 6:237, 1974.
191. Reuter, H.: Exchange of Calcium Ions in the Mammalian Myocardium: Mechanisms and Physiological Significance, *Circ. Res.,* 34:599, 1974.
192. Katz, A. M.: Congestive Heart Failure: Role of Altered Myocardial Cellular Control, *N. Engl. J. Med.,* 293:1184, 1975.
193. Dhalla, N. S., Tomlinson, C. W., Yates, J. C., et al.: Role of Mitochondrial Calcium Transport in Failing Heart, in N. S. Dhalla (ed.), "Recent Advances on Cardiac Structure and Metabolism," vol. 5, University Park Press, Baltimore, 1975, p. 177.
194. Katz, A. M., and Hecht, H. E.: The Early "Pump" Failure of the Ischemic Heart, *Am. J. Med.,* 47:497, 1969.
195. Wrogemann, K., and Nylen, E. G.: Mitochondrial Calcium Overloading in Cardiomyopathic Hamsters, *J. Mol. Cell. Cardiol.,* 10:185, 1978.
196. Langer, G. A.: Ionic Movements and the Control of Contraction, in G. A. Langer and A. J. Brady (eds.), "The Mammalian Myocardium," John Wiley & Sons, New York, 1974, p. 193.
197. Carafoli, E., Tiozzo, R., Lugli, G., Crovetti, F., and Kratzing, C.: The Release of Calcium from Heart Mitochondria by Sodium, *J. Mol. Cell. Cardiol.,* 6:361, 1974.
198. Van Winkle, W. B., and Schwartz, A.: Ions and Inotropy, *Ann. Rev. Physiol.,* 38:247, 1976.
199. Dock, W.: How Some Hearts Age, *JAMA,* 195:442, 1966.
200. Burch, G., and Giles, T.: Senile Cardiomyopathy, *J. Chronic Dis.,* 24:1, 1971.
201. Dock, W.: Cardiomyopathies of the Senescent and Senile, in G. E. Burch (ed.), "Cardiomyopathy," F. A. Davis Company, Philadelphia, 1972, p. 361.
202. Lakatta, E. G., Gerstenblith, G., Angell, C. S., Shock, N. W., and Weisfeldt, M. L.: Diminished Inotropic Response of Aged Myocardium to Catecholamines, *Circ. Res.,* 36:262, 1975.
203. Vincent, W. R., Buckberg, G. D., and Hoffman, J. E.: Left Ventricular Subendocardial Ischemia in Severe Valvular and Supravalvular Aortic Stenosis: A Common Mechanism, *Circulation,* 49:326, 1974.
204. Brazier, J. R., and Buckberg, G. D.: Effects of Tachycardia on the Adequacy of Subendocardial Oxygen Delivery in Experimental Aortic Stenosis, *Am. Heart J.,* 90:222, 1975.
205. Downey, J. M., and Kirk, E. S.: Inhibition of Coronary Blood Flow by a Vascular Waterfall Mechanism, *Circ. Res.,* 36:753, 1975.
206. Brazier, J., Cooper, M., and Buckberg, G.: The Adequacy of Subendocardial Oxygen Delivery: The Interaction of Determinants of Flow, Arterial Oxygen Content, and Myocardial Oxygen Need, *Circulation,* 49:968, 1974.
207. Honig, C. R., and Bourdeau-Martini, J.: Extravascular Component of Oxygen Transport in Normal and Hypertrophied Hearts with Special Reference to Oxygen Therapy, *Circ. Res.,* 35(suppl. 2):97, 1974.
208. Eckberg, D. L., Gault, J. H., Bouchard, R. L., Karliner, J. S., and Ross, J., Jr.: Mechanics of Left Ventricular Contraction in Chronic Severe Mitral Regurgitation, *Circulation,* 47:1252, 1973.
209. Mitchell, J. H., Gilmore, J. P., and Sarnoff, S. J.: The Transport Function of the Atrium: Factors Influencing the Relation between Mean Left Atrial Pressure and Left Ventricular End Diastolic Pressure, *Am. J. Cardiol.,* 9:237, 1962.
210. Braunwald, E.: Hemodynamic Significance of Atrial Systole, *Am. J. Med.,* 37:665, 1964.
211. Burchell, H. B.: A Clinical Appraisal of Atrial Transport Function, *Lancet,* 1:775, 1964.
212. Suga, H.: Importance of Atrial Compliance in Cardiac Performance, *Circ. Res.,* 35:39, 1974.
213. Ikram, H., Nixon, P. G. F., and Arcan, T.: Left Atrial Function after Electrical Conversion to Sinus Rhythm, *Br. Heart J.,* 30:80, 1968.
214. Brill, I. C., Rosenbaum, E. E., and Flanery, J. R.: Congestive Failure due to Auricular Fibrillation in an Otherwise Normal Heart, *JAMA,* 173, 784, 1960.
215. Borow, K. M., Green, L. H., Grossman, W., and Braunwald, E.: Left Ventricular End-Systolic Stress-Shortening and Stress-Length Relations in Humans: Normal Values and Sensitivity to Inotropic State, *Am. J. Cardiol.,* 50:1301, 1982.
216. Taylor, R. R., Covell, J. W., Sonnenblick, E. H., and Ross, J., Jr.: Dependence of Ventricular Distensibility on Filling of the Opposite Ventricle, *Am. J. Physiol.,* 213:711, ,1967.
217. Kelly, D. T., Spotnitz, H. M., Beiser, G. D., Pierce, J. E.,

and Epstein, S. E.: Effects of Chronic Right Ventricular Volume and Pressure Loading on Left Ventricular Performance, *Circulation,* 44:403, 1971.
218. Bemis, C. E., Serur, J. R., Borkenhagen, D., Sonnenblick, E. H., and Urschel, C.: Influence of Right Ventricular Filling Pressure on Left Ventricular Pressure and Dimension, *Circ. Res.,* 34:498, 1974.
219. Chidsey, C. A., Kaiser, G. A., Sonnenblick, E. H., Spann, J. F., Jr., and E. Braunwald: Cardiac Norepinephrine Stores in Experimental Heart Failure in the Dog, *J. Clin. Invest.,* 43:2386, 1964.
220. Buccino, R. A., Harris, E., Spann, J. F., Jr., and Sonnenblick, E. H.: Response of Myocardial Connective Tissue to Development of Experimental Hypertrophy, *Am. J. Physiol.,* 216:425, 1969.
221. Mitchell, J. H., Sarnoff, S. J., and Sonnenblick, E. H.: The Dynamics of Pulsus Alternans: Alternating End-Diastolic Fiber Length As a Causative Factor, *J. Clin. Invest.,* 42:55, 1963.
222. Hada, Y., Wolfe, C., and Craige, E.: Pulsus Alternans Determined by Biventricular Simultaneous Systolic Time Intervals, *Circulation,* 65:617, 1982.
223. Hess, O. M., Surber, E. P., Ritter, M., and Krayenbuehl, H. P.: Pulsus Alternans: Its Influence on Systolic and Diastolic Function in Aortic Valve Disease, *J. Am. Coll. Cardiol.,* 4:1, 1984.
224. Ross, J., Jr., Gault, J. H., Mason, D. T., Linhart, J. W., and Braunwald, E.: Left Ventricular Performance during Muscular Exercise in Patients with and without Cardiac Dysfunction, *Circulation,* 34:597, 1966.
225. Braunwald, E., Goldblatt, A., Harrison, D. C., and Mason, D. T.: Studies on Cardiac Dimensions in Intact, Unanesthetized Man: III. Effects of Muscular Exercise, *Circ. Res.,* 13:460, 1963.
226. Gorlin, R., Cohen, L. S., Elliott, W. C., Klein, M. D., and Lane, F. J.: Effect of Supine Exercise on Left Ventricular Volume and Oxygen Consumption in Man, *Circulation,* 32:361, 1965.
227. Gorlin, R., Krasnow, N., Levine, H. J., and Messer, J. V.: Effect of Exercise on Cardiac Performance in Human Subjects with Minimal Heart Disease, *Am. J. Cardiol.,* 13:293, 1964.
228. Braunwald, E.: The Control of Ventricular Function in Man, *Br. Heart J.,* 27:1, 1965.
229. Chapman, C. B. (ed.): Physiology of Muscular Exercise, *Circ. Res.,* 20(suppl. 2):1, 1967.
230. Bevegard, B. S., and Shepherd, J. T.: Regulation of the Circulation during Exercise in Man, *Physiol. Rev.,* 47:178, 1967.
231. Weissler, A. M., Harris, W. S., and Schoenfeld, C. D.: Systolic Time Intervals in Heart Failure in Man, *Circulation,* 37:149, 1968.
232. Astrand, P.-O., and Rodahl, K.: "Textbook of Work Physiology: Physiological Basis of Exercise," McGraw-Hill Book Company, New York, 1977.
233. Weissler, A. M., Lewis, R. P., and Leighton, R. F.: The Systolic Time Intervals as a Measure of Left Ventricular Performance in Man, in P. N. Yu and J. F. Goodwin (eds.), "Progress in Cardiology," vol. 1, Lea & Febiger, Philadelphia, 1972, p. 155.
234. Vatner, S. F., Franklin, D., Higgins, C. B., Patrick, T., and Braunwald, E.: Left Ventricular Response to Severe Exertion in Untethered Dogs, *J. Clin. Invest.,* 51:3052, 1972.
235. Horwitz, L. D., Atkins, J. M., and Leshin, S. J.: Role of the Frank-Starling Mechanism in Exercise, *Circ. Res.,* 31:868, 1972.
236. Guyton, A. C., Jones, C. E., and Coleman, T. G.: Cardiac Output in Muscular Exercise, in "Circulatory Physiology: Cardiac Output and Its Regulation," 2d ed., W. B. Saunders Company, Philadelphia, 1973, p. 436.
237. Vatner, S. F., and Pagani, M.: Cardiovascular Adjustments to Exercise: Hemodynamics and Mechanisms, *Prog. Cardiovasc. Dis.,* 19:91, 1976.
238. Bertrand, M. E., Carre, A. G., Ginestet, A. P., Lefebvre, J. M., Desplanque, L. A., and Lekieffre, J. P.: Maximal Exercise in Normal Subjects, *Eur. J. Cardiol.,* 5/6:481, 1977.
239. Schlant, R. C.: Physiology of Exercise, in G. F. Fletcher (ed.), "Exercise in the Practice of Medicine," Futura Publishing, Mount Kisco, N.Y., 1982, p. 1.
240. Christensen, N. J., and Galbo, H.: Sympathetic Nervous Activity during Exercise, *Ann. Rev. Physiol.,* 45:139, 1983.
241. Ludbrook, J.: Reflex Control of Blood Pressure during Exercise, *Ann. Rev. Physiol.,* 45:155, 1983.
242. Blomqvist, C. G., and Saltin, B.: Cardiovascular Adaptations to Physical Training, *Ann. Rev. Physiol.,* 45:169, 1983.
243. Brengelmann, G. L.: Circulatory Adjustments to Exercise and Heat Stress, *Ann. Rev. Physiol.,* 45:191, 1983.
244. Stone, H. L.: Control of the Coronary Circulation during Exercise, *Ann. Rev. Physiol.,* 45:213, 1983.
245. Mitchell, J. H., Kaufman, M. P., and Iwamoto, G. A.: The Exercise Pressor Reflex: Its Cardiovascular Effects, Afferent Mechanisms, and Central Pathways, *Ann. Rev. Physiol.,* 45:229, 1983.
246. Epstein, S. E., Robinson, B. F., Kahler, R. L., and Braunwald, E.: Effects of Beta-Adrenergic Blockage on the Cardiac Response to Maximal and Submaximal Exercise in Man, *J. Clin. Invest.,* 44:1745, 1965.
247. Robinson, B. F., Epstein, S. E., Kahler, R. L., and Braunwald, E.: Circulatory Effects of Acute Expansion of Blood Volume: Studies during Maximal Exercise and at Rest, *Circ. Res.,* 19:26, 1966.
248. Bristow, J. D., Kloster, F. E., Farrehi, C., Brodeur, M. T. H., Lewis, R. P., and Griswold, H. E.: The Effects of Supine Exercise on Left Ventricular Volume in Heart Disease, *Am. Heart J.,* 71:319, 1966.
249. Skelton, C. L., and Sonnenblick, E. H.: Physiology of Cardiac Muscle, in H. J. Levine (ed.), "Clinical Cardiovascular Physiology," Grune & Stratton, New York, 1976, p. 57.
250. LeJemtel, T. H., and Sonnenblick, E. H.: Should the Failing Heart Be Stimulated?, *N. Engl. J. Med.,* 310:1384, 1984.
251. Wilhelmsen, L.: Lung Mechanics in Rheumatic Valvular Disease, *Acta Med. Scand.,* 184(suppl. 489):1, 1968.
252. Fishman, A. P., and Hecht, H. H.: "The Pulmonary Circulation and Interstitial Space," The University of Chicago Press, Chicago, 1969.
253. Bates, D. V., MacKlem, P. T., and Christie, R. V.: "Respiratory Function in Disease," 2d ed., W.B. Saunders Company, Philadelphia, 1971, p. 585.
254. Rapaport, E.: Dyspnea: Pathophysiology and Differential Diagnosis, *Prog. Cardiovasc. Dis.,* 13:532, 1971.
255. Yu, P. N.: "Pulmonary Blood Volume in Health and Disease," Lea & Febiger, Philadelphia, 1969, p. 328.
256. Luepker, R., Liander, B., Korsgren, M., and Varnauskas, E.: Pulmonary Intervascular and Extravascular Fluid Volumes in Exercising Cardiac Patients, *Circulation,* 44:626, 1971.
257. Avery, W. G., Samet, P., and Sackner, M. A.: The Acidosis of Pulmonary Edema, *Am. J. Med.,* 48:320, 1970.
258. Aberman, A., and Fulop, M.: The Metabolic and Respiratory Acidosis of Acute Pulmonary Edema, *Ann. Intern. Med.,* 76:173, 1972.
259. Visscher, M. B., Haddy, F. J., and Stephens, G.: The Physiology and Pharmacology of Lung Edema, *Pharmacol. Rev.,* 8:389, 1956.
260. Greene, D. G.: Pulmonary Edema, in W. O. Fenn and H. Rahn (eds.): "Handbook of Physiology," American Physiological Society, Washington, 1965, p. 1585.
261. Staub, N. C., Nagano, H., and Pearce, M. L.: Pulmonary Edema in Dogs, Especially the Sequence of Fluid Accumulation in Lungs, *J. Appl. Physiol.,* 22:227, 1967.
262. Lee, G. de J.: Pulmonary Oedema, in P. N. Yu and J. F. Goodwin (eds.), "Progress in Cardiology," vol. 1, Lea & Febiger, Philadelphia, 1972, p. 261.
263. Fishman, A. P.: Pulmonary Edema: The Water-Exchanging Function of the Lung, *Circulation,* 46:390, 1972.
264. Robin, E. D., Cross, C. E., and Zells, R.: Pulmonary Edema, *N. Engl. J. Med.,* 288:239, 292, 1973.
265. Staub, N. C.: Pulmonary Edema, *Physiol. Rev.,* 54:678, 1974.

266. Schreiner, B. F., and Yu, P. N.: Pulmonary Circulation and Edema: Anatomic and Physiologic Considerations, in H. J. Levine (ed.), "Clinical Cardiovascular Physiology," Grune & Stratton, New York, 1976, p. 635.
267. Gaar, K. A., Jr., Taylor, A. E., Owens, L. J., and Guyton, A. C.: Development of Pulmonary Edema, *Am. J. Physiol.*, 213:79, 1967.
268. Robin, E. D., Carey, L. C., Grenvik, A., Glauser, F., and Gaudio, R.: Capillary Leak Syndrome with Pulmonary Edema, *Arch. Intern. Med.*, 130:66, 1972.
269. Uhley, H. N., Leeds, S. E., Sampson, J. J., and Friedman, M.: Right Duct Lymph Flow in Experimental Heart Failure following Acute Elevation of Left Atrial Pressure, *Circ. Res.*, 20:306, 1967.
270. Vasko, J. S., Henney, P., Oldham, H. N., Brawley, R. K., and Morrow, A. G.: Mechanisms of Action of Morphine in the Treatment of Experimental Pulmonary Edema, *Am. J. Cardiol.*, 18:876, 1966.
271. Ward, J. M., McGrath, R. L., and Weil, J. V.: Effects of Morphine on the Peripheral Vascular Response to Sympathetic Stimulation, *Am. J. Cardiol.*, 29:659, 1972.
272. Zelis, R., Mansour, E. J., Capone, R. J., and Mason, D. T.: The Cardiovascular Effects of Morphine: The Peripheral Capacitance and Resistance Vessels in Human Subjects, *J. Clin. Invest.*, 54:1247, 1974.
273. Vismara, L. A., Leaman, D. M., and Zelis, R.: Effects of Morphine on Venous Tone in Patients with Acute Pulmonary Edema, *Circulation*, 54:335, 1976.
274. Overland, E. S., and Severinghaus, J. W.: Noncardiac Pulmonary Edema, *Ann. Rev. Med.*, 23:307, 1978.
275. Hultgren, H. N., and Grover, R. F.: Circulation Adaptation to High Altitude, *Ann. Rev. Med.*, 19:119, 1968.
276. Roy, S. B., Guleria, J. S., Khanna, P. K., Manchanda, S. C., Pande, J. N., and Subba, P. S.: Haemodynamic Studies in High Altitude Pulmonary Oedema, *Br. Heart J.*, 31:52, 1969.
277. Viswanathan, R., Jain, S. K., and Subramanian, S.: Pulmonary Edema of High Altitude: III. Pathogenesis, *Am. Rev. Resp. Dis.*, 100:342, 1969.
278. Vogen, J. H. D. (ed.): Hypoxia, High Altitude and the Heart, in "Advance in Cardiology," vol. 5, S. Karger, Basel, 1970.
279. Severinghaus, J. W.: Transarterial Leakage: A Possible Mechanism of High Altitude Pulmonary Edema, in R. Porter and J. Knight (eds.), "High Altitude Physiology: Cardiac and Pulmonary Aspects," Churchill Livingstone, London, 1971, p. 61.
280. Kleiner, J. P., and Nelson, W. P.: High Altitude Pulmonary Edema: A Rare Disease? *JAMA*, 234:491, 1975.
281. Recavarren, S.: The Preterminal Arterioles in the Pulmonary Circulation of High Altitude Natives, *Circulation*, 33:177, 1966.
282. Hultgren, H., Robinson, M., and Wuerflein, R.: Over-perfusion Pulmonary Edema, *Circulation*, 34(suppl. 3):132, 1966. (Abstract.)
283. Duberstein, J. L., and Kaufman, D. M.: A Clinical Study of an Epidemic of Heroin Intoxication and Heroin-induced Pulmonary Edema, *Am. J. Med.*, 51:704, 1971.
284. Paranthaman, S. K., and Khan, F.: Acute Cardiomyopathy with Recurrent Pulmonary Edema and Hypotension following Heroin Overdosage, *Chest*, 69:117, 1976.
285. Kuida, H., Hinshaw, L. B., Bilbert, R. P., and Visscher, M.: Effect of Gram-negative Endotoxin on Pulmonary Circulation, *Am. J. Physiol.*, 192:335, 1958.
286. Theodore, J., and Robin, E. D.: Pathogenesis of Neurogenic Pulmonary Edema, *Lancet*, 2:749, 1975.

21

The Recognition and Management of Heart Failure

James F. Spann, Jr., M.D.

J. Willis Hurst, M.D.

When the patient thinks there is something amiss with his heart, he fears it may fail. It is therefore necessary that the doctor should understand what heart failure is, and the signs by which it is made manifest.

Sir James Mackenzie, 1916[1]

Heart failure is said to be present when the heart fails to function properly as a pump. The compensatory mechanisms of the body which ordinarily aid the failing heart are only useful up to a point, because they can, and often do, lead to the derangement of the function of other organs. In fact, it is the derangement of the function of other organs that causes many of the troublesome signs and symptoms that are associated with heart failure.

The clinical description of heart failure and its treatment will be discussed in this chapter. The details of the altered physiology that is responsible for heart failure and its signs and symptoms are discussed in Chap. 20 and later in this chapter.

Definition of Terms

Heart failure is a continuum which progresses in severity from normal ventricular overload or damage to ventricular dysfunction with or without continued overload to ventricular dysfunction and compensation with symptoms and signs of congestion with a normal cardiac output at rest to persistence of signs and symptoms of congestion with a low cardiac output at rest.

In practice we identify the following subsets of heart failure. Each subset may require a different therapeutic approach.

Ventricular Dysfunction

The patient exhibits signs of ventricular dysfunction such as a ventricular gallop rhythm but presents no evidence of pulmonary congestion such as dyspnea, rales, radiographic evidence of congestion, neck vein distension, or peripheral edema.

Congestive Heart Failure

The patient experiences dyspnea on effort, has evidence of ventricular dysfunction and pulmonary congestion on chest x-ray and may have peripheral edema. Mild congestive heart failure implies that moderate activity produces dyspnea [labeled New York Heart Association (NYHA) class II]. Moderate congestive heart failure implies that mild activity produces dyspnea (formerly labeled class III). Severe congestive heart failure implies that the patient is dyspneic at rest (labeled class IV).

Compensated Congestive Heart Failure

This term should imply that the heart and circulation utilize compensatory mechanisms (mechanisms which frequently result in the signs and symptoms that we recognize as the congestive syndrome) to prevent a fall in cardiac output below systemic requirements at rest and to optimally distribute the limited cardiac output during exercise. In practice, however, physicians refer to patients as having compensated congestive heart failure when, by appropriate treatment, they are able to eliminate the congestion that troubled the patient.

Intractable Heart Failure

Intractable heart failure is said to exist when the failure persists after the physician has made every effort to control it.

Abnormal Physiology

The details of altered physiology that is responsible for heart failure are discussed in Chap. 20. The altered physiology that is essential for recognition and management of heart failure is discussed below.

In the more common forms of heart failure the basic lesion is a depression of myocardial contractility with or without a continuing overload on the heart.[2–10] The myocardial lesion can result from direct damage, as in cardiomyopathy or coronary heart disease,[11] or can be related to chronic overload on the heart, as in valve disease[5,6,8] or systemic hypertension.[13,14,24] However, even when extensive depression of myocardial contractility is present, the heart's compensatory mechanisms can usually maintain a relatively normal resting cardiac output.[3,5] Not until relatively late in the usual clinical course of congestive failure are the patient's symptoms caused by reduced resting cardiac output. Before that time, the disturbing symptoms of heart failure are caused by the compensatory mechanisms which are striving to maintain cardiac output. Unfortunately, these undesirable secondary effects limit the utility of compensatory mechanisms.

The Frank-Starling mechanism, whereby diastolic cardiac dilatation causes increased force and volume of the subsequent systolic contraction and ejection, is vital for the maintenance of cardiac output but is also responsible for many congestive heart failure symptoms.[5,15,16] Figure 21-1 shows this principle. In these diagrams systolic events are shown as solid curves, and the corresponding diastolic events are shown as dashed curves. The vertical axis for systolic events (cardiac output) is on the left, and the vertical axis for diastolic events [left ventricular end-diastolic pressure (LVEDP)] is on the right. When heart muscle is damaged, the systolic muscle function falls from the upper systolic curve (solid line), at point A, to the lower systolic curve (solid line), at point B. However, at point B the systolic cardiac

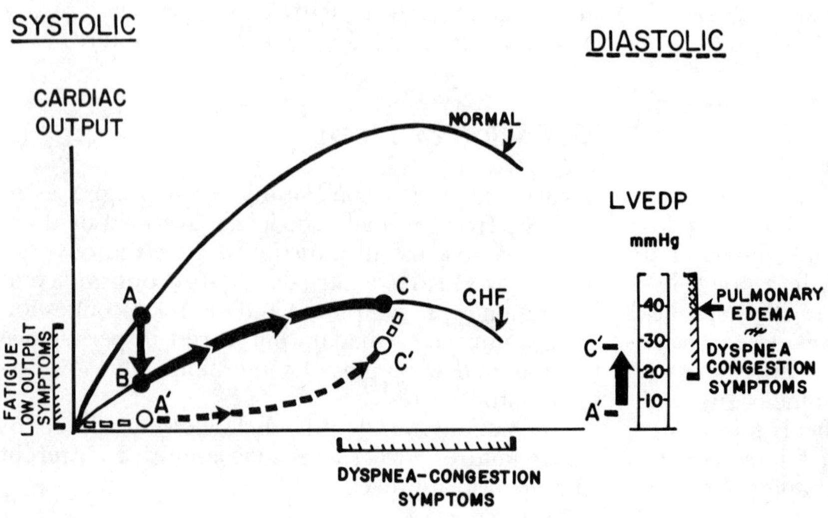

FIGURE 21-1 Compensated heart failure. Frank-Starling compensation for heart failure and how it causes congestive symptoms. (See text for explanation.) LVEDP = left ventricular end-diastolic pressure.

output would be too low to support systemic needs, and low-output symptoms such as fatigue, weakness, renal failure, and even confusion and stupor or death would ensue. Fortunately, the end-diastolic volume (shown in the dashed curve) increases, and this diastolic change results in improvement in the subsequent systole. Cardiac residual volume increases as a result of the low ejection fraction, venous constriction occurs, and salt and water are retained, which increases left ventricular end-diastolic volume from point A′ to point C′ along the diastolic curve (dashed line). At diastolic C′, the associated subsequent systole C is improved and ejects a greater stroke volume, resulting in a better cardiac output. However, as the heart increases its diastolic volume from point A′ to point C′, it has moved to the right and upward along the dashed curve relating passive ventricular diastolic distension to LVEDP. As LVEDP becomes elevated it causes dyspnea and other congestive symptoms. Thus, the symptoms of pulmonary congestion with dyspnea, orthopnea, and even pulmonary edema may occur as unfortunate side effects of the Frank-Starling mechanism, which has maintained cardiac output.

Other compensatory mechanisms include cardiac hypertrophy and changes in the sympathetic nervous system and renin-angiotensin-aldosterone system with resultant changes in peripheral venous and arterial circulation. In congestive heart failure, there is an increase in total sympathetic discharge and an abnormal augmentation of the norepinephrine blood level with exercise.[17,18] The failing heart has improved support of contractility and an increase in heart rate as a result of increased circulating catecholamines despite a reduction of intrinsic cardiac norepinephrine[17,19] and impairment of direct cardiac sympathetic nerve function.[20] The patient with heart failure has increased venous pressure and venous tone at rest, which is due to increased blood volume, venous tone, and tissue pressure.[21,22] The increased blood volume is caused by the renal retention of salt and water in response to the renin-angiotensin-aldosterone system.[23] With exercise the venous pressure and tone are further exaggerated by a sympathetically mediated constriction of the veins,[24,25] which aids the return of blood to the heart when heart failure is present. This increased venous return provides part of the increased preload which is used by the Frank-Starling compensation, but it heightens congestive symptoms such as dyspnea and edema.

Increased peripheral resistance and altered flow distribution are compensatory mechanisms provided by the systemic arterial system.[25,26] Three major factors appear to cause the increased peripheral resistance: first, increased sympathetic tone and circulating catecholamines to the peripheral resistance vessels;[18,27] second, increased local stiffness of resistance vessels that is thought to be caused by increased arterial sodium content and increased tissue pressure;[25,26] and third, increased angiotensin level.[23] Plasma renin often is increased in heart failure. The renin then converts a liver globulin into the inactive molecule, angiotensin I. Subsequently, the angiotensin-converting enzyme converts this molecule to active angiotensin II. Angiotensin II is a potent vasoconstrictor and stimulus to adrenal release of aldosterone. As angiotensin II is released and as circulating catecholamines increase, vascular resistance rises and blood flow is redistributed. The resistance vessels demonstrate an abnormal response to exercise, resulting in intense visceral vasoconstriction and subnormal dilatation of the arteries to exercising muscles, skin, and kidney.[28,29] In severe cases, this altered flow distribution is present at rest.[28] When the heart is severely failing and unable to maintain cardiac output, these changes in arterial resistance maintain central blood pressure and allocate the limited cardiac output, providing flow to vital areas such as the brain and heart while reducing flow to less essential areas such as the skin, renal system, and viscera and maintaining an intermediate level of flow to the exercising muscles.[30–34]

These arterial and venous compensations are diagramed in Fig. 21-2*A* and *B*. Figure 21-2*A* shows the normal circulation, in which preload is normal because venous capacitance and diastolic ventricular size are normal; therefore, ventricular end-diastolic pressure is normal and there are no congestive symptoms. Cardiac contractility is normal. The heart contracts from a normal end-diastolic volume (the outer concentric circle) to a normal end-systolic volume (the inner concentric circle). The ejection fraction, which is the ratio of end-systolic volume to end-diastolic volume, is normal at 0.60. Stroke volume, which is the volume of the shell of blood extruded when the outer diastolic circle constricts to the inner systolic circle, is also normal and moves as blood flows into the arteries, shown by the arrows in the figure. Systemic resistance and blood pressure (flow × resistance = blood pressure) are normal, cardiac output is normal, and there are no low-output symptoms. Figure 21-2*B* shows severe overt heart failure. Cardiac contractility is low, so less systolic contraction occurs from any diastolic volume and the ejection fraction is low. Venous constriction helps increase venous return, thus dilating the heart and allowing utilization of Frank-Starling compensation (also see Fig. 21-1).[22–24] However, the increased ventricular volume causes increased diastolic pressure with resultant congestive symptoms. Despite this venous compensation, stroke volume continues to be low and less blood flows into the arteries. With inadequate blood flow, the only way that blood pressure can be maintained is by increased peripheral arterial resistance.[26,27]

Here again, the compensation which is essential to life causes adverse symptoms and signs. Decreased skin flow is accompanied by an increase of arteriovenous oxygen extraction, and cool, bluish extremities result. In advanced situations, severely decreased skin flow impairs the ability of the body

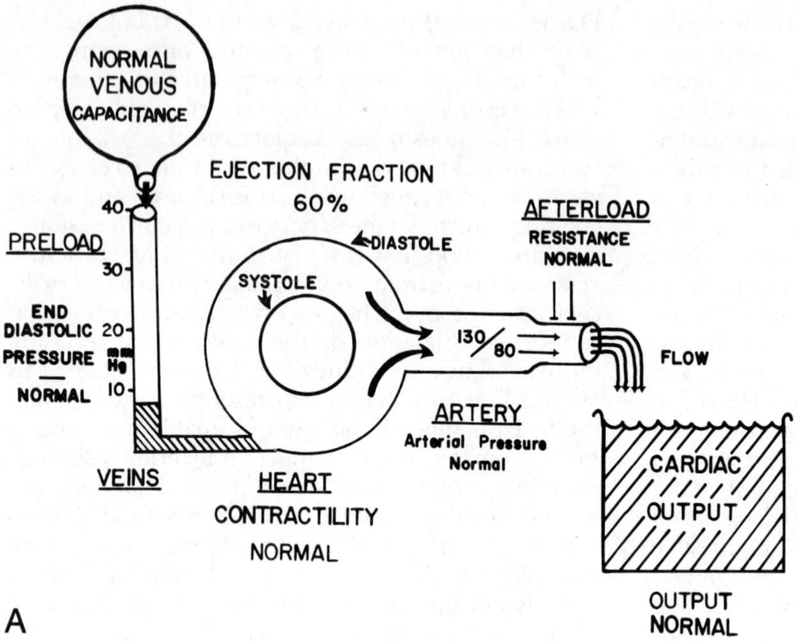

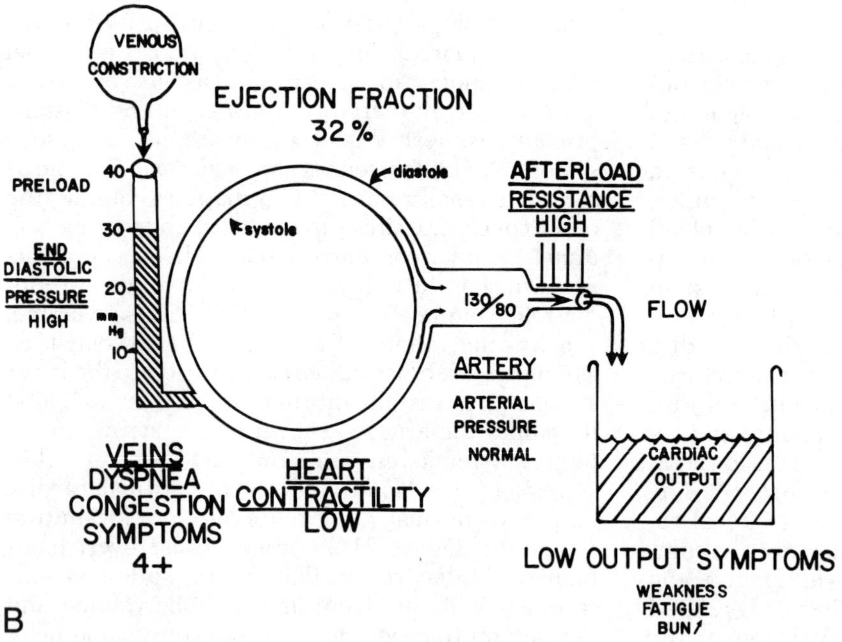

FIGURE 21-2 *A.* Diagram of normal heart and circulation. (See text for explanation.) *B.* Diagram of failing heart and circulation. (See text for explanation.)

to rid itself of heat. Decreased flow to the exercising muscles, while preventing hypotension, also causes fatigue and muscle weakness, which are prominent symptoms in advanced heart failure. The chronic increase in general arteriolar tone is an increased afterload on the heart that may result in a "vicious circle" or positive feedback loop. The increased afterload further decreases the diminished ejection fraction of the failing heart, which in turn further reduces cardiac output.[35] The natural history of severe congestive heart failure is to worsen, whether or not the inciting cause is worsening, because of this positive feedback loop. Arterial vasodilators and angiotensin-converting enzyme inhibitors attempt to break this vicious circle.

Therapy is often the selective removal of a portion of a compensation that has "gone too far" and is causing symptoms or has become part of a positive feedback loop. For example, dyspnea is the symptom caused by overuse of the Frank-Starling mechanism as it supports the cardiac output. Diuretics selectively remove some of the Frank-Starling mechanism and relieve dyspnea. Excessive removal of a compensation by therapy often causes undesirable side effects. For example, too extensive a diuresis removes too much of the Frank-Starling compensation, thus causing the cardiac output to fall. Excessive use of diuretics relieves the patient's dyspnea but causes new symptoms of low cardiac output such as fatigue and weakness.

Clinical Manifestations

History

The heart itself produces no symptoms when it fails to function as a pump. Symptoms are the result of the physiological derangement of the lungs, kidneys, liver, muscles, and other organ systems (see Chap. 20).

Dyspnea

The patient with heart failure may have dyspnea and complain of "breathlessness" or "shortness of breath." The rise in left atrial, pulmonary venous, and pulmonary capillary pressures (see Fig. 21-1) causes an increase in lung turgidity. Decreased compliance of the congested lungs increases the work of breathing, causing the subjective symptom of dyspnea.

Dyspnea on Effort

Dyspnea on effort is a common and relatively early symptom of left-sided heart failure. Certain patients may have heart failure with pulmonary congestion but not have dyspnea on effort because they either have very gradually decreased their activity level without noticing it, are very sedentary or bedridden, are stoic, or have abnormal mental acuity.

Patients with chronic lung disease may also have dyspnea. Decrease in exercise tolerance over a short period of time suggests heart failure, while gradually developing dyspnea suggests lung disease.

The patient with dyspnea caused by anxiety exhibits deep, sighing respiration, a feeling that the "breath does not go down," hyperventilation, fatigue, and other symptoms of anxiety, and may have dyspnea at rest but not during exercise (see Chap. 7).

Patients with severe anemia and thyrotoxicosis may become dyspneic with effort.

Orthopnea

The patient with orthopnea experiences dyspnea in a recumbent position and has less dyspnea in the upright position. Relief occurs in the upright position because of a decrease in venous return, a decrease in hydrostatic pressure in the upper portion of the lungs, and an increase in vital capacity.

The symptom of orthopnea is not specific for heart failure since it can also be caused by chronic lung disease.

A therapeutic trial for heart failure is occasionally justified to identify the contribution of heart failure to the dyspnea and orthopnea that occur in patients with lung disease.

Paroxysmal Nocturnal Dyspnea

A patient has paroxysmal nocturnal dyspnea when he or she suddenly awakens with dypsnea a few hours after retiring. Such patients may sit on the side of the bed, get up for a drink of water, or go to the window for a "breath of fresh air." The symptoms subside, and the patient returns to bed and usually sleeps the remainder of the night. If the symptoms recur, it usually is 2 to 3 h later.

This unique type of breathing difficulty is considered to be a very specific symptom of heart failure related to disease of the left side of the heart. However, patients with advanced pulmonary emphysema and chronic bronchitis may have paroxymsal nocturnal dyspnea because of increased wheezing and accumulation of bronchial secretions when lying flat.

Anxious patients may awaken from sleep, with or without recalling a nightmare, sit on the side of the bed, and have an episode of extreme hyperventilation. They may go to the window, searching for air, and finally return to bed. Such an episode may occur at any time after going to sleep. The patient usually has a history of anxiety and absence of signs of heart disease.

Cardiac Asthma

Cardiac asthma is wheezing due to bronchospasm produced by heart failure. Cardiac asthma is usually precipitated by effort or occurs during the night. Patients may or may not be aware of their wheezing, and occasionally such patients may complain only of a nocturnal cough. When there is no evidence of pulmonary disease in the patient above the age of 40, newly developed "asthma" should suggest heart failure.

Patients with bronchial asthma also experience increased wheezing and coughing with effort, but the long history of these symptoms usually will aid in identifying bronchial asthma. Clinical distinction is more difficult when chronic lung disease is associated with left-sided heart disease. Pulmonary function studies rarely help. Occasionally, the response of the patient to a trial treatment for heart failure may be necessary to clarify the problem.

Symptoms and Signs of Acute Pulmonary Edema

The sudden onset of suffocation due to acute pulmonary edema is terrifying to the patient. It may occur in patients with known heart failure which worsens. Acute myocardial infarction, acute myocardial ischemia, tight mitral stenosis, advanced aortic stenosis or regurgitation, severe hypertension, or rupture of the chordae tendineae may cause sudden pulmonary edema without antecedent clinical heart failure. Ectopic tachycardia or pulmonary embolism may also precipitate acute pulmonary edema in a person with a normal or diseased heart.

Patients with pulmonary edema may sit or may stand in the upright position. Usually, they are anxious, agitated, pale, and drenched with sweat. The skin may be cyanotic, cold, and clammy. The respiratory rate is rapid (30 to 40 per minute); the depth of respiration may be deep or shallow. The alae nasi may be dilated, the accessory muscles of respiration may be used, and retraction of intercostal supraclavicular areas is often present. There may be coughing, prolonged expiratory wheezing, and tracheal rattling sounds. Sputum may be profuse, frothy, watery, or blood-tinged. The pulse rate is rapid. If the pulse is not rapid, heart block should be suspected. The systolic and diastolic blood pressures may be elevated without previous systemic hypertension. If pulmonary edema is profound, blood pressure may drop to shock levels. The systemic venous pressure is usually very elevated. Bubbling rales, wheezing, and rhonchi may be heard throughout the lungs and may obscure the heart sounds, murmurs, and gallop sounds. The chest roentgenogram may show the characteristic pattern of pulmonary edema (Fig. 21-7).

Classic acute pulmonary edema is unmistakable. However, when the patient is too sick to give a history and the heart is not audible because of wheezing, it may be difficult to distinguish pulmonary edema from acute bronchial asthma. In that case, it is wise to avoid administering morphine, which is ordinarily used for pulmonary edema, or epinephrine, which is often used for bronchial asthma. Morphine may be fatal in severe lung disease, and epinephrine may be fatal in severe ischemic heart disease. Aminophylline, oxygen, rotating tourniquets, and/or sublingual nitroglycerin may be used, may help, and will not usually harm a patient with either diagnosis. A chest x-ray usually clarifies the diagnosis.

Cough

Cough due to chronic heart failure usually appears when the patient first lies down, may bother the patient throughout the night, and may produce no sputum. Cough due to heart failure may be present with or without rales, and the cardiac origin of the cough may be revealed by the pattern of interstitial pulmonary edema seen on the chest roentgenogram.

Insomnia

Patients with heart failure due to left-sided heart disease may complain of restlessness and inability to sleep. In some patients the insomnia is due to pulmonary congestion that has not progressed to dyspnea. In others, the insomnia is due to Cheyne-Stokes breathing.

Cheyne-Stokes Respiration[36,37]

Cheyne-Stokes breathing, which may be a dominant symptom of left-sided heart failure, tends to occur soon after the patient goes to sleep. The patient may awaken during the rapid, deep-breathing phase which follows a period of apnea and sleep. The breathing abnormality is increased by opiates and sedatives and may be prevented or relieved by aminophylline.

History of Weight Gain and Peripheral Edema

Patients with severe chronic heart failure usually gain weight because of abnormal retention of salt and water. Such patients may detect edema at the end of the day; however, a patient may gain 10 lb or more without development of edema. During the period of fluid retention the patient's urinary frequency and volume may decrease during the day and increase at night (nocturia). A weight loss of 5 lb or more in 24 to 36 h following a potent diuretic may indicate chronic heart failure. Edema is a late finding in left-sided heart failure since secondary pulmonary hypertension and resultant right-sided heart failure usually cause the elevation of systemic venous pressure necessary for the production of edema. Noncardiac causes of edema include varicose veins, obesity, phlebitis, pregnancy, liver disease, renal disease, cyclic edema, lymphedema, corticosteroid or calcium-channel-blocker administration, retroperitoneal tumor, or even prolonged periods of standing or sitting.

History of Increasing Body Girth

An increase in body girth as a result of ascites is another type of localized accumulation of extracellular fluid. Ascites is more likely to occur in patients with heart failure who have cirrhosis, constrictive pericarditis, restrictive cardiomyopathy, or tricuspid valve disease.

Weakness

Weakness on effort because of inadequate blood flow to the skeletal muscle during exertion (see Fig. 21-2*B*) may be a prominent symptom in advanced heart failure. Patients with advanced heart failure may have weakness, exhaustion, and even postural hypotension following excessive diuresis with associated fall in cardiac output (see Fig. 21-9 and section on diuretics in this chapter). Weakness may be due to potassium ion depletion. Weakness may be accentuated because of anorexia caused by drug toxicity or progressive heart failure.

Mental Symptoms of Confusion

Occasional patients with congestive heart failure may have emotional disorders when they find that, despite optimum therapy, their activity is severely limited by symptoms. When heart failure is severe or when overdiuresis decreases cardiac output, there may be a decrease in cerebral blood flow sufficient to evoke cerebral symptoms such as dizziness, somnolence, and confusion.

Gastrointestinal Symptoms

Patients with heart failure may exhibit anorexia, nausea, vomiting, abdominal distension, "fullness" after meals, constipation, and abdominal pain. These complaints may be due to venous engorgement and congestion of the gastrointestinal tract or to digitalis toxicity. Gangrene of the intestine may occur in severe heart failure due to intense splanchnic vasoconstriction. Protein-losing enteropathy may occur in some patients with severe chronic heart failure.[38]

Cardiac Cachexia

Cardiac cachexia may occur in the very late stages of chronic severe heart failure.[39] Hypermetabolism, protein-losing enteropathy, poor appetite as a result of congestion, drug toxicity, mental depression, and cellular hypoxia all contribute to this condition.

Liver Pain

Congestion of the liver in heart failure causes tension on the liver capsule, which may produce pain and tenderness in the right upper quadrant and occasionally hepatic pain on effort.

History of Cyanosis

Patients with severe heart failure may have a "dusky" appearance of their face and distal extremities. Arterial oxygen saturation is usually normal. Cyanosis occurs because the oxygen content of the venous blood is decreased as a result of increased oxygen extraction by the tissues, which are receiving a low blood flow.

History of Sweating

Some patients with heart failure have excessive sweating. Such patients need to lose body heat through sweating since it cannot be dissipated properly through the constricted skin circulation.

Physical Examination

Ventricular Gallop Sound

A ventricular gallop sound (protodiastolic gallop, third heart sound gallop, S_3 gallop; see Chap. 11) is the cardiac hallmark of ventricular failure. This sound occurs in early diastole and is the result of rapid ventricular filling into a noncompliant ventricle or a ventricle distended by the increased preload of the Frank-Starling compensation (see Fig. 21-1). This low-pitched sound is heard best when the bell of the stethoscope is applied with light pressure. A left ventricular gallop sound is heard best at the left ventricular apex. A right ventricular gallop sound is heard best over the right ventricle. The normal third sound of the child or adolescent is identical to the abnormal ventricular gallop sound and does not indicate heart failure. The normal adult rarely has a ventricular gallop sound.

The ventricular gallop sound becomes a very reliable sign of early myocardial failure when its appearance is documented in a patient with heart disease. A patient who is pregnant and patients with mitral regurgitation, aortic regurgitation, patent ductus arteriosus, interventricular septal defect, interatrial septal defect, or anemia may have a ventricular gallop sound in the absence of heart failure as a result of the excessive ventricular volume of these conditions. A patient with tricuspid stenosis cannot have a right ventricular gallop sound, and a patient with tight mitral stenosis cannot have a left ventricular gallop sound since rapid ventricular filling cannot occur. The patient with tight mitral stenosis and right-sided heart failure due to pulmonary hypertension can have a right ventricular gallop.

Atrial Gallop Sound

An atrial gallop sound (presystolic gallop, fourth heart sound gallop, S_4 gallop; see Chap. 11) is not a specific indicator of congestive heart failure.

Abnormal Precordial Movements

The precordial movements associated with audible or subaudible ventricular or atrial gallop sounds may be seen or felt (see Chap. 10).

In a patient with left-sided heart disease, a sustained systolic lift of the sternum as a result of right ventricular enlargement suggests heart failure. The right ventricle is large secondary to the elevation of pressure in the pulmonary circuit produced by prolonged failure to the left ventricle. The pulmonic component of the second sound may become louder as pulmonary hypertension develops.

Pulsus Alternans

Pulsus alternans of the peripheral arteries indicates heart failure due to disease of the left ventricle (see Chap. 9). It is a relatively uncommon finding and indicates severe ventricular dysfunction.

Abnormalities of the Neck Veins

The deep jugular veins can be thought of as tubes that are filled with blood and connected to the right atrium and that act as manometers. Measurement of the vertical distance in centimeters from the upper level of deep jugular vein pulsation to a horizontal line projected through the center of the right atrium estimates mean central venous pressure and right ventricular end-diastolic pressure. The upper limit of normal is 7 cm. High right end-diastolic pressure is usually present in right-sided heart failure, and right-sided heart failure is most commonly due to left-sided heart failure. Distension of the deep jugular veins are initially sought with the trunk of the body elevated 45° from the supine position. With very severe distension of the neck veins, pulsations cannot be seen at 45°. In such situations, it is important to examine the neck veins with the patient sitting up at 90°. A prominent early *v* wave, prominent sustained *a* and *v* waves with a rapid and deep *y* descent, and an abnormal hepatojugular reflux test also can be seen in heart failure. The hepatojugular reflux test involves determination of normal jugular venous pressure, then determination of jugular venous pressure after gentle compression of the liver. A positive test occurs when liver compression, with its attendant increase in central venous volume, causes an increase in jugular venous pressure as the failing heart is unable to adjust to the increased venous return. (See Chap. 9.)

Physical Examination of the Lungs
As left ventricular end-diastolic pressure rises in heart failure, the left atrial mean and pulmonary venous pressures also rise. Pulmonary congestion results. Moist rales may be heard at the lung bases or over the entire lung field. However, heart failure is often present without rales, and rales may be due to noncardiac disease.

Bronchial wheezing is often caused by heart failure and is frequently misinterpreted as being produced by bronchial asthma.

Hydrothorax may develop in patients with heart failure and is usually bilateral or present only on the right side.[40] (See Chap. 13.)

Physical Examination of the Subcutaneous Tissues
The location of edema is determined by local factors, the most important of which is increased hydrostatic pressure. The erect position favors collection of the fluid in the feet, ankles, and lower portion of the legs, whereas the recumbent position favors the accumulation of the fluid in the presacral region. Anasarca is generalized body edema, often with hydrothorax and ascites. (See Chap. 13.)

Physical Examination of the Abdomen
The liver may become large and tender with severe heart failure and high systemic venous pressure. Ascites may be due to chronic heart failure and always represents advanced disease.

The spleen may become enlarged as a result of chronic, passive congestion related to heart failure. Splenomegaly is usually encountered in patients who have hepatomegaly, and it may be associated with cardiac cirrhosis. (See Chap. 13.)

Physical Examination of the Eyes
Patients with long-standing severe heart failure may have a stare and slight exophthalmos because of an increase in venous pressure. Jaundice may be detected in a small percentage of patients, but the level of bilirubin is seldom greater than 2 mg/dl. Jaundice in patients with heart failure should suggest pulmonary infarction as well as centrilobular necrosis of the liver.

Chest Roentgenogram

Pulmonary congestion of heart failure can often be detected by x-ray examination before it becomes clinically apparent (see Chap. 15). An early hemodynamic change characteristic of failure of the left ventricle is pulmonary venous hypertension, which may occur without auscultatory abnormalities. When the pulmonary venous pressure becomes raised over the upper limit of normal (about 13 mmHg), the pulmonary veins become distended, and when the pressure approaches and exceeds the oncotic pressure of plasma proteins (25 to 30 mmHg), fluid may move from the capillary into the interstitial tissue of the lungs.

FIGURE 21-3 T. S., a 41-year-old male with mild mitral stenosis. The cause of his hemoptysis was initially diagnosed as bronchiectasis. *A.* Note the distension of superior pulmonary veins (large arrow) and costophrenic septal lines (small arrow). *B.* Note the antler-like appearance of the superior pulmonary veins.

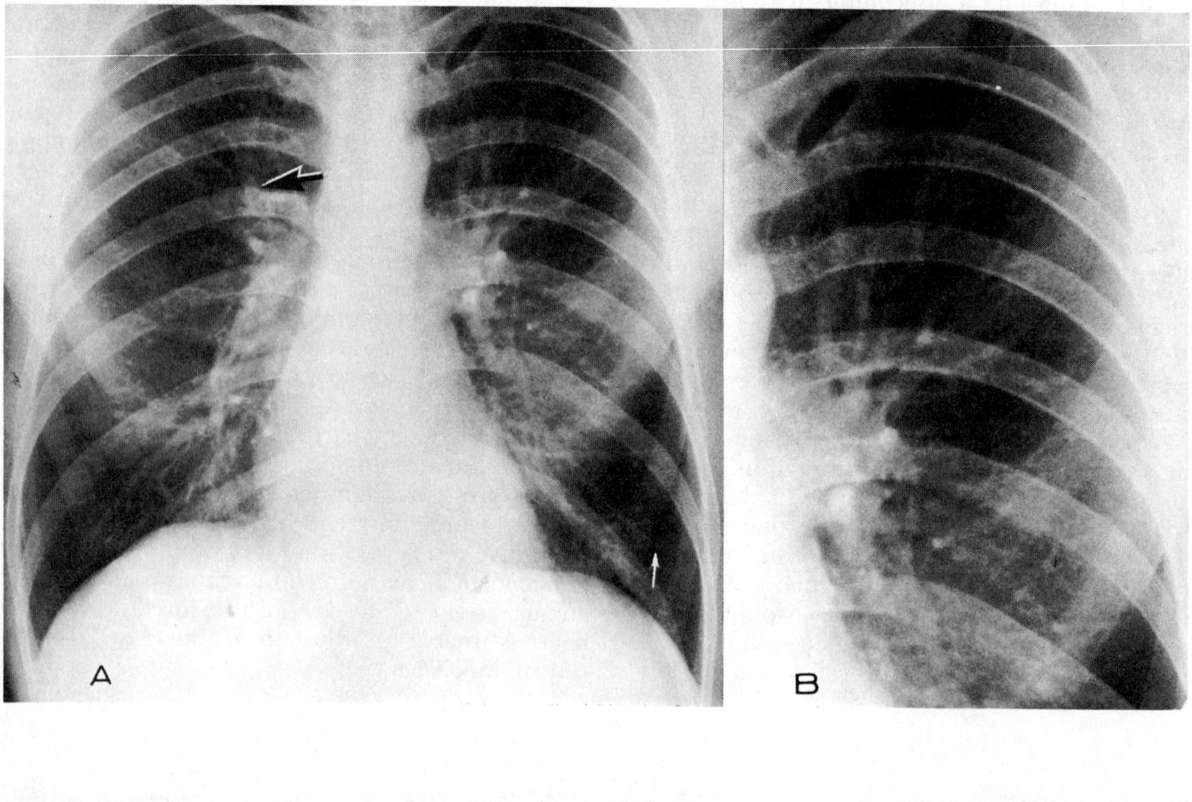

Dilatation of the Pulmonary Veins

In the normal lung, the veins to the lower portion of the lungs are more prominent when the individual is in the upright posture because of the effects of hydrostatic pressure. Thus, on an upright chest radiogram in the normal person there is relative prominence of the inferior vessels in relation to the vessels of the superior aspects of the lung. This relationship is altered when heart failure causes pulmonary venous hypertension. Then, there is generalized dilatation of the pulmonary veins and resultant prominence of the superior pulmonary veins in the upright chest radiograph (Fig. 21-3).

Dilatation of the Central Right and Left Pulmonary Arteries

Shortly after the pulmonary venous pressure becomes elevated in heart failure due to disease of the left side of the heart, the pulmonary artery pressure becomes elevated. On x-ray examination this may be noted as a dilatation of the central right and left pulmonary artery shadows (Fig. 21-3).

Pulmonary Clouding and Interstitial Pulmonary Edema

Interstitial pulmonary edema occurs when an excess amount of fluid enters the tissue which surrounds the pulmonary capillaries. Pulmonary clouding with increased interstitial density of the central lung markings occurs early in the course of interstitial pulmonary edema. The accumulation of edema fluid in the perivascular connective tissue causes haziness and loss of the sharp outline of the arteries and veins (Figs. 21-4 and 21-5).

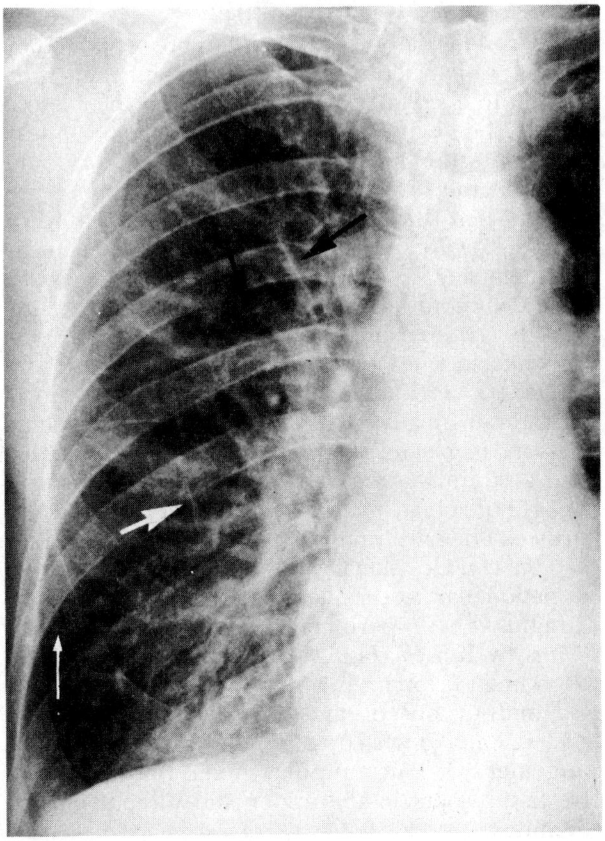

FIGURE 21-4 H. P., a 57-year-old male, suffered an acute myocardial infarction. Note A lines (large arrows) and B lines (small arrow), pulmonary clouding, and hilar engorgement.

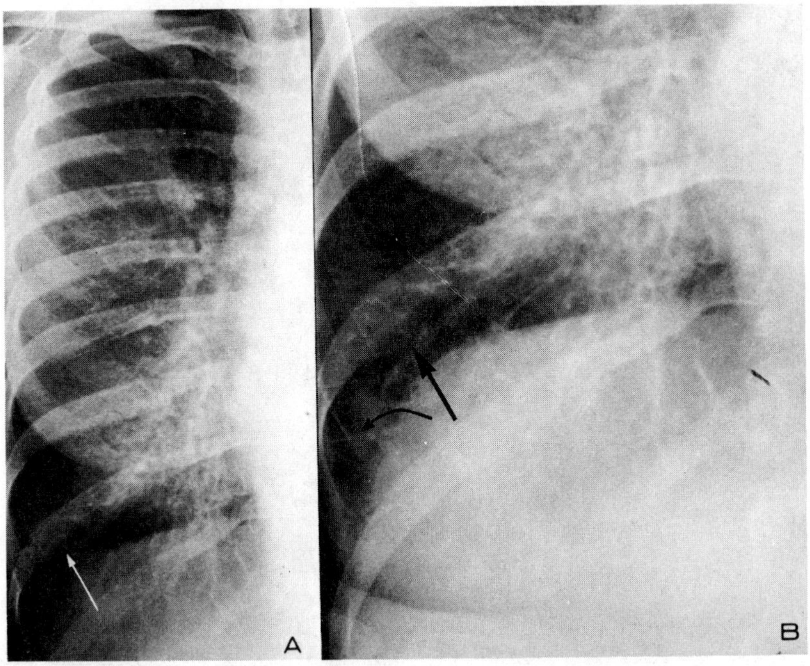

FIGURE 21-5 A. O., a 43-year-old male, had mitral stenosis. Note costophrenic septal lines, dilated superior pulmonary veins, and increased interstitial density (clouding) of the lungs.

Interlobar Fissure "Thickening"

The secondary lobules of the lungs are separated by fine interlobar septa, and, at the periphery of the lungs, these septa lie perpendicular to the pleural surface. These interlobular septa near the periphery of the lung are normally microscopic in size, and therefore they are not seen in the chest roentgenogram. When they are thickened by edema fluid or fibrosis, however, they become visible as sharp linear densities (see Fig. 21-6). These linear densities are more commonly seen in the lower portions of the lungs for two reasons: (1) the fibrous connective tissue septa in the lingula and middle lobes are well developed, vertically stacked, and located anteriorly and laterally in a visible area; and (2) the hydrostatic pressure is greater in the lower lungs, and edema fluid accumulates early. These thickened septa are usually horizontal, and they may extend to the pleural surface. They are rarely longer than 3 cm or wider than 0.2 cm. Occasionally they are vertical and project perpendicular to the pleural surface over the diaphragm. These peripheral markings are termed *B lines* by Kerley (Fig. 21-5*B*). Similar longer lines extending peripherally from the hilum in the upper and midportions of the lungs have been termed *A lines*. The A lines correspond to the anatomic arrangement of long unbroken interlobular connective tissue septa in the upper and midportions of the lungs.

Both types of septal lines may result from heart failure and any other condition which thickens the septa, for example, inflammation such as that produced by viral infection, hemochromatosis, infiltration by tumor, and fibrosis. When they are due to the edema fluid of heart failure, the left atrial mean pressure, pulmonary capillary pressure, and pulmonary artery diastolic pressure usually exceed 18 mmHg. When the lines result from brief pulmonary congestion, they are often transitory and leave no trace after the heart failure improves. Recurrent failure may cause the lines to become permanent.

Subpleural Fluid

Subpleural fluid may accumulate in the area of the costophrenic sulci and simulate free pleural fluid. When localized in the basal subpleural space, it may simulate the elevation of a leaf of the diaphragm.

Free Pleural Fluid

Free pleural fluid produces blunting of the costophrenic angles and is usually seen best in the lateral film. It is bilateral in 70 percent of cases, but when unilateral, it is more frequently located on the right side.[40]

Alveolar Pulmonary Edema

Advanced pulmonary alveolar edema is recognized without difficulty. Edema fluid fills alveolar spaces in the central area of the chest, giving a "butterfly" appearance to the chest roentgenogram. The heart makes the body of the butterfly, and the edema makes the wings. The radiographic picture of pulmonary edema may also occur from noncardiac causes of pulmonary edema. (See Fig. 21-7.)

FIGURE 21-6 T. G., a 74-year-old male, had coronary atherosclerotic heart disease with old myocardial infarctions. *A*. Typical changes of interstitial pulmonary edema. *B*. In the lateral film fluid is seen in the posterior costophrenic sulcus, which cannot be seen well in the posteroanterior view. There is also thickening of the interlobar fissures, which is usually more apparent in the lateral views.

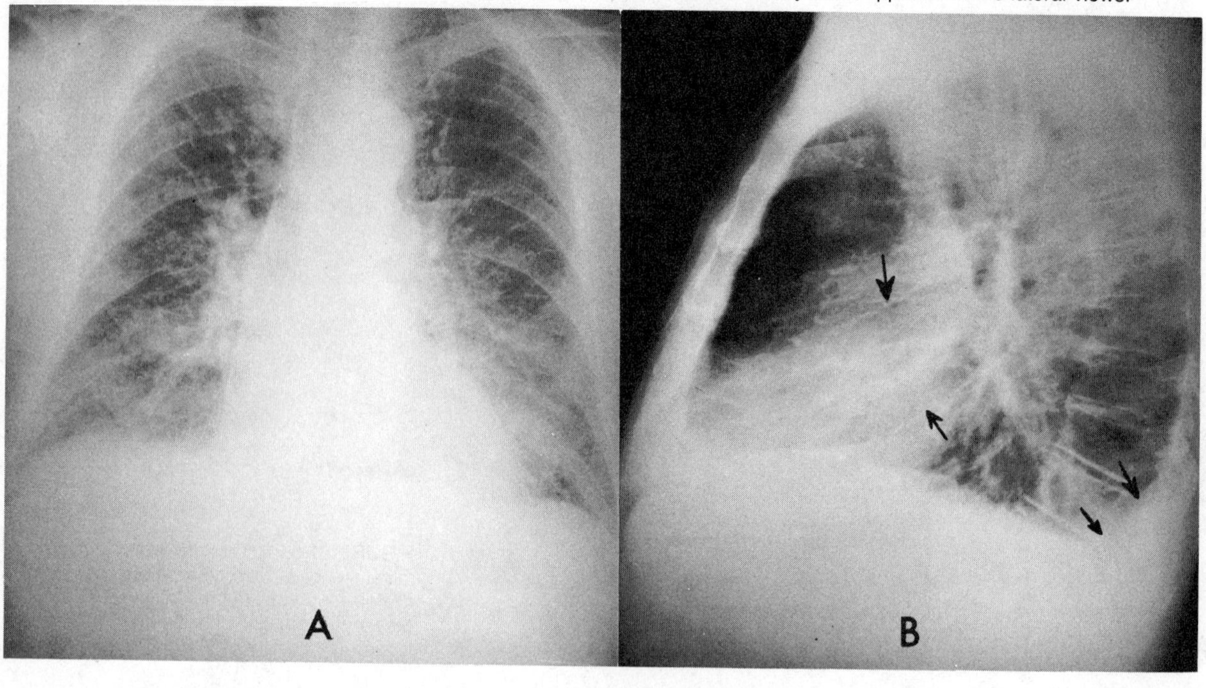

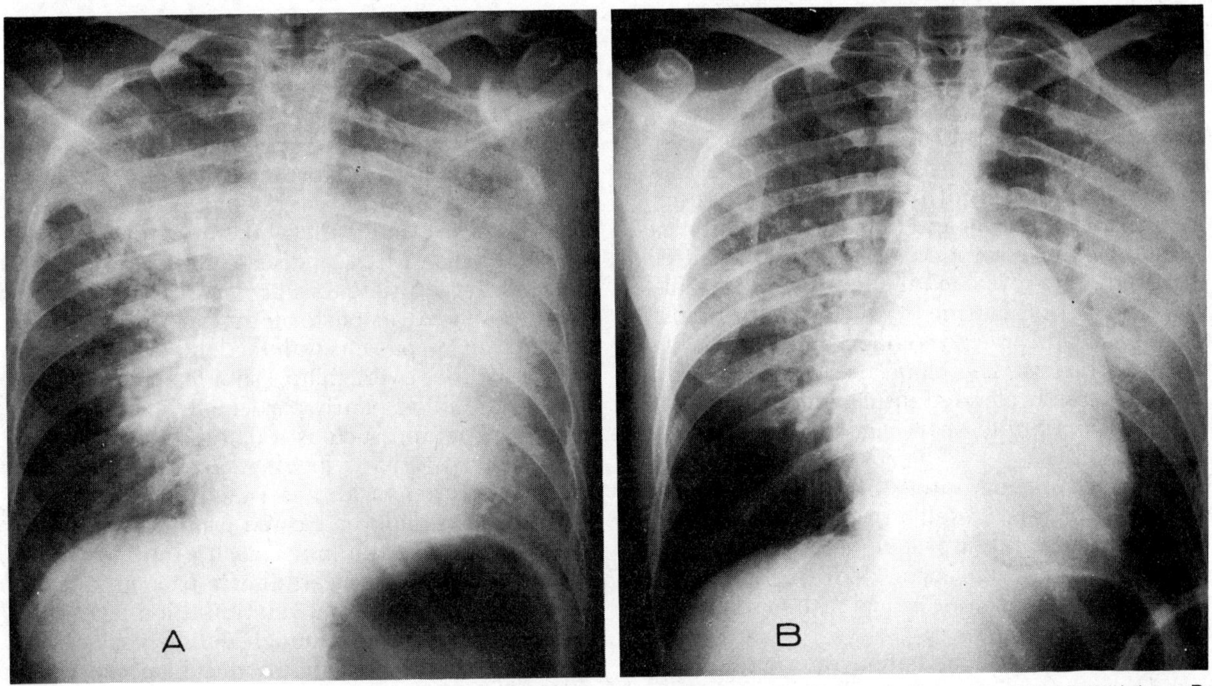

FIGURE 21-7 Roentgenogram of a 24-year-old male with tight mitral stenosis. *A.* Intraalveolar pulmonary edema. *B.* 24 h later. Partial clearing of the intraalveolar edema on the right side with persistent interstitial edema on the left side.

Pseudotumor

The localized accumulation of edema fluid in the interlobar spaces may simulate pneumonia, tumor, or infarction. It may disappear after treatment for heart failure.

Dilatation of the Superior Vena Cava and Azygos Veins

The superior vena cava and azygos veins often become dilated when there is right-sided heart failure in association with increases in blood volume and in systemic vasoconstriction.

Electrocardiogram

There are no electrocardiographic findings of heart failure itself. The electrocardiogram of patients with heart failure is usually abnormal because heart failure is a consequence of severe heart disease, which, as a rule, is associated with an abnormal electrocardiogram. (See Chap. 14.)

When correlated with other findings, it may give information regarding the etiology of heart failure.

Laboratory Studies

Special Cardiac Laboratory Studies

Swan-Ganz catheterization usually is not necessary to determine that a patient has heart failure (Chap. 124). This study can be helpful in documenting the presence of congestive heart failure by measurement of central venous, right ventricular end-diastolic, and pulmonary wedge pressures as well as cardiac output. These determinations can be especially helpful in some patients in the acute phase of a myocardial infarction and in some patients who may need vasodilator therapy for late-stage failure. However, Swan-Ganz catheterization is not needed in the vast majority of patients who are put on vasodilator therapy.

Radionuclide angiograms provide accurate, noninvasive measurement of ejection fraction (Chap. 109). This study is helpful in determining the etiology of congestive heart failure since, in the absence of large increases in ventricular afterload, a reduced ejection fraction indicates ventricular dysfunction. Large decreases in afterload may falsely increase the ejection fraction, for example, in mitral regurgitation.[6]

Echocardiography also can determine the ejection fraction, although limited areas of regional ventricular wall dysfunction can be misleading (Chap. 120). Echocardiography is of major use in determining the etiology of heart failure. This is especially true in mitral stenosis, aortic stenosis, idiopathic hypertrophic subaortic stenosis, ruptured mitral chordae, valvular endocardial vegetations, and left atrial myxoma.

In the patient with heart failure one or more of the following may be found on *cardiac catheterization:* an elevated end-diastolic pressure in the involved ventricle; a lower resting cardiac output as compared with that prior to the onset of failure; an inability to increase cardiac output in response to exercise; an abnormally high arteriovenous oxygen difference at rest or during exercise; or a reduced ventricular ejection fraction determined during angiography (Chap. 108). Usually, one does not subject a patient to cardiac catheterization to determine the presence or absence of heart failure; rather, this procedure is used to determine the cause or to grade the severity of the underlying heart disease.[41,42]

Routine Laboratory Tests

Dysfunction of the liver, kidneys, or brain may develop in the late stages of heart failure as a result of altered cardiac output and diminished organ perfusion, or as a result of increased venous pressure.

Urinalysis may reveal moderate proteinuria. The specific gravity of the urine may be high during the phases of salt and water retention and low during periods of diuresis. The blood urea nitrogen level may be moderately elevated, usually no higher than 50 mg/dl, secondary to heart failure (prerenal azotemia).

Hepatic dysfunction, often with structural damage to the liver, may result in slight elevations of serum bilirubin and aspartate aminotransferase (AST) levels and serum lactic dehydrogenase.[43,44] Hepatic necrosis may be associated with marked elevation of the serum AST.

The erythrocyte sedimentation rate may be retarded during congestive heart failure.

Natural History and Prognosis

In patients with mild heart failure the prognosis is often that of the underlying disease. For example, mild heart failure due to an old myocardial infarction in a patient with severe triple-vessel coronary artery disease has a relatively poor prognosis because of the coronary artery disease and infarction rather than the heart failure per se. Mild heart failure due to rheumatic mitral regurgitation has a relatively favorable and predictable long-term prognosis.

In patients with very severe chronic heart failure of any cause, the prognosis is poor, although the first carefully controlled statistical study is just now being conducted. It appears that sudden cardiac death is frequent and the average life span may be less than 18 months once a patient reaches late class III or class IV heart failure.[45]

Because of the vicious circle or positive feedback loops discussed earlier in this chapter, severe heart failure usually gets worse whether or not the inciting condition gets worse. Interrupting the positive feedback loops by therapy may stabilize a patient's condition and improve the patient's quality of life, but proof of increased longevity resulting from such therapeutic intervention is not available.

Management of Patients with Heart Failure

Prevention of Heart Failure

Since heart failure results from heart disease, preventing heart disease, when possible, should be the first step in our effort to prevent heart failure. For example, hypertension may produce heart disease and heart failure in the absence of other heart diseases, and control of the hypertension usually prevents heart failure.[12,13] At present, however, we do know how to modify or prevent many types of heart disease. Therefore, our next step in preventing heart failure is to prevent or delay the onset of heart failure in patients with heart disease. For some patients, it may be appropriate to suggest ways to reduce the effort expended in performing their job activities. However, many patients with moderately severe heart disease without overt failure should stay active and can and should regularly participate in a reasonable exercise program, such as walking. Beware of urging too much activity; jogging, for example, is not useful for patients with heart failure.

Infections should be treated promptly. Viral diseases that involve the lungs, such as influenza, are especially difficult for heart disease patients and may cause pulmonary edema. Immunization against influenza is important, although only partially effective. Streptococcal pharyngitis must be prevented or promptly treated in patients with rheumatic carditis and rheumatic heart disease (Chap. 62). Infective endocarditis likewise must be prevented or treated promptly (Chap. 56).

Excessive ingestion of salt should be avoided. Many patients with compensated heart disease eat more than average amounts of salt, and some go on sprees of eating salted foods. This precipitates heart failure. Sodium-retaining hormones should be used with caution, and sodium-containing intravenous fluid administered with care.

Patients with significant heart disease who could eventually develop heart failure must not smoke. Among environmental factors, high temperature, high humidity, and very high altitude without a pressurized cabin should be avoided by patients with heart disease (Chap. 84).

If thrombophlebitis, pulmonary emboli, or cardiac arrhythmias occur, they should be promptly treated and appropriate measures applied (Chaps. 27, 54, and 68). Prompt treatment should be instituted for renal disease or lower urinary tract obstructions; circulatory overload may develop in patients with these diseases even when heart disease is not present.

Very severe, chronic anemia and thyrotoxicosis may produce heart failure in some patients who do not have heart disease. More often, however, heart failure related to these conditions occurs in patients with additional heart disease (Chap. 24). However, sickle cell anemia is associated directly with severe depression of ventricular function and with heart failure without other heart disease.[46]

Special consideration must be given to patients with heart disease who undergo surgical procedures (Chaps. 79 and 80).

An issue of continuing concern is whether administering digitalis helps delay the onset of heart failure in heart disease patients. Digitalis may be given to patients with heart disease who have subtle signs of failure, but we do not recommend that it be routinely given to patients who have heart disease without evidence of heart failure. Digitalis should be given to patients with known heart disease or moderate to marked cardiomegaly who have even minimal symptoms and signs of failure when they must undergo stresses such as major surgical procedures. In such cases, the risk of digitalis toxicity can be reduced by giving only two-thirds of the usual doses, because toxicity usually occurs with higher doses.[47] Improvement in cardiac contraction is proportional to the size of the dosage.

Some recent studies have suggested the use of arterial vasodilator therapy such as hydralazine in patients with severe aortic regurgitation or mitral regurgitation but not heart failure.[48,49] The concept is to reduce the extent of regurgitation by producing a fall in afterload. Further clinical trial is needed before practical guidelines can be given.

Management Components[49a]

In this section, eight management components will be discussed in detail. In the next section, these components will be arranged in various combinations to describe the appropriate practical therapy for various degrees of heart failure. The management components will be related to the pathophysiology described earlier in this chapter and in Chap. 20. The specific overused compensation which is causing symptoms and which can be selectively withdrawn by the therapy will be identified. New symptoms which may be expected if the therapy is overapplied will be outlined, with suggestions for avoiding them. In-depth discussion of clinical pharmacology of digitalis, diuretics, and vasodilators will be provided in Chaps. 88, 92, and 94.

The eight management components for treatment of heart failure are:

- Identify and manage specific etiology when possible.
- Discover and manage precipitating causes so as to decrease the workload on the heart.
- Control heart rate.
- Increase myocardial contractility and increase cardiac output.
- Decrease congestion by reducing preload.
- Decrease afterload and increase cardiac output.
- Decrease workload by agents which alter preload and afterload.
- Manage surgically.

Identify and Manage Specific Etiology

Identification of a specific etiology is the important first step in heart failure treatment. Identification of the occasional curable patient justifies a reasonable search for a specific etiology in all patients.

We divide the possible etiologies into the following categories:

1. Direct myocardial damage: myocardial infarction, viral myocarditis, etc.
2. Ventricular overload
   a. volume overload including mitral or aortic regurgitation, systemic arteriovenous fistula, etc.
   b. Pressure overload including systemic hypertension, aortic stenosis, etc.
3. Restriction to diastolic filling: mitral stenosis, constrictive pericarditis, etc.

Patients who fit into the categories of direct myocardial damage and ventricular overload usually have enlarged hearts. Exceptions to this rule may include acute myocardial infarction, acute mitral or aortic regurgitation, and some cases of aortic stenosis and hypertension. Patients who fit into the category of restriction to diastolic filling generally have small hearts unless there is pericardial fluid. Patients with heart disease due to direct myocardial damage often have a weak apex impulse and low-amplitude carotid pulses. Patients in the subcategory of disease due to ventricular pressure overload often have diagnostic physical findings such as high systemic blood pressure or a diagnostic murmur of aortic stenosis. They usually have a forceful apical impulse. Patients in the volume overload subcategory may have increased amplitude of the carotid pulses (except mitral or tricuspid regurgitation); a marked displacement of the apical impulse during each heartbeat; and diagnostic murmurs of a shunt lesion or valvular regurgitation. Patients with ventricular overload without extensive cardiac muscle damage may have a normal ejection fraction. In patients who have direct myocardial damage, the ejection fraction will be reduced.

These three etiologic categories are also helpful in selecting therapy. For example, patients with the ventricular myocardial weakness associated with direct myocardial damage need the increase in ventricular contractility provided by digitalis, while patients with restriction to diastolic filling as a result of chronic constrictive pericarditis or pure mitral stenosis with normal sinus rhythm may receive little or no benefit from digitalis.

Discover and Manage Precipitating Causes so as to Decrease the Workload on the Heart

Precipitating and aggravating factors in heart failure may include: excessive activity, excessive salt intake, excess intravenous fluid administration, obesity, pulmonary infection, pulmonary embolism, cardiac arrhythmias, myocardial infarction, prostatic enlargement with lower genitourinary tract obstruction, renal disease, anemia, and thyrotoxicosis.

The desired level of physical activity of the patient with heart failure must be calculated to cause as little harm as possible while providing what the patient needs for a meaningful, productive, happy life. It is usually economically necessary as well as psychologically valuable to keep patients "on the job" or otherwise reasonably active as long as possible.

Some patients have advanced symptoms when they first seek medical help and require hospitalization and bed or chair rest in a trunk up–legs down position. After diuresis has occurred and symptoms have been relieved, the patient may gradually assume more activity.

A number of complications may result from prolonged bed rest, including poor muscle tone, poor cardiovascular activity (including postural hypotension and decreased cardiac output), venous stasis with thromboembolism, and mental depression. Complications are especially likely to occur in elderly patients. Passive exercises of the legs should be carried out in an effort to prevent venous stasis. Elastic stockings may also help decrease venous stasis by increasing the velocity of blood flow in the veins.

Congestive heart failure occurring under certain conditions such as pregnancy or acute rheumatic myocarditis may require more prolonged rest or complete inactivity until the pregnancy is terminated or the acute rheumatic myocarditis subsides (Chaps. 62 and 69).

Control Heart Rate

Specific abnormalities of heart rate or rhythm are distinct from the compensatory sinus tachycardia mediated by increased sympathetic activity.

Intermittent ectopic tachyarrhythmias can increase ventricular dysfunction in heart failure due to ischemic heart disease by increasing cardiac oxygen consumption and aggravating myocardial ischemia. The same is true for dilated cardiomyopathy. Such tachyarrhythmias are often so subtle that the patient is unaware of them. The therapy of tachyarrhythmias is discussed in Chap. 27. Frequent premature ventricular beats can enhance mitral regurgitation. If one suspects such occult arrhythmia as a contributing factor in the worsening of heart failure, continuous 24-h ambulatory monitoring should be done to make the diagnosis (Chap. 100). When the patient has serious arrhythmias coexisting with severe heart failure, and administration of an antiarrhythmic drug is considered, the ventricular contractile depressant effects of many antiarrhythmic drugs must be considered (Chap. 89). If cessation of the arrhythmia is a major benefit, any negative inotropic effect of the necessary antiarrhythmic drug may be counterbalanced by the benefit achieved by abolishing the arrhythmia. The potential for worsening latent heart failure by beta-blocking drugs is not as real as was previously thought, and the use of such drugs for angina or arrhythmias in patients with latent or mild congestive failure is now believed to be reasonably safe. Increases in diuretic drugs may be required to allow addition of beta-blocking drugs. In rare patients with an inappropriate degree of sinus tachycardia and heart failure and in some patients with cardiomyopathy, beta-blockade therapy may be helpful.[50]

In mitral stenosis, the natural history includes sudden appearance of intermittent atrial fibrillation, usually followed by persistence of this arrhythmia. When there is sudden atrial fibrillation with a rapid ventricular response, severe worsening of the degree of heart failure and even pulmonary edema are frequent. Digitalis is the usual therapy since it increases the atrioventricular refractory time, thereby decreasing the number of atrial impulses per minute reaching the ventricle (Chap. 92). Occasionally, propranolol or verapamil may also be used in this situation.

A very slow heart rate due to complete heart block can initiate or precipitate heart failure, especially in patients with preexisting heart disease. Pacemaker therapy may be required (Chap. 28).

Increase Myocardial Contractility and Increase Cardiac Output

The effect of administering a positive inotropic drug is shown in Fig. 21-8. An increase in myocardial contractility results, and the solid lower systolic curve of congestive heart failure (CHF) is increased to the intermediate solid curve of increased contractility with congestive heart failure at point F. On this improved curve, the required cardiac output can be achieved at point G. As the ejection fraction increases, cardiac output increases, cardiac size decreases, and the stimulus to retain salt and water decreases. The ventricle then has moved from point C′ to point G′ on the dashed diastolic pressure curve with resultant lower left ventricular end-diastolic pressure (LVEDP), and there is relief of congestive symptoms. If the original cardiac output had been low, then the positive inotropic drug would increase the cardiac output by this mechanism. All of the positive inotropic drugs, including digitalis, dopamine, dobutamine, amrinone, and milrinone affect the failing heart in this way, although the mechanism by which each works may vary.

Recent controversy surrounds the widely held clinical opinion that most patients with heart failure require digitalis. A number of investigators have discontinued long-term maintenance digitalis in elderly patients with normal sinus rhythm. A relatively low incidence of deterioration was observed. However, some of the studies are poorly designed, some patients were on small doses of digitalis, and some studies showed hemodynamic but not clinical deterioration.[51–53]

While it appears that some patients with heart failure do not require digitalis when they have normal sinus rhythm, the majority do benefit by chronic digitalis therapy. Arnold et al.[54] showed that long-term digitalis therapy improves left ventricular function in heart failure based upon invasive hemodynamic measurements. Other studies have shown

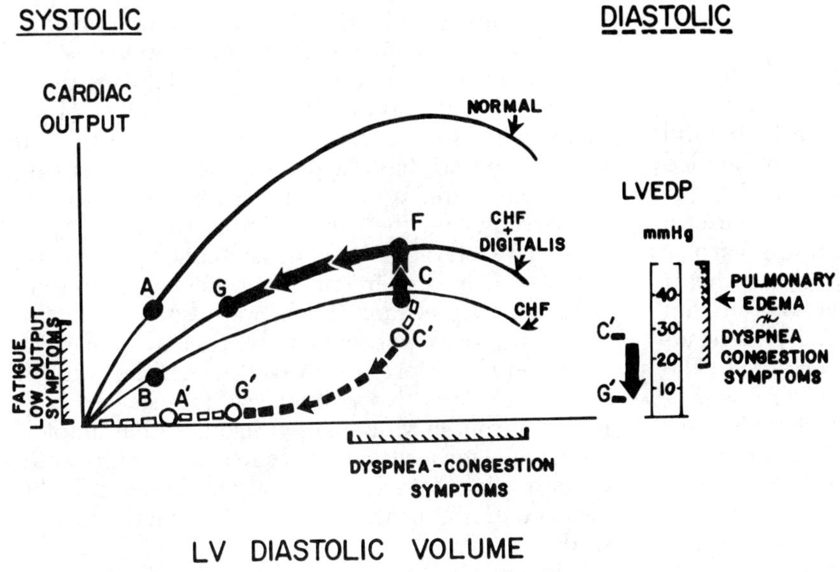

FIGURE 21-8 Heart failure and digitalis. Effect of digitalis on the Frank-Starling compensation, the cardiac output, and the congestive symptoms of heart failure. (See text for explanation.)

similar proof of the effectiveness of digoxin in chronic heart failure.[55]

The majority of patients with heart failure should receive digitalis. Clinically, the response to digitalis appears to vary with the disease responsible for the heart failure. A good response often occurs in patients with hypertensive heart disease, valvular aortic stenosis or regurgitation, rheumatic mitral regurgitation, chronic heart failure due to atherosclerotic coronary heart disease and old myocardial infarction, and congenital heart disease with left-to-right shunts. A less satisfactory or poor response may be noted in patients whose heart failure is due to acute myocardial infarction, cor pulmonale, myocarditis, constrictive pericarditis, primary pulmonary hypertension, Eisenmenger's syndrome, and congestive heart failure associated with thyrotoxicosis, beriberi, anemia, or acute glomerulonephritis. Pure mitral stenosis, a lesion of diastolic restriction to ventricular filling, is not helped by digitalis when there is normal sinus rhythm.

Digoxin (Lanoxin) may be given orally unless the clinical situation demands more rapid action. When administered orally, the onset of action occurs within 1 to 2 h, and the maximum effect is reached in 1½ to 5 h. The average half-life is 36 h. The drug's effect disappears in about 7 to 10 days. The usual oral loading dose for adults and children over 10 years of age is 1.0 mg. The usual oral maintenance dose is 0.25 mg (0.125 to 0.50 mg) each day. Smaller dosages may be effective for elderly patients.

When the clinical situation does not demand speed, in many patients it may be preferable to start therapy with an average maintenance daily dose, omitting the loading dose. The drug will slowly build up in the tissues until its metabolic and excretion rates match its administration rate, achieving gradually the same equilibrium that the loading dose would have achieved rapidly. This gradual method achieves an adequate steady-state plateau in about 7 days. It is especially desirable in the outpatient who does not require rapid maximum digitalis effect and who might become confused and suffer overdosage by failing to reduce the dosage to one tablet daily as directed.

The maximum speed which may be attained by oral dosage is accomplished by giving 0.5 to 0.75 mg followed by 0.25 to 0.5 mg every 5 to 8 h until the average total loading dose is given. If greater speed is demanded by the clinical condition of the patient, digoxin may be given intravenously. The dose given intravenously is only one-half to two-thirds of the oral dose, since only 50 to 70 percent of orally administered digoxin is absorbed and bioavailable. If no digitalis preparation has been given within the past 2 to 3 weeks, an initial dose of 0.25 to 0.5 mg may be given intravenously followed by 0.25 or 0.125 mg every 3 to 5 h, until the average loading dose is given. Intravenous digoxin begins to take effect within 15 to 30 min and reaches its peak in 1 to 5 h, which usually obviates the need for such preparations as ouabain or acetyl strophanthidin. The daily maintenance dose of digoxin given intravenously is 0.125 to 0.25 mg (usually 0.125 mg).

Digoxin is rarely given intramuscularly since a digoxin injection is painful and only 83 percent is bioavailable. Further, in patients with severe heart failure, edema, or poor tissue flow, the absorption of digoxin from the muscular site is not predictable.

When renal failure is present, the maintenance dose of digoxin must be decreased by one-third to one-half depending on the severity of renal impairment.

More specific and detailed information about digitalis dose, route of administration, preparation, and toxicity are discussed in Chap. 92.

Other Drugs Which Increase Myocardial Contractility

Certain sympathomimetic amines (epinephrine, isoproterenol, dopamine, dobutamine) increase contractility in appropriate dosages and may be helpful in certain acute situations but are not recommended for long-term use (Chaps. 88 and 93).

Isoproterenol infusion may be particularly useful in support of the very sick patient with low cardiac output during the first few hours after open heart surgery. With isoproterenol, however, the rhythm must be monitored constantly and the patient attended by specially trained nursing personnel. The excessive sinus tachycardia which isoproterenol produces in some patients may reduce rather than increase cardiac output. Afterload reduction using other drugs is often helpful in the immediate postoperative patient.

Dopamine has less of a chronotropic effect. It lowers renal vascular resistance but increases peripheral vascular resistance. Unfortunately, dopamine's positive inotropic action is partially effected through release of cardiac norepinephrine. Therefore the action of dopamine may be reduced in heart failure where cardiac stores of norepinephrine are low.

Dobutamine is a synthetic derivative of dopamine. It acts directly on the adrenergic receptors and does not depend on release of endogenous norepinephrine. Dobutamine has positive inotropic effects and increases cardiac output with little change in heart rate or blood pressure. Dobutamine appears to be the best of the currently available sympathomimetic amines. However, these amines are used only in extremely severe situations, and must be used with constant monitoring. Parenteral vasodilators are often preferred in these situations. At times, nitroprusside and dobutamine are infused simultaneously. Dobutamine may be of use in situations where critical heart failure requires treatment but severe hypotension prevents the use of nitroprusside.

Bipyridine agents are new drugs that increase cardiac contractility and cause arterial vasodilation. They decrease cardiac filling pressure and systemic vascular resistance, increase cardiac output, and improve symptoms in patients with heart failure.[56] They do not appear to act through the cellular mechanisms of either digitalis or catecholamines.

Amrinone, the first bipyridine to be studied, was useful for acute therapy of severe heart failure but lacked sustained effectiveness when administered orally.[56a] Furthermore, when the drug was administered orally for prolonged periods it produced a dose-related reversible thrombocytopenia in approximately 15 percent of patients. Therefore this drug is not clinically useful for chronic, oral administration. However, intravenous amrinone is available and useful for acute therapy of severe heart failure. When used in this manner, the hemodynamic effects are similar to those of intravenous infusion of dobutamine in maximum dosage.[57a]

Milrinone is a bipyridine derivative of amrinone which has approximately 20 times the inotropic potency of amrinone and has afterload reducing properties.[58] In acute studies in a limited number of patients with severe congestive heart failure, left ventricular end-diastolic pressure fell by 33 percent, pulmonary capillary wedge pressure was reduced by 38 percent, and the cardiac index rose by 53 percent. The elevated baseline systemic vascular resistance fell by 35 percent. All of these changes were statistically significant. There was also a 28 percent rise in the peak positive left ventricular *dP/dt*. The improvements were sustained during follow-up for 1 to 11 months. No patient was reported to have fever, thrombocytopenia, gastrointestinal intolerance, or aggravation of ventricular ectopy. Although it is too early to judge performance of this new agent, it appears promising and merits further study.[58]

Glucagon has minimal effect on cardiac contractility in the failing heart and now appears to be of no use in treating heart failure.

Decrease Congestion by Reducing Preload

Reducing excessive preload of the failing heart improves congestive symptoms (Fig. 21-9). As ventricular end-diastolic volume decreases, the ventricular end-diastolic pressure moves from C′ to D′ along the diastolic curve (the dashed curve). Since the dilated failing heart is on a relatively steep portion of the diastolic passive pressure-volume curve, the reduction in ventricular diastolic volume causes a large reduction in the elevated LVEDP. Simultaneously, because of the Frank-Starling mechanism, the systolic cardiac output is reduced from C to D on the systolic curve (the lower solid curve) of congestive heart failure (CHF). The movement from C to D on the solid curve of systole is in a relatively flat area of the curve, so the reduction in ventricular volume causes only modest reduction of cardiac output. Also, a decrease in cardiac volume may decrease wall stress (the law of Laplace, Chap. 20), and this decreases effective cardiac afterload.[59] Thus, congestive symptoms are relieved by the careful removal of a portion of the Frank-Starling compensation with minimal reduction of cardiac output. If overdiuresis occurs, cardiac output will fall greatly. Symptoms of low cardiac output will then occur as the congestive symptoms are relieved.[16,60]

There are three ways to reduce excessive preload: restrict dietary sodium intake, use diuretics to promote excretion of salt and water, or administer a venous-dilating drug to pool blood in the veins.

Dietary Sodium Restriction

An average diet in the United States contains about 10 g of sodium chloride daily. The excess is excreted in the urine when the kidneys and other organs are functioning normally. Heart failure causes the kidneys to function abnormally, increasing aldosterone, which leads to sodium and water retention as well as weight gain, edema, visceral congestion, and increased venous pressure (Chap. 20). The increased sodium and water retention can be partially controlled by decreasing the amount of salt ingested in the diet.

The usual patient with heart failure does not require rigid restriction of sodium. Diets with severe salt restriction are quite unpalatable for most patients, and potent oral diuretics have decreased the need for rigid restriction. Salt intake should be decreased to about 5 g daily by avoiding obviously salty foods and additional salt at the table. If congestive symptoms are not controlled by such a diet and reasonable diuretic therapy, restrict salt intake to 2 to 4 g daily by avoiding naturally salty foods and omitting salt during cooking and at the table. A strict low-salt diet containing only 0.5 to 1 g daily may be used if the less-restricted measures are not successful, but ingenuity is required to make this diet palatable and nutritious. Low-salt diet lists and booklets have been prepared by the American Heart Association and are available upon request.

Sodium-free salt substitutes are available, but they are not popular because of taste problems. Many salt substitutes contain potassium and may be toxic in patients with renal failure or patients who are taking aldosterone inhibitors. Since one of the effects of converting enzyme inhibition is suppression of aldosterone, potassium-containing salt substitutes should not be given with captopril or enalapril.

There is no need to restrict the water intake in the average patient with heart failure. Fluid intake may be decreased to 500 to 1000 ml daily when intractable heart failure is associated with dilutional hyponatremia.

Diuretics

Specific diuretic agents are discussed in detail in Chap. 94. Diuretics are eventually needed in most patients with heart failure.[61] Diuretics may prevent or reduce pulmonary congestion, other visceral congestion, and peripheral edema. Three frequently used drugs are hydrochlorothiazide (Esidrix, HydroDiuril, Oretic), ethacrynic acid (Edecrin), and furosemide (Lasix). The usual daily doses of these drugs are: hydrochlorothiazide, 50 to 150 mg; ethacrynic acid, 50 to 200 mg; furosemide, 40 to 200 mg.

A diuretic selectively reduces the excessively used Frank-Starling compensation. Congestive symptoms are relieved (Fig. 21-1). If this compensation is removed too much by overvigorous diuresis, cardiac output will fall to levels which cause symptoms. This is shown as moving too far to the left on the lower solid-line curve in Fig. 21-1. The Frank-Starling compensatory mechanism is lost and cardiac output and tissue perfusion suffer, producing complaints of weakness and even confusion and oliguria. The extreme effectiveness of current loop diuretics makes it possible to "overdiurese" even the most severe cases of congestive heart failure.

Many diuretics produce mild to severe electrolyte depletion, including potassium loss, which may produce weakness and arrhythmias. Other diuretics may cause potassium retention.

Determination of accurate daily body weight is the best way to monitor a diuresis. Each liter of lost fluid weighs 1 kg. Daily weight changes in excess of 0.25 kg are due to water loss or gain. Whether the fluid loss is beneficial or harmful is determined by other clinical observations.

Many diuretics produce electrolyte depletion; therefore, the serum electrolytes should be measured. It is frequently necessary to supplement the diuretic with potassium chloride or to use combinations of potassium-wasting with potassium-sparing diuretics. Potassium supplements should not be used together with potassium-sparing diuretics since hyperkalemia may result. Potassium supplementation and potassium-sparing drugs must be decreased or eliminated when renal failure or a rising blood urea nitrogen (BUN) level occurs.

Accurate measurement of fluid intake and urine output is essential during the early treatment days. These will help estimate the amount of diuresis.

We must monitor certain features of the clinical response to diuresis. The level of the jugular venous pressure should be determined to estimate right ventricular end-diastolic pressure. An increasing pulse rate may be a sign of hypovolemia and a low cardiac output. A moderate increase in pulse rate and reduction of systolic pressure immediately after leaving the recumbent position to stand for a minute or two may signal overdiuresis. Hypotension in the recumbent position is a clear sign of overdiuresis. Some patients will complain of thirst, dizziness, fatigue, and weakness as they are relieved of their dyspnea. In advanced overdiuresis, oliguria and progressive renal failure may occur.

It may be necessary for a drug to be given intravenously and while the patient is resting in bed to assure that it will reach the renal tubule. Severe heart failure may impair the absorption of oral or intramuscular doses.

Potassium depletion in patients with heart failure is usually due to the effects of diuretics. The thiazides, ethacrynic acid, bumethanide, and furosemide may produce severe potassium depletion. The depletion is accentuated when the patient has diarrhea, is given intravenous fluid without potassium, or has inadequate dietary potassium intake. The excessive loss of potassium may produce alkalosis, because the hydrogen ions may enter the cells, leaving the plasma alkaline. Potassium depletion may cause weakness and diminished reflexes and may also precipitate the cardiac dysrhythmias in the patient who is receiving digitalis. See Chap. 77 for details of diagnosis and therapy of potassium depletion. When potassium depletion requires prompt therapy, 40 meq of potassium chloride (3 g) dissolved in 250 ml of 5% glucose in water may be given intravenously in 4 h, and it may be necessary to repeat the dose in 12 to 24 h. Great care must be exercised when potassium chloride is given intravenously: a large vein or central venous catheter should be used; the serum potassium level should be known before potassium is given; the urine output should be adequate; and the heart rhythm should be monitored during the infusion. When oral medication is acceptable, 1 g of potassium chloride (13.4 meq) may be given in tomato juice three times a day. Preparations such as Kaon or Triplex, which contain potassium salts, may be used if the chloride ion is supplied from other sources. Some believe that chloride must be available in such patients. In the usual case when the thiazides or ethacrynic acid or furosemide must be continued, potassium chloride must be given continuously in order to prevent potassium depletion. One or two tablets of slow-K (8 meq per tablet) three times per day may be used, as may potassium chloride liquid for chronic therapy. Potassium-retaining diuretics such as triamterene (Dyrenium) or spironolactone (Aldactone) may be used in conjunction with the potassium-losing group, to offset the potassium depletion. Potassium supplements should not be used while potassium-retaining diuretics are being given, since dangerous hyperkalemia may develop. Potassium supplements should be decreased or discontinued and potassium level monitored when such patients are given captopril (Capoten) or enalapril.

Hyponatremia (serum sodium level is below 130 meq/liter) is a problem that is often of ominous significance. In congestive heart failure, hyponatremia is almost always associated with excess body water and dilutional hyponatremia. The body stores of sodium are usually increased, but, because of low-salt diets and diuretics, not as much as the total body water is increased. This is usually treated by reduction of fluid intake to 500 ml daily, cautious use of diuretics, and use of potassium supplements. Captopril, which will be discussed later, may be useful in treating detectional hyponatremia of heart failure. Sodium or hypertonic sodium chloride should not be given.

Hyperchloremic acidosis may develop in patients with heart failure who are given excessive amounts of ammonium chloride, L-lysine, L-arginine monohydrochloride, or acetazolamide (Diamox). These drugs are contraindicated in patients with renal disease, hepatic failure, and respiratory acidosis. The symptoms are hyperventilation, anorexia, nausea, vomiting, drowsiness, and even stupor. The serum chloride level is increased and the pH is decreased. Intravenous infusion of 5% sodium bicarbonate solution is the treatment.

Management of Excessive Diuresis As discussed above, diuresis may be used in patients to the point where the reduction of venous filling pressure reduces cardiac output (see Fig. 21-9). This is a very frequent complication of diuretics. The reduction of cardiac output is often detected by observing muscle weakness and fatigue, or by a rising blood urea nitrogen or a drop in arterial blood pressure and an increase in heart rate when the patient stands up. The elderly patient with marginal cerebral blood flow may become confused or have a subtle negative personality change. In some patients with very severely reduced myocardial contractility, constrictive pericarditis, cor pulmonale, or poor cardiac compliance, the cardiac output may fall even with venous pressure above normal and with some edema present.

Treatment requires removal of diuretics. If that does not work, removal of dietary sodium restriction for a day or two may help.

Venous-Vasodilating Drugs

There are three major categories of vasodilator drugs: those that act principally on the veins to increase venous pooling, those that act principally on the arteries to decrease systemic arterial resistance, and those that have combined venous-pooling and arterial-dilating effects. The angiotensin-converting

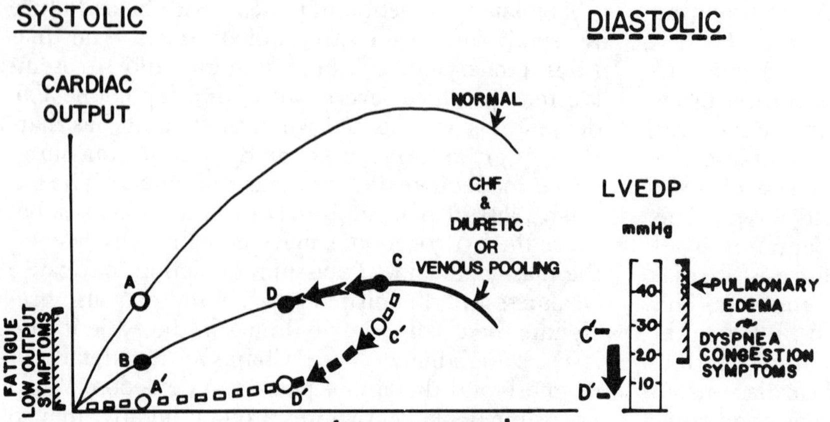

FIGURE 21-9 Heart failure and diuretics. Effect of diuretics on the Frank-Starling compensation, the cardiac output, and the congestive symptoms of heart failure. (See text for explanation.)

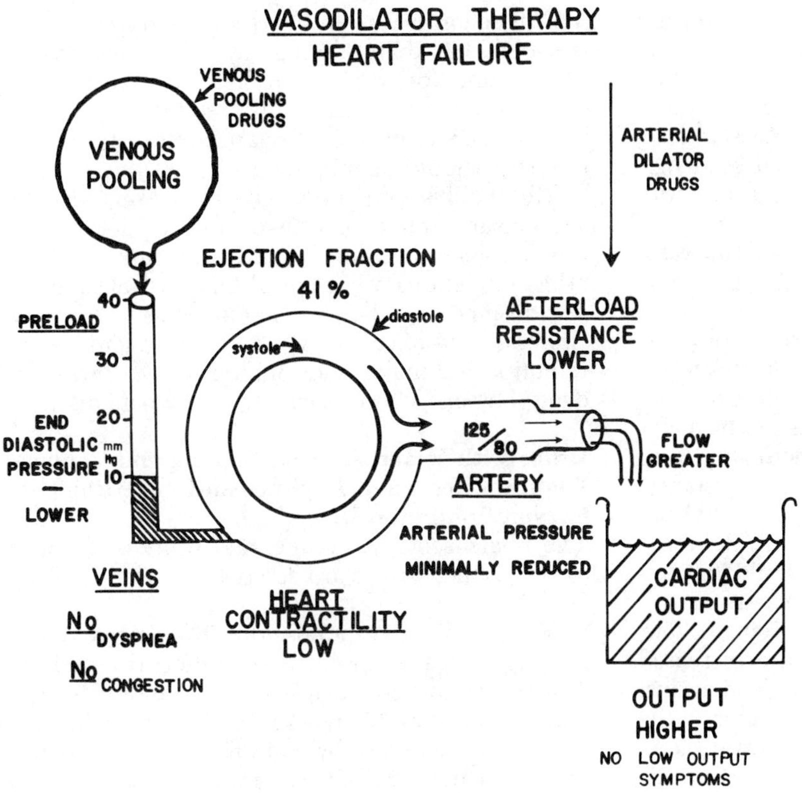

FIGURE 21-10 Diagram of effects of arterial dilator drugs and venous pooling drugs on the failing heart and circulation. (See text for explanation.)

enzyme inhibitors also produce combined reduction of systemic vascular resistance and preload. These drugs vary in method of administration, onset of action, duration of action, and specific toxic side effects and are discussed in Chap. 88. The venous-pooling drugs will be discussed here. The arterial-dilating drugs, the mixed venous-pooling and arterial-dilating drugs, and angiotensin-converting enzyme inhibitors will be discussed later in the section on afterload reduction.

When a drug works directly only to reduce venous tone and thereby increase venous pooling, it only reduces preload.[62] The effect of preload reduction is shown in Figs. 21-9 and 21-10. As venous pooling occurs, diastolic ventricular volume falls (just as it does with a diuretic) along the diastolic curve (dashed line) from C′ to D′ in Fig. 21-9. There is a large reduction in end-diastolic pressure and in congestive symptoms. Cardiac output falls from C to D along the systolic curve (solid lower curve) as preload is reduced. However, this output reduction may be small or may not be perceived at all in severe heart failure because of the flat systolic curve (solid lower curve) relating output to ventricular volume.

From the above description, it is clear that overuse of venous-vasodilating drugs can cause low-output symptoms or even shock in an improperly selected patient. For example, if cardiac output is very low and end-diastolic pressure is not high, perhaps as a result of previous extensive use of diuretics, then cardiac output may further deteriorate with venous vasodilatation.[16,60] It is therefore important to estimate reliably ventricular filling pressure before administering venodilator drugs. In occasional cases, right atrial mean pressure and pulmonary capillary wedge pressure must be actually measured.

Two of the major venous vasodilator drugs are nitroglycerin and isosorbide dinitrate.

Nitroglycerin causes relaxation of the smooth muscle in the systemic veins, which increases the capacitance of this reservoir. As blood pools in the veins, cardiac size is reduced and there is a direct reduction of ventricular preload.

The pharmacology, dosage, and route of administration of the nitrates are discussed in detail in Chap. 88.

Large doses of nitroglycerin have been used for emergency treatment of acute pulmonary edema.[4]

Isosorbide dinitrate (Isordil) relaxes the systemic venous smooth muscle and results in venous pooling and reduction of ventricular preload. Oral administration is an effective method of achieving relatively long-lasting, hemodynamically effective nitrate medication, but large doses must be given (Chap. 88). Often doses of 20 to 40 mg every 6 h orally must be used.

Decrease Afterload and Increase Cardiac Output

As discussed earlier, the chronic increase in arteriolar tone results in a vicious circle or positive feedback loop which worsens the heart failure (see Fig. 21-2*B*). While the increased arteriolar tone provides compensation by maintaining blood pressure and redistributing the limited cardiac output, it also results in an increased cardiac afterload, which itself further compromises the failing heart. Arterial vasodilator therapy of heart failure consists of selective, controlled reduction of afterload by drugs. Afterload reduction is often done in conjunction with preload reduction.

The effects of both arterial and venous vasodilators on heart failure are diagramed in Fig. 21-10, and the effects of afterload are shown in Figs. 21-2*A*, 21-2*B*, and 21-10. These figures depict cardiac output and three of the four major factors which determine it: preload, contractility, and afterload. The fourth major factor, heart rate, is not of major importance to this topic. As the vasodilator drug causes a reduction in peripheral arterial resistance, peripheral flow increases. If stroke volume did not increase, there would be depletion of central arterial volume and central blood pressure would fall, resulting in syncope and shock. Fortunately, as resistance falls, even though contractility remains low, stroke volume and ejection fraction are increased because it is easier for the heart to eject blood against a decreased afterload. Since blood pressure is the product of resistance times flow, the central blood pressure falls little, despite the decreased resistance, because of the simultaneous increase in flow. Cardiac output is increased and low-output symptoms are ameliorated. Congestive symptoms may be improved somewhat by the arterial vasodilators, because the end-systolic residual volume and consequently the end-diastolic volume both fall as the afterload falls (compare the size of the concentric circles in Fig. 21-10 with those in Fig. 21-2*B*). The fall in end-diastolic volume also lowers end-diastolic pressure [see also diastolic curve (dashed line) of Fig. 21-9], further relieving congestive symptoms.

Arterial vasodilator therapy has additional beneficial effects on severe heart failure patients with mitral or aortic regurgitation since it reduces the extent of valvular regurgitation.

No significant change in heart rate occurs when any of the current vasodilators are properly used to treat severe congestive heart failure. Instead, withdrawal of the excessive sympathetic stimulation of advanced heart failure decreases the heart rate, counterbalancing any tendency of the therapy to increase heart rate.

Specific Arterial Dilator Drugs

The pharmacology, dosage, and route of administration of the major arterial dilator drugs are described in detail in Chap. 88.

Hydralazine (Apresoline) is widely used for arterial vasodilator therapy in heart failure.[63] It acts to reduce afterload by direct relaxation of arterial smooth muscle and allows increased cardiac output (Fig. 21-10) with little or no venous-pooling effect. High-dose hydralazine causes a reversible lupus erythematosus-like (LE) syndrome in some patients. This reaction is rare in heart failure since the dose is usually less than 400 mg/day. The usual dose of hydralazine for therapy of heart failure is 50 to 75 mg four times a day. Fluid retention may occur in hydralazine therapy of heart failure. If it occurs, diuretics should be increased.

Minoxidil is a potent, direct arterial smooth-muscle relaxant, requiring only once-a-day dosage, and it is not associated with an LE syndrome. It has no effect on venous capacitance. Like hydralazine, minoxidil increases the cardiac output as it drops peripheral resistance in hypertensive patients. Fluid retention is a major and limiting problem with this drug. Hypertrichosis occurs in many patients.

Drugs with Mixed Arterial-Dilating and Venous-Pooling Effects and Angiotensin-Converting Enzyme Inhibition Drugs

The pharmacology, dosage, and route of administration of these drugs are described in detail in Chap. 88.

Some patients respond either to selected venous pooling or to arterial dilatation; others respond best to a combination of arterial dilatation and venous pooling (Figs. 21-2*B* and 21-10). The combined effect may be achieved by administering both hydralazine and nitrates, but also may be provided by a single drug.[64] Currently, there are two such drugs: nitroprusside, given intravenously, and prazosin, given orally. A third class of drugs, which inhibits angiotensin-converting enzyme (ACE) and affects both arteries and veins, is also given orally.

Nitroprusside relaxes the smooth muscle of arteries and veins. The peak effect occurs almost instantly and is gone in 5 min. It decreases left ventricular end-diastolic pressure, systemic vascular resistance, and venous tone. Arterial dilatation decreases afterload, increases ejection fraction, and tends to increase cardiac output.[65,66] The venous pooling reduces filling pressure to low levels, reducing use of the Frank-Starling mechanism (see Fig. 21-9), and may prevent an increase or cause a net reduction in cardiac output. The use of nitroprusside to treat a patient with relatively low filling pressure may cause a reduction in cardiac output, so it is very important to know that left ventricular filling pressure is elevated before administration of this drug. Swan-Ganz catheterization is often useful in this setting when nitroprusside is used.

Prazosin is an oral quinazoline derivative which increases the capacitance of the postcapillary venous vessel, increases cardiac output, decreases systemic vascular resistance, decreases arterial pressure, and diminishes pulmonary and systemic venous pressures.[101,106]

A large number of studies have shown beneficial clinical and hemodynamic effects of prazosin in heart failure.[67,68] The usual dose for heart failure is 2 to 7 mg four times per day. Cardiac index increases, pulmonary capillary wedge pressure falls, and patient symptoms are reduced. A subsequent study by

Packer et al.[69] noted a significant attenuation of effects by the third dose, and a randomized, double-blind, placebo-controlled study of prazosin showed no demonstrable subjective or objective improvement in patients with stable chronic class III (NYHA) heart failure.

Another carefully conducted double-blind, 8-week trial showed clear improvement in symptoms and objective measures of exercise duration, ejection fraction, and ventricular dimension after prazosin.[70] In this study, the dose was titrated up to initial effectiveness and to a maximum of 16 mg/day. After 4 weeks, the dose of prazosin was again titrated up to the effective dose and a new maximum of 24 mg/day. As therapy continued, the patients retained more sodium, which required increased dosages of diuretics. The sodium retention was thought to result from a prazosin-induced increase in plasma renin activity with subsequent stimulation of aldosterone secretion. The authors concluded that a decrease in responsiveness to prazosin can be overcome by an increased dosage of the drug with concomitant diuretic therapy.

Angiotensin-Converting Enzyme Inhibition

Much of the pathophysiology of congestive heart failure involves alterations of the renin-angiotensin-aldosterone system.[23,71] Symptoms of low output and congestion are due, in part, to overuse of this system. Inhibition of the conversion of inactive angiotensin I to active angiotensin II by angiotensin-converting enzyme blocks this system. Angiotensin-converting enzyme inhibitors are now available and are discussed in detail in Chap. 88. Captopril (Capoten) is an orally active angiotensin-converting enzyme inhibitor which has been widely studied and proved effective in the treatment of heart failure.[72–74] Maximal hemodynamic effects in congestive heart failure are generally seen with doses of 25 mg or less administered four times per day.

In the study by Ader et al.[73] the cardiac output increased 28 percent while pulmonary capillary wedge pressure and mean arterial pressure fell 40 percent and 23 percent respectively when captopril was given. Systemic vascular resistance was reduced by 41 percent. These results are typical of many other studies. As is the case with vasodilators, patients with the initially highest systemic vascular resistance have the largest improvement in cardiac output. The heart rate generally is reduced by approximately 10 percent.

Long-term effectiveness of captopril in heart failure has been shown in a recent multicenter, randomized, double-blind trial[74] which showed gradual and progressive improvement in exercise tolerance over 12 weeks. Eighty percent of the patients in the captopril group exhibited clinical improvement. Patients on captopril generally require lower doses of diuretics.

Captopril has been well tolerated in most patients. Blood pressure generally falls approximately 20 percent, although this reduction is rarely symptomatic and gradually returns to pretreatment values. Patients who have had overdiuresis with depletion of intravascular volume may have a sudden and severe drop in blood pressure when one simultaneously reduces both afterload and preload with captopril. This hypotensive effect can generally be avoided by selecting patients who have adequate or large preload and low cardiac output and who have not recently been overdiuresed. Patients with serum sodium below 130 and very high renin also are prone to hypotension.[75] Since the major effect of captopril occurs within $1\frac{1}{2}$ h, it is also helpful when initiating outpatient therapy to observe the patient's blood pressure in the office for 2 h. The initial dose of captopril should be 6.25 mg. If there is no hypotension within 2 h, the patient is allowed to leave and instructed to take 6.25 to 12.5 mg four times per day and to return in 1 week, when the dose may be increased further. Neutropenia was reported to occur in 38 of 6000 patients and was usually seen in patients with poor renal function or autoimmune disease.[72]

Another converting enzyme inhibitor, enalapril, was recently reported to be effective in nine patients on initial U.S. report.[76] After 1 month of therapy, the improvement persisted. Similar beneficial effects which persisted for 3 months were observed in a placebo-controlled, randomized, double-blind study of 36 patients.[76a] Enalapril requires dosing only every 12 h, and does not contain a sulfhydral group. This drug appears promising and additional studies will be necessary before the full effectiveness, side effects, dose, and patient selection for enalapril are well worked out.

The ability to block the renin-angiotensin-aldosterone system in congestive heart failure represents a very major advance in our therapy of these patients. It clearly improves the quality of life and decreases the symptomatology. Unfortunately, however, patients with class IV (NYHA) congestive heart failure have a mortality of approximately 50 percent within 15 months[72,77,78] on all types of therapy. It is not known whether earlier therapy with vasodilator drugs or angiotensin-converting-enzyme inhibitions could extend the life of patients with early heart failure.

Manage Surgically

If surgery is selected, the procedure employed must be safe compared with the untreated condition. Commissurotomy for noncalcified mitral stenosis with no associated mitral regurgitation has low risk and should be considered for patients who have relatively early symptoms of heart failure. Replacement of a chronically diseased valve with a prosthesis has a greater risk and therefore is usually reserved for patients who have moderately severe (class III) symptoms despite medical therapy. Patients with severe heart failure may choose to undergo a high-risk surgical procedure because their condition is otherwise intractable. For example, persistent heart failure caused by a large and resectable postinfarction aneurysm may warrant surgery. Cardiac transplantation has been used for certain patients who are dying of severe, intractable heart failure (Chap. 136). The availability of cyclosporin A for suppression of rejection has increased to approximately 70 percent the number of patients surviving 2 years following cardiac transplantation.

Practical Application of Management Components

In this section, we will discuss practical outlines for organizing the eight management components into combinations suitable for various types of patients.

Management of Mild Heart Failure

- Search for curable etiology.
- Decrease the physical activity slightly.
- Give an average loading dose of digitalis followed by an average maintenance dose, or start with an average maintenance dose.
- Omit obviously salty foods and salt during cooking or eating.

Management of Moderately Severe Heart Failure

- Search for curable etiology.
- Decrease physical activity to a moderate degree, increasing permitted activity after improvement occurs.
- Give an average loading dose of digitalis followed by an average maintenance dose, or start with an average maintenance dose.
- Give a thiazide diuretic 5 days per week.
- Give 1 g of liquid potassium chloride into tomato juice twice a day to prevent potassium depletion.
- If the above therapy does not produce the desired results, give the thiazide diuretic more often or change to furosemide or ethacrynic acid. Also, start a venous vasodilator if there is continued congestion and an arterial vasodilator if weakness or other low-output symptoms are present. If both congestion and weakness are present, begin prazosin or an angiotensin-converting enzyme inhibitor such as captopril.

Management of Severe Chronic Heart Failure

- Search for curable etiology.
- The physical activity of the patient should be restricted, but total bed rest should be avoided if possible.
- The patient with a history of severe nocturnal orthopnea should be given topical nitroglycerin at bedtime. If that does not relieve the nocturnal orthopnea, then small amounts of morphine sulfate may be given in the muscle 2 or 3 h before the expected episode. After the other therapeutic measures have had some effect (ordinarily 2 to 3 days), the narcotic may be discontinued and topical nitroglycerin used.
- A loading dose of digitalis should be given, followed by an average maintenance dose.
- Furosemide, ethacrynic acid, or bumetanide should be given. If this does not produce the desired results, a potassium-sparing diuretic may be added. If this combination of diuretics does not work, a thiazide diuretic may be added.
- If congestive symptoms predominate, use venous vasodilators. If low-output symptoms predominate, use arterial vasodilators. Many patients have both congestive and low-output symptoms and benefit from either a combination of arterial and venous vasodilator drugs, a drug with mixed arterial- and venous-dilating effects, or an angiotensin-converting enzyme inhibitor such as captopril. Many patients receiving long-term arterial or mixed arterial and venous vasodilators often require increased doses of diuretics. Patients receiving captopril often require reduction of diuretic dose.
- Surgical therapy should be considered if the etiologic lesion is surgically treatable, e.g., valve replacement.

Management of Acute Heart Failure and Acute Pulmonary Edema

Acute pulmonary edema is life-threatening and requires prompt measures, with many steps carried out simultaneously.

- The majority of patients are more comfortable in the trunk up–legs down position.
- From 5 to 10 mg of morphine sulfate should be given intravenously, with close scrutiny for respiratory depression. If it is not possible to be sure that pulmonary edema due to heart failure rather than primary respiratory failure is the patient's problem, morhpine should not be used until the heart failure diagnosis is certain. Morphine is contraindicated in the presence of severe pulmonary disease or myxedema.
- Oxygen should be given by mask, intranasal catheter, or rarely by intermittent positive pressure. If severe lung disease with carbon dioxide retention is a possible diagnosis, oxygen should be given in very low amounts.
- It is important to reduce preload so as to decrease dyspnea and pulmonary congestion, but the potentially deleterious effects of preload reduction must be considered. Sublingual nitroglycerin, 0.4 to 1.2 mg, may be given, or tourniquets (sufficiently tight to occlude venous return but not to impair arterial flow) may be applied to three extremities and rotated every 15 min. Tourniquets have the advantage of being immediately reversible.

- If response to other measures is not prompt or if bronchospasm and wheezing are prominent, aminophylline may be given intravenously. Generally, 250 mg diluted in 50 ml of dextrose and water is administered in a 30-min infusion.
- When the patient is not receiving digitalis, 0.75 mg of digoxin may be given intravenously, followed by additional doses as indicated. This drug is usually of secondary importance in comparison with morphine, oxygen, and preload reduction unless there is atrial fibrillation or a digitalis-responsive ectopic supraventricular tachycardia.
- When atrial fibrillation or supraventricular ectopic tachycardia does not respond to the usual therapy, in urgent cases, or when ventricular tachycardia is present, the rhythm may be reverted electrically with a direct current synchronized cardioverter.
- Diuretics, especially ethacrynic acid and furosemide, have been used extensively in the treatment of pulmonary edema. It appears that some diuretics may have acute vasodilator effects as well as renal effects. The exact place of diuretics in the early treatment of pulmonary edema is not clear,[85] although most patients with pulmonary edema need diuresis.
- Normotensive patients often develop paroxysmal hypertension early in an attack of pulmonary edema, but the blood pressure returns to normal when the symptoms are controlled. Routine use of arterial vasodilators in pulmonary edema is not recommended since the usual measures for treating pulmonary edema are generally successful.

Management of Intractable Heart Failure

In practice there are two types of intractable heart failure:

- There is heart failure that is not responsive to the simple methods of treatment, including the proper use of rest, diet, digitalis, diuretics, and vasodilators. Under these circumstances, the physician must survey the patient's condition and treatment in an attempt to develop a new approach to the seemingly intractable heart failure. The physician must ask questions such as: Is the diagnosis correct? Does the patient really have heart disease, or is it some other condition that mimics heart disease? Is there any clue to a correctable form of heart disease? Have any factors that might aggravate heart failure been overlooked? Has the proper combination of rest, diet, digitalis, diuretics, and vasodilators been used? Is this a suitable patient for vigorous vasodilator therapy? Have all the complications of treatment been identified and corrected? Should open heart surgery be undertaken for valve replacement or resection of a ventricular aneurysm? Should the new approach produce results, the patient's condition may be reclassified; it is no longer intractable heart failure.
- There is unrelenting heart failure in which every known form of therapy has been tried without success. The physician has considered all the points listed above and has modified the therapy to the utmost, but heart failure persists. This second definition of heart failure has a very personal meaning for each physician. It implies that the responsible physician has done all that he or she knows how to do, without success. Another opinion may yet be sought; a new observer may possibly identify an overlooked factor. Even so, there comes a time when no one can help, and perhaps the term *absolute refractory heart failure* should be applied to this clinical state. At this point, the wise physician's foremost concern is the comfort of the patient, which may justify using morphine in small doses, even on a daily basis, to relieve dyspnea, or using very powerful diuretics to reduce preload, so that the patient has more comfort and less dyspnea even though cardiac output and renal function are further reduced.

References

1. Mackenzie, J.: "Principles of Diagnosis and Treatment in Heart Affections," Henry Frowde, Oxford University Press, London, 1916, p. 38.
2. Spann, J. F., Jr., Buccino, R. A., and Sonnenblick, E. H.: Muscle Obtained from Cats with Experimentally Produced Ventricular Hypertrophy and Heart Failure, *Circ. Res.*, 21:341, 1967.
3. Spann, J. F., Jr., Covell, J. W., Eckberg, D. L., Sonnenblick, E. H., Ross, J., Jr., and Braunwald, E.: Contractile Performance of the Hypertrophied and Chronically Failing Cat Ventricle, *Am. J. Physiol.*, 223:1150, 1972.
4. Newman, W. H., and Webb, J. G: Pressure Overload Cardiac Hypertrophy: Length-Tension Curves, and Responses to Isoproterenol, Ca^{2+}, and Ouabain, *Am. J. Physiol.*, 238:134, 1980.
5. Spann, J. F., Bove, A. A., Natarajan, G., and Kreulen, T.: Ventricular Performance, Pump Function and Compensatory Mechanisms in Patients with Aortic Stenosis, *Circulation*, 62:576, 1980.
6. Carabello, B. A., Nolan, S. P., and McGuire, L. B.: Assessment of Preoperative Left Ventricular Function in Patients with Mitral Regurgitation: Value of the End-Systolic Wall Stress-End-Systolic Volume Ratio. *Circulation*, 64:1212, 1981.
7. Newman, W. H.: Volume Overload Heart Failure: Length-Tension Curves, and Response to Beta-Agonists, Ca^{2+}, and Glucagon. *Am. J. Physiol.*, 235(6):H690, 1978.
8. Osbakken, M., Bove, A. A., and Spann, J. F., Jr.: Left Ventricular Function in Chronic Aortic Regurgitation with Reference to End-Systolic Pressure, Volume and Stress Relations, *Am. J. Cardiol.*, 47:193, 1981.
9. Spann, J. F., Jr.: Functional Changes in Pathologic Hypertrophy, in R. Zak (ed.), "Growth of the Heart in Health and Disease," Raven Press, New York, 1984, p. 421.
10. Spann, J. F., Jr.: Contractile and Pump Function of the Pressure-Overloaded Heart, in N. R. Alpert (ed.), "Myocardial Hypertrophy and Failure," in A. M. Katz (series ed.), "Perspectives in Cardiovascular Research," vol. 7, Raven Press, New York, 1983, p. 19.
11. Gorlin, R.: "Coronary Artery Disease," W. B. Saunders Company, Philadelphia, 1976.
12. Kannel, W. B., Castelli, W. P., McNarmara, P. M., McKee, P. A., and Feinleib, M.: Role of Blood Pressure in the Development of Congestive Heart Failure, The Framingham Study, *N. Engl. J. Med.*, 287:781, 1972.

13. Veterans Administration Cooperative Study Group on Antihypertensive Agents: Effects of Treatment on Morbidity in Hypertension, *JAMA*, 202:1028, 1967.
14. Oparil, S.: Cardiac Hypertrophy and Hypertension, in R. Zak (ed.), "Growth of the Heart in Health and Disease," Raven Press, New York, 1984, p. 275.
15. Spann, J. F., and Hurst, J. W.: Vasodilator Therapy of Congestive Heart Failure, in J. W. Hurst (ed.), "Update I: The Heart," McGraw-Hill Book Company, New York, 1979, p. 167.
16. Spann, J. F., Jr., Mason, D. T., and Zelis, R. F.: Recent Advances in the Understanding of Congestive Heart Failure, Parts I and II, *Mod. Concepts Cardiovasc. Dis.*, 39:73, 1970.
17. Chidsey, C. A., Braunwald, E., and Morrow, A. G.: Catecholamine Excretion and Cardiac Stores of Norepinephrine in Congestive Heart Failure, *Am. J. Med.*, 39:442, 1965.
18. Chidsey, C. A., Harrison, D. C., and Braunwald, E.: Augmentation of the Plasma Norepinephrine Response to Exercise in Patients with Congestive Heart Failure, *N. Engl. J. Med.*, 267:650, 1962.
19. Spann, J. F., Chidsey, C. A., Pool, P. E., and Braunwald, E.: Mechanisms of Norepinephrine Depletion in Experimental Heart Failure Produced by Aortic Constriction in the Guinea Pig, *Circ. Res.*, 17:312, 1965.
20. Covell, J. W., Chidsey, C. A., and Braunwald, E.: Reduction of Cardiac Response to Postganglionic Sympathetic Nerve Stimulation in Experimental Heart Failure, *Circ. Res.*, 19:51, 1966.
21. Wood, J. E., Litter, J., and Wilkins, R. W.: Peripheral Venoconstriction in Human Congestive Heart Failure, *Circulation*, 13:524, 1956.
22. Zelis, R.: The Contribution of Local Factors to the Elevated Venous Tone of Congestive Heart Failure, *J. Clin. Invest.*, 54:219, 1974.
23. Cody, R. J., and Laragh, J. H.: The Role of The Renin-Angiotensin-Aldosterone System in The Pathophysiology of Chronic Heart Failure, in J. N. Cohn (ed.), "Drug Treatment of Heart Failure," Yorke Medical Books, New York, 1983, p. 35.
24. Wood, J. E.: The Mechanism of the Increased Venous Pressure with Exercise in Congestive Heart Failure, *J. Clin. Invest.*, 41:2020, 1962.
25. Zelis, R., and Flaim, S. F.: Peripheral Vascular Mechanisms Mediating Vasoconstriction, in E. Braunwald, M. B. Mock, and J. T. Watson (eds.): Congestive Heart Failure, Grune & Stratton, New York, 1982, p. 115.
26. Zelis, R., and Mason, D. T.: Compensatory Mechanisms in Congestive Heart Failure: The Role of the Peripheral Resistance Vessels, *N. Engl. J. Med.*, 282:962, 1970.
27. Zelis, R., Mason, D. T., and Braunwald, E.: A Comparison of the Effects of Vasodilator Stimuli on Peripheral Resistance Vessels in Normal Subjects and in Patients with Congestive Heart Failure, *J. Clin. Invest.*, 47:960, 1968.
28. Zelis, R., Mason, D. T., and Braunwald, E.: Partition of Blood Flow to the Cutaneous and Muscular Beds of the Forearm at Rest and during Leg Exercise in Normal Subjects and in Patients with Heart Failure, *Circ. Res.*, 24:799, 1969.
29. Higgins, C. B., Vatner, S. F., Franklin, D., and Braunwald, E.: Effects of Experimentally Produced Heart Failure on the Peripheral Vascular Response to Severe Exercise in Conscious Dogs, *Circ. Res.*, 31:196, 1972.
30. Zelis, R., Mason, D. T., and Braunwald, E.: Partition of Blood Flow to the Cutaneous and Muscular Beds of the Forearm at Rest and during Leg Exercise in Normal Subjects and Patients with Heart Failure, *Circ. Res.*, 24:799, 1969.
31. Epstein, S. E., Beiser, G. D., Stampfer, M., et al.: Characterization of the Circulatory Response to Maximal Upright Exercise in Normal Subjects and Patients with Heart Disease, *Circulation*, 35:1049, 1967.
32. Sparks, H. V., Kopald, H. H., Carriere, S., Chimoskey, J. E., Kinoshita, M., and Barger, A. C.: Intrarenal Distribution of Blood Flow with Chronic Congestive Heart Failure, *Am. J. Physiol.*, 223:840, 1972.
33. Cannon, P. J.: The Kidney in Heart Failure, *N. Engl. J. Med.*, 296:26, 1977.
34. Hollenberg, N. K.: Pathophysiology of Congestive Heart Failure: The Role of the Kidney, in J. N. Cohn (ed.), "Drug Treatment of Heart Failure," Yorke Medical Books, New York, 1983, p. 53.
35. Reeve, R., Sakai, F. J., Kennedy, J. W., Hood, W. P., Jr., Rackley, C. E., Alderman, E. L., and Lawson, W.: Ejection Fraction in Man: A Comparison of Methods, *Circulation*, 51:677, 1975.
36. Cheyne, J.: A Case of Apoplexy in which the Fleshy Part of the Heart Was Converted to Fat, Dublin Hospital Reports and Communications, *Med. Surg.*, 11:216, 1818.
37. Lange, R. L., and Hecht, H. H.: The Mechanisms of Cheyne-Stokes Respiration, *J. Clin. Invest.*, 41:42, 1962.
38. Davidson, J. D., Waldmann, T. A., Goodman, D. G., and Gordon, R. S., Jr.: Protein-Losing Enteropathy in Congestive Heart Failure, *Lancet*, 1:899, 1961.
39. Pittman, J. G., and Cohen, P.: The Pathogenesis of Cardiac Cachexia, *N. Engl. J. Med.*, 271(9):403, 1964.
40. Weiss, J. M., and Spodick, D. H.: Laterality of Pleural Effusions in Chronic Congestive Heart Failure, *Am. J. Cardiol.*, 53:951, 1984.
41. Grossman, W.: "Cardiac Catheterization and Angiography," Lea & Febiger, Philadelphia, 1974.
42. Kreulen, T. H., Bove, A. A., McDonough, M. T., Sands, M. J., and Spann, J. F., Jr.: The Evaluation of Left Ventricular Function in Man: A Comparison of Methods, *Circulation*, 51:677, 1975.
43. Fragge, R. G., Kopel, F. B., and Iglauer, A.: Serum Glutamic Oxalacetic Transaminase (SGOT) in Congestive Heart Failure: Clinical Study and Review of the Literature, *Ann. Intern. Med.*, 52:1042, 1960.
44. West, M., Pilz, C. G., and Zimmerman, H. J.: Serum Enzymes in Disease. III. Significance of Abnormal Serum Enzyme Levels in Cardiac Failure, *Am. J. Med. Sci.*, 241:350, 1960.
45. Romankiewicz, J. A., Brogder, R. N., Heel, R. C., et al.: Captopril: An Update Review of Its Pharmacologic Properties and Therapeutic Efficacy in Congestive Heart Failure. *Drugs*, 25:6, 1983.
46. Denenberg, B. S., Criner, G., Jones, R., and Spann, J. F., Jr.: Cardiac Function in Sickle Cell Anemia, *Am. J. Cardiol.*, 51:1674, 1983.
47. Williams, J. F., Jr., Klocke, F. J., and Braunwald, E.: Studies on Digitalis. XIII. Comparison of the Effects of Potassium on the Inotropic and Arrhythmia-Producing Actions of Ouabain, *J. Clin. Invest.*, 45:346, 1966.
48. Yoran, C., Yellin, E. L., Becker, R. M., et al.: Mechanism of Reduction of Mitral Regurgitation with Vasodilator Therapy, *Am. J. Cardiol.*, 43:773, 1979.
49. Greenberg, B. H., DeMots, H., Murphy, E., and Rahimtoola, S. H.: Mechanism for Improved Cardiac Performance with Arteriolar Dilators in Aortic Insufficiency, *Circulation*, 63:263, 1981.
49a. Cohn, J. N.: New Concepts in the Mechanisms and Treatment of Congestive Heart Failure, *Am. J. Cardiol.*, 55(no. 2):1A, 1985.
50. Waagstein, F., Hjalmarson, A., Varnauskas, E., and Wallentin, I.: Effect of Chronic Beta-Adrenergic Receptor Blockade in Congestive Cardiomyopathy, *Br. Heart J.*, 37:1022, 1975.
51. Dall, J. L. C.: Maintenance Digoxin in Elderly Patients. *Br. Med. J.*, 2:705, 1970.
52. Dobbs, S. M., Kenyon, W. I., and Dobbs, R. J.: Maintenance Digoxin after an Episode of Heart Failure: Placebo-Controlled Trial in Outpatients, *Br. Med. J.*, 1:749, 1977.
53. Fleg, J. L., Gottlieb, S. H., and Lakatta, E. G.: Is Digoxin Really Important in the Treatment of Compensated Heart Failure?: A Placebo-Controlled Crossover Study in Patients with Normal Sinus Rhythm, *Am. J. Med.*, 73:244, 1982.
54. Arnold, S., Byrd, R. C., Meister, W., et al.: Long-Term Digitalis Therapy Improves Left Ventricular Function in Heart Failure, *N. Engl. J. Med.*, 303:1443, 1980.
55. Doherty, J. E.: Conventional Drug Therapy in the Man-

agement of Heart Failure, in J. N. Cohn (ed.), "Drug Treatment of Heart Failure," Yorke Medical Books, New York, 1983, p. 91.

56. LeJemtel, T. H., Keung, E., Ribner, H. S., et al.: Sustained Beneficial Effect of Oral Amrinone on Cardiac and Renal Function in Patients with Severe Congestive Heart Failure, *Am. J. Cardiol.,* 45:123, 1980.

56a. DiBianco, R., Shabetai, R., Silverman, B. D., Lier, C. V., Benotti, J. R., with the Amrinone Multicenter Study: Oral Amrinone for the Treatment of Chronic Congestive Heart Failure: Results of a Multicenter Randomized Double-Blind and Placebo-Controlled Withdrawal Study, *J. Am. Coll. Cardiol.* 4:855, 1984.

57. Maskin, C. S., Forman, R., Klein, N. A., et al.: Long-Term Amrinone Therapy in Patients with Severe Heart Failure: Drug-Dependent Hemodynamic Benefits Despite Progression of the Disease, *Am. J. Med.,* 72:113, 1982.

57a. Klein, N. A., Siskind, S. J., Frishman, W. H., Sonnenblick, E. H., and LeJemtel, T. H.: Hemodynamic Comparison of Intravenous Amrinone and Dobutamine in Patients with Chronic Congestive Heart Failure, *Am. J. Cardiol.,* 48:170, 1981.

58. Baim, D. S., McDowell, A. V., Cherniles, J., et al.: Evaluation of a New Bipyridine Inotropic Agent—Milrinone—in Patients with Severe Congestive Heart Failure, *N. Engl. J. Med.,* 309:748, 1983.

59. Wilson, J. R., Reichek, N., Dunkman, W. B., and Goldberg, S.: Effect of Diuresis on the Performance of the Failing Left Ventricle in Man, *Am. J. Med.,* 70:234, 1981.

60. Stamfer, M., Epstein, S. E., Beiser, G. D., and Braunwald, E.: Hemodynamic Effects of Diuresis at Rest and during Upright Exercise in Patients with Impaired Cardiac Function, *Circulation,* 37:900, 1968.

61. Laragh, J. H.: Diuretics in the Treatment of Congestive Heart Failure, in E. Braunwald (ed.), "The Myocardium: Failure and Infarction," H. P. Publishing Company, New York, 1974.

62. Taylor, W. R., Forrester, J. S., Magnusson, P., Chatterjee, K., and Swan, H. J. C.: Hemodynamic Effects of Nitroglycerin Ointment in Congestive Heart Failure, *Am. J. Cardiol.,* 38:469, 1976.

63. Franciosa, J. A., Pierpont, G., and Cohen, J. N.: Hemodynamic Improvement after Oral Hydralazine in Left Ventricular Failure, *Am. Intern. Med.,* 86:388, 1977.

64. Massie, B., Chatterjee, K., Werner, J., Greenberg, B., Hart, R., and Parmley, W. W.: Hemodynamic Advantage of Combined Administration of Hydralazine Orally and Nitrates Nonparenterally in the Vasodilator Therapy of Chronic Heart Failure, *Am. J. Cardiol.,* 40:794, 1977.

65. Guiha, N. H., Cohn, J. N., Mikulic, E., Franciosa, J. A., and Limas, C. J.: Treatment of Refractory Heart Failure with Infusion of Nitroprusside, *N. Engl. J. Med.,* 291:587, 1974.

66. Awan, N. A., Miller, R. R., and Mason, D. T.: Comparison of Effects of Nitroprusside and Prazosin on Left Ventricular Function and the Peripheral Circulation in Chronic Refractory Congestive Heart Failure, *Circulation,* 57:152, 1978.

67. Chatterjee, K.: Vasodilator Therapy for Heart Failure, in J. N. Cohn (ed.), "Drug Treatment of Heart Failure," Yorke Medical Books, New York, 1983, p. 151.

68. Awan, N. A., Miller, R. R., DeMaria, A. N., Maxwell, K. S., Neumann, A., and Mason, D. T.: Efficacy of Ambulatory Systemic Vasodilator Therapy with Oral Prazosin in Chronic Refractory Heart Failure, *Circulation,* 56:346, 1977.

69. Packer, M. D., Meller, J., Gorlin, R., Herman, M. V.: Hemodynamic and Clinical Tachyphylaxis to Prazosin-Mediated Afterload Reduction in Severe Chronic Congestive Heart Failure, *Circulation,* 59:531, 1979.

70. Colucci, W. S., Wynne, J., Holman, B. L., and Braunwald, E.: Long-Term Therapy of Heart Failure with Prazosin: A Randomized Double Blind Trial, *Am. J. Cardiol.,* 45:337, 1980.

71. Curtiss, C., Cohn, J. N., Vrobel, T., and Franciosa, J. A.: Role of the Renin-Angiotensin System in the Systemic Vasoconstriction of Chronic Congestive Heart Failure, *Circulation,* 58:763, 1978.

72. Parmley, W. W.: Captopril for Heart Failure, in J. N. Cohn (ed.), "Drug Treatment of Heart Failure," Yorke Medical Books, New York, 1983, p. 179.

73. Ader, R., Chatterjee, K., Ports, T., Brundage, B., Hiramatsu, B., and Parmley, W.: Immediate and Sustained Hemodynamic and Clinical Improvement in Chronic Heart Failure by an Oral Angiotensin-Converting Enzyme Inhibitor, *Circulation,* 61:931, 1980.

74. Captopril Multicenter Study Group: A Placebo Trial of Captopril in Refractory Chronic Congestive Heart Failure, *J. Am. Coll. Cardiol.,* 2:755, 1983.

75. Packer, M., Medina, N., and Yushak, M.: Relation between Serum Sodium Concentration and the Hemodynamic and Clinical Responses to Converting Enzyme Inhibition with Captopril in Severe Heart Failure, *J. Am. Coll. Cardiol.,* 3:1035, 1984.

76. Levine, T. B., Olivari, M. T., Garberg, V., Sharkey, S. W., and Cohn, J. N.: Hemodynamic and Clinical Response to Enalapril, A Long-Acting Converting-Enzyme Inhibitor, in Patients with Congestive Heart Failure, *Circulation,* 69:548, 1984.

76a. Sharpe, D. N., Murphy, J., Coxon, R., and Hannan, S. F.: Enalapril in Patients with Chronic Heart Failure: A Placebo-controlled, Randomized, Double-blind Study, *Circulation,* 70:271, 1984.

77. Massie, B., Ports, T., Chatterjee, K., et al.: Long-Term Vasodilator Therapy for Heart Failure: Clinical Response and Its Relationship to Hemodynamic Measurements, *Circulation,* 63:269, 1981.

78. Walsh, W. F., and Greenberg, B. H.: Results of Long-Term Vasodilator Therapy in Patients with Refractory Congestive Heart Failure, *Circulation,* 64:499, 1981.

22

Pathophysiology of Hypotension and Shock

Francois M. Abboud, M.D.

Shock is a defect in the perfusion of tissues or a failure of the circulatory system to deliver the necessary substrates and remove metabolites. This hemodynamic abnormality may result in cellular death.

Early recognition and management of the abnormal circulatory state are essential for the reversal of shock before cellular membranes are damaged. This requires an understanding of circulatory physiology and the pharmacology of vasoactive drugs. The pathophysiology of hypotension and shock is presented in this chapter in two parts:

Part A: "Hemodynamic Abnormalities in Hypotension and Shock." Some of the basic concepts of circulatory adjustment are reviewed.

Part B: "Cellular and Biochemical Events in Shock." The cellular and biochemical events leading to irreversibility of shock and cellular death are discussed.

Part A. Hemodynamic Abnormalities in Hypotension and Shock

Perfusion of any organ depends on systemic arterial pressure and vascular resistance of that particular organ. Systemic arterial pressure is determined by cardiac output and total vascular resistance:

$$\text{Arterial pressure} = \text{cardiac output} \times \text{total systemic vascular resistance}$$

Vascular resistance is predominantly related to the radius of blood vessels, and the radius is influenced by the structure of the vessel wall and the degree of encroachment on the lumen as well as the tone of vascular smooth muscle. The tone of vascular muscle is regulated by neurogenic impulses, humoral factors, and intrinsic myogenic factors. Thus, the amount of blood flow to an organ depends on cardiac performance and total systemic vascular resistance, which determine arterial pressure, and on local vascular resistance in that organ:

$$\text{Organ blood flow} = \frac{\text{systemic arterial pressure}}{\text{organ vascular resistance}}$$

Exchange of substrates and metabolites depends not only upon the amount of blood flow reaching an organ, but also upon whether that flow perfuses the nutritional capillaries in the microcirculation. The capillary network is the critical interface between the blood and the cells. Thus, the basic abnormalities that would prevent blood and nutrients from reaching the tissues are:

1. The heart may fail to pump an adequate cardiac output.
2. Systemic vessels may dilate markedly and cause a fall in arterial pressure and physiologic arteriovenous shunts.
3. The arterioles and resistance vessels in a vascular bed may constrict sufficiently to prevent blood from reaching a particular organ.
4. The microcirculation of an organ may be occluded so that the blood reaching the organ does not perfuse the exchange capillaries.

Stages of Hypotension and Shock

The progress of the syndrome and its pathogenesis seem to occur in three stages that reflect the severity of the defect in tissue perfusion and the intensity of cellular damage.

Stage I: Compensated Hypotension

The fall in blood pressure may result from vasodilatation or reduced cardiac output. In the majority of situations, a fall in cardiac output rather than vasodilatation is responsible for the hypotension, except in septic shock, where cardiac output may be normal or increased but the increase does not meet the metabolic demands of tissues because of physiologic arteriovenous shunting. As soon as arterial blood pressure falls, there are compensatory mechanisms triggered by activation of baroreceptor reflexes that result in restoration of arterial blood pressure through an increase in cardiac output and in peripheral resistance. Blood flow to vital organs such as the brain and heart is preserved, and the symptoms and signs of this compensated state are minimal.[1]

Stage II: Decompensated Hypotension

The compensatory mechanisms in this phase are insufficient to maintain arterial blood pressure or perfusion of vital organs. There is evidence of cerebral, renal, and myocardial ischemia. There are signs of excessive sympathetic discharge, and the majority of patients in this stage should be treated aggressively to restore cardiac output and tissue perfusion and reverse the syndrome.[2]

Stage III: Irreversible Shock—Microcirculatory Failure and Cellular Membrane Injury

In this stage, severe ischemia, toxins, antigen-antibody reactions, or complement activation damage cellular membranes. The damage may involve the blood cellular elements, the capillary endothelium, the kidneys, the liver, the lungs, etc. Vasoconstriction, which takes place initially as a compensatory response to the hypotension, is intense and may result in aggregation and sludging of blood corpuscles in capillaries and venules. A progressive fall in arterial blood pressure below critical levels results in ischemia of all organs. Necrotic damage of the gastrointestinal mucosa leads to absorption of bacteria and toxins into the circulation, which, in turn, may have detrimental effects on other organs and may contribute to a generalized endothelial damage with potentially disseminated intravascular coagulation. Renal ischemia and hypotension may lead to acute tubular necrosis. Coronary ischemia in patients with coronary artery disease would lead to a depression of myocardial contractility, further hypotension, and a vicious cycle. Damage to the capillary endothelium increases permeability and transudation of fluids and proteins into the extracellular space, exacerbating the hypovolemia and hypotension. Neutrophils may release vasodilator peptides. Severe acidosis causes myocardial depression and vasodilatation. Finally, the release of lysosomal enzymes and the depletion of high-energy phosphates are associated with cellular destruction.

Major Determinants of Tissue Perfusion

Tissue perfusion is determined by cardiac and vascular properties which are regulated by neural, humoral, and metabolic factors.

Cardiac Output

Cardiac output is the product of heart rate and stroke volume. A normal output of approximately 5 liters/min delivers 250 ml of oxygen to the tissues, which meets our metabolic demands at rest. When cardiac output falls below 2 liters/min per square meter of body surface area the shock is severe.

A fall in blood pressure may result from a fall in cardiac output, and the latter may be caused by an abnormal heart rate or a low stroke volume.

Heart Rate Atrial or ventricular tachycardia (more than 140 beats per minute) may decrease cardiac output significantly, because a rapid heart rate limits cardiac filling time and lowers stroke volume, particularly in patients with limited myocardial reserve. Failure to correct the tachycardia may result in cardiogenic shock, whereas early treatment could restore heart rate and normal blood pressure. One has to be aware of the possibility that an increase in rate may be compensatory in some patients with anemia, fever, sepsis, or hemorrhage, in order to maintain cardiac output. Severe bradycardia (less than 40 beats per minute) may cause a fall in output. Sinus bradycardia and atrioventricular block are often seen immediately following myocardial infarction of the inferior wall of the ventricle and may cause hypotension. Bradycardia contributes significantly to the common faint syndrome or vasovagal syncope.

Stroke Volume Stroke volume is the amount of blood pumped out of the left or right ventricles with each contraction. At rest it equals 70 ml per beat and it may decrease because of a decrease in cardiac filling (preload) and in myocardial contractility, or because of an increased "afterload."

Decreased Cardiac Filling. In accordance with Starling's law of the heart, the blood remaining in the ventricles at the end of each diastole determines the end-diastolic pressure and wall tension, which in turn determine the force of the subsequent contraction. There are many factors that regulate filling pressure, such as heart rate, duration of filling, ventricular compliance, venous tone, and total blood volume as well as the posture of the patient. A reduction in total blood volume may result from external or internal bleeding, vomiting, diarrhea, diuretics, burns, or excessive perspiration.

A reduction in blood volume may also be relative rather than absolute when vascular tone decreases. This may occur with administration of anesthetics, ganglion blockers, or venodilators; after spinal cord injury; in patients with autonomic insufficiency; or in patients with septic shock. Excessive pooling of blood in the lower extremities may also cause a significant reduction in filling pressure.

Mechanical compression of the heart may also prevent its filling. This may be seen with pericardial tamponade, tension pneumothorax, positive pressure breathing or superior vena caval syndrome, particularly in hypovolemic individuals. Mechanical obstruction to blood flow occurs with extensive pulmonary embolism, occlusion of the large pulmonary vessels, atrial myxoma, or a ball-valve thrombus, all of which may cause severe hypotension and shock.

Decreased Myocardial Contractility. This is the major cause of shock in myocardial infarction and a contributing factor in many different types of shock, including septic and hemorrhagic shock. There are important reversible factors that depress contractility.

A fall in arterial P_{O_2} results from ventilation-perfusion abnormalities of the lung which occur early in shock. In late shock malignant hypoxia is associated with the pathologic entity of shock lung or ARDS (acute respiratory distress syndrome). Hypoxia has a direct vascular effect, causing vasodilatation, particularly in the coronary or cerebral circulations; and an indirect effect (through activation of chemoreceptors) that causes reflex vasoconstriction in vessels of skeletal muscle, skin, and splanchnic bed. The combination of a direct dilator effect and an indirect vasoconstrictor effect allows redistribution of blood flow to the organs that depend on aerobic metabolism. Despite the compensatory mechanisms that permit delivery of oxygen to the vital organs, myocardial contractility may be impaired as arterial

P_{O_2} declines. Often the severity of the decline in arterial P_{O_2} reflects the extent of myocardial infarction. Hypoxia is one of the reversible causes of myocardial depression and should be corrected aggressively.

There are three main reasons for *acidosis* in shock: anaerobic metabolism in ischemic tissue causes the release of lactate; decreased glomerular filtration and acute renal failure cause the retention of organic acids;[3] and severe hypoventilation causes hypoxia, CO_2 retention, and respiratory acidosis. The reduced pH of arterial blood which reflects tissue or intracellular pH causes myocardial depression, vasodilatation, and a decreased responsiveness to sympathomimetic amines. Correction of acidosis may restore arterial blood pressure in hypotensive patients and eliminate the need for more aggressive therapy.

It has often been stated that the main goal of therapy in shock is to restore cardiac output and perfusion of the organs without being too concerned about the level of arterial blood pressure. However, cardiac output depends on myocardial contractility and in acute myocardial infarction contractility depends on coronary blood flow through collateral vessels to the ischemic myocardium, which in turn depends on the level of arterial diastolic pressure.[4,5] Also, in patients with coronary artery disease without myocardial infarction, hemorrhagic or hypovolemic hypotension may be complicated by myocardial ischemia and depressed contractility. Therefore, although it is true that restoration of perfusion is the main goal of therapy, *maintenance of arterial pressure* is essential for myocardial flow and function, for an adequate cardiac output, and, consequently, for tissue perfusion. Unfortunately, the optimum level of arterial pressure is difficult to define and may vary from patient to patient, depending on the severity and degree of vascular narrowing in the coronary vessels. The pressure necessary to drive flow across an arterial narrowing or through collateral vessels in each patient is difficult to determine. For this reason, judicious restoration of arterial pressure to reasonable levels between 100 and 120 mmHg, guided by the clinical picture of the patient, should be the goal of therapy, assuming that the patients are normotensive before they go into shock.

Oxygen requirement of the myocardium varies and can influence cardiac performance, since an *increase in oxygen requirement without increase in oxygen supply means deterioration of function.*[6] The factors that increase myocardial oxygen demand are: increased heart rate, elevated arterial blood pressure, increased cardiac size, and increased myocardial wall tension. Hypotension, bradycardia, and reduced cardiac size decrease oxygen demand.

A slight reduction in arterial pressure may be beneficial but a significant reduction may be detrimental as it reduces myocardial perfusion. Vasodilator drugs, such as isoproterenol, may lower arterial blood pressure but paradoxically increase myocardial oxygen requirement because of the associated tachycardia and increased myocardial contractility. Conversely, propranolol causes bradycardia and reduces myocardial oxygen demand but it also depresses myocardial contractility in patients with cardiogenic shock.

The appropriate use of venodilators and diuretics causes a reduction in preload, cardiac size, and myocardial oxygen demand; however, an excessive reduction in preload is detrimental because it reduces cardiac output.

Several factors depress myocardial contractility and vascular tone, cause relative hypovolemia, and reduce cardiac filling pressure and consequently cardiac output. These include barbiturates, adrenergic blocking drugs (e.g., ganglion blockers, reserpine, guanethidine, beta blockers), high spinal anesthetics, spinal cord injury, intracranial lesions involving the medullary centers, and severe hypoglycemia.

Cellular damage from any type of shock may be associated with the release of factors that have a myocardial depressant effect.[7]

Increased Afterload. In order for the left ventricle to eject the stroke volume, it has to generate enough power to appose the ventricular distending force at the end of diastole, open the aortic valve, and move a column of blood from the aortic arch into the arterial tree against the diastolic arterial pressure and the impedance of the vasculature. The combination of resistances which have to be overcome by the left ventricle during systole is the "afterload." In severe heart failure with cardiomegaly, the end-diastolic tension in the left ventricle is elevated, peripheral vascular resistance is increased, and stroke volume and cardiac output are reduced. In this situation the "afterload" is excessive and may be reduced by giving a vasodilator which reduces vascular impedance, decreases the power needed during systole, and facilitates the ejection of a larger stroke volume. This in turn reduces cardiac size and ventricular wall tension. This beneficial effect would be offset if arterial pressure were reduced drastically and myocardial perfusion were impaired.

Vascular Factors

Blood vessels have five different functions which may be altered during shock.[8]

Large Arteries These provide an impedance function that dampens pulsatile flow and contributes to cardiac afterload. In shock, increased impedance may cause a significant afterload. In addition, intense constriction of large arteries may prevent the accurate estimation of arterial blood pressure by sphygmomanometry. This may result in undetectable blood pressure by sphygmomanometry when intraarterial pressure may be normal.[9] The effectiveness of vasodilator therapy may depend, in large part, on the reduction in arterial impedance and an associated decrease in afterload rather than on decreased arterial pressure.

Arterioles These vessels develop the critical resistance to blood flow. The tone of vascular muscle in the arterioles is controlled by neurogenic, humoral, and local metabolic factors. The relative degree of vascular resistance in an organ determines the amount of blood flow reaching that organ. Intense constriction in the splanchnic or renal circulation and relaxation of coronary arterioles allow a redistribution of flow to favor the coronary circulation. The effects of the sympathetic nervous system, vasoactive humoral agents, and drugs on arterioles in various vascular beds are not uniform, and this selectivity determines the blood flow between organs and is an important determinant of our choice of vasoactive drug.[1,8,10]

Arterioles are also important determinants of the distribution of flow *within* an organ. Adequate perfusion of any organ depends not only on the amount of blood reaching that organ but on the patency of the nutritional capillaries and vascular channels in which diffusion between blood and tissue occurs. Nonnutritional channels such as arteriovenous shunts, either anatomic or functional, reduce flow through nutritional or exchange capillaries. For example, in myocardial infarction some coronary vasodilators may be detrimental in redistributing coronary flow away from an ischemic region toward a nonischemic region, a phenomenon referred to as a *vascular steal.*

Another example of intraorgan redistribution of blood flow is the acute renal tubular necrosis associated with shock in which a localized increase in vascular resistance causes a reduction in glomerular filtration in the outer cortex and oliguria. Conversely, renal vasodilatation with furosemide may shunt blood preferentially toward the outer cortical nephrons, causing a diuresis.

Precapillary Sphincters The tone of precapillary sphincters determines the patency of exchange capillaries and capillary surface area and may be modulated by neurohumoral factors as well as local metabolites. Exchange of fluids between the intravascular compartment and the extracellular space depends on the hydrostatic pressure, the oncotic pressure, capillary surface area, and capillary permeability. During hypovolemia and hemorrhage, the fall in arterial pressure and constriction of arterioles and precapillary sphincters cause a fall in capillary hydrostatic pressure, and fluids move from the extracellular, extravascular space to the intravascular compartment. This causes a fall in plasma oncotic pressure which is partially corrected by rapid synthesis of new proteins. If shock persists and metabolic acidosis sets in, arterioles and precapillary sphincters tend to dilate, capillary surface area increases, and fluids may shift back to the extravascular space.

Capillaries The surface area of capillaries, their hydrostatic pressure, and their permeability determine intravascular volume, glomerular filtration, the presence of pulmonary edema, and the exchange of oxygen, substrates, and metabolites. Significant defects in capillary function may be present in shock.

Capillary Hydrostatic Pressure and Venules. The *venules* are postcapillary resistance vessels. They are important regulators of capillary hydrostatic pressure and filtration, and intravascular volume. The ratio of postcapillary over precapillary arteriolar resistance may increase in response to norepinephrine and epinephrine;[10] and late in shock, when acidosis prevails, the tone of precapillary sphincters is reduced, but venular resistance may remain elevated. The resulting increase in the ratio of postcapillary resistance to precapillary resistance exaggerates the hypovolemic state by increasing capillary hydrostatic pressure and filtration. An alpha-adrenergic receptor blocker, such as phentolamine, might reverse this detrimental imbalance between post- and precapillary resistance because of a preferential effect on postcapillary resistance vessels.

Capillary Permeability and Oncotic Pressure. Fluid flux across the capillaries is determined by a balance between transcapillary *colloidal osmotic pressure* and hydrostatic pressure; by capillary permeability; and by capillary surface area. *Capillary permeability* may increase in shock because of endothelial injury or the formation of vasoactive peptides. Protein leaks out, plasma oncotic pressure drops, and capillary filtration increases.[11] In addition to the fall in oncotic pressure, severe hypoproteinemia causes an increase in hydraulic conductivity across the capillary endothelium, exaggerating the loss of intravascular fluid.[12]

The balance between oncotic and hydrostatic pressure is also critical in the management of shock lung syndrome and the level of pulmonary edema.[13] Plasma oncotic pressure of normal adults is approximately 25 mmHg, whereas the pulmonary wedge pressure which parallels the pulmonary hydrostatic capillary pressure is 10 to 12 mmHg. Despite this imbalance, capillary filtration does take place because of the high *interstitial* oncotic pressure in the lung. Plasma oncotic pressure may fluctuate drastically; for example, it declines markedly after 12 h of bed rest and this may be a factor in pulmonary edema and orthopnea and paroxysmal nocturnal dyspnea. If oncotic pressure is significantly higher than pulmonary capillary hydrostatic pressure (by approximately 8 mmHg or more), the risk of pulmonary edema is negligible; but if oncotic pressure is low, the patient is at risk of pulmonary edema. This has implications concerning the choice of fluid for treatment of hypovolemia. Although the administration of saline solution or Ringer's lactate may be appropriate in many hypovolemic states, a more effective treatment, if there is protein loss, is the use of colloids such as human serum albumin, purified plasma protein, dextran, or hydroxyethyl starch. Colloids that stay longer in the circulation and increase oncotic pressure are necessary when patients have manifestations of extensive endothelial damage and interstitial or pulmonary edema, or when they are chronically ill or malnourished and have hypoalbuminemia.[13] When given intravenously, dextran and mannitol are excreted by the kidney and increase oncotic pressure in Bowman's capsule, creating a pressure gradient across the glomerulus that facilitates filtration even at low arterial pressure.[14] If, after dextran administration, arterial pressure is not restored and oliguria persists, despite administration of diuretics such as furosemide, then there might be danger of overexpansion of plasma volume and accentuation of pulmonary edema with further administration of colloids.

Anaphylactic shock or snake venom poisoning are characterized by severe reduction in plasma volume because of increased capillary permeability. This may be secondary to the release of histamine or other humoral factors from macrophages or the release of other cellular metabolites which alter endothelial integrity.[15] A similar capillary abnormality may complicate shock from sepsis or prolonged hypovolemic or cardiogenic shock.

Thus, loss of intravascular volume may result from several factors: increased ratio of post- to precapillary resistance, dilatation of precapillary sphincters, excessive capillary permeability, and loss of intravascular proteins. There may also be an increase in cellular permeability and a shift of fluids from extracellular to intracellular spaces.

Capillaries and Microaggregates. Erythrocytes, leukocytes, and platelets may aggregate to obstruct capillaries and venules in severe shock. Several factors may be involved: circulating catecholamines, thromboxane released from platelets, oxygen radicals released as a result of changes in cellular metabolism, vasoactive peptides and anaphylatoxins formed as a result of complement activation, endothelial damage and fibrin deposition with formation of microthrombi, and increased red blood cell rigidity as a result of hypoxia. This is exaggerated by the increase in capillary permeability, rise in microvascular hematocrit, and viscosity and sludging. Disseminated intravascular coagulation is a syndrome often seen in gram-negative septicemia and shock causing necrosis of several organs and consumption of coagulation factors with complicating hemorrhage.

The Large Veins These subserve a capacity function that can influence cardiac filling pressure and cardiac output.[16] In hypotension high levels of circulating catecholamines or vasopressin cause intense venoconstriction that maintains cardiac filling pressure and cardiac output. Conversely, the administration of a spinal anesthetic, sympathetic blockers, or a venodilator such as phentolamine or nitroprusside might precipitate a serious reduction in cardiac filling pressure if blood volume is reduced. For this reason, adequate replacement of blood volume is necessary before the administration of a venodilator.[2,16]

Mechanisms of Cardiovascular Adjustments in Shock

Hypotension and shock trigger acute circulatory adjustments to maintain perfusion of vital organs until the cause of shock is treated. The mechanisms by which these adjustments come into play to restore cardiac output, filling pressure, and arterial blood pressure may be discussed under three headings: neural and reflex mechanisms, humoral and metabolic factors, and autoregulatory adjustments of blood vessels.

Neural and Reflex Mechanisms

The autonomic control of the circulatory system is regulated by neurons in the medulla. Afferent neural impulses from various sensory receptors located in strategic areas around the body modulate the activity of these neurons.[1,17] Some of these receptors trigger impulses that suppress the sympathoadrenal drive and are called *inhibitory receptors,* e.g., arterial baroreceptors and left ventricular receptors. Other receptors generate impulses that stimulate the sympathoadrenal system and are called *excitatory receptors,* e.g., chemoreceptors.

Arterial Baroreceptors These are located in the adventitia and media of the arch of the aorta and in the adventitia of the carotid arteries in the carotid sinus regions. Increases in receptor activity are caused by their stretch or deformation during the rise in arterial pressure, and conversely, a fall in pressure results in decreased activity. When their activity decreases during hypotension and shock, the number of "inhibitory" nerve impulses reaching the vasomotor center declines, resulting in an excessive sympathetic discharge. Increased sympathetic discharge causes arteriolar constriction that is more predominant in the splanchnic and renal than in skeletal muscle beds and is negligible in the coronary and cerebral vascular beds. This preferential effect favors the distribution of blood flow to the vital organs.

There is also a reflex splanchnic constriction that mobilizes a large amount of blood from the splanchnic bed to the central veins, increases central venous pressure and cardiac filling pressure, and tends to restore cardiac output during hypotension.

Increased sympathetic drive to the heart causes tachycardia and increased contractility that may restore cardiac output. Increased sympathetic drive to the kidneys causes the release of renin and formation of angiotensin, which raises arterial blood pressure.

The integrity of this reflex may not be preserved in certain types of shock. We have recently found that after coronary occlusion the gain of the arterial baroreceptor reflex may be suppressed significantly. This means that a fall in arterial pressure is not effectively compensated by an appropriate increase in sympathetic activity.[17] It has also been shown that after endotoxin administration to dogs there is a shift in the baroreceptor discharge frequency of the carotid sinus nerve so that there is a greater frequency of discharge at the same level of distending pressure.[18] A higher level of carotid sinus nerve activity suppresses sympathetic drive and may contribute to hypotension in endotoxic shock.

Cardiac Receptors These are cardiac *sensory nerve endings,* mostly in the left ventricle, which initiate impulses that travel predominantly along unmyelinated fibers in the vagus, reach the vasomotor centers, and inhibit sympathetic discharge.[1] These sensory endings may be activated either mechanically, by distension of the left ventricle; or chemically, through the release in the myocardium of metabolites and chemicals such as bradykinin or prostaglandin. Their activity is reduced when cardiac filling pressure falls (e.g., hemorrhage or hypovolemia), and this triggers an increased sympathoadrenal drive.[19] The well-known cardiocirculatory inhibition with bradycardia, vasodilatation, and hypotension, described as the Bezold-Jarisch reflex, is ascribed to activation of these cardiac nerve endings with veratridine or other chemicals. The clinical counterpart of this chemical activation may be the bradycardia and hypotension seen following intracoronary injection of contrast medium. During myocardial infarction the release of metabolites or chemicals within the myocardium, such as prostaglandin and bradykinin, may activate these nerve endings. They may also be activated as a result of the dyskinesis and stretch of the ischemic region, and the reflex response is an inhibition of sympathoadrenal drive. Thus, in shock cardiac receptors may have decreased activity during hypovolemia or increased activity during myocardial infarction.

Activation of these cardiac afferents may cause the bradyarrhythmia and hypotension frequently seen immediately following acute myocardial infarction. The greater incidence of bradyarrhythmia and hypotension in posterior-inferior myocardial infarction in contrast to anterior myocardial infarction may be caused by a greater density of these nerve endings in the region of the posterior-inferior wall of the left ventricle.[17] It has been known that the hypotension associated with acute myocardial infarction in humans is rarely accompanied by acute renal failure, whereas the hypotension from hemorrhagic shock frequently causes acute renal failure. It is possible to ascribe the preservation of renal perfusion during myocardial infarction to activation of these cardiac nerve endings, which inhibit the sympathoadrenal drive, particularly to the renal circulation.[20] Because these receptors are sensitive to changes in cardiac size and blood volume, their regulatory effect on the renal sympathetic nerves is important in modulating urinary sodium and water excretion and thereby regulating blood volume.

These cardiac sensory endings, as well as the arterial baroreceptors, regulate the release of the antidiuretic hormone vasopressin from the posterior pituitary. Elevation of arterial pressure and cardiac distension from increased blood volume result in suppression of ADH release. Conversely, arterial hypotension and hypovolemia facilitate the release of ADH, which is a compensatory mechanism in the restoration of arterial pressure and blood volume through vasoconstriction and water retention.

Chemoreceptors Chemoreceptors provide a control system for oxygen conservation and for increasing oxygen delivery during hypoxic states.[1] The sensors are present in the carotid and aortic bodies and are particularly sensitive to reductions in arterial P_{O_2}, increases in P_{CO_2}, and decreases in pH. During shock, the hypoxia and acidosis activate the reflex that consists primarily of arteriolar constriction in the muscle and splanchnic circulation and arteriolar dilatation in the coronary vessels without a significant change in cerebral vascular resistance. This selective effect on the arterioles of various vascular beds favors a distribution of blood flow and oxygen delivery to the coronary and cerebral circulations. The reflex also includes venous constriction, primarily of the splanchnic veins, favoring a central shift of blood volume to increase cardiac filling pressure and cardiac output. If the hyperventilatory response to chemoreceptor stimulation is prevented, a pronounced reflex bradycardia may be seen. The bradycardia is beneficial in that it reduces myocardial oxygen demand, but if the ventilatory drive is suppressed and apnea and asphyxia coexist, the bradycardia may be excessive and lead to cardiac arrest.

Integrated Reflex Responses In a patient in shock, *several reflexes*[20] may be activated simultaneously because of hypovolemia, hypotension, and hypoxia. The net effect on the cardiovascular system is the result of a complex central integration of the various afferent signals. This may result in one set of afferent impulses overriding the effects of another. For example, during cardiogenic hypotension following myocardial infarction, the fall in arterial pressure unloads the arterial baroreceptors and triggers a reflex increase in sympathetic activity to the kidneys, but the cardiac sensory endings are activated simultaneously and cause a reflex inhibition of the sympathetic efferents to the kidneys. The net result of this interaction is generally a reduction in the sympathetic efferent impulses to the kidneys. In some situations, activation of two reflex mechanisms may be synergistic: for example, unloading of the arterial baroreceptors during hypotension increases sympathetic efferent activity; hypoxia also increases sympathetic activity through the stimulation of chemoreceptors, and the effect of combined hypotension and hypoxia is a pronounced sympathetic stimulus as hypotension *augments* the reflex response to chemoreceptor stimulation by hypoxia.

Humoral and Metabolic Factors

Various hormones or humoral factors such as renin, vasopressin, or the kinins may be released as a compensatory mechanism to bring about circulatory adjustments or as a result of direct and indirect cellular effects of toxins, ischemia, and antigens on various organs. There are vasodilator factors and vasoconstrictor factors.

Vasodilator Factors These include hypoxia, acidosis, and various humoral factors released from the tissues as a result of ischemia. Their vasodilator effects are potent, particularly in the coronary and cerebral circulations, where they override the vasoconstricting effect of the sympathoadrenal system and maintain perfusion of these vital organs.

Kinins. Kinins are vasodilator polypeptides resulting from proteolytes of inactive endogenous precursors. Bradykinin is the major active peptide and its major physiologic role is the local regulation of blood flow and function of such organs as the salivary gland, pancreas, kidney, and possibly the heart. Renal kinins may increase sodium and water excretion, and cardiac kinins may participate in the activation of cardiac receptors and may cause the perception of anginal pain by activation of sympathetic afferents. Kinins may play a part in the hyperemia associated with inflammation and the hypotension of anaphylactic reactions.

Prostacyclins. These are extremely potent vasodilator prostaglandins. Prostacyclin precursors, the endoperoxides, are formed in blood vessels from arachidonic acid and are pivotal in the synthesis of prostacyclin, mostly in the endothelial layers of blood vessels, where they cause vasodilatation and inhibit platelet aggregation. Some prostaglandin endoperoxides have opposite effects in platelets where they are converted to thromboxane A2, a potent vasoconstrictor which also causes platelet aggregation. In shock, the damaged endothelial cells may not synthesize prostacyclin, but the platelets may continue to release thromboxane A2 which enhances platelet aggregation, and vasoconstriction, causing additional endothelial damage.

Beta Endorphins. These are vasodilator peptides that appear to be released from the pituitary gland along with the adrenocorticotropic hormones during periods of stress. Recently it has been shown that the administration of naloxone, a beta-endorphin antagonist, is beneficial in the management of endotoxic shock in rats and dogs and hypovolemic shock in dogs. The effectiveness of naloxone raised the possibility that part of the hemodynamic failure in shock may be related to the release of endorphins.[21] Furthermore, endorphin receptors have been identified not only in the brain, but also in the heart, gastrointestinal tract, and various other organs. It is not known, however, whether the hypotensive effects of endorphins in shock are related to a central or a peripheral action of the compounds or some of their metabolites.

Vasoconstrictor Factors These include norepinephrine, epinephrine, dopamine, angiotensin, and vasopressin.[22]

Catecholamines. Catecholamines such as norepinephrine and epinephrine are released from the sympathetic terminals and from the adrenal medulla as a result of excessive sympathetic discharge during hypotension. Their effects on the circulation are mediated through adrenergic receptors. The adrenergic receptors may be classified as alpha or beta receptors with respect to their cardiovascular action. The alpha receptors are predominantly in blood vessels and mediate vasoconstriction. Postjunctional $alpha_1$ receptors (blocked by prazosin) and $alpha_2$ receptors (blocked by yohimbine) mediate the action of circulating catecholamines as well as neuronally released catechols. The beta receptors are present in blood vessels as well as in myocardium. Activation of the $beta_1$ receptors in myocardium causes an increase in myocardial contractility and heart rate, whereas activation of $beta_2$ receptors in blood vessels causes vasodilatation. The same catecholamine may activate both alpha and beta receptors, depending on the dose and the organ on which it is acting.

Norepinephrine. Norepinephrine increases myocardial contractility by activating $beta_1$ receptors and increases cardiac output in shock. In blood vessels it activates primarily alpha or vasoconstricting receptors. The magnitude of its effect on alpha receptors varies from one organ to another. It is a potent vasoconstrictor in skin, muscle, and splanchnic beds, whereas in the coronaries it activates $beta_2$ receptors as well as alpha receptors; but because there is a paucity of alpha receptors in the coronary vessels (in contrast to other vascular beds), the drug causes predominantly vasodilatation in the coronaries. The coronary dilatation is caused by direct stimulation of coronary vascular $beta_2$ receptors or indirectly through the release of metabolites during the increase in contractile activity of the heart. Norepinephrine offers several distinct advantages in the treatment of shock because it increases cardiac output and redistributes blood flow away from the extremities and toward the heart and brain and increases arterial pressure which, in turn, increases coronary flow to the ischemic myocardium.

Epinephrine. Released from the adrenal gland, epinephrine activates primarily myocardial $beta_1$ receptors and vasoconstrictor alpha receptors in most vessels except in skeletal muscle and coronary vessels, where it activates $beta_2$ receptors when administered in low doses. It increases cardiac output, but redistributes blood flow away from kidney and splanchnic circulation toward skeletal muscle. Its effect on redistribution of blood flow is not optimal, and its effect on arterial pressure is only modest because of its dilator influence in skeletal muscle. Two other effects of epinephrine should be mentioned. One is the potential role of epinephrine in releasing endogenous norepinephrine through stimulation of prejunctional $beta_2$ receptors. Prejunctional receptors are important in modulating the release of endogenous norepinephrine. Activation of prejunctional $alpha_2$ receptors inhibits release, whereas activation of prejunctional $beta_2$ receptors facilitates release. Epinephrine has a greater relative potency on prejunctional $beta_2$ receptors and may cause its effect through the release of endogenous norepinephrine. Another effect is related to its uptake by the noradrenergic terminal and its subsequent release as a transmitter.

Dopamine. This is another naturally occurring catecholamine.[23] It is the precursor of norepinephrine and has a different cardiovascular effect, depending on its dose level. When it is given in a low concentration, its dilator effect, mediated through $beta_2$ receptors and through specific dopaminergic receptors, is most apparent in the renal and mesenteric circulations. It also has a slight dilator effect in the cerebral and coronary circulations. When given in larger doses, it increases myocardial contractility and cardiac output through activation of $beta_1$ receptors, but in very large doses it causes vasoconstriction by activation of alpha receptors in both arterioles and veins. The drug may redistribute blood flow away from the extremities and toward the kidneys, gut, heart, and brain. However, it may be necessary to give large doses to maintain arterial pressure and coronary flow, particularly following myocardial infarction, and these large doses will then tend to oppose to some degree the advantageous vasodilator effect seen in some vascular beds.

Renin-Angiotensin. Circulating levels of renin-angiotensin are too low to cause significant circulatory effects in physiologic states, but angiotensin may traverse the blood-brain barrier in the area postrema where it affects medullary cardiovascular centers and causes the release of vasopressin. Hypotension and increased sympathetic activity to the kidneys cause the release of renin, the formation of angiotensin, and peripheral vasoconstriction, as well as sodium and water retention. Angiotensin constricts the coronary vessels as well as other vascular beds. This is in contrast to the catecholamines, which have a minimal constricting effect on the coronary vessels.

Vasopressin. This is a potent vasoconstrictor, water-retaining antidiuretic hormone, released from the posterior pituitary gland primarily in response to increased serum osmolality. Its release may be inhibited by neurogenic afferent impulses originating in cardiac receptors and arterial baroreceptors. Increased arterial pressure and stretch of the left ventricle and atrium inhibit the release of vasopressin. Conversely, during hemorrhage and systemic hypotension and in patients on cardiopulmonary bypass, vasopressin levels increase significantly because of a reduction in the cardiac and arterial baroreceptor afferent impulses. Vasopressin may be released also by a central nervous system action of angiotensin which simultaneously induces thirst. It is a vasoconstricting hormone with potent effects in the coronary circulation as well as several other vascular beds. This coronary vasoconstriction may explain in part the negative inotropic effect occasionally seen during its infusion.

Local Autoregulatory Adjustments of Blood Vessels

In addition to the regulation of blood flow to various organs through neurogenic and humoral factors, there is a mechanism by which the blood flow to various organs may be maintained constant despite significant fluctuations in arterial blood pressure. This mechanism is intrinsic to the vasculature and is independent of neural and humoral factors. It is referred to as the autoregulatory mechanism for blood flow. Autoregulation of blood flow is the capacity of a vascular bed to maintain a constant blood flow over a wide range of perfusion pressures. Organs such as the brain, the heart, and the kidney demand a sustained blood flow despite significant fluctuations in the arterial blood pressure which may occur over a range between 50 mmHg and 160 mmHg. A fall in arterial blood pressure from a mean of 100 mmHg to 50 mmHg would be associated with vasodilatation, and blood flow is maintained constant. Conversely, a rise in pressure from 100 mmHg to 160 mmHg would be associated with vasoconstriction, and blood flow also remains constant. Changes in pressure beyond this range would be associated with parallel changes in flow as these exceed the autoregulatory range. There are three factors which could explain the autoregulatory phenomenon and changes in vascular tone secondary to changes in perfusion pressure. These include (1) a myogenic response, which results in increased vascular tone as a rise in pressure causes stretching of the vascular muscle, and a decrease in vascular tone as a fall in pressure unloads the smooth muscle. (2) Another mechanism relates to the possible increase in tissue pressure during a rise in arterial pressure and capillary filtration which in turn creates a compressive force on the resistance vessels with an increase in resistance. (3) Finally, with a transient reduction in flow at the initiation of the fall in pressure, there may be accumulation of vasodilator metabolites which will tend to rapidly induce vasodilatation and restore flow at a lower arterial pressure. These metabolites could include the accumulation of adenosine, changes in pH, and increase in hydrogen ion concentration, increase in CO_2, increase in osmolality, accumulation of the Kreb's cycle intermediates, or a decrease in P_{O_2}. Conversely, a transient increase in flow associated with the initiation of a rise in pressure may cause a washout of these metabolites which would tend to increase vascular tone and increase resistance. It is possible that any or all of these three mechanisms may be active to various degrees in different vascular beds to bring about the phenomenon of local autoregulation.

Part B. Cellular and Biochemical Events in Shock

The terminal events in shock result from cellular damage. The factors which determine the delivery of oxygen to tissues, the generation of ATP, and membrane permeability or integrity are the most critical determinants of survival. In a recent monograph, *Molecular and Cellular Aspects of Shock and Trauma,* by Allan M. Lefer and William Schumer,[24] new concepts in cellular and metabolic aspects of shock and their therapeutic implications were reviewed. In the following paragraphs, several articles included in this monograph are referred to.

Metabolism of Various Organs in Shock

Cellular metabolism may be greatly altered in shock.[25] When oxygen and other substrates are not delivered to the tissues, there is an immediate reduction in the amount of ATP. Under aerobic conditions, 38 moles of ATP are produced from 1 mole of glucose, but under anaerobic states, the cell can produce a small fraction of that amount (only 2 moles of ATP/mole of glucose). This anaerobic glycolysis also leads to lactate production with severe consequences on the acidity of the blood and cells.

Skeletal Muscle

During severe circulatory deficiency, ATP production by the muscle proceeds first through utilization of glycogen stores and then muscle proteins. The catabolism of muscle mass leads to oxidation of leucine to carbon dioxide and conversion of aspartate, arginine, glutamine, isoleucine, and valine into Krebs cycle intermediates. The serum concentration of branched-chain amino acids and of lactic acid rises as they are released from the muscle in shock. Alanine and lactate are converted to glucose through gluconeogenesis in liver and returned to muscle for metabolism.

Gastrointestinal Function

Glucose and amino acid absorption are impaired because their active transport is dependent on ATP. Abnormalities in gastric mucosal membranes may lead to disturbances in proton or H^+ ion fluxes and in the maintenance of intracellular acid-base balance, which could lead to mucosal ulcerations. Studies on hemorrhagic shock in dogs indicate that the gastrointestinal tract contributes the largest release of lactate.

Renal Function

Sato et al.[26] reported minimal changes in glomeruli in human shock of various causes. The damage is predominantly in tubular epithelium where there is focal necrosis, accumulation of lysosomes, and distal tubular casts.

Active absorption of sodium and water depends on oxidative metabolism. In the early stages of shock (especially in septic shock), there may be polyuria and marked sodium loss. Subsequently, a reduction in glomerular filtration as a result of hypotension and constriction of preglomerular arterioles causes oliguria. Metabolic acidosis is worsened as a result of tubular damage because H^+ ion secretion and bicarbonate reabsorption, which are ATP-dependent, are impaired. Furthermore, ammonia formation via glutamine by renal tubular cells may also be impaired because glutamine deamination by glutaminase I is linked to the oxygen-requiring citric acid cycle.

Pulmonary Function

The process of gas exchange in the lung requires minimal energy; difficulty arises when there is alveolar membrane injury as well as injury to the capillary endothelium.

The alveoli are composed of two types of pneumocytes. Type I pneumocytes cover 97 percent of the alveolar surface, providing a thin barrier for oxygen diffusion. Type II pneumocytes produce surfactant, a lipoprotein complex responsible for preventing the collapse of the thin-walled alveoli. Surfactant coats the alveoli and decreases the surface tension of the air-tissue interface, thereby decreasing the tendency to collapse (dipolar effect of the fatty acid and its negative charges repelling each other).[27] Type II cells are very active metabolically and are dependent on ATP; thus, in shock the production of surfactant is reduced. Furthermore, damage to type I pneumocytes may cause leakage of interstitial fluid into the alveoli, washing out the surfactant, and thereby compounding the atelectasis which is part of the adult respiratory distress syndrome.

Pulmonary alveolar macrophages also reside in the alveoli and serve an important role in pulmonary defense and clearance mechanisms. A major part of the bactericidal activity of the macrophage results from its production of H_2O_2. The oxygen radicals may also expose the macrophage itself to destruction were it not for the sulfhydryl system (reduced glutathione) in erythrocytes which protects the macrophage from oxidant injury by reducing hydrogen peroxide. Reduced glutathione is replenished by the regeneration of nicotinamide adenine dinucleotide phosphate (NADPH) through the hexose-monophosphate pathway. In shock, the alveolar macrophage releases oxygen radicals because of a lack of NADPH and reduced glutathione. The released oxygen radicals may damage type I and type II pneumocytes, thus compounding the decrease in surfactant, fluid movement into the alveoli, and hypoxia.

In addition to the possible damage to alveolar membranes, there may also be significant *capillary damage* in the shock lung. The lungs of patients dying in shock may show marked capillary dilatation with microaggregates of platelets, polymorphonucleocytes, and red blood cells, alveolar hemorrhages, atelectasis, and possibly hyaline membrane. As a result of the pulmonary capillary damage, lymph flow is increased in the early stages of shock. This may explain the distended pulmonary lymphatic system filled with proteinaceous material seen in patients dying of hemorrhagic shock.[15]

Oxygen-Hemoglobin Affinity

The affinity of hemoglobin for oxygen may determine to a significant degree the availability of oxygen to the tissues. An increase in hydrogen ion concentration through the Bohr effect will reduce the affinity and facilitate the delivery of oxygen to the tissues. Conversely, the overcorrection of acidosis with bicarbonate may increase the affinity of hemoglobin for oxygen and reduce oxygen delivery to the tissues. An increase in CO_2, as well as an increase in 2,3-diphosphoglyceric acid (2,3-DPG), also reduced the affinity of hemoglobin for oxygen. The 2,3-DPG concentration in red blood cells is a by-product of glycolysis and may increase in chronic and acute hypoxic states, in anemia, and in acidosis.[28] The oxygen dissociation curve for hemoglobin which determines the hemoglobin-oxygen saturation at various levels of P_{O_2} will shift depending on the affinity of hemoglobin for oxygen. A shift of the hemoglobin-oxygen dissociation curve to the right occurs when the affinity of the hemoglobin for oxygen is reduced and results in a favorable increase in the delivery of oxygen to the tissues.[29] Conversely, a shift to the left increases the affinity of hemoglobin for oxygen. It is difficult for this reason to predict from the arterial P_{O_2} what the hemoglobin-oxygen saturation will be particularly in shock when the various factors which tend to alter affinity are predominant and are changing. If arterial oxygen saturation is less than what might be predicted from the P_{O_2}, one will have to assume that there is a shift of the dissociation curve to the right and vice versa.

Hepatic Function

The work of Williamson et al.[30] on gluconeogenesis in endotoxin-treated rats indicates that glucose-6-phosphate is consistently reduced in both the early and late phases of endotoxemia, suggesting that the other changes in the glycolytic intermediates in the liver may be secondary homeostatic readjustments of metabolic pool constituents. Glucose-6-phosphate is a central substrate leading to glycogen formation, to pentose shunt, toward glycolysis via fructose-6-phosphate, and back to glucose itself. If endotoxin directly or indirectly imposes a biochemical lesion on glucose-6-phosphate regulating enzymes, carbohydrate metabolism could be deranged at many sites.

Detoxification is another important function of the liver, which may be suppressed in shock. The allosteric enzymes involved in detoxification (glucuronidase, sulfatase, and hydroxylase) are NAD-dependent. Detoxification and excretion of various potent hormones such as serotonin, histamine, and various steroids are impaired. Furthermore, the detoxifying function in the reticuloendothelial system of the liver plays a significant role in the neutralization of bacterial exotoxins and endotoxins.

Damage to the liver will also reduce the deamination and transamination of amino acids, which need ATP to produce glucose or the various substrates that enter into the citric acid cycle. Decreased urea nitrogen in the blood of patients in shock reflects hepatic damage.

Cardiac Function

The heart generates high concentrations of ATP and metabolizes fatty acids, glucose, and lactic acid. During myocardial ischemia and anaerobic metabolism, the heart produces rather than consumes lactic acid. Spitzer et al.[32] demonstrated that in septic dogs there is a marked decrease in uptake and oxidation of free fatty acid which impairs myocardial energy metabolism. Glycogen stores are rapidly depleted, followed by depletion of creatine phosphate and later ATP stores.

The presence of myocardial depressant factors in the circulation contribute to myocardial depression in severe shock. These active peptides are presumably released by the pancreas during shock.

Rapid impairment of myocardial contractility is noted within seconds following occlusion of the coronary artery. It is unlikely that this acute phenomenon reflects depletion of high-energy phosphates and may be explained on the basis of failure of mobilization of intracellular Ca^{2+} pools. With reperfusion after transient occlusion and before any significant muscle damage occurs, the restoration of contractility is very gradual and occurs over the course of several hours. One may view the abrupt suppression of myocardial contractility in the ischemic segment of the heart as a "protective" effect which reduces myocardial oxygen in the face of sudden reduction in supply.

Brain Function

ATP requirements of brain cells are similar to those of other organs. The main substrate is glucose, metabolized through the glycolytic and Krebs cycles, and the hexose-monophosphate shunt. Lactate production increases markedly during anoxia, and is associated with a decline in phosphocreatine and ATP. Apparently glutamic acid is the only amino acid metabolized in brain tissue. It is formed by the transamination of ketoglutarate formed in the Krebs cycle from glucose. In the brain, ammonia combines with glutamic acid to form glutamine, which is released in plasma for liver metabolism. This may be the brain's defense against the anoxia, reduced perfusion, and the elevated ammonia from a hypoperfused liver. During shock, the brain is the last organ to be underperfused and it appears to retain the necessary enzymatic activity to support its major metabolic function.

Cellular Structure and Function in Shock[33,34]

Two major cellular functions may be seriously altered in shock. These include the synthesis of high-energy phosphates (adenosine triphosphate—ATP from adenosine diphosphate—ADP) in mitochondria which requires the largest amount of oxygen used by the cell (state III respiration). The availability of ATP is essential for cellular functions.

Another important cellular function is the availability of calcium for various intracellular processes and in particular muscular contraction. Calcium availability for intracellular function may also be significantly altered in shock.

Cellular Death

Two processes have been described. One is the result of depletion of ATP because of ischemia, lack of oxygen, and substrate in failure of the electron transport system. This results in suppression of membrane transport functions including calcium transport mechanisms.

Another type of cellular death is not caused by failure of synthesis of high-energy phosphate and ATP, but rather by an antigen-antibody type of reaction, activation of complement, or release of bacterial products such as antitoxin, phospholipases, or oxygen radicals. In this type of cellular death, calcium may be transported into the cell and precipitated in the mitochondria. Thus, one can differentiate the two types of cellular deaths from the appearance of the mitochondria. In the first situation, because of inhibition of the energy-dependent calcium transport mechanism in depletion of intracellular ATP, there is no calcium in the mitochondria, whereas in the other type of cell death the preservation of these transport mechanisms apparently allows the precipitation of calcium in the mitochondria.

The only structural changes include cellular swelling, clumping of nuclear chromatin, and dilatation of endoplasmic reticulum.[35] Subsequently, mitochondria begin to swell and appear flocculent. Calcium may or may not accumulate in mitochondria depending on the cause of cellular death, and in the late stages lysosomes begin to disappear from the cell, presumably associated with a release of lysosomal enzymes, which herald terminal and irreversible cellular death.

Cellular Membrane Damage

One of the earliest functional changes in the cell is an increased cellular permeability to sodium and water. This may then be associated with an increased sodium-potassium ATPase activity in an attempt to drive sodium out of the cell. Eventually, there is depletion of ATP and cyclic adenosine monophosphate (cyclic AMP) which results in alteration of the cellular response to various hormones which are dependent on the activation of cyclase and cyclic AMP for their action. For example, the reduced effect of insulin on glucose uptake by skeletal muscle in animals subjected to hemorrhagic shock may be the result of such membrane alteration. Similarly, the reduced cardiovascular responses to catecholamines in shock may be related to reductions in cyclic AMP and ATP. Significant reductions in ATP in various organs most certainly account for the rapid deterioration of various functions in shock, although the minimum level of ATP necessary for cellular function is not known. It is believed, however, that as long as ATP and oxygen can be made available and substrate is provided, ATP generation may be resumed within minutes as long as mitochondrial structure has not been damaged. In fact, it has been shown that, after a period of hypoxia, the rate of ATP generation is increased as soon as oxygen is made available.[33–38]

Mitochondrial Damage[36,37]

The rate of ATP synthesis may be significantly reduced by hypoxia but this does not result in significant mitochondrial damage unless the hypoxia is very severe and sustained. As soon as ADP and oxygen become available, ATP synthesis is restored. In contrast to hypoxia, ischemia as well as endotoxins may result in significant mitochondrial damage in addition to the reduced synthesis of ATP and reduced mitochondrial ATPase activity.[37] The cause of the mitochondrial damage is not known and may be related to the release of intracellular lysosomal enzymes, changes in intracellular pH, or changes in the cellular ionic milieu, as well as the accumulation of metabolites or intracellular oxygen radicals.

Lysosomal Enzymes

Lysosomal enzymes are contained in cytoplasmic granules called lysosomes which have relatively impermeable membranes.[39] Once the lysosomal membranes are damaged and lysosomal enzymes are released intracellularly, their potent hydrolytic activity digests all intra- and extracellular macromolecules and contributes very significantly to the pathogenesis of cellular injury and death. Several observations support their destructive role in shock. In several organs, the lysosomes have been described as enlarged and their granules reduced in density in the early stages of shock. This structural change has been associated with a decline in the lysosomal hydrolase activity in the tissues with an increase in the activity recovered from the soluble fraction of tissue homogenates.

Furthermore, several studies have established a good correlation between the hydrolase activity of blood, lymph, and serum and the severity of shock as well as the integrity of lysosomal membrane, particularly in endotoxic shock in animals. Furthermore, the lysosomes obtained from such animals in shock have an enhanced release of enzymes in vitro.

Goldfarb and Glenn[40] review data which suggest a change in the integrity of myocardial lysosomes during myocardial ischemia. They propose that stability of the lysosomes can be correlated with myocardial cyclic AMP/cyclic GMP ratio. Furthermore, cyclic AMP concentration in the myocardium was negatively correlated with prostaglandin A (PGA) and E (PGE) concentrations. In that study, treatment with indomethacin reduced myocardial PGA and PGE concentration approximately 60 percent following coronary artery ligation. One may propose that myocardial infarction induces synthesis and release of prostaglandins which in turn induce alterations in intramyocardial cyclic nucleotide ratio such that release of lysosomal enzymes is promoted.

Myocardial Depressant Factor

The presence of a myocardial depressant factor in shock is still controversial,[7] although there is evidence of a depressed myocardial contractility in a variety of types of shock without any obvious cause. It has been suggested that pancreatic ischemia causes the release of lysosomal and other intracellular enzymes which act on an endogenous substrate yielding a low-molecular-weight substance with myocardial depressant activity. The supporting evidence, though indirect, has been the demonstration that infusion of lysosomal hydrolases in animals reproduces the shock syndrome with myocardial depression and a fall in cardiac output. Experimentally induced pancreatitis as well as a variety of other types of shock are associated with a rise in plasma lysosomal hydrolases as well as a myocardial depressant activity. The responsiveness of animals in shock to large amounts of corticosteroids[41,42] and the associated reduction in circulating levels of lysosomal hydrolases coupled with the in vitro demonstration that corticosteroids may stabilize lysosomal membranes, preventing their lysis, provide indirect evidence of the presence of a myocardial depressant activity linked with lysosomal enzymes.

It has been proposed[43] that endotoxins release a lysosomal releasing factor (LRF) through the activation of complement pathways which triggers the release of lysosomal enzymes from human polymorphonuclear leukocytes. This LRF possesses several of the characteristics of C5a which has important chemotactic as well as anaphylatoxin activities.

Complement Activation in Shock[44–47]

Complements are the major humoral mediators of the antigen-antibody reaction. The complement system is plasma proteins which may be activated by limited proteolytic cleavage into very potent compounds. Antigen-antibody reactions which involve the IgG and IgM immunoglobulins, for example, and which could trigger an acute anaphylactic reaction depend on the activated complement to trigger the response. There are certain antigen-antibody reactions, however, that do not require complement, such as those involving an IgE antibody seen in the anaphylactic reaction to penicillin or to pollen antigen.

Complement may be activated in shock states by either of two mechanisms. One is the interaction of antigen-antibody complexes with proteins of the classic activation pathways; the second is the interaction of certain naturally occurring polysaccharides such as bacterial or fungal endotoxins with the proteins of the alternative activation pathway without the participation of any immunoglobulins. Activation by either mechanism leads to cleavage from the complement proteins of several low-molecular-weight, biologically active peptides with properties of enhancing local inflammation, stimulating phagocytosis, neutralizing viruses, killing microorganisms or normal cells, and modulating the immune response. These reactions can be beneficial, particularly if they tend to restrict and limit an inflammatory response but they may also be detrimental to the host if they lead to the release of vasoactive peptides which increase capillary permeability, cause intravascular cellular aggregation, induce a Schwartzman reaction, and release lysosomal enzymes from various cells, causing cellular destruction. Such a reaction may contribute significantly to the pathogenesis of shock in a variety of shock states, but most particularly in endotoxin and anaphylactic shock.

References

1. Abboud, F. M., Heistad, D. D., Mark, A. L., and Schmid, P. G.: Reflex Control of the Peripheral Circulation, *Prog. Cardiovasc. Dis.*, 18:371, 1976.
2. Abboud, F. M.: The Sympathetic Nervous System and Alpha Adrenergic Blocking Agents in Shock, *Med. Clin. North Am.*, 52:1049, 1968.
3. Williamson, J. R., Schaffer, S. W., Ford, C., and Safer, B.: Contribution of Tissue Acidosis to Ischemic Injury in the Perfused Rat Heart, *Circulation*, 53(suppl. 1):3, 1976.
4. Mueller, H., Ayres, S. M., Gregory, J. J., Giannelli, S., Jr., and Grace, W. J.: Hemodynamics, Coronary Blood Flow, and Myocardial Metabolism in Coronary Shock; Response to *l*-Norepinephrine and Isoproterenol, *J. Clin. Invest.*, 49:1885, 1970.
5. Mueller, H., Ayers, S. M., Giannelli, S., Jr., Conklin, E. F., Mozzara, J. T., and Grace, W. J.: Effect of Isoproterenol, *l*-Norepinephrine and Intraaortic Counterpulsation on Hemodynamics and Myocardial Metabolism in Shock Following Acute Myocardial Infarction, *Circulation*, 45:335, 1972.
6. Maroko, P. R., and Braunwald, E.: Effects of Metabolic and Pharmacologic Interventions of Myocardial Infarct Size Following Coronary Occlusion, *Circulation*, 53(suppl. 1):162, 1976.
7. Lefer, A. M., and Martin, J.: Origin of Myocardial Depressant Factor in Shock, *Am. J. Physiol.*, 218:1423, 1970.
8. Abboud, F. M.: Control of the Various Components of the Peripheral Vasculature, *Fed. Proc.*, 31:1226, 1972.
9. Cohn, J. N.: Blood Pressure Measurement in Shock, *JAMA.*, 199:972, 1967.
10. Abboud, F. M., and Eckstein, J. W.: Comparative Changes in Segmental Vascular Resistance in Response to Nerve Stimulation and to Norepinephrine, *Circ. Res.*, 18:263, 1966.
11. Brigham, K. L., Woolverton, W. C., Blake, L. H., and Staub, N. C.: Increased Sheep-Lung Vascular Permeability Caused by *Pseudomonas* Bacteremia, *J. Clin. Invest.*, 54:792, 1974.
12. Mason, J. C., Curry, F. E., and Michel, C. C.: The Effects of Proteins upon the Filtration Coefficient of Individually Perfused Frog Mesenteric Capillaries, *Microvasc. Res.*, 13:185, 1977.
13. Dawidson, I., Hadling, E., and Gelin, L. E.: Hemodilution and Oxygen Transport to Tissue in Shock, *Acta. Chir. Scand.*, 489(suppl.):245, 1979.

14. Wendling, M. G., Eckstein, J. W., and Abboud, F. M.: Effects of Mannitol on the Renal Circulation, *J. Lab. Clin. Med.*, 74:541, 1969.
15. Ayres, S. M.: The Shock Lung, in "The Organ in Shock," The Upjohn Company, Kalamazoo, Mich., April 1977, pp. 24–31.
16. Abboud, F. M., Schmid, P. G., and Eckstein, J. W.: Vascular Responses after Alpha Adrenergic Receptor Blockade. I. Responses to Capacitance and Resistance Vessels to Norepinephrine in Man, *J. Clin. Invest.*, 47:1, 1968.
17. Abboud, F. M.: Integration of Reflex Responses in the Control of Blood Pressure and Vascular Resistance, *Am. J. Cardiol.*, 44:903, 1979.
18. Trank, J. W., and Visscher, M. B.: Carotid Sinus Baroreceptor Modifications Associated with Endotoxin Shock, *Am. J. Physiol.*, 202:971, 1962.
19. Abboud, F. M., and Mark, A. L.: Cardiac Baroreceptors in Circulatory Control in Humans, in R. Hainsworth and R. Linden (eds.), "Cardiac Receptors," Cambridge University Press, Oxford, 1979, pp. 437–462.
20. Thames, M. D., and Abboud, F. M.: Reflex Inhibition of Renal Sympathetic Nerve Activity during Myocardial Ischemia Mediated by Left Ventricular Receptors with Vagal Afferents in Dogs, *J. Clin. Invest.*, 63:395, 1979.
21. Holaday, J. W., and Faden, A. I.: Naloxone Reversal of Endotoxin Hypotension Suggests Role of Endorphins in Shock, *Nature*, 275:450, 1978.
22. Abboud, F. M.: Vascular Responses to Norepinephrine, Angiotensin, Vasopressin and Serotonin, *Fed. Proc.*, 27:1391, 1968.
23. Goldberg, L. I.: Dopamine—Clinical Uses of Endogenous Catecholamine, *N. Engl. J. Med.*, 291:707, 1974.
24. Lefer, A. M., and Schumer, W. (eds.): "Molecular and Cellular Aspects of Shock and Trauma," Alan R. Liss, Inc., New York, 1983.
25. Schumer, W.: Overall Cell Metabolism, in A. M. Lefer and W. Schumer (eds), "Molecular and Cellular Aspects of Shock and Trauma," Alan R. Liss, Inc., New York, 1983, pp. 1–19.
26. Sato, T., Kamiyama, Y., Jones, R. T., Cowley, R. A., and Trump, B. F.: Ultrastructural Study on Kidney Cell Injury Following Various Types of Shock in 26 Immediate Autopsy Patients, in A. M. Lefer, T. M. Saba, and L. M. Mela (eds.), "Advances in Shock Research," vol. 1, Alan R. Liss, Inc., New York, 1979, pp. 55–69.
27. Clowes, G. H. A., Jr.: Pulmonary Abnormalities in Sepsis, *Surg. Clin. North Am.*, 54:993, 1974.
28. Lecompte, F., Aberkane, H., Axoulary, C., Muffat-Joly, M., and Pocidalo, J. J.: Blood Affinity for Oxygen in Experimental Hemorrhagic Shock with Metabolic Acidosis, *Pfluegers Arch.*, 359(1–2):147, 1975.
29. Thomas, H. M., 3d, Lefrak, S. S., Irwin, R. S., Fritts, H. W., Jr., and Coldwell, P. R. B.: The Oxyhemoglobin Dissociation Curve in Health and Disease. Role of 2,3-Diphosphoglycerate, *Am. J. Med.*, 37:331, 1974.
30. Williamson, J. R., Refino, C., and LaNoue, K.: Effects of *E. coli* Lipopolysaccharide B Treatment of Rats on Gluconeogenesis, in R. Porter and J. Knight (eds.), "Energy Metabolism in Trauma," A Ciba Symposium, J. and A. Churchill, London, 1970, pp. 145–154.
31. Nagler, A. L., Seifter, E., and Levenson, S. M.: Prevention of Shock by Glucose-Phosphate Therapy, *Circ. Shock*, (abstr. 51), 5:212, 1978.
32. Spitzer, J. A., Leach, G. J., and Palmer, M. A.: Some Metabolic and Hormonal Alterations in Adipocytes Isolated from Septic Dogs, in W. Schumer, J. J. Spitzer, and B. E. Marshall (eds.), "Advances in Shock Research," vol. 4, Alan R. Liss, Inc., New York, 1980, pp. 63–71.
33. Baue, A. E., Chaudry, I. H., Wurth, M. A., and Sayeed, M. M.: Cellular Alterations with Shock and Ischemia, *Angiology*, 25:31, 1974.
34. Trump, B. F.: The Role of Cellular Membrane Systems in shock, in "The Cell in Shock," The Upjohn Company, Kalamazoo, Mich., April 1976, pp. 16–29.
35. Laiho, K. Y., and Trump, B.: Relationship of Ionic, Water, and Cell Volume Changes in Cellular Injury of Ehrlich Ascites Tumor Cells, *Lab. Invest.*, 31:207, 1974.
36. Trump, B. F., Mergner, W. J., Kahng, M. W., and Saladino, A. J.: Studies on the Subcellular Pathophysiology of Ischemia, *Circulation*, 53(suppl. 1):17, 1976.
37. Mela, L., Bacalzo, L. V., Jr., and Miller, L. D.: Defective Oxidative Metabolism of Rat Liver Mitochondria in Hemorrhagic and Endotoxin Shock, *Am. J. Physiol.*, 220:571, 1971.
38. Ozawa, K.: Biological Significance of Mitochondrial Redox Potential in Shock and Multiple Organ Failure. Redox Therapy, in A. L. Lefer, and W. Schumer (eds.), "Molecular and Cellular Aspects of Shock and Trauma," Alan R. Liss, Inc., New York, 1983, pp. 39–66.
39. deDuve, C., and Wattiaux, R.: Functions of Lysosomes, *Ann. Rev. Physiol.*, 28:435, 1966.
40. Goldfarb, R. D., and Glenn, T. M.: Regulation of Lysosomal Membrane Stabilization via Cyclic Nucleotides and Prostaglandins—The Effects of Steroids and Indomethacin, in A. L. Lefer, and W. Schumer (eds.), "Molecular and Cellular Aspects of Shock and Trauma," Alan R. Liss, Inc., New York, 1983, pp. 147–166.
41. Nichijima, H., Weil, M. H., Shubin, H., and Cavanilles, J.: Hemodynamic and Metabolic Studies on Shock Associated with Gram Negative Bacteremia, *Medicine*, 52:287, 1973.
42. Altura, B. M., and Bella, T.: Peripheral Vascular Actions of Glucocorticoids and their Relationship to Protection in Circulatory Shock, *J. Pharmacol. Exp. Ther.*, 190:300, 1974.
43. Goldstein, I., Hoffstein, S., Gallin, J., and Weissman, G.: Mechanisms of Lysosomal Enzyme Release from Human Leukocytes: Microtubule Assembly and Membrane Fusion Induced by a Component of Complement (C5a/Chemotaxis Cytochalasin B/cAMP; cGMP Antagonism), *Proc. Nat. Acad. Sci. U.S.A.*, 70:2916, 1973.
44. Muller-Eberhard, H. J.: "Complement. Annual Review of Biochemistry," Annual Reviews, Inc., Palo Alto, Calif., 1975, pp. 607–724.
45. Muller-Eberhard, H. J.: The Significance of Complement Activity in Shock, in "The Cell in Shock," The Upjohn Company, Kalamazoo, Mich., April 1976, pp. 16–29.
46. Brown, E. J., and Frank, M. M.: Complement Activation. *Immunol. Today*, 2:129, 1981.
47. Jacob, H. S.: The Role of Activated Complement and Granulocytes in Shock States and Myocardial Infarction, *J. Lab. Clin. Med.*, 98:645, 1981.

23

The Recognition and Management of Shock

David W. Ferguson, M.D.   Francois M. Abboud, M.D.

Shock is a clinical syndrome which complicates a serious and sometimes catastrophic medical or surgical problem. It is an acute medical emergency requiring vigilance, early recognition, and vigorous management to avoid the irreversible complications of cellular damage and resultant death of the patient. For the appropriate management of shock, it is essential to have a thorough understanding of its pathophysiology, of the basic mechanisms which determine circulatory control, and of the pharmacology of vasoactive drugs.

The basic principles underlining the pathophysiology of hypotension and shock have been reviewed in the previous chapter. This chapter covers the recognition and management of the shock state.

Clinical Picture

The clinical syndrome may present in one of three stages. In stage I (*compensated hypotension*), there may be a fall in cardiac output or abnormal peripheral vasodilatation, but effective compensatory mechanisms restore arterial pressure and blood flow to vital organs, such as the brain, the kidney, and the heart. The symptoms and signs are consequently minimal and hence may require a strong degree of clinical suspicion to recognize, especially in the early stages. The only manifestation may be that of a patient who is anxious, may have a normal blood pressure, and have mild to moderate tachycardia. Some patients with early septic shock may present in stage I with warm hyperperfused extremities, a so-called warm shock due to abnormal peripheral vasodilatation. Recognition of this early stage of shock requires a high degree of clinical suspicion, but is rewarding, as appropriate intervention at this stage is most effective in reversing the shock state if the underlying disease process can be arrested or reversed.

In stage II (*decompensated hypotension*), the compensatory mechanisms that tend to maintain arterial pressure and perfusion of vital organs have failed and signs of decreased cerebral perfusion, renal perfusion, and even myocardial perfusion become apparent. The majority of patients with the "classic" picture of shock are recognized in this phase and should be treated aggressively.

Usually the clinical presentation is that of a patient who is hypotensive with a systolic blood pressure of 90 mmHg or less, hyperventilating, with cold and cyanotic skin. The mental status ranges from agitation to a dulled sensorium or stupor and coma. The pulse is rapid and thready and the patient is frequently oliguric with a urinary output of less than 20 ml/h. The patient may be hypoxic and acidotic. One must remember, however, that the level of blood pressure measurement alone does not define shock, as hypotension can be "relative" as well as "absolute."

Stage III (*irreversible shock*) occurs when excessive and prolonged reduction of tissue perfusion leads to significant alteration in cellular membrane function, sludging in the capillaries, intense vasoconstriction, severe acidosis, renal failure, and irreversible organ damage. Most of these patients require large doses of catecholamines when attempts to restore arterial pressure and urinary flow or attempts to correct the acidosis with volume expansion and lower doses of inotropes and vasopressors have failed. This late form of shock carries the worst prognosis as it reflects irreversible damage at the cellular level.

The clinical manifestations of the disease that caused or precipitated the shock state are an essential part of the syndrome and play important roles in its recognition and differential diagnosis.

Causes of Shock

There are four major etiologic categories.

Decreased Intravascular Volume

This is the most common cause of shock seen in clinical practice. The decreased intravascular volume may be absolute or relative. An *absolute* loss of intravascular volume occurs during acute hemorrhage such as with gastrointestinal bleeding, retroperitoneal bleeding, ruptured aortic aneurysm, severe hemoptysis, hemothorax, or trauma.

Intravascular volume may also be reduced by excessive fluid loss, such as is seen with vomiting from intestinal or pyloric obstruction, severe diarrhea, excessive sweating, and dehydration. Polyuria may contribute to hypovolemia as is sometimes seen in diabetes mellitus and diabetes insipidus, with excessive use of diuretics and during the diuretic phase of acute renal failure. Peritonitis, pancreatitis, splanchnic ischemia with intestinal obstruction, and gangrene cause extravasation of the intravascular volume to the interstitial space with so-called third spacing of large volumes of fluid, resulting in marked intravascular volume depletion. Similarly, trauma, extensive muscle injury, and burns reduce circulating intravascular volume.

A *relative* reduction in intravascular volume occurs from vasodilatation when the vascular capacity exceeds the intravascular volume. Neurogenic vasodilatation may be drug-induced as with anesthesia, ganglionic blockers, adrenergic blockers, overdose of barbiturates, or may result from spinal cord injury, cerebral vascular accidents, and severe dysautonomia.

Metabolic, toxic, or humoral vasodilatation may occur in septicemia, particularly with gram-negative endotoxemia, but also with gram-positive bacteremia, in acute adrenal insufficiency, and in anaphylactic reactions.

Decreased Cardiac Output

The most common cause in this category is acute myocardial infarction. Myocarditis and myocardial depression resulting from hypoxia, acidosis, septic shock, release of myocardial depressant factors, or severe hypoglycemia also cause or sustain a decreased cardiac output.

Acute valvular insufficiency may occur with bacterial endocarditis, or as a complication of underlying cardiovascular malformations (i.e., Marfan's syndrome, with acute aortic dissection). Myocardial rupture, left ventricular free wall and septal perforation, or acute papillary muscle dysfunction or rupture may complicate acute myocardial infarction and lead to acute regurgitant lesions.

Arrhythmias, either a severe bradycardia or a tachycardia, particularly if associated with depression of myocardial contractility, may cause hypotension and shock.

Myocardial compression or obstruction as seen with pericardial effusion or tamponade and with positive pressure ventilation, tension pneumothorax, pulmonary embolism, ball-valve thrombus, or atrial myxoma may all cause a significant reduction in cardiac output and consequently the development of a shock state.

Microcirculatory Failure

Diffuse endothelial injury with aggregation of corpuscles may be the primary event in certain types of shock such as anaphylaxis, which is often seen with septic shock and as a complication of burns or trauma.

Cellular Membrane Injury

This may result without a primary defect in the macro- or microcirculation, but rather through activation of the complement system, either through an antigen-antibody complex or by bacterial or fungal mucopolysaccharides. This results in cellular membrane defects, or the release of vasoactive peptides, and eventually the release of lysosomal enzymes, all of which would contribute to vascular endothelial injury in addition to injury of various tissue cells. This is seen in septic shock, anaphylactic shock, and with prolonged ischemia, hypoxia, and tissue injury.

The Approach to Management

The important steps in the management of shock include early recognition of the shock state, rapid correction of the initiating cause (for example, by defibrillation, hemostasis, or pericardiocentesis) correction of complicating factors such as hypoxia and acidosis, and maintenance of vital organ functions such as arterial pressure, cardiac output, urinary flow, and ventilation.

The prognosis of the patient depends to a large extent on the initiating cause of the shock and its duration. This in turn is related to the rapidity of recognition of the shock state and the appropriateness and aggressiveness of intervention. For example, hemorrhagic hypotension discovered early in a young individual before oliguria and acidosis carries a good prognosis, whereas an anterior wall myocardial infarction associated with extensive coronary artery disease and low output syndrome with cardiogenic shock generally carry a poor prognosis, despite aggressive management.

Perhaps the most important element in the management of patients in shock is the rapid recognition of those reversible factors that could perpetuate the decreased cardiac output and decreased perfusion. This can be facilitated most effectively by the appropriate use of hemodynamic monitoring.

Monitoring of Patients in Shock

Accurate, frequent, and continuous monitoring of several hemodynamic and respiratory functions is necessary. This includes measurements of heart rate and rhythm, respiratory rate, systemic arterial blood pressure, cardiac filling pressure, cardiac output, blood gases, and indexes of tissue perfusion such as urinary output, mental status, and liver function.

Recently, Wiedemann et al.[1] published a two-part review of the use of cardiopulmonary monitoring in the intensive care unit. This is a thorough review which describes in detail the procedures of hemodynamic monitoring, including a consideration of the potential risks and benefits.

The Electrocardiogram

This allows early recognition of serious arrhythmias and permits prompt management. In specific circumstances, serial 12-lead electrocardiograms will allow assessment of the progress of ischemic changes or the evolution of ventricular aneurysms or pericarditis.

Arterial Pressure Monitoring

Indwelling arterial catheters provide continuous assessment of systemic arterial pressure and provide rapid and repeated access for blood sampling. Arterial lines may be placed percutaneously or under limited surgical cutdown in the radial, brachial, or femoral arteries, depending on the clinical need and considerations of access and safety.

Urinary Catheter
A sterile indwelling venous catheter is necessary for routine hourly measurement of urinary output. A drop in urinary output below 20 ml/h is an indication of inadequate renal perfusion in patients in shock.

Central Venous Pressure
Measurement of central venous pressure has a limited role in monitoring patients in shock as it provides an indication of the adequacy of absolute blood volume or of the relative blood volume with respect to the capacity of the vascular system. It reflects the adequacy of fluid administration and replacement of blood volume, and represents the filling pressure of the right ventricle. Central venous pressure is measured from the superior vena cava and is normally between 5 and 8 mmHg. One should increase it to approximately 10 mmHg in patients in shock in an attempt to obtain an adequate cardiac output. These values assume that there is a negative intrapleural pressure and the patient is not receiving positive end-expiratory pressure therapy (PEEP).

However, in the majority of patients in shock, monitoring of central venous pressure alone is not sufficient, because many such patients have left ventricular pulmonary vascular disease or pulmonary hypertension. Under these conditions, there is frequently a discrepancy between the central venous pressure and the pulmonary artery wedge pressure (PAWP). The pulmonary artery wedge pressure best represents left atrial pressure and the filling of the left ventricle. The latter is of critical importance in managing hypotension and shock from the majority of initiating causes. If, however, it is difficult to obtain a pulmonary artery wedge pressure with a Swan-Ganz catheter, it is recommended that the central venous pressure be obtained and the factors which determine the discrepancy between right and left ventricular cardiac filling pressures be kept in mind. Young adults suffering from hemorrhagic, traumatic, or hypovolemic shock may, in the initial stages of management, have their central venous pressure monitored and may not require monitoring of PAWP.

Pulmonary Artery Catheterization and Monitoring of PAWP
Catheterization of the pulmonary artery at the bedside was introduced by Swan et al. in 1970[2] and is an essential part of the monitoring of patients in intensive care units. The special feature of this catheter is that it has an inflatable balloon at its tip which allows it to be directed by blood flow through the great veins and the right-sided cardiac chambers into proper position in a branch of the pulmonary artery. It can be used at the bedside, usually without the aid of a fluoroscope, in most patients.

The reader is referred to Chap. 124 written by Dr. H. J. C. Swan for a discussion of the technique of using the Swan-Ganz catheter, indications for its use, and complications of its use.

Monitoring of Cardiac Output
One of the most useful modifications of the Swan-Ganz catheter included the addition of a thermistor to the tip of the catheter along with the development of a triple lumen system. The thermistor can detect changes in temperature following injection of cold dextrose in the right atrium. This "temperature dilution curve" obtained with the temperature sensor provides an estimate of cardiac output. The distance between the injection site in the right atrium and the thermistor is fixed and one has to assume that blood flow is constant during the period of time necessary for the indicator (i.e., cold dextrose) to travel from the injection site to the sampling site at the catheter tip. One must remember that the thermodilution technique with the Swan-Ganz catheter provides an assessment of right-sided cardiac output. In most clinical circumstances, one assumes that the output of the right ventricle equals that of the left, but this is *not* always correct. Patients who have significant tricuspid insufficiency or intracardiac shunting have unreliable measurements of thermodilution cardiac output. Furthermore, respiratory variations in flow may affect the determination of the thermodilution output. At least three consecutive samples of thermodilution curves with less than 10 percent variation should be averaged.[3]

Within certain limitations and with various assumptions, the measurement of *mixed venous oxygen saturation* in the pulmonary artery may be used as an index of the effectiveness of total body perfusion. Of particular value is the change in mixed venous oxygen saturation during an intervention. One assumes that total body oxygen consumption and arterial oxygen content do not vary significantly during an intervention. An arteriovenous oxygen difference of $\geq$ 6 ml/dl of blood indicates poor tissue perfusion because a greater extraction than normal is needed to deliver oxygen to the tissues. Some of the problems that have to be taken into consideration relate to the need for a slow rate of blood withdrawal from the Swan-Ganz catheter while obtaining the mixed venous oxygen saturation in order not to contaminate the blood with pulmonary venous blood. Furthermore, the presence of a left-to-right intracardiac shunt will give an unreliable mixed venous sample. Although in most patients with simple cardiac failure a decreased mixed venous P_{O_2} does reflect a low cardiac output,[4] the correlation is poor in patients with adult respiratory distress syndrome (ARDS) or after cardiac surgery, or in patients with septic shock and significant shunting of blood in peripheral tissues.[5] Under some circumstances, the mixed venous P_{O_2} is a better indicator of the delivery of oxygen to the tissues than is the cardiac output, particularly in instances where arterial P_{O_2} is low or when arterial oxygen content is also low, as in anemia. When mixed venous P_{O_2} drops to a level of 27 to 30 mmHg (normal range is approximately 39 mmHg), there is an increase in blood lactate levels suggestive of tissue hypoxia.

A high mixed venous P_{O_2} with a high cardiac output often seen in septic shock may be the result of peripheral AV shunting. Under those circumstances a rise in lactate and drop in pH are the indications of decreased tissue oxygenation. It is important in considering the significance of a venous P_{O_2} measurement to appreciate the fact that P_{O_2} does not necessarily always relate to oxygen content. In patients with severe anemia, a P_{O_2} in the range of 40 mmHg may represent a significant reduction in oxygen content, indicative of poor tissue perfusion. Thus, although one is measuring P_{O_2}, one should be thinking in terms of oxygen content. Mixed venous oxygen content should be viewed in terms of the arterial oxygen content to define the adequacy of tissue oxygenation.

The sampling of pulmonary arterial blood can also be used as a "check-and-balance" system for assessing the accuracy and reproducibility of thermodilution cardiac output measurements. Simultaneous sampling of pulmonary arterial blood (from the Swan-Ganz catheter) and arterial blood (from an arterial line) allows the calculation of an arterial-venous O_2 content difference (AV Δ O_2C). By the Fick principle, AV Δ O_2C is inversely proportional to the cardiac output, assuming constancy of O_2 consumption. Thus, occasional cross-checking of the thermodilution cardiac output with determination of an AV O_2C allows one to have more confidence in the measurements being used to guide therapy.

Arterial Catheterization for Arterial Pressure Monitoring

In patients in shock this sphygmomanometric measurement of arterial blood pressure is often inaccurate and that may be why there is a discrepancy between intraarterial pressure and the cuff pressure. Often the pressure is too low or even undetectable by the cuff technique when intraarterial pressure recording with an intraarterial cannula shows normal or even slightly elevated arterial pressures.[6] This discrepancy may be related to intense peripheral vasoconstriction associated with a very low cardiac output. Under those circumstances palpation of the femoral artery at the groin may give some indication of the strength of the pulse even though the cuff pressure may be undetectable, suggesting the necessity for intraarterial cannulation before the use of various pressor agents. Another very practical value in using the intraarterial cannula is the rapid and easy access to arterial blood samples for monitoring of blood gases and various electrolytes.

The usual sites of insertion of the arterial cannula include the radial, brachial, and femoral arteries. The radial artery is recommended because of its easy accessibility; however, before introducing a catheter in the radial artery, one has to ascertain that there is good ulnar artery flow by performing the Allen's test. This is accomplished by occluding both the radial and ulnar arteries at the wrist and allowing the palm of the hand to blanch. Upon release of the ulnar artery compression one observes a rapid flush of the hand. If the flush occurs promptly, this indicates that there is adequate ulnar flow and cannulation of the radial artery is appropriate. Otherwise, cannulation of the brachial artery would be safer. In patients with severe hypotension on large doses of vasoactive drugs, cannulation of the brachial or femoral artery is generally preferable because the marked vasoconstriction makes it difficult to palpate the radial artery.

The major potential complications of arterial line placement are infection[7] and ischemia.[8] The risk of infection is increased if the insertion is by surgical cutdown rather than percutaneously, if the duration of cannulation exceeds 4 days, and if there is inflammation at the site of catheterization.

The risk of thrombosis is minimal (0.6 percent), but occasionally requires emergency thrombectomy.[9] A significant percentage of patients have reversible subclinical arterial occlusion.[9] Daily assessment of the adequacy of perfusion distal to the catheter is necessary by examining the color and temperature of the skin. The catheter should be flushed continuously with normal saline solution containing 2 units per milliliter of heparin at a rate of 3 ml/h. The cannulation should be limited to 4 or 5 days at any one site. Again, continuous monitoring of the arterial waveform pattern is essential to ensure proper placement and patency and as a guide to early thrombosis or occlusion.

Progress in Cardiovascular and Respiratory Monitoring

This is discussed in the article by Wiedemann et al.[1] and covers four areas.

Measurement of Extravascular Lung Water In the presence of a significant change in pulmonary capillary permeability, the measurement of PAWP is insufficient to provide an index of capillary filtration pressure, in view of the absence of an estimate of transcapillary oncotic pressure. A reliable method for measurement of extravascular lung water would be very helpful in noncardiogenic pulmonary edema and in ARDS. A combined thermal and dye dilution technique has been used recently to assess the magnitude of accumulation of extravascular lung water.[10] Using this double-indicator technique, one can obtain an estimate of the intravascular dilution volume with indocyanine green, since indocyanine is nondiffusible, and an estimate of both the intravascular space and the extravascular lung water with the thermal indicator which is "diffusible." Injection at the bedside, through the Swan-Ganz catheter or the central venous line, of a bolus consisting of 5 mg of indocyanine green dye in 10 ml of cold 5% dextrose solution, with sampling from the femoral artery, allow measurement of the two dilution curves. The equipment for processing the dilution curves is commercially available.[11]

Microvascular Injury The pulmonary vascular endothelium is an extremely active endothelium, releasing a number of vasoactive substances such as bradykinin, serotonin, prostaglandins, and angiotensin.[12,13] Endothelial abnormalities in various disease states, particularly in ARDS, may be assessed using a double-indicator dilution technique with indocyanine green as the reference tracer for intravascular volume and another tracer which is removed selectively by the intact endothelium (e.g., radioactive 14C-5-hydroxytryptamine, or ^{3}H-norepinephrine, or ^{3}H-prostaglandin E). Both are given through the Swan-Ganz catheter and the arterial sample collected from the radial artery. Many animal studies[13] suggest that this measurement would be valuable to assess a variety of types of endothelial damage in the lung. It is too early to predict their applicability to humans.

Assessment of Left Ventricular Function The noninvasive assessment of ventricular function using radionuclide angiography is now common, but is not used routinely in the intensive care unit. A recent modification of blood pool imaging referred to as the nuclear probe shows promise for repeated monitoring.[14] The nuclear probe does not provide an image of the whole ventricle, but instead a single hole detector-collimator system is analyzed. The curves are generated by the detection of the blood radionuclide label, with a miniature cadmium telluride detector placed directly on the chest wall. This allows a beat-to-beat measurement of left ventricular ejection fraction in the clinical setting. This detector has been used in a few ambulatory patients and has allowed serial monitoring of left ventricular ejection fraction with a single radionuclide injection for 6 to 24 hours.[14] From the measurement of cardiac output and heart rate, one can calculate the stroke volume and using the left ventricular ejection fraction, one can then estimate left ventricular end-diastolic volume noninvasively. By estimating left ventricular end-diastolic pressure and left ventricular end-diastolic volume, one can obtain an assessment of ventricular compliance.

Another method for assessing left ventricular volume and ejection fraction is the echocardiogram. Recent studies[15] suggest that the echocardiogram can allow an estimate of pulmonary artery wedge pressure.

Respiratory Muscles The onset of fatigue of respiratory muscles may be detected by evaluating the high- and low-frequency power spectra of the diaphragm using a surface electromyogram. A reduction in the high-to-low ratio often precedes the clinical manifestations of impending respiratory failure in patients who have been weaned from the respirator.[16,17]

An assessment of the respiratory muscle fatigue can also be predicted by measurements of respiratory work.[18] The work of breathing may be obtained by simultaneous recording of pressure and flow change with time. A calculated work of breathing between 1.3 and 1.8 kg·m/min is critical in deciding the necessity for ventilator support.[18] The clinical applicability of these measurements in patients requires further study.

The Specific Treatment of Shock

General Measures

Patients who are in shock are generally apprehensive, frightened, and often in pain. They should be reassured and placed in a comfortable supine position, preferably with the legs elevated if this does not exacerbate dyspnea.

Rapid intravenous access should be secured with at least two large-bore intravenous catheters, one of which is preferably central in location, i.e., subclavian, internal jugular, or femoral. Adequacy of the airway must be assured immediately and endotracheal intubation performed if the patient is unconscious or cannot protect his or her airway. Supplemental oxygen should be delivered, preferably by a high-flow delivery system if available, as arterial blood gases are obtained.

Rapid assessment of vital signs, including heart rate and rhythm, respiratory rate and pattern, blood pressure and vital organ function (mentation, urine flow, etc.) should be accomplished with a rapid but thorough physical exam. Initial samples for blood gases and hematologic and chemical profiles should be drawn. Other studies as indicated by the clinical setting (i.e., toxicology screen if poisoning is suspected) should be performed as well.

Relief of pain is important, but must be achieved judiciously without suppressing the patient's sensorium or respiratory activity. Morphine sulfate intravenously in 2- to 4-mg increments, or meperidine in 10- to 25-mg increments may be administered as needed with careful monitoring of vital signs. Intramuscular injection is less desirable due to inadequacy and unreliability of absorption.

Adequacy of circulation must be assessed rapidly and achieved with pharmacologic and/or mechanical means if needed. Use of vasopressor agents and volume expanders may be initially required during placement of hemodynamic monitoring lines.

A rapid and thorough search for any precipitating and reversible factors which may have induced the shock state or may be contributing to a decrease in cardiac output and hypotension (i.e., tension pneumothorax, cardiac tamponade, marked acidosis or alkalosis, tachyarrhythmias or bradyarrhythmias, rapid blood loss, hyperemia, and hypercarbia) should be undertaken. These should be promptly corrected if possible.

The treatment of shock is discussed under five general headings:

- Treatment of General Hemodynamic and Metabolic Abnormalities

- Treatment of Septic Shock
- Sympathomimetic Amines in Shock
- Vasodilator Therapy
- Surgical Treatment of Cardiogenic Shock

Treatment of General Hemodynamic and Metabolic Abnormalities

Treatment of Hypovolemia

Hypovolemia may be absolute or relative. Blood loss or loss of fluid from the intravascular to the extracellular space or excessive pooling of blood in the splanchnic circulation may account for significant reductions in intravascular volume and a reduction of cardiac filling pressure. This requires immediate restoration of circulating blood volume. An adequate cardiac filling pressure is essential to maintain cardiac output. The administration of cardiotonic drugs and catecholamines to increase the force of contraction would be ineffective and potentially deleterious if cardiac filling were suboptimal. An objective assessment of the adequacy of cardiac filling pressure and blood volume may be obtained by measurement of the pulmonary artery wedge pressure (PAWP) as indicated earlier.

In patients with myocardial infarction the ventricular compliance is decreased and an end-diastolic pressure of 20 mmHg may be necessary to achieve adequate cardiac performance. One may clinically perform an in vivo Starling function curve by measuring cardiac output at various levels of PAWP to define the optimal level of cardiac filling for the individual patient at that time. One has to be concerned, however, in patients who have ARDS because a high wedge pressure may contribute to an excessive capillary filtration in the presence of abnormalities in pulmonary capillary permeability. In general, if pulmonary artery diastolic pressure or pulmonary artery wedge pressure were below 15 mmHg, one should administer 100 ml of Ringer's lactate or saline solution every 10 to 15 min. This can be continued as long as the pulmonary artery wedge pressure is between 15 and 20 mmHg and there are steady indications that the tissue perfusion is improving. On the other hand, if pulmonary artery wedge pressure exceeds 20 mmHg and there are signs of pulmonary congestion or indications that the condition has worsened clinically, volume expansion should be stopped. Improvement of tissue perfusion may be indicated by the disappearance of cyanosis, a reduction in the clamminess of the skin, an increase in arterial blood pressure and in urinary output, improvement of the sensorium of the patient, and improvement of blood gases and pH.

Hemorrhagic hypotension should be treated with Ringer's lactate or saline solution, and, after typing and cross-matching, with blood. The effects of the crystalloids are only transient because these would rapidly leave the intravascular space. If blood is not available, a more effective volume replacement would be colloids, particularly in patients who have a low serum albumin and plasma oncotic pressure as a result of chronic illness. Colloids include dextran, mannitol, and albuminoplasma, which tend to remain in the intravascular space longer and maintain cardiac filling pressure and cardiac output.

Furthermore, dextran and mannitol are filtered by the glomeruli and increase oncotic pressure in Bowman's capsule, thus favoring glomerular filtration despite a fall in arterial blood pressure during hypotension and shock.

If, despite volume replacement and restoration of arterial pressure, oliguria persists, the use of a diuretic such as furosemide is appropriate because further expansion of blood volume with colloids may increase the potential for pulmonary edema. In some patients with ARDS and in the "shock lung syndrome," capillary endothelial damage in the lung may increase pulmonary interstitial oncotic pressure to such a degree that capillary filtration becomes excessive. In these patients, attempts to increase the intravascular oncotic pressure by administration of colloids may be only transiently successful since the colloid will also be lost in the pulmonary interstitial fluid across the injured pulmonary capillary endothelium.

Some side effects of fluid therapy should be kept in mind. Isotonic saline solution contains 140 meq sodium and 140 meq of chloride and if used in excessive amounts may tend to cause dilutional acidosis. This is avoided if Ringer's lactate is used. Ringer's lactate has 130 meq sodium, 108 meq chloride, 28 meq lactate, and 4 meq potassium. The lactate is readily converted to bicarbonate.

The intravenous administration of dextran, which has a high molecular weight and remains in the intravascular compartment, allows for a significant and stable expansion of the intravascular volume for several hours. Side effects occur if volumes exceeding 1 liter are given intravenously. These include primarily a bleeding tendency related to either platelet dysfunction or abnormalities in coagulation, the nature of which is not defined, and occasionally anaphylactoid reactions. Therefore, dextran should be avoided in patients who have bleeding tendencies and hypofibrinogenemia. Dextran is available in two molecular weights. One is dextran 40 (40,000 MW) which comes in a 10% solution, and dextran 70 (70,000 MW) which comes in a 6% solution. Dextran 40 is associated with an increased incidence of acute renal failure, possibly because its low molecular weight results in its rapid filtration, a high intratubular concentration with increased viscosity, and potentially tubular obstruction. In contrast, dextran 70 is filtered at a much slower rate. Hydroxyethyl starch or hetastarch is a more effective volume expander than dextran, has fewer side effects, and is less expensive.

Human serum albumin and purified plasma protein are two other compounds available for volume expansion, but they are expensive, costing up to $300 per 500 ml and represent a drain on the resources of most blood donor programs. Serum albumin comes in two concentrations, 5 g/dl and 25 g/dl. The latter is necessary only in the presence of severe hypoalbuminemia. The purified plasma protein, which is not contaminated with hepatitis virus, has some contamination with vasoactive substances.

Treatment of Hypoxia

Attempts should be made to maintain arterial P_{O_2} above 70 mmHg in patients who are hypotensive or in shock. The effectiveness with which this goal can be achieved will depend entirely on the underlying clinical condition. High-flow systems used to deliver a predetermined, fixed inspired oxygen concentration (FIO_2) are the preferred way to deliver oxygen. These systems, which include intubation with mechanical ventilation or T-tube devices or a tight-fitting face mask, allow careful titration of a fixed concentration of oxygen. Other systems such as nasal prongs or a simple face mask, which are low-flow systems, do not allow the delivery of a fixed FIO_2 but are more comfortable and less expensive.

Adequacy of the airway may be a limiting factor in restoring oxygenation in any patient in shock, and if the patient is obtunded, endotracheal intubation may be necessary. Under certain conditions, a positive pressure ventilator to improve gas exchange is necessary, such as in cases with pulmonary edema. However, one has to keep in mind the possibility that the use of positive pressure ventilation will tend to reduce venous return and cardiac output by increasing intrathoracic pressure. Appropriate measurement of cardiac filling pressure during mechanical ventilation of the patient in shock is therefore essential. One should also be concerned about giving 100% oxygen because of the possible toxic changes in the lung if such a high concentration of oxygen is sustained for more than several hours.

Frequent endotracheal suction and hyperinflation are necessary to maintain a high alveolar concentration of oxygen. Calculation of the A-a (Alveolar-arterial) oxygen gradient is possible when a high-flow system with a fixed FIO_2 is used and can provide an index of the adequacy of diffusion or perfusion of the lung as well as cardiac output.

Treatment of Acidosis

Acidosis is a very frequent metabolic abnormality in patients with hypotension or shock because of the accumulation of lactate as a result of failure of oxidative metabolism. Once respiratory acidosis is ruled out, the administration of sodium bicarbonate intravenously (a 50-ml vial has 44.6 meq) is indicated if the pH is less than 7.30. If the pH is less than 7.20, two vials may be necessary. The blood gases and pH should be measured every 15 to 30 min as a guide to further therapy. The correction of acidosis is imperative because it depresses myocardial function and inhibits responsiveness to catecholamines, thus perpetuating a state of circulatory failure and shock. One has to avoid overcorrection of metabolic acidosis because alkalosis shifts the oxygen dissociation curve to the left and reduces oxygen delivery to the tissues.

Treatment of Arrhythmias

Sinus bradycardia (heart rate of less than 40 beats per minute) may cause hypotension. It is often associated with inferior wall myocardial infarction and represents a reflex increase in parasympathetic tone to the heart and as such carries a reasonably good prognosis. It can be readily reverted with atropine sulfate, 0.4 to 1.0 mg (occasionally up to 2.0 mg is required) given intravenously. If bradycardia is associated with hypotension and other signs of decreased cardiac output, and is refractory to atropine, electrical pacing should be attempted. Complete AV block may also be seen following acute myocardial infarction. If the block is associated with inferior wall myocardial infarction, it is again most likely to be reflexly triggered by overactivity of the parasympathetic system and can be reversed readily with atropine intravenously. If, on the other hand, the block is associated with anterior wall myocardial infarction, it is more often caused by ischemic damage to the three fascicles of the conduction system and may reflect an extensive degree of necrosis and high mortality. These patients generally require immediate placement of a temporary transvenous pacemaker and may require permanent pacemaker implantation if they survive.

One has to be very careful in attempting to treat sinus tachycardia of a rate between 120 and 130 since this may be the natural hemodynamic response to hypotension, hypovolemia, or shock; this is particularly true in septic shock when there is a decreased peripheral resistance, a high output, and a high temperature. On the other hand, supraventricular arrhythmia, such as atrial tachycardia, atrial flutter, and atrial fibrillation may be associated with hypotension and may require treatment with digoxin unless one suspects a Wolff-Parkinson-White syndrome. If the rhythm persists after digoxin or if there is an associated hemodynamic deterioration, synchronized cardioversion should be utilized immediately.

A sustained ventricular tachycardia is often seen with myocardial infarction and requires a bolus of 50 to 100 mg of lidocaine and continuous lidocaine infusion with the dosage adjusted with regard to the degree of shock or heart failure present. If there is an associated hypotension or question of inadequate tissue perfusion, electroshock therapy should be used immediately. Patients with ventricular fibrillation should have the usual resuscitative procedures with closed chest massage, mouth-to-mouth respiration, and intravenous bicarbonate as well as defibrillation.

Recurrence of ventricular fibrillation or ventricular tachycardia despite adequate therapy with lidocaine may require the intravenous administration of procainamide or bretylium while attempts at defibrillation are repeated.

Treatment of Septic Shock

The characteristic hemodynamic abnormalities in septic shock include a marked decrease in total peripheral vascular resistance with a high cardiac output. Later, as the syndrome progresses, there may be a reduction in the cardiac output as myocardial depressant factors are released into the circulation or as hypoxia and acidosis complicate the clinical picture. Despite the high cardiac output, there is often a very significant relative hypovolemia because of peripheral vasodilatation and pooling of blood in the splanchnic circulation, requiring the prompt administration of significant amounts of fluids. Careful monitoring of hemodynamics, including pulmonary artery wedge pressure, is necessary for the proper management of this condition since it can become complicated with the acute respiratory distress syndrome with its attendant increased pulmonary capillary permeability, a situation which would require judicious replacement of fluids and thoughtful interpretation of the capillary wedge pressure as well as plasma oncotic pressure.

Organisms involved in the pathogenesis of septic shock may be gram-negative or gram-positive. Endotoxemia associated with gram-negative septicemia is a complication seen with *Escherichia coli,* which is the predominant organism, or with *Klebsiella–Aerobacter* groups. Gram-positive infections without endotoxemia may also cause the same shock syndrome and often complicate pneumococcal pneumonia, *Staphylococcus aureus* infection, or streptococcal bacteremias.

Patients recovering from surgical interventions involving the urinary tract or the biliary system may present with gram-negative septicemia. Chronic alcoholism is a commonly associated illness among patients who present with gram-positive bacteremias, and the more recently described toxic shock syndrome is a complication of *Staphylococcus aureus* infection most commonly associated with tampon usage in women.

In addition to vigorous fluid replacement, an aggressive approach to the use of antibiotics is essential in the treatment of septic shock. If a culture sensitivity is obtained, appropriate antibiotics should be used. If septic shock is diagnosed on the basis of the clinical picture and the precipitating organism not yet known, a rational approach to antibiotic therapy must be based on the use of broad-spectrum agents which will cover the most likely organisms involved.

Corticosteroids have been used extensively in the treatment of septic shock and their usage has been based primarily on experimental studies in animals and an understanding of their membrane-stabilizing properties. While some experimental studies suggest efficacy of corticosteroids for the therapy of septic shock, clinical use of such agents remains controversial at present, although recent studies in humans are encouraging.[19]

Steroids are also known to interact with biomembranes and confer a stabilizing effect in vitro, particularly on lysosomes. Lysosomes isolated from animals treated with corticosteroids appear to have a greater resistance to lysis in vitro. The glucocorticoid effect of corticosteroids does not appear to play a role in the protective effect in septic shock. Since membrane damage and injury are an important pathogenetic mechanism in different types of shock, particularly in septic and anaphylactic shock, the use of steroids has a very strong rationale in these conditions.

It has also been proposed that the release of beta endorphin by the pituitary may play a role in depressing the myocardium in shock states. Steroids may prevent the release of pituitary beta endorphins. Naloxon, a beta-endorphin antagonist, provides an impressive protective effect against endotoxin-mediated shock in animals and preliminary trials in humans.[20]

A dose of 30 mg/kg of methylprednisolone is recommended for use in patients as early as possible in the presence of septicemia and hypotension. The administration of corticosteroids in patients with cardiogenic shock is unwise because of the high incidence of malignant arrhythmias and the possibility that steroids may interfere with the process of healing and fibrosis of the ventricle, which could lead to ventricular aneurysms.

It had been suggested that corticosteroids may have a beneficial effect through their influence on the cardiovascular system, but most of the information available in this regard suggests that their effects on the circulation is minimal, particularly the suggested blockade of alpha receptors. If there is a beneficial effect, it will have to be primarily through their effects on membrane stabilization.

With prompt management of septicemia and hypotension, using a generous amount of fluids to obtain an adequate cardiac filling pressure, intravenous administration of antibiotics, and high doses of methylprednisolone in the early stage of shock, this syndrome can often be reversed. Sympathomimetic amines may be necessary to maintain a degree of vasoconstriction as well as to improve cardiac performance in the face of myocardial-depressing factors.

Sympathomimetic Amines in Shock

The purpose of sympathomimetic amines in shock is to maintain or reestablish an adequate blood pressure, increase cardiac output, and redistribute blood flow to the vital organs. This is achieved through a positive inotropic effect on the myocardium (a cardiotonic action mediated through $beta_1$ receptors in the heart) and a vasoconstricting effect (mediated through $alpha_1$ receptors) on blood vessels. The difference in effects of sympathomimetic amines is based on their respective potency with respect to activation of $beta_1$ receptors in the myocardium and the $alpha_1$ receptors in the blood vessels. Furthermore, the density of $alpha_1$ receptors and their affinity to the various sympathomimetic amines will determine the degree of vasoconstriction. In order to achieve a beneficial redistribution of blood flow to vital organs, one would have to induce significant vasoconstriction in nonvital organs (i.e., muscle, skin, splanchnic circulation) of sufficient magnitude to elevate blood pressure without any vasoconstriction in the vital organs, such as the brain and the myocardium. The density and affinity of $alpha_1$ adrenoreceptors to sympathomimetic amines are indeed such that a greater vasoconstriction is achieved in the cutaneous, splanchnic, and muscle circulation with very little or no vasoconstriction in the coronary and cerebral vessels.

Potential complications from the use of sympathomimetic amines include ventricular arrhythmia, seen with very potent $beta_1$ stimulants such as isoproterenol and epinephrine; and excessive elevation of arterial blood pressure, which is to be avoided, since an increase in arterial pressure significantly above normal levels will increase cardiac afterload. This is undesirable when shock is caused by myocardial infarction or is associated with significant myocardial depression. A moderate elevation of arterial pressure is desirable, however, to maintain coronary perfusion through collateral vessels. Another potential complication is intense vasoconstriction, particularly in the renal circulation, which could exaggerate oliguria and might induce ischemic necrosis in certain organs. One should mention, however, that ischemic necrosis in patients in shock may not only be the result of excessive administration of vasoconstricting sympathomimetic amines, but also the result of a natural progression of the clinical syndrome of shock with the excessive reduction in tissue perfusion.

Norepinephrine

Norepinephrine is the natural neurotransmitter. It increases myocardial contractility through activation of $beta_1$ receptors and causes vasoconstriction through activation of $alpha_1$ receptors in various regions of the circulation. It causes vasoconstriction in the cutaneous, splanchnic, and muscle circulation, where it reduces blood flow, while it can increase blood flow in the coronary circulation. This is due to both the paucity of $alpha_1$ receptors in the coronary vessels and because of the effect of norepinephrine on $beta_2$ vasodilator receptors in the coronary vessels and a metabolically mediated coronary vasodilation induced as the result of a positive inotropic effect. The resulting rise in arterial pressure will produce several beneficial effects. First, there is an increase of cerebral perfusion; second, there is an increase in myocardial perfusion through the coronary collateral circulation in patients who have had a coronary occlusion; and third, there is an increase in glomerular filtration.

Norepinephrine (Levophed R, 4 mg base per ampule) should be given intravenously through an indwelling catheter with care taken to avoid extravasation. When two ampules of Levophed are diluted in 500 ml glucose and water the final concentration of norepinephrine base is 16 μg/ml. The infusion should be started at a slow rate since some patients will respond to low doses (i.e., 4 to 16 μg/min). The goal is to attempt to achieve an arterial pressure ranging from systolic levels of 100 to 120 mmHg; depending, of course, on the patient's initial level of blood pressure. Occasionally, patients may require a higher dose (up to 40 μg/min). In general, if such doses are necessary to maintain arterial pressure or tissue perfusion, the prognosis is very poor. It is essential to remember that the effectiveness of sympathomimetic amines depends on the correction of acidosis, hypoxia, and hypovolemia. If these have been corrected and the patient is still unresponsive to norepinephrine, this is an indication that there has been a significant degree of myocardial damage, or that the shock state is irreversible.

Epinephrine

Epinephrine is another naturally occurring neurotransmitter which is released from the adrenal gland. It activates both $beta_1$ receptors in the myocardium and $alpha_1$ and $beta_2$ receptors in blood vessels. It has a vasoconstricting effect through $alpha_1$ receptors in cutaneous, splanchnic, and renal vessels, and a vasodilator effect through activation of $beta_2$ receptors in skeletal muscle when given in relatively low concentrations. The doses given range from 2 to 30 μg/min intravenously.

Dopamine

Another naturally occurring sympathomimetic amine, dopamine, is the precursor of norepinephrine. At present, it is probably the most commonly used inotropic and vasopressor agent in the clinical management of shock and hypotension. There are several differences in the action of dopamine and norepinephrine. First, the vasoconstricting effect of dopamine is a bit more restricted, involving the cutaneous and muscular circulations. In addition, dopamine stimulates dopaminergic receptors in the renal, splanchnic, and cerebral circulations and has a vasodilator effect in the splanchnic and renal circulations and a minimal vasodilator influence on the cerebral and coronary vessels. Dopamine also has a positive inotropic effect due to stimulation of $beta_1$ adrenoreceptors in the myocardium. The increase in cerebral and coronary blood flow is generally achieved by virtue of the rise in arterial pressure rather than by a direct dilator effect on these circulations.

Dopamine exerts dose-dependent hemodynamic effects. At doses of 2 to 5 μg/kg/min the vasodilator influences are most pronounced, with activation of dopaminergic receptors, while doses in excess of 20 μg/kg/min exert marked vasoconstricting effects due to activation primarily of $alpha_1$ adrenoreceptors in most vascular beds. Side effects of dopamine include nausea, vomiting, tachyarrhythmias, and in high doses include intense vasoconstriction. If the drug extravasates from the intravenous site of administration it may cause intense cutaneous vasoconstriction and skin necrosis. This potential side effect is common to all the major vasopressor agents and thus it is recommended that they be administered through a well-placed and secure large-bore intravenous line, preferably in a large central vein.

Dobutamine
This synthetic sympathomimetic amine produces a strong positive inotropic action through the activation of $beta_1$ receptors and, in contrast to dopamine, it has a lesser vasoconstricting effect and reportedly less tendency to cause ventricular arrhythmias. In models of myocardial infarction in dogs, it has been shown to decrease the infarct size as compared to dopamine. When given in equipotent inotropic doses, dobutamine tends to elevate the cardiac output to a similar extent, but without increasing pulmonary artery wedge pressure when compared to dopamine. Thus, in the setting of acute myocardial infarction without significant hypotension, dobutamine may be a preferred drug.

Isoproterenol
This is another synthetic sympathomimetic amine which activates primarily the $beta_1$ receptors in the myocardium, inducing its positive inotropic effect, and $beta_2$ vascular receptors in blood vessels, causing vasodilatation. The vasodilator response to isoproterenol in various vascular beds depends on the density and affinity of $beta_2$ receptors. Although it might be theoretically appealing to induce vasodilatation in a setting of myocardial depression in order to decrease afterload, the vasodilatation with isoproterenol tends to redistribute blood flow to nonvital organs such as skeletal muscle and skin. Furthermore, the vasodilatation at the microcirculatory level appears to be at sites which do not necessarily improve nutritional capillary flow. Thus, the net effect could be a reduction in oxygen delivery to the tissues and particularly the vital organs, despite the fact that both cardiac output and organ blood flow may be increased. It may be used only temporarily in situations where a severe bradycardia needs to be reversed after unsuccessful attempts to increase heart rate with atropine, pending placement of a temporary pacemaker.

Vasodilator Therapy

The goal of vasodilator therapy in shock is (1) to decrease preload, thereby decreasing cardiac size, myocardial wall tension, and myocardial oxygen demands, as well as reducing pulmonary congestive pressure and pulmonary edema; (2) to decrease afterload, thereby facilitating left ventricular ejection and increasing stroke volume by reducing arterial impedance and by causing peripheral vasodilatation; and (3) dilatation of microcirculatory vessels to increase nutritional capillary blood flow.

The best indication for vasodilator therapy is in patients who have a low cardiac output, a high pulmonary artery wedge pressure or end diastolic pressure, an enlarged heart, and signs of pulmonary edema, but who are not hypotensive.

Reduction in Preload
Preload or cardiac filling pressure is reduced by the venodilator effect of the vasodilator drugs. Not all vasodilator drugs have a venodilator action. For example, hydralazine dilates predominantly arterioles, whereas nitroprusside and especially nitroglycerin have significant venodilator influences. Because of these very potent venodilator effects, intravenous administration of nitroprusside or nitroglycerin should be accompanied by monitoring of both arterial pressure and pulmonary artery wedge pressure to avoid a precipitous drop in cardiac output resulting from a significant drop in cardiac filling pressure. Only if fluid administration has failed to improve tissue perfusion and if pulmonary artery wedge pressure is significantly elevated will the attempt to reduce preload be indicated.

Reduction in Afterload
Here the goal is not necessarily to reduce arterial pressure but to reduce vascular impedance. One often sees an improvement in cardiac output and ejection fraction without a significant change in mean arterial pressure. This is because the vasodilator effect is offset by an increase in cardiac output and arterial pressure remains constant. A drop in arterial pressure exceeding 10 mmHg should be avoided because one wishes to maintain diastolic arterial pressure at a significant level to achieve adequate perfusion of the coronary, cerebral, and renal circulations. Patients with cardiomyopathy but without coronary artery disease may be the best candidates for this therapy because the perfusion of coronary vessels is not necessarily as dependent on an adequate diastolic pressure as in those patients with significant coronary artery disease.

Reduction in afterload should be approached very cautiously in patients with cardiogenic shock and hypotension following myocardial infarction. If the patient has a myocardial infarction complicated by an *elevated* arterial blood pressure with continuing pain despite administration of morphine and nitroglycerin, the administration of nitroprusside to reduce arterial blood pressure would be indicated. The consequent reduction in afterload may be effective in controlling the symptoms and reducing myocardial oxygen consumption.

Microcirculatory Vasoconstriction and Alpha Receptor Blockers In some patients with severe shock, decreased tissue perfusion continues despite the high circulating levels of catecholamines and the attempt to improve perfusion by administering fluids and sympathomimetic amines. In these patients, failure to improve tissue perfusion may be due to intense constriction at the microcirculatory level which may be preventing perfusion of nutritional capillaries. The poor prognosis in these patients is generally the result of the advanced disease underlying the shock syndrome. Nevertheless, under these circumstances an attempt to use an alpha-adrenoreceptor blocker which specifically antagonizes the vasoconstricting action of circulating sympathomimetic amines without opposing their positive inotropic effect should be considered.

Phentolamine is a very potent alpha$_1$-receptor antagonist and may be used in an initial dose of 2 mg intravenously followed by 5 mg. One must attempt to carefully monitor the patient's hemodynamics and the amount given because of the possibility of a rapid hypotensive action resulting from venous relaxation and relative hypovolemia with a reduction in the effective blood volume. Phentolamine may also be added to the intravenous infusion containing norepinephrine to oppose the vasoconstricting effects of this drug and retain its positive inotropic action as well as its vasodilator effect through activation of beta$_2$ receptors. By mixing 4 ampules of phentolamine (20 mg) in 500 ml glucose and water, the final concentration of 40 μg/ml would be achieved, and a dose ranging from 20 to 80 μg/min may be necessary to restore perfusion of the microcirculation.

Although an extensive amount of animal experimentation supports the use of alpha$_1$-adrenoreceptor blockade with phentolamine in treating shock, there are no clinical studies that confirm these beneficial effects in patients. Thus, the use of phentolamine in such severe forms of shock is to be considered only experimental at the present time.

Nitroglycerin When given intravenously in doses of 15 to 100 μg/min, nitroglycerin can reduce preload through its vasodilator effect as well as afterload. Its effectiveness is most marked in patients who have congestive heart failure, particularly following myocardial infarction, when pulmonary artery wedge pressure is significantly elevated and arterial pressure is within the normal range. It can also cause coronary vasodilatation and improve subendocardial blood flow. Occasionally, in the presence of hypotension with elevated wedge pressure, a combination of intravenous nitroglycerin and dopamine may allow a reduction in preload with a reduction in cardiac size while simultaneously improving the inotropic response and maintaining some vasoconstriction and a redistribution of blood flow to vital organs with dopamine.

Vasodilator drugs which do not have a venodilator action such as hydralazine would not be effective in reducing cardiac size and myocardial oxygen demand and, in fact, could be detrimental in that a reflex increase in heart rate would increase myocardial oxygen consumption and the reduction in arterial pressure will tend to reduce coronary collateral flow.

Nitroprusside This is a very effective drug in reducing both preload and afterload. It has a significant venodilator action as well as an arteriolar dilatatory effect. A dose of ~ 16 μg/min should be attempted first and increases of up to 200 μg/min may be used while constantly monitoring arterial pressure and pulmonary artery wedge pressure. By also reducing arteriolar tone and arterial impedance, nitroprusside facilitates ventricular ejection and increases stroke volume.

Surgical Treatment of Cardiogenic Shock

Coronary artery bypass surgery as well as infarctectomy have been attempted in patients with shock from acute myocardial infarction. However, the results have not been uniformly encouraging so that these procedures should be considered still in the experimental stage. There are two complications of myocardial infarction, however, that are potentially amenable to surgery. These include rupture of a papillary muscle and ventricular septal perforation.

Sudden appearance of a pansystolic murmur accompanied by a thrill is very suggestive of acute perforation of the interventricular septum. However, it is sometimes very difficult to clinically differentiate a ruptured papillary muscle from a perforated interventricular septum. Patients with a perforated ventricular septum have a marked left-to-right shunt which can be initially diagnosed at the bedside by sampling blood from the right atrium, right ventricle, and pulmonary artery during the introduction of a Swan-Ganz catheter. The surgical treatment of an interventricular septal defect following myocardial infarction might best be delayed for several weeks to allow the formation of sufficient amounts of scar tissue to permit surgical closure and repair.

In both of these conditions, attempts to improve perfusion pressure with vasopressor drugs will increase mitral insufficiency or the left-to-right shunt due to increased afterload on the left ventricle, and the condition would likely worsen. The selective lowering of systolic pressure with intraaortic balloon counterpulsation is ideal in these circumstances, as it will reduce afterload and facilitate ventricular ejection. The reduced afterload will reduce the acute mitral regurgitation or decrease the left-to-right shunt of an acute ventricular septal defect. Although one may achieve a similar beneficial effect by giving a vasodilator drug such as nitroprusside or nitroglycerin to reduce afterload, the associated fall in diastolic pressure may extend myocardial ischemia. The balloon counterpulsation will increase diastolic pressure when the aortic valve is closed and thus improve coronary perfusion without subjecting the left ventricle to an increased afterload. The surgical correction of the defect should be carried out as soon as it is feasible and safe.

Ruptured papillary muscle or papillary muscle dysfunction may cause significant left ventricular failure. The posterior papillary muscle is more frequently involved than the anterior, and occasionally replacement of the mitral apparatus with a prosthetic valve has been effective, especially in patients whose myocardial infarction is limited and who have good myocardial function.

The use of intraaortic balloon counterpulsation has been a beneficial advance in the management of cardiogenic shock, particularly in those patients in whom surgery might be anticipated, such as for ventricular septal rupture or papillary muscle rupture. The balloon can be introduced into the aorta at the end of a catheter through the femoral artery, either by a surgical cutdown or percutaneously. The balloon is automatically inflated in diastole and deflated in systole. The sudden inflation of the balloon in the thoracic aorta increases diastolic pressure and its deflation decreases systolic pressure or afterload. By increasing diastolic pressure, coronary perfusion through collateral vessels is increased. The reduction in systolic pressure reduces afterload and myocardial work. Despite the theoretical advantages of the technique, its use in patients in shock has not given uniformly good results, but this is primarily due to the fact that the disease is advanced and the extent of the myocardial damage is significant in patients who do require balloon counterpulsation. This assistance is valuable, however, in sustaining the hemodynamics while the patients are being prepared for cardiac surgery whenever surgery is indicated, or as a temporizing measure in certain select patients in whom immediate surgery is not a feasible alternative to attempt to stabilize the patient with medication. However, cardiogenic shock complicating an acute infarction without a mechanical lesion (i.e., mitral regurgitation or ventricular septal defect) carries an extremely poor prognosis, even with the use of mechanical circulatory assist devices.

References

1. Wiedemann, H. P., Matthay, M. A., and Matthay, R. A.: Cardiovascular-Pulmonary Monitoring in the Intensive Care Unit (Part 1) and (Part 2), *Chest,* 85:537 and 656, 1984.
2. Swan, H. J. C., Ganz, W., Forrester, J. S., Marcus, H., Diamond, G., and Channette, D.: Catheterization of the Heart in Man with the Use of a Flow-Directed Balloon-Tipped Catheter, *N. Engl. J. Med.,* 283:447, 1970.
3. Jansen, J. R. C., Schreuder, J. J., Bogaard, J. M., van Rooyen, W., and Versprille, A.: Thermodilution Technique for Measurement of Cardiac Output During Artificial Ventilation, *J. Appl. Physiol.,* 51:584, 1981.
4. Wagner, P. D.: Interpretation of Arterial Blood Gases, *Chest,* 77:131, 1980.
5. Manny, J., Justice, R., and Hechtman, H. B.: Abnormalities in Organ Blood Flow and Its Distribution during Positive End-Expiratory Pressure, *Surgery,* 85:425, 1979.
6. Cohn, J. N.: Blood Pressure Measurement in Shock, *JAMA,* 199:972, 1967.
7. Shinozaki, T., Deane, R., Mazuzan, J. E., Hamel, A. J., and Hazelton, D.: Bacterial Contamination of Arterial Lines: A Prospective Study, *JAMA,* 249:223, 1983.
8. Shapiro, B. A.: Monitoring Gas Exchange in Acute Respiratory Failure, *Respir. Care,* 28:605, 1983.
9. Gardner, R. M., Schwartz, R., Wong, H. C., and Burke, J. P.: Percutaneous Indwelling Radial-Artery Catheters for Monitoring Cardiovascular Function, *N. Engl. J. Med.,* 290:1227, 1974.
10. Lewis, F. R., Elings, V. B., Hill, S. L., and Christensen, J. M.: The Measurement of Extravascular Lung Water by Thermal Green-Dye Indicator Dilution, *Ann. N.Y. Acad. Sci.,* 384:394, 1982.
11. Sibbald, W. J., Warshawski, F. J., Short, A. K., Harris, J., Lefcoe, M. S., and Holliday, R. L.: Clinical Studies of Measuring Extravascular Lung Water by the Therman Dye Technique in Critically Ill Patients, *Chest,* 83:725, 1983.
12. Stalcup, S. A., Turino, G. M., and Mellins, R. B.: Critical Issues in the Use of Vasoactive Substances to Assess Lung Microvascular Injury, *Ann. N.Y. Acad. Sci.,* 384:435, 1982.
13. Gillis, C. N., and Catravas, J. D.: Altered Removal of Vasoactive Substances in the Injured Lung: Detection of Lung Microvascular Injury, *Ann. N.Y. Acad. Sci.,* 384:458, 1982.
14. Hoffer, P. B., Berger, H. J., Steidley, J., Brendel, A. F., Gottschalk, A., and Zaret, B. L.: A Miniature Cadmium Telluride Detector Module for Continuous Monitoring of Left-Ventricular Function, *Radiology,* 138:477, 1981.
15. Askenazi, J., Koenigsberg, D. I., Ziegler, J. H., and Lesch, M.: Echocardiographic Estimates of Pulmonary Artery Wedge Pressure, *N. Engl. J. Med.,* 305:1566, 1981.
16. Cohen, C. A., Zagelbaum, G., Gross, D., Roussos, C. H., and Macklem, P. T.: Clinical Manifestations of Inspiratory Muscle Fatigue, *Am. J. Med.,* 73:308, 1982.
17. Gross. D., Grassino, A., Ross, W. R. D., and Macklem, P. T.: Electromyogram Pattern of Diaphragmatic Fatigue, *J. Appl. Physiol.,* 46:1, 1979.
18. Proctor, H. J., and Woolson, R.: Prediction of Respiratory Muscle Fatigue by Measurements of the Work of Breathing, *Surg. Gynecol. Obstet.,* 136:367, 1973.
19. Sheagren, J. N.: Septic Shock and Corticosteroids, *N. Engl. J. Med.,* 305:456, 1981.
20. Faden, A. J., and Holaday, J. W.: Experimental Endotoxic Shock: The Pathophysiologic Function of Endorphine and Treatment with Opiate Antagonists. *J. Infect. Dis.,* 142:229, 1980.

24

High-Cardiac-Output States

Noble O. Fowler, M.D.

In 1947, Burwell and Dexter[1] first demonstrated by the direct Fick method that the cardiac output was increased in a patient with acute beriberi and congestive heart failure. They stated:

> These observations supplement and confirm those of Hayasaka and Inawashiro, Weiss and Wilkins, and Porter and Downs in showing that cardiac failure in patients with beri-beri is associated with a cardiac output that is *increased*. . . . They are the first reported measurements of the pressure in the pulmonary artery and the right ventricle in beri-beri disease.
>
> . . . Since this method is preferable to those previously used, these are the most reliable measurements so far available of the cardiac output in heart failure due to beri-beri heart disease.*

The disorders discussed in this chapter are those in which the resting cardiac output is increased in adult humans beyond the normal range of 2.3 to 3.9 liters/min/m^2.

Contraction of ventricular muscle and thus cardiac output is controlled by four major factors[2] (Table 24-1).

Variations in cardiac filling pressure are not usually responsible for increasing cardiac output beyond normal values in resting human beings. The increased cardiac output of the hyperdynamic states usually does not result from increased cardiac contractility alone.

It is probable that a reduced afterload is a major mechanism in many human hyperdynamic states. Left ventricular afterload is defined as the resistance to ejection and further shortening encountered by the contracting muscle fibers at the end of isovolumetric systole. Reduced left ventricular afterload may occur when there is peripheral shunting of blood (systemic arteriovenous fistula), central shunting (patent ductus arteriosus), peripheral vasodilatation (thyrotoxicosis), or reduced blood viscosity (anemia).

*Reproduced with the permission from the publisher and author.

TABLE 24-1 Physiologic Mechanisms of Increased Cardiac Output

1. Increased preload (blood volume, venous compliance)
2. Decreased systemic vascular resistance
   a. Geometric; e.g., systemic AV fistula, metabolic, pregnancy, drugs such as hydralazine
   b. Rheologic; e.g., anemia
3. Increased cardiac contractility
   a. β_1 sympathetic stimulation
   b. Humoral factors; e.g., serotonin, thyroxin
   c. Drugs; e.g., amrinone, terbutaline, isoproterenol
4. Heart rate

Physical Findings in the Hyperdynamic States

When there is an increase in the cardiac output at rest, certain physical findings tend to appear. Thyrotoxicosis, liver disease, and severe anemia are by far the commonest clinical disorders associated with an increase of cardiac output at rest, if one excepts pregnancy, fever, and emotional excitement. The physical findings commonly associated with the hyperdynamic state in these disorders may be taken as a model for the physical findings to be expected when the resting cardiac output is increased.

Heart Rate

The tachycardia is usually moderate, and the heart rate at rest is likely to be in the range of 85 to 105 beats per minutes. Anemic patients with hyperdynamic states usually have a resting heart rate below 100 beats per minute unless there is acute blood loss.[3] In hyperthyroidism, the heart rate is seldom above 110 beats per minute unless there is severe thyrotoxicosis, bordering on thyroid storm, or complicating atrial fibrillation.

Systemic Veins

The systemic veins may display useful signs of an accelerated circulation. A cervical venous hum, heard over the deep internal jugular veins, more often on the right side, is a common finding in the hyperdynamic states. This continuous murmur with diastolic accentuation can be heard as a normal finding in children in the sitting position. When a cervical venous hum is readily heard in an adult, however, especially in the recumbent posture, a hyperdynamic state is likely. Uncommonly, there may be a venous hum over the femoral veins, especially in patients with sickle cell anemia.

Systemic Arteries

The systemic arteries may display signs related to the increased left ventricular stroke volume. The pulse tends to be bounding with a quick upstroke. The pulse pressure typically is wide, with a decrease of diastolic pressure and an increase of systolic blood pressure. Pistol-shot sounds, and Duroziez's murmur may be heard over the femoral arteries. A systolic bruit may be heard over the carotid arteries. In the absence of aortic regurgitation or patent ductus arteriosus, or other left-to-right extracardiac shunt, these signs are highly suggestive of an elevated left ventricular stroke volume owing to a hyperdynamic state and, if the heart rate is normal or rapid, of an increased cardiac output. It should be recalled that the pulse pressure may be high with a normal diastolic pressure where there is increased sclerosis of thoracic aorta—a finding usually restricted to the elderly. Further, the left ventricular stroke volume may be high but the cardiac output normal or low when there is complete AV block with a slow ventricular rate.

Precordial Auscultation

The increased rate of ventricular ejection commonly produces turbulence and causes a midsystolic murmur in the second and third left intercostal spaces. Decreased blood viscosity may contribute to increased turbulence of blood flow. Increased rate of ventricular filling may cause a third heart sound to be audible at the cardiac apex. An apical fourth heart sound is common in thyrotoxicosis if there is sinus rhythm, but its mechanism is uncertain. Diastolic aortic murmurs have been described in occasional patients with severe anemia or thyrotoxicosis, but are rare in the absence of associated aortic valvular disease except in uremic patients. Mitral diastolic murmurs are occasionally heard in patients with sickle cell anemia.

Systemic and Pulmonary Congestion in the Hyperdynamic States

Patients with one of the many high-cardiac-output states may develop the signs, symptoms, and physiologic evidence of pulmonary or systemic congestion or both. In these patients the cardiac output, although lower than before the onset of congestion, may remain above normal. Eichna suggested that these patients be designated by the term *noncardiac circulatory congestion*[4] rather than heart failure, since the cardiac output is above normal and these patients often have little or no response to digitalis. Since the symptoms and physical findings are similar to those of patients with the more common "low-output" congestive failure syndrome, however, we have used the more common label of *congestive failure* for the congestive state accompanying the hyperdynamic disorders. (See Chap. 21.)

Hyperthyroidism (Thyrotoxicosis)

Abnormal Physiology

Thyrotoxicosis, which has several different causes, is characterized by an increased cardiac output. The increased oxygen consumption raises the cardiac output to supply the metabolic needs of the body, yet in many patients there is an increase in cardiac output beyond this requirement. Tachycardia, which is usually found in this disorder, serves to increase the output of the heart while cardiac stroke volume is maintained or increased.[5] There are at least three major factors to consider in the increased cardiac output of thyrotoxicosis. There is probably a direct action of thyroid hormone upon the heart that causes it to beat more rapidly, even when devoid of adrenergic and cholinergic influences. Thyroid hormone has been thought to stimulate adenylate cyclase, to increase the number of β-adrenergic receptors, to increase contractility, heart rate, oxygen consumption, and protein synthesis.[6] Increased sensitivity to circulating epinephrine and norepinephrine has been demonstrated in thyrotoxicosis. This tends to increase cardiac stroke volume. Studies of subjects with spontaneous hyperthyroidism demonstrated that β-sympathetic receptor blockade reduced heart rate and lengthened the circulation time. The left ventricular preejection period and ejection times remained abbreviated, and oxygen consumption remained elevated.[6] The left ventricular preejection period/ejection time ratio (PEP/LVET) is decreased in hyperthyroidism and returns to normal when the patient becomes euthyroid.[7] In thyrotoxicosis there is decreased peripheral vascular resistance, which tends to increase cardiac output. When the systemic vascular resistance was increased in thyrotoxic subjects by infusion of phenylephrine, cardiac output was decreased.[8] This observation suggests that peripheral vasodilatation with decreased left ventricular afterload is important in the increased cardiac output of thyrotoxicosis.

Clinical Manifestations

Physical Findings

Most patients with thyrotoxicosis have evidence of increased cardiac output without congestive heart failure. It is postulated that most patients who have congestive heart failure with thyrotoxicosis have additional underlying heart disease, but in many instances neither the heart disease nor its nature can be clearly established. In patients under the age of 35 one occasionally observes cardiac decompensation without evident additional heart disease.[5] Most patients with thyrotoxicosis demonstrate the usual physical findings of stare; exophthalmos; enlarged and firm thyroid gland with or without nodule formation; fine tremor of the outstretched hands; warm, moist skin of salmon hue; and tachycardia. If the metabolic rate is considerably increased, there is usually a loud cervical venous hum. In this writer's experience, continuous murmurs over the thyroid gland in thyrotoxic patients have almost always been caused by a cervical venous hum rather than by dilated arteries within the gland. In thyrotoxicosis without heart failure, the cardiac rhythm is usually of normal sinus origin; approximately 10 percent of patients have atrial fibrillation, which is often paroxysmal. On the other hand, in patients with heart failure, atrial fibrillation is found more often. There is characteristically an increase of systolic blood pressure with a modest decrease of diastolic pressure, and the peripheral arterial pulse may be bounding. The heart is usually of normal size, unless there is complicating heart disease or congestive heart failure. The first heart sound is often of increased intensity and may at times suggest an incorrect diagnosis of mitral stenosis. Both presystolic and diastolic apical gallop sounds are common in hyperthyroidism.[9] In older patients with thyrotoxicosis and heart disease, the thyrotoxicosis may be masked; namely, the eye signs may be minimal or absent, and the thyroid enlargement and tachycardia may be inconspicuous. The possibility of thyrotoxic heart disease is often suggested by the observation of atrial fibrillation without obvious cause, some widening of the arterial pulse pressure, and an unusually alert patient with congestive heart failure. Studies for thyrotoxicosis should be made in patients with unexplained atrial fibrillation or atrial flutter. Thyrotoxicosis should be more strongly considered as a possibility in patients with atrial fibrillation whose ventricular rate fails to respond with an adequate decrease with adequate amounts of digitalis. Persistent unexplained sinus tachycardia, especially in elderly patients, should suggest the possibility of thyrotoxicosis.

Special Laboratory Studies

The diagnosis of thyrotoxicosis is made by demonstrating a raised plasma total (protein-bound and unbound) thyroxine (total T_4), together with a raised radioactive triiodothyronine uptake (rT_3U). The latter test is a measure of protein binding. It is necessary to obtain both tests, since the total T_4 may be elevated by increased levels of thyroxine-binding globulin in the absence of thyroid dysfunction, as in pregnancy, estrogen administration (including oral contraceptives), etc. The clinician should be familiar with the causes of euthyroid hyperthyroxinemia.[10] The free T_4 level (FT_4) is calculated from the total T_4 and the rT_3U, and gives the approximate level of unbound T_4. An elevated FT_4, therefore, also indicates thyrotoxicosis. The total plasma triiodothyronine (T_3) measures circulating T_3, and should not be confused with the rT_3U. The T_3 level is a sensitive indicator of thyrotoxicosis. In rare instances it may be elevated in the presence of a normal total T_4 and FT_4 (T_3 toxicosis). It is also affected somewhat by protein binding. Radioactive iodine uptake by the thyroid is now less commonly used for the diagnosis of thyrotoxicosis. In borderline cases, the T_3 TSH suppression test, or the response of TSH to intravenous thyrotropin-releasing hormone may be useful.

Catheterization Hemodynamic studies characteristically reveal an increase of the resting cardiac output and at times an increase of cardiac stroke volume with an arteriovenous oxygen difference decreased below the normal value of 4.5 ± 0.7* ml/dl of blood. The circulation time characteristically is shortened in the absence of heart failure. The central venous pressure and right atrial pressure are normal in the absence of congestive heart failure. When heart failure develops, the cardiac output is lower than before, but usually is still elevated above the normal range.[15]

Echocardiogram An echocardiogram study was made of 11 patients with hyperthyroidism.[10] Left ventricular end-diastolic diameter was not significantly altered. The mean velocity of circumferential fiber shortening and the maximum velocity of posterior wall motion were increased; these variables did not change with propranolol therapy, but became normal when the patients became euthyroid. The left ventricular systolic time intervals showed a decreased PEP/LVET ratio that was not changed with propranolol therapy. In a later study of 10 thyrotoxic patients, PEP/LVET ratios became significantly greater ($p < 0.01$) when the patients were euthyroid.[11] Another study reported increased left ventricular end-diastolic volume and ejection fraction in hyperthyroid patients.[12] The left ventricular ejection fraction may fail to rise further with exercise.[6]

Management

Treatment of younger patients under the age of 25 years usually consists of subtotal thyroidectomy preceded by adequate preparation with the combination of methimazole and Lugol's solution. In older patients, and especially in those with congestive heart failure or recurrent thyrotoxicosis after surgical treatment, the oral administration of radioactive iodine is usually preferred. In patients with a history of heart failure, oral antithyroid drugs, e.g., propylthiouracil, should be given before radioiodine treatment.[13] If there is severe thyrotoxicosis, propranolol may mitigate some of the adverse effects upon the heart until the thyrotoxicosis can be controlled. Propranolol, a β-adrenergic blocking agent, is often used in dosages of 10 to 40 mg orally four times daily. This agent decreases the heart rate and cardiac output in thyrotoxic patients, and thus appears useful until the effects of thyroidectomy or radioactive iodine can be assessed. There is some risk of a deleterious effect upon left ventricular function. In patients with hyperthyroidism and congestive failure, propranolol should probably not be used until digitalis and diuretics have been administered.[13]

Beriberi Heart Disease

Abnormal Physiology

Beriberi heart disease is a rare disorder in the United States and is apparently now even less common than it was 20 years ago. Blankenhorn collected 12 cases

*Standard deviation.

from 1940 to 1948 at the Cincinnati General Hospital,[14] and Akbarian and associates reported four instances from the Boston City Hospital.[15] Five cases were reported in 1981 from New Zealand; these patients were alcoholics.[16] Twenty-three cases in nonalcoholics were reported from Japan in 1980.[17] These patients, mostly teenagers, had a diet low in thiamine and high in polished rice, noodles, and soft drinks.

The mechanisms of increased cardiac output in beriberi are obscure. Some patients with beriberi have lesions of the sympathetic nuclei[15] that may decrease peripheral arterial resistance, thus increasing cardiac work and leading to congestive failure.

Clinical Manifestations

Physical Examination

In Blankenhorn's study made at a large city general hospital,[14] patients with beriberi heart disease were almost invariably chronic alcoholics. They demonstrated evidence of either peripheral neuritis or pellagra. Patients with advanced beriberi heart disease display the usual findings of biventricular congestive failure. These findings include elevation of the systemic venous pressure and pulmonary wedge pressure, edema, and hepatic engorgement. Characteristically, there are widening of the arterial pulse pressure and bounding peripheral arterial pulses. Pistol-shot sounds may be heard over the peripheral arteries. The heart is usually dilated, and apical diastolic gallop rhythm is characteristic.

Electrocardiogram

The electrocardiogram in patients with beriberi heart disease is usually normal except for sinus tachycardia and perhaps minor nonspecific ST-segment and T-wave changes.

Special Laboratory Studies

Catheterization

Hemodynamic studies in patients with heart failure due to beriberi have shown elevations of the right atrial and pulmonary wedge pressures, an increase in cardiac index,[1,15] and a decrease is arteriovenous oxygen difference. These abnormalities can be returned to normal after treatment with thiamine and other vitamins of the B-complex group. Left ventricular ejection fraction was below normal in one

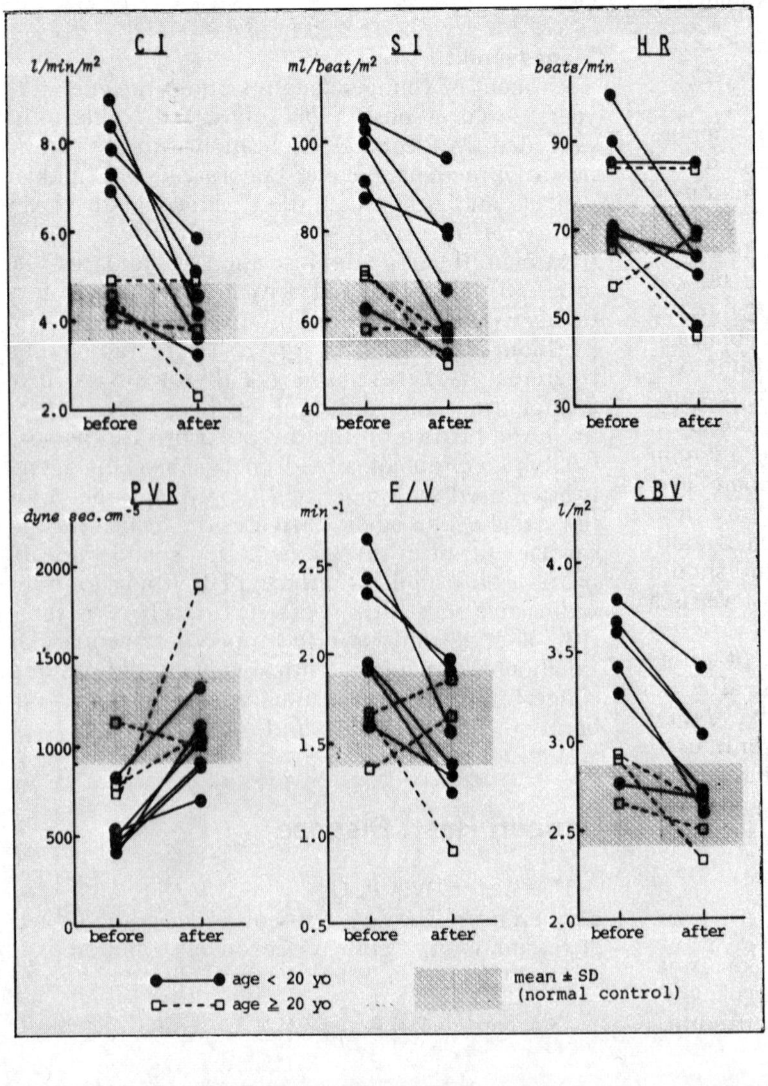

FIGURE 24-1 Changes of hemodynamic parameters before and after treatment in patients under and above 20 years of age. CI, cardiac index; SI, stroke index; HR, heart rate; PVR, peripheral vascular resistance; F/V, blood turnover rate; and CBV, circulatory blood volume. *(From C. Kawai, A. Wakabayashi, T. Matsumura, et al., Reappearance of Beriberi Heart Disease in Japan, Am. J. Med., 69:383, 1980. Reproduced with permission from the publisher and author.)*

TABLE 24-2 Berberi Heart Disease

	Dates of Catheterization		
	9/22	11/17	12/29
Pressures, mmHg:			
Right atrium	10	5*	3
Pulmonary artery	36/25(32)	25/8(17)	21/7(14)
Pulmonary wedge	22	8.5	8
Systemic arterial O_2 saturation, percent of capacity	87	93	94
Arteriovenous O_2 difference, ml/dl	3.4	4.5	3.1
Cardiac index, liters/min/m^2	6.1	4.9	4.5

*Right ventricular end-diastolic pressure.

Comment This patient was first studied 4 days after admission to the hospital while still in clinical heart failure. The catheterization data from the right side of the heart were consistent with biventricular failure. There was elevation of both right atrial and pulmonary wedge pressures, and the cardiac output was twice the average normal cardiac index of 3.1 liters/min/m^2. The arteriovenous oxygen difference was decreased. After the patient was treated with rest and thiamine, congestive heart failure was no longer present when she was studied on November 17 and December 29. The right atrial and pulmonary wedge pressures were normal at the time of the second and third studies. The cardiac output had decreased but remained above the normal range (cardiac index, 3.1 ± 0.4* liters/min/m^2).

of five cases studied by Ikram et al.,[16] and was not increased in the other four.[16]

Figure 24-1 shows hemodynamic data from nine young patients with cardiac beriberi who were studied by Kawai et al.[17]

Table 24-2 shows hemodynamic studies from one of our patients, a 28-year-old barmaid. The second and third studies were after treatment.

Diagnosis

The criteria for the diagnosis of beriberi heart disease were listed by Blankenhorn.[14] They include a history of a thiamine-deficient diet for 3 months or longer, absence of another cause of heart disease, elevation of systemic venous pressure, edema, enlarged heart, minor electrocardiographic changes, evidence of peripheral neuritis or pellagra, and a response to thiamine with a decrease in heart size, or autopsy findings consistent with the diagnosis. Akbarian and associates reported that elevation of the serum transketolase values was a useful laboratory test.[15] Kawai et al. found erythrocyte transketolase values to be low in beriberi heart disease.[17]

Management

These patients should be treated with bed rest. Because there is a tendency to syncope and sudden death, it is important that they receive treatment early. The optimum treatment is thiamine along with the remainder of the vitamin B complex. Thiamine may be given parenterally in doses of 50 mg daily.

Digitalis has been thought to be of little use,[4] but Akbarian and associates showed that ouabain might be beneficial.[15] Sodium restriction and diuretics are of some value. Lactic acidosis has been described, and cautious bicarbonate infusion may be of merit.[18]

*Standard deviation.

Anemia

Abnormal Physiology

The exact pathophysiology of anemia is not completely understood. The circulatory effects of anemia were reviewed.[3] Possible factors involved in the elevated cardiac output of anemia include variations in ventricular preload, ventricular contractility, and ventricular afterload. Blockade of β-adrenergic nerves does not prevent the increase of left ventricular performance with anemia.[19] Increased preload is not likely to be the major factor but may contribute to some degree. Decreased left ventricular afterload seems to be the most important mechanism.[19] Peripheral vasodilatation, arteriovenous shunts, and decreased blood viscosity may be important. Cardiac output did not rise in dogs when blood oxygen transport was reduced without lowering blood viscosity by means of transfusion of red blood cells containing methemoglobin. Fowler and Holmes showed that experimental anemia increased the cardiac output much less when blood viscosity was not allowed to fall.[20] These observations supported the concept that reduction of blood viscosity is an important mechanism in the increased cardiac output of anemia. In patients with chronic anemia, administration of methoxamine decreased the cardiac output an average of 20 percent.[21] This study is consistent with the concept that decreased peripheral resistance is important in the high cardiac output of anemia. Brannon and associates[22] found that the cardiac output was usually not increased by chronic iron-deficiency anemia until the hemoglobin is below 7 g/dl of blood, or about one-half the normal value. Patients who are anemic may develop congestive heart failure. As in thyrotoxicosis, most patients who develop congestive heart failure with anemia have underlying heart disease, and the anemia serves as an aggravating factor which increases the work of the heart.[3] On the other hand, congestive heart failure may occur from very severe anemia alone. This event is uncommon in the United States but apparently is more common in tropical countries. As a rule, it may be said that cardiac enlargement or congestive heart failure caused solely by chronic blood loss anemia is unlikely unless the hemoglobin is below 5 g/dl of blood. When anemia results from sickle cell disease or from thalassemia, cardiac enlargement may occur with lesser degrees of anemia. In sickle cell anemia this is perhaps a reflection of myocardial and pulmonary arterial disease and an altered oxyhemoglobin dissociation curve.

An echocardiographic study of 44 children with sickle cell anemia (average age 8.6 years) showed significantly depressed left ventricular performance.[23] Dyspnea, dependent edema, and reduction in vital capacity may result from anemia alone without added congestive heart failure.

Clinical Manifestations

Physical Examination

In patients with severe anemia (hemoglobin below 7 g/dl of blood) there is pallor of the skin and mucous membranes. Tachycardia is usually present. The peripheral arterial pulses may be bounding, and there may be a Duroziez's sign and pistol-shot sounds over the femoral artery. There may be "capillary" pulsations in the lips and nail beds. Cervical venous hums are common in these patients, and were described in the majority of patients receiving hemodialysis for renal failure.[24] Early systolic bruits are often found over both carotid arteries. There is commonly a pulmonary midsystolic murmur, presumably reflecting the increased blood flow and turbulence in this area. Murmurs of aortic regurgitation have been described in patients with severe anemia. This finding is extremely unusual in our experience at the University of Cincinnati Hospitals unless the patient is uremic, where hypertension may be a factor. Anemia may be associated with a vibratory or musical systolic Still's murmur. Patients with sickle cell anemia may display a wider variety of cardiac murmurs. A diastolic apical murmur may suggest mitral stenosis, and as a rule the diagnosis of mitral stenosis should be made with great caution in patients with sickle cell anemia. In children with sickle cell anemia, systolic murmurs are found almost invariably.[25] Most commonly these are loudest in the second left intercostal space. A prominent third heart sound in middiastole is common in sickle cell anemia. There is a tendency to expiratory splitting of the second heart sound,[25] and the auscultatory findings of atrial septal defect may be closely simulated. In sickle cell anemia, cor pulmonale may develop because of pulmonary arterial thrombosis, but this complication is uncommon. A 1982 review was able to document only six cases of cor pulmonale related to sickle hemoglobinopathy.[26]

Special Laboratory Studies

Catheterization and Noninvasive Studies

There is an increase of resting cardiac output usually with an additional increase of cardiac stroke volume.[27] With mild anemia (average hemoglobin 9.4 g) the cardiac output was normal at rest, but with exercise it rose more than normally.[27] With maximal treadmill exercise, the peak cardiac output and the exercise level achieved were little affected by anemia, but the oxygen debt was increased. In patients with anemia who develop congestive failure the cardiac output may fall from the peak value but tends to remain above the normal resting value.[27] When studied by echocardiography, patients with sickle cell anemia have increased left ventricular systolic and diastolic dimensions; evidence of ventricular dysfunction may be found.[23,28] In chronic anemia, systolic time intervals were generally normal when blood hemoglobin was above 7 g/dl. In severe anemia without heart failure, PEP was decreased and LVET was increased, with a decrease of PEP/LVET ratio. With severe anemia and heart failure, PEP/LVET ratio was increased.[29]

Management

The treatment of anemia depends on the underlying cause. It is generally believed that digitalis is of little or no benefit in congestive heart failure accompanied by severe anemia.[4] On the other hand, we found that ouabain was effective in anemia heart failure produced in the heart-lung preparation, since it lowered elevated atrial pressures and increased cardiac output. Anemia alone is seldom the cause of heart failure; hence it seems logical to use digitalis when heart failure occurs in an anemic patient. Bed rest, sodium restriction, and diuretics may be desirable. The anemia should be corrected gradually. In chronic anemia,[30] expansion of plasma volume tends to correct total blood volume almost to normal; hence rapid infusion of whole blood in the severely anemic patient may precipitate heart failure with pulmonary edema. When rapid improvement in anemia is necessary, slow infusions of one-half unit of packed red blood cells (125 ml) may be carried out over a period of 3 or 4 h, with careful examination of the patient for dyspnea and auscultation of the lungs for evidence of pulmonary edema. Monitoring pulmonary wedge pressure with the Swan-Ganz flow-directed catheter as a guide to sudden increments to left ventricular diastolic pressure may be desirable in patients with cardiac enlargement or previous congestive heart failure. At times it may be necessary to correct anemia quickly in this way in order to obtain satisfactory improvement in congestive heart failure. Too rapid correction of anemia by transfusing 1000 to 2000 ml of blood or packed red blood cells within 24 h may cause pulmonary edema; this occurs in our institution several times a year. It may be necessary to employ diuretics simultaneously with transfusion, or to use phlebotomy along with transfusion, to prevent a dangerous rise of pulmonary wedge pressure.

Systemic Arteriovenous Fistula

Abnormal Physiology

As a rule, increased cardiac output can be demonstrated only when there is a large fistula that involves a major artery such as the aorta, or such arteries as the subclavian artery, the femoral artery, the common carotid arteries, and the iliac vessels.

Multiple small arteriovenous fistulas may cause a rise of cardiac output. Pulmonary arteriovenous fistulas involve the low-resistance lesser circulation and seldom, if ever, lead to increased cardiac output, cardiac enlargement, or congestive heart failure. When there is an arteriovenous fistula, arterialized blood from a high-pressure artery is shunted into a low-pressure vein, thus decreasing the arterial blood flow to the tissue beyond the fistula and increasing the venous pressure distal to the fistula. The venous pressure proximal to the fistula and pressures in the right side of the heart are usually normal unless there is congestive heart failure. As a compensatory mechanism for the low systemic vascular resistance, the heart rate and stroke volume increase. The diastolic blood pressure falls, and the cardiac output rises. Obliteration of the arteriovenous fistula by compression results in a fall in cardiac output. There tends to be an increase of plasma volume in patients with systemic arteriovenous fistulas.

Physical Findings

If the examiner finds an increased systemic arterial pulse pressure when there is no evidence of aortic regurgitation, the possibility of a systemic arteriovenous fistula should be considered. If the patient has had an injury or a surgical operation, careful auscultation should be carried out over the site in order to look for the typical continuous murmur of arteriovenous fistula with a systolic accentuation. Manual compression of the fistula tends to produce slowing of the heart. This response is known as Branham's sign. Hepatic arteriovenous fistula was reported in two patients with hereditary hemorrhagic telangiectasia,[31] and we have studied two similar patients, each of whom had an elevated cardiac output. Patients with large arteriovenous fistulas may develop congestive heart failure. The onset of heart failure may be quite delayed. In one instance a 30-year-old man who was studied at the Cardiac Laboratory of the Cincinnati General Hospital developed congestive heart failure in 1951, 7 years following a gunshot wound involving the internal iliac artery and vein. In another instance, a 68-year-old patient developed congestive heart failure 57 years after a gunshot wound involving the femoral artery and vein. Presumably, in patients like the latter there is additional underlying heart disease; however, in such patients repair of the fistula may result in the return of heart size and function to normal.

Hepatic Hemangiomatosis

This rare condition has been studied by deLorimier et al.[32] Of 27 patients with hepatic hemangioendothelioma, 23 had cutaneous capillary hemangiomas and all but 2 had heart failure.[32] This lesion acts as an arteriovenous fistula between hepatic artery and veins. The congestive failure responds to hepatic artery ligation; however, in adults hepatic artery ligation might cause fatal hepatic necrosis.

Hemodialysis

Striking increases of cardiac output may be found in patients with subcutaneous arteriovenous fistulas constructed for later hemodialysis.[33] Anemia accompanying uremia usually contributes to the high cardiac output in such patients.

Special Laboratory Studies

Catheterization

Intracardiac pressures are normal unless congestive heart failure develops. If right-sided heart failure develops, right atrial and peripheral venous pressures rise. The cardiac output is above normal resting levels,[34] and may show a greater than normal increase with mild exercise in the absence of heart failure. Left ventricular ejection fraction was normal (0.64) in one recent case of systemic arteriovenous fistula with biventricular failure and an elevated cardiac output of 16 liters/min.[35] Heart failure may develop in patients with apparently normal hearts. The cardiac output may fall with exercise.[34] We have observed, however, that exercise evoked an increase in cardiac output in such patients when the heart was previously normal. The following description illustrates some of the hemodynamic features of a large systemic arteriovenous fistula:

A 57-year-old man was admitted to the hospital because of congestive heart failure for 4 years. Twenty-two years before admission, he had sustained a gunshot wound of the right supraclavicular area. Physical examination revealed signs of a right subclavian arteriovenous fistula. The results of catheterization of the right side of the heart during exercise and at rest are shown in Table 24-3.

Comment The data were consistent with biventricular failure. Both right atrial and pulmonary wedge pressures were above normal. The cardiac index was well above the normal range of 3.1 ± 0.4 liters/min/m^2. The increased cardiac output was associated with a narrow arteriovenous oxygen difference. Venous blood proximal to the fistula showed a step-up in oxygen content of 3.4 volumes per deciliter of blood. With exercise, there was a relatively normal increase of total cardiac output from 7.6 to 8.8 liters/min with an exercise-induced increment of oxygen consumption of 140 ml/min. Such response of cardiac output to exercise would be very unusual for patients with "low-output" heart failure.

TABLE 24-3 Systemic Arteriovenous Fistula

	Rest	Exercise
Pressures, mmHg:		
Right atrium	7	
Pulmonary artery	56/18(31)	64/28(43)
Pulmonary wedge	24	
Systemic arterial O_2 saturation, percent of capacity	92.5	94.4
Arteriovenous O_2 difference, ml/dl	3.3	4.4
O_2 consumption, ml/min	246	386
Cardiac index, liters/min/m^2	4.1	5.1

Diagnosis and Treatment

Systemic arteriovenous fistula should be considered in patients who have an increase in systemic arterial pulse pressure with bounding arterial pulses. When there is no obvious cause of heart failure or for a wide arterial pulse pressure, such as aortic regurgitation, patent ductus arteriosus, severe anemia, or thyrotoxicosis, careful auscultation should be carried out over all scars and major arteries. If the characteristic continuous murmur with systolic accentuation is found in an area of trauma or surgical operation, no further studies should be required to establish the diagnosis. When there is doubt, arteriography may be employed to demonstrate the lesion. In some instances the systemic arteriovenous fistula may become infected so that there is endarteritis. This complication in turn may lead to aortic valve involvement with aortic infective endocarditis. In dogs with large experimental arteriovenous fistulas, aortic, mitral or tricuspid endocarditis may develop with or without infection of the fistula. The treatment of a systemic arteriovenous fistula, when it is large enough to produce increased arterial pulse pressure, cardiac enlargement, or congestive heart failure, should be surgical repair or excision of the fistula.

Hepatic Disease

Resting cardiac output may be increased in patients with liver disease, especially in those with nutritional cirrhosis or infectious hepatitis. The mechanism is uncertain but has been attributed to increased blood volume, intrahepatic arteriovenous shunts, mesenteric arteriovenous shunts, and defects in inactivation of a circulating vasodilator.[36] In a few patients with nutritional cirrhosis or infectious hepatitis, the cardiac output may be considerably elevated and accompanied by the clinical evidence of a bounding pulse and wide pulse pressure. Congestive heart failure may develop,[37] but most patients in this group probably die of hepatic failure before heart failure can develop. One authority has described a cardiac output as high as 15 liters/min, or at least twice the normal, in a patient with infectious hepatitis.[37] Twenty-five cirrhotic patients with responsive ascites tended to have higher cardiac output and lower peripheral resistance than did eight with refractory ascites.[38] An echocardiographic study of 14 patients with liver cirrhosis found significant increases in cardiac index, left ventricular diastolic diameter, and in mean velocity of left ventricular wall contraction.[39]

Paget's Disease of Bone

In Paget's disease of the bone the more common circulatory effects are increased systemic arterial pulse pressure and increased cardiac output. Cor pulmonale and atrioventricular (AV) block may occasionally occur. Lequime and Denolin found evidence of increased blood flow to limbs involved by Paget's disease, but increase of resting cardiac output was unusual.[40] The cardiac output in patients with extensive bone involvement showed a greater than normal increase with exercise. The cardiac index can be correlated roughly with the percentage of skeletal involvement (Fig. 24-2).[41] The increased

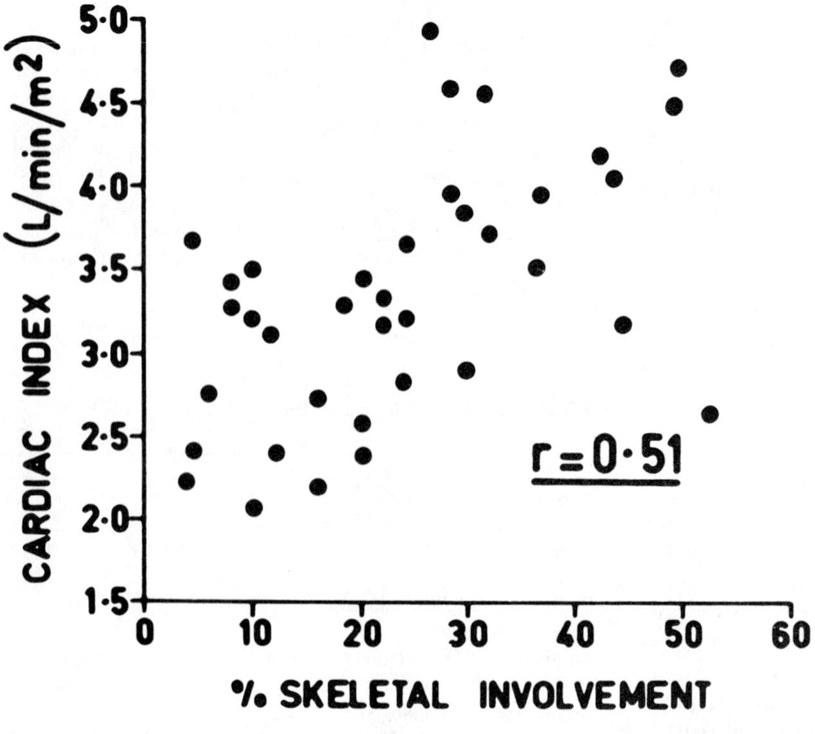

FIGURE 24-2 Scatter plot showing correlation between cardiac index and percentage of skeletal involvement in Paget's disease of bone. *(From J. W. Henley, R. S. Croxson, and H. K. Ibbertson, The Cardiovascular System in Paget's Disease of Bone and the Response to Therapy with Calcitonin and Diphosphonate, Aust. N.Z. J. Med., 9:390, 1979. Reproduced with permission from the publisher and author.)*

cardiac output is presumably related to multiple, small systemic arteriovenous fistulas in the bones involved by this disorder, especially in the lower extremities. No evidence of increased AV shunting in the lower extremities was found in one study.[42] The possibility of Paget's disease of the bone as a cause of an increased systemic arterial pulse pressure must be considered in a middle-aged or older patient who has enlargement of the skull, decreased stature, and bowing of the tibias. Radiologic studies of the skull, pelvis, and bones of the lower extremities will usually confirm the diagnosis. As a rule, serum alkaline phosphatase is increased. Calcitonin therapy may decrease the elevated cardiac output.

Hyperdynamic Heart Syndrome

Gorlin and associates[43] described a hyperkinetic syndrome of unknown cause which they found principally in young patients and in those of early middle age. In their report 24 patients were described. The majority of the patients had an increased cardiac output at rest. Others did not but had an increased rate of ventricular ejection. Bounding peripheral pulses were common. Heart failure developed in some patients observed for as long as 16 years. Electrocardiograms usually showed evidence of left ventricular enlargement. Systolic ejection clicks were common. Ejection and apical pansystolic murmurs were found. Nineteen of these 24 patients were observed for 11 to 25 years. Only two of eight reexamined were found to have a hyperkinetic heart on reexamination; ECG abnormalities and systolic hypertension tended to regress.[44] These patients are believed related to but different from Frolich's group with hyperdynamic β-adrenergic circulatory states.[45] The possibility that a common denominator of increased activity of the sympathetic nervous system exists in these two groups of patients must not be overlooked, since β-adrenergic receptor blockade may be of value in therapy.[45]

Cor Pulmonale (See Chap. 55)

The resting cardiac output may be above normal in some patients with chronic cor pulmonale associated with chronic obstructive airway disease. Increased cardiac output in cor pulmonale associated with obstructive airway disease is not found in the majority of patients.[46] A study of 50 patients with chronic obstructive airway disease found an increased cardiac index ($\geqslant$ 4.0 liters/min) in only two, and these had severe hypoxia and hypercapnia.[47] In our study, the cardiac output in patients with cor pulmonale caused by chronic obstructive lung disease was on the average higher during heart failure than in patients with hypertensive or coronary artery disease accompanied by congestive heart failure.[46]

Polyostotic Fibrous Dysplasia (Albright's Syndrome)

In patients with polyostotic fibrous dysplasia the cardiac output may be increased above normal. The cardiac index was 3.9 liters/min/m^2 or greater in five of six patients studied by McIntosh and associates.[48] Biopsy material from involved bones showed numerous thin-walled sinusoidal capillaries. The authors postulated that the lesions of polyostotic fibrous dysplasia act as minute arteriovenous fistulas, thus increasing cardiac output by lowering peripheral resistance.

Carcinoid Syndrome

The resting cardiac output may be increased in patients with metastatic carcinoid tumors.[49] The patients may have a lowered arteriovenous oxygen difference and decreased peripheral vascular resistance. Serotonin, known to be elaborated by carcinoid tumors, increases myocardial contractility by direct action. It seems likely that the increased cardiac output combined with tricuspid or pulmonary valve deformity, often found in patients with the carcinoid syndrome, may explain the high incidence of heart failure in this disease.

Warm and Humid Environment (See Chap. 84)

Burch and associates[50] studied 10 subjects in New Orleans during the summers of 1957 and 1958. The mean of their cardiac outputs when in an air-conditioned ward was 4.0 liters/min. When the subjects were exposed to environmental conditions with the room temperature of 30.5 to 33.3°C (87 to 92°F) and relative humidity 58 to 93 percent, the mean cardiac output rose 43 percent to 5.7 liters/min. Calculated ventricular work rose in some subjects, suggesting that an air-conditioned ward may reduce the workload of the heart in some patients with heart disease. Short periods of exposure to dry heat apparently had little effect on cardiac output. When whole-body hyperthermia was used to treat malignant neoplasms, however, a body temperature of 41.8°C (107.1°F) was associated with doubling of cardiac output.[51]

Cold Environment (See Chap. 84)

In healthy young men exposed to 5°C ambient temperature, cardiac output and total body oxygen consumption were increased.[52] Since the arteriovenous oxygen difference was also increased, the rise of cardiac output can be explained by the increased metabolic demands of the tissues.

Renal Disease

In acute glomerulonephritis, the cardiac output at rest may be normal (in other words, relatively high) when the right atrial pressure is elevated, and there are clinical features usually found in heart disease.[53] Some patients have hypervolemia, increased systemic venous pressure, enlargement of the heart, and pulmonary edema. Systemic atrial hypertension is common. The decreased glomerular filtration and increased aldosterone secretion lead to retention of sodium and water with resultant hypervolemia. Some such patients, when treated with intravenous digoxin, show no decrease of right atrial or venous pressure, no increase of cardiac output, and no sodium or water diuresis.[4] The authors concluded that some patients with edema and increased venous pressure with acute glomerulonephritis do not have heart failure.

An increase of resting cardiac index, not explained by fever or anemia, may be found in patients with acute renal failure associated with tubular necrosis. With chronic renal failure and anemia, the cardiac output is usually increased.[54] The cardiac output was found to return to normal when the anemia was corrected. Patients undergoing hemodialysis for the treatment of uremia tend to have an elevated cardiac output. In addition to anemia, the shunt used for dialysis and a uremic hypermetabolic state may contribute to the elevated cardiac output.[33]

Polycythemia Vera

The cardiac output and cardiac stroke index may be increased in patients with polycythemia vera.[55] The mechanism of increased cardiac output is uncertain but appears to be correlated with the degree of hypervolemia. Right atrial and pulmonary wedge pressures are not increased.

Pregnancy (See Chap. 69)

During normal pregnancy the cardiac output increases progressively until the seventh or eighth month. The increase averages 30 to 50 percent.

Certain Cutaneous Diseases

A significant increase in the resting cardiac output may occur in patients with "erythrodermic" skin disease. It is believed that increased blood flow to the skin might be at least partly responsible for the elevated cardiac output. Hecht and coworkers found high resting cardiac output in psoriasis and in exfoliative dermatitis and also demonstrated a hyperdynamic state in patients with Kaposi's sarcoma.[56]

Obesity (See Chap. 75)

In extreme obesity, the cardiac output tends to be increased, but only in proportion to the increased weight and oxygen consumption. The arteriovenous oxygen difference is not decreased.[57] Obese subjects ($\geqslant$ 150 percent ideal body weight) were found to have increased cardiac output, stroke volume and total blood volume, and decreased peripheral resistance.[58]

Systemic Arterial Hypertension (See Chap. 49)

The resting cardiac index has been found to be elevated in some patients with labile hypertension or borderline blood pressure elevation. The cardiac output tends to be higher in those patients with labile hypertension than in those with established hypertension. An increased cardiac output, however, may be found in some patients with severe hypertension.[59]

Drugs that Tend to Cause a High Cardiac Output

The cardiac output may be raised by certain drugs that have a positive cardiac inotropic effect (isoproterenol, dopamine, epinephrine) and by certain vasodilators (nitrates, calcium channel blocking agents, hydralazine). Seldom does the cardiac output in patients treated for congestive heart failure rise above normal levels as the result of vasodilator therapy, but this may occasionally happen with nifedipine[60] or hydralazine.[61] In some patients the clinical signs of hyperdynamic state are reproduced. We are reporting a recent instance in which cardiac output rose from 4.5 to 10.1 liters/min with appearance of wide arterial pulse pressure (194/85 mmHg) and systolic arterial bruits when nitroprusside was used intravenously to treat congestive heart failure.[62]

References

1. Burwell, C. S., and Dexter, L.: Beri-Beri Heart Disease, *Trans. Assoc. Am. Physicians,* 60:59, 1957.
2. Braunwald, E.: On the Difference between the Heart's Output and Its Contractile State, *Circulation,* 43:171, 1971 (editorial).
3. Varat, M. A., Adolph, R. J., and Fowler, N. O.: Cardiovascular Effects of Anemia, *Am. Heart J.,* 83:415, 1972.
4. Eichna, L. W., Farber, S. J., Berger, A. R., Rader, R., Smith, W. W., and Albert, R. E.: Non-cardiac Circulatory Congestion Simulating Congestive Heart Failure, *Trans. Assoc. Am. Physicians,* 68:72, 1954.
5. Graettinger, J. S., Muenster, J. J., Selverstone, L. A., and Campbell, J. A.: A Correlation of Clinical and Hemodynamic Studies in Patients with Hyperthyroidism with and without Congestive Heart Failure, *J. Clin. Invest.* 38:1316, 1959.

6. Klein, I., and Levy, G. S.: New Perspectives on Thyroid Hormone, Catecholamines, and the Heart, *Am. J. Med.*, 76:167, 1984.
7. Lewis, B. S., Ehrenfeld, E. N., and Lewis, N.: Echocardiographic LV Function in Thyrotoxicosis, *Am. Heart J.*, 97:460, 1979.
8. Theilen, E. O., and Wilson, W. R.: Hemodynamic Effects of Peripheral Vasoconstriction in Normal and Thyrotoxic Subjects, *J. Appl. Physiol.*, 22:207, 1967.
9. Leonard, J. J., and deGroot, W. J.: The Thyroid State and the Cardiovascular System, *Mod. Concepts Cardiovasc. Dis.*, 38:23, 1969.
10. Borst, G. C., Eil, C., and Burman, K. D.: Euthyroid Hyperthyroxinemia, *Ann. Intern. Med.*, 98:366, 1983.
11. Lien, E., and Aanderud, S.: Systolic Time Intervals in the Evaluation of Thyroid Dysfunction, *Acta Med. Scand.*, 211:265, 1982.
12. Merillon, J. P., Passa, P., Chastre, J., et al.: Left Ventricular Function and Hyperthyroidism, *Br. Heart J.*, 46:137, 1981.
13. Blonde, L., and Skelton, C. L.: Hyperthyroidism and Cardiovascular Disease: Concepts and Management, *Cardiovasc. Med.*, 1145, 1978.
14. Blankenhorn, M. A.: Effect of Vitamin Deficiency on the Heart and Circulation, *Circulation*, 11:288, 1955.
15. Akbarian, M., Yankopoulos, N. A., and Abelmann, W. H.: Hemodynamic Studies in Beriberi Heart Disease, *Am. J. Med.*, 41:197, 1966.
16. Ikram, H., Maslowski, A. H., Smith, B. L., et al.: The Haemodynamic, Histopathological, and Hormonal Features of Alcoholic Cardiac Beriberi, *Quart J. Med.*, 200:359, 1981.
17. Kawai, C., Wakabayashi, A., Matsumura, T., et al.: Reappearance of Beriberi Heart Disease in Japan, *Am. J. Med.*, 69:383, 1980.
18. Attas, M., Hanley, H. G., Stultz, D., Jones, M. R., and McAllister, R. G.: Fulminant Berberi Heart Disease with Lactic Acidosis: Presentation of a Case with Evaluation of Left Ventricular Function and Review of Pathophysiologic Mechanisms, *Circulation*, 58:566, 1978.
19. Fowler, N. O., and Holmes, J. C.: Ventricular Function in Anemia, *J. Appl. Physiol.*, 31:260, 1971.
20. Fowler, N. O., and Holmes, J. C.: Blood Viscosity and Cardiac Output in Acute Experimental Anemia, *J. Appl. Physiol.*, 39:453, 1975.
21. Duke, M., and Abelmann, W. H.: The Hemodynamic Response to Chronic Anemia, *Circulation*, 39:503, 1969.
22. Brannon, E. S., Merrill, A. J., Warren, J. V., and Stead, E. A., Jr.: The Cardiac Output in Patients with Chronic Anemia as Measured by the Techniques of Right Atrial Catheterization, *J. Clin. Invest.*, 24:332, 1945.
23. Rees, A. H., Stefadouros, M. A., Strong, W. B., Miller, M. D., Gilman, P., Rigby, J. A., and McFarlane, J.: Left Ventricular Performance in Children with Homozygous Sickle Cell Anaemia, *Br. Heart J.*, 40:690, 1978.
24. Danaly, D. T., and Ronan, J. A., Jr.: Cervical Venous Hums in Patients on Chronic Hemodialysis, *N. Engl. J. Med.*, 291:237, 1974.
25. Shubin, H., Kaufman, R., Shapiro, M., and Levinson, D. C.: Cardiovascular Findings in Children with Sickle Cell Anemia, *Am. J. Cardiol.*, 6:875, 1960.
26. Collins, F. S., and Orringer, E. P.: Pulmonary Hypertension in the Sickle Hemoglobinopathies, *Am. J. Med.*, 73:814, 1982.
27. Graettinger, J. S., Parsons, R. L., and Campbell, J. A.: A Correlation of Clinical and Hemodynamic Studies in Patients with Mild and Severe Anemia with and without Congestive Failure, *Ann. Intern. Med.*, 58:617, 1963.
28. Val-Mejias, J., Lee, W. K., Weisse, A. B., and Regan, T. J.: Left Ventricular Performance during and after Sickle Cell Crisis, *Am. Heart J.*, 97:585, 1979.
29. Abdullah, A. K., Siddiqui, M. A., and Tajuddin, M.: Systolic Time Intervals in Chronic Anemia, *Am. Heart J.*, 94:287, 1977.
30. Duke, M., Herbert, V. D., and Abelmann, W. H.: Hemodynamic Effects of Blood Transfusion in Chronic Anemia, *N. Engl. J. Med.*, 271:975, 1964.
31. Razi, B., Beller, B. M., Ghidoni, J., Linhart, J. W., Talley, R. C., and Urban, E.: Hyperdynamic States due to Intrahepatic Fistula in Osler-Weber-Rendu Disease, *Am. J. Med.*, 50:809, 1971.
32. deLorimier, A. A., Simpson, E. B., Baum, R. S., and Carlsson, E.: Hepatic Artery Ligation for Hepatic Hemangiomatosis, *N. Engl. J. Med.*, 277:333, 1967.
33. McMillan, R., and Evans, D. B.: Experience with Three Brescia-Cimino Shunts, *Br. Med. J.*, 3:781, 1968.
34. Muenster, J. J., Graettinger, J. S., and Campbell, A. J.: Correlation of Clinical and Hemodynamic Findings in Patients with Systemic Arteriovenous Fistulas, *Circulation*, 20:1079, 1959.
35. Johnson, R. A., and Boucher, C. A.: Normal Left Ventricular Ejection Fraction in Systemic A-V Fistula, *Chest*, 79:607, 1981.
36. Schlant, R. C.: Cardiovascular Effects of Hepatic Cirrhosis, in J. W. Hurst (ed.), "Update III: The Heart," McGraw-Hill Book Company, New York, 1980, p. 129.
37. Murray, J. F., Dawson, A. M., and Sherlock, S.: Circulatory Changes in Chronic Liver Disease, *Am. J. Med.*, 24:358, 1958.
38. Lebrec, D., Kotelanski, B., and Cohn, J. N.: Splanchnic Hemodynamic Factors in Cirrhosis with Refractory Ascites, *J. Lab. Clin. Med.*, 93:301, 1979.
39. Lewis, B. S., Tur-Kaspa, R., and Lewis, N.: Left Ventricular Function in Liver Cirrhosis: An Echocardiographic Study, *Isr. J. Med. Sci.*, 16:489, 1980.
40. Lequime, J., and Denolin, H.: Circulatory Dynamics in Osteitis Deformans, *Circulation*, 12:215, 1955.
41. Henley, J. W., Croxson, R. S., and Ibbertson, H. K.: The Cardiovascular System in Paget's Disease of Bone and the Response to Therapy with Calcitonin and Diphosphonate, *Aust. N.Z. J. Med.*, 9:390, 1979.
42. Rhodes, B. A., Grayson, N. D., Hamilton, C. R., Jr., White, R. I., Jr., Giargiana, F. A., Jr. and Wagner, H. N., Jr.: Absence of Arteriovenous Shunts in Paget's Disease of Bone, *N. Engl. J. Med.*, 287:686, 1972.
43. Gorlin, R.: The Hyperkinetic Heart Syndrome, *JAMA*, 182:823, 1962.
44. Gillum, R. F., Teichholz, L. E., Herman, M. V., et al.: The Idiopathic Hyperkinetic Heart Syndrome: Clinical Course and Long-Term Prognosis, *Am. Heart J.*, 102:728, 1981.
45. Frolich, E. D.: Beta Adrenergic Blockade in the Circulatory Regulation of Hyperkinetic States, *Am. J. Cardiol.*, 27:195, 1971.
46. Fowler, N. O., Westcott, R. N., Scott, R. C., and Hess, E.: The Cardiac Output in Chronic Cor Pulmonale, *Circulation*, 6:888, 1952.
47. Barrows, B., Kettel, L. J., Niden, A. H., et al.: Patterns of Cardiovascular Dysfunction in Chronic Obstructive Lung Disease, *N. Engl. J. Med.*, 286:912, 1972.
48. McIntosh, H. D., Miller, D. E., Gleason, W. L., and Goldner, J. L.: The Circulatory Dynamics of Polyostotic Fibrous Dysplasia, *Am. J. Med.*, 32:393, 1962.
49. Schwaber, J. R., and Lukas, D. S.: Hyperkinemia and Cardiac Failure in the Carcinoid Syndrome, *Am. J. Med.*, 32:846, 1962.
50. Burch, G. E., dePasquale, N., Hyman, A., and DeGraff, A. C.: Influence of Tropical Weather on Cardiac Output, Work, and Power of Right and Left Ventricles of Man Resting in Hospital, *A.M.A. Arch. Intern. Med.*, 104:553, 1959.
51. Bull, J. M., Lees, D., Schuette, W., Whang-Peng, J., Smith, R., Bynum, G., Atkinson, E. R., Gottdiener, J. A., Gralnick, H. R., Shawker, T. H., and DeVita V. T., Jr.: Whole Body Hyperthermia. A Phase-1 Trial of a Potential Adjuvant to Chemotherapy, *Ann. Intern. Med.*, 90:317, 1979.
52. Raven, P. B., Niki, I., Dahms, T. E., and Horvath, S. M.: Compensatory Cardiovascular Responses during Environmental Cold Stress, 5°C, *J. Appl. Physiol.*, 29:417, 1970.
53. Farber, S. J.: Physiologic Aspects of Glomerulonephritis, *J. Chronic Dis.*, 5:87, 1957.
54. Neff, M. S., Kim, K. E., Persoff, M., Onesti, G., and Swartz, C.: Hemodynamics of Uremic Anemia, *Circulation*, 43:876, 1971.
55. Cobb, L. A., Kramer, R. J., and Finch, C. A.: Circulatory

Effects of Chronic Hypervolemia in Polycythemia Vera, *J. Clin. Invest.*, 39:1722, 1960.
56. Hecht, H. H. (by invitation), Candiolo, B. M., Malkinson, F. D., Nair, K. G., and Saqueton, A. C.: On Cardio-cutaneous syndromes, *Trans. Assoc. Am. Physicians*, 80:91, 1967.
57. White, R. I., Jr., and Alexander, J. K.: Body Oxygen Consumption and Pulmonary Ventilation in Obese Subjects, *J. Appl. Physiol.*, 20:197, 1965.
58. Messerli, F. H., Sundgaard-Riise, K., Reisin, E., et al.: Disparate Cardiovascular Effects of Obesity and Arterial Hypertension, *Am. J. Med.*, 74:808, 1983.
59. Ibrahim, M. M., Tarazi, R. C., and Dustan, H. P.: Hyperkinetic Heart in Severe Hypertension: A Separate Clinical Hemodynamic Entity, *Am. J. Cardiol.*, 35:667, 1975.
60. Matsumoto, S., Ito, T., Sada, T., et al.: Hemodynamic Effects of Nifedipine in Heart Failure, *Am. J. Cardiol.*, 46:476, 1980.
61. Hindman, M. D., Slosky, D. A., Peter, R. H., et al.: Rest and Exercise Hemodynamic Effects of Oral Hydralazine in Patients With Coronary Artery Disease and Left Ventricular Dysfunction, *Circulation*, 61:751, 1980.
62. Fullin, K., and Fowler, N. O.: Clinical Hyperdynamic State in Congestive Heart Failure Treated with Vasodilator Drugs. (in preparation, 1984.)

25

Mechanisms of Arrhythmias and Conduction Abnormalities

Warren M. Smith, M.B. John J. Gallagher, M.D.

No fact is better established concerning the histological structure of cardiac muscle than that there exist connexions between the various portions or columns of cells. There exist therefore closed circuits in the myocardium. Supposing an excitation to be started in such a closed circuit and supposing that for some reason it travels in one direction but not in the other. If the rate of propagation is rapid as compared with the duration of the wave, the whole circuit will be in the excited state at the same time, and the excitation will die out. . . . But if, on the other hand, the wave is slower and shorter (and it is made slower and shorter by the conditions which produce fibrillation) the excited state will have passed off at the region where the excitation started before the wave of excitation reaches this point on the circle at the completion of its revolution. Not only so, but there will have been time for the excitability of the muscle to return to something near the value it had at the time of the first excitation. Under these circumstances, the wave of excitation may spread a second time over the same tract of tissue; once started in this way it will continue unless interfered with by some external stimulus arriving during that part of the cycle when the portion of the muscle stimulated is neither in the excited state nor in the condition of depressed excitability which outlasts it.

G. R. Mines, 1913[1,*]

The term *arrhythmia* implies a deviation beyond conventionally defined limits of the rate or regularity of the heartbeat or any disturbance in the normal sequence of cardiac activation. In the normal heart, impulses arise from the sinoatrial node because it has the fastest inherent rate of depolarization (i.e., the highest degree of automaticity—see Chap. 4). Arbitrarily, rates between 60 and 100 impulses per minute are defined as normal and result in atrial contraction followed shortly by ventricular contraction. Rhythm disturbances may be classified in a variety of ways, including rate, site of origin, and site of conduction delay or block.

In the early 1900s, Mines, Lewis, and other investigators of the day[1–8] attempted to identify the role of automaticity and reentry in cardiac arrhythmias. To this day we remain with a similar dilemma. With the advent of direct microelectrode recordings of cellular activity[9,10] and the voltage clamp technique,[11,12] a gap began to develop between our knowledge of in vitro cellular events and observed clinical arrhythmias. The application to patients of multiple catheter-electrode recordings from the atria, ventricles, and specialized conducting tissues (Chaps. 18, 101, and 102), together with the use of programmed stimulation, led to remarkable advances. Unfortunately, present methodology does not yet permit us to define precisely the mechanisms responsible for many clinical arrhythmias. Nor are we yet at the point where knowledge of a specific mechanism can be equated with specific therapy. Nevertheless the ability to reproduce experimentally disorders that resemble clinical arrhythmias often has led to hypotheses regarding the pathogenesis of these abnormalities in humans. While it remains difficult to get a total representation of any arrhythmia at the cellular level alone, realization of the complexity of the cellular basis of cardiac arrhythmias is a necessary first step to eventual effective clinical control.

In the following sections, the basic mechanisms of arrhythmias as they are presently understood are discussed, beginning with abnormalities of impulse formation (including automaticity and triggered au-

*Reproduced with permission from the publisher.

tomaticity), impulse conduction (including reentry and repolarization arrhythmias), and combinations of both these mechanisms.[13–26]

Mechanisms of Arrhythmias

Impulse Formation

This section will discuss (1) normal automaticity, (2) abnormal automaticity, and (3) triggered activity. These phenomena can all be demonstrated at a cellular level and are the result of impulse formation due to diastolic depolarization occurring during phase IV of the action potential.[13,18–20,22,24–38]

Normal Automaticity

The ability to develop slow diastolic depolarization allows some cells in the heart to reach threshold spontaneously and initiate action potentials. This property of self-initiation of excitation independently of any prior impulse is properly termed *automaticity*. This is evident in the sinus node, while additionally some specialized cells in the atria, distal atrioventricular (AV) node, bundle of His, bundle branches, and Purkinje network possess the latent ability to become pacemakers.

The two most important factors determining the rate of firing of automatic cells (see Fig. 4-9) are the slope of diastolic depolarization, which is more important, and the difference between maximum diastolic potential and threshold potential. Thus the normal hierarchy of pacemaker dominance in the heart reflects the gradual decrease of the slope of phase IV depolarization as one moves down the conducting system from the sinus node to the peripheral Purkinje network. The dominant pacemaker also suppresses the rate of firing of subsidiary pacemakers by overdrive,[25] as well as underdrive,[39] suppression.

The sinus node is under the tonal influence of the autonomic nervous system and can alter its rate of firing, resulting in sinus bradycardia or tachycardia. Enhanced vagal activity can inhibit sinus node automaticity but may have minimal effect on the automaticity of latent pacemakers in the atrium or His-Purkinje system, allowing a passive shift in the site of impulse formation to ectopic sites.

Usurpation of sinus node dominance by a subsidiary pacemaker may also occur if its rate of firing has been abnormally increased, a situation referred to as *enhanced automaticity*. Such enhanced automaticity is not observed in ordinary atrial or ventricular cells (Fig. 25-1), arises at high levels of maximum diastolic potential (i.e., greater than −60 mV), and is capable of being suppressed by overdrive pacing. It may occur in fibers exhibiting either a fast or a slow response.

There are probably several ionic mechanisms underlying spontaneous diastolic depolarization. The most obvious example is the difference in automaticity exhibited by fibers capable of the fast response compared with fibers with a slow response (see Chap.

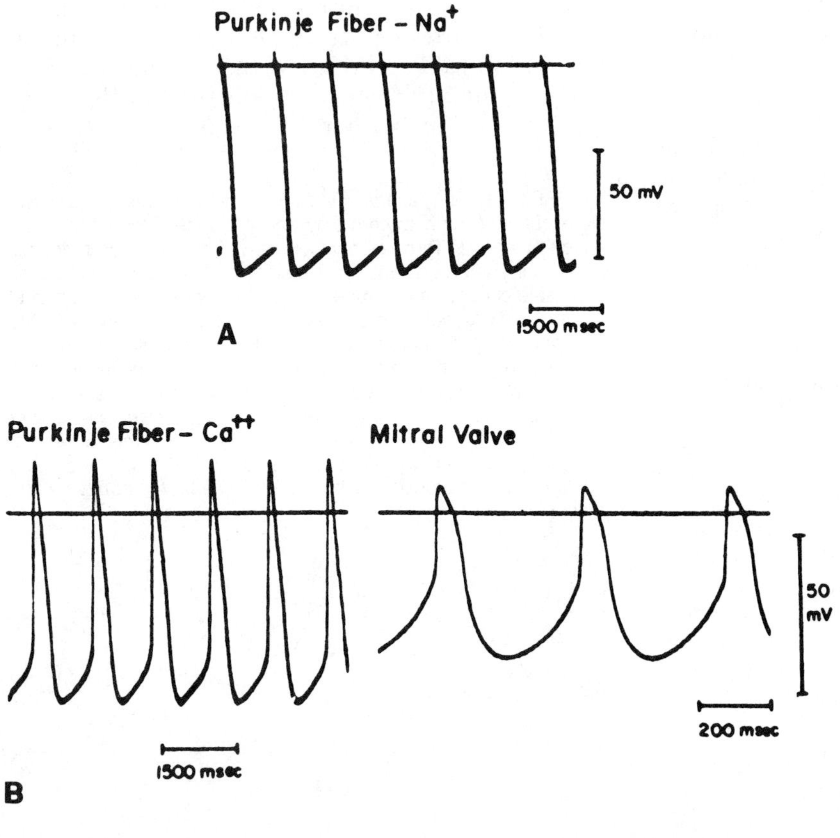

FIGURE 25-1 Automatic activity associated with the "fast" and "slow" response. *A.* Spontaneous diastolic depolarization and fast-response activity recorded from a canine Purkinje fiber with a maximum diastolic potential of −90 mV. *B.* On the left is shown a slow response recorded from a canine Purkinje fiber perfused with a sodium-free medium. Spontaneous diastolic depolarization is prominent, and the maximum diastolic potential is −65 mV. On the right is shown slow-response potentials recorded from a cardiac fiber in the mitral valve leaflet of a monkey. Prominent phase IV depolarization is present. The maximum diastolic potential in this fiber is −58 mV. (*From A. L. Wit, M. R. Rosen, and B. F. Hoffman, Electrophysiology and Pharmacology of Cardiac Arrhythmias: II. Relationship of Normal and Abnormal Electrical Activity of Cardiac Fibers to the Genesis of Arrhythmias: B. Reentry, Am. Heart J., 88:798, 1974. Reproduced with permission from the publisher and author.*)

4). Fast-response fibers in the atrium and specialized conduction system are capable of spontaneous depolarization that begins after repolarization to a maximum diastolic potential of greater than −60 mV and results from a time- and voltage-dependent decrease in membrane potassium (K^+) conductance and a coexisting steady inward sodium (Na^+) current. When the rate of spontaneous diastolic repolarization is rapid and the threshold is normal, the resulting action potential will have a fast Na^+-dependent depolarization phase or a so-called fast response (Fig. 25-1*A*). The slope of spontaneous diastolic depolarization in these circumstances will be enhanced by a fall and suppressed by a rise in extra cellular potassium. Under certain conditions, the upstroke and repolarization phases of the fast-fiber action potential can be converted to the slow response while the mechanism for spontaneous diastolic depolarization remains characteristic for fast fibers.[20]

A second mechanism of spontaneous diastolic depolarization probably exists only in slow-response fibers. It occurs at low maximum diastolic potentials of −60 mV or less (Fig. 25-1*B*) when the fast response is inactivated. The prototype for spontaneous diastolic depolarization in slow fibers is the sinus node, although this type of automaticity probably occurs in cardiac fibers of the mitral and tricuspid valves as well as the lower AV node (Fig. 25-1*B*).

Abnormal Automaticity

Under appropriate conditions, ordinary atrial and ventricular muscle cells, as well as specialized conducting tissue, may become capable of spontaneous impulse generation by phase IV depolarization if they are partially depolarized to the order of −50 or −60 mV.[40–44] Thus, the number of potential sites of disturbance that is due to impulse formation outside the sinus node is greatly expanded in the setting of disease. Such abnormal automaticity may be slowed by acetylcholine and accelerated by catecholamines, but does not necessarily suppress, and may in fact be accelerated by, overdrive pacing.

Triggered Activity

In contrast to normal and abnormal mechanisms of automaticity, where spontaneous diastolic depolarization occurs independently of any preceding impulse, triggered activity requires an initiating action potential (automatic or stimulated) before one or more additional abnormal impulses are generated. Thus cells exhibiting this mechanism may be quiescent in the absence of an excitatory stimulus, but once excited, they give rise to two or more action potentials or a long run of repetitive responses. Triggered activity results from depolarizing afterpotentials, which may be of two types: early and delayed afterdepolarization.[27–37]

Early afterdepolarizations occur when a fiber fails to repolarize completely after completion of the action potential upstroke (Fig. 25-2). Oscillatory depolarizations may occur at intermediate levels of membrane potential which may reach threshold and initiate one or more responses. Although they have been demonstrated experimentally in fibers perfused with Na^+-free solutions, they have also been induced when normal Purkinje fibers are exposed to very high concentrations of catecholamines.[45] Thus, early afterdepolarizations could be relevant in some clinical situations, although this is as yet unproven.

Delayed afterdepolarizations occur after completion of phase III repolarization, although the maximum diastolic potential is usually slightly reduced from normal (Fig. 25-3). These afterdepolarizations may attain threshold and initiate a premature response, and because of the tendency for the amplitude of the afterdepolarization to increase with decreasing preceding cycle length, repetitive firing is likely if one afterdepolarization reaches threshold (Fig. 25-4). Furthermore, there is a tendency for

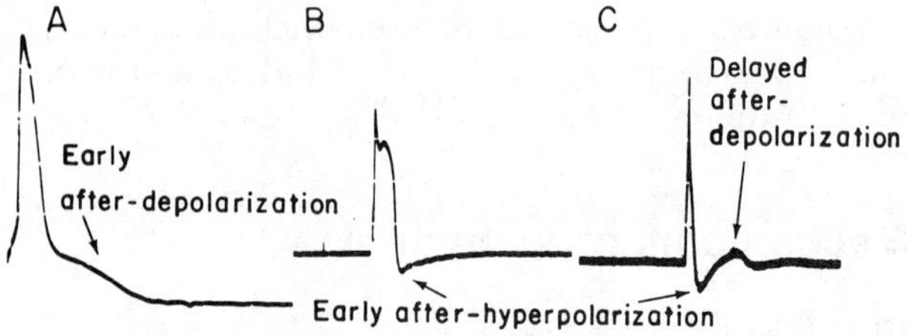

FIGURE 25-2 Various types of afterpotentials. The delay in repolarization shown in *A* is an early afterdepolarization; the swing in membrane potential during repolarization to a level more negative than the resting potential shown in *B* and *C* is an early afterhyperpolarization; in *C*, the early afterhyperpolarization is followed by a delayed afterdepolarization. (*From P. F. Cranefield, "The Conduction of the Cardiac Impulse," Futura Publishing Company, Mount Kisco, New York, 1975, p. 199. Reproduced with the permission from the publisher and author.*)

FIGURE 25-3 Early afterdepolarization. The action potentials shown were obtained by a rhythmically active canine Purkinje fiber exposed to normal Tyrode's solution. *A.* A normal action potential. *B.* An early afterdepolarization (arrow). *C.* Four nondriven action potentials occur at a membrane potential corresponding to that of the early afterdepolarization. Behavior of the kind seen in *B* and *C* is often seen in vitro in fibers usually regarded as having been slightly damaged during dissection or during mounting in the tissue bath. Time marks appears at 1-s intervals. (*From P. F. Cranefield, Does Spontaneous Activity Arise from Phase 4 Depolarization or from Triggering?, in F. Bonke (ed.), "The Sinus Node: Structure, Function and Clinical Relevance," Martinus Nijhoff, The Hague. 1978, p. 348. Reproduced with permission from the publisher and author.*)

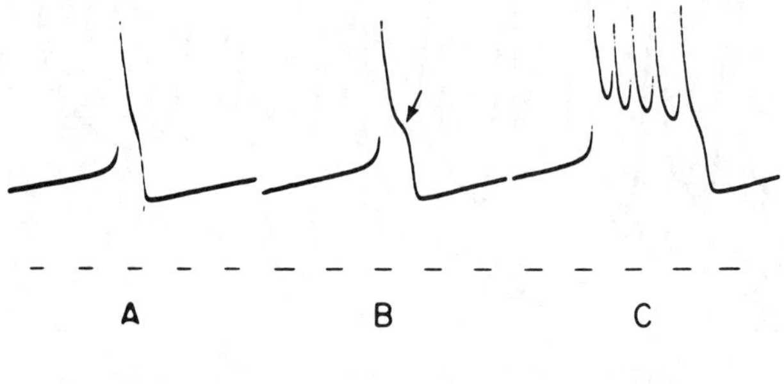

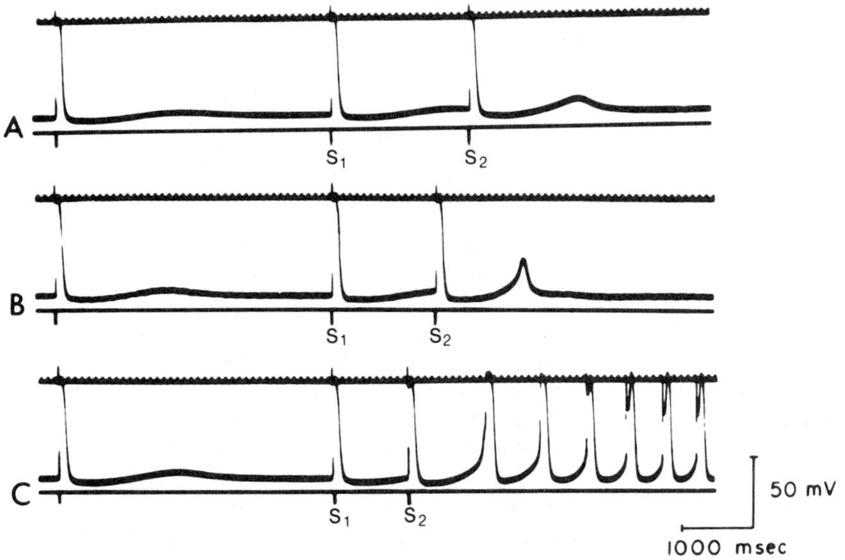

FIGURE 25-4 Afterdepolarization and triggered activity. The potentials shown were recorded from a canine coronary sinus. The transmembrane recording is shown on the middle trace of each panel, and the time of stimulation is indicated by a vertical marker on the bottom trace. The fiber is stimulated at a cycle length of 4000 ms for 10 cycles and is then stimulated prematurely; in each panel, the last cycle of the basic drive train is shown followed by a premature stimulus (S_2), which is delivered at increasing prematurity from *A* to *C*. *A*. At a coupling interval of 2000 ms, the afterdepolarization is 11 mV in amplitude and occurs long after the premature response. *B*. The coupling interval is decreased to 1400 ms. The afterdepolarization increases to 31 mV in amplitude and peaks relatively soon after the premature response. *C*. The coupling interval is 1000 ms. Triggered activity now arises from the peak of the afterdepolarization and is sustained. In addition note the "warm-up" in the rate of triggered activity. *(From A. L. Wit and P. F. Cranefield, Triggered Automatic Activity in the Canine Coronary Sinus, Circ. Res., 41:435, 1977. Reproduced with permission from the American Heart Association, Inc., and the author.)*

successive afterdepolarizations to occur earlier and earlier with respect to their predecessors, until a stable rate is reached, which may exceed the original driven rate. Delayed afterdepolarizations have been recorded from specialized atrial fibers, Purkinje fibers, and myocardial cells in the setting of digitalis intoxication.[36] The mechanism for delayed afterdepolarization is still uncertain, although it is likely that the extracellular sodium concentration or inward sodium current is important. Triggerable activity has been described in fibers from the atrial surface of the mitral and tricuspid valves in the normal dog and monkey,[27,31] the canine coronary sinus,[32] and the human mitral valve.[33] Thus, because sustained rhythmic activity due to this mechanism can be induced and terminated by stimulation, triggered activity exhibits behavior formerly reserved for reentry (see below). Nonetheless, other distinctive features are also present:

1. There is a tendency toward a gradual increasing rate or so-called warm-up effect.
2. The phenomenon is usually observed at fast basic rates (in contrast to reentry, which is more common at slow rates).
3. Overdrive pacing results in acceleration of the rate of activity (in contrast to reentry, which in general terminates or is unaffected by overdrive).
4. The number of triggered responses appears directly related to the basic cycle length of pacing (no such direct relation seen with reentry).
5. Triggered activity can be promptly suppressed by verapamil, whereas reentry (at least that confined to small regions in the ventricle) seems resistant to verapamil.

At present the role of triggered activity in the genesis of clinically observed arrhythmias is unknown, although some reports have alluded to this mechanism.[37,38]

Other less well-studied and defined mechanisms of abnormal automaticity have been recorded,[22,28,34] including oscillatory changes (prepotentials) in membrane potential, which gradually increase until an action potential is evoked, as well as slow and very gradual depolarization (in contrast to the usual phase IV depolarization) in markedly abnormal fibers.[28]

Impulse Conduction

Abnormalities of impulse propagation or conduction are probably more common as a basis for arrhythmias than abnormal impulse formation. In this section, the basis of conduction delay and block will be examined, followed by consideration of the concepts of reentry and reflection.

As previously noted, the cardiac fibers constitute a syncytium and may be likened to cylindrical conductors surrounded by an insulating membrane. This membrane has properties of capacitance and a high electrical resistance; in contrast, the intercalating disks that connect fibers end to end present a pathway of low resistance. These anatomic and electrophysiological properties liken cardiac fibers to a cable conductor, favoring longitudinal progression of current, although the complexities of fiber dimension and geometry of cells must be taken into account.[46]

In Chap. 4, the factors principally determining conduction velocity in cardiac fibers were noted to be (1) the action potential amplitude, (2) the rate of rise of the action potential in phase 0, (3) the threshold potential, and (4) the internal and external resistance. Action potential amplitude, by its influence on the flow of depolarizing current, determines the distance ahead that already depolarized tissue can initiate a propagated action potential. Increasing the magnitude of this depolarizing current allows excitation of quiescent tissue at a greater distance ahead. Similarly, increasing the rate of depolarization accelerates conduction because threshold can be reached more rapidly in more distant excitable tissues. Decreasing thresholds can enhance conduction velocity by decreasing the amount of current needed to initiate propagated action potentials ahead of a wave front. Finally, lower resistance to axial flow made possible by the presence of more numerous "tight" junctions favors longitudinal flow of current in the direction of the wave front, while an increase in sarcolemma resistance also favors longitudinal current flow by reducing the loss of depolarizing current across the membrane perpendicular to the wave front of activation.[24]

Changes in local properties along the route of conduction can influence conduction velocity, accounting for decremental conduction. This phenomenon was first recognized in the laboratory by Erlanger[6,7] during studies of conduction disorders caused by pressure and local application of potassium in the canine His bundle. Thus, if a normal action potential encounters a region of myocardium with slow conduction velocity, the amplitude of the propagating impulse gradually attenuates. In parallel with this loss of amplitude, the impulse constitutes a progressively less adequate stimulus to unexcited tissues in its path, so that successful conduction depends on the length of the abnormal segment, the amplitude and upstroke velocity of the action potential that penetrates the segment, and the threshold or responsiveness of the fibers beyond the abnormal segment. Severe decremental conduction results in block, after which impulse spread will be in accordance with the passive electrical properties of the zone (electrotonic spread). Slow decremental conduction may be mediated by either a depressed fast fiber response or a true slow fiber response. Thus, under abnormal conditions of ischemia and hypoxia cells such as Purkinje fibers can lose their fast response and revert to a slow-response mechanism similar to that in the AV node.[47–49] In such circumstances, the success of propagation is not as critically dependent on the length of the abnormal segment or on the rate of rise of the action potential that entered the abnormal segment. Nonetheless, the safety factor for conduction is low and block is not uncommon. A correlation has also been shown between the presence of atrial arrhythmias clinically and in vitro demonstration of slow responses in diseased atrial cells.[40,41,44]

Decremental conduction occurs in certain regions of the normal heart, such as the AV node, where contributing factors include both structural features such as loosely arranged small-diameter fibers, with a relative paucity of gap junctions, and membrane properties such as a decreased resting membrane potential and a low upstroke velocity in phase 0. Impulse propagation, already exceedingly slow, may be further impaired by cholinergic influences which further depress the rate of rise of phase 0, resulting in block. Early premature beats invading the AV node before recovery is complete may also show delay and block. Recovery of full excitability typically outlasts the duration of the action potential in the AV node, resulting in a time and voltage dependence of refractoriness. These properties of the AV node, therefore, normally prevent rapid impulse transmission from the atrium to the ventricles.

Undirectional Block and Reentry

The concept of reentry implies continuous impulse propagation: it requires a finite circuit, which need not, however, be static, unidirectional block, and sufficiently slow conduction such that the transit time around the circuit exceeds the longest effective refractory period of participating cells. However, it must be admitted that when propagation becomes exceedingly slow, it is probably impossible to distinguish between an active membrane response and purely passive electrotonic spread.

The closed loop of reentry may be formed by natural anatomic structures, such as branching Purkinje fibers, or in part by the presence of an accessory pathway, or may be a consequence of the temporal dispersion of recovery times in normal cardiac structures. In this latter regard, recent studies by Allessie have demonstrated that in certain circumstances the propagating impulse may circulate around a functionally inactive core, comprising normal tissue kept in a constant state of depolarization by random centripetal wavelets.[50]

Unidirectional block may arise as a consequence of impedance mismatch,[51,52] but, as Hoffman and Rosen have stressed,[26] this concept does not presuppose any particular anatomic format, but requires simply that fiber properties vary as a function of distance. In Fig. 25-5*A*, a situation is depicted whereby a proximal common pathway meets two divergent pathways (alpha and beta) converging upon a distal common pathway. Impulses originating after a normal diastolic interval propagate uniformly through both pathways. In Fig. 25-5*B*, a premature impulse encounters two divergent pathways with differing properties, and block occurs in an area of depressed conduction in the beta pathway, where recovery of excitability may be incomplete and where the premature impulse may constitute a less adequate stimulus compared with a normal action potential. Slow

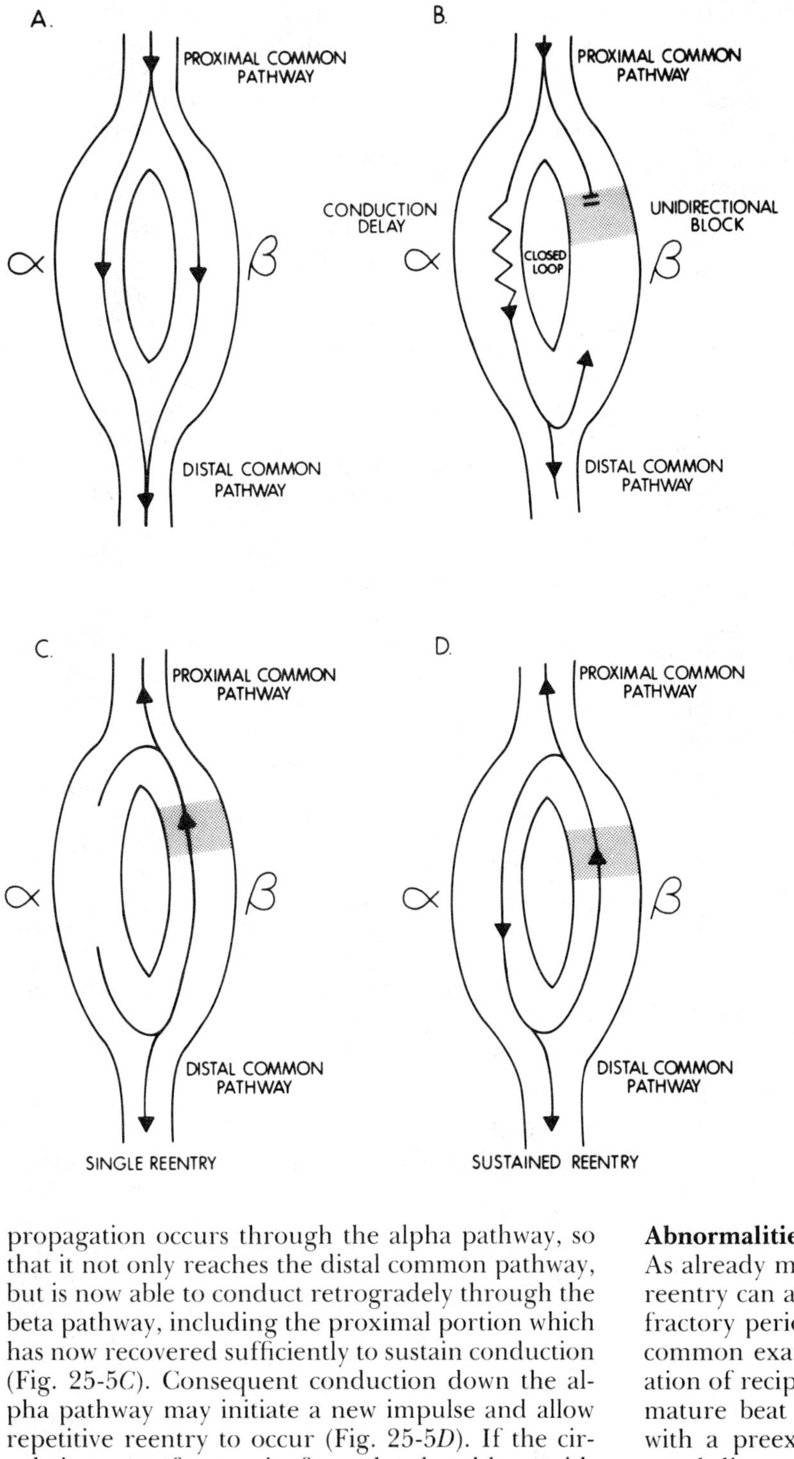

FIGURE 25-5 Mechanism of reentry. A hypothetical reentry circuit is demonstrated in which a proximal common pathway divides into two divergent paths, the alpha and beta pathways, before reuniting in the distal common pathway. *A.* Conduction proceeds equally in both the alpha and beta pathways under normal circumstances. *B.* A premature beat encounters an area of unidirectional block in the beta pathway. Conduction succeeds in the alpha pathway, but with considerable delay. *C.* The excitability of the beta pathway has recovered, allowing the impulse traveling down the alpha pathway to return up the beta pathway, resulting in reentry. *D.* Sustained reentry is present. (*From J. J. Gallagher, Cardiac Arrhythmias, in J. B. Wyngaarden and L. H. Smith (eds.), "Cecil Textbook of Medicine," W. B. Saunders, Philadelphia, 1982, p. 264. Reproduced with permission from the publisher, editor, and author.*)

propagation occurs through the alpha pathway, so that it not only reaches the distal common pathway, but is now able to conduct retrogradely through the beta pathway, including the proximal portion which has now recovered sufficiently to sustain conduction (Fig. 25-5*C*). Consequent conduction down the alpha pathway may initiate a new impulse and allow repetitive reentry to occur (Fig. 25-5*D*). If the circulating wave front exits from the closed loop with each cycle, activation of the surrounding cardiac tissue will result in a manifest arrhythmia.

Before the discovery of the slow response, many investigators felt it was unlikely that conduction which was sufficiently slow to allow a reentrant rhythm could occur outside the AV node. However, knowledge that very depressed fast responses or the slow response may be associated with exceedingly slow impulse propagation has made reentry feasible in very small areas of the myocardium.

Abnormalities of Repolarization

As already mentioned, the necessary conditions for reentry can also result from an inequality in the refractory periods of different parts of the circuit. A common example of this phenomenon is the initiation of reciprocating tachycardia by block of a premature beat in the accessory pathway of patients with a preexcitation syndrome (see below). Temporal dispersion of myocardial recovery times may also be due to disease when, following the passage of a single wave front of depolarization, excitability may recover in one region of the heart before an adjacent area has fully repolarized, allowing current to pass from the depolarized tissue to the recovered tissue, causing focal excitation.[53] This type of reentry may be observed for example when acute ischemia suddenly abbreviates the action potential in a focal area of the ventricle; the same mechanism can obviously occur when disease regionally prolongs the duration of the action potential or repolarization. Abnormalities of repolarization may be manifest on the electrocardiogram (ECG) as a prolonged QT interval. Marked prolongation of the QT interval is associated with electrical instability and susceptibility to ventricular tachycardia and fibrillation, and may be associated with asynchronous recovery of large portions of the ventricle.[54] In patients with congenital prolongation of the QT interval, imbalance in the sympathetic innervation of the heart is believed important.[55]

Aberrant Conduction

The duration of the action potential and recovery of excitability are nonuniform through the His-Purkinje system and ventricular myocardium so that a certain heterogeneity of repolarization and of the refractory periods of cardiac cells is physiologic in fibers that exhibit the fast response. In general, the action potential duration and refractoriness gradually increase from the proximal to the distal His-Purkinje system until an area of maximal refractoriness or "gate" is encountered near the junction of the Purkinje network with muscle; just beyond this gate the refractoriness markedly decreases at the level of the myocardium.[56] Alterations in QRS morphology of premature beats due to "physiologic" refractoriness in some part of the normal conduction system is called *aberrant conduction,* and because the gate for conducting tissues in the right ventricle exceeds those for the left ventricle, clinical right bundle branch block is the most common variety of aberration encountered.

The duration of the action potential and refractoriness is directly related to cycle length; thus longer cycle lengths augment subsequent refractoriness and shorter cycle lengths abbreviate refractoriness. Clinically, aberration is therefore probable when long cycle lengths are followed by short cycle lengths, as often occurs during atrial fibrillation.

Reflection

Another kind of reentry, called *reflection,* can be readily demonstrated in isolated bundles of cardiac tissue.[22,57] Thus an impulse may be propagated to an area where conduction is severely depressed. Passive electrotonic changes may occur in this area, and if there is sufficient delay, the electrotonic currents may sometimes reexcite the fibers that brought the impulse to the depressed segment, resulting in a recurrent response. The essence of this concept is the absence of active impulse generation in the depressed segment. Such a model of ectopic impulse formation has been suggested in some instances of parasystolic pacemaker activity.

Concealed Conduction

The disorders of conduction described thus far all result in some manifest change on the surface ECG, such as conduction delay or obvious block. The concept of concealed conduction, introduced by Langendorf in 1948,[58] referred to depolarization of fibers of the AV transmission system not accompanied by identifiable events on the surface ECG. Such phenomena were therefore concealed, but could be inferred by their effect on subsequent impulse formation and conduction.[59,60]

Combinations of Abnormal Impulse Formation and Conduction

It is not uncommon for conditions of abnormal impulse formation to coexist with abnormal impulse conduction. Thus as we have seen, under various abnormal conditions resulting in partial depolarization of cells with attendant slow conduction, pacemaker activity of abnormal cells is enhanced. Similarly, phase IV depolarization can reduce transmembrane potential, resulting in diminished ability of a fiber to generate a normal action potential. If phase IV depolarization is enhanced in some part of the specialized conducting system or if it proceeds for an unusually long period of time, the response to a propagated impulse will be abnormal. The latter is the most likely cause of abnormal impulse propagation observed with long diastolic intervals (so-called phase IV block).[61–63]

When abnormal automaticity coexists with abnormal conduction into (entrance block) and/or out of (exit block) the automatic focus, the phenomenon of parasystole is said to be present.[64,65] Experimentally, such "protected foci" are susceptible to modulation by the dominant rhythm across an area of depressed excitability, resulting in parasystolic rhythms that may show either fixed or variable coupling with sinus rhythm.[66,67] At the present juncture, therefore, the clinical criteria for the diagnosis of parasystole are subject to review.

Basis of Determination of Mechanisms of Arrhythmias in Humans

In the following section, some of the more common tachyarrhythmias and bradyarrhythmias will be discussed, with emphasis on those situations in which interrelationships between clinical electrophysiologic findings and basic electrophysiologic mechanisms are most apparent. Unfortunately, no clinical electrophysiologic criteria permit the unequivocal separation of reentry from automaticity.[68] Nonetheless, the use of programmed stimulation of the heart (see Chaps. 18 and 102) in concert with multiple catheter-electrode recordings of activity from the atria, ventricles, and specialized conduction system (see Chap. 101) has greatly advanced our understanding of many clinical arrhythmias. Thus reentry is said to be strongly favored when clinical electrophysiologic study finds the following:

1. The ability to initiate and terminate tachycardia by premature stimulation delivered within well-defined, reproducible coupling intervals.

2. The ability to demonstrate continuous excitation of elements of the proposed reentry circuit.
3. The ability to terminate tachycardia abruptly by overdrive pacing.
4. An inverse relation between the coupling interval of a premature beat that initiates tachycardia and the interval between the premature beat and the first beat of tachycardia.

In contrast, the diagnosis of automaticity is largely by exclusion, because of inability to induce and terminate tachycardia by programmed stimulation.[69] Characteristically also, overdrive pacing results in only a brief pause followed by reappearance of the tachycardia with a progressive increase in rate (warm-up phenomenon). The most recently discovered mechanism—triggered activity—remains a problem in terms of diagnostic criteria. While in vitro it can be induced and terminated by programmed stimulation, it tends to occur only at fast basic rates, is highly sensitive to verapamil, and exhibits an apparent direct relation between the coupling intervals of the drive beat to the initiating premature beat and from the premature beat to the first triggered impulse. The prevalence of triggered rhythms in clinical arrhythmias is still unknown.

Tachyarrhythmias

Sinus Tachycardia; Sinus Node Reentry

Sinus tachycardia is usually the consequence of excessive sympathetic drive and is mediated by an increased rate of diastolic depolarization as a result of an increased inward current. It is a result of altered activity of the autonomic nervous system rather than a primary disorder in function of the sinus node.

Allessie has demonstrated the ability of the sinus node to sustain reentry.[70] Possible clinical examples of sinus node reentry have been reported, in which episodes of supraventricular tachycardia have been initiated and terminated by programmed stimulation, with a P-wave morphology identical to that of sinus rhythm.[71–74] Such tachycardias are infrequent and unstable, and rarely present a problem.

Atrial Tachycardia

Atrial tachycardias may result from automaticity or reentry. Those resulting from digitalis excess appear to be caused by abnormal impulse formation, perhaps related to afterdepolarizations. The multifocal atrial tachycardias observed in patients with chronic lung disease are probably also related to abnormal automaticity. Goldreyer[75] first proposed the criteria that have come to be regarded as strongly suggestive of automaticity in the study of atrial tachycardia in humans. These included the following observations:

1. The P-wave morphology of tachycardia differed from that of the sinus P wave.
2. Atrial tachycardia was induced by premature atrial beats that did not result in conduction delay in the AV node.
3. During atrial tachycardia, the cycle length of tachycardia was not a function of conduction in the AV node.
4. A gradual acceleration of the rate of tachycardia, or warm-up, was observed following overdrive pacing or premature atrial stimulation.
5. The introduction of premature atrial beats during tachycardia resulted in reset of the tachycardia.
6. The tachycardia could not be terminated by pacing nor could it be initiated by programmed stimulation during periods of quiescence.

Evidence of atrial reentry as a mechanism for supraventricular tachycardia in humans has been summarized by Coumel.[76] Experimentally it has been demonstrated that reentry in the atrium can be determined by anatomically defined circuits as originally suggested by Mines[1] or solely by the functional properties of atrial tissue[77] (see "Atrial Flutter," below). The characteristics of these two types of circus movement are summarized in Fig. 25-6. The ability of the atrium to sustain reentry in the absence of an anatomically defined obstacle was shown by Allessie using the *leading circle concept.*[77] In this model, a premature stimulus was used to initiate a tachycardia in isolated left atrial tissue (Fig. 25-7). Recordings were made from approximately 100 sites, demonstrating a clockwise circus movement with a revolution time of 105 ms. In this model, the circus movement is the smallest possible circuit in which the stimulating efficacy of the circulating wave front

FIGURE 25-6 Circus movement. See text for discussion.

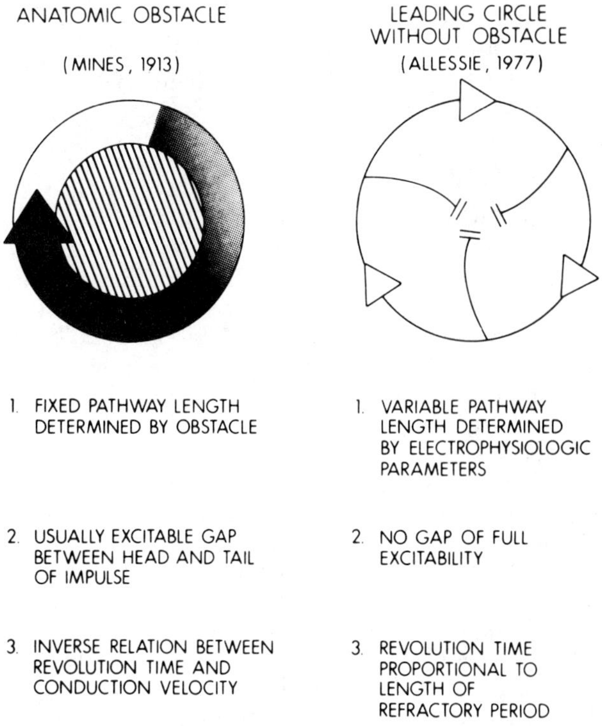

ANATOMIC OBSTACLE
(MINES, 1913)
LEADING CIRCLE WITHOUT OBSTACLE
(ALLESSIE, 1977)
1. FIXED PATHWAY LENGTH DETERMINED BY OBSTACLE
1. VARIABLE PATHWAY LENGTH DETERMINED BY ELECTROPHYSIOLOGIC PARAMETERS
2. USUALLY EXCITABLE GAP BETWEEN HEAD AND TAIL OF IMPULSE
2. NO GAP OF FULL EXCITABILITY
3. INVERSE RELATION BETWEEN REVOLUTION TIME AND CONDUCTION VELOCITY
3. REVOLUTION TIME PROPORTIONAL TO LENGTH OF REFRACTORY PERIOD

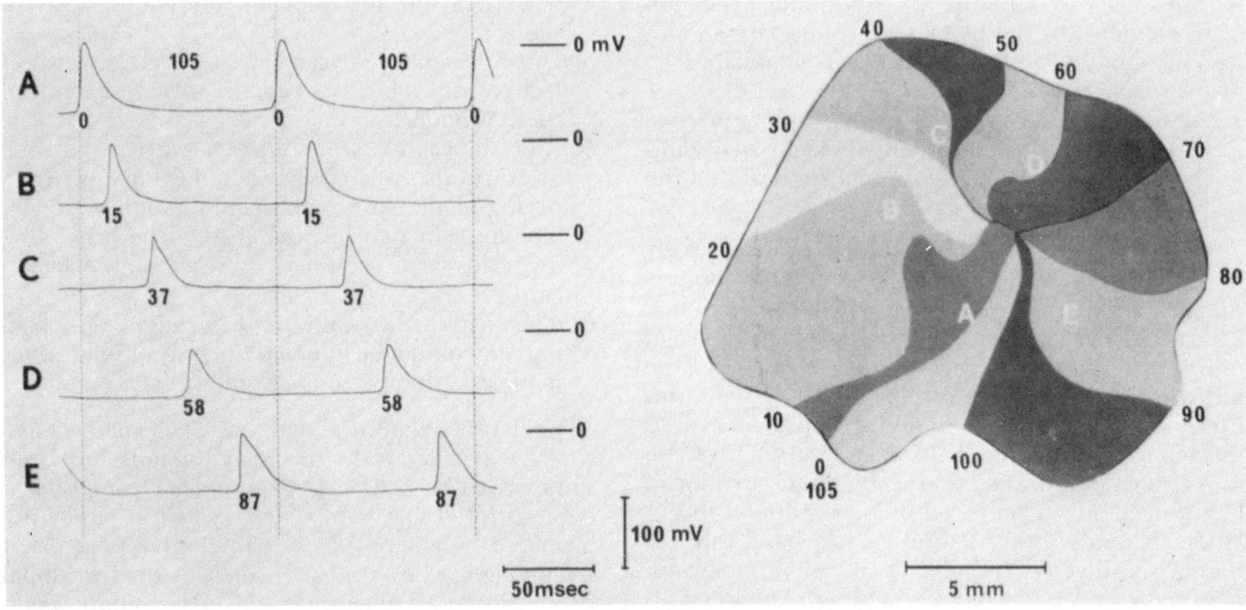

FIGURE 25-7 Atrial reentry in isolated left atrial muscle. *A* to *E*. The transmembrane potentials of five fibers which lie along the circular path. To the right, the isochronous map derived from recordings of action potentials from 94 different fibers is shown. The moments of depolarization in milliseconds are given together with the action potentials and the isochronic lines of the map. (*From M. A. Allessie, Circulating Excitation in the Heart, doctoral thesis, University of Limburg, Masstricht, 1977, p. 101. Also published in Circ. Res., 41:9, 1977. Reproduced with permission from the American Heart Association, Inc., and the author.*)

is sufficient to excite the relatively refractory tissue ahead. Thus the head of the circulating wave is continually traveling in the wake of its own refractoriness. From this leading circle, centripetal wavelets activate the area in the center of the circle but collide with each other. On the other hand, centrifugal wavelets readily activate the surrounding atrial tissues. Allessie was able to demonstrate sustained reentry in pieces of atrial muscle with a radius of 5 to 6 mm. Because the dimensions are so small, it would obviously be difficult to distinguish such a leading circle from a focus of spontaneously discharging atrial fibers.[78]

Atrial Flutter

The majority of available studies support the mechanism of circus rhythm and reentry as the most common basis for atrial flutter.[79] The idea that a circuitous activation process was responsible for atrial flutter was first popularized by Lewis in 1920 based on experiments in the dog, although he himself found it very difficult to initiate atrial flutter reproducibly.[80] Later, Rosenbleuth and Garcia Ramos[81] developed a model whereby they crushed a band of atrial tissue adjacent to the natural orifice of the inferior vena cava to provide a large anatomic obstacle. Following atrial stimulation, a regular tachycardia developed during which sequential activation could be recorded around the borders of the lesion. Subsequent studies established that experimental atrial flutter was possible without a physical obstruction. Pastelin[82] suggested that the preferential atrial pathways may form a loop through which flutter waves circulate, while the studies of Allessie in isolated rabbit left atria[77] and in the intact canine heart[83] have demonstrated reentry on the basis of the leading circle mechanism.

The majority of studies emphasize the importance of the association of a nonuniform distribution of atrial refractory periods and the presence of suitably located and timed premature atrial beats in the induction of atrial flutter, concepts demonstrated mathematically by Moe.[84] Slow conduction of the flutter wave is a natural consequence of the premature wave front encountering partially refractory tissue. However, Boineau[85] has suggested an additional factor, namely structural discontinuity of atrial bands to satisfactorily account for the slowness of observed propagation. These studies favor a reentry basis for atrial flutter. On the other hand, a potential role for abnormal automaticity is suggested by some microelectrode studies[86] and by the ability of aconitine to induce flutter via the mechanism of abnormal impulse formation.[87] In this latter instance, however, it is difficult to exclude rate-related conduction delay and block leading to functional reentry as a consequence of the rapid impulse formation.

Clinical studies in humans[88–94] have confirmed that atrial flutter may often be induced by premature beats, while termination of flutter has been achieved by overdrive pacing of 115 to 125 percent of the basic flutter rate. It has also been noted that termination is associated with entrainment,[93] whereby at critical rates of overdrive atrial pacing, the P-wave morphology changes from that present in flutter, suggesting that the reentrant pathway has been engaged. The fact that the "entrained" P-wave morphology is not identical to that obtained by pacing at the same site during sinus rhythm suggests that atrial fusion or rate-related atrial conduction disturbances are present during the period of entrainment.

Although reentry seems probable in most cases of atrial flutter, it is still impossible to exclude a role for abnormal automaticity in some instances.

Atrial Fibrillation

The physiologic mechanism of atrial fibrillation has not been conclusively established.[95] Experimental observations, however, suggest that while it may be induced by rapid atrial stimulation, it is sustained by a reentrant process. In dogs anesthetized by barbiturates, atrial fibrillation induced by rapid atrial pacing or the local application of aconitine[87] usually ceases when electrical stimulation is discontinued or the site of drug application is isolated from the remainder of the atria. In contrast, if the vagi are stimulated or an anesthetic that enhances vagal tone is used, a self-sustaining arrhythmia suggestive of atrial fibrillation persists after the initiating agent is removed.[96] Increased vagal tone abbreviates atrial refractory periods in a markedly inhomogenous manner,[97] and in such a situation, premature stimulation would result in markedly irregular propagation due to multiple areas of conduction delay and block. This would lead in turn to further disparities in local recovery times with the end result being multiple independent activation wave fronts or wavelets due to reentry. A mathematical model incorporating features of nonuniform refractory periods has confirmed the feasibility of this mechanism.[78,98]

The facts that a critical mass of tissue is necessary for atrial fibrillation and that the arrhythmia may be terminated by a single electric shock are readily explained by the reentry hypothesis, while the induction of atrial fibrillation by premature stimulation during the so-called vulnerable period of the cardiac cycle is similarly compatible with reentry assuming a critical degree of inhomogeneity exists during this interval. However, it has been shown that experimentally induced atrial fibrillation persists longer in the presence of an intact sinus node,[99] so that pacemaker activity may still have some role in the mechanism of sustained atrial fibrillation. In contrast to animal studies, relatively little information is available on atrial fibrillation in humans. It is known that the incidence of the arrhythmia increases with age, and it is commonly associated with atrial dilatation. Although a wide variety of anatomic abnormalities have been found in patients with atrial fibrillation, sinoatrial nodal muscle cell loss and fibrosis is a common finding in published studies,[100–102] as are focal lesions throughout the atrial walls and preferential pathways. Such lesions may both disrupt the normal sequence of atrial activation and repolarization and provide potential foci of abnormal automaticity. Whether pathologic changes in the autonomic innervation of the atria are also important is unknown at present.

In vitro electrophysiologic studies[40,44] performed on human atrial tissue removed from patients with atrial arrhythmias have shown large numbers of depolarized fibers, considerable variability in diastolic potential and action potential characteristics, decreased responsiveness in conductivity, and various types of oscillatory potentials. Such pathophysiologic observations suggest the simultaneous operation of multifocal pacemaker activity, reentry, and abnormal automaticity in the pathogenesis of atrial fibrillation.

The Preexcitation Syndromes

Ventricular preexcitation[103] is said to be present when, in relation to atrial events, the whole or part of the ventricular myocardium is activated by the impulse originating in the atrium *earlier* than would be expected if the impulse reached the ventricles by way of the normal specialized conducting system. This classic definition, of course, refers only to phenomena occurring during *anterograde* conduction. It is now well established that the accessory pathway underlying preexcitation syndromes can exhibit unidirectional block in the anterograde *or* retrograde direction. Thus, a more liberal definition would recognize preexcitation to be present whenever one cardiac chamber is activated in whole or part by an impulse originating in the other chamber *earlier* than would be expected if the impulse had proceeded over the normal conducting system.

The term *syndrome* is applied when electrocardiographic or electrophysiologic evidence of preexcitation is accompanied by clinical arrhythmias. A variety of potential anatomic substrates exist for which a new nomenclature has been suggested[104] (Fig. 25-8). These include fibers coursing directly from atrium to ventricle (accessory AV pathways or Kent bundles); fibers coursing from atrium to His bundle,

FIGURE 25-8 Substrates of preexcitation. A schematic representation of the junction in the region of the normal conduction system is shown. Atrio-Hisian (A-H) fibers insert directly into the His bundle, thus bypassing the area of physiologic delay; AV pathways or Kent bundles pass directly from atrium to ventricle; nodoventricular (NV) fibers (Mahaim fibers) pass directly from the AV node to the ventricle; fasciculoventricular (FV) fibers pass from the His bundle or bundle branches directly to the ventricle. AVN = atrioventricular node; BB = bundle branch.

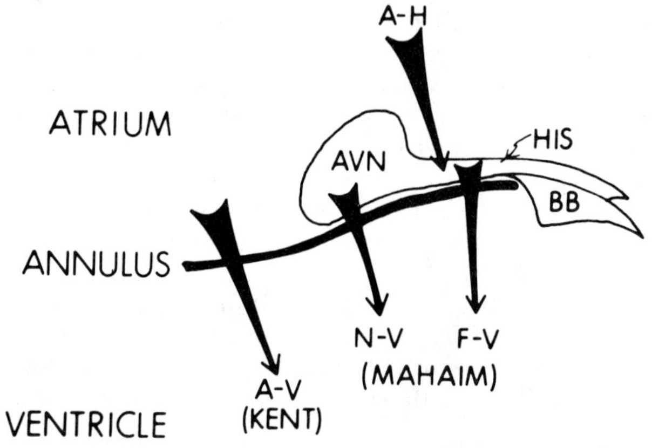

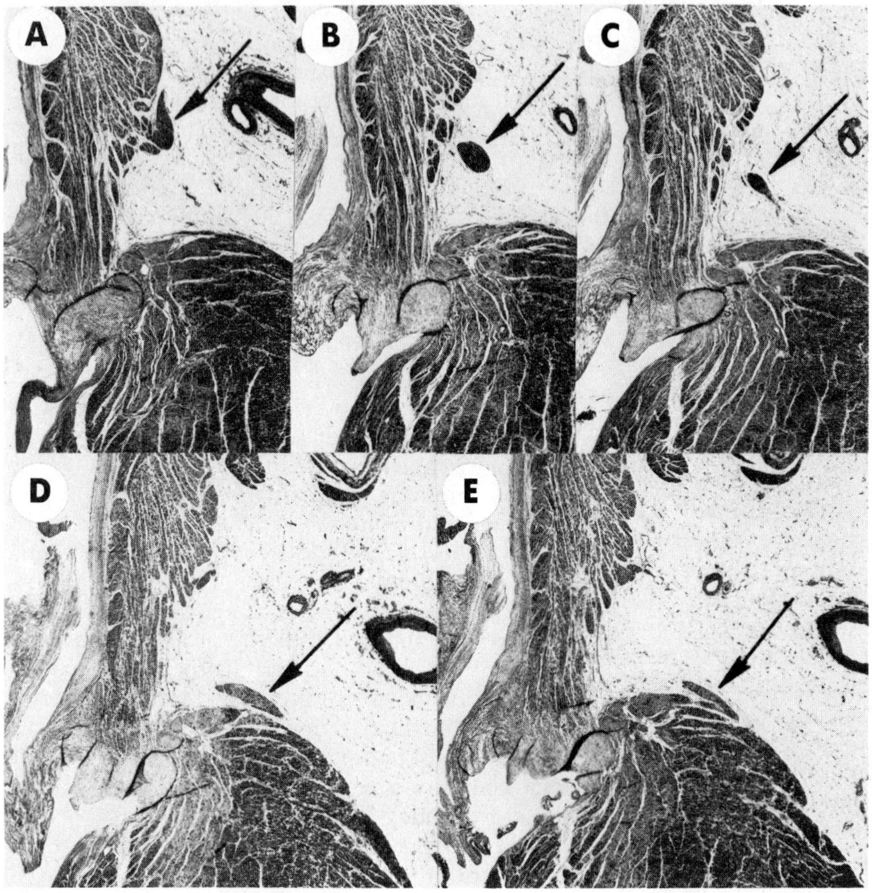

FIGURE 25-9 Accessory AV pathway (Kent bundle). *A* to *E*. Sequential steps taken from the left AV junction of a patient with WPW syndrome. Note the bridge passing from left atrium in *A* across epicardial fat in *B, C,* and *D* and joining the left ventricle in *E*. Epicardial fat is to the right; left atrial and left ventricular cavities are to the left. Masson's stain; ×9.5 (*From G. J. Klein, et al., Anatomic Substrate of Impaired Antegrade Conduction over an Accessory Atrioventricular Pathway in the Wolff-Parkinson-White Syndrome, Circulation, 61:1249, 1980. Reproduced with permission from the American Heart Association, Inc., and the author.*)

bypassing the physiologic delay of the AV node (atrio-Hisian fibers); and two varieties of Mahaim fibers: those passing from the AV node to the ventricle (nodoventricular fibers) and those arising in the His bundle–bundle branches and inserting in the ventricular myocardium (fasciculoventricular fibers).

The most common variety of preexcitation is the accessory AV pathway present in the Wolff-Parkinson-White (WPW) syndrome and some of its variants (Fig. 25-9). If it is assumed that the accessory pathway linking atrium to ventricle is capable of anterograde conduction, two parallel routes of conduction are possible, one subject to physiologic delay over the AV node and the other passing directly from atrium to ventricle. In general, ventricular activation in sinus rhythm will be the result of fusion of these two ventricular inputs, resulting in abbreviations of the PR interval and an anomalous QRS complex due to the abnormal sequence of ventricular activation that results from eccentric depolarization of the ventricles by the accessory pathway (Fig. 25-10).

The most common arrhythmia associated with the WPW syndrome is a reciprocating supraventricular tachycardia, which has become the model of reentrant rhythms. Initiation of a typical paroxysm of tachycardia (Fig. 25-10) results from a premature beat that blocks in the accessory pathway and conducts with delay down the normal conducting system (resulting in a normal QRS complex). Activation spreading through the ventricles finds the accessory pathway excitable in the retrograde direction (as a result of functional unidirectional block), allowing impulse propagation back to the atrium. Circus movement is then established by anterograde conduction over the normal conducting system and retrograde conduction over the accessory pathway. The typical conditions for reentry illustrated in Fig. 25-5 are thus all present: closed circuit, conduction delay, and unidirectional block. Detailed recordings of the sequence of atrial activation during reciprocating tachycardia provide information concerning the point in the atria where the retrograde impulse first penetrates and thus can be used to localize accessory pathways by catheter-electrode techniques (Fig. 25-11).

Patients with the WPW syndrome are also subject to a second symptomatic arrhythmia, that of a rapid ventricular response occurring in the setting of atrial fibrillation. During atrial fibrillation, rapid impulses in the atria are not subject to the usual decremental conduction of the AV node and thus can result in a malignant ventricular response, accounting for ventricular fibrillation in a small subset of these patients[105] (Fig. 25-12). Although atrial fibrillation could be a coincidental association with the WPW syndrome, in some patients the transition from reciprocating tachycardia to atrial fibrillation has been

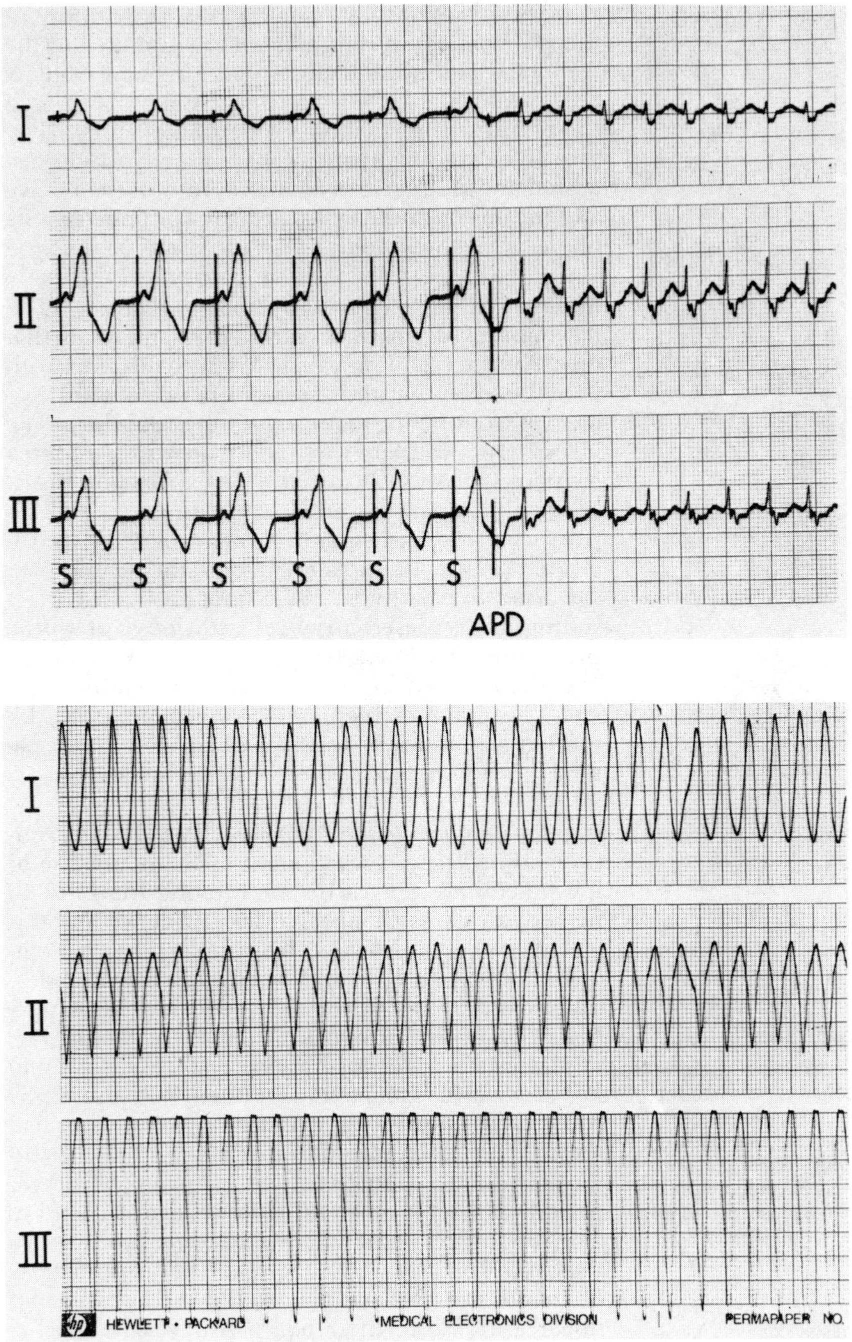

FIGURE 25-10 Arrhythmias associated with the WPW syndrome. The upper panel demonstrates induction of a supraventricular tachycardia in a patient with WPW syndrome. The atria are initially being paced, resulting in a short PR interval, wide QRS complex due to ventricular preexcitation over an accessory AV pathway. An atrial premature depolarization (APD) is introduced which blocks in the accessory pathway and initiates an episode of supraventricular tachycardia. The lower panel demonstrates an episode of atrial flutter in another patient with preexcitation, resulting in 1:1 AV conduction with an anomalous QRS complex. (*Upper panel from J. J. Gallagher, E. L. C. Pritchett, W. C. Sealy, J. Kasell, and A. G. Wallace, The Preexcitation Syndromes, Prog. Cardiovasc. Dis., 20(4): 288, 1978. Reproduced with permission from the publisher, editor, and author.*)

consistently observed,[103] possibly in part because of atrial distension.

The remaining varieties of preexcitation syndromes are considerably less common. As demonstrated in Fig. 25-13, both nodoventricular Mahaim fibers and atrio-Hisian fibers can sustain a normal QRS supraventricular tachycardia by providing a return limb for the reentry circuit, comparable to the situation described for Kent bundles.[106–109] Nodoventricular Mahaim fibers can also sustain anterograde conduction resulting in a wide QRS tachycardia[107] indistinguishable from ventricular tachycardia (see below).

Atrio-Hisian fibers may be one substrate of the Lown-Ganong-Levine syndrome, which comprises supraventricular tachyarrhythmias (both AV reciprocating tachycardias and atrial fibrillation and flutter) in association with a short PR interval, normal P-wave axis and narrow QRS complexes.[110,111] Such patients may be subject to a rapid ventricular response in the setting of atrial fibrillation because of the bypass of their AV node.

AV Junctional Tachycardia

In this section, the topic of narrow QRS supraventricular tachycardia (SVT) occurring in patients *without* overt evidence of preexcitation will be dis-

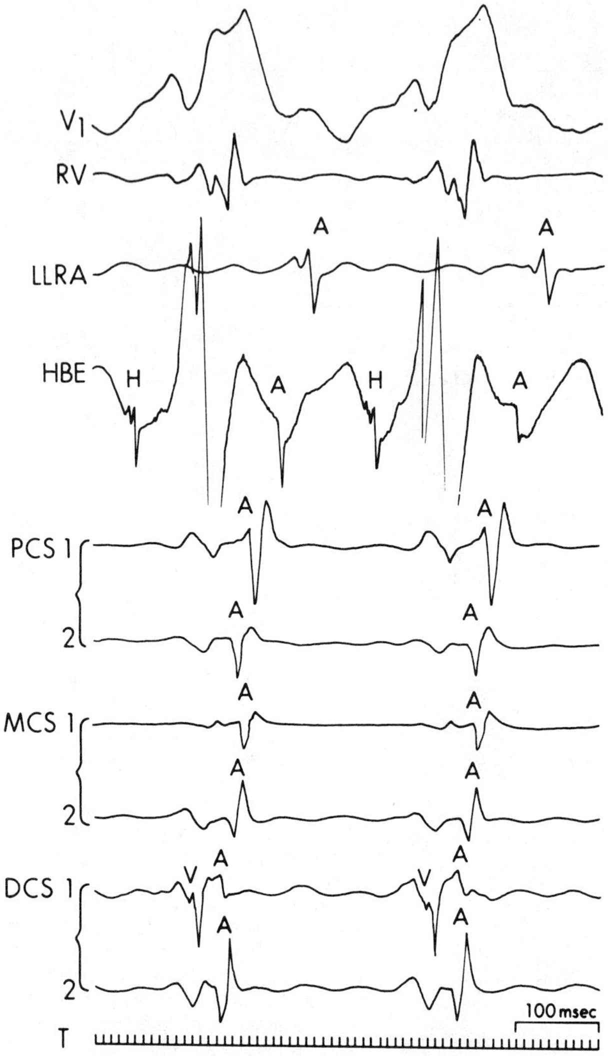

FIGURE 25-11 Atrial mapping during reciprocating tachycardia in a patient with WPW syndrome. The recordings from the top down include standard ECG leads V_1 and bipolar electrograms from the right ventricle (RV), the low lateral right atrium (LLRA), the region of the His bundle (HBE), and the proximal coronary sinus (PCS), midcoronary sinus (MCS), and distal coronary sinus (DCS). The recordings were obtained during reciprocating tachycardia using the normal AV conduction system as the antegrade limb and the accessory pathway as the retrograde limb of a reentrant circuit. The QRS complex demonstrates right bundle branch block. The sequence of retrograde atrial activation is eccentric, with earliest atrial activity recorded in the distal coronary sinus tracing, reflecting early activity of the lateral left atrium. *(From G. J. Klein et al., Anatomic Substrate of Impaired Antegrade Conduction over an Accessory Atrioventricular Pathway in the Wolff-Parkinson-White Syndrome, Circulation, 61:1249, 1980. Reproduced with permission from the American Heart Association, Inc., and author.)*

cussed. A variety of potential mechanisms exist which in general can be subdivided into paroxysmal and nonparoxysmal types, with or without 1:1 association of atrial and ventricular activity.

Paroxysmal AV Junctional Tachycardia with 1:1 AV Association

This term identifies a subset of patients with SVT most commonly due to three potential mechanisms: reentry utilizing a concealed accessory pathway of the AV type (Kent bundle), reentry confined to the AV node, and atrial tachycardia. This undoubtedly accounts for the variety of terms that have been used to describe the electrocardiographic entity (Fig. 25-14). Atrial tachycardia has already been discussed and is suggested by the contour of the P wave and the ability of the tachycardia to continue despite block in the AV node.

Reentry Utilizing a Concealed Accessory Pathway The mechanism of this tachycardia is identical to that described for SVT in classic WPW syndrome, with the exception that the accessory pathway is incapable of conducting anterogradely (unidirectional block). One wonders why such patients are not in a constant state of tachycardia. One explanation is that the atrium near the accessory pathway is still refractory from the sinus impulse when the retrograde impulse attempts to reexcite the atrium over the accessory pathway. With sinus tachycardia (resulting in decreased atrial refractoriness) or with a premature atrial beat (which results in AV conduction delay), recovery of the accessory pathway occurs, resulting in reentry. In our experience this mechanism accounts for 40 percent of SVT in patients with no overt evidence of preexcitation.

Reentry Confined to the AV Node SVT due to reentry confined to the AV node is a common cause of AV junctional tachycardia, accounting for 40 to 50 percent of cases in most series. Evidence for this mechanism was provided by Moe,[112,113] who demonstrated that SVT could be produced by longitudinal dissociation of the AV node into two functional pathways designated alpha and beta. The mechanism he proposed is essentially that shown in Fig. 25-5. He originally suggested that the alpha pathway was the slower-conducting pathway but had the shorter refractory period, while the beta pathway conducted faster but had a longer refractory period. Thus a premature atrial beat might tend to block in the beta pathway and conduct slowly down the alpha pathway. If sufficient conduction delay occurred, the beta pathway would recover, permitting reentry from the alpha pathway. The mechanism was subsequently confirmed using multiple microelectrode recordings in AV nodal preparations from rabbits demonstrating SVT.[114,115] The interrelationship of conduction and refractoriness has been validated in humans as well through the use of programmed premature stimulation.[14,69,116,117] Although a number of potential configurations for the reentry circuit in the AV node can be imagined (Fig. 25-15), in most cases atrial and ventricular activation occur almost simultaneously. This provides an easy method to differentiate SVT due to a concealed accessory pathway from reentry confined to the AV node (Fig. 25-16):[118] with a concealed accessory pathway, the propagating impulse must depolarize the ventricle *before* it can re-

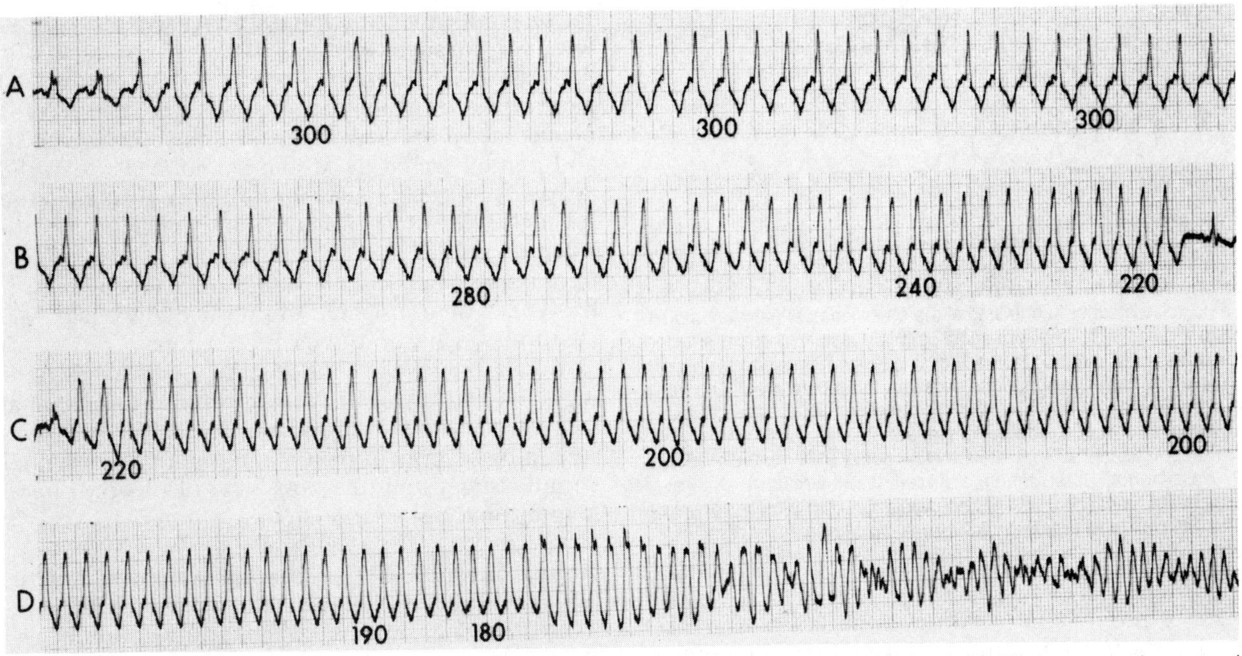

FIGURE 25-12 Induction of ventricular fibrillation in a patient with WPW syndrome by atrial pacing. *A* and *B*. These are continuous and demonstrate 1:1 AV conduction during rapid atrial pacing from cycle length 300 ms to 220 ms. *C*. After a resting period of sinus rhythm, pacing was reinstituted at a cycle length of 220 ms. *D*. Ventricular fibrillation appeared shortly after reaching a cycle length of 180 ms. The patient had a history of spontaneous ventricular fibrillation.

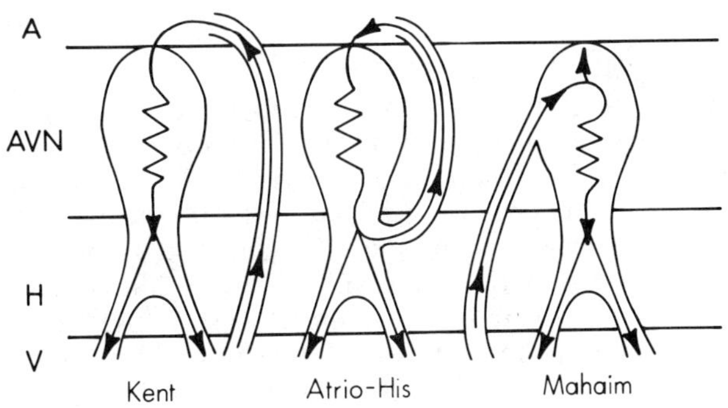

FIGURE 25-13 Extranodal mechanisms of supraventricular tachycardia. A schematic ladder diagram depicts some theoretical representations of reentry circuits involving accessory pathways. The return limb of the reentry circuit can be provided by retrograde conduction over a pathway between ventricle and atrium (Kent bundle), between the His bundle and atrium (atrio-Hisian fiber), or a fiber between the ventricle and the AV node (nodoventricular or Mahaim fiber).

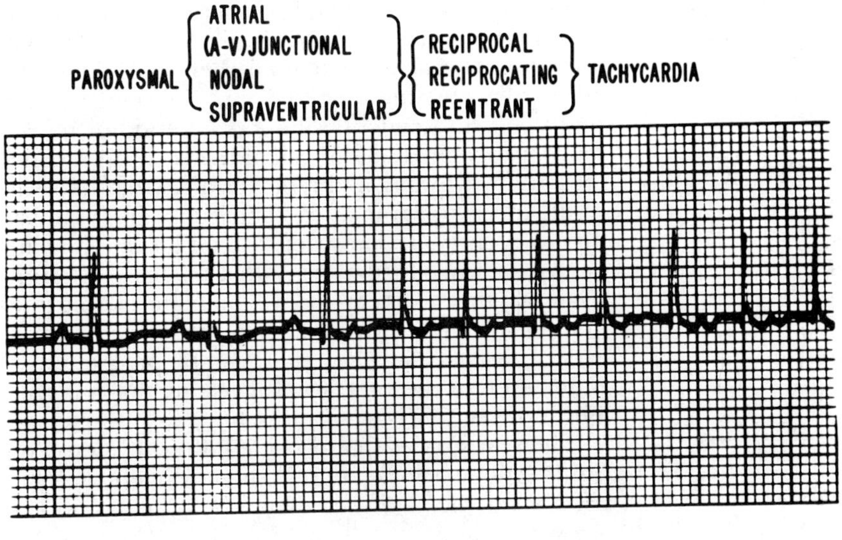

FIGURE 25-14 AV junctional tachycardia. A representative rhythm strip demonstrating the onset of AV junctional tachycardia is shown along with the variety of terms that have been used to describe this arrhythmia. After three sinus beats associated with a normal PR interval and normal QRS complex, there is sudden onset of a narrow-QRS tachycardia.

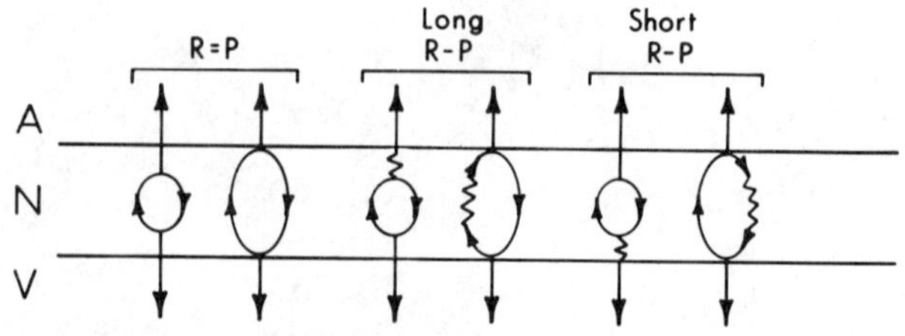

FIGURE 25-15 Mechanisms of reentry confined to the atrioventricular node. A schematic ladder diagram depicts theoretical representations of reentry circuits in the AV node. Areas of delay can be postulated either in one limb of the so-called dual-pathway model or in the initial or final common pathway issuing from a smaller microreentrant circuit. Depending on the location and magnitude of delay, a variety of relations between atrial (P waves) and ventricular (R waves) depolarization is possible. Thus atrial depolarization may precede, occur simultaneously with, or follow ventricular depolarizations. A = atrium; N = node; V = ventricle. *(From J. J. Gallagher, W. M. Smith, J. Kasell, W. M. Smith, A. O. Grant, and D. W. Benson, Use of Esophageal Lead in the Diagnosis of Mechanisms of Reciprocating Supraventricular Tachycardia, PACE, 3:440, 1980. Reproduced with permission from the publisher and author.)*

turn to the atrium, resulting in an obligatory relation of these events during tachycardia; with reentry in the AV node, the QRS complex and P wave can occur simultaneously. A simple examination of the relation of the P wave and QRS complex during SVT by electrocardiographic or esophageal lead recordings allows exclusion of a concealed accessory pathway if the P wave during tachycardia does not *follow* the QRS complex.

Recently, yet another mechanism of SVT has been discovered in which tachycardia occurs almost incessantly and the RP interval is long, exceeding the PR interval. This has been demonstrated to be due to either an accessory AV node,[119] a "fast-slow" configuration of the functional pathways in the AV node, or ectopic atrial tachycardia (Fig. 25-17).

FIGURE 25-16 Comparison of reentry confined to the AV node with reentry utilizing a Kent bundle. The most common variety of reentry confined to the AV node has been schematically depicted, with atrial and ventricular depolarization occurring almost simultaneously. In contrast, reentry utilizing an accessory pathway (Kent bundle) requires that ventricular depolarization precede retrograde atrial depolarization. *(From J. J. Gallagher, W. M. Smith, J. Kasell, W. M. Smith, A. O. Grant, and D. W. Benson, Use of Esophageal Lead in the Diagnosis of Mechanisms of Reciprocating Supraventricular Tachycardia, PACE, 3:440, 1980. Reproduced with permission from the publisher and author.)*

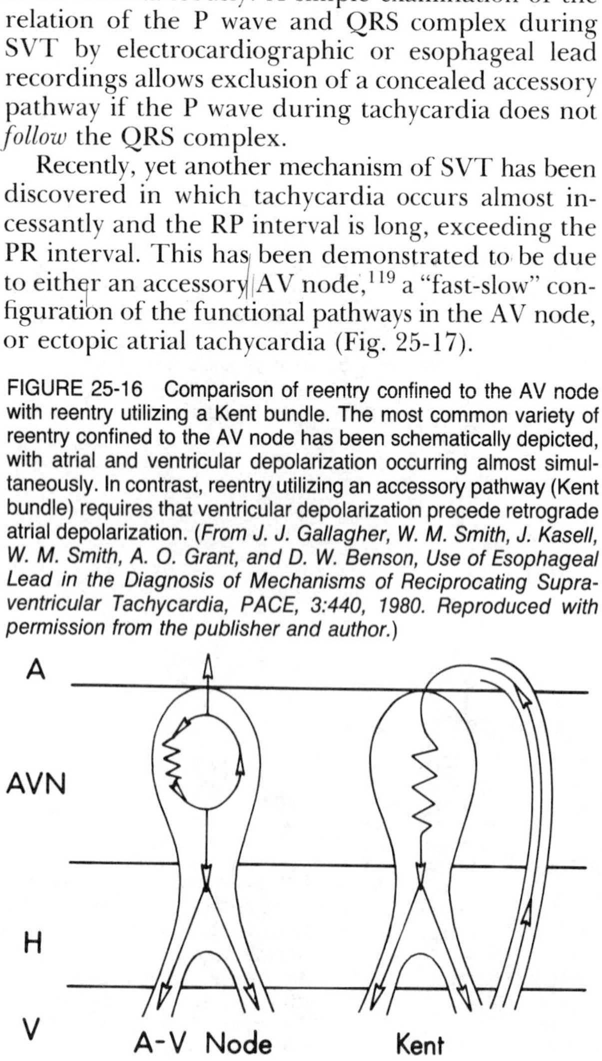

Paroxysmal AV Junctional Tachycardia with AV Dissociation

This is an uncommon variety of AV junctional tachycardia in which the atrium is not required for perpetuation of tachycardia. As shown in Fig. 25-16 and demonstrated by Mignone and Wallace,[120] the atrium is not necessarily required for reentry in the AV node to ensue, although this possibility is considered rare.

Mahaim fibers of the nodoventricular variety[107] have been demonstrated to produce this type of arrhythmia, again on the basis of reentry.

Brechenmacher[121] has described pathologic findings in a child who died from rapid AV junctional tachycardia with AV dissociation: the His bundle was split into several thin and longitudinally oriented strands, suggesting the possibility of reentry due to longitudinal dissociation.

Nonparoxysmal AV Junctional Tachycardia with AV Dissociation (Accelerated Junctional Rhythm)

This type of arrhythmia[122] generally occurs at relatively slow rates with gradual onset and offset and is likely to be observed in the setting of an acute diaphragmatic myocardial infarction or digitalis toxicity. Most reports suggest that this rhythm is due to abnormally enhanced automaticity of a pacemaker in the junctional region.

Ventricular Tachycardia

A variety of mechanisms of premature ventricular beats and sustained ventricular tachycardia have been proposed, including automaticity,[64,123–126] triggered activity,[37] micro reentry circuits in the ventricle,[127–137] macro reentry circuits confined to the specialized conduction system,[138–143] and Mahaim fibers.[107–109] Even in the same disease model (e.g., ischemia) the mechanism of the arrhythmia demonstrated in any given stage may vary, depending on the experimental conditions.[144–147] Immediately following coronary occlusion there is an initial arrhythmogenic period; this was formerly believed to be due solely to macro and micro reentry circuits in ischemic myocardium, but Janse has proposed a role for automatic activity in nonischemic Purkinje or myocardial tissue triggered by the injury current.[146,147] Subsequently there is a period of quiescence, probably due to block of the early-appearing reentrant pathways, and reperfusion at this time will result in reappearance of ventricular arrhythmias due to reentry. If, however, the occlusion is maintained, or reperfusion is gradual or delayed, automatic rhythms appear to predominate during the first 24 h. After several days to weeks, ventricular arrhythmias can again be initiated by programmed stimulation of the ventricle, suggesting that a mechanism of reentry is again present.

The first studies that provided direct evidence of unidirectional block and circus movement in ventricular muscle were carried out by Schmitt and Er-

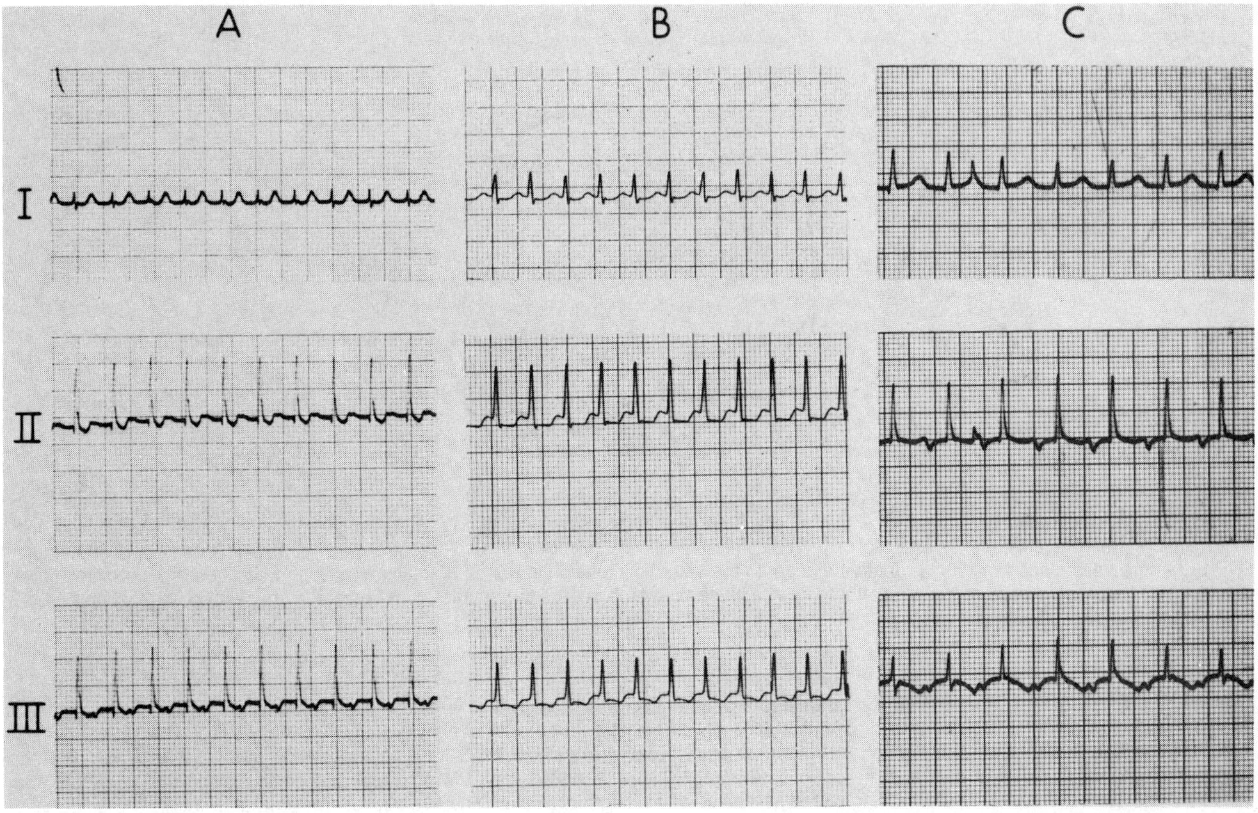

FIGURE 25-17 Three varieties of supraventricular tachycardia. *A.* Examination of lead III demonstrates that a P wave deforms the initial portion of the ST segment, which is compatible with tachycardia utilizing a Kent bundle. *B.* No P wave is visible because the P wave occurs simultaneously with the QRS complex, which is compatible with reentry in the AV node. *C.* P waves occur just after the T wave, and in fact are situated closer to the following QRS complex. This latter configuration is compatible with reentry utilizing an accessory AV node, with atrial tachycardia, or with an atypical form of reentry in the AV node. See text for discussion.

langer in 1929.[7] These workers used a multicompartmented model of turtle ventricle in which segmental areas of depressed function were induced by local pressure and the application of potassium chloride. Unidirectional block was frequently observed in the preparation, and multiple responses to a single stimulus could be elicited. Schmitt and Erlanger speculated that the particular arrangement of the specialized conducting tissues in the mammalian heart might favor reentry. The hypothetical microcircuit of a Purkinje twig anastomosing with ventricular muscle that they proposed had essentially the same features as the diagramatic representation of reentry shown in Fig. 25-5. For some time, however, there was reluctance to accept micro reentry in the ventricles as a mechanism of ventricular tachycardia because the postulated dimensions of such a reentry loop seemed unacceptably large. For example, assuming an area of unidirectional block in a tissue exhibiting a conduction velocity of 3 m/s and a refractory period of 300 ms, a reentry pathway of 0.09 m would be required to allow reexcitation. However, if conduction velocity could proceed at 0.01 m/s, a 3-mm pathway would satisfy the conditions for reentry. The subsequent discovery of the slow response or depressed fast response provided the appropriately low conduction velocity required for postulating this type of micro reentry.

The mechanism of the ubiquitous premature ventricular contraction remains uncertain.[126] Although the presence of fixed coupling has been adduced as evidence for reentry, Moe has demonstrated that a parasystolic focus operating under electronic influences could produce the same pattern of coupling.[64] The mechanism of chronic sustained tachyarrhythmias has been more thoroughly studied, and in the majority of instances a reentrant basis has been favored. Our clinical knowledge is largely the result of observations using catheter-electrode recordings together with programmed stimulation. As previously mentioned, the implicit hypothesis of this technique is that a reentry mechanism can be equated with the ability to initiate and terminate the tachycardia by premature beats. Unfortunately, no criteria exist for the diagnosis of triggered activity in the ventricle; in addition the technique of programmed stimulation has limitations which have recently been reviewed.[69] A representative example of this technique is shown in Figs. 25-18 and 25-19. Programmed stimulation may result in an initiation of reentry in an area of pathology, local reentry in nonpathologic myocardium, or macro reentry involving conduction in portions of the specialized conducting tissue. However, the technique has intrinsic false positive and false negative results. For example, with aggressive

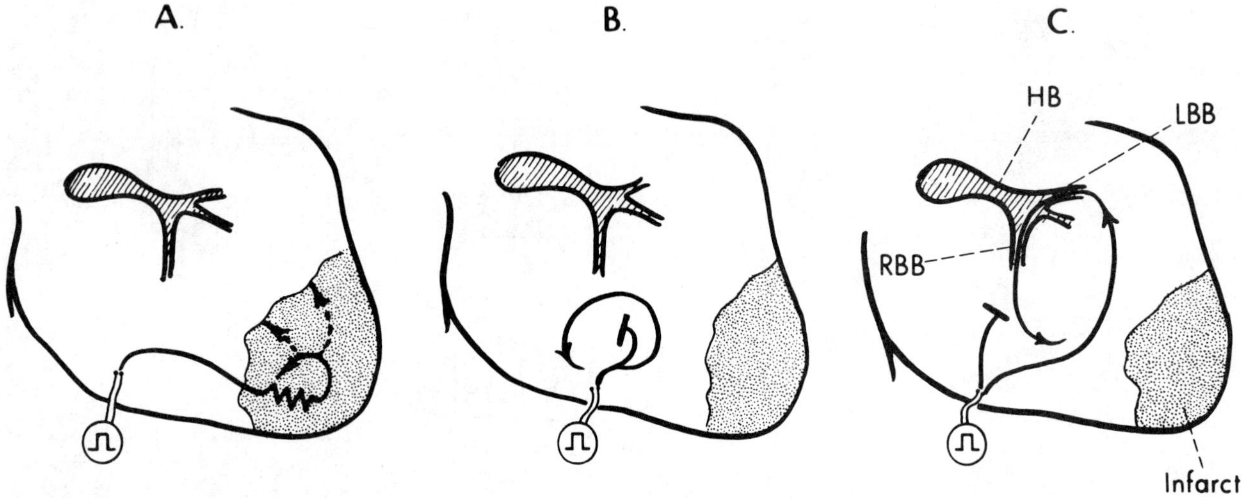

FIGURE 25-18 Mechanisms of ventricular arrhythmias induced by programmed stimulation. The figures demonstrate a stippled zone representing a theoretical area of infarction. *A.* Stimulation results in the creation of a reentrant arrhythmia in the area of infarction. *B.* Programmed stimulation results in reentry adjacent to the site of stimulation in nonpathologic myocardium. *C.* Programmed stimulation results in the induction of a macroreentrant ventricular tachycardia which utilizes the bundle branches of the specialized conduction tissues for its perpetuation.

FIGURE 25-19 Induction of ventricular tachycardia in a patient with chronic recurrent ventricular tachycardia. *A.* 12-lead ECG obtained in a patient during a spontaneous episode of ventricular tachycardia at a rate of 171 beats per minute. *B.* (*opposite*). Recordings during serial electrophysiologic studies. From top to bottom in each panel are surface ECG lead V_1, and intracardiac ECGs from the right ventricular apex (RV), the high lateral right atrium (RA), the His bundle (HBE), and the proximal and distal coronary sinus (PCS and DCS). In each panel, the ventricles are being paced at a basic cycle length of 550 ms and two successive premature beats are introduced (S_2 and S_3). In the top panel recording in the absence of drug, ventricular tachycardia is induced. Using the same coupling intervals, the administration of procainamide (*middle panel*) and quinidine (*bottom panel*) abolishes the ability to induce ventricular tachycardia. (*From D. G. Benditt et al., Recurrent Ventricular Tachycardia in Man: Evaluation of Antiarrhythmic Drug Therapy by Programmed Intracardiac Stimulation, in E. Sandoe (ed.), "Management of Ventricular Tachycardia—Role of Mexiletine," Excerpta Medica, Amsterdam, 1978, p. 507. Reproduced with permission from the publisher and author.*)

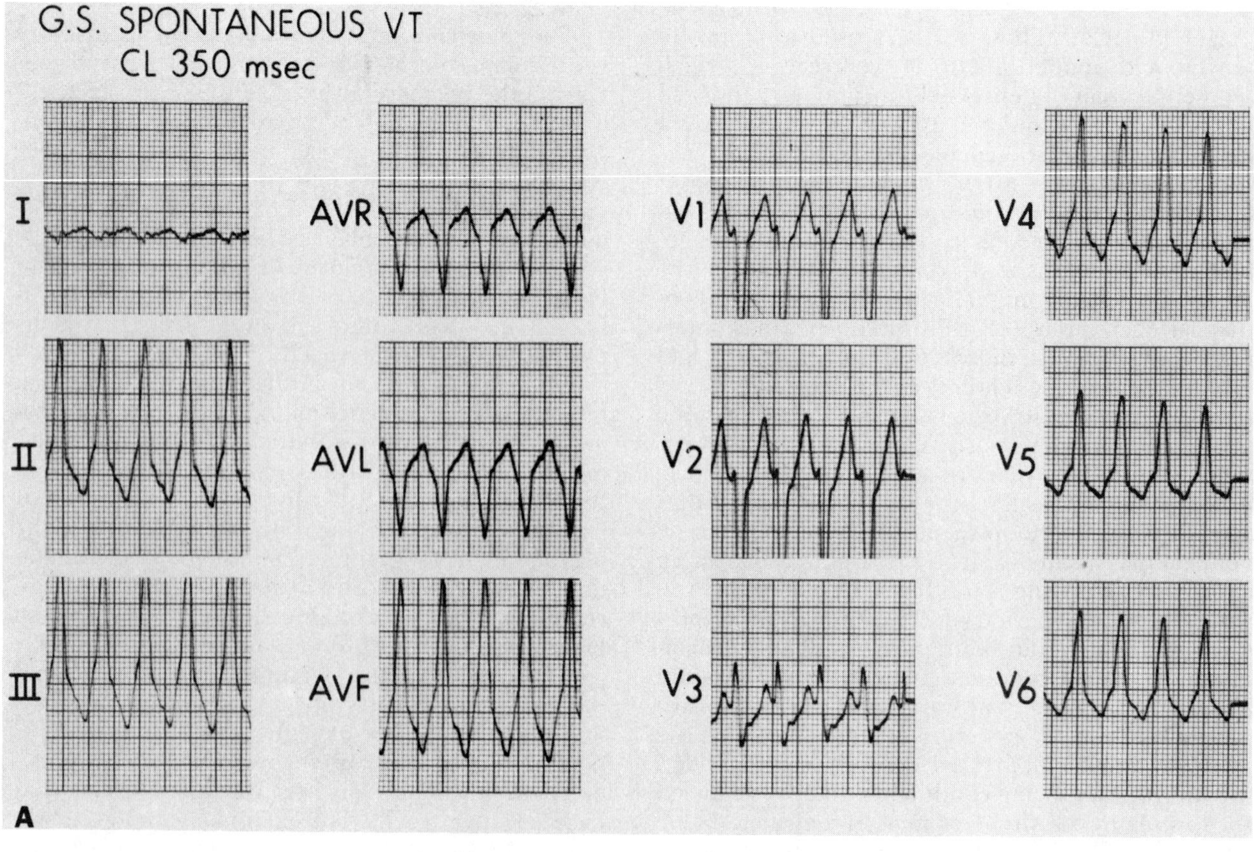

stimulation it is possible to induce so-called nonclinical ventricular tachycardias in patients who have not previously experienced such arrhythmias; this emphasizes the need to correlate the morphology and characteristics of arrhythmias induced by programmed stimulation with those occurring spontaneously. In practice, sustained ventricular tachycardia associated with coronary artery disease may be reproduced by programmed stimulation in the majority of cases, with less success in nonsustained ventricular tachycardia and ventricular tachycardia of non-coronary-related causes.[148,149] The results of catheter electrode studies together with cardiac mapping studies at the time of surgery suggest that in a majority of instances the reentrant process is confined to a relatively small area, although macro reentry has been observed (Fig. 25-20).[138–143] Investigations to date remain limited by the complex architecture of the ventricle, although the development of multiple electrode recording systems and the facility for online computer analysis should advance our understanding by allowing three-dimensional localization of the reentrant circuits involved.[150,151]

In general, it has not been possible to reproducibly initiate ventricular arrhythmias due to acute

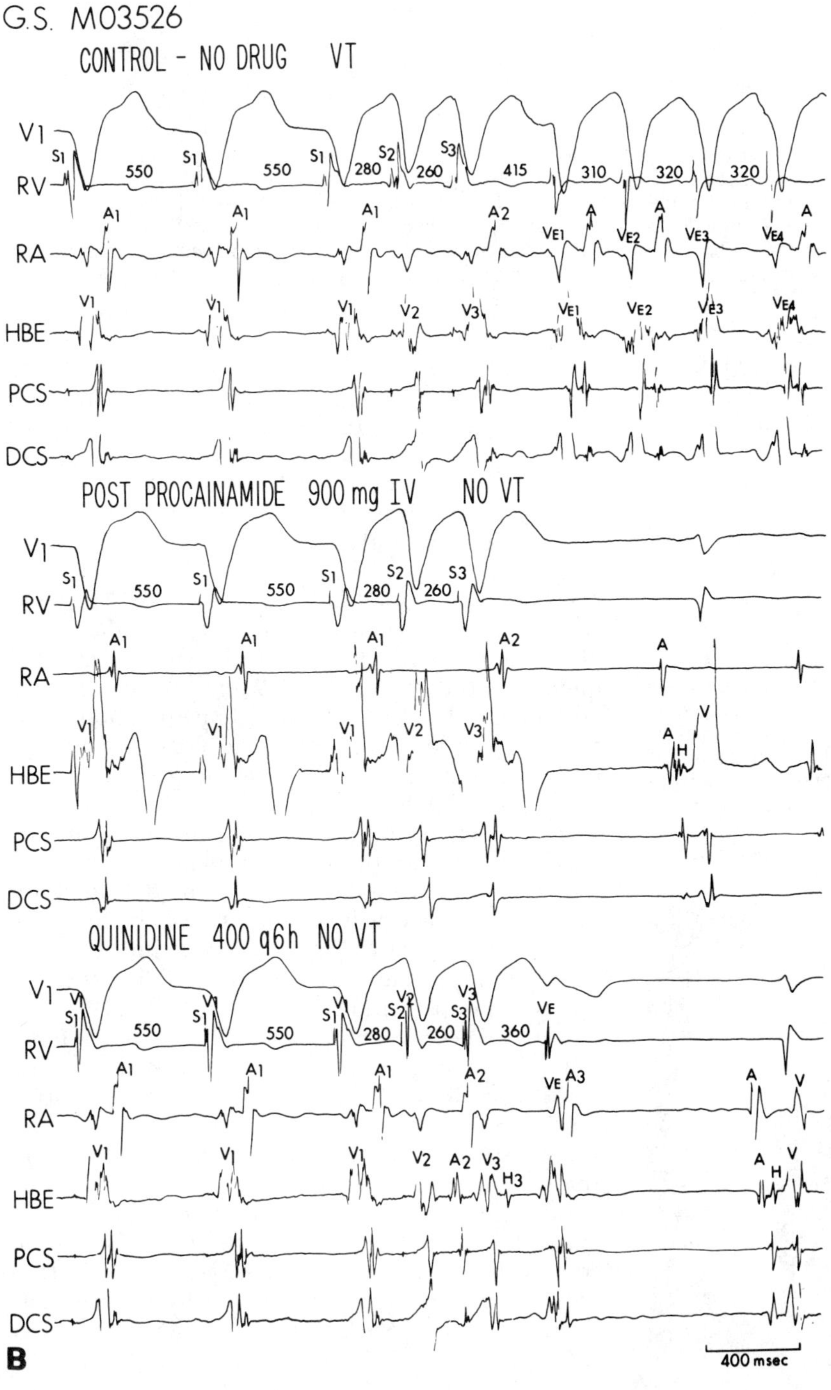

FIGURE 25-19 *Continued.*

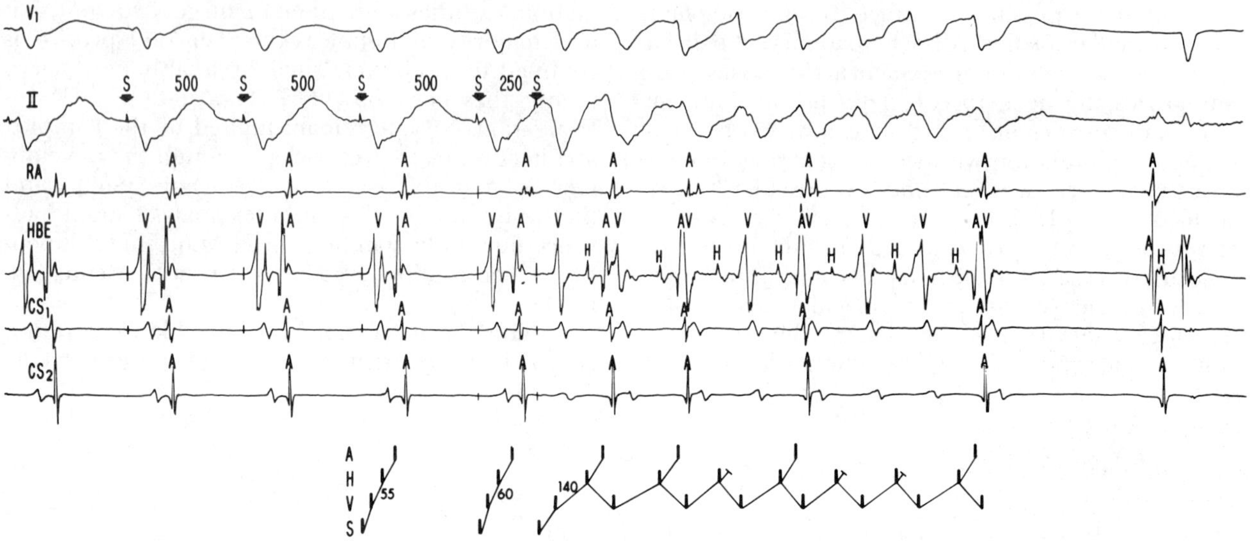

FIGURE 25-20 Induction of a macroreentrant ventricular tachycardia. This tracing was taken from the study of a patient with recurrent palpitations following a diaphragmatic myocardial infarction. The ventricles are being paced at a basic cycle length of 500 ms. During ventricular pacing, a retrograde His deflection is observed in the ventricular electrogram. The sequence of events is diagrammatically shown in a ladder diagram below the electrograms. Following a premature ventricular beat at a coupling interval of 250 ms, the interval between ventricular depolarization and the retrograde His bundle lengthens from 60 ms to 140 ms, initiating a rapid ventricular tachycardia with ventriculoatrial dissociation. Note that in this macroreentrant ventricular tachycardia, a His deflection precedes each QRS complex. This finding is typical of macroreentry in the ventricles.

ischemia, mitral valve prolapse, or the long QT syndrome. In some patients with exercise-induced ventricular tachycardia, the arrhythmia can also be induced by programmed stimulation, while in others catecholamine-sensitive automaticity appears responsible.[152] Ventricular tachycardia originating in the right ventricle, previously assumed to have a benign prognosis,[153] has been shown to be of heterogenous causation. Included are cases of right ventricular dysplasia (Fig. 25-21), which appear to be a cardiomyopathy of the right ventricle,[154,155] cases of the nodoventricular variety of Mahaim fibers,[107,156] (Figs. 25-22 and 25-23) patients following repair of tetralogy of Fallot,[157] and a residual group in whom no discernible hemodynamic or angiographic abnormality of the right ventricle is present.[158,159] In patients with ischemic heart disease, ventricular tachycardia with a left bundle branch block morphology has been shown to arise frequently in the ventricular septum.[160] Such diversity emphasizes the need for careful investigation of patients with a left bundle branch block morphology of ventricular tachycardia, including right ventricular angiography.

FIGURE 25-21 Angiogram of a patient with arrhythmogenic right ventricular dysplasia. A selected frame from a cineangiogram of the right ventricle is shown. An electrode catheter is present in the coronary sinus and an angiographic catheter has been positioned near the apex of the right ventricle. Note the abnormal appearance of the right ventricle with numerous thin-walled areas. These abnormal areas constitute the anatomic substrate of ventricular tachycardia in patients with this disorder. The disorder is notably marked at the apex, where contrast stagnated for 10 cardiac cycles.

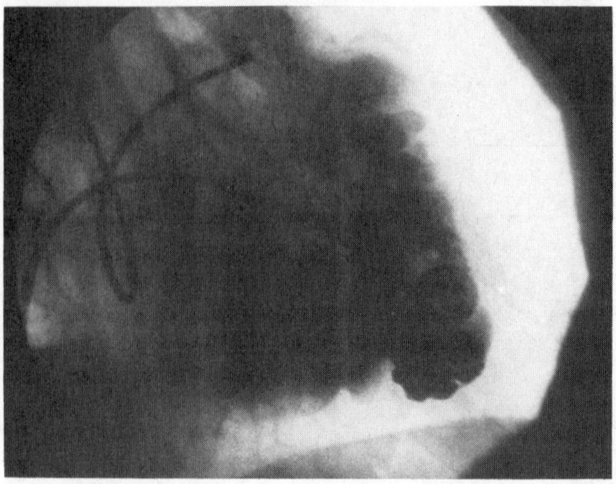

The mechanism(s) underlying the intriguing arrhythmia torsades de pointes remain uncertain, although recent work with a canine model suggested that the characteristic "spindles" which link morphologically distinct QRS complexes during the arrhythmia represent fusion of two colliding cycles of epicardial depolarization.[161]

The role of the autonomic nervous system in the initiation and maintenance of ventricular tachycardia as well as other arrhythmias deserves emphasis. There has been an unfortunate tendency to view the substrate of most arrhythmias as static rather than dynamic and subject to varying influences such as autonomic tone, stretch, and hypoxia.[162–164] For example, Waxman[165,166] recently showed that, contrary to popular opinion, enhanced vagal tone is capable of terminating ventricular tachycardia in some cases, presumably as a result of reflex sympathetic withdrawal.

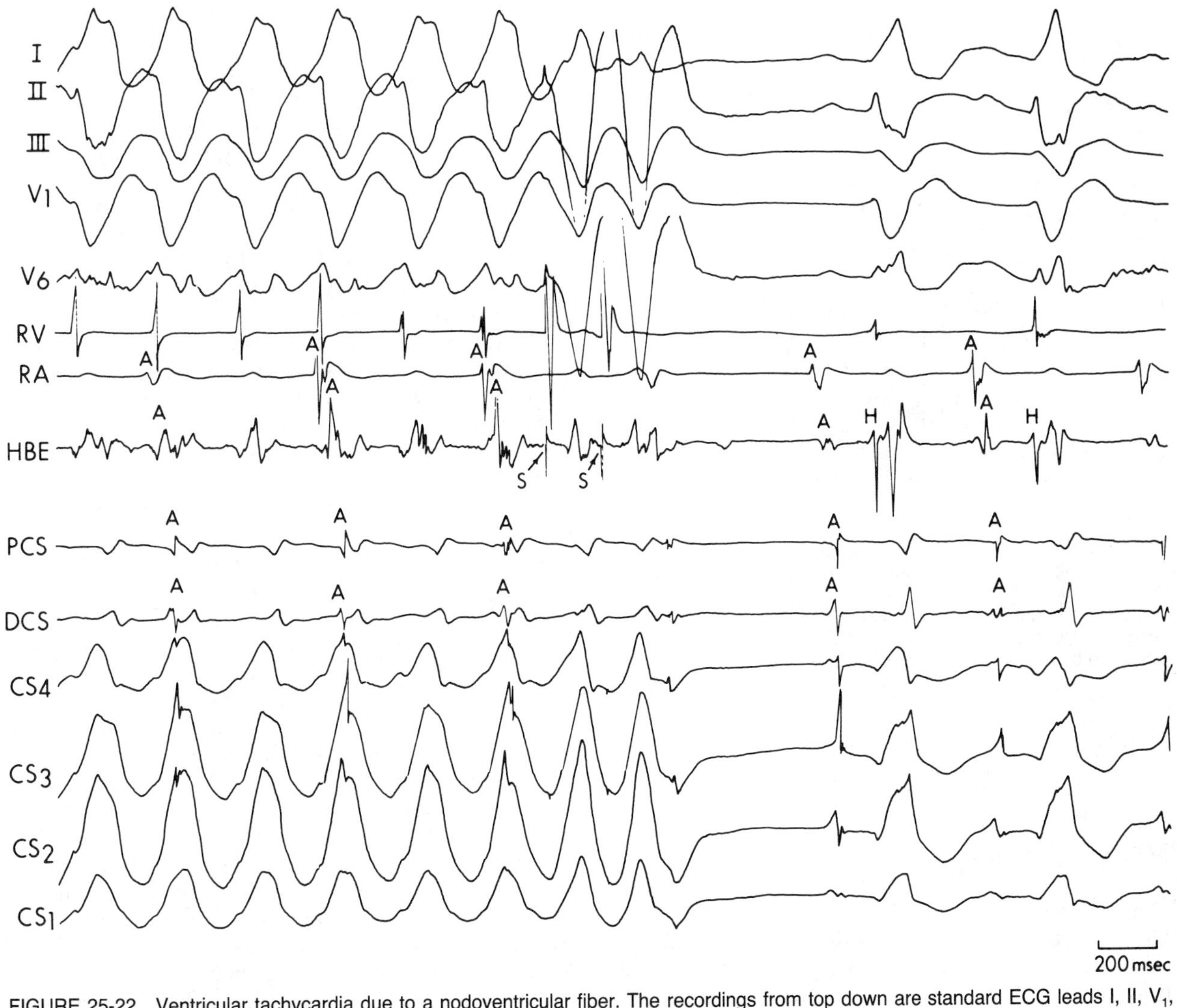

FIGURE 25-22 Ventricular tachycardia due to a nodoventricular fiber. The recordings from top down are standard ECG leads I, II, V_1, V_6, bipolar electrograms from the right ventricle (RV), the right atrium (RA), the region of the His bundle (HBE), the proximal coronary sinus (PCS) and distal coronary sinus (DCS), and unipolar electrograms recorded from the same coronary sinus catheter going from proximal (CS_4) to distal (CS_1) coronary sinus. Initially, a tachycardia with left bundle branch block morphology is present. Ventriculoatrial dissociation is apparent. No His deflections can be observed preceding the onset of the QRS complex. Following six beats of tachycardia, two successive premature depolarizations are introduced to the right ventricular apex during tachycardia, resulting in termination of tachycardia. Following the return to sinus rhythm, a normal PR interval is present associated with QRS complexes with left bundle branch block morphology. Note however that the His deflection occurs at the onset of the QRS complex. The latter combination of events was proved to be due to a nodoventricular fiber.

Ventricular Fibrillation

No single mechanism can be proposed to explain all types of spontaneous or induced ventricular fibrillation. As in the case of atrial fibrillation, however, the features of (1) critical mass of tissue, (2) critical interrelationship between conduction velocity and refractoriness required to initiate and maintain ventricular fibrillation, and (3) the ability to terminate the arrhythmia with a single shock all favor the role of multiple wavelets due to random reentry as the mechanism for sustaining this arrhythmia.[167] As with atrial flutter, however, it remains possible that in some instances the transition to ventricular fibrillation may be associated with a rapidly discharging automatic focus initiating conditions which subsequently sustain random reentry.[150]

Few clinical investigations of ventricular fibrillation have been reported.[168,169] In general, there appears to be a correlation between the ease of induction of ventricular fibrillation in laboratory studies and its clinical occurrence. The ability to induce sustained ventricular tachycardia in patients resuscitated from out of hospital ventricular fibrillation suggests that prodromal ventricular tachycardia may be the initiating cause of some instances of ventricular fibrillation.[169] It is possible that transient coronary artery spasm resulting in reperfusion arrhythmias[145] may be the cause of spontaneous ventricular fibrillation associated with ischemia in humans (Fig. 25-24).

Finally, the important role that the autonomic nervous system and neuropathology[164,170] plays in

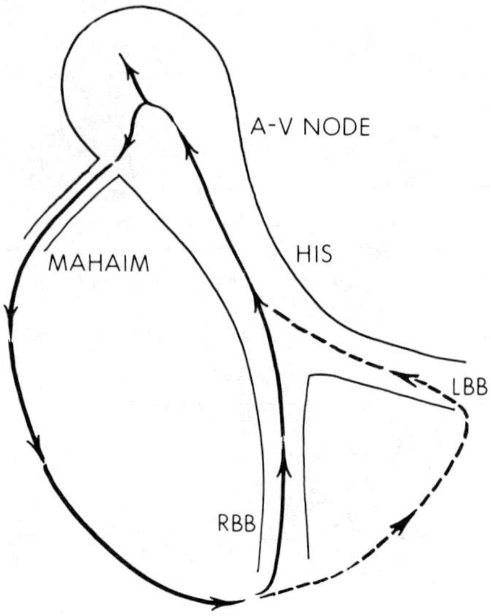

FIGURE 25-23 Schematic diagram of reentry utililzing a nodoventricular fiber. The proposed mechanism of arrhythmia demonstrated in Fig. 25-22 is illustrated. Conduction proceeds antegradely over a nodoventricular fiber from the AV node to the right ventricle and returns retrogradely up the right bundle (or left bundle branch) retrogradely over the His bundle. The reentrant loop is completed by a portion of the circuit located in the AV node.

the genesis of ventricular fibrillation in humans remains to be adequately defined.

Bradyarrhythmias

Sinus Node Dysfunction

Abnormalities of the sinus node may be caused by abnormal impulse formation within the sinus node itself or abnormal conduction of impulses propagating out of the sinus node. In many instances it is difficult to distinguish between abnormal automaticity and varying degrees of sinus node exit block. The recent ability to record the sinus node potential in humans using a catheter-electrode technique[74] promises to further our understanding of the mechanisms of atrial pauses.[171]

There are many similarities between the sinus node and the AV node: the sinus node lacks "fast" channels, and thus sinus node cells have a low resting membrane potential and a contour suggestive of a slow response. Surrounding the sinus node are perinodal fibers which have a normal resting membrane potential and upstroke velocity but whose refractory period exceeds that of cells of both the sinus node and contiguous atrium. We have previously seen that the safety margin with the slow response is low, and that block may appear at boundaries of dissimilar refractoriness; thus, it is not surprising that disorders of impulse formation in the sinus node as well as disorders due to delay and block at the sinoatrial junction (exit block) are observed clinically.[172–174] Relatively few histological studies have been published from patients with sinus node dysfunction.[100–102,175–179] From the available data and their own experience, Davies et al.[100] have defined four distinct morphological patterns comprising (1) amyloid deposition within the node and adjacent atrial musculature, (2) marked loss of nodal cells beyond the normal degree for age, (3) atrophy or hypoplasia of the node, and (4) a group in which there is no detectable morphological abnormality present. Alterations are usually also found in the atrial wall and perinodal nervous structures, although the sinus node artery itself is rarely involved. Furthermore, in many cases there is associated loss of conduction fibers in the more distal conduction

FIGURE 25-24 Ventricular fibrillation due to reperfusion. This tracing demonstrates femoral artery pressure and standard electrographic monitoring lead in a dog in whom the left anterior descending coronary artery was temporarily ligated. At the beginning of the tracing, the coronary artery was released, resulting within seconds in the onset of ventricular fibrillation and loss of blood pressure.

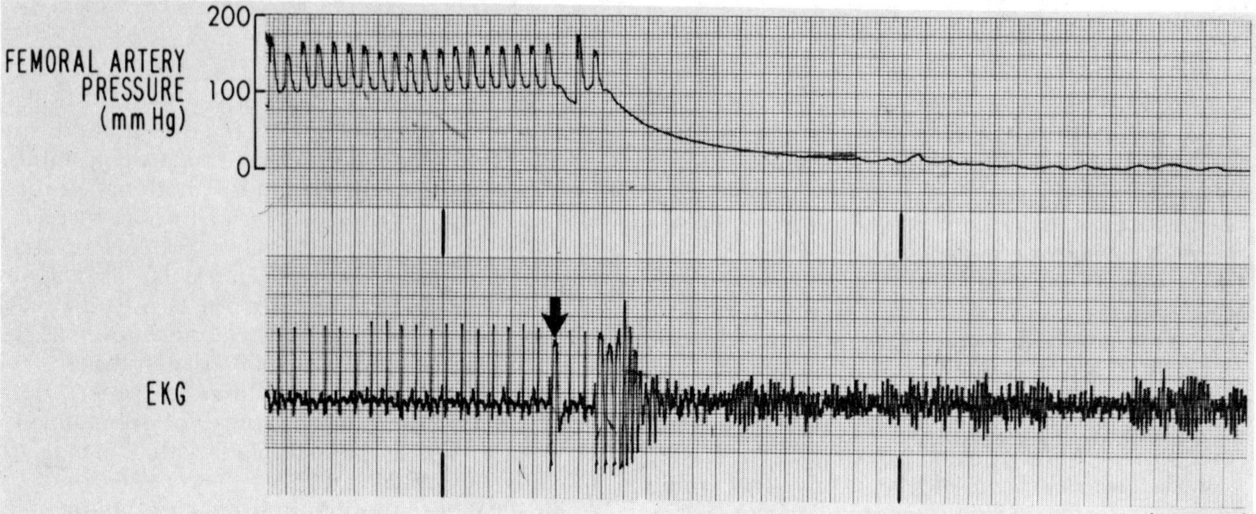

system, which may help to explain the multiple functional abnormalities of the conduction system demonstrated in patients with the sick sinus syndrome.[180,181]

AV Block (Including Bundle Branch Block)

A variety of factors may affect propagation of cardiac impulses, particularly in depressed tissues. Thus decremental conduction is likely to develop in the presence of a lower level of membrane potential and a slower rate of rise of phase 0 depolarization. These conditions can be seen in any fibers showing either incomplete repolarization, significant diastolic depolarization, or partial depolarization caused by various pathophysiologic factors.[182,183] Since the fibers in the N region of the AV node show the above characteristics even under physiologic conditions, decremental conduction is more commonly seen in this tissue than in other portions of the AV conduction system. Many factors known to impair AV conduction, such as acetylcholine, cardiac glycosides, low potassium, or ischemia, enhance the degree of decrement and usually result in conduction delay and block in the AV node. Disorders of conduction in the His-Purkinje system, on the other hand, appear more "all or none" in keeping with the low safety factor observed in fibers from the His-Purkinje system during experimental study of the slow response in these tissues. It is entirely possible that the pathophysiologic mechanisms of conduction delay and block are the same in the AV node and His-Purkinje system and the observed functional differences in these two sites of conduction disorders relate more to other factors such as tissue architecture, nature of intercellular connections, and nervous innervation.

Most of our information concerning the functional behavior of conduction disorders in humans is derived from catheter-electrode recordings of the specialized conducting tissues performed during stimulation of the heart (see Chap. 101). In the few studies published,[184–186] there has been a good correlation between electrophysiologic and pathologic findings in the setting of chronic AV and bundle branch block. In general, in cases of block distal to the recorded His deflection, bilateral lesions of the bundle branches have been present, whereas in cases of block proximal to the recorded His deflection, lesions were present in the penetrating and/or branching portion of the His bundle. The extent of pathologic change is often more diffuse than might have been predicted on clinical grounds; however, it is impossible to predict function completely from structural changes since it is not known how much structure must be retained for proper function. This is especially true of structures with wide cross-sectional areas, such as approaches to the AV node.

The ECG has frequently been used to suggest the presence of block in localized areas of the specialized conducting tissues. It must be stressed, however, that the ECG merely represents the summation of electric forces derived from myocardium. Thus intramural delay distal to the Purkinje myocardial junction can conceivably result in patterns of conduction delay and block normally attributable to lesions in the specialized conducting tissues.[187] Furthermore, although the term *block* is liberally applied, the same pattern can result from simple delay in a localized segment of the conduction system.

Catheter-electrode recordings have confirmed that complete AV block can result from interruption of conduction at the level of the AV node or the His bundle, or can be due to bilateral bundle branch block (see Chap. 101).

The pathology of established AV block shows the most frequent cause to be idiopathic bundle branch fibrosis, characterized by a slowly progressive loss of conduction fibers without demonstrable myocardial abnormality. Two subgroups have been distinguished in the literature, depending upon whether conduction fiber loss is maximal proximally (Lev's disease),[188] involving the branching AV bundle, or distally, involving the middle and distal portions of both bundle branches (Lenegre's disease).[189] However, these may well represent extremes of a continuous spectrum rather than distinct diseases.[190] Pathologic studies of chronic complete heart block due to bilateral bundle branch block generally show diffuse changes throughout the His-Purkinje system, undoubtedly accounting for the slow, capricious behavior of subsidiary pacemaker function in these cases.[191]

Disturbances of conduction accompanying ischemic heart disease can best be understood by referring to the vascular supply of the conduction system. In 90 percent of cases the AV node is supplied by the posterior descending coronary artery, accounting for the frequent association of conduction disturbance in the AV node with diaphragmatic myocardial infarction. The His bundle derives its blood supply from two sources: the AV nodal artery and the first septal perforator of the left anterior descending branch of the left coronary artery. In 50 percent of cases, the right bundle branch has a twofold blood supply: the AV nodal artery and the first septal perforator of the left anterior descending artery; in the other 50 percent, it derives its blood supply only from the first septal perforator or the left anterior descending artery. The anterior fascicle of the left bundle branch has the same blood supply as the right bundle branch, accounting for the frequent association of right bundle branch block with left anterior fascicular block during acute myocardial infarction. Finally, the left posterior fascicle derives its blood supply from the AV nodal artery in 50 percent of cases; in the remaining cases it has a dual blood supply: the first septal perforator of the left anterior descending artery and the AV nodal artery.[192] From the vascular distribution to the conduction system, it is apparent that conduction disturbances in the AV node and, rarely, in the His bundle might be expected following diaphragmatic myocardial infarction; right bundle branch block and left anterior fascicular block, possibly progressing to complete heart block, might be expected in the setting of anteroseptal myocardial infarction. Functional block may also result from local hyperkalemia secondary to potassium efflux from the infarcted myocardium.

Although one might logically expect that the cause of fatality in cases of complete heart block might be the appearance of asystole, it is well known that ventricular tachycardia and fibrillation constitute the fatal arrhythmia in approximately 50 percent of cases, emphasizing the importance of nonhomogeneous depolarization and repolarization that occur at slow heart rates.

References

1. Mines, G. R.: On Dynamic Equilibrium in the Heart, *J. Physiol.*, 46:349, 1913.
2. Mines, G. R.: On Circulating Excitations in Heart Muscles and Their Possible Relation to Tachycardia and Fibrillation, *Trans. R. Soc. Can.*, IV:43, 1914.
3. Lewis, T.: "The Mechanism and Graphic Registration of the Heart Beat," Shaw and Sons, London, 1925.
4. Mayer, A. G.: Rhythmical Pulsation in Scyphomedusae, Publication No. 47, The Carnegie Institution of Washington, 1906.
5. Mayer, A. G.: Rhythmical Pulsation in Scyphomedusae: II. Papers from the Marine Biological Laboratory at Tortugas, Washington, 1908, p. 115.
6. Erlanger, J.: Further Studies on the Physiology of Heart Block: The Effect of Extrasystoles upon the Dog's Heart and upon Strips of Terrapin's Ventricle in the Various Stages of Block, *Am. J. Physiol.*, 16:160, 1906.
7. Schmitt, F. O., and Erlanger, J.: Directional Differences in the Conduction of the Impulse through Heart Muscle and Their Possible Relation to Extrasystolic and Fibrillary Contractions, *Am. J. Physiol.*, 87:326, 1928–29.
8. Garrey, W. E.: The Nature of Fibrillary Contraction of the Heart: Its Relation to Tissue Mass and Form, *Am. J. Physiol.*, 33:397, 1914.
9. Ling, G., and Gerard, R. W.: The Normal Membrane Potential of Frog Sartorius Fibres, *J. Cell. Comp. Physiol.*, 34:383, 1949.
10. Fozzard, H. A.: Cardiac Muscle: Excitability and Passive Electrical Properties, *Prog. Cardiovasc. Dis.*, 29:343, 1977.
11. Cole, K. S., and Marmont, G.: The Effect of Ionic Environment upon the Longitudinal Impedance of the Squid Giant Axon, *Fed. Proc.*, 1:15, 1942.
12. Hodgkin, A. L., and Huxley, A. F.: A Quantitative Description of Membrane Current and Its Application to Conduction and Excitation in Nerve, *J. Physiol.*, 117:500, 1952.
13. Hoffmann, B. F., and Cranefield, P. F.: "Electrophysiology of the Heart," Futura Publishing Company, Mount Kisco, N.Y., 1976.
14. Wellens, H. J. J.: "Electrical Stimulation of the Heart in the Study and Treatment of Tachycardias," University Park Press, Baltimore, 1971.
15. Arnsdorf, M. F.: Membrane Factors in Arrhythmogenesis: Concepts and Definitions, *Prog. Cardiovasc. Dis.*, 29:413, 1977.
16. Pick, A.: Mechanisms of Cardiac Arrhythmias: From Hypothesis to Physiologic Fact, *Am. Heart J.*, 86:249, 1973.
17. Bigger, J. T., Jr.: Electrical Properties of Cardiac Muscle and Possible Causes of Cardiac Arrhythmias, in L. S. Dreifus and W. Lidoff (eds.), "Cardiac Arrhythmias," Grune & Stratton, Inc., New York, 1973, p. 13.
18. Cranefield, P. E., Wit, A. L., and Hoffman, B. F.: Genesis of Cardiac Arrhythmias, *Circulation*, 47:190, 1973.
19. Rosen, M. R., Wit, A. L., and Hoffman, B. F.: Electrophysiology and Pharmacology of Cardiac Arrhythmias: I. Cellular Electrophysiology of the Mammalian Heart, *Am. Heart J.*, 88:380, 1974.
20. Wit, A. L., Rosen, M. R., and Hoffman, B. F.: Electrophysiology and Pharmacology of Cardiac Arrhythmias: II. Relationship of Normal and Abnormal Electrical Activity of Cardiac Fibers to the Genesis of Arrhythmias: A. Automaticity, *Am. Heart J.*, 88:515, 1974.
21. Wit, A. L., Rosen, M. R., and Hoffman, B. F.: Electrophysiology and Pharmacology of Cardiac Arrhythmias: II. Relationship of Normal and Abnormal Electrical Activity of Cardiac Fibers to the Genesis of Arrhythmias: B. Reentry, *Am. Heart J.*, 88:798, 1974.
22. Cranefield, P. F.: "The Conduction of the Cardiac Impulse," Futura Publishing Company, Mount Kisco, N.Y., 1975, p. 199.
23. Hoffman, B. F., Rosen, M. R., and Wit, A. L.: Electrophysiology and Pharmacology of Cardiac Arrhythmias: III. Causes and Treatment of Cardiac Arrhythmias: Part A, *Am. Heart J.*, 89:115, 1975.
24. Katz, A. M.: "Physiology of the Heart," Raven Press, New York, 1977.
25. Vassalle, M.: Cardiac Automaticity and Its Control, *Am. J. Physiol.*, 223:H625, 1977.
26. Hoffman, B. F., and Rosen, M. R.: Cellular Mechanisms for Cardiac Arrhythmias, *Circ. Res.*, 49:1, 1981.
27. Cranefield, P. F., and Aronson, R. S.: Initiation of Sustained Rhythmic Activity by Single Propagated Action Potentials in Canine Purkinje Fibers Exposed to Sodium Free Solution or to Ouabain, *Circ. Res.*, 34:477, 1974.
28. Cranefield, P. F.: Does Spontaneous Activity Arise from Phase 4 Depolarization or from Triggering? in F. Bonke (ed.), "The Sinus Node: Structure, Function and Clinical Relevance," Martinus Nijhoff, The Hague, 1978, p. 348.
29. Cranefield, P. F.: Action Potentials, After-Potentials and Arrhythmias, *Circ. Res.*, 41:415, 1977.
30. Wit, A. L., Boyden, P. A., Gadsby, D. C., and Cranefield, P. F.: Triggered Activity as a Cause of Atrial Arrhythmias, in O. S. Narula (ed.), "Cardiac Arrhythmias, Electrophysiology, Diagnosis and Management," The Williams & Wilkins Company, Baltimore, 1979, p. 14.
31. Wit, A. L., and Cranefield, P. F.: Triggered Activity in Cardiac Muscle Fibers of the Simian Mitral Valve, *Circ. Res.*, 38:85, 1976.
32. Wit, A. L., and Cranefield, P. F.: Triggered and Automatic Activity in the Canine Coronary Sinus, *Circ. Res.*, 38:85, 1976.
33. Fenoglio, J. J., Reemtsma, K., Hordof, A. J., and Wit, A. L.: The Human Anterior Mitral Valve Leaflet As a Possible Site of Origin of Atrial Arrhythmias, *Am. J. Cardiol.*, 4:386, 1978.
34. Hauswirth, O., Noble, D., and Tsien, R. W.: The Mechanism of Oscillatory Activity at Low Membrane Potentials in Cardiac Purkinje Fibers, *J. Physiol.*, 200:255, 1969.
35. Ferrier, G. R.: Digitalis Arrhythmias: Role of Oscillatory Potentials, *Prog. Cardiovasc. Dis.*, 29:459, 1977.
36. Ferrier, G. R., and Moe, G. K.: Effect of Calcium on Acetylstrophanthidin-Induced Transient Depolarization in Canine Purkinje Tissue, *Circ. Res.*, 33:508, 1973.
37. Zipes, D. P., Foster, P. R., Troup, J., and Pedersen, D. H.: Atrial Induction of Ventricular Tachycardia: Reentry versus Triggered Automaticity, *Am. J. Cardiol.*, 44:1, 1979.
38. Rosen, M. R., Fisch, C., Hoffman, B., Danilo, P., Lovelace, E., and Knoebel, S. B.: Can Accelerated Atrioventricular Junctional Escape Rhythms Be Explained by Delayed After Depolarizations? *Am. J. Cardiol.*, 45:1272, 1980.
39. Loeb, J. M., Murdock, D. K., Randall, W. C., and Euler, D. E.: Supraventricular Pacemaker Underdrive in the Absence of Sinus Nodal Influences in the Conscious Dog, *Circ. Res.*, 44:329, 1979.
40. Ten Eick, R. E., and Singer, D. H.: Electrophysiological Properties of Diseased Human Atrium: I. Low Diastolic Potential and Altered Cellular Response to Potassium, *Circ. Res.*, 44:545, 1979.

41. Hordof, A. J., Edie, E. R., Malm, J. R., Hoffman, B. F., and Rosen, M. R.: Electrophysiologic Properties and Response to Pharmacologic Agents of Fibers from Diseased Human Atria, *Circulation,* 54:774, 1976.
42. Friedman, P. L., Stewart, J. R., Fenoglio, J. J., Jr., and Wit, A. L.: Survival of Subendocardial Purkinje Fibers after Extensive Myocardial Infarction in Dogs, *Circ. Res.,* 33:597, 1973.
43. Lazzara, R., El-Sherif, N., and Scherlag, B. J.: Electrophysiological Properties of Canine Purkinje Cells in One Day Old Myocardial Infarction, *Circ. Res.,* 33:722, 1973.
44. Singer, D. H., Ten Eick, R. E., and DeBoer, A. A.: Electrophysiologic Correlates of Human Atrial Tachyarrhythmias, in L. S. Dreifus and W. Likoff (eds.), "Cardiac Arrhythmias," Grune & Stratton, Inc., New York, 1973, p. 97.
45. Brooks, C. McC., Hoffman, B. F., Sucking, E. E., and Orias, O.: "Excitability of the Heart," Grune & Stratton, Inc., New York, 1955.
46. Roberts, D. E., Hersh, L. T., and Scher, A. M.: Influence of Cardiac Fiber Orientation Velocity and Tissue Resistivity in the Dog, *Circ. Res.,* 44:701, 1979.
47. Cranefield, P. F., Klein, H. O., and Hoffman, B. F.: Conduction of the Cardiac Impulse: I. Delay, Block, and One-Way Block in Depressed Purkinje Fibers, *Circ. Res.,* 28:199, 1971.
48. Cranefield, P. F., and Hoffman, B. F.: Conduction of the Cardiac Impulse: II. Summation and Inhibition, *Circ. Res.,* 28:220, 1971.
49. Wit, A. L., Cranefield, P. F., and Hoffman, B. F.: Slow Conduction and Reentry in the Ventricular Conducting System: II. Single and Sustained Circus Movement in Networks of Canine and Bovine Purkinje Fibers, *Circ. Res.,* 30:11, 1972.
50. Allessie, M. A., Bonke, F. M., and Schopman, F. J. G.: Circus Movement in Rabbit Atrial Muscle As a Mechanism of Tachycardia: III. The "Leading Circle" Concept, *Circ. Res.,* 41:9, 1977.
51. De la Fuente, D., Sasyniuk, B., and Moe, G. K.: Conduction through a Narrow Isthmus in Isolated Canine Atrial Tissue: A Model of the WPW Syndrome, *Circulation,* 44:803, 1971.
52. Downar, E., and Waxman, M. B.: Depressed Conduction and Unidirectional Block in Purkinje Fibers, in H. J. J. Wellens, K. I. Lie, and M. J. Janse (eds.), "The Conduction System of the Heart," Lea & Febiger, Philadelphia, 1976, p. 393.
53. Janse, M. J., Cinca, J., Morena, H., Fiolet, J. W. T., Klëber, A. G., de Vries, G. P., Becker, A. E., and Durrer, D.: The "Border Zone" in Myocardial Ischemia: An Electrophysiological, Metabolic and Histochemical Correlation in the Pig Heart, *Circ. Res.,* 44:576, 1979.
54. Smith, W. M., and Gallagher, J. J.: Les Torsades de Pointes, *Ann. Intern. Med.,* 93:578, 1980.
55. Schwartz, P. J.: The Long QT Syndrome, in H. E. Kulbertus and H. J. Wellens (ed.), "Sudden Death," Martinus Nijhoff, The Hague, 1980.
56. Myerburg, R. J., Stewart, J. W., and Hoffman, B. F.: Electrophysiological Properties of the Canine Peripheral AV Conducting System, *Circ. Res.,* 26:361, 1970.
57. Antzelevitch, C., Jalife, J., and Moe, G. K.: Characteristics of Reflection as a Mechanism of Reentrant Arrhythmias and Its Relationship to Parasystole, *Circulation,* 61:182, 1980.
58. Langendorf, R.: Concealed AV Conduction: The Effect of Blocked Impulses on the Formation and Conduction of Subsequent Impulses, *Am. Heart J.,* 35:542, 1948.
59. Watanabe, Y.: Terminology and Electophysiologic Concepts in Cardiac Arrhythmias: II. Concealed Conduction, *PACE,* 1:345, 1978.
60. Moore, E. N., Knoebel, S. B., and Spear, J. F.: Concealed Conduction, *Am. J. Cardiol.,* 28:406, 1971.
61. Rosenbaum, M. B., Lazzari, J. O., and Elinzari, M. V.: The Role of Phase 3 and Phase 4 Block in Clinical Electrocardiography, in H. J. J. Wellens, K. I. Lie, and M. J. Janse (eds.), "The Conduction System of the Heart," Lea & Febiger, Philadelphia, 1976, p. 126.
62. Watanabe, Y., and Nishimura, M.: Terminology and Electrophysiologic Concepts in Cardiac Arrhythmias: VI. Phase 3 Block and Phase 4 Block. Part II, *PACE,* 2:624, 1979.
63. Watanabe, Y., and Nishimura, M.: Terminology and Electrophysiologic Concepts in Cardiac Arrhythmias: V. Phase 3 Block and Phase 4 Block. Part I, *PACE,* 2:335, 1979.
64. Moe, G. K., Jalife, J., Mueller, W. J., and Moe, B.: A Mathematical Model of Parasystole and Its Application to Clinical Arrhythmias, *Circulation,* 56:968, 1977.
65. Pick, A.: The Electrophysiologic Basis of Parasystole and Its Variants, in H. J. J. Wellens, K. I. Lie, and M. J. Janse (eds.), "The Conduction System of the Heart," Lea & Febiger, Philadelphia, 1976, p. 143.
66. Rosenthal, J. E., and Ferrier, G. R.: Contribution of Variable Entrance and Exit Block in Protected Foci to Arrhythmogenesis in Isolated Ventricular Tissues, *Circulation,* 67:1, 1983.
67. Castellanos, A., and Myerburg, R. J.: The Electrophysiologic Manifestations of Abnormal Automatic Activity Arising in Depolarised Foci (Editorial), *Circulation,* 67:9, 1983.
68. Zipes, D. P., Heger, J. J., and Prystowsky, E. N.: Pathophysiology of Arrhythmias: Clinical Electrophysiology, *Am. Heart J.,* 106:812, 1983.
69. Wellens, H. J. J.: Value and Limitations of Programmed Electrical Stimulation of the Heart in the Study and Treatment of Tachycardias, *Circulation,* 57:845, 1978.
70. Allessie, M. A., and Bonke, F. I. M.: Direct Demonstration of Sinus Node Reentry in the Rabbit Heart, *Circ. Res.,* 44:557, 1979.
71. Wu, D., Amat-y-Leon, F., Denes, P., Dhingra, R., Pietras, R. J., and Rosen, K. M.: Demonstration of Sustained Sinus and Atrial Re-entry as a Mechanism of Paroxysmal Supraventricular Tachycardia, *Circulation,* 51:234, 1975.
72. Damato, A. N.: Clinical Evidence of Sinus Node Reentry, in F. I. M. Bonke (ed.), "The Sinus Node," Martinus Nijhoff, The Hague, 1978, p. 379.
73. Wellens, H. J. J.: Role of Sinus Node Reentry in the Genesis of Sustained Cardiac Arrhythmias, in F. I. M. Bonke (ed.), "The Sinus Node," Martinus-Nijhoff, The Hague, 1978, p. 422.
74. Hariman, R. J., Krongrad, E., Boxer, R. A., Weiss, M. B., Steeg, C. N., and Hoffman, B. F.: Method for Recording Electrical Activity of the Sinoatrial Node and Automatic Atrial Foci during Cardiac Catheterization in Human Subjects, *Am. J. Cardiol.,* 45:775, 1980.
75. Goldreyer, B. N., Gallagher, J. J., and Damato, A. N.: The Electrophysiological Demonstrations of Atrial Ectopic Tachycardia in Man, *Am. Heart J.,* 88:202, 1973.
76. Coumel, P., Flammang, D., and Attuel, P.: Intra-atrial Reentry Tachycardia, in P. Puech and R. Slama (eds.), "The Cardiac Arrhythmias," The Arrhythmia Working Group of the French Cardiac Society, Roussel UCLAF, Paris, 1979, p. 108.
77. Allessie, M. A., Bonke, F. I. M., and Schopman, F. J. G.: Circus Movement in Rabbit Atrial Muscle as a Mechanism of Tachycardia: III. The "Leading Circle" Concept: A New Model of Circus Movement in Cardiac Tissue without the Involvement of an Anatomical Obstacle, *Circ. Res.,* 41:9, 1977.
78. Moe, G. K., Pastelin, G., and Mendez, R.: Circus Movement Excitation of the Atria, in R. C. Little (ed.), "Physiology of Atrial Pacemakers and Conductive Tissues," Futura Publishing Company, Mount Kisco, N.Y., 1980, p. 207.
79. Rytand, D. A.: Circus Movement (Entrapped Circuit Wave) Hypothesis and Atrial Flutter, *Ann. Intern. Med.,* 65:125, 1966.
80. Lewis, T., Feil, H. S., and Stroud, W. D.: Observations on Flutter and Fibrillation. Part II: The Nature of Auricular Flutter, *Heart,* 7:191, 1920.
81. Rosenbleuth, A., and Garcia Ramos, J.: Studies on Flutter and Fibrillation, *Am. Heart J.,* 33:677, 1947.
82. Pastelin, G., Mendez, G. R., and Moe, G. K.: Participation of Atrial Specialized Conduction Pathways in Atrial Flutter, *Circ. Res.,* 42:386, 1978.
83. Allessie, M. A.: Mechanism of Atrial Flutter in the Isolated

Canine Heart, in "European Congress of Cardiology 1980 (Abstracts)," S. Karger A.G., Basel, 1980, p. 255.
84. Moe, G. K., Rheinboldt, W. C., and Abildskov, J. A.: A Computer Model of Atrial Fibrillation, *Am. Heart J.*, 67:200, 1964.
85. Boineau, J. P., Schuessler, R. B., Mooney, C. R., Miller, C. B., Wylds, A. C., Hudson, R. D., Borremans, J. M., and Brockus, C. W.: Natural and Evoked Atrial Flutter Due to Circus Movement in Dogs: Role of Abnormal Atrial Pathways, Slow Conduction, Nonuniform Refractory Period Distribution and Premature Beats, *Am. J. Cardiol.*, 45:1167, 1980.
86. Hogan, P. M., and Davis, L. D.: Evidence for Specialized Fibers in the Canine Right Atrium, *Circ. Res.*, 23:387, 1968.
87. Scherf, D.: Studies on Auricular Tachycardia Caused by Aconitine Administration, *Proc. Soc. Exp. Biol. Med.*, 64:233, 1967.
88. Puech, P., Latour, H., and Grolleau, R.: Le Flutter et ses limites, *Arch. Mal. Coeur*, 63:116, 1970.
89. Josephson, M. E., and Seides, S. F.: "Clinical Cardiac Electrophysiology: Techniques and Interpretations," Lea & Febiger, Philadelphia, 1979, p. 191.
90. Wellens, H. J. J., Janse, M. J., van Dam, R. T., and Durrer, D.: Epicardial Excitation of the Atria in a Patient with Atrial Flutter, *Br. Heart J.*, 33:233, 1971.
91. Watson, R. M., and Josephson, M. E.: Atrial Flutter. I. Electrophysiological Substrates and Modes of Initiation and Termination, *Am. J. Cardiol.*, 45:732, 1980.
92. Disertori, M., Inama, G., Vergara, G., Guarneno, M., Del Favero, A., and Furlanello, F.: Evidence of a Reentry Circuit in the Common Type of Atrial Flutter in Man, *Circulation*, 67:434, 1983.
93. Waldo, A. L., MacLean, W. A. H., Karp, R. B., Kouchoukos, N. T., and James, T. N.: Entrainment and Interruption of Atrial Flutter with Atrial Pacing: Studies in Man following Open Heart Surgery, *Circulation*, 56:737, 1977.
94. Waldo, A. L., Wells, J. L., Plumb, J. V., Cooper, T. B., and MacLean, W. A. H.: Characterization of Atrial Flutter: Studies in Patients following Open Heart Surgery, in O. S. Narula (ed.), "Cardiac Arrhythmias, Electrophysiology, Diagnosis and Management," The William & Wilkins Company, Baltimore, 1979, p. 257.
95. Abildskov, J. A., Miller, K., and Burgess, M. J.: Atrial Fibrillation, *Am. J. Cardiol.*, 28:263, 1971.
96. Moe, G. K., and Abildskov, J. A.: Atrial Fibrillation As a Self-Sustaining Arrhythmia Independent of Focal Discharge, *Am. Heart J.*, 58:59, 1959.
97. Moe, G. K.: Nonuniform Distribution of Vagal Effects on the Atrial Refractory Period, *Am. J. Physiol.*, 194:406, 1958.
98. Moe, G. K.: On the Multiple Wavelet Hypothesis of Atrial Fibrillation, *Arch. Int. Pharmacodyn. Ther.*, 140:183, 1962.
99. Nadeau, R. A., Roberge, F. A., and Billette, J.: Role of Sinus Node in the Mechanism of Cholinergic Atrial Fibrillation, *Circ. Res.*, 27:129, 1970.
100. Davies, M. J., Anderson, R. H., and Becker, A. E.: "Pathology of Atrial Arrhythmias," in the Conduction System of the Heart, Butterworth Scientific Publication, London, 1983.
101. Davies, M. J., and Pomerance, A.: Pathology of Atrial Fibrillation in Man, *Br. Heart J.*, 34:520, 1972.
102. Thery, C., Gosselin, B., Lekieffre, J., and Warembourge, H.: Pathology of Sino-atrial node-correlations with ECG in 111 patients, *Am. Heart J.*, 93:735, 1977.
103. Gallagher, J. J., Pritchett, E. L. C., Sealy, W. C., Kasell, J., and Wallace, A. G.: The Preexcitation Syndromes, *Prog. Cardiovasc. Dis.*, 20:285, 1978.
104. Anderson, R. H., Becker, A. E., Brechenmacher, C., Davies, M. J., and Rossi, L.: Ventricular Preexcitation Nomenclature for Its Substrates, *Eur. J. Cardiol.*, 3:27, 1975.
105. Klein, G. J., Bashore, T. M., Seller, T. D., Pritchett, E. L. C., and Gallagher, J. J.: Ventricular Fibrillation in the Wolff-Parkinson-White Syndrome, *N. Engl. J. Med.*, 301:1080, 1979.
106. Benditt, D. G., Pritchett, E. L. C., Smith, W. M., Wallace, A. G., and Gallagher, J. J.: Characteristics of Atrioventricular Conduction and the Spectrum of Arrhythmias in Lown-Ganong-Levine Syndrome, *Circulation*, 57:454, 1978.
107. Gallagher, J. J., Smith, W. M., Kasell, J. H., Benson, D. W., Sterba, R., and Grant, A. O.: Role of Mahaim Fibers in Cardiac Arrhythmias in Man, *Circulation*, 64:176, 1981.
108. Motte, G., Brechenmacher, C., Davy, J. M., and Belhassen, B.: Association de fibres nodoventriculaires et atrioventriculaires á l'origine de tachycardies réciproques: Confrontation électrophysiologique et anatomo-pathologique, *Arch. Mal. Coeur*, 73:737, 1980.
109. Bharati, S., Bauernfiend, R., Scheinman, M., Massie, B., Cheitlin, M., Denes, P., Wu, D., Lev, M., and Rosen, K. M.: Congenital Abnormalities in the Conduction System of Two Patients with Tachyarrhythmias, *Circulation*, 59:593, 1979.
110. Castellanos, A., Zaman, L., Moleio, F., Aranda, J. M., and Myerburg, R. J.: The Lown-Ganong-Levine Syndrome, *PACE*, 5:715, 1982.
111. Weiner, I.: Syndromes of Lown-Ganong-Levine and Enhanced Atrioventricular Nodal Conduction, *Am. J. Cardiol.*, 52:637, 1983 (Editorial).
112. Moe, G. K., Preson, J. B., and Burlington, H.: Physiologic Evidence for a Dual A-V Transmission System, *Circ. Res.*, 4:357, 1956.
113. Moe, G. K., and Mendez, C.: The Physiological Basis of Reciprocal Rhythm, *Prog. Cardiovasc. Dis.*, 8:461, 1966.
114. Janse, M. J., van Capelle, F. J. L., Freud, G. E., and Durrer, D.: Circus Movement within the AV Node As a Basis for Supraventricular Tachycardia As Shown by Multiple Microelectrode Recordings in the Isolated Rabbit Heart, *Circ. Res.*, 28:403, 1971.
115. Wit, A. L., Goldreyer, B. N., and Damato, A. N.: An in Vitro Model of Paroxysmal Supraventricular Tachycardia, *Circulation*, 43:862, 1971.
116. Akhtar, M.: Paroxysmal Atrioventricular Nodal Reentrant Tachycardia, in O. S. Narula (ed.), "Cardiac Arrhythmias," The Williams & Wilkins Company, Baltimore, 1979, p. 294.
117. Denes, P., Dhingra, R. C., Chuquima, R., and Rosen, K. M.: Demonstration of Dual A-V Nodal Pathways in Patients with Paroxysmal Supraventricular Tachycardia, *Circulation*, 43:549, 1973.
118. Gallagher, J. J., Smith, W. M., Kasell, J., Smith, W. M., Grant, A. O., and Benson, D. Woodrow: Use of Esophageal Lead in the Diagnosis of Mechanisms of Reciprocating Supraventricular Tachycardia, *PACE*, 3:440, 1980.
119. Gallagher, J. J., and Sealy, W. C.: The Permanent Form of Junctional Reciprocating Tachycardia: Further Elucidation of the Underlying Mechanism, *Eur. J. Cardiol.*, 8:413, 1978.
120. Mignone, R. J., and Wallace, A. G.: Ventricular Echoes: Evidence for Dissociation of Conduction and Reentry within the AV Node, *Circ. Res.*, 19:638, 1966.
121. Brechenmacher, C., Coumel, P., and James, T. N.: De Subitanis Mortibus, *Circulation*, 53:377, 1976.
122. Rosen, K. M.: Junctional Tachycardia: Mechanism, Diagnosis, Differential Diagnosis and Management, *Circulation*, 47:654, 1973.
123. Gallagher, J. J., Damato, A. N., and Lau, S. H.: Electrophysiologic Studies during Accelerated Idio-ventricular Rhythm, *Circulation*, 44:671, 1971.
124. Coumel, P., Fidelle, J., Jucet, V., Attuel, P., and Bouvrain, Y.: Catecholamine-Induced Severe Ventricular Arrhythmias with Adams-Stokes Syndrome in Children: Report of Four Cases, *Br. Heart J.*, 15(suppl.):28, 1978.
125. Benson, D. W., Gallagher, J. J., Sterba, R., Klein, G. J., and Armstrong, B. E.: Catecholamine Induced Double Tachycardia: Case Report in a Child, *PACE*, 3:96, 1980.
126. Kinoshita, S.: Mechanisms of Ventricular Arrhythmias: A Theoretical Model Derived from the Concepts of "Electrotonic Interaction" and "Longitudinal Dissociation," *Am. J. Cardiol.*, 52:1350, 1983 (Editorial).
127. Wellens, H. J. J., Schuilenburg, R. M., and Durrer, D.: Electrical Stimulation of the Heart in Patients with Ventricular Tachycardia, *Circulation*, 46:216, 1972.
128. Wellens, H. J. J., Lie, K. I., and Durrer, D.: Further Observations on Ventricular Tachycardia as Studied by Elec-

trical Stimulation of the Heart: Chronic Recurrent Ventricular Tachycardia and Ventricular Tachycardia during Acute Myocardial Infarction, *Circulation*, 49:647, 1974.
129. Wellens, H. J. J., Durrer, D., and Lie, K. I.: Observations on Mechanisms of Ventricular Tachycardia in Man, *Circulation*, 54:237, 1976.
130. Boineau, J. P., and Cox, J. L.: Slow Ventricular Activation in Acute Myocardial Infarction: A Source of Re-entrant Premature Ventricular Contractions, *Circulation*, 43:702, 1973.
131. Wellens, H. J. J., Farre, J., and Bar, F. W.: Ventricular Tachycardia: Value and Limitations of Stimulation Studies, in O. S. Narula (ed.), "Cardiac Arrhythmias," The Williams & Wilkins Company, Baltimore, 1979, p. 436.
132. Hope, R. R., Scherlag, B. J., and Lazzara, R: Excitation of Ischemic Myocardium: Altered Properties of Conduction, Refractoriness and Excitability, *Am. Heart J.*, 99:753, 1980.
133. Karagueuzian, H. S., Fenoglio, J. J., Weiss, M. R., and Wit, A. L.: Protracted Ventricular Tachycardia Induced by Premature Stimulation of the Canine Heart after Coronary Artery Occlusion and Reperfusion, *Circ. Res.*, 44:833, 1979.
134. Josephson, M. D., Horowitz, L. N., and Farshidi, A.: Continuous Local Electrical Activity: A Mechanism of Recurrent Ventricular Tachycardia, *Circulation*, 57:659, 1978.
135. Josephson, M. D.: Recurrent Sustained Ventricular Tachycardia: Mechanisms, *Circulation*, 57:431, 1978.
136. Touboul, P., Clavyrolas, R., Huerta, F., Porte, J., and Delahaye, J. P.: Tachycardie ventriculaire induite par des battements supraventriculaires prematures à complex QRS normal: Analyse d'une cas, *Arch. Mal. Coeur*, 68:969, 1975.
137. Vanderpol, C., Farshidi, A., Spielman, S. R., Greenspan, A. M., Horowitz, L. N., and Josephson, M. E.: Incidence of Clinical Significance of Induced Ventricular Tachycardia, *Am. J. Cardiol.*, 45:725, 1980.
138. Reddy, P. C., and Khoraschian, A.: Intraventricular Reentry with Narrow QRS Complex, *Circulation*, 61:641, 1980.
139. Lozano, J., Mandel, W. J., Hayakawa, H., Shine, K. I., and Eber, L. M.: Reentrant Tachycardia: Participation of the Distal A-V Conduction System, *Chest*, 63:23, 1972.
140. Reddy, P. C., and Slack, J. D.: Recurrent Sustained Ventricular: A Report of a Case with His-Bundle Branches Reentry as the Mechanism, *Eur. J. Cardiol.*, 11:23, 1980.
141. Spurrell, R. A. J., Sowton, E., and Deuchar, D. C.: Ventricular Tachycardia in 4 Patients Evaluated by Programmed Electrical Stimulation of the Heart and Treated in 2 Patients by Surgical Division of the Anterior Radiation of the Left Bundle Branch, *Br. Heart J.*, 35:1014, 1973.
142. Akhtar, M., Damato, A. N., Batsford, W. P., Ruskin, J. N., Ogunkelu, J. B., and Vargas, G.: Demonstration of Reentry within the His-Purkinje System in Man, *Circulation*, 50:1150, 1974.
143. Guerot, C. L., Vateri, P. A., Castello-Fenoy, A., and Tricot, R.: Tachycardie par réentre de branche à branche, *Arch. Mal. Coeur*, 67:1, 1975.
144. Karagueuzian, H. S., and Wit, A. L.: Studies on Ventricular Arrhythmias in Animal Models of Ischemic Heart Disease: What Can We Learn?, in H. E. Kulbertus and H. J. J. Wellens (eds.), "Sudden Death," Martinus Nijhoff, The Hague, 1980, p. 69.
145. Murdock, D. K., Loeb, J. M., Euler, D. E., and Randall, W. C.: Electrophysiology of Coronary Reperfusion: A Mechanism for Reperfusion Arrhythmias, *Circulation*, 61:175, 1980.
146. Janse, M. J., Van Capelle, J. L., Morsink, H., Kleber, A. G., Wilms-Schopman, F., Cardinal, R., D'Alnoncourt, C. N., and Durrer, D.: Flow of "Injury" Current and Patterns of Excitation during Early Ventricular Arrhythmias in Acute Regional Myocardial Ischemia in Isolated Porcine and Canine Hearts: Evidence for Two Different Arrhythmogenic Mechanisms, *Circ. Res.*, 47:151, 1980.
147. Janse, M. J., and Kleber, A. G.: Electrophysiological Changes and Ventricular Arrhythmias in the Early Phase of Regional Myocardial Ischemia, *Circ. Res.*, 49:1069, 1981.
148. Buxton, A. E., Waxman, H. L., Marchlinski, F. E., and Josephson, M. E.: Electrophysiologic Studies in Nonsustained Ventricular Tachycardia: Relation to Underlying Heart Disease, *Am. J. Cardiol.*, 52:985, 1983.
149. Naccarelli, G. B., Prystowsky, E. N., Jackman, W. M., Heger, J. J., Rahilly, J. J., and Zipes, D. P.: Role of Electrophysiologic Testing in Managing Patients Who Have Ventricular Tachycardia Unrelated to Coronary Artery Disease, *Am. J. Cardiol.*, 50:165, 1982.
150. Ideker, R. E., Klein, G. J., Smith, W. M., Harrison, L., Kasell, J., Wallace, A. G., and Gallagher, J. J.: Epicardial Activation Sequences during the Onset of Ventricular Tachycardia and Ventricular Fibrillation, in H. E. Kulbertus and H. J. J. Wellens (eds.), "Sudden Death," Martinus Nijhoff, The Hague, 1980, p. 165.
151. Wit, A. L., Allessie, M. A., Bonke, F. I. M., Lammers, W., Smeets, J., and Fenolio, J. J.: Electrophysiologic Mapping to Determine the Mechanism of Experimental Ventricular Tachycardia Initiated by Premature Impulses, *Am. J. Cardiol.*, 49:166, 1982.
152. Sung, R. J., Shen, E. N., Morady, F., Scheinman, M. M., Hess, D., and Botvinick, E. H.: Electrophysiologic Mechanism of Exercise-Induced Sustained Ventricular Tachycardia, *Am. J. Cardiol.*, 51:525, 1983.
153. Pietras, R. J., Mautner, R., Denes, P., Wu, D., Dhingra, R., Towne, W., and Rosen, K. M.: Chronic Recurrent Right and Left Ventricular Tachycardia: A Comparison of Clinical, Hemodynamic and Angiographic Findings, *Am. J. Cardiol.*, 40:32, 1977.
154. Fontaine, G. F., Guiraudon, G., and Frank, R.: Mechanism of Ventricular Tachycardia with and without Chronic Myocardial Ischemia: Surgical Management Based on Epicardial Mapping, in O. S. Narula (ed.), "Cardiac Arrhythmias," The Williams & Wilkins Company, Baltimore, 1979, p. 516.
155. Marcus, F. I., Fontaine, G. H., Guiradon, G., Frank, R., Laurenceau, J. L., Malergue, C., and Grosgogeat, Y.: Right Ventricular Dysplasia: A Report of 24 Adult Cases, *Circulation*, 65:384, 1982.
156. Reiter, M. J., Smith, W. M., and Gallagher, J. J.: Clinical Spectrum of Ventricular Tachycardia with Left Bundle Branch Block Morphology, *Am. J. Cardiol.*, 51:113, 1983.
157. Horowitz, L. N., Vetter, V. L., Harken, A. H., Josephson, M. E.: Electrophysiologic Characteristics of Sustained Ventricular Tachycardia Occurring after Repair of Tetralogy of Fallot, *Am. J. Cardiol.*, 46:446, 1980.
158. Pietras, R. J., Lam, W., Bauernfeind, R., Sheikh, A., Palileo, E., Strasberg, B., Swiryn, S., and Rosen, K. M.: Chronic Recurrent Right Ventricular Tachycardia in Patients without Ischemic Heart Disease: Clinical, Hemodynamic, and Angiographic Findings, *Am. Heart J.*, 105:357, 1983.
159. Palileo, E. V., Ashley, W. W., Swiryn, S., Bauernfeind, R. A., Strasberg, B., Petropoulus, T., and Rosen, K. M.: Exercise Provocable Right Ventricular Outflow Tract Tachycardia, *Am. Heart J.*, 104:185, 1982.
160. Josephson, M. E., and Seides, S. F.: "Clinical Cardiac Electrophysiology," Lea & Febiger, Philadelphia, 1979, p. 247.
161. Bardy, G. H., Ungerleider, R. M., Smith, W. M., and Ideker, R. E.: A Mechanism of Torsades de Pointes in a Canine Model, *Circulation*, 67:52, 1983.
162. Verrier, R. L.: Neural Factors and Ventricular Electrical Instability, in H. E. Kulbertus and H. J. J. Wellens (eds.), "Sudden Death," Martinus Nijhoff, The Hague, 1980, p. 137.
163. Coumel, P., LeClercq, J. F., Attuel, P., Levallee, J. P., and Flammang, D.: Autonomic Influences and the Genesis of Ventricular Arrhythmias, in O. S. Narula (ed.), "Cardiac Arrhythmias," The Williams & Wilkins Company, Baltimore, 1979, p. 457.
164. Lown, B., DeSilva, R. A., and Lenson, R.: Roles of Psychologic Stress and Autonomic Nervous System Changes in Provocation of Ventricular Premature Beats, *Am. J. Cardiol.*, 41:979, 1978.
165. Waxman, M. B., Downar, E., Berman, N. D., and Felder-

hof, C. H.: Phenylephrine (Neo-Synephrine) Terminated Ventricular Tachycardia, *Circulation,* 50:656, 1974.
166. Waxman, M. B., and Wald, R. W.: Termination of Ventricular Tachycardia by an Increase in Vagal Drive, *Circulation,* 56:385, 1977.
167. Surawicz, B.: Ventricular Fibrillation, *Am. J. Cardiol.,* 28:268, 1971.
168. Spielman, S. R., Farshidi, A., Horowitz, L. W., and Josephson, M. E.: Ventricular Fibrillation during Programmed Ventricular Stimulation: Incidence, and Clinical Implications, *Am. J. Cardiol.,* 42:913, 1978.
169. Ruskin, J., DiMarco, J. P., and Garan, H.: Out-of-Hospital Cardiac Arrest: Electrophysiologic Observations and Selection of Long-Term Antiarrhythmic Therapy, *N. Engl. J. Med.,* 303:607, 1980.
170. James, T. N.: Neural Pathology of the Heart in Sudden Death, in H. E. Kulbertus and H. J. J. Wellens (eds.), "Sudden Death," Martinus Nijhoff, The Hague, 1980, p. 49.
171. Asseman, P., Berzin, B., Desry, D., Vilarem, D., Durand, P., Delmotte, C., Sarkis, E. H., Lekieffre, J., and Thery, C.: Persistent Sinus Nodal Electrograms during Abnormally Prolonged Postpacing Atrial Pauses in Sick Sinus Syndrome in Humans: Sinoatrial Block vs. Overdrive Suppression, *Circulation,* 68:33, 1983.
172. Strauss, H. C., Prystowsky, E. N., and Scheinman, M.: Sino-Atrial Electrogenesis, *Prog. Cardiovasc. Dis.,* 29:385, 1977.
173. Brooks, McC. C., and Lu, H. H.: "The Sino-Atrial Pacemaker of the Heart," Charles C Thomas, Springfield, Ill., 1972.
174. Bonke, F. I. M.: "The Sinus Node," Martinus Nijhoff, The Hague, 1978.
175. Lev, M.: The Conduction System, in S. E. Gould (ed.), "Pathology of the Heart and Blood Vessels," 3d ed., Charles C Thomas, Springfield, Ill., 1968.
176. Kulbertus, H. E., DeLeval-Rutten, R., and Demoulin, J. C.: Sinoatrial Disease: A Report on 13 Cases, *J. Electrocardiol.,* 6:303, 1973.
177. Evans, R., and Shaw, D. B.: Pathological Studies in Sino-Atrial Disorder (Sick Sinus Syndrome), *Br. Heart J.,* 39:778, 1977.
178. Bharati, S., Nordenberg, A., Bauernfiend, R., Varghese, J. P., Carvalho, A. G., Rosen, K., and Lev, M.: The Anatomic Substrate for the Sick Sinus Syndrome in Adolescence, *Am. J. Cardiol.,* 46:163, 1980.
179. Kaplan, B. M., Langendorf, R., Lev, M., and Pick, A.: Tachycardia-Bradycardia Syndrome (So-called Sick Sinus Syndrome), *Am. J. Path.,* 31:497, 1973.
180. Rosen, J. M., Loeb, H. S., Sinno, M. Z., Rahimtoola, S. H., Gunnar, R. M.: Cardiac Conduction in Patients with Symptomatic Sinus Node Disease, *Circulation,* 43:836, 1971.
181. Kaplan, B. M., Langendorf, R., Lev, M., and Pick, A.: Tachycardia-Bradycardia Syndrome (so-called "Sick Sinus Syndrome"): Pathology, Mechanisms and Treatments, *Am. J. Cardiol.,* 31:497, 1973.
182. Childers, R.: The A-V Node: Normal and Abnormal Physiology, *Prog. Cardiovasc. Dis.,* 29:361, 1977.
183. Watanabe, Y., and Dreifus, L. S.: Arrhythmias: Mechanisms and Pathogenesis, in L. S. Dreifus and W. Likoff, "Cardiac Arrhythmias," Grune & Stratton, Inc., New York, 1973, p. 35.
184. Bharati, S., and Lev, M.: Histological and Electrophysiological Correlations in Atrioventricular Block and Bundle Branch Block, in O. S. Narula (ed.), "Cardiac Arrhythmias," The Williams & Wilkins Company, Baltimore, 1979, p. 164.
185. Ohkawa, S., Sugiura, M., Itoh, Y., Kitano, K., Hiraoka, K., Veda, K., and Murakami, M.: Electrophysiologic and Histologic Correlations in Chronic Complete Atrioventricular Block, *Circulation,* 64:215, 1981.
186. Rossi, Lino: His Bundle in Electrocardiographic Semantics of AV Block: Anatomicoclinical Considerations, *PACE,* 3:275, 1980.
187. Uhley, H. N.: The Concept of Trifascicular Intraventricular Conduction: Historical Aspects and Influence on Contemporary Cardiology, *Am. J. Cardiol.,* 43:643, 1979.
188. Lev, M.: The Pathology of Complete Atrioventricular Block, *Prog. Card. Dis.,* 6:317, 1964.
189. Lenégre, J.: Aetiology and Pathology of Bilateral Bundle Branch Fibrosis in Relation to Complete Heart Block, *Prog. Cardiovasc. Dis.,* 6:409, 1964.
190. Davies, M. J., Anderson, R. H., and Becker, A. E.: Permanent Atrioventricular Block in "The Conduction System of the Heart," Butterworth Scientific Publications, London, 1983, p. 231.
191. Kulbertus, H. E., and Demoulin, J. C.: The Conduction System: Anatomical and Pathological Aspects, in D. M. Krikler and J. F. Goodwin, "Cardiac Arrhythmias, the Modern Electrophysiological Approach," W. B. Saunders Company, Philadelphia, 1975, p. 25.
192. Roos, J. C., and Dunning, A. J.: Bundle Branch Block in Acute Myocardial Infarction, *Eur. J. Cardiol.,* 6:403, 1978.

26

Recognition of Arrhythmias and Conduction Abnormalities

Henry J. L. Marriott, M.D.   Robert J. Myerburg, M.D.

Glossary

atrial capture Retrograde conduction to the atria following a period of atrioventricular dissociation.
automatic beat A beat arising in an automatic focus, independent of the dominant rhythm.
automaticity The property of spontaneously generating impulses.
AV dissociation The independent beating of atria and ventricles.
block A pathological delay or interruption of impulse conduction.
bradyarrhythmia Any disturbance of rhythm resulting in a heart (or chamber) rate under 60 beats per minute.
bradycardia A heart (or chamber) rate under 60 beats per minute.
capture(d) beat A conducted beat following a period of AV dissociation.
coupling The relation of a premature beat to its preceding "forcing" beat.
coupling interval The interval between a premature beat and the beat preceding it.
ectopic beat A beat arising in any focus other than the normal sinus pacemaker.
escape beat An automatic beat occurring after an interval longer than the dominant cycle length.
extrasystole An ectopic beat, dependent on and coupled to the preceding beat, occurring before the next dominant beat.
idionodal rhythm An independent, relatively slow rhythm arising in the AV junction and controlling only the ventricles.
idioventricular rhythm A relatively slow rhythm arising in and controlling only the ventricles.
parasystole An independent, ectopic rhythm operating alongside the dominant rhythm; its pacemaking center is "protected" so that it cannot be discharged by the dominant pacemaker's impulses.
premature beat See extrasystole.
tachyarrhythmia Any disturbance of rhythm resulting in a heart (or chamber) rate over 100 beats per minute.
tachycardia A heart (or chamber) rate over 100 beats per minute.
ventricular capture Conduction to the ventricles following a period of AV dissociation.
ventricular preexcitation Activation of part of the ventricular myocardium by a descending atrial impulse earlier than expected with conduction via normal AV pathways.

Graphic Methods

Standard Electrocardiogram

The easiest test, and frequently the only one necessary, for the evaluation of a disturbance of rhythm or conduction remains the standard electrocardiogram. A long strip of leads carefully selected to yield the most informative QRS complexes and discrete P waves and which reflect direction of atrial propagation as well (usually leads II and V_1) will yield sufficient information in most instances to make the proper diagnosis.

The analysis of a rhythm strip may be facilitated by the use of *ladder diagrams.* These diagrams are useful for illustrating the mechanism of any rhythm, but they are especially valuable in elucidating complex arrhythmias. Sir Thomas Lewis used them freely; they are sometimes called *Lewis lines.* For most purposes they are constructed with only three tiers—A, AV, and V (Fig. 26-1*A*)—but for special arrhythmias an additional tier must be added: one above (Fig. 26-1*B*) to depict the mechanism of sinoatrial (SA) block, or one below (Fig. 26-1*C*) for the finer points of some ectopic ventricular rhythms.

The three main tiers, A, AV, and V, represent conduction through the atria, the AV junction, and the ventricles. The lines representing conduction are diagramed under the actual tracing and are accurately drawn so that the A line begins at the beginning of the P wave, and the V line at the beginning of the QRS complex. Passage of time is indicated by the slope of the line, and arrowheads are sometimes added to clarify direction of spread, but these are not necessary since the direction of the slope immediately tells which way the impulse is traveling. (Many authors use only vertical lines in A and V

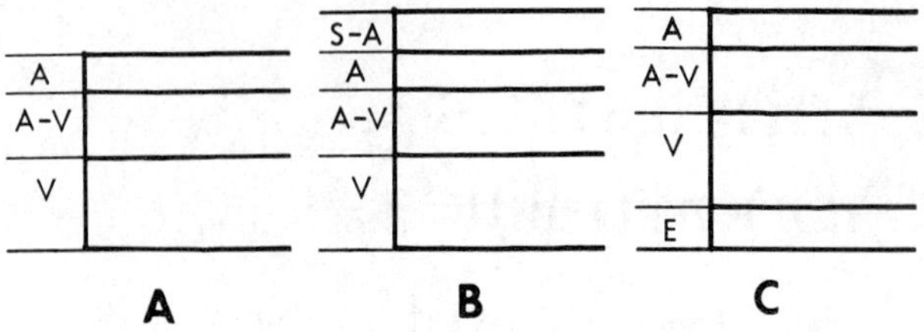

FIGURE 26-1 Skeletons of ladder diagrams used for illustrating the mechanisms of rhythm and conduction.

tiers, reserving the sloping lines to depict conduction in the AV junction.) The site of impulse formation may or may not be represented by a black dot. When an impulse is blocked, the block is indicated by a short bar at a right angle to the main line (Fig. 26-2*C* and *D*). A symbol we have adopted to indicate aberrant ventricular conduction is a pair of slightly divergent lines (Fig. 26-2*A*). A variety of arrythmic mechanisms are diagramed in Fig. 26-2.

In using the diagram for unraveling a difficult arrhythmia, the first rule is draw in only what you can see—do not fill the AV tier with guesses. Only after you have represented the atrial impulses in the A tier and the ventricular impulses in the V tier should you start trying to join them. These stages are illustrated in Fig. 26-3.

FIGURE 26-2 The following mechanisms are diagramed: *A.* Sinus beat with normal conduction (a); sinus beat with prolonged AV conduction (b); atrial premature beat with prolonged AV and aberrant ventricular conduction (c). *B.* AV beat with atrial-before-ventricular activation (a); AV beat with ventricular-before-atrial activation (b); AV beat with retrograde delay and reciprocal beating (c). *C.* Ventricular ectopic beat without retrograde conduction (a); ventricular ectopic beat with penetration into AV junction (b); ventricular ectopic beat with retrograde conduction to atria (c). *D.* AV dissociation between sinus and ventricular pacemakers (a); ventricular fusion beat (b); atrial fusion beat (c). *(From H. J. L. Marriott, "Armchair Arrhythmias," Tampa Tracings, 1966. Reproduced with permission from the publisher and author.)*

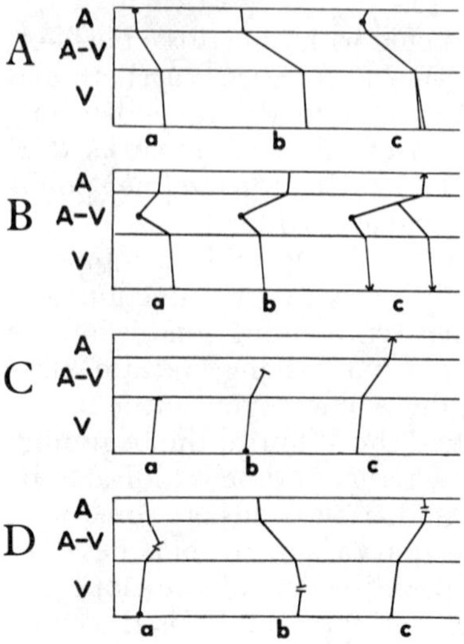

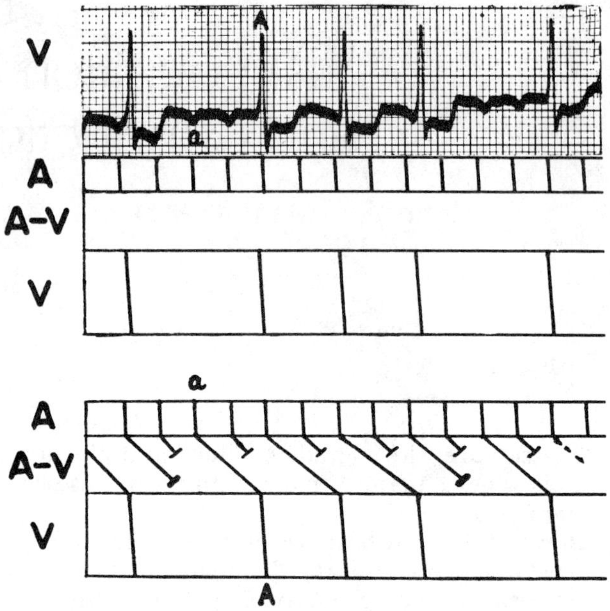

FIGURE 26-3 The proper use of ladder diagrams involves two stages. *Stage 1:* Draw in lines to represent the atrial flutter waves (seen and inferred by measurement) and the ventricular complexes. *Stage 2:* Since in flutter the FR interval usually ranges between 0.26 and 0.45 s, we start by connecting F wave *a* to the QRS A. As we proceed to diagram successive impulses, it quickly becomes plain that we have a basic 2:1 AV conduction with a Wenckebach period of the alternate cycles.[1] *(From H. J. L. Marriott, "Armchair Arrhythmias," Tampa Tracings, 1966. Reproduced with permission from the publisher and author.)*

Special Leads

When standard surface electrocardiography fails to yield sufficient information to make a diagnosis, special systems may be employed. Since failure of the standard techniques sometimes results from failure to identify atrial activity, some special systems are designed to amplify atrial activity in relation to ventricular activity. The unipolar or bipolar esophageal lead to record atrial activity and the unipolar or bipolar intraatrial lead to record right atrial activity are two systems commonly used. In either case, a surface electrocardiographic lead should be used simultaneously with the special lead if a two-channel recorder is available.

For constant monitoring in special care units, a right-sided chest lead takes advantage of precordial QRS morphology and is superior to the formerly popular modified lead II. Of right-sided bipolar leads, MCL$_1$ (modified CL$_1$)—in which the positive electrode is situated at the C$_1$ (V$_1$) position with the negative electrode at the left shoulder—has proved most satisfactory.

Intracardiac Electrography

Although in the great majority of cases, surface electrocardiography is adequate to make an accurate diagnosis of rhythm and conduction disturbances, in difficult cases intracardiac electrograms constitute the final court of appeal (Chap. 101). Together with intracardiac pacing techniques, they may be indispensable for determining the origin of wide QRS complexes, especially in differentiating ventricular tachycardia from supraventricular tachycardia with ventricular aberration; for identifying the precise pathways of reciprocating tachycardias, ventricular and supraventricular; for establishing the site of accessory pathways in the Wolff-Parkinson-White (WPW) syndrome; for ascertaining the level of AV block, whether above or below the bundle of His; for distinguishing genuine AV block from pseudoblock caused by concealed junctional extrasystoles; and for evaluating sinus nodal function.

TABLE 26-1 Range of Sinus Rates in Normal Populations

Population	Number	Maximum (Awake)	Minimum (Asleep)
Normal infants (< 10 days)[2]	134	220	42
Healthy children (7–11 years)[3]	92	195	37
Healthy boys (10–13 years)[4]	131	200	30
Healthy boys (14–16 years)[5]	100	200	23
Male medical students[7]	50	180	37
Young women (22–28 years)[6]	50	189	40
Healthy runners[9]	80	200	35
Middle-aged marathoners[11]	20	132	24

Arrhythmias in Normal Populations

The development of dynamic (Holter) monitoring has enabled us to determine the prevalence of rhythm disturbances in normal populations—necessary background information if we are to evaluate the significance of arrhythmias complicating disease—and the revealed incidence of "abnormal" rhythms in normal subjects of all ages has often been surprising.

The variation in sinus rates in normal children was largely unappreciated before continuous 24-h monitoring became available; the range between the fastest and slowest recorded rates is remarkably wide and indeed remains so in all age groups (Table 26-1).

The frequency of arrhythmias at all ages is no less surprising. Among 134 normal infants monitored for 24-h during the first 10 days of life, atrial premature beats were found in 19 (14 percent).[2] In a subgroup of 71 infants, sinus pauses of up to 1.8 s occurred in 72 percent.

Junctional escape, resulting from sinus slowing, occurred in no less than 45 percent of 92 healthy children aged 7 to 11 years; in one child the escape rhythm persisted for 25 min.[3] Nine of these children had first degree AV block with PR intervals up to 0.28 s. Three had Wenckebach periods, one of whom had over 50 episodes. Atrial and ventricular extrasystoles were found in 21 percent of the children.

First degree AV block was found in 8.4 percent and type I AV block in 10.7 percent of 131 healthy boys aged 10 to 13 years.[4] Single atrial extrasystoles were present in 13 percent and ventricular extrasystoles in 26 percent of these boys.

Among 100 healthy teenage boys, Holter monitoring uncovered the following arrhythmias:[5] ventricular extrasystoles in 41 (10 of which were multiform), short runs of ventricular tachycardia in 3, first degree AV block in 12, and type I second degree AV block in 11.

Atrial premature beats were found in 64 percent and ventricular premature beats in 54 percent of 50 young women, aged 22 to 28 years, without heart disease.[6] One woman had a 3-beat run of ventricular tachycardia, and two had periods of type I AV block.

One-half of 50 male medical students with no apparent heart disease had sinus arrhythmia sufficient to produce 100 percent change in consecutive cycle lengths, and 28 percent had sinus pauses lasting more than 1.75 s.[7] Three students had periods of type I AV block, and atrial extrasystoles were found in 56 percent and ventricular extrasystoles in 50 percent. Even among young athletes extrasystoles may be common: of 20 male long-distance runners, aged 19 to 29 years, all had atrial premature beats and 14 had ventricular premature beats.[8] Eight of these 20 athletes had intermittent type I AV block. Again, in 80 apparently healthy runners under the age of 40 years, atrial extrasystoles were recorded in 41 percent and ventricular extrasystoles in 51 percent during exercise; two had paired ventricular extrasystoles, and one had a 5-beat run of ventricular tachycardia.[9]

Among 98 active, healthy subjects between the ages of 60 and 85 years, whose normal health was confirmed by maximum exercise test and thallium scintigraphy, the following arrhythmias were found:[10] supraventricular premature beats in 88 percent, paroxysmal atrial tachycardia in 13 percent, atrial flutter in 1 percent, and accelerated junctional rhythm in 1 percent; ventricular premature beats in 80 percent (including multiform extrasystoles in 35 percent and pairs in 11 percent), ventricular tachycardia in 4 percent, and accelerated idioventricular rhythm in 1 percent.

An appreciation of the frequency with which the various disturbances of rhythm are found in normal, active subjects in all age groups enables us to approach more intelligently the patient with an arrhythmia.

Sinus Rhythms

Sinus or SA rhythm is the heart's normal mechanism, the controlling impulses arising regularly or almost regularly in the sinus node and driving the heart at a rate between 60 and 100 beats per minute. The node possesses inherent automaticity, but its rate of impulse formation is influenced by vagal and sympathetic tone. If the regularity of rate deviates from the defined standard, the sinus mechanism becomes arrhythmia, tachycardia, or bradycardia.

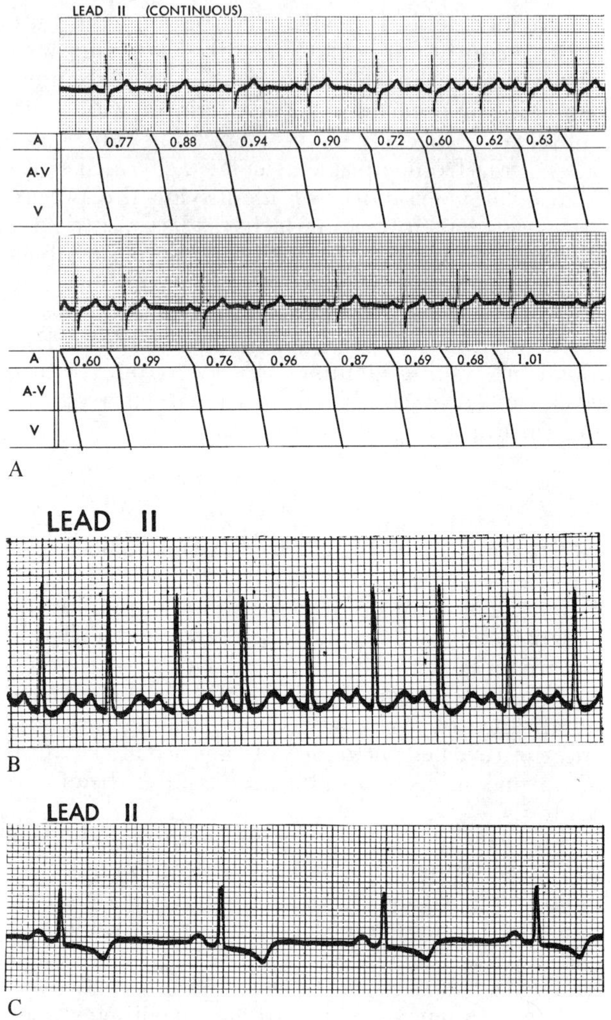

FIGURE 26-4 *A.* Sinus arrhythmia. The sinus cycles are indicated in seconds in the atrial (A) tier; they range from 0.60 to 1.01 s. Notice that as the sinus pacemaker accelerates, the P waves become more prominent. *B.* Sinus tachycardia. Note normally shaped and directed P waves, normal PQ (PR) interval, and a rate of almost 150. *C.* Sinus bradycardia. Note normally directed (but abnormally wide) P waves, normal PQ interval, and a rate of slightly more than 50.

Sinus Arrhythmia

Slight variation in the cycle length is a feature of normal sinus rhythm; if the variation exceeds 0.12 s between the longest and shortest cycles, sinus arrhythmia is present (Fig. 26-4*A*). A normal finding in children and young adults, it tends to diminish and disappear with advancing years. Its presence does *not* rule out organic heart disease.

Sinus arrhythmia occurs in two forms: phasic (respiratory) and nonphasic (nonrespiratory). In the more common phasic form, the heart accelerates with inspiration and slows with expiration; this is mainly owing to rhythmic fluctuations in vagal tone mediated through Bainbridge's reflex. In the nonphasic variety, the irregularity is unrelated to the phases of respiration. Either form may be induced or exaggerated by factors that increase vagal tone. Electrocardiographic features include a variation of at least 0.12 s between the longest and shortest PP intervals, with normal and constant P wave configuration and PR intervals unless associated with type I AV block.

Sinus Bradycardia

By the generally accepted definition, sinus bradycardia implies a rate of less than 60 beats per minute (Fig. 26-4*C*). In adult life, under basal conditions, *physiological* sinus bradycardia occurs much more often than tachycardia and is frequently associated with arrhythmia. Sinus bradycardia was found in 38 percent of 1000 healthy aviators in their twenties.[12] It also appeared in 15 to 28 percent of 6014 asymptomatic Air Force personnel.[13] Its frequency decreased with advancing age: it was present in 22 to 28 percent of subjects between the ages of 20 and 30, but in only 15 or 16 percent between the ages of 35 and 58. Nevertheless, in old age it is not uncommon to find a significant sinus bradycardia in persons with no signs of heart disease. Physiological sinus bradycardia is often found in well-trained athletes, especially those whose activities involve sustained effort (e.g., long-distance runners), and it may develop in other persons during sleep. It is part of the normal reaction to vagal stimulation, as by carotid sinus pressure or eyeball compression, or following Valsalva's maneuver. *Pharmacologic* sinus bradycardia may result from digitalis, morphine, reserpine, pressor amines, or beta blockers. *Pathological* sinus bradycardia may accompany the vagal stimulation produced by vomiting; it is also seen in convalescence from febrile illnesses (notably typhoid and influenza). It accompanies the hypometabolic state, including hypothermia and myxedema. It may be part of the clinical picture of obstructive jaundice, increased intracranial pressure, and depressed mental states. Sinus bradycardia may be the earliest or only manifestation of a "sick sinus." It is common in acute myocardial infarction, averaging 12.5 percent in several series. The incidence of sinus bradycardia is higher when the patient is seen in the early hours of infarction, and it is seen much more often in inferior than in anterior infarctions. The incidence of sinus bradycardia in patients with inferior infarction seen within 1 h of the onset was 41 percent.[14]

The development of sinus bradycardia in acute myocardial infarction, unless it is hemodynamically devastating, appears to presage a favorable outcome: pooled series indicate that the mortality rate among patients with infarctions and untreated sinus bradycardia was 13 percent compared with 28 percent in patients who developed no sinus bradycardia. In another series of 735 patients, the mortality among those with normal sinus rates between 60 and 100 beats per minute was 15 percent, in contrast with a mortality of only 6 percent in patients with sinus bradycardia.[15]

Sinus Tachycardia (Fig. 26-4*B*)

Although the range of normal sinus rates is generally set at 60 to 100 beats per minute, this does not imply that rates outside this range are abnormal. Graybiel found that 96 percent of 1000 healthy airmen between 20 and 30 years of age had basal heart rates between 40 and 85; only 3 (0.3 percent) had rates over 100, whereas 38 percent had rates below 60 beats per minute. Again, analysis of 6014 normal electrocardiograms (ECG) recorded from asymptomatic Air Force personnel between the ages of 16 and 58 years disclosed a rate range from 39 to 129 beats per minute. Accepted ranges of normal rates in infancy and childhood are indicated in Table 26-2.

The word *tachycardia* itself sometimes evokes argument. It is one of our basic arrhythmic terms and as such should be clearly defined; it usually is defined as a heart or chamber rate over 100 beats per minute. Though a heart rate of 140 beats per minute with a sinus mechanism is normal for an infant, it is nonetheless a tachycardia—a physiological tachycardia. Physiological sinus tachycardia also occurs during and after exercise and as a result of anxiety or other emotional stress. It is an integral part of the "fight-or-flight" adaptive response mediated through the sympathetic nervous system.

By definition, the lower limit of sinus tachycardia is 100 beats per minute. The upper reaches of the rate range vary. In infants, the sinus tachycardia rate may exceed 200 beats per minute; well-trained young athletes, driving themselves to the maximal effort, may sometimes attain a rate of 190 to 200. The maximum attainable with extreme exertion tends to decrease with advancing age and poorer conditioning. Most tachycardias induced by exercise or emotional stress in adults fall in the range of 100 to 150 beats per minute.

It is not always easy to distinguish between physiological, pharmacological, and pathological sinus tachycardia. Nevertheless, these three categories provide a useful framework. *Physiological* sinus tachycardia characterizes infancy and early childhood, occurs during and after exercise, and is produced by excitement, anxiety, and other everyday emotions. *Pharmacological* sinus tachycardia can result from medications such as atropine, epinephrine, ephedrine, amyl nitrite, isoproterenol, and thyroid extract, and from such social drugs as alcohol, nicotine, and caffeine. *Pathological* sinus tachycardia occurs with abnormal states such as fever, hypoxia, hemorrhage, hypotension, shock, infections, hyperthyroidism, anemia, beriberi, pulmonary embolism, and heart failure.

TABLE 26-2 Normal Heart Rate in Infancy and Childhood

Age	Minimum	Mean	Maximum
30 h	95	126	155
1 month	110	152	200
2–3 months	95	147	180
4–5 months	115	139	170
6–8 months	110	136	160
9–11 months	95	127	150
12–19 months	95	121	140
2–5 years	70	98	130
6–14 years	65	86	120

(*Source:* Based on data of Namin, E.P.: In B.M. Gasul, R.A. Arcilla, and M. Lev (eds.), "Heart Disease in Children: Diagnosis and Treatment," J.B. Lippincott Company, Philadelphia, 1966.)

Diagnosis

Clinically, sinus rhythms are assumed to be present when the regularity or pattern of irregularity is appropriate, with normally shaped and directed P waves preceding every ventricular complex by an adequate PR interval. Minor variations in the shape and size of the P waves do not exclude a consistent sinus mechanism, since normal P waves may be influenced by respiration and by fluctuations in autonomic tone. The rate and regularity obviously determine whether the mechanism is classified as sinus rhythm or as sinus arrhythmia (Fig. 26-4*A*), tachycardia (Fig. 26-4*B*), or bradycardia (Fig. 26-4*C*).

Supraventricular Arrhythmias

Atrial Extrasystoles

Premature beats (extrasystoles) arising in ectopic foci in the atria are common. They may or may not be conducted to the ventricles, depending on (1) their degree of prematurity and (2) the state of AV conduction. They occur at all ages (Fig. 26-5) and are often seen in the absence of heart disease; they were found in 0.4 percent of 122,000 apparently healthy male Air Force personnel between the ages of 16 and 50 years.[16] However, atrial disease obviously predisposes to them, and they in turn undoubtedly predispose to atrial tachyarrhythmias (tachycardia, flutter, and fibrillation).

Emotion, fatigue, alcohol, tobacco, or coffee may precipitate atrial premature beats in normal persons. They may result from digitalis, atrial distension (as in congestive failure), or ischemia. They are

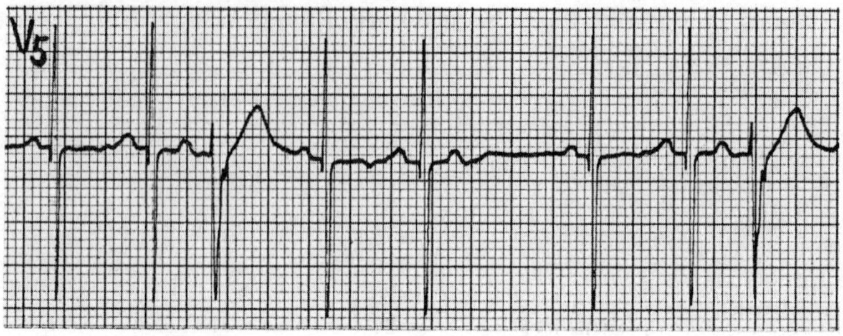

FIGURE 26-5 Atrial extrasystoles with aberrant ventricular conduction—from an infant on the first day of life.

reported in up to 50 percent of myocardial infarctions and are sometimes a sign of atrial infarction. When atrial extrasystoles are due to digitalis intoxication, they may forerun the development of atrial tachycardia with block.

The hallmark of the atrial premature beat is a premature abnormal P wave (P′). When followed by a ventricular complex, the P′R interval is usually normal though often somewhat prolonged. The P′ wave is often difficult to find when it is superimposed on the preceding T wave. Most atrial premature beats are conducted to the ventricles with a QRS-T configuration identical with that of the surrounding conducted sinus beats (Fig. 26-6*A*); but many are conducted with ventricular aberration (Fig. 26-6*B*), and then may closely simulate ventricular premature beats. The cycle following the atrial extrasystole is usually slightly longer than the dominant sinus cycle (Fig. 26-6*A*) but less than fully compensatory. At times it is exactly the same as the sinus cycle, and at other times the ectopic atrial impulse may so suppress the sinus pacemaker that the pause is fully compensatory or even longer. Nonconducted atrial extrasystoles are quite common (Fig. 26-6*C*) and are often overlooked if the premature P′ wave is inconspicuous. In fact, the nonconducted atrial premature beat is easily the most common cause of an abruptly lengthened cycle for which the reason is not apparent at first sight. Careful comparison of the T wave of the ventricular complex immediately preceding the pause with another nearby T wave will often reveal subtle distortion owing to the superimposition of an ectopic P wave. Nonconducted atrial bigeminy is of importance because, if the P′ waves are overlooked, it can simulate sinus bradycardia (Fig. 26-7) and invite erroneous treatment.

Atrioventricular Junctional Extrasystoles

Physiologists have been unable to find pacemaking cells in the AV node of the experimental animal, though they have found them at its junction with the His bundle and in the bundle itself. For this reason it has become the vogue to refer to beats arising in the AV junction as *junctional.* However, there is no conclusive evidence that the human AV node lacks automaticity,[17] and, so long as the matter remains unsettled, we, and others,[18] have no objec-

FIGURE 26-6 *A.* The fifth beat is an atrial premature beat: there is a premature P′ wave followed by a normal QRS-T complex, and the postextrasystolic pause is longer than the sinus cycle but less than compensatory. *B.* The fourth beat is an atrial premature beat with aberrant ventricular conduction: there is a premature P′ wave followed by an anomalous QRS-T complex; the postextrasystolic pause is less than compensatory. *C.* Nonconducted atrial premature beat. Following the third ventricular complex, a P′ wave negatively deforms the ST segment and is not followed by a ventricular response.

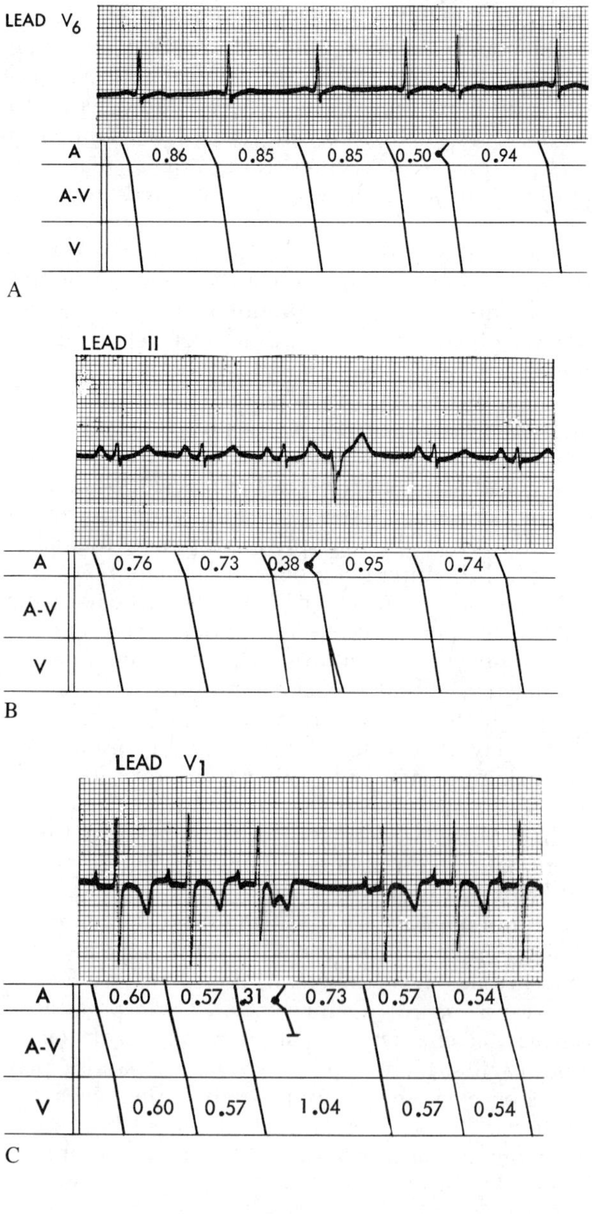

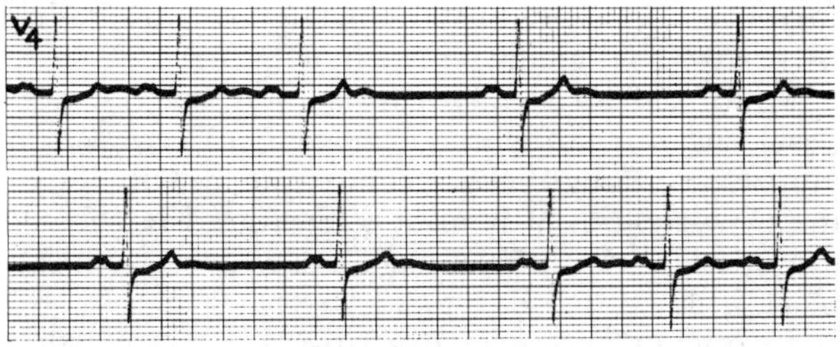

FIGURE 26-7 Atrial bigeminy, nonconducted. The strips are continuous. After three sinus beats, five nonconducted atrial bigeminal sequences simulate sinus bradycardia. *(From H. J. L. Marriott, "Workshop in Electrocardiography," Tampa Tracings, 1972. Reproduced with permission from the publisher and author.)*

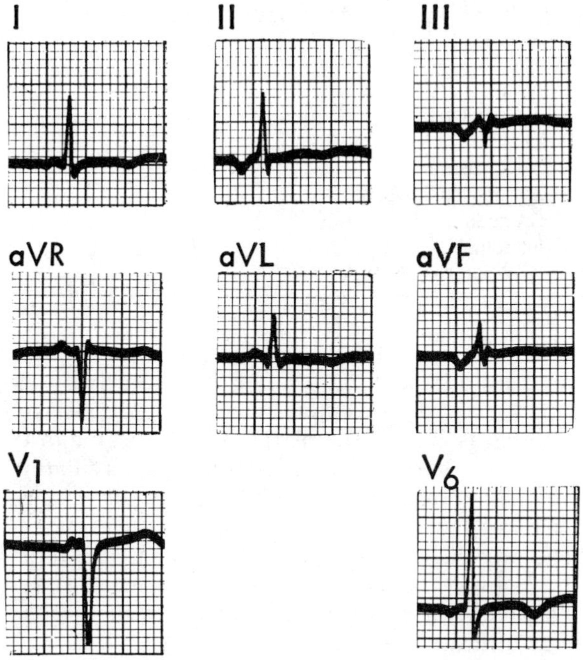

FIGURE 26-8 The short PQ (PR) interval and the polarity of retrograde P waves in key leads in AV (nodal) rhythms: inverted in leads II, III, aV_F, and V_6; upright in leads aV_R, aV_L, and V_1; almost isoelectric in lead I.

tion to the terms *AV nodal* or, simply, *nodal*. We shall use here the more noncommittal terms *junctional* or *AV* as used by Frank Wilson 60 years ago.

Impulses arising in the AV junction spread simultaneously upward to the atria and downward to the ventricles. Depending on the rate of spread in each direction, and perhaps to some extent on the level of origin within the AV junction, the atria may be activated before, after, or simultaneously with the ventricles.

AV premature beats are much less common than atrial or ventricular premature beats, both in health and disease. They were found in 0.2 percent of 122,000 apparently healthy Air Force personnel ranging in age from 16 to over 50 years.[16]

The "retrograde" P waves characteristic of AV rhythm are typified in Fig. 26-8. They are inverted in leads II, III, and aV_F and upright in leads aV_R and aV_L. They are nearly isoelectric in lead I (unless there is atrial hypertrophy); i.e., their frontal-plane axis is close to $-90°$. They are usually upright, or diphasic, in right precordial leads and shallowly inverted in left precordial leads. These P waves precede the QRS complex by less than 0.12 s, coincide with the QRS complex, or follow it.

The retrograde P′ waves of AV extrasystoles are usually associated with normal QRS-T complexes, but, as with atrial premature beats, ventricular aberration may complicate the picture (Fig. 26-9*A*). At times, no retrograde conduction to the atria occurs, so that the sinus rhythm is undisturbed and the postextrasystolic pause is fully compensatory (Fig. 26-9*B*). When the typical retrograde P-wave pattern is associated with a normal—rather than short—PR interval, the rhythm may arise in the junction and be conducted with delay below the junctional pacemaker; or it may arise in an ectopic atrial focus.

Supraventricular Tachycardia

The supraventricular tachycardias (SVT) include all the tachyarrhythmias whose site of impulse formation or reentry circuit is above the bifurcation of the His bundle. By strict definition this group includes sinus, atrial, and AV tachycardias as well as the tachycardias associated with atrial flutter and fibrillation. Sinus tachycardia, atrial flutter, and atrial fibrillation are dealt with elsewhere; this section deals with atrial and junctional tachycardia due either to reentry or to enhanced ectopic automaticity.

Up to about 1970, it was generally thought that the supraventricular tachycardias were due to en-

FIGURE 26-9 *A.* "Lower" AV extrasystole; the retrograde P wave follows the premature QRS complex, which shows some degree of ventricular aberration. *B.* The fourth beat is an AV premature beat without retroconduction to the atria, so that the sinus rhythm is undisturbed.

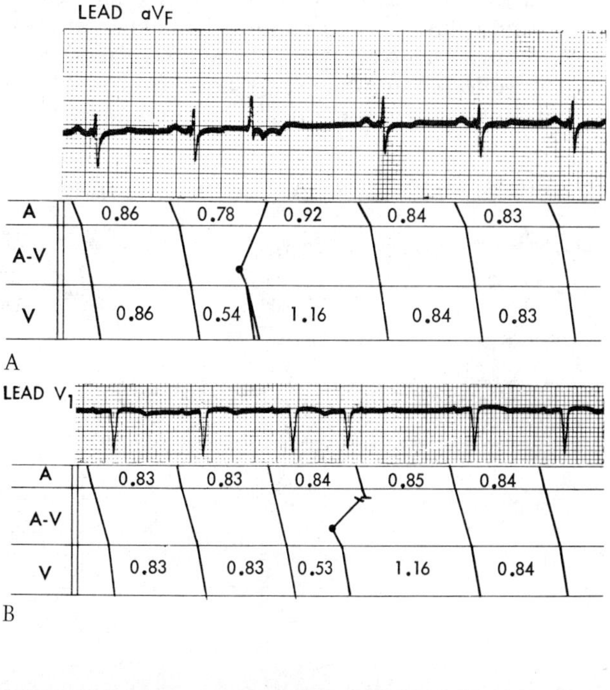

TABLE 26-3 The Supraventricular Tachycardias

1. Ectopic
   a. Atrial
   b. AV junctional
2. Reentrant
   a. AV junctional
   b. AV junctional bypass
   c. SA nodal
   d. Intraatrial
   e. Kent bundle (WPW)

hanced automaticity, i.e., rapid discharge from an ectopic pacemaking center; since then, the electrophysiologists have demonstrated that the majority of such tachycardias are in fact due to a circulating wave front (reentrant, reciprocating, or circus-movement tachycardia). The majority of these reciprocating tachycardias (RT) occupy a circuit within the AV junction. However, there are many other available circuits, and the SVTs have been reclassified as indicated in Table 26-3.

Ectopic Supraventricular Tachycardia

Ectopic atrial or junctional tachycardia may complicate such conditions as acute myocardial infarction, chronic or acute cor pulmonale, pneumonia, and pharmacological intoxications (alcohol, catechols, digitalis, etc.). Ectopic atrial tachycardia is commonly caused by digitalis intoxication, and then it is often associated with AV block, usually 2:1 but sometimes in varying ratios so that the ventricular rhythm is quite irregular. Occasionally the AV block is latent, becoming manifest only with carotid sinus stimulation. Atrial tachycardia with AV block has long been recognized as a common manifestation of digitalis toxicity. Although in the experience of some investigators as much as 75 percent of atrial tachycardias with AV block were due to digitalis toxicity,[19] others have found that only a small percentage of such atrial tachycardias were so caused and that most resulted from underlying heart disease which required digitalis in therapy.[20] The simultaneous occurrence of atrial and AV tachycardia is highly suggestive of digitalis intoxication.

Multifocal atrial tachycardia (also called *chaotic* atrial tachycardia) is unquestionably of ectopic origin, and, although it may complicate any disease of the myocardium, it is most often found in chronic lung disease. Multifocal atrial tachycardia with AV block is illustrated in Fig. 26-10.

Ectopic junctional tachycardia can be a devastating occurrence in children, in whom heredity and the trauma of nearby surgery appear to play causative roles.[21] It is most often seen either after surgical closure of a ventricular septal defect, or in the infant of less than 6 months in whom it precipitates congestive heart failure.[22]

Reentrant Supraventricular Tachycardias

These constitute the great majority of the SVTs; and of them, approximately two-thirds are due to reentry within the AV node and almost another third to reentry involving a bypass tract.[23] The percentage of SVTs that are due to reentry within the AV node as reported from three centers are listed in Table 26-4. A small number result from reentry within the sinus node or atrial myocardium. Reentrant supraventricular tachycardias occur in both the normal and diseased heart. If they are paroxysmal and not chronic or persistent, they are usually well tolerated. The healthy heart may tolerate them well for hours, days, or even weeks. On the other hand, the extremely rapid ventricular rates (300 to 400) sometimes achieved in infancy may cause even the normal heart to fail. Rarely, a paroxysm of supraventricular tachycardia precipitates shock or heart failure in an otherwise healthy youth. Even in the presence of myocardial infarction, short paroxysms of supraventricular tachycardia often require little or no therapy; on the other hand, when such a paroxysm attacks an already disabled heart, it may rapidly induce congestive heart failure, pulmonary edema, or shock. Supraventricualr tachycardia has been reported in 6 percent of patients with mitral valve prolapse.[24] Reentrant SVT can be precipitated by atropine.[25]

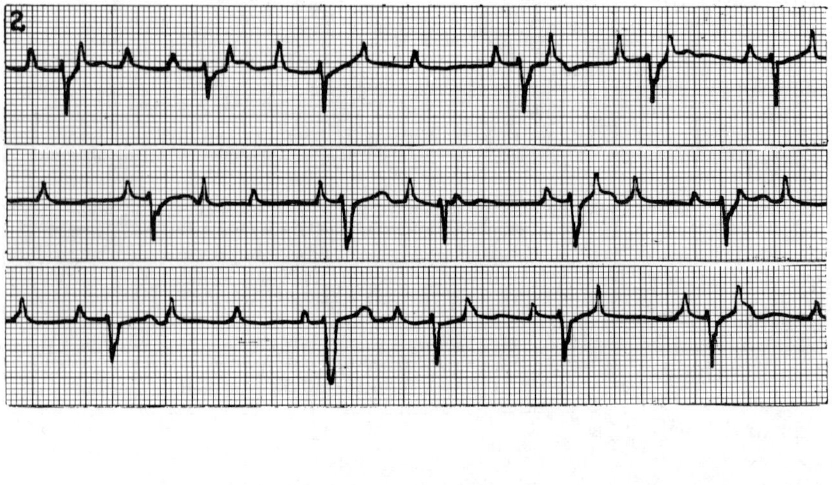

FIGURE 26-10 Multifocal (or "chaotic") atrial tachycardia with varying AV block (from a patient with chronic cor pulmonale). *(From H. J. L. Marriott, "Workshop in Electrocardiography," Tampa Tracings, 1972. Reproduced with permission from the publisher and author.)*

TABLE 26-4 Proportion of SVTs Due to AV Nodal Reentry (AVNR)

Authors	Total SVTs	AVNR	Percent
Wellens and Durrer (1975)[28a]	54	47	87
Wu et al. (1978)[27]	79	50	63
Farshidi et al. (1978)[28b]	60	40	67

Differentiation between Reentry and Ectopic Tachycardias

Since the mechanism and therapy differ, it is clearly desirable to distinguish between the SVT that is due to reentry and the SVT that is due to ectopic automaticity. Although their precise mechanisms can be identified only by invasive methods (Chap. 101), they can often be separated with a high degree of probability from features in the clinical (surface) tracing.[26–28]

The following features are suggestive of an ectopic mechanism: (1) the presence of "warm-up" (progressive acceleration for the first few beats; Fig. 26-11*A*); (2) sameness of all the P′ waves, including the first (Fig. 26-11*A*); and (3) the "resetting" of the tachycardia by a premature stimulus (Fig. 26-11*C*), just as an atrial premature beat resets the sinus. On the other hand, in a reentering tachycardia: (1) warm-up is absent; (2) the initial (ectopic) P′ wave differs from the subsequent (retrograde) P′ waves (Fig. 26-11*B*); (3) a premature stimulus does not reset but may terminate the tachycardia (Fig. 26-11*D*); and (4) prolongation of the first P′R interval is the rule (Fig. 26-11*B*).

The AV node that can host a reentrant tachycardia contains parallel pathways with differing properties: one that conducts slowly but usually has a shorter refractory period (slow, or alpha, pathway), and one that conducts rapidly but usually has a longer refractory period (fast, or beta, pathway). Most reentrant SVTs are initiated by a premature atrial impulse that arrives in the AV node before its pathway with the longer refractory period (usually the fast pathway) has recovered. The early impulse can descend, therefore, only the slow pathway; however, when it reaches the lower junction of the two pathways, the fast pathway has recovered so that the impulse can travel up to the atria rapidly. This "slow-fast" tachycardia thus starts with a prolonged P′R interval (slow downward path), but the RP′ interval is short or absent (P′ wave is lost inside the QRS) because of the rapid retrograde transit.

Much less often, the slow pathway has the longer refractory period and, in this case, the premature impulse travels down the fast pathway and up the slow pathway—a "fast-slow" tachycardia characterized by a long RP′ interval. However, when a reentrant tachycardia is characterized by RP′ > P′R, it is more likely that the reentry circuit incorporates a slowly conducting accessory pathway, often situated in the posterior part of the septum,[29–31] as its retrograde limb. Such tachycardias tend to be "incessant" and are markedly resistant to therapy.[32]

Several other clues point to specific mechanisms: If the P′ wave during the paroxysm is similar to the sinus P waves, there is a likelihood of sinus nodal reentry. If the P′ waves are neither of retrograde form and polarity nor like the sinus P waves, an ectopic atrial or reentrant atrial tachycardia is likely. The presence of AV dissociation or AV block rules out AV nodal bypass reentry; on the other hand, the presence of ventricular aberration tends to confirm the presence of an AV nodal bypass; and when the cycle length of the tachycardia increases (rate decreases) with the development of bundle branch block, it indicates that the bypass tract is on the same side as the bundle branch block. Alternation of the QRS, during a sustained narrow-QRS tachycardia, strongly suggests that the tachycardia is reentrant and that a retrograde accessory pathway is involved.[29] A negative P′ in lead I indicates a probably left-sided bypass.

Electrocardiographic Features of Supraventricular Tachycardias

Supraventricular tachycardia is recognizable in the electrocardiogram (1) if the ventricular complexes are normal or (2) if, in the presence of widened QRS complexes, either an ectopic P wave that is clearly *not* of retrograde form is related to each ventricular complex or the wide QRS complexes are morphologically typical of right bundle branch block. If the P′ waves *are* of retrograde form, ventricular tachycardia with 1:1 retrograde conduction may not be excludable. But P′ waves are often not distinguishable with certainty; if they are, one *may* be able to distinguish between atrial and AV junctional tachycardia (Fig. 26-12*A*). AV junctional tachycardia (Fig. 26-12*B* can be recognized with certainty only if either of the following occurs:

1. The beginning or end of a paroxysm is recorded and the first or last beat of the paroxysm is associated with an appropriately directed retrograde P′ wave that either follows or shortly precedes the QRS complex.
2. Independent atrial activity (independent P waves or atrial fibrillation) is evident (Fig. 26-12*C*).

Atrial tachycardia can be diagnosed with certainty only if abnormal P waves, *not* appropriately directed for retrograde impulses, are seen in recognizable relation to the QRS complexes. If in the presence of rapid normal ventricular complexes, P waves are not discernible or are of retrograde or uncertain form, one cannot usually tell whether the mechanism is atrial, AV, or reciprocating. The retrograde P wave that is closely associated with a QRS complex may "belong" to it (AV junctional tachycardia) or may represent the ectopic atrial impulse that is responsible for the *next* ventricular com-

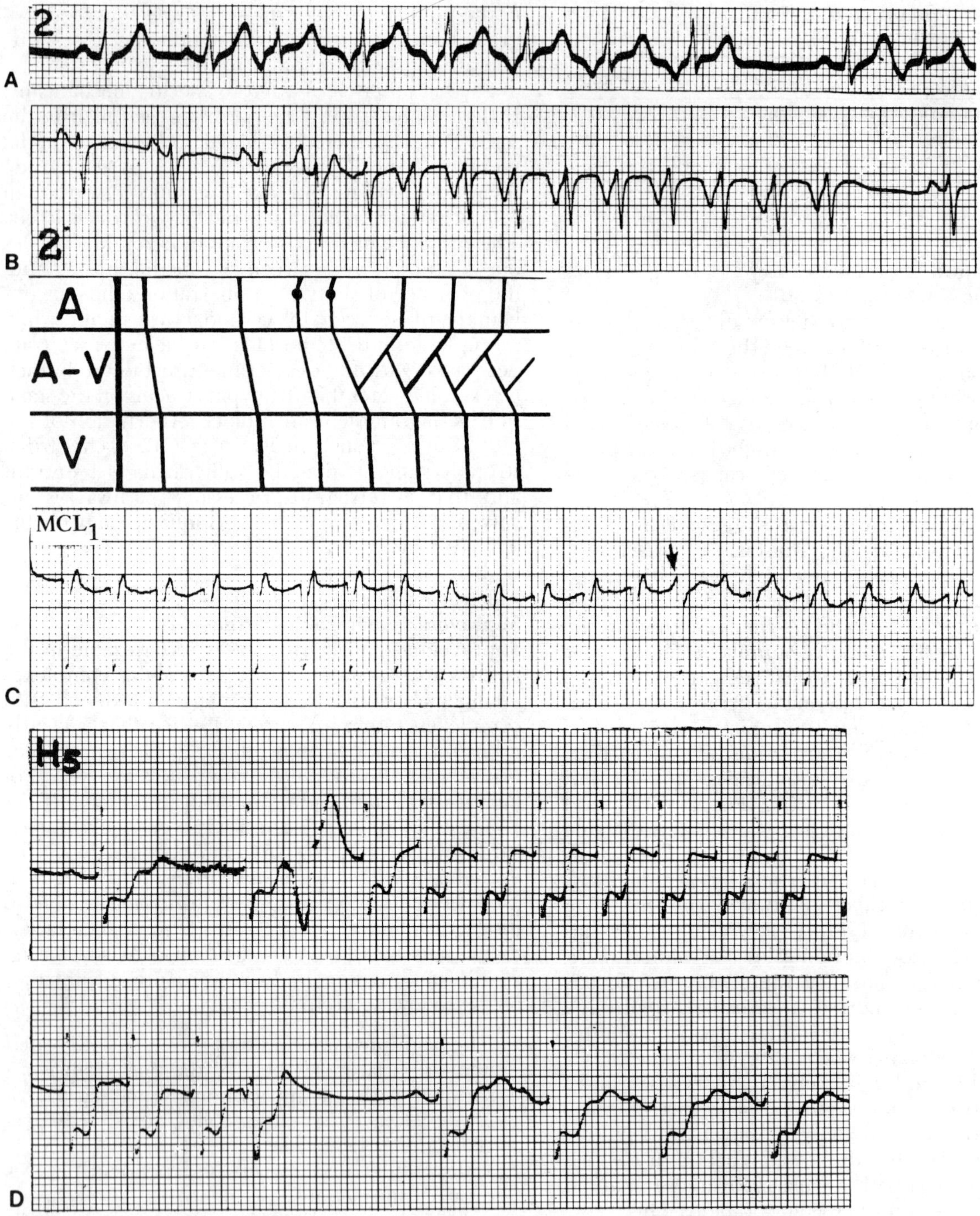

FIGURE 26-11 *A.* Ectopic atrial tachycardia: the inverted P′ waves are all identical and the first few atrial beats show gradual acceleration. *B.* Reciprocating tachycardia: the tachycardia is initiated by the second of two atrial extrasystoles (upright P′ wave) while all subsequent P′ waves are inverted (retrograde). *C.* Ectopic atrial tachycardia: the regular tachycardia is interrupted by a premature P′ wave (arrow) which "resets" the ectopic atrial pacemaker. *D.* Reciprocating tachycardia initiated by a ventricular extrasystole and terminated by another premature beat (from a Holter recording).

plex (atrial tachycardia). Complete invisibility of the P waves may mean that they are "lost" in the T wave or QRS complex; if lost in the QRS, they may be retrograde P waves of junctional origin, or, since PR intervals are frequently prolonged in atrial tachycardia, they may be ectopic atrial P waves responsible for the *following* QRS complex. When the P′ waves of atrial tachycardia are plainly visible, their important feature is that they are different from the dominant P of the sinus rhythm. Ectopic rhythms may have P waves with polarity similar to that of sinus P waves but different in shape, or they may be indistinguishable from retrograde P waves of AV origin. The P waves of atrial tachycardia caused by

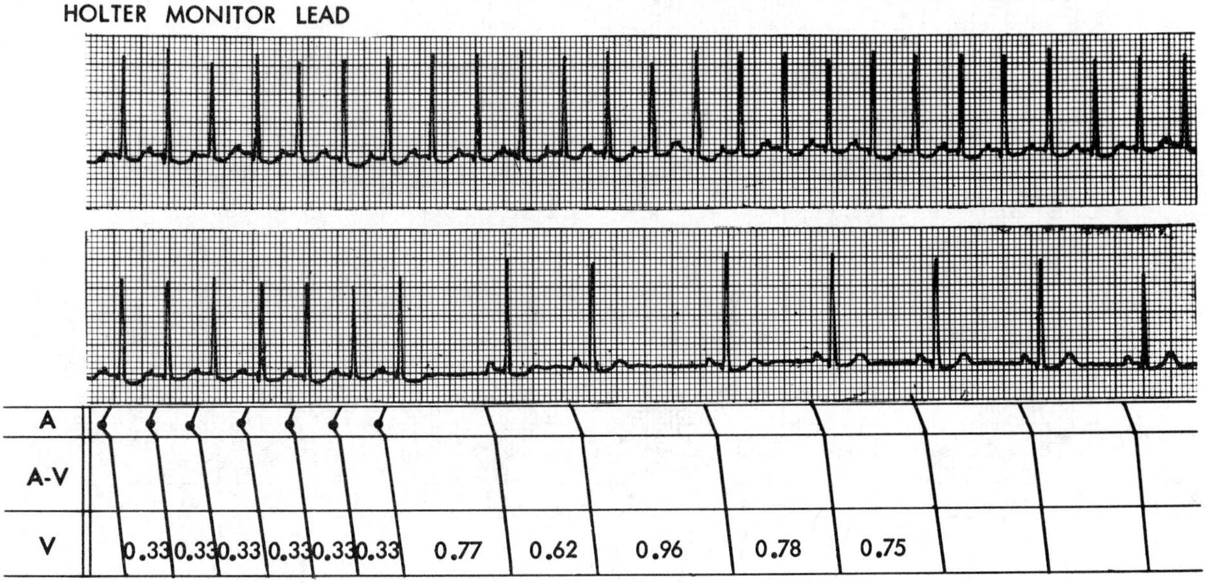

A

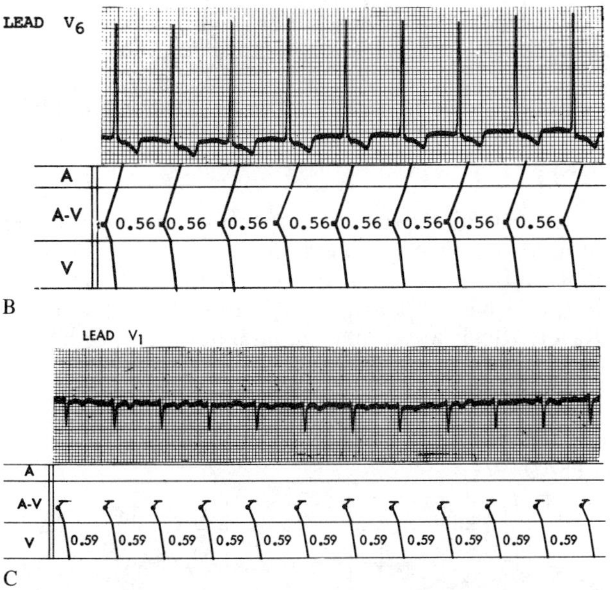

B

C

FIGURE 26-12 *A.* Atrial tachycardia. End of typical paroxysm. Note P′ wave preceding each normal QRS complex at the rate of 190; paroxysm abruptly stops in lower strip. *B.* AV tachycardia. Note retrograde P wave shortly following each QRS complex at the rate of 105. *C.* AV tachycardia at the rate of 102 in the presence of atrial fibrillation.

digitalis toxicity tend to be normally directed but of small amplitude (Fig. 26-13*A*; unlike the sturdy P waves of sinus tachycardia) and somewhat variable in form from beat to beat; the P′P′ intervals are often slightly irregular. Multifocal atrial tachycardia (also called chaotic atrial tachycardia) is diagnosed when the ectopic P waves vary in shape and the P′P′ intervals also vary (Fig. 26-13*B*).[33]

Atrial Flutter

Atrial flutter has never been satisfactorily defined. When an elderly person with heart disease develops an atrial rate of about 320 impulses per minute, with typical "sawtooth" waves in the electrocardiogram and 2:1 AV conduction, the term *flutter* is universally applied. When a healthy adolescent develops an atrial rate of about 180 beats per minute with abnormal P waves and 1:1 AV conduction, everyone calls it atrial tachycardia. But between these two classic pictures there is a shadowland of imprecision in which there are no sure signposts, and it is a moot point whether the boundaries between tachycardia and flutter can be set.

Mindful of the overlap with tachycardia, one can say that the typical example of atrial flutter occurs in a patient with heart disease, that the atrial rate is usually between 280 and 320 beats per minute, and that there is usually a 2:1 conduction ratio. It is wrong to call this 2:1 "block" because, at rates around 300, physiological refractoriness—not pathological block—prevents the 1:1 ventricular response.

Atrial flutter is rarely seen in normal subjects. It was found only once among the 67,000 Air Force personnel screened by Fosmoe.[34] It may occur at all ages, even in infancy, and in fact is more common than atrial fibrillation in the first few years of life.[35] However, flutter is most commonly encountered in persons with ischemic heart disease over the age of 40 years, and paroxysms complicate 2 to 5 percent of cases of acute myocardial infarction. It may rarely be caused by digitalis intoxication, and sometimes results from treatment of atrial fibrillation with quinidine or procainamide. Paroxysms of flutter may complicate any form of heart disease or be precipitated by many acute illnesses.

Electrocardiographic Features

The waves of flutter in the ECG are labeled F waves, and their rate is usually between 280 and 320 per minute. Their pattern is variable, but the most com-

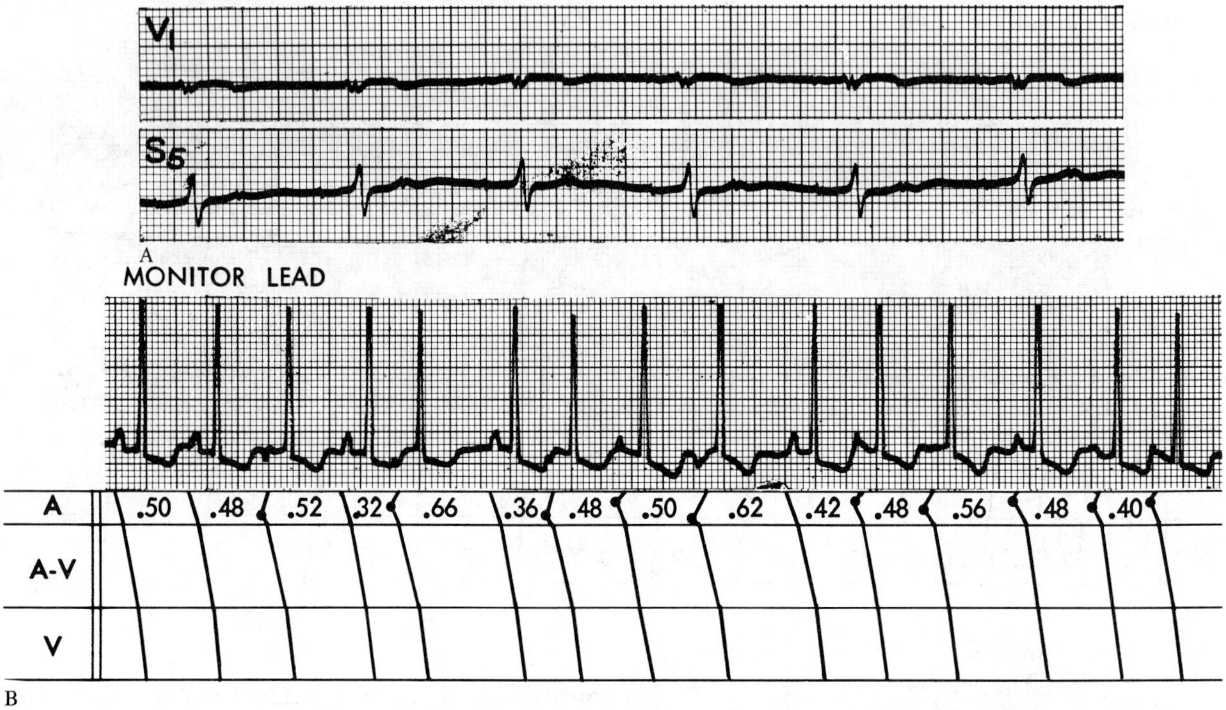

FIGURE 26-13 *A.* Atrial tachycardia with 2:1 AV block due to digitalis intoxication. Note the diminutive P waves, barely visible even in V_1. *B.* Multifocal (chaotic) atrial tachycardia. Note the constantly changing form of the ectopic P waves and the irregular rhythm at the rate of 122.

mon one presents the typical sawtooth waves in leads II, III, and aV_F, more discrete waves separated by isoelectric intervals in V_1 and other precordial leads, and poorly registered activity in lead I (Fig. 26-14). When the rate is slow enough, a definite isoelectric "shelf" appears even in the limb leads. Less commonly, atrial activity may not show up at all in the limb leads but may be evident only in right precordial leads; or again, it may be obvious in limb leads but relatively inconspicuous in right chest leads. Rarely the F waves may be notched or undulating, rather than serrated.

FIGURE 26-14 Atrial flutter. Note the "sawtooth" pattern in leads II and III with poorly registered atrial activity in leads I and V_6.

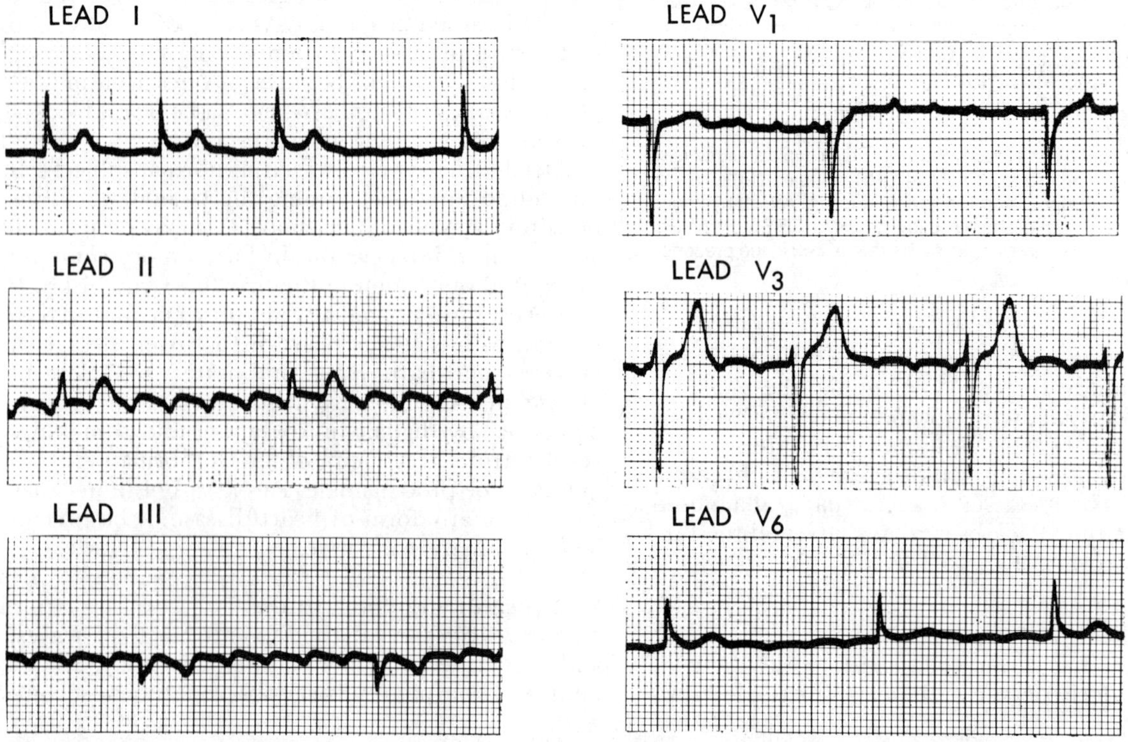

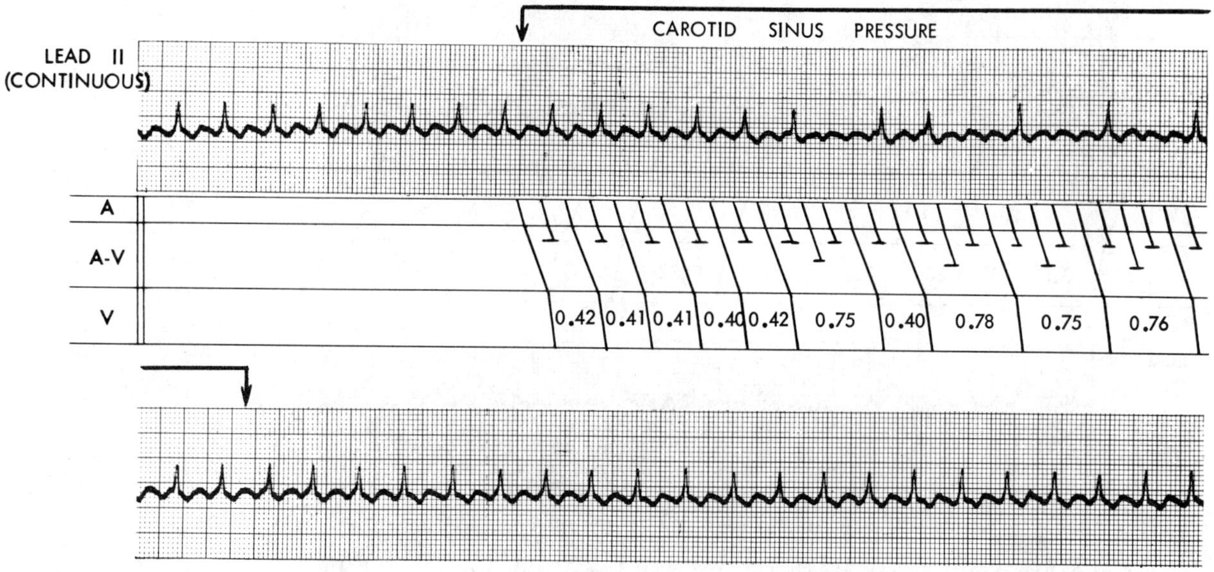

FIGURE 26-15 Atrial flutter. At the beginning of the strip there is the common 2:1 ratio, and flutter (F) waves can be suspected but not proved; however, after carotid sinus stimulation, the conduction ratio increases to 4:1 and the F waves are clearly exposed.

The commonest AV conduction ratio is 2:1; at this ratio it often happens that alternate F waves are lost in or merge with the QRS complex, so that the underlying mechanism may be overlooked. In this situation, when flutter is suspected, carotid sinus stimulation may prove the point by momentarily increasing AV blockade and so uncovering the lurking F waves (Fig. 26-15). The next most common ratio is 4:1, especially after therapy with digitalis or propranolol. Ratios of 5:1, 3:1, and 1:1 are rare. Atrial flutter with 1:1 AV conduction should always be suspected when a tachycardia with a rate in the neighborhood of 300 beats per minute is seen.

Atrial flutter with alternating 4:1 and 2:1 conduction is quite common and is a significant cause of bigeminal rhythm (Fig. 26-16). At times the ventricular complex ending the shorter RR interval shows aberration, and then ventricular bigeminy is simulated. This can be a dangerous situation if the patient is receiving digitalis to control the ventricular rate; often the simulation of ventricular bigeminy is thought to be due to digitalis intoxication and the drug is stopped, when, in fact, more digitalis may be indicated to increase the conduction ratio still further to a constant 4:1. A less common cause of bigeminal grouping is 3:2 conduction. Sometimes the AV ratio is variable (e.g., 2:1, 4:1, 5:1, and 3:1), and then the utter irregularity of atrial fibrillation is mimicked (Fig. 26-17*A*). Such bizarre irregularity is probably due to "multilevel" block in the AV junction.[36]

Wenckebach periods are common in atrial flutter. When 4:1 and 2:1 conduction alternate, the condition is generally attributed to a constant 2:1 transmission at an upper level in the AV junction with 3:2 Wenckebach periods at a lower level (Fig. 26-16).[1]

Atrial flutter may be associated with complete AV block, in which case the slow but regular ventricular complexes are seen to vary their relation to the preceding F wave (Fig. 26-17*B*).

Because of "concealed conduction" of the atrial impulses that are constantly bombarding and penetrating the AV junction to varying levels, the FR interval of conducted beats (measured from the nadir of the F wave to the beginning of the QRS complex) is believed to be constantly prolonged, ranging between 0.26 and 0.46 s.[1]

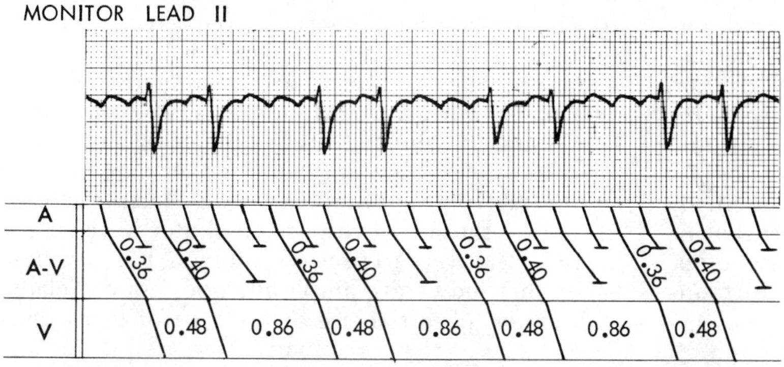

FIGURE 26-16 Atrial flutter with alternating 4:1 and 2:1 conduction. This common cause of bigeminal rhythm is almost always due to a basic 2:1 AV conduction high in the AV junction with 3:2 Wenckebach periods at a lower level (as diagramed).

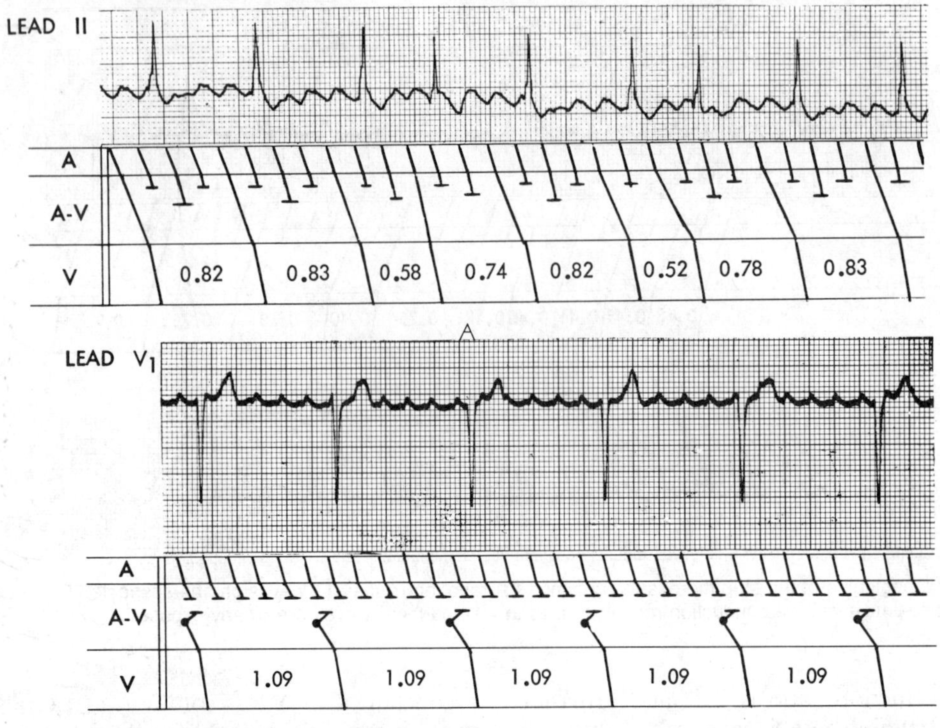

FIGURE 26-17 *A.* Atrial flutter with varying AV conduction, resulting in an irregular ventricular rhythm that mimics atrial fibrillation. *B.* Atrial flutter with AV block and resulting AV dissociation; note that the ventricular rhythm remains perfectly regular while the relation of the ventricular complexes to the F waves varies.

Atrial Fibrillation

Atrial fibrillation exacts two hemodynamic penalties: the ineffective writhing of atrial muscle deprives the heart of its atrial transport function, and the incessant and irregular bombardment of the AV junction with numerous impulses excites rapid and irregular ventricular responses. In the heart already compromised by disease, these handicaps may be critical. Atrial fibrillation also predisposes to peripheral or pulmonary emboli. Approximately 30 percent of all persons with long-standing chronic atrial fibrillation experience at least one embolic episode during the course of the fibrillation. Some studies have indicated that atrial fibrillation is present in 90 percent of patients with mitral stenosis who have peripheral emboli.

Atrial fibrillation is a relatively common arrhythmia and is much more common than the other atrial tachyarrhythmias. It may occur in sustained or paroxysmal form. Atrial fibrillation usually draws attention to one of four diseases: rheumatic mitral disease, hypertension, ischemic heart disease,[37] or thyrotoxicosis. It has a less common but well-recognized association with atrial septal defect, chronic lung disease, and constrictive pericarditis. The arrhythmia is reported in from 7 to 16 percent of continuously monitored patients with myocardial infarction. In susceptible persons with otherwise apparently normal hearts, the arrhythmia is occasionally precipitated by an alcoholic spree ("holiday heart").[38,39] Heart failure from any cause may initiate atrial fibrillation; on the other hand, the recent onset of fibrillation may precipitate failure in the diseased but otherwise well-compensated heart. It is occasionally found in apparently healthy persons, when it is called *lone fibrillation;* some of these may be due to occult thyrotoxicosis.[40]

Atrial fibrillation may be precipitated by an atrial extrasystole occurring in the vulnerable period of the atrial cycle; this is likely when the ectopic atrial impulse is so early that the PP′ cycle is less than half the preceding PP cycle. Factors which favor the development or perpetuation of fibrillation include an increased mass of atrial muscle, increased vagal tone, and asynchrony (temporal dispersion) in the recovery curves of adjacent myocardial fibers.

Electrocardiographic Features

The cardinal features of atrial fibrillation in the ECG are (1) fibrillatory (f) waves of atrial activity and (2) an irregular ventricular response. Of the routine 12 leads, the best for identifying atrial activity is V_1; next best are leads II, III, and aV_F, whereas leads I, aV_L, and the left chest leads often show little sign of atrial activity. The fibrillatory waves may vary in amplitude from nothingness (Fig. 26-18*A*) to irregular waves the size of respectable flutter waves (Fig. 26-18*B*). Contrary to previous opinion, it is now believed that the f-wave amplitude does not correlate with either left atrial size or the type of heart dis-

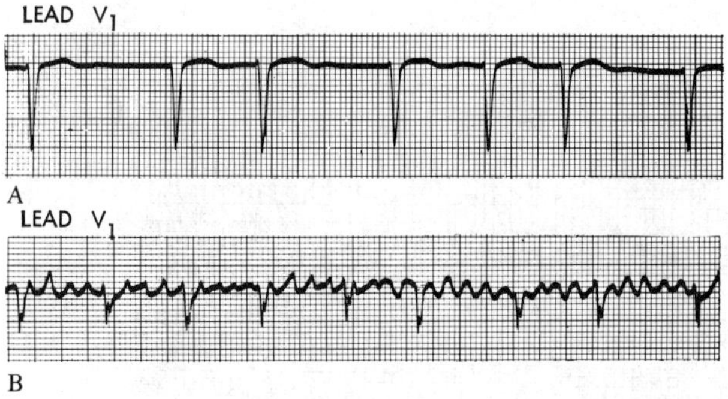

FIGURE 26-18 *A.* Atrial fibrillation leaving virtually no imprint on the baseline ("straight-line" fibrillation). *B.* Coarse atrial fibrillation; the fibrillatory (f) waves are the size of respectable flutter waves but irregular.

ease.[41] When there is no sign of atrial activity, even in right precordial leads, yet the ventricular response is characteristically irregular, one may reasonably infer the diagnosis of ("straight-line") atrial fibrillation.

In uncomplicated atrial fibrillation, the QRS complexes are of normal configuration, though irregular, testifying to normal intraventricular conduction. It is important, however, to appreciate the frequency of aberrant ventricular conduction. This is more difficult to identify in the presence of atrial fibrillation, since the diagnostic value of preceding atrial activity is lost. Its importance lies in the fact that aberrantly conducted beats may be mistaken for ectopic ventricular activity, and this may influence the physician to withhold digitalis when it is sorely needed or to give antiarrhythmic drugs when they are not needed and may even be contraindicated. Aberration is particularly likely to develop when a lengthening of the ventricular cycle is immediately followed by a short cycle; the beat ending the short cycle shows aberrant conduction (Fig. 26-19). This long cycle–short cycle sequence promoting aberration is often called *Ashman's phenomenon.*[42] Runs of consecutive aberrant beats may imitate ventricular tachycardia and so create a real therapeutic dilemma. Because the diagnostic assistance of a preceding P wave is obviated by fibrillating atria, in separating the aberration from ventricular ectopy special reliance has to be placed on the shape of the anomalous complexes.[43] Criteria that may be employed in differentiation, with their approximate relative values in differentiation, are summarized in Table 26-5.

FIGURE 26-19 Ashman's phenomenon. During atrial fibrillation, the beat ending a short cycle preceded by a relatively long cycle manifests aberrant ventricular conduction. In this example the aberrant beat shows typical right bundle branch block type aberration with rsR′ pattern and the initial deflection identical with that of the flanking conducted beats.

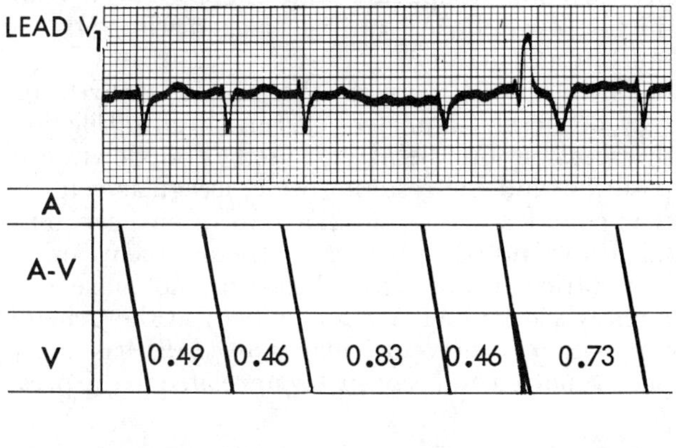

TABLE 26-5 Specificity Rating of Criteria for Aberration or Ectopy*

Criterion	Likelihood of Aberration	Likelihood of Ectopy
Right bundle branch block:		
rsR′ in V_1	4+	1+
R or qR in V_1		
With taller left peak	1+	4+
With taller right peak	2+	3+
qRs in V_6	3+	–
Left bundle branch block	2+	2+
Fixed coupling	1+	3+
Identical initial vector	3+	–
Long-short cycle sequence	4+	4+
Short-long cycle sequence	–	3+
Wide r in V_1	–	3+
Concordant positivity (V_1 to V_6)	+ (WPW)	3+
Concordant negativity (V_1 to V_6)	–	3+
Frontal axis −95 to −175	–	3+

**Notes:* 4+, highly likely; 3+, often seen; 2+, not uncommon; 1+, not characteristic, but seen; –, unlikely.

Arrhythmias Complicating Preexcitation[44]

Wolff-Parkinson-White Syndrome

The predisposition of people with the WPW syndrome to supraventricular arrhythmias is well known. There is evidence that atrial premature beats are seen more frequently in patients with WPW syndrome than in the general population, and there is no doubt that atrial flutter affects a significant minority of these patients. Indeed, atrial flutter with conduction down the accessory pathway (AP) was found to be the most common cause of a wide-QRS tachycardia in the WPW syndrome.[45] However, the most important supraventricular arrhythmias to complicate the syndrome are reciprocating (reentrant, circus-movement) tachycardia (RT) and atrial fibrillation. In Wellens's large series of 212 patients with WPW and tachyarrhythmias, 64 percent had only RT, 20 percent had only atrial fibrillation, and 16 percent had both.[46]

The WPW anatomy is ready-made for RT since there are two parallel AV pathways with different conductive characteristics. The tachycardia is usually initiated when a premature impulse finds one

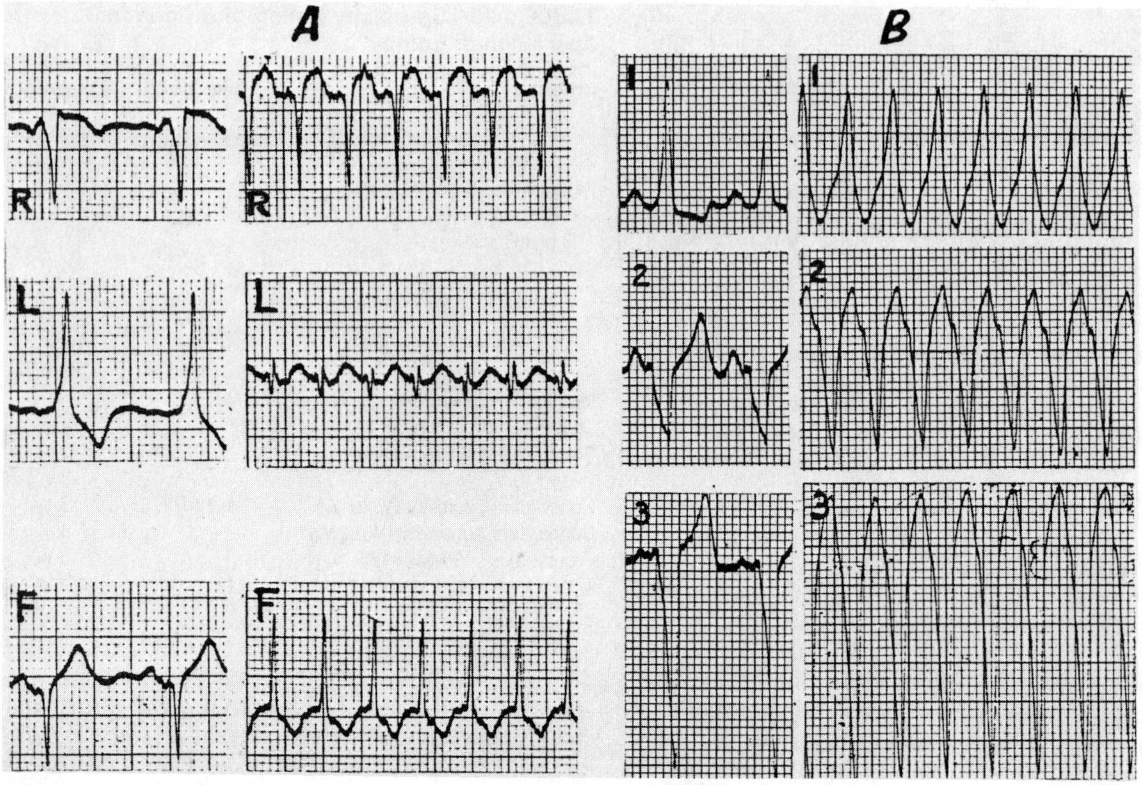

FIGURE 26-20 Wolff-Parkinson-White syndrome with reciprocating tachycardia. *A.* Before and after development of "orthodromic" tachycardia. *B.* From another patient, before and after developing "antidromic" tachycardia.

of the pathways still refractory after the other has recovered.[47] As the AP generally has a longer refractory period than the AV node, the early, initiating impulse travels anterogradely down the AV junction; by the time it reaches the ventricular end of the AP, this has recovered and can accommodate the impulse retrogradely—and so the stage is set for the wavefront to continue to circulate down the AV junction and up the AP ("orthodromic" tachycardia, Fig. 26-20*A*). Much less often, the circulating impulse uses the AP for its downward journey and returns retrogradely via the AV junction ("antidromic" tachycardia, Fig. 26-20*B*). The initiating impulse is usually an atrial extrasystole, but sometimes it is a retrogradely conducted premature ventricular impulse.

A few patients are endowed with more than one AP, and, ignoring the AV junction, the tachycardia may use one AP for the downward and the other for the retrograde journey.

Although most tachycardias make use of the anomalous pathway in one direction or the other, some reciprocal mechanisms are confined to the AV junction,[48] the atria, or the ventricle.[49] If surgical intervention is entertained, identification of the prevailing circuit obviously becomes crucial.

Some individuals have accessory pathways that will not conduct anterogradely so that they never manifest preexcitation during sinus rhythm; yet the accessory bundle may conduct retrogradely and provide a tailor-made circuit for a reentering tachycardia. This situation has been called *concealed WPW* syndrome and is being reported with increasing frequency.[50–52] Again, if surgery is considered, the implications are obvious. Occasionally an unsuspected, underlying WPW syndrome may be unmasked by vagal stimulation or isoproterenol.[53]

Atrial fibrillation may be life-threatening if the AP has a short refractory period and so conducts at an inordinately rapid rate. Obviously those at highest risk are those with the shortest refractory period in the AP; these may be recognized if, during atrial fibrillation, ventricular cycles are distressingly short (less than 0.25 s). On the other hand, lack of a dangerously short refractory period, and therefore absence of the highest risk, can be predicted if the preexcitation is intermittent,[54] if the evidence of preexcitation disappears with exercise, or if conduction over the AP can be blocked with intravenous procainamide.[46]

When the QRS is wide, ventricular tachycardia may be closely simulated. During atrial fibrillation the accessory bundle may be used as the downward pathway, and the resulting wide, irregular ventricular complexes (Fig. 26-21) have often been mistaken for and published as ventricular tachycardia.

Ventricular premature beats are no more frequently seen in WPW patients than in the general population. True ventricular tachycardia has rarely been reported and is probably unrelated to the pres-

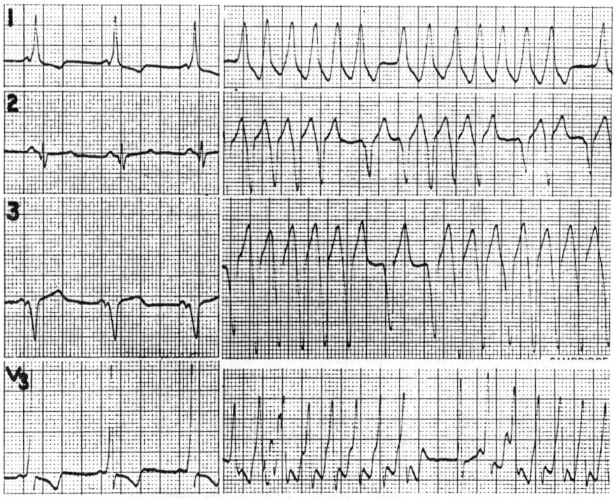

FIGURE 26-21 Atrial fibrillation with Wolff-Parkinson-White conduction. *Left,* sinus rhythm with a typical preexcitation pattern. *Right,* persistence of the preexcitation pattern, the QRS axis having shifted to the left (as it often does with the development of tachycardia); the ventricular rhythm is now irregular at a rate well over 200. *(Courtesy of Dr. Arland A. Adams. From H. J. L. Marriott and H. M. Rogers, Mimics of Ventricular Tachycardia Associated with the W-P-W Syndrome, J. Electrocardiol., 2:77, 1969. Reproduced with permission from the publisher and author.)*

ence of the preexcitation syndrome. Ventricular fibrillation sometimes eventuates and may be the cause of death in some cases; it may develop because a descending impulse invades the ventricles during their vulnerable period, or it may be secondary to the hypoxia engendered by a frenetic ventricular rate approaching 300 beats per minute.

Since the anatomic matrix for preexcitation and its arrhythmias is congenital, it follows that its manifestations may affect all ages. Fortunately, most infants with the anatomic trait "outgrow" their tendency to develop tachyarrhythmias;[55] in one series[56] only 4 of 46 infants retained their predisposition to tachyarrhythmias into childhood and adolescence.

Lown-Ganong-Levine Syndrome

All patients with a short PR interval and normal QRS complex do not have the Lown-Ganong-Levine (LGL) syndrome. The syndrome exists when the short PR–normal QRS combination is associated with supraventricular tachyarrhythmias. Many short PR intervals probably represent merely one extremity of the bell-shaped curve of the normal PR range; at other times the abbreviated PR may be due to conduction via an extranodal or intranodal bypass, or to excessive adrenergic tone as in the presence of a pheochromocytoma.[57]

The arrhythmias complicating the LGL syndrome have not been studied in the same detail as those of the WPW syndrome; but most tachycardias in the LGL syndrome are reentrant (slow-fast) in the AV node.[58] In one small series of 12 patients, 6 had supraventricular tachycardia (4 as a result of reentry in the AV node and 2 using a concealed bypass), 2 had atrial fibrillation, and 4 ventricular tachycardia.[59]

The term *enhanced AV nodal conduction* (EAVNC) has been applied both to the capability of the node to conduct at rapid rates, implying a short refractory period (e.g., 1:1 conduction at more than 200 beats per minute), and to a short AV nodal transit time (e.g., AH interval of less than 60 ms).[58] Subjects with the LGL syndrome may or may not enjoy EAVNC; and EAVNC is clearly not necessarily a member of the LGL clan.

Sick Sinus Syndrome

Under this catchy heading many authorities include any form of sinus nodal depression, including marked sinus bradycardia, prolonged sinus pauses, sinus arrest, or SA block (see next section); but the term is most often applied—although this application has been criticized as "inaccurate and inappropriate"—to the tachycardia-bradycardia syndrome, in which bursts of an ectopic atrial tachyarrhythmia, often atrial fibrillation, alternate with prolonged periods of sinus nodal inertia and often AV junctional inertia as well (Fig. 26-22). Apart from these florid signs of dysfunction, the syndrome may initially manifest itself as paroxysmal atrial fibrillation, as prolonged sinus inactivity following cardioversion or spontaneous reversion of atrial fibrillation, or as an inappropriate sinus rate, for instance in failure to develop adequate sinus acceleration with exercise or fever. Lone atrial fibrillation, at any age but particularly in youth, is most likely due to a sick sinus node, and intraatrial block or shifting atrial pacemaker may precede symptomatic sinus nodal disease by years. Although much more common in older age groups, the syndrome spares no decade, and it may be the cause of sudden death in young athletes.

Temporary and reversible manifestations of the syndrome may be induced by vagotonia, including that due to digitalis or subarachnoid hemorrhage, or by thyrotoxicosis, hyperpotassemia, quinidine, nicotine, beta blockers, lithium therapy,[61] or aerosol propellants. Such influences must always be excluded before diagnosing the chronic progressive syndrome, which may result from ischemic, rheumatic, or inflammatory disease; from involvement of the sinus node by pericarditis, one of the cardiomyopathies (especially amyloidosis), Friedreich's progressive muscular dystrophy, collagen disease, or metastatic disease; or from surgical injury. Apathy of the sinus node is sometimes familial and may accompany the prolonged QT syndrome. When it results from acute myocardial infarction, it is usually associated with occlusion of the right coronary or left circumflex artery. Some degree of dysfunction, usually an asymptomatic sinus bradycardia, complicates at least 50 percent of acute inferior infarctions. It is said that patients who develop serious sinus nodal dysfunction during myocardial infarction, de-

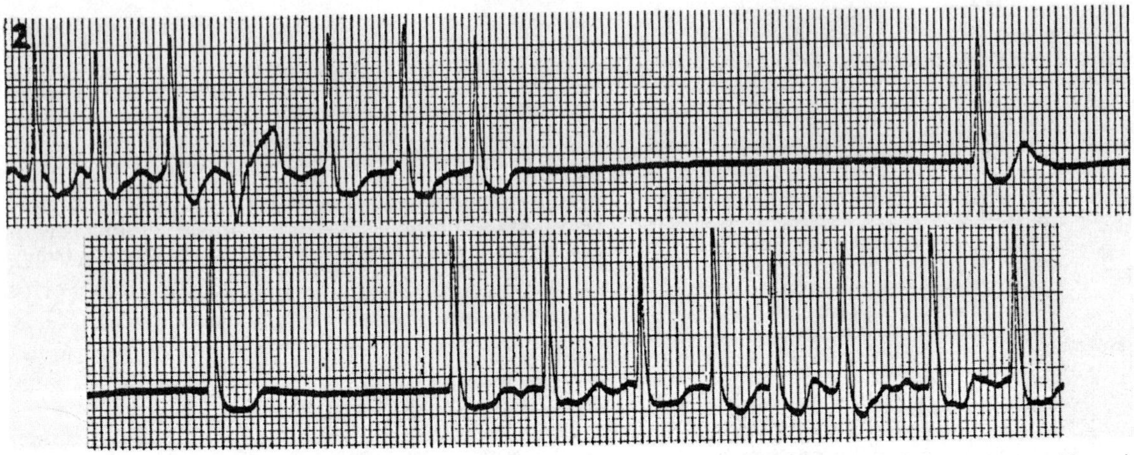

FIGURE 26-22 Tachycardia-bradycardia syndrome (often labeled sick sinus syndrome). Between the two runs of irregular supraventricular tachyarrhythmias (? atrial fibrillation) there is complete absence of all atrial activity, punctuated by junctional escape beats at long and erratic intervals. (The strips are continuous.)

spite complete recovery, should be followed indefinitely since later recurrence is not uncommon.[62]

Nevertheless, sinoatrial dysfunction appears to be a relatively benign malady. Shaw and coworkers[63] in a 10-year prospective survey found no significant difference in survival rates of patients with established or potential sick sinus syndromes, whether paced or not, when compared with the normal population.

Electrocardiographic Features

At the time of examination, the tracing may be entirely normal or may show signs of the associated ischemic or other cardiac disease. The rhythm may be normal, or there may be evidence of sinus bradycardia, intraatrial block, or shifting atrial pacemaker. Sinus bradycardia or prolonged sinus pauses may alternate with runs of atrial tachycardia, flutter, or fibrillation. Sinus arrest or patterns of SA block may be recognized, and coexisting AV and intraventricular blocks complicate the picture in a significant proportion of patients.

It is important to appreciate the fact that quite marked sinus bradycardia and prolonged sinus pauses (more than 1.75 s) are common occurrences in apparently healthy young adults.[7]

Diagnosis

Although the diagnosis of an ailing sinus node is sometimes easily made from the history, physical findings, and routine ECG, it often requires more sophisticated investigation. Continuous tape recording for 24 h by Holter monitor may be necessary, but this may also fail to record diagnostic stretches of sinus nodal dysfunction. At times the syndrome may be recognized only when evoked by provocative tests, such as failure to accelerate appropriately after an intravenous dose of 1 to 2 mg atropine or during titration with an intravenous drip of isoproterenol (1 to 2 mg per 500 ml). Atrial pacing at a rate of 120 to 140 beats per minute for 2 to 4 min may be necessary to demonstrate that the sinus node recovery time (SNRT), that is, the interval from the last paced P wave to the first returning sinus P wave, is inappropriately long.[64] A prolonged SNRT is good evidence of sinus dysfunction, but a normal SNRT by no means excludes a sick sinus. Sinoatrial conduction time (SACT) is an adjunctive but less sensitive test of sinus dysfunction. It is possible that determination of the sinus node's refractory period will prove to be a more dependable test.[65]

Ventricular Arrhythmias

Ventricular Extrasystoles

The mechanisms of production of premature (extrasystolic) beats are not certainly known; theories of their genesis are discussed in Chap. 25. Since they bear a more or less constant time relation (coupling interval) to the preceding beat, it is assumed that they are in some way "forced" by it; when the coupling interval is almost unvaried, the relation is called *fixed coupling.* The allowable variation is about 0.04 s, although some authors are much more lenient and permit—erroneously, we think—much greater variation (up to 0.12 s)[66] to qualify as "fixed."

Ventricular extrasystoles are the most common form of rhythm disturbance, both in health and in disease. Hiss[16] found them in 0.8 percent of 122,000 asymptomatic Air Force personnel ranging in age from 16 to over 50 years; they are recorded in the majority of continuously monitored patients with acute myocardial infarction, but they were also found in the majority (62 percent) of 300 actively employed middle-aged men monitored for a period of 6 h.[67] In some apparently normal persons, ventricular extrasystoles may persist, even in the form of bigeminy, for many years. On the other hand, they may result from any form of heart disease and are frequently due to overdigitalization. They commonly accompany heart failure; in this situation digitalis may eliminate them. Since potassium depletion also favors them, digitalis-induced extrasystoles are especially likely to appear after diuresis with kaliuretic preparations. They may result from hypocalcemia and from caffeine, tobacco, alcohol, and any of the sympathomimetic drugs—epinephrine, isoproterenol, and amphetamine (even in the form of nose drops, sprays, or inhalers). Hypoxia is a potent cause of ventricular extrasystoles, as in anesthesia, especially with cyclopropane. They may develop as a result of infectious diseases, visceral reflexes (e.g., from a diseased gallbladder), or psychic stimuli. In most individuals who are subject to ventricular extrasystoles, their incidence decreases during sleep; but in others, especially in the presence of neurological disease, the extrasystolic frequency may actually increase with sleep.[68] Vagal stimulation and exercise, even in some normal persons,[69] may elicit them. Ventricular extrasystoles are claimed to develop in about 33 percent of apparently healthy men and in about 15 percent of normal women with exercise.[70] Although ventricular premature beats may be evoked by exercise in the normal subject, it has been claimed that if the axis of the extrasystole is markedly superior it may furnish evidence of ischemic heart disease.[71] They have been reported in 45 percent of patients with mitral valve prolapse.[24] Total abstinence from smoking and caffeine with a reduction in alcohol intake and a program of physical conditioning failed to affect the frequency or occurrence of ventricular extrasystoles in apparently healthy men with persistent and frequent premature beats.[72]

Ventricular extrasystoles have prognostic implications for patients who have recovered from acute myocardial infarction. Of more than 2000 patients who had survived infarction by 3 months or more, 11.5 percent had ventricular premature beats in a resting ECG containing 50 beats.[73] The 3-year mortality was twice as great (22 percent) in those who had *any* ventricular extrasystoles than in those with none (11 percent). In another study[74] sudden cardiac death was six times more common in coronary patients who had frequent ventricular premature beats than in those who had few or none.

Electrocardiographic Features

Since the impulse of a ventricular extrasystole originates in one of the ventricles and spreads anomalously, the QRS complex is wide and bizarre as well as premature. If the focus of origin is in the septum near the bifurcation of the bundle, the QRS may be little widened and only slightly deformed. Rosenbaum postulates that such beats arise from proximal segments of the main intraventricular conduction fascicles (fascicular beats).[75] The ST-T segment usually points in a direction opposite to the terminal portion of the QRS. Most ventricular premature beats do not disturb the rhythm of the sinus node and are therefore followed by a compensatory pause or cycle (Fig. 26-23*A*); or they may be interpolated between two consecutive sinus beats (Fig. 26-23*B*). On the other hand, it is quite common for the ectopic impulse to be conducted retrogradely into the atria and to inscribe a retrograde P′ wave on the ST segment (Fig. 26-24), usually 0.12 to 0.20 s after the beginning of the QRS complex.[76] If the sinus node is discharged ahead of schedule by the retrograde

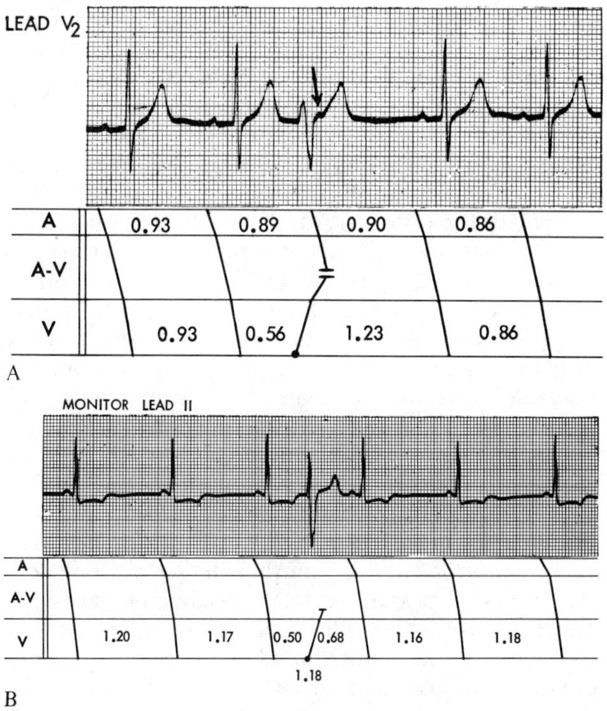

FIGURE 26-23 *A.* Ventricular premature beat. The third beat is wide and bizarre—quite unlike the QRS-T pattern of the sinus beats—and, since the sinus rhythm is undisturbed (next sinus P wave indicated by arrow), the postextrasystolic pause is compensatory. *B.* The fourth beat is an interpolated ventricular premature beat; it is sandwiched between two consecutive sinus beats.

FIGURE 26-24 Exceptions to the rules for compensatory pauses. *Top.* Ventricular extrasystole with less-than-compensatory pause. Retrograde conduction to the atria (retrograde P wave deforms first part of ST segment) discharges the sinus pacemaker early and so shortens the postextrasystolic cycle. *Middle.* Atrial premature beat followed by fully compensatory pause. The third and eighth beats are atrial extrasystoles but, presumably because they suppress the sinus pacemaker, are followed by compensatory pauses. *Bottom.* Ventricular extrasystoles with less-than-compensatory pauses. Each postextrasystolic cycle ends in an escape beat and so is slightly less than compensatory.

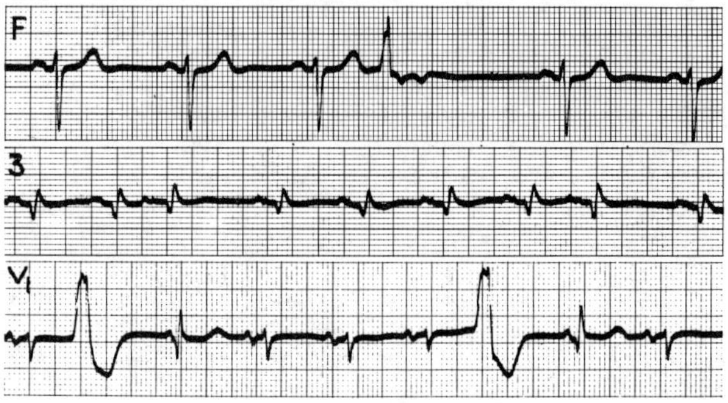

impulse, the following pause may be less than compensatory. Most ventricular extrasystoles maintain a constant coupling interval (fixed coupling), not varying by more than 0.04 s, in contrast with parasystolic beats, whose coupling intervals typically vary. Some ventricular premature beats, however, manifest marked variation in coupling, yet do not conform with the criteria for parasystole. Although ventricular extrasystoles are commonly found in normal hearts, when the ectopic QRS complex is unduly wide (more than 0.16 s) or splintered, it is presumptive evidence of heart disease. In the absence of evident heart disease, even frequent and complex ventricular premature beats are seemingly benign.[77]

In the majority of ventricular ectopic beats, the ventricle of origin can be inferred from the polarity of the ectopic complex in a right chest lead such as V_1 (predominantly positive = *left* ventricular, predominantly negative = *right* ventricular). For possible exceptions to this general rule, see under "Ventricular Tachycardia," below. It is claimed that organic heart disease is the rule in people with left ventricular extrasystoles, and that when extrasystoles affect persons without heart disease, they are almost invariably right ventricular.[78]

The contour of the QRS complex can be extremely helpful in recognizing ventricular ectopy and in distinguishing it from aberration: morphological clues are summarized in Tables 26-5 and 26-6.

If an impulse arises in the Purkinje network of, say, the anterior fascicle of the left bundle branch, it presumably reaches the myocardium supplied by that fascicle sooner than it can spread retrogradely to and down the posterior fascicle and the right bundle branch. Depending upon the respective distances involved and the rates of propagation anterogradely and retrogradely, it writes a QRS pattern resembling less or more complete right bundle branch block with left posterior hemiblock. Similarly, an impulse arising in the territory of the posterior fascicle writes a pattern resembling less or more complete right bundle branch block with left anterior hemiblock.[79] Such beats, usually somewhat narrower than full-fledged ectopic ventricular beats, are now often alluded to as *fascicular* beats.[80]

TABLE 26-6 Electrocardiographic Recognition of Ventricular Tachycardia*

V_1	V_6	Probability†
rsR′	Rs or qRs	AVC
rsR′	rS	AVC
qR or R	Rs or qRs	AVC
qR or R	rS or QS	Ect
qR or R	R	Ect (unless WPW)
QS	QS	Ect
QS or rS	R	Either

*Morphologic probabilities in V_1/V_6.
†*Notes:* AVC = aberrant ventricular conduction; Ect = ectopic ventricular.

The dangerous potential of early ventricular extrasystoles (R on T) has been frequently stressed. But in one series of 20 consecutive patients with ventricular fibrillation complicating acute myocardial infarction, 11 were initiated by "late" extrasystoles.[81] Moreover, it was found that pairs and runs of ventricular ectopic beats after myocardial infarction were initiated more often by late than by early beats.[82]

The morphology of the ectopic QRS may be helpful in recognizing myocardial infarction: the presence of a wide Q wave followed by a significant R wave is said to be evidence of an infarction, old or recent, with a specificity of 97 percent.[83,84,84a] Unfortunately, the QR pattern may also be present in hypertrophic cardiomyopathy.[85]

Ventricular Tachycardia

Three or more ectopic ventricular beats, occurring at a rate equivalent to more than 100 per minute, constitute a run of ventricular tachycardia (VT). Paroxysms of VT usually begin with a coupled (forced) ventricular premature beat—*extrasystolic* VT. Some of these may be perpetuated by rapid firing of a single ectopic focus; others, by a circulating wave front using a microscopic Purkinje circuit (microreentry) or a wider sweep involving fascicular pathways (macroreentry). The paroxysm may begin with an ectopic beat that is or is not closely coupled to the preceding beat; if there are repeated paroxysms beginning with variation in the initial coupling interval, and if the interectopic interval between the last beat of a paroxysm and the first beat of the next paroxysm is a multiple of the ventricular cycle during the tachycardia, it is a *parasystolic* VT.

It is well established, both experimentally and clinically, that an impulse reaching the ventricles in their "vulnerable" period can initiate a repetitive response in the form of VT, flutter, or fibrillation. The initiating impulse may be an endogenous ectopic ventricular impulse, a descending supraventricular impulse, or an artificial, extrinsic electric impulse of sufficient magnitude. Nevertheless, more recent studies have documented the fact that many, if not most, paroxysms of VT are initiated by late-coupled ventricular extrasystoles.[86] In one series, only 6 of 44 (14 percent) paroxysms began with R on T.[87] Others noted that many late-coupled extrasystoles that initiated VT fell on the P wave, suggesting that atrial contraction producing myocardial stretch might be the trigger.[88]

VT almost always affects a diseased heart, although it has rarely been described in apparently normal ones. Lesch was able to collect 34 such cases.[89] Only one three-beat burst was found among the more than 67,000 asymptomatic Air Force personnel screened by Hiss.[90] Six of seventeen young patients with VT had no recognizable heart disease.[91] In another small series, 10 percent of the patients had no demonstrable heart disease, while ischemia (71 percent) and rheumatic disorders (12 percent) were the most common pathological associations. VT has been reported in 6 percent of patients with mitral valve prolapse,[24] and indeed malignant refractory ventricular tachyarrhythmias have complicated this "syndrome."[92] Among continuously monitored patients with acute myocardial infarction, the reported incidence ranges from 6 to 28 percent. On the other hand, among 52 men Holter-monitored for 24 h during the first 2 days of an acute infarction, VT was detected in 24 (46 percent).[93]

Wide-QRS tachycardias, with mainly negative complexes in lead V_1 (left bundle branch block pattern), deserve special mention. Most such tachycardias originate in the right ventricle, and many are apparently benign.[94] However, in the presence of right ventricle disease, and even in some normal hearts,[95] such tachycardias may be life-threatening. Furthermore, in the sick ischemic heart, a tachycardia with this morphology may originate in the *left* side of the ventricular septum and, by "preferential septal activation," depolarize the right ventricle first.[96]

This pattern of tachycardia is seen in right ventricle dysplasia,[97] right ventricle dilatation,[98,99] and coronary[100] and congenital heart disease.[100,101] In any young person presenting with VT, the possibility of right ventricle dysplasia or dilatation should be entertained—especially in males, and especially if the 12-lead ECG during sinus rhythm is characterized by significant T-wave inversion in leads V_1 to V_3 or V_4.

A pattern originally described by Rosenbaum[79] that is probably diagnostic of right ventricle ectopy and is often seen in young athletic subjects is characterized by a left bundle branch block pattern in V_6, but with two features elsewhere in the 12-lead tracing that are quite unlike left bundle branch block: right axis deviation in the frontal plane and a wide (more than 0.04 s) initial r wave in V_1 (Fig. 26-25).

VT in youth should also prompt diagnostic consideration of the following possible causes: mitral valve prolapse, myocarditis, and hypokalemia, especially in dieting females.

Intractable VT sometimes complicates a ventricular aneurysm resulting from myocardial infarction. Undoubtedly the arrhythmia can complicate any form of heart disease; examples have been reported in sarcoidosis, hypertrophic cardiomyopathy,[102] and myxedema coma undergoing treatment. Numerous drugs, including digitalis, quinidine, procainamide, sympathetic amines, papaverine, potassium, intravenous mercurials, chloroform, and cyclopropane, have been incriminated. Runs of VT are frequently induced at cardiac catheterization and often follow in the wake of countershock; less often the arrhythmia may be caused by a malfunctioning ("runaway") artificial pacemaker or by one delivering its stimulus in the vulnerable phase of a competitive natural beat.

Runs of VT are sometimes initiated by a simple change of posture—standing up (orthostatic tachycardia) or lying down. Exercise or emotional excitement may bring one on. Vagal stimulation sometimes evokes a run of ectopic ventricular beats.

Electrocardiographic Features

The ventricular complex is wide and bizarre, recurs regularly at a rate of over 100 beats per minute (usually between 150 and 200 but may approach 300), and gives the appearance of a run of ventricular premature beats. If the onset is observed, the paroxysm may be seen to begin with a coupled ventricular extrasystole. In perhaps 20 percent of cases, independent P waves will be discernible (Fig. 26-26*A*), and in a smaller percentage retrograde P waves (Fig. 26-26*B*) may be found in the surface tracing. Occasionally retrograde conduction occurs with Wenckebach periodicity or in a 2:1 ratio. If it is important to record atrial activity, an esophageal

FIGURE 26-25 Right ventricular extrasystoles. Each lead contains a sinus beat and a coupled ventricular extrasystole of characteristic morphology: Left bundle branch pattern in V_6, wide initial r wave in V_1, and right axis deviation in the frontal plane.[79]

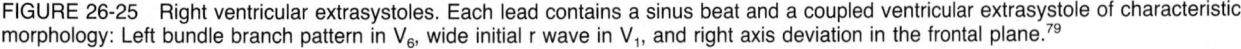

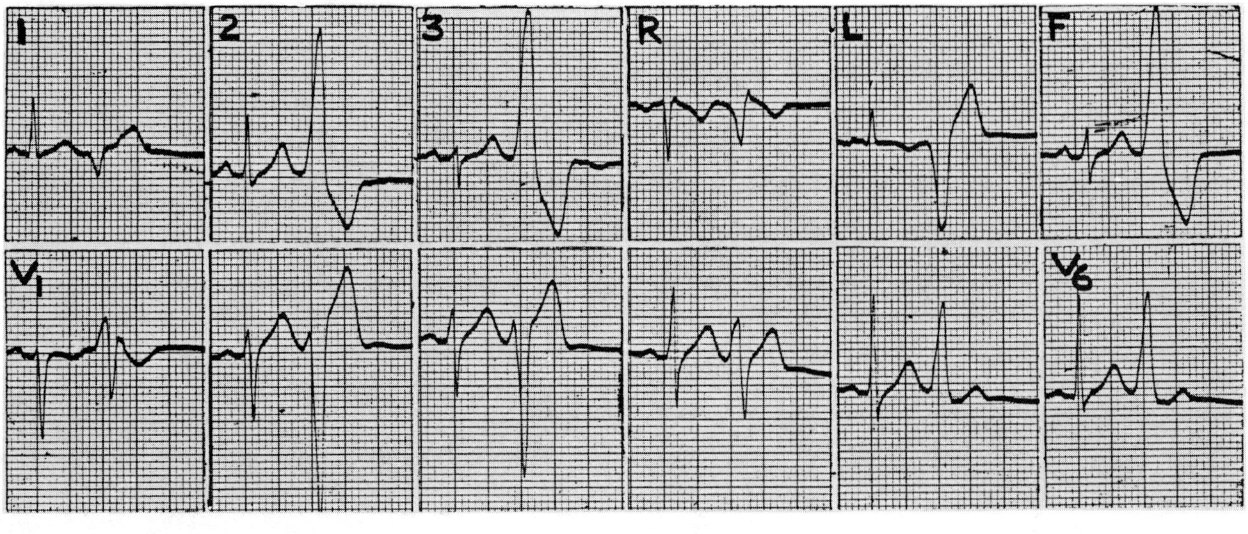

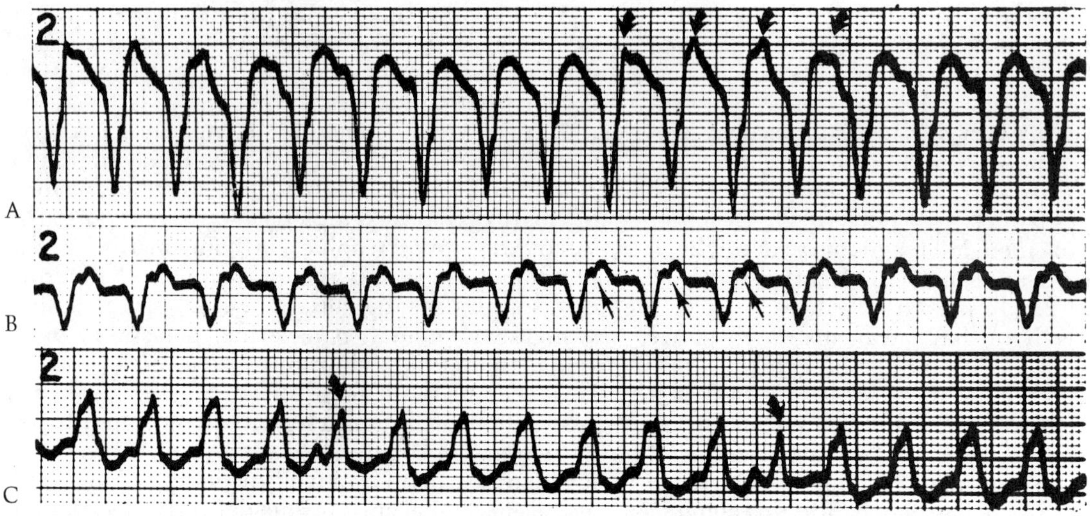

FIGURE 26-26 *A.* Ventricular tachycardia with regular independent P waves (indicated by arrows). *B.* Ventricular tachycardia with retroconduction to atria (retrograde P waves indicated by arrows). *C.* Ventricular tachycardia with fusion (Dressler's) beats—indicated by arrows. Note the sinus P wave preceding each fusion beat.

or intracardiac electrode will invariably capture it. With intracardiac recordings, independent atrial activity and retrograde conduction to the atria were each found in about half of 100 cases studied.[103,104] One should stress that independent atrial activity does *not* prove that the tachycardia is of ventricular origin, but it increases the probability.

The presence of fusion beats is helpful, but they are likely to be seen only if the rate is relatively slow (i.e., 150 or less). They are due to partial capture of the ventricles by an opportunistic sinus impulse (Fig. 26-26*C*). Such beats are always on time or slightly early—never late.

In recognition of the VT, the shape of the ventricular complexes is often helpful; the morphological probabilities are, of course, the same as for ventricular premature beats, which were described earlier in this chapter and are summarized in Table 26-6. If an rsR′ variant is present in V_1, the rhythm is probably not VT. On the other hand, a dominant monophasic R in all chest leads (Fig. 26-27*A*)—provided preexcitation can be excluded—or a totally negative (QS) complex in all chest leads (Fig. 26-27*B*) is much more likely to indicate an ectopic ventricular rather than an aberrant mechanism. One of the most common QRS patterns produced by left ventricular tachycardia in leads V_1 and V_6 is shown in Fig. 26-28.

FIGURE 26-27 Ventricular tachycardia with concordant QRS complexes across precordium: all upright in *A;* all negative in *B.*

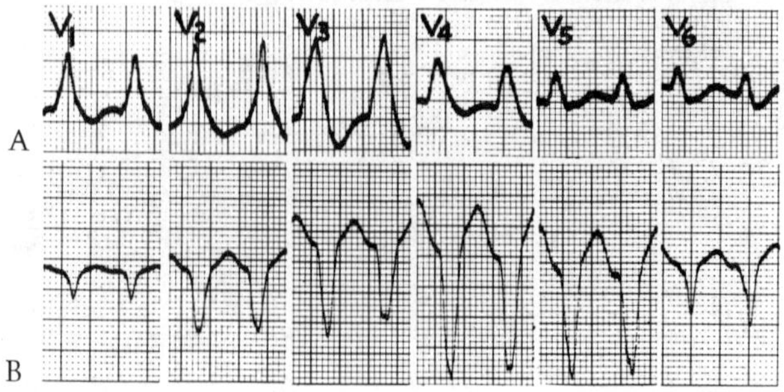

It may be impossible to distinguish ventricular tachycardia from "antidromic" reentrant tachycardia complicating the WPW syndrome. A clue to the latter is an abrupt change in the ventricular cycle length, without change in the morphology of the wide QRS, presumably due to a switch in the bundle branch included in the retrograde pathway.[105]

Until 1978, the morphologic clues in use for more than a decade were based only upon clinical observation and deduction. Wellens and coworkers[103,104] retrospectively examined the morphology of the ventricular complex in 200 patients with wide-QRS

FIGURE 26-28 Beginning of a run of left ventricular tachycardia showing classic morphology: Taller left peak ("rabbit-ear") in V_1, with rS configuration in V_6. Contrast with the triphasic right bundle branch block morphology in the conducted sinus beats. *(From H. J. L. Marriott, "Workshop in Electrocardiography," Tampa Tracings, 1972. Reproduced with permission from the publisher and author.)*

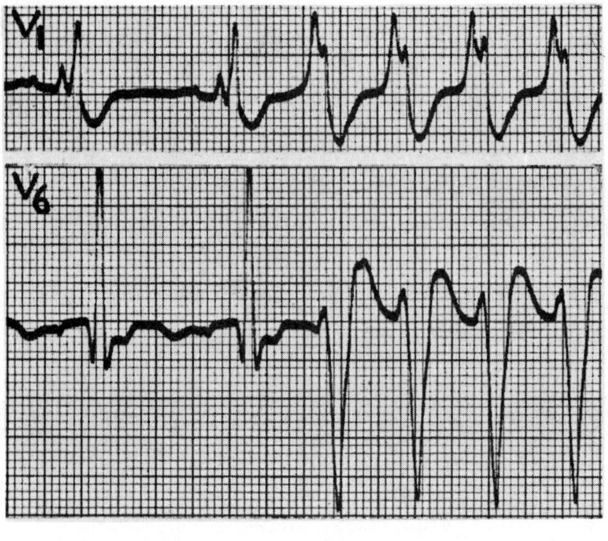

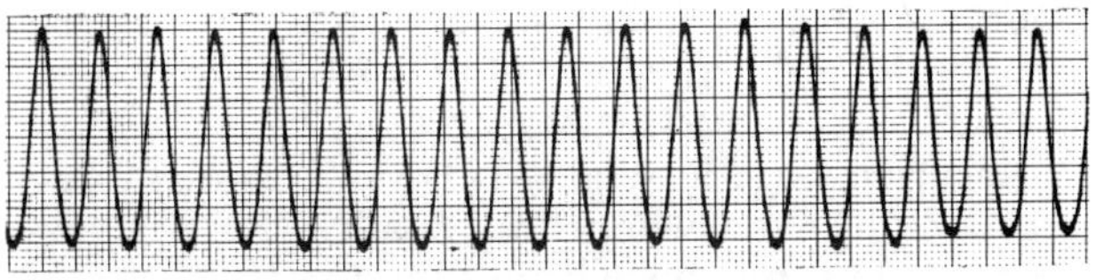

FIGURE 26-29 Ventricular flutter. Note the regular zigzag pattern without definite QRS-T formation at a rate of 172.

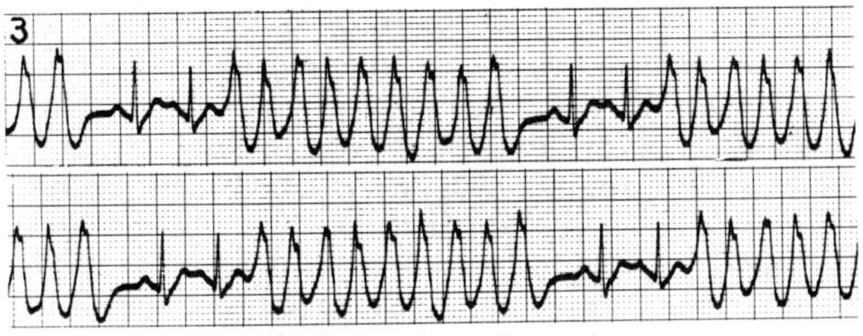

FIGURE 26-30 Repetitive ventricular tachycardia. The strips are continuous. Note that the tachycardia recurs in short nine-beat bursts separated by pairs of sinus beats.

tachycardias (100 with VT and 100 with supraventricular tachycardia with ventricular aberration proven by intracardiac recordings) and confirmed the validity of the clues just described. In an ongoing prospective study,[106] they have since been able to diagnose over 90 percent of wide-QRS tachycardias correctly from the clinical surface tracing *before* establishing the diagnosis with intracardiac recordings.

Several variants of VT are worth noting. When the rate is unusually rapid and the pattern a continuous regular zigzag without clear definition of QRS complexes and T waves (Fig. 26-29), the term *ventricular flutter* is sometimes applied; it is frequently an intermediary between tachycardia and fibrillation. Sometimes relatively brief runs of tachycardia (Fig. 26-30) are separated by one or two sinus beats, and the term *repetitive tachycardia* applies. This is usually a relatively benign form of the arrhythmia and is sometimes found in hearts without evident disease. *Bidirectional tachycardia* is the term used when the ventricular complexes alternate in polarity (Fig. 26-31*A*). It usually carries an ominous prognosis and is often associated with digitalis intoxication. When the ventricular complexes alternate in height but have the same polarity, some call it *alternating tachycardia.* The distinction between bidirectional and alternating tachycardia is far from complete, since in the same paroxysm in the same patient the contour is often "bidirectional" in one lead but "alternating" in another.

When the QRS complex in VT manifests many shapes, the terms *pleomorphic*[107] and *polymorphous*[108] have both been applied. Such paroxysms are most likely to develop in the presence of severe myocardial disease when the QT interval has been prolonged by drugs.[108] Despite their variegation, pleomorphic beats may be shown to arise from a single center.[107]

A form of polymorphous ventricular tachycardia that enjoys a "tantalizingly euphonious" title[109] is *torsades de pointes* (twisting of the points), so-called because the QRS axis shifts back and forth around the baseline (Fig. 26-31*B*). In addition to this morphological characteristic, most authors insist on an associated prolonged QT interval (more than 0.60 s) to make the diagnosis.[110,111] Although commonly regarded as an intermediary between uniform ventricular tachycardia and ventricular fibrillation, torsade has not quite found its niche in the gallery of ventricular arrhythmias: its mechanism is uncertain, although current evidence suggests reentry; and precise criteria for diagnosis are still debated.

Virtually any influence that prolongs the QT interval can cause torsade: quinidine, procainamide, disopyramide, aprindine, amiodarone, phenothiazines, and insecticides have all been implicated, as well as liquid protein diets, electrolyte disturbances

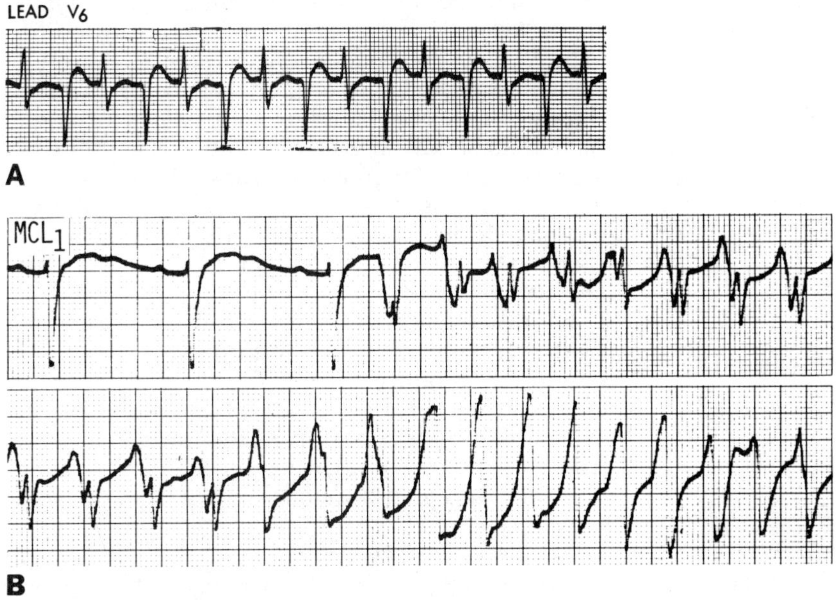

FIGURE 26-31 Bidirectional or alternating tachycardia. The tachycardia is regular at a rate of 160, but the form of the QRS-T complexes alternates. *B.* Torsades de pointes, a dangerous form of ventricular tachycardia in which the polarity of the ventricular complexes swings between positive and negative. Note the much prolonged QT interval.

(especially hypokalemia and hypomagnesemia),[112] intracranial lesions, and congenital QT prolongation. There is an unquestionable association with bradycardia, particularly when due to AV block, and with variant angina. Two or more factors are often recognizable in the same patient.[113]

The clinical importance of torsade lies in the facts that (1) it may degenerate into ventricular fibrillation and (2) it should not be treated with the usual QT-lengthening antiarrhythmic drugs, since most of these have been causally culpable and administering them will only make matters worse.

Accelerated Idioventricular Rhythm

When an ectopic ventricular pacemaker discharges at a rate of less than 100 beats per minute and controls only the ventricles, it is called *idioventricular.* When the idioventricular rate exceeds 45 to 50 but is less than 100 beats per minute (Fig. 26-32), it must be considered abnormal for that site of impulse formation. By definition, it is not a tachycardia and is best referred to as *accelerated idioventricular rhythm,* though such terms as *idioventricular tachycardia, nonparoxysmal ventricular tachycardia,* and *slow ventricular tachycardia* have been applied. Such rhythms received scant attention before the coronary care era, but are now recorded with surprising frequency in series of patients with acute myocardial infarction who are continuously monitored. These slower ventricular rhythms are, in fact, as common as true ventricular tachycardia, being recognized in 15 to 20 percent of patients after acute myocardial infarction, especially of the inferior wall.

The ectopic rate is often similar to the prevailing sinus rate, and these rhythms therefore usually appear because of slight slowing of the sinus pacemaker or slight acceleration of the ectopic center. They often begin with a fusion beat or two, produce a short run of isorhythmic dissociation,[114] and then surrender control once more to the sinus pacemaker. Occasionally, instead of dissociation, retrograde conduction to the atria develops. A few of these rhythms are parasystolic, but most are not.

FIGURE 26-32 Accelerated idioventricular rhythm, rate 85. After three sinus beats conducted with right bundle branch block, an ectopic left ventricular pacemaker gradually takes over—via three fusion beats—gaining full control of the ventricles by the end of the top strip. Note that the ectopic beats have a tall left peak ("rabbit ear") characteristic of left ventricular ectopy. In the bottom strip, the sinus pacemaker regains control. (The strips are continuous.)

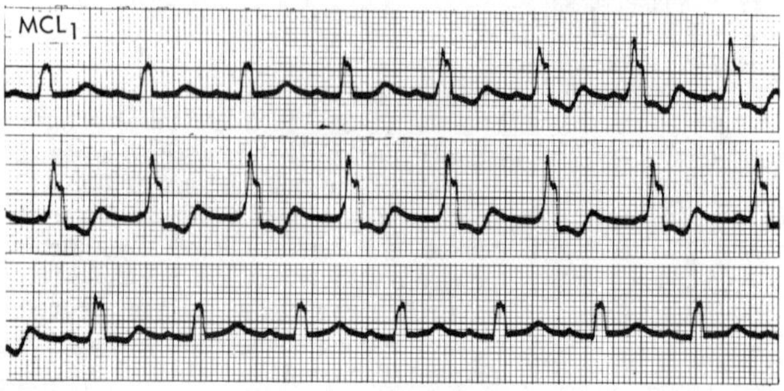

Some possibly represent an underlying ventricular tachycardia with exit block. Most runs are short-lived, lasting for only 3 to 30 beats.

As a rule, these accelerated idioventricular rhythms are benign, even when the ectopic QRS is multiform,[115] and they have been found even in healthy children.[116] They usually require no treatment, even after myocardial infarction, unless the loss of atrial transport function consequent to the AV dissociation compromises the patient's hemodynamic status. Rarely, accelerated idioventricular rhythm is associated with more serious ventricular arrhythmias.[117,118]

Parasystole

Parasystole (from the Greek *para,* "beside") is an independent, ectopic rhythm that operates alongside the primary rhythm and whose pacemaker enjoys neighborhood protection from invasion by outside impulses; its behavior is analogous to that of a fixed-rate artificial pacemaker. Because the ectopic pacemaking center is "protected," it is able to maintain its rhythm without interruption.

Parasystole is not as uncommon as used to be thought. In 1963 Scherf was able to collect only 51 examples of the arrhythmia, but many more cases have been reported since then. Most of the reported cases have been found in diseased hearts, but it is probable that parasystole, particularly the supraventricular varieties, may occur in normal persons. The parasystolic center is usually ventricular; it is atrial or AV junctional much less commonly.

Electrocardiographic Features

There are two cardinal features of the ectopic beats of parasystole: (1) variation in coupling intervals and (2) a common denominator in the interectopic intervals (Fig. 26-33). The variation in coupling is a sign that the beats represent an independent mechanism, i.e., they are not dependent beats; the mathematic relation of the interectopic intervals testifies to the protection, which prevents their rhythm from being interrupted. The steps in diagnosis are usually (1) noticing that the coupling interval is variable and (2) measuring the interectopic intervals and disclosing a common denominator. Fusion beats are commonly seen (Fig. 26-33). The *manifest* rate of most parasystolic pacemakers is slow, usually in the neighborhood of 20 to 60 beats per minute, but much faster rates are sometimes seen.

Because the manifest rate of parasystolic rhythms is often about half that of most sinus rhythms, parasystole may produce a form of ventricular bigeminy in which the coupling intervals progressively shorten or lengthen for a few couplets. On rare occasions a true extrasystolic ventricular bigeminy may alternate with runs of parasystolic rhythm from the same ectopic center.

In supraventricular parasystole, the P waves, or unchanged QRS complexes, manifest a changing re-

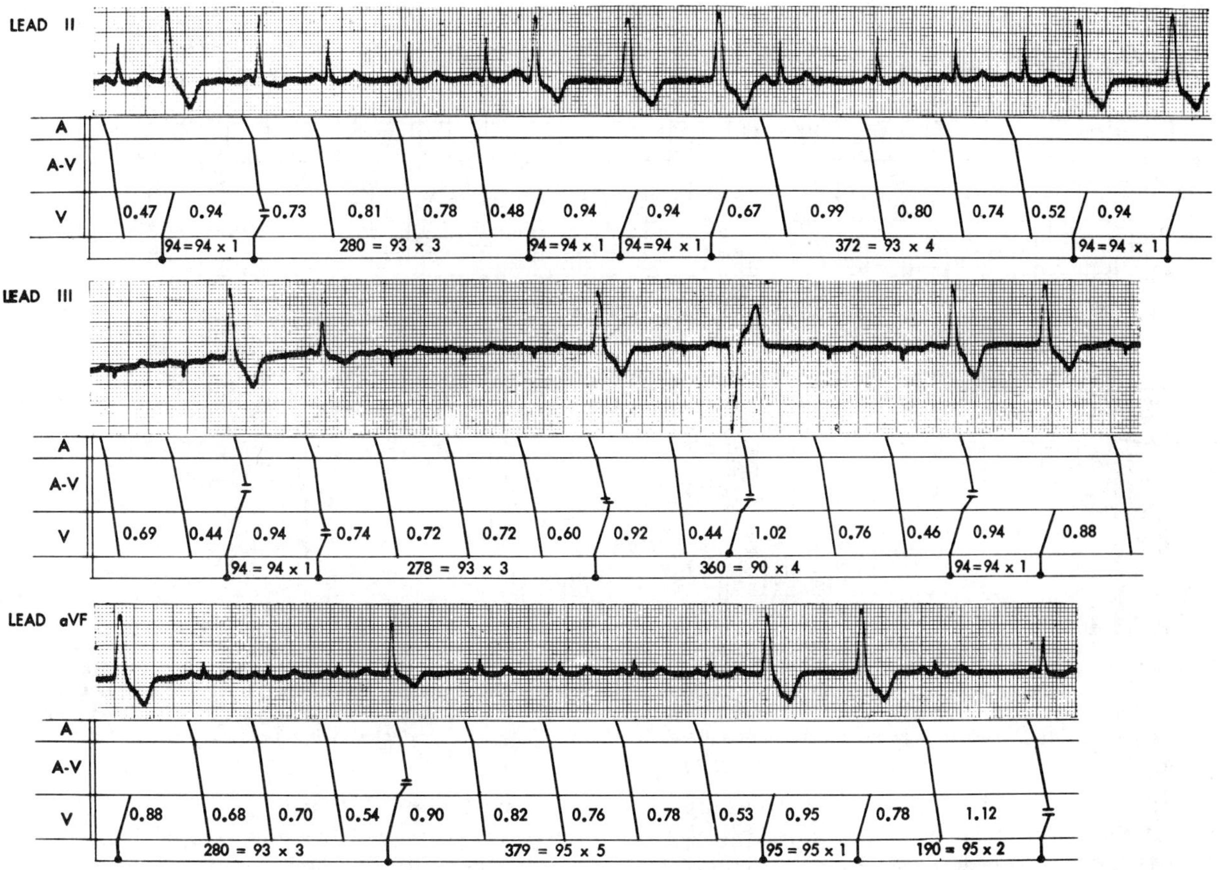

FIGURE 26-33 Ventricular parasystole. The strips are continuous. Note (1) that the interval between an ectopic beat and the preceding sinus beat varies; (2) that the interectopic intervals all have a common denominator of 0.90 to 0.95 s; and (3) occasional fusion beats (third beat in top strip; fourth beat in second strip; last beat in bottom strip). *(From J. W. Hurst and R. Myerburg, "Introduction to Electrocardiography," McGraw-Hill Book Company, New York, 1973. Reproduced with permission from the publisher and authors.)*

lationship to the beats of the dominant rhythm; and the interectopic intervals between consecutive parasystolic complexes demonstrate a common denominator.

Aberrant Ventricular Conduction[119]

Aberrant ventricular conduction (ventricular aberration or aberrancy), first described by Lewis in 1910, is the *temporary* abnormal intraventricular conduction of supraventricular impulses. There are three forms of aberration: the common form develops when a supraventricular impulse arrives at some point in the ventricular conduction system that is still refractory. This form is therefore associated with early impulses and is the form we are most concerned with in differentiating aberration from ventricular ectopy (Fig. 26-34*A*). It complicates supraventricular extrasystoles (and other causes of early beats, such as ventricular captures and reciprocal beats) and supraventricular tachycardias (Fig. 26-35); it can be a particularly treacherous mimic during atrial fibrillation (Fig. 26-36), when it is often called Ashman's phenomenon. This form occasionally occurs, not because the aberrant beat is early, but because the *previous* cycle has unexpectedly lengthened, thereby prolonging the ensuing refractory period of the conduction system. The most common form of aberration is right bundle branch block. By experimentally producing ventricular aberration with progressively premature atrial stimulations, Kulbertus[120] obtained the patterns listed in Table 26-7.

The second form of aberration is due to anomalous conduction above the ventricles, leading to maldistribution within the ventricles (Fig. 26-34*B*). Since this form of aberration is not dependent upon refractoriness, it is independent of cycle length and may be found in early, late, or punctual beats. The most obvious example of this form of aberration results from preexcitation in which the ventricular complex is distorted because anomalous conduction at a supraventricular level (accessory pathway) produces an unorthodox sequence of activation in the ventricles. This second form of aberration is frequently seen in AV junctional beats when they arise eccentrically in the junction and spread "preferentially," either via a Mahaim tract or asynchronously down the bundle branches.

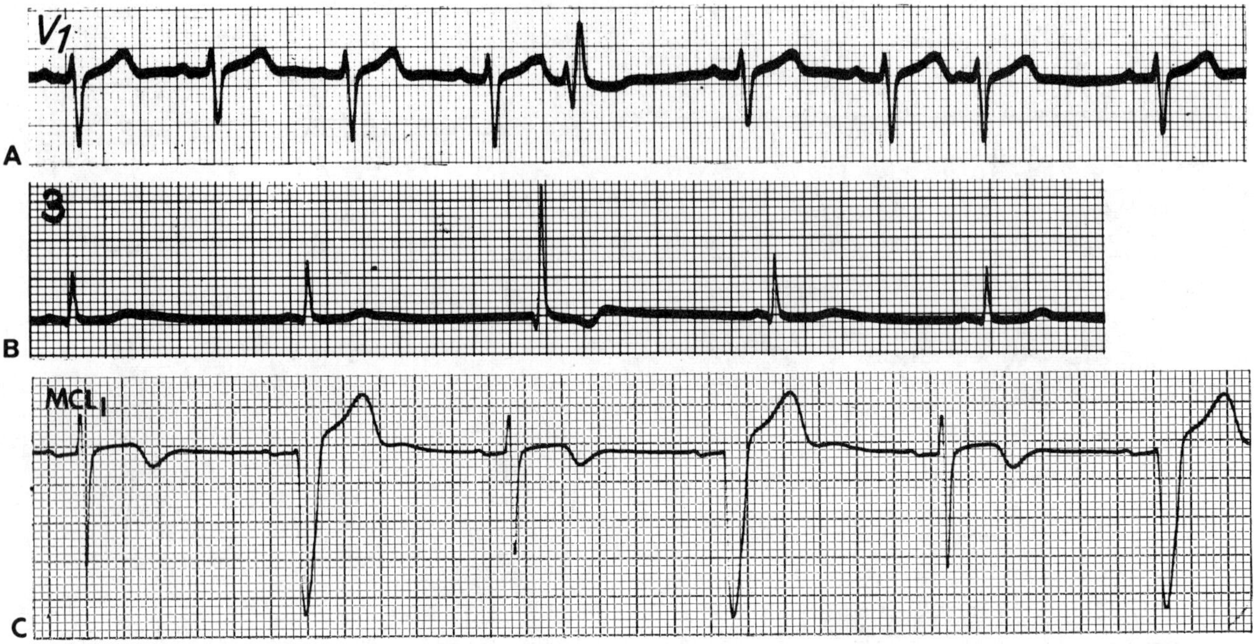

FIGURE 26-34 The three forms of ventricular aberration. *A.* The fifth beat is an atrial extrasystole with right bundle branch block aberration. This is the common form due to an early impulse finding a fascicle still refractory. *B.* The third beat, although one cannot exclude a "fascicular" origin, is probably a junctional beat conducted aberrantly because it arises from an eccentric focus. *C.* Paradoxical critical rate (?phase 4) aberration: only the beats that end the slightly *longer* cycles are conducted with left bundle branch block.

The third form of aberration results from lengthening of the ventricular cycle and may be due to (phase 4) spontaneous depolarization of a conducting fascicle. In this form, only late beats are aberrant (Fig. 26-34*C*), and the term *paradoxical critical rate* or *bradycardia-dependent bundle branch block* may be applicable.

Differentiation of Ventricular Premature Beats from Supraventricular Beats with Aberrant Ventricular Conduction

The ventricular extrasystole is often morphologically indistinguishable from an aberrant beat, but there are a number of clues that may serve to separate them.

FIGURE 26-35 The beginning of two paroxysms of atrial tachycardia with aberrant ventricular conduction simulating ventricular tachycardia. Each paroxysm starts with a telltale premature P′ wave (arrow).

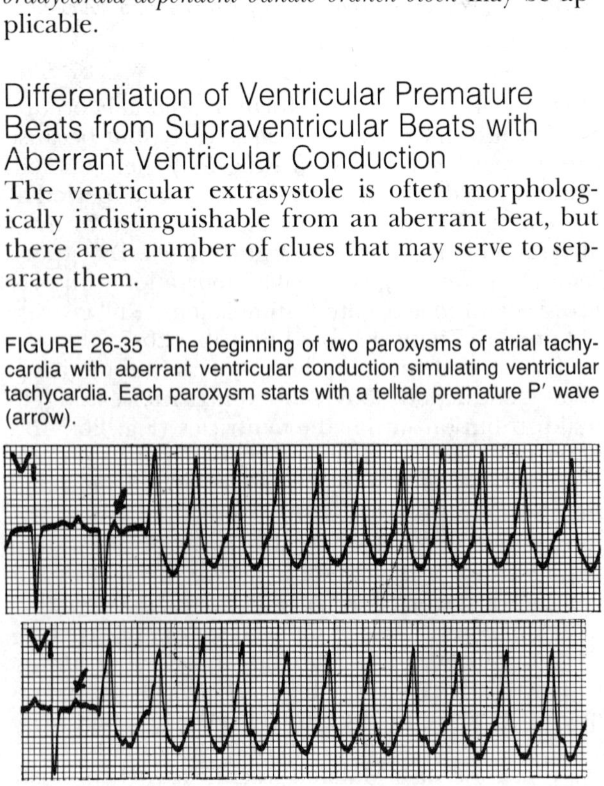

Preceding Ectopic P Wave

The presence of a preceding ectopic P (P′) wave (Figs. 26-34*A*, 26-35, and 26-37*A*) is excellent evidence favoring conduction with aberration, although one cannot always exclude the coincidence of simultaneous atrial and ventricular premature beats.

Postextrasystolic Pause

More often than not the postextrasystolic pause is fully compensatory after a ventricular premature beat (Fig. 26-23*A*) and less than compensatory after a supraventricular beat (Figs. 26-34*A* and 26-37*A*); but the postextrasystolic cycle length is not entirely reliable (see exceptions below).

FIGURE 26-36 Atrial fibrillation complicated by aberrant ventricular conduction. The beats that end the shortest ventricular cycles (0.28 to 0.32 s) present anomalous, widened complexes. These almost certainly represent a right bundle branch block type of ventricular aberration rather than ventricular ectopy. Note that the cycle preceding the onset of the salvos of anomalous beats is relatively long (0.54 and 0.50 s) in accordance with Ashman's phenomenon (see Fig. 26-19).

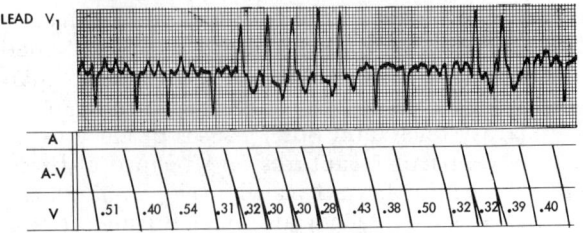

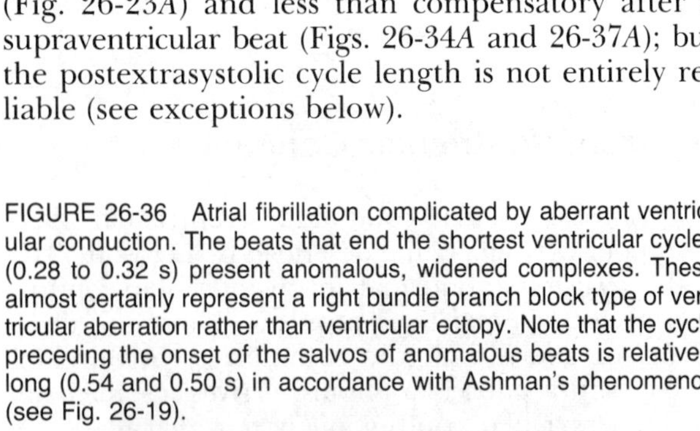

TABLE 26-7 Patterns of Induced Aberration*[75]

RBBB alone	28
RBBB + LAHB	21
RBBB + LPHB	12
LAHB alone	17
LPHB alone	10
LBBB	10
ILBBB	6
Unclassified	12
	116

i.e: RBBB = 53%
LAHB = 32%
LPHB = 19%
LBBB = 15 %
Unclassified = 10%

Note: RBBB = right bundle branch block; LAHB = left anterior hemiblock; LPHB = left posterior hemiblock; LBBB = left bundle branch block; ILBBB = incomplete left bundle branch block.

Second in the Row

When only the second in a row of rapidly consecutive beats is anomalous (Fig. 26-37*B*), it is more likely aberrant than an isolated ventricular ectopic beat; however, this eye-catching sequence can be imitated by a ventricular extrasystole that initiates a run of reentrant tachycardia in the AV junction.

QRS Morphology

Right ventricular ectopic beats simulate a *left* bundle branch block pattern, and indeed these two mutual mimics may be indistinguishable. However, there are a few clues that sometimes help: It is rare for supraventricular beats with left bundle branch block to be associated with right axis deviation, whereas right ventricular ectopic beats frequently have right axis deviation. In left bundle branch block, if there is an initial *r* wave in V_1, it is almost invariably narrow, whereas in right ventricular ectopic beats such an initial *r* wave is often wide (0.04 s or more). Finally, the deepest negative QRS complex in the precordial leads in left bundle branch block is almost always found between V_1 and V_3, whereas in right ventricular ectopic beats the deepest negative complex is frequently in V_4 or V_5.[121]

Left ventricular ectopic beats simulate a *right* bundle branch block[121] pattern, but there are several points that help to distinguish them.[122,123] In lead V_1 the ventricular ectopic beats are usually diphasic (qR) or monophasic (R), whereas the aberrant beat of right bundle branch block type is often triphasic and of rsR′ form (Fig. 26-37*A*). Moreover, when the aberrant beat *is* diphasic or monophasic, it almost always reaches its peak relatively late, whereas the ectopic beat often (in about 55 percent of cases) reaches an early peak (Fig. 26-37*C*).

The great majority of ventricular ectopic beats have an initial deflection that obviously differs from that of the conducted beats (Fig. 26-37*C*).

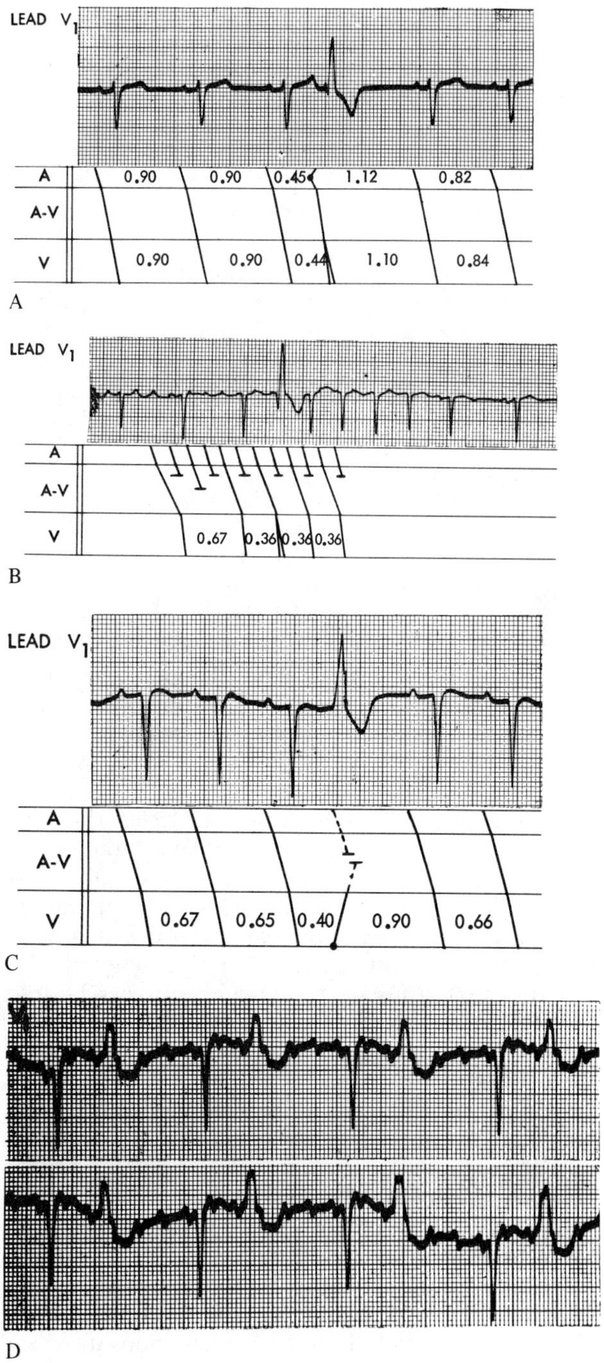

FIGURE 26-37 *A.* Atrial premature beat with ventricular aberration. Note the premature P′ wave peaking the T wave of the third beat and followed by a wide, triphasic (rsR′) complex; the ensuing cycle is less than compensatory. *B.* The fourth beat looks like a ventricular premature beat; but, since it is the second of a group of rapid beats, it is more likely aberrantly conducted than ectopic ventricular. (The basic rhythm is as diagramed: atrial flutter with 4:1 conduction changing to 2:1, with aberration of the beat that ends the first short cycle.) *C.* Ventricular premature beat. Note the monophasic R-wave pattern and compensatory pause. *D.* Atrial flutter with alternating 4:1 and 2:1 conduction; the beats ending the shorter cycles show ventricular aberration and so simulate ventricular bigeminy. *(D, from H. J. L. Marriott, Things Are Not Always What They Seem, Curr. Med. Digest, 25:60, 1958. Reproduced with permission from The Williams & Wilkins Co., Baltimore, and author.)*

Varying Degrees of the Same Bundle Branch Block Pattern

Differing degrees of the same bundle branch block pattern correlated with variations in the coupling intervals (the shorter the coupling, the greater the degree of block) undoubtedly favor aberration over ectopy.

Cycle Sequences

In the presence of atrial fibrillation, or other causes of ventricular irregularity, a study of cycle sequences[43] may be revealing: an anomalous beat that ends a cycle *longer* than cycles ending in normally conducted beats is more likely to be ectopic than aberrant.

Bigeminy in Atrial Flutter

Whenever apparent ventricular bigeminy complicates atrial flutter, one should always suspect that one of the conduction ratios that produce pairing of the ventricular complexes (3:2, or alternating 4:1 and 2:1) has developed and that there is aberrant ventricular conduction of the beats ending the shorter ventricular cycles (Fig. 26-37*D*). Proper distinction of this form of aberration from ectopic ventricular bigeminy is important and may be lifesaving.

The Compensatory Pause

When it begins and ends in the ventricles, the ventricular extrasystole does not disturb the sinus rhythm, and therefore the next sinus beat falls when expected and the pause is *compensatory*. On the other hand, if the premature beat arises in the atrium, it depolarizes the sinus node ahead of schedule, so that the next sinus beat is also ahead of schedule and the cycle is *less than compensatory*.

Unfortunately there are so many exceptions that the compensatory pause is rather a broken reed: ventricular ectopic impulses are often conducted backward to the atria;[76] these retrograde impulses may discharge the sinus node ahead of schedule and so result in a pause that is less than compensatory (Fig. 26-24, top). Because of the propensity of ectopic impulses to suppress pacemakers, an ectopic atrial impulse may so suppress the sinus pacemaker that the postextrasystolic cycle is fully compensatory (Fig. 26-24, middle). Two further situations in which a ventricular extrasystole is followed by a less than compensatory pause are when the postectopic cycle ends with an escape beat (Fig. 26-24, bottom) and when the premature beat interrupts a Wenckebach sequence.

Differentiation of Ventricular Tachycardia from Supraventricular Tachyarrhythmias with Aberration

Many of the points of differentiation between ventricular tachycardia and supraventricular tachyarrhythmias with aberrant ventricular conduction (Fig. 26-35) have already been touched upon. It remains to outline a systematic approach to the distinction.

When a rapid run of anomalous beats is seen, one should never take it for granted that it represents an ectopic ventricular mechanism. Instead, one should develop the habit of immediately recognizing the possibility that the mechanism is *either* ventricular ectopic *or* ventricular aberration, and then seek confirmation of one or the other.

1. Morphological features of the QRS complexes may be most helpful and are the same as for premature beats.
2. Fusion (Dressler) beats are strong evidence in favor of an ectopic ventricular origin, although fusion has been demonstrated to occur between two supraventricular impulses provided one of them travels aberrantly via a preferential pathway.
3. If independent atrial activity is discernible, atrial tachycardia with aberration is excluded; but the possibility of AV junctional tachycardia with aberration but without retroconduction (thus permitting independent atrial activity) remains (Fig. 26-38).

As indicated earlier, the differentiation between the various supraventricular tachycardias is often difficult, as is the distinction between ventricular tachycardia and supraventricular tachycardia with aberration. At times the diagnosis rests on uncovering causative atrial waves that are buried invisibly in the ventricular complexes. When the underlying mechanism is supraventricular with conduction to the ventricles, inhibiting AV conduction temporarily may bring the latent P waves to light and so reveal the true mechanism. Carotid sinus pressure or other means of vagal stimulation is the first maneuver to try. If this fails, intravenous procainamide may be tried; if the arrhythmia is a ventricular tachycardia,

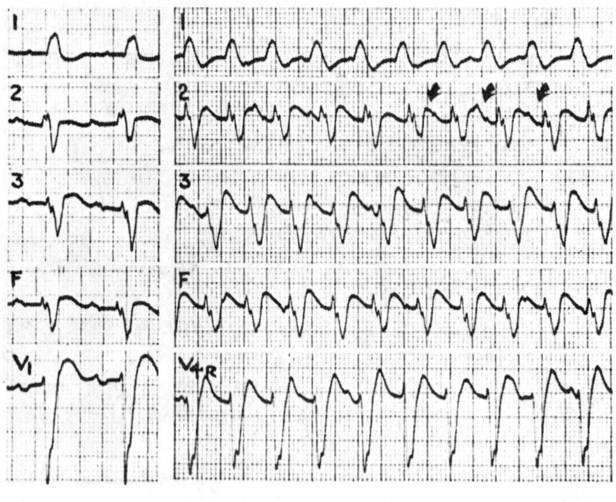

FIGURE 26-38 AV (nodal) tachycardia with left bundle branch block and without retrograde conduction to the atria. The strips on the right simulate ventricular tachycardia with their wide QRS complexes and independent P waves (arrows); but the pattern on another occasion during sinus rhythm (strips on left) shows that the ventricular pattern is not ectopic but represents a fixed left bundle branch block. The tachycardia therefore must have arisen above the bifurcation of the common bundle.

this drug is appropriate treatment, and if the underlying mechanism is supraventricular, the drug may induce AV block and so reveal the culpable atrial waves.

In the presence of atrial fibrillation, a run of aberrant beats simulating ventricular tachycardia can create a clinical problem of great importance. Differentiation may be difficult (Fig. 26-36), and considerable reliance must be placed on the structure of the anomalous complexes[122] if these are of the right bundle branch block type. Additional pointers of modest assistance are (1) the very presence of a right bundle branch block pattern gives a statistical edge in favor of aberrant conduction (but unfortunately a majority of ectopic beats arise in the left ventricle, which narrows this edge); (2) the presence of a longer cycle preceding the short cycle that initiates the run of anomalous beats favors aberrancy (but by the rule of bigeminy, a similar cycle sequence also favors the development of ventricular ectopy); (3) the presence of a considerably longer cycle immediately following the run of anomalous beats suggests an abortive compensatory pause and favors an ectopic ventricular mechanism (but it is not uncommon for aberrant conduction to be fortuitously followed by abrupt cycle lengthening); (4) obviously the presence in previous tracings of single beats of similar contour that can be identified with reasonable certainty as ectopic or aberrant may be of crucial aid in differentiation; (5) the persistence of the anomalous pattern despite adequate lengthening of the ventricular cycle obviously speaks against aberration; but even this is not foolproof since aberration, once established, sometimes persists in the face of cycle lengthening well beyond the measure of previous cycles that ended with normal intraventricular conduction.[43]

Another situation that requires special consideration is the presence of a supraventricular tachyarrhythmia complicated by WPW conduction. The error of mistaking atrial fibrillation with WPW conduction for ventricular tachycardia, and then investing the error with the sanctity of print, is one of the main reasons that ventricular tachycardia has acquired its undeserved reputation for irregularity. There are several clues that help us to avoid this mistake: (1) If the patient is known to have a WPW syndrome, even if the complexes during the tachycardia are different from his or her usual preexcitation pattern, the tachyarrhythmia is likely to be supraventricular; (2) an irregular tachycardia with bizarre complexes at a rate of 240 beats or more (Fig. 26-21) is said to be virtually diagnostic of atrial fibrillation with WPW conduction; and (3) the presence of slurred initial components (delta waves or equivalents) in the bizarre tachycardial complexes (Fig. 26-21) suggests, but does not prove, a WPW mechanism. Care must be taken not to mistake T waves "buttressing" the next QRS complex for delta waves.

Heart Block

Sinoatrial Block

If impulses fail to emerge or emerge tardily from the sinus node, SA block is present. If the impulse merely takes an undue length of time to enter the atrial muscle, first degree SA block is present, but it cannot be recognized in the clinical ECG. If one or more impulses fail to emerge, second degree block exists. If no impulses emerge, complete SA block is present.

SA block is relatively uncommon. Vagal stimulation can suppress SA nodal function in sensitive subjects, but most instances of SA block are due to structural disease or drug toxicity. Digitalis is a potent cause of SA block, often producing Wenckebach periods (see below). Quinidine, atropine, and salicylates are all reported to cause SA block. Block may result from myocardial ischemia or infarction; rheumatic fever, diphtheria, and other acute infections have produced SA block.

Electrocardiographic Features

SA block is recognized by the absence of an expected P wave. Since the sinus impulse is wanting, no ventricular response is provoked, and so the entire P-QRS-T sequence is missing—unless the sinus cycle is replaced by an escaped beat from a lower center. When a sinus beat is dropped, the resulting pause is equal to two sinus cycles (Fig. 26-39); if an existing sinus rate exactly halves, 2:1 SA block is diagnosed.

It is important to recognize SA Wenckebach periods because they invariably indicate an abnormality of the sinus node, yet they are usually overlooked and called *sinus arrhythmia*—a normal mechanism. Their recognition is discussed further on in this chapter. If P waves are entirely absent, complete SA block may be diagnosed, but it is well to keep in

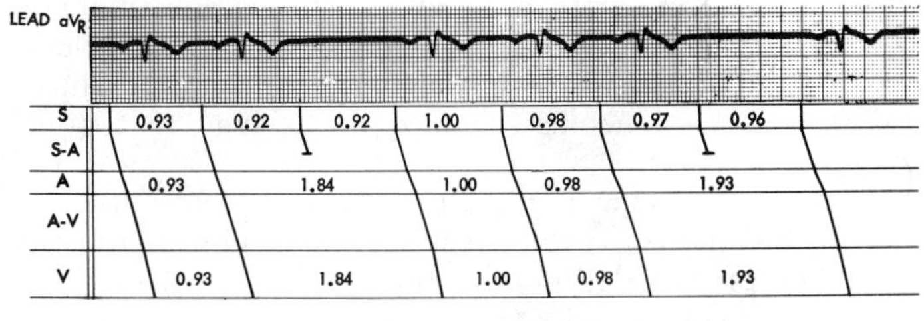

FIGURE 26-39 Sinoatrial (SA) block. In each pause the entire P-QRS-T sequence is missing, and the long cycle is approximately equal to two of the sinus cycles.

mind that there are four possible explanations for absent P waves: (1) failure of the sinus node to form impulses (generator failure); (2) failure of the impulse to emerge from the node (exit block): (3) atrial paralysis, as in potassium intoxication; and (4) a sinus impulse that is too weak to activate normally responsive atria (inadequate stimulus). Block should be diagnosed only when a mathematical relation can be demonstrated between the P waves or when the cycle sequence of Wenckebach conduction is recognized.

Any abrupt pause produced by failure of one or more sinus impulses to occur on time, and failure to satisfy the mathematic relations of recognizable block, may be called *sinus pause,* and its duration should be specified.

Atrioventricular Block

AV block is usually classified into three degrees (Table 26-8). In *first degree,* AV conduction time is prolonged, but all impulses are conducted to the ventricles. *Second degree* means that more or less frequent impulses are blocked and fail to reach the ventricles. This is usually subdivided into type I, type II, and high grade (or advanced). *Third degree* is complete block, in which no impulses can reach the ventricles.

The current classification of AV block has serious shortcomings because its categories fail to correlate with prognosis or with indicated therapy. This is because two decades ago there was no consistently effective treatment for AV block, and consequently it mattered little how blocks were graded. Pacemakers then entered the picture and revolutionized the therapy of block, while nothing was done to renovate its taxonomy. It is regrettable that, in the days before pacemakers muddied the prognostic waters, a careful assessment of the many and various patterns of AV conduction disturbance was not attempted. There is no doubt that, to correlate realistically with prognosis and the need for therapy, a classification expanded by several additions and subcategories is needed (Table 26-8, bottom).

TABLE 26-8 Classification of AV Block

Common Classification of AV Block
First degree (prolonged PR interval)
Second degree:
Type I (Wenckebach periodicity)
Type II
High grade (advanced)
Third degree (complete)
Categories of AV Block Requiring Consideration
Prolonged PR interval
Block/acceleration dissociation
Occasional "dropped" beats:
Type I (Wenckebach periodicity)
Type II
2:1 AV block:
Type I
Type II
High-grade block:
Type I
Type II
Complete block:
Junctional escape
Ventricular escape
Transient ventricular asystole:
Spontaneous
Phase 4 (?)
Vagal

One of the many factors that have helped to maintain the unsatisfactory status quo is the consistent failure of almost all authors to define terms such as complete, high-grade (or advanced), and type II AV block. An extreme example of the unfortunate result of not defining these terms is that disturbances as different as spontaneous ventricular asystole and AV dissociation, at least partly due to block but in the company of an independent junctional rhythm at a rate of 45 per minute or more—a combination which, for want of a better term, we have called *block/acceleration dissociation*—are often lumped under the heading of "complete AV block," Yet, in acute myocardial infarction transient spontaneous ventricular asystole (Fig. 26-40*A*) is associated with a mortality (whether paced or not) of about 90 percent, while block/acceleration dissociation (Fig. 26-40*B*) in our experience is associated with a mortality of less than 10 percent.

Another factor is that "degrees" as they are currently defined do not necessarily correlate with the severity of the conduction disturbance—definitions are predicated mainly on conduction ratios to the neglect of atrial rate. Thus 2:1 block, which some classify as high grade, may represent anything from a disaster (2:1 block at an atrial rate of 60) to a blessing (2:1 block at an atrial rate of 140). Again, if the sinus rate is 70 and, despite a slow independent ventricular rate of 30, no impulses are conducted to the ventricles, complete AV block can be diagnosed; but if the rate of an independent accelerated AV junctional pacemaker is 85, complete absence of AV conduction in these circumstances may represent only a minor degree of block. In fact, mere delayed AV conduction (prolonged PR interval) associated with an accelerated subsidiary pacemaker may be responsible for this form of complete AV dissociation. It is therefore obvious that in any meaningful consideration of AV block the respective rates of the involved pacemakers must be taken into account.

In fact, with definitions and misconceptions as they presently exist, a patient with "first degree block" may have a worse conduction disturbance than another erroneously labeled as having "high-grade block."

The recipe for confusion is complete if we add the following widespread misconceptions to the lack of precise definitions and the fact that "degrees"

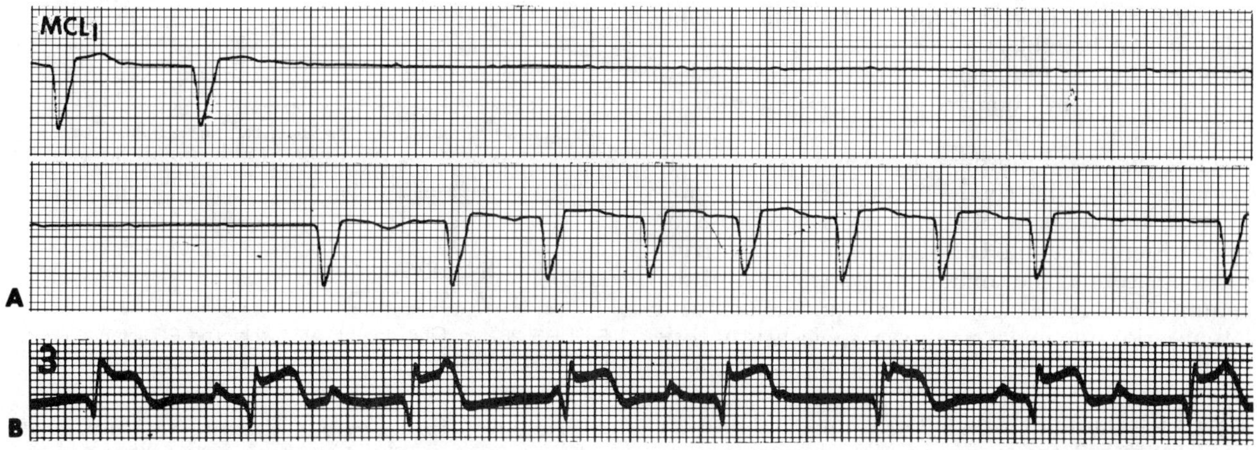

FIGURE 26-40 *A.* Spontaneous ventricular asystole lasting for over 7 s and due to the abrupt development of AV block at a time when no escaping pacemaker is active. From a patient with acute anteroseptal infarction. *B.* Complete AV dissociation due to a combination of some degree of AV block with an accelerated junctional rhythm (rate 68 per minute). From a patient with acute inferior infarction.

are not really degrees: 2:1 AV block is necessarily high-grade;[124] 2:1 AV block is necessarily type II block;[125,126] the block is necessarily high-grade when most, but not all, atrial impulses are not conducted to the ventricles;[127] and total absence of conduction, as in Fig. 26-40*B*, is necessarily evidence for complete block.[128] In view of these deficiencies in current usage, it seems desirable that the following three remedial measures be implemented: (1) "degrees," as presently used, should be eliminated or at least deemphasized; (2) the inclusion of stated atrial and ventricular rates should be an integral part of all diagnosis of AV conduction disorders; and (3) the AV blocks should be reclassified into a realistic set of sufficient and *defined* categories, including at least those listed in Table 26-8. Only then will the current confusion be remedied and indications for therapy clearly limned.

Since most reports concerned with AV block fail to define their terms, and since basic terms are variably used, some of the following observations on etiology and incidence must be accepted with appropriate reservation.

Prolonged PR intervals are occasionally found in apparently normal subjects.[3–5,7] In their survey of over 67,000 asymptomatic Air Force personnel, Johnson et al.[129] found 350 examples of first degree block (5.2 per 1000). Twenty percent of them had PR intervals that were over 0.24 s. Of 19,000 young aircrew applicants, 59 had PR intervals of 0.24 s or greater.[130]

In both normal and diseased hearts, standing, exercise, and use of atropine or isoproterenol tend to shorten the lengthened PR interval. There is a widespread belief that the PR interval tends always to shorten with an increase in heart rate. Though this is true in normal hearts with natural acceleration, when the rate is increased with artificial atrial pacing, the PR lengthens even in normal hearts; in diseased hearts a natural increase in rate is frequently associated with lengthening of the PR interval. AV block with Wenckebach periods may occur in normal hearts[3–5,7] and was found in 3 of the 67,000 Air Force personnel screened by Johnson.[129]

Prolonged AV conduction (PR interval) and dropped beats can be caused by vagal stimulation and by a variety of drugs, including digitalis, quinidine sulfate, procainamide, propranolol, verapamil, and potassium. Diseases that most commonly produce AV block are rheumatic fever, chronic ischemic heart disease, and myocardial infarction, especially inferior infarction. Any infectious disease that produces myocarditis may have this effect. Some patients with hyperthyroidism have prolonged PR intervals. Adrenocortical insufficiency tends to be associated with a prolonged PR interval, and congenital heart lesions, including atrial septal defect and Ebstein's disease, are sometimes associated with first degree AV block. Hypoxia from any cause (e.g., anesthesia, pulmonary embolism) may produce significant AV block.

Complete AV block may be congenital, occurring as an isolated finding; but in approximately half the congenital cases it is found in association with congenital malformations of the heart, viz., corrected transposition and ventricular septal defect (usually as part of a more complex defect). It is often thought that the most common cause of chronic complete AV block is ischemic heart disease, but there are a surprising number of cases with no clear-cut evidence of ischemic or any other sort of myocardial disease. Some authorities postulate that these are due to "primary" disease of the specialized conducting tissues; in one series,[131] these cases constituted the majority (59 percent against 23 percent ischemic).

Two lesions that involve the conduction fascicles and produce AV and intraventricular blocks in the absence of associated myocardial disease are Lenègre's disease and Lev's disease. Lenègre's disease[132] is an obscure sclerodegenerative process involving only the conduction system and is one of the most common causes of right bundle branch block and left anterior hemiblock in persons over the age of 50 years. The natural course of this disease is a slow progression toward complete heart block several years later.

Lev's disease,[133] on the other hand, is caused by an invasion of the conduction system from without—an involvement of the fascicles by fibrosis or calcification spreading from any of the fibrous structures adjacent to the conducting system. One of the common causes of right bundle branch block with left anterior hemiblock in elderly subjects is fibrosis of the summit of the muscular septum. Calcification of the aortic valve may cause right bundle branch block, left bundle branch block, bilateral bundle branch block, left anterior hemiblock, or complete AV block. Fibrosis or calcification of the central fibrous body or mitral ring is the most common cause of complete heart block with narrow QRS complex in the elderly. Among patients whose conduction is continuously monitored after myocardial infarction, 4.2 and 8.6 percent are said to develop complete block. In a series of personally observed 1001 consecutive acute myocardial infarctions, the incidence of complete block was only 2.1 percent. Most of these blocks complicate inferior infarction. Occasional cases are associated with calcific aortic stenosis, diphtheria, or syphilitic involvement of the His bundle. Digitalis and potassium intoxication may produce complete AV block. Rare causes of complete AV block include sarcoidosis, Hodgkin's disease, myeloma and other tumors of the heart, rheumatoid disease, dermatomyositis, Reiter's syndrome,[134] Paget's disease, hyperthyroidism, myxedema, amyloidosis, progressive muscular dystrophy, and trauma (penetrating and nonpenetrating). The surgical closure of ventricular septal defects and implantation of aortic valves have furnished new causes of traumatic complete block in recent decades. Myocardial bridging is an uncommon cause of paroxysmal AV block.[135]

Electrocardiographic Features

First degree AV block is diagnosed when the PR interval is prolonged to 0.21 s or beyond. The interval may be constant, or it may vary inversely with the RP interval during a sinus arrhythmia, a situation that the French have aptly called *floating PR*. Though most examples of first degree AV block have PR intervals between 0.21 and 0.35 s (Fig. 26-41), occasional intervals have been recorded up to 1.0 s or slightly greater.

In second degree AV block, some P waves are not followed by QRS complexes (dropped beats). The most common form, type I, is the Wenckebach period, in which, after progressively lengthening PR intervals, the final P wave is not followed by a ventricular response. The sequence of PR lengthening usually follows a recognizable pattern, at least for the first few beats: although the lengthening is progressive, the amount by which the PR interval increases over the previous PR interval (the increment) decreases (Fig. 26-42*A*). Since each ventricular cycle is determined by the basic sinus cycle and the current increment, an apparent paradox results, provided the sinus rhythm is regular: as the PR interval lengthens, the RR interval shortens. Thus the pause of the dropped beat is followed by slight but measurable ventricular acceleration (Fig. 26-42*A*). Since the pause of the dropped beat contains the shortest PR interval, it is equal to less than two of the shortest cycles. These features enable one to recognize the Wenckebach type of conduction even when no conduction intervals are available for measurement. An example of such conduction out of the sinus node is illustrated in Fig. 26-42*B*. In this tracing the P waves show the same type of periodicity that the QRS complexes showed in Fig. 26-42*A*: the longest PP interval is less than twice the shortest PP interval, and after the long interval there is measurable acceleration of the sinus P waves. It is important not to overlook sinus Wenckebach periods and mistake them for sinus arrhythmia, because sinus arrhythmia is a normal mechanism whereas the sinus Wenckebach period is almost invariably a sign of drug effect or disease.

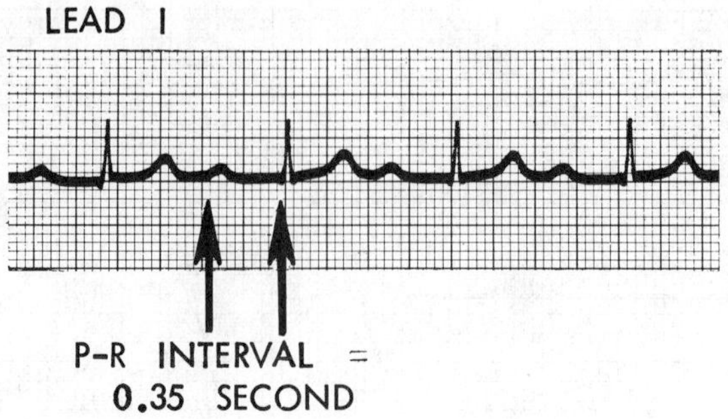

FIGURE 26-41 First degree AV block. The PR interval is prolonged to 0.35 s.

The most common Wenckebach ratio is 3:2, leaving the ventricular complexes grouped in pairs, but any $(x + 1){:}x$ ratio (e.g., 4:3, and 7:6) may be seen. In type II block, a beat is dropped after *consecutive* preceding atrial impulses have been conducted with a constant, usually normal, PR interval and with bundle branch block. His bundle electrography has demonstrated that type I AV block is almost always due to conduction delay in the AV node proper, whereas type II block occurs in or below the bundle of His;[136] in fact, Damato regards type II block as a manifestation of bilateral bundle branch block.[137] Type I block with Wenckebach periods usually develops in acute situations (myocardial infarction, rheumatic fever, or digitalis intoxication), is therefore temporary, and carries a relatively good prognosis. Type II block is usually permanent and often progresses to complete AV block.

In second degree AV block, either type I or type II, every alternate beat may be dropped so that there are two P waves to each QRS complex (2:1 block) (Fig. 26-43); or there may be several P waves to each

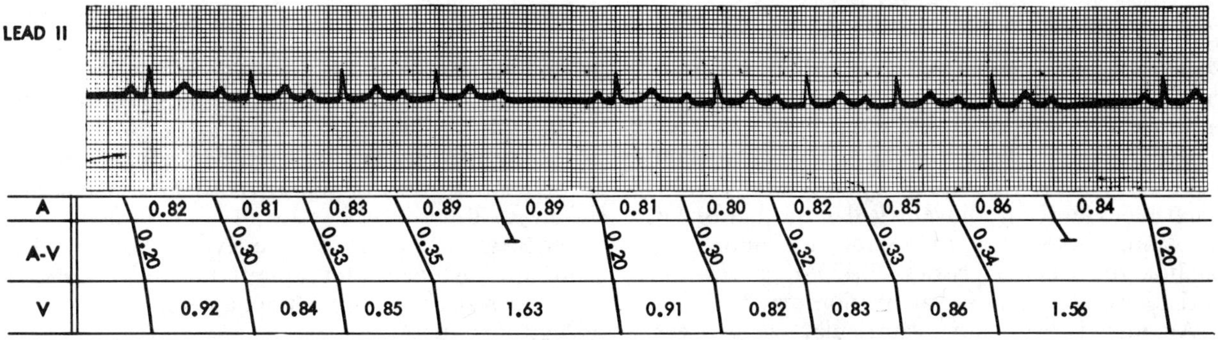

A

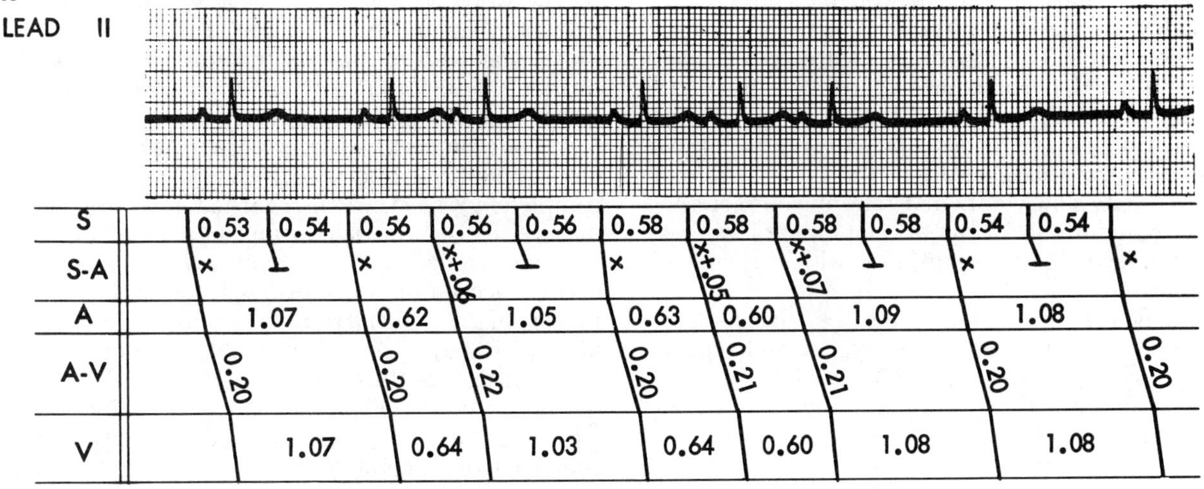

B

FIGURE 26-42 Wenckebach phenomenon. *A.* A 5:4 and 6:5 AV Wenckebach period. Note that the PQ interval progressively lengthens, but by a decreasing increment; therefore the ventricular cycle tends to shorten (at least for the first two cycles following the dropped beat). *B.* A 3:2 and 4:3 sinus Wenckebach period with 2:1 SA block at beginning and end of strip. *(From J. W. Hurst and R. Myerburg, "Introduction to Electrocardiography," McGraw-Hill Book Company, New York, 1973. Reproduced with permission from the publisher and author.)*

QRS complex (3:1, 4:1, etc.), in which case, provided the atrial rate is reasonable, a diagnosis of high-grade (or advanced) block is justified.

In complete (third degree) AV block the ventricular complexes occur independently at a slow rate, usually between 30 to 45 beats per minute, except in congenital heart block, in which the rate is somewhat faster. Usually regular but independent P waves constantly change their relation to the QRS complexes (Fig. 26-44). Despite complete anterograde block, retroconduction to the atria may occasionally produce retrograde P waves after the ventricular complex occurs. In a more recent series of 42 patients with "complete" block investigated with sophisticated electrophysiological techniques, retrograde conduction to the atria was detected in 36 percent, with concealed conduction as far as the AV junction in an additional 17 percent.[138]

The ventricular complex may be normal or anomalous. If the site of block is high in the AV

FIGURE 26-43 Second degree AV block. There are two P waves to each QRS—2:1 AV block (every alternate sinus impulse is blocked).

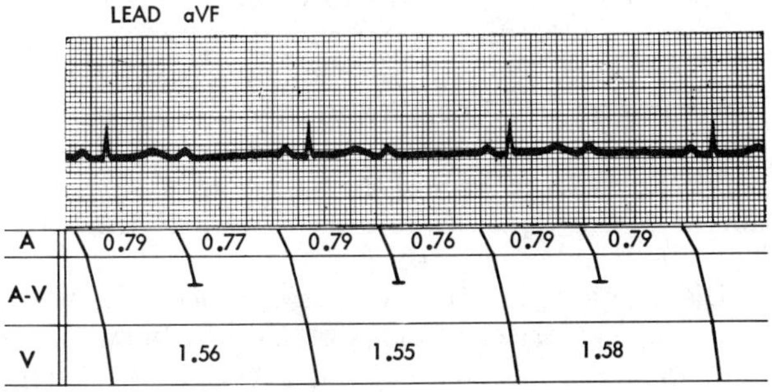

FIGURE 26-44 Complete (third degree) AV block. There is a regular idioventricular rhythm at rate 36, and the P waves indicate their independence by changing their relation to the QRS complexes.

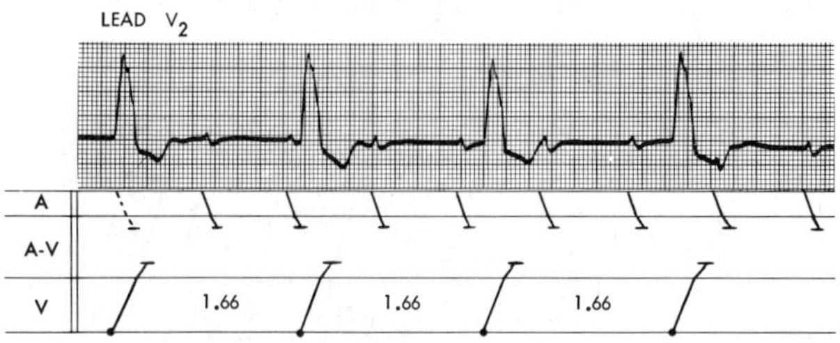

junction (monofascicular) and the pacemaker is situated above the bifurcation of the AV bundle, the QRS complex will be normal unless there is an associated bundle branch block. An abnormal QRS complex will also be written if the pacemaker is ectopic ventricular (idioventricular). The distinction between an AV (junctional) pacemaker with bundle branch block and an idioventricular mechanism is often impossible, but the same distinguishing morphological characteristics outlined earlier for ventricular ectopy and for aberration may be helpful. At times two or more ventricular pacemakers operate simultaneously or in sequence, often at remarkably similar rates, producing varying patterns of fusion beats. The picture of complete AV block is often preceded, sometimes for years, by a pattern of bundle branch block; and indeed many cases of complete block are in fact due to bilateral bundle branch block (bifascicular) or to multifascicular block.[139] The slow ventricular rates in complete AV block frequently favor the development of ventricular extrasystoles, in accordance with the rule of bigeminy.

In conclusion, one must remember that first degree AV block, second degree type I and type II block, and high-grade AV block can all be imitated by concealed junctional[140] or fascicular[141] extrasystoles or parasystole.[142]

Group Beating

This term is applied when bursts of similar ventricular complexes are separated by pauses. The most common cause is undoubtedly repetitive Wenckebach periods in the presence of sinus or atrial tachycardia (Fig. 26-45). The P waves often are difficult or impossible to discern, but the diagnosis can be confidently made from the cycle sequences (see "Wenckebach Phenomenon," above).

Other, less common causes are bursts of repetitive ventricular tachycardia and groups of agonal beats in the dying heart.

Atrioventricular Dissociation

AV dissociation, like jaundice, is not in itself a diagnosis. It is always a secondary result of a primary disturbance. Like jaundice, it may be the first sign

FIGURE 26-45 Group beating during atrial (sinus?) tachycardia as a result of 4:3 Wenckebach periods.

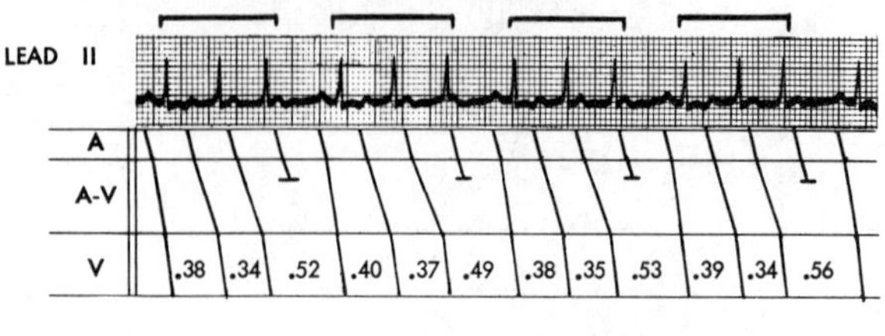

that catches the eye, but the underlying cause must then be uncovered.

The terminology of the subject has been unnecessarily confused. *AV dissociation* is commonly used in three different ways: as a synonym for complete AV block; in a quasi-specific sense for an arrhythmic sequence that was called *interference dissociation*; and simply to describe the state of independence between atria and ventricles whenever the normal AV sequence has been interrupted. This third sense—to characterize the independent state of affairs—is its legitimate usage.

The word *interference* has been so sinned against that, to avoid confusion, we prefer not to use it. For those who wish to pursue the semantic problems further, we draw your attention to an earlier review[143] and the pertinent references.

If the momentary dissociation occasioned by single ectopic beats and the dissociation secondary to complete AV block are disregarded, AV dissociation may result from atrial slowing (*default* of primary pacemaker; Fig. 26-46*A*); from AV nodal or ventricular acceleration (*usurpation* by secondary pacemaker; Fig. 26-46*B*); from reduction in the number of atrial impulses reaching the AV junction or ventricles because of SA or AV block (Fig. 26-46*C*); from the opportunism of an escaping pacemaker taking advantage of the pause provided by a premature beat; or from a combination of any of these conditions.

AV dissociation may affect the normal heart, as when it results from sinus bradycardia in an athlete. It may also result from sinus bradycardia induced by unnatural stimuli such as anesthesia or eye operations. Among its many other causes are (1) drugs, including digitalis, atropine, quinidine, and procainamide; (2) infections; (3) rheumatic fever; and (4) ischemic heart disease, especially acute inferior infarction.

Electrocardiographic Features

Since there are so many and such varied circumstances in which AV dissociation can arise, one cannot give a unified description of its electrocardiographic findings. But one cardinal electrocardiographic sign is common to all conditions in which dissociation in any form is sustained: a changing relation between atrial and ventricular complexes.

The dissociated sequence that earned the name *interference dissociation* from Mobitz in 1923 is illustrated in Fig. 26-46*B*. Because the automatic AV pacemaker is beating faster than the SA node, the P waves "overtake" and pass the QRS complex. Since there may be little or no disturbance in AV conduction, when the P wave has emerged far enough beyond the QRS complex, the atrial impulse is conducted to the ventricles to effect "capture" (captured beat, ventricular capture).

Dissociation does not necessarily occur between sinus and AV pacemakers; two AV junctional pacemakers may dissociate, the upper one controlling

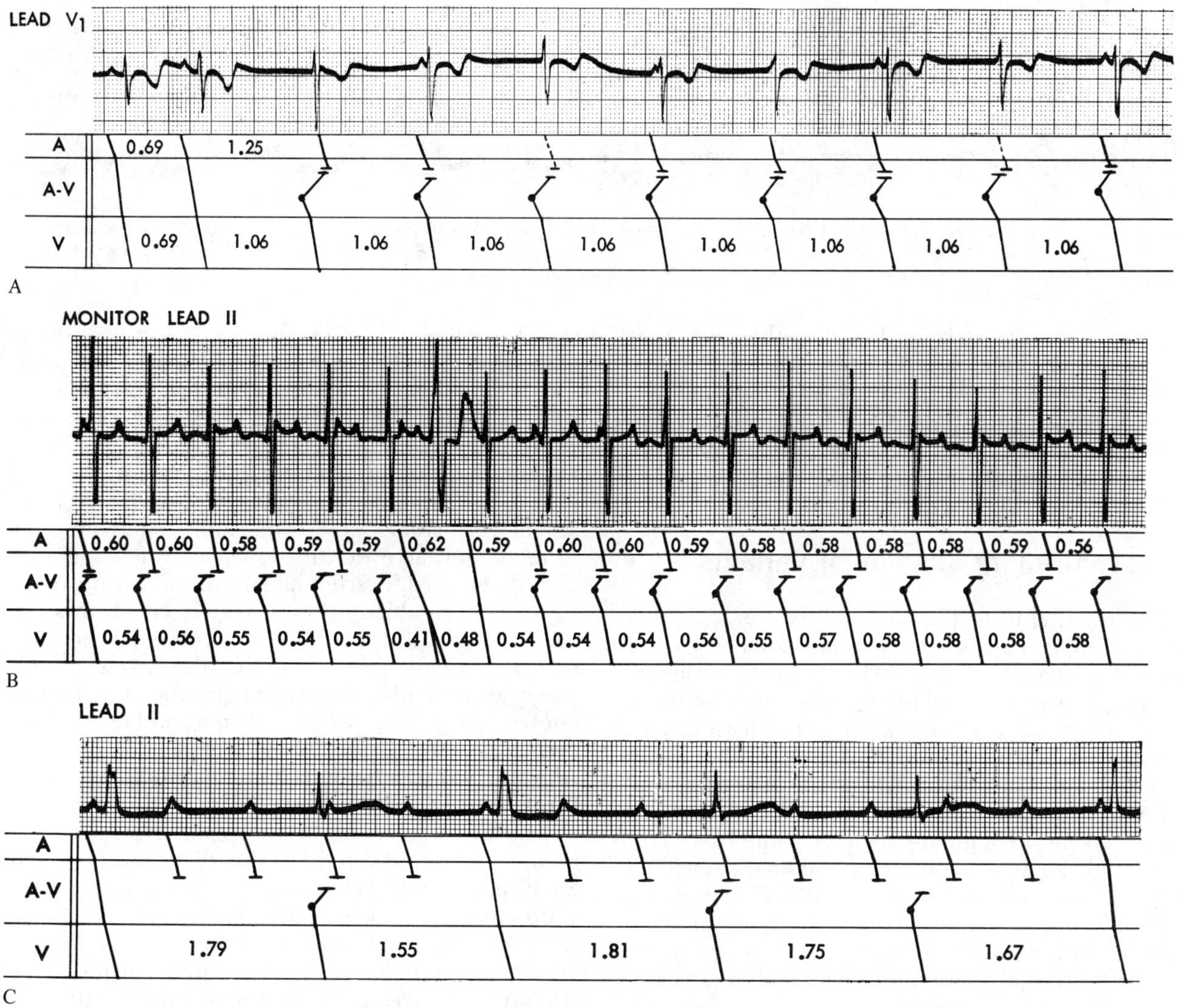

FIGURE 26-46 AV dissociation. *A.* Sinus arrhythmia: the bradycrotic phase enables the AV node to escape, with resulting dissociation. *B.* AV tachycardia: the tachycardia enables the AV pacemaker to usurp control of the ventricles, with resulting dissociation; the seventh and eighth beats are ventricular captures, the seventh, ending the shorter cycle, showing ventricular aberration. *C.* High-grade AV block permits the AV node to escape (second, fourth, and fifth beats), with resulting dissociation.

the atria, and the lower the ventricles. Or the ventricles may be controlled by a dissociated idioventricular pacemaker (Fig. 26-32). In such cases ventricular fusion beats frequently intervene between the runs of dissociation and the captured beats.

It is quite common for a heart to harbor two independent pacemakers with identical or nearly identical rates. It therefore sometimes happens that dissociated pacemakers may beat at similar rates for longer or shorter periods without the occurrence of conduction (capture). In the tracing, the P waves are seen to flirt with the QRS complexes, never leaving them far in front or behind, until a sufficient change in the rate of one of them restores AV conduction. This situation was called *isorhythmic dissociation* by French authors. The isorhythmicity may be the result of fortuitous identity of rates; or at times there may be evidence that the two pacemakers are held in phase by electrical or mechanical influences, a phenomenon called *synchronization* or *accrochage*.

Sometimes, when two pacemakers with similar rates are operative, the dissociated P wave approaches the QRS complex, disappears within it for several beats, then reappears again and recedes from the QRS complex until a normal PR interval is achieved and maintained for a few beats. It then once again approaches the QRS complex and repeats this sequence again and again (Fig. 26-47). Such behavior has been attributed to fluctuations in arterial blood pressure conditioned by changes in atrial transport function secondary to changes in the relation of atrial to ventricular contraction.

Just as ventricular fusion beats may occur between runs of dissociation and capture beats when the lower pacemaker is idioventricular, so atrial fusion beats can occur between runs of AV rhythm and dissociation if the atria are not protected by retrograde block from ascending AV impulses. Both forms of fusion represent *partial* dissociation: in the one case only a part of the ventricular moiety is dis-

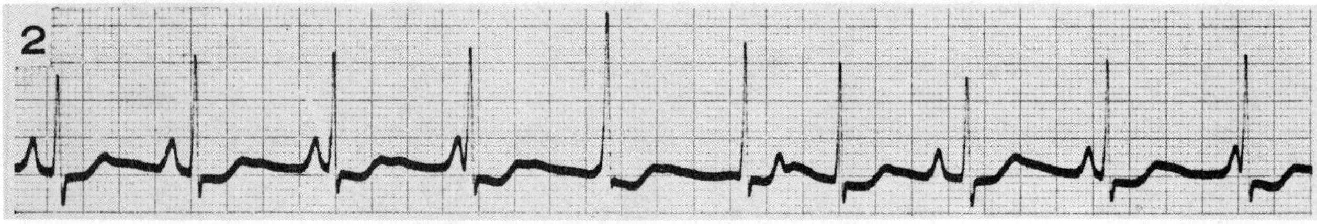

FIGURE 26-47 Accelerated idionodal rhythm producing AV dissociation. From a girl of 10 years with rheumatic heart disease and digitalis intoxication developing after mitral valvotomy. The seventh beat is a ventricular capture. *(From H. J. L. Marriott, "Armchair Arrhythmias," Tampa Tracings, 1966. Reproduced with permission from the publisher and author.)*

sociated from the atria, and in the other only part of the atria is dissociated. Thus, although AV dissociation can occur in the presence of normal anterograde and retrograde conduction, impairment of conduction in either direction favors the development and maintenance of dissociation.

Atrioventricular Junctional Variants

Accelerated Junctional Rhythm

Depending at least to some extent upon the level of the pacemaker,[17] junctional rhythms have an inherent rate between 30 and 60 beats per minute. If the rate exceeds 60 beats per minute, the rhythm is *accelerated.* Accelerated junctional rhythms may control both ventricles and atria, or the atria may continue to beat independently. Accelerated junctional rhythm is most commonly seen as a complication of acute inferior infarction, acute rheumatic fever, or digitalis intoxication. Figure 26-40*B* illustrates accelerated junctional rhythm complicating an acute inferior infarction, and Fig. 26-48 shows an accelerated junctional rhythm due to digitalis toxicity.

Reciprocal Rhythm

Reciprocal rhythms require the assumption of at least two functioning pathways in the AV junction with unequal refractory periods. In a reciprocal beat the impulse arises in the AV junction and travels both downward to the ventricles and upward into the atria. The impulse on its upward journey encounters a refractory path which it cannot penetrate and proceeds upward by another path to reach the atria. Higher in the AV junction, the impulse may find a level in the hitherto refractory path at which it is no longer refractory, "spill over" into it, and descend to reach and activate the ventricles. Such spillover and downward descent are favored by delay in retrograde conduction, since such delay affords the descending path more time for recovery. The phenomenon of the retrograde impulse reentering an anterograde path and reactivating the ventricles is known as *reciprocal rhythm* or *beating,* and the beat so produced is a *reciprocal* or *echo beat.* The point in the AV junction at which the impulse spills over and turns down is the *reflecting level.*

FIGURE 26-48 Accelerated idionodal rhythm with resulting isorhythmic AV dissociation. After four sinus beats, the sinus rate slows slightly, enabling the accelerated junctional pacemaker to escape at a rate of 94. After several seconds the sinus pacemaker accelerates and recapturers the ventricles. The same sequence is then repeated. (The strips are continuous.) *(From H. J. L. Marriott, "Workshop in Electrocardiography," Tampa Tracings, 1972. Reproduced with permission from the publisher and author.)*

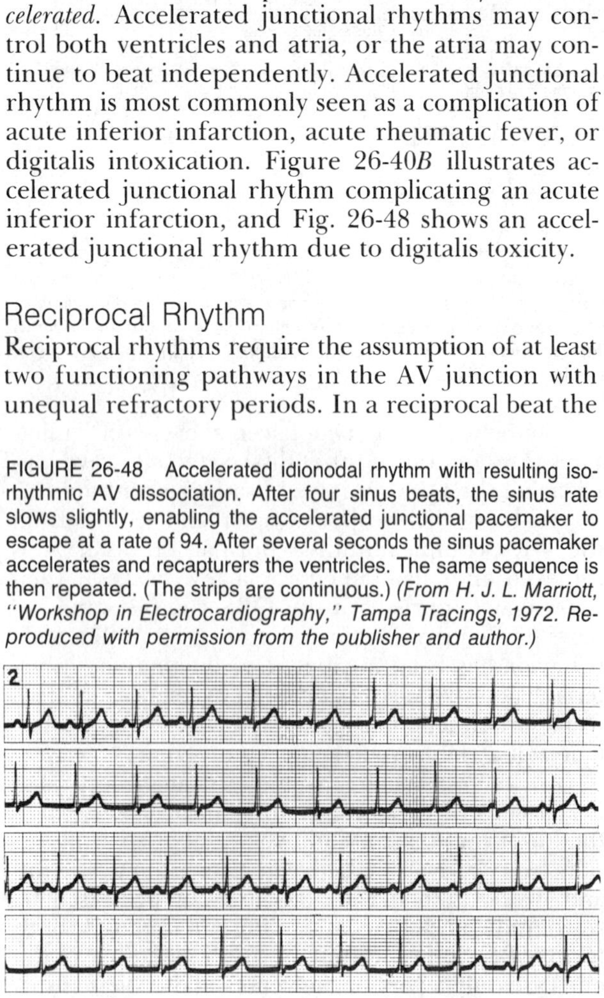

There are several variations on the reciprocal theme, as is indicated in the diagrams in Figs. 26-49 and 26-50. When the impulse begins in the ventricle as an ectopic beat and returns to reactivate the ventricles, it has been called a *return extrasystole.* When the impulse circulates rapidly around the AV junction, giving off daughter impulses to atria and ventricles at two reflecting levels, a *reciprocating tachycardia* results.

A reciprocal beat usually occurs at the end of a run of AV junctional rhythm with progressively lengthening retrograde conduction. Any of the factors that can produce AV junctional rhythm can contribute to the production of reciprocal beating; undoubtedly one of the commonest causes is digitalis excess.

Wandering or Shifting Pacemaker

These terms are applied when, as a result of suppression of one pacemaker, usually the sinus node,

FIGURE 26-49 Diagram of reciprocal mechanisms. *(From H. J. L. Marriott, "Workshop in Electrocardiography," Tampa Tracings, 1972. Redrawn and reproduced with permission from the publisher and author.)*

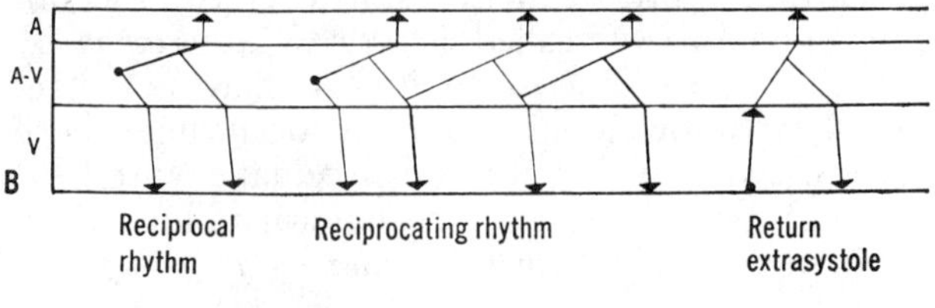

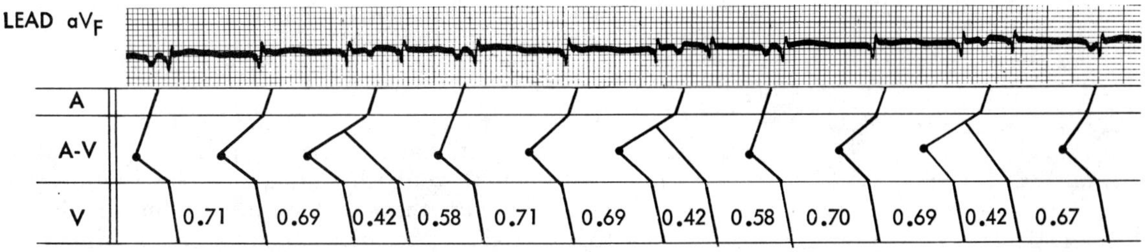

FIGURE 26-50 Reciprocal rhythm. AV nodal rhythm with progressively lengthening retrograde conduction until, with the third beat, there is enough retrograde delay for the impulse to find a nonrefractory downward path and be "reflected" back to the ventricles—the reciprocal beat.

another center takes over the role of pacemaking. Most commonly, pacemaking activity shifts back and forth between the sinus node and AV junction. The terms should not be applied when the pacemaking changes are due to premature beats. The mechanism may appear in normal hearts and may be a manifestation of fluctuating vagal tone; it obviously can be encouraged by any influence that enhances vagal activity.

In the ECG, a changing contour of the P waves is associated with changes in cycle length and in the PR interval. In the most typical case, sinus P waves are replaced after several beats by retrograde P′ waves, often with intermediate fusion P waves (Fig. 26-51*A*); then, after a few AV beats, pacemaking reverts to the sinus node. The characteristic feature of wandering pacemaker is that changes in the P waves occur, at least part of the time, with cycle *lengthening,* never with abrupt decrease in cycle length. A momentary shift of pacemaker often follows ectopic or retrograde atrial activation, the returning cycle showing an altered P wave (atrial escape; Fig. 26-51*B*).

Escape Rhythms

When a higher pacemaker defaults, a lower pacemaker may come to the rescue and "escape." Thus by definition an escape (or escaped) beat is a *late* beat occurring only after an interval longer than the dominant cycle. If the sinus pacemaker unduly slows or otherwise defaults, the most likely pacemaker to take over and escape is the AV junction. Less often, an ectopic ventricular pacemaker escapes. When the sinus pacemaker is suppressed by an atrial extrasystole or other ectopic atrial activity, the returning beat is often an atrial escape. If several junctional escape beats occur in succession, with the AV pacemaker controlling both atria and ventricles, a *junctional escape rhythm* is present. If a series of escape beats occurs but the atria continue to be controlled by their own sinus pacemaker, we have *AV dissociation.* If pacemaking switches back and forth between sinus and junctional pacemakers, the rhythm is called *shifting* or *wandering pacemaker.* If a junctional rhythm shows considerable retrograde delay of conduction to the atria, *reciprocal beating* may occur. There is thus an intimate interplay between escape, junctional rhythm, shifting pacemaker, reciprocal rhythm, and AV dissociation, so that to some extent they must be considered together.

Escape Beats

Escape occurs after an interval longer than the dominant cycle. It represents a safety mechanism; escape beats therefore should never be suppressed. Anything that provides a pause longer than the prevailing cycle may permit escape to occur: the slow

FIGURE 26-51 *A.* Wandering pacemaker. The first four beats are AV junctional, the next is an atrial fusion beat, and the next three are sinus. *B.* Shift of pacemaker induced by an atrial extrasystole (arrow); immediately following the premature beat, pacemaking shifts to the AV node and then returns, via several atrial fusion beats, to sinus rhythm.

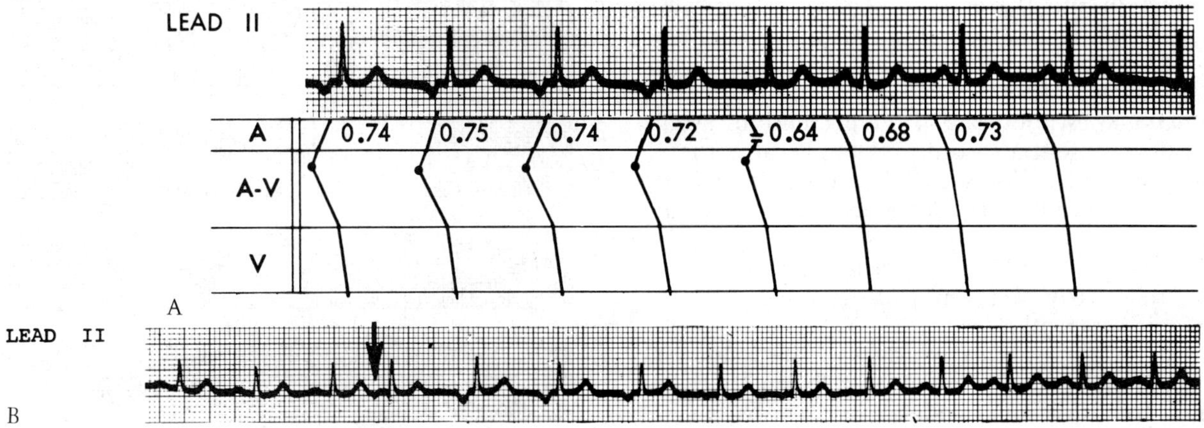

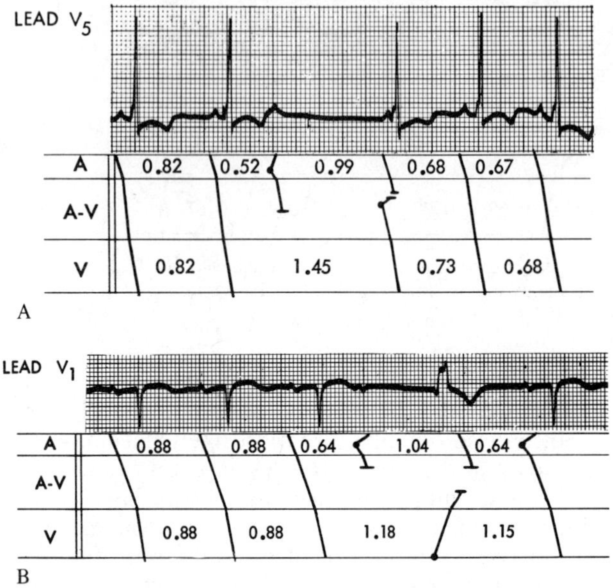

FIGURE 26-52 *A.* AV (nodal) escape beat. After two sinus beats there is a nonconducted atrial premature beat; the pause that follows this ends with an escape beat whose QRS-T pattern is similar to that of the sinus beats. *B.* Ventricular escape beat. After three sinus beats there is a nonconducted atrial premature beat; the pause that follows this ends with a bizarre beat of typical ectopic ventricular contour.

phase of sinus arrhythmia, SA block, AV block, extrasystoles, and the ending of a paroxysm of tachycardia each may provide an adequate pause to release an escaping beat.

In the ECG the junctional escape beat usually shows a QRS-T contour similar to that of the sinus beat, but it sometimes shows a slight variation from the dominant beats (Fig. 26-52*A*). Less often it can show quite marked distortion and widening (aberration) of the QRS complex and simulate an ectopic ventricular beat. This is contrary to what one would expect, since aberration classically develops with shortening of the cycle, not lengthening. This seeming paradox is explained by assuming that such escaping impulses travel by preferential pathways provided by paraspecific (Mahaim) fibers and so enter the ventricles by an unorthodox path. Or such AV impulses may arise from an eccentric focus in the AV junction and therefore spread asymmetrically down the bundle of His to enter one bundle branch before the other, and thus result in an anomalous ventricular complex.[144]

Junctional escape beats in the presence of atrial fibrillation present a special problem because there is no dominant cycle. Escape is usually diagnosed when the longest ventricular cycles are all equal in length.

Ventricular escapes are characterized by the late rather than early occurrence of the usual patterns of ectopic ventricular beats (Fig. 26-52*B*).

Atrial escape beats are seldom described and yet are common; they are often seen when there is suppression of the sinus node by atrial extrasystoles, by runs of atrial tachycardia, or by retrograde atrial activation (Fig. 26-12).

Atrioventricular Junctional Rhythm

In AV junctional rhythm a junctional pacemaker controls both ventricles and atria. This rhythm can result from anything that suppresses sinus node activity, such as physiological sinus bradycardia, any form of vagal stimulation, digitalis, the initial phase of atropine action, SA block, or congenital absence of the SA node, or from anything that enhances AV automaticity, such as digitalis intoxication, rheumatic fever, or inferior myocardial infarction. When the rhythm is due to default of the sinus pacemaker, the rate is usually between 30 and 60 beats per minute, and it is referred to as a *junctional escape rhythm.* When it results from enhanced junctional automaticity, the rate is faster (60 to 100 per minute) and the rhythm is best termed *accelerated junctional rhythm.* This is the preferred term because the rate is faster than the normal rate for this pacemaker site (30 to 60 per minute) but less than the necessary rate of more than 100 to meet the criterion for a tachycardia. When the rate exceeds 100, the term *junctional tachycardia* is appropriately employed.

In the ECG the P′ wave of retrograde atrial activation may be seen in front of the QRS complex (with short P′R interval) or following the QRS complex, or it may be lost within the ventricular complex. When the P′ waves are visible, they are narrow and usually inverted in leads II, III, aV_F, and often in the left chest leads; they are upright in aV_R and aV_L and often in V_1. The QRS-T pattern is usually normal but may be somewhat aberrant as a result of preferential pathway conduction or eccentric impulse origin.

Idioventricular Rhythm

When the ventricles operate independently under control of an ectopic ventricular pacemaker at slow or normal rates (20 to 100 beats per minute), the

FIGURE 26-53 *A, B,* and *C.* Deteriorating ventricular fibrillation. *D.* Ventricular standstill.

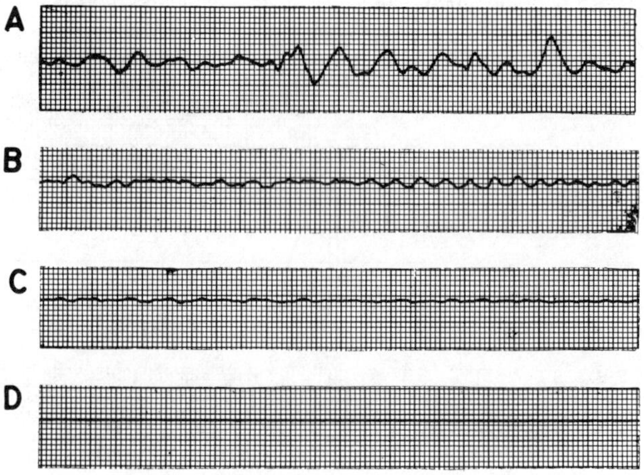

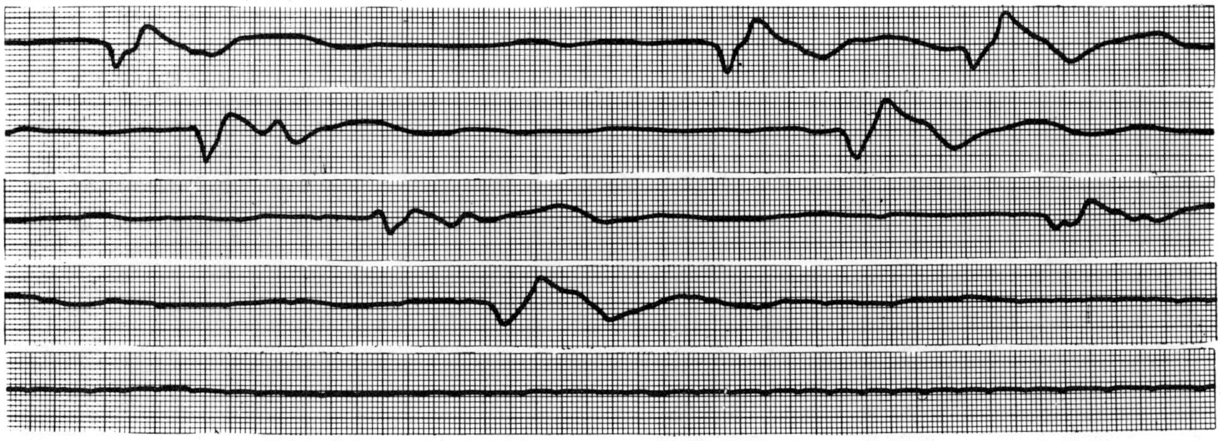

FIGURE 26-54 Agonal rhythm (continuous strips). Grossly widened and distorted ventricular complexes occur irregularly and slow to a standstill.

rhythm is called *idioventricular.* Three consecutive ventricular escape beats constitute the shortest run of idioventricular rhythm, and they may result from any of the causes of escape enumerated above. However, idioventricular rhythm is usually a manifestation of complete AV block, and the subject has been dealt with under that heading. Rarely it may result from complete SA block. If the idioventricular rate is between 50 and 100 beats per minute, the appropriate term is *accelerated idioventricular rhythm* (see discussion earlier in this chapter).

Cardiac Arrest

Cardiac arrest includes all conditions in which effective ventricular contraction has ceased. Thus it embraces (1) ventricular fibrillation (VF), the ultimate arrhythmia, in which the ventricular myocardium writhes in uncoordinated activity; (2) ventricular standstill or asystole, in which there is no mechanical or electrical ventricular activity; and (3) agonal rhythm, in which there are wide, distorted ventricular complexes but no associated mechanical activity.

Factors that may contribute to the development of cardiac arrest include hypotension, shock, anoxia, metabolic acidosis, bradycardia, or tachycardia. Autonomic influences, both vagal and sympathetic, may play a role. Fibrillation may be initiated by potassium depletion: drugs, such as digitalis, quinidine sulfate, procainamide, and disopyramide;[145] and anesthetic agents, such as chloroform and cylopropane. Atropine, administered intravenously for sinus bradycardia in acute myocardial infarction, has precipitated ventricular fibrillation.[146] An electric shock of appropriate voltage—as from household ac outlets or from lightning—will induce fibrillation. Other causes of arrest include anaphylaxis and drowning. VF sometimes complicates the WPW syndrome in the wake of atrial fibrillation with excessively rapid ventricular response.[147] Rarely, paroxysms of VF, starting and stopping spontaneously, may occur in otherwise apparently normal hearts.

In VF there are no formed ventricular complexes in the tracing; instead, there is an irregular zigzag pattern of variable amplitude (Fig. 26-53*A* to *C*). The pattern of fibrillation is of some importance, since the larger and better formed the zigzag contours, the easier is defibrillation. Ventricular standstill (Fig. 26-53*D*) is recognized by the complete absence of any sign of ventricular activity in the electrocardiogram. Agonal rhythm, which may appear in any heart approaching death, results in wide, bizarre complexes (Fig. 26-54) these are usually irregular and are often recorded at an extremely slow rate.

References

1. Besoin-Santander, M., Pick, A., and Langendorf, R.: A-V Conduction in Auricular Flutter, *Circulation,* 2:604, 1950.
2. Southall, D. P., Richards, J., Mitchell, P., Brown, D. J., Johnston, P. G. B., and Shinebourne, E. A.: Study of Cardiac Rhythm in Healthy Newborn Infants, *Br. Heart J.,* 43:14, 1980.
3. Southall, D. P., Johnston, F., Shinebourne, E. A., and Johnston, P. G. B.: A 24-Hour Electrocardiographic Study of Heart Rate and Rhythm Patterns in Population of Healthy Children, *Br. Heart J.,* 45:281, 1981.
4. Scott, O., Williams, G. J., and Fiddler, G. I.: Results of 24-Hour Ambulatory Monitoring of Electrocardiogram in 131 Healthy Boys Aged 10 to 13 Years, *Br. Heart J.,* 44:304, 1980.
5. Dickinson, D. F., Scott, O.: Ambulatory Electrocardiographic Monitoring in 100 Healthy Teenage Boys, *Br. Heart J.,* 51:179, 1984.
6. Sabotka, P. A., Mayer, J. H., Bauernfeind, R. A., Kanakis, C., and Rosen, K. M.: Arrhythmias Documented by 24-Hour Continuous Ambulatory Electrocardiographic Monitoring in Young Women without Apparent Heart Disease, *Am. Heart J.,* 101:753, 1981.
7. Brodsky, M., Wu, D., Denes, P., Kanakis, C., and Rosen, K. M.: Arrhythmias Documented by 24-Hour Continuous Electrocardiographic Monitoring in 50 Male Medical Students without Apparent Heart Disease, *Am. J. Cardiol.,* 39:390, 1977.
8. Talan, D. A., Bauernfeind, R. A., Ashley, W. W., Kanakis,

C., and Rosen, K. M.: Twenty-Four Hour Continuous ECG Recordings in Long-Distance Runners, *Chest,* 82:19, 1982.
9. Pilcher, G. F., Cook, A. J., Johnston, B. L., and Fletcher, G. F.: Twenty-Four Hour Continuous Electrocardiography during Exercise and Free Activity in 80 Apparently Healthy Runners, *Am. J. Cardiol.,* 52:859, 1983.
10. Fleg, J. L., and Kennedy, H. L.: Cardiac Arrhythmias in a Healthy Elderly Population: Detection by 24-Hour Ambulatory Electrocardiography, *Chest,* 81:302, 1982.
11. Zeppilli, P.: High-Grade Arrhythmias in Well-Trained Runners, *Am. Heart J.,* 106:775, 1983.
12. Graybiel, A., McFarland, F. A., Gates, D. C., and Webster, F. A.: Analysis of the Electrocardiograms Obtained from 1000 Young Healthy Aviators, *Am. Heart J.,* 27:524, 1944.
13. Hiss, R. G. Lamb, L. E., and Allen, M. F.: Electrocardiographic Findings in 67,375 Asymptomatic Subjects. X. Normal Values, *Am. J. Cardiol.,* 6:200, 1960.
14. Adgey, A. A. J., Geddes, J. S., Mulholland, H. C., Keegan, D. A. J., and Pantridge, J. F.: Incidence, Significance, and Management of Early Bardyarrhythmia Complicating Acute Myocardial Infarction, *Lancet,* 2:1097, 1968.
15. Norris, R. M., Mercer, C. J., and Yeates, S. E.: Sinus Rate in Acute Myocardial Infarction, *Br. Heart J.,* 34:901, 1972.
16. Hiss, R. G., and Lamb, L. E.: Electrocardiographic Findings in 122,043 Individuals, *Circulation,* 25:947, 1962.
17. Scherlag, B. J., Lazzara, R., and Helfant, R. H.: Differentiation of "A-V Junctional Rhythms," *Circulation,* 48:304, 1973.
18. Guntheroth, W. G., Selzer, A., and Spodick, D. H.: Atrioventricular Nodal Rhythm Reconsidered, *Am. J. Cardiol.,* 52:416, 1983.
19. Lown, B., Wyatt, N. F., and Levine, H. D.: Paroxysmal Atrial Tachycardia with Block, *Circulation,* 21:129, 1960.
20. Morgan, W. L., and Breneman, G. M.: Atrial Tachycardia with Block Treated with Digitalis, *Circulation,* 25:787, 1962.
21. Garson, A., and Gillette, P. C., Junctional Ectopic Tachycardia in Children: Electrocardiography, Electrophysiology and Pharmacologic Response, *Am. J. Cardiol.,* 44:298, 1979.
22. Gillette, P. C., Garson, A., Porter, J., Ott, D., McVey, P., Zinner, A., and Blair, H.: Junctional Automatic Ectopic Tachycardia: New Proposed Treatment by Transcatheter His Bundle Ablation, *Am. Heart J.,* 106:619, 1983.
23. Josephson, M. E., and Seides, S. F.: "Clinical Cardiac Electrophysiology: Techniques and Interpretations," Lea & Febiger, Philadelphia, 1979, pp. 148–176.
24. Swartz, M. H., Teichholz, L. E.,and Donoso, E.: Mitral Valve Prolapse: A Review of Associated Arrhythmias, *Am. J. Med.,* 62:377, 1977.
25. Akhtar, M., Damato, A. N., Batsford, W. P., Caracta, A. R., Ruskin, J. N., Weisfogel, G. M., and Lau, S. H.: Induction of AV Nodal Reentrant Tachycardia after Atropine, *Am. J. Cardiol.,* 36:286, 1975.
26. Josephson, M. E.: Paroxysmal Supraventricular Tachycardia: An Electrophysiologic Approach, *Am. J. Cardiol.,* 41:1123, 1978.
27. Wu, D., Denes, P., and Amat-y-Leon, F.: Clinical, Electrocardiographic and Electrophysiologic Observations in Patients with Paroxysmal Supraventricular Tachycardia, *Am. J. Cardiol.,* 41:1045, 1978.
28. Benditt, D. G. Pritchett, E. L. C., Smith, W. M., and Gallagher, J. J.: Ventriculo-atrial Intervals: Diagnostic Use in Paroxysmal Supraventricular Tachycardia, *Ann. Intern. Med.,* 91:161, 1979.
28a. Wellens, H. J. J., and Durrer, D.: The Role of an Accessory Atrioventricular Pathway in Reciprocal Tachycardia: Observations in Patients with and without the Wolff-Parkinson-White Syndrome, *Circulation,* 52:58, 1975.
28b. Farshidi, A., Josephson, M. E., and Horowitz, L. N.: Electrophysiologic Characteristics of Concealed Bypass Tracts: Clinical and Electrocardiographic Correlates, *Am. J. Cardiol.,* 41:1052, 1978.
29. Green, M., Heddle, B., Dassen, W., Wehr, M., Abdollah, H., Brugada, P., and Wellens, H. J. J.: Value of QRS Alternation in Determining the Site of Origin of Narrow QRS Supraventricular Tachycardia, *Circulation,* 68:368, 1983.
30. Brugada, P., Bär, F. W. H. M., Vanagt, E. J., Friedman, P. L., and Wellens, H. J. J.: Observations in Patients Showing A-V Junctional Echoes with a Shorter P-R than R-P Interval: Distinction between Intranodal Reentry or Reentry Using an Accessory Pathway with a Long Conduction Time, *Am. J. Cardiol.,*. 48:611, 1981.
31. Brugada, P., Farre, J., Green, M., Heddle, B., Roy, D., and Wellens, H. J. J.: Observations in Patients with Supraventricular Tachycardia Having a P-R Interval Shorter than the R-P Interval: Differentiation between Atrial Tachycardia and Reciprocating Atrioventricular Tachycardia Using an Accessory Pathway with Long Conduction Times, *Am. Heart J.,* 107:556, 1984.
32. Guarnieri, T., Sealy, W. C., Kasell, J. H., German, L. D., and Gallagher, J. J.: The Nonpharmacologic Management of the Permanent Form of Junctional Reciprocating Tachycardia, *Circulation,* 69:269, 1984.
33. Shine, K. I., Kastor, J. A., and Yurchak, P. M.: Multifocal Atrial Tachycardia: Clinical and Electrocardiographic Features in Thirty-two Cases, *Circulation,* 36(suppl. 2):236, 1967.
34. Fosmoe, R. J., Averill, K. H., and Lamb, L. E.: Electrocardiographic Findings in 67,375 Asymptomatic Subjects: II. Supraventricular Arrhythmias, *Am. J. Cardiol.,* 6:84, 1960.
35. Langendorf, R., and Pick A.: Cardiac Arrhythmias in Infants and Children, in B. M. Gasul, R. A. Arcilla, and M. Lev (eds.) "Heart Disease in Children," J. B. Lippincott Company, Philadelphia, 1966, p. 121.
36. Slama, R., Leclercq, J. F., Rosengarten, M., Coumel, P., and Bouvrain, Y.: Multilevel Block in the Atrioventricular Node during Atrial Tachycardia and Flutter Alternating with Wenckebach Phenomenon, *Br. Heart J.,* 42:463, 1979.
37. Kannel, W. B., Abbott, R. D., and Savage, D. D.: Coronary Heart Disease and Atrial Fibrillation: The Framingham Study, *Am. Heart J.,* 106:389, 1983.
38. Ettinger, P. O., Wu, D. F., De La Cruz, C., Weisse, A. B., Ahmed, S. S., and Regan, T. J.: Arrhythmias and the "Holiday Heart": Alcohol-Associated Cardiac Rhythm Disorders, *Am. Heart J.,* 95:555, 1978.
39. Engel, T. R., and Luck, J. C.: Effect of Whiskey on Atrial Vulnerability and "Holiday Heart," *J. Am. Coll. Cardiol.,* 1:816, 1983.
40. Forfar, J. C., Miller, H. C., and Toft, A. D.: Occult Thyrotoxicosis: A Correctable Cause of "Idiopathic" Atrial Fibrillation, *Am. J. Cardiol.,* 44:9, 1979.
41. Morganroth, J., Horowitz, L. N., Josephson, M. E., and Kastor, J. A.: Relationship of Atrial Fibrillatory Wave Amplitude to Left Atrial Size and Etiology of Heart Disease. An Old Generalization Re-examined, *Am. Heart J.,* 97:194, 1979.
42. Gouaux, J. L., and Ashman, R.: Auricular Fibrillation with Aberration Simulating Ventricular Paroxysmal Tachycardia, *Am. Heart J.,* 34:366, 1947.
43. Marriott, H. J. L., and Sandler, I. A.: Criteria, Old and New, for Differentiating between Ectopic Ventricular Beats and Aberrant Ventricular Conduction in the Presence of Atrial Fibrillation, *Prog. Cardiovasc. Dis.,* 9:18, 1966.
44. Gallagher, J. J., Pritchett, E. L. C., Sealty, W. C., Kasell, J., and Wallace, A. G.: The Preexcitation Syndromes, *Prog. Cardiovasc. Dis.,* 20:285, 1978.
45. Benditt, D. G., Pritchett, E. L. C., Gallagher, J. J.: Spectrum, of Regular Tachycardias with Wide QRS Complexes in Patients with Accessory Atrioventricular Pathways, *Am. J. Cardiol.,* 42:828, 1978.
46. Wellens, H. J. J.: Wolff-Parkinson-White Syndrome. Part I. Diagnosis, Arrhythmias, and Identification of the High Risk Patient. *Mod. Concepts Cardiovasc. Dis.,* 52:53, 1983.
47. Durrer, D., Schoo, L., Schuilenburg, R. M., and Wellens, H. J. J.: The Role of Premature Beats in the Initiation and the Termination of Supraventricular Tachycardia in the Wolff-Parkinson-White Syndrome, *Circulation,* 36:644, 1967.
48. Rosen, K. M.: A-V Nodal Reentrance: An Unexpected Mechanism of Paroxysmal Tachycardia in a Patient with Preexcitation, *Circulation,* 47:1267, 1973.
49. Wellens, H. J. J.: Contribution of Cardiac Pacing to Our

Understanding of the Wolff-Parkinson-White Syndrome, *Br. Heart J.*, 37:231, 1975.
50. Sung, R. J., Castellanos, A., Gelband, H., and Myerburg, R. J.: Mechanisms of Reciprocating Tachycardia during Sinus Rhythm in Concealed Wolff-Parkinson-White Syndrome, *Circulation*, 54:338, 1976.
51. Barold, S. S., and Coumel, P.: Mechanisms of Atrioventricular Tachycardia: Role of Reentry and Concealed Accessory Bypass Tracts, *Am. J. Cardiol.*, 39:97, 1977.
52. Gillette, P. C.: Concealed Anomalous Cardiac Conduction Pathways: A Frequent Cause of Supraventricular Tachycardia, *Am. J. Cardiol.*, 40:848, 1977.
53. Przybylski, J., Chiale, P. A., Halpern, M. S., Nau, G. J., Elizari, M. V., and Rosenbaum, M. B.: Unmasking of Ventricular Preexcitation by Vagal Stimulation or Isoproterenol Administration, *Circulation*, 61:1030, 1980.
54. Klein, G. J., and Gulamhusein, S. S.: Intermittent Preexcitation in the Wolff-Parkinson-White Syndrome, *Am. J. Cardiol.*, 52:292, 1983
55. Giardina, A. C. V., Ehlers, K. H., and Engle, M. A.: Wolff-Parkinson-White Syndrome in Infants and Children: A Long-Term Follow-Up Study, *Br. Heart J.*, 34:839, 1972.
56. Wolff, G. S., Han, J., and Curran, J.: Wolff-Parkinson-White Syndrome in the Neonate, *Am. J. Cardiol.*, 41:559, 1978.
57. Huang, S. K., Rosenberg, M. J., and Denes, P.: Short PR Interval and Narrow QRS Complex Associated with Pheochromocytoma: Electrophysiologic Observations, *J. Am. Coll. Cardiol.*, 3:872, 1984.
58. Wiener, I.: Syndromes of Lown-Ganong-Levine and Enhanced Atrioventricular Nodal Conduction, *Am. J. Cardiol.*, 52:637, 1983.
59. Benditt, D. G., Pritchett, E. L. C., Smith, W. M., Wallace, A. G., and Gallagher, J. J.: Characteristics of Atrioventricular Conduction and the Spectrum of Arrhythmias in Lown-Ganong-Levine Syndrome, *Circulation*, 57:454, 1978.
60. Kaplan, B. M., Langendorf, R., Lev, M., and Pick, A.: Tachycardia-Bradycardia Syndrome (So-Called "Sick Sinus Syndrome"), *Am. J. Cardiol.*, 31:497, 1973.
61. Palileo, E. V., Coelho, A., Westveer, D., Dhingra, R., and Rosen, K. M.: Persistent Sinus Node Dysfunction Secondary to Lithium Therapy, *Am. Heart J.*, 106:1443, 1983.
62. Ferrer, M. I.: "The Sick Sinus Syndrome," Futura Publishing Company, Mt. Kisco, N.Y., 1974.
63. Shaw, D. B., Holman, R. R., and Gowers, J. I.: Survival in Sinoatrial Disorder (Sick-Sinus Syndrome), *Br. Med. J.*, 1:139, 1980.
64. Strauss, H. C., Bigger, J. T., Jr., Saroff, A. L., and Giardina, E. G. V.: Electrophysiologic Evaluation of Sinus Node Function in Patients with Sinus Node Dysfunction, *Circulation*, 53:763, 1976.
65. Kerr, C. R., and Strauss, H. C.: The Measurement of Sinus Node Refractoriness in Man, *Circulation*, 68:1231, 1983.
66. Surawicz, B., and MacDonald, M. G.: Ventricular Ectopic Beats with Fixed Variable Coupling: Incidence, Clinical Significance and Factors Influencing the Coupling Interval, *Am. J. Cardiol.*, 13:198, 1964.
67. Hinkle, L. E., Carver, S. T., and Stevens, M.: The Frequency of Asymptomatic Disturbances of Cardiac Rhythm and Conduction in Middle-Aged Men, *Am. J. Cardiol.*, 24:629, 1969.
68. Rosenberg, M. J., Uretz, E., and Denes, P.: Sleep and Ventricular Arrhythmias, *Am. Heart J.*, 106:703, 1983.
69. Faris, J. V., McHenry, P. L., Jordan, J. W., and Morris, S. N.: Prevalence and Reproducibility of Exercise-Induced Ventricular Arrhythmias during Maximal Exercise Testing in Normal Man, *Am. J. Cardiol.*, 37:617, 1976.
70. Ekblom, B., Hartley, L. H., and Day, W. C.: Occurrence and Reproducibility of Exercise-Induced Ventricular Ectopy in Normal Subjects, *Am. J. Cardiol.*, 43:35, 1979.
71. Mardelli, T. J., Morganroth, J., and Dreifus, L. S.: Superior QRS Axis of Ventricular Premature Complexes: An Additional Criterion to Enhance the Sensitivity of Exercise Stress Testing, *Am. J. Cardiol.*, 45:236, 1980.
72. DeBacker, G., Jacobs, D., Prineas, R., Crow, R., Vilandre, J., Kennedy, H., and Blackburn, H.: Ventricular Premature Contractions: A Randomized Non-drug Intervention Trial in Normal Men, *Circulation*, 59:762, 1979.
73. Coronary Drug Project Research Group: The Prognostic Importance of Premature Beats following Myocardial Infarction: Experience in the Coronary Drug Project, *JAMA*, 223:1116, 1973.
74. Kotler, M. N., Tabatsnik, B., Mower, M. M., and Tominaga, S.: Prognostic Significance of Ventricular Ectopic Beats with Respect to Sudden Death in the Late Postinfarction Period, *Circulation*, 47:959, 1973.
75. Rosenbaum, M. B., Halpern, M. S., Nau, G. J., Elizari, M. V., and Lazzari, J. O.: The Mechanism of Narrow Ventricular Ectopic Beats, in "Symposium of Cardiac Arrhythmias," AB Astra, Sodertalje, Sweden, 1970, p. 223.
76. Kistin, A., and Landowne, M.: Retrograde Conduction from Premature Ventricular Contractions, a Common Occurrence in the Human Heart, *Circulation*, 3:738, 1951.
77. Montague, T. J., McPherson, D. D., MacKenzie, B. R., Spencer, C. A., Nanton, M. A., and Horacek, B. M.: Frequent Ventricular Ectopic Activity without Underlying Cardiac Disease: Analysis of 45 Subjects, *Am. J. Cardiol.*, 52:980, 1983.
78. Lewis, S., Kanakis, C., Rosen, K. M., and Denes, P.: Significance of Site of Origin of Premature Ventricular Contractions, *Am. Heart J.*, 97:159, 1979.
79. Rosenbaum, M. B.: Classification of Ventricular Extrasystoles According to Form, *J. Electrocardiol.*, 2:289, 1969.
80. Massumi, R. A., Hilliard, G., DeMaria, A., Fabregas, R., Lindsay, A. E., Amsterdam, E., and Mason, D. T.: Paradoxic Phenomenon of Premature Beats with Narrow QRS in the Presence of Bundle Branch Block, *Circulation*, 47:543, 1973.
81. Lie, K. I., Wellens, H. J. J., Downar, E., and Durrer, D.: Observations on Patients with Primary Ventricular Fibrillation (A Double-Blind Randomized Study of 212 Consecutive Patients), *N. Engl. J. Med.*, 291:1324, 1974.
82. Roberts, R., Ambos, H. D., Loh, C. W., and Sobel, B. E.: Initiation of Repetitive Ventricular Depolarizations by Relatively Late Premature Complexes in Patients with Acute Myocardial Infarction, *Am. J. Cardiol.*, 41:678, 1978.
83. Bisteni, A., Medrano, G. A., and Sodi-Pallares, D.: Ventricular Premature Beats in the Diagnosis of Myocardial Infarction, *Br. Heart J.*, 23:521, 1961.
84. Benchimol, A., Lasry, J. E., and Carvalho, F. R.: The Ventricular Premature Contraction: Its Place in the Diagnosis of Ischemic Heart Disease, *Am. Heart J.*, 65:334, 1963.
84a. Dash, H., and Ciotola, J. J.: Morphology of Ventricular Premature Beats as an Aid in the Electrocardiographic Diagnosis of Myocardial Infarction, *Am. J. Cardiol.*, 52:458, 1983.
85. Abdulla, A. M., Baute, A. V., Friedland, L. B., Canedo, M. I., Stefadouros, M. A., and Frank, M. J.: Value of Ventricular Premature Complex (VPC) Morphology in the Diagnosis of Hypertrophic Cardiomyopathy, *J. Electrocardiol.*, 16:73, 1983.
86. Winkle, R. A., Derrington, D. C., and Schroeder, J. S.: Characteristics of Ventricular Tachycardia in Ambulatory Patients, *Am. J. Cardiol.*, 39:487, 1977.
87. Chou, T-C, and Wenzke, F.: The Importance of R on T Phenomenon, *Am. Heart J.*, 96:191, 1978.
88. Tye, K-H, Samant, A., Desser, K. B., and Benchimol, A.: R on T or R on P Phenomenon? Relation to the Genesis of Ventricular Tachycardia, *Am. J. Cardiol.*, 44:632, 1979.
89. Lesch, M., Lewis, E., Humphries, J. O., and Ross, R. S.: Paroxysmal Ventricular Tachycardia in the Absence of Organic Heart Disease: Report of a Case and Review of the Literature, *Ann. Intern. Med.*, 66:950, 1967.
90. Hiss, R. G., Averill, K. H., and Lamb, L. E.: Electrocardiographic Findings in 67,375 Asymptomatic Subjects: III. Ventricular Rhythms, *Am. J. Cardiol.*, 6:96, 1960.
91. Pedersen, D. H., Zipes, D. P., Foster, P. R., and Troup, P. J.: Ventricular Tachycardia and Ventricular Fibrillation in a Young Population, *Circulation*, 60:988, 1979.
92. Wei, J. Y., Bulkley, B. H., Schaeffer, A. H., Greene, H. L., and Reid, P. R.: Mitral-Valve Prolapse Syndrome and Re-

current Ventricular Tachyarrhythmias: A Malignant Variant Refractory to Conventional Drug Therapy, *Ann. Intern. Med.*, 89:6, 1978.
93. de Soyza, N., Meacham, D., Murphy, M. L., Kane, J. J., Doherty, J. E., and Bissett, J. K.: Evaluation of Warning Arrhythmias before Paroxysmal Ventricular Tachycardia during Acute Myocardial Infarction in Man, *Circulation*, 60:814, 1979.
94. Buxton, A. E., Waxman, H. L., Marchlinski, F. E., Simson, M. B., Cassidy, D., and Josephson, M. E.: Right Ventricular Tachycardia: Clinical and Electrophysiologic Characteristics, *Circulation*, 68:917, 1983.
95. Holt, P., Curry, P. V. L., O'Keeffe, D. B., and Wainwright, R. J.: Ventricular Arrhythmias in Normal Heart, *Br. Heart J.*, 49:300, 1983.
96. Josephson, M. E., Horowitz, L. N., Waxman, H. L., Cain, M. E., Spielman, S. R., Greenspan, A. M., Marchlinski, F. E., and Ezri, M. D.: Sustained Ventricular Tachycardia: Role of the 12-Lead Electrocardiogram in Localizing Site of Origin, *Circulation*, 64:257, 1981.
97. Marcus, F. I., Fontaine, G. H., Guiraudon, G., Frank, R., Laurenceau, J. L., Malergue, C., and Grosgogeat, Y.: Right Ventricular Dysplasia: A Report of 24 Adult Cases, *Circulation*, 65:384, 1982.
98. Rowland, E., McKenna, W. J., Sugrue, D., Barclay, R., Foale, R. A., and Krikler, D. M.: Ventricular Tachycardia of Left Bundle Branch Block Configuration in Patients with Isolated Right Ventricular Dilation: Clinical and Electrophysiologic Features, *Br. Heart J.*, 51:15, 1983.
99. Fitchett, D. H., Sugrue, D. D., MacArthur, C. G., and Oakley, C. M.: Right Ventricular Dilated Cardiomyopathy, *Br. Heart J.*, 51:25, 1983.
100. Reiter, M. J., Smith, W. M., and Gallagher, J. J.: Clinical Spectrum of Ventricular Tachycardia with Left Bundle Branch Block Morphology, *Am. J. Cardiol.*, 51:113, 1983.
101. Horowitz, L. N., Vetter, V. L., Harken, A. H., and Josephson, M. E.: Electrophysiologic Characteristics of Sustained Ventricular Tachycardia Occurring after Repair of Tetralogy of Fallot, *Am. J. Cardiol.*, 46:446, 1980.
102. McKenna, W. J., Chetty, S., Oakley, C. M., and Goodwin, J. F.: Arrhythmia in Hypertrophic Cardiomyopathy. Exercise and 48-Hour Ambulatory Electrocardiographic Assessment with and without Beta Adrenergic Blocking Therapy, *Am. J. Cardiol.*, 45:1, 1980.
103. Wellens, H. J. J., Bar, F. W. H. M., and Lie, K. I.: The Value of the Electrocardiogram in the Differential Diagnosis of a Tachycardia with a Widened QRS Complex, *Am. J. Med.*, 64:27, 1978.
104. Wellens, H. J. J., Bär, F. W. H. M., Vanagt, E. J. D. M., and Brugada, P.: Medical Treatment of Ventricular Tachycardia; Considerations in the Selection of Patients for Surgical Treatment, *Am. J. Cardiol.*, 49:187, 1982.
105. Kuck, K.-H., Brugada, P., and Wellens, H. J. J.: Observations on the Antidromic Type of Circus Movement Tachycardia in the Wolff-Parkinson-White Syndrome, *J. Am. Coll. Cardiol.*, 2:1003, 1983.
106. Wellens, H. J. J.: Personal communication.
107. Josephson, M. E., Horowitz, L. N., Farshidi, A., Spielman, S. R., Michelson, E. L., and Greenspan, A. M.: Recurrent Sustained Ventricular Tachycardia: 4. Pleomorphism, *Circulation*, 59:459, 1979.
108. Sclarovsky, S., Strasberg, B., Lewin, R. F., and Agmon, J.: Polymorphous Ventricular Tachycardia: Clinical Features and Treatment, *Am. J. Cardiol.*, 44:339, 1979.
109. Kossman, C. E.: Torsade de Pointes: An Addition to the Nosography of Ventricular Tachycardia, *Am. J. Cardiol.*, 42:1054, 1978.
110. Smith, W. M., and Gallagher, J. J.: "Les Torsades de Pointes": An Unusual Ventricular Arrhythmia, *Ann. Int. Med.*, 93:578, 1980.
111. Tzivoni, D., Keren, A., and Stern, S.: Torsades de Pointes Versus Polymorphous Ventricular Tachycardia, *Am. J. Cardiol.*, 52:639, 1983.
112. Kay, G. N., Plumb, V. J., Arcinegas, J. G., Henthorn, R. W., and Waldo, A. L.: Torsade de Pointes: The Long-Short Initiating Sequence and Other Clinical Features: Observations in 32 Patients, *J. Am. Coll. Cardiol.*, 2:806, 1983.
113. Taboul, P.: Torsade de Pointes, in H. J. J. Wellens and H. E. Kulbertus (eds.), "What's New in Electrocardiography," Martinus Nijhoff, Boston, 1980, p. 229.
114. Massumi, R. A., and Ali, A.: Accelerated Isorhythmic Ventricular Rhythms, *Am. J. Cardiol.*, 26:170, 1970.
115. Sclarovsky, S., Strasberg, B., and Fuchs, J.: Multiform Accelerated Idioventricular Rhythm in Acute Myocardial Infarction: Electrocardiographic Characteristics and Response to Verapamil, *Am. J. Cardiol.*, 52:43, 1983.
116. Gaum, W. E., Biancaniello, T., and Kaplan, S.: Accelerated Ventricular Rhythm in Childhood, *Am. J. Cardiol.*, 43:162, 1979.
117. DeSoyza, N., Bissett, J. K., Kane, J. J., Murphy, M. L., and Doherty, J. E.: Ectopic Ventricular Prematurity and Its Relation to Ventricular Tachycardia in Acute Myocardial Infarction in Man, *Circulation*, 50:529, 1974.
118. Lichstein, E., Ribas-Meneclier, C., Gupta, P. K., and Chadda, D. K.: Incidence and Description of Accelerated Ventricular Rhythm Complicating Acute Myocardial Infarction, *Am. J. Med.*, 58:192, 1975.
119. Fisch, C.: Aberration: Seventy-Five Years after Sir Thomas Lewis, *Br. Heart J.*, 50:297, 1983.
120. Kulbertus, H. E., de Leval-Ruten, F., and Casters, P.: Vectorcardiographic Study of Aberrant Conduction. Anterior Displacement of QRS: Another Form of Intraventricular Block, *Br. Heart J.*, 38:549, 1976.
121. Swanick, E. J., LaCamera, F., and Marriott, H. J. L.: Morphologic Features of Right Ventricular Ectopic Beats, *Am. J. Cardiol.*, 30:888, 1972.
122. Marriott, H. J. L.: Differential Diagnosis of Supraventricular and Ventricular Tachycardia, *Geriatrics*, 25:91, 1970.
123. Sandler, I. A., and Marriott, H. J. L.: The Differential Morphology of Anomalous Ventricular Complexes of RBBB-Type in Lead V1: Ventricular Ectopy versus Aberration, *Circulation*, 31:551, 1965.
124. WHO/ISC Task Force: Definition of Terms Related to Cardiac Rhythm, *Am. Heart J.*, 95:796, 1978.
125. DePasquale, N. P.: The Electrocardiogram in Complicated Acute Myocardial Infarction, *Prog. Cardiovasc. Dis.*, 13:72, 1970.
126. Stock, R. J., and Macken, D. L.: Observations on Heart Block during Continuous Electrocardiographic Monitoring in Myocardial Infarction, *Circulation*, 38:993, 1968.
127. Scheinman, M., and Brenman, B.: Clinical and Anatomic Implications of Intraventricular Conduction Blocks in Acute Myocardial Infarction, *Circulation*, 46:753, 1972.
128. Beregovich, J., Fenig, S., Lasser, J., and Allen, D.: Management of Acute Myocardial Infarction Complicated by Advanced Atrioventricular Block: Role of Artificial Pacing, *Am. J. Cardiol.*, 23:54, 1969.
129. Johnson, R. L., Averill, K. H., and Lamb, L. E.: Electrocardiographic Findings in 67,375 Asymptomatic Subjects: VII. Atrioventricular Block, *Am. J. Cardiol.*, 6:153, 1960.
130. Manning, G. W., and Sears, G. A.: Postural Heart Block, *Am. J. Cardiol.*, 9:558, 1962.
131. Zoob, M., and Smith, K. S.: The Aetiology of Complete Heart-Block, *Br. Med. J.*, 2:1149, 1963.
132. Rosenbaum, M. B.: Intraventricular Trifascicular Block, *Heart Lung*, 1:216, 1972.
133. Lev, M.: Anatomic Basis for Atrioventricular Block, *Am. J. Med.*, 37:742, 1964.
134. Hassel, D., Heinsimer, J., Califf, R. M., Benson, A., Rice, J., and German, L.: Complete Heart Block in Reiter's Syndrome, *Am. J. Cardiol.*, 53:967, 1984.
135. DenDulk, K., Brugada, P., Braat, S., Heddle, B., and Wellens, H. J. J.: Myocardial Bridging as a Cause of Paroxysmal Atrioventricular Block, *J. Am. Coll. Cardiol.*, 1:965, 1983.
136. Damato, A. N., Lau, S. H., Helfant, R. H., Stein, E., Berkowitz, W. D., and Cohen, S. I.: A Study of Heart Block in Man Using His Bundle Recordings, *Circulation*, 39:297, 1969.
137. Damato, A. N., and Lau, S. H.: Clinical Value of the Elec-

trocardiogram of the Conducting System, *Prog. Cardiovasc. Dis.*, 13:119, 1970.
138. Khalilullah, M., Singhal, N., Gupta, U., and Padmavati, S.: Unidirectional Complete Heart Block, *Am. Heart J.*, 97:608, 1979.
139. Rosenbaum, M. B.: Intraventricular Trifascicular Block, *Heart Lung*, 1:216, 1976.
140. Fisch, C., Zipes, D. P., and McHenry, P. L.: Electrocardiographic Manifestations of Concealed Junctional Ectopic Impulses, *Circulation*, 53:217, 1976.
141. Castellanos, A., Befeler, B., and Myerburg, R. J.: Pseudo AV Block Produced by Concealed Extrasystoles Arising below the Bifurcation of His Bundle, *Br. Heart J.*, 36:457, 1974.
142. Lindsay, A. E., and Schamroth, L.: Atrioventricular Junctional Parasystole with Concealed Conduction Simulating Second Degree AV Block, *Am. J. Cardiol.*, 31:397, 1973.
143. Marriott, H. J. L., and Menendez, M. M.: A-V Dissociation Revisited, *Prog. Cardiovasc. Dis.*, 8:522, 1966.
144. Sherf, L., and James, T. N.: A New Electrocardiographic Concept: Synchronized Sinoventricular Conduction, *Dis. Chest*, 55:127, 1969.
145. Nicholson, W. J., Martin, C. E., Gracey, J. G., and Knoch, H. R.: Disopyramide-Induced Ventricular Fibrillation, *Am. J. Cardiol.*, 43:1053, 1979.
146. Cooper, M. J., and Abinader, E. G.: Atropine-Induced Ventricular Fibrillation: Case Report and Review of the Literature, *Am. Heart J.*, 97:225, 1979.
147. Wellens, H. J., and Durrer, D.: Wolff-Parkinson-White Syndrome and Atrial Fibrillation, *Am. J. Cardiol.*, 34:777, 1974.

27

Management of Arrhythmias and Conduction Abnormalities

Warren M. Smith, M.B.

Andrew G. Wallace, M.D.

I do not know what I may appear to the world: but to myself I seemed to have been only like a boy, playing on the seashore, and diverting myself and now and then finding a smoother pebble, or a prettier shell than ordinary, while the great ocean of truth lay all undiscovered before me.

Sir Isaac Newton[1]

In the mid-1980s the successful control of cardiac arrhythmias remains a meticulous and challenging issue for physicians. The mechanisms of arrhythmia causation have proved to be more complex than once imagined (see Chap. 25), and such knowledge has, as yet, been incompletely translated into improved clinical control. Thus, the treatment of most arrhythmias remains largely empirical: a measure of contemporary humility is still appropriate.

Treatment is generally recommended for sustained arrhythmias because symptoms are frequently present and there may be the potential for sudden death. It remains the responsibility of the treating physician to perform the clinical titration of the possible harmful effects of any given arrhythmia against the known toxicity and hazards of possible modes of treatment. Many factors may be relevant to the expression of an arrhythmia, including the severity of any associated heart disease, pulmonary disease,[2] endocrine or autonomic imbalance,[3] concurrent drug therapy,[4] QT prolongation,[5] psychologic stress,[6] excessive dieting,[7] and undue dependence on cigarettes, caffeine, or alcohol.[8] Electrolyte imbalance should always be excluded, especially hypokalemia, which not only exacerbates many arrhythmias[9] but also impairs the effectiveness of many standard drugs.

Although it is true that ventricular arrhythmias are prognostically more serious than supraventricular rhythms, this most likely reflects the greater probability of associated serious myocardial impairment with the former. The clinical import of any given arrhythmia therefore depends more upon the rate of the ventricular response and severity of any coexistent cardiovascular disease than upon the chamber of origin. Thus, rapid supraventricular tachycardia in the presence of impaired left ventricular function may precipitate left ventricular failure and ventricular fibrillation (VF), whereas slower ventricular tachycardia (VT) in the presence of apparently normal myocardium may be well tolerated for several days.

The elective treatment of an arrhythmia begins with a careful assessment of the patient by history and physical examination, evaluation of the serum electrolytes, and examination of a chest x-ray and 12-lead electrocardiogram (ECG). Ambulatory ECG monitoring is often helpful if symptoms are reasonably frequent, and treadmill testing may be appropriate if the history suggests exercise induction of symptoms. Selected patients will need referral for electrophysiologic testing, usually if the diagnosis or prognostic significance of the symptoms remains unclear after noninvasive measures, or to enable selection of a demonstrably effective treatment.

Treatment involves both general measures, including elimination or modification of associated factors as listed above, and specific measures, including pharmacologic, electrical, and surgical therapy. When antiarrhythmic drugs are prescribed, the physician must be familiar with the side effects, correct dosage, and appropriate intervals of administration (see Chap. 89). If a patient appears refractory to a particular drug, the plasma concentration (before a dose) should be measured. Careful documentation of the response to each drug given is essential, particularly if surgery or pacemaker therapy is being considered.

This chapter will discuss the treatment of specific arrhythmias and conduction disturbances, with emphasis on the pharmacologic and electrical control; the treatment of tachycardia by cardiac surgery is discussed in detail elsewhere (see Chap. 127).

Management of Tachyarrhythmias

Supraventricular Arrhythmias

Paroxysmal Atrial Tachycardia

Reentrant Supraventricular Tachycardia (SVT) Acute paroxysms may often be terminated by vagal maneuvers,[10] such as the Valsalva maneuver, or by carotid sinus massage. In resistant cases, intravenous verapamil[10,11] is the drug of choice, although diltiazem is also reportedly as effective[12,13] and may prove desirable in patients with left ventricular impairment because of its reportedly less negative inotropic effect. The usual dose of verapamil is 5 mg given over 2 min, which may be repeated. Great caution should be exercised if the patient is also on concurrent beta-adrenergic blocking drugs, as fatalities have occurred in this circumstance (see Chap. 89): no more than 5 mg should be given, and calcium chloride should always be available for immediate injection if hemodynamic collapse occurs. Intravenous propranolol[14] and amiodarone[15] are alternative treatments. Because of the potential for serious complications intravenous drug therapy for SVT should always be given in a hospital setting. Drug-resistant rhythms may require cardioversion or overdrive pacing for termination.

Oral verapamil may be effective for chronic prophylaxis,[16] with beta-blocking drugs or digoxin as alternative treatments. Type I antiarrhythmic drugs may also be useful, especially if tachycardia is mediated by a concealed atrioventricular (AV) accessory pathway, and oral amiodarone is also highly effective.[17] In a minority of patients resistant to or intolerant of drug therapy, either a radio-frequency pacemaker (patient activated) or a fully implantable antitachycardia pacemaker may be considered.[18] Tachycardia in such patients should be consistently responsive to overdrive pacing or programmed extra stimuli, without the induction of atrial fibrillation or flutter. In otherwise refractory cases, surgical section of an AV accessory pathway or ablation of the His bundle with permanent pacemaker implantation may be justified. Until recently this latter procedure was always surgical, but a catheter technique for closed chest His bundle ablation has now been successfully developed.[19,20] A rare subgroup of patients in whom tachycardia is virtually continuous appears to have an accessory AV node.[21] Such patients are characteristically refractory to medical management and usually require surgery.

Ectopic Supraventricular Tachycardia Persistent automatic supraventricular tachycardia is fortunately rare, but it is characteristically refractory to medical treatment. Several cases of successful surgical ablation of automatic atrial tachycardia have been published,[22] and junctional automatic tachycardia in children, which carries a high mortality, has recently been treated successfully by the transcatheter technique of His bundle ablation.[23]

Atrial Flutter

Paroxysmal atrial flutter is usually associated with the presence of heart disease and not infrequently follows acute myocardial infarction or open heart surgery. The aims of treatment are to control the ventricular rate and to restore and maintain sinus rhythm. When urgent control of the ventricular rate is required, direct current (dc) cardioversion using low energies (40 W·s) is often most appropriate, although carotid sinus massage may be temporarily effective by increasing the conduction ratio of the flutter waves over the AV node. Alternatively, intravenous verapamil,[11] diltiazem,[12] or propranolol[14] are usually effective if given slowly. In less urgent situations, oral digitalization will usually adequately control the ventricular rate, although occasionally persistent 2:1 AV conduction will require elective cardioversion.

Reversion to sinus rhythm may sometimes be achieved pharmacologically by infusion of type I antiarrhythmic drugs such as disopyramide,[24] although success is less often achieved than with atrial fibrillation. In the postoperative cardiac patient, in whom temporary atrial pacing wires are usually available, termination of flutter by rapid atrial pacing has been very successful.[25] In other circumstances reversion is more difficult and poorer success rates of 50 to 75 percent are usual.[26] A pacing rate slightly faster than the atrial flutter rate is usually required, and after atrial entrainment is attained, cessation of pacing may be followed by sinus rhythm directly or following transient atrial fibrillation. If atrial fibrillation persists as the predominant rhythm, slowing of the ventricular rate is usually observed because of concealed conduction into the AV node. Recently, atrial flutter has been successfully terminated by pacing via an esophageal catheter.[27] For chronic prophylaxis, quinidine and disopyramide remain standard drugs, although amiodarone may be effective for otherwise refractory cases.[28]

Atrial Fibrillation
Atrial fibrillation is usually managed in similar fashion to atrial flutter, although termination of the arrhythmia by rapid atrial pacing is not possible. Neither atrial flutter nor atrial fibrillation should be treated with quinidine or disopyramide without previous digitalization of the patient. In recent-onset atrial fibrillation, pharmacologic reversion by intravenous disopyramide[24] or procainamide[29] is often successful. Where atrial fibrillation is of longer duration, direct current cardioversion will usually restore sinus rhythm, although when atrial fibrillation has been longer than 1 year's duration, long-term maintenance of sinus rhythm is unlikely.[30] As with atrial flutter, long-term prophylaxis with quinidine or disopyramide is required after successful cardioversion, with amiodarone sometimes controlling otherwise resistant cases.[28] In established atrial fibrillation, treatment must be directed to controlling the ventricular response with digitalis, propranolol, or verapamil, singly or in combinations,[31] supplemented more recently by diltiazem and amiodarone.* Most patients in chronic atrial fibrillation will also require long-term anticoagulation provided the usual contraindications are observed. In a minority of patients in whom a satisfactory ventricular rate cannot be attained without toxic drug effects, ablation of the His bundle either surgically or by a closed chest catheter technique[19] with permanent pacemaker implantation is required.

Arrhythmias Complicating the Preexcitation Syndromes

Wolff-Parkinson-White Syndrome
The principal arrhythmias requiring treatment in patients with Wolff-Parkinson-White (WPW) syndrome are orthodromic reciprocating tachycardia (RT) and atrial flutter/fibrillation. Orthodromic reciprocating tachycardia may often be terminated by simple vagal maneuvers combined if necessary with intravenous edrophonium chloride (Tensilon) or phenylephrine hydrochloride (Neo-Synephrine). If these measures fail, intravenous verapamil and ajmaline* are the drugs of choice, although propranolol or procainamide are alternatives.[10] Drug-resistant tachycardias require atrial or esophageal overdrive pacing or elective cardioversion.

Rapid atrial fibrillation or flutter with 1:1 atrioventricular conduction is usually best treated by immediate cardioversion as VF may occur in patients whose accessory pathway has a short antegrade effective refractory period (ERP).[32] In patients with a more controlled response, agents blocking anterograde conduction over the accessory pathway, such as intravenous procainamide, disopyramide, or ajmaline, may be tried. Digitalis and verapamil are contraindicated in rapid atrial fibrillation as they may increase the rate of the ventricular response.[33,34]

Prophylaxis against Recurrent Arrhythmias While it is desirable to identify patients with a short antegrade refractory period of their accessory pathway, it is not appropriate to subject every patient with WPW syndrome to full electrophysiologic study. Certainly, patients who are known to have suffered an episode of atrial fibrillation with a rapid ventricular response, whose arrhythmias fail to respond to empiric drug treatment or are associated with hypotension, presyncope, or syncope, should be advised to undergo electrophysiologic study in order to select effective drug treatment and/or evaluate possible pacemaker or surgical therapy. Failure to achieve anterograde block in the accessory pathway following the infusion of intravenous procainamide in a dose of 10 mg/kg over 5 min during sinus rhythm has been advocated as strongly suggesting the presence of an accessory pathway with a short anterograde refractory period.[35] Such a method might be used to screen patients for referral for more detailed electrophysiologic study, although such rapid infusion of procainamide is not without risk of hypotension or complete heart block and should be under the supervision of suitably experienced physicians.

The long-term treatment of RT seeks both to reduce the number of premature beats that may initiate tachycardia and to lessen the disparity between the respective refractory periods of the normal and accessory pathways and thereby diminish the probability of reentry occurring. Drugs acting primarily on the AV node, such as beta blockers, may therefore constitute effective treatment for this arrhythmia. Quinidine and disopyramide are the main drugs used to prevent recurrences of atrial flutter/fibrillation, although where it is available, amiodarone has proved very effective.[36] Failure to medically control the ventricular response during atrial fibrillation is one indication for surgical section of the accessory pathway(s). Recently there have been preliminary communications of attempted accessory pathway ablation by the closed chest catheter technique,[37] although the future role, if any, of this intervention is as yet uncertain. (The role of surgery is discussed in Chap. 127.)

Other Forms of Preexcitation
A rapid ventricular response during atrial fibrillation may also be encountered with the Lown-Ganong-Levine syndrome when enhanced AV node conduction is present.[32] Such patients may be refractory to medical therapy and require ablation of the His bundle. RT may also occur in patients with nodoventricular Mahaim fibers, which has been responsive to medical management in the limited experience to date.[38]

*This drug has not been approved by the Food and Drug Administration of the United States at the time of publication.

Ventricular Arrhythmias

Ventricular Premature Beats

The risks versus benefits of treating asymptomatic ventricular premature beats in patients with organic heart disease remains a confused issue. Only beta-adrenergic blocking drugs have been shown to conclusively reduce mortality following treatment after acute myocardial infarction;[39] in all other circumstances, treatment of ventricular premature beats is of unproven value. Identification of patients at increased risk of sudden death is clearly desirable but also controversial: the Lown risk stratification[40] is open to substantial criticism,[41,42] and ambulatory ECG monitoring has not been shown to contribute independent prognostic information if ventricular function is accurately known.[43] Invasive electrophysiologic testing has provided conflicting results[44–46] and, while important as a research protocol, cannot be presently justified as a routine prognostic intervention. While the results of further multicenter trials with newer antiarrhythmic agents are awaited, it seems prudent to treat patients with frequent or "complex" ventricular premature beats who have associated impairment of left ventricular contractility, accepting that careful follow-up is necessary, as all drugs appear capable of a proarrhythmic effect in susceptible patients.[4]

Survivors of Out-of-Hospital Cardiac Arrest

The development of effective community resuscitation programs has resulted in increasing numbers of this hitherto rare patient subgroup. The natural history of a high propensity to a further episode within 2 years[47] may be favorably modified by either drug treatment guided by electrophysiologic testing[48,49] or empiric treatment with high-dose amiodarone.[50,51] The long-term comparability of these two approaches is not yet established, but clearly the latter is simpler.

Ventricular Tachycardia

The management of the patient with VT involves confirmation of the diagnosis whenever possible (see Chap. 26), treatment of the acute episode, and a strategy to prevent recurrence. Immediate cardioversion of a wide-QRS tachycardia, presumed to be ventricular, is always appropriate when there is serious associated hemodynamic compromise. Conversely, wide-QRS tachycardia which is hemodynamically and symptomatically well tolerated requires accurate diagnosis—passage of an esophageal catheter to record atrial activity and seek evidence of VA dissociation is strongly recommended to supplement morphological clues from the 12-lead ECG.[52]

Intravenous lidocaine is the initial treatment of choice for stable VT (see Chap. 89). VT resistant to lidocaine will often respond to intravenous procainamide or disopyramide, although elective cardioversion may be a safer option than subjecting the patient to potential drug-related myocardial depression or hypotension. If cardioversion is elected, very low energies (for example, 5 to 10 W·s) often prove sufficient.

Three treatment modes are available for the chronic prophylaxis of VT: pharmacologic therapy, use of implanted pacemakers or defibrillators, and surgery (see Chap. 127). Empirical treatment may still be successful if episodes of tachycardia recur frequently and drug administration is optimized to maintain therapeutic plasma levels. Furthermore, experience has shown that patients whose tachycardias are related to acute myocardial infarction, mitral valve prolapse, or QT prolongation are unlikely to profit by electrophysiologic study as initiation of the arrhythmia during catheterization is very uncommon. For the remainder, an electrophysiologic study is desirable to plan management.[53]

At electrophysiologic study, it is not unusual for tachycardias of more than one morphology to be induced,[54] some of which may not have been clinically documented. While the significance of polymorphic tachycardias induced by three or more extrastimuli is still controversial, some authorities state that in the majority of patients continued follow-up will eventually document spontaneous examples of all laboratory-induced rhythms.[53] The duration of serial drug testing and electrophysiologic study may be reduced by the use of procainamide as an index drug. Thus, several large studies have shown that both positive and negative responses to this agent are highly predictive of results with other type I antiarrhythmic agents.[53,55]

It is important to realize that some drugs may not be amenable to electrophysiologic testing. The most obvious example is amiodarone, for which most[56] but not all[57] investigators agree that electrophysiologic testing during drug therapy is not predictive of ultimate clinical outcome. It seems that further examples will be discovered as newer antiarrhythmic drugs become available for testing. For the conventional drugs presently used, the response to therapy during electrophysiologic study has been shown to be an independent predictor of patient survival.[58]

In patients refractory to or intolerant of antiarrhythmic drugs, patient-activated underdrive or overdrive (see below) pacemakers or fully automatic antitachycardia pacemakers may be suitable.[59] However, there is always some risk of acceleration of tachycardia with consequent degeneration into VF, requiring careful patient evaluation with protracted trials of pacemaker effectiveness both before and after implantation. Mirowski et al. have developed an automatic implantable defibrillator which is undergoing clinical evaluation.[60] At present it is expensive and requires surgical placement, but provisional results are encouraging. Other investigational devices that utilize low-energy defibrillation via a transvenous catheter are also being developed.[61] (The surgical management of VT is discussed in Chap. 127.)

In conclusion, the management of VT is an area of active clinical investigation with important issues such as the role of empiric high-dose amiodarone therapy versus guided electrophysiologic study presently unresolved. The attractive advantages of electrical treatment of arrhythmias over life-long medication with its associated therapeutic uncertainties promises to become increasingly important in the future.[62]

Delayed Repolarization Arrhythmias (Torsades de Pointes)

Delayed repolarization, which is usually manifest on the surface ECG by QT prolongation,[5] is frequently accompanied by vulnerability to ventricular arrhythmias, commonly torsades de pointes.[63,64] The treatment of such arrhythmias consists of correction of the underlying cause, where possible, and overdrive cardiac pacing. Hypokalemia, even of mild degree, should always be promptly corrected, and all drugs known to cause QT prolongation should be withheld, especially antiarrhythmic drugs such as quinidine or procainamide. Cardioversion may be necessary to terminate prolonged episodes. The treatment of choice is overdrive atrial or ventricular pacing,[63,64] although for emergency control an isoproterenol infusion has been recommended,[63] which shortens the QT interval both directly and via the resultant sinus tachycardia. Cardiac pacing can usually be discontinued after 24 to 48 h, by which time the underlying cause of delayed repolarization has often been corrected. Exceptions include patients with chronic AV block who require permanent pacing and patients with the long-QT syndrome who are best treated with beta-adrenergic blocking drugs and/or partial sympathectomy.[65]

Arrhythmias Associated with Digitalis Intoxication

Digitalis toxicity may be associated with bradyarrhythmias due to impaired AV conduction and/or tachyarrhythmias due to either reentry or enhanced automaticity. The decision whether a given arrhythmia requires more digitalis or signifies that toxicity is already present is not always obvious. Although serum digoxin levels may be very helpful, they are not always immediately available and there is a substantial overlap between therapeutic and toxic values.[66] The serum potassium should be promptly checked, as associated hypokalemia markedly increases the likelihood of toxicity being present. Once a diagnosis of digitalis toxicity has been made, the first step is to withhold digitalis.

In the absence of digitalis-related AV block, hypokalemia should be promptly corrected (intravenous potassium may be given up to 0.5 to 0.75 meq/min with ECG monitoring) and plasma concentrations maintained in the high normal range.[67] Special care is necessary when administering potassium to patients with atrial flutter and a fixed AV conduction ratio, as conduction may be improved, resulting in acceleration of the ventricular response. If drug therapy for digitalis-induced arrhythmias is required, diphenylhydantoin is effective for both supraventricular and ventricular arrhythmias, and lidocaine is effective for ventricular arrhythmias. Beta-adrenergic blocking drugs have also been recommended[68] and are theoretically attractive because the sympathetic nervous system appears, at least partly, to mediate the effects of digitalis toxicity. Cardioversion should be avoided, if at all possible, because of the increased incidence of postreversion arrhythmias, including refractory VF.[69] If cardioversion becomes essential, hypokalemia should be corrected and a preliminary infusion of diphenylhydantoin given. Initially, very low energy levels (for example, 10 W·s) should be used with subsequent gradual increases as necessary.

In the presence of digitalis-induced AV block, potassium and any antiarrhythmic drugs should be given very cautiously. If progression to complete AV block occurs, asystole may ensue because of drug-related suppression of subsidiary pacemakers. Therefore, if impairment of AV conduction beyond first degree block is present, placement of a temporary demand ventricular pacemaker is desirable before proceeding with drug therapy.

Newer approaches to treating digitalis toxicity include the use of intravenous purified Fab fragments of digoxin-specific antibodies[70] and potassium canrenoate, a specific aldosterone antagonist.[71]

Management of Bradyarrhythmias and Conduction Defects

The management of chronic conduction disturbances is largely a question of the indications for permanent cardiac pacing.

Sinus Bradycardia

Sinus bradycardia generally does not require treatment unless congestive heart failure, cerebral hypoperfusion, or exercise intolerance ensues. In doubtful cases, a trial of temporary pacing may be helpful, with permanent pacemaker implantation if unequivocal benefit is observed. In occasional patients with myocardial infarction and bradycardia-related suboptimal cardiac output, temporary pacing to speed the heart rate may improve the circulatory status during the early recovery phase.

The Sick Sinus Syndrome

Although sanctioned by common usage, the term *sick sinus syndrome*[72] focuses attention on only one aspect of what is now appreciated as a more pervasive disorder, with frequently associated impairment of atrioventricular conduction, atrial tachyarrhythmias, and suppression of subsidiary pacemakers.[73]

Most symptomatic patients require permanent cardiac pacing either for bradyarrhythmias or to enable effective drug treatment of associated atrial tachyarrhythmias without fear of precipitating complete AV block or sinus arrest. However, in a small group of adolescents and young adults with symptomatic bradyarrhythmias, oral theophylline therapy was reportedly an effective alternative treatment.[74]

When pacing is required, usually a ventricular or synchronous atrioventricular pacing mode is chosen because of the possible development of complete AV block in predisposed patients.[75] However, in some patients with intact VA conduction, ventricular pacing alone may be associated with decreased hemodynamic efficiency. Atrial pacing is therefore not unreasonable in selected patients without evidence of AV conduction impairment. In patients with a bradycardia-tachycardia syndrome, the development of permanent AF in one-half of the group may result in spontaneous "cure."

The role of digitalis in sick sinus syndrome is slightly controversial. Although digitalis has been shown not to exacerbate resting bradycardia or prolong the duration of overdrive suppression in some patients with sick sinus syndrome,[76] other patients definitely appear sensitive to the drug, with marked aggravation of postpacing asystole. Therefore pacemaker implantation is recommended before digitalization in symptomatic patients with sick sinus syndrome. Similarly, preliminary implantation is prudent in such patients before treating paroxysmal atrial fibrillation or atrial flutter with propranolol or type I antiarrhythmic drugs. Patients with the bradycardia-tachycardia syndrome appear to have a substantial risk of thromboembolism, and anticoagulation should be considered if paroxysmal atrial fibrillation or atrial flutter are not suppressed by drug medication. With treatment, the prognosis of sick sinus syndrome appears to be that of any associated coronary artery disease or congestive heart failure.[77]

Atrioventricular Block

As discussed in Chaps. 25 and 26, conduction disturbances are most usefully divided into those occurring proximal to the His bundle (usually in the AV node) and those occurring distal to the His bundle, intra-Hisian conduction disorders being uncommon. Thus escape pacemakers associated with a proximal level of block are situated in the region of the AV node–His bundle and result in stable, reliable rhythms of 40 to 60 per minute. In contrast, when block occurs below the His bundle, escape pacemakers arise in the distal His-Purkinje tissue and result in unstable rhythms of 20 to 40 per minute. Thus, cardiac pacing is likely to be much more important for distal than for proximal conduction disturbances.

First Degree Heart Block

This is virtually never an indication for permanent pacing, unless the prolongation is entirely at the expense of the HV interval and the patient is symptomatic, a situation discussed below.

Second Degree Heart Block

Type I second degree AV block (Wenckebach) is generally benign,[78] reflecting its usual localization to the AV node, although decremental responses may occur in severely diseased His-Purkinje tissue. It is the anticipated response to rapid atrial pacing and has been observed during resting sinus rhythm in some athletes.[79] Progression to complete AV block is unusual, and escape of a stable subsidiary rhythm may be anticipated. Therapy is therefore usually conservative and guided by the ventricular response. However, in patients with organic heart disease, the clinical course may be less favorable, although this probably reflects the extent and severity of the associated disease rather than the presence of AV nodal block and routine prophylactic pacing is not advised.[80]

In contrast, type II second degree AV block (Möbitz) is uncommon, is almost invariably localized to the His-Purkinje system, and frequently progresses to complete heart block with anticipated escape of a slow, unstable, idioventricular pacemaker. It is therefore almost always an indication for permanent cardiac pacing. An exception is the "pseudo" type II block that has been demonstrated in the laboratory in patients with enhanced AV node conduction when atrial pacing is begun early in diastole.[81] In these artificial circumstances, block is physiological and without prognostic significance. AV block with a fixed conduction ratio (for example, 2:1) cannot immediately be characterized as either a type I or a type II response, but the probable site of block may be judged by the attendant circumstances. Thus, if the QRS complex is wide and periods of sustained conduction are followed by sudden block, a distal site of block is probable and suggests that permanent pacing will be required. Conversely, if 2:1 block is interrupted by periods of typical type I Wenckebach cycle with narrow QRS complexes, block at the level of the AV node is probable with a favorable prognosis, although temporary pacing may be necessary if the ventricular rate is unduly slow. If doubt persists, recourse to direct recording of the His bundle deflection may be necessary (see Chap. 101).

Third Degree (Complete) Heart Block

Acute third degree heart block, whether arising from chronic conduction tissue disease or complicating normal sinus rhythm following acute myocardial infarction, is a medical emergency. Although the prompt institution of cardiac pacing is the anticipated response to acute heart block, considerable time may elapse before reliable ventricular capture is ensured with an electrode catheter. In the interim, the intrinsic rate of the escape pacemaker distal to the site of block may or may not be adequate to support the circulation. In the latter circumstance, and in the absence of acute myocardial infarction, an isoproterenol infusion should be started to accelerate the idioventricular pacemaker while arrangements for cardiac pacing are being made. An initial infusion rate of 0.5 μg/min is appropriate, increasing as necessary to a maximum rate of 4 μg/min providing hypotension or enhanced ventricular ectopy do not supervene. In the presence of acute myocardial infarction, the threshold for this intervention will be higher because of the deleterious effects of catecholamines upon the survival of injured myocardium. Nevertheless, if circulatory collapse is present in this setting, an isoproterenol infusion may be lifesaving until emergency cardiac pacing is achieved. Recently the feasibility of external cardiac pacing as an interim measure in emergencies has been reexamined and may ultimately have clinical relevance.[82]

In the majority of patients, temporary cardiac pacing will be succeeded by implantation of a permanent unit (see section on pacemakers later in this chapter). However, some children in whom congenital block apparently occurs at the level of the AV node have a sufficiently reliable junctional pacemaker to postpone at least the need for permanent pacing.

Atrioventricular Dissociation

AV dissociation is never a primary diagnosis, and treatment depends upon the underlying cause. When AV dissociation arises by "default" (as a result of slowing of a primary pacemaker) or because of AV block, with emergence of a subsidiary escape rhythm, treatment should never be directed toward suppression of the escape rhythm itself, which may be life-supporting. Temporary pacing may be required, depending upon the patient's hemodynamic status. Specific therapy should aim at counteracting factors responsible for depressing sinus node function and/or AV conduction, such as stopping beta-adrenergic blocking drugs or giving atropine. When AV dissociation is due to an enhanced subsidiary pacemaker, treatment should again be directed to the underlying cause, such as digitalis toxicity or hypokalemia. Suppression of the focus with antiarrhythmic therapy should be considered only if the tachycardia rate is rapid.

Indications for Prophylactic Cardiac Pacing

Temporary and Permanent Pacing

Complete AV block as a complication of myocardial infarction occurs in about 5 percent of patients, and opinions differ as to the indications for prophylactic pacing (see Chap. 28). In the majority of cases of inferior (posterior) infarction there is no significant conduction tissue damage and block is apparently due to a reversible process affecting the AV node.[83] Occasionally, inferior infarction alone, if it extends well forward into the interventricular septum, may involve both bundle branches at their origins, although the overall infarct size need not be large to achieve this result. In contrast, anterior infarction causes block by necrosis and destruction of the bundle branches in the middle and lower thirds of the septum and is usually very extensive. Thus, prognosis for complete AV block due to anterior infarction is poor, irrespective of cardiac pacing.

At present prophylactic pacing seems reasonable in patients with newly acquired right bundle branch block complicating acute myocardial infarction. Some clinicians require the additional presence of axis deviation greater than −60 to +90° (i.e., associated hemiblock) and advocate frequent 12-lead ECGs in the remaining patients with right bundle branch block in whom the cardiac axis has not exceeded these limits.[84] Prophylactic pacing is not recommended for acquired left bundle branch block or for preexisting left or right bundle branch block.

The indications for permanent pacemaker implantation in patients with bundle branch block complicating acute myocardial infarction are also not fully resolved. However, in a large multicenter study, Hindman et al.,[85] reported a significantly higher incidence of sudden death or recurrent high-degree AV block in patients with transient high-degree AV block during infarction who were not continuously paced, versus those who were so treated. Permanent pacemaker implantation in such patients with transient high-degree AV block would therefore seem reasonable.

Prophylactic Pacing in Patients with Bifascicular Block

The controversy over the wisdom of prophylactic pacing in patients with bifascicular block appears largely resolved. Several large studies[86,87] have shown that in asymptomatic patients with this finding, the risk of AV block is low, that the sensitivity and specificity of a prolonged HV interval is also likely to be low, and that prophylactic pacing is not justified. However, in subgroups known to be at high risk of AV block, such as patients with the Kearns-Sayre syndrome (ophthalmoplegia, retinitis pigmentosa, and distal conduction disease), the finding of a prolonged HV interval might be clinically valuable. Furthermore, in patients with transient unexplained neurologic symptoms, the finding of an HV interval greater than 70 ms was associated with a significantly greater progression to second or third degree AV block on follow-up, and prophylactic pacemaker implantation has been recommended in such patients.[88] Finally, prophylactic pacemaker insertion in a subgroup of symptomatic patients with chronic bundle branch block, important heart disease, and a prolonged HV interval did not protect against sudden death, which was presumably due to ventricular arrhythmias.[89]

Pacemakers and Pacing Modes in the Treatment of Cardiac Arrhythmias

A pacemaker is an electronic device that generates stimuli to be delivered to the endocardium or myocardium by electrodes (pacing leads). (See Chaps. 102, 104, and 105.) Pacemakers may be used on a temporary basis when reversible factors are present, or they may be permanently implanted. Transvenous pacing systems can be implanted under local anesthesia with minimal risk, and recent improvements, including the development of polyurethane leads and leads which passively ("tined") or actively ("screw in")[90] engage the endocardium, have favored a return to this approach. Direct placement of electrodes on the ventricles can also be achieved by transmediastinal exposure, which does not enter the pleural cavities, although this approach carries a slightly higher risk than the transvenous alternative. The most common indications for permanent pacing are the presence of complete heart block and the sick sinus syndrome.

Pacing systems have also been developed for the treatment of tachyarrhythmias. Radio-frequency pacemakers consisting of an implantable receiver and pacing leads and an external, patient-operated transmitter are useful in the treatment of infrequent but symptomatic supraventricular tachycardias and, to a lesser extent, ventricular tachycardias. However, concern over the possible induction of VF has limited this latter application. Implantable automatic antitachycardia pacemakers are now also available, which may interrupt tachycardia by coupled extra stimuli or a burst of overdrive pacing.[18]

In general, patients being considered for pacemaker therapy for tachycardia should have first proved to be unresponsive to medical treatment and should not be surgical candidates.[59] Before committing the patient to a pacing system, it is essential to reliably demonstrate during repeated trials efficacy of the proposed unit. Finally, various types of implantable defibrillating devices are being evaluated.[60]

Pacing Modes Available to Treat Arrhythmias

Cardiac Pacing

Until recently, all patients with complete heart block received a demand ventricular pacemaker, which senses spontaneous ventricular activity and generates a stimulus if this activity is not detected after a certain fixed interval. More complex units are now in use that are capable of sensing and pacing both atria and ventricles, enabling each atrial contraction (spontaneous or paced) to be followed at a preselected PR interval by a ventricular contraction (spontaneous or paced). This type of unit, termed an *AV sequential pacemaker,* preserves the atrial contribution to ventricular filling and, in a P tracking mode, the rate response to exercise (so-called physiologic pacing).[91,92] (See Chap. 28.)

Another major advance has been the development of external programming, making it possible to noninvasively change many of the pulse-generator parameters such as rate or pulse width. Judicious modulation of the pulse width and energy can enhance battery longevity, and reprogramming can sometimes avoid premature explantation.

Demand pacing of either the atria or the ventricles may also be used to suppress recurrent tachycardia. Here the underlying principle is that of overdrive suppression of ectopic beats due to either reentry or abnormal automaticity. Simple correction of bradycardia alone may prove sufficient, or faster pacing rates may be necessary.[92] Suppression of reentrant beats is achieved through direct effects upon conduction, refractoriness, and the temporal dispersion of recovery of excitability of cardiac cells.[93] Enhanced atrial pacemakers are suppressed primarily by the release of acetylcholine, while Purkinje pacemakers appear to be suppressed both by an increase in extracellular potassium and by electrogenic extrusion of sodium.[94]

Overdrive and Underdrive Cardiac Pacing

The principle common to both these modes of pacing is that penetration of a reentrant circuit by a paced beat will create refractoriness ahead of the circulating impulse, thereby terminating the tachycardia.[95] (See Chap. 102.) With underdrive pacing, a rate slower than the arrhythmia is chosen so that pacing stimuli fall randomly during tachycardia until, at a critical coupling interval, the reentrant circuit is invaded and reciprocation ended. Overdrive pacing employs a rate faster than the arrhythmia, so that rate-related shortening of refractoriness favors similar penetration of the reentrant circuit and extinction of tachycardia. The susceptibility of a reentrant tachycardia to termination is governed by the following factors: (1) the dimensions of the tachycardia circuit (with longer circuits the probability that paced beats will successfully interrupt reciprocation increases); (2) the distance separating the site of stimulation from the site of tachycardia (stimulation from the right ventricle may fail to terminate reentrant ventricular tachycardia arising from the left ventricle); (3) the heart rate during tachycardia (termination is difficult with very fast rates); (4) the electrophysiologic properties of the tissues between the site of stimulation and the tachycardia circuit (an intervening zone of depressed conduction may prevent paced beats from invading the reentrant circuit).[96] Occasionally overdrive pacing accelerates the rate of tachycardia, which may then require emergency cardioversion.

Other Pacing Modalities
Both paired depolarization of the heart and simultaneous atrial and ventricular stimulation have been used clinically. Paired stimulation may be achieved by driving the heart at a regular rate with two stimuli sufficiently close so that the second occurs early in the relative refractory period of the first complex and results only in electrical depolarization without mechanical contraction. A similar result may be achieved by coupling a single pacing stimulus to each atrial or ventricular complex. Although some success has been reported with this technique,[97] the risk of the second stimulus initiating VF limits its application to atrial arrhythmias. Simultaneous stimulation of the atrium and ventricle has been utilized in the treatment of patients with the permanent form of junctional tachycardia.[21] However, in addition to the hemodynamic disadvantages of this pacing mode, very premature atrial beats falling within the refractory period of the atrial pacemaker may still sometimes initiate tachycardia.

Cardioversion

Direct current cardioversion is a safe, reliable, and rapid treatment of reentrant arrhythmias in both elective and emergency situations. Conversely, although automatic rhythms may be briefly interrupted, resumption of tachycardia is to be expected as continued ectopic discharge resumes. The rationale underlying the method is the simultaneous depolarization of all cardiac tissue, with initial recovery of the dominant pacemaker, normally the sinus node.

Cardioversion has remained the definitive treatment of VF since its first successful use in 1947.[98] Because it is the current flow through the ventricles that actually defibrillates when pulse duration is held constant, a low-impedance pathway for defibrillation is very important.[99] Factors affecting impedance include the diameter of the paddle electrodes, the nature of the paddle-skin interface, the number of preceding dc shocks, and the time interval between any previous discharges.

Technique of Cardioversion
See Chap. 103 for further discussion of cardioversion and defibrillation.

Indications and Contraindications to Cardioversion
Cardioversion is indicated for any reentrant arrhythmia associated with circulatory collapse or severe symptoms. Elective cardioversion is commonly indicated to try and revert sustained AF to sinus rhythm, may be required for drug-resistant paroxysmal atrial tachycardia, and is often the preferred alternative to aggressive pharmacologic therapy for paroxysmal VT, especially when impaired ventricular function is present. Conversely, cardioversion should be avoided in situations where it is likely that the tachyarrhythmia will immediately recur or attempts at reversion may lead to more serious arrhythmias. These situations include long-standing atrial fibrillation (greater than 2 years), suspected digitalis toxicity, sick sinus syndrome, active inflammatory conditions of the heart (e.g., pericarditis), and the period following recent embolic episodes, when anticoagulation for 3 to 4 weeks is necessary prior to attempted cardioversion. Prior anticoagulation for any patient undergoing attempted reversion of chronic atrial fibrillation is also recommended.

Complications of Cardioversion
In the vast majority of cases, cardioversion may be carried out uneventfully if the precautions indicated above are observed. The complications of cardioversion relate chiefly to the induction of VF if the shock is not properly synchronized with the R wave, possible myocardial damage, and the appearance of postconversion arrhythmias.

At present the risk of myocardial damage with cardioversion employing conventional energies appears small. In anesthetized animals subjected to ten consecutive dc shocks of 400 W·s, subepicardial foci of myocardial necrosis were observed by 4 days and were more severe in animals in whom smaller paddle sizes had been used.[100] In humans, muscle-brain creatine kinase (MB-CPK) elevations have been reported in a minority of patients undergoing elective cardioversion who received a cumulative energy dose of greater than 425 W·s.[101] Increasing the size of the paddles used to deliver the charge both reduces the degree of myocardial damage and increases the effectiveness of defibrillation, although eventually, with very large paddle sizes, reduced current density decreases defibrillatory effectiveness.[99]

Postconversion arrhythmias may be partly due to myocardial injury, or partly related to the autonomic outflow associated with cardioversion. This autonomic outflow appears to include simultaneous cholinergic and adrenergic responses, the latter requiring an intact cardiac innervation, whereas cholinergic responses can still be elicited after surgical denervation of the heart.[102] Atrial arrhythmias are usually due to escape beats following transient overdrive suppression of the sinus node, increased atrial automaticity, or induction of atrial fibrillation. Cardiac standstill may occasionally occur in patients cardioverted from atrial fibrillation who are not recognized as having an underlying sick sinus syndrome. Ventricular arrhythmias are less common, though ventricular premature beats, VT, and even VF may occur. Postconversion arrhythmias are more likely to occur in digitalized patients, and the presence of digitalis toxicity is a contraindication to elective cardioversion.[103] VF following countershock in this situation has sometimes proved unresponsive to further shocks, possibly because the mechanism of fibrillation is now one of enhanced automaticity. Rarely, pulmonary edema or systemic embolism has followed the elective cardioversion of chronic atrial fibrillation to sinus rhythm.

References

1. Da Costa Andrade, E. N.: "Sir Isaac Newton," Doubleday & Company, Inc., Garden City, N.Y., 1958.
2. Senior, R. M., Lefrak, S. S., and Kleiger, R. E.: The Heart in Chronic Obstructive Pulmonary Disease. Arrhythmias, *Chest,* 75:1, 1979 (Editorial).
3. Zipes, D. P., Barber, M. J., Takahashi, N., and Gilmour, R. F.: Influence of the Autonomic Nervous System on the Genesis of Cardiac Arrhythmias, *PACE,* 6:1210, 1983.
4. Velebit, V., Podrid, P., Lown, B., Cohen, B. H., and Graboys, T. B.: Aggravation and Provocation of Ventricular Arrhythmias by Antiarrhythmic Drugs, *Circulation,* 65:886, 1982.
5. Reynolds, E. W., and Vander Ark, C. R.: Quinidine Syncope and the Delayed Repolarisation Syndromes, *Mod. Concepts Cardiovasc. Dis.,* 45:117, 1976.
6. Engel, G. L.: Sudden and Rapid Death during Psychological Stress, *Ann. Intern. Med.,* 74:771, 1971.
7. Isner, J. M., Sours, H. E., Paris, A. L., Ferrans, V. J., and Roberts, W. C.: Sudden Unexpected Death in Avid Dieters Using the Liquid-Protein-Modified-Fast Diet: Observations in 17 Patients and the Role of the Prolonged QT Interval, *Circulation,* 60:1401, 1979.
8. Ettinger, P. O., Wu, C. F., De La Cruz, C., Weisse, A. B., Ahmed, S. S., and Regan, T. J.: Arrhythmias and the "Holiday Heart." Alcohol-Associated Cardiac Rhythm Disorders, *Am. Heart J.,* 95:555, 1978.
9. Curry, P., Stubbs, W., Fitchett, D., and Krikler, D.: Ventricular Arrhythmias and Hypokalemia, *Lancet,* 2:231, 1976.
10. Wellens, H. J. J.: Wolff-Parkinson-White Syndrome. Part II. Treatment, *Mod. Concepts Cardiovasc. Dis.,* 52:57, 1983.
11. Singh, B. N., Ellrodt, G., and Peter, C. T.: Verapamil: A Review of Its Pharmacological Properties and Therapeutic Use, *Drugs,* 15:169, 1978.
12. Betriu, A., Chaitman, B. R., Bourassa, M. G., Brevers, G., Scholl, J-M., Bourassa, P., Gagne, P., and Chabot, M.: Beneficial Effect of Intravenous Diltiazem in the Acute Management of Paroxysmal Supraventricular Tachyarrhythmias, *Circulation,* 67:88, 1983.
13. Rowland, E., McKenna, W. J., Gulker, H., and Krikler, D. M.: The Comparative Effects of Diltiazem and Verapamil on Atrioventricular Conduction and Atrioventricular Re-entry Tachycardia, *Circ. Res.,* 52(suppl. 1):I-163, 1983.
14. Singh, B. N., and Jewitt, D. E.: β-Adrenergic Receptor Blocking Drugs in Cardiac Arrhythmias, *Drugs,* 7:426, 1974.
15. Wellens, H. J. J., Brugada, P., Abdollah, H., and Dassen, W. R.: A Comparison of the Electrophysiologic Effects of Intravenous and Oral Amiodarone in the Same Patient, *Circulation,* 69:120, 1984.
16. Pritchett, E. L. C., Hammill, S. C., Reiter, M. J., et al.: Life-Table Methods for Evaluating Antiarrhythmic Drug Efficacy in Patients with Paroxysmal Atrial Tachycardia, *Am. J. Cardiol.,* 52:1007, 1983.
17. Wellens, H. J. J., Brugada, P., and Abdollah, H.: Effect of Amiodarone in Paroxysmal Supraventricular Tachycardia with or without Wolff-Parkinson-White Syndrome, *Am. Heart J.,* 106:876, 1983.
18. Spurrell, R. A. J., Nathan, A. W., Bexton, R. S., Hellestrand, K. J., Nappholz, T., and Camm, A. J.: Implantable Automatic Scanning Pacemaker for Termination of Supraventricular Tachycardia, *Am. J. Cardiol.,* 49:765, 1982.
19. Gallagher, J. J., Svenson, R. H., Kasell, J. H., et al.: Catheter Technique for Closed-Chest Ablation of the Atrioventricular Conduction System: A Therapeutic Alternative for the Treatment of Refractory Supraventricular Tachycardia, *N. Engl. J. Med.,* 306:194, 1982.
20. Scheinman, M. M., Morady, F., Hess, D. S., and Gonzalez, R.: Catheter Induced Ablation of the Atrioventricular Conduction Junction to Control Refractory Supraventricular Arrhythmias, *JAMA,* 248:851, 1982.
21. Coumel, P., Attuel, P., and Mugica, J.: Junctional Reciprocating Tachycardia: The Permanent Form, in H. E. Kulbertus (ed.), "Re-entrant Arrhythmias," University Park Press, Baltimore, 1976.
22. Cox, J. L.: Surgery for Cardiac Arrhythmias, *Current Probl. Cardiol.,* 8:25, 1983.
23. Gillette, P. C., Garson, A., Coburn, J. P., et al.: Junctional Automatic Ectopic Tachycardia: New Proposed Treatment by Transcatheter His Bundle Ablation, *Am. Heart J.,* 106:619, 1983.
24. Campbell, J. J., and Morgan, J. J.: Treatment of Atrial Arrhythmias after Cardiac Surgery with Intravenous Disopyramide, *Aust. N.Z. J. Med.,* 10:644, 1980.
25. Waldo, A. L., Maclean, W. A. H., Karp, R. B., Kouchoukos, N. T., and James, T. N.: Entrainment and Interruption of Atrial Flutter with Rapid Atrial Pacing: Studies in Man following Open Heart Surgery, *Circulation,* 56:737, 1977.
26. Batchelder, J. E., and Zipes, D. P.: Treatment of Tachyarrhythmias by Pacing, *Arch. Intern. Med.,* 135:1115, 1975.
27. Kerr, C. R., Gallagher, J. J., Smith, W. M., et al.: The Induction of Atrial Flutter and Fibrillation and the Termination of Atrial Flutter by Esophageal Pacing, *PACE,* 6:60, 1983.
28. Graboys, T. B., Podrid, P. J., and Lown, B.: Efficacy of Amiodarone for Refractory Supraventricular Tachyarrhythmias, *Am. Heart J.,* 106:870, 1983.
29. Fenster, P. E., Comers, K. A., Marsh, R., Katzenberg, C., and Hager, W. D.: Conversion of Atrial Fibrillation to Sinus Rhythm by Acute Intravenous Procainamide Infusion, *Am. Heart J.,* 106:501, 1983.
30. Upton, A. R. M., and Honey, M.: Electroconversion of Atrial Fibrillation after Mitral Valvotomy, *Br. Heart J.,* 33:732, 1971.
31. Panidis, I. P., Morganroth, J., and Baessler, C.: Effectiveness and Safety of Oral Verapamil to Control Exercise-Induced Tachycardia in Patients with Atrial Fibrillation Receiving Digitalis, *Am. J. Cardiol.,* 52:1197, 1983.
32. Gallagher, J. J., Pritchett, E. L. C., Sealy, W. C., Kasell, J., and Wallace, A. G.: The Pre-excitation Syndromes, *Prog. Cardiovasc. Dis.,* 20:285, 1978.
33. Sellers, T. D., Bashore, T. M., and Gallagher, J. J.: Digitalis in the Pre-excitation Syndrome: Analysis during Atrial Fibrillation, *Circulation,* 56:260, 1977.
34. Gulamhusein, S., Ko, P., Carruthers, S. G., and Klein, G. J.: Acceleration of the Ventricular Response during Atrial Fibrillation in the Wolff-Parkinson-White Syndrome after Verapamil, *Circulation,* 65:348, 1982.
35. Wellens, H. J. J., Braat, S., Brugada, P., Gorgels, A. P. M., and Bar, F. W.: Use of Procainamide in Patients with the Wolff-Parkinson-White Syndrome to Disclose a Short Refractory Period of the Accessory Pathway, *Am. J. Cardiol.,* 50:1087, 1982.
36. Rosenbaum, M. B., Chiale, P. A., Ryba, D., and Elizan, M. V.: Control of Tachyarrhythmias Associated with Wolff-Parkinson-White Syndrome by Amiodarone Hydrochloride, *Am. J. Cardiol.,* 34:215, 1974.
37. Jackman, W. M., Friday, K. J., Scherlay, B. J., et al.: Direct Endocardial Recording from an Accessory Atrioventricular Pathway: Localization of the Site of Block, Effect of Antiarrhythmic Drugs, and Attempt at Nonsurgical Ablation, *Circulation,* 68:906, 1983.
38. Gallagher, J. J., Smith, W. M., Kasell, J. H., Benson, D. W., Jr., Sterba, R., and Grant A. O.: Role of Mahaim Fibers in Cardiac Arrhythmias in Man, *Circulation,* 64:176:1981.
39. May, G. S.: A Review of Long Term Beta-Blocker Trials in Survivors of Myocardial Infarction, *Circulation* 67(suppl. 1): I-46, 1983.

40. Lown, B., and Wolf, M.: Approaches to Sudden Death from Coronary Heart Disease, *Circulation,* 44:130, 1971.
41. Bigger, J. T., Jr., Wenger, T. L., and Heissenbuttel, R. H.: Limitations of the Lown Grading System for the Study of Human Ventricular Arrhythmias, *Am. Heart J.,* 93:727, 1977.
42. Engel, T. R., Meister, S. G., and Frankl, W. S.: The "R-on-T" Phenomenon—An Update and Critical Review, *Ann. Intern. Med.,* 88:221, 1978.
43. Califf, R. M., McKinnis, R. A., Burks, J., et al.: Prognostic Implications of Ventricular Arrhythmias during 24 hr Ambulatory Monitoring in Patients Undergoing Cardiac Catheterization for Coronary Artery Disease, *Am. J. Cardiol.,* 50:23, 1982.
44. Richards, D. A., Cody, D. V., Denniss, A. R., Russell, P. A., Young, A. A., and Uther, J. B.: Ventricular Electrical Instability: A Predictor of Death after Myocardial Infarction, *Am. J. Cardiol.,* 51:75, 1983.
45. Marchlinski, F. E., Buxton, A. E., Waxman, H. L., and Josephson, M. E.: Identifying Patients at Risk of Sudden Death after Myocardial Infarction: Value of the Response to Programmed Stimulation, Degree of Ventricular Ectopic Activity, and Severity of Left Ventricular Dysfunction, *Am. J. Cardiol.,* 52:1190, 1983.
46. Kowey, P. R., Folland, E. D., Parisi, A. F., and Lown, B.: Programmed Electrical Stimulation of the Heart in Coronary Artery Disease, *Am. J. Cardiol.,* 51:531, 1983.
47. Schaffer, W. A., and Cobb, L. A.: Recurrent Ventricular Fibrillation and Modes of Death in Survivors of Out-of-Hospital Ventricular Fibrillation, *N. Engl. J. Med.,* 293:259, 1975.
48. Ruskin, J. N., DiMasco, J. P., and Garan, H.: Out-of-Hospital Cardiac Arrest. Electrophysiological Observation and Selection of Long-Term Antiarrhythmic Therapy, *N. Engl. J. Med.,* 303:607, 1980.
49. Roy, D., Waxman, H. L., Kienzle, M. G., Buxton, A. E., Marchlinski, F. E., and Josephson, M. E.: Clinical Characteristics and Long-Term Followup in 119 Survivors of Cardiac Arrest: Relation to Inducibility at Electrophysiologic Testing, *Am. J. Cardiol.,* 52:969, 1983.
50. Morady, F., Sauve, M. J., Malone, P., Shen, E. N., et al.: Long-Term Efficacy and Toxicity of High-Dose Amiodarone Therapy for Ventricular Tachycardia or Ventricular Fibrillation, *Am. J. Cardiol.,* 52:975, 1983.
51. Nademanee, K., Singh, B. N., Cannom, D. S., Weiss, J., Feld, G., and Stevenson, W. G.: Control of Sudden Recurrent Arrhythmic Deaths: Role of Amiodarone, *Am. Heart J.,* 106:895, 1983.
52. Wellens, H. J. J., Bas, F. W. H. M., and Lie, K. I.: The Value of the Electrocardiogram in the Differential Diagnosis of a Tachycardia with a Widened QRS Complex, *Am. J. Med.,* 64:27, 1978.
53. Buxton, A. E., and Josephson, M. E.: Ventricular Tachycardia-1983, *PACE,* 7:96, 1984.
54. Josephson, M. E., Horowitz, L. N., Farshidi, A., Spielman, S. R., Michelson, E. L., and Greenspan, A. M.: Recurrent Sustained Ventricular Tachycardia 4. Pleomorphism, *Circulation,* 59:459, 1979.
55. Waxman, H. L., Buxton, A. E., Sadowski, L. M., and Josephson, M. E.: The Response to Procainamide during Electrophysiologic Study for Sustained Ventricular Tachyarrhythmias Predicts the Response to Other Medications, *Circulation,* 67:30, 1983.
56. Heger, J. J., Prystowsky, E. N., and Zipes, D. P.: Clinical Efficacy of Amiodarone in Treatment of Recurrent Ventricular Tachycardia and Ventricular Fibrillation, *Am. Heart J.,* 106:887, 1983.
57. Horowitz, L. N., Spielman, S. R., Greenspan, A. M., Webb, C. R., and Kay, H. R.: Ventricular Arrhythmias: Use of Electrophysiologic Studies, *Am. Heart J.,* 106:881, 1983.
58. Swerdlow, C. D., Winkle, R. A., and Mason, J. W.: Determinants of Survival in Patients with Ventricular Tachyarrhythmias, *N. Engl. J. Med.,* 308:1436, 1983.
59. Fisher, J. D., Kim, S. G., Furman, S., Matos, J. A.: Role of Implantable Pacemaker in Control of Recurrent Ventricular Tachycardia, *Am. J. Cardiol.,* 49:194, 1982.
60. Mirowski, M.: Management of Malignant Ventricular Tachyarrhythmias with Automatic Implanted Cardioverter-Defibrillators, *Mod. Concepts Cardiovasc. Dis.,* 52:41, 1983.
61. Zipes, D. P., Jackson, W. M., Heges, J. J., et al.: Clinical Transvenous Cardioversion of Recurrent Life Threatening Ventricular Tachyarrhythmias: Low Energy Synchronized Cardioversion of Ventricular Tachycardia and Termination of Ventricular Fibrillation in Patients Using a Catheter Electrode, *Am. Heart J.,* 103:789, 1982.
62. Zipes, D. P.: Electrical Therapy of Cardiac Arrhythmias, *N. Engl. J. Med.,* 309:1179, 1983 (Editorial).
63. Motte, G., Coumel, P., Abitol, G., Dessertenne, F., and Slama, R.: Le Syndrome QT long et syncopes pas "Torsades de Pointe," *Arch. Mal Coeur.,* 63:831, 1970.
64. Smith, W. M., and Gallagher, J. J.: Les Torsades de Pointes, *Ann. Int. Med.,* 93:578, 1980.
65. Schwartz, P. J., Periti, M., and Malliani, A.: The Long Q-T Syndrome, *Am. Heart J.,* 89:378, 1975.
66. Shapiro, W.: Correlative Studies of Seven Digitalis Levels and the Arrhythmias of Digitalis Intoxication, *Am. J. Cardiol.,* 41:852, 1978.
67. Fisch, C., and Knoebel, S. B.: Recognition and Treatment of Digitalis Toxicity, *Prog. Cardiovasc. Dis.,* 12:71, 1970.
68. Mason, D. T., Zelis, R., Lee, G., et al.: Current Concepts and Treatment of Digitalis Toxicity, *Am. J. Cardiol.,* 27:546, 1971.
69. Rabbino, M. D., Likoff, W., and Dreifus, L. S.: Complications and Limitations of Direct-Current Countershock, *JAMA,* 190:417, 1964.
70. Smith, T. W., Habes, E., Yeatman, L., and Butler, V. P.: Reversal of Advanced Digoxin Toxication with Fab Fragments of Digoxin Specific Antibodies, *N. Engl. J. Med.,* 294:797, 1976.
71. Yeh, B. K., Chiang, B. N., and Sung, P. K.: Antiarrhythmic Activity of Potassium Canrenoate in Man, *Am. Heart J.,* 92:308, 1976.
72. Ferrier, M. I.: "The Sick Sinus Syndrome," Futura Publishing Company, Inc., Mount Kisco, N. Y., 1974.
73. Dhingra, R. C.: Sinus Node Dysfunction, *PACE,* 6:1062, 1983.
74. Benditt, D. G., Benson, D. W., Kreitt, J., et al.: Electrophysiologic Effects of Theophylline in Young Patients with Symptomatic Bradyarrhythmias, *Am. J. Cardiol.,* 52:1223, 1983.
75. Rosen, K. M., Loeb, H. S., Sinno, M. Z., Rahimtoola, S. H., and Gunnar, R. M.: Cardiac Conduction in Patients with Symptomatic Sinus Node Disease, *Circulation,* 43:1836, 1971.
76. Engel, T. R., and Schaal, S. F.: Digitalis in the Sick Sinus Syndrome. The Effects of Digitalis on Sinoatrial Automaticity and Atrioventricular Conduction, *Circulation,* 48:1201, 1973.
77. Breivik, K., Ohm, O. J., and Segadal, L.: Sick Sinus Syndrome Treated with Permanent Pacemaker in 109 Patients, *Arch. Med. Scand.,* 206:153, 1979.
78. Zipes, D. P.: Current Topics. Second Degree Atrioventricular Block, *Circulation,* 60:465, 1979.
79. Zeppilli, P., Feniei, R., Sassara, M., Pisrami, M. M., and Caselli, G.: Wenckebach Second-Degree A-V Block in Top-Ranking Athletes: An Old Problem Revisited, *Am. Heart J.,* 100:281, 1980.
80. Strasbery, B., Amat-Y-Leon, F., Dhingra, R. C., et al.: Natural History of Chronic Second-Degree Atrioventricular Nodal Block, *Circulation,* 63:1043, 1981.
81. Damato, A. N., Varghese, P. J., Caracta, A. R., Akhtar, M., and Lau, S. H.: Functional 2:1 A-V Block within the His Purkinje System. Simulation of Type II A-V Block, *Circulation,* 47:534, 1973.
82. Falk, R. H., Zoll, P. M., and Zoll, R. H.: Safety and Efficiency of Noninvasive Cardiac Pacing. A Preliminary Report, *N. Engl. J. Med.,* 309:1166, 1983.
83. Davies, M. J., Anderson, R. H., and Becker, A. E.: Atrioventricular Conduction Disturbances in Acute Myocardial Infarction, in "The Conduction System of the Heart," Butterworth & Co., Ltd., London, 1983.

84. Lie, K. I., Wellens, H. J., and Schuilenburg, R. M.: Bundle Branch Block and Acute Myocardial Infarction, in H. J. Wellens, K. I. Lie, and M. J. Janse (eds.), "The Conduction System of the Heart," Lea & Febiger, Philadelphia, 1976.
85. Hindman, M. C., Wagner, G. S., and Jaro, M.: The Clinical Significance of Bundle Branch Block Complicating Acute Myocardial Infarction: 2. Indications for Temporary and Permanent Pacemaker Insertion, *Circulation*, 58:689, 1978.
86. Dhingra, R. C., Palileo, E., Strasberg, B., et al.: Significance of the HV Interval in 517 Patients with Chronic Bifascicular Block, *Circulation*, 64:1265, 1981.
87. McAnulty, J. H., Rahimtoola, D. H., Murphy, E. S., et al.: A Prospective Study of Sudden Death in High Risk Bundle Branch Block, *N. Engl. J. Med.*, 299:209, 1978.
88. Scheinman, M. M., Peters, R. W., Modin, G., Brennan, M., Mies, C., and O'Young, J.: Prognostic Value of Infranodal Conduction Time in Patients with Chronic Bundle Branch Block, *Circulation*, 56:240, 1977.
89. Peters, R. W., Scheinman, M. M., Modin, G., O'Young, J., Somelofski, C. A., and Mies, C.: Prophylactic Permanent Pacemaker for Patients with Chronic Bundle Branch Block, *Am. J. Med.*, 66:978, 1979.
90. Morse, D., Yankaskas, M., Johnson, B., Spagna, P., and Lemole, G. M.: Transvenous Pacemaker Insertion with a Zero Dislodgement Rate, *PACE*, 6:283, 1983.
91. Geddes, J. S.: Physiologic Pacing, *Br. Heart J.*, 50:109, 1983 (Editorial).
92. Levine, P. A., and Mace, R. C.: "Pacing Therapy. A Guide to Cardiac Pacing for Optimum Hemodynamic Benefit," Futura Publishing Company, Inc., Mount Kisco, N.Y., 1983.
93. Sowton, E., Leatham, A., and Carson, P.: The Suppression of Arrhythmias by Artificial Pacemaking, *Lancet*, 2:1098, 1964.
94. Vassalle, M.: The Relationship among Cardiac Pacemakers, *Circ. Res.*, 41:269, 1977.
95. Wellens, H. J. J., Bar, F. W., Gorgels, A. P., and Muncharaz, J. F.: Electrical Management of Arrhythmias with Emphasis on the Tachycardias, *Am. J. Cardiol.*, 41:1025, 1978.
96. Wellens, H. J. J.: "Electrical Stimulation of the Heart in the Study and Treatment of Tachycardias," University Park Press, Baltimore, 1971.
97. Braunwald, E., Ross, J., Jr., and Sonnenblick, E. H.: Clinical Observations on Paired Electrical Stimulation of the Heart, *Am. J. Med.*, 37:700, 1964.
98. Beck, C. S., Pritchard, W. H., and Feil, H.: Ventricular Fibrillation of Long Duration Abolished by Electric Shock, *JAMA*, 135:985, 1947.
99. Ewy, G. A.: Cardiac Arrest and Resuscitation: Defibrillators and Defibrillation, *Curr. Probl. Cardiol.*, II:8, 1978.
100. Warnes, E. D., Dahl, C., and Ewy, G. A.: Myocardial Injury from Transthoracic Defibrillator Countershock, *Arch. Pathol.*, 99:55, 1975.
101. Ehsani, A., Ewy, G. A., and Sobel, B. E.: Effects of Electrical Countershock on Serum Creatinine Phosphokinase (CPK) Isoenzyme Activity, *Am. J. Cardiol.*, 37:12, 1976.
102. Cobb, F. R., Wallace, A. G., and Wagner, G. S.: Cardiac Inotropic and Coronary Vascular Responses to Countershock. Evidence for Excitation of Intracardiac Nerves, *Circ. Res.*, 23:721, 1968.
103. Resnekov, L.: Present Status of Electroversion in the Management of Cardiac Dysrhythmias, *Circulation*, 47:1356, 1973.

28

Artificial Cardiac Pacemakers

Harry G. Mond, M.D.   J. Graeme Sloman, E.D.

I designed a machine by means of which direct stimulation to the heart's muscle may be applied. Voltage was used from 1.5 to 120 and it was found that somewhere about 16 volts was the pressure required.

The method was completely successful in a case of a stillborn infant. The needle was plunged into the ventricle and the heart responded to each impulse. At the end of ten minutes, the current was stopped and it was found that the heart would beat of its own accord. The child recovered completely.

M. C. Lidwill, 1929[1]

Entering its third decade, cardiac pacing continues to be a rapidly advancing and ever-changing specialty. The value of pacing in the treatment of a variety of brady- and tachyarrhythmias cannot be challenged. Recent advances in pacemaker technology include new electrode designs and lead insulators, miniature electronic circuitry, long-lived power sources, multiprogrammability, telemetry, and sophisticated dual-chamber pacing systems. Coupled to a manufacturing reliability and quality control unparalleled in any other industry, the indications for pacing, particularly in the pediatric age group, have broadened in recent years. Today, an estimated 1 million people throughout the world have benefited from implantation of a cardiac pacemaker.

Continued research and development in the 1980s will further improve pulse generator longevity, provide even more reliable lead systems, and incorporate into pulse generators new physiologic sensors able to alter the pacing rate according to patient requirements. Because of an insatiable physician demand, the highly sophisticated physiologic pacemaker of the fourth decade will be awesome, reflecting the brilliant adaptation of available technology by the electronic engineer.

Historical Aspects of Pacing

Although Hyman in 1932 has been credited with the design and use of the first pacemaker,[2] in his writings he does refer to a similar device developed in Sydney, Australia, during the mid-1920s.[3] This equipment was developed by an Australian physician, Mark C. Lidwill, who used it to successfully resuscitate a stillborn infant.[1,4] Unfortunately, apart from Lidwill's original description, little is known of the equipment and no photographs are known to exist. Because of the unavailability of electronic equipment, antiarrhythmic drugs, defibrillators, and thoracic surgery, almost no work was done on developing cardiac pacing techniques until Zoll, in 1952, demonstrated his high-voltage external pacemaker with plate electrodes strapped to the chest wall.[5] In 1957 Lillehei and others using epicardial leads, paced patients who developed heart block at cardiac surgery.[5] The following year Furman and Schwedel[5] developed a transvenous endocardial electrode for long-term use. External generators with pacing leads breaching the skin were a constant source of complications. By the late 1950s, the first transistors had become available, allowing for development of small, self-contained, implantable battery-operated pulse generators. Such a pulse generator using a rechargeable power source was implanted in Sweden by Senning and Elmquist in 1958.[5] In 1959, Greatbatch in the United States developed the first self-contained implantable pulse generator using zinc mercury batteries.[5] By 1968, QRS sensing circuits had been designed, allowing for development of "demand" pacemaker systems. The 1970s and early 1980s have seen remarkable developments in pulse generator and lead designs.

Indications for Permanent Cardiac Pacing

During the early 1960s, the only indication for permanent cardiac pacing was incapacitating Stokes-Adams attacks, usually resulting from complete heart block.[6] In such patients who remained unpaced, the incidence of sudden death was high and the morbidity from the bradycardia resulted in a poor quality of life which was often interspersed with frightening and debilitating syncopal episodes.[7] Experience with long-term pacing has shown a significant reduction in the incidence of sudden death and improvement in the quality of life in these elderly patients. Consequently, the indications for permanent pacing have now broadened. Within this group of indications, however, lie gray zones where controversy still exists, especially regarding permanent pacing in asymptomatic patients or following myocardial infarction.

Despite exhaustive cardiac investigations there still exists a small group of patients with serious syncope, often infrequent, presumably due to a cardiac bradyarrhythmia. In this group of patients, if syncope is regarded as more serious or life-threatening than the morbidity of the pacemaker procedure, then permanent pacing may be indicated on an empirical basis.

In most patients the decision for permanent pacing is made on assessment of the resting ECG, symptoms, predicted patient prognosis, and physical state. In more complex cases, the final decision depends on the results of ECG monitoring, electrophysiological studies, the continuing need for drugs such as cardiac glycosides or beta-adrenergic blockers, the state of the underlying myocardium, or even knowledge of the long-term follow-up with similar patients.

Relative contraindications to permanent pacing include debilitating general diseases, poor left ventricular function, dementia, and advanced cancer. However, patients with such contraindications should not necessarily be deprived of a pacemaker if the indications are significant and the management of these other problems simplified. In some countries, the cost of the pacing hardware is quoted as a relative contraindication to permanent pacing. In this situation refurbishing of pulse generators where practiced has been found to be safe and economic.[8] It is often forgotten that the cost of prolonged intensive nursing of patients with Stokes-Adams attacks, intractable cardiac failure, arrhythmias, or severe weakness is far greater than the cost of implanting a permanent pacemaker and transferring the patient to a less intensive nursing environment.

The two major indications for permanent cardiac pacing are failure of impulse formation and failure of cardiac conduction. These usually result from degenerative, fibrotic, or atherosclerotic processes which damage pacemaker cells, the surrounding tissue, and the conductive elements. Other etiologies include infective, rheumatic, vascular, infiltrative, or neoplastic processes.[9] At the time of clinical presentation, although ECG features are usually straightforward, the exact etiology is usually obscure. ECG disorders of the sinus node are called the *sick sinus syndrome,* whereas disorders of the atrioventricular (AV) node and distal conducting system are referred to as heart block. The term *high-degree AV block* will be used as a major heading for a variety of ECG patterns, including complete heart block, second degree AV block, bundle branch blocks, or combinations of these.

When evaluating ECG tracings, the sick sinus syndrome and high-degree AV block are frequently associated, and this is referred to as a panconduction defect. Both tend to occur in advanced age groups and may have similar pathological processes. Despite this, diseases of the components of the pacemaker and conducting system continue to be differentiated into separate clinical, pathological, and ECG entities, as outlined in Table 28-1.

TABLE 28-1 Indications for Permanent Cardiac Pacing

1. Symptomatic acquired high-degree AV block
   a. Complete heart block
   b. Second degree AV block
      (1) Proximal
      (2) Distal
   c. Bundle branch block configurations with intermittent bradyarrhythmias
2. Asymptomatic acquired high-degree AV block
   a. Complete heart block
   b. Bundle branch block configurations
3. Congenital high-degree AV block
4. High-degree AV block following acute myocardial infarction
   a. Inferior—persistent
   b. Anterior—bifascicular block associated with transient or persistent Mobitz II or complete heart block
5. Sick sinus syndrome
6. Other symptomatic bradyarrhythmias
7. Control, prevention, and reversion of tachyarrhythmias
8. Syncope without an ECG diagnosis

Symptomatic Acquired High-Degree Atrioventricular Block

Complete Heart Block

Patients with fixed, chronic, complete heart block with a slow ventricular response should be paced irrespective of symptoms. Although asymptomatic patients exist, careful history taking suggests that this is unusual. Often, asymptomatic patients attribute their slowing down to advancing age or factors other than the bradycardia and the results of permanent pacing in these patients can be very impressive.

Significant numbers of elderly patients with symptomatic complete heart block are receiving digitalis at the time of presentation. Although digitalis toxicity may be a contributing factor, cessation of the drug usually reveals underlying and unstable chronic conduction defects which frequently require permanent pacing.

Second Degree Atrioventricular Block

Second degree AV block is divided into two groups: Möbitz types I and II. Möbitz type I, or Wenckebach block, most frequently results from a conduction disturbance in the AV node. It is usually associated with a normal width QRS complex and progression to complete heart block with a marked symptomatic bradycardia is unusual. In Möbitz type II block, the conduction disturbance is distal and the QRS is widened unless the block is in the common His bundle. In general, Möbitz type II block is progressive, unpredictable, and likely to result in Stokes-Adams attacks. Permanent pacing is usually unnecessary for Möbitz type I block but frequently required for type II block.

Bundle Branch Blocks

Although the various types of bundle branch blocks are frequently and easily recognized on the ECG, the natural history and the progression of the lesions are not well understood. Electrophysiologic investigations of patients with bundle branch block on the ECG although helpful, cannot by themselves be used as accurate predictors of complete heart block. Therapeutic decisions require clinical data. Symptomatic patients with bifascicular block or intermittent complete heart block and a wide QRS will have a prolonged infranodal conduction time, and pacing is indicated without electrophysiological studies.

A more difficult clinical situation is chronic bifascicular block without demonstrable ECG evidence of disease in the third fascicle. Here, knowledge of the infranodal conduction time is of value. Narula[10] showed that patients with bifascicular block and a prolonged HV interval who are not permanently paced have a 23 percent mortality per year compared to those with a normal HV interval, whether symptomatic (8 percent) or asymptomatic (6 percent). The actual measured HV interval also appears important. Scheinman[11] et al. demonstrated that in patients with bifascicular block, the incidence of progression to higher degrees of heart block was much higher if the HV interval was equal to or greater than 70 ms. Patients who show alternating right and left bundle branch block have significant bilateral bundle branch disease and the clinical course is primarily determined by the severity of the underlying heart disease and not by the occurrence of AV block.

Congenital High-Degree Atrioventricular Block

First described in 1901,[12] this uncommon entity is present at birth. However, it must be remembered that complete heart block detected in the young may be acquired and result from myocarditis, rheumatic heart disease, trauma, vascular, neoplastic, or infiltrative disorders. If congenital cardiac malformations are also present, then the term *congenital heart block* can be applied even if not detected at birth. Congenital complete heart block as an isolated anomaly is usually well tolerated in childhood. The ventricular rate, although stable in each individual, may range from 40 to 90 beats per minute and often increases modestly with exercise. Most infants and children with isolated congenital complete heart block grow and develop normally and can lead active lives.

Permanent cardiac pacing is indicated in all symptomatic cases of congenital heart block irrespective of age. The asymptomatic child with complete heart block, whether congenital or acquired, may also require permanent pacing. In these cases, the prognosis must be considered. The site and particularly the stability of the ventricular pacemaker can be assessed by ambulatory monitoring and, if necessary, electrophysiological studies.[13] A single focus usually lies in the AV junctional tissue or His bundle. An additional ectopic ventricular focus may predispose to instability and consequently life-threatening ventricular tachyarrhythmias and Stokes-Adams attacks. Because of the small numbers of children with congenital or acquired complete heart block, the true incidence of sudden death in this group is hard to establish, and thus it is difficult to prove the value of permanent pacing. With the development of sophisticated physiologic pacing systems, it has become fashionable to recommend permanent pacing in all children with complete heart block if ambulatory monitoring reveals additional unstable ventricular ectopic foci.

High-Degree Atrioventricular Block following Acute Myocardial Infarction

A major controversy in cardiac pacemaker therapy is the role of prophylactic, temporary, or permanent pacing following an acute myocardial infarction. The physician is dealing with a difficult clinical situation involving both a myocardial conduction defect and a prognosis limiting myocardial contraction abnormality with a propensity for further acute infarction. Any attempt to evaluate the effects of pacing will be hampered by the myocardial dysfunction, manifested by congestive cardiac failure, reduced forward output, angina, arrhythmias, and sudden death.

In the early 1970s it became popular to pace on a temporary basis all patients who developed complete heart block following an acute inferior myocardial infarction. However, because of the transient nature of this complete heart block and its usual benign hemodynamic consequences, temporary pacing is now only performed when significant hemodynamic indications prevail.

High-degree AV block complicating an acute anterior myocardial infarction is only one-third as common but three times as lethal as the acute inferior type.[14] Unlike inferior myocardial infarction, it is advisable to predict which patients with anterior myocardial infarction will develop complete heart block and to institute prophylactic temporary pacing before this event. Patients most likely to require temporary pacing are those who develop a combination of a new right bundle branch block and a left hemiblock, or a pattern of alternating left and right bundle branch blocks.[15] Patients who survive Möbitz type II block or complete heart block during the course of an acute anterior myocardial infarction should be considered for permanent pacing even if the block was transient.[15]

Sick Sinus Syndrome

The sick sinus syndrome entails episodic or persistent sinus bradycardia together with periods of sinus arrest or sinoatrial block with or without an escape AV junctional rhythm and with varying degrees of AV block.[16] Paroxysmal tachyarrhythmias, such as atrial fibrillation, atrial flutter, paroxysmal atrial tachycardia, or even ventricular tachycardia and fibrillation may alternate with the bradycardia. Termination of the tachyarrhythmias may reveal a failure or slow recovery of sinus node function and the resultant profound bradycardia may manifest in Stokes-Adams attacks.

With regard to clinical presentation and prognosis, the sick sinus syndrome can be divided into three groups. Patients with the most benign course are those who present with sinus bradycardia. A second patient group exhibits sinus arrest or sinoatrial block. The most severe group is a combination of both bradyarrhythmias and paroxysmal tachyarrhythmias and is called the *tachycardia-bradycardia syndrome.* Pathologically, chronic sinoatrial block is associated with extensive degenerative lesions within and around the sinus node. The tachycardia-bradycardia syndrome, however, is also associated with lesions in atrial tissue.[17]

Patients with the sick sinus syndrome are usually elderly and form a group similar to those that present with complete heart block. However, sinus node dysfunction may occur in children and young adults.[18] The syndrome may be familial[19] and it may follow corrective congenital cardiac surgery.[20] Patients with sick sinus syndrome may present with syncope or dizziness resulting from a profound bradycardia or even a tachycardia with a reduced cardiac output. Other symptoms include palpitations, tiredness, lethargy, heart failure, angina, or even senility. The diagnosis of the sick sinus syndrome is dependent on documentation of the arrhythmias.

The asymptomatic patient with ECG features of the sick sinus syndrome usually does not require permanent pacing. There are, however, a number of clinical situations where permanent pacing may be recommended. These include severe sinus bradycardia and coronary artery disease requiring beta-adrenergic blockade or antiarrhythmic drugs. Pacemaker therapy is highly successful in patients with sick sinus syndrome and syncopal episodes.[17,21] In the majority of cases, the syncopal episodes are abolished with a marked physical and psychological improvement. Because of the atrial arrhythmias and frequent association of distal conduction tissue disturbances, simple ventricular rather than atrial pacing is usually recommended. In elderly patients with impaired left ventricular function, the atrial boost provided with atrial pacing may be invaluable for congestive cardiac failure. In these cases, provided atrial fibrillation is not present, dual chamber pacing is highly recommended.

Following implantation of a pacemaker system, it is not surprising to find the tachyarrhythmias improved or abolished. Antiarrhythmic drugs can often be reduced or withdrawn. The long-term prognosis of patients with sick sinus syndrome, whether paced or not, depends on the patient's age, the presence or absence of cardiac failure, and the nature of the underlying pathology.[22] Because of diffuse atrial disease, patients with tachycardia-bradycardia syndrome have the worst prognosis. Despite an overall high mortality in patients with the sick sinus syndrome, symptomatic patients, irrespective of the underlying myocardial pathology, should not be denied the benefits of permanent pacing.

Other Symptomatic Bradyarrhythmias

A number of other symptomatic bradyarrhythmias exist which occasionally require consideration for permanent pacing.

Patients with Hereditary Prolongation of the QT Interval

These patients are prone to syncope and sudden death. Permanent atrial pacing has been used together with beta-adrenergic blockade in an attempt to override the drug-induced bradycardia which may encourage ventricular ectopics.

Carotid Sinus Hypersensitivity

Carotid sinus hypersensitivity is a common problem in elderly males with coronary atherosclerosis and hypertensive heart disease. Syncope due to bradycardia and vasodilatation may be induced by shaving, micturition, sneezing, head turning, looking up, exercise, and tight neck collars.[23] Asymptomatic or mildly symptomatic patients with carotid sinus hypersensitivity do not require therapy apart from avoidance of any precipitating factors. Permanent ventricular or dual chamber pacing is usually successful in preventing syncope due to bradycardia. Atrial pacing is not recommended because of the high incidence of AV nodal block in these patients.

Atrial Inexcitability

Atrial inexcitability, where the atria cannot be stimulated by pacing, is a rare condition resulting from a diffuse abnormality of atrial muscle. Usually the etiology remains obscure although it has been reported with cardiomyopathies, amyloid heart disease, atherosclerotic heart disease, and muscular dystrophies.[24] On the ECG, there is no P wave, and electrophysiological studies show a complete lack of electrical and mechanical activity in the atrium. When symptomatic, ventricular pacing is indicated.

Slow Junction Rhythm

Slow junction rhythm is usually a manifestation of the sick sinus syndrome but can also occur in normal patients such as athletes. Symptomatic patients with failure of sinus node activity or an insignificant rise in pulse rate with exercise may require permanent pacing.

Slow Atrial Fibrillation or Flutter

This condition, without the influence of drugs such as digitalis or beta-adrenergic blockers, usually reflects extensive AV nodal block. When the ventricular response is regular and slow, complete heart block is usually present. Symptomatic patients may respond dramatically to ventricular pacing.

Recurrent Ventricular Standstill

When not due to drug toxicity, recurrent ventricular standstill reflects extensive pacemaker and conduction tissue degeneration and belongs to the panconduction disease group. Although pacing can successfully abolish symptoms, the prognosis depends on the underlying pathology.

Tachyarrhythmias

Atrial and ventricular pacing for the treatment of both supraventricular and ventricular tachyarrhythmias has been used for many years with limited success. Most earlier techniques were temporary, although permanent pacemakers occasionally were implanted for overdrive suppression. Recent developments in the field of clinical electrophysiology have resulted in marked progress in the understanding of tachyarrhythmias, especially with regard to the initiation and termination of reentry pathways. This information is now being applied to the treatment of tachyarrhythmias using sophisticated pacemakers.

Therapeutic indications for pacing tachyarrhythmias include termination of the arrhythmia, its control by reversion to a more acceptable arrhythmia, or prevention. The techniques used may be either temporary or permanent. Although the literature on the value of pacemakers in treating tachyarrhythmias is extensive, use has been limited to those patients who are resistant to drug therapy. Of the many systems described, only overdrive suppression, radio-frequency-induced rapid atrial pacing, and specialized complex automatic systems have been successful in treating tachyarrhythmias.[16]

The Pacemaker Pulse Generator

Modern pacemaker pulse generators are sophisticated power packs which are small, compact, reliable, long-lived, and multiprogrammable. Within the pulse generator lies the power source and electronics, hermetically sealed in a titanium or stainless steel can to protect the contents from the hostile environment of body tissues.

Pulse Generator Power Source

The original power source that sustained the pacemaker industry for 15 years was the zinc-mercury battery. This chemical battery had an unpredictable failure mode and an average life of only 2 to 3 years.

Consequently, by the mid-1970s the zinc-mercury battery was replaced by other power sources. Rechargeable power cells using a nickel-cadmium battery were introduced at this time and although reliable, patients resented having to regularly recharge their power source and the system lost favor. Nuclear power cells were first used in 1970, and have proven to be reliable and have projected longevities of 10 to 20 years. Unfortunately, because of expense, limited implant indications, nuclear radiation fear, strict nuclear regulatory controls, and failure of the companies to keep abreast of other technologies, nuclear-powered pulse generators are only rarely used today.

The lithium anode battery has within the last decade completely revolutionized the pacemaker industry. The original pulse generators utilizing this power source were large, thick, and heavy, but no more so than those using other power sources available during the early 1970s. The major advantages of the lithium battery are reliability and longevity. The main battery used for implantable pulse generators has been the lithium-iodine cell and numerous small long-lived models are now available. A feature of the power source is a gradual fall in voltage output as the lithium and iodine are consumed in the chemical reaction. A satisfactory voltage output is retained for 90 percent of the battery's life, and this voltage decline can be used by the manufacturer to monitor pulse generator progress and impending power source depletion. Other lithium cathode materials used in cardiac pulse generators include silver chromate, thionyl chloride, lead iodide, and copper sulfide.

Pulse Generator Circuitry

Three basic electronic circuits are necessary for a pulse generator. The timing circuit controls the pulse repetition rate or pacing interval, and the output circuit controls the charging and discharging of the impulse. The third major circuit is the sensing circuit, which is responsible for recognition of spontaneous intracardiac electrical signals. Pacing circuits are further complicated by a variety of other electronic accessories which include filtering and protective devices, voltage multipliers, reed switches and complex circuitry required for programmability, telemetry, memory, and dual chamber logic.

The incorporation of the sensing circuit into the pulse generator was the major pacing advance during the 1960s. This circuit analyzes the electrical signals that return to the pulse generator from the heart via the lead and can discriminate true intracardiac signals from false signals. There is a time constraint on the functioning of the timing circuit. During and for a set period after myocardial depolarization, whether it be paced or spontaneous, there is a period of non-sensing for about 300 to 400 ms called the *pulse generator refractory period.* This is to prevent T-wave or after-potential sensing.

In order to confirm pacing when the pulse generator output is inhibited, a reed switch is used to convert the pulse generator to the asynchronous mode. This switch, which is actuated by positioning a special test magnet over the implanted pulse generator, usually consists of two ferromagnetic strips sealed in a thin glass tube. Under the influence of a magnetic field, the two strips make contact, triggering asynchronous pacing. The removal of the magnetic field allows the reed switch to assume its base status and the pulse generator sensing circuit will respond in a synchronous manner.

The Pacemaker Lead

The pacemaker lead is responsible for delivery of the pulse generator charge to the myocardium and for conducting intracardiac potentials back to the sensing circuit of the pulse generator. Originally, epicardial or epimyocardial leads were used but because of the necessity for a thoracotomy, transvenous leads gradually became popular. During the 1970s sutureless epimyocardial leads implanted by a simplified thoracic technique became available but nevertheless continued to play only a minor role. In recent years, with improvements in transvenous leads, epimyocardial leads represent less than 10 percent of all permanent implants.

Bipolar and Unipolar Electrode Systems

There are two major types of lead systems. A unipolar lead has only one electrode—the cathode, or active lead. Current flows from the cathode, stimulates the heart, and must return to the anode on the casing of the pulse generator to complete the circuit. A bipolar lead has two poles on the lead a short distance from each other at the distal end, and both electrodes lie within the heart. Usually the tip electrode is the cathode, while behind it is the ring anode.

With modern pacemakers, there is very little difference between unipolar and bipolar lead systems. Both are reliable and consistent with long-term pacing. Currently, very thin unipolar leads with polyurethane insulators are popular. However, thin coaxial bipolar leads are now available.

The major difference between the two leads systems is the theoretical superiority of unipolar systems with sensing. Because of the larger distance between electrodes, the unipolar system has a larger area for sensing. In practice, however, sensing is only a problem with temporary rather than permanent bipolar systems, especially following an acute myocardial infarction. Because of the enhanced sensing capability of unipolar leads, such systems are more sensitive to extracardiac electrical potentials and especially skeletal myopotentials.

Another disadvantage of the unipolar system is the proximity of skeletal muscle to the indifferent plate. In this situation, skeletal muscle may be stimulated when the current is returning to the anode after myocardial stimulation. However, muscle-twitching can be prevented by having the indifferent plate on only one side of the pulse generator facing subcutaneous tissues. Traditionally bipolar pulse generators require two entry ports for the two lead connectors and consequently the pulse generator is slightly larger and thicker. Coaxial leads with a single connector have overcome this problem. It can be shown experimentally that the fibrillation threshold is lower for bipolar compared to conventional unipolar cathodal stimulation.[25] Consequently, if a stimulus artifact falls in the vulnerable period of an ischemic heart, then bipolar pacing is more likely to cause ventricular fibrillation than unipolar pacing.

The Electrode

Original pacing leads had large stimulating electrodes, usually with a surface area of 20 to 100 mm^2 (Fig. 28-1). However, by reducing the surface area, better current drain was achieved and the pacemaker system became more energy-efficient.[26] The electrode surface area of most current lead designs ranges from 6 to 12 mm^2. On a theoretical basis, the shape is also important because of the area of contact of the stimulating electrode with the myocardium. Designs currently used include doughnut, mushroom, or dish shapes.[26,27] The electrode may also incorporate the lead fixation device; these include screws, helifix coils, prongs, and springs.[26,27] Another important and successful design is the porous electrode, which has been used with endocardial leads.[26] This electrode has a small stimulating area but a large sensing surface area. By allowing tissue ingrowth, better anchoring is provided at the electrode–tissue interface. Porous designs include a fine wire mesh, an interconnecting network of pores, and a standard electrode with a series of laser-drilled holes or slits.[27] The materials used for the electrode include pure platinum, platinum-iridium alloy, Elgiloy carbon, and, more recently, titanium.[27]

Lead Conductor

The lead conductor is responsible for delivering current to the electrode–tissue interface. In the past, conductor fractures were responsible for a significant proportion of late lead complications. Marked improvements in recent years have overcome this problem, resulting in conductors with immense strength and flexibility as well as high fracture and corrosion resistance.

Modern transvenous lead conductors are composed of one or more strands of wire tightly coiled around a hollow core to allow removable stylets to pass all the way to the distal electrode. Materials used include stainless steel, platinum-iridium, Elgiloy or a nickel alloy material such as MP35N. Bipolar leads require two conductors. These can run parallel or in a coaxial design which results in small-diameter bipolar leads. Epimyocardial leads do not require a stylet and there is consequently more flexibility with lead conductor design.

Lead Insulator

The earliest insulating material was polyethylene, which had poor long-term insulation properties, particularly in wearing and biodeterioration. Silicone rubber was substituted, but because of its tendency to tear and cut, the insulation layer became thicker. More recently, a number of polyurethanes have been found to be suitable for pacemaker lead insulation. These polyurethanes are tougher and stiffer than silicone rubber and the insulation thickness can be reduced. There is, however, no long-term implantation data available on polyurethanes, and thus this material is still not universally accepted.

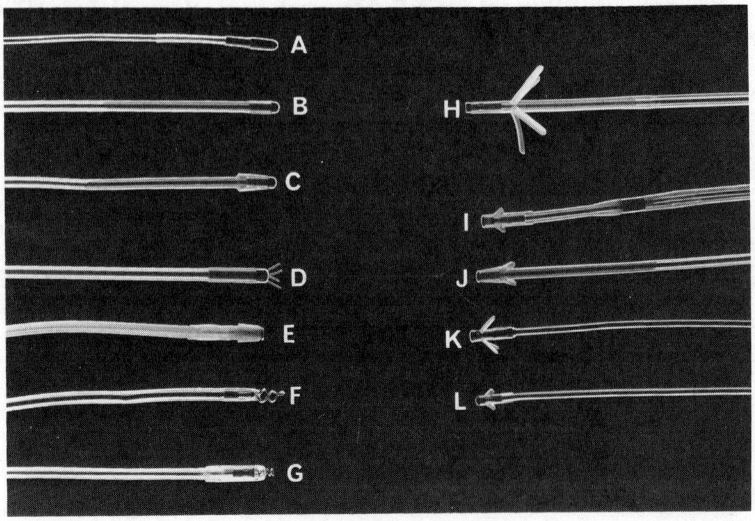

FIGURE 28-1 Transvenous ventricular leads—electrodes and fixation devices: *A,* Elema, no fixation device; *B,* Telectronics, no fixation device; *C,* Telectronics, wedge tip; *D,* Vitatron, four retractable nylon prongs; *E,* Elema, balloon and wedge tip (balloon not inflated); *F,* Vitatron, helifix electrode; *G,* Medtronic, screw-in (Bisping); *H,* Medtronic, large tines; *I–L,* variety of small tines. Only *D* and *G* are active fixation leads.

Lead Connector

The connector joins the lead to the pulse generator. The ideal connector is small, compact, reliable, and universal, allowing any unipolar lead to be attached to the pulse generator of any manufacturer. Similar principles apply to bipolar leads. Most pacemaker companies use one of two connector sizes; the larger Cordis "C" size and the smaller Medtronic "M" size. An M-size connector can be easily adapted to the C size with a sleeve.[27] A number of pulse generator companies have universal entry portholes which will accept both types of lead connectors. Bipolar leads have either two lead connectors, or the new coaxial lead designs have a single lead connector with both poles on the lead pin separated by an insulator.

Lead Fixation

A relatively recent innovation with endocardial lead systems is lead fixation. This may be active or passive. Active fixation leads invade the endomyocardium, whereas passive fixation leads promote fixation to the endocardium by indirect means. Passive fixation leads include the wedge or flange tip,[28] tines,[28] balloons,[29] and helifix designs[27] (Fig. 28-1). To date, the most successful results have been published with tined leads.[28] The most impressive of the active fixation leads has been the transvenous screw-in design, such as the Medtronic Bisping lead[30] (Fig. 28-1). Another active fixation lead has four nylon prongs which emerge from the electrode and penetrate the myocardium (Fig. 28-1).

Transvenous Atrial Leads

Because of unsuitable anatomy, long-term pacing of the atria has not, until recently, gained widespread acceptance. The right atrial appendage, however, is trabeculated and suitable for atrial pacing and sensing. A number of endocardial atrial J leads have been developed for use in this area (Fig. 28-2). Although clinically successful, the incidence of complications remains higher than with similar leads in the ventricle. Modern atrial J leads are thin and tined.[27] A number of authors prefer to use standard ventricular tined leads positioned in the atrial appendage using a J-shaped stylet.[31,32] Of the active fixation leads, the screw-in lead has been successfully placed in the right atrial appendage using either J leads or a preshaped stylet (Fig. 28-2). Another advantage of the screw-in lead is the ability to secure the electrode to almost any part of the right atrium, particularly for specialized automatic tachycardia reversion pacing systems where lead placement should be close to the reentry circuit to interrupt it.[30,33]

Another endocardial lead for atrial pacing is the coronary sinus lead with electrodes placed proximally so as to pace the atrium and not the ventricle.[34] Such leads are rarely used today for permanent pacing. A single-pass lead incorporates both the atrial and ventricular leads within a single body. For atrial pacing, the atrial electrode must make contact with the atrial wall. An electrode or electrodes lying within the chamber of the right atrium are only suitable for sensing. Single-pass leads have not been widely used and most implanters prefer to use two separate leads, one in the right atrium and the other in the right ventricle. Despite continuing problems with transvenous atrial leads, they are still favored over epimyocardial atrial leads, which in general remain unsuccessful despite new designs continually being assessed.[35]

Epimyocardial Leads

Direct suturing of the pacemaker lead to the epicardial surface was the original method of permanent lead implantation. As transvenous leads improved, they gradually began to dominate pacemaker implants, despite the initial success of the sutureless epimyocardial screw-in electrode introduced in 1971.[36] Today, epimyocardial lead implantation

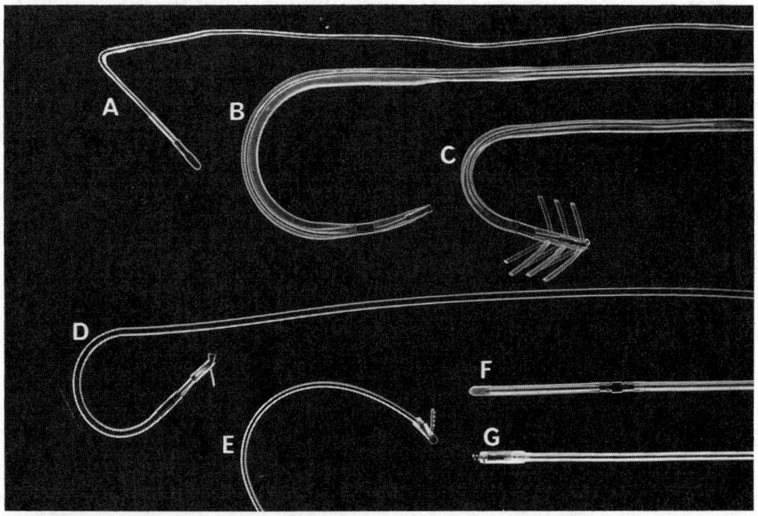

FIGURE 28-2 Transvenous atrial leads—electrodes and fixation devices. *A*, Elema J, no fixation device; *B*, Medtronic J, no fixation device; *C*, Medtronic J, X-mas tree design; *D*, Medtronic J, small tines; *E*, Cordis J, small tines and porous electrode; *F*, Cordis, unipolar coronary sinus lead; *G*, Medtronic, screw-in (Bisping). *A*, *B*, and *C* are obsolete.

should be relegated to those situations where the transvenous approach is technically impossible, not recommended, or has failed.

Pacemaker Electrocardiography

The Normal Ventricular Electrocardiogram

The normal ventricular pacemaker ECG is composed of three major components: a stimulus artifact followed by depolarization (QRS) wave and repolarization (T) wave (Fig. 28-3). The stimulus artifact as seen on the ECG represents about 5 V, delivered to the heart for approximately 0.5 ms. The suitably damped ECG machine will record a perpendicular, often biphasic, voltage deflection of about 2 to 3 mV. Following the initial spike, there is a voltage exponential decay curve which represents the dissipation of energy through body tissues (Fig. 28-3). This decay curve can cause marked distortion of the subsequent QRS and even ST segments. In this situation, QRS axis determination can be difficult and the first 40 to 60 ms of the QRS should be ignored.[27]

Vector analysis of the pacemaker QRS reveals typical characteristics when pacing is established from various parts of the heart. Ventricular pacing from the apex of the right ventricle, whether endocardial or epimyocardial, should give a left bundle branch block configuration and the frontal plane vector is to the extreme left (Fig. 28-4). If an endocardial pacing lead is dislodged toward the right ventricular outflow tract, then the pacing appearance still has a left bundle branch block configuration, but now the axis shift is toward the right.

Epicardial left ventricular pacing has a right bundle branch block configuration with an axis depending on the position of the lead on the left ventricular surface.

FIGURE 28-3 ECG leads I and II, simultaneous. Unipolar endocardial lead in the right ventricle. The pacemaker ECG consists of a stimulus artifact (S), depolarization (QRS), and repolarization (T). In lead I, the first complex, the stimulus artifact is followed by a small QRS and T wave. The second complex is composed of a stimulus artifact and no QRS or T wave, i.e., a failed paced beat. Note that the stimulus artifact is composed of the spike followed by an exponential decay curve and that this decay curve deforms the subsequent QRS. In lead I the decay curve could be confused with a small, almost isoelectric QRS. In lead II, however, the QRS and T waves are prominent and despite the decay curve there is no doubt about failed pacing.

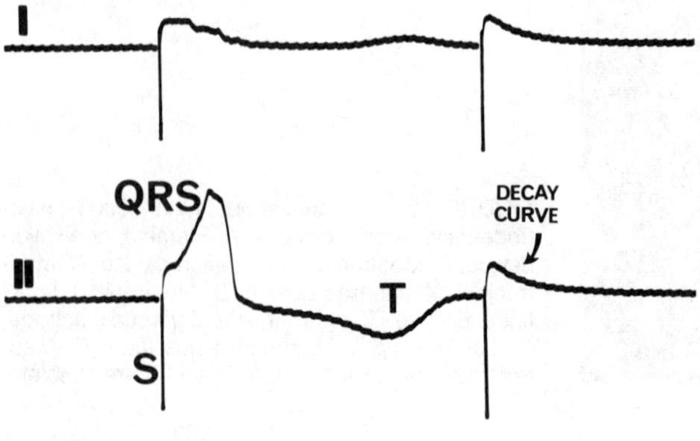

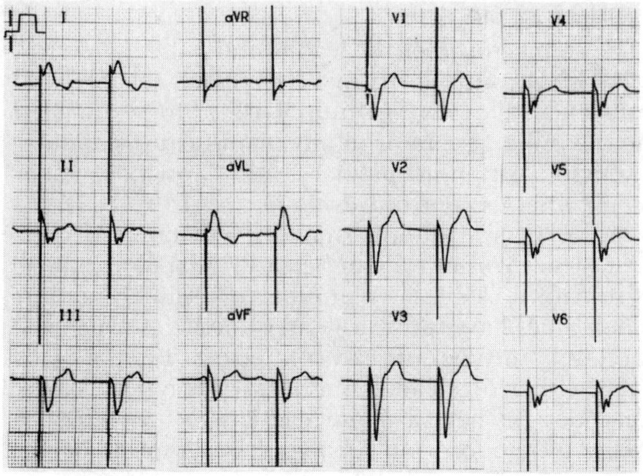

FIGURE 28-4 Twelve-lead ECG showing endocardial unipolar pacing from the apex of the right ventricle. There is a left bundle branch block configuration with only a small R wave in the lateral chest leads. The frontal plane axis is to the extreme left.

Fusion and Pseudofusion Beats

A true pacing fusion beat results from the simultaneous activation of the atrium or ventricle by a spontaneous impulse and a paced one. Both foci contribute in varying amounts to the total chamber depolarization. It is important to recognize that this is not a malfunction of the pacemaker system, but the spontaneous impulse occurs at a similar time as the paced one, leaving insufficient time for the spontaneous impulse to be sensed and for the pulse generator to respond appropriately (Fig. 28-5).

Pseudofusion beats are more complicated and can masquerade as pacemaker malfunction, which may lead to pulse generator replacement.[37] A ventricular pseudofusion beat results when there is electrocardiographic superimposition of a stimulus artifact on a QRS complex which is generated from a single nonpaced focus. The stimulus artifact does not contribute to ventricular depolarization. Like fusion, pseudofusion beats do not indicate failure of the sensing mechanism but constitute a normal manifestation of demand pacing.[27] Although the stimulus artifact is usually late, in some cases it occurs early within the spontaneous QRS, making it hard

FIGURE 28-5 ECG lead II showing normal ventricular inhibited (VVI) pacing. The first complex is sensed normally and there is pulse generator output inhibition. The last two complexes show normal ventricular pacing. Complexes 3 and 4 are fusion beats. Complex 3 is predominantly from a sinus origin and complex 4 is predominantly paced. Complex 2 is a pseudofusion beat. Although the stimulus artifact occurs early, nevertheless it does not appear to contribute to cardiac depolarization.

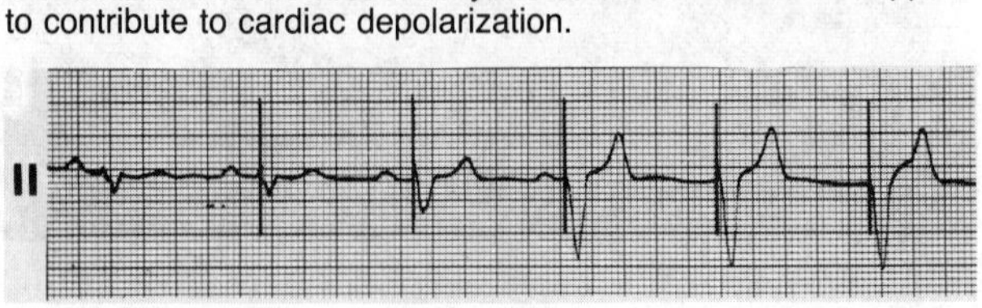

TABLE 28-2 Five-Position Pacemaker Code (ICHD)

Position	I	II	III	IV	V
Category	Chamber(s) Paced	Chamber(s) Sensed	Mode of Response(s)	Programmable Functions	Special Tachyarrhythmia Functions
Letters	V-ventricle	V-ventricle	T-triggered	P-programmable (rate and/or output)	B-bursts
	A-atrium	A-atrium	I-inhibited	M-multi programmable	N-normal rate competition
	D-double	D-double	D-double		S-scanning
		O-none	O-none	O-none	E-external

to understand why actual fusion does not occur (Fig. 28-5).

ECG Diagnosis of Acute Myocardial Infarction in Patients with Pacemakers

In pacemaker patients with suspected acute myocardial infarction, the diagnosis depends on the history, clinical findings, serial serum enzymes, and occasionally other more sophisticated investigations such as myocardial imaging. This is because a left bundle branch block configuration is seen on the electrocardiograph with most pacing rhythms. However, in atrial pacing, acute myocardial infarct changes may be seen as the QRS is not altered. With the sick sinus syndrome the pacing rhythm can be slowed or inhibited and the underlying rhythm then inspected. This is usually of no value if complete heart block is present, particularly with a bundle branch block configuration.

Despite these limitations, massive ST changes may occasionally be seen on the electrocardiograph of a pacing rhythm during the evolution of an acute myocardial infarction, and provided the changes are acute and transient, the diagnosis of an acute myocardial infarction can be made. With extensive anteroseptal transmural myocardial infarction and a left bundle branch block configuration on the electrocardiograph, Q waves may occur in leads I, aV_L, V_5 and V_6.[38] Similar reasoning can be applied to right ventricular pacing as leads V_5 and V_6 normally do not have an initial Q wave.[39] For inferior wall myocardial infarction the presence of a pacing qR pattern in leads II, III, and aV_F appears specific for infarction in this area.[40]

Modes of Cardiac Pacing

The original and traditional method of cardiac pacing is ventricular with or without sensing of spontaneous QRS complexes. Today, with sophisticated endocardial leads, reliable long-term sensing and pacing of both the atrium and ventricle can be achieved with a low incidence of complications.

With the development of complex pacing systems, difficulties with terminology became apparent. In the early 1970s, the Inter-Society Commission for Heart Disease Resources (ICHD) suggested a classification code which is now widely accepted.[41] The original nomenclature involved a three-letter identification code. The first position referred to the chamber paced and three letters were used: V (ventricle), A (atrium), and D (double-chamber). The second letter referred to the chamber sensed, and again the same three letters were used. In the situation where there was no sensing capability (asynchronous) the letter *O* was used. In the third position, the mode of response was documented and four letters were adopted: I (inhibited), T (triggered), O (asynchronous), and D (more than one response). During 1980 the code was extended to five positions[42] (Table 28-2). Position IV defined programmable functions and position V identified special pacing systems for treatment of tachyarrhythmias. These latter two positions can be deleted when not present.

Ventricular Pacing Systems

Ventricular Asynchronous—VOO

Other designation—ventricular fixed rate.

This was the original pacing mode and today is virtually obsolete, although available in mode programmable pulse generators. There is ventricular pacing but no sensing function (Fig. 28-6). Occasionally VOO pulse generators may be indicated for troublesome pulse generator inhibition due to skeletal myopotential or other extracorporeal oversensing. In this situation patients should be pacemaker-dependent and have no evidence of a competitive rhythm or ischemic heart disease.

FIGURE 28-6 ECG lead II, VOO pacing. There is no ventricular sensing and thus the stimulus artifact continues through the tracing at a regular repetition rate. Stimulus artifacts 1, 6, and 7 occur within the refractory period of the previous sinus beat and are ineffective. Stimulus artifacts 2, 3, and 4 are normal-paced beats. Stimulus artifact 5 occurs at the commencement of a QRS of sinus origin and results in a fusion beat.

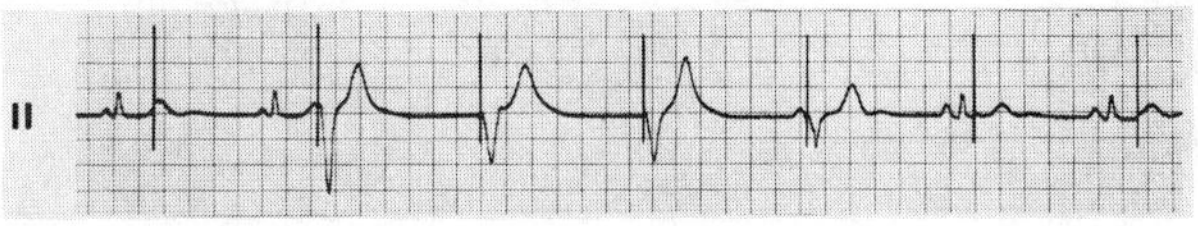

Ventricular Inhibited—VVI
Other designation—R-wave inhibited.

This is by far the most common pacing system used today. Spontaneous QRS potentials are sensed by the pacemaker and the subsequent pacing stimulus inhibited. The output circuit of the pulse generator is recycled and a pacing stimulus will then occur at a set pulse repetition rate unless further spontaneous QRS potentials fall within that period (Fig. 28-5). Compared with VOO pacing, the VVI system allows power source energy conservation in the presence of spontaneous rhythms and this system prevents competitive rhythms which may lead to lethal ventricular arrhythmias.

Ventricular Triggered—VVT
Other designation—R-wave triggered.

Although popular during the late 1960s, this system is rarely used today. The sensing mechanism is similar to the VVI system but the response is the reverse. Instead of inhibition, the full output of the pulse generator is delivered into and deforms the spontaneous QRS during the absolute refractory period (Fig. 28-7). Although energy-wasteful, this system was useful when sensing circuits were unreliable, particularly with oversensing. VVT pacing is today available in mode programmable pulse generators. It has limited use, although one application is symptomatic skeletal myopotential oversensing, especially in patients with ischemic heart disease where asynchronous pacing or changing the sensitivity may be contraindicated.

Atrial Pacing Systems

Atrial Asynchronous—AOO
Other designation—atrial fixed rate.

This system is virtually obsolete. There is atrial pacing, but no atrial sensing.

Atrial Inhibited—AAI
Other designation—P-wave inhibited.

Like its ventricular equivalent, this is the most common form of pure atrial pacing (Fig. 28-8). This useful form of pacing has not been widely utilized because of poor long-term results with atrial leads, the high incidence of AV conduction abnormalities, and atrial arrhythmias in patients with sick sinus syndrome requiring pacing. The advantage of AAI pacing is the maintenance of the atrial contribution to ventricular filling.

FIGURE 28-7 ECG lead II, VVT pacing. Following a normal-paced beat, there are two sinus complexes. Soon after the upstroke of the R wave is inscribed, the complex is sensed and the full output of the pulse generator is delivered into the QRS deforming it. This is seen again with complexes 6 and 7.

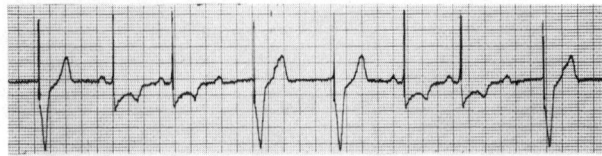

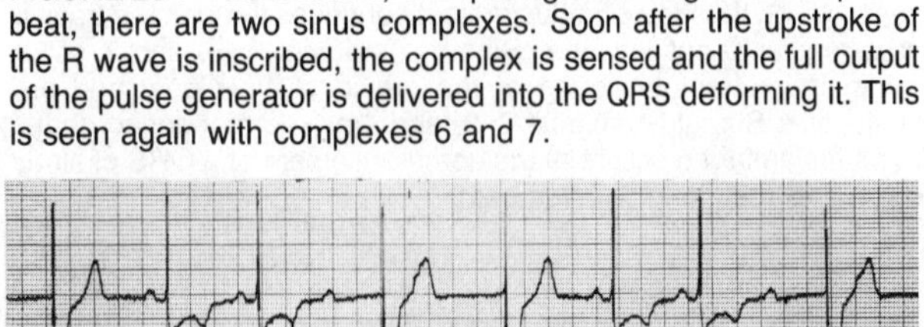

I

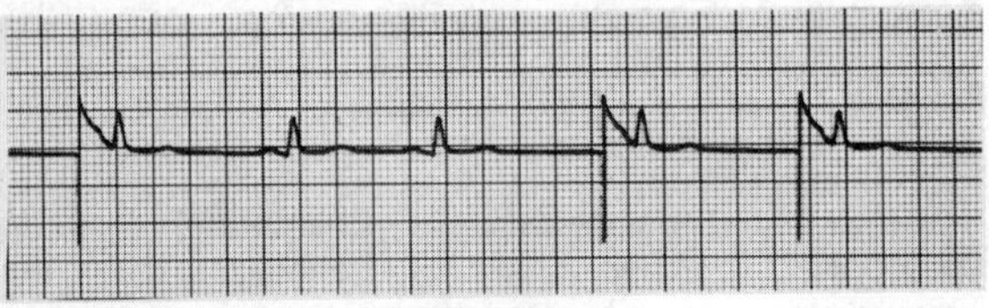

FIGURE 28-8 ECG lead I, AAI pacing. Complexes 1, 4, and 5 commence with a stimulus artifact and a prominent decay curve. Within this decay curve, there is a small convexity which represents the P wave. Almost 200 ms after the stimulus artifact there is a narrow QRS complex. Complexes 2 and 3 are of sinus origin and inhibit the atrial pulse generator output. Note that the QRS complexes, whether they be paced or of sinus origin, are identical.

Atrial Triggered—AAT
Other designation—P triggered.

This form of atrial pacing is of academic interest only.

Dual-Chamber Pacing Systems

At least five different pacing systems using both atrial and ventricular leads are available. All these modes of pacing can be incorporated into a single universal pulse generator. The systems to be described deal first with atrial and ventricular pacing, then with atrial sensing instead of pacing, and finally the ultimate combination of atrial and ventricular pacing and sensing. The order of presentation also represents the developmental and chronological order and reflects the changing state of the art as improvements in lead systems and microcircuitry evolved.

Atrioventricular Asynchronous Sequential—DOO
Other designation—AV fixed-rate sequential.

This was the earliest and most primitive form of sequential pacing and is now of academic interest only. The atrium is paced and after a set period, called the AV sequential interval or delay (AV delay), the ventricle is stimulated (Fig. 28-9).

There is no sensing in either chamber and competitive rhythms could be troublesome. On rare occasions, DOO pacing with a very short AV delay is

FIGURE 28-9 ECG lead II, AV sequential pacing (DOO, DVI, or DDD). There are two stimulus artifacts, atrial (A) and ventricular (V), which result in depolarization of the respective chambers. The interval between the two stimulus artifacts is fixed and is the AV delay.

II

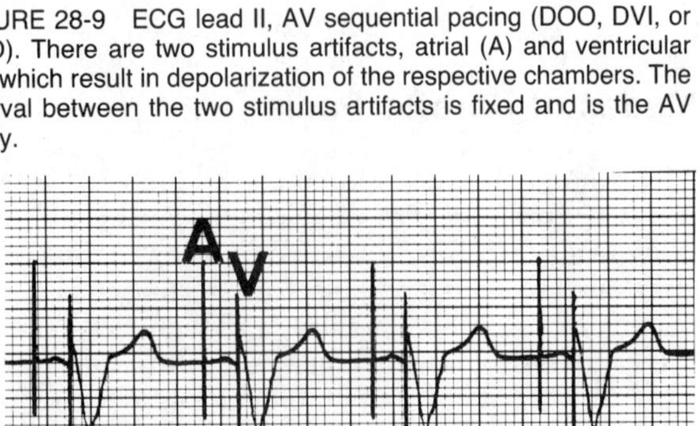

used for reversion and control of incessant supraventricular reentry tachyarrhythmias.

Atrioventricular Sequential—DVI
Other designation—bifocal sequential demand.

In this system, both chambers are paced but only the ventricle is capable of sensing and it responds in both a ventricular-inhibited and atrial-inhibited fashion. The atrial and ventricular pulse repetition rates are both identical and are separated by a fixed AV delay.

DVI pacemaker manufacturers initially found difficulties in designing the sensing circuit function during the AV delay because of inappropriate sensing of the atrial after-potential. For this reason, a number of manufacturers used a committed system. Once the atrial stimulus is delivered, the ventricular stimulus must follow asynchronously after a set AV delay. Spontaneous QRS complexes occurring during this period will not be sensed by the ventricular lead. This may make some pacing rhythms difficult to interpret, leading to the false diagnosis of pacing system malfunction.[43] Fortunately, most DVI pulse generators currently manufactured are noncommitted. In these systems, there is sensing during the AV delay but only after a very short ventricular blanking period at the time of the atrial stimulus. During most of the AV delay, spontaneous QRS complexes will be sensed and the ventricular output inhibited. There are variations between manufacturers. Spontaneous QRS complexes which occur prior to the atrial stimulus will also inhibit the atrial output (Fig. 28-10).

FIGURE 28-10 ECG lead II, normal noncommitted DVI pacing. There is sequential AV pacing and no atrial sensing. Ventricular sensing will inhibit the ventricular output and if early enough the atrial output. *Above:* The first two and last two complexes show normal sequential pacing. Complex 1 has a P wave prior to the atrial stimulus artifact. Because of intact AV conduction, a nonpaced QRS follows after a 200-ms delay. This is too late for ventricular sensing and a pseudofusion beat results. *Below:* The first two and the last complexes show normal sequential pacing. Complex 2 has a P wave prior to the atrial stimulus artifact. However, this occurs 40 ms later than with complex 1 and the nonpaced QRS is sensed normally. With complex 3, the nonpaced QRS occurs prior to the next atrial stimulus artifact and thus both atrial and ventricular outputs are inhibited.

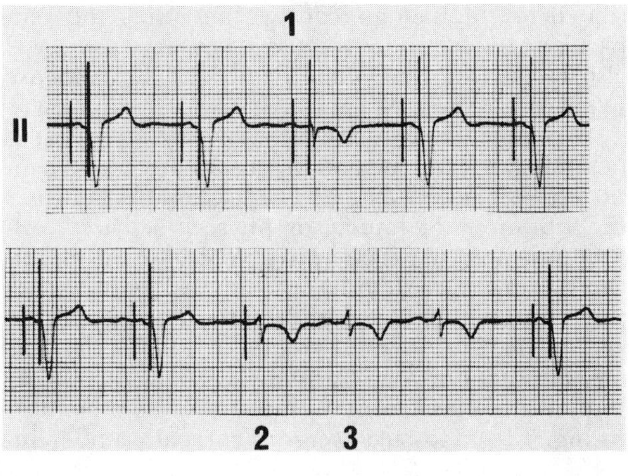

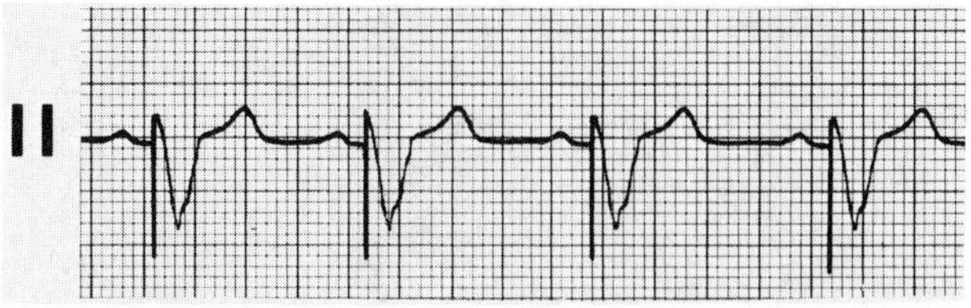

FIGURE 28-11 ECG lead II, VAT pacing. Prior to each ventricular paced complex there is a P wave. This P wave is sensed and triggers the ventricular output after an appropriate AV delay.

Atrial Synchronous—VAT
Other designation—P-wave synchronous.

With VAT pacing, there is atrial sensing but no atrial pacing. Once a P wave is recognized, ventricular pacing follows after a set AV delay (Fig. 28-11). In this rate-responsive system, AV synchrony is reestablished and the ventricular pacing rate varies according to the atrial rate and thus the physiologic needs of the patient. Because there is no ventricular sensing, the system is now obsolete.

Atrial Synchronous Ventricular Inhibited—VDD
Other designation—ASVIP (atrial synchronous ventricular inhibited pacing).

Like the VAT system, the atrial lead senses the P wave, triggering the ventricle. However, this system has the advantage of also being ventricular inhibited (Fig. 28-12). For the ICHD classification code, the third letter reads D and denotes that the mode of sensing response is triggered in the atrium and inhibited in the ventricle. VDD pacing is an ideal system for pacemaker management of complete heart block, provided sinus node function remains normal.

There are two important programmable functions with all VDD pacemakers. The first is the atrial upper rate limit the ventricle will respond to. This protects the ventricle from rapid atrial arrhythmias such as atrial flutter. The upper rate limit is usually set at 125, 150, or 175 beats per minute. The second programmable function is the atrial lower rate limit that the ventricle will respond to before escape ven-

FIGURE 28-12 ECG lead II, VDD pacing. Complexes 1, 2, 3, 7, and 8 show normal VDD pacing with sensing of the P wave and triggering of the ventricular output. Complex 4 (A), is premature ventricular pacing and may represent sensing of an atrial ectopic. This is followed by a ventricular ectopic beat (V) which is sensed and inhibits the ventricular output of the pulse generator. After a delay of 920 ms (the atrial lower rate limit), ventricular pacing (P) occurs. The P wave prior to this complex occurs too late to be sensed.

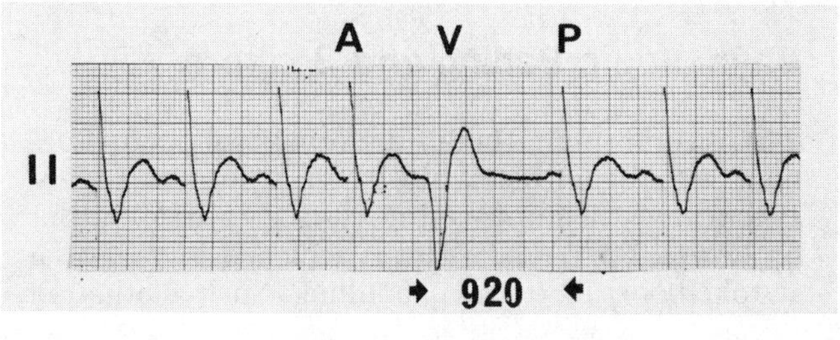

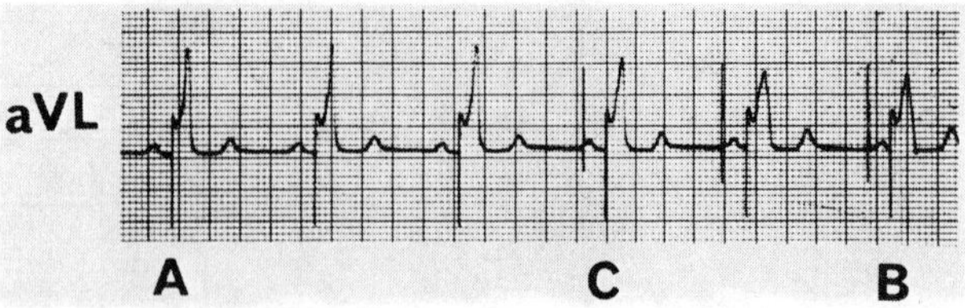

FIGURE 28-13 ECG lead aV_L, DDD pacing. There is both sensing and pacing of the atrium with ventricular pacing after a set AV delay. Complex A shows atrial sensing, B, atrial pacing, and C is an atrial fusion beat.

tricular pacing (VVI). This is important in the event of atrial sensing failure or atrial bradyarrhythmias. The lower rate limit is usually set at 50, 60, or 70 beats per minute.

A disadvantage to the VDD system is the establishment of VVI pacing in the event of sinus bradycardia because there is no atrial backup pacing. In patients with an intact atrioventricular node and distal conduction system, the VDD pacing system may be contraindicated because of retrograde conduction with possible sensing of these retrograde P waves leading to a pacemaker mediated reentry tachyarrhythmia.[44] This can be corrected by lengthening the atrial refractory period of the pulse generator.

Fully Automatic—DDD

Other designations—universal; optimal sequential; atrial synchronous, atrial demand, ventricular demand; atrial synchronous, atrial inhibited, ventricular inhibited.

This is the ultimate form of pacing. There is atrial sensing and pacing, together with ventricular sensing and pacing (Fig. 28-13). With the three-letter ICHD code, there are three modes of response and the letter is D. There is triggering of the ventricle, either as a result of atrial pacing or atrial sensing, together with an atrial inhibited and a ventricular inhibited response to spontaneous activity in those respective chambers. Programmable features include the mode of pacing, the AV delay, the maximum atrial rate which the ventricle will follow, and the minimum atrial rate for sensing at which atrial pacing commences. There is a wide range of indications for DDD pacing. It can be used for the sick sinus syndrome and for all degrees of heart block. There is, however, no added value over VVI pacing in atrial fibrillation. Like VDD pacing, DDD pacing may cause pacemaker-mediated reentry tachyarrhythmias in the presence of retrograde conduction. This can be prevented by pacing the atrium prior to the ventricle (DVI) or lengthening the atrial refractory period.

Physiologic Pacing and Sensors

There is no doubt that in the otherwise normal patient with heart block, the reestablishment of AV synchrony will improve the resting cardiac output by 15 to 20 percent.[45] This is achieved by the atrial systolic boost to ventricular filling. Such a situation can be seen clinically when comparing VVI pacing to DVI pacing at similar rates. The other, more important factor that physiologically aids the cardiac output is rate-responsiveness. The atrium via the sinus node pacemaker will alter its rate according to hemodynamic requirements and because of AV synchrony, the ventricular rate alters accordingly. Rate-responsive systems, which include VDD and DDD pacing, depend on the atrium as the physiologic sensor. The major advantage of such pacing is the ability in appropriate patients to increase the cardiac output by 200 to 300 percent under extreme stress. Under similar stress, patients with VVI and DVI pacing can only achieve a modest increase in cardiac output. A major deficiency of VDD and DDD pacing is the dependence on the atrium as the physiologic sensor. The majority of pacemaker patients are elderly and have clinical or subclinical atrial disease. Atrial tachyarrhythmias and particularly atrial fibrillation are common and these hinder the effectiveness of the atrial sensor.

In the study comparing rate-responsive pacing (VAT) with matched VVI pacing, Karlof[46] concluded that the increase in cardiac output at fast ventricular rates was limited by the end-diastolic volume. The atrial systolic contribution to ventricular filling was not important at fast ventricular rates. At rest, with both VAT and VVI pacing rate 72 beats per minute, the cardiac output not unexpectedly with VAT pacing was 15 percent greater than with VVI pacing. On exercise, the VAT pacing rate increased to 120 beats per minute with an appropriate 75 percent increase in cardiac output. However, by adjusting the VVI rate to 120 beats per minute and performing the same exercise, the cardiac output rose by greater than 100 percent to almost match the VAT cardiac output at the same rate. Santini[47] performed a similar study but only used VVI pacing. During exercise, at 70 beats per minute, the cardiac output rose to 10 liters/min. However, by increasing the VVI pacing rate to 115 beats per minute, the cardiac output rose to 17 liters/min and there was 100 percent improvement in exercise capacity.

From these studies it can be concluded that the atrial sensor as seen with atrial synchrony is not essential for physiologic pacing. Increasing the ventricular rate alone by the use of other sensors will also result in an adequate hemodynamic response to stress.

A number of new nonatrial or sinus-dependent hemodynamic or metabolic sensors are being considered for pacemaker use. The simplest device senses the vibrations of muscle or physical activity.[48] Although somewhat crude physiologically, this multiprogrammable system has the advantage of having the sensor within the pulse generator casing and no special lead system is required. Similarly, the measurement of the QT interval to vary the pacing rate also has its sensor within the pulse generator casing.[49] Intravascular sensors currently under investigation include pH,[50] central body temperature,[51] and mixed venous oxygen saturation.[52] Clinical experience is limited to the pH sensor which has been implanted for a number of years but technical problems have limited its use. The use of respiration rate as a determinant of the ventricular pacing rate also has been used clinically with encouraging results.[53] Other sensors under investigation include measurement of stroke volume and right ventricular pressure. Because of the nature of the patient population being treated, there is no doubt that hemodynamic and metabolic sensors will play a major role in physiologic pacing in the future.

Pacing Systems for Treatment of Tachyarrhythmias

Because of the complexities of the pacing systems available and the nature of the tachyarrhythmias themselves, there is no consensus of opinion of what is the ideal pacing system for the treatment of tachyarrhythmias. In general, the use of permanent pacing has been limited to those patients who have hemodynamically disabling tachycardias and who are resistant to or intolerant of drug therapy. There must be physiologic proof of repeated tachycardia interruption by the pacing method to be used. There must be no evidence of atrial fibrillation in patients in whom an atrial system has been considered, or ventricular fibrillation produced by ventricular stimulation in any patient. Consideration should also be given to the benefits of surgical cure of the tachyarrhythmia by other therapeutic modes such as open heart surgical mapping and section of reentrant or accessory pathways or surgical or catheter ablation of the His bundle.

An ideal tachycardia reversion, control, and prevention pacemaker system should have the following characteristics:

1. The system should be fully implantable. The leads and pulse generator should be reliable, the pulse generator small, compact, and long-lived.
2. The pacemaker should have automatic tachycardia recognition and should respond spontaneously to revert the arrhythmia.
3. The system must be versatile. If the delivered impulse or series of impulses are unsuccessful in reverting the tachycardia then the system should change automatically.
4. Automatic deactivation. The system must be able to recognize the tachycardia reversion and then inhibit its program.
5. The system must be multiprogrammable. Extrinsic adaptability is essential to cover the range of individual differences between different types of pacemakers.
6. The system should have a bradycardia standby system for either atrial, ventricular, or dual-chamber pacing.
7. There must be a system for external deactivation of the pulse generator output separate from the bradycardia standby.
8. The system should be safe.

Such an ideal and universal antitachycardia pacing system is not yet available. Multiprogrammability and highly complex circuits incorporated into fully implantable pulse generators are becoming available. These can be automatic and versatile. Typical examples are the PASAR (TELECTRONICS) and Cybertach-60 (INTERMEDICS).

The PASAR (*p*rogrammable *a*utomatic *s*canning *a*rrhythmia *r*eversion) pulse generator automatically detects the tachycardia by rate and then delivers one or two extra stimuli at a programmable time after a tachycardia QRS. If unsuccessful in reverting the tachycardia, four cycles of tachycardia are then remeasured and the next extra stimulus or extra stimuli are delivered this time 6 mm closer to the QRS. Where tachycardia reversion is unsuccessful the pulse generator will repeat the decremental cycle 16 times and then start the cycle again. If reversion occurs, the pulse generator turns itself off but the successful timing interval is retained in the pulse generator memory and on detection of another tachycardia this interval is the first to be delivered. The ECG in Fig. 28-14 shows two ventricular extra stimuli successfully reverting ventricular tachycardia.

The Cybertach-60 is a multiprogrammable bipolar pulse generator which is a standard AAI or VVI unit with the capability of automatically responding to tachycardia by rapid burst. There are 28 standard combinations of burst rates and durations of firing. The rate sensing of the arrhythmia is also programmable. Highly complex dual-chamber pacemakers may also have a programmable rapid burst function incorporated into some models.

FIGURE 28-14 ECG simultaneous leads I, II, and III showing ventricular tachycardia reverted to sinus rhythm by two ventricular extrasystoles delivered from a PASAR pulse generator with the bipolar lead at the apex of the right ventricle.

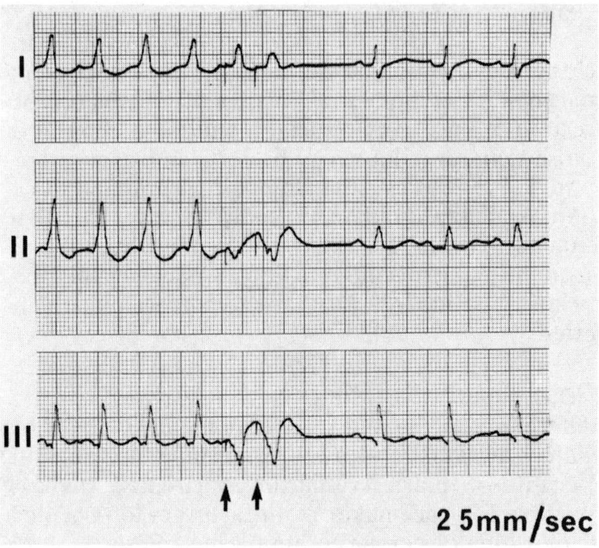

Despite the current emphasis on complex automatic pacing systems, a most effective permanent pacemaker system to terminate supraventricular tachycardia is simple patient-activated rapid atrial pacing by radiofrequency.[54] The atrial lead is attached to a receiver coil implanted in the subclavicular subcutaneous tissues. Appropriate radio frequency stimulation of this coil by a hand-held transmitter produces rapid atrial pacing at a preset rate. This rate is adjusted by the physician.

Pacemaker Programmability

Pacemaker programmability is a noninvasive, stable, reversible change in the operating parameter of an implanted pulse generator.[55] The majority of pulse generators manufactured (particularly in the United States) have one or more functions which are programmable. When three or more functions can be altered the system is called *multiprogrammable*. Recently, telemetry has been linked to programmability. Here the program change can be telemetered back to the programmer on interrogation of the pulse generator. Telemetry may also include pulse generator identification, battery status, lead impedance, threshold measurement, intracardiac electrogram, event marking, percentage pacing, arrhythmia documentation, and special data, such as patient details, which can be programmed into the pulse generator memory for later retrieval. The list of options is immense.

To reprogram an implanted pulse generator, a hand-held programmer is necessary. These programmers range from powerful magnets to highly sophisticated bench-top computers. For telemetry, printers are necessary, adding futher bulk and expense to the equipment. To reprogram an implanted pulse generator, the programmer must transmit a preselected coded message. Three systems are available; magnetic, radiofrequency, and ultrasonic. Radiofrequency is the easiest, most efficient, and most commonly used.

The major advantages of programmability include the selection of the most appropriate pacing parameters or mode, noninvasive diagnosis and correction of pacing malfunction, and the extension of pulse generator longevity by reducing energy output. Table 28-3 lists the major programmable functions available. To date, no company offers all these functions within a single pulse generator, and consequently if a specific function is required, the physician must make sure that the correct pulse generator is implanted.

TABLE 28-3 Programmable Functions

1. Rate
2. Output
   a. Pulse duration
   b. Voltage output
   c. Energy output
3. Sensitivity
4. Refractory period
5. Hysteresis
6. Mode of pacing
7. Polarity change
8. Conversion bipolar to unipolar pacing
9. Threshold function
   a. Voltage
   b. Pulse duration
10. Programmable functions of:
   a. Dual-chamber pulse generators
   b. Automatic tachycardia reverting pulse generators

Rate Reprogramming

Alteration of the pulse repetition rate is the most widely available and used programmable function. Because of quartz crystal timing circuits, it is now possible for pacemaker manufacturers to provide a wide range of very accurate pacing rates.

Fast pulse repetition rates may be indicated in the following situations:

Pediatric use
Following general surgery or open heart surgery
Toxemia
Overdrive suppression of ectopic beats or tachyarrhythmias
Improvement of cardiac output
Analysis of pacing rhythm problems and in particular fusion beats

Slow pulse repetition rates may be indicated in the following situations:

To permit sinus rhythm in patients with sick sinus syndrome
To prolong pulse generator life
To observe underlying rhythm
During bypass surgery

Output Reprogramming

The pulse generator output is dependent on the voltage and pulse duration. In multiprogrammable pulse generators, either or both of these may be programmable. The normal voltage output is 5 V. A number of programmable pulse generators provide a half-voltage output capability for patients with low chronic threshold leads. A high-voltage output capability of 7 to 10 V is also available for high threshold exit block. Pulse duration programmability is a common function of modern programmable pulse generators. Either a small number of predetermined pulse durations are available or a large range of 0.1-ms intervals can be programmed, although the latter is used for pulse duration threshold measurements.

The major indications for output reprogramming include:

Prolonging power source life
Treating high-voltage threshold (exit block)

Threshold testing
Correcting diaphragmatic pacing
Reduction of voltage to below threshold, such as at open heart surgery

Sensitivity Reprogramming

Multiprogrammable pulse generators generally have a range of sensitivity values useful for correcting sensing problems and allowing the pulse generator to be used for both atrial and ventricular pacing. A very sensitive setting will recognize small potentials as low as about 1 mV. Normal sensing is of the order of 2 mV. The major indication to increase the sensitivity is a failure to sense R or P waves. The major indication for decreasing the sensitivity is oversensing (discussed under "Pacemaker Malfunction").

Hysteresis Programming

In pacing, *hysteresis* refers to an escape interval which differs from the pulse repetition rate. The escape interval is the period from the sensed beat to the next paced beat. With hysteresis this escape interval is longer than the pulse repetition rate. Hysteresis is particularly useful for patients with sick sinus syndrome with a sinus rate just below the pacing rate. It is preferable to keep the patient in sinus rhythm but when pacing is required because of a bradyarrhythmia, this rate should be adequate to maintain a satisfactory cardiac output.

Dual-Chamber and Automatic Tachycardia Reverting Pulse Generator Programming

The newer complex dual-chamber and automatic tachycardia reverting pulse generators must be multiprogrammable. With dual-chamber systems, programmable features include minimum atrial sensed rate, AV delay, sensitivity, maximum ventricular rate, and ability to change the mode of pacing. With automatic tachycardia reverting pulse generators, the programmable functions are specific to the methods of reversion.

Pacemaker Malfunction

In devising a practical classification of pacemaker malfunction, the ECG appearances of pacing, both in the synchronous (demand) and asynchronous (magnet or test) modes, are used. Three principles must be fulfilled to establish normal pacing:

1. A normal stimulus artifact is produced regularly at the preset rate in the asynchronous mode.
2. The stimulus artifact is followed by ventricular depolarization (QRS) and repolarization (T).
3. The pacemaker senses normally.

Using these principles, a flow diagram has been constructed (Fig. 28-15). The first part investigates the stimulus artifact and the magnet must be applied. The second part investigates the QRS and T wave and magnet application is not essential. The third part investigates demand function and the magnet must be removed. Within each section of the flow diagram there are a number of endpoints. One is "normal," indicating that the pacemaker malfunction under investigation is not within this section, since the basic principle being examined has been fulfilled. The other endpoints represent pacemaker malfunction groups as identified by an ECG or electronic testing abnormality, and specific causes of each malfunction are tabulated (Tables 28-4 to 28-6). The tables are subdivided into true malfunctions and pseudomalfunctions. Pseudomalfunctions usually result from misinterpretation or faulty documentation of test data or from a poor understanding of the pacemaker system.

If the ECG and electronic testing is normal, then clinical features may suggest that the problem is not strictly pacemaker malfunction but rather physical or psychological side effects of pacing (Table 28-7). The symptoms may also suggest that the problem is not related to the pacemaker system or is of an uncertain origin and further investigation is warranted.

The Stimulus Artifact

The flow diagram (Fig. 28-15) recognizes four abnormalities of the stimulus artifact: absent, intermittent, deformed, and present and regular but at an altered rate.

Stimulus Artifact Absent—Inoperative Pacemaker System

There is no detectable stimulus artifact and no pulse generator output in the asynchronous mode. There are three major true malfunctions listed in Table 28-4. Diagnosis of the actual malfunction may be difficult by routine noninvasive testing because the stimulus artifact is absent. Chest radiography and fluoroscopy are usually diagnostic for lead conductor fractures with complete discontinuity. Treatment of all true malfunctions requires surgical intervention. Pseudomalfunctions are extremely important, because surgical intervention is not indicated.

Stimulus Artifact Intermittent

Here, intermittently in the asynchronous mode, the stimulus artifact is not recorded on the ECG or detected with electronic testing equipment (Table 28-4). The most important cause is an intermittent break in the pacemaker-patient electrical circuit, such as a fractured lead conductor in which the fractured ends intermittently make contact. Provocative maneuvers and prolonged ambulatory monitoring may be helpful in the diagnosis.

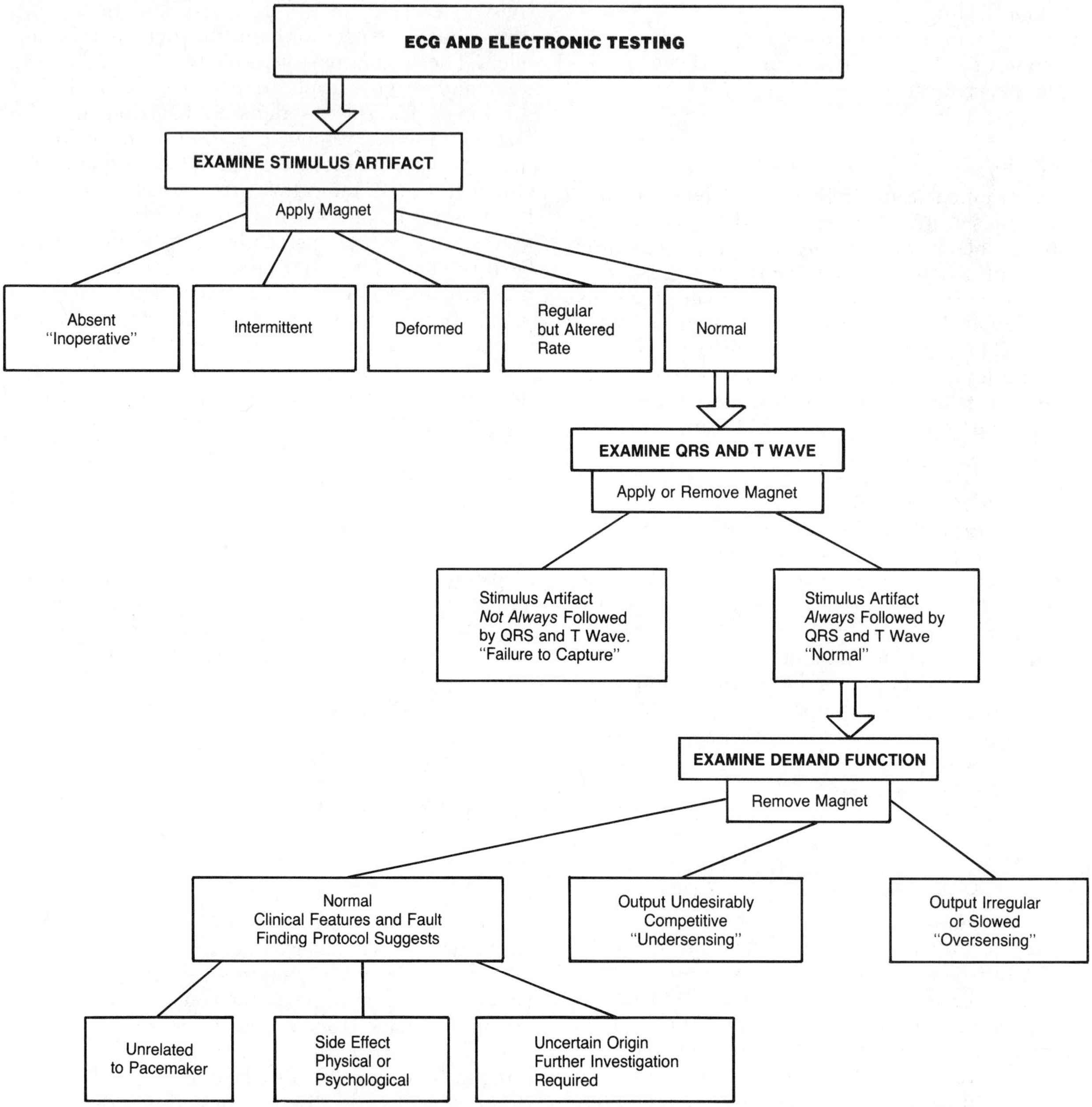

FIGURE 28-15 Flow diagram demonstrating the protocol for investigation of pacemaker malfunction using the ECG and electronic testing.

Stimulus Artifact Deformed

A deformed stimulus artifact may be attenuated or broad (Table 28-4). The attenuated stimulus artifact is usually subthreshold and represents reduced current reaching the heart. A common cause is a fractured lead conductor in which the ends make contact but result in a high lead impedance (Fig. 28-16). Pseudomalfunctions in this group are usually obvious and should be easily recognized. A broad stimulus artifact is rare and usually represents direct current (dc) leakage into the heart, due to a short circuit in the output circuit.

Stimulus Artifact Present but Altered Rate

True malfunctions are peculiar to the pulse generator (Table 28-4). A marked fall in rate suggests impending power source failure. The runaway pulse generator usually refers to an increase in pacing rate beyond 150 beats per minute with sufficient output to capture the heart.[56] Improved pacemaker technology has significantly decreased this probability in modern pulse generators.

The QRS and T Wave

Pacemaker malfunction can be recognized when *the stimulus artifact in the asynchronous or synchronous mode demonstrates intermittent or absent capture.* An example of intermittent capture is shown in Fig. 28-3 and the causes listed in Table 28-5. This malfunction is unrelated to demand function and sensing may be retained.[27] The problem of a lead incorrectly placed at implant should be overcome by good surgical

TABLE 28-4 Malfunctions Related to the Stimulus Artifact

I. Stimulus artifact absent (inoperative pacemaker system)
  A. True malfunction
    1. Power source failure
    2. Output circuit failure
    3. Pacemaker–patient electrical circuit incomplete, e.g., lead conductor fracture
  B. Pseudomalfunction
    1. Misinterpretation, ECG (e.g., pulse artifact overlooked)
    2. Testing equipment problem (e.g., equipment failure)
II. Stimulus artifact intermittent
  A. True malfunction
    1. Pacemaker–patient electrical circuit incomplete, intermittent
    2. Timing or output circuit, intermittent component failure
    3. Pacemaker–patient electrical short circuit, intermittent
  B. Pseudomalfunction
    1. As for stimulus artifact absent
III. Stimulus artifact deformed
  A. True malfunction
    1. Attenuated
      a. Lead fracture with some contact
      b. Loss of insulation
      c. Pacemaker–patient electrical short circuit
      d. Power source failure
      e. Lead dislodgment
    2. Broad
      a. Output capacitor short circuit
      b. Electrochemical potentials
  B. Pseudomalfunction
    1. Attenuated
      a. Respiratory effect
      b. Faulty ECG recorder
      c. Marker spikes
      d. Chest wall stimulation
    2. Broad
      a. ECG artifacts
IV. Stimulus artifact at altered rate
  A. True malfunction
    1. Power source failure (rate slow)
    2. Timing circuit
      a. Inadvertent reprogramming of programmable pulse generator
      b. Random component failure—runaway pulse generator; rate slow
  B. Pseudomalfunction
    1. Misinterpretation
      a. Lack of understanding of rate changes with temperature change, power source depletion, and activation of reed switch (magnet or test rate)
    2. Faulty ECG recording or testing equipment
      a. Asynchronous and synchronous testing confused
      b. ECG recorder—variable speed

technique. New lead designs, such as the incorporation of tines behind the electrode, have markedly reduced lead displacement.[28]

Demand Function

The two major abnormalities of sensing function are undersensing (output undesirably competitive) or oversensing (synchronous output slowed or irregular). These malfunctions are temporarily correctable by magnet conversion to the asynchronous mode.

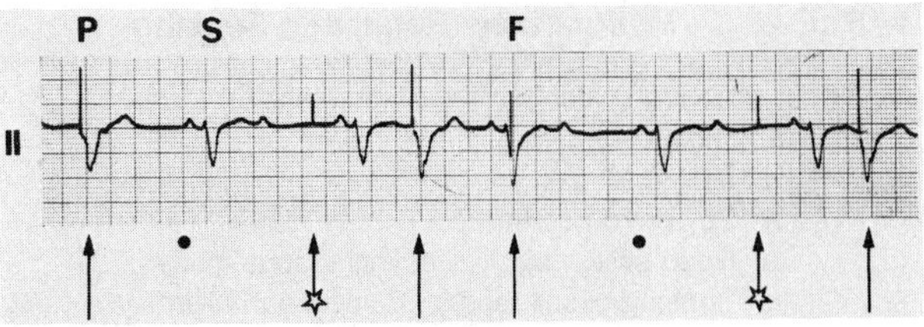

FIGURE 28-16 ECG, lead II. Fractured lead conductor with intermittent contact and loss of sensing. The underlying rhythm is sinus with 2:1 AV block. The QRS complex of sinus origin is labeled S, a paced beat P, and F represents a probable fusion beat with little if any contribution by the pacemaker. The long arrows indicate normal stimulus artifacts followed by ventricular depolarization. The small arrows with stars indicate attenuated subthreshold stimulus artifacts. Current is still reaching the heart along the lead but is limited by the high impedance at the fracture site. Prior to these subthreshold stimulus artifacts, there is no ECG evidence of pulse generator output because of complete lead discontinuity at the fracture site. This rhythmic variation of the stimulus artifacts probably represents a respiratory cycle with complete discontinuity with inspiration. There is an unexplained minor variation in the stimulus artifact repetition rate.

Undesirably Competitive Pulse Generator Output

Failure to sense the P or QRS waves may result either from a fault in the pulse generator or electrode lead system or from the size and type of potentials produced by the myocardium (Table 28-6). Chest wall stimulation (Chapter 105) is useful in differentiating a pulse generator defect from a myocardial cause of undersensing.

Slow or Irregular Pulse Generator Output in the Synchronous Mode

Slowing of the pulse generator output only in the synchronous mode implies oversensing. Intermittent oversensing produces an irregular output whereas persistent oversensing may appear as a decreased rate or total inhibition of the synchronous output. As seen in Table 28-6, oversensing may oc-

TABLE 28-5 Malfunctions Related to the QRS and T Wave

I. Capture intermittent or absent
  A. True malfunction
    1. Improper electrode-lead position
      a. Incorrectly placed at implant, e.g., coronary sinus displacement: dislodgment or perforation
    2. Pulse generator voltage output to heart below pacing threshold
      a. Power source failing
      b. Current leakage, loss of insulation
      c. Output circuit random component failure
    3. Increased pacing threshold
      a. Exit block—fibrosis?
      b. Myocardial infarction
      c. Severe metabolic imbalance
      d. Drug overdose, e.g., antiarrhythmics, antidepressants
    4. High resistance in electrode-lead system (e.g., lead conductor partial fracture)
  B. Pseudomalfunction
    1. Misinterpretation of ECG (e.g., threshold testing)

TABLE 28-6 Malfunctions Related to Sensing

- I. Output undesirably competitive (undersensing)
  - A. True malfunction
    - 1. Pulse generator
      - *a.* Power source failure
      - *b.* Reed switch stuck in asynchronous mode
      - *c.* Sensing circuit random component failure
      - *d.* Reprogramming sensitivity
    - 2. Electrode-lead system
      - *a.* Loss of insulation
      - *b.* Improper electrode-lead position
    - 3. Myocardium (size of QRS)
      - *a.* Broad QRS (poor slew rate)
      - *b.* Reduced size of QRS
  - B. Pseudomalfunction
    - 1. Misinterpretation ECG
      - *a.* Fusion beats
      - *b.* Ventricular triggered pacing
    - 2. Faulty recording
      - *a.* Magnet applied during test or synchronous mode
      - *b.* Asynchronous testing labeled as synchronous mode
- II. Synchronous output slowed or irregular (oversensing)
  - A. True malfunction
    - 1. Cardiac source: P wave, T wave, or concealed ventricular ectopics
    - 2. Pacemaker source: after-potentials, partial lead fracture, current leakage from pulse generator, loose connections, insulation break
    - 3. Skeletal source: muscle beneath implanted pulse generator
    - 4. Extracorporeal source: electromagnetic or radiofrequency
  - B. Pseudomalfunction
    - 1. Misinterpretation of ECG
      - *a.* Pulse generator inhibition owing to test magnet placement or removal
      - *b.* Hysteresis interpreted as oversensing
      - *c.* VVT interpreted as VVI
    - 2. Faulty recording
      - *a.* Monitoring equipment faulty
      - *b.* ECG recorder speed variable

cur from four sources: cardiac, pacemaker, skeletal, and extracorporeal. Myopotentials produced by contracting skeletal muscle represent a common cause of oversensing, but despite an apparent high incidence of this problem, significant clinical symptoms are unusual (Figure 28-17).

Extracorporeal pulse generator interference resulting in oversensing is a vast topic which has generated a great deal of interest and publicity. However, it is nevertheless only very occasionally a significant clinical problem today. Protection devices include electronic barriers, metal encapsulation of the pulse generator, and reversion to the asynchronous mode in the presence of recognized interference. A number of common potential problems appear unfounded. Microwave oven irradiation represents high-frequency interference that is easily rejected by modern pacemaker systems.[27] Airport security magnetometers do not affect conventional implanted pulse generators.[57] However, potential and documented interference may still occur with surgical diathermy,[27] arc welding,[27] radar installations,[27] telephone transformers,[27] and high-tension electric fields.[58]

FIGURE 28-17 ECG lead II demonstrating skeletal myopotential inhibition. The fine tremor represents isometric pectoral muscle contractions.

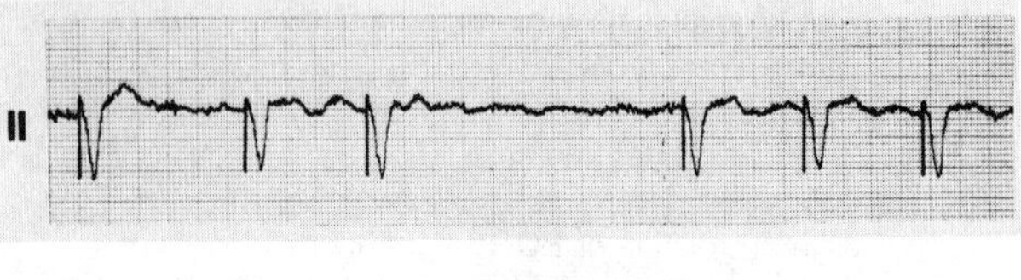

Normal Function of Pacemaker Systems

On occasion, investigation of apparent pacemaker system malfunction reveals no problem but the patient may have a side effect from the pacemaker system.

Pacemaker System Produces Side Effects

Pacemaker side effects can be divided into physical or psychologic (Table 28-7). The problems of pulse generator erosion and infection have diminished significantly in recent years. Preerosion can be diagnosed when an area of reddening develops, usu-

TABLE 28-7 Pacemaker Side Effects (Functioning Normally)

- I. Physical side effects
  - A. Placement of pacemaker system, causing
    - 1. Erosion or preerosion
    - 2. Infection
      - *a.* Local
      - *b.* Septicemia or endocarditis
    - 3. Failure to heal
    - 4. Pain
      - *a.* Local
      - *b.* Remote, anginal, or pericardial
    - 5. Venous thrombosis or stenosis
    - 6. Pulmonary emboli or lead migration into pulmonary artery
    - 7. Pacemaker twiddler's syndrome (lead dislodgment may occur)
    - 8. Allergy to components
    - 9. Pericardial tamponade owing to lead perforation
    - 10. Carcinoma of breast
  - B. Pacing causing undesirable stimulation
    - 1. Skeletal muscle stimulation
    - 2. Diaphragmatic, direct, or via phrenic nerve
    - 3. Ventricular fibrillation with asynchronous pacing
  - C. Defibrillation of electrosurgery, causing
    - 1. Pacemaker malfunction
    - 2. Cardiac burning or infarction at electrode site
  - D. Physiotherapy short-wave treatment with local heat production
  - E. Pacemaker syndrome
- II. Psychological side effects
  - A. Frequent self-detection of ectopic beats, distressing patient
  - B. Enforced reliance on pacing system by patient, causing psychologic disturbance
  - C. Attempted suicide using pacemaker system

ally on a corner of an implanted pulse generator site. Although bacterial endocarditis on an endocardial lead is rare, sustained bacteremia or septicemia can occur in 1 to 3 percent of patients; the usual organism is a *Staphylococcus*.[59] Clinical evidence of recurrent pulmonary emboli secondary to thrombosis around a permanent lead is surprisingly rare, even if the thrombotic material is infected. Symptomatic local venous thrombosis induced by pacemaker leads is also very uncommon.

The pacemaker-twiddler's syndrome is due to repeated turning of the implanted pulse generator under the skin, which results in lead retraction from the endocardium.[27] Skeletal muscle may be stimulated locally by the indifferent plate of the unipolar system or from a loss of lead insulation. Myocardial burning may occur with dc electrocardioversion or surgical diathermy and is due to the electric discharge transmitted along the lead. Physiotherapy short-wave treatment may result in local heat production, thus damaging the pulse generator or surrounding tissues.

The pacemaker syndrome is a physiologic disturbance caused by a normal ventricular-inhibited pacemaker system inserted in a patient with intact ventriculoatrial conduction. A retrograde P wave or ventriculoatrial conduction follows each ventricular complex. In some patients, this retrograde atrial conduction may have a negative effect on cardiac output. The result is vertigo, lightheadedness, syncope, and hypotension.[60] The problem is cured with a DVI pacemaker system.

Psychologic side effects following pacemaker system implantation can be minimized through careful explanation of the procedure to the patient and relatives beforehand. In the elderly age group, depression is common. The patient may fear that the inevitable battery failure will produce a further crisis in his or her life or that he or she is being run by an artificial device. There have been suicide attempts by patients endeavoring to damage the pacemaker system.

References

1. Lidwill, M. C.: Cardiac Disease in Relation to Anaesthesia, in Transactions of the Third Session, Australasian Medical Congress (British Medical Association), Sydney, Australia, September 2–7, 1929, p. 160.
2. Schechter, D. C.: Background of Clinical Cardiac Electrostimulation. V. Direct Electrostimulation of Heart without Thoracotomy, *N.Y. State J. Med.*, 72:605, 1972.
3. Hyman, A. S.: Resuscitation of the Stopped Heart by Intracardial Therapy: II. Experimental Use of an Artificial Pacemaker, *Arch. Intern. Med.*, 50:278, 1982.
4. Mond, H. G., Sloman, J. G., and Edwards, R. H.: The First Pacemaker, *PACE*, 5:278, 1982.
5. Schechter, D. C.: Background of Clinical Cardiac Electrostimulation. VII. Modern Era of Artificial Cardiac Pacemakers. *N.Y. State J. Med.*, 72:1166, 1972.
6. Pomerantz, B., and O'Rourke, R. A.: The Stokes-Adams Syndrome, *Am. J. Med.*, 46:941, 1969.
7. Penton, G. B., Miller, H., and Levine, S. A.: Some Clinical Features of Complete Heart Block, *Circulation*, 13:801, 1956.
8. Mond, H., Tartaglia, S., Cole, A., and Sloman, G.: The Refurbished Pulse Generator, *PACE*, 3:311, 1980.
9. Lev, M., and Bharati, S.: Atrioventricular and Intraventricular Conduction Disease, *Arch. Intern. Med.*, 135:405, 1975.
10. Narula, O. S.: Prognostic Value of H-V Interval and New Interpretations of Bundle Branch Block Patterns, in D. Kelly (ed.), "Advances in the Management of Arrhythmias," Telectronics Pty. Ltd., Sydney, Australia, 1978, p. 374.
11. Scheinman, M. M., Peters, R. W., Modin, G., Brennan, M., Mies, C., and O'Young, J.: Prognostic Value of Infranodal Conduction Time in Patients with Chronic Bundle Branch Block, *Circulation*, 56:240, 1977.
12. Morquio, L.: Sure une maladie infantile et familiale caracterisee par des modifications permanents du pouls des attaques syncopales et epileptiformes et al morte subite, *Arch. Med. Enf.*, 4:467, 1901.
13. Levy, A. M., Camm, A. J., and Keane, J. F.: Multiple Arrhythmias Detected during Nocturnal Monitoring in Patients with Congenital Complete Heart Block, *Circulation*, 55:247, 1977.
14. Brown, R. W., Hunt, D., and Sloman, J. G.: The Natural History of Atrioventricular Conduction Defects in Acute Myocardial Infarction, *Am. Heart J.*, 78:460, 1969.
15. Hinderman, M. C., Wagner, G. S., JaRo, M., Atkins, J. M., Scheinman, M. M., DeSanctis, R. W., Hutter, A. H., Yeatman, L., Rubenfire, M., Pujura, C., Rubin, M., and Morris, J. J.: The Clinical Significance of Bundle Branch Block Complication in Acute Myocardial Infarction: 2. Indications for Temporary and Permanent Pacemaker Insertion, *Circulation*, 58:689, 1978.
16. Mond, H. G.: Indications for Cardiac Pacing, in J. W. Hurst (ed.), "Update V. The Heart," McGraw-Hill, New York, 1981.
17. Kaplan, B. M., Langendorf, R., Lev, M., and Pick, A.: Tachycardia-Bradycardia Syndrome (so-called 'Sick Sinus Syndrome"), Pathology, Mechanisms and Treatment, *Am. J. Cardiol.*, 31:497, 1973.
18. Ferrer, M. I.: The Sick Sinus Syndrome, *Circulation*, 47:635, 1973.
19. Caralis, D. G., and Vanghese, P. J.: Familial Sinoatrial Node Dysfunction Increased Vagal Tone and Possible Aetiology, *Br. Heart J.*, 38:951, 1976.
20. Greenwood, R. D., Rosenthal, A., Sloss, L. J., LaCorte, M., and Nadas, A. S.: Sick Sinus Syndrome after Surgery for Congenital Heart Disease, *Circulation*, 52:295, 1975.
21. Chokshi, D. S., Mascarenhas, E., Samet, P., and Center, S.: Treatment of Sinoatrial Rhythm Disturbances with Permanent Cardiac Pacing, *Am. J. Cardiol.*, 32:215, 1973.
22. Wohl, A. J., Laborde, N. J., Atkins, J. M., Blomquist, C. G., and Mullens, C. B.: Prognosis of Patients Permanently Paced for Sick Sinus Syndrome, *Arch. Intern. Med.*, 136:406, 1976.
23. Walter, P. F., Crawley, I. S., and Dorney, E. R.: Carotid Sinus Hypersensitivity and Syncope, *Am. J. Cardiol.*, 42:396, 1978.
24. Amram, S. S., Vagueiro, M. C., Pimenta, A., and Machado, H. B.: Persistent Atrial Standstill with Atrial Inexcitability, *PACE* 1:80, 1978.
25. Merx, W., Han, J., and Yoon, M.: Effects of Unipolar Cathodal and Bipolar Stimulation on Vulnerability of Ischemic Ventricles to Fibrillation, *Am. J. Cardiol.*, 35:37, 1975.
26. Timmis, G. C., Helland, J., Westveer, D. C., Stewart, J., and Gordon, S.: The Evolution of Low Threshold Leads, *Clin. Prog. in Pacing and Electrophysiology*, 1:313, 1983.
27. Mond, H. G.: "The Cardiac Pacemaker: Function and Malfunction." Grune & Stratton, New York, 1983.
28. Kertes, P., Mond, H., Sloman, G., Vohra, J., and Hunt, D.: Comparison of Lead Complications with Polyurethane Tined, Silicone Rubber Tined and Wedge Tip Leads: Clinical Experience with 822 Ventricular Endocardial Leads, *PACE* 6:957, 1983.
29. Sloman, J. G., Mond, H. G., Bailey, B., Cole, A., and Duffield, A.: The Use of Balloon Tipped Electrodes for Permanent Cardiac Pacing, *PACE*, 2:579, 1979.
30. Bisping, H. J., Kreuger, J., Kirkenheier, H.: Three Years' Clinical Experience with a New Endocardial Screw-in Lead

with Introduction Protection for Use in the Atrium and Ventricle, *PACE* 3:424, 1980.
31. Kruse, I., Ryden, L., and Ydse, B.: A New Lead for Transvenous Atrial Pacing and Sensing, *PACE* 3:395, 1980.
32. Curzio, G., Alliengro, A., Santini, M., and Capriolo, V.: A New Passive Fixation Transvenous Atrial Lead: Clinical Experience, *PACE,* 4:A-39, 1981 (Abstract).
33. Kleinert, M.: Permanent Atrial Leads, *PACE,* 3:487, 1980.
34. Ellestad, M. H., Messenger, J., Greenberg, P., and Castellanet, J. M.: The Use of Coronary Sinus Pacing, in H. J. Th. Thalen and J. W. Harthorne (eds.), "To Pace or Not to Pace," Martinus Nijhoff, The Hague, 1978, p. 156.
35. Bognolo, D., Stoker, K., Wiebush, W., Vljayanager, R., Eckstein, P., and Cromastie, S.: Experimental and Clinical Study of a New Permanent Myocardial Atrial Sutureless Pacing Lead (abstr.), *PACE,* 4:A-35, 1981.
36. Mansour, K. A., Fleming, W. H., and Hatcher, C. R.: Initial Experience with a Sutureless Screw-in Electrode for Cardiac Pacing, *Ann. Thorac. Surg.,* 16:127, 1973.
37. Martin, C. M., and Kleid, J. J.: Pseudofusion Beats Masquerading as Pacemaker Failure, *J. Electrocardiol.,* 7(2):179, 1974.
38. Barold, S. S., Ong, L. S., and Heinle, R. A.: Electrocardiographic Diagnosis of Myocardial Infarction in Patients with Transvenous Pacemakers, *J. Electrocardiol.,* 9:99, 1976.
39. Castellanos, A., Zoble, R., Procacci, P. M., Myerburg, R. J., and Berkovitz, B. V.: St-qR Pattern: New Sign of Diagnosis of Anterior Myocardial Infarction during Right Ventricular Pacing, *Br. Heart J.,* 35:1161, 1973.
40. Barold, S. S., Ong, L. S., and Banner, R. L.: Diagnosis of Inferior Wall Myocardial Infarction during Right Ventricular Apical Pacing, *Chest,* 69:232, 1976.
41. Parsonnet, V., Furman, S., and Smyth, N. P. D.: Implantable Cardiac Pacemakers: Status Report and Resource Guideline. Report of the Inter-Society Commission for Heart Disease Resources, *Am. J. Cardiol.,* 34:487, 1974.
42. Parsonnet, V., Furman, S., and Smyth, N. P. D.: A Revised Code for Pacemaker Identification, *PACE* 4:400, 1981.
43. Barold, S. S., Falkoff, M. D., Ong, L. S., and Heinle, R. A.: Interpretation of Electrocardiogram Produced by a New Unipolar Multiprogrammable "Committed" AV Sequential Demand (DVI) Pulse Generator, *PACE* 4:692, 1981.
44. Tolentino, A. O., Javier, R. P., Byrd, C., and Samet, P.: Pacer-Induced Tachycardia Associated with an Atrial Synchronous Ventricular Inhibited (ASVIP) Pulse Generator, *PACE* 5:251, 1982.
45. Goldreyer, B. N.: Physiologic Pacing: The Role of AV Synchrony, *PACE* 5:613, 1982.
46. Karlof, I.: Haemodynamic Effect of Atrial Triggered Versus Fixed Rate Pacing at Rest and During Exercise in Complete Heart Block, *Acta. Med. Scand.,* 197:195, 1975.
47. Santini, M., MacCarter, D., Knudson, M., and Alliegro, A.: Automatic Atrial Rate Responsive VVI Pacing: A Simple Physiologic Approach, *PACE* 4:A-72, 1981.
48. Humen, D. P., Anderson, K., Brumwell, D., Huntley, S., and Klein, G. J.: A Pacemaker Which Automatically Increases Its Rate with Physical Activity. Cardiac Pacing, in K. Steinbach, D. Glogan, A. Lasykovics, W. Scheibelhofer, and H. Weber (eds.), Proceedings of the VIIth World Symposium on Cardiac Pacing. Steinkopff Verlag, Darmstadt, 1983, p. 259.
49. Rickards, A. F., Donaldson, R. M. and Thalen, H. J. Th.: The Use of QT Interval to Determine Pacing Rate: Early Clinical Experience, *PACE* 6:346, 1983.
50. Cammilli, L., Alcidi, L., Shapland, E., and Obino, S.: Results, Problems and Perspectives with the Autoregulating Pacemaker, *PACE* 6:488, 1983.
51. Griffin, J. C., Jutzy, K. R., Claude, J. P., and Knutti, J. W.: Central Body Temperature as a Guide to Optimal Heart Rate, *PACE* 6:498, 1983.
52. Wirtzfeld, A., Heinze, R., Liess, H. D., Stangl, K., and Alt, E.: An Active Optical Sensor for Monitoring Mixed Venous Oxygen Saturation for an Implantable Rate Regulating Pacing System, *PACE* 6:494, 1983.
53. Rossi, P., Plicchi, G., Canducci, G., Rognoni, G., and Aina, F.: Respiratory Rate as a Determinant of Optimal Pacing Rate, *PACE,* 6:502, 1983.
54. Waxman, M., Wald, R. W., Bonet, J. F., MacGregor, D. C., and Goldman, B. S.: Self Conversion of Supraventricular Tachycardia by Rapid Atrial Pacing, *PACE,* 1:35, 1978.
55. Furman, S.: Pacemaker Programmability, *PACE,* 1:161, 1978.
56. Runaway Protection of CPI Implantable Pacemakers, CPI. Tech. Issues, Number 11, Cardiac Pacemakers Incorporated, St. Paul, Minn.
57. Smyth, N. P. D., Keshishian, J. M., Hood, O. C., Hoffman, A. A., Baker, N. R., and Podolak, E.: Effect of an Active Magnetometer on Permanently Implanted Pacemakers, *JAMA,* 221:162, 1972.
58. Butrous, G. S., Bexton, R. S., Barton, D. G., Male, J. C., and Camm, A. J.: Interference with the Pacemakers of Two Workers at Electricity Substations, *Br. J. Ind. Med.,* 40:462, 1983.
59. Morgan, G., Ginks, W., Siddons, H., and Leatham, A.: Septicemia in Patients with an Endocardial Pacemaker, *Am. J. Cardiol.,* 44:221, 1979.
60. Miller, M., Fox, S., Jenkins, R., Schwartz, J., and Toonder, R. G.: Pacemaker Syndrome: A Non-invasive Means to Its Diagnosis and Treatment, *PACE,* 4:503, 1981.

29

Syncope: Pathophysiology and Differential Diagnosis

Arnold M. Weissler, M.D.   James V. Warren, M.D.

Syncope is a sudden and, by definition, transient disruption of consciousness which may occur in individuals under environmental stress or which may result from a wide range of underlying disease. Presyncope and near syncope are less well-defined entities, but probably represent lesser degrees of the same disorder. Diagnostically, syncope and presyncope must be differentiated from coma, narcolepsy, epilepsy, hysteria, sleep, and sudden death. Although at times laboratory studies are required to exclude such diagnoses, the nature of the episode is usually obvious. The physician's role then is to distinguish between the benign and relatively inconsequential forms of syncope and those which are ominous signals of serious underlying disease. This chapter deals with the broad range of causes of syncope and their mechanisms. Chapter 30 focuses on the particular problems in the recognition and evaluation of *cardiac* syncope.

The maintenance of a state of full consciousness depends on a normally active brain. Anything that disturbs brain function such as circulatory inadequacy, electrical dysfunction, metabolic deficiencies, or the influence of drugs may suddenly alter brain function.

The word *syncope* means "to cut short" and indeed that is exactly what happens to consciousness in the syncopal episode. At times there may be premonitory sensations and drifting off of consciousness, but more often the episode occurs with alarming rapidity. There may be associated manifestations such as convulsive movements, loss of bladder control, general pallor, and sweating.

Syncope, even the benign common faint, can be an alarming episode. The general picture may indicate to those observing that the patient has suddenly dropped dead. On the other hand, there may be much less sagging of the level of consciousness, with an episode of short duration which is quick to terminate (presyncope). Patients and their families are usually apprehensive about even minimal episodes. The physician can often supply great reassurance, which is itself a positive therapeutic influence, even while he or she is alert to the possibility of more ominous causes of the episode.

In the past, descriptions of syncope were largely restricted to a pathophysiologic analysis of the various types and a clinical description of their characteristics. This is still important, but in contemporary medicine the key issue for the physician is to make the fundamental distinction of whether the episode is a common faint or an indication of a serious underlying problem. Episodes of syncope should warn physicians that an extensive and detailed evaluation is in order. For example, an episode of syncope in a high school basketball player may indicate that the individual has some underlying abnormality such as a congenital anomaly of the coronary arteries or an obstructive cardiomyopathy which not only renders him susceptible to syncope, but also makes him a candidate for sudden death. A preventive approach in such an instance could avoid a mysterious sudden death on the gymnasium floor. Similarly, an episode of unconsciousness in an elderly individual may uncover serious disorders of the cardiac conduction system which might lead to sudden death. Today, the preventive use of cardiac pacemakers in persons identified with this type of disorder may again lead to the avoidance of sudden death. It can be seen, therefore, that it is imperative for the physician to recognize the various types of syncope and to be aware of the situations where a careful evaluation is indicated. This ability becomes the primary goal in a physician's study of the problems of syncope.

For the purpose of clinical analysis, it is convenient to classify syncope (or presyncope) into three major categories[1]: vasodepressor, cardiovascular, and noncardiovascular (Table 29-1). In the following discussion we will present a practical approach to the differential diagnosis of syncope, emphasizing a diagnostic evaluation based on the clinical picture and pathophysiologic mechanisms in these three basic subgroups.

Vasodepressor Syncope

Central to the large cluster of disorders causing transient unconsciousness is vasodepressor syncope (the common faint).[2] Approximately 15 to 25 percent of young individuals experience one or more

TABLE 29-1 Basic Diagnosis of Syncope

Vasodepressor syncope (common faint)
Cardiovascular syncope
Cardiac syncope
Obstructive
Arrhythmic
Vascular syncope
Noncardiovascular syncope

episodes of vasodepressor syncope at some time during early adolescence. Vasodepressor syncope usually occurs early in life and is rare after 35 years of age in otherwise normal individuals. The clinical characteristics are usually diagnostic. However, in the patient with recurrent vasodepressor syncope a careful history and physical examination should be obtained to rule out an underlying organic cause. Clinical recognition of the vasodepressor syncope syndrome can save unnecessary anxiety and expensive laboratory study. Thorough knowledge of the clinical picture of the common faint is critical in evaluating patients complaining of syncope.

Vasodepressor syncope may occur as a response to sudden emotional stress or in a setting of real, threatened, or fantasied injury.[3] The reaction is not infrequently brought on by venipuncture or the sight of blood and is also observed after a sudden, painful experience such as surgical manipulation or following severe tissue injury. It is particularly likely to occur in certain environmental settings, such as in a hot and crowded room, especially if the individual is fatigued, hungry, ill, or has recently experienced blood loss. The common faint usually occurs when the patient is upright or sitting, but may rarely occur while the patient is recumbent. Clinically it is characterized by a fall in arterial pressure associated with impairment or loss of consciousness and loss of postural tone accompanied by variable degrees of autonomic overactivity evidenced by pallor, sweating, nausea, mydriasis, hypotension, and bradycardia.

Less dramatic than the sudden collapse, but equally important in recognizing the clinical syndrome, are the premonitory symptoms of the fainting reaction. These changes occur gradually and may appear minutes before loss of consciousness and postural tone. Often pallor is noted first, accompanied by beads of perspiraton. The patient soon experiences epigastric discomfort, frequently likened to nausea, but often distinguished as a separate sensation. Close observation reveals pupillary dilation, and the individual reports the occurrence of visual blurring just prior to loss of consciousness. Although bradycardia is often present at the time of unconsciousness, the premonitory phase of the fainting reaction is most often associated with a relatively rapid heart rate. When the person suffering a syncopal reaction is allowed to rest head down, consciousness is rapidly regained, while the relative bradycardia persists. Of additional importance in the overall clinical picture of vasodepressor syncope are the postsyncopal findings of persistence of pallor, nausea, weakness, and sweating with a tendency toward recurrence of the reaction if the individual prematurely returns to an upright posture.

The hemodynamic mechanisms responsible for vasodepressor syncope have intrigued physicians for over a century. Although it was first thought that fainting might represent a severe depression of cardiac output, measurements have demonstrated little decline in cardiac output beyond that which occurs with assumption of the head-up posture. The entire reaction may develop in the absence of a diminution in cardiac output. It is rather the marked and consistent fall in total peripheral vascular resistance that is the essential hemodynamic factor responsible for the fall in arterial pressure and the diminished perfusion pressure to the brain in vasodepressor syncope. The peripheral hemodynamic factors responsible for the marked fall in arterial pressure were first suggested in observations by John Hunter in 1793, when he wrote, "I bled a lady but she fainted and while she continued in the fit the colour of the blood that came from the vein was a fine scarlet." This description of arterialization of venous blood was the first observation reflecting on the greatly increased skeletal muscle blood flow during fainting, a finding which has been confirmed repeatedly in studies employing plethysmographic techniques. From such studies it is apparent that vascular resistance in the skeletal muscle bed is markedly reduced. Resistance is reduced, as well, in other major vascular areas, such as the mesenteric, renal, and cerebral beds. Of particular relevance to the circulatory mechanisms underlying vasodepressor syncope is the fact that the fall in total peripheral resistance is not compensated by a rise in cardiac output, a phenomenon which occurs regularly in normal individuals in the presence of widespread vascular dilatation. Why the heart fails to respond to this stimulus is not entirely clear. Vagal inhibition may be a contributory factor. However, laboratory-induced vasodepressor syncope has been observed when the vagal-induced bradycardia is entirely blocked by atropine.

Present evidence favors the concept that the failure of the heart to respond to the fall in peripheral resistance results dominantly from postural shifts in blood volume to the lower extremities and abdomen. The shift in intravascular volume is sufficient to induce a diminution in the volume of the central venous reservoir with a resultant decrease in the rate of ventricular filling. Stroke volume and hence the cardiac output response is thus limited. Peripheral venodilatation which of itself could impair ventricular filling is not an important contributing factor. In fact, active venoconstriction appears to be the predominant response during vasodepressor syncope. The venoconstriction, however, does not provide sufficient restoration of central blood volume to permit an adequate cardiac output response. Thus, the failure of the cardiac output to increase in the presence of a profound fall in peripheral arterial resistance accounts for the marked decrease in arterial pressure and the diminished perfusion to the brain in vasodepressor syncope. Studies have demonstrated a diminished rise in plasma renin activity during upright tilt among subjects who are prone to posturally induced vasodepressor syncope. These observations suggest that the renin-angiotensin system may play a role in postural circulatory adjustments and may thus influence the development of vasodepressor syncope.

In a comprehensive study of a young woman with reproducible episodes of vasodepressor syncope, Goldstein and associates demonstrated that hypotension preceded the bradycardia and that cardiac pacing as well as atropine failed to reverse the hypotension.[4] The patient exhibited no increase in plasma norepinephrine during vasodepressor attacks. Between episodes, norepinephrine responses to standing, exercise, and pharmacologically induced vasodilation remained normal. These data corroborate evidence that bradycardia is not the primary basis for the hypotension in vasodepressor syncope. It would appear from this study that inhibition of sympathetic neural responsiveness to hypotension may be a factor contributing to the failure of the cardiac output to compensate for the fall in peripheral resistance in vasodepressor syncope. Of note was the finding that plasma renin activity doubled at the peak of an episode of vasodepressor syncope reflecting, most probably, a shunting of blood flow from the kidneys. A net increase in circulatory vasodilator substances in syncope were tested for by injecting the patient's plasma, obtained at rest and at the peak of a hypotensive episode, into a bilaterally nephrectomized pentolinium pretreated rat. No hypotensive response was elicited.

The onset of unconsciousness in syncope is associated with the sudden appearance in the electroencephalogram of large-amplitude slow-wave activity. This dramatic change in the electroencephalogram occurs only after severe diminution in mean arterial pressure (average mean arterial pressure of 25 mmHg at heart level) and is accompanied by a fall in cerebral blood flow to 50 to 70 percent of normal. Accompanying the common faint is usually a moderate-to-severe degree of hyperventilation, most probably the result of associated anxiety as well as the cerebral hypoxia. Associated with the hyperventilation is a fall in the arterial carbon dioxide content. The lowering of cerebral blood flow by hypocapnia may serve to accentuate the circulatory embarrassment in vasodepressor syncope.

An intriguing aspect of the fainting reaction is postsyncopal oliguria, which appears to be related to excessive secretion of antidiuretic hormone. The possible role of the posterior pituitary substance in inducing some of the other clinical manifestations in syncope, i.e., pallor and nausea, has been suggested by some investigators.

The precipitating event in vasodepressor syncope has been the subject of considerable speculation. Vasodepressor syncope often occurs in the normal person in the upright posture and under circumstances that he or she finds distasteful. The association between emotional factors and vasodepressor syncope was first described by Charles Darwin and in later years elaborated on by Engel and Romano.[3] A possible neurogenic mechanism connecting the emotional and cardiovascular changes in the syncopal responses has been suggested recently by Wallin and Sundlöff,[5] who were able to record sympathetic vasoconstrictor impulses with microelectrodes in peroneal muscle nerve fascicles during the induction of vasodepressor syncope in two normal subjects. After a premonitory period of increased nerve activity, syncope was associated with a sudden cessation of sympathetic nerve outflow. These data are consistent with the failure of norepinephrine plasma levels to increase in vasodepressor syncope and support the view that the fall in peripheral resistance during vasodepressor syncope may be caused or accentuated by a marked inhibition of sympathetic vasoconstrictor impulses. The mechanisms underlying the sudden attenuation of sympathetic nervous activity require further study.

Although vasodepressor syncope can often be observed in individuals with a normal circulation, the syncopal reaction is not uncommon in patients with certain cardiovascular diseases.[1] The hemodynamic mechanisms causing fainting under these circumstances may be similar to those in the normal person, and the fall in peripheral resistance is often precipitated by emotional arousal and exercise. This type of syncope may be observed in patients with aortic stenosis, various forms of congenital heart disease, and in primary pulmonary hypertension where the circulatory disorder offers a major impediment to cardiac responsiveness. Cardiac arrhythmias often contribute to the syncope in these conditions. Profound arterial hypoxia due to sudden increases in right-to-left shunting during the fall in peripheral arterial resistance (physiologic afterload reduction) in patients with cyanotic congenital heart disease (e.g., tetralogy of Fallot) may accentuate the cerebral hypoxia. Occasionally, vasodepressor syncope occurs early in the course of acute myocardial infarction (most commonly inferior myocardial infarction) or during a severe attack of angina pectoris (often associated with administration of nitrates or other vasodilators). In addition to vasodepressor syncope, fainting due to a complicating cardiac arrhythmia must always be considered in the patient with severe coronary artery disease. Vasodepressor syncope may be the presenting event in other cardiovascular catastrophes such as pulmonary embolism and aortic dissection. In the latter, obstruction to the brachiocephalic vessels by the aortic dissection may sensitize the patient to cerebral hypoxia and syncope.

Syncope is often noted in patients with acute or chronic anemia and in individuals who have received surgical or pharmacologic sympathectomies. Under these circumstances, the lowered blood volume or the diminished vascular responsiveness in the upright posture creates a hemodynamic setting predisposing to the fainting reaction. Vasodepressor syncope of an unusual type may occur in pregnancy. It is notable that this form of syncope may actually be precipitated by lying down and relieved by standing. Syncope has also been noted to occur following strenuous exercise, after the intake of vasodilating drugs, in patients receiving various tranquilizing agents, and in those receiving L-dopa for Parkinson's disease. Fainting is particularly likely to occur in the course of acute febrile infections and following prolonged recumbency in chronic illness. Normal persons at bed rest for several days have a propensity for fainting, particularly when they arise abruptly from the recumbent position. A problem of importance in aviation and space medicine is the vasodepressor syncope occurring during acceleration, particularly when centrifugal force is applied in the head-to-foot position. Vasodepressor syncope is probably the most frequent cause of cardiovascular collapse during dental manipulations.

Therapy for vasodepressor syncope consists of placing the patient in a recumbent position with the head lower than the body. When profound bradycardia persists, intravenous atropine may be required. Rarely, vasopressor therapy is needed to control prolonged hypotension associated with vasodepressor syncope.

The terms *vasodepressor* and *vasovagal syncope* are often used interchangeably in describing this syndrome. The former term emphasizes the fall in peripheral resistance and arterial pressure, the latter the associated vagal-induced bradycardia. We prefer the term *vasodepressor syncope,* since the vagal factors appear to result from the cerebral hypoxia and are not the primary cause for the syncope.

Cardiovascular Syncope

If a fainting episode is found not to be typical for vasodepressor syncope, then one must consider two additional general causes, cardiovascular and noncardiovascular (Table 29-1). Cardiovascular causes for syncope are conveniently considered in terms of two subgroups, cardiac and vascular syncope. Chapter 30 is devoted to a comprehensive discussion of cardiac syncope. The current discussion will hence focus on vascular syncope and syncope of noncardiovascular cause.

Vascular Syncope

Vascular syncope is conveniently divided into five major categories: orthostatic, cerebrovascular, carotid sinus, reflex, and less common forms of vascular syncope (Table 29-2). The following discussion will follow this classification.

TABLE 29-2 Vascular Syncope

Orthostatic syncope (orthostatic hypotension)
Syncope in cerebrovascular disease
Carotid sinus syncope
Reflex syncope
Less common forms of vascular syncope

Orthostatic Syncope (Orthostatic Hypotension)

When the normal individual assumes the upright posture, the attendant gravitational stresses on the circulation are compensated for by several mechanisms, including reflex arteriolar and venous constriction, acceleration of heart rate, and mechanical factors such as the venous valvular system, mechanical pumping of the leg muscles, and a decrease in intrathoracic pressure. The increased sympathetic activity during upright posture, mediated via pressor receptors in the carotid sinus and the aortic arch, and probably by receptors at the junction of the atria with the pulmonary veins and venae cavae, is reflected in an increase in plasma catecholamine levels. Delayed activation of the renin-angiotensin-aldosterone system and possibly the secretion of vasopressin serves to sustain the vasoconstriction initiated by the more immediate baroreceptor and mechanical responses. Orthostatic hypotension is a disorder in which assumption of the upright posture is associated with a prompt fall in arterial pressure, associated with lightheadedness, blurring of vision, and a sense of weakness and unsteadiness.[6,7] When individuals with chronic orthostatic hypotension are observed under laboratory conditions, the role of mechanical factors in maintaining arterial pressure in the upright posture is reflected in transient elevations in arterial pressure induced by leg motion, deep inspiration, or infusions of saline solution or blood volume expanders. Postural symptoms are often accentuated in the morning and are aggravated by heat, humidity, a heavy meal, and exercise. Hypotension is progressive over a period of seconds to minutes, depending upon the degree of loss in the adaptive processes, until perfusion pressure to the brain becomes insufficient to sustain cerebral blood flow, with consequent loss of consciousness. When the individual becomes recumbent, the arterial pressure rapidly returns to normal and consciousness is regained.

Orthostatic hypotension may result from two major physiologic disorders: (1) depletion of the total or central blood volume, and (2) loss or impairment of autonomic cardiovascular reflex activity. Clinically, both circumstances may coexist. In general, when total blood volume or central blood volume depletion through peripheral venous pooling is the primary cause of postural hypotension, in the presence of an intact autonomic nervous system, tachycardia, pallor, coldness of the extremities, and sweating are prominent accompaniments to the orthostatic hypotension. Because of the display of sympathetic nervous system activation, orthostatic hypotension in the presence of an intact autonomic nervous system is termed *hyperadrenergic orthostatic hypotension.*

Chronic orthostatic hypotension due to loss or impairment of autonomic reflexes is a manifestation of a profound deficiency in autonomic function. Among patients with orthostatic hypotension due to autonomic deficiency who are observed during the presyncopal period there is commonly little or no increase in heart rate and an absence of the marked pallor, sweating, and adrenergic manifestations which are usually observed during the hypotensive episode in vasodepressor syncope and hyperadrenergic orthostatic hypotension. Between episodes of fainting, patients with autonomic dysfunction and postural syncope often exhibit other evidence of defects in autonomic nervous system function (both sympathetic and parasympathetic), including impotence, disturbances of bladder and bowel function, heat intolerance, and loss of sweating. Urinary excretion of catecholamines and catecholamine metabolites are diminished and plasma catecholamine levels, which may be normal or diminished in the resting supine posture, fail to rise during head-up tilt or with exercise. Other manifestations of the autonomic imbalance include a decrease or absence of the arterial pressure overshoot in the Valsalva response, a drop in arterial pressure during supine exercise, increased pressor and cardiac responses to infused catecholamines, and increased sensitivity to catecholamine-induced mobilization of free fatty acids from adipose tissue. Whether secretion of renin and aldosterone upon assumption of the upright posture is consistently impaired in chronic autonomic nervous system deficiency remains controversial, although reduced plasma renin and aldosterone secretion have been observed in some patients with these disorders.

For purposes of differential diagnosis the causes of orthostatic hypotension are conveniently classified into three major categories: venous pooling and/or blood volume depletion, pharmacologically induced, and neurogenic (Table 29-3). Excessive venous pooling accounts for the postural hypotension accompanying prolonged bed rest, prolonged standing, pregnancy, marked venous varicosities, and a rare familial syndrome of hyperbradykinism due to deficient enzymatic degradation of bradykinin. Tall asthenic individuals with poorly developed musculature are particularly prone to postural hypotension. Blood volume depletion accounts for the orthostatic hypotension associated with dehydration, excessive diuresis, anemia, hemorrhage, excessive gastrointestinal fluid loss, third space sequestration, prolonged fever, renal dialysis, excessive perspiration, weightlessness, adrenal insufficiency, pheochromocytoma, and diabetes insipidus. Deconditioning of autonomic reflex vasoconstriction may add to the orthostatic hypotension associated with prolonged bed rest and following extended periods of weightlessness in astronauts.

TABLE 29-3 Basic Classification of Causes of Orthostatic Syncope*

Venous pooling and/or blood volume depletion
Pharmacologically induced
Neurogenic

*See text for detailed information.

Postural hypotension is a complicating side effect of a wide variety of pharmacologic agents including antihypertensives, diuretics, nitrates and other vasodilators, antidepressants, phenothiazines, other tranquilizers and antipsychotic agents, antiparkinsonian drugs, and CNS depressants.

Neurogenic postural hypotension has been observed in a wide variety of diseases affecting the autonomic nervous system, including peripheral neuropathies, spinal cord disease, intracranial tumors, parkinsonism, multiple cerebrovascular accidents, encephalopathies, paraneoplastic syndromes, and brainstem lesions.[8] Among specific disease entities in which postural hypotenson is not infrequently observed are diabetes mellitis, tabes dorsalis, syringomyelia, subacute combined sclerosis, polyneuropathy, Guillain-Barré syndrome, alcoholic neuropathy, Wernicke's encephalopathy, porphyria, amyloidosis, multiple sclerosis, Homes-Adie syndrome, familial dysautonomia (Riley-Day syndrome), traumatic and inflammatory myelopathies, posterior fossa and parasellar tumors, hydrocephalus, intramedullary and extramedullary tumors of the spinal cord, following multiple cerebrovascular accidents, primary aldosteronism with hypokalemia, pheochromocytoma, mitral valve prolapse, malignant hypertension, and after surgically induced sympathectomy.[9] Lesions of the spinal cord associated with autonomic failure sufficient to induce orthostatic hypotension are usually localized above the T6 level.

Elderly individuals are uniquely prone to episodes of postural hypotension.[10] It has been demonstrated that the elderly have diminished baroreceptor-mediated cardioacceleration in response to hypotensive stimuli and exhibit diminished cardiac slowing in response to increases in arterial pressure. Postprandial hypotension is frequently observed in the elderly.[11] The more frequent occurrence of disease states predisposing to postural hypotension and the common use of drugs affecting circulatory adaptation to postural stress, along with diminished autonomic responsiveness and postprandial postural hypotension, account for the high incidence of postural syncope in the aged.

Because of their pathophysiologic implications two syndromes in which orthostatic hypotension is the dominant manifestation have received considerable investigative attention in recent years. The first, an idiopathic form of chronic autonomic failure in which postural hypotension is accompanied by fixed heart rate, heat intolerance, anhidrosis, nocturnal polyuria, urinary and anal sphincter dysfunction, and impotency was reported in 1925 by Bradbury and Eggleston. The second, reported in 1960 by Shy and

Drager, is a syndrome of orthostatic hypotension accompanied by multiple neurologic manifestations of central nervous system disease. In recent years the former syndrome has been named *idiopathic orthostatic hypotension* (IOH) while the latter is termed *multiple system atrophy* (MSA).

Both IOH and MSA usually begin in middle age and occur more commonly in men than in women. In both forms of chronic autonomic dysfunction symptoms may appear gradually over a period of years. The central nervous system manifestations in MSA may be indistinguishable from idiopathic Parkinson's disease. The neurologic manifestations in MSA may appear several years after onset of orthostatic hypotension. In general, prognosis is worse in patients with MSA than IOH, death often resulting from general debilitation and its complications, pulmonary embolism, malnutrition, and pneumonia. Severe supine hypertension may complicate the presence of orthostatic hypotension in each of these entities. In IOH with isolated autonomic dysfunction the pathological process appears to be concentrated in the efferent sympathetic pathway. MSA appears to result from degenerative changes in the basal ganglia, substantia nigra, cerebellum, and other parts of the central nervous system including the dorsal nucleus of the vagus, pigmented brainstem nuclei, intermediate and lateral columns of the spinal chord, and sympathetic ganglia. Evidence for the differentiation of the site of autonomic degeneration in IOH and MSA is to be found in a host of pharmacologic, metabolic, and histochemical studies.[12–15] Thus, in the recumbent posture patients with IOH have low levels of plasma norepinephrine which fail to increase normally on assumption of the upright posture or with exercise. Patients with MSA tend to have normal plasma levels of norepinephrine in the recumbent posture which also fail to increase normally after standing or exertion. Both groups have low levels of plasma dopamine beta-hydroxylase. Patients with IOH demonstrate an absence of vasoconstriction in response to intraarterial administration of tyramine (an indirectly acting amine which releases norepinephrine), while patients with MSA syndrome show a significant vasoconstrictor response marked by a decrease in forearm blood flow in response to intraarterial tyramine. Patients with IOH have exaggerated vasoconstriction in response to intraarterial administration of norepinephrine, while patients with the MSA syndrome have normal vasoconstrictor responses to norepinephrine.

Urinary excretion of the major norepinephrine metabolites (3-methoxy-4-hydroxymandelic acid, 3-methoxy-4-hydroxy-phenylglycol, and normetanephrine) are decreased in parallel in patients with IOH. Patients with MSA excrete greater amounts of the deaminated metabolites than patients with IOH, while normetanephrine levels are diminished equivalent to that of patients with IOH.[16] Histochemical studies reveal the absence of catecholamine-specific fluorescence from perivascular nerve fibers in the walls of the blood vessels in muscle biopsies from patients with IOH.[13] Patients with MSA and moderate to severe autonomic failure also exhibit some reduction of catecholamine-specific fluorescence as well. However, electron microscopic studies suggest that patients with pure autonomic failure (IOH) have more extreme degeneration of adrenergic nerves than patients with MSA.[15]

The above studies are consistent with the hypothesis that patients with IOH have a primary defect in the efferent limb of the sympathetic nervous system resulting in loss of neurotransmitter norepinephrine from the nerve endings. The autonomic defect in patients with MSA, in contrast, appears to be located centrally or in part in the afferent pathways controlling the reflex adjustment to changes in posture. The occurrence of multiple degenerative lesions in the central nervous system supports a primary central nervous system defect. The peripheral adrenergic lesion in the MSA group would appear to be secondary to the central lesions. However, histochemical evidence favoring overlapping of the sites of the disorder (presynaptic versus postsynaptic) prompts caution in invoking a simple differentiation for all patients with IOH and MSA. The fact that some patients may present with isolated autonomic deficiency only to develop manifestations of central nervous system disease years later further complicates such a simple differentiation into central and peripheral loci of the disease. Further, in the population of patients with IOH there appear to be rare individuals with an isolated defect in peripheral noradrenaline release with otherwise intact peripheral autonomic nerves.[17] Other individuals with IOH may have isolated baroreceptor dysfunction with intact efferent sympathetic function. In general, the degree of deficiency in norepinephrine release, which is the ultimate basis for postural hypotension, is more profound when the nervous system defect is primarily peripheral than when it is central.

Multiple studies have suggested profound dysfunction of the parasympathetic system in patients with chronic autonomic dysfunction.[18] Studies on the effect of insulin-induced hypoglycemia in patients with IOH and MSA who retain diminished catecholamine responses reveal impaired release of pancreatic polypeptides. The response of pancreatic polypeptides, which in experimental studies is mediated via the vagus and is unaffected by splanchnic nerve section, lends strong evidence favoring parasympathetic involvement in IOH and MSA.[19,20]

The physiologic and metabolic characteristics of several other specific forms of postural hypotension have come under investigative analysis during the past decade. Recent evidence indicates that postural hypotension in diabetes may be associated with either exaggerated sympathetic responses related to a basic deficit in intravascular volume, specifically in erythrocyte mass, and/or a deficit in peripheral sympathetic arteriolar innervation.[21,22] Further, administration of insulin in the upright posture may lead to marked hypotension, in particular in patients with autonomic dysfunction.[23] The mechanism of the hypotension is presently unclear. In familial dysautonomia (Riley-Day syndrome), in which autonomic insufficiency becomes apparent at birth, postural hypotension is associated with hypersensitivity to intravenously infused catecholamines and normal resting catecholamines which fail to respond with upright posture.[24] With more detailed pharmacologic and metabolic studies among patients with orthostatic hypotension complicating other disease processes, it is expected that a clearer delineation of the nature of the autonomic disorders will evolve.

One cannot overemphasize the importance of a careful history and physical examination in the clinical evaluation of the patient with postural hypotension. In approaching the differential diagnosis the three fundamental clinical mechanisms for the causes of postural hypotension cited previously, venous pooling and/or blood volume depletion, pharmacologically induced, and neurogenic, should be kept in mind. The broad range of clinical entities which may induce orthostatic hypotension can promote a potentially extensive and costly laboratory evaluation. Thus, the laboratory evaluation should be highly selective and based on clinical impressions derived from a thorough basic clinical evaluation. In this regard, the diagnosis of autonomic dysfunction per se may now involve a host of laboratory studies designed to test the integrity of baroreceptor reflexes, vasomotor center responsiveness, efferent sympathetic fibers, efferent vagal fibers, cholinergic function, and extraadrenal stores of norepinephrine.[16–18] These tests should be applied in a stepwise analytic fashion and should be performed by individuals whose experience can ensure their critical interpretation.

Effective therapy in postural hypotension is closely linked to an accurate diagnosis. Primary emphasis must be based on treatable causes, in particular, pharmacologically induced postural hypotension, blood volume loss, venous pooling, and reversible disease entities. In patients with intractable orthostatic hypotension three major approaches are generally applied: (1) mechanical maneuvers, (2) volume expanders, and (3) pharmacologic agents. A summary of treatment modalities currently applied in chronic orthostatic hypotension is presented in Table 29-4. The wide variety of recommended approaches reflects the rather generally disappointing nature of the response in patients with chronic postural hypotension. Commonly, multiple maneuvers are necessary, each to be applied independently before using combinations. Undesirable side effects, including supine hypertension, frequently accompany responses to the potent pharmacologic agents that are applied so that close and continuous monitoring of blood pressure is essential. Of importance is the need to minimize factors that are known to accentuate postural hypotension—blood volume depletion, pharmacologic agents which may induce postural hypotension, and drugs that inhibit orthostatic adaptation. Each patient must be carefully evaluated for remediable accentuating factors. Frequent small feedings should be recommended for patients with marked postprandial orthostatic symptoms. Patients should be taught to rise slowly, to flex the calf muscles during assumption of the upright posture, and to remain as mobile as possible. The use of atrial tachypacing, at a rate of 100 in a patient with a fixed heart rate, has been reported to maintain effective symptomatic and hemodynamic improvement.[25] This novel form of therapy, designed to augment the cardiac response to postural stress in the patient without the normal postural acceleration of heart rate, merits additional trial.

TABLE 29-4 Treatment of Chronic Orthostatic Hypotension

1. Evaluate for reversible and accentuating disease entities.
2. Specific modalities for irreversible orthostatic hypotension:
   a. Mechanical measures:
      (1) Head-up position of bed
      (2) Lower body compression garment
      (3) Slow motion and calf muscle flexing on arising
   b. Volume expansion:
      (1) High-salt diet
      (2) Fludrocortisone acetate
   c. Pharmacologic agents:
      (1) Sympathomimetics
      (2) Vasoconstrictors
      (3) Beta-receptor blockers
      (4) Alpha$_2$-receptor agonists
      (5) Prostaglandin synthesis inhibitors
      (6) Antiserotonergics
      (7) Monoamine oxidase inhibitors and tyramine
      (8) Vasopressin
   d. Atrial pacing

Syncope in Cerebrovascular Disease

Cerebrovascular disease may manifest itself in symptoms of syncope and presyncope in two ways: (1) as a presenting symptom in patients with transient cerebral ischemic attacks (TIA), and (2) as a predisposing factor in individuals prone to syncope from other circulatory disorders. The most common disorder involving the major arteries to the brain is atherosclerotic disease, frequently manifested by recurrent transient cerebral ischemic attacks (TIAs). Syncopal episodes are most likely to occur when atherosclerotic disease involves the vertebro-basilar system wherein perfusion to the medullary arousal center may be affected. Syncope as a manifestation of TIA is uncommon in the presence of atherosclerotic disease in the carotid artery. In vertebro-basilar vascular insufficiency, syncope or presyncope is often associated with symptoms of vertigo, diplopia, dysarthria, and ataxia. These episodes appear to derive largely from microemboli arising from atherosclerotic plaques and/or thrombotic narrowing in the vertebro-basilar arterial system. Cerebral vasospastic episodes involving the carotid-vertebro-basilar arterial system may account for symptoms of presyncope and syncope through accentuation of the cerebral circulatory impairment due to existing atherosclerotic occlusive disease.

Small emboli originating from the cardiac chambers or the cardiac valves may be responsible for such episodes as well. Patients with mitral valve prolapse syndrome and those with intracardiac mural thrombi or intracardiac tumors are subject to such embolic episodes. Atrial fibrillation is a common predisposing cause. Cerebral emboli may arise from calcific and fibrotic disease of the mitral and aortic valve, and from infective or noninfective endocarditis. Emboli may arise as well from prosthetic mitral and aortic valves.

Impairment or loss of consciousness in relation to changing positions of the head, particularly hyperextension and lateral rotation, has been described in mechanical narrowing of the vertebral arteries. Such symptoms have been observed in patients with disease of the upper cervical spine such as Klippel-Feil deformity, cervical spondylosis, and in severe cervical osteoarthritis. Usually there is a lag between the head movement and the occurrence of syncope, since several seconds of reduction in cerebral blood flow are necessary to produce the cerebral ischemia in these disorders. Attacks may occur in any position but usually develop when the patient is upright or when the upright posture is suddenly assumed. Under these circumstances syncope may be preceded by vestibular symptoms. When vertigo is a prominent symptom, the syndrome of benign positional vertigo must be considered.

Syncope due to obstruction in the carotid-vertebro-basilar arterial system, be it atherosclerotic or mechanical in origin, may mimic carotid sinus syncope (described in the next section). In fact, among patients with major occlusive disease of the carotid-vertebro-basilar arterial system, manual compression of either carotid artery as a test for carotid sinus hypersensitivity may provoke syncope, at times associated with focal neurologic signs. One must hence be extremely cautious in applying carotid sinus massage in patients with suspected occlusive cerebral vascular disease. Indeed, the occurrence of a cerebrovascular accident following manual compression of the carotid sinus during diagnostic evaluation for carotid sinus hypersensitivity has been reported in patients with cerebrovascular disease.

In addition to the symptoms induced directly by cerebrovascular narrowing, partial or complete occlusion of the carotid-vertebro-basilar arterial system predisposes to syncope during transient falls in arterial pressure. With partial or complete occlusion of the major arteries of the neck, perfusion to the brain becomes a more direct function of the level of arterial pressure. The greater the degree of cerebral vascular involvement, the more likely it is that syncope will become a part of the clinical picture. Thus, in patients with extensive occlusive involvement of the origins of the brachiocephalic vessels, such as pulseless disease (aortic arch syndrome, Takayasu's arteritis), syncope occurs with a high degree of frequency. With lesser degrees of cerebral vascular occlusion, as in cerebrovascular atherosclerotic disease, transient lowering of arterial pressure, such as that immediately following the assumption of the upright posture, may be followed by vague symptoms suggesting impaired or marginal cerebral blood flow. In the presence of cerebrovascular arterial disease, transient falls in cardiac output as may occur during severe bradycardia or with episodes of supraventricular or ventricular tachycardia may induce syncope or presyncope at levels of arterial pressure which would be tolerated in the absence of a preexisting cerebral perfusion defect.

A unique form of syncope is known as *subclavian steal syndrome.* This syndrome is caused by major occlusive disease of the proximal subclavian artery. With the decrease in vascular resistance accompanying upper extremity exercise, blood flow is shunted via the circle of Willis retrograde from the vertebral artery to the distal subclavian artery on the affected side. The consequent loss of blood flow to the cerebral circulation induces symptoms of cerebral ischemia. The propensity for a patient with proximal subclavian arterial occlusive disease to develop cerebral ischemic symptoms is related not only to the severity of occlusion but to other factors such as the extent of existing cerebrovascular disease and the magnitude of exercise in the extremity. This syndrome is diagnosed by the findings of diminished brachial arterial pressure on the affected side, a bruit which is maximal over the supraclavicular area, and the induction of symptoms by exercise of the involved extremity.

The treatment for recurrent syncope in cerebrovascular disease is predicated on an accurate diagnosis. In this regard, it is essential to attempt to segregate the contributing role of cardiac and vascular factors in the presence of a cerebral perfusion defect. Anticoagulants alone or combined with platelet antiaggregant agents are recommended for the prevention of embolic disease originating in the cardiac chambers, i.e., emboli from prosthetic valves and intramural thrombi. The treatment of primary cerebrovascular disorders associated with transient alterations in consciousness remains controversial. Platelet antiaggregates, in particular aspirin, appear to be effective preventive therapy.[26] Some authorities advise transient anticoagulant therapy for recently developed TIAs due to carotid and vertebrobasilar arterial disease when antiaggregant therapy fails. Surgical endarterectomy is commonly applied in carotid vascular occlusive disease. Its overall effectiveness relative to medical management remains unestablished.

Carotid Sinus Syndrome

In the classical monograph on the hyperactive carotid sinus reflex Weiss and Baker quote the casual observation made in 1799 by Caleb H. Parry: "In patients whose hearts have been beating with undue quickness and force, I have often, in a few seconds, retarded their motions many pulsations by strong pressure on one of the carotid arteries."[27] This earliest of clinical observations on the possible role of reflexes originating in the carotid artery was amplified in 1862 by Waller,[28] who commented that slowing of the heart rate on carotid pressure was not caused by compression of the artery but rather by irritation of the vagus and sympathetic nerves. In 1866 Czermak[29] announced his "Vagusdruckversuch" (vagus pressure test), a test which consisted of pressing firmly on the skin of the upper part of the neck (as we now know over the carotid sinus) to induce cardiac slowing. Hering localized the afferent limb of the carotid sinus reflex to the carotid sinus nerve, a branch of the glossopharyngeal nerve which conveys impulses from the carotid sinus to the reticular formation of the medulla.[30] The regulatory role of the carotid sinus on the circulation of the mammal was documented in the now classical experiments of Heymans.[31] In humans, the afferent limb of the carotid sinus reflex may follow the glossopharyngeal nerve or alternate routes through the cervical sympathetics of the twelfth cranial nerve. The pressure-sensitive receptors responsible for the reflex are present in the adventitia of the carotid artery. The efferent limb of the carotid sinus reflex includes the vagus nerve and the sympathetics, the former accounting for the cardiac slowing while the latter, through inhibition of arteriolar vasoconstrictor activity and perhaps concomitant cholinergic vasodilator activity, accounts for the hypotensive components of the reflex.

Massage or compression of the carotid sinus in normal persons is often associated with transient slowing of the heart and mild hypotension. As a consequence of the activation of the carotid sinus reflex in some patients such stimulation is followed by marked slowing in heart rate, a profound fall in arterial pressure, or a combination of the two. This disorder is referred to as *carotid sinus syncope* or *carotid sinus syndrome*.[32,33] Stimulation of the carotid sinus by pressure or massage can produce syncope of three types: cardioinhibitory, manifested by profound bradycardia, sinus standstill, or atrioventricular block and prevented by atropine; vasodepressor, manifested by a profound hypotensive response with bradycardia and blocked by epinephrine but not by atropine; and a central type of syncope without bradycardia or hypotension, not influenced by atropine or epinephrine.[27]

Carotid sinus hypersensitivity is common in elderly patients, many of whom have diffuse atherosclerosis or other organic heart disease. Such carotid hypersensitivity has not been observed in men of similar age without heart disease. These considerations have led to the impression that it is the associated cardiac disease and not age per se which predisposes to carotid sinus hyperirritability and carotid sinus syncope in the aged. In patients with a hyperirritable carotid sinus reflex, symptoms of lightheadedness and impaired consciousness may be initiated by relatively minor stimulation of the carotid sinus, classically by head motion, shaving, or a tight collar. It is to be emphasized that not all patients with a hypersensitive response to carotid sinus massage experience recurrent syncope. The frequency of a hypersensitive response to carotid massage and the potential for marked bradycardia and hypotension enjoin caution whenever carotid massage is attempted, particularly in the elderly. Testing for carotid sinus syndrome by digital massage should first be done with gentle and very brief (2 to 4 s) maneuvers and always when the patient is supine. The administration of digitalis, beta-blocking agents and alpha methyldopa appears to accentuate carotid sinus hyperirritability.[10]

The cardioinhibitory type of carotid sinus syncope is associated primarily with slowing of the heart rate due to marked sinus bradycardia, sinoatrial block, and/or high-degree atrioventricular block. In these circumstances, syncope is related to the prolonged asystole rather than to a marked fall in peripheral vascular resistance.

The vasodepressor type of carotid sinus syncope is that form of the syndrome in which fainting or impaired consciousness occurs in the absence of profound bradycardia. Presyncopal signs such as nausea, sweating, and pallor are usually not observed and the fall in perfusion pressure to the brain may be precipitous. Carotid sinus syncope may occur as a result of combined cardioinhibitory and vasodepressor mechanisms. Often the vasodepressor component will not be evident until after atropine blockage or during cardiac pacing when carotid massage uncovers the hypotension without bradycardia.

In addition to the vasodepressor and cardioinhibitory types, Weiss and Baker described a third form in which loss of consciousness was unassociated with pulse rate or arterial pressure changes. In this type of carotid sinus syndrome, symptoms may occur with the patient in any position, and the loss of consciousness may be preceded or accompanied by focal neurologic manifestations. It has been suggested that inhibition of the center for regulation of consciousness by a reflex mechanism or by secondary focal circulatory disturbances may account for these rare episodes. In light of the occurrence of syncope during carotid sinus manipulation in patients with carotid-vertebro-basilar arterial insufficiency, questions have been raised as to whether some of these episodes are related directly to obstructive cerebrovascular disease. The possibility of hysterical syncope must also be considered when the diagnosis of the cerebral type of hypersensitive carotid sinus is entertained.

Carotid sinus syncope has been observed in patients with neoplasm and inflammatory masses in the neck.[34–36] The causes of carotid sinus hypersensitivity and syncope in the presence of head and neck tumors are not entirely clear. It has been observed that such tumors (malignant or benign) need not directly involve the carotid body or the carotid sinus nerve. It has been postulated that injury of adjacent nerve branches can induce spontaneous firing of the carotid sinus nerve, causing increased sensitivity of the carotid sinus reflex.

Therapy for carotid sinus syncope includes pharmacologic agents, surgical and radiotherapeutic maneuvers, and cardiac pacemaker therapy. Anticholinergic and sympathomimetic agents in addition to thorough patient education concerning avoidance of carotid sinus pressure may be effective in preventing syncopal episodes. However, inadequacy of drug therapy and the occurrence of side effects, including urinary retention, hypertension, and precipitation of glaucoma, may necessitate additional maneuvers. Surgical denervation of the carotid sinus nerve or radiotherapeutic ablation of the afferent reflex limb has been applied with some success. Periarterectomy in the area above the carotid bifurcation is an effective means of carotid sinus denervation. However, the presence of large tumors infiltrating the region of the carotid sinus often preempts adequate dissection for such denervation. The most aggressive form of surgical intervention for carotid sinus syncope involves intracranial section of the glossopharyngeal nerve, a procedure associated with the side effects of hypesthesia of the palate and base of the tongue and the morbidity of a craniotomy.

Implantation of a permanent transvenous ventricular demand pacemaker was the earliest form of pacemaker therapy for intractable carotid sinus syncope.[37] This therapy has been most effective for the cardioinhibitory type of carotid sinus syncope. In patients with the mixed form of cardioinhibitory and vasodepressor carotid sinus syncope or in those with a pure vasodepressor carotid sinus response, ventricular demand pacing may pose serious therapeutic problems. Thus, not only does the vasodepressor response and symptoms persist in such patients but it would appear that a significant hypotensive response may be induced by ventricular pacing (pacemaker syndrome). The hypotensive response to carotid sinus massage may actually be accentuated during such ventricular pacing. Atrioventricular sequential pacing appears to minimize the hypotensive effect of cardiac pacing and is hence considered to be the preferred treatment for patients with carotid sinus syndrome with combined cardioinhibitory and significant vasodepressor responses.[38] Prior to implementing pacemaker therapy it is necessary to evaluate the nature of the carotid sinus hypersensitivity (cardioinhibitory versus vasodepressor type) and to test for possible concomitant sinoatrial disease (sick sinus syndrome) and/or high-degree AV conduction disturbances. It is also essential that pacemaker effectiveness be verified objectively through observation of the effect of carotid sinus stimulation on cardiac rhythm and arterial pressure following pacemaker insertion.

Reflex Types of Syncope

Reflex suppression of atrial pacemaker activity or atrioventricular conduction by the vagus plays an important role in several forms of syncope. Thus, in the course of vasodepressor syncope, sinus bradycardia and various levels of incomplete heart block are often seen. Although the vagal mechanism may not be the primary cause of fainting under these circumstances, the slowing of the heart rate to critically low levels is certainly a contributing factor. Vagal influences may also play an important role in the course of atrial arrhythmias when sudden slowing or acceleration in ventricular rate due to vagal-induced variation in AV block occurs. Similarly, alterations in vagal tone may account for episodes of syncope in patients with heart block, when changes to high-degree or complete AV block are responsible for fainting. The role of the vagus in the carotid sinus syndrome has been discussed previously.

Syncope may occur in individuals without evidence of heart disease as a result of reflex-induced bradycardia. The term *vagovagal syncope* is applied to such episodes of syncope in which the entire reflex arc is located within the vagal system. Syncopal episodes associated with painful stimulation of the endobronchial, pharyngeal, laryngeal, or esophageal mucosa are most probably based on this mechanism. Vagally induced sinus bradycardia, sinus arrest, nodal bradycardia, or secondary AV block is responsible for the syncope or presyncope associated with these forms of vagovagal syncope. A similar mechanism for cardiac standstill has been attributed to syncope following distension of the viscera, fainting associated with irritation of the pleura or peritoneum, and the cardiac asystole associated with esophagoscopy or bronchoscopy.

Syncope induced by swallowing (swallow or deglutition syncope) has been reported in association with tumor, diverticulum, achalasia, stricture, and spasm of the esophagus. While no radiologically definable lesion could be identified in some patients, the patients commonly have symptoms of dysphagia or pain on swallowing food or beverages. Distension of the esophageal wall appears to activate the afferent limb of the reflex arc. Cardiac arrhythmias responsible for swallow syncope include sinus or nodal bradycardia, sinoatrial and AV block, ventricular tachycardia, and asystole.[39,40]

Glossopharyngeal neuralgia is an extremely painful syndrome which may occur as an isolated entity or with neoplasms of the oropharynx and base of the skull.[41,42] It is rarely associated with recurrent episodes of syncope due to sinus bradycardia, sinus arrest, or high-degree atrioventricular block associated with hypotension. The triggering mechanism is most commonly swallowing, and attacks may be provoked by tactile stimulation in the region of the tonsil. Severe lancinating pain in the neck, tonsillar area, ear, and jaw upon swallowing distinguish this form of syncope from deglutition syncope. The vagal inhibition of the heart and the hypotension are explained by "spillover" of glossopharyngeal impulses transmitted from the central tractus solitarius to the dorsal motor nucleus of the vagus or through the occurrence of false synapses between the glossopharyngeal nerve and the carotid sinus nerve. Interestingly, plasma catecholamines are not increased during the hypotensive episode in glossopharyngeal neuralgia, suggesting an inhibition of adrenergic vasoconstriction.[41] A similar inhibition of norepinephrine release has been noted to occur during the hypotension in vasodepressor syncope (see earlier discussion).

Reflex syncope usually occurs in the absence of underlying heart disease. However, the occurrence of intrinsic cardiac rhythm disturbances, in particular sick sinus syndrome, may accentuate the bradycrotic effects of vagal inhibition associated with reflex syncope. Associated cerebrovascular occlusive disease may be responsible for altered consciousness at levels of bradycardia or hypotension which would otherwise go unnoticed.

Treatment of recurrent vagovagal reflex syncope often necessitates interventions directed at the initiating mechanisms, i.e., esophageal tumor or stricture. Episodes of syncope can be prevented by anticholinergic drugs such as atropine. However, when episodes of bradycardia and syncope are uncontrolled by such maneuvers, cardiac pacemaker therapy may be necessary. In glossopharyngeal neuralgia, anticonvulsants (carbamazepine and diphenylhydantoin) have been effective in relieving episodes of neuralgia and syncope. However, thermocoagulation of the ganglion of the glossopharyngeal nerve or resection of the ninth nerve and rostral fibers of the vagus may be the only effective means of controlling the neuralgia and syncope in some patients. Pacemaker therapy has also been used in patients with uncontrolled syncopal episodes related to glossopharyngeal neuralgia.[42]

Less Common Forms of Syncope

Under less common forms of syncope are included a variety of syncopal or presyncopal episodes often defined by the circumstances which precipitate the event (i.e., cough, micturition, defecation, sneezing, Valsalva maneuver). The mechanism of syncope in these disorders is generally explained on the basis of mechanical factors. Recent observations suggest that, at least in part, reflexly induced sinus bradycardia, sinus arrest, or high-degree AV block may be an additional factor contributing to the syncope.[43,44] Further, impaction of the base of the brain in the foramen magnum with constriction of the subarachnoid space and compression of brainstem circulation has been suggested as a mechanism for syncope in patients with congenital bony malformations at the base of the brain (i.e., Arnold-Chiari malformation).[45,46]

Cough Syncope

In cough syncope (also called *laryngeal vertigo* and *tussive syncope*), loss of consciousness occurs following a paroxysm of vigorous coughing. It is often seen in robust men and children, rarely in women. This syndrome is particularly frequent among individuals with chronic bronchitis and a "hacking cough." The impairment in cerebral blood flow is related to the marked increase in intrathoracic pressure during the coughing episode. Several factors may be implicated in the mechanism of cough syncope, including an abrupt decrease in cardiac output, peripheral vasodilation following cough, a marked increase in cerebrospinal fluid pressure with resultant compression of the intracranial capillary and venous beds, an increase in cerebral vascular resistance induced by the hypocapnia of coughing, and a "concussive" effect caused by the sudden rise in intracranial pressure transmitted from the thorax and abdomen via the cerebrospinal fluid. Episodes of syncope following sneezing (sneeze syncope) most probably have a similar mechanism.

Syncope related to more prolonged increases in intrathoracic pressure may be observed during the sustained Valsalva maneuver (Valsalva syncope). With prolonged exhalation against a closed glottis, there is a progressive fall in arterial pressure and cardiac output. These hemodynamic changes may be sufficient to impair cerebral circulation. Associated post-Valsalva sinus bradycardia in sensitized patients (i.e., those with cerebral occlusive disease or carotid sinus hypersensitivity) adds to the impairment in cerebral blood flow. The "fainting lark," a trick indulged in by schoolchildren and consisting of sudden manual compression of the chest of the victim, made sensitive following a period of hyperventilation, is most probably caused by this mechanism. Syncope following a similar prank, in which the individual squats and hyperventilates and quickly stands and performs a Valsalva maneuver, has a similar mechanism.

The patient with cough syncope should be informed of the deleterious effects of vigorous coughing. Omission of smoking and therapy of associated bronchitis is mandatory in the treatment of cough syncope. Avoidance of sustained Valsalva maneuvers is essential in patients predisposed to syncopal episodes on this basis.

Micturition Syncope

Micturition syncope is often seen in adult men with nocturia. During or immediately following voiding, there is a sudden loss of consciousness, often without premonitory symptoms.[47] Many such persons report drinking large quantities of alcoholic beverage before retiring. A similar type of syncope may be observed following drainage of a distended bladder or after removal of large quantities of ascitic fluid. Some investigators suggest that the loss of consciousness in these circumstances is related to bradycardia and a sudden reflex decrease in peripheral vascular resistance induced by the precipitous fall in intraabdominal volume. Others have thought the loss of consciousness in postmicturition syncope to be related to typical vasodepressor syncope accentuated by such factors as the Valsalva maneuver and the peripheral vasodilation associated with a warm bed and recent alcohol consumption.

Defecation Syncope

Syncope during defecation occurs most commonly in the elderly, usually after arising from bed at night or with manual disimpaction of the rectum.[48] Syncope with defecation has been attributed to sudden decompression of the rectum. Valsalva-related syncope associated with high-degree AV block or profound sinus bradycardia could also explain defecation syncope. Syncope during defecation should suggest the possibility of pulmonary embolism.

Diver's Syncope

Unusual and poorly understood forms of loss of consciousness and even sudden death may occur in underwater diving. Some may be forms of vasodepressor syncope. Hypoxia may be a factor, and the bradycardia of the "diving reflex" may be involved.

In many instances, particularly in the elderly, several factors may be responsible for syncope. While each factor alone may be insufficient to produce syncope, a combination of contributing events, i.e., intrinsic cardiac or vascular disease, reflex bradycardia, and hypotension accentuated by adrenergic blocking or vasodilator drugs, may deplete cerebral blood flow sufficiently to induce loss of consciousness.

Noncardiovascular Syncope

The differential diagnosis of syncope often includes a group of disorders in which altered consciousness is not primarily related to changes in cardiac output, cardiac rhythm, or arterial pressure. These forms are referred to as syncope of noncardiovascular (or noncirculatory) origin and may be caused by primary disorders of cerebral function, profound alterations in cerebral metabolism, or psychologically induced behavioral mechanisms (Table 29-5).

TABLE 29-5 Noncardiovascular Syncope

Hypoxia
Hypoglycemia
Hyperventilation
Convulsive disorders
Vertigo
Hysteria
Syncopal migraine

Hypoxia

Fainting due to hypoxia may be related primarily to lack of oxygen or to an episode of vasodepressor syncope initiated during a period of oxygen lack. The effect of hypoxia alone is best observed in persons studied in altitude chambers. Though there is considerable individual variation, the onset of hypoxic symptoms depends on the level of altitude and the rate of ascent. With altitude exposure of 3000 m or greater, the point in the oxyhemoglobin dissociation curve is reached where an abrupt decrease in oxygen saturation occurs with further fall in oxygen tension. Oxygen saturation falls rapidly from approximatley 90 percent saturation at 3000 m to 80 percent at 4500 m, and 63 percent at 6100 m. At the time of impairment of consciousness one may note cyanosis; with severe oxygen deprivation, convulsive movements are seen. With cardiovascular disease, pulmonary insufficiency, and anemia, symptoms of hypoxia occur at lower levels of oxygen deprivation. The impairment of consciousness due to hypoxia is accompanied by sinus tachycardia while arterial pressure is preserved. The environmental setting in which impaired consciousness due to hypoxia occurs usually leaves little difficulty in differentiating it from other forms of syncope.

Hypoglycemia

Severe hypoglycemia is associated with weakness, sweating, a hunger sensation, confusion, and altered consciousness. The symptoms are unrelated to posture and usually respond promptly to food ingestion or intravenous glucose administration. Altered consciousness associated with overdosage of insulin, islet cell adenomas of the pancreas, retroperitoneal tumors, reactive hypoglycemia, and in the presence of advanced adrenal, pituitary, or hepatic disease may be explained on this basis. Impaired consciousness is associated with sinus rhythm and is rarely accompanied by hypotension; in contrast to syncope of circulatory origin, it is gradual in onset.

Hyperventilation

In normal persons, anxiety is regularly accompanied by varying degrees of hyperventilation. In the hyperventilation syndrome, anxiety is associated with an inordinate degree of hyperventilation. Symptoms of hypocapnia dominate the clinical picture under these circumstances and actually may replace the anxiety as the major discomfort. Early during the episode, the patient complains of a tightness in the chest and a feeling of suffocation. Later, there appears confusion, a sense of unreality, bewilderment, and a feeling of panic. Symptoms of palpitation, precordial oppression, and dyspnea may suggest an acute cardiac or pulmonary catastrophe. Associated with the above, there are sensations of numbness or coldness of the extremities and the circumoral areas. The symptoms may last as long as

30 min, and in the most severe episodes may occur in the sitting or recumbent posture. Often there is slight hypotension, but not a profound drop in arterial pressure, and the heart rate is rapid. The episode is usually terminated after the patient's anxiety is allayed and the hyperventilation ceases. One may assist the resolution of symptoms of hypocapnia by having the patient rebreathe in a paper or plastic bag. It is notable that although mentation is impaired, complete loss of consciousness usually does not occur. Typical vasodepressor syncope may be superimposed in the hyperventilation attack, making identification of the syndrome more difficult.

The pathogenesis of the syndrome is incompletely understood. Though an underlying emotional disorder is almost invariably present, the factors leading to hyperventilation remain undefined. Many of the chemical findings in the syndrome, particularly the lowering of arterial carbon dioxide tension and alkalosis, can be explained by the effects of hypocapnia. The induction of a typical episode by voluntary hyperventilation in patients with hyperventilation syndrome is a helpful diagnostic maneuver and can aid in educating the patient regarding the prevention and control of attacks.

Convulsive Disorders

Differentiation of the various forms of syncope of circulatory origin from the transitory loss of consciousness that occurs during a generalized convulsive seizure is often made on the basis of history alone. One form of epilepsy, the akinetic form of petit mal, offers particular difficulty in differentiation. Epilepsy as a cause of sudden loss of consciousness is suggested in the dramatic nature of the onset of the attack, which is often preceded by an aura. Other observations which aid in distinguishing the loss of consciousness in epilepsy are the absence of hypotension and cardiac arrhythmia (other than sinus tachycardia), the presence of tonic convulsive movements with upturning of the eyes, prolonged unconsciousness, urinary incontinence, postictal drowsiness, headache, and confusion. Although any of the above findings may occur in individual episodes of syncope of circulatory origin, the frequent combination of these events in epilepsy allows differentiation of the cause of the event. The finding of an abnormal electroencephalogram suggesting cerebral arrhythmia between episodes of unconsciousness is most helpful in this differentiation.

Vertigo

Though recurrent episodes of vertigo may first be described by the patient as a loss or impairment of consciousness, careful attention to the history will often reveal the true nature of this symptom. In true vertigo there is a keen sense of movement, either of the environment or of the patient. Falling may be abrupt; it is due not to weakness of postural muscles but to loss of balance. Nausea, pallor, and cold perspiration may suggest vasodepressor syncope, but the lack of true loss or impairment of consciousness, the increased distress with head movement, and the associated nystagmoid movements of the eyes, together with the finding of a normal arterial pressure and pulse, will help differentiate the syndrome.

Hysterical Syncope

Hysterical syncope is of particular importance because it may mimic altered consciousness of circulatory origin. Hysterical episodes occur most frequently in young adults, often with severe emotional illness. The episode usually occurs in the presence of an audience. The patient slumps gently, even gracefully, to the floor or in a convenient chair or sofa, typically without injury or awkwardness. The patient may be motionless at the time of the episode or may show symbolic and resistive movements. Episodes are of varying duration and may last as long as an hour or more. Although the patient is unresponsive to verbal stimulation, there is often evidence that consciousness is not lost, and there are no abnormalities in pulse, arterial pressure, or skin color. A distinctive characteristic is the calm emotional detachment with which the patient describes symptoms and the fact that there is no sharp reversal in his or her progress when the recumbent posture is assumed.

Syncopal Migraine

Symptoms suggesting syncope are rarely encountered in ordinary types of migraine. In rare instances in which the basal arterial system is involved (as opposed to the more usually affected carotid system), the premonitory aura of migraine terminates in a period of unconsciousness of several minutes' duration. The unconsciousness is slow in onset, never abrupt, and may be preceded by a dreamlike state. When the patient awakens, there is severe headache, typically in the occipital area. This form of migraine usually afflicts adolescent girls and has a strong menstrual association. In the original descriptions of the syndrome, the period of unconsciousness was apparently unassociated with circulatory alterations.[49] Many of the symptoms in syncopal migraine suggest hyperventilation and/or hysterical syncope. Brainstem ischemia from longstanding localized basilar artery spasm is the postulated mechanism of the syncope. Recently, hyperresponsiveness of dopamine receptors (tested via the administration of bromocriptine, a dopamine receptor agonist) with inhibition of the vasomotor center has been posed as an alternative explanation for syncope in patients with migraine.[50] Additional studies documenting electrocardiographic and arterial pressure responses in syncopal migraine are necessary to clarify the nature of the altered consciousness in this syndrome.

Diagnostic Evaluation of Syncope

Syncope or presyncope is among the most difficult of symptoms to evaluate. While in many patients syncope is not associated with severe circulatory disease, or a poor prognosis, in others it may be a harbinger of sudden death.

As an initial approach to the diagnosis it is essential to attempt to distinguish the underlying cause in terms of the three basic mechanisms previously outlined: vasodepressor, cardiovascular, and noncardiovascular syncope. This differentiation is accomplished in a majority of patients in whom a diagnosis could be established (85 percent by one estimate) through careful attention to the history and physical examination supplemented by the routine electrocardiogram.[51] Clearly the evaluation of syncope employing these basic clinical steps must be rooted in a thorough knowledge of the various causes of syncope. Based on these findings further evaluation is predicated on one's estimation of mortality and morbidity risk (high in cardiovascular syncope, low in noncardiovascular and isolated vasodepressor syncope). In patients considered at high risk, pursuit of the diagnosis via appropriate noninvasive and invasive testing should be introduced. While cost-effectiveness in diagnosis must be practiced, this should not dismiss the need for an assiduous search when lethal and life-limiting disease is suspected. Detailed discussions of those laboratory tests which pertain to the investigation of disease processes which may underly the symptom of syncope is described in Chapter 30 and elsewhere in the text.

References

1. Boudoulas, H., Weissler, A. M., Lewis, R. P., and Warren, J. V.: The Clinical Diagnosis of Syncope, *Curr. Prob. Cardiol.*, 7:1, 1982.
2. Weissler, A. M., and Warren, J. V.: Vasodepressor Syncope, *Am. Heart J.*, 57:786, 1959.
3. Engel, G. L., and Romano, J.: Studies of Syncope: IV. Biologic Interpretations of Vasodepressor Syncope, *Psychosom. Med.*, 9:288, 1947.
4. Goldstein, D. S., Spanarkel, M., Pitterman, A., et al.: Circulatory Control Mechanisms in Vasodepressor Syncope, *Am. Heart J.*, 104:1071, 1982.
5. Wallin, B. G., and Sundlöff, G.: Sympathetic Outflow to Muscles During the Vasovagal Syncope, *J. Auton. Nerv. Syst.*, 6:287, 1982.
6. Schatz, I. J.: Orthostatic Hypotension, *Arch. Intern. Med.*, 144:773 and 1037, 1984.
7. Thomas, J. E., Schirger, A., Fealey, R. D., and Sheps, S. G.: Orthostatic Hypotension, *Mayo. Clin. Proc.*, 56:117, 1981.
8. Johnson, R. H.: Orthostatic Hypotension in Neurological Disease, *Cardiology*, 61(suppl. 1):150, 1976.
9. Lindenfeld, J.: Syncope, in L. Horwitz (ed.), "Signs and Symptoms of Cardiology," J. B. Lippincott, Philadelphia, 1984.
10. Lipsitz, L. A.: Syncope in the Elderly, *Ann. Intern. Med.*, 99:92, 1983.
11. Lipsitz, L. A., Nyquist, R. P., Jr., Wei, J. Y., and Rowe, J. W.: Postprandial Reduction in Blood Pressure in the Elderly, *N. Engl. J. Med.*, 309:81, 1983.
12. Ziegler, M. G.: Postural Hypotension, *Ann. Rev. Med.*, 31:239, 1980.
13. Kontos, H. A., Richardson, D. W., and Norvell, J. E.: Norepinephrine Depletion in Idiopathic Orthostatic Hypotension, *Ann. Intern. Med.*, 82:336, 1975.
14. Ziegler, M. G., Lake, C. R., and Kopin, I. J.: The Sympathetic-Nervous-System Defect in Primary Orthostatic Hypotension, *N. Engl. J. Med.*, 296:293, 1977.
15. Bannister, R., Crowe, R., Eames, R., and Burnstock, G.: Adrenergic Innervation in Autonomic Failure, *Neurology*, 31:1501, 1981.
16. Kopin, I. J., Polinsky, R. J., Oliver, J. A., Oddershede, I. R., and Ebert, M. H.: Urinary Catecholamine Metabolites Distinguish Different Types of Sympathetic Neuronal Dysfunction in Patients with Orthostatic Hypotension, *J. Clin. Endocrinol. Metab.*, 57:632, 1983.
17. Nanda, R. N., Boyle, F. C., Gillespie, J. S., Johnson, R. H., and Keogh, H. J.: Idiopathic Orthostatic Hypotension from Failure of Noradrenaline Release in a Patient with Vasomotor Innervation, *J. Neurol. Neurosurg. Psychiatry*, 40:11, 1977.
18. Khurana, R. K., Nelson, E., Azzarelli, B., and Garcia, J. H.: Shy-Drager Syndrome: Diagnosis and Treatment of Cholinergic Dysfunction, *Neurology*, 30:805, 1980.
19. McGrath, B. P., Stern, A. I., Esler, M., and Hansky, J.: Impaired Pancreatic Polypeptide Release to Insulin Hypoglycaemia in Chronic Autonomic Failure with Postural Hypotension: Evidence for Parasympathetic Dysfunction, *Clin. Sci.*, 63:321, 1982.
20. Polinsky, R. J., Taylor, I. L., Chew, P., Weise, V., and Kopin, I. J.: Pancreatic Polypeptide Responses to Hypoglycemia in Chronic Autonomic Failure, *J. Clin. Endocrinol. Metab.*, 54:48, 1982.
21. Cryer, P. E., Silverberg, A. B., Santiago, J. V., et al.: Plasma Catecholamines in Diabetes. The Syndromes of Hypoadrenergic and Hyperadrenergic Postural Hypotension, *Am. J. Med.*, 64:407, 1978.
22. Hilsted, J., Parving, H. H., Christensen, N. J., Benn, J., and Galbo, H.: Hemodynamics in Diabetic Orthostatic Hypotension, *J. Clin. Invest.*, 68:1427, 1981.
23. Page, M. M., and Watkins, P. J.: Provocation of Postural Hypotension by Insulin in Diabetic Autonomic Neuropathy, *Diabetes*, 25:90, 1976.
24. Ziegler, M. G., Lake, C. R., and Koplin, I. J.: Deficient Sympathetic Nervous Response in Familial Dysautonomia, *N. Engl. J. Med.*, 294:630, 1976.
25. Moss, A. J., Glaser, W., and Topol, E.: Atrial Tachypacing in the Treatment of a Patient with Primary Orthostatic Hypotension, *N. Engl. J. Med.*, 302:1456, 1980.
26. Dyken, M. L.: Assessment of the Role of Antiplatelet Aggregating Agonists in Transient Ischemic Attacks, Stroke and Death, *Curr. Concepts Cerebrovasc. Dis.*, 14:9, 1979.
27. Weiss, S., and Baker, J. P.: The Carotid Sinus Reflex in Health and Disease, Its Role in the Causation of Fainting and Convulsions, *Medicine*, 12:297, 1933.
28. Waller, A.: Experimental Researches on the Functions of the Vagus and the Cervical Sympathetic Nerves in Man, *Proc. R. Soc. Med.*, 11:302, 1862.
29. Czermak, J. Ueber Mechanische Vagus Reizung Beim Menschen, *Jenaische Ztschr. f. Med. u. Naturwiss.*, 2:384, 1866.
30. Hering, H. E.: "Die Karotissinusreflexe auf Herz und Gefasse," T. R. Steinkoff, Dresden and Leipzig, 1927.
31. Heymans, C.: "Le Sinus Carotidien et les Autres Zones Vasosensibles Reflexogenes," H. K. Lewis & Co., London, 1929.
32. Poggi, L., Dijiane, P., Egre, A., et al.: Carotid Sinus Syndrome. Apropos of 6 Cases with the Cardio-Inhibitory Type, *Arch. Mal. Coeur*, 73:883, 1980.
33. Davies, A. B., Stephens, M. R., and Davies, A. G.: Carotid Sinus Hypersensitivity in Patients Presenting with Syncope, *Br. Heart J.*, 42:583, 1979.
34. Patel, A. K., Yap, V. U., Fields, J., et al.: Carotid Sinus Syncope Induced by Malignant Tumors in the Neck. Emergence of Vasodepressor Manifestations Following Pacemaker Therapy, *Arch. Intern. Med.*, 139:1281, 1979.
35. Matthew, T. K., et al.: Carotid Sinus Syncope as a Manifestation of Parotid Tumors, *Am. Heart J.*, 104:316, 1982.
36. Muntz, H. R., and Smith, P. G.: Carotid Sinus Hypersensi-

tivity: A Cause of Syncope in Patients with Tumors of the Head and Neck, *Laryngoscope,* 93:1290, 1983.
37. Peretz, D. W., Gerein, A. N., and Miyagishima, R. T.: Permanent Demand Pacing for Hypersensitive Carotid Sinus Syndrome, *Can. Med. Assoc. J.,* 108:1131, 1973.
38. Morley, C. A., Perrins, E. J., Grant, P., Chan, S. I., McBrien, D. J., and Sutton, R.: Carotid Sinus Syncope Treated by Pacing Analysis of Persistent Symptoms and Role of Atrioventricular Sequential Pacing, *Br. Heart J.,* 47:411, 1982.
39. Levin, B., and Posner, J. B.: Swallow Syncope, *Neurology,* 22:1086, 1972.
40. Bortolotti, M., Cirignotta, F., and Labo, G.: Atrioventricular Block Induced by Swallowing in a Patient with Diffuse Esophageal Spasm, *JAMA,* 248:2297, 1982.
41. Dykman, T. R., Montgomery, I. B., Gerstenberger, P. D., Zeigler, M. E., Clutter, W. E., and Cryer, P. E.: Glossopharyngeal Neuralgia with Syncope Secondary to Tumor, *Am. J. Med.,* 71:165, 1981.
42. St. John, J. N.: Glossopharyngeal Neuralgia Associated with Syncope and Seizures, *Neurosurgery,* 10:380, 1982.
43. Hart, G., Oldershaw, P. J., Cull, R. E., Humphrey, P., and Ward, D.: Syncope Caused by Cough-Induced Complete Atrioventricular Block, *PACE,* 5:564, 1982.
44. Saito, D., Matsuno, S., Matsushita, K., et al.: Cough Syncope Due to Atrio-Ventricular Conduction Block, *Jpn. Heart J.,* 23:1015, 1982.
45. Hampton, B., Williams, B., and Loizou, L.: Syncope as a Presenting Feature of Hindbrain Herniation with Syringomyelia, *J. Neurol. Neurosurg. Psychiatry,* 45:919, 1982.
46. Corbett, J. J., Butler, A. B., and Kaufman, B.: "Sneeze Syncope" Basilar Invagination and Arnold-Chiari Type I Malformation, *J. Neurol. Neurosurg. Psychiatry,* 39:381, 1976.
47. Godec, C. J., and Cass, A. S.: Micturition Syncope, *J. Urol.,* 126:551, 1981.
48. Pathy, M. S.: Defaecation Syncope, *Age Ageing,* 7:233, 1978.
49. Bickerstaff, E. R.: Impairment of Consciousness in Migraine, *Lancet,* 2:1057, 1961.
50. Sicuteri, F., Boccuni, M., Fanciullacci, M., D'Egidio, P., and Bonciani, M.: A New Nonvascular Interpretation of Syncopal Migraine, *Adv. Neurol.,* 33:199, 1982.
51. Day, S. C., Cook, E. F., Funkenstein, H., and Goldman, L.: Evaluation and Outcome of Emergency Room Patients with Transient Loss of Consciousness, *Am. J. Med.,* 73:15, 1982.

30

Cardiac Syncope: Diagnosis, Mechanism, and Management

Harisios Boudoulas, M.D. Richard P. Lewis, M.D.

Evaluation of a patient with suspected cardiac syncope is one of the truly difficult problems in clinical medicine. Recent studies underscore the alarming 1-year mortality of cardiac syncope while pointing out the low diagnostic yield of a traditional syncope workup.[1–5] The history and physical examination may well identify underlying cardiovascular disease, but they often are of limited value for establishing the cause of syncope per se.[6,7] Thus, suspected cardiac syncope usually requires more extensive laboratory evaluation than does syncope arising from most other causes.[6] Unfortunately many of these methodologies are not universally available, while other needed methodologies are still evolving.

Studies of large, hospital-based series of patients with syncope have suggested that in as many as half of such patients, definitive diagnosis is not established by the initial evaluation. Of those in whom a diagnosis is made, cardiac syncope is the cause in at least half of the patients. Ventricular tachycardia, often unsuspected, and sick sinus syndrome are the commonest causes. Obstruction of cardiac output, atrioventricular (AV) block, and rapid supraventricular tachycardia are the remaining major diagnostic categories. It is likely that as laboratory methods improve, many patients with syncope of undetermined cause will be shown to have arrhythmic syncope.

A high incidence of significant arrhythmias in asymptomatic individuals has been demonstrated by ambulatory monitoring in recent studies.[8] The incidence dramatically increases with age. Two-thirds of patients with suspected cardiac syncope are over 60 years of age, and establishing cause and effect between symptoms and arrhythmias is a major problem in this age group. The problem is compounded because older patients often have inadequate compensatory mechanisms for defending against syncope, increased sensitivity to cardioactive drugs, and a high incidence of underlying disease. Thus syncope may result from phenomena which would be benign in younger individuals.

Prognostic studies indicate that 1-year mortality for cardiac syncope is 20 to 30 percent, with sudden death as the major outcome. One-year mortality is only 5 percent for noncardiac syncope; it is as great as 10 percent for syncope of unknown cause.[1,3] In cardiac syncope, mortality is influenced largely by the underlying disease. Arrhythmic syncope, in the absence of evidence of underlying heart disease, rarely leads to a fatal outcome.

Presyncope, which is defined as light-headedness or transient loss of cerebral function without frank syncope, constitutes a major problem. Though presyncope is frequently mechanistically the same as syncope and the two coexist, presyncope is often a benign syndrome for which a precise cause is less likely to be found. Mild postural hypotension is probably the major cause. However, in certain high-risk patients (those having ischemic heart disease, cardiomyopathy, aortic stenosis, or pulmonary hypertension) presyncope may have an ominous mechanism.

Perhaps the most difficult clinical decision in patients with suspected syncope or presyncope is how aggressively to pursue the diagnosis. Because of the high 1-year mortality and the fact that effective therapy is available in many cases, this symptom cannot be lightly regarded. A reasonable general approach based upon current knowledge would be as follows: in patients with underlying heart disease (assuming it is not end-stage disease), the evaluation should be aggressive; in those without demonstrable heart disease in whom syncope is infrequent and not abrupt, a more conservative approach is justified.

Classification and Pathophysiology of Cardiac Syncope

Either severe obstruction of cardiac output or disturbances of cardiac rhythm can produce syncope of cardiac origin. Obstructive lesions and arrhythmias frequently coexist; indeed, one abnormality may accentuate the other.[6]

Cardiac Syncope—Obstructive

Obstruction of cardiac output may reflect lesions or structural abnormalities on either the left or the right side of the circulation (Table 30-1).

Syncope, particularly that occurring with effort, is a major symptom of aortic stenosis and often is the initial presentation. The mechanisms are unclear, but studies suggest a reflex fall in peripheral vascular resistance as the usual cause.[9] However, failure of cardiac output to increase adequately during exercise, while peripheral resistance decreases, may also play a role. Transient arrhythmias can also precipitate syncope in aortic stenosis. Syncope associated with effort (often occurring immediately after effort) is also observed in patients with hypertrophic cardiomyopathy. Nonexertional syncope related to acute decreases in preload, afterload, or inotropic stimulation or to transient arrhythmias also occurs with hypertrophic cardiomyopathy. Prosthetic valve malfunction can produce transient obstruction to blood flow which results in syncope.

A left atrial myxoma may obstruct left ventricular filling, leading to low cardiac output and syncope. The obstruction to left ventricular inflow in atrial myxoma may be posturally induced. Mitral stenosis can produce cardiac syncope but usually does so only when tachycardia or other arrhythmias supervene. Thus, in patients with physical signs of obstruction at the mitral valve level and recurrent episodes of syncope, left atrial myxoma should be considered.

TABLE 30-1 Common Causes of Cardiac Syncope

Obstructive Causes
Left side of heart
Aortic stenosis
Hypertrophic cardiomyopathy
Prosthetic valve malfunction
Left atrial myxoma
Mitral stenosis
Right side of heart
Eisenmenger's syndrome
Tetralogy of Fallot
Primary pulmonary hypertension
Pulmonary embolus
Pulmonary stenosis
Both sides of heart
Cardiac tamponade
Arrhythmic Causes
Bradycardia
Sinus bradycardia or SA block
AV block
AV node disease
His-Purkinje disease
Reflex bradycardia or AV block
Tachycardia
Ventricular tachycardia
Supraventricular tachycardia
Frequent premature ventricular beats
Pacemaker malfunction
Pacemaker-induced syndromes

Primary pulmonary hypertension and pulmonary hypertension secondary to congenital heart disease may both be complicated by syncope, particularly effort-related syncope. In these conditions limitation of right ventricular outflow markedly inhibits the cardiac output response during increased peripheral demand. The drop in peripheral resistance in the presence of limited cardiac output response may result in profound hypotension. A reflex drop in peripheral resistance similar to that which occurs with aortic stenosis may also play a role. In young patients without cardiac murmurs who present with syncope during or shortly after exertion, primary pulmonary hypertension should be considered.[10] In pulmonary stenosis and pulmonary embolism, similar mechanisms may account for syncope.

In tetralogy of Fallot the magnitude of flow through the right-to-left shunt increases with effort because the right ventricular outflow obstruction is usually fixed, while systemic resistance drops. This results in marked arterial hypoxia, which may precipitate a syncopal episode. Cardiac tamponade, which affects both the right side and the left side of the heart, can produce syncope. The likelihood of syncope is increased by concomitant arrhythmias.

Cardiac Syncope: Arrhythmic

Either extreme of ventricular rate—bradycardia or tachycardia—can depress cardiac output to the point of critical hypotension and syncope (Table 30-1). Cerebral blood flow is maintained in supine, healthy individuals over a wide range of heart rates—from approximately 35 to 190 beats per minute. Pulse rates outside these limits may reduce cerebral circulation and function.

The Stokes-Adams syndrome, with its characteristic abrupt syncope unrelated to posture, is usually due to episodic high-grade AV block with marked bradycardia or asystole. Marked sinus bradycardia, high-grade AV block, or cardiac asystole may be mediated vagally by reflex mechanisms; they have been observed in a variety of disease states (e.g., cough, neuralgias) and during a variety of diagnostic procedures (e.g., endoscopy, thoracentesis, cardiac catheterization).[11] Paroxysmal atrial tachycardias are an uncommon cause of syncope in young individuals but may cause syncope in elderly patients. Syncope may occur in younger individuals who have accessory AV pathways when supraventricular tachycardia is associated with very rapid ventricular response.

The common underlying disorders in which arrhythmia may be the major contributory factor of syncope are summarized in Table 30-2.

TABLE 30-2 Common Underlying Disorders Associated with Arrhythmic Syncope

Diffuse conduction system disease
- Sick sinus syndrome (including tachycardia-bradycardia syndrome)
- AV block
  - AV node disease
  - His-Purkinje disease

WPW syndrome

Lown-Ganong-Levine syndrome

Long-QT syndromes
- Congenital
- Acquired

Coronary artery disease
- Acute ischemic syndromes
- Chronic stable disease

Primary myocardial disease
- Congestive cardiomyopathy
- Hypertrophic cardiomyopathy

Mitral valve prolapse syndrome

Pharmacologic agents (antiarrhythmic agents, digitalis, beta-blocking agents, aminophylline, terbutaline, calcium blocking agents)

Metabolic derangements

Pacemakers
- Malfunction
- Pacemaker syndromes

Bradycardia in the sick sinus syndrome may result from a failure of sinus node impulse formation or failure of conduction of the impulse through the specialized atrial conduction system. A degenerative or fibrotic lesion in the sinus node and the specialized conduction tissue is the most frequent cause of the sick sinus syndrome. The sick sinus syndrome may be manifested by persistent or episodic sinus bradycardia, sinoatrial (SA) exit block, impaired junctional escape rhythm, and supraventricular tachycardias. The tachycardias are also related to the conduction system disease, which allows reentry mechanisms. The appearance of alternating atrial bradycardia with paroxysmal supraventricular tachycardia is quite common and is referred to as the *bradycardia-tachycardia syndrome.* Syncope often occurs after abrupt termination of a tachycardia, when there is overdrive suppression of the SA or junctional pacemakers or of AV conduction. A high incidence of AV block and intraventricular conduction defects may also be present in the sick sinus syndrome. Thus AV block, impaired junctional escape rhythm, or ventricular arrhythmias may actually be responsible for syncope in so-called sick sinus syndrome.[12]

High-grade AV block may be due to disease of the AV node or of the His-Purkinje system. It may be caused by degenerative disease or may be secondary to ischemic, myocardial, or valvular disease. Disease of the AV node is associated with an intact junctional pacemaker and a normal QRS complex, and often there is antecedent first degree AV block. Second degree block is usually of the Wenckebach type (Möbitz type I). AV block due to disease of the His-Purkinje system is usually associated with a wide, complex idioventricular escape rhythm, which may be quite slow. Second degree block is usually of Möbitz type II. Most of these patients have antecedent bifascicular block. If first degree AV block is present, it may be due to AV node disease, trifascicular block, or both.

Syncope due to high-grade AV block is most likely to occur when AV block is due to His-Purkinje disease. Progression to high-grade AV block in patients with bifascicular block and normal PR interval is rare. However, if bifascicular block is associated with a prolonged PR interval, the risk of developing high-grade AV block is substantially higher.

Wolff-Parkinson-White (WPW) syndrome and Lown-Ganong-Levine syndrome are often associated with supraventricular tachycardia, which may be the cause of syncope when the ventricular rate is rapid and/or when other abnormal conditions coexist. Both syndromes are produced by anomalous conduction tracts.

The long-QT-interval syndrome may be congenital or acquired. The recognition of long-QT syndromes depends on demonstration of QT prolongation and recurrent syncope, which is almost always due to ventricular arrhythmia. The ventricular arrhythmia is usually torsades de pointes ventricular tachycardia, which is characterized by a rapid rate and a gradually changing QRS morphology. The congenital long-QT syndrome may be associated with deafness (Jerell and Lange-Nielsen's syndrome) or may not be associated with deafness (Romano-Ward syndrome).

It is particularly important to recognize the acquired long-QT syndromes because they are a common and life-threatening side effect of many antiarrhythmic drugs and metabolic abnormalities.[13] The most frequent acquired long-QT syndromes are those due to class I antiarrhythmic drugs (most commonly quinidine and disopyramide), the tricyclic antidepressant drugs, and the phenothiazines. Additional causes are electrolyte abnormalities (hypokalemia and possibly hypomagnesemia), acute ischemia, myocarditis, cardiomyopathy, liquid protein diet, and, rarely, mitral valve prolapse syndrome. Torsade de pointes ventricular tachycardia has been described in patients with a QT interval that appears to be normal when corrected for heart rate. This may be related to weakness of the traditional Bazett formula in identifying patients with long-QT syndrome when the heart rate is slow. It has been shown that the QT interval is best corrected for heart rate by a linear correction. In ischemic heart disease, relating the QT interval to the duration of mechanical systole (QS_2) appears to be superior to correcting for heart rate.[14,15]

In patients with mitral valve prolapse syndrome, syncope may be related to arrhythmias. However, vasovagal or vasodepressor syncope is also common in patients with mitral valve prolapse, as is postural hypotension.

Digitalis may be responsible for ventricular or supraventricular arrhythmias or AV block in patients with AV node disease. Calcium channel blocking agents and beta-blocking agents may cause profound bradycardia and AV block, particularly in patients with conduction system disease. Aminophylline and beta agonists may precipitate or initiate ventricular or supraventricular arrhythmias. Therapy with diuretics often causes hypokalemia and resultant ventricular arrhythmias. Combined therapy with class I antiarrhythmic drugs and diuretics is a common cause of arrhythmias.

Pacemaker malfunction may cause syncope in patients who are dependent on a paced rhythm. This must be distinguished from the *pacemaker syndromes.*

The so-called pacemaker syndromes include syncope induced by two different mechanisms: (1) syncope due to pacemaker-induced arrhythmias, and (2) hemodynamic syncope due to a decrease in cardiac output or to a reflex decrease in peripheral vascular resistance. Some dual-chamber pacemakers can produce pacemaker-mediated tachycardias when there is retrograde conduction of the ventricular impulse to the atria. Improvements in technology should reduce the incidence of this complication. Cardiac output in patients with ventricular pacemakers may decrease owing to loss of the normal AV synchronism of contraction. Loss of the atrial contribution to ventricular filling is only part of the problem. When there is intact ventriculoatrial conduction of the impulse and an atrial contraction occurs during ventricular systole, mitral and tricuspid regurgitation may result. Finally, atrial contraction against closed AV valves may decrease the peripheral arterial resistance by a reflex mechanism, particularly in patients with carotid sinus hypersensitivity. These pacemaker-induced hemodynamic abnormalities may account for persistence of symptoms after placement of a permanent pacemaker.[16–18]

Diagnosis

The diagnosis of lesions producing obstruction to flow can usually be made by physical examination. The diagnosis of arrhythmias is more difficult because of their transient nature.

Cardiac Syncope: Obstructive

While the history and physical examination usually suggest the diagnosis of obstructive syncope, laboratory studies are usually required for the determination of the severity of the disorder. The routine ECG is often of diagnostic importance for detection of atrial or ventricular hypertrophy and to suggest the presence of conduction or rhythm disturbances. The chest roentgenogram may reveal dense calcifications at the aortic or mitral valve areas. Image-intensification fluoroscopy, an often neglected procedure, may define such valvular calcification when this finding is absent on the chest roentgenogram. The chest roentgenogram often reveals additional significant insight into the state of the central and peripheral pulmonary circulation, providing clues to the diagnosis of right-sided obstructive disease at either the cardiac or pulmonary vascular level. Clinical indications for the presence of congenital heart disease are often first detected on the chest roentgenogram. Image-intensification cinefluoroscopy is of special usefulness when prosthetic valve dysfunction is under consideration.

In the modern era, the echocardiogram has become of critical importance in the diagnosis of obstructive cardiac disease; it is also of great value in establishing a diagnosis of pericardial effusion (which may be associated with pericardial tamponade). The echocardiogram is also useful in the diagnosis of congenital heart disease as a cause of syncope.[6] Systolic time intervals are useful for evaluating left ventricular outflow obstruction. Thus, the finding of a prolonged left ventricular ejection time is consistent with significant aortic valvular stenosis or hypertrophic cardiomyopathy. The configuration of the carotid arterial pulse often is useful for differentiating valvular aortic outflow obstruction from that due to obstructive cardiomyopathy. Simultaneous recordings of an M-mode echocardiogram and a phonocardiogram are of great value in evaluating prosthetic valve function and may provide the definitive diagnosis. Arterial blood gases and combined ventilatory and perfusion radioisotope lung scanning are very useful in the diagnosis of pulmonary embolism. In obstructive cardiac disorders noninvasive tests are not always conclusive and cardiac catheterization is often required, especially if corrective open heart surgery is contemplated.

Cardiac Syncope: Arrhythmic

Diagnostic Studies for the Underlying Disease
Except for syncope due to reflex arrhythmias, arrhythmic cardiac syncope implies an abnormality in the specialized conduction tissue of the heart. In many cases the conduction disease is relatively isolated, but in others it is secondary to underlying heart disease. In these instances the prognosis is usually related to the underlying disease, and most fatalities occur in this group. Thus, in patients with syncope secondary to cardiac arrhythmia, diagnostic studies directed at the nature of the underlying cardiac disease should be pursued assiduously. After complete clinical examination, an ECG, and a chest roentgenogram, appropriate noninvasive evaluation (echocardiography, systolic time intervals, or nuclear studies) should be undertaken. These often establish a diagnosis. Exercise stress testing with myocardial nuclear perfusion studies or the determination of ejection fraction before and after exercise may be indicated when coronary artery disease is a serious consideration. However, coronary angiography is often indicated in patients in whom coronary artery disease is the major consideration.

Arrhythmia Detection
Many patients with cardiac conduction and/or rhythm disturbances leading to syncope are unaware of their arrhythmias. Hence, the evaluation of arrhythmic syncope is often a great diagnostic challenge. Furthermore, an unequivocal linkage between arrhythmia and the occurrence of syncope may be impossible to obtain. Presumption of a cause-and-effect relation based on the total clinical presentation is often all that can be done. However, studies of the efficacy of specific therapy for such arrhythmias indicate that this approach is reasonable.[19]

Laboratory methods used to evaluate arrhythmias include the routine ECG, exercise testing, ambulatory monitoring, patient-activated telephonic devices, and invasive electrophysiological studies.[6,20]

Because of the transient nature of most arrhythmias, the routine ECG is of limited value. However, it is useful in identifying patients having electrophysiologic abnormalities which may predispose them to syncopal episodes; these include the presence of a remote or recent myocardial infarction, WPW or Lown-Ganong-Levine syndrome, sinus and AV node disease, fascicular blocks, and a prolonged QT interval. At some time in the evaluation, careful carotid sinus massage with electrocardiographic and blood pressure monitoring should be performed, since many elderly patients, particularly when they are taking digitalis or antihypertensive drugs, may exhibit a hypersensitive response.

Exercise testing is a method for directly provoking cardiac arrhythmias in the patient with episodic rhythm disorders. It is useful for uncovering ventricular arrhythmias but of limited use for bradyarrhythmias[21] (Fig. 30-1). It should be performed in those with exertional symptoms when ventricular arrhythmia is suspected but not documented by ambulatory monitoring.

The chance of detecting arrhythmias is greater with prolonged ambulatory monitoring than with exercise. While such observation can be done in a hospital monitoring unit, particularly with telemetry, experience has shown that ambulatory monitoring is more efficacious in diagnosing transient arrhythmias when the patient is allowed to perform ordinary daily activities. Ambulatory monitoring for 24 h permits study of one diurnal wake-sleep cycle. The nature of the procedure permits an evaluation of the relation of symptoms to the presence of a cardiac rhythm disturbance. It is important to recognize that one 24-h monitoring period may not be sufficient for detecting transient rhythm disturbances. Indeed, the diagnostic yield significantly increases with up to four 24-h studies. In certain situations more prolonged monitoring is indicated.

When prolonged ambulatory monitoring does not document an arrhythmia, the use of a patient-activated transtelephonic electrocardiographic device may prove efficacious in making the diagnosis. For patients in whom this approach is not successful because of the transient nature of symptoms, a device with internal recording capabilities may establish the diagnosis.

FIGURE 30-1 Sensitivity of ambulatory monitoring and exercise testing in detecting arrhythmia in patients with syncope suspected to be arrhythmic in origin. Ordinate on left indicates number of patients who had cardiac arrhythmia recorded on 24-h ambulatory monitoring. Ordinate on right indicates those who had arrhythmia noted by exercise testing. Ambulatory monitoring was far superior to exercise testing. However, in a few patients, complex ventricular arrhythmias were detected only with exercise testing. SA = sinoatrial; AV = atrioventricular. *(From H. Boudoulas, P. Gleris, S. F. Schaal, C. V. Leier, and R. P. Lewis, Comparison between Electrophysiologic Studies and Ambulatory Monitoring in Patients with Syncope, J. Electrocardiol., 16:91, 1983. Reproduced with permission from the publisher and authors.)*

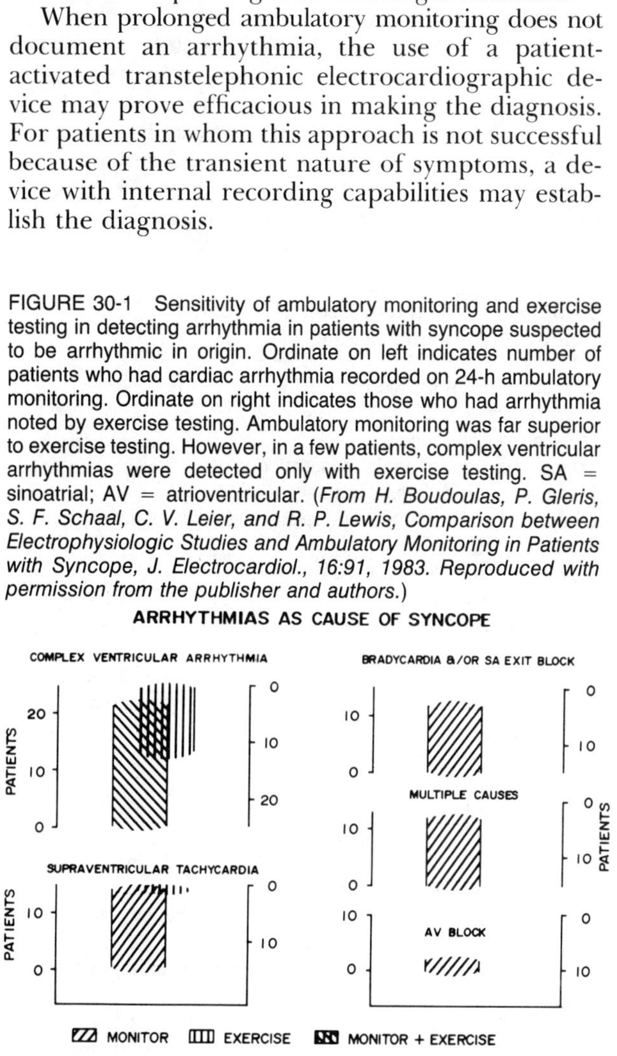

When ambulatory monitoring and exercise testing fail to reveal a clear-cut arrhythmic basis for syncope, invasive electrophysiologic studies employing direct intracardiac recordings and stimulation have been employed.[19,22] The clinical uses of such electrophysiologic studies are summarized in Table 30-3. Electrophysiologic studies may identify abnormalities within the conduction system and localize such abnormalities to various sites, such as the sinus node, atrium, AV node, His bundle, and Purkinje system. Sinus node and atrial function may be evaluated by measuring the SA recovery time, the SA conduction time, and interatrial and intraatrial conduction. AV conduction and automaticity are assessed both at rest and during atrial pacing during such studies. In patients with syncope due to suspected tachycardia, either supraventricular or ventricular, the arrhythmia may be provoked by programmed electrical stimuli with or without adrenergic stimulation. This approach may also define the mechanism of the tachycardia, though nonreentrant tachycardias cannot easily be reproduced. There is also debate over the significance of nonsustained tachyarrhythmias that require aggressive stimulation techniques. The hemodynamic consequences of an arrhythmia can also be measured by simultaneous measurements of arterial pressure and cardiac output. The effectiveness of antiarrhythmic drug therapy and of cardiac pacing in the control of cardiac rhythm disturbances can be directly tested. Potential adverse effects on sinus node function and AV conduction can also be documented. Electrophysiologic testing is a sophisticated technique which is rapidly evolving. Consequently, availability of the technique is still limited and completeness of study varies from one laboratory to another. These factors must be considered both in the decision to perform the study and in the interpretation of the results.

TABLE 30-3 Clinical Uses of Invasive Electrophysiologic Studies

Evaluation of SA function
- SA recovery time
- SA conduction time
- Interatrial and intraatrial conduction time

Evaluation of junctional pacemakers

Evaluation of AV conduction (before and during atrial pacing)
- Atrial to His interval
- His to ventricular depolarization interval
- Dual AV pathways

Evaluation of accessory pathways
- WPW syndrome

Induction and definition of the mechanisms of arrhythmias (Programmed electric stimulation with or without adrenergic stimulation)
- Atrial tachycardias
- Atrial flutter-fibrillation
- Ventricular tachycardia
- Ventricular flutter-fibrillation

Definition of the hemodynamic effects of arrhythmias

Termination of the arrhythmias

Evaluation of the effect of antiarrhythmic agents on arrhythmias, sinus node function, AV conduction

Evaluation of antiarrhythmic and hemodynamic effects of pacemaker therapy

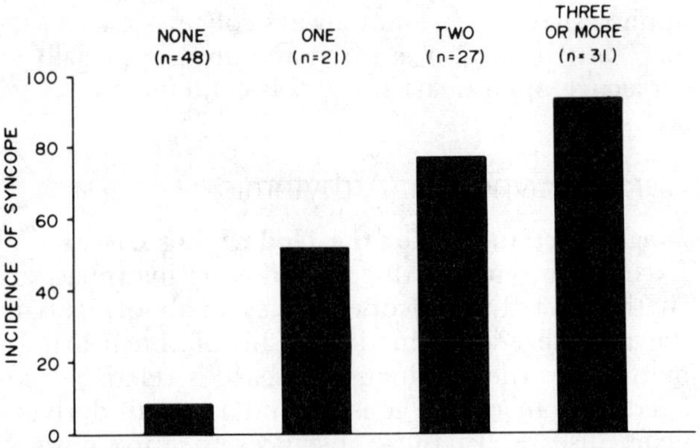

FIGURE 30-2 Relation between the number of electrophysiologic abnormalities and incidence of syncope. The frequency of syncope is plotted against the electrophysiologic abnormalities, which include SA recovery time, SA conduction time, atrial to His interval, His to ventricular depolarization interval, and AV block at slow rates during pacing. As the number of abnormalities increases, the likelihood of syncope increases. (*From H. Boudoulas, S. F. Schaal, and R. P. Lewis, Electrophysiologic Risk Factors of Syncope, J. Electrocardiol., 11:339, 1978. Reproduced with permission from the publisher and authors.*)

Studies in our laboratory have shown that when patients have syncope based on transient SA dysfunction or an AV conduction defect, there are usually at least two electrophysiologic abnormalities[22,23] (Fig. 30-2). The likelihood of syncope increases as the number of electrophysiologic abnormalities increases. Syncope is unlikely to be caused by SA dysfunction or AV conduction defects if these abnormalities are not detected during electrophysiologic studies.

In patients with no obvious cause of syncope or presyncope in whom arrhythmia is strongly suspected, a probable arrhythmic cause can be established in 70 to 80 percent by ambulatory monitoring, exercise testing, transtelephonic patient-activated devices, electrophysiologic studies, or a combination of these tests. For ventricular and supraventricular arrhythmias, electrophysiologic studies are the most helpful, followed by ambulatory monitoring and exercise testing. For detection of SA and AV conduction abnormalities, electrophysiologic studies and ambulatory monitoring are equally useful, whereas exercise testing is of little diagnostic aid (Table 30-4).

Since the yield of diagnostic information increases with more prolonged monitoring, the difficult question often arises as to how much is reasonable. Electrophysiologic studies possess the advantage that arrhythmia can be induced at the time of study. The appropriate diagnostic approach must depend on the perceived severity of the problem in the patient under consideration.

TABLE 30-4 Relative Diagnostic Usefulness of Laboratory Studies in Detection of Arrhythmias

Type of Arrhythmias	Ambulatory Monitoring	Electrophysiologic Studies	Exercise Testing
Ventricular	+ + +	+ + + +	+ +
Supraventricular	+ + +	+ + + +	+
Sinoatrial, atrioventricular	+ + + +	+ + + +	−

Source: H. Boudoulas, A. M. Weissler, R. P. Lewis, and J. V. Warren: The Clinical Diagnosis of Syncope, in W. P. Harvey, et al. (eds.), "Current Problems in Cardiology," Year Book Medical Publishers, Inc., Chicago, 1982, vol. 7, no. 7. Copyright © 1982 by Year Book Medical Publishers, Inc., Chicago. Reproduced with permission from the publisher, editors, and authors.

Combined Causes of Cardiac Syncope

The occurrence of syncope with either obstruction to cardiac output or arrhythmia frequently depends upon additional factors[6,24,25] (Fig. 30-3). Anatomic factors include cerebrovascular disease, ischemic heart disease, left ventricular dysfunction, and valvular heart disease. Physiologic factors include age, posture, wakefulness, state of hydration, medications which impair circulatory responses, arterial blood pressure, anemia, and the metabolic milieu.

Patients with normal cardiac function and normal cerebral circulation can tolerate the changes in heart rate accompanying most cardiac arrhythmias. If there is obstruction to cardiac output, a change in cardiac rhythm (e.g., frequent ventricular premature beats in obstructive cardiomyopathy) may produce a profound reduction in cardiac output. A given arrhythmia may not always produce symptoms, depending upon the setting in which it occurs (e.g., a burst of ventricular tachycardia with the patient in the supine position may not cause syncope).

Reflex bradycardia or vasodepressor response commonly occurs in patients with cardiac disease (e.g., acute inferior myocardial infarction or aortic stenosis). Patients with cardiac syncope often have cerebrovascular disease, so that syncope may present with focal neurologic symptoms. When cerebral blood flow and oxygen delivery are marginal, any minor stress or additional acute illness may cause syncope. Finally, the occurrence of a syncopal episode related to activity may depend not only on the kind of activity but also on its level of intensity. These important contributory factors are often not considered in a routine syncope evaluation. This is a major reason for failure to establish cause-effect relations in patients with cardiac syncope.[8]

FIGURE 30-3 Syncope often is the result of combined factors. Arrhythmia or obstruction to blood flow may or may not induce syncope, depending upon the contributory factors.

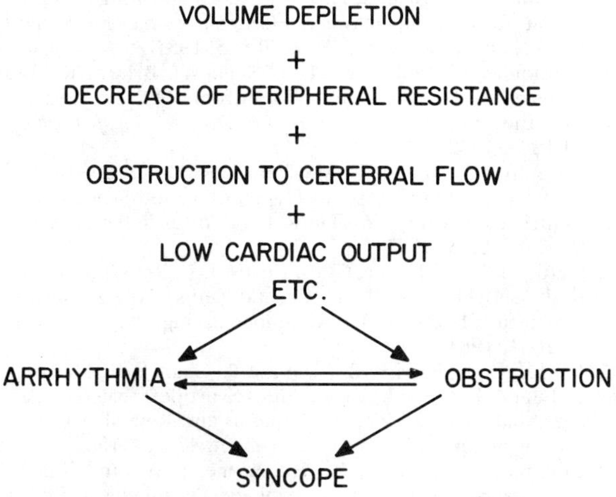

Cardiac Syncope and Sudden Death

Both obstructive and arrhythmic syncope are associated with a high incidence of sudden death.[1,3] Most causes of obstructive syncope can lead to sudden death. Ventricular arrhythmias in coronary artery disease (and possibly in primary myocardial disease) are risk-prognostic indicators independent of the status of left ventricular function and severity of underlying coronary artery disease. In such cases syncope is a manifestation of serious arrhythmias in a patient with severe cardiac disease and thus is a sign of poor prognosis. Syncope due to high-grade AV block can also lead to sudden death, but lesser manifestations of conduction disease such as the sick sinus syndrome or asymptomatic bilateral bundle branch block are not as likely to cause sudden death as has been supposed in the past.

Treatment

A detailed discussion of therapy will not be presented in this chapter since use of cardioactive drugs, pacemakers, and management of arrhythmias are described in Chaps. 27, 28, 89, 104, 105, and 106. A few general principles can, however, be stated. For the patient with syncope caused by obstructive heart disease, open heart surgery is often the treatment of choice (Fig. 30-4). Patients with hypertrophic cardiomyopathy and syncope may respond well to pharmacologic therapy; however, if the obstruction is severe and the patient is symptomatic, surgery is usually indicated. There is no satisfactory therapy for fixed pulmonary hypertension.

Syncope caused by arrhythmia often represents a very difficult therapeutic challenge. Management should be addressed first to any underlying cardiovascular disease and to precipitating or initiating factors. Caffeine or other stimulants should be in-

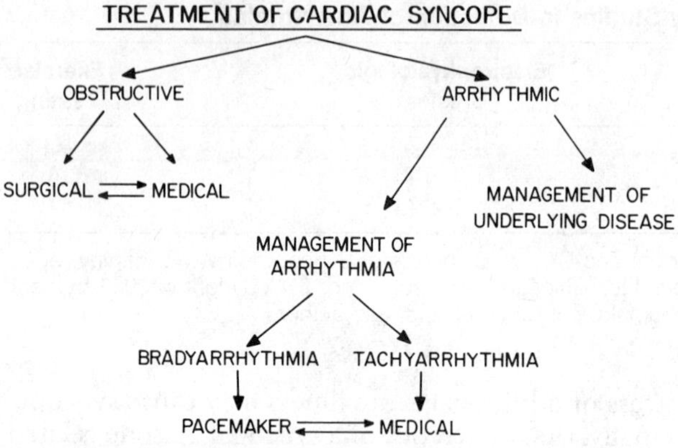

FIGURE 30-4 Treatment of cardiac syncope.

terdicted in patients with tachyarrhythmias. During therapy with antiarrhythmic drugs, efficacy always should be documented with objective criteria such as ambulatory monitoring, exercise testing, or electrophysiologic studies. In patients with tachycardia-bradycardia syndrome, antiarrhythmic drugs that suppress the tachyarrhythmia may aggravate the bradyarrhythmia. In this situation, the placement of a permanent transvenous pacemaker may be required to make it possible for appropriate antiarrhythmic agents to be administered (Fig. 30-4).

One of the most controversial areas of therapy is the use of pacemakers for bradycardic syndromes. In particular, this includes such treatment in older patients with sinus bradycardia, in patients with sick sinus syndrome, and in patients with bifascicular or trifascicular block. In general these disorders have low mortality; therefore pacemaker placement must be justified solely by reduction of symptoms. Although the results of pacemaker therapy in patients with syncope presumed to be due to conduction disease have been questioned, severe syncopal attacks are usually relieved. Care must be taken to avoid pacemaker syndromes, especially in those patients with carotid sinus hypersensitivity or postural hypotension.[18–20]

In patients with idiopathic long-QT syndromes and syncope, beta-blocking drugs usually control the symptoms.[26] If syncope persists despite therapy with beta-blocking drugs, left sympathetic stelectomy with or without beta-blockade therapy is indicated. In syncope due to drugs or metabolic disorders, simple discontinuation of the offending agent and restoration of the metabolic milieu is usually successful.

In patients with recurrent tachyarrhythmias that are refractory to antiarrhythmic drugs, different pacing techniques may be helpful. Pacemakers may be useful in preventing the occurrence of the arrhythmia or in terminating the arrhythmia. Cardiac surgery may play a role in patients with WPW syndrome and refractory supraventricular tachyarrhythmias.

Surgical myocardial revascularization may be helpful in a subgroup of patients with effort-related ventricular arrhythmias and severe proximal coronary artery stenoses. Ventricular aneurysmectomy with nondirected or directed myocardial resection or encircling myocardial ventriculotomy may play a role in a limited number of patients.[27] Finally, in selected patients, particularly those at risk for sudden death syndrome, automatic defibrillator implantation may play a role in controlling ventricular arrhythmias[28] (see Chap. 106).

References

1. Kapoor, W. N., Karpf, M., Wieand, S., Peterson, J. R., and Levey, G. S.: A Prospective Evaluation and Followup of Patients with Syncope, *N. Engl. J. Med.*, 309:197, 1983.
2. Kapoor, W. N., Karpf, M., Maher, Y, Miller, R. A., and Levey, G. S.: Syncope of Unknown Origin, *JAMA* 247:2687, 1982.
3. Silverstein, M. D., Singer, D. E., Mulley, A. G., Thibault, G. E., and Barnett, G. O.: Patients with Syncope Admitted to Medical Intensive Care Units, *JAMA*, 248:1185, 1982.
4. Kapoor, W., Karpf, M., and Levey, G. S.: Issues in Evaluating Patients with Syncope, *Ann. Intern. Med.*, 100:755, 1984. (Editorial.)
5. Morady F., Shen, E., Schwartz, A., et al.: Long-Term Follow-up of Patients with Recurrent Unexplained Syncope Evaluated by Electro-Physiologic Testing, *J. Am. Coll. Cardiol.*, 2:1053, 1983.
6. Boudoulas, H., Weissler, A. M., Lewis, R. P., and Warren, J. V.: The Clinical Diagnosis of Syncope, in W. P. Harvey, et al. (eds.), "Current Problems in Cardiology," Year Book Medical Publishers, Inc., Chicago, vol. 7, no. 7, 1982.
7. Medina, R. P., and Dreifus, L. S.: Syncope, in W. P. Harvey, et al. (eds.), "Current Problems in Cardiology," Year Book Medical Publishers, Inc., Chicago, vol. 8, no. 6, 1983.
8. Gibson, T. C., and Heitzman, M. R.: Diagnostic Efficacy of 24-Hour Electrocardiographic Monitoring for Syncope, *Am. J. Cardiol.*, 53:1013, 1984.
9. Schwartz, L. S., Goldfischer, J., Sprague, G. J., et al.: Syncope and Sudden Death in Aortic Stenosis, *Am. J. Cardiol.*, 23:647, 1969.
10. Dressler, W.: Effort Syncope as an Early Manifestation of Primary Pulmonary Hypertension, *Am. J. Med. Sci.*, 223:131, 1952.
11. Strauss, M. J., Longstreth, W. T., Jr., and Thiele, B. L.: Atypical Cough Syncope, *JAMA*, 251:1731, 1984.
12. Scarpa, W. J.: The Sick Sinus Syndrome, *Am. Heart J.*, 92:648, 1976.
13. Steinbrecher, U. P., and Fitchett, D. H.: Torsade de Pointes. A Cause of Syncope with Atrioventricular Block, *Arch. Intern. Med.*, 140:1223, 1980.
14. Boudoulas, H., Geleris, P., Lewis, R. P., and Rittgers, S. F.: Linear Relationship between Electrical Systole, Mechanical Systole, and Heart Rate, *Chest*, 80:613, 1981.
15. Boudoulas, H., Sohn, Y. H., O'Neill, W., Brown, R., and Weissler, A. M.: The QT QS2 syndrome: A New Mortality Risk Indicator in Coronary Artery Disease, *Am. J. Cardiol.*, 50:1229, 1982.
16. Alicandri, C., Fouad, F. M., Tarazi, R. C., Castle, L., and Morand, V.: Three Cases of Hypotension and Syncope with Ventricular Pacing: Possible Role of Atrial Reflexes, *Am. J. Cardiol.*, 42:137, 1978.
17. Madigan, N. P., Flaker, G. C., Curtis, J. J., Reid, J., Mueller, K. J., and Murphy, T. J.: Carotid Sinus Hypersensitivity: Beneficial Effects of Dual-Chamber Pacing, *Am. J. Cardiol.*, 53:1034, 1984.
18. Morley, C. A., Perrins, E. J., Grant, P., Chan, S. L., McBrien, D. J., and Sutton, R.: Carotid Sinus Syncope Treated by Pacing. Analysis of Persistent Symptoms and Role of Atrioventricular Sequential Pacing, *Br. Heart J.*, 47:411, 1982.
19. DiMarco, J. P., Garan, H., Harthorne, J. W., and Ruskin, J. N.: Intracardiac Electrophysiologic Techniques in Recur-

rent Syncope of Unknown Cause, *Ann. Intern. Med.*, 95:542, 1981.
20. Alpert, M. A.: Syncope: Clinical, Pathophysiologic, and Therapeutic Considerations (Part I & II), *Cardiovasc. Rev. Rep.*, 4:1119, 1983.
21. Boudoulas, H., Schaal, S. F., Lewis, R. P., et al: Superiority of 24-Hour Outpatient Monitoring over Multi-stage Exercise Testing for the Evaluation of Syncope, *J. Electrocardiol.*, 12:103, 1979.
22. Boudoulas, H., Geleris, P., Schaal, S. F., Leier, C. V., and Lewis, R. P.: Comparison between Electrophysiologic Studies and Ambulatory Monitoring in Patients with Syncope, *J. Electrocardiol.* 16:91, 1983.
23. Boudoulas, H., Schaal, S. F., and Lewis, R. P.: Electrophysiologic Risk Factors of Syncope, *J. Electrocardiol.*, 11:339, 1978.
24. Boudoulas, H., and Lewis, R. P.: Differential Diagnosis of Syncope, in H. F. Conn and R. B. Conn (eds.), "Current Diagnosis," W. B. Saunders Company, Philadelphia, 1980, p. 53.
25. Lipsitz, L. A.: Syncope in the Elderly, *Ann. Intern. Med.*, 99:92, 1983.
26. Locati, E., Moss, A. J., Schwartz, P. J., Crampton, R., and Carleen, E.: The Long QT Syndrome, *J. Am. Coll. Cardiol.*, 3:516, 1984. (Abstract.)
27. McGovern, B., DiMarco, J. P., Garan, H., and Ruskin, J. N.: New Concepts in the Management of Ventricular Arrhythmias and Sudden Death, in W. P. Harvey, et al. (eds.), "Current Problems in Cardiology," Year Book Medical Publishers, Inc., Chicago, vol. 7, no. 11, 1983.
28. Mirowski, M., Reid, P. R., Winkle, R. A., et al.: Mortality in Patients with Implanted Automatic Defibrillators, *Ann. Intern. Med.*, 98:585, 1983.

31

Pathology and Mechanisms of Sudden Death

Giorgio Baroldi, M.D.

The science of the precognition of sudden deaths is seen to be not merely useful but extremely necessary to physicians, since the Teacher of our Art [Hippocrates] clearly shows that man not only absolves himself from all blame, but acquires the name of and the admiration owed to a good physician, when he, unable to make everyone well, at least divines and foretells what is about to happen.

G. M. Lancisi, 1707[1]

For millennia, *mors subita,* as any unknown phenomenon, was interpreted in a mythical-religious sense. It took time to replace a voodoo death concept with a more objective approach. From the sudden death of Phidippides the marathon runner in 490 B.C., one of the first examples mentioned in history, we waited until 1707 to have the first objective clinicopathological report. In this year Lancisi[1] described an epidemic of sudden death which had occurred in Rome in 1705. The reader may recognize and translate into up-to-date medical language the close relationship that exists in many cases between cardiac disease and sudden death. Most were wealthy males living in a luxurious style. Common people were subsequently involved, but with less frequency. Females and people continent with respect to food, drink, and sexual life were preserved, a fact providing an early insight into risk factors and prevention. One of the more important contributions was the categorizing of different types of death. Among the three main categories of *natural, untimely,* and *violent,* the death was defined as "slow" or "sudden" and in turn as "foreseen" and "forefelt" or "unforeseen, unperceptible, and unexpected."

From the pathological standpoint, both expectancy and survival time are essential to correctly evaluate the morphologic changes. Accordingly, as a working definition for proper selection of cases, *sudden cardiac death* can be defined as clinical unexplained, rapid death occurring in apparently healthy people, during their normal activity, without a history of pertinent disease and not receiving therapy of any type (*unwarned* or *unexpected*); or as an unusual, unexplained event in the course of an acute or chronic manifest disease (*warned* or *expected*). The pathological findings are confined to the heart; the other organs are involved as a secondary phenomenon. In the present era of resuscitation, one point to be stressed is that at postmortem examination the pathological changes resulting from iatrogenic causes have to be distinguished from natural ones. Prospective studies in subjects dying without therapeutic interference of any type are required.

Pathological Findings in Sudden Cardiac Death

Sudden death may occur in any type of cardiac disease. The aim should be to know the exact frequency of both warned and unwarned events in each type. Generally, in the literature, we deal more with impressions than with figures, the expectancy being variously interpreted. This chapter attempts to list the more frequent pathological findings reported in sudden death, determining the frequency, when possible.

Coronary Arteries

Congenital Malformations

Sudden death is rarely observed in either minor (without abnormal connections) or major (with abnormal connections) coronary anomalies. Rare cases of persons with a single coronary artery or with severe hypoplasia of the right coronary artery dying suddenly after stressful exercise have been reported.[2] Only one variant of a minor abnormality, the dislocation of coronary ostia, shows a significantly higher frequency of sudden death. Among 51 subjects with this anomaly, both coronary arteries arose from the left sinus of Valsalva in 18, and from the anterior sinus of Valsalva in 33.[3] In the latter group, 8 (24.2 percent) subjects died suddenly and unexpectedly, while 1 died suddenly 4 months after a massive infarct. All subjects were young males (mean age 20.0 years, in contrast to 57.3 years in others dying from known causes), and death occurred during or after physical exercise. In contrast, there were no sudden deaths in the group where the coronary arteries originated from the left sinus of Valsalva. When the left coronary artery arises from the anterior sinus, it runs leftward, passing between the aorta and the pulmonary artery. In this anatomic disposition, the left ostium has a slitlike lumen due to its origin at an acute angle. It is postulated that increased physical activity with consequent aortic and pulmonary artery distension may induce a flaplike closure of the stretched anomalous artery, resulting in sudden, fatal ischemia.

Infectious-Immune and Thromboembolic Processes

In coronary arteritis, sudden death may ensue because of the rupture of an aneurysm (polyarteritis nodosa, benign mucocutaneous lymph node syndrome) or following secondary occlusive thrombosis.[4–7] Of 233 cases with luetic aortitis, 37 had mono- or bilateral obstruction of the coronary ostia and death was sudden in 17.[8] In 11 subjects with aortitis of various types (personally reviewed from the files of the Armed Forces Institute of Pathology), bilateral (sub)occlusion of the coronary ostia was associated with sudden and unexpected death in one instance.

Coronary embolism is frequently associated with sudden death. It has been reported in 60 percent of 74 cases. The underlying disorders were acute and subacute bacterial endocarditis (63.6 percent); thrombus of the heart chambers (10.9 percent); luetic aortitis (5.4 percent); ulcerated aortic plaque (4.1 percent); paradoxical emboli of various kinds (4.1 percent); aortic (2.7 percent) or proximal (2.7 percent) coronary thrombosis; pulmonary thrombus, caseous tuberculous material, neoplastic tissue, fragment of calcific valve (1.3 percent); or disorders of undetermined nature (1.3 percent). Frequent sites of embolization were the left main coronary trunk (32.4 percent), the left anterior descending branch (35.1 percent), the right coronary artery (12.2 percent), and the left circumflex (4.1 percent).[9]

Contradictory results have been reported regarding the frequency of platelet aggregates occluding the small intramural arterial vessels in sudden death. In one study[10] they were found with high frequency in sudden coronary deaths without acute coronary lesions, while in another study no difference was noted between sudden death cases and controls.[11]

Degenerative Processes

The atherosclerotic plaque is the most frequent postmortem finding in sudden death cases. This is the reason why, today, we speak of *sudden coronary death.* In a recent study of 208 selected cases (182 males, 26 females) of sudden and unexpected death (unrelated to physical effort), the maximal lumen/diameter reduction due to an atherosclerotic plaque was as follows: 28 cases (13.4 percent) with less than 50 percent, 23 cases (11.0 percent) between 50 and 69 percent, and 157 cases (75.4 percent) with more than 70 percent lumen reduction (29 cases between 70 and 79 percent, 53 between 80 and 89 percent, and 75 with more than 90 percent). In 53 cases only one main coronary vessel had a severe stenosis (≥70 percent); in 60 cases, two vessels had severe stenosis; and in 44 cases, three or more vessels were severely narrowed. Of 401 severe stenoses, 48 had a length of less than 2 mm, 139 were between 6 and 20 mm, and 214 were more than 20 mm long; most were concentric (345 concentric versus 56 semilunar). The structure of 216 plaques was mainly fibrous, while in 185 plaques atheromatous material prevailed. The right coronary artery, particularly its anterior segment, and the left anterior descending artery were the most compromised vessels. The left main trunk and the posterior descending branch only rarely showed severe stenosis (11 and 12 cases, respectively). In 32 cases (15.3 percent) an acute occlusive thrombus was located in an area of severe stenosis, generally longer than 20 mm and caused by a concentric atheromatous plaque. In 16 cases, the thrombus showed organization histologically, indicating that it antedated the sudden death by days. In 22 cases, a mural thrombus (thin, laminar, fibrin platelet deposition) was present, showing the same characteristics related to the plaque as the occlusive one.[12]

The rare primary dissecting aneurysm of coronary arteries is caused by an unknown "degenerative" process and leads to myocardial infarction and/or sudden death. The latter, if defined as unexpected, occurred in 18 (15 females, 3 males) of 24 cases reported in the literature.[13] Perhaps this is one of the few examples in which the frequency of sudden death is significantly higher in females than in males.

Heart Muscle and Cardiac Valves

Congenital Malformations

Among complications (heart failure, bacterial endocarditis, embolism, pulmonary hypertension, etc.) of congenital malformations of the heart,[14] sudden death seems to be a rare expected event. It is generally stated that it occurs more frequently in aortic stenosis, as well as in any condition producing obstruction of the left ventricular outflow tract. However, in a large series of children with congenital aortic stenosis, the frequency of sudden death was 1 percent (2 of 199 cases).[15]

Infectious-Immune Diseases

An inflammatory reaction in the myocardium during the course of an infectious or allergic disease may be the cause of sudden death.[16]

Of 45 human transplanted heart cases, 2 died suddenly and 2 had ventricular fibrillation which was successfully treated. In 72 percent there were atrial arrhythmias, and in 52 percent there were ventricular premature beats, frequently preceding episodes of acute rejection.[17]

On the other hand, foci of inflammatory reaction are frequently seen in the myocardium of people dying suddenly. In one of the first reports, sudden and unexpected death (three cases) was attributed to an "acute interstitial myocarditis." The latter consisted of rare microfoci of lymphocytes and occasional plasma cells, often associated with degenerative changes in myocardial cells.[18] Similar findings were observed in 81 percent of sudden death cases, in contrast to 33 and 31 percent of chronic coronary and noncoronary patients, respectively.[19] In our experience, microscopic foci of lymphocytes within "normal" myocardium were found in 66.8 percent of selected sudden death cases and in 53.6 percent of normal subjects. In the latter, however, the infiltrates were less numerous and extensive. Furthermore, lymphocytes and histiocytes were frequently associated with focal Zenker necrosis in a reparative stage.

Cardiomyopathies—Myocardial Necrosis

The *idiopathic* or *primary* cardiomyopathies, as well as the secondary cardiomyopathies, include a variety of conditions. Sudden death may occur in any of them. Among the four different morphofunctional categories (hypertrophic, congestive, obliterative, restrictive) into which they have been classified, hypertrophic cardiomyopathy shows the highest frequency of sudden death, even without prodromes. In two series of 119 and 190 patients, followed for 10 to 15 years, the frequency of sudden death was 15.9 and 13.6 percent, respectively.[20] Of 26 other cases who died suddenly and unexpectedly, 19 were male and 7 female. There was no left ventricular outflow tract gradient in 6 of 12 catheterized patients, and all 19 had abnormal electrocardiograms. A family history of sudden death was recorded in 9.[21]

The term *myocardial necrosis* is used in a very broad sense, as a common end result of many causes. However, the myocardial cell may die, not only for different reasons, but also in different ways. At present, at least three types of myocardial cell death may be recognized morphologically, each suggesting a different functional status of the cell: (1) *irreversible relaxation* (coagulation or infarct necrosis); (2) *irreversible hypercontraction* (myofibrillar degeneration, contraction band necrosis, or Zenker necrosis so-called because of its similarity to Zenker lesion in skeletal muscles); (3) *progressive failure* of relaxation-contraction coupling (colliquative myocytolysis or myocytolysis tout court).

In coronary atherosclerotic heart disease, all three types of necrosis can be seen, frequently together (Table 31-1).[22] Irrespective of the size of the coagulation necrosis, most infarcts show a more or less extensive associated Zenker necrosis in the surrounding normal myocardium. Also, in about 40 percent of cases, myocytolysis is observed in the noninfarcted subendocardial or perivascular myocardial layers. In sudden and unexpected coronary death cases, coagulation necrosis was found in 17 percent; Zenker necrosis was found in 86 percent, being the unique detectable acute lesion in 72 percent. In contrast, myocytolysis was seen in only 8 percent of the subjects. It was mainly associated with extensive myocardial fibrosis. It may be pertinent to emphasize that there was no relation between both coagulation and Zenker necrosis and cardiac hypertrophy; the latter was in general unrelated to sudden death.

A general consideration is that one lesion may have several causes, but each cause produces one type of lesion. Accordingly, the clear-cut morphology of the histologic changes (Fig. 31-1) suggests that both the underlying biochemical disorder and the etiopathogenesis are specific for each type of myocardial cell death.

Heart Tumors

The frequencies of both warned and unwarned sudden death according to clinical findings reported in a recent publication are summarized in Table 31-2.

In primary malignant tumors no sudden death was reported, but sudden death occurred in 2 of 39 patients with angiosarcoma and in 4 of 26 with rhabdomyosarcoma.[23] Sudden death may occur without any previous symptoms and signs, despite an extremely large tumor mass.

Conduction System

Examination of the conduction system should be mandatory in any subject dying suddenly. A serial

TABLE 31-1 Histologic Pattern in Different Types of Myocardial Necrosis in Coronary Heart Disease

Myocardium	Coagulation Necrosis (Infarct Necrosis)	Coagulative Myocytolysis (Zenker Necrosis)	Colliquative Myocytolysis (Myocytolysis)
Functional status	Irreversible relaxation (atonic death) + stretching by intraventricular pressure	Irreversible contraction (tetanic death)	Progressive loss of function (failing death)
Muscle fiber	Early thinning	Normal or swollen	Increasing edema, vacuolization
Nucleus	Elongation, pyknosis, progressive fading	Normal	Normal
Myofibrils	Elongated sarcomeres in normal registered order, even in late stage	Rhexis, anomalous irregular crossband formations (coagulation of hypercontracted sarcomeres)	Progressive disappearance
Vessels	Secondary wall degeneration and thrombosis	Normal	Normal
Infiltration	Massive polymorphonuclear exudation	No early infiltrates, possible late lymphocytes	No infiltrates
Extension-location	In general single massive focus of different size, internal to transmural	Multiple (mono- or pluri-cellular) disseminated or confluent foci of different size in any muscular layer	Focal subendocardial and perivascular, progressively spreading
Irreversible within	At least 20–60 min	Few minutes	?
Healing	Removal by macrophages; collagenization of empty sarcolemmal tubes	Removal by macrophages; collagenization of empty sarcolemmal tubes	Removal by macrophages; collagenization of empty sarcolemmal tubes
Frequency in coronary heart disease:			
Acute infarct	100% pathognomonic	100% external layer of infarct 77% in normal myocardium	43%
Sudden death	17% histologically demonstrated	72% only demonstrable lesion 86% including cases with coagulation necrosis	8%
Other conditions	——	Pheochromocytoma, "stone heart," transplanted human heart, Chagas heart disease, exp. infusion of catecholamines	Cardiomyopathies with low-output syndrome

Source: G. Baroldi, G. Falzi, and F. Mariani, Sudden Coronary Death. A Post-mortem Study in 208 Selected Cases Compared to 97 "Control" Subjects, *Am. Heart J.*, 98:20, 1979. Reprinted with permission from the publisher and authors.

section study is required for the correct evaluation of this anatomic structure, and this requirement has limited our source of information. A major contribution has been made in a series of 30 clinicopathological reports ("De Subitaneis Mortibus") published in *Circulation* from August 1973 to June 1978.[24,25] The conduction system was examined by serial sections in a total of 77 sudden death cases (43 males and 34 females), excluding one instance of coronary embolism in a 20-week-old fetus (spontaneous abortion). In 60 cases the underlying diseases were asymmetric septal hypertrophy (22 cases), scleroderma (8 cases), long QT syndromes (8 cases), rupture of an infarcted interventricular septum (5 cases), pheochromocytoma (3 cases), type A Wolff-Parkinson-White syndrome (2 cases), persistent superior vena cava (2 cases), rheumatoid arthritis (2 cases), Pickwickian syndrome, homocystinuria, familial congenital heart block, Whipple's disease, ankylosing spondylitis, sarcoidosis, coarctation of aorta, and metastatic hypernephroma (1 case each). Most of the 60 cases presented with arrhythmias, while conduction disturbances (varying degrees of heart block, paroxysmal atrial fibrillation, premature ventricular beats, etc.) were the only signs in 7 cases. In 10 cases the history contributed nothing. In these cases, as well as in 17 cases with hypertrophic cardiomyopathy, the sudden death occurred without warning. The main pathological findings within the conduction system were:

1. Benign tumor (fibroma compressing His bundle, polycystic tumor of the AV node, multifocal Purkinje cell tumor) was found in 4 cases.
2. Focal neuritis and neural degeneration occurred in the cases with long QT syndromes.
3. Structural anomalies (persistent fetal dispersion of AV node and His bundle in central fibrous body, loop or unusual connections, malformation of AV node and His bundle, venous lacunae, etc.) occurred in 25 cases.
4. Focal degeneration and/or fibrosis was found in more than half of the cases.
5. Focal or diffuse replacement by adipose tissue was found in 12 cases.
6. "Fibromuscular medial dysplasia" obstructing the sinus and AV node arterial vessels was an isolated finding in 6 patients and was frequently observed

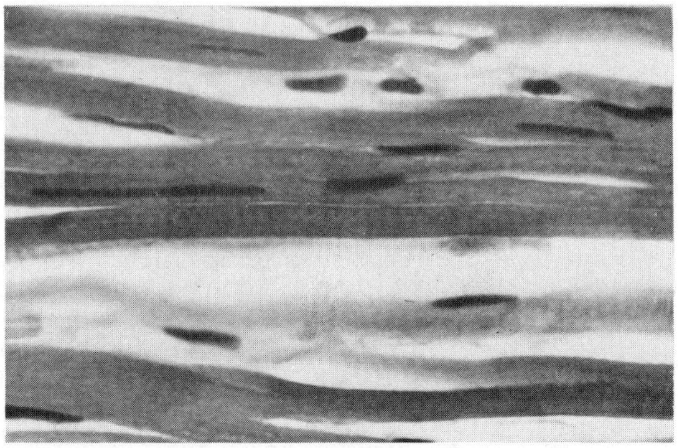

A

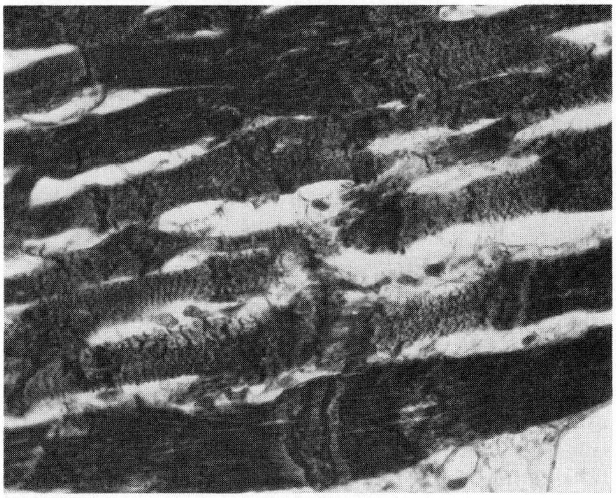

B

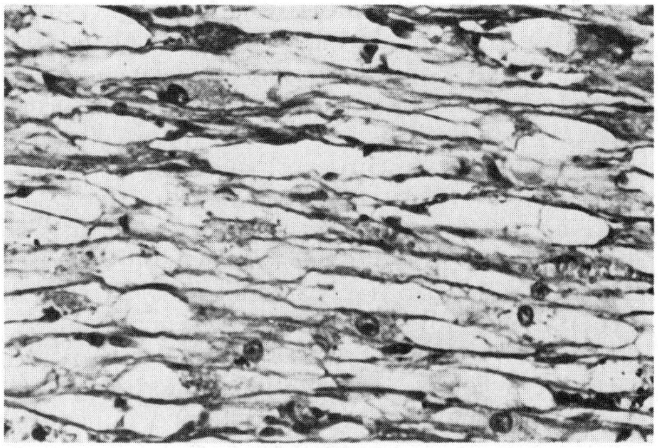

C

FIGURE 31-1 Early changes in different types of myocardial necrosis in coronary heart disease. *A.* Coagulation necrosis (atonic death). Thinning of the myocardial cells and elongation of the nuclei due to stretching by intraventricular pressure. The myofibrillar apparatus is undamaged. H&E; × 314. *B.* Zenker necrosis or coagulative myocytolysis (tetanic death). Hypercontraction with myofibrillar rhexis and anomalous crossband formation. PTAH; × 431. *C.* Myocytolysis or colliquative myocytolysis (failing death). Disappearance of the myofibrils secondary to progressive vacuolization of the muscle fibers. H&E; × 216.

in cases with underlying diseases (7 with scleroderma, 13 with asymmetric hypertrophy, all 3 cases of pheochromocytoma, 3 cases with rupture of interventricular septum, 1 case with homocystinuria, rheumatoid arthritis, ankylosing spondylitis, sarcoidosis, coarctation of aorta, extensive acute myocarditis).

7. Other vascular lesions were panarteritis in the Whipple's disease case, disseminated intravascular coagulation in a pregnant woman with paroxysmal atrial fibrillation, platelet aggregates in the pheochromocytoma and homocystinuria cases, and occlusion of a normal sinus node artery by a fibromuscular polypoid mass. In only 10 of these 77 cases was there a severe obstruction of the main subepicardial coronary arteries. In one instance it was located proximally to the origin of the AV node artery (case with Pickwickian syndrome), while in another (acute extensive myocarditis in a 19-year-old male with a history of atrial fibrillation) atresia of the left main trunk was observed.

In another serial section study[26] done on 49 cases of sudden death associated with severe coronary atherosclerosis with or without demonstrable myocardial infarction, no specific findings were noted in the conduction system. Intimal thickening with significant luminal narrowing was present in the sinus node or an AV node artery in 25 and 50 percent, respectively. In only two instances with massive interventricular septal infarction was the AV node necrotic. Other nonspecific findings, such as a marked degree of fibrosis or fatty replacement, were found in the sinus node (9 cases), AV node (21 cases), His bundle (22 cases), and right (4 cases), left (14 cases), or both (7 cases) bundle branches.

Main Pathogenetic Mechanisms in Sudden Cardiac Death

In about 90 percent of sudden death cases occurring out of a hospital, as well as in all but one of the reported patients who died suddenly while undergoing electrocardiographic monitoring, ventricular fibrillation (preceded by heart rate acceleration and ventricular ectopic activity) is the terminal cardiac disorder. Asystole, idioventricular rhythm, or electromechanical dissociation was observed in the remaining subjects (see Chap. 32). Despite this limited information confined to a selected group of sudden death patients with coronary atherosclerosis, ventricular fibrillation seems to be the leading cause of a cardiac arrest. The general belief is that the latter may be triggered by ischemia due to obstructive coronary vascular changes (absolute or coronarogenic ischemia) leading to electrical instability of the myocardium. Any other condition (anemia, hypertrophy of the heart, aortic stenosis, strenuous exercise, hypotension, hyperthyroidism, etc.) thought

TABLE 31-2 Sudden Death in Primary Benign Cardiac Tumors*

Type	Number of Cases	Sudden Death Unwarned	Sudden Death Warned	Annotations
Myxoma	130	5	–	
Papillary fibroelastoma	42	3	–	13 aortic cusps (occl. cor. ostium)
Rhabdomyoma	36	?	–	
Fibroma, IV septum	10	6	–	Compression bundle branches
Fibroma, free wall	7	–	–	
Lipomatous hypertrophy, atrial septum	32	2	–	
Lipoma, heart/pericardium	5	–	1	
Hemangioma	15	–	–	
Mesothelioma, AV node	12	2	5	Symptoms lasted 5 months to 37 years
Teratoma	14	2	–	
Bronchogenic/pericardial cysts	89	–	–	

*From data of H. A. McAllister and J. J. Fenoglio.[23]

able to reduce either the oxygen supply or the coronary flow or to increase the metabolic demand may be responsible for inducing the fatal arrhythmias (relative or noncoronarogenic ischemia or relative coronary insufficiency).

From the pathological standpoint, most people who died suddenly can be included in the ischemic group. In the small percentage of nonischemic cases, particularly those who died without warning, little is known as to the type of the terminal disorder. What they show are (1) extracardiac complications of a primary cardiac disease and/or dysfunction (cardiogenic embolism, pulmonary lesions, cerebral anoxia, etc.) causing sudden death by extracardiac damage or possibly by nervous reflexes affecting cardiac function; or (2) myocardial or conduction system changes (microfocal degenerative and/or inflammatory processes, structural abnormalities, neoplastic growth) associated or not associated with a specific disease. Both ischemic and nonischemic lesions may be present in combination in particular conditions, as in hypertrophic cardiomyopathy (compression of the intramural vessels, obstruction of the outflow tract, inflow resistance due to impaired relaxation, abnormal arrangement of the myocardial cells, deep clefts of the septum, vascular narrowing, fibrosis of the sinus node, cystic central fibrous body, etc.).

The basic question concerns the significance of the various lesions found in cases of sudden death in terms of their cause-effect relations. Apart from situations in which the latter seems evident (e.g., cardiac tamponade following rupture of a necrotic cardiac wall, of a coronary aneurysm, or of the ascending aorta; of the 208 cases of sudden coronary death, wall rupture was observed in three with coagulation necrosis and in one with transmural Zenker necrosis), most, if not all, lesions are nonspecific and mainly reported in single case reports without a controlled study of their frequency in the general population, in which normal subjects and noncardiac patients have to be included. With but few exceptions and despite the need of more accurate prospective studies, it may be stated that, in general, these nonspecific lesions in the majority of cases are not associated with sudden death. Why then does sudden death occur?

Pathogenetic Significance of the Pathological Findings in Sudden Cardiac Death

At present the true linkage between the pathological findings and the fatal cardiac disorders is still unclear and often questionable; sudden death remains for the majority of the cases an unanswered question. In an attempt to review this point we may distinguish primary vascular and myocardial lesions, both acute and chronic.

Vascular Lesions

Among *acute vascular lesions,* dissecting aneurysm and embolism of the main subepicardial coronary arteries appear as the lesions more frequently linked with sudden death. These rare events may be compared with an experimental acute occlusion of a normal coronary artery which is frequently followed by ventricular fibrillation. However, since the latter may be prevented by beta-adrenergic blocking drugs, the possibility arises that a mechanism other than ischemia could promote the cardiac disorders (see "Myocardial Lesions"). Subepicardial coronary thrombus is another acute event seen in a small percentage of sudden death cases associated with coronary atherosclerosis. Its significance in terms of blood flow reduction has been questioned, since the thrombus is always found at the site of a severe stenosis already bypassed by compensatory collateral flow; this concept is supported by finding organizing occlusive thrombi without associated infarction and by the lack of any cardiac changes paralleled by a dramatic increase in collaterals after occlusion of an experimental stenosis which had lasted a few days.[27,28]

Platelet aggregates formed in situ or embolized from major vessels into the intramural circulation are frequently reported as a cause of ischemic sudden death. In our experience, sudden death and control cases showed no difference in the frequency and number of vessels involved. Platelet aggregates appear to be linked with a protracted terminal type of blood stasis with separation of the blood elements. On the other hand, thrombotic thrombocytopenic purpura (TTP) looks like an experimental pooling in human beings of several ischemic and hypoxic factors (extremely severe hemolytic anemia and obstructive microangiopathy, hemorrhagic diathesis, neurologic convulsive disorders, coma). If each factor was a true cause of absolute or relative ischemia, any TTP patient should be a "coronary" patient. In our 39 cases, and 200 reviewed from the literature no one had angina or infarction and only two died suddenly in the course of manifest disease. Finally, ischemic heart disease is a chronic pattern in which a continuous shower of platelet aggregates might be expected. Consequently, a TTP-like microangiopathy should also be expected in ischemic heart disease; but this is a finding never shown, as it was impossible to show any type of so-called small-vessel disease which could be considered responsible for sudden death.[11]

The previous example of TTP raises questions about many of the other proposed mechanisms of sudden death (anemia, disseminated intravascular coagulation, hypotension), as well as any other cause which implies an increased metabolic demand of the myocardium. Embolism of atheromatous material originating from a ruptured atherosclerotic plaque deserves a few words. This is a hypothesis often quoted but never demonstrated. Extensive examination of several hundred hearts (an average of 30 total wall samples per heart), both with acute infarction and from subjects dying suddenly, showed only one instance of chronic "cholesterol" embolus found in a septal branch surrounded by normal myocardium.

Among the *chronic vascular lesions,* the obstructive atherosclerotic plaque is thought to be a major culprit in causing sudden death. However, three main facts question this point of view. First, there is a very high frequency of severe, multiple atherosclerotic obstructions found in normal subjects dying by accident and in atherosclerotic noncardiac patients dying in hospitals of diseases not involving the heart. Second, there is apparently no relationship between the degree of atherosclerotic damage and ischemic heart disease. In other words, one may have a first infarction or die suddenly without warning with no or minimal coronary stenosis or with one severe (lumen/diameter reduction greater than 70 percent) or three 90 percent stenoses, all or most of the main vessels being involved; there is apparently no critical degree of damage which causes ischemia. Third, severe atherosclerosis must be a very chronic process existing for a long time before the first clinical episode. This means that candidates for clinically overt disease are handling a normal, often stressful lifestyle despite severe coronary lesions. Marathon runners dying suddenly are a good example. All these facts suggest that the increase in the number of enlarged collaterals (proportional to the number of stenoses, without relation to sex, age, and sudden death) demonstrated postmortem by tridimensional coronary casts is capable of maintaining an adequate compensatory flow to the myocardium. No proof exists that sudden death or infarction is due to an acute failure of this compensatory mechanism. The concept of spasm of the collaterals cannot be accepted since, in human beings, the collaterals lack a muscular tunica. The same can be stated in the cases with bilateral occlusion of the coronary ostia where extracoronary collaterals are present, even in the presence of a greatly hypertrophied heart, but without signs of ischemia in most cases.[28]

The same criticism seems appropriate for the chronic obstructive lesions occasionally seen in the intramural vessels. We were unable to demonstrate any cause-effect relations between these lesions (intimal or medial hyperplasia obliterans) and sudden death, their frequency being the same in sudden death, infarction, and control cases. Furthermore, it has been demonstrated in human beings and experimentally that proliferative medial and intimal thickening is a phenomenon which occurs in the intramural arterial vessels surviving myocardial coagulation necrosis, or infarction. To find them around a scar means that they are a consequence and not the cause of the infarction.[28] In contrast, TTP is a good example, in this regard, to show that a severe microangiopathy does not induce ischemic heart disease.

Only a very small percentage of cases with aortic stenosis and/or cardiac hypertrophy die suddenly. The microfocal fibrosis seen in these conditions has been interpreted as ischemic. However, they may have a different nature (see "Myocardial Lesions"). In evaluating the possible ischemic effect of cardiac hypertrophy, there is an extreme example worthy of mention. In cor pulmonale, the right ventricle increases its muscular mass dramatically, approximating that of the left ventricle. In the hypertrophic right ventricle, even in the presence of severe obstruction of the right coronary artery, a primitive infarction has never been demonstrated in our material, and the patients died of congestive heart failure.

Myocardial Lesions

Scars of the myocardium found in sudden death cases are the anonymous end result of several degenerative processes and obviously have preceded the sudden death by a long time. Tumors of the heart may also exist for many years before being associated with sudden death. Their meaning in relation to the pathogenesis of the latter is still unclear, as are the microfocal lymphocytic infiltrates frequently found in sudden death cases but also present with a relatively high frequency in the normal controls. The nature of these infiltrates is totally unknown. One is reluctant to accept them as "foci of irritability" leading to ventricular fibrillation when found within a normal myocardium. On the other hand, lymphocytes and macrophages are often found as a secondary response to an acute lesion, namely Zenker necrosis found in the majority of sudden death cases associated with coronary atherosclerosis.

This necrosis, however, is unrelated to the degree of the coronary damage, showing the same incidence in subjects with absent or minimal atherosclerosis. Therefore those studies which excluded subjects with less than 50 percent stenosis may not be representative of the so-called sudden coronary death. In discussing this lesion, four main facts seem pertinent: (1) its identity with the necrosis induced by catecholamines;[29] (2) its constant presence around an infarct; (3) its relation to ventricular fibrillation, both being prevented by beta blockers;[30] and (4) the increasing evidence that a sympathetic overactivity acts in sudden death as well as in acute infarct.[31,32] These facts suggest the following two pathogenic possibilities. The first is a sympathetic overstimulation of the normal myocardium to compensate for the loss of contraction of a large, overdistended, infarcted area, damage similar to that shown to produce cardiac hypertrophy in the early phase of experimental aortic stenosis. The second is a congenital or acquired sympathetic overactivity, since the same lesion, even an extensive one, can be seen in small infarcts which cannot mechanically affect the function of the pump. Coincidentally, the occurrence of Zenker necrosis may assume two possible meanings. It may be the hallmark (this necrosis is already visible in a few minutes) of a nondemonstrable large infarct (for unequivocal histologic demonstration of an infarct, 6 to 8 h of survival are needed, all other methods proposed for an earlier recognition being untenable), or it may be the histologic hallmark of a primitive metabolic disorder due to catecholamines or catecholamine-like agents. The cases of sudden death without myocardial infarction, in which different stages of organization of Zenker foci are shown, indicate that this may be the case,[33] a view further supported by the fact that 81 percent of subjects successfully resuscitated by defibrillation do not show evidence of an infarct, and 62 percent do not present lactic acid dehydrogenase isoenzymes (see Chap. 32). Keep in mind that enzymes may be released by Zenker necrosis and not necessarily by the coagulation necrosis of an infarct.

Myocardial Infarct in Relation to Sudden Death

From the previous data it seems possible to say that a patient with an infarct may die suddenly and that most of the sudden death subjects do not die because of an infarct. In the present terminological confusion in which terms such as *coronary thrombosis* (or *atherosclerosis, insufficiency, occlusion*), *cardiac infarct, sudden coronary death,* and *myocardial necrosis* are all used without discrimination, it is time for a more precise definition according to the morphofunctional significance of the lesions found.

A cause-effect relation means that any time a cause acts the expected effect has to occur. Most, if not all, of the proposed causes of sudden death do not follow this basic law. The related pathological findings or associated processes are too frequently present in controls. At the most they may be regarded as morphologic predisposing or risk factors. One may speculate that in a heart with such a jeopardizing handicap—how could the person survive so long?—any stimulus increasing function may lead to a fatal arrhythmia, taking into consideration the different types of myocardial necrosis and their different possible meanings. In this context, myocardial infarction and sudden death can be considered two different aspects of a unique entity in which various pathogenic mechanisms appear to interact, leading to different types of death.

In this era of the coronary spasm, the pathologist also has to consider what he or she cannot see. Cineangiography has demonstrated that spasm is a fact, and that it occurs in angina and myocardial infarction. It still remains unknown if it is the cause of these events or if it is an associated, secondary phenomenon. Nevertheless, it is a provocative concept even for sudden death, both as an occlusive cause per se and as a cause of temporary occlusion. We know that reflow after a certain period of time induces contraction band necrosis and extensive interstitial hemorrhage, often associated with ventricular fibrillation. Contraction band necrosis, alias Zenker necrosis, is typical in sudden coronary death; however, no interstitial hemorrhage is found.

References

1. Lancisi, G. M.: "De Subitaneis Mortibus", Buegni, Roma, 1707. (Translated by P. D. White and A. V. Boursey, St. John's University Press, New York, 1971.)
2. Blake, H. A., Manion, W. C., Mattingly, T. W., and Baroldi, G.: Coronary Artery Anomalies, *Circulation,* 30:927, 1964.
3. Cheitlin, M. D., De Castro, C. M., and McAllister, H. A.: Sudden Death as a Complication of Anomalous Left Coronary Origin from the Anterior Sinus of Valsalva. A Not-So-Minor Congenital Anomaly, *Circulation,* 50:780, 1974.
4. Sinclair, W., Jr., and Nitsch, E.: Polyarteritis Nodosa of the Coronary Arteries. Report of a Case with Rupture of an Aneurysm and Intrapericardial Hemorrhage, *Am. Heart J.,* 38:898, 1949.
5. Kegel, S. M., Dorsey, T. J., Rowen, M., and Taylor, W. F.: Cardiac Death in Mucocutaneous Lymph Node Syndrome, *Am. J. Cardiol.,* 40:282, 1977.
6. Burns, C. J., and Manion, W. C.: Sudden Unexpected Death of a Two-Year-Old Child from Thrombosis of Both Coronary Arteries with Aneurysmal Dilatation of the Vessels, *Med. Ann. D. C.,* 38:381, 1969.
7. Ahronheim, J. H.: Isolated Coronary Periarteritis: Report of a Case of Unexpected Death in a Young Pregnant Woman, *Am. J. Cardiol.,* 40:287, 1977.
8. Scharfman, W. B., Wallach, J. B., and Angrist, A.: Myocar-

dial Infarction due to Syphilitic Coronary Ostial Stenosis, *Am. Heart J.*, 40:603, 1950.
9. Wenger, N. K., and Bauer, S.: Coronary Embolism. Review of the Literature and Presentation of Fifteen Cases, *Am. J. Med.*, 25:549, 1958.
10. Haerem, J. W.: Platelet Aggregates in Intramyocardial Vessels of Patients Dying Suddenly and Unexpectedly of Coronary Artery Disease, *Atherosclerosis*, 15:199, 1972.
11. Baroldi, G., Falzi, G., Mariani, F., and Baroldi, L. A.: Morphology, Frequency and Significance of Intramural Arterial Lesions in Sudden Coronary Death, G. *Ital. Cardiol.*, 10:644, 1980.
12. Baroldi, G., Falzi, G., and Mariani, F.: Sudden Coronary Death. A Post-mortem Study in 208 Selected Cases Compared to 97 "Control" Subjects, *Am. Heart J.*, 98:20, 1979.
13. Claudon, D. G., Claudon, D. B., and Edwards, J. E.: Primary Dissecting Aneurysm of Coronary Artery. A Cause of Acute Myocardial Ischemia, *Circulation*, 45:259, 1972.
14. Edwards, J. E.: Congenital Malformations of the Heart and Great Vessels, in S. E. Gould (ed.), "Pathology of the Heart and Blood Vessels," 3d ed., Charles C Thomas, Publisher, Springfield, Ill., 1968, p. 262.
15. Glew, R. H., Varghese, J. P., Krovetz, J. L., Dorst, J. P., and Rowe, R. D.: Sudden Death in Congenital Aortic Stenosis. A Review of Eight Cases with an Evaluation of Premonitory Clinical Features, *Am. Heart J.*, 78:615, 1969.
16. Gore, I., and Kline, I. K.: Pericarditis and Myocarditis. B Myocarditis, in S. E. Gould (ed.), "Pathology of the Heart and Blood Vessels," 3d ed., Charles C Thomas, Publisher, Springfield, Ill., 1968, p. 731.
17. Schroeder, J. S., Berke, D. K., Graham, A. F., Rider, A. K., and Harrison, D. C.: Arrhythmias after Cardiac Transplantation, *Am. J. Cardiol.*, 33:604, 1974.
18. Helwig, F. C., and Wilhelmy, E. W.: Sudden and Unexpected Death from Acute Interstitial Myocarditis: A Report of Three Cases, *Am. Intern. Med.*, 13:107, 1939.
19. Haerem, J. W.: Myocardial Lesions in Sudden Unexpected Coronary Death, *Am. Heart J.*, 90:562, 1975.
20. Goodwin, J. F., and Krikler, D. M.: Sudden Death in Cardiomyopathy, in V. Manninen and P. I. Halonen (eds.), "Sudden Coronary Death," *Adv. Cardiol.*, 25:98, 1978.
21. Maron, B. J., Roberts, W. C., Edward, J. E., McAllister, H. A., Jr., Foley, D. D., and Epstein, S. E.: Sudden Death in Patients with Hypertrophic Cardiomyopathy: Characterization of 26 Patients without Functional Limitation, *Am. J. Cardiol.*, 41:803, 1978.
22. Baroldi, G.: Different Morphologic Types of Myocardial Cell Death in Man, in A. Fleckstein and G. Rona (eds.) "Pathophysiology and Morphology of Myocardial Cell Alteration," vol. 6: "Recent Advances in Studies on Cardiac Structure and Metabolism," University Park Press, Baltimore, 1975, p. 383.
23. McAllister, H. A., and Fenoglio, J. J.: Tumors of the Cardiovascular System, in W. H. Hartmann and W. H. Cowan (eds.), "Atlas of Tumor Pathology," Armed Forces Institute of Pathology, Washington, D.C., 1978.
24. James T. N., Carson, D. J. L., and Marshall, T. K.: De Subitaneis Mortibus: I. Fibroma Compressing His Bundle, *Circulation*, 48:428, 1973.
25. James, T. N., Froggatt, P., Atkinson, W. J., Jr., Lurie, P. R., McNamara, D. G., Miller, W. W., Schloss, G. T., Carroll, J. F., and North, R. L.: De Subitaneis Mortibus: XXX. Observations on the Pathophysiology of the Long QT Syndromes with Special Reference to the Neuropathology of the Heart, *Circulation*, 57:1221, 1978.
26. Lie, J. T.: Histopathology of the Conduction System in Sudden Death from Coronary Heart Disease, *Circulation*, 51:446, 1975.
27. Silver, M. D., Baroldi, G., and Mariani, F.: The Relationship between Acute Myocardial Infarction Studied in 100 Consecutive Patients, *Circulation*, 61:219, 1980.
28. Baroldi, G.: Diseases of Coronary Arteries, in M. D. Silver (ed.) "Cardiovascular Pathology," Churchill Livingstone Inc., New York, 1983, p. 317.
29. Todd, G. L., Baroldi, G., Pieper, G. M., Clayton, F., and Eliot, R. S.: Experimental Cathecholamine-Induced Myocardial Necrosis. I. Morphology, Quantification and Regional Distribution of Acute Contraction Band Lesions, *J. Mol. Cell Cardiol.*, 17, 1985.
30. Baroldi, G., Silver, M. D., Lixfield, W., and McGregor, D. C.: Irreversible Myocardial Damage Resembling Catecholamine Necrosis Secondary to Acute Coronary Occlusion in Dogs: Its Prevention by Propranolol, *J. Mol. Cell. Cardiol.*, 9:687, 1977.
31. Raab, W.: Preventive Myocardiology, Fundamentals and Targets, in N. I. Kugelmass (ed.), "Bannerstone Division of American Lectures in Living Chemistry," Charles C Thomas, Publisher, Springfield, Ill., 1970.
32. Lown, B.: Sudden Cardiac Death: The Major Challenge Confronting Contemporary Cardiology, *Am. J. Cardiol.*, 43:313, 1979.
33. Baroldi, G.: Different Types of Myocardial Necrosis in Coronary Heart Disease: A Pathophysiological Review of Their Functional Significance, *Am. Heart J.*, 89:742, 1975.

32

Predictors and Prevention of Sudden Cardiac Death

Leonard A. Cobb, M.D. Jeffrey A. Werner, M.D.

The readiness with which the ventricles are thrown into the fibrillar condition varies remarkably in different conditions of the cardiac tissues. In a normally contracting and vigorous heart it usually requires a faradic current of considerable strength to produce the result in question. But in certain changed conditions of the organ it becomes extremely easy to throw the ventricles into the fibrillar movement.

J. A. MacWilliam, 1887[1]

Definition of Sudden Cardiac Death

Several definitions of sudden cardiac death have been proposed. For epidemiologic reasons and for practical purposes this disorder is commonly defined as unexpected cardiac death occurring without symptoms or with symptoms of less than an hour's duration. When this or similar definitions are used, the majority of episodes occur outside of hospital, usually without acute prodromal symptoms.[2–5]

Community Impact of Sudden Cardiac Death

Approximately one-half to two-thirds of deaths from coronary atherosclerotic heart disease can be classified as sudden cardiac death, and in the United States the incidence of sudden cardiac death approximates 400,000 per year, an estimated 80 percent due to coronary atherosclerotic heart disease. Although most victims have had prior signs or symptoms of cardiovascular disease, in 20 to 25 percent of cases cardiac arrest is the first such manifestation. There is a distinct predominance of males, whose average age approximates 60 years.[5,6] Sudden cardiac death most often occurs during the routine activities of daily life.[7,8] However, in patients with recognized heart disease there appears to be an additional risk for sudden cardiac death during physical exertion.[9,10] The magnitude of this additional hazard is unknown but is probably not great.

Arrhythmias Underlying Sudden Cardiac Death: Importance of Ventricular Fibrillation

The majority of sudden cardiac deaths are thought to be precipitated by ventricular fibrillation.[6,7,10] Although the electrical events immediately prior to sudden cardiac death have been recorded and reported in only a small number of patients, ventricular fibrillation has usually (but not always) been confirmed.[11,12] On the other hand, asystole, complete heart block, and electromechanical dissociation are commonly seen in the setting of cardiovascular collapse in which there has been substantial delay in initiating emergency care or in situations where collapse has terminated a complicated systemic illness.[7,13]

Persons at Risk for Sudden Cardiac Death

More than three-fourths of sudden cardiac deaths are due to coronary atherosclerotic heart disease, usually with major obstruction of two or three coronary arteries.[2,14] However, many other cardiac lesions are occasionally responsible for sudden cardiac death.[15] In the absence of structural heart disease or evident conduction abnormalities, sudden cardiac death due to an arrhythmia is unusual.

Significance of Coronary "Risk Factors"

In view of the very high proportion of sudden deaths due to coronary atherosclerotic heart disease, it is to be expected that established coronary risk factors would be prevalent in patients at risk for sudden cardiac death. And indeed, hypertension, hypercholesterolemia, and/or a history of cigarette smoking are commonly present in sudden cardiac death victims.[3,16] An important point in the Framingham experience was an association with cigarette smoking: every one of the men who died before age 65 of coronary atherosclerotic heart disease, but without prior cardiovascular stigmas, was a cigarette smoker.[3]

Arterial Hypertension

Hypertension warrants special comment because it may be the sole recognized manifestation of cardiovascular disease prior to sudden cardiac death. In the Framingham cohort, high blood pressure was the only recognized cardiovascular abnormality in nearly one-fourth of sudden deaths due to coronary atherosclerotic heart disease in men aged 65 and younger. Furthermore, left ventricular hypertrophy on ECG was present (in the absence of symptomatic heart disease) in an additional 19 percent.[3]

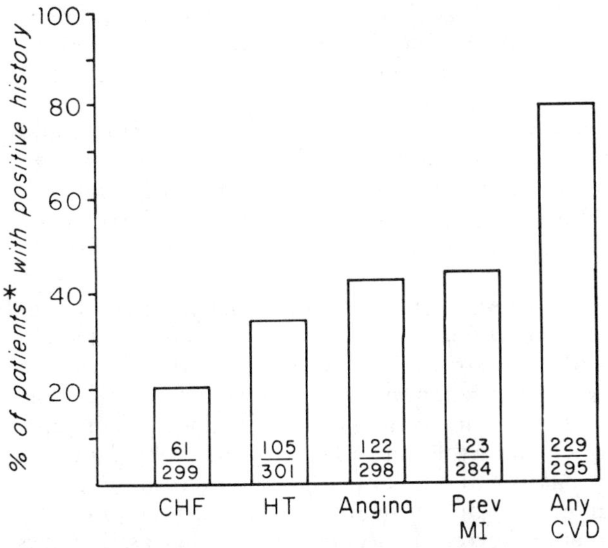

FIGURE 32-1 Manifestations of cardiovascular disease prior to cardiac arrest. * = 305 patients with coronary atherosclerotic heart disease resuscitated from out-of-hospital ventricular fibrillation. CHF = congestive heart failure; HT = hypertension; Prev MI = history of previous myocardial infarction. *(From L. A. Cobb, A. P. Hallstrom, W. D. Weaver, M. K. Copass, and R. E. Haynes, Clinical Predictors and Characteristics of the Sudden Cardiac Death Syndrome, in "Proceedings of the U.S.A.–U.S.S.R. First Joint Symposium on Sudden Death." DHEW Publ. 78-1470, U.S. Government Printing Office, Washington, 1978.)*

Cardiovascular Manifestations Prior to Sudden Cardiac Death

As shown in Fig. 32-1, patients successfully resuscitated from out-of-hospital ventricular fibrillation usually have had some manifestation of cardiovascular disease prior to cardiac arrest. Histories of remote heart attack, angina, congestive heart failure, or hypertension were present in 78 percent of patients who experienced an aborted episode of sudden cardiac death due to coronary atherosclerotic heart disease. In the remaining 22 percent, out-of-hospital cardiac arrest was the first indication of cardiovascular disease. Comparable data were reported in the Framingham study: of 59 men who died suddenly, sudden cardiac death was the first manifestation of cardiovascular disease in 20 percent of men younger than 65 years.[3]

Recognition of High-Risk Patients

In patients with clinically evident coronary atherosclerotic heart disease and/or hypertension, four major characteristics have been shown to be associated with enhanced risk for sudden cardiac death: (1) ventricular electrical instability, (2) extensive coronary arterial narrowing, (3) abnormal left ventricular function, and (4) electrocardiographic conduction and repolarization abnormalities. Although the data in support of these predictors are of necessity limited by the special populations studied, a remarkable similarity has been shown in several subgroups. Although these predictors have unquestioned statistical significance in identifying groups of patients at risk for sudden cardiac death, they are less than satisfactory in both sensitivity and specificity. This is perhaps a reflection of the seemingly erratic manner in which sudden cardiac death occurs.

Ventricular Electrical Instability Since sudden cardiac death is predominately due to ventricular fibrillation, substantial attention has been directed to manifestations of myocardial electrical instability as harbingers. Several studies have shown that ventricular ectopic activity in patients with coronary atherosclerotic heart disease is predictive of sudden cardiac death.[17–19] In particular, so-called complex forms of ventricular ectopy, i.e., multiform beats, repetitive forms, bigeminy, or early (R-on-T) ventricular premature depolarizations, have usually been recognized as statistical predictors of patients at high risk. When large numbers of patients with coronary atherosclerotic heart disease have been examined, ventricular premature depolarizations have commonly been found in ambulatory patients likely to develop sudden cardiac death, even when evaluated with a single resting 12-lead ECG.[20,21] An additional group in whom ventricular ectopic activity has been shown to be a harbinger of sudden cardiac death are patients in the recovery phase of acute myocardial infarction. Moss and colleagues reported that complex ventricular premature depolarizations noted on a predischarge 6-h monitoring carried a significant risk for sudden cardiac death during 1 to 5 years of follow-up. However, in that study mortality due to nonsudden cardiac death was also greater in those with complex forms of ventricular ectopy.[17]

Clearly, complex ventricular premature depolarizations are predictors of sudden cardiac death *in patients with known coronary atherosclerotic heart disease.* In persons without demonstrable heart disease, ventricular ectopic activity by itself appears to have little, if any, prognostic import.[17] At one time it was hoped that ventricular premature depolarizations detected by ambulatory ECG monitoring or during exercise might prove to be sensitive and specific markers of patients at risk for sudden cardiac death. However, ventricular premature depolarizations in patients with recognized coronary atherosclerotic heart disease are ubiquitous, and even high grades of ventricular premature depolarizations fall short in their predictive value to discriminate among patients. For example, in a carefully performed study by Ruberman et al.,[18] complex ventricular ectopy was clearly a predictor of sudden cardiac death in ambulatory patients after myocardial infarction. However, 51 percent of sudden cardiac deaths occurred in patients who *did not* have complex ventricular premature depolarizations during 1 h of monitoring. Furthermore, only 15 percent of those with complex ventricular premature depolarizations developed sudden cardiac death during 4 years of observation.

Coronary Arterial Narrowing Patients who develop sudden cardiac death on the basis of coronary atherosclerotic heart disease typically have severe obstruction (70 percent or greater diameter narrowing) in two or three coronary arteries.[2,14,22] Although some reports have described sudden cardiac death victims as having most involvement in the left anterior descending coronary artery,[23] others have indicated that all three of the major coronary arterial systems appear to be equally affected.[14,22] Severe obstruction of the left main coronary artery, in our experience, is infrequently encountered in both survivors and nonsurvivors of out-of-hospital cardiac arrest.[14,22]

The extent of coronary artery narrowing, independent of other clinical findings, is not a specific predictor of sudden cardiac death.[24] However, there is probably a gradient for risk within clinical subgroups.[22,25] In ambulatory patients who had been resuscitated from an episode of out-of-hospital ventricular fibrillation, recurrences of the sudden cardiac death syndrome were reported in nearly 50 percent of patients (9 of 19) with triple vessel narrowing, compared to only 10 percent of patients (2 of 20) with single vessel narrowing.[22]

Abnormal Ventricular Function It is well recognized that there is an association between left ventricular aneurysms and malignant ventricular arrhythmias, particularly recurrent ventricular tachycardia. In patients who had been resuscitated from ventricular fibrillation, Ritchie el al. reported a high incidence of left ventricular wall motion abnormalities—particularly in patients who later developed recurrences of the sudden cardiac death syndrome.[26] Also in that study there was a striking correlation of worsening left ventricular ejection fraction and subsequent recurrent cardiac arrest. Another example of the association between impaired ventricular function and sudden cardiac death is found in the posthospital phase of acute myocardial infarction, where there is a relatively high mortality, commonly from sudden cardiac death, during the first year after infarction.[27]

Because of the association between ventricular ectopic activity and abnormal ventricular function, it is uncertain whether complex ventricular premature depolarizations are *independent* predictors of sudden cardiac death or whether they are merely reflective of myocardial dysfunction. Ruberman and colleagues reported that the predictive value of complex ventricular premature depolarizations in identifying patients who later developed sudden cardiac death was independent of clinical manifestations of heart failure.[18] On the other hand, Schulze et al. followed 81 patients for an average of 7 months after acute myocardial infarction; they observed that each of the 8 patients who developed sudden cardiac death had *both* impaired left ventricular ejection fraction (less than 40 percent) and complex ventricular premature depolarizations.[27] In a multivariate analysis of survivors of the sudden cardiac death syndrome, ventricular ectopy was shown to be a relatively weak, but nevertheless independent, predictor of recurrences whereas left ventricular ejection fraction was a considerably more powerful predictor.[26] Although there is clearly an interaction between ventricular premature depolarizations and ventricular dysfunction, their ability to predict sudden cardiac death appears additive.

Electrocardiographic Abnormalities of Conduction and Repolarization Resting ECG markers of patients with coronary atherosclerotic heart disease who are at greater than average risk for sudden cardiac death include abnormalities of conduction, prolongation of QT intervals, and ST-T changes.[16,20,21] However, it has yet to be shown that these are independent markers which provide additional prognostic information beyond that obtained by other assessments.

Lessons Learned from Survivors of the Sudden Cardiac Death Syndrome

If patients with ventricular fibrillation are treated with early initiation of cardiopulmonary resuscitation and promptly defibrillated, a substantial proportion can be resuscitated with good functional recovery.[10,28]

Experience in Treating Ventricular Fibrillation

Experience in the management of out-of-hospital ventricular fibrillation in Seattle is represented in Fig. 32-2. That city's emergency care system operates with a tiered response, providing both basic and advanced life support. The major goal of such a service is to deliver care comparable to that which a well-trained physician would provide on the scene. Paramedics are trained in such skills as tracheal intubation, use of common emergency drugs, arrhythmia recognition, and defibrillation. The response time from dispatch until arrival of the first fire department unit averages 3 min, and the advanced life-support (medic) units arrive on the scene approximately 4 min later. Except for cardiac arrest and hypovolemic shock, all therapy is carried out in conjunction with a physician who is in communication by radio or telephone with the paramedics.[28]

Each year the fire department paramedics have treated approximately 300 patients who were in cardiac arrest with ventricular fibrillation when first examined—about 6 cases per 10,000 population per year. (An additional 40 to 50 patients typically develop ventricular fibrillation after arrival of the mobile units.) In the initial years of the Seattle experience, 10 to 12 percent of patients found in ventricular fibrillation were ultimately discharged home; more recently, this figure has approximated 30 percent.[28]

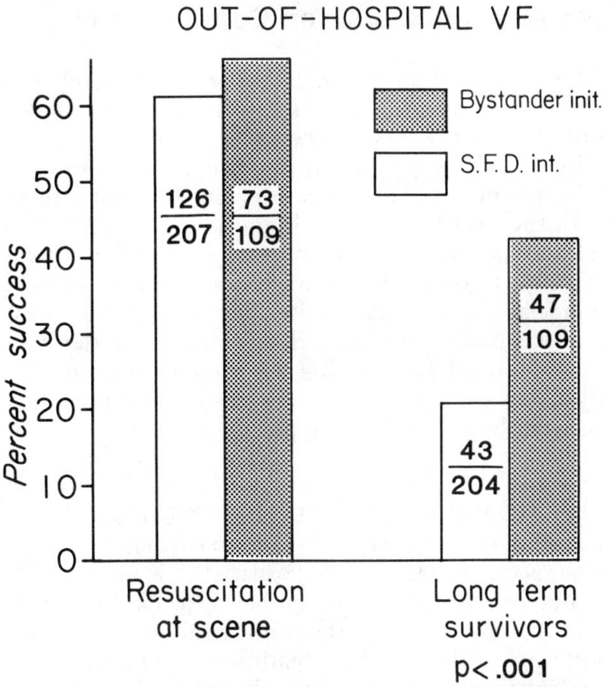

FIGURE 32-2 Outcomes in 316 consecutive patients treated for out-of-hospital ventricular fibrillation. Victims are grouped according to the presence or lack of bystander-initiated cardiopulmonary resuscitation. (*From R. G. Thompson, A. P. Hallstrom, and L. A. Cobb, Bystander-Initiated Cardiopulmonary Resuscitation in the Management of Ventricular Fibrillation, Ann. Intern. Med., 90:737, 1979. Adapted and reproduced with permission from the publisher and authors.*)

Bystander-Initiated Cardiopulmonary Resuscitation

The involvement of the general public in the initiation of cardiopulmonary resuscitation (CPR) is a useful adjunct to an emergency care system.[29] In Seattle, for example, approximately 225,000 persons of high school age and older have received CPR training during the past 13 years. More than one-third of resuscitations in that city are initiated by bystanders prior to arrival of the fire department, and survival in such cases is twice that of patients for whom initiation of CPR is delayed until arrival of fire department personnel (Fig. 32-2).[29] Similarly improved survival rates have been reported in several other communities.[29]

Acute Myocardial Infarction and Sudden Cardiac Death

Although coronary atherosclerotic heart disease is responsible for most episodes of out-of-hospital ventricular fibrillation, a minority of resuscitated patients appear to have developed ventricular fibrillation as a consequence of *acute* myocardial infarction. In the days following resuscitation, new Q waves of transmural myocardial infarction developed in only 19 percent of patients (Fig. 32-3). The majority of patients had ST and/or T wave changes or no appreciable electrocardiographic changes during the postresuscitation hospitalization. Lactate dehydrogenase isoenzyme patterns of myocardial necrosis were found in 38 percent of patients. The disparity between the incidence of electrocardiographically determined acute transmural infarction and the occurrence of isoenzyme evidence for necrosis may be explained by either acute nontransmural infarction or, perhaps more likely, by enzymatic elevation secondary to cardiac arrest and resuscitation. In either case, it is apparent that the majority of patients developed ventricular fibrillation without acute myocardial infarction as a precipitating event.[28,30] This is in accord with the observation that most victims of sudden cardiac death syndrome do not have antecedent chest pain[4] and is also in accord with previously reported autopsy series.[2,14]

Recurrence of the Sudden Cardiac Death Syndrome

During the first year following resuscitation, there has been an approximate 30 percent mortality rate at the end of 1 year, with three-fourths of the deaths due to recurrences of the sudden cardiac death syndrome.[31] When cardiac rhythms were recorded during the recurrent episodes, ventricular fibrillation was usually present if patients were monitored shortly after collapse.[7]

Predictors of Recurrent Sudden Cardiac Death Syndrome

Using easily obtained information from survivors of out-of-hospital ventricular fibrillation, multivariate risk profiles have been developed and validated. As

FIGURE 32-3 ECG changes during the days following resuscitation from out-of-hospital ventricular fibrillation. Acute transmural myocardial infarction (ATMI) was identified by the development of new Q waves in 19 percent of 305 patients with coronary atherosclerotic heart disease. NO CH = no change; UNK = unknown. (*From L. A. Cobb, J. A. Werner, and G. R. Trobaugh, Sudden Cardiac Death: I. A Decade's Experience with Out-of-Hospital Resuscitation, Mod. Concepts Cardiovasc. Dis., 19:31, 1980. Reproduced with permission from the American Heart Association, Inc., and authors.*)

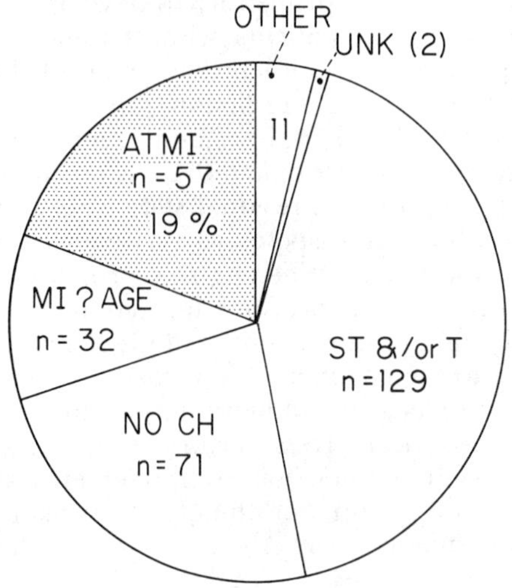

TABLE 32-1 One-Year Risk of Recurrent SCD Syndrome in 425 VF Survivors with Coronary Atherosclerotic Heart Disease

Type of Survivor	Recurrence
ATMI	2% (2 of 85 patients)
No ATMI	22% (75 of 340 patients)
History of remote MI	30%
No history of remote MI	14%
With CHF	30%
Without CHF	11%

Notes: VF = ventricular fibrillation; ATMI = acute transmural myocardial infarction associated with VF; MI = myocardial infarction; CHF = history of congestive heart failure.

Source: L. A. Cobb, J. A. Werner, and G. B. Trobaugh: Sudden Cardiac Death: I. A Decade's Experience with Out-of-Hospital Resuscitation, *Mod. Concepts Cardiovasc. Dis.*, 19:31, 1980. Reproduced with permission from the American Heart Association, Inc., and authors.

shown in Table 32-1, recurrences of the sudden cardiac death syndrome were predominantly in patients whose initial episode of ventricular fibrillation was *not* associated with acute transmural myocardial infarction. Historical factors associated with recurrences included remote myocardial infarction and congestive heart failure prior to the episode of ventricular fibrillation. Other predictors of recurrence were gender (males), abnormal left ventricular function, extensive coronary artery narrowing, and complex ventricular premature depolarizations.[22,26,32]

Vulnerability to Recurrent Ventricular Fibrillation

The contrasting rates of sudden cardiac death syndrome recurrence in patients stratified according to the presence of acute transmural myocardial infarction (Table 32-1) are striking and warrant comment. First, this information provides a simple and useful prognostic indicator in resuscitated patients. Second, this comparison emphasizes a concept of continuing myocardial propensity to develop ventricular fibrillation. In patients with acute myocardial necrosis, there is a transient likelihood of their developing ventricular fibrillation during the initial hours or days. On the other hand, when ventricular fibrillation is not precipitated by acute infarction, there appears to be a residual state of electrical instability which predisposes to recurrences of ventricular fibrillation. Whether this propensity is related to scars from previous infarction, to chronic ischemia, or to intermittent acute ischemia is often difficult to determine. Other factors which may modulate myocardial vulnerability include physical and psychological "stress," arousal of the autonomic nervous system, metabolic derangements such as potassium depletion, and the effects of many pharmacologic agents.

Prevention of Sudden Cardiac Death

The control of sudden cardiac death ultimately lies with the prevention, slowing, or reversal of the atherosclerotic process. However, until that can be attained, efforts to reduce mortality, once coronary atherosclerotic heart disease is present, rest largely with the prevention of sudden cardiac death and to a lesser extent in the treatment of symptomatic complications, particularly myocardial infarction and congestive heart failure. Because ventricular fibrillation is usually the immediate cause of sudden cardiac death, it follows that attempts to prevent this disorder should be directed to the treatment and prevention of ventricular fibrillation.

The Treatment of Ventricular Fibrillation

In the majority of victims, sudden cardiac death appears to represent a primary arrhythmic event which is potentially responsive to electrical defibrillation. Unfortunately, the difficulties in aborting an episode of sudden cardiac death are compounded by the inherent nature of this disorder—first, by the location of the incident, which is most often removed from a usual site of medical care, and second, by the lack of warning symptoms in 70 percent or more of cases.[4] Nevertheless, as discussed previously in this chapter ("Experience in Treating Ventricular Fibrillation"), the development of systems to provide advanced-level prehospital emergency care has resulted in the resuscitation of many persons who otherwise would clearly have died.

The effectiveness of emergency medical systems in managing cardiac arrest depends in large part on the speed in responding. Since logistic considerations often preclude a rapid response, other means of providing defibrillation have been proposed. Simple, portable defibrillators placed, under medical supervision, in the homes of "high-risk" patients or in public places have been considered.[33] Additionally, Mirowski and colleagues[34] have developed an implantable defibrillator which provides electronic sensing of fibrillation and appropriate delivery of a defibrillatory current through implanted electrodes. While these latter approaches offer the potential for reversion of ventricular fibrillation moments after its onset, their use is limited, at least for the time being, to patients at very high risk for developing recurrent cardiac arrest.

Prevention of Ventricular Fibrillation

Ventricular fibrillation can be prevented in experimentally induced myocardial ischemia or infarction, and studies have shown that the propensity to develop ventricular fibrillation may be modified by several measures including psychological adaptations, beta-adrenergic blocking agents, and antiarrhythmic drugs. Furthermore, clinical studies in patients with acute myocardial infarction have shown that the prophylactic use of lidocaine, in some circumstances, may prevent the development of ventricular fibrillation.[35]

In view of the association between complex ventricular ectopic activity and sudden cardiac death (see "Recognition of High-Risk Patients," above), attention has been directed to the possibility of preventing sudden cardiac death through the reduction of ventricular premature depolarizations. Although it is possible that rigorous efforts to suppress complex ventricular premature depolarizations may prevent ventricular fibrillation, that issue remains unsettled. The paradox of an acute lethal event arising in the setting of long-standing ventricular dysfunction and chronic ventricular ectopy has stimulated a search for precipitating factors. Current knowledge suggests that the events leading to ventricular fibrillation may be electrical or mechanical, both of which are likely mediated at the cellular level and modulated by neural traffic. Several investigators have attempted to address the problem of detecting myocardial electrical instability by utilizing provocative cardiac pacing techniques.[36,37] This approach, first proposed by Lown and coworkers, is noteworthy in that it defines a state of electrical instability which may be related to the susceptibility to development of ventricular fibrillation. Such techniques also have potential therapeutic implications since the provoked ventricular arrhythmias may be modified by pharmacologic interventions. Recent studies in survivors of out-of-hospital cardiac arrest point to a reduction in the rate of recurrent cardiac arrest in those patients in whom ventricular tachycardia can no longer be induced.[37]

Clinical Trials to Prevent Sudden Cardiac Death

Clinical trials aimed at the reduction of sudden cardiac death have predominantly been carried out in ambulatory patients who had recently sustained an acute myocardial infarction. Although such studies have an important bearing on the problem of sudden cardiac death, the characteristics of patients in the postinfarction period may not be representative of the large number of patients with chronic coronary atherosclerotic heart disease who are at risk for sudden cardiac death. It is noteworthy that in patients resuscitated from out-of-hospital ventricular fibrillation in Seattle, only 15 percent had sustained a recognized acute myocardial infarction in the year preceding the episode of ventricular fibrillation, and 60 percent had no history of *ever* having an acute myocardial infarction. Hence, one should be somewhat circumspect in the extrapolation of interventions in this group to the broader clinical spectrum of patients with coronary atherosclerotic heart disease.

Beta-Adrenergic Blocking Agents Studies carried out in Europe in the 1970s indicated that two beta-blocking drugs, alprenolol and practolol, appeared to lower the incidence of sudden cardiac death during the first year or two following myocardial infarction. Subsequently, these observations were confirmed in several large-scale and well-controlled trials.[38,39] Thus the chronic administration of currently available beta blockers can be expected to prolong the survival of perhaps 2 to 4 percent of patients 1 year after myocardial infarction. A major proportion of this benefit is in the reduction of sudden cardiac death. Although the mechanisms underlying this protection are not known, it is important to note that the incidence of recurrent, nonfatal myocardial infarction is also reduced by the use of beta blockers.

Antiarrhythmic Drug Therapy It is of interest that ventricular ectopic activity was not used as a major endpoint in the trials of beta-blocking drugs cited above. This is in contrast to the approaches of others who have vigorously investigated and treated patients with advanced grades of ventricular ectopy who were considered to be at increased risk for sudden cardiac death. As reported by Graboys et al.,[40] the virtual abolition of high grades of ventricular arrhythmias was attempted using acute drug testing and multidrug regimens—and was accomplished in 98 of 123 patients who had recurrent ventricular tachycardia and/or cardiac arrest. In these "controlled" patients the annual incidence of sudden cardiac death was 2.3 percent. In contrast, 44 percent of the 25 patients who could not be "controlled" died suddenly in 1 year. Although these results appear promising, they should be interpreted cautiously in view of the lack of a concomitant control population and of the heterogeneous population studied. Other investigators have focused interest on suppression of recurrent, symptomatic ventricular tachycardia (see Chap. 27). However, it remains to be shown that observations in these patients can be extended to the very large numbers of patients at risk for sudden cardiac death.

Myerburg and colleagues[41] have also advocated the use of antiarrhythmic agents in patients at high risk for sudden cardiac death. These investigators studied the long-term use of quinidine or procainamide in 32 patients who had survived at least one episode of prehospital cardiac arrest and found no correlation between the suppression of ventricular ectopy and the recurrence of cardiac arrest. On the other hand, there were fewer recurrences in those patients in whom relatively stable drug levels were maintained than in those who had unstable plasma levels, often below what was considered the therapeutic range. These observations suggested that attainment of adequate plasma levels of antiarrhythmic drugs, rather than suppression of ventricular premature depolarizations per se, may be of importance in preventing the emergence of ventricular fibrillation.

Unfortunately, the use of antiarrhythmic agents to reduce the incidence of sudden cardiac death is hampered not only by unacceptable and sometimes dangerous side effects[37,42] but also by the uncertainty of therapeutic guidelines.

Other Drug Therapy Several other interventions have been proposed to reduce the likelihood of sudden cardiac death following myocardial infarction; these include anticoagulants, hygienic measures, lipid-lowering drugs, and antiplatelet agents. To date, none of these measures has shown a clear-cut effect on mortality.[43]

Heart Surgery Since most victims of sudden cardiac death have atherosclerotic coronary artery obstruction, it might follow that improvement in coronary blood flow would enhance the survival of these patients, particularly by preventing or forestalling sudden death. Since coronary bypass surgery is performed on about 100,000 patients each year in the United States, it is proper to ask if this operation will prevent sudden cardiac death. Randomized, prospective trials of coronary artery bypass grafting have been carried out in patients with stable angina pectoris. In spite of appreciable symptomatic relief from angina, the effects on overall long-term mortality have not consistently favored the surgically treated groups, except for patients with left main coronary artery obstruction (see Chap. 45). In the European Coronary Surgery Study Group trial, there was improved survival in a major subgroup of surgically treated patients who had triple vessel disease—with reduction in total deaths and sudden cardiac deaths[44] (see Chap. 45). In the Coronary Artery Surgery Study carried out in the United States,[24] survival following coronary artery bypass grafting was not significantly different in the patients treated surgically or medically. However, it is important to point out that the medically treated patients in this study had excellent survival rates, and the life-extending effect of any intervention, regardless of its value, would have been most difficult to recognize in those selected patients. This probably occurred because patients at high risk, for a variety of reasons, were not entered in this study (see Chap. 45). Although uncertainties remain, evidence to date suggests that sudden death may be forestalled or prevented in subgroups of symptomatic patients with significant left main and triple vessel coronary artery obstruction. However, available evidence indicates that ventricular ectopy remains unaffected by coronary artery bypass grafting.[45]

Coronary bypass surgery is rarely employed in patients without a history of, or symptoms of, coronary artery disease. Therefore that operation has not been performed in asymptomatic patients prior to sudden cardiac death, and its status in preventing sudden cardiac death in such persons is unknown. Although there are encouraging preliminary reports concerning the efficacy of myocardial surgery for patients with recurrent, drug-resistant ventricular tachycardia, the strategy in managing patients with symptomatic, recurrent ventricular tachycardia is usually not relevant to the very large proportion of patients who develop sudden cardiac death without previously recognized cardiac arrhythmias.

Sudden Cardiac Death in Patients with Cardiac Disease Other Than Coronary Atherosclerotic Heart Disease

Approximately 20 percent of sudden cardiac death victims have cardiac diagnoses other than coronary atherosclerotic heart disease. Uncommon causes of sudden cardiac death, such as congenital anomalies of the coronary arteries and Marfan's syndrome, are discussed in Chap. 47. For the purposes of this section, three major classifications are briefly considered: (1) cardiomyopathic syndromes, (2) valvular lesions, and (3) primary electrical disturbances.

Cardiomyopathic Syndromes

Virtually any cardiomyopathy may on occasion result in sudden cardiac death. However, sudden cardiac death plays a particularly prominent role in the natural history of hypertrophic cardiomyopathy, including so-called idiopathic hypertrophic subaortic stenosis. Indeed sudden cardiac death, probably due to ventricular fibrillation, is the most common mode of death in patients with that diagnosis. It is not clear if treatment, particularly with beta blockade, has an effect on either the arrhythmias or sudden cardiac death in these disorders.[46] (See also Chap. 58.)

Valvular Lesions

Aortic valvular lesions and mitral valve prolapse syndromes have been indicted specifically as causes of sudden cardiac death. (See Chaps. 37, 38, and 39.)

Primary Electrical Disturbances

Of the primary electrical syndromes responsible for sudden cardiac death, sinoatrial disorders, ventricular preexcitation, and prolonged QT syndromes are most commonly described. While such syndromes are frequently associated with other cardiac or metabolic abnormalities, the congenitally prolonged QT syndromes are worthy of note. Drug therapy in the form of beta-blocking agents and also excision of the left stellate ganglion (high thoracic left sympathectomy) have been reported to be effective in preventing sudden cardiac death and recurrent syncope in patients with idiopathic QT prolongation.[47] (See also Chaps. 14 and 25.)

Summary

Most deaths from coronary atherosclerotic heart disease are sudden, unexpected events which occur outside the hospital. In approximately 80 percent of instances, there have been prior manifestations of heart disease or arterial hypertension or both. In patients at risk for sudden cardiac death, cessation of cigarette smoking and treatment of high blood pressure are prudent, albeit unproven, preventive measures. In patients with recognized cardiovascular disease, the presence of complex ventricular premature depolarization has a statistical relation to sudden cardiac death. However, it is not clear that these markers are completely independent of the severity of myocardial dysfunction, which is probably the most useful predictor of sudden cardiac death.

Following acute myocardial infarction, beta-blocking drugs have been shown to prevent or forestall sudden cardiac death in the initial 2 years, and the use of antiarrhythmic drugs to prevent sudden cardiac death is undergoing intense study. This latter approach has its advocates, but the issue at this time is unsettled. The essential purpose of drug therapy for control of sudden cardiac death is to prevent the emergence of ventricular fibrillation—with or without alteration of frequency of ventricular premature depolarization.

The application of emergency medical services represents a major advance is preventing sudden cardiac death. Further steps to facilitate prompt initiation of cardiopulmonary resuscitation and rapid defibrillation will likely continue the trend of steadily improved rates of resuscitation and survival.

In symptomatic patients with left main or triple vessel coronary atherosclerosis, there is reason for optimism in anticipating a reduction in the incidence of sudden cardiac death if transient myocardial ischemia can be relieved by coronary artery bypass grafting. On the other hand, asymptomatic patients or those with mild symptoms of angina are unlikely to derive a life-extending effect by surgical revascularization (see Chap. 45).

References

1. MacWilliam, J. A.: Fibrillar Contraction of the Heart, *J. Physiol. (London)*, 8:296, 1887.
2. Kuller, L. H.: Sudden Death—Definition and Epidemiologic Considerations, *Prog. Cardiovasc. Dis.*, 23:1, 1980.
3. Gordon, T., and Kannel, W. B.: Premature Mortality from Coronary Heart Disease, *JAMA*, 215:1617, 1971.
4. Gillum, R. F., Reinleid, M., Margolis, J. R., Fabsitz, R. R., and Brasch, R. D.: Delay in the Prehospital Phase of Acute Myocardial Infarction, *Arch. Intern. Med.*, 136:649, 1976.
5. Baum, R. D., Alvarez, H., and Cobb, L. A.: Survival after Resuscitation from Out-of-Hospital Ventricular Fibrillation, *Circulation*, 50:1231, 1974.
6. Lown, B.: Sudden Cardiac Death: The Major Challenge Confronting Contemporary Cardiology, *Am. J. Cardiol.*, 43:313, 1979.
7. Schaffer, W. A., and Cobb, L. A.: Recurrent Ventricular Fibrillation and Modes of Death in Survivors of Out-of-Hospital Ventricular Fibrillation, *N. Engl. J. Med.*, 293:260, 1975.
8. Wikland, B.: Medically Unattended Fatal Cases of Ischemic Heart Disease in a Defined Population, *Acta Med. Scand. Suppl.*, 524, 1971.
9. Burchell, H. B.: Patients with Coronary Artery Disease Should Avoid Strenuous Physical Exertion, in E. Rapaport (ed.), "Current Controversies in Cardiovascular Disease," W. B. Saunders, Co., Philadelphia, 1980, pp. 139–149.
10. Hossack, K. F. and Hartwig, R.: Cardiac Arrest Associated with Supervised Cardiac Rehabilitation, *J. Cardiac Rehabil.*, 2:402, 1982.
11. Nikolic, G., Bishop, R. L., and Singh, J. B.: Sudden Death Recorded During Holter Monitoring, *Circulation*, 66:218, 1982.
12. Pratt, C. M., Francis, M. J., Luck, J. C., Wyndham, C. R., Miller, R. R., and Quinones, M. A.: Analysis of Ambulatory Electrocardiograms in 15 Patients during Spontaneous Ventricular Fibrillation with Special Reference to Preceding Arrhythmic Events, *J. Am. Col. Cardiol.*, 2:789, 1983.
13. Iseri, L. T., Humphrey, S. B., and Sinner, E. J.: Prehospital Bradyasystolic Cardiac Arrest, *Ann. Intern. Med.*, 88:741, 1978.
14. Reichenback, D. D., Moss, N. S., and Meyer, E.: Pathology of the Heart in Sudden Cardiac Death, *Am. J. Cardiol.*, 39:865, 1977.
15. Goldstein, S.: "Sudden Death Coronary Heart Disease," Futura Publishing Company, Inc., Mt. Kisco, N.Y., 1974, p. 22.
16. Friedman, G. D., Klatsky, A. L., and Siegelaub, A. B.: Predictors of Sudden Cardiac Death, *Circulation*, 51, 52(suppl 3):164, 1975.
17. Moss, A. J.: Clinical Significance of Ventricular Arrhythmias in Patients with and without Coronary Artery Disease, *Prog. Cardiovasc. Dis.*, 23:33, 1980.
18. Ruberman, W., Weinblatt, E., Goldberg, J. D., Frank, C. W., Chaudhary, B. S., and Shapiro, S.: Ventricular Premature Complexes and Sudden Death After Myocardial Infarction, *Circulation*, 64:297, 1981.
19. Weaver, W. D., Cobb, L. A., and Hallstrom, A. P.: Ambulatory Arrhythmias in Resuscitated Victims of Cardiac Arrest, *Circulation*, 66:212, 1982.
20. The Coronary Drug Project Research Group: Prognostic Importance of Premature Beats Following Myocardial Infarction, *JAMA*, 223:1116, 1973.
21. Haynes, R. E., Hallstrom, A. P., and Cobb, L. A.: Repolarization Abnormalities in Survivors of Out-of-Hospital Ventricular Fibrillation, *Circulation*, 57:652, 1978.
22. Weaver, W. D., Lorch, G. S., Alvarez, H. A., and Cobb, L. A.: Angiographic Findings and Prognostic Indicators in Patients Resuscitated from Sudden Cardiac Death, *Circulation*, 54:895, 1976.
23. Liberthson, R. R., Nagel, E. L., Hirschman, J. C., Nussenfield, J. D., Blackbourne, B. D., and Davis, J. D.: Pathophysiologic Observations in Prehospital Ventricular Fibrillation and Sudden Cardiac Death, *Circulation*, 49:790, 1974.
24. CASS principal investigators: Coronary Artery Surgery Study (CASS): A Randomized Trial of Coronary Artery Bypass Surgery Survival Data, *Circulation*, 68:939, 1983.
25. Oberman, A., Ray, M., Turner, M. E., Barnes, G., and Grooms, C.: Sudden Death in Patients Evaluated for Ischemic Heart Disease, *Circulation*, 51, 52(suppl. 3):170, 1975.
26. Ritchie, J. L., Hallstrom, A. P., Trobaugh, G. B., and Cobb, L. A.: Out-of-Hospital Sudden Death Syndrome: Post-exercise Radionuclide Angiography and Holter Monitoring, *Circulation*, 66(suppl 2):26, 1982. (Abstract.)
27. Schulze, R. A., Strauss, H. W., and Pitt, B.: Sudden Death in the Year Following Myocardial Infarction, *Am. J. Med.*, 62:192, 1977.
28. Cobb, L. A., Werner, J. A., and Trobaugh, G. B.: Sudden Cardiac Death: I. A Decade's Experience with Out-of-Hospital Resuscitation, *Mod. Concepts Cardiovasc. Dis.*, 19:31, 1980.
29. Cobb, L. A., and Hallstrom, A. P.: Community-Based Cardiopulmonary Resuscitation: What Have We Learned?, *Ann. N. Y. Acad. Sci.*, 382:330, 1982.
30. Liberthson, R. R., Nagel, E. L., Hirschman, J. C., and Nussenfeld, S. R.: Prehospital Ventricular Fibrillation: Prognosis and Follow-Up Course, *N. Engl. J. Med.*, 291:317, 1974.

31. Cobb, L. A., Baum, R. S., Alvarez, H., and Schaffer, W. A.: Resuscitation from Out-of-Hospital Ventricular Fibrillation: 4 Year Follow-Up, *Circulation*, 51, 52(suppl. 3):223, 1975.
32. Cobb, L. A., Werner, J. A., and Trobaugh, G. B.: Sudden Cardiac Death: II. Outcome of Resuscitation: Management, and Future Directions, *Mod. Concepts Cardiovasc. Dis.*, 49:37, 1980.
33. Friedberg, C. K.: Symposium—Myocardial Infarction 1972, Part I, *Circulation*, 45:179, 1972.
34. Mirowski, M.: Management of Malignant Ventricular Tachyarrhythmias with Automatic Implanted Cardioverter-Defibrillators, *Mod. Concepts Cardiovasc. Dis.*, 52:41, 1983.
35. Lie, K. I., Wellens, H. J., Van Capelle, F. J., and Durrer, D.: Lidocaine in the Prevention of Primary Ventricular Fibrillation. A Double-Blind Randomized Study of 212 Consecutive Patients, *N. Engl. J. Med.*, 291:1324, 1974.
36. Greene, H. L., Reid, P. R., and Schaeffer, A. H.: The Repetitive Ventricular Response in Man: A Predictor of Sudden Death, *N. Engl. J. Med.*, 399:729, 1978.
37. Ruskin, J. N., McGovern, B., Garan, H., DiMarco, J. P., and Kelly, E.: Antiarrhythmic Drugs: A Possible Cause of Out-of-Hospital Cardiac Arrest, *N. Engl. J. Med.*, 309:1302, 1983.
38. Norwegian Multicenter Study Group: Timolol-Induced Reduction in Mortality and Reinfarction in Patients Surviving Acute Myocardial Infarction, *N. Engl. J. Med.*, 304:801, 1981.
39. Frishman, W. H., Furberg, C. D., and Friedewald, W. T.: Beta-Adrenergic Blockade for Survivors of Acute Myocardial Infarction, *N. Engl. J. Med.*, 310:830, 1984.
40. Graboys, T. B., Lown, B., Podrid, P. J., and DeSilva, R.: Long-Term Survival of Patients with Malignant Ventricular Arrhythmia Treated with Antiarrhythmic Drugs, *Am. J. Cardiol.*, 50:437, 1982.
41. Myerburg, R. J., Kessler, K. M., Zaman, L., Conde, C. A., and Castellanos, A.: Survivors of Prehospital Cardiac Arrest, *JAMA*, 247:1485, 1982.
42. Velebit, V., Podrid, P., Lown, B., Cohen, B. H., and Graboys, T. B.: Aggravation and Provocation of Ventricular Arrhythmias by Antiarrhythmic Drugs, *Circulation*, 65:886, 1982.
43. May, G. S., Eberlein, K. A., Furburg, D. D., Passamoni, E. R., and Mets, D. L.: Secondary Prevention after Myocardial Infarction: A Review of Longterm Trials, *Prog. Cardiovasc. Dis.*, 24:331, 1982.
44. European Coronary Surgery Study Group. Long-Term Results of Prospective Randomized Study of Coronary Artery Bypass Surgery in Stable Angina Pectoris, *Lancet*, 2:1173, 1982.
45. Tilkian, A. G., Pfeifer, J. F., Barry, W. J., Lipton, M. J., and Hultgren, H. N.: The Effect of Coronary Bypass Surgery on Exercise-Induced Ventricular Arrhythmias, *Am. Heart J.*, 92:707, 1976.
46. Maron, B. J., Roberts, W. C., Edwards, J. E., McAllister, H. A., Foley, D. D., and Epstein, S. E.: Sudden Death in Patients with Hypertrophic Cardiomyopathy: Characterization of 26 Patients without Functional Limitation, *Am. J. Cardiol.*, 41:803, 1978.
47. Moss, A. M., and Schwartz, P. J.: Delayed Repolarization (QT or QTU Prolongation) and Malignant Arrhythmias, *Mod. Concepts Cardiovasc. Dis.*, 51:85, 1982.

33

Cardiopulmonary Resuscitation and the Subsequent Management of the Patient

Myron L. Weisfeldt, M.D. Nisha Chibber Chandra, M.D.

Then he went up and lay upon the child, putting his mouth upon his mouth, his eyes upon his eyes, and his hands upon his hands and he stretched himself upon him; the flesh of the child became warm.

2 Kings 4:34[1]

Since biblical times, humans have attempted to restore life to the dead or nearly dead individual. In the eighteenth century, it was a common practice in Europe to throw unconscious persons over the back of trotting horses or to roll them over barrels in an attempt to move air in and out of their chests. Bellows were also used to inflate the lungs. One technique that gained broad use in this century was the Schafer prone pressure method of artificial respiration, in which the lower back was pressed cyclically, thus forcing air from the lungs.[2]

Although at the time all these methods were viewed as a means for providing lung ventilation, recent research suggests that circulation of blood might also have concurrently occurred. For example, pressure on the chest with the airway at least partially obstructed in the prone position would be an ideal way to increase intrathoracic pressure and thereby circulate blood (see below).

In 1954 Elam and his colleagues[3] showed that mouth-to-mouth or mouth-to-nose resuscitation was superior to the Schafer method in terms of efficacy of ventilation. The importance of circulation of blood was also recognized, and direct or internal cardiac massage became an accepted technique as early as 1916. Despite proven efficacy,[4] internal massage remains fraught with complications and should only be employed by trained personnel.

It was not until 1960 that Kouwenhoven, Jude, and Knickerbocker developed the present technique of external chest compression in the supine position and coupled this with artificial respiration.[5] These investigators proposed that during chest compression in the arrested state, the heart was squeezed or massaged between the sternum and vertebral column, resulting in the forward flow of blood. This technique of cardiopulmonary resuscitation (CPR) gained rapid popularity and was shown to be effective,[6] although it now appears that the mechanism of blood flow during external chest compression is usually related to the rise in intrathoracic pressure rather than to direct cardiac compression.

Mechanisms of Movement of Blood during CPR

The original hypothesis, as mentioned above, suggested that blood flow to the periphery during external chest compression resulted from direct compression of the heart between the sternum and the vertebral column.[5] According to this concept, chest compression (*systole*), similar to internal cardiac massage, resulted in blood being squeezed from both ventricles into the great arteries as the pulmonary and aortic valves opened. Retrograde flow of blood was prevented by closure of the atrioventricular valves. During the release phase of chest compression (*diastole*), the ventricles recoiled to their original shape and filled by a suction effect, while elevated arterial pressure was thought to close both the pulmonic and aortic valves.

This widely held concept is not, however, consistent with a number of observations in animal models[7] and humans[8] that suggest a correlation between the rise in intrathoracic pressure during chest compression and the apparent magnitude of carotid flow and pressure. The importance of fluctuations in intrathoracic pressure, as a means for generating blood flow, is further supported by the observations of Criley et al. that by the continuous and early initiation of coughing, patients in ventricular fibrillation can maintain consciousness as long as cough is continued.[9] The critical ingredient of the cough is clearly a rise in intrathoracic pressure and, likely, no cardiac compression.

Criley's observations strongly suggest that a rise in intrathoracic pressure is a potent mechanism for the movement of blood to the brain, in human beings, following cardiac arrest.

Experimental Observations

For blood flow to occur in a fluid-filled system (such as the circulation) a pressure gradient must be present, and if a structure functions as a pump (as the heart does in the normal circulation), then a pressure gradient must be present across the pump (that is, the normal arteriovenous pressure gradient between the aorta and the central veins). In large animals, chest compression during CPR results in an essentially equal rise in central venous, right atrial, pulmonary artery, aortic, esophageal, and lateral pleural space pressures, with no transcardiac gradient being developed (Fig. 33-1).[10]

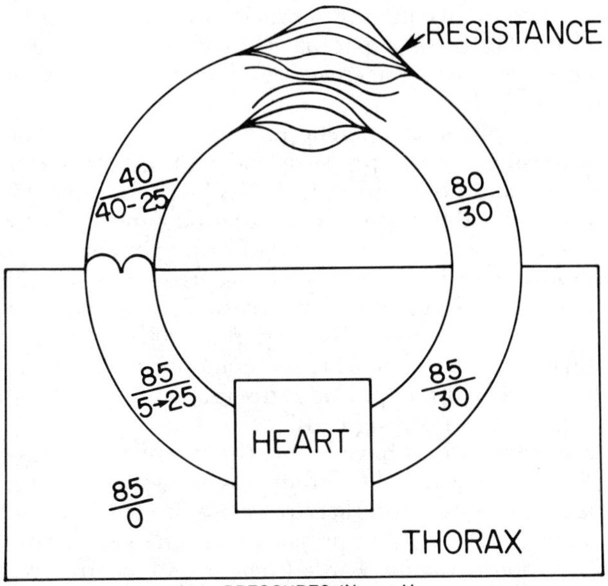

FIGURE 33-1 Representative pressures recorded during conventional cardiopulmonary resuscitation with forward carotid flow. Pressures are those recorded during compression. Intrathoracic pressures were indexed from esophageal pressures. There is no significant pressure gradient across the heart. The extrathoracic arterial pressure is similar to the intrathoracic aortic pressure. The extrathoracic venous pressure is markedly lower than the intrathoracic venous (right atrial) pressure. There is an extrathoracic arteriovenous pressure gradient which results in forward flow.

In such animals, aortic pressure is transmitted efficiently to the carotid arteries, but retrograde transmission of intrathoracic venous pressure into the jugular veins is prevented by valves at the thoracic inlet and also by venous collapse. Thus, during chest compression (systole) a peripheral arteriovenous pressure gradient appears, and blood flow occurs consequent to this gradient. In such a system, there is no pressure gradient across the heart and therefore the heart cannot be the pump responsible for generating blood flow during CPR. In fact the heart functions merely as a passive conduit. When chest compression is released (diastole), intrathoracic pressures fall toward zero and venous flow into the right heart and lungs occurs. Retrograde flow into the aorta from extrathoracic arteries also occurs but is limited by the relatively low capacitance of the intrathoracic arterial bed and closure of the aortic valve.

Studies of vital organ perfusion indicate that during CPR cerebral flow is dependent on the gradient between the carotid artery and the intracranial pressure during systole, with myocardial flow being dependent on the gradient between the aorta and right atrium during diastole.[11]

Building on these concepts, maneuvers and techniques have been developed to increase intrathoracic pressure and hence arterial pressure during chest compression. One such technique, simultaneous compression-ventilation CPR, allows safe cyclical increments in intrathoracic pressure to 70 to 90 mmHg during external chest compression and has been shown to increase significantly cerebral flow during CPR.[11,12]

Epinephrine is a potent pharmacologic means for increasing arterial pressure and both cerebral and myocardial flow during CPR. Its hemodynamic effects are additive to those of other maneuvers. With simultaneous compression-ventilation CPR and epinephrine infusion, 60 percent of prearrest cerebral flow and 29 percent of prearrest myocardial flow can be achieved (versus 43 percent and 5 percent during conventional CPR and epinephrine infusion, Fig. 33-2).[13] Epinephrine is discussed in detail later ("Drugs Used during CPR").

Recent studies have shown that there are two aspects of external chest compression alone that can be manipulated and that are critical in determining vital organ perfusion pressures. (1) Greater sternal force augments myocardial perfusion but often results in greater tissue injury. (2) Adequate compression duration during each chest compression-release cycle is critical for maintaining maximal myocardial and cerebral flow during resuscitation. Myocardial and brain flow are optimal at chest compression durations of 50 percent of cycle length. Short-duration, low-force chest compression cycles are undesirable as they result in a considerable reduction in both cerebral and myocardial flow. It is important to note that at optimal chest compression force and duration, vital organ perfusion is not greatly influenced by compression rate.

Unlike the hemodynamic pattern described above, in small animals and rarely in large dogs, intrathoracic vascular pressures are much higher than pleural pressure. It is likely that in such animals the rise in vascular pressures is a result of compression of the heart during chest compression and is not principally due to a rise in intrathoracic pressure. The classic mechanism of direct cardiac compression is likely operating in these animals, and under these conditions higher compression rates should augment blood flow. As discussed below, the frequency of direct cardiac compression in human beings is unclear. Fortunately both mechanisms for blood flow during CPR (i.e., manipulation of intrathoracic pressure and direct cardiac compression) have certain physiological similarities. Even during cardiac compression, venous valves at the thoracic inlet remain essential for establishing a peripheral arteriovenous pressure gradient which facilitates peripheral flow. Also, vital organ perfusion is governed by the same hemodynamic principles. Thus, pharmacologic interventions such as epinephrine and phys-

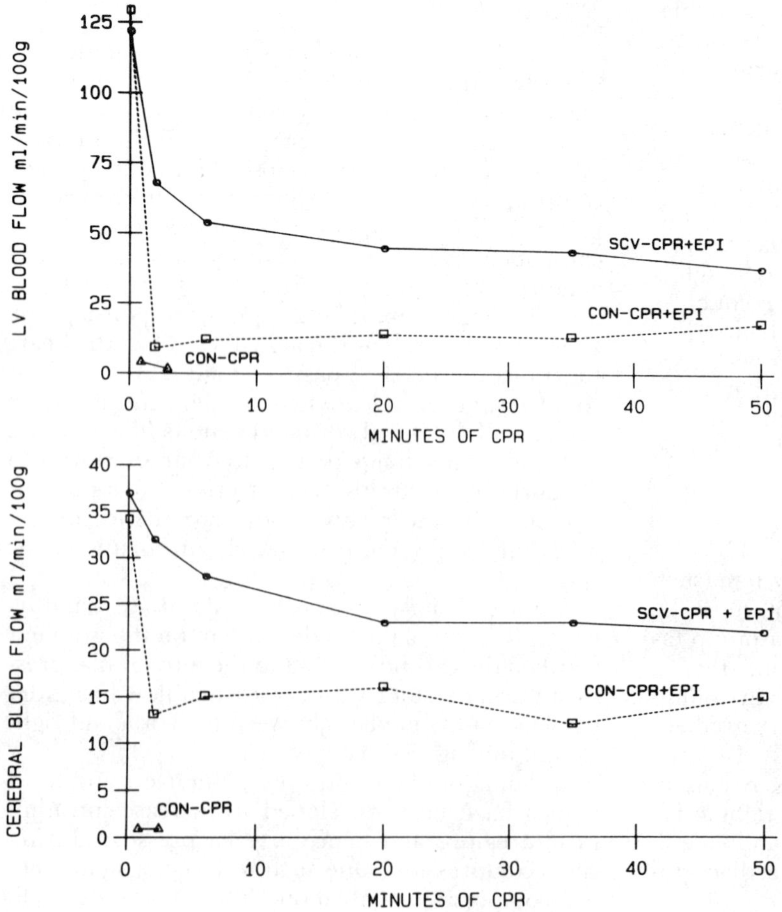

FIGURE 33-2 Left ventricular and cerebral blood flow before arrest and during three types of CPR: conventional CPR (CON-CPR), conventional CPR with epinephrine infusion (CON-CPR + EPI), and simultaneous compression-ventilation CPR with epinephrine infusion (SCV-CPR + EPI). The values for percentage of prearrest flow for CON-CPR are similar to those for CON-CPR + EPI. During SCV-CPR + EPI, 60 percent of prearrest cerebral flow and 29 percent of prearrest myocardial flow can be achieved as compared to 43 percent and 5 percent, respectively, during CON-CPR + EPI and less than 5 percent and less than 2 percent, respectively, during CON-CPR.

ical interventions such as increased sternal force will similarly increase arterial systolic and diastolic pressure and therefore increase regional flow during CPR. Both of the mechanisms for blood flow are also additive.

Observations in Human Beings

Unfortunately, at this point we can draw no final conclusion as to the frequency or importance of the two mechanisms (chest compression and generalized increase in intrathoracic pressure) during conventional cardiopulmonary resuscitation in human beings.

In a number of patients comparable arterial and right atrial pressures have been observed as well as the presence of a pressure gradient at the thoracic inlet upon withdrawing intravascular catheters from the superior vena cava to the extrathoracic internal jugular vein.[10] This hemodynamic picture favors the concept of forward flow of blood through manipulation of intrathoracic pressure. This concept is further strengthened by the observation that maneuvers designed to increase intrathoracic pressure during chest compression, such as prolonged compression duration, abdominal binding, and simultaneous compression-ventilation CPR, are rewarded by a significant increase in peripheral arterial pressure.[14,15]

Two-dimensional echocardiographic studies obtained during CPR further support this mechanism. These studies show that during chest compression both mitral and aortic valves are open with little deformity of the left ventricular chamber cavity itself.[16] On the other hand, in some patients (about 30 percent), who are usually thin-chested with cardiomegaly, extremely high arterial pressures are generated with conventional cardiopulmonary resuscitation. In a few of these patients we have monitored simultaneous arterial and central venous pressures and have found venous pressure to be lower than radial arterial pressure—a hemodynamic picture that suggests cardiac compression. In some patients, however, this higher arterial pressure may reflect higher generalized intrathoracic pressure during chest compression as a result of functional airway obstruction due to pulmonary congestion and/or bronchospasm. In the majority of the patients in whom we have measured radial artery pressure during cardiopulmonary resuscitation, the arterial pressure has been relatively low and similar to that seen in the dog during conventional cardiopulmonary resuscitation.

In human beings it is not essential to think about these mechanisms in an exclusive fashion. We can consider direct cardiac compression as useful, when possible. Where this mechanism is not potent enough to maintain cerebral and myocardial perfusion, it would not be surprising to see that manipulation of intrathoracic pressures would have a favorable additive effect on carotid blood flow.[17]

Diagnosis and Identification of Cardiac Arrest

Cardiac arrest is defined as the sudden cessation of effective cardiac pumping function as a result of either ventricular asystole (electrical or mechanical) or ventricular fibrillation. Rapid diagnosis is essential because (1) more than a few minutes of total cardiac arrest results in permanent cerebral anoxic damage and (2) the success of resuscitative measures is related to the rapidity with which they are instituted following arrest.[18]

Cardiac arrest should be considered in the differential diagnosis of sudden collapse in any patient. It can be clinically confirmed by pulseless major vessels and absent heart sounds. Although respirations may continue for a minute or two, the patient with cardiac arrest becomes rapidly cyanotic and unconscious.

If available, an electrocardiogram can confirm the diagnosis and identify asystole, ventricular fibrillation, or electromechanical dissociation as the mechanisms of arrest. Cardiopulmonary resuscitation, however, should be initiated immediately once the clinical diagnosis is made without delaying to obtain this information. If a defibrillator but not an electrocardiogram is immediately available, a 200-J countershock should be administered without delay.

Respiratory Arrest

Respiratory arrest is the cessation of effective respiratory effort. It can result from airway obstruction (due to a foreign body or other causes), drug overdose, head trauma, cerebrovascular accident, or suffocation. When respiratory arrest occurs suddenly (as with foreign body obstruction), the patient rapidly becomes cyanotic, though a palpable pulse with blood pressure, consciousness, and ineffective respiratory efforts may be maintained for several minutes. All that is necessary to resuscitate such a patient may be opening the airway and/or rescue breathing.

Three manual maneuvers are recommended for relieving foreign body airway obstruction:

- Manual removal. Open the victim's mouth and manually attempt to dislodge any obvious foreign body with a finger.
- Back blows. Deliver four sharp blows with the heel of the hand high on the spine between the shoulder blades.
- Heimlich maneuver. Deliver a series of sharp thrusts to the upper abdomen with a closed fist while standing behind the victim.[19] Abdominal thrusts can also be used directly in the unconscious supine patient to help mechanically dislodge a foreign body. If incorrectly administered, this maneuver can lead to visceral damage.[20]

Ventilation during Cardiopulmonary Resuscitation

Clearing the airway is of the utmost importance. Foreign bodies, loose dentures, and any other oral obstruction should be removed. Next, the head tilt–chin lift technique, which causes the tongue to move anteriorly, is used to open the airway. The chin is lifted forward, with the fingers of one hand supporting the jaw and the head tilted back by the other hand on the forehead of the patient.[21] The head tilt–neck lift method of opening the airway is also commonly employed and is an acceptable technique. Here the head is tilted back with one hand on the forehead; the other hand is placed behind the neck, lifting it upward to open the airway. If no spontaneous respirations are present, mouth-to-mouth ventilation is immediately initiated, with adequacy being judged by the rise and fall of the patient's chest with each breath.

Equipped rescuers will use a bag-mask technique of ventilation together with a small plastic oral "airway" which moves the tongue anteriorly. Adequate ventilation is difficult with this method, and gastric distension and aspiration are common. An esophageal obturator with balloon obstruction of the esophagus and ventilation through proximal ports in the mouth avoids aspiration and appears to provide some, but not optimal, ventilation.[22] Skill is needed in placing and using this device properly. After successful resuscitation, balloon deflation frequently results in regurgitation of gastric contents.

In skilled hands endotracheal intubation is the ideal procedure, but much valuable time can be wasted by repeated unskilled attempts at intubation. If this technique is used, cardiopulmonary resuscitation should be discontinued for no more than 20 s while the tube is being passed into the airway. If more than 20 s elapse without successful intubation, the laryngoscope should be withdrawn and cardiopulmonary resuscitation reinstituted. Whenever possible a nasogastric tube should be inserted to drain the stomach and thus decrease the chances of aspiration.

Chest Compression during Cardiopulmonary Resuscitation

In 1974 and 1980 (revised) the American Heart Association published "Standards for Cardiopulmonary Resuscitation and Emergency Cardiac Care."[23] In reference to external chest compression, they advised (1) 60 sternal compressions per minute, (2) 50 percent of each compression-relaxation cycle to be compression, and (3) one ventilation for every five compressions.

The importance of prolonged chest compression duration is further supported by recent data that suggest that longer compression cycles result in increased myocardial and cerebral flow. Therefore, while performing CPR, operators should consciously pause at peak chest compression in order to ensure prolonged compression duration.

In addition to these recommendations, it is critical when performing chest compression to use sufficient force to depress the sternum by 2 to $2\frac{1}{2}$ in. As this is usually difficult to gauge, sufficient chest compression force should be used to generate a palpable femoral or carotid arterial pulse.

Definitive Therapy

During cardiac arrest the electrocardiogram will usually show rapid ventricular tachycardia or fibrillation, asystole, or heart block; however, it may be near normal.

Ventricular Tachycardia or Fibrillation

With ventricular fibrillation an attempt at electrical defibrillation should be made as quickly as possible. Direct-current defibrillation is employed, with one electrode paddle placed at the right upper sternal edge and the other placed left of the cardiac apex. The paddles, coated with low-resistance gel, should be applied firmly to the chest and then discharged with 200 J, which should be repeated if the first shock is unsuccessful. Prospective studies by Adgey, Pantridge, Gascho and colleagues[24–26] have shown 85 to 90 percent successful defibrillation using only 200 J in patients weighing up to 90 kg. Some advocate higher-energy defibrillation,[27] but few currently use more than 400 J. High-energy defibrillation may cause more cardiac injury and there is no clear evidence that it increases the frequency of successful resuscitation.[28]

When the electrocardiogram shows "fine" fibrillation waves, such defibrillation efforts are often unsuccessful. The administration of epinephrine (5 to 10 ml of 1:10,000) intravenously (IV) results in a more vigorous and coarse fibrillation which is more responsive to defibrillation. This effect is probably due to improved coronary flow following epinephrine administration (see below). If defibrillation fails, it is likely that marked acidosis or hypoxemia is present. Emphasis should be on optimal ventilation with supplemental oxygen to correct both hypoxemia and acidosis.[29] Sodium bicarbonate should then be administered (1 meq/kg) to aid in the management of acidosis, and defibrillation should be repeated with 400 J.

For recurrent ventricular fibrillation, the administration of 75 to 100 mg of lidocaine IV followed by repeat defibrillation may increase the likelihood of returning to a stable rhythm. Bretylium tosylate, a quaternary ammonium compound, is the only available drug that may terminate ventricular fibrillation without electric shock. It has recently been recommended as an additional first line drug for recurrent ventricular fibrillation to be used either in addition to or as an alternative to lidocaine. Haynes et al. have shown comparable survival from ventricular fibrillation in patients receiving either lidocaine or bretylium.[30] Initially, 5 mg/kg of bretylium is given IV followed by electrical defibrillation. The dose can be increased to 10 mg/kg and repeated at 15- to 30-min intervals until a maximum dose of 30 mg/kg has been given. Procainamide can be used in patients failing lidocaine and bretylium therapy. For recurrent ventricular fibrillation, propranolol is another effective drug. It seems particularly helpful in the setting of primary ventricular fibrillation complicating acute myocardial infarction.

Hyperkalemia is a readily treated condition which can cause AV block and impaired intraatrial and intraventricular conduction and which occasionally leads to ventricular fibrillation or, less commonly, asystole. It can be recognized by the development of tall, peaked T waves with a normal QT interval and sine-wave-like ventricular tachycardia. Life-threatening hyperkalemia responds most readily to calcium infusion; 10 to 30 ml of 10% calcium gluconate is infused intravenously over 1 to 5 min under constant electrocardiographic monitoring. Calcium counteracts the adverse effects of potassium on the neuromuscular membranes but does not alter plasma potassium. Its effect, though immediate, is transient. Hyperkalemia should subsequently be treated by either glucose-insulin infusion or sodium bicarbonate and/or ion-exchange resins.

With ventricular tachycardia, cough[31] and/or chest blows may revert the arrhythmia without defibrillation, and repeated cough will maintain the conscious state as a result of the rise in intrathoracic pressure.[9]

Asystole or Heart Block

Asystole due to vagal stimulation is the commonest cause of cardiac arrest associated with anesthesia induction and surgical procedures. Asystole also occurs as a result of heart block or sinus node disease (see Chaps. 25 and 26). Atropine (0.5 mg) given IV and repeated in 5 min can be used acutely to prevent or reverse severe bradycardia in many of these settings.

If asystole is diagnosed, vigorous blows to the precordium are sometimes sufficient to restart the heart. Rhythmic chest blows may be continued if needed, while the femoral or carotid pulse is palpated, until other treatment is available. If the chest blows fail, CPR should be initiated and intravenous epinephrine (5 to 10 ml of 1:10,000) given. If that fails, intracardiac epinephrine should be administered. Efforts should be made to correct acidosis and hypoxemia by ventilation and sodium bicarbonate administration. Resuscitation measures may result in a slow ventricular rhythm returning, which can subsequently be supported with atropine (1 to 2 mg IV) or isoproterenol until a temporary pacemaker is placed.

Temporary pacing is the optimal treatment for asystole or profound bradycardia. Obviously considerable skill and training are required for temporary transvenous pacemaker placement. External pacing has been developed as a noninvasive and simple pacing technique that can be used by paramedical personnel. The technique uses external surface electrodes with a high-voltage pacing source. Higher voltages are required to overcome transthoracic resistance, and it is therefore painful and used mainly on unconscious patients. The energy delivered to the heart by this technique is unclear, as is its efficacy. Recently pacing sources with longer pacing stimulus duration have been developed and may offer less painful but effective pacing. Transesophageal pacing is an alternative technique for noninvasive pacing but its clinical use has been limited.

Electromechanical Dissociation

In electromechanical dissociation there is evidence of organized electrical activity on the electrocardiogram at a reasonable rate but failure of effective perfusion (no pulse or blood pressure). The most treatable causes of this condition are (1) hypovolemia due to severe hemorrhage, (2) pericardial tamponade, and (3) tension pneumothorax. Signs of these problems should be sought and definitive therapy undertaken with fluids and/or blood replacement, pericardiocentesis, or placement of a pleural needle or tube. These conditions should also be strongly considered if cardiopulmonary resuscitation results in no palpable pulse or evidence of perfusion. Unfortunately, many patients with electromechanical dissociation have primary myocardial failure. After optimizing ventilation, epinephrine and calcium (5 to 7 mg/kg calcium chloride repeated every 10 min if necessary) may be helpful but are often ineffective. In acute myocardial infarction sudden electromechanical dissociation is a sign of myocardial rupture. In such cases pericardiocentesis and surgical repair rarely result in survival.

Establishment of an Intravenous Route

While external chest compression and artificial ventilation are continued, a plastic catheter should be inserted into a large peripheral vein. If a peripheral vein cannot be cannulated, a cutdown should be attempted or a central venous line placed by a percutaneous route. If cardiopulmonary resuscitation is properly performed, drugs administered through a peripheral line will reach the arterial circulation within 15 to 30 s.[29] Intracardiac injections are unnecessary except when there is no intravenous access or in asystole after failure of peripherally administered epinephrine. If an intravenous route is unavailable, epinephrine (dose, 1 to 2 mg in 10 ml of sterile distilled water) and lidocaine (dose, 50 to 100 mg in 10 ml of sterile distilled water) can be administered via the endotracheal tube into the bronchial tree.

Major Drugs Used during Cardiopulmonary Resuscitation

Drugs which are used for the treatment of various arrhythmias are mentioned above.

Catecholamines

Catecholamines are used in cardiac arrest to (1) increase arterial and coronary perfusion during and following cardiopulmonary resuscitation, (2) stimulate spontaneous contraction during asystole, (3) make fine ventricular fibrillation more responsive to defibrillation, and (4) act as an inotropic agent.

Epinephrine is effective in achieving all these goals. Recent studies have extensively evaluated the hemodynamic effects of epinephrine during resuscitation and have clearly shown it to be the single most important drug for common use during CPR.

Animal studies show that during conventional CPR, cerebral and myocardial perfusion pressures are low. Epinephrine increases brain and heart flow by two mechanisms:

- It prevents carotid artery collapse and raises arterial pressure during both chest compression and the release phase of chest compression (i.e., systole and diastole, respectively) thus resulting in higher carotid arterial systolic and aortic diastolic pressures. This in turn is reflected in higher cerebral perfusion and myocardial perfusion pressures and flow.[13]
- It preferentially reduces blood flow to the external carotid, renal, and splanchnic beds, thereby redirecting flow toward the brain and heart.

Arterial collapse at the thoracic inlet has been shown to be the critical limiting factor for cerebral perfusion pressure and flow during prolonged CPR. Arterial collapse results from high extravascular intrathoracic pressures, low intravascular volumes, and loss of arterial tone. Collapse results in a precipitous fall in carotid arterial and hence cerebral perfusion pressure. Epinephrine during CPR not only can reverse arterial collapse but can also prevent arterial collapse from developing. With the frequent administration of epinephrine during conventional CPR in the dog, cerebral blood flow can be maintained at more than 33 percent and myocardial flow at more than 10 percent of prearrest values for 50 min (see Fig. 33-2). If the experimental technique of simultaneous compression-ventilation CPR is used along with the frequent administration of epinephrine in dogs, cerebral flow can be maintained at more than 60 percent and myocardial flow at more than 30 percent of prearrest values (Fig. 33-2).[13]

These data strongly support the early and frequent use of epinephrine during CPR in an effort to optimize vital organ perfusion. Hence, once the diagnosis of cardiac arrest is established and CPR initiated, epinephrine should be administered as soon as possible. The recommended dose is 0.5 to 1 mg IV, and this dose should be repeated at approximately 5-min intervals unless effective cardiac activity is restored. If an intravenous route is not available, epinephrine can be administered down the endotracheal tube. The dose should be 10 ml of a 1:10,000 solution, and it too can be repeated every 5 min.

Norepinephrine is a potent vasoconstrictor and generally produces a rise in blood pressure; it is also an inotropic agent. Its disadvantage is that it causes renal and mesenteric vasoconstriction, and it should not be used in the initial phase of resuscitation. This agent is most useful where severe hypotension is present but where the chronotropic effects of epinephrine are not desirable (as in acute myocardial infarction or severe ischemia). This agent should be cautiously administered since severe tissue injury results from extravasation around an intravenous site.

Similarly, dopamine (a chemical precursor of norepinephrine) and dobutamine (a synthetic catecholamine) are preferred for use as inotropic agents because of their lesser chronotropic effect. Both these drugs, however, have little use in the initial phases of resuscitation when peripheral vasoconstriction is of primary importance. Isoproterenol (a synthetic catecholamine) is a pure beta-adrenergic agonist and is useful for treatment of bradycardia due to heart block or asystole until a temporary pacemaker is placed. Since it is a peripheral vasodilator its use is contraindicated in CPR.

Sodium Bicarbonate

Recent studies have shown that much less sodium bicarbonate should be used than previously advocated for acid-base control during cardiac arrest. As with other types of metabolic acidosis, if adequate alveolar ventilation is achieved, the metabolic acidosis of arrest is partially corrected through CO_2 excretion. Ideally, sodium bicarbonate should be given according to the results of measurement of arterial blood pH, P_{CO_2} determination, and calculation of the base deficit. Routinely, 1 meq/kg of sodium bicarbonate is administered after cardiopulmonary resuscitation is initiated, and no more than half this dose is repeated every 15 min. Excessive use of sodium bicarbonate can result in metabolic alkalosis, hypernatremia, and hyperosmolality.

Calcium chloride (5 to 7 mg/kg) enhances the contractile state of the heart and is indicated in treating severe hypotension and electromechanical dissociation refractory to catecholamines.

Calcium Channel Blockers

Calcium channel blockers inhibit calcium influx into smooth muscle and myocardial cells. They are principally vasodilators and negative inotropic agents and, under certain circumstances, antiarrhythmic agents with primary supraventricular effects. It has also been proposed that these agents may directly reduce ischemic injury to the brain. By virtue of these properties, some have suggested their use during resuscitation and in the immediate postresuscitation period in an effort to improve vital organ flow and reduce reperfusion tissue injury. Initial animal studies have shown improved brain blood flow post arrest with the administration of a calcium blocker during the arrest period. These studies must be interpreted with caution since in these animals myocardial function and flow following the administration of the calcium channel blocker were not evaluated. Several other factors must be considered before these agents are evaluated for use during resuscitation. The only calcium channel blocker that is currently available for intravenous use, verapamil, is a potent negative inotropic agent and therefore undesirable in the immediate postresuscitative period. Also, because of their vasodilatory properties, calcium channel blockers may reduce peripheral flow by counteracting the clearly beneficial effects of epinephrine-induced peripheral vasoconstriction, as discussed above. Use of these agents during resuscitation should await further studies.

Termination of Cardiopulmonary Resuscitation

Despite resuscitative efforts, the patient in cardiac arrest may not regain spontaneous circulation. The decision to end cardiopulmonary resuscitation should be based on a physician's assessment of the cerebral, cardiovascular, and general status of the patient. Failure is likely if there is absence of organized ventricular electrocardiographic activity and/or peripheral perfusion after 10 to 15 min of adequate cardiopulmonary resuscitation and appropriate therapy. Persistent deep unconsciousness and absence of respiration, reflex response, or pupillary reaction suggest cerebral death, and resuscitative efforts are usually unproductive. These guidelines, however, should be altered in patients with hypothermia, barbiturate overdose, and perhaps following electrocution, where recovery has been seen even after hours of resuscitation.[32]

Postarrest Care

Patients who have been successfully resuscitated usually require monitoring in an intensive care setting. These patients are prone to cardiac arrhythmias, hemodynamic and ventilatory instability, and ischemic encephalopathy. Ventilatory support with a respirator may well be necessary initially. Serial arterial blood gas determinations should be made to identify hypoxemia and assess the rapidly changing acid-base status.

The treatment of post-cardiac-arrest encephalopathy involves the prevention of further anoxia and hypotension. For cerebral edema after cardiac arrest methylprednisolone (60 to 100 mg) or dexamethasone sodium phosphate (12 to 20 mg IV every 6 h) has been recommended, but there is no conclusive evidence that these agents are beneficial. High-dose barbiturates, in animal studies, have also been shown to reduce postarrest brain injury;[33] the value of this therapy in human beings is uncertain. The prognosis of the patient with anoxic encephalopathy is related to the depth and continued duration of cerebral dysfunction.

Other potential life-threatening problems in the postarrest period include acute renal failure, bowel infarction, infection, and sepsis. Patients regaining consciousness may have postarrest amnesia or may develop psychotic behavior.

Outcome of Resuscitation

No discussion of resuscitation is complete without commenting on the outcome of resuscitation. In their initial study, Jude, Kouwenhoven, and Knickerbocker reported a 24 percent successful resuscitation and discharge rate from the hospital.[6] Recent studies have shown that with a paramedical response system a near 40 percent successful out-of-hospital resuscitation rate can be achieved. The critical factors for successful out-of-hospital resuscitation include less than 7 min total duration of CPR, less than 4 min from collapse to the initiation of CPR, and less than 10 min to successful delivery of first countershock. It is important to point out that the quality of life for such resuscitated patients is often good, with most discharged patients being able to return home to gainful employment.[34]

References

1. Holy Bible, King James version, 2 Kings 4:34.
2. Comroe, J. H.: Retrospectroscope, ". . . In Comes the Good Air," *Am. Rev. Respir. Dis.*, 119:803, 1979.
3. Elam, J. O., Brown, E. S., and Elder, J. D.: Artificial Respiration by Mouth-to-Mask Method, *N. Engl. J. Med.*, 250:749, 1954.
4. Turell, D. J., and Husni, E. A.: Cardiac Resuscitation after Documented Myocardial Infarction, *Am. J. Cardiol.*, 7:736, 1961.
5. Kouwenhoven, W. B., Jude, J. R., and Knickerbocker, G. G.: Closed Chest Cardiac Massage, *JAMA*, 173:1064, 1960.
6. Jude, J. R., Kouwenhoven, W. B., and Knickerbocker, G. G.: Cardiac Arrest: Report of Application of External Cardiac Massage on 118 Patients, *JAMA*, 178:1063, 1961.
7. Weale, F. E., and Rothwell-Jackson, R. L.: The Efficiency of Cardiac Massage, *Lancet*, 1:990, 1962.
8. MacKenzie, G. J., Taylor, S. H., McDonald, A. H., and Donald, K. W.: Hemodynamic Effects of External Cardiac Compression, *Lancer*, 1:1342, 1964.
9. Criley, J. M., Blaufuss, A. N., and Kissel, G. L.: Cough-Induced Cardiac Compression, *JAMA*, 236:1246, 1976.
10. Rudikoff, M. T., Maughan, W. L., Effron, M., Freund, P., and Weisfeldt, M. L.: Mechanisms of Flow during Cardiopulmonary Resuscitation, *Circulation*, 61:345, 1980.
11. Koehler, R. C., Chandra, N., Guerci, A. D., Tsitlik, J., Traystman, R. J., Rogers, M. C., and Weisfeldt, M. L.: Augmentation of Cerebral Perfusion by Simultaneous Chest Compression and Lung Inflation with Abdominal Binding Following Cardiac Arrest in Dogs, *Circulation*, 67:266, 1983.

12. Chandra, N., Weisfeldt, M. L., Tsitlik, J., Vaghaiwalla, F., Snyder, L., Hoffecker, M., and Rudikoff, M.: Augmentation of Carotid Flow During CPR in Dogs by Ventilation at High Airway Pressures Simultaneous with Chest Compression, *Am. J. Cardiol.*, 48:1053, 1981.
13. Michael, J. R., Guerci, A. D., Koehler, R. C., Shi, A. Y., Tsitlik, Jr., Chandra, N., Niedermeyer, E., Rogers, M. C., Traystman, R. J., and Weisfeldt, M. L.: Mechanisms by which Epinephrine Augments Cerebral and Myocardial Perfusion during Cardiopulmonary Resuscitation in Dogs, *Circulation*, 69:822, 1984.
14. Chandra, N., Snyder, L. D., and Weisfeldt, M. L.: Abdominal Binding during CPR in Man, *JAMA*, 246:351, 1981.
15. Chandra, N., Rudikoff, M., and Weisfeldt, M. L.: Simultaneous Chest Compression and Ventilation at High Airway Pressure during Cardiopulmonary Resuscitation, *Lancet*, 1:175, 1980.
16. Werner, J. A., Greene, H. L., Janko, C. L., and Cobb, L. A.: Visualization of Cardiac Valve Motion in Man during External Chest Compression Using Two-Dimensional Echocardiography. Implications Regarding the Mechanism of Blood Flow, *Circulation*, 63:1417, 1981.
17. Chandra, N., Snyder, L., Tsitlik, J., and Weisfeldt, M. L.: Non-invasive Assisted Circulation by Synchronized Cyclical High Intrathoracic Pressure Support, *Clin. Res.*, 28:161A, 1980.
18. Chazen, J. A., Stenson, R., and Kurland, G. S.: The Acidosis of Cardiac Arrest, *N. Engl. J. Med.*, 278:360, 1968.
19. Heimlich, H. J.: A Life Saving Maneuver to Prevent from Choking, *JAMA*, 234:398, 1975.
20. Visintine, R. E., and Baick, C. H.: Ruptured Stomach after Heimlich Maneuver, *JAMA*, 234:415, 1975.
21. Greene, D. G., Elam, J. O., Dobkin, A. B., and Studley, C. L.: Cinefluorographic Study of Hyperextension of the Neck and Upper Airway Patency, *JAMA*, 176:570, 1961.
22. Bryson, T. K., Kenvmof, J. F., and Ward, C. F.: The Esophageal Obturator Airway, A Clinical Comparison to Ventilation with a Mask and Oralpharnygeal Airway, *Chest*, 74:537, 1978.
23. American Heart Association: Standards and Guidelines for Cardiopulmonary Resuscitation (CPR) and Emergency Cardiac Care (ECC), *JAMA*, 244:453, 1980.
24. Adgey, A. A. J., Patton, J. N., Campbell, N. P. S., and Webb, S. W.: Ventricular Defibrillation: Appropriate Energy Levels, *Circulation*, 60:219, 1979.
25. Pantridge, J. F., Adgey, A. A. J., Webb, S. W., and Anderson, J.: Electrical Requirements for Ventricular Defibrillation, *Br. Med. J.*, 2:313, 1975.
26. Gascho, J. A., Crampton, R. S., Cherwek, M. L., Sipes, J. N., Hustert, P., and O'Brien, W. M.: Determinants of Ventricular Defibrillation in Adults, *Circulation*, 60:231, 1979.
27. Tacker, W. A., and Ewy, G. A.: Emergency Defibrillation Dose, Recommendation and Rationale, *Circulation*, 60:233, 1979.
28. Weaver, W. D., Cobb, L. A., Copass, M. K., and Hallstrom, A. P.: Ventricular Defibrillation—A Comparative Trial Using 175-J and 320-J Shocks, *N. Engl. J. Med.*, 307:1101, 1982.
29. Bishop, R. L., and Weisfeldt, M. L.: Sodium Bicarbonate Administration during Cardiac Arrest. Effect of Arterial pH, PCO_2 and Osmolality, *JAMA*, 235:506, 1976.
30. Haynes, R. E., Copass, M. K., Chinn, T. L., and Cobb, L. A.: Randomized Comparison of Bretylium and Lidocaine in Resuscitation of Patients from Out-of-Hospital Ventricular Fibrillation, *Circulation*, 58(suppl. 2-686): 177, 1978.
31. Wei, J. Y., Greene, H. L., and Weisfeldt, M. L.: Cough-Facilitated Conversion of Ventricular Tachycardia, *Am. J. Cardiol.*, 45:174, 1980.
32. Ravitch, M. M., Lane, R., Safar, P., Steichen, F. M., and Knowles, P.: Lightning Stroke. Report of a Case with Recovery after Cardiac Massage and Prolonged Artificial Respiration, *N. Engl. J. Med.*, 264:36, 1961.
33. Bleyaert, A. L., Nemoto, E. M., Safar, P., Stezoski, S. W., Michell, J. J., Moossy, J., and Rao, G.: Thiopental Amelioration of Brain Damage after Global Ischemia in Monkeys, *Acta Neurol. Scand.*, 56(suppl. 64):144, 1977 and *Anesthesiology*, 49:390, 1978.
34. Eisenberg, M. S., Hallstrom, A., Bergner, L.: Long-Term survival After Out-of-Hospital Cardiac Arrest, *N. Engl. J. Med.*, 306:1340, 1982.

PART V

Diseases of the Heart and Blood Vessels

The purpose of Part V, "Diseases of the Heart and Blood Vessels," is to present a discussion of the *disease processes* that can affect the heart and blood vessels. The reader should review the preface to Part IV in order to understand the distinction we have made between a *disease process* and a *disorder*. Briefly, we define a *disease process* as a basic abnormality that exists in the tissue. The cause of the abnormality may be known or unknown. The pathologist can usually identify an abnormal disease process at autopsy when he or she examines the heart and blood vessels. A *disorder* is defined as a consequence of a disease process. A disorder is the derangement of function due to the disease process. A disorder is the final common pathway by which many different diseases make the patient ill. The pathologist may not be able to state that a patient had a disorder such as chest pain, ventricular dysfunction, a hyperdynamic circulation, arrhythmia, or syncope by examining the heart and blood vessels.

Whenever a physician identifies a disease process in a patient, he or she must ask: *"Are any of the known consequences (disorders) of the disease process present in my patient?"*

34

Incidence, Prevalence, and Mortality of Cardiovascular Diseases

William B. Kannel, M.D. Thomas J. Thom, B.A.

When meditating over a disease I never think of finding a remedy for it but instead a means of preventing it.
Louis Pasteur, 1884[1]

Life expectancy has never been higher in the United States than at present, largely as a result of the improved standard of living and quality of life. The death rate is now declining at a rate of 2 percent per year, suggesting that today's leading causes of death, cardiovascular diseases, are amenable to preventive and therapeutic management.

Cardiovascular Diseases as a Major Health Hazard

General Morbidity and Mortality

Despite recent improvements, cardiovascular disease continues to be the most serious threat to life and health. One in every three men in the United States can expect to develop some major cardiovascular disease before reaching age 60; the odds for women are one in ten.[2] Coronary heart disease is the major cause of death after the age of 40 in men and after the age of 50 in women.[3] An estimated 43 million persons, or 19 percent of the U.S. population, have heart disease or hypertension, causing limitation of activity in about 8.5 million persons (Fig. 34-1). Almost two-thirds of the 43 million persons are under 65 years of age. The most common cardiovascular diseases are hypertension and the arteriosclerotic-related diseases: coronary heart disease, cerebrovascular disease, and peripheral vascular disease. Heart conditions and hypertension rank third and fourth, respectively, among the leading chronic diseases causing disability. Each year the cardiovascular diseases account for an estimated 600 million days of restricted activity, 170 million bed days, and 45 million work-loss days.[4] Most of these disability days are due to heart disease and hypertension. There are about 50 million days in short-stay hospitals each year and 50 million visits to physicians' offices for these diseases. In 1979, over 115,000 workers with cardiovascular disease were allowed Social Security disability benefits, which amounted to 32 percent of all such benefits.[5]

Cardiovascular diseases account for one-half of all deaths in the United States. Of the 979,000 deaths from these diseases in 1982, most were due to atherosclerosis, and 20 percent occurred before 65 years of age.[6] About 77 percent of the cardiovascular disease deaths are caused by heart disease, 16 percent by stroke. Compared with other major diagnostic groups, cardiovascular disease is the leading cause of death, of short-stay hospital days, and of worker disability allowances, and it is the second leading cause of bed days.[4]

Because cardiovascular disease accounts for one-half of the nation's mortality and much of the nation's morbidity, its cost to the nation's economy is by far the largest for any diagnostic group; an estimated $96.9 billion in 1981 (Fig. 34-2). For cardiovascular disease patients that year, the nation spent $37.9 billion for hospital care, physician and other professional services, drugs, and nursing home care, or 1 percent of the GNP. The economy lost $59 billion in productivity due to illness ($11 billion) and premature death ($48 billion) attributed to these diseases. Included in the $48 billion is the value of future productivity that would have occurred if those who died from cardiovascular diseases in 1981 had lived to normal life expectancy.

Reliable incidence data for the cardiovascular diseases are scarce. Data from the Framingham (Massachusetts) Heart Study provide reliable estimates for 26 years of follow-up of a defined population sample of 5209 men and women aged 35 to 84. Average annual rates of first major cardiovascular events rose from 4.7 per 1000 men at ages 35 to 44

FIGURE 34-1 Estimated prevalence of the major cardiovascular diseases, United States, 1981. (*Unpublished estimates from the Health Interview Survey obtained by personal communication from the National Center for Health Statistics.*)

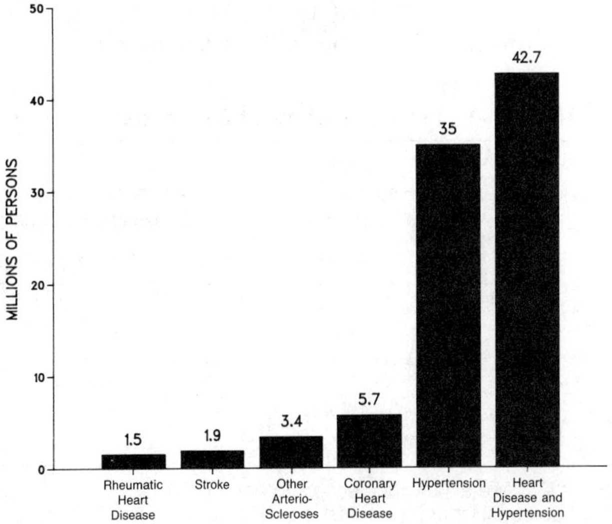

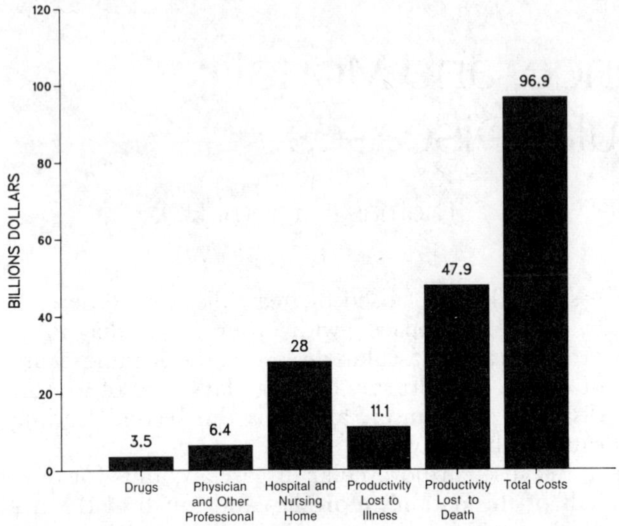

FIGURE 34-2 Estimated economic costs in billions of dollars for cardiovascular diseases, United States, 1981. (*From National Heart, Lung and Blood Institute.*)

years to 51 per 1000 at ages 75 to 84 (Table 34-1). For women, comparable rates are achieved 10 years later in life, with the gap closing with advancing age. This 10-year lag in incidence applies for coronary heart disease, occlusive peripheral arterial disease, and cardiac failure but not for stroke.

Secular Trends

The trend in mortality from the cardiovascular diseases as a group has been downward since about 1940, with long-term declines for the three subgroups, rheumatic, cerebrovascular, and hypertensive diseases, and a recent decline for coronary heart disease (Fig. 34-3).[4,7] The decline antedates effective antibiotic and antihypertensive treatment. Prior to 1940 cardiovascular mortality increased and became the predominant cause of death because of control of infectious and parasitic diseases and an epidemic increase in fatal coronary attacks. Cardiovascular mortality declined just under 1 percent per year in the 1950s and 1960s. The decline became more precipitous in the 1970s, with the rate falling 2.7 percent per year since then.[4] Over one-half of the decline between 1950 and 1982 occurred in the 10 years after 1972. For stroke, the rate of decline since 1972 has exceeded 5 percent per year.

A striking feature of the recent decline in cardiovascular mortality has been its universal nature—it has declined in all races, both sexes, all age groups, and all geographic areas in the United States. However, greatest improvements have been noted in females, blacks, young adults, and the higher socioeconomic subgroups, and there are geographic differences in the rate of decline.[4] The largest percent declines are noted for hypertension and cerebrovascular diseases, and in recent years the largest absolute decline has been in coronary heart disease. Except for lung cancer and chronic obstructive pulmonary diseases, mortality from other natural causes has also been declining. But because cardiovascular diseases account for one-half of all deaths, declines in these diseases are largely responsible for a recent major improvement of average life expectancy, now at 74.1 years.[6]

The decline in coronary heart disease mortality reverses the earlier epidemic rise persisting into the 1960s; it coincides with improvements in the major cardiovascular risk factors, more vigorous and effective treatment of the acute episode, and greater efforts at secondary prevention.[8] The decline in coronary heart disease mortality in the United States exceeds that observed elsewhere in the world. Many Western countries are still experiencing a rising trend in coronary heart disease mortality.[9]

The proportionately greater gains in life expectancy in adults relative to newborns in recent decades suggests that cardiovascular health problems are being dealt with effectively. The decline in cardiovascular mortality indicates that the major force of mortality is controllable. Whether attributable more to changes in disease-promoting life-style or to better medical care of those already afflicted, it is clear that cardiovascular disease is not an inevitable burden of aging or genetic makeup. Although the cause of the decline in cardiovascular mortality is uncertain, it has been substantial, sustained, and real. The decline has coincided with increased efforts to achieve

TABLE 34-1 Incidence of Major Cardiovascular Events: Framingham Study, 26-Year Follow-up*

	Cardiovascular Diseases (All Types)		Coronary Heart Disease		Cerebrovascular Accident		Peripheral Arterial Disease		Cardiac Failure	
Age	**Men**	**Women**	**Men**	**Women**	**Men**	**Women**	**Men**	**Women**	**Men**	**Women**
35–44	47	15	42	7	2	4	4	2	5	4
45–54	141	54	108	33	20	12	20	9	20	9
55–64	264	144	202	99	40	26	53	24	44	27
65–74	336	211	227	136	92	80	69	40	86	57
75–84	511	402	247	236	196	112	61	27	188	119
35–84	193	119	144	73	39	30	36	22	40	26

*Average annual incidence rate per 10,000.
Source: Unpublished rates from Framingham Heart Study, personal communication.

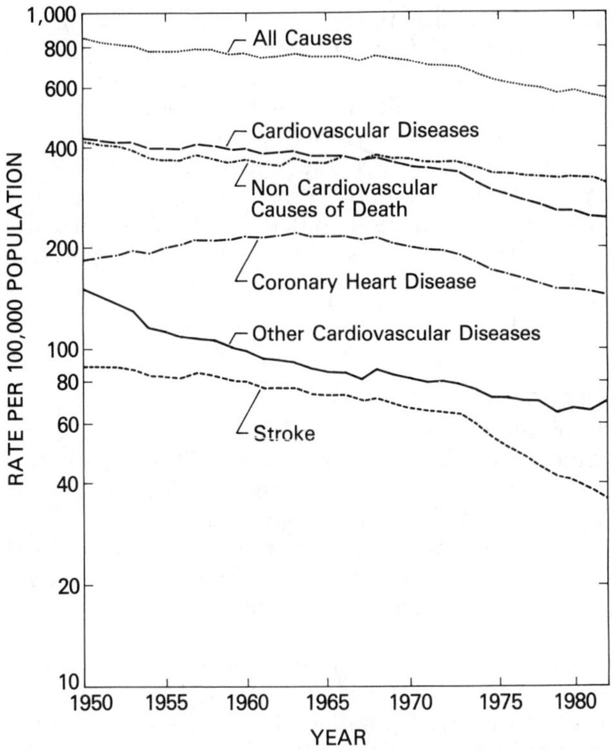

FIGURE 34-3 Death rates: for all causes of death, for total cardiovascular disease and its subgroups, and for total deaths not caused by cardiovascular disease; United States, 1950 to 1982. (*From Vital Statistics of The United States, National Center for Health Statistics.*)

healthier living habits and with improvements in the ambient burden of cardiovascular risk factors.

Unfortunately, there are very little data on trends in morbidity. This is important because reduction in mortality without a decline in the attack rate would indicate better medical care was responsible, while a reduction in both would suggest environmental influences.

Coronary Heart Disease

Coronary heart disease kills and disables people in their most productive years and accounts for $8.6 billion of the $37.9 billion spent in 1981 for medical care of cardiovascular disease patients. Coronary disease is the third most frequent cause of short-stay hospitalizations, after complications of pregnancy and accidents, and the per admission hospital costs for this disease are the highest. Coronary heart disease is the leading cause of premature permanent disability in the American labor force, accounting for 19 percent of disability allowances by the Social Security Administration.[5]

Prevalence

Estimates from the National Health Interview Survey indicate that 2.5 percent of Americans (5.7 million) have coronary heart disease, 42 percent of whom are limited in activity because of it. For men the prevalence rises from 3.5 per 1000 population at ages 17 to 44 to 75.5 at ages 45 to 64 and 145.1 at ages 65 and over. For women the estimates by age are 1.1, 34.3, and 96.1 per 1000, respectively.

Incidence

Coronary heart disease causes about 800,000 new heart attacks each year and an additional 450,000 recurrences.[4] The chance of an American male developing this disease before age 60 is one in five. Incidence in women lags by 10 years for total coronary heart disease and by 20 years for more serious clinical manifestations such as myocardial infarction and sudden death (Table 34-2). Male predominance is least striking for uncomplicated angina pectoris.

The presenting coronary complaint for women is more likely to be angina, whereas in men it is more likely to be myocardial infarction or sudden death. More angina in men occurs after infarction than afresh. Only 20 percent of coronary attacks are preceded by long-standing angina, less if the infarction is silent or unrecognized. Serious manifestations of coronary heart disease such as infarction or sudden death are rare in the premenopausal female. The incidence and severity of coronary heart disease increase precipitously after the menopause, with coronary heart disease rates in postmenopausal women two to three times that of women the same age who remain premenopausal. This applies whether the menopause is natural or surgical, and, in the latter, whether the ovaries are removed or not and whether or not estrogen replacement therapy is prescribed.[10] The gap in incidence between the sexes narrows progressively with advancing age.

Unrecognized myocardial infarctions are common, numbering at least one in five.[11] Half are silent, and the rest are atypical so that neither the patient nor the physician entertains the possibility. More than half of these subjects eventually develop some overt clinical manifestations of coronary heart disease and hence come under medical care. Angina

TABLE 34-2 Incidence of Specified Clinical Manifestations of Coronary Heart Disease; Framingham Study, 26-Year Follow-up*

	Angina Pectoris†		Myocardial Infarction		Sudden Death	
Age	Men	Women	Men	Women	Men	Women
35–44	8	5	21	2	4	0
45–54	30	21	54	9	11	3
55–64	74	54	91	25	21	6
65–74	52	51	119	51	31	13
75–84	25	94	168	90	43	32
35–84	42	37	71	22	16	6

*Average annual incidence rate per 10,000.
†Uncomplicated by myocardial infarction.
Source: Unpublished rates from Framingham Heart Study, personal communication.

is less frequent in such subjects than in those with recognized symptomatic myocardial infarction, but the risk of subsequent mortality is nearly the same.

Although about two-thirds of myocardial infarction patients do not make a complete recovery, 88 percent under age 65 are able to return to their usual occupations.[10] Within 5 years after an initial infarction 13 percent of the men and almost 40 percent of the women develop a second infarction.[12] While the case-fatality rate is 30 percent for initial infarctions and 50 percent for recurrences, 10-year survival is 50 percent for men and 30 percent for women.[10]

Mortality

Coronary heart disease is the leading cause of death in American adults, accounting for one-third of deaths in persons over age 35. It is estimated that a 30-year-old American male would survive to age 79 rather than 73 if coronary heart disease could be eliminated. In 1982 there were 552,000 coronary deaths. In the age range 35 to 64 about 75 pecent of all cardiac deaths—including deaths from hypertensive, rheumatic, and pulmonary causes and deaths from other heart diseases such as heart failure, endocarditis, and cardiomyopathy—are attributed to this cause. Mortality from coronary heart disease increases with age, but coronary heart disease is also a prominent cause of death in adults at the peak of their productive lives.

In a substantial number of cases of coronary heart disease mortality, the progression from inapparent clinical disease to death is rather swift. Much of the premature mortality from coronary heart disease comes on with little warning in a population prone to this disease. Sudden, unexpected, out-of-hospital coronary deaths that occur too rapidly to allow arrival at the hospital while the patient is still alive account for more than one-half of all coronary fatalities. Sudden deaths are less likely in women than men and less likely in the elderly than in the young.

About 80 percent of coronary mortality in persons under age 65 occurs during the initial coronary attack. Thus, despite a higher risk of death with a prior coronary attack, most coronary deaths arise from the population still free of symptomatic coronary heart disease. Hence, primary prevention appears to offer more to society than secondary prevention. The first year following an attack is especially dangerous, with 20 percent of men and 45 percent of women with myocardial infarction succumbing. After myocardial infarction, sudden deaths occur at nine times the rate of the general population.

Hypertension

Hypertension is the most prevalent cardiovascular disease, and it is one of the most powerful contributors to cardiovascular morbidity and mortality. It is the most important factor contributing to the 500,000 cases of stroke which occur each year and is a major factor in the estimated 1.25 million annual coronary events. Each year it is the underlying cause of 32,000 deaths classified as due to hypertensive disease, and it is the main contributor to all 159,000 deaths from stroke, the 27,000 deaths from cardiac failure, many of the 550,000 deaths from coronary heart disease, and many of the 18,000 deaths from kidney disease. This amounts to an estimated 250,000 deaths per year.

Prevalence

Preliminary data from the National Health and Nutrition Examination Survey for 1976 to 1980 indicated a hypertension prevalence of 30.7 percent for persons 25 to 74 years of age in the United States.[13] For that estimate hypertension is defined as blood pressure equal to or greater than 140/90 mmHg. When the data include persons below that level but on antihypertensive medication, and the data are extrapolated to all ages, prevalence is about 60 million: 26 percent of the total population and 36 percent of the adult population.[4] For persons with hypertension greater than 160/95 mmHg or who are on medication, prevalence is about 35 million persons: 15 percent of the total population and 21 percent of the adult population. Prevalence of mild hypertension, defined as a diastolic blood pressure of 90 to 104 mmHg, is about 24 million persons, or 40 percent of the 60 million with hypertension. Prevalence of isolated systolic hypertension, defined as systolic blood pressure over 160 mmHg and diastolic under 95 mmHg, is about 4 million persons, comprised mostly of the elderly.

Percent prevalence increases with age and is highest among blacks and the elderly. Isolated systolic hypertension is a common and distinctly hazardous condition in the elderly. Persons with hypertension face serious excess risks of cardiovascular sequelae, and since much of this excess risk is attributable to mild hypertension, there is need for intervention through preventive life-style modification if not through drug treatment. Because of the higher prevalence of milder hypertension, almost 60 percent of the excess mortality attributable to hypertension comes from this blood pressure range. Risks of cardiovascular sequelae are proportional to the blood pressure level at any age, in either sex, whether the elevation is systolic or diastolic. Approximately one-half of the persons who suffer a first heart attack and two-thirds who suffer a first stroke have blood pressures above 160/95 mmHg.

Although in most affluent populations there is a rise in blood pressure with age in both sexes, this is not universal and it does not mean that blood pressure must inevitably rise with age or that in those whose pressures do rise it reflects a normal aging process. There is about a 20 mmHg systolic and 10 mmHg diastolic rise from age 30 to age 64. Systolic pressures continue to rise into the eighties in women and into the seventies in men. Diastolic pressures level off earlier and, in men, decline precipitously beyond age 55. The pressures start lower in women and rise more steeply, so that they equal those of men in the fifties and then progressively exceed those of men in later life; this crossover is observed for both systolic and diastolic pressure. In some populations in the world, blood pressure does not rise with age.

The percent of persons 25 to 74 years of age with blood pressures equal to or greater than 160/95 mmHg declined from 17.7 in 1960 to 1962 to 14.5 in 1976 to 1980. There have been big improvements in the percent of hypertensives aware of it (from 54 to 73 percent), on antihypertensive medication (from 36 to 56 percent), and under control (from 16 to 34 percent) during that time (Fig. 34-4). "Under control" in this case means on medication and having blood pressures below 160/95 mmHg.

Incidence

Longitudinal observation of blood pressures as people age reveals a different pattern than do cross-sectional data. The reason for this difference is obscure. Diastolic pressures are essentially parallel in the sexes, with women's pressures consistently below those of men. Systolic pressures in women, initially lower than those in men, rise more steeply to converge at age 60 with those of men but never to exceed them. A progressive and disproportionate rise in systolic pressure with advancing age is presumed to result from loss of arterial elasticity.

Black persons have higher blood pressures than do white persons in most Western cultures. The crossover in blood pressures in the sexes appears to occur 10 years earlier in blacks than whites.

Mortality

Only 3 percent of cardiovascular deaths in 1982 were nominally attributed to hypertensive disease, a gross underestimate of its impact on mortality. Hypertensive disease mortality is largely due to atherosclerotic sequelae such as coronary disease, stroke, and cardiac failure. Renal failure due to necrotizing arteriolar disease is uncommon, and malignant hypertension is vanishing as a cause of death. In 1979 only 6 percent of deaths directly attributed to hypertension were ascribed to malignant hypertension. The marked downward trend in mortality attributed to hypertensive disease and stroke strongly suggests that mortality resulting from hypertension is on the decline. The rate of decline accelerated from 2 percent per year in the 1940s to 4 percent per year in the 1950s to 7 percent per year in the 1970s, coinciding with more vigorous antihypertensive treatment and earlier detection of hypertension subjects. The rate of decline in mortality for stroke accelerated from a 1 percent per year decline in the 1940s and 1950s, to a 2 percent per year decline in the 1960s, to a 5 percent per year decline since 1970.

Determinants

While genetic susceptibility plays a large role, this may be only permissive, requiring one or more environmental cofactors such as salt intake, alcohol, or weight gain to bring on hypertension. New underlying causes of hypertension are discovered every decade, but the causes of the vast majority of cases remain undetermined. Of the identifiable causes, chronic renal diseases, renovascular disease, and hypertension induced by oral contraceptives head the list. Routine search for underlying causes not suggested by signs or symptoms is usually unrewarding and often counterproductive.

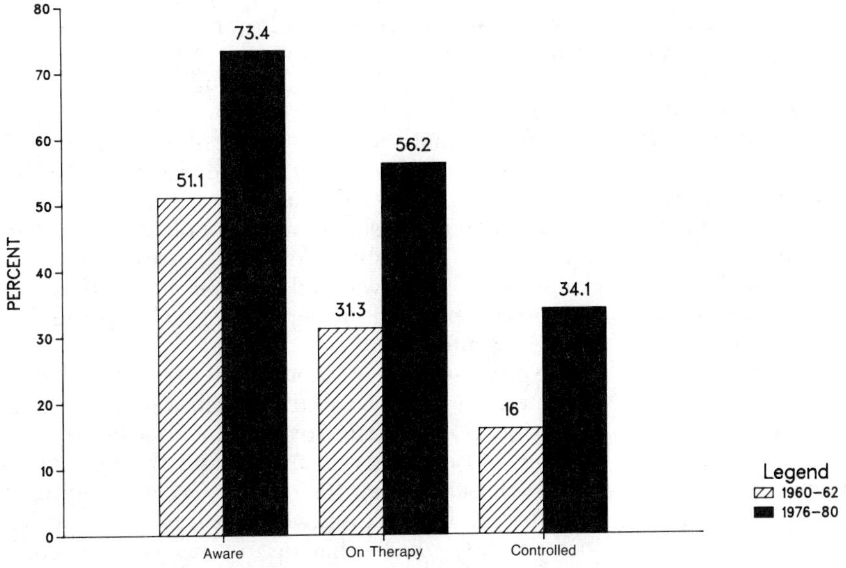

FIGURE 34-4 Percent of hypertensive persons by aware, therapy, and control status, ages 25 to 74, United States, 1960 to 1962 and 1976 to 1980. (*Derived by the National Heart, Lung, and Blood Institute primarily from data from the National Center for Health Statistics.*)

Stroke

Prevalence

There are about 8 stroke patients per 1000 population in the United States, a total of 1.9 million persons, according to the National Health Interview Survey of 1981. An estimated 45 percent are limited in their usual activity because of this disease. An additional 200,000 residents of nursing homes suffer from cerebrovascular disease. Prevalence rises from less than 2 per 1000 adults under age 45 to 13 per 1000 at ages 45 to 64 and to 45 per 1000 over age 65. The most common variety of stroke is atherothrombotic brain infarction, which accounts for 59 percent of all strokes. Next most common are cerebral embolus (14 percent), subarachnoid hemorrhage (10 percent), and intracerebral hemorrhage (5 percent). Intracerebral hemorrhage has apparently declined most in recent decades.

Incidence

The chance of having a stroke before age 70 in the United States is 1 in 20 for either sex.[14] However, incidence rates vary depending on the age of the study sample, whether the sample is derived from the general population or from some select subgroup such as hospitalized patients, and whether recurrent strokes are included. In 1972 the Joint Committee for Stroke Facilities estimated that stroke incidence increased from 1 per 1000 at ages 45 to 54 to 9 per 1000 at ages 65 to 74.[15] These figures are similar to those in the Framingham Study. Although strokes occur most frequently late in life, 20 percent occur under age 65. The incidence reaches substantial proportions only after age 55. Unlike other hypertension- and atherosclerosis-related disease, there is no clear male predominance for stroke, except under age 55. In the Framingham Study, brain infarctions occurred in men at one-third the rate of myocardial infarctions in the age range 45 to 74. For women, the incidence of brain and myocardial infarction is similar at all ages.

Disability

Strokes rank high on the list of crippling diseases because many of the estimated 250,000 Americans who survive a stroke each year remain disabled by paralysis, speech disorders, and incontinence. According to the National Hospital Discharge Survey, there were an estimated 825,000 hospital discharges (alive or dead) from stroke in 1982, not including strokes as a secondary cause of admission. Residual disability is often substantial. In the Framingham Study, 31 percent of stroke survivors needed assistance in self-care, 20 percent required help in ambulation, and 71 percent had an impaired vocational capacity when examined an average of 7 years after their stroke.[16] Of the 2 million persons afflicted by stroke in the United States, 40 percent require special services and 10 percent total care.

Cerebrovascular disease need not be a result of aging. Modifiable contributing factors offer the possibility of prevention by identifying stroke candidates for corrective measures. Stroke prevention requires early treatment of persons with hypertension, cardiac disorders, and transient cerebral ischemic attacks.

Mortality

In 1973, cerebrovascular diseases were responsible for about 214,000 deaths. In 1982, the yearly toll had declined to 159,000, or 8 percent of total mortality. Although 86 percent of stroke deaths occur in persons over age 65, premature deaths are not uncommon. This is particularly true among black adults under age 65. The stroke death rate in this group is three times that in whites, largely as a result of the higher prevalence and increased severity of hypertension. Stroke remains the third leading cause of death behind heart disease and cancer.

Cardiac Failure and Cardiomyopathy

Heart failure is the end stage of cardiac disease after the myocardium has used all its reserve and compensatory mechanisms. Once overt signs appear, half of the patients will be dead within 5 years despite modern medical management.[17] Cardiac failure is a tragic consequence of a variety of heart diseases, particularly hypertensive, coronary, rheumatic, and congenital heart disease. The dominant cause is hypertension, which precedes failure in 75 percent of cases. Coronary heart disease, generally accompanied by hypertension, is responsible in 39 percent of cases.[18] Precursive rheumatic heart disease, noted in 21 percent of cases of cardiac failure, is also often accompanied by hypertension.

Over 2 million Americans have heart failure and at least 250,000 new cases occur each year, requiring 500,000 to 1,000,000 hospitalizations annually. Reports of the incidence of cardiac failure in the United States vary from 0.05 to 2 per 1000 per annum.[19] From physician surveys, Gibson et al. estimated the occurrence at 3.8 to 5.0 per 1000 persons age 45 and over per year.[20] The Framingham Study estimated the rate at 2.3 per 1000 for men and 1.4 per 1000 for women 30 to 79 years of age. Incidence increases with age, so that by the sixth decade the rate among men is five times that of the fourth decade. With an increasing geriatric population, cardiac failure is a formidable problem. If preventive programs are to be developed, identification of factors that predispose and influence the course of the disease is essential.

Despite early recognition and more sophisticated treatment of cardiac failure, its clinical course and prognosis remain grim for the chief causes, hypertension and coronary heart disease; the outlook is not much better than for cancer. Greater emphasis must be given to preventive measures instituted before the heart has exhausted its reserve and compensatory mechanisms. Since hypertension is such an important predisposing factor, early and sustained treatment would seem a key to the prevention of most cardiac failure.

Arrhythmias

An arrhythmia is a disturbance of the cardiac impulse. It is a manifestation of most major cardiac diseases, a major cause of morbidity in rheumatic heart disease, and a contributor to half of the mortality from coronary heart disease. Many such victims die suddenly, without warning. Together with cardiac failure, arrhythmias are the final common pathways in heart disease.

Although the frequency of arrhythmias is not known, in 1982 there were an estimated 2 million hospital discharges with arrhythmias listed as one of the diagnoses. In about one-quarter of these cases arrhythmia was the primary diagnosis. There are about 2 million physician office visits a year due to this condition, larger than the number due to stroke. It is not known how many deaths are attributed to arrhythmias each year because it is the immediate cause, not the underlying cause, of much cardiac mortality.

Rheumatic Fever and Rheumatic Heart Disease

Rheumatic fever is the chief cause of serious valvular heart disease. Acute rheumatic fever and subsequent rheumatic heart disease remain one of the important cardiovascular problems in the tropical and subtropical developing countries in South America, Africa, the Middle East, and Asia.[21] It occurs there with a frequency seen in the United States and Europe a century ago.[22] Although preventable, this disease occurs because of overcrowding, the deceptive self-limited nature of streptococcal pharyngitis, and the mild and often clinically inapparent nature of streptococcal infections. The availability of penicillin to treat these infections and living conditions that are less crowded than formerly have made rheumatic fever uncommon in the United States, although incidence remains high in disadvantaged subgroups such as blacks, Puerto Ricans, Mexican-Americans, and American Indians. Because this disease has not been eradicated in this country, there is need to better define its incidence and prevalence and the infective endocarditis which follows, as well as to better define those at risk.

The estimated prevalence in 1981 of active rheumatic fever and chronic rheumatic heart disease is 1.5 million persons, 6.5 per 1000 persons of all ages, 12 per 1000 above age 45. About 18 percent of these persons are limited in activity because of the resulting chronic carditis. Incidence, generally thought to be about 100,000 new cases per year, may be overestimated; there are no good national estimates. Occurrence is concentrated in the lower socioeconomic subgroups. Rheumatic fever is rare before age 3, occurring most frequently between 5 and 15 years of age, when streptococcal infections are most frequent. During epidemics of streptococcal pharyngitis, the rheumatic fever attack rate is 3 percent, whereas in endemic situations it is only 0.3 percent. There are about ½ million physician office visits per year for this disease and about 50,000 annual hospital discharges where this disease is the primary diagnosis. Many of the 37,000 annual open heart operations on cardiac valves are performed on rheumatic heart disease patients.

With decline in rheumatic fever in the United States, its clinical manifestations have also moderated so that carditis is detected in less than 20 percent of acute patients.[23] Annual mortality has declined to about 7000 deaths per year, which reflects an 85 percent decline in the age-adjusted death rate from 1950 to 1982. But because the cardiac sequelae of rheumatic fever are still seen in adults and adequate treatment can reduce attacks by 90 percent, rheumatic fever and rheumatic heart disease are still the two most preventable serious cardiovascular disorders.

Other Valvular Disease

In the two decades since mitral valve prolapse was described, the syndrome has changed from a curiosity to the most frequently diagnosed valvular deformity. The exact prevalence is not clear. It appears to occur in 6 to 10 percent of presumably normal young women[24] and is reported in about 4 percent of healthy young men.[25] Although the condition may become manifest at any age, it is reported most frequently in young women aged 14 to 30, where it may reach a prevalence exceeding 10 percent. Echocardiographic studies indicate that it may be even more common, with 10 to 15 percent of the population possibly afflicted; however, many diagnosed by echocardiography exhibit neither clinical nor angiographic evidence of the syndrome. The fact that 6 to 10 percent of asymptomatic young women have this syndrome is prima facie evidence that it is generally a benign condition. The natural history is not well established. Limited follow-up suggests that few cases progress to a severe form, and initial reports of sudden-death risk appear to have been overstated. The major importance may be the threat of endocarditis, which must be rare, and arrhythmias, which may be common.

Congenital Heart Disease

The prevalence of congenital heart disease at birth as determined during the infant's brief stay in the hospital is likely to be underestimated, and recognition of specific lesions may be inaccurate. Most data are deficient for congenital heart disease diagnosed after the first week of life. Prevalence data based on autopsy findings are unreliable because they reflect a fraction of the deaths and relate only to fatal lesions. Most information comes from retrospective studies based extensively on referral practices.

Structural abnormalities of the heart or intrathoracic great vessels seem to affect 8 to 10 of every 1000 infants born alive in the United States. About 1 newborn per 1000 live births has a cardiac birth defect which cannot be managed medically or surgically. Most infants who previously would have died now survive to adult life because of improved treatment, but 5 to 6 per 1000 live births require frequent medical or surgical attention.

Except for the recent unexplained twofold increase in ventricular septal defects and the threefold increase in patent ductus arteriosus, the incidence of most congenital heart diseases has remained stable. Rubella vaccine has reduced rubella-caused congenital heart disease, and congenital heart defects associated with Down's syndrome are less common because older women are having fewer babies. Preventive strategies are impeded by lack of knowledge of the cause of most congenital heart disease, although we have learned that alcohol, trimethadione, and lithium can cause cardiac defects. The majority of congenital heart defects may involve complex genetic-environmental interactions which remain to be elucidated.

About 72 of each 1000 live births in the United States are premature, with the infants weighing less than 2500 g. Almost half of premature infants weighing less than 1750 g will maintain patency of the ductus arteriosus, possibly because their immature lungs do not properly metabolize prostaglandins, which cause the ductus to remain open.[26] The growing number of teratogens identified appears to account for only 5 percent of all human malformations. However, single mutant genes are said to be responsible for only 3 percent of cases.[27]

In all evaluations of mortality from congenital heart disease, death in infancy predominates at 1.3 to 2.8 per 1000 live births. Later mortality is more speculative, about 0.4 per 1000 live births over the subsequent 3 years. About 25 percent of infants with congenital heart disease have a malformation incompatible with life beyond the first year; possibly half of these can be treated surgically to improve the quality of life if not to produce a cure. About 2.5 per 1000 live-born infants require specialized services for diagnosis and treatment of congenital heart disease shortly after birth, and another 2.5 per 1000 will need these resources later in childhood.

Pulmonary Thromboembolism

Estimates of mortality from pulmonary embolism vary widely, depending on the source and accuracy of data. It is probably directly responsible for 50,000 deaths annually in the United States and contributes to an equal number of deaths. It is the most common lethal pulmonary disease. If it is untreated, recurrent episodes are frequent, and more than 25 percent will be fatal. Mortality is probably underreported since more than half of cases found at autopsy were overlooked before death. More than 60 percent of fatalities occur within 1 h of onset; hence, pulmonary embolism is likely to be confused with sudden coronary death.

The incidence of pulmonary embolism is even more uncertain than is mortality. Only 10 percent of cases occur in normal persons without predisposing factors such as chronic cardiopulmonary and malignant disease, estrogen therapy, orthopedic trauma, immobilization, operative procedures, obesity, pregnancy, or blood dyscrasias. The elderly are more vulnerable.

Postoperative pulmonary emboli alone produce 4000 to 8000 deaths annually. It is a major cause of death post partum and in patients hospitalized for orthopedic conditions. Evidence from Britain suggests that the annual mortality from pulmonary embolism has been increasing for several decades despite anticoagulant drugs. More than 5 million persons over age 40 undergo major surgery each year in the United States; one or two of each 1000 will die postoperatively from pulmonary embolism. The recent advent of low-dose heparin prophylaxis may substantially reduce this risk.[28]

Preventive Implications

Examination of the incidence, prevalence, mortality, and natural history of cardiovascular disease suggests the need for a preventive approach. It is not likely that any recent innovations in diagnosis and therapy for cardiovascular disease, impressive as they have been, or any advances in the foreseeable future can have a major impact on the continuing epidemic of cardiovascular disease. Only a preventive approach involving correction of predisposing factors in advance of the overt clinical expression of the disease can be expected to make a sizable impact. When the heart or brain is infarcted, no therapy can be expected to restore full function.

Coronary heart disease often strikes without warning. One in five coronary attacks presents as sudden death, and two-thirds of the deaths occur in the community too precipitously to be brought under medical attention.

While some strokes may give warning by transient ischemic attacks, most do not. Even when they do, intervention at that stage may not necessarily greatly delay a permanently damaging stroke or prolong life.

Heart valves damaged by rheumatic heart disease and infective endocarditis can be surgically repaired or replaced by prosthetic appliances; this approach often requires anticoagulants to prevent emboli, and valve failure and hemolysis are distressingly common. Although such patients live longer, more comfortable lives than formerly, their survival does not approach that of patients with rheumatic fever kept from progressing to severe valve damage by antibiotic prophylaxis against recurrent disease.

Hypertension which progresses to target organ involvement is less manageable than if it is vigorously treated prior to such manifestations. The first sign of target organ involvement is too often a stroke, myocardial infarction, or sudden death. Half such cardiovascular catastrophes occur before evidence of organ involvement can be discovered on biennial examination.

Awaiting overt signs and symptoms of cardiovascular disease is no longer justified. In some respects, the occurrence of symptoms may be more properly regarded as a medical failure rather than as the initial indication for treatment.

A major impact on cardiovascular morbidity and mortality should derive from the practice of preventive medicine, from public health measures to alter life-style to one more favorable to cardiovascular health, and from health education to inform people of what they must do to protect their cardiovascular health.[8,29] Recent expansion and improvements have occurred in these measures, conceivably contributing significantly to the dramatic 37 percent decline in cardiovascular mortality during the past two decades, which contributed to 73 percent of the decline in overall mortality. To continue these measures would seem not only desirable but efficacious. Reliance on therapeutic measures alone is not enough.

References

1. Pasteur, L.: Address to the Fraternal Association of Former Students of the Ecole Centrale de Arts et Manufactures, Paris, May 15, 1884, in M. B. Strauss (ed.), "Familiar Medical Quotations," Little, Brown, and Company, Boston, 1968.
2. Gordon, T., and Kannel, W. B.: Premature Mortality from Coronary Heart Disease: The Framingham Study, *JAMA*, 215:1617, 1971.
3. National Center for Health Statistics: "Vital Statistics of the United States, 1978," 1983, vol. 2, pt. A.
4. National Heart, Lung, and Blood Institute: "Tenth Report of the Director, National Heart, Lung, and Blood Institute," vol. 2, "Heart and Vascular Diseases. 2. Magnitude of the Problem," Oct., 1982.
5. U.S. Department of Health and Human Services, Social Security Administration: "Characteristics of Social Security Disability Insurance Beneficiaries," SSA Publ. 13-11947, Nov. 1983.
6. National Center for Health Statistics: "Monthly Vital Statistics Report," 1983, vol. 13, no. 13.
7. Moriyama, I., Krueger, D. E., and Stamler, J.: "Cardiovascular Disease in the United States," Harvard University Press, Cambridge, 1971.
8. Kannel, W. B., and Thom, T. J.: Implications of the Recent Decline in Cardiovascular Mortality, *Cardiovasc. Med.*, 4:983, 1979.
9. Pisa, Z., and Uemura, K.: Trends of Mortality from Ischaemic Heart Disease and Other Cardiovascular Diseases in 27 Countries, 1968–1977. *World Health Statistics Quart.*, 35:11, 1982.
10. Kannel, W. B.: "The Natural History of Myocardial Infarction: The Framingham Study." Leiden University Press, Leiden, The Netherlands, 1973.
11. Margolis, J. R., Kannel, W. B., Feinleib, M., Dawber, T. R., and McNamara, P. M.: Clinical Features of Unrecognized Myocardial Infarction—Silent and Symptomatic: Eighteen Year Follow-up: The Framingham Study. *Am. J. Cardiol.*, 32:1, July 1973.
12. Kannel, W. B., Sorlie, P., and McNamara, P. M.: Prognosis after Initial Myocardial Infarction: The Framingham Study. *Am. J. Cardiol.*, 44:53, July, 1979.
13. National Center for Health Statistics: Blood Pressure Levels and Hypertension in Persons Ages 6–74 Years: United States, 1976–80, *Advance Data,* no. 84, Oct. 8, 1982.
14. Kannel, W. B., Wolf, P. A., and Dawber, T. R.: An Evaluation of the Epidemiology of Atherothrombotic Brain Infarction. *Milbank Mem. Fund Quart.*, p. 405, Fall, 1975.
15. Report of the Joint Committee for Stroke Facilities, *Stroke,* 3:351, May–June, 1972.
16. Gresham, G. E., Fitzpatrick, T. E., Wolf, P. A., McNamara, P. M., Kannel, W. B., and Dawber, T. R.: Residual Disability in Survivors of Stroke: The Framingham Study, *N. Engl. J. Med.*, 293:954, 1975.
17. McKee, P. A., Castelli, W. P., McNamara, P. M., and Kannel, W. B.: The Natural History of Congestive Heart Failure: The Framingham Study, *N. Engl. J. Med.*, 285:1441, 1974.
18. Kannel, W. B., Castelli, W. P., McNamara, P. M., McKee, P. A., and Feinleib, M.: Role of Blood Pressure in the Development of Congestive Heart Failure: The Framingham Study, *N. Engl. J. Med.*, 287:781, 1972.
19. Klainer, L. M., Gibson, T. C., and White, K. L.: The Epidemiology of Cardiac Failure, *J. Chronic Dis.* 18:797, 1965.
20. Gibson, T. C., White, K. L., and Klainer, L. M.: The Prevalence of Congestive Heart Failure in Two Rural Communities, *J. Chronic Dis.*, 19:141, 1966.
21. Bisno, A. L.: World Wide Control of Rheumatic Fever, *Ann. Intern. Med.*, 91:918, 1979. (Editorial.)
22. Elkholy, A., Rotta, J., Wannamaker, L. W., et al.: Recent Advances in Rheumatic Fever Control and Future Prospects: A World Health Organization Memorandum, *Bull. WHO* 56:887, 1978.
23. Persellin, R. H.: Acute Rheumatic Fever: Changing Manifestations, *Ann. Intern. Med.*, 89:1002, 1978. (Editorial.)
24. Procacci, P. M., Savran, S. V., Schreiter, S. L., and Bryson, A. L.: Prevalence of Clinical Mitral Valve Prolapse in 1969 Young Women, *N. Engl. J. Med.*, 294:1086, 1976.
25. Sbarbara, J. A., Mehlman, D. J., Wu, L., and Brooks, H. L.: A Prospective Study of Mitral Valvular Prolapse in Young Men, *Chest,* 75(5):555, May, 1979.
26. Department of Health, Education, and Welfare: "Proceedings of the Second Conference on the Epidemiology of Aging," DHEW Publ. 80-969, July, 1980, p. 65.
27. Michaelson, M.: "Report on a Study of Congenital Cardiovascular Malformations—Etiology, Incidence, Natural History and Organization of Diagnostic and Therapeutic Services," World Health Organization, Regional Office for Europe, May 1979.
28. Council on Thrombosis of the American Heart Association: Prevention of Venous Thromboembolism in Surgical Patients With Low Dose Heparin, *Circulation,* 55:423A, 1977.
29. Havlik, R. J., and Feinleib, M. (eds.): "Proceedings of the Conference on Decline in Coronary Heart Disease Mortality." National Institutes of Health, Washington, 1979.

35

Genetics and the Cardiovascular System

W. Jape Taylor, M.D.

If two plants which differ constantly in one or several characters be crossed, numerous experiments have demonstrated that the common characters are transmitted unchanged to the hybrids and their progeny.

G. Mendel, 1865[1]

Segregation of phenotypic characters was used by Mendel and geneticists of the next century to deduce inheritance patterns of organisms. Now the genes themselves are being analyzed. In a startling role reversal it is now possible to learn the structure of a polypeptide, which defies isolation and analysis, by first studying the deoxyribonucleic acid (DNA) which directs its production. Biologically active genes have been manufactured and inserted in bacteria to transform them into factories for the production of human insulin and other biological polypeptides.[2] The chromosomes can be sorted with great precision, and the localization of genes on specific chromosomes is proceeding at a rapid pace.[3] But mysteries still await unraveling, particularly the relation between the expressed regions (exons) and the much longer, but not directly expressed, portions (introns) of our genes.[4] One cannot help facing the future with great anticipation—and a tinge of apprehension.

New techniques of cell biology have led to the recognition of new diseases and an increased understanding of old ones. An increasing number of disorders can be diagnosed early in pregnancy. Prospects for the prevention of disease or for its amelioration with specific replacement therapy are bright. In this chapter, emphasis is placed on entities in which genetic determinants have a prominent role, particularly those for which fundamental mechanisms are known.

Congenital Heart Disease

The incidence of congenital heart disease in the industrialized societies is between 5 and 10 per 1000 live births; it is quite possibly higher if entities such as bicuspid aortic and prolapsing mitral valves are included. Numerous studies have demonstrated that the incidence of congenital cardiac lesions in the siblings of individuals with congenital heart defects approximates 2 percent, significantly higher than the expected rate.[5] When multiple cases of congenital heart disease are found in one family, they are generally identical or similar defects. The familial risk of certain types of congenital heart disease was emphasized by Nora et al., who found that when one parent has an atrial septal defect, 2.6 percent of the children have the same defect, an incidence which is 37 times the control expectancy. For ventricular septal defect, the risk was 21 times that of the population at large.[6]

Evidence from twin studies regarding the genetic contribution to congenital heart disease has been controversial. It has been pointed out that monozygotic twins are frequently not concordant for congenital heart disease, in that one member of these single-egg twins would have a cardiac anomaly and the other would be normal. Still, it is clear that concordance for congenital heart lesions is much higher in identical than in fraternal twins, supporting the concept of a significant genetic contribution to the genesis of congenital heart disease.[7] The lack of a higher rate of concordance for congenital heart disease in monozygotic twins emphasizes the importance of an interaction between genetic and environmental factors. Striking examples of this concept are monozygotic twins with Down's syndrome, clearly a disorder of primary genetic causation, who are discordant for congenital heart disease.[8]

Environmental stimuli clearly influence the manifestations of various genetic disorders after birth, and the interaction between genes and their milieu undoubtedly begins in utero. The response of experimental animals to teratogens such as alcohol, thalidomide, and various drugs varies with different genetic strains. This interplay between genetic and environmental forces is often referred to as multifactorial, a useful concept in considering potential etiologies of disorders such as congenital heart disease when only a minority of cases are due to isolated genetic or teratogenic effects.[9] However, it should not obscure the fact that in a given patient the causation may be fundamentally either genetic or environmental.

Chromosomal Aberrations

Aside from mitochondrial DNA, the entire genetic complement of mammals is packaged as nuclear DNA in chromosomes. For this reason and the fact that chromosomal aberrations produce an important minority of patients with congenital heart disease, a discussion of abnormalities related to defects of chromosomes is appropriate. Some 50,000 structural genes and a 50- to 100-fold quantity of DNA in excess, whose function is not entirely certain, are divided among the 22 pairs of autosomes and single pair of sex chromosomes. With each chromosome containing many genes, major chromosomal anomalies produce multiple defects and are often incompatible with life. Failure of both physical and mental development and defects which involve multiple organ systems are the rule with such aberrations.

The remarkable process of meiosis generally is successful in providing each ovum or sperm with 22 autosomes and either the X or Y sex chromosome so that the fertilized egg contains its full complement of 46 chromosomes. Still, chromosome mishaps appear to outnumber gene mutations by far; in a study of approximately 14,000 newborn infants, Hamerton et al. found chromosome abnormalities of varying severity in 2 percent; 0.46 percent of these were major.[10] If the 25 percent of spontaneous abortions and the 5 percent of stillbirths with chromosome defects are also considered, approximately 20 percent of fetuses bear such a problem. In the report of Hoffman and Christianson, clinically diagnosed chromosomal abnormalities were found in 0.26 percent of live births and these accounted for some 8 percent of the infants with congenital heart disease.[11]

In relation to cardiac disease, as well as historically, Down's syndrome is the most important of these disorders. In individuals with Down's syndrome, there is a very high incidence of congenital heart disease, particularly ventricular septal defect and common atrioventricular canal, as well as other complex malformations. The early development of severe pulmonary hypertension with left to right shunts or of primary pulmonary hypertension are striking features in Down's syndrome.[12] Although patients with this disease have upper airway and other respiratory problems which may contribute to the development of pulmonary hypertension, the possibility of a genetic link to pulmonary vascular reactivity exists.

Shortly after the correct chromosome constitution for human beings was determined by Tijio and Levan in 1956, Lejeune, Gautier, and Turpin found that one of the smallest of chromosomes (no. 21) was present in triplicate in a patient with Down's syndrome.[13,14] Nondisjunction of a chromosome during meiosis is the genesis of the extra chromosome in the trisomy syndromes. With this mishap, a gamete is produced which has two of the particular chromosomes while the other gamete from that meiotic division is devoid of that chromosome. In Down's syndrome, an egg containing two of chromosome 21 is fertilized by a normal sperm, resulting in a triplication of this small acrocentric chromosome. More frequent nondisjunction in the ovarian tissues of aging mothers is responsible for the increased incidence of Down's syndrome in babies born to older mothers. The precise mechanism by which such triploidy produces the clinical picture remains unknown.

Trisomy of autosomes other than 21, most notably 18 and 13, are much rarer, but with them, predictably, multiple defects of many organ systems are present, including complicated congenital heart disease. The major autosomal defects often have characteristic external abnormalities and are lethal early in life.[15]

In contrast to the widespread somatic disturbances due to major autosomal abnormalities, disordered sex chromosomes are generally not associated with such disastrous effects. Gonadal dysgenesis (Turner's syndrome) is of particular interest to the cardiologist; as a result of meiotic nondisjunction only one sex chromosome—an X—is present, giving a total complement of 45. The individual develops as a female without ovarian function and with variable webbing of the neck, hypertelorism, minor skeletal defects, and congenital heart disease. Coarctation is a frequent cardiac component of this entity, but by no means the only one.[16] Other systemic effects become apparent in older patients with Turner's syndrome, particularly hypertension and atherosclerosis.[17] Most males with the Turner phenotype have normal karyograms, although chromosomal aberrations have been described and congenital heart disease is common.[18]

Families in which Down's syndrome was present in several members of succeeding generations cannot be explained by nondisjunction. Subsequent observations indicate that one parent of some affected children has a translocation of chromosome 21 to another chromosome, most commonly 15.[19] Accordingly, this parent has only 45 chromosomes and is monosomic for chromosomes 15 and 21, so that the total genetic composition and phenotype of the carrier are normal. Half of the children will have the equivalent of trisomy 21 and will have Down's syndrome when a gamete containing the abnormal chromosome is fertilized.

The number and array of known chromosomal abnormalities have expanded greatly in the last decade because of banding stains, which permit the more accurate identification not only of the chromosomes, but of various segments of them. Deletions of portions of chromosomes, abnormal forms, mosaics, and similar defects are routinely diagnosed; with a number of these, specific syndromes, including congenital heart disease, are seen. Although routine surveys for chromosome defects of patients with congenital heart disease are not rewarding, defects of multiple organ systems should prompt chromosome analysis. Cytogenetic studies may be indicated for prenatal diagnosis and for identification of carrier states.

Recessive Inheritance of Congenital Heart Disease

Single gene defects make a minimal quantitative contribution to congenital heart disease. In an autosomal recessive disorder, an affected offspring receives the mutant gene from each heterozygous parent, who bears no overt evidence of the trait. Classically, the occurrence of multiple affected members of a single generation with normal preceding and following generations has suggested recessive inheritance. If large groups are analyzed, the mathematical ratio of one homozygous recessive person demonstrating the trait to three phenotypically normal individuals is found. However, in relatively small families, now the rule in the United States and Europe, the number of isolated cases will outnumber those with a familial cluster.

Common ancestry can increase the likelihood that recessive genes may be present in both marriage partners, and evaluation of consanguinity has been widely applied to the study of recessive inheritance. Working with the Amish people of Lancaster County, Pennsylvania, McKusick et al. detected more individuals with the Ellis–van Creveld syndrome than had been reported in the entire earlier literature.[20] From the cardiovascular viewpoint, the recessive gene—which is responsible for dwarfism, syndactyly, and chondroectodermal dysplasia—also produces a single atrium or other congenital cardiac defects.

Only the heart disease of Ellis–van Creveld syndrome and probably that of complete transposition of the viscera seem established as congenital cardiac disorders which are due to the effects of a single recessive gene. However, the higher incidence of congenital heart disease in siblings of affected patients without a striking increase in more distant kin suggests a recessive genetic trait. That recessive diseases may rarely produce infants with familial congenital heart disease via alteration of the maternal environment is strikingly illustrated in the children of phenylketonuric mothers in whom the blood levels of phenylalanine are elevated.[21]

Dominant Inheritance of Congenital Heart Disease

Because reproductive capacities of patients with the more severe cardiac anomalies were limited before the era of surgery, it seems unlikely that a dominant gene could be responsible for many such lesions. On the other hand, a defect well tolerated through early adult life, such as the secundum atrial septal defect, could have this mode of inheritance. Several kinships involving marriages between individuals with this defect and normal mates have produced atrial septal defects in approximately half of the children. Involved offspring have had at least one parent with an atrial septal defect, except in a few instances in which incomplete expression of the gene may be present (possibly a patent foramen ovale). These findings do not indicate the proportion of atrial septal defects which are the result of genetic influence, but indicate that a gene transmitted in classic autosomal dominant fashion produces this defect. In such a family the odds are virtually 50:50 that further children from the affected members will be involved, rather than the lower and much less precise estimate which is derived from studying groups of all types of congenital cardiac anomalies.[22]

Patients with congenital heart disease have a greatly increased incidence of noncardiovascular defects, whether the disease is genetic or not. The dominant inheritance of atrial septal defect and bony abnormalities of the upper extremities is often called the *Holt-Oram syndrome*. This term has been expanded to include an array of associated cardiac and upper-extremity anomalies.[23]

The dominant inheritance of supravalvular aortic stenosis was reviewed by Kahler et al.[24] In contrast with sporadic cases of supravalvular aortic stenosis, mental retardation and a readily identifiable facial appearance are not seen in the familial disorder.

The billowing, or prolapsing, mitral valve is a common lesion which is often congenital and in which a dominant genetic transmission is frequent, although many cases are sporadic.[25] The billowing valve is also seen in other disorders of genetic origin, such as Marfan's and Ehlers-Danlos syndromes and osteogenesis imperfecta.

The Cardiomyopathies

The cardiomyopathies encompass a large and diverse group of disorders; for most of them the etiology is unknown and treatment is not specific. Generally they have been classified as either primary or secondary (i.e., associated with another disease), or by clinical presentation. The best known of the latter schemes is that of Goodwin, which divides patients who present primarily with heart failure into congestive, obliterative, and restrictive groups; in another major category, hypertrophy, with or without ventricular outflow gradients, predominates.[26] I have suggested that derangements of heart muscle can be categorized as being due to abnormalities in (1) energy supply; (2) structure; or (3) activation-contraction coupling.[27] Numerous genetically determined examples of the first two divisions exist, but the third remains conjectural. Although some of these diseases are quite rare, they may provide clues for further understanding of the idiopathic cardiomyopathies.

Defective Energy Supply

The syndromes of *carnitine deficiency* are prototypes of myopathies due to energy deprivation. In concert with two transferases, carnitine facilitates the transport of fatty acids into mitochrondria; its absence deprives the heart of its dominant substrate. At least two recessively inherited causes of carnitine deficiency exist with systemic carnitine deficiency being characterized by low serum and tissue levels and the muscle carnitine deficiency by normal serum concentrations and low muscle values. A peripheral myopathy which is often lethal at an early age characterizes both disorders, but cardiac involvement may predominate. Muscle carnitine deficiency appears to be due to defective tissue uptake; systemic deficiency was originally considered to be caused by inadequate synthesis, but excessive renal losses of carnitine have recently been demonstrated.[28] Dramatic reversal of cardiomyopathy by oral administration of large quantities of carnitine has been achieved.[29]

Cardiac involvement is virtually a sine qua non for the diagnosis of Friedreich's ataxia. Since the striking clinical abnormalities are neurological rather than dystrophic, the genesis of the cardiomyopathy has been puzzling. Biochemical studies have delineated a subset of patients with Friedreich's ataxia who have a decrease in lipoamide dehydrogenase activity in cultured fibroblasts or in platelet-enriched blood.[30] Although heterogeneity of the clinical picture still exists, in these patients the disease is inherited as an autosomal recessive trait and carriers have an intermediate degree of enzyme deficiency. Lipoamide dehydrogenase is involved in the last step of pyruvate oxidation and occupies a critical role in several metabolic pathways. Although the enzyme has not been assayed in the hearts of patients with Friedreich's ataxia, a deficiency in the heart may be responsible for the cardiomyopathy. It is not clear how commonly cardiac disease is found in other hereditary ataxias.

Mitochondrial myopathies include a galaxy of fascinating myopathies with abnormal mitochondrial structure and function that have been described since Luft's classical description of a young woman with hypermetabolism without hyperthyroidism.[31] Most of these have clustered in siblings and consanguinity has been frequent, indicating autosomal recessive inheritance, but a sex-linked recessive pattern has also been described. The myopathic symptoms vary in this group, which is unified by abnormal mitochondria that are increased in number, enlarged, or bizarre in structure. The ultrastructural abnormalities can often be predicted by light microscopy because the modified trichrome stain gives a "ragged-red" appearance due to increased numbers of mitochondria and lipid deposits. These syndromes are rare, but probably more common than recognized. The heart is usually hypertrophied, sometimes with obstructive physiology, which is a common pattern of response to excess metabolic demand. Abnormal mitochrondria are as striking in cardiac tissue as in skeletal muscle.[32,33]

External ophthalmoplegia, ptosis, retinal pigmentation, and heart block constitute an unusual syndrome in which mitochondrial abnormalities are found frequently. None of the early cases were familial, and debate has ensued about the entity because individuals with the major determinants may also have varying degrees of hearing loss, pharyngeal paralysis, or mental retardation. Recently familial cases have been described, but the genetics remain unclear.[34] The reason for the common vulnerability of ophthalmic and heart muscles and the cardiac conduction system is unknown.

Predominantly maternal transmission of mitochondrial myopathy to children of both sexes led Egger and Wilson to suggest that this disorder is transmitted by mitochondrial rather than nuclear DNA.[35] The entire sequence of human mitochondrial genes, which code for metabolic enzymes, is known and the predominant contribution of the maternal line to the overall energetics of the organism is fascinating to contemplate.

Structural Abnormalities of the Heart

Hypertrophic Obstructive Cardiomyopathy

Hypertrophic obstructive cardiomyopathy is an entity with distinctive gross and ultrastructural morphology. Angina, syncope, and sudden death are the dominant symptoms; when these are combined with a loud systolic murmur and left ventricular hypertrophy, aortic stenosis is mimicked. The genetics of this disorder make it immediately suspected in any patient with apparent aortic stenosis and a dominant history of cardiac disease. Although a familial incidence was emphasized in some early reports, in others isolated cases appeared to be common, leading to the designation of idiopathic hypertrophic subaortic stenosis.[36] Brock, who first recognized obstructive cardiomyopathy, suggested that it might develop secondary to hypertension.[37] Debate about its being an acquired or heritable disorder was largely laid to rest by echocardiographic evidence indicating autosomal dominant transmission. Asymmetrical septal hypertrophy was found in almost 50 percent of first degree relatives, although many had no clinical evidence of disease.[38] A broader spectrum of the disorder is now recognized; within the same family some members may present with a nonobstructive hypertrophic cardiomyopathy while others have the typical obstructive findings.

The gross pathology of this entity, with its massive ventricular hypertrophy and, disproportionately, hypertrophy of the septum is quite distinctive (Fig. 35-1). The ultrastructural architecture of the outflow tract has extreme muscle-cell and myofibrillar disorganization, so that some myofibrils are perpendicular to the long axes of cells or may insert into the Z bands of contiguous myofibrils.[39] This arrangement suggests that the genetic defect involves an autosomal dominant gene which regulates the organization of embryonic heart cells.

Infiltrative Cardiomyopathy

A variety of genetically determined diseases result in myocardial deposits which greatly alter the structure and function of the heart. In many of these, cardiovascular involvement is diffuse with depositions in blood vessels, heart valves, and even pericardium, but myocardial involvement often predominates. It is recognized that the abnormal morphology may be accompanied by metabolic derangements, but it is considered that structural changes are more important in this group. The cardiac presentation is usually heart failure, but rhythm disturbances are common also.

In *systemic amyloidosis,* aggregates of immunoglob-

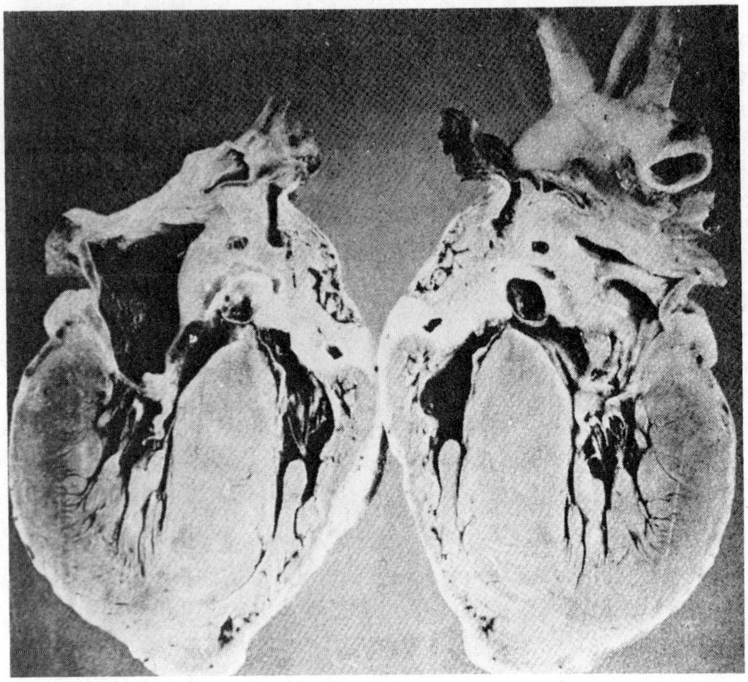

FIGURE 35-1 The extreme hypertrophy of the interventricular septum and the bulk of the entire heart with mild deformity of the mitral valve characterize muscular subaortic stenosis. Angina had been alleviated by propranolol in this 32-year-old man who died abruptly.

ulin chains encase myocardial fibers, thereby reducing contractility and, if extensive enough, producing restriction of ventricular filling. Many types of autosomal dominant amyloidosis occur and cardiac involvement is usual; in some families, it dominates the clinical picture.[40] Generally neuropathic, renal, or ophthalmologic disturbances, in varying combinations, are cardinal features of the inherited amyloidoses.[41] A rare arrhythmia, atrial standstill, has also been produced by infiltration with amyloid.[42]

In phytanic acid storage disease, unlike in amyloidosis, the accumulation of an exogenous compound of dietary origin is due to a deficiency of the required α-hydroxylase. This autosomal recessive disease is seen primarily in individuals of Norwegian ancestry and is characterized by retinitis pigmentosa, peripheral neuropathy, and cerebellar ataxia, but cardiac enlargement, conduction delays and arrhythmias are common. Exclusion from the diet of vegetables which contain phytol and phytanic acid attenuates the progression of this disease.[43]

In type II glycogen storage disease (Pompe's disease), heart failure is a common cause of death in infancy, although myopathic symptoms usually precede cardiac ones. Pathological effects are produced primarily by accumulation of massive amounts of glycogen, although a component of energy deprivation may be present as well. The cardiomyopathy is hypertrophic, with striking electrocardiographic evidence of this, and occasionally an obstructive hemodynamic picture.[44] Deficiency of acid α-1,4-glucosidase (acid maltase) is responsible for this lethal disease of early life. Pompe's disease is inherited as an autosomal recessive trait, and partial enzyme deficiency can be demonstrated in heterozygotes and in amniotic-fluid cells. Less severe varieties of acid maltase deficiency become symptomatic later in life and may be due to ineffective enzyme variants or a mutation affecting the rate of production or degradation of the enzyme. Cardiac involvement in the other enzymatic defects of glycogen metabolism is not as prominent, but an ineffective debrancher enzyme, amylo-1,6-glucosidase, results in deposition of large quantities of an abnormal glycogen in the liver and heart, producing hepatomegaly and a cardiomyopathy. This type III glycogenesis is an autosomal recessive disorder with an increased incidence in Jewish immigrants from North Africa to Israel.[45] Peripheral muscle phosphorylase deficiency (McArdle's disease, type IV glycogenesis) does not produce cardiac disease because of separate cardiac phosphorylases. A fatal infantile form of myophosphorylase deficiency has been described; electrophoresis revealed that two of the usual three cardiac enzymes were missing.[46]

In *hemochromatosis,* or iron storage disease, a genetically determined disorder of variable expression, myocardial iron deposits lead to cardiac fibrosis and congestive failure. Serum iron levels and liver biopsies can detect asymptomatic individuals with increased iron stores. Transmission of abnormal iron metabolism through multiple generations has been studied in conjunction with specific HLA (human histocompatibility leukocyte antigen) linkage to indicate recessive inheritance with partial expression in heterozygotes.[47]

Inflammatory Cardiomyopathies

The myocarditis of *Lyme disease* makes a meager quantitative contribution to inflammatory heart disease but illuminates some aspects of genetically determined host interactions with a specific infectious vector. Lyme disease is an acute illness caused by a spirochete which is harbored by ixodid ticks.[48] A delayed immune-mediated carditis follows the acute illness in a small percentage of patients, primarily those with the alloantigen DRw_2.

No clear-cut genetic marker for *rheumatic fever* has been identified.

In *systemic lupus erythematosus* both vertical and horizontal grouping with families have been reported, and concordance is high in identical twins.[49] Some heritable defects in the complement system are also associated with lupus erythematosus, additionally suggesting a strong genetic contribution. Impaired suppressor-cell function occurs in first degree relatives of individuals with lupus erythematosus as well as the patients themselves.[50] An association of specific HLA type with lupus erythematosus has been noted, as well as a perplexing increase in antinuclear antibodies in both relatives and household contacts of individuals with this disease.[51] The development of active lupus erythematosus appears to require an environmental agent acting on a genetically prepared host.

Transmission of *endocardial fibroelastosis* from generation to generation has been reported infrequently, but multiple occurrences in siblings and concordance in monozygotic twins is evidence for a recessive inheritance in some families. The disorder is more than 700 times as common in the siblings of affected patients as in the public at large.[52] Fibroelastosis, usually combined with complete heart block, has been reported in the children of mothers with systemic lupus erythematosus and may be familial.[53] This is a clear warning that *familial* and *genetic* are not synonymous terms.

Tuberous sclerosis is characterized by malformations of the brain which result in mental deficiency and epilepsy. It is associated with rhabdomyomas of the myocardium. Adenoma sebaceum of the skin leads to its recognition early in life. The gene for tuberous sclerosis may have a relatively high mutation rate since the reproductive capacity of affected patients is reduced, which, in the absence of new mutations, should lead to its extinction.

Muscular Dystrophies

As information has accumulated about the peripheral muscular dystrophies, it has become apparent that cardiomyopathy is a feature of virtually all of them although their clinical manifestations and age of onset are variable. Neither the precise biochemical defect nor the site of primary cellular abnormality is known. A variety of membrane and intracellular biochemical abnormalities has been described but it is uncertain if these are primary or secondary. Evidence for a structural defect (other than cell necrosis and fibrosis), inadequate energy supply, or deficient activation-contraction coupling is lacking, although the association with certain types of arrhythmias suggests the latter possibility—at least in some of them. A variety of animal models with both peripheral and cardiac dystrophies is the subject of extensive research.[27]

X-Linked Muscular Dystrophies The Duchenne type of muscular dystrophy is the most common of this group; it is characterized by early age of onset, rapid progression, pseudohypertrophy, elevated levels of serum creatine kinase (CK), and late occurrence of heart failure. It is a sex-linked recessive trait, and is transmitted to males by apparently healthy mothers. The phenotypically normal female carries the abnormal gene on one X chromosome but does not manifest the disease because of the normal gene on the other X chromosome. One-half of her male progeny receive the X chromosome bearing the abnormal gene and develop the disorder, since their only other sex chromosome is a Y; the remaining male offspring are normal genetically and phenotypically. Half of the daughters of heterozygous females are also carriers, and many can be detected by mild elevations in serum CK levels.

Milder sex-linked recessive types of muscular dystrophy of a later age of onset and slower progression are sometimes referred to as the Becker type of dystrophy. Linkage data indicate that the Becker gene is near the glucose-6-phosphate dehydrogenase (G6PD): deutan color-blindness cluster, while the Duchenne gene is not, indicating that the two genes are not alleles and the diseases are separate.[54] More than one type of benign X-linked dystrophy exists, but the cardiac findings, usually subclinical, have not been clearly defined; rarely, severe heart failure is seen relatively early.

Myotonia Dystrophica This is an autosomal dominant disorder with appearance in both sexes and transmission through consecutive generations, since the onset of symptoms is relatively late. Cataracts, testicular atrophy, baldness, and varying degrees of mental retardation combine with involvement of skeletal and cardiac muscle as symptoms of this disease. Variation in age of onset suggests considerable genetic heterogenicity, but no biochemical markers or linked traits permit clear distinction of subgroups, and cardiac involvement has been common in all types.[55] Rarely, patients with myotonia dystrophica die of heart failure, but electrocardiographic abnormalities are more usual, with a high incidence of atrioventricular and bundle branch conduction delays.

X-Linked Recessive Disorder In one X-linked recessive neuromuscular disorder, proximal upper extremity and distal leg involvement dominate the skeletal muscle symptoms, while arrhythmias, including arrest and sudden death, characterize the cardiac presentation.[56] In both peripheral muscle and heart, electrophysiological studies demonstrated a defect in electromechanical coupling. This may lead to persistent atrial standstill, sometimes preceded by atrial fibrillation or atrioventricular (AV) conduction delays.

Miscellaneous The peroneal muscular atrophies have a variable inheritance and clinical picture, but arrhythmias, including atrial standstill and third degree AV block, are common. In the Kugelberg-Welander syndrome (juvenile progressive muscular atrophy), some cases are probably autosomal recessive disorders.[57]

Systemic Diseases with Diffuse Cardiovascular Involvement

Mucopolysaccharidoses

The mucopolysaccharidoses constitute a large and diverse group of disorders relative to inheritance, age of symptomatic onset, and severity, but are unified by their underlying pathogenesis and sites of organ involvement.[58] Since they are due to deficiencies in the degradative lysosomal enzymes which catalyze dermatan sulfate and heparin sulfate (keratan sulfate in type IV), mucopolysacchariduria and widespread involvement of connective tissue cells and the musculoskeletal, cardiovascular, and central nervous systems are predictable.

Valvular and myocardial disease are characteristic in patients with *Hurler's syndrome* (Fig. 35-2). Increased consanguinity and involvement of multiple siblings of both sexes from normal parents provide the typical features of autosomal recessive inheritance, now proved by biochemical studies on the obligatory heterozygous carriers. This disorder is due to an α-L-iduronidase deficiency; this is also defective in the much less severe Scheie's syndrome, in which intelligence is normal and life span is preserved. In both syndromes the same diffusible factor corrects the abnormal accumulation of mucopolysaccharides in cultured fibroblasts, indicating that Hurler's and Scheie's syndromes are due to mutations at the same gene locus.

FIGURE 35-2 The dwarfism, facial features, and bodily configuration of this child are characteristic of Hurler's syndrome, a heritable disease of mucopolysaccharide metabolism. (*Courtesy of Dr. L. J. Krovetz.*)

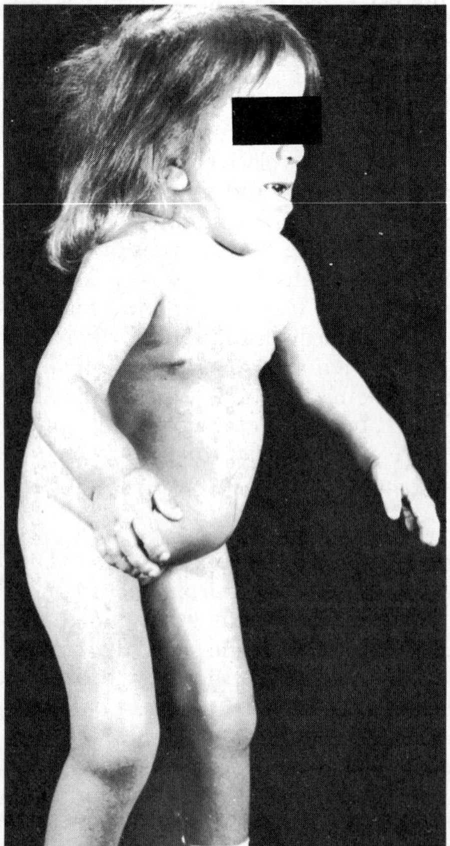

The severity of the cardiovascular manifestations parallels that of the generalized disease. Mucopolysaccharide accumulation may produce cardiac failure early in Hurler's syndrome, while more indolent valvular disease, most commonly aortic, is found in the less severe syndromes.

The use of cell cultures has permitted identification of enzyme defects in at least 12 distinct entities, most of which are autosomal recessive defects; two, including the classic Hurler's syndrome, are X-linked mutants. Although effective enzyme replacement therapy is not available, intrauterine diagnosis with cultured amniotic fluid cells is now routine. Heterozygote detection is feasible with the use of enzyme detection in various tissues, including hair roots.[59]

Mucolipidoses

The phenotypic expressions of the mucolipidoses resemble those of the mucopolysaccharidoses, leading to considerable confusion before biochemical differences were defined. Only type II (formerly called I-cell disease because of inclusions in cultured fibroblasts) and type III are properly classified as mucolipidoses. Both myocardial and valvular tissues are infiltrated in these autosomal recessive diseases. They differ from other lysosomal storage diseases in that only a modest deficiency of lysosomal hydrolases is found in cultured fibroblasts, while these enzymes are greatly increased in body fluids. It has been suggested that the defect is in packaging of the enzymes into lysosomes, perhaps because of a defect in a recognition site on the hydrolase.[60]

Fabry's Disease

Angiokeratoma corporis diffusum (Fabry's disease) is a rare sex-linked recessive disorder in which deficiency of α-galactosidase leads to deposition of glycolipids in blood vessels, heart muscle, and other viscera.[61] Cardiac failure, hypertension, and angina are seen. Carrier females may have evidence of less severe clinical disease.

Glycoproteinoses

Cardiovascular manifestations have not been as clearly defined in the enzyme deficiencies which lead to defective catabolism of glycoproteins. Lysosomal storage of the compounds is diffuse, and cardiovascular involvement will undoubtedly be found in some of them as biochemical definition permits more accurate diagnosis.[58]

Gaucher's Disease

Gaucher's disease was the first heritable disorder in which an attempt was made to administer the deficient enzyme.[62] Constrictive pericarditis and severe pulmonary hypertension may accompany the recessively inherited deficiency of glucocerebrosidase.

Mulibrey Nanism

Myocardial fibrosis, pericardial constriction accompanied by calcification, in the context of multiple organ pathology is inherited in an autosomal fashion.[63] Mulibrey nanism was the name devised to indicate involvement of *mu*scle, *li*ver, *br*ain and *ey*e. To date, this entity has been described only in Finland, and it may be quite isolated in its occurrence.

Connective Tissue Disorders

Research into the biochemical structure of connective tissue has confirmed the heterogeneity of Ehlers-Danlos syndrome, Marfan's syndrome, and osteogenesis imperfecta. Ehlers-Danlos syndrome has at least seven variants, with differing skin fragility, joint hypermobility, and visceral involvement. Specific enzyme deficiencies have been demonstrated in three variants, while type III collagen is deficient in the threatening Sack variety, which leads to rupture of major arteries.[64] The latter is usually inherited as a dominant disease, while sex-linked or autosomal recessive modes are found in other variants.

Aortic dilatation and dissecting aneurysm are dominant cardiac features of *Marfan's syndrome* (Fig. 35-3). Although the severity of expression varies, a pattern of dominant inheritance is usual.

The cardiovascular manifestations in osteogenesis imperfecta include a billowing mitral valve and aortic dilatation; this is also a heterogeneous group.[65]

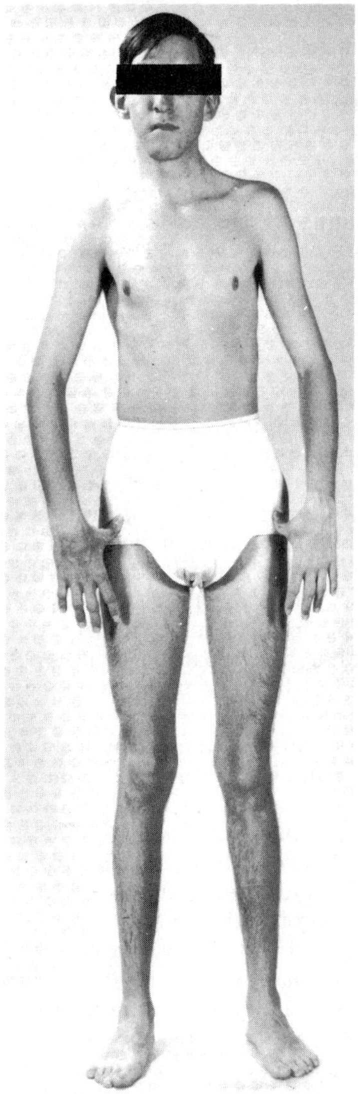

FIGURE 35-3 Absence of subcutaneous tissue, frail musculature, and scoliosis in this young man with aortic insufficiency and a cleft palate are hallmarks of Marfan's syndrome.

Vascular Disorders

Atherosclerosis

Persuasive evidence from studies of relatives of index patients with coronary artery disease confirms the clinical impression that it is a familial disorder. Slack and Evans reported that the incidence of coronary atherosclerosis in first degree relatives of women who died of the disease before the age of 65 years was seven times that of the population at large.[66] The male relatives of men who died of coronary disease under the age of 55 years had a fivefold higher risk, and female relatives had an increased risk of over twofold. Similarly, twin studies have implicated heredity in susceptibility to atherosclerosis. Knowledge of the structure of the carrier apoproteins and the membrane receptors which interact in the regulation of lipid transport and metabolism has expanded greatly in recent years, giving promise of greater understanding of the genetic-environmental interactions of this multifactorial disease.

The Arterial Wall

Many factors which contribute to the development of atherosclerosis are subject to genetic variability. Increased susceptibility of the arterial wall is one factor which has been difficult to study and is considered significant only in rare disorders such as pseudoxanthoma elasticum, an autosomal dominant disease, and Werner's syndrome;[67] premature atherosclerosis and valve calcification with balding, cataracts, and atrophy of the skin produce a picture of precocious senility in this latter recessive disorder.

Some data suggest that atherosclerotic plaques have a monoclonal origin.[68] Electrophoretic variants of G6PD are common in blacks, and random inactivation of either X chromosome in a given cell (Lyon hypothesis) produces black women who are mosaics for this enzyme. Plaques from women heterozygous for G6PD were reported to contain only one enzyme type, suggesting that mutational events produced these monoclonal lesions. This concept has been challenged by workers who demonstrated that a higher number of samples from aortic plaques reveals increasingly more with both G6PD variants.[69] Monotypism for G6PD in some plaques was considered due to differences in growth potential.

Hyperlipidemia

Familial hyperlipidemia is discussed in Chapter 42.

The otherwise insoluble lipids are linked to eight or more distinct apoproteins to facilitate their transport in blood.[70] Specific receptors, which bind the lipoproteins, augment the transfer of lipids into cells, thereby modulating the production or degradation of intracellular cholesterol.[71] The structures of the low-density-lipoprotein (LDL) receptor, a glycoprotein, and of some of the apoproteins have been defined to a degree. As anticipated, pathological structural variants of some of these proteins have been defined.

Familial hypercholesterolemia (type II hyperlipoproteinemia) is a group of closely related dominant disorders which, in the usual heterozygous individual, produce a serum cholesterol level of 350 to 450 mg/dl, normal triglyceride levels, corneal arcus, tuberous and tendinous xanthoma, and accelerated atherosclerosis. Homozygotic children, sometimes produced by consanguineous parents, exhibit extreme hypercholesterolemia (600 to 1000 mg/dl); death from vascular involvement is common in the first and second decades of life. The primary structure of the high-affinity receptors which bind LDL is abnormal—and functionally absent—in these extremely hypercholesterolemic individuals. Without functional LDL receptors, transfer of LDL into cells is deficient, leading to a lack of catabolism in the liver and continuing cholesterol synthesis in other cells.

Familial hypercholesterolemia is not the homogeneous entity which it once appeared to be. Individuals with a less marked deficiency of LDL binding are known, as well as an intriguing variant in which LDL binding is normal but transfer of LDL cholesterol into the cells is impaired. The genes for LDL binding and internalization are alleles, suggesting that the LDL receptor is a bifunctional molecule with at least two active sites.[72] A mutation in the β-apoprotein of LDL has been suggested as another etiology of familial hypercholesterolemia because of the finding that LDL from a hypercholesterolemic father and daughter did not suppress 3-hydroxy-3-methylglutaryl coenzyme A reductase (HMG-CoA reductase) activity in either their own or normal leukocytes.[70]

The Watanabe rabbit is a strain of LDL-receptor-deficient animals which mimic very precisely the anatomic and biochemical features of familial hypercholesterolemia.[73] This animal model confirms that endogenous hypercholesterolemia per se is a sufficient cause of florid atherosclerosis. In addition to the genetic determinants of LDL binding in man and rabbit, environmental factors may alter receptor number or affinity. Further exploration of these genetic-environmental interactions should lead to more effective regulation of cholesterol metabolism.

Familial dysbetalipoproteinemia (type III HLP) is characterized by elevated cholesterol and triglyceride levels, which are unusually responsive to dietary manipulations, and a broad (electrophoretically) or floating (ultracentrifugally) β-lipoproteinemia; plantar xanthoma and premature atherosclerosis are the usual clinical manifestations. Deficient clearance of very low density lipoprotein (VLDL) remnants is the cause of the elevated lipid levels. Like familial hypercholesterolemia, it is of special interest because of the insights it provides regarding lipoprotein regulation. Apoproteins E (apo E) are the major apoprotein determinants of this lipoprotein class and are determined by three alleles at a single gene locus.[74] The type III phenotype is most commonly due to homozygosity of the ϵ2 allele. Another mechanism for the production of the type III phenotype was detected in a family in which no apo E could be found, indicating that apo E is critical to the degradation of chylomicron remnants.[75]

High levels of high-density lipoproteins (HDL) and the HDL/LDL ratio are negatively related to atherosclerosis. Serum concentrations of HDL are to a degree regulated by genetic factors with an increased level segregating in an autosomal dominant fashion in some families. Higher HDL levels are found in American blacks than whites and may contribute to the lesser susceptibility of blacks to atherosclerosis despite a high incidence of hypertension.[76]

Studies of a family from Tangier Island in Chesapeake Bay, in which two children had marked hypocholesterolemia and deposition of lipids in reticuloendothelial tissues, led to the definition of familial α-lipoprotein deficiency;[77] the major apoprotein of HDL is the apo A-I, which appears to be important in the transport of cholesterol from tissues, so that it is logical that atherosclerosis is a component of a deficiency state. The primary structure of apo A-I, which is also a cofactor for the esterification of cholesterol by lecithin-cholesterol-acetyltransferase (LCAT) is known, and it has been shown that its production is normal in Tangier's disease, so that a posttranslational event is responsible for its afunctionality.[78] The actual DNA clone which codes for apo A-I has been isolated.

Other familial lipid abnormalities are more frequent than hypercholesterolemias, which have a heterozygote frequency of 0.1 to 0.2 percent.[79] In relatives of survivors of myocardial infarction, the most common familial hyperlipidemia was an entity in which serum cholesterol and triglycerides were elevated individually or together;[80] this was termed *combined hyperlipidemia* and is considered to be the result of a single dominant gene effect. The lipoprotein phenotypes in this disorder can be either IIa, IIb, or IV, and precise characterization of a lipid disorder requires family studies.

Familial hypertriglyceridemia is an autosomal dominant trait with a frequency between that of familial hypercholesterolemia and combined hyperlipidemia.[80] By electrophoretic classification, most of these individuals would be classified as type IV hyperlipoproteinemia.

Antigenic polymorphisms have evolved among the lipoproteins, and two separate systems, the Ag and Lp, have been described in human beings. Increased vascular disease with specific alleles in each system has been reported.[81]

Other rare abnormalities of lipid metabolism associated with an atherogenic diathesis include familial lecithin: α-cholesterol acetyl-transferase deficiency, cerebrotendinous xanthomatosis, β-sitosterolemia and xanthomatosis, Wolman's disease, and cholesterol ester storage disease.

Many individuals with elevation of serum lipid concentrations cannot be fitted into one of the single-gene disorders of lipid metabolism. In general population studies, a marked resemblance of cholesterol values within family groups is found, particularly for siblings below 16 or above 40 years of age.[82]

Diabetes Mellitus

Diabetes mellitus is one of the major genetic determinants of atherosclerosis. Although a familial predisposition to diabetes mellitus was noted early, a melding of classic genetic approaches and new immunochemistry has been required for more precise interpretations of the genetics of the disease.[83,84]

Twin studies have confirmed genetic heterogeneity in diabetes; virtually all identical-twin pairs are concordant for adult-onset insulin-insensitive diabetes, whereas only half of the juvenile insulin-dependent twins are both diabetics.

HLA antigens have provided a powerful tool for the study of genetic segregation in diabetes. No linkage is present between HLA-type and non-insulin-dependent diabetes, but juvenile insulin-dependent diabetes is related to specific HLA phenotypes. The current consensus is that a gene (or genes) closely associated with the HLA-DRw3 and HLA-DRw4 genes conveys increased susceptibility to viruses which, directly or through autoimmune responses, destroy the beta cells of the pancreatic islets and produce insulin-dependent diabetes.[84] Recent studies in monozygotic twins have demonstrated that islet cell antibodies and progressive beta-cell dysfunction may precede clinical diabetes for an extended period.[85] Debate continues as to whether more than one gene locus is involved and, assuming a single gene site, if it transmits diabetes in a dominant or recessive manner. An examination of the incidence of diabetes in American blacks, a racial outcross between Africans with no insulin-dependent diabetes and Caucasians, in which the disease is prevalent, reveals that the incidence of diabetes is comparable to the degree of genetic admixture, indicating a dominant inheritance.[86] About 20 percent of the American black gene pool (including the HLA diabetes-associated genes) is of Caucasian origin, and if a single recessive gene were responsible for diabetes, the frequency in American blacks should be approximately one-twenty-fifth $[(\frac{1}{5})^2]$ of the white incidence. An alternative proposal is that two susceptibility alleles interact with a normal gene in a codominant fashion.[87]

Non-insulin-dependent diabetes is heterogeneous. In some families a dominant inheritance is suggested by pedigree analysis. In one such family the secretion of an abnormal insulin was identified by direct structural analysis of the insulin and of the insulin gene.[88] It has also been suggested that a restriction fragment polymorphism adjacent to the insulin gene on chromosome 11 may serve as a genetic marker for non-insulin-dependent diabetes.[89] Evidence has been presented that a specific allele in the polymorphic region adjacent to the insulin gene may also confer a 2.5-fold risk for the development of atherosclerosis, even in nondiabetics.[90] Recessive inheritance of non-insulin-dependent diabetes may be related to an abnormal insulin release in some families.[91]

Systemic Hypertension

The arterial blood pressure is regulated by a host of interacting neural and humoral elements, some of which have pressor and others depressor effects. These various agents and their receptors are under genetic control but are modifiable by various stimuli; this multifactorial regulation results in a unimodel distribution of blood pressure in population surveys. However, in experimental animals hypertensive and normotensive strains have been produced by only a few generations of selective breeding, indicating that only a few, possibly linked, gene loci are of major import in producing hypertension.[92]

A familial clustering of blood pressure levels is found in population surveys, and the hypertension-prone individual can be identified quite early in life.[93] Aggregation of blood pressure in siblings and a high concordance rate for identical twins are well known. Ethnic differences in frequency and severity of hypertension have been recognized for many years. Comparisons of the renal responsiveness to sodium loading and of plasma renin levels of black and white subjects demonstrate more sodium retention in blacks, which may relate to their increased incidence of hypertension.[94] The ethnic susceptibility, the familial clustering of blood pressure, and the twin studies all support a significant influence of genetic factors in the production of hypertension.

In uncommon forms of hypertension, single-gene

influences have been recognized. Pheochromocytoma may occur in association with neurofibromatosis, a disorder with well-known genetic transmission. More commonly familial pheochromocytoma, which may account for 10 percent of the total, is a component of the multiple endocrine tumor syndrome and carcinoma of the thyroid.[95] Hypertension is also present in the rarest of adrenogenital syndromes, an enzymatic defect in 11-hydroxylation of the steroid molecule, inherited as an autosomal recessive characteristic.[96]

Pulmonary Hypertension

Generally, hypertension in the lesser circulation is secondary to elevations of pulmonary venous pressure, left-to-right shunts, or alterations in the vascular bed due to intrinsic lung disease. However, the rise in pulmonary vascular resistance which causes this pulmonary hypertension is not uniform from individual to individual in response to apparently identical stimuli. A genetic basis for primary pulmonary hypertension, which develops without a known stimulus, suggests that the response to an abnormal load may be governed, in part, by inheritance. This infrequent illness is familial in about one-third of cases; autosomal dominant inheritance is suggested.[97]

Pulmonary hypertension is seen in a variety of inherited diseases including cystic fibrosis, α_1-antitrypsin deficiency, Gaucher's disease, and tuberous sclerosis (Fig. 35-4). With the exception of the latter dominant illness, these are all autosomal recessive diseases.

Arrhythmias

The presence of conduction disturbances in multiple members of certain families indicates a genetic basis. Usually autosomal dominant transmission is present, although the age of onset of complete heart block varies from intrauterine to midadult life.[98] Advanced AV block is often preceded by sinus bradycardia and varying degrees of fascicular block. Familial congenital heart block is not as benign as isolated congenital heart block.[99] In a few families conspicuous freckling has been noted as an associated hallmark.

Multiple siblings with heart block in infancy have been reported in a pattern which suggests an autosomal recessive inheritance. However, in some cases the mother had systemic lupus erythematosus; a variety of tissue antibodies can cross the placenta and damage the fetal conduction system and also produce other cardiac anomalies.[53]

Familial tachycardias have been noted less frequently, but Gould reported a five-generation pedigree with 22 members in whom atrial fibrillation without other evidence of heart disease was well tolerated.[100] A similar suggestion of dominant inheritance of nodal rhythm has been made.[101] The preexcitation (Wolff-Parkinson-White) syndrome may

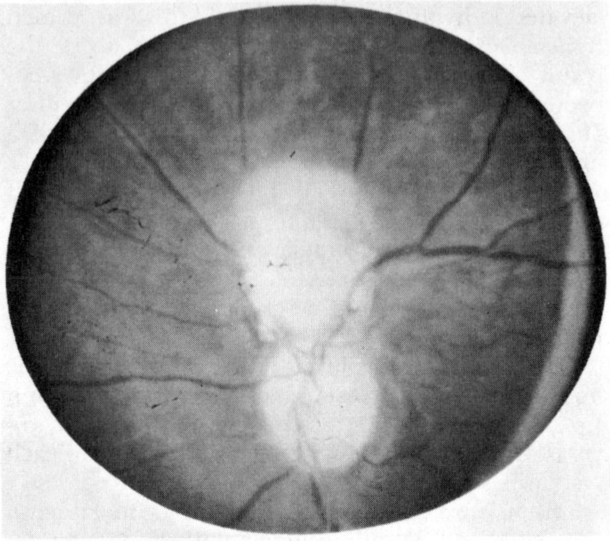

A

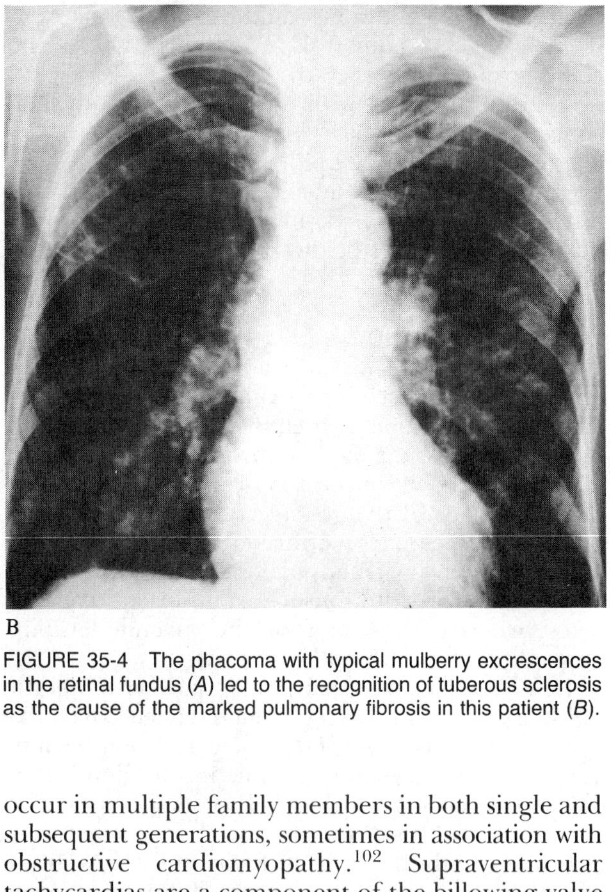

B

FIGURE 35-4 The phacoma with typical mulberry excrescences in the retinal fundus (*A*) led to the recognition of tuberous sclerosis as the cause of the marked pulmonary fibrosis in this patient (*B*).

occur in multiple family members in both single and subsequent generations, sometimes in association with obstructive cardiomyopathy.[102] Supraventricular tachycardias are a component of the billowing valve syndrome, sometimes inherited in an autosomal dominant fashion.

Prolongation of the QT interval of the electrocardiogram was described by Jervell and Lange-Neilsen as a part of a syndrome with recessive inheritance.[103] Congenital deafness and sudden death are other features; other investigators have reported dominant inheritance of QT interval prolongation without deafness.[104] The same ominous clinical implications are present in both syndromes.

Familial sudden death with minimal physical or psychic stimulation was described in apparently healthy teenaged siblings; unexpected death, often heralded by fainting episodes, appeared due to an autosomal dominant gene. Defects in the AV node and bundle were present, but no electrocardiographic or other clinical evidences of cardiac diseases were noted.[105]

References

1. Mendel, G.: Experiment in Plant Hybridization, *Proceedings of the Natural History Society of Brunn,* 1865 (English translation).
2. Riggs, A. D., and Itakura, K.: Synthetic DNA and Medicine, *Am. J. Hum. Genet.,* 31:531, 1979.
3. McKusick, V. A.: The Human Genome through the Eyes of a Clinical Geneticist, *Cytogenet. Cell Genet.,* 32:7, 1982.
4. Gilbert, W.: DNA Sequencing and Gene Structure, *Science,* 214:1305, 1981.
5. Anderson, R. C.: Fetal and Infant Death, Twinning and Cardiac Malformations in Families of 2,000 Children with and 500 without Cardiac Defects, *Am. J. Cardiol.,* 38:218, 1976.
6. Nora, J. J., Dodd, P. F., McNamara, D. G., Hattwick, M. A. W., Leachman, R. D., and Cooley, D. A.: Risk to Offspring of Parents with Congenital Heart Defects, *JAMA,* 209:2052, 1969.
7. Anderson, R. S.: Congenital Cardiac Malformations in 109 Sets of Twins and Triplets, *Am. J. Cardiol.,* 39:1045, 1977.
8. Telfer, M. A., Baker, D., and Bergman, M.: Twins, Probably Monozygotic, Displaying Down's Syndrome, Physical and Functional Mirror-Imaging, and Discordance for Congenital Heart Disease, *Am. J. Ment. Defic.,* 76:391, 1972.
9. Nora, J. J., and Nora, A. H.: Genetic Epidemiology of Congenital Heart Diseases, in A. G. Steinberg, A. G. Bearn, A. G. Motulsky, and B. Childs (eds.), "Progress in Medical Genetics. Genetics of Cardiovascular Disease," W. B. Saunders Company, Philadelphia, 1983, vol. 5, p. 91.
10. Hamerton, J. L., Canning, N., Ray, M., and Smith, S.: A Cytogenetic Survey of 14,069 Newborn Infants: I. Incidence of Chromosome Abnormalities, *Clin. Genet.* 8:223, 1975.
11. Hoffman, J. I. E., and Christianson, R.: Congenital Heart Disease In a Cohort of 19,502 Births with Long-Term Follow-up, *Am. J. Cardiol.,* 42:641, 1978.
12. Laursen, H. B.: Congenital Heart Disease in Down's Syndrome, *Br. Heart J.,* 38:32, 1976.
13. Tijio, J. H., and Levan, A.: The Chromosome Number of Man, *Hereditas,* 42:1, 1956.
14. Lejeune, J., Gautier, M., and Turpin, R.: Etude des Chromosomes Somatiques de Neuf Enfants Mongoliens, *Acad. Sci.,* 248:1721, 1959.
15. Gorlin, R. J.: Classical Chromosome Disorders, in J. J. Yunis (ed.), "New Chromosomal Syndromes," Academic Press, New York, 1977, p. 59.
16. Nora, J. J., Torres, A. K., Sinha, A. K., and McNamara, D. G.: Characteristic Cardiovascular Anomalies of XO Turner Syndrome, XX and XY Phenotype and XO/XX Turner Mosaic, *Am. J. Cardiol.,* 25:639, 1970.
17. Engle, E., and Forbes, A. P.: Cytogenetic and Clinical Findings in 48 Patients with Congenitally Defective or Absent Ovaries, *Medicine,* 44:135, 1965.
18. Chaves-Carballo, E., and Hayles, A. B.: Ullrich-Turner Syndrome in the Male, *Mayo Clin. Proc.,* 41:843, 1966.
19. Carter, C. O., Hamerton, J. L., Polani, P. E., Gunalp, A., and Weller, S. D. W.: Chromosome Translocation as a Cause of Familial Mongolism, *Lancet,* 2:679, 1970.
20. McKusick, V. A., Egeland, J. A., Eldridge, R., and Krusen, D. E.: Dwarfism in the Amish: I. The Ellis–van Creveld Syndrome, *Bull. Johns Hopkins Hosp.,* 115:306, 1964.
21. Lenke, R. R., and Levy, H. L.: Maternal Phenylketonuria and Hyperphenylalaninemia. An International Survey of the Outcome of Untreated and Treated Pregnancies, *N. Engl. J. Med.,* 303:1202, 1980.
22. Lynch, H. T., Bachenberg, K., Harris, R. E., and Becker, W.: Hereditary Atrial Septal Defect. Update of a Large Kindred, *Am. J. Dis. Child.,* 132:600, 1978.
23. Kaufman, R. L., Rimoin, D. L., McAlister, W. H., and Hartmann, A. F.: Variable Expression of the Holt-Oram Syndrome, *Am. J. Dis. Child.,* 127:21, 1974.
24. Kahler, R. L., Braunwald, E., Plauth, W. H., Jr., and Morrow, A. G.: Familial Congenital Heart Disease: Familial Occurrence of Atrial Septal Defect with A-V Conduction Abnormalities; Supravalvular Aortic and Pulmonic Stenosis; and Ventricular Septal Defect, *Am. J. Med.,* 40:384, 1966.
25. Shell, W. E., Walton, J. A., Clifford, M. E., and Willis, P. W.: The Familial Occurrences of the Syndrome of Mid-Late Systolic Click and Late Systolic Murmur, *Circulation,* 39:327, 1969.
26. Goodwin, J. F.: The Congestive and Hypertrophic Cardiomyopathies—A Decade of Study, *Lancet,* 1:733, 1970.
27. Taylor, W. J.: Genetic Aspects of the Cardiomyopathies, in A. G. Steinberg, A. G. Bearn, A. G. Motulsky, and B. Childs (eds.), "Progress in Medical Genetics. Genetics of Cardiovascular Disease," W. B. Saunders Company, Philadelphia, 1983, vol. 5, p. 163.
28. Hart, Z. H., Chang, C-H., DiMauro, S., Farooki, Q., and Ayyar, R.: Muscle Carnitine Deficiency and Fatal Cardiomyopathy, *Neurology (Minneap.),* 28:147, 1978.
29. Waber, L. J., Valle, D., Neill, C., DiMauro, S., and Shug, A.: Carnitine Deficiency Presenting as Familial Cardiomyopathy: A Treatable Defect in Carnitine Transport, *J. Pediatr.,* 101:700, 1982.
30. Kark, R. A. P., Rodriguez-Budelli, M., Perlman, S., Gulley, W. F., and Toron, K.: Preclinical Diagnosis and Carrier Detection in Ataxia Associated with Abnormalities of Lipoamide Dehydrogenase, *Neurology (Minneap.),* 30:502, 1980.
31. Luft, R., Ikkos, D., Palmieri, G., Ernster, L., and Arzelius, B.: A Case of Severe Hypermetabolism of Nonthyroid Origin with a Defect in the Maintenance of Mitochondrial Respiratory Control: A Correlated Chemical, Biochemical, and Morphological Study, *J. Clin. Invest.,* 41:1776, 1962.
32. Stumpf, D. A.: Mitochrondrial Multisystem Disorders: Clinical, Biochemical, and Morphologic Features, in H. R. Tyler and D. M. Dawson (eds.), "Current Neurology," Houghton Mifflin Professional Publishers, Medical Division, Boston, 1979, vol. 2, p. 117.
33. Mackay, E. H., Brown, R. S., and Pickering, D.: Cardiac Biopsy in Skeletal Myopathy: Report of a Case with Myocardial Mitochondrial Abnormalities, *J. Pathol.,* 120:35, 1976.
34. Schnitzler, E. R., and Robertson, W. C., Jr.: Familial Kearns-Sayre Syndrome, *Neurology (Minneap.),* 29:1172, 1979.
35. Egger, J., and Wilson, J.: Mitochrondrial Inheritance in a Mitochrondrially Mediated Disease, *N. Engl. J. Med.,* 309:142, 1983.
36. Brent, L. B., Aburano, A., Fisher, D. L., Moran, T. J., Myers, J. D., and Taylor, W. J.: Familial Muscular Subaortic Stenosis: An Unrecognized Form of "Idiopathic Heart Disease" with Clinical and Autopsy Observations, *Circulation,* 21:167, 1960.
37. Brock, R. C.: Functional Obstruction of the Left Ventricle, *Guy's Hosp. Reports,* 106:221, 1957.
38. Clark, C. E., Henry, W. L., and Epstein, S. E.: Familial Prevalence and Genetic Transmission of Idiopathic Hypertrophic Subaortic Stenosis, *N. Engl. J. Med.,* 289:709, 1973.
39. Ferrans, V. J., Morrow, A. G., and Roberts, W. C.: Myocardial Ultrastructure in Idiopathic Hypertrophic Subaortic Stenosis. A Study of Operatively Excised Left Ventricular Outflow Tract Muscle in 14 Patients, *Circulation,* 45:769, 1972.
40. Frederiksen, T., Gotzche, H., Harloe, N., Kiser, W., and Mellemgaard, K.: Familial Primary Amyloidosis with Severe Amyloid Heart Disease, *Am. J. Med.,* 33:328, 1962.
41. Benson, M. D., and Cohen, A. S.: Generalized Amyloid in a Family of Swedish Origin. A Study of 426 Family Mem-

bers in Seven Generations of a New Kinship With Neuropathy, Nephropathy, and Central Nervous System Involvement, *Ann. Intern. Med.*, 86:419, 1977.
42. Allensworth, D. C., Rice, G. J., and Lowe, G. W.: Persistent Atrial Standstill in a Family with Myocardial Disease, *Am. J. Med.*, 47:775, 1969.
43. Steinberg, D.: Elucidation of the Metabolic Error in Refsum's Disease: Strategy and Tactics, in R. A. P. Kark, R. N. Rosenberg, and L. J. Schut (eds.), "Advances in Neurology," Raven Press, New York, 1978, vol. 21 p. 113.
44. Hohn, A. R., Lowe, C. V., Sokal, J. E., and Lambert, E. C.: Cardiac Problems in the Glycogenesis with Specific Reference to Pompe's Disease, *Pediatrics*, 35:313, 1965.
45. Levin, S., Moses, S. W., Chayoth, R., Jagoda, N., and Steinitz, K.: Glycogen Storage Disease in Israel. A Clinical, Biochemical, and Genetic Study, *Isr. J. Med. Sci.*, 3:397, 1967.
46. Miranda, A. F., Nette, E. G., Hartlage, P. L., and DiMauro, S.: Phosphorylase Isoenzymes in Normal and Myophosphorylase-Deficient Human Heart, *Neurology (Minneap.)*, 29:1538, 1979.
47. Kravitz, K., Skolnick, M., Cannings, C., Carmelli, D., Baty, B., Amos, B., Johnson, A., Mendell, N., Edwards, C., and Cartwright, G.: Genetic Linkage Between Hereditary Hemochromatosis and HLA, *Am. J. Hum. Genet.*, 31:601, 1979.
48. Steere, A. C., Grodzicki, R. L., Kornblatt, A. N., Craft, J. E., Barbour, A. G., Burgdorfer, W., Schmid, G. P., Johnson, E., and Malawista, S. E.: The Spirochetal Etiology of Lyme Disease, *N. Engl. J. Med.*, 308:733, 1983.
49. Arnett, F. C., and Shulman, L. E.: Studies in Familial Systemic Lupus Erythematosus, *Medicine*, 55:313, 1976.
50. Miller, K. B., and Schwartz, R. S.: Familial Abnormalities of Suppressor-Cell Function in Systemic Lupus Erythematosus, *N. Engl. J. Med.*, 301:803, 1979.
51. Cleland, L. G., Bell, D. A., Williams, M., and Saurino, B. C.: Familial Lupus. Family Studies of HLA and Serologic Findings, *Arthritis Rheum.*, 21:183, 1978.
52. Singh, A., Doyle, E. F., Danilowicz, D. A., and Finegold, J.: Familial Nonobstructive Cardiomyopathy with Endocardial Fibroelastosis beyond Infancy, *Pediatrics*, 61:410, 1978.
53. McCue, C. M., Mantakas, M. E., Tingelstad, J. B.., and Ruddy, S.: Congenital Heart Block in Newborns of Mothers with Connective Tissue Disease, *Circulation*, 56:82, 1977.
54. Zatz, M., Itskan, S. B., Sanger, R., Frota-Pessoa, O., and Saldanha, P. H.: New Linkage Data for the X-Linked Types of Muscular Dystrophy and G6PD Variants, Colour Blindness, and Xg Blood Groups, *J. Med. Genet.*, 11:321, 1974.
55. Bundery, S., and Carter, C. D.: Genetic Heterogeneity for Dystrophia Myotonica, *J. Med. Genet.*, 9:311, 1972.
56. Waters, D. D., Nutter, D. O., Hopkins, L. C., and Dorney, E. R.: Cardiac Features of an Unusual X-Linked Humeroperoneal Neuromuscular Disease, *N. Engl. J. Med.*, 293:1017, 1975.
57. Tanaka, H., Vemura, N., Toyama, Y., Kudo, A., Okkatsu, Y., and Kanehisa, T.: Cardiac Involvement in the Kugelberg-Welander Syndrome, *Am. J. Cardiol.*, 38:528, 1976.
58. Pyeritz, R. E.: Cardiovascular Manifestations of Heritable Disorders of Connective Tissue, in A. G. Steinberg, A. G. Bearn, A. G. Motulsky, and B. Childs (eds.), "Progress in Medical Genetics. Genetics of Cardiovascular Disease," W. B. Saunders Company, Philadelphia, 1983, vol. 5, p. 191.
59. Nwokoro, N., and Neufeld, E. F.: Detection of Hunter Heterozygotes by Enzymatic Analysis of Hair Roots, *Am. J. Hum. Genet.*, 31:42, 1979.
60. Neufeld, E. F., and McKusick, V. A.: Disorders of Lysosomal Enzyme Synthesis and Localization: I-Cell Disease and Pseudo-Hurler Polydystrophy, in J. B. Stanbury, et al. (eds.), "The Metabolic Basis of Inherited Disease," 5th ed., McGraw-Hill Book Company, New York, 1983, p. 778.
61. Ferrans, V. J., Hibbs, R. C., and Burda, C. D.: The Heart in Fabry's Disease: A Histochemical and Electronmicroscopic Study, *Am. J. Cardiol.*, 24:95, 1969.
62. Brady, R. O.: Glucosyl Ceramide Lipidosis: Gaucher's Disease, in J. B. Stanbury, J. B. Syngaarden, D. S. Fredrickson (eds.), "The Metabolic Basis of Inherited Disease," 4th ed., McGraw-Hill Book Company, New York, 1978, p. 731.
63. Perheentupa, J., Aurio, S., Leisti, S., Raitta, C., and Tuuteri, L.: Mulibrey Nanism, Autosomal Recessive Syndrome with Pericardial Constriction, *Lancet*, 1:351, 1973.
64. Pinnel, S. R.: Disorders of Collagen, in J. B. Stanbury, J. B. Wyngaarden, and D. S. Fredrickson (eds.), "The Metabolic Basis of Inherited Disease," 4th ed., McGraw-Hill Book Company, New York, 1978, p. 1366.
65. Sillence, D. O., Senn, A., and Danks, D. M.: Genetic Heterogeneity in Osteogenesis Imperfecta, *J. Med. Genet.*, 16:101, 1979.
66. Slack, J., and Evans, K. A.: The Increased Risk of Death from Ischaemic Heart Disease in First Degree Relatives of 121 Men and 96 Women with Ischaemic Heart Disease, *J. Med. Genet.*, 3:239, 1966.
67. Epstein, C. J., Martin, G. M., Schultz, A. L., and Motulsky, A. G.: Werner's Syndrome, *Medicine*, 45:177, 1966.
68. Benditt, E. P., and Benditt, J. M.: Evidence for a Monoclonal Origin of Human Atherosclerotic Plaques, *Proc. Natl. Acad. Sci., U.S.A.*, 70:1753, 1973.
69. Thomas, W. A., Reiner, J. M., Jonakidevi, K., Florentin, R. A., and Lee, K. T.: Population Dynamics of Arterial Cells During Atherogenesis: X. Study of Monotypism in Atherosclerotic Lesions of Black Women Heterozygous for Glucose-6-Phosphate Dehydrogenase (G-6-PD), *Exp. Mol. Pathol.*, 31:367, 1979.
70. Galton, D. J., Stocks, J., and Rees, A.: Molecular Variants of the Lipoproteins, *Clin. Sci.*, 64:559, 1983.
71. Goldstein, J. L., Kita, T., and Brown, M. S.: Defective Lipoprotein Receptors and Atherosclerosis. Lessons from an Animal Counterpart of Familial Hypercholesterolemia, *N. Engl. J. Med.*, 309:288, 1983.
72. Goldstein, J. L., Brown, M. S., and Stone, N. J.: Genetics of the LDL Receptor: Evidence That the Mutations Affecting Binding and Internalization Are Allelic, *Cell*, 12:629, 1977.
73. Steinberg, D.: Lipoproteins and Atherosclerosis. A Look Back and a Look Ahead, *Atherosclerosis*, 3:283, 1983.
74. Breslow, J. L., Zannis, V. I., SanGiacomo, T. R., Third, T. L. H. C., Tracy, T., and Glueck, C. J.: Studies of Familial Type III Hyperlipoproteinemia Using as a Genetic Marker the Apo E Phenotype E2/2, *J. Lipid Res.* 23:1224, 1982.
75. Ghiselli, G., Schaefer, E. J., Gascon, P., and Brewer, H. B., Jr.: Type III Hyperlipoproteinemia Associated with Apolipoprotein E Deficiency. *Science*, 214:1239, 1981.
76. Srinivasan, S. R., Frerichs, R. R., Webber, L. S., and Berenson, G. S.: Serum Lipoprotein Profile in Children from a Biracial Community. The Bogalusa Heart Study, *Circulation*, 54:309, 1976.
77. Herbert, P. N., Gotto, A. M., and Fredrickson, D. S.: Familial Lipoprotein Deficiency (Abetalipoproteinemia, Hypobetalipoproteinemia, and Tangier Disease), in J. B. Stanbury, J. B. Wyngaarden, and D. S. Fredrickson (eds.), "The Metabolic Basis of Inherited Disease," 4th ed., McGraw-Hill Book Company, New York, 1978, p. 544.
78. Breslow, J. L., Ross, D., McPherson, J., Williams, H., Kurnit, D., Nussbaum, A. L., Karathanasis, S. K., and Zannis, V. I.: Isolation and Characterization of cDNA Clones for Human Apolipoprotein A-I, *Proc. Natl. Acad. Sci. U.S.A.*, 79:6861, 1982.
79. Berg, K.: Genetics of Coronary Heart Disease, in A. G. Steinberg, A. G. Bearn, A. G. Motulsky, and B. Childs (eds.), "Progress in Medical Genetics. Genetics of Cardiovascular Disease," W. B. Saunders Company, Philadelphia, 1983, vol. 5, p. 35.
80. Goldstein, J. L., Schrott, H. G., Hazzard, W. R., Bierman, E. L., and Motulsky, A. G.: Hyperlipidemia in Coronary Heart Disease: II. Genetic Analysis of Lipid Levels in 176 Families and Delineation of a New Inherited Disorder, Combined Hyperlipidemia, *J. Clin. Invest.*, 52:1544, 1973.
81. Rapacz, J.: Lipoprotein Immunogenetics and Atherosclerosis, *Am. J. Med. Genet.*, 1:377, 1978.

82. Deutscher, S., Epstein, F. H., and Kjelsberg, M. D.: Familial Aggregation of Factors Associated with Coronary Heart Disease, *Circulation*, 33:911, 1966.
83. Cudworth, A. G.: Type I Diabetes Mellitus, *Diabetologia*, 14:281, 1978.
84. Craighead, J. E.: Current Views on the Etiology of Insulin-Dependent Diabetes Mellitus, *N. Engl. J. Med.*, 299:1439, 1978.
85. Srikanta, S., Ganda, O. P., Jackson, R. A., Gleason, R. E., Kaldany, A., Garovoy, M. R., Milford, E. L., Carpenter, C. B., Soeldner, J. S., and Eisenbarth, G. S.: Type I Diabetes Mellitus in Monozygotic Twins: Chronic Progressive Beta Cell Dysfunction, *Ann. Intern. Med.*, 99:320, 1983.
86. MacDonald, M. J.: The Frequencies of Juvenile Diabetes in American Blacks and Caucasians Are Consistent with Dominant Inheritance, *Diabetes*, 29:110, 1980.
87. Rotter, J. I., and Hodge, S. E.: Racial Differences in Juvenile-Type Diabetes Are Consistent with More than One Mode of Inheritance, *Diabetes*, 29:115, 1980.
88. Haneda, M., Polonsky, K. S., Bergenstal, R. M., Jaspan, J. B., Shoelson, S. E., Blix, P. M., Chan, S. J., Kwok, S. C. M., Wishner, W. B., Zeidler, A., Olefsky, J. M., Friedenberg, G., Tager, H. S., Steiner, D. F., and Rubenstein, A. H.: Familial Hyperinsulinemia Due to a Structurally Abnormal Insulin. Definition of an Emerging New Clinical Syndrome, *N. Engl. J. Med.*, 310:1288, 1984.
89. Rotwein, P. S., Chirqwin, J., Province, M., Knowler, W. C., Pettitt, D. J., Cordell, B., Goodman, H. M., and Permutt, M. A.: Polymorphism in the 5′ Flanking Region of the Human Insulin Gene: A Genetic Marker for Non-Insulin-Dependent Diabetes, *N. Engl. J. Med.*, 308:65, 1983.
90. Mandrup-Poulsen, T., Owerbach, D., Mortensen, S. A., Johansen, K., Meinertz, H., Sorensen, H., and Nerup, J.: DNA Sequences Flanking the Insulin Gene on Chromosome 11 Confer Risk of Atherosclerosis, *Lancet*, 1:250, 1984.
91. Iselius, L., Lindsten, J., Morton, N. E., Efendic, J., Cerasi, E., Haegermark, A., and Luft, R.: Evidence for an Autosomal Recessive Gene Regulating the Persistence of the Insulin Response to Glucose in Man, *Clin. Genet.*, 22:180, 1982.
92. Childs, B.: Causes of Essential Hypertension, in A. G. Steinberg, A. G. Bearn, and A. G. Motulsky (eds.), "Progress in Medical Genetics. Genetics of Cardiovascular Disease," W. B. Saunders Company, Philadelphia, 1983, vol. 5, p. 1.
93. Kass, E. H., Rosner, B., Zinner, S. H., Margolius, H. S., and Lee, Y-H.: Studies on the Origin of Human Hypertension, *Postgrad. Med. J.*, 53(suppl. 2):145, 1977.
94. Luft, F. C., Grim, C. E., Higgins, J. T., Jr., and Weinberger, M. H.: Differences in Response to Sodium Administration in Normotensive White and Black Subjects, *J. Lab. Clin. Med.*, 90:555, 1977.
95. Gagel, R. F., Melvin, K. E. W., Tashjian, A. J., Jr., Miller, H. H., Feldman, Z. T., Wolfe, H. J., DeLellis, R. A., Cervi-Skinner, S., and Reichlin, S.: Natural History of the Familial Medullary Thyroid Carcinoma-Pheochromocytoma Syndrome and the Identification of Pre-neoplastic States by Screening Studies: A Five-Year Report, *Trans. Assoc. Am. Physicians*, 88:177, 1975.
96. Wilkins, L.: Adrenal Disorders: II. Congenital Virilizing Adrenal Hyperplasia, *Arch. Dis. Child.*, 37:231, 1962.
97. Melmon, K. L., and Braunwald, E.: Familial Pulmonary Hypertension, *N. Engl. J. Med.*, 269:770, 1963.
98. Hodgson, C. H., Curchell, H. B., Good, C. A. II, and Claggett, O. T.: Hereditary Hemorrhagic Telangiectasia and Pulmonary Arteriovenous Fistula: Survey of a Large Family, *N. Engl. J. Med.*, 261:625, 1959.
99. Sarchek, N. S., and Leonard, J. J.: Familial Heart Block and Sinus Bradycardia: Classification and Natural History, *Am. J. Cardiol.*, 29:451, 1972.
100. Gould, W. L.: Auricular Fibrillation: Report on a Study of a Familial Tendency, 1920–1956, *A.M.A. Arch. Intern. Med.*, 100:916, 1957.
101. Bacos, J. M., Eagar, J. T., and Orgain, E. S.: Congenital Familial Nodal Rhythm, *Circulation*, 22:887, 1960.
102. Morrooka, S., Kato, A., Murao, S., and Ohsuzu, H.: A 17-Year Follow-up Study of a Family with Idiopathic Hypertrophic Cardiomyopathy and WPW Syndrome, *Jpn. Heart J.*, 19:332, 1978.
103. Jervell, A., and Lange-Neilsen, F.: Congenital Deaf-Mutism, Functional Heart Disease with Prolongation of the Q-T Interval and Sudden Death, *A. Heart J.*, 54:59, 1957.
104. Garza, L. A., Vick, R. L., Nora, J. J., and McNamara, D. G.: Heritable Q-T Prolongation without Deafness, *Circulation*, 41:39, 1970.
105. Green, J. R., Jr., Krovetz, L. J., Shanklin, D. R., DeVito, J. J., and Taylor, W. J.: Sudden Unexpected Death in Three Generations, *A.M.A. Arch. Intern. Med.*, 124:359, 1969.

Section A

Congenital Heart Disease

36

The Pathology, Abnormal Physiology, Clinical Recognition, and Medical and Surgical Treatment of Congenital Heart Disease*

Elizabeth W. Nugent, M.D.
William H. Plauth, Jr., M.D.
Jesse E. Edwards, M.D.
Robert C. Schlant, M.D.
Willis H. Williams, M.D.

Incidence and Etiology

Fetal Circulation and the Transition to Neonatal and Adult Circulation
Persistence of Fetal Circulation

Complications of Congenital Heart Disease
Congestive Heart Failure
Cyanosis
Pulmonary Arterial Hypertension and Pulmonary Vascular Obstructive Disease
Retardation of Growth and Development
Exertional Intolerance and Restrictions

Intracardiac Communications between the Systemic and Pulmonary Circulations, Usually without Cyanosis
Ventricular Septal Defect
Atrial Septal Defect
Partial Anomalous Pulmonary Venous Connection
Common Atrioventricular Canal Defects
Single Atrium
Left Ventricular–Right Atrial Communication

Extracardiac Communications between the Systemic and Pulmonary Circulations, Usually without Cyanosis
Patent Ductus Arteriosus
Aorticopulmonary Septal Defect (Window)
One Pulmonary Artery from the Ascending Aorta
Sinus of Valsalva Fistula
Anomalous Systemic Arterial Supply to the Lung
Coronary Arteriovenous Fistula

Valvular and Vascular Malformations of the Left Side of the Heart with Right-to-Left, Bidirectional, or No Shunt
Aortic Arch Anomalies
Coarctation of the Aorta
Interruption of the Aortic Arch
Valvular Aortic Stenosis
Subvalvular Aortic Stenosis
Supravalvular Aortic Stenosis
Bicuspid Aortic Valve
Congenital Aortic Regurgitation
Aortic–Left Ventricular Tunnel
Aortic Atresia
Mitral Atresia
Mitral Stenosis
Mitral Regurgitation
Cor Triatriatum
Stenosis of Pulmonary Veins and Venules
Endocardial Fibroelastosis

Valvular and Vascular Malformations of the Right Side of the Heart with Right-to-Left, Bidirectional, or No Shunt
Valvular Pulmonary Stenosis with Intact Ventricular Septum
Subvalvular Pulmonary Stenosis
Supravalvular Pulmonary Stenosis and Peripheral Pulmonary Arterial Coarctations
Pulmonary Atresia with Intact Ventricular Septum
Tetralogy of Fallot
Absent Pulmonary Valve
Absence of Anatomic Origin of Pulmonary Arterial System from the Heart: With and without Confluence of Right and Left Pulmonary Arteries.

*The editor-in-chief wishes to thank Dr. John Kirklin for his past contributions to this chapter. He has led the way for our profession, and the patients with congenital heart disease receive better care today because of his work.

Tricuspid Atresia
Tricuspid Regurgitation
Ebstein's Anomaly
Uhl's Malformation
Pulmonary Arteriovenous Fistula
Unilateral Absence of a Pulmonary Artery

Abnormalities of the Pulmonary Venous Connections
Total Anomalous Pulmonary Venous Connection
Partial Anomalous Pulmonary Venous Connection

Abnormalities of Systemic Venous Connections
Union of Superior or Inferior Vena Cava with Left Atrium
Persistent Left Superior Vena Cava
Continuity of Inferior Vena Cava with Azygous Venous System

Malpositions of the Cardiac Structures
Definition and Terminology
The Segmental Approach to Diagnosis
Levocardia, Dextrocardia, and Mesocardia
Asplenia and Polysplenia Syndromes
Dextro Transposition of the Great Arteries
Double-Outlet Right Ventricle
Double-Outlet Left Ventricle
Corrected Transposition of the Great Arteries
Single Ventricle
Crisscross Heart
Ectopia Cordis

Congenital Abnormalities of the Coronary Arterial Circulation
Coronary Arteriovenous Fistula
Origin of the Left Coronary Artery from the Pulmonary Artery
Origin of the Right or Both Coronary Arteries from the Pulmonary Artery
Origin of the Left Coronary Artery from the Right Aortic Sinus
Origin of the Circumflex Coronary Artery from the Right Aortic Sinus or Right Coronary Artery
Atresia of the Left Coronary Ostium
Aneurysm of Coronary Artery

Congenital Abnormalities of the Coronary Venous Circulation
Coronary Sinus Malformations

Congenital Abnormalities of the Pericardium
Deficiency
Cysts and Diverticula

Incidence and Etiology

The incidence of congenital heart disease in the United States is approximately 8 per 1000 live births. The incidence among stillborns is higher, but cardiac malformations are not accorded a significant role in fetal death.[1,2] Most of the infants born alive with cardiac defects will have anomalies that do not represent a threat to life, at least during infancy. Almost one-third, or 2.6 per 100 live births, however, will have *critical disease,* defined as a malformation severe enough to result in cardiac catheterization, cardiac surgery, or death within the first year of life.[3] In the past, the majority of these infants died within the first year of life, almost two-thirds of the deaths occurring within the first 4 weeks.[4] Today, with early detection, prompt referral, and remarkable advances in management, 60 percent of infants with critical disease can be expected to survive the first year of life.[3]

Estimates of the incidence of specific lesions vary depending upon whether the data are drawn from infants or older children and upon whether the diagnosis is based on clinical, catheterization, surgical, or postmortem studies (Table 36-1). Hoffman has reviewed the problems of assessing incidence and natural history of congenital heart disease.[5] In a collaborative prospective study of 56,109 total births at 12 medical centers in the United States,[1] the diagnosis was verified by autopsy, surgery, or cardiac catheterization in 56 percent. In another prospective study of 19,502 births among members of a health plan in the United States,[2] the diagnosis was made by these methods in 48 percent, with cumulative incidence increasing from 3.3 per 1000 at birth to 7.8 at 1 year of age and to 9.1 at 5 years of age. The New England study was also prospective, but it included only symptomatic infants to 1 year of age.[3] Diagnosis was established by catheterization, surgery, or postmortem examination in all except 0.7 percent, who died before any intervention and did not have autopsies performed. In the large series of 10,624 reported by Nadas,[4] 76 percent were diagnosed by catheterization, surgery, or postmortem examination. Incidence in other countries is remarkably similar to that reported for the United States.[6]

Despite these differences in case material, except for bicuspid aortic valve when older patients are included, it is apparent that ventricular septal defect is the most common malformation, occurring in about 30 percent of all patients with congenital heart disease (Table 36-1). Pulmonary stenosis, patent ductus arteriosus, atrial septal defect, tetralogy of Fallot, aortic stenosis, coarctation of the aorta, and transposition of the great arteries are also relatively common. These eight defects constitute approximately 75 percent of all congenital heart disease in infants and children.

Of 2251 infants with critical congenital heart disease in the New England study,[3] 53.7 percent were male. Certain defects, however, are considerably more common in one sex than the other. The incidence among blacks does not differ significantly from that among white patients.[1] A seasonal influence on the incidence of certain defects has been demonstrated.[7]

The most popular concept regarding etiology is that cardiac defects are due to a combination of genetic and environmental interactions. This multifactorial etiology requires a genetic predisposition, probably polygenic, and an environmental terato-

TABLE 36-1 Incidence of Specific Lesions of Congenital Heart Disease

	Percent of Cases of Congenital Heart Disease				
Lesion	Keith[6]	Nadas[4]	Collaborative Study[1]	Hoffman[2]	New England Study[3]
VSD	28.3	19.4	29.5	31.3	16.6
PS	9.9	7.5	8.6	13.5	3.5
PDA	9.8	15.5	8.3	5.5	6.5
ASD, secundum	7.0	4.5	7.4	6.1	3.1
VSD with PS*	9.7	10.5	6.4	3.7	9.4
AS	7.1	5.7	3.8	3.7	2.0
AO atresia	1.5	NL	3.1	0.6	7.9
AVC†	3.4	2.7	3.6	3.7	5.3
Coarctation AO	5.1	8.1	2.6	5.5	8.0
Peripheral PS	NL	1.0	3.6	NL	NL
EFE	0.9	NL	2.4	NL	NL
TGA	4.9	4.0	2.6	3.7	10.5
Truncus arteriosus	0.7	0.8	1.7	2.5	1.5
TAPVC	1.4	1.3	NL	0.6	2.8
Tricuspid atresia	1.2	1.0	1.2	NL	2.7
DORV	0.5	0.2	1.0	0.6	1.6
Pulmonary atresia without VSD	0.7	0.3	0.01	0.6	3.3
Number of patients	15,104	10,624	56,109	19,502	2,251

*Includes tetralogy of Fallot.
†Includes partial and complete.
Notes: NL = not listed; VSD = ventricular septal defect; PS = pulmonary stenosis; PDA = patent ductus arteriosus; ASD = atrial septal defect; AS = aortic stenosis; AVC = atrioventricular canal; AO = aorta; EFE = endocardial fibroelastosis; TGA = transposition of great arteries; TAPVC = total anomalous pulmonary venous connection; DORV = double-outlet right ventricle.

gen to which the susceptible fetus is exposed in a critical or vulnerable period.[8,9] The incidence among siblings of patients with congenital heart disease has been reported as 17 per 1000, as compared to an incidence in the general population in the same series of only 7.6 per 1000 live births.[10] Genetic and environmental counseling for families with congenital heart disease is now a reality[9,11] (see Chap. 35).

Some examples of congenital heart disease have a primarily genetic basis. An increased incidence of cardiac defects is associated with major chromosomal abnormalities such as trisomy, deletion, and mosaicism. Down's syndrome is a well-known example. Mendelian inheritance can be demonstrated in a few families with repeated occurrences of specific cardiac abnormalities, such as atrial septal defect, which may be associated with other noncardiac anomalies.

Environmental factors can cause certain defects. Congenital heart disease, predominantly patent ductus arteriosus and peripheral pulmonary stenosis in association with noncardiac abnormalities can occur as a consequence of intrauterine rubella.[6] On the other hand, the aggressive management of very small premature infants, with a resultant increase in survival, has led to new and serious problems with patent ductus arteriosus, particularly when associated with respiratory distress.

Fetal Circulation and the Transition to Neonatal and Adult Circulation[12–21]

The fetus obtains all of its nutritional requirements, including oxygen, via the placental circulation. Consequently, there is a need for a high blood flow to the placenta, but there is no need to pass most of the blood through the uninflated fetal lungs. The fetal circulation accomplishes its special function with the aid of the following three vascular channels: (1) the *foramen ovale* in the atrial septum allows blood to pass from the right to the left atrium; (2) the *ductus arteriosus* connects the pulmonary artery to the aorta distal to the origin of the left subclavian artery and enables most of the blood reaching the pulmonary artery to bypass the uninflated lungs; and (3) the *ductus venosus* shunts blood returning from the placenta through the umbilical cord to the inferior vena cava to bypass the liver.

In the developed fetus, the total return of blood to the heart by the inferior vena cava is equal to 65 to 70 percent of the combined ventricular output (CVO); of this volume an amount equal to 25 to 28 percent of CVO passes through the foramen ovale to the left atrium, where it is joined by 5 to 10 percent of CVO returning from the lungs. The left ventricle thus receives and ejects only 33 percent of the CVO of the fetal heart. The remaining 38 to 42 percent of CVO returning in the inferior vena cava mixes with most of the 22 to 25 percent of CVO that returns in the superior vena cava and goes into the right ventricle, which thus receives and ejects about 66 percent of the CVO of the fetal heart. About 85 to 90 percent of the blood ejected by the right ventricle, or about 60 percent of the CVO, is diverted from the lungs through the ductus arteriosus to the aorta. The remainder passes through the pulmonary circulation.[17] About 40 to 50 percent of the CVO goes to the placenta for the exchange of carbon dioxide, oxygen, and other metabolites. The CVO of the fetal lamb near term is about 5000 ml/kg/min; after birth the CVO decreases about 25 percent.[13]

Umbilical venous blood has a P_{O_2} of about 30 to 35 mmHg and an oxygen saturation of about 80 percent. As the result of the various mechanisms described above, fetal arterial blood in the ascending aorta has a P_{O_2} of about 26 to 28 mmHg and an oxygen saturation of 55 to 60 percent.

During the delivery of the fetus, the umbilical cord is usually somewhat compressed and the placenta may begin to separate. Simultaneously, the newborn baby is suddenly exposed to a cold, strange environment. Both asphyxia and cold are strong respiratory stimuli, and the baby usually begins to breathe soon after birth. Within seconds after expansion of the lungs with air, the tremendous increase in blood flow to the lungs takes over the function of gas exchange from the placental circulation. The removal of the placenta from the circulation markedly increases arterial resistance and decreases blood return from the inferior vena cava.

The calculated fetal pulmonary vascular resistance is very high, about 6 mmHg/min/ml at 0.4 gestation, but it falls progressively to 0.35 to 0.3 mmHg/min/ml at term. The marked decrease is probably due mainly to the growth of new pulmonary blood vessels.

The initial fall in pulmonary vascular resistance after birth is produced by two mechanisms. The first of these is a mechanical reduction due to the physical expansion of the lungs with air, with a resultant decrease in the kinking and compression of the pulmonary vessels. The second and main mechanism is a marked diminution in the pulmonary arterial vasoconstriction related to the increased alveolar and interstitial P_{O_2}. Bradykinin may be involved as a supplementary mechanism in the immediate pulmonary vasodilatation after birth. There is suggestive evidence that prostacycline (PGI_2) is involved in the fall in pulmonary vascular resistance associated with ventilation and distention of the lungs of the newborn.[15] In addition, the fetal pulmonary circulation is influenced by the autonomic nervous system, and it is possible that reflex autonomic effects contribute to the changes in pulmonary vascular resistance.

After birth, the pulmonary vascular resistance initially falls very rapidly, and it reaches adult levels by about 6 to 8 weeks after birth. During this time, there is a rapid regression of the medial muscle layer of the pulmonary arteries and arterioles. There is a further decrease in total pulmonary vascular resistance associated with growth of the lungs for several years.

Prior to birth the foramen ovale is held open by the large flow of blood from the inferior vena cava to the left atrium. After birth, the left atrial pressure increases due to the increase in pulmonary flow and the increase in systemic arterial resistance; the right atrial pressure decreases. These changes in left and right atrial pressures produce functional closure of the foramen ovale by the apposition of the valve of the foramen ovale, the septum primum, against the edge of the crista dividens. The septum primum usually becomes adherent, with permanent closure, in several months. In 15 to 20 percent of normal adults, however, a small opening or potential opening may persist.

Prior to delivery, patency of the ductus arteriosus is probably an active condition produced by a prostaglandin formed intramurally. A likely candidate for this role is PGE_2, which is mainly degraded in the lungs; its action may be complemented by that of PGI_2.

The ductus arteriosus usually is functionally closed 10 to 15 h after birth in a normal full-term infant, with complete closure within 10 to 21 days. The trigger for closure of the ductus arteriosus after birth is the postnatal rise in arterial P_{O_2} or oxygen tension. It is not clear, however, whether the effect of oxygen is exerted directly on the smooth-muscle cells of the ductus or whether other vasoactive agents are involved. Prostaglandins are probably involved, although the exact mechanism is not known. Several possible mechanisms have been suggested.[22]

Prior to birth, the pulmonary and systemic circuits are in communication through the relatively large ductus arteriosus. Consequently, the systolic pressures in both of the ventricles, the aorta, and the pulmonary artery are almost identical. The pressures are approximately 30 mmHg above amniotic cavity pressure at 0.4 gestation and increase progressively to about 50 mmHg at term.[23] In association with the abrupt fall in pulmonary vascular resistance shortly after birth and the closure of the ductus arteriosus, the pulmonary artery pressure decreases, at first rather abruptly, to a mean pressure of about 20 to 30 mmHg; thereafter it decreases more slowly until it reaches normal childhood values in a few weeks.[13]

Although the right and the left ventricles are about the same thickness at birth, the markedly increased load on the left ventricle after birth causes it to increase rapidly in thickness and weight during the first few weeks after birth. The increase in left ventricular mass at this age is predominantly due to hyperplasia, with an increase in the number of cells, rather than to hypertrophy of individual cells. Since the right ventricular mass remains stable during this period, the ratio of left to right ventricular weights increases rapidly for 1 to 2 weeks and then increases more slowly.

Persistence of Fetal Circulation

Persistent fetal circulation,[21,22] or persistent pulmonary hypertension, in the newborn results in right-to-left shunting through the patent foramen ovale and/or patent ductus arteriosus. It most commonly occurs in full-term infants. Severe hypoxia is usually manifested in the first few hours of life with tachypnea, acidosis, and a chest roentgenogram that shows diminished vascular flow but no evidence of pulmonary parenchymal disease. Physical examination may reveal a parasternal heave, a loud second heart sound, and a systolic murmur.

Polycythemia, transient myocardial ischemia from hypoglycemia, and cyanotic congenital cardiac defects must be excluded. A greater oxygen level in the right radial artery than in the umbilical artery confirms right-to-left shunting through the ductus. Contrast echocardiography from a vein draining the upper segment of the body will demonstrate the right-to-left shunt at atrial level.

Initial treatment[22] includes an increase in the inspired oxygen level and correction of acidosis with sodium bicarbonate. Frequently, artificial ventilation is required. Hyperventilation to diminish the partial pressure of carbon dioxide is often successful in lowering the pulmonary pressure and diminishing the right-to-left shunt. Intravenous infusion of tolazoline either into the upper segment of the body, to enhance flow to the lungs, or directly into the pulmonary artery may be beneficial. Successful treatment of severe disease with an extracorporeal membrane oxygenator has been reported.[23]

Untreated, a majority of these infants will die of problems related to the hypoxia. Survival is greatly improved by medical treatment.

Similar hemodynamic alterations may also be seen in premature infants with respiratory distress syndrome and other newborns with parenchymal lung disease.

Complications of Congenital Heart Disease

Congestive Heart Failure

Congestive heart failure occurs at one time or another in one child in five with congenital heart disease. It occurs in over 80 percent of infants who have malformations severe enough to produce death or require cardiac catheterization or surgery within the first year of life.[24]

The onset usually is a phenomenon of the first 6 months of life. Although it may persist for many months or even years, its onset after 1 year of age is rare without a serious intercurrent problem such as infective endocarditis.

Heart failure within the first 12 to 18 h of life is usually due to malformations that involve volume overload independent of pulmonary flow, as occurs with severe valvular regurgitation. Rarely, endocardial fibroelastosis or myocarditis may produce failure from the time of birth, as may congenital complete heart block or supraventricular tachycardia. To be distinguished from primary cardiac disease in this age group is the volume overload from a systemic arteriovenous fistula or severe polycythemia and the depressed myocardial contractility from neonatal asphyxia, hypocalcemia, hypoglycemia, anemia, or sepsis.

The majority of full-term infants presenting with severe heart failure during the remainder of the first week have critical obstruction to systemic arterial flow which, in many cases, has been unmasked by narrowing or closure of the ductus arteriosus. Examples are aortic atresia, coarctation of the aorta, interruption of the aortic arch, and critical aortic stenosis. During the second week of life aortic atresia and coarctation remain the most common causes of heart failure, but ventricular septal defect, transposition of the great arteries with a ventricular septal defect, and truncus arteriosus make their appearance. These are malformations which require a pulmonary vascular bed with a reduced vascular resistance for full expression of their severity. Thereafter ventricular septal defect is the primary cause of congestive failure, followed by transposition, coarctation, complete atrioventricular canal, and patent ductus arteriosus.[3]

Congestive failure in the infant may be fulminant and often is associated with respiratory tract infections. The most common symptom is difficulty in breathing, with rapid, grunting, or gasping breathing or breathlessness with feeding, except in those rare instances of isolated right ventricular failure. Observation of the undisturbed infant will reveal dyspnea, the signs of which are nasal flaring and sub- or intercostal retractions. A respiratory rate consistently above 60 is abnormal, and rates in the range of 90 to 100 are not uncommon when failure is present. Poor weight gain is the rule. Cool, moist skin, a subdued and rapid arterial pulse, and hepatic enlargement are common accompanying signs. A gallop rhythm, pulmonary rales, and expiratory wheezes may be present. It may be difficult to distinguish the pulmonary findings of heart failure from those of pneumonia or bronchiolitis, and, indeed, many infants have both heart failure and pulmonary infection. Edema, if present, usually is found in the periorbital area and on the dorsa of the feet and hands. Cardiac enlargement will be confirmed by chest roentgenogram. Infants with malformations such as coarctation of the aorta and total anomalous pulmonary venous connection, abnormalities usually not characterized by an impressive murmur, sometimes are referred only after weeks of tachypnea and failure to thrive, after a chest roentgenogram, taken to explore the possibility of lung disease, has revealed cardiac enlargement.

When a sizable systemic-to-pulmonary communication exists in the premature infant, usually a patent ductus, signs of heart failure may be recognized as early as the first day or two of life and usually are associated with signs of ventilatory failure.

Hospitalization is recommended for all infants with congestive failure. Elevation of the head and chest to an angle of approximately 30° and administration of humidified oxygen by techniques that do not disturb the infant will help relieve dyspnea and cyanosis. Arterial P_{O_2} levels should be monitored in the newborn, particularly the premature, to avoid the risk of retrolental fibroplasia. Rest, aided by sedation, is beneficial. With severe failure oral feedings should be temporarily suspended and fluid intake restricted to 65 ml/kg/day intravenously for at least the first 24 h. Abnormalities such as anemia, acidosis, hypoxia, hypercarbia, hypoglycemia, or hypocalcemia should be sought and corrected; serum sodium, potassium, BUN, and creatinine concentrations should be monitored. Because of the difficulty of recognizing the presence of infection in these very sick infants, a low threshold for the administration of antibiotics is appropriate.

Digitalis remains the most important medication for the management of congestive failure in infants and children. Digoxin is recommended because of its excellent absorption when given orally, rapid onset of action, relatively rapid excretion, and convenience of administration. The recommended doses for daily oral maintenance therapy are given in Table 36-2. The total digitalizing dose is three times the daily maintenance dose. Half of the digitalizing dose may be given initially, followed by the remaining two quarters at 4-, 8-, or 12-h intervals depending upon the desired speed of total digitalization. Maintenance therapy should be started 8 to 12 h after the last digitalizing dose. In the severely ill infant, who has decreased perfusion and unpredictable absorption, digitalization by the intravenous route is recommended. The parenteral doses of digoxin are approximately 75 percent of the oral doses for digitalization and maintenance. Impaired renal function will lead to digoxin accumulation and toxicity, so the initial and maintenance doses should be adjusted accordingly.[25] Toxicity, if it is to occur, usually occurs within the first week of therapy. If anorexia, nausea or vomiting, or electrocardiographic evidence of either atrial or ventricular ectopy or atrioventricular block appear, digoxin should be stopped and the serum digoxin level determined. Toxicity is probable if the level exceeds 3.0 ng/ml in the infant below 6 months of age or 2.0 ng/ml in the older infant or child. We try to keep serum digoxin levels near but below these levels. Written instructions including signs of toxicity should be given to the parents so that there is no confusion. Warning should be given to prevent accidental ingestion of the medication by the patient or other children. If the need for digoxin continues, the dose is adjusted as the patient grows and gains weight.

TABLE 36-2 Recommended Doses for Digoxin

Age	Daily Oral* Maintenance Dose,† mg/kg/day‡	Total Oral Digitalizing Dose, mg/kg
Premature:		
<1250 g	0.006	0.018
>1250 g	0.010	0.030
Newborn:	0.015	0.045
2 days–2 years	0.020	0.060
2–5 years	0.020–0.015	0.060–0.045
5–10 years	0.015–0.010	0.045–0.030
10–15 years	0.010–0.005	0.030–0.015
Adult	0.004–0.005	0.012–0.015

*Parenteral dose is 75 percent of the oral dose.

†Digitalizing dose is three times daily maintenance dose.

‡It is recommended that the daily dose be divided into two equal doses given every 12 h in the hospital and twice daily at home with approximately 12 h between doses, depending upon the family schedule.

The diuretics furosemide or ethacrynic acid, used intravenously in doses of 1.0 mg/kg or orally in doses of 2.0 mg/kg, are very effective in the acute management of congestive failure. With severe congestive failure, the dose of either drug may be increased by 1.0 mg/kg increments intravenously if no urinary response has been achieved after 45 min. For long-term oral diuretic therapy, 2.0 mg/kg once daily or (if necessary) twice daily is recommended. Chlorothiazide, a slightly less potent diuretic but one with a longer duration of action, may be given orally in a dose of 20 to 40 mg/kg/day. Hypokalemia and hypochloremia can be induced with these potent diuretics, and a daily oral supplement of potassium chloride in the range of 1.0 to 1.5 meq/kg, with adjustment depending upon the serum level, is recommended. The serum potassium should not be allowed to fall below 3.5 meq/liter. Spironolactone, an aldosterone antagonist, has proved useful in supplementing the diuresis and in preventing the hypokalemia induced by the diuretics described above. It may be given orally in a single daily dose of 2 to 3 mg/kg. A regimen of spironolactone, 2 mg/kg given every day, and chlorothiazide, 20 mg/kg given on alternate days, has been our preference for long-term diuretic therapy in most infants. This regimen is adequate for all but the most severe degrees of heart failure and does not require potassium supplementation. With more severe heart failure, chlorothiazide may be given daily, the dose of both diuretics may be increased, or furosemide may be added. Under these circumstances potassium supplementation is usually necessary.

In emergency situations it may be necessary to

provide an immediate inotropic stimulus to the heart. This may be accomplished by the intravenous administration of sympathomimetic amines by constant infusion pump. Isoproterenol, in a dose of 0.1 μg/kg/min, exerts a powerful inotropic effect, but its usefulness may be limited by induced tachycardia and peripheral vasodilatation, sometimes to the detriment of renal perfusion. Epinephrine in a dose of 0.1 to 1.0 μg/kg/min or dobutamine or dopamine in a dose of 5 to 15 μg/kg/min generally have been more helpful, with dopamine providing more adequate renal flow. Systemic arterial blood pressure, urinary output, and the electrocardiogram should be monitored continuously. Vasodilator therapy in the form of intravenous sodium nitroprusside may be of considerable help in patients with severe congestive failure not associated with large left-to-right shunts (see also Chaps. 20 and 21). The infusion rate at the start should be no greater than 0.5 μg/kg/min, but it may be increased gradually to 4.0 μg/kg/min to achieve the desired effect. Systemic arterial pressure should be monitored continuously to detect serious hypotension. Two oral vasodilators, hydralazine in a dose of 0.25 to 0.50 mg/kg four times daily for children with normal or only mildly elevated ventricular filling pressure or prazosin in a dose of 0.05 to 0.10 mg/kg four times daily if ventricular filling pressures are elevated, have proved beneficial in selected patients.[26]

Infants with potentially exhausting respiratory effort or with hypoxia or hypercapnea secondary to pulmonary edema or respiratory failure will benefit from endotracheal intubation and ventilation on a volume-controlled, positive pressure respirator, usually with the addition of positive end-expiratory pressure. These measures may permit additional therapy, cardiac catheterization, and surgical intervention with a much greater margin of safety.

Finally, infants or children in whom medical therapy is clearly inadequate or only temporarily successful may require prompt surgical intervention for control of their heart failure. As a rule, the earlier the onset of congestive failure the more likely will be the need for surgery.

Cyanosis

Cyanosis is one of the more frequent initial signs of congenital heart disease in the infant, but it may also be an early sign of pulmonary, central nervous system, or metabolic disease or of methemoglobinemia. The advent of nonsurgical palliation with prostaglandin,[27] as well as the rapid development of surgical techniques, particularly for infants, makes prompt distinction between cardiac and noncardiac cyanosis even more important.

Respiratory distress syndrome of the newborn occurs most frequently in the premature infant, the infant of a diabetic mother, or the infant delivered by cesarean section. The cyanosis is almost invariably preceded by tachypnea and retraction of the chest wall, frequently with grunting respirations. The infant with cyanosis due to congenital heart disease may be tachypneic but otherwise appears comfortable unless the cyanosis is severe and prolonged, with development of acidosis. In the infant with respiratory distress syndrome, there may be a striking parasternal lift, hepatomegaly, rales, and a systolic murmur, and cardiomegaly may develop later. Chest roentgenograms may show the characteristic reticulogranular appearance of the lungs and "air bronchograms" due to hypoaeration. Right-to-left shunting can occur through the foramen ovale and ductus arteriosus as well as in the lungs.

The infant with cyanosis secondary to disease of the central nervous system will have other neurological manifestations. Periodic breathing and peripheral vasomotor instability found in the normal newborn may be accentuated. In methemoglobinemia, blood exposed to air will retain a brownish color instead of becoming a normal bright red. The syndrome of persistent fetal circulation is very important since it may be the most difficult to distinguish from cyanotic forms of congenital heart disease. Two-dimensional echocardiography is very helpful in distinguishing cyanotic heart disease[28] from other causes of cyanosis.

Cyanosis in congenital heart disease may be due to heart failure with pulmonary edema rather than to intracardiac right-to-left shunting. Measurement of the partial pressure of oxygen with the infant breathing 100 percent oxygen can help in diagnosis, since the hypoxia due to heart failure or lung disease with intrapulmonary shunting[29] will usually respond dramatically to oxygen administration, whereas that due to cyanotic defects will not. Low cardiac output and peripheral vasoconstriction can cause a grayish discoloration due to the underlying pallor, rather than typical cyanosis.

The normal full-term newborn infant has a hemoglobin concentration of 17 to 21 g/dl. This drops to 10.4 to 12.2 g/dl by 3 months of age and then slowly rises to 12 to 13 g/dl by 2 years.[30] Systemic arterial desaturation will result in polycythemia with a higher hemoglobin level after the newborn period.

Cyanosis will lead to clubbing, which appears after the age of 3 months, initially as fullness at the base of the thumbnail with obliteration of the normal concavity. Tachypnea and dyspnea may be due to desaturation and are exaggerated with exercise. Squatting may also occur. Paroxysms of increased cyanosis, as seen in tetralogy of Fallot, can occur, with an increase in the rate and depth of respiration, without obstruction to airflow. Failure to gain weight is usually an indication of heart failure and not of cyanosis alone, unless the hypoxia is extreme.[31]

To a large extent, the complications of cyanosis result from polycythemia and paradoxical embolism. In patients with prolonged polycythemia, the resultant hyperuricemia can precipitate a secondary form of gout.[32] Most frequently the central nervous system is the target organ, with cerebrovascular accidents and brain abscesses occurring[6] as a result of the effects of polycythemia and paradoxical embolism, especially in the setting of dehydration or febrile states. Paradoxical embolism is a potential complication whenever a right-to-left shunt exists. An infected venous thrombus or ulfiltered blood during a bacteremia can cause a cerebral abscess. Brain abscess is rare under 2 years of age. The incidence and mortality are directly related to the degree of hypoxia.[33] Thrombosis, embolism, and hemorrhage can cause cerebrovascular accidents. Venous thrombosis is a common finding at autopsy, particularly in tetralogy of Fallot or transposition of the great arteries. A majority of instances occur in infants up to 1 year of age, with relatively few after 4 or 5 years of age. The younger patients very frequently have iron deficiency anemia, relative to the degree of desaturation, whereas the older patients have polycythemia.[34] Rheological studies in cyanotic patients have demonstrated impaired deformability of microcytic erythrocytes.[35]

Disturbances in hemostasis also occur with polycythemia.[6] Coagulation factors are commonly abnormal in patients with hematocrits in excess of 60 percent.[36] Actual platelet counts may be normal, but they can be increased initially in some patients, with subsequent decreases related to persistent and worsening desaturation.[37] There is evidence of shortened platelet survival time in patients with cyanotic heart disease.[38] Laboratory evaluation of coagulation status requires that to avoid false results, correction be made for the diminished volume of plasma and for the volume of anticoagulant used in the blood samples.

The major consequences of cyanosis can be avoided in many instances. Prevention of iron deficiency by dietary supplementation in infants and of excessive polycythemia by surgical intervention should decrease the number of cerebrovascular accidents and help prevent the occurrence of brain abscess.

Pulmonary Arterial Hypertension and Pulmonary Vascular Obstructive Disease

Pulmonary arterial hypertension (PAH) and pulmonary vascular obstructive disease (PVOD) are serious and feared complications of congenital heart disease. PAH usually is the result of direct transmission of systemic arterial pressure to the right ventricle or pulmonary artery via a large communication. Less frequently, it is due to severe obstruction to blood flow through the left side of the heart at the pulmonary venous level or beyond. *PVOD* refers to a process involving structural and developmental changes in the smaller muscular arteries and arterioles of the lung that gradually diminishes and eventually destroys the ability of the pulmonary vascular bed to transport blood from the larger pulmonary arteries to the pulmonary veins without an abnormal elevation of the proximal pulmonary arterial pressure.

Pulmonary resistance (R_p) may be as high as 8 to 10 units/m^2 immediately after birth but falls rapidly throughout the first week; by 6 to 8 weeks it usually has reached the normal adult levels (1 to 3 units/m^2).[4] The pulmonary arterial pressure is free to vary independently of the systemic arterial pressure following spontaneous closure of the ductus, usually within 10 to 15 h after birth; it normally declines rapidly, in the face of the diminishing pulmonary resistance, reaching normal adult levels by about 7 days of age. These changes are accompanied by a gradual dilatation of first the smaller and then the larger muscular pulmonary arteries and then, in the weeks and months that follow, a thinning of their muscular walls, an extension of muscle more peripherally into the acinus, growth of existing arteries, and the development of new arteries and arterioles. The latter process contributes over 90 percent of the smaller or intraacinar pulmonary arterial vessels present in the older child and adult.[39]

Increased pulmonary arterial pressure has an adverse effect on the normal maturation of the pulmonary vascular bed. This encourages a persistence of the thick muscular medial layer present in the smaller pulmonary arteries of the term newborn, stimulates an extension of smooth muscle into smaller and more peripheral arteries than normal for age and, lastly, retards the growth of existing and the development of new acinar arteries.

In the presence of a large systemic-to-pulmonary communication, pulmonary arterial pressures tend to remain at or near systemic levels, with the result that the diminution in pulmonary muscle mass and pulmonary resistance is less rapid and of less magnitude than it is in the normal infant. Nevertheless, the diminution is usually sufficient to permit a large pulmonary blood flow and, as a result, to cause congestive failure by the end of the first month. Exceptions are found among those infants with a large systemic-to-pulmonary communication but with alveolar hypoxia, a stimulus for pulmonary vasoconstriction, in whom there is less than normal involution of the medial musculature and diminution in pulmonary vascular resistance. Clinically, this is expressed by the lower incidence of congestive failure observed among infants with large ventricular septal defects born and living at high altitude and by the increase in pulmonary blood flow and the appearance of congestive failure in such infants if they are transported from high altitude to sea level.[40] Rarely an infant will maintain a very high pulmonary vascular resistance in the face of an anatomically large systemic-to-pulmonary communication, without evidence of significant hypoxia or acidemia, and remain free of the signs and symptoms of congestive failure. In the premature infant, in whom the medial muscle mass is less at birth than it is in the full-term infant, the fall in pulmonary vascular resistance usually is much more rapid than normal and, in the face of a large systemic-to-pulmonary communication, congestive failure may become severe within a matter of days.

Chronic PAH or increased flow, or both, produce a characteristic series of histological and morphometric changes, described by Heath and Edwards[41] and refined and extended by Rabinovitch and colleagues,[42] which consist of the following:

- Grade I—increased medial thickness of the small pulmonary arteries and proximal pulmonary arterioles with extension of smooth muscle into smaller and more peripheral arteries than is normal for age. The latter appears related to increased flow rather than pressure.[42] These changes, noted as early as 4 to 6 weeks of age among infants with a ventricular septal defect,[41] probably are completely reversible. Assessment of the degree of extension of muscle and percent wall thickness of the muscular pulmonary arteries permits a further subdivision and refinement of this stage which has proved valuable for analysis of lung biopsy tissue.[42]
- Grade II—concentric or eccentric cellular intimal proliferation and thickening within the smaller pulmonary arteries and arterioles capable, in the extreme, of producing vascular occlusion. Increased shearing stresses, induced by increased velocity of blood flow within the narrowed muscular arteries resulting in internal injury and smooth muscle proliferation, are considered to play a role in the production of these lesions. Whether or not these changes are completely reversible is uncertain; if the changes are mild, it seems unlikely that significant residual obstruction will result even if complete regression does not occur. A reduction in the number of new arteries and a retardation of growth of existing arteries, recognized as early as 5 months of age in some instances, can be demonstrated in most, if not all, infants beyond 2 years of age with significant PAH. When grade II lesions are present, the arterial concentration, expressed as an alveolar/arterial ratio, can be recognized as being reduced and the R_p usually is greater than 3.5 units/m^2.[39]
- Grade III—relatively acellular intimal fibrosis with accumulation of concentric or eccentric masses of fibrous tissue leading to widespread occlusion of the smaller pulmonary arteries and arterioles. Grade III changes may be seen as early as 2 months of age in patients with transposition of the great arteries along with a large ventricular septal defect or patent ductus arteriosus and as early as 10 to 12 months of age in patients with complete atrioventricular canal. Grade III changes are seldom seen before 1 year of age in the infant with a small, isolated ventricular septal defect.[41] The arterial concentration, expressed as an alveolar/arterial ratio, is generally half normal with Grade III changes, and R_p is often greater than 6 units/m^2. It is unlikely that grade III changes are reversible.
- Grade IV—progressive, generalized dilatation of the muscular arteries and the appearance of plexiform lesions, complex vascular structures composed of a network or plexus of proliferating endothelial tissue, frequently accompanied by thrombus, within a dilated thin-walled sac. Whether these are the result of aneurysms of the media, of vasculitis, or of thrombosis is unclear, but their appearance signifies very severe PVOD. Grade IV changes may be seen as early as 2 to 4 months among patients having transposition with ventricular septal defect and by 10 to 12 months among infants with complete atrioventricular canal. They are rare before 2 years of age with isolated ventricular septal defect. Grade IV changes are considered irreversible.[41]
- Grade V—thinning and fibrosis of the media superimposed upon the formation of numerous complex dilatation lesions.
- Grade VI—necrotizing arteritis within the media and necrosis of muscle accompanied by surrounding areas of inflammatory reaction and granulation tissue. This form of PVOD is extremely rare among patients with congenital heart disease and is found more commonly among patients with primary pulmonary hypertension.

Estimation of pulmonary vascular resistance from data obtained at cardiac catheterization remains the most widely used means of assessing the state of the pulmonary vascular bed. Hypoxia from oversedation, atelectasis, or pneumonia at the time of study should be scrupulously avoided. If pulmonary vascular resistance is elevated, its responsiveness to vasodilatation induced by the inhalation of 100 percent oxygen or the intravenous administration of tolazoline, or both, should be tested.

Values of R_p values of 3 units/m^2 or less are considered normal, although in an infant with a large ventricular septal defect and high pulmonary blood flow a resistance of 2 units undoubtedly reflects an increase in vascular tone, since the normal pulmonary vascular bed responds to such a high flow with a reduction of R_p to levels of 0.5 units/m^2 or less. R_p may also be expressed as a ratio of pulmonary vascular resistance to systemic vascular resistance (R_p/R_s). Pulmonary/systemic resistance ratios of less than 0.2:1 are considered normal.

As pulmonary vascular resistance increases, pulmonary blood flow generally decreases. Eventually a point is reached where surgical closure of the defect will produce only a small diminution of blood flow, a proportionately small decrease in pulmonary arterial pressure, and no significant change in the factors contributing to the progression of the vascular disease. Patients in this category are considered prohibitive risks for surgery because of the increased mortality associated with the procedure and the early postoperative period. An R_p/R_s ratio of 0.7:1 or greater, or an R_p of 11 units/m^2 or more with a pulmonary/systemic blood flow ratio of less than 1.5:1 are the criteria generally used to define this situation. Without surgery, these patients survive as examples of the *Eisenmenger syndrome,* where pulmonary vascular resistance is equal to or greater than systemic vascular resistance and in whom at least some right-to-left shunting occurs at rest or with exercise. These patients may survive for several decades, leading productive lives, with relatively mild symptoms and few limitations.[43]

The decision regarding surgery for patients with less severe PVOD is a clinical one. The higher the resistance at any given age, or the older the patient with any given level of elevated resistance, the less likely it is that the outcome will be satisfactory. Data compiled by Blackstone and colleagues[44] indicate that the chances of a 2 year old having a satisfactory outcome (defined as the patient surviving the operation and having a mean pulmonary arterial pressure of less than 25 mmHg 5 years or more later) are 90 percent if the R_p is 4 units/m^2, 75 percent if R_p is 8 units/m^2, and only 55 percent if the R_p is 12 units/m^2, provided that the pulmonary/systemic blood flow ratio is greater than 1.3:1. By the same token, a satisfactory outcome with R_p of 8 units/m^2 would be in the range of 75 percent for a 2 year old, 65 percent for a 3 year old, and only 50 percent for a 4 year old.[44] Open lung biopsy[42] or magnification pulmonary wedge angiography[39] are of value in judging the severity of pulmonary vascular disease in this group of patients.

The prevention of PVOD is of far greater service to the patient than is an accurate estimate of the degree of its severity once established. For prevention one needs first to identify those patients at risk, namely all patients with a systemic-to-pulmonary communication and a pulmonary arterial systolic pressure greater than half the systemic arterial systolic pressure. Also included would be all patients with transposition, regardless of pressure or flow, with the possible exception of those with severe pulmonary stenosis or pulmonary arterial banding with documented pulmonary arterial pressures in the normal range. Ideally all patients at risk should undergo correction or pulmonary arterial banding unless there is proof that the pulmonary arterial systolic pressure has fallen to or is less than half the systemic systolic pressure before the end of the first year of life. Among patients with transposition with a large ventricular septal defect, action must be taken within the first 6 months of life; among those with normally related great arteries, correction or banding by the end of the first year probably is acceptable.

Retardation of Growth and Development

On a standard growth chart the third percentile line represents two standard deviations below the mean. Children with mild congenital abnormalities of the heart tend to grow normally. Those with more severe malformations frequently have evidence of serious growth abnormality, namely, height and weight measurements near or below the third percentile or weight measurements 20 percentile points or more below those for height.[45]

Growth retardation is most severe among those children with overt cyanosis and those with large left-to-right shunts causing heart failure. Cyanosis tends to produce a rather parallel retardation of both height and weight, while heart failure tends to cause a greater retardation of weight than height. Skeletal retardation, reflected by bone age, usually occurs along with height and weight retardation, and among children with cyanotic heart disease, it can be correlated with the severity of hypoxia. In general girls are more resistant than boys to factors producing growth retardation.

Other factors may play a serious role in the growth retardation. Insufficient caloric intake is caused by anorexia, dyspnea, frequent infections or psychological disturbances, malabsorption, and hypermetabolism. Among infants with severe congenital heart disease recognized within the first year of life, there is a significantly increased incidence of subnormal birth weight, intrauterine growth retardation (6.1 percent), and major extracardiac anomalies (19.9 percent).[46] Finally, a relatively small number of children will have associated syndromes known to be characterized by growth retardation, such as rubella and Noonan's, Turner's, or Down's syndromes.

Growth retardation related primarily to the congenital heart disease usually responds to surgical correction or palliation of the malformation, with an impressive acceleration of growth and a return to or toward normal measurements. Acceleration tends to be greatest in children operated upon in the first year or two of life, with weight showing a more abrupt change than height. Girls tend to experience a more complete return to normal than boys do. If the acceleration of weight gain and linear growth is small, such factors as additional unrecognized heart disease or inadequate repair or palliation should be considered.

While cardiac surgery seldom is recommended on the basis of growth failure alone, this undesirable trend should be recognized early and, until proved otherwise, considered an index of the severity of heart disease. In general the earlier and the more successful the surgery the less will be the retardation of growth and development, with its sequelae of physical, psychological, and intellectual problems.[45]

Exertional Intolerance and Restrictions

Certain infants and children with congenital heart disease may manifest exertional intolerance that is clinically overt. The infant with heart failure frequently demonstrates intolerance with feeding, since this is a major form of exercise for the infant. The child with a significant degree of cyanosis may squat or breathe more deeply and rapidly during play. Increased need for sleep or rest can parallel the increase in motor activity seen with increasing age. In general, infants and children with such overt manifestations of intolerance to exercise will restrict their own activities on the basis of their physical capacities so that there is usually no need for parental or other external restrictions.

For the less severely restricted or asymptomatic child, the questions of parents usually revolve around the potential harm of exercise. How much a child can do and how the heart responds to exercise should be used as guides when making recommendations concerning the need for external restrictions of activity. Exercise testing with measurement of work capacity and electrocardiographic and cardiorespiratory responses are useful in evaluating these children.

Data on the responses of normal children to exercise, measured using bicycle and treadmill protocols,[47–49] and that of children with specific defects are available.[6,47,48] In general terms, exertional endurance is commonly affected in those children with heart disease,[50] but usually it is adequate for participation in childhood activities. Only children with cyanosis or other severe disease have consistently reduced exercise capacity. Individual variability is expected. Radionuclide angiography can be combined with exercise to assess reserve more definitively in selected patients.[51]

Restrictions other than those due to limited physical capacity exist for young people with congenital heart disease. Problems with insurability[52] and employment are recognized, and efforts to minimize these are ongoing.

Intracardiac Communications between the Systemic and Pulmonary Circulations, Usually without Cyanosis

When a communication exists between the two circulations, it usually takes the form of a septal defect or a communication between the aorta, on one hand, and the pulmonary arterial system, on the other. In the uncomplicated state, such communications are responsible for left-to-right shunts. Cyanosis is absent unless pulmonary vascular obstructive disease appears.

Shunts may be divided into those which are *intracardiac* and those which are *extracardiac*. The intracardiac shunts result from defects in either the atrial or the ventricular septum. In some cases the lesion is an isolated one; in others it is part of a complex anomaly, as in common atrioventricular canal. Because a partial anomalous pulmonary venous connection may resemble an atrial septal defect functionally and clinically, the former condition will also be considered in this section. Conditions in which a shunt begins in an extracardiac structure and leads to the right atrium or to the ventricle or pulmonary vascular system are considered under "Extracardiac Communications."

Ventricular Septal Defect

Definition

Ventricular septal defect represents an opening in that part of the ventricular septum that separates the two ventricles. (Left ventricular–right atrial communication is a special type and is discussed separately.)

Pathology

A defect of the ventricular septum represents the most common alteration among malformed hearts. In some this is the only condition, while in others it is part of a complex malformation.

Anatomic Types Three-fourths of all defects are paramembranous and lie in the outflow portion of the right ventricle immediately below the crista supraventricularis and posterior to the papillary muscle of the conus. Less common are the conal or supracristal defects (8 percent), posterior defects lying beneath the septal leaflet of the tricuspid valve in the region of the atrioventricular canal (4 percent), and, finally, defects toward the apex of the right ventricle in the muscular septum (15 percent).[53] (See Fig. 36-1.)[54]

Defects lying in the wall of the right ventricular outflow tract are, from the left ventricular aspect, closely related to the aortic valve and may be overhung by it (Fig. 36-2). Multiplicity of muscular defects is characteristic, the defects being represented by tortuous channels within the septum.

FIGURE 36-1 Types of ventricular septal defects. *1.* A high defect immediately under the pulmonary valve. 2. The typical high ventricular septal defect. 3. The atrioventricular canal type of ventricular septal defect. *4.* A defect in the muscular portion of the septum. (*From J. W. Kirklin, H. G. Harshbarger, D. E. Donald, and J. E. Edwards, Surgical Correction of Ventricular Septal Defect: Anatomic and Technical Considerations, J. Thorac. Cardiovasc. Surg., 33:45, 1957. Reproduced with permission from the publisher and authors.*)

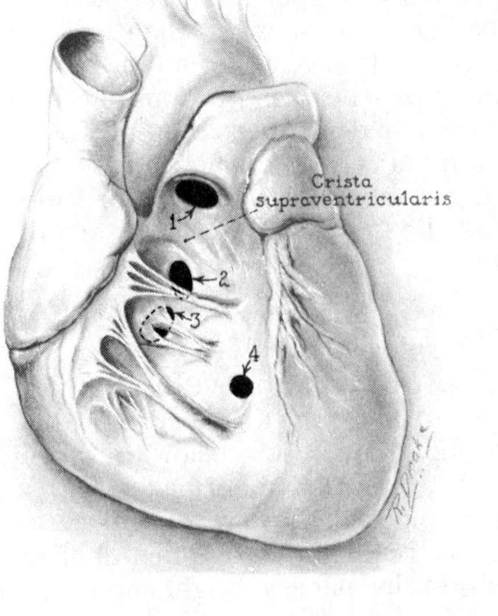

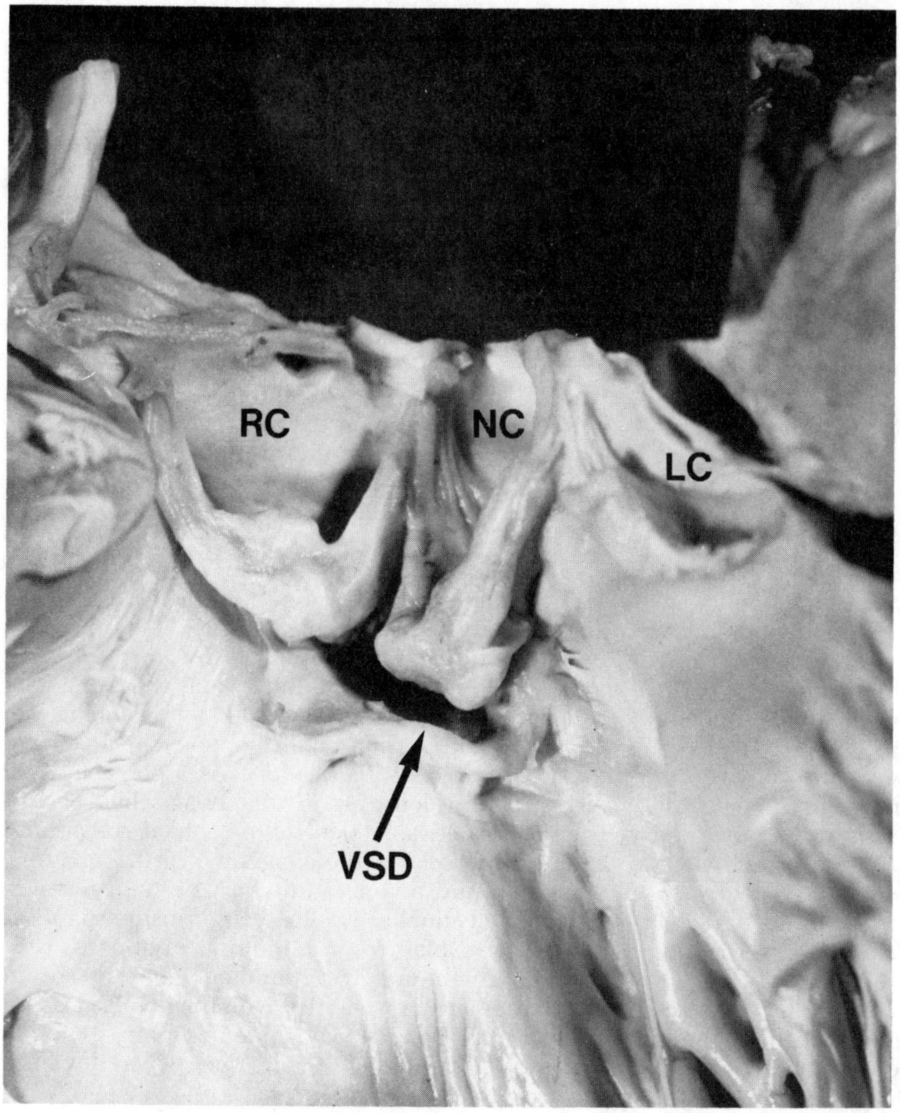

FIGURE 36-2 Necropsy specimen of aortic valve (viewed from left ventricular aspect) from a patient with ventricular septal defect (VSD) and aortic valve regurgitation. Note prolapse of noncoronary cusp (NC) with elongated, pendulous free edge of leaflet. RC = right coronary cusp; LC = left coronary cusp. (*This illustration appeared originally in the first edition of "The Heart," in 1966, and in all subsequent editions. It is reproduced here by courtesy of Dr. John W. Kirklin, Birmingham, Alabama.*)

The major conduction tissue is most closely related to the infracristal defect. The bundle of His and the left bundle branches lie close to the posteroinferior and inferior rim of the defect and favor the left side of the edge of the defect.

The Cardiac Chambers Because the blood flows through the small ventricular septal defect in a jetlike fashion, it may cause focal fibrous deposits or jet lesions on the anterior wall of the right ventricle and the tricuspid valve.

In the large defect, jet lesions are not present. The pulmonary trunk is considerably wider than the aorta, and the right ventricle is about as thick as the left. The left atrial and left ventricular cavities tend to be enlarged in instances with large left-to-right shunts. After complicating occlusive pulmonary vascular lesions develop and the volume of left-to-right shunt flow falls, there is some regression in size of the chambers, notably of the left ventricle, which may assume a normal size.

Aortic regurgitation may develop in childhood or adolescence as a consequence of lack of support of the aortic root. It is seen typically in supracristal defects (Fig. 36-2) and in some infracristal defects.[55]

Associated Conditions The most common malformations found associated with ventricular septal defect among postmortem specimens have been, in order of decreasing frequency, as follows: (1) obstructive anomalies of the aorta, of which coarctation was the most common; (2) additional shunts, most commonly atrial septal defect of the fossa ovalis type and patent ductus arteriosus; (3) intracardiac obstructions such as subaortic stenosis, mitral stenosis, and anomalous muscle bundle of the right ventricle; and (4) incompetent valves.

Abnormal Physiology

The physiology of ventricular septal defect is largely dependent upon the size of the defect and the reaction of the pulmonary vasculature. Patients with isolated ventricular septal defect may be divided into three groups, depending on the size of the defect. In the first the defect is small, probably less than 0.5 cm^2/m^2, and, consequently, the defect itself offers a large resistance to flow. There is no elevation of pulmonary arterial pressure. The left-to-right shunt may be so small that it is not detected by oxygen analysis of blood samples from the right side of the heart and pulmonary artery, but it can be detected by special indicator techniques. This type of defect imposes little burden on the heart except for the danger of infective endocarditis.

In the second group of patients, the defect is moderate in size, probably 0.5 to 1.0 cm^2/m^2 in effective cross-sectional area, but it permits a separation of right and left ventricular systolic pressures with the right ventricular systolic pressure generally being 80 percent or less of the left ventricular systolic pressure. A large left-to-right shunt may be present, with resulting left atrial hypertension and dilatation and serious left ventricular volume overload. Usually the right ventricular and pulmonary arterial pressures are only mildly or moderately elevated. The development of pulmonary vascular disease among these patients is unusual but possible.

In the third group of patients, the effective area of the defect is approximately equal to or greater than the aortic valve orifice, or at least 1.0 cm^2/m^2. This defect offers virtually no resistance to the flow of blood; consequently, the systolic pressures in both ventricles, the aorta, and the pulmonary artery are essentially the same. The relative proportion of blood going to the two circulations is directly governed by the relative resistance of the two vascular beds.

At birth, the pulmonary vasculature has high resistance and there is little if any left-to-right shunt despite the presence of a large defect. After birth, the usual decrease in pulmonary vascular resistance begins. This decrease continues over the first few weeks of life, although the rate of decrease is somewhat less rapid than it is in the normal newborn. This permits a progressively greater amount of blood to flow through the defect, the lungs, and back to the left atrium and left ventricle. The high-volume work of the left ventricle produces an increase in its end-diastolic volume and pressure, which increases the stroke volume by the Frank-Starling mechanism. In some infants, the left ventricle "fails" and develops markedly elevated left ventricular end-diastolic pressure and left atrial pressure, producing pulmonary edema.

Other factors that may influence left ventricular performance include the degree of maturation of the myocardial contractile mechanism, the sympathetic innervation of the myocardium, the time available to increase ventricular mass by hyperplasia and hypertrophy, and the presence of additional stress due to anemia, fever, or infection. In addition, left ventricular function may be impaired by a decrease in left ventricular coronary blood flow secondary to elevation of left ventricular diastolic pressure or to tachycardia.

As a result of the above changes, clinical pulmonary congestion may occur at any time from about 3 to 12 weeks after birth in term infants born at sea level with a large ventricular septal defect. In premature infants, in whom the less well developed pulmonary vasculature regresses more rapidly, failure is frequently noted at 1 to 4 weeks. Among infants born at altitude with large ventricular septal defects, the lower partial pressure of inspired oxygen significantly delays and lessens the normal decrease in pulmonary vascular resistance and, as a result, heart failure is less common, less severe, and of later onset.

The harmful effects of continued high flow and elevated pressures upon the pulmonary vascular bed have been discussed in the preceding section "Pulmonary Arterial Hypertension and Pulmonary Vascular Obstructive Disease."

Clinical Manifestations

Ventricular septal defect is a common form of congenital heart disease, second only to a bicuspid aortic valve. It occurs as an isolated defect in approximately 23 percent of infants and children with congenital heart disease and occurs in combination with other important malformations in an additional 26 percent.[6] Its incidence is 2 per 1000 live births, its prevalence among school-age children has been estimated as 1 per 1000,[56] and it constitutes about 10 percent of the congenital cardiac malformations found among adults.[57] Males and females are affected equally. The mode of transmission usually is best explained on a multifactorial basis. It is the most common defect found among infants with chromosomal abnormalities, with the notable exceptions being Down's syndrome (trisomy 21) and Turner's syndrome (XO genotype), where it ranks second.

History Infants or children with a small isolated defect are asymptomatic. The murmur is usually detected at the first routine office examination following discharge from the hospital. The murmur of a small defect may actually be present within the first 24 to 36 h of life, since the very restrictive opening permits the normal rapid fall in pulmonary arterial pressures and resistance. Characteristically, infants with larger defects present between 3 to 12 weeks of age with congestive failure, frequently with associated lower respiratory tract infections. Parents describe tachypnea, grunting respirations, and fatigue, particularly with feedings. Weight gain is slow, and excessive sweating is common.

Physical Examination The child with a small defect is comfortable. A systolic thrill at the lower left sternal border is common, although with very small defects this may not be present. The second heart sound is normal. The systolic murmur along the lower left sternal border is characteristically holosystolic, but may be decrescendo and limited to early or midsystole. These latter features would suggest a defect in the muscular rather than the membranous ventricular septum.

Infants with large defects, large flow, and pulmonary arterial hypertension tend to be restless, irritable, and underweight. Linear growth is usually fairly well preserved, but weight is seldom above the third percentile. Moderate respiratory distress, with flaring of the nostrils and intercostal retractions, may be present, and respiratory rates of 80 to 100 are not unusual in such infants under 3 or 4 months of age. Both the right and left ventricular systolic impulses are impressively hyperdynamic to palpation. A thrill at the lower left sternal border is the rule. The second heart sound is narrowly split, with a loud, frequently palpable pulmonary component. Third heart sound gallops at the apex are common. Characteristically, the systolic murmur is holosystolic at the lower left sternal border and is accompanied by a middiastolic rumble of grade 2 to 3 intensity at the apex, the latter indicating a pulmonary/systemic blood flow ratio (Q_P/Q_S) of 2:1 or greater. Hepatic enlargement, a helpful guide to the severity of congestive heart failure, can be identified below the right costal margin. Pulmonary rales are common with severe failure.

With the passage of time one may observe signs of a diminishing left-to-right shunt with an improved rate of weight gain, less dyspnea, a diminution of the precordial hyperactivity, and disappearance of the apical diastolic flow rumble. This clinical improvement may be the result of the defect becoming smaller, the development of subvalvular pulmonary stenosis with little or no appreciable change in the size of the defect, or, most worrisome, the development of pulmonary vascular obstructive disease with continued severe pulmonary arterial hypertension. As the defect narrows, the lower sternal systolic murmur usually becomes more localized and softer and occasionally shortens in duration. The second heart sound splits easily with respiration, and the pulmonary component returns to normal intensity. With developing subpulmonary stenosis, the systolic murmur radiates more and more impressively to the upper left sternal border and the second heart sound becomes more widely split, with a progressive diminution in the intensity of the pulmonary component. Decreased flow due to pulmonary vascular disease is characterized by a gradual reduction in the intensity and duration of the systolic murmur, more narrow splitting of the second heart sound, and marked accentuation of the pulmonary component.

The clinical picture of advanced pulmonary vascular disease, or *Eisenmenger syndrome,* is that of a relatively comfortable older child, adolescent, or young adult with mild cyanosis and clubbing in whom one finds a prominent *a* wave in the jugular venous pulse. Prominence of the left anterior precordium may suggest cardiac enlargement during early childhood. Palpation usually reveals a mild right ventricular lift, a second heart sound which is narrowly split or virtually single with a very loud, usually palpable pulmonary component. An early pulmonary systolic ejection sound, reflecting dilatation of the main pulmonary artery, may be heard, and the systolic murmur is usually confined to early systole; with dominant right-to-left shunting, there may be no systolic murmur at all. In older adolescents and adults, the early diastolic murmur of pulmonary regurgitation (Graham Steell murmur) or a holosystolic murmur of tricuspid regurgitation may appear.[43]

Chest Roentgenogram In the presence of a small defect the heart size and shape are barely altered. The pulmonary blood flow may appear to be at the upper limits of normal. With large defects there will be moderate to marked enlargement of the heart with prominence of the main pulmonary arterial segment and impressive overcirculation in the peripheral lung fields. The left atrium is dilated in the absence of an associated atrial septal defect, and partial or complete atelectasis of the left lower lobe of the lung from bronchial compression is not unusual. With increasing pulmonary vascular disease, there is diminution in heart size toward normal while the central pulmonary arteries remain dilated. The peripheral pulmonary arterial markings become attenuated and a "pruned" effect is produced in the outer third of the lung fields (Fig. 36-3).

Electrocardiogram With a small defect, one can expect the normal progression of the mean QRS axis from right to left and the normal gradual diminution of the prominent right ventricular voltages

FIGURE 36-3 Frontal view of the chest roentgenogram of a 12 year old with a large ventricular septal defect and Eisenmenger syndrome. The main and central pulmonary arteries are markedly dilated while the peripheral segmental branches appear attenuated.

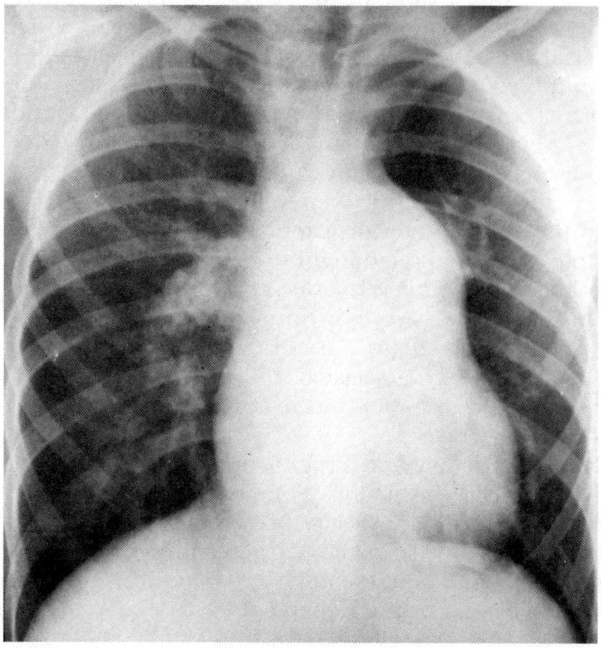

characteristic of the newborn. The left ventricular forces will either remain within normal limits or become slightly augmented as a reflection of the mild left ventricular volume overload. With large defects, the mean QRS axis tends to remain oriented to the right and there is little or no regression in right ventricular voltage. The left ventricular forces gradually increase, resulting in a pattern of biventricular hypertrophy within the first few weeks of life. Left atrial hypertrophy is usually present, and frequently right atrial hypertrophy is present as well. With the development of pulmonary vascular disease or significant pulmonary stenosis, the mean QRS axis progresses even further to the right, while the evidence of left ventricular and left atrial hypertrophy lessens or even disappears. Right ventricular and right atrial hypertrophy remain.

Echocardiogram M-mode and two-dimensional imaging provide valuable information concerning the position and orientation of the ventricular septum and can distinguish the uncomplicated ventricular septal defect from more complex malformations. Two-dimensional echocardiography is capable of imaging the defect directly when multiple transducer positions are used.[58]

Cardiac Catheterization An increase in oxygen saturation at the right ventricular level reflects the left-to-right shunt via the ventricular septal defect. With small defects, the right ventricular and pulmonary arterial systolic pressures are normal. With large defects, these pressures are at or near systemic levels and the mean left atrial pressure may be elevated to the 10- to 15-mmHg range. Left-to-right shunting also may be present at the atrial level due to a stretched foramen ovale when pulmonary blood flow is very large and the left atrium is hypertensive and dilated.

It is wise to obtain the following in addition to the routine right heart, pulmonary, and systemic arterial pressures and blood samples: (1) left atrial or pulmonary arterial wedge pressures or both; (2) left atrial or pulmonary arterial wedge pressures and left ventricular end-diastolic pressures in a manner that permits assessment of possible mitral valve obstruction; (3) selective left ventricular angiography in the anteroposterior, lateral, and oblique views to note the spatial relations of the great arteries to each other and to the ventricles and also to determine the exact site, size, and number of septal defects (Fig. 36-4); and (4) aortography to eliminate the possibility of an associated ductus arteriosus or unsuspected coarctation of the aorta.

Natural History and Prognosis

Fortunately, the majority of ventricular septal defects are small and do not present a serious clinical problem. Approximately 24 percent of these small defects close spontaneously by 18 months, 50 percent by 4 years, and 75 percent by 10 years.[59] Even large defects tend to become smaller and many eventually close.[44]

Congestive failure is a threatening and almost inevitable complication of large ventricular septal defects. Approximately 35 percent of infants with large defects will be symptomatic enough to warrant hospitalization by 4 weeks of age, and almost 80 percent will have required hospitalization by the age of 4 months.[3] The onset of failure beyond the age of 8 months is unusual and suggests additional complications. The risk of death with congestive failure is in the range of 11 percent, with slightly more than half of the deaths being among those infants with major noncardiac malformations and very low birth weights (under 2000 g).[3] Significant subvalvular pulmonary stenosis develops in approximately 3 percent of these individuals and may progress even to the point of severe tetralogy of Fallot. Pulmonary vascular obstructive disease is seldom severe and rarely irreversible in the first 12 months of life, but thereafter it becomes progressively more common and less likely to regress.[44] At risk of this complication are those infants and children with a pulmonary systolic pressure in excess of 50 percent of the systemic arterial systolic pressure beyond the first year of life.[60] Pulmonary vascular obstructive disease accounts for virtually all of the deaths in medically managed patients beyond infancy.[60] A very small number of the infants with large ventricular septal defects will maintain a relatively high level of pulmonary vascular resistance throughout the first year of life and will remain almost entirely free of symptoms and congestive heart failure. Irreversible

FIGURE 36-4 Left anterior oblique view of the left ventricular angiogram from a 5 year old child with a small, membranous ventricular septal defect (arrow). RV = right ventricle; LV = left ventricle; Ao = ascending aorta; PA = pulmonary artery.

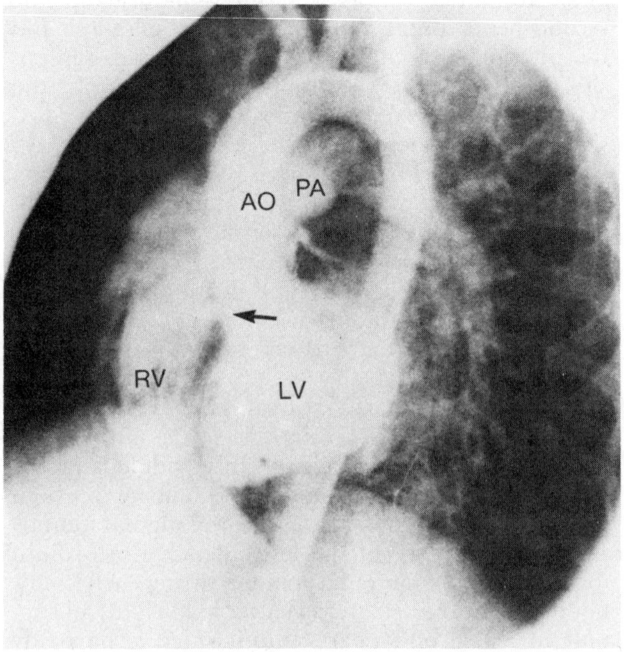

pulmonary vascular disease may develop in these patients without the usual and expected clinical signs and symptoms described above.[61]

A small number of children, 0.6 percent in a large group of carefully followed patients, will develop aortic regurgitation as a result of prolapse of the right, the posterior, or both aortic valve leaflets into the defect.[60] This complication is more prevalent among males, in a ratio of 2:1, and seems particularly likely to occur with defects in the supracristal or conal septum region (Fig. 36-2). Shunt size appears unrelated to the development of this complication. The characteristic aortic diastolic murmur may appear at any time between the ages of 12 months and 20 years. Regurgitation is usually progressive, sometimes rapidly so, and appears to predispose these individuals to infective endocarditis. The risk of infective endocarditis in patients with an uncomplicated ventricular septal defect managed medically is approximately 10 percent for the first 30 years of life, with the risk being some six times greater for the interval between 20 and 30 years than that from birth to 20 years.[60]

Medical Management

It is important to identify as early as possible those patients in whom the size of the defect is moderate or large, since these are the patients at special risk of developing congestive failure, pulmonary vascular disease, or serious pulmonary stenosis. The newborn should be reexamined at 1- and then 2-week intervals for the first 4 to 6 weeks in order to detect early signs of increasing cardiac volume overload. The electrocardiogram, repeated frequently in the early weeks, is particularly helpful in identifying those infants in whom the right ventricular systolic pressure is remaining at or near systemic levels. Heart failure is treated with digoxin and, if necessary, oral diuretics. Anemia is prevented or corrected and respiratory infections are treated promptly. The success of medical management depends so heavily upon the accuracy of the diagnosis and a knowledge of the pulmonary arterial pressure that it is appropriate to adopt a relatively low threshold for the recommendation of cardiac catheterization and angiography in these infants. At present we recommend cardiac catheterization for all infants who develop overt congestive heart failure or who retain impressive right ventricular or biventricular voltage in the electrocardiogram, or both. If the pulmonary arterial systolic pressure is greater than half the systemic systolic pressure and congestive failure is difficult to manage medically, the defect should be closed surgically. Exceptions would be those infants with multiple septal defects or large defects in the muscular septum for whom pulmonary arterial banding is recommended. If congestive failure is not severe, medical management is continued with the hope that spontaneous narrowing of the defect will occur. This trial of medical management is limited to no longer than 6 months; at that point, with or without clinical improvement, the patient undergoes repeat cardiac catheterization. If the pulmonary arterial systolic pressure is still greater than half of the systemic systolic pressure, the defect should be closed without delay. If the pulmonary pressure has fallen to less than half the systemic pressure, the infant may be managed medically into the second year of life with the expectation that the size of the defect will continue to diminish and that the pulmonary arterial pressure will continue its fall to normal levels.[60] This course must be supported by diminishing right ventricular potentials in the electrocardiogram and continued clinical improvement. If, by the second birthday, the pulmonary arterial pressure has not returned to normal (a mean pulmonary arterial pressure of less than 20 mmHg), as judged by persistent right or biventricular hypertrophy or direct measurement at catheterization, the defect should be closed. A few children will remain symptomatic or continue to have cardiac enlargement beyond the second year of life due to a large left-to-right shunt despite a normal pulmonary arterial pressure. At present, surgical closure is recommended before the child enters school if the pulmonary/systemic blood flow ratio (Q_P/Q_S) is above 1.8:1 or if symptoms or cardiac enlargement persist with the Q_P/Q_S above 1.4:1. Finally, closure of a defect in an adult is usually recommended if the flow ratio is above 1.4:1 and severe pulmonary vascular disease is not present.

Unfortunately, not all patients with a large defect are encountered during the first or even the second year of life, when it would be possible to prevent injury to the pulmonary vascular bed. If significant pulmonary arterial hypertension is allowed to persist, one can expect progression to irreversible pulmonary obstructive disease. For this reason prompt surgical closure of defects is recommended in all individuals beyond the age of 2 years if the pulmonary arterial systolic pressure is greater than half the systemic arterial systolic pressure, the mean pulmonary pressure exceeds 20 mmHg, or the pulmonary/systemic vascular resistance ratio exceeds 0.2:1. With severe pulmonary vascular obstructive disease, a point is reached eventually where the risks of death at operation or in the months or years immediately following operation due to progressive vascular disease more than offset the possible benefits from surgical closure. At present, surgery is recommended if the calculated pulmonary vascular resistance is less than 11 units/m^2 or if the ratio of the pulmonary/systemic vascular resistance is less than 0.7:1, provided the Q_P/Q_S ratio is still 1.5:1 or greater. In adults, the upper limit of pulmonary vascular resistance for surgery is approximately 800 dyn·s·cm^{-5}.

Those patients in whom the defect is judged clinically to be small at 2 or 3 months of age may be reexamined at 1- or 2-month intervals through the age of 6 months to be certain that the initial impression is supported by a normal weight gain, lack of symptoms, and a normal regression of the right ventricular forces in the electrocardiogram. Periodic examinations after that, at 1- or 2-year intervals, are advisable to reassure the patient and family, to reemphasize the importance of antibiotic protection against infective endocarditis, to document the further narrowing or closure of the defect, and (in a very small number of patients) to detect the first signs of aortic valve prolapse.

In those individuals with *Eisenmenger's complex*,[43] stamina is limited by systemic arterial hypoxia and, in some, right-sided heart failure. Complications to be anticipated include syncope, hemoptysis, brain abscess, hyperuricemia, and congestive failure. Pregnancy, with a mortality of 27 percent, and oral contraceptives are contraindicated. Transient symptomatic relief from extreme polycythemia may be achieved by careful erythropheresis. Travel to or living at high altitude is poorly tolerated, and supplemental oxygen should be provided and used in commercial airlines if the cabin pressure is permitted to decrease below pressure at sea level. The average age of death for individuals with Eisenmenger's complex is 33 years, with sudden death being the mode of exitus in the majority.[43]

Individuals with preoperative pulmonary arterial hypertension or elevated pulmonary vascular resistance should be restudied by cardiac catheterization 1 or 2 years following surgery. Earlier restudy is indicated if there is a persistent loud murmur, unexplained cardiac enlargement, or congestive failure. Following surgical repair, precautions against infective endocarditis are continued for at least 1 year in all patients and indefinitely in patients with any residual murmur. Symptoms suggesting an arrhythmia, particularly in a setting of postoperative right bundle branch block and left anterior hemiblock, should be evaluated by 24-h ambulatory monitoring of the electrocardiogram.[62]

The risk of congenital heart disease for a subsequent sibling of a single affected child is in the order of 3 to 4 percent. The risk to the child having one parent with ventricular septal defect is estimated at 4 percent. Pregnancy in the presence of a small defect and normal pulmonary vascular resistance does not appear to carry an increased risk to the patient or infant, although precautions against infective endocarditis should be observed.

Finally, when a patient with a residual defect or one who has undergone corrective surgery leaves the pediatric age group, arrangements should be made with an adult cardiologist for future care.[63]

Surgical Management

Although reduction of pulmonary blood flow by pulmonary arterial banding played an important role in management of ventricular septal defect prior to predictably successful open heart surgery in the infant, banding is now used only for complex and uncorrectable defects.[64,65] Complications of pulmonary arterial banding include deformity of the pulmonary arteries and the pulmonary valve, unpredictable palliation, progressive right ventricular hypertrophy, and subaortic left ventricular outflow tract obstruction. Early primary closure of ventricular septal defects is preferred, usually during the first two or three years of life.[66–68]

Ventricular septal defects in children weighing more than 10 kg are closed on total cardiopulmonary bypass with cardioplegia and moderate hypothermia (25 to 28°C). For smaller infants we prefer to use total circulatory arrest with profound hypothermia (18 to 20°C), cardioplegia, and considerable hemodilution (hematocrit 15 to 18 percent by volume).[69] Cardiopulmonary bypass with a single right atrial cannula for venous drainage and direct cannulation of the ascending aorta is used for cooling and rewarming.

Closure of the ventricular septal defect is usually accomplished through the right atrium and tricuspid valve orifice (Fig. 36-5).[70] This approach is particularly useful in patients having elevated pulmonary vascular resistance, where it is desirable to avoid injury to the right ventricle. The septal leaflet of the tricuspid valve can be incised near the annulus to facilitate exposure.[71] The outflow tract of the right ventricle can be incised transversely or longitudinally, avoiding major coronary arteries, for adequate exposure of high defects, particularly supracristal (type I) defects where a prolapsing aortic valve leaflet may be encountered.[55,72]

Care is required to avoid injury to the atrioventricular node near the ostium of the coronary sinus and to the bundle of His as it courses inferiorly near the tricuspid annulus, passing to the left side of the ventricular septum near the posterocaudal margin of the septal defect.[73] A Dacron patch is secured over the septal defect, using a series of fine, interrupted mattress sutures buttressed with Teflon felt pledgets.[74] Sutures are placed in fibrous tissue, well away from the inferior rim on the right side of the septum and parallel to the axis of the conduction system to avoid complete heart block. The portion of the patch adjacent to the tricuspid valve is anchored to the fibrous tricuspid annulus. Small septal defects with firm fibrous margins can be closed by direct suture without a patch.

Defects in the muscular septum (type IV) are frequently multiple and form the so-called Swiss cheese septum. They are usually small and can be closed by direct suture, but they may be difficult to locate through either the tricuspid orifice or a right ventriculotomy.[75] Exposure of muscular defects through an apical or posterior left ventriculotomy facilitates closure; care is required to avoid trauma to coronary arteries and mitral papillary muscles.[76]

The results achieved by primary closure of ventricular septal defects are generally excellent. Operative risk is 1 to 2 percent in older children with normal pulmonary vascular resistance. When growth retardation exists preoperatively in a young child, an acceleration of growth can be anticipated postoperatively. The pulmonary vasculature responds favorably when a left-to-right shunt is eliminated prior to the age of 2 years.

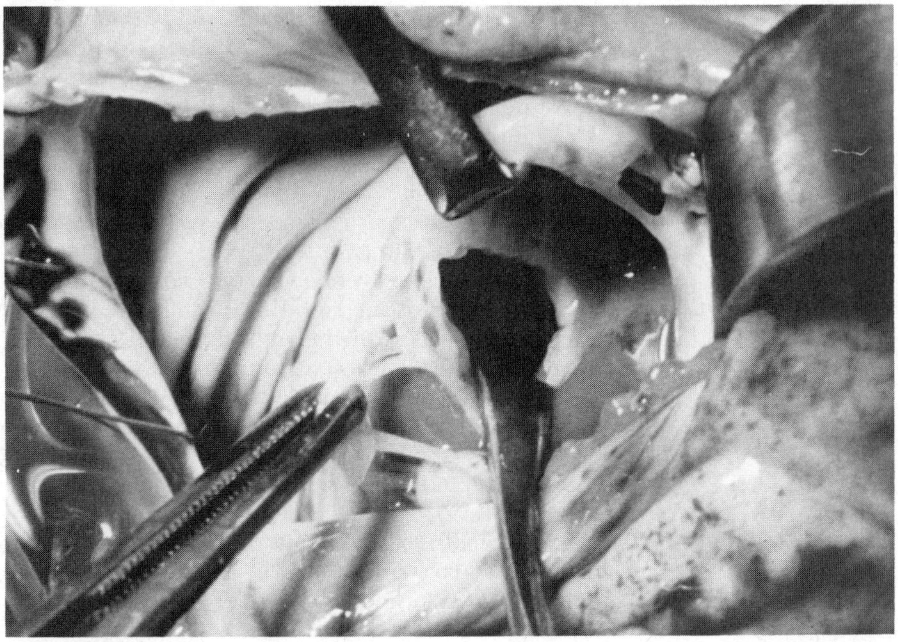

FIGURE 36-5 Exposure of the usual high perimembranous ventricular septal defect through the right atrial approach on cardiopulmonary bypass with hypothermic circulatory arrest. The defect is exposed through the retracted leaflets of the tricuspid valve. (*Courtesy of Dr. S. Bert Litwin, Milwaukee, Wisconsin.*)

Suboptimal postoperative results are largely due to preexisting pulmonary vascular obstructive disease, technical error producing complete heart block or a significant residual shunt, the development of left ventricular outflow tract obstruction in a patient having a previous pulmonary arterial band, or the presence of anatomically complex or multiple ventricular septal defects.

Rein and colleagues,[66] in a review of their experience with primary closure of ventricular septal defects in 50 infants during the first year of life for control of intractable congestive heart failure and failure to thrive, described only three hospital deaths (6 percent)—all in the second month of life. There were no late deaths. Only one of the 24 children subjected to repeat cardiac catheterization had a significant residual shunt. These good results in high-risk infants suggest the excellent prognosis to be expected in older children having normal pulmonary vascular resistance.

Atrial Septal Defect

Definition

An atrial septal defect is a through-and-through communication between the atria at the septal level. The condition is to be distinguished from the valvular-competent foramen ovale, a condition that is a potential opening. The latter is common in the adult population (approximately 35 percent).[77]

Pathology

Atrial septal defects are usually sufficiently large to allow free communication between the atria. They may be subdivided according to anatomic location (Fig. 36-6).[78,79]

FIGURE 36-6 Types of interatrial communications. *A.* Large ostium secundum type of atrial septal defect. *B.* So-called sinus venosus type of defect—one high in the atrial septum associated with anomalous connection of the right superior pulmonary vein to the junctional area of the superior vena cava and right atrium. *C.* Very large ostium secundum type of atrial septal defect with absence of the posterior rim. *D.* Partial form of common atrioventricular canal with cleft mitral valve. SVC = superior vena cava; RPVs = right pulmonary veins; IVC = inferior vena cava. (*From F. J. Lewis, P. Winchell, and F. A. Bashour, Open Repair of Atrial Septal Defects: Results in Sixty-Three Patients, JAMA, 165:922, 1957. Copyright 1957, American Medical Association. Reproduced with permission from the publisher and authors.*)

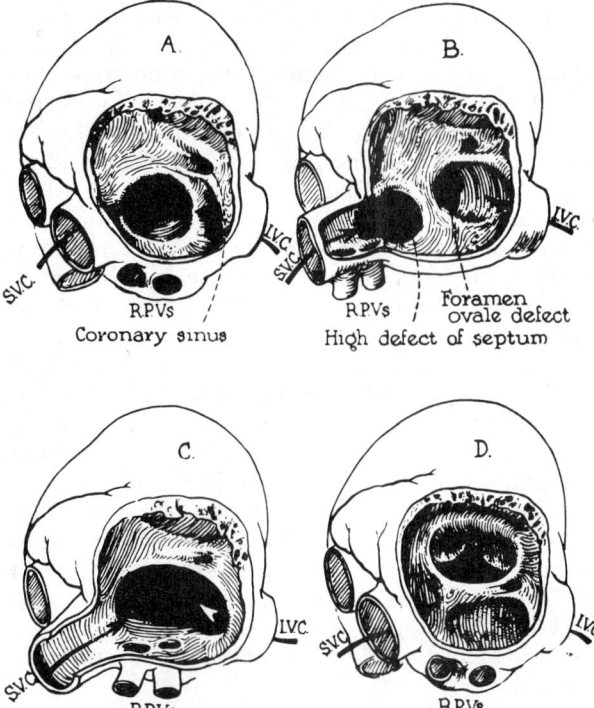

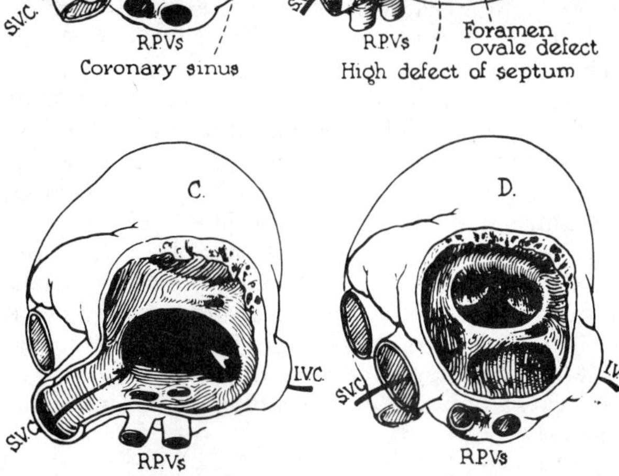

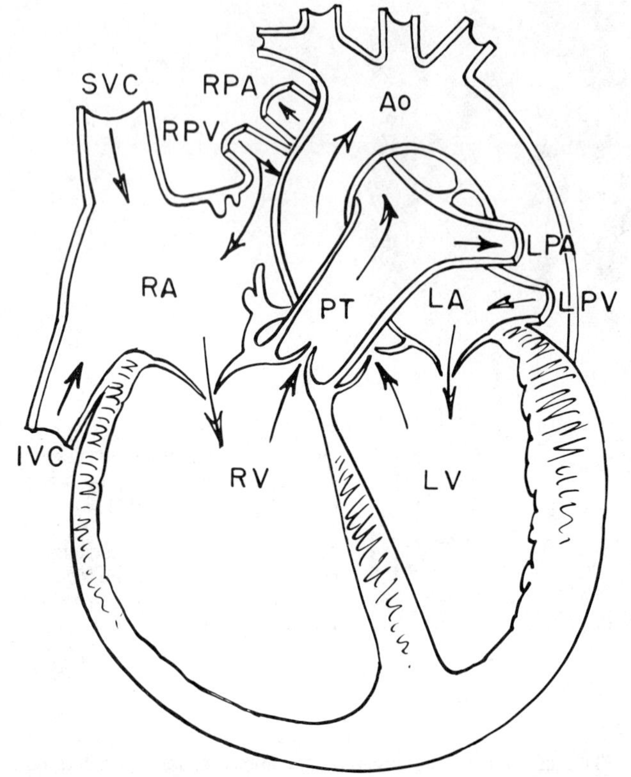

FIGURE 36-7 Atrial septal defect at fossa ovalis, with left-to-right shunt. SVC = superior vena cava; IVC = inferior vena cava; RA = right atrium; RV = right ventricle; PT = main pulmonary arterial trunk; RPA = right pulmonary artery; LPA = left pulmonary artery; RPV = right pulmonary vein; LPV = left pulmonary vein; LA = left atrium; LV = left ventricle; Ao = aorta. (*From J. E. Edwards, Classification of Congenital Heart Disease in the Adult, in W. C. Roberts (ed.), "Congenital Heart Disease in Adults," Cardiovasc. Clin. Series 10/1, F. A. Davis Company, Philadelphia, 1979, p. 1. Reproduced with permission from the publisher, editor, and author.*)

Anatomic Types *Defect at the Fossa Ovalis (Ostium Secundum).* This defect classically involves the region of the fossa ovalis and is the most common type (Fig. 36-6*A* and *C* and Fig. 36-7).[78,80] Its posterior border may be so deficient that the posterior atrial wall forms a boundary for the defect. Separating the inferior edge of the defect from the atrioventricular valves is atrial septal tissue. By virtue of its position, the defect has its posteroinferior zone in close proximity to the right atrial orifice of the inferior vena cava.

Various causes of left or right atrial enlargement may cause tensions or disproportions at the site of an initially valvular-competent foramen ovale so as to yield a septal defect. Removal of the underlying condition may result in spontaneous closure of this opening. Mitral stenosis and mitral valve prolapse are unusual but important associated defects.

Defect Inferior to the Fossa Ovalis. Defects of the atrial septum which lie inferior to the fossa ovalis usually are part of a complex malformation known as common atrioventricular canal defect (Fig. 36-6*D*).[78] This type of defect will be considered later in this section under "Common Atrioventricular Canal Defects."

Defect Superior to the Fossa Ovalis (Sinus Venosus Type). Some atrial septal defects lie superior to the fossa ovalis in close relation to the right atrial ostium of the superior vena cava (Figs. 36-6*B* and 36-8).[78,80] Such defects are but one of two parts of an entity in which the second element involves anomalous termination of right-sided pulmonary veins, either into the superior vena cava or into the right atrium near the junction of the two. Most often the anomalous connection is made by one vein or several veins from the upper lobe of the right lung, while the veins of the remaining part of the right lung and of the entire left lung join the left atrium normally. Less commonly, the venous system of the entire right lung is involved in the anomalous connection.[81]

Defect Posteroinferior to the Fossa Ovalis. This uncommon type of atrial septal defect is located in the posteroinferior angle of the atrial septum in the position normally occupied by the right atrial ostium of the coronary sinus (Fig. 36-6*C*).[78] This defect is part of a developmental complex consisting of this type of atrial septal defect with (1) absence of the coronary sinus and (2) entry of the left superior vena cava into the left atrium.[82] This type of atrial septal defect may also be associated with persistent common atrioventricular canal. Under this circumstance the atrial septal defects are continuous, resulting in a large defect involving the lower part of the atrial septum. This phenomenon commonly occurs in the

FIGURE 36-8 Sinus venosus type of atrial septal defect with anomalous termination of right pulmonary veins to the right atrium or to the superior vena cava. RUPV = right upper pulmonary vein; RLPV = right lower pulmonary vein; LUPV = left upper pulmonary vein; LLPV = left lower pulmonary vein. (*From J. E. Edwards, Classification of Congenital Heart Disease in the Adult, in W. C. Roberts (ed.), "Congenital Heart Disease in Adults," Cardiovasc. Clin. Series 10/1, F. A. Davis Company, Philadelphia, 1979, p. 1. Reproduced with permission of the publisher, editor, and author.*)

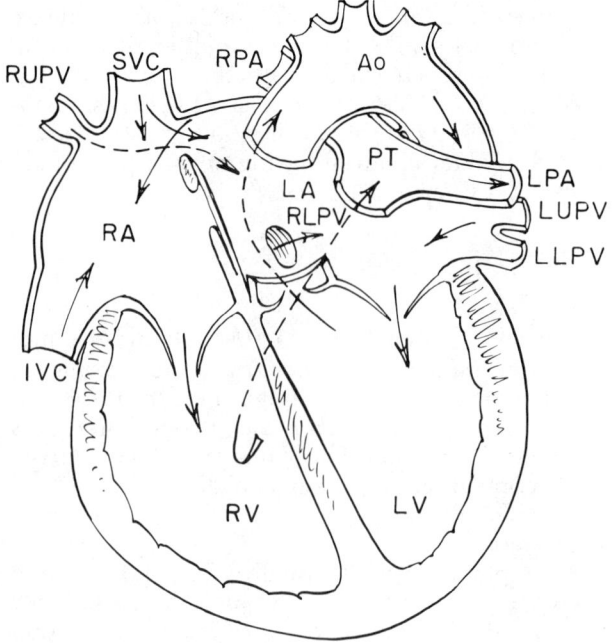

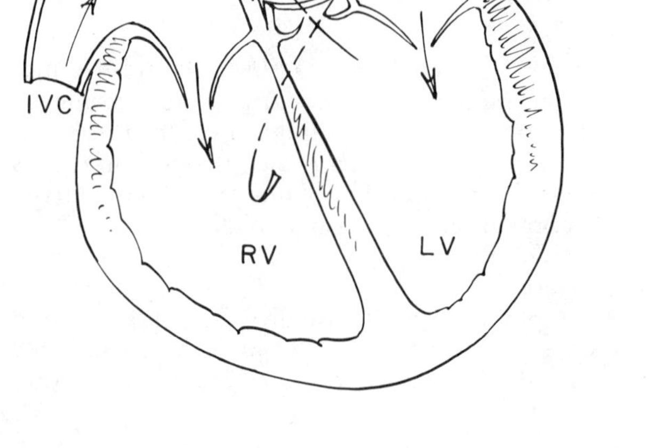

syndrome of asplenia with congenital cardiac disease, but it may be seen in cases in which the spleen is present.

Conditions Common to All Anatomic Types *The Cardiac Chambers.* The right atrial and ventricular chambers become grossly enlarged, but their walls are not hypertrophied. The left atrium has a tendency not to become enlarged. When atrial septal defect becomes complicated by pulmonary hypertension, the right ventricular wall becomes hypertrophied, but the right atrial and ventricular enlargement remain.

Pulmonary Vasculature. In uncomplicated atrial septal defect, the major pulmonary arteries are dilated and the pulmonary trunk is considerably wider than the aorta. The absolute caliber of the latter vessel may be less than normal.

When pulmonary hypertension is a complication, atherosclerosis occurs in the major pulmonary arteries. Saccular aneurysm and thrombosis with dissecting aneurysm or rupture may occur.

Pulmonary hypertension may develop, but usually not before the third decade. The earliest lesion appears to be characterized by cellular fibrous intimal thickening in the proximal segments of arterioles. The pulmonary arterial pressure then rises; this is followed by the development of medial hypertrophy of muscular arteries and the appearance of plexiform lesions. In the final state, the pulmonary vascular bed may be difficult to distinguish from that in ventricular septal defect with pulmonary vascular obstructive disease.[83]

Abnormal Physiology

The mean left atrial pressure may be slightly higher, usually by less than 3 mmHg, than that in the right atrium, but usually there is no resistance to blood flow across the defect and no significant pressure difference between the two atria. Most of the blood from the functional common atrial chamber will go to the right ventricle (Fig. 36-7), producing a left-to-right shunt of blood, because (1) the right atrial system is more distensible than the left, (2) the tricuspid valve is normally more capacious than the mitral valve, and (3) the thinner-walled right ventricular chamber will more readily accommodate a larger volume of blood at the same filling pressure than will the left ventricle after a few months of age. In about 70 percent of cases, a very small amount of blood passes from right atrium to left atrium, but this is so slight that it usually does not lower systemic arterial saturation below normal.

It has usually been assumed that there is little or no left-to-right shunt in atrial septal defects immediately after birth and before the rapid increase in left ventricular mass decreases the compliance of the left ventricle relative to that of the right ventricle. Subsequent studies, however, have shown that large left-to-right shunts can sometimes occur in this period and during infancy.[84]

In patients with secundum atrial septal defect the pulmonary arterial system undergoes normal maturation after birth, with most patients tolerating the tremendous volume load on the right ventricle and pulmonary circuit quite well for many years. With the development of pulmonary vascular disease and pulmonary arterial hypertension, the left-to-right shunt decreases, largely because of the increased thickness and decreased compliance or distensibility of the right ventricle. In some patients the process continues until there is eventually shunt reversal with arterial desaturation and cyanosis. It is not known why some patients with atrial septal defect have a progressive course and develop pulmonary vascular disease while other patients with the same apparent hemodynamics do not suffer the same fate.

Atrial Septal Defect Associated with Mitral Stenosis Atrial septal defect associated with mitral stenosis, referred to as *Lutembacher's syndrome,* has varying hemodynamic patterns, depending mainly on the size of the atrial septal defect and the severity of the mitral stenosis. If the atrial septal defect is large, there will be a large flow into the right ventricle and pulmonary artery.

Clinical Manifestations

Atrial septal defect is a relatively common cardiac malformation. It is found in approximately 10 percent of children surviving beyond the first year of life with congenital heart disease,[4] and if one excludes the congenitally bicuspid aortic valve, it is the most common form of congenital heart disease among adults. Between 20 and 25 percent of interatrial communications are of the ostium primum type, the partial form of the atrioventricular canal malformation, and are discussed below. The remainder, about 75 to 80 percent of atrial septal defects, are considered clinically to be of the secundum type. When these defects are identified surgically, approximately 70 percent prove to be limited to the central portion of the atrial septum (Fig. 36-6*A* and *C* and Fig. 36-7), 20 percent extend to the posterior atrial wall and inferior vena cava, and about 6 percent are found to be the sinus venosus type of defects adjacent to the superior vena cava (Fig. 36-6*B* and Fig. 36-8).[85] The remaining 3 or 4 percent are identified as multiple defects or other rare forms of interatrial communication, such as the coronary sinus defect.

Atrial septal defects are more common among females, with a female/male ratio of approximately 2:1. The mode of transmission is best explained in most instances on a multifactorial basis, where the risk would be approximately 2.5 percent for first degree relatives of a single affected family member. However, examples of autosomal dominant transmission are recognized either as an isolated entity, associated with severe atrioventricular conduction disturbances, or with upper extremity malformations as in the Holt-Oram syndrome. Examples of

Mendelian autosomal recessive transmission are found in the Ellis–van Creveld and thrombocytopenia–absent radius syndromes.[86]

History The majority of children are considered asymptomatic by themselves and by their parents. Probably most have some mild diminution of stamina, since it is not unusual for the patient or the parents to comment on the increased endurance that follows surgical correction. Symptoms of mild fatigue and dyspnea tend to be recognized in the late teens and early twenties, and approximately three-quarters of individuals will be definitely symptomatic as adults. Congestive heart failure is rare in childhood, but a few infants, perhaps 5 percent, will have heart failure in the first year of life. Failure becomes more common again in the fourth and fifth decades, usually associated with the onset of arrhythmias. Approximately 40 percent of adults develop severe symptoms such as easy fatigue, dyspnea, orthopnea, chest pain, and syncope.[87]

Physical Examination Many children have a slender habitus, but normal growth and development are the rule. Color, breathing, and the jugular venous pulse are normal in the absence of failure or severe pulmonary arterial hypertension. Prominence of the left anterior chest is common, and a hyperdynamic right ventricular systolic lift can usually be felt. The first heart sound may be slightly accentuated at the lower left sternal border. The two components of the second heart sound are characteristically widely split, with the interval of splitting relatively fixed despite expiration or the Valsalva maneuver. The pulmonary component of the second heart sound may be slightly to moderately accentuated, even in the absence of pulmonary arterial hypertension. With increasing pulmonary arterial pressure and resistance, the interval between the aortic and pulmonary components of the second heart sound narrows and the pulmonary component becomes louder, but the lack of respiratory influence on the interval between the two components persists. A midsystolic spindle-shaped murmur of grade 2 to 3 intensity at the left upper sternal border, reflecting increased right ventricular stroke volume, is to be expected. A low- to medium-pitched early diastolic murmur over the lower left sternal border, denoting increased diastolic flow across the tricuspid valve, is present in most individuals with large shunts. Findings of mitral valve prolapse, mitral stenosis, or mitral regurgitation occasionally occur. Adults with other causes of left atrial hypertension may have pulmonary rales, jugular venous distension, and hepatomegaly. Cyanosis and clubbing reflect right-to-left shunting. In this setting, the murmurs of tricuspid and pulmonary regurgitation are not uncommon.

Chest Roentgenogram Mild-to-moderate cardiac enlargement and prominence of the main and branch pulmonary arteries are characteristic. The ascending aorta is inconspicuous. The absence of left atrial displacement of the barium-filled esophagus in the lateral view helps to distinguish atrial septal defect from other large left-to-right shunts (Fig. 36-9). With advanced pulmonary vascular disease the findings are as with ventricular septal defect.

Electrocardiogram An rsR′ pattern over the right precordium, indicating mild right ventricular conduction delay or mild right ventricular hypertrophy,

FIGURE 36-9 *A.* Frontal and *B.* lateral chest roentgenograms of a 4-year-old child with a secundum atrial septal defect, a large left-to-right shunt, and normal pulmonary arterial pressures. Right ventricular enlargement (seen in the lateral view) accompanies prominence of the main pulmonary arterial segment and increased blood flow. No left atrial dilatation is present.

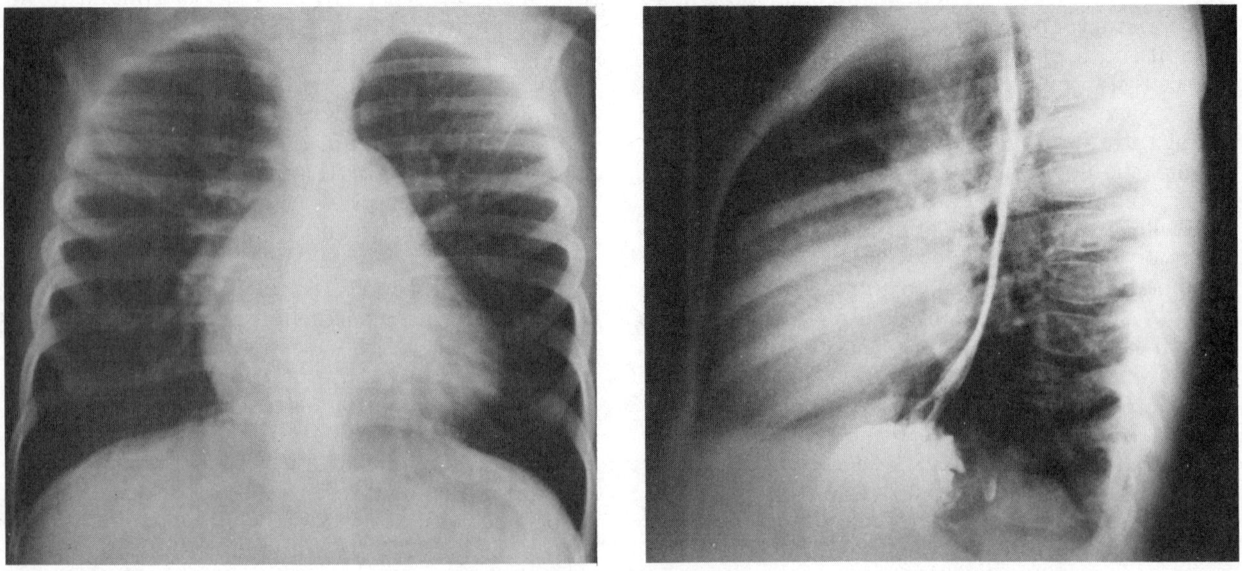

A B

is characteristic. The PQ interval is slightly prolonged in approximately 20 percent of patients. The mean QRS axis in the frontal plane is 90° or greater in 60 percent of patients, while a few (a little over 2 percent) will have a superior QRS axis lying between −10 and −160°. About half of these will have apparently uncomplicated secundum defects, while the remainder will be found to have a variety of unusual features such as mitral valve prolapse, hypertrophic cardiomyopathy, Noonan's syndrome, or single coronary artery. Serious arrhythmias are usually, though not invariably, limited to adults; atrial fibrillation and atrial flutter are the most common.

Echocardiogram Echocardiographic studies reflect the volume overload of the right side of the heart by showing an increase in right atrial and right ventricular dimensions as well as paradoxical ventricular septal motion (Fig. 36-10). Two-dimensional echocardiographic visualization of the atrial septum, preferably from the subcostal approach, permits identification of the secundum type of defects with a sensitivity approaching 90 percent. Two-dimensional contrast and Doppler studies enhance this sensitivity. Sinus venosus defects are more difficult to demonstrate, the success rate being in the range of 50 percent.[88]

Cardiac Catheterization There will be a significant increase in oxygen saturation in the blood samples drawn from the right atrium, right ventricle, and pulmonary artery compared with those from the superior or inferior venae cavae. Pulmonary arterial and right ventricular systolic pressures usually are normal or only slightly elevated. A systolic pressure gradient of up to 20 mmHg across the right ventricular outflow tract is accepted as secondary to flow rather than to organic obstruction. The right and left atrial mean and phasic pressures will be virtually identical, with little if any elevation above normal. A mean pressure gradient of 3 mmHg or more between the two atria should alert the operator to the possibility that the oxygen step-up at atrial level is due to a left ventricular–right atrial communication or to partial anomalous pulmonary venous connection, or that the interatrial opening is a stretched foramen ovale associated with left atrial hypertension. The cardiac catheter, if passed from the inferior vena cava, usually crosses a central interatrial opening easily. Passage across a sinus venosus defect may be difficult or impossible from this route. The site of connection of pulmonary veins can often be established by selective injections of contrast material in the individual veins or by dye-dilution studies.

Natural History and Prognosis

Defects of the secundum type usually go undetected in the first year or two of life because of the lack of symptoms and unimpressive auscultatory findings. A soft systolic murmur, perhaps considered innocent initially, is the usual reason for referral. A small number of infants have congestive heart failure in the first year, but most children and adolescents lead a normal life. In the late teens and twenties, symptoms become more common, and by age 40 the majority of individuals are symptomatic, some severely so.[87] Though rare in childhood,[89] pulmonary vascular disease with serious pulmonary hypertension

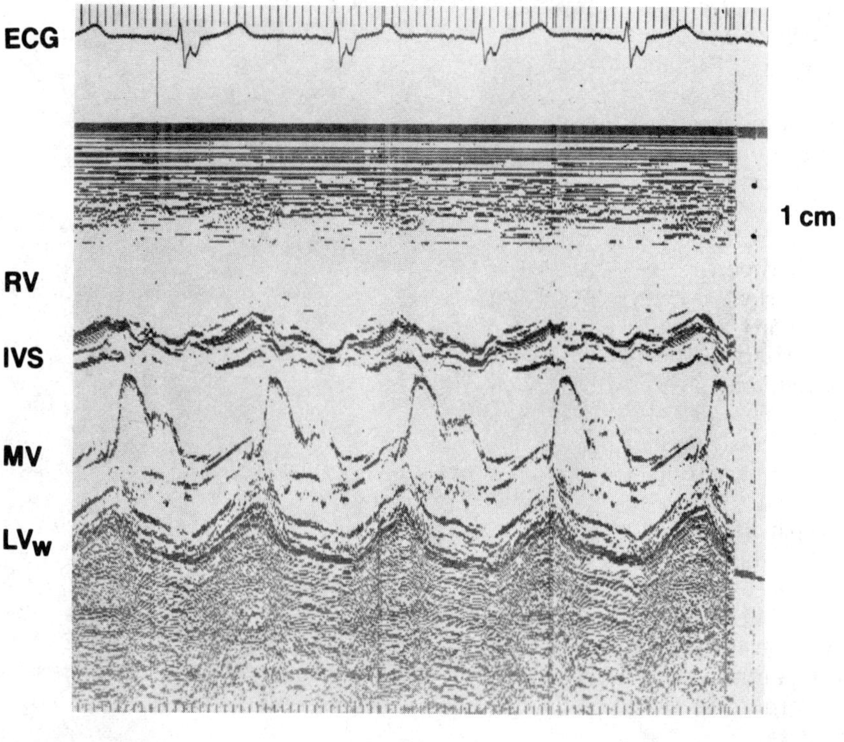

FIGURE 36-10 M-mode echocardiogram from a child with a secundum atrial septal defect demonstrating the increased right ventricular cavity dimension (2.4-cm end-diastolic diameter) and anterior systolic motion of the interventricular septum (IVS) characteristic of right ventricular diastolic overload. ECG = electrocardiogram; RV = right ventricle; MV = mitral valve; LV_w = posterior left ventricular wall.

begins to make its appearance in the early twenties. It affects approximately 15 percent of young adults with this defect, particularly women, and may be rapidly progressive, especially with pregnancy. The incidence of atrial fibrillation or flutter also increases with each decade and is closely linked to the onset of congestive failure. Mitral valve prolapse is detected in some, though usually a minority. Echocardiographic evidence of disappearance or diminution of prolapse following surgery suggests that a reversible distortion of the left ventricular cavity may be responsible for this abnormality rather than an intrinsic anatomic deformity of the mitral valve itself.[90] Spontaneous closure of secundum defects is rare beyond the first year of life. Although longevity is possible in the absence of closure, it is clear that the passage of time, certainly after adolescence, is associated with a steady increase in the frequency and the severity of symptoms, a higher prevalence of pulmonary arterial hypertension and pulmonary vascular disease, a greater number of individuals with important right ventricular dilatation and hypertrophy, a greater frequency of arrhythmias and congestive failure, and a higher mortality and morbidity with and following corrective surgery.[87] Congestive failure is the most common cause of death among patients with unoperated atrial septal defects. Other causes of death include pulmonary embolism or thrombosis, paradoxical emboli, brain abscess, and infection.

Medical Management
Asymptomatic infants and children are usually followed at yearly intervals and surgery recommended just prior to their entry into school or shortly thereafter. Restrictions on activity or exercise are usually unnecessary. If the physical, laboratory, and echocardiographic findings are completely characteristic, preoperative catheterization is not necessary; if there is any suspicion about the accuracy or completeness of the diagnosis, however, catheterization is indicated. Surgery is recommended if the pulmonary/systemic blood flow ratio is 1.7:1 or greater, provided no serious malfunction of the left side of the heart is present. Surgical closure is also recommended for those patients with ratios between 1.5:1 and 1.7:1 if right ventricular volume overload is evident on clinical examination or pulmonary arterial hypertension is documented by catheterization. Closure would seem prudent prior to pregnancy or to the use of contraceptives, in view of the tendency of a few individuals to develop rapidly progressive pulmonary vascular obstructive disease in this setting. Postoperative follow-up is recommended to determine the completeness of surgical repair, to document the extent of return to normal of the clinical and laboratory abnormalities, to manage arrhythmias dating from before or after the time of surgery, and to be certain that no previously undetected heart disease (particularly of the mitral valve) is present. Genetic counseling is in order. In the absence of a syndrome transmitted dominantly or recessively in a Mendelian pattern and if the patient is the only first degree relative affected, the risk of the next sibling or offspring of the patient having congenital heart disease is on the order of 2.5 percent.[91] Infective endocarditis is rare, but antibiotic coverage at times of possible bacteremia is recommended if associated mitral valve disease is suspected.

Surgical Management
Defects of the interatrial septum are closed by direct suture or placement of a pericardial or Dacron patch, depending upon the location and size of the defect and the integrity of the margins (Fig. 36-11). The operation is usually performed through a median sternotomy. A bilateral submammary skin incision or a right thoracotomy can be used in females and offers a much better cosmetic result. Total cardiopulmonary bypass with moderate hypothermia (30 to 32°C) and minimal hemodilution is used to pro-

FIGURE 36-11 *A.* Large atrial septal defect in the secundum position. *B.* Same defect, now closed by a knitted Dacron patch. (*Courtesy of Dr. S. Bert Litwin, Milwaukee, Wisconsin.*)

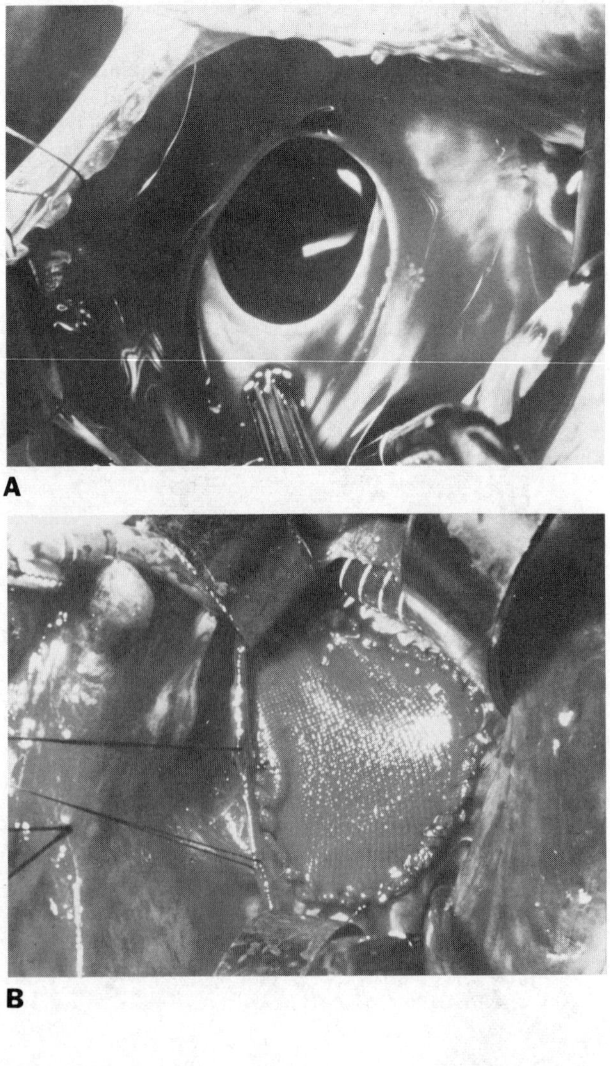

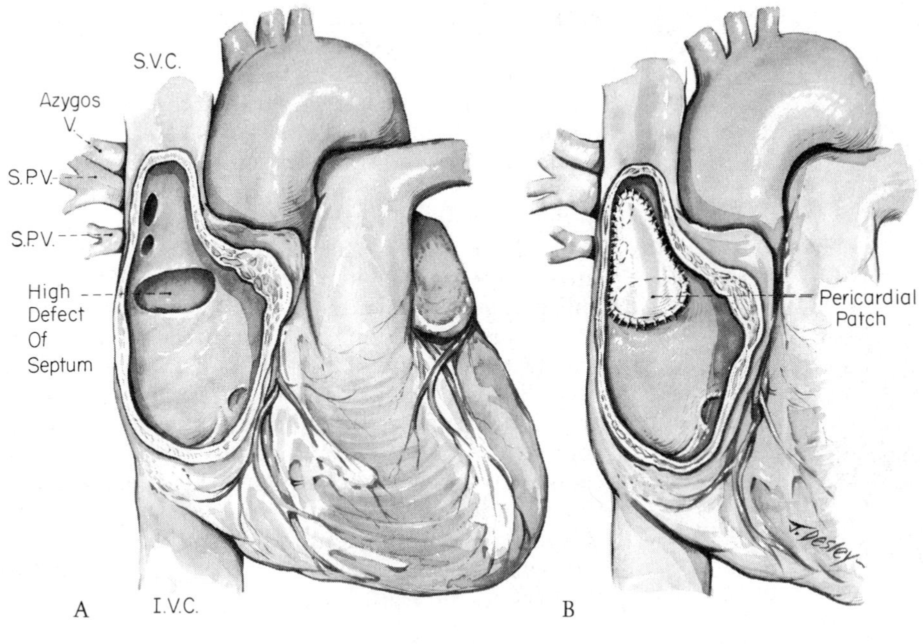

FIGURE 36-12 *A.* Sinus venosus type of atrial septal defect, with its constantly accompanying anomalous pulmonary venous connection of superior pulmonary vein (SPV) to superior vena cava (SVC). *B.* Repair is effected with a pericardial patch, so placed as to divert pulmonary venous blood across the defect into the left atrium and to divert superior vena caval blood to the right atrium. (*This illustration appeared originally in the first edition of "The Heart," in 1966, and in all subsequent editions. It is reproduced here by courtesy of Dr. John W. Kirklin, Birmingham, Alabama.*)

vide excellent visualization and protection from cerebral and myocardial ischemia. The risk of air embolization is reduced when this technique is combined with temporary aortic occlusion with or without cardioplegia. Operative mortality and morbidity have been virtually eliminated.

Foramen ovale defects are closed by simple suture during intracardiac repair of complex defects such as tetralogy of Fallot. Ostium secundum defects can be closed by direct suture if the margins are firm. If the membranous atrial septum has multiple fenestrations and tenuous margins, closure will require placement of a patch of pericardium or Dacron.

High atrial septal defects of the sinus venosus type are often associated with anomalous drainage of one or more right pulmonary veins into the superior vena cava. These defects are corrected by placement of a pericardial or tubular Dacron patch from above the abnormally draining vein down to and around the atrial septal defect (Fig. 36-12).[92] Pulmonary venous blood is thus diverted through the defect into the left atrium.[93,94] Pericardial gusset enlargement of the superior vena cava at the atrial junction may be required to avoid obstruction. Alternatively, the superior vena cava can be divided cephalad to the orifice(s) of high anomalous pulmonary vein(s) and anastomosed to the right atrial appendage; a patch in the right atrium diverts pulmonary venous blood through the atrial septal defect into the left atrium.[95]

Closure of ostium primum atrial septal defect is described as part of the repair of partial atrioventricular canal.

Consequences of an atrial septal defect in older patients include right atrial dilatation and hypertrophy, supraventricular arrhythmias, chronic congestive heart failure, tricuspid and mitral valvular incompetence secondary to ventricular and annular dilatation, and mild-to-moderate pulmonary vascular obstructive disease. Although clinical improvement can be anticipated following closure of atrial septal defects in adults with these complications, mortality is higher than it is in children and the degree of improvement uncertain.[96] Mortality in patients over 40 years of age may be as high as 5 percent.[97,98] The frequency of complications in adults and the low risk of surgical closure in the young child mandates operation in the preschool or preadolescent years.[99] The possibility that even earlier operation, at about 2 years of age, would avoid late and persistent right ventricular dysfunction encourages consideration of surgical intervention when the child is quite young.[100]

While life-threatening complications following closure of atrial septal defects in children are rare, transient postoperative atrial arrhythmias are relatively common. Long-term prognosis is excellent for patients undergoing closure of an uncomplicated atrial septal defect.

Partial Anomalous Pulmonary Venous Connection

Pathology

In partial anomalous pulmonary venous connection one or more, but not all, of the pulmonary veins enter the right atrium or its venous tributaries. The atrial septum may be intact, but an atrial septal defect is usually present. There are many patterns of anomalous pulmonary venous connection, but the four most common, in order of decreasing frequency, are (1) pulmonary veins from the right upper and/or middle lobe to the superior vena cava, usually with a sinus venosus atrial septal defect;

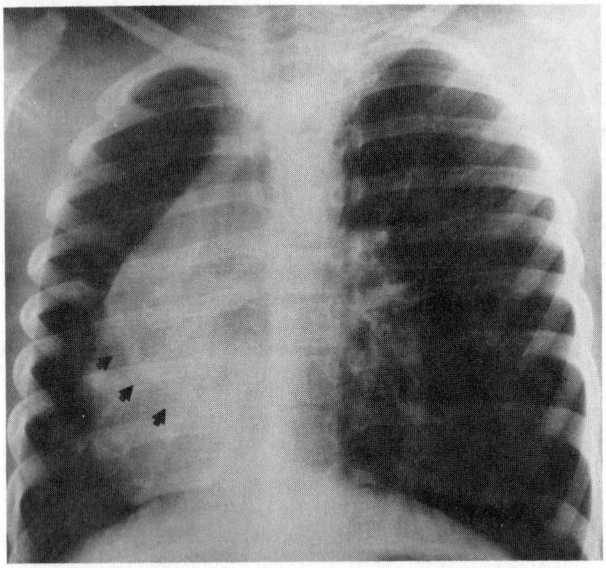

FIGURE 36-13 Frontal view of the chest roentgenogram of an 8 year old boy with scimitar syndrome. The crescent-shaped curve of the right common pulmonary vein (arrows) lies behind the heart, which is rotated into the right hemithorax due to hypoplasia of the right lung.

(2) all of the right pulmonary veins to the right atrium, usually in the polysplenia syndrome; (3) all of the right pulmonary veins to the inferior vena cava, entering the systemic vein just above or below the diaphragm; and (4) the left upper or both left pulmonary veins to an anomalous vertical vein draining to the left brachiocephalic vein.

When the right pulmonary veins are connected to the inferior vena cava, the atrial septum may be intact. This venous anomaly may be isolated or may be part of the *scimitar syndrome.* The latter includes hypoplasia of the right lung, bronchial abnormalities, anomalous systemic pulmonary arterial supply to the right lung from branches of the descending thoracic and/or the abdominal aorta, and dextroposition of the heart (Fig. 36-13). The right pulmonary artery, as well as the left, is present.

Clinical Manifestations

This malformation occurs in approximately 1 in every 160 individuals, or 0.6 percent of the population.[101] There is no sex predilection. Most examples are found in association with atrial septal defects. Approximately 15 percent of all atrial septal defects have this coexisting anomaly; however, in the case of the sinus venosus type of defect the association is in the range of 85 percent. Anomalous connection of a single pulmonary vein also may be discovered, usually accidentally at the time of catheterization, in combination with more complex cardiac malformations. The remaining examples are found as an isolated abnormality with an intact atrial septum. In the latter situation abnormal connections from the right lung outnumber those from the left in a ratio of approximately 3:1.

History When partial anomalous pulmonary venous connection coexists with an atrial septal defect, the symptoms, as well as the electrocardiographic and, usually, the roentgenographic findings are indistinguishable from those of an isolated atrial septal defect. Isolated, uncomplicated anomalous connection of a single pulmonary vein usually goes undetected clinically, since in this circumstance only about 20 percent of the pulmonary venous flow returns to the right atrium or its tributaries. When the entire venous return from one lung or two pulmonary veins are connected anomalously, approximately 65 percent of the pulmonary venous flow returns to the right side of the heart and symptoms are similar to those of an atrial septal defect with a comparable increase in pulmonary blood flow. Easy fatigue, dyspnea, and occasionally heart failure, particularly during early infancy, may be present.[102] Respiratory symptoms in individuals with the scimitar syndrome may, at least in part, be due to hypoplasia of the right lung.

Physical Examination The findings are the same as those in patients with an atrial septal defect with the notable exception that the two components of the second heart sound, though usually widely split, move normally with respiration if the atrial septum is intact.

Chest Roentgenogram Right ventricular enlargement, pulmonary arterial dilatation, and increased pulmonary blood flow in the lung fields are characteristic when more than one pulmonary vein connects anomalously. Only occasionally can one detect dilatation of the superior vena cava, azygous vein, or a left vertical vein, which would suggest anomalous pulmonary venous connection to that vessel. An exception, however, is found with anomalous connection of the right pulmonary veins to the inferior vena cava, where the pulmonary venous pattern assumes a crescent-shaped or scimitar curve in the right lower lung field along the right lower heart border. This syndrome usually is associated with varying degrees of hypoplasia of the right lung and right hemithorax with displacement of the heart toward the midline or into the right chest (Fig. 36-13).

Electrocardiogram The electrocardiogram is either normal (in the case of anomalous connection of a single pulmonary vein) or reflects volume overload of the right side of the heart.

Echocardiogram If more than one pulmonary vein drains anomalously, the volume usually is sufficient to produce the characteristic pattern of right ventricular diastolic overload. Failure to visualize an atrial septal opening with two-dimensional imaging should arouse suspicion of an intact atrial septum.

Cardiac Catheterization Anomalously connected pulmonary veins may be entered directly with the venous catheter. Selective biplane angiograms in these vessels will document their site of connection. A large step-up in oxygen saturation at the atrial level favors the presence of an atrial septal defect, since left-to-right shunting with partial anomalous pulmonary venous connection and an intact atrial septum is usually small or moderate. The presence of anomalous connection of a single, isolated pulmonary vein may go undetected by oximetry techniques unless multiple blood samples are drawn and a localized increase in oxygen saturation can be demonstrated. Even with drainage of the entire right lung to the inferior vena cava, as in the case of scimitar syndrome, the increase in oxygen saturation within the right atrium may be unimpressive because of hypoplasia and diminished volume of the right pulmonary vascular bed and the normal relatively high saturation of the inferior vena cava samples due to blood contributed by the renal veins. In these situations selective indicator-dilution curves in the right and left pulmonary arteries with systemic arterial sampling can detect the lung with the anomalous pulmonary venous connection, and selective biplane angiograms in the pulmonary artery branches will visualize these connections.

Natural History and Prognosis
Patients with partial anomalous pulmonary venous connection with atrial septal defect appear to follow a course similar to, if not identical with, that of patients with an isolated atrial septal defect. When the atrial septum is intact, the course depends primarily upon the volume of pulmonary venous blood returning to the right side of the heart. Rarely, pulmonary vascular obstructive disease may be found even in the presence of a single anomalously connected pulmonary vein and in intact atrial septum.[103] Finally, increasing left atrial pressure, due either to mitral valve disease or diminishing left ventricular compliance, will, in the course of time, encourage a greater redistribution of pulmonary arterial blood flow to that portion of the lung drained by the more compliant right atrium. Thus, patients who are initially asymptomatic and have a very modest volume of anomalous pulmonary venous return in youth may become symptomatic and even develop congestive failure in adult life.

Medical Management
Medical management does not differ significantly from that of the patient with atrial septal defect. Asymptomatic patients with small shunts require no treatment, while those with symptoms, larger pulmonary blood flows, congestive failure, or pulmonary arterial hypertension require surgical correction. With an intact atrial septum, precise preoperative identification of the site of the anomalous venous connection is essential. Long-term follow-up in patients who have not had surgery is indicated to detect increasing flow or the appearance of pulmonary arterial hypertension. A relatively low threshold for postoperative cardiac catheterization is appropriate in view of the subtle, but important effects on the pulmonary vascular bed of either persistent pulmonary venous hypertension or pulmonary arterial volume overload.

Surgical Management
Anomalous connection of right pulmonary vein(s) to the superior vena cava is usually associated with a sinus venosus atrial septal defect (Fig. 36-12). See "Atrial Septal Defect, Surgical Management."

Anomalous connection of right inferior pulmonary vein(s) to the right atrium or to the inferior vena cava above or below the diaphragm is corrected by placement of a contoured intracardiac patch to divert the anomalous pulmonary venous blood into the left atrium through a surgically created atrial septal defect.[104] Cardiopulmonary bypass, moderate hypothermia, and possibly a brief period of circulatory arrest allow placement of the patch within the inferior vena cava.

Individual left pulmonary veins draining into the brachiocephalic venous system usually have sufficient length for transplantation to the left atrial appendage without cardiopulmonary bypass.[105]

Rare cases of bilateral partial anomalous pulmonary venous connection require combined operative approaches. As with cases of atrial septal defect, operative mortality and morbidity are low in patients without other complications. Long-term prognosis is excellent.[93,94]

Common Atrioventricular Canal Defects

Definition
The condition called atrioventricular (AV) canal, persistent common AV canal, and endocardial cushion defect is characterized by an atrial septal defect in the lowermost part of the atrial septum, a cleft condition of the mitral valve (either alone or in combination with cleft of the tricuspid valve), and deficiency of ventricular septal tissue. The condition appears to result from incomplete growth of the AV endocardial cushions.[106]

Pathology
The *ostium primum type* of atrial septal defect is characterized by a crescent-shaped upper border, and no septal tissue forming the lower border. The lower aspect of the defect is bounded by the atrial surfaces of the AV valves and in the complete type (see below) in part by the upper edge of the ventricular septum. A small amount of septal tissue separates the defect from the posterior atrial wall.

Anatomic Types Variations occur with respect to the nature of the AV valves. The terms *partial* and *complete* were first introduced to describe these types.[107]

Partial Type. The so-called ostium primum atrial septal defect with cleft mitral valve is characterized

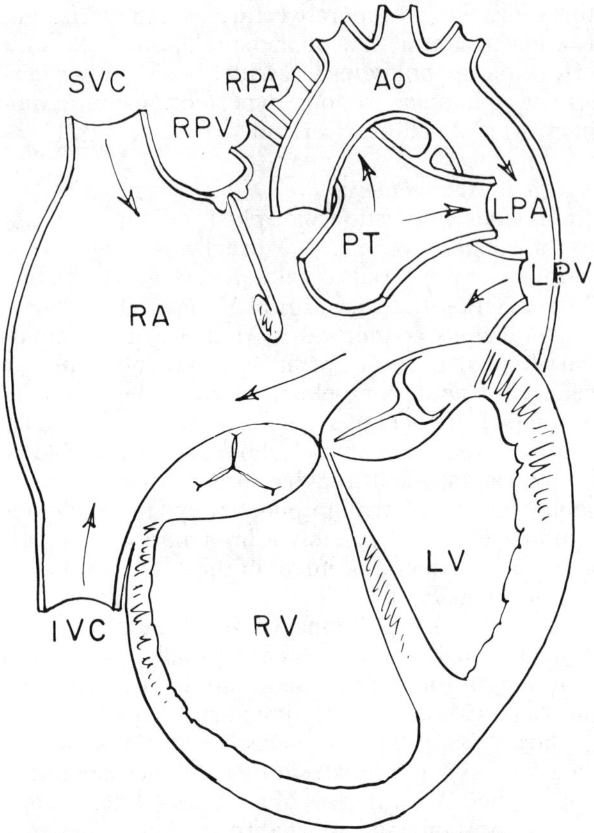

FIGURE 36-14 Common AV canal of the partial type. The mitral valve shows a cleft in its anterior leaflet, while the tricuspid valve is undisturbed. SVC = superior vena cava; IVC = inferior vena cava; RA = right atrium; RV = right ventricle; PT = main pulmonary arterial trunk; RPA = right pulmonary artery; LPA = left pulmonary artery; RPV = right pulmonary vein; LPV = left pulmonary vein; LV = left ventricle; AO = aorta. (*From J. E. Edwards, Classification of Congenital Heart Disease in the Adult, in W. C. Roberts (ed.), "Congenital Heart Disease in Adults," Cardiovasc. Clin. Series 10/1, F. A. Davis Company, Philadelphia, 1979, p. 1. Reproduced with permission from the publisher, editor, and author.*)

by a cleft in the anterior mitral leaflet and an ostium primum atrial septal defect (Figs. 36-6*D* and 36-14).[80] The tricuspid valve either is not cleft or shows minor central deficiency. The ventricular aspects of the anterior mitral valve elements are usually fused to the upper edge of the deficient ventricular septum, precluding an interventricular communication. The characteristics of the chambers are like those in classic atrial septal defect.

Complete Type. The complete type of *common AV canal* is characterized by failure of partitioning of the primitive canal into separate AV orifices. The orifice between the atria and the ventricles is guarded by a common valve, of which the anterior leaflet is derived from the ventral AV endocardial cushion and represents the anterior halves of the anterior mitral and septal tricuspid leaflets. The posterior leaflet is derived from the dorsal AV endocardial cushion and represents the posterior halves of the anterior mitral and septal tricuspid leaflets.

Usually, considerable space exists between the anterior and posterior leaflets, above, and the ventricular septum, below, so that in most cases of the complete type there is free communication between the ventricles. Accordingly, the various anatomic characteristics of a large ventricular septal defect are present. Included in these are congestive pulmonary changes.

Rastelli and associates[108] subdivided the complete variety into three subgroups as follows:

- *Type A.* The anterior common leaflet is subdivided into mitral and tricuspid halves; both halves are attached in the midline to the ventricular septum by short chordae, with chordae from the edges of the leaflets inserting into appropriate ventricles. Spaces between chordae allow free communication between the ventricles.
- *Type B.* As in type A, the anterior leaflet is subdivided. Chordae from the mitral side insert into a papillary muscle in the right ventricle, however, and there are no chordal attachments to the ventricular septum.
- *Type C.* There is no subdivision of the anterior common leaflet and no chordae run from this leaflet to the ventricular septum. The anterior common leaflet may be said to be free-floating.

With regard to the posterior common leaflet, there is variation among the three foregoing types as to presence or absence of subdivision, and as to whether the posterior leaflet is attached to the ventricular septum by chordae or an imperforate membrane.

Variations from the classic types of common AV canal defects are recognized; the most often occurring of these is the AV canal type of isolated ventricular septal defect. Other variations include isolated ostium primum atrial septal defect without malformed AV valves, and isolated cleft of the anterior mitral or septal tricuspid valve leaflets.

Associated Conditions In the asplenic syndrome the complete variety is almost universal; with polysplenia it occurs in about one-quarter of cases. An atrial septal defect of the fossa ovalis type is present in about half of the cases. Double orifice of the mitral valve and tetralogy of Fallot may also be associated with the complete type.[109] The association of double-outlet right ventricle with common AV canal defects is usually also attended by pulmonary stenosis.

Abnormal Physiology

If the communication at the ventricular level is large, the right ventricular and pulmonary artery pressures will be elevated. These patients are similar to those with large ventricular septal defects. Patients with a communication at the atrial level only usually have normal pressures in the right side of the heart and a large pulmonary blood flow, as in the secundum type of atrial septal defect. Defects in the tricuspid or mitral valve, or both, may result in severe regurgitation or direct shunting of blood from the left ventricle to the right atrium.

Clinical Manifestations

Approximately 3 percent of infants and children with congenital heart disease have AV canal defects. Fortunately, the majority, some 60 to 70 percent, have the partial or incomplete form.[4] The female/male ratio is approximately 1.3:1. Well over half of the patients with the complete form have associated Down's syndrome.[3] Among children with Down's syndrome, 45 percent have some form of congenital heart disease. Malformations of the AV canal type, usually of the complete variety, comprise 25 to 36 percent of these abnormalities.[86]

History Only if the mitral valve is incompetent do the symptoms of patients with partial AV canal differ from those associated with a secundum type of atrial septal defect. Mild mitral regurgitation may be tolerated quite well, but moderate or severe regurgitation is associated with poor weight gain, easy fatigue, dyspnea, repeated respiratory infections, and congestive heart failure. Those patients with complete AV canal are almost invariably very sick. Heart failure appears early and is severe. Almost 40 percent of infants with this malformation will require hospitalization within the first month of life; with medical therapy only, death can be expected in approximately 60 percent within the first year. A small number of infants will maintain an elevated pulmonary vascular resistance throughout the first months of life, will gain weight acceptably, and will have surprisingly few symptoms.

Physical Examination The findings on inspection, palpation, and auscultation among patients with the partial defect are those of an atrial septal defect, unless the cleft anterior mitral leaflet is incompetent. In this event the murmur of mitral regurgitation will be heard, and if regurgitation is severe, this murmur will be accompanied by a diastolic filling sound, a middiastolic flow rumble at the apex, and a hyperdynamic apical impulse.

The physical findings with the complete canal are those of a very large ventricular septal defect usually with full-blown congestive failure. The murmur of mitral regurgitation may not be heard or recognized as such, but fixed splitting of the second heart sound would suggest the presence of an associated atrial septal defect and hence the possibility of complete canal. With the development of pulmonary vascular obstructive disease the examination is virtually indistinguishable from that of a patient with a large ventricular septal defect and a similar elevation of the pulmonary vascular resistance, with the exception of the second heart sound which remains split and fixed. In some patients the murmurs of tricuspid and mitral regurgitation may also be present.

Chest Roentgenogram Overall cardiac enlargement, out of proportion to the degree of pulmonary plethora, or a cardiac silhouette suggesting combined ventricular dilatation may serve to distinguish the uncomplicated secundum atrial septal defect from the primum defect with significant mitral regurgitation. Marked cardiac enlargement with severe pulmonary overcirculation are features of the complete canal. Absence of impressive left atrial dilatation with the clinical and radiological features of a very large left-to-right shunt and congestive failure would suggest the presence of an atrial septal defect and the suspicion of complete AV canal.

Electrocardiogram The most helpful diagnostic feature in distinguishing individuals with AV canal defects from those with isolated atrial or ventricular septal defects is the characteristic superior orientation of the mean QRS axis in the frontal plane (Fig. 36-15). Between 92 and 95 percent of both types of canal have a QRS axis lying between 0 and −150°. The axis also is of value within the canal family, since 70 percent of patients with a partial canal will have an axis between 0 and −90° and only 22 percent between −91 and −150°. On the other hand, 70 percent of patients with complete canal will have an axis between −91 and −150° and only 23 percent between 0 and −90°. About 3 percent of both forms of canal defect will have right axis deviation, i.e., +91 to +180°.[110] The PQ interval is slightly prolonged in the majority of both partial and complete defects. Mild right ventricular hypertrophy is characteristic of partial canal. The presence of associated left ventricular hypertrophy reflects moderate or severe mitral regurgitation. With complete AV canal, biatrial hypertrophy, and biventricular hypertrophy are characteristic (Fig. 36-15). In the presence of severe pulmonary vascular obstructive

FIGURE 36-15 Electrocardiogram from an infant with complete AV canal, a large left-to-right shunt, and severe pulmonary arterial hypertension. The superior mean QRS axis (−70°) is accompanied by first degree heart block, biatrial hypertrophy, and biventricular hypertrophy.

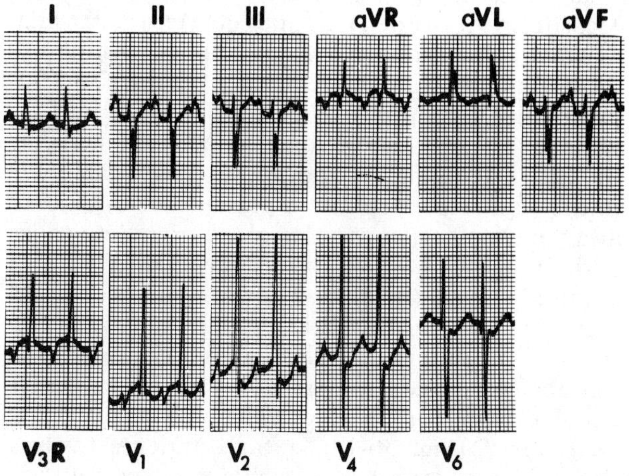

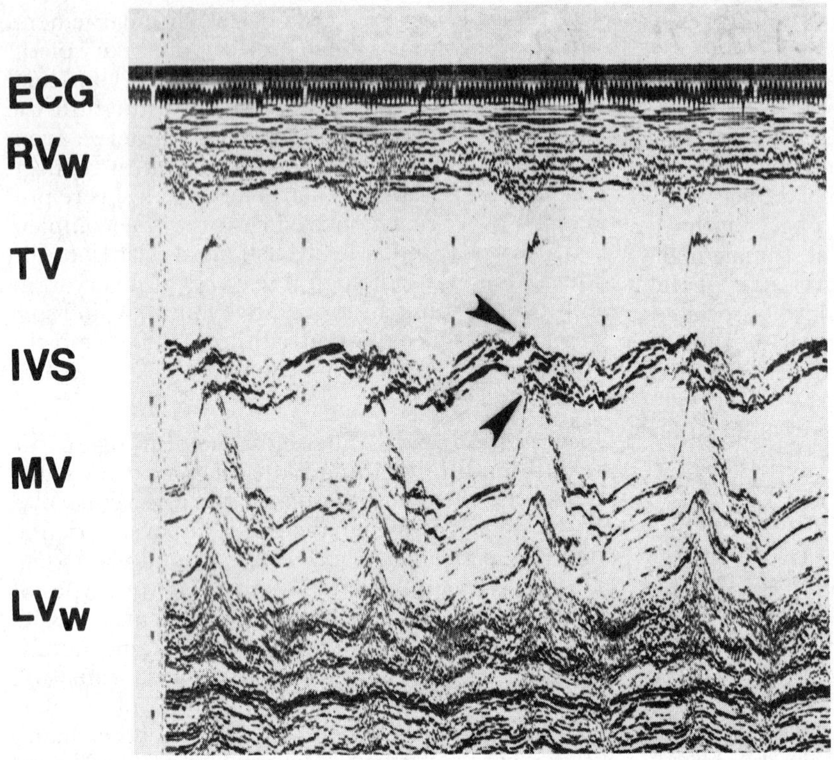

FIGURE 36-16 M-mode echocardiogram from a child with a primum atrial septal defect. The increased right ventricular cavity dimension and anterior systolic motion of the interventricular septum (IVS) are characteristic of diastolic overload of the right ventricle, while diastolic apposition of the anterior mitral valve (MV) leaflet (lower arrowhead) to the interventricular septum and near continuity of the anterior mitral and tricuspid valve (TV) echoes (lower and upper arrowheads) without absence of interventricular septum echoes are characteristic of a partial AV canal defect. ECG = electrocardiogram; RV_w = anterior right ventricular wall; LV_w = posterior left ventricular wall.

disease or important pulmonary stenosis, the pattern is one of right atrial and right ventricular hypertrophy.

Echocardiogram M-mode study of the partial defect will demonstrate the increased right ventricular dimensions and anterior systolic movement of the ventricular septum consistent with the diastolic volume overload of an atrial septal defect. Features characteristic of AV defects include prolonged diastolic apposition of the anterior mitral valve leaflet to the interventricular septum, multiple anterior leaflet systolic echoes, narrowing of the left ventricular outflow tract, and the appearance of the tricuspid valve opening from within the ventricular septal echoes (Fig. 36-16). Ventricular septal motion usually is normal in the presence of a complete canal. Measurement of the right and left ventricular end-diastolic dimensions and their ratio will distinguish those patients with serious and perhaps surgically prohibitive hypoplasia of either ventricle.[111] Two-dimensional sector scanning is capable of visualizing the atrial septal defect and mitral valve attachment to the ventricular septum in partial canal, the atrial and ventricular components of the complete canal, and the cleft anterior mitral valve leaflet with or without an associated atrial or ventricular septal defect (Figs. 36-17 and 36-18).[112] The anatomic features of the anterior AV leaflet and its connections may be visualized with sufficient clarity to permit subdivision of complete AV canal defects into types A, B, or C (Fig. 36-19).[113] Straddling AV valves, double-orifice mitral valve, single papillary muscles, and hypoplasia or outflow obstruction of the right or left ventricles can be determined with this technique.[112,114]

Cardiac Catheterization A significant increase in oxygen saturation between the superior vena cava and the right atrium is present in both the uncomplicated incomplete and complete forms of AV canal. Serious right ventricular and pulmonary arterial systolic hypertension are unusual with a partial defect, and a right ventricular or pulmonary arterial systolic pressure in excess of 60 percent of the systemic systolic pressure favors the presence of a complete canal. With a large communication between the two ventricles below the AV valves, the right ventricular, pulmonary arterial, and systemic arterial systolic pressures are virtually identical. Left ventricular angiography in the frontal view demonstrates the gooseneck deformity of the left ventricular outflow tract characteristic of AV canal malformations (Fig. 36-20) and allows a semiquantitative assessment of the degree of mitral regurgitation and shunting from left ventricle to right atrium. The left anterior oblique view with craniocaudal angulation is recommended for visualizing the interventricular defect and judging the extent of ventricular septal deficiency.[115] Aortography is essential to eliminate the possibility of a patent ductus arteriosus.

Natural History and Prognosis

Partial defects without significant mitral regurgitation follow a course similar to that described for the secundum type of septal defects. An exception would

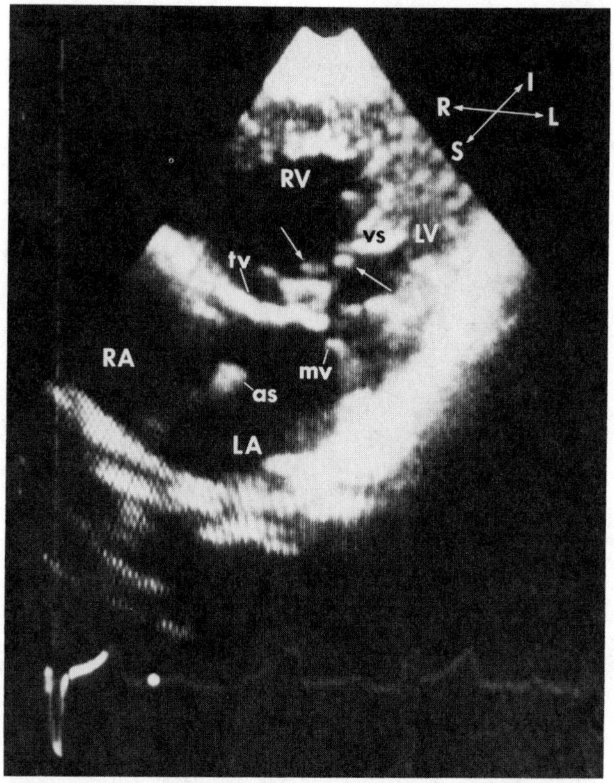

FIGURE 36-17 Two-dimensional echocardiogram in the apex view from a child with type A complete AV canal. The common anterior leaflet to the tricuspid (tv) and mitral (mv) valves appears to be attached to the crest of the ventricular septum (vs) by multiple chordae (arrows). The area of the ostium primum atrial septal defect lies between the lowermost edge of the atrial septum (as) and the mitral valve (mv). R = right; S = superior; I = inferior; L = left; RV = right ventricle; LV = left ventricle; RA = right atrium; LA = left atrium. (*From D. J. Hagler, A. J. Tajik, J. B. Seward, D. D. Mair, and D. G. Ritter, Real-Time Wide-Angle Sector Echocardiography: Atrioventricular Canal Defects, Circulation, 59:140, 1979. Reproduced by permission of the American Heart Association, Inc., and the authors.*)

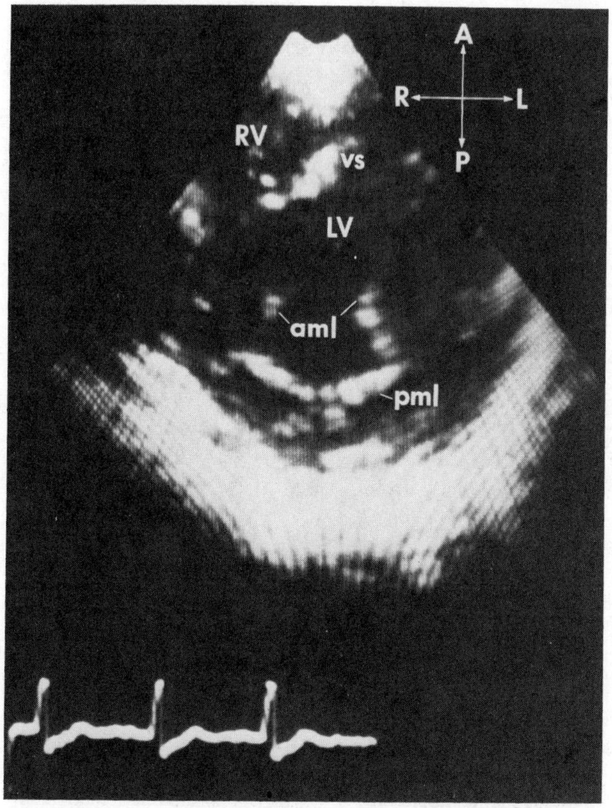

FIGURE 36-18 Two-dimensional echocardiogram in the parasternal short-axis view of a child with an AV-canal type of ventricular septal defect, intact atrial septum, and mitral valve cleft. The cleft in the anterior mitral valve leaflet (aml) is noted during diastole. R = right; A = anterior; P = posterior; L = left; RV = right ventricle; LV = left ventricle; vs = ventricular septum; pml = posterior mitral valve leaflet. (*From D. J. Hagler, A. J. Tajik, J. B. Seward, D. D. Mair, and D. G. Ritter, Real-Time Wide-Angle Sector Echocardiography: Atrioventricular Canal Defects, Circulation, 59:140, 1979. Reproduced by permission of the American Heart Association, Inc., and the authors.*)

be the greater likelihood of infective endocarditis because of the mitral valve deformity. Moderate or severe mitral regurgitation produces heart failure with the resulting symptoms and growth retardation. Infants with a complete AV canal without protective pulmonary stenosis quickly develop and continue in congestive failure until the course is altered by death, the development of pulmonary vascular obstructive disease, or surgical intervention in the form of pulmonary arterial banding or complete repair. Spontaneous narrowing or closure of the atrial or ventricular portion of a complete AV canal defect does not seem to occur.

Medical Management

Children with an uncomplicated partial defect are managed in the same manner as children with uncomplicated atrial septal defect. Those who are symptomatic with or without mitral regurgitation should undergo surgical closure of their primum atrial septal defect and plication of the cleft of the anterior mitral valve leaflet. Those few patients with significant residual mitral regurgitation following surgery are managed medically until such time as mitral valve replacement is appropriate.

The clinical approach to the infant with complete AV canal is the same as described for infants with a large ventricular septal defect but is tempered by the knowledge that spontaneous improvement is very unlikely except at the expense of the pulmonary vascular bed. For very tiny infants, under 3 or 4 months of age, in severe congestive heart failure with a documented large interventricular defect and little or no mitral regurgitation, banding of the pulmonary artery is still recommended. In the older infant, or in the presence of moderate or severe mitral regurgitation, complete correction is recommended. For those infants in whom failure is more manageable and pulmonary arterial pressure somewhat lower, perhaps because of a smaller interventricular communication, the indications for recatheterization and surgery are the same as those for a ventricular septal defect.

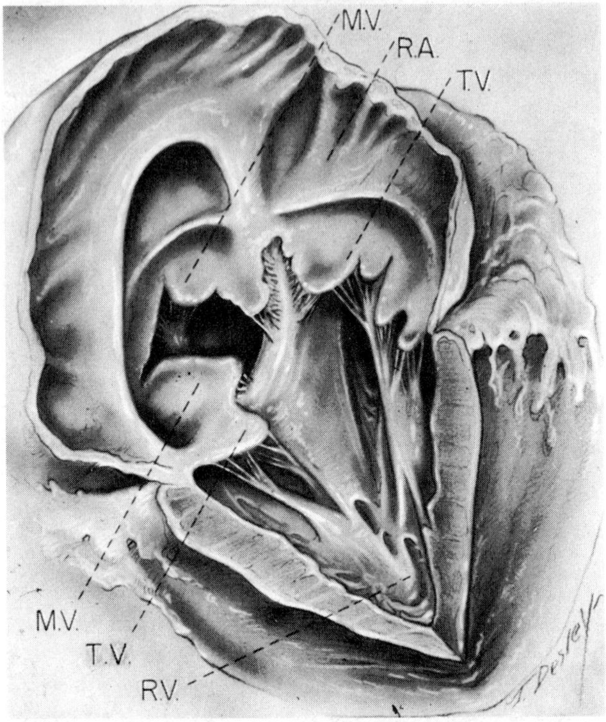

FIGURE 36-19 Complete form of common AV canal, type A. The common anterior leaflet has a recognizable mitral component, MV, and tricuspid component, TV. In type B, not illustrated, those components are attached by chordae to a papillary muscle in the right ventricle. In type C, not illustrated, the common anterior leaflet is a single unit without any attachment to the underlying ventricular septum. Type A is most amenable to repair. RV = right ventricle; RA = right atrium. (*From G. C. Rastelli, P. A. Ongley, J. W. Kirklin, and D. C. McGoon, Surgical Repair of the Complete Form of Persistent Common Atrioventricular Canal, J. Thorac. Cardiovasc. Surg., 55:299, 1968. Reproduced with permission from the publisher and authors.*)

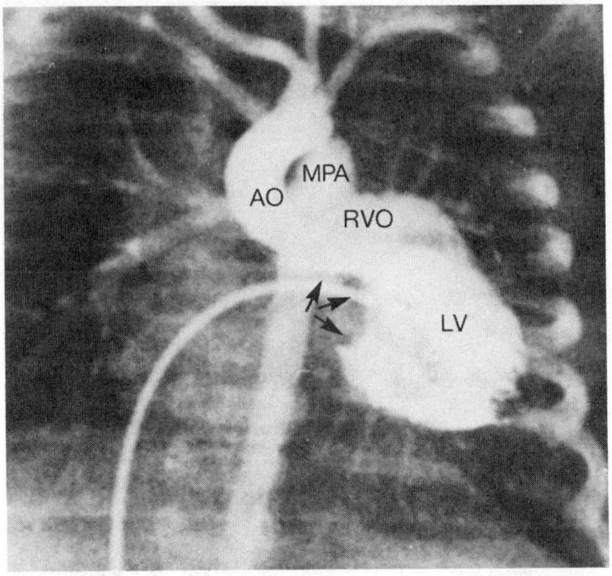

FIGURE 36-20 Posteroanterior view of the left ventricular angiogram, from a child with complete AV canal, demonstrating the characteristic gooseneck deformity (arrows) of the outflow tract of the left ventricle (LV). Opacification of the right ventricular outflow tract (RVO) and main pulmonary artery (MPA) before, or in the absence of, atrial opacification reflects the presence of the interventricular communication. AO = aorta.

Complete heart block, an uncommon complication of surgical correction today, carries the same serious consequences whether it is induced during correction of the partial or complete form of AV canal or whether it develops months or years following surgery. Permanent ventricular pacing is indicated.

Antibiotic coverage at times of special risk of bacteremia is indicated indefinitely for all forms of AV canal, operated or unoperated, in view of the complexity of the lesion and the mitral valve deformity which must persist.

With regard to genetic counseling, the risk of a subsequent sibling having heart disease in the presence of a single affected family member is in the range of 2 percent; it is probably the same for the offspring of an affected parent. Concordance for AV canal defects among affected siblings or offspring is much higher than with other forms of congenital heart disease and approaches 90 percent.[116]

Surgical Management

The excellent results achieved following anatomic repair of complete common AV canal defects in infancy encourage early correction.[117–124] Banding of the pulmonary artery still deserves consideration in the critically ill infant having a large interventricular communication and markedly increased pulmonary blood flow rather than AV valvular regurgitation.[117,119,125] When associated right ventricular outflow tract obstruction is severe, a palliative anastomosis of systemic artery to pulmonary artery will reduce hypoxemia and its complications and promote pulmonary arterial growth prior to anatomic correction.

Specifics of repair are dictated by anatomic detail;[121,122,126] individual variation is considerable (Fig. 36-19).[113] The interior of the heart is exposed through a generous right atriotomy during hypothermic extracorporeal circulation. Hypothermic (18°C) circulatory arrest allows precise repair in the infant weighing less than 10 kg.[117,126] One or both of the common bridging leaflets may require division to create separate mitral and tricuspid components (Fig. 36-21).[113] Construction of a competent mitral valve is crucial.

A Dacron patch is sutured to the right side of the ventricular septum to obliterate the interventricular communication. The anterior and posterior components of the mitral valve are sutured to the Dacron patch at an appropriate level. Mitral valve competence is assessed by gentle distension of the left ventricle with saline solution. The "cleft" created between the anterior and posterior components of the mitral apparatus can be closed by suture if approximation of these edges appears to increase competence. Annuloplasty may further improve competence in older patients having annular dilatation.

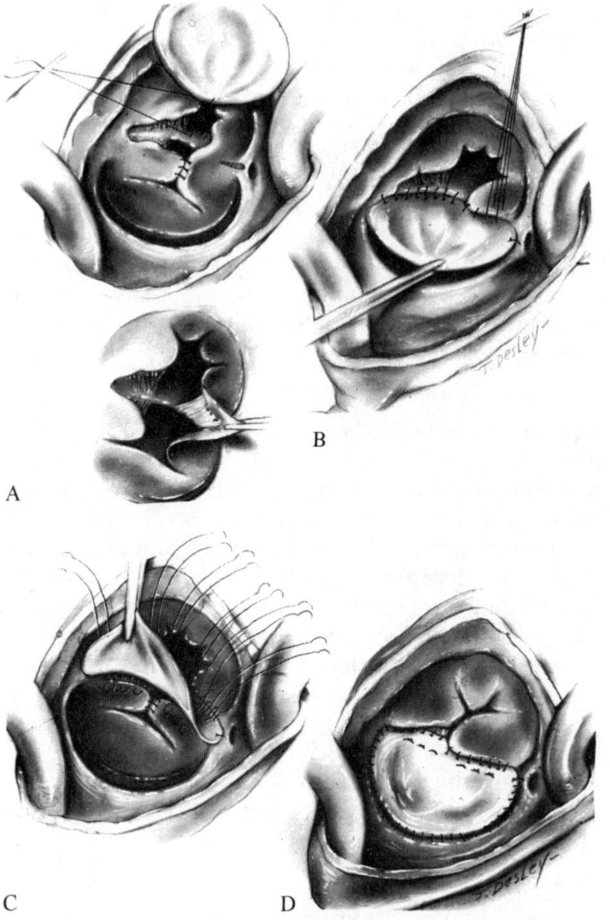

FIGURE 36-21 Steps in the repair of the complete form of common AV canal, type A. *A* and *B*. A pericardial patch is sutured to the ventricular septum. *C* and *D*. The anterior leaflet of the mitral valve is reconstructed and attached to the patch. A portion of the tricuspid leaflet is attached to the patch. *(From G. C. Rastelli, P. A. Ongley, J. W. Kirklin, and D. C. McGoon, Surgical Repair of the Complete Form of Persistent Common Atrioventricular Canal, J. Thorac. Cardiovasc. Surg., 55:299, 1968. Reproduced with permission from the publisher and authors.)*

Residual mitral regurgitation may require subsequent mitral valve replacement, but prosthetic valve insertion is rarely required at primary anatomic repair.[117,121] The tricuspid apparatus is similarly reconstructed.

The interatrial communication is closed using the remainder of the septal patch or a separate piece of pericardium, which appears to minimize hemolysis in the presence of residual mitral incompetence. Associated right ventricular outflow tract obstruction and previous palliative pulmonary arterial bands or anastomoses of systemic arteries to pulmonary arteries are eliminated during cooling and warming.

Reported hospital mortality for total correction of complete AV canal in infancy ranges from zero to 27 percent, the highest mortality being encountered during the first few months of life and in those infants with severe AV valve regurgitation or elevated pulmonary vascular resistance.[117–124] Survival to the age of 5 years without operation occurs in only 4 percent.[127] A 5-year survival of 91 percent for patients discharged from the hospital following total correction has been reported by Berger.[127] The likelihood for "surgical cure" (alive 5 years later with a mean pulmonary arterial pressure of 25 mmHg or less) was greatest (73 percent) if correction was performed when the child was about 14 months old. Operation may be required before this age if symptoms dictate.

Successful corrections of complete AV canal associated with common ventricle,[128] tetralogy of Fallot, double-outlet right ventricle,[129] and other complex anomalies[130–132] have been reported.

Studer and colleagues at the University of Alabama[133] have reviewed the determinants of early and late results of repair of atrioventricular canal defects in 310 consecutive patients undergoing repair. The magnitude of preoperative AV valvular regurgitation is a significant prognostic factor.

Ostium primum atrial septal defect with or without mitral valve incompetence secondary to a cleft in the anterior (aortic) leaflet, partial AV canal, is repaired through a right atriotomy. A cleft in the anterior mitral leaflet is closed with a few simple interrupted sutures. The atrial septal defect is closed by placement of a pericardial patch. Dacron is avoided to reduce hemolysis in the presence of residual mitral regurgitation. Care is exercised to avoid injury to the bundle of His and the atrioventricular node in the area of contiguous mitral and tricuspid valves by confining the sutures to fibrous tissue to the left of the annulus and on the left atrial side of the atrial septum, away from the medial rim of the coronary sinus.

Severe mitral regurgitation is difficult to correct even by closure of the cleft between the anterior and posterior portions of the anterior mitral valve leaflet. Annuloplasty may be of benefit in older patients having a dilated annulus. Excessive or inaccurate closure of the cleft may produce mitral stenosis. A leaflet may be deficient, fenestrated, or severely deformed, and abnormal papillary muscle position or associated left ventricular outflow tract obstruction may further complicate repair.[134,135] If the interventricular septum is deficient, with consequent downward displacement of the mitral valve leaflets, the leaflets may require detachment from the septum and attachment at a higher point on a septal patch to assure competence and relief of left ventricular outflow tract obstruction.

McMullan and associates of the Mayo Clinic[136] reviewed 232 patients between the ages of 3 months and 50 years operated upon between 1955 and 1972. Hospital mortality was 6 percent; risk of death was greater in patients having severe preoperative disability, those having a cardiothoracic ratio exceeding 0.60, and infants under 1 year of age. Of 210 patients for whom follow-up data were available 8 (3.8 percent) required mitral valve replacement 3 months to 14 years after the initial operation. Permanent complete heart block contributed substantially to early mortality and morbidity but is now extremely rare. A low operative mortality and good late results can be anticipated from correction of partial AV canal in all but those few patients having severe mitral valvular incompetence, in whom mitral valve replacement may be required. Patients undergoing repair of partial AV canal should be observed for the possible development of subaortic left ventricular outflow tract obstruction.

Single Atrium

Definition and Pathology

Single atrium (cor triloculare biventriculare) refers to the condition in which either no atrial septal tissue is present or the atrial septum is so rudimentary as to yield a common chamber involving both atria.

Its secondary effects are essentially like those in atrial septal defect. The great vessels are usually normally related. There is a strong tendency for the atrioventricular valves to be characteristic of the common atrioventricular canal defects.[110]

The form of single atrium present in the syndrome of asplenia is commonly associated with other malformations, including pulmonary stenosis, malposed great vessels, and anomalous pulmonary venous return.

Clinical Manifestations

The clinical features of this malformation are those of a very large atrial septal defect of the atrioventricular canal variety. Though rare, it is the characteristic malformation described among patients with the autosomal recessive Ellis–van Creveld syndrome.

History Symptoms of shortness of breath and easy fatigue usually appear within the first year of life. Mild cyanosis is commonly observed with crying. Weight gain tends to be slow and lower respiratory tract infections frequent.

Physical Examination Mild tachypnea, mild cyanosis, and clubbing of the fingers and toes are characteristic. Prominence of the right precordium, a hyperdynamic right ventricular lift, and fixed splitting of the second heart sound reflect the right ventricular volume overload and the unobstructed interatrial opening. A holosystolic regurgitant murmur at the apex would indicate mitral regurgitation, a common feature of this malformation.

Laboratory Mild to moderate polycythemia reflects the mild systemic arterial oxygen desaturation usually found with this lesion.

Chest Roentgenogram Cardiac enlargement is usual, with prominence of the main and branch pulmonary arteries and an impressive increase in pulmonary blood flow but little, if any, left atrial enlargement. Dextrocardia, mesocardia, or levocardia with situs ambiguus also may be present.

Electrocardiogram The mean QRS axis is superior, as with other varieties of atrioventricular canal defect. Mild first degree atrioventricular block, a mild to moderate right ventricular conduction delay, and right ventricular hypertrophy complete the picture. Ectopic atrial rhythms and junctional escape rhythms are frequent.

Echocardiogram Both M-mode and two-dimensional studies show the characteristic features of an atrioventricular canal defect with absence of atrial septal echoes.

Cardiac Catheterization Complete or nearly complete mixing of systemic venous and pulmonary venous blood is found at the atrial level, and mild systemic arterial oxygen desaturation is the rule. Pulmonary arterial hypertension is common, with a mild to moderate increase in the pulmonary vascular resistance in some cases. Selective angiography with injections in both systemic and pulmonary veins is recommended to define abnormalities of venous return. Left ventricular angiography will assess the presence and degree of mitral regurgitation, assess the presence of an associated ventricular septal defect, establish the relations of the great arteries, and demonstrate the gooseneck deformity characteristic of atrioventricular canal defects.

Natural History, Prognosis, and Medical Management

The natural history, management, and indications for surgery are the same as those for the ostium primum type of atrioventricular canal defects. Abnormalities of pulmonary and systemic venous return may add considerably to the complexity of the surgery, however.

Surgical Management

The common atrial chamber is partitioned with a pericardial or Dacron patch placed to divert pulmonary venous blood to the mitral orifice. Superior and inferior caval flow is directed to the tricuspid orifice. Hepatic veins may enter the atrium directly and should be placed on the systemic side of the atrial partition. The coronary sinus may be placed in either atrium. Anomalies of the atrioventricular valves are repaired and coexisting ventricular septal defects are closed.

Care is required to avoid injury to the atrioventricular node near the coronary sinus. Conduction disturbances and supraventricular dysrhythmias are common preoperatively in patients with single atrium, but postoperative complete heart block can usually be avoided.

Long-term outcome is generally good but depends upon the severity of associated anomalies and competence of the atrioventricular valves.

Left Ventricular–Right Atrial Communication

Definition

A left ventricular–right atrial communication is a defect that allows direct communication between the two chambers named. The defect is usually small.

Pathology

In this uncommon condition one of several anatomic arrangements may be observed; the most common is an infracristal ventricular septal defect associated with a cleft in the septal leaflet of the tricuspid valve (Fig. 36-22).[80] The edges of the valvular cleft are attached to the edges of the defect, thereby committing the left ventricle to communicate with the right atrium. Less commonly there is a defect in that part of the membranous septum that normally separates the two chambers involved. The left and right ventricles may be somewhat dilated. The right atrium is enlarged.

Associated conditions that have been observed are complete transposition, Ebstein's malformation of the tricuspid valve, and subaortic stenosis.[137]

FIGURE 36-22 Left ventricular–right atrial communication. SVC = superior vena cava; IVC = inferior vena cava; RA = right atrium; RV = right ventricle; PT = main pulmonary arterial trunk; RPA = right pulmonary artery; LPA = left pulmonary artery; RPV = right pulmonary vein; LPV = left pulmonary vein; LA = left atrium; LV = left ventricle; Ao = aorta. *(From J. E. Edwards, Classification of Congenital Heart Disease in the Adult, in W. C. Roberts (ed.), "Congenital Heart Disease in Adults," Cardiovasc. Clin. Series 10/1, F. A. Davis Company, Philadelphia, 1979, p. 1. Reproduced with permission from the publisher, editor, and author.)*

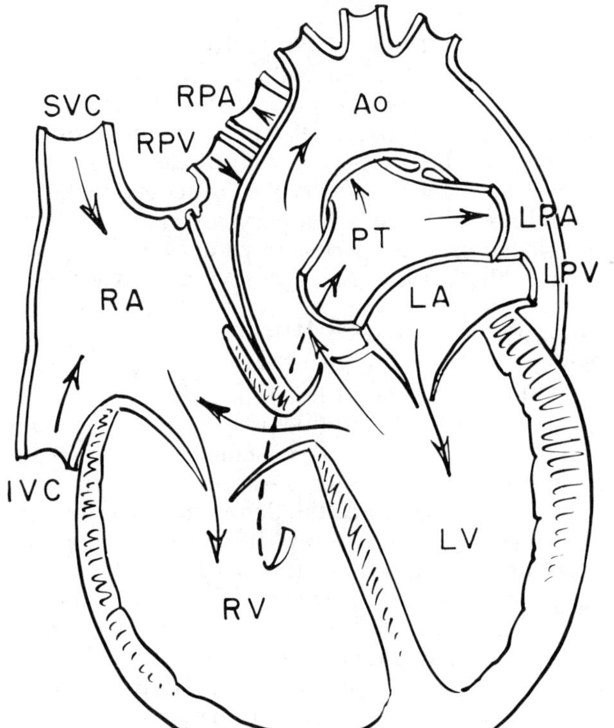

Clinical Manifestations

This malformation makes up somewhat less than 1 percent of all congenital cardiac defects. Females are slightly more commonly affected than males.

History The murmur frequently is detected within the first day of life, since flow through the defect is not dependent upon a reduced pulmonary vascular resistance. Slow weight gain, tachypnea, repeated lower respiratory infections, and congestive failure appearing within the first few months of life are typical if the defect is large, but many individuals with small defects are entirely asymptomatic.

Physical Examination A holosystolic murmur typical of a ventricular septal defect is present at the lower left sternal border but may radiate unusually well to the right midsternal border area. A diastolic flow rumble at the apex is common with large shunts. A hyperdynamic left parasternal lift, with or without an early diastolic flow murmur at the lower left sternal border, reflects the right ventricular volume overload one might expect from an associated atrial septal defect; however, normal movement of the aortic and pulmonary components of the second heart sound indicates an intact atrial septum.

Chest Roentgenogram The pulmonary vascular engorgement, cardiac enlargement, and left atrial dilatation support the diagnosis of ventricular septal defect. Impressive right atrial enlargement, best seen in the frontal view, an unexpected finding with typical ventricular septal defect, should suggest this variant malformation.

Electrocardiogram The QRS axis in the frontal plane may be superior if the septal defect is in the canal position, but in the majority of patients the QRS axis is normal. Left ventricular hypertrophy and usually right ventricular hypertrophy are present unless the shunt is small. Tall, peaked P waves are not uncommon in this setting and provide a valuable clue to the correct diagnosis.

Echocardiogram M-mode studies have demonstrated high-frequency systolic fluttering of the anterior tricuspid leaflet, coinciding in time with the holosystolic murmur, at least in those patients where the stream of left ventricular blood must traverse the tricuspid leaflets to reach the right atrium.

Cardiac Catheterization A step-up in oxygen saturation will be found at the right atrial level together with mean and phasic pressure differences between the left and right atria, which indicate an intact interatrial septum. The diagnosis may be made by selective left ventricular angiography in the frontal view, where immediate opacification of the dilated right atrium will be seen.

Natural History and Prognosis
The clinical course is similar to that described for ventricular septal defect.

Medical Management
The management of congestive failure, the indications for operation, and the other features of management are as described for ventricular septal defect.

Surgical Management
The left ventricular–right atrial communication is exposed through a right atriotomy. The defect is usually near or actually within the tricuspid annulus, lying just superior to the septal leaflet of the tricuspid valve in the atrioventricular septum. The edges of a cleft in the septal leaflet of the tricuspid valve may be fused to the edges of the defect.

Closure is accomplished by direct suture approximation of the fibrous margins or placement of a small Dacron patch after the tricuspid leaflet edges are freed, sutures being placed carefully to avoid injury to the atrioventricular node near the orifice of the coronary sinus and to the bundle of His. If present, the cleft in the septal leaflet of the tricuspid valve is sutured. Hemodynamic results are excellent. Morbidity and mortality are low.

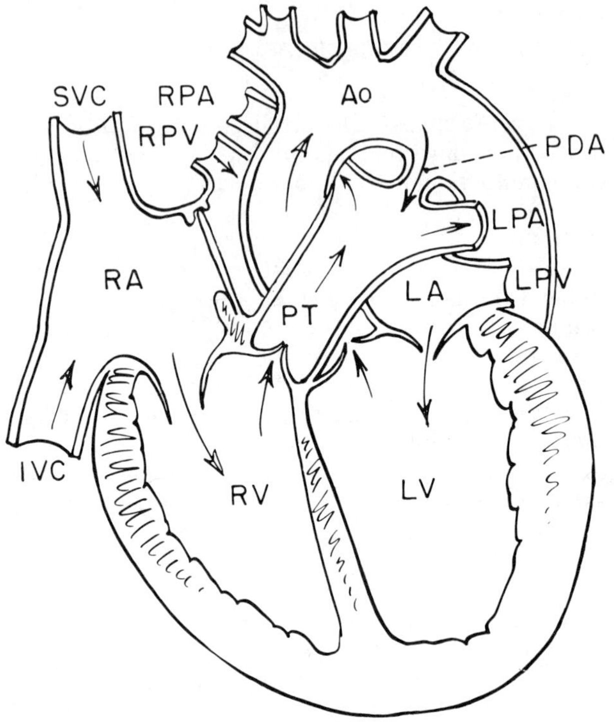

FIGURE 36-23 Patent ductus arteriosus (PDA). SVC = superior vena cava; IVC = inferior vena cava; RA = right atrium; RV = right ventricle; PT = main pulmonary arterial trunk; RPA = right pulmonary artery; LPA = left pulmonary artery; RPV = right pulmonary vein; LPV = left pulmonary vein; LA = left atrium; LV = left ventricle; Ao = aorta. [*From J. E. Edwards, Classification of Congenital Heart Disease in the Adult, in W. C. Roberts (ed.), "Congenital Heart Disease in Adults," Cardiovasc. Clin. Series 10/1, F. A. Davis Company, Philadelphia, 1979, p. 1. Reproduced with permission from the publisher, editor, and author.*]

Extracardiac Communications between the Systemic and Pulmonary Circulations, Usually without Cyanosis

Patent Ductus Arteriosus

Definition
Patent ductus arteriosus, the most common type of extracardiac shunt, represents persistent patency of the vessel that normally connects the pulmonary arterial system and the aorta in the fetus (Fig. 36-23).[80]

Pathology
The ductus arteriosus usually closes within 2 or 3 weeks after birth and becomes the ligamentum arteriosum,[138] but it may remain patent as long as 8 weeks postnatally.[139] It runs from the origin of the left pulmonary artery, below, to the lower aspect of the aortic arch just beyond the level of origin of the left subclavian artery, above. The recurrent branch of the left vagus nerve hooks around its lateral and inferior aspects.

The hearts of subjects with patent ductus arteriosus show varying degrees of enlargement of the left atrium and ventricle. The character of the right ventricle depends upon the state of the ductus—whether it is narrow (obstructive) or wide (so-called hypertensive ductus). In the former the right ventricle is normal; in the latter its wall is hypertrophied.

Associated Conditions Many cardiovascular anomalies may be associated with a patent ductus, the more common being coarctation of the aorta and ventricular septal defect. Patent ductus arteriosus is an integral part of interruption of the aortic arch. In certain anomalies (so-called ductus-dependent conditions such as pulmonary atresia with intact ventricular septum) persistent patency of the ductus is desirable, but it tends to close at a normal rate.

Abnormal Physiology[140–143]
Patients with patent ductus arteriosus may be divided into groups according to whether the vascular resistance through the ductus itself is small, moderate, or large. Since the resistance of the ductus is related not only to its cross-sectional area but also to its length, it is difficult to define the anatomic size of the ductus in each group. In patients with a ductus of high resistance, the flow across the ductus will be relatively small. The extra volume of work on the left ventricle is tolerated well and the pulmonary pressure and resistance are not elevated. Patients with only moderate resistance in the ductus have some increase in pulmonary artery pressure with a moderately greater volume of shunting across the ductus.

In patients with a large patent ductus which offers minimal resistance to blood flow, the aorta and pulmonary artery are essentially in free communication; the systolic pressure in the pulmonary artery will be nearly equal to that in the aorta. In patent ductus, the volume load is on the left ventricle, which may "fail." Pulmonary congestion results from left ventricular failure with increased pressure in the left atrium and pulmonary capillaries and the failure of the pulmonary vasculature to "protect" the pulmonary capillaries from the high pulmonary artery pressure and flow. With time, the left ventricle compensates with dilatation and hypertrophy to carry the volume load, and the pulmonary vasculature responds to the high pressure. (See preceding section on pulmonary arterial hypertension and pulmonary vascular obstructive disease.)

In patients with a moderate or large ductus, the right ventricle is burdened mainly by a pressure load in the pulmonary circuit caused largely by pulmonary vasoconstriction.

If the pulmonary resistance equals or exceeds the resistance of the systemic circulation, there is shunting of unsaturated blood from pulmonary artery to aorta. This causes the arterial oxygen saturation to be higher in the arms, especially the right arm, than in the legs.

Clinical Manifestations

History The history of the mother's pregnancy and of perinatal events may provide clues that are associated with a high incidence of patent ductus arteriosus.[6] Exposure to rubella in the first trimester by a nonimmunized mother is an example. Patent ductus is also more common in the premature infant, especially those with birth asphyxia or respiratory distress syndrome.[141,144–146] There is a much higher incidence in females, except in rubella syndrome where the sexes are affected equally.[147] An extensive review of the literature[6] and a report on a large number of patients[147] can be referred to for more detail.

Symptoms are usually restricted to patients with large shunts that produce heart failure or with other complicating problems such as respiratory distress in the premature infant. The symptoms related to heart failure were discussed earlier. Heart failure is most likely to develop in the first few weeks or months of life. If it does not appear during infancy, it is unlikely to occur before the third decade. Growth may be affected in those with large shunts and failure. The clinical presentation in the premature infant is usually very different from that in the full-term infant. This is particularly true in those with a birth weight under 1.5 kg, who are more likely to have moderate to severe respiratory distress. In these infants, the clinical features of respiratory distress often blend over the course of several days into those of heart failure. Increasing ventilatory or oxygen requirements with carbon dioxide retention or episodic apnea and bradycardia are often the first signs that a patent ductus may be complicating the picture.

Physical Examination In the full-term infant or child with patent ductus arteriosus, there is frequently a systolic thrill over the pulmonary artery and in the suprasternal notch. The peripheral pulses are generally brisk and bounding, especially with the larger shunts. Blood pressure measurement in older patients with significant shunts will frequently demonstrate a pulse pressure of 45 mmHg or more.[147] Diffuse cyanosis may be present if there is pulmonary edema. The patient with elevated pulmonary vascular resistance and shunt reversal will have cyanosis, clubbing of the toes, and occasionally clubbing of the fingers on the left. The apex impulse may be increased or displaced in those with large shunts. The right ventricular impulse is increased in the premature infant with respiratory distress and in infants and children with significant pulmonary hypertension. Auscultatory findings will vary with age, size of the shunt, and the pulmonary vascular status. The typical murmur is a continuous or machinery murmur that is best heard at the left upper sternal border and below the left clavicle. It is usually a rough murmur with eddy sounds that are helpful in making the diagnosis, and it peaks at or near the second heart sound. The murmur may have an abbreviated diastolic component, especially in newborns and those with very small shunts or pulmonary hypertension. A nonspecific systolic murmur is present in a small percentage of patients, more commonly the premature or very young infants. Uncommonly, the murmur may vary widely[148] or be absent.[149] In patients with at least a moderate shunt, there is a middiastolic rumble at the apex. The second heart sound may be difficult to hear due to the continuous murmur, but it is usually normal. The pulmonary component will be accentuated in those with pulmonary hypertension. Other causes of continuous murmurs, such as aorticopulmonary septal defect and sinus of Valsalva fistula, are extremely uncommon. They are discussed later in this chapter.

Chest Roentgenogram Findings on chest roentgenogram are also dependent on the magnitude of the shunt. In patients with a small shunt, the chest roentgenogram is normal, or the contour produced may suggest that the aorta and pulmonary artery are dilatated. With larger shunts, the left atrium is enlarged with posterior indentation on a barium-filled esophagus or elevation of the left mainstem bronchus. The left ventricle is also enlarged. Increases in pulmonary arterial flow parallel the magnitude of the shunt. In the presence of heart failure, there are signs of pulmonary edema. In older patients who have developed Eisenmenger's physiology, the only abnormality may be marked prominence of the central pulmonary arteries with rapid tapering to the periphery of the lung fields.

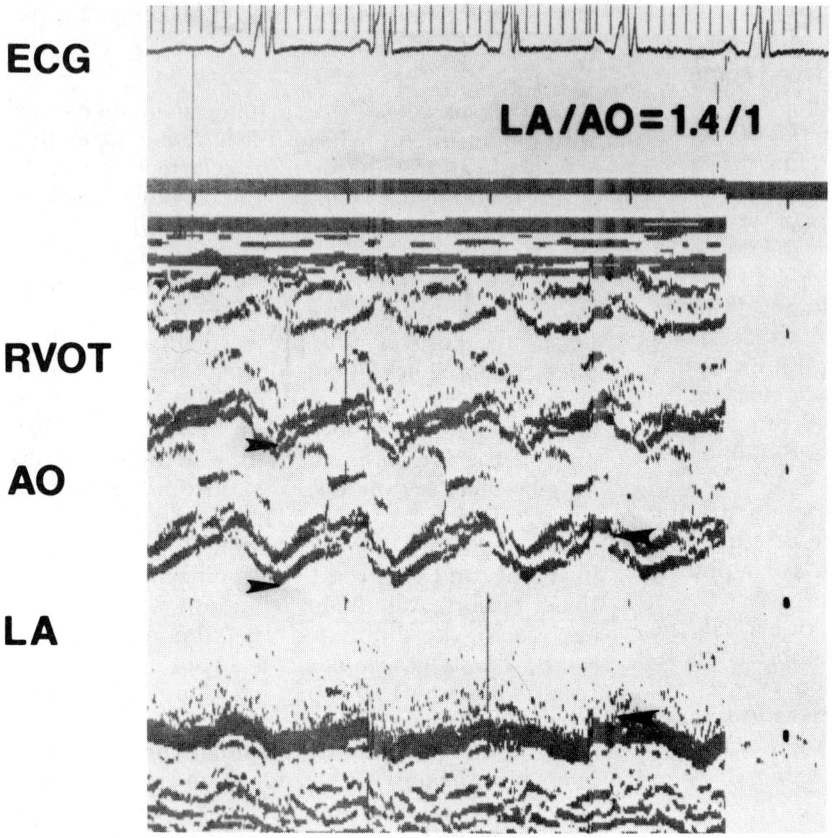

FIGURE 36-24 M-mode echocardiogram of a premature infant with a large patent ductus arteriosus. Aortic and left atrial dimensions (arrows) yield increased ratio due to left atrial enlargement. ECG = electrocardiogram; RVOT = right ventricular outflow tract; AO = aortic root; LA = left atrium.

Electrocardiogram With a small shunt, the electrocardiogram is normal. The QRS axis is usually normal, but it may be deviated to the left in some patients. Left atrial hypertrophy is probably the most common abnormality found, but left ventricular hypertrophy of the volume overload type, with deep Q waves and increased R-wave voltage in the left precordial leads, is also common. Right ventricular hypertrophy is seen with pulmonary hypertension.

Echocardiogram M-mode echocardiography is a noninvasive method for detection of left atrial enlargement, although it is not specific for patent ductus (Fig. 36-24). The ratio of left atrial diameter to aortic diameter, with its internal correction for body size, and left atrial dimension corrected for body surface area have been used.[150,151] There are rapid changes to normal after surgical ligation, and serial measurements are of value. The left ventricular end-diastolic dimension and mean velocity of circumferential fiber shortening are significantly increased.[152] The percentage shortening of the internal diameter of the left ventricle is increased until myocardial performance deteriorates, and it then decreases.[153] Pulsed Doppler ultrasonography offers a sensitive method[154] of detection of patent ductus, and continuous wave Doppler allows quantitation of flow.[155]

Cardiac Catheterization In those with typical, uncomplicated patent ductus, cardiac catheterization is not a necessity for diagnosis. When catheterization is performed, the catheter usually passes quite easily from the pulmonary artery to the descending aorta, except when the ductus is too small. The saturation will be increased in the pulmonary artery to a degree relative to the size of the shunt. The systemic arterial saturation is normal in the absence of pulmonary edema. The pulmonary arterial and right ventricular pressures are usually normal, but they are elevated in those with a large ductus. The pulmonary vascular resistance is almost always normal in infants and young children. It will be elevated in older patients who have developed changes in the pulmonary vascular bed. These patients will also have diminished saturation in the descending aorta once the pulmonary resistance reaches a level that will reverse the shunt. Aortography will opacify the ductus and pulmonary arteries. Radionuclide angiography is an alternative method.[156]

Natural History and Prognosis[6,140]

The complications related to patent ductus include infective endarteritis, heart failure, and pulmonary hypertension with vascular damage. Infection of the ductus is a risk regardless of its size. The risk increases with length of survival. This can lead to development of a mycotic aneurysm with the potential of compressing the recurrent laryngeal nerve, embolizing septic material to the lungs, or rupturing.

In patients with large shunts, heart failure can cause significant morbidity and mortality, particularly in the premature and young infant, and sudden death can occur. Progressive damage to the pulmonary vascular bed can occur in some, but it rarely occurs to an irreversible degree in the first year or two of life. Once irreversible damage occurs, premature death in late adolescence or early adulthood can be anticipated. Calcification of the ductal wall is common in adults.

Medical Management

Primary prevention results from obstetrical measures that decrease the incidence of prematurity. Primary prevention by widespread immunization of children has already been largely successful in reducing the number of those born with rubella syndrome. For women who are immunologically unprotected and exposed during the first trimester of pregnancy, abortion offers a controversial form of prevention.

Medical management centers around the symptomatic patients and the prevention of infection of the ductus. For prevention and treatment of infection refer to Chap. 56. This is important regardless of the size of the ductus and can be accomplished most effectively in the older infant and child by surgical ligation.

For symptomatic patients, usually premature and young infants, standard medical measures for treatment of heart failure are initiated. Management will be more successful if anemia is also prevented. In the premature infant, attempts to improve oxygenation can promote spontaneous ductal closure. A relation of volume of fluid administration to the incidence of ductus in premature infants has been demonstrated.[157] Reported differences in incidence of the clinically significant ductus may be iatrogenic.[158]

For those who do not respond to this type of management, alternatives to surgery have been sought, particularly for the higher-risk patients. Methods of transfemoral catheter closure using an Ivalon plug[159] and a foam-covered prosthesis with hooks[160] have been used successfully in selected patients. Such techniques are not in widespread clinical use at the present time. Successful pharmacologic closure of the ductus in premature infants using inhibitors of prostaglandin synthesis, aspirin and indomethacin, was first reported in 1976.[142,143] Subsequent reports include further assessment of responses[161] as well as of significant side effects such as changes in renal function[162] and other complications.[163] In addition, since anatomic closure is delayed beyond functional closure, the ductus may be a recurrent problem in these infants. From a national collaborative study of newborns with birth weights under 1750 g, administration of indomethacin appears to be indicated when other medical treatment fails.[164] Surgical ligation and/or division is an alternative, since accumulated experience here is great.[165,166]

The current indications for surgery include uncontrollable heart failure in the newborn and young infant, failure to grow properly in association with signs of a significant shunt in the infant, and continued patency with any size of shunt beyond the first year or so of life. Recommended age for elective surgical ligation is usually 1 to 2 years of age. The tendency in the premature has been toward earlier intervention in attempts to decrease incidence of chronic pulmonary disease. The presence of irreversible pulmonary vascular disease is a contraindication to surgery.

Intraoperative and postoperative management require special care with a team approach for the ill newborn. Most patients demonstrate increases in the systemic pressure in the immediate postoperative period. In a few patients, this rise can produce significant hypertension that is sustained[6] and may require medical treatment.

Surgical Management

Operation for patent ductus arteriosus has been pivotal in the historical development of surgery for congenital heart disease.[167]

The ductus is exposed through a subscapular left thoracotomy in the fourth intercostal space and is carefully mobilized, to avoid injury to the recurrent laryngeal nerve as it passes around the inferior margin. Details of the operation are described by Jones.[168]

Ductus obliteration is accomplished by division or ligation. A short, broad, or thin-walled ductus is usually divided between vascular clamps. The ends are closed with continuous suture (Fig. 36-25).[92] A long, narrow, thick-walled ductus can be divided or ligated with two or three sutures spaced a few millimeters apart. The suture ligatures at each end are superficially anchored in the ductus wall to avoid migration and to assure thrombosis and obliteration.

The fragile and thin-walled patent ductus arteriosus of the premature infant is obliterated by gentle ligation with a thick suture to minimize disruption or, if small, by occlusion using two metallic surgical hemostatic clips.

Closure of a patent ductus arteriosus in an adult requires particular caution because of possible calcification and rigidity of the ductus wall. Placement of a Dacron patch over the aortic orifice of the ductus from within the aorta may be advisable.[169]

Mortality for elective closure of uncomplicated patent ductus arteriosus by experienced surgeons is now virtually zero. Hemodynamics improve immediately; stroke volume and heart rate fall to nearly normal. In children showing growth retardation, acceleration can be anticipated following ductus obliteration. Long-term results are excellent, with very few late complications. The risk of ductus closure remains somewhat higher in adults and in those patients with elevated pulmonary vascular resistance. In fact, the risk of operation in patients with severe elevation of pulmonary vascular resistance is pro-

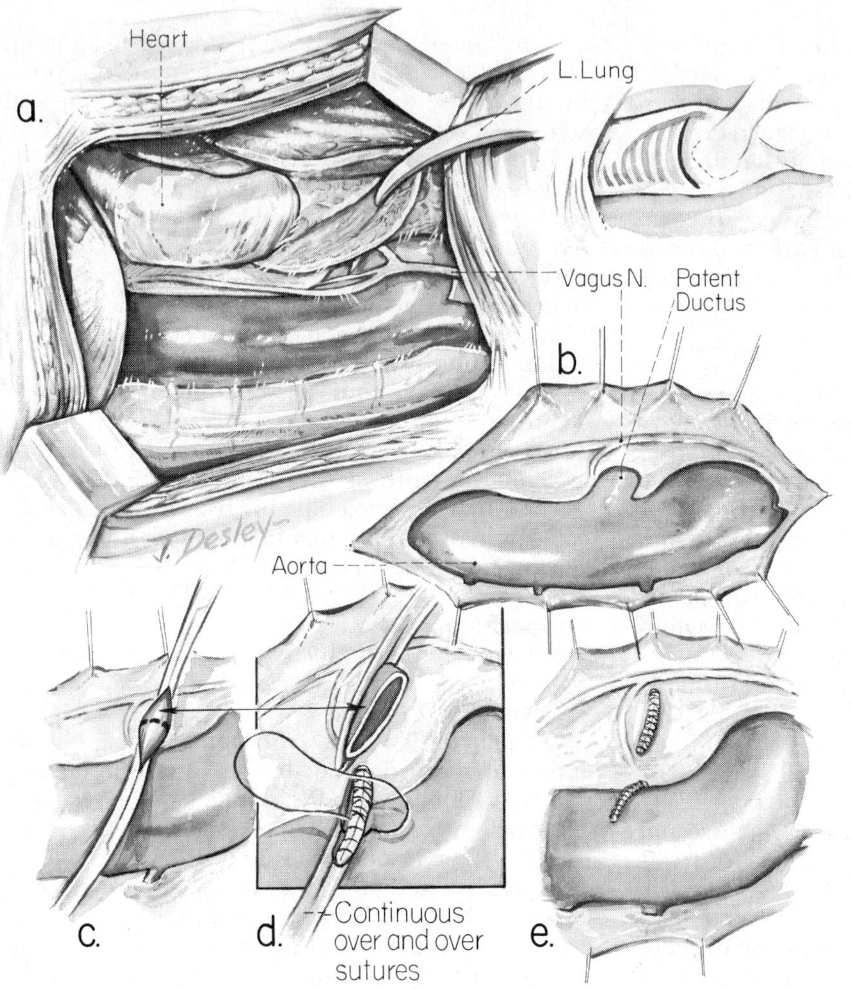

FIGURE 36-25 Division of patent ductus arteriosus. *a.* Mediastinal pleura is opened over the upper part of the descending thoracic aorta, and pleural flaps are retracted with fine silk sutures. *b.* Ductus arteriosus is nicely exposed as the vagus and recurrent laryngeal nerves are reflected medially. *c* and *d.* Ductus is appropriately clamped. *e.* Aortic and pulmonary ends are oversewn with two rows of continuous no. 5-0 silk sutures. (*This illustration appeared originally in the first edition of "The Heart," in 1966, and in all subsequent editions. It is reproduced here by courtesy of Dr. John W. Kirklin, Birmingham, Alabama.*)

hibitive; death even after closure is likely within 1 or 2 years.[170] Those patients with moderately elevated pulmonary vascular resistance will be helped but not cured by this operation.

Ductus obliteration offers clinical improvement in infants weighing as little as 600 g, with minimal operative risk, a reduced incidence of necrotizing enterocolitis, reduced duration of intubation, and improvement in late survival.[171] The influence of early ductus ligation upon the development of bronchopulmonary dysplasia and other sequelae of respiratory distress syndrome in prematurity remains to be established.

Aorticopulmonary Septal Defect (Window)

Definition

An aorticopulmonary septal defect is a communication between the ascending aorta and the pulmonary trunk.

Pathology

The condition is usually represented by a solitary opening between the left side of the ascending aorta and the right side of the main pulmonary trunk close to the origin of the right pulmonary artery. Classically, the defect is wide and unobstructive.[172] Uncommonly, it is narrow.

The condition results from focal deficiency in the septum that divides the primitive truncus arteriosus.

Associated conditions are relatively uncommon and include patent ductus arteriosus and ventricular septal defect.[173]

Clinical Manifestations

Clinical manifestations are dependent on the size of the communication. Those with the unusual small defect are similar to those with a small patent ductus and will not be discussed further.

When the defect is large, the clinical picture is similar to that of a large patent ductus with heart failure and pulmonary hypertension. Only the differences will be discussed. The presence of associated defects may be confusing.[173] The murmur is usually systolic, harsh, and heard lower at the left sternal border than is the case for a patent ductus. A systolic ejection click at the left sternal border may be heard.[174]

The findings on chest roentgenogram are also similar to those for a large patent ductus, although the aortic knob is not enlarged. A right aortic arch is occasionally associated.[173] On the electrocardiogram, there is usually biventricular hypertrophy similar to that in large ventricular septal defects. Isolated right ventricular hypertrophy occurs in very young infants and in older patients with severe pulmonary vascular disease.[174]

At catheterization, the venous catheter may cross the defect and enter the ascending aorta. Aortography will elucidate the diagnosis and demonstrate associated defects.[174]

Natural History and Prognosis

Unfortunately, the diagnosis of aorticopulmonary septal defect may not be suspected until the time of surgery or at autopsy, since it mimics the clinical picture of patent ductus so closely and is uncommon in comparison. Performance of catheterization and aortography is recommended in patients suspected of having a patent ductus with any atypical findings or evidence of pulmonary hypertension, and in all patients with ventricular septal defect.

Since most defects are large, the complications of heart failure and pulmonary vascular disease are very common.[174] Death occurs frequently in patients with failure managed medically. Most others will succumb in childhood with complications resulting from pulmonary vascular disease. There is also a risk of infective endarteritis.

Medical Management

Medical management is similar to that for a large patent ductus. Although reported surgical risk is high,[174] repair should be recommended because of the poor prognosis otherwise. Irreversible pulmonary vascular disease is a contraindication to surgery.

Surgical Management

Although historically aorticopulmonary septal defects were obliterated by division between vascular clamps or by ligation without the use of cardiopulmonary bypass, these methods are generally unsatisfactory and ill-advised. Ligation often resulted in recurrence, incomplete closure, intraoperative hemorrhage, deformity of the great vessels, or obstruction of the coronary arteries or the branch pulmonary arteries.[175]

Transaortic obliteration of the aortic orifice of the aorticopulmonary septal defect using a Dacron patch placed during cardiopulmonary bypass or hypothermic circulatory arrest is safe, precise, and effective (Fig. 36-26).[176,177] No dissection is required outside the aorta. The aortic valve leaflets, the coronary arterial ostia, and the orifices of the branch pulmonary arteries are identified and protected.

Survival of about 90 percent should be anticipated following closure of uncomplicated aorticopulmonary septal defects.[175–178] The relatively high incidence of complex associated defects complicates repair and increases risk. Early development of pulmonary vascular obstructive disease is common. Long-term outcome is excellent for young children with uncomplicated defects corrected early; it is equivalent to that achieved following obliteration of patent ductus arteriosus.

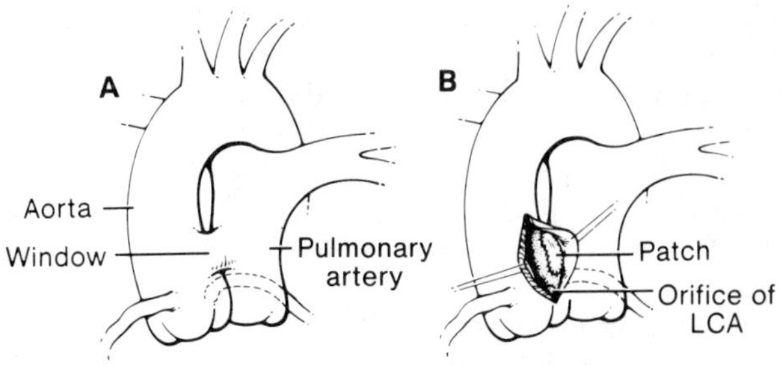

FIGURE 36-26 Technique for repair of aorticopulmonary window. *A.* External anatomy. *B.* Closure by patch. Note the proximity of the orifice of the left coronary artery (LCA).

One Pulmonary Artery from the Ascending Aorta

Pathology[179]

The origin of one pulmonary artery from the ascending aorta and one from the right ventricle, sometimes called *hemitruncus,* is a rare anomaly. The anomalous pulmonary artery is usually on the side opposite the aortic arch. The more commonly associated defects are patent ductus in approximately 75 percent, tetralogy of Fallot in 12 percent, and ventricular septal defect in 8 percent.

Clinical Manifestations

The clinical picture is similar to that of a large patent ductus.[179] Heart failure occurs within the first weeks or months of life. Cyanosis is associated in over half of the patients. The pulses are usually increased. Auscultation commonly reveals a nonspecific systolic murmur and an accentuated pulmonary closure sound caused by pulmonary hypertension. The clinical picture may be further confused by the presence of associated defects.

The electrocardiogram shows right ventricular hypertrophy in most and biventricular hypertrophy in some. Chest roentgenogram demonstrates cardiomegaly, and unilaterally increased pulmonary flow is frequent on the side of the anomalous pulmonary artery. Pulmonary flow may be increased bilaterally, particularly in the presence of a patent ductus. Lung scans show uptake on the side supplied by the normally arising pulmonary artery, usually the left, if there is no right-to-left intracardiac shunt. Cardiac catheterization reveals pulmonary hypertension on both sides, with diagnosis confirmed by angiograms in the aorta and right ventricle.

Natural History and Prognosis

Deaths frequently occur in early infancy due to heart failure or complications thereof, although associated defects may contribute. Histological examination of the lungs at autopsy[179] has not revealed significant obstructive changes in most of the infants dying at less than 6 months of age, but these are common and predominant in the lung supplied by the anomalous artery beyond 6 months. Thus, the natural history is a rapidly progressive one with death occurring in infancy or young childhood for most of those untreated or managed medically.

Medical Management

Medical treatment of heart failure after prompt diagnosis may temporarily improve the status of the patient. This should be followed by surgical correction as soon as possible, except in patients with severe pulmonary vascular disease.

Surgical Management

The orifice of the anomalous pulmonary artery is excised from the ascending aorta with a small button of aortic wall, unless ductus-like tissue requiring exclusion is present near the aortic end of the pulmonary artery. The aortic wall defect is repaired by direct suture. Continuity is established between the pulmonary artery from the right ventricle and the anomalous pulmonary artery by direct anastomosis or interposition of a small segment of polytetrafluoroethylene graft or free segment of subclavian artery. Cardiopulmonary bypass is usually not required but should be available if the partially occlusive vascular clamps are poorly tolerated.

Palliation, including banding of the aberrant pulmonary artery, ligation of a patent ductus arteriosus and the anomalous pulmonary artery, and ligation of a patent ductus alone, has failed.[179]

Early operation is required to prevent the development of pulmonary vascular obstructive disease.[180]

Sinus of Valsalva Fistula

Pathology

The condition is uncommon and also referred to as aortic sinus aneurysm. Because of an assumed intrinsic weakness at the union of the aorta with the heart, the aortic media may separate from the aortic annulus and retract upward. The structure that lies between becomes aneurysmal and may rupture[181] to form a fistula. The usual sites of the defects are the posterior (noncoronary) sinus aneurysms that rupture through the atrial septal wall into the right atrium (Fig. 36-27*A*) and those of the right sinus that rupture into the right ventricular infundibulum (Fig. 36-27*B*).[80,182,183] The aneurysm is represented by a gray pouch with multiple perforations in the wall. The principal associated condition is that of

FIGURE 36-27 Sinus of Valsalva fistula. *a.* Aneurysm involves the posterior sinus and ruptures into the right atrium. *b.* Aneurysm involves right aortic sinus and ruptures into the right ventricle. A ventricular septal defect is commonly associated, as illustrated. SVC = superior vena cava; IVC = inferior vena cava; RA = right atrium; RV = right ventricle; PT = main pulmonary arterial trunk; RPA = right pulmonary artery; LPA = left pulmonary artery; RPV = right pulmonary vein; LPV = left pulmonary vein; LA = left atrium; LV = left ventricle; Ao = aorta. (*From J. E. Edwards, Classification of Congenital Heart Disease in the Adult, in W. C. Roberts (ed.), "Congenital Heart Disease in Adults," Cardiovasc. Clin. Series 10/1, F. A. Davis Company, Philadelphia, 1979, p. 1. Reproduced with permission from the publisher, editor, and author.*)

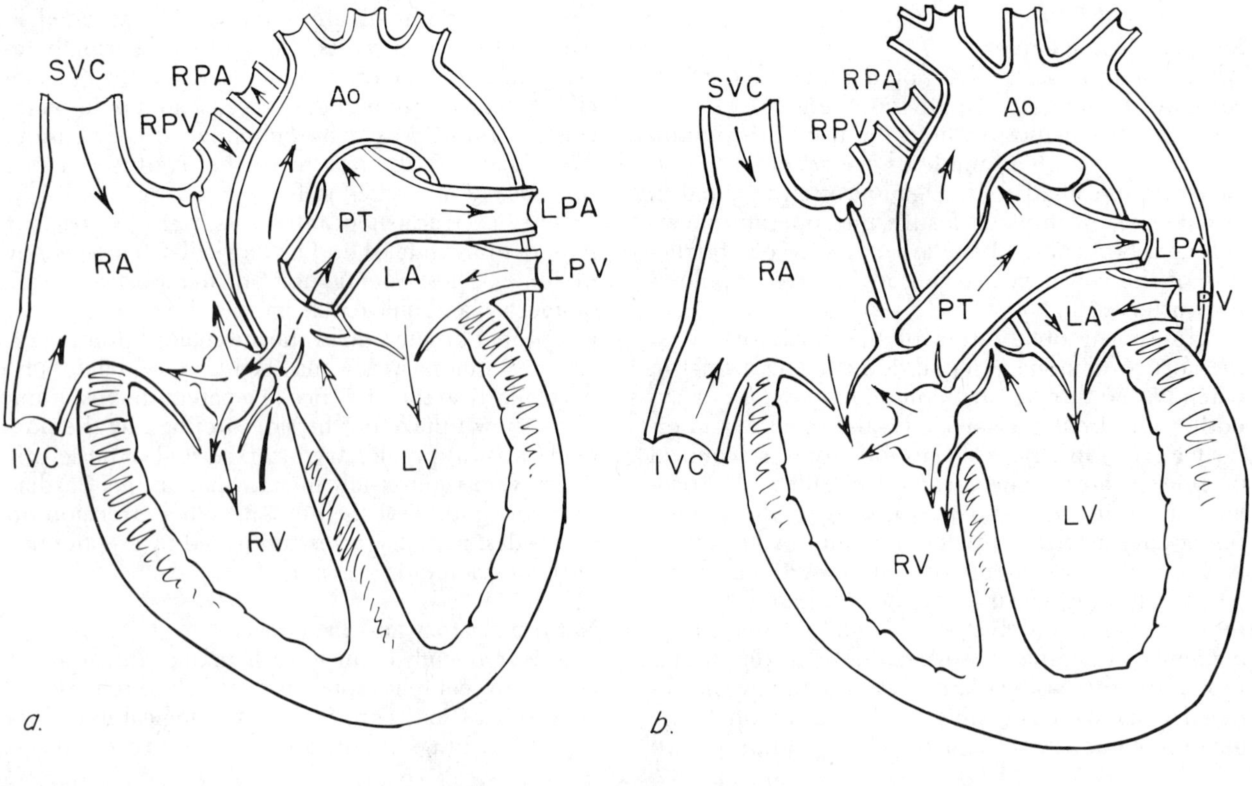

supracristal ventricular septal defect in cases with aneurysms of the right sinus (about 50 percent).

Clinical Manifestations

Sinus of Valsalva fistulas are most common in adults. When the rupture is secondary to bacterial endocarditis,[184] evidence of preceding infection is found. If the rupture occurs slowly, a small fistulous tract into the right atrium or ventricle will develop and present recent-onset findings of a small left-to-right shunt. With sudden rupture, there is usually a tearing pain in the midchest associated with dramatically rapid development of pulmonary congestion due to the sudden onset of a large shunt. Characteristically the murmur is loud and continuous but heard lower on the chest than the murmur of a patent ductus. A to-and-fro murmur rather than a continuous one may be heard at times. The apex impulse is hyperdynamic and the pulse pressure is widened. Ventricular septal defect may complicate the clinical picture. The chest roentgenograms are similar to those of patent ductus and are dependent on the magnitude of the shunt. The electrocardiogram may show biventricular diastolic overload patterns.

Cardiac catheterization will confirm the level of the shunt. Aortography is necessary for confirmation of the diagnosis. A pressure difference across the right ventricular outflow tract may be present if the right sinus is involved.

Natural History and Prognosis

With slow rupture and a small shunt, the major risk is infective endocarditis or extension of the rupture with an increasing shunt. With a large shunt, the heart failure is usually rapidly progressive and may result in death very quickly. A few patients seem to stabilize in this situation.[185]

Medical Management

Appropriate cultures should be drawn and antibiotics begun if endocarditis is suspected. Treatment of heart failure should be instituted rapidly. Because of the natural history, all patients should be corrected surgically.[186]

Surgical Management

Ruptured or unruptured aneurysms of the noncoronary or right coronary sinuses are usually repaired through an aortotomy which allows precise visualization of the aortic valve leaflets, the margin of the aneurysm, and the coronary arterial orifices. Aneurysms of the noncoronary sinus can be repaired through the right atrium; those arising from the right coronary sinus are accessible through the right ventricle. When the origin of the aneurysm is small and the margin is firm, the orifice can be obliterated by direct suture of the distal media to the proximal aortic annulus. Larger orifices are obliterated by a Dacron patch.

A supracristal (type I) ventricular septal defect must be sought and closed through either the aortic valve or the right ventricular outflow tract when an aneurysm of the right coronary sinus extends into the right ventricle. If the ventricular septal defect extends to the tricuspid valve, it should be approached through the right ventricle or right atrium to avoid injury to the conduction system. Associated right ventricular outflow tract obstruction requires resection of hypertrophic infundibular myocardium. Aortic valve replacement was required to correct aortic regurgitation in 24 of the 45 patients reported by Meyer.[186]

Nowicki[187] reviewed 176 cases of aortic fistula to the heart published in the English literature between 1839 and 1972. Of these, 126 underwent operative repair, which was successful in 108 (86 percent). Pan-Chih[188] reported correction of ruptured aneurysm of the aortic sinuses by exposure through the cardiac chamber into which rupture occurred in 51 patients with 88 percent survival. There were no hospital deaths in a group of 21 patients operated upon at the Mayo Clinic and reviewed in 1971,[189] although 3 patients required another operation to correct dehiscence of the repair. Congestive heart failure is controlled by successful closure of the fistula.

Anomalous Systemic Arterial Supply to the Lung

Pathology[190,191]

Anomalous systemic arterial supply to the lung originates from the descending thoracic or abdominal aorta. Commonly, sequestration of a portion of the lung, usually one of the lower lobes, is an associated condition. In this situation, there is no communication with the tracheobronchial tree and no supply from the pulmonary arterial system is present.

Clinical Manifestations

Clinical manifestations vary with the anatomic spectrum of associated defects.[190] About one-half are diagnosed by 10 years of age.[192] If sequestration of a portion of the lung is associated with this defect, there may be no symptoms or (more frequently) there may be pulmonary symptoms with recurrent infections.[191] If the anomalous systemic arterial supply is to a portion of the lung in communication with the tracheobronchial tree, there are usually no symptoms. Rarely, the arterial supply is large and high output can result in congestive heart failure in infancy.[192,193] This situation is emphasized in the following discussion.

The clinical picture may be similar to that of a large patent ductus, but there may be no precordial murmur or a nonspecific systolic murmur. The peripheral pulses are increased. This is distinguished from pulmonary arteriovenous fistula by the fact that there is no cyanosis unless pulmonary edema is severe. The chest roentgenogram will show cardiomegaly and pulmonary edema if there is heart failure,[193] and a density in the right or left lower lobe if there is sequestration. The electrocardiogram may reveal left ventricular hypertrophy with a volume overload pattern if the shunt is large. Cardiac catheterization will exclude left-to-right intracardiac shunts. Pulmonary hypertension is rare.[193] Aortography will demonstrate the anomalous vessel from the descending aorta with pulmonary venous return to the left atrium. If sequestration is present, pulmonary arteriography will show no branch to the involved area of the lung.[191]

Natural History and Prognosis
Although the complications of recurrent infection and heart failure do occur, asymptomatic adults are reported.[192]

Medical Management
Medical management consists of vigorous treatment of infection and heart failure if they occur. Surgery is indicated for those who are symptomatic.

Surgical Management
Angiographic or CT (computer-assisted tomographic) demonstration of the anomalous systemic arteries is required. The descending thoracic aorta is exposed through a thoracotomy, usually on the left. The anomalous systemic arteries to the lung are mobilized and ligated or divided.[193] A vessel may pass upward through the diaphragm or inferior pulmonary ligament from the abdominal aorta. When anomalous systemic arteries are associated with pulmonary sequestration, nonventilated pulmonary tissue is excised.[190] When recurrent pulmonary infections have damaged the pulmonary parenchyma, lobectomy is performed.

Descriptions of obliteration of anomalous arteries by embolization (silicone balloons, bucrylate adhesive) through intravascular catheters are provocative,[194,195] but the minimal morbidity and the definitiveness of ligation remain appealing.[196] Dramatic clinical improvement is usual after elimination of the anomalous vessels.

Coronary Arteriovenous Fistula
See the section on congenital abnormalities of the coronary arterial circulation, below.

Valvular and Vascular Malformations of the Left Side of the Heart with Right-to-Left, Bidirectional, or No Shunt

Aortic Arch Anomalies
Aortic arch anomalies encompass all of the variations of the aortic arch with regard to its position and branching. Some are sufficiently common and unimportant functionally as to be considered *variations.* A common origin for the innominate and left common carotid arteries is seen in about 10 percent of individuals. In a like proportion, the left vertebral artery arises from the arch just proximal to the left subclavian origin. Others cause compression of the esophagus and trachea with the potential for disturbance in function of these tubes. Such anomalies are often broadly grouped under the heading of *vascular rings.* Still others, although not functioning as vascular rings, may simply incite interest from their nature alone, or may be responsible for peculiar circulatory derangements. For details as to the variety of patterns and the developmental bases for these, the reader is referred to the literature.[197]

The following will identify the morphologic highlights of the more common variations and significant anomalies of the aortic arch system.

Aberrant Subclavian Artery
Pathology In about 0.5 percent of persons with a left aortic arch, the right subclavian artery arises as the fourth branch of the aortic arch. From the aorta it runs behind the esophagus to reach the position normally occupied by the right subclavian artery.

Aberrant left subclavian artery may be associated with a right aortic arch. Further discussion of this subject will be given under "Right Aortic Arch."

Clinical Manifestations Though occasionally implicated in instances of dysphagia, it would appear that an aberrant right subclavian artery with an otherwise normal left aortic arch seldom if ever produces symptoms. It may be found in association with the rare vascular ring created by a left aortic arch that crosses the midline and descends on the right of the spine. This is referred to as a *circumflex aortic arch.* In this instance the aberrant right subclavian artery is connected by a persistent ductus or ligamentum arteriosum to the right pulmonary artery, but the symptoms and radiological features are due primarily to the retroesophageal position of the aorta itself.[198] An aberrant left subclavian artery arising from a right aortic arch almost invariably is part of a loose, but complete, vascular ring by virtue of its connection with the left pulmonary artery via a persistent left patent ductus arteriosus or ligamentum arteriosum. This is the most common of vascular rings but only rarely produces symptoms. Atresia or stenosis of the origin of a subclavian artery appears to be more common if its origin is aberrant.

On chest roentgenogram the aberrant right subclavian artery creates a shallow, oblique, posterior indentation of the barium-filled esophagus, slanting upward from left to right. The aberrant left subclavian artery associated with right aortic arch and tetralogy of Fallot creates a similar shallow, oblique indentation, slanting upward from right to left. In contrast, the aberrant left subclavian artery either not associated with heart disease or associated with heart disease other than tetralogy of Fallot arises from the right arch via an aortic diverticulum of relatively large diameter. It creates a larger posterior esophageal indentation and assumes a more horizontal course from right to left.

Medical Management Infants or children with persistent symptoms of respiratory obstruction and evidence of an aberrant subclavian artery should undergo bronchoscopy and, if external compression is demonstrated, aortography. Those who are asymptomatic may be followed medically. Individuals with either atresia or stenosis of an aberrant subclavian artery are at risk of developing the subclavian steal syndrome.

Surgical Management The retroesophageal subclavian artery rarely causes symptoms or requires surgical intervention,[199,200] although we have operated upon one patient in whom a large aneurysm of such a vessel produced both respiratory distress and dysphagia. The artery is divided through a left thoracotomy after mobilization of the retroesophageal segment to allow the vessel to retract into the right hemithorax. Development of the subclavian steal syndrome is a potential complication of subclavian artery division for which reconstitution of flow can be accomplished using a graft from the ascending aorta placed through a right thoracotomy.[201]

Right Aortic Arch

Pathology Right aortic arch is characterized by the aortic arch passing over the right, rather than the left, bronchus. Mirror-image branching of the vessels is the most common pattern, with the left innominate artery being the first branch. No retroesophageal aortic segment is present under these circumstances. The ductus arteriosus may be absent, right-sided, or left-sided.

Less common than mirror-image branching is that in which the left subclavian artery is aberrant and, in effect, represents a mirror image of the common aberrant right subclavian artery. The aberrant left subclavian artery or the diverticulum from which it arises indents the posterior aspect of the esophagus; this is accentuated if a left ductus is present as this structure runs between the origins of the left subclavian and the left pulmonary arteries. Occasionally, with this pattern of aortic malformation, the aortic arch, after passing over the right bronchus, turns to the left behind the esophagus. At the left aspect of the junction of the right arch with the descending thoracic aorta a diverticulum is present. The left subclavian artery arises from the upper aspect of the diverticulum, and the aortic end of the ductus arteriosus or ligamentum arteriosum inserts into the lower aspect of the diverticulum. Compression of the trachea and esophagus results from a complexity of vascular structures oriented around these tubes. The vascular structures are as follows: anteriorly, the bifurcation of the pulmonary trunk; on the right, the right aortic arch; posteriorly, the retroesophageal segment of the aorta; and on the left, the ductus arteriosus or ligamentum arteriosum.[197]

Isolation of the left subclavian artery forms the third and least common pattern of branching in right aortic arch without retroesophageal segment.

Clinical Manifestations This anomaly occurs in approximately 0.1 to 0.14 percent of the population. Its importance lies in its use as a predictor of the presence or absence of congenital disease in general and its association with several important cardiac malformations in particular. In addition, its connection with a left patent ductus or ligamentum arteriosum creates the possibility of a complete and symptomatic vascular ring. When there is mirror-image branching, the incidence of congenital heart disease is 98 percent, with the majority of patients having tetralogy of Fallot. In the presence of an aberrant left subclavian artery the incidence of cardiac anomalies is estimated at only 10 percent. A right aortic arch is found in approximately 53 percent of patients with pulmonary atresia and ventricular septal defect, 31 percent of patients with tetralogy of Fallot, 31 percent of patients with truncus arteriosus, 20 percent of patients with double-outlet right ventricle, and 5 percent of patients with tricuspid atresia.[6] The incidence may also be slightly higher among individuals with transposition of the great arteries associated with a ventricular septal defect and pulmonary stenosis. In the absence of heart disease or with a nonrestrictive vascular ring, individuals with a right aortic arch are asymptomatic.

On the chest roentgenogram, the right aortic arch is seen as a prominent vascular shadow to the right of the esophagus and trachea in the frontal view. The lateral margin of the descending aorta is usually seen to the right of the thoracic spine as well. There is no vascular shadow on the left to suggest a left aortic arch or left descending aorta. When these structures are obscured by the thymus, one may still see a slight deviation of the air-filled trachea to the left, leaving little or no room for a normal left aortic arch within the mediastinal shadow. Similarly, the barium-filled esophagus will show the aortic indentation on the right and reveal the presence or absence of a retroesophageal vascular structure in the form of an aberrant left subclavian artery, ductus, or ligamentum arteriosum, or the aorta itself. Two-dimensional echocardiography from the suprasternal view can identify the right aortic arch with a high degree of reliability.[202]

Surgical Management A right aortic arch assumes surgical significance when tracheal and esophageal compression exists[200] or when creation of a shunt from the systemic arterial to the pulmonary arterial system is required for palliation of an associated congenital heart defect in which pulmonary blood flow is inadequate. Angiography allows selection of the appropriate vessel for a shunt, usually the left subclavian artery in patients having a right aortic arch with mirror-image brachiocephalic branching.

In symptomatic patients having a right aortic arch with a retroesophageal segment and a left ligamentum arteriosum, tracheoesophageal compression caused by the tethered bifurcation of the pulmonary artery is relieved by division of the ligamentum arteriosum through a left thoracotomy.

Double Aortic Arch

Pathology Double aortic arch is characterized by persistence of two aortic arches. Arising from the ascending aorta and after passing over the respective bronchi, the left and right arches join at a level posterior to the esophagus to form the descending thoracic aorta. Each common carotid and subclavian artery arises independently from its respective aortic arch. Usually, the right aortic arch is wider than the left.[197]

The relatively narrow state of the left arch compared to the right varies from minor differences to atresia of a segment of the left arch. The ductus arteriosus or ligamentum is left-sided.

Clinical Manifestations Double aortic arch is the most common type of symptomatic vascular ring. Approximately one-fifth of patients will have associated congenital heart disease, with ventricular septal defect and tetralogy of Fallot being the most frequent malformations.[6] About 75 percent of affected individuals are symptomatic, with symptoms ranging from mild to life-threatening respiratory obstruction and apnea. A few individuals remain asymptomatic and are detected accidentally as older children and young adults. Inspiratory stridor, dyspnea, and wheezing, which are accentuated with feeding, crying, or respiratory infections, are characteristic. Fluids are usually better tolerated than are solids. A brassy cough may be described.

Suprasternal and intercostal retractions, bilateral rhonchi, and even cyanosis may be found with severe obstruction. The head and neck may be held in hyperextension, and ill-advised flexion by the examiner may completely obstruct the airway and precipitate a respiratory crisis. A heart murmur and other features of associated heart disease may be present.

Since the right arch is the larger of the two arches in between 75 and 85 percent of patients, the usual picture on the chest roentgenogram is that of a vascular shadow to the right of the esophagus and trachea simulating an isolated right aortic arch. A barium swallow or esophagram will reveal, in the frontal view, bilateral compression of the esophagus with the larger and more superior indentation indicating the dominant arch. In the lateral view, a large posterior esophageal indentation will be seen as the dominant arch crosses the midline. Emphysema, atelectasis, or pneumonia may also be present. Aortography is recommended to evaluate the relative sizes and the patency of the two arches and to identify the brachiocephalic arterial branches. Approximately 16 percent will have atresia of the left arch, usually just distal to the origin of the left subclavian artery.[6] If associated heart disease is suspected, complete cardiac catheterization is always indicated.

Natural History, Prognosis, and Medical Management A few patients remain asymptomatic and require no therapy. The majority present within the first month or two of life with symptoms that may have been present since birth. Once present, symptoms persist and usually progress.

For symptomatic patients, a brief period of stabilization for treatment of pneumonia and diagnostic studies is justified, but surgical relief of the constricting ring is recommended as soon as possible. Preoperative bronchoscopy adds little in these particular patients. Despite the immediate and dramatic diminution in symptoms, mild degrees of respiratory obstruction may persist for weeks and even months before disappearing completely.

Surgical Management The double aortic arch is exposed through a left thoracotomy. The left or anterior component is usually the smaller of the two arches and is the one most often divided to break the compressing ring.[200,203,204] An atretic or stenotic segment in the smaller arch may determine the optimum point for division. The recurrent laryngeal nerve must be protected as it passes beneath the ligamentum arteriosum. The surgeon should verify the persistence of carotid or temporal arterial pulses while the arch is temporarily occluded at the point of anticipated division. The arch is then divided between vascular clamps and the ends are sutured (Fig. 36-28). The anterior arch can usually be pulled forward, away from the trachea, and sutured to the posterior periosteum of the sternum to assure relief of tracheal compression. This maneuver is particularly beneficial in the infant with secondary tracheomalacia or when the anterior arch is larger and remains intact after division of a smaller posterior arch.[205]

Isolation of Subclavian Artery

Pathology Isolation of a subclavian artery is an uncommon condition. It is usually observed in subjects with other cardiovascular anomalies, the most common being tetralogy of Fallot and interruption of the aortic arch. The condition is characterized by the involved subclavian artery not having connection with the aorta. Instead, it arises from the homolateral pulmonary artery by way of the ductus arteriosus or ligamentum arteriosum of that side.

Cases with normally arising arteries but with atresia of origin of a subclavian artery or the innominate artery have sometimes been designated as examples of "isolation." However, from a developmental viewpoint, such cases are different from that described above.

The isolated subclavian artery is always on the side opposite the aortic arch. Isolation of the left subclavian artery is about four times more common than is isolation of the right artery. The periphery of the isolated artery is fed by systemic collaterals, including the vertebral arteries that arise from the contralateral subclavian artery.

Clinical Manifestations This malformation does not cause symptoms; it is usually detected at the time of

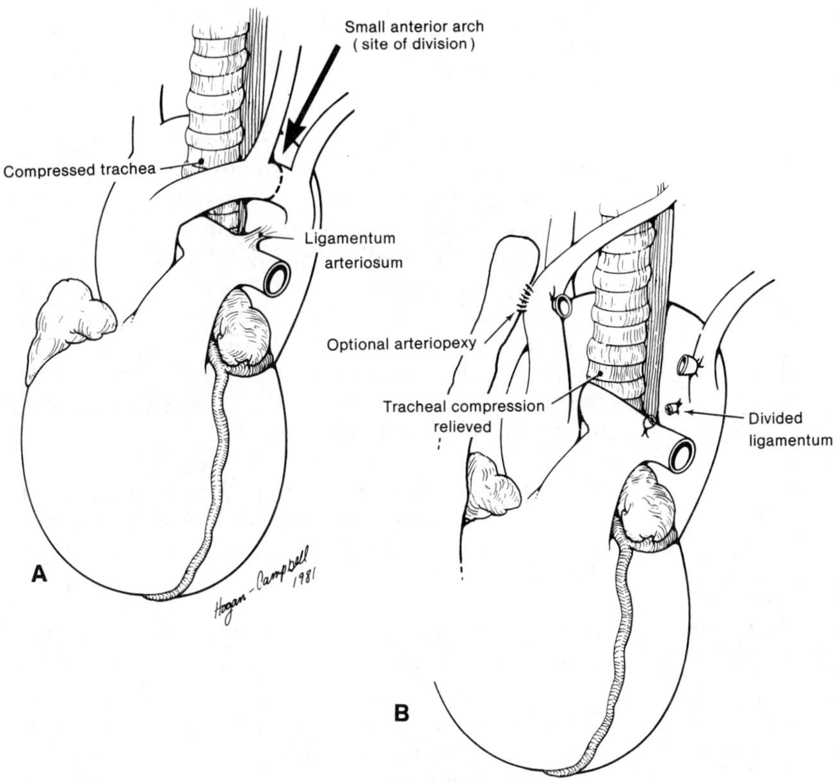

FIGURE 36-28 Relief of tracheal compression caused by double aortic arch (vascular ring). The great vessels are exposed through a left thoracotomy. *A.* The anatomy must be assessed carefully prior to division of vessels. *B.* In this case, the smaller, anterior arch is divided between the left carotid and the left subclavian arteries. The ligamentum arteriosum is divided. The anterior arch may be sutured to the posterior sternal periosteum to pull the vessels away from the trachea. Fibrous attachments between vessels and trachea are not divided.

aortography and catheterization for intracardiac malformations, particularly tetralogy of Fallot. Since the blood supply of the isolated subclavian artery may be derived from the pulmonary artery via a patent ductus or from systemic arterial collaterals, subdued and delayed pulses and diminution of blood pressure readings in the affected arm would be expected.

The chest roentgenogram usually reveals the aortic arch on the side opposite the arm with the delayed, diminished, or absent pulses. The esophogram will not demonstrate the posterior indentation characteristic of an aberrant subclavian artery to that arm.

Aortography will fail to opacify the subclavian artery arising from either the innominate artery or as the fourth branch of the aortic arch. Later frames usually will reveal opacification of the isolated subclavian artery by collateral circulation or retrograde flow in the ipsilateral vertebral artery.[206]

Natural History, Prognosis, and Medical Management Isolation precludes use of the involved subclavian artery for a Blalock-Taussig anastomosis, and, over the course of time, individuals with this malformation are candidates for the subclavian steal syndrome.

Surgical Management If a clinically significant subclavian steal syndrome exists as a consequence of isolation of the subclavian artery, the artery can be exposed through a thoracotomy, detached from the pulmonary artery and ligamentum arteriosum, and anastomosed to the aorta or another brachiocephalic vessel.

Pulmonary Arterial Sling

Pathology In this condition, after the usual site of origin of the ductus arteriosus, the pulmonary trunk continues simply as the right pulmonary artery. The left pulmonary artery arises to the right of the midline from the right pulmonary artery just proximal to the normal branching of the latter. The left pulmonary artery then arches over the origin of the right main bronchus and proceeds leftward behind the trachea and anterior to the esophagus to reach the left lung. The anterior aspect of the esophagus is indented.[207] A bronchus suis (independent origin of the right upper bronchus from the trachea) is commonly associated with this defect. If a bronchus suis is present, the left pulmonary artery arches over the origin of the intermediate bronchus (Fig. 36-29).[208]

As the left pulmonary artery passes over the right main bronchus or the intermediate bronchus, the pertinent structure is indented by the artery.

Pulmonary arterial sling may be an independent gross malformation or may be associated with congenital heart disease such as tetralogy of Fallot, ventricular septal defect, persistent truncus arteriosus, or interruption of the aortic arch.

Tracheomalacia and complete cartilaginous encirclement of the trachea have been described.

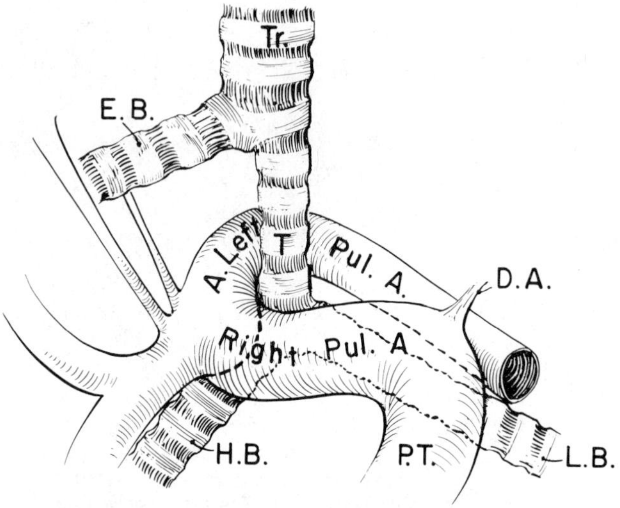

FIGURE 36-29 Vascular sling associated with bronchus suis. In bronchus suis, as illustrated, the eparterial bronchus (E.B.) arises from the trachea (Tr.). The vascular sling consists of the anomalous left pulmonary artery (A. Left Pul. A.) arising from the right pulmonary artery (Right Pul. A.) and arching over the right bronchus in a situation of normal tracheal bifurcation. When bronchus suis is present, as shown, the left pulmonary artery arches over the origin of the hyparterial bronchus (H.B.) from the trachea (T) and causes compression of the origin of that airway. P.T. = main pulmonary arterial trunk; D.A. = ductus arteriosus; L.B. = left bronchus. (*From K. L. Jue, G. Raghib, K. Amplatz, P. Adams, and J. E. Edwards, Anomalous Origin of the Left Pulmonary Artery from the Right Pulmonary Artery, Am. J. Roentgenol., 95:598, 1965. Reproduced with permission from the publisher and authors.*)

Clinical Manifestations Between 60 and 80 percent of patients with this rare cause of respiratory distress have associated cardiovascular disease, and almost 50 percent have associated tracheobronchial abnormalities as well. The male/female ratio is 1:1.[207] The majority present with symptoms of respiratory obstruction and distress either at birth or within the first 6 months of life. Symptoms tend to be progressive and consist of expiratory wheezing, stridor, apneic episodes, and cyanosis. Signs of unequal aeration and mediastinal shift are characteristic. A few individuals are asymptomatic.

Unilateral obstructive emphysema characteristically is present on the chest roentgenogram, and although either lung may be involved, hyperaeration of the right lung with mediastinal shift to the left is the more common pattern. The left hilar shadow is displaced inferiorly, and the esophagram will usually, although not invariably, demonstrate an anterior indentation of the esophagus at the level of the carina.

Bronchoscopy will demonstrate posterior compression of the distal trachea by a pulsatile mass and, in addition, will identify complicating tracheobronchial abnormalities. Selective pulmonary angiography in the frontal view with craniocaudal angulation will demonstrate the vascular deformity and is the definitive diagnostic procedure. If there is any suggestion of associated congenital disease, complete cardiac catheterization is warranted, since palliative or corrective surgical procedures may be possible at the time of the surgical approach to the aberrant left pulmonary artery.

Natural History and Prognosis Death from airway obstruction is the fate of untreated patients with severe symptoms. Symptoms of respiratory obstruction may persist for weeks and months after vascular surgery before finally clearing. If those symptoms are due to associated anomalies of the trachea or bronchi such as major segments of hypoplasia or stenosis, they will tend to persist. Hemoptysis, the result of extensive compensatory collateral circulation to the left lung with a thrombosed pulmonary artery, may be a late complication.

Medical Management Prompt diagnosis and surgery are indicated for symptomatic infants. Postoperative pulmonary arteriography is recommended.

Surgical Management In 1954 Potts[209] described dramatic reduction of dyspnea and cyanosis in a 5-month-old infant following ligation, division, and reimplantation of an anomalous left pulmonary artery into the main pulmonary artery. Twenty-four years following the operation this patient had normal exercise tolerance but minimal perfusion of the left lung.[210] Other approaches to this difficult problem have included division and repositioning of the trachea, left main stem bronchus division, and division of a patent ductus arteriosus. Results of operation have been disappointing, with surgical mortality approaching 50 percent.[207] Left pulmonary arterial patency has rarely persisted following anastomosis of the left pulmonary artery to the main pulmonary artery.[211]

Management of pulmonary arterial sling is often complicated by associated cardiovascular abnormalities. Deformity of the right main stem bronchus and trachea present prior to surgical intervention may not be relieved by reimplantation of the left pulmonary artery; symptoms of airway obstruction commonly persist following the operation.[211] Asymptomatic older children having a pulmonary arterial sling should not be subjected to surgery unless there is bronchoscopic evidence of tracheobronchial compression.

Cervical Aortic Arch

Pathology In cervical aortic arch the right or left aortic arch lies at a higher level than normal and may be evident in the supraclavicular area. The branches are usual for the type of arch. No significant pathological processes result from this condition. It has been suggested that cervical aortic arch is due to persistence of the right second or third aortic arches of the embryo, but it seems more likely that the condition represents an arrest in downward migration of the structures that form the normal aortic arch.

Clinical Manifestations This anomaly is usually recognized during childhood when attention is drawn to a pulsating mass in either the right or left supraclavicular area, usually the right. Most patients are asymptomatic. A few will have symptoms of stridor or dysphagia, suggesting the presence of a vascular ring. A murmur and thrill usually are present over the mass but not over the precordium. Occasionally a delay in arterial pulse transmission can be appreciated by simultaneous palpation of the radial and femoral arterial pulses. Digital compression of the mass may produce a discernible diminution in femoral arterial pulses.

The chest roentgenogram will reveal widening of the upper mediastinum, reflecting the vascular shadow of the aortic arch on the side of the supraclavicular mass. The trachea may be displaced to the opposite side. Posterior indentation of the barium-filled esophagus at the level of a normal aortic arch will be seen if the descending aorta crosses the midline.

Aortography will demonstrate the cervical aortic arch, establish the pattern of branching of the great vessels to the head, neck, and arms, and eliminate other possible alternative diagnoses such as carotid arterial aneurysm or arteriovenous fistula.

Natural History, Prognosis, and Medical Management This developmental anomaly is considered benign and is very infrequently associated with cardiac malformations. In the absence of signs or symptoms of vascular ring, medical or surgical intervention is unnecessary.[197,212]

Tracheal Compression by the Innominate Artery or Left Carotid Artery

Pathology Either of these two great arteries can, in rare instances, produce anterior compression of the trachea and severe symptoms of respiratory obstruction. No diagnostic indentation of the esophagus is present. In the case of compression of the trachea by the innominate artery, the more common of the two situations, the innominate artery appears to arise in a position more posterior or "later" than usual from the normal aortic arch. On its course back to the right, the innominate artery compresses the trachea anteriorly. The left carotid artery, arising either more to the right than usual from the aortic arch or arising as a third branch of the innominate artery, crosses the trachea from right to left and may have a similar compressing effect.

Clinical Manifestations The symptoms of stridor, wheezing, and apneic episodes may be no different from those seen with complete vascular rings or double aortic arch and usually begin within the first month or two of life. A series of lateral chest roentgenograms will show a constant anterior indentation of the tracheal air shadow just below the thoracic inlet. A similar indentation is present in normal infants but will be seen to vary in depth from film to film, depending on the phase of breathing.

Aortography is of limited help, since the variation in the vascular pattern of the symptomatic patient usually falls within the wide range of normal seen among asymptomatic individuals. Bronchoscopy will reveal significant pulsatile anterior compression of the trachea in symptomatic infants.

Natural History, Prognosis, and Medical Management The majority of infants with mild symptoms can be managed conservatively with the expectation of gradual improvement as tracheal rigidity increases with age. Those infants with severe symptoms will benefit dramatically from surgery.[6]

Surgical Management When anterior tracheal compression is suspected clinically and by air tracheograms or CT, confirmatory bronchoscopy is performed under light general anesthesia. Corrective surgery follows immediately if pulsatile anterior tracheal compression is present. The endotracheal tube is placed lower than usual with the tip near the carina to temporarily stent the compressed tracheal segment.

The ascending aorta and innominate artery are exposed through a right anterior submammary thoracotomy. The right lobe of the thymus is excised and the pericardium is opened longitudinally well anterior to the phrenic nerve. Pledget-reinforced mattress sutures of nonabsorbable monofilament material are placed in the adventitia and media of the ascending aorta and innominate artery and then passed through the posterior periosteum of the manubrium and the sternum. Fibrous tissue between arteries and trachea is not divided. The sutures are tightened and tied, pulling the vessels anteriorly toward the sternum. The remaining fibrous attachments to the trachea tend to pull the anterior tracheal wall forward, opening the lumen.[205] Tracheal compression is relieved; symptomatic improvement is dramatic; complications are minimal.

Abnormalities of left carotid arterial origin producing tracheal compression are managed by a similar operation conducted through a left thoracotomy. Detachment of the carotid artery with subsequent anastomosis in a different location has been suggested, but we have found this unnecessary.

Coarctation of the Aorta

Pathology

Coarctation of the aorta is a discrete narrowing of the distal segment of the aortic arch. The characteristic lesion is a deformity of the media of the aorta. The deformity, involving the anterior, superior, and posterior walls, is represented by a curtain-like infolding of the wall which causes the lumen to be narrowed and eccentric.[213]

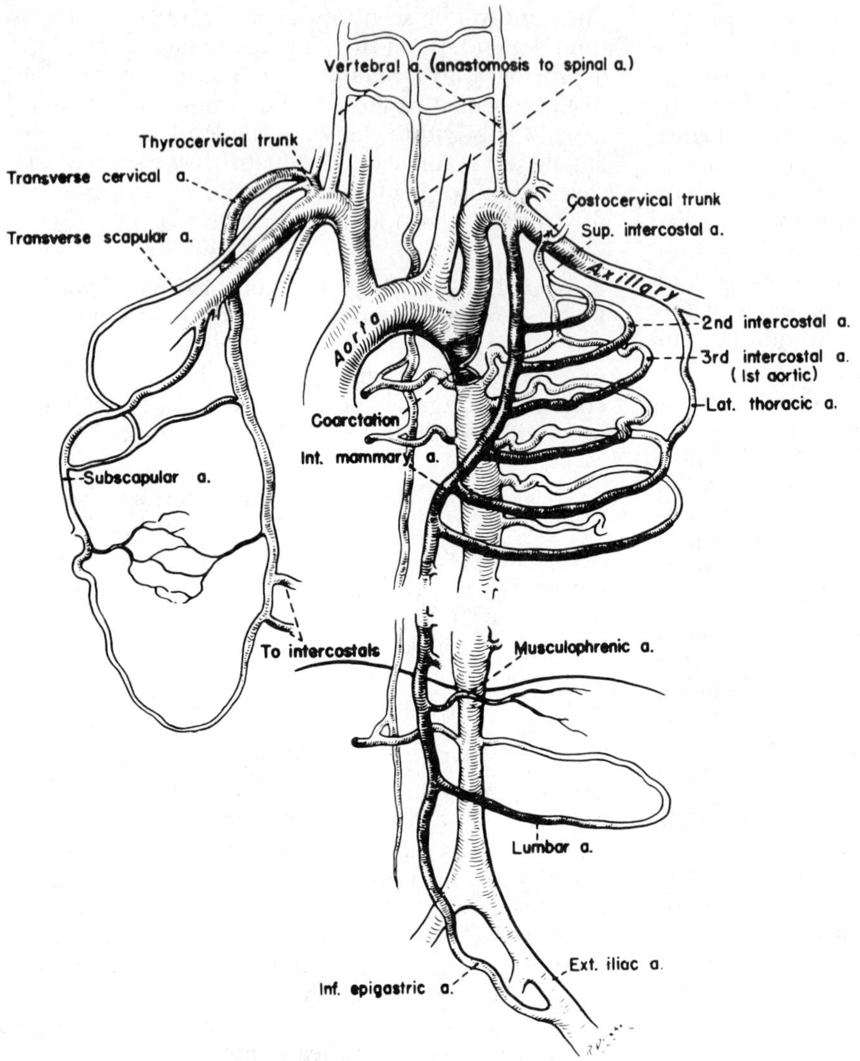

FIGURE 36-30 Collateral circulation in coarctation of the aorta. (*From J. E. Edwards, O. T. Clagett, R. L. Drake, and N. A. Christensen, The Collateral Circulation in Coarctation of the Aorta, Mayo Clin. Proc., 23:333, 1948. Reproduced with permission from the publisher and authors.*)

In symptomatic infants the lesion lies either opposite the ductus or in a preductal location. In adolescents and adults it is usually distal to the ligamentum arteriosum. In rare cases the lesion lies proximal to the origin of the left common carotid artery.

The principal cardiac abnormality is left ventricular hypertrophy. In some infants left ventricular endocardial fibroelastosis may be associated. Proximal to the obstruction, the aorta may show moderate degrees of cystic medial necrosis. Beyond the coarctation the lining may show a localized jet lesion.[213]

Prominent collaterals are evident anatomically, especially in the adolescent and adult (Fig. 36-30).[214] The collaterals may be divided into anterior and posterior systems, the source for each being the subclavian arteries.[214] The anterior system originates with the internal mammary arteries and makes use of the epigastric arteries in the abdominal wall to supply the lower extremities. The posterior system involves parascapular arteries which are connected with the posterior intercostal arteries and carry blood to the distal aortic compartment principally for supply of the abdominal viscera. The anterior spinal artery, receiving branches from the proximal and distal compartments of the aorta, is also dilated and tortuous.

Associated Conditions Becker and associates[215] reviewed 100 specimens from patients with coarctation of the aorta, the majority of whom were infants. Associated conditions, in order of decreasing frequency, were the following: *tubular hypoplasia of the aortic arch* (a narrow segment but with histologically normal characteristics); abnormal communications, mainly ventricular septal defect and patent ductus; left ventricular outflow obstruction, mainly subaortic stenosis; left ventricular inflow obstruction; and a variety of transpositions of the great vessels. A bicuspid aortic valve was present in 46 percent of the cases. Aberrant right subclavian artery may be associated. In about one-half of such cases the vessel arises proximal to the coarctation; it is distal to the coarctation in the other half.

Rosenquist[216] studied the mitral valves in 53 specimens from subjects with aortic coarctation. Abnormalities present in 31 were (1) fused or closely related chordae, (2) underdevelopment in the space

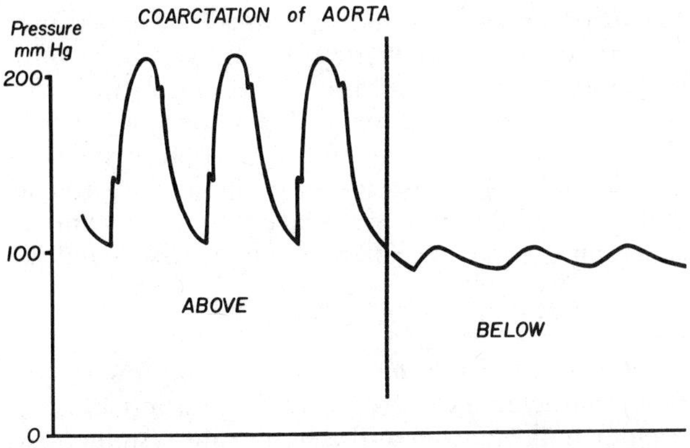

FIGURE 36-31 Characteristic tracings above and below a coarctation of the aorta. The arterial pressure pulse below the coarctation is damped by the coarctation and is characterized by a slow rate of rise of pressure and a delayed peak pressure.

between the papillary muscles and ventricular wall, and (3) parachute mitral valve (one case).

Abnormal Physiology

In most instances both the systolic and the diastolic arterial pressures above the coarctation are elevated above normal levels. Below the coarctation, the systolic pressure is lower than that in the upper extremities, and the diastolic pressure usually is near or only slightly below the normal range (Fig. 36-31). The mechanism of the hypertension in the upper limbs appears to involve mechanical factors (the increased resistance to aortic flow produced by the coarctation and the decreased capacity and distensibility of the vessels into which the left ventricle ejects its contents during systole) and probably humoral factors as well.[217] Once the pressure is increased by other mechanisms, it is also probable that the hypertension is maintained, in part, by an increased capability of the blood vessels to respond to increased intraluminal pressure secondary to increased tone and muscular hypertrophy. As a result of the damping effect of the coarctation on the transmission of the pulse wave, the onset of the femoral pulse wave is delayed about 0.03 s beyond that of the radial pulse wave and the femoral pulse wave has a prolongation of the systolic upstroke time.

Clinical Manifestations

This malformation accounts for approximately 8 percent of congenital heart disease in infants and children, ranking behind only ventricular septal defect and patent ductus arteriosus in frequency.[4] Of all individuals born with coarctation, approximately half will present within the first months of life with varying degrees of heart failure, usually severe. Of these infants, 60 percent will require hospitalization by the end of 2 weeks and the majority of the rest will require similar management in the next few weeks.[3] About 22 percent of infants so admitted will have uncomplicated coarctation, and a similar proportion will have a patent ductus. Almost half will have an associated ventricular septal defect.[3] The timing of ductal tissue constriction, both in terms of ductal closure and, perhaps, aortic constriction as well, appears to play a decisive role in the onset or worsening of symptoms in some of these patients.[218] The male/female ratio is approximately 3:1 for isolated coarctation but is only 1.1:1 for complicated coarctation. Approximately 45 percent of children with Turner's syndrome will have coarctation. Familial occurrence has been described.[219]

History The clinical picture in the symptomatic infant is one of dyspnea, difficulty in feeding, and poor weight gain. Older children are for the most part asymptomatic, although a few will complain of mild fatigue, dyspnea, or symptoms of claudication in their legs when running. Without surgery, symptoms again appear in the patient in the twenties, with congestive heart failure being a major complication after the age of 40.

Physical Examination In the symptomatic infant, signs of congestive heart failure are characteristic. Right and left ventricular impulses are hyperdynamic. A gallop rhythm is common, and a murmur from associated defects or from the coarctation itself (posteriorly in the interscapular area) may be heard. Frequently, these murmurs are either inaudible or nondescript on admission and become characteristic only when congestive failure is brought under control. In the older, usually asymptomatic child, disproportionate development of the arms, chest, and shoulder girdle compared to that of the legs may be noted. Prominent arterial pulses may be visible in the suprasternal notch and carotid arteries, and the left ventricular impulse is forceful. The aortic component of the second heart sound frequently is accentuated. An early systolic ejection click at the apex suggests the presence of a bicuspid aortic valve. The murmur from the coarctation is medium-pitched, systolic, and blowing in quality. It is best heard posteriorly in the interscapular area, usually with some degree of radiation to the left axilla, apex, and anterior precordium. Low-pitched, continuous murmurs of collateral circulation may be heard over the chest wall, particularly posteriorly, but seldom before adolescence. Murmurs consistent with mitral or aortic regurgitation or stenosis may be heard in a few patients. A short middiastolic rumble at the apex without clinical evidence of mitral disease is relatively common.

The characteristic clinical feature of coarctation, namely, a significant systolic blood pressure difference between the upper and lower extremities, may be difficult to appreciate or measure in infants with severe congestive failure or with a large ventricular septal defect or ductus. With improved compensation, pulses in the upper extremities become readily palpable. The femoral pulses remain weak, delayed, or absent. In these very young infants, it is important that the pulses in both brachial and carotid arteries be assessed. Weak or absent pulses in all sites are characteristic of critical aortic stenosis or aortic atresia. A normal pulse in one or both carotids would raise the possibility of coarctation or interruption of the aortic arch with one or both subclavian arteries arising below the coarctation or interruption.

In older children and adults, the radial arterial pulses typically are strong while those in the femoral arteries are either diminished, delayed, or absent. A measured systolic pressure difference between the upper and lower extremities is diagnostic. The pulse pressure in the leg is reduced, and in some patients no pressure can be measured by auscultation. Approximately one-third of children have little or no hypertension. Two-thirds have mild to severe hypertension, with the latter defined here as a systolic pressure above 150 mmHg, a diastolic pressure above 100 mmHg, or both. A systolic pressure difference between the two arms suggests that the origin of one subclavian artery is at or below the obstruction. It is useful to measure the blood pressure difference between the arms and legs before and after exercise in order to evaluate patients with only mild pressure differences at rest.

Chest Roentgenogram For the symptomatic infant, the pattern will be one of impressive cardiac enlargement, venous congestion, and, in the presence of ventricular septal defect or patent ductus, pulmonary arterial overperfusion. In the older and asymptomatic child, the heart size is generally at the upper limits of normal with a left ventricular prominence. A figure-three configuration of the left margin of the aorta at the level of the coarctation may be seen in overpenetrated films, with the upper curve formed by the slightly dilated aorta just above the coarctation, the central indentation by the coarctation itself, and the lower curve by the poststenotic dilatation below the coarctation. The mirror image of this, or *E sign,* may be outlined by the barium-filled esophagus along the right margin of the aorta. Notching of the inferior margin of the ribs by tortuous intercostal arteries acting as collaterals is seldom present before 7 or 8 years of age. Notching signifies clinically important coarctation and localizes the obstruction to the thoracic aorta. Prominent enlargement of the left ventricle and dilatation of the left atrium are not uncommon in older individuals with coarctation without operation.

Electrocardiogram The electrocardiogram of the symptomatic infant will show right-axis deviation, right atrial hypertrophy, and right ventricular or biventricular hypertrophy during the first 3 months of life. Isolated left ventricular hypertrophy is rare. T-wave inversion in the left precordial leads is common. Among older children, the electrocardiogram is usually normal or may indicate mild left ventricular and left atrial hypertrophy. Among older individuals there is a higher incidence than normal of conduction abnormalities, including left anterior hemiblock and ventricular bigeminy.

Echocardiogram M-mode echocardiography is useful in assessing left ventricular function. Two-dimensional echocardiographic imaging of the aortic arch from the suprasternal notch permits visualization of the coarctation and prediction of such anatomic variations as isthmic hypoplasia. The precordial and subxiphoid views are of great value in assessing the presence and severity of associated defects.[220]

Cardiac Catheterization Study of symptomatic infants characteristically reveals left atrial and left ventricular hypertension and a significant systolic pressure difference between the left ventricle and the femoral artery, particularly if the coarctation is isolated. In the presence of a large ventricular septal defect or patent ductus, the left ventricular hypertension and the systolic pressure difference between the left ventricle and femoral artery is less impressive and may not exist at all. Every attempt should be made to define the nature and severity of associated defects. Aortography is recommended in older children to demonstrate the exact site and length of the coarctation as well as to show unusual features of the collateral circulation that may be of importance to the surgeon.

Natural History and Prognosis

Approximately one-fifth of those infants admitted with heart failure within the first weeks of life will have coarctation without significant associated defects. The majority, though not all, of these infants will respond well to medical management and, usually, reach a stage at 2 or 3 years of age where they are indistinguishable from those asymptomatic children of the same age whose coarctation is first detected on a routine physical examination. Upper-extremity hypertension usually increases during the first several months of life and then tends to diminish again as collateral circulation improves. Cardiac enlargement, tachypnea, and other signs of failure diminish at the same time, and digitalis can usually be discontinued during the second year of life. For infants with severe failure and any serious associated defects, surgery provides virtually the only chance of survival despite the most vigorous and skillful medical management. These patients, and those few with isolated coarctation in whom the response to medical management has been marginal, require prompt relief of the coarctation and simultaneous correction or palliation of associated defects. These patients generally do extremely well, although some may require correction of residual significant associated defects at some point in the future. The incidence of recoarctation over the course of the next several years in very young infants undergoing end-to-end anastomosis of the aorta in the first year of life is in the order of 38 percent.[221] In a small number of patients this generally optimistic postoperative course will be complicated by rapidly recurrent coarctation or the development of moderate or severe mitral stenosis or regurgitation.

Without surgery, older children on the whole do well. The consequences of persistent hypertension may appear in the second and third decades in the form of aortic rupture or intracranial hemorrhage from an aneurysm of the circle of Willis. They appear in the fourth decade in the form of congestive heart failure often complicated by mitral or aortic valve disease, dissecting aneurysm of the aorta, or atherosclerosis. The risk of endocarditis on the aortic or mitral valves or endarteritis at the site of coarctation appears spread relatively evenly over the course of years. The median age of death of patients surviving childhood with coarctation without surgery is 31 years.[222] Among older adults with congestive failure, the results of surgery, though less dramatic, are decidedly beneficial in most instances.

Normal blood pressures are achieved in at least 80 percent of patients if surgery is performed during childhood and if those individuals with recurrent coarctation are excluded.[222] All postoperative patients, particularly those in whom the blood pressure has not returned to normal following surgery, should be assessed by arm and leg blood pressure measurement at rest and at exercise.[223]

Residual or recurrent hypertension among patients without demonstrable recurrent coarctation, renal disease, or significant aortic regurgitation appears related to the duration of hypertension prior to surgery. This complication seems rare among individuals operated upon before the age of 6 years but becomes progressively more common as surgery is delayed and may be present in from 20 to 50 percent of individuals operated upon at 20 years of age or beyond.[224] Similarly, the risk of premature death from cardiovascular disease in the form of aortic or cerebral arterial rupture, congestive heart failure, or myocardial infarction is increased if surgical correction is delayed into the third decade.[224] Finally, survivors of surgery frequently carry with them residual congenital heart disease primarily in the form of aortic and mitral valve malformations. While some 60 to 70 percent of patients fall in this category, in only a small proportion will these lesions prove hemodynamically significant.

Medical Management

Vigorous medical treatment with digitalis, intravenous diuretics, oxygen, and sedation are indicated for those infants with severe heart failure. Cardiac catheterization, usually after 24 h of medical management, is recommended to detect and assess the severity of associated lesions. An occasional infant will require intravenous infusion of prostaglandin E_1 to reopen the closing ductus; pulmonary edema is thereby controlled and the patient is stabilized sufficiently to permit catheterization and operation.[225] Prompt surgical correction of the coarctation is recommended for those infants in whom there is one or more associated defects and for infants with isolated coarctation as well, unless the response to medical management has been dramatic and sustained. The role of balloon dilation angioplasty in infants and older children, whether or not surgery has been performed, is yet to be determined.[226] Infants should be followed closely after the operation to detect the occasional patient with rapid redevelopment of coarctation or with continuing or progressive symptoms related to severe aortic or mitral stenosis or insufficiency. Infants not requiring surgery generally improve steadily despite impressive hypertension in the first months of life. The persistence of failure or its appearance for the first time beyond the age of 6 months suggests a complication or an associated lesion.

Elective correction of coarctation is now recommended between the ages of 4 and 6 years in order to avoid the relatively high rate of recoarctation found among patients with coarctation corrected under 1 year of age and the complication of persistent or recurrent hypertension, without demonstrable recoarctation, among those individuals having surgery after 6 years of age. Increasing fatigue or dyspnea, progression of hypertension with or without symptoms suggesting impending encephalopathy or cerebral vascular accident, significant cardiac enlargement, or severe left ventricular hypertrophy shown by the electrocardiogram would indicate a need for earlier correction. Restriction from strenuous sports or exercise is recommended prior to correction.

Older children and adults should undergo correction without delay. Even older adults who are symptomatic with hypertension and associated lesions usually benefit significantly from repair.

Patients who have had coarctation should be followed indefinitely. For those with significant recoarctation, expressed as a systolic pressure gradient of 30 mmHg or more at rest between the upper and lower extremities, angiography and, if feasible, reoperation is recommended.[221] Postoperative patients, with or without resting hypertension, who have insignificant or small resting gradients but who manifest abnormal upper-extremity hypertension and significant gradients with exercise probably should undergo reoperation as well. Patients with persistent hypertension without gradients either at rest or with exercise and those patients described above in whom reoperation seems unjustified or unduly hazardous will probably benefit from restricted activity and antihypertensive medication. Pregnancy carries a mortality rate of approximately 10 percent and a complication rate of 90 percent among women with uncorrected coarctation. With correction the mortality rate does not differ significantly from the normal, while complications are on the order of 15 percent.[227] The risk of congenital heart disease in the offspring of one affected parent or in a sibling of a single affected family member is estimated at 2 percent, with about a 50 percent chance of the defect being coarctation.[116]

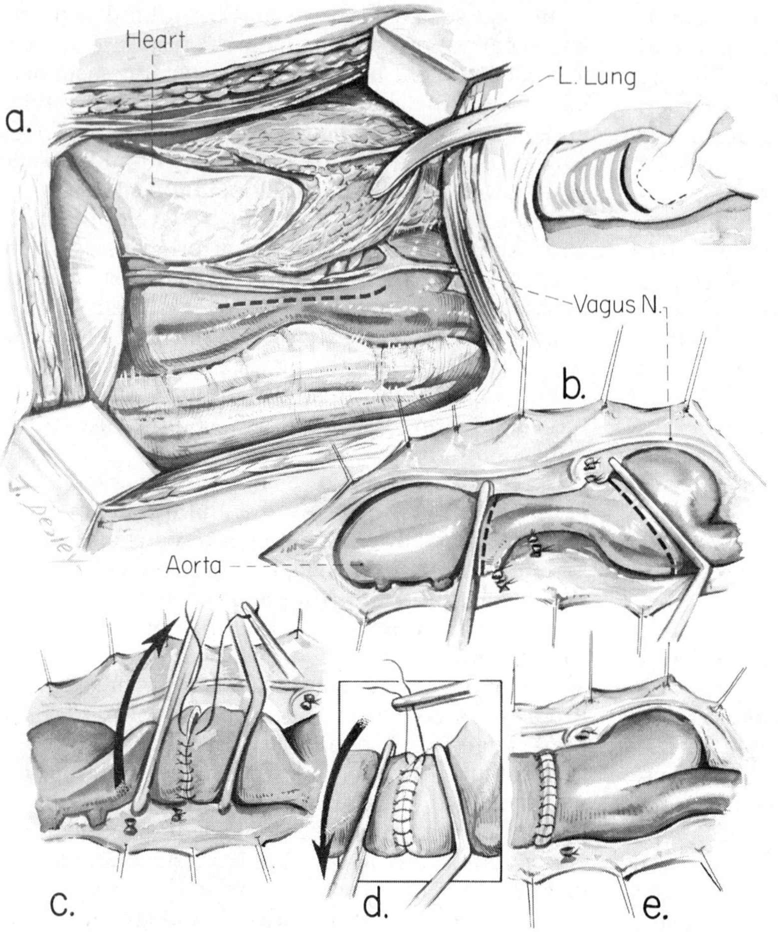

FIGURE 36-32 Steps in operative repair of coarctation of aorta. *a.* Mediastinal pleura is opened over the upper part of the descending thoracic aorta. *b.* After appropriate mobilization of the coarctate area and division of ligamentum arteriosum, appropriate clamps are placed above and below the stricture. At times the distal clamp must be placed farther downstream than is shown here, and then the intercoastal arteries are temporarily controlled with bulldog clamps. *c, d,* and *e.* End-to-end anastomosis is made with interrupted simple sutures of no. 5-0 silk. (*This illustration appeared originally in the first edition of "The Heart," in 1966, and in all subsequent editions. It is reproduced here by courtesy of Dr. John W. Kirklin, Birmingham, Alabama.*)

Surgical Management

Coarctation of the aorta should be corrected in all symptomatic infants and in asymptomatic children between the age of 4 and 6 years.[228,229] Repair by subclavian flap aortoplasty in the first year of life probably offers the greatest likelihood of long-term cure.

The coarctation is exposed and mobilized through a posterolateral left thoracotomy. It is usually possible to resect the narrow segment and restore continuity by direct end-to-end anastomosis[230,231] (Fig. 36–32).[92] Occasionally a tubular vascular prosthesis is required to bridge the gap between the two ends of the aorta when the coarctation is unusually long, the aortic isthmus is hypoplastic, or there is an associated aneurysm. In adults with a relatively nonelastic or calcified aorta and in secondary repairs, a tubular vascular prosthesis can be used to bypass the unresected coarctation.[232] The child having Turner's syndrome appears to be at greater risk of perioperative hemorrhage and suture-line complications because of the friability of the thin-walled aorta.[233] Tension-free suture lines are essential.

The infant and small child with coarctation pose unique problems. While early repair is desirable, growth of a circular suture line at the site of an end-to-end anastomosis will probably not be adequate; recurrent stenosis will develop as the child grows,[234] and hypertension is likely, particularly during exercise. Techniques offering promise of reducing the incidence of recoarctation include the Dacron patch aortoplasty,[235] the subclavian arterial flap aortoplasty,[236,237] (Fig. 36–33)[238] and the use of absorbable sutures.[239] Transluminal angioplasty has been applied in the management of coarctation and restenosis, but the effectiveness of this technique remains to be established.[226]

If a significant ventricular septal defect is also present, distal pulmonary arterial pressure is reduced to about one-third of the systemic arterial pressure by placement of a pulmonary arterial band at coarctation repair during infancy. The ventricular septal defect is closed if required and the band removed during the second 6 months of life. If the ventricular septal defect is of an anatomically complex form and adequate palliation has been achieved, repair is deferred until the child is about 2 years old. Tiraboschi[240] has reported excellent results, however, with simultaneous repair of coarctation and closure of the ventricular septal defect in a few older infants. Others prefer not to band the pulmonary artery at all, closing the ventricular septal defect at a subsequent early date if required by the child's clinical course.[241]

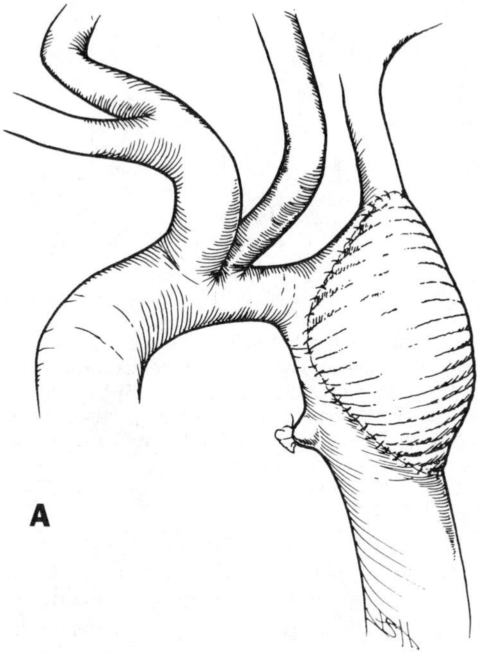

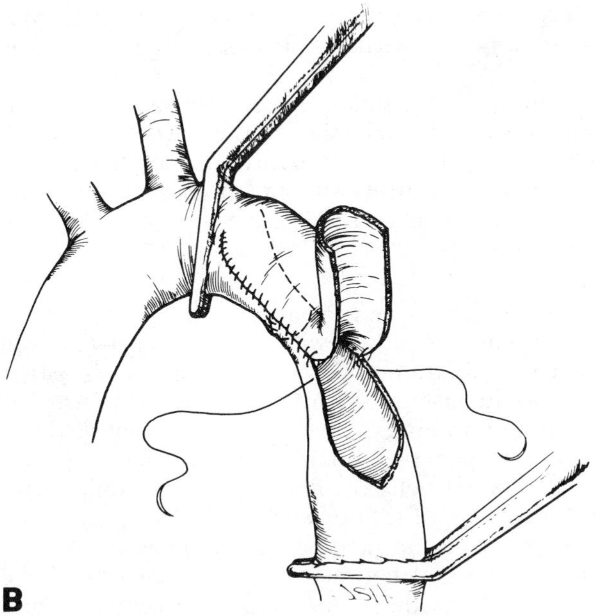

FIGURE 36-33 *A.* Coarctation repair using Dacron patch angioplasty. A longitudinal incision extends from the normal aorta below the coarctation to a point well above the coarctation on the subclavian artery. A relatively large patch is cut from a Dacron tube graft and is sutured across the coarctation after excision of any intraluminal membrane. Circular suture lines are thus avoided. The patch is large, allowing for growth. *B.* Repair of coarctation of the aorta by subclavian arterial flap angioplasty. The subclavian artery is divided in the apex of the left pleural cavity. The lateral wall of the artery is incised downward, the incision continuing across the coarctation onto normal aorta below. The flap thus created is sutured across the coarctation, after excision of intraluminal membrane, using fine, continuous monofilament suture. Circular suture lines are avoided. The viable flap should grow as the child and aorta grow, minimizing recurrent coarctation. *(From V. M. Herrmann, H. Laks, L. Fagan, D. Terschluse, and V. L. William, Repair of Aortic Coarctation in the First Year of Life, Ann. Thorac. Surg., 25:57, 1978. Reproduced with permission of the publisher and authors.)*

Adequacy of collateral circulation is crucial for safe repair of coarctation. A rise in proximal systemic arterial pressure of more than 20 mmHg when the aorta is clamped above the coarctation suggests marginal collaterals. Pressure in the descending aorta can be measured, and, if necessary, cardiopulmonary bypass or a shunt can be used to provide distal perfusion.[242] Aortic occlusion time should obviously be kept to a minimum. Monitoring of somatosensory cortical evoked potentials may warn of impending ischemic insult to the spinal cord.[243]

Postoperative paradoxical hypertension is common between the second and tenth postoperative day[244] and may contribute to the postcoarctation syndrome in which ileus, abdominal pain, mesenteric vasculitis, and even visceral infarction may occur. We have not encountered this syndrome in patients in whom we have maintained the postoperative diastolic blood pressure within normal range for age with sodium nitroprusside, propranolol, or reserpine, and in whom nasogastric tube decompression of the gastrointestinal tract has been maintained postoperatively for 48 h.

Williams reviewed the cases of 191 infants less than 1 year old who underwent repair of coarctation of the aorta during a recent 14-year period.[245] Operative mortality was 4 percent for infants with isolated coarctation and 25 percent when other cardiovascular defects were present. There were no subsequent deaths in hospital survivors with isolated coarctation, but the 5-year mortality for those having coarctation with other defects was 25 percent. Recurrent coarctation, suggested by a gradient between arm and leg blood pressures at rest, occurred in 54 percent of survivors within 7 years. Hypertension was present in 27 percent of children followed more than 5 years after repair. Bergdahl demonstrated that very small size of the infant, the presence of major associated cardiac anomalies other than ventricular septal defect, and failure to use the subclavian flap aortoplasty were incremental risk factors for hospital death following coarctation repair in infancy.[246]

Maron reported data from 248 older patients (over 2 years) followed 11 to 15 years after correction of coarctation.[247] Of these patients 12 percent had died and 78 percent had persistent evidence of cardiovascular disease. Premature death was believed to correlate with the duration of hypertension present preoperatively.

Sehested reviewed the cases of 182 patients undergoing repair of coarctation between the ages of 3 weeks and 60 years.[228] Four operative deaths occurred in children less than 14 months old, all having other cardiac defects. Two patients sustained lower limb paralysis. There were no operative or late deaths in patients with uncomplicated coarctation, but about one-third of the patients remained hypertensive on follow-up.

Early correction of coarctation in infancy is suggested[229] by the dismal prognosis for untreated

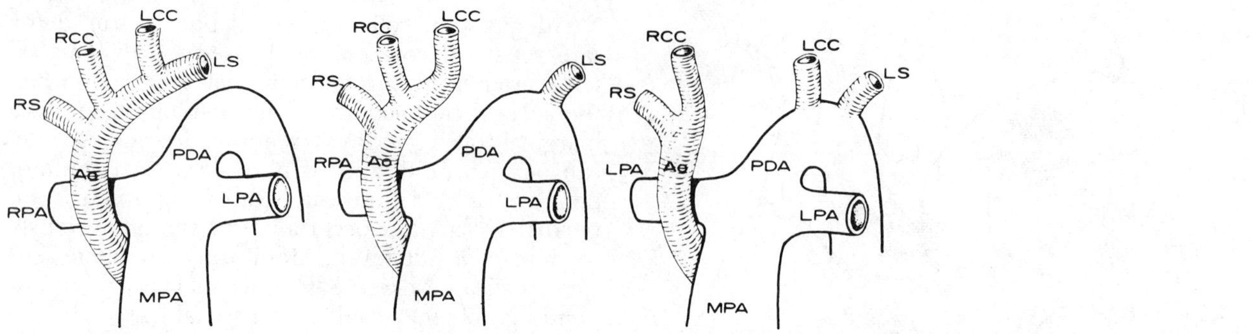

FIGURE 36-34 Classification of interrupted aortic arch. Type A is interruption distal to left subclavian artery (LS); type B is interruption distal to left common carotid artery (LCC); type C is interruption distal to the innominate or right common carotid artery (RCC). Ao = ascending aorta; LPA = left pulmonary artery; MPA = main pulmonary artery; PDA = patent ductus arteriosus; RPA = right pulmonary artery; RS = right subclavian artery. (*From E. L. Jones, W. H. Plauth, Jr., and C. R. Hatcher, Jr., A Palliative Operation for All Types of Aortic Arch Interruption in the Neonate, J. Thorac. Cardiovasc. Surg., 69:581, 1975, p. 581. Reproduced with permission from the publisher and authors.*)

coarctation, the excellent hemodynamic results achieved by aortoplasty, and the relatively low mortality and incidence of restenosis now anticipated.[236–237]

Interruption of the Aortic Arch

Definition and Pathology

Interruption of the aortic arch is characterized by lack of a channel between the aortic arch and the descending aorta. The descending aorta is connected to the pulmonary arterial system by the ductus arteriosus. Classically, the ductus is left-sided, as is the descending aorta.

Variations occur in the origin of branches of the arch.[248] In over half of the cases (53 percent) the left subclavian artery arises from the descending aorta (type B). In about 42 percent all of the branches of the arch arise proximal to the interruption (type A) (Fig. 36–34).[249] Less common patterns are (1) origin of both subclavian arteries from the descending aorta, (2) origin of the right subclavian artery from the descending aorta, (3) isolation of the subclavian artery on the side opposite the descending aorta, and (4) very rarely, origin of the left common carotid and left subclavian arteries from the distal compartment (type C). Ventricular septal defect is present in over 90 percent of patients. Less commonly associated anomalies are aorticopulmonary septal defect, complete transposition, persistent truncus arteriosus, and origin of both great vessels from the right ventricle.

Clinical Manifestations

This very rare malformation accounts for about 4 percent of the deaths among infants with congenital heart disease in the first month of life.[3] Without surgery, the median age of death is 4 days.[248] There is no sex predilection. The clinical picture is the same as that of the newborn with severe complicated coarctation, except that in approximately half of these infants the left subclavian arterial pulse is weak or absent. If both subclavian arteries arise below the interruption, pulses in all extremities will be weak or absent. Preservation of a right carotid pulse will distinguish these patients from those with aortic atresia or critical aortic stenosis. Two-dimensional echocardiographic studies will distinguish infants with interruption or coarctation from those with aortic atresia.[250]

The pressure and oxygen saturation data at catheterization will be similar to those of infants with severe coarctation, ventricular septal defect, and patent ductus arteriosus, but high-quality biplane angiography will reveal the absence of an aortic isthmus.

Natural History and Prognosis

Rarely, an individual with this malformation will survive to adulthood. In these instances either (1) the ductus and the intracardiac or supracardiac communication remained patent and a marked elevation of the pulmonary vascular resistance prevented overwhelming flooding of the pulmonary vascular bed, or (2) ductal closure was delayed long enough to permit compensatory collateral circulation to develop between the two segments of the aorta.[251] Individuals in the latter group are candidates for correction.

Medical Management

Intensive therapy to control congestive failure usually is futile without intravenous infusion of prostaglandin E_1 to maintain ductal patency. Cardiac catheterization and surgery may then be carried out under less critical conditions.

Surgical Management

All forms of interrupted aortic arch require for survival (1) the establishment of descending aortic blood flow that is not ductus-dependent, (2) relief of excessive left ventricular afterload, and (3) normalization of pulmonary blood flow.

Gradual spontaneous closure of the patent ductus arteriosus and development of collateral vascularization to the distal aorta occasionally allow survival to childhood. Repair is then accomplished either by the interposition of a prosthetic vascular graft between the ascending aorta and the descending aorta or by direct aortic anastomosis. A significant ventricular septal defect is rarely present in these older children.

Palliation has been accomplished by creation of a "permanent" patent ductus arteriosus by using a prosthetic vascular graft between the main pulmonary artery and the descending aorta.[252] The main pulmonary artery is banded distal to the origin of the vascular graft. Results have been poor.

The left subclavian artery and the left common carotid artery have been used to bridge the gap between the ascending aorta and descending aorta.[253,254] Obstruction due to the small size of these vessels and the circular suture lines required usually persists or evolves as the child grows.

A two-stage repair is generally preferred for those infants having an associated large ventricular septal defect.[254–256] Temporary ductal patency is assured by a prostaglandin E_1 infusion. Aortic continuity is established through a left thoracotomy by direct anastomosis or interposition of an expanded polytetrafluoroethylene (PTFE, Gore-Tex) graft. The ductus is ligated or divided and, if a large ventricular septal defect is present, a pulmonary arterial band is placed. The ventricular septal defect is closed and the band removed through a median sternotomy a few months later.

Although the initial risk of primary total correction in these critically ill infants is high, this approach may well offer the greatest likelihood for long-term survival free of pulmonary vascular obstructive disease. Moulton[257] described the management of 6 infants (7 days to 5 months old) by mobilization of the descending aorta through a median sternotomy, excision of ductus tissue, anastomosis of the end of the descending aorta to the side of the ascending aorta, and closure of associated ventricular or atrial septal defects during hypothermic circulatory arrest. Of the 6 infants, 5 survived more than 30 days. Norwood[258] reported primary total correction in 13 infants having interrupted aortic arch with ventricular septal defect; 10 infants (77 percent) survived. Complications included perioperative hypocalcemia and the development of severe subaortic stenosis.

Valvular Aortic Stenosis

Definition

Aortic stenosis is defined as subtotal obstruction of varying severity in the channel of left ventricular outflow. In order of decreasing frequency, the sites of obstruction are (1) valvular, (2) subvalvular, and (3) supravalvular.

Pathology

Most commonly the aortic valve is bicuspid with two commissures, one or both of which are fused to varying degrees. A third rudimentary commissure or raphe frequently is present in the larger of the leaflets. The valve opening is eccentric. Less frequently encountered is the unicuspid, unicommissural, or noncommissural valve in which the orifice is often slitlike, at first glance suggesting a bicuspid valve. Two shallow raphes lie opposite and equidistant from the commissure. Uncommonly a true dome is present, resembling the valve of congenital isolated pulmonary stenosis. Rarely the valve will be tricuspid with fusion of one or more of the three commissures.[259] When survival to adult life occurs, varying degrees of calcification may appear in the valvular tissue, leading to major rigidity of the valve. In the majority of patients manifesting cardiac dysfunction in infancy, the left ventricular wall is hypertrophied, but the chamber is small and significant degrees of endocardial fibroelastosis may occur.

Some patients with valvular stenosis in which the left ventricular cavity is of normal dimension reach adult life. Other cases become complicated by mitral insufficiency as a consequence of infarction of the left ventricular wall, including the papillary muscles. In all cases, poststenotic dilatation of the ascending aorta occurs to some degree. Coarctation of the aorta is the most common associated anomaly.

Abnormal Physiology

The hemodynamics of congenital valvular aortic stenosis are similar to those of acquired aortic stenosis (see Chap. 37) except that a persistent ductus arteriosus or stretched foramen ovale in the immediate postnatal period may lessen the severity of pulmonary edema by decreasing left atrial pressure.

Clinical Manifestations

About 7 percent of infants and children with clinically identified congenital heart disease will have aortic stenosis in one of its several forms. Approximately 80 percent of these patients will have valvular aortic stenosis. Valvular aortic stenosis is much more common among males than females, in a ratio of 4:1. Severity usually is judged by the peak systolic pressure gradient across the aortic valve and the calculated aortic valve area. In the presence of a normal cardiac output, a gradient of 80 mmHg or more or an aortic valve area of less than 0.5 cm^2/m^2 is considered severe; a gradient between 50 and 79 mmHg or a valve area between 0.5 and 0.8 cm^2/m^2 is considered moderate; a gradient of less than 50 mmHg or a valve area greater than 0.9 cm^2/m^2 is considered mild.[260]

History The detection of a systolic murmur leads to the discovery of this malformation in most patients. Although it may be heard within the first 24 to 48 h of life, the murmur is detected within the first year in slightly less than half of the patients. Growth and development usually are normal and the vast majority of children are asymptomatic. Easy fatigue, dyspnea, syncope, or angina suggest severe obstruction, but severe obstruction may exist in the absence of any symptoms. Sudden death may occur from this malformation, but in most such cases death is preceded by symptoms or electrocardiographic changes. Infants with critical stenosis from birth will present with congestive failure within the first week or two of life, and these patients represent true medical emergencies. A similar small number of patients with less critical but still very severe obstruction are detected over the course of the next 4 to 6 months. Dyspnea, easy fatigue with feedings, and slow weight gain usually are present.

Physical Examination The arterial blood pressure and the quality of the peripheral arterial pulses of the older infant and child usually are normal. A measured pulse pressure of less than 20 mmHg suggests severe stenosis. The heart is usually not detectably enlarged to palpation or percussion, but the cardiac apex impulse may be heaving and sustained. A systolic thrill along the right upper sternal border and over the carotid arteries is present in about 90 percent of patients. The absence of such a thrill at the right upper sternal border suggests a systolic pressure gradient of 30 mmHg or less. Paradoxical splitting of the second heart sound is rare and is associated either with very severe obstruction or with coexisting myocardial disease. A fourth heart sound heard in patients between 12 and 40 years of age usually signifies severe obstruction. (See Chap. 37.) An early systolic ejection click at the apex is characteristic and serves to distinguish valvular aortic stenosis from other forms of left ventricular outflow tract obstruction. The classic auscultatory finding is a harsh systolic spindle-shaped murmur, loudest at the right upper sternal border with radiation into the carotid arteries and down the left sternal border to the apex. Among infants with critical obstruction there may be no palpable peripheral pulses and no distinctive murmur, with a return of weak pulses and typical murmur only after decongestive therapy. Marked respiratory distress, pulmonary rales, and a gallop rhythm are characteristic. A systolic ejection click may also appear with improved compensation. Occasionally, the murmur of mitral regurgitation may be present or appears later.

Chest Roentgenogram The overall heart size usually is normal, but the left ventricle may appear prominent. Cardiac enlargement indicates severe disease in most instances. Poststenotic dilatation of the ascending aorta is characteristic. Calcification of the valve is not seen during childhood but appears with increasing frequency after adolescence. Infants with failure will have generalized cardiac enlargement, left atrial dilatation, and varying degrees of pulmonary edema.

Electrocardiogram The QRS axis usually is normal regardless of severity. Left ventricular hypertrophy, as indicated by voltage criteria in the left precordial leads, seldom is helpful in distinguishing those patients with severe obstruction from those with mild to moderate obstruction. However, diminished anterior forces in the right precordial leads and a deep SV_1 of 30 mm or more suggest severe stenosis, as does absence of the Q wave in V_6. Virtually all patients with pressure gradients of less than 50 mmHg will have a normal, upright T wave in V_6, while 20 percent of patients with moderate and 50 percent with severe obstruction will have a flat, biphasic, or inverted T wave in V_6. It should be noted, however, that T wave is normal in the other 50 percent of patients with severe stenosis. A superior T-wave vector in the frontal plane between 270 and 359° favors severe obstruction (Fig. 36-35). Severe and even critical obstruction may be present with none of the electrocardiographic abnormalities mentioned above.[261] Monitoring of the ST segment in leads V_5 through V_7 during exercise appears to be a reliable method of detecting those children in whom a significant pressure gradient (greater than 50 mmHg) has developed and in whom that gradient might represent a threat of sudden death if the obstruction were not relieved.[262] Symptomatic infants may show right, left, or biventricular hypertrophy, frequently with T-wave inversion over the left precordium.

Echocardiogram M-mode technique may show abnormally eccentric closure of the aortic cusps and multiple nonmoving echoes may fill the aortic root in those infants with critical aortic stenosis and a unicuspid valve. With this exception, diminished valve movement is not a distinctive feature of valvular aortic stenosis in children. The magnitude of left ventricular hypertrophy appears dependent upon left ventricular wall stress, and this in turn is dependent upon left ventricular systolic pressure and cavity dimensions:

$$\text{Wall stress} = \text{pressure} \times \left(\frac{\text{cavity diameter}}{\text{wall thickness}}\right)$$

An estimate can therefore be made of the left ventricular peak systolic pressure if the wall stress and the cavity dimensions remain relatively constant.[263] An estimate of the peak systolic pressure gradient may be obtained by subtracting the arterial systolic pressure obtained by cuff at the time of the echocardiographic recording from the estimated left ventricular peak systolic pressure. Unfortunately, these estimates are not valid in the postoperative patient. Continuous wave Doppler echocardiography guided by two-dimensional echocardiographic imaging appears to predict very accurately the systolic pressure gradient across discrete forms of left ventricular outflow tract obstruction.[264] Two-dimensional echocardiography can distinguish valvular from supravalvular or subvalvular obstruc-

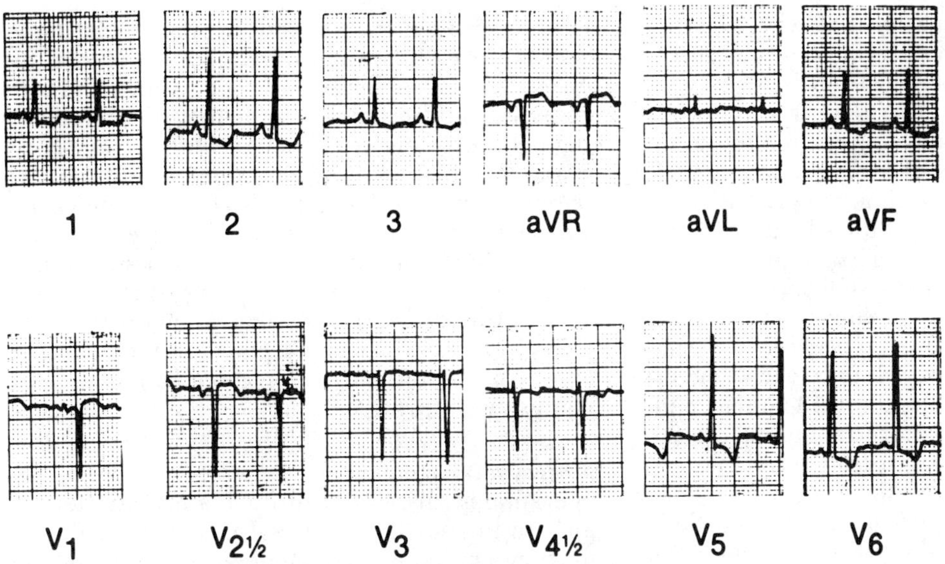

FIGURE 36-35 Electrocardiogram from an 8 year old boy with valvular aortic stenosis and a 94-mmHg peak systolic pressure gradient. The small anterior QRS forces (rV_1, rV_2, and rV_3), abnormally large posterior QRS forces (SV_2), absent Q waves in leads V_5 and V_6, and abnormal T waves and ST segments reflect severe left ventricular systolic pressure overload with ischemia.

tion. Both M-mode and two-dimensional techniques are capable of identifying those critically ill infants in whom the left ventricular cavity dimensions and aortic root diameter are hypoplastic to a degree that would preclude survival in the first weeks of life.[265]

Cardiac Catheterization In infants who are symptomatic with severe aortic obstruction there often is a left-to-right shunt at the atrial level through a stretched foramen ovale. Pulmonary arterial and right ventricular hypertension are the rule, and there may be also a right-to-left shunt through a patent ductus arteriosus which temporarily provides adequate systemic arterial perfusion and relieves some of the burden on the already congested pulmonary venous bed. A marked increase in left ventricular end-diastolic pressure usually is present. The systolic pressure gradient between the left ventricle and the central aorta or femoral artery should be documented whenever possible. If left ventricular output is markedly diminished, this gradient may be relatively small, even in the presence of severe obstruction. Left ventricular angiography will confirm the site of obstruction and outline the size of the left ventricular cavity. Mitral stenosis, mitral regurgitation, and fibroelastosis are common complicating features.

In older infants and children pressures on the right side of the heart usually are normal, although the pulmonary arterial wedge or left atrial pressures may be elevated. Simultaneous recording of central aortic and left ventricular pressures or a pressure tracing upon catheter withdrawal from the left ventricle to the aorta, coupled with an accurate estimate of cardiac output, is necessary for reliable assessment of severity. Left ventricular angiography will document the site of obstruction. The aortic leaflets typically will be thickened and domed, with a central or eccentric jet of contrast material entering the ascending aorta. Poststenotic dilatation is characteristic. Supravalvular aortography is recommended to assess the presence and severity of aortic regurgitation and, again, the degree of the aortic valve deformity.

Natural History and Prognosis

About half of the infants born with severe valvular aortic stenosis are symptomatic enough to require hospitalization within the first week of life.[9] The remainder develop congestive failure over the course of the next 6 months. Not uncommonly, the murmur is mistaken for that of a ventricular septal defect. Failure beyond infancy and before adolescence is not usually seen without the presence of complicating factors. Symptomatic infants require prompt surgery, but the mortality remains significant. Endocardial fibroelastosis, papillary muscle necrosis, associated intracardiac and extracardiac deformities, and a small left ventricular cavity contribute to this mortality. From 30 to 90 percent of survivors will have significant aortic regurgitation, but the majority can be managed medically until such time as valve replacement is feasible.

Among the infants and children with milder degrees of aortic valvular stenosis, a gradual progression in the severity of the systolic pressure gradient during childhood can be documented in about a third. Similarly the appearance of symptoms, cardiac enlargement, or the development of a left ventricular strain pattern in the electrocardiogram can be expected in about 40 percent of children followed over a 4- to 8-year period, including some with mild gradients at the outset. Sudden unexpected death is a very uncommon but definite threat to those with at least a moderate gradient.[260] Infective endocarditis on the aortic valve poses an extremely serious threat in the form of systemic arterial emboli, the production of serious chronic aortic regurgitation, or the appearance of sudden catastrophic regurgitation with congestive failure, shock, and death. Surgical mortality, except for those infants in the first 2 months of life, is relatively low, being in the range of 2 percent among the 179 patients operated on in the Joint Study.[260] Six percent of survivors developed serious aortic regurgitation. One-third of the survivors had systolic pressure gradients of less than 25 mmHg, while another third had residual gradients ranging between 25 and 50 mmHg. The final third were found to have either recurrent or residual gradients above 50 mmHg, and half of these were in the severe range. Of the 26 patients undergoing two postoperative catheterizations, it could be documented that 6 (about 20 percent) were developing significant restenosis. Surgery, then, while reducing the risk of sudden death and relieving symptoms, is palliative in most if not all instances. Despite evidence of improved myocardial perfusion, persistent elevation of left ventricular end-diastolic pressures and left ventricular hypertrophy indicate that the heart seldom returns to a completely normal state.

Medical Management

Infants with the characteristic murmur detected in the first weeks of life should be observed very carefully to be certain the obstruction is not severe. Those who develop failure should be operated upon without delay. Beyond infancy yearly reexaminations usually are adequate. Careful questioning regarding symptoms, a thorough cardiac examination including recording of blood pressure, yearly electrocardiograms, periodic echocardiograms and exercise testing, and less frequent chest roentgenograms should prevent progression from going unrecognized. Indications for cardiac catheterization include the appearance of symptoms, an arterial pulse pressure of less than 20 mmHg on physical examination, cardiac enlargement shown by chest roentgenogram, small anterior forces with an SV_1 of 30 mm or more or flattening or inversion of the T wave in V_6 in the resting electrocardiogram, abnormal ST-T segments on exercise testing, or an estimated peak systolic pressure gradient of 50 mmHg or greater by echocardiographic techniques. At present we recommend surgical relief of valvular aortic stenosis if there is a peak systolic pressure gradient of 75 mmHg or more or if the calculated aortic valve area is 0.5 cm^2/m^2 or less. We would recommend surgery for a systolic pressure gradient as low as 40 mmHg if the patient were clearly symptomatic or the heart enlarged or if the electrocardiogram showed ST-T wave changes. Children with more than mild aortic stenosis are restricted from strenuous organized athletics, isometric exercises, and activities that require a good deal of stamina and produce shortness of breath. Since stenosis is usually progressive, and since at least some degree of left ventricular obstruction persists in most children into adult life, even following surgery, it would seem reasonable to counsel the parents of a young child with moderate and perhaps even mild aortic stenosis to channel the youngster's energies into activities and sports that do not require strenuous exercise or stamina and that will not need to be forbidden later. For genetic counseling, the risk of congenital heart disease is estimated at 2 percent for a subsequent sibling and 4 percent for offspring of an affected parent. Aortic stenosis, alone or in conjunction with such defects as ventricular septal defect, patent ductus, or coarctation, is found in about half of affected siblings or offspring.

Surgical Management

Operation is carried out through a median sternotomy. In infancy the aortic valve is exposed during low-flow perfusion with moderate hypothermia or during brief inflow occlusion with a circulatory arrest.[265,266] Standard cardiopulmonary bypass, mild hypothermia, and cardioplegia are used for older children.[267,268] A transverse oblique aortotomy is made just above the aortic valve and right coronary arterial orifice. Appropriate retractors, traction sutures, and an ear canal speculum permit careful inspection of the valve prior to division of fused commissures. The surgeon must discriminate between true commissures and abortive raphes, incision of the latter producing intolerable aortic valvular incompetence. Relief of aortic valvular stenosis is accomplished by a carefully placed incision in the middle of each fused but well-supported true commissure (Fig. 36-36).[269]

FIGURE 36-36 Types of valvular deformities in patients with congenital valvular aortic stenosis. (*From F. H. Ellis, Jr., and J. W. Kirklin, Congenital Valvular Aortic Stenosis: Anatomic Findings and Surgical Technique, J. Thorac. Cardiovasc. Surg., 43:199, 1962. Reproduced with permission from the publisher and authors.*)

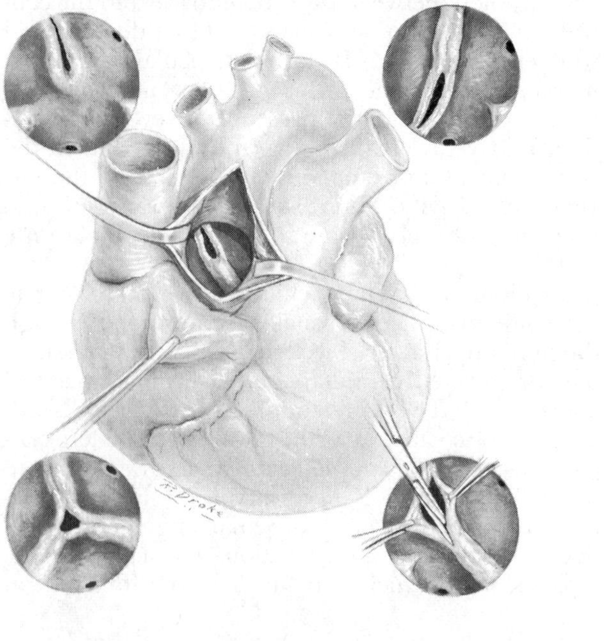

A conservative attitude is essential during operation for aortic stenosis in the infant or small child. Moderate residual stenosis is preferable to intolerable aortic valvular incompetence in infants, in whom prosthetic aortic valve implantation is technically difficult and associated with substantial morbidity and mortality. Mild valvular incompetence almost always occurs consequent to commissurotomy but is usually well tolerated. In fact, the left ventricular cavity may develop somewhat more normally in the presence of slight valvular regurgitation.

Secondary valvotomy for recurrent or residual stenosis can be attempted,[270] but eventual aortic valve replacement because of calcification and restenosis should be anticipated in all children requiring surgical relief of aortic stenosis.[271] We prefer to salvage the child's own valve for as long as possible; an ideal valve substitute for pediatric use does not exist.[272–275] (See "Congenital Aortic Regurgitation" for further discussion of aortic valve replacement.)

Complications of aortic valvotomy in the older child are rare; results are good.[267,276,277] Risk of the operation is much higher in the critically ill infant[265,266] in whom the natural history of aortic stenosis is also dismal. Systemic acidosis and marginal cardiac output are usually present at the time of operation in these infants. Late deaths are usually secondary to a small left ventricle causing low cardiac output and congestive heart failure, endocardial fibroelastosis, or dysrhythmias.

Survival and eventual outcome depend upon the degree to which stenosis can be relieved without the creation of intolerable valvular regurgitation. If the aortic valve has a tricuspid configuration, a good result can be anticipated. Satisfactory results with some reduction in left ventricular pressure are usually obtained when the valve is bicuspid, but moderate aortic insufficiency is usually present postoperatively. A unicommissural valve orifice can rarely be enlarged surgically without the creation of severe valvular incompetence.

A small aortic annulus limits severely the degree to which left ventricular hypertension can be relieved without resorting to radical operations in which the annulus is divided, a ventricular septal defect is created, the anterior leaflet of the mitral valve is incised, and a prosthetic aortic valve is implanted[278,279] or a valve-containing conduit is placed between the left ventricular apex and the descending aorta.[280,281]

The role of percutaneous balloon aortic valvuloplasty remains to be established, but preliminary data are promising.[282]

Subvalvular Aortic Stenosis

Pathology

Three classic varieties of subvalvular aortic stenosis involve the left ventricular outflow tract primarily. These are the membranous, the tunnel, and the muscular types. The membranous type is characterized by a localized fibrous encirclement of the left ventricular outflow tract a short distance below the aortic valve. The anterior leaflet of the mitral valve is involved in receiving attachment to this membrane. The tunnel type shows hypoplasia of the aortic annulus and a channel with a fibrous lining in the subjacent left ventricular outflow tract.[259,283]

The muscular type is variously known as *asymmetric septal hypertrophy* (ASH), *hypertrophic obstructive cardiomyopathy* (HOCM), or *idiopathic hypertrophic subaortic stenosis* (IHSS) and is discussed in Chap. 58.

Other forms of subvalvular stenosis result from abnormalities of the mitral valve, including accessory tissue and abnormal adhesions to the ventricular septum of either the anterior mitral leaflet or ectopic chordae emanating from it, as in certain instances of the atrioventricular canal malformation.[135]

Clinical Manifestations

Discrete subvalvular aortic stenosis is present in about 9 percent of children with left ventricular outflow tract obstruction.[6] It is more frequent among males, with a male/female ratio of approximately 2.5:1. The majority of patients are referred because of the detection of a murmur which, not uncommonly, is mistaken initially for that of a ventricular septal defect. Symptoms of fatigue, dyspnea, angina, and syncope have the same implications as they do for valvular aortic stenosis.

The physical examination is similar to that of valvular aortic stenosis with the two exceptions than an early systolic ejection click is not heard at the apex and an early diastolic murmur of aortic regurgitation is present in approximately one-half of these patients. In patients with mild obstruction, the murmur may be best heard at the mid left sternal border and may have musical overtones.

The roentgenographic features and electrocardiogram will be similar to those of valvular aortic stenosis except for absence of poststenotic dilatation of the ascending aorta.

Echocardiogram M-mode studies document what appears to be a characteristic narrowing of the left ventricular outflow tract. Systolic fluttering and early systolic partial closure of the aortic leaflets are seen in most patients. The membrane itself is very infrequently demonstrated. Two-dimensional studies (Fig. 36-37) permit excellent visualization of the obstructing membrane or fibromuscular ridge.[284] Estimation of the left ventricular peak systolic pressure and left ventricular–aortic systolic pressure gradient from M-mode and Doppler echocardiographic studies, as described for valvular aortic stenosis, appear valid.[263,264]

Cardiac Catheterization As with valvular aortic stenosis, a careful pullback pressure tracing across the left ventricular outflow tract is important to document the severity of the gradient and establish the site of the obstruction. Left ventricular biplane an-

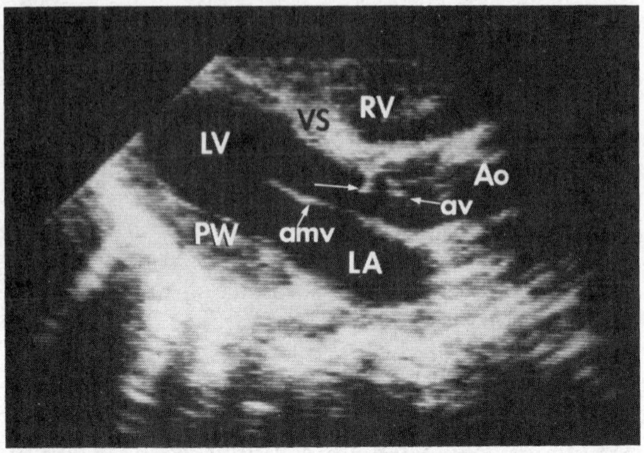

FIGURE 36-37 Two-dimensional echocardiogram in the parasternal long-axis view from a patient with discrete, fibrous subvalvular aortic stenosis. A thin, discrete membrane (unlabeled arrow) is seen attached to the interventricular septum (VS) in the left ventricular (LV) outflow tract immediately below the aortic valve (av). RV = right ventricle; Ao = ascending aorta; PW = posterior left ventricular wall; amv = anterior leaflet of the mitral valve; LA = left atrium.

giography, usually in angled as well as conventional views, will visualize the subvalvular ridge or membrane, its extent, and the presence or absence of associated diffuse outflow tract, annular, or supravalvular narrowing. Since over half of the patients with subvalvular obstruction will have associated intra- or extracardiac malformations, it is important that a careful and complete right-sided and left-sided heart catheterization be performed with appropriate angiography. Supravalvular aortography is recommended to evaluate the degree of aortic regurgitation.

Natural History and Prognosis

Severe congestive failure in infancy is unusual with subvalvular aortic stenosis and, if present, is almost invariably associated with complicating defects such as patent ductus, ventricular septal defect, or coarctation. Cardiac catheterization and corrective surgery for the associated lesions may have been carried out prior to the discovery of subvalvular aortic obstruction.[283] Obstruction is progressive in most instances, sometimes rapidly so. The associated aortic regurgitation also tends to be progressive and appears to result, at least in part, from prolonged turbulence with secondary thickening and deformity of the valve leaflets. Sudden unexpected death has been described but, fortunately, is rare. Results of surgery depend on the extent of involvement of the entire left ventricular outflow tract, with the best results being obtained in patients with a thin, discrete subvalvular membrane. The least satisfactory results, in terms of residual gradient or recurring obstruction, occur in patients with tunnel obstruction.[283]

Medical Management

The medical treatment and indications for surgery are similar to those for patients with valvular aortic stenosis. Surgery usually is recommended for patients with a considerably lower pressure gradient, however, because of the possibility of rapid progression of obstruction, the likelihood of progressive aortic valvular deformity and increasing aortic regurgitation with time, and the likelihood of complete and lasting relief if the membrane can be removed entirely. At present surgery is recommended for those patients with discrete subvalvular obstruction with systolic pressure gradients of 30 mmHg or more.

Continued follow-up for assessment of reobstruction and progression of aortic regurgitation, and for reemphasis of the precautions against infective endocarditis, is essential in all patients.

Surgical Management

Subvalvular fibromuscular (membranous) left ventricular outflow tract obstruction is exposed through the aortic root as described for aortic valvular stenosis (Fig. 36-38).[285] A nasal speculum, an ear speculum, and small flat retractors protect the aortic valve leaflets. Small sutures or hooks are placed in the abnormal fibromuscular tissue, pulling it into view for precise excision from the ventricular septum and the anterior leaflet of the mitral valve. The area of the bundle of His, usually just beneath the commissure between the right and noncoronary leaflets, is avoided.[286,287] An additional septal myectomy or myotomy beneath the right coronary leaflet may be required if secondary hypertrophy is significant. If present, an associated ventricular septal defect is closed with a Dacron patch or, if it is small and has fibrous margins, by buttressed sutures.[288] Immediate and early operative outcome is generally good, but residual, recurrent, and progressive subaortic obstruction is well documented, demanding continued assessment.[283,289]

Diffuse tunnel obstruction in the left ventricular outflow tract poses a difficult technical problem re-

FIGURE 36-38 Localized subvalvular aortic stenosis. Obstruction is immediately upstream from the aortic valve. (*From J. W. Kirklin, and F. H. Ellis, Jr., Surgical Relief of Diffuse Subvalvular Aortic Stenosis, Circulation, 24:739, 1961. Reproduced by permission of the American Heart Association, Inc., and the authors.*)

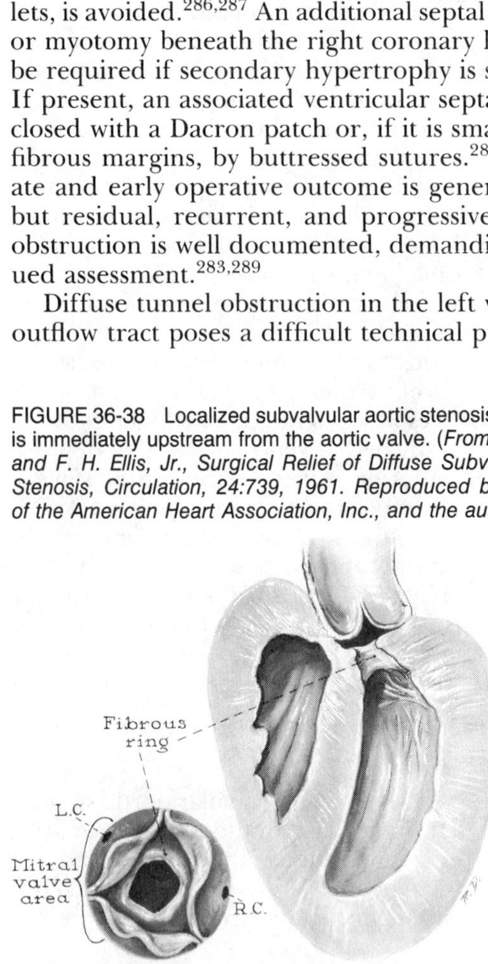

quiring aortoseptoplasty or insertion of a valve-containing conduit from the apex of the left ventricle to the lower thoracic or abdominal aorta.[281,289–291]

Treatment of idiopathic hypertrophic subaortic stenosis (IHSS), or asymmetric septal hypertrophy (ASH), by septal myotomy and myectomy is discussed elsewhere.[292]

Supravalvular Aortic Stenosis

Pathology

The obstruction is in the ascending aorta downstream from the coronary ostia. The three types are (1) hourglass, (2) hypoplastic, and (3) membranous obstructions. The process may be viewed as more widespread than the valvular or subvalvular types, as it tends to be associated with obstruction in the pulmonary trunk, peripheral pulmonary arteries, and branches of the aortic arch; valvular abnormalities, including myxomatous mitral valve; deformities of the mandible; and mental retardation.[293] The hourglass type may be associated with coronary arterial stenosis or atresia of the left coronary artery. Among the complications specific to this type of aortic stenosis are hypertrophy of the coronary arterial walls and premature coronary atherosclerosis.

Clinical Manifestations

Supravalvular stenosis may be familial, associated with characteristic facies and mental retardation, sporadic, or (rarely) the result of congenital rubella. All forms may be, and usually are, associated with varying degrees of peripheral or branch pulmonary arterial stenosis. The familial form is transmitted as an autosomal dominant trait with variable expression. Mental retardation is not present and there are no characteristic facial features. Supravalvular aortic stenosis associated with mental retardation, frequently called *Williams' syndrome,* is sporadic and associated with a high and prominent forehead, epicanthal folds, underdevelopment of the bridge of the nose and mandible, and a broad, overhanging upper lip. It has been linked with idiopathic hypercalcemia of infancy, but in the majority of patients recognized beyond infancy hypercalcemia is not present.

History The symptoms of supravalvular aortic stenosis are similar to those of valvular and subvalvular aortic stenosis, although critical obstruction with congestive failure in the neonatal period is exceedingly rare.[3] Those with characteristic facies and mental retardation usually have a history of irritability, vomiting, and hypotonia in early life, an observation lending support to the hypothesis of hypercalcemia in these infants. Those with the familial form usually have a distinctive family history, but one which seldom emerges in its entirety on initial questioning.

Physical Examination A systolic thrill, frequently very prominent, can be felt over the carotid arteries, in the suprasternal notch, and, to a lesser degree, at the right upper sternal border area. The midsystolic murmur is maximal in the same areas and somewhat less well heard along the right upper sternal border. The murmur of mitral regurgitation may also be present. Usually no systolic ejection click is heard. A systolic blood pressure difference may be recorded between the two arms on occasion. The characteristic facies are described above.

Chest Roentgenogram No dilatation of the ascending aorta will be seen.

Electrocardiogram The findings are similar to those of other forms of aortic stenosis with the exception that right ventricular hypertrophy may be present if associated pulmonary arterial stenosis is severe.

Echocardiogram M-mode technique may demonstrate the narrowed diameter of the aortic lumen just distal to the aortic valve. However, two-dimensional technique visualizes this much more clearly and permits an estimation of the degree of severity in terms of both the narrowing of the aortic lumen and the extent of ascending aortic involvement.[294]

Cardiac Catheterization A systolic pressure gradient can be demonstrated just above the aortic valve by careful pullback pressure tracings from the left ventricular cavity to the aortic arch. Supravalvular aortography or left ventricular angiography will visualize the supravalvular narrowing. Pressure recordings in the branch pulmonary arteries should be obtained and right ventricular or pulmonary arterial angiography performed in the presence of any significant right ventricular systolic pressure elevation, in order to rule out associated stenoses of the pulmonary arteries.

Natural History and Prognosis

The sequence of progressive obstruction, the appearance of symptoms and electrocardiographic changes, and the possibility of sudden death appears to apply for supravalvular aortic stenosis as well as for valvular aortic stenosis. Infective endocarditis represents a threat to these patients throughout life. Surgical relief of the obstruction may be complicated by marked hypoplasia and diffuse thickening of a considerable length of the ascending aorta. In addition a few patients will have severe pulmonary arterial stenoses which may or may not be amenable to repair, the presence of which may increase the risk of aortic surgery considerably.

Medical Management

The indications for cardiac catheterization and sur-

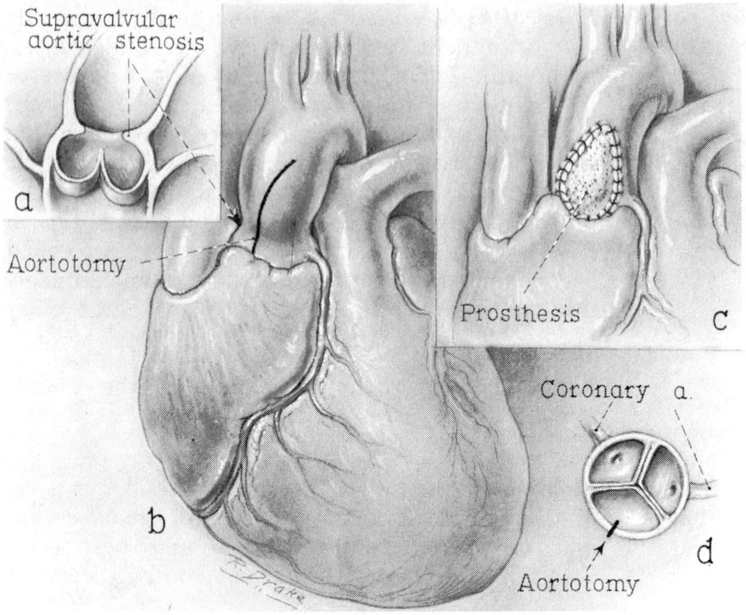

FIGURE 36-39 *a* to *d*. Supravalvular aortic stenosis and its repair. Obstruction is almost diaphragmatic in nature (*a*) and is not easily recognized externally (*b*). The complete repair is shown (*c*). (*From D. C. McGoon, H. T. Mankin, P. Vlad, and J. W. Kirklin, The Surgical Treatment of Supravalvular Aortic Stenosis, J. Thorac. Cardiovasc. Surg., 41:125, 1961. Reproduced with permission from the publisher and authors.*)

gery are the same as for valvular aortic stenosis. The patient and the parents of the patient with the familial variety of supravalvular aortic stenosis will need genetic counseling. The parents of the child with mental retardation will also benefit from genetic counseling, from referral to resources which aid in the care and training of these children, and, eventually, from advice regarding contraception for the retarded adolescent female.

Surgical Management
Discrete supravalvular aortic stenosis is relieved by one or more incisions through the narrow segment of the ascending aorta, usually at the level of the sinotubular ridge at the top of the commissures. Incisions are extended well down into the aortic sinuses (Fig. 36-39).[295] Ridges of obstructing fibrous tissue are excised. The aorta is enlarged by the insertion of a gusset of prosthetic vascular graft material or pericardium to increase the circumference.[296] Rigidity and fibrous thickening of the aortic wall may prevent the aorta from opening up adequately even after insertion of the usual oval gusset in the noncoronary sinus of Valsalva. An extended aortoplasty in which the fibrous ring is incised at two points and the aorta augmented with a pants-shaped tailored Dacron prosthesis is useful in this difficult problem.[297] A favorable outcome can be anticipated postoperatively in most patients having discrete supravalvular aortic stenosis.

Diffuse tubular hypoplasia of the descending aorta is a technically challenging problem associated with a high mortality and poor postoperative hemodynamic results.[298,299] Use of a conduit from the apex of the left ventricle to the descending or abdominal aorta is appealing,[300] although most attempts at repair have used an extensive prosthetic enlargement of the ascending aorta.[301]

Aortic valvular regurgitation and/or stenosis may coexist with supravalvular stenosis. Fusion of commissures and tethering of leaflets should be relieved at the time of aortoplasty. Treatment of valvular insufficiency, unless massive, should await postoperative reassessment before valve replacement. Intimal obstruction of the coronary arterial ostia may require debridement, dilatation, or even saphenous vein bypass grafting.[299]

Bicuspid Aortic Valve

Pathology
Classically, the two cusps are oriented anteriorly and posteriorly, the anterior or conjoined cusp being the larger; from its sinus the two coronary arteries arise. A raphe, or ridge, is present along the aortic aspect of the larger cusp. The ridge runs from the aortic wall toward or to the free edge of the cusp.

Associated Conditions The most common associated conditions of significance are coarctation of the aorta and interruption of the aortic arch. The most common complication is calcification of the valve. In about 85 percent of cases of calcific aortic stenosis, the fundamental valve is congenitally bicuspid. Aortic regurgitation from prolapse of the larger cusp is a less common complication and usually is not evident until adolescence or adult life.

Clinical Manifestations
The incidence of this malformation in the general population approaches 2 percent; therefore it is the most common congenital abnormality of the heart or great vessels. Its importance lies in its frequent association with other forms of congenital heart disease, the predisposition of the valve to become ste-

notic as a result of fibrosis and deposition of calcium over the course of years, the tendency of the valve to become regurgitant, and, finally, in the susceptibility of the valve to infective endocarditis.[302] A bicuspid aortic valve is found among patients with coarctation of the aorta, primary endocardial fibroelastosis, isolated ventricular septal defect, and atrioventricular canal malformations.[6] It is also found among patients with valvular aortic stenosis, where bicuspid aortic valve is the underlying malformation in some 60 percent of patients between the ages of 15 and 65 years,[302] patients with isolated or dominant aortic regurgitation,[303] patients with infective endocarditis with or without a history of predisposing heart disease, and, probably most frequently, among otherwise normal individuals who come to the physician's attention because of unrelated illnesses. The incidence among males is approximately 2.5 times that among females. Patients with uncomplicated bicuspid aortic valve are asymptomatic, while those with aortic stenosis, aortic regurgitation, or infective endocarditis have symptoms related to these complications.

Physical Examination The characteristic feature is auscultatory and consists of an early systolic, loud, high-pitched ejection sound or click which is best heard at the apex and which does not vary with respiration. This sound follows the first heart sound by 43 to 91 ms and can be demonstrated to coincide with the halting of the opening movement of the aortic valve cusps. The aortic component of the second heart sound is usually accentuated at the apex unless the leaflets are fibrotic or calcified. A soft, early, or midsystolic murmur of no greater than grade 3 intensity frequently is present at the right upper sternal border. Less commonly, a soft murmur of aortic regurgitation may be heard. In patients with a demonstrated pressure difference between the left ventricle and aorta, the aortic ejection sound occurs slightly earlier, about 30 to 65 ms after the first heart sound.[304]

Echocardiogram Two-dimensional echocardiography, with adequate images, can identify the bicuspid valve with a sensitivity of 78 percent and a diagnostic accuracy of 96 percent. The M-mode technique is less reliable.[305]

Natural History and Prognosis

The majority of congenitally bicuspid aortic valves are nonobstructive at birth, but with the passage of time a few of these valves will become fibrotic, stiffer, and more obstructive and will eventually be the site of calcium deposition. Uncommonly, this process of fibrosis, deformity, and stenosis may be rapid enough to produce severe obstruction during childhood; however, it is primarily among individuals between the ages of 15 and 65 that one finds the bicuspid valve as the cause of serious aortic valvular obstruction. Important calcium deposition is unusual before the age of 30, whereas large, grossly visible deposits of calcium are present in the valves of virtually all patients with severe stenosis beyond that age. A much smaller number of individuals born with a bicuspid aortic valve will develop isolated aortic regurgitation.[303] In approximately one-third, this will be the result of fibrosis, prolapse, or retraction of one or both of the leaflets, and in the remainder regurgitation will be the result of infective endocarditis on an apparently functionally normal bicuspid valve. Why one individual with a bicuspid valve will develop stenosis, another regurgitation, and still others live a functionally normal life is not known. It is estimated that among individuals with an aortic ejection sound but no evidence of aortic stenosis or regurgitation, the passage of a decade will find about 12 percent to have developed aortic stenosis. The majority of these will be beyond the age of 45 at that point and will have evidence of calcium deposition. Mild aortic regurgitation will have been developed in 6 percent, 8 percent will have experienced infective endocarditis, 8 percent will have died of unrelated causes, and a little over 60 percent will have remained without complications.[306] (See Chap. 37.)

Medical Management

Patients suspected of having a bicuspid aortic valve should be followed expectantly, without restrictions but with particular attention paid to the prevention of infective endocarditis.

Surgical Management

Operation is required only when significant aortic stenosis or incompetence is present. (See "Valvular Aortic Stenosis" and "Congenital Aortic Regurgitation.")

Congenital Aortic Regurgitation

Definition

This section describes conditions in which aortic regurgitation results from a primary anomaly of the aortic valve. Aortic regurgitation resulting from complications of congenital disease is not included.

Pathology

The principal anomalies underlying the uncommon condition of aortic regurgitation as defined are congenital bicuspid aortic valve; rudimentary, dysplastic, or tethered individual cusps; and cystic medial necrosis of the aorta, as in Marfan's syndrome.[307]

In the first condition, prolapse of the larger of the two cusps is the cause of regurgitation.[303] In extensive cystic medial necrosis of the aorta, incompetence of the valve results from dilatation of the aorta, associated floppy aortic valve, or the two together.

Associated Conditions Some, but not all, cases of bicuspid aortic valve with primary regurgitation are associated with coarctation of the aorta. With Marfan's syndrome features of associated mitral valve prolapse may be present.

Clinical Manifestations

Aortic valvular regurgitation as an isolated entity is unusual among children and particularly unusual among infants. Occasionally, the diastolic murmur of pulmonary regurgitation, particularly in the presence of pulmonary arterial hypertension, may be confused with that of aortic regurgitation. The diastolic murmurs heard with a coronary arterial fistula or even patent ductus arteriosus may also simulate aortic regurgitation in individual patients. In the newborn, the diastolic murmurs of aortic–left ventricular tunnel and truncal valve insufficiency with truncus arteriosus may simulate that of isolated aortic regurgitation. The history, physical, and laboratory findings are characteristic of valvular aortic regurgitation in adults. (See Chap. 37.)

Natural History, Prognosis, and Medical Management

Mild and even moderate isolated aortic regurgitation usually is well tolerated during childhood, with slow or barely detectable progression in most patients. Catastrophic acceleration of this course may be associated with complicating infective endocarditis. Medical management of isolated valvular aortic regurgitation may include, as necessary, restriction of activity, digitalis, diuretics, and vasodilators. Careful assessment of ventricular function is important in order to avoid permanent left ventricular injury. Valve replacement is recommended for patients with symptoms or ventricular dysfunction.

Surgical Management

Surgical correction of congenital aortic regurgitation almost always requires prosthetic valve implantation. Occasionally a conservative salvage procedure such as suspension valvuloplasty, advocated for the management of aortic regurgitation associated with a supracristal (type I) ventricular septal defect, can be accomplished.[308,309]

Children tolerate aortic regurgitation poorly; symptomatic deterioration of left ventricular function occurs relatively quickly, necessitating aortic valve replacement long before full annular growth is achieved. Small prosthetic valves are intrinsically obstructive. The need for a larger valve and an annulus-enlarging procedure must be anticipated if the child survives and grows following initial valve replacement. As experience with aortoseptoplasty has accumulated, a more aggressive approach toward enlargement of the annulus at the time of primary valve implantation has been adopted.[279,310,311]

Choice of a valve substitute for implantation in children remains a major problem.[312] The porcine heterografts deteriorate quickly in children,[274,313,314] although the reduced incidence of thromboembolic complications in the absence of anticoagulation was initially appealing. Mechanical prostheses require anticoagulation, or certainly antiplatelet agents.[315] Ball-in-cage prostheses require more space than is usually available in the heart of a small child, and eccentric tilting-disk prostheses are subject to impingement against the walls of cardiac chambers and vessels. The St. Jude prosthesis with double tilting-disk and central orifice has a low incidence of thromboembolic complications and a relatively large effective orifice.[316,317] Experience to date with this valve in children has been satisfactory, and it is currently our valve substitute of choice.

Aortic regurgitation secondary to cystic medial necrosis may require composite replacement of the aortic valve and the ascending aorta; the coronary arteries are usually reimplanted into the aortic graft.[318] Echocardiographic evidence of progressive aortic root dilatation to about 5.5 cm and moderate aortic regurgitation have been considered indications for surgical intervention to replace the ascending aorta and usually the valve.[319] Unfortunately, replacement of the aortic valve in children having severe aortic regurgitation does not usually result in normalization of left ventricular performance.[320]

Aortic–Left Ventricular Tunnel

Definition

An aortic–left ventricular tunnel is a channel beginning in the ascending aorta, proceeding into the epicardium, and then penetrating the ventricular septum to empty into the subaortic region of the left ventricle.

Pathology

The aortic aspect of the anomalous channel lies in the anterior wall of the aorta, slightly above the levels of the origins of the coronary arteries. At its beginning, and while in the epicardium, the channel has an arterial structure. While in the ventricular septum, it exhibits a sinusoidal structure. In the septum, the tunnel lies in the posterior wall of the right ventricular infundibulum and may distort the structure of the latter. In the same position it lies close to the aortic valve. In its epicardial segment the tunnel may develop a saccular aneurysm.

Complications The principal complications are those associated with excessive diastolic volume of the left ventricle and are comparable to those of classic aortic regurgitation. Incompetence of the aortic valve may also occur.[321] A fibrotic, sometimes bicuspid, aortic valve may be associated.

Clinical Manifestations
This very rare malformation, which characteristically presents in very early infancy, is amenable to correction and is seldom associated with other defects.

The majority of infants are only mildly symptomatic in the first week or two after birth, presumably due to compensatory myocardial hypertrophy developed in utero. A few develop congestive heart failure within the first day or two of life, and the majority develop symptoms of dyspnea, easy fatigue with activity, and growth failure as the weeks and months go by.

Physical findings are those of gross aortic regurgitation. Bounding arterial pulses, sometimes visible, a wide pulse pressure, and a hyperdynamic left ventricular lift are characteristic. The murmur usually is to-and-fro, but the diastolic component is almost invariably louder than the systolic, is inclined to be harsh, and is frequently associated with a thrill at the left sternal border.

The chest roentgenogram will show an enlarged heart with a left ventricular configuration, and the ascending aorta is impressively dilated.

Left ventricular hypertrophy is present in the electrocardiogram from birth in the majority of patients. ST-segment and T-wave changes of myocardial ischemia may be present at the outset or may develop with time. Two-dimensional echocardiographic visualization of the tunnel is possible.[322]

Cardiac Catheterization The characteristic abnormality is visualized best with selective aortography in the ascending aorta. Marked ascending aortic dilatation and left ventricular dilatation are characteristic.

Natural History and Prognosis
In most instances, the characteristic murmur is heard within the first 3 months of life, frequently within the first few days. Although the hemodynamic burden is tolerated reasonably well in most patients initially, the course appears to be one of progressive paravalvular regurgitation and progressive dilatation of the aortic root and left ventricle. Rapid onset of congestive failure and sudden death have been described.

Medical Management
Prompt cardiac catheterization and early repair of aortic–left ventricular tunnel are recommended before the deformities of the ascending aorta, aortic ring, and aortic valve produce permanent aortic valvular regurgitation. Long-term follow-up of these patients is indicated to monitor any residual aortic regurgitation or stenosis and to reemphasize the precautions against infective endocarditis.

Surgical Management
This rare anomaly should be repaired as soon as the diagnosis is established in order to avoid progressive dilatation of the tunnel and left ventricle, deformity of the aortic valve and annulus, and elevation of the posterior wall of the right ventricle (septum) with subsequent right ventricular outflow tract obstruction.[323,324]

The aortic orifice of the tunnel is exposed and distinguished from the nearby coronary arterial orifices through an aortotomy while the child is supported on hypothermic cardiopulmonary bypass. A small Dacron patch is sutured over the orifice.[321,322] The aortic valve leaflets, coronary arterial orifices, and area of the subaortic conduction system are protected from deformity and trauma. The ventricular end of the tunnel can usually be closed using pledget-reinforced sutures placed through the aortic valve orifice, but care must be exercised to avoid distortion of the aortic cusps and subsequent valvular incompetence. Of 26 surgically treated patients reviewed by Levy, 21 (80.5 percent) survived,[321] while all 12 patients treated medically died.

Aortic Atresia

Definition
In aortic atresia the region of the aortic valve shows no patency.

Pathology
Usually the ventricular septum is intact and the aorta is normally related to the pulmonary trunk and the left ventricle. The atretic segment lies proximal to the coronary arterial origins. The left ventricle shows major hypertrophy of its wall, but the cavity is tiny and the mitral valve, although formed, is hypoplastic (Fig. 36-40). The right-sided heart chambers are enlarged and the ventricle hypertrophied. The usual route of escape of blood from the left side of the heart is at the foramen ovale. Rarely, when the foramen ovale is sealed or narrow, alternate routes for the flow of blood are present. Among these are (1) connection between a pulmonary vein and a systemic vein and (2) prominent sinusoids in the left ventricular wall which connect the left ventricular cavity with coronary arteries. The ductus arteriosus is wide and the ascending aorta is hypoplastic.[325]

Associated Conditions Coarctation of the aorta manifesting varying degrees of stenosis is common both when aortic atresia appears alone and when it occurs in association with mitral atresia.[326] When atresia of the mitral valve is associated, the left ventricle is a tiny, blind, endocardium-lined cavity in the wall of the right ventricle; it usually requires microscopic study for identification.[325] In exceptional cases a ventricular septal defect is present. In such cases the left ventricular cavity and the mitral valve are near normal size.

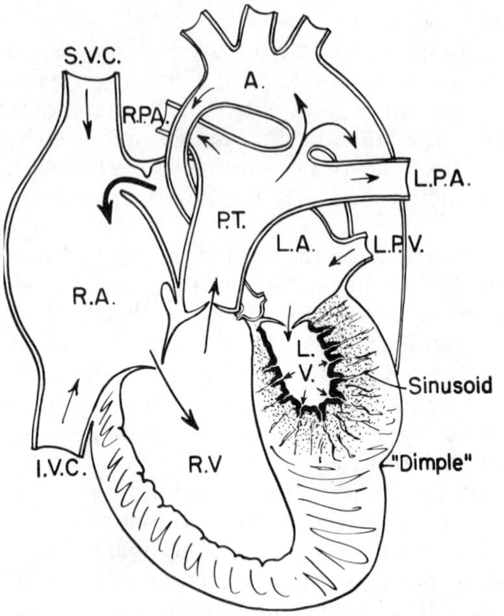

FIGURE 36-40 The central circulation in aortic atresia. The mitral valve is hypoplastic, as is the left ventricle (L.V.). The aortic channel (A.) is supplied from the right ventricle (R.V.) through the ductus arteriosus. Blood flows in a retrograde fashion in the ascending aorta. The only outlet for blood from the left side of the heart is a communication between the left atrium (L.A.) and right atrium (R.A.) at the level of the fossa ovalis (bold arrow). S.V.C. = superior vena cava; I.V.C. = inferior vena cava; P.T. = main pulmonary arterial trunk; R.P.A. = right pulmonary artery; L.P.A. = left pulmonary artery; L.P.V. = left pulmonary vein.

Clinical Manifestations

Aortic atresia is an uncommon cardiac malformation but it is the leading cause of death among children with heart disease in the first 2 weeks of life.[3] Males are more commonly affected than females in a ratio of 1.8:1. Familial occurrence has been reported, with the transmission apparently on a multifactorial basis. The recurrence risk in siblings for this specific defect is approximately 0.5 percent and for all types of congenital heart disease is 2.2 percent.[116]

History The clinical situation usually is that of a 1- to 3-day-old infant, considered entirely well until then, who develops the sudden onset of severe respiratory distress and slate-gray cyanosis.

Physical Examination Signs of aortic atresia are those of systemic arterial hypoperfusion and congestive failure. Pulses are weak or absent in all areas, including the carotids, but may wax and wane initially as the ductus opens and closes. The disparity between the forceful heart action felt on palpation and the weak arterial pulses is striking. The second heart sound is single and loud, and a gallop rhythm is frequent. Murmurs, if present at all, usually are soft and nondistinctive. Moist rales and severe hepatomegaly complete the clinical picture.

Chest Roentgenogram Moderate to marked cardiac enlargement is seen, with a combination of pulmonary arterial and pulmonary venous engorgement.

Electrocardiogram Right axis deviation and marked right ventricular hypertrophy, frequently with a qR pattern in the right precordial leads, are characteristic.

Echocardiogram Both M-mode and two-dimensional studies usually are diagnostic. In both, the aortic root echoes are small or absent and the mitral valve echoes are small, distorted, or absent. The posterior ventricle is small or nondemonstrable, while the anterior ventricular chamber is large. Easily identifiable anterior tricuspid valve echoes can be seen.[327] Rarely, in the presence of a sizable ventricular septal defect, the left ventricular chamber size and mitral valve echoes may be normal or near normal.

Cardiac Catheterization A large left-to-right shunt will be found at the atrial level with virtually complete mixing of systemic and pulmonary venous blood within the right atrium. Right ventricular and pulmonary arterial systolic pressures will be equal to or, in the case of a closing ductus, greater than those in the systemic circuit. Pulmonary arterial or aortic angiography will demonstrate a greatly dilated main pulmonary artery with patent ductus supplying the descending aorta and, in a retrograde fashion, the brachiocephalic vessels and the extremely hypoplastic ascending aorta.

Natural History and Prognosis

This malformation is almost invariably fatal, with 80 percent of affected infants dying within the first week and only 6 percent surviving beyond the first month. The mean age of death, related directly to ductal closure and deprivation of flow to the systemic arterial circulation, is 5 days.[325]

Medical Management

In the past, treatment of aortic atresia has been symptomatic and palliative surgery has not been recommended. Recently developed surgical techniques, designed to afford a two-stage physiologic correction, have proved successful albeit at a relatively high risk to date.[328] Intravenous prostaglandin E_1 infusion will maintain ductal patency until cardiac catheterization and surgery can be accomplished. Emotional support and genetic counseling for the parents are particularly important in this devastating situation.

Surgical Management
Successful palliation and physiologic repair of aortic atresia and the hypoplastic left heart syndrome have recently been described by Norwood.[328] Palliation includes division of the pulmonary artery, anastomosis of the proximal main pulmonary arterial stump to the side of the diminutive ascending aorta, obliteration of the patent ductus arteriosus, enlargement of the interatrial communication, and creation of a small shunt from the proximal pulmonary arterial–aortic trunk to the distal pulmonary arteries. The right ventricle thus serves as the systemic ventricle while perfusing the lungs via the shunt, usually a polytetrafluoroethylene (PTFE, Gore-Tex) tube. Physiologic correction utilizes the Fontan concept. Right atrial–to–pulmonary arterial continuity provides pulmonary blood flow while the right ventricle functions as the systemic ventricle after closure of the extracardiac shunt and diversion of pulmonary venous blood through the atrial septal defect to the tricuspid valve. Experience is limited to only a few infants and follow-up is brief but encouraging.

Mitral Atresia

Pathology
In mitral atresia, in most instances, there is a depression at the anticipated location of the mitral valve but no opening or valvular tissue are present. Uncommonly, valvular tissue with or without an orifice exists (in so-called membranous mitral atresia or imperforate membrane).[329] In about half the cases, mitral atresia coexists with aortic atresia, a condition that has been discussed under "Aortic Atresia," above.

The balance of this discussion relates to those cases of mitral atresia with a patent aortic valve.

In about one-half of the cases in which only the mitral valve is atretic, the great vessels are normally related. Two ventricles are present, of which the left is relatively hypoplastic, as is the ascending aorta. The ventricular septum shows one or, usually, multiple defects. When the great vessels are malposed, the ventricular portion of the heart exhibits features of a single ventricle.[330]

The usual route for exit of blood from the left atrium is through the foramen ovale. When the foramen ovale is sealed or narrow, alternate routes exist; for example, a vein may connect the left atrium to a systemic vein (levoatrial cardinal vein) or a vein may connect a pulmonary vein to a systemic vein.[331] Coarctation of the aorta and double-outlet right ventricle are fairly common.

Clinical Manifestations
The clinical features of this uncommon malformation are determined by the presence or absence of significant pulmonary stenosis and the presence or absence of adequate left atrial decompression. There is no sex predilection.

The majority of patients are detected within the first 2 weeks of life. Those without significant pulmonary stenosis usually present with severe respiratory distress and other symptoms of serious congestive failure and pulmonary edema. Infants with pulmonary stenosis or pulmonary atresia usually present with severe cyanosis.

Without pulmonary stenosis, the findings are those of dyspnea, a hyperdynamic right ventricular lift, a nonspecific systolic murmur, and a diastolic flow rumble at the lower left sternal border. Pulmonary rales may be present and cyanosis usually is minimal. In rare instances, a low-pitched continuous murmur may be heard at the left sternal border due to flow from the left to the right atrium through an incompetent and restrictive foramen ovale. With pulmonary stenosis, the findings are similar to those of patients with tetralogy of Fallot. With pulmonary atresia, there is usually no murmur and cyanosis is intense.

On chest roentgenogram cardiac enlargement, the degree of pulmonary arterial overperfusion, and the severity of pulmonary venous congestion will reflect the presence or absence of pulmonary stenosis and the size of the interatrial opening. Left atrial dilatation rarely is present.

Right axis deviation in the electrocardiogram and right atrial and right ventricular hypertrophy are the rule. Left atrial hypertrophy may or may not be present.

M-mode and two-dimensional echocardiographic techniques will demonstrate absence of mitral valve echoes and will permit estimation of the size of the aortic root and the left ventricular cavity.[332]

There will be a step-up in oxygen saturation at the right atrial level at cardiac catheterization, with complete mixing of systemic venous and pulmonary venous blood at that site and beyond. Varying degrees of left atrial hypertension will be present, depending upon the adequacy of left atrial decompression and the volume of pulmonary arterial blood flow. Balloon atrial septostomy should be attempted in all patients under 1 month of age.

Natural History and Prognosis
In mitral atresia, rapid deterioration and death within the first few weeks of life from either pulmonary edema or hypoxia is characteristic unless a fortuitous balance of pulmonary stenosis and adequate left atrial decompression exists. Such a natural balance is rare, but if pulmonary blood flow can be adjusted to a near-normal level and adequate left atrial runoff ensured by balloon septostomy or surgical atrial septectomy, survival beyond infancy is possible.[333]

Medical Management
Early recognition combined with prompt surgical palliation is essential. Among survivors there will be

a continuing need to maintain pulmonary arterial blood flow at an optimal level and to reassess the adequacy of the interatrial opening, either by repeat cardiac catheterization or by two-dimensional echocardiography.

Surgical Management

Repair of mitral atresia has not been accomplished. Palliation, including (1) decompression of the left atrium and pulmonary veins by enlargement of the interatrial communication and (2) adjustment of pulmonary blood flow by ligation of the patent ductus arteriosus, banding of the pulmonary artery, or creation of a systemic-to-pulmonary arterial shunt, offers a chance for survival and an improved quality of life.[333]

Mitral Stenosis

Pathology

The stenotic lesion may be at the inlet to the mitral valve (it is then called the *supravalvular ring*), at the valve, or below the valve.

The supravalvular ring is a fibrous encirclement at the inlet to the mitral valve, the lesion lying downstream from the left atrial appendage. Varying degrees of this condition may exist. It may appear as an isolated condition or it may be associated with the parachute mitral valve and the other two conditions associated with the parachute valve, namely, coarctation of the aorta and subaortic stenosis (Fig. 36-41).[334,335] Stenotic lesions at or below the valve are of two principal types, the *dysplastic mitral valve* and the *parachute mitral valve*.

In the dysplastic valve the leaflets are nodular and the chordae are poorly developed and unusually short, causing the papillary muscles to be held close to the valvular orifice. Valvular commissures are poorly developed. Dysplasia of all or any of the other valves and supravalvular aortic and pulmonary arterial stenosis may coexist.[336]

In the parachute mitral valve only one papillary muscle is present in the left ventricle, and the chordae of the two leaflets converge to insert into this single muscle (Fig. 36-41).[334,335] Blood must flow in the interchordal spaces to reach the left ventricle.

Clinical Manifestations

This is a rare malformation found in only 0.42 percent of children with congenital heart disease. Approximately 75 percent of patients so affected have important associated cardiac malformations, and in these situations it is not uncommon for mitral stenosis to be detected for the first time at cardiac catheterization, operation, or postmortem examination. A male/female ratio of 2.2:1 is estimated.[334]

Although symptoms may appear during the neonatal period, they are, on the average, most commonly detected in the second year of life. Symptoms consist of exertional dyspnea, cyanosis, episodes of respiratory distress suggesting pulmonary edema, repeated and persistent lower respiratory tract infections, and poor weight gain.

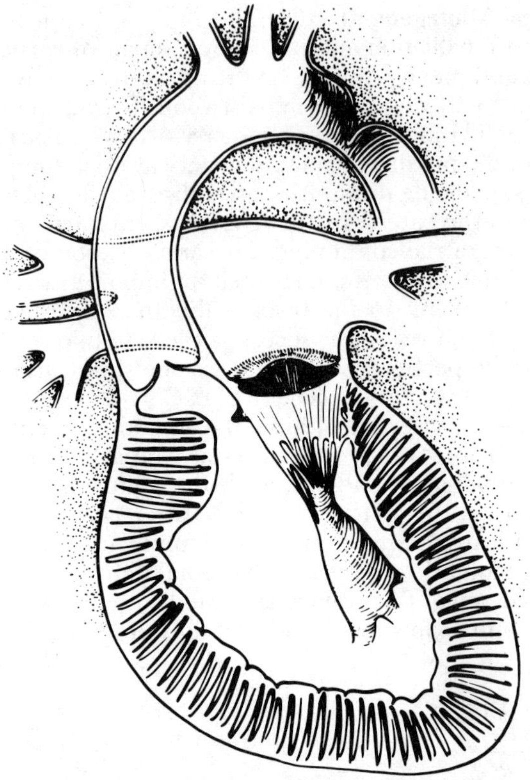

FIGURE 36-41 The four obstructive anomalies in the complex described by Shone and associates: *1.* Stenosing ring of the left atrium. *2.* Parachute deformity of mitral valve. *3.* Subaortic stenosis. *4.* Coarctation of aorta. (*From J. D. Shone, R. D. Sellers, R. C. Anderson, P. Adams, Jr., C. W. Lillehei, and J. E. Edwards, The Developmental Complex of "Parachute Mitral Valve," Supravalvular Ring of Left Atrium, Subaortic Stenosis, and Coarctation of the Aorta, Am. J. Cardiol., 11:714, 1963. Reproduced with permission from the publisher and authors.*)

On physical examination the first heart sound usually is loud at the apex, and an opening snap can be detected in a few patients. The characteristic murmur is a relatively harsh, well-localized, low-pitched diastolic murmur at the apex with presystolic accentuation. The presystolic component helps to distinguish this murmur from that of increased diastolic flow across the mitral valve. A thrill on palpation is relatively common. On initial examination, this murmur frequently is mistaken for a systolic murmur, particularly if no systolic murmur is present to aid with timing. Soft murmurs of mitral, pulmonary, or tricuspid regurgitation may be heard. In some patients, particularly those with diminished pulmonary blood flow, as with tetralogy of Fallot, no murmur is audible.

Mild to moderate cardiac enlargement on chest roentgenogram is not unusual and generally reflects right ventricular dilatation. Pulmonary venous engorgement, Kerley B lines, and prominence of the left atrium and left atrial appendage are characteristics of important obstruction.

Varying degrees of normal or right axis deviation are present in the electrocardiogram with left atrial, right ventricular, and right atrial hypertrophy.

M-mode echocardiogram can detect the signs of left ventricular inflow obstruction, namely, anterior motion of the posterior valve leaflet during diastole and a markedly decreased EF slope, diminished excursion, and a reduced rate of diastolic closure of the anterior leaflet. It is of limited value, however, in defining the precise structural malformation or providing an estimate of severity.[337] Two-dimensional echocardiography appears capable of distinguishing the parachute mitral valve deformity with a single papillary muscle from valvular mitral stenosis and supravalvular stenosis in the form of an obstructing membrane. The distinction between a supravalvular membrane or ring and the membrane of cor triatriatum is less secure.[338]

Cardiac Catheterization A diastolic pressure gradient between the left ventricle and the left atrium is diagnostic of mitral stenosis. Left atrial or pulmonary arterial wedge hypertension is present in most patients, but in circumstances of reduced pulmonary blood flow or a sizable interatrial opening, this hypertension and the mitral diastolic pressure gradient may be only relative and their significance may go unrecognized. Pulmonary arterial hypertension and elevation of the pulmonary vascular resistance also are characteristic. Left atrial angiography will show left atrial size and may demonstrate a supravalvular chamber created by a supravalvular ring, restriction of mitral leaflet motion, or a subvalvular funnel converging on a single papillary muscle, which is characteristic of parachute mitral valve. Left ventricular angiography will permit identification of the papillary muscles, evaluation of mitral valve leaflet motion, and an estimate of the breadth and width of the column of unopacified blood entering the ventricle from the left atrium.

Natural History and Prognosis

In general, the outlook for symptomatic infants and young children with mitral stenosis is poor, since the congenitally malformed mitral apparatus usually does not lend itself to successful palliative or corrective surgery. Exceptions are found among patients with a supravalvular ring, where removal of the ring, usually with additional valvulotomy, may produce excellent and permanent relief of obstruction. Those children able to survive to an age and size when mitral valve replacement is feasible also can expect relief of symptoms and the return of the pulmonary arterial pressure and vascular resistance to normal or near-normal levels. Without surgery the course is one of progressive stenosis with increasing pulmonary venous congestion.

Medical Management

The physician must be alert to the possibility of mitral obstruction in any patient with an apical diastolic murmur or a disproportionate elevation of left atrial pressure as judged by unusual dyspnea, radiological evidence of pulmonary venous congestion, or by direct measurement at catheterization. This is particularly true among patients with coarctation of the aorta and valvular or subvalvular aortic stenosis, but it also is true for patients in whom the mitral orifice has not yet been subjected to normal or increased flow, as with tetralogy of Fallot or atrial septal defect. Medical therapy includes the use of digitalis, diuretics, restriction of activity, prompt treatment of respiratory infections, and protection against infective endocarditis. With the exception of those patients with a supravalvular mitral ring, who make up about 20 percent of individuals with congenital mitral obstruction and in whom palliative or even corrective surgery might be possible, management consists of supportive measures to permit survival until valve replacement is feasible or necessary.

Surgical Management

The spectrum of congenital mitral valve stenosis (hypoplastic annulus, commissure fusion, the "hammock valve," the parachute valve, and the funnel-shaped valve) requires individualized operations.[334–339] Fused commissures are incised, thickened chordae are excised, and obstructing subvalvular tissue is fenestrated or excised when possible. Results achieved by these difficult valvuloplasties are variable; surgical mortality approaches 25 percent.[334]

Mitral valve replacement may be required for relief of obstruction without intolerable mitral regurgitation. The small child requiring mitral valve replacement must undergo insertion of a larger prosthetic valve as growth occurs. A valve-containing conduit from the left atrium to the left ventricular apex has been used successfully for relief of congenital mitral stenosis with a small annulus.[340]

Mitral Regurgitation

Pathology

Mitral regurgitation resulting from congenital disease may be a consequence of a primary anomaly of the valve, or it may be secondary to either a systemic condition or a primary anomaly in a nonvalvular structure. The most common cause is the mitral deformity that is part of the common atrioventricular canal defect. (See preceding discussion.) In addition, a variety of rare primary malformations have been implicated, including isolated clefts of the anterior or posterior leaflet,[341] absence of leaflet tissue, fenestration, and duplication of the mitral orifice as well as malformations and ectopic insertions of the papillary muscles and chordae tendineae.[336] In cases of corrected transposition (see later section), inversion of the ventricles and atrioventricular valves places the tricuspid valve on the left side of the heart, where it functions as a "mitral" valve. The inverted tricuspid valve has a strong tendency to be associated with an Ebstein-like malformation, and incompetence of the valve may occur. Secondary causes include infarction of the papillary muscles associated with endocardial fibroelastosis, aortic stenosis, coarctation of the aorta, and anomalous origin of the left coronary artery from the pulmonary trunk.

Systemic diseases associated with mitral regurgitation include mucopolysaccharidosis[342] and Marfan's syndrome.

Clinical Manifestations

Isolated mitral regurgitation is uncommon during childhood. Easy fatigue, dyspnea with exertion, excessive sweating, numerous episodes of lower respiratory tract infection, and slow weight gain are symptoms of significant mitral regurgitation.

The patient is usually a slender, dyspneic infant or child, frequently with cool and clammy skin and a prominent left precordial bulge. The left ventricular lift is hyperdynamic, diffuse, and sustained. The second heart sound is widely split but varies normally with respiration. The pulmonary component is accentuated in the presence of pulmonary arterial hypertension. A third heart sound at the apex is common. The characteristic holosystolic blowing murmur is loudest at the apex with radiation to the axilla. In the presence of leaflet fenestration, the murmur may radiate to the base of the heart and simulate aortic stenosis. A middiastolic rumble at the apex accompanies significant regurgitation.

Both left ventricular and left atrial enlargement are present on the chest roentgenogram. The left mainstem bronchus may be displaced upward and left lower lobe atelectasis is not uncommon.

Left ventricular and left atrial hypertrophy with deep Q waves in leads aV_L, V_5, and V_6 are characteristic in the electrocardiogram. Flattening and inversion of the T waves over the left precordium usually reflect severe regurgitation.

Echocardiogram M-mode echocardiographic technique will demonstrate the nonspecific findings of a slightly hyperkinetic left ventricle, as well as enlargement of the left ventricle and atrium. Regurgitation associated with left atrium myxoma, prolapse, or flail mitral valve leaflet can be distinguished. Two-dimensional echocardiography, in addition, permits identification of an isolated cleft of the mitral leaflet,[343] displacement of the left atrioventricular valve associated with corrected transposition of the great arteries, and the single papillary muscle associated with parachute mitral valve deformity.[344]

Cardiac Catheterization With severe mitral regurgitation, there will be elevation of the left ventricular end-diastolic, left atrial, and pulmonary arterial wedge pressures. Left ventricular angiography documents the regurgitation and the degree of left ventricular and left atrial dilatation and provides a semiquantitative estimate of severity. A measured regurgitant volume of 50 percent or more of the left ventricular stroke volume is considered indicative of severe mitral regurgitation in children.

Natural History and Prognosis

While mild and even moderate isolated mitral regurgitation may be tolerated well for many years, the clinical course among patients with severe regurgitation usually is one of increasing dyspnea, frequent respiratory infections, recurrent left lower lobe atelectasis, and marked retardation of growth. There will be clinical and laboratory evidence of increasing left ventricular and left atrial dilatation as well as pulmonary congestion and pulmonary arterial hypertension. Arrhythmias may appear in late childhood but are uncommon in infancy. The response to successful valve annuloplasty or valve replacement in children usually is dramatic.

Medical Management

With severe regurgitation, decongestive measures in the form of digitalis, diuretics, vasodilator agents, and restriction of activity are indicated. Prompt and vigorous therapy for respiratory infections, including postural drainage, is important to avoid pulmonary complications. Protection against infective endocarditis is emphasized. Every attempt should be made to remove or relieve complicating associated cardiac lesions. Fortunately, medical therapy is sufficient in most instances to permit the infant or young child to reach a size sufficient to allow mitral valve replacement if necessary. Finally, it should be emphasized that rheumatic fever is still a cause of isolated mitral regurgitation during childhood. Unless it can be established that the regurgitation is congenital or the result of some well-documented disorder or disease, antibiotic prophylaxis against streptococcal infections and recurrent rheumatic fever is indicated.

Surgical Management

Incompetence of the mitral apparatus caused by annular dilatation, clefts, fenestrations, agenesis of leaflets or chordae, elongation of chordae, and papillary muscle abnormalities requires individualized surgical management.[339] Simple clefts are closed by suture. A dilated annulus can be constricted by suture or prosthetic annuloplasty.[345] Results of complex plastic procedures for subvalvular causes of incompetence have been generally unsatisfactory.[339]

Significant mitral regurgitation not correctable by reconstruction requires mitral valve replacement. A larger valve must be inserted as the child grows;

unfortunately, no good method exists for surgical enlargement of the mitral annulus. Injury to the bundle of His with subsequent complete heart block is more likely to occur in mitral valve replacement for congenital abnormalities than for rheumatic disease. (See discussions of aortic regurgitation and surgery for valvular heart disease for details regarding choices of valve substitutes, management and surgical technique, and complications of prosthetic valves.)

Cor Triatriatum

Definition

Cor triatriatum is characterized by the presence in the left atrium of a perforated muscular membrane which separates the atrium into upper and lower chambers.

Pathology

The dividing membrane of cor triatriatum lies horizontally above the level of the atrial appendage. Its structure is that of cardiac muscle covered on its superior and inferior aspects by endocardial tissue. The pulmonary veins enter the upper chamber, and blood must pass through the opening in the membrane to reach the lower aspect of the left atrium. The caliber of the perforation in the membrane determines the degree of obstruction to pulmonary venous flow. With severe degrees of obstruction right ventricular hypertrophy and pulmonary venous hypertensive vascular changes are present. The mitral valve is intrinsically normal.

Associated Conditions A defect in the atrial septum is uncommonly present and may allow communication between the upper left atrial compartment and the right atrium. A pulmonary vein may connect anomalously with a systemic vein. Tetralogy and pulmonary stenosis have been observed uncommonly.[101,346]

Clinical Manifestations

This malformation is one of the rarest congenital cardiac deformities. In most instances it lends itself to complete surgical correction, but the absence of a heart murmur (and certainly lack of a distinctive murmur) frequently leads to an initial diagnosis of primary pulmonary vascular or parenchymal disease. Almost invariably patients are considered normal at birth and in the immediate neonatal period. Symptoms are those of pulmonary venous congestion and include dyspnea, orthopnea, difficulty with feeding, poor weight gain, and frequent lower respiratory tract infections. Episodes of pulmonary edema, particularly associated with exertion, may occur.

Signs of pulmonary arterial and right ventricular hypertension are present, with a forceful right ventricular lift, accentuated pulmonary second sound, and, occasionally, the soft early diastolic murmur of pulmonary regurgitation. Dyspnea, orthopnea, and basal lung rales reflect the pulmonary venous congestion. Right-sided heart failure is usually severe. Murmurs described with this malformation usually are soft and nondescript. An apical diastolic murmur is extremely rare. Occasionally, a soft, continuous murmur is present and is most likely due to continuous flow across the small aperture in the obstructing membrane.[6]

On chest roentgenogram, at least mild cardiac enlargement is the rule, with prominence of the pulmonary arterial segment and evidence of pulmonary venous congestion. The latter may include Kerley B lines and the "ground-glass" pattern of acute pulmonary edema in the hilar areas. Left atrial dilatation rarely is present.

The characteristic electrocardiogram pattern is one of right axis deviation and right atrial and right ventricular hypertrophy.

Echocardiogram Two-dimensional echocardiography offers a definitive view of this intraatrial membrane.[347]

Cardiac Catheterization Severe elevation of the pulmonary arterial wedge pressure is characteristic and usually is associated with severe pulmonary arterial hypertension as well. A normal left ventricular diastolic pressure places the obstruction at the mitral, left atrial, or pulmonary venous level. Occasionally it is possible to enter the distal, low-pressure, left atrial chamber via a patent foramen ovale. Pulmonary arterial angiography usually will permit visualization of the obstructed dorsal chamber, with its delayed emptying and lack of contraction, as well as the diminutive ventral chamber with its characteristic crescent shape and left atrial appendage. In the frontal view, the membrane may be seen as a thin, oblique, radiolucent line slanted from an inferior medial to a superior lateral position. Since a little over 10 percent of patients will have partial anomalous venous return, angiography also will be helpful in distinguishing this variant.

Natural History and Prognosis

The course of cor triatriatum is one of progressive pulmonary venous hypertension and congestion with pulmonary edema and right-sided heart failure. The majority of patients are recognized during childhood, while a few become symptomatic in early infancy. A rare patient may develop symptoms for the first time as a young adult. Surgical removal of the membrane results in relief of symptoms and, usually, a return of the pulmonary arterial pressure and vascular resistance to normal.

Medical Management

Prompt diagnostic studies are indicated to identify this curable cause of serious pulmonary venous and pulmonary arterial hypertension. Surgical removal of the obstructing membrane should be carried out with dispatch. Digitalis and diuretics may be indicated in the circumscribed preoperative management and in the immediate postoperative period until the pulmonary vascular resistance returns to normal.

Surgical Management
The obstructive accessory septum is excised on cardiopulmonary bypass or during hypothermic circulatory arrest in infants. Exposure of coronary sinus, mitral valve, pulmonary veins, and the accessory septum is accomplished through the right atrium and interatrial septum or through the left atrium.[348–350] After excision of the membranous accessory septum and visual confirmation of free communication between mitral orifice and pulmonary veins, the interatrial communication is closed with a small patch. Clinical improvement is dramatic. Mortality and morbidity are low in the absence of associated complex anomalies if excision is performed before the development of pulmonary vascular obstructive disease and right ventricular failure. Of 25 patients described by Oglietti, 21 (84 percent) survived correction.[348]

Stenosis of Pulmonary Veins and Venules

Definition
Obstruction in major pulmonary veins is usually designated as *stenosis of individual pulmonary veins,* while obstruction in the venules and small veins is designated as *pulmonary venocclusive disease.*

Pathology
Stenosis of individual pulmonary veins may be characterized either by hypoplasia of involved veins or, more commonly, by a fibrous intimal lesion at the junction of a vein with the left atrium. All or only some of the veins may be involved in a given case. Stenosis of individual pulmonary veins may be an isolated condition, but in the few reported cases atrial septal defect was common.

In pulmonary venocclusive disease, venules and small veins are obstructed by vascular connective tissue. This picture suggests an acquired process, namely, organized thrombosis.[351] Pulmonary venocclusive disease characteristically is not associated with cardiovascular anomalies.

Clinical Manifestations
Stenosis of the individual pulmonary veins and pulmonary venocclusive disease are both very rare conditions and both, particularly the latter, carry an extremely poor outlook for survival.

Symptoms are those of dyspnea, easy fatigue, frequent lower respiratory tract infections, and poor weight gain. Venous stenosis tends to occur somewhat earlier in life, frequently within the first year, while venocclusive disease has a somewhat wider age distribution. Hemoptysis may occur in both, but syncope, cough, and chest pain are more typical of venocclusive disease.

Both tend to show evidence of central cyanosis, and in both the physical findings are those of severe pulmonary arterial hypertension and pulmonary venous congestion. There are no distinctive murmurs.

A diffuse pattern of pulmonary venous congestion may be seen on the chest roentgenogram. The central pulmonary arteries will be enlarged, and there is usually mild cardiac enlargement due to right ventricular dilatation. No left atrial enlargement is present.

Echocardiographic studies are helpful in excluding mitral stenosis and cor triatriatum.

Cardiac catheterization in both conditions is characterized by severe pulmonary arterial hypertension and varying degrees of systemic arterial oxygen desaturation. With stenosis of the individual pulmonary veins, the corresponding pulmonary arterial wedge pressures are elevated, whereas in pulmonary venocclusive disease, the pulmonary arterial wedge pressures usually are normal. Left atrial pressures are normal. Stenosis of the individual pulmonary veins may be visualized by high-quality pulmonary arterial angiography, but selective pulmonary venous angiography is preferable.

Natural History and Prognosis
In the case of stenosis of the individual pulmonary veins, the course is usually relatively short, ending in death within a year or two. The average age of death is estimated to be 4 years, with a range from 5 months to 10 years.[101] Among children with pulmonary venocclusive disease, the course also is one of rapid deterioration, with an average survival of 20 months from the onset of symptoms.[352]

Medical Management
At least temporary control of right-sided heart failure and relief of pulmonary edema can be achieved with digitalis, diuretics, and restricted activity. Oxygen therapy in the acute situation is helpful. Among patients with discrete stenosis limited to one or two relatively large veins, surgery may be recommended. As yet, there is no specific therapy for pulmonary venocclusive disease and only supportive measures can be offered.

Surgical Management
Discrete stenosis of pulmonary veins has seldom been relieved by operation or balloon dilatation.[353] Stenosis of the orifice or of the extraparenchymal vein can be widened by pericardial patch angioplasty or by excision and anastomosis of a proximal dilated segment to the left atrium. Rarely, a membranous diaphragm can be excised.[354]

When attempts to relieve obstruction have failed or when there appears little hope of providing adequate venous drainage to a relatively small area of lung, the affected pulmonary tissue should be resected to prevent intrapulmonary hemorrhage and pneumonitis.

Endocardial Fibroelastosis

Pathology

Endocardial fibroelastosis is characterized by a proliferation of elastic and collagenous fibers within the endocardium. Grossly, the endocardium is abnormally thickened and has a smooth, glistening, milky white or "porcelain" appearance. The left ventricle is involved either exclusively or, less commonly, along with the right ventricle. In the left ventricle two types are recognized, the dilated, which is more common, and the contracted.

In the dilated type, the left ventricular cavity is enlarged and the wall thick. The condition may be said to be primary or secondary (Fig. 36-42). The secondary type is associated with a variety of conditions, principally aortic valvular stenosis, coarctation of the aorta, and anomalous origin of the coronary artery from the pulmonary trunk, while lesser degrees may be observed with left-to-right shunts, such as ventricular septal defect and patent ductus arteriosus.[355] It may follow primary myocardial disease. Mitral insufficiency is a common complication.

The contracted type is characterized by the presence of a smaller than normal left ventricular cavity. The most severe forms of left ventricular hypoplasia are seen in association with aortic atresia. An unusual variety of the contracted type appears as an isolated condition.

FIGURE 36-42 Endocardial fibroelastosis. Interior of left ventricle shows hypertrophy of wall, enlargement of chamber, and marked endocardial fibrous thickening.

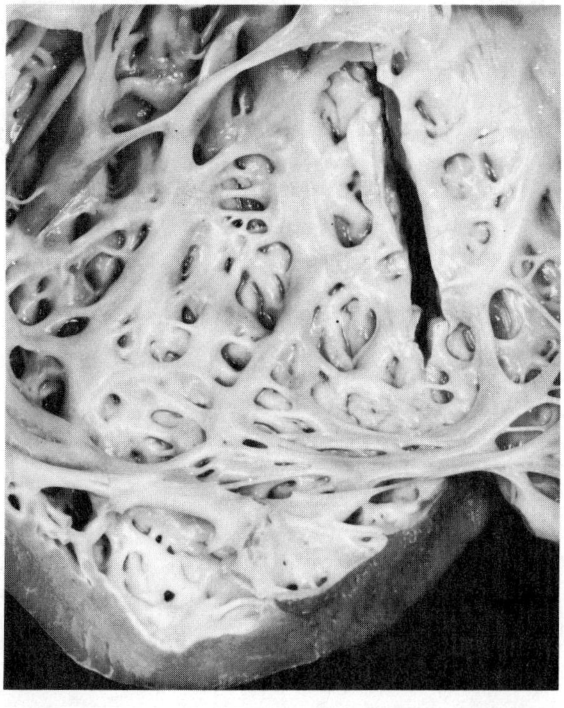

Clinical Manifestations

Primary fibroelastosis is a disease chiefly of infants, with approximately 80 percent of affected patients being symptomatic by 10 months of age. When related to a total clinical population of infants and children affected with congenital heart disease, its incidence is slightly less than 1 percent. It would appear that this incidence is distinctly less today than in years past. The female/male ratio lies between 1.3:1 and 1.6:1. Familial occurrence is uncommon but well described. The risk of fibroelastosis for a sibling of an affected infant is estimated at 4 percent by Nora,[116] although the risk to later-born siblings may be higher.[356]

History Patients are almost always in heart failure when first seen, but they generally have normal growth and development until that time. Approximately 10 percent of patients are symptomatic from birth. The onset is rapid, with dyspnea, grunting respirations, cough, irritability, weakness, and pallor being the most common observations. In over half the infants, the onset of congestive failure is linked with an immediately preceding respiratory infection.

Physical Examination Respiratory distress, with flaring of the nostrils and intercostal retractions, is evident. Fine, moist rales are frequent in the lung fields, the heart is enlarged, and a gallop rhythm is almost invariably present. A soft systolic murmur of mitral regurgitation may be heard, but characteristically no significant murmur is present early in the illness.

Chest Roentgenogram The heart is massively enlarged, usually with left atrial dilatation. Left lower lobe atelectasis due to bronchial compression is frequent.

Electrocardiogram The electrocardiogram indicates isolated left ventricular hypertrophy in almost all instances with tall R waves in leads V_5 and V_6 and a small rS ratio and deep S wave in V_1. Flat or inverted T waves over the left precordium are characteristic. Left atrial or biatrial hypertrophy usually is present as well. Tall, peaked T waves in the midprecordial leads should raise the question of systemic carnitine deficiency, which may present as familial fibroelastosis.[357] Rarely, one finds a low-voltage pattern more typical of myocarditis.

Echocardiogram M-mode echocardiography will demonstrate a markedly dilated left ventricle, a thin free wall, and greatly diminished contractility.

Cardiac Catheterization A wide difference in systemic arteriovenous oxygen content, a diminished cardiac output, and elevated left ventricular end-diastolic, left atrial, and pulmonary arterial wedge pressures are the usual findings. Left ventricular angiography reveals a markedly dilated chamber with prolonged opacification and little change in chamber size from systole to diastole.

Natural History and Prognosis
This disease formerly was considered almost invariably fatal, but there is now reason to believe that early recognition and prompt, diligent, and prolonged therapy may salvage as many as 60 percent of affected infants and children. Eighty percent of deaths occur in the first year of life. The course in these infants usually is one of recurrent episodes of congestive failure with persistent cardiac enlargement and electrocardiographic abnormalities. Death is from congestive heart failure or tachyarrhythmias in most instances. Systemic or pulmonary emboli from mural thrombi occur in approximately 10 percent of patients. Early recognition, a prompt response to decongestive measures, a rapid return of heart size to normal, disappearance of abnormal T waves, and a gradual resolution of left ventricular hypertrophy are favorable signs. Survival to the fifth birthday suggests continued survival with little or no handicap. Unfortunately, deaths have been described in a few children several years after an excellent initial clinical response. The diagnosis of fibroelastosis is documented by postmortem examination in those who succumb. Whether the same disease process existed and then resolved or became tolerable in the survivors is open to question.

Medical Management
Prompt, vigorous, and sustained treatment of heart failure with adequate amounts of digitalis and diuretics is essential. Carnitine levels should be determined in the plasma and skeletal muscle, and if they are reduced, treatment with L-carnitine should be begun.[357] Rest, with sedation if necessary, and restriction of activity are advised. Anemia should be corrected promptly and recurrence prevented. Complicating congenital cardiac lesions should be corrected or relieved if possible. The value of steroids in patients with fibroelastosis is unproved, but since a few patients with inflammatory myocarditis appear to benefit from their use early in the course of the illness, a trial of therapy should be considered. Full medical support, including administration of digitalis and diuretics, should be continued at least until the electrocardiogram and chest roentgenogram have returned to normal and probably considerably longer. The aim of such therapy is to control congestive failure, reduce heart size, and extend life with the hope that the disease will resolve and permit long-term survival. In selected patients, mitral valve replacement for mitral regurgitation may be indicated.

Valvular and Vascular Malformations of the Right Side of the Heart with Right-to-Left, Bidirectional, or No Shunt

Valvular Pulmonary Stenosis with Intact Ventricular Septum

Pathology
Valvular pulmonary stenosis with intact ventricular septum is usually characterized by the so-called *dome-shaped stenosis of the pulmonary valve* and only uncommonly by dysplasia of the valve (Fig. 36-43).[80] In dome-shaped stenosis, the valvular tissue is represented by a cone or dome-shaped structure perforated at its distal end, with the opening representing the effective orifice of the pulmonary valve.[358] The pulmonary trunk exhibits poststenotic dilatation. In adult patients, calcification of the valve may appear.[359]

In pulmonary valvular dysplasia, the annulus of the valve may be abnormally narrow, but the most dramatic changes are related to the cusps, of which three are identifiable. The cusps are exceedingly thickened by mucoid and dense connective tissue.[360]

FIGURE 36-43 Congenital pulmonary valvular stenosis with intact ventricular septum. SVC = superior vena cava; IVC = inferior vena cava; RA = right atrium; RV = right ventricle; PT = main pulmonary arterial trunk; RPA = right pulmonary artery; LPA = left pulmonary artery; RPV = right pulmonary vein; LPV = left pulmonary vein; LA = left atrium; LV = left ventricle; Ao = aorta. *[From J. E. Edwards, Classification of Congenital Heart Disease in the Adult, in W. C. Roberts (ed.), "Congenital Heart Disease in Adults," Cardiovasc. Clin. Series 10/1, F. A. Davis Company, Philadelphia, 1979, p. 1. Reproduced with permission from the publisher, editor, and author.]*

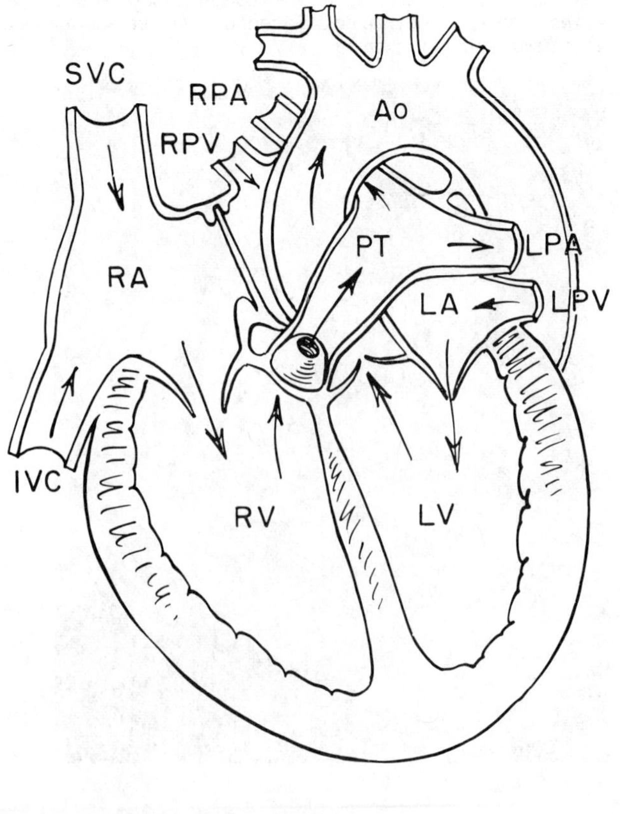

Concentric hypertrophy of the right ventricle is present, its degree reflecting the degree of obstruction at valve level. The hypertrophy, as it affects the infundibular musculature, may cause secondary muscular infundibular stenosis.

The tricuspid valve may show fibrous thickening with secondary contracture of leaflets and chordae. The atrial septum varies. In some instances, the foramen ovale is anatomically sealed, in others it is patent. In cases of dome-shaped stenosis with patent foramen ovale or atrial septal defect, the term *trilogy of Fallot* is applied by some.

Associated Conditions Among conditions associated with valvular pulmonary stenosis are anomalous muscle bundle of the right ventricle[361] and focal stenosis of the pulmonary arteries. Among family members of patients with pulmonary valvular dysplasia, dome-shaped valvular pulmonary stenosis has been observed.[360]

Abnormal Physiology[362–365]

There is a pressure difference during systole between the main right ventricular cavity and the pulmonary artery. The area of the pulmonary valve orifice is normally 2 cm^2/m^2; it is about 0.5 cm^2 at birth and increases in size with body growth. In general, the effective valve area must be decreased by about 60 percent before there is hemodynamically significant obstruction to flow.

In patients with severe valvular stenosis, the pulmonary artery pressure is usually lower than normal and has a pulse wave which is less distinct than normal. Just distal to the stenotic valve, there may be negative systolic waves referred to as *Venturi waves.* The right ventricular pressure pulse typically has a rapid rate of increase in pressure to a delayed but sharp peak pressure and then a rapid fall in pressure. The peak systolic pressure difference may reach 150 to 240 mmHg; rarely, it may be higher. The degree of obstruction is assessed by the mean systolic pressure gradient and the amount of flow across the valve. Severe stenosis may be associated with a relatively small pressure difference if the flow is very low as a result of right ventricular failure. If pulmonary flow is normal, most patients with peak pressure differences at rest of less than 50 mmHg have mild stenosis, and patients with a pressure difference over 100 mmHg have severe stenosis.

When the pulmonary stenosis is severe, the right ventricle may fail and the cardiac output may be decreased, even at rest; this is associated with elevation of both the right ventricular end-diastolic pressure and the right atrial mean pressure. This may cause the foramen ovale to open and allow shunting of blood from the right to the left atrium. Arterial oxygen unsaturation and cyanosis result. In addition, with decreased cardiac output, "peripheral" or "stagnant" cyanosis may result from the low flow to the peripheral tissues. This may occur in severe pulmonary stenosis even without a patent foramen ovale. In such a situation the arterial oxygen saturation is normal.

In most adolescent or adult patients with significant pulmonary stenosis, the resting cardiac output is within normal limits but it usually does not increase normally during exercise. In contrast, children may be able to increase cardiac output during exercise.[362] Since a doubling of flow across a stenotic valve requires a *fourfold* increase of pressure, and since the peak pressure in either ventricle rarely exceeds 320 mmHg, flow through a severely stenotic valve is limited.

Trilogy of Fallot[359] Atrial septal defect associated with pulmonary stenosis presents a wide spectrum of hemodynamic alterations, depending mainly on the severity of the pulmonary stenosis. If the stenosis is mild, the shunt may be predominantly left-to-right, although it seldom has the "torrential" volume found in uncomplicated atrial septal defect. If the stenosis is more severe or the right ventricle "fails," the shunting of blood may be predominantly right-to-left.

Clinical Manifestations

Pulmonary stenosis is one of the most common congenital heart defects and account for about 10 percent of patients in most large study populations (see Table 36-1). The stenosis is at the level of the pulmonary valve in most instances, but it can occur within the right ventricle or in the pulmonary arteries. Distinguishing clinical features will be discussed separately, although combinations occur in some patients. Approximately one-quarter of patients with stenosis of the pulmonary valve also have an atrial shunt,[366] but this frequency is probably dependent on the age group studied.

History Most infants and children are asymptomatic, but a small percentage with very severe obstruction will manifest symptoms. The most common symptoms are mild fatigue or shortness of breath with exertion. Young infants with critical obstruction present with symptoms related to heart failure and may have cyanosis if there is a patent foramen ovale or atrial septal defect.[367] Squatting and syncope are rare in childhood. Growth and development are normal. There is no sex preference, and familial transmission is reported,[368] especially when the valve is dysplastic[360] and associated with certain dysmorphisms described by Noonan.[369]

Physical Examination Only patients with a dysplastic valve have consistent noncardiac abnormalities. These patients frequently have short stature, hypertelorism, ptosis, low-set ears, and mental retardation.[369]

In patients with valvular pulmonary stenosis, cyanosis is uncommon, except with severe obstruction and an atrial communication.[361] Tachypnea, hepatomegaly, and the murmur of tricuspid regurgitation may be present in infants with severe obstruction. In those with at least moderate obstruction, a prominent *a* wave is seen on examination of the jugular venous pulse. A systolic thrill in the suprasternal notch and at the left upper sternal border is present. The right ventricular parasternal impulse becomes increasingly forceful with more severe obstruction. On auscultation an early systolic click, accentuated with expiration, is heard at the left upper sternal border unless the obstruction is severe or the valve is dysplastic. As obstruction increases in severity, the pulmonary component of the second heart sound becomes progressively softer and more delayed. As the right ventricular pressure reaches systemic levels or greater, it becomes inaudible. A fourth heart sound is heard if obstruction is severe. The characteristic systolic murmur is harsh, crescendo-decrescendo in shape, and best heard at the left upper sternal border with radiation toward the left clavicle. The duration of the murmur and the timing of peak intensity correlate well with the severity of obstruction. With mild to moderate stenosis, the murmur peaks in midsystole and ends at or before the aortic component of the second heart sound. In patients with severe stenosis, the murmur peaks late in systole and extends beyond the aortic component (A_2) of the second heart sound.

Chest Roentgenogram Most patients have a normal or only slightly increased heart size. Significant enlargement is seen with critical obstruction and is an ominous sign. Characteristically, the main and proximal left pulmonary arteries are prominent owing to poststenotic dilatation. This finding may be absent with very severe obstruction, with a dysplastic valve, or in very young infants. The pulmonary vascular pattern is normal in most but is diminished in those with right-to-left shunt at atrial level.

Electrocardiogram Right ventricular forces in the anterior precordial leads correlate reasonably well with the degree of obstruction.[370] They will be normal or demonstrate mild hypertrophy with an rsR′ pattern if there is mild obstruction. With severe stenosis, there is right axis deviation, right atrial hypertrophy, and very tall R waves in the anterior precordial leads. The presence of a qR pattern in these leads is almost always a sign of very severe obstruction. Those with a dysplastic valve frequently have a superior QRS axis.[360]

Vectorcardiogram The Frank vectorcardiogram provides an estimate of peak right ventricular systolic pressure by the use of the right maximum spatial voltage in a regression equation.[371] Estimation from physical and electrocardiographic data has been shown to be nearly as accurate as this method.[370,372]

Echocardiogram With moderate or severe pulmonary valvular stenosis, there is exaggeration of the maximal *a* wave depth of the pulmonary valve recorded with inspiration; when echocardiograms of the anterior and posterior leaflets are recorded, presystolic opening of the valve is seen to occur. The latter finding is probably the more specific.[373] Absence of these findings does not exclude the diagnosis, particularly if the stenosis is mild.

Cardiac Catheterization There is elevated right ventricular systolic pressure with a distinct systolic pressure difference across the valve, which can be shown by slow withdrawal of the catheter from the pulmonary artery to the right ventricle. If critical obstruction is suspected, it may be wise not to attempt to advance the catheter into the pulmonary artery due to the risk of compromising an already marginal opening. Simultaneous measurement of systemic arterial and right ventricular pressures with measurement of flow is necessary to assess severity accurately. The right ventricular end-diastolic pressure and right atrial *a* wave may be elevated. Systemic oxygen saturation will be diminished only in those with more severe obstruction and a patent foramen ovale or, less commonly, a true septal defect. A left-to-right shunt at atrial level is detected in some patients with mild to moderate obstruction.[366] Right ventricular angiography will demonstrate thickened and doming valve leaflets and a jet of contrast material entering the dilated pulmonary artery (Fig. 36-44). Doming is not characteristic of the dysplastic valve (Fig. 36-45).[360] Secondary infundibular subvalvular narrowing due to muscular hypertrophy may be seen. Studies of ventricular volume characteristics have demonstrated depressed ventricular function in those with right-to-left shunts.[365] Percuta-

FIGURE 36-44 Lateral view of a right ventricular (RV) angiogram demonstrating the typical features of valvular pulmonary stenosis with doming of the pulmonary valve (arrow) and a narrow jet of contrast entering the dilated main pulmonary artery (MPA).

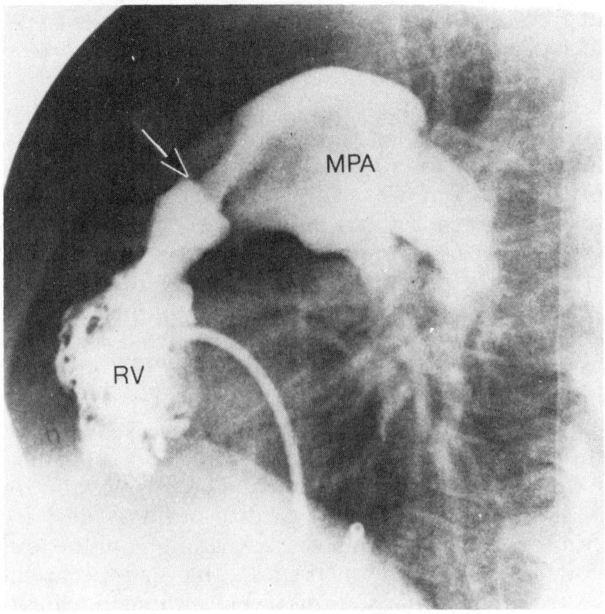

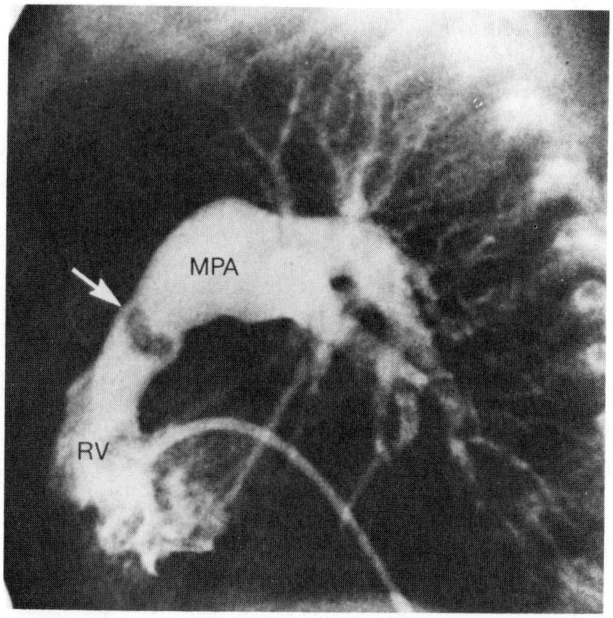

FIGURE 36-45 Lateral view of a right ventricular (RV) angiogram with very thickened dysplastic pulmonary valve (arrow) and mild poststenotic dilatation of the main pulmonary artery (MPA).

neous transluminal balloon valvuloplasty has been used successfully.[374]

Natural History and Prognosis

The clinical course is favorable in most patients with mild to moderate obstruction. In a national cooperative study,[372] 86 percent of patients had no significant increase in their pressure gradients over a 4- to 8-year interval. Those with a significant increase were less than 4 years of age and had at least moderate stenosis intitially. Progression during the period of growth seems the likely explanation for most of the increases, but a few developed subvalvular muscular hypertrophy, which increased the obstruction. Even mild obstruction may progress significantly in some infants during the first year of life.[364] The prognosis of those with severe obstruction is poor, especially for infants with critical obstruction. With severe obstruction, right ventricular damage and dysfunction can ensue over the years and heart failure or arrhythmias can cause premature death in adults.[364] Tricuspid regurgitation may also result. Brain abscess can occur if a right-to-left shunt is present. Infective endocarditis with vegetations on the valve, pulmonary arterial wall, or infundibular region is also a risk.

Medical Management

Management will obviously depend on the severity of obstruction. For those with mild to moderate valvular pulmonary stenosis, periodic reexamination and electrocardiograms are indicated to detect any evidence of progression, with more frequent evaluation for those under 1 year of age. Measures to treat heart failure should be instituted in the infant with critical stenosis, but prompt surgical intervention is mandatory. Cyanosis or a right ventricular systolic pressure well above systemic levels also are indications for prompt surgery. In asymptomatic older infants and children, elective surgery is usually recommended when the right ventricular systolic pressure is near 70 mmHg or the gradient is near or over 50 mmHg. For those beyond infancy, there is some suggestion that surgery gives better overall results, even in the group with pressures somewhat less than this.[372] Exercise studies[362] during catheterization have demonstrated that altered cardiac function observed in some children is reversible by surgery. This does not appear to be true for adults, so the best results are likely if surgery is done relatively early in childhood. Prophylaxis against infective endocarditis is recommended for all patients whether or not surgery is done.

Surgical Management

The stenotic pulmonary valve is exposed during normothermic cardiopulmonary bypass through a short incision in the main pulmonary artery. Fused commissures are incised to the annulus and each leaflet is detached slightly from the annulus to improve mobility.[375,376] Hypertrophic subvalvular muscle bundles are divided and excised through the annulus without a ventriculotomy. A thickened, im-

FIGURE 36-46 Pulmonary valvotomy in the infant using brief circulatory arrest with inflow occlusion. Tourniquets around the inferior and superior venae cavae interrupt blood flow into the heart, allowing exposure and excision or incision of the obstructing valve or membrane in the right ventricular outflow tract. Operation can be accomplished in 60 to 90 s of circulatory arrest. Resuscitation usually requires no more than release of the tourniquets to restore blood flow through the heart. Air is aspirated from the ascending aorta as forward flow is resumed. MPA = main pulmonary artery; Ao = aorta.

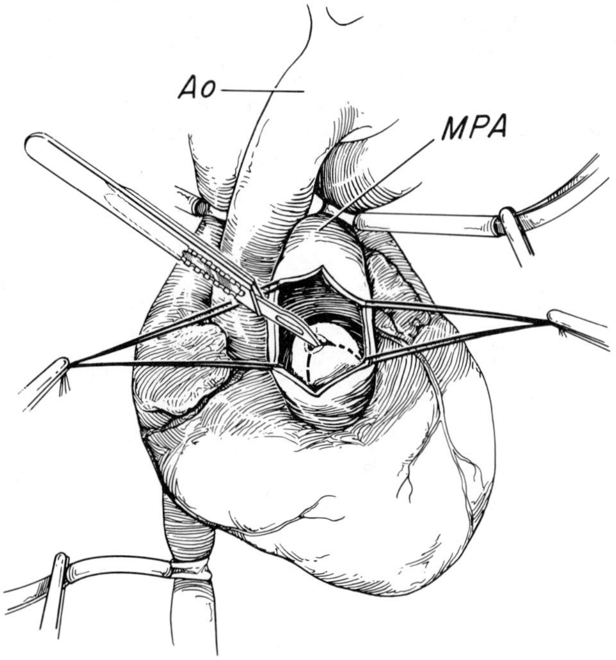

mobile, dysplastic pulmonary valve is completely excised (valvectomy), and a small annulus is augmented with a pericardial or Dacron gusset.[377]

In infants with life-threatening valvular pulmonary stenosis and hypoxemia, valvotomy or valvectomy can be accomplished during about 90 s of venous inflow occlusion and circulatory arrest (Fig. 36-46). Resuscitation usually requires only the restoration of cardiac filling by release of caval tourniquets.[378,379] Closed transventricular valvotomy using a valvulotome without inflow occlusion is preferred by others.[380] Further valve resection or annular augmentation may be required as the child grows.[381]

Beyond the first few months of life mortality is virtually nil; morbidity is low. Nearly normal right ventricular pressures can be expected.

Subvalvular Pulmonary Stenosis

Pathology

Subvalvular pulmonary stenosis is commonly at the infundibular level and is characterized by a fibrous collar that encircles the inlet to the right ventricular infundibulum. The obstruction less frequently is due to an anomalous muscle bundle across the middle of the chamber. In both instances, an intact ventricular septum is rare. The right ventricular hypertrophy is limited to that part of the right ventricle proximal to the obstruction.

In some cases of hypertrophic obstructive cardiomyopathy, the asymmetrical hypertrophy of the ventricular septum may cause infundibular stenosis.

Abnormal Physiology

Typically, as the catheter is withdrawn from the pulmonary artery across the pulmonary valve into the infundibular chamber, it is seen that systolic pressure stays the same but diastolic pressure decreases to right ventricular level. When the catheter is further withdrawn to the main right ventricular cavity, the systolic pressure is seen to be significantly higher than it is in the infundibular chamber or pulmonary artery. The physiology is otherwise similar to valvular pulmonary stenosis.

Clinical Manifestations

Isolated subvalvular pulmonary stenosis in the infundibular area or from an anomalous muscle bundle is uncommon.[382] The clinical picture varies with the associated defects, the most common of which are ventricular septal defect, valvular pulmonary stenosis, and tetralogy of Fallot. The reader is referred to sections of this chapter describing these specific defects.

Patients with the isolated form of this anomaly have a clinical picture similar to that of valvular pulmonary stenosis, but a thrill in the suprasternal notch is usually not present and the systolic murmur is best heard lower along the left sternal border. There is no ejection click. The electrocardiogram is similar to that of valvular stenosis, but the chest roentgenogram shows no poststenotic dilatation of the pulmonary artery. The echocardiogram usually shows fluttering of the pulmonary valve leaflets,[373] but this is not specific for this defect. It is helpful in distinguishing this defect from valvular obstruction.

Cardiac catheterization will show a pressure difference as the catheter is slowly withdrawn as described above. Right ventricular angiography will further define the nature of the obstruction. Since an associated ventricular septal defect is common, even a small defect should be excluded by sensitive methods such as hydrogen electrode study, reverse dye curves, or selective left ventricular angiography.

The muscular hypertrophy and severity of obstruction frequently increase with time. Otherwise, the clinical course, medical management, and indications for surgery are the same as those described for valvular stenosis.

Surgical Management

Subvalvular pulmonary stenosis is relieved through a right ventriculotomy, a main pulmonary arteriotomy, or a right atriotomy (Fig. 36-47). Hypertrophic

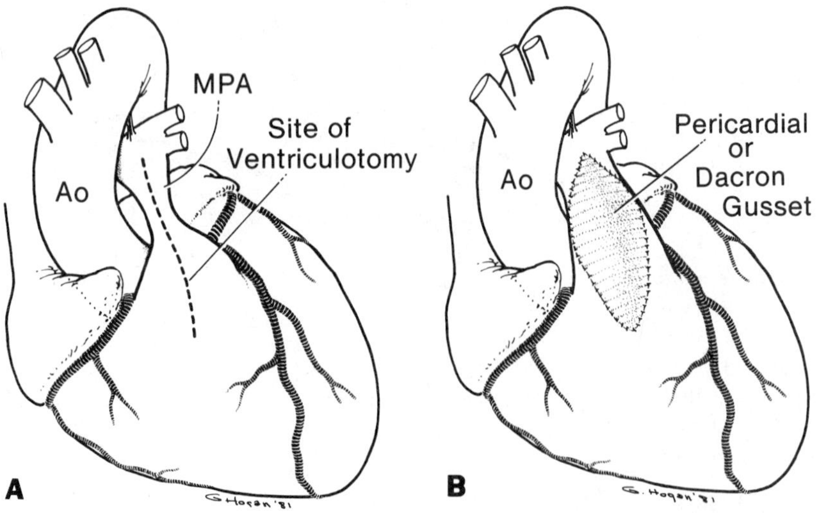

FIGURE 36-47 *A.* Site of incision for enlargement of the right ventricular outflow tract. Major coronary arteries are avoided. The incision is carried well out onto the main pulmonary artery to the bifurcation when the annulus and main pulmonary artery are small. The ventricular septal defect in tetralogy of Fallot is exposed through the caudal right ventricular portion of this incision. *B.* Pericardial or Dacron gusset used to widen the restrictive right ventricular outflow tract. Pericardial patches have become aneurysmal when elevated pulmonary vascular resistance or distal obstruction has resulted in persistent elevation of right ventricular pressures postoperatively.

parietal and septal muscle bands constituting the fibrous orifice of the os infundibulum and obstructing moderator bands or muscle bundles within the body of the right ventricle are excised. The right ventriculotomy can usually be closed by direct suture, but a small oval patch of pericardium or Dacron can be used to prevent constriction of the outflow tract (Fig. 36-47). Right ventricular function is minimally compromised by a small patch which does not extend across the annulus; larger patches to the pulmonary arterial bifurcation probably impair ventricular performance but may be necessary when there is associated annular or main pulmonary arterial hypoplasia. When possible, excision from the pulmonary artery or the right atrium is preferred to avoid ventricular injury.

Excellent relief of right ventricular outflow tract obstruction can be expected following resection. Mortality and significant morbidity are rare. Repair during childhood reduces the likelihood of complications related to severe right ventricular hypertrophy, diminished ventricular compliance and function, subendocardial ischemia, tricuspid regurgitation, and supraventricular dysrhythmias associated with right atrial hypertrophy.

Supravalvular Pulmonary Stenosis and Peripheral Pulmonary Arterial Coarctations

Pathology

From angiographic studies, D'Cruz and associates[383] classified the anomalies into four types: (1) localized stenosis with poststenotic dilatation, (2) segmental stenosis, (3) diffuse hypoplasia, and (4) multiple peripheral stenoses. The stenosis may be localized to any segment of the pulmonary arterial system. The process is unilateral in about one-third of the cases and bilateral in two-thirds. Pulmonary arterial stenosis is commonly (about 75 percent), *though not universally,* associated with other cardiovascular anomalies, among which are ventricular septal defect and pulmonary stenosis, supravalvular aortic stenosis, coarctation of the aorta, and tetralogy of Fallot. Pulmonary arterial stenosis has been identified in some as one of the sequelae of maternal rubella.[384]

Clinical Manifestations

There are many clinically associated abnormalities that give some clues to the causes.[6] It can occur as part of the syndrome described by Noonan, which was discussed under valvular stenosis, and it is a frequent abnormality in rubella syndrome,[6,384] along with cataracts, sensorineural deafness, microcephaly, and other cardiac anomalies, most commonly patent ductus. It may be found in patients with Williams' syndrome or idiopathic hypercalcemia in association with characteristic facies, dental anomalies, mental retardation, and supravalvular aortic stenosis. There is also a familial occurrence associated with supravalvular aortic stenosis but not with the other characteristics of Williams' syndrome.

Manifestations are similar to those of valvular stenosis—only the differences are discussed here. The stigmata of the above-mentioned syndromes should be looked for and careful histories of the pregnancy, neonatal period, and familial abnormalities obtained. The second heart sound is usually normal and there is no ejection click. A spindle-shaped midsystolic murmur is heard at the left upper sternal border, the axillae, and the back. It may be heard unilaterally if only one side has significant obstruction. A similar murmur may be heard during the first weeks of life in premature infants, but this will disappear.[385] Occasionally, a continuous murmur is heard in those with severe stenosis in whom a diastolic gradient is demonstrable.[6] There is usually no poststenotic dilatation on chest roentgenogram. Cardiac catheterization will reveal a systolic pressure difference or differences with careful exploration of the entire pulmonary arterial tree. A widened pulse pressure in the proximal main pulmonary artery with a low dicrotic notch and low diastolic pressure reflecting distal pressure are typical of the more severe obstructions when they are bilateral.[9] Angiography will demonstrate the sites of obstruction in the main pulmonary artery and branches (Fig. 36-48). Study of the left side of the heart should also be done because of the frequency of associated supravalvular aortic stenosis or abnormalities of the left ventricular morphology and function.

Natural History and Prognosis

Although natural history[6] is not well defined, available information suggests that there is little change in severity with time. Those with severe obstructions may thrombose or rupture the thin-walled distal vessels, with hemoptysis resulting.

Medical Management

Medical management is the same as with valvular stenosis but should include special attention to the noncardiac handicaps in many of these patients. Surgical relief is possible for those with severe stenosis in whom the stenoses are proximal and relatively discrete. Balloon dilation may be palliative in selected patients, especially when surgery has been unsuccessful.[386]

Surgical Management

Stenoses of main or extraparenchymal branch pulmonary arteries can be widened by pericardial or synthetic patch angioplasty if poststenotic dilatation is present. Proximal coarctations in the larger portion of the arterial tree are more readily corrected than those located in smaller distal branches beyond the bifurcation of either the right or left pulmonary artery, where results are poor.[387] Tubular conduits can be placed to bypass obstructions but are usually not needed unless there is absence of confluence of the arteries centrally. An artery treated by excision of a discrete stenosis with repair by primary anastomosis is subject to restenosis as the child grows.

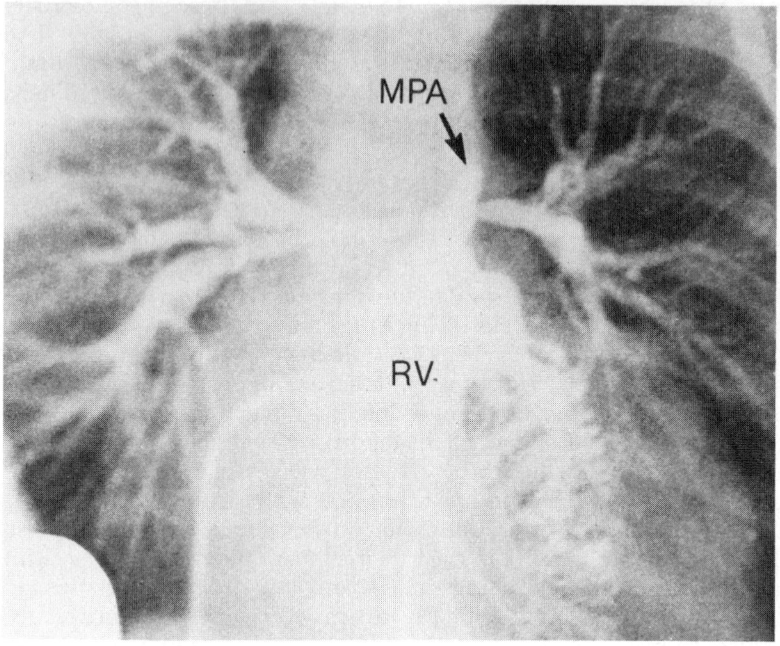

FIGURE 36-48 Posteroanterior view of a right ventricular (RV) angiogram showing diffuse hypoplasia of the main pulmonary artery (MPA) and proximal branches.

Pulmonary Atresia with Intact Ventricular Septum

Pathology

The pulmonary valve is an atretic membrane with either a horizontal fibrous plate or a dome-shaped structure without an opening.[388] Three equidistant raphes of varying length are present along the arterial aspect of the valve. Cases tend to fall into two groups, depending on the size of the right ventricular chamber.[389] In one, the chamber is smaller than normal, in some instances even diminutive (Fig. 36-49). In the other, the chamber of the right ventricle is either of normal size or grossly enlarged. The difference in size of the chamber among patients with this valvular anomaly appears to depend on the state of the tricuspid valve. When the tricuspid valve is incompetent, the right ventricular cavity develops to a normal size or is even enlarged and is grossly hypertrophied. Patients with a functionally competent (although hypoplastic) tricuspid valve tend to have a smaller than normal right ventricular cavity. Also, in patients with the small right ventricle, large sinusoids, present in the wall of the ventricle, communicate with the coronary arteries.[390] Vital channels for the flow of blood are the foramen ovale and the ductus arteriosus.

Associated Conditions Ebstein's deformity of the tricuspid valve is common in cases of pulmonary atresia, both with small and large right ventricles.

Clinical Manifestations

History Although pulmonary atresia with intact ventricular septum is uncommon, it is one of the most frequent causes of cyanosis and death in the neonatal period.[3] Cyanosis and tachypnea appear soon after birth. Since these infants are dependent on an atrial communication and patency of the ductus, progressive cyanosis or hypoxic attacks occur as the ductus undergoes spontaneous closure. Acidosis and death will ensue if there is no intervention.

Physical Examination These infants are usually extremely cyanotic; tachypnea is associated. The precordium is quiet. The second heart sound is single. There may be no murmur, but the continuous or abbreviated murmur of a ductus may be heard intermittently. In some infants a blowing holosystolic murmur of tricuspid regurgitation is heard at the lower sternal border.[9] Progressive hepatomegaly and a prominent *a* wave in the jugular venous pulse may appear later.

Chest Roentgenogram Diminished pulmonary flow is invariably seen on the chest roentgenogram. The heart size may be near normal to grossly enlarged. The latter is primarily due to right atrial enlargement, particularly if there is tricuspid regurgitation.

Electrocardiogram The findings on electrocardiogram vary to a large extent, depending on the size of the right ventricle, although this is not completely reliable as an indicator of cavity size. In those with a hypoplastic right ventricle, which is the most common type, the QRS axis is normal to slightly leftward for age and there is absence of the usual right ventricular dominance for age. Right atrial hypertrophy is common. Less commonly there is a large right ventricle with right axis deviation and right ventricular hypertrophy similar to that seen with severe valvular stenosis.[9]

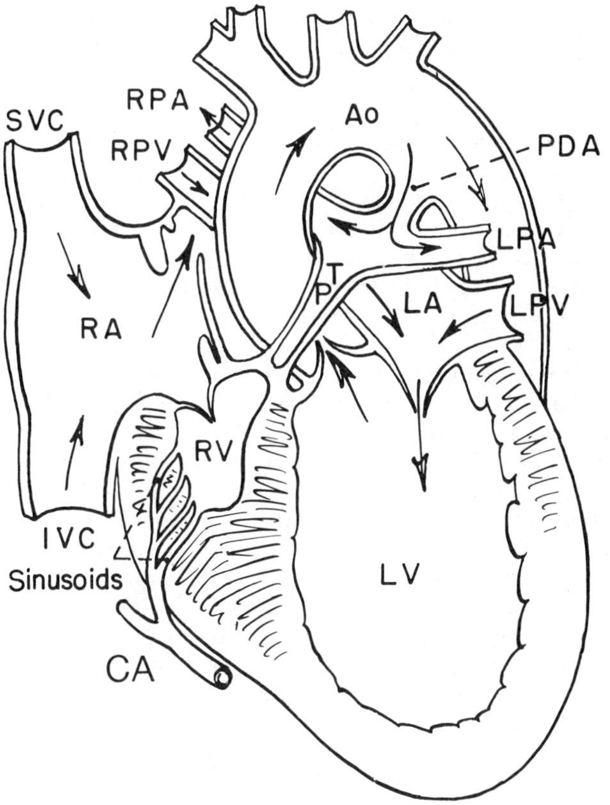

FIGURE 36-49 Pulmonary valvular atresia with intact ventricular septum and with small right ventricle (RV). CA = coronary arterial branches; SVC = superior vena cava; IVC = inferior vena cava; RA = right atrium; PT = main pulmonary arterial trunk; RPA = right pulmonary artery; LPA = left pulmonary artery; RPV = right pulmonary vein; LPV = left pulmonary vein; LA = left atrium; LV = left ventricle; Ao = aorta; PDA = patent ductus arteriosus.

Echocardiogram The echocardiographic findings will also depend on cavity size. Commonly, there are delayed and diminished tricuspid excursion, diminished right ventricular dimension, no demonstrable pulmonary valve, and normal to slightly increased left heart diameter.[391] Less commonly, the right ventricular size is increased and the pulmonary valve can be recorded with only presystolic motion or *a* dip.[392]

Cardiac Catheterization Immediate cardiac catheterization is indicated if the diagnosis of pulmonary atresia is suspected, since rapid deterioration can occur. The right atrial pressure is elevated and there is a right-to-left shunt at atrial level. Right ventricular pressure is markedly elevated, frequently above left ventricular pressure. Occasionally, only a damped diphasic pressure can be recorded if the right ventricle is extremely diminutive. Arterial oxygen saturations are usually very low and acidosis may be present. Right ventricular angiography will demonstrate cavity size, shape of the infundibulum, and any pinpoint opening in the pulmonary valve that might exist. Enlarged sinusoids are frequent and may opacify the coronary arteries and aortic root. The degree of tricuspid regurgitation can be estimated. Volume studies may be performed for prognostic implications.[393,394] Aortography with simultaneous right ventricular injection can help to define the length of the atretic segment more accurately.[395] Left ventricular or aortic angiogram is needed to assess the size of the pulmonary arteries filled via the ductus.

Natural History and Prognosis
The natural history generally follows the course of events outlined. Most infants will die as the ductus closes in the first month of life. An occasional survivor to a slightly older age is noted if the ductus remains open long enough for development of a collateral circulation. Without surgery, the patient inevitably dies in the first year, but even with surgery in competent centers, only one of four infants will survive to 1 year of age.[3] The postoperative course is largely dependent on right ventricular size. Growth of the cavity has been reported, and eventual outcome is better for those with a large right ventricle who have had continuity established between the right ventricle and pulmonary arteries.[394]

Medical Management
Medical management of pulmonary atresia includes supportive measures. Once the diagnosis is established, prostaglandin infusion will usually result in ductal dilatation so that oxygenation is improved and acidosis can be corrected.[396] This should be continued until surgery can be done, to keep the infant in optimal condition and to diminish surgical risks. Surgery is recommended for all. The type of surgery is largely dependent on the anatomic variations[388] of right ventricular and tricuspid size, length of atresia, and size of the pulmonary arteries.

Surgical Management
Survival and quality of life depend largely upon the size, growth, and function of the right ventricle and the appropriateness of pulmonary blood flow. A shunt from systemic artery to pulmonary artery, usually the Blalock-Taussig subclavian arterial–to–pulmonary arterial anastomosis, must be constructed before the ductus arteriosus closes (Fig. 36-54). A pulmonary valvectomy is performed at the same operation or a short time later to decompress the noncompliant right ventricle, promote forward flow, and stimulate growth of the ventricular cavity (Fig. 36-46). Decompression of the ventricle probably reduces the frequency and severity of dysrhythmias caused by subendocardial ischemia. Tricuspid regurgitation and the right-to-left shunt through the foramen ovale complicate the initial surgical palliation.[397]

Subsequent correction of the adequately palliated infant requires augmentation or reconstruction of the right ventricular outflow tract (Fig. 36-47) and closure of the atrial septal defect and the surgically created shunt.[398,399] If the right ventricle remains tiny, a direct right atrial–to–pulmonary arterial anastomosis can be created; this is the Fontan concept (Fig. 36-65). Reports of physiologic correction of this anomaly are insufficient to allow significant conclusions regarding long-term prognosis.

Tetralogy of Fallot

Definition

Tetralogy of Fallot is characterized by biventricular origin of the aorta above a large ventricular septal defect, right ventricular hypertrophy, and obstruction to pulmonary flow. When the obstruction is complete (pulmonary atresia), the term *pseudotruncus arteriosus* is applied. This will be discussed separately.

Pathology

The aorta straddles the ventricular septum and arises partly from each ventricle with varying degree, usually about two-thirds from the left ventricle and one-third from the right (Fig. 36-50).[80] In uncommon cases the aorta arises almost exclusively from the right ventricle (extreme dextroposition).[400] Yet fibrous continuity of the aortic origin and the anterior mitral valve is maintained, as in all cases of tetralogy. Uncommonly there is also fibrous continuity of the aorta and the tricuspid valve.[401]

FIGURE 36-50 Classic tetralogy of Fallot. There is infundibular and pulmonary valvular stenosis. SVC = superior vena cava; IVC = inferior vena cava; RA = right atrium; RV = right ventricle; RPA = right pulmonary artery; LPA = left pulmonary artery; RPV = right pulmonary vein; LPV = left pulmonary vein; LA = left atrium; LV = left ventricle; Ao = aorta. [*From J. E. Edwards, Classification of Congenital Heart Disease in the Adult, in W. C. Roberts (ed.), "Congenital Heart Disease in Adults," Cardiovasc. Clin. Series 10/1, F. A. Davis Company, Philadelphia, 1979, p. 1. Reproduced with permission from the publisher, editor, and author.*]

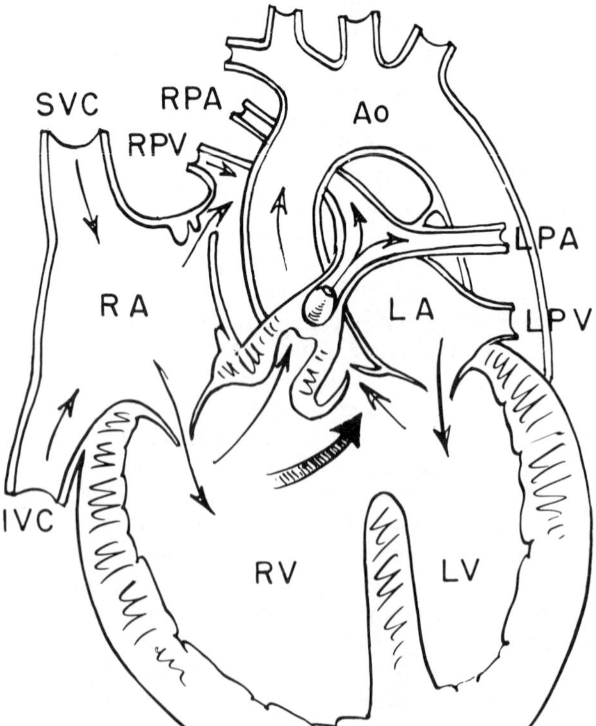

The right ventricular infundibulum lies anterior to the position of the ventricular septal defect and is bounded by the anterior and septal walls anteriorly and medially, while the posterior wall is said to be a vertical crista supraventricularis or displaced conus septum.[402] The right ventricular infundibulum is a distinctive channel that has been termed a third ventricle. The caliber of the channel varies. Uncommonly, it is only mildly obstructive. Usually, it exhibits a significant degree of stenosis and is the dominant site of the obstruction to pulmonary flow characteristic of tetralogy. In the young, the lining of the infundibulum is normal, but in adolescents and adults it shows varying degrees of endocardial fibroelastosis, especially at its inlet.

The pulmonary valve is often malformed, usually being either bicuspid or unicuspid. The valve may contribute to pulmonary stenosis, but only uncommonly will it be the only site of significant obstruction to pulmonary flow.[403] Characteristically, the pulmonary trunk is thin-walled and its lumen is more narrow than normal, but usually it is wider than either the right ventricular infundibulum or the orifice of the pulmonary valve. The aorta is wider than normal, its change in caliber roughly opposite to that of the pulmonary trunk. The foramen ovale is usually patent in patients of all ages. In all cases of tetralogy with significant pulmonary obstruction, collateral branches to the lungs arise from the aorta.

Associated Conditions The condition most commonly associated with tetralogy of Fallot is right aortic arch (about 30 percent).[403] It is usually of the type that does not have a retroesophageal segment (see "Aortic Arch Anomalies"). A double aortic arch occurs uncommonly. A persistent left superior vena cava has been described in 10.6 percent of cases. When an associated atrial septal defect exists, this anomaly is referred to as *pentalogy (pentad) of Fallot.* The ductus arteriosus may be absent, present unilaterally on either the right or left side, or bilateral. Common atrioventricular canal malformations as well as isolated anomalies of the tricuspid or mitral valves may be associated. A particular type of tricuspid anomaly is that of an accessory flap on the septal leaflet. This flap may serve to obstruct the ventricular septal defect.[404] Coronary arterial anomalies, characterized by a major artery crossing the infundibulum, are seen in some cases.

Abnormal Physiology[405–408]

Since the ventricular septal defect is usually large, with an area about as large as that of the aortic valve, both ventricles and the aorta have essentially the same systolic pressures. The basic hemodynamic factor that determines how well these patients tolerate their disease is the ratio between the resistance to flow into the aorta and the resistance to flow across the stenotic right ventricular infundibulum and/or the stenotic pulmonary valve. If the resistances to right ventricular outflow are not large, the pulmonary flow may be twice the systemic flow and the arterial oxygen saturation may be normal (this is so-called acyanotic tetralogy of Fallot). On the other hand, the resistance to the pulmonary flow may be markedly increased, causing right-to-left shunting, arterial unsaturation, and subsequent polycythemia. When the pulmonary stenosis is very severe, much or most of the pulmonary blood flow may be by way of collateral blood flow. The infundibular obstruction, which is very dynamic, is increased by drugs, maneuvers, or activities that increase myocardial contractility or heart rate or that decrease right ventricular volume. In addition, the infundibular hypertrophy may gradually increase.[409] Since the systolic pressure in the right ventricle cannot exceed that in the left ventricle because of the large ventricular septal defect, the right ventricle is "protected" from excessive pressure-work, although exercise tolerance may be limited.

The precise mechanism by which squatting relieves breathlessness and faintness after exercise in patients with tetralogy of Fallot is unknown. It is known that the arterial saturation returns to its resting value more rapidly if the patient squats after exercise. In normal subjects, it is probable that squatting also produces an increase in systemic arterial blood pressure, an increase in venous return to the heart, and an increase in systemic cardiac output. Presumably squatting produces these same changes in patients with tetralogy. It is possible that in these patients the increase in arterial saturation produced by squatting is also related to an increase in peripheral resistance by compression and kinking of the femoral arteries. Squatting does not obstruct the return of markedly unsaturated blood from the legs. Actually, it usually increases venous return to the heart with increases in right ventricular stroke volume, pressure, and pulmonary blood flow.

Hypercyanotic episodes in patients with tetralogy are of uncertain origin. It is possible that some episodes are caused by periods of unusual hyperactivity of muscular fibers in the right ventricular outflow tract producing, or exaggerating, the infundibular stenosis. Some spells may be caused by a decrease in peripheral resistance and systemic arterial pressure, which cause the right ventricular pressure and pulmonary blood flow to decrease. Cyanosis is also often much worse during crying, presumably due to decreased pulmonary blood flow from a combination of performing a Valsalva maneuver, breath holding, and sympathetic excitation.

Clinical Manifestations

Tetralogy of Fallot is one of the most common congenital cardiac defects causing cyanosis. Of cyanotic patients over age 2 years and not yet requiring surgery, approximately three-fourths have tetralogy of Fallot.[6] Tetralogy with an associated atrial septal defect, or *pentalogy of Fallot,* is not distinguishable clinically. The reader is referred to the section on cyanosis and its complications earlier in this chapter.

History The majority of patients are first seen by 6 months of age because of cyanosis. If the right ventricular outflow obstruction is very severe, marked cyanosis is present at birth or as soon as the ductus closes. Other patients slowly develop progressively more severe obstruction and cyanosis and will present later in infancy, childhood, or even in adulthood. Some patients with a large ventricular septal defect and left-to-right shunt in early infancy may acquire infundibular pulmonary stenosis and become clinically indistinguishable from the usual patient with tetralogy of Fallot. Dyspnea with exertion occurs commonly. Attacks of suddenly increasing cyanosis associated with hyperpnea, or hypoxic spells,[410,411] are common between the ages of 2 months and 2 years. There are many precipitating events, including infection, exertion, and summer heat. They occur most often in the morning, and the infant is usually irritable. Frequency and duration vary widely, but prolonged episodes can lead to syncope, seizures, and death. Squatting with exercise is common from $1\frac{1}{2}$ to 10 years of age and is almost pathognomonic of this diagnosis.

Physical Examination Growth is usually normal unless cyanosis is extreme.[31] Clubbing occurs after 3 months of age and is proportional to the level of cyanosis. Signs of congestive heart failure do not appear in tetralogy of Fallot during childhood unless there is a superimposed illness such as anemia or infective endocarditis.

On physical examination, increased right ventricular activity is observed. A systolic thrill is frequently palpable at the left midsternal border, with a harsh midsystolic murmur in this location. Softer murmurs signal more severe obstruction and are common when presentation is in the newborn period or during hypoxic spells. The murmur ends before the second heart sound, which is characteristically single. A continuous murmur is heard if a patent ductus or large bronchial collateral vessels are present. An early systolic ejection sound at the left sternal border and apex is common.

Chest Roentgenogram The total heart size is usually normal on chest roentgenogram, but right ventricular enlargement is present in the lateral projection. The aorta arches to the right in 25 percent or more of cases.[412] Pulmonary flow is diminished. The pulmonary segment is concave and the apex elevated, giving the coeur en sabot (boot-shaped) contour (Fig. 36-51). The very young infant may have only diminished pulmonary flow.

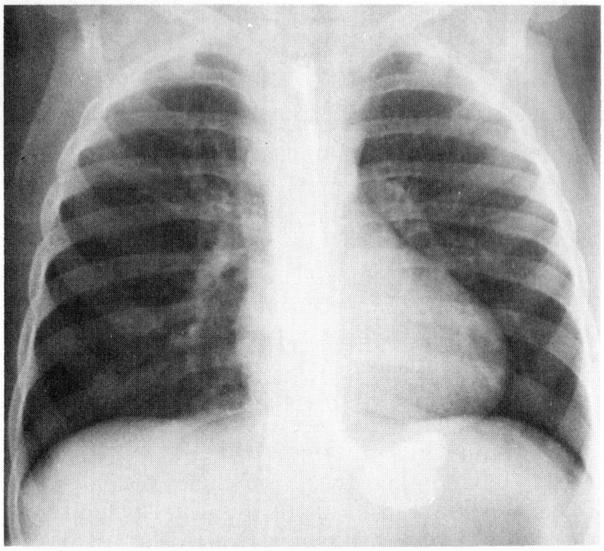

FIGURE 36-51 Chest roentgenogram in a 3-year-old boy with tetralogy of Fallot, demonstrating a "boot-shaped" heart with a right aortic arch and mildly diminished pulmonary flow.

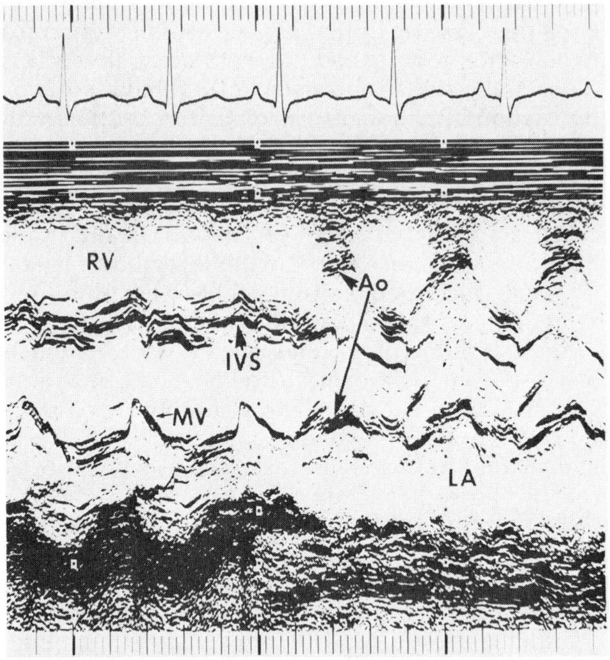

FIGURE 36-52 M-mode echocardiogram in a child with tetralogy of Fallot, demonstrating aortic (Ao) override of the interventricular septum (IVS) and aortic (Ao)-mitral (MV) continuity. LA = left atrium; RV = right ventricle.

Electrocardiogram In tetralogy of Fallot, the mean QRS axis of the electrocardiogram is usually to the right, between +90 and +210°. If the axis is superior, endocardial cushion defects, single ventricle, or double-outlet right ventricle with pulmonary stenosis should be suspected. There is right ventricular hypertrophy with a tall R wave in the right precordial leads and a deep S wave in the left. Some patients have right atrial hypertrophy.

Echocardiogram M-mode echocardiography[413] will show abrupt ending of the septal echoes just below the overriding aorta (Fig. 36-52). Frequently, right ventricular enlargement and hypertrophy, narrowing of the outflow tract, and aortic dilatation also occur. The pulmonary valve may be difficult to record; if this attempt is unsuccessful, truncus arteriosus and ventricular septal defect with pulmonary atresia are not excluded. The left atrium is usually small in tetralogy and normal to enlarged in truncus arteriosus. Continuity of the anterior mitral leaflet and posterior aortic wall excludes double outlet of the right ventricle with pulmonary stenosis.[414] Associated endocardial cushion defect can be excluded. False overriding of the aorta can be created by a transducer position that is too high along the sternal border. Cross-sectional echocardiography[28,415] is extremely helpful in delineating the anatomy and is more specific for definitive diagnosis.

Hematologic and Other Laboratory Studies (Refer to section on cyanosis, earlier in this chapter.) Measurement of hemoglobin and hematocrit should be done in all patients at initial evaluation and periodically thereafter, both for determination of the degree of polycythemia and the early detection of anemia relative to the degree of cyanosis. The latter is common, especially in those under 2 years of age and in those in this age group with cerebrovascular accidents. Platelet counts and clotting studies may be advisable in patients with marked polycythemia, particularly if a surgical procedure is planned. Serum uric acid levels should be measured in older children and adults with severe polycythemia.

Cardiac Catheterization The right ventricular systolic pressure is equal to that in the left ventricle and aorta. The right atrial pressure is almost always normal. If the pulmonary artery can be entered, the pressure will be normal or low. The level(s) of obstruction can be evaluated by careful pullback to the right ventricle. Caution should be observed if the pulmonary artery is entered, as the catheter may critically reduce the pulmonary flow and cause a hypoxic episode. It is unnecessary to attempt to enter the pulmonary artery in those with severe cyanosis or with a history of severe hypoxic spells. Systemic arterial oxygen saturation is low because of right-to-left shunting from the right ventricle. If a patent foramen ovale or atrial septal defect is present, there will be an additional right-to-left or bidirectional shunt at the atrial level. Selective biplane right ventricular angiography (Fig. 36-53) is extremely valuable to demonstrate levels of obstruction, size of the pulmonary arteries, size and position of the ventricular defect, and opacification of the left ventricular outflow tract and aorta, which will frequently demonstrate the aortic-mitral relation. Left ventricular angiography may be necessary at times to aid in exclusion of double outlet of the right ventricle.

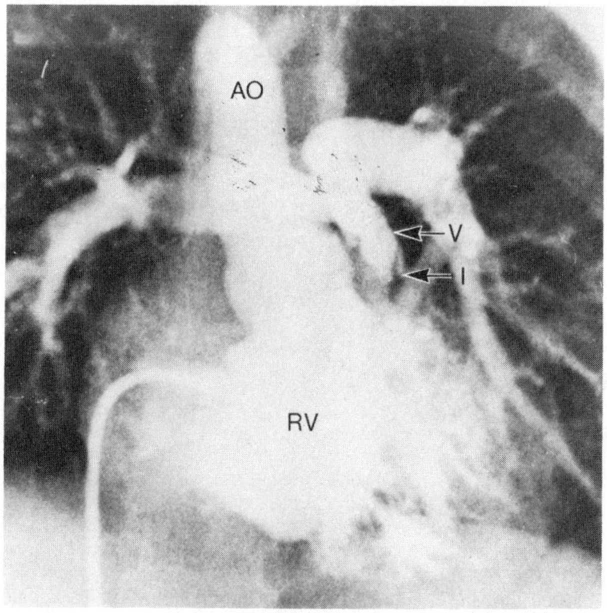

FIGURE 36-53 Posteroanterior view of a right ventricular (RV) angiogram in a child with tetralogy of Fallot, with severe infundibular (I) and valvular (V) narrowing creating an outflow chamber (between arrows) and with right-to-left shunting into the aorta (AO), which arches to the right.

Aortography should be done on all patients preoperatively to demonstrate the coronary arterial pattern. Selective coronary angiography can be done if necessary for better delineation.[416,417]

Natural History and Prognosis

Prognosis is poorest in very young infants who present with severe cyanosis, because of the severity of obstruction and the size of the pulmonary arteries, which are usually very small.[406] Hypoxic spells offer a poor prognosis if they are allowed to continue untreated. Obstruction to pulmonary flow tends to progress even to atresia[409] with increasing cyanosis and polycythemia. The complications of polycythemia, including cerebrovascular accident and brain abscess, were discussed in a previous section. With polycythemia and decreased flow, multiple thrombi in small pulmonary vessels can occur.[418] Pulmonary vascular disease occurs with large systemic-to-pulmonary shunts. The risk of infective endocarditis is high. Without surgery, approximately one-third die by age 1 year, one-half by age 3 years, and three-quarters by age 10 years, with less than 5 percent surviving beyond age 30 years.[419]

Medical Management

The medical management in tetralogy of Fallot is directed primarily toward prevention and treatment of complications. Iron deficiency anemia should be promptly treated with iron supplementation. Fever or other common pediatric illness that would lead to dehydration and possible thrombotic complications should also be treated promptly. Hypoxic spells in infants should be treated initially by placing the infant in the knee-chest position. Parental education will help in prevention or management of all three of these problems. Further treatment of hypoxic spells includes administration of a high concentration of oxygen and morphine sulfate. If acidosis is present and does not correct spontaneously and promptly, intravenous sodium bicarbonate should be given. Propranolol is useful in the acute treatment and prevention of prolonged hypoxic spells.[420] Propranolol, a beta-adrenergic blocker, should be given orally for prevention and intravenously only for severe hypoxic spells. If for some reason the hematocrit should reach a level of 70 to 75 percent, erythropheresis is recommended, using fresh frozen plasma or a colloid equivalent. This will temporarily diminish viscosity, but more definitive surgical treatment is indicated. Early and vigorous treatment should be given for intercurrent infections. Prophylactic antibiotics are recommended for prevention of infective endocarditis.

For the severely cyanotic newborn, prostaglandin administration may be of benefit, as with pulmonary atresia,[27,396] to open the ductus until surgery can be done. Prompt surgical intervention is indicated. Surgical correction is recommended in children for progressive symptoms or polycythemia with hematocrit approaching 65 percent. Elective surgical correction should be done in early childhood, since further delay offers no advantage and the continuing risks of complications of cyanosis are significant.

The infant who is symptomatic may be treated in three ways: palliation with propranolol and delayed correction, palliation with a shunt from systemic artery to pulmonary artery and delayed correction, or early correction. There is currently much debate on this issue. Clearly, certain anatomic variables, such as tiny pulmonary arteries or a coronary arterial abnormality, make early correction less attractive. Otherwise, early correction seems desirable if risk is no more than the total risk of other choices and outcome is equally favorable. There are centers where this is possible in selected patients. One group has reported a method of looking at results in a statistical manner.[421] They found that propranolol and delayed correction were the best choice at their center, but that early correction is probably best at centers where early operative mortality is 10 percent or less. This type of analysis seems warranted. Additional variables, such as anatomic characteristics, should also be included to offer a firmer basis for recommendation of mode of treatment in the symptomatic infant.

Surgical Management

"Ideally, the surgical treatment of the tetralogy of Fallot is primary repair, done whenever signs and symptoms become important or in any event in the first several years of life, performed so that the ventricular septal defect (VSD) is completely closed, sinus rhythm is preserved, no residual right ventricular outflow obstruction is present, and the patient's pulmonary valve remains competent."[422] The presence of small pulmonary arteries or pulmonary atresia in the symptomatic infant with tetralogy of Fallot encourages two-stage management, a Blalock-Taussig shunt or modification thereof[423,424] followed by secondary repair during the first few years of life.[425,426]

Technical details of shunt creation and repair are illustrated in Figs. 36-54, 36-55, and 36-56.[427] The variable surgical anatomy of tetralogy of Fallot has been detailed by Anderson and colleagues.[428] Decision regarding the need for transannular patch augmentation of the right ventricular outflow tract at the time of repair is based upon measurement of pulmonary annular diameter and the ratio of right ventricular to left ventricular systolic pressure after closure of the ventricular septal defect and excision of obstructive muscle bundles. This latter ratio should probably be less than 0.7:1 for optimum outcome[422] and can be predicted with reasonable accuracy by preoperative angiography and intraoperative annular measurements.[422,429]

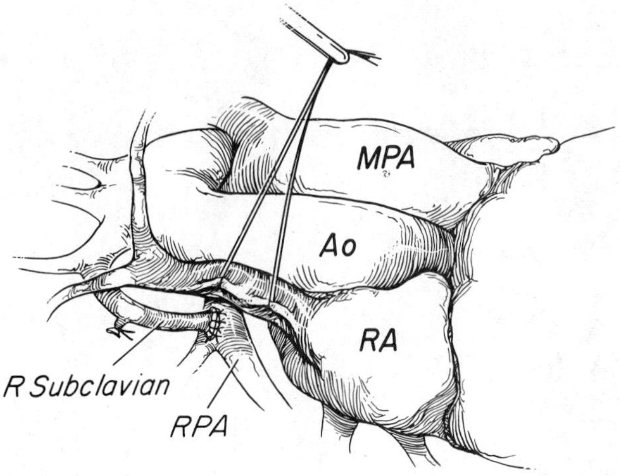

FIGURE 36-54 The Blalock-Taussig shunt. The divided end of the subclavian artery, usually on the side opposite the aortic arch, is anastomosed to the cephalad side of the ipsilateral pulmonary artery. This was the first, and is still the preferred, method for increasing pulmonary blood flow. Complications are rare, and closure at the time of subsequent total correction of the intracardiac defect is relatively simple.

FIGURE 36-55 Relief of infundibular stenosis in a patient with tetralogy of Fallot. *A.* The septal band has been resected, and the parietal band is being mobilized. *B.* The parietal band has been excised and the free wall of the right ventricle is being mobilized. (*From J. W. Kirklin and R. B. Karp, "The Tetralogy of Fallot," W. B. Saunders Company, Philadelphia, 1970, p. 71. Reproduced with permission from the publisher and authors.*)

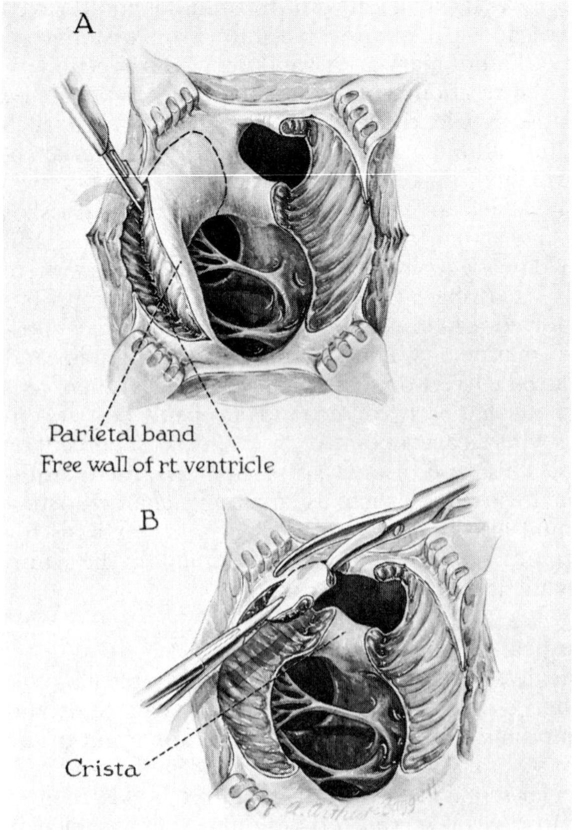

FIGURE 36-56 Repair of the ventricular septal defect in a patient with tetralogy of Fallot. A patch of knitted Dacron is sewn into place with continuous sutures, with the stitches placed so as to avoid the area occupied by the bundle of His. (*From J. W. Kirklin and R. B. Karp, "The Tetralogy of Fallot," W. B. Saunders Company, Philadelphia, 1970, p. 71. Reproduced with permission from the publisher and authors.*)

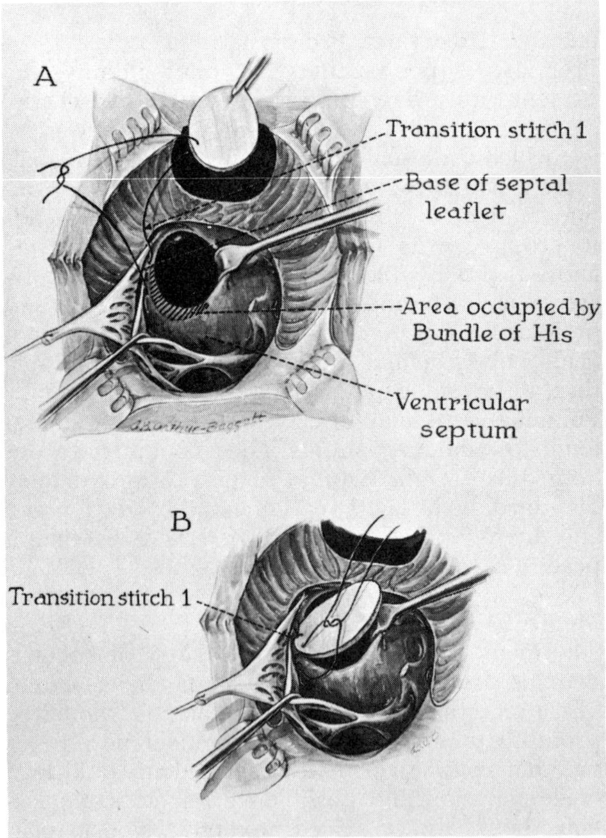

Long-term prognosis of patients benefiting from correction of tetralogy of Fallot is quite good; there is no adverse effect upon life expectancy up to 10 to 22 years following operation[430] and near-normal exercise tolerance in those free of significant residual abnormalities.[431] Preliminary data suggest that early primary repair in infancy yields excellent survival and improved long-term left ventricular function.[432]

Absent Pulmonary Valve

Pathology

All vestiges of the pulmonary valve may be absent, or only remnants of tissue at valve level may be identifiable.[433] The right ventricular infundibulum is wider than normal. The pulmonary arteries are distinctly enlarged, and bronchial compression may result. The basic features of tetralogy are usually present. In only a rare case are there no intracardiac anomalies.

Clinical Manifestations

Although absent pulmonary valve is an uncommon defect, in the infant it can cause significant problems with cyanosis and heart failure.[433] In the newborn, pulmonary hypertension, which is normally present, can lead to marked pulmonary regurgitation, since valve tissue is very deficient. Commonly, the pulmonary valve ring is small and causes obstruction to pulmonary flow and there is an associated ventricular septal defect. Thus, some compare this entity to tetralogy of Fallot, but there are notable distinctions in the hemodynamics and the clinical picture. Aneurysmal dilatation of the central pulmonary arteries occurs and causes bronchial compression with obstructive emphysema and resulting atelectasis. Respiratory symptoms[434] frequently dominate the clinical picture and can lead to impressive respiratory distress in infants. Superimposed infection causes recurrent and episodic increases in the respiratory symptoms. Congestive heart failure can occur if the pulmonary regurgitation is great, especially in the newborn, or if the annulus is not very restrictive so that significant left-to-right shunting through an associated ventricular septal defect occurs. Cyanosis can occur with heart failure but is more frequently due to some right-to-left shunting across the ventricular defect in cases where a restrictive pulmonary valve annulus exists.

A hyperdynamic left parasternal impulse and harsh systolic and diastolic murmurs with a to-and-fro quality are found. The second heart sound is single. The electrocardiogram usually shows right axis deviation and right ventricular hypertrophy. The chest roentgenogram shows cardiomegaly and aneurysmal dilatation of the central pulmonary arteries. There are frequently signs of hyperinflation, atelectasis, or pneumothorax.

Cardiac catheterization will reveal associated shunts. Difficulty may be encountered in entering the pulmonary arteries, but assessment of the annular pressure difference is important. Angiography (Fig. 36-57) demonstrates the massive size of the pulmonary arteries and the pulmonary valve anatomy, particularly the annular size as little leaflet tissue is usually present.

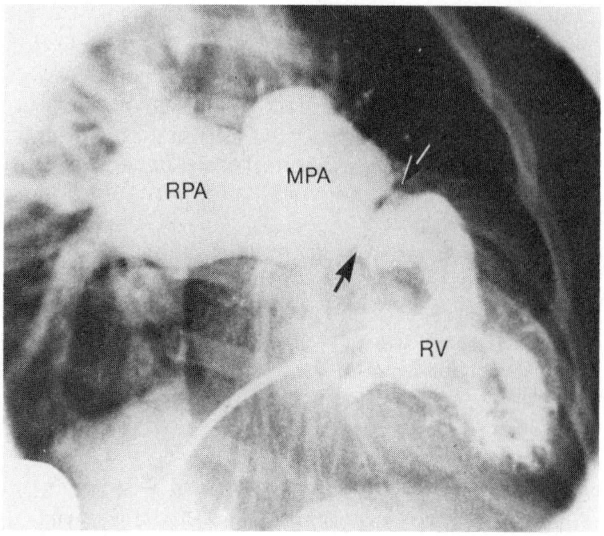

FIGURE 36-57 Right anterior oblique view of right ventricular (RV) angiogram in a child with absent pulmonary valve with narrowing of the pulmonary annulus (arrows) and aneurysmal dilatation of the main (MPA) and proximal (RPA) pulmonary arteries.

Natural History and Prognosis

The natural history is not well defined due to the small number of patients.[433] The newborn with heart failure may respond to medical management as the pulmonary vascular resistance decreases. Infants can succumb to severe hypoxia, rarely, or pulmonary complications, more commonly.

Medical Management

Infants with mild or no symptoms should be managed conservatively.[433] Medical management includes treatment of heart failure and pulmonary complications in addition to prevention of infective endocarditis. For infants who are severely symptomatic or older children with milder symptoms, surgical palliation or correction of intracardiac defects and relief of bronchial compression should be attempted.[435]

Surgical Management

Absence of the pulmonary valve in infants with tetralogy of Fallot remains a difficult surgical problem. We prefer to create a shunt from a systemic artery to the left pulmonary artery through a left thoracotomy, using polytetrafluoroethylene (Gore-Tex), or to create a modification of the Blalock-Taussig anastomosis. The main pulmonary artery is then tightly banded or ligated just beyond the pulmonary valve. The pulmonary arterial aneurysmal dilatation will regress; bronchial compression is relieved.[436,437] When the child is older, larger, less critically ill, and free of tracheobronchial compression, the ventricular septal defect can be closed and the right ventricular outflow tract and main pulmonary artery can be reconstructed in the way required for a child having tetralogy of Fallot with pulmonary atresia.

A more aggressive approach, involving ventricular septal defect closure during hypothermic circulatory arrest with plication of the dilated pulmonary artery in infancy, has been advocated but is almost certainly associated with a greater overall risk.[438]

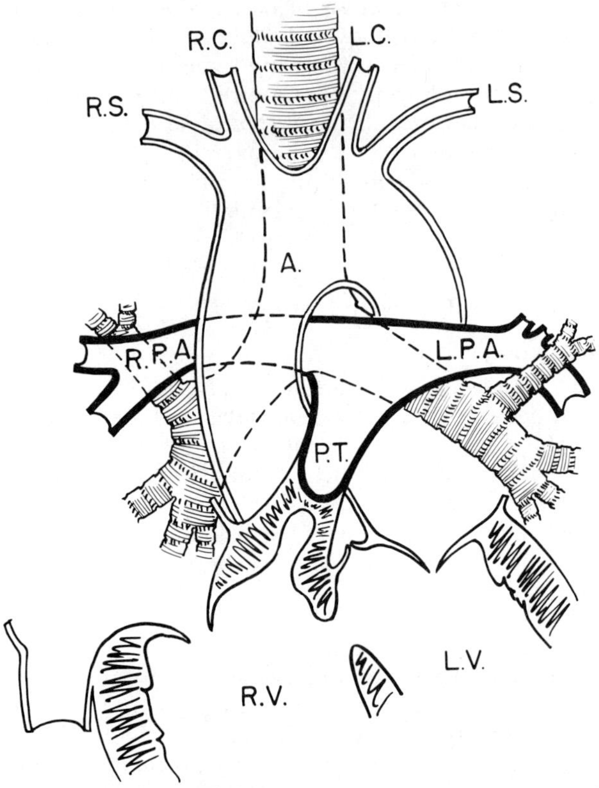

FIGURE 36-58 Tetralogy of Fallot with pulmonary atresia at the valve level, sometimes referred to as pseudotruncus arteriosus. There is confluence of the two pulmonary arteries. R.V. = right ventricle; L.V. = left ventricle; P.T. = main pulmonary arterial trunk; R.P.A. = right pulmonary artery; L.P.A. = left pulmonary artery; A. = aorta; R.S. = right subclavian artery; R.C. = right carotid artery; L.C. = left carotid artery; L.S. = left subclavian artery. *(From J. E. Edwards and D. C. McGoon, Absence of Anatomic Origin from Heart of Pulmonary Arterial Supply, Circulation, 47:393, 1973. Reproduced by permission of the American Heart Association, Inc., and the authors.)*

Absence of Anatomic Origin of Pulmonary Arterial System from the Heart: With and without Confluence of Right and Left Pulmonary Arteries

Classification

Among some patients two conditions occur together—ventricular septal defect and lack of direct connection of the pulmonary arterial supply with the heart. From the surgical point of view, one of the crucial points is whether the arterial supply to one lung is connected with that to the other *(confluence)*, or whether each supply is independent of the other *(nonconfluence)*. With this pivotal point in mind, the following classification is modified from that of Edwards and McGoon.[439]

1. Confluent origin of pulmonary arteries
   a. Remnant of pulmonary trunk present (pseudotruncus)
      (1) Proximal atresia and distal patency (pseudotruncus with patent pulmonary trunk) (Fig. 36-58)
      (2) Uniform cordlike atresia (pseudotruncus with atretic pulmonary trunk) (Fig. 36-59*A*)
   b. No remnant of pulmonary trunk present (isolated confluent pulmonary arteries) (Fig. 36-59*B*)
   c. Persistent truncus arteriosus present, types I and II (Fig. 36-60)
2. Nonconfluent origin of pulmonary arterial supply
   a. True pulmonary arteries present
      (1) Arising from persistent truncus arteriosus, type III
      (2) Arising from ductus arteriosus
      (3) Arising from bronchial arteries
   b. True pulmonary arteries absent. Pulmonary blood supply from bronchial arteries (truncus arteriosus, type IV)

This classification will be rearranged into three clinical groups for ease of discussion concerning the clinical manifestations, natural history, and management.

FIGURE 36-59 Pseudotruncus arteriosus with confluent pulmonary arteries. *A.* The pulmonary trunk is identified but atretic. *B.* The pulmonary trunk is not identifiable. R.V. = right ventricle; L.V. = left ventricle; R.P.A. = right pulmonary artery; L.P.A. = left pulmonary artery; A. = aorta; R.S. = right subclavian artery; L.S. = left subclavian artery; R.C. = right carotid artery; L.C. = left carotid artery. *(From J. E. Edwards and D. C. McGoon, Absence of Anatomic Origin from Heart of Pulmonary Arterial Supply, Circulation, 47:393, 1973. Reproduced by permission of the American Heart Association, Inc., and the authors.)*

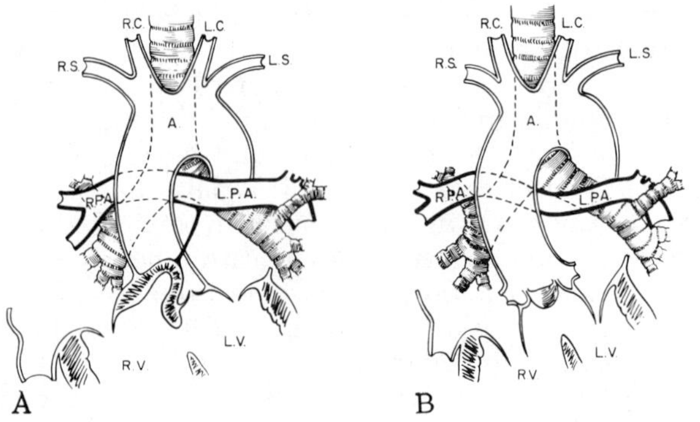

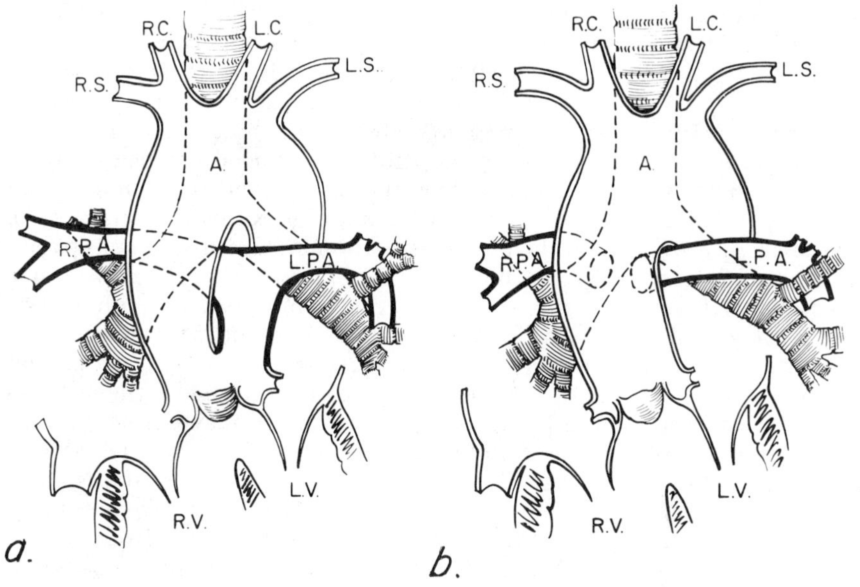

FIGURE 36-60 Persistent truncus arteriosus. *a.* Type I. *b.* Type II. R.V. = right ventricle; L.V. = left ventricle; R.P.A. = right pulmonary artery; L.P.A. = left pulmonary artery; A. = aorta; R.S. = right subclavian artery; R.C. = right carotid artery; L.C. = left carotid artery; L.S. = left subclavian artery. (*From J. E. Edwards and D. C. McGoon, Absence of Anatomic Origin from Heart of Pulmonary Arterial Supply, Circulation, 47:393, 1973. Reproduced by permission of the American Heart Association, Inc., and the authors.*)

Pathology
In all cases of this anomaly there is a ventricular septal defect. Usually the ventricles are not inverted, and the aorta or truncus arteriosus shows biventricular origin and fibrous continuity with the mitral valve. Uncommonly, the aorta or truncus arteriosus arises entirely from the right ventricle, as in double-outlet right ventricle.

Rarely, the ventricles are inverted, with the aorta (and theoretically the truncus arteriosus) arising from the inverted right ventricle. Such cases may be viewed as variants of corrected transposition.

Confluence and Origin of Pulmonary Arteries When confluence of pulmonary arterial supply is present, several variations are possible.

With Remnant of Pulmonary Trunk. When there is an identifiable remnant of a pulmonary trunk, its origin is from the right ventricle. The atresia may involve simply the valve level and a short segment of the pulmonary trunk, while the more distal part of the pulmonary trunk is patent and of varying width. In other cases the pulmonary trunk is represented by a cordlike structure leading to confluence of the right and left pulmonary arteries. The ductus arteriosus may be present or absent. Cases with a remnant of a pulmonary trunk are usually considered variants of tetralogy of Fallot and may be so termed along with the qualification of *with pulmonary atresia,* or they may simply be termed *pseudotruncus arteriosus.*

Without Remnant of Pulmonary Trunk. This type of condition may be referred to as *isolated confluent pulmonary arteries.* The patent aspects of the pulmonary arterial system are like those in pseudotruncus arteriosus with atretic pulmonary trunk except for the absence of any vestige of a pulmonary trunk. As with the foregoing condition, a patent ductus may lead to the pulmonary arterial confluence, although this is not necessarily so.

Persistent Truncus Arteriosus, Types I and II. The condition referred to as persistent truncus arteriosus is characterized by one arterial vessel leaving the heart above a ventricular septal defect. From this vessel the coronary and pulmonary arteries, as well as the aorta, arise. There are several subdivisions of this condition, according to the classification of Collett and Edwards.[440] Relevant to the condition discussed in this section are the types referred to as *persistent truncus arteriosus types I and II.* Type I is characterized by partial septation of the truncus so that a pulmonary trunk of varying length, usually very short, arises from the truncus and, in turn, the pulmonary arteries arise from the vestigial pulmonary trunk. The pulmonary arteries originate usually from the left side of the truncus, and only rarely from the right. In persistent truncus arteriosus type II, the two pulmonary arteries arise separately from the posterior wall of the truncus.

Defects associated with all of the types of truncus arteriosus are fairly numerous.[441] A right aortic arch is present in about 20 percent of the cases. Single coronary artery is fairly common (about 5 percent). Unusually high origin of the coronary arteries is about twice as common; the most significant feature of this condition is that branches of the right coronary artery have a tendency to cross the anterior wall of the right ventricle.[442] Interruption of the aortic arch is present in about 10 percent of cases. So-called absence of a pulmonary artery occurs in about 2 percent, more commonly on the side of the aortic arch than contralateral to it.

In these, as in other types of persistent truncus arteriosus, the truncal semilunar valve may show a variety of alterations characterized by thickening of the cusps with mucoid connective tissue. This process, if severe, may be responsible for either stenosis or insufficiency.[443]

Nonconfluent Origin of Pulmonary Arteries When nonconfluence of pulmonary arterial supply is present, a number of variations are possible, the simplest being persistent truncus arteriosus, type III.

Origin from Persistent Truncus Arteriosus, Type III. In rare instances of persistent truncus arteriosus, each pulmonary artery arises independently from the lateral aspects of the truncus; this is called truncus arteriosus type III.

Origin from Ductus Arteriosus. When pulmonary arteries originate from the ductus, two basic patterns exist: (1) bilateral origin of the pulmonary arteries from ductus arteriosi and (2) origin of one pulmonary artery from the homolateral ductus, while the other pulmonary artery has a normal site of origin; however, there is atresia of the pulmonary trunk and/or of the normally arising pulmonary artery.[444]

Origin from the Descending Aorta through Bronchial Arteries. Hypothetically, a situation may occur in which true pulmonary arteries may arise from the descending thoracic aorta, the stems of origin for the vessels being bronchial arteries.

Pulmonary Arterial Supply from Bronchial Arteries (Truncus Arteriosus, Type IV); Pulmonary Arteries Absent. As the description implies, this condition is characterized by no true pulmonary arterial system being present, while the arterial supply to the lung is by way of bronchial arteries. A name for this condition, *persistent truncus arteriosus type IV,* was contributed by Collett and Edwards.[440]

While such a condition may exist, some cases considered to be examples of truncus type IV are, in fact, examples either of confluent or nonconfluent origin of the pulmonary arteries associated with atresia of these vessels in the mediastinum. Dissection of the pulmonary hili in cases thought to be examples of truncus type IV usually reveals patent pulmonary arteries of varying caliber at the hili.[444]

Pulmonary Atresia with Ventricular Septal Defect with and without Pulmonary Arterial Confluence

The anatomic types[439] of the preceding classification considered here are those with:

1. Confluence of pulmonary arteries originating from the pulmonary trunk with patency of some portion of the pulmonary trunk (pseudotruncus) or isolated confluence without remnant of pulmonary trunk
2. Nonconfluence of pulmonary arteries with origin of true pulmonary arteries through bilateral ductus arteriosi or bronchial arteries

Clinical Manifestations[445] These defects create a clinical picture very similar to that of severe tetralogy of Fallot. The size of the pulmonary arteries and ductus and/or bronchial collateral vessels determines the clinical manifestations. In the large majority of patients, these vessels are small, so that pulmonary blood flow is diminished. Marked cyanosis is then present from birth or shortly thereafter. Most patients are dependent on ductal patency for their pulmonary flow, therefore rapid deterioration can occur as the ductus undergoes spontaneous closure. For the minority in whom the ductus remains patent or who have adequate bronchial supply, the course in the newborn period is more stable. With growth of the infant and increasing physical activity, the cyanosis progresses gradually. In the rare patient with numerous large collateral vessels, the cyanosis will be mild and heart failure may ensue from increased pulmonary flow.

On auscultation, the second heart sound is single and there may be no murmur. Soft, continuous murmurs from the ductus or collateral vessels may be heard. The electrocardiogram and chest roentgenogram are indistinguishable from those in tetralogy of Fallot. Approximately 50 percent will have a right aortic arch.[445] In the rare patient with large collateral flow, biatrial and biventricular hypertrophy may be present on the electrocardiogram, and the chest roentgenogram will show cardiomegaly and increased pulmonary flow. The M-mode echocardiogram is similar to that in tetralogy of Fallot, which can be distinguished from this defect only if the pulmonary valve can be recorded. Two-dimensional echocardiography is very helpful.

Findings at cardiac catheterization are similar to findings in tetralogy of Fallot, except that the pulmonary artery cannot be entered from the right ventricle. The combination of aortography and selective arteriography in collateral vessels will usually demonstrate the origin of pulmonary flow, the size of the pulmonary arteries, and the presence or absence of confluence between the right and left pulmonary arteries.[446] Pulmonary vein wedge angiography may be necessary for this in some patients.[447]

Natural History and Prognosis[445] Outlook is, in general, much worse than prognosis for tetralogy of Fallot. Without intervention, only those with large collateral vessels are likely to survive beyond infancy. The complications of cyanosis and endocarditis were discussed earlier in this chapter.

Medical Management These patients are managed in the same way as patients with severe tetralogy of Fallot, except that propranolol is not useful. Prostaglandin infusion has been extremely helpful in newborns with critical cyanosis and acidosis.[27,396] If there are pulmonary arteries of adequate size, surgery can be done.[448] This usually consists of palliation by a shunt with correction deferred until the child's body is larger.

Surgical Management Systemic bronchial collateral vessels or the patent ductus arteriosus often allow early survival. Prostaglandin E_1 infusion has improved survival, in association with palliation in those infants requiring surgical intervention. Palliation has traditionally consisted of the creation of a systemic arterial–to–pulmonary arterial anastomosis.[449] We prefer the Blalock-Taussig shunt or a modification in which a segment of polytetrafluoroethylene (PTFE, Gore-Tex) is placed between the side of the subclavian artery or the aorta and the pulmonary artery. In the presence of nonconfluence of the pulmonary arteries centrally, bilateral shunts are required to maintain pulmonary arterial patency and to promote growth of the arteries. In some cases large systemic-to-pulmonary arterial collateral vessels provide sufficient pulmonary blood flow without the need for palliative surgical intervention.[449] Recently palliation has been achieved by patch or conduit reconstruction of the right ventricular outflow tract, the ventricular septal defect being deliberately left open or even enlarged surgically.[450,451]

If pulmonary arterial growth occurs, physiologic correction is possible by (1) closure of the ventricular septal defect and atrial septal defect, (2) obliteration of surgically created extracardiac shunts and, if significant, naturally occurring systemic-to-pulmonary arterial collateral vessels from the descending aorta, and (3) the establishment of continuity from right ventricle to pulmonary artery using valve-containing conduits or aortic homografts.[452,453] In cases lacking central confluence of the pulmonary arteries, a Y- or T-shaped conduit is required. Early survival has been excellent, but late conduit and valve deterioration or obstruction has proved a significant complication.[452] Persistent large bronchial collateral arteries complicate repair and cause significant postoperative right ventricular hypertension and congestive heart failure; these must be controlled surgically[454] or by embolization techniques.[455]

Truncus Arteriosus Types I, II, and III

Clinical Manifestations These defects are grouped together whether there is (types I and II) or is not (type III) pulmonary arterial confluence, since clinical distinction is impossible. Clinical manifestations depend on the size of the pulmonary arteries and thus on the amount of pulmonary flow. Most patients with truncus arteriosus have increased pulmonary flow and mild cyanosis with heart failure. Severe congestive failure and poor growth are observed in the first few weeks of life. If the pulmonary arteries are small, cyanosis will predominate and heart failure will be absent or mild. A prominent left parasternal lift and apical impulse are palpated. A loud, constant systolic click and a single second heart sound are common. Elevated jugular venous pulsations, hepatomegaly, tachypnea, and rales are frequent. There are bounding pulses and a wide pulse pressure. After the first month of life, 70 percent of patients will have a systolic murmur, occasionally accompanied by a thrill, in the third and fourth left intercostal spaces.[4,6] A continuous murmur may be heard over the lung fields if pulmonary resistance is low. Approximately one-third of these patients[443] will have a decrescendo diastolic murmur of truncal valvular regurgitation at the left sternal border and apex. If this is severe, a more rapid downhill course with heart failure occurs.

The electrocardiographic findings are nonspecific, with a mean QRS axis within normal range and biventricular hypertrophy. The chest roentgenogram will show moderate-to-severe cardiomegaly with increased pulmonary flow. The "aorta" may be enlarged, and a right arch is frequently present. The latter finding is a helpful clue in distinguishing this from other large left-to-right shunts. In the rare patient with small pulmonary arteries, the heart size is less impressive and pulmonary flow is normal to diminished. The M-mode echocardiographic findings are similar to those in tetralogy of Fallot, except that two semilunar valves can never be recorded and the left atrium is more commonly enlarged. Two-dimensional echocardiography is very helpful.

Cardiac catheterization will demonstrate bidirectional shunting, with more severe systemic arterial desaturation in those with small pulmonary arteries or pulmonary vascular disease. Initially, the diagnosis may not be apparent, since the catheter may advance easily from the right ventricle into the pulmonary trunk with a near-normal appearance of the catheter course. There is usually pulmonary hypertension at or near systemic pressure levels. Attempts to enter both right and left pulmonary arteries should be made, to evaluate the pulmonary vascular resistance completely, especially in those patients beyond the newborn period. Right ventricular angiography will demonstrate the ventricular septal defect. Angiography in the proximal truncus will show the severity of any truncal regurgitation and usually is necessary to visualize the origin of the pulmonary arteries. Biplane angiography is particularly useful in this defect.

Natural History and Prognosis[4,6,456] The majority of patients die before 1 year of age from congestive heart failure and its complications. Severe pulmonary vascular disease occurs early in these patients. It is usually present to some degree by 6 months of age and progresses thereafter. The majority of children surviving to age 5 years have severe pulmonary vascular disease, although a teenager with only mild to moderate disease may be rarely seen. Those who have small pulmonary arteries that restrict pulmonary flow survive somewhat longer, although survival to early adulthood is extremely rare. The complications of cyanosis (discussed earlier in this chapter) can occur, but polycythemia is usually not as marked as it is in patients with obstruction to pulmonary flow until pulmonary vascular disease becomes severe. Infective endocarditis also occurs.

Medical Management Medical management is primarily directed toward treatment of heart failure and prevention of the complications of cyanosis and endocarditis. Numerous anatomic features delineated by angiography are important when surgery is being considered.[457] Infants with severe heart failure should have surgical intervention in the first few months of life. Early primary correction, with anticipated replacement of the outflow tract conduit at a later age, is done in small infants with reasonable mortality and comparable outcome at some centers. In other centers, banding is still performed in early infancy and correction is delayed until the patient is several years of age because of differences in risk and outcome.[458,459] In those patients with restricted flow and very small pulmonary arteries, systemic-to-pulmonary arterial anastomosis may be necessary. Severe pulmonary vascular disease is a contraindication to surgery. Patients with severe truncal valve regurgitation may require valve replacement in the aortic position early or late after initial correction. This is associated with all of the problems attendant to valve replacement in children and should not be done unless the degree of regurgitation allows no medical alternative.

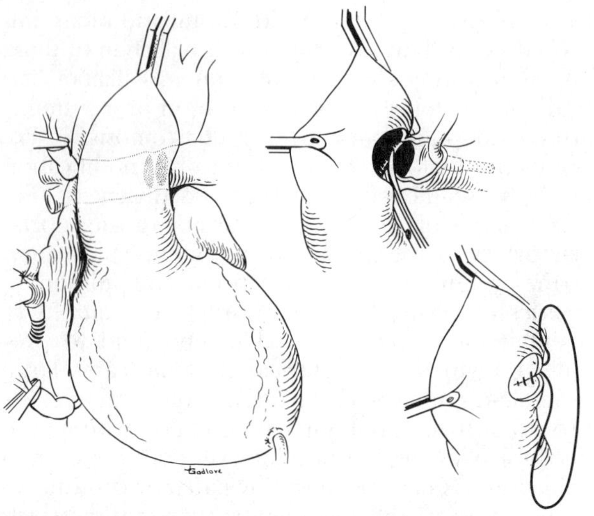

FIGURE 36-61 Steps in the repair of truncus arteriosus. After cardiopulmonary bypass has been established and the aorta cross-clamped, the pulmonary arteries are disconnected from the common arterial trunk. The defect in the trunk is repaired. (*From D. C. McGoon, G. C. Rastelli, and P. A. Ongley, An Operation for the Correction of Truncus Arteriosus, JAMA, 205:69, 1968. Copyright 1968, American Medical Association. Reproduced with permission from the publisher and the author.*)

Surgical Management Until recently, palliation for infants having persistent truncus arteriosus was attempted by placement of separate bands on the right and left pulmonary arteries or around the common origin of the branches from the aorta. Benefit was unpredictable and deformity of the pulmonary arteries complicated subsequent repair.

The excellent results achieved from physiologic correction of this anomaly in infancy by Ebert,[460,461] extending concepts developed earlier in older children by McGoon,[462] have encouraged a more aggressive approach before congestive heart failure and the development of pulmonary vascular obstructive disease have taken their toll.

Under conditions of profound hypothermia and circulatory arrest, the ventricular septal defect is closed with a patch placed through a right ventriculotomy. The truncal valve is placed on the left side of the patch to divert left ventricular blood to the aorta. The pulmonary arteries and a portion of adjacent aortic wall are excised from the posterolateral aorta; the defect thus created in the aortic wall is repaired by direct suture or a small patch (Fig. 36-61 and 36-62).[463] Right ventricular–pulmonary arterial continuity is established using a valve-containing conduit, either a corrugated Dacron tube containing a gluteraldehyde-preserved porcine heterograft or a fresh aortic homograft stored in antibiotic solution.[453,460,464]

Truncal valvular regurgitation reduces the likelihood of a favorable operative outcome. Replacement of the truncal valve with a mechanical prosthesis can, of course, be incorporated into the repair or carried out subsequently if required.

FIGURE 36-62 Steps in the repair of truncus arteriosus. The ventricular septal defect is repaired with a patch. An aortic homograft with its valve is used to connect the right ventricle to the previously disconnected pulmonary arteries. (*From D. C. McGoon, G. C. Rastelli, and P. A. Ongley, An Operation for the Correction of Truncus Arteriosus, JAMA, 205:69, 1968. Copyright 1968, American Medical Association. Reproduced with permission from the publisher and the author.*)

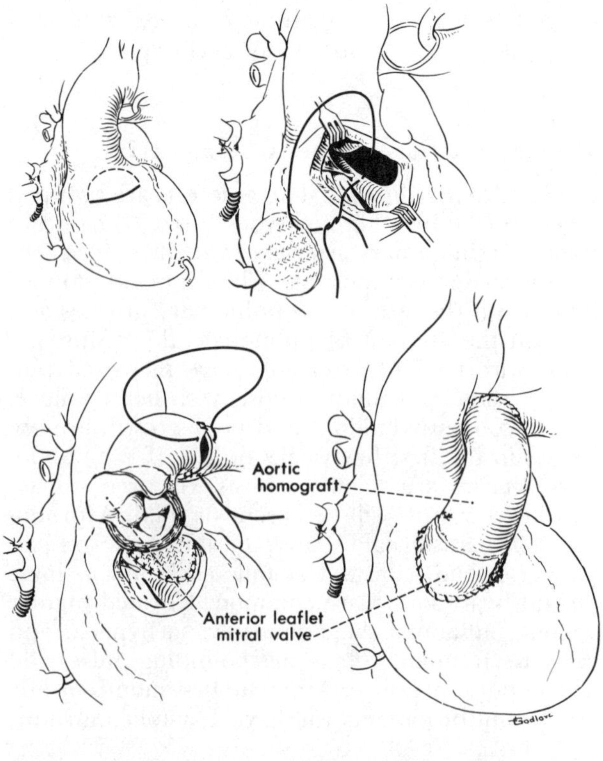

Hospital survival of 80 percent has been achieved following total correction in infancy; 90 percent of older children, appropriately selected, should survive.[464] Small conduits implanted during infancy will require replacement as the child grows and as the conduits become restrictive or degenerate; these revisions have been accomplished with less difficulty and morbidity than one would have expected.

Truncus Arteriosus Type IV
The clinical picture is similar to that described above for ventricular septal defect and pulmonary atresia with pulmonary arteries. With selective angiography, no true pulmonary arteries and only bronchial collateral circulation to the lungs can be seen. These patients are usually severely hypoxic and die early in life. Occasionally, with larger collateral flow, survival to older age is possible. If there are no true pulmonary arteries, there is no effective surgical treatment; however, surgical exploration is usually recommended because pulmonary arteries may be found.[444]

Tricuspid Atresia

Pathology
Classically, in tricuspid atresia there is neither a tricuspid orifice nor valvular tissue. A dimple lies in the floor of the right atrium at the anticipated location of the tricuspid orifice.

The great arteries may be normally related or, less commonly, malpositioned (Fig. 36-63).[465] In a study of 45 specimens, Tandon and Edwards found that in 25 the great vessels were normally related (one had pulmonary atresia as well).[465] Malposition of the great vessels was found in the remaining 19 cases. In 16 of these there was a single (subaortic) conus (the malposition was dextrotype in 12 of these, levotype in 4), and 3 cases had double (subaortic and subpulmonary) coni. Persistent truncus arteriosus was present in one case.

Pulmonary valvular atresia or stenosis may occur with either of the major configurations of the great vessels. When the great vessels are normally related, there is a greater tendency for pulmonary stenosis than there is when malposition occurs, the basis for the stenosis being the narrow state of the ventricular septal defect. In particular, when the great vessels are not malpositioned, the ventricular septal defect may, over time, narrow or close.[466] In cases with malposition the ventricular configuration is like that in single or common ventricle, the aorta arising from the infundibulum of that chamber. An interatrial communication of varying caliber, usually a patent foramen ovale, is present in all cases.

A modification of this classification[465] has been recommended for a more unified approach with surgical considerations.[467]

A condition fairly commonly associated with malposition of the great vessels is *juxtaposition of the atrial appendages.*[468] This condition is characterized by both atrial appendages lying to one side, more commonly the left side, of the great vessels.

Coarctation of the aorta and patent ductus arteriosus has been described as occurring in about 25 percent of cases with tricuspid atresia and dextromalposition.[13]

Clinical Manifestations[6,469]

History The clinical picture varies with associated defects. The most common combination occurring with tricuspid atresia is normally related great arteries, a small ventricular septal defect, a small right ventricle, and pulmonary stenosis. The predominant problem in these infants is cyanosis, which usually presents quite early in the newborn period. When the ventricular septal defect is large, the right ventricle is large, and there is no pulmonary stenosis or, more commonly, when there is transposition of the great arteries without pulmonary stenosis, the pulmonary flow is higher and clinical manifestations are due to congestive heart failure with only very mild cyanosis. These patients may present at a few weeks to months of age. Patients with pulmonary atresia with or without transposition are ductal-dependent and frequently will present with severe cyanosis immediately after birth. Growth failure may occur, particularly in those with large pulmonary flow. Paroxysmal hypoxic spells similar to those in tetralogy of Fallot can occur. Squatting occurs at a later age. When transposition is present, subaortic obstruction can occur if the ventricular septal defect is small.

Physical Examination In patients with predominant cyanosis, tachypnea and even hypoxic episodes may be seen. Clubbing is not seen until later in infancy. A prominent *a* wave is noted in the jugular venous pulse, and the liver may be moderately enlarged. The apex impulse is prominent. The second heart sound is single. Murmurs will depend on associated defects. If a ductus is present, a soft systolic or continuous murmur may be heard. If the pulmonary stenosis is not extremely severe, there may be a midsystolic murmur at the left sternal border. With pulmonary atresia or severe stenosis, there may be no murmur. In those with increased pulmonary flow, the parasternal and apical impulses are hyperdynamic and the second heart sound is usually split. There is a systolic thrill with a long systolic murmur at the lower left sternal border, similar to that of a ventricular septal defect. A middiastolic rumble may be audible at the apex. Signs of heart failure are also found. A pulse discrepancy should be looked for, since coarctation or aortic interruption has been reported to be common in patients with transposition.[470]

Chest Roentgenogram Total heart size shown by chest roentgenogram is usually normal, but it may be at least moderately increased in those with increased

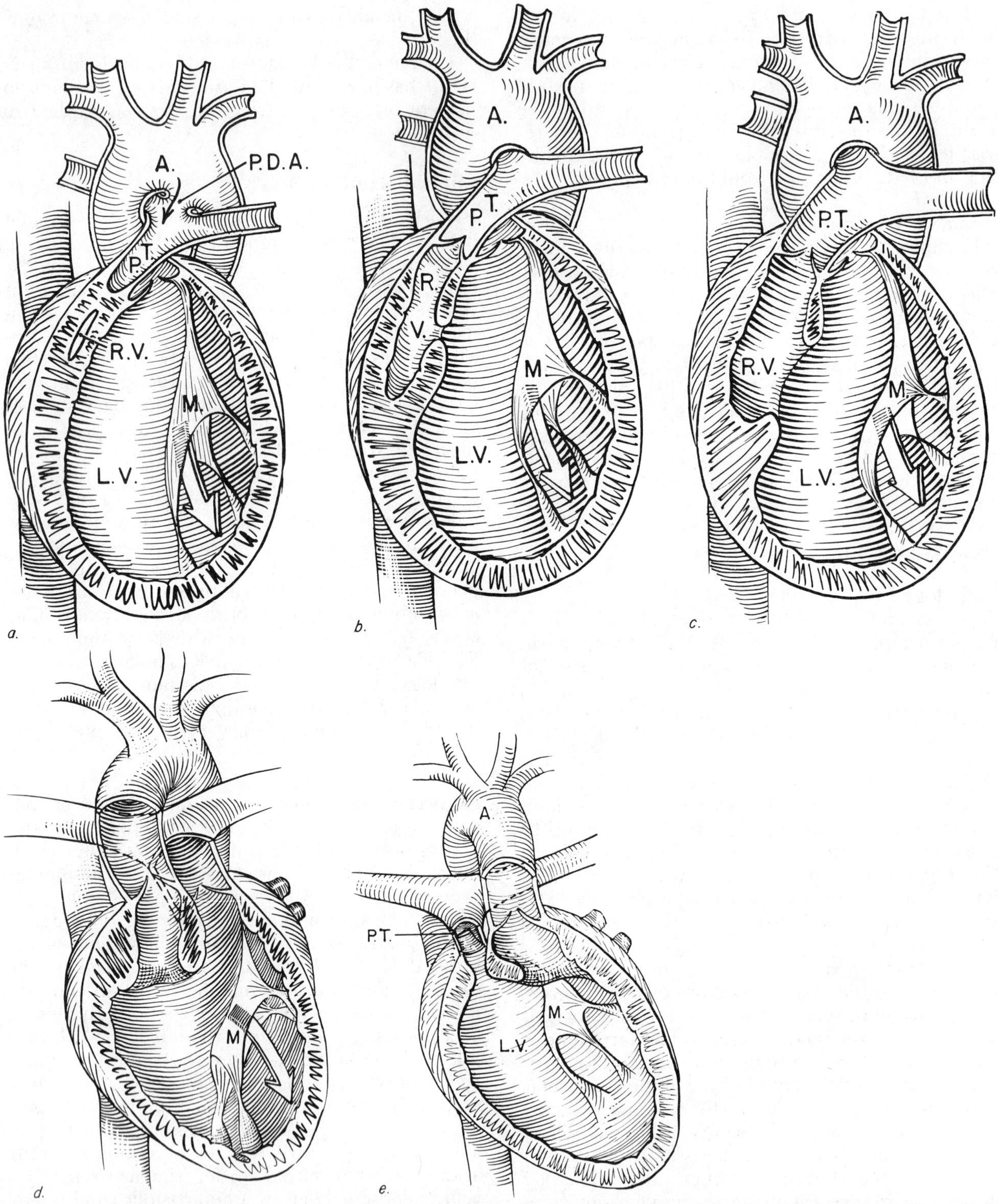

FIGURE 36-63 Tricuspid atresia: *a, b, and c,* with normally related great vessels; *d* and *e,* with malposition of great vessels. *a.* Type Ia. Pulmonary atresia is associated. *b.* Type Ib. Subpulmonary stenosis by virtue of small ventricular septal defect. *c.* Type Ic. No pulmonary stenosis. *d.* Type IIa. Associated with dextro-malposition of the great vessels. *e.* Type IIb. Associated with levo-malposition of the great vessels. Pulmonary stenosis is also present. R.V. = right ventricle; L.V. = left ventricle; M. = mitral valve; P.T. = main pulmonary arterial trunk; A. = aorta; P.D.A. = patent ductus arteriosus. (*From R. Tandon and J. E. Edwards, Tricuspid Atresia. A Re-evaluation and Classification, J. Thorac. Cardiovasc. Surg., 67:530, 1974. Reproduced with permission from the publisher and the author.*)

flow. A straight border of the right side of the heart is considered characteristic. Commonly, the pulmonary segment and flow are markedly diminished. The opposite is true in the minority with increased flow, described above.

Electrocardiogram[471] The electrocardiographic manifestations generally show diminished right ventricular forces for age and left ventricular hypertrophy with ST and T changes. Right atrial hypertrophy is frequently present. In those without transposition, the mean QRS axis is between 0 and $-90°$ in three-fourths of the cases. It is usually between 0 and $+90°$ in those with transposition.[469]

Echocardiogram The common findings on M-mode echocardiography[391] are those of a hypoplastic right side of the heart (Fig. 36-64). There is failure to record the tricuspid valve, but in those patients with pulmonary stenosis, the pulmonary valve also may not be recorded. In this case, the diagnosis is not distinguishable from that of pulmonary atresia with intact ventricular septum. Cross-sectional echocardiography[28] offers clearer distinction and better evaluation of such associated abnormalities as transposition.

Cardiac Catheterization There is usually a mean pressure difference between the atria, with the right atrial pressure being the higher, because at least two-thirds of the patients have a patent foramen ovale rather than an atrial septal defect.[6] The mean gradient and height of the *a* wave in the right atrium correspond to the size of the atrial communication. There is always desaturation throughout the left side of the heart, with the degree dependent on the pulmonary flow. With the help of flow-directed catheters, the right ventricle and great vessels can be entered from the left ventricle except in the unusual case where there is no ventricular septal defect and pulmonary flow is by a ductus or collaterals. Measurement of pulmonary pressure in this manner is most important in those with increased pulmonary flow. There is frequently pulmonary stenosis or obstruction created by the restrictive size of the ventricular septal defect or right ventricle. Right atrial angiography will demonstrate a flow pattern with a triangular nonopacified area in the usual region of the inflow portion of the right ventricle. Left ventricular biplane angiography will demonstrate the relations of ventricular sizes, the ventricular septal defect, and the great vessels. Studies of left ventricular function may be of prognostic significance.[472]

FIGURE 36-64 M-mode echocardiogram from a patient with tricuspid atresia demonstrates the tiny right ventricular size in comparison to the left ventricular size. ECG = electrocardiogram; RV = right ventricle; IVS = interventricular septum; MV = mitral valve; LVW = posterior left ventricular wall.

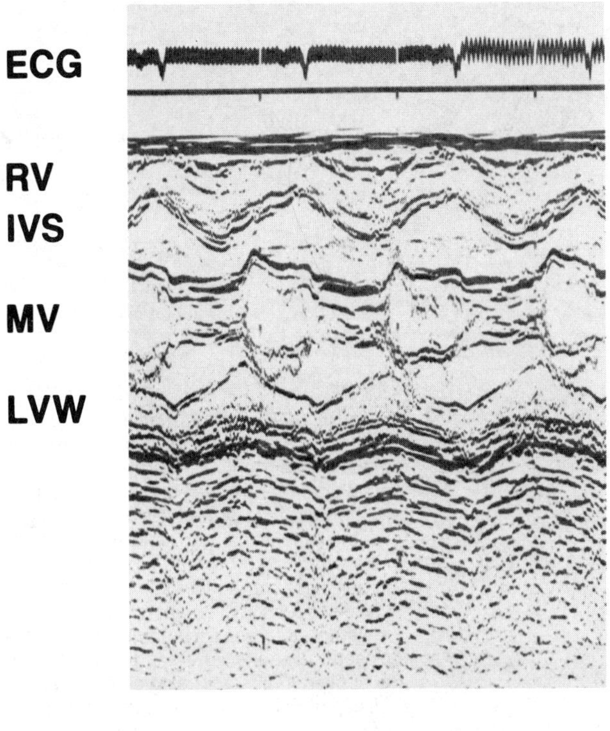

Natural History and Prognosis

Over 50 percent of patients present with cyanosis on the first day of life.[469] Cyanosis is usually progressively severe due to ductal closure, increasing pulmonary stenosis, or spontaneous diminution or closure of the ventricular defect.[466]

The overall prognosis[6] is poor, with an average life expectancy of less than 3 months in infants with pulmonary atresia. Overall, one-half die by 6 months of age, two-thirds by 1 year, and 90 percent by 10 years. The best-tolerated combination, with an average life expectancy of over 7 years, is that of transposition with pulmonary stenosis. Hypoxia is the most common cause of death, but death can result from congestive heart failure or pulmonary vascular disease.

Medical Management

Medical management of cyanosis and heart failure have been discussed previously. Prostaglandin is of temporary help in the critically cyanotic newborn.[27] Hypoxic spells should be treated as discussed for tetralogy of Fallot.[473] Prompt and vigorous treatment of intercurrent infections and prophylaxis against endocarditis is recommended.

Occasionally there is evidence for an inadequate opening between the two atria—extremely tall P waves on electrocardiogram, a progressively enlarging liver, and a large pressure difference between the atria measured at catheterization. In a very young infant, balloon atrial septostomy may help. Commonly, the atrial septum is thickened in this situation, and in older infants it is normally too thick for this procedure to be performed safely. An atrial defect can then be created surgically.

For infants with severe hypoxia, prompt surgical intervention with creation of a systemic-to-pulmonary arterial shunt is indicated. For those who have uncontrollable heart failure and poor growth, the pulmonary artery should be banded. This should be done only after an adequate trial of medical therapy, since some of these patients will have a progressive decrease in pulmonary flow over a few months such that the failure may spontaneously resolve and surgery can be avoided. Such patients should be recatheterized before 6 months of age to evaluate pulmonary pressure and resistance. Overall, surgery definitely increases life expectancy.[469] Right atrial–pulmonary arterial anastomosis[473] is done on selected patients with encouraging results.

Surgical Management

Palliation should be consistent with eventual physiologic correction. Factors dictating palliation include magnitude of pulmonary blood flow and adequacy of the interatrial communication.[474,475] Palliation may include: (1) a systemic-to-pulmonary arterial shunt, usually the Blalock-Taussig subclavian arterial–to–pulmonary arterial anastomosis or a modification thereof, (2) a systemic venous–to–pulmonary arterial shunt or the Glenn superior vena caval–to–right pulmonary arterial anastomosis, (3) pulmonary arterial banding and, (4) balloon atrial septostomy or surgical atrioseptectomy.

Fontan first accomplished physiologic correction of tricuspid atresia in 1968 by diverting right atrial blood directly to the pulmonary artery, using a valve-containing conduit.[473] If the pulmonary vascular resistance is low, left ventricular function is good, and the pulmonary arteries are of adequate size, valves can be omitted from the right-sided circulation. Direct atriopulmonary anastomosis without the use of prosthetic material (Fig. 36-65) probably offers the greatest opportunity for improved survival and quality of life.[476,477]

Morbidity following physiologic correction includes dysrhythmias; systemic venous hypertension with visceral and hepatic manifestations, pleural effusions and chylothorax; low cardiac output; and deterioration of allograft valves used in conduits with significant conduit obstruction.

Fontan's recently reported hospital mortality for physiologic correction is about 4 percent. Of 100 patients undergoing repair since 1968, 82 survived; 94 percent of these are in New York Heart Association class I or II (old classification).[478]

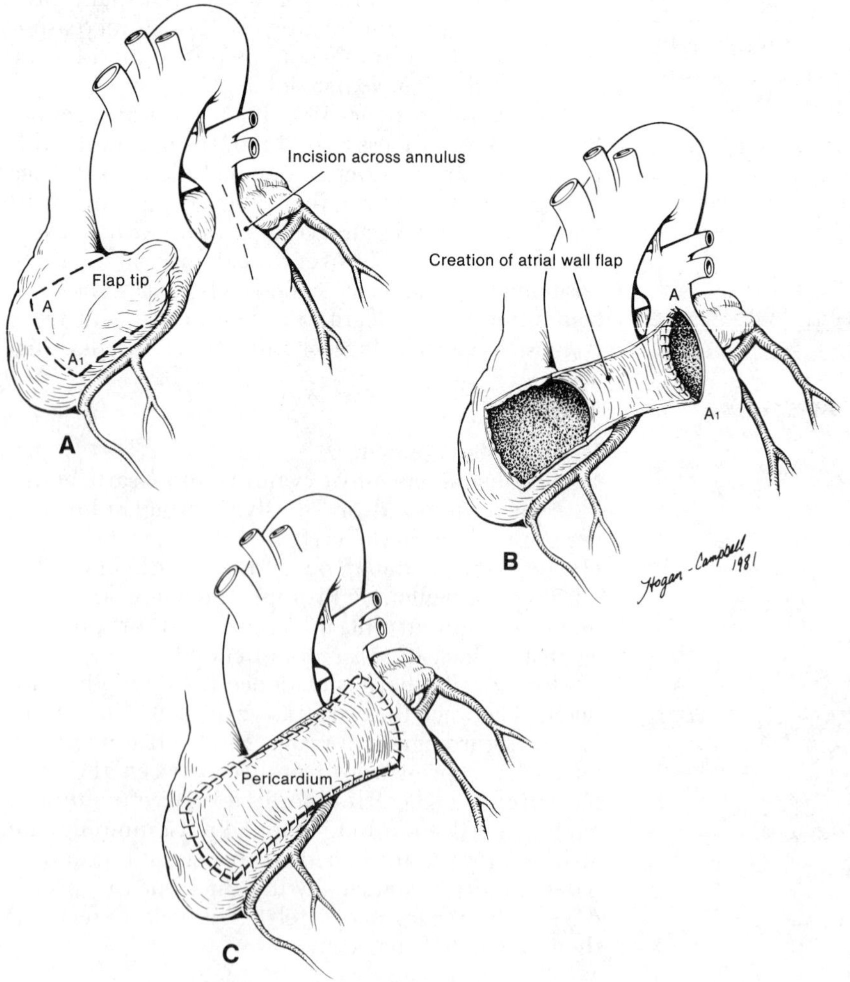

FIGURE 36-65 Bjork modification of the Fontan operation, or right atrium to pulmonary artery shunt. A large flap of right atrial anterolateral wall is created, sutured to the right side of an incision in the right ventricular outflow tract and main pulmonary artery, and covered anteriorly with a large piece of pericardium to create a valveless conduit of entirely autologous material. Interatrial communications are closed with a patch. When this procedure is applied in cases of single ventricle, the tricuspid orifice is closed with a patch.

Tricuspid Regurgitation

Pathology

Tricuspid regurgitation based upon intrinsic anomalies of the valve is uncommon as an isolated entity. It may be part of Ebstein's anomaly or may be observed in cases of multiple dysplasia of valves.[479] The usual basis for regurgitation caused by an anomalous condition involving the tricuspid valve other than Ebstein's anomaly is dysplasia of the valve. This is characterized by poor differentiation of the leaflets and the chordae.[480] A patent foramen ovale is usually present regardless of the reason for the tricuspid regurgitation.

Clinical Manifestations

Clinical manifestations vary somewhat depending on the cause of tricuspid regurgitation, since there are primary and secondary forms. (Endocardial cushion defects and Ebstein's anomaly are discussed in separate sections of this chapter.)

In reports on a small number of cases[481,482] that identify those with isolated tricuspid valvular dysplasia, most presented with cyanosis at less than 1 day of age and all within the first week. Failure occurred in most. Prenatal history and delivery were uncomplicated. There is tachypnea, hepatomegaly, a prominent left parasternal impulse with a thrill, and loud holosystolic murmur in this area. Occasionally, a middiastolic murmur at the lower left sternal border or a ductal murmur is also heard. Chest roentgenograms show extreme cardiomegaly, and pulmonary flow, when visible, is diminished. The electrocardiogram shows right axis deviation, right atrial enlargement, and right bundle branch block or right ventricular hypertrophy. The right ventricle is dilated as shown by echocardiogram. Cardiac catheterization demonstrates a right-to-left shunt at the atrial level and right ventricular pressures that are normal to moderately elevated, but lower than systemic pressure in all patients. The pulmonary artery is occasionally not entered, but there is no pressure difference across the pulmonary valve when it is. The right atrial pressure shows a large regurgitant (*r* or *cv*) wave during systole consistent with tricuspid regurgitation. Intracavitary electrocardiograms exclude tricuspid displacement. Right ventricular angiography demonstrates an enlarged chamber with massive tricuspid regurgitation. Opacification of the pulmonary artery is late and faint or may not be visible.

Pulmonary atresia with intact ventricular septum, in which there is a large right ventricle with severe tricuspid regurgitation,[481] must be excluded. When the pulmonary artery cannot be entered and is not visualized by angiography, catheterization does not distinguish between the atretic valve and the normal valve that does not open. Aortography has been reported to be valuable, since patients with primary tricuspid abnormality have associated pulmonary regurgitation.[483]

The clinical distinction may be possible in some patients with secondary forms of tricuspid regurgitation. There are numerous causes of persistently elevated pulmonary resistance in newborns that may cause this murmur. (See persistent fetal circulation discussed earlier in this chapter.) In a number of infants, transient tricuspid regurgitation has been found to be due to myocardial dysfunction.[484] These infants have a birth history of asphyxia, and hypoglycemia has occurred in many. The electrocardiographic abnormalities include ST depression in the midprecordial leads with T-wave inversion in the left precordial leads. Thus this cause can be strongly suspected on clinical grounds alone. Diseases such as myocarditis are clinically distinguishable from primary tricuspid regurgitation due to additional findings related to the left-sided involvement.

Natural History and Prognosis

The courses of patients with an isolated tricuspid valvular abnormality seem to be widely divergent. They may die of hypoxia and related problems in the first week of life;[481] if they survive this critical period,[482] the cardiovascular abnormalities may improve dramatically. They continue to have a soft murmur of tricuspid regurgitation with or without mild cardiomegaly and right ventricular hypertrophy. This is to some extent due to the normal decrease in pulmonary resistance at this age.

Medical Management

Medical management of those with primary tricuspid abnormalities includes administration of oxygen, assisted ventilation when necessary, and treatment of congestive heart failure. Potentially additive problems such as hypoglycemia must be prevented. Surgery for the mistaken diagnosis of pulmonary atresia should be avoided whenever possible.[481] There is no surgical management for this in the newborn.

Surgical Management

Correction of tricuspid regurgitation associated with endocardial cushion defects and Ebstein's anomaly is described with that of these anomalies.

Most infants with tricuspid regurgitation secondary to dysplasia of the valve are too small, hypoxic, and acidotic to allow successful operative intervention. In the rare child who survives with unresolved tricuspid regurgitation, suture annuloplasty, prosthetic ring annuloplasty, commissural plication, or tricuspid valve replacement should be considered. An atrial septal defect or patent foramen ovale, if present, should be closed at the same operation.[485]

Ebstein's Anomaly

Pathology

In Ebstein's anomaly, the anterior leaflet of the tricuspid valve is attached normally to the annulus, while varying portions of the posterior and the septal leaflets are displaced downward, being attached

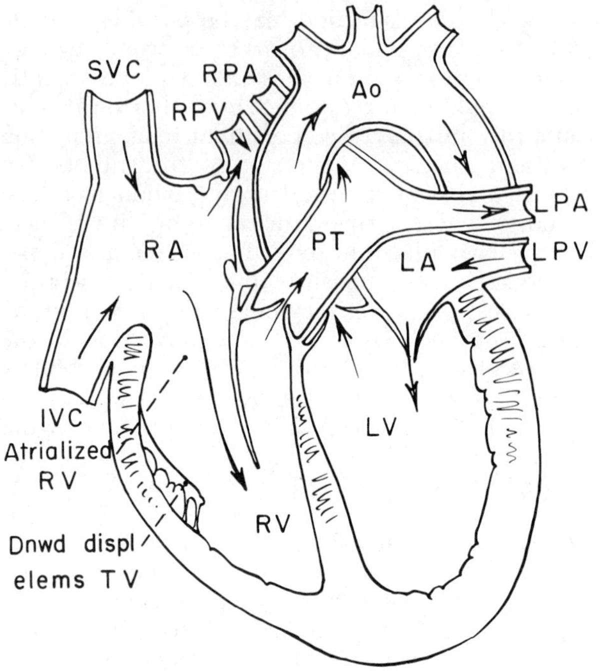

FIGURE 36-66 Ebstein's malformation of the tricuspid valve. The low attachment of elements of the tricuspid valve (TV) functions in such a way that part of the right ventricle (RV) is common with the right atrium (RA). SVC = superior vena cava; IVC = inferior vena cava; PT = main pulmonary arterial trunk; RPA = right pulmonary artery; LPA = left pulmonary artery; RPV = right pulmonary vein; LPV = left pulmonary vein; LA = left atrium; LV = left ventricle; Ao = aorta. [*From J. E. Edwards, Classification of Congenital Heart Disease in the Adult, in W. C. Roberts (ed.), "Congenital Heart Disease in Adults," Cardiovasc. Clin. Series 10/1, F. A. Davis Company, Philadelphia, 1979, p. 1. Reproduced with permission from the publisher, editor, and author.*]

to the ventricular wall below the annulus. The proximal part of the right ventricle is thin-walled and continuous with the right atrium. The functional right ventricle is small and made up of the apical and infundibular portions of the right ventricle[486] (Fig. 36-66).[80] An additional common finding is that the papillary muscles and chordae are highly malformed, so that great variation occurs in the manner of attachment of the two involved leaflets to the right ventricular wall. Commonly, multiple direct attachments of valvular tissue to the right ventricular mural endocardium occur.[480]

An interatrial communication is present in most cases, usually taking the form of a patent foramen ovale. Continuity of right atrial and right ventricular myocardial tissues, in addition to the usual connections by way of the main conduction pathways, has been observed. Atrophy of right ventricular myocardium is common, principally in that part proximal to the tricuspid valve.

Abnormal Physiology[487]

Ebstein's anomaly results in obstruction to right ventricular filling because of a decrease in size of the right ventricle, part of which is incorporated into the huge right atrium. The deformed tricuspid valve also frequently allows tricuspid regurgitation. As a consequence, there is usually a large right-to-left shunt through the foramen ovale.

Clinical Manifestations

History Approximately one-half of reported cases develop symptoms of cyanosis and right-sided heart failure in early infancy. The remainder present because of a murmur or abnormal chest roentgenogram with no symptoms in early childhood or because of gradual progression of symptoms through late childhood or adult life.[488] Those with associated defects may be more symptomatic. The most common symptom is dyspnea on exertion at all ages.[488] Growth and development are usually normal.[489] Palpitations due to supraventricular tachyarrhythmias occur.[487] Occasionally, syncope occurs due to arrhythmia or low cardiac output if the atrial septum is intact.

Physical Examination The newborn with elevated pulmonary vascular resistance has severe cyanosis. In older infants and children, cyanosis and clubbing are mild. Only a small percentage do not have an atrial septal defect or patent foramen ovale and thus are not cyanotic. The precordium is generally quiet even in those with striking cardiomegaly. The liver is frequently enlarged, and the jugular venous pulse may be elevated. The murmur of tricuspid regurgitation is heard at the lower left sternal border and may be accompanied by a "scratchy" diastolic murmur of tricuspid stenosis. The first heart sound is split and loud, and the second heart sound is widely and persistently split. Loud third and fourth heart sounds are usual in older patients.

Chest Roentgenogram Heart size by chest roentgenogram varies, but it is ordinarily very large, predominantly owing to a very dilated right atrium (Fig. 36-67). In those with cyanosis, pulmonary blood flow is diminished correspondingly.

Electrocardiogram Giant, peaked P waves are common, along with a prolonged PQ interval and right ventricular conduction delay or complete right bundle branch block. Electrophysiologic correlates of these abnormalities have been reported.[490] In approximately 10 percent, the pattern of Wolff-Parkinson-White syndrome (with a short PQ interval and delayed conduction of initial QRS forces, or a delta wave) is seen.[488]

Echocardiogram A large tricuspid valve is recorded widely by echocardiogram, but the most specific finding is that of delayed closure as compared to the mitral valve.[491] Two-dimensional echocardiography is very helpful.[489]

Cardiac Catheterization There is a higher risk than usual associated with cardiac catheterization because

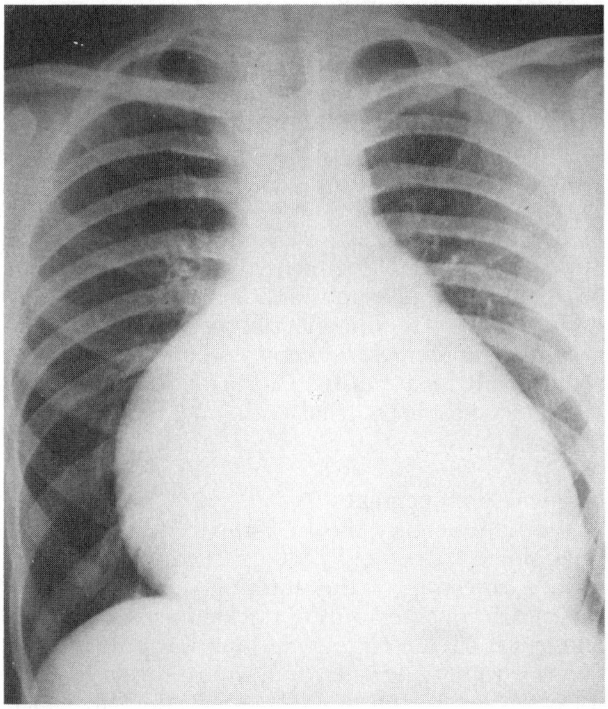

FIGURE 36-67 Chest roentgenogram in a 12-year-old boy having Ebstein's anomaly with marked cardiomegaly and diminished pulmonary flow.

of the frequency of rhythm disturbances. Proper precautions and prompt use of cardioversion when necessary will minimize this risk. There is usually right-to-left shunting at atrial level. Right atrial hypertension can occur with a prominant *v* or regurgitant *r* wave if there is tricuspid regurgitation. The characteristic right ventricular pressure recording is not obtained until the catheter is advanced to the apex or outflow tract. An intracardiac electrocardiogram[492] will demonstrate, on pullback from the right ventricle, an area where the electrocardiogram is ventricular but the pressure is atrial in contour. This method is not infallible, but it is good evidence of tricuspid displacement with an "atrialized" portion of the right ventricle. The pulmonary artery may be difficult to enter, but it is very important in the cyanotic newborn to exclude associated pulmonary atresia. (See section on tricuspid regurgitation for further discussion of methods.) Right ventricular angiography will demonstrate tricuspid regurgitation and the right ventricular morphology. Definitive diagnosis of mild forms is difficult. Frequent abnormalities of the left ventricle and mitral valve are reported;[487] therefore, left ventricular angiography should be considered.

Natural History and Prognosis

Natural history varies greatly with the severity of the abnormality. Fifty percent of those diagnosed in infancy die early, whereas late survival is reported into the ninth decade.[489] Significant associated cardiac defects will lead to a worse prognosis; almost one-half of an autopsy series fell in this group.[486]

Symptomatically, most patients tend to progress. In one study,[489] mortality was highly correlated with one or more of these factors: severe symptoms, cardiothoracic ratio greater than 0.65 by chest roentgenogram, cyanosis, and diagnosis in infancy. Premature deaths can result from heart failure, complications of cyanosis, arrhythmias, and low cardiac output if the atrial septum is intact.

Medical Management

Medical management involves treatment of heart failure and arrhythmias and prevention and treatment of complications of cyanosis and endocarditis. Surgical success has varied, so a conservative approach toward surgery is recommended. Surgical results may offer lower morbidity and mortality for older patients with severe disease.[489]

Surgical Management

Experience with surgical palliation of Ebstein's anomaly has been poor. Recently, both plastic reconstruction of the tricuspid valve and valve replacement have proved effective in the management of the symptomatic patient (New York Heart Association classes III and IV) or in those having significant cyanosis, paradoxical emboli, or associated right ventricular outflow tract obstruction.[493,494] The case for plication of the atrialized portion of the right ventricle remains unsettled, but the procedure seems desirable when this chamber contracts poorly or paradoxically (Fig. 36-68).[495] Accessory conduction pathways associated with the Wolff-Parkinson-White syndrome can be interrupted surgically at the time of repair, and atrial septal defects should be closed.

FIGURE 36-68 Plication for Ebstein's malformation. The atrialized aneurysmal portion of right ventricle is obliterated by the placement of Teflon felt reinforced mattress sutures between the spiral line attachment of the inferiorly displaced tricuspid valve and the true annulus fibrosus. Tricuspid valve replacement may be required. Associated atrial septal defects are closed.

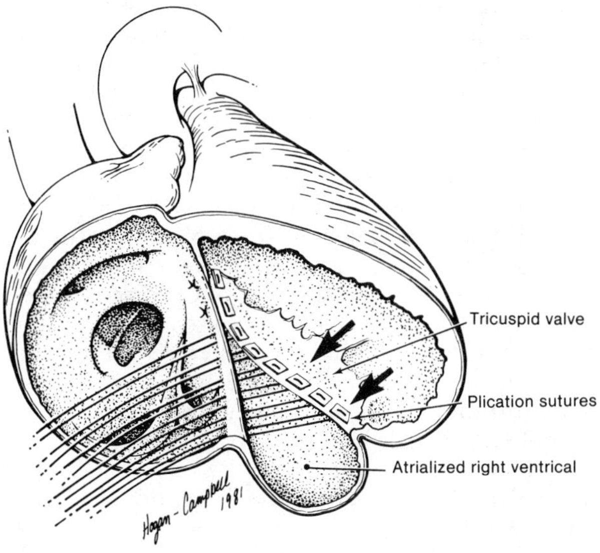

Dysrhythmias are not considered an indication for operation unless associated with significant functional impairment and cardiomegaly. Persistent atrial and ventricular dysrhythmias remain a major source of postoperative morbidity and mortality.[495] Complete heart block, historically associated with tricuspid valve replacement, occurred in only 1 of 16 patients undergoing valve replacement reported by Westaby[493] and did not occur in 42 patients reported by Danielson and Fuster[494] in which 34 (81 percent) has nonprosthetic reconstructions of the valve. There were 3 hospital deaths (7.1 percent) among this group of 42 patients, with 2 late deaths, both of whom had preoperative ventricular arrhythmias and cardiomegaly. Tricuspid valve replacement, for which long-term valve-related complications may be significant, should probably be reserved for the severely symptomatic patient in whom anatomic considerations do not allow plastic reconstruction of the valve. The Fontan concept of direct right atrial–to–pulmonary arterial anastomosis with closure of the atrial septal defect and tricuspid orifice has also been applied successfully in the management of Ebstein's anomaly.[496]

Uhl's Malformation

This rare malformation, also called *parchment heart,* is characterized by a normal tricuspid valve while the right ventricular wall is atrophic and the chamber is noticeably dilated. Histologically, much of the right ventricular wall is fibrotic, with irregular distribution of islands of myocardial tissue.[497]

Clinical Manifestations

Eighteen cases[498] have been reviewed. In many ways, Uhl's malformation is similar to Ebstein's anomaly. The age of presentation is 1 day to 57 years of age with progressive cyanosis, dyspnea, and fatigue with exercise. Chest pain and syncope related to exertion are common. Growth and development are normal.

Physical examination shows a quiet precordium, cyanosis, prominent *a* wave in the jugular venous pulse, widely split and soft second heart sound, and a nonspecific systolic murmur. The chest roentgenogram usually shows significant cardiomegaly. The electrocardiogram shows diminished right ventricular forces, some with a Qr pattern in midprecordial leads, and very tall, peaked P waves. The echocardiogram[499] demonstrates right ventricular dilatation, delayed tricuspid closure, and diastolic opening of the pulmonary valve. Cardiac catheterization reveals an atrial pressure wave with predominant *a* wave throughout the right side of the heart, since the atrium is the driving force. A right-to-left shunt through a patent foramen ovale or atrial septal defect is usually found. Intracardiac electrocardiography and angiography exclude Ebstein's anomaly and demonstrate the large, noncontractile right ventricle.

Natural History and Prognosis

Of the 18 cases reviewed,[498] only one 14-year-old was alive. Cause of death was heart failure in the majority and otherwise was similar to those discussed under Ebstein's anomaly. Right ventricular thrombi have been found on postmortem examination.

Medical Management

Supportive therapy for heart failure and treatment of cyanotic complications and arrhythmias are necessary. Surgery is not generally recommended. Surgical intervention with systemic-to-pulmonary shunts is uniformly unsuccessful. Closure of the atrial septal defect has been tried with one reported survivor.[498]

Surgical Management

A recent report of the first apparently successful physiologic correction[500] of this rare anomaly described resection of the anterior right ventricular wall which consisted only of thickened endocardium and epicardial fat. No myocardium was present. The anterior right ventricular wall was reconstructed using pericardium buttressed with Teflon, to which the tricuspid papillary muscle was reattached. A tricuspid annuloplasty using a Carpentier ring reduced tricuspid regurgitation.

Although not to our knowledge reported, patch closure of the tricuspid valve orifice and interatrial communication and establishment of right atrial–pulmonary arterial continuity applying Fontan's concept (Fig. 36-65) might offer relief of cyanosis, congestive heart failure, and dysrhythmias in patients having Uhl's malformation.

Pulmonary Arteriovenous Fistula

Pathology

In this anomaly, a direct connection between a pulmonary arterial branch and a pulmonary vein is present. The process, which tends to involve the subpleural part of the lung, may occur in any segment of either lung; however, the right middle and both lower lobes seem most commonly involved. Classically, the site of communication is represented by a thin-walled, aneurysm-like structure into which is fed one or more arterial branches and from which one or several veins leave. Among 63 cases of classic pulmonary arteriovenous fistula studied by Dines and associates[501] there were single lesions in 41 cases and multiple lesions in 22 cases. Among the latter, bilateral involvement was present in 5 cases.

A familial tendency has been observed with Rendu-Osler-Weber syndrome.[501]

Clinical Manifestations

Clinical manifestations depend on the size of the connecting vessels between the pulmonary artery and the pulmonary vein. Large defects present in early infancy[502] with cyanosis and heart failure. Smaller ones may go undetected into the adult years. Those with pulmonary arteriovenous fistula due to hereditary hemorrhagic telangiectasia[503] have angioma of the skin and mucous membranes and a positive family history. These fistulas are usually multiple small defects that increase in number with age; the patient does not have frank cyanosis or failure in childhood. There are commonly no precordial murmurs, but a continuous murmur may be heard over the area of the fistula. Chest roentgenogram will show a mass or multiple masses in the lung fields in the larger fistulas. The heart is frequently enlarged, and the mediastinum may be shifted due to the space-occupying mass. Pulmonary arteriography will establish the diagnosis except in very small defects.

Medical Management
Medical management is aimed at treatment of heart failure and prevention of bacterial infection. Prompt diagnosis can be followed by surgery[502] to prevent complications of cyanosis[504] if the lesion is single or if multiple lesions are confined to one area. Continued support with particular attention to respiratory care is important postoperatively.

Surgical Management
The potential for life-threatening complications in the natural history of pulmonary arteriovenous fistulas justifies early conservative excision when the fistula or aneurysm is localized by angiography, even when presenting symptoms are minimal.[501] Occasionally the thin-walled subpleural saccular aneurysms can be dissected free of adjacent pulmonary parenchyma and excised after ligation of the artery and vein. Segmental resection or lobectomy is usually required.[505] Morbidity is low; improvement is dramatic. Embolization may be useful, but experience is limited.[506]

Unilateral Absence of a Pulmonary Artery[507]

Pathology
In this anomaly there is no branch from the main pulmonary trunk to the affected side, which is usually on the side opposite the aortic arch. Blood flow to the affected lung is through bronchial collaterals or a ductus arteriosus. It may be an isolated anomaly or it may be associated with intracardiac defects, particularly tetralogy of Fallot.

Clinical Manifestations and Natural History
The majority of patients are asymptomatic until late childhood or adult life. Symptoms are usually related to bronchiectasis or other malformations of the affected lung, with repeated pulmonary infections and hemoptysis occurring. The cardiovascular examination is normal except for a nonspecific ejection murmur at the left upper sternal border. About 20 percent of those with the isolated anomaly develop pulmonary hypertension in the overperfused lung. In this group, the findings are those of pulmonary hypertension.

The clinical manifestations in those with intracardiac defects are dominated by the other defects. If there is a left-to-right shunt, over 85 percent will develop pulmonary hypertension.

The chest roentgenogram shows diminished flow with a smaller than normal lung on the affected side and increased flow to the opposite side. Ventilation-perfusion studies are helpful. Angiography is diagnostic.

Medical Management
Prompt treatment of infection is important. Associated cardiac defects should be surgically corrected, especially if a left-to-right shunt exists, to prevent pulmonary vascular disease. Pneumonectomy should be considered for those with severe pulmonary disease.

Abnormalities of the Pulmonary Venous Connections

Pulmonary veins terminating anomalously may involve either all of the pulmonary veins or some of them (partial anomalous connection; see earlier section of this chapter on "Intracardiac Communications between the Systemic and Pulmonary Circulations").

Total Anomalous Pulmonary Venous Connection

Pathology
When all pulmonary veins fail to join the left atrium, but instead terminate in a systemic vein or the right atrium, the term *total anomalous pulmonary venous connection* is applied (Fig. 36-69). Synonyms include *anomalous pulmonary venous drainage or anomalous pulmonary venous return.* The usual veins leave the lung and then join a chamber-like confluence. The latter lies superior to the left atrium and inferior to the tracheal bifurcation. From the confluence of veins, one vessel leads to the anomalous termination. Less commonly, two or more vessels lead to multiple sites of termination.

Sites of supradiaphragmatic termination, in order of decreasing frequency, are the left innominate vein, the coronary sinus, the right atrium, the superior vena cava and the azygous vein.[508] Usually supradiaphragmatic termination is not associated with pulmonary venous obstruction, but exceptions occur. The most common of these relates to total anomalous pulmonary venous connection to the left innominate vein. The vein that ascends from the confluence of pulmonary veins to the brachiocephalic vein commonly runs anterior to the left pulmonary hilus. Less commonly, the ascending vein runs between the left pulmonary artery and the left

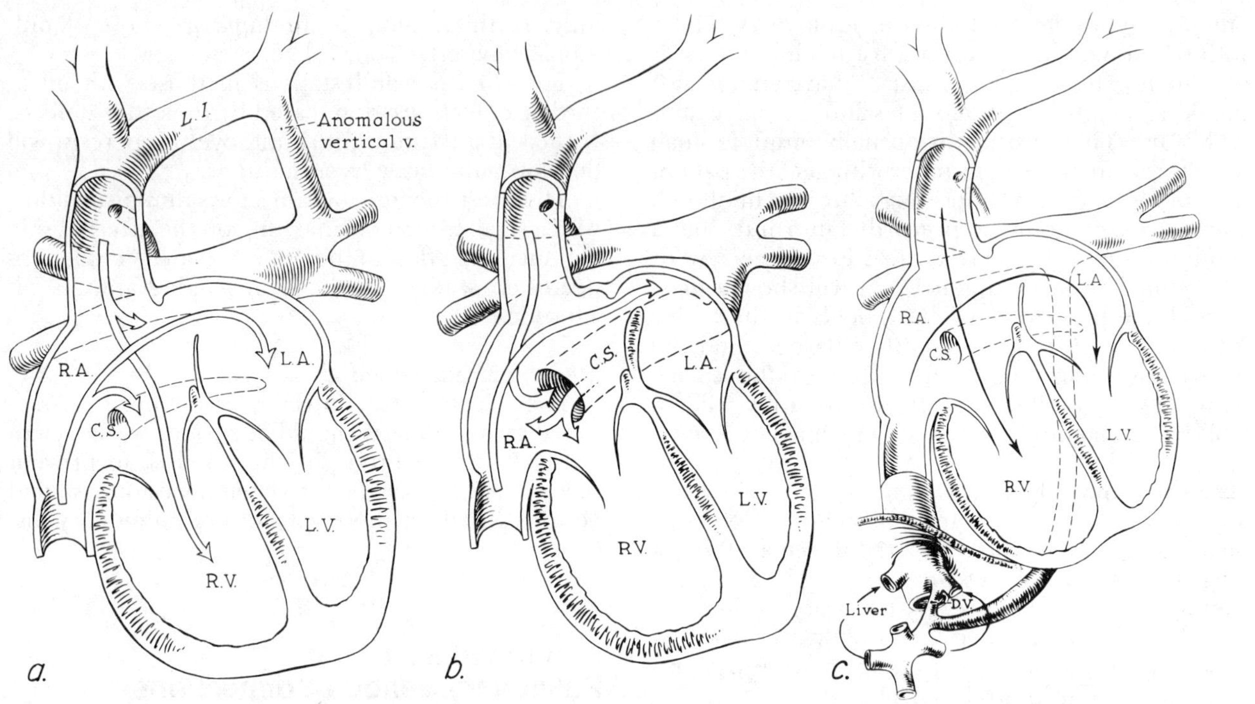

FIGURE 36-69 Three common types of total anomalous pulmonary venous connection. *a.* Total anomalous pulmonary venous connection to the left brachiocephalic (innominate) vein (L.I.). *b.* Total anomalous pulmonary venous connection to the coronary sinus (C.S.). *c.* Total anomalous pulmonary venous connection of the infradiaphragmatic type to the ductus venosus (D.V.). R.A. = right atrium; R.V. = right ventricle; L.A. = left atrium; L.V. = left ventricle.

main bronchus. In this position the ascending anomalous vein is compressed in what has been called a *hemodynamic vise*,[509] and pulmonary venous obstruction occurs. When there is total anomalous connection of pulmonary veins to the coronary sinus, the latter is markedly dilated.

The site of termination may also be infradiaphragmatic, with connection to the portal venous system. The anomalous vein leaves the confluence of pulmonary veins and descends into the abdomen along the esophagus. The veins that receive the anomalous vein include one of the following: the ductus venosus, the portal vein, or the left gastric vein. Pulmonary venous obstruction characteristically is manifested in all cases of infradiaphragmatic connection.[510]

A particular type of total anomalous pulmonary venous connection has been termed *atresia of the common pulmonary vein.* There is a chamberlike confluence of the pulmonary veins leaving the lungs, but there is no gross channel of exit from the confluence of veins. Small veins running from the confluence enter the esophageal wall.

In all cases of total anomalous pulmonary venous connection, there is a patent foramen ovale. The atrium and ventricle of the left side are small in comparison with the right-sided chambers but are within normal limits as to absolute size.

In the absence of asplenia or polysplenia, associated anomalies are not common. When present, there is usually asplenia or polysplenia and the various cardiovascular anomalies of that syndrome (refer to later discussion).

Abnormal Physiology[511]

In this anomaly all the blood from both pulmonary and systemic circulations returns to the right atrium. It is compatible with life only if there is a communication between the right and left sides of the heart. In most situations the pulmonary resistance is low, and a large volume of blood from the right atrium flows to the pulmonary circuit. Consequently, a large volume of fully saturated blood returns to the right atrium, where it mixes with a smaller volume of unsaturated blood returning from the systemic circulation. Since systemic arterial blood comes from this mixture of blood in the right atrium, the systemic arterial saturation may remain high. The systemic arterial saturation will be low if pulmonary blood flow is decreased because of either increased pulmonary vascular resistance or obstruction to pulmonary venous flow.

Clinical Manifestations[511]

History Male predominance, particularly of the subdiaphragmatic type of total anomalous pulmonary venous connection, has been noted in some reports; familial instances are very unusual. Almost all patients are cyanotic, with over one-half presenting with cyanosis in the first month of life. Most also have congestive heart failure, including all of those with and two-thirds of those without pulmonary hypertension. The symptoms of congestive heart failure occur in almost two-thirds before 3 months of age. All patients who present in the first year of life are thin and most gain little weight after birth.

In the few who gain weight, there is no pulmonary hypertension.

Physical Examination These infants are dusky, tachypneic, and diaphoretic. The jugular venous pulse is elevated and hepatomegaly appears early. There is a diffuse and hyperdynamic right ventricular impulse. The second heart sound is split and relatively fixed. The pulmonary component is usually increased. There is usually a grade 2 to 3 midsystolic murmur at the left sternal border. At the lower sternal border, there is a middiastolic rumble and prominent third and fourth heart sounds. Rales may be heard over the lung fields, and periorbital edema is frequent. A continuous murmur may be heard over the common venous channel.

If there is significant obstruction to pulmonary venous flow, the cyanosis is more marked. The heart is not as hyperkinetic, and auscultation may reveal little or no murmur with a very loud second heart sound.

Chest Roentgenogram With the unobstructed types of anomalous connection, the heart is enlarged and the pulmonary flow is increased. Pulmonary edema may be seen. In those patients with return to the left innominate vein, there may be a characteristic bulging of the superior mediastinum bilaterally, producing a "snowman," or figure-of-eight, contour.[6] With obstructed types, the heart size is near normal; there is very marked pulmonary edema, which may give a granular appearance to the lungs.

Electrocardiogram There is right axis deviation and right atrial and right ventricular hypertrophy. Commonly, there is a qR pattern in the right precordial leads.

Echocardiogram The M-mode echocardiogram[512] usually shows volume overload of the right side of the heart in the unobstructed types. The only abnormality in obstructed types may be abnormal right ventricular systolic time intervals caused by pulmonary hypertension. Occasionally, an echo-free space, thought to be the common pulmonary venous channel, is seen behind the left atrium. Cross-sectional echocardiography is more specific and may outline the site of drainage.[513]

Cardiac Catheterization There will be an increase in oxygen saturation at the level of the abnormal connection, with similar saturations in the remainder of the chambers on the right and left sides of the heart. Right atrial, right ventricular, and pulmonary arterial pressures are elevated to a variable degree. Pulmonary pressure may be above systemic pressure if there is marked pulmonary venous or pulmonary vascular obstruction. Pulmonary capillary wedge pressures are elevated in proportion to the degree of venous obstruction. The atrial communication may rarely be obstructive.[511] Pulmonary arteriography will usually show the anomalous venous connection. Angiography directly in the common venous channel, if it is entered, will outline its course and any sites of obstruction optimally. Left ventricular angiography will demonstrate its volume[514] and also detect an associated ventricular septal defect or, more commonly, a patent ductus. Balloon atrial septostomy may be helpful in the uncommon case where significant obstruction is demonstrated at the atrial level.[515]

Natural History and Prognosis

The clinical course is commonly that of progressive congestive heart failure, with death in the first year of life.[511] There are significant differences among patients with varying degrees of pulmonary hypertension. The majority of those with severe pulmonary hypertension and pulmonary vascular obstruction die by the age of 3 months, whereas those with significant pulmonary hypertension alone may survive to 1 year of age. The best clinical course is seen in those with pulmonary pressures lower than one-half of systemic pressure. The majority of these patients survive to 1 year, and some do not develop congestive heart failure. Severe growth failure occurs in all but a few of this latter group. At postmortem examination, structural changes in the pulmonary vascular bed are present to some degree at all ages, but changes are more severe in those with venous obstruction.[516]

Medical Management

Medical management involves vigorous treatment of congestive heart failure and intercurrent respiratory infections and prevention of endocarditis.

Initial surgical success in the 1960s was followed by numerous reports outlining the high risk involved. Surgical mortality for the early 1970s was still high[515]; therefore, a conservative attitude toward surgical correction continued except in the very ill infant. Some of the factors contributing to this high risk, particularly in the subdiaphragmatic type,[517] have been examined. More recent reports indicate that a lower risk, 13 percent, can now be achieved[518] with improvements in surgical technique and intensive postoperative care. In this series, age did not appear to be a major factor in survival. Because of this success and the poor outlook with medical management alone, surgery is being recommended at even younger ages. Any newborn or young infant with severe obstruction or pulmonary edema should have prompt surgical correction. Surgery may be delayed for a few months in those without critical obstruction. Failure to grow usually occurs in patients with pulmonary hypertension, and surgery should be done at a few months of age. For infants with less than one-half systemic pressure in the pulmonary artery who grow, surgery may be deferred until the latter half of the first year.

Surgical Management

Correction of total anomalous pulmonary venous connection[519] requires (1) creation of a large com-

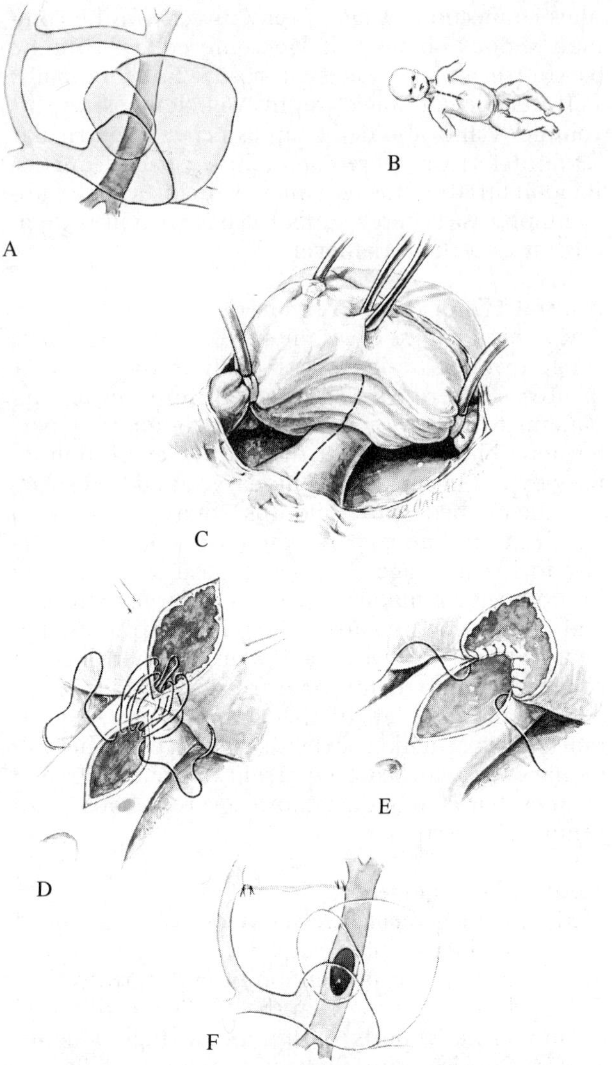

FIGURE 36-70 Correction of total anomalous pulmonary venous connection draining to a left vertical vein. *A.* Schematic representation of anatomy, as seen from surgeon's side, of total anomalous pulmonary venous connection to left brachiocephalic vein. *B.* Median sternotomy incision. *C.* Appearance after posterior pericardial attachments are cut. Retraction forcep is on right atrium. Proposed incisions in posterior wall of left atrium and in anterior wall of common pulmonary venous sinus are shown. *D.* The two incisions are made, and the first few stitches of a double-armed monofilament suture are placed. *E.* These have been snugged up and the suturing continued. *F.* Final result. [*From J. W. Kirklin, Surgical Treatment for Total Anomalous Pulmonary Venous Connection in Infancy, in B. G. Barratt-Boyes (ed.), "Heart Disease in Infancy: Diagnosis and Surgical Treatment," Churchill Livingstone, Edinburgh, 1973. Reproduced with permission from the publisher, editor, and author.*]

munication between the left atrium and the pulmonary venous system, (2) obliteration of the anomalous pulmonary venous connection to the systemic circulation, and (3) closure of the associated interatrial communications (Fig. 36-70).[520]

Supracardiac anomalous connection to the left brachiocephalic (vertical) vein and infracardiac connections to the portal venous system or the inferior vena cava are corrected by the creation of a wide anastomosis between the posterior aspect of the left atrium and the common transverse pulmonary venous sinus (Fig. 36-70).[520] The stretched foramen ovale or associated atrial septal defect is closed. The ascending or descending anomalous pulmonary venous connection to the systemic circulation is ligated.

Anomalous pulmonary venous connection to the coronary sinus is repaired by creation of a large fenestration in the common wall between the coronary sinus and the left atrium (Fig. 36-71). The coronary sinus is diverted into the left atrium by placement of an intracardiac patch which also closes the interatrial communication.

Total anomalous pulmonary venous connection to the right atrium is repaired by excision of the atrial septum and placement of a patch diverting the opening of the anomalous pulmonary venous connection into the left atrium.

Mixed forms of total anomalous pulmonary venous connection pose particular technical difficulties requiring individualized operations.

Katz reviewed 51 cases of repair of total anomalous pulmonary venous connection.[521] Seven patients (14 percent) died in the hospital. Late results were excellent. Operative survival is poor in infants having significant pulmonary venous obstruction, particularly those with infradiaphragmatic drainage.[518]

Corrective operative intervention is indicated when the diagnosis is established for infracardiac and other obstructed types of anomalous drainage and within the first year of life for those who have no significant pulmonary venous obstruction. Long-term prognosis is good for those patients surviving correction.

Partial Anomalous Pulmonary Venous Connection

(See section on "Intracardiac Communications between the Systemic and Pulmonary Circulations" above.)

Abnormalities of Systemic Venous Connections

Union of Superior or Inferior Vena Cava with Left Atrium

When a vena cava joins the left atrium, it is rare that the inferior vena cava is involved.[522] More commonly, the situation is one in which a left superior vena cava is present. The union of the left superior vena cava with the left atrium lies just posterior to the base of the atrial appendage. In this condition, the coronary sinus is not formed. Union of a left superior vena cava with the left atrium is usually observed in association with one of three phenomena: (1) asplenia, (2) polysplenia, or (3) presence of an atrial septal defect in the posteroinferior angle of the atrial septum. The frequently associated defects of either the asplenia or the polysplenia syndrome and atrial septal defect are discussed in other sections of this chapter.

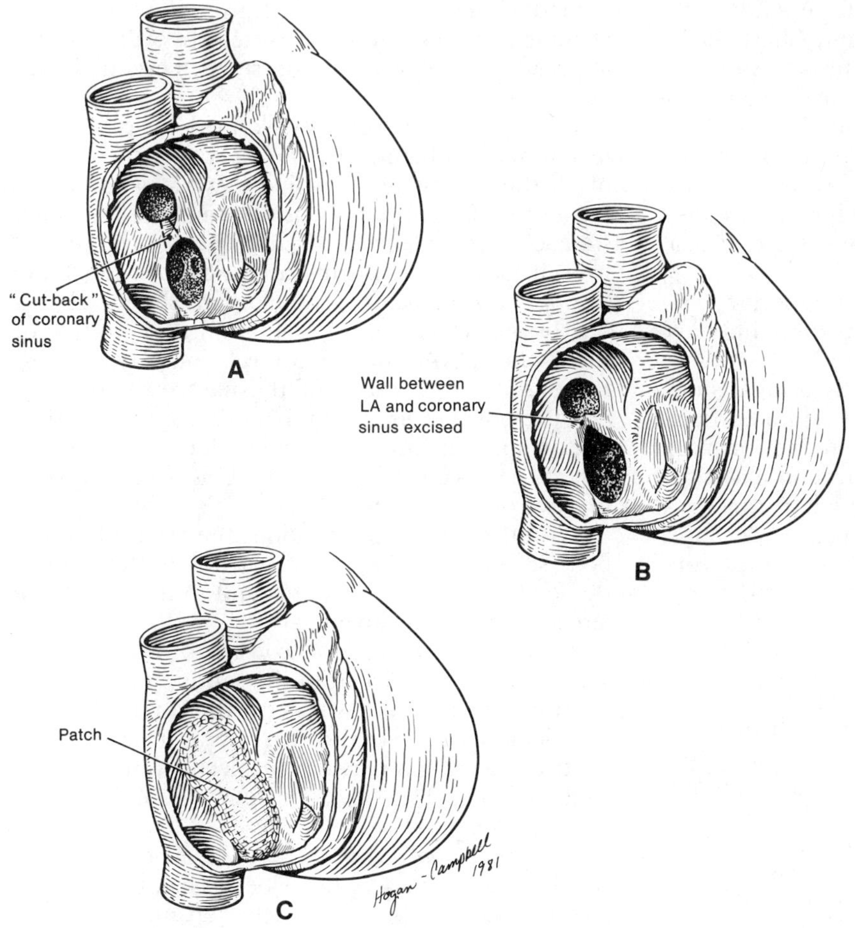

FIGURE 36-71 Correction of total anomalous pulmonary venous drainage to the coronary sinus. The tissue between the coronary sinus and the interior of the left atrium is excised, cutting back the coronary sinus orifice well away from the area of the atrioventricular node. A Dacron patch is then sutured over the orifice of the coronary sinus and the associated atrial septal defect, with pulmonary venous and coronary venous blood being diverted to the left atrium. The patch must be anchored in areas remote from the atrioventricular node to avoid conduction disturbances.

In the rare isolated case, cyanosis is usually detected. Cardiac catheterization and venous angiography will establish the diagnosis. If all systemic venous return is to the left atrium, there is hypoplasia of the right side of the heart. Medical treatment is directed toward the prevention and management of the complications of cyanosis. Surgical treatment is recommended to prevent these complications.[523]

A pericardial or Dacron patch baffle is placed to divert the desaturated systemic venous blood from the left atrial orifices of the anomalous venae cavae to the right atrium and tricuspid valve, avoiding injury to the conduction system near the orifice of the coronary sinus. Residual atrial septum is excised and patched as necessary to allow unobstructed flow of pulmonary venous blood to the mitral orifice. Occasionally the hepatic veins enter the inferior aspect of the atrium directly rather than entering the inferior vena cava; this, too, is corrected by individualized baffle placement. Cannulation of the venae cavae for cardiopulmonary bypass may be more difficult than usual. Hypothermic circulatory arrest (18 to 20°C) facilitates repair of these rare anomalies of systemic venous return, especially in the small infant. Reports of repair are limited, but results in general are good.[524–526]

Persistent Left Superior Vena Cava

Usually, malformations of the systemic intrathoracic veins are of incidental significance. Persistent left superior vena cava, the most common of these malformations, may occur either as an isolated condition or in association with other cardiovascular malformations. The left brachiocephalic vein is formed by its usual tributaries and descends as the left superior vena cava. It passes ventrally to the aortic arch and root of the left lung to become continuous with the coronary sinus. The latter, because of carrying the additional blood it receives through the anomalous connection, is wider than normal. The coronary sinus terminates in the right atrium.

Winter, who presented an extensive review on the subject of persistent left superior vena cava,[527] found that in about 60 percent of cases studied a bridge connected the two brachiocephalic veins. Usually, the *hemiazygous vein* joins the left superior vena cava after arching over the left main bronchus to form a mirror image of the normal arrangement of the azygous vein and superior vena cava on the right. In rare cases the venous system in the neck is essentially a mirror image of the normal, but the left superior vena cava terminates in the coronary sinus.

The presence of a persistent left superior vena cava is hemodynamically insignificant. Chest roentgenogram may show fullness of the left superior mediastinum. Technical difficulties may be encountered if cardiac catheterization is done from the left arm. Identification is made by catheter course to the left brachiocephalic vein through the coronary sinus, or by angiography. Recognition is of importance only if open heart surgery is anticipated, since special bypass techniques are required.[528]

The presence of a persistent left superior vena cava complicates cannulation for cardiopulmonary bypass in some operations within the heart. A large left vena cava can be drained directly using a small right-angle cannula, or blood can be aspirated from the open right atrium as it drains from the coronary sinus. When an adequate communication exists between right and left venae cavae, the left vena cava can be clamped. The persistent left vena cava causes no additional problems during operations conducted under hypothermic circulatory arrest.

Continuity of Inferior Vena Cava with Azygous Venous System

In this condition, the hepatic portion of the inferior vena cava is absent. Under this circumstance, the inferior vena cava remains a posterior structure and joins either the azygous or hemiazygous vein and subsequently the right or left superior vena cava. The hepatic veins converge to form a relatively narrow trunk which joins the right atrium at the usual location of junction of the inferior vena cava with this cardiac chamber. This venous pattern has also been termed the *candy cane* deformity or *absence of hepatic segment of inferior vena cava*. Polysplenia is usually associated.[529]

This abnormality is of clinical significance in those with congenital heart disease only because of the technical problems it poses during cardiac catheterization or during cannulation for cardiopulmonary bypass. On chest roentgenogram, there may be fullness of the right or left superior mediastinum, depending on whether the drainage is via the azygous or hemiazygous system. On the lateral view, absence of the shadow of the inferior vena cava below the atrium posteriorly may also be a clue to the diagnosis. Superior orientation of the mean P axis on the electrocardiogram is frequently associated. Venous angiography from the leg will demonstrate the anomaly. In small infants, it may be safer and easier to approach cardiac catheterization from the arm if this anomaly is strongly suspected clinically.[530]

Malpositions of the Cardiac Structures

Definition and Terminology

The segmental approach to the diagnosis of complex congenital heart disease[531] provides an orderly, effective method for determining the anatomic and hemodynamic interrelationships of the cardiac chambers, valves, and great vessels. In order for this approach to be better understood, certain definitions will be helpful.

Positioning of viscera is described as situs solitus, inversus, or ambiguus. In *situs solitus*, (S) distribution of all the organs is according to what is generally recognized as normal, as, for example, a left-sided stomach and spleen, a predominantly right-sided liver, a trilobed right lung and a bilobed left lung. In *situs inversus (totalis)*, (I) the organs show a perfect mirror image, as regarding left and right, to that of situs solitus. Anteroposterior relations are not disturbed. When, because of the nature of the atria and the position of abdominal organs, neither situs solitus nor situs inversus can be identified, *situs ambiguus* (A) is said to be present. This usually applies in cases of asplenia or polysplenia.

With the rarest of exceptions the atria follow the body situs (morphologic right atrium to the right of the left atrium in situs solitus and to the left of the left atrium in situs inversus).

The atrioventricular canal consists of the tricuspid valve, the mitral valve, and the septum of the atrioventricular canal and connects the atrial with the ventricular portion of the heart. As a rule each atrioventricular valve is part of the specific ventricle into which it leads. The valve situs may be solitus, inversus, or ambiguus.

Atrioventricular alignment, via the atrioventricular canal structure, may be described as being *concordant* (right atrium to right ventricle, left atrium to left ventricle) or *discordant* (right atrium to left ventricle, left atrium to right ventricle). The mode of atrioventricular connection may be normal, stenotic, atretic, straddling, overriding, with double inlet or with common inlet.

The position of the ventricles is described by the terms *d loop and l loop.* When the morphologic right ventricle lies to the right of the morphologic left ventricle, the ventricular portion of the heart is said to exhibit a *d loop* (D). The ventricles are said to be *noninverted* or in the solitus position. When the ventricular relations are reversed, l loop is said to be present (L). The ventricles are *inverted* or in the inversus position. These designations are independent of visceral or visceroatrial situs.

The *infundibulum* (conus) connects the ventricles with the great arteries and may be subpulmonic, subaortic, bilateral, very deficient, or absent. Although normally incorporated into the right ventricle, the infundibulum is not an intrinsic part of the true right ventricle.[531]

The great arteries may deviate from the usual with respect to both their anteroposterior and their lateral (left to right) relationships.

In *solitus, normally related great arteries* (NRGA), the aortic origin lies to the right of and posterior to the position of the pulmonary valve. In *inversus, normally related great arteries,* the anteroposterior relationships are not disturbed but the aortic origin lies to the left of the pulmonary arterial origin. In *transposition of the great arteries* (TGA), the aorta arises from the anatomic right ventricle and the pulmonary artery from the anatomic left ventricle. Usually, the aortic origin is more anterior than that of the pulmonary artery.

In transposition of the great arteries, when the aortic origin is to the right of the pulmonary origin, the transposition is called dextro transposition (dTGA) (see discussion of complete transposition of great arteries below). When the reverse is the case, levo transposition (lTGA) is present (see the section on corrected transposition, below). When the transposed aorta lies directly anterior to the pulmonary artery, the anomaly is designated as aTGA.

When the abnormal relation of the great arteries is neither complete nor corrected transposition, the term *malposition of the great arteries* (MGA) is used. Malposition may be designated as dMGA, lMGA, or aMGA, depending on the laterality in the relation between the origins of the two great arteries.[531] Two specific types of malposition have been described. The first is characterized by one artery arising from the appropriate ventricle while the other artery also arises from the same (or inappropriate) ventricle, yielding a situation either of *double-outlet right ventricle* (DORV) or *double-outlet left ventricle* (DOLV).[531] The second type of malposition has been termed *anatomically corrected malposition* (ACM). This is characterized by the great arteries having the same laterality as the ventricles from which they arise. The reader should not confuse the rare condition of anatomically corrected malposition with the condition commonly called corrected transposition. In the latter condition the course for the flow of blood is normal. In anatomically corrected malposition, the route for the flow of blood may be normal or abnormal, depending upon the atrioventricular connections.

The terms *concordance* and *discordance* refer to the alignments of the atria with the ventricles (see above) and alignment of the ventricles with the great arteries; these terms are applied regardless of body situs. When the anatomic right ventricle is aligned with the pulmonary artery and the anatomic left ventricle with the aorta, *ventriculoarterial concordance* exists. *Ventriculoarterial discordance* is present when the morphologic right ventricle is aligned with the aorta and the left ventricle with the pulmonary trunk.

The Segmental Approach to Diagnosis

The segmental or step-by-step approach is a valuable tool for arriving at the correct diagnosis in patients with complex congenital heart disease. This approach is independent of cardiac position and as such can be applied equally well to hearts in the normal position or to those with dextrocardia, mesocardia, or levocardia. In order, one determines:

1. The locations of the right and left atria and their venous connections
2. The situs and mode of connection of the atrioventricular valves
3. The location of the right and left ventricles and their alignment with the atria
4. The location and connections of the infundibulum
5. The position of the great arteries and their alignment with the ventricles

In addition, one must search for associated malformations between and within each of these segments.[531]

Determining atrial situs can be accomplished in most instances by taking advantage of the high degree of abdominal visceroatrial concordance. With abdominal situs solitus (S), the liver is on the right and the right atrium will almost invariably be on the right as well; with abdominal situs inversus (I), the liver is on the left and the right atrium will almost invariably be on the left. With abdominal situs ambiguus (A), the liver may be almost symmetrically placed across the midline and the atria may be normally located or inverted or both atria may have morphologic characteristics of either the right or the left atrium. When both atria have the characteristics of a right atrium (i.e., bilateral superior venae cavae and no pulmonary venous connections), *dextroisomerism* or "bilateral right-sidedness" is said to be present. This situation is usually, though not invariably, accompanied by asplenia. When both atria have characteristics of a left atrium (i.e., pulmonary venous drainage from the ipsilateral lung) *levoisomerism* or "bilateral left-sidedness" is said to exist. This usually, but again not invariably, is accompanied by polysplenia. Unfortunately a symmetrical liver, a good predictor of situs ambiguus, is found in only a little over one-third of patients with situs ambiguus. Lateralization of the liver, evident in the remainder, may simulate either situs solitus or situs inversus.

Bronchial situs, determined by overpenetrated chest roentgenogram or bronchial tomography, has proved to be a more accurate predictor of atrial situs than is abdominal situs. The longer of the two main bronchial lengths, measured from the carina to the proximal wall of the upper lobe bronchus, is divided by the shorter. A value of 2.0 or greater indicates lateralization of the bronchi, and hence the atria, with the longer being the anatomic left bronchus. A value of 1.5 or less indicates bronchial situs ambiguus with either dextro- or levoisomerism.[532]

Of all the techniques for determining atrial situs, the most accurate appears to be identification of the hepatic portion of the inferior vena cava, which almost always enters the morphologic right atrium. The location can be determined by catheter position, angiography, or two-dimensional echocardiography.[533]

Additional clues to atrial situs may be provided. A superiorly oriented P-wave vector in the electrocardiogram and absence of the suprarenal and infrahepatic portion of the inferior vena cava with azygous extension to the superior vena cava are characteristics of levoisomerism and polysplenia and the presence of Howell-Jolly bodies in the peripheral blood smear is a characteristic of dextroisomerism and asplenia. Selective atrial angiography at the time of catheterization may permit visualization of the triangular right atrium with its broad, pyramidal atrial appendage or the elliptical left atrium with its narrow, "crooked-finger" appendage.

For determination of the atrioventricular and ventricular relations, high-quality, selective biplane ventricular angiography is essential. The right ventricle, with its globular shape, blunt apex, coarse trabeculations, and (usually) semilunar-atrioventricular valve discontinuity, may be distinguished from the left ventricle, with its footlike shape in diastole and tail-like shape in systole and its fine trabeculations and two papillary muscles. Two-dimensional echocardiography is capable of permitting recognition of these morphologic features and other, more distinctive features as well.[534]

Finally, the ventriculoarterial relationships or connections and the type of conus must be established, again either angiographically or echocardiographically.

The symbols used to designate the combination or sequence of segments are arranged in order as follows: (1) the visceroatrial or bronchoatrial situs, (2) the ventricular loop, and (3) the relations of the great arteries. These are included within parentheses and are preceded by words or abbreviations which indicate the ventriculoarterial alignment, for example, TGA, DORV, or single ventricle (SV). Associated malformations such as ventricular septal defect, pulmonary stenosis, and straddling tricuspid valve are listed after the parentheses. Thus, the typical or usual transposition of the great arteries with situs solitus, d-ventricular loop, and aorta arising from the right ventricle and to the right of the pulmonary artery, with an intact ventricular septum (IVS), would be designated TGA (SDD) IVS. The designation for typical corrected transposition with situs solitus, l-ventricular loop, and aorta arising from the morphologic right ventricle and lying to the left of the pulmonary artery, also with ventricular septal defect and pulmonary stenosis, would be TGA (SLL), VSD, PS. These designations apply to these particular transpositions with situs solitus, whether the heart lies in the right or left chest (dextrocardia or levocardia, respectively). It should be noted that the description of the position of the heart within the chest would offer no additional information referable to the intracardiac anatomy or great-vessel alignment.[531]

Levocardia, Dextrocardia, and Mesocardia

The position of the cardiac apex indicates a condition of levocardia, dextrocardia, or mesocardia. Most attention is directed to a right-sided apex (dextrocardia). When the heart is shifted to the right because of other intrathoracic abnormalities, the situation has been termed *dextroposition.* Rotation of the heart to the right about a superoinferior axis but with normally related atria, ventricles, and great arteries has been referred to as *dextroversion.*

If situs inversus is present, the heart may be normal fundamentally except for total inversion in keeping with the status of the other organs. Dextrocardia of this type has been called *mirror-image dextrocardia.* Unfortunately, within this category one finds frequent examples of ventricular noninversion, complete transposition of the great arteries, or double-outlet right ventricle.[531] When the other organs of the body are normally oriented, yet the heart lies in the right chest, the term *isolated dextrocardia* has been applied. While the cardiac chambers and great arteries are frequently normally related though rotated to the right (the *dextroversion* described above), transposition of the great arteries with atrial and ventricular inversion is at least as common a finding in this arrangement.[531]

The trend today is to discard the terms *dextroposition, dextroversion, mirror-image dextrocardia,* and *isolated dextrocardia* because they do not provide any significant information beyond what is already known, namely, that the cardiac apex is in the right chest, and to use the broad term *dextrocardia* for all right-sided hearts, followed by a description of the visceroatrial situs. In the case of those patients in whom the heart appears to have been pulled or pushed into the right chest by massive atelectasis, hypoplasia of the right lung, diaphragmatic hernia, eventration of the diaphragm, pleural effusion, obstructive emphysema, or pneumothorax, an appropriate descriptive phrase should be added. The term *isolated levocardia* is applied to all left-sided hearts with situs inversus or situs ambiguus, and a description of the visceroatrial situs should follow.

Dextrocardia with complete situs inversus occurs in approximately 2 per 10,000 live births. The incidence of congenital heart disease is relatively low among these individuals and is estimated to be about 3 percent. Dextrocardia with situs solitus or situs ambiguus is considerably less common and occurs in perhaps 1 per 20,000 live births. The incidence of congenital heart disease is extremely high in this situation, however, and is probably in the range of 90 percent or greater.[6] From these figures one could project that approximately 12 percent of individuals found to have dextrocardia and congenital heart disease would have complete situs inversus. This estimate compares favorably with the figure of 18 percent observed in large autopsy series.[9] About 50 percent of patients with dextrocardia and heart disease have situs solitus, and the remainder have situs ambiguus.[531] An l-ventricular loop is found in the majority of patients with dextrocardia regardless of situs but is most common, as one might expect, among those patients with situs inversus, where it approaches 80 percent. Cardiac malformations usually, although not invariably, are severe and complex.

The most common lesions and their approximate frequency are as follows: transposition of the great arteries, 50 to 75 percent; double-outlet right ventricle, 10 to 18 percent; ventricular septal defect, 60 to 80 percent; single ventricle, 15 to 40 percent; and pulmonary stenosis or atresia, 70 to 80 percent.[6,9] Aproximately three-quarters of the transposed great arteries will have the segmental arrangement of corrected transposition. Tetralogy of Fallot is distinctly uncommon. Polysplenia or asplenia is found in about one-third of patients with dextrocardia and almost invariably with situs ambiguus. *Kartagener's syndrome,* the triad of situs inversus, sinusitis, and bronchiectasis, is present in approximately 20 percent of patients with dextrocardia and situs inversus totalis.[535] The incidence of *isolated levocardia* is estimated at approximately 0.6 per 10,000 live births. It is estimated that over 90 percent of affected individuals will have associated heart disease.[9] Situs inversus is present in approximately 15 percent while the remainder have situs ambiguus, with the ratio of asplenia to polysplenia or accessory spleens being from 2.5:1 to 1.5:1. Regardless of situs, the ventricular loop is most frequently a d loop. Transposition of the great arteries and double-outlet right ventricle are present in the majority and are of about equal frequency. The associated defects are comparable in complexity and severity to those associated with dextrocardia.[531] *Mesocardia* may exist either as a variant position of the normal heart or as a variant position of dextrocardia or isolated levocardia.

Medical and Surgical Management

Medical management of patients with cardiac malposition is similar to that of patients with normally located hearts, with the exceptions of continuous daily antibiotic coverage and pneumococcal vaccine for patients with asplenia and the particular attention to detail that is necessary to establish the correct diagnosis in those individuals with unusual and complex malformations.

Surgical management differs in the technical considerations imposed by the malposition of the heart itself, the frequency of occurrence of the l-ventricular loop, and the variability of the intracardiac conduction system.

Asplenia and Polysplenia Syndromes

The association of congenital heart disease, usually severe, with thoracic or abdominal visceral heterotaxia is well documented. Abdomoinal visceral heterotaxia (Greek: *heteros,* other; *taxis,* arrangement) is characterized by varying degrees of malposition of the liver and stomach, varying degrees of malrotation of the gastrointestinal tract, and, usually, abnormalities of the spleen. The latter includes absence of the spleen (asplenia) and the presence of multiple small masses of splenic tissue (polysplenia). In the case of the bronchopulmonary viscera, heterotaxia usually takes the form of isomerism with the presence of either (1) bilateral right or eparterial bronchi (above the pulmonary artery) and trilobed lungs or (2) bilateral left or hyparterial bronchi (below the pulmonary artery) and bilobed lungs. These abdominal and thoracic anomalies appear to represent an abnormal persistence of the embryonal pattern of symmetry, which gives way to lateralization between the thirtieth and thirty-sixth day of fetal life. This state of heterotaxia, lying between situs solitus and its mirror image, situs inversus, has been termed *situs ambiguus* by Van Mierop and is the situs found in approximately one-third of patients with dextrocardia and over 80 percent of those with isolated levocardia.[536] From this picture of visceral heterotaxia or situs ambiguus has emerged at least two rather distinct syndromes, namely, the asplenia syndrome and the polysplenia syndrome.

The *asplenia syndrome* is characterized by duplication or persistence of right-sided structures and absence or displacement of left-sided structures. This situation has been termed *dextroisomerism* or "bilateral right-sidedness," a name which, although unsound from an embryological viewpoint, provides a helpful reminder of the features of the asplenia syndrome. These include an abnormally symmetrical liver placed across both sides of the upper abdomen, a stomach displaced to the right side in approximately half of the patients, and bilateral trilobed lungs with eparterial bronchi. The inferior vena cava may lie to the right or left of the spine and, in the abdomen, is almost invariably on the same side of the spine as the abdominal aorta. Both atria frequently have the morphologic characteristics of a right atrium, with bilateral superior venae cavae, absence of the coronary sinus, and total anomalous pulmonary venous return. The characteristic cardiovascular malformations are presented in Table 36-3.[537] Note should be taken of the high incidence of dextrocardia, transposition of the great arteries, pulmonary atresia or stenosis, total anomalous pulmonary venous connection, complete atrioventricular canal, and single ventricle. Males are more commonly affected than females in a ratio of 1.7:1.

The usual clinical picture is that of a very young male infant with severe cyanosis and a symmetrical liver. The P-wave axis in the electrocardiogram is normal, while the QRS axis is superior in most instances, reflecting the presence of a malformation of the atrioventricular canal. On chest roentgenogram, pulmonary blood flow is usually seen to be diminished and an abnormal position of the stomach may be recognized. An overpenetrated chest roentgenogram may permit identification of bilateral eparterial bronchi. Howell-Jolly and Heinz bodies may be seen on the stained smear of peripheral blood, and no splenic tissue will be demonstrated by radioisotope scanning.

Approximately one-third of these infants will die within the first week of life, and only a very small number, perhaps 15 to 20 percent, will survive to

TABLE 36-3 Cardiovascular Abnormalities in Asplenia and Polysplenia Syndromes

	Asplenia, %	Polysplenia, %
Cardiac position:		
Dextrocardia	41	42
Levocardia	59	58
Great arteries:		
Normal relation	19	84
Transposition	72	8
Double-outlet RV	9	8
Pulmonary valve:		
Normal	22	58
Pulmonary stenosis	34	33
Pulmonary atresia	44	9
Great veins:		
Normal	16	50
TAPVC	72	0
PAPVC	6	42
Absent infrahepatic/suprarenal IVC	0	84
Bilateral SVC	53	33
Atrial septum:		
Intact	0	16
Primum ASD	100	42
Secundum ASD	66	26
Single atrium	0	16
Atrioventricular valves:		
Two	13	50
Single or common	87	16
Ventricular septum:		
Intact	6	25
Single ventricle	44	8
Atrioventricular canal	50	33
Other VSD	3	33
Coronary arteries:		
Single	19	0
Coronary sinus:		
Absence	85	42

Note: RV = right ventricle; TAPVC = total anomalous pulmonary venous connection; PAPVC = partial anomalous pulmonary venous connection; IVC = inferior vena cava; SVC = superior vena cava; ASD = atrial septal defect; VSD = ventricular septal defect.

Source: V. Rose, T. Izukawa, and C. A. F. Moes, Syndromes of Asplenia and Polysplenia. A Review of Cardiac and Non-cardiac Malformations in 60 Cases with Special Reference to Diagnosis and Prognosis, *Br. Med. J.*, 37:840, 1975. Reproduced with permission from the publisher and authors.

the end of the first year. Shunting procedures to increase pulmonary blood flow are necesssary for survival in most instances. Renal and gastrointestinal malformations are present in some 10 to 15 percent of patients. Sudden, overwhelming bacterial sepsis is a constant hazard for patients with asplenia. The most common offending organisms for children below 6 months of age are *Klebsiella* and *Escherichia coli;* for those beyond 6 months of age, pneumococcus and *Haemophilus influenzae.* Continuous daily oral antibiotic coverage is recommended for all individuals with this syndrome, with the antibiotics of choice being amoxicillin for children under the age of 10 years and penicillin for those older than 10 years.

Polysplenia, defined as two or more splenic masses and usually consisting of two somewhat larger spleens accompanied by a number of smaller splenules, tends to be characterized by levoisomerism or "bilateral left-sidedness." The liver is abnormally symmetrical in about one-quarter of patients, and the stomach is on the right in about two-thirds of patients. Isomerism of the lungs is not nearly as frequent as it is in asplenia, but bilateral hyparterial bronchi and bilobed lungs are found in perhaps two-thirds of these patients. Partial, rather than total, anomalous pulmonary venous connection is frequent; the most frequent pattern is that of pulmonary venous drainage of each lung to the corresponding atrium. The other characteristic cardiovascular malformations are listed in Table 36-3.[537] Despite the relatively high incidence of cardiac malposition, it can be seen that the anomalies, in general, are less severe than those associated with asplenia. More patients have normally related great arteries and fewer have transposition, pulmonary atresia, complete atrioventricular canal, or single ventricle. From 50 to 85 percent of patients have absence of the infrahepatic to suprarenal portion of the inferior vena cava, with azygous or hemiazygous vein continuation of the suprarenal inferior vena cava to the ipsilateral superior vena cava. A superior and leftward P-wave vector in the frontal plane, falling between -30 and $-90°$, is extremely common among these patients and warns of difficulties that might be encountered with catheter passage from the femoral vein to the cardiac chambers at the time of cardiac catheterization. A superior QRS axis is present in one-third of patients. Chest roentgenogram tends to show increased pulmonary blood flow. Splenic tissue may be demonstrated in the dorsal mesogastrium on both sides of the abdomen when radioisotope scanning is used. Renal and gastrointestinal anomalies are present in approximately 15 percent of patients. Survival of patients with polysplenia is considerably better than that of patients with asplenia, with almost 40 percent living into and beyond the second year of life.

Exceptions to and overlap between these two syndromes have been identified. Bilateral eparterial bronchi with trilobed lungs, situs ambiguus, and cardiac malformations characteristic of asplenia have been described in the presence of a normal spleen. Bilateral eparterial bronchi with bilobed lungs and bilateral hyparterial bronchi with trilobed lungs have also been described.[532] Asplenia with bilateral bilobed lungs does occur rarely, but, to our knowledge, asplenia with bilateral hyparterial bronchi has not been reported. At present it appears that bronchial situs and the location of the hepatic portion of the inferior vena cava are the most accurate predictors of dextro- or levoisomerism, with their characteristic cardiac malformations, and of atrial situs, respectively.[532] The state of the spleen is a less accurate predictor but remains of importance in terms of the possibility of lethal sepsis and as a colorful reminder of the different patterns of cardiovascular and visceral abnormalities.

Dextro Transposition of the Great Arteries

Definition

In this condition, the aorta and the pulmonary artery are misplaced in relation to the ventricular septum, with the aorta arising from the right ventricle and the pulmonary artery arising from the left ventricle.

Pathology

In the majority of cases there is situs solitus of the atria and viscera (S) and atrioventricular concordance, the right ventricle lying to the right of the left ventricle (d loop, D). (Fig. 36-72) The aorta lies to the right of the pulmonary arterial origin (d transposition, D) and is anterior. Of the communications between the two sides of the circulation, a narrow patent foramen and patent ductus are common in very young infants. The ventricular septum is intact in the majority of patients. (Fig. 36-72*A*) A ventricular septal defect of significant size and varying location occurs in somewhat over one-third of cases[538] (Fig. 36-72*B*).

The incidence of associated pulmonary stenosis varies with the state of the ventricular septum; incidence is about 4 percent in patients with intact ventricular septum is 20 percent in those with ventricular septal defect.[538] Anatomic causes of pulmonary stenosis include the presence of bilateral coni with a narrow state of the subpulmonary conus, presence of a membranous collar encircling the left ventricular outflow tract, anomalous adhesion of the anterior mitral leaflet to the ventricular septum, stenotic deformity of the pulmonary valve, rarely an aneurysm at the site of a ventricular septal defect and, in cases of intact ventricular septum, a bulging of the ventricular septum into the left ventricular outflow area.

The coronary arteries usually arise from the left and posterior sinuses, the right artery arising from the latter location.

Hypertensive pulmonary vascular disease may occur at an inordinately early age and may even occur with intact ventricular septum.

Three-quarters or more of those patients with d transposition, situs solitus, and d loop [TGA (SDD)], either have no significant associated cardiac defects or have relatively simple malformations in the form of ventricular septal defect, atrial septal defect, patent ductus arteriosus, or pulmonary stenosis. The remainder generally have more complicated lesions.[3] The more common and relatively uncomplicated form of transposition is the subject of this section.

Abnormal Physiology

The systemic and pulmonary circulations are arranged so that the systemic venous return is conducted back to the systemic arterial system and the pulmonary venous return back to the pulmonary arterial system, with no obligatory mixing or inter-

FIGURE 36-72 Complete transposition of the great arteries. *a.* With intact ventricular septum. A patent foramen ovale and enlarged bronchial arteries (Br. Art.) are present. *b.* With ventricular septal defect and without pulmonary stenosis. SVC = superior vena cava; IVC = inferior vena cava; RA = right atrium; RV = right ventricle; Ao = aorta; LA = left atrium; LV = left ventricle; PT = main pulmonary arterial trunk; RPA = right pulmonary artery; LPA = left pulmonary artery; RPV = right pulmonary vein; LPV = left pulmonary vein.

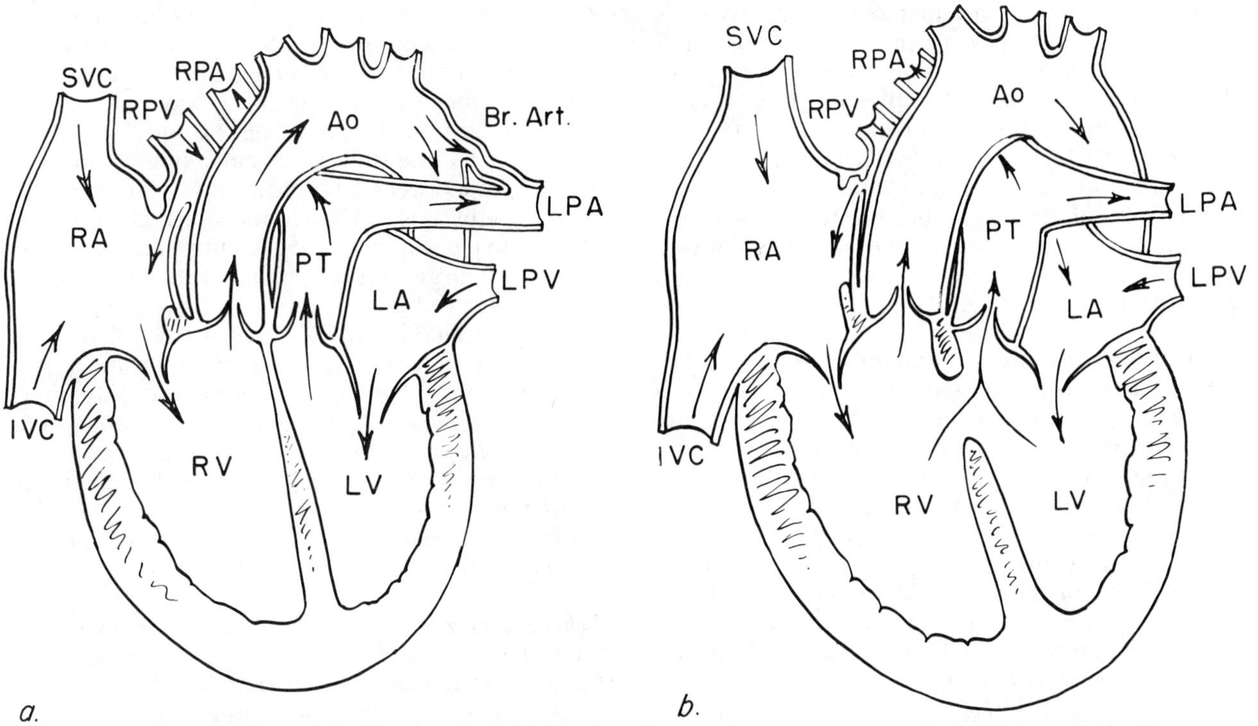

change. For survival there must be communication between the two circulations in the form of a patent foramen ovale, a patent ductus arteriosus, or a ventricular septal defect. The hemodynamics are dependent on the combination of defects present and particularly on the amount of mixing between the systemic and pulmonary circulations. The right ventricle is the systemic ventricle and its systolic pressure will be the same as systemic arterial pressure.

Clinical Manifestations

Approximately 9 percent of children with recognized congenital heart disease will have transposition of the great arteries,[6] an extremely serious malformation with a mortality rate, untreated, of 30 percent within the first week.[538] Transposition, almost always with an intact ventricular septum, is the most common diagnosis among infants admitted to the hospital with heart disease within the first week of life and ranks second only to ventricular septal defect in frequency among infants with heart disease serious enough to produce death or to require cardiac catheterization or cardiac surgery within the first year of life. Males are more commonly afflicted than females in a ratio between 2:1 and 3:1.

History More than half of the infants with transposition will have an intact ventricular septum, and very early, severe, and progressive cyanosis is the presenting symptom or sign in this group. Approximately 60 percent require transfer to a cardiac center within the first 2 days of life, 75 percent within the first week. In a very few, a patent ductus in combination with an incompetent foramen ovale or a small ventricular septal defect will permit survival for several weeks, but narrowing or closure of any of the three will produce critical hypoxia. Those infants with a sizable ventricular septal defect present with severe congestive failure and only mild or barely detectable cyanosis toward the middle or latter part of the first month of life. Tachypnea, dyspnea, and failure to thrive are characteristic. Those infants or children with large ventricular septal defects and significant pulmonary stenosis may present within the first days of life with cyanosis if stenosis is severe; with more moderate stenosis, they may present with cyanosis and little if any congestive failure somewhat later within the first year.

Physical Examination Among infants with an intact ventricular septum, the most prominent feature is intense cyanosis. Tachypnea and mild dyspnea are present. Arterial pulses are easily felt. The right ventricular lift is forceful, and the first sound is usually loud at the lower left sternal border. In most patients the second heart sound may be heard to be split narrowly, confirming the presence of two semilunar valves. Murmurs are seldom impressive or distinctive. Signs of congestive failure are uncommon unless the infant is beyond the first week of life and a large ductus is present. Among infants with a large ventricular septal defect, slenderness and mild cyanosis or a grayish pallor are apparent. Breathing is labored, and both right and left ventricular impulses are hyperactive. A thrill is uncommon. A systolic murmur at the lower left sternal border usually is present, but it is seldom loud or completely holosystolic. A gallop rhythm and a diastolic flow rumble at the apex are typical. Infants and children with ventricular septal defect and significant pulmonary stenosis generally are severely cyanotic. The possibility of transposition is suggested by a forceful or hyperdynamic right ventricular lift, an audible sound of pulmonary closure, or a stenotic murmur of greater intensity and duration than one might expect in tetralogy of Fallot with a similar degree of cyanosis.

Chest Roentgenogram With an intact ventricular septum, the heart size and pulmonary vascularity appear normal or at the upper limits of normal during the first week. A narrow base due to the displaced pulmonary artery may give rise to the characteristic "egg-on-side" contour. Impressive cardiomegaly, pulmonary plethora, and this characteristic contour are more common during the second week and beyond. With a large ventricular septal defect, marked cardiac enlargement involving all chambers, impressive pulmonary plethora, and the egg-on-side contour are present. With significant pulmonary stenosis, the heart resembles that of tetralogy of Fallot, but it is usually slightly larger and the pulmonary vascularity less diminished than one would expect for a comparable degree of clinical cyanosis. A right aortic arch is present in 4 to 16 percent of patients.[538]

Electrocardiogram If the ventricular septum is intact, the electrocardiogram may reveal tall or peaked P waves by the second or third day of life; however, clearly abnormal right ventricular forces are not usually apparent until the latter part of the first week. The persistence of an upright T wave in leads V_1 and V_3R beyond 4 days of age would provide an early clue that the right ventricular systolic pressure is at systemic levels. The older infant will have abnormal right axis deviation and marked right ventricular hypertrophy. A large ventricular septal defect with a large pulmonary blood flow usually will produce biatrial and biventricular hypertrophy. If pulmonary blood flow is reduced toward normal, whether by significant pulmonary stenosis, by pulmonary arterial banding, or by severe pulmonary vascular obstructive disease, the pattern becomes one of right ventricular and right atrial hypertrophy. Diminutive right ventricular forces or isolated left ventricular hypertrophy suggests right ventricular hypoplasia, frequently associated with overriding of the tricuspid valve.

Echocardiogram Two-dimensional study can document the fact that the pulmonary artery arises from the left ventricle and the aorta from the right ventricle; it also provides information regarding asso-

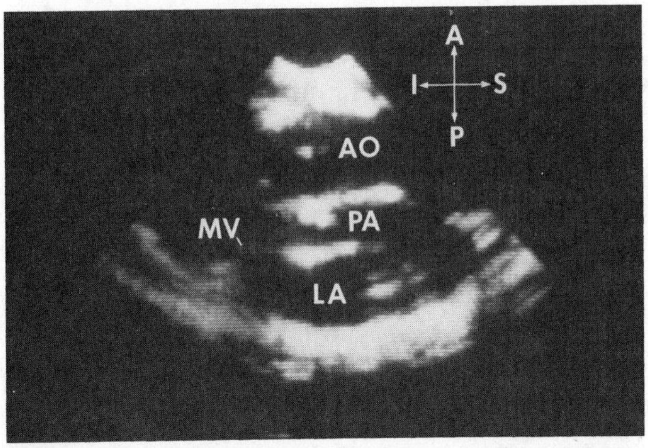

FIGURE 36-73 Two-dimensional echocardiogram in the parasternal long-axis view from a patient with transposition of the great arteries and intact ventricular septum. Both great arteries are visualized, with the pulmonary artery (PA) identified as posterior to the aorta (AO) by the sharp posterior angulation of the pulmonary artery around the superior aspect of the left atrium (LA). MV = mitral valve; A = anterior, I = inferior; S = superior; P = posterior. *(From D. J. Hagler, A. J. Tajik, J. B. Seward, D. D. Mair, and D. G. Ritter, Wide-Angle Two-Dimensional Echocardiographic Profiles of Conotruncal Abnormalities, Mayo Clin. Proc., 55:73, 1980. Reproduced with permission from publisher and authors.)*

ciated anomalies[539] (Fig. 36-73).[415] The success of balloon septostomy or surgical septectomy can be judged by visualizing the atrial septal opening directly using the subxiphoid approach.[540] The ratio of left ventricular pre-ejection period to left ventricular ejection time, determined by the M-mode technique, can be used to estimate pulmonary arterial pressure in the weeks and months beyond the newborn period in the absence of bundle branch block, atrioventricular dissociation, or arrhythmias.[541]

Cardiac Catheterization Systemic arterial oxygen desaturation will be present in all patients, with saturation values ranging from 18 to 70 percent among those with an intact ventricular septum and from 70 to 90 percent in those with a large ventricular septal defect without pulmonary stenosis. The pulmonary arterial oxygen saturation invariably is higher than the systemic arterial saturation. The right ventricular systolic pressure will be at systemic levels; the left ventricular pressure will also be at systemic levels if a large ventricular septal defect, ductus arteriosus, or significant pulmonary stenosis is present. A wide pressure difference between the two ventricles or between the two atria indicates an intact or virtually intact ventricular or atrial septum, but the lack of such a gradient certainly does not guarantee the presence of an adequate opening at either level. Selective ventricular angiography will document the anteriorly located aorta arising from the right ventricle with the aortic valve displaced superiorly and anteriorly by the subaortic conus. The pulmonary artery will arise from the left ventricle posteriorly and to the left (Fig. 36-74). The presence of a ventricular septal defect, patent ductus, and pulmonary stenosis should be noted, as well as the morphology

FIGURE 36-74 *A.* Posteroanterior view of the right ventricular angiogram from a patient with d-transposition of the great arteries and intact ventricular septum. The aorta (AO) arises from the heavily trabeculated right ventricle (RV) above a subaortic conus (arrow). *B.* The left ventricular angiogram. The main pulmonary artery (MPA) arises from the smooth-walled left ventricle (LV).

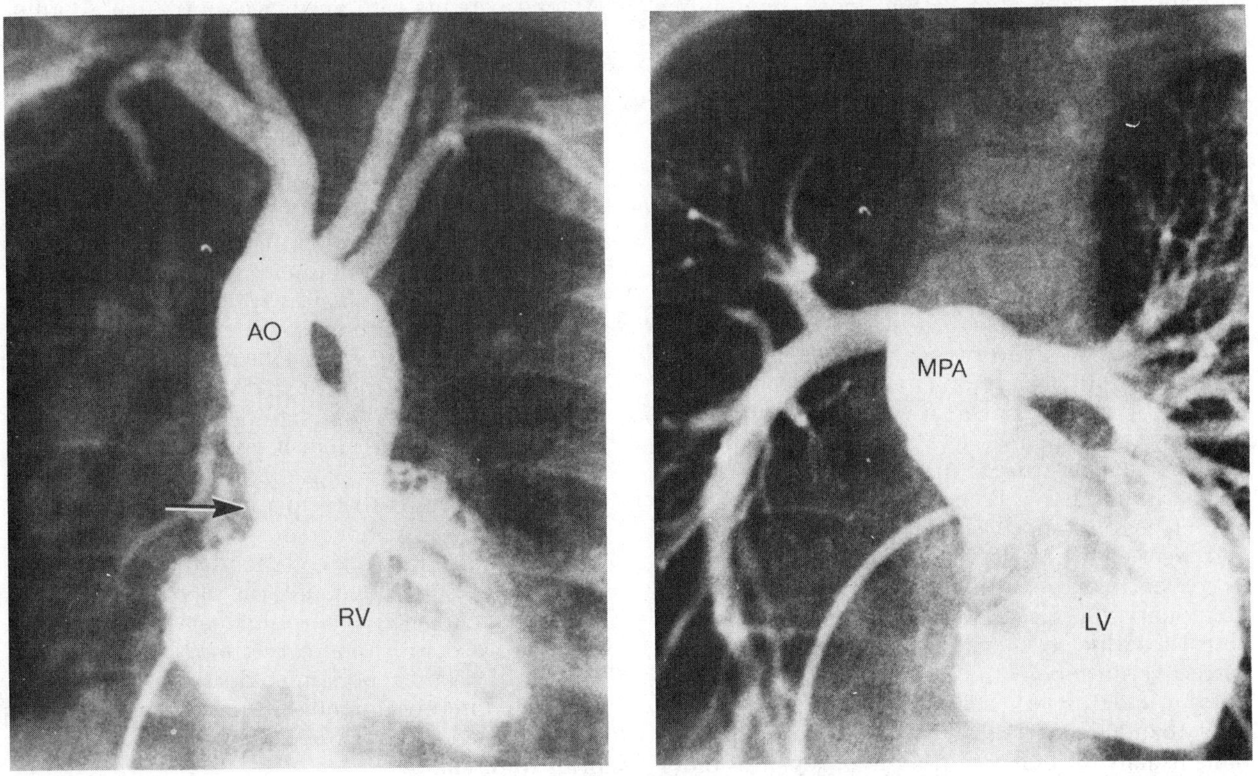

and size of both ventricular chambers. The pulmonary artery can and should be entered using a balloon-guided catheter in all patients with transposition, with the possible exception of very small infants with critical hypoxia and those with extremely severe pulmonary stenosis. All newborns with transposition will benefit from balloon atrial septostomy at initial catheterization by virtue of the increased mixing of the pulmonary and systemic venous circulations and the decompression of the left atrium that will result.

Natural History and Prognosis
Without balloon septostomy or surgical intervention, 50 percent of infants with transposition will die within the first month and 90 percent within the first year of life. Those with an intact ventricular septum die very early from hypoxia. Those with a large ventricular septal defect usually live somewhat longer, but the majority die in the first months of congestive failure, while the few survivors will have severe pulmonary vascular obstructive disease. Those with a large ventricular septal defect and pulmonary stenosis have the best outlook, but the average life expectancy is barely 5 years even with this combination of defects. With an adequate interatrial opening, whether it be natural, balloon-induced, or surgically created, infants with an intact ventricular septum do relatively well during the first year. Easy fatigue and slow weight gain are common, and mild to moderate cyanosis is present, but congestive failure is seldom troublesome. Continuing significant failure following atrial septal defect creation in patients with documented absence of a ventricular septal defect indicates a complicating lesion, most commonly a persistent ductus. Documented spontaneous closure of small ventricular septal defects occurs in perhaps 10 percent of patients; subvalvular pulmonary stenosis develops in approximately one out of seven patients. Increasing cyanosis during the first year in these patients may be due to a gradual diminution of the size of the atrial septal opening, narrowing or closure of a persistent patent ductus or small ventricular septal defect, the gradual development of subvalvular pulmonary stenosis, or the development of pulmonary vascular obstructive disease. Below the age of 2 years, cerebrovascular accidents are a hazard to these hypoxic infants and occur, almost invariably, in a setting of relative anemia rather than extreme polycythemia. The appearance of pulmonary vascular obstructive disease is unusual, but can occur within the first 12 months of life;[542] it becomes more frequent, approaching 10 percent, in the second year of life and thereafter.[543] Infants with a large ventricular septal defect and no significant pulmonary stenosis will develop pulmonary vascular obstructive disease; they become prohibitive risks for corrective surgery by the end of the first year of life unless the defect has been closed or the pulmonary artery banded. After a banding procedure, these infants usually do well and await total repair as older children. Those with a ventricular septal defect and severe pulmonary stenosis usually become progressively more cyanotic and require systemic-to-pulmonary arterial shunting procedures.

Corrective surgery, whether by intraatrial techniques or by a variety of other ingenious surgical interventions, has enabled a relatively large group of patients to survive beyond infancy and early childhood. Among these survivors will be found such residual abnormalities as pulmonary stenosis or pulmonary vascular obstructive disease, as well as complications that are the result of surgery or a consequence of the greater longevity. A small number of patients will develop serious pulmonary or systemic venous obstruction following intraatrial repair and will require appropriate corrective surgery. Whether the result of injury to the sinus node or its artery or to interruption of internodal pathways, postoperative arrhythmias, consisting of tachyarrhythmias, sinus node dysfunction with slow junctional escape rhythms, or atrioventricular conduction abnormalities, occur at one time or another in perhaps 40 percent of patients. While the majority of these arrhythmias are not clinically troublesome, late sudden death has been described in about 3 percent of survivors and is very possibly the result of these or related arrhythmias. Finally, right ventricular dysfunction with or without tricuspid regurgitation has been documented in many of the somewhat older survivors and raises the question of whether the right ventricle can function adequately as the systemic arterial ventricle beyond adolescence and early adult life.[544]

Medical Management
Among patients with an intact ventricular septum, the first step is to establish an adequate interatrial opening. Balloon septostomy should be performed without delay. The adequacy of this opening can be determined by whether there is a sustained increase in the systemic arterial oxygen saturation above 60 percent or P_{O_2} above 30 mmHg; it can also be verified by direct visualization with two-dimensional echocardiography. If the relief of hypoxia is unsatisfactory and the interatrial opening is judged by echocardiography to be small, we recommend surgical atrial septectomy without delay. Another alternative would be to proceed directly with corrective surgery, although the risk of the Mustard or Senning procedures appears to be significantly greater under the age of 4 months than beyond that age.[3] If the response to balloon septostomy is unsatisfactory but the size of the interatrial opening is judged by echocardiography to be adequate, a trial of intravenous prostaglandin E_1 is recommended.[538] If the response is still not adequate, the alternatives would be to create a systemic-to-pulmonary arterial shunt or to proceed with total correction. In the circumstances of a large, persistent ductus arteriosus, an adequate interatrial opening should be created and the ductus closed with indomethacin or operation prior to discharge.

Once an adequate atrial septal defect has been

created, infants with transposition may be followed during the first year of life with the expectation of corrective surgery sometime between 4 and 12 months. Care is taken to prevent anemia or infective endocarditis. Echocardiographic assessment of pulmonary arterial pressure at intervals is recommended. Increasing hypoxia or a suspicion of increasing pulmonary arterial pressure is an indication for prompt recatheterization. Even if the course is uncomplicated, these infants are recatheterized electively at 4 or 10 months of age and the defect repaired shortly thereafter using an intraatrial technique. Experience with direct arterial correction is limited to date but appears encouraging in selected patients.[538] Careful observation for development of pulmonary venous or systemic venous obstruction and arrhythmias following corrective surgery is important, as are the continued precautions against infective endocarditis. Whether or not digitalis should be continued indefinitely in view of the possibility of existing or potential right ventricular dysfunction is unknown, but we have set a very low threshold for its use. Postoperative catheterization a year or two following corrective surgery is appropriate to assess pressure gradients, residual intracardiac shunting, pulmonary vascular resistance, and ventricular function.

Infants with transposition, a large ventricular septal defect, and pulmonary arterial hypertension should either be repaired or undergo banding of the pulmonary artery within the first 4 to 6 months of life if severe pulmonary vascular obstructive disease is to be prevented. Our preference has been pulmonary arterial banding because of the high mortality associated to date with correction of this group during infancy. Children with banding or shunting procedures will require correction at an older age but may benefit from the increased medical and surgical experience that will be available at that time. Finally, the severe hypoxia present in those children with a large ventricular septal defect and severe pulmonary vascular obstructive disease may be reduced, in selected patients, by an intraatrial repair performed as a palliative procedure with no attempt at closure of the ventricular septal defect.[538]

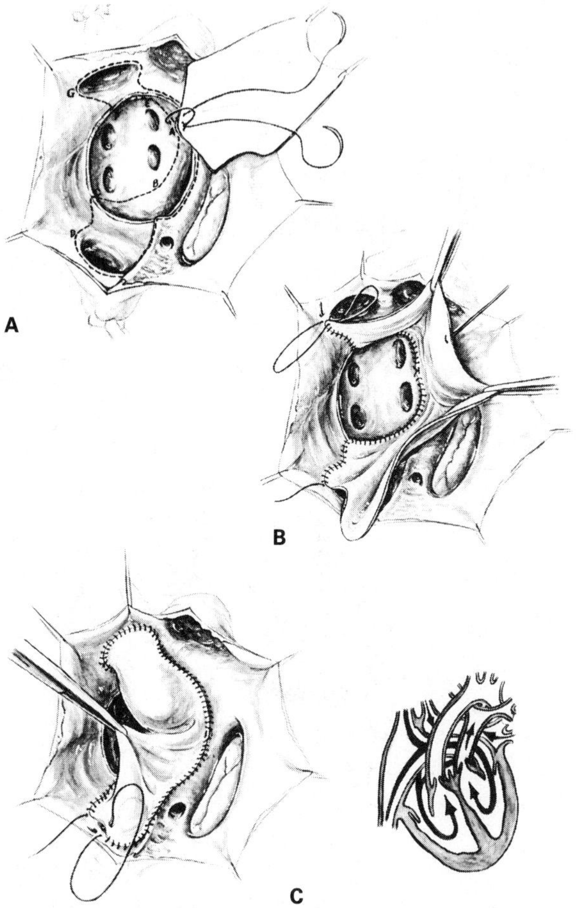

FIGURE 36-75 The Mustard operation with interatrial baffle to invert venous return to correct transposition of the great arteries. *A*, *B*, and *C*. The patch is sutured into place so as to divert systemic venous return to the mitral valve. Pulmonary and coronary venous blood pass to the tricuspid valve. [*From J. W. Kirklin, Surgery for Transposition of the Great Arteries and Other Types of Malpositions of the Great Arteries, in B. G. Barratt-Boyes (ed.), "Heart Disease in Infancy: Diagnosis and Surgical Treatment," Churchill Livingstone, Edinburgh, 1973. Reproduced with permission from the publisher, editor, and author.*]

Surgical Management

Balloon atrial septostomy[545] at initial catheterization is followed by elective physiologic correction during the first year of life using modifications of the interatrial baffle or venous transposition techniques of Mustard[546,547] (Fig. 36-75)[548] or Senning[549,550] (Fig. 36-76). The prosthetic material or pericardium used to construct the baffle in Mustard's operation has produced late caval and pulmonary venous obstruction.[551] This complication prompted the revival of Senning's operation in which viable autogenous atrial septum, appendage, and free wall are used in an effort to minimize fibrosis and growth-related problems.[552]

Both the Mustard and the Senning operations leave the right ventricle to function as the systemic ventricle and the tricuspid valve to contend with systemic systolic pressure. Arterial "switch" operations[553] have recently evolved as an appealing physiologic alternative, restoring the left ventricle and mitral valve to the role of systemic ventricle and systemic atrioventricular valve. These operations are complicated by the need for an adequately prepared left ventricle capable of supporting cardiac output against systemic vascular resistance, the technical challenge of coronary arterial translocation in the infant, and uncertainty pertaining to growth of circular suture lines in the aorta, pulmonary artery, and around the coronary orifices. Recent early and intermediate follow-up is encouraging.[552–555] Accumulation of operative experience and careful follow-up in a few centers is required before arterial switching should be universally adopted.

Early physiologic or anatomic correction has superseded staged palliation in most centers, but excision of the interatrial septum by the Blalock-

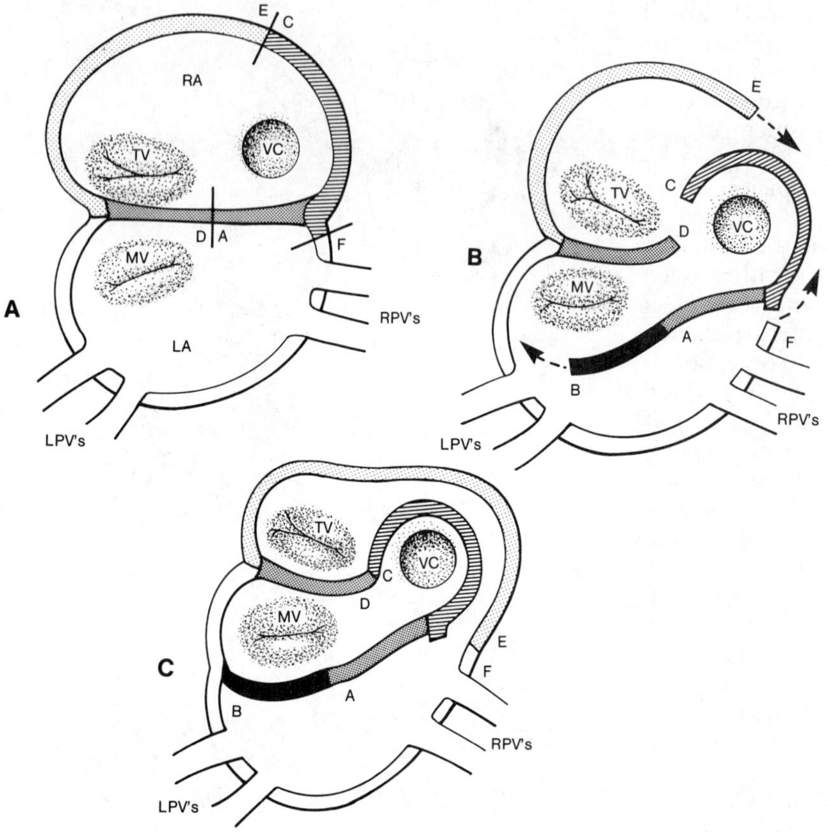

FIGURE 36-76 Senning operation for interatrial transposition of venous return to correct transposition of the great arteries. Incisions in the right atrium (E/C) and left atrium just anterior to the right pulmonary veins (F) combined with detachment of the atrial septum (D/A) allow the creation of an interatrial baffle directing systemic venous blood from the venae cavae (VC) through the mitral valve (MV) while pulmonary venous blood is directed through the tricuspid orifice (TV). The atrial septum is sutured anteriorly and to the left of the left pulmonary veins (B). When deficient, the atrial septum is augmented with a small prosthetic patch (solid dark line). The posterior edge of the right atrial wall is attached to the atrial septum between the mitral and tricuspid orifices (D). Right and left atria are approximated just anterior to the right pulmonary veins (E/F) to create the pulmonary venous atrium. Enlargement of this chamber with a small pericardial patch is occasionally required. In many cases the use of prosthetic material can be avoided entirely, a possible advantage of the Senning operation over the Mustard procedure. RPV = right pulmonary vein; LPV = left pulmonary vein.

Hanlon[556] or inflow occlusion[557] technique remains an acceptable alternative for initial management of the infant having persistent hypoxemia after balloon atrial septostomy. Intracardiac correction can then be performed when the child is older, larger, and metabolically stable. Repair should probably not be delayed beyond 12 to 18 months however; increasing pulmonary vascular resistance will compromise the outcome.[558]

Repairs of complex forms of transposition of the great arteries, including those with associated ventricular septal defect[550] and subpulmonic left ventricular outflow tract obstruction[559] or double-outlet right ventricle (the Taussig-Bing heart),[560] are beyond the scope of this discussion. Combinations of patch closure of ventricular septal defects, resection of obstruction, extracardiac conduits, interatrial baffle procedures, and arterial switch operations are being evaluated in small groups of appropriately palliated patients. Initial management of infants having these complex defects consists of provision of adequate intracardiac mixing of systemic and pulmonary venous blood by atrial septostomy or surgical septectomy and the adjustment of pulmonary blood flow by pulmonary arterial banding or the creation of a systemic arterial–to–pulmonary arterial shunt. Complex anatomic repairs are accomplished later, when risk of injury to the conduction system and growth-related problems imposed by the repair are less significant.

Double-Outlet Right Ventricle

Pathology

In this malformation more than 90 percent of both great arteries arise from the morphologic right ventricle. Situs solitus (S) is usual. In most cases the ventricles display a d loop (D), and the pulmonary arterial origin is normally positioned, arising from a conus above the right ventricle. The aorta also arises from the right ventricle above a second conus. The two semilunar valves are at about the same level and there is no fibrous continuity between the semilunar and mitral valves (Fig. 36-77).

In most cases the aortic origin is to the right (d malposition) of the pulmonary arterial origin, the two vessels usually displaying a side-by-side relationship. Uncommonly, the aortic origin is distinctly anterior to the pulmonary origin or the aorta arises to the left (l malposition) of the pulmonary artery.[561]

With rare exceptions, there is a ventricular septal defect. The condition may be further subdivided on the basis of the position of the ventricular septal defect with regard to the arterial origins. The ventricular septal defect will be subaortic in approximately two-thirds of patients, subpulmonary (*Taussig-Bing heart*) in 20 percent, related to both great arteries (*doubly committed*) in 3 percent, and remote or unrelated to either great artery in about 7 percent.[561]

When in situs solitus there is ventricular inversion (atrioventricular discordance) and double-outlet right

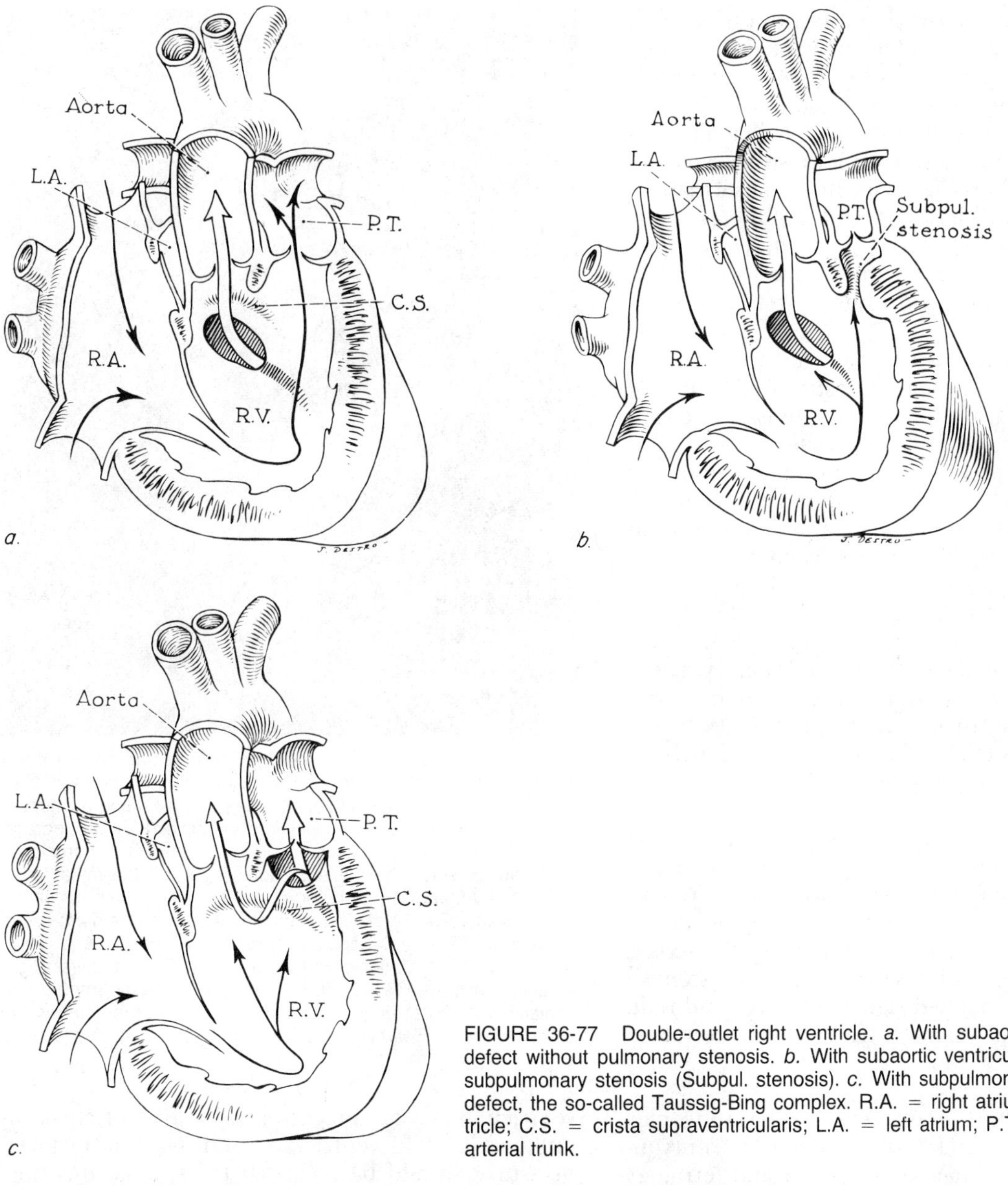

FIGURE 36-77 Double-outlet right ventricle. *a.* With subaortic ventricular septal defect without pulmonary stenosis. *b.* With subaortic ventricular septal defect and subpulmonary stenosis (Subpul. stenosis). *c.* With subpulmonary ventricular septal defect, the so-called Taussig-Bing complex. R.A. = right atrium; R.V. = right ventricle; C.S. = crista supraventricularis; L.A. = left atrium; P.T. = main pulmonary arterial trunk.

ventricle, both great vessels arise from the left-sided anatomic right ventricle. Such cases should not be confused with double-outlet left ventricle.

Associated Conditions Pulmonary stenosis occurs in over half of cases, the condition usually resulting from a narrow subpulmonary conus. Atrial septal defect, subaortic stenosis, and coarctation of the aorta are also relatively common, with the latter particularly associated with the subpulmonary defect. Obstruction at the mitral valve may be observed in about one-fifth of cases of double-outlet right ventricle. Mitral valve straddling of the ventricular septal defect and varying degrees of left ventricular hypoplasia also are encountered.[561,562]

Clinical Manifestations

Double-outlet right ventricle, or origin of both great arteries from the right ventricle, is a relatively rare malformation found in only 0.5 percent of patients with congenital heart disease.[6] It is of considerable importance, however, because its clinical and laboratory features frequently resemble those of more common and more easily correctable malformations. The incidence among males and females is equal, except in the presence of pulmonary stenosis where two-thirds are male.[3] An association with trisomy 18 syndrome has been described. The clinical picture depends almost entirely upon the presence or absence of pulmonary stenosis and the relation of the ventricular septal defect to the aortic and pulmonary valves.

History and Physical Examination Patients with a subaortic ventricular septal defect without pulmonary stenosis (Fig. 36-77*A*) have the same findings on examination as do patients with a large isolated ventricular septal defect. Congestive failure appears within a few weeks of birth, and cyanosis is seldom described. Those with a subaortic ventricular septal defect and pulmonary stenosis (Fig. 36-77*B*) usually present after the newborn period and follow a course similar to patients with tetralogy of Fallot. Patients with a subpulmonary defect without pulmonary stenosis (Fig. 36-77*C*), the Taussig-Bing malformation, resemble patients with transposition of the great arteries and a large ventricular septal defect without pulmonary stenosis. The findings are those of severe congestive failure and impressive cyanosis.

Chest Roentgenogram Cardiomegaly with pulmonary overperfusion is characteristic of all types of this anomaly without pulmonary stenosis. The similarity of double-outlet right ventricle with subaortic ventricular septal defect and pulmonary stenosis to tetralogy of Fallot extends to a 30 percent incidence of right aortic arch. However, in double-outlet right ventricle the cardiac contour is seldom boot-shaped and heart size tends to be somewhat larger than it is in patients with classic tetralogy of Fallot. If the patient has subpulmonary ventricular septal defect without pulmonary stenosis, the pulmonary artery usually lies beside rather than posterior to the aorta; this clearly visible, dilated main pulmonary artery may permit distinction of this malformation from transposition, which it mimics so closely.

Electrocardiogram Right axis deviation and right atrial and right ventricular hypertrophy are characteristic of double-outlet right ventricle. Among patients with subaortic ventricular septal defect without pulmonary stenosis, a superior QRS axis is relatively common. Patients with pulmonary stenosis usually have more marked right ventricular and right atrial hypertrophy than do patients with tetralogy of Fallot.

Echocardiogram M-mode echocardiography may distinguish double-outlet right ventricle from uncomplicated ventricular septal defect and tetralogy of Fallot by demonstrating a lack of continuity between the anterior mitral leaflet and the posterior aortic annulus. Two-dimensional echocardiography is capable of demonstrating the commitment of both great arteries to the right ventricle as well as mitral-semilunar discontinuity (Fig. 36-78),[563] left ventricular hypoplasia, and important atrioventricular valvular anomalies.[563]

Cardiac Catheterization In double-outlet right ventricle, there will be an increase in oxygen saturation at the right ventricular level. The pulmonary arterial saturation usually is lower than that of the aorta in patients with a subaortic ventricular septal defect and is invariably higher than that of the aorta in those with a subpulmonary septal defect. Aortic and right ventricular and left ventricular systolic pressures usually are equal, but the left ventricular systolic pressure may be higher than the right if the ventricular septal defect is small and restrictive. Simultaneous left ventricular and systemic arterial pressures should be recorded to evaluate this possibility. The possibility of mitral valve abnormalities and of pulmonary or aortic stenosis should be determined. Selective right and left ventricular biplane angiography is recommended to determine the size of the ventricular septal defect and its relation to the great arteries, the presence of conal tissue beneath both semilunar valves, and the spatial relation of the great arteries. Lack of mitral-aortic continuity can be seen in the lateral view. An aortogram is recommended to exclude a persistent ductus and anomalies of the coronary arterial distribution that might interfere with the surgical approach.

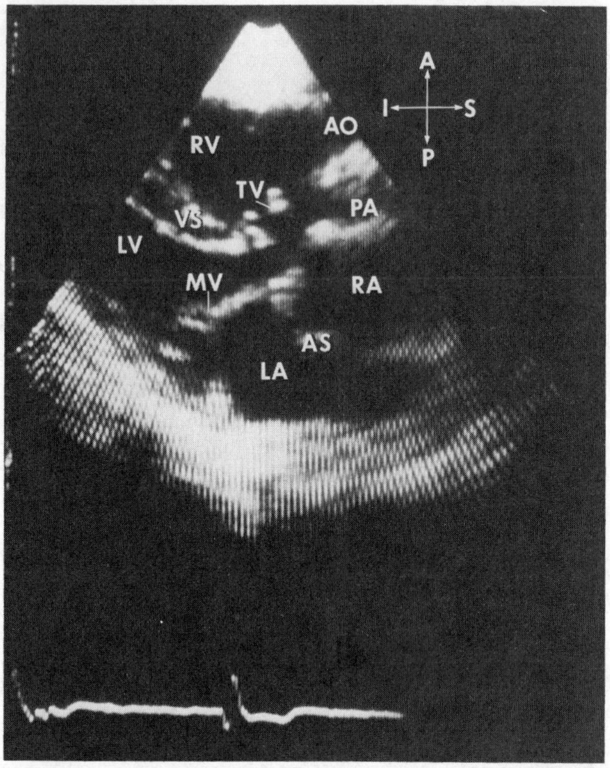

FIGURE 36-78 Two-dimensional echocardiogram in the parasternal long-axis view from a patient with double-outlet right ventricle and ventricular septal defect. The aorta (AO) and pulmonary artery (PA) both arise from the right ventricle (RV) in a parallel orientation anterior to the ventricular septum (VS). There is no continuity between the posterior aortic wall and the mitral valve (MV). A = anterior; I = inferior; S = superior; P = posterior; TV = tricuspid valve; LV = left ventricle; RA = right atrium; LA = left atrium; AS = atrial septum. (*From D. J. Hagler, A. J. Tajik, J. B. Seward, D. D. Mair, and D. G. Ritter, Double-Outlet Right Ventricle, Wide-Angle, Two-Dimensional Echocardiographic Observations, Circulation, 63:419, 1981. Reproduced by permission of the American Heart Association, Inc., and the authors.*)

Natural History and Prognosis

The clinical course of each variety of double-outlet right ventricle is determined by the associated defects. Without surgical intervention, those with an unguarded pulmonary artery either die in infancy with congestive failure or develop pulmonary vascular obstructive disease. Spontaneous narrowing or closure of the ventricular septal defect may indeed occur and is life-threatening. Increasing dyspnea, increasing intensity of the systolic murmur, and progressive left ventricular hypertrophy suggest this complication. Patients with pulmonary stenosis tend to have progresssive obstruction and cyanosis.

Medical Management

The defects in the majority of patients with double-outlet right ventricle can be corrected surgically. Until recently it has been our recommendation to band the pulmonary artery of all infants with double-outlet right ventricle who have increased pulmonary blood flow and significant pulmonary arterial hypertension. Selected infants with these findings and a subaortic ventricular septal defect are probably best managed today by total correction between the age of 3 and 12 months. Infants with Taussig-Bing malformation have been managed with a combination of pulmonary arterial banding and atrial septal defect creation, with corrective surgery postponed until the age of 5 or 6 years. Systemic-to-pulmonary arterial shunts are performed in those patients with cyanosis and diminished pulmonary blood flow, with correction postponed until the patient is large enough to accept, if necessary, an external valved conduit. Whether or not corrective surgery has been performed, all patients in whom the left ventricular output must pass through the ventricular septal defect should be observed continuously for the possibility of spontaneous narrowing and obstruction at that site.

Surgical Management

Great variability exists in the morphologic spectrum of double-outlet right ventricle.[564–566] Surgical correction requires (1) closure of the ventricular septal defect, (2) relief of pulmonary stenosis in about 20 percent of cases, (3) diversion of pulmonary venous blood through the ventricular septal defect to the aorta, and (4) diversion of systemic venous blood to the pulmonary artery.[566] When the ventricular septal defect is committed to the aorta, a Dacron semiconduit or tunnel-shaped patch is placed to obliterate the interventricular communication while diverting the left ventricular blood through the ventricular septal defect to the aorta (Fig. 36-79).[567] Pulmonary stenosis is corrected by a valvotomy with excision of obstructing muscle bundles and placement of a transannular patch when necessary. Otherwise, an extracardiac conduit is placed between the systemic venous ventricle and the pulmonary artery.[564,568]

Consideration of repair of double-outlet right ventricle associated with atrioventricular discordance, situs ambiguus, d malposition of the aorta, and other complex subsets is beyond the scope of this discussion.[564–566,569]

Palliation (pulmonary arterial banding, atrial septal excision, and creation of systemic arterial–to–pulmonary arterial shunts) still plays a significant role in the management of complex variants of double-outlet right ventricle in infancy.[564]

In a 10-year review of repair of classic double-outlet right ventricle in 62 patients,[569] early mortality was 15 percent. Among the 53 survivors of the operation, 11 late deaths (21 percent) occurred, 10 of which were attributable to arrhythmias. All but one of the surviving patients were in New York Heart Association class I or II.

Double-Outlet Left Ventricle

Pathology

Rarely, both great vessels arise entirely, or predominantly, above the morphologic left ventricle.

The aorta may lie either to the left or the right

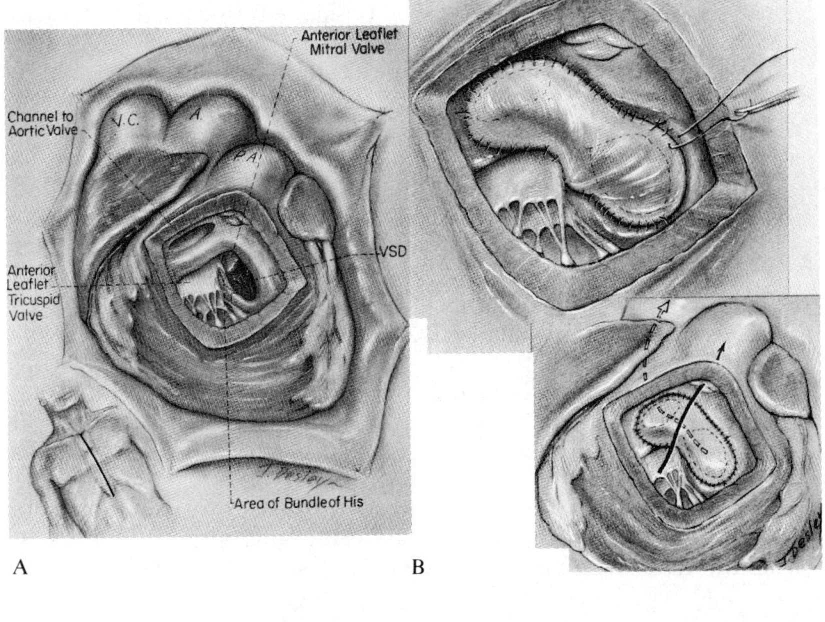

FIGURE 36-79 *A.* The anatomy of double-outlet right ventricle with subaortic ventricular septal defect as viewed through the right ventriculotomy incision. Note that there is no continuity between atrioventricular valves and semilunar valves and that the ventricular septal defect is in a subaortic position. *B.* The patch has been sutured into place so as to close the interventricular communication and to conduct blood from the ventricular septal defect to the aorta. (*From J. W. Kirklin, R. A. Karp, and D. C. McGoon, Surgical Treatment of Origin of Both Vessels from Right Ventricle, Including Cases with Pulmonary Stenosis, J. Thorac. Cardiovasc. Surg., 48:1026, 1964. Reproduced with permission from the publisher and authors.*)

of the pulmonary artery. A ventricular septal defect and pulmonary stenosis are usually associated.[570]

Clinical Manifestations

The clinical manifestations of this extremely rare anomaly are similar to those of tricuspid atresia, tetralogy of Fallot, or transposition of the great arteries with ventricular septal defect. Most patients, then, are cyanotic. The diagnosis depends upon high-quality selective biplane angiography with special attention paid to the location of the ventricular septal defect (if such exists), the relation of the great arteries to the septal defect, and the interrelations and origin of the great arteries themselves. Tricuspid valve abnormalities are common, as are varying degrees of right ventricular hypoplasia. This malformation is correctable in some patients.[570]

Surgical Management

Significant pulmonary stenosis or pulmonary arterial hypoplasia and a ventricular septal defect may require palliation by the creation of a systemic arterial–to–pulmonary arterial shunt prior to consideration of total anatomic or physiologic repair of double-outlet left ventricle. Few corrections have been accomplished;[571–574] the first successful repair utilized an intraventricular baffle to close the ventricular septal defect and to direct systemic venous blood to the pulmonary artery.[574] This approach is probably less generally applicable than simple closure of the ventricular septal defect, closure of the proximal pulmonary artery, and establishment of right ventricular–to–pulmonary arterial continuity by use of an extracardiac conduit. When repair is complicated by right ventricular hypoplasia or right atrioventricular valve abnormalities, the Fontan concept of direct right atrial–to–pulmonary arterial anastomosis with closure of the atrial septal defect and tricuspid valve orifice is applicable if the pulmonary arteries are anatomically adequate and the pulmonary vascular resistance is low.

Corrected Transposition of the Great Arteries

Definition

Atrioventricular discordance and ventriculoarterial discordance form the characteristics of corrected transposition.

Pathology

Usually situs solitus is present (S), but the ventricles are inverted (an l loop) (L). The great vessels are transposed and in the l position so that the pulmonary artery arises from the right-sided morphologic left ventricle and the anterior, l-transposed aorta arises from the left-sided right ventricle, yielding an SLL pattern (Fig. 36-80). Along with the ventricular inversion there is atrioventricular valve inversion. The mitral valve is on the right and shows fibrous continuity with the pulmonary valve, while the tricuspid valve is on the left. If situs inversus is present, the segmental pattern is IDD.

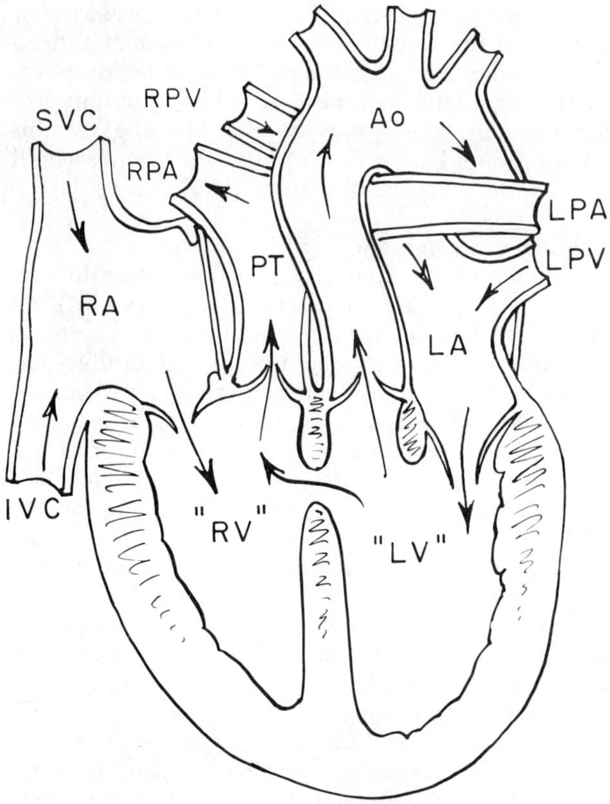

FIGURE 36-80 Corrected transposition with ventricular septal defect, "RV" and "LV" represent the right-sided and left-sided ventricles, respectively. Anatomically, "RV" is the morphologic left ventricle, and "LV" is the morphologic right ventricle. SVC = superior vena cava; IVC = inferior vena cava; RA = right atrium; PT = main pulmonary arterial trunk; RPA = right pulmonary artery; LPA = left pulmonary artery; RPV = right pulmonary vein; LPV = left pulmonary vein; LA = left atrium; Ao = aorta.

The aortic arch usually is left-sided. The anterior of the three aortic sinuses in the noncoronary one, while the two coronary arteries arise from the right and left (posteriorly positioned) sinuses. The courses of the arteries are inverted. The cardiac apex points to the right in about 25 percent of cases.

Associated Conditions Rarely, no associated conditions are present and the circulation is normal.[575] In the majority of cases of corrected transposition of the great arteries (about 80 percent) a ventricular septal defect is present. Two types of ventricular septal defect have been described, one lies beneath both semilunar valves and the other lies beneath the pulmonary valve but is remote from the aortic valve.[576]

In about half the cases, whether or not a septal defect is present, the inverted left-sided tricuspid valve shows some degree of an Ebstein-like malformation. It may be incompetent.

Pulmonary atresia or stenosis, the latter sometimes with an intact ventricular septum, is present in about 70 percent of cases.[577] The obstruction is usually subvalvular, being a mirror image of membranous subaortic stenosis or resulting from accessory tissue of the anterior mitral leaflet. Patent ductus, atrial septal defect, coarctation of the aorta, mitral stenosis, and single ventricle are less common abnormalities.

Clinical Manifestations

Corrected transposition is an uncommon malformation, occurring in slightly less than 1 percent of children with congenital heart disease. Males are slightly more commonly affected than females, in a 1.4:1 ratio.[6] The importance of this anomaly lies in its frequent association with serious atrioventricular conduction disturbances and intracardiac malformations, and in the medical and surgical implications of the ventricular inversion. The clinical picture is determined primarily by the associated anomalies. In addition to the structural abnormalities described above, about 15 percent will have either second degree or third degree atrioventricular block. The clinical manifestations described below will pertain to those patients with left atrioventricular valve regurgitation or atrioventricular block, ventricular septal defect without pulmonary stenosis, and ventricular septal defect with significant pulmonary stenosis.

History A slow, irregular heart rate is often detected in utero, and 10 percent of patients with congenital complete block will prove to have corrected transposition. Those patients with a large ventricular septal defect without pulmonary stenosis usually present within the first month or so of life with symptoms which are indistinguishable from those of infants with a large septal defect alone. Patients with ventricular septal defect and pulmonary stenosis generally present with symptoms of cyanosis and resemble patients with tetralogy of Fallot.

Physical Examination The murmur of left atrioventricular valve regurgitation may be best heard either at the apex or at the lower left sternal border and is described as not radiating so well to the axilla as does the murmur of rheumatic mitral regurgitation. Occasionally an inordinately accentuated second heart sound at the upper left sternal border will suggest the presence of pulmonary arterial hypertension, although in reality it represents the sound of aortic valve closure augmented to auscultation by the anterior and superior displacement of the aorta. Dyspnea, a hyperdynamic precordium, a pansystolic murmur, and an apical middiastolic rumble are characteristic of the patient with a large ventricular septal defect. Those with a ventricular septal defect and associated pulmonary stenosis have the physical findings of tetralogy of Fallot except for the accentuated second heart sound. In a few patients, the murmur of pulmonary stenosis may be louder to the right of the sternum than to the left.

Chest Roentgenogram The usual, slightly convex shadow of the ascending aorta along the upper right border of the heart will be absent in corrected transposition. The right pulmonary artery, angled upward slightly and emerging at the same level as the left pulmonary artery, may create a "waterfall" appearance as it curves inferiorly. Among those patients with increased pulmonary blood flow or pulmonary arterial hypertension, the absence of the expected pulmonary arterial dilatation in the usual location should suggest a displaced main pulmonary artery. A straight or gently curved convex upper left heart border, representing the contour of the transposed ascending aorta, is characteristic and is seen most frequently in those patients with a ventricular septal defect and pulmonary stenosis, in whom there is a mild dilatation of the ascending aorta.

Electrocardiogram Varying degrees of atrioventricular conduction delay are present in almost a third of patients, with half of these having second or third degree block. The initial forces of ventricular depolarization are oriented anteriorly and to the left, with Q waves in the right precordial leads and not in leads I, V_5, and V_6. Absence of left precordial Q waves is not invariable, however.[578] With normal or near normal pressure in the systemic venous or morphologic left ventricle, a QS pattern in the right and an RS pattern in the left precordial leads is usual. Similarly upright T waves in the right precordial leads and somewhat flattened T waves in the left are a frequent pattern.

Echocardiogram With the M-mode technique, it may be difficult or impossible to record ventricular septal echoes since the long axis of the septum lies nearly perpendicular to the anterior chest wall. There is no continuity between the left atrioventricular valve and a semilunar valve, but there is continuity between the right atrioventricular valve and the posterior semilunar valve. Two-dimensional echocardiography permits identification of the characteristic morphology of the ventricles, identification of the aorta and pulmonary artery, and recognition of important associated anomalies.[579]

Cardiac Catheterization From the right atrium the morphologic left ventricle is entered, and, in the presence of a ventricular septal defect, the catheter may cross the defect, traverse the morphologic right ventricle, and enter the ascending aorta in the position normally occupied by the pulmonary artery. Entry into the medially placed pulmonary artery may be much more difficult, but the use of flow-guided catheters will permit successful entry for measurement of pressure in most instances. Selective angiography in the right-sided morphologic left ventricle will reveal the characteristic "sock" shape and smooth walls, as well as the medially placed main pulmonary artery with its almost symmetrical right and left branches. Angiography in the left-sided

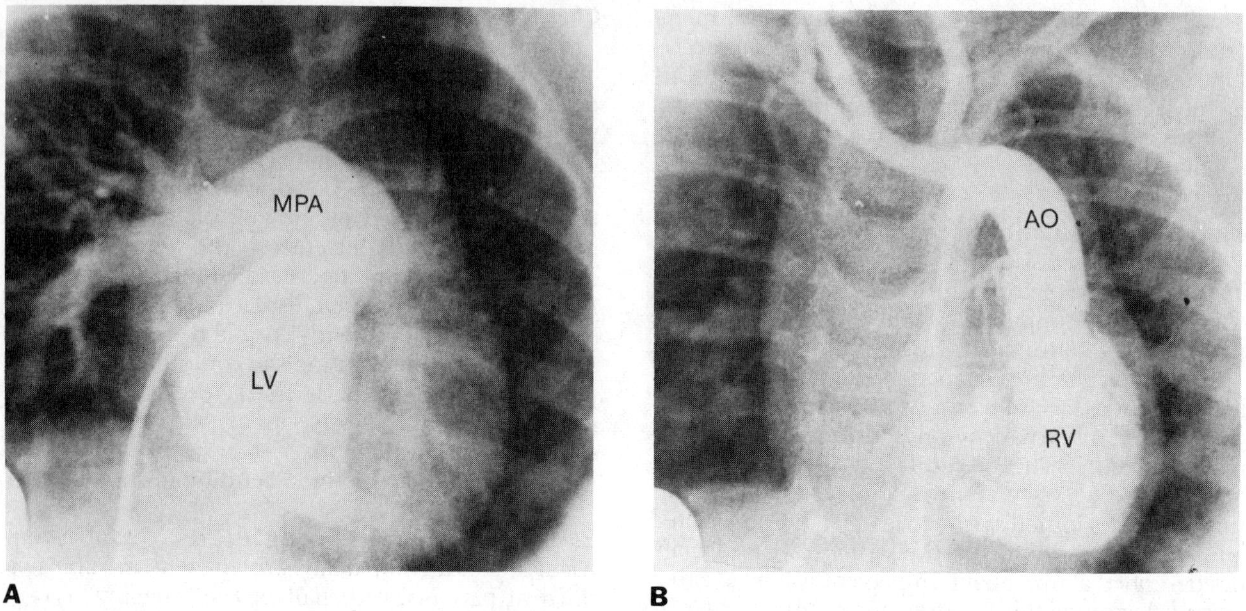

FIGURE 36-81 *A.* Posteroanterior view of the left ventricular (LV) angiogram in a child with corrected transposition of the great arteries. The main pulmonary artery (MPA) arises from the smooth-walled left ventricle, which receives the systemic venous blood. *B.* Posteroanterior view of the right ventricular angiogram (RV). The ascending aorta (AO) arises to the left of the pulmonary artery from the more heavily trabeculated right ventricle, which receives the pulmonary venous blood. The ventricular septum, seen here perpendicular to the frontal plane, is intact.

morphologic right ventricle permits assessment of chamber size and competency of the left atrioventricular valve. The ventricular septum usually lies in the anteroposterior plane, and a ventricular septal defect may be seen best in the frontal view (Fig. 36-81). Gentle manipulation of the catheter within the heart is indicated, since the production of varying degrees of transient atrioventricular block is not uncommon and, in a rare instance, may prove permanent.

Natural History and Prognosis

The clinical course is determined primarily by the severity of the associated defects. It is estimated that only about 1 percent of individuals with corrected transposition have an otherwise normal heart. Even with complicating anomalies, survival to adulthood is possible, with one-quarter of the patients in a large clinical series being over 16 years of age.[578] Congestive heart failure associated with a large ventricular septal defect has been the most common cause of death, with most fatalities occurring within the first year of life. Atrioventricular conduction abnormalites tend to be progressive and complete atrioventricular block may appear at any age. Similarly left atrioventricular valve regurgitation may present at any age, but in the majority this is detected in infancy and early childhood. Even without associated malformations, or following correction of these abnormalities, the question remains as to whether the morphologic right ventricle is capable of sustaining adequate cardiac output over a normal life span.

Medical Management

Management of corrected transposition includes the treatment of congestive failure and the prevention of infective endocarditis. Patients with large ventricular septal defects and severe pulmonary hypertension or congestive heart failure should undergo early banding of the pulmonary artery or repair of the defect. Similarly those patients with a ventricular septal defect, severe pulmonary stenosis, and cyanosis will benefit from systemic-to-pulmonary artery shunting procedures or total correction. The vulnerability of the ventricular conduction system, and the difficulty in visualization of the septal defect and the subpulmonary region of the morphologic left ventricle, have influenced us to recommend the palliative approach in both groups of patients, especially during infancy. The incidence of surgically induced atrioventricular block has been reduced substantially, although not eliminated, with intraoperative mapping of the conduction system. This system arises from an anterior atrioventricular node, crosses anterior to the pulmonary artery, and descends along the anterior and superior aspect of the ventricular septal defect in patients with situs solitus. Patients with complete atrioventricular block induced surgically should be managed, without exception, by the insertion of a permanent pacemaker. Those with congenital block may require pacemaker therapy if they are symptomatic. Patients symptomatic with left atrioventricular valve regurgitation will require valve replacement. Regularly scheduled follow-up examinations are recommended for all patients with corrected transposition of the great arteries, with or without associated anomalies, in order to detect progressive atrioventricular conduction disorders and the late appearance of left atrioventricular valve incompetence.

Surgical Management

Ventricular septal defect closure and relief of pulmonary stenosis are often required in patients having congenital corrected transposition of the great arteries.[580,581] The specialized electrical conduction system is particularly at risk in these patients because of its right-sided location and abnormal anatomic course. Approach to the ventricular septal defect through an incision in the left-sided ventricle,[582] placement of sutures through the septal defect on the left side of the septum, and the use of intracardiac mapping[580] appear to reduce the incidence of complete heart block.

Of 17 patients undergoing intracardiac repair of defects associated with congenital corrected transposition of the great arteries,[581] all had large ventricular septal defects requiring closure; 8 had associated pulmonary stenosis for which surgical intervention was required. A valve-containing extracardiac conduit was implanted in 4 of the patients having obstruction to pulmonary blood flow. Left atrioventricular valve incompetence required tricuspid valve replacement in 3. There were 4 hospital deaths (23.5 percent), 2 late deaths (11.8 percent), 6 instances of atrioventricular dissociation (37.5 percent), and 6 cases of postoperative tricuspid valvular incompetence. A more recent review of 18 patients[580] revealed similar outcomes.

Repair of intracardiac defects in those individuals having congenital corrected transposition of the great arteries is clearly associated with a greater than usual operative risk and the likelihood of residual defects, but repair is probably indicated because of the potential for increased longevity and improved quality of life.

Single Ventricle

Definition

As used here, *single ventricle*,[583] also called *common ventricle* or *univentricular heart*, is characterized by the entire flow from the two atria being carried directly through the mitral and tricuspid valves into the same ventricular chamber. This *double-inlet* type of atrioventricular connection may take the form of either one common or two separate atrioventricular valves.[584] As used here, cases of either mitral or tricuspid atresia are excluded. The ventriculoarterial connections may be *concordant* (pulmonary artery from the right ventricle and aorta from left ventricle), *discordant* (pulmonary artery from left ventricle and aorta from right ventricle), *double-outlet* (both great arteries from either the left or right ventricle), or *single-outlet* (atresia of one great artery).

Pathology

The most common type (65 to 75 percent of cases)[585] is that in which the dominant ventricular chamber has the trabecular pattern of a left ventricle and communicates through an opening, the bulboventricular foramen, with an infundibulum or rudimentary right ventricle. The ventriculoarterial connection is discordant (transposition of the great arteries) in about 90 percent of patients (Fig. 36-82).[584] The uncommon concordant connection is referred to as the *Holmes heart*.[586] In about 20 percent of cases the dominant ventricle shows the trabecular features of a right ventricle and the rudimentary chamber those of a left ventricle. The majority of these patients have a double-outlet ventriculoarterial connection from the main chamber, and a smaller number have a single-outlet connection, with pulmonary atresia.[587] In 10 to 14 percent neither ventricular sinus can be identified; this is the so-called primitive ventricle.[584,585]

In about 80 percent of cases of single ventricle the great vessels are malposed (about equally levo and dextro in position), the aorta arising from the infundibulum or rudimentary right ventricle when one is present. The position of the infundibulum usually corresponds to the position of the aorta.

Associated Conditions Pulmonary stenosis or atresia may be observed in about 25 percent of cases when the single ventricle is not associated with asplenia. If the latter condition is present, total obstruction to pulmonary flow occurs in most cases. Subaortic stenosis may result from a narrow bulboventricular foramen. The main tendency for as-

FIGURE 36-82 Common ventricle with dextro-malposition and without pulmonary stenosis. T = tricuspid valve; M = mitral valve.

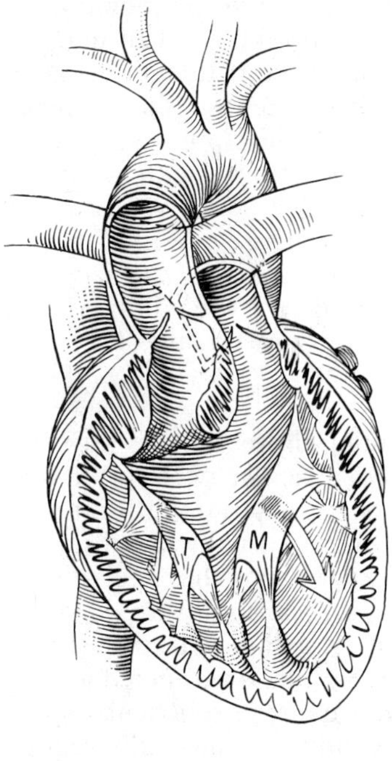

sociated cardiovascular abnormalities is observed when asplenia is present.

Clinical Manifestations

This complex and challenging malformation is relatively rare and is found in only 1.5 percent of individuals with congenital heart disease.[6] Males are slightly more commonly afflicted than females, in a 1.6:1 ratio.[3] Interestingly, 70 percent of patients reported with single ventricle of the left ventricular type, pulmonary stenosis, and normally related great arteries have been female.[588] The clinical picture is determined largely by the associated defects, of which pulmonary stenosis, present in a little over half of the patients, is the most important.

History All patients will have some degree of systemic arterial oxygen desaturation, although cyanosis, appreciated clinically, may range from barely detectable to severe. Infants without significant pulmonary stenosis will present with little or no cyanosis but with features of congestive failure. Those with severe pulmonary stenosis or atresia will be hypoxic and resemble patients with tetralogy of Fallot. Approximately 60 percent of all patients with single ventricle will require hospitalization within the first month of life.[3]

Physical Examination The findings on palpation and auscultation are not distinctive of single ventricle but mimic those of patients with a large ventricular septal defect, tetralogy of Fallot, or transposition. The presence of a left-sided or symmetrical liver should arouse suspicion of a more complicated lesion.

Chest Roentgenogram Almost all patients with single ventricle have at least some degree of cardiac enlargement. Those with little or no pulmonary stenosis generally have very large hearts with marked pulmonary plethora. Only those patients with atresia or very severe pulmonary stenosis show a near-normal heart size and diminished pulmonary arterial blood flow. Those few patients with normally related great arteries will have a clearly visible or prominent pulmonary arterial segment. The remainder will either have the narrow cardiac base characteristic of d transposition or the mildly convex left upper cardiac border characteristic of l transposition.

Electrocardiogram Among those patients with single ventricle of the left ventricular type and d-ventricular loop, the pattern usually is one of left ventricular hypertrophy. Q waves usually are absent in all precordial leads. The QRS axis characteristically lies between 0 and +90°. A superior QRS axis would suggest the presence of an associated atrioventricular canal malformation, but this is also noted among those few patients with the above ventricular morphology, pulmonary stenosis, and normally related great arteries. Patients with single ventricle of the left ventricular type but with an l-ventricular loop generally have a pattern of right or biventricular hypertrophy. These patients may also show evidence of significant atrioventricular block. The characteristic pattern of single ventricle of the right ventricular type is less well defined, but a superior QRS axis is present in the majority and right ventricular hypertrophy appears to be the rule.[587] A few patients with single ventricle will have an rS pattern across the entire precordium.

Echocardiography M-mode echocardiography may establish the diagnosis by simultaneous recording of two atrioventricular valves without interposing septal echoes on a base-to-apex scan. An anterior outflow chamber, if present, usually can be identified anterior to both atrioventricular valves.[589] Two-dimensional echocardiography can identify most of the anatomic abnormalities with a very high degree of accuracy.[584,585]

Cardiac Catheterization An increase in oxygen saturation will be found at the ventricular level and frequently at the atrial level as well. A degree of systemic arterial oxygen desaturation will be present in all patients. Preferential streaming of pulmonary venous blood to either the aorta or the pulmonary artery may vary, but the level of systemic arterial saturation appears to be related more to the volume of pulmonary blood flow than to the orientation of the great arteries or the type of single ventricle. Careful recording of intracardiac and arterial pressures is essential in order to detect significant or potentially significant obstruction to blood flow across either atrioventricular valve, across the atrial septum, or between the single ventricle and the aorta or pulmonary artery. The mode of atrioventricular connection is of particular importance. The presence of two atrioventricular valves or the presence of a single atrioventricular valve in the form of a common orifice can be confirmed by a combination of selective catheter passage and visualization of the common or separate orifices as negative-contrast areas following ventricular angiography. The morphologic features of the ventricle, relation of the aorta and pulmonary artery, and other features can be established by high-quality selective ventricular angiography using specially angled views to supplement conventional views.[584,587,590]

Natural History and Prognosis

Patients with single ventricle usually present within the first month or two of life with cyanosis, congestive failure, or a combination of both. Almost half of these patients expire before the age of 1 year as a result of these complications or attempted surgical palliation.[3] Those in whom the pulmonary arterial pressure and blood flow are increased require surgical banding of the pulmonary artery to avoid death from congestive heart failure or progressive pulmonary vascular obstructive disease. Those patients with severe pulmonary stenosis and serious hypoxia will require systemic-to-pulmonary arterial shunting procedures. Among patients with single ventricle there is a propensity for the development of subaortic obstruction, usually in the form of progressive narrowing of the bulboventricular foramen between the single ventricle and the outflow chamber. In addition survivors are subject to the threats of infective endocarditis, brain abscess, and progressive pulmonary vascular obstructive disease. Longevity, nevertheless, is possible with this condition. Of 18 patients who survived systemic-to-pulmonary arterial anastomoses during the early years of experience with that procedure, 11 were alive at the end of 15 years and 8 alive at the end of 20 years. In all, some 33 patients are described as having survived beyond the age of 15 years, the eldest being 56 years old.[591]

Medical Management

Early recognition and identification of patients with a single ventricle are important if successful palliative surgical procedures are to be carried out for the relief of congestive failure or cyanosis. Digitalis and diuretics may be necessary for those patients with continuing heart failure. Care is taken that anemia or severe polycythemia does not develop and that these patients are adequately protected against infective endocarditis. If surgical correction in the future is to be considered, the pulmonary vascular bed must be preserved with confirmation by catheterization and direct pressure measurements if possible. The long-term outlook for the survivors has yet to be determined.

Surgical Management

Palliation for patients with univentricular heart requires adjustment of pulmonary blood flow as appropriate, either with a pulmonary arterial band or by the creation of a systemic arterial–to–pulmonary arterial shunt—usually a Blalock-Taussig subclavian arterial–to–pulmonary arterial anastomosis (Fig. 36-54) or a modification utilizing a segment of polytetrafluoroethylene graft (PTFE, Impra, Gore-Tex). Unfortunately, palliation of the child with univentricular heart is often less effective than that achieved for other defects. Presumably the single ventricle is more susceptible to the increased work load imposed by the necessity to perfuse both the systemic and the pulmonary circulations, even if these loads are relatively well balanced.[592]

Physiologic correction of selected patients has been accomplished by (1) septation or partitioning of the single ventricle using a woven Dacron patch placed to separate the pulmonary and systemic outflow through semilunar valves and the systemic and pulmonary venous inflow through individual atrioventricular valves[593,594] (Fig. 36-83), and (2) complete exclusion of the pulmonary circulation from the sys-

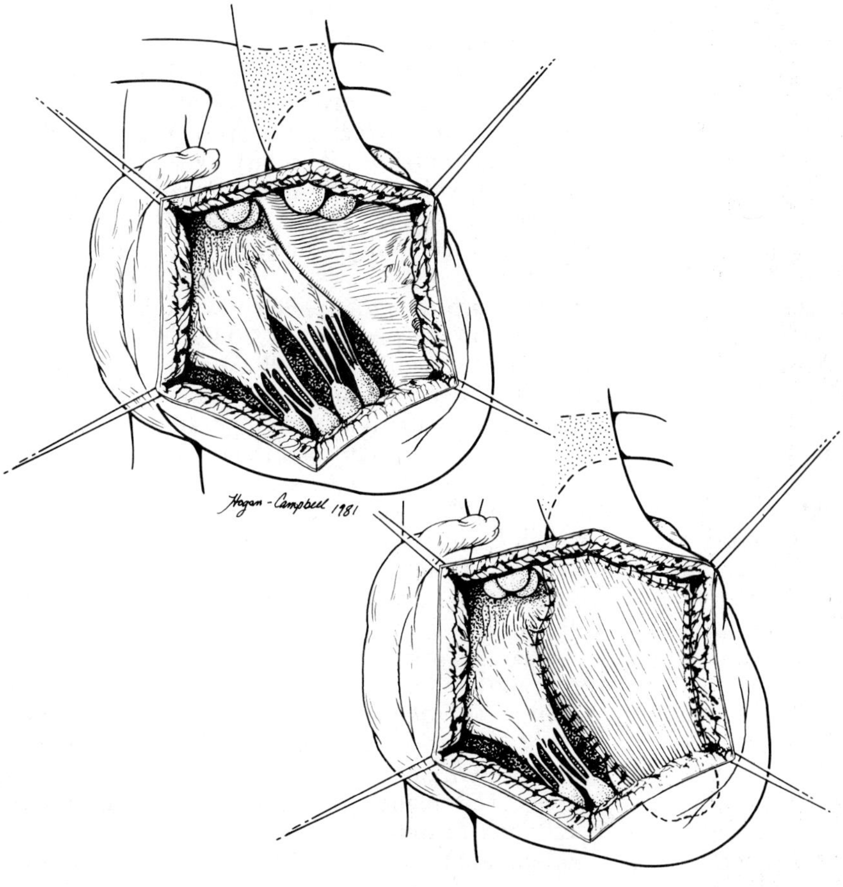

FIGURE 36-83 Septation of the univentricular heart. A large Dacron or Teflon patch is placed in the ventricle so that systemic venous blood from the tricuspid orifice is directed to the pulmonary artery, while pulmonary venous blood from the mitral orifice is directed to the aorta. Knowledge of the course of the conduction system, facilitated by intracardiac electrophysiologic mapping during the operation, is required to avoid heart block. The bulboventricular foramen must usually be enlarged surgically in cases having a subaortic outflow chamber. Injury to major coronary arteries must be avoided.

temic ventricular outflow applying the Fontan concept of direct right atrial–to–pulmonary arterial anastomosis.[595–597] With atriopulmonary anastomosis, the atrial septal defect and right atrioventricular valve, if present, are closed (Fig. 36-65). The single ventricle is thus relieved of the burden of the pulmonary circulation and is required only to provide systemic cardiac output.

Early mortality has been relatively high for both septation and atriopulmonary anastomosis (40 to 50 percent), but experience and patient selection appear to yield improved survival in more recently corrected patients.[592] Early survival has been better with the Fontan atriopulmonary anastomosis but morbidity is significant, exercise tolerance is limited, and long-term prognosis—especially if significant arrhythmias occur—remains uncertain. Early mortality and the incidence of complete heart block have been higher in those patients managed by septation, but those surviving appear to have good exercise tolerance and a better overall quality of life.

Only continued surgical experience in a few centers and careful analysis of surviving patients with univentricular heart will establish the operation of choice and the optimum time for surgical intervention.

Crisscross Heart

Definition

This very rare malformation is characterized by an atrioventricular spatial relation that places or appears to place each ventricle in a contralateral position relative to its associated atrium.

Pathology

Among individuals with crisscross heart having situs solitus and atrioventricular concordance (d loop), the major portion of the right ventricular chamber occupies a left and superior position, while the left ventricle lies in a right and inferior position. This relationship also has been called the "upstairs downstairs" heart or the superoinferior heart.[598] This situation, with a virtually horizontal ventricular septum, appears to result from underdevelopment of the inflow or sinus portion of the right ventricle, which, in turn, permits a greater than normal clockwise ventricular rotation among patients with a d-ventricular loop and counterclockwise rotation among those with an l-ventricular loop along the longitudinal axis of the heart as seen from the apex. In the case of situs solitus and d-ventricular loop (atrioventricular concordance), a normally located right atrium is connected to and supplies, via a superiorly and anteriorly displaced tricuspid valve, a right ventricle whose major portion, the infundibulum, is positioned anteriorly, superiorly, and to the left in relation to the left ventricle. The normally positioned left atrium supplies a left ventricle, which, by virtue of the clockwise rotation and diminutive right ventricular sinus, now occupies the posterior and inferior portion of the heart, at times extending almost to the right side of the heart border. With situs solitus and an l-ventricular loop (atrioventricular discordance), a normally located right atrium is connected to and supplies a left ventricle which lies posteriorly, inferiorly, and to the left. The normally located left atrium supplies a right ventricle whose dominant infundibular portion is located anteriorly, superiorly, and to the right by virtue of counterclockwise rotation. Atrioventricular discordance has been present in almost one-third of recorded cases to date. The connections of the ventricles with the great arteries are almost invariably abnormal. A very few patients have ventriculoarterial concordance, in which case the basic circulation may be normal. The majority have ventriculoarterial discordance, in which case the circulation has been that of d transposition, l transposition, or double-outlet right ventricle. A ventricular septal defect, usually large, is present in the majority of patients, and pulmonary stenosis, either valvular or subvalvular, is found in about half of the patients with this anomaly. Straddling of either of the atrioventricular valves, particulary the right-sided mitral valve in the presence of l-ventricular loop, is common. The tricuspid valve displays varying degrees of hypoplasia, reflecting the right ventricular inflow underdevelopment, and may override the ventricular septum as well. With l-ventricular loop, the tricuspid valve is almost invariably abnormal with resultant tricuspid regurgitation, stenosis, or both.

Clinical Manifestations

The history and physical examination appear to be indistinguishable from those of patients with d transposition, corrected transposition, or double-outlet right ventricle with a large ventricular septal defect and with or without significant pulmonary stenosis. The presentation, then, is dominated by cyanosis or heart failure or both.[599]

Cardiac Catheterization Selective right atrial angiography in the presence of situs solitus and atrioventricular concordance will demonstrate a right atrium aligned with and filling a contralateral left-sided right ventricular chamber, hence the term *crisscross atrioventricular connection.* However, the inflow portion of the right ventricle, diminutive and less obvious than the enlarged infundibular portion, can still be seen to arise on the right and will still demonstrate the right-to-left sequence which identifies it as a right ventricle and part of a d-ventricular loop; i.e., the right-to-left sequence is from tricuspid valve to right ventricular inflow or sinus region, to septal and moderator bands, and then to the infundibulum. This sequence is right-to-left in the presence of a d-ventricular loop and from left-to-right in the presence of an l-ventricular loop. High-quality selective biplane angiography in both ventricles is essential to define the precise ventriculoarterial relations and connections. The coronary arterial distribution should be established by aortography in those patients being considered for corrective surgery.[600]

Natural History, Prognosis, and Management
Palliative rather than corrective surgical procedures are recommended in infants unless associated complicating malformations can be excluded with reasonable certainty and the corrective surgery performed in a center with particular interest and experience with this malformation. Among older children, the principal limiting factors would appear to be the size of the right ventricular chamber and the presence of atrioventricular valve overriding.

Ectopia Cordis

Definition
Ectopia cordis is the condition in which the heart lies in some location outside of the thorax.

Pathology and Clinical Manifestations
This condition is an extremely rare malformation but one easily recognized, particularly in its thoracic form. The heart, almost invariably lacking any covering, lies on the anterior chest wall with its apex pointing cephalad and, at times, touching the infant's chin. The great arteries and veins exit and enter the heart through a cleft of variable size in the sternum. The thoracic cavity has no provision for the heart, and thus a return of the heart to its usual position is precluded. Ravitch, in 1977, described 20 patients with true thoracic ectopia cordis in whom a surgical attempt had been made to position the heart within the chest or to provide a protective covering of skin.[601] There was only one survivor. Death was due to kinking of the great arteries or veins, to tamponade of the heart itself as a result of repositioning, or to associated intracardiac defects. The latter consisted of ventricular septal defect in nine, single ventricle in three, transposition in one, and coarctation in two. In two patients only a patent ductus was noted, and in three the internal structure of the heart was not known. Among those patients with a ventricular septal defect, three had pulmonary atresia and four severe pulmonary stenosis. There are, then, a few patients with intracardiac anomalies that would permit survival if the malposition of the heart could be managed successfully. True abdominal ectopic cordis appears to be rarer still, with only 1 or 2 reported instances of the heart lying completely within the abdomen.[531,601]

Patients with thoracic ectopia cordis are to be distinguished from those with an *isolated cleft of the sternum,* either of the superior portion or of the entire sternum except for the xiphoid process. In this situation, the heart can be seen to pulsate beneath a covering of skin or cutaneous tissue which has the appearance of scar tissue. The heart may protrude anteriorly and superiorly with crying, but true ectopia, or displacement of the heart from the thorax, does not exist. There does not appear to be a propensity for intracardiac malformations with this condition, and the sternal defect lends itself to surgical repair.[601]

Finally, both thoracic and abdominal ectopia cordis are to be distinguished from the syndrome consisting of five associated defects referred to as *Cantrell's pentalogy.*[602] In its complete form this syndrome consists of (1) a midline supraumbilical abdominal wall defect, (2) a defect of the lower sternum, (3) a deficiency of the anterior diaphragm, (4) a defect of the diaphragmatic pericardium, and (5) a congenital intracardiac malformation, usually a ventricular septal defect.[602] The ventral abdominal defect may take the extreme form of an omphalocele, covered by a translucent membrane and containing liver, bowel, and the cardiac apex; in other patients it may merely be an area of wrinkled, hyperpigmented skin overlying a wide supraumbilical diastasis. Similarly, the sternal defect may be either quite striking or inconspicuous. Mesocardia usually is present, with the heart appearing to have undergone a counterclockwise rotation as seen from below, but the heart is not totally displaced from the thoracic cavity. Approximately 80 percent of patients with this syndrome will have a ventricular septal defect, particularly in the form of tetralogy of Fallot, but isolated instances of other defects have been described.[531] In addition, almost two-thirds will have a muscular diverticulum of the apical portion of the left ventricle which may present along with an omphalocele or as a small, pulsating, frequently tubular midline mass in the epigastrium. The diverticulum may be enclosed by pericardium or may extend through a defect in the pericardium.

Congenital Abnormalities of the Coronary Arterial Circulation

Coronary Arteriovenous Fistula

Pathology
A coronary arteriovenous fistula is represented by a gross communication between a coronary artery, on one hand, and a cardiac chamber, the coronary sinus, or the pulmonary trunk, on the other (Fig. 36-84).

The site of origin may involve any of the epicardial coronary arteries. The right coronary artery is the site of origin in somewhat over half of the cases, and the two most common sites into which the fistula feeds are a cardiac vein (usually the coronary sinus) and the right ventricle. Although solitary communication is the rule, rare cases may show multiple sites of termination into the involved site of reception.[603]

A fistula into the pulmonary trunk is usually characterized by one or more vessels opening into the pulmonary trunk and making connection with branches of each of the two main coronary arteries. The artery or arteries feeding the fistula are grossly

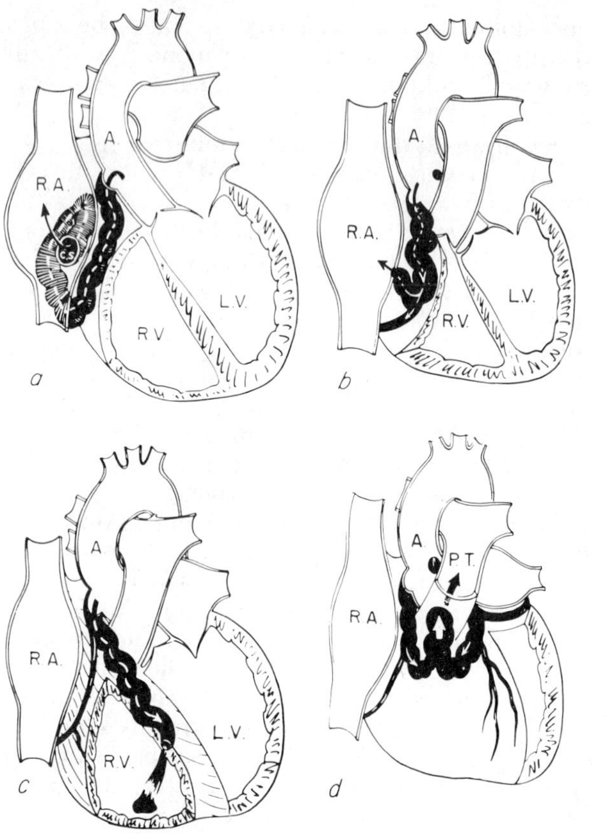

FIGURE 36-84 Anomalous communications of coronary arteries. *a.* Right coronary artery communicates with coronary sinus. *b.* Right coronary artery communicates with right atrium (RA). *c.* Anomalous communication of right coronary artery with right ventricle (RV). *d.* Two coronary arteries arise from the aorta (A) and make collateral communication with accessory coronary artery arising from pulmonary trunk (PT). LV = left ventricle.

enlarged and tortuous. Saccular aneurysms may develop in segments of dilated vessels; such aneurysms are usually observed in the adult and frequently show calcification of the wall.

Clinical Manifestations[604,605]

Many patients with a coronary arteriovenous fistula are asymptomatic. In some, the magnitude of the shunt into the right side of the heart is great enough to cause congestive heart failure, with a tendency for this to occur in early infancy or after 40 years of age. The classic finding is that of a continuous murmur with an unusual location, since it is loudest over the fistula. It may have a louder diastolic component, especially if communication is with the right ventricle. In those with large shunts, there may be cardiomegaly and increased pulmonary flow shown by chest roentgenogram and right ventricular hypertrophy shown by electrocardiogram. At cardiac catheterization, an increase in oxygen saturation may be encountered, usually in the right atrium or right ventricle, if the shunt is large enough. Pressures are normal. Aortography or selective coronary arteriography will demonstrate the involved coronary artery and site of entry of the fistula.[416] The most common complication is infective endocarditis, but thrombosis, myocardial ischemia, and rupture may occur.

Medical Management

Medical management involves treatment and prevention of the complications. Surgical closure is recommended.[606]

Surgical Management

Closure of coronary arteriovenous fistulas requires obliteration of the fistula at its point of entry into the atrium, ventricle, coronary sinus, or pulmonary trunk while preserving continuity of the coronary artery. In some cases this can be accomplished without the use of cardiopulmonary bypass by lateral arteriorrhaphy, the placement of obliterating mattress sutures across the fistula beneath the coronary artery as it passes over the surface of the heart.[607] Cardiopulmonary bypass is preferred for safe exposure of large or multiple fistulas such as those entering the right atrium near the junction of the superior vena cava and right atrium and arising from the artery to the sinus node. The orifice of the fistula is obliterated from within the heart by direct suture or placement of a Dacron patch. Coronary arterial aneurysms, common when the artery to the sinus node arises from a branch of the left coronary artery, are mobilized and resected or obliterated with multiple sutures. Fistulas have been closed from within the opened coronary artery, the artery then being repaired by direct suture or venous patch angioplasty.

Only 4 deaths occurred in 116 reported cases of coronary arteriovenous fistulas which were closed surgically.[606] Operation is safe, relatively simple, and effective.

Origin of the Left Coronary Artery from the Pulmonary Artery

In this anomaly, the right coronary artery arises from the aorta, while the left coronary artery arises from the left anterior pulmonary arterial sinus (Fig. 36-85). This is also known as the Bland-White-Garland syndrome. The course and branching of the vessel are normal. In the young, the coronary arteries are of normal size, but if the patient survives beyond infancy, there is noticeable dilatation of these vessels. In cases of infant death from this condition, the left ventricle is dilated and may show sites of infarction with calcification of affected myocardium. In subjects surviving infancy, there is often scarring of the left ventricular papillary muscles and of the left ventricular wall, particularly in the distribution of the left coronary artery. The left ventricular cavity is dilated and the chamber shows endocardial fibroelastosis. The mitral valve may become incompetent.[608,609] Associated conditions are uncommon.

An extensive literature review helped elucidate the clinical spectrum and mode of presentation in

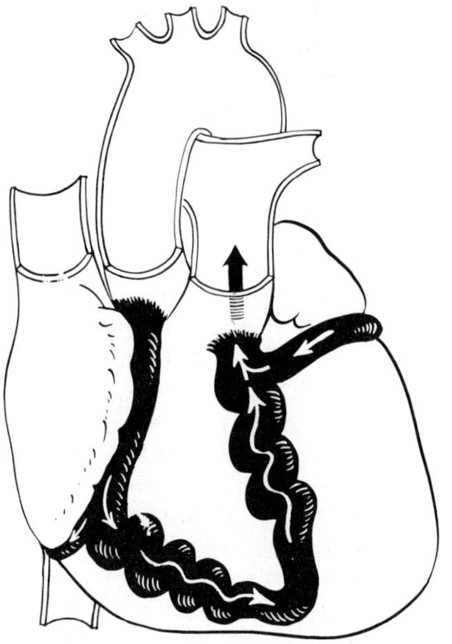

FIGURE 36-85 Anomalous origin of the left coronary artery from the pulmonary trunk. With time, wide collaterals develop between the two coronary systems, so that right coronary arterial blood is shunted into the left coronary system and thence into the pulmonary trunk.

patients with this abnormality.[610] The majority of patients present at a few months of age. Acute episodes of irritability, profuse cold sweating, pallor, and respiratory distress occur, with evidence of heart failure. Less often the patients present at any age with mitral regurgitation and heart failure. A few reach adolescence or adulthood with relatively few symptoms other than occasional exertional angina or palpitations. Sudden death may be the first and only sign of this diagnosis.

On physical examination, the heart is enlarged with an abnormal left ventricular apex impulse. Other signs of failure are usually present. Pallor and clammy skin are common. In some, a soft continuous murmur is heard at the upper left sternal border. This murmur is more prominent in the older patients, presumably due to development of a more extensive collateral circulation. The murmur of mitral regurgitation may be heard at the apex, radiating to the axilla; however, in young infants with heart failure there can be a surprising degree of regurgitation without a distinctive murmur.

The chest roentgenogram typically shows marked enlargement of the heart with posterior displacement of the esophagus by a large left atrium. There is pulmonary edema, and there may be atelectasis of the left lower lobe due to bronchial compression.

The electrocardiogram demonstrates the pattern of anterolateral infarction (Fig. 36-86) with a deep Q wave in leads I and aV_L and abnormal R-wave progression across the precordium. Arrhythmias are frequent. The horizontal loop of the vectorcardiogram is clockwise and posteriorly oriented. The echocardiogram shows marked enlargement of the left atrium and ventricle with little or no left ventricular wall motion. Myocardial perfusion imaging with ^{201}Tl can help distinguish this from congestive cardiomyopathy.[611]

At cardiac catheterization, there may be an increase in saturation in the pulmonary artery if there is enough retrograde flow. There is usually some pulmonary hypertension with very elevated pulmonary wedge pressure. Left ventricular angiography will delineate the left ventricular volume and function as well as the degree of mitral regurgitation. Aortography or selective right coronary arteriography[416] will demonstrate the collateral circulation filling the left coronary artery retrogradely with at least faint opacification of the main pulmonary artery.

FIGURE 36-86 Twelve-lead electrocardiogram in an infant having origin of the left coronary artery from the pulmonary artery, demonstrating the pattern of anterolateral infarction. Chest leads are recorded at one-half standard voltage.

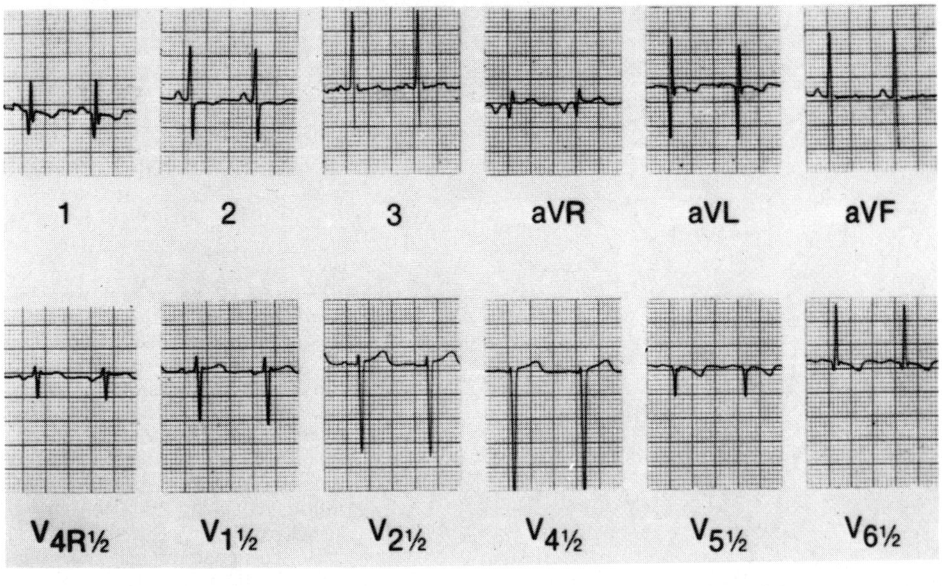

Natural history and prognosis are indicated by the modes of presentation. Most patients will die in infancy. Medical management is aimed at control of congestive heart failure and arrhythmias. Surgical anastomosis to the aorta should be attempted to improve myocardial blood flow and prevent further myocardial damage.[612] The optimum age for operation has not been decided. Clearly the risk is greater for infants, but this may also be the group who have the poorest natural prognosis.[613]

Ligation of the anomalous left coronary artery near its pulmonary arterial orifice reduces the "steal" or "run-off" of coronary arterial blood into the low-resistance pulmonary vascular bed, but does not provide a dual myocardial blood supply.[614]

Antegrade left coronary arterial flow can be established by interposition of autologous vein or synthetic grafts between the aorta and the anomalous left coronary artery, with subsequent ligation of the artery near its pulmonary arterial orifice.[615] Alternative methods for perfusion of the left coronary arterial system after ligation include internal mammary or subclavian arterial anastomosis. Direct perfusion of the left coronary arterial orifice without ligation is accomplished by creation of a synthetic or autogenous tissue conduit from the aorta within the pulmonary artery or excision of the orifice from the pulmonary artery with subsequent anastomosis to the ascending aorta (Fig. 36-87).[615]

Assuming appropriate intraoperative myocardial protection, mortality is largely attributable to preexisting left ventricular infarction and failure, ventricular arrhythmias, and mitral regurgitation secondary to papillary muscle dysfunction and annular dilatation. These problems are most prevalent in critically ill infants requiring urgent operation. Improvement in severely impaired left ventricular function following operation has been reported.[616] Low mortality and a good hemodynamic result should be anticipated in older patients.[617]

Origin of the Right or Both Coronary Arteries from the Pulmonary Artery

Origin of the right coronary artery from the pulmonary artery while the left arises from the aorta is highly uncommon. Some infants and, more commonly, adults manifest evidence of inadequate perfusion of the myocardium.[618] Origin of both coronary arteries from the pulmonary trunk is rare,[619] as is the case when there is a single coronary artery and this vessel arises from the pulmonary trunk.[620] In anomalous origin of the right coronary artery, sudden death has been described.[621] If both coronary arteries arise from the pulmonary artery, early death commonly occurs.[620]

Since anomalous origin of the right coronary artery from the pulmonary artery has been associated with sudden death, operative correction is justified even in the asymptomatic patient. Normal coronary arterial circulation is established by excision of the right coronary artery from the pulmonary artery followed by direct implantation of the coronary artery, with a cuff of surrounding pulmonary artery, into the ascending aorta.[622] (Alternative methods are described in the discussion of surgical management in the section "Origin of the Left Coronary Artery from the Pulmonary Artery".)

Origin of both coronary arteries from the pulmonary artery has not been corrected surgically; a

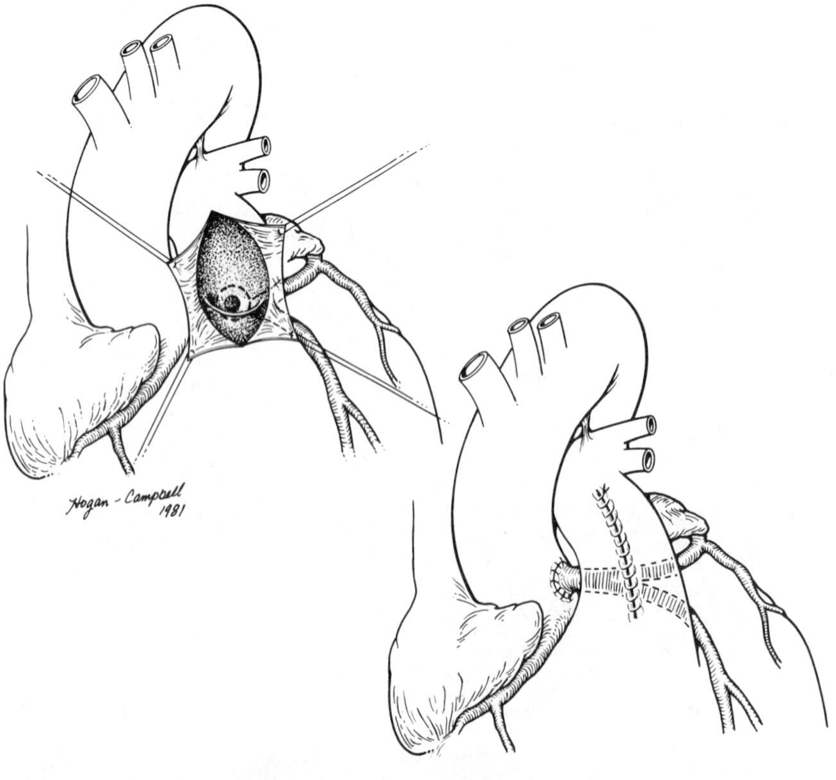

FIGURE 36-87 Transposition of anomalous left coronary artery from the pulmonary artery to the aorta. The orifice of the left coronary artery is excised from within the opened pulmonary artery (on cardiopulmonary bypass). The proximal segment of the left coronary artery and its branches, the circumflex and the left anterior descending branches, are mobilized to provide sufficient length for a tension-free anastomosis of the orifice, with a surrounding cuff of pulmonary arterial wall, to the left posterolateral wall of the aorta.

recent report describes two unsuccessful surgical attempts to establish antegrade coronary flow in critically ill infants.[623]

Origin of the Left Coronary Artery from the Right Aortic Sinus

In this condition both coronary arteries arise from the right aortic sinus from one or two ostia. The left coronary artery takes a sharp turn to the left and, after passing behind the pulmonary artery, courses and branches in a normal manner.[624] Sudden death during exercise has been reported in such patients.[624,625] If the patient is symptomatic and the anomaly has been demonstrated angiographically, surgery should be recommended.

Origin of the left coronary artery from the right sinus with a course anterior to the right ventricular outflow tract, or similar origin of the left anterior descending branch alone, is not clinically significant. In patients such as those with tetralogy of Fallot,[626] preoperative diagnosis is important to avoid incision of a coronary artery at the time of surgery (see section in this chapter on "Tetralogy of Fallot").

In symptomatic patients with angiographic confirmation of this anomaly, surgical intervention using an internal mammary artery or a saphenous vein bypass graft[627] or a left coronary arterial ostioplasty[628] should be strongly considered.

Origin of the Circumflex Coronary Artery from the Right Aortic Sinus or Right Coronary Artery

In less than 0.5 percent of the general population, the left circumflex coronary artery arises either from the proximal segment of the right coronary artery or from the right aortic sinus just posterior to the origin of the right artery. From either site of origin the vessel courses along the posterior aspect of the aorta to reach the proximal part of the left atrioventricular sulcus.

In the absence of coronary atherosclerosis, this anomaly probably has no clinical significance.

Atresia of the Left Coronary Ostium

Atresia of the origin of the left coronary artery is an unusual basis for ischemic heart disease in the young. Each coronary artery has a normal site of origin. The atresia usually affects the entire length of the main left coronary artery, and various degrees and lengths of stenosis may involve the proximal segments of the anterior descending and left circumflex arteries. There is an association with a forme fruste of supravalvular aortic stenosis, wherein the media of this vessel may histologically show a mosaic pattern. The mitral valve may show features of prolapse.

This rare abnormality has been recently reviewed with the addition of another case.[629] The clinical picture is identical to that of anomalous left coronary artery arising from the pulmonary artery. The diagnosis can be suspected by angiography if it is noted that there is no filling of the pulmonary artery once the main left coronary fills via collaterals. Successful coronary bypass grafting has been reported in a 14-year-old boy.[630]

Aneurysm of Coronary Artery

Localized congenital aneurysms are uncommon; they tend to favor the male and to be located in the right coronary artery. The basis for the defect is probably a dysplastic condition of the arterial media. The potential danger is thrombosis with either occlusion of the parent artery or embolism downstream. Rupture may occur. In cases with coronary arterial fistula, saccular aneurysms may be of an acquired nature. Multiple aneurysms have been reported in the young. While some of these may be of congenital origin, some are probably secondary to Kawasaki disease.[631]

In general, the diagnosis of congenital aneurysm of the coronary arteries[632] has been made at postmortem examination. Some patients are apparently asymptomatic, but the usual clinical picture is one of angina and myocardial infarction. It may be suspected clinically if these findings occur in a very young person. A systolic murmur or systolic and diastolic murmurs may be heard. The chest roentgenogram may show cardiomegaly with an unusual round shadow at the cardiac margin, particularly common along the distribution of the right coronary artery. Patterns of ischemia or infarction will be evident on the electrocardiogram. The diagnosis is made by coronary arteriography (Fig. 36-88).[633]

Coronary artery bypass grafting[634] and, if possible, resection of the aneurysm are recommended.

FIGURE 36-88 Right anterior oblique view of a selective right coronary arteriogram in a patient with multiple saccular aneurysms. *(From D. E. McMartin, A. J. Stone, and R. H. Franch, Multiple Coronary-Artery Aneurysms in a Child with Angina Pectoris, N. Engl. J. Med., 290:669, 1974. Reprinted by permission of The New England Journal of Medicine and the authors.)*

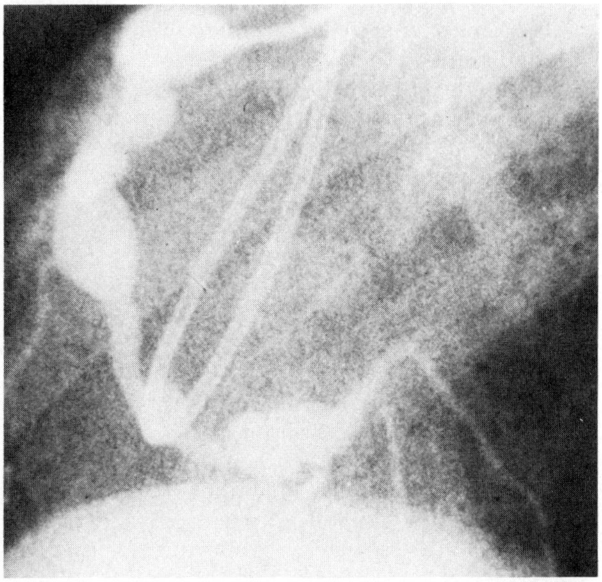

Both early and long-term patency rates for grafts in these patients appear poor compared to grafts performed for atherosclerotic occlusive disease, perhaps because of the small size of the distal vessels or the presence of an inflammatory process in the mucocutaneous lymph node syndrome.[635]

Congenital Abnormalities of the Coronary Venous Circulation

Coronary Sinus Malformations

A comprehensive review of anomalies involving the coronary sinus has been presented by Mantini and associates.[636] These relate to enlargement of the sinus, absence of the sinus, atresia of its right ostium, and hypoplasia.

Delivery of blood foreign to the coronary sinus into the channel results in *enlargement* of the coronary sinus. Persistent left superior vena cava joining the coronary sinus is the most common cause. Less common is that in which the inferior vena cava is continuous with the left superior vena cava by way of the hemiazygous vein.

Absence of the coronary sinus occurs when there is direct communication of the left superior vena cava with the left atrium or with the left side of a common atrium.

Atresia of the right atrial ostium of the coronary sinus may occur as an independent abnormality or may be associated with other conditions. Cardiac venous blood may leave the coronary sinus through a persistent left superior vena cava or, more commonly, through multiple connections between the coronary sinus and the atria.

The clinical importance of coronary sinus malformations is mainly limited to the technical aspects of cardiac catheterization and cardiac surgery in those who have associated defects. Abnormalities resulting in enlargement of the coronary sinus were discussed in preceding sections of this chapter.

In the absence of the coronary sinus[637] or atresia of the ostium, there may be minimal desaturation of systemic arterial blood if the coronary venous blood returns to the left side of the heart. The magnitude of flow is usually not sufficient to cause cyanosis which is clinically apparent, unless there is a contribution from a persistent left superior vena cava.

Congenital Abnormalities of the Pericardium

Deficiency

Moore[638] classified pericardial defects into three groups: (1) heart and left lung in a common cavity, 60 percent; (2) foramen between the pericardial and left pleural sacs, 21 percent; and (3) pericardium absent or rudimentary, 19 percent.

Nasser and associates[639] reported six cases of pericardial defect, two with partial absence and two with complete absence, each condition involving the left side of the pericardium.

Defects are three times more common in males than females. Commonly associated conditions involve the heart, lungs, pleural cavities, peritoneum, or kidneys. Two of Nasser's six patients had atrial septal defect. Other associated defects reported by Hipona and associates[640] included patent ductus arteriosus in four patients, bifid heart in two, tetralogy of Fallot in two, and bronchogenic cysts in six. Bronchial cysts and enterogenous thoracic cysts have been reported as associated defects. Diaphragmatic pericardial defects may be combined into a pentalogy with abdominal wall defects, lower sternal defects, deficiency of the anterior diaphragm, and congenital intracardiac defects.[641]

Congenital pericardial deficiency[5,638,639,642] may not produce symptoms. Associated cardiac defects and defects of the thoracoabdominal wall can occur and dominate the clinical picture. A partial defect on the right can produce symptoms of obstruction of the superior vena cava due to herniation of the lung into the pericardium. The chest radiograph is diagnostic.

Partial defects on the left are rare causes of chest pain. The pain may be related to position. The left atrial appendage and ventricle can herniate and strangulate. Sudden death has been reported with left ventricular strangulation. There is also an increased risk of infection because of the communication between the pleural and pericardial cavities.

On physical examination with defects on the left, the apex impulse is displaced to the left, and even posteriorly in some. The chest roentgenogram will demonstrate this leftward displacement and prominence of the pulmonary arterial segment. An unusual convexity on the left is seen with herniation of the left atrial appendage. Fluoroscopy is helpful. In those with defects on the left, the electrocardiogram may show right axis deviation and, less commonly, right ventricular hypertrophy. Echocardiographic study in patients with large defects on the left may mimic the findings of volume overload of the right ventricle.[643]

Surgery is usually recommended to remove any constrictive, or potentially constrictive, portions of the pericardium in symptomatic patients and in those with partial defects on the left, in whom left ventricular strangulation is a risk.

Cysts and Diverticula

A true diverticulum communicates with the pericardial cavity; a cyst does not. These abnormalities were classified by Loehr[644] into the following three varieties:

1. Congenital true cysts: coelomic (mesodermal), lymphangiomatous, bronchial, or teratomatous cysts

2. Acquired cysts: secondary to hematoma, neoplasm, or parasitic disease
3. Pseudocysts: pericardial diverticula encapsulating pericardial exudate

Pericardial cysts and diverticula are not rare. The cysts may be congenital pericardial coelomic cysts, which are usually not connected with the pericardium except by loose connective tissue. Lymphangiomatous cysts may arise from the pericardium and are usually multilocular. When the fibrous structure of the pericardium is weak, the serosa may herniate to form a diverticulum. When the diverticulum loses its connection with the pericardial sac, a pericardial cyst is formed.

A pericardial cyst or diverticulum[644] does not usually cause symptoms but is commonly discovered when a chest roentgenogram is obtained for an unrelated reason. A mass is then noted, usually in the right anterior cardiophrenic angle. Computed tomographic (CT) scans can usually differentiate a pericardial cyst or diverticulum from more ominous lesions. Surgical exploration may be required to exclude other diagnoses, such as tumors or a Morgagni hernia.

References

1. Mitchell, S.C., Korones, S. B., and Berendes, H. W.: Congenital Heart Disease in 56,109 Births: Incidence and Natural History, *Circulation*, 43:323, 1971.
2. Hoffman, J.I.E., and Christianson, R.: Congenital Heart Disease in a Cohort of 19,502 Births with Long-Term Follow Up, *Am. J. Cardiol.*, 42:641, 1978.
3. Fyler, D. C.: Report of the New England Regional Infant Cardiac Program, *Pediatrics*, 65(suppl. 2):375, 1980.
4. Nadas, A. S., and Fyler, D. C.: "Pediatric Cardiology," 3d ed., W.B. Saunders Company, Philadelphia, 1972.
5. Hoffman, J. I. E.: Natural History of Congenital Heart Disease: Problems in Its Assessment with Special Reference to Ventricular Septal Defects, *Circulation*, 37:97, 1968.
6. Keith, J. D., Rowe, R. D., and Vlad, P.: "Heart Disease in Infancy and Childhood," 3d ed., The Macmillan Company, New York, 1978.
7. Miettinen, O. S., Reiner, M. L., and Nadas, A. S.: Seasonal Incidence of Coarctation of the Aorta, *Br. Heart J.*, 32:103, 1970.
8. Jaffee, O. C. (ed.): "Cardiac Development with Special Reference to Congenital Heart Disease" (proceedings, international symposium), University of Dayton Press, Dayton, Ohio, 1968.
9. Moss, A. J., Adams, F. H., and Emmanouilides, G. C.: "Heart Disease in Infants, Children, and Adolescents," 2d ed., The Williams & Wilkins Company, Baltimore, 1977.
10. Anderson, R. C.: Fetal and Infant Death, Twinning and Cardiac Malformations in Families of 2,000 Children with and 500 without Cardiac Defects, *Am. J. Cardiol.*, 38:218, 1976.
11. Nora, J. J., and Nora, A. H.: The Evolution of Specific Genetic and Environmental Counseling in Congenital Heart Diseases, *Circulation*, 57:205, 1978.
12. Comline, K. S., Cross, K. W., Dawes, G. S., and Nathanielze, P. W. (eds.): "Fetal and Neonatal Physiology" (proceedings, Sir Joseph Barcroft Centenary Symposium), Cambridge University Press, Cambridge, 1973.
13. Rudolph, A. M.: "Congenital Diseases of the Heart. Clinical-Physiologic Considerations in Diagnosis and Management," Year Book Medical Publishers, Inc., Chicago, 1974.
14. Rudolph, A. M., and Heymann, M. A.: Neonatal Circulation and Pathophysiology of Shunts, in H. J. Levine (ed.), "Clinical Cardiovascular Physiology," Grune & Stratton, Inc., New York, 1976, p. 597.
15. Young, M.: The Fetal and Neonatal Circulation, in W. F. Hamilton and P. Dow (eds.), "Handbook of Physiology," sec. 2: "Circulation," vol. 2, American Physiological Society, Washington, D. C., 1963, p. 1619.
16. Dawes, G. S.: "Foetal and Neonatal Physiology," Year Book Medical Publishers, Inc., Chicago, 1968.
17. Rudolph, A. M.: The Changes in the Circulation after Birth: Their Importance in Congenital Heart Disease, *Circulation*, 41:343, 1970.
18. Heymann, M. A., and Rudolph, A. M.: Effects of Congenital Heart Diseases on Fetal and Neonatal Circulation, *Prog. Cardiovasc. Dis.*, 15:115, 1972.
19. Coceani, F., and Olley, P. M.: Role of Prostaglandins, Prostacyclin, and Thromboxanes in the Control of Prenatal Patency and Postnatal Closure of the Ductus Arteriosus, in M. A. Heymann (ed.), "Prostaglandins in the Perinatal Period," Grune & Stratton, Inc., New York, 1980, p. 109.
20. Rudolph, A. M.: Fetal and Neonatal Pulmonary Circulation, *Ann. Rev. Physiol.*, 41:383, 1979.
21. Levin, D. L., Heymann, M. A., Kitterman, J. A., Gregory, G. A., Phibbs, R. H., and Rudolph, A. M.: Persistent Pulmonary Hypertension of the Newborn Infant, *J. Pediatr.*, 89:626, 1976.
22. Fox, W. W., and Duara, S.: Persistent Pulmonary Hypertension in the Neonate: Diagnosis and Management, *J. Pediatr.*, 103:505, 1983.
23. Kirkpatrick, B. V., Krummel, T. M., Mueller, D. G., Ormazabal, M. A., Greenfield, L. J., and Salzberg, A. M.: Use of Extracorporeal Membrane Oxygenation for Respiratory Failure in Term Infants, *Pediatrics*, 72:872, 1983.
24. Talner, N. S.: Heart Failure, in F. H. Adams and G. C. Emmanouilides (eds.), "Moss' Heart Disease in Infants, Children, and Adolescents," The Williams & Wilkins Company, Baltimore, 1983, p. 708.
25. Jelliffe, R. W., and Brooker, G.: A Nomogram for Digoxin Therapy, *Am. J. Med.*, 57:64, 1974.
26. Beekman, R. H., Rocchini, A. P., Dick, M., II, Crawley, D. C., and Rosenthal, A.: Vasodilator Therapy in Children: Acute and Chronic Effects in Children with Left Ventricular Dysfunction or Mitral Regurgitation, *Pediatrics*, 73:43, 1984.
27. Olley, P. M.: Nonsurgical Palliation of Congenital Heart Malformations, *N. Engl. J. Med.*, 292:1292, 1975.
28. Houston, A. B., Gregory, N. L., and Coleman, E. N.: Two-Dimensional Sector Scanner Echocardiography in Cyanotic Congenital Heart Disease, *Br. Heart J.*, 39:1076, 1977.
29. Shannon, D. C., Lusser, M., Goldblatt, A., and Bunnell, J. B.: The Cyanotic Infant—Heart Disease or Lung Disease, *N. Engl. J. Med.*, 287:951, 1972.
30. Avery, G. B.: "Neonatology. Pathophysiology and Management of the Newborn," J. B. Lippincott Company, Philadelphia, 1975.
31. Danilowicz, D. A.: Delay in Bone Age in Children with Cyanotic Congenital Heart Disease, *Radiology*, 108:655, 1973.
32. Somerville, J.: Gout in Cyanotic Congenital Heart Disease, *Br. Heart J.*, 23:31, 1961.
33. Fischbein, C. A., Rosenthal, A., Fisher, E. G., Nadas, A. S., and Welch, K.: Risk Factors for Brain Abscess in Patients with Congenital Heart Disease, *Am. J. Cardiol.*, 34:97, 1974.
34. Phornphutkul, C., Rosenthal, A., Nadas, A. S., and Berenberg, W.: Cerebrovascular Accidents in Infants and Children with Cyanotic Congenital Heart Disease, *Am. J. Cardiol.*, 32:329, 1973.
35. Linderkamp, O., Klose, H. J., Betke, K., et al.: Increased Blood Viscosity in Patients with Cyanotic Congenital Heart Disease and Iron Deficiency, *J. Pediatr.*, 95:567, 1979.
36. Henriksson, P., Varendh, G., and Lundstrom, N.: Hemostatic Defects in Cyanotic Congenital Heart Disease, *Br. Heart J.*, 41:23, 1979.
37. Gross, S., Keefer, V., and Liebman, J.: The Platelets in Cyanotic Congenital Heart Disease, *Pediatrics*, 42:651, 1968.

38. Waldman, J. D., Czapek, E. E., Paul, M. H., Schwartz, A. D., Levin, D. L., and Schindler, S.: Shortened Platelet Survival in Cyanotic Heart Disease, *J. Pediatr.*, 87:77, 1975.
39. Rabinovitch, M.: Pulmonary Hypertension, in F. H. Adams and G. C. Emmanouilides (eds.), "Moss' Heart Disease in Infants, Children, and Adolescents," The Williams & Wilkins Company, Baltimore, 1983, p. 669.
40. Blount, S. G., Jr.: Comparison of Patients with Ventricular Septal Defect at High Altitude and Sea Level, in A. S. Nadas (ed.), Report from the Joint Study on the Natural History of Congenital Heart Defects, *Circulation,* 56(suppl. 1): 79, 1977.
41. Heath, D., and Edwards, J. E.: The Pathology of Hypertensive Pulmonary Vascular Disease. A Description of Six Grades of Structural Changes in the Pulmonary Arteries with Special Reference to Congenital Cardiac Septal Defects, *Circulation,* 18:533, 1958.
42. Rabinovitch, M., Haworth, S. G., Casteneda, A. R., Nadas, A. S., and Reid, L. M.: Lung Biopsy in Congenital Heart Disease: A Morphometric Approach to Pulmonary Vascular Disease, *Circulation,* 58:1107, 1978.
43. Graham, T. P., Jr.: The Eisenmenger Reaction and Its Management, in W. C. Roberts (ed.), "Congenital Heart Disease in Adults," F. A. Davis Company, Philadelphia, 1979, p. 531.
44. Blackstone, E. H., Kirklin, J. W., Bradley, E. L., DuShane, J. W., and Applebaum, A.: Optimal Age and Results in Repair of Large Ventricular Septal Defects, *J. Thorac. Cardiovasc. Surg.*, 72:661, 1976.
45. Rosenthal, A., and Castaneda, A. R.: Growth and Development after Cardiovascular Surgery in Infants and Children, *Prog. Cardiovasc. Dis.,* 18:27, 1975.
46. Levy, R. J., Rosenthal, A., Fyler, D. C., and Nadas, A. S.: Birthweight of Infants with Congenital Heart Disease, *Am. J. Dis. Child.*, 132:249, 1978.
47. Godrey, S.: "Exercise Testing in Children: Applications in Health and Disease," W. B. Saunders Company, London, 1974.
48. James, F. W., Kaplan, S., Glueck, C. J., Tsay, J., Knight, M. J. S., and Sarwar, C. J.: Responses of Normal Children and Young Adults to Controlled Bicycle Exercise, *Circulation,* 61:902, 1980.
49. Riopel, D. A., Taylor, A. B., and Hohn, A. R.: Blood Pressure, Heart Rate, Pressure-Rate Product and Electrocardiographic Changes in Healthy Children during Treadmill Exercise, *Am. J. Cardiol.*, 44:697, 1979.
50. Cumming, G. R.: Maximal Exercise Capacity of Children with Heart Defects, *Am. J. Cardiol.*, 42:613, 1978.
51. Reduto, L. A., Berger, H. J., Johnstone, D. E., et al.: Radionuclide Assessment of Right and Left Ventricular Exercise Reserve after Total Correction of Tetralogy of Fallot, *Am. J. Cardiol.*, 45:1013, 1980.
52. American Heart Association, Ad Hoc Committee of the Council on Cardiovascular Disease in the Young: Guidelines for Insurability of Patient with Congenital Heart Disease, *Circulation,* 62:1419A, 1980.
53. Graham, T. P., Jr., Bender, H. W., and Spach, M. S.: Ventricular Septal Defect, in F. H. Adams and G. C. Emmanouilides (eds.), "Moss' Heart Disease in Infants, Children, and Adolescents," The Williams & Wilkins Company, Baltimore, 1983, p. 134.
54. Kirklin, J. W., Harshbarger, H. G., Donald, D. E., and Edwards, J. E.: Surgical Correction of Ventricular Septal Defect: Anatomic and Technical Considerations, *J. Thorac. Surg.*, 33:45, 1957.
55. Karpawich, P. P., Duff, D. F., Mullins, C. E., Cooley, D. E., and McNamara, D. G.: Ventricular Septal Defect with Associated Aortic Valve Insufficiency. Progression of Insufficiency and Operative Results in Young Children, *J. Thorac. Cardiovasc. Surg.*, 82:182, 1981.
56. Hoffman, J. I. E., and Rudolph, A. M.: The Natural History of Isolated Ventricular Septal Defect, *Adv. Pediatr.*, 17:57, 1970.
57. Engle, M. A., and Kline, S. A.: Ventricular Septal Defect in the Adult, in W. C. Roberts (ed.), "Congenital Heart Disease in Adults," F. A. Davis Company, Philadelphia, 1979, p. 279.
58. Copelli, H., Andrade, J. L., and Somerville, J.: Classification of the Site of Ventricular Septal Defect by 2-Dimensional Echocardiography, *Am. J. Cardiol.*, 51:1474, 1983.
59. Alpert, B. S., Cook, D. H., Varghese, P. J., and Rowe, R. D.: Spontaneous Closure of Small Ventricular Septal Defects: 10 Year Follow-up, *Pediatrics,* 63:204, 1979.
60. Weidman, W. H., Blount, S. G., Jr., DuShane, J. W., Gersony, W. M., Hayes, C. J., and Nadas, A. S.: Clinical Course in Ventricular Septal Defect, *Circulation,* 56(suppl. 1):56, 1977.
61. Blount, S. G., Jr.: Comparison of Patients with Ventricular Septal Defect at High Altitude and Sea Level, *Circulation,* 56(suppl. 1):1, 1977.
62. Blake, R. S., Chung, E. E., Wesley, H., and Hallidie-Smith, K. A.: Conduction Defects, Ventricular Arrhythmias, and Late Death after Surgical Closure of Ventricular Septal Defect, *Br. Heart J.*, 47:305, 1982.
63. Jablonsky, G., Hilton, J. D., Liu, P. P., et al.: Rest and Exercise Ventricular Function in Adults with Congenital Ventricular Septal Defects, *Am. J. Cardiol.*, 51:293, 1983.
64. Muller, W. H., Jr., and Dammann, J. F., Jr.: The Treatment of Certain Congenital Malformations of the Heart by the Creation of Pulmonic Stenosis to Reduce Pulmonary Blood Flow: A Preliminary Report, *Surg. Gynecol. Obstet.*, 95:213, 1952.
65. Hallman, G. L., Cooley, D. A., and Bloodwell, R. D.: Two-Stage Surgical Treatment of Ventricular Septal Defect: Results of Pulmonary Artery Banding in Infants and Subsequent Open-Heart Repair, *J. Thorac. Cardiovasc. Surg.*, 52:476, 1966.
66. Rein, J., Freed, M. D., Norwood, W. I., and Castaneda, A. R.: Early and Late Results of Closure of Ventricular Septal Defect in Infancy, *Ann. Thorac. Surg.*, 24:19, 1977.
67. Barratt-Boyes, B. G., Neutze, J. M., Clarkson, P. M., Shardey, G. C., and Brandt, P. W. T.: Repair of Ventricular Septal Defect in the First Two Years of Life Using Profound Hypothermia–Circulatory Arrest Techniques, *Ann. Surg.*, 184:376, 1976.
68. Kirklin, J. W., and DuShane, J. W.: Repair of Ventricular Septal Defect in Infancy, *Pediatrics,* 27:961, 1961.
69. Barratt-Boyes, B. G., Simpson, M., and Neutze, J. M.: Intracardiac Surgery in Neonates and Infants Using Deep Hypothermia with Surface Cooling and Limited Cardiopulmonary Bypass, *Circulation,* 43/44(suppl. 1):25, 1971.
70. Cartmill, T. B., DuShane, J. W., McGoon, D. C., and Kirklin, J. W.: Results of Repair of Ventricular Septal Defect, *J. Thorac. Cardiovasc. Surg.*, 52:486, 1966.
71. Frenckner, B. P., Olin, C. L., Bomfim, V., Bjarke, B., Wallgren, C. G., and Bjork, V. O.: Detachment of the Septal Tricuspid Leaflet during Transatrial Closure of Isolated Ventricular Septal Defect, *J. Thorac. Cardiovasc. Surg.*, 82:773, 1981.
72. Trusler, G. A., Moes, C. A. F., and Kidd, B. S. L.: Repair of Ventricular Septal Defect with Aortic Insufficiency, *J. Thorac. Cardiovasc. Surg.*, 66:394, 1973.
73. Milo, S., Ho, S. Y., Wilkinson, J. C., and Anderson, R. H.: Surgical Anatomy and Atrioventricular Conduction Tissues of Hearts with Isolated Ventricular Septal Defects, *J. Thorac. Cardiovasc. Surg.*, 79:244, 1980.
74. Doty, D. B., and McGoon, D. C.: Closure of Perimembranous Ventricular Septal Defect, *J. Thorac. Cardiovasc. Surg.*, 85:781, 1983.
75. Breckenridge, I. M., Stark, J., Waterston, D. J., and Bonham-Carter, R. E.: Multiple Ventricular Septal Defects, *Ann. Thorac. Surg.*, 13:128, 1972.
76. Aaron, B. L., and Lower, R. R.: Muscular Ventricular Septal Defect Repair Made Easy, *Ann. Thorac. Surg.*, 19:568, 1975.
77. Sweeny, L. J., and Rosenquist, G. C.: The Normal Anatomy of the Atrial Septum in the Human Heart, *Am. Heart J.*, 98:194, 1979.

78. Lewis, F. J., Winchell, P., and Bashour, F. A.: Open Repair of Atrial Septal Defects: Results in Sixty-Three Patients, *J. Am. Med. Assoc.*, 165:922, 1957.
79. Edwards, J. E.: The Pathology of Atrial Septal Defect, *Semin. Roentgenol.*, 1:24, 1966.
80. Edwards, J. E., Classification of Congenital Heart Disease in the Adult, in W. C. Roberts (ed.), "Congenital Heart Disease in Adults," *Cardiovasc. Clin.* Series 10/1, F. A. Davis Company, Philadelphia, 1979, p. 1.
81. Lee, M. E., and Sade, R. M.: Coronary Sinus Septal Defect: Surgical Considerations, *J. Thorac. Cardiovasc. Surg.*, 78:563, 1979.
82. Raghib, G., Ruttenberg, H. D., Anderson, R. C., Amplatz, K., Adams, P., Jr., and Edwards, J. E.: Termination of Left Superior Vena Cava in Left Atrium, Atrial Septal Defect, and Absence of Coronary Sinus: A Developmental Complex, *Circulation*, 31:906, 1965.
83. Heath, D., and Edwards, J. E.: The Pathology of Hypertensive Pulmonary Vascular Disease. A Description of Six Grades of Structural Changes in the Pulmonary Arteries with Special Reference to Congenital Cardiac Septal Defects, *Circulation*, 18:533, 1958.
84. Hoffman, J. I. E., Rudolph, A. M., and Danilowicz, D.: Left to Right Atrial Shunts in Infants, *Am. J. Cardiol.*, 30:868, 1972.
85. Bedford, D. E.: The Anatomical Types of Atrial Septal Defect: Their Incidence and Clinical Diagnosis, *Am. J. Cardiol.*, 6:568, 1960.
86. Noonan, J. A.: Syndromes Associated with Cardiac Defects, in M. A. Engle and A. N. Brest (eds.), "Pediatric Cardiovascular Disease," F. A. Davis Company, Philadelphia, 1981, p. 97.
87. Hamilton, W. T., Haffajee, C. E., Dalen, J. E., Dexter, L., and Nadas, A. S.: Atrial Septal Defect Secundum: Clinical Profile with Physiologic Correlates in Children and Adults, in W. C. Roberts (ed.), "Congenital Heart Disease in Adults," F. A. Davis Company, Philadelphia, 1979, p. 267.
88. Shub, C., Dimopoulos, I. N., Seward, J. B., et al.: Sensitivity of Two-Dimensional Echocardiography in the Direct Visualization of Atrial Septal Defect Utilizing the Subcostal Approach: Experience with 154 Patients, *J. Am. Coll. Cardiol.*, 3:127, 1983.
89. Haworth, S. G.: Pulmonary Vascular Disease in Secundum Atrial Septal Defect in Childhood, *Am. J. Cardiol.*, 51:265, 1983.
90. Schreiber, T. L., Feigenbaum, H., and Weyman, A. E.: Effect of Atrial Septal Defect Repair on Left Ventricular Geometry and Degree of Mitral Valve Prolapse, *Circulation*, 61:888, 1980.
91. Nora, J. J., and Fraser, F. C.: "Medical Genetics: Principles and Practice," Lea & Febiger, Philadelphia, 1974.
92. Plauth, W. H., Jr., Nugent, E. W., Schlant, R. C., Edwards, J. E., Williams, W. H., and Kirklin, J. W.: The Pathology, Abnormal Physiology, Clinical Recognition, and Medical and Surgical Treatment of Congenital Heart Disease, in J. W. Hurst (ed.), "The Heart," McGraw-Hill Book Company, New York, 1982, p. 643.
93. Trusler, G. A., Kazenelson, G., Freedom, R. M., Williams, W. G., and Rowe, R. D.: Late Results following Repair of Partial Anomalous Pulmonary Venous Connection with Sinus Venosus Atrial Septal Defect, *J. Thorac. Cardiovasc. Surg.*, 79:776, 1980.
94. Kyger, E. R., III, Frazier, O. H., Cooley, D. A., et al.: Sinus Venosus Atrial Septal Defect: Early and Late Results following Closure in 109 Patients, *Ann. Thorac. Surg.*, 25:44, 1978.
95. Williams, W. H., Zorn-Chelton, S., Raviele, A. A., et al.: Extracardiac Atrial Pedicle Conduit Repair of Partial Anomalous Pulmonary Venous Connection to the Superior Vena Cava in Children, *Ann. Thorac. Surg.*, 38:345, 1984.
96. St. John Sutton, M. G., Tajik, A. J., and McGoon, D. C.: Atrial Septal Defect in Patients Ages 60 Years or Older: Operative Results and Long-Term Postoperative Follow-Up, *Circulation*, 64:402, 1981.
97. Daicoff, G. R., Brandenburg, R. O., and Kirklin, J. W.: Results of Operation for Atrial Septal Defect in Patients Forty-Five Years of Age and Older, *Circulation*, 35/36(suppl. 1):143, 1967.
98. Bryer, R. H., Monson, D. O., Ruggie, N. T., Weinberg, M., Jr., and Najafi, H.: Atrial Septal Defect: Repair in Patients Over Thirty-Five Years of Age, *J. Cardiovasc. Surg.*, 20:583, 1979.
99. Kolbjorn, F., Simonsen, S., Anderson, A., and Efskind, L.: Atrial Septal Defect of Secundum Type in the Middle-Aged: Clinical Results of Surgery and Correlations between Symptoms and Hemodynamics, *Am. Heart J.*, 94:44, 1977.
100. Meyer, R. A., Korfhagen, J. C., Covitz, W., and Kaplan, S.: Long-Term Follow-up Study after Closure of Secundum Atrial Septal Defect in Children: An Echocardiographic Study, *Am. J. Cardiol.*, 50:143, 1982.
101. Lucas, R. V. Jr.: Anomalous Venous Connections, Pulmonary and Systemic, in F. H. Adams and G. C. Emmanouilides (eds.), "Moss' Heart Disease in Infants, Children, and Adolescents," The Williams & Wilkins Company, Baltimore, 1983, p. 458.
102. Rowe, R. D.: Anomalies of Venous Return, in J. D. Keith, R. D. Rowe, and P. Vlad (eds.), "Heart Disease in Infancy and Childhood," The Macmillan Company, New York, 1978, p. 554.
103. Saalouke, M. G., Shapiro, S. R., Perry, L. W., and Scott, L. P.: Isolated Partial Anomalous Pulmonary Venous Drainage Associated with Pulmonary Vascular Obstructive Disease, *Am. J. Cardiol.*, 39:439, 1977.
104. Murphy, J. W., Kerr, A. R., and Kirklin, J. W.: Intracardiac Repair for Anomalous Pulmonary Venous Connection of Right Lung to Inferior Vena Cava, *Ann. Thorac. Surg.*, 11:38, 1971.
105. Geraci, J. E., and Kirklin, J. W.: Transplantation of Left Anomalous Pulmonary Vein to Left Atrium: Report of a Case, *Proc. Staff Meetings Mayo Clin.*, 28:472, 1953.
106. Becker, A. E., and Anderson, R. H.: Atrioventricular Septal Defects: What's in a Name? *J. Thorac. Cardiovasc. Surg.*, 83:461, 1982.
107. Rogers, H. M., and Edwards, J. E.: Incomplete Division of the Atrioventricular Canal with Patent Interatrial Foramen Primum (Persistent Common Cardioventricular Ostium). Report of Five Cases and Review of the Literature, *Am. Heart J.*, 36:28, 1948.
108. Rastelli, G. C., Kirklin, J. W., and Titus, J. L.: Anatomic Observations on Complete Form of Persistent Common Atrioventricular Canal with Special Reference to Atrioventricular Valves, *Mayo Clin. Proc.*, 41:296, 1968.
109. Nath, P. H., Soto, B., Bini, R. M., Bargeron, L. M., Jr., and Pacifico, A. D.: Tetralogy of Fallot with Atrioventricular Canal. An Angiographic Study, *J. Thorac. Cardiovasc. Surg.*, 87:421, 1984.
110. Feldt, R. H., Edwards, W. D., Puga, F. J., Seward, J. B., and Weidman, W. H.: Atrial Septal Defects and Atrioventricular Canal, in F. H. Adams and G. C. Emmanouilides (eds.), "Moss' Heart Disease in Infants, Children, and Adolescents," The Williams & Winkins Company, Baltimore, 1983, p. 118.
111. Mehta, S., Hirschfeld, S., Riggs, T., and Liebman, J.: Echocardiographic Estimation of Ventricular Hypoplasia in Complete Atrioventricular Canal, *Circulation*, 59:888, 1979.
112. Hagler, D. J., Tajik, A. J., Seward, J. B., Mair, D. D., and Ritter, D. G.: Real-Time Wide-Angle Sector Echocardiography: Atrioventricular Canal Defects, *Circulation*, 59:140, 1979.
113. Rastelli, G. C., Ongley, P. A., Kirklin, J. W., and McGoon, D. C.: Surgical Repair of the Complete Form of Persistent Common Atrioventricular Canal, *J. Thorac. Cardiovasc. Surg.*, 55:299, 1968.
114. Chin, A. J., Bierman, F. Z., Sanders, S. P., Williams, R. G., Norwood, W. I., and Castaneda, A. R.: Subxyphoid 2-Dimensional Echocardiographic Identification of Left Ventricular Papillary Muscle Anomalies in Complete Common Atrioventricular Canal, *Am. J. Cardiol.*, 51:1695, 1983.

115. Soto, B., Bargeron, L. M., Pacifico, A. D., Vanini, V., and Kirklin, J. W.: Angiography of Atrioventricular Canal Defects, *Am. J. Cardiol.*, 48:492, 1981.
116. Nora, J. J., and Nora, A. H.: "Genetics and Counseling in Cardiovascular Diseases," Charles C Thomas, Publisher, Springfield, Ill., 1978.
117. Williams, W. H., Guyton, R. A., Michalik, R. E., et al. Individualized Surgical Management of Complete Atrioventricular Canal, *J. Thorac. Cardiovasc. Surg.*, 86:838, 1983.
118. Berger, T. J., Kirklin, J. W., Blackstone, E. H., Pacifico, A. D., and Kouchokos, N. T.: Primary Repair of Complete Atrioventricular Canal in Patients Less than 2 Years Old, *Am. J. Cardiol.*, 41:906, 1978.
119. Kirklin, J. W., and Blackstone, E. H.: Management of the Infant with Complete Atrioventricular Canal, *J. Thorac Cardiovasc. Surg.*, 78:32, 1979.
120. Mair, D. D., and McGoon, D. C.: Surgical Correction of Atrioventricular Canal during the First Year of Life, *Am. J. Cardiol.*, 40:66, 1977.
121. Abbruzzese, P. A., Livermore, J., Sunderland, C. O., et al.: Mitral Repair in Complete Atrioventricular Canal, *J. Thorac. Cardiovasc. Surg.*, 85:388, 1983.
122. Mavroudis, C., Weinstein, G., Turley, K., and Ebert, P. A.: Surgical Management of Complete Atrioventricular Canal, *J. Thorac. Cardiovasc. Surg.*, 83:670, 1982.
123. Bender, H. W., Hammon, J. W., Jr., Hubbard, S. G., Muirhead, J., and Graham, T. P.: Repair of Atrioventricular Canal Malformation in the First Year of Life, *J. Thorac. Cardiovasc. Surg.*, 84:515, 1982.
124. Chin, A. J., Keane, J. F., Norwood, W. I., and Casteneda, A. R.: Repair of Complete Common Atrioventricular Canal in Infancy, *J. Thorac. Cardiovasc. Surg.*, 84:437, 1982.
125. Epstein, M. L., Moller, J. H., Amplatz, K., and Nicoloff, D. M.: Pulmonary Artery Banding in Infants with Complete Atrioventricular Canal, *J. Thorac. Cardiovasc. Surg.*, 78:28, 1979.
126. Danielson, G. K.: Endocardial Cushion Defects, in M. M. Ravitch, K. J., Welch, C. D. Benson, E. Aberdeen, and J. G. Randolph (eds.), "Pediatric Surgery," Year Book Medical Publishers, Inc., Chicago, 1979, p. 720.
127. Berger, T. J., Blackstone, E. H., Kirklin, J. W., Bargeron, L. M., Jr., Hazelrig, J. B., and Turner, M. E., Jr.: Survival and Probability of Cure without and with Operation in Complete Atrioventricular Canal, *Ann. Thorac. Surg.*, 27:104, 1979.
128. Danielson, G. K., Guiliani, E. R., and Ritter, D. G.: Successful Repair of Common Ventricle Associated with Complete Atrioventricular Canal, *J. Thorac. Cardiovasc. Surg.*, 67:152, 1974.
129. Pacifico, A. D., Kirklin, J. W., and Bargeron, L. M., Jr.: Repair of Complete Atrioventricular Canal Associated with Tetralogy of Fallot or Double-Outlet Right Ventricle: Report of 10 Patients, *Ann. Thorac. Surg.*, 29:351, 1980.
130. Danielson, G. K., Tabry, I. F., Ritter, D. G., and Maloney, J. D.: Successful Repair of Double-Outlet Right Ventricle, Complete Atrioventricular Discordance Associated with Dextrocardia and Pulmonary Stenosis, *J. Thorac. Cardiovasc. Surg.*, 76:710, 1978.
131. Danielson, G. K., McMullan, M. H., Kinsley, R. H., and DuShane, J. W.: Successful Repair of Complete Atrioventricular Canal Associated with Dextroversion, Common Atrium, and Total Anomalous Systemic Venous Return, *J. Thorac. Cardiovasc. Surg.*, 66:817, 1973.
132. Alfieri, O., and Plokker, M.: Repair of Common Atrioventricular Canal Associated with Transposition of the Great Arteries and Left Ventricular Outflow Obstruction, *J. Thorac. Cardiovasc. Surg.*, 84:872, 1982.
133. Studer, M., Blackstone, E. H., Kirklin, J. W., et al.: Determinants of Early and Late Results of Repair of Atrioventricular Septal (Canal) Defects, *J. Thorac. Cardiovasc. Surg.*, 84:523, 1982.
134. Ilbawi, M. N., Idriss, F. S., DeLeon, S. Y., et al.: Unusual Mitral Valve Abnormalities Complicating Surgical Repair of Endocardial Cushion Defects, *J. Thorac. Cardiovasc. Surg.*, 85:697, 1983.
135. Lappen, R. S., Muster, A. J., Idriss, F. S., et al.: Masked Subaortic Stenosis in Ostium Primum Atrial Septal Defect: Recognition and Treatment, *Am. J. Cardiol.*, 52:336, 1983.
136. McMullan, M. H., McGoon, D. C., Wallace, R. B., Danielson, G. K., and Weidman, W. H.: Surgical Treatment of Partial Atrioventricular Canal, *Arch. Surg.*, 197:705, 1973.
137. Riemenschneider, T. A.: Left Ventricular–Right Atrial Communication, in F. H. Adams and G. C. Emmanouilides, (eds.), "Moss' Heart Disease in Infants, Children, and Adolescents," The Williams & Wilkins Company, Baltimore, 1983, p. 154.
138. Wells, H. G.: Persistent Patency of the Ductus Arteriosus, *Am. J. Med. Sci.*, 136:381, 1908.
139. Christie, A.: Normal Closing Time of the Foramen Ovale and the Ductus Arteriosus, *Am. J. Dis. Child.*, 40:323, 1930.
140. Campbell, M.: Natural History of Persistent Ductus Arteriosus, *Br. Heart J.*, 30:4, 1968.
141. Kitterman, J. A., Edmonds, H., Jr., Gregory, G. A., Heymann, M. A., Tooley, W. H., and Rudolph, A. M.: Patent Ductus Arteriosus in Premature Infants, Incidence, Relation to Pulmonary Disease and Management, *N. Engl. J. Med.*, 287:473, 1972.
142. Friedman, W. F., Hirschklau, M. J., Printz, M. F., Pitlick, P. T., and Kirkpatrick, S. E.: Pharmacologic Closure of Patent Ductus Arteriosus in the Premature Infant, *N. Engl. J. Med.*, 295:526, 1976.
143. Heymann, M. A., Rudolph, A. M., and Silverman, N. H.: Closure of the Ductus Arteriosus by Prostaglandin Inhibition, *N. Engl. J. Med.*, 295:530, 1976.
144. Neal, W. A., Bessinger, F. B., Jr., Hunt, C. E., and Lucas, R. V., Jr.: Patent Ductus Arteriosus Complicating Respiratory Distress Syndrome, *J. Pediatr.*, 86:127, 1975.
145. Thibeault, D. W., Emmanouilides, G. C., Nelson, R. J., Lachman, R. S., Rosengart, R. M., and Oh, W.: Patent Ductus Arteriosus Complicating the Respiratory Distress Syndrome in Preterm Infants, *J. Pediatr.*, 86:120, 1975.
146. Siassi, B., Blanco, C., Cabal, L. A., and Coran, A. G.: Incidence and Clinical Features of Patent Ductus Arteriosus in Low-Birthweight Infants: A Prospective Analysis of 150 Consecutiviely Born Infants, *Pediatrics*, 57:347, 1976.
147. Krovetz, L. J., and Warden, H. E.: Patent Ductus Arteriosus: An Analysis of 515 Surgically Proven Cases, *Dis. Chest*, 42:46, 1962.
148. Thapar, M. K., Rao, P. S., Rogers, J. H., Jr., Moore, H. V., and Strong, W. B.: Changing Murmur of Patent Ductus Arteriosus, *J. Pediatr.*, 92:939, 1978.
149. McGrath, R. L., McGuinness, G. A., Way, G. L., Wolfe, R. R., Nora, J. J., and Simmons, M. A.: The Silent Ductus Arteriosus, *J. Pediatr.*, 93:110, 1978.
150. Silverman, N. H., Lewis, A. B., Heymann, M. A., and Rudolph, A. M.: Echocardiographic Assessment of Ductus Arteriosus Shunt in Premature Infants, *Circulation*, 50:821, 1974.
151. Baylen, B. G., Meyer, R. A., Kaplan, S., Ringenburg, W. E., and Korfhagen, J.: The Critically Ill Premature Infant with Patent Ductus Arteriosus and Pulmonary Disease—An Echocardiographic Assessment, *J. Pediatr.*, 86:423, 1975.
152. Sahn, D. J., Vaucher, Y., Williams, D. E., Allen, H. D., Goldberg, S. J., and Friedman, W. F.: Echocardiographic Detection of Large Left to Right Shunts and Cardiomyopathies in Infants and Children, *Am. J. Cardiol.*, 38:73, 1976.
153. Baylen, B., Meyer, R. A., Korfhagen, J., Benzing, G. III, Bubb, M. E., and Kaplan, S.: Left Ventricular Performance in the Critically Ill Premature Infant with Patent Ductus Arteriosus and Pulmonary Disease, *Circulation*, 55:182, 1977.
154. Wilcox, W. D., Carrigan, T. A., Dooley, K. J., et al.: Range-Gated Pulsed Doppler Ultrasonographic Evaluation of Carotid Arterial Blood Flow in Small Preterm Infants with Patent Ductus Arteriosus, *J. Pediatr.*, 102:294, 1983.
155. Serwer, G. A., Armstrong, B. E., and Anderson, P. A. W.: Continuous Wave Doppler Ultrasonographic Quantitation of Patent Ductus Arteriosus Flow, *J. Pediatr.*, 100:297, 1982.
156. Vick, G. W., Satterwhite, C., Cassady, G., Philips, J., Yester, M. V., and Logic, J. R.: Radionuclide Angiography in the

Evaluation of Ductal Shunts in Preterm Infants, *J. Pediatr.*, 101:264, 1982.
157. Stevenson, J. G.: Fluid Administration in the Association of Patent Ductus Arteriosus Complicating Respiratory Distress Syndrome, *J. Pediatr.*, 90:257, 1977.
158. Krovetz, L. J., and Rowe, R. D.: Patent Ductus, Prematurity and Pulmonary Disease, *N. Engl. J. Med.*, 287:513, 1972.
159. Porstmann, W., Wierny, L., Warnke, H., Gerstberger, G., and Romaniuk, P. A.: Catheter Closure of Patent Ductus Arteriosus: 62 Cases Treated without Thoracotomy, *Radiol. Clin. North Am.*, 9:203, 1971.
160. Rashkind, W. J., and Cuasco, C. C.: Transcatheter Closure of Patent Ductus Arteriosus: Successful Use in a 3.5 Kilogram Infant, *Pediatr. Cardiol.*, 1:3, 1979.
161. Merritt, T. A., White, C. L., Jacob, J., et al.: Patent Ductus Arteriosus Treated with Ligation or Indomethacin: A Follow-up Study, *J. Pediatr.*, 95:588, 1979.
162. Yeh, T. F., Wilks, A., Singh, J., Betkerur, M., Lilien, L., and Pildes, R. S.: Furosemide Prevents the Renal Side Effects of Indomethacin Therapy in Premature Infants with Patent Ductus Arteriosus, *J. Pediatr.*, 101:433, 1982.
163. Halliday, H. L., Hirata, T., and Brady, J. P.: Indomethacin Therapy for Large Patent Ductus Arteriosus in the Very Low Birth Weight Infant: Results and Complications, *Pediatrics*, 64:154, 1979.
164. Gersony, W. M., Peckham, G. J., Ellison, R. C., Miettinen, O. S., and Nadas, A. S.: Effects of Indomethacin in Premature Infants with Patent Ductus Arteriosus: Results of a National Collaborative Study, *J. Pediatr.*, 102:895, 1983.
165. Gay, J. H., Daily, W. J. R., Meyer, B. H. P., Trump, D. S., Cloud, D. T., and Moltham, M. E.: Ligation of the Patent Ductus Arteriosus in Premature Infants: Report of 45 Cases, *J. Pediatr. Surg.*, 8:677, 1973.
166. Lewis, C. E., Jr., Coen, R. W., Talbot, W., and Edwards, W. S.: Early Surgical Intervention in Premature Infants with Respiratory Distress and Patent Ductus Arteriosus, *Am. J. Surg.*, 128:829, 1974.
167. Castaneda, A. R.: Patent Ductus Arteriosus: A Commentary, *Ann. Thorac. Surg.*, 31:92, 1981.
168. Jones, J. C.: Twenty-Five Years' Experience with Surgery of Patent Ductus Arteriosus, *J. Thorac. Cardiovasc. Surg.*, 50:149, 1965.
169. Bell-Thomson, J., Jewell, E., Ellis, F. H., and Schwaber, J. R.: Surgical Technique in the Management of Patent Ductus Arteriosus in the Elderly Patient, *Ann. Thorac. Surg.*, 30:80, 1980.
170. Ellis, F. H., Jr., Kirklin, J. W., Callahan, J. A., and Wood, E. H.: Patent Ductus Arteriosus and Pulmonary Hypertension: Analysis of Patients Treated Surgically, *J. Thorac. Cardiovasc. Surg.*, 31:268, 1956.
171. Mikhail, M., Lee, W., Toews, W., et al.: Surgical and Medical Experience with 734 Premature Infants with Patent Ductus Arteriosus, *J. Thorac. Cardiovasc. Surg.*, 83:349, 1982.
172. Neufeld, H. N., Lester, R. G., Adams, P., Jr., Anderson, R. C., Lillehei, C. W., and Edwards, J. E.: Aorticopulmonary Septal Defect, *Am. J. Cardiol.*, 9:12, 1962.
173. Tandon, R., daSilva, C. L., Moller, J. H., and Edwards, J. E.: Aorticopulmonary Septal Defect Coexisting with Ventricular Septal Defect, *Circulation*, 50:188, 1974.
174. Blieden, L. C., and Moller, J. H.: Aorticopulmonary Septal Defect. An Experience with 17 Patients, *Br. Heart J.*, 36:630, 1974.
175. Doty, D. B., Richardson, J. V., Falkovsky, G. E., Gordonova, M. I., and Burakovsky, V. I.: Aortopulmonary Septal Defect: Hemodynamics, Angiography, and Operation, *Ann. Thorac. Surg.*, 32:244, 1981.
176. Clarke, C. P., and Richardson, J. P.: The Management of Aortopulmonary Window. Advantages of Transaortic Closure with a Dacron Patch, *J. Thorac. Cardiovasc. Surg.*, 72:48, 1976.
177. Deverall, P. B., Aberdeen, E., Bonham-Carter, R. E., and Waterston, D. J.: Aortopulmonary Window, *J. Thorac. Cardiovasc. Surg.*, 57:479, 1969.
178. Lau, K. C., Calcaterra, G., Miller, G. A. H., et al: Aortopulmonary Window, *J. Cardiovasc. Surg.*, 23:21, 1982.
179. Keane, J. F., Maltz, D., Bernhard, W. F., Corwin, R. D., and Nadas, A. S.: Anomalous Origin of One Pulmonary Artery from the Ascending Aorta: Diagnostic, Physiologic, and Surgical Considerations, *Circulation*, 50:588, 1974.
180. Matsuda, H., Zavanella, C., Lee, P., and Subramanian, S.: Aortic Origin of the Right Pulmonary Artery, *Ann. Thorac. Surg.*, 24:374, 1977.
181. Edwards, J. E., Burchell, H. B., and Christensen, N. A.: Specimen Exhibiting the Essential Lesion in Aneurysm of the Aortic Sinus, *Mayo Clin. Proc.*, 31:407, 1956.
182. Edwards, J. E., and Burchell, H. B.: Pathologic Anatomy of Deficiencies Between the Aortic Root and the Heart Including Aortic Sinus Aneurysms, *Thorax*, 12:125, 1957.
183. Sakakibara, S., and Konno, S.: Congenital Aneurysm of the Sinus of Valsalva. Anatomy and Classification, *Am. Heart J.*, 63:405, 1962.
184. Shumaker, H. B., Jr.: Aneurysms of the Aortic Sinuses of Valsalva Due to Bacterial Endocarditis with Special Reference to Their Operative Management, *J. Thorac. Cardiovasc. Surg.*, 63:896, 1972.
185. Kakos, G. S., Kilman, J. W., Williams, T. E., and Hosier, D. M.: Diagnosis and Management of Sinus of Valsalva Aneurysm in Children, *Ann. Thorac. Surg.*, 17:474, 1974.
186. Meyer, J., Wukasch, D. C., Hallman, G. L., and Cooley, D. A.: Aneurysm and Fistula of the Sinus of Valsalva: Clinical Considerations and Surgical Treatment in 45 Patients, *Ann. Thorac. Surg.*, 19:170, 1975.
187. Nowicki, E. R., Aberdeen, E., Friedman, S., and Rashkind, W. J.: Congenital Left Aortic Sinus–Left Ventricle Fistula and Review of Aortocardiac Fistulas, *Ann. Thorac. Surg.*, 23:378, 1977.
188. Pan-Chih, Ching-Heng, T., Chen-Chun, and Chieh-Fu, L.: Surgical Treatment of the Ruptured Aneurysm of the Aortic Sinuses, *Ann. Thorac. Surg.*, 32:162, 1981.
189. Bonfils-Roberts, E. A., DuShane, J. W., McGoon, D. C., and Danielson, G.: Aortic Sinus Fistula—Surgical Considerations and Results of Operation, *Ann. Thorac. Surg.*, 12:492, 1971.
190. Sade, R. M., Clouse, M., and Ellis, R. H., Jr.: The Spectrum of Pulmonary Sequestration, *Ann. Thorac. Surg.*, 18:644, 1974.
191. Telander, R. L., Lenox, C. C., and Sieber, W.: Sequestration of the Lung in Children, *Mayo Clin. Proc.*, 51:578, 1976.
192. Ransom, J. M., Norton, J. B., and Williams, G. D.: Pulmonary Sequestration Presenting as Congestive Heart Failure, *J. Thorac. Cardiovasc. Surg.*, 76:378, 1978.
193. Litwin, S. B., Plauth, W. H., Jr., and Nadas, A. S.: Anomalous Systemic Arterial Supply to the Lung Causing Pulmonary-Artery Hypertension, *N. Engl. J. Med.*, 283:1098, 1970.
194. White, R. I., Jr., Kaufman, S. L., Barth, K. H., DeCaprio, V., and Strandberg, I. D.: Embolo-therapy with Detachable Silicone Balloons: Technique and Clinical Results, *Radiology*, 131:619, 1979.
195. Zuberbuhler, J. R., Dankner, E., Zoltun, R., Burkholder, J., and Bahnson, H. T.: Tissue Adhesive Closure of Aortopulmonary Communications, *Am. Heart J.*, 88:41, 1974.
196. Thurer, R. J.: Communication between the Pulmonary and Systemic Circulation, *Ann. Thorac. Surg.*, 21:114, 1976.
197. Sissman, N. J.: Anomalies of the Aortic Arch Complex, in F. H. Adams and G. C. Emmanouilides (eds.), "Moss' Heart Disease in Infants, Children, and Adolescents," The Williams & Wilkins Company, Baltimore, 1983, p. 199.
198. Berman, W., Jr., Yabek, S. M., Dillon, T., Neal, J. F., Akl, B., and Burstein, J.: Vascular Ring Due to Left Aortic Arch and Right Descending Aorta, *Circulation*, 63:458, 1981.
199. Gross, R. E.: Surgical Treatment for Dysphagia Lusoria, *Ann. Surg.*, 124:532, 1946.
200. Arciniegas, E.: Vascular Anomalies Compressing the Trachea and Esophagus, in M. M. Ravitch, K. J. Welch, C. D. Benson, E. Aberdeen, and J. G. Randolph, (eds.), "Pediatric Surgery," Year Book Medical Publishers, Inc., Chicago, 1979, p. 649.
201. Hallman, G. L., and Cooley, D. A.: Congenital Aortic Vascular Ring: Surgical Considerations, *Arch. Surg.*, 88:666, 1964.

202. Celano, V., Pieroni, D. R., Gingell, R. L., and Roland, J. M. A.: Two-Dimensional Echocardiographic Recognition of the Right Aortic Arch, *Am. J. Cardiol.*, 51:1507, 1983.
203. Richardson, J. V., Doty, D. B., Rossi, N. P., and Ehrenhaft, J. L.: Operation for Aortic Arch Anomalies, *Ann. Thorac. Surg.*, 31:426, 1981.
204. Roesler, M., De Leval, M., and Chrispin, A.: Surgical Management of Vascular Ring, *Ann. Surg.*, 197:139, 1983.
205. Gross, R. E.: Vascular Anomalies of the Thorax Producing Compression of the Trachea and Esophagus, in "The Surgery of Infancy and Childhood," W. B. Saunders Company, Philadelphia, 1952, p. 913.
206. Rodriguez, L., Izukawa, T., Moes, C. A. F., Trusler, G. A., and Williams, W. G.: Surgical Implications of Right Aortic Arch with Isolation of Left Subclavian Artery, *Br. Heart J.*, 37:931, 1975.
207. Gumbiner, C. H., Mullins, C. E., and McNamara, D. G.: Pulmonary Artery Sling, *Am. J. Cardiol.*, 45:311, 1980.
208. Jue, K. L., Raghib, G., Amplatz, K., Adams, P., and Edwards, J. E.: Anomalous Origin of the Left Pulmonary Artery from the Right Pulmonary Artery, *Am. J. Roentgenol.*, 95:598, 1965.
209. Potts, W. C., Holinger, P. H., and Rosenblum, A. H.: Anomalous Left Pulmonary Artery Causing Obstruction to the Right Mainstem Bronchus, *JAMA* 155:1409, 1954.
210. Campbell, C. D., Wernly, J. A., Koltip, P. C., Vitullo, D., and Replogle, R. L.: Aberrant Left Pulmonary Artery (Pulmonary Artery Sling): Successful Repair and 24 Year Follow-up Report, *Am. J. Cardiol.*, 45:316, 1980.
211. Sade, R. M., Rosenthal, A., Fellows, K., and Castaneda, A. R.: Pulmonary Artery Sling, *J. Thorac. Cardiovasc. Surg.*, 69:333, 1975.
212. McCue, C. M., Mauck, H. P., Jr., Tingelstad, J. B., and Kellett, G. N., Jr.: Cervical Aortic Arch, *Am. J. Dis. Child.*, 125:738, 1973.
213. Clagett, O. T., Kirklin, J. W., and Edwards, J. E.: Anatomic Variations and Pathologic Changes in 124 Cases of Coarctation of the Aorta, *Surg. Gynecol. Obstet.*, 98:103, 1954.
214. Edwards, J. E., Clagett, O. T., Drake, R. L., and Christensen, N. A.: The Collateral Circulation in Coarctation of the Aorta, *Mayo Clin. Proc.*, 23:333, 1948.
215. Becker, A. E., Becker, M. J., and Edwards, J. E.: Anomalies Associated with Coarctation of Aorta. Particular Reference to Infancy, *Circulation*, 41:1067, 1970.
216. Rosenquist, G. C.: Congenital Mitral Valve Disease Associated with Coarctation of the Aorta. A Spectrum That Includes Parachute Deformity of the Mitral Valve, *Circulation*, 49:985, 1974.
217. Parker, F. B., Jr., Streeten, D. H. P., Farrell, B., Blackman, M. S., Sondheimer, H. M., and Anderson, G. H., Jr.: Preoperative and Postoperative Renin Levels in Coarctation of the Aorta, *Circulation*, 66:513, 1982.
218. Ho, S. Y., and Anderson, R. H.: Coarctation, Tubular Hypoplasia, and the Ductus Arteriosus, Histological Study of 35 Specimens, *Br. Heart J.*, 41:268, 1979.
219. Simon, A. B., Zloto, A. E., Perry, B. L., and Sigmann, J. M.: Familial Aspects of Coarctation of the Aorta, *Chest*, 66:687, 1974.
220. Smallhorn, J. F., Huhta, J. C., Adams, P. A., Anderson, R. H., Wilkinson, J. L., and Macartney, F. J.: Cross-Sectional Echocardiographic Assessment of Coarctation in the Sick Neonate and Infant, *Br. Heart J.*, 50:349, 1983.
221. Beekman, R. H., Rocchini, A. P., Behrendt, D. M., and Rosenthal, A.: Reoperation for Coarctation of the Aorta, *Am. J. Cardiol.*, 48:1108, 1981.
222. Liberthson, R. R., Pennington, D. G., Jacobs, M. L., and Daggett, W. M.: Coarctation of the Aorta: Review of 234 Patients with Clarification of Management Problems, *Am. J. Cardiol.*, 43:835, 1979.
223. Freed, M. D., Rocchini, A., Rosenthal, A., Nadas, A. S., and Castaneda, A. R.: Exercise Induced Hypertension after Surgical Repair of Coarctation of the Aorta, *Am. J. Cardiol.*, 43:253, 1979.
224. Maron, B. J.: Coarctation of the Aorta in the Adult, in W. C. Roberts (ed.), "Congenital Heart Disease in Adults," F. A. Davis Company, Philadelphia, 1979, p. 311.
225. Heymann, M. A., Berman, W., Rudolph, A. M., and Whitman, V.: Dilatation of the Ductus Arteriosus by Prostaglandin E-1 in Aortic Arch Abnormalities, *Circulation*, 59:169, 1979.
226. Lock, J. E., Bass, J. L., Amplatz, K., Fuhrman, B. P., and Castaneda-Zuniga, W.: Balloon Dilation Angioplasty of Aortic Coarctations in Infants and Children, *Circulation*, 68:109, 1983.
227. Barash, P. G., Hobbins, J. C., Hook, R., Stansel, H. C., Jr., Whittemore, R., and Hehre, F.: Management of Coarctation of the Aorta during Pregnancy, *J. Thorac. Cardiovasc. Surg.*, 69:781, 1975.
228. Sehested, J.: Evaluation of Optimum Time for Surgical Repair of Coarctation of the Aorta, *Surg. Gynecol. Obstet.*, 146:593, 1978.
229. Kirklin, J. W., and Nadas, A. S.: Editorial Comments, in W. P. Harvey, W. M. Kirkendall, J. W. Kirklin, A. S. Nadas, O. Paul, and E. H. Sonnenblick (eds.), "The Year Book of Cardiology—1979," Year Book Medical Publishers, Inc., Chicago, 1979, p. 286.
230. Hallman, G. L., and Cooley, D. A.: Coarctation of Thoracic Aorta, in G. L. Hallman and D. A. Cooley (eds.), "Surgical Treatment of Congenital Heart Disease," Lea & Febiger, Philadelphia, 1975, p. 28.
231. Harlan, B. J., Starr, A., and Harwin, F.: Coarctation, in B. J. Harlan, A. Starr, and F. Harwin (eds.), "Manual of Cardiac Surgery," Springer-Verlag, New York, 1981, p. 170.
232. Morris, G. C., Cooley, D. A., DeBakey, M. E., and Crawford, E. S.: Coarctation of the Aorta with Particular Emphasis upon Improved Techniques of Surgical Repair, *J. Thorac. Cardiovasc. Surg.*, 40:705, 1960.
233. Ravelo, H. R., Stephenson, L. W., Friedman, S., et al: Coarctation Resection in Children with Turner's Syndrome: A Note of Caution, *J. Thorac. Cardiovasc. Surg.*, 80:427, 1980.
234. Conners, J. P., Hartmann, A. F., and Weldon, C. S.: Considerations in the Surgical Management of Infantile Coarctation of Aorta, *Am. J. Cardiol.*, 36:489, 1975.
235. Reul, G. J., Jr., Kabbani, S. S., Sandiford, F. M., Wukasch, D. C., and Cooley, D. A.: Repair of Coarctation of the Thoracic Aorta by Patch Graft Aortoplasty, *J. Thorac. Cardiovasc. Surg.*, 68:696, 1974.
236. Pierce, W. S., Waldhausen, J. A., Berman, W., Jr., and Whitman, V.: Late Results of the Subclavian Flap Procedure in Infants with Coarctation of the Thoracic Aorta, *Circulation*, 58(suppl. 1):78, 1978.
237. Moulton, A. L., Brenner, J. I., Roberts, G., et al: Subclavian Flap Repair of Coarctation of the Aorta in Neonates—Realization of Growth Potential?, *J. Thorac. Cardiovasc. Surg.*, 87:220, 1984.
238. Herrmann, V. M., Laks, H., Fagan, L., Terschluse, D., and William, V. L.: Repair of Aortic Coarctation in the First Year of Life, *Ann. Thorac. Surg.*, 25:57, 1978.
239. Myers, J. L., Waldhausen, J. A., Pae, W. E., Abt, A. B., Prophet, G. A., and Pierce, W. S.: Vascular Anastomoses in Growing Vessels: The Use of Absorbable Sutures, *Ann. Thorac. Surg.*, 34:529, 1982.
240. Tiraboschi, R., Alfieri, O., Carpentier, A., and Parenzan, L.: One-Stage Correction of Coarctation of the Aorta Associated with Intracardiac Defects in Infancy, *J. Cardiovasc. Surg. (Torino)*, 19:11, 1978.
241. McNicholas, K. W., Stafford, M., and Malm, J. R.: Surgical Repair of Coarctation of the Aorta, *J. Thorac. Cardiovasc. Surg.*, 82:642, 1981. (Letter.)
242. Moreno, N. N., deCampo, T., Kaiser, G. A., and Pallares, V. S.: Technical and Pharmacologic Management of Distal Hypotension During Repair of Coarctation of the Aorta, *J. Thorac. Cardiovasc. Surg.*, 80:182, 1980.
243. Coles, J. G., Wilson, G. J., Sima, A. F., Klement, P., and Tait, G. A.: Intraoperative Detection of Spinal Cord Is-

chemia Using Somatosensory Cortical Evoked Potentials during Thoracic Aortic Occlusion, *Ann. Thorac. Surg.*, 34:299, 1982.
244. Fox, S., Pierce, W. S., and Waldhausen, J. A.: Pathogenesis of Paradoxical Hypertension after Coarctation Repair, *Ann. Thorac. Surg.*, 29:135, 1980.
245. Williams, W. G., Shindo, G., Trusler, G. A., Dische, M. R., and Olley, P. M.: Results of Repair of Coarctation of the Aorta During Infancy, *J. Thorac. Cardiovasc. Surg.*, 69:603, 1980.
246. Bergdahl, L. A. L., Blackstone, E. H., Kirklin, J. W., Pacifico, A. D., and Bargeron, L. M.: Determinants of Early Success in Repair of Aortic Coarctation in Infants, *J. Thorac. Cardiovasc. Surg.*, 83:736, 1982.
247. Maron, B. J., Humphries, J. O., Rowe, R. D., and Mellits, E. D.: Prognosis of Surgically Corrected Coarctation of the Aorta: A 20-Year Postoperative Appraisal, *Circulation*, 47:119, 1973.
248. Collins-Nakai, R. L., Dick, M., Paresi-Buckley, L., Fyler, D. C., and Castaneda, A. R.: Interrupted Aortic Arch in Infancy, *J. Pediatr.*, 88:959, 1976.
249. Celoria, G. C., and Patton, R. B.: Congenital Absence of the Aortic Arch, *Am. Heart J.*, 58:407, 1959.
250. Riggs, T. W., Berry, T. E., Aziz, K. U., and Paul, M. H.: Two-Dimensional Echocardiographic Features of Interruption of the Aortic Arch, *Am. J. Cardiol.*, 50:1385, 1982.
251. Dische, M. R., Tsai, M., and Baltaxe, H. A.: Solitary Interruption of the Arch of the Aorta. Clinicopathologic Review of Eight Cases, *Am. J. Cardiol.*, 35:271, 1975.
252. Jones, E. L., Plauth, W. H., and Hatcher, C. R., Jr.: A Palliative Operation for All Types of Aortic Arch Interruption in the Neonate, *J. Thorac. Cardiovasc. Surg.*, 69:579, 1975.
253. Copeland, J. G., Record, J. A., Salomon, N. W., Sahn, D. J., Allen, H. D., and Goldberg, S. J.: Successful Palliation Using Partial Cardiopulmonary Bypass in a Two-Day-Old Infant with Type B Interruption of the Aortic Arch, *J. Thorac. Cardiovasc. Surg.*, 76:495, 1980.
254. Kron, I. L., Rheuban, K. S., Carpenter, M. S., and Nolan, S. P.: Interrupted Aortic Arch—A Conservative Approach for the Sick Neonate, *J. Thorac. Cardiovasc. Surg.*, 86:37, 1983.
255. Fowler, B. N., Lucas, S. K., Razook, J. D., Thompson, W. M., Jr., Williams, G. R., and Elkins, R. C.: Interruption of the Aortic Arch: Experience in 17 Infants, *Ann. Thorac. Surg.*, 37:25, 1984.
256. Braunlin, E. A., Lock, J. E., and Foker, J. E.: Repair of Type B Interruption of the Aortic Arch—Results and Follow-up, *J. Thorac. Cardiovasc. Surg.*, 86:920, 1983.
257. Moulton, A. L., and Bowman, F. O., Jr.: Primary Definitive Repair of Type B Interrupted Aortic Arch, Ventricular Septal Defect, and Patent Ductus Arteriosus, *J. Thorac. Cardiovasc. Surg.*, 82:501, 1981.
258. Norwood, W. I., Lang, P., Casteneda, A. R., and Hougen, T. J.: Reparative Operations for Interrupted Aortic Arch with Ventricular Septal Defect, *J. Thorac. Cardiovasc. Surg.*, 86:832, 1983.
259. Roberts, W. C.: Valvular, Subvalvular, and Supravalvular Aortic Stenosis: Morphologic Features, in *Cardiovasc. Clin.* Series 5/1, F. A. Davis Company, Philadelphia, 1973, p. 98.
260. Wagner, H. R., Ellison, R. C., Keane, J. F., Humphries, J. O., and Nadas, A. S.: Clinical Course in Aortic Stenosis, in A. S. Nadas (ed.), "Pulmonary Stenosis, Aortic Stenosis, Ventricular Septal Defect: Clinical Course and Indirect Assessment" (report from the Joint Study on the Natural History of Congenital Heart Defects), *Circulation*, 55(suppl. 1): 47, 1977.
261. Wagner, H. R., Weidman, W. H., Ellison, R. C., and Miettinen, O. S.: Indirect Assessment of Severity in Aortic Stenosis, in A. S. Nadas (ed.), "Pulmonary Stenosis, Aortic Stenosis, Ventricular Septal Defect: Clinical Course and Indirect Assessment" (report from the Joint Study on the Natural History of Congenital Heart Defects), *Circulation*, 55(suppl. 1):20, 1977.
262. Whitmer, J. T., James, F. W., Kaplan, S., Schwartz, D. C. and Knight, M. J. S.: Exercise Testing in Children before and after Surgical Treatment of Aortic Stenosis, *Circulation*, 63:254, 1981.
263. Gewitz, M. H., Werner, J. C., Kleinman, C. S., Hellenbrand, W. E., and Talner, N. S.: Role of Echocardiography in Aortic Stenosis: Pre and Post Operative Studies, *Am. J. Cardiol.*, 43:67, 1979.
264. Lima, C. O., Sahn, D. J., Valdescruz, L. M., et al: Prediction of the Severity of Left Ventricular Outflow Tract Obstruction by Quantitative Two-Dimensional Echocardiographic Doppler Studies, *Circulation*, 68:348, 1983.
265. Sink, J. D., Smallhorn, J. F., Macartney, F. J., Taylor, J. F. N., Stark, J., and de Leval, M. R.: Management of Critical Aortic Stenosis in Infancy, *J. Thorac. Cardiovasc. Surg.*, 87:82, 1984.
266. Keane, J. F., Bernhard, W. F., and Nadas, A. S.: Aortic Stenosis Surgery in Infancy, *Circulation*, 52:1138, 1975.
267. Ankeney, J. L., Tzeng, T. S., and Liebman, J.: Surgical Therapy for Congenital Aortic Valvular Stenosis: A 23 Year Experience, *J. Thorac. Cardiovasc. Surg.*, 85:41, 1983.
268. Sandor, G. G. S., Olley, P. M., Trusler, G. A., Williams, W. G., Rowe, R. D., and Morch, J. E.: Long-Term Follow-up of Patients after Valvotomy for Congenital Valvular Aortic Stenosis in Children, *J. Thorac. Cardiovasc. Surg.*, 80:171, 1980.
269. Ellis, F. H., Jr., and Kirklin, J. W.: Congenital Valvular Aortic Stenosis: Anatomic Findings and Surgical Technique, *J. Thorac. Surg.*, 43:199, 1962.
270. Fulton, D. R., Hougen, T. J., Keane, J. F., Rosenthal, A. R., Norwood, W. I., and Bernhard, W. F.: Repeat Aortic Valvotomy in Children, *Am. Heart J.*, 106:60, 1983.
271. Lawson, R. M., Bonchek, L. I., Menashe, V., and Starr, A.: Late Results of Surgery for Left Ventricular Outflow Tract Obstruction in Children, *J. Thorac. Cardiovasc. Surg.*, 71:334, 1976.
272. Smith, J. M., III, Cooley, D. A., Ott, D. A., Ferrerira, W., and Reul, G. J., Jr.: Aortic Valve Replacement in Preteenage Children, *Ann. Thorac. Surg.*, 29:512, 1980.
273. Sade, R. M., Ballenger, J. F., Hohn, A. R., Arrants, J. E., Riopel, D. A., and Taylor, A. B.: Cardiac Valve Replacement in Children: Comparison of Tissue with Mechanical Prostheses, *Ann. Thorac. Surg.*, 28:123, 1979.
274. Sanders, S. P., Levy, R. J., Freed, M. D., Norwood, W. I., and Castaneda, A. R.: Use of Hancock Porcine Xenografts in Children and Adolescents, *Am. J. Cardiol.*, 46:429, 1980.
275. Williams, W. G., Pollock, J. C., Geiss, D. M., Trusler, G. A., and Fowler, R. S.: Experience with Aortic and Mitral Valve Replacement in Children, *J. Thorac. Cardiovasc. Surg.*, 81:326, 1981.
276. Dobell, A. R. C., Bloss, R. S., Gibbons, J. E., and Collins, G. F.: Congenital Valvular Aortic Stenosis: Surgical Management and Long-Term Results, *J. Thorac. Cardiovasc. Surg.*, 81:916, 1981.
277. Chiariello, L., Agosti, J., Vlad, P., and Subramanian, S.: Congenital Aortic Stenosis—Experience with 43 Patients, *J. Thorac. Cardiovasc. Surg.*, 72:182, 1976.
278. Rastan, H., and Koncz, J.: Aortoventriculoplasty, *J. Thorac. Cardiovasc. Surg.*, 71:920, 1976.
279. Misbach, G. A., Turley, K., Ullyot, D. J., and Ebert, P. A.: Left Ventricular Outflow Enlargement by the Konno Procedure, *J. Thorac. Cardiovasc. Surg.*, 84:696, 1982.
280. Ergin, M. A., Cooper, R., LaCorte, M., Golinko, R., and Griepp, R. B.: Experience with Left Ventricular Apicoaortic Conduits for Complicated Left Ventricular Outflow Obstruction in Children and Young Adults, *Ann. Thorac. Surg.*, 32:369, 1981.
281. Norman, J. C., Cooley, D. A., Hallman, G. L., and Nihill, M. R.: Left Ventricular Apical–Abdominal Aortic Conduits for Left Ventricular Outflow Tract Obstructions, *Circulation*, 56:62, 1977.
282. Lababidi, Z., Wu, J., and Walls, J. T.: Percutaneous Balloon Aortic Valvuloplasty: Results in 23 Patients, *Am. J. Cardiol.*, 53:194, 1984.

283. Wright, G. B., Keane, J. F., Nadas, A. S., Bernhard, W. F., and Castaneda, A. R.: Fixed Subaortic Stenosis in the Young: Medical and Surgical Course in 83 Patients, *Am. J. Cardiol.*, 52:830, 1983.
284. Motro, M., Schneeweiss, A., Shem-Tov, A., et al: Two-Dimensional Echocardiography in Discrete Subaortic Stenosis, *Am. J. Cardiol.*, 53:896, 1984.
285. Kirklin, J. W., and Ellis, F. H., Jr.: Surgical Relief of Diffuse Subvalvular Aortic Stenosis, *Circulation*, 24:739, 1961.
286. Bjork, V. O., Holtquist, G., and Lodin, H.: Subaortic Stenosis Produced by Abnormally Plated Anterior Mitral Leaflet, *J. Thorac. Cardiovasc. Surg.*, 41:659, 1961.
287. McKay, R., and Ross, D. N.: Technique for the Relief of Discrete Subaortic Stenosis, *J. Thorac. Cardiovasc. Surg.*, 84:917, 1982.
288. Vogel, M., Freedom, R. M., Brand, A., Trusler, G. A., Williams, W. G., and Rowe, R. D.: Ventricular Septal Defect and Subaortic Stenosis: An Analysis of 41 Patients, *Am. J. Cardiol.*, 52:1258, 1983.
289. Moses, R. D., Barnhart, G. R., and Jone, M.: The Late Prognosis after Localized Resection for Fixed (Discrete and Tunnel) Left Ventricular Outflow Tract Obstruction, *J. Thorac. Cardiovasc. Surg.*, 87:410, 1984.
290. Reis, R. L., Peterson, L. M., Mason, D. T., Simon, A. L., and Morrow, A. G.: Congenital Fixed Subvalvular Aortic Stenosis: An Anatomical Classification and Correlations with Operative Results, *Circulation*, 43/44(suppl. 1):11, 1971.
291. De Vivie, E. R., Koncz, J., Rupprath, G., Vogt, J., and Beuren, A. J.: Aortoventriculoplasty for Different Types of Left Ventricular Outflow Tract Obstructions, *J. Cardiovasc. Surg.*, 23:6, 1982.
292. Morrow, A. G.: Hypertrophic Subaortic Stenosis: Operative Methods Used to Relieve Left Ventricular Outflow Obstruction, *J. Thorac. Cardiovasc. Surg.*, 76:423, 1978.
293. Friedman, W. F., and Benson, L. N.: Aortic Stenosis, in F. H. Adams and G. C. Emmanouilides (eds.), "Moss' Heart Disease in Infants, Children, and Adolescents," The Williams & Wilkins Company, Baltimore, 1983, p. 171.
294. Weyman, A. E., Caldwell, R. L., Hurwitz, R. A., et al: Cross-Sectional Echocardiographic Characterization of Aortic Obstruction: I. Supravalvular Aortic Stenosis and Aortic Hypoplasia, *Circulation*, 57:491, 1978.
295. McGoon, D. C., Mankin, H. T., Vlad, P., and Kirklin, J. W.: The Surgical Treatment of Supravalvular Aortic Stenosis, *J. Thorac. Cardiovasc. Surg.*, 41:125, 1961.
296. Rastelli, G. C., McGoon, D. C., Ongley, P. A., Mankin, H. T., and Kirklin, J. W.: Surgical Treatment of Supravalvular Aortic Stenosis: Report of 16 Cases and Review of Literature, *J. Thorac. Cardiovasc. Surg.*, 51:873, 1966.
297. Doty, D. B., Polansky, D. B., and Jenson, C. B.: Supravalvular Aortic Stenosis: Repair by Extended Aortoplasty, *J. Thorac. Cardiovasc. Surg.*, 74:362, 1977.
298. Keane, J. F., Fellows, K. E., LaFarge, C. G., Nadas, A. S., and Bernhard, W. F.: Surgical Management of Discrete and Diffuse Supravalvular Aortic Stenosis, *Circulation*, 54:112, 1976.
299. Landes, R. G., Zavoral, J. H., Emery, R. W., Moller, J. H., Lindsay, W. G., and Nicoloff, D. M.: The Surgical Management of Vascular Abnormalities Associated with Supravalvular Aortic Stenosis, *J. Thorac. Cardiovasc. Surg.*, 75:80, 1978.
300. Norman, J. C., Cooley, D. A., Hallman, G. L., and Nihill, M. R.: Left Ventricular Apical–Abdominal Aortic Conduits for Left Ventricular Outflow Tract Obstructions, *Circulation*, 56:62, 1977.
301. Thevenet, A.: Symmetric Enlargement of the Ascending Aorta in Supravalvular Aortic Stenosis of the Diffuse Type (An Alternative to Apico-Aortic Conduit), *J. Cardiovasc. Surg.*, 22:1, 1981.
302. Roberts, W. C.: Congenital Cardiovascular Abnormalities Usually "Silent" until Adulthood: Morphologic Features of the Floppy Mitral Valve, Valvular Aortic Stenosis, Discrete Subvalvular Aortic Stenosis, Hypertrophic Cardiomyopathy, Sinus of Valsalva Aneurysm and the Marfan's Syndrome, in W. C. Roberts (ed.), "Congenital Heart Disease in Adults," F. A. Davis Company, Philadelphia, 1979, p. 407.
303. Roberts, W. C., Morrow, A. G., McIntosh, C. L., Jones, M., and Epstein, S. E.: Congenitally Bicuspid Aortic Valve Causing Severe, Pure Aortic Regurgitation without Superimposed Infective Endocarditis, *Am. J. Cardiol.*, 47:206, 1981.
304. Leech, G., Mills, P., and Leatham, A.: The Diagnosis of a Non-stenotic Bicuspid Aortic Valve, *Br. Heart J.*, 40:941, 1978.
305. Brandenburg, R. O., Jr., Tajik, A. J., Edwards, W. D., Reeder, G. S., Shub, C., and Seward, J. B.: Accuracy of Two-Dimensional Echocardiographic Diagnosis of Congenitally Bicuspid Aortic Valve: Echocardiographic Anatomic Correlation in 115 Patients, *Am. J. Cardiol.*, 51:1469, 1983.
306. Mills, P., Leech, G., Davies, M., and Leatham, A.: The Natural History of Non-stenotic Bicuspid Aortic Valve, *Br. Heart J.*, 40:951, 1978.
307. Hashimoto, R., Miyamura, H., and Eguchi, S.: Congenital Aortic Regurgitation in a Child with a Tricuspid Non-stenotic Aortic Valve, *Br. Heart J.*, 51:358, 1984.
308. Spencer, F. C., Bahnson, H. T., and Neill, C. A.: The Treatment of Aortic Regurgitation Associated with a Ventricular Septal Defect, *J. Thorac. Cardiovasc. Surg.*, 43:222, 1962.
309. Murphy, D. A., and Poirier, N.: A Technique of Aortic Valvuloplasty for Aortic Insufficiency with Ventricular Septal Defect, *J. Thorac. Cardiovasc. Surg.*, 64:800, 1972.
310. Konno, S., Imai, Y., Nakajima, M., and Tatsuno, K.: New Method of Prosthetic Valve Replacement in Congenital Aortic Stenosis Associated with Hypoplasia of the Aortic Valve Ring, *J. Thorac. Cardiovasc. Surg.*, 70:909, 1975.
311. Manouguian, S., and Seybold-Epting, W.: Patch Enlargement of the Aortic Ring by Extending the Aortic Incision into the Anterior Mitral Leaflet, New Operative Technique, *J. Thorac. Cardiovasc. Surg.*, 78:402, 1979.
312. Geha, A. S.: Valve Replacement in Children, *Ann. Thorac. Surg.*, 29:500, 1980.
313. Rocchini, A. P., Weesner, K. M., Heidelberger, K., Keren, D., Behrendt, D., and Rosenthal, A.: Porcine Xenograft Valve Failure in Children: An Immunologic Response, *Circulation*, 64(suppl. 2):162, 1981.
314. Williams, D. B., Danielson, G. K., McGoon, D. C., Puga, F. J., Mair, D. D., and Edwards, W. D.: Porcine Heterograft Valve Replacement in Children, *J. Thorac. Cardiovasc. Surg.*, 84:446, 1982.
315. Weinstein, G. S., Mavroudis, C., and Ebert, P. A.: Preliminary Experience with Aspirin for Anticoagulation in Children with Prosthetic Cardiac Valves, *Ann. Thorac. Surg.*, 33:549, 1982.
316. Bonchek, L. I.: Current Status of Cardiac Valve Replacement: Selection of a Prosthesis and Indications for Operation, *Am. Heart J.*, 101:96, 1981.
317. Chaux, A., Gray, R. J., Matloff, J. M., Feldman, H., and Sustaita, H.: An Appreciation of the New St. Jude Valvular Prosthesis, *J. Thorac. Cardiovasc. Surg.*, 81:202, 1981.
318. Mayer, J. E., Lindsay, W. G., Wang, Y., Jorgensen, C. R., and Nicoloff, D. M.: Composite Replacement of the Aortic Valve and Ascending Aorta, *J. Thorac. Cardiovasc. Surg.*, 76:816, 1978.
319. Sisk, H. E., Zahka, K. G., and Pyeritz, R. E.: The Marfan Syndrome in Early Childhood: Analysis of 15 Patients Diagnosed at Less than 4 Years of Age, *Am. J. Cardiol.*, 52:353, 1983.
320. Bisset, G. S., III, Meyer, R. A., Hirschfeld, S. S., James, F. W., Schwartz, D. C., and Kaplan, S.: Aortic Valve Replacement in Childhood: Evaluation of Left Ventricular Function by Electrocardiography, Echocardiography and Graded Exercise Testing, *Am. J. Cardiol.*, 52:568, 1983.
321. Levy, M. J., Schachner, A., and Blieden, L. C.: Aortico–Left Ventricular Tunnel. Collective Review, *J. Thorac. Cardiovasc. Surg.*, 84:102, 1982.
322. Turley, K., Silverman, N. H., Teitel, D., Mavroudis, C., Snider, R., and Rudolph, A.: Repair of Aortico–Left Ventricular Tunnel in the Neonate: Surgical, Anatomic, and Echocardiographic Considerations, *Circulation*, 65:1015, 1982.

323. Bjork, V. O., Eklof, O., Wallgren, G., and Zetterquist, P.: Successful Surgical Treatment of an Aortico–Left Ventricular Tunnel in a Four-Month-Old Infant, *J. Thorac. Cardiovasc. Surg.*, 78:35, 1979.
324. Bernhard, W. F., Plauth, W., and Fyler, D.: Unusual Abnormalities of the Aortic Root or Valve Necessitating Surgical Correction in Early Childhood, *N. Engl. J. Med.*, 282:68, 1970.
325. Roberts, W. C., Perry, L. W., Chandra, R. S., Myers, G. E., Shapiro, S. R., and Scott, L. P.: Aortic Valve Atresia: A Study of 73 Necropsy Patients, *Am. J. Cardiol.*, 37:753, 1976.
326. Freedom, R. M.: Hypoplastic Left Heart Syndrome, in F. H. Adams and G. C. Emmanouilides (eds.), "Moss' Heart Disease in Infants, Children, and Adolescents," The Williams & Wilkins Company, Baltimore, 1983, p. 411.
327. Lange, L. W., Sahn, D. J., Allen, H. D., Ovitt, T. W., and Goldberg, S. J.: Cross-Sectional Echocardiography in Hypoplastic Left Ventricle: Echocardiograhic-Angiographic-Anatomic Correlations, *Pediatr. Cardiol.*, 1:287, 1980.
328. Norwood, W. I., Lange, P., and Hansen, D. D.: Physiologic Repair of Aortic Atresia—Hypoplastic Left Heart Syndrome, *N. Engl. J. Med.*, 308:23, 1983.
329. Gittenberger-de Groot, A. C., and Wenink, A. C. G.: Mitral Atresia. Morphological Details, *Br. Heart J.*, 51:252, 1984.
330. Shore, D., Jones, O., Rigby, M. L., Anderson, R. H., and Lincoln, C.: Atresia of Left Atrioventricular Connection. Surgical Considerations, *Br. Heart J.*, 47:35, 1982.
331. Beckman, C. B., Moller, J. H., and Edwards, J. E.: Alternate Pathways to Pulmonary Venous Flow in Left-Sided Obstructive Anomalies, *Circulation*, 52:509, 1975.
332. Rigby, M. L., Gibson, D. G., Joseph, M. C., et al.: Recognition of Imperforate Atrioventricular Valves by Two-Dimensional Echocardiography, *Br. Heart J.*, 47:329, 1982.
333. Mickell, J. J., Mathews, R. A., Park, S. C., Lenox, C. C., and Fricker, F. J.: Left Atrioventricular Valve Atresia: Clinical Management, *Circulation*, 61:123, 1980.
334. Collins-Nakai, R. L., Rosenthal, A., Castaneda, A. R., Bernhard, W. F., and Nadas, A. S.: Congenital Mitral Stenosis: A Review of 20 Years' Experience, *Circulation*, 56:1039, 1977.
335. Shone, J. D., Sellers, R. D., Anderson, R. C., Adams, P., Jr., Lillehei, C. W., and Edwards, J. E.: The Developmental Complex of "Parachute Mitral Valve," Supravalvular Ring of Left Atrium, Subaortic Stenosis, and Coarctation of the Aorta, *Am. J. Cardiol.*, 11:714, 1963.
336. Baylen, B. G., and Criley, J. M.: Diseases of the Mitral Valve, in F. H. Adams and G. C. Emmanouilides (eds.), "Moss' Heart Disease in Infants, Children, and Adolescents," The Williams & Wilkins Company, Baltimore, 1983, p. 516.
337. Driscoll, D. J., Gutgesell, H. P., and McNamara, D. G.: Echocardiograhic Features of Congenital Mitral Stenosis, *Am. J. Cardiol.*, 42:259, 1978.
338. Snider, A. R., Roge, C. L., Schiller, N. B., and Silverman, N. H.: Congenital Left Ventricular Inflow Obstruction Evaluated by Two-Dimensional Echocardiography, *Circulation*, 61:848, 1980.
339. Carpentier, A., Branchini, B., Cour, J. C., et al.: Congenital Malformation of the Mitral Valve in Children, *J. Thorac. Cardiovasc. Surg.*, 72:854, 1976.
340. Lansing, A. M., Elbl, F., Solinger, R. E., and Rees, A. H.: Left Atrial–Left Ventricular Bypass for Congenital Mitral Stenosis, *Ann. Thorac. Surg.*, 35:667, 1983.
341. Segni, E. D., and Edwards, J. E.: Cleft Anterior Leaflet of the Mitral Valve with Intact Septa. A Study of 20 Cases, *Am. J. Cardiol.*, 51:919, 1983.
342. Krovetz, L. J., Lorincz, A. E., and Schiebler, G. L.: Cardiovascular Manifestations of the Hurler Syndrome. Hemodynamic and Angiocardiographic Observations in 15 Patients, *Circulation*, 31:132, 1965.
343. Segni, E. D., Bass, J. L., Lucas, R. V., Jr., and Einzig, S.: Isolated Cleft Mitral Valve: A Variety of Congenital Mitral Regurgitation Identified by 2-Dimensional Echocardiography, *Am. J. Cardiol.*, 51:927, 1983.
344. Mintz, G. S., Kotler, M. N., Segal, B. L., and Parry, W. R.: Two-Dimensional Echocardiographic Evaluation of Patients with Mitral Insufficiency, *Am. J. Cardiol.*, 44:670, 1979.
345. Kahn, D. R., Stern, A. M., Sigmann, J. M., Kirsh, M. M., Lennox, S., and Sloan, H.: Long-Term Results of Valvuloplasty for Mitral Insufficiency in Children, *J. Thorac. Cardiovasc. Surg.*, 53:1, 1967.
346. Van Praagh, R., and Corsini, I.: Cor Triatriatum: Pathologic Anatomy and a Consideration of Morphogenesis Based on 13 Post-mortem Cases and a Study of Normal Development of the Pulmonary Vein and Atrial Septum in 83 Human Embryos, *Am. Heart J.*, 78:379, 1969.
347. Ostman-Smith, I., Silverman, N. H., Oldershaw, P., Lincoln, C., and Shinebourne, E. A.: Cor Triatriatum Sinistrum. Diagnostic Features on Cross-Sectional Echocardiography, *Br. Heart J.*, 51:211, 1984.
348. Oglietti, J., Cooley, D. A., Izquierdo, J. P., et al.: Cor Triatriatum: Operative Results in 25 Patients, *Ann. Thorac. Surg.*, 35:415, 1983.
349. Arciniegas, E., Farooki, Z. Q., Hakimi, M., Perry, B. L., and Green, E. W.: Surgical Treatment of Cor Triatriatum, *Ann. Thorac. Surg.*, 32:571, 1981.
350. Richardson, J. V., Doty, D. B., Siewers, R. D., and Zuberbuhler, J. R.: Cor Triatriatum (Subdivided Left Atrium), *J. Thorac. Cardiovasc. Surg.*, 81:232, 1981.
351. McDonnell, P. J., Summer, W. R., and Hutchins, G. M.: Pulmonary Veno-occlusive Disease. Morphologic Changes Suggesting a Viral Cause, *JAMA*, 246:667, 1981.
352. Rosenthal, A., Vawter, G., and Wagenvoort, C. A.: Intrapulmonary Veno-occlusive Disease, *Am. J. Cardiol.*, 31:78, 1973.
353. Driscoll, D. J., Hesslein, P. S., and Mullins, C. E.: Congenital Stenosis of Individual Pulmonary Veins: Clinical Spectrum and Unsuccessful Treatment by Transvenous Balloon Dilation, *Am. J. Cardiol.*, 49:1767, 1982.
354. Sade, R. M., Freed, M. D., Matthews, E. C., and Castaneda, A. R.: Stenosis of Individual Pulmonary Veins, *J. Thorac. Cardiovasc. Surg.*, 67:953, 1974.
355. Maron, B. J.: Cardiomyopathies, in F. H. Adams and G. C. Emmanouilides (eds.), "Moss' Heart Disease in Infants, Children, and Adolescents," The Williams & Wilkins Company, Baltimore, 1983, p. 757.
356. Chen, S., Thompson, M. W., and Rose, V.: Endocardial Fibroelastosis: Family Studies with Special Reference to Counseling, *J. Pediatr.*, 79:385, 1971.
357. Tripp, M. E., Katcher, M. L., Peters, H. A., et al.: Systemic Carnitine Deficiency Presenting as Familial Endocardial Fibroelastosis. A Treatable Cardiomyopathy, *N. Engl. J. Med.*, 305:385, 1981.
358. Currens, J. H., Kinney, T. D., and White, P. D.: Pulmonary Stenosis with Intact Interventricular Septum: Report of Eleven Cases, *Am. Heart J.*, 30:491, 1945.
359. Hardy, W. E., Gnoj, J., Ayres, S. M., Giannelli, E., and Christianson, L. C.: Pulmonic Stenosis and Associated Atrial Septal Defects in Older Patients. Report of Three Cases, Including One with Calcific Pulmonic Stenosis, *Am. J. Cardiol.*, 24:130, 1969.
360. Koretzky, E. D., Moller, J. H., Korns, M. E., Schwartz, C. J., and Edwards, J. E.: Congenital Pulmonary Stenosis Resulting from Dysplasia of Valve, *Circulation*, 40:43, 1969.
361. Lucas, R. V., Jr., Varco, R. L., Lillehei, C. W., Adams, P., Jr., Anderson, R. C., and Edwards, J. E.: Anomalous Muscle Bundle of the Right Ventricle. Hemodynamic Consequences and Surgical Considerations, *Circulation*, 25:443, 1962.
362. Stone, F. M., Bessinger, F. B., Jr., Lucas, R. V., Jr., and Moller, J. H.: Pre- and Postoperative Rest and Exercise Hemodynamics in Children with Pulmonary Stenosis, *Circulation*, 49:1102, 1974.
363. Danilowicz, D., Hoffman, J. I. E., and Rudolph, A. M.: Serial Studies of Pulmonary Stenosis in Infancy and Childhood, *Br. Heart J.*, 37:808, 1975.
364. Mody, M. R.: The Natural History of Uncomplicated Valvular Pulmonic Stenosis, *Am. Heart J.*, 90:317, 1975.
365. Nakazawa, M., Marks, R. A., Isabel-Jones, J., and Jarmakani, J. M.: Right and Left Ventricular Volume Character-

istics in Children with Pulmonary Stenosis and Intact Ventricular Septum, *Circulation,* 53:884, 1976.
366. Roberts, W. C., Shemin, R. J., and Kent, K. M.: Frequency and Direction of Interatrial Shunting in Valvular Pulmonic Stenosis with Intact Ventricular Septum and without Left Ventricular Inflow or Outflow Obstruction, *Am. Heart J.,* 99:142, 1980.
367. Freed, M. D., Rosenthal, A., Bernhard, W. F., Litwin, S. B., and Nadas, A. S.: Critical Pulmonary Stenosis with Diminutive Right Ventricle in Neonates, *Circulation,* 48:875, 1973.
368. Campbell, M.: Factors in the Aetiology of Pulmonary Stenosis, *Br. Heart J.,* 24:625, 1962.
369. Noonan, J. A.: Hypertelorism with Turner Phenotype: A New Syndrome with Associated Congenital Heart Disease, *Am. J. Dis. Child.,* 116:373, 1968.
370. Cayler, C. G., Ongley, P., and Nadas, A. S.: Relation of Systolic Pressure in the Right Ventricle to the Electrocardiogram, *N. Engl. J. Med.,* 258:979, 1958.
371. Hugenholtz, P. G., and Gamboa, R.: Effect of Chronically Increased Ventricular Pressure on Electrical Forces of the Heart: A Correlation between Hemodynamic and Vectorcardiographic Data (Frank System) in 90 Patients with Aortic or Pulmonic Stenosis, *Circulation,* 30:511, 1964.
372. Nadas, A. S. (ed.): Pulmonary Stenosis, Aortic Stenosis, Ventricular Septal Defect: Clinical Course and Indirect Assessment (Report from the Joint Study on the Natural History of Congenital Heart Defects), *Circulation,* 56(suppl. 1):1, 1977.
373. Weyman, A. E., Dillon, J. C., Fiegenbaum, H., and Chang, S.: Echocardiograhic Differentiation of Infundibular from Valvular Pulmonary Stenosis, *Am. J. Cardiol.,* 36:21, 1975.
374. Kan, J. S., White, R. I., Jr., Mitchell, S. E., Anderson, J. H., and Gardner, T. J.: Percutaneous Transluminal Balloon Valvuloplasty for Pulmonary Valve Stenosis, *Circulation,* 69:554, 1984.
375. Hallman, G. L., and Cooley, D. A.: Pulmonary Stenosis, in G. L. Hallman and D. A. Cooley (eds.), "Surgical Treatment of Congenital Heart Disease," Lea & Febiger, Philadelphia, 1975, p. 45.
376. Harlan, B. J., Starr, A., and Harwin, F. M.: Pulmonary Valve Stenosis, in B. J. Harlan, A. Starr, and F. M. Harwin (eds.), "Manual of Cardiac Surgery," Springer-Verlag, New York, 1981, p. 78.
377. Vancini, M., Roberts, K. D., Silove, E. D., and Singh, S. P.: Surgical Treatment of Congenital Pulmonary Stenosis Due to Dysplastic Leaflets and Small Valve Annulus, *J. Thorac. Cardiovasc. Surg.,* 79:464, 1980.
378. Litwin, S. B., Williams, W. H., Freed, M. D., and Bernhard, W. F.: Critical Pulmonary Stenosis in Infants: A Surgical Emergency, *Surgery,* 74:880, 1973.
379. Mistrot, J., Neal, W., Lyons, G., et al.: Pulmonary Valvulotomy under Inflow Stasis for Isolated Pulmonary Stenosis, *Ann. Thorac. Surg.,* 21:30, 1976.
380. Srinivasan, V., Konyer, A., Broda, J. J., and Subramanian, S.: Critical Pulmonary Stenosis in Infants Less than Three Months of Age: A Reapparisal of Closed Transventricular Pulmonary Valvotomy, *Ann. Thorac. Surg.,* 34:46, 1982.
381. Awariefe, S. O., Clarke, D. R., and Pappas, G.: Surgical Approach to Critical Pulmonary Valve Stenosis in Infants Less than Six Months of Age, *J. Thorac. Cardiiovasc. Surg.,* 85:375, 1983.
382. Li, M. D., Coles, J. C., and McDonald, A. C.: Anomalous Muscle Bundle of the Right Ventricle: Its Recognition and Surgical Treatment, *Br. Heart J.,* 40:1040, 1978.
383. D'Cruz, I. A., Agustsson, M. H., Bicoff, J. P., Weinberg, M., Jr., and Arcilla, R. A.: Stenotic Lesions of the Pulmonary Arteries. Clinical and Hemodynamic Findings in 84 Cases, *Am. J. Cardiol.,* 13:441, 1964.
384. Rowe, R. D.: Cardiovascular Disease in the Rubella Syndrome, *Cardiovasc. Clin.,* 5:62, 1972.
385. Dunkle, L. M., and Rowe, R. D.: Transient Murmur Simulating Pulmonary Artery Stenosis in Premature Infants, *Am. J. Dis. Child.,* 124:666, 1972.
386. Lock, J. E., Castaneda-Zuniga, W. R., Fuhrman, B. P., and Bass, J. L.: Balloon Dilatation Angioplasty of Hypoplastic and Stenotic Pulmonary Arteries, *Circulation,* 67:962, 1983.
387. McGoon, M. D., Fulton, R. E., Davis, G. D., Ritter, D. G., Neill, C. A., and White, R. I., Jr.,: Systemic Collateral and Pulmonary Artery Stenosis in Patients with Congenital Pulmonary Valve Atresia and Ventricular Septal Defect, *Circulation,* 56:473, 1977.
388. Zuberbuhler, J. R., and Anderson, R. H.: Morphological Variations in Pulmonary Atresia with Intact Ventricular Septum, *Br. Heart J.,* 41:281, 1979.
389. Davignon, A. L., Greenwold, W. E., DuShane, J. W., and Edwards, J. E.: Congenital Pulmonary Atresia with Intact Ventricular Septum: Clinicopathologic Correlation of Two Anatomic Types, *Am. Heart J.,* 62:591, 1961.
390. Freedom, R. M., and Harrington, D. P.: Contributions of Intramyocardial Sinusoids in Pulmonary Atresia and Intact Ventricular Septum to a Right-Sided Circular Shunt, *Br. Heart J.,* 36:1061, 1974.
391. Solinger, R., Elbl, F., and Minhas, K.: Echocardiography: Its Role in the Severely Ill Infant, *Pediatrics,* 57:543, 1976.
392. Lewis, B. S., Amitai, N., Simcha, A., Merin, G., and Gotsman, M. S.: Echocardiograhic Diagnosis of Pulmonary Atresia with Intact Ventricular Septum, *Am. Heart J.,* 97:92, 1979.
393. Graham, T. P., Jr., Bender, H. W., Atwood, G. F., Page, D. L., and Sell, C. G. R.: Increase in Right Ventricular Volume following Valvulotomy for Pulmonary Atresia or Stenosis with Intact Ventricular Septum, *Circulation,* 50(suppl. 2):69, 1974.
394. Patel, R. G., Freedom, R. M., Moes, C. A. F., et al.: Right Ventricular Volume Determination in 18 Patients with Pulmonary Atresia and Intact Ventricular Septum: Analysis of Factors Influencing Right Ventricular Growth, *Circulation,* 61:428, 1980.
395. Freedom, R. M., White, R. I., Jr., Ho, C. S., Gingell, R. L., Hawker, R. E., and Rowe, R. D.: Evaluation of Patients with Pulmonary Atresia and Intact Ventricular Septum by Double Catheter Technique, *Am. J. Cardiol.,* 33:892, 1974.
396. Heymann, M. A., and Rudolph, A. M.: Ductus Arteriosus Dilatation by Prostaglandin E_1 in Infants with Pulmonary Atresia, *Pediatrics,* 59:325, 1977.
397. De Leval, M., Bull, C., Stark, J., Anderson, R. B., Taylor, J. F. N., and Macartney, F. J.: Pulmonary Atresia and Intact Ventricular Septum: Surgical Management Based on a Revised Classification, *Circulation,* 66:272, 1982.
398. Freedom, R. M., Wilson, G., Trusler, G. A., Williams, W. G., and Rowe, R. D.: Pulmonary Atresia and Intact Ventricular Septum, *Scand. J. Thorac. Cardiovasc. Surg.,* 17:1, 1983.
399. Moulton, A. L. Bowman, F. O., Jr., Edie, R. N., et al.: Pulmonary Atresia with Intact Ventricular Septum: Sixteen-Year Experience, *J. Thorac. Cardiovasc. Surg.,* 78:527, 1979.
400. Lev, M., and Eckner, F. A. O.: The Pathologic Anatomy of Tetralogy of Fallot and Its Variations, *Dis. Chest,* 45:251, 1964.
401. Rosenquist, G. C., Sweeney, L. J., Stemple, D. R., Christianson, S. D., and Rowe, R. D.: Ventricular Septal Defect in Tetralogy of Fallot, *Am. J. Cardiol.,* 31:749, 1973.
402. Becker, A. E., Connor, M., and Anderson, R. H.: Tetralogy of Fallot: A Morphometric and Geometric Study, *Am. J. Cardiol.,* 35:402, 1975.
403. Rao, B. N. S., Anderson, R. C., and Edwards, J. E.: Anatomic Variations in the Tetralogy of Fallot, *Am. Heart J.,* 81:361, 1971.
404. Neufeld, H. N., McGoon, D. C., DuShane, J. W., and Edwards, J. E.: Tetralogy of Fallot with Anomalous Tricuspid Valve Simulating Pulmonary Stenosis with Intact Septum, *Circulation,* 22:1083, 1960.
405. Higgins, C. B., and Mulder, D. G.: Tetralogy of Fallot in the Adult, *Am. J. Cardiol.,* 28:837, 1972.
406. Bonchek, L. I., Starr, A., Sunderland, C. O., and Menashe, V. D.: Natural History of Tetralogy of Fallot in Infancy: Clinical Classification and Therapeutic Implications, *Circulation,* 48:386, 1973.
407. Ruzyllo, W., Nihill, M. B., Mullins, C. E., and McNamara,

D. G.: Hemodynamic Evaluation of 221 Patients after Intracardiac Repair of Tetralogy of Fallot, *Am. J. Cardiol.*, 34:565, 1974.
408. Taussig, H. B., Kallman, C. H., Nagel, D., Baumgardner, R., Momberger, N., and Kirk, H.: Long-Time Observations on the Blalock-Taussig Operation: VIII. 20- to 28-Year Follow-up on Patients with a Tetralogy of Fallot, *Johns Hopkins Med. J.*, 137:13, 1975.
409. Roberts, W. C., Friesinger, G. C., Cohen, L. S., Mason, D. T., and Ross, R. S.: Acquired Pulmonary Atresia. Total Obstruction to Right Ventricular Outflow after Systemic to Pulmonary Arterial Anastomoses for Cyanotic Congenital Cardiac Disease, *Am. J. Cardiol.*, 24:335, 1969.
410. Morgan, B. C., Guntheroth, W. G., Bloom, R. S., and Fyler, D. C.: A Clinical Profile of Paroxysmal Hyperpnea in Cyanotic Congenital Heart Disease, *Circulation*, 31:66, 1965.
411. Guntheroth, W. G., Morgan, B. C., and Mullins, G. L.: Physiologic Studies of Paroxysmal Hyperpnea in Cyanotic Congenital Heart Disease, *Circulation*, 31:70, 1965.
412. Knight, L., and Edwards, J. E.: Right Aortic Arch. Types and Associated Cardiac Anomalies, *Circulation*, 50:1047, 1974.
413. Morris, D. C., Felner, J. M., Schlant, R. C., and Franch, R. H.: Echocardiographic Diagnosis of Tetralogy of Fallot, *Am. J. Cardiol.*, 36:908, 1975.
414. Story, W. E., Felner, J. M., and Schlant, R. C.: Echocardiograhic Criteria for the Diagnosis of Mitral-Semilunar Valve Continuity, *Am. Heart J.*, 93:575, 1977.
415. Hagler, D. J., Tajik, A. J., Seward, J. B., Mair, D. D., and Ritter, D. G.: Wide-Angle Two-Dimensional Echocardiographic Profiles of Conotruncal Abnormalities, *Mayo Clin. Proc.*, 55:73, 1980.
416. Formanek, A., Nath, P. H., Zollikofer, C., and Moller, J. H.: Selective Coronary Arteriography in Children, *Circulation*, 61:84, 1980.
417. Dabizzi, R. P., Caprioli, G., Aiazzi, L., et al.: Distribution and Anomalies of Coronary Arteries in Tetralogy of Fallot, *Circulation*, 61:95, 1980.
418. Ferencz, C.: The Pulmonary Vascular Bed in Tetralogy of Fallot: I. Changes Associated with Pulmonary Stenosis, *Bull. Johns Hopkins Hosp.*, 106:81, 1960.
419. Bertranaou, E. G., Blackstone, E. H., Hazelrig, J. B., Turner, M. E., Jr., and Kirklin, J. W.: Life Expectancy without Surgery in Tetralogy of Fallot, *Am. J. Cardiol.*, 42:458, 1978.
420. Ponce, F. E., Williams, L. C., Webb, H. M., Riopel, D. A., and Hohn, A. R.: Propranolol Palliation of Tetralogy of Fallot: Experience with Long-Term Drug Treatment in Pediatric Patients, *Pediatrics*, 52:100, 1973.
421. Garson, A., Jr., Gorry, G. A., McNamara, D. G., and Cooley, D. A.: The Surgical Decision in Tetralogy of Fallot: Weighing Risks and Benefits with Decision Analysis, *Am. J. Cardiol.*, 45:108, 1980.
422. Kirklin, J. W., and Blackstone, E. H.: Editorial on Papers by Naito, Wessel, and their Colleagues, *J. Thorac. Cardiovasc. Surg.*, 80:594, 1980.
423. Guyton, R. A., Owens, J. E., Waumett, J. D., Dooley, K. J., Hatcher, C. R., Jr., and Williams, W. H.: The Blalock-Taussig Shunt: Low Risk, Effective Palliation, and Pulmonary Artery Growth, *J. Thorac. Cardiovasc. Surg.*, 85:917, 1983.
424. Kirklin, J. W., Bargeron, L. M., Jr., and Pacifico, A. D.: The Enlargement of Small Pulmonary Arteries by Preliminary Palliative Operations, *Circulation*, 56:612, 1977.
425. Arciniegas, E., Farooki, Z. Q., Hakimi, M., and Green, E. W.: Results of Two-Stage Surgical Treatment of Tetralogy of Fallot, *J. Thorac. Cardiovasc. Surg.*, 79:876, 1980.
426. Puga, F. J., DuShane, J. W., and McGoon, D. C.: Treatment of Tetralogy of Fallot in Children Less than 4 Years of Age, *J. Thorac. Cardiovasc. Surg.*, 64:247, 1972.
427. Kirkin, J. W., and Karp, R. B.: "The Tetralogy of Fallot," W. B. Saunders Company, Philadelphia, 1970, p. 71.
428. Anderson, R. H., Allwork, S. P., Ho, S. Y., Lenox, C. C., and Zuberbuhler, J. R.: Surgical Anatomy of Tetralogy of Fallot, *J. Thorac. Cardiovasc. Surg.*, 81:887, 1981.
429. Naito, Y., Fujita, T., Manabe, H., and Kawashima, Y.: The Criteria for Reconstruction of Right Ventricular Outflow Tract in Total Correction of Tetralogy of Fallot, *J. Thorac. Cardiovasc. Surg.*, 80:574, 1980.
430. Fuster, V., McGoon, D. C., Kennedy, M. A., Ritter, D. B., and Kirklin, J. W.: Long-Term Evaluation (12 to 22 Years) of Open Heart Surgery for Tetralogy of Fallot, *Am. J. Cardiol.*, 46:635, 1980.
431. Wessel, H. U., Cunningham, W. J., Paul, M. H., Bastanier, C. K., Muster, A. J., and Idriss, F. S.: Exercise Performance in Tetralogy of Fallot after Intracardiac Repair, *J. Thorac. Cardiovasc. Surg.*, 80:582, 1980.
432. Borow, K. M., Green, L. H., Castaneda, A. R., and Keane, J. F.: Left Ventricular Function after Repair of Tetralogy of Fallot and Its Relationship to Age at Surgery, *Circulation*, 61:1150, 1980.
433. Lakier, J. B., Stanger, P., Heymann, M. A., Hoffman, J. I. E., and Rudolph, A. M.: Tetralogy of Fallot with Absent Pulmonary Valve. Natural History and Hemodynamic Considerations, *Circulation*, 50:167, 1974.
434. Pinsky, W. W., Nihill, M. R., Mullins, C. E., Harrison, G., and McNamara, D. G.: The Absent Pulmonary Valve Syndrome: Considerations of Management, *Circulation*, 57:159, 1978.
435. Litwin, S. B., Rosenthal, A., and Fellows, K.: Surgical Management of Young Infants with Tetralogy of Fallot, Absence of the Pulmonary Valve, and Respiratory Distress, *Am. J. Thorac. Cardiovasc. Surg.*, 65:552, 1973.
436. Byrne, J. P., Hawkins, J. A., Battiste, C. E., and Khoury, A. H.: Palliative Procedures in Tetralogy of Fallot with Absent Pulmonary Valve: A New Approach, *Ann. Thorac. Surg.*, 33:499, 1982.
437. Opie, J. C., Sandor, G. C. S., Ashmore, P. G., and Patterson, M. W. H.: Successful Palliation by Pulmonary Artery Banding in Absent Pulmonary Valve Syndrome with Aneurysmal Pulmonary Arteries, *J. Thorac. Cardiovasc. Surg.*, 85:125, 1983.
438. Stellin, G., Jonas, R. A., Goh, T. H., Brawn, W. J., Venables, A. W., and Mee, R. B. B.: Surgical Treatment of Absent Pulmonary Valve Syndrome in Infants: Relief of Bronchial Obstruction, *Ann. Thorac. Surg.*, 36:468, 1983.
439. Edwards, J. E., and McGoon, D. C.: Absence of Anatomic Origin from Heart of Pulmonary Arterial Supply, *Circulation*, 47:393, 1973.
440. Collett, R. W., and Edwards, J. E.: Persistent Truncus Arteriosus: A Classification according to Anatomic Types, *Surg. Clin. North Am.*, 29:1245, 1949.
441. Calder, L., Van Praagh, R., Van Praagh, S., et al.: Truncus Arteriosus Communis. Clinical, Angiocardiographic, and Pathologic Findings in 100 Patients, *Am. Heart J.*, 92:23, 1976.
442. Anderson, K. R., McGoon, D. C., and Lie, J. T.: Surgical Significance of the Coronary Arterial Anatomy in Truncus Arteriosus Communis, *Am. J. Cardiol.*, 41:76:1978.
443. Gelband, H., Van Meter, S., and Gersony, W. M.: Truncal Valve Abnormalities in Infants with Persistent Truncus Arteriosus. A Clinicopathologic Study, *Circulation*, 45:397, 1972.
444. Sotomora, R. F., and Edwards, J. E.: Anatomic Identification of So-Called Absent Pulmonary Artery, *Circulation*, 57:624, 1978.
445. Miller, W. W., Nadas, A. S., Bernhard, W. F., and Gross, R. E.: Congenital Pulmonary Atresia with Ventricular Septal Defect, *Am. J. Cardiol.*, 21:673, 1968.
446. Jefferson, K., Simon, R., and Somerville, J.: Systemic Arterial Supply to the Lungs in Pulmonary Atresia and Its Relation to Pulmonary Artery Development, *Br. Heart J.*, 34:418, 1972.
447. Nihill, M. R., Mullins, C. E., and McNamara, D. G.: Visualization of the Pulmonary Arteries in Pseudotruncus by Pulmonary Vein Wedge Angiography, *Circulation*, 58:140, 1978.
448. Doty, D. B., Kouchoukos, N. T., Kirklin, J. W., Barcia, A., and Bargeron, L. M., Jr.: Surgery for Pseudotruncus Arteriosus with Pulmonary Blood Flow Originating from Upper Descending Thoracic Aorta, *Circulation*, 45(suppl. 1):121, 1972.

449. Somerville, J.: Management of Pulmonary Atresia, *Br. Heart J.*, 32:641, 1970.
450. Piehler, J. M., Danielson, G. K., McGoon, D. C., Wallace, R. B., Rulton, R. E., and Maier, D. D.: Management of Pulmonary Atresia with Ventricular Septal Defect and Hypoplastic Pulmonary Arteries by Right Ventricular Outflow Construction, *J. Thorac. Cardiovasc. Surg.*, 80:552, 1980.
451. Freedom, R. M., Pongiglione, G., Williams, W. G., Trusler, G. A., and Rowe, R. D.: Palliative Right Ventricular Outflow Tract Construction for Patients with Pulmonary Atresia, Ventricular Septal Defect, and Hypoplastic Pulmonary Arteries, *J. Thorac. Cardiovasc. Surg.*, 86:24, 1983.
452. Puga, F. J., McGoon, D. C., Julsrud, P. R., Danielson, G. K., and Mair, D. D.: Complete Repair of Pulmonary Atresia with Nonconfluent Pulmonary Arteries, *Ann. Thorac. Surg.*, 35:36, 1983.
453. Moore, C. H., Martelli, V., and Ross, D. N.: Reconstruction of Right Ventricular Outflow Tract with a Valved Conduit in 75 Cases of Congenital Heart Disease, *J. Thorac. Cardiovasc. Surg.*, 71:11, 1976.
454. McGoon, D. C., Baird, D. K., and Davis, G. D.: Surgical Management of Large Bronchial Collateral Arteries with Pulmonary Stenosis or Atresia, *Circulation,* 52:109, 1975.
455. Szarnicki, R., Krebber, H. J., and Wack, J.: Wire Coil Embolization of Systemic-Pulmonary Artery Collaterals following Surgical Correction of Pulmonary Atresia, *J. Thorac. Cardiovasc. Surg.*, 81:124, 1981.
456. Marcelletti, C., McGoon, D. C., and Mair, D. D.: The Natural History of Truncus Arteriosus, *Circulation,* 54:108, 1976.
457. Mair, D. D., Ritter, D. G., Davis, G. D., Wallace, R. B., Danielson, G. K., and McGoon, D. C.: Selection of Patients with Truncus Arteriosus for Surgical Correction: Anatomic and Hemodynamic Considerations, *Circulation,* 49:144, 1974.
458. Parker, R. K., McGoon, D. C., Danielson, G. K., Wallace, R. B., and Mair, D. D.: Repair of Truncus Arteriosus in Patients with Prior Banding of the Pulmonary Artery, *Surgery,* 78:761, 1975.
459. Appelbaum, A., Bargeron, L. M., Jr., Pacifico, A. D., and Kirklin, J. W.: Surgical Treatment of Truncus Arteriosus, with Emphasis on Infants and Small Children, *J. Thorac. Cardiovasc. Surg.*, 71:436, 1976.
460. Ebert, P. A., Robinson, S. J., Stanger, P., and Engle, M. A.: Pulmonary Artery Conduits in Infants Younger than Six Months of Age, *J. Thorac. Cardiovasc. Surg.*, 72:351, 1976.
461. Ebert, P. A.: Truncus Arteriosus, in W. L. Glenn, A. E. Baue, A. S. Geha, G. L. Hammond, and H. Laks (eds.), "Thoracic and Cardiovascular Surgery," Appleton-Century-Crofts, Norwalk, Conn., 1983, p. 785.
462. McGoon, D. C., Rastelli, G. C., and Ongley, P. A.: An Operation for Correction of Truncus Arteriosus, *JAMA*, 205:69, 1968.
463. McGoon, D. C., Rastelli, G. C., and Ongley, P. A.: An Operation for the Correction of Truncus Arteriosus, *JAMA*, 205:69, 1968.
464. Marcelletti, C., McGoon, D. C., Danielson, G. K., Wallace, R. B., and Mair, D. D.: Early and Late Results of Surgical Repair of Truncus Arteriosus, *Circulation,* 55:636, 1977.
465. Tandon, R., and Edwards, J. E.: Tricuspid Atresia. A Reevaluation and Classification, *J. Thorac. Cardiovasc. Surg.*, 67:530, 1974.
466. Rao, P. S.: Natural History of the Ventricular Septal Defect in Tricuspid Atresia and Its Surgical Implications, *Br. Heart J.*, 39:276, 1977.
467. Rao, P. S.: A Unified Classification for Tricuspid Atresia, *Am. Heart J.*, 99:799, 1980.
468. Charuzi, Y., Spanos, P. K., Amplatz, K., and Edwards, J. E.: Juxtaposition of the Atrial Appendages, *Circulation,* 47:620, 1973.
469. Dick, M., Fyler, D. C., and Nadas, A. S.: Tricuspid Atresia: Clinical Course in 101 Patients, *Am. J. Cardiol.*, 36:327, 1975.
470. Marcano, B. A., Riemenschneider, T. A., Ruttenberg, H. D., Goldberg, S. J., and Gyepes, M.: Tricuspid Atresia with Increased Pulmonary Blood Flow: An Analysis of 13 Cases, *Circulation,* 40:399, 1969.
471. Davachi, F., Lucas, R. V., Jr., and Moller, J. H.: The Electrocardiogram and Vectorcardiogram in Tricuspid Atresia: Correlation with Pathologic Anatomy, *Am. J. Cardiol.*, 25:18, 1970.
472. La Corte, M. A., Dick, M., Scheer, G., LaFarge, C. G., and Fyler, D. C.: Left Ventricular Function in Tricuspid Atresia: Angiographic Analysis in 28 Patients, *Circulation,* 52:996, 1975.
473. Fontan, F., and Baudet, E.: Surgical Repair of Tricuspid Atresia, *Thorax,* 26:240, 1971.
474. Weinberg, P. M.: Anatomy of Tricuspid Atresia and Its Relevance to Current Forms of Surgical Therapy, *Ann. Thorac. Surg.*, 29:306, 1980.
475. Trusler, G. A., and Williams, W. G.: Long-Term Results of Shunt Procedures of Tricuspid Atresia, *Ann. Thorac. Surg.*, 25:312, 1978.
476. Bjork, V. O., Olin, C. L., Bjarke, B. B., and Thoren, C. A.: Right Atrial–Right Ventricular Anastomosis for Correction of Tricuspid Atresia, *J. Thorac. Cardiovasc. Surg.*, 77:452, 1979.
477. Kreutzer, G. O., Vargas, F. J., Schlichter, A. J., et al.: Atriopulmonary Anastomosis, *J. Thorac. Cardiovasc. Surg.*, 83:427, 1982.
478. Fontan, F., Deville, C., Quaegebeur, J., et al.: Repair of Tricuspid Atresia in 100 Patients, *J. Thorac. Cardiovasc. Surg.*, 85:647, 1983.
479. Bharati, S., and Lev, M.: Congenital Poly-valvular Disease, *Circulation,* 47:575, 1973.
480. Becker, A. E., Becker, M. J., and Edwards, J. E.: Pathologic Spectrum of Dysplasia of the Tricuspid Valve. Features in Common with Ebstein's Malformations, *Arch. Pathol.*, 91:167, 1971.
481. Barr, P. A., Celermajer, J. M., Bowdler, J. D., and Cartmill, T. B.: Severe Congenital Tricuspid Incompetence in the Neonate, *Circulation,* 49:962, 1974.
482. Boucek, R. J., Graham, T. P., Jr., Morgan, J. R., Atwood, G. F., and Boerth, R. C.: Spontaneous Resolution of Massive Congenital Tricuspid Insufficiency, *Circulation,* 54:795, 1976.
483. Freedom, R. M., Culham, G., Moes, F., Olley, P. M., and Rowe, R. D.: Differentiation of Functional and Structural Pulmonary Atresia: Role of Angiography, *Am. J. Cardiol.*, 41:914, 1978.
484. Bucciarelli, R. L., Nelson, R. M., Egan, E. A., II, Eitzman, D. V., and Gessner, I. H.: Transient Tricuspid Insufficiency of the Newborn: A Form of Myocardial Dysfunction in Distressed Newborns, *Pediatrics,* 59:330, 1977.
485. Barr, P. A., Celermajer, J. M., Bowdler, J. D., and Cartmill, T. B.: Severe Congenital Tricuspid Incompetence in the Neonate, *Circulation,* 49:962, 1974.
486. Lev, M., Liberthson, R. R., Joseph, R. H., et al.: The Pathologic Anatomy of Ebstein's Disease, *Arch. Pathol.*, 90:334, 1970.
487. Kumar, A. E., Fyler, D. C., Miettinen, O. S., and Nadas, A. S.: Ebstein's Anomaly. Clinical Profile and Natural History, *Am. J. Cardiol.*, 28:84, 1971.
488. Watson, H.: Natural History of Ebstein's Anomaly of the Tricuspid Valve in Childhood and Adolescence: An International Cooperative Study of 505 Cases, *Br. Heart J.*, 36:417, 1974.
489. Giuliani, E. R., Fuster, V., Brandenburg, R. O., and Mair, D. D.: Ebstein's Anomaly: The Clinical Features and Natural History of Ebstein's Anomaly of the Tricuspid Valve, *Mayo Clin. Proc.*, 54:163, 1979.
490. Kastor, J. A., Goldreyer, B. N., Josephson, M. E., et al.: Electrophysiologic Characteristics of Ebstein's Anomaly of the Tricuspid Valve, *Circulation,* 52:987, 1975.
491. Farooki, Z. Q., Henry, J. G., and Green, E. W.: Echocardiographic Spectrum of Ebstein's Anomaly of the Tricuspid Valve, *Circulation,* 53:63, 1976.
492. Hernandez, F. A., Rochkind, R., and Cooper, H. R.: The Intracavitary Electrocardiogram in the Diagnosis of Ebstein's Anomaly, *Am. J. Cardiol.*, 1:181, 1958.
493. Westaby, S., Kary, R. B., Kirklin, J. W., Waldo, A. L., and Blackstone, E. H.: Surgical Treatment in Ebstein's Malformation, *Ann. Thorac. Surg.*, 34:388, 1982.

494. Danielson, G. K., and Fuster, V.: Surgical Repair of Ebstein's Anomaly, *Ann. Surg.*, 196:499, 1982.
495. Danielson, G. K.: Ebstein's Anomaly: Editorial Comments and Personal Observations, *Ann. Thorac. Surg.*, 34:396, 1982.
496. Marcelletti, C., Duren, D. R., Schuilenburg, R. M., and Becker, A. E.: Fontan's Operation for Ebstein's Anomaly, *J. Thorac. Cardiovasc. Surg.*, 79:63, 1980.
497. Gasul, B. M., Lendrum, B. L., and Arcilla, R. A.: Congenital Aplasia or Marked Hypoplasia of the Myocardium of the Right Ventricle (Uhl's Anomaly), *Circulation*, 22:752, 1960.
498. Vecht, R. J., Carmichael, D. J. S., Gopal, R., and Philip, G.: Uhl's Anomaly, *Br. Heart J.*, 41:676, 1979.
499. French, J. W., Baum, D., and Popp, R.: Echocardiographic Findings in Uhl's Anomaly. Demonstration of Diastolic Pulmonary Valve Opening, *Am. J. Cardiol.*, 36:349, 1975.
500. Child, J. S., Perloff, J. K., Francoz, R., et al.: Uhl's Anomaly (Parchment Right Ventricle): Clinical, Echocardiographic, Radionuclear, Hemodynamic, and Angiocardiographic Features in 2 Patients, *Am. J. Cardiol.*, 53:635, 1984.
501. Dines, D. E., Arms, R. A., Bernatz, P. E., and Gomes, M. R.: Pulmonary Arteriovenous Fistulas, *Mayo Clin. Proc.*, 49:460, 1975.
502. Crosby, I. K., Tompkins, D. G., and Carpenter, M. A.: Pulmonary Arteriovenous Fistula and Patent Ductus Arteriosus in the Newborn Infant, *J. Pediatr.*, 86:986, 1975.
503. Hodgson, C. H., Burchell, H. B., Good, C. A., and Clagett, O. T.: Hereditary Hemorrhagic Telangiectasia and Pulmonary Arteriovenous Fistula, *N. Engl. J. Med.*, 261:65, 1959.
504. Sisel, R. J., Parker, B. M., and Bahl, O. P.: Cerebral Symptoms in Pulmonary Arteriovenous Fistula. A Result of Paradoxical Emboli (?), *Circulation*, 41:123, 1970.
505. Mattila, S., Meurala, H., Jarvinen, A., and Ketonen, P.: Pulmonary Arteriovenous Fistulas, *Scand. J. Thorac. Cardiovasc. Surg.*, 16:165, 1982.
506. Terry, P. B., Barth, K. H., Kaufman, S. L., and White, R. I., Jr.: Balloon Embolization for Treatment of Pulmonary Arteriovenous Fistulas, *N. Engl. J. Med.*, 302:1189, 1980.
507. Pool, P. E., Vogel, J. H. K., and Blount, S. G., Jr.: Congenital Unilateral Absence of a Pulmonary Artery, *Am. J. Cardiol.*, 10:706, 1962.
508. Blake, H. A. R., Hall, J., and Manion, W. C.: Anomalous Pulmonary Venous Return, *Circulation*, 32:406, 1965.
509. Elliott, L. P., and Edwards, J. E.: The Problem of Pulmonary Venous Obstruction in Total Anomalous Pulmonary Venous Connection to the Left Innominate Vein, *Circulation*, 25:913, 1962.
510. Lucas, R. V., Jr., Adams, P., Jr., Anderson, R. C., Varco, R. L., Edwards, J. E., and Lester, R. G.: Total Anomalous Pulmonary Venous Connection to the Portal Venous System: A Cause of Pulmonary Venous Obstruction, *Am. J. Roentgenol.*, 86:561, 1961.
511. Gathman, G. E., and Nadas, A. S.: Total Anomalous Pulmonary Venous Connection. Clinical and Physiologic Observations of 75 Pediatric Patients, *Circulation*, 42:143, 1970.
512. Paquet, M., and Gutgesell, H.: Echocardiograhic Features of Total Anomalous Pulmonary Venous Connection, *Circulation*, 51:599, 1975.
513. Sahn, D. J., Allen, H. D., Lange, L. W., and Goldberg, S. J.: Cross-Sectional Echocardiographic Diagnosis of the Sites of Total Anomalous Pulmonary Venous Drainage, *Circulation*, 60:1317, 1979.
514. Mathew, R., Thilenius, O. G., Replogle, R. L., and Arcilla, R. A.: Cardiac Function in Total Anomalous Pulmonary Venous Return before and after Surgery, *Circulation*, 55:361, 1977.
515. Galioto, F. M., Jr., Fyler, D. C., and Chameides, L.: Total Anomalous Pulmonary Venous Drainage (TAPVD): A 5 Year Review in New England, *Am. J. Cardiol.*, 35:138, 1975.
516. Newfeld, E. A., Wilson, A., Paul, M. H., and Reisch, J. S.: Pulmonary Vascular Disease in Total Anomalous Pulmonary Venous Drainage, *Circulation*, 61:103, 1980.
517. Duff, D. F., Nihill, M. R., and McNamara, D. G.: Infradiaphragmatic Total Anomalous Pulmonary Venous Return: Review of Clinical and Pathological Findings and Results of Operation in 28 Cases, *Br. Heart J.*, 39:619, 1977.
518. Turley, K., Tucker, W. Y., Ullyot, D. J., and Ebert, P. A.: Total Anomalous Pulmonary Venous Connection in Infancy: Influence of Age and Type of Lesion, *Am. J. Cardiol.*, 45:92, 1980.
519. Harlan, B. J., Starr, A., and Harwin, F. M.: Total Anomalous Pulmonary Venous Connection, in B. J. Harlan, A. Starr, and F. M. Harwin (eds.), "Manual of Cardiac Surgery," Springer-Verlag, New York, 1981, vol. 2, p. 333.
520. Kirklin, J. W.: Surgical Treatment for Total Anomalous Pulmonary Venous Connection in Infancy, in B. G. Barratt-Boyes (ed.), "Heart Disease in Infancy: Diagnosis and Surgical Treatment," Churchill Livingstone, Edinburgh, 1973, p. 89.
521. Katz, N. M., Kirklin, J. W., and Pacifico, A. D.: Concepts and Practices in Surgery for Total Anomalous Pulmonary Venous Connection, *Ann. Thorac. Surg.*, 25:479, 1978.
522. Gardner, D. L., and Cole, L.: Long Survival with Inferior Vena Cava Draining into Left Atrium, *Br. Heart J.*, 17:93, 1955.
523. Roberts, K. D., Edwards, J. M., and Astley, R.: Surgical Correction of Total Anomalous Systemic Venous Drainage, *J. Thorac. Cardiovasc. Surg.*, 64:803, 1972.
524. Crenshaw, R., Okies, J. E., Phillips, S. J., Bonchek, L. I., and Starr, A.: Partial Anomalous Systemic Venous Return, Report of Surgical Treatment in Two Cases, *J. Thorac. Cardiovasc. Surg.*, 69:3, 1975.
525. Gueron, M., Hirsh, M., and Borman, J.: Total Anomalous Systemic Venous Drainage into the Left Atrium, *J. Thorac. Cardiovasc. Surg.*, 58:570, 1969.
526. Alpert, B. S., Rao, S., Moore, V., and Covitz, W.: Surgical Correction of Anomalous Right Superior Vena Cava to the Left Atrium, *J. Thorac. Cardiovasc. Surg.*, 82:301, 1981.
527. Winter, F. S.: Persistent Left Superior Vena Cava: Survey of World Literature and Report of Thirty Additional Cases, *Angiology*, 5:90, 1954.
528. Fraser, R. S., Dvorkin, J., Rossall, R. E., and Eidem, R.: Left Superior Vena Cava: A Review of Associated Congenital Heart Lesions, Catheterization Data, and Roentgenologic Findings, *Am. J. Med.*, 31:711, 1961.
529. Freedom, R. M., and Ellison, R. C.: Coronary Sinus Rhythm in the Polysplenia Syndrome, *Chest*, 63:952, 1973.
530. Merrill, W. H., Pieroni, D. R., Freedom, R. M., and Ho, C. S.: Diagnosis of Infrahepatic Interruption of the Inferior Vena Cava, *Johns Hopkins Med. J.*, 133:329, 1973.
531. Van Praagh, R., Weinberg, P. M., Matsuoka, R., and Van Praagh, S.: Malpositions of the Heart, in F. H. Adams and G. C. Emmanouilides (eds.), "Moss' Heart Disease in Infants, Children, and Adolescents," The Williams & Wilkins Co., Baltimore, 1983, p. 422.
532. Anderson, R. H., and Shinebourne, E. A. (eds.): "Paediatric Cardiology 1977," Churchill Livingstone, Edinburgh, 1978.
533. Huhta, J. C., Smallhorn, J. F. and Macartney, F. J.: Two Dimensional Echocardiograhic Diagnosis of Situs, *Br. Heart J.*, 48:97, 1982.
534. Foale, R., Stefanini, L., Richards, A., and Somerville, J.: Left and Right Ventricular Morphology in Complex Congenital Heart Disease Defined by Two Dimensional Echocardiography, *Am. J. Cardiol.*, 49:94, 1982.
535. Miller, R. D., and Divertie, M. B.: Kartagener's Syndrome, *Chest*, 62:130, 1972.
536. Van Mierop, L. H. S., Gessner, I. H., and Schiebler, G. L.: Asplenia and Polysplenia Syndromes, *Birth Defects*, 8:36, 1972.
537. Rose, V., Izukawa, T., and Moes, C. A. F.: Syndromes of Asplenia and Polysplenia. A Review of Cardiac and Noncardiac Malformations in 60 Cases with Special Reference to Diagnosis and Prognosis, *Br. Med. J.*, 37:840, 1975.
538. Paul, M. H.: Transposition of the Great Arteries, in F. H. Adams and G. C. Emmanouilides (eds.), "Moss' Heart Disease in Infants, Children, and Adolescents," The Williams & Wilkins Co., Baltimore, 1983, p. 296.
539. Bierman, F. Z., and Williams, R. G.: Prospective Diagnosis of D-Transposition of the Great Arteries in Neonates by Subxiphoid Two-Dimensional Echocardiography, *Circulation*, 60:1496, 1979.

540. Bierman, F. Z., and Williams, R. G.: Subxiphoid Two-Dimensional Imaging of the Interatrial Septum in Infants and Neonates with Congenital Heart Disease, *Circulation,* 60:80, 1979.
541. Gutgesell, H. P.: Echocardiographic Estimation of Pulmonary Artery Pressure in Transposition of the Great Arteries, *Circulation,* 57:1151, 1978.
542. Gutgesell, H. P., Garson, A., and McNamara, D. G.: Prognosis for the Newborn with Transposition of the Great Arteries, *Am. J. Cardiol.,* 44:96, 1979.
543. Newfeld, E. A., Paul, M. H., Muster, A. J., and Idriss, F. S.: Pulmonary Vascular Disease in Transposition of the Great Vessels and Intact Ventricular Septum, *Circulation,* 59:525, 1979.
544. Ramsay, J. M., Venables, A. W., Kelly, M. J., and Kalff, V.: Right and Left Ventricular Function at Rest and with Exercise after the Mustard Operation for Transposition of the Great Arteries, *Br. Heart J.,* 51:364, 1984.
545. Rashkind, W. J., and Miller, W. W.: Creation of an Atrial Septal Defect without Thoracotomy: A Palliative Approach to Complete Transposition of the Great Arteries, *JAMA,* 196:173, 1966.
546. Mustard, W. T.: Successful Two-Stage Correction of Transposition of the Great Vessels, *Surgery,* 55:469, 1964.
547. Piccoli, G. P., Wilkinson, J. L., Arnold, R., Musumeci, F., and Hamilton, D. I.: Appraisal of the Mustard Procedure for the Physiological Correction of "Simple" Transposition of the Great Arteries, *J. Thorac. Cardiovasc. Surg.,* 82:436, 1981.
548. Kirklin, J. W.: Surgery for Transposition of the Great Arteries and Other Types of Malpositions of the Great Arteries, in G. B. Barratt-Boyes (ed.), "Heart Disease in Infancy: Diagnosis and Surgical Treatment," Churchill Livingstone, Edinburgh, 1973, p. 253.
549. Senning, A.: Surgical Correction of Transposition of the Great Vessels, *Surgery,* 45:966, 1959.
550. Penkoske, P. A., Westerman, G. R., Marx, G. R., et al.: Transposition of the Great Arteries and Ventricular Septal Defect: Results with the Senning Operation and Closure of the Ventricular Septal Defect in Infants, *Ann. Thorac. Surg.,* 36:281, 1983.
551. Cobanoglu, A., Abbruzzese, P. A., Freimanis, I., Garcia, C. E., Grunkemeier, G., and Starr, A.: Pericardial Baffle Complications following the Mustard Operation, *J. Thorac. Cardiovasc. Surg.,* 87:371, 1984.
552. Weldon, C. S., Hartmann, A. F., Jr., and Kelly, J. P.: Current Management of Transposition of the Great Arteries: Immediate Septostomy, Occasional Prostaglandin Infusion, and Early Senning Operations, *Ann. Thorac. Surg.,* 36:10, 1983.
553. Jatene, A. D., Fontes, V. F., Souza, L. C. B., Paulista, P. P., Neto, C. A., and Sousa, J. E. M. R.: Anatomic Correction of Transposition of the Great Arteries, *J. Thorac. Cardiovasc. Surg.,* 83:20, 1982.
554. Borow, K. M., Arensman, F. W., Webb, C., Radley-Smith, R., and Yacoub, M. H.: Assessment of Left Ventricular Contractile State after Anatomic Correction of Transposition of the Great Arteries, *Circulation,* 69:106, 1984.
555. Pacifico, A. D., and McKay, R.: Advances in the Surgical Management of Congenital Heart Disease in Infants and Children, in D. C. McGoon (ed.), "Cardiac Surgery," *Cardiovasc. Clin.* (no. 12/3), F. A. Davis Co., Philadelphia, 1982, p. 127.
556. Blalock, A., and Hanlon, C. R.: Surgical Treatment of Complete Transposition of the Aorta and Pulmonary Artery, *Surg. Gynecol. Obstet.,* 90:1, 1950.
557. Litwin, S. B., Plauth, W. H., Jr., Jones, J. E., and Bernhard, W. F.: Appraisal of Surgical Atrial Septectomy for Transposition of the Great Arteries, *Circulation,* 43/44(suppl. 1):7, 1971.
558. Stark, J.: Primary Definitive Cardiac Operations in Infants: Transposition of the Great Arteries, in J. W. Kirklin (ed.), "Advances in Cardiovascular Surgery," Grune & Stratton, Inc., New York, 1973, p. 101.
559. Wilcox, B. R., Henry, G. W., and Anderson, R. H.: The Transmitral Approach to Left Ventricular Outflow Tract Obstruction, *Ann. Thorac. Surg.,* 35:288, 1983.
560. Abe, T., Sugike, K., Izumiyama, O., and Komatsu, S.: A Successful Procedure for Correction of the Taussig-Bing Malformation, *J. Thorac. Cardiovasc. Surg.,* 87:403, 1984.
561. Hagler, D. J., Ritter, D. G., and Puga, F. J.: Double-Outlet Right Ventricle, in F. H. Adams and G. C. Emmanouilides (eds.), "Moss' Heart Disease in Infants, Children, and Adolescents," The Williams & Wilkins Company, Baltimore, 1983, p. 351.
562. Zamora, R., Moller, J. H., and Edwards, J. E.: Double-Outlet Right Ventricle. Anatomic Types and Associated Anomalies, *Chest,* 68:672, 1975.
563. Hagler, D. J., Tajik, A. J., Seward, J. B., Mair, D. D., and Ritter, D. G.: Double-Outlet Right Ventricle, Wide-Angle Two-Dimensional Echocardiographic Observations, *Circulation,* 63:419, 1981.
564. Piccoli, G., Pacifico, A. D., Kirklin, J. W., Blackstone, E. H., Kirklin, J. K., and Bargeron, L. M., Jr.: Changing Results and Concepts in the Surgical Treatment of Double-Outlet Right Ventricle: Analysis of 137 Operations in 126 Patients, *Am. J. Cardiol.,* 52:549, 1983.
565. Anderson, R. H., Becker, A. E., Wilcox, B. R., Macartney, F. J., and Wilkinson, J. L.: Surgical Anatomy of Double-Outlet Right Ventricle—A Reappraisal, *Am. J. Cardiol.,* 52:555, 1983.
566. Stewart, S.: Double-Outlet Right Ventricle: A Collective Review with Surgical Viewpoint, *J. Thorac. Cardiovasc. Surg.,* 71:355, 1976.
567. Kirklin, J. W., Karp, R. A., and McGoon, D. C.: Surgical Treatment of Origin of Both Vessels from Right Ventricle, Including Cases with Pulmonary Stenosis, *J. Thorac. Cardiovasc. Surg.,* 48:1026, 1964.
568. Gomes, M. M. R., Weidman, W. H., McGoon, D. C., and Danielson, G. K.: Double-Outlet Right Ventricle with Pulmonary Stenosis, *Circulation,* 43:889, 1971.
569. Judson, J. P., Danielson, G. K., Puga, F. J., Mair, D. D., and McGoon, D. C.: Double-Outlet Right Ventricle, Surgical Results, 1970–1980, *J. Thorac. Cardiovasc. Surg.,* 85:32, 1983.
570. Van Praagh, R., and Weinberg, P. M.: Double-Outlet Left Ventricle, in F. H. Adams and G. C. Emmanouilides (eds.), "Moss' Heart Disease in Infants, Children, and Adolescents," The Williams & Wilkins Company, Baltimore, 1983, p. 370.
571. Bharati, S., Lev, M., Stewart, R., McAllister, H. A., and Kirklin, J. W.: The Morphologic Spectrum of Double Outlet Left Ventricle and Its Surgical Significance, *Circulation,* 58:558, 1978.
572. Pacifico, A. D., Kirklin, J. W., Bargeron, L. M., Jr., and Soto, B.: Surgical Treatment of Double-Outlet Left Ventricle, *Circulation,* 47/48(suppl. 3):19, 1973.
573. Villani, M., Lipscombe, S., and Ross, D. N.: Double Outlet Left Ventricle: How Should We Repair It? *J. Cardiovasc. Surg.,* 20:413, 1979.
574. Sakakiara, S., Takao, A., Arai, T., Hashimoto, A., and Nogi, M.: Both Great Vessels Arising from the Left Ventricle, *Bull. Heart Inst. Jpn.,* 66, 1967.
575. Mosden, R. R., and Franch, R. H.: Isolated Congenitally Corrected Transposition of the Great Arteries, in J. W. Hurst (ed.), "Update III, The Heart," McGraw-Hill Book Co., New York, 1980.
576. Okamura, K., and Konno, S.: Two Types of Ventricular Septal Defect in Corrected Transposition of the Great Arteries: Reference to Surgical Approaches, *Am. Heart J.,* 85:483, 1973.
577. Ruttenberg, H. D.: Corrected Transposition (L-Transposition) of the Great Arteries and Splenic Syndromes, in F. H. Adams and G. C. Emmanouilides (eds.), "Moss' Heart Disease in Infants, Children, and Adolescents," The Williams & Wilkins Company, Baltimore, 1983, p. 333.
578. Friedberg, D. Z. and Nadas, A. S.: Clinical Profile of Patients with Congenital Corrected Transposition of the Great Arteries. A Study of Sixty Cases, *N. Engl. J. Med.,* 282:1053, 1970.

579. Hagler, D. J., Tajik, A. J., Seward, J. B., Edwards, W. D., Mair, D. D., and Ritter, D. G.: Atrioventricular and Ventriculoarterial Discordance (Corrected Transposition of the Great Arteries). Wide-Angle Two-Dimensional Echocardiographic Assessment of Ventricular Morphology, *Mayo Clin. Proc.*, 56:591, 1981.
580. Hwang, B., Bowman, F., Malm, J., and Krongrad, E.: Surgical Repair of Congenitally Corrected Transposition of the Great Arteries: Results and Follow-up, *Am. J. Cardiol.*, 50:781, 1982.
581. Fox, L. S., Kirklin, J. W., Pacifico, A. D., Waldo, A. L., and Bargeron, L. M., Jr.: Intracardiac Repair of Cardiac Malformations with Atrioventricular Discordance, *Circulation*, 54:123, 1976.
582. Nagai, I., Kawashima, Y., Fujita, T., Mori, T., and Manabe, H.: Successful Closure of Ventricular Septal Defect Through a Left-Sided Ventriculotomy in Corrected Transposition of the Great Arteries, *Ann. Thorac. Surg.*, 21:491, 1976.
583. Van Praagh, R., David, I., and Van Praagh, S.: What Is a Ventricle? The Single-Ventricle Trap, *Pediatr. Cardiol.*, 2:79, 1982.
584. Elliott, L. P., Anderson, R. H., Bargeron, L. M., Jr., and Kirklin, J. W.: Single or Univentricular Heart, in F. H. Adams and G. C. Emmanouilides (eds.), "Moss' Heart Disease in Infants, Children, and Adolescents," The Williams & Wilkins Company, Baltimore, 1983, p. 386.
585. Sahn, D. J., Harder, J. R., Freedom, R. M., et al.: Cross-Sectional Echocardiographic Diagnosis and Subclassification of Univentricular Hearts: Imaging Studies of Atrioventricular Valves, Septal Structures and Rudimentary Outflow Chambers, *Circulation*, 66:1070, 1982.
586. Anderson, R. H., Lenox, C. C., Zuberbuhler, J. R., Ho, S. Y., Smith, A., and Wilkinson, J. L.: Double-Inlet Left Ventricle with Rudimentary Right Ventricle and Ventriculo-arterial Concordance, *Am. J. Cardiol.*, 52:573, 1983.
587. Shinebourne, E. A., Lau, K., Calcaterra, G., and Anderson, R. H.: Univentricular Heart of the Right Ventricular Type: Clinical, Angiographic and Electrocardiographic Features, *Am. J. Cardiol.*, 46:439, 1980.
588. Saalouke, M. G., Perry, L. W., Okoroma, E. O., Shapiro, S. R., and Scott, L. P.: Primitive Ventricle with Normally Related Great Vessels and Stenotic Subpulmonary Outlet Chamber. Angiographic Differentiation from Tetralogy of Fallot, *Br. Heart J.*, 40:49, 1978.
589. Seward, J. B., Tajik, A. J., Hagler, D. J., Guiliani, E. R., Gau, G. T., and Ritter, D. G.: Echocardiograms in Common (Single) Ventricle: Angiographic-Anatomic Correlation, *Am. J. Cardiol.*, 39:217, 1977.
590. Soto, B., Pacifico, A. D., Disciascio, G.: Univentricular Heart: An Angiographic Study, *Am. J. Cardiol.*, 49:787, 1982.
591. Graham, T. P., Jr., and Friesinger, G. C.: Complex Cyanotic Congenital Heart Disease in Adults, in W. C. Roberts (ed.), "Congenital Heart Disease in Adults," F. A. Davis Co., Philadelphia, 1979, p. 383.
592. McGoon, D. C., Danielson, G. K., and Puga, F. J.: Univentricular Heart, in W. W. L. Glenn, A. E. Baue, A. E. Geha, G. L. Hammond, and H. Laks (eds.), "Thoracic and Cardiovascular Surgery," Appleton-Century-Crofts, Norwalk, Conn., 1983, p. 770.
593. McKay, R., Pacifico, A. D., Blackstone, E. H., Kirklin, J. W., and Bargeron, L. M., Jr.: Septation of the Univentricular Heart with Left Anterior Subaortic Outlet Chamber, *J. Thorac. Cardiovasc. Surg.*, 84:77, 1982.
594. Feldt, R. H., Mair, D. D., Danielson, G. K., Wallace, R. B., and McGoon, D. C.: Current Status of the Septation Procedure for Univentricular Heart, *J. Thorac. Cardiovasc. Surg.*, 82:93, 1981.
595. Moreno-Cabral, R. J., Miller, C., Oyer, P. E., Stinson, E. B., Reitz, B. A., and Shumway, N. E.: A Surgical Aproach for S,L,L Single Ventricle Incorporating Total Right Atrium–Pulmonary Artery Division, *J. Thorac. Cardiovasc. Surg.*, 79:202, 1980.
596. Doty, D. B., Marvin, W. J., Jr., and Lauer, R. M.: Single Ventricle with Aortic Outflow Obstruction, *J. Thorac. Cardiovasc. Surg.*, 81:636, 1981.
597. Gale, A. W., Danielson, G. K., McGoon, D. C., and Mair, D. D.: Modified Fontan Operation for Univentricular Heart and Complicated Congenital Lesions, *J. Thorac. Cardiovasc. Surg.*, 78:831, 1979.
598. Van Praagh, S., La Corte, M., Fellows, K. E., et al.: Superoinferior Ventricles: Anatomic and Angiographic Findings in Ten Post Mortem Cases, in R. Van Praagh and A. Takao (eds.), "Etiology and Morphogenesis of Congenital Heart Disease," Futura Publishing Co., Mount Kisco, N.Y., 1980.
599. Atie, F., Munoz-Castellanos, L., Ovseyevitz, J., et al.: Crossed Atrioventricular Connections, *Am. Heart J.*, 99:163, 1980.
600. Schneeweiss, A., Shem-Tov, A., Blieden, L. C., Deutsch, V., and Neufeld, H. N.: Criss-Cross Heart—A Case with Horizontal Septum, Complete Transposition, Pulmonary Atresia and Ventricular Septal Defect, *Pediatr. Cardiol.*, 3:325, 1982.
601. Ravitch, M. M.: "Congenital Deformities of the Chest Wall and Their Operative Correction," W. B. Saunders Company, Philadelphia, 1977.
602. Cantrell, J. R., Haller, J. A., and Ravitch, M. M.: A Syndrome of Congenital Defects Involving the Abdominal Wall, Sternum, Diaphragm, Pericardium, and Heart, *Surg. Gynecol. Obstet.*, 107:602, 1958.
603. McNamara, J. J., and Gross, R. E.: Congenital Coronary Artery Fistula, *Surgery*, 65:59, 1969.
604. Liberthson, R. R., Sagar, K., Berkoben, J. P., Weintraub, R. M., and Levine, F. H.: Congenital Coronary Arteriovenous Fistula: Report of 13 Patients, Review of the Literature and Delineation of Management, *Circulation*, 59:849, 1979.
605. Jaffee, R. B., Glancy, D. L., Epstein, S. E., Brown, B. G., and Morrow, A. G.: Coronary Arterial–Right Heart Fistula: Long-Term Observations in Seven Patients, *Circulation*, 47:133, 1973.
606. Oldham, H. N., Jr., Ebert, P. A., Young, W. G., and Sabiston, D. C., Jr.: Surgical Management of Congenital Coronary Artery Fistula, *Ann. Thorac. Surg.*, 12:503, 1971.
607. Urrutia-S, C. O., Falaschi, G., Ott, D. A., and Cooley, D. A.: Surgical Management of 56 Patients with Congenital Coronary Artery Fistulas, *Ann. Thorac. Surg.*, 35:300, 1983.
608. Noren, G. H., Raghib, G., Moller, J. H., Amplatz, K., Adams, P., Jr., and Edwards, J. E.: Anomalous Origin of the Left Coronary Artery from the Pulmonary Trunk with Special Reference to the Occurrence of Mitral Insufficiency, *Circulation*, 30:171, 1964.
609. Burchell, H. B., and Brown, A. L., Jr.: Anomalous Origin of Coronary Artery from Pulmonary Artery Masquerading as Mitral Insufficiency, *Am. Heart J.*, 63:388, 1962.
610. Wesselhoeft, H., Fawcett, J. S., and Johnson, A. L.: Anomalous Origin of the Left Coronary Artery from the Pulmonary Trunk: Its Clinical Spectrum, Pathology, and Pathophysiology Based on a Review of 140 Cases with 7 Further Cases, *Circulation*, 38:403, 1968.
611. Gutgesell, H. P., Pinsky, W. W., and DePuey, E. G.: Thallium-201 Myocardial Perfusion Imaging in Infants and Children: Value in Distinguishing Anomalous Left Coronary Artery from Congestive Cardiomyopathy, *Circulation*, 61:596, 1980.
612. Wilson, C. L., Dlabal, P. W., and McGuire, S. A.: Surgical Treatment of Anomalous Left Coronary Artery from Pulmonary Artery: Follow-up in Teenagers and Adults, *Am. Heart J.*, 98:440, 1979.
613. Driscoll, D. J., Nihill, M. R., Mullins, C. E., Cooley, D. A., and McNamara, D. G.: Management of Symptomatic Infants with Anomalous Origin of the Left Coronary Artery from the Pulmonary Artery, *Am. J. Cardiol.*, 47:642, 1981.
614. Shrivastava, S., Castaneda, A. R., and Moller, J. H.: Anomalous Left Coronary Artery from Pulmonary Trunk: Long-Term Follow-up after Ligation, *J. Thorac. Cardiovasc. Surg.*, 76:130, 1978.
615. Arciniegas, E., Farooki, Z. Q., Hakimi, M., and Green, E. W.: Management of Anomalous Left Coronary Artery from the Pulmonary Artery, *Circulation*, 62(suppl. 1):180, 1980.

616. Levitsky, S., van der Horst, R. L., Hastreiter, A. R., and Fisher, E. A.: Anomalous Left Coronary Artery in the Infant: Recovery of Ventricular Function following Early Direct Aortic Implantation, *J. Thorac. Cardiovasc. Surg.*, 79:598, 1980.
617. Moodie, D. S., Fyfe, D., Gill, C. C., Cook, S. A., et al.: Anomalous Origin of the Left Coronary Artery from the Pulmonary Artery (Bland-White-Garland Syndrome) in Adult Patients: Long-Term Follow-up after Surgery, *Am. Heart J.*, 106:381, 1983.
618. Tingelstad, J. B., Lower, R. R., and Eldredge, W. J.: Anomalous Origin of the Right Coronary Artery from the Main Pulmonary Artery, *Am. J. Cardiol.*, 30:670, 1972.
619. Blake, H. A., Manion, W. C., Mattingly, R. W., and Baroldi, G.: Coronary Artery Anomalies, *Circulation*, 30:927, 1964.
620. Feldt, R. H., Ongley, P. A., and Titus, J. L.: Total Coronary Arterial Circulation from Pulmonary Artery with Survival to Age Seven: Report of a Case, *Mayo Clin. Proc.*, 40:539, 1965.
621. Neufeld, H. N., and Blieden, L. C.: Coronary Artery Disease in Children, *Prog. Cardiol.*, 4:119, 1975.
622. Lerbery, D. B., Ogden, J. A., Zuberbuhler, J. R., and Bahnson, H. T.: Anomalous Origin of the Right Coronary Artery from the Pulmonary Artery, *Ann. Thorac. Surg.*, 27:87, 1979.
623. Goldblatt, E., Adams, A. P. S., Ross, I. K., Savage, J. P., and Morris, L. L.: Single-Trunk Anomalous Origin of Both Coronary Arteries from the Pulmonary Artery, *J. Thorac. Cardiovasc. Surg.*, 87:59, 1984.
624. Cheitlin, M. D., De Castro, C. M., and McAllister, H. A.: Sudden Death as a Complication of Anomalous Left Coronary Origin from the Anterior Sinus of Valsalva. A Not-So-Minor Congenital Anomaly, *Circulation*, 50:780, 1974.
625. Liberthson, R. R., Dinsmore, R. E., and Fallon, J. T.: Aberrant Coronary Artery Origin from the Aorta: Report of 18 Patients. Review of Literature and Delineation of Natural History and Management, *Circulation*, 59:748, 1979.
626. Fellows, K. E., Freed, M. D., Keane, J. F., Van Praagh, R., Bernard, W. F., and Castaneda, A. R.: Results of Routine Preoperative Coronary Angiography in Tetralogy of Fallot, *Circulation*, 51:561, 1975.
627. Moodie, D. S., Gill, C., Loop, F. D., and Sheldon, W. C.: Anomalous Left Main Coronary Artery Originating from the Right Sinus of Valsalva, *J. Thorac. Cardiovasc. Surg.*, 80:198, 1980.
628. Mustafa, I., Gula, G., Radley-Smith, R., Durrer, S., and Yacoub, M.: Anomalous Origin of the Left Coronary Artery from the Anterior Aortic Sinus: A Potential Cause of Sudden Death, *J. Thorac. Cardiovasc. Surg.*, 82:297, 1981.
629. Byrum, C. J., Blackman, M. S., Schneider, B., Sondheimer, H. M., and Kavey, R. W.: Congenital Atresia of the Left Coronary Ostium and Hypoplasia of the Left Main Coronary Artery, *Am. Heart J.*, 99:354, 1980.
630. Mullins, C. E., El-Said, G., McNamara, D. G., Cooley, D. A., Treistman, B., and Garcia, E.: Atresia of the Left Coronary Ostium: Repair by Saphenous Vein Graft, *Circulation*, 46:989, 1972.
631. Onouchi, Z., Shimazu, S., Kiyosaua, N., Takamatsu, T. and Hamaoka, K.: Aneurysms of the Coronary Arteries in Kawasaki Disease: An Angiographic Study of 30 Cases, *Circulation*, 66:6, 1982.
632. Wilson, C. S., Weaver, W. F., Zeman, E. D., and Forker, A. D.: Bilateral Nonfistulous Congenital Coronary Arterial Aneurysms, *Am. J. Cardiol.*, 35:319, 1975.
633. McMartin, D. E., Stone, A. J., and Franch, R. H.: Multiple Coronary-Artery Aneurysms in a Child with Angina Pectoris, *N. Engl. J. Med.*, 290:669, 1974.
634. Tibbits, P., Stanton, K., Ashworth, H., and Baker, W.: Congenital Coronary Aneurysms Nine Years following Saphenous Vein Bypass Graft Surgery, *Ann. Thorac. Surg.*, 32:411, 1981.
635. Suma, K., Takeuchi, Y., Shiroma, K., et al.: Early and Late Postoperative Studies in Coronary Arterial Lesions Resulting from Kawasaki's Disease in Children, *J. Thorac. Cardiovasc. Surg.*, 84:224, 1982.
636. Mantini, Ed., Grondin, C. M., Lillehei, C. W., and Edwards, J. E.: Congenital Anomalies Involving the Coronary Sinus, *Circulation*, 33:317, 1966.
637. Foale, R. A., Baron, D. W., and Richards, A. F.: Isolated Congenital Absence of Coronary Sinus, *Br. Heart J.*, 42:355, 1979.
638. Moore, R. L.: Congenital Deficiencies of the Pericardium, *Arch. Surg.*, 11:765, 1925.
639. Nasser, W. K., Helmen, C., Tauel, M. E., Feigenbaum, H., and Fisch, C.: Congenital Absence of the Left Pericardium, *Circulation*, 41:469, 1970.
640. Hipona, F. A., and Crummy, A. J., Jr.: Congenital Pericardial Defect Associated with Tetralogy of Fallot, *Circulation*, 29:132, 1964.
641. Spitz, L., Bloom, F., Milner, S., and Levin, S. E.: Combined Anterior Abdominal Wall, Sternal, Diaphragmatic, Pericardial, and Intracardiac Defects: A Report of 5 Cases and Their Management, *J. Pediatr. Surg.*, 10:481, 1975.
642. Ellis, K., Leeds, N. E., and Himmelstein, A.: Congenital Deficiencies of the Parietal Pericardium, *Am. J. Roentgenol. Radium Ther. Nucl. Med.*, 82:125, 1959.
643. Payvandi, M. N., and Kerber, R. E.: Echocardiography in Congenital and Acquired Absence of the Pericardium, *Circulation*, 53:86, 1976.
644. Loehr, W. M.: Pericardial Cysts, *Am. J. Roentgenol.*, 68:584, 1952.

Section B

Valvular Heart Disease

37

Aortic Valve Disease

Charles E. Rackley, M.D.
Jesse E. Edwards, M.D.
Robert B. Wallace, M.D.
Nevin M. Katz, M.D.

Aortic Stenosis*

Strong action of the left ventricle; extremely loud and musical murmur at the extent of the arterial tree; the heart's action generally regular.

William Stokes, 1854[1]

Etiology

Aortic stenosis can be caused by a congenital unicuspid or bicuspid valve, rheumatic fever (see Chap. 62), or valve calcification in the elderly. The incidence and prevalence of aortic stenosis have been modified by reinterpretation of pathological studies, a significant decline in rheumatic fever, and an increase in the life span of the adult population. Pathological studies during the early part of the century attributed aortic stenosis to inflammation or valvular sclerosis, but a series in 1947 suggested rheumatic valvulitis as the major cause.[2,3] More recent studies indicated congenital valvular stenosis as the most common cause with the recognition of a bicuspid valve as a major cause of aortic stenosis.[4,5]

If aortic stenosis is detected in a patient under the age of 30 years, a congenitally stenotic aortic valve is the most likely etiology.[6] From ages 30 to 70 years, rheumatic disease plays a role and beyond 70 years, calcification of the aortic valve is the usual cause.[8] If the aortic stenosis is an isolated lesion, 6 to 24 percent of affected individuals may reveal a rheumatic basis, but aortic stenosis in combination with mitral valve disease increases the likelihood of a rheumatic basis.[9,10]

Pathology

Acquired stenosis results primarily either from commissural fusion, yielding the fibrous type of stenosis, or from calcification of the cusps of the valve. While a rheumatic etiology may underlie each of these types, calcific stenosis is most commonly engrafted upon nonrheumatic valves, either congenitally bicuspid valves, or, commonly, on a tricuspid valve.

The Fibrous Type

Recurrent rheumatic endocarditis causes fibrous contracture with shortening of cusps and a tendency for fusion of adjacent cusps at commissures. When commissural adhesion occurs only at one aortic commissure, the valve becomes bicuspid (acquired bicuspid valve). In a valve so affected, the orifice is somewhat reduced, but usually not measurably. Such valves offer (as do congenital bicuspid valves) the tendency for acquired calcification of the cusps.

If there is fusion at two or three commissures the cusps are sufficiently restrained so as to cause obstruction at the valve level. The valve that is stenotic because of commissural fusion may show varying degrees (sometimes heavy) of calcification, but the primary basis for stenosis resides in adhesions of one cusp to another, yielding the fibrous type of aortic stenosis.[11] This is usually of rheumatic origin.

*The editor-in-chief wishes to thank John W. Kirklin, M.D., and Robert B. Karp, M.D., for their contribution to the chapter on this subject that appeared in the fifth edition of *The Heart*.

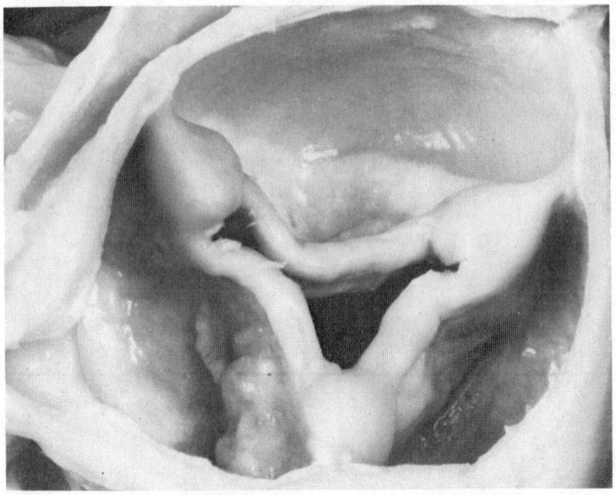

FIGURE 37-1 Fibrous (rheumatic) aortic stenosis. There is fusion of all three commissures. (*From J. E. Edwards, Pathology of Acquired Valvular Disease of the Heart, Semin. Roentgenol., 14:96, 1979. Reproduced with permission from the publisher and author.*)

Because of associated shortening of cusps, this type of aortic stenosis is usually accompanied by some degree of aortic insufficiency (Fig. 37-1). Also, it is common that some degree of rheumatic change be present in the mitral valve and, in some cases, the tricuspid valve also.

The Calcific Type

Aortic stenosis resulting primarily from rigidity of cuspid tissue incident to calcification usually occurs in a bicuspid valve, and relatively uncommonly in a tricuspid or unicuspid aortic valve.[7,12] There are two etiologies for the bicuspid state, either acquired through rheumatic disease (Fig. 37-2*A*) or congenital (Fig. 37-2*B*). In instances of the calcific type of aortic stenosis, the congenital bicuspid valve is more common than the acquired bicuspid valve by a ratio of about 4:1. Classically, the aortic valve is competent and, in instances of the congenital bicuspid valve, no other valve of the heart is diseased.

In the congenital bicuspid valve, the large, conjoined cusp as a rule lies anteriorly, and the two coronary arteries arise from its sinus. In acquired bicuspid valve the conjoined cusp may occupy the same position or be oriented toward the right or left. It is common for some degree of calcification to appear in the normal aortic valves of persons 70 years and older.[13] Usually, the calcification is inadequate to cause stenosis, although it may be responsible for a murmur. In exceptional cases, each of the three cusps is highly calcified, making the valve stenotic. This uncommon type of aortic stenosis may be called the senile type of calcific aortic valvular sclerosis (Fig. 37-2*C*).

Miscellaneous Types

Aortic stenosis observed from infancy to adolescence is usually of congenital origin, the valve displaying the unicommissural, unicuspid character. Occasionally, individuals with such valves may reach adulthood before they display significant signs of aortic stenosis. This phenomenon may result from calcification with secondary incompetence (regurgitation) of a congenitally deformed but intrinsically mildly stenotic valve (Fig. 37-2*D*). The resultant effects of the incompetence (aortic regurgitation) may then serve to bring the element of stenosis into evidence.

Uncommonly, aortic stenosis may result from the presence of a congenital papillary mass or flap of endocardial tissue that obstructs an otherwise normal valve. Extensive thrombosis at the valve site has been a cause of aortic stenosis in lupus erythematosus.[14] The secondary effects of aortic stenosis include left ventricular hypertrophy and poststenotic dilatation of the ascending aorta.

Numbered among the common complications of aortic stenosis are sudden death and congestive cardiac failure. Other complications include embolism, including coronary embolism of valvular fragments in calcific aortic stenosis.[15] In aortic stenosis, as in aortic regurgitation, as the left ventricle enlarges downward there may be undue restraint upon the mitral chordae, and secondary mitral insufficiency may result.[16] Mitral insufficiency may also result from congenital aortic stenosis through fibrosis of papillary muscles and related left ventricular free wall.[17] Dissecting or saccular aneurysm of the aorta may occur as a consequence of the cystic medial necrosis of the aorta that may accompany aortic stenosis.[18]

Although aortic stenosis has been claimed as protective against coronary atherosclerosis, studies indicate that the average degree of coronary atherosclerosis among patients with aortic stenosis is not materially different from that in persons with normal aortic valves.[19]

Abnormal Physiology

Stenosis of the aortic valve creates resistance to ejection, and a pressure gradient during systole develops between the left ventricle and the systemic arterial tree. The size of the aortic orifice is normally 2 to 3 cm^2, and a reduction is accompanied by a progressive increase in the left ventricular systolic pressure. Elevation of the systolic pressure produces a pressure overload on the left ventricle, which adapts by an increase in thickness of the left ventricular wall and left ventricular mass or hypertrophy of the myocardium (Figs. 37-3 and 37-4).[20] This concentric hypertrophy without chamber dilatation normalizes the systolic force or wall stress and preserves ventricular function as estimated by normal cardiac output and ejection fraction.[21] Dilatation of the left ventricle does not occur until the contractile state of the myocardium is significantly depressed. The increase in wall thickness and cross-sectional area of the left ventricular myocardium normalizes the distribution of the elevated systolic chamber pressure

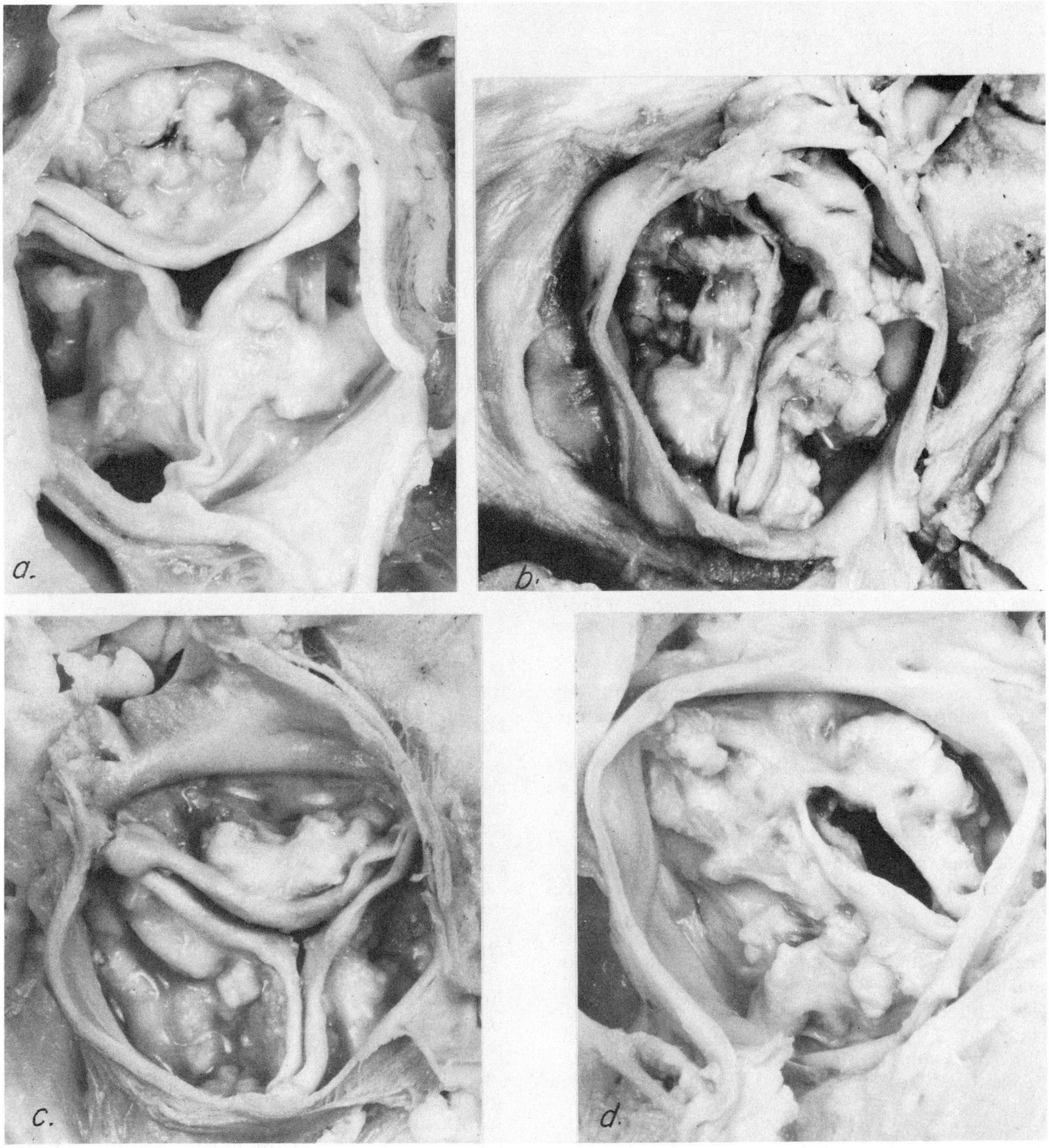

FIGURE 37-2 Four types of calcific aortic stenosis. In each, the unopened aortic valve is viewed from above. *a.* Acquired bicuspid aortic valve with secondary calcification. At the center of the conjoined cusp (lower center) are elements of two preexisting cusps, now fused. *b.* Congenital bicuspid valve. The characteristic raphe of the congenital bicuspid aortic valve appears at the lower portion of the illustration. *c.* Senile type. None of the commissures are fused, but there is major intrinsic calcification of the three cusps. *d.* Unicuspid, unicommissural congenital aortic stenosis with secondary calcification. (*From J. E. Edwards, Pathology of Acquired Valvular Disease of the Heart, Semin. Roentgenol., 14:96, 1979. Reproduced with permission from the publisher and author.*)

throughout the cardiac cycle until the inotropic state is depressed and the ventricle dilates.[22]

The compensatory hypertrophy and increase in left ventricular mass in aortic stenosis result in an elevation of the left ventricular end-diastolic pressure, which is further raised by atrial systole. Atrial systole contributes significantly to the percent of systolic volume ejected in aortic stenosis compared to the normal ventricle.[23] Although the Frank-Starling mechanism has been proposed to explain the contribution of atrial systole in aortic stenosis, end-diastolic wall stress or preload is usually normal in the hypertrophied left ventricle of aortic stenosis.[24] Left ventricular compliance decreases, which contributes

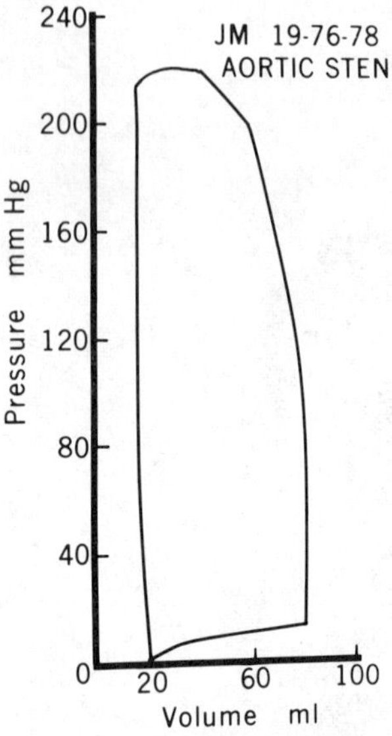

FIGURE 37-3 Left ventricular pressure-volume diagram in compensated aortic stenosis and left ventricular pressure overload. The significant abnormality is the abnormally elevated systolic pressure, but end-diastolic volume, end-systolic volume, and ejection fraction remain normal. [*From C. E. Rackley, Value of Ventriculography in Cardiac Function and Diagnosis: Diagnostic Methods in Cardiology, in N. O. Fowler (ed.), "Cardiovascular Clinics," F. A. Davis Company, Philadelphia, 1975. Reproduced with permission from the publisher and author.*]

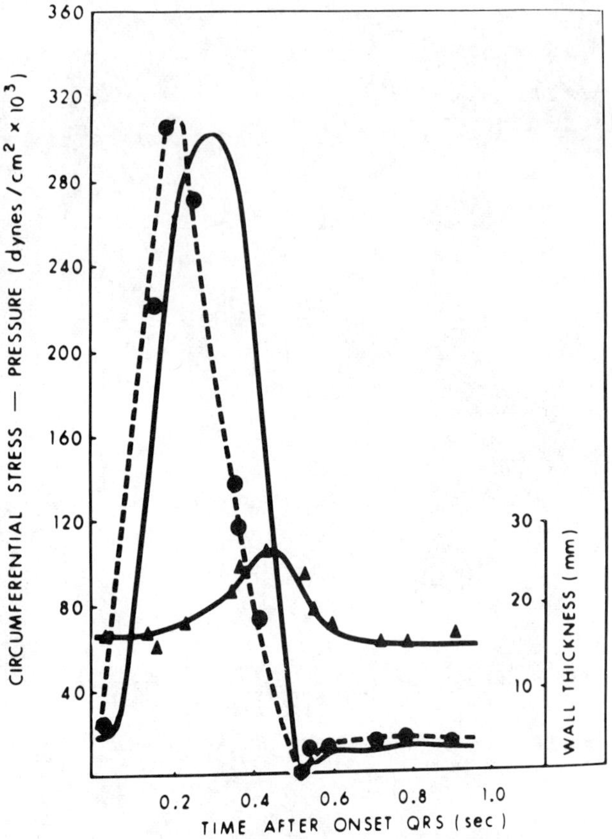

FIGURE 37-4 Left ventricular pressure, circumferential wall stress, and wall thickness in compensated aortic stenosis and pressure overload. Diastole wall thickness is abnormally increased, and further thickening occurs during systolic ejection which results in a rapid decline of circumferential wall stress. (– · –, stress; ——, pressure; ▲ —— ▲, wall thickness.) [*From C. E. Rackley and W. P. Hood Jr., Aortic Valve Disease, in H. J. Levine (ed.), "Clinical Cardiovascular Physiology," Grune & Stratton, Inc., New York, 1976. Reproduced with permission from the publisher and author.*]

to the elevation of the left ventricular end-diastolic pressure after atrial systole, and left atrial enlargement results.

The sustained pressure overload on the myocardium in chronic aortic stenosis eventually leads to depression of the contractile state.[25] Declining mechanical performance is attended by dilatation of the left ventricle in order to maintain forward cardiac output. Although the systolic wall stress remains within the normal range during the compensated concentric hypertrophy phase of aortic stenosis, chamber dilatation will eventually result in abnormal elevation of systolic wall stress attended by a rising left ventricular end-diastolic pressure, a decline in ejection fraction, reduction in cardiac output, and eventual pulmonary hypertension.

Clinical Manifestations

The characteristic clinical manifestations of aortic stenosis are chest pain, syncope, and heart failure.[26] The patient's age at the recognition of the murmur can be helpful in attributing the lesion to a congenital, rheumatic, or calcific basis. The symptoms of aortic stenosis tend to occur late in the course of the disease when a critical reduction in valve size has developed. In adults, presentation of the usual manifestations of aortic stenosis may be complicated by underlying coronary artery disease.

Angina pectoris is the most frequent symptom of aortic stenosis and occurs in 50 to 70 percent of affected individuals.[27,28] Life expectancy has been estimated at an average of 5 years after the development of chest discomfort. Special features of the chest discomfort in aortic stenosis include the development of pain after physical exertion and a higher incidence of nitroglycerin-induced syncope.[29] Coronary arteriography has demonstrated that anatomical coronary disease is frequently present in adults with aortic stenosis, whether they have experienced chest pain or not.[30] The difference in myocardial oxygen demand and oxygen availability has been proposed as the mechanism for the chest pain. Myocardial oxygen consumption in aortic stenosis is greater than normal due to an increase in left ventricular mass and diminished oxygen availability at the subendocardial level.[31] Systolic wall stress is a major determinant of myocardial oxygen consumption and in the hypertrophied myocardium wall stress is the highest at the subendocardium.[32] Calcific emboli have been incriminated as a rare mechanism for impaired coronary blood flow.[33]

Effort syncope is a frequent symptom of aortic stenosis and often occurs following physical exertion.[27] Survival has been estimated at 3 to 4 years with syncope due to aortic stenosis.[26] One proposed mechanism for the syncope is left ventricular failure with an abrupt fall in cardiac output.[34] Arrhythmias may also contribute to the syncope of aortic stenosis, but some investigators have contended that the arrhythmia develops in the late stages of the circulatory impairment.[35] Exercise-induced peripheral vasodilatation may also aggravate the systolic pressure gradient and further reduce perfusion pressure of the myocardium. In older patients with calcific aortic stenosis, transient cerebral ischemia with underlying cerebrovascular disease may also be a mechanism.

Left ventricular failure is the third symptomatic presentation of severe aortic stenosis. Dyspnea may be described quite differently by children and adults and is influenced by the amount of exercise in the different age groups.[36] The symptoms of left ventricular failure may herald a shorter survival in older patients than in the younger age group. In adults with aortic stenosis, survival has been estimated at 2 years after symptoms of heart failure develop.[26,36]

Additional symptoms attributed to severe aortic stenosis include palpitations, fatigue, and visual defects. Fatigue is an early symptom in children. In the elderly, calcific aortic stenosis and carotid and cerebrovascular disease may produce additional symptoms in the central nervous system. Visual field defects from calcific emboli from the aortic valve can be rare but presenting manifestations.[33,37]

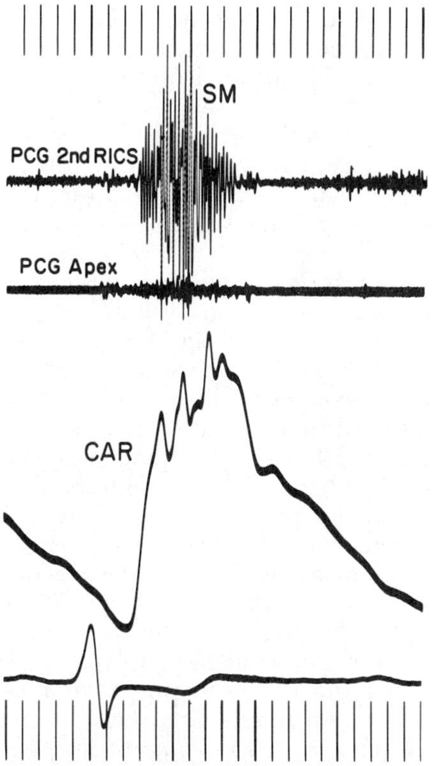

FIGURE 37-5 Phonocardiogram and carotid pulse recording in aortic stenosis. A loud crescendo-decrescendo, diamond-shaped systolic murmur is recorded in the aortic area and the carotid pulse shows the delayed upstroke with a jagged appearance corresponding with the vibrations of a thrill. PCG = phonocardiogram; RICS = right intercostal space; SM = systolic murmur; CAR = carotid artery. (*Courtesy of Dr. Ernest Craige.*)

Physical Examination

The *pulse pressure is narrowed* in significant aortic stenosis with a reduction in systolic pressure and maintenance of the diastolic level. Although a systemic systolic pressure above 200 mmHg is rarely encountered in severe aortic stenosis, elderly patients with calcific aortic stenosis and loss of arterial elasticity can sometimes present pressures above 180 mmHg with significant pressure gradients across the aortic valve.[27,38] The characteristic delay in upstroke and decline in the slope of the pulse contour can be detected in the carotid artery, but the examiner should be cautious in vigorously palpating the carotid arteries to recognize these waveform abnormalities (Fig. 37-5). In elderly patients carotid sinus sensitivity and cerebral ischemia can result in sudden bradycardia and loss of consciousness. The brachial artery is a much more accessible artery to palpate and evaluate arterial waveform abnormalities in aortic stenosis. Occlusion of the brachial artery with a single finger and gradual release of the pressure permits recognition of an anacrotic notch.[27] The anacrotic notch is attributed to peak turbulence across the aortic valve, and as the stenosis becomes more severe the notch is detected earlier on the initial upstroke. The delayed peak of the pulse, diminished amplitude, and gradual downslope are described by the term *pulsus parvus et tardus* (see Chap. 9).

Even with severe left ventricular hypertrophy, the apical impulse may remain focal and within the midclavicular line (see Chap. 10). A *palpable systolic murmur* should be sought, particularly over the aortic area in the right second interspace. This maneuver is facilitated by using the palm of the hand over the primary aortic valve area while the patient leans forward in full respiratory expiration. If palpable vibrations can be detected during systolic ejection, the gradient across the aortic valve usually exceeds 40 mmHg. Rarely, systolic vibrations can accompany the ejection murmur of relative aortic stenosis in severe aortic regurgitation.

The auscultatory findings in aortic stenosis include an *ejection click,* the *diamond-shaped crescendo-decrescendo systolic murmur, delayed closure of the aortic valve,* and a detectable *diastolic blow of aortic regurgitation* along the left sternal border (see Chap. 11). The ejection sound is high-pitched and is usually heard at the apex along the left sternal border shortly after the first heart sound.[39] The ejection sound occurs with the systolic elevation of the central aortic pulse and probably originates from the aortic valve leaflets. The ejection click is related to the mobility of the valve and not the severity of the gradient. Intensity of the click often correlates with the prominence of the aortic second sound.

Characteristics of the systolic murmur include a harsh crescendo-decrescendo or diamond-shaped pattern of the vibrations. An interval between the first heart sound and onset of the murmur can usually be appreciated, and the murmur terminates before the second sound. If the aortic second sound is sufficiently diminished, pulmonic closure sound may be identified as the aortic second sound and the murmur interpreted as holosystolic. The aortic second sound is often delayed in severe aortic stenosis and can produce paradoxical splitting of the second sound (see Chap. 11). Rather than the normal inspiratory splitting of the second heart sound, delayed closure of the aortic valve may coincide with the pulmonic sound during inspiration. With expiration, the pulmonic second sound will migrate toward the first heart sound, and the delayed aortic second sound can produce paradoxical splitting.[27] As the aortic valve becomes calcified and loses mobility, intensity of the second sound diminishes. One-third to one-half of individuals with isolated aortic valve stenosis reveal a high-pitched diastolic blow of aortic regurgitation along the left sternal border.[40] This murmur is attributed to fixed stenosis of the aortic valve which remains open during the diastole.

Calcific aortic stenosis in the elderly can produce different auscultatory features of the murmur.[41] Since calcification occurs in a nodular fashion at the base of the aortic cusps and root with preservation of leaflet mobility, the murmur is often musical and prominent at the apex as well as along the left sternal border. Detection of the murmur at the apex may raise the possibility of mitral annulus calcification and regurgitation across the mitral valve. The murmur of aortic stenosis may be higher-pitched at the apex and this, too, may lead one to think of separate mitral regurgitation. The murmur of aortic stenosis that is heard at the apex rarely radiates beyond that point as does the murmur of mitral regurgitation. In addition to the auscultatory variations of calcific aortic stenosis in the elderly, sclerosis and loss of compliance in peripheral arteries can obscure the characteristic pulse deformities.

Chest Roentgenogram

Since aortic stenosis imposes a pressure overload on the left ventricle, radiographic heart size will *initially remain within normal limits.*[42] The curvature of the apex may be prominent or bulging, suggesting concentric hypertrophy. *Poststenotic dilatation of the ascending aorta* is a common feature of aortic stenosis. Detection of *calcification in the aortic valve* usually requires fluoroscopy and cannot always be identified on plain films. Calcification is commonly encountered in significant aortic stenosis in patients over the age of 40 years. *Enlargement of the left atrium* can occur secondary to decreasing compliance of the left ventricle, but excessive dilatation should raise other possibilities, such as mitral stenosis or idiopathic hypertrophic subaortic stenosis. (See Chaps. 15 and 107.)

Electrocardiogram

Abnormalities in the electrocardiogram in aortic stenosis are produced by left ventricular hypertrophy and reflected in increased amplitude of the QRS complex and ST-T wave alterations.[27,43] Systolic overload, left ventricular strain, or left ventricular hypertrophy consist of increased size of the S waves in right precordial leads, increased size of the R waves in left precordial leads coupled with depression of the ST segment and inversion of the T waves. Conduction defects are frequent and range from first degree heart block to left bundle branch block. (See Chap. 14.)

Special Laboratory Studies

Echocardiogram Echocardiography can delineate structure and mobility in valvular as well as nonvalvular forms of aortic stenosis.[44] The characteristic echocardiographic changes are thickening, calcification, and reduced mobility of the aortic leaflet.[45] Left ventricular dimensions of septal wall thickness can demonstrate the extent of left ventricular hypertrophy as well as asymmetrical septal hypertrophy in idiopathic subaortic stenosis. Left ventricular function can be determined from chamber dimensions and estimates of end-diastolic and end-systolic volumes and ejection fraction. A bicuspid aortic valve can be recognized in the asymmetry of the two leaflets and used to calculate an eccentricity index.[46] A long-axis systolic aortic cusp separation less than 8 mm by two-dimensional echo is highly predictive of severe aortic stenosis.[47] (See Chap. 120.)

Cardiac Catheterization Cardiac catheterization in aortic stenosis can measure the gradient across the valve, estimate the stenosis, evaluate left ventricular function, and delineate coronary artery anatomy (Fig. 37-6). The normal systolic valve area is 2 to 3 cm^2, and calculations have revealed that reduction of 75 percent or more with an orifice size less than 0.8 cm^2 is necessary for significant impairment to flow and maintenance of cardiac output.[48] This degree of stenosis of the valve is usually accompanied by a gradient exceeding 50 mmHg, but a reduction in cardiac output will reduce the gradient across the valve (Fig. 37-7).[49]

Quantitative angiography can provide measurements of end-diastolic and systolic volume, ejection fraction, and left ventricular mass (Fig. 37-8).[50] Chamber dimensions, pressure, and wall thickness permit calcification of wall stress at end-systole (preload), at systolic valve opening (afterload), and at end-systole (Fig. 37-8). End-systolic indexes for pressure volume, wall thickness, and stress can be obtained.

Coronary arteriography in aortic stenosis has revealed a 50 percent incidence of underlying coronary artery disease whether patients describe a history of previous exertional chest pain or not (Fig. 37-9).[30] Findings on physical examination suggestive of aortic stenosis warrant coronary arteriography for both diagnostic and therapeutic reasons, since coronary artery surgery should be performed at the time of aortic valve replacement. (See Chap. 108.)

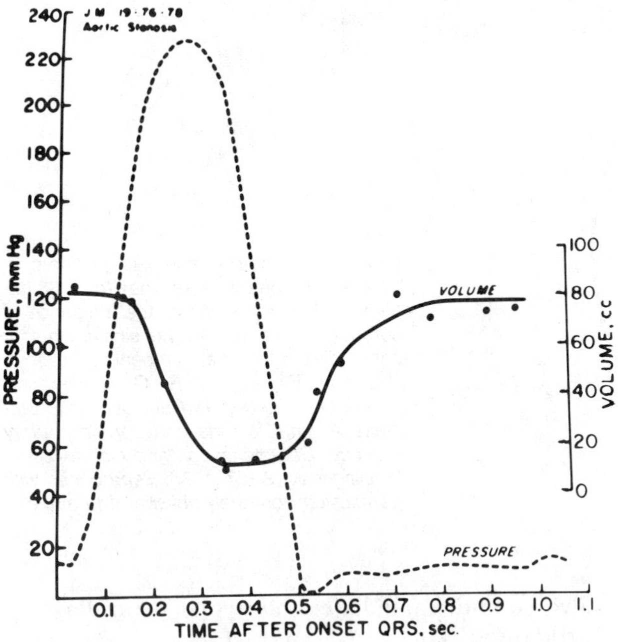

FIGURE 37-6 Left ventricular pressure and volume in compensated aortic stenosis. The end-diastolic volume is normal, the ejection fraction slightly higher than normal, and left ventricular mass significantly increased. These measurements indicate concentric hypertrophy of the ventricle in response to a pressure overload. End-diastolic volume (EDV) = 78; end-systolic volume (ESV) = 13; stroke volume (SV) = 65; ejection fraction (EF) = 65/78 = 0.83; left ventricular weight (LVwt) = 270; left ventricular end-diastolic pressure (LVedp) = 13. [*From C. E. Rackley and W. P. Hood, Jr., Measurements of Ventricular Volume, Mass and Ejection Fraction, in W. Grossman (ed.), "Cardiac Catheterization and Angiography," Lea & Febiger, Philadelphia. Reproduced with permission of the publisher and author.*]

FIGURE 37-7 Left ventricular pressure and volume in decompensated aortic stenosis. The stroke volume has remained normal, but end-diastolic and end-systolic volumes are significantly increased with a reduced ejection fraction. End-diastolic pressure is elevated, and there is a marked increase in left ventricular mass. EDV = 238; ESV = 163; SV = 75; EF = 75/238 = 0.31; LVwt = 557; LVedp = 34. [*From C. E. Rackley and W. P. Hood, Jr., Aortic Valve Disease, in H. J. Levine (ed.), "Clinical Cardiovascular Physiology," Grune & Stratton, Inc., New York, 1976. Reproduced with permission from the publisher and author.*]

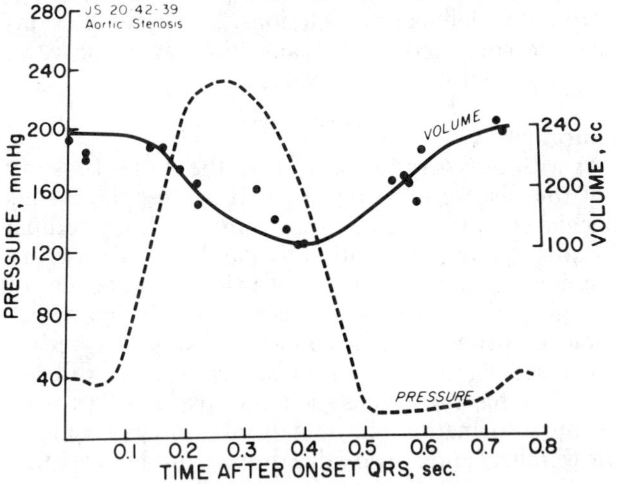

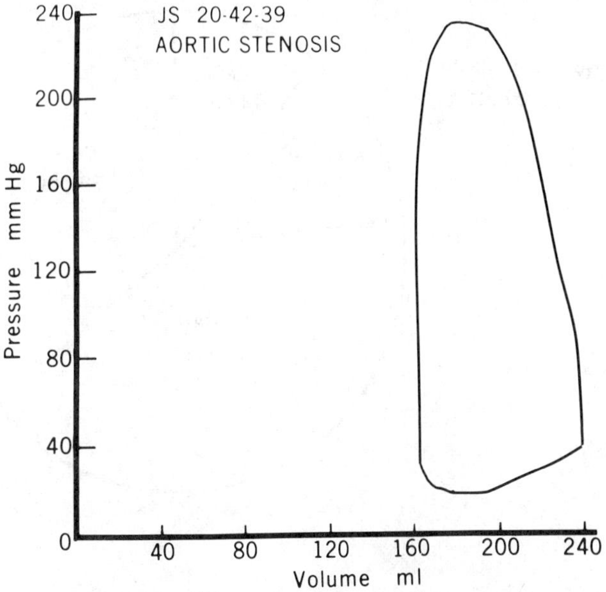

FIGURE 37-8 Left ventricular pressure-volume diagram in decompensated aortic stenosis. The systolic pressure remains abnormally elevated, but left ventricular stroke volume is maintained by abnormal increases in end-diastolic and end-systolic volume. The left ventricular end-diastolic pressure is also abnormally elevated. [*From C. E. Rackley and W. P. Hood, Jr., Aortic Valve Disease, in H. J. Levine (ed.), "Clinical Cardiovascular Physiology," Grune & Stratton, Inc., New York, 1976. Reproduced with permission from the publisher and author.*]

Radionuclide Studies Radionuclide scans can be used to assess ventricular function and myocardial perfusion in aortic stenosis.[51] Left ventricular ejection fraction at rest and during exertion may reveal deterioration of left ventricular function before clinical symptoms have developed. Impaired radioisotope myocardial perfusion may raise the possibility of underlying coronary artery disease in addition to aortic valve stenosis. (See Chap. 109.)

Exercise Studies Under carefully monitored conditions, the exercise test can be combined with the radionuclide studies to assess ventricular function as well as the clinical response.[51] However, exercise should be performed with caution, particularly in those patients with a history of syncope.

Natural History and Prognosis

The incidence of bicuspid aortic valve has been estimated at 4 out of 1000 live births with a 4-to-1 predominance of males to females.[4] Leaflets may thicken by age 40 and almost invariably by age 50, with calcium deposits rarely detected before 40 years of age. Although symptoms generally occur late in the course of aortic stenosis, 3 to 5 percent of patients may be subject to sudden death during the asymptomatic period, presumably due to an arrhythmia.[26,52] Any symptom of angina pectoris, syncope, or heart failure heralds a significant reduction in life expectancy. Adults with aortic stenosis have an average mortality of 9 percent per year. In one

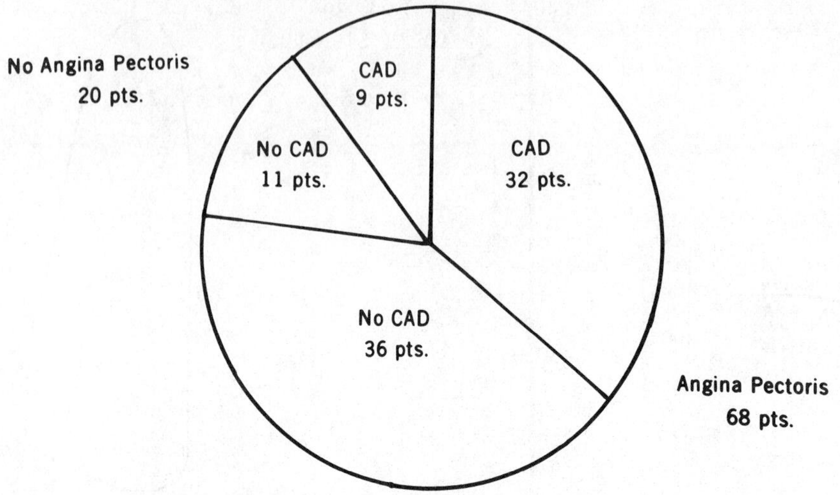

FIGURE 37-9 Aortic stenosis, angina pectoris, and coronary artery disease. In 88 patients with aortic stenosis the incidence of coronary artery disease was similar whether chest discomfort was present or absent. *(From R. E. Moraski, R. O. Russell, Jr., J. A. Mantle, and C. E. Rackley, Aortic Stenosis, Angina Pectoris, and Coronary Artery Disease, Catheterization and Cardiovascular Diagnosis, 2:157, 1976. Reproduced with permission from the publisher and author.)*

large series, the average age at clinical presentation was 48 years, whereas the average age at death was 63 years.[53] Once the patient has developed symptoms, survival is often less than 5 years, and the incidence of sudden death in symptomatic patients increases to 15 to 20 percent.[54] Exertional chest pain is associated with an average life expectancy of 5 years, and less than 5 percent of patients survive 10 to 20 years.[27] The prognosis after syncope is usually 3 to 4 years and patients generally survive less than 2 years after left ventricular failure develops.[26,36] Aortic stenosis progresses more rapidly in patients with a degenerative etiology than in those with congenital or rheumatic disease.[55] Thus, symptoms in aortic stenosis carry a much worse long-term prognosis than any other lesion affecting the aortic or mitral valve.

Treatment

Medical

The medical management of aortic stenosis prior to development of symptoms is generally prophylactic to prevent bacterial endocarditis, with elective dental and surgical procedures as described in detail in the mitral stenosis section (see Chap. 56). In patients with aortic and mitral involvement, rheumatic prophylaxis should be continued until age 35 years. With exertional chest pain, nitrates should be used with extreme caution and patients fully informed about orthostatic hypotension and possible syncope. Although digitalis and diuretics are indicated in left ventricular failure, the mechanical obstruction will not be altered by medical therapy, and surgical replacement of the valve is indicated.

Physicians should appreciate that depression of the contractile state and reduction of the cardiac output will diminish the intensity of the systolic murmur. Rarely, the patient with aortic stenosis may present in advanced heart failure or cardiogenic shock without an audible systolic murmur. Fluoroscopic detection of calcium in the area of the aortic valve should immediately alert one to underlying aortic stenosis.

Although criteria for early valve replacement in the asymptomatic patient have not been delineated, echocardiography and radionuclide angiography can provide data on ventricular dimensions and function, in addition to the standard radiographic estimates of heart size. Heart size in aortic stenosis may not increase until significant depression of the left ventricle has developed. The increased incidence of sudden death after development of symptoms, as well as the increased operative mortality with myocardial failure, emphasizes the need for the physician to proceed with surgery early in the patient's course.

In preparation for aortic valve replacement, elective surgery or dental work should be completed to reduce the postoperative incidence of endocarditis. Electrolyte abnormalities should be corrected if the patients have been on diuretics. In elderly patients with calcific aortic stenosis, radiation of the murmur into the carotid vessels may sometimes *obscure underlying carotid vascular lesions.* Therefore, noninvasive studies to detect disparity in carotid flow should be performed and if necessary, carotid arteriography for delineation of lesions. The carotid lesions can be corrected at the same time as aortic valve replacement if such is needed.

Surgical

As with any surgical procedure the natural history of the disease must be weighed against the results achieved by surgical intervention. Longitudinal studies of patients with valvular heart disease are limited to studies carried out prior to the advent of surgery for valve replacement and in many instances prior to the availability of objective means of assessing the degree of severity of the disease. Natural history studies such as Rapaport's[56] provide some information on the natural history of patients with mitral and aortic valve disease and indicate that patients with aortic stenosis have the poorest prognosis. Approximately 50 percent of patients diagnosed clinically as having severe stenosis with or without symptoms will die within 5 years of the time of diagnosis. If only those patients who are symptomatic are considered, the prognosis is much worse. The majority of patients with aortic stenosis develop symptoms of congestive failure, angina, or syncope. Angina may result from inadequate blood supply to hypertrophied myocardium with or without the presence of coronary artery disease. Exertional syncope is probably secondary to cerebral ischemia. Sudden death, usually due to arrhythmia, may occur in 3 to 5 percent of asymptomatic patients and a significantly higher percentage of symptomatic patients.[26,52]

Aortic stenosis, being a ventricular pressure-overload condition as opposed to aortic regurgitation, which is a volume-overload condition, usually results in well-maintained ventricular function except in far advanced situations, thus allowing for significant improvement in the patient's clinical status and longevity following surgery.

Indications for Operation Patients with congestive heart failure, angina, or exertional syncope in the presence of significant aortic valvular stenosis should undergo aortic valve replacement promptly. Asymptomatic patients with significant aortic valvular stenosis should be advised to have surgery. Although clinical assessment, including the presence of left ventricular hypertrophy and strain on the electrocardiogram will allow for identification of most patients with severe aortic valvular stenosis, certain patients may be missed by clinical assessment alone. For this reason we prefer that patients with suspected aortic stenosis undergo cardiac catheterization to assess the severity of obstruction as well as to define the coronary anatomy. The pressure gradient between the left ventricle and aorta and the cardiac output allow determination of the peak systolic pressure gradient as well as the valve orifice area. We rely mainly on the peak-to-peak systolic pressure gradient as the major determinant of the severity of obstruction, recognizing that in the presence of low cardiac output a low gradient may not reflect the severity of obstruction. Patients with a peak systolic gradient greater than about 50 mmHg are considered to have severe aortic valvular stenosis. If significant lesions are found in the coronary arteries, these should be bypassed at the time of valve replacement.

Operation In young patients with congenital aortic valvular stenosis a commissurotomy will usually relieve obstruction, but it is likely that most of these patients will ultimately require valvular replacement. In rare instances, relief of obstruction in patients with acquired aortic stenosis can be achieved by commissurotomy and calcium debridement; however, in most, valve replacement is required.

Two general types of valve replacements are available; namely, a mechanical prosthesis and a tissue prosthesis. There are several kinds of mechanical prostheses, such as the ball valve (Starr-Edwards), the tilting disk (Bjork-Shiley or Lillihi-Caster), and the central flow disk (St. Jude). There are also several tissue prostheses, including preserved homographs[57,58] and stent-mounted porcine heterographs (Hancock and Carpentier-Edwards). The primary advantage of the mechanical prosthesis is durability, whereas the disadvantage is a requirement that patients be on anticoagulant therapy to reduce the risk of thromboembolic complications. The advantage of the tissue prosthesis is a very low risk of thromboembolic complications without anticoagulant therapy; however, there is a tendency for tissue valves to degenerate, thus causing concern regarding durability.[59,60] This degenerative process appears to occur more rapidly in younger patients.[61] Certain other minor differences exist between the two general types of valves and specific valves of each type, but these have not been sufficient to establish clear superiority of any one valve or valve type.

The operation is performed through a median sternotomy incision utilizing cardiopulmonary bypass. Most surgeons vent the left heart by a vent introduced into the left atrium or left ventricle via the right superior pulmonary vein. Moderate hypothermia is employed, and the heart is further cooled and arrested by local external cooling and perfusion of the coronary arteries with cold cardioplegic solution. The aorta is cross-clamped and opened. The valve is excised and calcium carefully debrided from the valve ring. The prosthetic valve is then sutured in place (Fig. 37-10). The aortotomy is closed, being careful to evacuate all air from the heart before completing the closure. The aortic cross-clamp is then released while suction is applied to a vent in the ascending aorta as a further precaution against air embolus. When normothermia is achieved, extracorporeal circulation is terminated and the operation completed. When concomitant coronary artery bypass is done, the distal graft anastomoses are performed prior to valve replacement so that cold cardioplegic solution can be infused via the grafts distal to the areas of coronary artery obstruction. The proximal graft anastomoses are then performed after replacing the valve. (See Chaps. 131 and 132.)

Postoperative Management

Patients are kept in the intensive care unit 24 to 28 h postoperatively where arterial pressure, the left atrial pressure via a small catheter placed through the pulmonary vein at the time of operation, and cardiac rhythm are monitored. Hypertension, which is frequently present, is treated by nitroprusside infusion. Serum potassium is maintained at a level of about 4 meq/liter, and ventricular arrhythmias are treated by lidocaine infusion. When the cardiac rate is low, atrial pacing via small-wire epicardial electrodes placed at the time of surgery is initiated to augment cardiac output and may also be employed

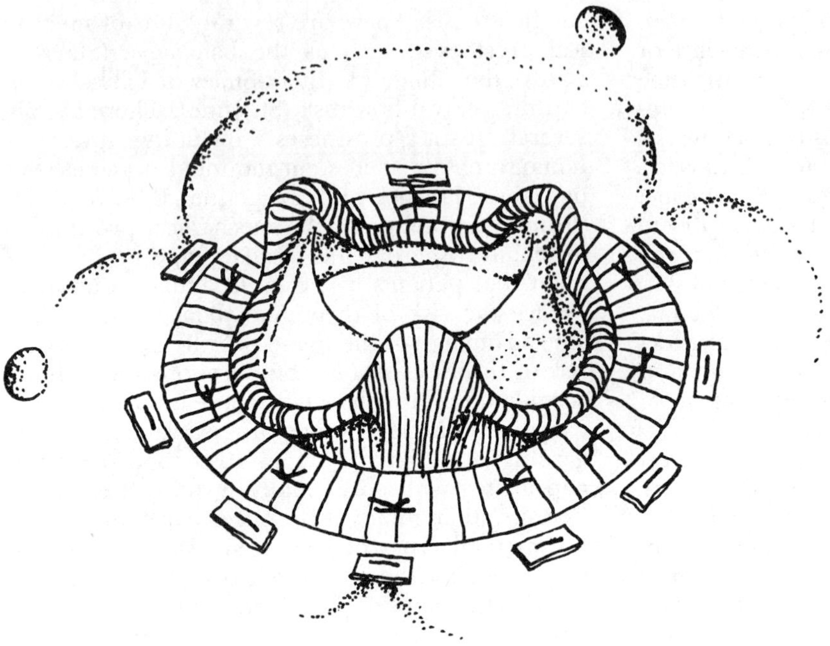

FIGURE 37-10 Technique for insertion of aortic xenograft using interrupted pledgeted mattress sutures. (*Courtesy of Dr. Robert Karp.*)

to suppress ventricular ectopy in patients with a slow heart rate. Prophylactic antibiotics which are started preoperatively are discontinued the third postoperative day. All patients were started on Coumadin (see Chap. 95) to rapidly achieve a prothrombin deficiency approximately two times normal. Generally, Coumadin is discontinued after 6 weeks in patients with tissue prostheses, but continued indefinitely in patients with mechanical prostheses. Dipyridamole (see Chap. 95) combined with Coumadin has been shown to decrease the incidence of thromboembolic complications compared to patients in whom Coumadin alone is used, and thus dipyridamole is started preoperatively and continued in patients with mechanical prostheses.[62] Digitalization is generally carried out only for the treatment of supraventricular arrhythmias. Following dismissal from the intensive care unit, the cardiac rhythm is monitored an additional 2 to 3 days. If significant ventricular ectopy is noted, antiarrhythmic therapy is initiated and maintained for approximately 6 weeks. Prophylactic antibiotics (see Chap. 56) are indicated during periods of increased susceptibility to bacteremia in all patients with any type of prosthetic valve. Patients with an uncomplicated postoperative course are usually discharged from the hospital 6 to 8 days following operation.

Early Results The current operative mortality for primary isolated aortic valve replacement is less than 3 to 4 percent in most centers and is most closely related to the degree of left ventricular failure, most deaths occurring in patients with end-stage disease. Concomitant coronary artery bypass has not been shown to have a significant influence on early mortality,[63] nor has sufficient data accumulated to determine an absolute effect on late mortality. It seems reasonable and advisable that in the presence of critical coronary artery stenosis that coronary artery bypass be performed at the time of aortic valve replacement in anticipation that further experience will show a beneficial effect.

Late Results The late results of patients surviving aortic valve replacement are generally satisfactory. Actuarial survival at 5 years with various types of valve prostheses is approximately 80 percent[64] (Fig. 37-11). Left ventricular dysfunction is a significant determinant of late results[65] (Fig. 37-12). Late deaths are most commonly due to heart failure, thromboembolism, myocardial infarction, and cardiac arrhythmia. Late complications are more closely re-

FIGURE 37-11 Actuarial survival for operative survivors with several current aortic prostheses. (*From Q. McManus, G. L. Grunkemeier, L. E. Lambert, J. F. Teply, B. J. Harland, and A. Starr, Year of Operation as a Risk Factor in the Late Results of Valve Replacement, J. Thorac. Cardiovasc. Surg., 80:834–840, 1980. Reproduced with permission from the publisher and author.*)

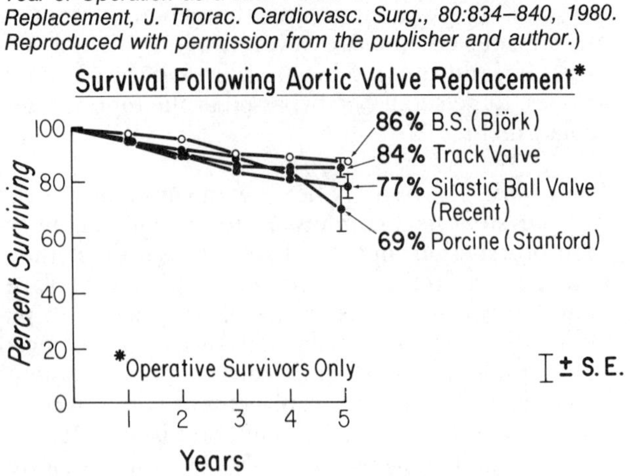

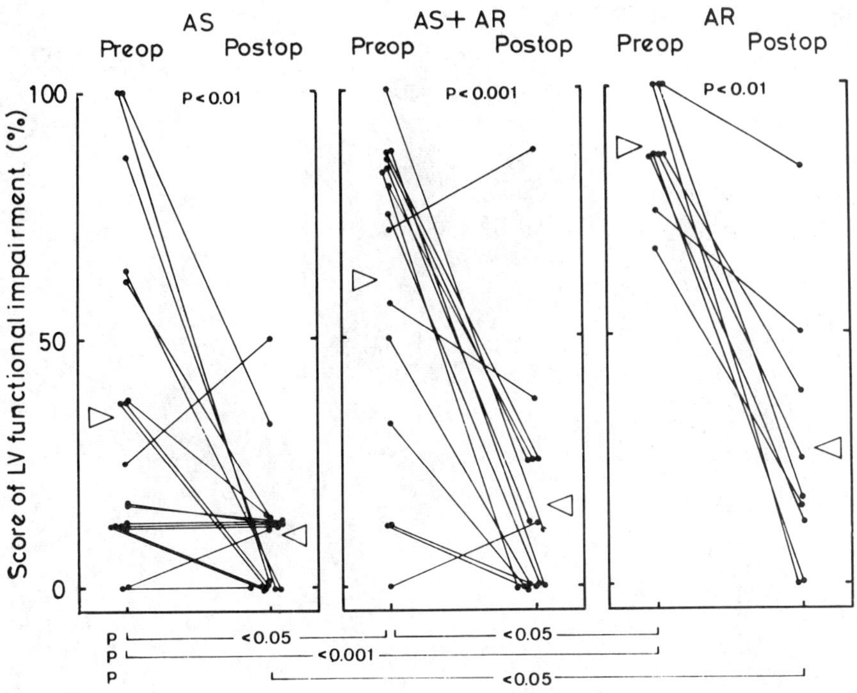

FIGURE 37-12 Change in multiple parameters of left ventricular impairment after aortic valve replacement in patients with aortic stenosis, mixed lesion, and aortic incompetence. *(From H. P. Krayenbuehl, M. Lurina, O. Hess, M. Rothlin, and A. Senning, Pre- and Postoperative Left Ventricular Contractile Function in Patients with Aortic Valve Disease, Br. Heart J., 41:204, 1979. Reproduced with permission from the publisher and author.)*

lated to the type of prosthesis used; mechanical prostheses being associated with a 2 to 3 percent per year incidence of thromboembolic complications, and tissue prostheses associated with valve failure requiring reoperation in approximately 20 percent of patients within 8 years.[60] Tissue valve degeneration is time-related, and thus the incidence will progressively increase with increasing time. Patients surviving aortic valve replacement with good left ventricular function experience good symptomatic results.

Cost Analysis

The excellent clinical results in patients having aortic valve replacement prior to the development of left ventricular dysfunction suggest that patients should be operated on before left ventricular dysfunction occurs. This has to be balanced against the mortality and morbidity associated with currently available prostheses. Currently available technology, such as echocardiography and radionuclide scanning, provides means of assessing left ventricular function and should provide assistance in determining the optimal time for intervention in patients with aortic valve disease, providing the maximum in longevity and productivity and the minimum in continuing medical costs.

Aortic Regurgitation

But when the semilunar valves, from any of the causes enumerated, became incapable of closing the mouth of the ventricle, a portion of the blood just sent into the aorta greater or less, according to the degree of the inadequacy of the valves turns back into the ventricle.

D. J. Corrigan, 1832[66]

Etiology

Although aortic regurgitation has been a long-recognized valvular mechanism for disturbed cardiac function, a gradual change has occurred in the incidence of diseases that affect the competence of the aortic valve. In decades past, rheumatic fever and syphilis were major causes of aortic regurgitation, but the incidence of these diseases has diminished in recent years.[67–69] With the decline in these two infectious conditions, connective tissue diseases and anatomic abnormalities of the aortic valve have increased. Marfan's syndrome can produce aortic dilatation with incompetence of the valve, and myxomatous transformation of the aortic valve may be a predisposing abnormality.[70] Osteogenesis imperfecta, ankylosing spondylitis, Reiter's syndrome, and even rheumatoid arthritis can produce aortic regurgitation.[71–74] A congenital defect in the ventricular septum with a sinus of Valsalva aneurysm can result in aortic regurgitation.[75] Chronic vascular disorders such as hypertension and arteriosclerosis can create mild incompetence of the aortic valve.[76] (See Table 37-1.)

Acute disturbances of a normal or diseased aortic valve can produce sudden aortic regurgitation. Dissection of the aorta, bacterial endocarditis, and acute rheumatic fever can create sudden regurgitation across the aortic valve.[77,78] Aortic dissection can distort the annulus of the aortic valve, bacterial endocarditis can perforate the leaflet or cause paravalvular incompetence, and acute rheumatic fever can lead to eversion of the aortic cusp.

Pathology

Aortic insufficiency results either from intrinsic disease of the cusps or from primary diseases of the

TABLE 37-1 Etiology of Chronic and Acute Aortic Regurgitation*

- Chronic aortic regurgitation
  - Rheumatic
  - Syphilis
  - Aortitis (Takayasu)
  - Heritable disorders of connective tissue
    - Marfan's syndrome
    - Ehlers-Danlos syndrome
    - Osteogenesis imperfecta
  - Congenital heart disease
    - Bicuspid aortic valve
    - Interventricular septal defect
    - Sinus of Valsalva aneurysm
  - Arthritic diseases
    - Ankylosing spondylitis
    - Reiter's syndrome
    - Rheumatoid arthritis
    - Lupus erythematosis
  - Cystic medial necrosis of aorta
  - Hypertension
  - Arteriosclerosis
  - Myxomatous degeneration of valve
  - Infective endocarditis
  - Following prosthetic valve surgery
  - Associated with aortic stenosis
- Acute aortic regurgitation
  - Rheumatic fever
  - Infective endocarditis
  - Congenital (rupture of sinus of Valsalva)
  - Acute aortic dissection
  - Following prosthetic valve surgery
  - Trauma

*Please note that certain disorders are capable of producing acute and chronic aortic regurgitation.

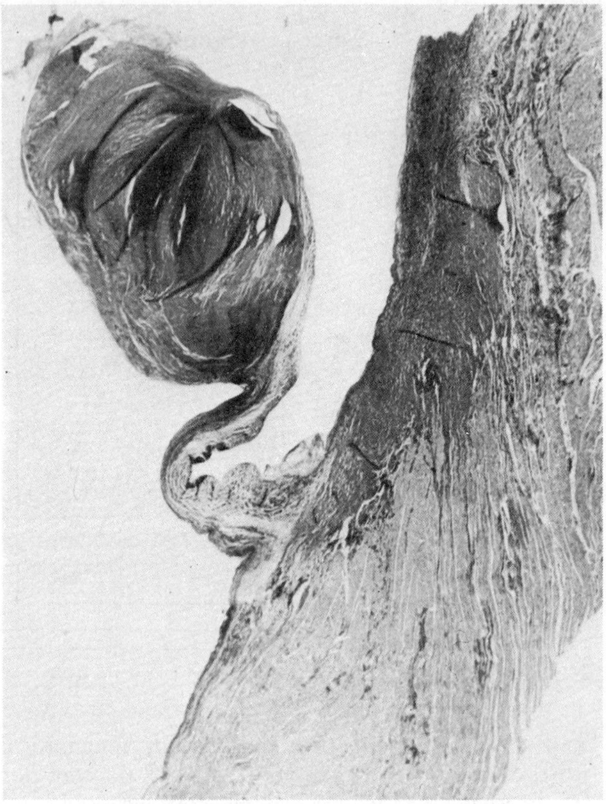

FIGURE 37-13 Low-power photomicrograph of an aortic cusp in chronic rheumatic aortic insufficiency. The distal one-half of the cusp is grossly thickened by fibrous tissue. Elastic tissue stain; ×5.

ascending aorta. Additionally, shunts originating in the aorta may simulate aortic insufficiency.

Intrinsic Disease of Aortic Valve

Aortic regurgitation from acquired intrinsic diseases of the valve is most commonly of rheumatic or of bacterial inflammatory origin. Less common changes are those associated with rheumatoid arthritis, lupus erythematosus, and trauma.[79] The principal congenital disease is the congenital bicuspid aortic valve. In arachnodactyly, wherein the primary basis for aortic insufficiency usually is in the aorta, there may be an intrinsically prolapsed condition of the aortic cusps.

Rheumatic Disease

Rheumatic diseases of the aortic valve may cause pure aortic incompetence or incompetence may be associated with some degree of stenosis (see section on aortic stenosis). Pure aortic insufficiency of rheumatic origin results from fibrosis and contracture of the cusps.[76] The cusps become shorter than normal (Fig. 37-13). This may be of equal severity among the cusps or unequal so that one cusp undergoes greater contracture than the other two. The result is a malalignment of the cusps, allowing for incompetence of the valve. In pure rheumatic aortic incompetence, commissural fusion is either absent or minimal. If contracture is coupled with fusion of two or three commissures, the effect is a combination of aortic stenosis and insufficiency.

Ankylosing Spondylitis

Aortic regurgitation may occur in patients with ankylosing spondylitis.[79a] Patients with this condition may also develop complete heart block.

Infective Endocarditis

Infective endocarditis of the aortic valve may involve a tricuspid aortic valve, but often the valve is bicuspid, either congenitally or acquired. The usual basis for incompetence is destruction of cusp tissue (Fig. 37-14). There may either be perforation of one or more cusps or detachment of a cusp at its aortic attachment. Atrioventricular conduction defects may be associated with aortic insufficiency caused by infective endocarditis as the infectious process extends to the nearby conduction tissue.[80]

Trauma

Deceleration external blunt trauma may cause rupture of a cusp, but only rarely.[81] The usual basis for post-traumatic aortic insufficiency is a laceration of the aorta (see below).

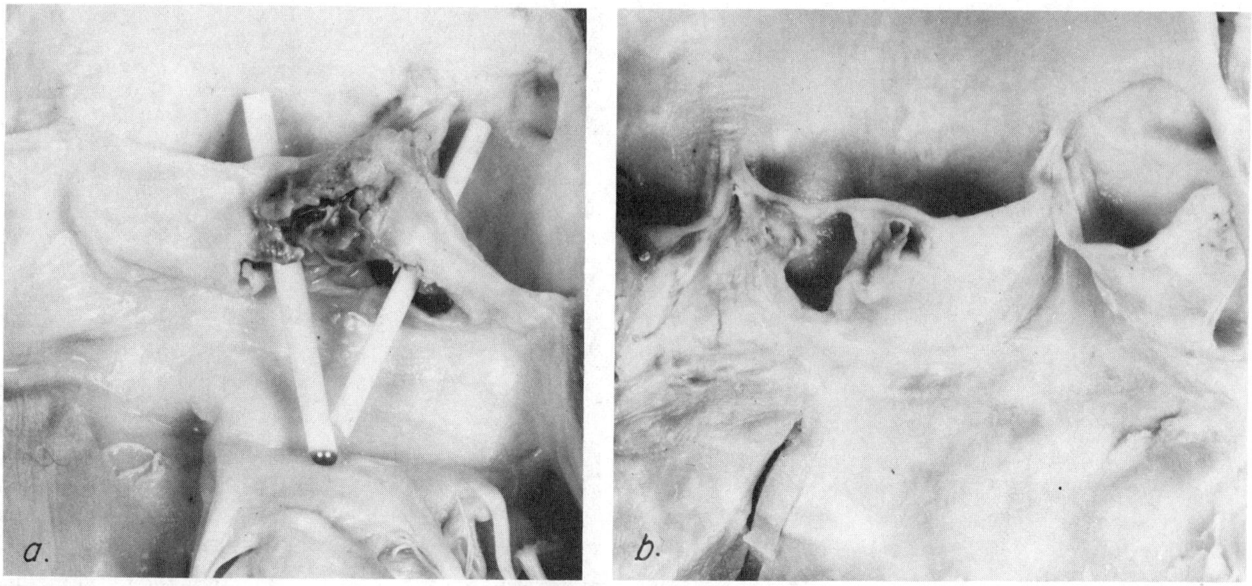

FIGURE 37-14 Bacterial endocarditis. *a.* Each of two cusps of the aortic valve shows perforation (probes) as part of active bacterial endocarditis. *b.* Perforation in an aortic cusp as a manifestation of bacteriologically healed bacterial endocarditis. (*From J. E. Edwards, Lesions Causing or Simulating Aortic Insufficiency, Cardiovasc. Clin., 5:128, 1973. Reproduced with permission from the publisher and author.*)

Congenital Anomalies

There are two principal causes of aortic regurgitation associated with congenital disease, namely congenital bicuspid aortic valve and ventricular septal defect. Fenestration of aortic cusps, while common, is a rare cause of aortic regurgitation.[82] Myxomatous change may also be a cause of aortic incompetence.

In the congenital bicuspid aortic valve with aortic regurgitation the larger cusp is redundant and prolapsed beyond the opposite cusp. Usually, aortic regurgitation due to a congenital bicuspid valve is not apparent until early adult life. In an uncommon type of congenital bicuspid valve the raphe is represented by a thin strand of tissue running from near the free aspect of the larger cusp, on one hand, to the aortic wall, on the other. Rupture of the strand causes the larger cusp to lose much of its support so that it prolapses. This may account for the sudden appearance of major aortic regurgitation.[83]

In aortic regurgitation associated with ventricular septal defect, the defect is closely related to the aortic root and valve. More commonly, the defect is of the supracristal type; it is less commonly infracristal.[84] The cause of the aortic incompetence appears to be an inadequate attachment of the aortic root to the cardiac skeleton. The aorta deviates to the right and the related cusp or cusps (usually the right, less commonly the left) are carried laterally with the displaced aorta and "tip." The result is malalignment of the cusps.

Myxomatous alteration of the aortic cusps ("floppy aortic valve") is usually associated with extensive cystic medial necrosis of the aorta. If aortic regurgitation is present, its cause lies principally in the aorta. Nevertheless, an element of prolapse of a cusp may be the only cause or a contributing one.

Primary Disease of Ascending Aorta

Primary disease of the aorta leading to aortic valvular regurgitation takes the form either of dilatation or laceration of the vessel.

Primary Dilatation Dilatation of the ascending aorta creates tension upon the individual cusps, causing them to be relatively short for closure of the dilated aortic root. One cause of this condition is aortitis, of which syphilitic aortitis is the classic example (Fig. 37-15).[85] Aortic changes associated with rheumatoid spondylitis[86] yield a similar picture, as do various types of aortitis of unknown etiology. In rheumatoid arthritis, the root of the aortic may be affected, and inflammatory and fibrotic changes of the valve cusps may also be associated.[72] Unusually, in a person of advanced age the natural process of aortic dilatation with age may be of such proportion as to be responsible for aortic incompetence.

Extensive cystic medial necrosis of the aorta, either of the idiopathic type or associated with Marfan's syndrome, even in the absence of laceration of the aorta, is another cause of aortic regurgitation (Fig. 37-16). In this condition a contributing factor to aortic regurgitation may be the intrinsic changes of the cusps that allow the cusps to prolapse (Fig. 37-17) or, rarely, rupture.[70]

Laceration of the Aorta Laceration of the ascending aorta may complicate hypertension, extensive cystic medial necrosis, external blunt trauma, or, uncommonly, aortitis. It may be a localized process or lead to dissecting aneurysm.[87] If the primary laceration occurs near a commissural attachment of two cusps, the secondary retraction of aortic tissue causes prolapse of the cusps at the related commissure[83] (Fig. 37-18*A* and 37-18*B*). The consequent malalignment

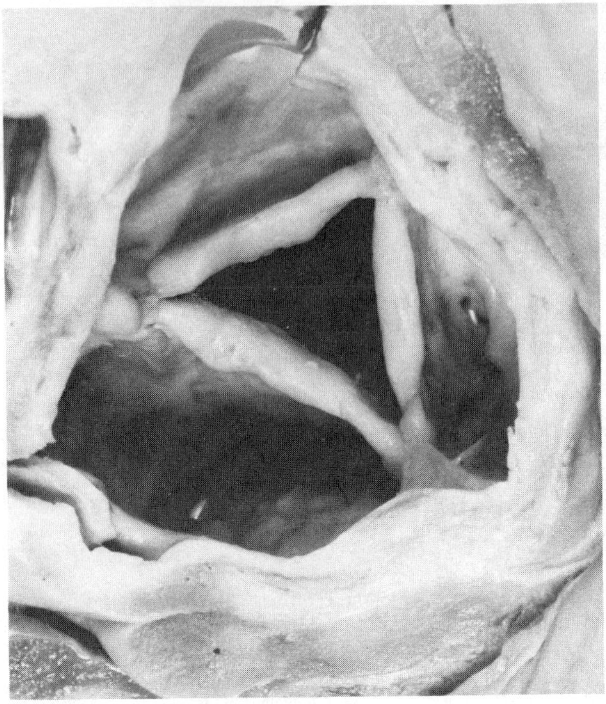

FIGURE 37-15 Aortic valve viewed from above in aortitis. Bowing of the cusps incident to dilatation of the aorta leaves a triangular defect through which regurgitation occurs. The commissures are not fused.

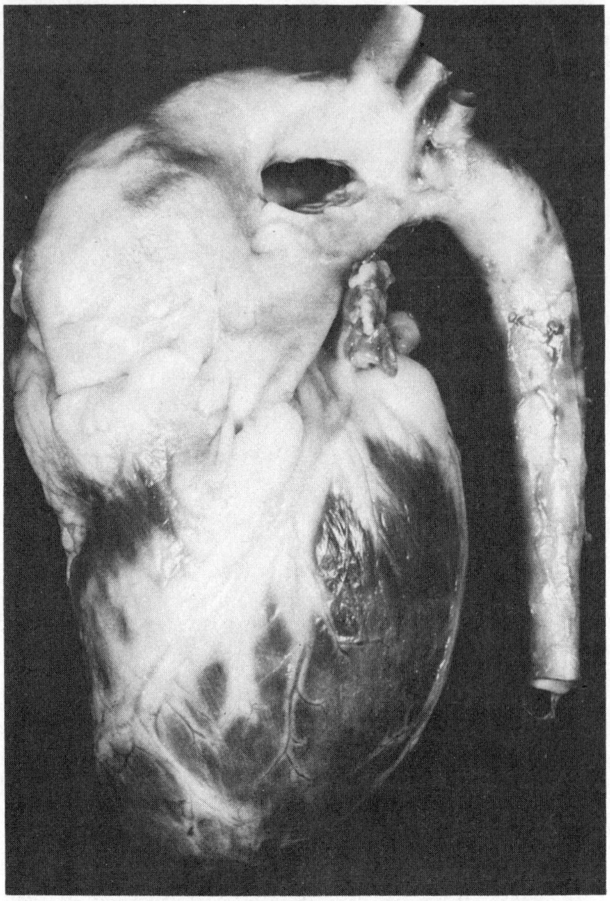

FIGURE 37-16 Cystic medial necrosis of aorta in Marfan's syndrome. Exterior view of heart and aorta viewed from the left side. Marked dilatation of the ascending aorta. (*From J. E. Edwards, Lesions Causing or Simulating Aortic Insufficiency, Cardiovasc. Clin., 5:128, 1973. Reproduced with permission from the publisher and author.*)

of the cusps underlies the appearance of aortic insufficiency, which may appear suddenly.

In some cases of aortic laceration, the laceration lies below the upper aspect of a commissure and there is, additionally, the chance of tearing related cusps by retraction of the edges of the laceration[88] (Fig. 37-18*C*). Abnormal escape of blood from the aorta as occurs in various types of shunts may simulate aortic insufficiency, even though the valve is normal.[88]

Abnormal Physiology

The diastolic flow (aortic regurgitation) across the incompetent aortic valve increases filling of the left ventricle and imposes a volume overload on the myocardium. The size of the regurgitant area, the diastolic pressure gradient across the valve, and the duration of systole influence the regurgitant volume (Fig. 37-19).[89,90] The magnitude of the volume overload depends on the chronicity and the severity of the incompetence and even a small incompetent area of the valve can eventually lead to significant aortic regurgitation over a period of time.[91]

Chronic aortic regurgitation causes a gradual increase in the end-diastolic volume of the left ventricle, since filling of the chamber derives from both the left atrium and the aorta. Total left ventricular stroke volume is increased to maintain the forward or effective stroke volume to the systemic circulation. The increased end-diastolic volume, or compensatory dilatation of the left ventricle, is accompanied by minimal elevation in the left ventricular end-diastolic pressure.[24] The diastolic compliance of the volume-overloaded left ventricle is increased due to slippage of myocardial fibers and other mechanisms such as stress relaxation and creep.[92] Forces within the ventricular wall are maintained within the normal range by a compensatory increase in wall thickness and left ventricular mass, or hypertrophy.[22] Compensatory left ventricular hypertrophy normalizes systolic wall stress or afterload.[21]

During the early stage of chronic aortic regurgitation, the increase in left ventricular stroke volume maintains a normal forward cardiac output during rest and exercise. The ratio of the left ventricular stroke volume to the end-diastolic volume or the ejection fraction remains within or near the normal range. In the late stage of chronic aortic regurgitation, primary myocardial factors or secondary lesions such as underlying coronary artery disease can depress the contractile state of the ventricular myocardium and produce an increase in end-systolic volume with a decline in ejection fraction (Fig. 37-20). During this phase, left ventricular end-diastolic

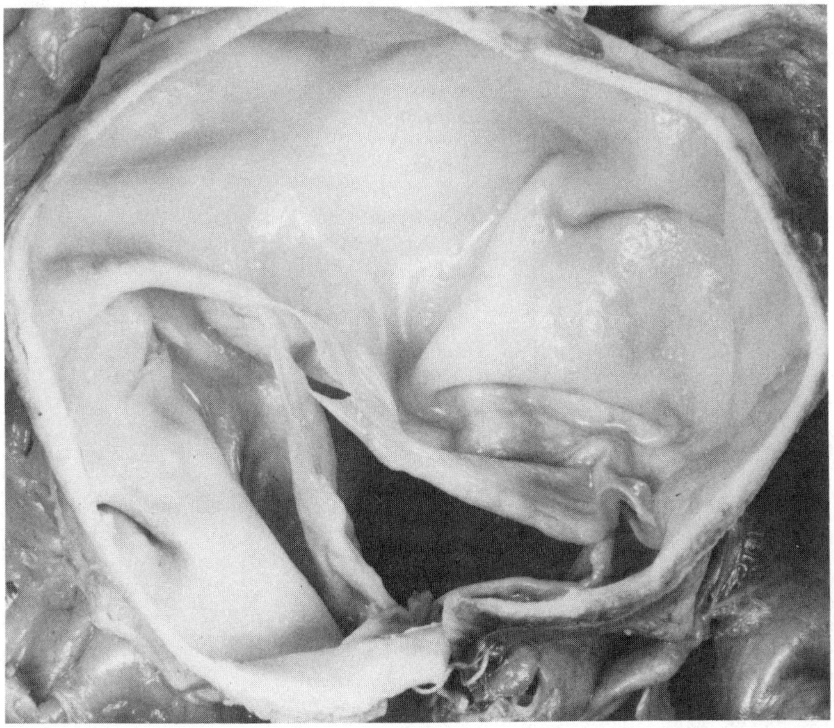

FIGURE 37-17 Interior of ascending aorta and aortic valve viewed from above in a case with extensive cystic medial necrosis of the aorta. Marked dilatation of aorta. The aortic cusps have been stretched and also show some features of prolapse. (*From J. E. Edwards, Lesions Causing or Simulating Aortic Insufficiency, Cardiovasc. Clin., 5:128, 1973. Reproduced with permission from the publisher and author.*)

pressure will increase as the compliant properties or elasticity of the ventricle further diminish. The increased end-systolic volume and decrease in diastolic compliance elevate left atrial pressure and eventually create pulmonary venous hypertension. When appropriate increases in systolic wall thickness fail to accompany further dilatation of the left ventricular chamber, systolic wall stress will rise abnormally.[21]

The hemodynamic changes of acute aortic regurgitation differ from the chronic condition if damage to the aortic apparatus occurs on a previously normal aortic valve. Under these circumstances, the regurgitation and volume overload will be suddenly imposed on a left ventricular chamber, which is unable to dilate acutely and adapt to the increased diastolic filling. Acute left ventricular dilatation is limited by the thickness of the ventricular myocardium. Thus, marked elevation in left ventricular end-diastolic pressure and minimal ventricular dilatation accompany acute aortic regurgitation. Left ventricular end-diastolic pressure may

FIGURE 37-18 Diagrammatic portrayal of consequences of laceration of the aorta in relation to an aortic commissure. *A.* Laceration without dissecting aneurysm. Retraction of the edges of the laceration allows for commissural prolapse and aortic incompetence. *B.* The process shown in *A* with regard to the aortic valve is the same, but there is the additional feature of classical dissecting aneurysm. *C.* Laceration of the aorta has been at a level just below the upper level of the commissure causing attenuation of one aortic cusp and rupture of the other. (*From J. E. Edwards, Pathology of Acquired Valvular Disease of the Heart, Semin. Roentgenol., 14:96–115, 1979. Reproduced with permission from the publisher and author.*)

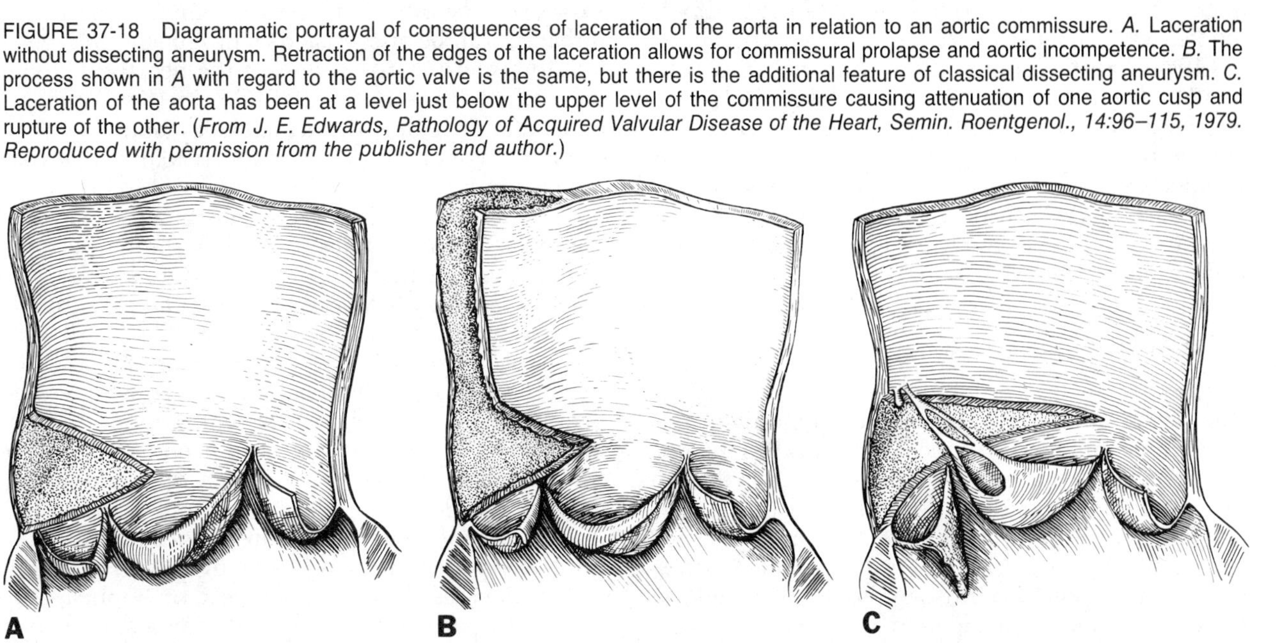

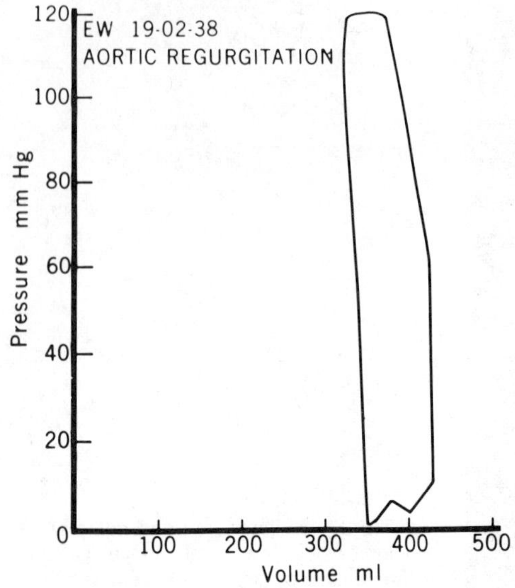

FIGURE 37-19 Left ventricular pressure-volume diagram in decompensated aortic regurgitation. The abnormal features of the loop are extreme displacement to the right due to an increase in end-diastolic volume and increased end-systolic volume indicative of depression of myocardial contractility. The isovolumic relaxation phase on the left-hand side of the pressure-volume loop is shortened due to early diastolic filling of the left ventricle from the aorta. The end-diastolic pressure is also abnormally elevated. [*From C. E. Rackley and W. P. Hood, Jr., Aortic Valve Disease, in H. J. Levine (ed.), "Clinical Cardiovascular Physiology," Grune & Stratton, Inc., New York, 1976. Reproduced with permission from the publisher and author.*]

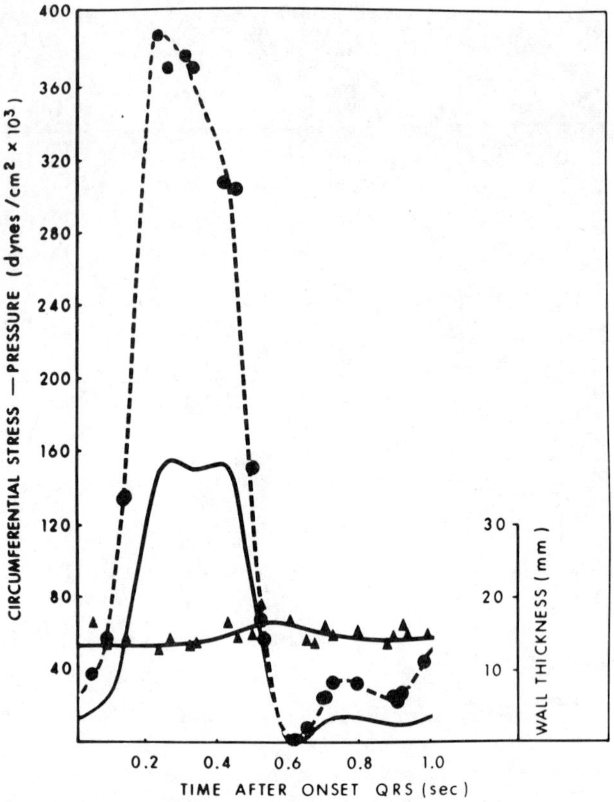

FIGURE 37-20 Left ventricular pressure, wall stress, and wall thickness in decompensated aortic regurgitation. Although the diastolic wall thickness is increased, there is a marked decrease in systolic wall thickening. This results in sustained elevation of the systolic wall stress, even though the left ventricular systolic pressure remains within the normal range. (———, stress; – · –, pressure; ▲ —— ▲, wall thickness.) [*From C. E. Rackley and W. P. Hood, Jr., Aortic Valve Disease, in H. J. Levine (ed.), "Clinical Cardiovascular Physiology," Grune & Stratton, Inc., New York, 1976. Reproduced with permission from the publisher and author.*]

approach, or even exceed, left atrial pressure and prematurely close the mitral valve. These sudden hemodynamic changes lead to pulmonary venous hypertension and acute pulmonary edema. If acute regurgitation is superimposed on a chronically diseased and incompetent aortic valve, the hemodynamic alterations will depend on the extent of preexisting left ventricular dilatation and subsequent changes in the end-diastolic pressure and pulmonary capillary pressure.

Chronic aortic regurgitation with severe left ventricular dilatation can result in the largest left ventricular stroke volume of any diseases affecting the left ventricle.[93] The largest left ventricular stroke volume will increase the mechanical pressure-volume work of the ventricle and together with compensatory hypertrophy will significantly increase myocardial oxygen consumption.[31]

Clinical Manifestations

History

The slowly developing aortic regurgitation and the attendant compensatory mechanisms of the left ventricle enable the patient to remain asymptomatic for many years. However, the abnormalities of the aortic valve tend to be progressive and provide a potential site for bacterial endocarditis with further structural damage. Prior to symptoms of limited exercise performance, patients may be aware of palpitations and the circulatory sensation of a large stroke volume with rapid diastolic runoff. These disturbances can be appreciated as prominent neck vein pulsations and an awareness of the heartbeat when the patient turns on the left side.[67] If ventricular irritability develops, the patient may notice the occasional augmentation in left ventricular stroke volume.

Patients with severe aortic regurgitation may experience exertional chest pain, but angina pectoris is less frequent than reported in some studies.[69,94] The chest discomfort is atypical compared to angina pectoris and can occur at rest as well as persist for a longer duration than coronary artery disease. Flushing, sweating, and palpitations sometimes accompany chest pain in aortic regurgitation.[95] Rest angina and nocturnal pain have been attributed to the deleterious effects of bradycardia with severe aortic regurgitation.

The common clinical manifestations of aortic regurgitation include symptoms of left ventricular failure, increased fatigue, dyspnea, orthopnea, and eventually paroxysmal nocturnal dyspnea. Left ventricular failure develops late in the course of aortic regurgitation, unless acute valvular destruction is imposed on a chronic lesion.

Unusual cardiac symptoms can also be experienced in severe aortic regurgitation and include neck and abdominal pain, postural dizziness, and excessive sweating on the trunk.[95] The stretching of the carotid sheath from the large left ventricular stroke volume may contribute to the neck discomfort, and a similar mechanism may explain the abdominal pain. The dizziness is attributed to disturbances in cerebral circulation with marked pressure changes in the rapid diastolic runoff.[69]

Physical Examination

Physical findings in chronic aortic regurgitation can produce the most marked alterations in the peripheral circulation of any lesion affecting the heart. These changes result from the large systolic stroke volume and rapid diastolic runoff. Although the characteristic diastolic murmur along the left sternal border may be unaccompanied by other physical findings, the most striking changes occur in severe aortic regurgitation. The peripheral pulse is quick in onset with a rapid rise in the upstroke followed by a peripheral collapse of the diastolic pulse known as Corrigan's pulse (see Chap. 9). The systolic blood pressure may be slightly increased and attended by an abnormally low diastolic pressure. The Korotkov sounds may be audible to a zero reading on the sphygmomanometer. If the pulse pressure does not exceed 50 percent of the peak systolic pressure or if the diastolic pressure is above 70 mmHg, the aortic regurgitation will not be hemodynamically severe unless left ventricular failure has developed.[96]

Physical examination may reveal abnormalities associated with the underlying mechanism for the aortic regurgitation. Yellowish linear streaks in the skin can be seen in the Ehlers-Danlos syndrome. The asthenic body habitus, long extremities, and arachnodactyly of the fingers are features of Marfan's syndrome. A bluish discoloration of the sclera is seen with osteogenesis imperfecta, and subluxation of the lens occurs in Marfan's syndrome. Retinal artery pulsations suggest significant hemodynamic aortic regurgitation. Hemorrhages and exudates in the fundus can be seen with bacterial endocarditis. Oral examination in Marfan's syndrome may reveal a high, arched palate.

DeMusset first described bobbing of the head with each cardiac pulsation. Neck veins will not be distended unless right ventricular failure has developed, but carotid vessels often display the exaggerated pulsatile motion caused by the large stroke volume. Aneurysmal dilatation of the aortic arch may sometimes cause the tracheal tug with each heartbeat. Pectus excavatum of the chest is another skeletal manifestation of Marfan's syndrome.

Cardiac findings depend on the severity of aortic regurgitation, and heart size can range from normal

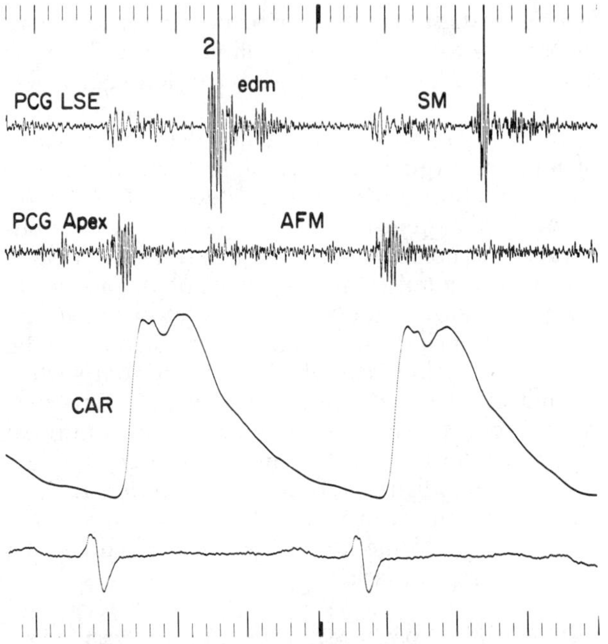

FIGURE 37-21 Phonocardiogram and carotid pulse recording in aortic regurgitation. At the left sternal edge a decrescendo diastolic murmur following the second sound (S_2) is recorded. At the cardiac apex there is a low-frequency middiastolic and presystolic murmur (Austin Flint) culminating at the time of the first heart sound. The carotid arterial tracing shows a bisferious pattern in the absence of the dicrotic notch. *(Courtesy of Dr. Ernest Craige.)*

to extreme dilatation. If the heart size and apical impulse are normal, mild aortic regurgitation is usually found (Fig. 37-21).[68] Severe regurgitation and dilatation of the ventricle will displace the apical impulse laterally and inferiorly.[97] The first heart sound at the apex is preserved in aortic regurgitation but can be diminished if the PR interval on electrocardiogram is prolonged or the heart rate is slow.[67] Sudden distension of the aorta can sometimes produce a systolic ejection click along the left sternal border. With significant aortic regurgitation, a systolic ejection murmur is invariably audible along the left sternal border as well as at the apex and in the primary aortic area.[67,69] In the late stages, scarring of the leaflet margins may diminish the aortic component of the second heart sound.

The characteristic auscultatory finding is the high-pitched diastolic blow along the left sternal border (see Chap. 11). This murmur can be heard best with the patient in the sitting position during full expiration. The duration of the diastolic blow correlates better with the hemodynamic abnormality than the intensity of the murmur.[69] Characteristically, the murmur is a high-pitched diastolic blow, but eversion of a cusp can produce a musical or cooing quality to the murmur.[98] Laceration of a leaflet or separation from the annulus due to aortic dissection may generate a loud, coarse vibrating sound. An early diastolic sound or ventricular gallop is frequently heard in aortic regurgitation (see Chap. 11). Although the third heart sound may reflect exaggerated early diastolic filling, patients usually reveal an increase in the end-systolic volume and a decrease in the contractile state as evidence of left ventricular dysfunction.[99,100]

In addition to the high-pitched diastolic murmur of aortic regurgitation, a rumbling diastolic murmur may be audible at the apex, as described by Austin Flint. This diastolic murmur can be presystolic, mid-diastolic, or holodiastolic[69] (see Chap. 11). The murmur is attributed to impingement of the aortic regurgitant flow on the anterior leaflet of the mitral valve, producing functional mitral stenosis. The middiastolic component of the murmur occurs when the mitral valve closes quickly after rapid ventricular filling from the aorta and left atrium.[101] Continued antegrade flow across the mitral valve creates turbulence which is responsible for the murmur. The Austin Flint murmur may reflect the severity of the aortic regurgitation, since such a murmur is not heard with mild regurgitation.

If acute aortic regurgitation is imposed on a normal left ventricle, the diastolic blow is distinctively different from the chronic condition.[102] Musical, cooing, or coarse vibrating qualities of the diastolic murmur suggest leaflet laceration, eversion, or separation from the aortic annulus (Fig. 37-22). With acute aortic regurgitation, the mitral leaflet may close prematurely, and the first heart sound becomes diminished or absent. Rarely, the diastolic murmur extends into early systole, since diastolic filling from the aorta continues after electrical depolarization of the ventricle. A systolic thrill can sometimes accompany the ejection murmur in acute aortic regurgitation.

Peripheral circulatory manifestations of aortic regurgitation are due to the large stroke volume and rapid diastolic runoff. The Corrigan's pulse is the abruptly rising and collapsing pulsation which can also be seen in any high-output condition with a large left ventricular stroke volume. Mueller's sign

FIGURE 37-22 Phonocardiogram and echocardiogram in aortic regurgitation. *A.* The murmur is loudest at the left sternal edge with high-frequency and diminuendo configuration. The musical quality of the murmur is indicated by the pattern of the vibrations and suggests an everted cusp as the cause of the valvular incompetence. *B.* At slower paper speed the contrast in phonocardiographic appearance of the murmur at different precordial locations is evident. At left sternal edge (LSE) the early diastolic murmur has a diminuendo silhouette, and at the apex the murmur is of lower frequency and becomes accentuated prior to the next systole owing to the addition of an Austin Flint murmur. The vibrations of the anterior leaflet of the mitral valve coincide with the early diastolic murmur and not the Austin Flint murmur. (*Courtesy of Dr. Ernest Craige.*)

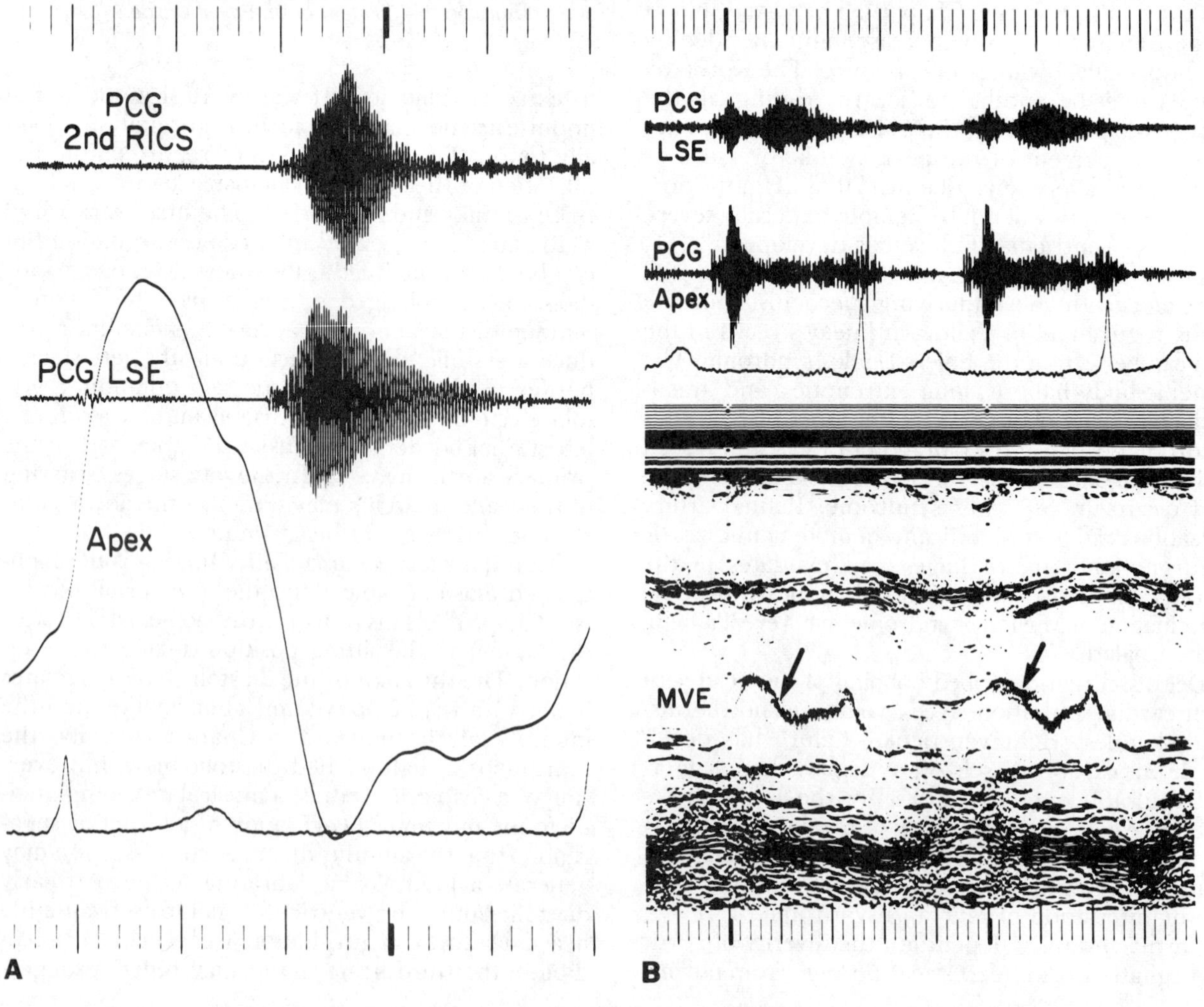

is the rhythmic pulsation of the uvula, and Quincke's sign is arterial pulsation of the nail beds, with alternating redness and blanching during each cardiac contraction. Duroziez's murmur is the systolic and diastolic murmur over the femoral artery, and a disproportionate elevation in femoral artery diastolic pressure has been designated Hill's sign.

Chest Roentgenogram

Cardiac enlargement due to dilatation of the left ventricle is the most common radiographic abnormality in aortic regurgitation. As the volume overload on the left ventricle increases, there is elongation of the apex of the ventricle inferiorly and posteriorly. Left atrial enlargement may also develop and pulmonary venous congestion indicates cardiac decompensation. Prominent dilatation of the ascending aorta is a feature of Marfan's syndrome and syphilitic aortitis. Calcification of the valve does not usually occur and should raise the possibility of combined aortic stenosis. With acute aortic regurgitation, heart size may remain normal despite the development of pulmonary venous congestion and pulmonary edema. (See Chap. 15.)

Electrocardiogram

Electrocardiographic changes reflect left ventricular dilatation and hypertrophy, manifested by increased QRS amplitude and ST-T wave depression.[67,69] The rhythm is usually normal sinus but prolonged AV conduction can occur in the late stages of aortic regurgitation.[103] A left ventricular volume overload pattern has been attributed to the early electrocardiographic changes of QRS prominence and tall precordial T waves.[104] (See Chap. 14.)

Special Laboratory Studies

Echocardiography The echocardiogram can provide anatomical information on the aortic valve apparatus, the aortic root, and measurements of ventricular function. Disturbances in mitral valve motion created by the regurgitant flow across the aortic valve can also be recognized.[105,106] Sometimes vegetations of bacterial endocarditis can be identified on the aortic leaflets.[107,108] Increased aortic dimensions suggest a chronic basis for the regurgitation.[109] Echocardiographic end-diastolic and end-systolic dimensions permit calculation of chamber volume and left ventricular stroke volume.[110] The ejection fraction can be obtained by relating the total left ventricular stroke volume to the end-diastolic volume. Mitral valve abnormalities include diastolic fluttering of the anterior mitral valve leaflet, rapid diastolic closure rate of the mitral leaflet, premature closure of the mitral valve before onset of the QRS complex, and thickening of mitral leaflets (Fig. 37-22*B*).[105,106] Echocardiographic assessment of left ventricular function during supine exercise can detect early left ventricular dysfunction in symptom-free patients with aortic regurgitation.[111]

In acute aortic regurgitation, diastolic oscillations in the aortic root or ventricular outflow tract can be seen with a flail leaflet.[112] Aortic dissection can be recognized by a double lumen in the ascending aorta.[109]

Pre- and postoperative echocardiographic studies have suggested that a left ventricular end-systolic dimension greater than 55 mmHg can identify a high-risk group for surgery or congestive heart failure.[113] The aortic valve replacement should be undertaken before irreversible left ventricular dilatation has developed and the echocardiogram may provide an objective technique for early recommendation of valve surgery. (See Chap. 120.)

Cardiac Catheterization Cardiac catheterization is indicated in aortic regurgitation to document the presence of aortic incompetence and assess its severity, to evaluate left ventricular function, and to identify additional abnormalities in the aorta, mitral valve, and coronary artery anatomy (Fig. 37-23). Although the traditional angiographic method for assessing aortic regurgitation is the aortic root injection during cineangiography, inconsistencies and disparities have been shown by this system when compared to quantitative angiocardiography.[114] Quantitative angiocardiography provides accurate measurements of end-diastolic and end-systolic volume. Left ventricular stroke volume can be related to the forward stroke volume, determined by the Fick or indicator dilution technique to quantitate the regurgitant flow per beat across the aortic valve.[115] A dilated left ventricular chamber may dilute the contrast material and give the impression of minimal regurgitation across the valve, whereas regurgitation into a normal-size left ventricular chamber can create the impression of severe aortic regurgitation.

Left ventricular end-diastolic pressure has been used as a hemodynamic index of ventricular function, but the end-diastolic pressure may remain normal in chronic aortic regurgitation.[24] Increased diastolic compliance in chronic volume overload is achieved by a slippage of myocardial fibers as well as stress relaxation and creep.[116] With moderate elevations of the left ventricular end-diastolic pressure, compensatory increases in wall thickness and hypertrophy can still result in a normal end-diastolic wall stress or preload. The ejection fraction remains a useful index of mechanical performance, but this value is artificially preserved in the volume overload of aortic incompetence since systolic ejection begins at a lower left ventricular pressure than normal. Contractile function measured as peak systolic stress/end-diastolic volume and end-systolic pressure/volume curves is more depressed in chronic aortic regurgitation patients with congestive heart failure than in asymptomatic patients.[117]

Coronary arteriography should be performed in adults with aortic regurgitation whether chest pain has been a symptom or not. Underlying coronary

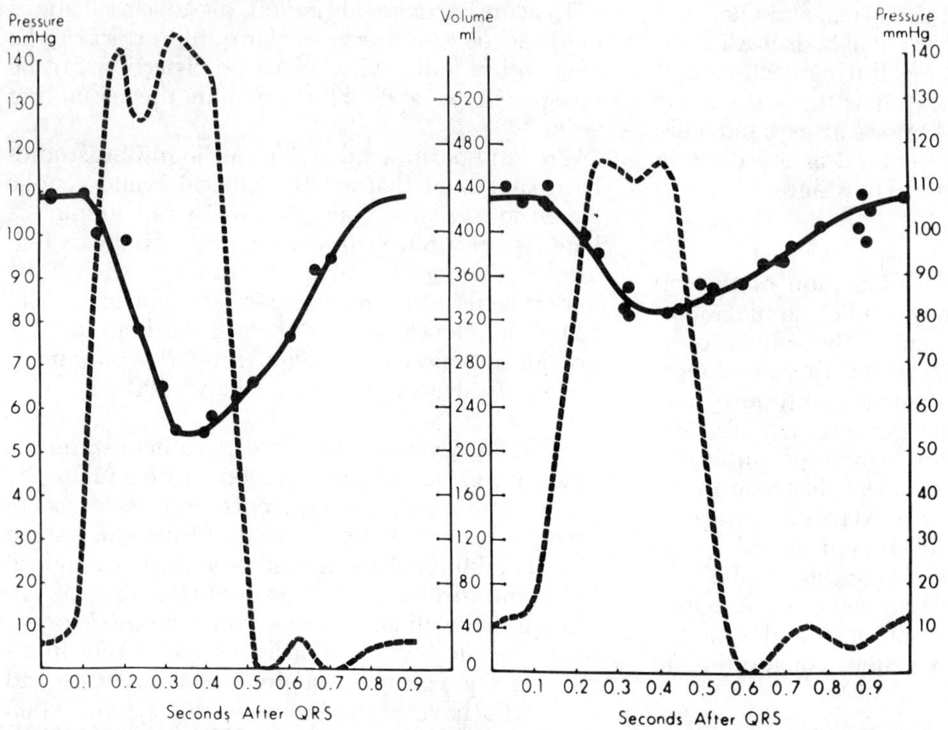

FIGURE 37-23 Left ventricular pressure and volume in two patients with aortic regurgitation. The patient on the left enjoyed unrestricted activity without symptoms, whereas the patient on the right was extremely limited with left ventricular failure. For the patient on the left, end-diastolic volume (EDV) = 436; end-systolic volume (ESV) = 219; left ventricular stroke volume (LVSV) = 217; forward stroke volume (FSV) = 97; aortic regurgitation (AR) = 120; ejection fraction (EF) = 217/436 = 0.50; left ventricular weight (LVwt) = 474; left ventricular end-diastolic pressure (LVedp) = 8. For the patient on the right, EDV = 430; ESV = 329; LVSV = 101; FSV = 67; AR = 34; EF = 101/430 = 0.23; LVwt = 561; LVedp = 13. [*From C. E. Rackley, W. P. Hood, Jr., B. R. Wilcox, and R. M. Peters, Quantitation of Myocardial Function in Valvular Heart Disease, in L. A. Brewer III (ed.), "Prosthetic Heart Valves," Charles C Thomas, Springfield, Ill., 1969. Reproduced with permission from the author. Courtesy of Charles C Thomas, Publisher, Springfield, Ill.*]

disease can contribute to abnormal left ventricular function and should be considered at the time of aortic valve replacement.

In acute aortic regurgitation the major hemodynamic change is marked elevation of the left ventricular end-diastolic pressure, since the end-diastolic volume can remain normal or slightly increased.[102] Severe elevation of end-diastolic pressure can prematurely close the mitral valve and abnormally elevate left atrial and pulmonary capillary pressures. (See Chap. 108.)

Radionuclide Studies Radionuclide angiography can be used to assess left ventricular function at rest and during exercise.[118–120] Blood pool imaging is useful for quantitation of regurgitant flow and valvular incompetence. Exercise studies in aortic regurgitation suggest that deterioration or decline of the ejection fraction with exercise is an index of myocardial decompensation prior to development of clinical symptoms. Preservation of the contractile state is associated with an increase in ejection fraction with exercise. Thallium scintigraphy can identify perfusion defects in the myocardium and would raise the possibility of underlying coronary artery disease.[121,122] However, exercise-induced wall motion abnormalities with radionuclide angiography are not reliable for the detection of underlying coronary disease, since such abnormalities can occur with normal coronary anatomy.[123] (See Chap. 109.)

Graded Exercise Testing Exercise testing can document physical endurance and evaluate atypical features in aortic regurgitation.[124] Patients can be followed with exercise testing in combination with radionuclide studies.

Natural History and Prognosis

The volume overload imposed on the left ventricle in chronic aortic regurgitation is usually well tolerated for long periods before the development of heart failure.[125] Three-fourths of patients with significant aortic regurgitation may survive 5 years, and 50 percent have been shown to live for 10 years after the diagnosis.[56] As many as 85 to 95 percent of patients with mild to moderate aortic insufficiency will survive for 10 years. Once symptoms develop in aortic regurgitation, there is fairly rapid deterioration. Patients developing congestive heart failure often expire within 2 years after onset of symptoms, and the average survival after the onset of angina pectoris is approximately 5 years. Late survival after valve replacement is better predicted by left ventricular systolic pump function variables. A preoperative ejection fraction above 45 percent and a cardiac index greater than 2.5 liters/min/m^2 are associated with higher postoperative survival than an ejection fraction less than 45 percent and a cardiac index below 2.5 liters/min/m^2.[126] Acute aortic regurgitation is associated with an extremely high mortality, progressing from acute pulmonary edema to rapid refractory heart failure and cardiogenic shock.

Treatment

Medical

Prophylaxis against bacterial endocarditis remains the primary responsibility in the care of the asymptomatic patient with aortic regurgitation (see Chap. 56). Antibiotics are indicated, not only for dental care but also surgical instrumentation of the gastrointestinal or genitourinary tract. Although left ventricular failure requires standard treatment with digitalis, diuretics, and vasodilating agents, hydralazine can reduce the aortic regurgitant volume and improve mechanical pump function by reducing the end-diastolic volume and raising the ejection fraction.[127] The physician must remember that the primary defect is mechanical and medical therapy alone cannot restore the impaired defect in the valve.

An important clinical consideration in the management of aortic regurgitation is selection of the optimal time for valve replacement. Ideally, surgery should be performed before clinical symptoms of heart failure develop. Echocardiographic evaluation of asymptomatic patients with aortic regurgitation suggests that an end-systolic dimension less than 50 mm should be followed at yearly intervals. When the end-systolic dimension is between 50 and 54 mm, the echocardiogram should be repeated every 4 to 6 months and surgery advised when the dimension exceeds 55 mm, even in the absence of symptoms.[113] Late survival after aortic valve replacement is better predicted preoperatively by left ventricular systolic pump variables of ejection fraction and cardiac index than LV diastolic parameters and clinical status.[126] A decline in the exercise-induced radionuclide ejection fraction may be an additional index for advising valve replacement before the development of symptoms of heart failure.[118] Therefore, noninvasive and invasive techniques can detect early deterioration of left ventricular function in chronic aortic regurgitation before the onset of symptoms and provide a basis for valve replacement in these patients.

The preparation of the patient undergoing aortic valve surgery involves stabilization of left ventricular function, control of arrhythmias, and correction of electrolyte abnormalities. However, vigorous measurements to improve cardiac function with digitalis and diuretics preoperatively should be avoided since these agents can present difficulties during anesthesia and the postoperative surgical period. The patient should have dental repair and other elective procedures performed prior to valve replacement to reduce the potential for future sources of bacterial endocarditis. In Marfan's syndrome, prophylactic resection should be considered when aortic root diameter exceeds 5.5 cm.[128] Acute aortic regurgitation from bacterial endocarditis will require valve replacement under intensive antibiotic coverage if heart failure develops.[129]

Surgical

The natural history of aortic valve regurgitation as reviewed earlier in this chapter indicates that chronic aortic regurgitation may be well tolerated for several years before causing evidence of left ventricular dysfunction and symptoms.[67] Patients with chronic aortic regurgitation may develop left ventricular dysfunction in the absence of any symptoms. Such dysfunction may be irreversible and compromise both early and late results of valve replacement.[113] It is therefore important that asymptomatic patients be identified prior to the onset of left ventricular dysfunction. Objective assessment of left ventricular function, both at rest and with exercise, is increasingly important in determining the appropriate time for surgical intervention in asymptomatic patients with aortic regurgitation. Acute aortic regurgitation resulting from bacterial endocarditis, acute dissection of the ascending aorta, and tearing of the aortic cusps is poorly tolerated and usually requires urgent or emergency surgical intervention.

Indications for Operation Patients with chronic aortic regurgitation who are symptomatic are advised to have surgery. Asymptomatic patients who show evidence of left ventricular dysfunction at rest as measured by radionuclide ventriculography or echocardiography should be advised to have surgery. Those patients who demonstrate left ventricular dysfunction only with exercise as evidenced by a decrease in ejection fraction should probably be operated upon. End-systolic left ventricular dimensions have been used to help determine the optimal time for valve replacement. It is apparent that patients with an end-systolic dimension greater than 55 mm have a poorer result in terms of longevity and function than those operated before this degree of left ventricular enlargement occurs.[113] However, this measurement probably will prove less helpful in decision making for individual patients than studies that assess left ventricular function.

Acute aortic regurgitation most frequently associated with dissection of the ascending aorta or infective endocarditis generally is an indication for prompt surgery. The major threat in patients with acute dissection is rupture of the aorta, and thus surgery is indicated regardless of the degree of aortic regurgitation. In most instances valve competency can be restored without valve replacement. Infective endocarditis may cause acute aortic regurgitation and congestive heart failure. Early oper-

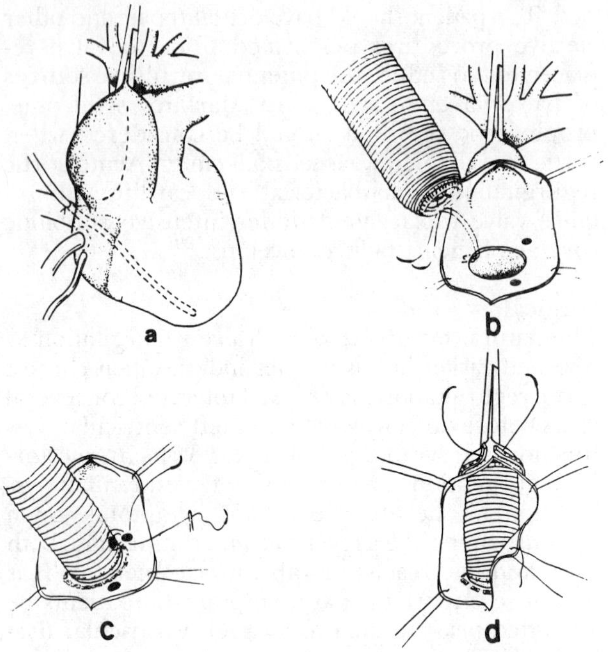

FIGURE 37-24 Technique for replacing the aortic valve and the proximal ascending aorta using a valved internal conduit. Modified from Kouchoukos. (*From N. T. Kouchoukos, R. B. Karp, and W. A. Lell, Replacement of the Ascending Aorta and Aortic Valve with a Composite Graft: Results in 25 Patients, Ann. Thorac. Surg., 24:140, 1977. Reproduced with permission from the publisher and author.*)

ation in these patients with even mild congestive failures offers a better prognosis than delayed surgery.[130,131]

Operation The type of operation used for aortic regurgitation depends primarily on the etiology. In patients with disease limited to the valve the operation is essentially as described in the previous section on aortic stenosis. In patients with infective endocarditis aortic root destruction may necessitate alterations in the described technique. Debridement and obliteration of abscessed cavities of the aortic ring and the use of alternate methods of valve fixation may be required.[132,133]

In cases of acute aortic dissection producing aortic regurgitation, resuspension and fixation of the leaflets will usually restore valvular competence.[134] Patients with aortic annular extasia and aneurysms of the sinuses of Valsalva usually require replacement of the aorta with a prosthetic graft in addition to valve replacement. In many instances this is accomplished by insertion of a separate valve and graft, retaining small cuffs of aorta about the coronary ostia. An alternate technique indicated when there is significant involvement of the sinuses involves the use of a composite Dacron tube–prosthetic valve replacement of the ascending aorta and aortic valve. Coronary ostia are then attached to the Dacron tube[135] (Fig. 37-24).

The type of prosthetic valve used for aortic valve replacement should be determined after considering the patient's age, the need for anticoagulants, and the durability of the prosthetic valve. In general, mechanical prostheses require long-term anticoagulation; tissue prostheses do not, but these prostheses will probably prove less durable than most mechanical prostheses. When a valved conduit is used, it is preferable to use a low-profile mechanical prosthesis for durability and ease of attachment of the coronary ostia to the conduit.

Patients with significant stenosis of the coronary arteries should undergo coronary artery bypass grafting at the time of valve replacement.

Results The *early mortality* for aortic valve replacement for patients with aortic regurgitation is generally about the same as those having the operation for aortic stenosis and is approximately 2 to 3 percent (Fig. 37-25). The risk is slightly increased in those patients requiring replacement of the ascend-

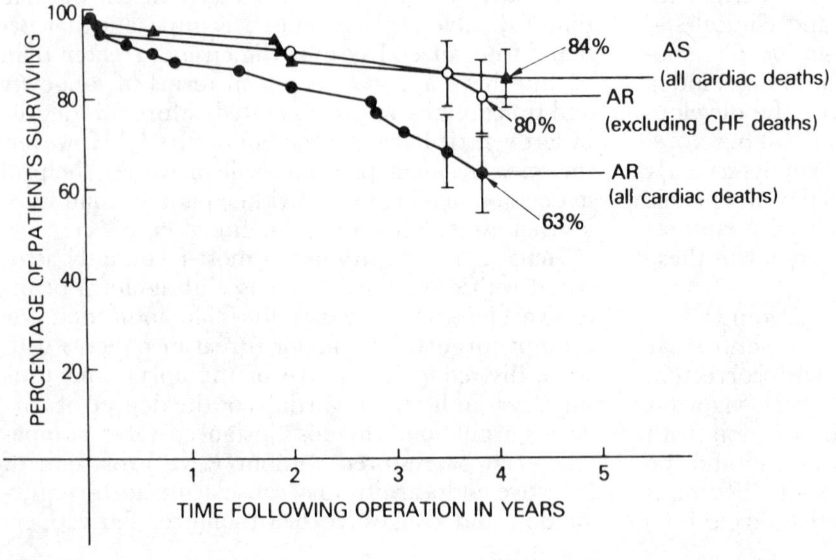

FIGURE 37-25 Actuarial survival following aortic valve replacement: aortic stenosis compared to aortic incompetence. (*From W. L. Henry, R. O. Bonow, D. R. Rosing, and S. E. Epstein, Observations on the Optimum Time for Operative Intervention for Aortic Regurgitation: II. Serial Echocardiographic Evaluation of Asymptomatic Patients, Circulation, 61:484, 1980. Reproduced with permission from the American Heart Association, Inc., and the author.*)

ing aorta and in patients with endocarditis, causing marked destruction of the aortic root. *Late results* are in part related to the etiology of the aortic regurgitation, but are most importantly related to the functional status of the left ventricle.[136] Results are somewhat less favorable than the results of valve replacement for aortic stenosis, a major cause of poor late results being congestive heart failure.

Postoperative Care
Postoperative management is similar to that described in the section on aortic stenosis. Anticoagulation is determined by the valve type used. Prophylactic antibiotics are indicated during periods of increased susceptibility to bacteremia. Antiarrhythmic therapy may be required to suppress ventricular ectopy. Patients should be followed at regular intervals to assess prosthetic valve function.

Cost Analysis
Cost-effectiveness will be most favorably influenced by optimal timing of operation. The use of noninvasive studies to determine left ventricular function should provide added information on the most appropriate time for valve replacement to achieve optimal longevity and productivity and minimal expenditures for continued medical care. The serious consequences in terms of morbidity and mortality of prosthetic valve infection mandate a long-term program of antibiotic prophylaxis.

References

1. Stokes, W.: "The Diseases of the Heart and the Aorta," Hodges and Smith, Dublin, 1854, p. 139.
2. Monckeberg, J. G.: Der normale histologische Bau und die sklerose der aorenklappen, *Virchows Arch. (Pathol. Anat.),* 176:472, 1904.
3. Karsner, H. T., and Koletsky, S.: "Calcific Disease of Aortic Valves," J. B. Lippincott, Philadelphia, 1947.
4. Campbell, M., and Kauntze, R.: Congenital Aortic Valvular Stenosis, *Br. Heart J.,* 15:179, 1953.
5. Roberts, W. C.: The Congenitally Bicuspid Aortic Valvular Stenosis, *Br. Heart J.,* 15:179, 1953.
6. Glancy, D. L., Epstein, S. E.: Differential Diagnosis of Type and Severity of Obstruction to Left Ventricular Outflow, *Prog. Cardiovasc. Dis.,* 14:153, 1971.
7. Roberts, W. C.: The Structure of the Aortic Valve in Clinically Isolated Aortic Stenosis: An Autopsy Study of 162 Patients over 15 Years of Age, *Circulation,* 42:91, 1970.
8. Roberts, W. C., Perloff, J. K., and Costantino, T.: Severe Valvular Aortic Stenosis in Patients over 65 Years of Age: A Clinicopathologic Study, *Am. J. Cardiol.,* 27:497, 1971.
9. Roberts, W. C.: Anatomically Isolated Aortic Valvular Disease: The Case Against Its Being of Rheumatic Etiology, *Am. J. Med.,* 49:151, 1970.
10. Pomerance, A.: Pathogenesis of Aortic Stenosis and Its Relation to Age, *Br. Heart J.,* 34:569, 1972.
11. Edwards, J. E.: Pathology of Acquired Valvular Disease of the Heart, *Semin. Roentgenol.,* 14:96, 1979.
12. Edwards, J. E.: On the Etiology of Calcific Aortic Stenosis, *Circulation,* 26:817, 1962.
13. Pomerance, A.: Cardiac Pathology and Systolic Murmurs in the Elderly, *Br. Heart J.,* 30:687, 1968.
14. Pritzker, M. R., Ernst, J. D., Caudill, C., Wilson, C. S., Weaver, W. F., and Edwards, J. E.: Acquired Aortic Stenosis in Systemic Lupus Erythematosus, *Ann. Intern Med.,* 93:434, 1980.
15. Kavanaugh, G. J., Pruitt, R. D., and Edwards, J. E.: Coronary Embolism and Cystic Medical Necrosis of Ascending Aorta Associated with Calcific Aortic Stenosis, *Proc. Mayo Clin.,* 33:222, 1958.
16. Levy, M. J., and Edwards, J. E.: Anatomy of Mitral Insufficiency, *Prog. Cardiovasc. Dis.,* 5:119, 1962.
17. Moller, J. H., Nakib, A., and Edwards, J. E.: Infarction of Papillary Muscles and Mitral Insufficiency Associated with Congenital Aortic Stenosis, *Circulation,* 34:87, 1966.
18. Fukuda, T., Tadavarthy, S. M., and Edwards, J. E.: Dissecting Aneurysm of Aorta Complicating Aortic Valvular Stenosis, *Circulation,* 53:169, 1976.
19. Nakib, A., Lillehei, C. E., Edwards, J. E.: The Degree of Coronary Atherosclerosis in Aortic Valvular Disease, *Arch. Pathol.,* 80:517, 1965.
20. Kennedy, J. W., Twiss, R. D., Blackmon, J. R., and Dodge, H. T.: Quantitative Angiocardiography. III. Relationships of Left Ventricular Pressure, Volume and Mass in Aortic Valve Disease, *Circulation,* 38:838, 1968.
21. Hood, W. P. Jr., Rackley, C. E., and Rolett, E. L.: Wall Stress in the Normal and Hypertrophied Human Left Ventricle, *Am. J. Cardiol.,* 22:550, 1968.
22. Rackley, C. E., and Hood, W. P., Jr.: Aortic Valve Disease, in H. J. Levine (ed.), "Clinical Cardiovascular Physiology," Grune & Stratton, New York, 1976, p. 493.
23. Stott, D. K., Marpole, D. G., Bristow, J. D., Kloster, F. E., and Griswold, H. E.: The Role of Left Atrial Transport in Aortic and Mitral Stenosis, *Circulation,* 41:1031, 1970.
24. Rackley, C. E., Hood, W. P., Jr., Rolett, E. L., and Young, D. T.: Left Ventricular End-Diastolic Pressure in Chronic Heart Disease, *Am. J. Med.,* 48:310, 1970.
25. Dodge, H. T., and Baxley, W. A.: Left Ventricular Volume and Mass and Their Significance in Heart Disease, *Am. J. Cardiol.,* 23:528, 1969.
26. Ross, J., Jr., and Braunwald, E.: Aortic Stenosis, *Circulation,* 38(suppl. 5): 61, 1968.
27. Wood, P.: Aortic Stenosis, *Am. J. Cardiol.,* 1:553, 1958.
28. Rotman, M., Morris, J. J., Behar, V. W., Peter, R. H., and Kong, Y.: Aortic Valvular Disease: Comparison of Types and Their Medical and Surgical Management, *Am. J. Med.,* 51:241, 1971.
29. Kumpe, C. W., and Bean, W. B.: Aortic Stenosis: Study of the Clinical and Pathological Aspects of 107 Proved Cases. *Medicine (Baltimore),* 27:139, 1948.
30. Moraski, R. E., Russell, R. O., Jr., Mantle, J. A., and Rackley, C. E.: Aortic Stenosis, Angina Pectoris, Coronary Artery Disease, *Catheterization and Cardiovasc. Diag.,* 2:157, 1976.
31. Baxley, W. A., Dodge, H. T., Rackley, C. E., Sandler, H., and Pugh, D.: Left Ventricular Mechanical Efficiency in Man with Heart Disease, *Circulation,* 55:564, 1977.
32. Hood, W. P., Jr., Thompson, W. J., Rackley, C. E., and Rolett, E. L.: Comparison of Calculations of Left Ventricular Wall Stress in Man from Thin-Walled and Thick-Walled Ellipsoidal Models, *Circ. Res.,* 24:575, 1969.
33. Holley, K. E., Bahn, R. C., McGoon, D. C., and Mankin, H. T.: Spontaneous Calcific Embolization Associated with Calcific Aortic Stenosis, *Circulation,* 27:197, 1963.
34. Flamm, M. D., Braiff, B. A., Kimball, R., and Hancock, E. W.: Mechanism of Effort Syncope in Aortic Stenosis, *Circulation,* 36(suppl. 2):II–109, 1967.
35. Schwartz, L. S., Goldfischer, J., Sprague, G. J., and Schwartz, S. P.: Syncope and Sudden Death in Aortic Stenosis, *Am. J. Cardiol.,* 23:647, 1969.
36. Baker, C., and Sommerville, J.: Clinical Features and Surgical Treatment of Fifty Patients with Severe Aortic Stenosis, *Guys Hosp. Rep.,* 108:101, 1959.
37. Brockmeier, L. B., Adolph, R. J., Gustin, B. W., Holmes, J. C., and Sacks, J. G.: Calcium Emboli to the Retinal Artery in Calcific Aortic Stenosis, *Am. Heart J.,* 101:32, 1981.
38. Andersen, J. A., Hansen, B. F., and Lyngborg, K.: Isolated Valvular Aortic Stenosis, *Acta Med. Scand.,* 197:61, 1975.
39. Hancock, E. W.: The Ejection Sound in Aortic Stenosis, *Am. J. Med.,* 40:569, 1966.
40. Crawley, I. S., Morris, D. C., and Silverman, B. D.: Valvular Heart Disease, in J. W. Hurst, R. B. Logue, R. C. Schlant,

and N. K. Wenger (eds.), "The Heart," 4th ed., McGraw-Hill Book Company, New York, 1978, p. 992.
41. Davison, E. T., and Friedman, S. A.: Significance of Systolic Murmurs in the Aged, *N. Engl. J. Med.,* 279:225, 1968.
42. Klatte, E. C., Tampas, J. P., Campbell, J. A., and Lurie, P. R.: The Roentgenographic Manifestations of Aortic Stenosis and Aortic Valvular Insufficiency, *Am. J. Roentgenol. Radium Ther. Nucl. Med.,* 88:57, 1962.
43. Myler, R. K., and Sanders, C. A.: Aortic Valve Disease and Atrial Fibrillation: Report of 122 Patients with Electrographic, Radiographic and Hemodynamic Observations, *Arch. Intern. Med.,* 121:530, 1968.
44. Reigenbaum, H.: "Echocardiography," Lea & Febiger, Philadelphia, 1976.
45. Johnson, M. L., Kisslo, J., Habersberger, P. G., and Wallace, A. G.: Echocardiographic Evaluation of Aortic Valvular Disease, *Circulation,* 47(suppl. 4):IV–46, 1973.
46. Radford, D. J., Bloom, K. R., Izukawa, T., Moes, C. A. F., and Rowe, R. D.: Echocardiographic Assessment of Bicuspid Aortic Valves: Angiographic and Pathological Correlates, *Circulation,* 53:80, 1976.
47. Godley, R. W., Green, D., Dillon, J. C., Rogers, E. W., Feigenbaum, H., and Weyman, A. E.: Reliability of Two-Dimensional Echocardiography in Assessing the Severity of Valvular Aortic Stenosis, *Chest,* 79:657, 1981.
48. Hancock, E. W., and Fleming, P. R.: Aortic Stenosis, *Q. J. Med.,* 29:209, 1960.
49. Braunwald, E., Goldbatt, A., Aygen, M. M., Rockoff, D. S., and Morrow, A. G.: Congenital Aortic Stenosis. I. Clinical and Hemodynamic Findings in 100 Patients; Morrow, A. G., Goldbatt, A., Braunwald, E.: Congenital Aortic Stenosis. II. Surgical Treatment and the Results of Operation, *Circulation,* 27:426, 1963.
50. Rackley, C. E.: Quantitative Evaluation of Left Ventricular Function by Radiographic Techniques, *Circulation,* 54:862, 1976.
51. Borer, J. S., Bacharach, S. L., Green, M. V., Kent, K. M., Rosing, D. R., Seides, F., McIntosh, C. L., Conkle, D., Morrow, A. G., and Epstein, S. E.: Left Ventricular Function in Aortic Stenosis: Response to Exercise and Effects of Operation, *Am. J. Cardiol.,* 41:382, 1978.
52. Takeda, J., Warren, R., and Holzman, D.: Prognosis of Aortic Stenosis, *Arch. Surg.,* 87:931, 1963.
53. Dexter, L.: Evaluation of the Results of Cardiac Surgery, in A. M. Jones (ed.), "Modern Trends in Cardiology," Appleton-Century-Crofts, New York, 1969, vol. 2, p. 311.
54. Frank, S., Johnson, A., and Ross, J., Jr.: Natural History of Valvular Aortic Stenosis, *Br. Heart J.,* 35:41, 1973.
55. Wagner, S., and Selzer, A.: Patterns of Progression of Aortic Stenosis: A Longitudinal Hemodynamic Study, *Circulation,* 65:709, 1982.
56. Rapaport, E.: Natural History of Aortic and Mitral Valve Disease, *Am. J. Cardiol.,* 35:221, 1975.
57. Thompson, R., Knight, E., Ahmed, M., Somerville, W., Towers, M., and Yacoub, M.: The Use of "Fresh" Unstented Homograft Valves for Replacement of the Aortic Valve: Analysis of 6½ Years Experience, *Circulation,* 56:837, 1977.
58. Barratt-Boyes, B. G., Roche, A. H. G., and Whitlock, R. M. L.: Six Year Review of the Results of Freehand Aortic Valve Replacement Using an Antibiotic Sterilized Homograft Valve, *Circulation,* 55:353, 1977.
59. Wallace, R. B., Londe, S. P., and Titus, J. L.: Aortic Replacement with Preserved Aortic Valve Homografts, *J. Thorac. Cardiovasc. Surg.,* 67(1):44–52, 1974.
60. Gallo, I., Ruiz, B., and Duran, C. M. G.: Five to Eight Year Follow-up of Patients with the Hancock Cardiac Prosthesis, *J. Thorac. Cardiovasc. Surg.,* 86:897–902, 1983.
61. Geha, A. S., Laks, H., Stanel, H. C., Cornhill, J. F., Kilman, J. W., Buckley, M. J., and Roberts, W. C.: Late Failure of Porcine Valve Heterografts in Children, *J. Thorac. Cardiovasc. Surg.,* 78:351, 1979.
62. Chesebro, J. H., Fuster, V., Elveback, L. R., McGoon, D. C., Pluth, J. R., Puga, F. J., Wallace, R. B., Danielson, G. K., Orszulak, T. A., Piehler, J. M., and Schaff, H. V.: Trial of Combined Warfarin Plus Dipyridamole or Aspirin Therapy in Prosthetic Heart Valve Replacement: Danger of Aspirin Compared with Dipyridamole, *Am. J. Cardiol.,* 45:1537–1541, 1983.
63. Reed, G. E., Sanoudos, G. M., Pooley, R. W., Moggio, R. A., McClung, J. A., Somberg, E. D., and Praeger, P. I.: Results of Combined Valvular and Myocardial Revascularization Operations, *J. Thorac. Cardiovasc. Surg.,* 85:422–426, 1983.
64. McManus, Q., Grunkemeir, G. L., Lambert, L. E., Tepley, J. F., Harlan, B. J., and Starr, A.: Year of Operation as a Risk Factor in the Late Results of Valve Replacement, *J. Thorac. Cardiovasc. Surg.,* 80:834, 1980.
65. Schwarz, F., Llameng, W., Langebartels, F., Sesto, M., Walter, P., and Schlepper, M.: Impaired Left Ventricular Function in Chronic Aortic Valve Disease: Survival and Function After Replacement by Bjork-Shiley Prosthesis, *Circulation,* 60:48, 1979.
66. Corrigan, D. J.: On Permanent Patency of the Mouth of the Aorta or Inadequacy of the Aortic Valves, *Edinburgh Med. Surg. J.,* XXXVII:225, 1832.
67. Segal, J., Harvey, W. P., and Hufnagel, C. L.: A Clinical Study of One Hundred Cases of Severe Aortic Insufficiency, *Am. J. Med.,* 21:200, 1956.
68. Stapleton, J. F., and Harvey, W. P.: A Clinical Analysis of Aortic Incompetence, *Postgrad. Med.,* 46:156, 1969.
69. Angloff, E.: Aortic Incompetence: Clinical Haemodynamic and Angiocardiographic Evaluation, *Acta Med. Scand.,* 193(suppl. 538):3, 1972.
70. Read, R. C., Thal, A. P., and Wendt, V. E.: Symptomatic Valvular Myxomatous Transformation (The Floppy Valve Syndrome): A Possible Forme Frust of the Marfan Syndrome, *Circulation,* 32:897, 1965.
71. Roberts, W. C., Hollingworth, J. F., Bulkley, B. H., Jaffe, R. B., Epstein, S. E., and Stinson, E. B.: Combined Mitral and Aortic Regurgitation in Ankylosing Spondylitis: Angiographic and Anatomic Features, *Am. J. Med.,* 56:237, 1974.
72. Bulkley, B. H., and Roberts, W. C.: Ankylosing Spondylitis and Aortic Regurgitation: Description of the Characteristic Cardiovascular Lesion from Study of Eight Necropsy Patients, *Circulation,* 48:1014, 1973.
73. Paulus, H. E., Pearson, C. M., and Pitts, W., Jr.: Aortic Insufficiency in Five Patients with Reiter's Syndrome: A Detailed Clinical and Pathologic Study, *Am. J. Med. J.,* 53:464, 1972.
74. Roberts, W. C., Kehoe, J. A., Carpenter, D. F., and Golden, A.: Cardiovascular Valvular Lesions in Rheumatoid Arthritis, *Arch. Intern. Med.,* 122:141, 1968.
75. Sakakibara, S., and Konno, S.: Congenital Aneurysm of the Sinus of Valsalva Anatomy and Classification, *Am. Heart J.,* 63:405, 1962.
76. Puchner, T. C., Huston, J. H., and Hellmuth, G. A.: Aortic Valve Insufficiency in Arterial Hypertension, *Am. J. Cardiol.,* 5:758, 1960.
77. Karp, R. B., and Carlson, D. E.: "Dissection of Aorta," F. A. Davis, Philadelphia, Cardiovascular Clinics, 1981, pp. 209–219.
78. Wilcox, B. R., Procter, H. J., Rackley, C. E., and Peters, R. M.: Early Surgical Treatment of Valvular Endocarditis, *JAMA,* 200:820, 1967.
79. Oh, W. M. C., Taylor, T. R., and Olsen, E. G. J.: Aortic Regurgitation in Systemic Lupus Erythematosus Requiring Aortic Valve Replacement, *Br. Heart J.,* 36:413, 1974.
79a. Roberts, W. C., Hollingsworth, J. F., Bulkley, B. H., Jaffe, R. B., Epstein, S. E., and Stinson, E. B.: Combined Mitral and Aortic Regurgitation in Ankylosing Spondylitis. Angiographic and Anatomic Features, *Am. J. Med.,* 56:237, 1974.
80. Wang, K., Gobel, F., Gleason, D. F., and Edwards, J. E.: Complete Heart Block Complicating Bacterial Endocarditis, *Circulation,* 46:939, 1972.
81. Spurny, O. M., and Hara, M.: Rupture of the Aortic Valve Due to Strain, *Am. J. Cardiol.,* 8:125, 1961.
82. Symbas, P. N., Walter, P. F., Hurst, J. W., and Schlant,

R. C.: Fenestration of Aortic Cusps Causing Aortic Regurgitation, *J. Thorac. Cardiovasc. Dis.,* 57:464, 1969.
83. Carter, J. B., Sethi, S., Lee, G. B., and Edwards, J. E.: Prolapse of Semilunar Cusps as Causes of Aortic Insufficiency, *Circulation,* 43:922, 1971.
84. Tatsuno, K., Konno, S., and Sakakibara, S.: Ventricular Septal Defect with Aortic Insufficiency, *Am. Heart J.,* 85:13, 1973.
85. Heggtveit, H. A.: Syphilitic Aortitis. A Clinicopathologic Autopsy Study of 100 Cases, 1950 to 1960, *Circulation,* 29:346, 1964.
86. Eversmeyer, W. H., Rosenstock, D., and Biundo, J. J., Jr.: Aortic Insufficiency with Mild Ankylosing Spondylitis in Black Men, *JAMA,* 240:2652, 1978.
87. Murray, C. A., and Edwards, J. E.: Spontaneous Laceration of Ascending Aorta, *Circulation,* 47:848, 1973.
88. Edwards, J. E.: Lesions Causing or Simulating Aortic Insufficiency, *Cardiovasc. Clin.,* 5:128, 1973.
89. Brawley, R. K., and Morrow, A. G.: Direct Determination of Aortic Blood Flow in Patients with Aortic Regurgitation: Effects of Alterations in Afterload, and Isoproterenol, *Circulation,* 35:32, 1967.
90. Judge, T. P., Kennedy, J. W., Bennett, L. J., Willis, R. E., Murray, J. A., and Blackman, J. R.: Quantitative Hemodynamic Effects of Heart Rate in Aortic Regurgitation, *Circulation,* 44:355, 1971.
91. Morrow, A. G., Brawley, R. K., and Braunwald, E.: Effects of Aortic Regurgitation on Left Ventricular Performance: Direct Determination of Aortic Blood Flow Before and After Valve Replacement, *Circulation,* 31(suppl. 1):80, 1965.
92. Lingback, A. J.: Heart Failure from the Point of View of Quantitative Anatomy, *Am. J. Cardiol.,* 5:370, 1960.
93. Dodge, H. T., Kennedy, J. W., and Petersen, J.: Quantitative Angiographic Methods in the Evaluation of Valvular Heart Disease, *Prog. Cardiovasc. Dis.,* 16:1, 1973.
94. Basta, L. L., Raines, D., Najjar, S., and Kioschos, J. M.: Clinical, Hemodynamic, and Coronary Angiographic Correlates of Angina Pectoris in Patients with Severe Aortic Valve Disease, *Br. Heart J.,* 37:150, 1975.
95. Harvey, W. P., Segal, J. P., and Hufnagel, C. A.: Unusual Clinical Features Associated with Severe Aortic Insufficiency, *Ann. Intern. Med.,* 47:27, 1957.
96. Cohn, L. H., Mason, D. T., Ross, J., Jr., Morrow, A. G., and Braunwald, E.: Preoperative Assessment of Aortic Regurgitation in Patients with Mitral Valve Disease, *Am. J. Cardiol.,* 19:177, 1967.
97. Conn, R. D., and Cole, J. S.: The Cardiac Apex Impulse: Clinical and Angiographic Correlations, *Ann. Intern. Med.,* 75:185, 1971.
98. Groom, D., and Boone, J. A.: The Dove-Coo Murmur and Murmurs Heard at a Distance from the Chest Wall, *Ann. Intern. Med.,* 42:1214, 1955.
99. Porter, C. M., Baxley, W. A., Eddleman, E. E., Jr., Frimer, M., and Rackley, C. E.: Left Ventricular Dimensions and Dynamics of Filling in Patients with Gallop Heart Sounds, *Am. J. Med.,* 50:721, 1971.
100. Abdulla, A. M., Frank, M. J., Erdin, R. A., and Canedo, M. I.: Clinical Significance and Hemodynamic Correlates of the Third Heart Sound Gallop in Aortic Regurgitation: A Guide to Optimal Timing of Cardiac Catheterization, *Circulation,* 64:464, 1981.
101. Fortuin, N. J., and Craige, E.: On the Mechanism of the Austin Flint Murmur, *Circulation,* 45:558, 1972.
102. Wigle, E. D., and Labross, C. J.: Sudden, Severe Aortic Insufficiency, *Circulation,* 32:708, 1965.
103. Herbert, W. A.: Prolonged Atrioventricular Conduction and Aortic Insufficiency, *Thorax,* 25:577, 1970.
104. Selzer, A., Naruse, D. Y., York, E., Kahn, K. A., and Matthew, H. B.: Electrocardiographic Findings in Concentric and Eccentric Left Ventricular Hypertrophy, *Am. Heart J.,* 63:320, 1962.
105. Winsberg, F., Gabor, G. E., Hernberg, J. H., and Weiss, B.: Fluttering of the Mitral Valve in Aortic Insufficiency, *Circulation,* 41:225, 1970.
106. Pridie, R. B., Benham, M. B., and Oakley, C. M.: Echocardiography of the Mitral Valve in Aortic Valve Disease, *Br. Heart J.,* 33:296, 1971.
107. Wray, T. M.: The Variable Echocardiographic Features in Aortic Valve Endocarditis, *Circulation,* 52:658, 1975.
108. Stewart, J. A., Silimperi, D., Harris, P., Wise, N. K., Fraker, T. D., and Kisslo, J. A.: Echocardiographic Documentation of Vegetative Lesions in Infective Endocarditis: Clinical Implications, *Circulation,* 61:374, 1980.
109. Gramiak, R., and Shah, P. M.: Echocardiography of the Normal and Diseased Aortic Valve, *Radiology,* 96:1, 1970.
110. Pombo, J. F., Troy, B. L., and Russell, R. O., Jr.: Left Ventricular Volumes and Ejection Fraction by Echocardiography, *Circulation,* 43:480, 1971.
111. Paulsen, W., Boughner, D. R., Persaud, J., and Devries, L.: Aortic Regurgitation: Detection of Left Ventricular Dysfunction by Exercise Echocardiography, *Br. Heart J.,* 46:380, 1981.
112. Whipple, R. L., Morris, D. C., Felner, J. M., Merrill, A. J., and Miller, J. I.: Echocardiographic Manifestations of the Flail Aortic Valve Leaflet Syndrome, *J. Clin. Ultrasound,* 5:417, 1977.
113. Henry, W. L., Bonow, R. O., Borer, J. S., Ware, J. H., Kent, K. M., Redwood, D. R., McIntosh, C. L., Morrow, A. G., and Epstein, S. E.: Observations on the Optimum Time for Operative Intervention for Aortic Regurgitation. I. Evaluation of the Results of Aortic Valve Replacement in Symptomatic Patients, *Circulation,* 61:471, 1980.
114. Hunt, D., Baxley, W. A., Kennedy, J. W., Judge, T. P., Williams, J. E., and Dodge, H. T.: Quantitative Evaluation of Cineaortography in the Assessment of Aortic Regurgitation, *Am. J. Cardiol.,* 31:696, 1973.
115. Sandler, H., Dodge, H. T., Hay, R. E., and Rackley, C. E.: Quantitation of Valvular Insufficiency in Man by Angiocardiography, *Am. Heart J.,* 65:501, 1963.
116. Rackley, C. E., Dalldorf, F. G., Hood, W. P., Jr., and Wilcox, B. R.: Sarcomere Length and Left Ventricular Function in Chronic Heart Disease, *Am. J. Med. Sci.,* 259:90, 1970.
117. Osbakken, M., Bove, A. A., and Spann, J. F.: Left Ventricular Function in Chronic Aortic Regurgitation with Reference to End-Systolic Pressure, Volume and Stress Relations, *Am. J. Cardiol.,* 47:193, 1981.
118. Borer, J. S., Bacharach, S. L., Green, M. V., Kent, K. M., Henry, W. L., Rosing, D. R., Seides, S. F., Johnston, G. S., and Epstein, E. S.: Exercise-Induced Left Ventricular Dysfunction in Symptomatic and Asymptomatic Patients with Aortic Regurgitation: Assessment with Radionuclide Cineangiography, *Am. J. Cardiol.,* 42:351, 1978.
119. Borer, J. S., Bacharach, S. L., and Green, M. V.: Radionuclide Cineangiography at Rest and During Exercise in the Evaluation of Patients with Heart Disease, *Cardiovasc. Review & Repeats,* 1:31, 1980.
120. Baxter, R. H., Becker, L. C., Alderson, P. O., Rigo, P., Wagner, H. N., and Weisfeldt, M. L.: Quantification of Aortic Valvular Regurgitation in Dogs by Nuclear Imaging, *Circulation,* 61:404, 1980.
121. Ritchie, J. L., Zaret, B. L., Strauss, H. W., Pitt, B., Berman, D. S., Schelbert, H. R., Ashburn, W. L., Berger, H. J., and Hamilton, G. W.: Myocardial Imaging with Thallium-201: A Multicenter Study in Patients with Angina Pectoris or Acute Myocardial Infarction, *Am. J. Cardiol.,* 42:345, 1978.
122. Turner, J. D., Schwartz, K. M., Logic, J. R., Sheffield, L. T., Kansal, S., Roitman, D. I., Mantle, J. A., Russell, R. O., Jr., Rackley, C. E., and Rogers, W. J.: Detection of Residual Jeopardized Myocardium Three Weeks after Myocardial Infarction by Exercise Testing with Thallium-201 Myocardial Scintigraphy, *Circulation,* 61:729, 1980.
123. Hecht, H. S., and Hopkins, J. M.: Exercise-Induced Regional Wall Motion Abnormalities in the Presence of Valvular Heart Disease, *Am. J. Cardiol.,* 47:861, 1981.
124. Sheffield, L. T., and Roitman, D. I.: Stress Testing Methodology, *Prog. Cardiovasc. Dis.,* 19:33, 1976.
125. Goldschlager, N., Pfeifer, J., Cohn, K., Popper, R., and Sel-

zer, A.: The Natural History of Aortic Regurgitation: A Clinical and Hemodynamic Study, *Am. J. Med.*, 54:577, 1973.
126. Greves, J., Rahimtoola, S. H., McAnulty, J. H., DeMots, H., Clark, D. G., Greenberg, B., and Starr, A.: Preoperative Criteria Predictive of Late Survival Following Valve Replacement for Severe Aortic Regurgitation, *Am. Heart J.*, 101:300, 1981.
127. Greenberg, B. H., DeMots, H., Murphy, E., and Rahimtoola, S. H.: Mechanism for Improved Cardiac Performance with Arteriolar Dilators in Aortic Insufficiency, *Circulation*, 63:263, 1981.
128. McDonald, G. R., Schaff, H. V., Pyeritz, R. E., McKusick, V. A., and Gott, V. L.: Surgical Management of Patients with the Marfan Syndrome and Dilatation of the Ascending Aorta, *J. Thorac. Cardiovasc. Surg.*, 81:180, 1981.
129. Dismukes, W. E.: Management of Infective Endocarditis, in C. E. Rackley and A. N. Brest (eds.), "Critical Care Cardiology," F. A. Davis, Philadelphia, Cardiovascular Clinics, 1981, pp. 189–208.
130. Croft, C. H., Woodward, W., Elliott, A., Commerford, P. J., Barnard, C. N., and Beck, W.: Analysis of Surgical versus Medical Therapy in Active Complicated Native Valve Infective Endocarditis, *Am. J. Cardiol.*, 51:1650, 1983.
131. Richardson, J. V., Karp, R. B., Kirklin, J. W., and Dismukes, W. E.: Treatment of Infective Endocarditis: A 10 Year Computer Analysis, *Circulation*, 58:589, 1978.
132. Danielson, G. K., Titus, J. L., and Dushane, J. W.: Successful Treatment of Aortic Valve Endocarditis and Aortic Root Abscess by Insertion of Prosthetic Valve in Ascending Aorta and Placement of Bypass Grafts to Coronary Arteries, *J. Thorac. Cardiovasc. Surg.*, 67:443, 1974.
133. Symbas, P. N., Vlasis, S. E., Zacharopoulos, L., and Lutz, J. F.: Acute Endocarditis: Surgical Treatment of Aortic Regurgitation and Aortico-Left Ventricular Discontinuity, *J. Thorac. Cardiovasc. Surg.*, 84:291, 1982.
134. Applebaum, A., Karp, R. B., and Kirklin, J. W.: Ascending vs. Descending Aortic Dissections, *Ann. Surg.*, 183:296, 1976.
135. Bentall, H., and deBono, A.: A Technique for Computer Replacement of the Ascending Aorta, *Thorax*, 23:338, 1968.
136. Cunha, C. L. P., Giuliani, E. R., Fuster, V., Seward, J. B., Brandenberg, R. O., and McGoon, D. C.: Preoperative M-mode Echocardiography as a Predictor of Surgical Results in Chronic Aortic Insufficiency, *J. Thorac. Cardiovasc. Surg.*, 79: 256, 1980.

38

Mitral Valve Disease*

Charles E. Rackley, M.D.
Jesse E. Edwards, M.D.
Robert B. Karp, M.D.

Mitral Stenosis

In examining the extraordinary dilatation of the body of the pulmonary vein, and its common openings, I perceived that the mouth of the left ventricle appeared very small and that it had an oval oblong shape.

Raymond Vieussens, 1715[1]

Etiology

Reduced diastolic flow across the mitral valve can result from rheumatic valvulitis, congenital stenosis, thrombus formation, atrial myxoma, bacterial vegetation, and calcification in the valve as well as in the annulus.[2–6] Rheumatic fever remains the most common cause of mitral stenosis and in temperate zones outside the United States, severe mitral stenosis can occur in children and adolescents.

*The editor-in-chief wishes to thank John W. Kirklin, M.D., for his previous contribution to the chapter on this subject that appeared in the fifth edition of *The Heart*.

Pathology

Mitral stenosis usually is the result of recurrent rheumatic endocarditis. The valvular leaflets and the chordae tendineae are affected by scarring with concomitant contracture (Fig. 38-1). An additional feature is that at each of the two junctional areas (the commissures) between the two major leaflets there is interadhesion between the two leaflets. This process, along with concomitant shortening of the chordae, causes the two interadherent leaflets to be held downward. The entire process is manifested by the leaflets' forming a funnel-shaped structure. The inlet to the funnel is at the level of the left atrial floor and is wider than the apex, which presents in the ventricular cavity.

In the normal heart, blood flows freely through the mitral valve. It may flow through the principal orifice, that part of the opening which lies between the papillary muscles, or through multiple secondary orifices, which are the spaces between the chordae[7] (Fig. 38-2). In rheumatic mitral stenosis,

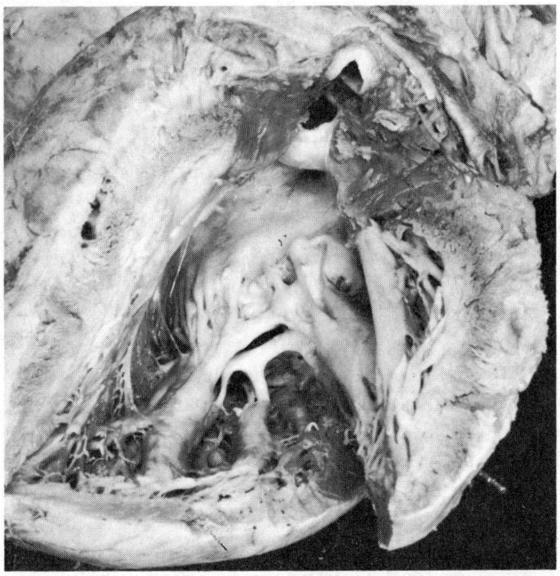

FIGURE 38-1 Mitral valve viewed from below in a case of mitral stenosis. The valve is converted into a funnel-shaped structure, the apex of which is in the left ventricle and is narrow.

because of interchordal fusion the secondary orifices are narrowed or obliterated and, by virtue of commissural fusion, the principal orifice is reduced in size. The anterior leaflet of the stenotic mitral valve frequently exhibits a deformity. Near its basal aspect the leaflet is convex toward the left atrium. It is possible that in early left ventricular diastole the deformity is buckled in the opposite direction and that this may account for the "opening snap" of mitral stenosis. Such movement does not affect the caliber of the effective orifice, which lies at a lower level. The deformity may contribute to closure of the valve as the prominence of the anterior leaflet is pressed against the base of the opposite leaflet during ventricular systole. Secondary effects of mitral stenosis include calcification of leaflet tissue, left atrial enlargement, and signs of pulmonary venous hypertension, including right ventricular hypertrophy.[8]

FIGURE 38-2 Diagrammatic portrayal of the normal mitral valve viewed from below. The principal orifice of the valve lies bounded anteriorly by the anterior leaflet, posteriorly by the posterior leaflet, and laterally by each papillary muscle and its related chordae. *A.* Secondary orifices lie in the spaces between the chordae tendineae and, for the most part, blood flowing through these orifices enters the left ventricle lateral to the respective papillary muscles. *B.* Diagrammatic portrayal of the stenotic mitral valve viewed from below. The principal orifice is narrow and, on the basis of commissural and chordal fusion, the secondary orifices are obliterated. *(From R. V. Bonnabeau, Jr., J. E. Stevenson, and J. E. Edwards, Obliteration of the Principal Orifice of the Stenotic Mitral Valve: A Rare Form of Restenosis, J. Thorac. Cardiovasc. Surg., 49:265, 1965. Reproduced with permission from the publisher and author.)*

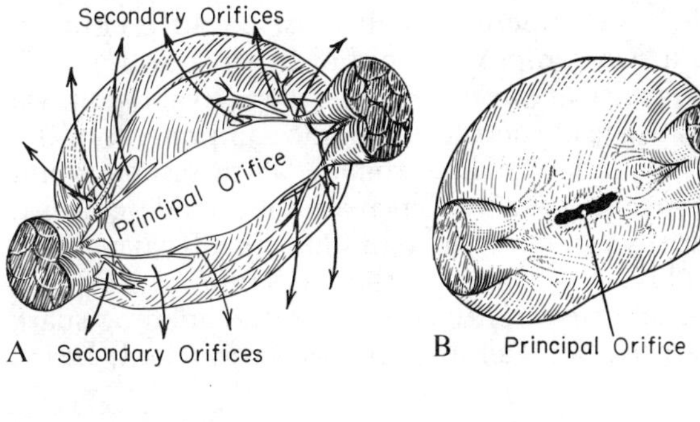

Fragmentation of leaflet tissue at calcific foci may lead to thrombosis upon the valvular surfaces and/or embolism of calcific material. Among the complications, thrombosis of the left atrial appendage and varying portions of the main left atrium is common, as is secondary systemic embolism.[9] Episodes of acute pulmonary edema and protracted right ventricular failure are common lethal complications.

Nonrheumatic mitral stenosis is rare in the adult. In the infant and child mitral stenosis results either from dysplasia of the valve or from the "parachute" deformity. Uncommonly, subjects with parachute mitral valve survive to adult life.[10,11]

Abnormal Physiology

Obstruction to flow across the mitral valve during the diastolic filling period of the left ventricle produces a pressure gradient between the left atrium and the left ventricular chamber. The pressure gradient is related to orifice size and diastolic flow through the mitral valve, which is determined by the cardiac output and the duration of diastole. The obstruction to flow increases the left atrial pressure and volume, which are further reflected to the pulmonary veins, capillaries, and eventually the pulmonary arteries. Chronic elevation of left atrial pressure will cause hyperplasia and hypertrophy of the pulmonary vessels, including the veins, capillaries, and arteries. Eventually, right ventricular hypertrophy results from the pulmonary arterial pressure. When noncompliant changes develop in the pulmonary veins, a redistribution of the flow pattern changes from the base to the apex of the lungs. Chronic mitral stenosis imposes a pressure overload on the left atrium, the pulmonary vascular tree, and the right ventricle.[12] Left ventricular function can deteriorate as a result of diminished diastolic filling from the left atrium, but analyses of the contractile state of the ventricular myocardium demonstrate preservation even with severe mitral stenosis.[13,14] Right ventricular function may remain normal even with moderate pulmonary hypertension.[15]

Clinical Manifestations

History

Approximately 50 percent of patients with recognized mitral stenosis recall a history of acute rheumatic fever[16] (see Chap. 62). The most frequent complaints in symptomatic patients with mitral stenosis are dyspnea, fatigue, palpitations, and hemoptysis.[17,18] Less frequently, hoarseness, chest pain, seizures, or a cerebrovascular accident from an embolus may be the initial symptom. The most prominent complaint in mitral stenosis is dyspnea due to pulmonary venous hypertension.[17]

In the early stage of mitral valve obstruction, conditions such as sudden development of atrial fibrillation with a rapid ventricular response, physical exertion, fever, emotional upsets, and pregnancy can increase mitral valve flow during diastole and elevate left atrial and pulmonary venous pressures and produce *pulmonary edema.*[18,19] *Fatigue* is another clinical manifestation of mitral stenosis and occasionally can be more severe than dyspnea. Right ventricular overload can result in hepatic congestion and peripheral edema. *Hemoptysis* caused by pulmonary venous hypertension is a significant symptom in mitral stenosis. On rare occasions, the bleeding can be massive and require emergency measures.[20] *Palpitations* in mitral stenosis are usually due to atrial fibrillation which can be paroxysmal or sustained.[18] A rapid ventricular response can aggravate pulmonary congestion and cause dyspnea and fatigue.

Less frequent symptoms in mitral stenosis include *chest pain,* which can be due to "pulmonary hypertension," underlying coronary artery disease, or a pulmonary embolism.[21] *Hoarseness* can result from enlargement of the left atrium and compression of the recurrent laryngeal nerve. Systemic emboli to the central nervous system can cause a stroke or seizure.[22]

Physical Examination

In the early stages of mitral stenosis, the characteristic *apical diastolic rumble* may not be recognized on routine cardiac auscultation unless the patient is exercised, and auscultation performed in the left lateral decubitus position. (See Chap. 11.) In more advanced obstruction to mitral valve flow, a resting tachycardia, often with atrial fibrillation, is present. The patient may reveal the mitral facies with *malar flush* and peripheral cyanosis. The *neck veins will be distended* if right ventricular failure is present. The venous pulsation should be examined closely for presence of a *v wave indicating tricuspid regurgitation* or, rarely, an *a* wave which may be due to concomitant tricuspid stenosis. On cardiac examination, the typical findings of mitral stenosis are the *accentuated first heart sound,* an *opening snap,* and a *diastolic rumble at the apex.* If pulmonary hypertension and right ventricular hypertrophy have developed, a right ventricular lift may be palpated along the left sternal border.[23] In advanced mitral stenosis, palpation may detect the accentuated first sound at the apex and vibration from the diastolic rumble. If significant right ventricular enlargement or severe left atrial dilatation have developed, there may be dullness to the right of the sternum.

Characteristically, auscultation at the apex reveals an accentuated first sound and an opening snap followed by a diastolic rumble. Accentuation of the first heart sound in mitral stenosis is due to sudden cessation of the upward motion of the valve which has been depressed in the left ventricular chamber during diastolic filling due to the gradient across the valve.[24–26] The mobility of the valve leaflets, the diastolic gradient across the valve, and the PR interval of the electrocardiogram all contribute to the intensity of the first sound.[27] Shortening of the PR interval by tachycardia, fever, or thyrotoxicosis can all accentuate the first heart sound. When mitral valve mobility is diminished due to calcification of the leaflet, as well as associated mitral regurgitation, the first sound diminishes in intensity.

The opening snap is considered the most important physical sound of mitral stenosis[17] (Fig. 38-3). The sound is produced during maximum excursion of the anterior leaflet of the mitral valve. The opening snap can occur from 0.03 to 0.14 s after the second heart sound.[28] The higher the left atrial pressure, the shorter will be the interval between aortic valve closure and the opening snap (2-OS). Critical mitral stenosis produces a 2-OS time less than 0.08 s. The time-interval expression (Q-1)-(2-OS) time has been used to estimate the severity of mitral stenosis.[29] The time from the onset of the QRS complex on the electrocardiogram to the first heart sound (Q-S1) is delayed in mitral stenosis and the 2-OS reflects the level of the left atrial pressure. Additional factors such as valve mobility, calcification, cardiac output, left ventricular systolic pressure, and relaxation of the left ventricle can influence the (Q-1)-(2-OS) time.[30,31] Opening snaps have also been recognized in other conditions, such as mitral regurgitation, ventricular septal defect, second and third degree heart block, tricuspid atresia with a large atrial septal defect, and tetralogy of Fallot after a Blalock-Taussig procedure.[32,33] An atrial myxoma can also produce an early diastolic sound similar to the opening snap.[3] Finally, a tricuspid origin must be considered in the differential diagnosis of an opening snap, since these sounds can also be generated by the tricuspid valve with tricuspid stenosis, atrial septal defect, or Ebstein's anomaly.[34–36]

The opening snap is best heard with the diaphragm of the stethoscope at the apex, but sometimes it is audible along the left sternal border, at the base of the heart, and rarely, in the suprasternal notch.[37] The opening snap must be differentiated from a two-component second heart sound as well as a ventricular protodiastolic gallop. Inspiration will separate the aortic and pulmonic components of the second sound. The time from the aortic second sound to the opening snap will increase with standing, which decreases venous return and lowers left atrial pressure.[38] Exercise shortens the 2-OS time by elevating left atrial pressure. In contrast to the opening snap, the ventricular gallop sound is low-pitched, heard

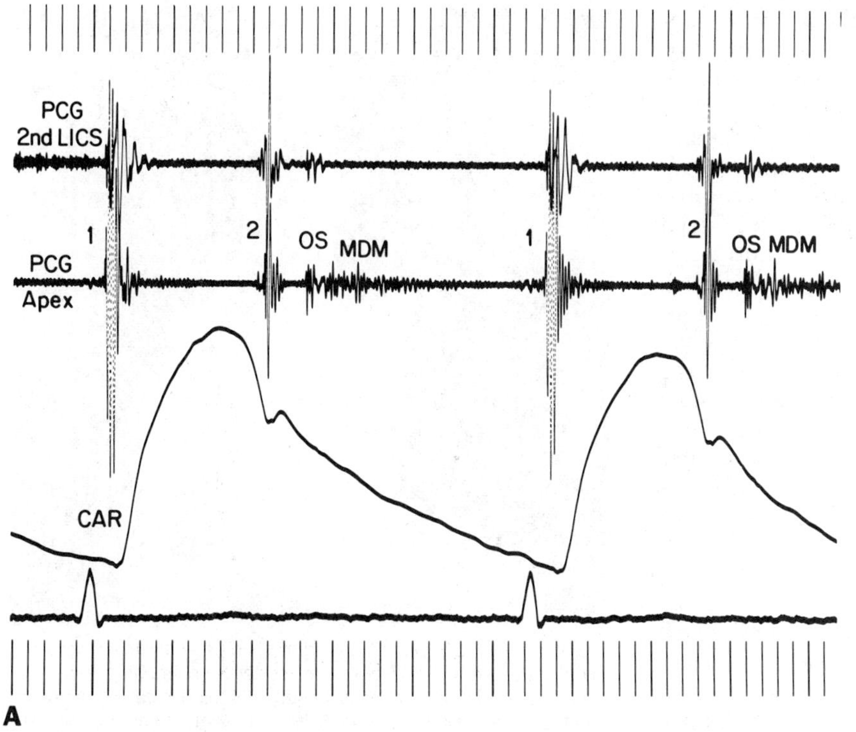

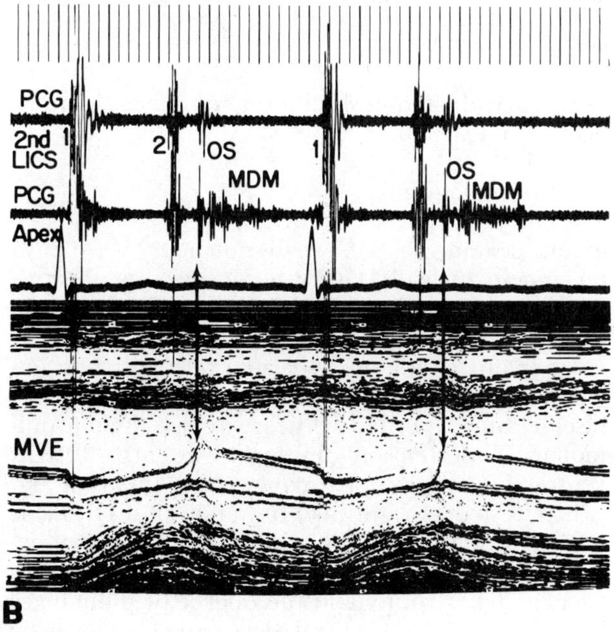

FIGURE 38-3 Phonocardiogram and carotid pulse recording in mitral stenosis and atrial fibrillation. *A.* A loud first sound (1), opening snap of the mitral valve occurs 0.11 s after the second heart sound, which is in turn followed by a low-frequency mid-diastolic murmur at the cardiac apex. *B.* The phonocardiogram on the same patient at a slower paper speed (50 mm/s) shows a relation between the first heart sound and completion of closing movement of the mitral valve and, similarly, the opening snap accompanying the termination of the opening movement of the valve. (*Courtesy Dr. Ernest Craige.*)

best with the bell of the stethoscope, and occurs 0.12 s or later after the second sound. If right ventricular failure has developed, the right ventricular gallop sound may be audible in the area of the apex.

A diastolic rumble is usually present in mitral stenosis but can be difficult to detect at rest during the early stages of the disease or diminished in the late stages with a decrease of mitral valve flow (Fig. 38-3). The murmur is low-pitched, best heard with the bell of the stethoscope placed lightly on the chest wall, and becomes crescendo in the latter phase of diastole with atrial contraction. Echocardiographic valve motion has revealed that the middiastolic rumble occurs as the mitral leaflets return toward the closed position despite continued flow.[39] Although the presystolic component of the rumble is augmented by atrial contraction, rarely this phase of the murmur will increase with atrial fibrillation.[40,41]

The diastolic rumble may be localized to a small area of the apex and becomes audible only after the patient turns to the left lateral decubitus position or following exercise. The intensity of the murmur does not necessarily relate to the severity of mitral stenosis. A rumble which starts with the opening snap and continues to the first heart sound suggests more severe impairment to flow across the valve. The rumble may diminish or disappear in the late stages of the disease when the cardiac output declines. Other conditions associated with a mitral diastolic rumble include a left atrial myxoma, a Blalock-to-left atrial shunt, cor triatriatum, calcification of the mitral annulus, pericardial constriction of the AV groove around the mitral apparatus, and the Carey-Coombs murmur in acute rheumatic fever.[3,42–44] Aortic regurgitation impinging on the anterior leaflet of the mitral valve can produce the Austin Flint rumble across the mitral valve. Sometimes the Graham Steell murmur of pulmonic insufficiency may be similar to that associated with aortic insufficiency, but peripheral signs may be helpful in differentiating an aortic or pulmonic origin.[45]

Chest Roentgenogram

The radiographic changes (see Chap. 15) of mitral stenosis (Fig. 38-4) are produced by left atrial hypertension and result in left atrial enlargement, alterations in pulmonary venous pattern, prominence of the pulmonary arteries, and right ventricular enlargement. Since the appendage occupies a position between the pulmonary artery segment and the left ventricle, left atrial enlargement can often be detected on the standard posteroanterior chest film and contributes to straightening of the left cardiac border.[46] The left atrium also enlarges to the right of the spine and can be recognized as a double density along the right cardiac border. A barium swallow will often demonstrate left atrial impingement on the esophagus.

In chronic pulmonary venous hypertension, there is not only prominence of the vessels but also a redistribution of the flow toward the apices of the lung. When the elevated pulmonary capillary pressure exceeds the oncotic pressure of the plasma proteins, which usually ranges from 20 to 25 mmHg, fluid will accumulate in the interstitial space of the lungs.[47] The interlobular septal changes and the linear shadows perpendicular to the pleura at the bases of the lungs were described by Kerley, and the Kerley B lines are frequently identified with elevated capillary pressure at the costophrenic angle.[48] Although pulmonary venous hypertension can redistribute blood flow to the upper lobes, acute elevation of the pulmonary venous pressure will cause pulmonary edema with interstitial and alveolar extravasation of fluid.[49,50] Pulmonary arterial hypertension in mitral stenosis will enlarge the pulmonary arteries. Eventually, right ventricular dilatation and hypertrophy result from the pressure overload on the right ventricle and can be detected on the lateral chest roentgenogram. The radiographic features of left atrial enlargement, redistribution of pulmonary venous flow, interstitial edema, enlargement of pulmonary arteries, and right ventricular dilatation should suggest mitral stenosis, but are not specific.

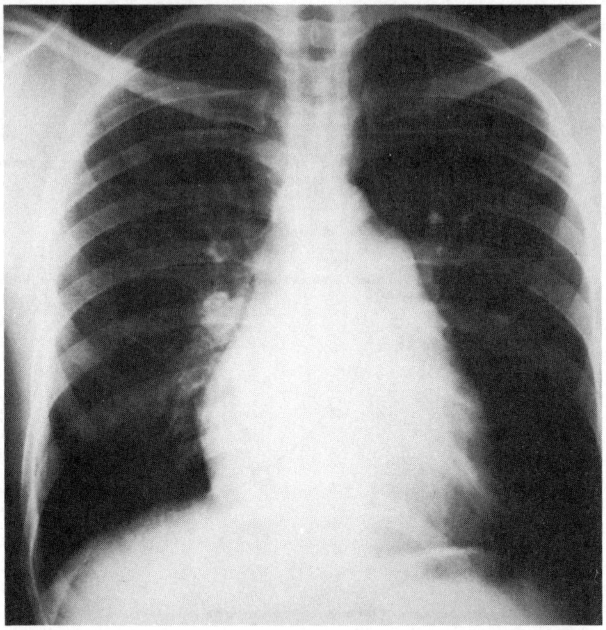

FIGURE 38-4 Chest roentgenogram of a patient with a calculated mitral valve area of 0.7 cm^2 and moderate pulmonary hypertension. Tricuspid regurgitation is evident on the physical examination, and the increase in the cardiac silhouette is due to right ventricular dilatation. Left atrial enlargement contributes to the heart shadow to the right of the spine and the left atrial appendage is seen along the left cardiac border. (*Courtesy of Dr. I. Sylvia Crawley.*)

Electrocardiogram

The characteristic electrocardiographic abnormality in mitral stenosis is the broad, notched P wave most prominent in lead II with a conspicuous negative terminal deflection in lead V_1 (Fig. 38-5).[51] Atrial fibrillation is common in mitral stenosis but can develop in any condition associated with left atrial enlargement as well as in the course of coronary artery disease and hypertensive heart disease. When pulmonary hypertension develops, evidence of right ventricular hypertrophy may become apparent and is manifested as rightward deviation of a QRS axis in the frontal plane. Unfortunately, correlation between electrocardiographic evidence of right ventricular hypertrophy and the degree of pulmonary hypertension of the mitral valve area has not been a predictable one.[52,53]

Special Laboratory Studies

Echocardiography (see Chap. 120) Echocardiography has become one of the most reliable noninvasive techniques in the detection of mitral valve stenosis.[54–56] A characteristic alteration is a decrease in the EF slope of the anterior leaflet of the mitral valve, which results in a characteristic square-wave configuration on the echocardiogram. Other abnormalities include abnormal posterior leaflet movement, decreased mitral valve motion, and thick echoes

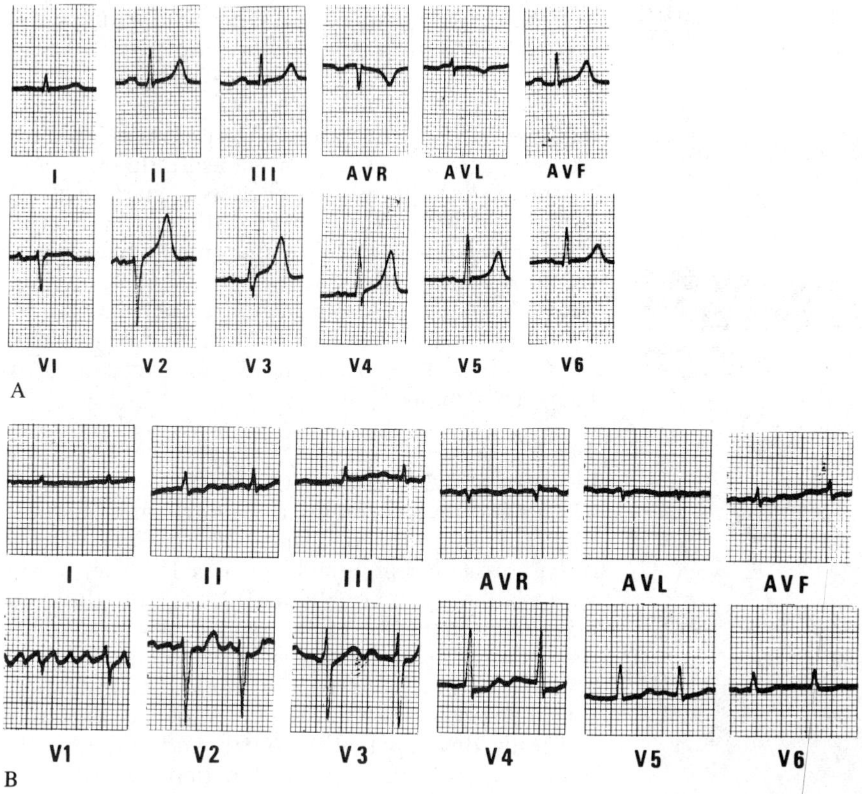

FIGURE 38-5 Electrocardiograms of a patient with mitral stenosis. The tracings were made 7 years apart, in which time the patient's symptoms and hemodynamic findings progressed. *A.* Left atrial abnormality and a +60° frontal QRS axis. *B.* Atrial fibrillation with coarse fibrillatory waves in a +85 percent frontal QRS axis. (*Courtesy of Dr. I. Sylvia Crawley.*)

around the valve suggesting calcification. The EF slope has been quantitated and a value less than 10 mm/s is usually associated with severe mitral stenosis.[56] Additional information on left atrial enlargement, right ventricular enlargement, and left ventricular dimensions can be obtained from the echocardiogram.

Another valuable contribution of the echocardiogram is detecting nonrheumatic mitral valve obstruction such as left atrial myxoma[57–59] (Fig. 38-6). Multiple echoes from a tumor are characteristic and there is usually displacement of the anterior leaflet.[57] Echocardiography has also improved detection of left atrial thrombi and can sometimes outline the nidus of infection in bacterial endocarditis on the mitral valve.[60] Vegetations and calcification on the leaflets can be delineated by the echoes. The clinical course of patients with mitral stenosis can be followed with serial echocardiograms before and after surgery.

Cardiac Catheterization (see Chap. 108) Cardiac catheterization in mitral stenosis can provide a recording of the gradient across the mitral valve, data for calculation of the mitral valve area, response of pulmonary artery pressure to exercise, recognition of other valvular lesions, assessment of ventricular function, and delineation of coronary artery anatomy.

The gradient across the mitral valve is obtained by simultaneously recording the pulmonary capillary wedge pressure or the direct left atrial pressure and the left ventricular pressure. Cardiac output is obtained at the time of mitral valve gradient recording and these measurements can be utilized in the Gorlin hydraulic formula to calculate mitral orifice size.[61–63] Mitral valve area is directly proportional to the diastolic flow across the valve and inversely related to the square root of the diastolic pressure gradient. The normal mitral valve area is 4 to 6 cm^2 and hemodynamic abnormalities develop when the valve is reduced to 1.5 to 2.5 cm^2. Pulmonary congestion often occurs when the valve size is reduced to 1.1 to 1.5 cm^2. With a mitral valve area less than 1.0 cm^2 pulmonary hypertension, right ventricular failure, and reduced cardiac output are generally present.

Symptomatic patients with mitral stenosis usually present a capillary wedge pressure greater than 15 to 20 mmHg.[64] Pulmonary artery pressure in severe mitral stenosis can approach systemic blood pressure due to severe arteriolar vasoconstriction and capillary hyperplasia. If the pulmonary artery diastolic pressure greatly exceeds the capillary wedge pressure, an increase in pulmonary vascular resistance will be calculated. In severe pulmonary hypertension, wedging the catheter may be technically difficult and transseptal puncture into the left atrium becomes necessary. Excessive elevations of pulmonary artery pressure may be attended by a reduction in cardiac outpout. If the patient is symptomatic and wedge pressure does not exceed 15 to 20 mmHg, some form of exercise should be performed in the catheterization laboratory. A striking rise in pul-

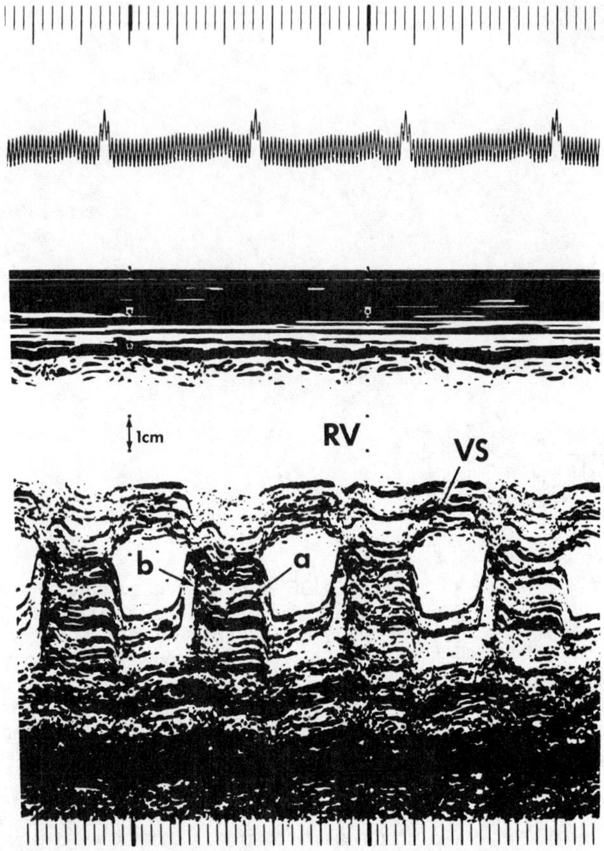

FIGURE 38-6 Echocardiogram of a left atrial myxoma. Arrow *a* points to the tumor, and arrow *b* points to the clear space, which is the time required for the tumor to move from the left atrium to the left ventricle. RV = right ventricle; VS = ventricular septum. (*Courtesy of Dr. Joel M. Felner.*)

monary artery pressure may be noted with a subnormal response of the cardiac output to exercise. However, right ventricular function has been shown angiographically to remain normal even with moderate pulmonary hypertension.

Left ventricular dysfunction has also been documented in isolated mitral stenosis, and segmental as well as global wall motion abnormalities have been described.[13–15,65–67] Left ventricular angiography is usually performed to detect concomitant mitral regurgitation and in the adult patient over 40 years, coronary arteriography should be done to delineate anatomy.[68]

Radionuclide Studies (see Chap. 109) Radionuclide techniques can assess left ventricular function for measurements of ejection fraction, end-diastolic volume, stroke volume, cardiac output, and diastolic filling rate before and after bicycle exercise.[69] The assessment of right ventricular function in patients with mitral or aortic valve disease can provide additional information which cannot be obtained from right-sided pressure measurements alone. Perhaps the greatest contribution of the radiographic techniques in mitral stenosis is the opportunity to obtain measurements before and during follow-up periods after corrective surgery which can document the course of the disease as well as improvement after mitral valve surgery.

Exercise Testing In the early clinical phase of mitral stenosis, exercise testing can be useful in evaluating symptomatic response as well as assessing functional capacity. A reduced response of the cardiac output of exercise has been the hemodynamic hallmark of mitral stenosis.[64] Exercise can be useful to demonstrate hemodynamic abnormalities should they be found normal at rest and to document the benefit of drugs such as propranolol for the control of tachyarrhythmias.[70–72]

Natural History and Prognosis

Rheumatic fever remains the most common cause of mitral stenosis worldwide. The average age of onset for acute rheumatic fever is 12 years of age with a latent period of about 19 years from the acute episode to detection of a murmur of mitral stenosis.[17] Thus, a patient experiencing rheumatic fever at age 12 could be expected to exhibit findings of mitral stenosis at about age 31. Cardiac symptoms generally develop in the fourth and fifth decade. Approximately 50 percent of patients will develop symptoms gradually while remaining individuals experience precipitation of symptoms from complications such as atrial fibrillation.[18]

Dyspnea and fatigue are the most common symptoms and can be attributed to pulmonary hypertension and right ventricular failure. Atrial fibrillation, fever, emotion, or pregnancy can increase the cardiac and abruptly elevate the pulmonary capillary pressure with the production of pulmonary edema. Longstanding elevation of pulmonary capillary pressure can generate levels of pulmonary arterial hypertension that approach systemic values. Severe pulmonary hypertension will gradually reduce the cardiac output and the pressure overload will lead to dilatation of the right ventricle. The typical picture of right-sided heart failure thus follows, with neck vein distension, hepatic enlargement, ascites, and peripheral edema. Physical findings are those of pulmonary hypertension, right ventricular failure, and venous congestion with *v* waves in the jugular veins reflecting tricuspid incompetence. The electrocardiogram and the chest x-ray will demonstrate evidence of pulmonary hypertension, right ventricular hypertrophy, and failure. The prognosis at this stage is poor but still may be improved with surgical intervention.

Atrial fibrillation develops in 40 to 50 percent of patients with mitral stenosis, particularly in those over the age of 40. The chronic left atrial pressure overload, as well as histologic changes that take place in the atrial wall, contributes to the development of atrial fibrillation. The left atrium may further dilate with the onset of fibrillation. The hemodynamic abnormality imposed on the left ventricle in mitral stenosis with atrial fibrillation is a rapid ventricular response, shortening of the diastolic filling period, elevation of left atrial pressure, and loss of the atrial contraction contribution to ventricular filling. These disturbances reduce cardiac output. Initially, atrial fibrillation may be paroxysmal or readily respond to pharmacologic agents or cardioversion. As the atrial fibrillation becomes more chronic, there is resistance to cardioversion.

One of the most serious complications of mitral stenosis is systemic embolization, and the incidence ranges from 9 to 20 percent.[73] The history of atrial fibrillation as well as the age of the patient appear associated with a high incidence of systemic embolization. However, the severity of the stenosis, size of the left atrium, and the development of heart failure do not consistently correlate with embolic complications. Systemic embolization may develop either pre- or postoperatively in the course of mitral stenosis, and mitral stenosis should always be considered as a possible mechanism in systemic embolization, especially in a young female.[74] Neurological symptoms from a cerebral embolus can sometimes be the presenting manifestation of mitral stenosis.

Bacterial endocarditis is infrequent in isolated mitral stenosis, but a prolonged fever should always raise this possibility. A left atrial myxoma should be considered in the presence of fever, arthralgias, anemia, and systemic embolization.

The prognosis of patients with mitral stenosis depends on the presence or absence of symptoms at the first examination. In Rapaport's series of randomly selected patients, 80 percent were alive at 5 years and 60 percent survived 10 years[75] (Fig. 38-7). The average age at the time of death in patients with medically managed mitral stenosis is 48 years.[76]

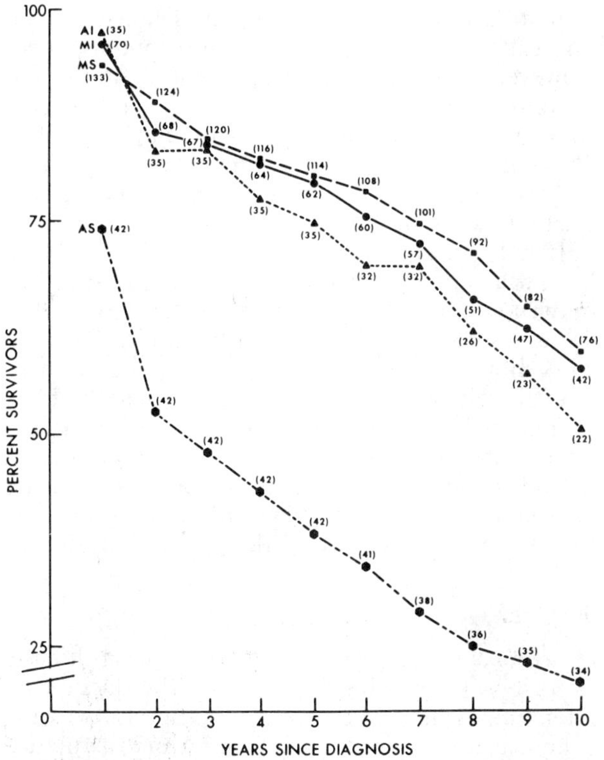

FIGURE 38-7 Actuarial survival in valvular heart disease treated medically, from time of diagnosis. AI = aortic insufficiency; MI = mitral insufficiency; MS = mitral stenosis; and AS = aortic stenosis. (*From E. Rapaport, Natural History of Aortic and Mitral Valve Disease, Am. J. Cardiol., 35:221, 1975. Reproduced with permission from the publisher and author.*)

Treatment

Medical

Medical management of mitral stenosis cannot relieve the obstruction of flow through the valve; therefore, efforts are directed at prevention of rheumatic fever and bacterial endocarditis. Rheumatic fever prophylaxis should continue until age 30 years (see Chap. 56). For dental procedures and bronchoscopy, adults should be given 600,000 units procaine penicillin G mixed with 1,000,000 units aqueous penicillin G intramuscularly 30 to 60 min before the procedure and 500 mg penicillin V orally q 6 h for 2 days.[77] If the patient is allergic to penicillin, erythromycin 1 g orally 1 to 2 h before the procedure and 500 mg q 6 h for 2 days should be given. With a prosthetic mitral valve, penicillin as described intramuscularly plus streptomycin 1 g intramuscularly should be given 30 to 60 min before the procedure and followed by penicillin V 500 mg orally every 6 h for 2 days. For gastrointestinal and genitourinary surgery 2,000,000 units of aqueous penicillin G intramuscularly or intravenously, or 1 g ampicillin intramuscularly or intravenously plus gentamycin 1.5 mg/kg (not to exceed 80 mg) intramuscularly or intravenously, or streptomycin 1 g intramuscularly should be given 30 to 60 min before the procedure. If gentamycin is used, it should be repeated every 8 h for 2 additional doses, or if streptomycin is used, every 12 h for 2 additional doses. If the patient is allergic to penicillin, vancomycin plus streptomycin should be substituted.

Digitalis can slow the ventricular response to atrial fibrillation, and in paroxysmal atrial fibrillation the drug may prevent recurrence of atrial irritability. Propranolol (Inderal) may also be needed to control the ventricular response. Quinidine can also be added to suppress atrial irritability and convert the rhythm to normal sinus rhythm. Should symptoms of pulmonary congestion develop with atrial fibrillation and a rapid ventricular response, cardioversion should be considered. With chronic atrial fibrillation, elective anticoagulation should be instituted 2 weeks prior to electrical cardioversion. Following successful cardioversion, digitalis and quinidine are continued to prevent recurrence of atrial irritability. After 3 months, the quinidine may be discontinued if the patient remains in sinus rhythm.

Systemic embolization requires anticoagulation treatment, usually for an indefinite period. If the embolus is to an extremity or the mesenteric system, surgical consideration should be contemplated. However, a systemic embolus is not an indication for mitral valve surgery, since the embolic phenomena can occur in milder forms of mitral stenosis. Symptoms of dyspnea and fatigue due to pulmonary venous congestion require evaluation for surgical intervention in mitral stenosis.

If mitral valve surgery is planned, dental repair as well as any minor surgery should be corrected under antibiotic coverage on an elective basis. Medications such as digitalis, diuretics, and anticoagulants should be reviewed and possibly discontinued immediately prior to surgery. Electrolytes should be examined for possible potassium depletion. If the patient has been on anticoagulants for a prolonged period, Coumadin should be discontinued several days before surgery and heparin can be substituted until the patient is taken to the operating room.

Surgical

Indications for Surgery For valvular heart disease, as in most other disease processes, the decision to intervene surgically is based on an appraisal of what is known concerning the natural history of the disease untreated or treated medically compared to the early and late results of surgical intervention. Analysis of the prognosis of patients with valvular heart disease treated medically depends on the stage of the disease at which the patient is first seen.[75] Three decades ago Olesen[76] reported that 20 percent of patients with mitral stenosis died within 1 year from the time that they were first seen. Within 10 years, 60 percent were dead. In the survivors there was progressive cardiac disability. This disability is usually gradual, although temporary plateaus of remarkable exercise tolerance occur. More recently, Rapaport[75] reported an 80 percent 5-year survival of patients followed from the time of first diagnosis (Fig. 38-7). It is apparent that the decision to intervene surgically must be based on the state of the disease process in any individual patient, and the New York Heart Association (NYHA) classification for functional disability is a convenient way to stratify these patients.

Because valve replacement is associated with more late complications than are reconstructive procedures, the decision to intervene surgically in mitral stenosis is partially based on the anticipated necessity of valve replacement versus reconstruction. In general, if there is a high probability of a reconstructive procedure, earlier operation is justified. In pure mitral stenosis, mitral commissurotomy is the procedure of choice. The commissurotomy can be done closed (without cardiopulmonary bypass) or open. In areas such as the Middle East and Far East where there is a relatively large group of patients with juvenile or third-decade pure mitral stenosis, closed commissurotomy remains the favored procedure. With certain exceptions, open commissurotomy has replaced the less precise closed method in the United States. At the present time, a mitral commissurotomy is offered to patients in functional classes II-B, III, and IV. These classes include the development of symptoms which interfere with a patient's productivity and enjoyment of life such as dyspnea, effort intolerance, and then, later, fluid retention, orthopnea, paroxysmal dyspnea, and, finally, weight loss. It is well known that the onset of atrial fibrillation in patients with mitral stenosis causes increased symptomatic distress. Thus, if atrial fibrillation becomes established or recurs after drug therapy or cardioversion, and the patient becomes increasingly symptomatic, operation is indicated. The occurrence of arterial thromboembolism in a patient with mitral stenosis is in general an indication for mitral commissurotomy. Perhaps the one clear-cut indication in the United States, at the present time, for closed commissurotomy is the presence of a pliable valve in a female with mitral stenosis who is pregnant and developing cardiac disability.

The feasibility of a mitral reconstructive procedure in mitral stenosis is based on preoperative assessment indicating a pliable mitral valve. Pliability is suggested by the presence of an opening snap, little or no calcification noted on echocardiography or cinefluoroscopy, and absent or mild mitral insufficiency. These patients are usually less than 50 years old and are most often in functional class II-B or III.

Preoperative evaluation usually includes typical findings on the electrocardiogram (in some cases) of P mitrale and right ventricular hypertrophy, chest roentgenogram changes suggestive of pulmonary venous hypertension along with left atrial and right ventricular enlargement, and an echocardiogram showing an EF slope typical of mitral stenosis. If these noninvasive studies point clearly to isolated mitral stenosis, and if the patient is less than 40 or 50 years old and angina is not present, it is entirely feasible to proceed to operation without cardiac catheterization.

Operation A median sternotomy incision is used routinely for the operation. The heart and the patient are cooled by the perfusate at the start of cardiopulmonary bypass. The aorta is cross-clamped and the heart is protected by multidose hypothermic potassium cardioplegia.[78] Thereafter, the left atrium is opened, with a flaccid heart and a clamped aorta, avoiding air and particulate embolization.

The mitral valve is studied for its suitability for mitral commissurotomy. If it is judged suitable, silk sutures are placed on the anterior and posterior leaflets for traction. An incision is made into the anterior lateral commissure just short of the edge of the valve ring. The chordae beneath the commissures go to both anterior and posterior leaflets and can be used as a guide to the commissures. When fused chordae exist beneath the commissure these may be separated carefully by sharp dissection to enlarge the orifice. A similar procedure is carried out at the posterior medial commissure. At times, when the chordae are short and the papillary muscles are scarred, the papillary muscle may be split between chordae to enlarge the orifice. Only if the leaflets are immobile or heavily calcified, or if the valve is found to be seriously incompetent after discontinuing cardiopulmonary bypass, is valve replacement utilized. At times, a larger mitral valve area can be achieved by incising areas within scarred commissures and making a secondary orifice for the valve. The degree of residual incompetence can be assessed moderately well by filling the left ventricle with a cold saline solution. Should there be major incompetence, further reconstruction of the valve may be effected by using a remodeling procedure such as that suggested by Carpentier[79] or Duran[80] with excision of certain chordal or leaflet structures and insertion of a flexible annular ring (see below). Any thrombi present within the left atrium are removed, and the left atrial appendage is oversewn before discontinuing cardiopulmonary bypass. Strict precautions are taken to avoid air embolization as the aortic clamp is removed and the heart is refilled with blood. After cardiopulmonary bypass is discontinued, palpation of the left atrium at its roof and at the left posterior AV groove is used to assess any degree of residual mitral valve incompetence.

Postoperative Care The postoperative course of patients undergoing open mitral commissurotomy is similar to that of other patients undergoing cardiac operations.[81] When cardiac performance is suboptimal, infusion of blood or blood substitutes is used to maintain the mean left atrial pressure at levels of about 14 mmHg. If arterial blood pressure is higher than normal, reduction of left ventricular afterload is accomplished by the continuous intravenous infusion of nitroprusside. Efforts are made to maintain a sinus rhythm when possible, including the use of atrial pacing at a rate of about 110 beats per minute. Should these procedures fail to optimize cardiac performance as judged by indicator dilution measurement of cardiac output, small doses of inotropic agents such as dopamine, isoproterenol, or epinephrine can be used.

If the hemodynamic state is good, the patient is usually extubated a few hours after operation. If cardiac output has been low, a nasotracheal tube is utilized, and the patient is maintained on intermittent mandatory ventilation with moderate positive end-expiratory pressure. In any event, extubation is usually possible between 12 and 48 h after operation. Urine flow is monitored, and when less than 15 ml/h, interventions to optimize cardiac performance are utilized or a diuretic such as furosemide or mannitol is employed.

Generally, patients having mitral commissurotomy are given anticoagulation treatment for 10 days to 6 weeks postoperatively, using warfarin sodium begun about 48 h postoperatively.

Hospital Morbidity and Mortality The hospital mortality following open mitral commissurotomy is as low as that for closed commissurotomy and is approximately 1 percent. Morbidity is minimal and includes an occasional patient with an atrial or ventricular arrhythmia.

Late Results A number of patients may require reoperation from 5 to 20 years after commissurotomy. This deterioration has been estimated to be at a rate of 5 percent of patients per year.[82] Heger, Wann et al.,[83] studied 18 patients 10 to 14 years after successful commissurotomy. At early restudy, mitral valve area increased from 0.9 cm^2 to 2.7 cm^2. Only 5 of the 18 patients had significant restenosis (average mitral valve area decreased from 2.7 cm^2 to 1.3 cm^2). This was associated with increased symptomatology. According to Higgs et al.,[84] symptoms recurrent after commissurotomy more often result from factors other than restenosis. These include residual stenosis, mitral regurgitation, or other associated valvular or cardiac abnormalities.

Clearly, most patients experience marked symptomatic improvement after mitral commissurotomy and at 5 years the clinical status for the majority is the old (NYHA) functional class I or II.

Postoperative Treatment

Patients will require digitalis or propranolol after mitral valve surgery to prevent a rapid ventricular response if atrial fibrillation persists. If a prosthetic valve has been inserted, long-term anticoagulation will be required. Long-term anticoagulation is not used after a porcine valve has been inserted unless the left atrium is large or atrial fibrillation is present. Infective endocarditis prophylaxis should be continued whether a commissurotomy was performed or prosthetic valve inserted. Since the patient may not fully achieve optimal return of function for 3 to 6 months after mitral valve surgery, noninvasive studies such as echocardiography and radionuclide exercise testing can be performed during the first 6 months after surgery to document the hemodynamic improvement as well as the patient's functional reserve.

Cost Analysis

In the asymptomatic patient with mitral stenosis, diligent rheumatic and endocardial prophylaxis can be most beneficial in retarding progression of the stenosis and preventing bacterial endocarditis. The goal of follow-up visits once or twice each year is to detect early symptoms as well as to gather noninvasive evidence of hemodynamic deterioration of the mitral lesion. Class II cardiac patients with symptoms on more than normal activity should be considered surgical candidates. An important consideration for mitral valve surgery can arise in the young female during her childbearing period when the stress of pregnancy produces symptoms of pulmonary congestion. In these individuals, careful thought has to be given to continued medical follow-up, a simple mitral commissurotomy, or the risk of mitral valve replacement with the need for long-term follow-up. If the patient remains asymptomatic, a conservative approach is probably justified, particularly in the younger individual; but for long-term benefits mitral valve surgery must be considered in a young woman with children who needs to perform physical tasks in properly caring for her youngsters. Thus, the cost consideration and risk/benefit ratio of continued medical therapy and surgical treatment must be directed toward preservation of function and prevention of heart failure and future complications.

Mitral Regurgitation

I have found perceptible purring tremor to be produced more frequently by regurgitation through the mitral valve than by any other valvular lesion—especially when the ventricle was hypertrophous and dilated by which the refluent current was rendered stronger.

James Hope, 1839[85]

Etiology

Although rheumatic fever remains an etiologic factor in mitral regurgitation, clinically and surgically mitral valve prolapse and coronary artery disease have become major mechanisms for incompetence of the mitral valve.[86] Prolapse of the mitral valve is probably the most common cause of mitral regurgitation in the adult population.[87] As shown in Table 38-1, causes for chronic mitral regurgitation result from rheumatic fever, mitral valve prolapse, coronary artery disease, and left ventricular dilatation due to several conditions which can alter the anatomy and histology of the mitral apparatus.[88,89] Less common etiologies of chronic mitral regurgitation include calcification of the annulus and connective tissue disorders such as Marfan's syndrome, Ehlers-Danlos syndrome, and pseudoxanthoma.[90–92] Papillary muscle dysfunction can result from coronary artery disease, infiltrative diseases, endocardial disorders, and inflammatory and myocardial diseases.[93-95] Congenital heart disease, such as corrected transposition of the great arteries, endocardial fibroelastosis, partial atrioventricular canal, and isolated cleft of the mitral valve often have associated mitral regurgitation.[96]

TABLE 38-1 Etiology of Chronic and Acute Mitral Regurgitation

Chronic regurgitation
Mitral leaflet prolapse (congenital; myxomatous degeneration)
Coronary artery disease
Left ventricular dilatation (numerous causes)
Rheumatic fever
Calcified mitral annulus
Heritable disorders of connective tissue (Marfan's, Ehlers-Danlos, osteogenesis imperfecta)
Papillary muscle dysfunction (infarction)
Congenital heart disease
Lupus erythematosus
Acute regurgitation
Rupture of chordae tendineae (myxomatous, endocarditis, trauma)
Rupture of papillary muscle (infarction, trauma)
Perforation of leaflet (endocarditis)

Acute mitral regurgitation can result from mechanical disturbances such as disruption of the chordae, rupture of the papillary muscle, or perforation of the mitral valve leaflet. Bacterial endocarditis, mitral valve prolapse, trauma, and spontaneous rupture can disrupt the chordae.[97,98] Rupture of papillary muscle is most commonly produced by acute myocardial infarction, and perforation of the mitral valve usually results from bacterial endocarditis.

Pathology

Mitral insufficiency may result from rheumatic endocarditis, bacterial endocarditis, myxomatous change, cardiomyopathy, heart failure, myocardial infarction, trauma, or undue restraint upon leaflets or chordae.[99,100]

Rheumatic Endocarditis

The same fundamental processes which result in rheumatic mitral stenosis may cause mitral insufficiency. (See Chap. 62.) The differences depend, in part, on fortuitous differences in physical orientation of the leaflets. Changes which tend to maintain the valve in a closed position cause mitral stenosis; those which cause the valve to be held open are associated with incompetence of the valve. The following structural patterns are found among cases of mitral insufficiency of rheumatic origin: (1) calcification of commissures (Fig. 38-8), (2) fibrous contracture of leaflet tissue, and (3) minor intrinsic valvular shortening with secondary distortion of the valve by the enlarged left atrium[101,102] (Fig. 38-9). The calcification which causes mitral insufficiency extends from one leaflet into the other across one or both of the commissures, keeping the two leaflets apart at the involved commissure or commissures. Fibrous contracture as a cause of mitral insufficiency is usually dominant at one commissure, but without fusion, shortening of valvular tissue is so great that the two leaflets cannot make complete contact.

Secondary distortion of the valvular tissue as a cause of major mitral insufficiency results from progressive enlargement of the left atrium from mitral insufficiency without commissural fusion. As the left atrium enlarges it causes the posterior leaflet to be displaced posteriorly. At the same time, the leaflet is restrained at the opposite end by the tensor apparatus. The result is that the posterior leaflet may lose its capacity to move as it becomes hamstrung over the base of the left ventricular wall. The progression leads to the situation wherein "mitral insufficiency begets mitral insufficiency."[103]

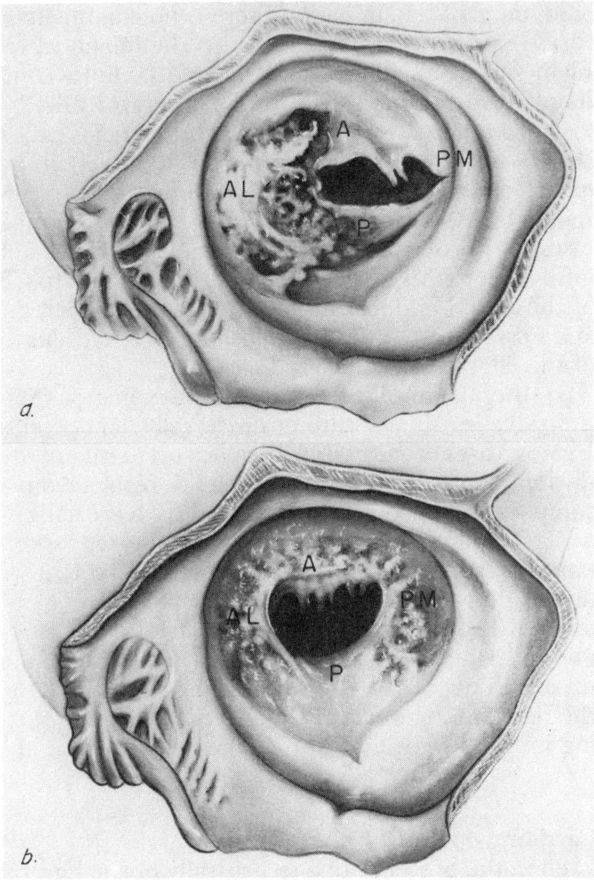

FIGURE 38-8 Anatomic types of rheumatic mitral insufficiency. Each unopened mitral valve viewed from above. In each, A = anterior, P = posterior leaflets of mitral valve, respectively; AL, PM = anterolateral and posteromedial commissures of mitral valve. *A.* Calcification and fusion of anterolateral commissure giving rise to the teardrop type of mitral insufficiency. *B.* Calcification of the leaflets and commissures in continuity, yielding a wedding-ring type of mitral insufficiency. Some restriction of the orifice is present, but incompetence is predominant. [*From J. E. Edwards, Pathology of Mitral Incompetence, in M. D. Silver (ed.), "Cardiovascular Pathology," Churchill Livingstone Inc., New York, 1983. Reproduced with permission from the publisher and author.*]

Bacterial Endocarditis

Bacterial endocarditis (Figure 38-10) as a cause of mitral insufficiency is usually through its destructive effects leading to erosion or perforation of leaflets and/or rupture of chordae (see Chap. 56). Either of these processes may result from primary infection of the valve or secondarily from primary bacterial endocarditis of the aortic valve.[104] A less common cause of incompetence from bacterial endocarditis is through healing of those vegetations in the angle between the posterior leaflet and the left ventricular wall. This process results in immobilization of the posterior leaflet.[99]

Myxomatous Change

The myxomatous mitral valve (Figs. 38-11 through 38-14), variously known as "floppy" or "billowing" valve and mid- or mid-late systolic click syndrome, among others, is common in the population and,

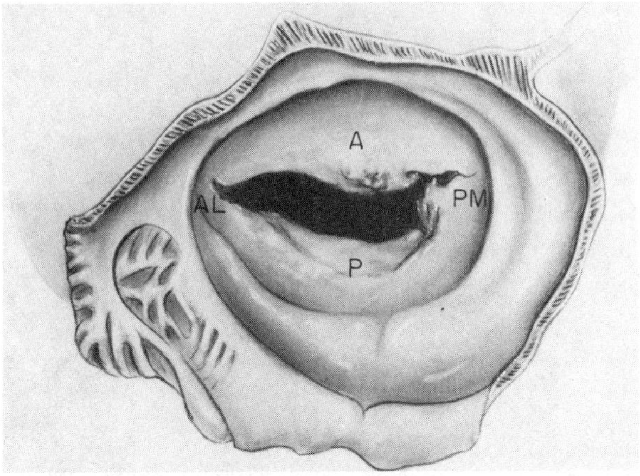

FIGURE 38-9 Rheumatic mitral insufficiency. Mitral valve viewed from above. Intrinsically short leaflets. Commissures essentially unaffected. (Abbreviations as in Figure 38-8.) [*From J. E. Edwards, Pathology of Mitral Incompetence, in M. D. Silver (ed.), "Cardiovascular Pathology," Churchill Livingstone Inc., New York, 1983. Reproduced with permission from the publisher and author.*]

through its various characteristics, may be the most common cause of mitral insufficiency that results from intrinsic disease of the valve. (The true incidence will evolve as pathologists desist in calling examples of this condition "rheumatic" simply because some fibrotic changes are observed.) The myxomatous valve is common in Marfan's syndrome, but in the vast majority of cases that syndrome is not identified.[105]

The basic process is an increase in size of the normally present mucinous layer of the valve, the

FIGURE 38-10 Healed bacterial endocarditis. Left side of heart shows major erosion of mitral valvular tissue and disappearance of many chordae.

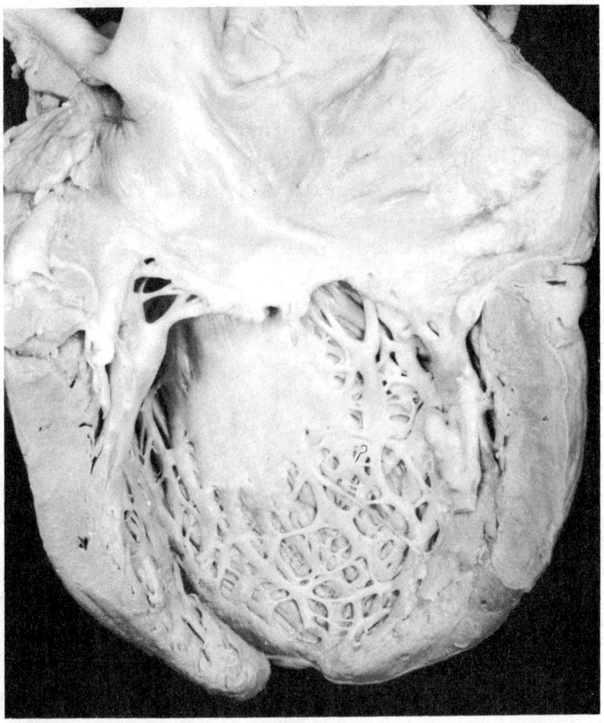

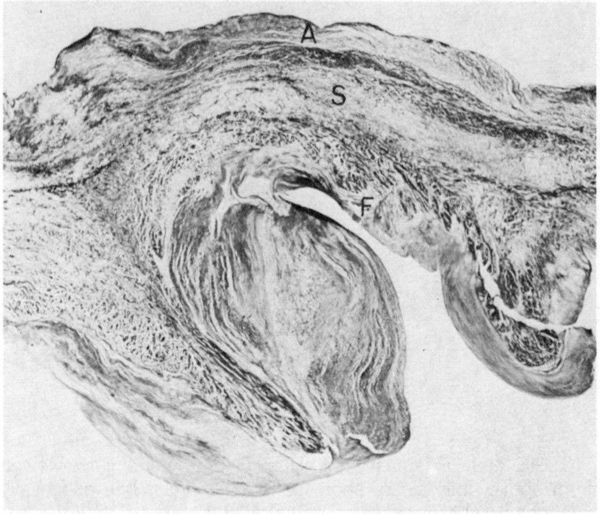

FIGURE 38-11 Photomicrograph of posterior mitral leaflet from a 29-year-old man with myxomatous mitral valve. The spongiosa layer (S) is increased in thickness and invades and interrupts the fibrosa (F). There is fibrous thickening on the atrial aspect of the leaflet (A), as well as fibrous pad on the ventricular aspect under the fibrous layer. Elastic tissue stain; ×15. (*From R. B. Guthrie and J. E. Edwards, Pathology of the Myxomatous Mitral Valve. Nature, Secondary Changes and Complications, Minnesota Med., 59:637, 1976. Reproduced with permission from the publisher and author.*)

so-called spongiosa[106] (Fig. 38-11). The mucinous layer invades and interrupts the continuity of the supporting fibrous layer of the leaflet, the fibrosa. From the resulting weakness of the leaflets, segments of the valve which lie between chordal insertions prolapse or hood abnormally toward the left atrium during ventricular systole. Part of the process of prolapse may result from weakness of chordae, which in some instances are elongated.

Secondary fibrotic changes of the leaflets occur in characteristic locations. There is fibroelastic thickening of the contact aspect of the leaflet. Fibrous tissue, predominantly collagenous, is deposited on the under aspect of prolapsing segments. The ultimate effect is that initially delicate, translucent leaflets may become opaque, thickened, and deformed[106] (Fig. 38-12). In spite of the fibrotic changes, the histologically identifiable intrinsic elements of the leaflet are maintained. This is one of the distinguishing characteristics from deforming rheumatic disease. Also, on gross examination there is no commissural fusion, a process common in the rheumatic valve. Elements of the posterior leaflet are more commonly involved than those of the anterior leaflet.[107]

A common secondary effect of myxomatous change of the mitral valve is fibrous deposits on the mural endocardium of the left ventricle as a response to friction by chordae[108] (Fig. 38-13). In some cases the fibrotic process may be extensive and result in incorporation of chordae into the fibrous tissue of the mural endocardium, as described by Salazar and Edwards.[108] If this happens, the effective length of the chordae becomes reduced.

In the uncomplicated state the myxomatous mitral valve is usually, but not universally, competent. In most cases of mitral insufficiency occurring in the myxomatous valve, the incompetence results from a complication of this process, such as bacterial endocarditis, and, most commonly, noninfected "spontaneous" rupture of the chordae (Fig. 38-14). It is now widely accepted that the usual basis for spontaneous rupture of the mitral chordae (to be distinguished from rupture of a papillary muscle) is the myxomatous valve.[106-109] When chordae rupture, the the ones most commonly involved are those inserting into the central scallop of the posterior leaflet.

Cardiomyopathy

Even in the presence of a structurally normal mitral valve, incompetence may result from left ventricular failure for any reason, including congestive cardiomyopathy. The mechanical factors leading to the valvular malfunction include enlargement of the valvular orifice and distortion of the alignment of the tensor apparatus.[103] The primary form of the dilated type of endocardial fibroelastosis is comparable to the congestive cardiomyopathies in regard to its cause of mitral insufficiency.[110]

Obstructive cardiomyopathy (muscular subaortic stenosis) may be associated with mitral insufficiency. This association is probably caused by the systolic anterior motion of the anterior mitral leaflet that occurs in this condition (see section on subaortic stenosis). The anatomic counterpart is fibrous thickening of the mural endocardium of the septal wall of the left ventricular outflow tract. Such thickening

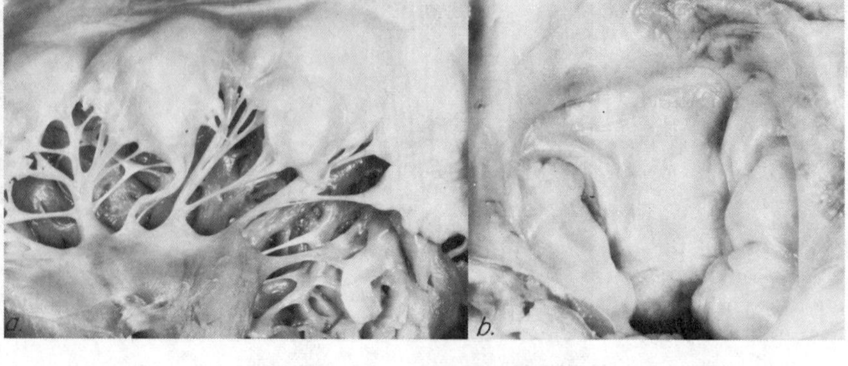

FIGURE 38-12 Photographs of the gross specimen from the case illustrated in Figure 38-11 (myxomatous mitral valve). *a.* The opened mitral valve shows characteristic interchordal hooding of the leaflets. *b.* The unopened mitral valve viewed from above showing unusual degrees of scalloping characteristic of the myxomatously altered mitral valve, the so-called floppy valve. (*From R. B. Guthrie and J. E. Edwards, Pathology of the Myxomatous Mitral Valve. Nature, Secondary Changes and Complications, Minnesota Med., 59:637, 1976. Reproduced with permission from the publisher and author.*)

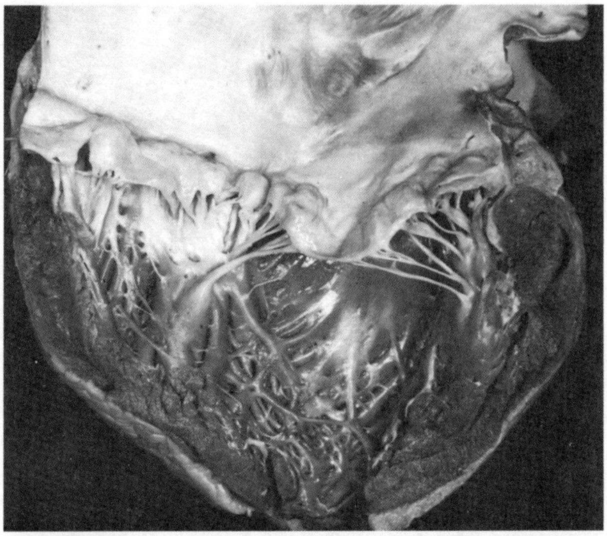

FIGURE 38-13 Left atrium and left ventricle in a case of myxomatous alteration of the mitral valve in a patient with Marfan's syndrome. Friction lesions upon the left ventricular endocardium have caused incorporation and functional shortening of the related chordae of the posterior mitral leaflet. (*From A. E. Salazar and J. E. Edwards, Friction Lesions of Ventricular Endocardium. Relation to Chordae Tendineae of Mitral Valve, Arch. Pathol., 90:364, 1970. Reproduced with permission from the publisher and author.*)

results from injury by contact of the anterior mitral leaflet with the mural endocardium.

Myocardial Infarction

Myocardial infarction may underlie mitral insufficiency in one of several ways, namely, (1) dilatation of the left ventricle in cases of extensive healed, myocardial infarction (so-called ischemic congestive cardiomyopathy); (2) rupture of a papillary muscle complicating acute myocardial infarction; and (3) infarction of a nonruptured papillary muscle.

Rupture of a papillary muscle involves the posteromedial set of muscles more commonly than the anterior set by a ratio of 4:1.[111] The intensity of mitral insufficiency resulting from rupture of a papillary muscle depends upon whether an entire set or only isolated heads are involved.[112]

Infarction of a nonruptured papillary muscle with mitral insufficiency is usually associated with infarction of the adjacent free wall of the left ventricle (Fig. 38-15). According to clinical and experimental evidence, incompetence of the valve depends not only upon intrinsic dysfunction of the papillary muscle but also upon distortion of the papillary muscular function by asynergic contraction of the related free wall.[113]

Trauma

A traumatic cause of mitral insufficiency is rupture of a papillary muscle. It is extremely rare that traumatic rupture of a papillary muscle is an isolated cardiac injury. Accompanying lesions often are rupture of the ventricular septum and/or the wall of a chamber.

Undue Restraint upon Leaflets or Chordae

Undue restraint upon leaflets or chordae is a cause of mitral insufficiency. Most of the conditions contributing to this process have been covered in foregoing parts of this section (bacterial endocarditis and myxomatous mitral valve with extensive friction lesions). Among conditions not mentioned are Loeffler's endomyocardial fibrosis and lupus erythematosus.[114,115] In either of these conditions, but more commonly in the former, the posterior mitral leaflet may become immobilized by its adhesions to the left ventricular endocardium.

Calcification of the Mitral Ring

Calcification of the mitral ring is a common state in the elderly, particularly in the elderly female.[116] In

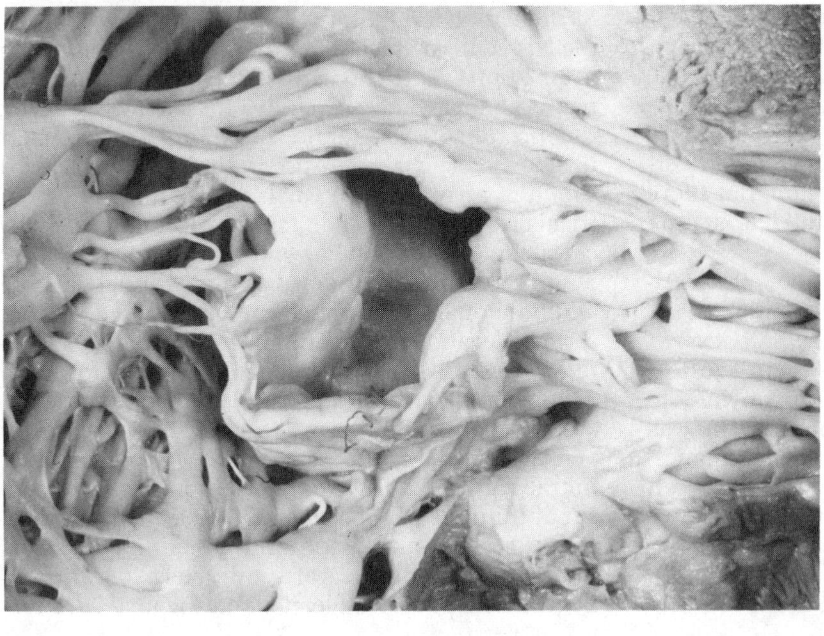

FIGURE 38-14 Myxomatous alteration of mitral valve with rupture of chordae to the posterior leaflet. The unopened mitral valve viewed from below. The central part of the posterior leaflet (lower center) shows fragments of ruptured chordae. The intact chordae are elongated and the leaflet tissue as seen through the orifice shows some prolapse and fibrous thickening as evidence of a preexisting myxomatous state. [*From J. E. Edwards, Pathology of Mitral Incompetence, in M. D. Silver (ed.), "Cardiovascular Pathology," Churchill Livingstone Inc., New York, 1983. Reproduced with permission from the publisher and author.*]

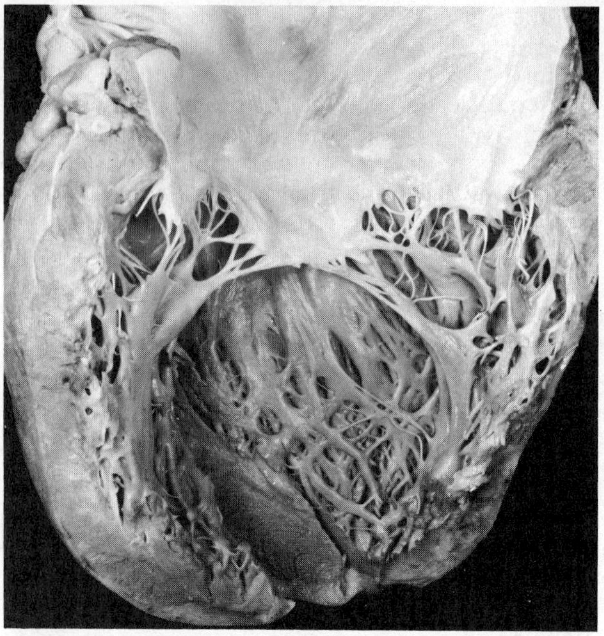

FIGURE 38-15 Healed myocardial infarction involving the inferior wall of the left ventricle and related papillary muscles. The inferior wall of the left ventricle and papillary muscle are atrophic on the basis of coexistent infarction.

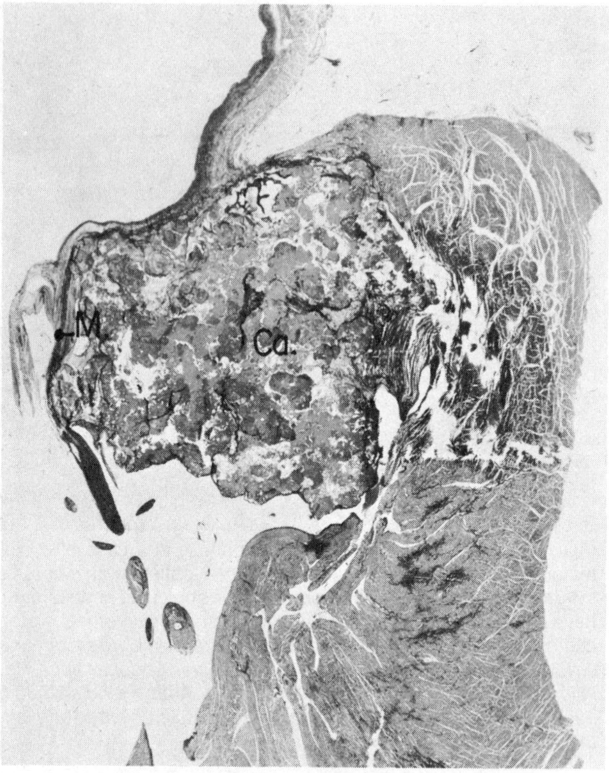

FIGURE 38-16 Calcification of mitral ring. Low-power photomicrograph showing calcific mass (CA) at the junction of the left atrium and left ventricle. The posterior mitral leaflet (M) is in part adherent to the calcified mass, a process leading to its immobilization. Elastic tissue stain; ×4.

the majority of instances it does not cause recognizable valvular dysfunction. When valvular malfunction results it usually takes the form of incompetence. This results from adhesions of the posterior mitral leaflet to the calcific mass (Fig. 38-16).

Abnormal Physiology

Mitral regurgitation results from improper coaptation of the mitral leaflets during left ventricular systolic ejection. The burden imposed on the left ventricle and left atrium will be determined by the etiology, severity, and duration of the mitral regurgitation. In chronic regurgitation, the amount of the left ventricular stroke volume ejected into the left atrium will determine the extent of left atrial enlargement as well as left ventricular dilatation.[117] The systolic regurgitant flow of blood produces a characteristic prominent *v* wave in the left atrium.[118] Chronic mitral regurgitation causes a volume overload on the left ventricle and left atrium, but there will also be elevation of pressure in the left atrium, pulmonary veins, and capillaries.

The compensatory mechanism of the left ventricle to chronic mitral regurgitation is dilatation of the chamber to accommodate the increased left ventricular stroke volume necessary to maintain the forward or systemic stroke volume. Accompanying dilatation of the left ventricle is an increase in wall thickness and hypertrophy to maintain mechanical function.[119,120] The extent of the increase in left ventricular wall thickness is determined by the force developed within the wall, and the myocardium hypertrophies to normalize systolic wall stress.[121] In addition, distensibility or compliance of the left ventricle and left atrium increases in chronic mitral regurgitation, and thereby reduces the extent of pulmonary venous hypertension.

Diastolic filling of the left ventricle in chronic mitral regurgitation consists of the normal systolic output of the right ventricle plus the amount of previously regurgitated volume into the left atrium from the prior cardiac cycle (Fig. 38-17). The elastic recoil of the left atrium and the increased distensibility of the left ventricle facilitate rapid early diastolic filling of the left ventricle without significant hemodynamic abnormalities.[122] Under these circumstances, the protodiastolic gallop sound possesses similar hemodynamic characteristics to the physiologic third sound in a young individual.[123] The increased ventricular compliance maintains a normal or mildly elevated left ventricular end-diastolic pressure.[124] Systolic regurgitation emptied into the left atrium and pulmonary venous bed can be tolerated without severe elevation of the pulmonary capillary or arterial pressure in chronic mitral regurgitation.

In the mitral leaflet prolapse syndrome, the anatomic changes in the valve and abnormalities in ventricular wall motion can influence the degree of mitral regurgitation.[125,126] These abnormalities consist of thinning of the leaflet, elongation of the chordae, excessive valve tissue, and sometimes dilatation of the mitral annulus. Abrupt deceleration of blood beneath the prolapsed leaflet and the increased ten-

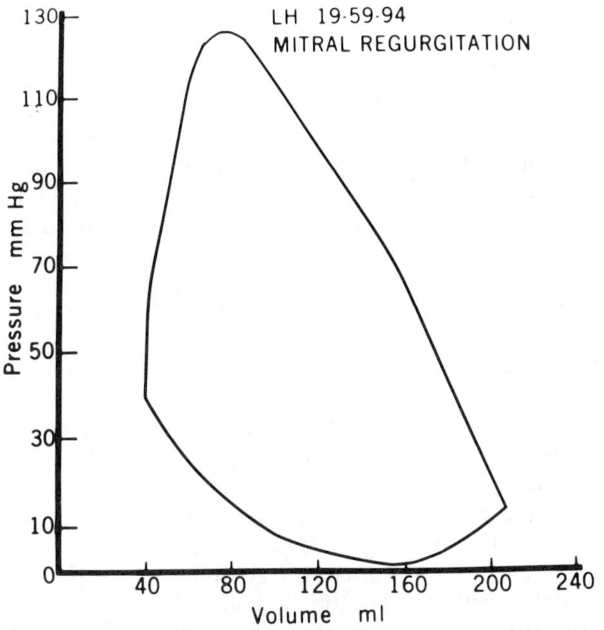

FIGURE 38-17 Pressure-volume diagram in a patient with mitral regurgitation. There is a loss of the isovolumic contraction phase on the right side of the pressure-volume loop due to the mitral valve incompetence, and the early diastolic filling is initiated by the 40 mmHg *v* wave in the left atrium. [*From C. E. Rackley, Value of Ventriculography in Cardiac Function and Diagnosis, in N. O. Fowler (ed.), "Diagnostic Methods in Cardiology," F. A. Davis Company, Philadelphia, 1975, p. 283. Reproduced with permission from the publisher and author.*]

sion on the chordae produce the systolic click. Abnormal systolic contraction patterns of the ventricle range from hyperkinesis of localized areas and cavity obliteration to hypokinesis and akinesis.[126-128] However, the end-diastolic pressure, end-diastolic volume, and left ventricular mass are usually normal in this condition.

Additional pathophysiologic mechanisms include myocardial ischemia, coronary spasm, and neurogenic mechanisms. Exercise-induced left ventricular dysfunction has been related to underlying coronary artery disease and not to mitral valve prolapse alone.[129] Chest discomfort, arrhythmias, and electrocardiographic abnormalities suggest a role for myocardial ischemia, and prolapse is a frequent finding in patients with angiographic coronary artery disease.[130,131] Positive ergonovine tests for coronary spasm are infrequently positive in this condition.[132] In symptomatic patients, plasma catecholamine and plasma norepinephrine levels have been found elevated in both supine and standing positions while the heart rate may be lower in supine positions.[133] Of the disturbed mechanisms in mitral leaflet prolapse, the abnormality of leaflet position appears most related to the degree of mitral regurgitation.

In coronary artery disease, mitral regurgitation can result from impaired papillary muscle function, abnormal ventricular wall motion, and significant dilatation of the ventricular chamber. A significant degree of mitral regurgitation requires not only papillary muscle dysfunction but also abnormal motion of the posterior ventricular wall.[88] Circumflex and right coronary artery lesions are most frequently associated with significant mitral regurgitation. Loss of 17 percent or greater ventricular wall motion after myocardial infarction will result in chronic dilatation of the left ventricle.[134] When the end-diastolic volume exceeds 50 percent of the normal value, secondary mitral regurgitation can occur in chronic coronary artery disease due to dilatation of the chamber.[88]

Dilatation of the left ventricle secondary to any intrinsic or extrinsic impairment of ventricular function can eventually cause secondary mitral regurgitation.[89] In dilated cardiomyopathy, functional mitral regurgitation is determined by the altered leaflet area and mitral annulus size, whereas left ventricular size appears a less important factor.[135] Echocardiographic studies have demonstrated dilatation of the mitral valve annulus with left ventricular enlargement, but annular dilatation does not occur proportionally to the degree of left ventricular dilatation.[136] Additional disturbances include loss of sphincteric action of the annulus and malalignment of the papillary muscles. The dilated left ventricle may further undergo changes from the ellipsoid to the spheroid configuration, which creates additional regurgitation.[120]

The hemodynamic disturbances in acute mitral regurgitation differ from chronic forms, and the valvular incompetence is often imposed on a previously normal ventricle. Sudden regurgitation of blood into the left atrium and pulmonary veins is not accompanied by immediate dilatation of the left atrium or ventricle.[137] These abrupt hemodynamic alterations result in marked elevation of the left ventricular end-diastolic pressure, the left atrial pressure, and pulmonary capillary pressure. The large *v* wave in the left atrium is reflected to the pulmonary veins, capillaries, and even to the pulmonary arteries. The lack of acute dilatation of the left ventricle and atrium without changes in compliance to accommodate the regurgitant volume, creates a pressure overload on the pulmonary vascular bed and produces acute pulmonary edema.

Clinical Manifestations

History

Mitral regurgitation can be tolerated for many years without cardiac symptoms.[138] *Dyspnea and fatigue* are often the initial symptoms which can gradually progress to orthopnea, paroxysmal nocturnal dyspnea, and peripheral edema.[139,140] In mitral valve prolapse symptoms are frequently palpitations, chest discomfort, fatigue, and anxiety.[125] Although 50 percent of patients may complain of palpitations with the mitral prolapse syndrome, monitoring may not confirm these complaints.[141] Atypical *chest discomfort* may be difficult to distinguish from angina pectoris, and other psychological complaints are often present. More than two-thirds of the patients are female, and a family incidence may be striking in some individuals.[87]

In coronary artery disease, mitral regurgitation is usually accompanied by symptoms of angina pectoris or develops with an acute myocardial infarction.[94,142] Chronic coronary artery disease with left ventricular dilatation and depressed ventricular function is often attended by dyspnea, fatigue, orthopnea, and fluid retention. Chest pain may be minimal or absent in this stage of coronary disease, sometimes referred to as ischemic cardiomyopathy. When mitral regurgitation is secondary to left ventricular dilatation and alterations in mitral valve function, the symptoms are generally those with left ventricular failure. In these circumstances systemic emboli can create additional vascular and neurologic symptoms.

In acute mitral regurgitation from sudden disruption of mitral valve integrity, the symptoms are often those of congestive heart failure or *acute pulmonary edema*. Chordal rupture has been observed in 11 percent of patients with echocardiographic evidence of mitral valve prolapse but some patients experience mild symptoms or remain asymptomatic.[143]

Physical Examination

The chronic volume overload for mitral regurgitation may be tolerated for long periods before development of heart failure and symptoms, but atrial fibrillation frequently occurs in the course of left atrial enlargement. The cardiac examination (see Chap. 11) in chronic mitral regurgitation will generally reveal displacement of the apical impulse with the hyperdynamic motion over a diffuse area (see Chap. 10). A lifting hyperactive apical impulse can be palpated lateral to the third left interspace along the sternal border.[144] The characteristic murmur is a high-pitched *holosystolic murmur beginning with the first heart sound* and extending to the second sound.[145] The intensity of the murmur is usually constant throughout the systolic ejection period and usually radiated into the axilla. The respiratory cycle does not influence the intensity of the mitral regurgitation murmur nor is there a variation in atrial fibrillation.[146]

The *first heart sound is diminished* in chronic mitral regurgitation, and the duration of systole shortened, resulting in premature closure of the aortic valve.[147] This can produce *splitting of the second heart sound* (see Chap. 11).[148] A protodiastolic or a *ventricular gallop* is frequently heard in mitral regurgitation, and rarely an *opening snap* can be detected in pure mitral regurgitation.[147] If the protodiastolic gallop sound is accompanied by a harsh mitral regurgitant murmur, ventricular function may be preserved.[123] When the gallop sound accompanies a regurgitant murmur of grade II or less, ventricular function is depressed. With the large diastolic volume across the mitral valve, a *diastolic flow rumble* may be created in early diastole.[149]

Additional physical findings in mitral leaflet prolapse involve *anomalies of the habitus and chest wall* along with the *systolic click and mid- or late systolic murmur*.[150] Patients are frequently asthenic, the majority are female, and orthostatic hypotension may be present.[151] The anteroposterior diameter of the chest may be decreased, and pectus excavatum, scoliosis, or kyphosis may also be present. A systolic retraction or dip synchronous with the systolic click may sometimes be palpated.[152] The characteristic auscultatory findings are the early, mid-, or late systolic click and the late systolic murmur[87,125,150,152,153] (Fig. 38-18). In 10 percent of patients the systolic murmur may be holosystolic and the auscultatory features can be influenced by changes in posture, the Valsalva maneuver, and pharmacologic agents to alter blood pressure. A diastolic sound and murmur can occur when the prolapsed valve returns from the left atrial position and coapts with the anterior leaflet.[154] Any maneuver which reduces the chamber size of the left ventricle will migrate the click and the onset of the murmur close to the first sound, and likewise a click and murmur will occur late in systole if ventricular size is increased[155] (Fig. 38-19).

In coronary artery disease, mitral regurgitation may be present in the patient without pain, during an episode of angina pectoris, with acute infarction, and in severe left ventricular failure.[88,94,142] The murmur may occur in early, mid-, or late systole, or be holosystolic with underlying coronary disease.[156,157] In contrast to other conditions, atrial gallops are common when mitral regurgitation is produced by underlying coronary artery disease. A ventricular gallop indicates significant depression of ventricular function and can be audible during an episode of angina, with acute infarction, or in chronic left ventricular failure.

Dilatation of the left ventricular chamber can produce secondary mitral regurgitation due to loss of sphincteric action of the annulus as well as malalignment of the papillary muscles. Since the dilatation results from depression of the inotropic state of the myocardium, a ventricular gallop is often audible. Mitral regurgitation can also result from connective tissue disorders, calcification of the mitral annulus, and congenital heart disease.

The findings on physical examination of acute mitral regurgitation are often those of acute pulmonary edema and left ventricular failure.[158,159] The heart may be normal in size with a hyperactive apical motion, and a systolic thrill can sometimes be palpated at the apex.[160] Rarely, the thrill will radiate over the primary aortic area if the posterior leaflet has prolapsed due to anterior direction of the regurgitant jet impinging on the atrial septum and the aorta. In acute regurgitation the murmur is harsh, over the back of the neck, vertebrae, and sacrum, and holosystolic. It radiates over the precordium into the axilla, back and along the left sternal border. Atrial and ventricular gallops may be present or there may be a summation gallop with tachycardia. If acute myocardial infarction has resulted in papillary mus-

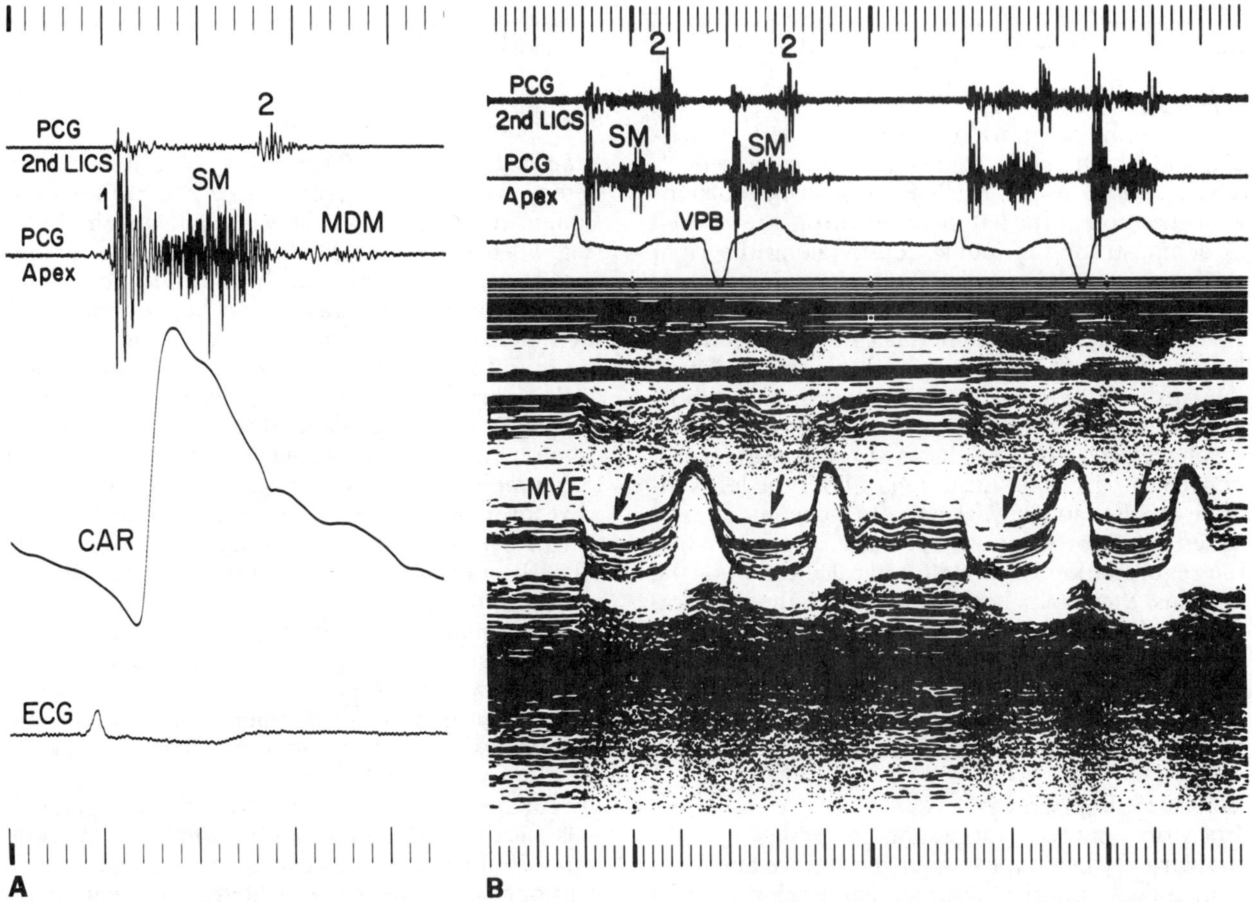

FIGURE 38-18 Mitral valve prolapse. *A.* The phonocardiogram demonstrates an intense high-frequency pansystolic murmur with accentuation in late systole. There is also a minimal middiastolic murmur (MDM). *B.* The echocardiogram demonstrates the hammock-shaped appearance of the valve leaflets (arrows), which coincides with the pansystolic murmur. The rhythm is atrial fibrillation with bigeminy. (*Courtesy of Dr. Ernest Craige.*)

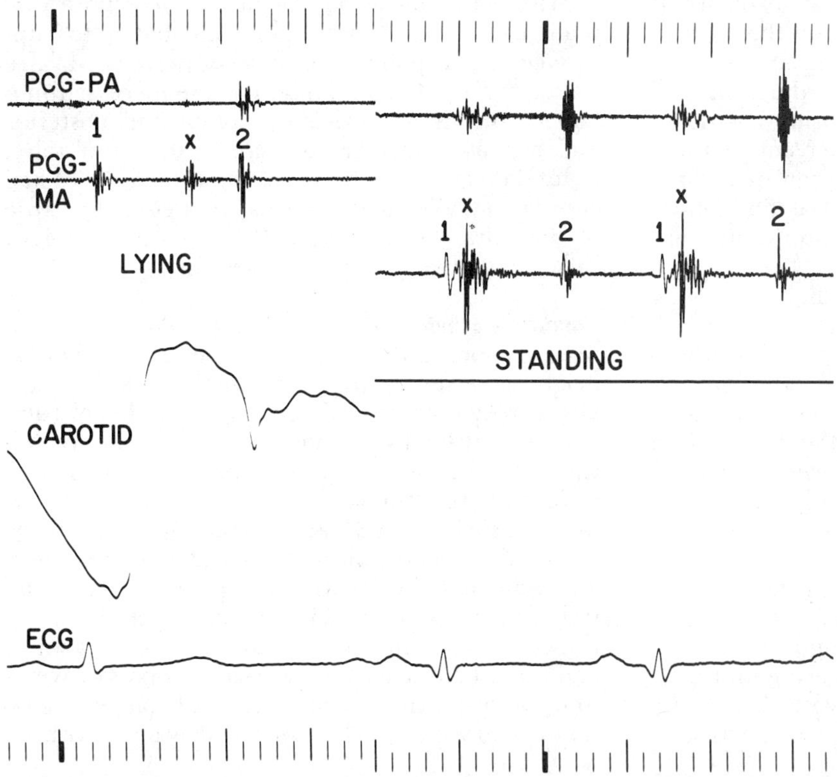

FIGURE 38-19 Mitral valve prolapse. A late systolic click (x) moves to a position early in systole with standing. (*Courtesy of Dr. Ernest Craige.*)

cle rupture, the murmur may be loudest either at the apex or along the left sternal border.

Chest Roentgenogram

In long-standing mitral regurgitation, left ventricular and left atrial enlargement are usually present.[139] The left atrium can reach enormous proportions with elevation of the left mainstem bronchus, as well as demonstrating a double density along the right cardiac border.[161] Cardiac fluoroscopy may reveal calcification in the region of the mitral valve, and systolic pulsations can sometimes be detected in the left atrium. (See Chap. 15.) In mitral valve prolapse, the cardiac silhouette is often normal, and abnormalities may be confined to the chest wall.[162,163] In coronary artery disease, heart size can range from normal to significant dilatation of both the left ventricle and left atrium. Calcium can sometimes be detected on fluoroscopy in coronary arteries. When the regurgitation is secondary to calcification of the annulus, there may be prominence of the calcification on the plain chest film and fluoroscopy will reveal conspicuous motion of the atrioventricular calcified groove. Acute mitral regurgitation due to disruption of the valve apparatus can present with pulmonary edema and a normal cardiac size.[94,95]

Electrocardiogram

In chronic mitral regurgitation, left atrial and ventricular enlargement can alter the P wave and QRS amplitude.[164] If atrial fibrillation has developed, atrial enlargement is suggested by a coarse fibrillatory pattern.[165] In mitral valve prolapse, electrocardiographic abnormalities are often manifested as ST-T wave changes, QT prolongation, and rhythm disturbances.[125] The most common abnormality is T-wave negativity in inferior leads and the ST segment may be slightly depressed as well. Arryhthmias are frequent on the resting electrocardiogram, and in such patients ambulatory monitoring has documented ventricular ectopy in 60 percent of these patients.[141,166] Other rhythm disturbances include sinus arrhythmias, sinus arrest, atrial fibrillation, premature ventricular contractions, and ventricular tachycardia.

If coronary artery disease is the underlying mechanism for the mitral regurgitation, there will often be Q-wave abnormalities of a previous infarction usually inferior or posterior in location. Although ST-segment changes have been attributed to papillary muscle dysfunction, these are often nonspecific and can occur with left ventricular hypertrophy, conduction defects, and digitalis.[167]

If the regurgitation is caused by ventricular dilatation, there will usually be voltage criteria for hypertrophy and secondary ST-T wave changes. If an infiltrative cardiomyopathy is present, there may also be loss of precordial R waves indistinguishable from a previous myocardial infarction. If acute mitral regurgitation is due to underlying myocardial infarction, there will be a higher incidence of electrocardiographic changes in inferior leads than in the anterior leads.[94]

Special Laboratory Studies

Echocardiogram (see Chap. 120) The noninvasive detection of mitral leaflet prolapse is one of the most significant contributions of echocardiography[168–170] (Fig. 38-18). Specific features include early to midsystolic posterior motion of the mitral leaflet, or holosystolic prolapse of the leaflet. These deviations of the mitral leaflet are related to the C and D line of the mitral valve echo, produced by systolic motion of the mitral apparatus. Suggestive features such as sagging of the mitral leaflet during systole, multiple echoes parallel to the mitral leaflet, and exaggerated leaflet mobility are not necessarily specific for mitral valve prolapse. Echocardiographic evidence of mitral prolapse has been recorded in approximately 10 percent of patients in the absence of auscultatory abnormalities.[37]

In coronary artery disease with mitral regurgitation, posterior wall motion abnormalities can be recorded which are involved in the mechanism of mitral regurgitation.[171] Segmental wall motion abnormalities can be recognized more readily by two-dimensional echocardiography. In mitral regurgitation with diffuse ventricular enlargement, diastolic dimensions, decreased systolic wall motion, and mitral valve motion can be assessed with echocardiography. The echocardiographic demonstration of moderate to severe annular calcification is significantly associated with mitral regurgitation, congestive heart failure, and left atrial enlargement.[172]

With acute mitral regurgitation, the echocardiogram can detect abnormalities attributed to ruptured chordae, papillary muscle, or perforated valve leaflet[173] (Fig. 38-20). These include increased motion of the interventricular septum and posterior wall, increased diastolic excursion of the mitral valve, redundant systolic echoes, echoes at the level of flail chordae, systolic atrial expansion, systolic prolapse of the mitral leaflets, and densities on the mitral valve suggestive of vegetative lesions.

Cardiac Catheterization (see Chap. 108) In mitral regurgitation, cardiac catheterization can confirm the diagnosis, assess ventricular function, identify certain etiologic mechanisms, recognize other cardiac lesions, and finally evaluate coronary anatomy. Mitral regurgitation is the most common cause of large v waves in the pulmonary wedge pressure recording, but such v waves can be associated with mitral obstruction, heart failure, ventricular septal defect, and a decrease in left atrial compliance without mitral regurgitation.[174,175] Pulmonary arterial v waves can be recorded in patients with high wedge v waves and are usually associated with acute onset of symptoms on a nonrheumatic basis.[176] Mitral regurgitation is confirmed by left ventriculography with in-

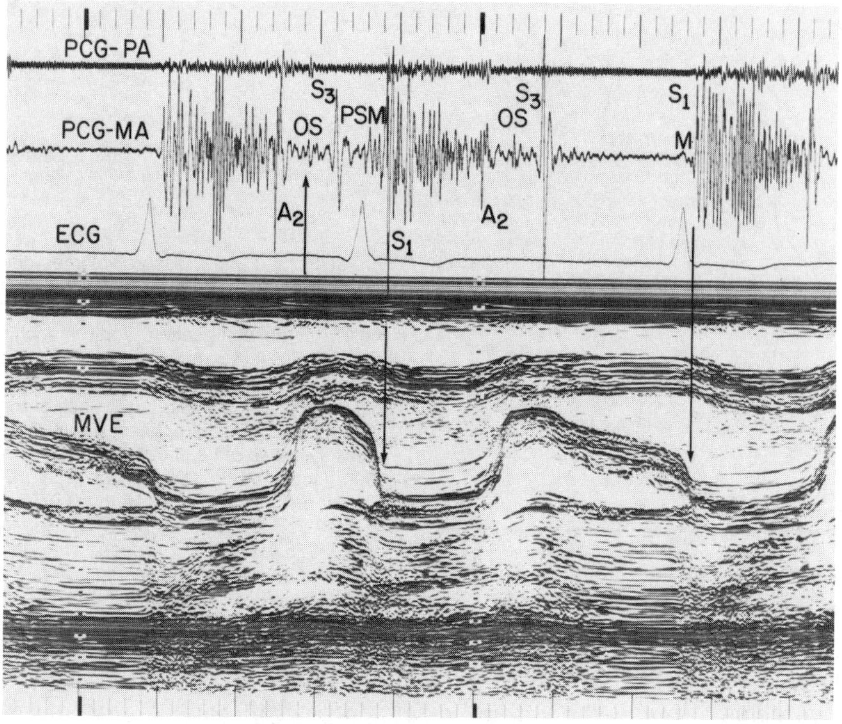

FIGURE 38-20 Phonocardiogram and echocardiogram in a patient with rheumatic heart disease, mitral regurgitation and stenosis, and atrial fibrillation. The echocardiogram is consistent with mitral stenosis. However, the pansystolic murmur is due to mitral regurgitation. There is a prominent presystolic murmur (PSM) after the short diastoles. Cardiac catheterization in 1968 showed moderate mitral regurgitation but no stenosis. Repeat catheterization in 1978 showed severe mitral regurgitation, and mean left atrial pressure 28 mmHg and a *v* wave of 42 mmHg. (*Courtesy of Dr. Ernest Craige.*)

jection into the chamber and documentation of regurgitation into the left atrium.

Left ventricular function is evaluated by measurement of the ventricular end-diastolic pressure, calculation of the ejection fraction, and quantitation of the regurgitant volume[120] (Fig. 38-21). Quantitative angiography permits determination of the left ventricular stroke volume as the difference between end-diastolic and end-systolic volumes (Fig. 38-22). The difference in the left ventricular stroke volume and the forward stroke volume determined by the Fick or indicator dilution technique will yield the regurgitant volume per beat into the left atrium.[177] This calculation assumes no regurgitation across the aortic valve. The end-diastolic volume in chronic mitral regurgitation may be significantly increased but the ejection fraction may remain within or near the normal range until severe myocardial depression develops. At the advanced stage, further elevation of the left ventricular end-diastolic and left atrial pressure will increase pulmonary venous, capillary, and arterial pressures.[138,139] Rarely, mitral regurgitation and a giant left atrium can develop with a normal end-diastolic and left atrial pressure due to increased compliance of the left atrium and ventricle.[178]

Quantitative angiography also permits calculation of left ventricular mass, a measure of hypertrophy of the ventricle.[179] Using the Laplace relationship and measurements of chamber pressure, volume, and wall thickness, left ventricular wall stress can be calculated throughout the cardiac cycle. End-diastolic wall stress is equated to the preload on the left ventricle, and wall stress at the time of aortic valve opening is equivalent to afterload.[124] The ratio

FIGURE 38-21 Left ventricular pressure and volume in a patient with mitral regurgitation. End-diastolic volume = 208; end-systolic volume = 42; left ventricular stroke volume = 166; forward stroke volume = 30; regurgitant stroke volume = 136; ejection fraction = 166/208 = 0.80; left ventricular weight in grams = 247; and left ventricular end-diastolic pressure = 14.

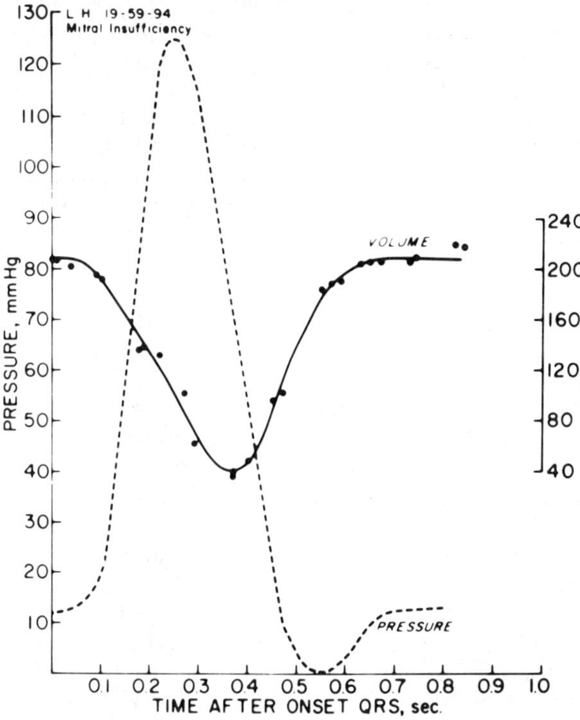

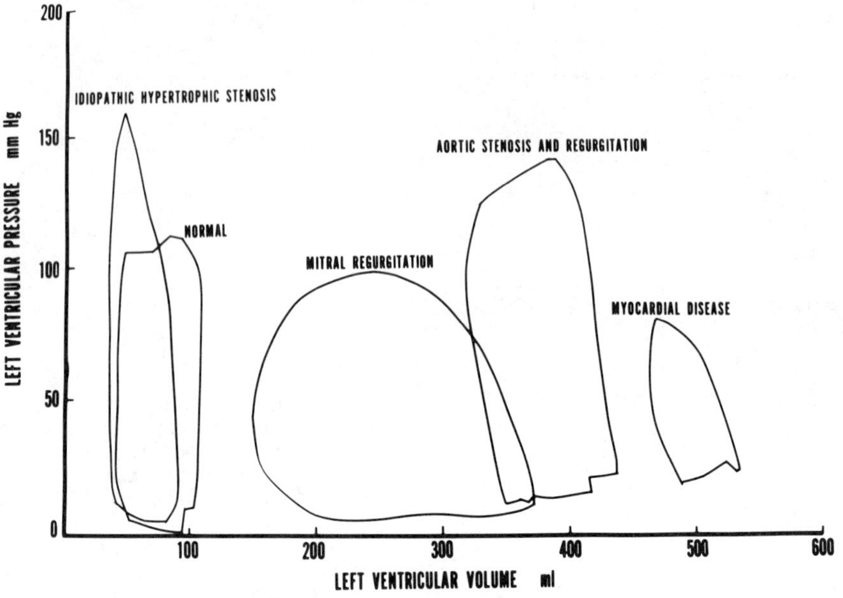

FIGURE 38-22 Pressure-volume diagrams for a normal subject and patients with idiopathic hypertrophic subaortic stenosis, mitral regurgitation, aortic stenosis and insufficiency, and a cardiomyopathy. Mitral regurgitation is present in all cardiac disease states as illustrated by loss of the isovolumic contraction phase. [*From C. E. Rackley, Value of Ventriculography in Cardiac Function and Diagnosis, in N. O. Fowler (ed.), "Diagnostic Methods in Cardiology," F. A. Davis Company, Philadelphia, 1975, p. 283. Reproduced with permission from the publisher and author.*]

of end-systolic wall stress to end-systolic volume index as a measure of left ventricular function has been shown to predict postoperative clinical improvement or survival in mitral regurgitation better than the ejection fraction.[180,181]

In mitral valve prolapse, hemodynamic measurements are often normal and mitral regurgitation minimal.[126,182] Left ventricular angiography does provide an optimal view of the mitral apparatus and the characteristic prolapse scallops of the posterior leaflet. Although abnormalities of left ventricular function can sometimes be assessed from the ventriculogram, mitral leaflet prolapse occurs commonly without detectable abnormalities in wall motion.[126,128,182] Coronary arteriography should also be performed in patients with mitral valve prolapse even though no specific relationship has been established between these two common diseases.[125,130,131,182]

When mitral regurgitation is associated with coronary artery disease, there is usually abnormal motion of the posterior wall and chamber dilatation (Fig. 38-23). Wall motion abnormalities, particularly at the base of the papillary muscle, play an important role in the development of mitral regurgitation with coronary disease.[88]

With acute mitral incompetence, left ventricular angiography will demonstrate massive regurgitation into the left atrium and pulmonary veins. Ventricular contraction is vigorous with systolic regurgitation into the left atrium and pulmonary vessels.[137] A large *v* wave in the left atrium can be recorded from the pulmonary capillary wedge position, and the Swan-Ganz catheter can be utilized to confirm this condition in acute myocardial infarction.[183] If a prominent *v* wave cannot be recorded from the pulmonary wedge position in a patient with acute infarction and suspected mitral incompetence, blood samples for oxygen saturation may have to be compared from the pulmonary artery and right atrium to exclude rupture of the ventricular septum.

Radionuclide Studies (see Chap. 109) Radionuclide techniques can measure the ejection fraction in both the left and right ventricles of patients with mitral regurgitation. Left ventricular diastolic and systolic volumes can be estimated, and radionuclide angiograms have shown normal left ventricular function in many subgroups with mitral regurgitation and diminished left ventricular reserve.[184–186] Since myocardial disease may also be present in adult forms of mitral regurgitation, myocardial perfusion studies can also be used to identify areas of abnormal fusion during exercise and rest.

Other Studies Exercise testing can quantitate functional reserve in patients without symptoms or at the earliest suspicion of cardiac deterioration in chronic mitral regurgitation. Holter monitoring can be employed to document the presence and frequency of arrhythmias, particularly in the mitral leaflet prolapse syndrome.[166]

Natural History and Prognosis

With the multiple etiologies and mechanisms, the prognosis of patients with mitral regurgitation will depend on the underlying cause and the state of left ventricular function.[138] In chronic mitral regurgitation volume overload may be tolerated for many years before early symptoms of failure develop. The ejection fraction is often normal due to regurgitation into the low-impedance area of the left atrium and pulmonary veins, and, therefore, early symptoms of decompensation may be questioned. Left atrial enlargement disposes to development of atrial fibrillation, which can be further complicated by embolization, but embolization is somewhat less frequent in mitral regurgitation than in mitral stenosis.[140,164] Patients remain susceptible to endocarditis, and survival of patients with chronic mitral regurgitation in a study of randomly selected patients re-

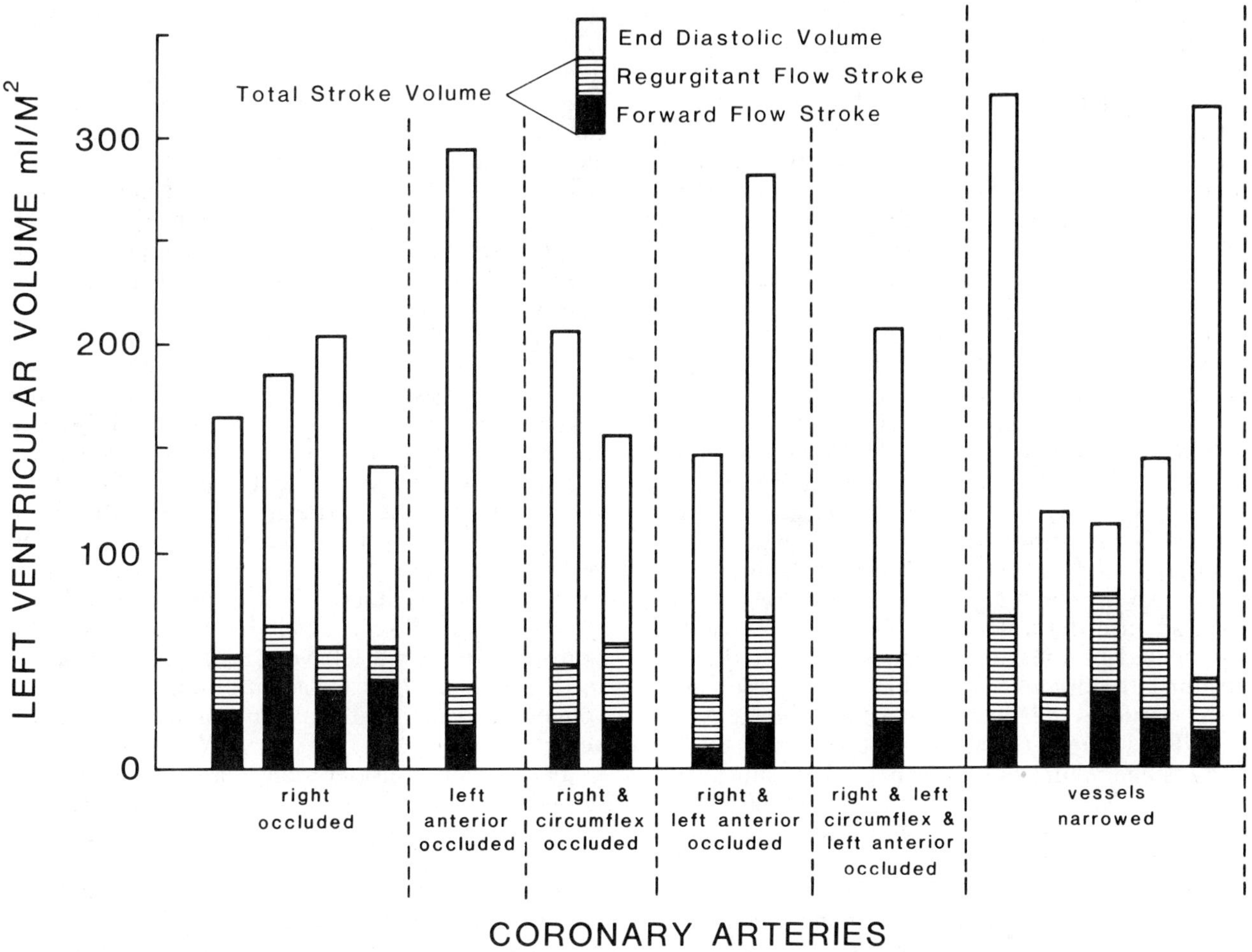

FIGURE 38-23 The left ventricular volume and coronary lesions in patients with mitral regurgitation. The total height of the bar is the end-diastolic volume, and the solid and slashed portion is the total left ventricular stroke volume. The mitral regurgitant stroke volume is indicated by the slashed area. (*From C. E. Rackley, H. D. Dear, W. A. Baxley, W. B. Jones, and H. T. Dodge, Left Ventricular Chamber Volume, Mass and Function in Severe Coronary Artery Disease, Circulation, 41:605, 1970. Reproduced with permission from the American Heart Association, Inc., and the author.*)

vealed that 80 percent were alive at 5 years and 60 percent survived 10 years.[75]

The majority of patients with mitral valve prolapse are asymptomatic. Chest pain and palpitations often cannot be related to any anatomic abnormalities even when prolapse is demonstrated. However, mitral valve prolapse in patients 60 years and older is frequently associated with chest pain, arrhythmias, and heart failure.[187] Although the prognosis remains good in the majority of patients with mitral valve prolapse, sudden death, endocarditis, rupture of chordae, and progressive mitral regurgitation remain infrequent complications. Operatively excised mitral valves for severe chronic mitral regurgitation revealed mitral prolapse as the mechanism in 62 percent of patients.[188] In several series of patients with prolapse, sudden death was recorded in 4 out of 387 patients.[150]

When coronary artery disease is the mechanism for mitral regurgitation, the extent of the anatomic disease and the state of left ventricular performance are the primary prognostic determinants. Complicating events are sudden death or acute myocardial infarction.

In acute mitral regurgitation, regardless of the mechanism, the course is often complicated by acute pulmonary edema and sometimes cardiogenic shock. In these conditions, the operative mortality may approach 60 to 80 percent. However, an occasional patient with a ruptured chordae may develop minimal or no symptoms, and prognosis is much more favorable.

Treatment

Medical

Prophylaxis for rheumatic fever (see Chap. 62) is recommended until age 30 years and coverage for prevention of infective endocarditis (see Chap. 56) is warranted for all etiologies for chronic mitral regurgitation as described in the section on mitral stenosis. The development of atrial fibrillation will require administration of digitalis to slow the ventricular response. With the incidence of embolism from 10 to 20 percent in chronic atrial fibrillation, anticoagulation should also be entertained. With the early development of atrial fibrillation, consideration should be given to electrical cardioversion.

Dyspnea, fatigue, and orthopnea suggest impaired left ventricular function and require digitalis and diuretics. It must be remembered that chronic mitral regurgitation is a form of high-output left ventricular failure, since total left ventricular output may greatly exceed the forward cardiac output. Optimal treatment of symptoms related to mitral incompetence requires correction of the mechanical defect rather than efforts to support the failing myocardium. Preload- and afterload-reducing agents can also be used in the early symptomatic treatment of mitral regurgitation. Long-acting nitrates as well as vasodilating agents such as hydralazine, prazosine, and captopril have demonstrated hemodynamic improvement and symptomatic relief.[180,188,189]

The optimal time for surgical replacement of the incompetent mitral valve remains a major challenge in the care of this condition. Surgery should be performed before clinical evidence of impaired contractility of the left ventricle becomes manifest, but the spuriously elevated ejection fraction can be misleading since the unloading of the left ventricle is augmented by the low-impedance area of the left atrium and pulmonary veins. Recent studies on end-systolic indexes of left ventricular function have suggested that the ratio of end-systolic wall stress to end-systolic volume index can predict clinical improvement and survival after surgery for mitral valve regurgitation more accurately than a measurement of the ejection fraction.[180,190]

The majority of patients with the mitral leaflet prolapse syndrome are asymptomatic and merely need reassurance. Propranolol has been effective in the management of palpitations, but treatment of asymptomatic ectopy is still not recommended. Nitrates, beta-blocking agents, and the calcium blocking agents may be required in patients with chest pain even though coronary anatomy is normal.

Mitral regurgitation complicating left coronary artery disease requires the standard therapy when heart failure develops, with digitalis, diuretics, and vasodilators. If the regurgitation is due to ventricular dilatation, calcification of the annulus, or connective tissue disorders, specific treatment is required only when heart failure develops.

Preoperative Management

The preoperative management of patients undergoing surgery for mitral regurgitation requires optimal control of cardiac rhythm, ventricular response, electrolytes, and anticoagulation. Digitalis should be discontinued before surgery, and electrolytes, particularly potassium, should be closely supervised. Any elective surgery or dental work should be completed before cardiac surgery, since this can eliminate future sources for infective endocarditis.

Surgical

Presently, there are two areas of very active discussion relative to surgery for mitral valve incompetence. The first is consideration of earlier operation to improve hospital mortality and lengthen long-term survival. Creating a competent mitral valve in a patient with severe mitral valve incompetence significantly increases left ventricular wall stress and myocardial oxygen consumption, and may decrease ejection fraction. The presumed mechanism for this is an abrupt change in resistance to ejection. In fact, there are two resistances in parallel in a patient with mitral incompetence; one, the usual impedance imposed by systemic arterial resistance, and the second, the factor associated with retrograde ejection through the incompetent mitral valve into a compliant left atrium. The mathematical characterization of two resistances in parallel suggests that following operative elimination of the low-resistance circuit (i.e., retrograde ejection), there is imposed a greater impedance to left ventricular ejection.[191,192] In cases where the mitral incompetence has been allowed to progress, restoration of mitral valve competency may cause the volume-overloaded ventricle to face a marked increase in impedance and wall stress. Indexes of contractility such as ejection fraction may drop, and left ventricular failure characterized early by low cardiac output and later by the congestive heart failure syndrome may supervene.[193]

The second consideration is associated with renewed interest in reconstructive rather than valve replacement procedures for a large number of patients with mitral valve incompetence. Pure rheumatic mitral valve incompetence, or incompetence associated with floppy or myxomatous valve which is mild to moderate in severity, may be well tolerated for a long time. The onset of more severe symptoms may be associated with rupture of chordae tendinae or a head of a papillary muscle, or increasing mitral annular dilatation, or left ventricular dysfunction. The natural history of medically treated rheumatic mitral incompetence is similar to that for mitral stenosis or aortic valve incompetence. The long-term survival of patients operated upon with mitral valve incompetence is very significantly related to their preoperative functional class, which to some degree is determined by the state of the left ventricular myocardium. Thus, it has been suggested that earlier operation would be appropriate in patients with mitral valve incompetence, particularly in those where a reconstructive procedure is feasible.[194]

Surgical Treatment A reparative procedure is done whenever the pathologic condition of the valve permits it. Examples are some cases of myxomatous degeneration, some cases secondary to ischemic heart disease, those cases where a combination of commissurotomy and annuloplasty can be done for mixed mitral stenosis and incompetence, and some cases where there is a degenerative process localized to a portion of one or the other mitral leaflets. Reparative procedures have the advantage of avoiding the long-term risk of devices used to replace the mitral valve and the need for long-term anticoagulant therapy inherent in many of them. Disadvantages of a reparative procedure include some lack of certainty that total competence will be established and the difficulty in knowing before starting the repair whether sufficient valvular competence can be established to avoid valve replacement. We employ valve repair (rather than replacement) in about 20 percent of patients with pure incompetence.

Carpentier and his associates have made major contributions to the treatment of mitral incompetence by reparative techniques. Their careful studies of the pathology of mitral incompetence have generated various procedures required for its care. Like others,[195] Carpentier has stressed that annuloplasty is the basic technique required for most patients in whom mitral incompetence is repaired. Rather than a narrowing procedure, this is a plastic reconstruction of the leaflets and the annulus, using multiple-point fixation to a flexible ring (Fig. 38-24). Procedures on the leaflets themselves are indicated in certain circumstances, particularly in ruptured chordae to the central portion of the posterior leaflet, wherein one uses a quadrangular excision of that portion of the leaflet and combines it with ring annuloplasty (Fig. 38-25). Less frequently, in some lesions involving the anterior leaflet, similar excisions can be used, and occasionally a solitary perforation of either leaflet from bacterial endocarditis can be repaired.

Calcification and immobility of the leaflets are indications for replacement. Replacement of the mitral valve is required in cases of rheumatic involvement leading to severe mitral regurgitation, mitral stenosis with loss of pliability of the leaflets, and various other causes of mitral regurgitation, such as infective endocarditis and in some cases of ischemic heart disease. Also, in occasional situations associated with idiopathic hypertrophic subaortic stenosis mitral valve replacement is needed for relief of left ventricular outflow tract obstruction or associated severe mitral regurgitation.

Surgical Technique The general technique for the operation is the same as described for mitral commissurotomy. The mitral valve is exposed after cooling the heart, cross-clamping the aorta, and introducing cold potassium cardioplegic solution. The valve is excised, with care being taken to leave sufficient residual valvular tissue for valve seating. Replacement is done, inserting the device using either interrupted suture or continuous monofilament suture (Fig. 38-26). If there is associated coronary artery disease, saphenous vein grafts are used to bypass the obstructive lesion.

The Device A number of artificial and biological devices have been used to replace the mitral valve. Since most of those presently in use have been in patients for less than 10 years, the final evaluation of each is not yet possible. Most are durable and

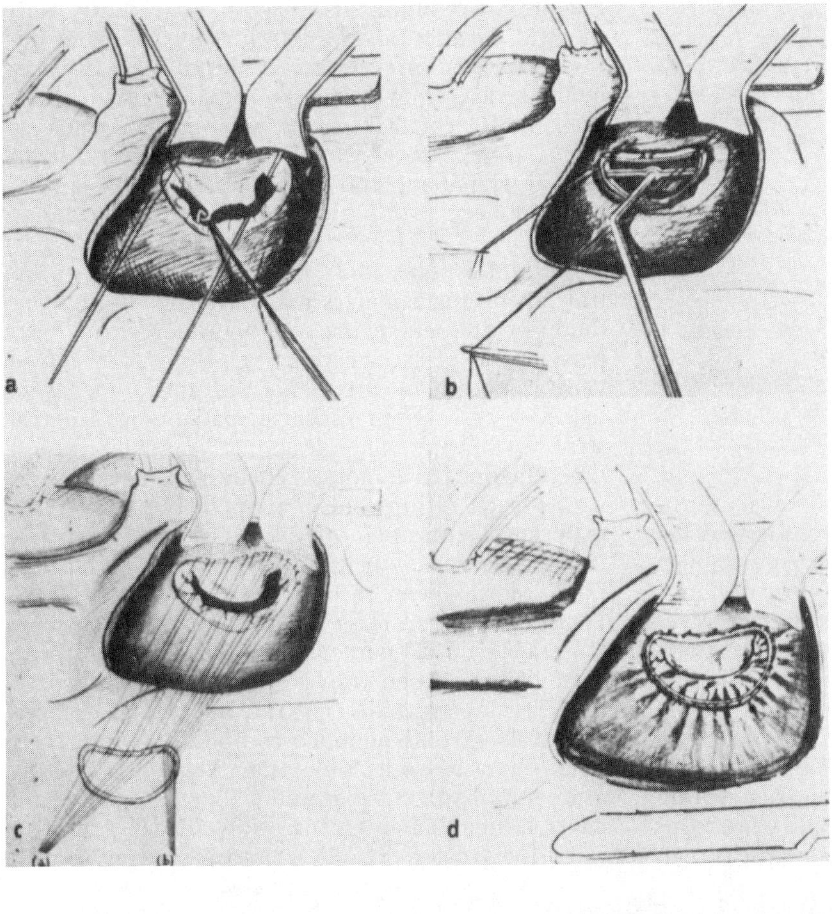

FIGURE 38-24 Repair of mitral insufficiency using the Carpentier ring for remodeling of the mitral annulus. [*From A. Carpentier, Plastic and Reconstructive Mitral Valve Surgery, in D. Kalmanson (ed.), "The Mitral Valve: A Pluridisciplinary Approach," Publishing Sciences Group, Inc., Littleton, Mass., 1976, p. 257, Reproduced with permission from the publisher and author.*]

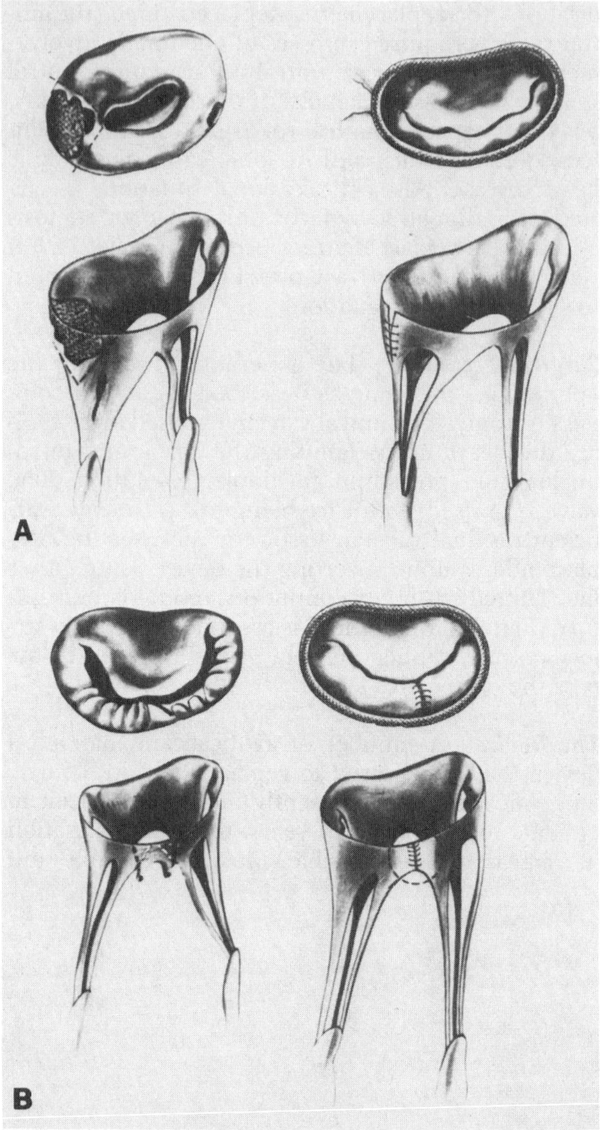

FIGURE 38-25 Repair of mitral insufficiency—Carpentier's methods. *A.* Resection of calcification. *B.* Quadrangular resection of prolapsed posterior leaflet secondary to ruptured chordae tendineae. Each repair is accompanied by ring annuloplasty. [*From A. Carpentier, Plastic and Reconstructive Mitral Valve Surgery, in D. Kalmanson (ed.), "The Mitral Valve: A Pluridisciplinary Approach," Publishing Sciences Group, Inc., Littleton, Mass., 1976, p. 534. Reproduced with permission from the publisher and author.*]

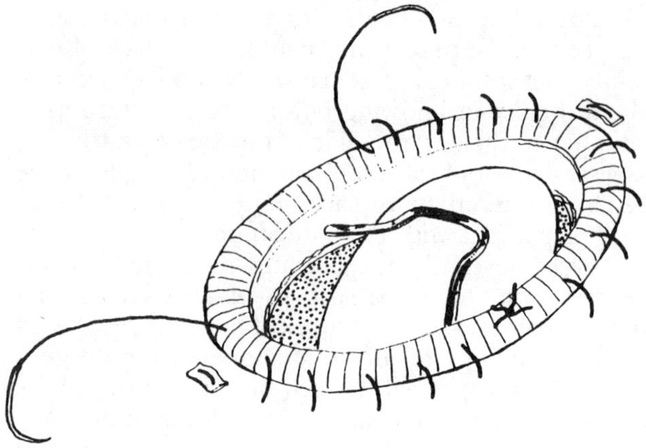

FIGURE 38-26 Insertion of Bjork-Shiley mitral prosthesis using continuous monofilament suture.

have given good long-term results. At present, unless anticoagulants are strongly contraindicated for the patient in question, we favor the Bjork-Shiley tilting disk valve prosthesis with a pyrolite occluder (Fig. 38-26). Long-term anticoagulant therapy is required. With less than optimal anticoagulation therapy, episodes of thromboembolism and occasionally thrombosis of the device have been reported (see below).

When anticoagulation therapy is contraindicated or particularly undesirable, as in children, young adult females, patients over 70 years old, or persons with a history of bleeding peptic ulcer disease, an alternative is the glutaraldehyde-preserved, stent-mounted porcine aortic valve xenograft. In contrast to the Bjork-Shiley prosthetic device, there is some question as to the long-term durability of the biological devices, and also the orifice size is not as large in relation to outside diameter as in the disk prosthesis. The incidence of thromboembolism has been low, but not totally absent. In some patients in whom there is chronic atrial fibrillation, anticoagulation therapy may be indicated on that basis alone; thus the xenograft loses its advantage.

There have been equally good results with the Starr-Edwards Silastic ball valve series 6300, the Lillehi-Caster tilting disk valve, and recently with the SJM bileaflet prosthesis. Although a further period of evaluation is necessary for all these replacement devices, they certainly are superior to those available 10 years ago. Therefore, there is some reason to move forward in the natural history of an individual patient and recommend valve replacement sooner.

Hospital Morbidity and Mortality The risk of mitral valve replacement is related to the clinical condition of the patient prior to operation. In our experience, as of several years ago the risk of mitral valve replacement in patients with mitral incompetence was greater than that in patients with mitral stenosis or in the mixed lesion.[196,197] At the present time, the operative mortality seems very nearly similar in each group and is about 3 percent. In an experience with open operations in general for mitral valve disease, including replacement, the hospital risk has been zero for patients in New York Heart Association class II, 1.3 percent for patients in class III, but 24 percent in patients with advanced disability associated with New York Heart Association class IV. Morbidity in surviving patients is modest. Early thromboembolic complications are rare. There may be some pulmonary dysfunction early after mitral valve replacement, but prolonged tracheal intubation and ventilation are seldom indicated for greater than 24 h postoperatively.

Anticoagulation treatment is begun on the second day with Coumadin, and in patients with porcine xenografts it is continued for 6 weeks and indefinitely if the left atrium is large or atrial fibrillation is present. In patients with prosthetic devices it is maintained indefinitely. Before hospital discharge, attempts are made to convert atrial fibrillation to a normal sinus mechanism either by drug therapy or electrical cardioversion. This is more successful in patients not having preoperative chronic atrial fibrillation of greater than 1-year duration.[198]

Late Results Thromboembolic complications were common with the early models of prosthetic mitral valves, but with currently used devices are much lower[199] (Fig. 38-27). We have found that the presence of atrial fibrillation, previous operation, advanced age, and double valve replacement each contribute some hazard to late postoperative thromboembolism. The survival rates for patients with presently available prosthetic or biological valves in the mitral position are also considerably higher than with devices that were initially available (Fig. 38-28). However, the results continue to be dependent on the degree of disability prior to operation, with nearly 90 percent of patients with class III disability preoperatively having a good long-term result, and only about 50 percent of patients with class IV disability having good long-term results. Again, this emphasizes the importance for advising operation before left ventricular dysfunction becomes advanced and irreversible. This concept has been documented recently by Schuler, Peterson, and colleagues in a small number of patients studied after mitral valve replacement for mitral incompetence.[193] In those patients with postoperatively normal ejection fractions (0.70), the ejection fraction fell only slightly 6 months after operation and hypertrophy regressed. However, in those patients with some element of left ventricular dysfunction preoperatively (ejection fraction, 0.57), left ventricular function progressively deteriorated after surgery, and left ventricular hypertrophy did not regress. The authors concluded that left ventricular shortening likely had become partially dependent on systolic afterload reduction through a load impedance leak in the latter group. After a valve replacement, ejection fraction became markedly impaired and chamber dilatation and myocardial hypertrophy persisted in some patients.

Postoperative Management
If the patient remains in atrial fibrillation after hospital discharge, chronic digitalis administration will be required to control the ventricular response. Antibiotic coverage for dental work and elective surgical procedures remains important for prevention of endocarditis. Depending on the prosthetic valve inserted, long-term anticoagulation therapy may be necessary. Endocardiographic and radionuclide studies can be obtained every 6 to 12 months to evaluate ventricular size and function. Recurrence of symptoms or change in prosthetic valve sounds warrants cinefluorography of the valve, which can be compared to films taken before hospital discharge.

Cost Analysis
Patients with chronic mitral regurgitation require periodic evaluations to assess cardiac function and to adjust medications. Emphasis on prophylaxis for rheumatic fever and bacterial endocarditis can obviously minimize these costly complications. The physician should be aware of noninvasive techniques to monitor ventricular size and performance, since many patients will eventually require mitral valve replacement, and the optimal time should be selected before heart failure and severe myocardial depression develop. Thus, prolonged medical treatment for symptoms of heart failure and mitral regurgitation can be costly, not only in terms of ex-

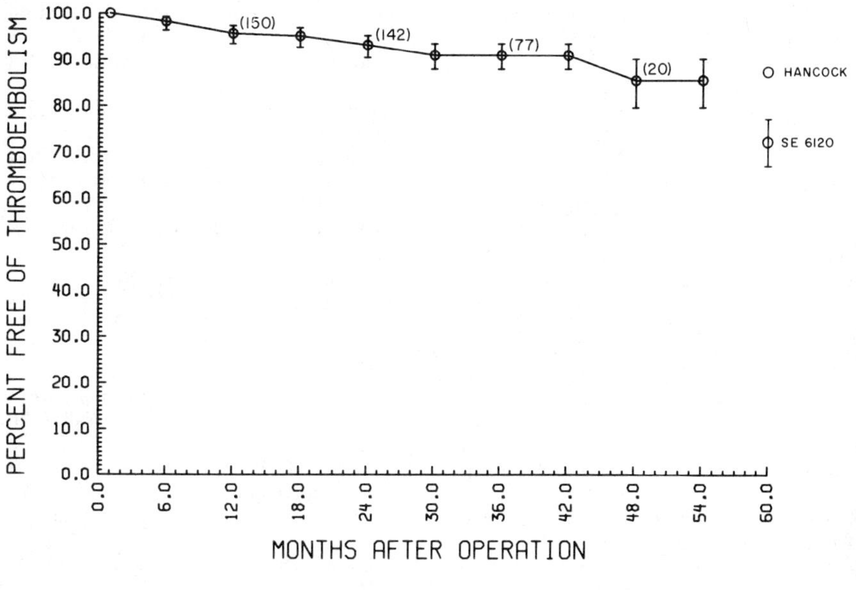

FIGURE 38-27 Actuarial freedom from thromboembolism in patients receiving Bjork-Shiley mitral prostheses at the University of Alabama in Birmingham. Data are compared to 5-year freedom from thromboembolism in patients with the Hancock xenografts (from Davila) and the Starr-Edwards (SE) valve (from Macmanus). (*The data regarding the Hancock valve and Starr-Edwards valve are from J. C. Davila, D. J. Magilligan, and J. W. Lewis, Is the Hancock Porcine Valve the Best Cardiac Valve Substitute Today? Ann. Thorac. Surg., 26:303, 1978; and Q. Macmanus, G. Grunkemeier, L. E. Lambert, and A. Starr, Non-Cloth-Covered Caged-Ball Prostheses: The Second Decade, J. Thorac. Cardiovasc. Surg., 76:788, 1978. Reproduced with permission from the publishers and authors.*)

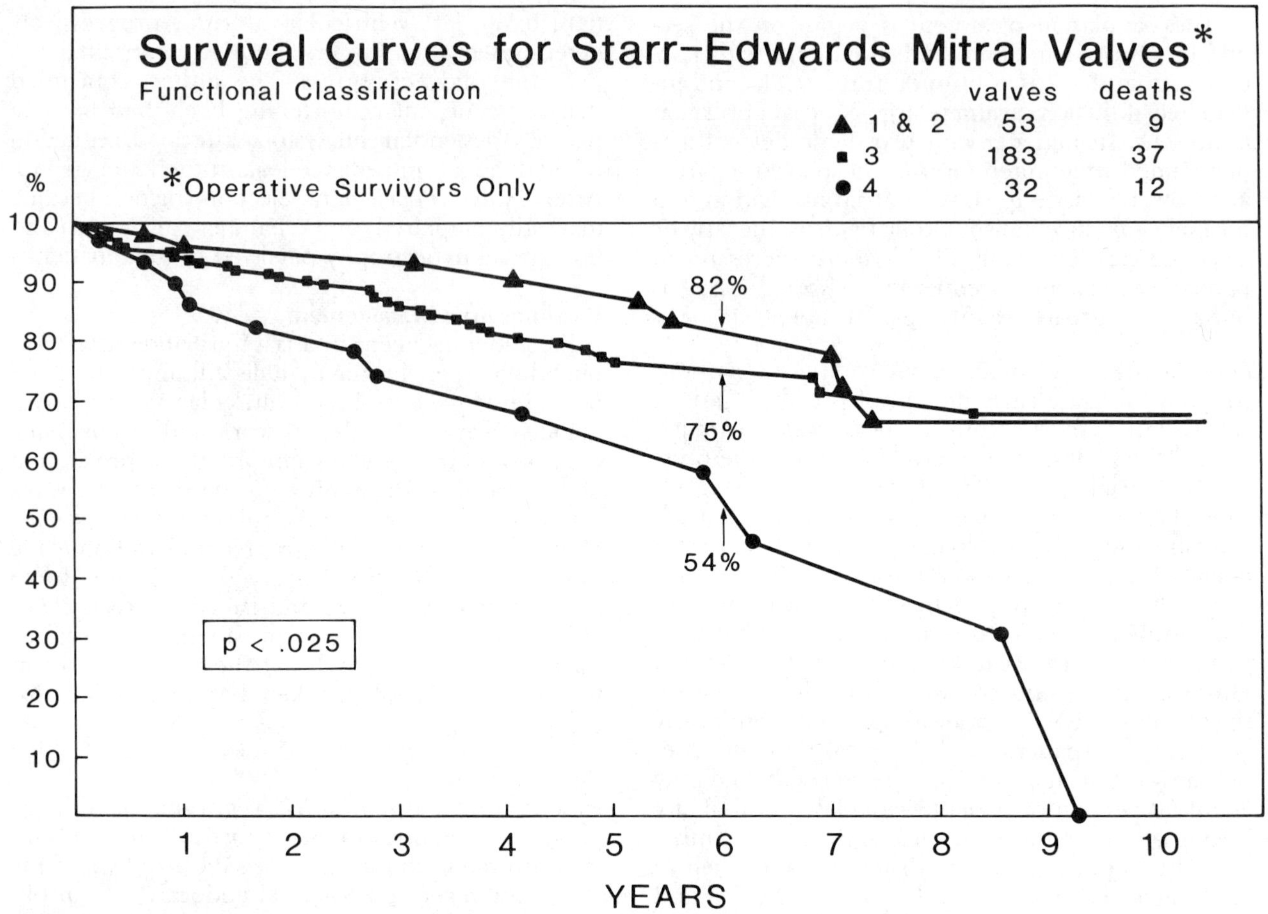

FIGURE 38-28 Actuarial survival according to preoperative functional class over a 10-year period for patients having mitral valve replacement. (*From A. Starr, G. Grunkemeier, L. Lambert, J. E. Okies, and D. Thomas, Mitral Valve Replacement: A 10-Year Following of Non-Cloth vs. Cloth-Covered Caged-Ball Prostheses, Circulation, 54:111–147, 1976. Reproduced with permission from the American Heart Association, Inc., and the author.*)

pense to patients, but also in minimizing the eventual surgical benefit from valve replacement. Periodic evaluation of ventricular size and function can be beneficial in cost and health economy to the patient.

References

1. Vieussens, R.: "Traite nouveau de la structure et des causes du mouvement naturel du coeur," Toulouse Guillemette, 1715, p. 101.
2. Perloff, J. K., and Roberts, W. C.: The Mitral Apparatus. Functional Anatomy of Mitral Regurgitation, *Circulation,* 46:227, 1972.
3. Nasser, W. K., Davis, R. H., Dillon, J. C., Tavel, M. E., Helmen, C. H., Feigenbaum, H., and Fisch, C.: Atrial Myxoma. I. Clinical and Pathologic Features in Nine Cases, *Am. Heart J.,* 83:694, 1972.
4. Buchbinder, N. A., and Roberts, W. C.: Left-Sided Valvular Active Infective Endocarditis. A Study of Forty-Five Necropsy Patients, *Am. J. Med.,* 53:20, 1972.
5. Hammer, W. J., Roberts, W. C., and de Leon, A. C., Jr.: "Mitral Stenosis" Secondary to Combined "Massive" Mitral Annular Calcific Deposits and Small, Hypertrophied Left Ventricles, Hemodynamic Documentation in Four Patients, *Am. J. Med.,* 64:371, 1978.
6. Osterberger, L. E., Goldstein, S., Khaja, F., and Lalsier, J. B.: Functional Mitral Stenosis in Patients with Massive Mitral Annular Calcification, *Circulation,* 64:472, 1981.
7. Bonnabeau, R. V., Jr., Stevenson, J. E., and Edwards: J. E.: Obliteration of the Principal Orifice of the Stenotic Mitral Valve: A Rare Form of "Re-Stenosis," *J. Thorac. Cardiovasc. Surg.,* 49:264, 1965.
8. Wooley, C. F., Baba, N., Kilman, J. W., and Ryan, J. M.: Thrombotic Calcific Mitral Stenosis. Morphology of the Calcific Mitral Valve, *Circulation,* 49:1167, 1974.
9. Jordan, R. A., Scheifley, C. H., and Edwards, J. E.: Mural Thrombosis and Arterial Embolism in Mitral Stenosis. A Clinicopathologic Study of Fifty-One Cases, *Circulation,* 3:363, 1951.
10. Shone, J. D., Sellers, R. D., Anderson, R. C., Adams, P., Jr., Lillehei, C. W., and Edwards, J. E.: The Developmental Complex of "Parachute Mitral Valve," Supravalvular Ring of Left Atrium, Subaortic Stenosis and Coarctation of Aorta, *Am. J. Cardiol.,* 11:714, 1963.
11. da Silva, C. L., and Edwards, J. E.: Parachute Mitral Valve in an Adult, *Arq. Bras. Cardiol.,* 26:149, 1973.
12. Kennedy, J. W., Yarnall, S. R., Murray, J. A., and Figley, M. M.: Quantitative Angiocardiography. IV. Relationships of Left Atrial and Ventricular Pressure and Volume in Mitral Valve Disease, *Circulation,* 41:817, 1970.
13. Curry, G. C., Elliott, L. P., and Ramsey, H. W.: Quantitative Left Ventricular Angiocardiographic Findings in Mitral Stenosis; Detailed Analysis of the Anterolateral Wall of the Left Ventricle, *Am. J. Cardiol.,* 29:621, 1972.
14. Silverstein, D. M., Hansen, D. P., Ojiambo, H. P., and Griswold, H. E.: Left Ventricular Function in Severe Pure Mitral Stenosis as Seen at the Kenyatta National Hospital, *Am. Heart J.,* 99:727, 1980.
15. Wrobleroski, E., James F., Spann, J. F., and Bore, A. A.:

Right Ventricular Performance in Mitral Stenosis, *Am. J. Cardiol.*, 47:51, 1981.
16. Rowe, J. C., Bland, E. F., Sprague, H. B., and White, P. D.: The Course of Mitral Stenosis without Surgery: Ten and Twenty Year Perspectives, *Ann. Intern. Med.*, 52:741, 1960.
17. Wood, P.: An Appreciation of Mitral Stenosis, *Br. Med. J.*, 1:1051, 1954.
18. Selzer, A., and Cohn, K. E.: Natural History of Mitral Stenosis: A Review, *Circulation*, 45:878, 1972.
19. Szekely, P., Turner, R., and Snaith, L.: Pregnancy and the Changing Pattern of Rheumatic Heart Disease, *Br. Heart J.*, 35:1293, 1973.
20. Schwartz, R., Meyerson, R. M., Lawrence, L. T., and Nichols, H. T.: Mitral Stenosis, Massive Pulmonary Hemorrhage and Emergency Valve Replacement, *N. Engl. J. Med.*, 272:755, 1966.
21. Ross, R. S.: Right Ventricular Hypertension as a Cause of Precordial Pain, *Am. Heart J.*, 61:134, 1961.
22. Baker, C. G., and Finnegan, T. R. L.: Epilepsy and Mitral Stenosis, *Br. Heart J.*, 19:159, 1957.
23. Mounsey, J. P. D.: Inspection and Palpation of the Cardiac Impulse, *Prog. Cardiovasc. Dis.*, 10:187, 1967.
24. Thompson, M. E., Shaver, J. A., Heidenreich, F. P., Leon, D. F., and Leonard, J. J.: Sound, Pressure and Motion Correlates in Mitral Stenosis, *Am. J. Med.*, 49:436, 1970.
25. Luisada, A. A., MacCanon, D. M., Kumar, S., and Feigen, L. P.: Changing Views on the Mechanism of the First and Second Heart Sounds, *Am. Heart J.*, 88:503, 1974.
26. Wooley, C. F., Klassen, K. P., Leighton, R. F., Goodwin, R. S., and Ryan, J. M.: Left Atrial and Left Ventricular Sound and Pressure in Mitral Stenosis, *Circulation*, 38:295, 1968.
27. Dack, S., Bleifer, S., Grishman, A., and Donoso, E.: Mitral Stenosis: Auscultatory and Phonocardiographic Findings, *Am. J. Cardiol.*, 5:815, 1960.
28. Mounsey, P.: The Opening Snap of Mitral Stenosis, *Br. Heart J.*, 15:135, 1953.
29. Wells, B.: The Assessment of Mitral Stenosis by Phonocardiography, *Br. Heart J.*, 16:261, 1954.
30. Rackley, C. E., Craig, R. J., McIntosh, H. D., and Orgain, E. S.: Phonocardiographic Discrepancies in the Assessment of Mitral Stenosis, *Arch. Intern. Med.*, 121:50, 1968.
31. Ebringer, R., Pitt, A., and Anderson, S. T.: Haemodynamic Factors Influencing Opening Snap Interval in Mitral Stenosis, *Br. Heart J.*, 32:350, 1970.
32. Nixon, P. G., Wooler, G. H., and Radigan, L. R.: The Opening Snap in Mitral Incompetence, *Br. Heart J.*, 22:395, 1960.
33. Millward, D. K., McLaurin, L. P., and Craige, E.: Echocardiographic Studies to Explain Opening Snaps in Presence of Non-stenotic Mitral Valves, *Am. J. Cardiol.*, 31:64, 1973.
34. Leatham, A., and Gray, I.: Auscultatory and Phonocardiographic Signs of Atrial Septal Defect, *Br. Heart J.*, 18:193, 1956.
35. Vacca, J. B., Bussman, D. W., and Mudd, J. G.: Ebstein's Anomaly: Complete Review of 108 Cases, *Am. J. Cardiol.*, 2:210, 1958.
36. Perloff, J. K., and Harvey, W. P.: Clinical Recognition of Tricuspid Stenosis, *Circulation*, 22:346, 1960.
37. Crawley, I. S., Morris, D. C., and Silverman, B. D.: Valvular Heart Disease, in J. W. Hurst, R. B. Logue, R. C. Schlant, and N. K. Wenger (eds.), "The Heart," 4th ed., McGraw-Hill Book Co., New York, 1978, p. 992.
38. Surawicz, B.: Effect of Respiration and Upright Position on the Interval Between the Two Components of the Second Heart Sound and that Between the Second Sound and Mitral Opening Snap, *Circulation*, 16:422, 1957.
39. Fortuin, N. J., and Craige, E.: Echocardiographic Studies of Genesis of Mitral Diastolic Murmurs, *Br. Heart J.*, 35:75, 1973.
40. Lakier, J. B., Pocock, W. A., Gale, G. E., and Barlow, J. B.: Haemodynamic and Sound Events Preceding First Heart Sound in Mitral Stenosis, *Br. Heart J.*, 34:1152, 1972.
41. Bonner, A. J., Jr., Stewart, J., and Travel, M. E.: "Presystolic" Augmentation of Diastolic Heart Sounds in Atrial Fibrillation, *Am. J. Cardiol.*, 37:427, 1976.
42. McGuire, L. B., Nolan, T. B., Reeve, R., and Dammann, J. F., Jr.: Cor Triatriatum as a Problem of Heart Disease, *Circulation*, 31:263, 1965.
43. Korn, D., DeSanctis, R. W., and Sell, S.: Massive Calcification of the Mitral Annulus, *N. Engl. J. Med.*, 267:900, 1962.
44. Spodick, D. H.: "Chronic and Constrictive Pericarditis," Grune & Stratton, Inc., New York, 1964.
45. McArthur, J. D., Sukumar, I. P., Munsi, S. C., Krishnaswami, S., and Cherian, G.: Reassessment of Graham Steell Murmur Using Platinum Electrode Technique, *Br. Heart J.*, 36:1023, 1974.
46. Chen, J. T. T., Behar, V. S., Morris, J. J., Jr., McIntosh, H. D., and Lester, R. G.: Correlation of Roentgen Findings with Hemodynamic Data in Pure Mitral Stenosis, *Am. J. Roentgenol. Radium Ther. Nucl. Med.*, 102:280, 1968.
47. Grainger, R. G.: Interstitial Pulmonary Edema and Its Radiographic Diagnosis: Signs of Pulmonary Venous and Capillary Hypertension, *Br. J. Radiol.*, 31:201, 1958.
48. Felson, B.: "Chest Roentgenology," W. B. Saunders Company, Philadelphia, 1973.
49. Chait, A.: Interstitial Pulmonary Edema, *Circulation*, 45:1323, 1972.
50. Meszaros, W. T.: Lung Changes in Left Heart Failure, *Circulation*, 47:859, 1973.
51. Saunders, J. L., Calatayud, J. B., Schulz, K. J., Maranhao, V., Gooch, A. S., and Goldberg, H.: Evaluation of ECG Criteria for P-Wave Abnormalities, *Am. Heart J.*, 74:757, 1967.
52. Lee, Y. C., Scherlis, L., and Singleton, R. T.: Mitral Stenosis: Hemodynamic, Electrocardiographic and Vector Cardiographic Studies, *Am. Heart J.*, 69:559, 1965.
53. Walston, A., Harley, A., and Pipberger, H. V.: Computer Analysis of the Orthogonal Electrocardiogram and Vectorcardiogram in Mitral Stenosis, *Circulation*, 50:472, 1974.
54. Duchak, J. M., Chang, S., and Feigenbaum, H.: The Posterior Mitral Valve Echo and the Echocardiographic Diagnosis of Mitral Stenosis, *Am. J. Cardiol.*, 29:6289, 1972.
55. Teicholz, L. E.: Echocardiography in Valvular Heart Disease, *Prog. Cardiovasc. Dis.*, 17:283, 1975.
56. Cope, G. D., Kisslo, J. A., Johnson, M. L., and Behar, V. S.: A Reassessment of the Echocardiogram in Mitral Stenosis, *Circulation*, 52:664, 1975.
57. Wolfe, S. B., Popp, R. L., and Feigenbaum, H.: Diagnosis of Atrial Tumors by Ultrasound, *Circulation*, 39:615, 1969.
58. McLarin, L. P., Gibson, T. C., Waider, W., Grossman, W., and Craige, E.: An Appraisal of Mitral Valve Echocardiograms Mimicking Mitral Stenosis in Conditions with Right Ventricular Pressure Overload, *Circulation*, 48:801, 1973.
59. Quinones, M. A., Gaash, W. H., Waisser, E., and Alexander, J. K.: Reduction in the Rate of Diastolic Descent of the Mitral Valve Echogram in Patients with Altered Left Ventricular Diastolic Pressure-Volume Relations, *Circulation*, 49:246, 1974.
60. Stewart, J. A., Silimperi, D., Harris, P., Wise, N. K., Fraker, T. D., and Kisslo, J. A.: Echocardiographic Documentation of Vegetative Lesions in Infective Endocarditis: Clinical Implications, *Circulation*, 61:374, 1980.
61. Gorlin, R., and Gorlin, S. G.: Hydraulic Formula for Calculation of the Area of the Stenotic Mitral Valve, Other Cardiac Valves and Central Circulatory Shunts, *Am. Heart J.*, 41:1, 1951.
62. Cohen, M. V., and Gorlin, R.: Modified Orifice Equation for the Calculation of Mitral Valve Area, *Am. Heart J.*, 84:839, 1972.
63. Hakki, A., Iskandrian, A. S., Bemis, C. E., Kimbiris, D., Mintz, G. S., Segal, B. L., and Brice, C.: A Simplified Valve Formula for the Calculation of Stenotic Valve Areas, *Circulation*, 63:1050, 1981.
64. Hungenholtz, P. G., Ryan, T. J., Stein, S. W., and Abelmann, W. H.: The Spectrum of Pure Mitral Stenosis: Hemodynamic Studies in Relation to Clinical Disability, *Am. J. Cardiol.*, 10:773, 1962.
65. Bolen, J. L., Lopes, M. G., Harrison, D. C., and Alderman, E. L.: Analysis of Left Ventricular Function in Response to Afterload Changes in Patients with Mitral Stenosis, *Circulation*, 52:894, 1975.

66. Heller, S. J., and Carleton, R. A.: Abnormal Left Ventricular Contraction in Patients with Mitral Stenosis, *Circulation,* 42:1099, 1970.
67. Hildner, F. J., Javier, R. P., Cohen, L. S., Samet, P., Nathan, M. J., Yahr, W. Z., and Greenberg, J. J.: Myocardial Dysfunction Associated with Valvular Heart Disease, *Am. J. Cardiol.,* 30:319, 1972.
68. Chun, P. K., Gertz, E., Davia, J. E., and Cheitlin, M. D.: Coronary Atherosclerosis in Mitral Stenosis, *Chest,* 81:36, 1982.
69. Newman, G. E., Bounous, P. W., Jones, R. H., and Saliston, D. C.: Noninvasive Assessment of Hemodynamic Effects of Mitral Valve Commissurotomy during Rest and Exercise in Patients with Mitral Stenosis, *J. Thorac. Cardiovasc. Surg.,* 78:750, 1979.
70. Bhathia, M. L., Shriuastava, S., and Roy, S. B.: Immediate Haemodynamic Effects of a Beta Adrenergic Blocking Agent, Propranolol, in Mitral Stenosis at Fixed Heart Rates, *Br. Heart J.,* 34:638, 1972.
71. Meister, S. G., Engel, T. R., Feitosa, G. S., Helfant, R. H., and Frankl, W. S.: Propranolol in Mitral Stenosis During Stress Rhythm, *Am. Heart J.,* 94:685, 1977.
72. Giuffrida, G., Bonzani, G., Betocchi, S., Piscione, F., Giudice, P., Miceli, D., Mazza, F., and Condorelli, M.: Hemodynamic Response to Exercise after Propranolol in Patients with Mitral Stenosis, *Am. J. Cardiol.,* 44:1076, 1979.
73. Abernathy, W. S., and Willis, P. W., III: Thromboembolic Complications of Rheumatic Heart Disease, *Cardiovasc. Clin.,* 5:131, 1973.
74. Kellogg, F., Lui, C. K., Fishman, W., and Larson, R.: Systemic and Pulmonary Emboli before and after Mitral Commissurotomy, *Circulation,* 24:263, 1961.
75. Rapaport, E.: Natural History of Aortic and Mitral Valve Disease, *Am. J. Cardiol.,* 35:221, 1975.
76. Olesen, K. H.: The Natural History of 271 Patients with Mitral Stenosis under Medical Treatment, *Br. Heart J.,* 24:349, 1962.
77. Kaplan, E. L., Anthony, B. F., Bisno, A., Durack, D., Houser, H., Millard, H. D., Sanford, J., Shulman, S. T., Stillerman, M., Taranta, A., and Wengar, N.: Prevention of Bacterial Endocarditis, *Circulation,* 56:7, 1977.
78. Kirklin, J. W., Conti, V. R., and Blackstone, E. H.: Prevention of Myocardial Damage during Cardiac Operations, *N. Engl. J. Med.,* 301:135, 1979.
79. Carpentier, A., Chauvaud, S., Fabiani, J. N., Deloche, A., Relland, J., Lessana, A., d'Allaines, C., Blondeau, P., Piwnica, A., and Dubost, C. H.: Reconstructive Surgery of Mitral Valve Incompetence, *J. Thorac. Cardiovasc. Surg.,* 79:338, 1980.
80. Duran, C. G., Pomar, J. L., Revuelta, J. M., Gallo, I., Poveda, J., Ochoteco, A., and Ubago, J. L.: Conservative Operation for Mitral Insufficiency: Critical Analysis Supported by Postoperative Hemodynamic Studies of 72 Patients, *J. Thorac. Cardiovasc. Surg.,* 69:326, 1980.
81. Kouchoukos, N. T., and Karp, R. B.: Management of the Postoperative Cardiovascular Surgical Patient, *Am. Heart J.,* 92:513, 1976.
82. Ellis, L. B., Singh, J. B., Morales, D. D., and Harken, D. E.: Fifteen to Twenty Year Study of One Thousand Patients Undergoing Closed Mitral Valvuloplasty, *Circulation,* 48:357, 1973.
83. Heger, J. J., Wann, L. S., Weyman, A. E., Dillon, J. C., and Feigenbaum, H.: Long-Term Changes in Mitral Valve Area after Successful Mitral Commissurotomy, *Circulation,* 59:443, 1979.
84. Higgs, L. M., Glancy, D. L., O'Brien, K. P., Epstein, S. E., and Morrow, A. G.: Mitral Restenosis an Uncommon Cause of Recurrent Symptoms Following Mitral Commissurotomy, *Am. J. Cardiol.,* 26:34, 1970.
85. Hope, J.: Signs of Disease of the Mitral Valve, in "A Treatise on the Diseases of the Heart," Churchill, London, 1839, p. 387.
86. Silverman, M. E., and Hurst, J. W.: The Mitral Complex, *Am. Heart J.,* 76:399, 1968.
87. Barlow, J. B., and Pocock, W. A.: The Problem of Nonejection Systolic Clicks and Associated Mitral Systolic Murmurs: Emphasis on the Billowing Mitral Leaflet Syndrome, *Am. Heart J.,* 90:636, 1975.
88. Rackley, C. E., Dear, H. D., Baxley, W. A., Jones, W. B., and Dodge, H. T.: Left Ventricular Chamber Volume, Mass and Function in Severe Coronary Artery Disease, *Circulation,* 41:605, 1970.
89. Perloff, J. K., and Roberts, W. C.: The Mitral Apparatus: Functional Anatomy of Mitral Regurgitation, *Circulation,* 46:227, 1972.
90. Rytand, D. A., and Lipsitch, L. S.: Clinical Aspects of Calcification of the Mitral Annulus Fibrosus, *Arch. Intern. Med.,* 78:544, 1946.
91. Roberts, W. C., Dangel, J. C., and Bulkley, B. H.: Nonrheumatic Valvular Cardiac Disease: A Clinicopathologic Survey of 27 Different Conditions Causing Valvular Dysfunction, in W. Likoff (guest ed.), "Valvular Heart Disease," *Cardiovasc. Clin.,* 5(2):333, 1973.
92. McKusick, V. A.: "Heritable Disorders of Connective Tissue," The C. V. Mosby Company, St. Louis, 1972.
93. Burch, G. E., DePasquale, N. P., and Phillips, J. H.: Clinical Manifestation of Papillary Muscle Dysfunction, *Arch. Intern. Med.,* 112:112, 1963.
94. Heikkila, J.: Mitral Incompetence Complicating Acute Myocardial Infarction, *Br. Heart J.,* 29:162, 1967.
95. DeBusk, R. F., and Harrison, D. C.: The Clinical Spectrum of Papillary-Muscle Disease, *N. Engl. J. Med.,* 281:1458, 1969.
96. Fowler, N. O., and Van der Mel-Kahn, J. M.: Indications for Surgical Replacement of the Mitral Valve; with Particular Reference to Common and Uncommon Causes of Mitral Regurgitation, *Am. J. Cardiol.,* 44:148, 1979.
97. Selzer, A., Kelly, J. J., Jr., Vannitamby, M., Walker, P., Gerbode, F., and Kerth, W. J.: The Syndrome of Mitral Insufficiency Due to Isolated Rupture of the Chordae Tendineae, *Am. J. Med.,* 43:822, 1967.
98. Sanders, C. A., Armstrong, P. W., Willerson, J. T., and Dinsmore, R. E.: Etiology and Differential Diagnosis of Acute Mitral Regurgitation, *Prog. Cardiovasc. Dis.,* 14:129, 1971.
99. Edwards, J. E.: Pathology of Acquired Valvular Disease of the Heart, *Semin. Roentgenol.,* 14:96, 1979.
100. Perloff, J. K., and Roberts, W. C.: The Mitral Apparatus. Functional Anatomy of Mitral Regurgitation, *Circulation,* 46:227, 1972.
101. Burchell, H. B., and Edwards, J. E.: Rheumatic Mitral Insufficiency, *Circulation,* 7:747, 1953.
102. Levy, M. J., and Edwards, J. E.: Anatomy of Mitral Insufficiency, *Prog. Cardiovasc. Dis.,* 5:119, 1962.
103. Edwards, J. E., and Burchell, H. B.: Pathologic Anatomy of Mitral Insufficiency, *Proc. Mayo Clin.,* 33:497, 1958.
104. Edwards, J. E.: Mitral Insufficiency Secondary to Aortic Valvular Bacterial Endocarditis, *Circulation,* 46:623, 1972.
105. Pomerance, A.: Ballooning Deformity (Mucoid Degeneration) of Atrioventricular Valves, *Br. Heart J.,* 31:343, 1969.
106. Guthrie, R. G., and Edwards, J. E.: Pathology of the Myxomatous Mitral Valve. Nature, Secondary Changes and Complications, *Minnesota Med.,* 59:637, 1976.
107. Ranganathan, N., Silver, M. D., Robinson, T. I., Kostuk, W. J., Felderhof, C. H., Patt, N. L., Wilson, J. K., and Wigle, E. D.: Angiographic Morphologic Correlation in Patients with Severe Mitral Regurgitation Due to Prolapse of the Posterior Mitral Leaflet, *Circulation,* 48:514, 1973.
108. Salazar, A. E., and Edwards, J. E.: Friction Lesions of Ventricular Endocardium. Relation to Chordae Tendineae of Mitral Valve, *Arch. Pathol.,* 90:364, 1970.
109. Goodman, D., Kimbiris, D., and Linhart, J. W.: Chordae Tendineae Rupture Complicating the Systolic Click-Late Systolic Murmur Syndrome, *Am. J. Cardiol.,* 33:681, 1974.
110. Moller, J. H., Lucas, R. V., Jr., Adams, P., Jr., Anderson, R. C., Jorgans, J., and Edwards, J. E.: Endocardial Fibroelastosis. A Clinical and Anatomic Study of 47 Patients with Emphasis on Its Relationship to Mitral Insufficiency, *Circulation,* 30:759, 1964.
111. Vlodaver, Z., and Edwards, J. E.: Rupture of Ventricular Septum or Papillary Muscle Complicating Myocardial Infarction, *Circulation,* 55:815, 1977.
112. Lee, K. S., Johnson, T., Karnegis, J. N., Quattlebaum,

F. W., and Edwards, J. E.: Acute Myocardial Infarction with Long-Term Survival Following Papillary Muscle Rupture, *Am. Heart J.*, 79:258, 1970.
113. Tsakiris, A. G., Rastelli, G. C., Amorim, D., Titus, J. L., and Wood, E. H.: Effect of Experimental Papillary Muscle Damage on Mitral Valve Closure in Intact Anesthetized Dogs, *Proc. Mayo Clin.*, 45:275, 1970.
114. Hall, S. W., Jr., Theologides, A., From, A. H. L., Gobel, F. L., Fortuny, I. E., Lawrence, C. J., and Edwards, J. E.: Hypereosinophilic Syndrome with Biventricular Involvement, *Circulation*, 55:217, 1977.
115. Bulkley, B. H., and Roberts, W. C.: Systemic Lupus Erythematosus as a Cause of Severe Mitral Regurgitation. New Problem in an Old Disease, *Am. J. Cardiol.*, 35:305, 1975.
116. Pomerance, A.: Pathological and Clinical Study of Calcification of the Mitral Valve Ring, *Br. J. Clin. Pathol.*, 23:354, 1970.
117. Braunwald, E.: Mitral Regurgitation: Physiologic, Clinical and Surgical Considerations, *N. Engl. J. Med.*, 281:425, 1969.
118. Ross, J., Jr., Braunwald, E., and Morrow, A. G.: Clinical and Hemodynamic Observations in Pure Mitral Insufficiency, *Am. J. Cardiol.*, 2:11, 1958.
119. Dodge, H. T., and Baxley, W. A.: Left Ventricular Volume and Mass and Their Significance in Heart Disease, *Am. J. Cardiol.*, 23:528, 1969.
120. Rackley, C. E., and Hood, W. P., Jr.: Quantitative Angiographic Evaluation and Pathophysiologic Mechanisms in Valvular Heart Disease, in E. J. Sonnenblick and M. Lesch (eds.), "Valvular Heart Disease," Grune & Stratton, Inc., New York, 1975, p. 109.
121. Hood, W. P., Jr., Rackley, C. E., and Rolett, E. L.: Wall Stress in the Normal and Hypertrophied Human Left Ventricle, *Am. J. Cardiol.*, 22:550, 1968.
122. Rackley, C. E.: Value of Ventriculography in Cardiac Function and Diagnosis, in A. N. Brest (ed.), "Diagnostic Methods in Cardiology," *Cardiovasc. Clin.*, 6:3:283, 1975.
123. Porter, C. M., Baxley, W. A., Eddleman, E. E., Jr. Frimer, M., and Rackley, C. E.: Left Ventricular Dimensions and Dynamics of Filling in Patients with Gallop Heart Sounds, *Am. J. Med.*, 50:721, 1971.
124. Rackley, C. E., Hood, W. P., Jr., Rolett, E. L., and Young, D. T.: Left Ventricular End-Diastolic Pressure in Chronic Heart Disease, *Am. J. Med.*, 48:310, 1970.
125. Jeresaty, R. M.: Mitral Valve Prolapse-Click Syndrome, *Prog. Cardiovasc. Dis.*, 15:623, 1973.
126. Nutter, D. O., Wickliffe, C., Gilbert, C. A., Moody, C., and King, S. A.: The Pathophysiology of Idiopathic Mitral Valve Prolapse, *Circulation*, 52:297, 1975.
127. Bulkley, B. H., and Roberts, W. C.: Dilatation of the Mitral Annulus, *Am. J. Med.*, 59:457, 1975.
128. Gooch, A. D., Vicencio, E., Maranchao, V., and Goldberg, H.: Arrhythmias and Left Ventricle Asynergy in the Prolapsing Mitral Leaflet, *Am. J. Cardiol.*, 29:611, 1972.
129. Newman, G. E., Gibbons, R. J., Jones, R. H.: Cardiac Function During Rest and Exercise in Patients with Mitral Valve Prolapse, *Am. J. Cardiol.*, 47:14, 1981.
130. Aranda, J. M., Befeler, B., Lazzara, R., Embi, A., and Marchado, H.: Mitral Valve Prolapse and Coronary Artery Disease, *Circulation*, 52:245, 1975.
131. Verani, M. S., Carroll, R. J., and Falsetti, H. L.: Mitral Valve Prolapse in Coronary Disease, *Am. J. Cardiol.*, 37:1, 1976.
132. Sabom, M. V., Curry, R. C., Jr., Pepine, C. J., Christie, L. G., and Conti, C. R.: Ergonovine Testing for Coronary Artery Spasm in Patients with Angiographic Mitral Valve Prolapse, *Cath. Cardiovasc. Diag.*, 4:265, 1978.
133. Pasternac, A., Tubau, J. F., Puddu, P. E., Krol, R. B., and De Champlain, J.: Increased Plasma Catecholamine Levels in Patients with Symptomatic Mitral Valve Prolapse, *Am. J. Med.*, 73:783, 1982.
134. Rackley, C. E., Russell, R. O., Jr., Mantle, J. A., and Rogers, W. J.: Modern Approach to the Patient with Acute Myocardial Infarction, in W. P. Harvey (ed.), "Current Problems in Cardiology," vol. 1, Yearbook Medical Publishers, Chicago, 1977, p. 10.
135. Boltwood, C. M., Tei, C., Wong, M., and Shah, P. M.: Quantitative Echocardiography of the Mitral Complex in Dilated Cardiomyopathy: The Mechanism of Functional Mitral Regurgitation, *Circulation*, 68:498, 1983.
136. Chandraratna, P. A. N., and Aronow, W. S.: Mitral Valve Ring in Normal vs. Dilated Left Ventricle: Cross-Sectional Echocardiography Study, *Chest*, 79:151, 1981.
137. Klughaupt, M., Flamm, M. D., Hancock, E. W., and Harrison, D. C.: Nonrheumatic Mitral Insufficiency: Determination of Operability and Prognosis, *Circulation*, 39:307, 1969.
138. Selzer, A., and Katayama, F.: Mitral Regurgitation: Clinical Patterns, Pathophysiology and Natural History, *Medicine (Baltimore)*, 51:337, 1972.
139. Bentivoglio, L., Urichio, J., and Goldberg, H.: Clinical and Hemodynamic Features of Advanced Rheumatic Mitral Regurgitation, *Am. J. Med.*, 30:372, 1961.
140. Ellis, L. B., and Ramirez, A.: The Clinical Course of Patients with Severe "Rheumatic" Mitral Insufficiency, *Am. Heart J.*, 78:406, 1969.
141. Winkle, R. A., Lopes, M. G., Fitzgerald, J. W., Goodman, D. J., Schroeder, J. S. and Harrison, D. C.: Arrhythmias in Patients with Mitral Valve Prolapse, *Circulation*, 52:73, 1975.
142. Brody, W., and Criley, J. M.: Intermittent Severe Mitral Regurgitation, *N. Engl. J. Med.*, 283:673, 1970.
143. Grenadier, E., Pan, G. A., Keidar, S., and Palant, A.: The Prevalence of Ruptured Chordae Tendineae in the Mitral Valve Prolapse Syndrome, *Am. Heart J.*, 105:603, 1983.
144. Basta, L. L., Wolfson, P., Eckberg, D. L., and Abboud, F. M.: The Value of Left Parasternal Impulse Recordings in the Assessment of Mitral Regurgitation, *Circulation*, 48:1055, 1973.
145. Reichek, N., Shelburne, J. C., and Perloff, J. K.: Clinical Aspects of Rheumatic Valvular Disease, *Prog. Cardiovasc. Dis.*, 15:491, 1973.
146. Karliner, J. S., O'Rourke, R. A., Kearney, D. J., and Shabetai, R.: Haemodynamic Explanation of Why the Murmur of Mitral Regurgitation Is Independent of Cycle Length, *Br. Heart J.*, 35:397, 1973.
147. Perloff, J. K., and Harvey, W. P.: Auscultatory and Phonocardiographic Manifestations of Pure Mitral Regurgitation, *Prog. Cardiovasc. Dis.*, 5:172, 1962.
148. Perloff, J. K., and Harvey, W. P.: Mechanisms of Fixed Splitting of the Second Heart Sound, *Circulation*, 18:998, 1958.
149. Bleifer, S., Dack, S., Grishman, A., and Donoso, E.: The Auscultatory and Phonocardiographic Findings in Mitral Regurgitation, *Am. J. Cardiol.*, 5:836, 1960.
150. Devereux, R. B., Perloff, J. K., Reichek, N., and Josephson, M.E.: Mitral Valve Prolapse, *Circulation*, 54:3, 1976.
151. Santos, A. D., Puthenpurakal, M. K., Ahmad, H., and Wallace, W. A.: Orthostatic Hypotension: A Commonly Unrecognized Cause of Symptoms in Mitral Valve Prolapse, *Am. J. Med.*, 71:746, 1981.
152. Epstein, E. J., and Coulshed, N.: Phonocardiogram and Apex Cardiogram in Systolic Click-Late Systolic Murmur Syndrome, *Br. Heart J.*, 35:260, 1973.
153. O'Rourke, R. A., and Crawford, M. H.: The Systolic Click-Murmur Syndrome: Clinical Recognition and Management, *Curr. Probl. Cardiol.*, 1(1):1, 1976.
154. Wei, J., and Fortuin, N. J.: Diastolic Sounds and Murmurs Associated with Mitral Valve Prolapse, *Circulation* 63:559, 1981.
155. Fontana, M. E., Wooley, C. G., Leighton, R. F., and Lewis, R. P.: Postural Changes in Left Ventricular and Mitral Valvular Dynamics in the Systolic Click-Late Systolic Murmur Syndrome, *Circulation*, 51:165, 1975.
156. Shelburne, J. C., Rubenstein, D., and Gorlin, R.: A Reappraisal of Papillary Muscle Dysfunction, *Am. J. Med.*, 46:862, 1969.
157. Holmes, A. M., Logan, W. F., and Winterbottom, T.: Transient Systolic Murmurs in Angina Pectoris, *Am. Heart J.*, 76:680, 1968.
158. Sanders, C. A., Austen, W. G., Harthorne, J. W., Dinsmore, R. E., and Scannell, J. G.: Diagnosis and Surgical Treatment of Mitral Regurgitation Secondary to Ruptured Chordae Tendineae, *N. Engl. J. Med.*, 276:943, 1967.

159. Ronan, J. A., Jr., Steelman, R. B., de Leon, A. C., Jr., Waters, T. J., Perloff, J. K., and Harvey, W. P.: The Clinical Diagnosis of Acute Severe Mitral Insufficiency, *Am. J. Cardiol.*, 27:284, 1971.
160. Sleeper, J. C., Orgain, E. S., and McIntosh, H. D.: Mitral Insufficiency Simulating Aortic Stenosis, *Circulation*, 26:428, 1962.
161. Priest, E. A., Finlayson, J. K., and Short, D. S.: The X-Ray Manifestations in the Heart and Lungs of Mitral Regurgitation, *Prog. Cardiovasc. Dis.*, 5:219, 1962.
162. BonTempo, C. P., Ronan, J. A., de Leon, A. C., and Twigg, H. L.: Radiographic Appearance of the Thorax in Systolic Click, Late Systolic Murmur Syndrome, *Am. J. Cardiol.*, 36:27, 1975.
163. Solomon, J., Shab, P. M., and Heinkle, R. A.: Thoracic Skeletal Abnormalities in Idiopathic Mitral Valve Prolapse, *Am. J. Cardiol.*, 36:32, 1975.
164. Bentivoglis, L. G., Uricchio, J. F., Waldow, A., Likoff, W., and Goldberg, H.: An Electrocardiographic Analysis of Mitral Regurgitation, *Circulation*, 18:572, 1956.
165. Peter, R. H., Morris, J. J., Jr., and McIntosh, H. D.: Relationship of Fibrillatory Waves and P Waves in the Electrocardiogram, *Circulation*, 33:599, 1966.
166. DeMaria, A. N., Amsterdam, E. A., Vismara, L. A., Neumann, A., and Mason, D. T.: Arrhythmias in the Mitral Valve Prolapse Syndrome, *Ann. Intern. Med.*, 84:656, 1976.
167. Burch, G. E., DePasquale, N. P., and Phillips, J. H.: The Syndrome of Papillary Muscle Dysfunction, *Am. Heart J.*, 75:399, 1968.
168. Popp, R. L., Brown, O. R., Silverman, J. F., and Harrison, D. C.: Echocardiographic Abnormalities in the Mitral Valve Prolapse Syndrome, *Circulation*, 49:428, 1974.
169. Burgess, J., Clark, R., Kamigaki, M., and Cohen, K.: Echocardiographic Findings in Different Types of Mitral Regurgitation, *Circulation*, 48:97, 1973.
170. DeMaria, A. N., King, J. F., Bogren, H. G., Lies, J. E., and Mason, D. T.: The Variable Spectrum of Echocardiographic Manifestations of the Mitral Valve Prolapse Syndrome, *Circulation*, 50:33, 1974.
171. Rackley, C. E., Russell, R. O., Jr., and Ratshin, R. A.: Hemodynamics of Acute Myocardial Infarction: Invasive and Noninvasive Studies. Proceedings of the William Likoff Symposium, New York, Dec. 14–16, 1973, in Henry I. Russek (ed.), "New Horizons in Cardiovascular Practice," University Park Press, Baltimore, 1975, p. 197.
172. Mellino, M., Salcedo, E. E., Lever, H. M., Vasudevan, G., and Kramer, J. R.: Echographic Quantified Severity of Mitral Annulus Calcification: Prognostic Correlation to Related Hemodynamic Valvular, Rhythm and Conduction Abnormalities, *Am. Heart J.*, 103:222, 1982.
173. Sweatman, T., Selzer, A., Kamageki, M., and Cohn, K.: Echocardiographic Diagnosis of Mitral Regurgitation Due to Ruptured Chordae Tendineae, *Circulation*, 46:580, 1972.
174. Fuchs, R. M., Heuser, R. R., Yin, F. C. P., and Brinker, J. A.: Limitations of Pulmonary Wedge V Waves in Diagnosing Mitral Regurgitation, *Am. J. Cardiol.*, 49:849, 1982.
175. Pichard, A. D., Kay, R., Smith, H., Rentrop, P., Holt, J., and Gorlin, R.: Large V Waves in the Pulmonary Wedge Pressure Tracing in the Absence of Mitral Regurgitation, *Am. J. Cardiol.*, 50:1044, 1982.
176. Grose, R., Strain, J., and Cohen, M. V.: Pulmonary Arterial V Waves in Mitral Regurgitation: Clinical and Experimental Observations, *Circulation*, 69:214, 1984.
177. Sandler, H., Dodge, H. T., Hay, R. E., and Rackley, C. E.: Quantitation of Valvular Insufficiency in Man by Angiocardiography, *Am. Heart J.*, 65:501, 1963.
178. Braunwald, E., and Awe, W. C.: The Syndrome of Severe Mitral Regurgitation with Normal Left Atrial Pressure, *Circulation*, 27:29, 1963.
179. Rackley, C. E., Dodge, H. T., Coble, Y. D., and Hay, R. E.: A Method for Determining Left Ventricular Mass in Man, *Circulation*, 29:666, 1964.
180. Mantle, J. A., Russell, R. O., Jr., Rogers, W. J., and Rackley, C. E.: Advances in the Treatment of Heart Failure, in C. E. Rackley and A. N. Brest (eds.), "Critical Care Cardiology," F. A. Davis, Philadelphia, Cardiovascular Clinics, 1981, pp. 49-64.
181. Carabello, B. A., and Spann, J. F.: The Uses and Limitations of End-Systolic Indexes of Left Ventricular Function, *Circulation*, 69:1058, 1984.
182. Scampardonis, G., Yang, S. S., Maranhao, V., Goldberg, H., and Gooch, A. S.: Left Ventricular Abnormalities in Prolapsed Mitral Leaflet Syndrome, *Circulation*, 48:287, 1973.
183. Rackley, C. E., Russell, R. O., Jr., Mantle, J. A., and Rogers, W. J.: Recognition of Acute Myocardial Infarction, in C. E. Rackley and R. O. Russell, Jr. (eds.), "Coronary Artery Disease: Recognition and Management," Futura Publishing Company, Mount Kisco, New York, 1979, p. 315.
184. Slutsky, R., Karliner, J., Ricci, D., Kaiser, R., Pfisterer, M., Gordon, D., Peterson, K., and Ashburn, W.: Left Ventricular Volumes by Gated Equilibrium Radionuclide Angiography: A New Method, *Circulation*, 60:556, 1979.
185. Dehmer, G. J., Lewis, S. E., Hillis, L. D., Twieg, D., Falkoff, M., Parkey, R. W., and Willerson, J. T.: Nongeometric Determination of Left Ventricular Volumes from Equilibrium Blood Pool Scans, *Am. J. Cardiol.*, 45:293, 1980.
186. Gottdiener, J. S., Borer, J. S., Bacharach, S. L., Green, M. V., and Epstein, S. E.: Left Ventricular Function in Mitral Valve Prolapse: Assessment with Radionuclide Cineangiography, *Am. J. Cardiol.*, 47:7, 1981.
187. Kokibash, A. J., Bush, C. A., Fontana, M. B., Ryan, J. M., Kilman, J., and Wooley, C. F.: Mitral Valve Prolapse Syndrome: Analysis of 62 Patients Aged 60 Years and Older, *Am. J. Cardiol.*, 52:534, 1983.
188. Greenberg, B. H., Masie, B. M., Brundage, B. H., Botvinick, E. H., Parmley, W. W., and Chatterjee, K.: Beneficial Effects of Hydralazine in Severe Mitral Regurgitation, *Circulation*, 58:273, 1978.
189. Miller, R. R., Awan, N. A., Maxwell, K. S., and Mason, D. T.: Sustained Reduction of Cardiac Impedance and Preload in Congestive Heart Failure with the Antihypertensive Vasodilator Prazosin, *N. Engl. J. Med.*, 297:303, 1977.
190. Carabello, B. A., and Spann, J. F.: The Uses and Limitations of End-Systolic Indexes of Left Ventricular Function, *Circulation*, 69:1058, 1984.
191. Mantle, J. A., Hood, W. P., Jr., Kouchoukos, N. T., Karp, R. B., Zisserman, D., and Rackley, C. E.: Physiologic Basis for Afterload Reduction Following Mitral Valve Replacement, *Am. J. Cardiol.*, 41:420, 1978.
192. Eckberg, D. L., Gault, J. H., Bouchard, R. L., Karliner, J. S., and Ross, J., Jr.: Mechanics of Left Ventricular Contraction in Chronic Severe Mitral Regurgitation, *Circulation*, 47:1252, 1973.
193. Schuler, G., Peterson, K. L., Johnson, A., Francis, G., Dennish, G., Utley, J., Ashburn, W., and Ross, J., Jr.: Temporal Response of Left Ventricular Performance to Mitral Valve Surgery, *Circulation*, 59:1218, 1979.
194. Kirklin, J. W.: Replacement of Mitral Valve for Mitral Incompetence, *Surgery*, 72:827, 1972.
195. Reed, G. E., Tice, D. A., and Clauss, R. H.: Asymmetric Exaggerated Mitral Annuloplasty: Repair of Mitral Insufficiency with Hemodynamic Predictability, *J. Thorac. Cardiovasc. Surg.*, 49:752, 1965.
196. Allen, W. B., Karp, R. B., and Kouchoukos, N. T.: Mitral Valve Replacement, *Arch. Surg.*, 109:642, 1974.
197. Kirklin, J. W., and Pacifico, A. C.: Surgery for Acquired Valvular Heart Disease, *N. Engl. J. Med.*, 288:133, 1973.
198. Hansen, J. F., Anderson, E. D., Olesen, K. H., Steiness, E., Lyngborg, K., Andersen, J. D., Efsen, F., Henningsen, P., and Wennevold, A.: DC Conversion of Atrial Fibrillation after Mitral Valve Operation, *Scand. J. Thorac. Cardiovasc. Surg.*, 13:267, 1979.
199. Williams, J. B., Karp, R. B., Kirklin, J. W., Kouchoukos, N. T., Pacifico, A. C., Zorn, G. L., Jr., Blackstone, E. H., Brown, R. N., Piantadose, S., and Bradley, E. L.: Considerations in Selection and Management of Patients Undergoing Valve Replacement with Glutaraldehyde-Fixed Porcine Bioprostheses, *Ann. Thorac. Surg.*, 30:247, 1980.

39

Combined Aortic and Mitral Valve Disease*

Charles E. Rackley, M.D.
Jesse E. Edwards, M.D.
Robert B. Karp, M.D.

Nature searching for the greatest brevity in her operations has found briefer expedients to shut such gate of the heart with the pannicles than with the substance of the heart.

Leonardo da Vinci, 1513[1]

Etiology

Rheumatic fever remains an important cause of combined disease of the mitral and aortic valves. Roberts reported a high incidence of anatomic lesions involving two or more valves when the characteristic Aschoff body was identified at necropsy.[2] In recent years, connective tissue diseases have been recognized as affecting not only the aortic but also the mitral valve. In the aging patient, calcification can develop in the aortic valve apparatus and the mitral annulus. Finally, the inflammatory process of bacterial endocarditis can extend from the aortic or mitral valve to involve the adjacent valve apparatus.

In an autopsy series of 996 patients with rheumatic fever, combined aortic and mitral valve disease was observed in 32 percent.[3,4] In a clinical follow-up of 1042 children with a history of rheumatic fever followed for a 30-year period, multiple valve involvement became apparent in 50 percent of the children.[5] In the 20-year follow-up of Bland and Jones, of 699 patients with cardiac involvement due to rheumatic fever, 99 percent of the patients exhibited aortic and mitral valve involvement.[6]

Pathology

Pathological conditions that affect both the aortic and mitral valves include rheumatic fever, myxomatous degeneration and prolapse, calcification in the aging, and endocarditis. Rheumatic fever damages valve leaflets with thickening and scarring which lead to fusion, fibrosis, and calcification (Fig. 39-1). Early pathological series reported that one-third of rheumatic hearts exhibited involvement of mitral and aortic valves, but Roberts later observed that histological confirmation of rheumatic fever as the Aschoff body at necropsy was frequently associated with anatomic lesions in two or more valves.[2]

Myxomatous degeneration and valvular prolapse has been observed in the aortic as well as the mitral valve (Fig. 39-2). In Marfan's syndrome fusiform aneurysms of the aortic sinus and ascending aorta also occur with mitral valve changes of dilated annulus prolapse, ruptured chordae, and annular calcification (Fig. 39-3). Annular dilatation with and without prolapse is a major cause of mitral regurgitation in Marfan's syndrome.[7]

Calcification in aging patients can involve the aortic and mitral valves. Stenosis of the aortic valve is common, whereas regurgitation usually results from mitral annular calcification (Fig. 39-4).

Finally, infective endocarditis can extend from either the aortic or mitral valve to involve the adjacent valve through an inflammatory process (Fig. 39-5).

Abnormal Physiology

Mechanical disturbances of the mitral and aortic valves can produce a pressure overload on the left ventricle, a volume overload, or gradations of the two.[8] A pressure overload will result in concentric hypertrophy of the left ventricle even if left ventricular myocardial failure develops.[9] Aortic and mitral regurgitation produce a volume overload on the left ventricle, which may further dilate with the development of heart failure.[10] The combination of mitral stenosis and aortic insufficiency usually results in a predominant volume overload on the ventricle with chamber dilatation. The pressure and volume overloads of aortic and mitral valve diseases increase left ventricular pressure-volume work and myocardial oxygen consumption.[11,12] Development of heart failure will reduce the mechanical efficiency of the left ventricle.

An important physiological factor in combined valve disease is the predominance of a single valve and possibly the concealment of involvement of the second valve. The presence of mitral stenosis will lead to left atrial and pulmonary venous hypertension and eventual pulmonary hypertension with right ventricular hypertrophy. Mitral stenosis may obscure concomitant aortic stenosis, but a pressure overload and hypertrophy will still develop in the left ventricle. When aortic stenosis is attended by mitral insufficiency, the pressure and volume loads on the left ventricle produce dilatation and hypertrophy. Left atrial enlargement and elevation of pul-

*The editor-in-chief wishes to thank John W. Kirklin, M.D., for his previous contribution to the chapter on this subject that appeared in the fifth edition of *The Heart*.

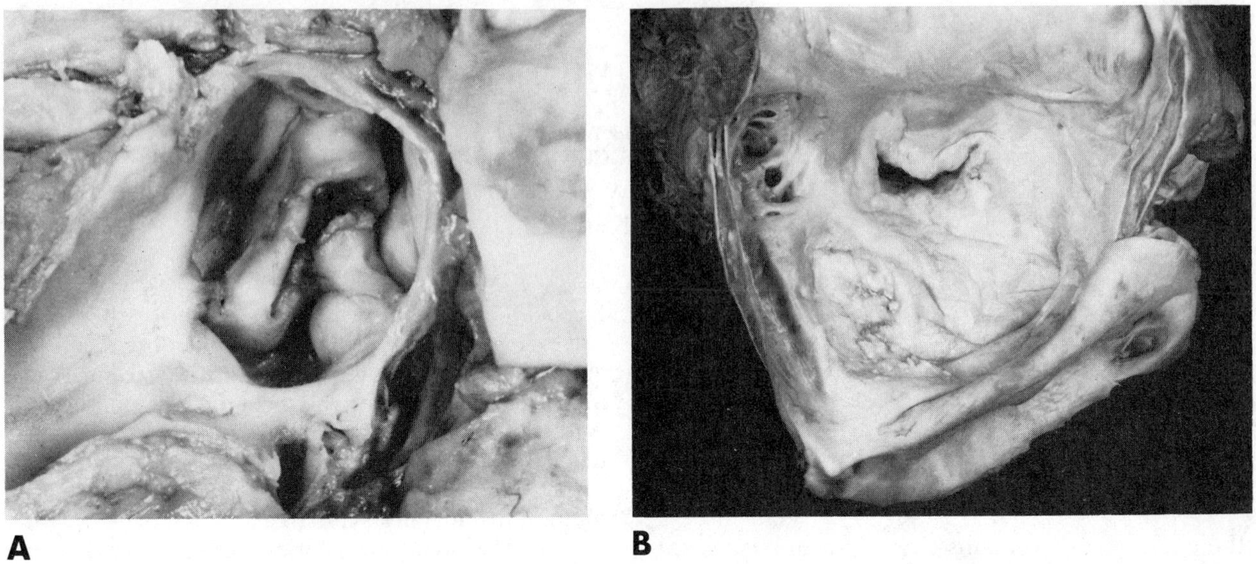

FIGURE 39-1 Rheumatic aortic stenosis and insufficiency and rheumatic mitral stenosis—specimens from a 57-year-old woman. *A.* Aortic valve, unopened and viewed from above. Fusion of each of the three aortic valvular commissures, causing reduction in caliber of the orifice of the aortic valve, is apparent. The associated shortening of the cusps results in aortic regurgitation. *B.* Mitral valve, unopened and viewed from above, and opened left atrium. The mitral valve shows fusion at each of the commissures. The orifice is reduced in caliber. The left atrium is large, and calcification of the posterior part of the left atrial wall is present (lower part of illustration).

monary artery pressures often accompany this combination. In mitral and aortic regurgitation, there is usually severe dilatation of the left ventricle with compensatory hypertrophy.[13] The compliant properties of the ventricle may be initially increased, resulting in smaller elevations of end-diastolic pressure of the left ventricle and of mean left atrial pressure for larger end-diastolic volumes.[14] In valvular regurgitation, abnormalities in early diastolic filling are likely related to impaired left ventricular relaxation.[15]

Regardless of the combinations of aortic or mitral valve lesions, pulmonary congestion with elevated capillary pressure usually develops when the contractile state of the left ventricle declines. Left atrial enlargement, due either to stenosis or insufficiency of the mitral valve, frequently leads to atrial fibrillation. Alterations in pulmonary flow and cardiac rhythm frequently attend the pressure or volume overload imposed on the left ventricle in combined mitral and aortic valve disease.

Clinical Manifestations

History

The most common complaint of patients with mitral and aortic valve disease is dyspnea.[16] In combined mitral and aortic stenosis chest pain, palpitations, and syncope are the most frequent clinical manifestations. Symptoms of heart failure due to pulmo-

FIGURE 39-2 Prolapsed mitral valve and prolapsed aortic valve. *A.* Specimen of aortic valve from a 61-year-old man. The aortic valve shows redundancy or prolapse of its right cusp (R). *B.* Specimen of mitral valve from a 73-year-old woman. The mitral valve shows prominent evidence of prolapse involving the posterior leaflet (right) and the posterior half of the anterior leaflet (A).

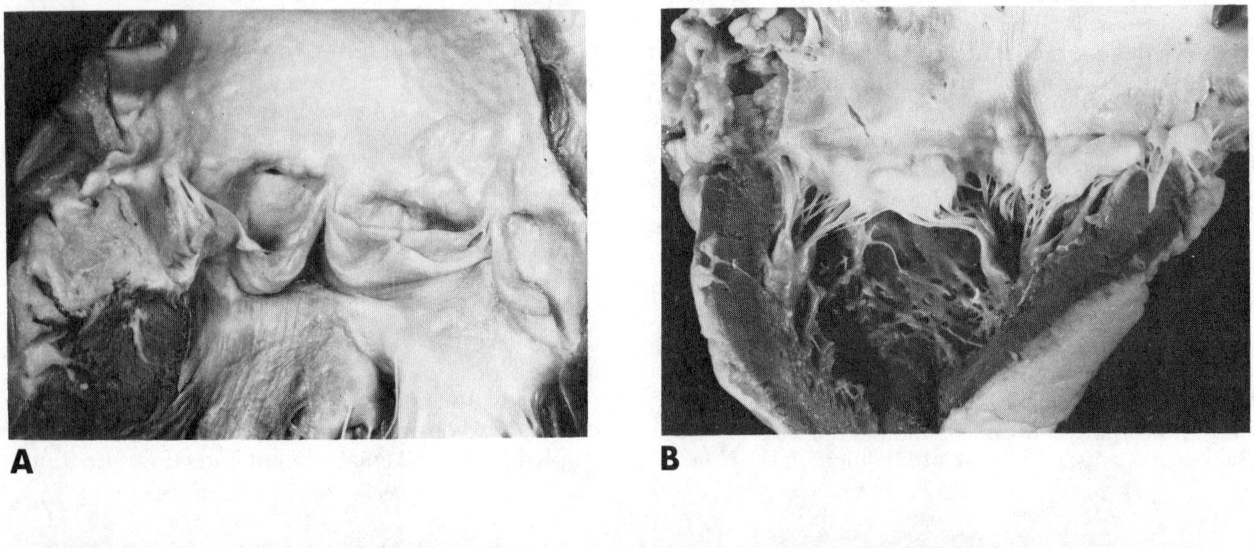

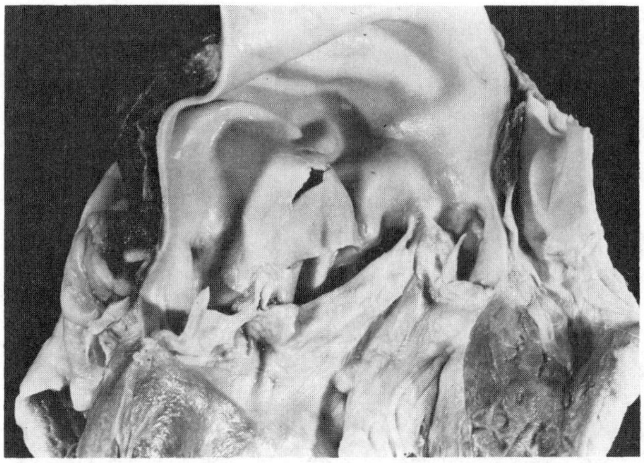

A

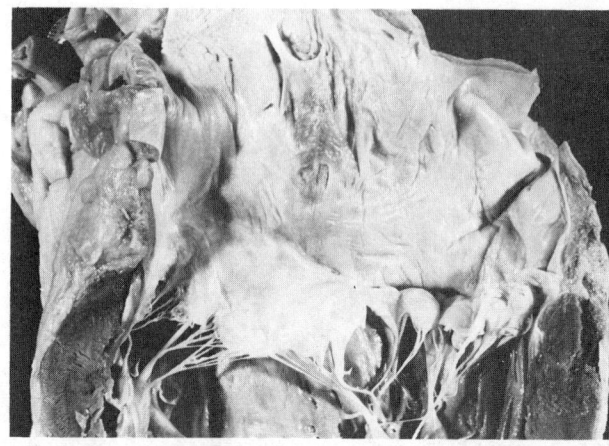

B

FIGURE 39-3 Floppy mitral valve and limited dissecting aneurysm of ascending aorta leading to aortic insufficiency—specimen from a 60-year-old man. *A.* Ascending aorta and aortic valve. The ascending aorta exhibits a laceration leading to a false channel within the aortic wall in which a hematoma is present (seen on each side of the opened aorta). Secondary distortion of the aortic valvular mechanism caused aortic insufficiency. *B.* Mitral valve, left atrium, and a portion of the left ventricle. The posterior leaflet of the mitral valve (right) shows several areas of prolapse.

FIGURE 39-4 Senile calcific aortic stenosis and calcification of the mitral ring—specimens from two different individuals. *A.* Aortic valve. Classic example of senile calcific aortic stenosis in unopened aortic valve viewed from above. *B.* Left atrium, mitral valve, and lateral wall of left ventricle. Sagittal section through left atrial (LA) and left ventricular (LV) walls reveals a calcified mass at the junction of the atrium, the left ventricle, and the posterior mitral leaflet (PM).

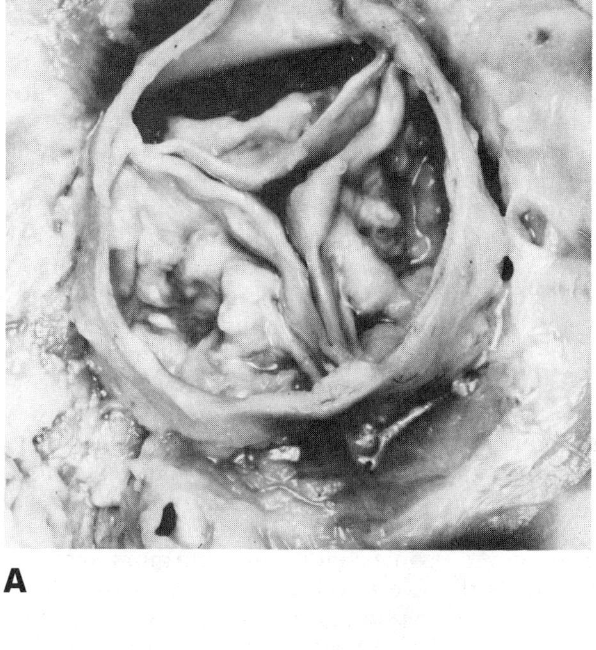

A

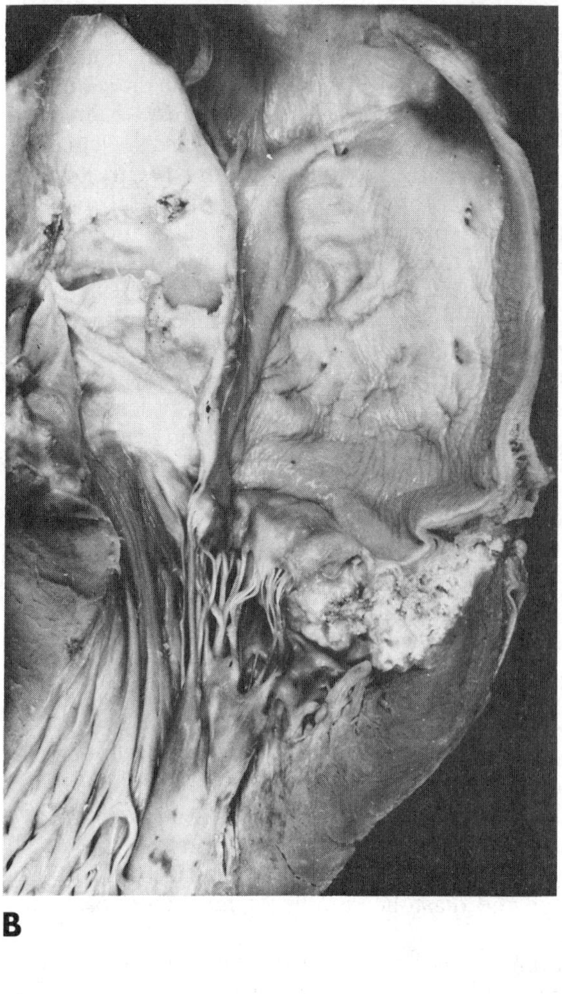

B

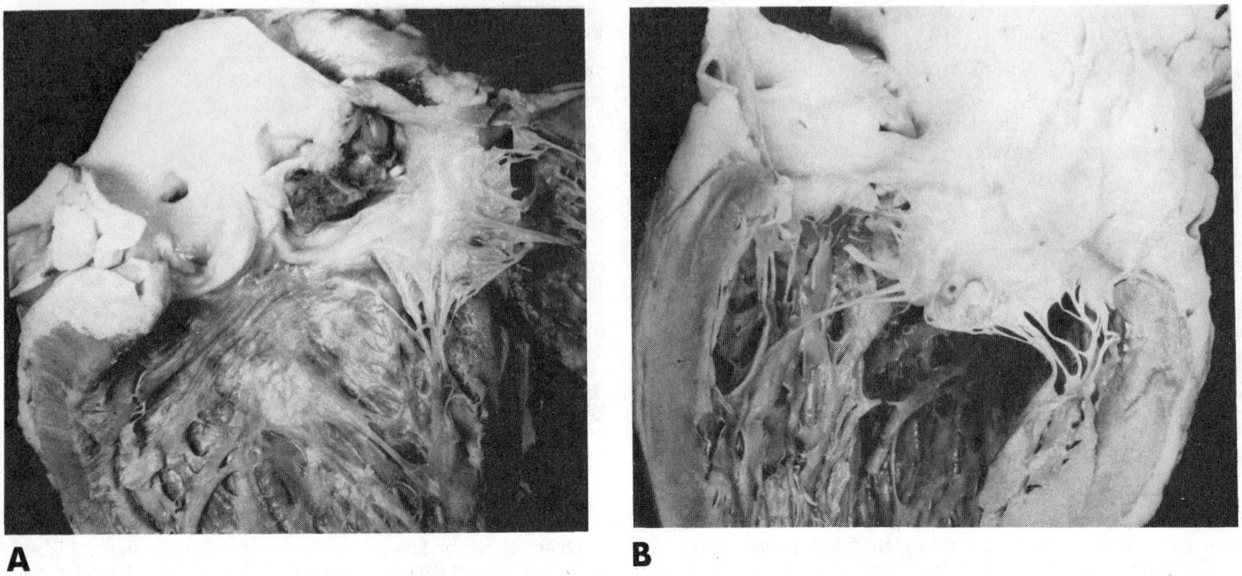

FIGURE 39-5 Bacterial endocarditis—specimens from a 36-year-old man. *A.* Aortic valve. The base of the aortic valve shows major destruction of a cusp with extension of inflammation onto the subjacent mitral valve. Near the free edge of the mitral valve, its ventricular aspect shows an ostium of a nonruptured mycotic aneurysm. *B.* Mitral valve, left atrium, and left ventricle. The lobulated mycotic aneurysm of the mitral valve lies near its free edge (area of aneurysm included within circle).

nary congestion and peripheral edema are frequently present. Angina pectoris usually does not occur in patients with predominant mitral regurgitation but may be a frequent symptom with incompetence of both aortic and mitral valves. Syncope may be experienced when significant regurgitation is present in both valves; it is rare if mitral incompetence is the predominant lesion. Palpitations may be present in the majority of patients, and symptoms of heart failure occur with similar frequency.

When aortic stenosis is accompanied by mitral insufficiency, angina and syncope are frequent symptoms, as are palpitations. When aortic insufficiency and mitral stenosis are the predominant lesions, angina remains a frequent complaint along with symptoms related to pulmonary congestion and heart failure.

Physical Examination

In mitral and aortic stenosis, an exaggerated left ventricular apex impulse and a palpable right ventricular heave can often be appreciated. A mitral diastolic rumble is appreciated in the majority of patients but can vary from grade III intensity down to a minimum of I to II intensity (on a scale from I to VI). The aortic ejection murmur is usually of high intensity, but a few patients may have a low-intensity aortic systolic murmur. A mitral opening snap can be detected in a minority of patients; in a small percentage the diastolic rumble of mitral stenosis will not be heard.

In mitral and aortic insufficiency the systemic arterial diastolic blood pressure is usually less than 70 mmHg. However, as many as 40 percent of patients with combined regurgitant lesions may exhibit a diastolic blood pressure above 70 mmHg. A loud mitral holosystolic murmur is present in the majority of patients. The early diastolic murmur is loud when aortic regurgitation is the predominant lesion but may be less intense when mitral regurgitation prevails. A mitral diastolic flow murmur can be heard in the majority of patients with mitral and aortic regurgitation. If the aortic regurgitation is predominant, there will be an audible aortic systolic flow murmur.

In patients with aortic stenosis and mitral insufficiency, an exaggerated left ventricular impulse is usually present. A loud mitral holosystolic murmur may be heard in the majority of patients, and a diastolic flow murmur across the mitral valve is frequently present.

When aortic insufficiency and mitral stenosis are both present, the left ventricular apical thrust is usually accentuated, but the early diastolic murmur at the apex may be faint or prominent.

Although the low-pitched, rumbling diastolic murmur of mitral stenosis and the systolic ejection murmur of aortic regurgitation are reliable diagnostic findings, neither is definitive when the two lesions are coexistent. Similarly, when mitral and aortic incompetence occur together, as many as 40 percent of patients may have a diastolic blood pressure above 70 mmHg in spite of severe aortic regurgitation. Mitral regurgitation may diminish aortic regurgitation by the increased left ventricular diastolic filling from the large left atrium. With mild regurgitation of both valves loud murmurs may be encountered; conversely, faint murmurs may be present with severe valvular regurgitation. Similarly, when severe regurgitation is present in both the mitral and the aortic valves, an aortic systolic murmur or mitral diastolic murmur does not necessarily indicate stenosis but may be due to relative stenosis secondary to the large flow of blood.

With the combination of aortic stenosis and mitral insufficiency a mitral holosystolic murmur is good evidence of associated mitral incompetence, but the intensity of the murmur is not reliable in judging severity. When aortic insufficiency is combined with mitral stenosis, the systemic pulse pressure may be helpful but not indicative of the severity of aortic incompetence. The presence of a prominent left ventricular impulse in pure mitral stenosis may suggest the possibility of associated aortic incompetence but will not indicate its severity. Finally, the intensity of the aortic diastolic murmur is of little value in predicting the severity of the aortic regurgitation in the presence of mitral stenosis.

Chest Roentgenogram

In mitral stenosis and aortic stenosis, the left atrium is always significantly enlarged and there is usually an overall increase in heart size with an increase in both left and right ventricular dimensions. Quite commonly the mitral and aortic valves are calcified. In regurgitation of both mitral and aortic valves, marked cardiomegaly and left atrial and left ventricular enlargement are usually present. Valvular calcification of either site is relatively infrequent. In aortic stenosis and mitral incompetence heart size is generally increased with both left ventricular and left atrial enlargement. In mitral stenosis with aortic insufficiency there is often marked left ventricular enlargement. (See Chap. 15.)

Electrocardiogram

With stenosis of the mitral and aortic valves, there is generally electrocardiographic evidence of left ventricular hypertrophy, left atrial enlargement, and accompanying atrial fibrillation. Similar findings are observed in mitral and aortic regurgitation, with a high incidence of left atrial and left ventricular enlargement and atrial fibrillation. In aortic stenosis and mitral regurgitation there is left ventricular hypertrophy with a moderate incidence of atrial fibrillation. Mitral stenosis with significant aortic regurgitation is also attended by left ventricular hypertrophy on the electrocardiogram. (See Chap. 14.)

Special Laboratory Studies

Echocardiogram

The echocardiogram can provide subjective information concerning valve anatomy, chamber dimensions, and ventricular function in combined lesions of the mitral and aortic valve. Characteristic echoes are generated by mitral stenosis and aortic stenosis. Prolapse of mitral, aortic, and tricuspid valves can be recognized with echocardiography.[17] The number of aortic cusps can be identified, as can calcium in either aortic or mitral valve apparatus. Dimensions of the left atrium, left ventricle, and right ventricle can be useful in determining the extent of volume and pressure overload along with left ventricular wall thickness measurements. The new two-dimensional echocardiographic techniques can even assess the orifice size of the aortic and mitral valves and can detect thrombus formation in the left atrium. (See Chap. 120.)

Radionuclide Studies

Radionuclide techniques can provide information on left ventricular function at rest and during exercise and can give a semiquantitative estimate of valvular regurgitation when only one valve is incompetent. The radionuclide techniques can quantitate segmental wall motion at rest and during exercise and can assist in the detection of subclinical coronary artery disease if such abnormalities become manifest. Since combined lesions of the aortic and mitral valves often create pulmonary hypertension and right ventricular dysfunction, the radionuclide techniques may be superior in estimating right ventricular ejection fraction and performance.[18] (See Chap. 109.)

Exercise Studies

In combined valvular disease, exercise studies can be useful in quantitating symptoms as well as the patient's functional capacity. The electrocardiographic changes are often difficult to interpret when left ventricular hypertrophy is present; therefore ischemic changes cannot be appreciated. The exercise test can be used to follow the course of patients and their disease before and after surgery.

Cardiac Catheterization

Cardiac catherization is described in detail in Chap. 108. In patients with aortic and mitral stenosis, systolic and diastolic gradients can be demonstrated across both valves, but the orifice size will be influenced by the cardiac output, which is often reduced. Pulmonary hypertension is invariably present in these patients, and the left ventricular end-diastolic pressure is often elevated despite the presence of mitral stenosis.

In mitral and aortic regurgitation, the left ventricular end-diastolic pressure will be abnormally elevated in the majority of patients and the central aortic pulse pressure will be greater than 40 mmHg in virtually all individuals. However, the central aortic diastolic pressure may be above 70 mmHg in 30 to 40 percent of these individuals. The *v* wave of mitral regurgitation can be recorded in the wedge position in the majority, and pulmonary capillary wedge and arterial pressures are abnormally elevated in most of these patients.

In aortic stenosis and mitral regurgitation, the left ventricular end-diastolic and pulmonary pressures are usually elevated, but the extent of the elevation does not reflect the severity of the mitral incompetence. When the mitral regurgitation is significant, the forward cardiac output may be reduced; thus a spuriously small pressure gradient across the aortic valve may be recorded.

In mitral stenosis and aortic regurgitation, left

ventricular end-diastolic pressure will be abnormally elevated in a majority of individuals and the central aortic diastolic pressure is usually less than 70 mmHg.

In these combined valve lesions, measurement of total left ventricular stroke volume is useful in estimating the regurgitant volume across each valve. When both valves are incompetent, quantitative techniques are unable to identify the regurgitant volume across each valve.[10]

Assessment of ventricular function is important in combined valve lesions, but the ejection fraction may be falsely elevated in regurgitation of the mitral valve and to a lesser extent in aortic regurgitation. Measurements of end-systolic pressure, volume, and wall thickness can be used to calculate the end-systolic wall stress, and this can be useful, particularly in pressure and volume overload conditions.[19]

Finally, coronary arteriography should be performed in patients above the age of 40 years since underlying disease can be present without symptoms and may contribute to left ventricular dysfunction.

Natural History and Prognosis

When combined aortic and mitral valve disease is the result of rheumatic fever, patients generally experience a 10-year period before the development of significant murmurs and an additional decade of time before symptoms may develop. If lesions of the aortic and mitral valves are due to degenerative collagen changes, symptoms may develop somewhat later in life. If combined lesions are due to calcific changes in the aortic valve and annulus as well as the mitral valve annulus, symptoms often develop much later in life.

Treatment

Medical Treatment

When a rheumatic basis is a reasonable cause of combined aortic and mitral valve disease, prophylactic penicillin should be continued until age 30 years (see Chap. 62). Dental prophylaxis with antibiotic coverage, using either penicillin or erythromycin, should be provided in all patient groups prior to dental maneuvers (see Chap. 56). For genitourinary or other abdominal procedures, gram-negative antibiotic coverage should be provided, as described in the section on mitral stenosis in Chap. 56.

The development of atrial fibrillation warrants anticoagulation since the incidence of systemic and cerebral emboli is estimated at 10 to 20 percent.

Early development of atrial fibrillation associated with hemodynamic deterioration warrants initial trial at medical and later electrical cardioversion. Digitalis as well as quinidine preparations should be administered thereafter for prophylaxis. Chronic atrial fibrillation must be controlled with digitalis (see Chap. 27). The development of symptoms, particularly dyspnea, limitations of exercise activity, and class III symptoms (or in some selected situations, class II symptoms) warrants consideration for surgery.

Surgical Treatment

A number of patients with severe and progressing symptoms exhibit evidence of disease at both mitral and aortic valves.[20] Our experience indicates that both valves can be replaced with a hospital mortality that is now between 5 and 10 percent—considerably less than the 22 percent reported for an earlier period.

Frequently in the presence of aortic and mitral valve disease, repair, rather than replacement, of the stenotic or regurgitant mitral valve can be accomplished. The aortic valve usually demands replacement. The combination of aortic valve replacement with mitral valve repair probably decreases early mortality and improves long-term survival. There has been marked subjective and objective improvement in surviving patients. When tricuspid replacement is added, the risk of the operation has been higher (about 20 percent), but even here the long-term results are considerably better than the life history of surgically untreated patients with triple valve disease. The increased use, when possible, of tricuspid annuloplasty rather than replacement has greatly improved the early results of operation in this group of patients.

Indications for Operation

Indication for operation in patients with involvement of aortic and mitral valves is usually the New York Heart Association (NYHA) class III status, but a number of patients present at a later stage of their disease. Atrial fibrillation is usually present, and tricuspid involvement is somewhat more frequent than it is in left-sided, isolated valvular disease.

There may be a place for surgical intervention in patients who have volume overload of the left ventricle when they remain in functional class II. Thus, in severe aortic regurgitation with moderate mitral valve involvement, or in important mitral regurgitation together with moderate aortic stenosis and regurgitation, operation may be advised to avert progressive and poorly reversible left ventricular dysfunction associated with dilatation.

Operation

Techniques of valvular surgery are described in Chap. 131. When hemodynamic derangement is significant at both valves, the decision to repair both is easily made, and the principles of surgical treatment are the same as they are when one valve alone requires attention. Median sternotomy is performed. With present techniques of myocardial preservation, using cold potassium cardioplegia, the operation can be done in an unhurried, precise manner with expectation of a quite low incidence of less than optimal cardiac performance. On cardiopulmonary bypass, the heart is cooled by the perfusate and by external cardiac cooling. The aorta is cross-clamped. The aorta is opened and cardioplegic solution is infused into each coronary orifice to attain a myocardial temperature of between 10 and 15°C (50 to 59°F). Reinfusion of the cardioplegic solution is done every 20 to 30 min, or when the myocardial temperature reaches 19 or 20°C (66 or 68°F). The aortic valve is resected and then attention is turned to the mitral valve. The left atrium is opened from the right side and the mitral valve is assessed and resected, if necessary, or repaired. The mitral prosthesis is inserted, and the left atrium is left open while the aortic valve is then sutured into place. If there is also tricuspid valve disease, the right atrium is opened at this time and either annuloplasty or replacement is done. The aortotomy is then closed and reperfusion with the perfusate is allowed while the left atriotomy and right atriotomy are closed. The usual procedures are followed for removing all air from the heart and preventing air embolization as the heart begins to eject.

Occasionally, when the aortic valve is severely diseased and only about class II mitral regurgitation (on a scale of I to VI) is evident, it is not necessary to replace the mitral valve. This is true even if left atrial pressure preoperatively was very high, since such pressure can result solely from severe pressure or volume overload of the left ventricle. After repair of the aortic valve disease, incompetence of the mitral valve usually regresses. However, when there is about class II regurgitation of the aortic valve in the presence of severe disease at the mitral valve, the aortic valve incompetence often appears to be of greater magnitude after repair of the mitral valve and may contribute to poor postoperative performance. In these situations, therefore, replacement of both the mitral and aortic valves seems indicated.

Results

Long-term survival after replacement of either the aortic or the mitral valve, or both, is only partially related to factors having to do with the device. Other factors more related to the preoperative condition of the patient, intraoperative events, and early postoperative events also have statistically significant association with late mortality.[21] In particular, patients having had previous valve replacement who need a second replacement, because of xenograft degeneration, paraprosthetic leak, or other complications, do less well than patients having primary valve replacement. In our series patients who have had left ventricular aneurysmectomy along with valve replacement have had less satisfactory long-term survival. However, there was no deleterious influence of ischemic heart disease in general, as suggested by the lack of any negative effect on long-term survival associated with coronary artery bypass grafting. Patients having lengthy periods of ischemic arrest had poorer survival when the operation was done without potassium cardioplegia. It is anticipated that use of potassium cardioplegia will mute this effect. Finally, patients in whom treatment of ventricular arrhythmias was necessary in the early postoperative course were found to have less satisfactory survival than the group as a whole. This suggests that long-term antiarrhythmic therapy would be prudent in that group.

References

1. Keele, K. D.: "Leonardo da Vinci on Movement of the Heart and Blood," J. B. Lippincott, Philadelphia, 1952, p. 87.
2. Roberts, W. C., and Virmani, R.: Aschoff Bodies at Necropsy in Valvular Heart Disease, *Circulation*, 57:803, 1978.
3. Clausen, B. J.: Rheumatic Heart Disease: An Analysis of 796 Cases, *Am. Heart J.*, 20:454, 1940.
4. Cooke, W. T., and White, P. D.: Tricuspid Stenosis: With Particular Reference to Diagnosis and Prognosis, *Br. Heart J.*, 3:147, 1941.
5. Wilson, M. G., and Lubschez, R.: Longevity in Rheumatic Fever, *JAMA*, 121:1, 1948.
6. Bland, E. F., and Jones, T. D.: Rheumatic Fever and Rheumatic Heart Disease: A Twenty Year Report on 1000 Patients Followed Since Childhood, *Circulation*, 4:836, 1951.
7. Roberts, W. C., and Honig, H. S.: The Spectrum of Cardiovascular Disease in the Marfan's Syndrome. A Clinico-Pathologic Study of 18 Necropsy Patients and Comparison to 151 Previously Reported Patients, *Am. Heart J.*, 104:115, 1982.
8. Rackley, C. E., Hood, W. P., Jr., Rolett, E. L., and Young, D. T.: Left Ventricular End-Diastolic Pressure in Chronic Heart Disease, *Am. J. Med.*, 48:310, 1970.
9. Hood, W. P., Jr., Rackley, C. E., and Rolett, E. L.: Wall Stress in the Normal and Hypertrophied Left Ventricle, *Am. J. Cardiol.*, 22:550, 1968.
10. Sandler, H., Dodge, H. T., Hay, R. E., and Rackley, C. E.: Quantitation of Valvular Insufficiency in Man by Angiocardiography, *Am. Heart J.*, 65:501, 1963.
11. Rackley, C. E., Behar, V. S., Whalen, R. E., and McIntosh, H. D.: Biplane Cineangiographic Determinations of Left Ventricular Function: Pressure-Volume Relationships, *Am. Heart J.*, 74:766, 1967.
12. Baxley, W. A., Dodge, H. T., Rackley, C. E., Sandler, H., and Pugh, D.: Left Ventricular Mechanical Efficiency in Man with Heart Disease, *Circulation*, 55:564, 1977.
13. Jones, J. W., Rackley, C. E., Bruce, R. A., Dodge, H. T., Cobb, L. A., and Sandler, H.: Left Ventricular Volumes in Valvular Heart Disease, *Circulation*, 29:887, 1964.
14. Dodge, H. T., Hay, R. E., and Sandler, H.: Pressure-Volume Characteristics of the Diastolic Left Ventricle in Man with Heart Disease, *Am. Heart J.*, 64:503, 1962.
15. Rousseau, M. F., Pouleur, H., Charlier, A. A., and Brasseur, L. A.: Assessment of Left Ventricular Relaxation in Patients with Valvular Regurgitation, *Am. J. Cardiol.*, 50:1028, 1982.
16. Terzaki, A. K., Cokkinos, D. V., Leachman, R. D., Meade, J. B., Hollman, G. L., and Cooley, D. A.: Combined Mitral and Aortic Valve Disease, *Am. J. Cardiol.*, 25:588, 1970.
17. Ogawa, S., Hayashi, J., Sasaki, H., Tani, M., Akaishi, M., Mitamoura, H., Sang, M., Hoshino, T., Handa, S., and Nakamura, Y.: Evaluation of Combined Valvular Prolapse Syndrome by 2-Dimensional Echocardiography, *Circulation*, 65:174, 1982.
18. Winzelberg, G. G., Boucher, C. A., Pohost, G. M., McKusick, K. A., Bingham, J. B., Okada, R. D., and Strauss, H. W.: Right Ventricular Function in Aortic and Mitral Valve Disease. Relation of Gated First-Pass Radionuclide Angiography to Clinical and Hemodynamic Findings, *Chest*, 79:520, 1981.

19. Rackley, C. E.: Quantitative Evaluation of Left Ventricular Function by Radiographic Techniques, *Circulation*, 54:862, 1976.
20. Stephenson, L. W., Edie, R. N., Harken, A. H., and Edmunds, L. H.: Combined Aortic and Mitral Valve Replacement: Changes in Practice and Prognosis, *Circulation*, 69:640, 1984.
21. Williams, J. B., Karp, R. B., Kirklin, J. W., Kouchoukos, N. T., Pacifico, A. C., Zorn, G. L., Blackstone, E. H., Brown, R. N., Piantadose, S., and Bradley, E. L.: Considerations in Selection and Management of Patients Undergoing Valve Replacement with Glutaraldehyde-Fixed Porcine Bioprosthesis, *Ann. Thorac. Surg.*, 30:247, 1980.

40

Tricuspid and Pulmonary Valve Disease*

Charles E. Rackley, M.D.
Jesse E. Edwards, M.D.
Robert B. Wallace, M.D.
Nevin M. Katz, M.D.

I wish to plead for the admission among the recognized auscultatory signs of disease of a murmur due to pulmonary regurgitation occurring independently of disease or deformity of the valve, and as the result of long-continued excess of blood pressure in the pulmonary artery.

Graham Steell, 1888[1]

Etiology

Tricuspid stenosis is most commonly caused by rheumatic fever and is often associated with mitral stenosis. Stenosis of the tricuspid valve has been observed with the carcinoid syndrome (see Chap. 61), endocardial fibroelastosis, endomyocardial fibrosis, and systemic lupus erythematosus. A right atrial myxoma, metastases from tumors, and thrombi can obstruct the tricuspid orifice and produce the hemodynamic abnormalities of tricuspid stenosis.[2,3] (Congenital tricuspid stenosis is discussed in Chap. 36.)

Regurgitation of the tricuspid valve is often functional and secondary to right ventricular dilatation and failure.[4] Left ventricular failure and/or pulmonary hypertension can eventually produce tricuspid regurgitation. The most common cause of isolated tricuspid regurgitation is infectious endocarditis in drug addiction.[5] Less common mechanisms include trauma, myocardial infarction, carcinoid, prolapsed leaflet, and congenital abnormalities such as atrial septal defect and Ebstein's anomaly (see Chap. 36).

Acquired lesions of the pulmonic valve generally lead to regurgitation; rarely, an inflammatory process produces stenosis and regurgitation of the valve. Pulmonary hypertension can produce pulmonary regurgitation as encountered in mitral stenosis, chronic lung disease, and pulmonary emboli. Inflammatory lesions such as endocarditis, rheumatic fever, and tuberculosis can, on very rare occasions, result in pulmonary regurgitation.[6,7] Sarcomas and myxomas can also extend to the valve.[8] Pulmonary incompetence can result from previous cardiac surgery on a congenital pulmonary valvular lesion. The pulmonary valve may be slightly stenotic, and there may be regurgitation due to carcinoid heart disease.[9] A mediastinal lesion such as a tumor, aneurysm, or constrictive pericarditis can compress the pulmonary artery and simulate stenosis of the valve. (See Table 40-1.)

Pathology

Rheumatic Disease

The most common cause of tricuspid stenosis is rheumatic disease.[10] The changes in the tricuspid valve are characterized by fibrosis with contracture of the leaflets and commissural fusion; the former leads to tricuspid regurgitation, the latter to stenosis (Fig. 40-1). It should be emphasized that the stenotic element of the rheumatic tricuspid valve is intrinsically minor and would usually go undetected were it not for the high flow across the valve incident to the coexistent regurgitation. In our view, whenever the tricuspid valve is involved by rheumatic disease, there is always coinvolvement of the left-sided valves, an observation in agreement with that of Clawson.[11]

Flammang and associates found that 9.5 percent of cases requiring surgical replacement of both the mitral and aortic valves exhibited rheumatic involvement of the tricuspid valve.[12] Among cases having mitral commissurotomy, the incidence of clinically

*The editor-in-chief wishes to thank John W. Kirklin, M.D., and Robert B. Karp, M.D., for their previous contribution to the chapter on this subject that appeared in the fifth edition of *The Heart*.

TABLE 40-1 Acquired Lesions of the Pulmonary Valve

- Pulmonary hypertension with pulmonary regurgitation
  - Mitral stenosis
  - Chronic lung disease
  - Pulmonary emboli
- Inflammatory lesions
  - Endocarditis
  - Rheumatic fever
  - Tuberculosis
- Tumors
  - Sarcoma
  - Myxoma
- Previous surgery for congenital lesions
- Mediastinal lesions
  - Tumor
  - Aneurysm
  - Constrictive pericarditis

evident tricuspid disease was 3 percent. In a series of 217 autopsied cases of rheumatic heart disease, Cooke and White found 47 cases (22 percent) in which the tricuspid valve was also involved by rheumatic disease.[13]

Carcinoid Tumor

See Chap. 61 for a discussion of neoplastic heart disease. In about 10 percent of cases of malignant carcinoid tumor (usually primary in the ileum) with extensive metastases, the tricuspid and pulmonary valves may be affected (Fig. 40-2). The changes are those of deposits of fibrous tissue on the surfaces of these valves. Fibrous plaques may also develop on the endocardial surfaces of the right atrium and ventricle and on the intima of the coronary sinus and pulmonary artery.[14] The hemodynamic effects result from the rigidity and contracture of the fibrous tissues deposited on the valves. In the tricuspid valve, the major functional effect is regurgitation; the pulmonary valve, if affected, may be both stenotic and incompetent. Hurst et al. have recently reported a patient with carcinoid heart disease who had both the tricuspid and pulmonary valves involved. The carcinoid tumor was in the ovary. She had successful removal of the tumor and replacement of the pulmonary and tricuspid valves with porcine valves.[14a]

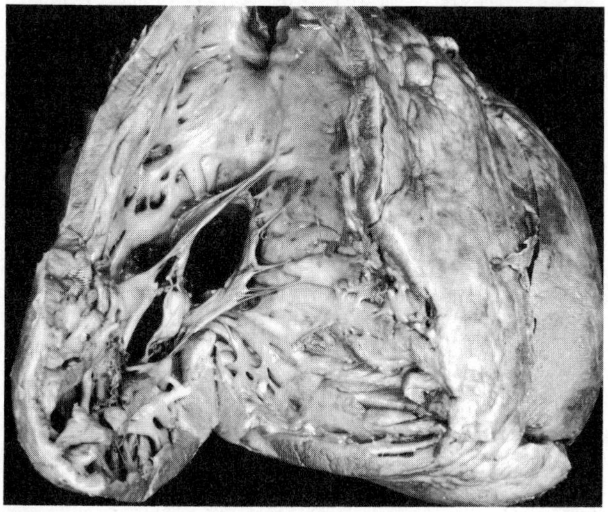

FIGURE 40-1 Tricuspid valve seen from below in chronic rheumatic endocarditis. Although the chordae are relatively uninvolved, there is fusion of the leaflets at the commissures, creating a narrowed and fixed orifice. The valve is both stenotic and incompetent.

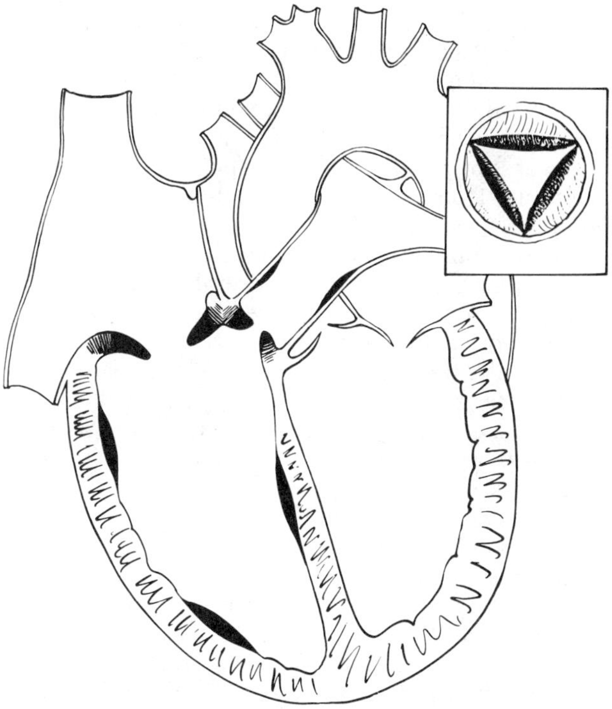

FIGURE 40-2 Carcinoid heart disease. Insert shows pulmonary stenosis. The leaflets of the tricuspid valve are thickened. The valve is predominantly incompetent and causes pulmonary regurgitation. Fibrous plaques are deposited on the lining of the right ventricle and pulmonary trunk. *(From J. E. Edwards, Effects of Malignant Noncardiac Tumors upon the Cardiovascular System, Cardiovasc. Clin., 4:282, 1971. Reproduced with permission from the publisher and author.)*

Congestive Cardiac Failure

The most common type of tricuspid regurgitation is the so-called secondary type resulting from enlargement of the orifice incident to congestive cardiac failure with right ventricular dilatation due to left ventricular disease. The tricuspid regurgitation may vanish when the heart failure is successfully treated. It may, however, be permanent with longstanding dilatation of the right ventricle.[15,16]

Infective Endocarditis

In infective endocarditis the cause of tricuspid regurgitation may, in part, be improper apposition of the leaflets because of interposed vegetations. Major degrees of tricuspid regurgitation may be due to rupture of chordae tendineae of the right ventricle.

Trauma

The classic background for traumatic tricuspid regurgitation is external blunt trauma (including sudden deceleration), most commonly occurring in an automobile accident. Gerry and associates described two cases of rupture of a tricuspid papillary muscle resulting from external cardiopulmonary resuscitation.[17]

The main cause of traumatic tricuspid regurgitation is rupture of one or several elements of the tensor apparatus, with rupture of a papillary muscle being more common than rupture of chordae. Less commonly, there is laceration of leaflet tissue and, in an occasional case, more than one of the anatomic elements of the valve are affected.[18,19] Stephenson and associates described an uncommon case in which traumatic tricuspid regurgitation and ruptured ventricular septum coexisted.[20]

Tolerance of tricuspid regurgitation of traumatic origin varies, with tolerance for 39 years reported.[21–24] Those patients with rupture of a papillary muscle tend to tolerate the tricuspid regurgitation less well than do those in which the trauma resulted in rupture of chordae.[22] Among cases of tricuspid regurgitation resulting from rupture of chordae, a traumatic background is more common than is bacterial endocarditis.[25]

Myocardial Infarction and Prolapse

Except for cases involving chronic congestive cardiac failure, myocardial infarction is not a common cause of tricuspid regurgitation.[26] Direct results of myocardial infarction causing tricuspid insufficiency are uncommon, but have been described as caused by aneurysmal dilatation of the right ventricle. A rare case arose from rupture of a right ventricular papillary muscle.[26–29]

Varying degrees of prolapse of the tricuspid valve are commonly present and usually associated with identified prolapse of the mitral valve. Nevertheless, instances of tricuspid insufficiency from this cause, though described, are uncommon.[30]

Congenital Abnormalities

Among the primary congenital lesions of the tricuspid valve that cause incompetence are Ebstein's malformation and valvular dysplasia. These are discussed in detail in Chap. 36.

Acquired diseases of the pulmonary valve are uncommon, while abnormalities in or near this valve are among the common types of congenital heart disease (see Chap. 36).

Pathophysiology

Stenosis of the tricuspid valve decreases diastolic flow across the valve, elevates the right atrial pressure, and reduces the cardiac output.[31,32] The normal area of the tricuspid valve is 7 cm^2, and impairment of right ventricular filling occurs when the valve area is reduced below 1.5 cm^2. Elevation of the mean right atrial pressure above 10 mmHg usually produces peripheral edema. In tricuspid stenosis, a higher mean right atrial pressure develops with atrial fibrillation than is present with sinus rhythm and normal atrial contraction. Hemodynamic abnormalities in tricuspid stenosis can be further influenced by the frequently coexisting mitral stenosis. The reduced right ventricular flow in tricuspid valve obstruction has been proposed as a mechanism for protection against severe pulmonary hypertension.

In tricuspid regurgitation the systolic regurgitation into the right atrium elevates the right atrial pressure.[33] The regurgitant flow produces a prominent v wave reflected throughout the venous system.

Pulmonary regurgitation is the most frequent acquired lesion of the valve. The incompetence may be secondary to pulmonary hypertension or may be caused by a primary abnormality in the leaflets. Pulmonary regurgitation imposes a volume overload on the right ventricle, and if pulmonary hypertension is preexistent, the overload is superimposed on a hypertrophied myocardium. Isolated pulmonary valvular insufficiency can be tolerated for a long period without cardiac decompensation.[34]

Clinical Manifestations

History

The most frequent symptoms in tricuspid stenosis are dyspnea and fatigue. In mitral stenosis, the development of significant tricuspid stenosis can diminish the paroxysmal symptoms of dyspnea, pulmonary edema, and hemoptysis by preventing increase in pulmonary congestion and hypertension.[2,3] Patients with tricuspid stenosis occasionally complain of prominent pulsations of the neck veins, which may precede the development of peripheral edema.

Since tricuspid regurgitation usually accompanies left ventricular failure or mitral stenosis, symptoms are those of dyspnea, orthopnea, and peripheral edema.[35] Paroxysmal nocturnal dyspnea may be surprisingly infrequent. Tricuspid regurgitation in these conditions may ameliorate the pulmonary symptoms and provide a physiological basis for the alleviation of left-sided heart failure by the development of right-sided heart failure. Some of the patients, however, probably have less pulmonary edema because of the development of pulmonary arteriolar diseases. If the tricuspid regurgitation is caused by bacterial endocarditis, symptoms of a febrile illness may be attended by fatigue and peripheral edema.

The clinical manifestations of acquired pulmonary valvular lesions depend on the severity of the impairment of the valve as well as the extent of the underlying disease. Isolated pulmonary regurgitation can be tolerated without symptoms. Severe pulmonary hypertension may cause not only dyspnea and fatigue but also syncope. With inflammatory lesions of the valve, febrile manifestations and pulmonary infections may be present. The carcinoid syndrome is characterized by episodes of facial flushing, increased intestinal activity, diarrhea, and bronchospasm. Tumors involving the pulmonary valve may exert pressure from expansion and metastases which affects the lungs and heart.

Physical Examination

Tricuspid stenosis is frequently associated with lesions of the mitral and aortic valves. The internal jugular veins will display the prominent *a* wave indicative of impaired right ventricular diastolic filling with atrial systole. The *a* wave in the neck will be of moderate height and sometimes may reach the mandible.[2,3] Auscultation of the heart may be necessary to document that the rise of the venous *a* wave is simultaneous with the first heart sound. The *v* wave is small, and the *y* descent is insignificant.

The finding of right ventricular hypertrophy on physical examination renders tricuspid stenosis less likely. Respiratory variation in splitting of the second heart sound may be absent in tricuspid stenosis, since right ventricular filling remains fairly constant throughout the respiratory cycle. The characteristic auscultatory finding in tricuspid stenosis is the diastolic rumble, heard best at the left lower sternal border.[2,3,36] With sinus rhythm, the murmur will be presystolic; with atrial fibrillation, the murmur may be early or middiastolic. The most effective differentiation of the murmur from that of mitral stenosis is the influence of respiration, since the diastolic rumble of tricuspid stenosis is markedly accentuated during the inspiratory phase (Fig. 40-3). The augmentation of the rumble of tricuspid stenosis with inspiration is designated *Carvallo's sign* and is due to the augmented venous return to the right atrium as well as to an increase in right ventricular filling.[37] An opening snap in tricuspid stenosis is rarely detected with clinical auscultation but can sometimes be recorded with intracardiac phonocardiography.

Atrial fibrillation is quite common in tricuspid regurgitation, and the internal jugular veins reveal a prominent *v* wave produced by the regurgitant flow into the right atrium.[35] The *v* wave and the jugular pulse are more gradual in upstroke than is the sharp rise of the *a* wave. Simultaneous auscultation of the first heart sound remains the best method for timing venous pulsations. The characteristic auscultatory finding is a holosystolic murmur at the left sternal border which increases during inspiration. Although the murmur of mitral regurgitation may also be present, respiration exerts a predominant influence on tricuspid regurgitation with little alteration in the intensity of a mitral regurgitation murmur.

If right ventricular failure and tricuspid regurgitation have developed as a result of pulmonary regurgitation, a prominent *v* wave will be present in the deep jugular pulse. Increased right ventricular activity can be palpated along the left sternal border, and if pulmonary hypertension is present, the second sound will be markedly accentuated over the pulmonary area. The pulmonary regurgitation murmur may be difficult to distinguish from the murmur of aortic regurgitation, but the systemic blood pressure and peripheral pulse findings of aortic regurgitation can be useful in the differentiation.

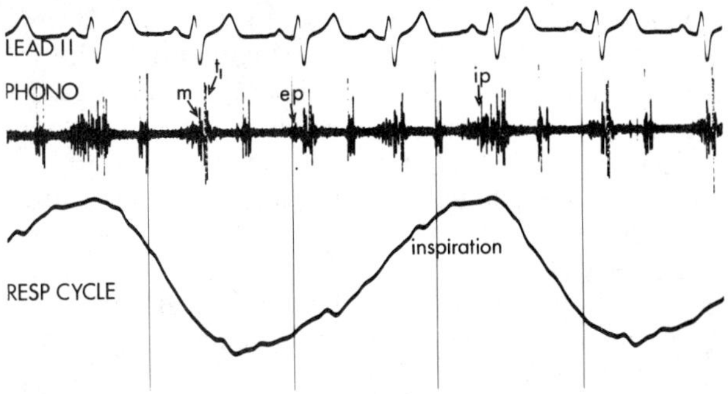

FIGURE 40-3 Phonocardiogram of a patient with tricuspid stenosis. Striking features are the prominent tricuspid component of the first sound (T_1), in comparison with the mitral component (m), and the late diastolic murmur which increases during the inspiratory phase (ip) of respiration. (*Courtesy of Dr. I. Sylvia Crawley.*)

Chest Roentgenogram

In tricuspid stenosis, the most characteristic finding is prominence of the right atrium without significant pulmonary arterial enlargement or changes due to pulmonary hypertension.[2] Tricuspid regurgitation will produce some degree of right atrial enlargement, but there will usually be accompanying right ventricular enlargement.[35] If the pulmonary valve is insufficient, the pulmonary artery may be prominent.[34] (See Chap. 15.)

Electrocardiogram

The characteristic electrocardiographic finding in tricuspid stenosis is a large P wave of right atrial enlargement in the absence of right ventricular hypertrophy.[2,36] Atrial fibrillation is quite common in patients with tricuspid regurgitation.[35] There are no characteristic changes with pulmonary valvular lesions other than preexisting pulmonary hypertension, P mitrale, and right axis deviation with mitral stenosis. (See Chap. 14.)

Special Laboratory Studies

Echocardiography

The characteristic pattern of stenosis of the tricuspid valve can sometimes be recorded with the echocardiogram. With tricuspid regurgitation systolic prolapse can occasionally be identified, as well as a vegetative lesion on the valve.[38] Increased right ventricular dimensions indicate impaired right ventricular function and the likelihood of secondary tricuspid regurgitation. Contrast echocardiography with peripheral venous injection can identify back-and-forth movement across the tricuspid valve.[39] M-mode echocardiography is superior to the two-dimensional technique in detection of contrast in the inferior vena cava in patients with tricuspid regurgitation.[40] If the pulmonary valve can be identified, leaflet motion, a vegetative lesion, or a tumor can sometimes be delineated in the pulmonary valve area. (See Chap. 120.)

Pulsed Doppler appears superior to M-mode echocardiography in the detection of pulmonary regurgitation and the prediction of pulmonary hypertension.[41] (See Chap. 121.)

Cardiac Catheterization

Simultaneous pressures must be recorded in the right atrium and the right ventricle in order to confirm the presence of tricuspid stenosis at cardiac catheterization.[31] Since the normal gradient across the tricuspid valve is less than 1 mmHg, small gradients will not be detected if a pullback pressure is recorded from the right ventricle to the right atrium. The area of the tricuspid valve in significant stenosis is less than 1.5 cm^2; in severe stenosis, it is less than 1 cm^2.

Angiographic documentation of tricuspid regurgitation is difficult to obtain, since the catheter overrides the tricuspid valve and ventricular irritability with a right ventricular injection can often induce tricuspid regurgitation. A prominent *v* wave in the right atrium suggests tricuspid regurgitation, and an intracardiac phonocardiogram may detect tricuspid regurgitation in the absence of Carvallo's sign.[42] Indicator-dilution curves have been used, with simultaneous injection into the right ventricle and sampling in the right atrium and femoral artery, to demonstrate early appearance in the right atrium. Pulmonary regurgitation cannot be easily demonstrated angiographically, but an aortic root injection can be helpful in the elimination of aortic regurgitation as the cause of the diastolic murmur. Intracardiac phonocardiography has been used to detect the diastolic murmur in the right ventricular outflow tract.

Natural History and Prognosis

In tricuspid stenosis the symptoms are primarily those of mitral stenosis, but absence of pulmonary congestion in the presence of peripheral edema should raise the possibility of coexistent tricuspid stenosis. Tricuspid stenosis may also hinder the development of the characteristic symptoms of mitral stenosis and result in an underestimation of the severity of mitral stenosis.

In tricuspid regurgitation the symptoms and course are primarily related to the left-sided heart conditions which produce a pressure-volume overload on the right ventricle. The development of tricuspid regurgitation would indicate severe right ventricular failure. In acute bacterial endocarditis of the tricuspid valve the type of organism will significantly influence the course and response to therapy.

In pulmonary valve lesions, the course will be more prolonged if there is chronic pulmonary hypertension due to mitral stenosis or chronic lung disease. Inflammatory conditions and tumors which affect the valve usually result in a much shorter clinical course.

Treatment

Medical Treatment

In tricuspid stenosis the usual precautionary measures for antibiotic coverage and prevention of endocarditis apply as described in Chap. 56. Peripheral edema may not respond to the usual administration of digitalis and diuretics, and this emphasizes the clinical importance of recognizing underlying tricuspid stenosis with mitral stenosis.

In tricuspid regurgitation, the treatment of right ventricular failure requires digitalis, diuretics, or vasodilating agents for management of left ventricular failure. If failure of the right side of the heart is caused by mitral stenosis, early surgical intervention is the best management.

In pulmonary lesions, antibiotic prophylaxis is required; if pulmonary emboli are present, anticoagulation is indicated. The treatment of pulmonary hypertension will require management of failure of the left side of the heart, correction of mitral stenosis, or the use of vasodilating agents, which can lower pulmonary artery pressure. Vasodilating agents are, however, not very effective in treating primary pulmonary hypertension.

Surgical Treatment

The decision to proceed with valvular heart surgery is usually based on the severity of the aortic and mitral valve disease, rather than on the severity of the disease of the tricuspid valve. The usual decisions to be made regarding the tricuspid valve are (1) whether a procedure should be added to the mitral and/or aortic valve procedures, and, if so, (2) which procedure, annuloplasty or valve replacement, should be performed. Patients may present with mild mitral valve disease and severe tricuspid dysfunction. Such patients may require an operation on the tricuspid valve.

Indications for Surgery

The severity of the symptoms and clinical signs of tricuspid valve disease are used to determine whether or not to perform tricuspid valve surgery. If there are signs of tricuspid stenosis and, particularly, if stenosis is demonstrated by cardiac catheterization and two-dimensional echocardiography, the tricuspid valve is directly visualized at operation with the anticipation of performing commissurotomy or valve replacement.

When there are signs of significant tricuspid regurgitation secondary to mitral stenosis, it is important to document the duration of the regurgitation and the severity and duration of pulmonary artery hypertension because these features of the condition are helpful in planning tricuspid valve surgery. If the tricuspid regurgitation is severe and of long standing and there is chronic pulmonary artery hypertension, it is unlikely that the tricuspid regurgitation will resolve in the early postoperative period after mitral valve surgery alone. In this circumstance, tricuspid valve surgery is usually indicated. In contrast, if the tricuspid regurgitation and pulmonary artery hypertension are of short duration, mitral valve replacement usually will reduce pulmonary artery pressure in the early postoperative period, and this will be followed by a decrease in the tricuspid valve regurgitation. In this circumstance we prefer to wait until discontinuation of bypass following mitral valve surgery to decide whether a procedure to reduce tricuspid regurgitation is indicated. Occasionally, severe tricuspid regurgitation will be present with only modest elevation of pulmonary artery pressure. In this circumstance the tricuspid valve leaflets are usually deformed and valve replacement is necessary.

The appearance of the heart at the time of surgery is helpful in assessing the severity of tricuspid valve disease. A thinned-out right atrial wall together with moderate to marked enlargement of the right atrium and venae cavae are indications of important disease. The degree of stenosis and regurgitation can be estimated by palpation through the right atrial appendage. If tricuspid valve surgery is not performed as the initial surgical approach, examination through the right atrial appendage can be performed after discontinuation of bypass for mitral valve surgery to assess residual tricuspid regurgitation.

Operation

Tricuspid stenosis may be well treated by commissurotomy. This is usually performed under direct vision. The procedure may be combined with annuloplasty to correct valve regurgitation. Valve replacement occasionally is necessary if the changes in the leaflets and subvalvular mechanism are advanced or if severe regurgitation cannot be relieved by annuloplasty.

For tricuspid regurgitation, three basic reconstructive techniques have been described (Fig. 40-4). The first procedure is widely used and consists of plication of the posterior leaflet.[43,44] This technique, which can be accomplished quickly, converts the tricuspid valve into a functionally bicuspid valve. De Vega[45] described a second type of annuloplasty which narrows the annulus along the anterior and posterior leaflets with a purse string suture. Carpentier[46] described the third major technique—placement of a carefully sized flexible ring along the anterior and posterior aspects of the annulus. It draws in and supports the tissue evenly. Studies have shown that the annular dilatation occurs in these areas rather than along the septal leaflet.[47]

When the leaflets and subvalvular mechanism are deformed as a result of rheumatic fever, reconstruction may not be feasible. In such a case, replacement is performed with either a mechanical or tissue valve. Anticoagulation with warfarin (Coumadin) is generally advisable in patients with tricuspid valve replacement, and therefore the major advantage of a bioprosthetic valve is negated. Nevertheless, the bioprosthetic valve has been the prosthesis of first choice of a number of surgeons. If a mechanical valve is preferred and the cavity of the right ventricle is not capacious, a low-profile prosthesis, such as the Bjork-Shiley tilting disk valve or the St. Jude bileaflet valve, seems advisable. Usually, however, if the degree of tricuspid incompetence is severe, a ball-cage prosthesis is accommodated well.

Results

Mild tricuspid regurgitation does not seem to increase the risk of surgery involving the mitral valve or both aortic and mitral valves. When the tricuspid disease is moderate to severe, the risk of operation is significantly increased. Though long-term improvement in tricuspid regurgitation after mitral valve replacement alone has been documented,[48] a tricuspid procedure is generally employed in the setting of moderate to severe tricuspid regurgitation to enhance cardiac function in the critical early days after operation. Mitral valve replacement alone does not invariably decrease tricuspid regurgitation even several months after operation.[49]

In general, the early and late results of tricuspid annuloplasty have been superior to those of valve replacement, and therefore the trend of surgical practice has been to avoid valve replacement when possible. There is an important incidence of thrombosis with tricuspid prostheses,[50] and the long-term functional results have been less favorable than those of aortic and mitral valve replacements. The less favorable results may be related to more advanced disease in these patients but also may be a function of the less favorable position of the prosthesis in relation to the ventricular outflow tract. The risk of annuloplasty in combination with aortic and mitral valve surgery is about 10 percent. Good early results have been obtained with all three methods of annuloplasty.[51–56] The ring annuloplasty probably gives the best long-term results. When tricuspid valve replacement is necessary, the 30-day operative risk increases to 15 to 20 percent. A variety of prostheses have been used for tricuspid valve replacement with variable results.[57–60] The valve of choice remains a topic of controversy. Early experience with the relatively new St. Jude prosthesis has been favorable in the tricuspid position.[61]

Tricuspid Valve Surgery for Infective Endocarditis

Though uncommon, infective endocarditis of the tricuspid valve is seen more frequently today because of drug abuse. In general the treatment of tricuspid valve endocarditis is medical. When septic

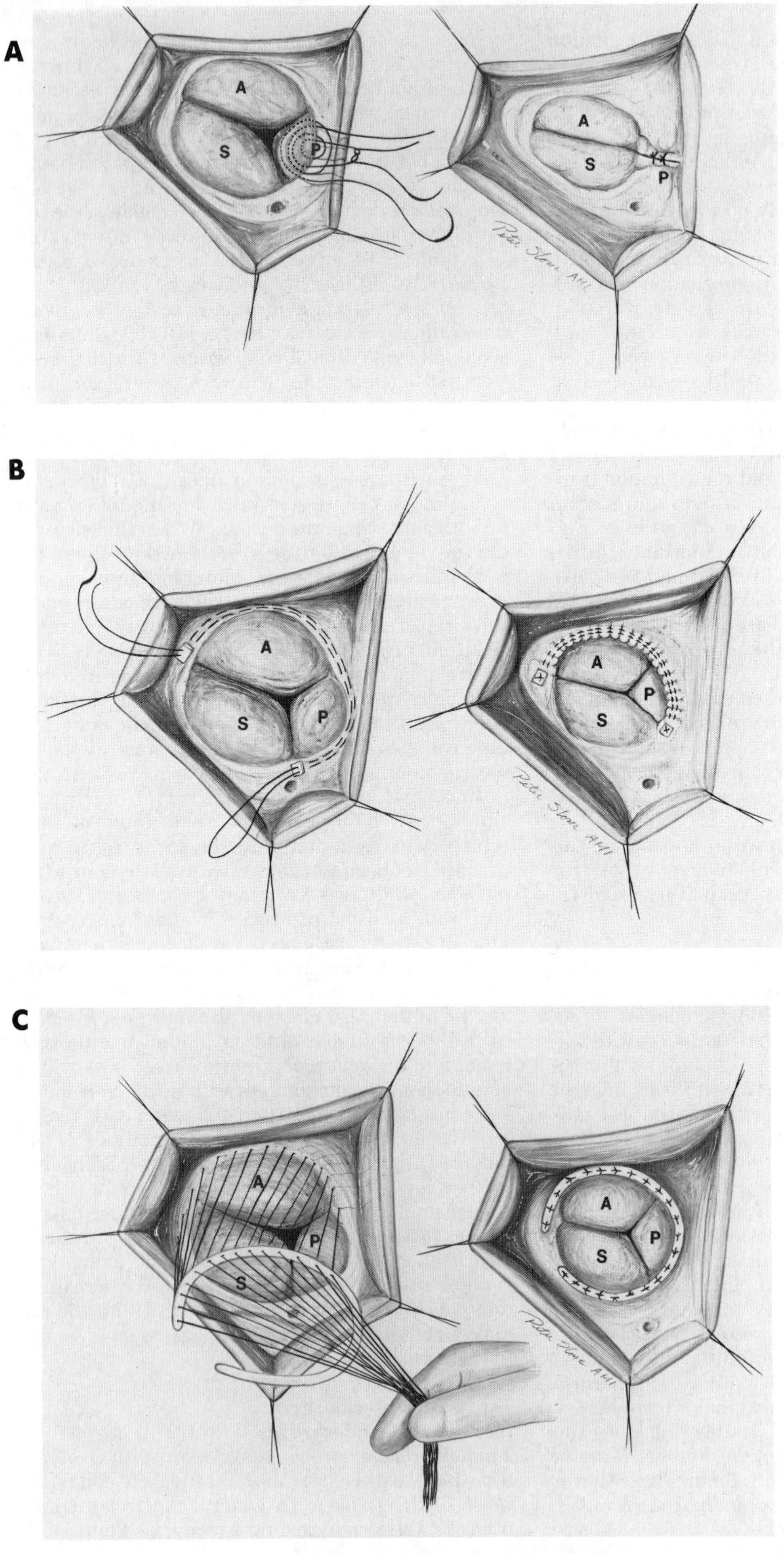

FIGURE 40-4 Three major types of tricuspid annuloplasty have been employed. *A.* The posterior leaflet may be plicated, with production of a bileaflet valve as described by Kay.[43] *B.* The annulus may be narrowed by a purse string suture as described by De Vega.[45] *C.* The annulus may also be narrowed by a prosthetic ring as described by Carpentier.[46] (*Drawing by Peter Stone, medical illustrator. Georgetown University, Washington, D.C.*)

pulmonary embolization occurs despite intensive antibiotic treatment, tricuspid valve surgery is indicated. In general, excision of the valve without replacement is the procedure performed. Results of this approach have been recently reported.[62]

Postoperative Management for Tricuspid Valve Surgery

It is relatively common for the cardiac output to be marginal after tricuspid valve surgery. This is usually a reflection of persistent pulmonary arterial hypertension and long-standing right ventricular dysfunction. Measurements of cardiac output and pulmonary artery pressure are used to guide postoperative care. If annuloplasty is performed, a Swan-Ganz catheter can be used for such measurements. If valve replacement has been performed, a cardiac output thermistor can be placed through the right ventricular outflow tract into the pulmonary artery along with a pulmonary artery catheter. It has been our experience that nitroglycerin infused via a central venous catheter is a valuable adjunct in reducing pulmonary artery pressure. Intravenous dopamine and dobutamine are used to enhance myocardial contractility. If cardiac output remains marginal, an intraaortic balloon pump may be used to reduce left-sided pressures (see Chap. 129). Pulmonary artery balloon counterpulsation has been employed for acute right ventricular failure.[63]

Digitalis and diuretics are usually employed for several months after tricuspid valve surgery. For patients with tricuspid valve replacement, warfarin (Coumadin) and dipyridamole (see Chap. 95) are used as anticoagulants. The use of antiplatelet agents in this setting may improve the long-term results.[64] Prophylaxis against infective endocarditis is also required (see Chap. 56).

Surgery for Pulmonary Valve Disease

Pulmonary valve surgery for acquired disease is performed infrequently. Pulmonary valve stenosis on an acquired basis is rare. Though there are a variety of causes of pulmonary valve regurgitation, this hemodynamic condition is relatively well tolerated if pulmonary vascular resistance is normal. Pulmonary valve replacement may be performed for acquired conditions such as carcinoid heart disease and infective endocarditis,[65] but it generally has been limited to cases where right ventricular dysfunction has become severe after congenital heart disease surgery.[66] Though pulmonary regurgitation is generally well tolerated for several years after correction of malformations such as tetralogy of Fallot, the regurgitation may become hemodynamically significant, especially if pulmonary artery hypertension is present or develops. In such a case the placement of a pulmonary valve prosthesis may importantly improve the patient's functional status. In general, bioprosthetic valves have been preferred because of the tendency for mechanical valve thrombosis in this position. In the future, pulmonary valve surgery probably will be performed more frequently, as studies indicate right ventricular dysfunction may be present in asymptomatic postoperative patients with pulmonary incompetence.[67]

References

1. Steell, G.: The Murmur of High-Pressure in the Pulmonary Artery, *Medical Chronicle,* IX:182, 1888.
2. Perloff, J. K., and Harvey, W. P.: Clinical Recognition of Tricuspid Stenosis, *Circulation,* 22:346, 1960.
3. Kitchin, A., and Turner, R.: Diagnosis and Treatment of Tricuspid Stenosis, *Br. Heart J.,* 26:354, 1964.
4. McMichael, J., and Shillingford, J. P.: The Role of Valvular Incompetence in Heart Failure, *Br. Med. J.,* 1:537, 1957.
5. Glancy, D. L., Marcus, F. I., Cuadra, M., Ewy, G. A., and Roberts, W. C.: Isolated Organic Tricuspid Valvular Regurgitation, *Am. J. Med.,* 46:989, 1969.
6. Espino Vela, J., Contreras, R., and Rustrian Sosa, F.: Rheumatic Pulmonary Valve Disease, *Am. J. Cardiol.,* 23:12, 1969.
7. Roberts, W. C., and Buchbinder, N. A.: Right Sided Valvular Infective Endocarditis, *Am. J. Med.,* 53:7, 1972.
8. Seymour, J., Emaneul, R., and Patterson, N.: Acquired Pulmonary Stenosis, *Br. Heart J.,* 30:776, 1968.
9. Rossignol, B., Machecourt, J., Denis, B., Roche, J., N'Golet, A., Morena, H., and Martin-Nobel, P.: Cardiopathie carcinoide secondaire a une tumeur du grele. A propos dun cas associat insuffisace tricuspidienne et insuffisance pulmonaire, *Arch. Mal. Coeur,* 70:1221, 1977.
10. Edwards, J. E.: The Spectrum and Clinical Significance of Tricuspid Regurgitation, *Practical Cardiol.,* 6:86, 1980.
11. Clawson, B. J.: Rheumatic Heart Disease. An Analysis of 796 Cases, *Am. Heart J.,* 20:454, 1940.
12. Flammang, D., Juamin, P., and Kremer, R.: Organic Tricuspid Pathology in Rheumatic Valvulopathies, *Acta Cardiol.,* 30:155, 1975.
13. Cooke, W. T., and White, P. D.: Tricuspid Stenosis: With Particular Reference to Diagnosis and Prognosis, *Br. Heart J.,* 3:147, 1941.
14. Ludwig, J.: Cardiac Vein Involvement in Carcinoid Syndrome. Possible Evidence of Retrograde Blood Flow in Cardiac Veins in Tricuspid Insufficiency, *Am. J. Clin. Pathol.,* 55:617, 1971.
14a. Hurst, J. W., Whitworth, H. B., O'Donoghue, S., et al.: Heart Disease Due to Ovarian Carcinoid: Successful Replacement of the Pulmonary and Tricuspid Valves with Porcine Heterografts and Removal of the Tumor, in J. W. Hurst (ed.), "Clinical Essays on the Heart," McGraw-Hill Book Company, New York, vol. 5, 1985.
15. McMichael, J., and Shillingford, J. P.: The Role of Valvular Incompetence in Heart Failure, *Br. Med. J.,* 1:537, 1957.
16. Boucek, R. J., Jr., Graham, T. P., Morgan, J. P., Atwood, G. F., and Boerth, R. C.: Spontaneous Resolution of Massive Congenital Tricuspid Insufficiency, *Circulation,* 54:795, 1976.
17. Gerry, J. L., Jr., Bulkley, B. H., and Hutchins, G. M.: Rupture of the Papillary Muscle of the Tricuspid Valve. A Complication of Cardiopulmonary Resuscitation and a Rare Cause of Tricuspid Insufficiency, *Am. J. Cardiol.,* 40:825, 1977.
18. Jahnke, E. J., Jr., Nelson, W. P., Aaby, G. V., and FitzGibbon, G. M.: Tricuspid Insufficiency. The Result of Nonpenetrating Cardiac Trauma, *Arch. Surg.,* 95:880, 1967.
19. VanGilder, J. E., Jain, A. C., Weiss, R. B., Bowyer, A. F., and Tarnay, T. J.: Traumatic Right Ventricular Aneurysm Presenting as Tricuspid Regurgitation, *W. Va. Med. J.,* 75:93, 1979.
20. Stephenson, L. W., MacVaugh, H., III, and Kastor, J. A.: Tricuspid Valvular Incompetence and Rupture of the Ventricular Septum Caused by Nonpenetrating Trauma, *J. Thorac. Cardiovasc. Surg.,* 77:768, 1979.
21. Brandenburg, R. O., McGoon, D. C., Campeau, L., and Giuliani, E. R.: Traumatic Rupture of the Chordae Tendineae of the Tricuspid Valve. Successful Repair Twenty-Four Years Later, *Am. J. Cardiol.,* 18:911, 1966.
22. Morgan, J. R., and Forker, A. D.: Isolated Tricuspid Insufficiency, *Circulation,* 43:559, 1971.

23. Marvin, R. F., Schrank, J. P., and Nolan, S. P.: Traumatic Tricuspid Insufficiency, *Am. J. Cardiol.*, 32:723, 1973.
24. Croxson, M. S., O'Brien, K. P., and Lowe, J. B.: Traumatic Tricuspid Regurgitation. Long-Term Survival, *Br. Heart J.*, 33:750, 1971.
25. Grubier, M., Denis, B., and Martin-Noel, P.: Les Ruptures de cordages tricuspidiens, *Coeur Med. Int.*, 15:215, 1976.
26. Collins, R., and Daly, J. J.: Tricuspid Incompetence Complicating Acute Myocardial Infarction, *Postgrad. Med. J.*, 53:51, 1977.
27. Zone, D. D., and Botti, R. E.: Right Ventricular Infarction with Tricuspid Insufficiency and Chronic Right Heart Failure, *Am. J. Cardiol.*, 37:445, 1976.
28. McAllister, R. G., Jr., Friesinger, G. C., and Sinclair-Smith, B. C.: Tricuspid Regurgitation following Inferior Myocardial Infarction, *Arch. Intern. Med.*, 136:95, 1976.
29. Eisenberg, S., and Suyemoto, J.: Rupture of a Papillary Muscle of the Tricuspid Valve following Acute Myocardial Infarction. Report of a Case, *Circulation,* 30:558, 1964.
30. Maranhao, V., Gooch, A. S., Yang, S. S., Sumathisena, D. R., and Goldberg, H. H.: Prolapse of the Tricuspid Leaflets in the Systolic Murmur-Click Syndrome, *Cath. Cardiovasc. Diag.*, 1:81, 1975.
31. Killip, T., and Lukas, D. S.: Tricuspid Stenosis: Physiologic Criteria for Diagnosis and Hemodynamic Abnormalities, *Circulation,* 16:3, 1957.
32. El-Sherif, N.: Rheumatic Tricuspid Stenosis: A Haemodynamic Correlation, *Br. Heart J.*, 33:16, 1971.
33. Hansing, C. E. and Rowe, G. G.: Tricuspid Insufficiency: A Study of Hemodynamics and Pathogenesis, *Circulation,* 45:793, 1972.
34. Holmes, J. C., Fowler, N. O., and Kaplan, S.: Pulmonary Valvular Insufficiency, *Am. J. Med.*, 44:851, 1968.
35. Salazar, E., and Levine, H. D.: Rheumatic Tricuspid Regurgitation: The Clinical Spectrum, *Am. J. Med.*, 33:111, 1962.
36. Killip, T., and Lukas, D. S.: Tricuspid Stenosis: Clinical Features in Twelve Cases, *Am. J. Med.*, 24:836, 1958.
37. Rivero-Carvallo, J. M.: El Diagnostica de la estenosis tricuspides, *Arch. Inst. Cardiol. Mex.*, 20:1, 1950.
38. Chandraratna, P. A., Lopez, J. M., Fernandex, J. J., and Cohen, L. S.: Echocardiographic Detection of Tricuspid Valve Prolapse, *Circulation,* 51:823, 1975.
39. Lieppe, W., Behar, V. S., Scallion, R., and Kisslo, J. A.: Detection of Tricuspid Regurgitation with Two-Dimensional Echocardiography and Peripheral Vein Injections, *Circulation,* 57:128, 1978.
40. Meltzer, R. S., VanHoogenhuyze, D., Serruys, P. W., Haalebos, M. M. P., Hugenholt, P. G., and Roelandt, J.: Diagnosis of Tricuspid Regurgitation by Contrast Echocardiography, *Circulation,* 63:1093, 1981.
41. Waggoner, A. D., Quinones, M. A., Young, J. B., Brandon, T. A., Shah, A. A., Verani, M. S., and Miller, R. R.: Pulsed Doppler Echocardiographic Detection of Right-Sided Valve Regurgitation: Experimental Results and Clinical Significance, *Am. J. Cardiol.*, 47:279, 1981.
42. Cha, S. D., Gooch, A. S., and Maranhao, V.: Intracardiac Phonocardiography in Tricuspid Regurgitation: Relation to Clinical and Angiographic Findings, *Am. J. Cardiol.*, 48:578, 1981.
43. Kay, J. H., Maselli-Campagna, G., and Tsuji, H. K.: Surgical Treatment of Tricuspid Insufficiency, *Ann. Surg.*, 162:53, 1965.
44. Boyd, A. D., Engelman, R. M., Isom, O. W., Reed, G. E., and Spencer, F. C.: Tricuspid Annuloplasty: Five and One-Half Years' Experience with 78 Patients, *J. Thorac. Cardiovasc. Surg.*, 68:344, 1974.
45. De Vega, N. F.: La Annuloplastia selectiva, reguable y permanente, *Rev. Esp. Cardiol.*, 25:6, 1972.
46. Carpentier, A., Deloche, A., Hanania, G., Forman, J., et al.: Surgical Management of Acquired Tricuspid Valve Disease, *J. Thorac. Cardiovasc. Surg.*, 67:53, 1974.
47. Deloche, A., Gierinon, J., Fabiani, J. N., Morillo, F., et al.: Etude anatomique des valvulopathies rhumatismales tricuspidiennes, *Ann. Chir. Thorac. Cardiovasc.*, 4:32, 1973.
48. Braunwald, N. S., Ross, J., and Morrow, A. G.: Conservative Management of Tricuspid Regurgitation in Patients Undergoing Mitral Valve Replacement, *Circulation* 35 (suppl. 1):1, 1967.
49. Simon, R., Oelert, H., Borst, H. G., and Lichtlen, P. R.: Influence of Mitral Valve Surgery on Tricuspid Incompetence Concomitant with Mitral Valve Disease, *Circulation,* 62:1, 1980.
50. Thorburn, C. W., Morgan, J. J., Shanahan, M. X., and Chang, V. P.: Long-Term Results of Tricuspid Valve Replacement and the Problem of Prosthetic Valve Thrombosis, *Am. J. Cardiol.*, 51:1128, 1983.
51. Carpentier, A., Deloche, A., Hanania, G., Forman, J., et al.: Surgical Management of Acquired Tricuspid Valve Disease, *J. Thorac. Cardiovasc. Surg.*, 67:53, 1974.
52. Grondin, P., Meere, C., Limet, R., Lopez-Bescos, L., Delcan, J. L., and Rivera, R.: Carpentiers Annulus and De Vega's Annuloplasty: The End of the Tricuspid Challenge, *J. Thorac. Cardiovasc. Surg.*, 70:852, 1975.
53. Kay, J. H., Mendez, A. M., and Zubiate, P.: A Further Look at Tricuspid Annuloplasty, *Ann. Thorac. Surg.*, 22:498, 1976.
54. Peterffy, A., Jonasson, R., Szamosi, A., and Henze, A.: Comparison of Kay's and De Vega's Annuloplasty in Surgical Treatment of Tricuspid Incompetence, *Scand. J. Thorac. Cardiovasc. Surg.*, 14:249, 1980.
55. Rabago, G., De Vega, N. G., Castillon, L., Moreno, T., et al.: The New De Vega Technique in Tricuspid Annuloplasty: Results in 150 Patients, *J. Cardiovasc. Surg.*, 21:231, 1980.
56. Reed, G. E., Boyd, A. D., Spencer, F. C., Engelman, R. M., et al.: Operative Management of Tricuspid Regurgitation, *Circulation,* 54 (suppl. 3):III-96, 1976.
57. Breyer, R. H., McClenathan, J. H., Michaelis, L. L., McIntosh, C. L., and Morrow, A. G.: Tricuspid Regurgitation: A Comparison of Nonoperative Management, Tricuspid Annuloplasty, and Tricuspid Valve Replacement, *J. Thorac. Cardiovasc. Surg.*, 72:867, 1976.
58. Jugdutt, B. I., Fraser, R. S., Lee, S. J. K., Rossal, R. E., and Callaghan, J. C.: Long-Term Survival after Tricuspid Valve Replacement: Results with Seven Different Prostheses, *J. Thorac. Cardiovasc. Surg.*, 74:20, 1977.
59. Kouchoukos, N. T., and Stephenson, L. W.: Indications for and Results of Tricuspid Valve Replacement, *Adv. Cardiol.*, 17:199, 1976.
60. Sanfelippo, P. M., Giuliani, E. R., Danielson, G. K., Wallace, R. B., et al.: Tricuspid Valve Prosthetic Replacement: Early and Late Results with the Starr-Edwards Prosthesis, *J. Thorac. Cardiovasc. Surg.*, 71:441, 1976.
61. Singh, A. K., Christian, F. D., Williams, D. O., Georas, C. S., et al.: Follow-Up Assessment of St. Jude Medical Prosthetic Valve in the Tricuspid Position: Clinical and Hemodynamic Results, *Ann. Thorac. Surg.*, 37:324, 1984.
62. Arbulu, A., Asfaw, I.: Tricuspid Valvulectomy without Prosthetic Replacement: Ten Years of Clinical Experience, *J. Thorac. Cardiovasc. Surg.*, 82:684, 1981.
63. Miller, D. D., Moreno-Cabral, R. J., Stinson, E. B., Shinn, J. A., and Shumway, N. E.: Pulmonary Artery Balloon Counterpulsation for Acute Right Ventricular Failure, *J. Thorac. Cardiovasc. Surg.*, 80:760, 1980.
64. Chesebro, J. H., Fuster, V., Elveback, L. R., McGoon, D. C., et al.: Trial of Combined Warfarin Plus Dipyridamole or Aspirin Therapy in Prosthetic Heart Valve Replacement: Danger of Aspirin Compared with Dipyridamole, *Am. J. Cardiol.*, 51:1537, 1983.
65. DePace, N. L., Iskandrian, A. S., Morganroth, J., Ross, J., Mattleman, S., and Neotico, P. F.: Infective Endocarditis Involving a Presumably Normal Pulmonic Valve, *Am. J. Cardiol.*, 53:385, 1984.
66. Misbach, G. A., Turley, K., Ebert, P. A.: Pulmonary Valve Replacement for Regurgitation after Repair of Tetralogy of Fallot, *Ann. Thorac. Surg.*, 36:684, 1983.
67. Wessel, H. U., Cunningham, W. J., Paul, M. H., Bastanier, C. K., et al.: Exercise Performance in Tetralogy of Fallot after Intracardiac Repair, *J. Thorac. Cardiovasc. Surg.*, 80:582, 1980.

Section C

Coronary Heart Disease

41

Factors Influencing Atherogenesis

Russell Ross, Ph.D.

The Lesions of Atherosclerosis

Atherosclerosis is not a single disease entity. The lesions of atherosclerosis take different forms, depending upon their anatomic site; the age, genetic and physiological status of the affected individual; and, presumably, upon the so-called risk factors to which each individual may have been exposed. Examination of atherosclerotic lesions with modern techniques of cell and molecular biology has revealed that each lesion contains significant elements of three cellular phenomena. These are smooth-muscle proliferation; formation by the proliferated cells of large amounts of connective tissue matrix including collagen, elastic fibers, and proteoglycans; and accumulation of intracellular and extracellular lipid.[1] In each instance, the relative degree to which each of the cells responds to different atherogenic stimuli determines the unique combination that defines the type and extent of the resulting lesion.

The lesions of atherosclerosis occur principally within the innermost layer of the artery wall, the intima. They include the fatty streak, the fibrous plaque, and the so-called complicated lesions.[2] (See Chap. 43.) Secondary changes have been noted in the media of the artery underlying the lesion, principally in association with the more advanced lesions of atherosclerosis (Fig. 41-1).

The Fatty Streak

The process of atherosclerosis begins in childhood with the development of flat, lipid-rich lesions called *fatty streaks* (see Chap. 43). These lesions consist of variable numbers of lipid-laden macrophages together with variable numbers of lipid-laden smooth-muscle cells within the arterial intima. Both of these cell types contain deposits of cholesterol and cholesterol oleate. Fatty streaks can be found in the aorta shortly after birth and appear in increasing numbers between the ages of 8 and 18 years. Fatty streaks appear in the coronary arteries at about age 15 and continue to increase in amount in these vessels through the third decade of life.[3]

The lesions are yellowish and sessile in appearance and cause little to no obstruction of the affected artery and no clinical sequelae. The fatty streak is ubiquitous in young people and even in those populations that do not appear to develop severe atherosclerosis. This observation suggests that lipid deposition does not inevitably lead to the advanced lesions of atherosclerosis, but that a number of other factors, as yet largely hypothetical, are associated with the progression of the lesions and with the development of the more complex form of atherosclerosis, the fibrous plaque.

The Fibrous Plaque

More advanced lesions begin to develop around the age of 25 in those populations in which there is a high incidence of atherosclerosis and its clinical sequelae. The fibrous plaque is grossly white in appearance and becomes elevated so that it may protrude into the lumen of the artery (see Chap. 43). If this lesion progresses sufficiently, it can occlude the lumen and compromise the vascular supply of the involved tissue. The principal change that occurs within the arterial intima during the development of the fibrous plaque consists of proliferation of smooth-muscle cells. These cells usually form a fibrous cap owing to the deposition by the cells of new connective tissue matrix and to the accumulation of intracellular and extracellular lipids. This fibrous cap covers a deeper deposit of varying amounts of extracellular lipid and cell debris[4] (Fig. 41-2).

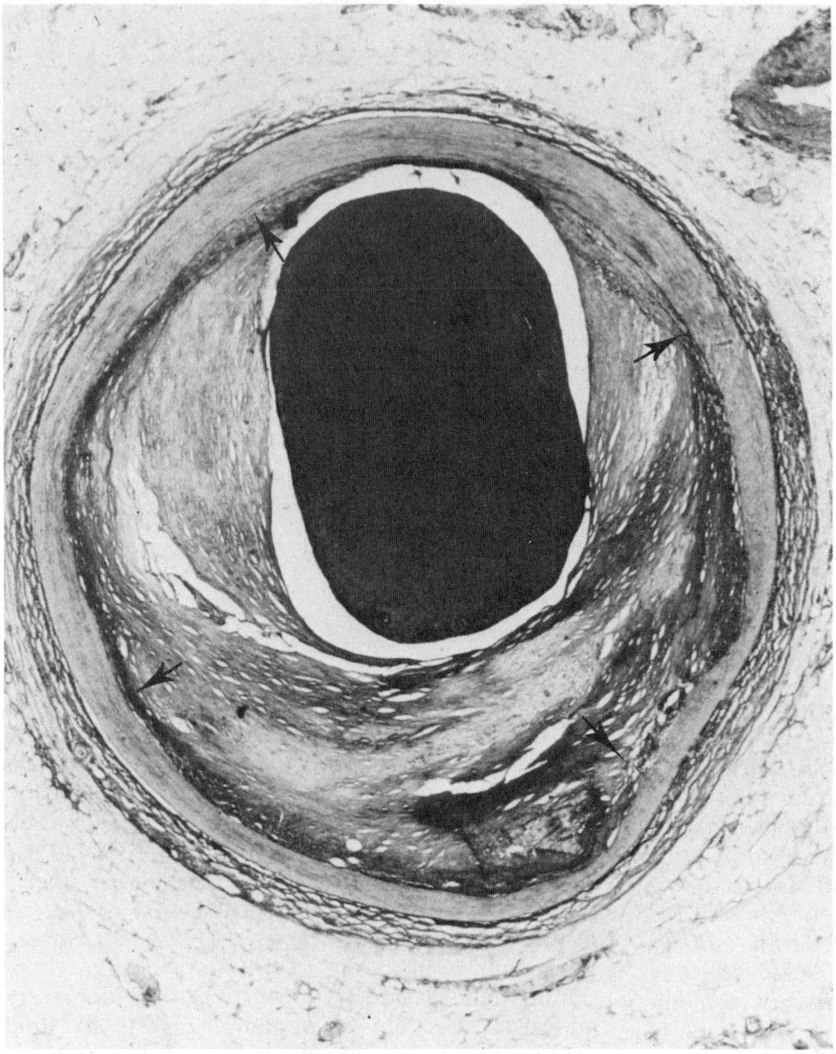

FIGURE 41-1 This is a classical light micrograph of a cross section of a coronary artery that contains a large atherosclerotic lesion. The lumen of the artery is relatively small. The original lumen is indicated by the arrows. In this preparation, it is virtually impossible to see cellular detail and, in particular, to determine the type of cells involved in the formation of the lesion.

It has been suggested that fibrous plaques are derived from fatty streaks that continue the process of cell proliferation, lipid accumulation, and connective tissue formation, and that the deep core of lipid and cell debris results from inadequate blood supply and cell necrosis. Such a relation has not been proved but has been questioned, since although fatty streaks in young individuals are often found in the same anatomic location in the coronary and extracranial cerebral arteries as fibrous plaques in older individuals, fatty streaks can also occur in anatomic sites that are different from those in which fibrous plaques appear. The reasons for these differences are not understood. It has been suggested that in those instances where their location is different, the fatty streaks may have simply regressed and disappeared, whereas in the instances where the anatomic location is the same, lesion progression has occurred. This remains a matter of controversy. There is a lesion that is generally accepted as a forerunner of the fibrous plaque. This is known as the *fibromusculoelastic lesion* of the intima, which consists of proliferated smooth-muscle cells surrounded by connective tissue which contains little to no lipid.[5]

The Advanced (Complicated) Lesion

The complicated lesions of atherosclerosis (see Chap. 43) occur in increasing frequency with increasing age. The fibrous plaque can become vascularized both from the luminal as well as its medial aspects. In the complicated lesion, the necrotic "lipid-rich core" increases in size and often becomes calcified. The lesions may become increasingly complex as a result of hemorrhage and calcification, and the intimal surface may disintegrate and ulcerate and become involved with thrombotic episodes that may lead to occlusive disease. Such thrombi may then organize and further increase the thickness of the plaque while progressively reducing the size of the arterial lumen. It is not uncommon that as the intimal lesions progress, the number of smooth-muscle cells in the underlying media decreases and the media undergoes atrophy, which can sometimes result in aneurysmal changes rather than lead to thrombotic occlusion of the artery.

There is quite a range of variability in the degree of severity of the lesions of atherosclerosis in different arteries. Recognition that the components of smooth-muscle proliferation, connective tissue for-

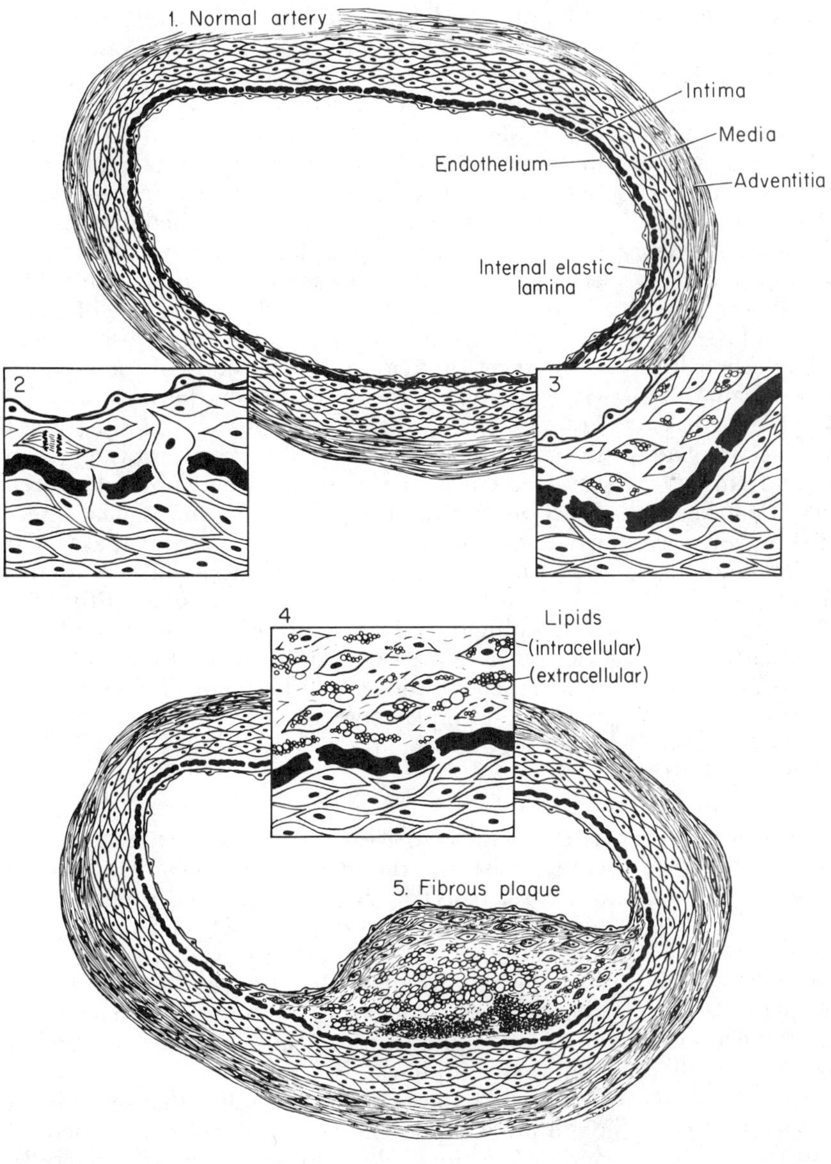

FIGURE 41-2 A series of possible stages in the development of the various lesions of atherosclerosis. (1) The appearance of a normal muscular artery and its component layers: the intima bounded by endothelium and internal elastic lamina, the media, and adventitia. In children and young adults the intima is thin and contains only an occasional smooth-muscle cell; with age it slowly and uniformly increases in thickness and cell content. It is important to note that there are no fibroblasts present in either the intima or the media of mammalian arteries. Fibroblasts are found only in the adventitia. (2) The first phase of a developing lesion in atherosclerosis; a focal thickening of the intima consists of an increase in smooth-muscle cells and extracellular matrix. Smooth-muscle cells are shown proliferating within the intima; two are in the process of migrating through fenestrae of the internal elastic lamina. Subsequent to or possibly concomitant with intimal smooth-muscle proliferation, accumulation of intercellular lipid deposits (3) or extracellular lipid (4), or both, occur resulting in a fatty streak. A fibrous plaque (5) may result from a continued accumulation of a connective tissue cap covering increased numbers of smooth-muscle cells laden with lipids, extracellular lipid, and cell debris overlying a deeper extracellular pool of lipid. A complicated lesion may form as a result of continuing cell degeneration, ingress of blood constituents, and calcification superimposed upon the elements present in the fibrous plaque. Observations made at necropsy and experiments such as those described in the text suggest that this may represent the sequence of events that occurs in humans. (*From J. A. Glomset and R. Ross, Atherosclerosis and the Arterial Smooth Muscle Cell, Science, 180:1332, 1973. Copyright 1973 by the American Association for the Advancement of Science. Reproduced with permission from the publisher and authors.*)

mation, and lipid accumulation represent the key elements of the developing lesions of atherosclerosis has led to the utilization of a number of models of experimentally induced atherosclerosis to study this process in different animal species.

Experimentally Induced Atherosclerosis

Four species have been widely used in studying atherogenesis: rabbits, chickens, swine, and nonhuman primates. Most early work was performed in rabbits; however, swine and nonhuman primates are generally considered to develop lesions that correspond more closely with those that occur in human beings. A great deal of new information has been gained from studies of swine and primates, although rabbits continue to provide important data in terms of understanding a number of cellular phenomena. Atherosclerosis has been induced in most animal models by a high-fat, high-cholesterol diet. A principal shortcoming of this approach, however, is that to produce more advanced lesions, it is necessary to maintain animals on such diets for years. Even though it is possible to induce the lesions in a relatively short period (1 to 3 years in the monkey), it is not clear that the lesions produced in this manner actually simulate those that may require 20 to 30 years to form in human beings. On the other hand, the rate at which lesions form in humans is not entirely clear, since some may progress more rapidly than had heretofore been considered to be possible.[6]

Other approaches to studying the smooth-muscle proliferative changes associated with atherosclerosis have included endothelial injury resulting from mechanical injury from varying types of intraarterial catheters,[7,8] chemically induced injury (from sources such as chronic hypercholesterolemia[9] or chronic homocystinemia[10]), immune-type injuries[11] (from exposure to antigen-antibody complexes), and, more recently, virally induced injury in diseases such as Marek's disease.[12] In a recent study of diet-induced hypercholesterolemia in nonhuman primates, Faggiotto et al.[13,14] have described the changes that led to fatty streak development and the manner in which some fatty streaks progress to become more complicated fibrous plaques. Within 12 days after induction of high levels of plasma cholesterol (approximately 700 to 1000 mg/dl), numerous monocytes were observed attached to the surface of the endothelium throughout the arterial tree. These monocytes probe between junctional complexes of the endothelium, migrate, and localize subendothelially, where they accumulate lipid and become foam cells to establish the initial fatty streak. These fatty streaks form at branches and bifurcations and accumulate increasing numbers of macrophages and smooth-muscle cells; in the process they create a markedly uneven surface contour and stretch the overlying endothelium exceedingly thin. After about 5 months, breaks occur between endothelial cells, exposing the lipid-filled macrophages, some of which appear to enter the circulation. Many of the exposed macrophages serve as sites where platelets adhere and form mural thrombi. In these monkeys, these sites of platelet-macrophage interactions were first observed in the iliac arteries, and, after longer periods of hypercholesterolemia, similar changes occurred at higher levels in the abdominal and thoracic aorta. Interestingly, the anatomic sites that were previously involved with platelet-macrophage interactions are the same sites that 1 to 2 months later contain proliferative smooth-muscle lesions of atherosclerosis. These studies further support observations that endothelial injury and platelet and macrophage interactions may be important in atherogenesis. This causal relation is exceedingly difficult to establish, however. It is also possible that some fatty streaks go on to progress directly to fibrous plaques. If the latter proves to be correct, the cellular and molecular base for this progression must be established.

Each animal model has its shortcomings; however, important new information has been obtained from these approaches, particularly when they can be studied in correlation with in vitro models using cell culture techniques. The latter have permitted in-depth studies of endothelium, smooth muscle, macrophages, and platelets. The interrelationships among these cells and among observations resulting from in vivo studies of atherogenesis and cell culture are discussed later in this chapter.

Hypotheses of Atherogenesis

Historical View of Atherogenesis

Atherosclerosis has been recognized in humans for thousands of years. Lesions of atherosclerosis were identified in Egyptian mummies as early as the fifteenth century B.C. Long[15] has discussed the development of clinical-pathological correlations that evolved during the era when autopsy examination permitted the development of an understanding between the degree of atherosclerosis and the incidence of myocardial infarction and stroke. In the mid-nineteenth century, Virchow[16] proposed the idea that some form of injury to the artery wall associated with an inflammatory response resulted in what was then considered to be a degenerative lesion of atherosclerosis. This idea was subsequently modified by Anitschkow[17] and further included the role of platelets and thrombogenesis in atherosclerosis, as expanded by Duguid[18] in 1948. Many of the modern views of atherogenesis stem from the work of John French,[19] who noted that the structural integrity of the endothelial lining of the artery represented a key element in the maintenance of normal arterial function, and that alterations in endothelial integrity might precede a sequence of events that would lead to the various forms of the lesions of atherosclerosis. Thus, over the years a number of theories concerning the etiology and pathogenesis of atherosclerosis have been developed. At least three of these deserve elaboration and comment. These are the response-to-injury hypothesis, the monoclonal hypothesis, and the lipogenic hypothesis.

The Response-to-Injury Hypothesis

One basis for the *response-to-injury hypothesis* of atherosclerosis[1,9,20] lies in the marked similarity observed by many investigators between the ubiquitous fibromusculoelastic lesions noted at autopsy and a similar lesion that can be induced in a number of animal species, including nonhuman primates, rabbits, and swine, after different forms of arterial endothelial injury.

The hypothesis (Fig. 41-3) states that some form of "injury" to the endothelium results in structural and/or functional alterations in the endothelial cells. Factors such as chronic hypercholesterolemia;[9] increased shear stress from the flow of blood over the endothelial cells, as may occur at branch points or bifurcations in arteries in hypertension;[21] and dysfunction induced by toxins or other injurious agents may lead to changes in the nature of the permeability barrier established by the endothelial cells. In the normal artery, the endothelial cells form a continuous monolayer that regulates the passage of substances from the plasma to the underlying artery wall. Injury to the endothelial cells may alter their permeability characteristics and change endothelial cell-cell or endothelial cell–connective tissue relations, permitting hemodynamic forces to induce focal endothelial cell detachment and thus permit interactions to occur between elements from the blood and the wall of the artery.

Not only do the endothelial cells play an important role as a permeability barrier but they also form a thromboresistant surface that promotes the continuous flow of blood throughout the vascular tree.

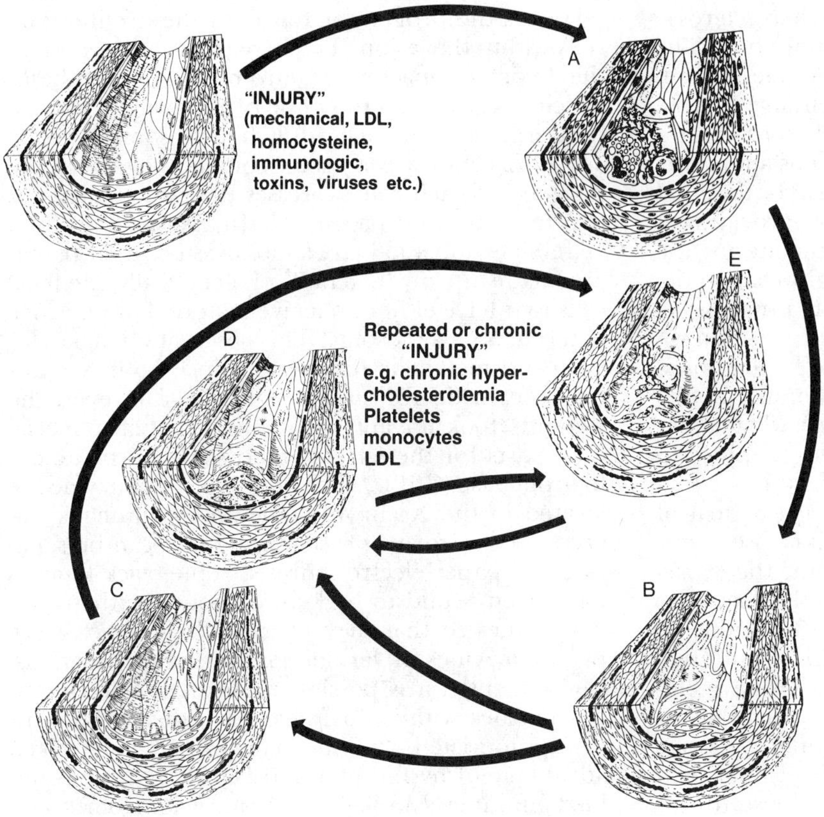

FIGURE 41-3 A version of the response-to-injury hypothesis of atherosclerosis. A series of events are postulated to occur in which endothelial injury results in exposure of the subendothelium (*A*) with interactions between monocytes, macrophages, and platelets. The endothelial injury represented in this diagram represents the maximal response in which cell-cell detachment and cell–connective tissue detachment leads to subendothelial denudation. Platelet interactions with the connective tissue or with macrophages lead to the possible deposition of growth factor such as platelet-derived growth factor, which can then induce migration and proliferation of smooth-muscle cells derived from the media of the artery into the intima (*B*). If the injury ceases and the endothelium regenerates, it is postulated that the lesion may be reversible and the resultant effect would be that of a slightly thickened intima (*C*). On the other hand, if the injury is continuous for a prolonged period of time, there may be a sequence of injury and repair, followed by reinjury and repair, leading to proliferative lesions that may compromise the vascular supply (*D* and *E*). (*From R. Ross, Atherosclerosis: A Problem of the Biology of the Arterial Wall Cells and Their Interactions with Blood Components, Arteriosclerosis, 1:293, 1981. Modified and reproduced with permission from the American Heart Association, Inc., and the author.*)

The thromboresistant character of the endothelium appears to be due principally to two factors produced by the cells. Both of these have been identified, but their physiological roles are relatively poorly understood. They are the cell surface glycoproteins and proteoglycans that form the surface coat of the endothelial cells, and a prostaglandin derivative, prostacycline (PGI_2).[22] Prostacycline is one of the most potent vasodilatory agents thus far isolated and is a potent inhibitor of platelet aggregation. Both endothelial cells and smooth-muscle cells are capable of synthesizing prostacycline: this is discussed in greater detail below.

Injury to the endothelium that results in alterations in permeability would permit plasma constituents such as lipoproteins to have more ready access to the artery wall. Such injury, and others that affect endothelial function, may not result in any changes in the morphology of the endothelial monolayer that lines the artery. Endothelial dysfunction could also alter the thromboresistant character of the lumen of the artery so that platelets could interact directly at sites of endothelial injury. If the injury were sufficiently severe, the endothelial cells might desquamate and be lost into the bloodstream, leading to exposure of the underlying connective tissue to platelets and to other elements in the circulation. The response-to-injury hypothesis suggests that the interaction between constituents in the plasma, platelets and monocyte/macrophages, and the endothelium or the connective tissue, principally collagen, results in platelet adherence, aggregation, and release of contents normally stored within the granules of the platelets or released from activated intimal macrophages, or foam cells. The exposure of the artery wall at sites of injury to factors derived from the platelets and/or macrophages, together with components from the plasma such as lipoproteins and hormones, would then lead to focal proliferation of arterial smooth-muscle cells. According to the hypothesis, this smooth-muscle proliferation would be derived from two sources: preexisting intimal smooth-muscle cells and medial smooth-muscle cells that are attracted to, and migrate and proliferate within, the intima at sites of "injury." Such a local stimulus could also lead to the formation of new connective tissue matrix constituents by the proliferating smooth-muscle cells and to the deposition of lipids both within and around the proliferated cells.

According to this hypothesis, if the injury to the endothelium were a self-limited event and endothelial integrity were restored, the proliferative lesions might be capable of regressing. If this were the case, the lesions would be reversible, and if they had not reached a critical size, would be clinically silent. There is evidence both in experimental animals and in human beings that the lesions of atherosclerosis can, under certain conditions, regress.[23]

On the other hand, if the injury at focal sites in the artery wall is either long-standing or chronically repeated over periods of many years, the lesions could continue to progress, become increasingly complex in terms of their composition, and eventually lead to the principal clinical sequelae of atherosclerosis, myocardial infarction, and cerebral infarction. The capacity of the endothelium to regenerate and restore endothelial integrity at sites of injury may be critical in determining whether the lesions of atherosclerosis enlarge, remain relatively constant in size, or regress. The superimposition of risk factors that might possibly affect this balance by providing a chronic source of injury, or by somehow altering the normal tissue response to injury, might change the balance so that lesions would be slowly progressive. As an example, the increased levels of plasma low-density lipoproteins associated with hypercholesterolemia may provide a source of injury to the endothelial cells and may also convert what might otherwise be a limited tissue response to injury to frank progressive lesions of atherosclerosis.

This hypothesis has stimulated a great deal of experimental work that has led to an increase in our understanding of factors that determine the capacity of the endothelial cells to maintain themselves as an integral continuous cell layer, and to studies of those factors that control the growth of endothelium. Of equal importance, many studies have elucidated the factors that modify the capacity of arterial smooth-muscle cells to form connective tissue proteins, to synthesize and metabolize lipids and lipoproteins, and to proliferate in response to different mitogenic factors.

One of the more important observations that has resulted from examination of this hypothesis is the discovery that platelets contain a potent mitogen, the platelet-derived growth factor, that is stored in the platelets.[24] It has been suggested that this factor may play an important role in inducing the intimal smooth-muscle proliferative response seen in experimentally induced atherosclerosis and in atherosclerosis in human beings. This is discussed in greater detail below.

A number of important questions have arisen concerning the factors that promote proliferation of smooth-muscle and endothelial cells and the mechanisms whereby lesions of atherosclerosis may regress. Relatively little is known concerning the factors responsible for the turnover of connective tissue matrix within the artery wall or concerning the mechanisms responsible for removing either this matrix or cholesterol from lesions. The response-to-injury hypothesis has provided explanations for some of these phenomena. However, much remains to be learned, for example, with respect to the capacity of endothelium and smooth muscle to bind and to metabolize the different types of lipoproteins. These will be discussed below.

The Monoclonal Hypothesis

The *monoclonal hypothesis* of atherosclerosis was proposed by Benditt and Benditt.[25] This hypothesis suggests that each lesion of atherosclerosis is derived from a single smooth-muscle cell and that this cell serves as the progenitor for all of the proliferating cells within the lesion. The hypothesis is based upon the Lyon, or inactive X chromosome, hypothesis, which suggests that only one of the two X chromosomes present in each adult female somatic cell is active. Except for early stages of embryogenesis, the progeny of each cell expresses the same inactive X chromosome as its parent cell. In a sense, therefore, all female individuals are a mosaic, since their tissues are made up of "patches" of genetically identical cells that have either an active maternal or an active paternal X chromosome. This observation makes little to no metabolic difference, since both X chromosomes code for similar enzymes. However, the Benditts took advantage of the fact that a special case exists for the enzyme glucose-6-phosphate dehydrogenase (G6PD). The genes for this enzyme are located in the X chromosome and in humans can occur in two forms of isoenzyme that can be separated by paper electrophoresis. Some black females have been found to be heterozygous for these two isoenzymes so that they represent a mosaic of the two isoenzymes in various somatic cell populations. Consequently, it is possible to distinguish different cell patches within this mosaic by identification of the appropriate isoenzyme. This was originally taken advantage of by Lindner and Gartler,[26] who examined multiple samples of uterine leiomyomas and found that they were composed of cells that contained the same active X chromosome, whereas comparable samples of normal myometrium contained a mixture of cells derived from both types of progenitor cells. Studies of some other tumors have demonstrated similar phenomena, and in some cases there are data supporting the notion that all the cells of a given tumor originate from a single cell and are therefore monoclonal.[27]

More recently, Benditt and others have referred to this character of lesions as *monotypic*. Additional research has produced data that both support and negate this hypothesis. Pearson et al.[28] observed that the majority of atherosclerotic lesions examined from a series of autopsied black females contained either one or the other of the two isoenzymes of G6PD, but that fatty streaks from these individuals and the noninvolved, or normal, arterial tissue contained both isoenzymes and therefore did not appear to be monotypic. Thomas et al. examined the lesion and nonlesion areas of arteries from black females at autopsy in a slightly different manner and obtained data that are at variance with the data supporting the hypothesis and which have been interpreted differently.[29] Thomas et al. examined multiple samples of lesions versus nonlesion areas and found a much higher percentage of both isoenzymes within lesions than had been reported in the earlier studies.

The Benditts[30] have interpreted their data to signify that since each lesion of atherosclerosis is monotypic and is presumably derived from a single smooth-muscle cell, each lesion is a benign neoplasm that may have occurred as a result of cell transformation by agents such as viruses or chemicals. These are interesting possibilities that deserve to be tested further. Fialkow[27] has pointed out that the observation of a single enzyme phenotype in a lesion does not necessarily imply a clonal origin for such a lesion. He stresses that each lesion could arise from a population of genetically identical cells that contained the same isoenzyme rather than from a single cell. These two possibilities could not be distinguished from one another using the single technique of paper electrophoresis. In the artery wall, the possibility of a monoclonal origin would presumably depend on the mosaic composition of the artery wall and therefore the distribution of cells with one or the other isoenzyme within the normal intima or media. Unfortunately, relatively little is known concerning the distribution of isoenzymes within the artery, and the possibility that sparsely distributed, single progenitor cells in the normal intima could give rise to smooth-muscle cell patches that are appreciably larger than those in the media deserves to be explored. If lesion development were characterized by repeated cycles of cell death and growth, according to Fialkow, "repetitive sampling could lead to a single enzyme phenotype, despite multicellular origin."[27] It is therefore possible that under those circumstances, clonal selection with evolution toward a single enzyme phenotype within the lesion could conceivably occur in some kinds of hyperplastic responses. Therefore it is likely that the lesions of atherosclerosis are derived not from a single cell, but rather from a population of cells of identical phenotype, or some combination of these events. It is probable that the bulk of the lesions of atherosclerosis are hyperplastic rather than neoplastic, which provides further reason for developing means of intervention and treatment leading to lesion regression.

The Lipogenic Hypothesis

Both lesion initiation and lesion progression in atherosclerosis appear somehow to be associated in many individuals with markedly increased elevations of plasma low-density lipoproteins (LDL). The accumulation of lipid within proliferated smooth-muscle cells, within macrophages in the lesions, and within the extracellular connective tissue matrix are common findings, particularly in the lesions of atherosclerosis.[31] The presence of elevated levels of LDL suggest that cholesterol internalization and esterification by cells may be accelerated to such a degree that proliferated smooth-muscle cells within lesions become filled with cholesterol oleate. Many of the cells may go on to become necrotic and may release their lipid into the extracellular spaces. In the presence of excess plasma LDL, which is relatively rich in cholesterol linoleate, the debris may be a mixture of both types of cholesteryl esters.

Some studies have suggested that there are factors present in LDL in hyperlipemic animals that, in themselves, may promote proliferation from smooth-muscle cells and the production of new connective tissue components by these cells.[32] Thus, a sequence of events involving injury to the endothelium by chronic elevated levels of LDL and continuing progression of lesions of atherosclerosis by exposure to elevated levels of LDL, and presumably, by decreased levels of high-density lipoproteins (HDL), could provide a sequence of events leading to the development of advanced lesions of atherosclerosis. This hypothesis might explain how some fatty streaks could progress to become fibrous plaques but fails to take into account many of the other components of the lesions of atherosclerosis, in particular, the basis for explaining, in addition to the proliferative response of smooth-muscle cells, other phenomena such as the stimulation of new connective tissue formation.

It is possible that the different lesions of atherosclerosis may occur by any of the mechanisms suggested in these different hypotheses or by different combinations of them. It is also clear that, as many aspects of our understanding of the biology of smooth muscle and endothelium continue to be expanded, new factors that have not been anticipated may be revealed that may play a role in the pathogenesis of atherosclerosis.

The Role of Risk Factors

A number of risk factors of atherosclerosis have become reasonably well established on the basis of their relation in epidemiologic studies to the incidence of clinically manifest disease. Unfortunately, there is no basis for comparison between risk factors and the severity or extent of the lesions of atherosclerosis. Among many factors that are considered to be important are hyperlipidemia, hypertension, cigarette smoking, male sex, and diabetes mellitus. These have in general been associated with an increased incidence of fibrous plaques and their sequelae. The associations are relatively strong when they are made on a group comparison basis, although all of the studies have demonstrated a high degree of variability among individuals within even the most homogeneous of groups.[33]

Hyperlipidemia

Dietary lipids are considered to be one of the most important environmental agents responsible for severe atherosclerosis and for the high frequency of atherosclerotic disease in industrially developed parts of the world. Saturated fats became associated with increased incidence of atherosclerosis when it was found that they elevated the concentration of plasma cholesterol; however, the specific contributions of cholesterol, saturated fats, polyunsaturated fats, and total fats in atherosclerosis are still unclear. It has recently become possible to demonstrate an unequivocal association between ingestion of dietary cholesterol and plasma cholesterol levels and the incidence and prevalence of coronary disease within population groups. The recently published results of the Lipid Research Clinics Trial[34,35] have demonstrated for the first time a direct association between the plasma lipoprotein profile, cholesterol levels, and morbidity and mortality from coronary atherosclerosis. By means of the combination of diet and cholestyramine, a decrease in plasma cholesterol of 8 percent was obtained, which led to a decrease in the incidence of myocardial infarction and in the need for coronary bypass surgery. Thus, for the first time, there are unequivocal data demonstrating that lowering of plasma cholesterol in humans will have beneficial effects in reducing the incidence of atherosclerosis and its sequelae. Unfortunately, there is a great deal of variation from individual to individual in terms of dietary intake of fats and plasma cholesterol levels on a daily basis. There is also intrinsic variation in plasma cholesterol levels among individuals who consume the same diet but respond differently to it.

There is little question that dietary cholesterol directly affects the levels of plasma cholesterol.[36] However, only recently has it been suggested that dietary cholesterol may affect the incidence of atherosclerosis by altering the profile of plasma lipoproteins and possibly by changing the structural or functional properties of these lipoproteins.[37] Increased dietary cholesterol generally results in an increase in LDL cholesterol with a lesser increase in HDL cholesterol. The role of these two lipoproteins in atherogenesis is not clear, although it has been suggested that elevated HDL may be protective, whereas the reverse is true for elevated LDL.

Unfortunately, there are many differences in the ways in which animals and humans respond to dietary cholesterol, and there are limits to the extent to which information concerning responses in experimental animals to dietary intake can be applied to human beings. Nevertheless, the epidemiologic association between the increased intake of fat is very strong. The means by which these fats affect the incidence of atherosclerosis at the cellular and molecular levels remain to be elucidated, as indicated in the discussions of the various hypotheses of atherogenesis.

Hypertension

Hypertension has been established unequivocally as an associated risk factor in that individuals with elevated blood pressure show accelerated atherogenesis, an increased incidence of coronary heart disease, and in particular, increased incidence of cerebrovascular disease. The effects of hypertension appear to be independent of other risk factors in an epidemiologic sense; however, it does not appear to be a primary cause of advanced atherosclerosis in those populations in which the incidence of clinically manifest atherosclerosis is less than average.

The means by which hypertension induces atherogenesis are not clear, although there are many humoral mediators of blood pressure which may participate in this process. For example, renin and other hypertensive agents may induce cellular changes that lead to atherogenesis. Fry[21] and his colleagues, as well as others, have suggested that the increased shear stress of the flow of blood, particularly in hypertensive individuals, at selected anatomic sites within the arterial tree may result in focally altered endothelium and in the development of atherosclerotic lesions very much as suggested in the response-to-injury hypothesis discussed earlier.

Cigarette Smoking

Cigarette smoking provides perhaps the strongest and most consistent correlation with the increased incidence of atherosclerotic disease and appears to be a major contributor to increased risk of disease, generally in combination with other risk factors. Unfortunately, there is relatively little information concerning the means by which cigarette smoking exerts an impact at the cellular level. Early studies suggested that carbon monoxide might be a causative agent; however, these have not been confirmed. Becker[38] has recently identified agents derived from cigarette smoke that may be injurious to the artery wall. It has also been suggested that inhalation of cigarette smoke may result in the exposure of arterial cells to mutagens that transform the smooth-muscle cells and result in the stimulation of their proliferation. Apparently, cessation of cigarette smoking decreases the risk for development of the clinical sequelae of atherosclerosis and possibly may augment regression of lesions. Further research is clearly required to identify the factors in cigarette smoke that are responsible for its cardiovascular effects and for determining the mechanisms by which it alters cellular metabolism.

Male Sex

Perhaps one of the best-documented and most consistent risk factors for coronary atherosclerosis is male sex. This differential is accentuated in non-white populations, and it has been suggested that females have a decreased incidence because of a protective function exerted by estrogens. Paradoxically, unfortunately, large doses of estrogenic hormones appear to increase cardiovascular mortality in men who have had one myocardial infarct and among men under treatment for prostatic cancer. Consequently, the reason for the sex difference is not understood and remains to be elucidated.

Diabetes

Another risk factor known to be associated with increased incidence of atherosclerosis and myocardial infarction is diabetes mellitus. The mechanisms involved are poorly understood. There is, unfortunately, no consistency in the evidence related to whether elevated concentrations of plasma cholesterol and lipoproteins occur in diabetics whose concentrations of blood and urine glucose are carefully regulated. There does appear to be some evidence suggesting a decreased concentration of HDL cholesterol in diabetics and a high prevalence of hypertension associated with hyperglycemia. The basic mechanisms associated with the proliferation of smooth-muscle-type cells in the mesangium of the kidney in renal complications of diabetes and in increased thickness of capillary basement membrane in diabetics with microvascular disease may bear some similarity to smooth-muscle proliferation in atherogenesis. However, the alterations in the arterial tree in diabetics that precede the lesions of atherogenesis are not well documented and are poorly understood.

Although a great deal of new information, to be discussed below, has evolved concerning our understanding of endothelial cells, smooth-muscle cells, and platelets and the interactions among these cells, the specific role of each of the risk factors that are associated with increased incidence of atherosclerosis on an epidemiologic basis remains, for the most part, to be investigated and elucidated. This information will be critical if we are to proceed with the development of improved means of diagnosis, prevention, and intervention in this disease process.

Cellular Modulations in Atherosclerosis

Endothelium

The Barrier Role

Endothelial cells provide a selective permeability barrier, a blood-compatible interface, and a thromboresistant lining to the artery wall, and are metabolically active. A number of studies of endothelial permeability using various tracer molecules have demonstrated the presence of pinocytotic vesicles, transendothelial channels, and intracellular clefts in different kinds of endothelium. The junctional complexes between endothelial cells and the artery wall appear to be functionally dynamic structures that can respond to stimuli such as changes in blood pressure and pharmacologic agents. The surface components, at the molecular level, of the endothelial cells appear to influence the selective permeability of the endothelium.[39,40] Endothelial cells have been shown by the Steins[41] to be capable of transporting plasma lipoproteins of given sizes into the artery wall via vesicles. Thus, molecules like HDL would be transported, but larger lipoproteins the size of very low density lipoproteins (VLDL) or chylomicrons would have difficulty in crossing the endothelial barrier without some kind of alteration of these lipid-rich particles.

The disruption of this barrier has been shown, in a number of experimental animals, to result in opportunities that permit interactions between platelets and the artery wall at sites of endothelial injury resulting in the formation of an intimal smooth-muscle proliferative response. Stemerman and Ross[7] observed that if endothelial cells were removed by abrasion with an intraarterial catheter, sites of exposure of the subendothelial connective tissue were quickly coated with a "carpet" of degranulated platelets (Fig. 41-4). The interaction of products released from the platelets and plasma constituents at such sites of endothelial injury precedes a sequence of events that begins with focal smooth-muscle mi-

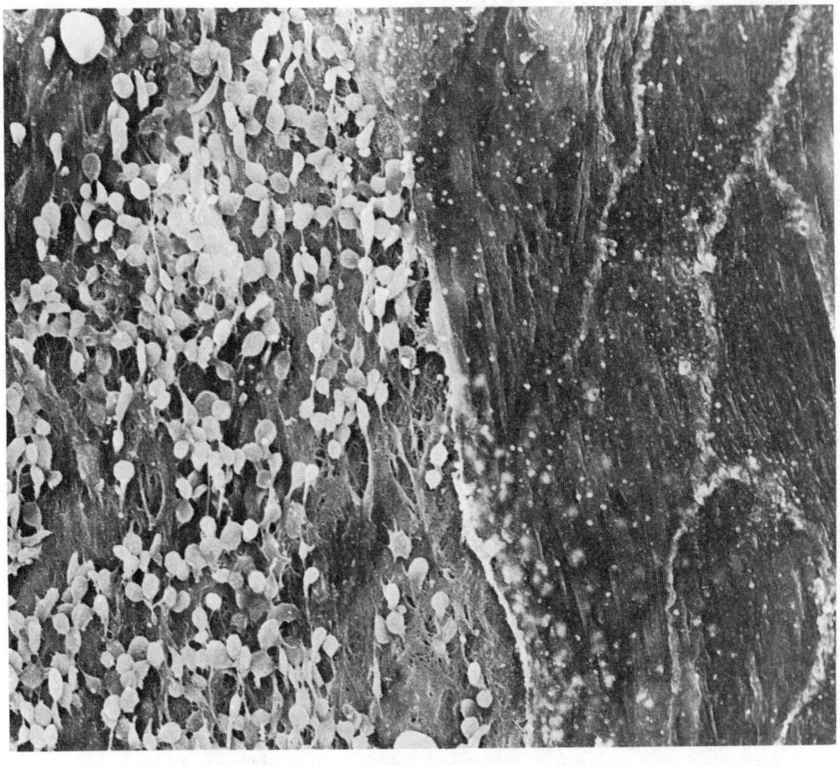

FIGURE 41-4 A scanning electron micrograph presenting a surface view of an artery in which the endothelial cells shown on the right have been removed with a catheter in the left portion of the micrograph. This scanning electron micrograph demonstrates platelets, seen as the small ovoid bodies which have attached to the subendothelial connective tissue that was exposed upon injury to the endothelium. These platelets tend to adhere to the exposed connective tissue and to one another, and in the process of doing so, release their intracellular contents.

gration and proliferation and that eventually leads to the development of a fibromusculoelastic lesion. If this mechanical injury is modified by the addition of a high-fat, high-cholesterol diet to the experiment, then the hyperlipemic animals whose endothelium has been mechanically injured develop intimal proliferative lesions essentially identical to fibrous plaques. In the normocholesterolemic animals, such endothelial injury leads to a fibromusculoelastic proliferative lesion that, over a period of 6 months, may undergo regression, whereas in hypercholesterolemic animals, the lesions become slowly progressive and show no signs of regression (Figs. 41-5 and 41-6).

Ross and Harker[9] observed that monkeys that received no mechanical injury but that were only fed a high-fat, high-cholesterol diet for a year or longer showed signs of endothelial injury as determined morphologically and by measurements of endothelial cell turnover at selected sites in the arterial tree.

Recently, as referred to earlier in this chapter, Faggiotto et al.[13,14] have observed a sequence of events in chronic hypercholesterolemic monkeys that culminates in dysjunction of endothelium overlying foam cells in fatty streaks that are derived from blood monocytes. Exposure of the foam cells leads to platelet interactions with both the macrophages and the exposed connective tissues. These interactions occur at the same anatomic sites that 1 to 2 months later are occupied by extensive smooth-muscle proliferative lesions of atherosclerosis.

Thus, the intimal smooth-muscle proliferation seen to accompany disruption of the endothelial cell barrier has been shown to be associated with the interaction between platelets and the exposed subendothelium at such sites of injury. This will be discussed below.

Endothelial Cell Culture

Arterial endothelial cells have been successfully cultured from a number of species, including the cow, rabbit, swine, nonhuman primate, and human being.[42,43] Endothelial cells from each of these species demonstrate a number of common characteristics. They grow, as they do in vivo, in a unique, continuous monolayer, and unlike cells such as smooth muscle or fibroblasts, appear to be truly "contact inhibited." That is, the cells become quiescent when they remain in contact and become confluent. If the monolayer is disrupted, for example,

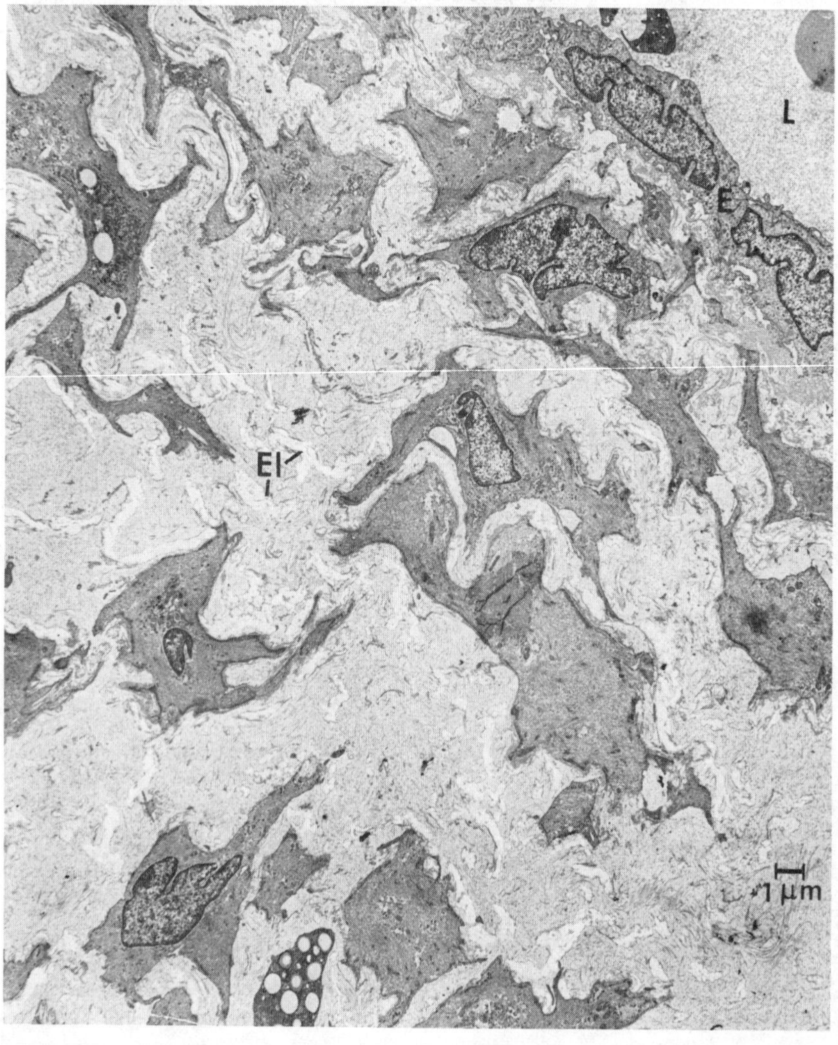

FIGURE 41-5 Electron micrograph of part of the intima from the right iliac artery of a macaque 3 months after the endothelium was removed with an intravascular balloon catheter. The lumen (L) is to the upper right. Endothelial cells cover the markedly thickened intima which contains large numbers of smooth-muscle cells surrounded by a matrix of small elastic fibers (El), collagen, and proteoglycan.

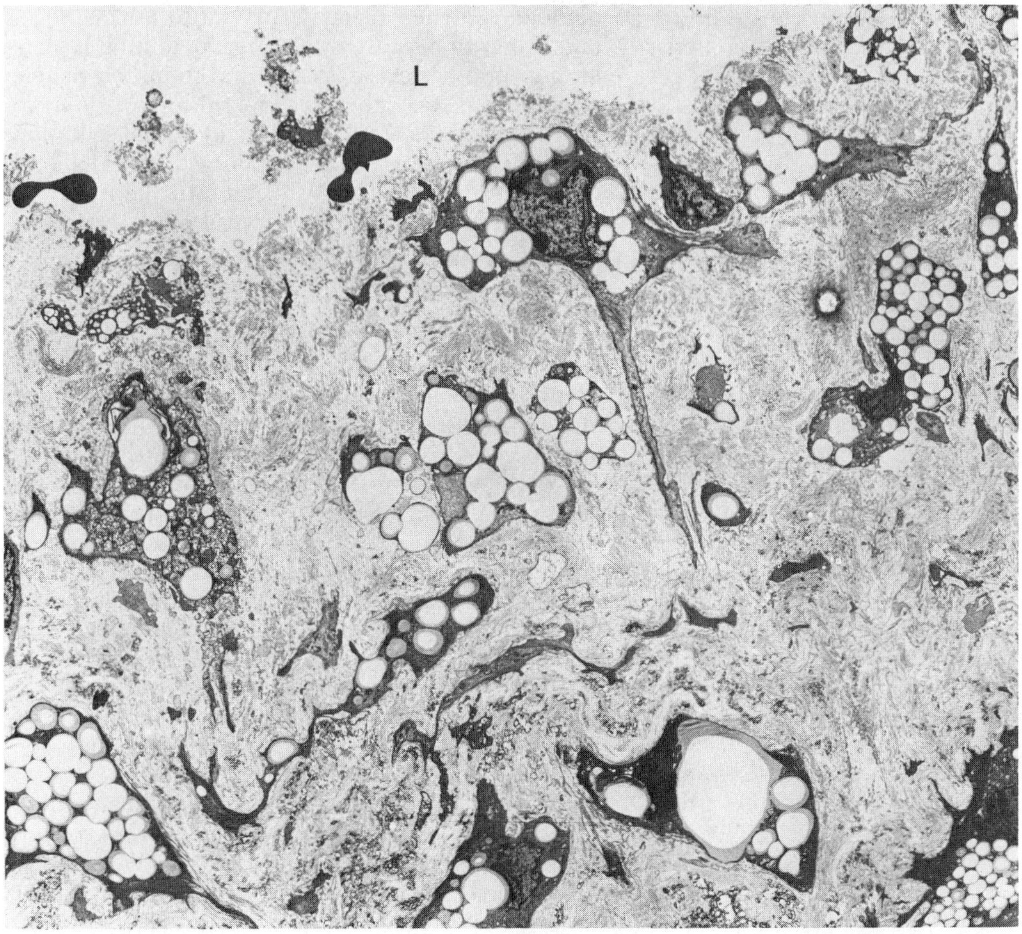

FIGURE 41-6 Electron micrograph of a portion of an intimal lesion in the iliac artery of a monkey on a hyperlipidemic diet 6 months after balloon injury. Most of the smooth-muscle cells in the lesion contain large lipid deposits. The cells are surrounded by small globular membranous deposits in the connective tissue. An endothelial cover is lacking at the luminal surface (L) at the crest of the lesion.

by wounding, the cells are stimulated to synthesize new DNA and to proliferate and restore the continuity of the monolayer. Only those cells in the culture next to the margins of the wound appear to undergo DNA synthesis and proliferation, whereas those in the monolayer at a distance from the wound appear to remain relatively quiescent. This peculiar characteristic of the growth of endothelium is so strikingly different from that of smooth-muscle cells that it has been suggested that these two different cell types are under different sets of controls of their growth and that somehow cell-cell contact appears to be important in determining the state of quiescence of endothelial cells. Endothelial cells grown in culture have been shown to be capable of forming a number of connective tissue matrix macromolecules including particular types of collagen;[44] of transporting lipids; of synthesizing prostacycline,[45] factor VIII,[46] and angiotensin-converting enzyme,[47] and in maintaining many aspects of their differentiated phenotype through several passages.

Endothelial-Derived Growth Factor

Recently, endothelial cells have been shown to be capable of forming a mitogen or growth factor in culture. This substance, termed the *endothelial-derived growth factor,* appears to be a potent molecule in terms of its capacity to stimulate cells such as fibroblasts and smooth muscle to proliferate.[48] Endothelial cells in culture release this factor into the medium after they have been exposed to plasma or to serum-free medium. Thus far, studies of this factor show that it appears to have a number of characteristics identical with those of the platelet-derived growth factor[65] (to be discussed below). It is not as yet known whether it is formed by endothelial cells in vivo. This observation could have potential importance in atherogenesis; however, the studies are too early in their development for this to be clear.

Smooth Muscle

Smooth-Muscle Proliferation

Smooth-muscle cells have long been recognized to possess a number of features important to normal arterial function, including their capacity to contract, to maintain arterial tonus, and to synthesize connective tissue proteins. Perhaps the most important phenomenon associated with the smooth-muscle cell is the process of cell proliferation in atherogenesis. Since intimal smooth-muscle proliferation is an important early feature in atherogenesis, the factors responsible for this proliferative response are under intensive investigation in vivo and in vitro. In cell culture, it is well known that serum provides all of the factors necessary for smooth-muscle proliferation. Arterial smooth-muscle cells from a large number of species can be grown in culture and are able to maintain their differentiated phenotype under these conditions.[49,50]

Ross and coworkers,[24] together with several other laboratories,[51,52] have demonstrated that the principal mitogenic component present in whole blood serum and missing in cell-free plasma-derived serum and responsible for the proliferation of arterial smooth-muscle cells in culture is a mitogen derived from the platelet, the *platelet-derived growth factor.* The observation that smooth-muscle proliferation in culture is stimulated principally by this mitogen led to a series of studies to examine the role of platelets in smooth-muscle proliferation induced in vivo.

As described above, several forms of endothelial injury result in adherence of platelets at sites of injury. Platelet adherence is followed by degranulation and release into the artery wall of material stored in the platelet granules. Together with plasma constituents, these platelet products have far-reaching effects upon the smooth-muscle cells of the artery wall.

Harker et al.[10] demonstrated that in homocystinuria, a genetic disease of childhood commonly associated with marked increased incidence of arteriosclerosis, platelets appear to interact at sites where the endothelium has somehow been injured by increased levels of plasma homocysteine. Harker et al.[10] demonstrated this association by measuring the survival of autologous ^{51}Cr-labeled platelets in homocystinuric children and observed that the greater the levels of plasma homocysteine, the greater the decrease in platelet survival. As a result of these observations, they developed an animal model of homocystinuria by chronically infusing homocysteine in baboons. In this model they showed a similar correlation between elevated levels of plasma homocysteine and decreased levels of platelet survival (or increased platelet utilization). When they maintained the baboons on a homocystinemic regimen for 3 months, they observed an increased incidence of missing endothelial cells by morphometric examination of whole-mount preparations of the aorta. Their studies established a correlation between the amounts of injured endothelium, decrease in platelet survival, and the formation of proliferative smooth-muscle atherosclerotic lesions at the sites of endothelial injury. Harker and his colleagues[10] went on to demonstrate that if they administered to the homocystinemic baboons one of two pharmacologic agents that could inhibit platelet interactions with the injured artery wall, they could prevent the intimal smooth-muscle proliferative lesions that otherwise developed. One of these agents, dipyridamole, returned platelet survival to normal levels and is known because of its capacity to inhibit platelet phosphodiesterase activity and to inhibit platelet adherence. The other agent, sulfinpyrazone, appeared to somehow protect the endothelial cells, since the sulfinpyrazone-treated homocystinemic baboons demonstrated fewer areas of endothelial injury. In both approaches, platelet survival levels were normalized, and the proliferative lesions of atherosclerosis were prevented. These were the first data to correlate a requirement for platelet function with experimentally induced atherosclerosis.

Other approaches to examining these same phenomena were taken by Moore and his colleagues[53] and by Friedman et al.[54] In both of their studies, atherosclerosis was induced in rabbits by injuring the endothelium with an intraarterial catheter. In each case, the investigators induced a thrombocytopenia by administration of a specific antiplatelet antiserum. The animals made thrombocytopenic in this manner had no proliferative atherosclerotic lesions, whereas the control animals had extensive lesions.

Using a different approach, Fuster and his colleagues[55] examined the incidence of atherosclerosis in the aortas of swine fed a high-fat, high-cholesterol diet. They were able to study the role of platelets in these swine by trying to induce atherosclerosis with a high-cholesterol diet in a group of swine that were homozygous for von Willebrand's disease, as compared with a group of normal swine. The swine with severe von Willebrand's disease contained essentially no factor VIII—von Willebrand's factor—in their plasma. Normally this factor is required for platelet adherence and release. The control animals on the high-lipid diet developed extensive proliferative lesions of atherosclerosis, whereas the von Willebrand's swine developed intimal infiltrates of lipid but no smooth-muscle proliferative lesions. In the absence of the von Willebrand's factor, platelet interactions may be somewhat inhibited in the hypercholesterolemic von Willebrand swine.

All of these studies point to the importance of platelet interactions at sites of endothelial alterations that precede the formation of experimentally induced proliferative lesions of atherosclerosis.

Lipid Metabolism

Since lipids are essential components of all cells, it is not surprising that they are involved in a number of cell functions and metabolic processes, as they represent the principal constituent of all cell membranes. Both the plasma membrane and the internal membranous compartments of all cells, including smooth muscle, are composed of phospholipids, proteins, and cholesterol, principally unesterified cholesterol. Esterified cholesterol is found in smooth muscle only under abnormal conditions. Accumulations of cholesteryl ester in smooth-muscle cells and macrophages lead to the development of foam cells found in the lesions of atherosclerosis. Some experiments have shown that smooth-muscle cells can acquire cholesterol both by de novo synthesis[56] and from an exogenous source of cholesterol-carrying lipoproteins.[57] Such a dual mechanism may help the cell to protect itself against possible deficits in cholesterol.

Smooth-muscle cells and many other cells can also protect themselves against excess cholesterol. The mechanism that has evolved for this purpose is the surface-located, high-affinity LDL receptor.[58,59] These receptors bind LDL, and the cell then internalizes the bound LDL by the process of endocytosis and transports it to lysosomes where the LDL is degraded and free cholesterol is liberated for use by the cell. If the cell is exposed to excess LDL, there is a feedback inhibitory pathway in the cell that inhibits the synthesis of LDL receptors. In addition, the presence within the cell of excess cholesterol provides a signal that inhibits cholesterol synthesis by the rate-limiting intracellular enzyme, hydroxymethylglutarylcoenzyme A reductase (HMG-CoA reductase).

Under normal circumstances, sterol balance in the cell maintains a given receptor level for LDL at the cell surface. In this way the requirements for extracellular cholesterol are met by concentrations of plasma LDL that are not atherogenic. Increased concentrations of plasma LDL may alter the endothelial barrier and bring large amounts of LDL in direct contact with the smooth-muscle cell, which may ingest much of the LDL by bulk-phase endocytosis, bypassing the high-affinity receptor mechanism, and leading to increased esterification and storage of cholesteryl esters and the development of foam cells.

LDL has been said to play a mitogenic role for smooth-muscle cells in culture. Wissler and his colleagues[32] have observed that LDL derived from hyperlipemic monkeys was mitogenic in explant cultures of aorta as compared to LDL from normolipemic monkeys. The means by which this LDL acts as a mitogen is not clear; however, there do appear to be differences between LDL from normolipemic versus hyperlipemic donors in terms of their effects on smooth muscle and endothelium. The elucidation of the effects of hyperlipemic LDL may be important in understanding the basis of the atherogenic effect of hyperlipidemia.

Evidence is accumulating in favor of the notion that HDL, in contrast to LDL, is a negative factor in the development of atherosclerosis. Two mechanisms have been proposed to explain how HDL might be a deterrent against atherosclerosis. The first suggests that HDL augments the removal of cholesterol from cells such as smooth muscle. The second mechanism involves the apparent ability of HDL to influence the binding and absorption of LDL by cells such as smooth muscle. However, neither of these mechanisms has been shown to be responsible for control of cellular cholesterol. Further information concerning the nature of the lipoproteins and their effects on cells and potential roles in atherogenesis is discussed in Chap. 42.

The Macrophage

Macrophages are commonly found in early lesions of atherosclerosis as well as in advanced lesions like the fibrous plaque. In their studies of hypercholesterolemia in nonhuman primates, Faggiotto et al.[13,14] found that monocyte-derived macrophages were a major component of the fatty streaks in these animals and were found in abundance in fibrous plaques as well. A new observation made in those studies was the exposure of subendothelial lipid-laden macrophages (foam cells) that sometimes became the foci for platelet adherence and formation of mural thrombi. Such cellular interactions were often found at anatomic sites (branches and bifurcations) that 1 to 2 months later were sites of advanced proliferative smooth-muscle lesions. The expansion of the macrophage-rich fatty streaks appeared to possibly predispose to rupture of endothelial junctions of overlying, thinly stretched endothelium. This established the conditions for macrophage exposure and for macrophage-platelet interactions. Macrophages could conceivably play several roles in lesion progression and possibly in regression as well. In tissue culture, macrophages have been shown to release a mitogen as potent as that derived from platelets into the culture medium.[60] Such a growth factor, if formed in vivo, could conceivably be important in lesion progression.

Macrophages have long been known to be largely responsible for tissue debridement. There is increasing evidence in experimental studies and in human beings[23] that some lesions of atherosclerosis are capable of regression. The potential role of the macrophage in this phenomenon remains to be elucidated.

Platelets

The Platelet-Derived Growth Factor

The platelet-derived growth factor is a mitogen that is stored in the alpha granule of the platelets and that has been purified to homogeneity. It has a molecular weight of approximately 32,000 and is a highly cationic (pI 9.8), stable, disulfide-bonded protein. This growth factor is extremely potent, as it will cause proliferation of all susceptible cells in culture at a level of 5 ng/ml of culture medium (equivalent to addition of 5% whole blood serum). As discussed earlier in this chapter, platelet-derived growth factor is the principal mitogen in whole blood serum to which cells characteristically respond by cell proliferation. Exposure of susceptible cells to this factor results in a sequence of events that includes binding of the molecule to the surface of the cells. This then causes the cell to undergo cell cycle traverse leading to DNA synthesis and cell multiplication.

The platelet-derived growth factor stimulates a

number of phenomena upon exposure to smooth-muscle cells in addition to DNA synthesis. It causes increases in pinocytosis, protein synthesis, RNA synthesis, and lipid metabolism. Chait et al.[57] have observed that exposure of arterial smooth-muscle cells to this growth factor results in increased binding of LDL to the cells due to the formation of an increased number of high-affinity receptors for LDL at the cell surface. This increased binding of LDL permits the cells to utilize exogenous sources of cholesterol for cell multiplication more effectively. Habenicht et al.[56] have demonstrated that this mitogen also stimulates increased cholesterol synthesis by cells if an exogenous source of cholesterol is not available to them. Davies and Ross[61] observed that smooth-muscle cells exposed to the platelet-derived growth factor undergo a marked increase in the rate of endocytosis of tracer molecules. In other words, exposure to this mitogen results in an increase in a number of cellular activities, many of which are associated with cell proliferation and with new protein synthesis, and therefore with connective tissue formation.[62] Thus, exposure to this factor could potentially provide the trigger that results in the initiation of all of the components of a proliferative lesion. This factor is clearly operative in cell culture, and now there are data in experimentally induced lesions of atherosclerosis that indicate that proliferative lesions can be prevented or reduced by administering appropriate levels of an antibody, anti-platelet-derived growth factor IgG, in vivo. These are the first definitive data for the role of this mitogen in vivo, and thus in atherosclerosis. The role of functional platelets in inducing experimental atherosclerosis in vivo is unquestioned. The role of the platelet-derived growth factor in stimulating mitogenesis in cell culture is clear in vivo and is rapidly becoming clarified.

Prostaglandins

A great deal has been learned during the past 10 years about a new category of substances, the prostaglandins, that may play critical roles in the metabolism of platelets, endothelium, and smooth muscle. All three cell types are capable of converting the fatty acid, arachidonic acid, into prostaglandin endoperoxides. Studies of these endoperoxides identified a number of unstable intermediates in the metabolic pathway of arachidonic acid that lead to the formation of two important end products: thromboxane A_2 (formed by platelets) and prostacycline (formed by endothelium and smooth muscle). Understanding these two end products has greatly expanded our view of the role potentially played by platelets in thrombosis and by endothelium and smooth muscle in prevention of thrombosis and potentially atherosclerosis.

Arachidonic acid is derived either from linoleic acid, an essential fatty acid in the membranes of cells, or from arachidonic acid in the diet. Thromboxane A_2 is a powerful vasoconstrictor and, therefore, is capable of stimulating smooth-muscle contraction and platelet aggregation. It has a short half-life (30 s) and breaks down spontaneously into a stable substance, thromboxane B_2. A number of inhibitors of thromboxane synthesis markedly reduce platelet aggregation. These include aspirin and indomethacin.[63,64]

Prostacycline (PGI_2) is the principal product of cycloxygenase activity in the walls of arteries and veins. Endothelium and smooth muscle synthesize PGI_2 from arachidonic acid and may also be able to synthesize this prostaglandin derivative from endoperoxides released from platelets. PGI_2 is also unstable and is an extremely potent vasodilator, as well as an inhibitor of platelet aggregation.

It is possible that an imbalance in the relative amounts of thromboxane A_2 versus PGI_2 may provide part of the explanation of the involvement of platelets in cardiovascular diseases. Since platelets contain thromboxane synthetase, the enzyme responsible for synthesis of thromboxane A_2, and since inhibition of the activity of this enzyme does not interfere with cycloxygenase activity, it has been speculated that platelets could potentially donate endoperoxides to endothelial cells which can then use them as substrates for PGI_2 production. Therefore, attempts are being made to develop specific inhibitors of thromboxane synthesis that would not affect PGI_2 production by cells of the blood vessel wall.

Prostaglandin biosynthesis may be important not only in thrombosis (in terms of platelet adherence and aggregation) but also in prevention of atherogenesis (by formation of PGI_2). This has led to speculation that alterations in the contents of fatty acids in the diet might offer some protection against the development of atherosclerosis. Populations that consume diets principally composed of marine animals often replace arachidonic acid, the normal substrate for prostaglandin synthesis, with eicosapentaenoic acid. This fatty acid is not completely metabolized by platelets and, instead, produces a relatively inert form of thromboxane, thromboxane A_3. Eicosapentaenoic acid appears to inhibit the capacity of platelets to metabolize arachidonic acid. When eicosapentaenoic acid is exposed to cells of the blood vessel, they will form an analogue of prostacycline, PGI_3. PGI_3 appears to be as effective as PGI_2 in preventing platelet aggregation and in inducing vasodilatation. Thus, further studies of the role of this fatty acid derived from marine animals could have implications for individuals who consume a marine diet in terms of being protected against atherogenesis. Clearly, there is much to be learned in prostaglandin metabolism before the agents that have thus far been discovered, and those that are yet undiscovered, can be understood, both in atherogenesis and in protection against this disease process.

The Role of Research at the Cellular Level in Diagnosis, Treatment, and Prevention

The field of atherosclerosis research has changed dramatically within the last decade. The emphasis in our understanding the pathogenesis of this disease process has shifted to probing the fundamental roles of the cells of the artery wall as well as those in the blood, particularly the platelet. The development of cell biology, experimental pathology, and immunology has provided tools that should lead to new approaches to diagnosis, intervention, and prevention.

If, for example, it can be demonstrated unequivocally that the platelet-derived growth factor plays a role in the initiation of the lesions of atherosclerosis and/or in their progression, and if it can be demonstrated that there are higher levels of this factor in the circulation in individuals who are actively forming lesions or who are at increased risk, then the development of a radioimmunoassay to detect the presence of this factor in the plasma would be significant in that it could be used in the diagnosis of patients who are at increased risk. Similarly, the efficacy of different pharmacologic agents or other modes of intervention could be determined with the use of such a radioimmunoassay. Other approaches to understanding the role of platelets in atherogenesis involve the use of radiolabeled platelets or the development of means to maintain endothelial integrity. As a consequence, future research at the cellular and molecular levels could provide important diagnostic tools that may be of use clinically.

The process of atherogenesis is a highly complex one, involving many cellular interactions as well as interactions between cells and constituents in the fluid phase of the blood, the plasma. The importance of these interactions will undoubtedly be modified by the genetic makeup of each individual. Consequently, the differences in susceptibility from individual to individual to each of the risk factors and at the cellular level to the different various components considered to be important in atherogenesis, will have to be understood if we are to make further progress, not only in diagnosis and treatment, but ultimately in prevention.

References

1. Ross, R., and Glomset, J. A.: The Pathogenesis of Atherosclerosis, *N. Engl. J. Med.*, 295:369, 420, 1976.
2. McGill, H. C., Jr.: Atherosclerosis: Problems in Pathogenesis, *Atherosclerosis Rev.*, 2:27, 1977.
3. Bierman, E. L., and Ross, R.: Aging and Atherosclerosis, *Atherosclerosis Rev.*, 2:79, 1977.
4. Geer, J. C., and Haust, M. D.: "Monographs on Atherosclerosis," S. Karger, Basel, Switzerland, 1972, vol. 2, p. 1.
5. "Arteriosclerosis: A Report by the National Heart and Lung Institute Task Force on Arteriosclerosis," DHEW Publication (NIH) 72-219, vol. 2, 1971.
6. Debakey, M. E.: "Atherosclerosis Reviews," Raven Press, New York, 1976, vol. 3, p. 1.
7. Stemerman, M. B., and Ross, R.: Experimental Atherosclerosis. I. Fibrous Plaque Formation in Primates, an Electron Microscope Study, *J. Exp. Med.*, 136:769, 1972.
8. Bjorkerud, S., and Bondjers, G.: Arterial Repair and Atherosclerosis after Mechanical Injury: I. Permeability and Light Microscopic Characteristics of Endothelium in Non-atherosclerotic and Atherosclerotic Lesions, *Atherosclerosis*, 13:355, 1971.
9. Ross, R., and Harker, L.: Hyperlipidemia and Atherosclerosis, *Science*, 193:1094, 1976.
10. Harker, L., Ross, R., Slichter, S., and Scott, C.: Homocystine-Induced Arteriosclerosis: The Role of Endothelial Cell Injury and Platelet Response in Its Genesis, *J. Clin. Invest.*, 58:731, 1976.
11. Minick, C. R., and Murphy, G. E.: Experimental Induction of Atheroarteriosclerosis by the Synergy of Allergic Injury to Arteries and Lipid-Rich Diet: II. Effect of Repeatedly Injected Foreign Protein in Rabbits Fed a Lipid-Rich, Cholesterol-Poor Diet, *Am. J. Pathol.*, 73:265, 1973.
12. Fabricant, C. G., Fabricant, J., Litrenta, M. M., and Minick, C. R.: Virus-Induced Atherosclerosis, *J. Exp. Med.*, 148:335, 1978.
13. Faggiotto, A., Ross, R., and Harker, L.: Studies of Hypercholesterolemia in the Nonhuman Primate: I. Changes That Lead to Fatty Streak Formation, *Arteriosclerosis*, 4:323, 1984.
14. Faggiotto, A., and Ross, R.: Studies of Hypercholesterolemia in the Nonhuman Primate: II. Fatty Streak Conversion to Fibrous Plaque, *Arteriosclerosis*, 4:341, 1984.
15. Long, E. R.: "Arteriosclerosis. A Survey of the Problem," The Macmillan Company, New York, 1933, p. 19.
16. Virchow, R.: "Gesammelte Adhandlungen zur Wissenschaftlichen Medicin," Meidinger Sohn and Company, Frankfurt-am-Main, 1856, p. 458.
17. Anitschkow, H. H.: "Cowdry's Arteriosclerosis," 2d ed., The Macmillan Company, New York, 1967, p. 21.
18. Duguid, J. B.: Thrombosis as a Factor in the Pathogenesis of Coronary Atherosclerosis, *J. Pathol. Bacteriol.*, 58:207, 1948.
19. French, J. E.: Atherosclerosis in Relation to the Structure and Function of the Arterial Intima, with Special Reference to the Endothelium, *Int. Rev. Exp. Pathol.*, 5:253, 1966.
20. Ross, R., and Glomset, J.: Atherosclerosis and the Arterial Smooth Muscle Cell, *Science*, 180:1332, 1973.
21. Fry, D. L.: "Cerebrovascular Diseases," Raven Press, New York, 1976, p. 77.
22. Moncada, S., Higgs, H. A., and Vane, J. R.: Human Arterial and Venous Tissue Generate Prostacycline, a Potent Inhibitor of Platelet Aggregation, *Lancet*, 2:18, 1977.
23. Wissler, R. W., and Vesselinovitch, D.: Studies of Regression of Advanced Atherosclerosis in Experimental Animals and Man, *Ann. N.Y. Acad. Sci.*, 275:363, 1976.
24. Ross, R., Glomset, J., Kariya, B., and Harker, L.: A Platelet-Dependent Serum Factor That Stimulates the Proliferation of Arterial Smooth Muscle Cells in Vitro, *Proc. Natl. Acad. Sci. U.S.A.*, 71:1207, 1974.
25. Benditt, E. P., and Benditt, J. M.: Evidence for a Monoclonal Origin of Human Atherosclerotic Plaques, *Proc. Natl. Acad. Sci. U.S.A.*, 70:1753, 1973.
26. Lindner, D., and Gartler, S. M.: Glucose-6-Phosphate Dehydrogenase Mosaicism: Utilization as a Cell Marker in the Study of Leiomyomas, *Science*, 150:67, 1965.
27. Fialkow, P.: The Origin and Development of Human Tumors Studied with Cell Markers, *N. Engl. J. Med.*, 291:26, 1974.
28. Pearson, T. A., Wang, A., Solez, K., and Heptinstall, R. H.: Clonal Characteristics of Fibrous Plaques and Fatty Streaks from Human Aortas, *Am. J. Pathol.*, 81:379, 1975.
29. Thomas, W. A., Reiner, J. M., Janakidevi, K., and Lee, K. T.: Population Dynamics of Arterial Cells during Atherogenesis: X. Study of Monotypism in Atherosclerotic Lesions

of Black Women Heterozygous for Glucose-6-Phosphate Dehydrogenase, *Exp. Mol. Pathol.*, 31:327, 1979.
30. Benditt, E. P.: "Atherosclerosis Reviews," Raven Press, New York, 1978, vol. 3, p. 77.
31. Geer, J. C., McGill, H. C., Jr., and Strong, J. P.: The Fine Structure of Human Atherosclerotic Lesions, *Am. J. Pathol.*, 38:263, 1961.
32. Wissler, R. W.: "Biochemistry of Atherosclerosis," Marcel Dekker, New York, 1979, vol. 7, p. 345.
33. McGill, H.: Risk Factors for Atherosclerosis, *Adv. Exp. Med. Biol.*, 104:273, 1977.
34. The Lipid Research Clinics Program: The Lipid Research Clinics Coronary Primary Prevention Trial Results: I. Reduction in Incidence of Coronary Heart Disease, *JAMA*, 251:351, 1984.
35. The Lipid Research Clinics Program: The Lipid Research Clinics Coronary Primary Prevention Trial Results: II. The Relationship of Reduction in Incidence of Coronary Heart Disease to Cholesterol Lowering, *JAMA*, 251:365, 1984.
36. Grundy, S. M.: "Nutrition, Lipids, and Coronary Heart Disease," Raven Press, New York, 1979, p. 89.
37. McGill, H. C., Jr.: The Relationship of Dietary Cholesterol to Serum Cholesterol Concentration and to Atherosclerosis in Man, *Am. J. Clin. Nutr.*, 32(suppl.):2664, 1979.
38. Becker, C. G., Dubin, T., and Widemann, H. P.: Hypersensitivity to Tobacco Antigen, *Proc. Natl. Acad. Sci. U.S.A.*, 73:1712, 1976.
39. Simionescu, N., Simionescu, M., and Palade, G. E.: Permeability of Muscle Capillaries to Small Heme-Peptides. Evidence for the Existence of Patent Transcendothelial Channels, *J. Cell Biol.*, 64:586, 1975.
40. Renkin, E. M.: Multiple Pathways of Capillary Permeability, *Circ. Res.*, 41:735, 1977.
41. Stein, Y., and Stein, O.: "Biochemistry of Atherosclerosis," Marcel Dekker, New York, 1979, vol. 7, p. 313.
42. Gimbrone, M. A., Jr.: "Progress in Hemostasis and Thrombosis," Grune & Stratton, Inc., New York, 1976, vol. 3, p. 1.
43. Jaffe, E. A., Nachman, R. L., Becker, C. G., and Minick, C. R.: Culture of Human Endothelial Cells Derived from Umbilical Veins, *J. Clin. Invest.*, 52:2745, 1973.
44. Jaffe, E. A., Adelman, B., and Minick, C. R.: Synthesis of Basement Membrane by Cultured Human Endothelial Cells, *Circulation*, 51(suppl. 2):11, 1975.
45. Moncada, S., Higgs, E. A., and Vane, J. R.: Human Arterial and Venous Tissue Generate Prostacyclin, a Potent Inhibitor of Platelet Aggregation, *Lancet*, 2:18, 1977.
46. Jaffe, E. A., Hoyer, L. W., and Nachman, R. L.: Synthesis of Antihemophilic Factor Antigen by Cultured Human Endothelial Cells, *J. Clin. Invest.*, 52:2757, 1973.
47. Gimbrone, M. A., Jr., and Alexander, R. W.: Angiotensin II Stimulation of Prostaglandin Production in Cultured Human Vascular Endothelium, *Science*, 189:219, 1975. (Abstract.)
48. Gajdusek, C., DiCorleto, P., Ross, R., and Schwartz, S.: An Endothelial Cell Derived Growth Factor, *J. Cell Biol.*, 85:467, 1980.
49. Ross, R., and Kariya, B.: Morphogenesis of Vascular Smooth Muscle in Atherosclerosis and Cell Culture, in D. F. Bohr, A. P. Somlyo, and H. V. Sparks (eds.), "Handbook of Physiology—Circulation, Vascular Smooth Muscle," American Physiological Society, Bethesda, Maryland, 1980, vol. 2, sec. 3, p. 69.
50. Chamley-Campbell, J., Campbell, G. R., and Ross, R.: The Smooth Muscle Cell in Culture, *Physiol. Rev.*, 59:1, 1979.
51. Kohler, N., and Lipton, A.: Platelets as a Source of Fibroblast Growth-Promoting Activity, *Exp. Cell Res.*, 87:297, 1974.
52. Heldin, C.-H., Wasteson, A., and Westermark, B.: Partial Purification and Characterization of Platelet Factors Stimulating the Multiplication of Normal Human Glial Cells, *Exp. Cell Res.*, 109:429, 1977.
53. Moore, A., Friedman, R. J., Singal, D. P., Gauldie, J., and Blajchman, M.: Inhibition of Injury Induced Thromboatherosclerotic Lesions by Antiplatelet Serum in Rabbits, *Thromb. Diath. Haemorr.*, 35:70, 1976.
54. Friedman, R. J., Stemerman, M. B., Wenz, B., Moore, S., Gauldie, J., Gent, M., Tiell, M. L., and Spaet, T. H.: The Effect of Thrombocytopenia on Experimental Atherosclerotic Lesion Formation in Rabbits. Smooth Muscle Cell Proliferation and Reendothelialization, *J. Clin. Invest.*, 60:1191, 1977.
55. Fuster, V., Bowie, E. J. W., Lewis, J. C., Fass, D. N., Owen, C. A., Jr., and Brown, A. L.: Resistance to Arteriosclerosis in Pigs with von Willebrand's Disease. Spontaneous and High Cholesterol Diet-Induced Arteriosclerosis, *J. Clin. Invest.*, 61:722, 1978.
56. Habenicht, A., Glomset, J., and Ross, R.: Relation of Cholesterol and Mevalonic Acid to the Cell Cycle in Smooth Muscle and Swiss 3T3 Cells Stimulated to Divide by Platelet-Derived Growth Factor, *J. Biol. Chem.*, 255:5134, 1980.
57. Chait, A., Ross, R., Albers, J., and Bierman, E.: Platelet Derived Growth Factor Stimulates Low Density Lipoprotein Receptor Activity, *Proc. Natl. Acad. Sci. U.S.A.*, 77:4084, 1980.
58. Brown, M. S., Faust, J. R., and Goldstein, J. L.: Role of the Low Density Lipoprotein Receptor in Regulating the Content of Free and Esterified Cholesterol in Human Fibroblasts, *J. Clin. Invest.*, 55:783, 1975.
59. Goldstein, J. L., and Brown, M. S.: The Low-Density Lipoprotein Pathway and Its Relation to Atherosclerosis, *Ann. Rev. Biochem.*, 46:879, 1977.
60. Leibovich, S. J., and Ross, R.: A Macrophage-Dependent Factor That Stimulates the Proliferation of Fibroblasts in Vitro, *Am. J. Pathol.*, 84:501, 1976.
61. Davies, P. F., and Ross, R.: Mediation of Pinocytosis in Cultured Arterial Smooth Muscle and Endothelial Cells by Platelet-Derived Growth Factor, *J. Cell Biol.*, 79:663, 1978.
62. Burke, J., and Ross, R.: "International Review of Connective Tissue Research," Academic Press, Inc., New York, 1979, vol. 8, p. 119.
63. Moncada, A., and Vane, J. R.: Arachidonic Acid Metabolites and the Interactions between Platelets and Blood-Vessel Walls, *N. Engl. J. Med.*, 300:1142, 1979.
64. Moncada, S., and Vane, J. R.: Mode of Action of Aspirin-like Drugs, *Adv. Intern. Med.*, 24:1, 1979.
65. Dicorleto, P. E., and Bowen-Pope, D. F.: Cultured Endothelial Cells Produce a Platelet-Derived Growth Factor-like Protein, *Proc. Natl. Acad. Sci. U.S.A.*, 80:1919, 1983.

42

Prevention of Coronary Atherosclerosis

Nanette Kass Wenger, M.D.   Robert C. Schlant, M.D.

In earlier times, starvation consigned languishing bodies to death; now, on the other hand, prosperity plunges them into the grave.

Lucretius, ca. 50 B.C.[1]

Although atherosclerotic coronary heart disease is among the most serious and costly health problems in industrialized nations, there is substantial evidence from basic and clinical research that atherosclerosis can be prevented and that progression of atherosclerosis can be retarded. This chapter summarizes the delineation of coronary risk factors, reviews the results of risk modification, and provides recommendations for risk modification in apparently healthy individuals and populations (primary prevention) as well as in persons known to have atherosclerotic coronary heart disease (secondary prevention).

Intervention in Populations

The World Health Organization recommends a population or community approach to altering the life-style and environmental characteristics that appear to be underlying causes of coronary heart disease.[2] Coronary heart disease remains the leading cause of death in the United States; because coronary disease often is associated with life-styles and habits of the population, the Intersociety Commission for Heart Disease Resources[3] and the American Heart Association[4] recommend that the general population (1) eliminate cigarette smoking, (2) control hypertension by diet and/or medication, (3) reduce serum cholesterol levels by reducing dietary saturated fat and cholesterol, (4) adjust calories to achieve ideal body weight, (5) exercise moderately, and (6) control diabetes mellitus.

Intervention in High-Risk Individuals

The recommendations of the World Health Organization[2] are based on identification and assessment of an individual's coronary risk from data available at a routine medical examination: age, sex, weight, family history, plasma cholesterol level, blood pressure, cigarette smoking history, oral contraceptive use, hyperglycemia, habitual physical activity, and electrocardiographic abnormalities. Although multiple factors are more predictive of risk in younger persons, the risk profile of elderly individuals is also predictive of coronary events.[5] The *Coronary Risk Handbook*,[6] based on Framingham Study data,[7] aids in multivariate risk assessment and is reasonably accurate in predicting cardiovascular prevalence and events in other populations in the United States.[8,9] In the Coronary Artery Surgery Study (CASS), the coronary risk factors correlated highly with angiographic evidence of coronary atherosclerosis in the total group of patients, although the association was much weaker for *individual* patients.[10] In selected patients identified as being at increased risk, exercise testing, with or without thallium scintigraphy, can further identify patients with evidence of myocardial ischemia (see Chaps. 98 and 109).

Although the concept of coronary risk factors is now widely accepted and risk reduction seems reasonable and desirable, there are no *absolute* data to support or refute the assumption that risk modification can avert or delay coronary atherosclerosis or its clinical manifestations in an *individual.*

The Basis for Prevention by Coronary Risk Reduction

Natural History of Atherosclerotic Coronary Heart Disease

Current theories of atherogenesis indicate a period of several decades of development in human beings (see Chap. 41) prior to the appearance of clinical manifestations. Since advanced atherosclerosis may be present before symptoms appear and many patients die within the first hours of myocardial infarction, atherosclerosis must be prevented if survival is to be improved.

The substantial decline (25 percent) in coronary heart disease mortality in both middle-aged and elderly patients in the United States between 1968 and 1976, with a comparable concomitant reduction in coronary mortality in some other countries,[11] is due, at least in part, to primary and secondary preventive efforts for coronary heart disease.[11a] Because this favorable trend has occurred in the United States while coronary mortality continued to increase in some other countries,[11] it has been suggested that the public-health approach to coronary risk factor control, with resultant favorable changes in life-style, is a major factor in reducing cardiovascular mortality in the United States.[11–15,15b] Much of the U.S. population has marginal abnormalities of multiple risk factors. It is not possible to attribute the dramatic reduction in cardiovascular mortality to modification of a single factor, despite the favorable dietary alterations and concomitant decline in plasma cholesterol levels in the population, the major advances in hypertension detection and control,[12] the decline in cigarette smoking (most prominent among middle-aged men), and the alterations in life-style, particularly the adoption of leisure-time physical activity. Whereas it is likely that coronary risk modification has had a major impact, other possible contributions to the decline in coronary mortality include widespread citizen training in cardiopulmonary resuscitation, the application of advanced life-support techniques by emergency personnel, advances in the medical treatment of angina, arrhythmias, and heart failure, the introduction of coronary care units, availability of cardiac pacemakers, and increasing application of coronary artery bypass surgery. The contribution of each remains uncertain.[11,13] Thus, it is reasonable that multifactorial considerations be addressed in prevention, with an emphasis on multifaceted risk intervention as early in life as feasible for primary prevention and a clinically appropriate comprehensive modification of coronary risk once manifestations of coronary disease are identified.

It is not known whether a reduction in the incidence of coronary events, an improvement in survival following a coronary event, or a combination of these changes best explains the decline in coronary mortality in the United States.

Pediatric Beginnings of Atherosclerosis

Despite the onset of clinical manifestations of coronary atherosclerosis in middle age or older, atherosclerosis begins in childhood. Some risk-prone behaviors are also acquired at a young age,[16,17] and some are easier to prevent than to alter. Diet and other risk-related behaviors are more a family than an individual characteristic and are often best addressed in a family context.[16] Studies suggest that it is possible to identify high-risk individuals in childhood.[18]

Primary and Secondary Prevention: Concepts and Problems in Validation

Primary prevention involves modification of atherogenic risk factors prior to clinical evidence of atherosclerotic coronary heart disease. Secondary prevention includes measures instituted to prevent recurrences or delay progression in patients with clinically manifest coronary heart disease.

It is difficult to validate the efficacy of either primary or secondary prevention. Most primary prevention trials, to be reasonably cost-effective, have involved sizable numbers of well persons who had an increased likelihood of sustaining an early coronary event; however, whether or not the data derived from studies of this high-risk population are applicable to the population at large is controversial. Positive results from intervention involving one risk factor would provide the strongest scientific basis for recommending its control; however, because of the complex etiology of atherosclerosis, it may be that single-factor risk alteration is inadequate. On the other hand, the challenge of altering multiple risk factors in a free-living apparently healthy population, with limited motivation for life-style alterations, limits the likelihood of compliance to such alterations. Furthermore, other changes in the population over the time of the study become confounding variables. For example, in the Multiple Risk Factor Intervention Trial (MRFIT), a study designed to assess the effect on mortality of intensive, multiple risk modifications in high-risk persons, a sizable but unexpected risk reduction in the control population occurred during the conduct of the study.[19] This reduction in risk factors was associated with a mortality in the control group substantially lower than anticipated, as a consequence of which no significant difference in total mortality was detected between the groups receiving usual care and those receiving special care.

The results of secondary prevention trials[20] are also confounded by a number of factors that are unrelated to alteration of the atherosclerotic process, but that may reduce mortality and decrease recurrent myocardial infarction. For example, drugs that improve cardiac rhythm, myocardial ischemia, ventricular function, vascular tone, or platelet function may improve longevity and limit morbidity following myocardial infarction independent of any basic effects on atherosclerosis. On the other hand, in patients with extensive atherosclerosis, limitation of the progression (or even modest regression) of atherosclerosis by substantial risk modification may not be able to produce significant differences in survival.

A World Health Organization collaborative study of rehabilitation and secondary prevention after acute myocardial infarction was unable to demonstrate a definite reduction in morbidity or mortality, or improvement in the quality of life, among patients assigned randomly to 3 years of multidisciplinary interventions, despite the trend in many centers that favored the patients enrolled in comprehensive care programs.[21] The enormous challenges of this type of study are evident by problems due to poor adherence, lack of standardization of intervention methods and assessments, imprecise delineation of baseline prognostic variables and thus unknown comparability of patients in the intervention and control populations, limited information about the control population and incomplete reporting about patients who dropped out of the study, and the impact of socioeconomic conditions, dietary habits, medical care systems, and health-related legislation in different countries. The Belgian group, however, showed a definite decrease in coronary incidence, although the reduction in coronary mortality was not significant.[22]

The difficulties of documenting benefit are apparent; however, most approaches to risk modification are simple, inexpensive, and carry little risk. Enthusiasm for this approach to secondary prevention for the estimated 7 million survivors of myocardial infarction in the United States is reinforced by experimental data suggesting that regression of atherosclerotic lesions can be induced by modification of coronary risks (see below).

Evidence for Atherosclerotic Risk Factors

Population versus Individual Data[7]

Prospective epidemiologic data[23–28] and studies in experimental animals have repeatedly established an association between specific factors and the development of coronary atherosclerosis. Despite this reproducible independent association, causation cannot be implied; prospective randomized intervention trials in human beings were and ultimately are necessary.[19,29–31] Further, the risk associated with a single factor varies with the presence or absence of other risk factors. For several risk factors, however, current data appear to be adequate to warrant recommendations both for individual patients and for the population as a whole.[2,4] Because of the multifactorial nature of atherosclerosis and the varying importance of these factors in an individual patient, however, physicians must use judgment in applying epidemiologic and investigative data to the care of an individual patient.

Alterable and Unalterable Risk Factors

Unalterable factors in atherogenesis include age, sex, and a family history of premature atherosclerosis.[32] A family history of angina pectoris, myocardial infarction, or cardiac death is statistically significant only if it occurred prior to 55 to 60 years of age, and it appears most predictive in young men.[33] The risk associated with family history may be important in individuals otherwise at low risk.[33a] In a small subset of the population with familial hypercholesterolemia, the clinical manifestations may be modified and the rate of progression of atherosclerosis retarded, although this trait cannot be presently altered. Because of the excessive risk of premature atherosclerosis in persons with familial hypercholesterolemia (type II hyperlipoproteinemia) or with type III hyperlipoproteinemia, intensive specific dietary management, often with concomitant drug therapy, is warranted.

The three major alterable coronary risk factors are an elevated plasma cholesterol level, hypertension, and cigarette smoking.

Evidence That Atherosclerosis Can Be Delayed or Reversed

Regression of Atherosclerosis in Experimental Animals[34–41]

A diet high in saturated fat and cholesterol has been shown to induce atherosclerosis in nonhuman primates, swine, and other animals;[36,37] hypertension has been shown to accelerate this atherogenesis. Reduction of dietary saturated fat and cholesterol produces regression of the atherosclerosis.[34,36,38–41] Achieving plasma cholesterol levels below 150 to 160 mg/dl through dietary changes and/or lipid-lowering drug therapy seems necessary for atherosclerosis to regress.[35,36,38–42] Extrapolation to human atherosclerosis suggests that regression of atherosclerosis is likely with dietary or drug therapy that reduces plasma cholesterol to about 150 mg/dl, with retardation of atherosclerosis likely at cholesterol levels of 150 to 180 mg/dl.

Regression of atherosclerosis in animal models has also been achieved with exercise, drug therapy, and ileal bypass surgery. Exercise substantially reduced overall coronary atherosclerosis in monkeys fed an atherogenic diet,[37] and calcium-antagonist drugs had comparable effects in rabbits.[43]

Regression of Atherosclerosis in Human Beings

The evidence for regression of human atherosclerosis[35,44] in response to risk reduction is fragmentary.[45–49] Human atherosclerosis is acquired more gradually than that induced in animal models; thus the rapidity of regression may not be comparable. In a few individuals with type III hyperlipoproteinemia, increased leg blood flow was documented after dietary and drug control of lipid abnormalities.[49] In some patients with types II and IV hyperlipoproteinemia, femoral angiographic evidence of regression was apparent after 1 year of therapy; this was more likely to occur in individuals with significant improvement in blood lipids and control of hypertension.[45,48,49]

Preliminary data suggest that regression of coronary atherosclerosis may occur in some patients treated by partial ileal bypass surgery, an investigative procedure that lowers plasma cholesterol level by about 40 percent.[50,50a] Plasma exchange[51,52] and portacaval shunts[53] have also been used to treat extreme hyperlipidemia in small numbers of patients, but the results to date are inconclusive. One patient with familial hypercholesterolemia has been treated with combined heart and liver transplantation.[54]

Community Approach to Coronary Prevention

Community adoption of a healthy life-style appears feasible.[2,55–58] The World Health Organization recommendations[2] are for communitywide progressive alteration of the habitual diet in order to lower plasma cholesterol levels in countries with a high incidence of coronary disease.

Community efforts to decrease sodium intake, to control or prevent obesity, to encourage regular exercise as part of daily life-style, and to decrease alcohol consumption may also lessen the problem of hypertension. Nonsmoking should be encouraged as normal behavior. Preventive efforts should be extended to young people, as many habits that increase risk characteristics are acquired early in life.

The strategies for achieving risk reduction include professional education, community leader education, public education, mass media education, community organization, and environmental change.[2,59] Developing countries should prevent the increase of coronary risk factors that appear to be occurring together with the clinical manifestations of coronary atherosclerosis.[11]

The Role of Unalterable Coronary Risk Factors

Although age, sex, and hereditary characteristics are unalterable, they indicate potential high-risk individuals for whom early risk assessment and appropriate intervention may be warranted. These include, for example, the middle-aged man with a strong family history of premature atherosclerosis (below age 55 to 60) and a history of cigarette smoking.

Primary Prevention: Modifiable Risk Factors

Diet; Plasma Cholesterol, Lipoproteins, and Triglycerides; and Coronary Heart Disease

Many studies throughout the world have provided convincing evidence of the relation of plasma cholesterol to the development of atherosclerotic coronary heart disease and to coronary mortality.[15] Coronary risk is a continuum; i.e., the higher the plasma cholesterol, the greater the coronary risk.[28,60] Plasma cholesterol is also a powerful independent risk predictor for individuals; persons whose plasma cholesterol levels are below 175 mg/dl have less than half the risk of infarction of those with levels of 250 to 275 mg/dl. However, the predictive value of this factor diminishes with increasing age. The predictive value of plasma cholesterol is increased when other coronary risk factors are present. Several studies have also shown a relation between lipoprotein levels and the presence and extent of coronary artery disease determined angiographically.[61–63]

When populations with minimal coronary disease and low plasma cholesterol levels, such as native Japanese with an ethnic diet, move to Hawaii and then to the U.S. mainland, the progressive change in diet is associated with a progressive increase in plasma cholesterol concentration and in coronary disease.[64]

Individuals with high cholesterol levels who have a genetic deficiency of receptors for low-density lipoprotein (LDL) (see Chaps. 35 and 41) are a special subset at extreme risk for atherosclerosis. By definition, most persons in the United States have plasma cholesterol levels within the "normal" range, although there is a twofold difference in cardiovascular morbidity between the high and low ends of this so-called normal range. A desirable level for plasma cholesterol is less than 180 to 200 mg/dl. Levels of 200 to 260 mg/dl are considered nonoptimal; those greater than 260 mg/dl, dangerously elevated.[2,4] The current age-adjusted mean cholesterol level of middle-aged men in the United States is 211 mg/dl, as compared with 213 mg/dl in the mid-1970s and 217 to 235 mg/dl in the 1950s and 1960s; comparable changes are described in women.[65] The plasma cholesterol levels of most individuals who are in the nonoptimal range can be lowered by dietary modification. Dietary recommendations should emphasize a decrease in both saturated fat and cholesterol.

Although the influence of habitual diet on plasma cholesterol has long been debated, some relations are well established.[66] There is a definite correlation between the habitual dietary intake of saturated fat and cholesterol in a given population and both the mean plasma cholesterol concentration of that population[67] and their coronary morbidity and mortality.[68] Weight reduction decreases plasma cholesterol and triglyceride levels, at least in part because of decreased dietary fat intake. There is an associated decrease in coronary events when the mean plasma cholesterol concentration of a population decreases. Although changes in mean plasma cholesterol level with dietary modification can be reasonably well predicted in populations by multifactorial equations,[69,70] this change is far less predictable for individuals.

Failure to document a definite alteration of coronary risk by dietary intervention has engendered considerable controversy about the so-called diet-heart hypothesis,[70a] although plasma cholesterol level, a powerful predictor of coronary risk in a population, is strongly correlated with the saturated fat and cholesterol content of that population's habitual diet. The diet-heart hypothesis may never be tested as a sole intervention in human beings because of the enormous cost and limited chance of success.[71] In most prior studies, lowered lipid levels were not associated with a decrease in total mortality, although coronary mortality decreased in some studies.[72,73] A limitation of many interventions may be the selection of subjects of middle age or older with advanced atherosclerotic lesions, the small sample sizes, and the short duration of intervention; alternatively, the usual dietary saturated fat and cholesterol intake may be so high that modest modifications are inadequate. Additionally, total dietary fat was not appreciably decreased in some studies that substituted polyunsaturated for saturated fat. In the Los Angeles Veterans Administration Study[72] and the Finnish Mental Hospital Study,[73] administration of a diet high in unsaturated fat and low in saturated fat to middle-aged or older patients decreased plasma cholesterol level by 10 to 15 percent and decreased coronary mortality; however, these studies failed to effect a statistically significant change in total mortality. In the Oslo Heart Study, the combination of reduction of dietary saturated fat and cholesterol and cessation of cigarette smoking significantly decreased the incidence of fatal and nonfatal cardiovascular events.[74] Of interest is that in the U.S. Coronary Artery Surgery Study (CASS), the same two risk factors, cigarette smoking and cholesterol level, best indicated increased risk, particularly among younger women.[10]

Although several drugs can lower plasma cholesterol concentration by a variety of mechanisms, a multinational primary prevention trial of clofibrate in 10,000 men at increased risk because of hyperlipidemia not only did not prevent infarction but was associated with an increase in mortality from all causes, as well as coronary mortality, both during and after the period of drug administration.[75] The benefits and hazards of other lipid-lowering drugs in primary prevention are uncertain, and no recommendations are yet warranted for the general population (see below).

Several studies provide additional information, although only one specifically addressed the diet-heart hypothesis. The Coronary Primary Prevention Trial (CPPT) compared the effect of modifying serum cholesterol level in almost 4000 hyperlipidemic men (cholesterol level at least 265 mg/dl) by diet and placebo versus diet and cholestyramine therapy.[31] There was a 24 percent decrease in coronary mortality and a 19 percent decrease in nonfatal myocardial infarction associated with the addition of drug therapy. Administration of cholestyramine over a 7-year period resulted in increased lowering of total cholesterol level by 8.5 percent and of LDL cholesterol level by 12.6 percent. In a small sample of these patients, coronary arteriography performed before and after 5 years of treatment suggested that cholestyramine administration retarded the rate of progression of angiographic lesions. Whereas these results support the importance of plasma cholesterol in coronary morbidity and mortality and document the benefit of therapy in men with cholesterol levels of at least 265 mg/dl, it is premature to extrapolate the results of this study to subjects with lower cholesterol levels, to persons of all ages, or to women.

The Multiple Risk Factor Intervention Trial investigated the effect of education for diet alteration, hypertension control, and intensive antismoking counseling on almost 13,000 middle-aged men at high coronary risk (upper 10 percent) because of combinations of three risk factors: elevated plasma cholesterol level, hypertension, and cigarette smoking.[19] Persons with high cholesterol levels in excess of 350 mg/dl or with diastolic blood pressures over 115 mmHg were excluded. Although cardiovascular events decreased in the special intervention group, there was an unexpected simultaneous decrease in cholesterol levels and in coronary events in the control (usual care) group. Thus, the study could not document benefit from the special intervention; the decrease in mean plasma cholesterol level at 6 years in the special intervention group was 12.1 mg/dl; in the usual care population it was 7.5 mg/dl.

The Type II Coronary Intervention Study was a randomized clinical trial designed to test the hypothesis that lowering LDL cholesterol level could arrest or retard the progression of coronary artery disease in patients who had elevated LDL levels that did not respond to dietary therapy. The 71 patients assigned at random to a regimen of cholestyramine plus diet had a significantly greater decrease in total cholesterol and LDL cholesterol levels than did the 72 patients who received daily placebo therapy and an identical diet. The rate of progression of angiographically evaluated coronary artery disease was lower in the cholestyramine-treated patients than in the control patients. In both groups the lower rate of progression appeared to be related to lower levels of LDL and total cholesterol, to higher levels of high-density lipoprotein (HDL) cholesterol, and to an increased ratio of HDL to either LDL or total cholesterol. In general, the risk of angiographic coronary progression was two to three times greater for individuals who had a less favorable lipid response than for those who had a more favorable lipid response.[76,77]

There is sufficient evidence[77a] to recommend the American Heart Association Diet[4] for most of the U.S. population; this diet is comparable to dietary changes recommended by the World Health Organization for high-coronary-incidence populations.[2] Individuals with optimal (desirable) plasma cholesterol levels need not alter their diet. Dietary management involves the limitation of dietary fat to 30 percent or less of calories, with fewer than 10 percent of calories from saturated fats, 10 percent or more from monounsaturated fats, and up to 10 percent from polyunsaturated fats; cholesterol intake is limited to less than 300 mg daily; and no salt is added.[3,4] There should be correction or avoidance of overweight and an increase in consumption of complex carbohydrates. A challenge to this approach is that this diet has not been formally tested in a general population; however, it is a safe diet, widely used in many countries with a low prevalence of atherosclerosis. Free-living subpopulations in the United States who habitually consume vegetarian diets, such as members of a commune in Boston[78] and Seventh-Day Adventists,[79] also have lowered plasma cholesterol levels. The American Cancer Society has also recommended a decrease in the dietary intake of fat in an attempt to decrease the occurrence of certain malignancies, e.g., breast and colon cancers.

Although there is an association of increased triglyceride levels with vascular disease, most epidemiologic data do not show fasting hypertriglyceridemia to be an independent coronary risk factor.[60,80,81] Many individuals with hypertriglyceridemia are obese; obesity is associated with an increased incidence of systemic hypertension. The obesity may contribute to both the hypertriglyceridemia and the hypertension, with the latter a proven independent risk factor for atherogenesis. Control of hypertriglyceridemia involves weight reduction, exercise, and the avoidance of excessive alcohol use and estrogen-containing drugs.[82] Reduction of triglyceride levels by drug therapy has not decreased coronary risk.[81]

The risk imparted by elevated cholesterol concentrations appears to be prominently related to elevation of the LDL cholesterol level.[84] Epidemiologic and research data also demonstrate an inverse relation of HDL cholesterol level[83] to individual coronary risk,[85,86] even when risk status is adjusted for LDL cholesterol and triglyceride levels.[87] A decrease in HDL concentration from 60 to 30 mg/dl[87] is associated with a doubled prevalence of coronary disease. The ratio of HDL to LDL may also better predict coronary risk;[85] decreased HDL level predicts coronary risk in the elderly, whereas total cholesterol level does not.[5,85] The predictive value of HDL cholesterol concentration in individuals with a nonoptimal total cholesterol concentration is not known. Studies have suggested that the HDL_2 subfraction may be a better index of risk than is total HDL,[88] and that quantitative analysis of apo A-1 and apo B may provide an even more precise prediction of coronary risk.[84,89,90]

HDL concentration is high in children and premenopausal women, groups with low coronary risk. The salutory effects of certain HDL subfractions may be due to their transport of cholesterol from tissues to the liver for excretion and their effect on lipoprotein lipase to help clear atherogenic very low density lipoprotein (VLDL) remnants from the circulation. Despite the epidemiologic association of low HDL level with increased coronary risk, there is no evidence that increasing HDL will lessen an individual's coronary risk. It is noteworthy, however, that other favorable risk alterations, including exercise,[91,92] decrease in obesity, and the discontinuation of cigarette smoking,[93,94] also elevate total plasma HDL concentrations. Although some epidemiologic data suggest that moderate alcohol consumption may also raise HDL level,[93] alcohol is not recommended because of multiple other adverse systemic effects and the risk of alcohol abuse. Further studies are needed to identify the HDL subfraction(s) influenced by all of these changes.

Despite the fact that all dietary trials to date designed to alter cholesterol levels have had negative or equivocal results, the strong epidemiologic association of elevated plasma cholesterol level and atherosclerotic coronary heart disease indicates that physicians should determine the coronary risk status of most individual patients, preferably at 20 to 25 years of age. In patients with a high-risk or nonoptimal profile, an attempt should be made to modify alterable risk factors, dependent on age and general health. The initial approach to the management of hyperlipidemia is dietary modification[3,4] (Prudent diet), including reducing caloric intake to attain ideal body weight. An increase in dietary fiber of vegetable origin may potentiate the lipid-lowering effect. Because different persons eating comparable diets may have different cholesterol levels, the Prudent diet may not change cholesterol levels in some persons. If necessary, progressive reduction of fat calories and dietary cholesterol[3,4] is subsequently recommended.

Weight reduction and reduced alcohol and sugar consumption are recommended for patients with significant hypertriglyceridemia (greater than 250 mg/dl).[81]

Because most hypolipidemic drugs have significant side effects and/or potential toxicity, they should generally be reserved for patients with familial hyperlipidemia or others at high risk for whom nonpharmacologic management has been unsuccessful.[95,96] A cholesterol-binding resin should usually be the initial drug used. Orally administered anion exchange resins lower plasma cholesterol by binding to bile acids in the gastrointestinal tract, thus preventing their reabsorption and causing them to be excreted in the feces.[97–99] There is an increase in the hepatic synthesis of bile salts, in the cell surface receptors for LDL, and in the de novo synthesis of cholesterol.[100–102] The net result, however, is a decrease in plasma LDL cholesterol level and in total cholesterol level.[102–104] The two currently available bile acid–sequestering resins, cholestyramine (Questran) and colestipol (Colestid), usually produce a 15 to 25 percent decrease in plasma cholesterol concentration in excess of that achieved by diet alone.[104–106] Resins are taken at mealtime, with the total daily dose gradually increased to a level of 24 g/day of cholestyramine or 30 g/day of colestipol. Both cholestyramine and colestipol[99] have relatively low patient acceptability due to significant gastrointestinal symptoms; they also interfere with the absorption of digoxin, thiazide diuretics, warfarin, and the like but otherwise have little apparent risk. Cholestyramine has produced regression of atherosclerosis in hypercholesterolemic nonhuman primates.[39–41]

Nicotinic acid lowers LDL cholesterol level by decreasing the hepatic synthesis of VLDL, the precursor of LDL, and perhaps by increasing the excretion of neutral steroids in bile;[107] it may also increase HDL levels.[108] The initial dose of nicotinic acid is 50 mg three times daily; this is gradually increased to 1 g three times daily. If the plasma LDL level has not decreased sufficiently, a dose of up to 2.5 g three times daily may be used. The marked flushing produced by nicotinic acid can be reduced by gradually increasing the dose and by concomitant administration of aspirin. Contraindications to nicotinic acid include peptic ulcer, liver disease, hyperuricemia, and cardiac arrhythmias.

Probucol (Lorelco) lowers plasma cholesterol level in association with increased clearance of LDL and excretion of cholesterol in bile.[109,110] Unlike nicotinic acid, it may decrease HDL levels.[111,112] In general, probucol is less effective than resins or nicotinic acid in reducing plasma cholesterol or LDL levels. The usual dose is 500 mg twice daily with meals. The major side effects are diarrhea and abdominal discomfort. The long-term effects of probucol are unknown, and the drug is slowly eliminated from fat stores in the body.[113]

Oral administration of neomycin, 2 g/day at bedtime, lowers LDL cholesterol level by 20 to 30 percent by increasing the fecal excretion of bile salts, decreasing cholesterol absorption, and decreasing total cholesterol and LDL synthesis.[114,115] It may produce nausea, abdominal cramps, and diarrhea; it has potential ototoxicity and nephrotoxicity[116] and may interfere with the absorption of digitalis compounds and potentiate the efficacy of warfarin.[117]

Nicotinic acid, probucol, and neomycin have each been successfully used together with a resin (cholestyramine or colestipol) in the therapy of hypercholesterolemia that fails to respond adequately to dietary therapy or to single drug therapy, particularly in patients with familial hypercholesterolemia.[104,118–122]

Compactin and mevinolin are experimental drugs that inhibit hydroxy-methylglutaryl CoA reductase, the rate-limiting enzyme in cholesterol synthesis.[123–126] They have reduced by 20 to 30 percent the plasma cholesterol levels of patients with familial hypercholesterolemia.

The fibric acid derivatives, clofibrate (Atromid-S), gemfibrozil (Lopid) and fenofibrate, reduce plasma triglyceride and VLDL levels. They have only a limited effect in lowering LDL level and occasionally produce a significant increase in LDL. Clofibrate tends to lower HDL level, but gemfibrozil may raise HDL cholesterol level.[127] Although these drugs are of questionable value in the treatment of patients with hypercholesterolemia or elevated LDL cholesterol levels, they are effective in reducing plasma VLDL and triglyceride levels in patients with dysbetalipoproteinemia (type III hyperlipoproteinemia).[96] Chronic clofibrate therapy appears to be associated with an increase in cardiac arrhythmias, sudden death, and cholelithiasis. The usual dose of clofibrate is 1 g twice daily, and of gemfibrozil, 600 mg twice daily. Fenofibrate has been used in Europe but is not approved for use in the United States.

Alternatives to the drug therapy of hypercholesterolemia that are currently being evaluated include partial ileal bypass,[50,50a] repeated plasma exchange,[51,52] and portacaval shunt.[53]

Cigarette Smoking[128]

Epidemiologic studies have firmly established that cigarette smoking independently predisposes to myocardial infarction and sudden cardiac death in populations with mean plasma cholesterol levels in excess of 180 mg/dl. The risk of infarction for both men and women correlates with the number of cigarettes smoked daily.[129] Young men smoking more than 40 cigarettes daily[130] and women taking oral contraceptive drugs who smoke cigarettes are most vulnerable; the relative risk may not be as great with increasing age.[131,132] Cigarette smoking also increases total mortality, lung cancer, and the likelihood of peripheral and cerebrovascular disease. The risk of cigarette smoking is additive, and probably synergistic, to that of other atherosclerotic risk factors; even moderate cigarette smoking may double or triple the vulnerability associated with other coronary risk factors. Pipe and cigar smokers have a coronary risk less than that of cigarette smokers, possibly because they are less likely to inhale; however, cigarette smokers who change to pipe or cigar smoking usually do inhale and do not reduce risk. There is no evidence that smoking low-tar low-nicotine cigarettes lessens coronary risk. Smokers who use these cigarettes may inhale more; smoking fewer cigarettes appears preferable.[129]

The prevalence of cigarette smoking in the United States has significantly decreased, particularly among the high-risk population for atherosclerotic coronary disease—middle-aged men. The decrease is more prominent among better-educated persons. This contrasts with the dramatic increase in teenagers who smoke, especially teenage girls. A particular problem for women is that oral contraceptive drugs potentiate the risk of vascular disease related to smoking; this is accentuated in women over age 35.[133]

Cigarette smoking may induce atherosclerosis by a number of mechanisms,[133a] some of which appear related to inhalation.[128] Cigarette smoking also unfavorably alters lipid levels; men and women who smoked more than 15 cigarettes daily were found to have lower HDL levels and higher LDL cholesterol and triglyceride levels.[134] An increase in myocardial electrical instability and a predisposition to sudden death have been documented in animal models. In addition, oxygen transport and utilization are impaired and myocardial oxygen demand is increased.

Randomized trials of discontinuation of cigarette smoking have shown an insignificant decrease in all-cause mortality in association with smoking cessation.[74,135] On the other hand, former smokers have a significantly lower risk of myocardial infarction and coronary death than do subjects who continue to smoke.[132,136] After smoking is discontinued, the coronary risk decreases rapidly, with a decrease in risk of about 50 percent within 1 year. Therefore, the risk approaches that of nonsmokers in from 2 to 10 years, as reported in different studies.[94,131–136] The cessation of cigarette smoking increases the HDL/LDL ratio.[93,94]

Community and individual preventive approaches should be designed to lessen smoking in adults and decrease the adoption of smoking by teenagers.

Hypertension

Many epidemiologic studies have established that an elevation of either systolic or diastolic blood pressure is a powerful, independent contributor to coronary risk in populations with elevated cholesterol levels. On the other hand, it does not appear important in populations with mean plasma cholesterol levels lower than 160 mg/dl. Systolic blood pressure levels appear slightly more predictive of risk, particularly in older age; both fixed and labile hypertension increase risk. The risk is a continuum; the higher the pressure, the greater the risk. Hypertension has an especially strong impact when there is coexistent hypercholesterolemia, and hypertension remains a risk factor in the elderly.[5] Although hypertension is a powerful risk factor for coronary atherosclerosis, the beneficial effects of blood pressure control on coronary events are less clearly proved, possibly because of the brief duration of the studies and the small number of events in the intervention trials.

Perhaps one-third of the U.S. population over age 60 has hypertension, predominantly mild hypertension, and hypertension is more prevalent among blacks, obese persons, and users of oral contraceptives. A genetic component in many individuals appears triggered by dietary salt intake;[137] in predisposed individuals or populations, restriction of dietary salt to less than 5 g/day (i.e., 2 g of sodium daily) may prevent the development of hypertension. Hypertension rarely occurs in populations with a habitual intake of salt below 2 g daily.[3] In addition to increased dietary sodium, other factors predisposing to hypertension include obesity, a sedentary life-style, excessive alcohol intake,[138] and oral contraceptive drug use (see also Chap. 49). A brief trial of alteration of these risk characteristics may be the initial approach in some patients with mild hypertension. Hypertension may predispose to atherogenesis by a variety of pathogenetic mechanisms[139] (see Chap. 41).

The early antihypertensive therapy trials conclusively demonstrated that control of moderate and severe hypertension decreased total mortality and the risk of heart failure and stroke; however, these trials did not demonstrate a statistically significant effect of control of hypertension on coronary events, possibly because of the small numbers of patients and events.[140–142] A decrease in coronary death and nonfatal infarction was evident in the treated hypertensive men in the Goteberg Study;[143] however, since most patients were treated with beta-blocking drugs, it is uncertain whether the improved coronary status represented the effect of hypertension control or of beta blockade. The U.S. Hypertension Detection and Follow-up Program (HDFP) involved about 11,000 men and women with mild and moderate hypertension. A standardized "stepped-care" regimen, designed to attain normal blood pressure levels, reduced 5-year cardiovascular mortality by 26 percent and all-cause mortality by 17 percent, as compared with the usual community treatment of hypertension (control group).[29,30,144] The greatest benefit of the stepped-care approach occurred in patients with mild hypertension, possibly because mild elevation of blood pressure was not routinely treated in the community prior to publication of the HDFP data. The Australian Therapeutic Trial in Mild Hypertension also demonstrated improved survival in the intervention group[145] but without a statistically significant decrease in coronary events, despite a favorable trend. In general, these studies reinforce the reported contribution of hypertension to coronary risk and study data suggest that control of hypertension appears to decrease coronary events and coronary mortality, especially for patients with diastolic blood pressures over 95 mmHg.

The therapy[146] of hypertension is discussed in Chap. 51. Thiazide diuretic therapy may elevate blood glucose, uric acid, and cholesterol concentrations and reduce potassium levels; some beta-blocking drugs may also elevate cholesterol levels. The MRFIT data[19] raised the question of potential adverse effects of thiazide therapy, especially in patients with baseline electrocardiographic changes; this issue is currently being addressed in the British Medical Research Council Hypertension Trial. Further analysis of the HDFP data did not find an increased mortality in patients with baseline electrocardiographic abnormalities treated with the stepped-care approach, a finding different from MRFIT results.[146a]

Genetic Factors

A small number of persons in the general population, perhaps 3 to 5 percent, have a genetic predisposition to hyperlipidemia (see Chaps. 35 and 41). A significantly higher percentage appears to have a genetic predisposition to hypertension; some may be more sensitive to high sodium intake (see Chaps. 35 and 49). Many subsets of diabetes appear to have a strong genetic basis. Other genetically determined disorders that may predispose to premature coronary atherosclerosis include the following: Hunter's syndrome (type II mucopolysaccharidosis), Hurler's syndrome (type I-H mucopolysaccharidosis), Fabry's disease, homocystinuria, alkaptonuria, pseudoxanthoma elasticum, Werner's syndrome, arterial calcification of infancy, and cholesteryl ester storage disease.[147]

Obesity

The association between obesity and premature atherosclerotic coronary heart disease, increased angina pectoris, and an increase in mortality, particularly by sudden death, is well known. The predominant rationale for control of obesity is that obesity adversely affects the risk profile and appears to accentuate atherosclerosis by predisposing to hypertension, impaired glucose tolerance, hyperinsulinemia, hyperlipidemia with elevated LDL and decreased HDL levels, and hyperuricemia;[93,148] it may also further lessen physical activity. Data suggest that the degree of obesity may be an independent risk factor, especially in women.[149] The mechanisms by which obesity predisposes to hypertension are not known; glucose intolerance may reflect the relative insensitivity of large fat cells to insulin.

Perhaps over one-third of the U.S. adult population is overweight. Weight reduction by a diet low in saturated fat and cholesterol lowers the risk of coronary events by decreasing most of the important atherogenic risk factors, except for smoking.[150] Although no confirmatory evidence from intervention studies is available, dietary management of obesity is recommended because there are no apparent adverse effects and because weight reduction has many systemic benefits. Exercise and behavior-modification techniques may aid in weight control. Prevention of obesity, beginning early in life, may be even more valuable.

Diabetes Mellitus and Impaired Glucose Tolerance

Diabetes mellitus increases the susceptibility to coronary heart disease. Glucose intolerance doubles the occurrence of coronary disease in men, and triples to quadruples the incidence in women, particularly prior to age 50.[151] The diabetic woman has atherosclerosis comparable to that of a nondiabetic male, thus losing the relative immunity of premenopausal women to coronary atherosclerosis.[23] A young woman with atherosclerotic disease typically has diabetes mellitus, hypertension, or hypercholesterolemia or smokes cigarettes.[10,152] Obesity worsens the risk profile of diabetic patients. Diabetic women also have an excess of both cardiovascular mortality and heart failure. Impaired glucose tolerance also independently increases coronary risk,[151] and hyperinsulinemia has also been implicated in imparting risk. Diabetes may predispose to atherosclerotic coronary heart disease by a variety of mechanisms[153–157] (see Chap. 41). Increased lipid levels, hypertension, and obesity do not appear to be adequate explanations for the adverse cardiovascular outcome.[156] Control of hyperglycemia alone does not eliminate coronary risk; substantial multifactorial risk reduction appears necessary.[158] A fat-modified diet may improve control of glucose levels.

Sedentary Living and Physical Activity

Data from several epidemiologic studies suggest that populations with habitual vigorous physical activity have decreased mortality from atherosclerotic coronary heart disease;[159] coronary disease is known to be more prevalent in highly industrialized societies. Some of the methodologic problems with these data, which were often collected retrospectively, involve the lack of standardization of diagnosis of coronary events, the unknown prevalence of associated risk factors, the difficulty in quantifying occupational and recreational physical activity, and the medical or other reasons for initiating and altering activity.[160] These problems also limit the assessment of relations between habitual activity levels and coronary risk as well; thus, it remains uncertain whether or not moderate exercise can confer the benefits alleged for strenuous physical activity. Although physical fitness is usually associated with a more favorable risk profile, the effect of the institution of physical activity in altering the severity of outcome of atherosclerotic coronary disease or in increasing the development of coronary collateral vessels in human beings has not been systematically examined or established. A favorable effect of physical activity could relate to the following: increased HDL levels and lipoprotein lipase levels, reduction in weight, increased cardiovascular functional capacity and decreased myocardial oxygen demand, decreased platelet adhesiveness and improved fibrinolysis, and improved electrical stability of the myocardium. Trials of exercise for primary prevention have never been deemed feasible, however, and data from epidemiologic studies have served as the basis for recommendations. Some epidemiologic data[161–163] suggest that contemporary occupational and recreational physical activity is associated with decreased coronary risk, independent of other major risk factors.[161–163] Morris's data on British civil servants,[163] Paffenbarger's study of Harvard alumni,[164] and Garcia-Palmieri's report of rural versus urban Puerto Rican men[165] demonstrate an apparent protective effect of vigorous physical activity. On the other hand, concerns about preselection and other uncontrolled factors are relevant to each of these studies.

Exercise may reduce blood pressure, decrease smoking, improve carbohydrate metabolism, and favorably alter psychological status; it is recommended as an adjunct to dietary modification in the control of obesity. A study showed that the level of physical fitness in women was independently associated with a more favorable lipid profile, lower blood pressure, and less cigarette smoking;[166] this relation had previously been demonstrated in men. Exercise is an inexpensive and often pleasurable social intervention with few adverse effects.

Oral Contraceptive Drugs; Menopause

Oral contraceptive drugs may increase coronary risk by altering a number of physiological and metabolic variables. Their use may increase body weight and blood pressure, elevate plasma triglyceride concentration, reduce glucose tolerance, and reduce HDL cholesterol concentration. In addition, oral contraceptive agents alter blood coagulation, platelet function, and fibrinolytic activity and may adversely affect the integrity of vascular endothelium. Nevertheless, the mechanisms that promote atherosclerosis need further elaboration. The varying estrogen and progesterone contents of oral contraceptive drugs variably influence lipoprotein levels.[82]

Although, in general, women using oral contraceptives have an increased mortality from myocardial infarction, cerebrovascular disease,[167,168] and other thromboembolic events, these drugs are relatively safe for women younger than age 35 who do not smoke cigarettes, are normotensive, and have no prior evidence of venous thromboembolism or arterial disease. Women over age 35 who use oral contraceptives are at increased risk; risk is magnified at any age by cigarette smoking,[133] hypertension, glucose intolerance, and other coronary risk factors. An alternative method of contraception should be recommended for women with these characteristics as well as for women with prior venous thromboembolism. Although low-dose estrogen oral contraceptives impart less risk than do those with higher doses, none are risk-free. Coronary risk may not be as great in developing countries where there is a low incidence of coronary disease in the population.

An increase in coronary events appears to follow either natural or surgical menopause in women;[169] the excess risk is evident whether or not the ovaries are removed. The reasons for the resistance of women in their reproductive years to coronary atherosclerosis remain poorly understood, as are the reasons for loss of this advantage after menopause. At present, there is no agreement as to whether or not estrogen administered to postmenopausal women increases the risk of a coronary event.[169,170] One study failed to identify a causal relation between noncontraceptive estrogen use and the occurrence of myocardial infarction in postmenopausal women;[171] another study suggested potential benefit of estrogen therapy for women.[172] (See also Chaps. 41 and 72.)

Psychosocial and Behavioral Factors[173]

Certain personality characteristics and behavior attributes appear to be associated with coronary risk in high-incidence populations.[25,174,175] Friedman[175a] and Rosenman describe type A behavior as characterized by time urgency, hostility, aggression, ambition, competitiveness, impatience, and frustration. The pathogenetic mechanism is unknown, but increased circulating catecholamines may cause hypertension, abnormal platelet function, increased fatty acid mobilization, and resultant elevation of free fatty acids. On the other hand, there is no conclusive evidence that modification of type A behavior alters coronary risk. An expert panel, convened by the National Heart, Lung, and Blood Institute, agreed that a causal link had not yet been established between behavior and coronary risk and that it was premature to recommend interventions designed to alter behavior and stress.[176]

Stressful life events, limited social support, and excessive social mobility have also been described as associated with increased coronary risk.[174] Psychosocial factors have not been well studied in black populations in the United States.[176a] Recommendations of the World Health Organization warn that misconceptions about stress in the genesis of coronary disease may distract from appropriate primary prevention.[2]

Alcohol[177]

More than moderate alcohol use (in excess of two to three average drinks per day) should be discouraged because of its correlation with an increase in coronary risk factors;[178] it may increase body weight, triglyceride levels, and systolic blood pressure[138] and may impair left ventricular function and induce arrhythmias. The prevalence of myocardial infarction was higher among heavy drinkers than nonheavy drinkers younger than age 60, after controlling for differences in cigarette smoking and angiographic severity of atherosclerosis.[178a] In most patients, these negative effects outweigh any potential beneficial effects on HDL levels.[179] There is no strong evidence to date of a causal relation between decreased coronary risk and the use of alcohol, which has numerous adverse systemic and social consequences.

Other Risk Factors

Many postulated associations with increased coronary risk have not been substantiated; these include mineral content (hardness) of drinking water, trace elements, blood groups, coffee drinking, climate, noise, and air pollution[180–182] (see Chap. 41).

Asymptomatic cervical bruits, probably as evidence of systemic atherosclerosis, are associated with increased cardiovascular and cerebrovascular events in men.[183] Although hyperuricemia has a modest association with the development of atherosclerotic coronary heart disease, the association of elevated serum uric acid level with other coronary risk factors makes it impossible to confirm or deny the independent effect of elevation of the serum uric acid level.[184] Both a decreased vital capacity and evidence of left ventricular hypertrophy on the ECG are associated with an increased coronary risk.[23,28]

Sociological variables[174,176a] that have an increased association with coronary events include excessive sociocultural mobility, urban environment, major socioeconomic changes, and loss of social support systems.[181] Both men and women whose spouses develop coronary disease are at significantly increased coronary risk.[185] Husbands whose wives are college-educated and hold white-collar jobs appear to be at increased risk, regardless of their social status or other coronary risk factors;[186] wives with a college education and wives working outside the home appear to impose a greater coronary risk on type A husbands than on type B husbands.[187] The implications of these studies are not clear. In some studies, educational level is inversely related both to those risk factors that are determined by life-style and to coronary and cardiac mortality.[188]

Role of the Physician in Primary Prevention: Multiple Risk Intervention

Since many adult Americans have marginal abnormalities of multiple coronary risk factors, recommendations for *individuals* should be based on that person's coronary risk status. Most adults should have an evaluation of personal risk attributes performed, preferably at age 20 to 25. The *Coronary Risk Handbook* of the American Heart Association provides a simple way to quantify the probability of developing coronary heart disease, based on the interaction of multiple factors and taking into account their synergistic effects.[6,7] Risk assessment may help to motivate selected individuals by estimating the risk reduction achievable by control of one or more risk factors. A family history of high coronary risk is an indication for risk assessment in the pediatric age group.

Communitywide education can reduce risk levels in a population.[189] The substantial decline in coronary risk and mortality in the control group of the MRFIT[19] suggests that public education may be an effective approach to emphasizing the multifactorial approach early in adult life. Diastolic blood pressure in this "control" group decreased 8 percent, plasma cholesterol was lowered 13 mg/dl, and 29 percent of smokers had discontinued cigarette use during the 6 years of the study.

A comprehensive risk intervention strategy as outlined can reasonably be expected to favorably influence outcome and can be accomplished without major disruption of life-style, with little risk, and with only modest costs and requirements for health care resources.

Secondary Prevention of Atherosclerotic Coronary Heart Disease

Secondary prevention refers to interventions designed to lessen the morbidity and mortality of patients with such clinical evidence of atherosclerotic coronary heart disease as angina pectoris or myocardial infarction, and of patients after coronary artery bypass surgery or angioplasty. In the past, the modification of traditional coronary risk factors has been evaluated and implemented most extensively in survivors of myocardial infarction. Because epidemiologic data suggest that risk for patients with angina pectoris is somewhat comparable to that of patients after myocardial infarction,[190] this subgroup of coronary patients also warrants attention. The increasing attention devoted to risk reduction in patients following coronary angioplasty or coronary bypass surgery is appropriate, since most of these patients are known to have accelerated atherosclerosis.

Secondary prevention includes not only those measures designed to retard the progression or induce regression of the atherosclerotic disease (traditional secondary prevention) but also the identification of patients at increased risk of recurrent coronary events (due to factors unrelated to the atherosclerotic process per se) and the institution of therapies to lessen these risks. During the past decade, there has been considerable refinement of the clinical and noninvasive prognostic indexes for patients recovered from myocardial infarction. The features associated with increased risk and the approaches to risk stratification after myocardial infarction and coronary bypass surgery are considered in Chap. 45. Since the early mortality following a coronary event is dominated by the extent of continuing myocardial ischemia,[191] left ventricular dysfunction, and complex ventricular ectopy,[191–193] it is unlikely that the effects of traditional coronary risk reduction can play a major role in the early months after infarction; the secondary preventive benefits of coronary bypass surgery are addressed in Chap. 45. Pharmacological approaches that may lessen the risk of early reinfarction or sudden death, particularly the use of beta-adrenergic blocking drugs and possibly platelet-active drugs, are important advances in management and are also discussed in Chap. 45.

The continuing acquisition of information from many research disciplines and from results of controlled clinical trials of cardiovascular therapies[20] help to define those interventions likely to improve prognosis. These are considered in recommendations for the secondary prevention of coronary heart disease recently compiled by the Scientific Councils of the International Society and Federation of Cardiology.[194] Although the traditional coronary risk factors appear to exert a less-powerful role in determining the prognosis following myocardial infarction, and the benefits of secondary prevention are less well established, secondary preventive efforts are particularly appropriate for younger patients in an attempt to arrest or delay their subsequent development of atherosclerosis. The impact of the three major risk factors—cigarette smoking, blood pressure, and cholesterol concentration—may be greater in the presence of myocardial ischemia.[195,196] This problem may be accentuated in patients with nontransmural infarction.[197] Among men surviving a first myocardial infarction, data from the Health Insurance Plan of New York identified that cigarette smoking, hypertension, and diabetes mellitus contribute to increased risk.[198] Traditional coronary risk factors—cigarette smoking and hypercholesterolemia—also increased the risk of coronary events in men recovered from myocardial infarction and enrolled in the Coronary Drug Project;[191] patients who were able to return to moderate or vigorous physical activity appeared to have less mortality; there was an inverse linear relationship between the level of HDL cholesterol and 5-year mortality.[199]

Cessation of Cigarette Smoking

Avoidance of cigarette smoking has the best documentation of benefit and may be the most effective single risk-factor intervention following myocardial infarction.[200] It substantially improves the prognosis in patients of all ages with angina and in survivors of myocardial infarction; it lowers the risk of fatal reinfarction, sudden death, and total mortality by 20 to 50 percent; it reduces nonfatal reinfarction, particularly in the first 5 years after infarction.[200–202] Survival of patients who smoked cigarettes at the time of myocardial infarction correlates best with their reduction or cessation of smoking; the greatest impact is observed in patients with an otherwise favorable prognosis.[203] Cigar and pipe smoking appear associated with continued increased risk in former cigarette smokers.[204]

Cigarette smoking may damage vascular endothelium and adversely affect ventricular arrhythmias and platelet adhesiveness. Heart rate and blood pressure increase, increasing myocardial oxygen demand, whereas there may be a decrease in oxygen transport. Cigarette smoking has been reported to increase coronary tone at the site of coronary obstruction, particularly with severe proximal stenosis, decreasing coronary blood flow.[205] Passive or involuntary smoking by patients with angina placed in the same room as cigarette smokers decreased the duration of exercise they were able to perform before the occurrence of angina and increased their ventricular ectopy.[206]

There is no evidence of harm from sudden cessation of cigarette smoking. The potential adverse effect of increase in weight often can be limited by dietary counseling. In some studies, as many as 70 percent of cigarette smokers have discontinued cigarette use, at least for the short term, after myocardial infarction, and benefits appear to persist with long-term discontinuation of smoking.[201,202] Since the adverse effects of continued cigarette smoking appear dose-related,[203] even a decrease in smoking may be of value.

Hypertension[207]

In patients with coronary heart disease, including survivors of myocardial infarction, elevated diastolic blood pressure is reported in some studies as an independent contributor to an adverse prognosis. It was not a significant factor in the placebo group of the Coronary Drug Project.[191] Proper control of hypertension may decrease angina pectoris and lessen the likelihood of cerebrovascular accident and congestive heart failure. Excessive lowering of blood pressure may, however, produce myocardial or cerebral ischemia (see Chaps. 45 and 51). In the Hypertension Detection and Follow-up Program, only a small percentage of patients had a history of myocardial infarction prior to entry into the study.[29,30] There was a trend that suggested that the control of blood pressure decreased recurrent infarction and coronary death in these patients, but the differences were not statistically significant.

In previously hypertensive patients, a decrease in blood pressure after myocardial infarction carries a poor prognosis, as it presumably reflects ventricular dysfunction;[208] it carried a twofold increase in mortality in the Framingham study.[209] This may explain the lack of correlation in some studies between blood pressure following myocardial infarction and subsequent survival.

Hygienic Measures[210,211]

Control of hypertension should initially involve the safest means possible, including weight reduction by dietary caloric restriction if needed, weight control, dietary sodium restriction, limitation of excessive alcohol consumption, and a program of regular physical activity of moderate intensity as appropriate for physical work capacity. Despite these measures, pharmacological therapy is required for most patients with systemic arterial hypertension; however, the drug dosage may be lessened, with potential reduction in adverse drug effects (see Chap. 51).

Antihypertensive Drugs

Hypertension is a major indication for pharmacotherapy in secondary prevention. Antihypertensive therapy and adverse effects of drug therapy are discussed in Chap. 51.

Diet, Lipoproteins, and Obesity

Since progression of atherosclerosis both in the native circulation and in graft vessels following coronary bypass surgery adversely affects prognosis, hypercholesterolemia, especially with raised LDL cholesterol levels, warrants modification, particularly in younger patients. This is despite the fact that no trial of lipid-lowering therapy by diet or drugs to date has prolonged life;[20] however, the reduction of cholesterol levels in previous trials were usually modest, and the studies did not selectively involve patients with hypercholesterolemia. Although hypercholesterolemia appears less predictive of recurrent infarction than of initial myocardial infarction, an elevated serum cholesterol concentration is a moderately strong independent risk factor for death in survivors of myocardial infarction[191] and is associated with increased coronary mortality in the presence of myocardial ischemia.[196] Lipid-lowering may also retard atherosclerosis in other vascular beds.

Dietary Lipid Alteration

The initial treatment of hyperlipidemia, as in primary prevention, is dietary (see above), including calorie restriction in obese patients to achieve near-ideal body weight, because of its greater safety[212,213] and lower cost than pharmacological therapy. Appropriate regular exercise is helpful in weight control. A low-fat, low-calorie diet has been reported to have a beneficial effect on myocardial energy metabolism in patients with exertional angina pectoris.[214]

Lipid-Lowering Drugs[96]

Drug therapy of hyperlipidemia may decrease lipoprotein synthesis or increase lipoprotein catabolism or excretion. Many hypolipidemic drugs have significant side effects, including cardiovascular complications, and other potential toxicity as well; some drugs cause significant problems with drug interactions. A design defect of most drug trials is that a differential effect has not been ascertained in patients who did or did not obtain cholesterol lowering from therapy.

In the Coronary Drug Project, administration of one of four lipid-lowering drugs for 8 years to over 8000 men who had recovered from myocardial infarction showed that they altered plasma cholesterol levels but did not improve survival.[215] The potential benefits of lipid lowering may have been offset by the increased mortality in patients treated with estrogen and *d*-thyroxine, which required premature termination of use of these drugs. Although neither nicotinic acid nor clofibrate altered total or coronary mortality, nicotinic acid therapy was associated with a decrease in nonfatal reinfarction. Both drugs, however, produced significant adverse symptoms and cardiac and noncardiac morbidity.

Two small studies of clofibrate in the United Kingdom demonstrated a decrease in nonfatal infarction and improvement in survival in patients with preexisting angina, but no effect on prognosis was evident in patients with a history of myocardial infarction alone. The effect was independent of plasma cholesterol level or cholesterol lowering.[216,217]

No sizable secondary prevention clinical trials of bile acid–sequestering resins or other antilipidemic drugs are available to provide information about efficacy and adverse responses.

In view of these considerations, the *routine* use of any lipid-lowering drug cannot be recommended for patients with clinical evidence of coronary disease because there is no documentation of decreased mortality, the costs of long-term therapy are considerable, and there is significant multisystem drug toxicity and drug interaction. In patients with very elevated cholesterol levels, the decision to institute drug therapy must be individualized; the younger the patient, the greater the hypercholesterolemia, the greater the burden of concomitant risk factors, and the smaller the response to dietary intervention, the greater the indication for drug therapy.

Partial ileal bypass,[50] repeated plasma exchange,[51,52] and portacaval shunts[53] remain experimental approaches.

Weight Control

Weight reduction lessens cardiac work and thereby decreases angina pectoris; it improves exercise tolerance; and it exerts a favorable effect on blood pressure, glucose intolerance, plasma uric acid level, and hyperlipidemia and improves the HDL/total cholesterol ratio. It is therefore an effective approach to correcting multiple atherogenic risk factors. Despite the documentation that obesity is a predictor of reinfarction,[197] however, conclusive evidence is lacking that weight loss lessens reinfarction or cardiac death.

Diabetes Mellitus and Impaired Glucose Tolerance

The management of diabetes mellitus in coronary patients is comparable to that in patients without clinical manifestations of coronary atherosclerosis. Specific features require attention, however, because of the increased coronary risk and poorer prognosis[217a] associated with diabetes. Dietary control of obesity in persons with maturity-onset diabetes should involve a diet restricted in saturated fat and high in complex carbohydrates. Dietary sodium restriction is indicated, especially when hypertension or heart failure is present. Pharmacologic therapy of hypertension with thiazide and other diuretic drugs may increase plasma levels of glucose and lipids, as well as lowering potassium concentration. Some beta-blocking drugs also raise lipid levels. Therapy with nonselective beta-adrenergic blocking drugs may alter insulin release and mute the sympathetic-mediated components of hypoglycemic reactions; beta-1-selective drugs are advised for patients with insulin-dependent diabetes. Particular care must be directed toward avoiding hypoglycemia, which may be especially dangerous in coronary patients (see also Chap. 72).

Coronary risk modification is also indicated for persons with impaired glucose tolerance.[218] Fasting hyperglycemia of equal to or greater than 140 mg/dl predicted recurrent myocardial infarction in the Coronary Drug Project.[191,219]

Oral Contraceptive Drugs; Estrogen Therapy

Oral contraceptive drugs are inadvisable for women with atherosclerotic coronary heart disease because they may increase the risk of hypertension and are associated with an increased occurrence of cerebrovascular accident and myocardial infarction. The risk is accentuated in older women and in those who smoke cigarettes. There is inadequate information to make recommendations about postmenopausal estrogen administration for women with coronary heart disease (see Chap. 72).

Physical Activity

Dynamic exercise can be recommended for selected patients with angina, after myocardial infarction, and after coronary bypass surgery in order to limit the deleterious effects of immobilization and to improve physical work capacity and cardiocirculatory performance. The decreased heart rate and blood pressure responses to submaximal workloads that occur with training allow individuals to function farther from their ischemic threshold in daily activities. Improvements in psychosocial functioning include a decrease in depression, fear, and dependency and an increase in self-confidence and self-esteem.[220] Exercise facilitates renouncing the sick role and encourages return to the preillness life-style,[221] including return to work. Favorable metabolic changes that occur with regular exercise include an improved HDL/LDL ratio, a decrease in triglyceride levels, and an increased sensitivity to insulin. Although there is little evidence from intervention studies that exercise training improves survival, lessens reinfarction, or increases the development of coronary collateral vessels,[220,222,223] a 24 to 32 percent favorable trend in survival that was not satisfactorily significant was evident in exercising patients in several studies. The data in most studies have been confounded by problems with compliance to the exercise regimen, as well as by exercise undertaken by patients in the control group. Regular physical activity is safe if sensibly regulated. Additional beneficial effects include weight control and increased joint mobility, stability, and neuromuscular coordination; exercise may also encourage modification of other coronary risk factors. Although exercise training may decrease exercise-induced ventricular ectopy,[224] unaccustomed or excessively vigorous physical activity may be hazardous for coronary patients, mandating medical clearance and individualized exercise recommendations. Exercise recommendations for coronary patients are discussed in Chap. 48.

Psychosocial Status

Although type A behavior pattern is associated with an increased risk of initial coronary events, the effect of coronary-prone and/or type A behavior on the risk of recurrent coronary events is controversial.

Return to Work

Return to work, as reasonable for functional capacity, can be recommended for economic, social, and emotional benefits. A recent report describes the patient's perception of his physical capabilities and the expectation of return to work as powerful predictors of the actual return to work after myocardial infarction.[225] Attitudes and expectations likewise were major determinants of return to work after coronary bypass surgery.[226]

Risk Reduction Unrelated to Conventional Coronary Risk Factors

Beta-Adrenergic Receptor-Blocking Drugs

There is compelling evidence from several clinical trials that beta-adrenergic blocking drugs, administered on a long-term basis to men and women after myocardial infarction, with therapy begun prior to discharge from the hospital, reduce mortality by 26 to 39 percent; a reduction in nonfatal infarction was also evident,[227–229] and the favorable effect persisted at least for 3 years. This improved prognosis was evident in patients with and without complications of infarction, and with both initial and recurrent infarctions. Therefore, institution of beta blockade is recommended for all survivors of myocardial infarction, in the absence of contraindications, until one can reliably select those patients most likely to benefit from therapy. Subgroup analysis suggests an increased benefit in patients with electrical and mechanical complications of infarction during the initial hospitalization; patients with arrhythmias derived the greatest benefit from beta blockade, whereas patients with abnormalities of pump function had moderate benefit but more adverse effects. These observations require confirmation.[230] In one study, therapy was as effective in patients aged 65 to 75 as in those younger than 65 years;[231] other reports described increased side effects in elderly patients.

Beta-adrenergic blocking drugs favorably alter the balance between myocardial oxygen supply and demand and thereby decrease exertional angina; they are also valuable in treating ventricular ectopy and may decrease exercise-induced ventricular arrhythmias, either by reducing sympathetic stimulation of the heart or by limiting myocardial ischemia. They are also valuable in the control of systemic arterial hypertension. Which, if any, of these mechanisms explains their favorable impact on survival after infarction remains speculative. Nevertheless, the reduced mortality after a first myocardial infarction in Goteborg, Sweden, between 1968 and 1977 seems best explained by treatment with beta-blocking drugs.[232] (See also Chaps. 45 and 90.)

Calcium-Antagonist Drugs and Nitrate Drugs

Although these classes of compounds effectively limit angina and myocardial ischemia, and are currently undergoing evaluation in patients after myocardial infarction, there is no evidence to date of alteration in morbidity or mortality. (See also Chaps. 45, 88, and 91.)

Antiarrhythmic Agents

Ventricular ectopic activity, particularly when frequent and of complex forms, increases the likelihood of mortality in patients after myocardial infarction. Although it is frequently associated with left ventricular dysfunction, the presence of ventricular ectopy may confer independent risk.[192]

To date there is no satisfactory documentation[233] that any antiarrhythmic agent (excluding beta-blocking drugs) studied in a randomized clinical trial has been effective in decreasing sudden death; however, most studies included all patients recovered from infarction, not solely those demonstrating ventricular ectopy. In a study of patients recovered from myocardial infarction, all of whom had complex ventricular ectopy, there was a trend for aprindine therapy to increase total survival.[234] The results of several randomized trials of antiarrhythmic agents, currently in progress, may delineate the appropriate antiarrhythmic therapy, if any, for these high-risk coronary patients. In one study,[235] adequate antiarrhythmic drug levels seemed associated with an improved survival in patients resuscitated from sudden death, even in the absence of control of ventricular ectopy. (See also Chaps. 27, 45, and 89.)

Platelet-Active Drugs

A number of drugs that inhibit various components of platelet function have been studied in survivors of myocardial infarction[236] to evaluate their effect in reducing reinfarction and sudden and total coronary death (see also Chap. 95). Major difficulties in secondary prevention trials of aspirin are the variability of the daily dose considered appropriate (300 to 1500 mg) and the differing times after infarction of initiation of therapy. Nevertheless, although no statistically significant reduction in *mortality* has been achieved in any trial,[237–239] nonsignificant trends favored the aspirin-treated groups in most studies. In the largest of the trials, the Aspirin Myocardial Infarction Study (AMIS), which involved over 4000 patients, only a nonsignificant trend to fewer nonfatal reinfarctions within the first 2 years[240] was seen in the aspirin-treated patients. Important unwanted effects include gastrointestinal symptoms and mild elevations of systolic blood pressure and of plasma urea nitrogen and uric acid concentrations.

Studies of dipyridamole (Persantine) are likewise inconclusive. A nonsignificant trend in the Persantine-Aspirin Reinfarction Study (PARIS) favored patients treated with dipyridamole-aspirin and aspirin alone, with a suggestion of greater benefit in patients treated within 6 months after infarction.[241] PARIS II is currently evaluating the effects of dipyridamole and aspirin versus a placebo, instituted early in the postinfarction period.[242] The endpoints are recurrent myocardial infarction, sudden death, coronary death, and death from all causes.

Although sulfinpyrazone administration was described as reducing sudden death in the early months following infarction, major controversies[243] regarding patient selection, diagnostic criteria, and study endpoints limit the value of these data in guiding clinical care. The Anturan Reinfarction Italian study showed a decrease in recurrent myocardial infarction, but no significant effect on total mortality.[244]

Although the results of a number of individual randomized clinical trials of platelet-active drugs have been inconclusive to date, an 8 to 10 percent reduction in total mortality and a decrease in nonfatal infarction are seen in the combined data from six randomized trials during the first year of daily aspirin use.[245] The potential benefit is further suggested by the documentation of a favorable effect of low-dose aspirin (325 mg daily) in patients with unstable angina pectoris[246] and following coronary angioplasty,[247] and of dipyridamole and aspirin in reducing graft occlusion in patients after coronary bypass surgery.[248] Yet to be documented is whether or not the mechanism of action is an antithrombotic effect. Although many physicians commonly prescribe these drugs for patients recovering from infarction,[249] these data are not decisive enough to permit routine recommendations for the use of platelet-active drugs.

Anticoagulant Drugs[250,251]

The early trials of long-term oral anticoagulant administration to patients after myocardial infarction suggested a decreased 2-year mortality in men, particularly those after recurrent infarction or with a long history of angina pectoris.[252] Concerns about adherence to therapy posed major problems.

A randomized study in an older population showed a highly significant benefit of anticoagulation in decreasing recurrent infarction over 2 years.[253] Data from another clinical trial showed no difference in cardiovascular morbidity or survival after infarction in patients randomly assigned to oral anticoagulation or to 0.5 g of aspirin three times daily; no control group was available for comparison.[254]

Despite the burden and risks of oral anticoagulant therapy, a number of studies show a trend favoring patients given anticoagulants; therapy is indicated in selected patients at increased risk of thromboembolic complications. (See also Chap. 95.)

Recommendations for Secondary Prevention: Multifactorial Intervention

A comprehensive approach to coronary risk management appears prudent for patients with a variety of manifestations of symptomatic atherosclerotic coronary artery disease, with the most intensive intervention reserved for younger patients with good residual myocardial function. In patients after myocardial revascularization by coronary bypass surgery or angioplasty, secondary prevention is a logical component of long-term care to prevent recurrence of the previous accelerated atherosclerosis. Despite these generalizations, there is a paucity of data regarding multifactorial risk intervention.

Multifactorial risk intervention in Finland significantly lowered 3-year mortality and morbidity in a small group of patients recovered from myocardial infarction.[255] Benefits were most evident in the first 6 months after infarction. Comprehensive medical care and attempts at multiple risk reduction in the intervention group effected a decrease in weight, a lowering of plasma lipid levels, and a reduction of systolic and diastolic blood pressures. This is comparable to Blankenhorn's approach to patients with hyperlipidemia—multiple interventions, including diet, weight loss, hypertension control, and drug therapy, produced regression of femoral atherosclerotic lesions.[45,48]

The initial emphasis involves healthful alterations of life-style, including avoidance of cigarette smoking; reduction of dietary intake of saturated fat, cholesterol, sodium, and calories (if needed to achieve optimal body weight); and institution of a program of regular moderate-intensity physical activity. Cessation of cigarette smoking and long-term adherence to hypertension control regimens have been shown to improve prognosis. Reasonable levels of physical activity can improve exercise capacity and favorably alter emotional status.

Blood pressure control decreases myocardial oxygen demand, and hypertension should be treated as in the general population. Pharmacological intervention designed to alter blood lipid levels, cardiac arrhythmias, or platelet function have not shown conclusive advantage and may have considerable adverse effects; the risk/benefit ratio of each intervention, particularly for patients with a favorable outlook, must be assessed in the individual patient. Beta-adrenergic blocking drugs appear to improve prognosis. The use of behavioral treatment strategies may encourage and improve adherence to the varied components of secondary prevention.[256]

References

1. Lucretius: "De Rerum Natura" chap. 5, 1.1007, ca. 50 B.C.
2. Report of a WHO Expert Committee, Prevention of Coronary Heart Disease, "Technical Report Series 678, World Health Organization, Geneva, 1982.
3. Inter-Society Commission for Heart Disease Resources: Optimal Resources for Primary Prevention of Atherosclerotic Diseases, *Circulation,* 70:153A, 1984.
4. AHA Special Report: A Joint Statement of the Nutrition Committee and the Council on Arteriosclerosis. Recommendations for Treatment of Hyperlipidemia in Adults, *Circulation,* 69:1065A, 1984.
5. Kannel, W. B., and Gordon, T.: Evaluation of Cardiovascular Risk in the Elderly: The Framingham Study, *Bull. N.Y. Acad. Med.,* 54:573, 1978.
6. "Coronary Risk Handbook. Estimating Risk of Coronary Heart Disease in Daily Practice," American Heart Association, New York, 1973.
7. Gordon, T., and Kannel, W. B.: Multiple Risk Functions for Predicting Coronary Heart Disease: The Concept, Accuracy, and Application, *Am. Heart J.,* 103:1031, 1982.
8. McGee, D., and Gordon, T.: The Results of the Framingham Study Applied to Four Other U.S.-Based Epidemiologic Studies of Cardiovascular Disease, in W. B. Kannel and T. Gordon (eds.), "The Framingham Study. An Epidemiological Investigation of Cardiovascular Disease," Section 31, U.S. Department of Health, Education, and Welfare, Public Health Service, National Institutes of Health, DHEW Publ. NIH-76-1083, 1976.
9. Salel, A. F., Fong, A., Zelis, R., Miller R. R., Borhani, N. O., and Mason, D. T.: Accuracy of Numerical Coronary Profile. Correlation of Risk Factors with Arteriographically Documented Severity of Atherosclerosis, *N. Engl. J. Med.,* 296:1447, 1977.
10. Vlietstra, R. E., Frye, R. L., Kronmal, R. A., Sim, D. A., Tristani, F. E., and Killip, T., III, and Participants in the Coronary Artery Surgery Study: Risk Factors and Angiographic Coronary Artery Disease: A Report from the Coronary Artery Surgery Study (CASS), *Circulation,* 62:254, 1980.
11. Havlick, R. J., and Feinleib, M. (eds): "Proceedings of the Conference on the Decline in Coronary Heart Disease Mortality," U.S. Department of Health, Education, and Welfare, Public Health Service, National Institutes of Health, DHEW Publ. NIH-79-1610, 1979.

11a. Pyörälä, K., Epstein, F. H. and Kornitzer, M. (eds.): Changing Trends in Congenital Heart Disease Mortality. Possible Explanations, *Am. J. Cardiol.,* 72:1, 1985.

12. Walker, W. J.: Changing United States Life-Style and Declining Vascular Mortality: Cause or Coincidence, *N. Engl. J. Med.,* 297:163, 1977.
13. Gillum, R. F., Folsom, A. R., and Blackburn, H.: Decline in Coronary Heart Disease Mortality. Old Questions and New Facts, *Am. J. Med.,* 76:1055, 1984.
14. Steinberg, D.: Lipoproteins and Atherosclerosis. A Look Back and a Look Ahead, *Arteriosclerosis,* 3:283, 1983.
15. Stamler, J.: Primary Prevention of Coronary Heart Disease. The Last 20 Years, *Am. J. Cardiol.,* 47:722, 1981.

15a. Goldman, L., and Cook, E. F.: The Decline in Ischemic Heart Disease Mortality Rates. An Analysis of the Comparative Effects of Medical Interventions and Changes in Lifestyle, *Ann. Intern. Med.,* 101:825, 1984.

15b. Levy, R. I. (Chm.): The Decline in Coronary Heart Disease Mortality. Status and Perspectives on the Role of Cholesterol, *Am. J. Cardiol.,* 54:1C, 1984.

16. Lauer, R. M., and Shekelle, R. B. (eds.), "Childhood Prevention of Atherosclerosis and Hypertension," Raven Press, New York, 1980.
17. Strong, W. B.: Atherosclerosis: Its Pediatric Roots, in N. M. Kaplan and J. Stamler (eds.), "Prevention of Coronary Heart Disease. Practical Management of the Risk Factors," W. B. Saunders Company, Philadelphia, 1983, p. 20.
18. Berenson, G. S., Blonde, C. V., Farris, R. P., et al.: Cardiovascular Disease Risk Factor Variables during the First Year of Life, *Am. J. Dis. Child.,* 133:1049, 1979.
19. Multiple Risk Factor Intervention Trial Research Group: Multiple Risk Factor Intervention Trial. Risk Factor Changes and Mortality Results, *JAMA,* 248:1465, 1982.
20. May, G. S., Eberlein, K. A., Furberg, C. D., Passamani, E. R., and DeMets, D. L.: Secondary Prevention after Myocardial Infarction: A Review of Long-Term Trials, *Prog. Cardiovasc. Dis.,* 24:331, 1982.
21. World Health Organization: "Rehabilitation and Comprehensive Secondary Prevention after Acute Myocardial Infarction. Report on a Study, EURO Reports and Studies 84 (document ICP/CVD 005). WHO Regional Office for Europe, Copenhagen, 1983.
22. Kornitzer, M., DeBacker, G., Dramaix, M., et al.: Belgian Heart Disease Prevention Project: Incidence and Mortality Results, *Lancet,* 1:1066, 1983.
23. Shurtleff D.: Some Characteristics Related to the Incidence of Cardiovascular Disease and Death: Framingham Study, 18-Year Follow-Up, in W. B. Kannel and T. Gordon (eds.), "The Framingham Study. An Epidemiological Investigation of Cardiovascular Disease," Section 30, U.S. Department of Health, Education, and Welfare, Public Health Service, National Institutes of Health, DHEW Publ. NIH-74-599, 1974.
24. Keys, A. (ed.): Coronary Heart Disease in Seven Countries, *Circulation,* 41(suppl. 1):1, 1970.
25. Rosenman, R. H., Brand, R. J., Jenkins, C. D., Friedman, M., Straus, R., and Wurm, M.: Coronary Heart Disease in the Western Collaborative Group Study. Final Follow-Up Experience of $8\frac{1}{2}$ Years, *JAMA,* 233:872, 1975.
26. Epstein, F. H., Napier, J. A., Block, W. D., et al.: The Tecumseh Study. Design, Progress, and Perspectives, *Arch. Environ. Health,* 21:402, 1970.
27. Kleinbaum, D. G., Kupper, L. L., Cassel, J. C., and Tyroler, H. A.: Multivariate Analysis of Risk of Coronary Heart Disease in Evans County, Ga., *Arch. Intern. Med.,* 128:943, 1971.
28. The Pooling Project Research Group: Relationship of Blood Pressure, Serum Cholesterol, Smoking Habit, Relative Weight and ECG Abnormalities to Incidence of Major

Coronary Events: Final Report of the Pooling Project, *J. Chron. Dis.*, 31:201, 1978.
29. Hypertension Detection and Follow-Up Program Cooperative Group: Five Year Findings of the Hypertension Detection and Follow-Up Program: I. Reduction in Mortality of Persons with High Blood Pressure, Including Mild Hypertension, *JAMA*, 242:2562, 1979.
30. Hypertension Detection and Follow-Up Program Cooperative Group: Five Year Findings of the Hypertension Detection and Follow-Up Program: II. Mortality by Race-Sex and Age, *JAMA*, 242:2572, 1979.
31. Lipid Research Clinics Program: The Lipid Research Clinics Coronary Primary Prevention Trial Results: I. Reduction in Incidence of Coronary Heart Disease. II. The Relationship of Reduction in Incidence of Coronary Heart Disease to Cholesterol Lowering, *JAMA*, 251:351, 365, 1984.
32. Chesebro, J. H., Fuster, V., Elveback, L. R., and Frye, R. L.: Strong Family History and Cigarette Smoking as Risk Factors of Coronary Artery Disease in Young Adults, *Br. Heart J.*, 47:78, 1982.
33. Barrett-Connor, E., and Khaw, K.: Family History of Heart Attack as an Independent Predictor of Death due to Cardiovascular Disease, *Circulation*, 69:1065, 1984.
33a. Shea, S., Ottman, R., Gabrieli, C., Stein, Z., and Nichols, A.: Family History as an Independent Risk Factor for Coronary Artery Disease, *J. Am. Coll. Cardiol.*, 4:793, 1984.
34. St. Clair, R. W.: Atherosclerosis Regression in Animal Models: Current Concepts of Cellular and Biochemical Mechanisms, *Prog. Cardiovasc. Dis.*, 26:109, 1983.
35. Schettler, G., Strange, E., and Wissler, R. W. (eds.): "Atherosclerosis—Is It Reversible?" Springer-Verlag, New York, 1978.
36. Armstrong, M. L.: Regression of Atherosclerosis, in R. Paoletti and A. M. Gotto, Jr., (eds.), "Atherosclerosis Reviews," Raven Press, New York, vol. I, 1976, p. 137.
37. Kramsch, D. M., Aspen, A. J., Abramowitz, B. M., Kreimendahl, T., and Hood, W. B., Jr.: Reduction of Coronary Atherosclerosis by Moderate Conditioning Exercise in Monkeys on an Atherogenic Diet, *N. Engl. J. Med.*, 305:1483, 1981.
38. Fritz, K. E., Augustyn, J. M., Jarmolych, J., Daoud, A. S., and Lee, K. T.: Regression of Advanced Atherosclerosis in Swine. Chemical Studies, *Arch. Pathol. Lab. Med.*, 100:380, 1976.
39. Wissler, W. R., and Vesselinovitch, D.: Combined Effect of Cholestyramine and Probucol on Regression of Atherosclerosis in Rhesus Monkey Aortas, *Appl. Pathol.*, 1:89, 1983.
40. Vesselinovitch, D., Wissler, R. W., Schaffner, T., Hughes, R., and Borensztajn, J.: Reversal of Advanced Atherosclerosis in Rhesus Monkeys by Prudent Diet with and without Cholestyramine, *Circulation*, 55, 56 (suppl. 3):144, 1977.
41. Armstrong, M. L., and Megan, M. B.: Arterial Fibrous Proteins in Cynomolgus Monkeys after Atherogenic and Regression Diets, *Circ. Res.*, 36:256, 1975.
42. Hauss, W. H., Wissler, R. W., and Lehmann, R. (eds.): "International Symposium. State of Prevention and Therapy in Human Arteriosclerosis and in Animal Models," Westdeutscher Verlag, Opladen, Germany, 1978.
43. Rouleau, J.-L., Parmley, W. W., Stevens, J., et al.: Verapamil Suppresses Atherosclerosis in Cholesterol-Fed Rabbits, *J. Am. Coll. Cardiol.*, 1:1453, 1983.
44. Malinow, M. R.: Atherosclerosis: Progression, Regression, and Resolution, *Am. Heart J.*, 108:1523, 1984.
45. Blankenhorn, D. H.: The Prevention, Deceleration, and Possible Regression of Coronary Atherosclerosis, in J. W. Hurst (ed.): "Update III: The Heart," McGraw-Hill Book Company, New York, 1980, p. 23.
46. Blankenhorn, D. H.: Studies of Regression/Progression of Atherosclerosis in Man, in G. W. Manning and M. D. Haust (eds.), "Atherosclerosis: Metabolic, Morphologic, and Clinical Aspects," *Adv. Exp. Biol. Med.*, vol. 82, Plenum Press, New York, 1977, p. 453.
47. Buchwald, H., Moore, R. B., and Varco, R. L.: The Partial Ileal Bypass Operation in Treatment of the Hyperlipidemias, in D. Kritchevsky, R. Paoletti, and W. Holmes (eds.), "Atherosclerosis: Metabolic, Morphologic, and Clinical Aspects," *Adv. Exp. Biol. Med.*, vol. 63, Plenum Press, New York, 1975, p. 221.
48. Barndt, R., Jr., Blankenhorn, D. H., Crawford, D. W., and Brooks, S. H.: Regression and Progression of Early Femoral Atherosclerosis in Treated Hyperlipoproteinemic Patients, *Ann. Intern. Med.*, 86:139, 1977.
49. Zelis, R., Mason, D. T., Braunwald, E., and Levy, R. I.: Effects of Hyperlipoproteinemias and Their Treatment on the Peripheral Circulation, *J. Clin. Invest.*, 49:1007, 1970.
50. Moore, R. B., Buchwald, H., Varco, R. L., and the Participants in the Program on the Surgical Control of the Hyperlipidemias: The Effect of Partial Ileal Bypass on Plasma Lipoproteins, *Circulation*, 62:469, 1980.
50a. Koivisto, P., and Miettinen, T. A.: Long-term Effects of Ileal Bypass on Lipoproteins in Patients with Familial Hypercholesterolemia, *Circulation*, 70:290, 1984.
51. King, M. E. E., Breslow, J. L., and Lees, R. S.: Plasma-Exchange Therapy of Homozygous Familial Hypercholesterolemia, *N. Engl. J. Med.*, 302:1457, 1980.
52. Stoffel, W., Borberg, H., and Greve, V.: Application of Specific Extracorporeal Removal of Low Density Lipoprotein in Familial Hypercholesterolaemia, *Lancet*, 2:1005, 1981.
53. Starzl, T. E., Putnam, C. W., and Koep, L. J.: Portacaval Shunt and Hyperlipidemia, *Arch. Surg.*, 113:71, 1978.
54. Starzl, T. E., Bahson, H. T., Hardesty, R. L., et al.: Heart-Liver Transplantation in a Patient with Familial Hypercholesterolaemia, *Lancet*, 1:1382, 1984.
55. Farquhar, J. W.: The Community-Based Model of Life Style Intervention Trials, *Am. J. Epidemiol.*, 108:103, 1978.
56. Puska, P., Tuomilehto, J., Salonen, J., et al.: Changes in Coronary Risk Factors during Comprehensive Five-Year Community Programme to Control Cardiovascular Diseases (North Karelia Project), *Br. Med J.*, 2:1173, 1979.
57. Ehnholm, C., Huttunen, J. K., Pietinen, P., et al.: Effect of Diet on Serum Lipoproteins in a Population with a High Risk of Coronary Heart Disease, *N. Engl. J. Med.*, 307:850, 1982.
58. Miettinen, T. A., Huttunen, J. K., Naukkarinen, V., Mattila, S., Strandberg, T., and Kumlin, T.: Multifactorial Primary Prevention of Cardiovascular Diseases, *Circulation*, 64(suppl. 4):IV–80, 1981. (Abstract.)
59. Working Group on Arteriosclerosis of the National Heart, Lung, and Blood Institute: "Arteriosclerosis 1981," U.S. Department of Health and Human Services, Public Health Service, National Institutes of Health, NIH Publ. 82-2035, Sept. 1981, vol. 2.
60. Kannel, W. B., Castelli, W. P., and Gordon, T.: Cholesterol in the Prediction of Atherosclerotic Disease. New Perspectives Based on the Framingham Study, *Ann. Intern. Med.*, 90:85, 1979.
61. Holmes, D. R., Jr., Elveback, L. R., Frye, R. L., Kottke, B. A., and Ellefson, R. D.: Association of Risk Factor Variables and Coronary Artery Disease Documented with Angiography, *Circulation*, 63:293, 1981.
62. Swanson, J. O., Pierpont, G., and Adicoff, A.: Serum High Density Lipoprotein Cholesterol Correlates with Presence but Not Severity of Coronary Artery Disease, *Am. J. Med.*, 71:235, 1981.
63. Maciejko, J. J., Holmes, D. R., Kottke, B. A., Zinsmeister, A. R., Dinh, D. M., and Mao, S. J. T.: Apolipoprotein A-1 as a Marker of Angiographically Assessed Coronary-rtery Disease, *N. Engl. J. Med.*, 309:385, 1983.
64. Robertson, T. L., Kato, H., Gordon, T., et al.: Epidemiologic Studies of Coronary Heart Disease and Stroke in Japanese Men Living in Japan, Hawaii, and California. Coronary Heart Disease Risk Factors in Japan and Hawaii, *Am. J. Cardiol.*, 39:244, 1977.
65. Abraham, S., Rifkind, B. M., Feinleib, M., et al.: Decline in Serum Cholesterol Levels among Adults in the United States, *Circulation* 68(suppl. 3):III–179, 1983. (Abstract.)

66. Grundy, S. M.: Absorption and Metabolism of Dietary Cholesterol, *Ann. Rev. Nutr.,* 3:71, 1983.
67. McGill, H. C., Jr.: The Relationship of Dietary Cholesterol to Serum Cholesterol Concentration and to Atherosclerosis in Man, *Am. J. Clin. Nutr.,* 32:2664, 1979.
68. Shekelle, R. B., Shryock, A. M., Paul, O., et al.: Diet, Serum Cholesterol, and Death from Coronary Heart Disease. The Western Electric Study, *N. Engl. J. Med.,* 304:65, 1981.
69. Keys, A., Anderson, J. T., and Grande, F.: Prediction of Serum-Cholesterol Responses of Man to Changes in Fats in the Diet, *Lancet,* 2:959, 1957.
70. Hegsted, D. M., McGandy, R. B., Myers, M. L., and Stare, F. J.: Quantitative Effects of Dietary Fat on Serum Cholesterol in Man, *Am. J. Clin. Nutr.,* 17:281, 1965.
70a. Blackburn, H., and Jacobs, D.: Sources of the Diet-Heart Controversy: Confusion over Population versus Individual Correlations, *Circulation,* 70:775, 1984.
71. National Diet-Heart Study Research Group: The National Diet-Heart Study Final Report, *Circulation,* 37(suppl. 1):1, 1968.
72. Dayton, S., Pearce, M. L., Hashimoto, S., Dixon, W. J., and Tomiyasu, U.: A Controlled Clinical Trial of a Diet High in Unsaturated Fat in Preventing Complications of Atherosclerosis, *Circulation,* 40(suppl. 2):1, 1969.
73. Turpeinen, O.: Effect of Cholesterol-Lowering Diet on Mortality from Coronary Heart Disease and Other Causes, *Circulation,* 59:1, 1979.
74. Hjermann, I., Holme, I., Velve Byre, K., and Leren, P.: Effect of Diet and Smoking Intervention on the Incidence of Coronary Heart Disease. Report from the Oslo Study Group of a Randomised Trial in Healthy Men, *Lancet,* 2:1303, 1981.
75. Report of the Committee of Principal Investigators: W.H.O. Cooperative Trial on Primary Prevention of Ischaemic Heart Disease Using Clofibrate to Lower Serum Cholesterol: Mortality Follow-Up, *Lancet,* 2:379, 1980.
76. Brensike, J. F., Levy, R. I., Kelsey, S. F., et al.: Effects of Therapy with Cholestyramine on Progression of Coronary Atherosclerosis: Results of the NHLBI Type II Coronary Intervention Study, *Circulation,* 69:313, 1984.
77. Levy, R. I., Brensike, J. F., Epstein, S. E., et al.: The Influence of Changes in Lipid Values Induced by Cholestyramine and Diet on Progression of Coronary Artery Disease: Results of the NHLBI Type II Coronary Intervention Study, *Circulation* 69:325, 1984.
77a. Consensus Conference: Lowering Blood Cholesterol to Prevent Heart Disease, *JAMA,* 253:2080, 1985.
78. Sacks, F. M., Castelli, W. P., Donner, A., and Kass, E. H.: Plasma Lipids and Lipoproteins in Vegetarians and Controls, *N. Engl. J. Med.,* 292:1148, 1975.
79. Walden, R. T., Schaefer, L. A., Lemon, F. R., Sunshine, A., and Wynder, E. L.: Effect of Environment on the Serum Cholesterol-Triglyceride Distribution among Seventh-Day Adventists, *Am. J. Med.,* 36:269, 1964.
80. Hulley, S. B., Rosenman, R. H., Bawol, R. D., and Brand, R. J.: Epidemiology as a Guide to Clinical Decisions. The Association between Triglyceride and Coronary Heart Disease, *N. Engl. J. Med.,* 302:1383, 1980.
81. NIH Consensus Development Conference Summary: Treatment of Hypertriglyceridemia, *Arteriosclerosis,* 4:296, 1984.
82. Bradley, D. D., Wingerd, J., Petitti, D. B., Krauss, R. M., and Ramcharan, S.: Serum High-Density-Lipoprotein Cholesterol in Women Using Oral Contraceptives, Estrogens and Progestins, *N. Engl. J. Med.,* 299:17, 1978.
83. DiGirolamo, M. and Schlant, R. C.: High-Density Lipoproteins, in J. W. Hurst (ed.), "Update IV: The Heart," McGraw-Hill Book Company, New York, 1981, p 153.
84. Kesaniemi, Y. A., and Grundy, S. M.: Overproduction of Low Density Lipoprotein Associated with Coronary Heart Disease, *Arteriosclerosis,* 3:40, 1983.
85. Gordon, T., Castelli, W. P., Hjortland, M. C., Kannel, W. B., and Dawber, T. R.: High Density Lipoprotein as a Protective Factor against Coronary Artery Disease. The Framingham Study, *Am. J. Med.,* 62:707, 1977.
86. Gotto, A. M., Jr., (ed.): Symposium on High-Density Lipoproteins and Coronary Artery Disease: Effects of Diet, Exercise, and Pharmacologic Intervention, *Am. J. Cardiol.,* 52:1B, 1983.
87. Castelli, W. P., Doyle, J. T., Gordon, T. et al.: HDL Cholesterol and Other Lipids in Coronary Heart Disease. The Cooperative Lipoprotein Phenotyping Study, *Circulation,* 55:767, 1977.
88. Miller, N. E., Hammett, F., Saltissi, S., et al.: Relation of Angiographically Defined Coronary Artery Disease to Plasma Lipoprotein Subfractions and Apolipoproteins, *Br. Med. J.,* 282:1741, 1981.
89. Thompson, G.: Apoproteins: Determinants of Lipoprotein Metabolism and Indices of Coronary Risk, *Br. Heart J.,* 51:585, 1984.
90. Brunzell, J. D., Sniderman, A. D., Albers, J. J., and Kwiterovich, P. O., Jr.: Apoproteins B and A-1 and Coronary Artery Disease in Humans, *Arteriosclerosis,* 4:79, 1984.
91. Wood, P. D., and Haskell, W. L.: The Effect of Exercise on Plasma High Density Lipoproteins, *Lipids,* 14:417, 1979.
92. Hartung, G. H., Foreyt, J. P., Mitchell, R. E., Vlasek, I., and Gotto, A. M., Jr.: Relation of Diet to High-Density-Lipoprotein Cholesterol in Middle-Aged Marathon Runners, Joggers, and Inactive Men, *N. Engl. J. Med.,* 302:357, 1980.
93. Tyroler, H. A. (ed.): Epidemiology of Plasma High-Density Lipoprotein Cholesterol Levels. The Lipid Research Clinics Program Prevalence Study, *Circulation,* 62(suppl. 4, part 2):1, 1980.
94. Garrison, R. J., Kannel, W. B., Feinleib, M., Castelli, W. P., McNamara, P. M., and Padgett, S. J.: Cigarette Smoking and HDL Cholesterol. The Framingham Offspring Study, *Atherosclerosis,* 30:17, 1978.
95. Gotto, A. M., Jr., and Jones, P.: How to Lower the Serum Cholesterol, in J. W. Hurst (ed.), "Clinical Essays on The Heart," McGraw-Hill Book Company, New York, 1983, p. 233.
96. Brown, V. W., Goldberg, I. J., and Ginsberg, H. N.: Treatment of Common Lipoprotein Disorders, *Prog. Cardiovasc. Dis.,* 27:1, 1984.
97. Grundy, S. M., Ahrens, E. H., Jr., and Salen, G.: Interruption of the Enterohepatic Circulation of Bile Acids in Man: Comparative Effects of Cholestyramine and Ileal Exclusion on Cholesterol Metabolism, *J. Lab. Clin. Med.,* 78:94, 1971.
98. Moutafis, C. D., Simons, L. A., Myant, N. B., Adams, P. W., and Wynn, V.: The Effect of Cholestyramine on the Faecal Excretion of Bile Acids and Neutral Steroids in Familial Hypercholesterolaemia, *Atherosclerosis,* 26:329, 1977.
99. Door, A. E., Gunderson, K., Schneider, J. C., Jr., Spencer, T. W., and Martin, W. B.: Colestipol Hydrochloride in Hypercholesterolemic Patients—Effect on Serum Cholesterol and Mortality, *J. Chron. Dis.,* 31:5, 1978.
100. Goldstein, J. L., and Brown, M. S.: The LDL Receptor Defect in Familial Hypercholesterolemia. Implications for Pathogenesis and Therapy, *Med. Clin. North Am.,* 66:335, 1982.
101. Shepherd, J., Packard, C. J., Bicker, S., Lawrie, T. D. V., and Morgan, H. G.: Cholestyramine Promotes Receptor-Mediated Low-Density-Lipoprotein Catabolism, *N. Engl. J. Med.,* 302:1219, 1980.
102. Grundy, S. M.: Treatment of Hypercholesterolemia by Interference with Bile Acid Metabolism, *Arch. Intern. Med.,* 130:638, 1972.
103. Miller, N. E., Clifton-Bligh, P., and Nestel, P. J.: Effects of Colestipol, a New Bile-Acid-Sequestering Resin, on Cholesterol Metabolism in Man, *J. Lab. Clin. Med.,* 82:876, 1973.
104. Goodman, D. S., Noble, R. P., and Dell, R. B.: The Effects of Colestipol Resin and of Colestipol plus Clofibrate on the Turnover of Plasma Cholesterol in Man, *J. Clin. Invest.,* 52:2646, 1973.
105. Levy, R. I., Fredrickson, D. S., Stone, N. J., et al.: Choles-

tyramine in Type II Hyperlipoproteinemia. A Double-Blind Trial, *Ann. Intern. Med.,* 79:51, 1973.
106. Blum, C. B., Havlik, R. J., and Morganroth, J.: Cholestyramine: An Effective, Twice-Daily Dosage Regimen, *Ann. Intern. Med.,* 85:287, 1976.
107. Grundy, S. M., Mok, H. Y. I., Zech, L., and Berman, M.: Influence of Nicotinic Acid on Metabolism of Cholesterol and Triglycerides in Man, *J. Lipid Res.,* 22:24, 1981.
108. Shepherd, J., Packard, C. J., Patsch, J. R., Gotto, A. M., Jr., and Taunton, O. D.: Effects of Nicotonic Acid Therapy on Plasma High Density Lipoprotein Subfraction Distribution and Composition and on Apolipoprotein A Metabolism, *J. Clin Invest.,* 63:858, 1979.
109. Nestel, P. J., and Billington, T.: Effects of Probucol on Low Density Lipoprotein Removal and High Density Lipoprotein Synthesis, *Atherosclerosis,* 38:203, 1981.
110. McCaughan, D.: The Long-Term Effects of Probucol on Serum Lipid Levels, *Arch. Intern. Med.,* 141:1428, 1981.
111. Miettinen, T. A., and Toivonen, I.: Treatment of Severe and Mild Hypercholesterolaemia with Probucol and Neomycin, *Postgrad. Med. J.,* 51(suppl. 8):71, 1975.
112. Mellies, M. J., Gartside, P. S., Glatfelter, L., et al.: Effects of Probucol on Plasma Cholesterol, High and Low Density Lipoprotein Cholesterol, and Apolipoproteins A-1 and A-2 in Adults with Primary Familial Hypercholesterolemia, *Metabolism,* 29:956, 1980.
113. Heel, R. C., Brogden, R. N., Speight, T. M., and Avery, G. S.: Probucol: A Review of its Pharmacological Properties and Therapeutic Use in Patients with Hypercholesterolaemia, *Drugs,* 15:409, 1978.
114. Sedaghat, A., Samuel, P., Crouse, J. R., and Ahrens, E. H., Jr.: Effects of Neomycin on Absorption, Synthesis and/or Flux of Cholesterol in Man, *J. Clin. Invest.,* 55:12, 1975.
115. Miettinen, T. A.: Effects of Neomycin Alone and in Combination with Cholestyramine on Serum Cholesterol and Fecal Steroids in Hypercholesterolemic Subjects, *J. Clin. Invest.,* 64:1485, 1979.
116. Jones, P., and Gotto, A. M., Jr.: Drug Treatment of Hyperlipidemia, *Mod. Conc. Cardiovasc. Dis.,* 53:53, 1984.
117. Samuel P: Treatment of Hypercholesterolemia with Neomycin—A Time for Reappraisal, *N. Engl. J. Med.,* 301:595, 1979.
118. Kane, J. P., Malloy, M. J., Tun, P., et al.: Normalization of Low-Density-Lipoprotein Levels in Heterozygous Familial Hypercholesterolemia with a Combined Drug Regimen, *N. Engl. J. Med.,* 304:251, 1981.
119. Kuo, P. T., Kostis, J. B., Moreyra, A. E., and Hayes, J. A.: Familial Type II Hyperlipoproteinemia with Coronary Heart Disease. Effect of Diet-Colestipol-Nicotinic Acid Treatment, *Chest,* 79:286, 1981.
120. Illingworth, D. R., Phillipson, B. E., Rapp, J. H., and Connor, W. E.: Colestipol plus Nicotinic Acid in Treatment of Heterozygous Familial Hypercholesterolaemia, *Lancet,* 1:296, 1981.
121. Hunninghake, D.: Drug Treatment of Type II Hyperlipoproteinemia. Effects on Plasma Lipid and Lipoprotein Levels, in A. Gotto, Jr., L. C. Smith, and B. Allen (eds.), "Atherosclerosis V" Springer-Verlag, New York, 1980, p. 74.
122. Dujovne, C. A., Krehbiel, P., Decoursey, S., et al.: Probucol with Colestipol in the Treatment of Hypercholesterolemia, *Ann. Int. Med.,* 100:477, 1984.
123. Mabuchi, H., Sakai, T., Sakai, Y., et al.: Reduction of Serum Cholesterol in Heterozygous Patients with Familial Hypercholesterolemia. Additive Effects of Compactin and Cholestyramine, *N. Engl. J. Med.,* 308:609, 1983.
124. Kovanen, P. T., Bilheimer, D. W., Goldstein, J. L., Jaramillo, J. J., and Brown, M. S.: Regulatory Role for Hepatic Low Density Lipoprotein Receptors *in Vivo* in the Dog, *Proc. Natl. Acad. Sci. U.S.A.,* 78:1194, 1981.
125. Pangburn, S. H., Newton, R. S., Chang, C.-M., Weinstein, D. B., and Steinberg, D.: Receptor-Mediated Catabolism of Homologous Low Density Lipoproteins in Cultured Pig Hepatocytes, *J. Biol. Chem.,* 256:3340, 1981.
126. Bilheimer, D. W., Grundy, S. M., Brown, M. S., and Goldstein, J. L.: Mevinolin and Colestipol Stimulate Receptor-Mediated Clearance of Low Density Lipoprotein from Plasma in Familial Hypercholesterolemia Heterozygotes, *Proc. Natl. Acad. Sci. U.S.A.,* 80:4124, 1983.
127. Lewis, J. E.: Long-Term Use of Gemfibrozil (Lopid) in the Treatment of Dyslipidemia, *Angiology,* 33:603, 1982.
128. Libow, M. and Schlant, R. C.: Smoking and Heart Disease, in P. N. Yu and J. F. Goodwin (eds.), "Progress in Cardiology," Lea & Febiger, Philadelphia, vol. 11, 1982, p. 131.
129. Kaufman, D. W., Helmrich, S. P., Rosenberg, L., Miettinen, O. S., and Shapiro, S.: Nicotine and Carbon Monoxide Content of Cigarette Smoke and the Risk of Myocardial Infarction in Young Men, *N. Engl. J. Med.,* 308:409, 1983.
130. "Smoking and Health. A Report of the Surgeon General," U.S. Department of Health, Education, and Welfare, Public Health Service, Office on Smoking and Health, DHEW Publ. (PHS) 79-50066, 1979.
131. Doyle, J. T., Dawber, T. R., Kannel, W. B., Kinch, S. H., and Kahn, H. A.: The Relationship of Cigarette Smoking to Coronary Heart Disease. The Second Report of the Combined Experience of the Albany, N.Y., and Framingham, Mass., Studies, *JAMA,* 190:886, 1964.
132. Gordon, T., Kannel, W. B., and McGee, D.: Death and Coronary Attacks in Men after Giving up Cigarette Smoking. A Report from the Framingham Study, *Lancet,* 2:1345, 1974.
133. "The Health Consequences of Smoking for Women. A Report of the Surgeon General," U.S. Department of Health and Human Services, Public Health Service Office on Smoking and Health, 1980.
133a. Klein, L. W.: Cigarette Smoking, Atherosclerosis and the Coronary Hemodynamic Response: A Unifying Hypothesis, *J. Am. Coll. Cardiol.,* 4:972, 1984.
134. Brischetto, C. S., Connor, W. E., Connor, S. L., and Matarazzo, J. D.: Plasma Lipid and Lipoprotein Profiles of Cigarette Smokers from Randomly Selected Families: Enhancement of Hyperlipidemia and Depression of High-Density Lipoprotein, *Am. J. Cardiol.,* 52:675, 1983.
135. Rose, G., Hamilton, P. J. S, Colwell, L., and Shipley, M. J.: A Randomised Controlled Trial of Anti-Smoking Advice: 10 Year Results, *J. Epidemiol. Comm. Health,* 36:102, 1982.
136. Hammond, E. C.: Smoking in Relation to Mortality and Morbidity. Findings in First Thirty-Four Months of Follow-up in a Prospective Study Started in 1959, *JNCI.,* 32:1161, 1964.
137. Freis, E. D.: Salt, Volume and the Prevention of Hypertension, *Circulation* 53:589, 1976.
138. Arkwright, P. D., Beilin, L. J., Rouse, I., Armstrong, B. K., and Vandongen, R.: Effects of Alcohol Use and Other Aspects of Lifestyle on Blood Pressure Levels and Prevalence of Hypertension in a Working Population, *Circulation,* 66:60, 1982.
139. Chobanian, A. V.: The Influence of Hypertension and Other Hemodynamic Factors in Atherogenesis, *Prog. Cardiovasc. Dis.,* 26:177, 1983.
140. Veterans Administration Cooperative Study Group on Antihypertensive Agents: Effects of Treatment on Morbidity in Hypertension. Results in Patients with Diastolic Blood Pressures Averaging 115 through 129 mm Hg, *JAMA,* 202:1028, 1967.
141. Veterans Administration Cooperative Study Group on Antihypertensive Agents: Effects of Treatment on Morbidity in Hypertension: II. Results in Patients with Diastolic Blood Pressure Averaging 90 through 114 mm Hg, *JAMA,* 213:1143, 1970.
142. Smith, W. M.: Treatment of Mild Hypertension. Results of a Ten-Year Intervention Trial. U.S. Public Health Service Hospitals Cooperative Study Group, *Circ. Res.,* 40(suppl. 1):I-98,, 1977.
143. Berglund, G., Sannerstedt, R., Andersson, O., et al.: Coronary Heart-Disease after Treatment of Hypertension, *Lancet,* 1:1, 1978.
144. The Hypertension Detection and Follow-Up Program Co-

operative Research Group: Five Year Findings of the Hypertension Detection and Follow-Up Program. Effect of Stepped Care Treatment on the Incidence of Myocardial Infarction and Angina Pectoris, *Hypertension,* 6(supp. I): I–198, 1984.
145. Report by the Management Committee: The Australian Therapeutic Trial in Mild Hypertension, *Lancet,* 1:1261, 1980.
146. The Joint National Committee on Detection, Evaluation, and Treatment of High Blood Pressure: The 1984 Report of the Joint National Committee on Detection, Evaluation, and Treatment of High Blood Pressure, *Arch. Intern. Med.,* 144:1045, 1984.
146a. The Hypertension Detection and Follow-Up Program Cooperative Research Group: The Effect of Antihypertensive Drug Treatment on Mortality in the Presence of Resting Electrocardiographic Abnormalities at Baseline: The HDFP Experience, *Circulation,* 70:996, 1984.
147. Feinleib, M.: Genetics, in N. M. Kaplan and J. Stamler (eds.), "Prevention of Coronary Heart Disease. Practical Management of the Risk Factors," W. B. Saunders Company, Philadelphia, 1983, p. 120.
148. Keys, A.: Coronary Heart Disease–The Global Picture, *Atherosclerosis,* 22:149, 1975.
149. Hubert, H. B., Feinleib, M., McNamara, P. M., and Castelli, W. P.: Obesity as an Independent Risk Factor for Cardiovascular Disease: A 26-Year Follow-Up of Participants in the Framingham Heart Study, *Circulation,* 67:968, 1983.
150. Ashley, F. W., Jr., and Kannel, W. B.: Relation of Weight Change to Changes in Atherogenic Traits: The Framingham Study, *J. Chronic Dis.,* 27:103, 1974.
151. Kannel, W. B., and McGee, D. L.: Diabetes and Cardiovascular Risk Factors: The Framingham Study, *Circulation,* 59:8, 1979.
152. Waters, D. D., Halphen, C., Theroux, P., David, P.-R., and Mizgala, H. F.: Coronary Artery Disease in Young Women: Clinical and Angiographic Features and Correlation with Risk Factors, *Am. J. Cardiol.,* 42:41, 1978.
153. Ruderman, N. B., and Haudenschild, S.: Diabetes as an Atherogenic Factor, *Prog. Cardiovasc. Dis.,* 26:373, 1984.
154. Dortimer, A. C., Shenoy, P. N., Shiroff, R. A., et al.: Diffuse Coronary Artery Disease in Diabetic Patients. Fact or Fiction? *Circulation,* 57:133, 1978.
155. Vigorito, C., Betocchi, S., Bonzani, G., et al.: Severity of Coronary Artery Disease in Patients with Diabetes Mellitus. Angiographic Study of 34 Diabetic and 120 Nondiabetic Patients, *Am. Heart J.,* 100:782, 1980.
156. Garcia, M. J., McNamara, P. M., Gordon, T. and Kannel, W. B.: Morbidity and Mortality of Diabetics in the Framingham Population. Sixteen Year Follow-Up Study, *Diabetes,* 23:105, 1974.
157. Orchard, T. J., Becker, D. J., Kuller, L. H., Wagener, D. K., La Porte, R. E., and Drash, A. L.: Age and Sex Variations in Glucose Tolerance and Insulin Responses: Parallels with Cardiovascular Risk, *J. Chron. Dis.* 35:123, 1982.
158. Stamler, R., Stamler, J., Lindberg, H. A., et al.: Asymptomatic Hyperglycemia and Coronary Heart Disease in Middle-Aged Men in Two Employed Populations in Chicago, *J. Chron. Dis.,* 32:805, 1979.
159. Froelicher, V. F., and Oberman, A.: Analysis of Epidemiologic Studies of Physical Inactivity as a Risk Factor for Coronary Artery Disease, *Prog. Cardiovasc. Dis.,* 15:41, 1972.
160. Eichner, E. R.: Exercise and Heart Disease. Epidemiology of the "Exercise Hypothesis," *Am. J. Med.,* 75:1008, 1983.
161. Paffenbarger, R. S., Jr., and Hale, W. E.: Work Activity and Coronary Heart Mortality, *N. Engl. J. Med.,* 292:545, 1975.
162. Kannel, W. B., and Sorlie, P.: Some Health Benefits of Physical Activity. The Framingham Study, *Arch. Intern. Med.,* 139:857, 1979.
163. Morris, J. N., Everitt, M. G., Pollard, R., Chave, S. P. W., and Semmence, A. M.: Vigorous Exercise in Leisure-Time: Protection Against Coronary Heart Disease, *Lancet,* 2:1207, 1980.
164. Paffenbarger, R. S., Jr., Wing, A. L., and Hyde, R. T.: Physical Activity as an Index of Heart Attack Risk in College Alumni, *Am. J. Epidemiol.,* 108:161, 1978.
165. Garcia-Palmieri, M. R., Costas, R. Jr., Cruz-Vidal, M., Sorlie, P. D., and Havlik, R. J.: Increased Physical Activity: A Protective Factor against Heart Attacks in Puerto Rico, *Am. J. Cardiol.,* 50:749, 1982.
166. Gibbons, L. W., Blair, S. N., Cooper, K. H., and Smith, M.: Association between Coronary Heart Disease Risk Factors and Physical Fitness in Healthy Adult Women, *Circulation,* 67:977, 1983.
167. Hennekens, C. H., and MacMahon, B.: Oral Contraceptives and Myocardial Infarction, *N. Engl. J. Med.,* 296:1166, 1977.
168. Stadel, B. V.: Oral Contraceptives and Cardiovascular Disease, *N. Engl. J. Med.,* 305:612, 1981.
169. Gordon, T., Kannel, W. B., Hjortland, M. C., and McNamara, P. M.: Menopause and Coronary Heart Disease. The Framingham Study, *Ann. Intern. Med.,* 89:157, 1978.
170. Barrett-Conner, E., Brown, W. V., Turner, J., Austin, M., and Criqui, M. H.: Heart Disease Risk Factors and Hormone Use in Postmenopausal Women, *JAMA,* 241:2167, 1979.
171. Bain, C., Willett, W., Hennekens, C. H., Rosner, B., Belanger, C., and Speizer, F. E.: Use of Postmenopausal Hormones and Risk of Myocardial Infarction, *Circulation,* 64:42, 1981.
172. Bush, T. L., Cowan, L. D., Barrett-Connor, E., et al.: Estrogen Use and All-Cause Mortality. Preliminary Results from the Lipid Research Clinics Program Follow Up Study, *JAMA,* 249:903, 1983.
173. Herd, J. A., and Weiss, S. M.: "Behavior and Arteriosclerosis," Plenum Press, New York, 1983.
174. Jenkins, C. D.: Recent Evidence Supporting Psychologic and Social Risk Factors for Coronary Disease, *N. Engl. J. Med.,* 294:987, 1033, 1976.
175. Haynes, S. G., Feinleib, M., and Kannel, W. B.: The Relationship of Psychosocial Factors to Coronary Heart Disease in the Framingham Study: III. Eight-Year Incidence of Coronary Heart Disease, *Am. J. Epidemiol.,* 3:37, 1980.
175a. Friedman, M., Thoresen, C. E., and Gill, J.: Type A Behavior: Its Possible Role, Detection, and Alteration in Patients with Ischemic Heart Disease, in J. W. Hurst (ed.), "Update V: The Heart," McGraw-Hill, New York, 1981, p. 87.
176. The Review Panel on Coronary-Prone Behavior and Coronary Heart Disease: Coronary-Prone Behavior and Coronary Heart Disease: A Critical Review, *Circulation,* 63:1199, 1981.
176a. Kasl, S. V.: Social and Psychologic Factors in the Etiology of Coronary Heart Disease in Black Populations: An Explanation of Research Needs. *Am. Heart J.,* 108:660, 1984.
177. Hennekens, C. H.: Alcohol, in N. M. Kaplan, and J. Stamler (eds.), "Prevention of Coronary Heart Disease. Practical Management of the Risk Factors," W. B. Saunders Company, Philadelphia, 1983, p. 130.
178. Dyer, A. R., Stamler, J., Paul, O., et al.: Alcohol, Cardiovascular Risk Factors and Mortality: The Chicago Experience, *Circulation,* 64(suppl. 3):III-20, 1981.
178a. Deutscher, S., Rockette, H. E., and Krishnaswami, V.: Evaluation of Habitual Excessive Alcohol Consumption on Myocardial Infarction Risk in Coronary Disease Patients, *Am. Heart J.,* 108:988, 1984.
179. Gordon, T., and Kannel, W. B.: Drinking Habits and Cardiovascular Disease: The Framingham Study, *Am. Heart J.,* 105:667, 1983.
180. Dawber, T. R., Kannel, W. B., and Gordon, T.: Coffee and Cardiovascular Disease. Observations from the Framingham Study, *N. Engl. J. Med.,* 291:871, 1974.
181. Harlan, W. R., Sharrett, A. R., Weill, H., Turino, G. M., Borhani, N. O., and Resnekov, L.: Impact of Environment

on Cardiovascular Disease. Report of the American Heart Association Task Force on Cardiovascular Disease, *Circulation,* 63:242A, 1981.
182. Garrison, R. J., Havlick, R. J., Harris, R. B., Feinleib, M., Kannel, W. B., and Padgett, S. J.: ABO Blood Group and Cardiovascular Disease. The Framingham Study, *Atherosclerosis,* 25:311, 1976.
183. Heyman, A., Wilkinson, W. E., Heyden, S., et al.: Risk of Stroke in Asymptomatic Persons with Cervical Arterial Bruits. A Population Study in Evans County, Georgia, *N. Engl. J. Med.,* 302:838, 1980.
184. Beard, J. J., II: Serum Uric Acid and Coronary Heart Disease, *Am. Heart J.,* 106:397, 1983.
185. Kannel, W. B.: Some Lessons in Cardiovascular Epidemiology from Framingham, *Am. J. Cardiol.,* 37:268, 1976.
186. Haynes, S. G., Eaker, E. D., and Feinleib, M.: Spouse Behavior and Coronary Heart Disease in Men: Prospective Results from the Framingham Heart Study: I. Concordance of Risk Factors and the Relationship of Psychosocial Status to Coronary Incidence, *Am. J. Epidemiol.,* 118:1, 1983.
187. Eaker, E. D., Haynes, S. G., and Feinleib, M.: Spouse Behavior and Coronary Heart Disease in Men: Prospective Results from the Framingham Heart Study: II. Modification of Risk in Type A Husbands according to the Social and Psychological Status of Their Wives, *Am. J Epidemiol.,* 118:23, 1983.
188. Liu, K., Cedres, L. B., Stamler, J., et al.: Relationship of Education to Major Risk Factors and Death from Coronary Heart Disease, Cardiovascular Diseases and All Causes. Findings of Three Chicago Epidemiologic Studies, *Circulation* 66:1308, 1982.
189. Farquhar, J. W., Maccoby, N., Wood, P. D., et al.: Community Education for Cardiovascular Health, *Lancet,* 1:1192, 1977.
190. Kannel, W. B., and Feinleib, M.: Natural History of Angina Pectoris in the Framingham Study. Prognosis and Survival, *Am. J. Cardiol.,* 29:154, 1972.
191. Schlant, R. C., Forman, S., Stamler, J., and Canner, P. L., for the Coronary Drug Project Research Group: The Natural History of Coronary Heart Disease: Prognostic Factors after Recovery from Myocardial Infarction in 2789 Men. The 5-Year Findings of the Coronary Drug Project, *Circulation,* 66:401, 1982.
192. The Multicenter Postinfarction Research Group: Risk Stratification and Survival after Myocardial Infarction, *N. Engl. J. Med.,* 309:331, 1983.
193. Rapaport, E., and Remedios, P.: The High Risk Patient after Recovery from Myocardial Infarction: Recognition and Management, *J. Am. Coll. Cardiol.,* 1:391, 1983.
194. Pyorala, K., Rapaport, E., Konig, K., Schettler, G., and Diehm, C. (eds.): "Secondary Prevention of Coronary Heart Disease." Workshop of the International Society and Federation of Cardiology, Titisee, 21–24 Oct. 1983, Georg Thieme Verlag, Stuttgart and New York, Thieme-Stratton, Inc., New York, 1983.
195. Heliovaara, M., Karvonen, M. J., Punsar, S., and Haapakoski, J.: Importance of Coronary Risk Factors in the Presence or Absence of Myocardial Ischemia, *Am. J. Cardiol.,* 50:1248, 1982.
196. Rose, G., Reid, D. D., Hamilton, P. J. S., McCartney, P., Keen, H., and Jarrett, R. J.: Myocardial Ischaemia, Risk Factors and Death from Coronary Heart-Disease, *Lancet,* 1:105, 1977.
197. Marmor, A., Geltman, E. M., Schechtman, K., Sobel, B. E., and Roberts, R.: Recurrent Myocardial Infarction: Clinical Predictors and Prognostic Implications, *Circulation,* 66:415, 1982.
198. Weinblatt, E., Shapiro, S., Frank, C. W., and Sager, R. V.: Prognosis of Men after First Myocardial Infarction: Mortality and First Recurrence in Relation to Selected Parameters, *Am. J. Public Health,* 58:1329, 1968.
199. Berge, K. G., Canner, P. L., and Hainline, A., Jr., and the Coronary Drug Project Research Group: High-Density Lipoprotein Cholesterol and Prognosis after Myocardial Infarction, *Circulation,* 66:1176, 1982.
200. Mulcahy, R.: Influence of Cigarette Smoking on Morbidity and Mortality after Myocardial Infarction, *Br. Heart J.,* 49:410, 1983.
201. Aberg, A., Bergstrand, R., Johansson, S. et al.: Cessation of Smoking after Myocardial Infarction. Effects on Mortality after 10 Years, *Br. Heart J.,* 49:416, 1983.
202. Daly, E., Mulcahy, R., Graham, I. M., and Hickey, N.: Long-Term Effect on Mortality of Stopping Smoking after Unstable Angina or Myocardial Infarction, *Br. Med. J.,* 287:324, 1983.
203. Salonen, J. T.: Stopping Smoking and Long-Term Mortality after Acute Myocardial Infarction, *Br. Heart J.,* 43:463, 1980.
204. Hickey, N., Mulcahy, R., Daly, L., Graham, I., O'Donoghue, S., and Kennedy, C.: Cigar and Pipe Smoking Related to Four Year Survival of Coronary Patients, *Br. Heart J.,* 49:423, 1983.
205. Klein, L. W., Ambrose, J., Pichard, A., Holt, J., Gorlin, R., and Teichholz, L. E.: Acute Coronary Hemodynamic Response to Cigarette Smoking in Patients with Coronary Artery Disease, *J. Am. Coll. Cardiol.,* 3:879, 1984.
206. Aronow, W. S.: Effect of Passive Smoking on Angina Pectoris, *N. Engl. J. Med.,* 299:21, 1978.
207. Lutz, J. F., and Hall, W. D.: The Influence of Systemic Arterial Hypertension on the Course of Patients with Coronary Atherosclerosis, in J. W. Hurst (ed.), "Clinical Essays on the Heart," vol. 3, McGraw-Hill, New York, 1984, p. 25.
208. Forman, S., Furberg, C., Wenger, N. K., and Stamler, J., for the Coronary Drug Project Research Group: Blood Pressure in Survivors of Myocardial Infarction, *J. Am. Coll. Cardiol.,* 4:1135, 1984.
209. Kannel, W. B., Sorlie, P., Castelli, W. P., and McGee, D.: Blood Pressure and Survival after Myocardial Infarction: The Framingham Study, *Am. J. Cardiol.,* 45:326, 1980.
210. Stamler, J., Farinaro, E., Mojonnier, L. M., Hall, Y., Moss, D., and Stamler, R.: Prevention and Control of Hypertension by Nutritional-Hygienic Means. Long-Term Experience of the Chicago Coronary Prevention Evaluation Program, *JAMA,* 243:1819, 1980.
211. Frumkin, K., Nathan, R. J., Prout, M. F., and Cohen, M. C.: Nonpharmacologic Control of Essential Hypertension in Man: A Critical Review of the Experimental Literature, *Psychosom. Med.,* 40:294, 1978.
212. Levy, R. I.: Hyperlipoproteinemia and Its Management, *J. Cardiovasc. Med.,* 5:435, 1980.
213. Leren, P.: The Oslo Diet-Heart Study. Eleven Year Report, *Circulation,* 42:935, 1970.
214. Thuesen, L., Thomassen, A., Nielsen, T. T., Bagger, J. P., and Henningsen, P.: Beneficial Effect of a Low-Fat Low-Calorie Diet on Myocardial Energy Metabolism in Patients with Angina Pectoris, *Lancet,* 2:59, 1984.
215. The Coronary Drug Project Research Group: Clofibrate and Niacin in Coronary Heart Disease, *JAMA,* 231:360, 1975.
216. Five-Year Study by a Group of Physicians of the Newcastle upon Tyne Region: Trial of Clofibrate in the Treatment of Ischaemic Heart Disease, *Br. Med. J.,* 4:767, 1971.
217. Report by a Research Committee of the Scottish Society of Physicians: Ischaemic Heart Disease: A Secondary Prevention Trial Using Clofibrate, *Br. Med J.,* 4:775, 1971.
217a. Smith, J. W., Marcus, F. I., and Serokman, R. with the Multicenter Postinfarction Research Group: Prognosis of Patients with Diabetes Mellitus after Acute Myocardial Infarction, *Am. J. Cardiol.,* 54:718, 1984.
218. "Diabetes Mellitus: Second Report of the WHO Expert Committee," WHO Technical Report Series, No. 646, World Health Organization, Geneva, 1980.
219. Coronary Drug Project Research Group: The Prognostic Importance of Plasma Glucose Levels and the Use of Oral Hypoglycemic Drugs after Myocardial Infarction in Men, *Diabetes,* 26:453, 1977.

220. Shaw, L. W.: Effects of a Prescribed Supervised Exercise Program on Mortality and Cardiovascular Morbidity in Patients after a Myocardial Infarction. The National Exercise and Heart Disease Project, *Am. J. Cardiol.,* 48:39, 1981.
221. Stern, M. J., and Cleary, P.: National Exercise and Heart Disease Project. Psychosocial Changes Observed during a Low-Level Exercise Program, *Arch. Intern. Med.,* 141:1463, 1981.
222. Wilhelmsen, L., Sanne, H., Elmfeldt, D., Grimby, G., Tibblin, G., and Wedel, H.: A Controlled Trial of Physical Training after Myocardial Infarction. Effects on Risk Factors, Nonfatal Reinfarction, and Death, *Prev. Med.,* 4:491, 1975.
223. Palatsi, I.: Feasibility of Physical Training after Myocardial Infarction and Its Effect on Return to Work, Morbidity, and Mortality, *Acta. Med. Scand.* (Suppl. 599–602), 1976, p. 1.
224. Blackburn, H., Taylor, H. L., Hamrell, B., Buskirk, E., Nicholas, W. C., and Thorsen, R. D.: Premature Ventricular Complexes Induced by Stress Testing. Their Frequency and Response to Physical Conditioning, *Am. J. Cardiol.,* 31:441, 1973.
225. Diederiks, J. P. M., van der Sluijs, H., Weeda, H. W. H., and Schobre, M. G.: Predictors of Physical Activity One Year after Myocardial Infarction, *Scand. J. Rehabil. Med.,* 15:103, 1983.
226. Stanton, B. A., Jenkins, C. D., Denlinger, P., Savageau, J. A., Weintraub, R. M., and Goldstein, R. L.: Predictors of Employment Status after Cardiac Surgery, *JAMA,* 249:907, 1983.
227. The Norwegian Multicenter Study Group: Timolol-Induced Reduction in Mortality and Reinfarction in Patients Surviving Acute Myocardial Infarction. *N. Engl. J. Med.,* 304:801, 1981.
228. Hjalmarson, A., Elmfeldt, D., Herlitz, J., et al.: Effect on Mortality of Metoprolol in Acute Myocardial Infarction. A Double-Blind Randomised Trial, *Lancet,* 2:823, 1981.
229. β-Blocker Heart Attack Research Group: A Randomized Trial of Propranolol in Patients with Acute Myocardial Infarction: I. Mortality Results, *JAMA,* 247:1707, 1982.
230. Furberg, C. D., Hawkins, C. M., and Lichstein, E., for the Beta-Blocker Heart Attack Trial Study Group: Effect of Propranolol in Postinfarction Patients with Mechanical or Electrical Complications, *Circulation,* 69:761, 1984.
231. Gundersen, T., Abrahamsen, A. M., Kjekshus, J., Ronnevik, P. K., for the Norwegian Multicentre Study Group: Timolol-Related Reduction in Mortality and Reinfarction in Patients Ages 65–75 Years Surviving Acute Myocardial Infarction, *Circulation,* 66:1179, 1982.
232. Aberg, A., Bergstrand, R., Johansson, S., et al.: Declining Trend in Mortality after Myocardial Infarction, *Br. Heart J.,* 51:346, 1984.
233. Furberg, C. D.: Effect of Antiarrhythmic Drugs on Mortality after Myocardial Infarction, *Am. J. Cardiol.,* 52:32C, 1983.
234. Van Durme, J. P., Hagemeijer, F., Bogaert, M., Glaser, B., and Hugenholtz, P. G.: Chronic Antidysrhythmic Treatment after Myocardial Infarction. Design of the Ghent-Rotterdam Aprindine Study, in J. P. Boissel and C. R. Klimt (eds.), "Multicenter Controlled Trials: Principles and Problems," INSERM, 76:43, 1977.
235. Myerburg, R. J., Conde, C., Sheps, D. S., et al.: Antiarrhythmic Drug Therapy in Survivors of Prehospital Cardiac Arrest: Comparison of Effects on Chronic Ventricular Arrhythmias and Recurrent Cardiac Arrest, *Circulation,* 59:855, 1979.
236. Braunwald, E., Friedewald, W. T., and Furberg, C. D., (eds.): Proceedings of the Workshop on Platelet-Active Drugs in the Secondary Prevention of Cardiovascular Events, *Circulation,* 62(suppl. 5, part II)V-1, 1980.
237. The Coronary Drug Project Research Group: Aspirin in Coronary Heart Disease, *J. Chron. Dis.,* 29:625, 1976.
238. Elwood, P. C., and Sweetnam, P. M.: Aspirin and Secondary Mortality after Myocardial Infarction, *Lancet,* 2:1313, 1979.
239. Breddin, K., Loew, D., Lechner, K., Uberla, K., and Walter, E.: Secondary Prevention of Myocardial Infarction. Comparison of Acetylsalicylic Acid, Phenprocoumon and Placebo. A Multicenter Two-Year Prospective Study, *Thromb. Haemost.,* 41:225, 1979.
240. Aspirin Myocardial Infarction Study Research Group: A Randomized, Controlled Trial of Aspirin in Persons Recovered from Myocardial Infarction, *JAMA,* 243:661, 1980.
241. The Persantine-Aspirin Reinfarction Study Research Group: Persantine and Aspirin in Coronary Heart Disease, *Circulation,* 62:449, 1980.
242. The Persantine-Aspirin Reinfarction Study Research Group: Persantine and Aspirin in Coronary Heart Disease, PARIS II, submitted for publication.
243. The Anturane Reinfarction Trial Research Group: Sulfinpyrazone in the Prevention of Sudden Death after Myocardial Infarction, *N. Engl. J. Med.,* 302:250,1980.
244. Report from the Anturan Reinfarction Italian Study: Sulphinpyrazone in Post-Myocardial Infarction, *Lancet,* 1:237, 1982.
245. Canner, P. L.: Aspirin in Coronary Heart Disease. Comparison of Six Clinical Trials, *Isr. J. Med. Sci.,* 19:413, 1983.
246. Lewis, H. D., Jr., Davis, J. W., Archibald, D. G. et al.: Protective Effects of Aspirin against Acute Myocardial Infarction and Death in Men with Unstable Angina. Results of a Veterans Administration Cooperative Study, *N. Engl. J. Med.,* 309:396, 1983.
247. Thornton, M. A., Gruentzig, A. R., Hollman, J., King, S. B., III, and Douglas, J. S.: Coumadin and Aspirin in Prevention of Recurrence after Transluminal Coronary Angioplasty: A Randomized Study, *Circulation,* 69:721, 1984.
248. Chesebro, J. H., Clements, I. P., Fuster, V. et al.: A Platelet-Inhibitor-Drug Trial in Coronary-Artery Bypass Operations. Benefit of Perioperative Dipyridamole and Aspirin Therapy on Early Postoperative Vein-Graft Patency, *N. Engl. J. Med.,* 307:73, 1982.
249. Wenger, N. K., Hellerstein, H. K., Blackburn, H., and Castranova, S. J.: Physician Practice in the Management of Patients with Uncomplicated Myocardial Infarction: Changes in the Past Decade, *Circulation,* 65:421, 1982.
250. Mitchell, J. R. A.: Anticoagulants in Coronary Heart Disease—Retrospect and Prospect, *Lancet,* 1:257, 1981.
251. Chalmers, T. C., Matta, R. J., Smith, H., Jr., and Kunzler, A.-M.: Evidence Favoring the Use of Anticoagulants in the Hospital Phase of Acute Myocardial Infarction, *N. Engl. J. Med.,* 297:1091, 1977.
252. An International Anticoagulant Review Group: Collaborative Analysis of Long-Term Anticoagulant Administration after Acute Myocardial Infarction, *Lancet,* 1:203, 1970.
253. Report of the Sixty Plus Reinfarction Study Research Group: A Double-Blind Trial to Assess Long-Term Oral Anticoagulant Therapy in Elderly Patients after Myocardial Infarction, *Lancet,* 2:989, 1980.
254. The E.P.S.I.M. Research Group: A Controlled Comparison of Aspirin and Oral Anticoagulants in Prevention of Death after Myocardial Infarction, *N. Engl. J. Med.,* 307:701, 1982.
255. Kallio, V., Hamalainen, H., Hakkila, J., and Luurila, O. J.: Reduction in Sudden Deaths by a Multifactorial Intervention Programme after Acute Myocardial Infarction, *Lancet,* 2:1091, 1979.
256. Blumenthal, J. A., Califf, R., Williams, R. S., and Hindman, M.: Cardiac Rehabilitation: A New Frontier for Behavioral Medicine, *J. Cardiac Rehabil.,* 3:637, 1983.

43

Pathology of Coronary Atherosclerotic Heart Disease*

Bernadine Healy Bulkley, M.D.

Those who have dissected or inspected many (bodies), have at least learned to doubt; when others, who are ignorant of anatomy, and do not take the trouble to attend to it, are in no doubt at all.

John Baptist Morgagni, 1682–1771

Despite a declining mortality from cardiovascular disease, these disorders still remain the leading cause of death in the western world.[1] Given an aging population and a degenerative disease that is more prevalent with age, atherosclerosis will only increase as a source of morbidity in our population at large. Understanding the pathology of atherosclerosis is useful in understanding and treating its consequences.

The large and medium-sized arteries are susceptible to atherosclerosis. In the largest vessel, the aorta, atherosclerosis manifests itself by degeneration of the vascular wall leading to aneurysm formation, mural thrombosis with risk for embolism, and at times aortic dissection or rupture. In the medium-sized vessels which branch off the aorta, including the coronary, carotid, renal, and iliac arteries, luminal narrowing by atheroma leads to compromised and at times complete interruption of blood supply.

Coronary Anatomy

Coronary arteries have some features which distinguish them from the other medium-sized arteries, both in health and disease.[1] They are the first and among the smallest in caliber of the vessels leading off directly from the aorta. They have a unique pulsatile flow pattern with peak flow in diastole rather than systole. They course across and encircle the organ they supply, sending off small, right-angle penetrating vessels into the myocardium, from the outside in. Since collateral blood flow is poorly developed in the normal human heart, these vessels can behave like end arteries. In the setting of chronic coronary obstructions and ischemia, collateral connections develop via subendocardial, subepicardial, transseptal, and transatrial vascular connections, and the vascular beds become variably interdependent.

There are three major coronary arteries, two left and one right. Shortly after its origin from the aorta, the left main coronary artery gives rise to two branches: the anterior descending and the left circumflex coronary arteries (Fig. 43-1). The left anterior descending coronary (LAD) courses over the anterior surface of the heart near the interventricular septum and turns around the apex of the heart, the latter often serving as a marker for identifying the LAD angiographically. The LAD gives off many branches to the right, including several septal perforators and one or more diagonal vessels to the left. The LAD supplies the anterior wall of the left ventricle, including the anterior interventricular septum. At times a large left diagonal may originate almost directly from the left main coronary artery and be called a *left main diagonal.* The left circumflex artery, the second branch vessel off the left main coronary artery, originates almost at a right angle to the LAD, and courses to the left in the atrioventricular (AV) groove around to the posterior surface of the heart. It gives off several branches called *marginal vessels* which supply the lateral wall and part of the posterior wall of the left ventricle.

In about 10 percent of hearts, there is left dominance, i.e., the left circumflex artery provides the posterior descending artery. In this situation the left circumflex takes a right-angle downward turn when it reaches the crux of the heart—or that site in the posterior AV groove where the interatrial and interventricular septum meet—to become the posterior descending coronary artery. In 90 percent of instances the posterior descending artery arises from the terminal portion of the right coronary artery, i.e., "right dominance." The right coronary artery arising from the aorta behind the right cusp of the aortic valve courses over the right ventricle, producing atrial and right marginal branches. As it courses around the heart in the AV groove it ends in the posterior descending artery.

In general terms, the left anterior descending coronary artery supplies about 40 percent of the heart, including the anterior wall of the left ventricle

*Note from the editor-in-chief: Dr. Bernadine Healy Bulkley's chapter, "Pathology of Coronary Atherosclerotic Heart Disease," emphasizes the type of pathology a clinician should know. She highlights the pathology of the coronary artery and myocardium as related to clinical problems. Accordingly, her discussion overlaps with Chaps. 2, 3, 19, 31, and 41–47. There is considerable overlap of this and Chapter 44, "Pathophysiology of Myocardial Ischemia," written by Drs. Kirk and Factor. This duplication has been permitted because the subject is extremely important, much progress has been made in the field; and it is useful to review the opinions of different experts on a similar subject. The views discussed here, however, are very similar.

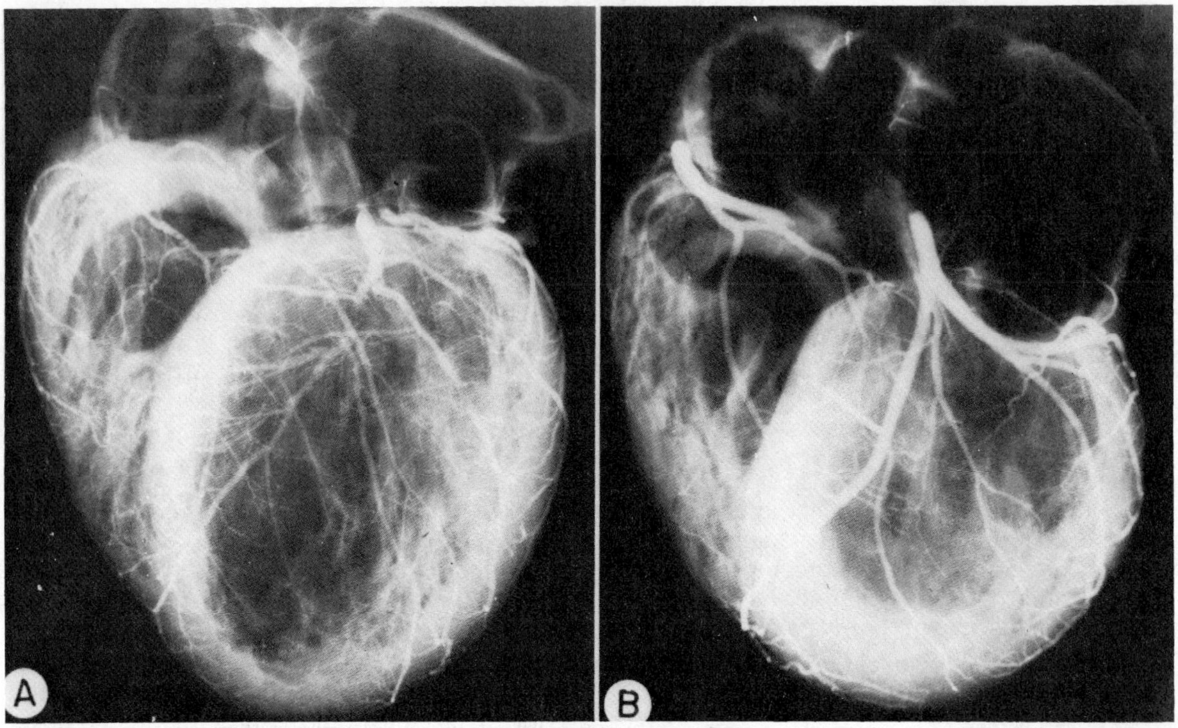

FIGURE 43-1 Shown are postmortem angiograms of two hearts with diseased (*A*) and normal (*B*) coronary anatomy. Shown in *B* is the left coronary artery as it bifurcates into the left anterior descending artery coursing down and across the left ventricle and interventricular septum; and the left circumflex artery which wraps around the basal part of the left ventricle, giving off several marginal vessels. The right coronary artery can be seen running in the atrioventricular groove at the base of the right ventricle. Shown in *A* are the same major vessels which contain extensive atherosclerotic disease. The left anterior descending artery is totally obstructed but collateral vessels are well formed in this heart and the left anterior descending artery has been opacified by retrograde filling. Both hearts are dilated; in *A* due to an ischemic cardiomyopathy, and in *B* due to an idiopathic dilated cardiomyopathy. (*From E. H. Schuster and B. H. Bulkley: Ischemic Cardiomyopathy: A Clinicopathologic Study of Fourteen Patients, Am. Heart J., 100:506, 1980. Reproduced with permission from the publisher and authors.*)

and more than half of the interventricular septum. The left circumflex coronary artery supplies the lateral wall and a variable amount of the posterior left ventricle. The right coronary artery supplies the right ventricle, up to half of the interventricular septum, and a variable amount of the posterior left ventricular wall. The AV node and sinus node are supplied by the right coronary artery most of the time, but the main portion of the conduction system, including the bundle branches which course near the surface of the anterior interventricular septum, are supplied by the left anterior descending coronary artery. The anterior papillary muscle gets its blood supply from the LAD and left circumflex coronary artery, and blood supply of the posterior papillary muscle is from the right coronary artery in most instances. The anatomic relation between coronary vasculature and the myocardium being supplied is important to understand since it can explain many of the clinical manifestations of the localized coronary artery narrowings or occlusions which typify atherosclerotic disease.

Coronary Arteries in Disease

When coronary artery abnormalities lead to clinical disease it is virtually always because of coronary artery narrowings or complete occlusions. It is generally accepted that a tubular conduit—whether it be a valve, blood vessel, or lead pipe—develops restriction to ordinary flow if the lumen is narrowed by 75 to 80 percent or more. Under conditions of "extraordinary" flow—as occurs during stress of exercise or tachycardia—a milder obstruction may become flow-limiting. In the human heart with the added complexities of collateral retrograde flow, and variable transmural perfusion pressure resulting from differing wall thickness and left ventricular end-diastolic pressures, an anatomic lesion narrowing vessel lumen by a designated amount does not always have a predictable functional effect. Studies using Doppler flow probes have shown that greater than 75 percent narrowing in one setting may be associated with no loss of coronary reserve, whereas in another heart an anatomically measured lesion of less narrowing may have severe coronary reserve limitation.[2] Nevertheless, despite these variations, which often can be taken into account on a case-by-case basis, it is important to recognize the broad general applicability of the relation of critical arterial lesions (greater than 75 percent narrowing) to ischemia, and the predictability of finding such critical stenosis in most instances when ischemia is clinically manifest.

The causes of coronary artery narrowing are many, although atherosclerosis is the leading and overwhelming cause of coronary obstruction in the adult population. Coronary atherosclerosis accounts for the majority of adult cardiovascular disease, and for more than 90 percent of ischemic heart disease. Other causes of coronary artery luminal narrowing include thrombosis, spasm, embolism, coronary dissection, and aneurysm formation. The first three of these may occur as isolated occurrences but most often are in combination with atherosclerotic coronary disease.

Pathology of Atherosclerosis

Atherosclerosis affects arteries. Regardless of the artery involved, the anatomy of the disease has certain characteristic features. Atherosclerotic plaques are generally classified into three types: fatty streaks, fibrous plaques, and complicated plaques.[3–5] *Fatty streaks* are focal accumulations of lipid-laden myointimal cells which are seen particularly at branch points of vessels, and can be identified in the vessels of humans of any age or sex. Fatty streaks tend to be shallow, small, and focal, and are thought to be benign by themselves. As possible precursors of advanced atheromatous lesions, however, they take on more interest. *Fibrous plaques* are white atherosclerotic lesions which are also composed of lipid-laden myointimal cells but are predominantly composed of fibrous tissue. The fibrous plaque is viewed as a more advanced atherosclerotic lesion and one that can and does progress to a more advanced lesion with potential for luminal narrowing and degeneration. The fibrous plaque is a proliferative lesion which is believed to be formed by smooth muscle cells which migrate up into the intima and secrete a protein which becomes the collagen matrix. What incites these events is not known. The third and most advanced atheroma is the *complicated plaque,* which is a degenerative lesion composed of fibrous tissue, fibrin, calcium, intracellular and extracellular lipid, and often extravasated blood. Necrotic debris may often form the core of the plaque, which is encapsulated and contained by a fibrous tissue cap (Fig. 43-2). The complicated plaque may enlarge acutely because of hemorrhage or degeneration within its core, and due to fibrin and platelet mural thrombus formation on its surface.

Origin of the Atheroma

There are three major pathogenetic theories of atheroma formation: the lipogenic theory, the thrombogenic theory, and the monoclonal theory. The *lipogenic* or *insudation theory* implicates lipids in the initiation and progression of atherosclerosis. Lipids are known to infiltrate the vessel wall by an interaction of lipids from the blood with smooth muscle cells migrating up to the intimal surface. Low-density lipoprotein (LDL) cholesterol in particular is thought to interact with specific receptor sites and lead to proliferation of the lipid-laden cells and the secretion of an extracellular matrix.[6] The lesion progresses via insudation of lipids from the bloodstream. Metabolic abnormalities within the cells of the arterial wall which interact with lipids in the bloodstream are thought to be important in this process and explain why lipids circulating in the blood are not necessarily the primary cause of the ather-

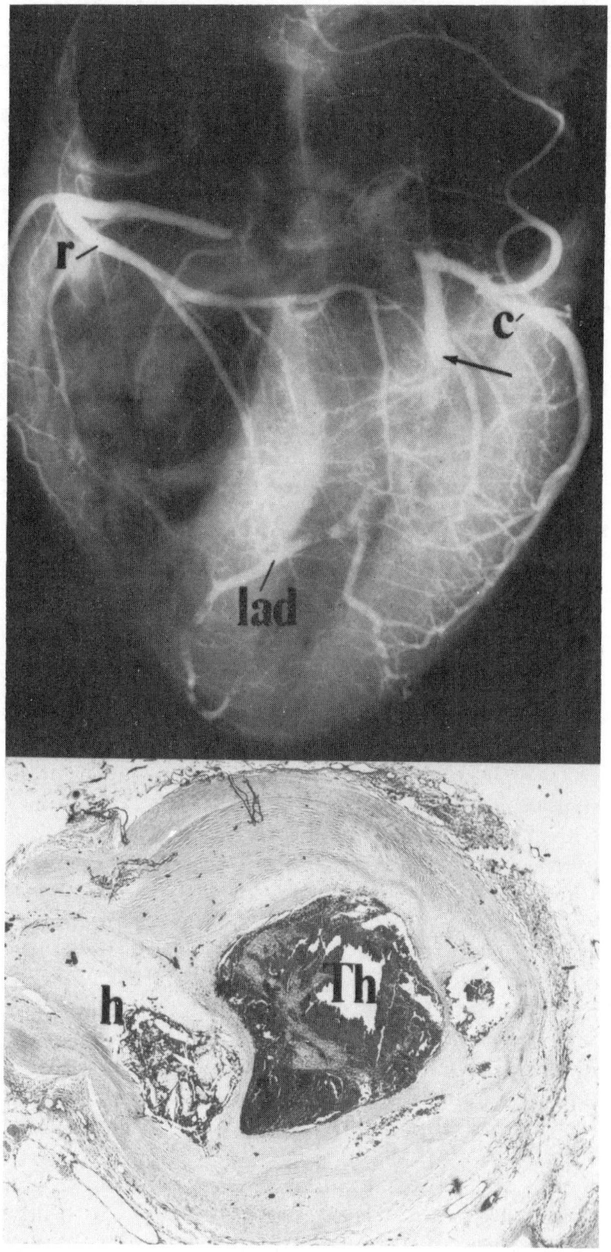

FIGURE 43-2 Acute myocardial infarction: Shown is a postmortem angiogram (*top*) from a patient who died with a fatal acute myocardial infarction. The left anterior descending coronary artery (lad) is totally occluded at the arrow. A transverse histologic section of the coronary artery at that site is shown in the lower panel. The artery is totally occluded by thrombus (Th) superimposed on a complicated atherosclerotic plaque. Hemorrhage (h) into the plaque is also present. r = right coronary artery; c = left circumflex coronary artery. (*From E. H. Schuster, L. S. C. Griffith, and B. H. Bulkley, Preponderance of Acute Proximal Left Anterior Descending Coronary Lesions in Fatal Myocardial Infarction: A Clinicopathologic Study, Am. J. Cardiol., 47:1189, 1981. Reproduced with permission from the publisher and authors.*)

oma. The nature of the abnormalities of the vessel wall and of the smooth muscle cell is only now beginning to be understood.

The second major theory of atherosclerosis is the *thrombogenic* or *encrustation theory* of atherosclerosis.[7] The role of thrombosis in the initiation of the atherosclerotic plaque is not at all certain, but there is general acceptance that recurrent mural thrombosis overlying an existing plaque is an important mechanism in the progression of the atheroma. Most animal models of atherosclerosis in nonprimates combine intimal erosion causing mural platelet fibrin thrombosis with a high-cholesterol diet. Virtually any type of naturally occurring intimal injury—as might be seen with an enlarging plaque stretching a fibrous cap, or vascular spasm—would result in platelet fibrin deposition at the site of intimal erosion. The mural thrombus would, within a matter of weeks, become organized into a fibrous intimal lesion, representing plaque progression. How or why intima of an existing plaque would develop recurrent erosion with mural thrombosis is not known.

The third and most recently proposed theory of atheroma formation is the *monoclonal hypothesis*. First advanced by Benditt and Benditt,[8] this theory proposes that atherosclerotic plaques develop from single precursor cells that proliferate like a tumor. The single-cell origin of a given plaque suggests that some transforming agent such as a virus, a chemical, a physical event, or a preexisting genetic defect is responsible for the initiation of the atheroma.

To believe that these three notions of pathogenesis of atherosclerosis are mutually exclusive is unnecessary, and controversy over which is "correct" reflects more the uncertainty and incompleteness of our knowledge about each hypothesis. Clearly, lipids are important and may play a central role and may also explain some of the intimal injury leading to vascular thrombosis and plaque proliferation. Proliferating thrombi have been shown to have monoclonal properties under certain conditions. The many risk factors known to be associated with atherosclerosis, including elevated blood lipids, hypertension, cigarette smoking, and diabetes, may be incitive or promoting factors which alter intimal cells and affect lipid metabolism or thrombogenesis, or both.

Atherosclerotic Heart Disease

When atherosclerosis affects the coronary arteries it causes manifestations of disease by virtue of chronic and/or acute luminal narrowings and compromise of blood flow. Coronary lesions develop over many years but typically do not manifest themselves as heart disease unless and until one of two things happens: The chronic stenosis exceeds 75 or 80 percent of the vessel lumen and compromises flow, especially with increased flow demand; or the atheroma erodes acutely, develops superimposed thrombosis, and causes an abrupt diminution or even total loss of blood supply. The former is the major pathologic substrate of angina pectoris; the latter, of acute myocardial infarction.

Pathology of Angina Pectoris

Angina pectoris is the clinical equivalent of myocardial ischemia. Ischemic precordial chest pain typically occurs in the setting of increased oxygen demand such as exercise, tachycardia, or other cardiovascular stress. The increased demand requires an increase in myocardial blood flow which an obstructed coronary vasculature cannot accommodate. Most often the obstruction is related to luminal narrowing by atherosclerosis. The atherosclerotic lesions usually occur in the proximal portion of the coronary tree and tend to be focal. Multiple focal, high-grade lesions often occur. A predilection for proximal disease and the focal nature of the obstructions are important anatomic features; it is in their combination that coronary bypass surgery and balloon angioplasty has been feasible and generally successful. In about 10 percent of patients, atherosclerosis occurs diffusely, and is severe in the distal portion of the coronary tree, making these procedures difficult if not ineffective. Fortunately, however, the nature of the disease allows palliation in the majority of patients.

Unstable or preinfarction angina describes angina at rest with no apparent increase in myocardial demand. Almost by definition its cause must relate to an abrupt alteration in supply. Coronary spasm, mostly superimposed on fixed critical anatomic obstruction, appears to be the cause in many of these patients.[9] Also called *preinfarction syndrome,* it is now clear that in some patients rest angina results from abrupt diminution in blood supply resulting from plaque swelling, erosion, and transient thrombosis which do not go on to acute infarction, either because of spontaneous thrombolysis or other means of restoring the abruptly reduced flow.

Angina pectoris is a disease of coronary arteries and not of myocardium. Although during ischemic episodes there may be transient myocardial dysfunction with aneurysmal bulging of the ischemic myocardial segment or transient papillary muscle dysfunction leading to valvular incompetence, the myocardium for the most part is structurally normal. There is evidence from experimental studies of myocardium that transient ischemia may cause high-energy phosphate depletion and subcellular alterations, including myofibrillar disarray and mitochondrial swelling which may persist for days, but that these subtle changes correlate with significant impairment in myocardial function has not been shown.

Acute Myocardial Infarction

The Acute Coronary Event

Acute myocardial infarction is the end result of prolonged, unrelieved ischemia. It is caused by total interruption in blood supply to a segment of myocardium and is largely unrelated to myocardial demand. The cause of the abrupt interruption in blood supply is usually an acute disruptive event within an atherosclerotic coronary segment; that event is most often thrombosis over a complicated atheroma which had previously narrowed the lumen by 75 to 80 percent[10,11] (Fig. 43-2). Plaque rupture, hemorrhage into the plaque, or erosion of the intima over the fibrous cap are the likely events which incite the thrombus formation which converts a critical narrowing into a total occlusion. Spasm or an acute alteration in vascular resistance leading to turbulent flow across a critical narrowing might be promoters of this acute event. The acute thrombotic episode which develops at a site of advanced atheroma formation seems to be totally occlusive initially, but with time luminal patency of some degree is restored spontaneously, either by clot lysis or by retraction of a wall which had been in spasm.

Angiographic and pathologic studies[11,12] have shown that thrombotic occlusions are almost always present when transmural infarction has occurred. In the setting of nontransmural infarction approximately two-thirds of hearts show thrombi as the cause of an abrupt flow reduction in the coronary tree. The recognition of the role of thrombosis in the pathogenesis of acute myocardial infarction has been an important step in leading to application of thrombolytic therapy to this condition. The next major understanding of the pathophysiology of acute myocardial infarction which might have therapeutic value would be knowing exactly why atherosclerotic plaques erode or rupture, and why thrombi abruptly form in what has been for months to years seemingly a stable atherosclerotic plaque.

The Coronary Risk Region

When an acute occlusion occurs in a segment of the coronary tree, leading to ischemia and then infarction, the myocardium at risk for damage is that tissue downstream from the occluded vessel. The area of myocardial infarction almost always lies within the anatomic risk region, and in most instances is smaller than the region at risk. Exactly how much of the region at risk undergoes infarction varies from patient to patient. The variables which determine the amount of myocardium that undergoes necrosis are to a limited extent oxygen demands on the myocardium but to a greater extent the amount of blood which gets into the ischemic zone after the abrupt occlusive coronary event. Flow can get into the risk region after a thrombotic occlusion by one of two paths—either *retrograde,* via collateral vessels from distant coronary beds; or *antegrade,* via restored patency of the thrombotic occlusion. To a large extent the major determinants of how much of the myocardium at risk undergoes necrosis is the *amount* of blood supply which is restored after abrupt occlusion, and the *time* period within which flow is returned.[13,14] In the most favorable circumstances, flow at least as great as that prior to occlusion would be restored within a period of 20 to 30 min. Data from animals suggest that collateral flow can at most supply flow to the level of about 30 percent of basal antegrade flow, and that near-peak collateral flow levels can be achieved in a zone of profound ischemia within 20 min of occlusion. In humans there is much uncertainty about the anatomy and physiology of collateral blood flow. It does appear, however, that there is substantial variability from patient to patient on the extent of collateral development. At least one stimulus for collateral formation is ischemia; other factors such as exercise have been suggested as possible promoters of collateral vessel development.

The importance of coronary collaterals in atherosclerotic heart disease was recognized many years ago by Herman Blumgart and his colleagues.[15] From their clinicopathologic studies of coronary collaterals they concluded that collaterals are important in keeping myocardium alive in the setting of a critical reduction in antegrade supply, but that collaterals were not sufficient to keep myocardium free of ischemia under conditions of increased demand. Thus, well-developed collaterals may be of less value in protecting against angina than they are in limiting the amount of myocardium which undergoes necrosis after an acute coronary occlusion.

Thrombolytic Therapy in Acute Myocardial Infarction

It is widely recognized that a major determinant of outcome after acute myocardial infarction is the amount of myocardium which undergoes necrosis. When more than 25 percent of left ventricular myocardium is lost, left ventricular dysfunction is common, and when more than 40 percent of left ventricle is lost, intractable heart failure and cardiogenic shock are likely to occur. This recognition of the relation between infarct size, left ventricular dysfunction, and mortality has provided the intellectual basis for pursuing measures to preserve ischemic myocardium with the goal of reducing infarct size.[16–18]

Over the past decade many therapies have been proposed with the hope that they would limit the extent of myocardial injury after acute coronary occlusion. Many of these interventions were directed toward limiting the demands on the heart undergoing infarction, such as reducing blood pressure, heart rate, and end-diastolic volume. Recently, therapies directed at an early restoration of flow have been attempted and appear to hold the greatest promise for limiting the amount of myocardium within a region at risk which is undergoing necrosis. The approach which has attracted the most attention recently is thrombolytic therapy in which the acute obstructing thrombus is dissolved by one of three methods: by administration of intracoronary streptokinase or urokinase,[19,20] by administration of these thrombolytic agents in substantially higher doses intravenously, or more recently by intravenous administration of human tissue plasminogen activator,[21] which is a thrombus-specific lytic agent. These approaches obviously vary in their methodology with regard to risk of systemic bleeding and the need for coronary angiography, but they are all directed toward the same common endpoint, namely thrombolysis and rapid restoration of antegrade flow. The extent to which this approach will limit infarct size, preserve function, and decrease mortality is still under investigation but the approach holds continued promise.

There is little doubt that if antegrade flow could be restored early enough and in sufficient amount and without recurrent loss, that myocardium could be saved. The factors which will determine the success of this approach in a given patient are variable. The extent to which retrograde collateral coronary blood flow can sustain life in the myocardium at risk after antegrade occlusion is one major variable in determining the time window within which antegrade flow must be restored to salvage myocardium. In a heart with virtually no source of adjunct blood supply, absence of blood under physiologic basal body conditions is likely to result in a completed infarct within an hour. In the setting of a well-developed collateral system time from occlusion to infarction may be extended to several hours. At present, we are unable to rapidly and noninvasively measure retrograde blood supply after coronary occlusion and therefore cannot identify precisely that subset of patients who have a chance of benefiting from this therapy.

A second important anatomic variable determining the value of thrombolytic therapy is the state of the anatomic vascular lesion which has led to the thrombosis. If the fixed lesion is sufficiently occlusive, and the residual stenosis so great that only a small amount of flow can pass through, adequate blood flow may not be able to be delivered to salvage the downstream ischemic myocardium. Since ischemia results in vasodilation, the downstream vascular bed will be maximally dilated and will have a capacity for greater flow than it had prior to the abrupt occlusion. The functional severity of the residual stenosis will be increased, therefore, and may limit the efficacy of restoring patency.

Another variable also linked to the underlying atherosclerotic lesion is whether the reopened artery undergoes restenosis. Restenosis occurs in approximately 30 percent of patients after thrombolysis, and mostly in the setting of a residual tight stenosis. In this setting, an approach which offers promise for preventing restenosis is combining thrombolysis with balloon angioplasty or coronary artery bypass surgery. With regard to angioplasty it is likely that balloon dilation of the stenotic plaque should be readily accomplished, as the plaque underlying the obstructing thrombus has already undergone fibrous cap rupture. Alternatively, if the critical lesion persists, and the patient shows signs of persistent ischemia or reocclusion, time should be available to perform coronary revascularization and in a controlled setting.

Pathology of Reperfused Myocardium

It is likely that thrombolytic therapy will almost never completely prevent at least some myocardial necrosis from occurring. Reperfusion of lethally ischemic myocardium therefore will have the effect of altering the pathologic feature of the infarct. Reperfusion or contraction band necrosis will become the predominant pattern of necrosis in this setting (Fig. 43-3). Whether there are functional or physiologic differences between the reperfusion infarct and the more usual coagulative infarct is not known (see below).

Thrombolytic therapy for acute myocardial infarction combines understanding of the pathology of the acute coronary event and the nature of the evolution of the myocardial insult. It is a logical therapy. The ultimate goal, however, salvage of myocardium, smaller infarcts, better function, and reduced mortality, awaits validation.

Pathology of the Myocardium

After several hours of acute interruption of blood flow, the myocardium undergoes irreversible injury. There are three types of irreversible cell injury that can be identified pathologically (Fig. 43-4).

Coagulation Necrosis *Coagulation necrosis* is the pattern of necrosis observed when blood flow is permanently interrupted, as occurs typically in the core of an infarct after a thrombotic occlusion. This pattern of necrosis was first described over 40 years ago by Mallory et al.[22] The coagulation infarct is pale or white in color, as it is devoid of blood. Within 6 to 12 h a thin, wavy fiber pattern can be seen microscopically in which the irreversibly injured cells become thin and stretched out, with sarcomeres fixed in a relaxed state. Thereafter, the fibers take on a hypereosinophilic pattern histologically, and during the next 72 h polymorphonuclear leukocytes infil-

FIGURE 43-3 Infarct after thrombolytic therapy. Transverse section of a heart from a patient who died after a large anteroseptal myocardial infarct which had been treated with thrombolytic therapy. The infarct is unusual in that it is a diffusely hemorrhagic infarct and distinct from the pale white infarct usually seen with acute coronary occlusion.

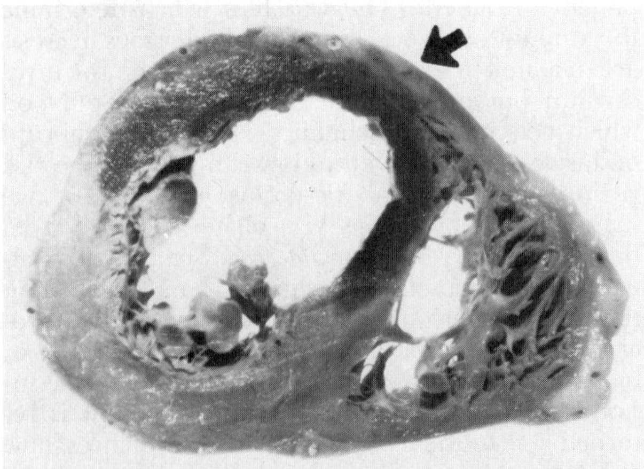

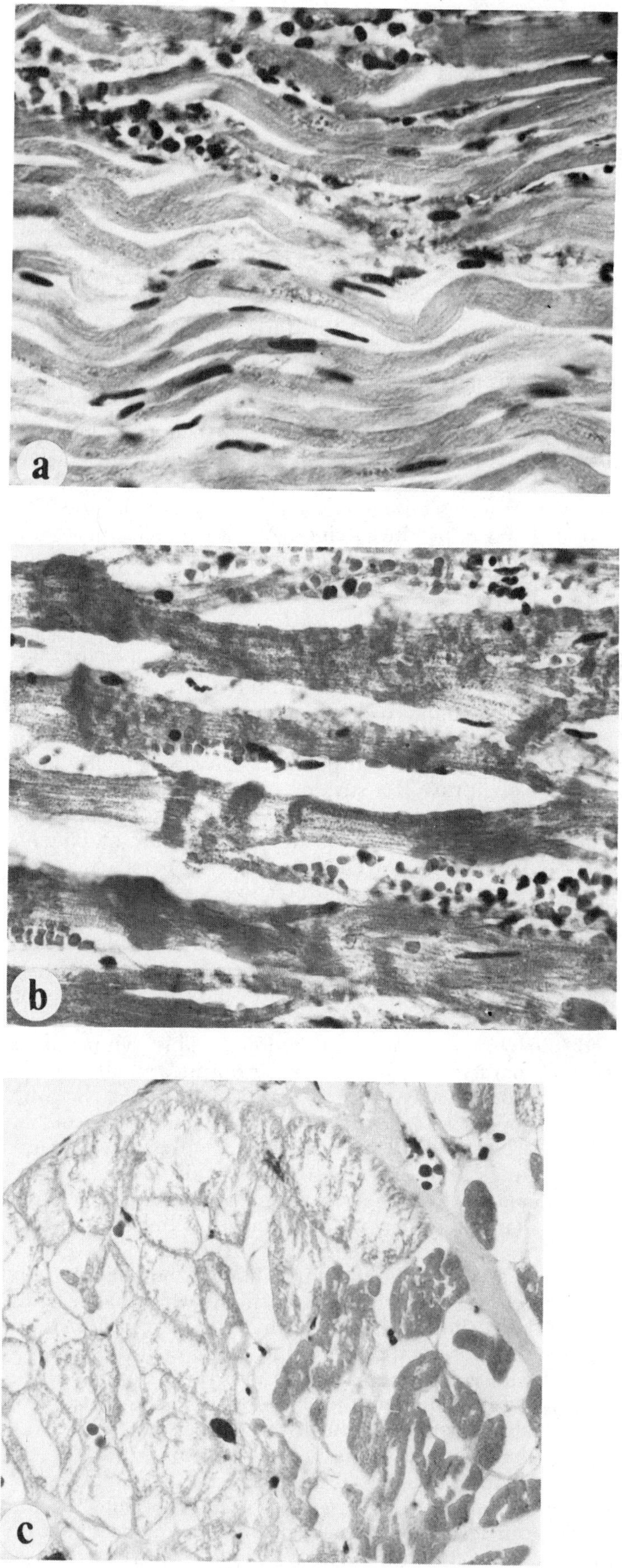

FIGURE 43-4 Three forms of ischemic myocardial cell damage. On the top (*a*) is coagulation necrosis, the injury associated with permanent coronary occlusion. The thin wavy fiber change is evident and leukocytic infiltration of the 2-day-old infarct is evident in the upper left portion of the photomicrograph. The middle panel (*b*) shows contraction band necrosis with the characteristic transverse eosinophilic bands, and myofiber separation and disruption characteristic of reperfusion injury. A hemorrhagic as well as leukocytic infiltrate is present. Shown in panel *c* are cells in the subendocardium which have undergone myocytolysis. The balloon-like degeneration of the myocardial cells is particularly evident in the left-hand portion of the photomicrograph. All hematoxylin and eosin, about ×400.

trate the infarct, and myocyte nuclei drop out. After a week, macrophages enter the infarct from its outer edges and collagen begins to form as dead myocytes are resorbed. The newly formed granulation tissue replaces the necrotic cells over the course of the next several weeks and finally by 4 to 6 weeks a largely healed infarct is present. The completeness of healing at any given point in time is in part a function of the size of the infarct and its type: A large transmural infarct takes at least 6 weeks to heal; a small nontransmural infarct may be healed in 3 to 4 weeks. The early healed infarct is comprised of loose cellular connective tissue with a rich supply of small newly formed blood vessels. In time, the infarct becomes less cellular and less vascular and within a year evolves into a dense collagen scar.

Contraction Band Necrosis A second type of ischemic necrosis which occurs in the heart is *contraction band necrosis*.[23,24] Contraction band necrosis is the type of cell death which occurs when a period of lethal myocardial ischemia is followed by reperfusion. Contraction band necrosis may develop in a variety of circumstances in which myocardial blood flow is temporarily interrupted. Grossly, contraction band necrosis appears as a red infarct since blood has been restored to the necrotic zone, and in the setting of vascular necrosis the reflow causes frank hemorrhage into the extracellular spaces (Figs. 43-3, 43-4). As a distinct pathologic lesion, this type of necrosis was first identified in humans in the hearts of patients who died after cardiac surgery with cardiopulmonary bypass in which there had been an obligatory interruption of flow to the heart. This type of necrosis may occur in patients with coronary spasm[24] and may also be seen commonly on the margins of an acute myocardial infarct which is predominantly coagulation necrosis. In the latter setting reflow related to retrograde collateral blood flow is the presumed cause of marginal contraction band necrosis. This pattern of necrosis can be produced experimentally by interrupting flow for 40 min and then reperfusing the vessel.[23]

Although the bulk of most acute infarcts which occur spontaneously in the setting of coronary atherosclerosis are of the coagulative type as noted above, with interventions causing early reperfusion, the pattern of necrosis will be altered toward infarcts with more contraction band injury.

Myocytolysis A third type of necrosis which occurs in focal nests of cells mainly on the border of infarcts or in the subendocardium is called *myocytolysis*. In this form of ischemic injury, there is subcellular damage with loss of organelles and myofibers, but the cells survive for a time and take on the appearance of a balloon-like degeneration. The ultimate fate of these damaged cells is not clear, but at least some of them die and are replaced by scar tissue. Focal subendocardial or perivascular myofibrillar degeneration can be seen at times in patients with angina without infarction, and may be a cause of the small scars sometimes observed in hearts of these patients at autopsy.

Site of Necrosis
Although infarct size is a major determinant of left ventricular function and mortality after acute myocardial infarction, site or location of the myocardial injury is also an important factor in determining outcome.[17] Anterior wall infarcts which result from occlusion of the left anterior descending coronary artery tend to be larger, associated with greater left ventricular dysfunction, are more apt to cause permanent complete heart block, develop mural thrombosis and late aneurysms, and carry a higher mortality. Occlusion of the left circumflex coronary artery causes infarction of the lateral wall of the left ventricle. Infarcts in this location are typically smaller than those due to occlusion of the right or left anterior descending coronary artery, and are the least likely to produce hemodynamic complications. With a less common left dominant circulation, a left circumflex occlusion can lead to a more extensive posterior wall infarct.

Occlusion of the right coronary artery typically causes an infarct of the posterior wall of the left ventricle and may lead to infarction of the right ventricle. Right coronary occlusions are also the ones typically associated with ischemia or infarction of the posteromedial papillary muscle. Papillary muscle rupture is a striking example of how *site* of infarction at times can be even more important than *size* of infarction. In an autopsy study of patients dying of cardiogenic shock due to papillary muscle rupture the mean infarct size was 11 percent, far less than the size of injury which is usually seen in hearts with fatal infarction and cardiogenic shock.[25]

Infarcts associated with right coronary occlusions involve the inferoposterior wall of the left ventricle and may also be associated with the syndrome of right ventricular infarction.[26] This syndrome is characterized by low cardiac output and often a typical clinical picture of cardiogenic shock but with little or no left ventricular dysfunction, a normal or even low pulmonary artery wedge pressure, and clear lungs. It is not clear that this syndrome can be adequately explained by the extent of anatomic right ventricular necrosis or damage. Rather, it may be a reflection of ischemic dysfunction of right ventricular myocardium, or possibly may be related to the release of a natriuretic hormone which has recently been shown to occur in the right atrium. Whatever the cause of this syndrome, it almost always resolves with volume replacement in one or two days' time.

The relation of location of necrosis to outcome is also illustrated in the difference between transmural and nontransmural infarcts.[12] Transmural infarcts, defined as those that involve the full thickness of the left ventricular wall, have a poorer outcome and can lead to certain negative consequences that do not occur in nontransmural infarcts, regardless of amount of necrosis. Transmural infarcts are the ones most likely to be associated with infarct expansion, cardiac dilation, cardiac rupture, mural thrombosis, and late aneurysm formation[27–31] (Figs. 43-5 to 43-8). A preserved epicardial rim of myocardium which is present in the nontransmural infarct appears to protect against the shape change of expansion and aneurysms and protects against rupture.[32,33]

It should be noted, however, that many clinical studies have suggested that nontransmural infarcts carry as high a mortality as transmural insults.[12] This similarity in the "bottom line" is because the two different forms of infarction carry different possible complications. Nontransmural infarcts may occur in patients with longer term and more severe ischemic coronary disease, as the epicardial salvage is also a marker of a better-developed collateral blood supply. Also, some studies of patients with subendocardial infarction have shown that they are more susceptible to sudden death because of recurrent ischemia and arrhythmias of the "incomplete" infarct.

Consequences of Acute Myocardial Infarction

Infarct Expansion If one focuses on the pathologic consequences of myocardial necrosis on the left ventricular structure per se it is clear that the transmural infarct is the one which most strikingly distorts structure. The pathophysiology of most of this structural deterioration is the fixed bulging, thinning, and dilatation of the infarct zone, which occur within 24 h of transmural necrosis. Expansion causes early global dilation of the heart which may not yet be evident by chest radiograph, since most of the early restructuring is in the internal contour of the left ventricle.[34] This shape change can be detected early by two-dimensional echocardiogram.[28] Serial echocardiographic studies have shown not only an early regional dilatation, but a late global dilatation in hearts that have undergone early expansion, suggesting a phenomenon well recognized in conditions of valvular regurgitation, namely, that dilatation begets dilatation.

Factors which prevent or aggravate this early shape change are not fully known but it does appear that limiting the extent of transmural infarction limits infarct expansion.[33] This may be of particular note if it can be shown that early reperfusion by thrombolytic agents preserves an epicardial rim of muscle and decreases the extent of transmurality. If that is the case, thrombolytic therapy should also hold some promise for reducing the development of infarct rupture and late aneurysm formation.

Infarct Rupture Cardiac rupture occurs in up to 20 percent of patients with fatal acute myocardial infarction coming to autopsy. After cardiogenic shock and arrhythmias cardiac rupture is the most common cause of death after acute infarction. Cardiac rupture tends to occur in hearts with first infarcts, and often infarcts of only small to moderate size, suggesting that most of these patients might have had a favorable course had the rupture not occurred. Risk factors for rupture include transmural infarct, and the presence of hypertrophy. In a recent autopsy study of 110 patients with fatal infarcts, of which 24 had cardiac rupture,[32] patients with rupture had a higher incidence of hypertension and transmural infarction, had smaller infarcts, and a greater incidence and severity of infarct expansion (Fig. 43-8). That the combination of regional dilatation and thinning of the infarct zone correlated well with rupture is not surprising in that dilatation increases wall tension and the increased tension is exerted on both a thinned and weakened wall.

Aneurysm Formation Aneurysms are a later consequence of acute infarction, but represent a complication which is initiated early after infarction. Aneurysms of the heart are defined as convex protrusions composed of mature scar of the full thickness of the left ventricular wall. Late aneurysms develop in about 20 percent of hearts that develop transmural infarcts. Although most left ventricular aneurysms usually come to attention late because of arrhythmias, embolism, or heart failure, the genesis of the aneurysm occurs during the early postinfarct period. In an experimental model of transmural infarction, early expansion of the acute infarct zone occurred within the first few days after coronary occlusion. This suggests that were we ever able to prevent or limit aneurysm formation, interventions would have to be imposed during the early hospital course.

Pathologically, aneurysms have two general forms.[31] The major difference among aneurysms has to do not with external contour but rather with endocardial pathology. One type of aneurysm has extensive endocardial fibroelastosis that appears as a dense white collagen peel overlying the infarct site (Fig. 43-7). The second type of aneurysm contains little or no endocardial fibroelastosis but often contains a large amount of layered thrombus. The amount of mural thrombus which develops is variable but often may be so great as to nearly reconstitute the internal cavity contour (Fig. 43-6). Hochman et al.[31] showed that these pathologic types correlated with clinical complications, as aneurysms with the dense white peel were more apt to develop ventricular arrhythmias, whereas aneurysms with mural thrombosis had a higher incidence of systemic embolism. The importance of endocardial pathology in the pathogenesis of left ventricular arrhythmias is also suggested by recent endocardial stripping procedures which seem to decrease ventricular arrhythmias associated with left ventricular aneurysms.

Congestive heart failure occurs with both forms of aneurysms, although pathophysiology in each may differ. In the ventricular aneurysm with endocardial

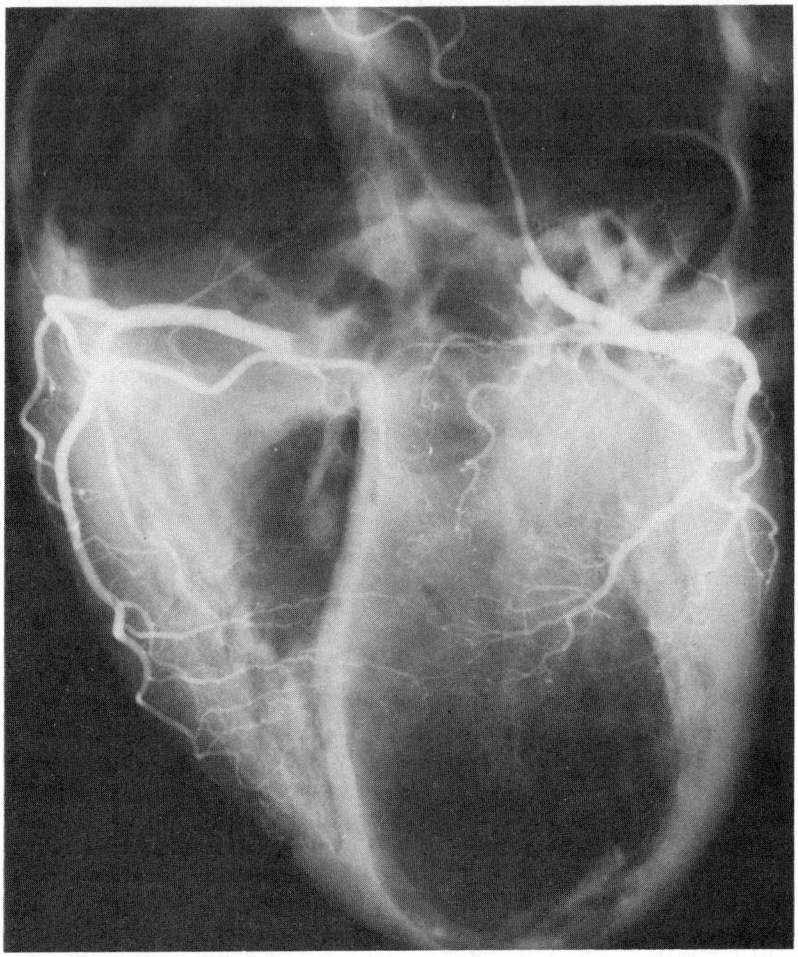

A

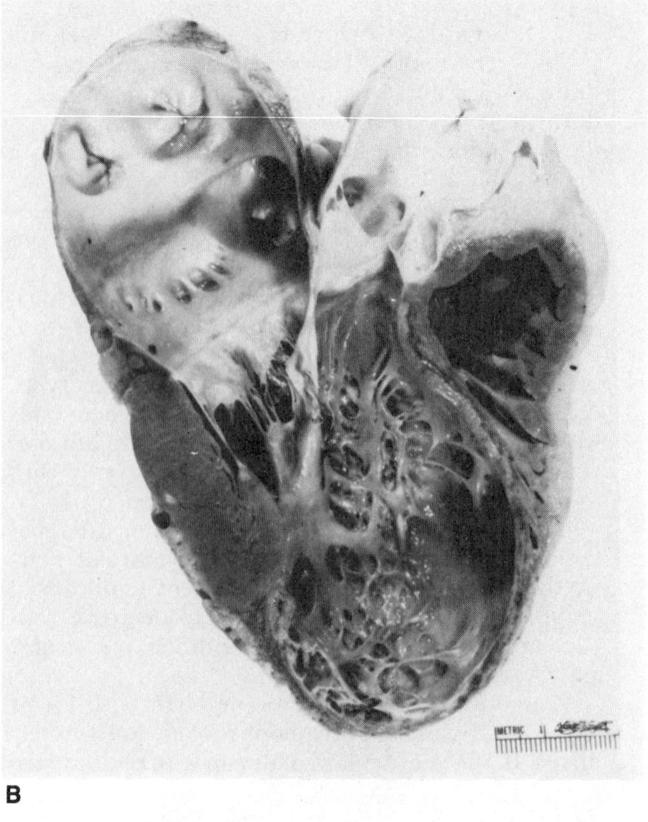

B

FIGURE 43-5 Acute myocardial infarct. *A*. A heart with a transmural myocardial infarct which has undergone expansion. The transmural infarct in the anteroseptal wall is both thinned and regionally dilated. *B*. The shape change is also apparent on the postmortem angiogram. A total occlusion of the left anterior descending coronary artery is present; only the left circumflex and right coronary arteries are opacified.

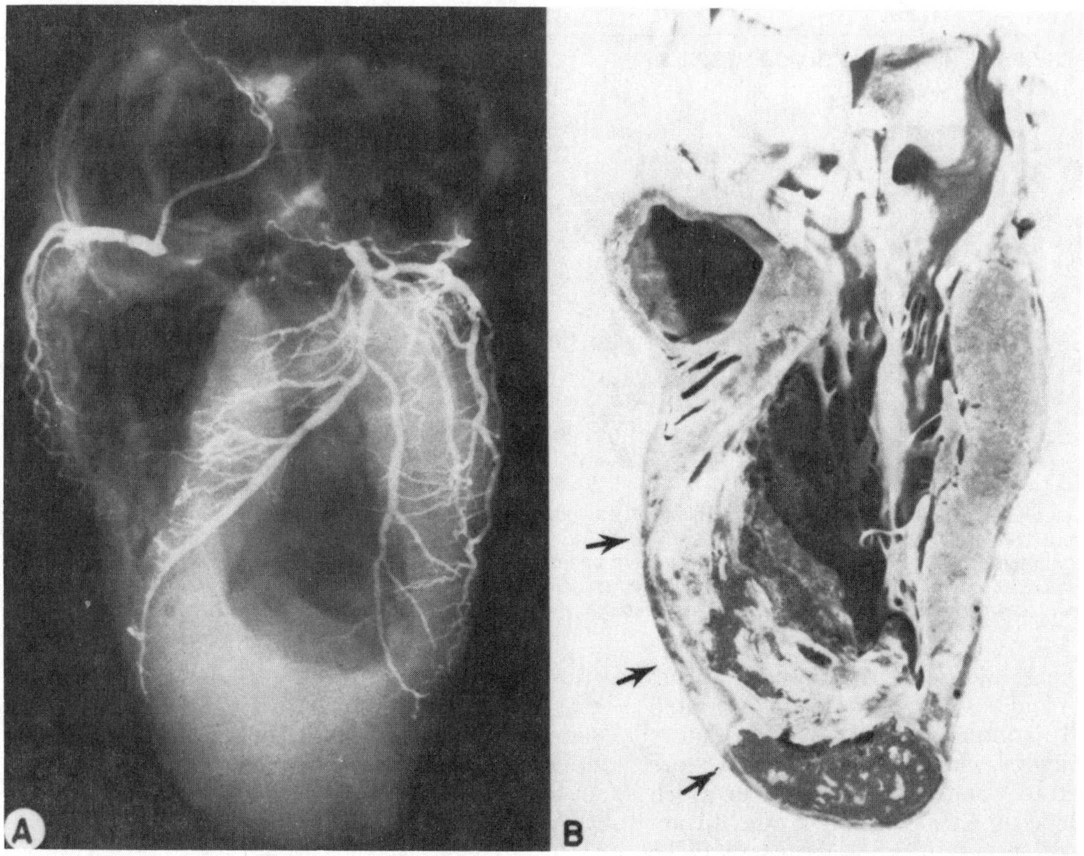

FIGURE 43-6 Healed myocardial infarct. Shown is a myocardial infarct which has formed a left ventricular aneurysm (arrows). The aneurysm is layered with thrombus. The postmortem angiogram (*A*) demonstrates filling of the left anterior descending coronary artery but a proximal high-grade stenosis of the vessel. It is likely that the artery had been totally occluded at the time of the large transmural infarct but has subsequently recanalized. (*From E. H. Schuster and B. H. Bulkley, Ischemic Cardiomyopathy: A Clinicopathologic Study of Fourteen Patients, Am. Heart J., 100:506, 1980. Reproduced with permission from the publisher and authors.*)

FIGURE 43-7 Left ventricular aneurysm with a thick fibroelastotic endocardial peel (arrows). There is no mural thrombus in this type of LV aneurysm. LV = left ventricle. (*From B. H. Bulkley, Baylor College of Medicine, Cardiology Series, 6:5, 1983. Reproduced with permission from the publisher and author.*)

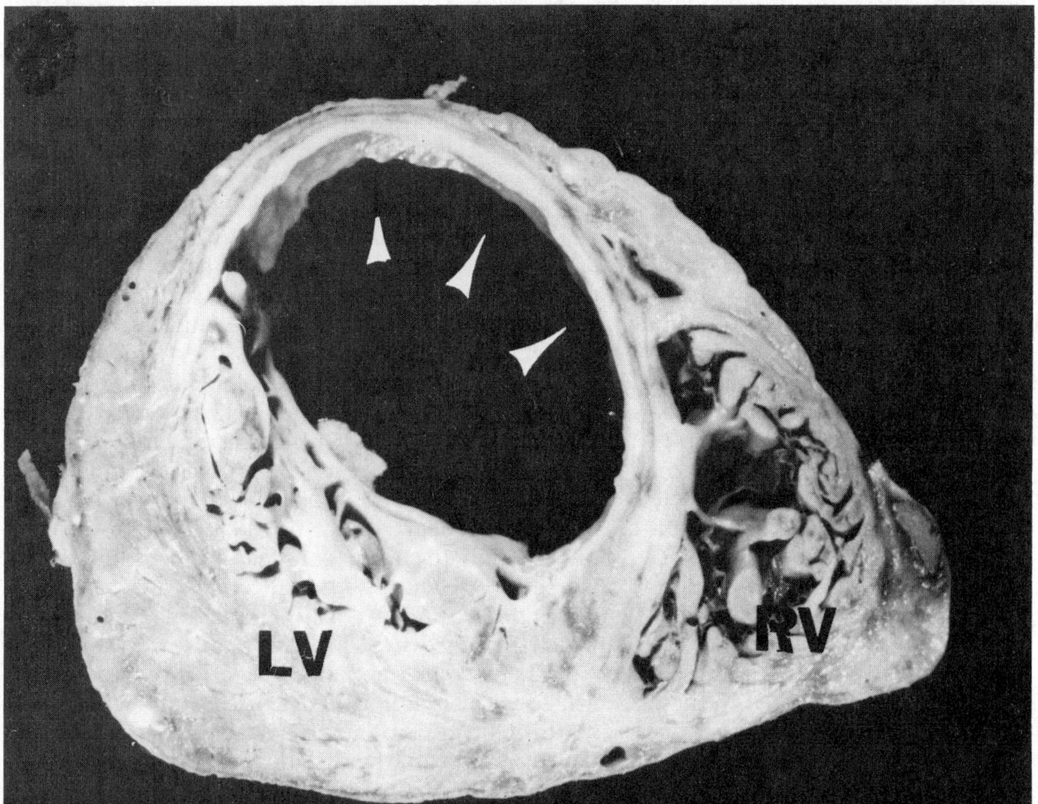

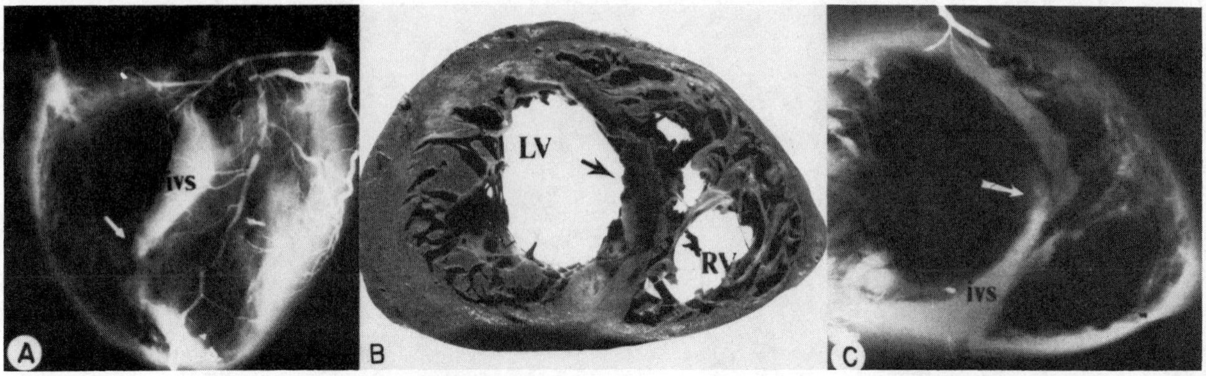

FIGURE 43-8 Rupture after acute myocardial infarction. This heart has undergone rupture of the interventricular septum (IVS) after an anteroseptal infarct. Shown are the postmortem angiograms (*A, C*) and a transverse section through right (RV) and left (LV) ventricles (*B*). Rupture occurs in the setting of transmural infarcts which have undergone expansion. (*From E. H. Schuster and B. H. Bulkley, Expansion of Transmural Myocardial Infarction: A Pathophysiologic Factor in Cardiac Rupture. Circulation, 60:1532, 1979. Reproduced with permission from the American Heart Association, Inc., and authors.*)

fibroelastosis, heart failure is likely related to net cavity dilatation and to volume overload aggravated by dyskinesis. In contrast, congestive heart failure in the heart heavily layered with thrombus is more apt to be related to a noncompliant chamber which is difficult to fill because it is "stented" by the thrombus. In this setting the infarct is more apt to be akinetic rather than dyskinetic.

Pathology of Sudden Cardiac Death

Most sudden death in the adult population is of cardiac origin, and most sudden cardiac death is due to coronary disease. Sudden death is one of the major clinical manifestations of ischemic heart disease, one that often comes as the first sign of coronary artery stenosis, and accordingly, often without warning or benefit of treatment.

The pathology associated with sudden cardiac death is reasonably predictable. Multiple coronary artery atherosclerotic lesions producing critical narrowings of the vessels are almost always present. The variables are whether an acute obstructing thrombus is also present, and whether the myocardium is structurally normal. With regard to the former, fresh thrombi overlying atherosclerotic plaque are identifiable in about 20 percent of patients, with sudden death suggesting that in these patients death occurred during the first few hours of an acute myocardial infarct, and due to profound myocardial ischemia. As it takes 6 to 12 h of flow interruption to identify necrosis pathologically, and since sudden death occurs by definition within minutes of the acute event, it is impossible to be sure whether or not myocardial infarction or myocardial ischemia had occurred. When a fresh obstructing thrombus is identified, however, an acute ischemic event seems clearly to be the cause. In the majority of patients severe atherosclerosis is present but without a fresh thrombosis, suggesting that sudden death occurred in these patients because of a lethal arrhythmia likely triggered by an episode of ischemia.[35,36] Clinical studies of survivors of sudden cardiac death indicate that a substantial number of them do not evolve myocardial infarction, but are prone to recurrent episode of sudden death, findings which support the notion of a primary ischemia leading to lethal arrhythmias.[43]

Ischemic Cardiomyopathy

A moderately frequent, although not well-appreciated, manifestation of chronic coronary artery disease is ischemic cardiomyopathy (Fig. 43-9). That a cardiomyopathy could be caused by severe coronary artery disease per se was first proposed about a decade ago.[37,38] The condition describes a heart which is enlarged, dilated, has hypodynamic function and is associated with congestive failure, but the state is induced by coronary disease per se rather than myocardial necrosis and fibrosis. In fact, anatomic study of hearts with ischemic cardiomyopathy show hearts with little or no myocardial destruction.

That dilatation and dysfunction of the heart could occur with only a small amount of ischemic destruction suggests that diffuse multivessel ischemia might be the mechanism of the hypodynamic function and of progressive cardiac dilatation. Severe ischemia can produce transient myocardial dysfunction,[39] expansion, and dilatation of the left ventricle, and these abnormalities may persist even after ischemia is reversed by full restoration of blood flow. Repetitive multivessel ischemia would have the potential for producing global left ventricular dilatation which, if persisting long enough, would be a stimulus to hypertrophy and eventually a permanent restructuring of the heart. Chronic dilation in a severely oxygen-limited heart can lead to continued and worsened ischemia. Thus, a cycle of ischemia begetting dilatation aggravating ischemia is created, in which a progressive cardiomyopathy may ensue.

Ischemic cardiomyopathy is a less common clinical form of ischemic heart disease and it also may be difficult to recognize because of potential misdiagnosis as an idiopathic dilated congestive cardiomyopathy. Chest pain commonly occurs in the latter

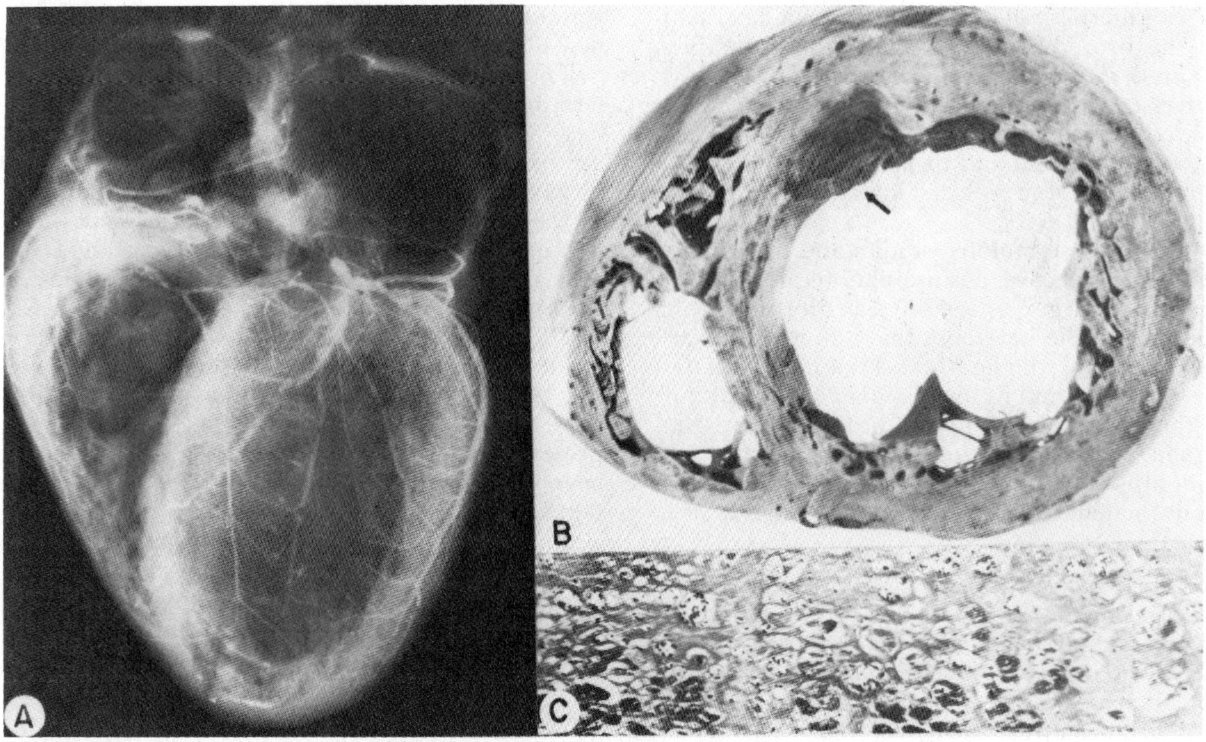

FIGURE 43-9 Ischemic cardiomyopathy. Diffuse dilatation of the heart and severe coronary artery disease are features of the heart with ischemic cardiomyopathy, illustrated in the postmortem angiogram (*A*) and also in the transverse section through both ventricles shown in *B*. Focal areas of scarring were present grossly and histologically (*C*) throughout myocardium. (*From E. H. Schuster and B. H. Bulkley, Ischemic Cardiomyopathy: A Clinicopathologic Study of Fourteen Patients, Am. Heart J., 100:506, 1980. Reproduced with permission from the publisher and authors.*)

condition, and up to 20 percent of patients with idiopathic dilated cardiomyopathy may have Q waves on electrocardiography. On the other hand, many patients who develop ischemic cardiomyopathy may have silent ischemia. Patients with diabetes mellitus, for example, appear to have an increased prevalence of silent myocardial ischemia and infarction, and may be at special risk to develop ischemic cardiomyopathy. Some of the so-called diabetic cardiomyopathy which has been recognized clinically may also be of ischemic etiology. Holter monitor studies in patients with known angina have also documented the presence of frequent episodes of silent ischemia. Thus, when considering the diagnosis of idiopathic cardiomyopathy in an adult, particularly one with risk factors for atherosclerosis, the possibility of ischemic etiology should be considered as it would alter the approach to patient management and therapy.

The Pathology of Coronary Artery Intervention for Atherosclerosis

The past decade has seen an explosion in therapies and interventions available or attempted to deal with problems of atherosclerotic coronary artery disease. The many interventions, successful or otherwise, which have been tried or hold promise are discussed in detail elsewhere in this book. What should be recognized, however, is that many of these interventions, even if not preventive or curative, do alter the structure and natural history of the disease, sometimes substituting a new pathology of less dire consequence for the older, more serious one. Such is clearly the case when a diseased valve is replaced by one that is prosthetic, or when a bland white infarct is replaced by a hemorrhagic, hopefully smaller, reperfused infarct. The main coronary interventions currently in use that alter the pathology of coronary artery disease are coronary artery bypass surgery and coronary angioplasty.

Coronary Bypass Surgery

In 1967 the era of coronary artery bypass surgery as we know it today began. Since then, the procedure has become a near-routine next step in the management of severe coronary atherosclerotic heart disease. At present, more than 170,000 patients per year undergo this procedure in the United States, and by now well over 1 million people have had bypass surgery at least once. This is a population in which the natural history of coronary artery disease has been altered significantly. We have known almost from the outset that this procedure dramatically relieves angina in the majority of patients, and that for the most severe form of coronary disease, that associated with critical narrowing of the left main coronary artery, the procedure prolongs life.[40–42] Recent clinical trials have suggested not surprisingly that for clinically *mild* forms of ischemic heart disease the procedure does not lengthen life when compared to current medical therapy.[43] But, for multivessel disease associated with objective evidence of myocardial ischemia (i.e., positive treadmill test), evidence continues to point toward a benefit for prevention of myocardial infarction and lengthening of life.[44]

To keep these multiple studies and their varied results in perspective, it is useful to recall that coronary bypass surgery offers a means for improving blood flow to the heart, but that a number of variables determine whether the risks of infarction (less than 5 percent) and death (less than 2 percent) during the acute phase of the procedure are outweighed by the longer-term benefit of improved blood supply to the heart. Variables which affect overall "benefit" to a given patient include:

1. The severity of the coronary lesions and ischemia before bypass, which determines the potential for improvement.
2. The anatomy of the native vessels downstream from the occlusion, including caliber and extent of atherosclerosis, which determine amount of blood flow improvement achieved.
3. The overall health of the myocardium, which contributes to acute and chronic mortality.
4. The overall status of the patient, including age, sex, and coexisting diseases.
5. Certain elements of the postoperative environment of the grafts, which may determine graft atherosclerosis. Many of these are not yet understood but likely include conventional risk factors such as smoking and hyperlipemia, and other less well-understood factors such as blood coagulability.
6. The skill of the surgeon and the hospital organization, which is the most subjective variable, but is important in that a tenfold or more range of operative mortality exists among institutions for patients of comparable risk.

Understanding the pathologic anatomy of the heart at each point in time is part of understanding at least five of these six variables. The cardiac pathology associated with coronary bypass surgery should be viewed in three phases: the preoperative, the perioperative, and the late follow-up phase.

The Acute Phase of Coronary Bypass Surgery

The preoperative state of the heart is important to outcome. Fortunately, coronary atherosclerosis occurs almost always as discrete focal narrowings having a predilection for a proximal location, sparing the distal arteries and intramural vessels. Furthermore, the coronary arteries and their lesions are conveniently situated on the surface of the heart just inside the pericardium, and are reasonably accessible without violating the myocardium. The caliber of the artery downstream from a critical narrowing, and the extent of atherosclerosis in the downstream or branch vessels are major determinants of runoff when a new blood supply is brought in.

The other major preoperative variable which determines outcome is the status of the ventricle. A heart which has been substantially damaged by prior infarction or one which has developed an ischemic cardiomyopathy is at greater operative risk. For hearts with ejection fractions of less than 20 percent there is limited if any benefit from revascularization, however favorable the vessels are for bypass, unless a discrete aneurysm can be resected.[41,42]

The perioperative phase of coronary bypass surgery is one which has undergone considerable change in the past decade. The techniques of creating the anastomoses, of performing multiple bypasses, and preserving the myocardium during the process have been vastly improved (Fig. 43-10). More than 90 percent of grafts are patent early after operation.[45–48] Early graft failure is usually due to a thrombotic occlusion at the distal anastomosis site.[47] Griffith et al.[47] showed that early graft failures are often related to small internal diameter of the native vessel into which the bypass is placed. Not surprisingly, a study by Chesebro et al.[48] showed that anticoagulant therapy with the platelet-active agents aspirin and persantine during the early postoperative phase is associated with a significantly greater graft patency. This study also confirmed earlier autopsy studies from patients who died early after surgery that thrombosis was the major cause of graft failure.[49,50]

The state of the myocardium before bypass surgery is important to outcome, but the condition of the myocardium coming out of surgery is equally important. Myocardial injury which occurs in the setting of bypass surgery reflects the pathophysiology of the insult. If severe ischemia during the period of cardiopulmonary bypass and aortic cross-clamp leads to cell necrosis, the pattern of injury which evolves after revascularizations and reflow is hemorrhagic contraction band necrosis. If the perioperative infarct results from occlusion of the coronary artery bypass graft or thrombosis of the native coronary artery, the pattern of injury is coagulation necrosis.

The past decade of coronary surgery has seen much success in preventing myocardial injury. The application of the concept of preservation of ischemic myocardium has seen no greater value than in cardiac surgery utilizing cardiopulmonary bypass.[41] Normothermic anoxic arrest necessary to create a quiet operative site for surgery has been replaced by hypothermia combined with chemical cardioplegia as a healthier means to still the heart during operation. In this operative setting the preservation technique of maximal reduction in oxygen demand can be accomplished prior to interruption in blood flow. The dramatic improvement in mortality and decrease in perioperative infarction seen in recent years is in large part due to cold chemical cardioplegia. Moreover, it might be said that the

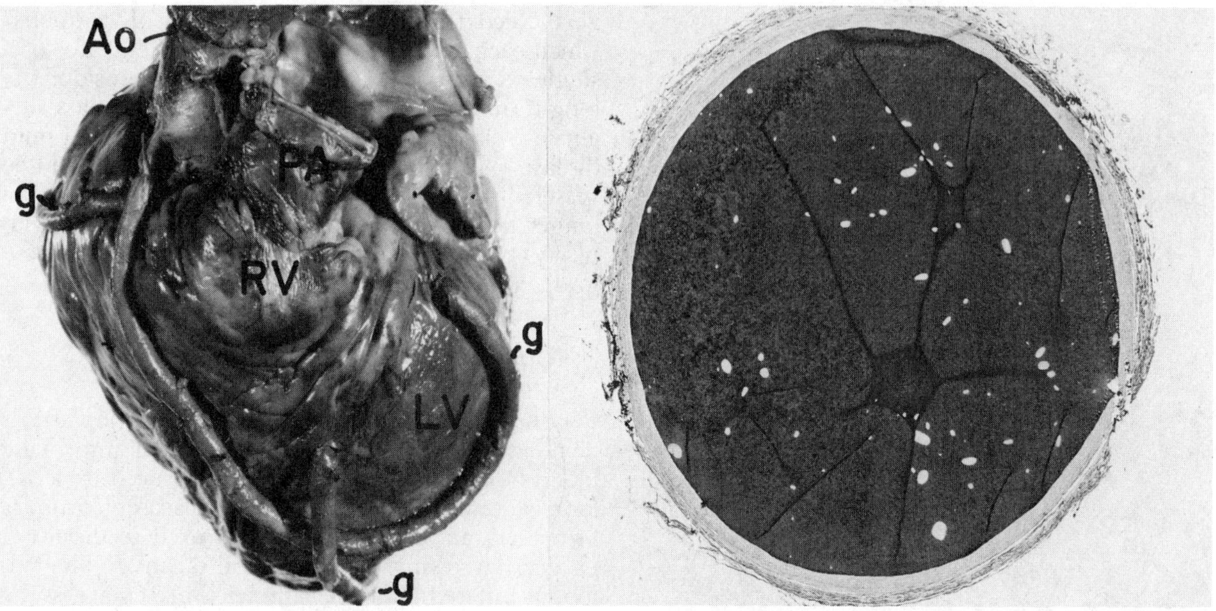

FIGURE 43-10 Shown is the surface of a postmortem heart which has undergone coronary artery bypass surgery. Multiple bypasses of coronary stenosis have been accomplished by implanting the three vein grafts (g). A histologic section of a vein graft which has been distended postmortem by a barium gel is shown on the right. The normal vein is thinner than the native artery and has a greater diameter. Ao = aorta; LV = left ventricle; RV = right ventricle.

concept of preservation of ischemic myocardium may have found its best application in the operating room, despite the fact that the approach was popularized in the coronary care unit.

Chronic Phase of Coronary Bypass Graft Surgery
With these improvements in techniques most patients undergo coronary bypass surgery with a low risk of mortality, a successfully revascularized heart, and well-preserved myocardium. What primarily determines ultimate long-term benefit in the chronic phase after operation is the subsequent course of the coronary pathology. Specifically, changes will occur both in the native coronary vasculature and within the implanted grafts which will dictate much of the long-term result of the procedure. Coronary bypass surgery does not arrest the underlying atherosclerotic process in the native coronary arteries, although full recognition of the disease and its consequences may at times lead patients to modify risk factors that may ultimately delay the progression of atherosclerosis. Additionally, the saphenous veins implanted into the coronary arterial system become subject to an atherosclerotic degeneration which leads to failure of approximately half of implanted vessels after 10 years of implantation.[51] The implanted veins undergo certain predictable changes, some of which represent normal repair (Figs. 43-10 and 43-11). Some amount of vein trauma occurs as a result of explanting and reimplanting the vessel into a higher pressure system, and though difficult to quantitate, it is likely that the amount of damage varies with ease of dissection and technique.

Virtually all grafts early after implantation show loss of endothelium and deposition of fibrin and platelet mural thrombi.[49] The intimal thrombi organize and by 4 weeks histologic study of these grafts shows a loosely organized fibrous tissue plaque overlying the luminal surface of the graft. In some patients for uncertain reasons this circumferential intimal plaque continues to proliferate in the ensuing months and in some cases leads to significant narrowing of the graft lumen. This process proceeds at a variable rate in patients and in some may lead to graft occlusion in 6 to 18 months, but in others not for a decade or more. That the occlusive lesion represents a true atherosclerotic process was initially questioned. Studies on late grafts, however, have now demonstrated complicated atheromas composed of extracellular lipid and necrotic debris covered by fibrous caps, capable of erosion and acute thrombosis, recreating in the implanted graft the same pattern of evolution of atherosclerotic change that occurs in native coronary arteries (Fig. 43-11).

The reasons for vein graft degeneration are not known. One factor may be exposure of the vein to a relatively hypertensive arterial environment. The latter may be a source of endothelial trauma leading to continued mural thrombus deposition and a thrombogenic progression of atherosclerosis. It is also likely that the same risk factors important in arterial atherosclerosis are important in the development of saphenous vein atherosclerosis, particularly hyperlipemia and smoking.

Use of the *internal mammary artery* as a means of bringing in arterial blood to the myocardium should be given special attention.[41] The internal mammary arteries may be implanted into virtually any of the anterior and lateral ventricular wall vessels. Although we know that the intermediate durability of

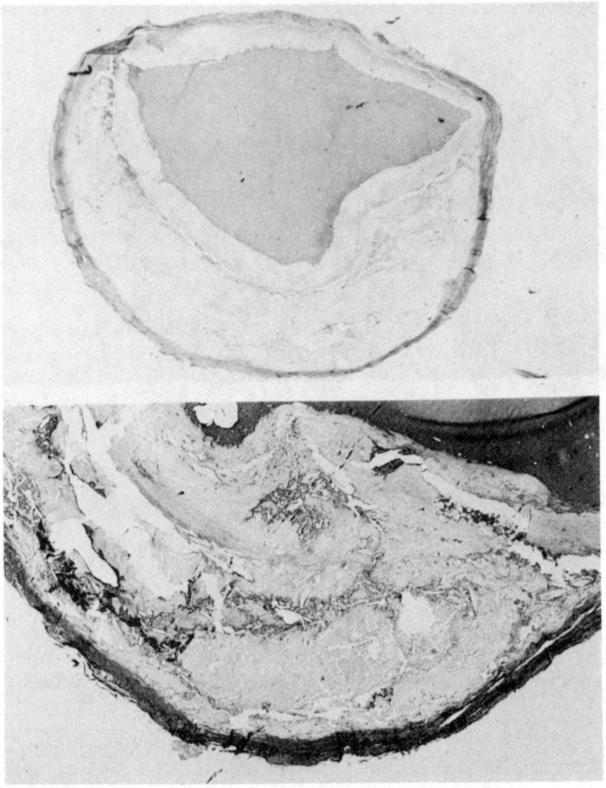

FIGURE 43-11 Atherosclerosis of a saphenous vein bypass graft. Shown here is a histologic section at low and higher power magnification of a coronary artery bypass vein graft which had been implanted in a patient for 9 years. A complicated atherosclerotic plaque developed in the graft. The patient died of an acute infarct due to thrombotic occlusion of this diseased graft. Thus the natural history of coronary atherosclerosis can be replayed in these veins implanted in the heart.

vein implants is poor, preliminary studies of long-term internal mammary grafts suggest that they may be sturdier and less susceptible to graft atherosclerosis. If this proves to be the case, internal mammary implantation may be preferable for first bypass procedures whenever possible.

Coronary Artery Bypass Reoperations

More than 1 million people have undergone coronary artery bypass surgery over the past 15 years and the number is growing. As a palliative procedure with limited durability, it is to be expected that we will continue to face a growing population of candidates who might need reoperation because of recurrence of stenoses and symptoms. Reoperations bring with them their own challenges. First, the pericardial space has been violated and epicardial scarring of the surface of the heart overlying the native vessels and their grafts makes the procedure more difficult technically. Also, the amount of autologous graft material is limited for each patient, and to date no synthetic material has proven satisfactory as a bypass conduit. Thus, options for reoperations are limited and at the present time most patients have only two and, under some circumstances, possibly three opportunities for bypass surgery. Recognizing the limited number of "coupons" which each patient holds, and the limited "life" of a single coupon, it makes great sense to consider the long-term outlook at the time coronary bypass surgery is selected for therapy. For patients with mild disease, particularly those who are young with single vessel disease, and who might be managed for a longer time with medical therapy or balloon angioplasty, the limited long-term durability of the vein grafts should be at least considered.

Percutaneous Transluminal Coronary Angioplasty

Percutaneous transluminal coronary angioplasty is a more recently developed method of improving blood flow to the heart.[52] With this procedure a balloon catheter introduced into the diseased coronary artery via an arterial catheter is used to disrupt a critical narrowing by mechanical means.[52] The balloon is inflated after the catheter is placed across the critical narrowing and the enlarging balloon stretches and splits the atherosclerotic lesion. Loss or diminution of the gradient across the lesion can usually be documented as well as angiographic improvement in the lesion. The mechanical disruption appears to split the fibrous cap over the atherosclerotic plaque, but because of treatment with coronary antispasmodics and anticoagulants concurrently, thrombosis is usually prevented. In approximately 30 percent of patients restenosis likely due to thrombotic occlusion occurs in the dilated vessel and the procedure carries with it a mortality in the range of 1 to 2 percent, despite the milder nature of the disease usually treated.*

Percutaneous transluminal angioplasty has created yet another variation in the natural history of the pathology of atherosclerotic heart disease. The full value of this procedure in the long term and its value relative to coronary bypass surgery in settings ranging from single to multivessel disease remain to be determined.

Summary

The pathology of atherosclerotic heart disease is varied with regard to the range of coronary lesions and the effect of these lesions on the myocardium. Most patients do not come to medical attention until they are well along in the course of their disease, and most of our therapies, whether medical or surgical, are often directed toward the end stage of the disease. It must be appreciated as well that the many therapies alter the natural history of the disease, mostly for the better, and their impact on the anatomy and pathology of atherosclerotic heart disease

*Note from editor-in-chief: The risk of balloon angioplasty by Gruentzig and his colleagues at Emory University Hospital in Atlanta is 0.1 to 0.2 percent.

need be considered. Ultimately, we would hope to understand the pathophysiology of coronary artery disease in its earliest stages so as to interrupt or attenuate its course early in its development. Nevertheless, atherosclerosis is linked to the aging process, and as our population lives longer atherosclerotic heart disease is likely to increase as a disease of major prevalence, offering continued diagnostic and therapeutic challenges.

References

1. Fulton, W. F. M.: "The Coronary Arteries," Charles C Thomas, Publisher, Springfield, Ill., 1965.
2. White, C. W., Wright, C. B., and Doty, D. B., et al.: Does Visual Interpretation of the Coronary Arteriogram Predict the Physiologic Importance of Coronary Stenosis? *N. Engl. J. Med.*, 310:819, 1984.
3. Bulkley, B. H.: Pathophysiology of Coronary Heart Disease, Baylor College of Medicine, Cardiology Series 6:5, 1983.
4. Ross, R., and Blomset, J. A.: The Pathogenesis of Atherosclerosis, *N. Engl. J. Med.*, 295:369, 1976.
5. Panganamala, R. V., Geer, J. C., Sharma, H. A., and Cornwell, D. G.: The Gross and Histologic Appearance and the Lipid Composition of Normal Intima and Lesions from Human Coronary Arteries and Aorta, *Atherosclerosis*, 20:93, 1974.
6. Smith, E. B., Slater, R. S., and Chu, P. K.: The Lipids in Raised Fatty and Fibrous Lesions in Human Aorta: A Comparison of Changes at Different Stages of Development, *J. Athero. Res.*, 8:399, 1968.
7. Mustard, J. F., Murphy, E. A., Rowsell, H. C., et al.: Platelets and Atherosclerosis, *J. Athero. Res.*, 4:1, 1964.
8. Benditt, E. P., and Benditt, J. M.: Evidence for a Monoclonal Origin of Human Atherosclerotic Plaques, *Proc. Natl. Acad. Sci. USA*, 70:1753, 1973.
9. Maseri, A., Mimmo, R., and Chierchio, S., et al.: Coronary Artery Spasm as a Cause of Acute Myocardial Ischemia in Man, *Chest*, 68:625, 1975.
10. Chapman, I.: The Cause-Effect Relationship between Recent Coronary Artery Occlusion and Acute Myocardial Infarction, *Am. Heart J.*, 87:267, 1974.
11. DeWood, A., Spores, C. R. N. A., Notske, R., et al.: Prevalence of Total Coronary Occlusion during the Early Hours of Myocardial Infarction, *N. Engl. J. Med.*, 303:897, 1980.
12. Freifeld, A. G., Schuster, E. H., and Bulkley, B. H.: Nontransmural Versus Transmural Myocardial Infarction: A Morphologic Study, *Am. J. Med.*, 75:423, 1983.
13. Reimer, K. A., Lowe, J. E., Rassmussen, M. M., et al.: The Wavefront Phenomenon of Ischemic Cell Death: Myocardial Infarct Size Vs. Duration of Coronary Occlusion in Dogs, *Circulation*, 56:786, 1977.
14. Herdson, P. B., Sommers, H. M., and Jennings, R. B.: A Comparative Study of the Fine Structure of Normal and Ischemic Dog Myocardium with Special Reference to Early Changes following Temporary Occlusion of a Coronary Artery, *Am. J. Pathol.*, 46:367, 1965.
15. Blumgart, H. L., Schlesinger, M. J., and Zoll, P. M.: Angina Pectoris, Coronary Failure and Acute Myocardial Infarction: The Role of Coronary Occlusion and Collateral Circulation, *JAMA*, 116:91, 1941.
16. Alonso, D. R., Scheidt, S., Post, M., and Killip, T.: Pathophysiology of Cardiogenic Shock, Quantification of Myocardial Necrosis, Clinical, Pathological and Electrocardiographic Correlations, *Circulation*, 48:588, 1973.
17. Bulkley, B. H.: Site and Sequelae of Myocardial Infarction, *N. Engl. J. Med.*, 305:337, 1981.
18. Hillis, L. D., and Braunwald, E.: Myocardial Ischemia, *N. Engl. J. Med.*, 296:1034, 1093, 1977.
19. Ganz, W., Buchbinder, N., Marcus, H., et al.: Intracoronary Thrombolyses in Evolving Myocardial Infarction, *Am. Heart J.*, 101:4, 1981.
20. Rentrop, P., Blancke, H., Karsch, K. R., et al.: Selective Intracoronary Thrombolysis in Acute Myocardial Infarction and Unstable Angina, *Circulation*, 63:307, 1981.
21. Topol, E. J., Shapiro, E. P., Brinker, J. A., Bulkley, B. H., Brin, K. P., Gottlieb, S. O., Gerstenblith, B., Flaherty, J. T., Chandra, N., Ouyang, P., Gottlieb, S. H., and Weiss, J. L.: Regional Wall Motion Improvement after Coronary Thrombolysis with Recombinant Tissue Plasminogen Activator, *Circulation*, 70(suppl. II):323, 1984.
22. Mallory, G. K., White, P. D., and Salcedo-Salgar, J.: The Speed of Healing of Myocardial Infarction: A Study of the Pathologic Anatomy in Seventy-Two Cases, *Am. Heart J.*, 18:647, 1939.
23. Reichenbach, D. D., and Benditt, E. P.: Myofibrillar Degeneration: A Response of the Myocardial Cell to Injury, *Arch. Pathol.*, 85:189, 1968.
24. Bulkley, B. H., Ridolfi, R. L., Salyer, W. R., et al.: Myocardial Lesions of Progressive Systemic Sclerosis: A Cause of Cardiac Dysfunction, *Circulation*, 53:483, 1976.
25. Wei, J. Y., Hutchins, G. M., and Bulkley, B. H.: Papillary Muscle Rupture in Fatal Acute Myocardial Infarction: A Potentially Treatable Form of Cardiogenic Shock, *Ann. Intern. Med.*, 90:149, 1979.
26. Lorell, B., Leinbach, R. C., Pohost, G. M., et al.: Right Ventricular Infarction, *Am. J. Cardiol.*, 43:465, 1979.
27. Hutchins, G. M., and Bulkley, B. H.: Infarct Expansion Versus Extension: Two Different Complications of Acute Myocardial Infarction, *Am. J. Cardiol.*, 41:1127, 1978.
28. Eaton, L. W., and Bulkley, B. H.: Expansion of Acute Myocardial Infarction: Its Relationship to Infarct Morphology in a Canine Model, *Circ. Res.*, 49:80, 1981.
29. Hochman, J. S., and Bulkley, B. H.: Expansion of Acute Myocardial Infarction: An Experimental Study, *Circulation*, 65:1446, 1982.
30. Hochman, J. S., and Bulkley, B. H.: The Pathogenesis of Left Ventricular Aneurysms: An Experimental Study in the Rat Model, *Am. J. Cardiol.*, 50:83, 1982.
31. Hochman, J. S., Platia, E. V., and Bulkley, B. H.: Differences in LV Aneurysms by Endocardial Pathology: Relationship to Ventricular Tachycardia in a Surgical Population, *Ann. Intern. Med.*, 100:29, 1983.
32. Schuster, E. H., and Bulkley, B. H.: Expansion of Transmural Myocardial Infarction: A Pathophysiologic Factor in Cardiac Rupture, *Circulation*, 60:1532, 1979.
33. Weisman, H. F., Bush, D. E., Mannisi, J. A., and Bulkley, B. H.: Effect of Extent of Transmurality on Infarct Expansion, *Clin. Res.*, 32:477A, 1984.
34. Weisman, H. F., Udvarhelyi, S., Bush, D. E., and Bulkley, B. H.: Cardiac Remodeling in Infarct Expansion: Differential Distortion of the Inner Wall, *Circulation*, 68(suppl III):195, 1983.
35. Spain, D. M., and Brades, V. A.: Sudden Death from Coronary Heart Disease, *Chest*, 58:107, 1970.
36. Warren, J. V.: Critical Issues in the Sudden Death Syndrome, in H. D. McIntosh (ed.), Baylor College of Medicine, Cardiology Series, vol. 5, no. 5, 1982.
37. Burch, G. E., Giles, T. D., and Cololough, H. L.: Ischemic Cardiomyopathy, *Am. Heart J.*, 79:291, 1970.
38. Schuster, E. H., and Bulkley, B. H.: Ischemic Cardiomyopathy: A Clinicopathologic Study of Fourteen Patients, *Am. Heart J.*, 100:506, 1980.
39. Braunwald, E., and Kloner, R. A.: The Stunned Myocardium: Prolonged Post-Ischemic Ventricular Dysfunction, *Circulation*, 66:1146, 1982.
40. European Coronary Surgery Study Group: Coronary Artery Bypass Surgery in Stable Angina Pectoris: Survival at Two Years, *Lancet*, 1:889, 1979.
41. Loop, F. D.: Progress in Surgical Treatment of Coronary Atherosclerosis, *Chest*, 84:611, 740, 1983.
42. Cosgrove, D. M., Loop, F. D., Lute, B. W., et al.: Primary Myocardial Revascularization: Trends in Surgical Mortality, *J. Thorac. Cardiovasc. Surg.* (in press).
43. CASS Principal Investigators and Their Associates: Coronary Artery Surgery Study (CASS): A Randomized Trial of

Coronary Artery Bypass Surgery. Survival Data, *Circulation,* 68:939, 1983.
44. Weiner, D. A., McCabe, C. H., Ryan, T. J., et al.: Value of Exercise Testing in Identifying Patients with Improved Survival after Coronary Bypass Surgery (CASS Registry), *Circulation,* 70(Suppl. II):20, 1984.
45. Kouchoukos, N. T., Karp, R. B., Oberman, A., et al.: Long-Term Patency of Saphenous Veins for Coronary Bypass Grafting, *Circulation,* 58(suppl. I):96, 1978.
46. Campeau, L., Lesperance, J., Corbara, F., et al.: Aortocoronary Saphenous Vein Bypass Graft Changes 5 to 7 Years after Surgery, *Circulation,* 58(suppl. I):170, 1978.
47. Griffith, L. S. C., Bulkley, B. H., Hutchins, G. M., et al.: Occlusive Changes at the Coronary Artery-Bypass Graft Anastomosis: Morphologic Study of 95 Grafts, *J. Thorac. Cardiovasc. Surg.,* 73:668, 1977.
48. Chesebro, J. H., Clements, I. P., Fuster, V., et al.: A Platelet-Inhibitor Drug Trial in Coronary Artery Bypass Operations: Benefit of Perioperative Dipyridamole and Aspirin Therapy on Early Postoperative Vein Graft Patency, *N. Engl. J. Med.,* 307:73, 1982.
49. Bulkley, B. H., and Hutchins, G. M.: Accelerated "Atherosclerosis": A Morphologic Study of 97 Saphenous Vein Coronary Artery Bypass Grafts, *Circulation,* 55:163, 1977.
50. Bulkley, B. H.: Morphologic Consequences of Myocardial Revascularization, in J. M. Moran and L. L. Michaelis (eds.), "Surgery for the Complications of Myocardial Infarction," Chicago, Grune & Stratton, 1980.
51. Campeau, L., Enjalbert, M., Lesperance, J., et al.: Atherosclerosis and Late Closure of Aortocoronary Saphenous Vein Grafts: Sequential Angiographic Studies at Two Weeks, One Year, Five to Seven Years, and Ten to Twelve Years after Surgery, *Circulation,* 68(suppl. II):1, 1983.
52. Gruentzig, A. R., Senning, A., and Siegenthaler, W. E.: Non-operative Dilation of Coronary Artery Stenosis: Percutaneous Transluminal Coronary Angioplasty, *N. Engl. J. Med.,* 301:61, 1979.

44

Pathophysiology of Myocardial Ischemia*

Stephen M. Factor, M.D.   Edward S. Kirk, Ph.D.

Besides, if the blood could permeate the substance of the septum, or could be imbibed from the ventricles, what use were there for the coronary artery and vein, branches of which proceed to the septum itself, to supply it with nourishments.

William Harvey, 1628[1]

Myocardial ischemia is the result of a deficiency of arterial blood supply to the heart muscle. This deficiency must be evaluated in terms of the requirements of the heart muscle for oxygen and nutrients. Severe deficiencies of arterial blood flow of the magnitude which leads to myocardial infarction are evident from direct measurements of myocardial blood flow, but it is not possible to predict the critical levels of flow and/or metabolic requirements which produce ischemia, even with the most sophisticated measurements of blood flow and cardiac function. However, the consequences of even mild ischemia are usually evident and include pain, electrophysiological and metabolic changes, cessation of contraction, and sometimes left ventricular failure. A detailed discussion of these events is beyond the scope of this chapter, but the underlying condition in each case, a defect in the energy production in the myocardium, is discussed in some detail below. These events take on added significance when irreversible injury is threatened. Accordingly, pathophysiological mechanisms that apply when the threshold of myocardial ischemia is approached are reviewed in the first part of this chapter. Subsequently, the pathogenesis and pathology of myocardial infarction will be discussed.

*Note from the editor-in-chief: Drs. Kirk and Factor's chapter, "Pathophysiology of Myocardial Ischemia," overlaps with Chapter 43 "Pathology of Coronary Atherosclerotic Heart Disease" by Dr. Bernadine Healy Bulkley. This overlap has been permitted because: the subject is extremely important; much progress has been made in the field; and it is useful to review the different opinions of experts on a similar subject.

Primary Causes of Myocardial Ischemia

The most frequently recognized cause of myocardial ischemia is obstructive coronary atherosclerosis, which either occludes or narrows the vessel lumen primarily, or may secondarily induce a coronary thrombus. Myocardial ischemia may also be caused by aortic valve disease; hypertrophic cardiomyopathy; stenosis of the coronary ostia secondary to primary disease of the aorta; coronary embolism; inflammatory disease of the coronary arteries, including periarteritis and mucocutaneous lymph node syndrome (Kawasaki's disease); and congenital states such as anomalous origins of coronary arteries from the pulmonary artery. Recently vasoconstriction of the larger coronary vessels (spasm), whether or not it occurs in an area of an atherosclerotic plaque, has been implicated as a cause of myocardial ischemia;[1a] although the relative importance of this cause has not been fully determined, vasospasm may also lead to the development of a coronary thrombosis. The overwhelming impression is that myocardial ischemia results from partial or complete obstruction of the coronary arterial system. This impression, although largely correct, tends to obscure the factors which influence the normal balance between myocardial blood flow (supply) and the metabolic requirements of the heart muscle (demand). This balance must be understood to evaluate the contributory causes of myocardial ischemia.

Under normal circumstances, metabolic demands are closely paralleled by myocardial blood flow despite wide variations in oxygen consumption of the heart.[2] Myocardial ischemia occurs when supply is insufficient for demand, and ischemia is normally avoided by a careful matching of blood flow to metabolism. The alternative strategy of having arterial flow excessive at all times, as in the kidneys, is not employed. On the other hand, cardiac metabolism appears unable to outstrip its supply in normal individuals, even at the extreme limits of activity,[3,4] so that excessive demand is never a primary cause of ischemia.

In the presence of coronary artery disease, however, increases in cardiac metabolism can place demands for increased blood flow that cannot be met, and myocardial ischemia can be avoided only by limiting the metabolism of the heart. Since the mechanical function of the heart is closely coupled to its metabolism, this strategy of avoiding ischemia restricts the permissible range of cardiac function; moreover, with severe reductions in coronary blood flow, this would require levels of cardiac function incompatible with life. Following acute coronary occlusion, local areas of ischemia of this degree generally cannot be avoided. For the purpose of this discussion, we will consider these as two different situations: one is characterized by incipient myocardial ischemia with ischemia absent at rest, in which frank ischemia only occurs transiently when metabolic demands are increased and/or blood flow is reduced; the other is characterized by persistent myocardial ischemia which ultimately may lead to necrosis. The determinants of myocardial metabolism are quite different under these two conditions.

Myocardial Blood Flow

A limited myocardial blood supply is common to both mild or incipient ischemia and severe ischemia, so that factors which determine blood flow will be a constant feature of myocardial ischemia. For this reason, as well as the fact that the primary cause of myocardial ischemia is invariably a deficiency in supply, it is useful to place primary emphasis on the blood flow aspect of the supply/demand ratio. We will therefore begin by reviewing the features of the normal regulation of coronary blood flow.

Autoregulation of Coronary Blood Flow

One of the most striking features of the regulation of the coronary circulation is the almost complete independence of coronary blood flow on changes in coronary perfusion pressure. This can be shown experimentally by isolating the coronary arterial system from the systemic circulation and measuring coronary blood flow as perfusion pressure is varied. If cardiac function and the composition of arterial blood remain constant, steady-state values of coronary blood flow are remarkably constant. For example, Mosher et al.[5] observed an average change in flow of only ± 7 percent over a range of pressures from 70 to 150 mmHg (Fig. 44-1). The twofold change in coronary vascular resistance that occurs is thought to be the result of an intrinsic, or autoregulatory, mechanism of the heart.

Coronary perfusion pressure normally is identical to aortic pressure, and aortic pressure is maintained within narrow limits by powerful baroreceptor reflexes. Moreover, any change in aortic pressure would produce a change in metabolic requirements of the heart and thus would have an indirect role in determining coronary blood flow. This is shown in Fig. 44-1: a lower level of coronary flow is maintained when cardiac effort is reduced by bleeding. Pressure-independent autoregulation of coronary blood flow, as shown in Fig. 44-1, is not normally manifest. However, *autoregulation is the primary adaptive response to coronary artery disease.* Thus, when an atheroma progressively narrows a large coronary artery, pressure distal to the obstruction is reduced by the resistance of the obstruction but ischemia is

FIGURE 44-1 Steady-state coronary arterial flow as a function of coronary perfusion pressure at a control level (solid circles) and at a decreased level of cardiac effort (open circles). The peak transient flow following a sudden increase of perfusion pressure from 40 mmHg has been drawn through triangles. At 40 mmHg the coronary vessels are nearly maximally vasodilated. Thus the instantaneous pressure-flow curve represents the maximal flow that can occur at each coronary perfusion pressure. (*From P. Mosher, P. J. Ross, Jr., P. A. McFate, and R. F. Shaw, Control of Coronary Blood Flow by an Autoregulatory Mechanism, Circ. Res., 14:250, 1964. Reproduced with permission from the American Heart Association, Inc., and the authors.*)

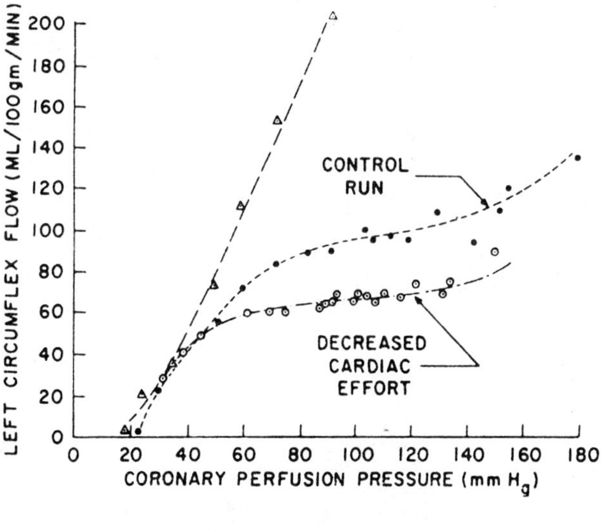

avoided by a progressive decrease in resistance in the distal coronary arteriolar bed. As long as the obstruction is limited to the large coronary vessels, the coronary circulation autoregulates its blood flow. Under these conditions the effective coronary perfusion pressure (*x* axis in Fig. 44-1) is the pressure distal to the obstruction, and flow will be maintained until this pressure falls below the "flat" portion of the autoregulatory curve.

The mechanism which causes coronary flow to be independent of perfusion pressure is probably identical to the mechanism which adjusts the tone of the coronary vessels relative to the metabolic needs of the myocardium. In this view, the plateau of the autoregulatory curve is indicative of the precision of this control. A change in the energy requirements of the heart causes coronary flow to change in the same direction to a new level, where flow is again autoregulated. The precise relation between coronary blood flow and myocardial metabolism suggests that the mechanism of coronary autoregulation involves a metabolite. Attention has been directed toward chemicals that induce relaxation of coronary vascular smooth muscle. When flow is insufficient, a metabolite may accumulate in the myocardium, reduce vascular tone, and thus restore normal flow. The most carefully documented model for this type of negative feedback for coronary autoregulation is the hypothesis presented by Berne and his colleagues[6] that adenosine is the mediator of metabolic regulation of tone (Fig. 44-2).

This hypothesis proposes that adenosine, a powerful vasodilator of the coronary vasculature, is continuously released into the interstitial fluid by the myocardial cells, and its release is enhanced in response to either an increase in myocardial metabolism or a reduction in arterial supply. An increase in the interstitial fluid concentration of adenosine decreases the resistance of the coronary vessels, augments flow, and thus restores the balance between supply and demand. The adenosine concentration in the interstitial fluid is determined by its net rate of release by the myocardial cells, balanced by the washout and inactivation by the deaminases of red cells in perfusing blood. When myocardial release of adenosine is constant, any decrease in coronary blood flow would increase the interstitial fluid concentration of adenosine and thereby reduce coronary vascular resistance. This negative feedback mechanism would account for pressure-independent autoregulation of coronary blood flow, while a change in myocardial release of adenosine would result in the autoregulation of a new level of flow.

Effect of Myocardial Contraction on Coronary Blood Flow

The beating heart inhibits its own supply. Sabiston and Gregg[7] clearly demonstrated this extravascular component of coronary resistance in a canine heart by showing that with perfusion pressure held constant, coronary blood flow increased immediately upon temporary stoppage of the heart by vagal stimulation. Under resting conditions, this throttling effect accounts for approximately 25 percent of the total resistance to coronary blood flow and increases to 35 percent with tachycardia.[8] If systole completely inhibited coronary flow, the component of total coronary resistance due to extravascular compression would be greater, and equal to the proportion of time spent in systole. Thus flow in the myocardium during systole is greatly reduced, but not totally absent.

Systole appears to inhibit blood flow in the layers nearer the endocardium more than in epicardial layers. Kirk and Honig[9] first demonstrated this in a preparation similar to that used by Sabiston and Gregg. Under conditions of constant coronary flow, vagal arrest caused the blood flow in the superficial myocardium to be redistributed to the deep layers. A more quantitative picture of this redistribution is obtained from the local myocardial uptake of a blood flow tracer when perfusion is limited to the period of systole.[10] Perfusion pressure can be alternated between normal aortic pressure during systole and near zero throughout diastole by perfusing the cannulated coronary artery with left ventricular pres-

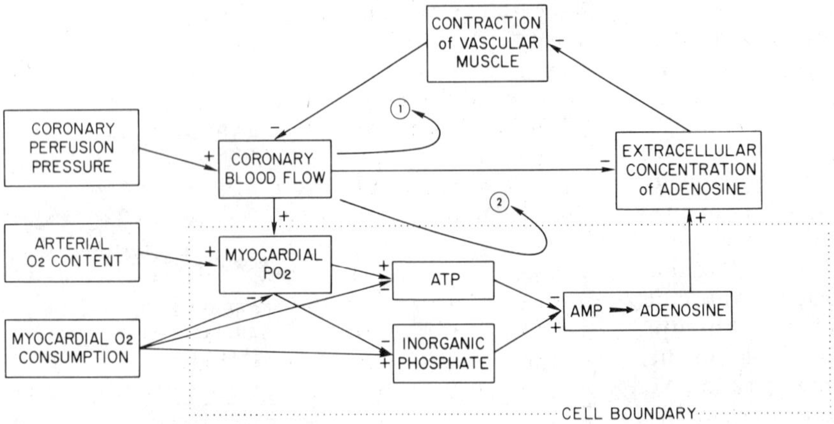

FIGURE 44-2 Diagram of feedback mechanism of regulation of coronary blood flow by adenosine.[6] Each variable is characterized as to its effect, that is, whether it increases (+) or decreases (−) the variable it acts on. In this type of diagram, negative feedback is characterized by having an odd number of negative signs in the feedback loop. Two negative feedback loops involving coronary blood flow are indicated: (1) one involving only extracellular variables and (2) one involving intracellular variables. In this diagram the balance between supply and demand is represented in terms of delivery and utilization of oxygen.[6]

sure. Under these conditions, a significant gradient in the distribution of myocardial blood flow during systole favoring the outer layers is observed.[10] A gradient across the wall of extravascular compression during systole would be expected to cause such a gradient of blood flow.

The magnitude of the forces which impede coronary flow during systole remains in doubt. Some confusion stems from an imprecise use of the term *intramyocardial pressure* for these forces.[11] A greater series of problems occurs when probes which distort and injure myocardial fibers are inserted into the myocardium to measure intramyocardial pressure.[12] There is general agreement, however, on the existence of a gradient of forces across the heart wall during systole with lesser forces in the epicardial layers than in the endocardial layer. This is sufficient to predict that a gradient of blood flow occurs across the heart wall during systole.

Blood vessels are collapsible tubes, and flow in collapsible tubes is inhibited in direct proportion to the magnitude of external forces compressing the vessels.[13] This phenomenon has been termed a *vascular waterfall* and results in significant inhibition of myocardial flow in the deeper layers during systole, even if the compressive forces are less than systolic ventricular pressure. Application of the vascular waterfall model also predicts that the extravascular component of coronary resistance is independent of vasomotor changes.[14] Thus, even under conditions of maximal coronary vasodilatation, the extravascular component of coronary resistance remains 25 to 35 percent of the total resistance. These estimates of extravascular resistance are averages of a gradient across the heart wall and underestimate the effect on the deeper layers. With maximal coronary vasodilatation, systolic compression in the deeper layers becomes one of the principal determinants of myocardial blood flow and may significantly influence the balance of supply and demand in the subendocardium.

Systole does not normally inhibit the blood supply to the right ventricle to the same extent that it does to the left ventricle. Right coronary flow occurs throughout the cardiac cycle, and the rate of systolic flow approximates diastolic flow. In right ventricular hypertension, however, systolic blood flow is reduced and may even be absent.[15] In acute pulmonary artery obstruction, increased myocardial impingement on right coronary artery flow during systole may be an important factor leading to ischemia of the right ventricular myocardium.[16]

Subendocardial Ischemia

Under normal hemodynamic conditions the distribution of coronary blood flow across the heart wall is uniform.[17,18] Apparently, the gradient in the distribution of flow during systole is compensated for by a reverse gradient during diastole. Since the amount of coronary blood flow which occurs during diastole is usually several times greater than that during systole, the diastolic gradient favoring flow in the deep layers is less than the reverse systolic gradient.

Satisfactory regulation of the transmural distribution of coronary blood flow can occur until the vessels become maximally dilated. Even under these conditions, uniform flow can occur if the resistance of the maximally dilated vessels allow a greater flow in the deep layers during diastole. This might be possible in some hemodynamic conditions. However, subendocardial ischemia usually occurs when the regulation of the distribution of blood flow changes from one of active vasomotor control (autoregulation) to one of passive dependence on coronary perfusion pressure and extravascular compression. This is especially true in coronary artery disease. With progressive obstruction of a large coronary artery, autoregulation maintains adequate flow throughout the heart wall, but the limit of this adaptation is reached first in the subendocardial layers. At the threshold of myocardial ischemia, blood flow becomes insufficient only in the inner layers of the heart, while the outer layers remain normal and can even recruit additional flow by vasodilatation.[19] Under these conditions myocardial flow in the epicardial layers characteristically exceeds flow in endocardial layers, so that the existence of a transmural gradient of myocardial blood flow favoring the epicardial layers is often identified as a sign of myocardial ischemia. The vulnerability of the subendocardial layers to ischemia in coronary artery disease reveals a limitation of the autoregulatory mechanism, which is not able to adapt completely to the stress imposed by the combination of extravascular compression and reduced coronary pressure. Whatever the cause, the important feature for this discussion is that *the onset of myocardial ischemia depends on physiological and pathological mechanisms in the subendocardial layers.*

Subendocardial ischemia following coronary occlusion was first carefully studied by Griggs and Nakamura,[20] who proposed a "coronary-ventricular pressure index" to predict transmural gradients of coronary blood flow. Later, Buckberg et al.[21] extended the use of this index to several other hemodynamic conditions characterized by subendocardial ischemia and identified the events affecting subendocardial flow more clearly. Subendocardial flow is predominantly diastolic and depends on the coronary driving pressure during diastole. If the opposition to flow of diastolic extravascular compression can be approximated by ventricular diastolic pressure, the factors determining perfusion of subendocardial layers when the vessels are maximally dilated should be represented by the area between the coronary pressure and left ventricular pressure curves in diastole. Buckberg et al.[21] termed this area the *diastolic pressure-time index* (DPTI) and identified it

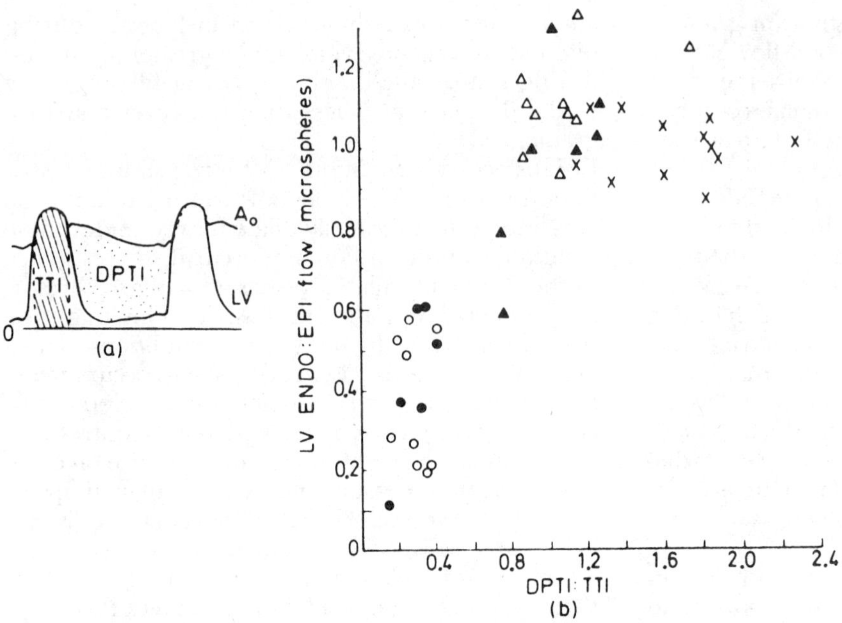

FIGURE 44-3 *a*. Method of calculating the diastolic pressure-time index (DPTI) and the tension-time index (TTI). The tension-time index[50] was used to indicate demand for flow. The DPTI/TTI ratio is therefore a pressure index which decreases when demand exceeds supply in the deeper layers. In some cases left atrial pressure or pulmonary wedge pressure was used to approximate left ventricular diastolic pressure. *b*. Relation of DPTI/TTI ratio to transmural distribution of coronary blood flow. Radioactive microspheres were used to measure myocardial blood flow. The flow in the endocardial half (ENDO) of the left ventricular (LV) wall is approximately equal to the flow in the epicardial half (EPI) when DPTI/TTI is greater than 0.8. When DPTI/TTI falls below 0.8, the ratio of ENDO to EPI flows falls below 1.0, indicating relative underperfusion of the subendocardium. X = control; ● = AV fistula; o = supravalvular aortic constriction; ▲ = ventricular pacing; △ = distal aortic construction. (*From G. D. Buckberg, D. E. Fixler, J. P. Archier, and J. I. E. Hoffman, Experimental Subendocardial Ischemia in Dogs with Normal Coronary Arteries, Circ. Res., 30:67, 1972. Reproduced with permission from the American Heart Association, Inc., and the authors.*)

with the factors responsible for supply of the subendocardial layers (see Fig. 44-3).

The DPTI was originally used to analyze conditions in which coronary pressures were equal to aortic pressures, but if coronary pressures distal to the obstruction are used in the calculation, the index is equally valid for coronary artery obstruction. Modified in this way the DPTI is a useful device for analyzing the factors which determine myocardial blood flow at the threshold of ischemia.

Three separate factors contribute to a reduction in DPTI; they will be discussed below.

Ventricular Systole Ventricular systole causes flow to cease in the subendocardial layers. DPTI is decreased in direct proportion to the systolic time per minute and consequently decreases with tachycardia and prolongation of systole. Shortening of systole only partially offsets the effects of increased heart rate, while depression of cardiac contractility will prolong systole and independently reduce DPTI.[22] The relative effect of systole on DPTI is independent of the other factors that determine myocardial blood flow and will always be an important determinant of blood flow in subendocardial layers, if unopposed by autoregulation.

Ventricular Diastolic Pressure Ventricular diastolic pressure inhibits flow in subendocardial layers in direct proportion to its magnitude;* however, the relative effect on DPTI depends on coronary pressure. Ventricular diastolic pressures are normally negligible compared to coronary perfusion pressure (i.e., aortic pressure), and even in congestive heart failure, perfusion of subendocardial layers will be sufficient if the coronary arteries are normal. With severe proximal coronary obstruction, the difference between ventricular diastolic pressure and coronary perfusion pressure, i.e., pressure distal to the obstruction, can be small and in some cases even negative. Under these circumstances small changes in ventricular diastolic pressure will greatly influence

*A phenomenon of "critical closing" has been described for coronary vessels in which blood flow ceases when perfusion pressure decreases below a critical level.[23,24] At the critical pressure the vessels are thought to close as the result of an external pressure or activity of vascular smooth muscle. Critical closing pressures greater than normal ventricular diastolic pressures are observed in the coronary circulation even with maximal coronary vasodilatation. Therefore, it may be necessary to modify the calculation of DPTI to include the effect of critical closing, but at the present time, the correct values of critical pressure at normal ventricular pressures are unresolved.[25] At higher ventricular-filling pressures critical closing pressures in ischemic subendocardial layers are likely to be similar to ventricular diastolic pressure and have the effect on DPTI as described here.

DPTI and become one of the primary determinants of flow in subendocardial layers.

Coronary Perfusion Pressure Coronary perfusion pressure is reduced by proximal coronary obstruction and also can be reduced by decreases in aortic pressure. The reduction of coronary perfusion pressure is determined by the severity of the obstruction, but even an 80 percent decrease in the cross-sectional area of the lumen of a coronary artery may not reduce coronary perfusion pressure below the range in which autoregulation will maintain sufficient myocardial flow in all layers of the heart wall under resting conditions.[26,27] With severe obstruction, however, vasodilatation may still be possible in epicardial layers, and the resultant increase in flow will cause an increased pressure drop across the obstruction and will further decrease coronary perfusion pressure.[19] Thus DPTI will be decreased by flow increases that may be caused by increased myocardial oxygen content as well as by increases caused by vasodilatation unrelated to cardiac metabolism.

If coronary flow remains constant, the pressure drop across the obstruction is constant, and thus changes in aortic pressure and coronary pressure are equal. This is an important consideration when the balance between changes in coronary perfusion pressure and ventricular diastolic pressure is considered. For example, a systemic vasodilator may reduce both aortic pressure and ventricular filling pressure, and if the changes are equal, the opposing effects on DPTI will be nullified.

Phasic flow in a normal coronary artery may cease or actually reverse during systole, which gives the impression that coronary blood flow is primarily a diastolic event. This is certainly true for flow in the subendocardial layers. Greater emphasis is therefore placed on aortic diastolic pressure than on systolic pressure as a determinant of myocardial perfusion, but this distinction is not as valid with coronary obstruction. Flow in an obstructed artery becomes less phasic as pressure distal to the obstruction decreases, and aortic systolic pressure becomes relatively more important in determining myocardial perfusion.[21] With severe coronary stenosis, the high resistance of the obstruction and the compliance of the arterial bed distal to the obstruction tend to damp out the oscillations in pressure so that diastolic pressures in the distal vessels, and consequently flow in the subendocardial layers, reflect, in part, flow through the obstruction during systole.

Myocardial Oxygen Supply

The DPTI summarizes the factors which determine blood flow in endocardial layers when autoregulation is exhausted, but under normal conditions *oxygen is the substrate which is critically limited in arterial blood, and its availability to the myocardium determines the adequacy of supply.* Decreases in arterial oxygen content (which can result from a variety of causes including anemia, pulmonary hypoxia, arterial hypoxia secondary to pulmonary disease, and carbon monoxide poisoning) reduce myocardial supply and would precipitate ischemia if not compensated for by an increase in flow. Myocardial oxygen supply can be approximated by the product of myocardial flow and arterial oxygen content.

Precise evaluation of myocardial oxygen supply, however, must be made at the level of the myocardial capillary bed. Oxygen diffuses from the capillaries to the mitochondria within the myocardial cells, where it is utilized. At this level, ischemia occurs when the concentration of oxygen, which is proportional to its partial pressure (P_{O_2}), falls below a critical level at the mitochondria. In broad terms, this level is equal to that required to rephosphorylate the adenosine triphosphate (ATP) load being produced by all kinds of myocardial work. In vitro experiments have shown that the critical level of P_{O_2} at the mitochondria is much less than the lowest levels of P_{O_2} obtained in coronary venous blood.[28] Nevertheless, the heart makes efficient use of oxygen delivery and extracts 70 to 80 percent of the oxygen reaching it, which is more than most other organs do. Moreover, myocardial oxygen extraction is relatively constant over a wide range of myocardial oxygen requirements and cannot be increased significantly without provoking ischemia. The discrepancy between critical levels of intracellular P_{O_2} and coronary venous P_{O_2} suggests that the diffusion of oxygen from the capillary has a decisive role in myocardial oxygen supply.

Anatomic evidence of closed metarterioles and precapillary sphincters indicates that myocardial capillaries are not all functional at all times.[29] These ideas are supported by physiological evidence[30] and by direct microscopic observation of in situ rat hearts[31] and suggest a control of precapillary sphincters by an autoregulation mechanism similar to the control of coronary resistance. Analysis of these findings in terms of a diffusion model for myocardial P_{O_2} suggests that changes in the number of open capillaries may be as important an adjustment in maintaining myocardial P_{O_2}, the mean tissue P_{O_2}, as changes in coronary vascular resistance.[32] For example, consider the effect on myocardial P_{O_2} were the capillary density fixed and myocardial oxygen utilization doubled. A corresponding doubling of coronary blood flow would maintain coronary venous P_{O_2} constant. Since the diffusion of oxygen from each capillary would also be doubled, the gradient for P_{O_2} from the capillary to the tissue would have to increase and, for the same capillary P_{O_2}, the mean tissue-value would decrease. Although proportional increments in myocardial oxygen utilization and blood flow will maintain the venous P_{O_2} constant, a fall in mean tissue P_{O_2} will occur unless compensated for by a decrease in intercapillary distance.

With myocardial ischemia and maximal vasodilatation, all of the available capillaries are likely to be recruited and the diffusion of oxygen will be limited by the anatomic capillary density. Myocardial capillaries parallel myocardial fibers, and viewed in cross section there is about one capillary for each fiber,[33] which places each fiber in contact with three to four capillaries. This ratio of one capillary per fiber remains constant in adults and is unchanged with cardiac hypertrophy.[33,34] Consequently the anatomic capillary density decreases when the diameter of myocardial fibers enlarges in hypertrophy, and this may contribute to the onset of myocardial ischemia (Fig. 44-4). Other factors that limit exchange between blood and myocardium, such as cardiac edema, cardiac fibrosis, capillary obstruction by microemboli, or precapillary vasoconstriction, could also be contributing factors in myocardial ischemia.

Coronary Vasoconstriction

Coronary vessels are invested with both alpha- and beta-adrenergic receptors, and with appropriate pharmacologic blockade, direct control of coronary resistance by sympathetic and parasympathetic nerves can be demonstrated.[2] However, autonomic nerve stimulation usually causes changes in myocardial compression which may obscure the direct effects on coronary vessels. For example, following beta-adrenergic blockade, carotid artery occlusion in the dog causes reflex increases in coronary resistance which result from stimulation of alpha-adrenergic receptors in the coronary vessels.[35] In contrast, carotid occlusion normally causes reflex tachycardia, increased cardiac contractility, and systemic hypertension; the increased cardiac metabolism which ensues is accompanied by coronary vasodilatation and increased coronary blood flow. Thus, coronary autoregulation appears to override neurally mediated coronary vasoconstriction. Moreover, maximum stimulation of cardiac nerves produces an increase in coronary resistance of only 30 percent, and the effect cannot be maintained.[35,36] In contrast, a sixfold increase in resistance can be elicited in skeletal muscle by neurogenic vasoconstriction.[37] Thus, alpha-adrenergic coronary vasoconstriction may "compete" with metabolic autoregulation;[38] under experimental conditions in which microspheres are embolized into precapillary vessels, it has been shown that an alpha-adrenergic mechanism can even override metabolic autoregulation sufficient to produce myocardial necrosis.[39] Whether this effect occurs in human resistance vessels is as yet unknown.

FIGURE 44-4 Relation of myocardial capillaries and muscle fibers in normal (*left*) and hypertrophied (*right*) hearts. There is about one capillary for each muscle fiber in both cases. Consequently, the distance between capillaries increases with cardiac hypertrophy, and diffusion of oxygen into the fibers may be impeded. [*After rendition by R. L. Van Citters of concept of J. T. Wearn, in T. C. Ruch and H. D. Patton (eds.), "Physiology and Biophysics," 19th ed., W. B. Saunders Company, Philadelphia, 1965, p. 692. Reproduced with permission from the publisher, editors, and authors.*]

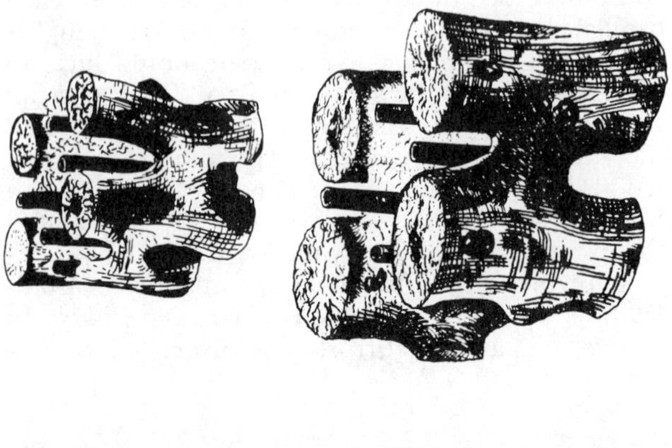

Neurogenic vasoconstriction and autoregulation can interact in vessels exposed to the mediators of metabolic regulation, but in large coronary vessels, vasoconstriction may go unopposed by the consequences of myocardial ischemia. This appears to be the situation in coronary artery spasm, where large-vessel constriction can completely block coronary flow and cause myocardial ischemia and even ultimate infarction.[1] *The negative feedback mechanism for coronary autoregulation, which normally prevents myocardial ischemia, is simply unable to dilate the large coronary vessels.*[40] Under normal conditions the vessels which do not participate in autoregulation contribute only a small portion of the total coronary resistance and can undergo large relative changes in resistance without significantly affecting coronary blood flow. Coronary artery disease removes increasing portions of the total coronary resistance from the control of autoregulation. Contraction of vascular smooth muscle, which might be benign in a large normal coronary artery, may significantly diminish coronary blood flow when the lumen is nearly obstructed by disease. It has become increasingly clear in recent years that vasoconstriction, i.e., spasm, in large vessels plays a significant role in myocardial ischemia, but the actual causes of large vessel constriction are, at present, not fully understood.[41] Alpha-adrenergic responses may be only one of several mechanisms involved. In addition, vasoconstriction or spasm in small vessels may contribute to myocardial ischemia[39,42] and potentially may cause necrosis of small volumes of myocardial cells.

Coronary Collateral Blood Flow

Thus far, we have considered the factors which contribute to an insufficiency of blood flow in subendocardial layers of the heart and which are involved when subtotal obstruction of a coronary artery develops. These considerations include many of the conditions characterized by myocardial ischemia being absent at rest and developing on effort. With total occlusion of a major coronary artery, severe ischemia and infarction will occur unless alternative arterial pathways exist. Although the normal heart has preexisting connections between distal branches of large coronary arteries, these anastomoses or collaterals are usually insufficient to prevent infarction following sudden occlusion of a major vessel. However, gradual obstruction of a coronary artery may result in the development of a collateral circulation with maintenance or reestablishment of an adequate coronary blood flow to the jeopardized region.[43,44]

There is considerable evidence that collateral development provides protection against myocardial ischemia in humans.[45] This evidence includes postmortem studies, measurements obtained during coronary bypass surgery, and angiograph studies. Although significant collateral development may indicate potential regional ischemia, the protection afforded by collaterals against myocardial infarction is indisputable. Thus, *development of a collateral circulation represents a long-range adaptation to coronary artery disease.*

If this adaptation is successful, ischemia will be absent at rest, but the capacity of the blood supply to increase on demand will usually be significantly limited[46] so that the myocardium supplied by collaterals will be vulnerable to ischemia in much the same way as a region supplied by a partially obstructed coronary artery. Moreover, the potential for ischemia is often compounded by disease in the coronary artery supplying the collateral vessels. Thus, all of the factors previously discussed which determine myocardial perfusion at the threshold of ischemia can be applied to a region supplied by collaterals. Change in heart rate, left ventricular diastolic pressure, or aortic pressure could precipitate the onset of ischemia in the subendocardial layers of this region.

Coronary collaterals appear to function strictly as an alternative arterial supply which effectively delivers flow to the arterial system immediately distal to the coronary obstruction. This concept is summarized diagrammatically in Fig. 44-5, which shows the myocardial blood flow distribution after acute occlusion of a coronary artery. Although severe ischemia and ultimately infarction occur with sudden occlusion, several of the important characteristics of the collateral circulation are more clearly revealed by the large differences in myocardial blood flows that occur under these conditions. Sudden obstruction of a major coronary artery in the dog does not result in an equal reduction of flow throughout the region at risk. Collateral flow entering the region through preexisting arterial anastomoses is distributed preferentially to the epicardial layers of the ischemic region as a result of the physical factors described above (see "Subendocardial Ischemia"). A transmural gradient of ischemia results, and, depending on the capacity of the preexisting collateral vessels, myocardial blood flow within the region at risk can vary from near-zero in the endocardial layers to nearly normal levels in the epicardial layers. This transmural gradient from severe ischemia to mild ischemia has significant consequences which are described below ("Patterns of Acute Myocardial Infarction").

Coronary Steal

Under special conditions an increase in myocardial blood flow in one region can reduce flow in another region. This phenomenon is termed *a coronary steal* and may have a role in myocardial ischemia. The simplest conditions necessary for a coronary steal include (1) a common coronary vessel having some resistance to flow which supplies two myocardial regions in parallel, and (2) vasodilatation in only one of the two parallel regions. The key to interpreting a coronary steal is the coronary pressure at the point where the common vessel branches into the parallel circulations. Any decrease in pressure at this point will decrease flow in the passive circulation. This is

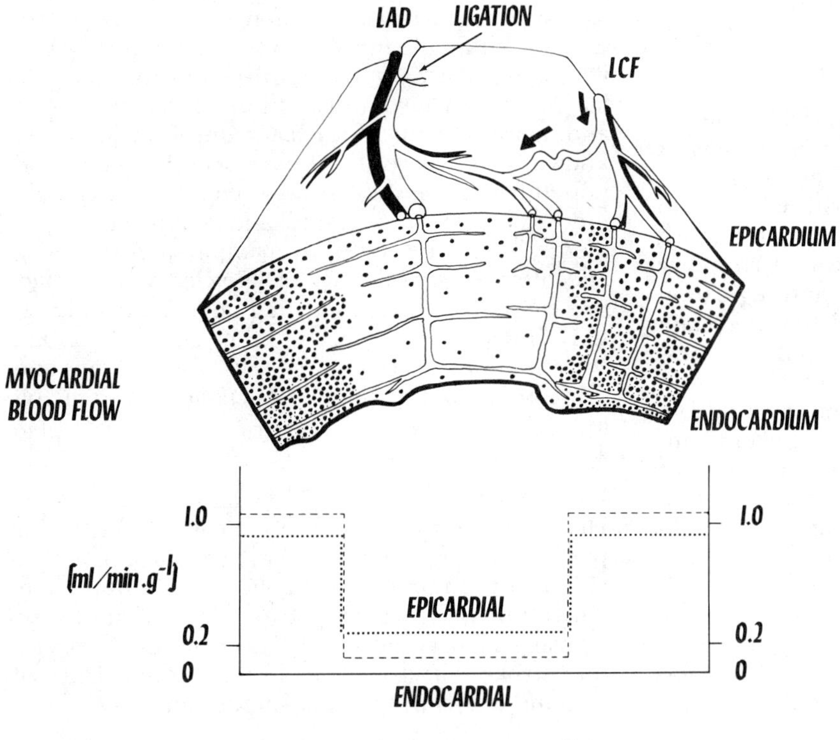

FIGURE 44-5 Myocardial blood flow after acute coronary artery ligation in the dog. The density of dots corresponds to local myocardial blood flow and indicates the deposition of microspheres injected into the left atrium shortly after coronary ligation. Representative flow values are given in the lower graph. Following coronary occlusion, collateral flow (indicated by arrows) enters the distal left anterior descending artery (LAD) via interarterial anastomoses. Although lateral borders are irregular, flow is uniform at each level of the ischemic region. A transmural gradient of flow exists with more severe ischemia in endocardial layers. LCF = left circumflex artery.

what happens when flow increases through the common vessel as a result of vasodilatation in the active circulation. The increase in total coronary flow accounts for most of the increase to the vasodilating region, however, and only a small portion of the increase to the active circulation is actually "stolen" from the passive one.

The resistance of the common supply vessel is a critical determinant of the potential for coronary steal.[47] With minimal resistance, large increases in flow would cause only minor decreases in pressure at the branch point, while with an increased common resistance, autoregulation will recruit increasing portions of the vasodilatory reserve in both branches and diminish the potential for a steal. Thus, there appears to be an optimal degree of common coronary resistance corresponding to some degree of partial coronary obstruction. However, identification of this condition would require physiological measurements not available except under the conditions of a laboratory experiment. Although vasodilatation in one of two parallel regions is often used as the sign of a coronary steal, small concomitant decreases in resistances in the common vessel or in the other parallel vascular bed could completely offset the tendency for a flow reduction. This possibility may be difficult to rule out whenever a coronary steal mechanism is considered as part of the action of a coronary vasodilator drug. In fact, some drugs such as nitroglycerin appear to elicit a selective long-acting vasodilatation in larger coronary vessels[40] and would therefore tend to prevent a coronary steal. The drugs with the greatest potential for eliciting a coronary steal are those which override the normal autoregulatory mechanisms; even so, examples such as the calcium-blocking agents (for instance nifedipine), appear to relax vasoconstriction in larger vessels (spasm) and, in fact, may have an important therapeutic role in this respect.[48]

Since autoregulation will recruit nearly all the reserve of vasodilatation before a region becomes ischemic, the conditions for a coronary steal suggest that the passive region is on the verge of or is actually ischemic, while the region which is able to vasodilate is normal. There are two situations in which this might occur: (1) critical reduction of coronary supply to the point of exhaustion of autoregulation in endocardial layers while epicardial layers retain some vasodilatory reserve, and (2) supply of an ischemic region via collateral vessels branching from a vessel supplying a nonischemic region. A steal from deep to superficial layers is likely to occur only under a narrow set of conditions and, with a small shift in supply and/or demand, all or none of the myocardial layers will become ischemic and the conditions for a steal will be diminished. Moreover, at the critical point the reserve of vasodilatation in epicardial layers is likely to be very small. Nevertheless, coronary vasodilator drugs can cause a coronary steal under these conditions.[19] Since vasodilator drugs also tend to lower aortic blood pressure, this effect may often be more important in causing ischemia in subendocardial layers.

In contrast, the conditions governing collateral blood flow are frequently well suited for a coronary steal. Collateral blood flow to an ischemic region always occurs in parallel with flow to an adjacent region, and often the adjacent region has a large vasodilatory reserve.[49] In fact, a steal of collateral blood can be ruled out following a stimulus for coronary vasodilatation only if both regions are ischemic or if the collateral vessels are so well developed that no ischemia occurs. On the other hand, with a critical level of collateral blood flow which results in a region balanced on the verge of ischemia, changes in demand and/or effective coronary perfusion pressure could be more significant determinants of myocardial ischemia than changes in supply caused by a coronary steal mechanism. Therefore, *it is doubtful whether a steal mechanism by itself ever precipitates myocardial ischemia,* but the potential for increasing the intensity of ischemia in a region supplied by collaterals is clear.

Determinants of Myocardial Oxygen Consumption

Although the primary cause of myocardial ischemia is a defect in arterial blood supply, ischemia does not occur until the tissue's demand for oxygen to support energy generation outstrips its supply of oxygen. Thus the determinants of myocardial oxygen consumption play a decisive role in setting the threshold for ischemia. The normal heart is completely dependent on aerobic metabolism for continued contractile function; thus oxygen consumption closely parallels energy production. The assessment of cardiac function versus energy production within the myocytes is related to certain easily measurable parameters. Although the exact relation between myocardial mitochondrial respiration and measurements of cardiac pump function is not known, good correlations have been frequently reported between myocardial oxygen consumption and indexes based on pressure and volume measurements.[50,51] At the risk of oversimplifying a complex and often empirical body of knowledge, three factors can be identified as having important, and possibly independent, effects on myocardial oxygen consumption: heart rate, systolic wall tension, and myocardial contractility. A discussion of each follows.

Heart Rate

Heart rate is the most easily measured of all the parameters and is likely to have the most direct relation to the rate of myocardial energy utilization. The effect of heart rate can be factored out by expressing myocardial oxygen consumption per cardiac stroke, but it is easier to relate the balance of demand and supply in per minute units.

Systolic Wall Tension
Systolic wall tension is proportional to ventricular systolic pressure and, according to the Laplace relation, is also proportional to ventricular radius. Systolic wall tension cannot be measured directly, however, and therefore various approximations derived from ventricular systolic pressure are used. Usually the important effect of the ventricular radius is neglected, with the result that the relation is imprecise.

The uncertainty surrounding systolic wall tension does not minimize its importance in determining myocardial oxygen consumption but does caution against a strict quantitative interpretation of changes in parameters. This may be of no great consequence if the effects of presumed changes in wall tension are not opposed by other factors. For example, a systemic vasodilator will reduce systolic ventricular pressure (afterload) and also ventricular filling pressure (preload); both effects tend to reduce systolic wall tension and consequently myocardial oxygen consumption. On the other hand, there is no precise way to balance an accompanying increase in heart rate against these changes.

Wall tension is inversely proportional to wall thickness and consequently decreases with cardiac hypertrophy caused by pressure overload. Under these conditions oxygen consumption per 100 g of myocardium will be decreased relative to a nonhypertrophied heart developing the same pressure and the same inner wall radius, but total myocardial oxygen consumption will be similar and the supply/demand ratio will be improved only if the coronary circulation hypertrophies as well.

Myocardial Contractility
Myocardial contractility is a concept with general utility but for which there is no agreed upon or easily obtained measure. There is no unique index that can be derived from pressure and/or volume measurements which quantitates changes in myocardial contractility. Nevertheless, indexes which rely on the rapidity of the contractile process, such as the rate of rise of pressure during isovolumic contraction, *dP/dt,* have been widely used and are helpful in estimating change in myocardial oxygen consumption.[52]

These three factors, *heart rate, systolic wall tension, and contractility, can be used to estimate directional changes in myocardial oxygen consumption, but it is impractical to balance quantitatively the factors determining myocardial blood flow against the factors determining demand.* Exact relations are not known, and the measurements available are seldom equal to the task. Under favorable conditions, changes in the determinants of oxygen demand and myocardial blood flow may not oppose each other, and the change in the balance of supply and demand can be clearly interpreted.

With *severe ischemia* aerobic metabolism of the myocardium rapidly decreases and anaerobic glycolysis becomes the predominant form of energy production. In the absence of adequate oxygen, contractile failure ensues and electrical inexcitability may ultimately follow. Under these conditions the determinants of myocardial need are likely to be unrelated to the mechanical function of normal myocardium.

Supply and Demand Considerations in the Therapy of Coronary Artery Disease

The preceding analysis of the physiological and pathological mechanisms that apply at the onset of myocardial ischemia are summarized diagrammatically in Fig. 44-6. This diagram is a model which can be used to evaluate the effect of an intervention on the balance of myocardial supply and demand. Based on the preceding analysis, the three underlying conditions of the model are that (1) the critical region to analyze is the subendocardial layers in segments of the heart supplied by obstructed arteries, (2) the

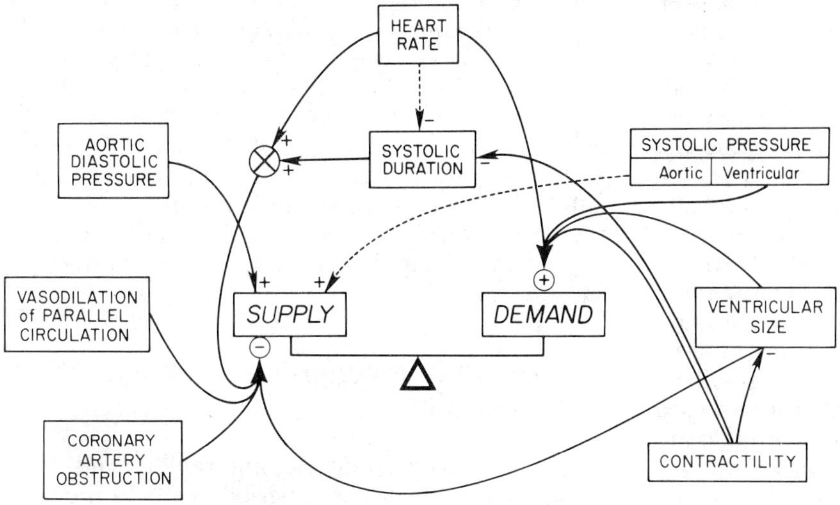

FIGURE 44-6 Diagram summarizing the factors in the balance of oxygen supply and demand in ischemic subendocardium. An increase in each variable is characterized as to its effect in increasing (+) or decreasing (−) the variables it acts on. The product (×) of heart rate and systolic duration decreases the relative diastolic time and thereby decreases supply. Interactions of secondary importance are shown by dotted lines. Some interactions have direct effects on the balance of oxygen supply and demand (e.g., effect of aortic diastolic pressure on supply), while other interactions have a secondary effect on supply or demand (e.g., contractility effect on ventricular size).

availability of oxygen to the myocardium determines the adequacy of supply, and (3) the ischemic myocardium is maximally vasodilated as a result of autoregulation.

In the model the effects of each of the factors on the balance of oxygen supply and demand in the ischemic subendocardium are shown by arrows. An increase in each variable is characterized as to its effect to increase (+) or decrease (−) the variable or variables it acts on, which, depending on the side of the equation affected, either raises or lowers the balance in favor of oxygen supply. Several factors, such as aortic pressure and coronary artery obstruction, act only on one side of the balance and therefore have a predictable effect on myocardial ischemia. Other variables affect both supply and demand and tend to shift the balance in an additive manner; examples of these are ventricular size and heart rate. Contractility has by far the most complex interaction with the factors determining supply and demand, and its effect on the balance is not easily predicted. Although contractility has a direct effect on myocardial oxygen consumption, the end result on demand of a positive inotropic intervention could be offset, particularly in the failing dilated ventricle, by a reduction of ventricular size and, consequently, of wall tension. In addition, increased contractility tends to increase blood supply by reducing both systolic and diastolic compression of the subendocardial layers, by shortening systole with a resultant increase in relative diastolic time, and by decreasing ventricular size. To further complicate the analysis, many interventions have effects on more than one variable in the model. Therefore, the purpose of the model is, in part, to emphasize the complexity of the balance between oxygen supply and demand and to caution against oversimplified interpretations of the effect of an intervention. This can be illustrated by analyzing a few specific examples.

Beta-Adrenergic Blocker

Beta-adrenergic blockers, which lower heart rate and contractility, relieve the symptoms of myocardial ischemia. It is tempting to identify the benefit of these drugs with the reduction in myocardial oxygen demand, but examination of the model shown in Fig. 44-6 suggests that other factors should be considered. As indicated above, lowering contractility has an ambiguous effect on myocardial supply and demand and could, under such circumstances as ventricular dilatation, actually increase ischemia. A decrease in heart rate is clearly beneficial, however, since heart rate has additive effects on both supply and demand. Thus, the capacity of beta-blocking drugs to increase cardiac performance in coronary artery disease is likely to be caused by lowered heart rates. Apparently physiological heart rates are not as well adapted for balancing myocardial oxygen supply and demand when supply is restricted as are the slower rates obtained by pharmacologic intervention.

Vasodilating Drugs

Vasodilating drugs decrease ventricular systolic pressure (afterload) and ventricular filling (preload) and consequently decrease myocardial oxygen demand. However, decreased coronary blood flow as a result of decreased aortic pressure could offset the benefit on the balance of supply and demand. Since afterload reduction has opposing effects on supply and demand, its net effect is unpredictable. In a normal heart with normal diastolic filling pressures, a reduction in coronary pressure and afterload will reduce supply more than demand. Moreover, a reflex tachycardia is response to afterload reduction will further worsen the balance. In the presence of failure, preload reduction exerts beneficial effects on both sides of the balance and is therefore the key factor in the potential benefit of vasodilating drugs on myocardial ischemia.[53]

A direct effect of vasodilatory drugs on the coronary circulation could also have either beneficial or detrimental effects. Vasodilatation in a parallel nonischemic vascular bed could worsen the balance (by coronary steal), while vasodilatation in the portions of the coronary bed unresponsive to autoregulation, i.e., large coronary vessels or collateral vessels, could improve myocardial perfusion.

Severe Ischemia

With severe ischemia resulting from sudden coronary occlusion in the absence of substantial collateral vessels, a balance of supply and demand cannot be achieved by a simple readjustment of the factors shown in Fig. 44-6. Moreover, Fig. 44-6 may not be an appropriate model for evaluating the balance of factors in severe ischemia. Two important points should be considered: (1) Myocardial need for oxygen under conditions of severe reduction of flow may not be of primary or singular importance, nor are the factors that determine the needs of severely ischemic myocardium likely to be the same as the determinants of oxygen demand in normal myocardium. Metabolism and function of severely ischemic myocardium is not normal, and the need is not to contract, but rather to survive. (2) Several of the factors affecting supply in Fig. 44-6 apply to the endocardial layers, whereas the epicardial layers often are the only layers likely to survive. Specifically, heart rate and ventricular diastolic size may have much less influence on the supply of the epicardial layers and thus on the ultimate extent of infarction. In this latter circumstance, when blood flow in the ischemic region is severely reduced, the factors determining the balance of supply and demand cannot effect tissue survival.

Pathology of Myocardial Ischemia and Infarction

Coronary ischemia, developing rapidly and then persisting for a sufficient period, leads to the evolution of characteristic morphologic features of tissue necrosis known as *myocardial infarction.* A myocardial infarction is both a spatial and temporal event, whose size and histopathology are dependent on the availability of coronary collateral blood supply and the metabolic demands of the tissue. As discussed in previous sections of this chapter the primary determinant of myocardial necrosis is blood flow; a diminution of coronary supply below a critical but often not predictable threshold leads to cell death. However, it is clear from studies on brief transient coronary occlusion,[54] as well as from observations in animals and patients subjected to complete cessation of coronary flow during open heart surgery, that myocardial necrosis is not inevitable if blood flow is restored within a finite period of time. The complex pathophysiological interrelationships between the underlying coronary anatomy, the development of transient or permanent coronary occlusion leading to myocellular necrosis, and the identification and evolution of the infarction process will be explored in the succeeding sections.

Coronary Artery Anatomy

If the coronary circulation was *diffusely* interconnected at all levels, sudden obstruction of any one major vessel or a smaller branch would theoretically not cause myocardial ischemia or necrosis. Even if myocardial infarction did develop because of *inadequate* collateral supply, the pattern of tissue necrosis would likely be irregular and patchy, with indistinct borders possibly representing ischemic but surviving myocardium. These pathological features are predicated on the supposition that at the level where cell necrosis is determined (i.e., the microcirculation), diffuse capillary interconnections, with the branches derived from both occluded and patent stem vessels, could provide oxygenated blood to some myocardial cells at the border between two circulatory fields. Two hypothetical capillary patterns are illustrated in Fig. 44-7, either of which could account for ischemic and surviving myocells at the lateral border of an infarct, i.e., *a lateral border zone.* A gradual but progressive diminution of blood flow could then extend from the periphery of the perfusion field of an obstructed coronary artery toward the center, until the ischemic threshold was reached and the myocardial cells necrosed. Thus multiple layers of ischemia would exist in a continuum from the lateral to the central zone thereby giving rise to a "bull's-eye" pattern of infarction. This, in fact, is the commonly accepted view of myocardial ischemia,[55] one which also provides a rationale for therapeutic interventions which may preserve *lateral* border zone tissue before it undergoes necrosis.

Is such a view consistent with objective data? Certainly, a number of investigators have identified indirect markers of ischemia in the lateral border zone which are quantitatively intermediate between those in the normal and those in the central necrotic

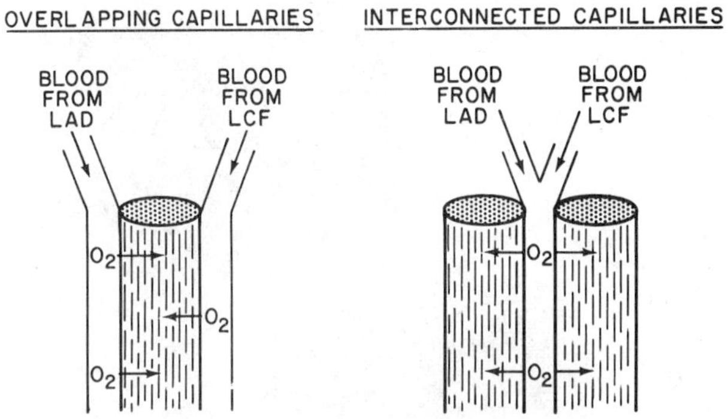

FIGURE 44-7 Two hypothetical capillary anatomic patterns that could explain the existence of surviving but ischemic myocardium at the lateral border of an acute myocardial infarction. On the left, each myocardial cell is intimately associated with interdigitating or overlapping capillaries derived from separate large coronary arteries. Occlusion of one main vessel would allow the cell to be supplied by oxygenated blood from the patent artery, in diminished amounts as compared with normal. On the right, capillaries derived from two major vessels are interconnected, so that occlusion of one coronary artery would allow cells to be partially supplied by the patent vessel. With both patterns, enough substrate might be provided from the nonoccluded vascular bed to keep the myocardial cells viable, though ischemic. LAD = left anterior descending coronary artery; LCF = left circumflex artery. (*From S. M. Factor, E. M. Okun, T. Minase, and E. S. Kirk, The Microcirculation of the Human Heart: End-Capillary Loops with Discrete Perfusion Fields, Circulation, 66:1241, 1982. Reproduced with permission from the American Heart Association, Inc., and the authors.*)

regions.[56–60] Absolute uncorrected blood flows measured with microspheres, when sampled across the border, also display a gradual falloff toward the central infarct.[61] Yet markers of ischemia, derived from gross tissue sampling at the border or indirect measures of myocardial injury such as the electrocardiogram, fail to take account of an alternative explanation for intermediate levels: that tissue at the border of an infarct is discretely necrotic or normal, and is so interdigitated that bulk analysis cannot be employed to separate the two cell populations. Thus gross sampling at the lateral margins invariably gives intermediate marker levels because it averages the two tissue types which comprise this region.

A number of sensitive techniques that can distinguish ischemic tissue recently have been used to study the nature of the lateral border; they have shown that there is a sharp transition between normal and ischemic myocardium.[62–67] Serial section analysis of completed infarcts with three-dimensional reconstruction has revealed that infarcts are remarkably complex along their lateral borders, with numerous interdigitating *peninsulas* of histologically normal or necrotic myocardium.[68] Routine two-dimensional histological sections tend to give a false impression of the spatial characteristics of an infarct; i.e., small regions of normal or necrotic myocardium appear as "islands," separated from homologous tissue. Reconstruction, however, demonstrates that this impression is caused by an artifact of examining a three-dimensional structure in two dimensions and that the border between normal and necrotic tissue is very sharp (Fig. 44-8).

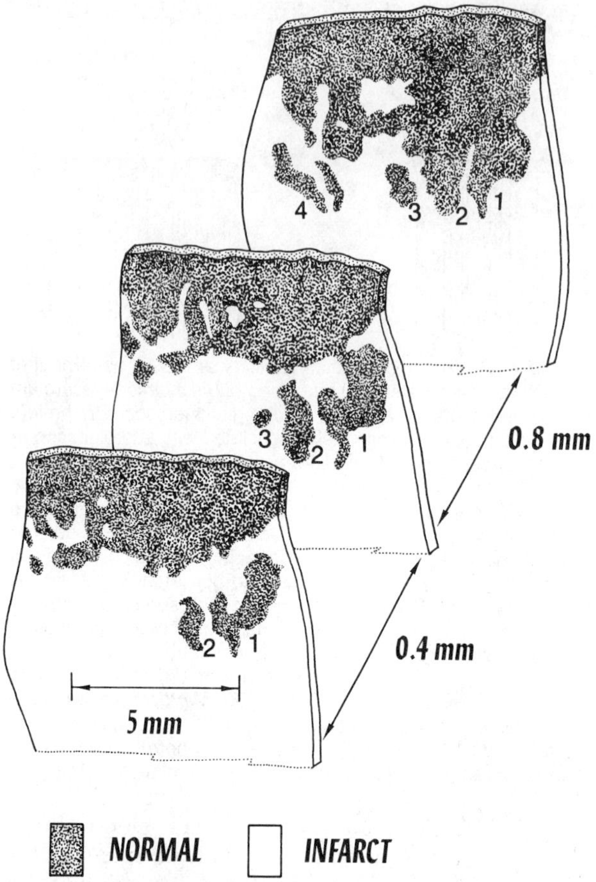

FIGURE 44-8 Composite illustration, based on original drawings of three myocardial sections. Intervening sections have been omitted for clarity. Preserved subepicardial normal myocardium (shaded area) can be seen at the top of each section. In the foreground, two islands of normal tissue (1 and 2) are completely separated from the subepicardial normal zone. Two sections deeper within the block, island number 2 is still isolated. At the same level, a new island (3) becomes apparent. The last drawing, four sections away, shows complete continuity between islands number 1 and 2 and the overlying subepicardial myocardium. Island number 3 is larger at this level and becomes attached in subsequent sections. Several islands on the left (4) progressively enlarge and eventually become peninsulas. Additionally, the islands of necrotic tissue (unshaded) within the subepicardial zone demonstrate continuity with the infarct region at various levels and therefore are also peninsulas. The reconstruction illustrates that the border region consists of numerous interdigitated peninsulas which may appear as islands of normal or necrotic tissue when any one section is viewed. *(From S. M. Factor, E. H. Sonnenblick, and E. S. Kirk, The Histologic Border Zone of Acute Myocardial Infarction: Islands or Peninsulas? Am. J. Pathol., 92:111, 1978. Reproduced with permission from the publisher and authors.)*

An anatomic explanation for this discrete separation of tissue is revealed by perfusion studies of the myocardial microcirculation. Normal dog[69] and human[70] hearts do not have microvascular connections at the boundaries between regions perfused by separate large coronary arteries. This discrete pattern of supply is illustrated by the specimen in Fig. 44-9, prepared from a human heart, which reveals that where two microcirculations abut, separately derived capillaries do not anastomose. Terminal homologous capillaries form loops instead of interconnecting with heterologous capillaries. As a result of these end-capillary loops, the coronary circulation is a functional end-artery system, in which the significant collateral vessels are proximal interarterial anastomoses located in the epicardial layers.

One important consequence of the end-artery circulation in the heart is that the *region of myocardium at risk following obstruction of a coronary artery is sharply delineated by the anatomic limit of the capillary bed supplied by the artery.* Tissue outside the artery bed is not made ischemic and is therefore not directly jeopardized. The concept of a region at risk determined by the arterial anatomy is emphasized by finding a close correlation between the size of an infarct and the size of the occluded artery bed.[71] Its relevance to humans is demonstrated by a recent autopsy study showing that transmural infarcts involve essentially the entire region of the occluded artery bed, with minimal surviving tissue at lateral margins of the area at risk.[72] When the cellular histology of infarcted or normal myocardium is correlated with the microvascular supply, there is an extremely close relation between the microcirculation derived from the occluded artery and the necrotic tissue.[73] Discordance at the lateral border (i.e., nonnecrotic tissue within the region at risk) extended over a distance of only 30 to 50 μm, suggesting that this myocardium may have survived by diffusion of oxygenated substrate from the normally perfused zone. Further analysis also demonstrated that the highly complex, interdigitated histological border resulted from an equally complex, interdigitated microvascular supply.

One can conclude from these observations that the preexisting coronary anatomy organized into an end-vessel system determines the *area at risk* of infarction if the supply vessel becomes occluded. Although preformed collaterals may mitigate the consequences of coronary occlusion, they are predominantly epicardial vessels which, as previously discussed, are affected by intraventricular and intramural pressures that limit their perfusion of the subendocardium. In addition, since they are located proximal to the terminal capillary loops their distal effects may be attenuated where they are most required to keep tissue viable. The result of this anatomic arrangement of the coronary circulation is the presence of numerous areas at risk progressing from the subendocardium to the subepicardium, and potentially involving the tissue supplied by a single arteriolar-capillary unit up to the largest stem coronary vessel.

Coronary Artery Occlusion

Previous sections have emphasized that the primary determinant of myocardial tissue viability is blood flow. Abrupt coronary occlusion in an experimental animal such as a dog leads to a transmural gradient of ischemia within the myocardium with lowest blood flows in the subendocardial zone and relatively higher

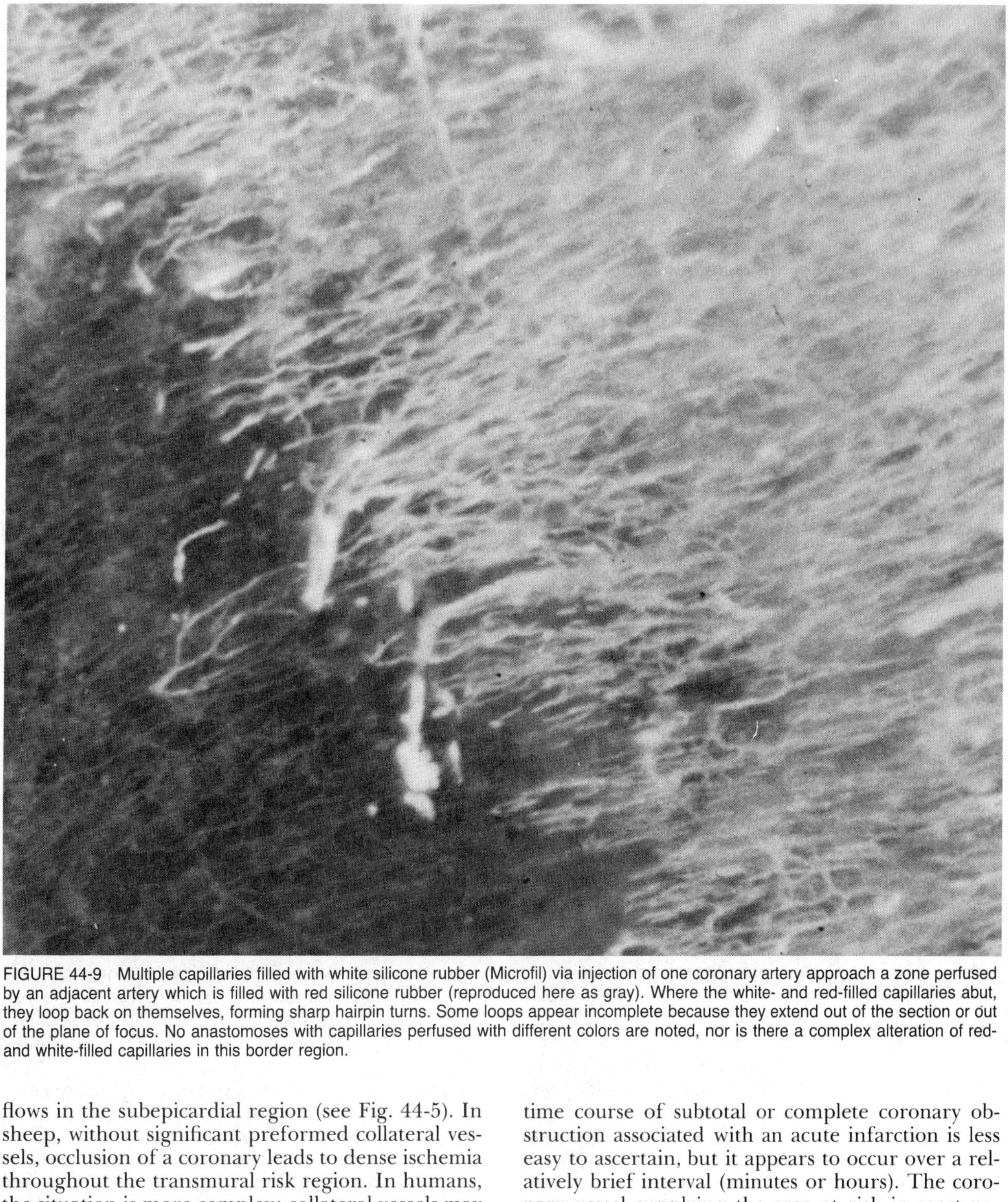

FIGURE 44-9 Multiple capillaries filled with white silicone rubber (Microfil) via injection of one coronary artery approach a zone perfused by an adjacent artery which is filled with red silicone rubber (reproduced here as gray). Where the white- and red-filled capillaries abut, they loop back on themselves, forming sharp hairpin turns. Some loops appear incomplete because they extend out of the section or out of the plane of focus. No anastomoses with capillaries perfused with different colors are noted, nor is there a complex alteration of red- and white-filled capillaries in this border region.

flows in the subepicardial region (see Fig. 44-5). In sheep, without significant preformed collateral vessels, occlusion of a coronary leads to dense ischemia throughout the transmural risk region. In humans, the situation is more complex: collateral vessels may or may not be present, several coronary arteries may have multiple areas of partial or complete occlusion, and the arteries supplying the collaterals may themselves be diseased. Thus the risk region may be more difficult to ascertain, and the beneficial effect of collateral supply may not be predictable.

In experimental animals myocardial infarcts generally are produced by *sudden* occlusion of an anatomically normal coronary artery. In humans, the time course of subtotal or complete coronary obstruction associated with an acute infarction is less easy to ascertain, but it appears to occur over a relatively brief interval (minutes or hours). The coronary vessel supplying the area at risk in most patients with transmural infarction reveals characteristic atherosclerosis with luminal narrowing.[74] Yet atherosclerosis is a chronic process which takes months or years to evolve. If slowly progressing atherosclerosis causes ischemia, collateral development also may be stimulated to provide alternative blood flow to the region, thus preventing tissue necrosis. Since atherosclerosis and infarction occur over different time frames, their frequent association is not reasonable proof of causation. Accordingly, in most instances the atherosclerotic coronary artery must have an acute, superimposed occlusive lesion to account for the development of a myocardial infarction. Recent observations support this conclusion.

Coronary Thrombosis

There has been considerable controversy and cyclical interest in the role played by coronary thrombosis in the causation of acute myocardial infarction.[75] A number of autopsy studies during the last two decades[76–78] suggested that coronary thrombi were secondary to infarction, primarily because they were rare in the early hours after infarct development and increased in frequency with temporal evolution of the myocardial necrosis. Although these investigations were carefully performed unavoidable problems with postmortem studies including biased patient selection, inability to diagnose myocardial infarction in the early hours after onset (see below), and lysis of an occlusive thrombus after it has caused infarction, may account for the discrepancy with recent data from living patients.

Rapid patient triage, because of the potential for interventions which may salvage acutely infarcting myocardium, have led a number of groups to perform coronary angiography during the early period after infarct onset. These studies have generally reported frequencies of occlusive coronary thrombosis to be greater than 70 to 80 percent in patients studied during the first 6 h after onset of symptoms. DeWood et al.[79] evaluated patients in the first 4 h and found 87 percent thrombotic occlusion, whereas this percentage decreased to 65 percent when patients were studied 12 to 24 h after onset. These data suggest that thrombi may undergo spontaneous thrombolysis, fragmentation, and distal embolization with infarct evolution to account for their diminished frequency in older infarcts.

Additional evidence that coronary thrombosis is involved in infarct development comes from intervention studies where either intracoronary streptokinase alone[80] or a combination of streptokinase and percutaneous transluminal coronary recanalization[81] have been employed in early myocardial infarction. The ability to reestablish coronary flow with these techniques is predicated on the concept that the coronary occlusion is due to an intraluminal thrombus. The rationale for such therapy is to preserve myocardium by preventing necrosis of jeopardized tissue. Although this goal is laudable, beneficial effects are difficult to demonstrate unequivocally in a clinical trial. Improvement of left ventricular function[82,83] and in-hospital mortality[83,84] supports the efficacy of these procedures and suggests that reperfusion occurred by clot lysis. On the other hand, even where reperfusion was obtained, some studies have not demonstrated objective benefits.[85] Although these negative results could be interpreted to indicate that coronary thrombosis is not a primary cause of myocardial infarction, it is more likely that they reflect already completed infarction or insensitive markers of functional improvement.

Even if it is accepted that coronary thrombosis is a primary cause of sudden coronary obstruction, it is clear that the thrombus occurs most often in a diseased vessel with subtotal atherosclerotic luminal compromise.[74] Although alterations of blood flow, including diminished velocity and turbulence, and direct atherosclerotic injury to the vessel intima may induce platelet adherence to subendothelial collagen with subsequent initiation of the coagulation process, other dynamic mechanisms may be involved. It is beyond the scope of this chapter to review the complex interrelationships between cellular, humoral, and coagulability parameters which may be associated with coronary thrombosis. Equally complex, but somewhat easier to study, plaque rupture and coronary artery spasm are two possibly related pathophysiological events which also have attained recent prominence because of their potential role in thrombus development.

Atherosclerotic Plaque Rupture

The human coronary atherosclerotic plaque is a complex structure composed of connective tissue, calcium, lipid, and inflammatory cells in proportions differing from patient to patient. Thin-walled vessels may enter the plaque and be potential sources of mural hemorrhage. Plaques may be eccentric (localized primarily along one segment of the wall), or they may be concentric (localized circumferentially); regardless of their orientation, some intact smooth muscle usually is present in the residual medial layer which may be a source of vessel vasomotion or vascular spasm under the appropriate stimulus. The consistency of plaques depends on the proportion of their component elements: a heavily calcified and fibrotic plaque is hard, while a plaque composed predominantly of cholesterol ester and lipid-containing macrophages is soft. Not infrequently, this soft lipid core of a plaque may be covered by a relatively thin cap of fibrous connective tissue separating the plaque material from the luminal blood flow (Fig. 44-10).

A number of studies have associated acute coronary thrombosis with rupture or cracks of the thin fibrous cap and release of the plaque material into the vascular lumen. Reports have found between 78 and 93 percent[86–88] of acute coronary thrombi at postmortem could be identified as secondary to plaque rupture. This work essentially confirms the findings of Friedman,[89] an early proponent of this concept, who found 98 percent concordance between thrombi and plaque rupture. Plaque rupture may induce thrombosis by any or a combination of several mechanisms: (1) contact of platelets with exposed collagen leading to thrombocyte adherence and the buildup of a platelet plug, (2) release of tissue thromboplastin from the plaque material in-

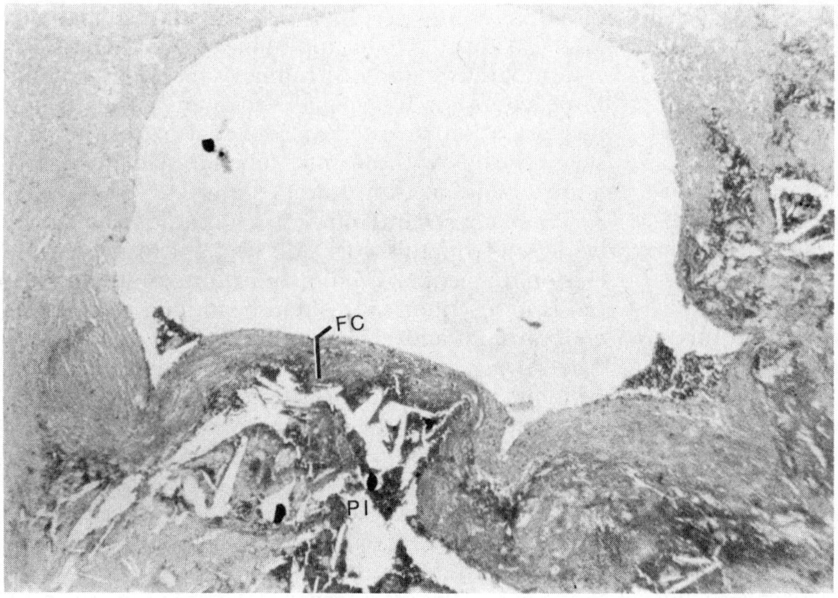

FIGURE 44-10 A segment of right coronary artery from a patient with an acute transmural myocardial infarction in the distribution of this vessel, associated with recent coronary thrombosis. The vessel was serially sectioned. At this level, there is a thin fibrous cap (FC) overlying a bulging atherosclerotic plaque (PI) composed of cholesterol crystals (empty spaces), hemorrhage, and debris. A subsequent section revealed complete rupture of the plaque into the lumen with occlusive thrombus admixed with the plaque material. (×60.)

ducing the initiation of the clotting cascade, and (3) mechanical obstruction of the vessel lumen by the plaque components.

An unanswered question is what causes the thin-walled fibrous cap to crack or rupture leading to release of the plaque debris. There have been suggestions that intraplaque hemorrhage related to rupture of the attenuated vessels in the atheroma may produce sufficient pressure to "blow-out" the surface cap. Although evidence of plaque hemorrhage even in unruptured plaques can be found with serial section investigations, hemodynamically it is not likely that sufficient pressure could be built up to overcome the intraluminal pressure acting in an opposite direction. Several investigators, including Friedman[89] and Horie,[87] believe that plaque hemorrhage, disruption of the fibrous cap, and eventual release of plaque material are related to entry of luminal blood into the plaque. Since luminal thrombosis and plaque rupture studied at postmortem are static processes, whereas in vivo they are likely to be dynamic, another potential mechanism—coronary spasm—may initiate the process but may not be identifiable at autopsy. It is conceivable that vasospasm or increased coronary tone, secondary to contraction of the residual medial smooth muscle of the vessel wall, may disrupt or crack the fibrous cap and/or lead to rupture of the blood vessels within the plaque provoking the onset of an acute coronary thrombus. The absence of a good animal model of coronary spasm makes this a difficult hypothesis to confirm.

Coronary Artery Spasm

Recent evidence linking coronary thrombosis to the pathogenesis of acute myocardial infarction has been developed in parallel with evidence which resurrected an old idea, i.e., that ischemic syndromes could be produced by coronary artery spasm. Originally proposed by Latham[90] over a century ago, and subsequently elaborated on by Sir William Osler[91] in 1910, there are now firm data that support the view that coronary artery spasm plays a major role in classic and variant angina pectoris as well as in acute myocardial infarction.[92–94] Angiographic studies performed while patients had clinical symptomatology or during provoked attacks have provided direct evidence that vasospasm can cause partial or complete coronary obstruction. Led by the pioneering efforts of Maseri in Europe[95] and Oliva[96] in the United States, there is now general acceptance for this view. What induces the vasospasm in most instances remains unknown;[94] however, preventive therapy with calcium channel blocking agents and nitrates has now entered the standard armamentarium for the treatment and prevention of the ischemic syndromes. Whether spasm due to a pathological contraction of medial smooth muscle in one or several segments of a vessel and lasting for a brief or indeterminate period is *solely* responsible for dynamic coronary obstruction is also not known. It has been suggested that normal coronary vasomotion occurring in an area of subtotal occlusion by atherosclerotic plaque may cause complete coronary obstruction and give the appearance of a spastic event.[97]

Though coronary artery spasm may occlude a vessel without any other associated vascular pathological conditions, most often the spasm occurs in the setting of coronary atherosclerosis. If the occlusion is of sufficient duration (see below), then tissue injury or necrosis may supervene before vascular relaxation restores blood flow. It is also conceivable that coronary vasospasm is the initiating event in the development of an acute thrombus.[98] Support for this concept comes from experimental studies demonstrating that arterial constriction induced with noreprinephrine[99] or nonocclusive ligation[100] can lead to vessel wall damage including endothelial injury and subsequent thrombosis. As suggested in the preceding section, coronary vasospasm may also be implicated in the frequent plaque ruptures associated with thrombi. Finally, and in somewhat of a more speculative vein, a hypothetical role for increased coronary tone and vasospasm has been proposed as a stimulus for smooth-muscle proliferation related to the development of atherosclerosis.[101]

With the latter hypothesis, we have now come full circle. Myocardial ischemia and infarction require a diminution of blood flow below a critical level before they occur. This process develops relatively suddenly but, in most instances, in the setting of chronically developing atherosclerosis. A significant body of evidence now has provided data suggesting that temporally abrupt coronary occlusion is related to thrombosis, plaque rupture, and vasospasm. It appears increasingly apparent that these pathophysiological processes are not mutually exclusive but may be intimately related. Thus plaque rupture can induce thrombosis which could be caused by vasospasm, and platelet adherence to an atherosclerotic vessel wall could lead to the release of vasoactive substances causing vasospasm and plaque rupture. Both vasospasm and nonocclusive thrombosis may even be implicated in the development or enlargement of an atherosclerotic plaque. It is the interplay of complex static and dynamic events in the coronary vessel which produces obstructive vascular changes intimately associated with the pathogenesis and pathophysiology of myocardial ischemia.

Patterns of Acute Myocardial Infarction

The onset of abrupt coronary obstruction, induced by the mechanisms discussed in the previous sections, leads to the development of transmural ischemia, within the area at risk, which is determined by the coronary anatomy. At least partially because collateral flow increases from the deepest subendocardial layers to the subepicardium, the jeopardized myocardium within the risk region dies in a transmural pattern beginning in the subendocardium. This progression of necrosis has been termed *wave front* by Jennings and coworkers.[102,103] They showed that in the open-chest anesthetized dog a 40-min occlusion of the left circumflex coronary artery, followed by 2 to 4 days of reperfusion, resulted in subendocardial necrosis involving 38 percent of the transmural dimension.[102] Subsequent occlusions of 3 or 6 h duration followed by reperfusions produced transmural infarcts of 57 and 71 percent respectively; 6-h reperfused infarcts did not differ from a 24-h infarct produced by permanent occlusions.[102] These observations have been confirmed by several laboratories,[104,105] which strongly indicate that this temporal and spatial progression of necrosis across the ventricular wall represents a fundamental pathophysiological phenomenon. This phenomenon also appears to be applicable to human infarcts. A comparative study of human subendocardial infarct extension following permanent coronary artery occlusion revealed an identical pattern to that seen in dogs with 40-min subendocardial infarcts and subsequent transmural extension.[105]

There are several important implications that can be drawn from this work. Most significant is the conclusion that jeopardized myocardium undergoes necrosis in a sequential fashion beginning in the subendocardium and extending toward the epicardium. The salvage of tissue in the epicardial layers is dependent either on the restoration of blood flow to this zone through the transiently occluded coronary artery or the presence of sufficient collateral supply to this area to prevent necrosis. By inference then, *subendocardial infarctions in humans are likely to be secondary to intermittent coronary artery occlusions.* This may occur because of coronary artery spasm with spontaneous or drug-induced relaxation or because of luminal thrombosis with clot lysis; in either case, the restoration of blood flow most likely must occur within a narrow time frame of several hours. Studies have also shown that the transmural progression of necrosis also involves the lateral subendocardial regions within the area at risk and occurs within 40 and 90 min,[103,104] thereby confirming that a significant lateral border zone does not exist even with evolving infarcts. A border zone does exist in the subepicardium; it can be preserved by restoration of flow within several hours.

Because of the complexity of atherosclerotic coronary disease in humans, and the unpredictability of collateral supply, it is difficult to know whether the relatively short time course available for reperfusion and salvage of subepicardial myocardium demonstrated experimentally also applies to clinical subjects. If transmural necrosis is essentially completed within 3 to 6 h, then there is little time available for institution of measures which will restore blood flow to the area at risk. Early reperfusion in animals has been shown to salvage myocardial function[106] and to have positive effects on survival even when infarct size did not significantly differ from that produced by permanent coronary occlusion.[107] In contrast, early reperfusion may lead to preservation of increased numbers of myocytes in the immediate subendocardial zone;[105] it has been suggested that these cells may be responsible for ventricular arrhythmias which may have adverse consequences in the postinfarction period.[108,109] Thus, although it seems logical to believe that reperfusion is invariably beneficial, the preservation of jeopardized tissue otherwise destined to die may have unanticipated results.

Morphologic Effects of Reperfusion

Myocardial infarction secondary to *complete* obstruction of a coronary artery is not entirely devoid of blood flow if collateral vessels are present, but the

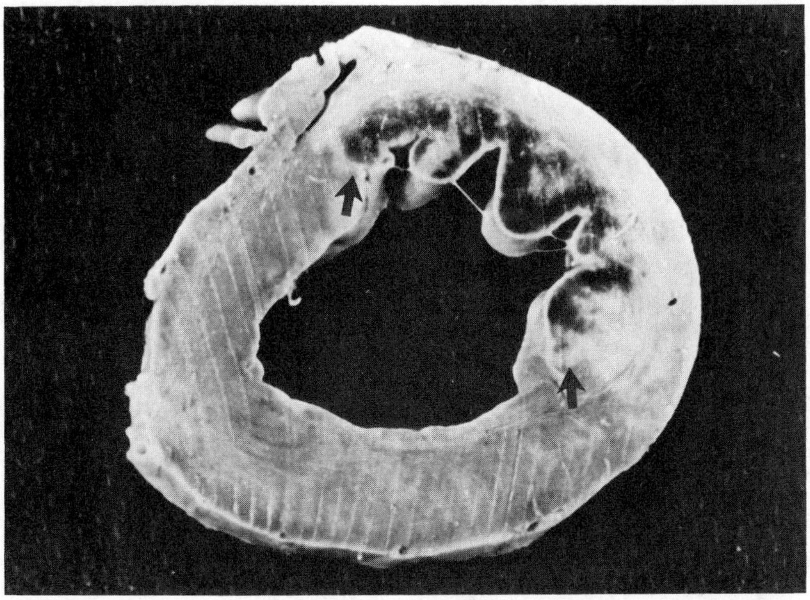

FIGURE 44-11 The left ventricle of a dog following a 40-min occlusion of the left anterior descending coronary artery (LAD) with 24 h of reperfusion. The region at risk has been delineated by perfusing the LAD with white silicone rubber. Note the dark subendocardial hemorrhage which was histologically verified to be within the necrotic zone. Laterally, the hemorrhage and necrosis closely approach the lateral extent of the risk region (arrows).

flows are below the threshold required to maintain viability. Despite this insufficient circulation, an infarct in which minimal reperfusion occurs evolves into a relatively pale, yellow-white zone of necrotic muscle over several days, with demarcation from the normal muscle by a rim of hyperemia. Mottling and hemorrhage may be present focally, but it is only due to residual flow and stasis. In contrast, a reperfused infarct is hemorrhagic (Fig. 44-11), with the hemorrhage localized within the necrotic tissue in the subendocardium. There has been considerable debate over whether reperfusion and the elicited intramyocardial hemorrhage have immediate or more chronic adverse consequences. The weight of evidence now strongly supports the view that although reperfusion may alter morphological parameters, it does not affect the ultimate evolution and healing of the infarct. This is a point of considerable practical importance because of the clinical application of techniques to reestablish blood flow to infarcting myocardium during the active phase of necrosis.

Studies by Kloner[110] and Fishbein[111] have shown that hemorrhage develops *within* the infarct region when reperfusion occurs at a point after the tissue can no longer be preserved. This hemorrhage is due to microvascular injury, which may follow[111] or precede[112] irreversible myocyte injury. Regardless of the time course of vascular damage, the localization of the hemorrhage within the infarct zone lends support to the concept that reperfusion and hemorrhage after 3 to 6 hours of ischemia do not damage tissue which would have been salvaged had no reperfusion occurred. Comparison of infarct size in a canine model in which similar-sized coronary vessels were selected for occlusion or reperfusion after 3 or 6 h of ischemia did not show any differences.[113] Similarly, though reperfusion produces accelerated damage to cells, these cells were destined to die regardless of the intervention.[114]

Reperfusion has a number of other consequences which may be related primarily to cell membrane damage.[115] The pathogenesis of the membrane damage remains in dispute, although the involvement of free oxygen radicals following reoxygenation of ischemic tissue has been supported by work of Lucchesi and associates.[116] Regardless of the cause, reperfusion leads to development of myocardial cell swelling,[117] accumulation of calcium in mitochondria,[118] accelerated washout of cellular enzymes,[119] and the presence of characteristic contraction bands.[120] These contraction bands are the morphological marker of reperfusion injury, indicating that myocardial cells were ischemically damaged and then subsequently supplied with oxygenated blood. For example, they are seen in acute subendocardial infarction throughout the necrotic zone, and they have been described following coronary bypass grafting of patients with acute myocardial ischemia, where they are thus secondary to surgical reperfusion.[121] They may also be observed along the periphery of transmural infarctions, often associated with focal mitochondrial calcification (Fig. 44-12). In this location, they are not likely to be related to collaterally determined perfusion of the microcirculation because of the absence of interconnections;[69,70] rather, their spatial extent is within the range consistent with diffusion of oxygenated substrate from the normally perfused tissue.[73] The presence of calcification at the periphery of infarcts corresponds to the localization of ^{99m}Tc-labeled pyrophosphate identified in nuclear imaging of acute infarcts.[122]

Contraction band necrosis is not necessarily the consequence only of large-vessel reperfusion (Fig. 44-13). Even transient obstruction of precapillary

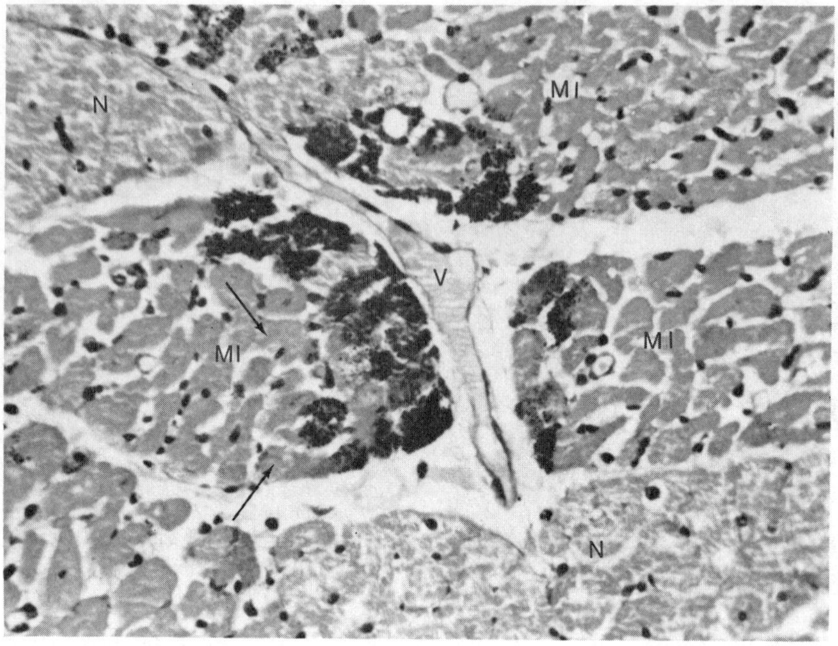

FIGURE 44-12 The histological border of a 24-h canine transmural infarction. The darker, hypereosinophilic necrotic myocardial cells (MI) are sharply delimited from peninsulas of normal myocardium (N). In the region surrounding a thin-walled patent vessel (V), the necrotic cells contain finely granular calcium precipitate (black in this photomicrograph), which extends 2 to 3 cells away from the vessel. A few contraction bands are observed in the same area (arrows). The spatial orientation of the calcification and contraction bands suggests that they were secondary to diffusion of substrate from the noninfarcted zone or the patent vessel. (×150.)

arteriole with a 25-μm microsphere, which induces spasm of this vessel through an alpha-adrenergic mechanism, causes a microscopic zone of contraction band necrosis.[39] The size of this lesion provides further evidence for the absence of interconnection at the microvascular level in the heart, since diffuse collateralization at this level should prevent necrosis.

Morphology of Nonreperfused Infarcts

There are several characteristic features of predominantly nonreperfused infarctions which permit histological identification and approximate dating. These features were outlined by Mallory et al.[123] in a classic paper in 1939, and they were verified recently by Fishbein and colleagues.[124] The major limitation of histology is the insensitivity of light microscopy in early infarctions; morphological alterations are not clearly defined in the first 12 h of infarct development. A variety of histochemical and ultrastructural methods have been employed to circumvent these problems, but light microscopy with hematoxylin-eosin staining still remains the "gold standard" for infarcts older than 12 to 24 h. The primary advantage of histology, particularly when compared with ultrastructure, is the ability to examine large regions of myocardium and to correlate the changes with vascular markers which can identify the area at risk. For early infarcts of less than 6 h duration, however, other methods are required.

The most significant histological marker of in-

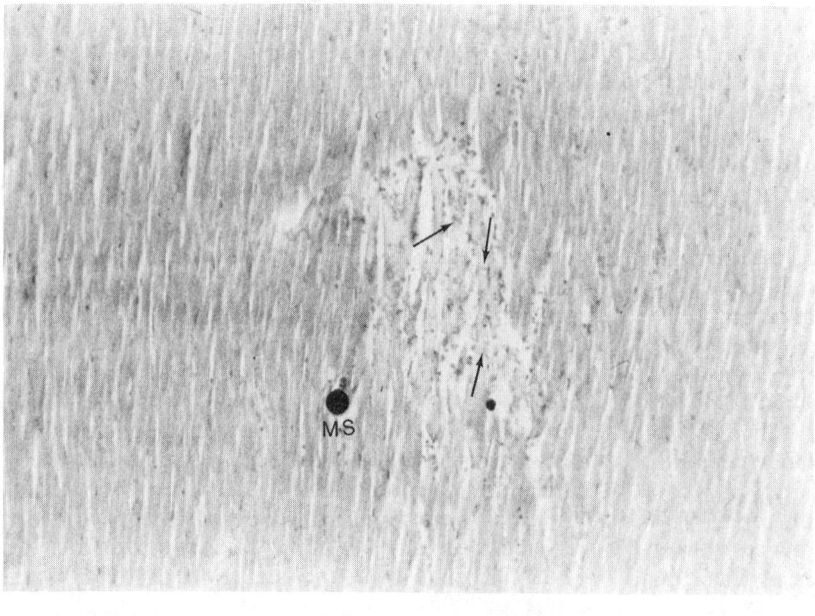

FIGURE 44-13 A 25-μm microsphere (MS), presumably within a precapillary arteriole, is spatially associated with a microscopic focus of contraction band necrosis measuring approximately 150 by 300 μm in maximum dimensions. Several contraction bands can be seen at the arrows. Other studies[39] have shown this type of necrotic lesion to be secondary to microvascular spasm, which can be prevented with alpha-adrenergic blocking drugs. (×120.)

farction is the presence of increased sarcoplasmic eosinophilia, or hypereosinophilia, characteristic of coagulation necrosis which can be appreciated within the first 24 h (Fig. 44-12). Myocytes at this stage also may be attenuated, and be aligned in parallel bundles of wavy fibers,[125] but this is not a constant finding. The waviness is related to stretching of the necrotic tissue by the surrounding viable myocardium, with subsequent relaxation post mortem. Because of stretching, cross striations are less prominent but they are still present with increased sarcomeric spacing. Nonreperfused infarcts may have congested vessels and interstitial edema, but prominent intercellular hemorrhage is usually absent. Even without reperfusion, however, some blood flow is usually present in the infarct zone unless collaterals are absent; because of this, some viable myocytes may be seen surrounding vessels deep within the necrotic tissue. Focal contraction bands and myocytolytic changes typical of reperfusion are usually seen along the periphery of the infarction. Whether this is related to reperfusion through collaterals, diffusion from the noninfarcted zone, or is caused by the effects of catecholamines is not known. As previously noted, this is also the region where focal cellular calcification can be identified.

Within the first 12 h polymorphonuclear leukocytes (PMNs) marginate in vessels and begin to migrate into the interstitial spaces; by 24 to 48 h, all infarcts have infiltrates of PMNs at variable depths within the necrotic tissue moving from the periphery toward the center. The variability probably reflects the extent of local blood flow, which may not be sufficient to keep the myocardium viable but may be capable of bringing inflammatory cells into the area and carrying away cellular proteins and enzymes which leak through damaged membranes, and which may be measured systemically as markers of necrosis. Serial sectioning of acute infarcts demonstrates that the PMN collections are not homogeneous but, rather, are discontinuous.[68] Absent blood flow related to microcirculatory damage (no-reflow phenomenon[126]), vascular thrombi within the infarct region, or inadequate collaterals may account for this discontinuity.

By 2 to 4 days of age the degree of PMN inflammation has increased and inflammatory cells begin to undergo necrosis and fragment. Centripetal degeneration of necrotic myocytes is observed, and the peripheral infarct begins to demonstrate admixtures of mononuclear inflammatory cells including lymphocytes, mast cells, and macrophages. The macrophages often contain lipofuscin pigment from the breakdown of myocytes. Eosinophils are an inconstant feature, but they may be observed in this early period.

Within the first 4 to 7 days, although PMNs are still present, the more chronic inflammatory infiltration increases. At the periphery of the infarct, progressing toward the central zone, fibroblasts and new capillaries can be identified. By one week, this granulation tissue is well defined, and loose collagen is being deposited in the interstitium. This process of scar formation progresses for weeks until a densely collagenized healed infarct is present. In very large infarctions, presumably where there is complete absence of blood flow in the center of the risk region, mummified necrotic myocytes surrounded by scar may be seen months or years after healing is complete. For most infarctions, scarring is generally completed within 6 to 8 weeks.

Alterations in the Postinfarct Period

Although we have stressed that myocyte necrosis secondary to ischemia is a temporal event that takes a minimum of several hours for completion across the ventricular wall, it is equally true that once the infarct has developed fully there may be associated changes with time, in the immediate and distant regions of the ventricle, which have adverse con-

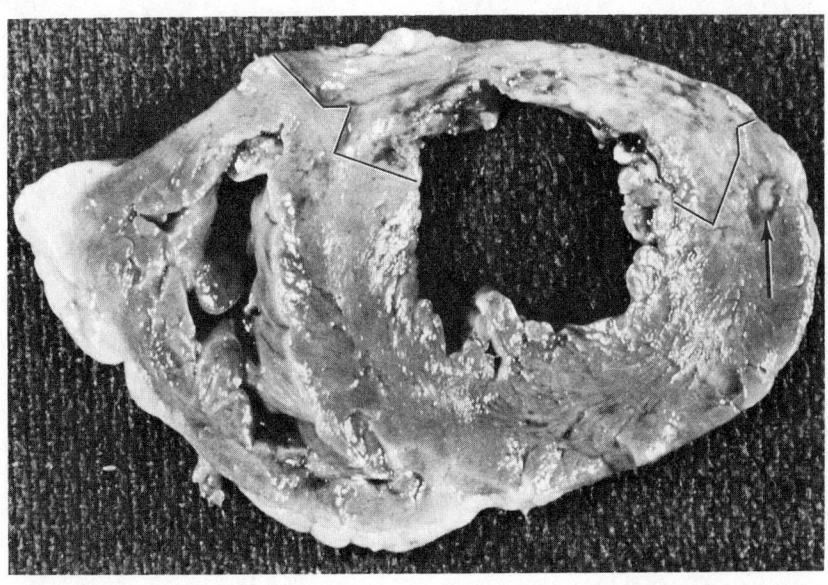

FIGURE 44-14 There is marked thinning of the posterior free wall secondary to a transmural acute myocardial infarction (approximately 72 h old). There was ventricular rupture present at another level. The infarct is demarcated at its gross lateral borders; a region of acute necrosis (arrow) is present peripheral to the main infarct.

sequences for the heart. There has been recent popularization of this concept by Bulkley and her colleagues, in descriptions of infarct expansion and extension. *Expansion* refers to the dilatation and thinning of the infarct without superimposed new myocyte necrosis. In one study, Hutchins and Bulkley[127] identified infarct expansion in 59 percent of 76 consecutive acute myocardial infarcts, with severe expansion occurring in infarcts greater than 5 days old. We have observed marked infarct thinning within the first 3 days (Fig. 44-14), and even as early as 1 day after onset, particularly if the infarct results in ventricular rupture. The pathogenesis of this pronounced thinning is unknown. Although it may be related to attenuation and disruption of myocardial fibers, recent observations suggest that it may be secondary to disruption or destruction of the connective tissue framework of the heart. Myocardial cells are surrounded by a complex connective tissue skeleton which serves to attach myocytes to each other and to other structures in the heart.[128] This skeleton is not observable with the commonly used staining procedures for connective tissue, and therefore it has not been evaluated routinely in myocardial infarction. It appears, however, that even in very early infarction there is absent staining of this skeleton, which suggests profound alterations in its composition and integrity (Fig. 44-15). Disruption of the framework holding myocardial cells to each other may account for their slippage during infarction, leading to wall thinning, ventricular aneurysm formation, or myocardial rupture. It should be noted, however, that expansion of experimental infarction also has been described following

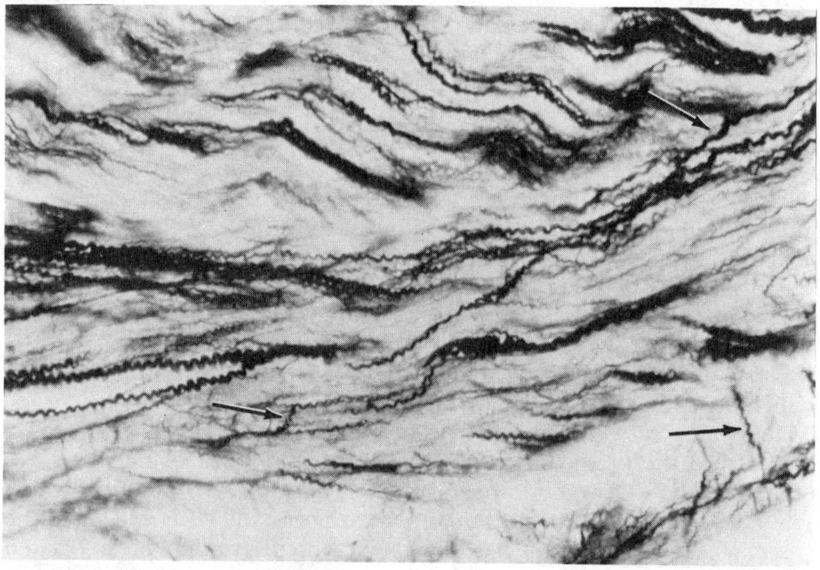

A

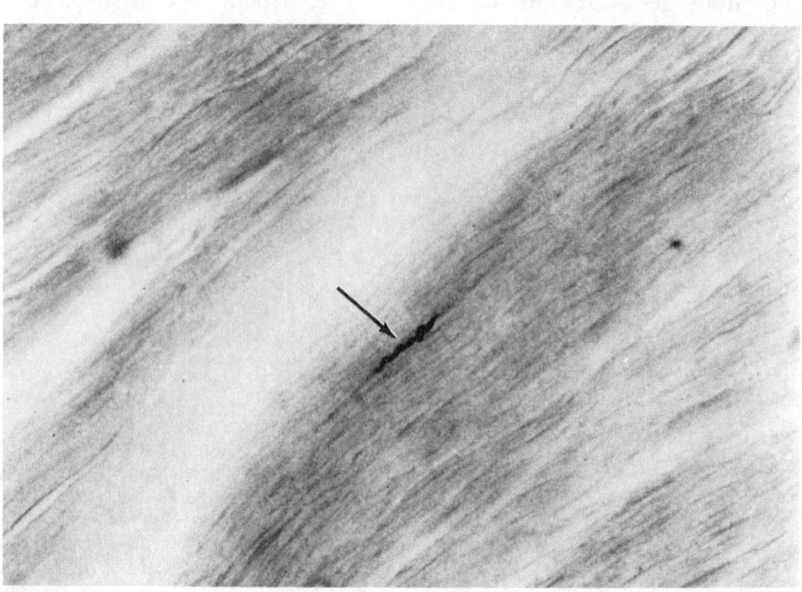

B

FIGURE 44-15 *A.* A section of normal myocardium from a patient with a 27-h-old rupture infarct has been reacted with the del Rio y Hortega silver stain to demonstrate the extent of the extracellular skeletal framework in this specimen.[128] Note the dark silver-positive collagen fibers in the extracellular space, some of which (arrows) act as struts between myocardial cells. (×150.) *B.* A section from the same heart taken from the myocardial rupture site. With the exception of a single silver-positive fiber (arrow), none of the skeletal framework is apparent in this area. (×150.)

treatment with indomethacin, without obvious alterations of hydroxyproline concentrations,[129] which suggest the collagen content was not changed. Because of the potential for adverse consequences in patients with expanded infarcts, this subject will require further investigation in the future.

In contrast to infarct thinning without new necrosis, the term *extension* refers to the development of additional myocardial necrosis adjacent to the initial infarct.[127] In the histological study reported by Hutchins and Bulkley, they described relatively small zones of contraction band necrosis in 17 percent of 76 acute infarctions and ascribed their occurrence to transient hypoperfusion.[127] Because of the small volume of myocardium involved, they believed that this process was probably hemodynamically insignificant. However, a clinical study by Fraker et al.[130] identified acute extension in 13 percent of 458 patients with acute infarction and observed a fourfold increase of in-hospital mortality and decreased 1-year survival. Although the mechanism for extension is unknown, experimental infarcts in which the risk region is precisely defined reveal that extension can occur in the normal nonrisk zone.[131] The contraction band morphology of the necrosis and its localization suggest that catecholamines and/or microvascular spasm may be implicated.

Identification of the vascular area at risk, with histological infarct extension into the normal region, links this phenomenon to the development of new necrosis at a distance from the initial infarct. This necrosis may represent a second myocardial infarction due to transient or complete obstruction of a main coronary artery with features of a subendocardial or transmural infarction. However, not infrequently new necrosis is identified with contraction band or myocytolytic morphology, in the epicardium or midventricular wall (Fig. 44-14), and thus is not in the vascular distribution expected with main coronary artery occlusion. The pathogenesis of this necrosis is unknown, but it may be similar to that proposed for acute extension.

Methods for Morphological Infarct Identification

Studies of myocardial infarction, particularly in regard to its modification, have been characterized by significant controversy during the past decade. It is fair to say that much of the disagreement between experienced investigators represents problems with methodology. Although major advances have been made in our understanding of the pathogenesis and pathophysiology of myocardial necrosis, its temporal and spatial characteristics, and its relation to a blood-flow-determined area at risk, differences still exist. No method currently available has all of the characteristics necessary for universal acceptability and for comparison of results between laboratories. The only unequivocal test of infarction is to allow necrosed myocardial cells to progress to the point of replacement and scarring. Clearly, however, this test is inadequate for studying the early stages of infarction and the efficacy of interventions designed to salvage myocardium.

As noted previously, the histological parameters of infarction are well defined after 12 to 24 h in hematoxylin-eosin stained sections, with hypereosinophilia the primary criterion of necrosis. Paraffin-embedded sections can be serially reconstructed for a three-dimensional analysis, and tissue alterations can be correlated with markers of the area at risk. However, these advantages, although significant, are not helpful in studying infarct modification by therapeutic interventions, since the infarction is already completed after 6 h. A method sensitive in the early period, such as electron microscopy, has the disadvantage that it is tedious, that only small volumes of tissue can be examined, and that correlation with a vascular risk region is difficult. Accordingly, a number of techniques have been developed for relatively simple, sensitive, and specific tissue evaluation in the early stages of necrosis.

Two popular approaches are the use of histochemical markers for evaluation at either the light microscopic or macroscopic levels. Histochemical analyses of mitochondrial oxidative enzymes,[56] glycogen depletion,[132,133] or lipid accumulation[132] have been extrapolated to indicate the metabolic state of the tissue and whether the tissue is viable or necrotic. However, these techniques are inconsistent and nonquantitative, and are reflections of tissue metabolism at only one point in time. Rapid alterations in the oxidative state of the tissue associated with ischemia[63,64] do not necessarily indicate that the tissue is destined to die. Similarly, periodic acid Schiff and oil red O identification of glycogen depletion or lipid accumulation, respectively, may occur in jeopardized ischemic tissue which will survive if blood flow is restored. This approach must be correlated with other indicators of tissue injury before it can be accepted as a useful method for diagnosing necrosis in an early stage.

A more popular method employed by many laboratories because of its simplicity and ease is the use of tetrazolium dyes on macroscopic slices of fresh myocardium. Both nitro-blue tetrazolium (NBT) and triphenyl tetrazolium chloride (TTC) stain normal myocardium and produce particulate formazan pigment visible as either a blue or red color. Although it is generally accepted that the color reaction is secondary to reduction of the dye by dehydrogenase enzymes,[134] recent evidence suggests that loss of reduced coenzymes (particularly, nicotinamide adenine dinucleotides) in the ischemic region accounts for the discrimination between ischemic and normal tissue.[135] Regardless of the mechanism, the major question is whether this macroscopic histochemical technique indicates tissue necrosis. Validation of tetrazolium staining at 24 or 48 h after coronary occlusion reveals a close correlation with histological parameters of infarction.[136] However, Fishbein et al.[134] have claimed that the TTC stain can be used as early as 3 to 6 h after coronary occlusion to diagnose myocardial necrosis before it becomes manifest histologically. This is more problematic, because it is difficult to verify that there is unequivocal necrosis throughout the unstained region at this stage.

In general, studies designed to validate the TTC technique have focused on determining whether the region of absent formazan pigment corresponds to morphological evidence of tissue necrosis. The region with formazan pigment is usually sampled either without regard to a vascular risk region or well within the normal zone. This may not be the appropriate approach, particularly if TTC is being used to evaluate tissue preservation by some therapeutic intervention. The significant question is not whether absent TTC staining reflects tissue necrosis, but whether positive staining indicates tissue viability. When TTC-positive staining was correlated with the vascular risk region in 6-h-old infarctions, or was correlated directly with histological infarction at 24 h, formazan pigment was associated focally with necrotic tissue in the infarct zone.[137] In addition, gross determination of TTC staining is subjective, and is generally thought to be an all-or-none phenomenon. The eye is probably incapable of discriminating subtle alterations in TTC staining which may occur as the tissue undergoes irreversible damage. When 6-h globally ischemic heart muscle was reacted with TTC, gross observation demonstrated a positive reaction; yet ultrastructure showed that the myocardium was necrotic and quantitation of the "positive" formazan pigment deposition revealed a 50 percent decline.[137] Therefore, gross evaluation using TTC as a marker, particularly in the early stages of infarction, may underestimate the extent of necrosis. If the area at risk is not carefully delineated, and TTC is used as the sole criterion of tissue viability or necrosis, inappropriate conclusions may be drawn concerning the efficacy of a therapeutic intervention.[138]

At the present time, all of the conventional morphological markers of infarction have disadvantages. No single method may be appropriate for different experimental protocols. The ideal marker, one which can discriminate between normal and necrotic, or jeopardized and condemned, myocardium at an early stage of ischemia does not exist.

Future Trends

The last decade has seen a significant increase in our understanding of the pathophysiology of myocardial ischemia. Concepts related to area at risk, temporal progression of necrosis, and dependency of cell survival on the availability of blood flow are generally accepted. Clinical and pathological investigations have established transient or thrombotic occlusion of an atherosclerotic coronary vessel as a primary cause of acute myocardial infarction. Accordingly, efforts to restore blood flow within the relatively brief period of time before jeopardized myocardium undergoes infarction have become a major clinical endeavor. Whether these efforts will have a significant impact on the morbidity and mortality of myocardial ischemia cannot be predicted at this date; however, it is likely that this approach will be actively pursued in the future. Current efforts to develop therapeutic interventions to delay necrosis until blood flow can be restored remain experimental. It is expected that this work will continue; however, until some generally accepted marker to identify early myocardial necrosis is developed, optimism must be tempered before we can be certain that a treatment has had a positive effect. Recent interest in the evolution of the infarcted tissue once the necrosis is completed suggests that there may be limits on how much can be done to prevent the loss of myocardium. Modification of the healing response in attempts to limit the development of infarct expansion or rupture may be an active field of investigation in the near future.

References

1. Laennec, R. T. H.: "Traité de l'auscultation médiate," 2d ed., Brosson et Chaude, Paris, 1826, vol. 1, p. 5.
1a. Maseri, A., Chierchia, S., and L'Abbate, A.: Pathogenetic Mechanisms Underlying the Clinical Events Associated with Atherosclerotic Heart Disease, *Circulation,* 62(suppl. 5): V-3, 1980.
2. Berne, R. M., and Rubio, R.: Coronary Circulation, in R. M. Berne and S. Sperelakis (eds.), "Handbook of Physiology," sec. 2: "The Cardiovascular System," vol. 1: "The Heart," American Physiological Society, Bethesda, 1979, p. 873.
3. Sanders, M., White, F. C., and Bloor, C. M.: Myocardial Blood Flow Distribution in Miniature Pigs during Exercise, *Basic Res. Cardiol.,* 72:326, 1977.
4. Barnard, R. J., Duncan, W. H., Livesay, J. J., and Buckberg, G. D.: Coronary Vasodilator Reserve and Flow Distribution During Near-Maximal Exercise in Dogs, *J. Appl. Physiol: Respir. Environ. Exercise Physiol.,* 43:988, 1977.
5. Mosher, P., Ross, J., Jr., McFate, P. A., and Shaw, R. F.: Control of Coronary Blood Flow by an Autoregulatory Mechanism, *Circ. Res.,* 14:250, 1964.
6. Berne, R. M.: The Role of Adenosine in the Regulation of Coronary Blood Flow, *Circ. Res.,* 47:807, 1980.
7. Sabiston, D. C., and Gregg, D. E.: Effects of Cardiac Contraction on Coronary Blood Flow, *Circulation,* 15:14, 1957.
8. Lewis, F. B., Coffmann, J. D., and Gregg, D. E.: Effect of Heart Rate and Intracoronary Isoproterenol, Levarterenol, and Epinephrine on Coronary Flow and Resistance, *Circ. Res.,* 9:89, 1961.
9. Kirk, E. S., and Honig, C. R.: Non-Uniform Distribution of Blood Flow and Gradients of Oxygen Tension within the Heart, *Am. J. Physiol.,* 207:661, 1964.
10. Downey, J. M., and Kirk, E. S.: Distribution of the Coronary Blood Flow across the Canine Heart Wall during Systole, *Circ. Res.,* 34:251, 1974.
11. Brandi, G., and MacGregor, M.: Intramural Pressure in the Left Ventricle of the Dog, *Cardiovasc. Res.,* 3:472, 1969.
12. Gregg, D. E., and Eckstein, R. W.: Measurements of Intramyocardial Pressure, *Am. J. Physiol.,* 132:781, 1941.
13. Holt, J. P.: Flow through Collapsible Tubes and through in Situ Veins, *IEEE Trans. Biomed. Eng.,* BME-16:274, 1969.
14. Downey, J. M., and Kirk, E. S.: Inhibition of Coronary Blood Flow by a Vascular Waterfall Mechanism, *Circ. Res.,* 36:753, 1975.
15. Lowensohn, H. S., Khouri, E. M., Gregg, D. E., Pyle, R. L., and Patterson, R. E.: Phasic Right Coronary Artery Blood Flow in Conscious Dogs with Normal and Elevated Right Ventricular Pressures, *Circ. Res.,* 36:760, 1976.

16. Brooks, H. L., Kirk, E. S., Vokonas, P. S., Urschel, C. W., and Sonnenblick, E. H.: Performance of the Right Ventricle under Stress: Relation to Right Coronary Flow, *J. Clin. Invest.*, 50:2176, 1971.
17. Cutarelli, R., and Levy, M. N.: Intraventricular Pressure and the Distribution of Coronary Blood Flow, *Circ. Res.*, 12:322, 1963.
18. Domenech, R. J., Hoffman, J. I. E., Noble, M. I. M., Saunders, K. B., Henson, J. R., and Subijanto, S.: Total and Regional Coronary Blood Flow Measured by Radioactive Microspheres in Conscious and Anesthetized Dogs, *Circ. Res.*, 25:581, 1969.
19. Forman, R., Kirk, E. S., Downey, J. M., and Sonnenblick, E. H.: Nitroglycerin and Heterogeneity of Myocardial Blood Flow. Reduced Subendocardial Blood Flow and Ventricular Contractile Force, *J. Clin. Invest.*, 52:905, 1973.
20. Griggs, D. M., Jr., and Nakamura, Y.: Effects of Coronary Constriction on Myocardial Distribution of Iodoantipyrine-I^{131}, *Am. J. Physiol.*, 215:1082, 1968.
21. Buckberg, G. D., Fixler, D. E., Archie, J. P., and Hoffman, J. I. E.: Experimental Subendocardial Ischemia in Dogs with Normal Coronary Arteries, *Circ. Res.*, 30:67, 1972.
22. Braunwald, E., Ross, J., Jr., and Sonnenblick, E. H.: "Mechanisms of Contraction of the Normal and Failing Heart," 2d ed., Little, Brown and Company, Boston, 1976, p. 122.
23. Rouleau, J., Boerboom, L. E., Surjadhana, A., and Hoffman, J. I. E.: The Role of Autoregulation and Tissue Diastolic Pressures in the Transmural Distribution of Left Ventricular Blood Flow in Anesthetized Dogs, *Circ. Res.*, 45:804, 1979.
24. Bellamy, R. F.: Diastolic Coronary Artery Pressure-Flow Relations in the Dog, *Circ. Res.*, 43:92, 1978.
25. Eng, C., Jentzer, J. H., and Kirk, E. S.: Coronary Capacitive Effects on the High Estimates of Coronary Critical Closing Pressures, *Circulation*, 62(suppl. 3):254, 1980.
26. Gould, K. L., and Lipscomb, K.: Effects of Coronary Stenoses on Coronary Flow Reserve and Resistance, *Am. J. Cardiol.*, 34:48, 1974.
27. Wusten, B.: Biophysics of Coronary Artery Narrowing, in W. Schaper (ed.), "The Pathophysiology of Myocardial Perfusion," Elsevier/North-Holland Biomedical Press, Amsterdam/New York/Oxford, 1979, p. 285.
28. Chance, B.: Pyridine Nucleotide as an Indicator of the Oxygen Requirements for Energy-Linked Functions of Mitochondria, *Circ. Res.*, 38(suppl. 1):1, 1976.
29. Provenza, D. V., and Scherlis, S.: Coronary Circulation in Dog's Heart: Demonstration of Muscle Sphincters in Capillaries, *Circ. Res.*, 7:318, 1959.
30. Winbury, M. M., and Gabel, L. P.: Effect of Nitrates on Nutritional Circulation of Heart and Hindlimb, *Am. J. Physiol.*, 212:1062, 1967.
31. Martini, J., and Honig, C. R.: Direct Measurement of Intercapillary Distance in Beating Rat Heart in Situ under Various Conditions of O_2 Supply, *Microvascular Res.*, 1:244, 1969.
32. Myers, W. W., and Honig, C. R.: Number and Distribution of Capillaries as Determinants of Myocardial Oxygen Tension, *Am. J. Physiol.*, 207:653, 1964.
33. Wearn, J. T.: Morphological and Functional Alterations of the Coronary Circulation, *Harvey Lect.*, 35:243, 1940.
34. Henquell, L., Odoroff, C. L., and Honig, C. R.: Intercapillary Distance and Capillary Reserve in Hypertrophied Rat Hearts Beating in Situ, *Circ. Res.*, 41:400, 1977.
35. Feigl, E. O.: Carotid Sinus Reflex Control of Coronary Blood Flow, *Circ. Res.*, 23:223, 1968.
36. Williams, D. O., and Most, A. S.: Responsiveness of the Coronary Circulation to Brief vs. Sustained Alpha-Adrenergic Stimulation, *Circulation*, 63:11, 1980.
37. Mellander, S.: Comparative Studies on the Adrenergic Neuro-Hormonal Control of Resistance and Capacitance Vessels in the Cat, *Acta Physiol. Scand.*, 50(suppl. 176), 1960.
38. Mohrmon, D. E., and Feigl, E. O.: Competition between Sympathetic Vasoconstriction and Metabolic Vasodilation in the Canine Coronary Circulation, *Circ. Res.*, 42:79, 1978.
39. Eng, C., Cho, S., Factor, S. M., Sonnenblick, E. H., and Kirk, E. S.: Myocardial Micronecrosis Produced by Microsphere Embolization. Role of an Alpha Adrenergic Tonic Influence on the Coronary Microcirculation, *Circ. Res.*, 54:74, 1984.
40. Cohen, M. V., and Kirk, E. S.: Differential Response of Large and Small Coronary Arteries to Nitroglycerin and Angiotensin, *Circ. Res.*, 33:445, 1973.
41. d'Hemecourt, A., and Detar, R.: Possible Physiological Basis for Locally Induced "Spasm" of Large Coronary Arteries, in A. Maseri, G. A. Klassen, and M. Lesch (eds.), "Primary and Secondary Angina Pectoris" (proceedings, international symposium, Pisa, Italy, June 15–17, 1976), Grune & Stratton, Inc., New York, 1978, p. 1977.
42. Factor, S. M., Minase, T., Cho, S., Dominitz, R., and Sonnenblick, E. H.: Microvascular Spasm in the Cardiomyopathic Syrian Hamster: A Preventable Cause of Focal Myocardial Necrosis, *Circulation*, 66:342, 1982.
43. Gregg, D. E.: The Natural History of Collateral Development, *Circ. Res.*, 35:335, 1974.
44. Schaper, W.: "The Collateral Circulation of the Heart," Elsevier/North-Holland Publishing Company, Amsterdam, 1971.
45. Gregg, D. E., and Patterson, R. E.: Functional Importance of the Coronary Collaterals, *N. Engl. J. Med.*, 303:1406, 1980.
46. Schaper, W., Flameng, W., Winkler, B., Wusten, B., Turschmann, W., Neugebauer, G., and Carl, M.: Quantification of Collateral Resistance in Acute and Chronic Experimental Coronary Occlusion in the Dog, *Circ. Res.*, 39:371, 1976.
47. Becker, L. C.: Conditions for Vasodilator-Induced Coronary Steal in Experimental Myocardial Ischemia, *Circulation*, 57:1103, 1978.
48. Muller, J. E., and Gunther, S. J.: Nifedipine Therapy for Prinzmetal Angina, *Circulation*, 57:137, 1978.
49. Schaper, W.: Influence of Chronic Coronary Occlusion on Maximal Blood Flow to Normal Areas, in W. Schaper (ed.), "The Pathophysiology of Myocardial Perfusion," Elsevier/North-Holland Biomedical Press, Amsterdam/New York/Oxford, 1979, p. 444.
50. Sarnoff, S. J., Braunwald, E., Welch, G. H., Jr., Case, R. B., Strainsby, W. N., and Macruz, R.: Hemodynamic Determinates of Oxygen Consumption of the Heart with Special Reference to the Tension Time Index, *Am. J. Physiol.*, 192:148, 1958.
51. Baller, D., Bretschneider, H. J., and Hellige, G.: Validity of Myocardial Oxygen Consumption Parameters, *Clin. Cardiol.*, 5:317, 1979.
52. Braunwald, E., Graham, T. P., Jr., Covell, J. W., Sonnenblick, E. H., and Ross, J., Jr.: Control of Myocardial Oxygen Consumption: Relative Influence of Contractile State and Tension Development, *J. Clin. Invest.*, 47:375, 1968.
53. Kirk, E. S., LeJemtel, T. H., Nelson, G. R., and Sonnenblick, E. H.: Mechanisms of Beneficial Effects of Vasodilators on Inotropic Interventions in the Failing Ischemic Heart, *Am. J. Med.*, 65:189, 1978.
54. Jennings, R. B., Sommers, H. M., Smyth, G. A., Flack, H. A., and Linn, H.: Myocardial Necrosis Induced by Temporary Occlusion of a Coronary Artery in the Dog, *Arch. Pathol.*, 70:68, 1960.
55. Edwards, J. E.: Correlations in Coronary Arterial Disease, *Bull. N.Y. Acad. Med.*, 33:199, 1957.
56. Cox, J. L., McLaughlin, V. W., Flowers, N. C., and Horan, L. G.: The Ischemic Zone Surrounding Acute Myocardial Infarction. Its Morphology as Detected by Dehydrogenase Staining, *Am. Heart J.*, 76:650, 1968.
57. Kjekshus, J. K., and Sobel, B. E.: Depressed Myocardial Creatine Phosphokinase Activity Following Experimental Myocardial Infarction in Rabbit, *Circ. Res.*, 27:403, 1970.
58. Kjekshus, J. K., Maroko, P. R., and Sobel, B. E.: Distribution of Myocardial Injury and Its Relation to Epicardial ST-Segment Changes after Coronary Artery Occlusion in the Dog, *Cardiovasc. Res.*, 6:490, 1972.
59. Lie, J. T., Pairolero, P. C., Holley, K. E., McCall, J. T., Thompson, H. K., Jr., and Titus, J. L.: Time Course and Zonal Variations of Ischemia-Induced Myocardial Cationic Electrolyte Derangements, *Circulation*, 51:860, 1975.
60. Ross, J., Jr.: Electrocardiographic ST-Segment Analysis in

the Characterization of Myocardial Ischemia and Infarction, *Circulation,* 53(suppl. 1):73, 1976.

61. Hirzel, H. O., Sonnenblick, E. H., and Kirk, E. S.: Absence of a Lateral Border Zone of Intermediate Creatine Phosphokinase Depletion Surrounding a Central Infarct 24 Hours after Acute Coronary Occlusion in the Dog, *Circ. Res.,* 41:673, 1977.
62. Marcus, M. L., Kerber, R. E., Ehrhardt, J., and Abboud, F. M.: Three Dimensional Geometry of Acutely Ischemic Myocardium, *Circulation,* 52:254, 1975.
63. Barlow, C. H., and Chance, B.: Ischemic Areas in Perfused Rat Hearts: Measurement by NADH Fluorescence Photography, *Science,* 193:909, 1976.
64. Harken, A. M., Barlow, C. H., and Chance, B.: Two- and Three-Dimensional Display of Myocardial Ischemic "Border Zone" in Dogs, *Am. J. Cardiol.,* 42:954, 1978.
65. Janse, M. J., Cinca, J., Morena, H., Fiolet, J. W. T., Kleber, A. G., DeVries, G. P., Becker, A. E., and Durrer, D.: The "Border Zone" in Myocardial Ischemia. An Electrophysiological, Metabolic, and Histochemical Correlation in the Pig Heart, *Circ. Res.,* 44:576, 1979.
66. Harken, A. H., Simson, M. B., Haselgrove, J., Wetstein, L., Harden, W. R. III, and Barlow, C. H.: Early Ischemia after Complete Coronary Ligation in the Rabbit, Dog, Pig, and Monkey, *Am. J. Physiol.,* 241:H202, 1981.
67. Yellon, D. M., Hearse, D. J., Crome, R., Grannel, J., and Wyse, R. K. H.: Characterization of the Lateral Interface between Normal and Ischemic Tissue in the Canine Heart during Evolving Myocardial Infarction, *Am. J. Cardiol.,* 47:1233, 1981.
68. Factor, S. M., Sonnenblick, E. H., and Kirk, E. S.: The Histologic Border Zone of Acute Myocardial Infarction: Islands or Peninsulas? *Am., J. Pathol.,* 92:111, 1978.
69. Okun, E. M., Factor, S. M., and Kirk, E. S.: End-Capillary Loops in the Heart: An Explanation for Discrete Myocardial Infarctions without Border Zones, *Science,* 206:565, 1979.
70. Factor, S. M., Okun, E. M., Minase, T., and Kirk, E. S.: The Microcirculation of the Human Heart: End-Capillary Loops with Discrete Perfusion Fields, *Circulation,* 66:1241, 1982.
71. Lowe, J. E., Reimer, K. A., and Jennings, R. B.: Experimental Infarct Size as a Function of the Amount of Myocardium at Risk, *Am. J. Pathol.,* 90:363, 1978.
72. Lee, J. T., Ideker, R. E., and Reimer, K. A.: Myocardial Infarct Size and Location in Relation to the Coronary Vascular Bed at Risk in Man, *Circulation,* 64:526, 1981.
73. Factor, S. M., Okun, E. M., and Kirk, E. S.: The Histologic Border of Acute Canine Myocardial Infarction: A Function of Microcirculation, *Circ. Res.,* 48:640, 1981.
74. Brosius, F. C., III, and Roberts, W. C.: Significance of Coronary Arterial Thrombus in Transmural Acute Myocardial Infarction. A Study of 54 Necropsy Patients, *Circulation,* 63:810, 1981.
75. Muller, J. E.: Coronary Artery Thrombosis: Historical Aspects, *J. Am. Coll. Cardiol.,* 1:893, 1983.
76. Erhlich, J. C., and Shinohara, Y.: Low Incidence of Coronary Thrombosis in Myocardial Infarction. A Restudy by Serial Block Technique, *Arch. Pathol.,* 78:432, 1964.
77. Roberts, W. C., and Buja, L. M.: The Frequency and Significance of Coronary Arterial Thrombi and Other Observations in Fatal Acute Myocardial Infarction: A Study of 107 Necropsy Patients, *Am. J. Med.,* 52:425, 1972.
78. Silver, M. D., Baroldi, G., and Mariani, F.: The Relationship between Acute Occlusive Coronary Thrombi and Myocardial Infarction Studied in 100 Consecutive Patients, *Circulation,* 61:219, 1980.
79. DeWood, M. A., Spores, J., Notske, R., Mouser, L. T., Burroughs, R., Golden, M. S., and Lang, H. T.: Prevalence of Total Coronary Occlusion During the Early Hours of Transmural Myocardial Infarction, *N. Engl. J. Med.,* 303:897, 1980.
80. Ganz, W., Ninomiya, K., Hashida, J., Fishbein, M. D., Buchbinder, N., Marcus, H., Mondkar, A., Maddahi, J., Shah, P. K., Berman, D., Charuzi, Y., Geft, I., Shell, W., and Swan, H. J. C.: Intracoronary Thrombolysis in Acute Myocardial Infarction: Experimental Background and Clinical Experience, *Am. Heart J.,* 102:1145, 1981.
81. Rutsch, W., Schartl, M., Mathey, D., Kuck, K., Merx, W., Dorr, R., Rentrop, P., and Blanke, H.: Percutaneous Transluminal Coronary Recanalization: Procedure, Results, and Acute Complications, *Am. Heart J.,* 102:1178, 1981.
82. Anderson, J. L., Marshall, H. W., Bray, B. E., Lutz, J. R., Frederick, P. R., Yanowitz, F. G., Datz, F. L., Klausner, S. C., and Hagan, A. D.: A Randomized Trial of Intracoronary Streptokinase in the Treatment of Acute Myocardial Infarction, *N. Engl. J. Med.,* 308:1312, 1983.
83. Smalling, R. W., Fuentes, F., Mathews, M. W., Freund, G. C., Hicks, C. H., Reduto, L. A., Walker, W. E., Sterling, R. P., and Gould, K. L.: Sustained Improvement in Left Ventricular Function and Mortality by Intracoronary Streptokinase Administration during Evolving Myocardial Infarction, *Circulation,* 68:131, 1983.
84. Merx, W., Dorr, R., Rentrop, P., Blanke, H., Karsch, K. R., Mathey, D. G., Kremer, P., Rutsch, W., and Schmutzler, H.: Evaluation of the Effectiveness of Intracoronary Streptokinase Infusion in Acute Myocardial Infarction: Post Procedure Management and Hospital Course in 204 Patients, *Am. Heart J.,* 102:1181, 1981.
85. Khaja, F., Walton, J. A., Jr., Brymer, J. F., Lo, E., Osterberger, L., O'Neill, W. W., Colfer, H. T., Weiss, R., Lee, T., Kurian, T., Goldberg, A. D., Pitt, B., and Goldstein, S.: Intracoronary Fibrinolytic Therapy in Acute Myocardial Infarction. Report of a Prospective Randomized Trial, *N. Engl. J. Med.,* 308:1305, 1983.
86. Ridolfi, R. L., and Hutchins, G. M.: The Relationship between Coronary Artery Lesions and Myocardial Infarcts: Ulceration of Atherosclerotic Plaques Precipitating Coronary Thrombosis, *Am. Heart J.,* 93:468, 1977.
87. Horie, T., Sekiguchi, M., and Hirosawa, K.: Coronary Thrombosis in Pathogenesis of Acute Myocardial Infarction, *Br. Heart J.,* 40:153, 1978.
88. Falk, E.: Plaque Rupture with Severe Pre-Existing Stenosis Precipitating Coronary Thrombosis. Characteristics of Coronary Atherosclerosis Plaques Underlying Fatal Occlusive Thrombi, *Br. Heart J.,* 50:127, 1983.
89. Friedman, M., and Van den Bovenkamp, G. J.: The Pathogenesis of Coronary Thrombus, *Am. J. Pathol.,* 48:19, 1966.
90. Latham, P. M.: Lecture 37, in "Collected Works," in New Sydenham Society, London, 1876, vol. 1, p. 445.
91. Osler, W.: Lumleian Lectures on Angina Pectoris, *Lancet,* 1:839, 1910.
92. Buja, L. M., Hillis, L. D., Petty, C. S., and Willerson, J. T.: The Role of Coronary Arterial Spasm in Ischemic Heart Disease, *Arch. Pathol. Lab. Med.,* 105:221, 1981.
93. Gorlin, R.: Role of Coronary Vasospasm in the Pathogenesis of Myocardial Ischemia and Angina Pectoris, *Am. Heart J.,* 103, 598, 1982.
94. Yasue, H., Omote, S., Takizawa, A., and Nagao, M.: Coronary Arterial Spasm in Ischemic Heart Disease and Its Pathogenesis. A Review, *Circ. Res.,* 52(suppl. 1):147, 1983.
95. Maseri, A., L'Abbate, A., Baroldi, G., Chierchia, S., Marzilli, M., Ballestra, A. M., Severi, S., Parodi, O., Biagini, A., Distante, A., and Pesola, A.: Coronary Vasospasm as a Possible Cause of Myocardial Infarction. A Conclusion Derived from the Study of "Preinfarction" Angina, *N. Engl. J. Med.,* 299:1271, 1978.
96. Oliva, P. B., and Breckenridge, J. C.: Arteriographic Evidence of Coronary Arterial Spasm in Acute Myocardial Infarction, *Circulation,* 56:366, 1977.
97. MacAlpin, R. N.: Relation of Coronary Arterial Spasm to Sites of Organic Stenosis, *Am. J. Cardiol.,* 46:143, 1980.
98. Dalen, J. E., Ockene, I. S., and Alpert, J. S.: Coronary Spasm, Coronary Thrombosis, and Myocardial Infarction: A Hypothesis concerning the Pathophysiology of Acute Myocardial Infarction, *Am. Heart J.,* 104:1119, 1982.
99. Joris, I., and Majno, G.: Endothelial Changes Induced by Arterial Spasm, *Am. J. Pathol.,* 102:346, 1981.
100. Gertz, S. D., Uretsky, G., Wajnberg, R. S., Navot, N., and Gotsman, M. S.: Endothelial Cell Damage and Thrombus Formation after Partial Arterial Constriction: Relevance to the Role of Coronary Artery Spasm in the Pathogenesis of Myocardial Infarction, *Circulation,* 63:476, 1981.
101. Marzilli, M., Goldstein, S., Trivella, M. G., Palumbo, C., and

Maseri, A.: Some Clinical Considerations regarding the Relation of Coronary Vasospasm to Coronary Atherosclerosis: A Hypothetical Pathogenesis, *Am. J. Cardiol.*, 45:882, 1980.

102. Reimer, K. A., Lowe, J. E., Rasmussen, M. M., and Jennings, R. B.: The Wavefront Phenomenon of Ischemic Cell Death: I. Myocardial Infarct Size vs. Duration of Coronary Occlusion in Dogs, *Circulation*, 56:786, 1977.
103. Reimer, K. A., and Jennings, R. B.: The "Wavefront Phenomenon" of Myocardial Ischemic Cell Death: II. Transmural Progression of Necrosis Within the Framework of Ischemic Bed Size (Myocardium at Risk) and Collateral Flow, *Lab. Invest.*, 40:633, 1979.
104. Schaper, W., Frenzel, H., Hort, W., and Winkler, B.: Experimental Coronary Artery Occlusion: II. Spatial and Temporal Evolution of Infarcts in the Dog Heart, *Basic Res. Cardiol.*, 74:233, 1979.
105. Forman, R., Cho, S., Factor, S. M., and Kirk, E. S.: Acute Myocardial Infarct Extension into a Previously Preserved Subendocardial Region at Risk in Dogs and Patients, *Circulation*, 67:117, 1983.
106. Lavellee, M., Cox, D., Patrick, T. A., and Vatner, S. F.: Salvage of Myocardial Function by Coronary Artery Reperfusion 1, 2, and 3 Hours after Occlusion in Conscious Dogs, *Circ. Res.*, 53:235, 1983.
107. Baughman, K. L., Maroko, P. R., and Vatner, S. F.: Effects of Coronary Artery Reperfusion on Myocardial Infarct Size and Survival in Conscious Dogs, *Circulation*, 63:317, 1981.
108. Fenoglio, J. J., Karagueuzian, H. S., Friedman, P. L., Albala, A., and Wit, A. L.: Time Course of Infarct Growth toward the Endocardial Surface During the First 24 Hours after Coronary Occlusion, *Am. J. Physiol.*, 236:H356, 1979.
109. Karagueuzian, H. S., Fenoglio, J. J., Weiss, M. B., and Wit, A. L.: Coronary Occlusion and Reperfusion: Effects on Subendocardial Cardiac Fibers, *Am. J. Physiol.*, 238:H581, 1980.
110. Roberts, C. S., Schoen, F. J., and Kloner, R. A.: Effect of Coronary Reperfusion on Myocardial Hemorrhage and Infarct Healing, *Am. J. Cardiol.*, 52:610, 1983.
111. Fishbein, M. C., Y-Rit, J., Lando, U., Kanmatsuse, K., Mercier, J. C., and Ganz, W.: The Relationship of Vascular Injury and Myocardial Hemorrhage to Necrosis After Reperfusion, *Circulation*, 62:1274, 1980.
112. Kloner, R. A., Ganote, C. E., Whalen, D. A., Jr., and Jennings, R. B.: Effect of a Transient Period of Ischemia on Myocardial Cells: II. Fine Structure during the First Few Minutes of Reflow, *Am. J. Pathol.*, 74:399, 1974.
113. Hofmann, M., Hofmann, M., Genth, K., and Schaper, W.: The Influence of Reperfusion on Infarct Size after Experimental Coronary Artery Occlusion, *Basic Res. Cardiol.*, 75:572, 1980.
114. Schaper, J., and Schaper, W.: Reperfusion of Ischemic Myocardium: Ultrastructural and Histochemical Aspects, *J. Am. Coll. Cardiol.*, 1:1037, 1983.
115. Frame, L. H., Lopez, J. A., Khaw, B. A., Fallon, J. T., Haber, E., and Powell, W. J., Jr.: Early Membrane Damage during Coronary Reperfusion in Dogs. Detection by Radiolabeled Anticardiac Myosin, *J. Clin. Invest.*, 72:535, 1983.
116. Jolly, S. R., Kane, W. J., Bailie, M. B., Abrams, G. D., and Lucchesi, B. R.: Canine Myocardial Reperfusion Injury. Its Reduction by the Combined Administration of Superoxide Dismutase and Catalase, *Circ. Res.*, 54:277, 1984.
117. Whalen, D. A., Hamilton, D. G., Ganote, C. E., and Jennings, R. B.: Effect of a Transient Period of Ischemia on Myocardial Cells. Effects on Cell Volume Regulation, *Am. J. Pathol.*, 74:381, 1974.
118. Shen, A. C., and Jennings, R. B.: Myocardial Calcium and Magnesium in Acute Ischemic Injury, *Am. J. Pathol.*, 67:417, 1972.
119. Hearse, D. J.: Reperfusion of the Ischemic Myocardium, *J. Mol. Cell. Cardiol.*, 9:605, 1977.
120. Sommers, H. M., and Jennings, R. B.: Experimental Acute Myocardial Infarction, Histologic and Histochemical Studies of Early Myocardial Infarcts Induced by Temporary or Permanent Occlusion of a Coronary Artery, *Lab. Invest.*, 13:1491, 1964.
121. Bulkley, B. H., and Hutchins, G. M.: Myocardial Consequences of Coronary Artery Bypass Graft Surgery: The Paradox of Necrosis in Areas of Revascularization, *Circulation*, 56:909, 1981.
122. Buja, L. M., Parkey, R. W., Dees, J. H., Stokely, E. M., Harris, R. A., Jr., Bonte, F. J., and Willerson, J. T.: Morphologic Correlates of Technetium-99m Stannous Pyrophosphate Imaging of Acute Myocardial Infarcts in Dogs, *Circulation*, 52:596, 1975.
123. Mallory, G. K., White, P. D., and Salcedo-Salgar, J.: The Speed of Healing of Myocardial Infarction: A Study of the Pathologic Anatomy in 72 Cases, *Am. Heart J.*, 18:647, 1939.
124. Fishbein, M. C., MacLean, D., and Maroko, P. R.: The Histopathologic Evolution of Myocardial Infarction, *Chest*, 73:843, 1978.
125. Bouchardy, B., and Majno, C.: Histopathology of Early Myocardial Infarcts: A New Approach, *Am. J. Pathol.*, 74:301, 1974.
126. Kloner, R. A., Ganote, C. E., and Jennings, R. B.: The "No-Reflow" Phenomenon after Temporary Coronary Occlusion in the Dog, *J. Clin. Invest.*, 54:1496, 1974.
127. Hutchins, G. M., and Bulkley, B. H.: Infarct Expansion Versus Extension: Two Different Complications of Acute Myocardial Infarction, *Am. J. Cardiol.*, 41:1127, 1978.
128. Robinson, T. F., Cohen-Gould, L., and Factor, S. M.: Skeletal Framework of Mammalian Heart Muscle. Arrangement of Inter- and Pericellular Connective Tissue Structures, *Lab. Invest.*, 49:482, 1983.
129. Hammerman, H., Schoen, F. J., Braunwald, E., and Kloner, R. A.: Drug-Induced Expansion of Infarct: Morphologic and Functional Correlations, *Circulation*, 69:611, 1984.
130. Fraker, T. D., Jr., Wagner, G. S., and Rosati, R. A.: Extension of Myocardial Infarction: Incidence and Prognosis, *Circulation*, 60:1126, 1979.
131. Factor, S. M., Okun, E. M., and Kirk, E. S.: Microextension of Acute Myocardial Necrosis into the Normal Zone of 7 Day Canine Infarcts, *Circulation*, 60(suppl.2):114, 1979.
132. Fishbein, M. C., Hare, C. A., Grissen, S. A., Spadaro, J., MacLean, D., and Maroko, P. R.: Identification and Quantification of Histochemical Border Zones during the Evolution of Myocardial Infarction in the Rat, *Cardiovasc. Res.*, 14:41, 1980.
133. Mitsunami, K., Fukuhara, T., Kato, S., Bito, K., Kinoshita, M., and Kawakita, S.: The Border Zone in Acute Myocardial Ischemia in the Dog. A Histochemical, Biochemical and Ultrastructural Study, *Jpn. Circ. J.*, 48:18, 1984.
134. Fishbein, M. C., Meerbaum, S., Rit, J., Lando, U., Kanmatsuse, K., Mercier, J. C., Corday, E., and Ganz, W.: Early Phase Acute Myocardial Infarct Size Quantification: Validation of the Triphenyl Tetrazolium Chloride Tissue Enzyme Staining Technique, *Am. Heart J.*, 101:593, 1981.
135. Klein, H. H., Puschmann, S., Schaper, J., and Schaper, W.: The Mechanism of the Tetrazolium Reaction in Identifying Experimental Myocardial Infarction, *Virchows Arch. Pathol. Anat.*, 393:287, 1981.
136. Schaper, W., Frenzel, H., and Hort, W.: Experimental Coronary Artery Occlusion: I. Measurement of Infarct Size, *Basic Res. Cardiol.*, 74:46, 1979.
137. Factor, S. M., Cho, S., and Kirk, E. S.: Non-Specificity of Triphenyl Tetrazolium Chloride for the Gross Diagnosis of Acute Myocardial Infarction, *Circulation*, 66(suppl. 2):84, 1982.
138. Kirk, E. S., Eng, C., Cho, S., and Factor, S. M.: Failure to Demonstrate Salvage of Myocardium at 6 Hours with Ibuprofen using Triphenyl Tetrazolium Chloride, *Circulation*, 66(suppl. 2):84, 1982.

45

Atherosclerotic Coronary Heart Disease: Recognition, Prognosis, and Treatment

J. Willis Hurst, M.D.
Spencer B. King III, M.D.
Gottlieb C. Friesinger, M.D.
Paul F. Walter, M.D.
Douglas C. Morris, M.D.

Historical Benchmarks
- Recognition of Angina Pectoris
- Etiology of Angina Pectoris
- Pathophysiology of Angina Pectoris
- Recognition of Coronary Thrombosis
- Electrocardiography—The First Diagnostic Tool Used to Diagnose Coronary Disease
- Clinical-Anatomic Correlations
- "In Between" Syndromes
- Variant Angina
- Cardiac Enzymes—The First Chemical Tests Used to Diagnose Coronary Disease
- Cardiac Catheterization as a Tool to Diagnose Coronary Disease
- Application of Nuclear Medicine to the Recognition of Coronary Disease
- Use of Sonar Techniques to Diagnose Certain Problems Due to Coronary Disease
- Prognosis (Natural History)
- Management
- Prevention

Clinical Recognition of Subsets
- The Clinical Spectrum
- Methods Used to Identify Subsets
- Echocardiography
- Other Laboratory Tests

Reminder

Conditions Simulating Atherosclerotic Coronary Heart Disease
- "Emotional" Causes of Chest Discomfort
- Noncoronary Cardiovascular Causes of Chest Discomfort
- Gastrointestinal Causes of Chest Discomfort
- Pulmonary Causes of Chest Discomfort
- Neuromuscular-Skeletal Causes of Chest Discomfort

Prognosis of Atherosclerotic Coronary Heart Disease
- Background and Principles
- Coronary Atherosclerosis without Angina or Other Evidence of Ischemia
- Coronary Atherosclerosis with Reversible Ischemia
- Coronary Atherosclerosis with Irreversible Myocardial Ischemia and Necrosis
- Sudden Death
- Ischemic Cardiomyopathy

Recognition, Classification, and Treatment of Patients with Atherosclerotic Coronary Heart Disease
- General Considerations
- Classification
- Medical Management (General Discussion)
- Percutaneous Transluminal Coronary Angioplasty
- Surgical Treatment—Coronary Bypass Surgery and Other Surgical Techniques

Treatment of Specific Subsets
- Coronary Atherosclerosis without Angina or Other Evidence of Ischemia
- Coronary Atherosclerosis with Reversible Myocardial Ischemia—Stable Subsets
- Coronary Atherosclerosis with Reversible Myocardial Ischemia—Unstable Subsets
- Coronary Atherosclerosis with Irreversible Myocardial Ischemia and Necrosis
- Sudden Death
- Syncope
- Cardiac Arrhythmias
- Ischemic Cardiomyopathy
- Atherosclerotic Coronary Heart Disease in Combination with Other Conditions

Reasons for Different Strategies

But there is a disorder of the breast marked with strong and peculiar symptoms, considerable for the kind of danger belonging to it, and not extremely rare, which deserves to be mentioned at length. The seat of it, and sense of strangling and anxiety with which it is attended, may make it not improperly be called angina pectoris.

William Heberden, M.D., 1802[1,*]

*Angina pectoris was originally discussed by Heberden in a lecture at a meeting of the Royal College of Physicians of London in July 1768 and published in their *Medical Transactions* in 1786 in an article entitled "Some Account of a Disorder of the Breast."[2] This quotation is from "Pectoris Dolor," a chapter in *Commentaries on the History and Cure of Diseases,* London, 1802.[1]

Obstruction of a coronary artery or of any of its large branches has long been regarded as a serious accident. Several events contributed toward the prevalence of the view that this condition was almost always suddenly fatal. . . . But there are reasons for believing that even large branches of the coronary arteries may be occluded—at times acutely occluded—without resulting death, at least without death in the immediate future. Even the main trunk may at times be obstructed and the patient live. It is the object of this paper to present a few facts along this line, and particularly to describe some of the clinical manifestations of sudden yet not immediately fatal causes of coronary obstruction.

James Herrick, M.D., 1912[3]

"Acute coronary insufficiency" is a syndrome of a more severe myocardial ischemia and is associated with myocardial damage. It is associated with a precipitating factor which decreases coronary flow or which increases the work of the heart and oxygen requirement of the heart muscle.

Arthur M. Master, M.D., 1944[4,†]

The purpose of this chapter is to discuss some of the *historical benchmarks, recognition, prognosis,* and *treatment* of atherosclerotic coronary heart disease. The factors that are known to influence atherogenesis are discussed in Chap. 41. The prevention of atherosclerosis is discussed in Chap. 42. The pathology of atherosclerosis is discussed in Chap. 43. The pathophysiology of myocardial ischemia is discussed in Chap. 44. Coronary artery spasm is discussed in Chap. 46, and nonatherosclerotic causes of coronary artery disease are discussed in Chap. 47. The rehabilitation of patients with symptomatic atherosclerotic coronary heart disease is discussed in Chap. 48.

Historical Benchmarks‡

Our current knowledge regarding the recognition, prognosis, and treatment of atherosclerotic coronary artery disease is considerable. It is, at the same time, grossly deficient. Our knowledge is considerable because it has developed over a span of several centuries and has accelerated enormously during the last three decades. Our knowledge is deficient because we know so little about the prevention of the disease or how to treat all the sequelae of it. These inadequacies assume even more importance, despite the evidence that the mortality rate of coronary heart disease has declined in the United States,[5,6] because the disease continues to be the leading cause of death in this country and many others as well.

Recognition of Angina Pectoris

Many people contributed to our ability to identify patients with atherosclerotic coronary heart disease. Only a few will be mentioned here. For further historical accounts of the recognition of angina pectoris and coronary disease the reader is referred to Benson,[7] Herrick,[8] and Proudfit.[9,10]

William Heberden, M.D. (1710–1801)

Heberden originally mentioned angina pectoris in a lecture before the Royal College of Physicians in London in 1768.[2] His observations were published in their *Medical Transactions* in 1786.[2] The following excerpts are from the 1802 account of the disorder:[1]

> They who are afflicted with it, are seized while they are walking, (more especially if it be up hill, and soon after eating) with a painful and most disagreeable sensation in the breast, which seems as if it would extinguish life, if it were to increase or to continue; but the moment they stand still, all this uneasiness vanishes.
>
> In all other respects, the patients are, at the beginning of this disorder, perfectly well, and in particular have no shortness of breath, from which it is totally different. The pain is sometimes situated in the upper part, sometimes in the middle, sometimes at the bottom of the os sterni, and often more inclined to the left than to the right side. It likewise very frequently extends from the breast to the middle of the left arm. The pulse is, at least sometimes, not disturbed by this pain, as I have had opportunities of observing by feeling the pulse during the paroxysm. Males are most liable to this disease, especially such as have past their fiftieth year.
>
> After it has continued a year or more, it will not cease so instantaneously upon standing still; and it will come on not only when the persons are walking, but when they are lying down, especially if they lie on the left side, and oblige them to rise up out of their beds. In some inveterate cases it has been brought on by the motion of a horse, or a carriage, and even by swallowing, coughing, going to school, or speaking, or any disturbance of mind.
>
> Such is the most usual appearance of this disease; but some varieties may be met with. Some have been seized while they are standing still, or sitting, also upon first waking out of sleep: and the pain sometimes reaches to the right arm, as well as to the left, and even down to the hands, but this is uncommon: in a very few instances the arm has at the same time been numbed and swelled. In one or two persons, the pain has lasted some hours, or even days; but this has happened when the complaint has been of long standing, and thoroughly rooted in the constitution: once only the very first attack continued the whole night.
>
> I have seen nearly a hundred people under this disorder, of which number there have been three women, and one boy twelve years old. All the rest were men near, or past the fiftieth year of their age.[1]

Heberden did not attribute angina pectoris to a decreased blood flow through obstructed coronary arteries. He actually did not know what disease his patients had. He recognized this shortcoming of his work and wrote the following:

> An useful addition might have been made to these papers by comparing them with the current doctrine of diseases and remedies, as also with what is laid down in practical writers, and with the accounts of those who treat of the dissections of morbid bodies; but at my advanced age it would be to no purpose to think of such an undertaking.[1]

He discussed only one autopsy:

> On opening the body of one, who died suddenly of this disease, a very skillful anatomist could discover no fault in the heart, in the valves, in the arteries, or neighbouring veins, excepting small rudiments of ossification of the aorta.[1]

It is highly likely *most* of his patients had atherosclerotic coronary heart disease, but it is almost certain *all* of the patients did not. Some of them prob-

†Reproduced with permission of the publisher.

‡*Note:* The interested reader is referred to *History of Cardiology* by H. A. Snellen, published by Donker Academic Publications, Rotterdam, The Netherlands, 1984.

ably had aortic valve disease, idiopathic hypertrophic subaortic stenosis, coronary spasm, and anxiety (neurocirculatory asthenia). Therefore, it is unwise to think of "classic" Heberden's angina as being pathognomonic of atherosclerotic coronary artery disease.

John Hunter, M.D. (1728–1793)

John Hunter recorded his observations on himself. He, more than anyone, emphasized that angina pectoris was precipitated by emotional turmoil. He said his life was in the hands of any rascal who chose to annoy or tease him. The following passage was written by Everard Home, who was Hunter's brother-in-law:[11]

> Although evidently relieved from the violent attacks of spasm by the gout in his feet, yet he was far from being free from the disease, for he was still subject to the spasms, upon exercise or agitation of mind; the exercise that generally brought it on, was walking, especially on an ascent, either of stairs or rising ground, but never on going down either the one or the other; the affections of the mind that brought it on were principally anxiety or anger: it was not the cause of the anxiety, but the quantity that most affected him; the anxiety about the hiving of a swarm of bees brought it on; the anxiety lest an animal should make its escape before he could get a gun to shoot it, brought it on; even the hearing of a story in which the mind became so much engaged as to be interested in the event, although the particulars were of no consequence to him, would bring it on; anger brought on the same complaint and he could conceive it possible for that passion to be carried so far as totally to deprive him of life; but what was very extraordinary, the more tender passions of the mind did not produce it; he could relate a story which called up all the finer feelings, as compassion, admiration for the actions of gratitude in others, so as to make him shed tears, yet the spasm was not excited; it is extraordinary that he ate and slept as well as ever, and his mind was in no degree depressed; the want of exercise made him grow unusually fat.
>
> In the autumn 1790, and in the spring and autumn 1791, he had more severe attacks than during the other periods of the year, but of not more than a few hours duration; in the beginning of October, 1792, one, at which I was present, was so violent that I thought he would have died. On October the 16th, 1793, when in his mind, and not being perfectly master of the circumstances, he withheld his sentiments, in which state of restraint he went into the next room, and turning around to Dr. Robertson, one of the physicians of the hospital, he gave a deep groan, and dropt down dead.[11]

Etiology of Angina Pectoris

Caleb Hillier Parry (1755–1822) and Edward Jenner (1749–1823)

Parry and Jenner are usually given the credit for recognizing that angina pectoris can be caused by coronary artery disease. Allan Burns wrote the following about their contribution to the subject:[12]

> To Drs. Heberden, Jenner, and Parry, we owe most of our information respecting this most fatal complaint. After the very able treatise which Dr. Parry has published on this subject, very little can now be added to the information he has communicated regarding the pathology of Syncope Anginosa. By a series of well related cases, he establishes the regular history of the disease, and by fair induction from a series of accurately performed dissections, he confirms his opinions respecting the cause of this affection; which I think, he has incontrovertibly proved to originate from some organic laesion of the nutrient vessels of the heart. In all patients who have died of Syncope Anginosa, where the body has been carefully examined, the coronary arteries have either been found ossified or cartilaginous.[12]

In addition to Parry and Jenner, Herrick writes[7] that we should also credit John Fothergill (1712–1780) for following Heberden's suggestions and identifying that angina was due to coronary disease.

Pathophysiology of Angina Pectoris

Allan Burns (1781–1813)

This creative genius was an anatomist and not a physician. He died at age 31. No one has contributed more in such a short time. Osler credited him for the belief that coronary arteries can undergo spasm.[13] Burns understood that the decreased blood flow that resulted from obstructed arteries caused angina pectoris. He wrote:

> It has been long known, that although the heart is always full of blood, yet it cannot appropriate to its own wants a single particle of fluid contained in its cavities. On the contrary, like every other part, it has peculiar vessels set apart for its nourishment. In health, when we excite the muscular system to more energetic action than usual, we increase the circulation in every part, so that to support this increased action, the heart and every other part has its power augmented. If, however, we call into vigorous action, a limb, round which, we have with a moderate degree of tightness applied a ligature, we find that then the member can only support its action for a very short time; for now its supply of energy and its expenditure, do not balance each other; consequently, it soon, from a deficiency of nervous influence and arterial blood, fails and sinks into a state of quiescence. A heart, the coronary vessels of which are cartilaginous or ossified, is in nearly a similar condition; it can, like the limb, be girt with a moderately tight ligature, discharge its functions so long as its action is moderate and equal. Increase however the action of the whole body, and along with the rest, that of the heart, and you will soon see exemplified, the truth of what has been said; with this difference, that as there is no interruption to the action of the cardiac nerves, the heart will be able to hold out a little longer than the limb.
>
> If a person walks fast, ascends a steep, or mounts a pair of stairs, the circulation in a state of health is hurried, and the heart is felt beating more frequently against the ribs than usual. If, however, a person, with the nutrient arteries of the heart diseased in such a way as to impede the progress of the blood along them, attempts to do the same, he finds, that the heart is sooner fatigued than the other parts are, which remain healthy. When, therefore, the coronary arteries are ossified, every

agent capable of increasing the action of the heart, such as exercise, passion, and ardent spirits, must be a source of danger.[12]

Recognition of Coronary Thrombosis

James Herrick (1861–1954)[3,14]
Herrick described the clinical features of coronary thrombosis (myocardial infarction) and stressed the fact that coronary thrombosis did not always lead to death as was believed at the time (see quotation at the beginning of this chapter).

He also stressed the need for a classification of the numerous clinical syndromes that resulted from coronary disease. He saw the need to link the subsets of the disorder to specific treatment.[3]

> All attempts at dividing these clinical manifestations into groups must be artificial and more or less imperfect. Yet such an attempt is not without value, as it enables one the better to understand the gravity of an obstructive accident, to differentiate it from other conditions presenting somewhat similar symptoms, and to employ a more rational therapy that may, to a slight extent at least, be more efficient.[3]

Electrocardiography—The First Diagnostic Tool Used to Diagnose Coronary Disease

Electrocardiography (see Chaps. 14 and 98)[15,16]
While many people were responsible for the invention of the electrocardiograph machine, Einthoven receives the credit.[17] The evolution of the instrument and discipline, however, was made possible by Lippmann,[18] Marey,[19] Ader,[20] and especially Waller.[21] Lewis,[22] Wilson,[23,24] and Grant[25] stand out as people who applied the instrument to the recognition of cardiac disease.

Bonsfield, in 1918, is credited with publishing the first electrocardiogram (ECG) of a patient with aortic regurgitation who was having a paroxysm of angina pectoris.[26] Herrick in his 1919 publication entitled *Thrombosis of the Coronary Arteries* described the ECG during the acute phase and late phase of the condition. Furthermore, he pointed out the similarity of the changes to ligation of the coronary artery in the dog.[27] Wood and Wolferth (1931), however, were among the first to explain the effect of ischemia due to coronary disease on the ECG.[28] Master should be credited as the physician who developed exercise stress testing using the ECG.[29]

The profession's problem has been to learn that a patient may have life-threatening coronary disease and the resulting ECG may be normal and that every electrocardiographic abnormality does not indicate serious heart disease (see quotation from Frank Wilson[30] at the beginning of Chap. 83).

Clinical-Anatomic Correlations

Blumgart, Schlesinger, and Zoll[31]
These men correlated elegant autopsy studies with the clinical course of patients. They used a new technique to inject coronary arteries after death and reported:[31]

> A detailed clinical and pathologic study of 355 consecutive cases examined post mortem has been made with particular reference to the role of coronary occlusion and the collateral circulation in angina pectoris, coronary failure and acute myocardial infarction.

They introduced many new concepts and laid the groundwork for understanding the disease so that coronary arteriography, which was introduced much later, was immediately appreciated.

"In Between" Syndromes

Arthur Master (1885–1973)
Master recognized that Heberden's angina was at one extreme of the clinical spectrum and that Herrick's acute coronary thrombosis (myocardial infarction) was at the other extreme of the clinical spectrum.[4] He emphasized that some patients exhibited a syndrome that was in between the two extremes. In 1944 he labeled this subset of patients as having "coronary insufficiency" (see the third quotation at the beginning of the chapter). Many physicians recognized this syndrome. Notable among them was Blumgart, who called the syndrome "*coronary failure*" and Grabiel, who used the term *intermediate coronary syndrome.*

Variant Angina

Myron Prinzmetal (1908–)
Prinzmetal's variant angina may occur in patients who have coronary spasm with normal coronary arteries, but it more commonly occurs in patients with obstructive coronary disease plus coronary spasm (see Chap. 46). Prinzmetal and his associates described variant angina in *The American Journal of Medicine* in 1959.[32] A portion of the summary is reproduced here with the permission of the publisher and author.*

> A variant form of angina pectoris is described. This syndrome differs from classic angina pectoris in several aspects.
>
> The pain is not brought on by increased cardiac work, is usually more severe and of longer duration, often waxes and wanes in cyclic fashion, often occurs at about the same time each day, and is not relieved by rest. Arrhythmias, often ventricular, occur in about 50 percent of cases during the peak of the pain. The pain usually disappears immediately after infarction. The variant form of angina exhibits the following electrocardiographic features which are in contrast to those found in the classic form of angina pectoris: (1) The ST segments are elevated transiently and often considerably during an attack, although there may be ST changes with a mild attack or at the onset of a severe attack. (2) Reciprocal ST depression occurs in standard leads. (3) ST and T wave changes during an attack

*We wish to thank Dr. Prinzmetal's son for his assistance and kindness in obtaining the permission to use this important quotation.

occasionally may seem to improve a previously abnormal electrocardiogram. (4) Areas of myocardium giving rise to ST elevation correspond to the distribution of a large coronary artery. (5) The area of myocardium giving rise to ST segment elevation during anginal pain often is the site of future infarction. (6) Exercise does not produce ST elevation. (7) The R wave may become taller and broader during an attack.

The clinical diagnosis of the variant form of angina is possible in typical cases even without the use of the electrocardiogram.

Temporary increased tonus of a large narrowed coronary artery is suggested as the cause of attacks of pain in the variant form of angina. Chemical changes in the myocardium differ from those occurring in classic angina pectoris.[32]

Prinzmetal postulated that the condition was caused by "temporary hypertonus of a large atherosclerotic artery" (Fig. 45-1).

See discussion regarding Prinzmetal's angina (variant) below and in Chap. 46.

Cardiac Enzymes—The First Chemical Tests Used to Diagnose Coronary Disease

Cardiac Enzymes

LaDue, Wroblewski, and Karmen described a rise in the level of serum glutamic oxaloacetic transaminase (SGOT) when myocardial cells are injured.[33] This discovery, reported in 1954, heralded the entrance of chemical testing into the diagnostic workup of patients with possible myocardial infarction due to atherosclerotic coronary heart disease. Later, other cardiac enzymes such as lactic dehydrogenase (LDH), creatine phosphokinase (CPK), and myocardial creatine kinase (MB-CK) were identified so that the physician's ability to diagnose myocardial infarction was improved even further (see discussion below regarding enzymes).

Cardiac Catheterization as a Tool to Diagnose Coronary Disease

Coronary Arteriography (see Chap. 108)

Sones "accidentally" performed the first coronary arteriogram in 1958.[34] His "accident" would not have occurred had not many others preceded him and developed cardiac catheterization and angiography. Among them were Forssmann,[35] who performed catheterization of the right side of the heart on himself in 1929 and Castellanos[36] and Robb and Steinberg[37] who performed angiography. Sones recognized the value of his "accident" and developed coronary arteriography, which will, without question, be recorded as one of the great advances in medical history.

Prior to coronary arteriography there was no way to identify the presence and location of the obstructing lesions except by postmortem examination. The physician's ability to diagnose atherosclerotic coronary heart disease in a living patient took a giant step forward with the development of modern coronary arteriography. The procedure also set the stage for coronary bypass surgery and percutaneous transluminal coronary angioplasty. With the advent of coronary arteriography, the concepts learned from the autopsy studies of Schlesinger, Blumgart, and Zoll[31] could be applied in the practice of medicine.

Coronary arteriography is discussed below and in Chap. 108.

Application of Nuclear Medicine to the Recognition of Coronary Disease

Nuclear Cardiology (see Chap. 109)

Nuclear cardiology came into its own in the 1970s, and new and improved equipment is brought forward each year. It is currently possible to measure

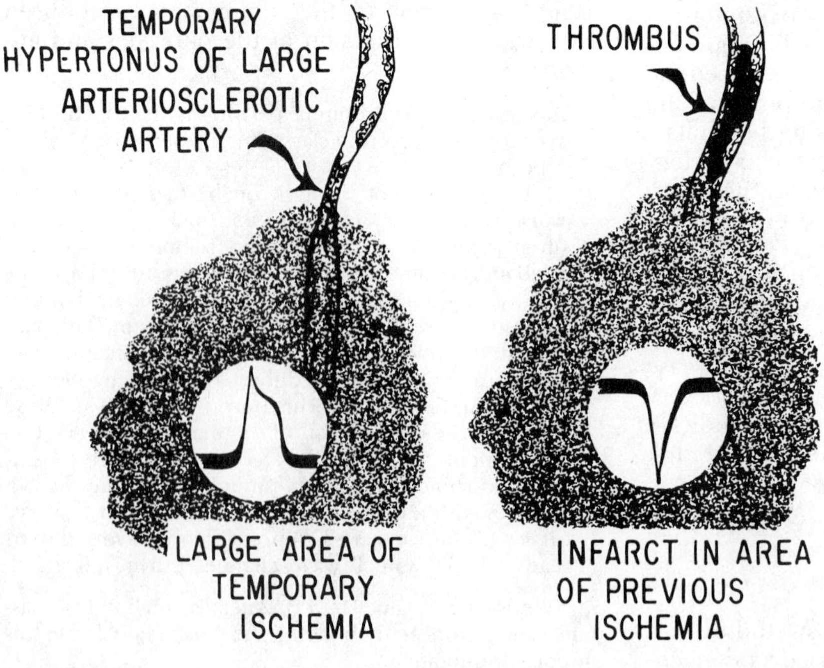

FIGURE 45-1 Theory of location of infarction. If myocardial infarction occurs, the area involved is the same as that which became ischemic during previous attacks of pain. The location of possible future infarction can thus be predicted. (*Legend and illustration from M. Prinzmetal, R. Kennamer, R. Merliss, T. Wada, and N. Bor. Angina Pectoris: I. A Variant Form of Angina Pectoris. Preliminary Report, Am. J. Med., 27:382, 1959. Reproduced with permission from the publisher and author. We wish to thank Dr. Prinzmetal's son for his assistance and kindness in obtaining permission to use this important figure.*)

the ejection fraction, identify areas of poor contractility, identify dead cardiac muscle, identify ischemic areas, and establish the prognosis of certain patients.

Use of Sonar Techniques to Diagnose Certain Problems Due to Coronary Disease

Echocardiography (see Chap. 120)
This technique was developed during the 1970s. It can be used to determine the ejection fraction and areas of poor myocardial contractility, and to identify left ventricular thrombi. It may be used for the diagnosis of certain subsets of patients with atherosclerotic coronary heart disease.

Prognosis (Natural History)

The prognosis of atherosclerotic heart disease could not be accurately determined as long as diagnostic methods were inadequate. A rough approximation of the natural history of angina pectoris and myocardial infarction was appreciated and taught by Paul White.[38,39] This knowledge permitted him to return Dwight Eisenhower to the presidency and permitted one of us (J.W.H.) to indicate that Lyndon Johnson could return to the Senate, and later run for the vice presidency and presidency.

In the past the prognosis was determined by following a group of patients with angina pectoris, infarction, or electrocardiographic abnormalities for several years. Paul White was a master at this type of study and taught that if a patient had no symptoms several years after a definite coronary event, the prognosis could be determined more accurately than if a patient had experienced a recent event.

Modern treadmill testing (Chap. 98), Holter monitoring (Chap. 100), coronary arteriography and left ventriculography (Chap. 108), and techniques using radionuclides (Chap. 109) have made it possible to determine the prognosis of the patients with coronary atherosclerosis more accurately than was possible in the past. Friesinger also addresses this problem later in this chapter.

Management

It is highly likely that the first form of treatment was discovered by patients themselves. They simply learned to walk more slowly or not to walk at all in an attempt to decrease or prevent angina pectoris produced by effort. This approach to relieving patients is still recommended today, particularly for those patients who have not responded to modern drugs, coronary angioplasty, or surgical therapy.

Amyl Nitrate (see Chap. 88)
Brunton (1844–1916) was the first to report that amyl nitrate would relieve angina pectoris. His work was far from being scientific and would not be accepted for publication today. He wrote:[40]

> On pouring from five to ten drops of the nitrite on a cloth and giving it to the patient to inhale, the physiological action took place in from thirty to sixty seconds; and simultaneously with the flushing of the face the pain completely disappeared, and generally did not return till its wonted time next night.

Nitroglycerin was not used for some years after Brunton used amyl nitrate. Murrell deserves the credit for discovering its beneficial effect on angina pectoris. He reported his discovery in 1879.[41]

Tinsley Harrison popularized the use of nitroglycerin ointment over 25 years ago. It was then abandoned but has recently enjoyed a return to the forefront with pharmaceutical houses making a new skin "patch" every few years. Intravenous nitroglycerin was introduced a few years ago as an effective treatment of myocardial ischemia.

Long-acting nitrates were used for many years but were, for the most part, ineffective. Dinitro isosorbide has stood the test of time and is effective.

More than 100 years passed after Brunton's discovery before we understood how nitrates relieved angina pectoris and before effective long-acting preparations were developed (see discussion later in this chapter).

Beta-Adrenergic Blocks (see Chap. 90)
Ahlquist deserves the credit for setting the stage for the development of the beta-adrenergic blockers.[42] He characterized the beta-adrenergic receptors, and this led to the discovery of drugs that block the receptors. Now there are many beta-blocking drugs which are used in the treatment of angina pectoris, hypertension, and cardiac arrhythmias. They are very effective and represent the first great advance since the discovery that nitroglycerin relieved angina pectoris. There is some evidence that certain of these drugs will prolong the lives of patients with myocardial infarction (see discussion later in this chapter).

Calcium Antagonists (see Chap. 91)
Fleckenstein deserves the credit for discovering the drugs named by him as calcium antagonists.[43] Now there are many such drugs, each with different pharmacological action, and more are being developed. Some of these excellent drugs are useful in the treatment of angina pectoris, especially Prinzmetal's angina, arrhythmias, hypertension, and other vasospastic disorders (see discussion later in this chapter).

Streptokinase, Anticoagulants, and Platelet Inhibitors (see Chaps. 95 and 118)
Streptokinase was discovered by Tillet and Garner in 1933.[44] Johnson and McCarty reported their results using streptokinase for thrombolysis in 1959.[45] Anticoagulants and platelet inhibitors are being used to prevent thrombosis, and streptokinase and other drugs are being investigated for the treatment of early infarction (see discussion later in this chapter).

Surgical Treatment (see Chap. 132)
Many surgical approaches have been used to treat angina pectoris (see discussion later in this chapter). Lawrie and Morris[46] point out that Alex Carrel wrote the following in 1910:[47]

> In certain cases of angina pectoris, when the mouth of the coronary arteries is calcified, it would be useful to establish a complementary circulation for the lower part of the arteries.

Carrel actually anastomosed a homograft (carotid artery) from the aorta to the left coronary artery in a dog to show that such a procedure could be done.

Coronary bypass surgery was first used by Sabiston in 1962.[48] He performed an end-to-end anastomosis. Garret, Dennis, and DeBakey reported the first use of the end-to-side technique in 1964.[49] Favaloro and Effler at the Cleveland Clinic and Johnson, Cooley, Spencer, Kirklin, Austin, and others deserve the credit for developing the technique that is widely used today (see discussion later in this chapter).

Now it is possible to surgically repair the complications of myocardial infarction including rupture of the interventricular septum; rupture of the papillary muscle; rupture of the ventricular wall; and a ventricular aneurysm (Chap. 132).

Percutaneous Transluminal Coronary Angioplasty (see Chap. 117)
Dotter was the first to use arterial dilatation for the treatment of obstructive atherosclerotic disease of the lower extremities.[50] Gruentzig, now at Emory University, was the first to dilate an obstructing lesion in the coronary arteries.[51–53] He has invented many new catheters for this purpose and has carefully refined the technique. He has shown that it is possible to work safely inside the coronary arteries (see discussion later in this chapter).

Prevention (see Chap. 42)
We have made some progress in the prevention of atherosclerotic coronary heart disease.[54] We still do not know all the factors involved in the etiology of the disease and because of this can address only those factors that are known. Even in the area of known factors such as tobacco smoking and undesirable blood lipids we are far from successful in leading the public at large to correct these "risk factors." More research is needed before we can place this disease into a category of preventable disease as has occurred with smallpox and poliomyelitis.

Clinical Recognition of Subsets

Herrick recognized in 1912 that there were many clinical manifestations of coronary disease and urged the creation of subsets that could be linked to a "more rational therapy."[3] Accordingly, it is proper to discuss the subsets that make up the clinical spectrum and the methods used to identify them.

The Clinical Spectrum
The disease, atherosclerotic coronary heart disease, has many manifestations. Various combinations of these manifestations can be used to establish the characteristics of the subsets (subgroups) that make up the clinical spectrum of the disease (Table 45-1). Note that some of the subsets are listed in the *reversible myocardial ischemia* group and other subsets are listed in the *irreversible myocardial ischemia* group.

The subsets of the clinical spectrum shown in Table 45-1 have been identified with four objectives in mind:

- The subsets are designed to reflect our most recent understanding of the pathophysiological processes which are responsible for them.
- The subsets are titled and organized so that the initial identification can be accomplished using

TABLE 45-1 The Clinical Spectrum of Atherosclerotic Coronary Heart Disease*

Coronary atherosclerosis without angina or other evidence of ischemia
Coronary atherosclerosis with reversible myocardial ischemia
  Stable subsets
    Stable angina pectoris
    Positive exercise test
    Angina equivalents
Coronary atherosclerosis with reversible myocardial ischemia
  Unstable subsets
    Unstable angina pectoris and equivalents
    Postinfarction angina pectoris
    Prinzmetal's angina pectoris
    Prolonged myocardial ischemia without objective evidence of infarction
Coronary atherosclerosis with irreversible myocardial ischemia and necrosis
    Very early profound ischemia
    Early evolving infarction
    Uncomplicated completed infarction
    Complicated infarction
Sudden death†
Syncope†
Cardiac arrhythmias†
Ischemic cardiomyopathy‡
Atherosclerotic coronary heart disease in combination with other conditions

*This classification of atherosclerotic coronary heart disease permits the linkage of pathophysiology, clinical syndromes, prognosis, and specific treatment. Clear definitions of the syndromes and their treatment are discussed in the text.

†Sudden death may occur in patients with reversible myocardial ischemia. It may also occur in patients who have had infarction due to irreversible myocardial ischemia. The mechanism for syncope may be similar to the mechanism for sudden death. Cardiac arrhythmias occurring in patients with coronary atherosclerotic heart disease may be, but are not always, due to myocardial ischemia.

‡The hearts of patients with ischemic cardiomyopathy have areas of infarction due to irreversible ischemia. The same patients may also experience episodes of reversible ischemia.

simple diagnostic methods but prepares the physician to consider additional noninvasive and invasive methods in order to create additional subsets within a subset.

- The subsets, with their subdivisions, are titled and organized so that the physician can link treatment, be it medical therapy, angioplasty, or coronary bypass surgery, to the patients who make up the subsets. By doing this we have followed the advice given by Herrick in 1912 (see above).[3]
- The subsets are carefully defined and titled so that physicians can communicate with each other. Without clear definitions it is not possible to engage in scientific studies or communicate accurately.

Any perceptive physician can recognize that many of the subsets which make up the clinical spectrum of atherosclerotic heart disease overlap with other subsets. In other words, the division between the subsets is not always a sharp one. Despite this problem it seems useful to identify subsets, imperfect as they are, and link them to the performance of procedures and treatment.

The definitions of the subsets are discussed later in this chapter. At this point it is sufficient simply to call attention to the clinical spectrum of atherosclerotic coronary heart disease (Table 45-1). *This initial introduction (and table) has been devised to serve as a road map for the remainder of the chapter.*

Methods Used to Identify Subsets

In practice the clinical setting, the history, the physical examination, the resting ECG, and the chest x-ray are used routinely to identify subsets. The vectorcardiogram (rarely used), the determination of the blood level of cardiac enzymes, exercise stress ECG and the long-term monitoring for arrhythmias, radionuclide scanning, coronary arteriography and ventriculography, Swan-Ganz catheterization, echocardiography, and other laboratory tests are not used routinely. One or more of these latter methods are used to identify subsets within subsets.

Each of these methods of data collection is *valuable,* but each method has its imperfections and *limitations.* Accordingly, the value and limitations of each method will be discussed.

The Clinical Setting

There is abundant information to indicate that certain individuals have a greater chance of developing atherosclerotic coronary heart disease than others (Chap. 42).[54] Such high-risk individuals include those who are male; are in a certain age range; smoke tobacco;[55] are hypertensive; have hyperlipidemia; are obese;[56] have a carotid artery bruit, abdominal aneurysm, or severe peripheral arterial disease due to atherosclerosis have carbohydrate intolerance (diabetes mellitus); are inactive;[57] are female and take a contraceptive pill (see Chap. 72); have hyperuricemia;[58] have certain electrocardiographic abnormalities; have a certain type of personality (type A); have a family history of premature atherosclerotic coronary heart disease; or have xanthoma. Obesity, formerly believed to be an associated risk factor, is considered by Hubert to be an independent risk factor.[56] There are data suggesting that the relatives of wives of myocardial infarct survivors have an increased frequency of coronary heart disease.[59] These attributes have been called "risk factors." The risk of a coronary event occurring within the years ahead in an individual with two or more predisposing factors is not the simple sum of the individual risk factors, but rather a much higher risk. The Gas Company study[54] and the Framingham study[60] showed the progressive and synergistic effect of the presence of two, three, or four risk factors (hypertension, cigarette smoking, overweight, and an elevated serum cholesterol level).

Mediastinal irradiations for neoplastic disease, such as Hodgkin's disease, have led to precocious coronary atherosclerosis as well as pericardial and myocardial disease.[61] Myocardial infarction may occur following irradiation of the chest in teenage patients and in patients in their early twenties.[62,63] Stewart and Fajardo have concluded that radiation predisposes patients to atherosclerosis by enhancing the aging process or by producing vascular injury with secondary vascular damage in the injured area.[64–66]

Certain patients receiving modern medical therapy may have an increased risk of developing atherosclerotic coronary heart disease. For example, patients receiving dialysis[67] for renal failure may have an increased incidence of atherosclerotic coronary heart disease.

Limitations Whereas the risk factor concept is a good one, it is proper to add a word of caution regarding its use in the diagnosis of an individual patient. Many patients without known risk factors have atherosclerotic coronary heart disease and many patients with the risk factors do not have atherosclerotic coronary heart disease. The presence of risk factors simply implies that the patient is more likely to develop overt signs of atherosclerotic heart disease in the years ahead than is an individual who does not have such markers. Many diagnostic errors are made when the risk factor concept is improperly used in individual patients.

The History: Symptoms and Other Historical Data Related to Coronary Disease

The *symptoms* of myocardial ischemia include those labeled as *angina pectoris, prolonged chest discomfort due to myocardial ischemia, palpitation, acute dyspnea at rest or with effort, and exhaustion.* The first two of these, angina pectoris and prolonged chest discomfort due to myocardial ischemia, deserve considerable emphasis since they are considered to be the most specific symptoms produced by atherosclerotic coronary heart disease. Chest pain, however, occurs in patients with other types of heart disease and in patients without heart disease. Accordingly, considerable diagnostic skill is needed to diagnose the etiology of chest pain. Episodes of dyspnea at rest or with effort, and exhaustion at rest or with effort, and cardiac arrhythmias have many causes but may be caused by atherosclerotic coronary heart disease. When these symptoms are due to coronary disease, they are called *angina equivalents* (see discussion later in this chapter).

It seems appropriate to present a generic discussion of the characteristics of angina pectoris and prolonged chest discomfort due to myocardial ischemia at this point and to define the characteristics of the subsets later in this chapter.

Angina pectoris, or "strangling in the chest,"[1] is identified by analyzing the symptoms related by the patient. Heberden's description of angina is the historical benchmark, and Proudfit has emphasized the variations on Heberden's theme.[68]

The recognition of angina pectoris requires that the physician establish the quality of the chest discomfort; the location of the discomfort; the duration of the discomfort; the size of the area of discomfort; what provokes the discomfort; what relieves the discomfort; and the actions taken by the patient during the episode. It is also necessary to seek out every detail of angina pectoris in order to classify the patient into the proper clinical subset (see Table 45-1 and discussion later in this chapter).

- It is always necessary to ascertain the *quality or characteristics* of the discomfort. Accordingly, the physician should not merely inquire about pain, since pain is often denied by the patient. The physician must ask about strangling, constriction, tightness, aching, squeezing, pressure, heaviness, expanding sensation, choking in the throat, indigestion, or burning. One patient referred to the chest discomfort as a "shoebox in the chest," while another patient stated it was like "pulling a pea on a string through a needle hole." Another patient referred to his discomfort as "only a faint, fuzzy, funny feeling—a softly spoken sternal word." The patient further advised us to pay attention to "any sternal feeling not normally there." Episodes of shortness of breath occurring at rest or produced by effort may be the complaint (see further discussion below). In the past this complaint was thought to be due to the patient's difficulty in describing sensations to the physician. We now know that transient myocardial ischemia may produce transient heart failure. Accordingly, some patients without angina pectoris may experience episodes of dyspnea at rest or with effort due to an acute decrease in left ventricular compliance secondary to myocardial ischemia. Dyspnea of this sort, when due to atherosclerotic heart disease, is called an *angina equivalent.* Exhaustion and palpitation at times may also be angina equivalents (see discussion later in this chapter).

  A patient may be unable to describe his or her condition in terms the physician can recognize. For example, the patient may say, "It bothers me here," while pointing to the anterior portion of the chest. It is necessary to allow the patient to use his or her own words to describe the feeling. The terms patients use are determined by their schooling, culture, occupation, and perceptiveness. The patient will often place the blame for the discomfort on the gastrointestinal tract. On the other hand, discomfort that is not due to heart disease may often be blamed on the heart.
- The *location of discomfort* due to myocardial ischemia, in the overwhelming majority of patients, is the retrosternal region. Although the term *angina pectoris* refers to sensations in the chest (pectoris), it is now used to include sensations that are located in the upper part of the body and upper extremities. Thus, the discomfort may be confined to the chest, or there may be associated aching in one or both arms, more often the left. Pain due to myocardial ischemia may be located in the mandible, maxilla, or teeth. Pain or a burning sensation in the tongue or hard palate, induced by effort or emotional tension and relieved by rest or nitroglycerin, may be angina pectoris. Pain in the front or back of the neck may trip the unwary. Aching in the left interscapular region may occur. The distress may rarely be noted in the right side of the chest or axillary region. Aching confined to the shoulder, wrist, elbow, or forearm may be due to myocardial ischemia.

  In the natural history of coronary atherosclerotic heart disease, the location of angina pectoris may occasionally change.
- It is helpful to have the patient localize the *site of distress* by circumscribing the area with his or her finger. As a result of this action the *size* of the area of discomfort can be accurately determined. The size of the area of discomfort is usually about the size of the fist. In fact, patients will often attempt to communicate the feeling they have by "making a fist" and holding it in front of the midsternal area. (This sign is attributed to Sam Levine.) Myocardial ischemia is seldom the cause of discomfort that is no larger than a fingertip.
- The *duration* of the pain or discomfort must be carefully determined. Angina pectoris lasts only a short time, usually 1 to 5 min if the precipitating factor is relieved. When it is precipitated by emotional stress, it may last 5 to 15 min. Discomfort that lasts no longer than the time it takes for one to snap one's fingers is not due to myocardial ischemia and should not be called angina pectoris. Discomfort that persists continuously for days at a time is not due to myocardial ischemia. Discomfort that lasts longer than 15 to 20 min may be due to myocardial ischemia. When it is due to myocardial ischemia, it should not be labeled as angina pectoris. It should be labeled *prolonged myocardial ischemia* (see discussion later in this chapter).

- The attacks of angina pectoris are commonly *provoked by effort or emotional distress* but may occur at rest, after eating, with exposure to cold weather, and with smoking.

When attacks are *provoked by effort,* the discomfort occurs during, rather than after, the exertion. A frequent story is that the discomfort first occurred while the patient was hurrying to catch a plane or bus or while he or she was carrying a bag to the plane. Parking a car in a tight place, driving in heavy traffic, eating, shaving, bathing, painful stimuli, sexual intercourse, micturition, or straining at stool may produce the discomfort. There is a small group of patients who develop symptoms during effort whose distress disappears while activity is continued. This condition is called "second wind" angina pectoris. Work utilizing the arms above shoulder level may precipitate angina pectoris in patients in whom walking produces no discomfort. One or more episodes of angina pectoris may occur upon arising in the morning. The discomfort may occur when the patient stands. Other morning activities that precipitate angina including shaving, stooping over, drying oneself with a towel, etc. This "early morning syndrome" may surprise the patient and the physician, since the patient may be able to engage in more strenuous effort during the remainder of the day and have no symptoms. In a rare patient, talking or singing may induce angina pectoris, whereas physical effort may not. Angina pectoris may be precipitated when the patient lies down. When this occurs, the gastrointestinal system is often blamed for the discomfort. Occasionally, eating or the postprandial state may induce angina pectoris. Exertion following meals is particularly likely to produce discomfort, and the sedentary individual may experience discomfort only after meals.

Of great importance is the intimate relation of *emotional tension* and angina pectoris.[11] Disturbing thoughts, stressful life situations, worry, anger, hurry, excitement, and nightmares commonly precipitate angina pectoris. The tragic story of John Hunter, "the thunderbolt of surgery," makes the point. Hunter had said that his life was "in the hands of any rascal who chose to annoy and tease" him.[11] Everard Home, who was John Hunter's brother-in-law, described Hunter's angina in unforgettable terms of 1796.[11]

Exposure to cold weather, cold wind (especially on the face), cold bed sheets, or cold drinks may precipitate angina pectoris. The patient may walk less far in cold weather before angina pectoris occurs than he or she can walk in warm weather. Snowstorms precipitate angina pectoris in climes where such occur. Shoveling snow, which combines effort and exposure to cold, commonly provokes angina.

Smoking tobacco may precipitate angina pectoris in some patients. This occurs because nicotine stimulates the release of adrenaline, which increases the work of the heart. Smoking also precipitates coronary artery spasm.[69] The relationship of smoking tobacco to coronary spasm is discussed in Chap. 46.

Angina pectoris may *occur at rest,* and no precipitating cause may be identified. When this occurs, however, it is proper to consider that the ischemia has been precipitated by an alteration of the supply end of the supply-demand myocardial perfusion system. The patient may be awakened at night with angina pectoris, which is occasionally precipitated by a *nightmare.*

- The factors responsible for the *relief of angina pectoris,* must be identified. Angina pectoris that is provoked by effort usually subsides in 1 to 5 min if the patient discontinues the effort. Angina pectoris provoked by emotional tension sometimes lasts longer than angina pectoris provoked by effort because one cannot control emotions as easily as one can control physical activity.

Nitroglycerin usually produces prompt, dramatic relief of angina pectoris within 1 to 2 min. The patient is able to walk farther after using nitroglycerin in a prophylactic manner. A physician may be misled if he or she accepts too easily that the discomfort under discussion is truly relieved by nitroglycerin. The pain could be noncoronary in origin and might last for only 2 min even if nitroglycerin were not used. Occasionally angina pectoris due to idiopathic hypertrophic subaortic stenosis is made worse by the use of nitroglycerin. It is important to remember that esophageal spasm may be relieved by nitroglycerin.

Carotid sinus massage applied during an attack of angina pectoris may give prompt relief of the discomfort if the heart rate is slowed. *We do not recommend this test* because of the neurological complications that may occasionally result from carotid sinus pressure.

The *Valsalva maneuver* may slow the heart rate and relieve angina pectoris. Some patients learn to use the maneuver with considerable success.* This maneuver slows the heart rate.

- *The action taken by a patient* during an episode is always interesting and may have some diagnostic value. Some patients with angina pectoris produced by effort will merely slow their pace in order to achieve relief, while others will stop and act nonchalantly as if they are observing a building or will stop to talk with those who are walking with them. The patient who has angina pectoris in the recumbent position may sit up in order to obtain relief. Patients with prolonged episodes of myocardial ischemia often walk the floor "searching" for relief.

The preceding discussion deals with the characteristics of chest discomfort due to myocardial ischemia. Several points must be made regarding the discussion.

*Taught to J.W.H. by William Dock, M.D.

- Whereas coronary atherosclerosis is the most common cause of myocardial ischemia, it is not the only cause. For example, coronary spasm without atherosclerosis may cause myocardial ischemia (see Chap. 46). There are several noncoronary causes of myocardial ischemia such as valve disease (see Chaps. 37 and 38) and cardiomyopathy (see Chap. 58).
- A generic discussion of the characteristics of myocardial ischemia has been offered at this point. The specific definition of the subsets of angina and prolonged myocardial ischemia will be given later in this chapter (see discussion later in this chapter).
- Angina equivalents (cardiac arrhythmias, dyspnea, and exhaustion) due to myocardial ischemia will be defined and discussed later in this chapter (see discussion later in this chapter).
- Other historical data may be useful. An effort should be made to determine the illnesses and cause of death of the patient's parents and siblings; obtain the records of former visits to physicians or hospitals; ascertain the habits and life-style of the patient; identify drug intolerance; and perceive therapeutic wishes and aversions to certain forms of therapy. It is very helpful to talk with the spouse or close relative about the patient's chest discomfort since many patients minimize their complaints when they discuss them with their physician.

Limitations of the History The limitations of the history as a diagnostic method must be highlighted. For centuries, the history has been considered to be the best arrow in the physician's diagnostic quiver and even to hint that it did not reveal everything bordered on heresy. We must point out, however, that Heberden described angina pectoris before coronary atherosclerosis had been discovered.[1] There was only one autopsy in his series of patients and it showed "normal arteries." The fact is, we do not know what diseases Heberden's patients had. It is likely that most of his patients had coronary disease. It is also likely that all of them did not. Accordingly, it is improper to consider "angina" as pathognomonic of coronary disease. It follows, too, that it is improper to refer to angina as "classic" or "atypical" of a specific disease process.

The history does not always reveal all of the answers. To begin with it is important to realize that patients can have objective signs of myocardial ischemia and even infarction without having symptoms. Cohn has labeled these patients as having a "defective warning system."[70] Many others have presented data supporting the concept that myocardial ischemia may occur without the patient being aware of it.[71–76] Kannel and Abbott have recently reported on 708 myocardial infarctions among 5127 participants in the Framingham study. Of the 708 infarcts 25 percent were discovered in the routine biennial ECGs recorded on the subjects. About one-half of the subjects identified as having infarction by the ECG had no symptoms of infarction, and the remaining patients had atypical symptoms. They concluded that infarction was often not recognized.[77] Then, too, we physicians are not equally skilled at history taking though all of us undoubtedly view ourselves as good historians. The way a question is asked may lead the patient to answer incorrectly, or we may fail to listen when the "clues" are pouring out from the patient. Some patients with angina during effort may walk more slowly and have fewer symptoms. Some patients may deny symptoms of angina pectoris. Denying symptoms because of some deep-seated emotional reason is vastly different from withholding information. Many patients who withhold information about symptoms believe it is to their advantage to deny the existence of symptoms. For example, the employees of some professions lose their positions if they have symptoms of angina pectoris. On the other hand, some patients may exaggerate their symptoms for self-gain in order to receive disability insurance or to win psychological battles at home. Other patients, depending upon their cultural background and emotional maturity, deny symptoms because they are simply more stoic than others. Some patients deny symptoms because they cannot cope with the consequences of recognizing the presence of a serious condition. The individual who has this type of denial should not be viewed in the same manner as the patient who withholds information for personal gain.

Everyone is aware of false-positive and false-negative laboratory tests, but few physicians appreciate false-positive and false-negative histories. For example, an asymptomatic 40-year-old female may be found to have a positive exercise ECG. The physician will then return to the patient, as one should, to "go over the history" again. The physician may emerge with a history of angina pectoris. Was the first history a false-negative history, or was the second history a false-positive history?

Symptoms depend upon: the presence of a disease process, the sensitivity of the patient's nervous system, the patient's intellectual capacity, and the patient's psychological makeup. The physician's ability to elicit and interpret the symptoms depends upon his or her skill and perception. It is a wonder that we do as well as we do with the analysis of symptoms. The recent Coronary Artery Surgery Study (CASS) reports revealed that 28.3 percent of 16,626 patients who had coronary arteriography for suspected coronary disease had normal or minimally diseased coronary arteries.[78,79]

This concept must be understood, or else diagnostic errors will be made. Accordingly, other data supporting this concept are presented here: Unfortunately, diagnostic errors may be made when the history-taking ability is excellent and a "clear-sounding" story is related by the patient. For example, when a middle-aged man gives a history of anterior chest discomfort produced by effort and relieved by rest, it is wise to think of angina pectoris. But the diagnostic error rate with this type of history is 6 to 10 percent.[80,81] When the story is difficult to obtain and the physician is less certain of all the attributes of the symptoms, the diagnostic error rate may be as high as 20 to 30 percent. When the anterior chest pain is prolonged and occurs intermittently at rest over a period of weeks, the physician's ability to analyze the symptoms correctly is alarmingly poor. The diagnostic error rate in this situation is 11 to 13 percent.[80,81] If the prolonged pain *is* due to myocardial ischemia, it is quite serious, but there is a greater chance that it is not due to myocardial ischemia than when substernal pain is produced by effort. The recognition of angina pectoris in women is more difficult than it is in men. The diagnostic error rate is 48 to 57 percent.[80,81] The predictive value of all angina subsets in males is 82 to 87 percent, and the predictive value of all angina subsets in females is 42 to 70 percent.[80,81] The point is, different types of chest pain have different predictive values. *It follows that physicians must know the predictive value of the history they obtain from each patient.* This perception, along with other data, assists the physician in establishing the pretest likelihood of coronary disease.

Now that we can correlate chest pain with the results of coronary arteriography, we are all learning a great deal. We now see patients, whom we would have labeled as having atherosclerotic coronary heart disease a few years ago, who have normal coronary arteriograms. We also see patients whose chest pain is not diagnostic of angina pectoris but is sufficiently worrisome to justify a coronary arteriogram. We are no longer surprised to find obstructive coronary disease delineated by coronary arteriography in some of these patients. Coronary arteriography and left ventriculography yield diagnostic and prognostic test results with the highest predictive value, but exercise electrocardiography and radionuclide studies may, at times, be used to avoid coronary arteriography. When the history has been completed, it is proper to ask if an exercise ECG, radionuclide study, or coronary arteriogram should be performed in the individual patient whose chest pain is being investigated.

The Physical Examination (see Chaps. 8 through 13)

Most patients with coronary atherosclerosis exhibit no abnormal physical abnormalities. Atherosclerotic coronary heart disease *may* be associated with abnormal physical signs, but few, if any, of the signs are pathognomonic for coronary disease.

One should search for the clues that indicate a noncoronary artery cause of myocardial ischemia. Aortic stenosis, aortic regurgitation, mitral stenosis, cardiomyopathy, idiopathic hypertrophic subaortic stenosis, and mitral valve click-murmur syndrome (Barlow's syndrome) can cause angina pectoris. These conditions can usually be identified by performing a careful physical examination on the heart.

Hypertension, xanthoma, and xanthelasma are well-known risk factors that stimulate one to consider coronary atherosclerosis, but they are not pathognomonic of obstructive coronary disease.

A patient with a carotid artery bruit,[82,83] atherosclerotic aortic aneurysm,[84] or atherosclerotic peripheral artery disease[85] is more likely to have atherosclerotic coronary heart disease than is a patient without such conditions. Therefore, any patient with a carotid bruit or other atherosclerotic conditions should be carefully examined for atherosclerotic coronary artery disease.

One may appreciate abnormal precordial movements, gallop sounds, new murmurs, a pericardial rub, abnormal neck veins, rales in the lungs, etc., since they may accompany certain complications of atherosclerotic coronary heart disease. A new systolic murmur at the apex may be due to papillary muscle rupture or dysfunction secondary to myocardial infarction. A new systolic murmur near the midsternal area or medial to the apex may be due to rupture of the septum secondary to infarction. A pericardial rub may be due to myocardial infarction or the postinfarction syndrome of Dressler. A systolic murmur due to an obstructed coronary artery may be heard on rare occasions. One should study the precordial movements and auscultate the heart when the patient has an episode of chest pain, since gallop sounds and an apical systolic murmur may be heard during the episode but not between episodes.

Limitations The limitations of the physical examination as a method of recognizing atherosclerotic coronary heart disease must be emphasized. The patient with angina pectoris due to atherosclerotic coronary heart disease often, in fact, usually, exhibits *no* abnormalities on physical examination. Even the patient with prolonged myocardial ischemia and infarction may have a normal physical examination. Gallop sounds are not specific for atherosclerotic coronary heart disease, and abnormal precordial pulsations, which are not present in most patients, may be due to cardiomyopathy rather than to infarction caused by atherosclerotic coronary heart disease.

The patient with heart failure secondary to myocardial infarction may not display physical abnormalities, and the pulmonary congestion may be detected only on the chest roentgenogram.

Abnormal physical findings may not be interpreted properly. For example, a newly developed systolic murmur at the apex may be thought to be due to a ruptured papillary muscle due to myocardial infarction, whereas it may actually be due to rupture of one of the mitral valve chordae tendineae secondary to myxomatous degeneration of the chordae. The patient with prolonged chest pain suggesting myocardial ischemia who exhibits a loud systolic murmur near the center of the sternum may be misdiagnosed as having myocardial infarction and septal rupture when, in reality, the diagnosis is hypertrophic cardiomyopathy.

The Chest Roentgenogram and Cardiac Fluoroscopy (see Chaps. 15 and 107)

The roentgenogram of the chest may reveal several important abnormalities that may be directly or indirectly related to atherosclerotic coronary heart disease and its complications. The heart size as determined by x-ray of the chest is usually normal in patients who have one of the varieties of angina pectoris due to coronary atherosclerosis. The heart size is usually normal in patients who have prolonged chest pain and objective evidence of muscle necrosis (myocardial infarction) even when acute heart failure is evident. The chest x-ray may reveal cardiac enlargement in patients with chronic heart failure due to atherosclerotic coronary heart disease. Signs of pulmonary congestion due to left ventricular dysfunction are commonly detected on the chest x-ray in patients with fresh myocardial infarction even when other signs of heart failure are absent. A portable x-ray cannot be used to determine heart size but may be used to assess the degree of pulmonary congestion. A myocardial bulge (aneurysm) secondary to myocardial infarction may be detected on x-ray of the chest. The size of a myocardial aneurysm is usually underestimated when this technique is used as compared to left ventriculography. Calcification of a myocardial infarction may be seen on the chest x-ray, and, rarely, calcification of the coronary arteries may be detected.

Cardiac fluoroscopy may reveal pericardial fluid (poor cardiac pulsations and an epicardial fat line) or localized areas of abnormal cardiac movement that may be related to myocardial infarction.

An abnormal expansion of the left atrium due to mitral valve regurgitation secondary to papillary muscle dysfunction may be detected by cardiac fluoroscopy.

Calcification of the coronary arteries may be detected on the chest x-ray, at fluoroscopy, or by cinefluoroscopy. The latter technique offers great advantages over the other techniques in detecting coronary calcification. Coronary calcification is virtually diagnostic of coronary atherosclerosis. Chen has emphasized that patients with fluoroscopic evidence of coronary artery calcification have a high prevalence of coronary artery disease and a low survival rate (see Chap. 15). Langou et al. have reported that the combination of coronary artery calcification and a positive exercise ECG stress test has great predictive value for diagnosing coronary artery disease in asymptomatic men.[86]

Limitations The greatest limitation of the chest x-ray and cardiac fluoroscopy in diagnosing atherosclerotic coronary heart disease is that the predictive value of a normal x-ray and fluoroscopic examination in excluding coronary disease is extremely poor. Since most patients with atherosclerotic coronary heart disease have a normal chest x-ray and fluoroscopy, it follows that they are not very useful in detecting coronary artery disease prior to the development of considerable cardiac muscle damage. Even then the abnormalities can often be due to other causes.

The Resting Electrocardiogram (see Chap. 14)

Every physician knows that the information gained from the ECG made on a *resting* patient is very valuable and that a cardiac examination is incomplete without it. The value of electrocardiography is discussed in Chap. 14 and in standard textbooks on electrocardiography.

Limitations The resting ECG is often normal in patients with atherosclerotic coronary heart disease. Excluding the diagnosis of angina pectoris or myocardial infarction because of a normal electrocardiogram is as great an error as inferring a diagnosis of atherosclerotic coronary heart disease from the incorrect interpretation of nonspecific electrocardiographic abnormalities.

The ECG may reveal QRS-complex, ST-segment, or T-wave abnormalities, arrhythmias, and conduction disturbances as a result of atherosclerotic coronary heart disease, but many of these abnormalities may occur in other conditions.

Approximately 50 to 70 percent of patients with stable angina pectoris have normal resting ECGs. Abnormalities in the ECG that may be present include nonspecific ST-T wave abnormalities, changes in intraventricular conduction, and arrhythmias. Left ventricular hypertrophy is usually due to associated aortic valve disease, hypertension, or hypertrophic cardiomyopathy rather than coronary atherosclerosis alone. Downsloping ST-segment displacement of 1 mm or greater which is characteristic of myocardial ischemia may be recorded during an episode of angina pectoris in some patients. On the other hand, Haiat et al. have reported that ST-T changes may not even occur during angina pectoris.[87] When ST-segment change does occur, it is due to the mean ST vector being directed away from the subendocardium of the left ventricle. This type of ST-segment shift has a relatively high degree of specificity for coronary artery disease when it occurs during chest pain that is characteristic of angina pectoris. It is important to remember that ST-segment displacement due to myocardial ischemia can occur in a patient with coronary disease and not be associated with angina. In other words, painless ischemia is common in such patients.[71,72,74]

Episodes of prolonged chest pain due to myocardial ischemia without elevation of cardiac enzyme levels may be associated with T-wave inversion, ST-segment displacement, or no change in the ECG.[88,89] Some of the patients with this clinical syndrome will have pathological evidence of myocardial infarction. This indicates that the routine ECG does not reveal all infarcts.

The syndrome of "variant" angina pectoris (Prinzmetal's angina) differs from the usual type in that the pain may not be associated with an increase in the heart rate or systolic blood pressure, two major determinants of myocardial oxygen consumption. Coincident with the pain, ST-segment displacement occurs. The mean ST-segment vector is directed toward a region of the left ventricle and produces ST-segment elevation in the ECG.[32] When the chest pain subsides, the ST-segment changes disappear. Transient Q waves and atrioventricular (AV) block may also occur during the pain.[32] This syndrome is due to coronary artery spasm with or without associated obstructive coronary disease (Chap. 46).

The electrocardiographic diagnosis of acute myocardial infarction is beset with many problems. When new and typical QRS-complex, ST-segment, and T-wave changes are present, a definite diagnosis can be made. (For a discussion of the electrocardiographic changes that accompany myocardial infarction, the reader is referred to Chap. 14.) Unfortunately, these characteristic changes are often absent.

Zarling et al. reported their concern that myocardial infarction was not diagnosed in a surprisingly large percentage of patients. They urge physicians not to disregard a clinical diagnosis of infarction because the enzymes and ECG do not confirm its presence.[90]

A single normal ECG is worthless in ruling out acute myocardial infarction since changes may never occur or may be delayed.[91] Minor ST-segment changes or T changes may be overlooked or may not stimulate the physician to consider myocardial infarction. Abnormal Q waves may not appear if the infarction is small.[91] Infarction of certain anatomic sites of the left ventricle, notably the laterobasal zone and apex,[92] may not deform the QRS complex with characteristic Q-wave abnormalities. Movahed and Becker compared the electrocardiographic abnormalities of lateral wall infarction with the abnormalities of Tl imaging. They discovered that no patient with lateral infarction had Q waves in the leads usually considered to represent the lateral left ventricular wall (I, aV_L, and V_6).[93] If there has been a previous infarction, a new infarct that involves a diametrically opposite wall of the ventricle may cancel the effects of the first infarction and the tracing may return toward normal. Third and fourth infarcts rarely produce further deformity of the QRS complex, but ST-segment and T-wave changes may accompany the new ischemic event. Complete left bundle branch block often prevents the inscription of diagnostic Q waves.[91]

There is poor agreement regarding the criteria that should be used to diagnose subendocardial infarction. Accordingly, there is much confusion about the diagnosis of subendocardial infarction. Pruitt's classic article on this subject should be reviewed by all interested readers.[94]

Studies of serial electrocardiographic changes correlated with pathological findings indicate that the ECG affords about 80 percent accuracy in diagnosing acute myocardial infarction. The electrocardiographic detection of an old, healed myocardial infarction is even less precise. Abnormal Q waves either disappear or revert to borderline significance in 30 percent of patients by 18 months.[95] In a large autopsy series, Horan et al. found that abnormal Q waves had a sensitivity of 61 percent.[96]

The electrocardiographic signs of right ventricular infarction are often overlooked or are not present. Elevation of the ST-segment in lead V_3R suggesting right ventricular infarction has been appreciated in the past. Geft et al. have suggested that elevation of the ST segment in leads V_1 to V_5 without Q waves may also be a clue.[97] Despite these clues we undoubtedly miss small right ventricular infarcts. The insensitivity of Q waves as a marker of myocardial infarction has also been confirmed by studies in which Q waves recorded on the surface ECG were correlated with the left ventriculogram and direct epicardial electrocardiographic recordings.[98] These studies show that the surface ECG underestimates the presence of both left ventriculographic abnormalities and abnormal Q waves recorded from the epicardium.

Transient Q waves have been produced by active myocardial ischemia alone in both experimental animals and human beings. Patients with Prinzmetal's angina pectoris may exhibit transient Q waves as well as the characteristic ST-segment shift. In a few patients with preoperative electrocardiographic findings of anterior wall myocardial infarction, anterior QRS forces may appear after coronary bypass surgery. This observation raises the intriguing possibility that chronically ischemic myocardium may, on rare occasions, produce Q waves.

Recently much has been said about reciprocal changes in the ECG. The "new view" is that some information about distant ischemia can be detected by analyzing the reciprocal changes. This is probably a poor concept since the extent and location of reciprocal electrocardiographic changes are determined by the location and extent of the primary cardiac damage.[99] The reciprocal changes in the ECG are not due to new and different electrical forces. They are the same forces that are generated by the primary abnormality. They appear different simply because the leads in which they are recorded "views" them from a different vantage point.

Many disorders may alter the ECG in such a way that myocardial infarction may be mistakenly diagnosed. QRS-complex changes mimicking myocardial infarction may be produced by the Wolff-Parkinson-White syndrome, chronic lung disease, pulmonary embolism, left ventricular hypertrophy, cardiomyopathy (hypertrophic and dilated), neuromuscular disease, and complex forms of congenital heart disease. ST-segment elevation produced by acute pericarditis and rarely by hyperkalemia is occasionally mistaken for acute epicardial injury due to myocardial infarction. Deeply inverted T waves, sometimes found in patients with subarachnoid hemorrhage or other cerebral lesions, are easily confused with the electrocardiographic changes of myocardial ischemia.

The Exercise Electrocardiogram (see Chap. 98)

One must judge the normality of the heart in relation to effort. It is not surprising that the ECG may reveal abnormalities *during and after exercise* that it does not reveal when the patient is at rest.

To interpret the exercise ECG as being simply normal or abnormal is passé. The presence and severity of coronary disease are predicted more accurately by additional findings. Multivessel coronary disease or left main coronary disease is suggested by the onset of ST-segment depression within the first 3 min of exercise, the persistence of ST-segment depression 8 min after exercise, downsloping ST-segment depression of 2 mm or greater, or a low maximum heart rate–blood pressure product.

Several investigators have examined the prognostic value of exercise testing (see Chap. 98). In fact, interest has shifted from using the exercise ECG solely as a diagnostic tool to using it as a prognostic tool. Exercise testing may identify a low-risk group among patients with chronic stable coronary artery disease.[100] A negative exercise test, a maximum heart rate greater than 160 beats per minute, and a duration of exercise that exceeds stage III (protocol of Bruce) suggest a good prognosis. Patients with ischemic ST-segment changes at stage I or stage II have a much less favorable outlook.[101]

Patients with recurrent angina pectoris after myocardial infarction should have a coronary arteriogram, and if conditions are found to be favorable, should be considered for coronary bypass surgery. Patients without complications of infarction should have a submaximal exercise stress test, a radionuclide test, or a coronary arteriogram (see later discussion). Most patients who perform poorly during the stress test several weeks after myocardial infarction should have a coronary arteriogram, because their prognosis is poorer than patients who perform well on the treadmill.[103]

Finally, we wish to emphasize that an exercise ECG stress test is usually contraindicated in patients who are thought to have unstable angina pectoris or in patients who have prolonged bouts of chest discomfort when myocardial ischemia is considered to be a possible cause.

Limitations The limitations of the exercise electrocardiogram as a tool for the recognition of atherosclerotic coronary heart disease need emphasis.[104] The predictive value of any electrocardiographic change for detecting atherosclerotic coronary heart disease is determined by the prevalence of the disease in the population being studied. When the exercise ECG is used to screen an asymptomatic population, there is a high prevalence of false-positive responses. Various forms of heart disease, including valvular disease, hypertension, and myocardial disease, may influence the response of the ST-segment to exercise. Left ventricular intraventricular conduction defects, hyperventilation, Wolff-Parkinson-White syndrome, hypokalemia, anemia, and vasoregulatory asthenia are among the many conditions that may produce a false-positive exercise test. It is well known that digitalis causes abnormalities of the ST segment at rest and after exercise. Young women are particularly prone to have a false-positive response.

When middle-aged adult male patients are studied because of chest pain, a positive response in the exercise ECG has a predictive value of approximately 70 percent for detecting the presence of atherosclerotic coronary heart disease. The predictive value of the test improves with increasing severity of coronary artery disease. Less than 50 percent of patients with single-vessel coronary disease have abnormal tests, but the incidence of abnormal tests exceeds 80 percent in patients with triple-vessel disease. A positive response in the exercise ECG in young women has a predictive value of about 50 percent. The predictive value of the exercise ECG may be enhanced by the use of multiple unipolar V leads connected to a central Wilson terminal.[105]

Quyyumi et al. have recently emphasized that the ST segment/heart rate slope did not accurately predict the severity of coronary artery disease.[106]

The Long-Term Monitoring of the Electrocardiogram (see Chap. 100)

The Vectorcardiogram (see Chap. 96)

The vectorcardiogram (VCG) has been used to identify myocardial infarction. It has the advantages of simultaneously recording two perpendicular axes and affording a better resolution of the initial QRS forces.

Limitations Despite the useful features described above, the vectorcardiogram is infrequently used because of the following limitations:

- The complexity of lead systems and the lack of uniform criteria for the diagnosis of myocardial infarction cause confusion.
- As compared to the scalar ECG, the vectorcardiogram offers only a modest increase in diagnostic sensitivity and little improvement in the frequency of false-positive diagnoses of infarction.
- The diagnostic accuracy of the vectorcardiogram in identifying myocardial infarction is impaired by ventricular hypertrophy and intraventricular conduction abnormalities.
- Most importantly, the vectorcardiogram rarely provides a conclusive answer when the diagnosis of myocardial infarction is questionable, and it does not obviate the need for more definitive studies such as stress electrocardiography, radionuclide stress testing, or coronary arteriography.
- Finally, it is cumbersome to use the vectorcardio-

gram, and this plus the reasons listed, has almost eliminated it as a diagnostic tool.

Cardiac Enzymes and Other Macromolecular Markers of Myocardial Injury (by Burton E. Sobel)*

Diagnostic enzymology began with the recognition in 1908 of elevated amylase as a sign of pancreatitis.[107] Cardiac applications were delayed until the 1950s, when LaDue, Worblewski, and Karmen reported elevated serum glutamic oxaloacetic transaminase (SGOT) and lactic dehydrogenase (LDH) in plasma after myocardial infarction.[33] Creatine kinase (CK) elevations were recognized soon thereafter.[108] Determination of SGOT, LDH, and CK activity rapidly became a cornerstone of the diagnosis of acute myocardial infarction. Numerous other macromolecules including aldolase, malic dehydrogenase, isomerase, lysosomal enzymes,[109] and components of myosin[110] appear in plasma after infarction as well. With such a panoply, principles are needed for selection of markers best suited for general diagnostic purposes.[111]

Since elevation of plasma enzymes after infarction reflects release of enzyme from irreversibly injured tissue, plasma profiles reflect the cardiac enzyme complement.[33,112] Onset of elevation correlates with onset of depletion of enzyme from myocardium,[113–115] but plasma time-activity curves are influenced by the release rate of enzyme from tissue, the volume of distribution of enzyme released from tissue, lymphatic transport,[116] clearance of enzyme from the circulation,[117] modification or conversion to subforms of enzymes in plasma,[118] and the presence or absence of reperfusion.[119] Thus, peak plasma activity may not correlate closely with infarct size.

Because most enzymes are present in tissues besides the heart, specificity for cardiac injury is far from complete. Sensitivity, however, is excellent because of the sensitivity of available assays and the rich endowment of myocardium with enzymes. Thus, necrosis of even milligram quantities of myocardium can be detected.

Plasma enzyme determinations must be interpreted in the context of factors that may modify catalytic activity, the amount of enzyme protein in the circulation, the nature of the assay employed, the dependence of "normal values" on age, gender,[120] and physical activity,[121,122] and the log-normal distribution of values typical of some enzymes.[111] *Unfortunately, clinical habit frequently results in the needless ordering of assays of multiple enzymes.* Relative sensitivities are not sufficiently different to justify this practice. The most specific and conventionally measured plasma enzyme indicative of myocardial infarction is the so-called myocardial (MB) isoenzyme of CK (see below).

In a typical patient with acute myocardial infarction, SGOT activity becomes elevated within 6 to 12 h after the onset of symptoms, peaks at 2- to 10-fold above normal within 18 to 36 h, and returns to normal within 3 to 4 days.[111] Even when the source of enzyme is the heart, elevations are not specific for infarction. They occur with myocarditis, cardiac trauma, and electrical conversion.[123,124] SGOT is less organ-specific than CK in part because the liver is so well endowed with the enzyme. Elevations are therefore common with congestive heart failure.[125]

In a typical patient with myocardial infarction plasma LDH activity increases relatively late, generally exceeding the normal range within 24 to 48 h, peaks 2- to 10-fold above normal within 3 to 6 days, and returns to normal within 8 to 14 days.[111] The delayed elevation reflects the origin of much of the LDH, released from erythrocytes and cellular elements involved in the local, cardiac inflammatory response to infarction, rather than from myocardium alone. Overall LDH appearing in plasma exceeds by far that present in myocardium undergoing necrosis. Like SGOT, LDH is a relatively nonspecific marker of myocardial injury.[126] Plasma elevations occur in 30 percent of patients with congestive heart failure, and although isoenzyme profiles may permit differentiation of hepatic from cardiac sources under these conditions,[127] nonspecificity is considerable.

In a typical patient with infarction plasma CK exceeds normal within 4 to 6 h, peaks at 2- to 10-fold above normal within 24 h, and declines to normal within 3 to 4 days after the onset of symptoms.[111] As with all macromolecular markers, organ specificity is not complete. In addition to the heart, skeletal and vascular smooth muscle and brain are richly endowed with CK. Specificity is better than that for SGOT and LDH, but plasma CK increases in patients with processes affecting skeletal muscle, including alcoholic intoxication and trauma,[128] and with pulmonary embolism.[129] Because of comparable sensitivity but better specificity, plasma CK determinations are generally replacing alternative, conventional enzyme determinations for the diagnosis of myocardial infarction.

Diagnostic specificity is enhanced with the use of isoenzymes. Isoenzymes are physically distinguishable molecular species which catalyze the same chemical reaction. Total plasma LDH activity generally reflects contributions from five individual LDH isoenzymes,[127] each composed of four subunits of either H (named for heart) or M (muscle) type.[127] LDH_1, composed of four H subunits, migrates most rapidly in conventional electrophoretic assay systems; LDH_5, with four M subunits, migrates most slowly; and isoenzymes with intermediate subunit combinations (LDH_2, LDH_3, and LDH_4) migrate at intermediate rates. Heart muscle contains predominantly LDH_1, but different proportions of the five isoenzymes are

*Dr. Burton E. Sobel, Professor of Medicine, Director of the Cardiovascular Division of the Department of Medicine, Washington University School of Medicine and Cardiologist-in-Chief at Barnes Hospital in St. Louis, Missouri, has kindly written this section.

found in many tissues. Thus, LDH_1 predominates in plasma after myocardial injury and LDH_5 after hepatic injury.

Isoenzymes of CK are dimers composed of M (muscle) or B (brain) subunits. The MM dimer predominates in skeletal muscle (MM) and the BB dimer in brain (BB).[130–137] Human myocardial CK includes approximately 14 percent as the MB isoenzyme, a species represented only minimally in human tissues other than the heart.[138] Thus, with rare exceptions, marked elevation of plasma MB-CK reflects irreversible myocardial injury. Release of CK from the heart is tantamount to cell death. It is not seen with ischemia insufficient to produce infarction.[139]

All "cardiac enzymes" may increase in plasma after cardiac surgery, electrical cardioversion, cardiac trauma, or pericarditis, presumably because of the concomitant epicardial inflammation. Although plasma MB-CK does not increase after cerebral vascular accidents, intramuscular injections, or gastrointestinal tract surgery, it may increase with massive injury to skeletal muscle.

In the setting of ischemic injury, myocardial CK depletion *correlates with infarct size estimated morphometrically* and with radiolabeled microspheres.[113,140–143] Although enzymes can be released from viable cells under some conditions unrelated to ischemia (such as perfusion of isolated hearts with calcium-free media), extensive clinical and experimental observations indicate that release from myocardium subjected to ischemia occurs only when irreversible injury has been induced. Plasma CK time-activity curves reflect myocardial CK depletion.[115,141–147] Infarct size can be estimated by analysis of these curves with consideration of enzyme clearance rates, the release/local degradation ratio, enzyme distribution volume, and enzyme concentration in myocardium. Estimates based on serial changes in plasma MB rather than total CK are more specific.[147–149] Enzymatic estimates of infarct size are paralleled by the severity of ventricular arrhythmia early and late after acute myocardial infarction, impaired ventricular performance, dyskinesis delineated by ventriculography, limited recovery of exercise tolerance, morphologically defined necrosis, and mortality rate.[133,138,140–143,145–156]

When evolution of infarction is modified by coronary thrombolysis or coronary artery bypass grafting, enzyme release rates from the heart may be altered.[119,157] Interpretation of plasma time-activity curves may therefore require modification with respect to these and other factors such as drugs that can influence the clearance or the distribution volume of enzyme. Despite these provisos, however, such curves provide information useful for assessing prognosis and planning management.

The timing of the onset of infarction can be based on the analysis of isoforms of individual isoenzymes of CK. Moieties derived from the same isoenzymes but exhibiting slightly different isoelectric points (isoforms) are formed from circulating CK isoenzymes released from the heart.[118,158] Since the time course of conversion is predictable when nondenaturing, quantitative methods are used;[158] the chronology of infarction can be delineated by determining fractional contributions of each isoform to overall CK isoenzyme activity in a small sample. This approach facilitates prospective selection of patients suitable for coronary thrombolysis and retrospective delineation of the duration of infarction in studies designed to evaluate potentially therapeutic interventions such as thrombolysis, percutaneous transluminal coronary angioplasty (PTCA), or laser-catheter angioplasty.

There are other macromolecular markers of myocardial injury. Elevation of plasma enzyme activity is a cornerstone of the diagnosis of myocardial infarction because of the simplicity, precision, and accuracy of assays, their low cost, and the extensive experience available facilitating their interpretation. Although other moieties such as myoglobin or myosin light chains exhibit attributes for clinical research, they do not presently offer distinct clinical advantages for the early diagnosis of initial or recurrent myocardial infarction.

Limitations Despite their intrinsic value, results of assays of plasma enzymes require intelligent interpretation by the physician. Apparent lack of elevation may occur despite definite myocardial infarction if the infarct is modest, the peak small, or the frequency of sampling insufficient. Elevations may be unrecognized because absolute values remain within the "normal" range—defined in terms of a presumed statistical distribution in the population. Enzymes such as CK in fact exhibit a log-normal distribution. Errors in interpretation can be avoided by serial sampling, which may reveal increases of several fold even though absolute activity does not become markedly high. False-positive elevations with respect to infarction can occur when tissues other than the heart liberate enzyme, particularly skeletal muscle, liver, or brain. They may result also from artifacts affecting assays. Hemolysis, liberating moieties such as ATP into the plasma sample, or drugs circulating in plasma that affect assay systems are two potential causes.

Interpretation of true-positive elevations may not be straightforward. Comparable elevations in a patient with initial compared with repeat infarction may have different biological significance. Obviously, the overall impairment of cardiac function and increased risk of death are greater with repeat infarction despite comparable tissue injury and hence comparable elevation of plasma enzymes.

Peak enzyme activity is of course related to the rate of release of enzyme from injured myocardium, the distribution volume into which the enzyme is released, and the rate of clearance, among other factors. Thus, no simple relation exists between peak activity and overall myocardial injury.

Clinicians often cogitate unnecessarily about patients with severe, prolonged chest pain without frank enzymatic criteria of infarction. It is probably true that the lack of detection of enzyme elevations despite frequent serial sampling of plasma excludes completed infarction. *However, the biological implications of severe coronary insufficiency may be as great or greater in patients with crescendo angina pectoris compared with those sustaining infarcts of minute or modest magnitude.* The issue is not simply whether the patient has had an infarct. Rather it is whether or not the patient is at risk because of the coronary insufficiency giving rise to the pain regardless of the presence or absence of concomitant elevation of plasma enzymes.

Radionuclide Imaging (by George Beller)*

With increasing experience with exercise stress testing for coronary artery disease (CAD) detection, concern has arisen regarding the sensitivity of the stress ECG for identifying patients with CAD among those whose initial complaint was chest pain. The predictive value of a negative stress ECG (the percentage of patients without coronary artery disease among all patients having a negative test result) is in the range of only 60 percent.[159] This is because the sensitivity of an ischemic electrocardiographic response (> 1.0 mm of horizontal or downsloping ST depression) ranges from 47 to 81 percent among predominantly symptomatic patients referred for chest pain evaluation.[159] This rather high prevalence of false-negative results yields a poor predictive value of a negative response.

The goals of exercise radionuclide imaging are to (1) enhance the sensitivity, specificity, and predictive value of CAD detection; (2) noninvasively assess the extent and severity of functionally significant CAD; (3) determine prognosis in order that specific therapeutic strategies can be more rationally implemented, such as improved selection of patients needing coronary artery bypass surgery or identification of low-risk patients who do not require further invasive evaluation or surgical intervention; (4) evaluate the response to therapeutic interventions aimed at enhancing coronary blood flow such as bypass surgery, percutaneous transluminal angioplasty, and thrombolytic therapy.

Two major radionuclide techniques have emerged as approaches to evaluating patients with suspected or known CAD during exercise testing. These are myocardial perfusion imaging with *thallium* (^{201}Tl) and *radionuclide angiography* performed after the administration of technetium (^{99m}Tc).

^{201}Tl The initial myocardial uptake of ^{201}Tl immediately after intravenous administration of the radionuclide is the result of both blood flow delivery to the heart and the extraction of ^{201}Tl by the myocardium.[160] ^{201}Tl does not remain fixed in myocardial cells after the initial extraction phase. After intravenous injection, there is a continuous exchange of myocardial ^{201}Tl recirculating from the systemic blood pool. After initial distribution, ^{201}Tl that washes out of the myocardium is replaced by recirculating ^{201}Tl originating from extracardiac compartments. This process of continuous exchange explains the phenomenon of "redistribution" which is observed after transient hypoperfusion such as occurs with exercise stress.[161] Redistribution implies that total or partial resolution of defects imaged 5 to 20 min after ^{201}Tl administration has occurred. Exercise ^{201}Tl scintigraphy is performed in the following manner: A dose of 1.5 to 2.0 mCi of ^{201}Tl is administered at symptom-limited endpoints during treadmill or bicycle exercise stress testing. Postexercise images are obtained at 10 min, 1 h and 2½ h later and are obtained in the anterior, 45° and 70° left anterior oblique projections. Areas of diminished ^{201}Tl activity on the early postexercise images are abnormal and represent areas of stress-induced ischemia or myocardial scar. To differentiate between these abnormal findings, delayed images are obtained in order to determine if the initial postexercise defect persists or demonstrates redistribution. Areas of previous infarction or scar usually appear as persistent defects over time, whereas areas of exercise-induced ischemia show the redistribution pattern.

The *value of exercise ^{201}Tl* scintigraphy is summarized in Table 45-2. ^{201}Tl scintigraphy is valuable as an adjunct to exercise electrocardiographic testing for detecting CAD in patients presenting with chest pain. The overall sensitivity and specificity of qual-

TABLE 45-2 Value of Exercise ^{201}Tl Scintigraphy

- Detecting coronary artery disease (CAD) in patients presenting with chest pain
- Predicting the extent of CAD by identifying defects in two or more vascular regions
- Differentiating between true- and false-positive abnormal ST-segment responses to exercise
- Evaluating chest pain in patients with resting ECG abnormalities
- Assessing physiological significance of known CAD (e.g., Does a given "50 percent stenosis" produce hypoperfusion?)
- Distinguishing ischemic from infarcted myocardium (redistribution versus persistent defects)
- Assessing prognosis in patients with stable angina and in patients with uncomplicated myocardial infarction
- Evaluating efficacy of therapeutic interventions aimed at enhancing myocardial blood flow (e.g., coronary bypass surgery, percutaneous transluminal coronary angioplasty, thrombolytic therapy)

*Dr. George Beller, Head, Division of Cardiology and Professor of Medicine, University of Virginia School of Medicine, Charlottesville, Virginia, has kindly written this section.

itative ^{201}Tl exercise scintigraphy for CAD detection are reported to be in the range of 85 percent and 90 percent, respectively.[162] Sensitivity and specificity values are reported to be in the 90 percent and above range when images are analyzed quantitatively utilizing computer-assisted techniques.[163]

^{201}Tl scintigraphy is of particular value in evaluating patients with chest pain who fail to reach 85 percent of maximum predicted heart rate on a symptom-limited stress test and who have a normal ST-segment response.[164] Such a test is considered to be nondiagnostic. It has been shown that patients with underlying CAD whose stress ECGs are nondiagnostic have a greater than 80 percent prevalence of an abnormal ^{201}Tl scintigram. Myocardial ^{201}Tl imaging is also useful in the evaluation of patients with abnormal resting ECGs in which ST-segment changes during exercise are uninterpretable.[165] Such patients may have complete left or right bundle branch block, left ventricular hypertrophy and strain, digitalis effect, conduction abnormalities, or Wolff-Parkinson-White syndrome. ^{201}Tl scintigraphy may also be valuable in distinguishing between true- and false-positive ST-segment responses to exercise stress in patients with a low pretest likelihood of coronary artery disease.[166] On the basis of age, absence of symptoms, and a normal resting ECG, these patients should be considered to have a low likelihood of significant underlying CAD prior to testing. The demonstration of a normal perfusion scan would lend strong support to the inference that the observed exercise-induced ST-segment depression did not indicate ischemia. On the other hand, if both the exercise ECG and ^{201}Tl scintigram were abnormal, then the diagnosis of underlying CAD would be more probable.

Exercise ^{201}Tl scintigraphy may aid in identifying patients with high-risk coronary artery anatomy. Patients with underlying two- and three-vessel disease by angiography have a 50 percent or more prevalence of multiple defects in the distribution of two or more major coronary arteries on scintigraphy.[167] Approximately two-thirds of patients with left main coronary artery stenosis will demonstrate multiple ^{201}Tl defects in the distribution of both anterior and posterior myocardial walls.[167] Recent evidence suggests that patients with multiple perfusion abnormalities, particularly of the redistribution type, have a worse prognosis than patients with comparable coronary angiographic findings who only exhibit a single defect in the distribution of the risk area of only one coronary vessel.[168]

^{201}Tl exercise scintigraphy performed prior to hospital discharge may provide important prognostic information in patients with a recent myocardial infarction. Figure 45-2 shows the exercise ^{201}Tl scintigrams performed 10 days after a nontransmural myocardial infarction in a patient with an uncomplicated hospital course. The scan demonstrates abnormal ^{201}Tl uptake and washout in two vascular regions. The majority of postinfarction patients who either die or experience a reinfarction or unstable angina during the first year after an acute myocardial infarction demonstrate exercise-induced ischemia characterized by redistribution defects elicited at a submaximal workload.[169] Also, patients who demonstrate increased lung ^{201}Tl uptake on exercise scintigraphy, indicating increased lung water, have a higher event rate than patients with normal lung ^{201}Tl distribution.

^{201}Tl scintigraphy can be employed for assessing regional myocardial perfusion and viability in patients undergoing revascularization surgery. Improved regional myocardial perfusion postoperatively is demonstrated in those patients who are successfully revascularized with patent grafts.[170] Areas perfused by occluded or stenosed grafts will often show persistent perfusion abnormalities in a postoperative scintigraphic study.

The *limitations of ^{201}Tl scintigraphy* are as follows. Several factors may adversely influence the results of ^{201}Tl imaging. Foremost, the technique requires a great attention to proper methodology. A knowledge of image artifacts is necessary in order to decrease false-positive interpretation. Overlying breast shadows, altered position of inflow and outflow tracks of the left ventricle, or greater than normal degree of apical thinning will produce local diminutions in ^{201}Tl activity which may be misinterpreted as reflecting underlying CAD.

Although ^{201}Tl scintigraphy is more sensitive than the exercise ECG at lower levels of exercise, the sensitivity of the scintigraphic technique does diminish at levels below 60 percent of maximum predicted heart rate. Patients with isolated stenoses of diagonal branches of the left anterior descending or marginal branches of the circumflex system may demonstrate normal ^{201}Tl uptake on scintigraphy. The overall sensitivity for detecting left circumflex disease is lower than that for identifying left anterior descending or right coronary obstructions. Some patients with three-vessel disease and "balanced" coronary stenoses may demonstrate uniform ^{201}Tl distribution on the immediate postexercise scintigram, which may be misread as a normal. However, if quantitative approaches to image interpretation are employed, abnormal ^{201}Tl clearance from these vascular regions will often be observed. Another limitation of ^{201}Tl scintigraphy is the inability to derive absolute measurements of myocardial blood flow in millimeters per gram of myocardium. This is because the attenuation of ^{201}Tl is inversely proportional to the depth of the activity from the camera. Also, unless tomographic imaging is undertaken, quantitation of the volume of ischemic or infarcted myocardium cannot easily be ascertained.

***Radionuclide Angiography* (^{99m}Tc)** Both first pass and equilibrium gated exercise radionuclide angiography using ^{99m}Tc are valuable in the detection of CAD in patients presenting with chest pain. In addition to measurement of left ventricular ejection

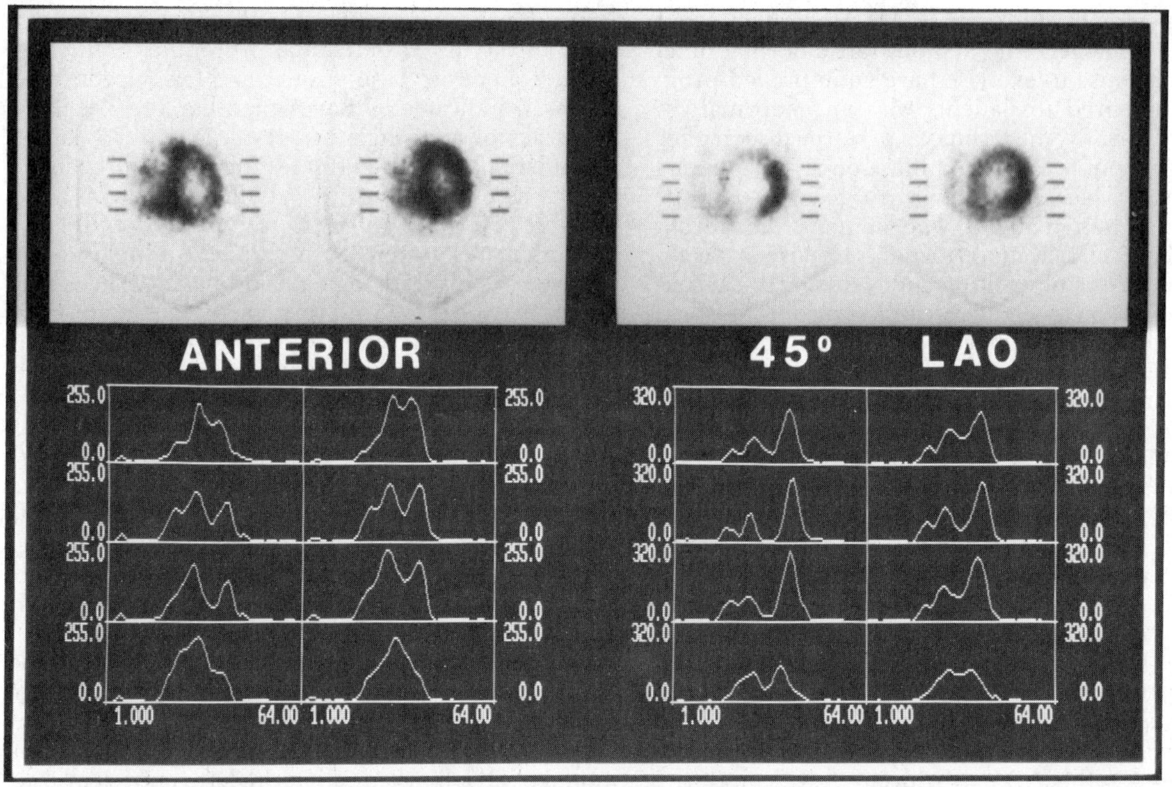

FIGURE 45-2 Submaximal exercise ^{201}Tl scintigram in a patient with a nontransmural myocardial infarction 10 days earlier. The quantitative count profiles are shown below each image and correspond to the planes indicated by the dashed lines. The initial anterior view image (*left*) demonstrates perfusion defects in the anterolateral wall and apex. The delayed images obtained at $2\frac{1}{2}$ h show Tl redistribution with normalization of the defects. There is abnormal washout from the high inferior wall as well. The postexercise 45° left anterior oblique (LAO) image (*right*) in this patient shows a marked anteroseptal defect with partial redistribution noted on the delayed image. Tl uptake in the posterolateral wall is homogeneous and shows a normal washout pattern which is confirmed by the quantitative count profiles shown below the scintigram. At cardiac catheterization, the patient had a 99 percent left anterior descending stenosis and a 90 percent right coronary narrowing. (*From R. S. Gibson, D. D. Watson, G. B. Craddock, et al., Prediction of Cardiac Events after Uncomplicated Myocardial Infarction: A Prospective Study Comparing Predischarge Exercise Thallium-201 Scintigraphy and Coronary Angiography, Circulation, 68(2):327, 1983. Reproduced with permission from the American Heart Association, Inc. and the author.*)

fraction and assessment of regional wall motion, other variables of ventricular systolic and diastolic function can be derived (Chap. 109). On the basis of studies of subjects without evidence of underlying cardiac or pulmonary disease, the normal ventricular response to exercise has been defined as an absolute increment of at least 5 percent in the left ventricular ejection fraction without the development of regional wall motion abnormalities.[171] When the end-systolic volume is shown to increase by 5 percent or more during exercise stress, this would also be considered an abnormal response.

The *value of exercise radionuclide angiography* is similar to that described for ^{201}Tl scintigraphy. The technique can be utilized for detection of CAD in patients presenting with chest pain. The sensitivity has been reported to be in the range of 85 to 90 percent,[172] but when the ejection fraction response is solely evaluated, the specificity of the technique diminishes. Failure to increase the left ventricular ejection fraction with exercise by 5 percent or more has a sensitivity of 88 percent but a somewhat lower specificity of 76 percent, as indicated from reports in the literature.[159] Patients with multivessel CAD and those with proximal left anterior descending stenoses have a more profound fall in ejection fraction in response to exercise than do patients with less high-risk anatomy.

Exercise radionuclide angiography, like ^{201}Tl scintigraphy, is useful in evaluating the results of therapy. In individual patients the efficacy of coronary artery bypass graft surgery,[173] percutaneous transluminal coronary angioplasty, and thrombolytic therapy with streptokinase can be evaluated with resting and/or exercise radionuclide angiography. Perioperative infarction in patients undergoing bypass surgery is characterized by a new resting wall motion abnormality and a fall in the resting ejection fraction. Following successful revascularization, the abnormal ejection fraction response to exercise is often reversed. After successful PTCA, the resting ejection fraction is usually unchanged, but the exercise ejection fraction increases significantly. Approximately 90 percent of patients with wall motion abnormalities during exercise prior to PTCA show improvement following the dilatation.

An important application of exercise radionuclide angiography is the determination of prognosis in patients with known CAD. Medically treated patients with CAD who demonstrate a normal functional response to exercise have an improved prognosis compared to patients with an abnormal response. Similarly, the technique performed soon after recovery from myocardial infarction at submaximal heart rates has been shown to have prognostic value.[174] Those patients who demonstrate an abnormal exercise ejection fraction response or an abnormal end-systolic volume index during a submaximal bicycle ergometer exercise test prior to hospital discharge have a higher prevalence of subsequent cardiac event than patients demonstrating a normal functional response.[174]

The limitation of radionuclide angiography with ^{99m}Tc is as follows. The response of the left ventricular ejection fraction to exercise appears to be age-dependent. Certain normal subjects over the age of 60 may not show the normal increase in ejection fraction with exercise, and in some instances it may actually diminish. Inadequate stress secondary to physical disabilities may result in normal responses despite the presence of underlying CAD. Conversely, beta-blocker therapy in normal patients may blunt the normal rise in ejection fraction during exercise.[175] Pretreatment with nitroglycerin or nitrates in patients with CAD may prevent exercise-induced ischemia and concomitant left ventricular dysfunction, yielding a false-negative result. Exercise radionuclide angiography provides less diagnostic information in women than in men. Almost one-third of women with chest pain and a normal resting ejection fraction and normal coronary arteries demonstrate a fall in ejection fraction during exercise. Patients with a very high resting ejection fraction (> 75 percent) and normal coronary arteries will be unable to further increase the ejection fraction by 5 percent or more in response to exercise. These patients have hyperdynamic resting function and cannot be expected to further decrease their end-systolic volume with exercise. The ejection fraction during exercise is a complex response influenced by many variables. Loading conditions during stress must be taken into account when interpreting the change in ejection fraction at various exercise workloads. The exercise radionuclide angiogram will also tend to be more sensitive in patients who demonstrate an ischemic ST-segment response and who have multivessel CAD.

Patients Who Benefit from Radionuclide Exercise Testing The patients who benefit from radionuclide exercise testing must be kept in mind. As previously indicated, radionuclide stress testing can be used either to detect CAD or to determine its extent and severity. Thus, one must be cognizant of the purpose of performing the test. Is it to diagnose the cause of chest pain, to evaluate functional status, or to identify high-risk patients and determine prognosis? When selecting either of these radionuclide tests (^{201}Tl scintigraphy or radionuclide angiography with ^{99m}Tc) for detecting CAD, it is vitally important to remember that the likelihood of disease in the tested individual profoundly influences the frequency of false-positive and false-negative results. As indicated by Bayes' theorem, the predictive accuracy of any single test result is poor in patient populations at both extremes for pretest probability of disease. In patients with an intermediate or a low pretest probability of CAD, the most cost-effective means of assessment is to employ multiple noninvasive tests for deriving CAD probability. These patients may be those with certain risk factors for CAD but who have atypical chest pain or asymptomatic ST-segment depression during exercise. Another example might be a patient who had a negative ST response to exercise but was not able to achieve 85 percent or more of maximum predicted heart rate with exercise. The level of exercise may have been too low to produce ischemic ST depression on the exercise ECG. In patients with a high pretest likelihood of disease, such as middle-aged men with typical angina and a positive ST-segment response during exercise, radionuclide testing would not be used solely for further enhancing the posttest likelihood of CAD, but to estimate prognosis. Patients with high-risk CAD are those who demonstrate during exercise (1) multiple ^{201}Tl defects with or without lung uptake, (2) a marked fall in the left ventricular ejection fraction, (3) multiple wall motion abnormalities, and (4) more than 2 mm of ischemic ST depression at a low workload.

Summary The development of exercise nuclear cardiology techniques for evaluating patients suspected of or diagnosed as having CAD has enhanced the clinical value of noninvasive exercise testing. Tests should be ordered with a sound understanding of the principle of Bayes' theorem and of conditional probability analysis. In most instances, the radionuclide test of choice should be performed in conjunction with conventional stress testing for detection of ischemia. High-risk patients can be identified by the magnitude of the functional disturbance in myocardial perfusion or ventricular performance in response to exercise stress.

Coronary Arteriography and Left Ventriculography[176] (see Chap. 108)

This section will deal with the value of coronary arteriography both as a diagnostic tool and as a necessary step in planning and evaluating the results of therapeutic interventions. The limitations of the technique will also be discussed.

Despite the impressive contributions of coronary arteriography over the past two decades, the decision to perform the examination on a given patient must always be subjected to a *risk-benefit* analysis.

Risks There are certain inherent dangers in placing catheters in the cardiac chambers and coronary arteries. The most feared complications are the formation and dislodgment of thrombotic material, which may cause obstruction of the coronary or cerebral vessels, and the production of potentially lethal arrhythmias. Fortunately, the incidence of acute myocardial infarction, stroke, and arrhythmia requiring defibrillation has declined; the review of Adams et al. in 1973 showed a 0.61 percent incidence of acute myocardial infarction, a 0.23 percent incidence of cerebral embolism, and a 1.2 percent incidence of severe arrhythmias.[177] The overall mortality rate of coronary arteriography was reported to be 0.45 percent. The femoral artery approach led to a higher incidence of these complications than the brachial approach. Later, Abrams and Adams showed that with additional experience in avoiding the thromboembolic complications, this difference in life-threatening complications between the two techniques disappeared.[178] Local complications of arterial thrombosis and dissection remain higher with the brachial approach than with the femoral technique, in which these complications are extremely rare. The registry of the Society for Cardiac Angiography contained data on 53,581 patients from 66 medical centers in 1980 demonstrating no difference in mortality between the brachial (0.1 percent) and femoral (0.12 percent) techniques.[179] The mortality associated with diagnostic catheterization of ambulatory patients at Emory University is almost zero. Patients with left main coronary artery obstruction;[180] unstable angina; fresh infarction; or hypotension from septal or papillary muscle rupture have a higher mortality rate. The risk of coronary arteriography for this group of patients is usually justified since they are at high risk unless operative intervention is possible.

Benefits The information to be gained is (1) an accurate map of the coronary circulation, (2) the degree of stenosis of the various segments, (3) the size and quality of the vessel beyond the stenosis, (4) the presence of collateral channels, and (5) the status of the left ventricle as a total contractile unit and of its regional contraction abnormalities. The value of coronary arteriography and left ventriculography has increased as these determinations have become more accurate. New technical developments have improved image quality, and new techniques of obtaining cranial and caudal angle views have increased the level of confidence in the results of the arteriography.[181] Experienced arteriographers using modern equipment can now obtain reliable and reproducible results.

The value of coronary arteriography and left ventriculography in the management of individual patients depends on the clinical problem confronting the physician. Even though coronary atherosclerosis can be quite advanced without clinical manifestations, these techniques have not been recommended in the absence of a clinical problem that should be solved. The true value of the test should not be determined just by its ability to accurately measure some parameter but should also be determined by the ability of the physician to use the knowledge to alter the course of the patient in a favorable way. Therefore those patients who can be symptomatically improved with coronary bypass surgery or angioplasty and those patients in whom life expectancy can be prolonged can benefit most from arteriography. A normal coronary arteriogram in a patient thought to have atherosclerotic coronary heart disease can be of great value in reducing anxiety, in reducing medical costs from repeated hospitalizations and emergency room visits, in eliminating chronic medications, and in returning patients to work and enjoyable leisure activity.

Indications for Coronary Arteriography With the preceding points in mind, certain indications for coronary arteriography can be established.

The indications for coronary arteriography in patients with *stable angina pectoris* are as follows: Patients with stable angina pectoris do not require coronary arteriography as urgently as patients with unstable angina. Those patients with stable angina whose symptoms interfere with their desired lifestyle are, however, candidates for surgery. Therefore, they must have coronary arteriography. What about those patients with stable angina who can be controlled medically? Should they have arteriography? We must not forget that about 25 percent of patients suspected of having angina do not have it.[78–81] Since it is important to make an accurate diagnosis in most patients with stable angina pectoria, a coronary arteriogram may be needed. Many patients with stable symptoms have severe obstructive coronary disease. Surgical consideration in these patients depends on the physician's attitude toward the value of surgery in avoiding major complications, and extending life in mildly symptomatic patients with severe obstructive disease. Randomized studies of patients with stable angina show improved survival rates for those with three-vessel coronary disease[101] and left main coronary disease[101,182] who are treated surgically compared to the medically treated group. Other data support an improved rate of survival for symptomatic patients with stable angina who have double-vessel disease when one of the obstructions is located in the proximal portion of the left anterior descending coronary artery.[101] Since many patients with stable angina have these conditions, we feel that these patients should be identified by catheterization. Additionally, patients with stable angina pectoris may be prevented from performing gainful and pleasurable work because of their chest discomfort. Some patients with stable angina pectoris, especially those with single-vessel coronary disease, are candidates for percutaneous coronary angioplasty and, of course, these patients cannot be identified without coronary arteriography.

Coronary arteriography is usually indicated in patients with unstable angina pectoris or prolonged chest pain due to myocardial ischemia without objective signs of infarc-

tion. A change in anginal pattern may signify an increase in the obstructive lesions or an increase in myocardial oxygen demand (usually the former). These conditions are (1) recent onset of angina; (2) progression of anginal symptoms occurring with less and less effort; (3) the occurrence of angina during rest; and (4) prolonged chest pain which is characteristic of myocardial ischemia without evidence of infarction. When possible, the patient should be stabilized with vigorous medical treatment prior to proceeding with catheterization. Because these syndromes often herald severe obstruction and multivessel disease which may precede acute myocardial infarction, we believe coronary arteriography should be performed. In those patients who continue to have pain at rest in the hospital, early catheterization is carried out in order to plan surgical intervention if anatomic conditions are found to be favorable.

Patients in the early phase of acute myocardial infarction may be candidates for thrombolytic therapy. If intracoronary thrombolysis is used, it is necessary to perform coronary arteriography. If intravenous thrombolysis is used, then coronary arteriography is usually performed a few days later (see discussion below and Chaps. 95 and 118).

Patients with myocardial infarction who continue to have repeated bouts of chest pain due to myocardial ischemia despite intensive medical treatment should have coronary arteriography. These patients are usually in the coronary intensive care unit, and most of them have coronary arteriography by the third or fourth day. Dead myocardium does not hurt, and therefore recurrent pain indicates that more muscle is at jeopardy. The operative risk of these carefully selected patients at Emory University Hospital is low.[183]

Patients with myocardial infarction who have a recurrence of chest discomfort due to myocardial ischemia after discharge from the intensive care unit or hospital should have coronary arteriography. Certain precautions are necessary in these brittle patients. These are discussed in Chap. 108.

Asymptomatic patients following acute myocardial infarction are frequently catheterized to establish the prognosis and guide therapy. Recently the exercise ECG and radionuclide studies have been used to stratify such patients into low- and high-risk groups for short-term survival (see discussion below and Chap. 98). Longer follow-up of such patients will be required to determine if such tests are as accurate as arteriography in predicting which asymptomatic patients will do well after acute myocardial infarction. The available data suggest that the noninvasive tests will adequately stratify such patients.

The indications for coronary arteriography in patients with complications of infarction are as follows: Those patients with myocardial infarction who develop ventricular septal rupture or papillary muscle rupture should undergo coronary arteriography. Most of these patients have pulmonary edema and are in cardiogenic shock. Use of the balloon counterpulsation device prior to catheterization has been helpful in temporarily stabilizing these patients. Catheterization should be done immediately, however, with plans to move toward surgery if feasible, because most of these patients deteriorate rapidly.

The indications for diagnostic coronary arteriography in patients with unusual presentations are as follows. As indicated earlier, coronary arteriography for purely diagnostic purposes can be extremely helpful. A relatively young patient carrying a false diagnosis of atherosclerotic coronary heart disease can be severely disabled. Some of the situations commonly diagnosed as angina pectoris are (1) hyperventilation syndrome, (2) gastroesophageal reflux, (3) chest wall pain, and (4) anxiety and depression. Most of the time these conditions should be identified and treated without coronary arteriography. If, however, the diagnosis of atherosclerotic coronary heart disease has been made, it is difficult to treat the patient without proving that the coronary arteries are normal. Even in patients suspected of having angina pectoris about 25 percent will have normal, minimally diseased coronary arteries as determined by arteriography.[78,80,81] This figure reaches 30 to 50 percent in women.[184,185] Diagnostic coronary arteriography is also important in certain high-risk professionals such as airline pilots and in clarifying the diagnosis for employment or insurance purposes. Coronary arteriography can be recommended in such situations because of the very low risk and the significant benefit to the patient if the findings are negative. This is not to say that all patients with any type of chest discomfort should have coronary arteriography. Many patients with low pretest probability of coronary disease can be reassured with a negative response to electrocardiographic and radionuclear stress testing. If, however, the patient and physician cannot be reasonably assured that the patient does not have coronary artery disease, then coronary arteriography should be done.

The indications for coronary arteriography in currently asymptomatic patients with other evidence of atherosclerotic coronary heart disease are as follows: The most controversial application of coronary arteriography and left ventriculography is in patients who are currently without symptoms but who have been identified as having other evidence of coronary artery disease. This arises primarily in patients who previously had angina or infarction, or who exhibit an abnormal exercise tolerance test. Coronary disease exists in most patients with previous angina or infarction and in a significant percentage of patients with a positive exercise ECG test. Why, then, the controversy? Relief of angina, one of the two major goals of therapy for coronary artery disease, is, of course, impossible to achieve in the asymptomatic patient. Natural history studies of survival have been constructed using data from patients who are symptomatic,[185] but no one knows whether asymptomatic patients with left main coronary disease are at less jeopardy than those with symptoms.

There are many patients, however, who have had

no symptoms preceding myocardial infarction or sudden death. Does objective evidence of ischemia, such as significant ST-segment depression or ^{201}Tl defects on exercise, in the absence of symptoms have the same prognostic significance as it does in symptomatic patients? This question has not been adequately studied but remains a very important one. In some patients with advanced coronary artery disease, eliciting a history of angina is sometimes difficult because the patient has already adapted to self-imposed limits or because he or she does not recognize the symptoms as being significant. Exercise stress testing of such patients frequently precipitates symptoms not previously recognized. We usually recommend bypass surgery for the following groups of asymptomatic patients with severe obstructive coronary disease in a manner similar to the way we treat symptomatic patients: those with left main coronary artery disease; three-vessel coronary disease with poor exercise performance; two-vessel coronary disease when there is obstruction of the proximal portion of the left anterior descending artery and poor exercise performance; and severe obstruction (greater than 90 percent of cross-sectional area) of vessels supplying very large areas of myocardium and poor exercise performance. The objective of surgery in these patients is to prolong life. Accordingly, patients who are suspected of having severe disease because of a previous infarction or who have a positive exercise ECG or radionuclide stress test, and are in the age group in which surgery would be recommended if severe disease were found, are candidates for coronary arteriography even when they are asymptomatic.

Although the Coronary Artery Surgery Study (CASS) showed good survival rates in both the medically and surgically treated groups with class I and II stable angina (Canadian Cardiovascular Society classification), it must be remembered that all of the patients had coronary arteriograms before they were entered in the study, and many patients with the most severe disease were excluded from the study.[78] It is incorrect to infer that patients with mild or no symptoms have mild disease. One should not give an opinion regarding prognosis in such patients without an exercise ECG or radionuclide stress test or a coronary arteriogram.

In older patients, more symptoms and disability are required to justify arteriography than are required in young patients. Identification of severe obstruction in the young patient holds the promise of prolongation of life, and because of this, the younger patient has more to gain from improved exercise tolerance. In addition, the surgical risk is higher in the older patient than it is in the young patient.

Contraindications Patients with *severe left ventricular dysfunction* usually are not suitable for coronary artery bypass grafting, and therefore it is desirable to identify them without catheterization. Patients with severe congestive heart failure secondary to infarction would ordinarily not be catheterized except to rule out aneurysm or mitral regurgitation. The history, physical examination, chest x-ray, ECG, echocardiogram, or nuclear angiogram are usually adequate to establish the presence of severe left ventricular dysfunction or ventricular aneurysm.

Other disabling or terminal diseases are usually considered to be contraindications to coronary arteriography. At times the disability and discomfort of the ischemic disease are such that catheterization is recommended even in these patients. The presence of treatable malignant disease is not a contraindication to catheterization, but the patient's overall outlook should be considered prior to making the decision for catheterization.

Important Factors in the Interpretation of Coronary Arteriograms Several technical advances have led to an improvement in the reliability of coronary arteriography. Most important has been the improvement in image intensification so that the arteries and their obstructions can be more adequately assessed. An equally important advance has been the use of new views of the arteries which are provided through angles outside the transverse plane. These views, with the x-ray beam angled toward the head or feet, have helped solve the problem of coronary arteries that overlap each other, and have eliminated the problem of foreshortening of vessels since each arterial segment can be viewed on its side.

In addition to excellent x-ray equipment, extensive experience in coronary arteriography by the arteriographer is essential in obtaining reliable results. The following items are of interest to the arteriographer in interpreting films:

Identification of Vessels. Multiple views and the assessment of the motion of adjacent epicardial vessels help to correctly identify coronary arteries.

Degree of Stenosis. The stenotic area should be viewed in multiple projections and compared to adjacent normal-appearing arterial segments. The arteriographer should make clear in his or her report whether the percent of stenosis is being expressed in diameter reduction or cross-sectional area reduction. A hemodynamically significant lesion is one that narrows the lumen diameter by 50 percent. This degree of narrowing represents a cross-sectional area narrowing of 75 percent. This magnitude of stenosis is consistent with normal coronary blood flow in the resting state but usually limits flow during significant exercise.

The Amount of Myocardium Served by the Artery Affected by the Stenosis. More important than the location of the lesion in a particular artery is the effect a particular obstruction has on the myocardial blood supply. Of course left main coronary lesions uniformly affect massive areas of myocardium and are therefore very significant. Other lesions, however, vary in their significance depending on the variation in coronary anatomy. A lesion of the left anterior descending artery in its most proximal part may affect over 50 percent of the left ventricular myocardium. Infarction caused by these lesions can lead to massive left ventricular damage and congestive heart failure or cardiogenic shock. Lesions of the left anterior descending artery after the takeoff of the first or second septal perforating branch and a large diagonal branch may jeopardize only 20 percent of the left ventricular myocardium. Stenosis of the circumflex artery which gives rise to the posterior descending artery also affects a massive amount of myocardium. Some circumflex systems supply only small lateral areas and are less important. A lesion of one marginal branch of the circumflex artery is less important if there are two or three other branches of similar size than if the circumflex terminates in one large marginal branch. The right coronary artery, if large and dominant, can supply the entire inferior surface and a large amount of the lateral surface of the left ventricle. A small nondominant right coronary artery may, on the other hand, supply only a portion of the right ventricle, and lesions of this artery are therefore less important. It is very important to determine whether there are one or two or three vessels involved and to estimate the amount of myocardium in jeopardy during periods of ischemia.

Effect of Total Occlusion on Collaterals. If a coronary artery becomes totally occluded, infarction occurs or collateral vessels develop and maintain viability of the affected segment. The arteriographer must have extensive knowledge of the variations of the coronary circulation so as not to miss a total occlusion. Late opacification almost always indicates collateral filling from the distal segments except in cases of relatively acute occlusion. Total occlusion does not usually engender the same concern as a 90 percent occluded lesion. Even with angiographically extensive collaterals, however, the collateral blood flow may be inadequate to supply the needed myocardial perfusion, and the heart may be significantly ischemic.

Spasm. Since coronary artery spasm is a transient event, it may or may not be discovered at coronary arteriography. One is more likely to identify spasm if one suspects its occurrence. The clinical syndrome of pain occurring principally at rest, especially if episodic and repetitive and associated with ST-segment elevation and/or arrhythmias, should lead one to suspect coronary spasm. When spasm is suspected, certain steps should be taken in performing the coronary arteriogram (these are enumerated in Chap. 108). Atropine sulfate, nitrites, and calcium channel blockers may block coronary spasm and therefore are avoided when this condition is suspected. Ergonovine maleate has been used to stimulate coronary spasm.[186] This is a very potent agent and may, on occasion, result in intense and prolonged coronary spasm. When it is suspected that spasm involves the artery supplying the AV node, a temporary pacemaker should be inserted prior to the use of the ergonovine. Nitrites should be available both in sublingual form and for parenteral use by either intravenous or intracoronary routes if necessary. Nifedipine is also helpful in relieving coronary spasm and should be available when provocative tests are used.[187] It is our belief that ergonovine should not be administered outside the cardiac laboratory and that all precautions should be taken when it is used.[188]

Myocardial Bridging. Systolic bridging of the artery produces an apparent lesion in systole, but further observation will show that the vessels are widely patent in diastole when the vast majority of coronary flow is occurring. It has been suggested that this may be a mechanism for coronary ischemia; however, in most cases bridging is probably only a curiosity.

Coronary Osteal Variations. The coronary arteries may originate from atypical locations. This is important to the angiographer, but it should not lead to confusion in the interpretation of these studies if proper filling of every artery is obtained.

Left Ventricular Function. This is one of the most important, if not the most important, feature in determining prognosis and operability. Measurements are made of the overall ventricular function by use of volume determinations and calculation of ejection fraction, and by indexes of left ventricular compliance such as end-diastolic pressure measurements. Regional wall motion is also assessed and expressed as decreased motion (hypokinesis), no motion (akinesis), or paradoxical wall motion (dyskinesis). Hypokinetic wall segments represent either active ischemia of either an entirely viable myocardium or a partially infarcted myocardium. Wall segments that are akinetic are more likely to represent scar tissue; however, ischemia can sometimes produce akinesis as well. Dyskinetic segments are almost always due to completed infarction. Various maneuvers such as the use of nitrites to decrease the preload and afterload and postextrasystolic potentiation of ventricular contraction have been used to assess wall motion. The beat following a premature ventricular contraction or the beats following unloading with nitrites augment the wall motion and may identify some motion in segments which appear akinetic during normal sinus rhythm. These are helpful maneuvers when making judgments about the viability of myocardium in surgical planning. When the overall ejection fraction falls below 20 percent, the opportunity for improvement postoperatively diminishes and the risk of surgery is significantly increased.[189,190] Patients with this severe degree of left ventricular dysfunction are ordinarily not referred for surgery.

Limitations of Coronary Arteriography and Left Ventriculography Despite impressive improvements in coronary arteriography, significant limitations remain.

Interobserver Variability. Coronary arteriograms read by different arteriographers may be interpreted differently. Careful measuring of lesions and interpretations by more than one observer help minimize these differences. The study of Trask et al. found that interobserver assessment was the same 93 percent of the time. They found the greatest interobserver disagreement occurred in the interpretation of lesions in the circumflex artery and diagonal branches.[191] White et al. discussed the interobserver and intraobserver variation in the interpretation of coronary arteriograms and also emphasized that it was difficult for the arteriographer to determine the functional significance of many coronary artery obstructions.[192]

Correlation with Flow. Lesions in the midrange of obstruction may or may not influence flow. *It is here that the information gained from other techniques such as radionuclide imaging may augment the information found by coronary arteriography.*

Progression of Disease. The arteriogram shows disease at one point in time. There is no way to predict the rate of progression of lesions. Less expensive ways of serial assessment of changes in coronary obstructions are needed.

Swan-Ganz Catheterization The value and limitation of Swan-Ganz catheterization is discussed later in this chapter and in Chap. 124.

Echocardiography (see Chap. 120)

Echocardiography can be used to identify pericardial effusion, mitral stenosis, mitral valve prolapse, mitral valve annulus calcification, aortic stenosis, aortic regurgitation, cardiac tumors, vegetations, left ventricular thrombi, right ventricular thrombi, myocardial wall motion, and ejection fractions.

Limitations

Echocardiography cannot give definitive answers to questions regarding the vast majority of patients with atherosclerotic coronary heart disease prior to the development of complications of the disease.

Other Laboratory Tests

Other laboratory tests may be needed to evaluate the patient with atherosclerotic coronary heart disease. They include the measurements of blood glucose and lipids.

Reminder

The evaluation of the clinical setting, history, physical examination, resting ECG, and chest x-ray are performed on all patients. The other procedures discussed in this section are not performed on all patients. They are used to answer specific questions a physician might have about a patient who has, or is thought to have, atherosclerotic coronary heart disease or any of its complications. The specific procedure(s) that is used is selected to answer the specific question(s) being asked.

Conditions Simulating Atherosclerotic Coronary Heart Disease

There are several conditions that simulate the clinical features of atherosclerotic coronary heart disease, and it is essential to remember that two or more conditions can coexist in the same patient. The physician may make an incorrect diagnosis of atherosclerotic coronary heart disease by misinterpreting a patient's chest discomfort or by misinterpreting the ECG.

"Emotional" Causes of Chest Discomfort[193–195]

Anxiety States

The symptoms associated with anxiety states are commonly confused with angina pectoris (see Chaps. 81 and 82). Patients with chest discomfort due to anxiety often have multiple complaints, such as weakness, giddiness, breathlessness, and palpitation.

There are several types of chest discomfort associated with anxiety. The pain may be sharp, intermittent, lancinating, or *stabbing* and located in the region of the left breast. The area of pain is often no larger than the tip of a finger, and it is often associated with a local area of hyperesthesia of the chest wall. The pain may last only a brief moment—no longer than it takes to snap the fingers. *Precordial aching* pain that lasts for hours or days and is unrelated to effort is also a common complaint in such patients. The area of discomfort is often the size of the hand. Substernal tightness of variable duration may occur, unrelated to exercise, and this sensation may be impossible to separate from myocardial ischemia. Some patients with anxiety may have a choking sensation in the throat due to *globus hystericus.* There may be associated hyperventilation, but this is not always the case. Discomfort in the upper portion of the chest, neck, and left arm may occur unrelated to effort. In earlier times the radiation of chest discomfort to the neck or left arm was considered to be diagnostic of atherosclerotic coronary heart disease. Now, stress electrocardiography, radionuclear stress testing, and coronary arteriography are employed to clarify such problems, and it has become evident that chest discomfort which is located in the upper part of the chest and radiates to the left arm and neck may occur in patients with normal coronary arteriograms.

Patients with anxiety may complain of palpitation, claustrophobia, and the occurrence of symptoms in crowded places. The quiet environment of church may precipitate the *hyperventilation syndrome.* Hyperventilation occurs in patients with and without heart disease and may mislead the physician.[196] Such patients have numbness and tingling of the hands and lips, feel as if they are going to "pass out," have chest discomfort, and are convinced they are dying. The patients often complain that they cannot get a satisfying breath and are, therefore, short of breath. The physician may notice deep sighing respiration that occurs several times each minute.

It is often impossible to detect chronic hyperventilation. Exact reproduction of the patient's symptoms with voluntary hyperventilation may permit identification of the nature of the complaints. Voluntary hyperventilation for 2 min is usually sufficient to produce symptoms since many patients with chronic hyperventilation become symptomatic after a few deep breaths. One cannot invariably reproduce the symptoms by forced hyperventilation, perhaps because the physician's presence produces a sense of security in contrast to the fear and terror engendered when the patient awakens at night with an attack.

The patient with anxiety may complain of persistent *weakness* and an *unpleasant awareness* of the heartbeat.

The patient with anxiety often feels certain that he or she has heart disease, and the symptoms of anxiety may be the major disabling symptoms in the patient with known atherosclerotic coronary heart disease. On the other hand, the symptoms of anxiety may stimulte a patient to see a physician, and a careful history may then reveal the presence of angina pectoris.

Patients with anxiety often exhibit a junctional-type ST-segment displacement in the ECG taken at rest or during exercise, and this accentuates the diagnostic problem. Furthermore, inversion of the T waves may be produced after 30 s of overbreathing. Friesinger et al. studied 14 patients with chest pain who were believed to have anxiety with false-positive ECGs.[197] The ECGs actually showed classic "injury" changes, with "square wave" ST-segment depressions of 1.0 mm or more during or following exercise. Eleven of the patients were subjected to coronary arteriography, and all were normal. One patient was given 5 mg propranolol orally, which prevented the electrocardiographic changes when the tracing was repeated 1 h later (see later discussion). Marcomichaelakis et al.[198] and others[199,200] also found that beta blockade prior to exercise testing improved the specificity and predictive value in detecting coronary disease.

The clinical features associated with anxiety may, at times, simulate myocardial ischemia so closely that the physician may find it necessary to admit the patient to a coronary care unit. If the ECG shows ST-segment displacement or if the serum CK level rises as a result of an intramuscular injection of an opiate, a misdiagnosis of infarction can be made. This unfortunate coincidence occurs sufficiently often to recommend that every physician should be on the alert for it. A coronary arteriogram is often needed to clarify the problem.

Depression[195]

Patients with mental depression may have chest pain that simulates myocardial ischemia. In this setting, it is very difficult to diagnose heart disease with certainty. The chest discomfort may be prolonged, and the patient may have a feeling of despair, be agitated, be unable to concentrate, and may have insomnia and loss of sexual interest and potency.

Cardiac Psychosis

Cardiac psychosis is far more complex than anxiety and emotional disturbances. Fortunately, it is rare. The patient is obsessed with the idea that his or her heart is seriously diseased despite adequate evidence to the contrary. These patients will usually dismiss a normal coronary arteriogram as being improperly performed or interpreted.

Self-Gain

Informed persons who have various reasons for self-gain, including those seeking sympathy or financial benefit from pensions or insurance, and narcotic addicts, can mislead the most experienced physicians. This is especially true of patients with chest pain who have had well-documented myocardial infarctions. Often the physician has a feeling that the patient's discomfort is not due to ischemia, but he or she may not be able to translate this impression into effective management in such an emotionally disturbed patient. Radionuclide imaging and coronary arteriography are useful in the diagnosis of such patients, but the techniques do not clarify every problem.

Combination of Problems

Patients with proven atherosclerotic coronary heart disease who also have symptoms due to anxiety or depression are difficult to diagnose and manage.

Noncoronary Cardiovascular Causes of Chest Discomfort

Premature Beats (see Chap. 26)

This arrhythmia may be accompanied by sharp, stabbing, or lancinating pain or brief duration. At times the complaint may be one of transient tightness or fullness. The uncomfortable feeling is usually experienced in the precordial area. An unpleasant sensation may be felt in the neck of patients with certain arrhythmias when the right atrium contracts against the closed tricuspid valve or when the stroke volume is increased by the contraction following a long diastole. A feeling of giddiness or faintness may occur. Extrasystoles commonly occur at rest, after meals, while reading the paper, or on retiring. Under these circumstances, activity may accelerate the heart rate and eliminate the premature beats. Sometimes exercise accelerates the heart rate and decreases the premature beats only to result in a flurry of extrasystoles during deceleration of the pulse at the end of exercise. The anxiety engendered may produce dyspnea and hyperventilation; accordingly, the patient may complain of pain and dyspnea related to exertion. If extrasystoles and symptoms occur fortuitously during the examination and during the recording of a routine ECG, recognition of the disorder may be simplified. At times an exercise ECG is needed in order to determine whether extrasystoles or other arrhythmias are produced during exercise or occur after exercise. The long-term monitoring of the heart rhythm with a Holter monitor is necessary to solve some of the problems (see Chap. 100).

Some sensitive patients are so alarmed by the feeling produced by premature beats and other arrhythmias that they feel as though they are dying. This feeling may continue all of their lives despite their own experience of many years, which should prove to them that their rhythm disturbance is benign. Other patients, of course, do not feel their premature beats or any other arrhythmia.

Acute Pericarditis (see Chap. 59)

This condition may produce precordial and substernal pain that is characteristically aggravated by deep inspiration, change of body position, and occasionally by swallowing. Pericarditis may be idiopathic in origin or may be due to viral or bacterial infection, rheumatic fever, collagen disease, neoplastic disease, trauma, or uremia, or may be secondary to myocardial infarction or cardiac surgery. Stimulation of sensory fibers involving the pericardium and diaphragmatic pleura produces radiation of pain to the precordium, the trapezius muscle area, the back of the neck, or the upper part of the abdomen. Confusion occurs when the discomfort is confined to the neck, shoulder, left pectoral region, or abdomen, unless there is a clear relation to breathing and turning. The pain of pericarditis may diminish if the breath is held. The pain tends to be sharp or cutting and may recur in intermittent bursts that are usually precipitated by a change of body position. At times the patient may become comfortable when he or she assumes the upright position and leans forward.

The early appearance of fever and a pericardial friction rub suggests pericarditis rather than myocardial ischemia and necrosis, in which these signs are usually delayed for several days. This rule is not always true, since an occasional patient with myocardial infarction will have a painless infarct and experience the pain of pericarditis a few days later.

A pericardial friction rub due to pericarditis may be present without pain, and the typical pain of pericarditis is often present without a pericardial friction rub.

Mediastinal drainage tubes (used after cardiac surgery) can stimulate the phrenic nerves and produce pain on the top of the shoulders and also produce a "pericardial rub." The rub and the pain may subside when the tubes are removed.

The aortic balloon pump produces a sound when gas goes in and out of the balloon. This is heard over the entire chest and usually surprises the individual who first encounters the noise in such patients.

The electrocardiographic abnormalities of pericarditis are confined to the ST segment, T waves, and PR segment. Abnormalities of the QRS complex do not occur except for occasional lowering of amplitude due to pericardial effusion. In general, the mean ST-segment vector due to epicardial injury is located between +30° and +90° in the frontal plane and is often directed slightly posteriorly, so that ST-segment elevation is recorded in leads I, II, III, aV_F, and in V_4, V_5, and V_6. The T wave represented as a mean vector tends to point in a direction opposite to the direction of the mean ST vector. As a rule, the mean ST vector decreases in magnitude before the mean T vector reaches its greatest size. The ST-T abnormalities of apical infarction may simulate pericarditis when significant Q waves are absent. T-wave inversion of considerable magnitude may occur with infarction, while the T-wave inversion associated with pericarditis tends to be slight. Occasionally, acute pericarditis produces depression of the PR segment. Pericarditis may produce no alterations in the electrocardiogram, even when a pericardial friction rub is present.

The echocardiogram may reveal pericardial fluid. A small pleural effusion that obscures the left costophrenic angle may be detected in the roentgenogram of the chest in some patients with pericarditis.

Modest elevation of the serum transaminase (SGOT) level may occasionally occur as a result of pericarditis. This is especially likely to happen when pericardial effusion produces venous hypertension and hepatic congestion. The serum level of CK usually remains normal in patients with pericarditis.

The clinical differentiation between pericarditis and myocardial infarction depends on the total synthesis of the information found in the history, physical examination, serial ECGs, serum enzyme determinations, and echocardiograms.

The reader is referred to Spodick for additional information regarding pitfalls in the recognition of pericarditis.[201]

Post-Myocardial Infarction Syndrome (see Chap. 59)

Post-myocardial infarction syndrome[201] (Dressler's syndrome) is discussed in Chap. 59 and later in this chapter.

Cardiomyopathy (see Chap. 58)

Patients with *hypertrophic cardiomyopathy* and left ventricular outflow tract obstruction may have angina pectoris, syncope, and dyspnea. The pathophysiology of the angina is multifactorial. We have reported patients with hypertrophic cardiomyopathy who experienced prolonged chest discomfort that is characteristic of myocardial ischemia.[202]

Pulsus bisferiens is usually present, and a systolic murmur is commonly heard in the aortic area, along the left sternal border and apex.

The ECG usually shows left ventricular hypertrophy, which is not usually seen in patients who have atherosclerotic coronary heart disease. The ECG, however, commonly shows ST and T-wave change and abnormal Q waves that simulate myocardial infarction due to coronary disease.

Patients with *dilated cardiomyopathy* may have angina pectoris and heart failure. They may also exhibit abnormal ECGs that suggest myocardial infarction.

Valve Disease (see Chap. 37)

Patients with *aortic stenosis or aortic regurgitation* may have angina pectoris. They often have coronary atherosclerosis in addition to the valve disease, but the coronary arteries may be normal. The etiology of angina pectoris occurring in patients with aortic valve disease cannot be clarified without a coronary arteriogram.

Right Ventricular Hypertension

Patients with *right ventricular hypertension* may have angina pectoris. Such has been observed in patients with pulmonary hypertension due to mitral stenosis, idiopathic pulmonary hypertension, and even severe pulmonary valve stenosis. The pain may be due to right ventricular myocardial ischemia.

Dissecting Aneurysm of the Aorta (see Chap. 64)

This condition is a less common cause of chest pain than myocardial infarction. A history of angina pectoris or prolonged myocardial ischemia due to coronary atherosclerosis always suggests that the patient's most recent chest discomfort is more of the same, but such a history does not exclude dissecting aneurysm of the aorta.

The chest pain of dissecting aneurysm is usually maximum at the outset, whereas there is a gradual buildup of pain in most patients with prolonged myocardial ischemia. Although back pain may occur with prolonged myocardial ischemia, wide radiation of the pain to the back, flank, abdomen, or legs suggests dissecting aneurysm.

A small percentage, perhaps 5 to 10 percent, of patients with dissection of the aorta have no chest pain.

If the patient appears to be in shock, but hypertension is present, dissection should be considered.

The diagnosis of dissecting aneurysm is suggested in a patient with chest pain who has any of the following signs and symptoms: syncope, weakness or transient paralysis of legs, hemiplegia, aortic regurgitation, pulsation of the sternoclavicular joint, differences in pulses or in blood pressure between the arms or legs, a decrease in pulsation of one or both carotid arteries, left pleural effusion, and significant widening of the aortic shadow as seen on the roentgenogram. Pericarditis may occur with both myocardial infarction and dissecting aneurysm and is of little differential value.

Since systemic hypertension is frequently associated with dissecting aneurysm, the ECG commonly reveals the pattern of left ventricular hypertrophy. The demonstration of serial electrocardiographic changes assists in the diagnosis of myocardial infarction due to coronary atherosclerosis. It should be recalled, however, that a myocardial infarction may be due to dissection of the coronary arteries.

The serum enzyme levels are not helpful since modest elevations may occur in both dissection and infarction.

An echocardiogram may reveal an abnormality of the proximal aorta, but in our experience this technique does not yield a test result that has a satisfactory predictive value.

Aortographic studies are usually necessary to confirm the presence of dissecting aneurysm. The procedure should not be done simply because the ECG does not show abnormal Q waves or ST-T waves suggesting myocardial necrosis and ischemia, since myocardial infarction may occur without electrocardiographic changes. The decision to perform an aortogram should be based on the total clinical picture.

Superficial Thrombophlebitis of the Precordial Veins

Superficial thrombophlebitis of the veins of the precordial area may occur rarely and produce a confusing clinical picture (Mondor's syndrome).[203] The tender, cordlike veins are often palpable in the precordial area and are the clue to the diagnosis.

Pulmonary Embolism

This condition is discussed in Chap. 54 and later in this chapter in the section entitled "Pulmonary Causes of Chest Discomfort."

Vasoregulatory Asthenia

Vasoregulatory asthenia is a disturbance of the autonomic nervous system and is characterized by a hyperdynamic circulation. The patients may have difficulty retaining a state of physical fitness. The arteriovenous oxygen difference does not increase with exercise as it should, and some observers believe that blood is shunted away from the muscles during exercise. In the pure form there need be no chest discomfort. Many patients with vasoregulatory asthenia develop some of the same symptoms as patients with anxiety.

This condition may be responsible for a false-positive exercise test and should be suspected when there is liability of the T waves and ST segments of the ECG. The T waves may become inverted in the lateral precordial leads or in leads II, III, and aV_F. These abnormalities may develop on standing, with hyperventilation, or with the administration of amyl nitrite or other nitrite preparations. Junctional ST displacement commonly occurs after exercise, but at times a classic ischemic response may occur. The inversion of the T waves and ST-segment changes can be prevented in whole or in part by the Valsalva maneuver or by the administration of propranolol.[198–200]

The symptoms and electrocardiographic abnormalities associated with anxiety (neurocirculatory asthenia), vasoregulatory asthenia, and mitral valve prolapse (click-murmur syndrome of Barlow) clearly overlap, and theoretically the three conditions may be present in the same patient.

Paroxysmal Hepatic Engorgement

Patients with severe heart failure may have pain in the right upper quadrant during exercise. This discomfort is due to paroxysmal hepatic engorgement and is rarely confused with angina pectoris.

Gastrointestinal Causes of Chest Discomfort[204] (by Theodore Hersh)*

Reflux Esophagitis and Hiatal Hernia[205]

Reflux esophagitis is caused by failure of the lower-esophageal sphincter to prevent the regurgitation of gastroduodenal secretions. The failure of the esophagus to clear the acid from its distal portion results in esophageal mucosal inflammation with consequent symptoms of *heartburn* or *indigestion.* The severity of the esophagitis depends on the concentration of the injurious agents, the pH of the gastric contents and pepsin, the persistent nature of the reflux, the length of time the esophagus is in contact with the offending acid, and mucosal barriers. In some patients, the esophagitis results from reflux of alkaline secretions containing bile and pancreatic enzymes. This entity is called alkaline or bile reflux esophagitis. The aberrations may be attributable to a loss of the high resting pressure at the gastroesophageal junction, the so-called lower-esophageal sphincter, which is readily detected on esophageal manometric studies as a zone of 2 to 4 cm in length which maintains a resting pressure of 12 to 30 mmHg. Competence of the sphincter may also be affected by mechanical, anatomic, and hormonal factors. Adrenergic, cholinergic, and purinergic nerve fibers are also participants. In the past it was postulated that a hiatus hernia played a major role in production of reflux, but recent studies indicate that reflux occurs independent of the radiological demonstration of the presence or absence of a hiatal hernia. More likely, the physiological sphincter in the gastroesophageal junction is the main barrier preventing reflux. The lower-esophageal sphincter maintains high pressure in the resting state and relaxes in response to swallowing. It also adapts to changing physiological conditions and thus maintains gastrosphincter pressure gradients that prevent reflux. Patients with reflux esophagitis have low or absent resting lower-esophageal sphincter pressures when compared with normal subjects.

Chest pains, "heartburn" or "indigestion," are the most prominent symptoms of reflux esophagitis. Patients describe the discomfort as a burning sensation located in the retrosternal area between the xiphoid and the suprasternal notch. Some patients become symptomatic and more intolerant of certain foods, such as chocolate, because they lower the resting pressure of the sphincter. Coffee, tomato and orange juice, and cocktails also cause heartburn not only by their lower pH, but by other mechanisms to be elucidated. Not infrequently, regurgitation of sour, bitter fluid, and occasionally food, is also described in association with the heartburn. Antacids and milk frequently relieve these symptoms. Belching may also alleviate this discomfort. The "heartburn" and regurgitation often occur after meals or ingestion of coffee, or following postural changes; the patient is often awakened by discomfort due to free acid reflux which occurs in the recumbent position. Another symptom is "water brash," the sensation that the mouth is filled with fluid from the esophagus. Delayed gastric emptying may contribute to the syndrome of gastroesophageal reflux with esophagitis. Patients may also describe their esophagitis as a localized pressure or squeezing pain across the middle portion of the chest which may radiate to the back. In some cases, nocturnal reflux leads to pulmonary symptoms secondary to aspiration and thus progression to chronic obstructive pulmonary disease. Patients with long-standing symptoms may develop distal esophageal stricture. Persistent dysphagia following the ingestion of solid foods also suggests development of a stricture.

The diagnosis is suggested by a history of heartburn, particularly in relation to meals, posture, and relief by antacids. The esophagogram and upper-gastrointestinal x-ray may demonstrate hiatal hernia, but the presence of a hiatal hernia alone does not establish a diagnosis of reflux or of esophagitis. The important information regarding the lower-esophageal sphincter is relayed by the fluoroscopist, who describes the reflux of barium from the stomach into the esophagus. The cineesophagogram may more vividly record this abnormality. Esophagoscopy and esophageal biopsy may demonstrate mucosal lesions, including superficial ulceration, diffuse hemorrhagic lesions with exudate, deep esophageal ulcers, and stricture. The histological studies show acute and chronic inflammatory changes. Esophagoscopy assesses the severity of the esophagitis and ensures, along with the pathological studies, the absence of malignancy, particularly in those cases with esophagitis and stricture. Sphincter incompetence may be further documented by use of esophageal manometry. Most normal subjects have

*Theodore Hersh, M.D., Professor of Medicine (Digestive Diseases), Emory University School of Medicine, kindly prepared the discussion on reflux esophagitis and hiatal hernia, diffuse esophageal spasm, esophageal rupture, cholecystitis, and peptic ulcer.

a resting lower-esophageal sphincter pressure higher than 15 mmHg; patients with an incompetent sphincter will experience an increase in esophageal sphincter pressure secondary to abdominal compression or leg raising. In patients with severe esophagitis, the body of the esophagus may show varying degrees of motor incoordination and feeble contractions, which also contribute to the failure in acid clearance by the involved distal esophagus. This mechanism of acid clearance then allows for greater contact time between the acid contents and the esophageal mucosa.

Intraesophageal pH may help demonstrate gastroesophageal reflux. The gastrointestinal pH gradient may be measured by inserting a pH electrode into the stomach and then gradually removing it. Acid reflux is determined with the electrode 5 cm above the lower-esophageal sphincter. Instruments are now being developed to measure changes in the pH of the distal esophagus over a 24-h period. The acid infusion (Bernstein) test records a patient's esophageal sensitivity to perfusion with acid.[206] In this technique, performed with the patient sitting up, the tip of a nasogastric tube is placed 30 cm from the nose; at different times normal saline and 0.1 *N* HCl are dripped at a rate of 100 to 125 drops per minute. Patients with reflux esophagitis will experience substernal burning pain or their original chest pain during the acid drip.

The gamma camera scintiscan utilizes radioactive substances as a means of quantifying and observing gastroesophageal reflux.

Medical management of reflux esophagitis is designed to prevent the reflux of gastric contents into the esophagus and to bind the acid with antacids. Therapy also includes elevation of the head of the bed (15 to 20 cm), avoidance of bending over, weight reduction, and elimination of acid foods including citrus juice, coffee, and excess fat from the diet, since the latter retard gastric emptying. Bethanechol chloride and metoclopramide may increase the lower-esophageal sphincter tone and prevent reflux. Metoclopramide also enhances gastric emptying. The H_2 antagonists, cimetidine (Tagamet) and ranitidine (Zantac), reduce the elaboration of acid by the stomach, while antacid therapy neutralizes refluxed acid. Antispasmodics do not help. When medical treatment fails or when a stricture has formed, surgical repair may be necessary.

Diffuse Esophogeal Spasm[207–209]

Diffuse esophageal spasm is a neuromuscular motor disorder of the esophagus characterized by chest pain and difficulty in swallowing. It produces various clinical, radiological, and manometric findings. The patients may have thickened esophageal muscles, up to 2 cm in thickness, from the aortic arch to the distal end of the esophagus. Although there are no apparent defects in the ultrastructure of the esophageal smooth muscle, the adjacent vagal fibers exhibit degenerative changes. Diffuse spasm may be related to achalasia in that both conditions have positive methacholine tests, indicating a sensitivity of denervated structures (Cannon's law), common manometric features, and case reports of transition from one to the other condition. Vigorous achalasia combines the features of both entities—failure of relaxation of the lower sphincter, as in achalasia, and vigorous disordered contractions in the body of the esophagus, as in diffuse spasm.

Patients with diffuse spasm may have symptoms suggestive of coronary artery disease, and the chest pain in both conditions may respond to nitroglycerin. Of course, the two diseases may coexist. Esophageal spasm may occur in any age group, but it is more common in individuals in the fifth decade. Retrosternal chest pain with radiation to the back, arms, and jaw is the most frequent symptom. It can last minutes or persist for hours. The pain may be dull or sharp and squeezing. It characteristically appears during or after a meal, particularly in association with the ingestion of cold liquids. Pain as a result of swallowing (odynophagia) is associated with difficulty in propelling the bolus of food to the stomach due to the spasm. Dysphagia without chest pain may also occur in patients with diffuse spasm. Many of these patients experience severe nocturnal chest pain and are awakened from their sleep. Exertion does not precipitate the pain, but anxiety and stress are common precipitating factors. The physical examination in such patients is unremarkable.

The diagnosis is based on the history, the exclusion of cardiopulmonary and musculoskeletal causes of chest pain, plus the verification of esophageal spasm on radiological and manometric studies. During the esophagogram, a peristaltic wave is initiated by the swallow, but it travels only to the aortic arch. Isolated and incoordinated movements of the lower two-thirds of the esophagus are noted by the fluoroscopist and are described as curling, corkscrew esophagus, or pseudodiverticula. When the lumen of the esophagus is full, the barium can be seen to be propelled by the contracting, spastic esophagus both orad and into the stomach. Esophageal manometric studies may confirm the radiological observations. The peristaltic contractions of the normal esophagus are replaced after most swallows by simultaneous, repetitive contractions. Contractions may be not only of large amplitude but also of abnormal duration. Chest pain may be reported at this time. The methacholine test may be positive. Gravino et al.[210] and others[211,212] have pointed out that esophageal spasm can simulate myocardial ischemia. They emphasize that ergonovine, which is used to provoke coronary spasm, can precipitate esophageal spasm as well as coronary spasm. The implications of this observation are obvious.

A variant of esophageal spasm has recently been described and called "nutcracker esophagus." Patients with this problem present with chest pain. Their manometry shows the presence of peristaltic contractions which are of greater amplitude and longer duration than normal contractions.[213]

Symptoms of diffuse esophageal spasm may respond to sublingual nitroglycerin or isosorbide dinitrate, probably as a result of their relaxing effect on smooth muscle. Nitroglycerin may be used before meals in patients with odynophagia or at the time of an episode of dysphagia. One of the calcium antagonists may relieve the spasm, but more studies are needed to declare them to be useful.[214] The beneficial symptomatic effect of nitroglycerin in both angina pectoris and diffuse esophageal spasm must alert the physician that other features must be present in order to make the appropriate diagnosis. Less often, diffuse esophageal spasm requires dilatation with bougies or pneumatic dilators. Occasionally, a long myotomy of the thickened muscle may afford symptomatic relief of the chest pain and dysphagia.

Esophageal Rupture[215]

Esophageal perforation or rupture is a serious and often rapidly lethal problem. The mortality has now been reduced to 30 percent with prompt surgical therapy. *Esophageal instrumentation* accounts for over 75 percent of the cases of esophageal rupture.

Spontaneous perforation of the esophagus may be the result of retching and vomiting following a heavy meal. This is associated with epigastric pain which may radiate to the interscapular area. The patient then becomes dyspneic, diaphoretic, and cyanotic. The symptoms may vary in location depending on the site of perforation (cervical, thoracic, or abdominal). Pallor, tachycardia, and shock ensue, followed by signs of the presence of mediastinal air in the form of palpable crepitus in the chest wall, neck, or supraclavicular fossa. Auscultation over the heart reveals a mediastinal auscultatory crunch (*Hamman's sign*).[216] Mediastinal air may be detected in the chest x-ray.

Iatrogenic instrumental perforations result from endoscopic procedures, from attempts at esophageal dilatation, or from balloon tamponade tubes. Perforations of either a diseased or a normal esophagus may occur. Endoscopic perforations usually occur at the junction of the pharynx and esophagus, particularly in patients with osteoarthritic bony spurs. Bougies or pneumatic dilators usually perforate the lower esophagus. Esophageal ruptures may also follow pressure necrosis caused by foreign bodies or indwelling tubes, blunt or penetrating trauma, peptic ulcerations, or carcinoma of the esophagus wall.

The diagnosis of esophageal rupture is based on symptoms and signs following vomiting or following esophageal instrumentation. A chest x-ray made with the patient in the upright position is helpful in the initial evaluation. Absence of free air under the diaphragm distinguishes esophageal rupture from a perforated intraabdominal viscus. The chest x-ray may reveal mediastinal air and pleural effusion. The rupture can be confirmed by barium swallow roentgenologic study; the site of perforation may also become evident. Since the perforation may have sealed and is therefore not detected by the esophagogram, aspiration of fluid with an acid pH from the thorax may provide further evidence of rupture.

Treatment of esophageal perforation is usually surgical. Drainage of the mediastinum is also done. If the perforation occurs in a diseased esophagus (benign stricture or carcinoma), resection of the esophagus with creation of a bypass using a segment of colon may be necessary.

Cholecystitis and Cholelithiasis[217]

Cholecystitis is characterized by varying degrees of inflammation of the gallbladder wall. In most patients, cholelithiasis is a concomitant feature, although acalculous cholecystitis may indeed occur. Gallstones should be suspected when the patient has attacks of cholecystitis or has symptoms of obstruction of the common duct, as manifested by onset of jaundice in a patient with clinical findings of biliary colic or cholecystitis. Pigment stones (calcium bilirubinate) are usually radiopaque and are often associated with hemolytic anemias. In Japan, *Escherichia coli* is invariably grown from these stones. Cholesterol gallstones (radiolucent stones) are more common in the United States and occur when bile contains high concentrations of cholesterol relative to the concentrations of bile acids and phospholipids. This phenomenon—lithogenic bile—has been shown to precede cholesterol crystal or stone formation.

Cholecystitis presents as discrete attacks of epigastric or right upper quadrant pain, associated with nausea, vomiting, and fever and chills. The pain has an abrupt onset, is either steady or intermittent, and is associated with tenderness to palpation in the right upper quadrant. The pain may be referred to the back and right scapular area. Rarely, left upper quadrant and anterior chest pain occur. Dark urine and jaundice indicate that the stone has obstructed the common duct. Symptoms of dyspepsia, flatulence, indigestion, and intolerance to fatty and spicy foods often lead to the discovery of gallstones, yet the gallbladder is often not responsible for these symptoms.

The diagnosis of gallbladder disease is suspected from the history and the presence of right subcostal tenderness. Radiological examination of the gallbladder and biliary tract leads to the demonstration of cholelithiasis or choledocholithiasis. Calcified calculi are seen on x-rays of the abdomen made with the patient in the supine position. The oral cholecystogram may reveal the presence of radiolucent gallstones, but often the diseased gallbladder will not concentrate the contrast agents. Such nonvisualization also occurs when the calculus has obstructed the cystic duct. However, care must be taken in interpreting nonvisualization, because impaired absorption of the dye or disease of the liver may be responsible rather than a diseased gallbladder. Abdominal ultrasound is a very sensitive procedure for detecting gallstones. Since it does not depend on prior administration of a contrast agent, it may be used in the acutely ill patient as well as in the routine evaluation of patients suspected of gallstone disease. Ultrasonography may also detect aberrations of the biliary tract, such as duct dilatation and disease of the pancreas. In the acutely ill patient suspected of cholecystitis, injection of radiolabeled substance, so-called HIDA or PIPODA scans, may be suggestive of cholecystitis with cystic duct obstruction by demonstrating the isotope in the common duct and clearance into the duodenum, but no uptake is detected in the gallbladder. Duodenal drainage may be undertaken for detection of cholesterol crystals or for determination of cholesterol, bile acid, and phospholipid concentrations in order to determine whether lithogenic bile is present.

The recommended treatment of cholecystitis resulting from cholelithiasis is surgery, with cholecystectomy as the procedure of choice. Cholecystectomy with common bile duct exploration is mandatory in those patients with a history of jaundice or the current presence of hyperbilirubinemia and/or elevated serum alkaline phosphatase values and concomitant pancreatitis with elevated serum amylase values. There is less agreement regarding the therapy when the patient is asymptomatic or when the disease is associated with nonspecific gastrointestinal symptoms without cholecystitis. In less than 3 percent of patients gallstones may disappear; more than 30 percent may become asymptomatic with no attacks of cholecystitis within 5 years. Few patients with gallstone disease become symptomatic when followed for years after diagnosis. Treatment with chenodeoxycholic acid will return cholesterol into solution in bile so that bile is no longer lithogenic.[218] Early reports indicated that up to 70 percent of patients with cholesterol gallstone achieved dissolution with chenodeoxycholic acid therapy. The National Cooperative Gallstone Study, however, recorded complete dissolution in only 14 percent of patients and partial dissolution in 40 percent.[219] Chenodeoxycholic acid has recently been approved for use in selected cases of cholelithiasis. Lithogenic bile, however, reportedly tends to recur on cessation of chemotherapy, suggesting long-term treatment may be required. Another related bile acid, ursodeoxycholic acid, is available abroad and is being tested in this country for dissolution of cholesterol gallstones. Ursodeoxycholic acid appears to be as effective as chenodeoxycholic acid, but has reportedly fewer side effects in that it does not induce diarrhea, abnormalities in the liver tests, or alterations in serum cholesterol levels.

Peptic Ulcer[220]

The discomfort associated with a peptic ulcer is usually located in the epigastric region. The pain is relieved by food and is not produced by effort. It lasts longer than angina pectoris. The diagnosis is usually simple and is usually made by finding the ulcer on the x-ray of the stomach and duodenum. At times, the discomfort of myocardial ischemia may be located a bit lower in the chest than usual or the pain of peptic ulcer may be felt a bit higher than usual, causing a diagnostic problem. The physician must be aware of this problem and obtain the proper x-rays and confirm the presence of ulcer with gastroscopy. One must remember, too, that both conditions may be present in the same patient. Ulcer pain is often immediately relieved by use of antacids or ingestion of food, such as milk or bland foodstuffs. Treatment of ulcer disease to reduce acid secretion may be accomplished by the use of H_2 antagonists such as cimetidine (Tagamet) or ranitidine (Zantac).

Perforation of a peptic ulcer may occur without previous symptoms. The pain is usually confined to the epigastrium or upper-abdominal region and is associated with tenderness and muscle spasm. An x-ray of the abdomen made with the patient sitting usually demonstrates air under the diaphragm.

Acute bleeding from a peptic ulcer may produce hypotension, syncope, or shock. Tachycardia is usually present, but some patients at the onset have a slow pulse that simulates that seen in occlusion of the right coronary artery. Depression of the ST segment secondary to shock may cause confusion. The reduction of hematocrit, demonstration of blood in the stools, and abnormalities found on the gastrointestinal roentgenogram identify the cause of the problem.

The long-term use of a diet containing large amounts of milk and cream by patients with ulcers is associated with an increase in the incidence of atherosclerotic coronary heart disease.

Acute Pancreatitis[221,222]

Acute pancreatitis may occasionally simulate myocardial infarction or dissecting aneurysm. This disease may be associated with biliary tract disease, alcohol intake, peptic ulcer, mumps, viral hepatitis, chlorothiazide intake, glucocorticoid intake, hypercalcemic states, hyperlipidemic states, and trauma. Pancreatitis is thought to occur when the proteolytic and lipolytic enzymes of the pancreas are activated.

Acute pancreatitis causes pain in the upper part of the abdomen which radiates to the back (at the level of tenth thoracic to second lumbar vertebrae) and may spread out over the lower chest. Severe pancreatitis may produce a shocklike state. A fever may develop in a day or so. The degree of pain is out of proportion to the amount of abdominal tenderness. There may be a boardlike abdomen, and ileus may occur. Pleural fluid, pericarditis, and gastrointestinal bleeding may occur.

The white blood cell count may be as high as 20,00 to 50,000 per cubic millimeter. The hematocrit rises because of hemoconcentration due to subscapular, peripancreatic edema and because of the "peritoneal burn" produced by the enzymes. Hyperglycemia and jaundice may develop. The serum amylase level rises in 8 h in most cases and exceeds 280 Somogyi units. This elevation tends to return to normal in 48 h. The serum calcium level usually falls. Hyperlipidemia may be present and usually antedates the acute attack.

The ECG may show ST-T depression and T-wave change. These may occur as the result of hypotension and myocardial ischemia. The ST-T change of pericarditis may occur. On rare occasions the QRS changes of infarction may occur. This is probably due to hypotension in a patient with severe coronary atherosclerosis.

An x-ray of the abdomen may show paralytic ileus, distended loops of intestine, calcification in the pancreas, and ascites. An x-ray of the chest may show elevation of the left leaf of the diaphragm and pleural fluid, which, if tapped, has an amylase level higher than that found in the serum.

This serious disease is managed by treating the shock, maintaining an adequate blood volume, decreasing pancreatic secretion, and treating complications. Surgical drainage is no longer used. The mortality rate is high and ranges from 5 to 80 percent depending on the degree of pancreatic edema, necrosis, and hemorrhage.

The "Café Coronary"

The dramatic and frightening occurrence of a café coronary must be recognized in order to execute specific treatment. When a person aspirates food, usually meat and sometimes peanut butter[223] or bubble gum, he or she may clutch the chest, become cyanotic, and die. The condition is not rare. Since these signs and symptoms may mimic an acute bout of myocardial ischemia, the event is referred to as a café coronary. The usual setting is that of a man eating steak at a restaurant. He has had a few drinks of alcohol and is enjoying the evening. He suddenly aspirates the meat and develops the symptoms. The victim is unable to talk and may rush to the restroom with food in his mouth. We have also observed the condition in psychotic patients who hold food in their mouths. If a victim is conscious but cannot talk and clutches his or her throat under the circumstances being discussed, one should consider the possibility of a café coronary. A blow over the back may produce expulsion of the bolus of food. Heimlich devised a new treatment for this condition.[224] He recommends that the rescuer stand behind the victim; wrap his or her arms around the victim's waist; grasp one fist with the other hand placing the thumb side of the fist against the victim's abdomen just above the navel and below the rib cage; press the fist into the victim's abdomen with a quick thrust; and repeat until the food is dislodged and expelled. The maneuver may not dislodge peanut butter.[223]

Distension of the Splenic Flexure of the Colon[225]

This condition may give rise to pain in the left hypochondrium and precordial region with referred pain to the left arm. The pain is not induced by effort and may be relieved by bowel movements or passage of flatus. It can be reproduced by distension of the colon through use of a colon tube. The splenic flexure syndrome is more common in patients who swallow air, have "irritable" colons, and are bowel-conscious.

Pulmonary Causes of Chest Discomfort

"Pulmonary Hypertensive Pain"

In the opinion of the authors, pulmonary hypertensive pain is not due to distension of the pulmonary artery, nor is it critically related to the height of the pulmonary arterial pressure. This pain may occur with lesions such as mitral stenosis, Eisenmenger's syndrome due to left-to-right shunt, primary pulmonary hypertension, pulmonary embolism, and cor pulmonale due to chronic lung disease. It may occur in the presence of low pulmonary arterial pressure, i.e., severe valvular pulmonary stenosis with right ventricular hypertension. The pain is believed to be caused by inadequate myocardial perfusion due to a limitation in cardiac output, reduced coronary flow during systole as a result of right ventricular systolic hypertension, and an increase in right ventricular oxygen demand. Therefore, the discomfort may be due to myocardial ischemia. It is not clear whether the ischemia is confined to the right or left ventricle, but logic dictates that the right ventricle may be more affected than the left. Since an attack of the discomfort may be self-limited and disappear within a few minutes without therapy, the response to nitroglycerin may be difficult to evaluate. When pain can be reproduced by a given amount of exercise and can be prevented by the prophylactic administration of nitroglycerin, associated coronary atherosclerosis is the most likely cause. Many patients with pulmonary hypertension develop ST-segment displacement in the ECG during or after exercise.

A coronary arteriogram may be the only way to evaluate the coronary arteries in such patients and should be done if cardiac catheterization is performed to identify mitral stenosis, congenital shunt, primary pulmonary hypertension, or pulmonary emboli. Some patients with pulmonary emphysema who have chest discomfort should have a coronary arteriogram, since carefully selected patients may be candidates for coronary bypass surgery despite the lung disease.

Pulmonary Embolism[226] (see Chap. 54)

The syndrome of massive pulmonary embolism without infarction of the lung may closely simulate myocardial ischemia due to coronary atherosclerosis, since myocardial ischemia is present in both conditions. The diagnosis of pulmonary embolism is favored by the presence of cyanosis, profound dyspnea, and tachypnea that occurs simultaneously with the chest pain. Syncope may be the initial or sole complaint of the patient with pulmonary embolism. The clinical setting of the patient may furnish a clue to the diagnosis. Pulmonary embolism is more likely to occur in the postoperative or postpartum period; after a long automobile or plane trip; following trauma, fractures, or amputation; in patients with congestive heart failures; and in patients with thrombophlebitis.

The development of acute tricuspid regurgitation, which may be recognized by observing a regurgitant systolic jugular venous pulse wave in addition to prominent *a* waves, may be noted following a pulmonary embolism. The diagnosis of pulmonary embolism is favored by the following physical signs: fixed, wide splitting of a second heart sound; a new systolic murmur at the second and third left intercostal spaces; a contact sound in systole due to dilation of the pulmonary artery, simulating a pericardial friction rub; right atrial and ventricular gallop sounds; and rarely a systolic bruit, which may be heard in the back or over the lateral thorax, due to a partially obstructed pulmonary artery. A systolic impulse over the pulmonary artery area or a systolic lift of the sternum or parasternal area may occur.

Sinus tachycardia, atrial tachycardia, atrial fibrillation, or atrial flutter may develop in patients with pulmonary embolism. ECG may exhibit evidence of myocardial ischemia and intraventricular conduction abnormalities. Sinus tachycardia with ST-segment displacement of variable degree is common. The terminal portion of the QRS complex may be altered as a result of acute cor pulmonale so that an S wave appears in leads I and V_6, and a terminal R wave appears in aV_R and V_1. Along with these changes, Q waves may appear in leads II, III, and aV_F, suggesting inferior myocardial infarction. In other patients anterior myocardial ischemia with inverted T waves and transient loss of R waves in the right precordial leads may occur and simulate anterior myocardial infarction. On occasion myocardial infarction may actually be precipitated by pulmonary embolism.

Cardiac enzyme levels (MB-CK) are usually normal in patients with pulmonary embolism.

The chest roentgenogram associated with pulmonary embolism may reveal the following: no abnormality; an increase in radiolucency in an area of the lung; dilation of the proximal portion of the pulmonary artery with an abrupt decrease in size of a branch of the artery; or elevation of the hemidiaphragm. It should be reemphasized that less than 10 percent of pulmonary emboli produce infarction of the lung; however, the detection of an area of infarction by x-ray may clinch the diagnosis. Conventional pulmonary infarcts with pleuritic pain and pleural rub offer little diagnostic problem, but many do not have these features and therefore are difficult to identify.

Selective pulmonary angiography or pulmonary scanning using radioactive substances may confirm the diagnosis (see Chap. 113). An excellent sign that pulmonary embolism has occurred is the combination of a normal chest roentgenogram and an abnormal lung scan. Pulmonary embolism may produce an alteration in blood gases which includes a decrease in P_{O_2} and a normal-to-low P_{CO_2}.

Post-Myocardial Infarction Syndrome (see Chap. 59)

This syndrome is listed here because pleurisy and pleural fluid occur. Pericarditis related to this condition is discussed in Chap. 59 and later in this chapter.

Mediastinal Emphysema (Hamman's Disease)[216]

Mediastinal emphysema develops when the pulmonary alveoli rupture, thereby permitting air to dissect along periarterial tissue spaces.

Mediastinal emphysema produces chest pain, mediastinal crepitation which is often noticed by the patient, air in the mediastinum and left pleural space, and occasionally subcutaneous emphysema of the neck and upper part of the thorax.

The mediastinal crunch heard on auscultation is characteristic even to the inexperienced observer.

The diagnosis may be established by detecting air in the mediastinum on the lateral chest roentgenogram.

Spontaneous Pneumothorax[227]

Pneumothorax may produce pain over the lateral portion of the thorax and is usually associated with dyspnea. The condition may or may not be suspected from physical findings but is confirmed by x-ray examination of the chest (if the examiner looks carefully).

Neuromuscular-Skeletal Causes of Chest Discomfort

Thoracic Outlet Syndrome[228–231] (by Robert B. Smith)*

Thoracic outlet syndrome refers to compression of the neural and vascular structures that exit from, or pass over, the superior rim of the thoracic cage. A variety of different names have been given to the condition, including first thoracic rib, cervical rib, scalenus anticus, costoclavicular, and hyperabduction syndrome, according to the presumed site of major neurovascular compression. Pressure may occur at the interscalene triangle, in the costoclavicular space, or at the coracoid process as the vessels pass under the pectoralis minor tendon. Identifiable abnormalities of bone such as anomalous cervical ribs, bifid first rib, fusion of the first and second ribs, or clavicular deformities contribute to compression in 30

*Dr. Robert B. Smith III, Professor of Surgery, Emory University School of Medicine, kindly prepared the discussion on thoracic outlet syndrome.

percent of the patients. Symptoms may be related to occupational activities, to poor posture, to sleeping with arms elevated over the head, or to acute injuries such as cervical whiplash. Most patients become symptomatic in the third or fourth decades. Women are affected three times more often than men. The differential diagnosis includes any condition that can produce chronic, recurrent pain in the upper extremity; carpal tunnel syndrome, cervical arthritis, cervical disk syndrome, cervical cord lesions, superior sulcus tumor, peripheral neuropathy, causalgia, shoulder-hand syndrome, angina pectoris, arterial occlusive disease, and Raynaud's syndrome.

Most individuals with thoracic outlet syndrome experience pain in the upper extremity resulting from somatic nerve compression, usually in the distribution of the ulnar nerve. Paresthesias and hypesthesia are common, but anesthesia and motor weakness are reported in only 10 percent. While the pain almost always involves the hand and arm, it may also radiate into the neck, the shoulder region, the scapula, or the axilla. In a few individuals the pain is experienced mainly in the anterior chest wall and may occur in episodes suggestive of coronary heart disease. Vascular compression is thought to be responsible for symptoms in only a few patients and is manifest as more diffuse pain in the limb, with associated fatigue and weakness. With more severe arterial compromise the patient may describe coolness, pallor, cyanosis, or symptoms of Raynaud's phenomenon. Rarely the arterial impingement is sufficient to produce poststenotic dilatation of the subclavian artery. A mural thrombus may form and give rise to emboli and result in focal necrosis of the skin or gangrene of a part. Venous compression symptoms infrequently result from thoracic outlet conditions but may present as episodic edema and plethora of the extremity; major venous thrombosis on this basis is rare.

The diagnosis of thoracic outlet syndrome can be confirmed in many patients by careful physical and neurological examination. Palpation of the supraclavicular space may elicit tenderness or may define a prominence indicative of cervical rib syndrome; firm palpation at the root of the neck may reproduce the patient's symptoms. If nerve compression is suggested by the history, the examiner may detect confirmatory hypesthesia, anesthesia, paresis, or muscle atrophy in the appropriate distribution. Nerve conduction velocity studies are seldom confirmatory of thoracic outlet compression but should be performed in order to identify nerve compression at other sites in the arm, such as at the carpal tunnel, and thus allow surgical treatment at the correct level. Chest and cervical spine roentgenograms are obtained on all patients. Cervical myelography and neurological consultation may be indicated if the diagnosis remains uncertain after the above studies have been completed. In patients with anterior chest pain as a major component, an exercise stress test and coronary arteriography should be considered as part of the complete workup.

If the history indicates that compression of the subclavian artery is mainly responsible for the patient's discomfort, the examiner may find obliteration or significant diminution in the radial or the brachial pulses when the patient assumes a position that produces symptoms. The effect of *Adson's maneuver* (deep inspiration with the neck fully extended and the head rotated toward the side of symptoms), *the hyperabduction test* (arm extended overhead), and the *costoclavicular test* (exaggerated military attention posture) should be compared in both arms. Any changes in pulse amplitude should be confirmed by a decrease in blood pressure in that extremity, as measured by using a stethoscope or a Doppler ultrasound instrument. A bruit also may be detectable along the course of the subclavian artery when the extremity is moved through the range of test positions. Interpretation of the results of these vascular studies, however, must include an awareness that false-positive results occur with considerable frequency among asymptomatic and presumably normal individuals. If symptoms or physical findings suggest vascular involvement, it is desirable to obtain subclavian arteriograms, done with the extremity in both the neutral and the symptomatic positions. Venograms are useful only in the rare patient with evidence of impaired venous flow.

Although some forms of thoracic outlet syndrome have been recognized and treated surgically for more than 100 years, it is only recently that the problem has been accurately diagnosed and appropriately treated. A trial of nonoperative therapy is desirable for several weeks in most patients and will be successful in many. The subject should be instructed to avoid the posture or activity known to provoke symptoms. Shoulder-girdle exercises are prescribed along with the application of local heat, muscle relaxants, and analgesic medications. Surgical intervention should be recommended if conservative treatment fails or if, at the time of initial evaluation, the patient has advanced physical signs such as motor weakness, muscle atrophy, or significant arterial ischemia. Successful surgical management consists of elimination of all constricting forces on the neurovascular structures. This goal is achieved most reliably and with the least functional impairment by resection of the first rib via a transaxillary or supraclavicular approach. Removal of the first rib releases the floor of the interscalene triangle allowing the brachial plexus and the subclavian artery to drop away from any impingements. During the same procedure, associated cervical ribs or constricting fibrous bands are excised and any necessary vascular repair or cervical sympathectomy accomplished. The rate of morbidity and mortality associated with surgery should be quite low, and the long-term results are generally very satisfactory in properly selected patients. The few individuals who have poor results should be reevaluated carefully for the possibility of incorrect diagnosis or underlying psychogenic factors, including self-gain.

Tietze's Syndrome[232,233]

Local pain and swelling of costochondral or chondrosternal joints or of the xiphisternal joint may occur for unknown reasons (Tietze's syndrome). The second costocartilage on either side is the most common area of involvement, but any of the costochondral articulations can be involved. Pain and tenderness may be reproduced by palpation of the local areas. The condition may persist for months without fever or systemic symptoms.

The usual laboratory tests are normal.

The patient may not appreciate the superficial and local nature of the involvement and may wrongly attribute these sensations to heart disease. The condition runs its course, but local procaine infiltration and local infiltration of corticosteroids may be needed for severe cases.

Herpes Zoster[234]

This condition may simulate myocardial ischemia. The preeruptive stage of herpes zoster is characterized by discomfort over one or more dermatomes. The skin is frequently sensitive over the involved area. The patient may complain of malaise, headache, and fever. The condition is commonly missed until the skin eruption develops, which may not occur for 4 to 5 days. The vesicles and pain are confined to the somatic distribution of one of the spinal nerves, and because of this distribution the condition may be confused with myocardial ischemia. Treatment should be directed toward the relief of pain.

Chest Wall Pain and Tenderness[235]

Chest wall pain and tenderness may occur for unknown reasons. The pain may be reproduced by palpating the area and by movements of the thoracic cage such as bending, stooping, twisting, turning, or swinging the arms while walking. In contrast to angina pectoris, the pain may last for seconds or for hours, and prompt relief is not afforded by nitroglycerin. As a rule, no therapy is required. Salicylates may be needed on occasion.

Many types of chest discomfort occur after cardiac surgery. The mediastinal tubes may stimulate the phrenic nerves and cause pain to be felt on top of the shoulders. Other causes of chest pain include angina pectoris, pericarditis, and chest wall pain. The latter may be noted in the region of the incision. When there has been a sternal split, the patient may complain of discomfort at the superior portion of the incision especially when the neck is hyperextended. Intercostal muscle pain is common following cardiac surgery. Cartilages or ribs may be fractured due to rib spreading at surgery, and pain associated with a "popping" sensation may be experienced by the patient. Numbness of the ring and small finger and the ulnar aspect of the hand and forearm may also result from compression of the brachial plexus following spreading of the rib cage at surgery.

Prognosis of Atherosclerotic Coronary Heart Disease (by Gottlieb C. Friesinger)*

The capacity to make effective use of today's diagnostic, therapeutic, or preventive technology depends in large measure on the accuracy with which the physician can perceive the dangers to the patient at that particular moment. In a real sense, therefore, prognosis *is a master technology that determines the momentary value of each of the others. The ability to forecast with reasonable accuracy is one of the most important things a doctor can do.*

Walsh McDermott†

Background and Principles

Establishing prognosis with reasonable confidence is particularly difficult in atherosclerotic coronary heart disease. The principal factors contributing to difficulties are the inherent complexity of the condition, its propensity to pursue a long and relapsing course, and the lack of fully satisfactory, easily available techniques to obtain objective data in many patients. A large number of patients will follow a course of many years (often greater than 10) with long periods of stability interrupted by apparently unpredictable (sometimes catastrophic) intercurrent events. These intercurrent events and the propensity for sudden death, which is present in all groups with atherosclerotic coronary heart disease, provide a disconcerting element and add an emotional feature to prognosis not present in most diseases.

Our ability to judge prognosis has greatly improved during recent years as we have obtained better objective data on large numbers of patients, and developed a clearer understanding of the most important determinants of prognosis. The most useful approach in assessing prognosis is to place patients into subsets using multiple factors, clinical descriptors, and laboratory data, which have independent importance.[236,237] Objective and quantitative data are superior to subjective qualitative data. Since silent myocardial ischemia is common, the duration of treadmill exercise and degree of ST-segment depression are of greater value than merely eliciting the patient's complaint of chest discomfort. An es-

*This section on prognosis was kindly written by Dr. Gottlieb C. Friesinger, Professor of Medicine and Director of the Division of Cardiology, Vanderbilt University School of Medicine, Nashville, Tennessee.

†The quotation by Walsh McDermott appeared in the final issue of the *Johns Hopkins Medical Journal* (December 1982, vol. 151, no. 6). It is reproduced here with the permission of the Johns Hopkins University Press. Permission was also obtained from David Rogers, M.D., who was coauthor of the article "Social Ramifications of Control of Microbial Disease" that appeared in that issue.

timate of left ventricular function is a more powerful prognostic item than eliciting a history of breathlessness and fatigue. However, the clinical and symptomatic evaluation is important and additive to the objective data.

Table 45-3 lists the principal prognostic determinants in patients whose symptoms are stable. Although the order of importance for the factors listed will differ from patient to patient, the *degree of left ventricular dysfunction* tends to be the most powerful predictive item in most subsets.

The most important clinical factor is a *change in the patient's symptoms.* When a patient with stable angina pectoris presents a change in symptoms, and so is judged to have entered the unstable phase, his prognosis worsens for a period of months. Similarly, a patient who has experienced a myocardial infarction has a worsened prognosis in the 6 to 9 months following that infarct as compared to a time more remote from the event. The patient may be considered to be in a "transition zone"; a situation depicted in Fig. 45-3.

The physician should assume that most patients with atherosclerotic coronary heart disease, even those patients who express no curiosity, have concern about their prognosis. Denial and/or fear may prevent patients from asking the physician about outcome. The physician's willingness to discuss prognosis in a realistic and sympathetic manner, with as much optimism as is warranted, at the appropriate time, and under proper circumstances, is important to the overall management of patients with atherosclerotic coronary heart disease.

The popularity of aortocoronary bypass surgery has augmented the importance of estimating prog-

TABLE 45-3 Principal Prognostic Determinants of Stable Subsets

Degree of left ventricular dysfunction
Objective severity of ischemia
Duration of treadmill
Degree of ST shift
Extent of coronary atherosclerosis
Recent (6–12 month) intercurrent ischemic events
Myocardial infarction
Unstable angina
Sudden cardiac death with resuscitation
Additional factors
Hypertension
Cardiomegaly
Congestive failure
Electrocardiographic abnormalities
Ventricular arrhythmias
Conduction defects
Remote infarction
Smoking

FIGURE 45-3 The hypothetical course of three patients (A,B,C) with atherosclerotic coronary heart disease. The slope of the lines is related to risk factors and other unknown items which determine the progression of coronary atherosclerosis. All three patients enter the transition zone, a time when they develop new manifestations. Patient A died with acute myocardial infarction, or suffered sudden cardiac death. Patient B continued at a slope unchanged after having experienced a period of unstable angina pectoris but without myocardial necrosis. Patient C had a large myocardial infarction with considerable myocardial necrosis resulting in reduced ventricular function which made the slope of his line steeper and the severity of his disease worse. A patient is in the transition zone for a variable period, probably 3 or 4 months on the basis of data available for unstable angina pectoris and perhaps 6 to 12 months for the patient who has survived acute myocardial infarction. MI = myocardial infarction; UAP = unstable angina pectoris; SCD = sudden cardiac death. (*From G. C. Friesinger, Prognosis in Ischemic Heart Disease, Trans. Assoc. Am. Phys., 93:98, 1981. Reproduced with permission from the author.*)

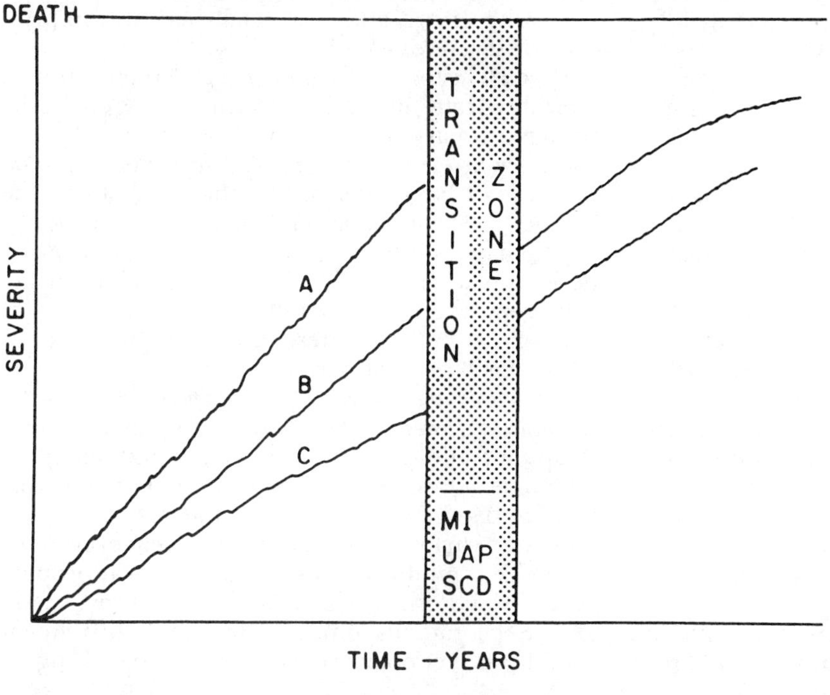

nosis in each patient. The indications for surgery include relief of symptoms, prevention of complications, improvement of quality of life, and prolongation of life, but the most objective and important is prolongation of life. Because of the long course many patients pursue and since grafts may fail, the timing of the first procedure is a critical issue.

In the subsequent sections, a brief résumé of how these principles can be utilized in assessing prognosis in a variety of subsets of patients with atherosclerotic coronary heart disease is given. Although numbers and probabilities are cited, it should be emphasized that it is unwise to take a rigid statistical approach. Within the context of the probabilities given, an individualized approach is desirable. In addition, our knowledge of prognosis is continuing to improve, and our ability to influence prognosis favorably by a variety of interventions, including drug therapy and behavioral modifications, significantly alters this situation. *Finally, prognosis in each patient needs to be continually reassessed since important changes may occur in the extent of coronary atherosclerosis, exercise tolerance, frequency of arrhythmia, and status of left ventricular function without change in symptoms or complaints.*

Coronary Atherosclerosis without Angina or Other Evidence of Ischemia

The natural history of asymptomatic coronary atherosclerosis is unknown. The studies of Zoll, Blumgart, and Edwards and others[31,238–240] demonstrate that moderately severe or severe coronary atherosclerosis is common in our population, particularly with increasing age in males, but frequently is not associated with symptoms. This asymptomatic population contains two major subsets.[241,242] One group of patients has never been symptomatic and cannot produce ischemia, in the form of ST-segment shift or ventricular functional abnormalities, when stressed with exercise. This group has coronary atherosclerosis without ischemia. The second group of asymptomatic patients contains multiple subsets. Included are patients who are free of complaints because they never participate in enough exercise to produce symptoms, those who have truly silent myocardial ischemia and can be shown to have asymptomatic electrocardiographic and ventriculographic abnormalities on exercise when stressed, and patients who have had previous symptoms of myocardial ischemia but who are totally free of symptoms and/or functional abnormalities when evaluated on no medications. This latter group contains a substantial number of patients, and symptom-free periods may last for many years. The prognosis of all these subsets is different. Those patients who are currently asymptomatic but have past manifestations of myocardial ischemia fit into prognostic subsets discussed in subsequent paragraphs.

We have no useful and/or systematic prognostic information about patients with coronary atherosclerosis without current or past ischemia. The history of this group has assumed greater importance in recent years because of the widespread use of coronary arteriography, which has identified patients in this subset. It is suspected that many physicians currently do not make a distinction in reference to clinical decision making between these asymptomatic subjects. It is important to do so since all available data suggest coronary atherosclerosis without current or past ischemia carries a better prognosis than other subsets.

Coronary Atherosclerosis with Reversible Ischemia

Stable Subsets

The key feature in this large group of patients is the relationship between an increase in myocardial oxygen demand and the development of ischemia. These subsets have fixed coronary arteriosclerotic lesions, usually multiple and severe, which result in the rather predictable appearance of ischemia when a certain myocardial oxygen demand is exceeded. Apparent variability in the stress required to produce ischemia can often be related to the presence of several factors combining to produce the increased myocardial oxygen demand or, possibly, variable threshold from time to time related to changes in coronary arterial tone. Many patients with stable angina also have *silent myocardial ischemia* as manifested by electrocardiographic ST-segment shifts and/or alteration in left ventricular function during exercise. These objective manifestations of ischemia as well as the symptoms must be considered when estimating prognosis. Some patients with reversible myocardial ischemia have *angina equivalents* rather than angina. They experience exhaustion or dyspnea with effort, and this usually signals the presence of severe disease.

Given a history of *stable angina pectoris,* the annual mortality rate in patients with angiographically proven coronary atherosclerosis but without left main coronary artery obstruction is 3 to 4 percent. The presence of hypertension and abnormalities on the resting electrocardiogram, such as nonspecific ST-T changes and/or Q waves, worsens the prognosis. If neither hypertension nor ECG abnormality is present, the mortality rate is as low as 2 percent per year. If both are present, the mortality may be as high as 8 percent per year.[243–246]

Estimating the severity of the symptoms is of limited assistance in assessing prognosis. Although profound symptoms and symptoms of long duration (more than 5 years) worsen prognosis, there is a poor correlation between prognosis and the patient's symptoms since many patients can effectively prevent or minimize symptoms by using nitroglycerin prophylactically and/or avoiding activities that provoke angina. Such patients appear to have mild infrequent complaints, yet objective data, such as exercising on the treadmill, indicate marked diminution in exercise tolerance.

Ambient ventricular ectopy, as a separate diagnosis factor, is controversial since it tends to be associated with ventricular dysfunction and other prognostic factors. However, it is probable that ectopy, per se, worsens prognosis.[247]

The widespread use of exercise testing and angiographic study has greatly enhanced our ability to understand the determinants of prognosis and has provided more reliable predictions in individual patients.

The single most important item is exercise tolerance. Multiple studies confirm the striking relationship between exercise tolerance and the 5-year outcome.[248–250] Patients with superb exercise tolerance, as judged by the heart rate achieved or exercise duration, have an excellent prognosis with steadily worsening prognosis as exercise tolerance lessens. Achieving a heart rate of 160 or reaching stage 4 in the Bruce protocol is associated with a short-term annual mortality rate of not more than 1 or 2 percent. Failure to achieve stage 2 on the Bruce protocol because of cardiac limitation is accompanied by an annual mortality rate as high as 6 to 10 percent, depending on other features, especially left ventricular function. These estimates are independent of the presence or degree of ST-segment depression, since the failure of ST-segment depression to occur does not necessarily denote a good prognosis. Conversely, a study of 220 patients, all of whom had 2-mm ST-segment depression with exercise, demonstrated an excellent correlation between 5-year outcome and duration of exercise on the treadmill. It is suspected that the occurrence of pain accompanying ST-depression during exercise testing is an independent additive prognostic factor. However, critical large studies which allow a close intercorrelation among onset of pain, extent of ST-segment depression, duration of exercise on the treadmill, heart rate achieved, and reasons for stopping the exercise have not been done. No systematic data concerning the importance of exercise-induced arrhythmias as an independent prognostic factor are available. It is suspected that exercise-induced ventricular ectopy, in contrast to ambient ectopy, is not an independent prognostic feature. The appearance of significant exercise-induced hypotension is a powerful adverse prognostic factor since it indicates that the ischemic process and/or scarring from past infarction is so severe that the stress exceeds the left ventricle's ability to meet the demand. *Exercise testing is more valuable and more easily interpreted if used to estimate prognosis in patients with manifest stable ischemic heart disease than it is in establishing the diagnosis of the condition.* The extensive data available can be summarized by stating that the functional capacity of patients with stable disease is a powerful prognostic factor and is additive to any other prognostic factor, including anatomic abnormalities.

The use of angiographic information, extent of coronary atherosclerosis and left ventricular contractile patterns, in estimating prognosis in patients with reversible stable myocardial ischemia has been studied since 1970,[251–254] but the most extensive and valuable information reported has been accumulated through the National Heart, Lung, and Blood Institute Coronary Artery Surgical Study (CASS)[78,255,256] (see Fig. 45-4). Data on 25,000 patients have been collected and submitted to sophisticated statistical analyses. The criteria utilized to define a significant coronary arterial narrowing is important. The CASS study utilized 70 percent or more reduction in internal diameter of the epicardial vessels, excepting for the left main coronary artery, where 50 percent or more reduction in internal diameter was judged significant. Other studies have utilized a 50 percent reduction in internal diameter (75 percent cross-sectional area reduction) as significant. Although, in general, findings related to outcome are similar, since the measurements have a subjective element and other items such as the length of the narrowing, the presence of collaterals, and overall extent of disease in a given vessel can usually not be taken into account, prognosis worsens when more severe narrowings are used. Even allowing for the interobserver differences which occur,[257,258] the simplified classification of patients with stable reversible myocardial ischemia into single-, double-, and triple-vessel disease is useful and widespread. However, data do exist to indicate that lesions of less than 50 percent narrowing contribute to prognosis.[259]

So-called single-vessel disease carries a mortality rate of 1 to 3 percent per year for the 5 years following presentation with stable angina. Two-vessel disease, when the left anterior descending (LAD) artery is involved, has an annual mortality of 6 to 9 percent, but significantly less when no LAD disease is present. Three-vessel disease probably carries a slightly higher mortality rate than two-vessel disease, but when arteriographic disease is extensive, the multiple factors listed in Table 45-3 have great importance in individual patients and need to be assessed carefully.

The presence of significant left main coronary arterial narrowing is shown to be the most powerful arteriographic prognostic item. Ordinarily, left main disease is accompanied by extensive disease in other trunks. Regardless, this lesion carries the poorest prognosis, as high as 15 to 20 percent annual mortality rate in some reports. There is a spectrum of rates of survival even in patients with left main disease, depending on its association with other factors such as ventricular function and exercise tolerance. One-year survivorship as high as 97 percent and as low as 59 percent have been reported; 3-year figures were 74 percent and 25 percent.[260]

An estimate of ventricular function is a more valuable prognostic factor than extent of arteriographic narrowing.[78,250,254] In the CASS study (see

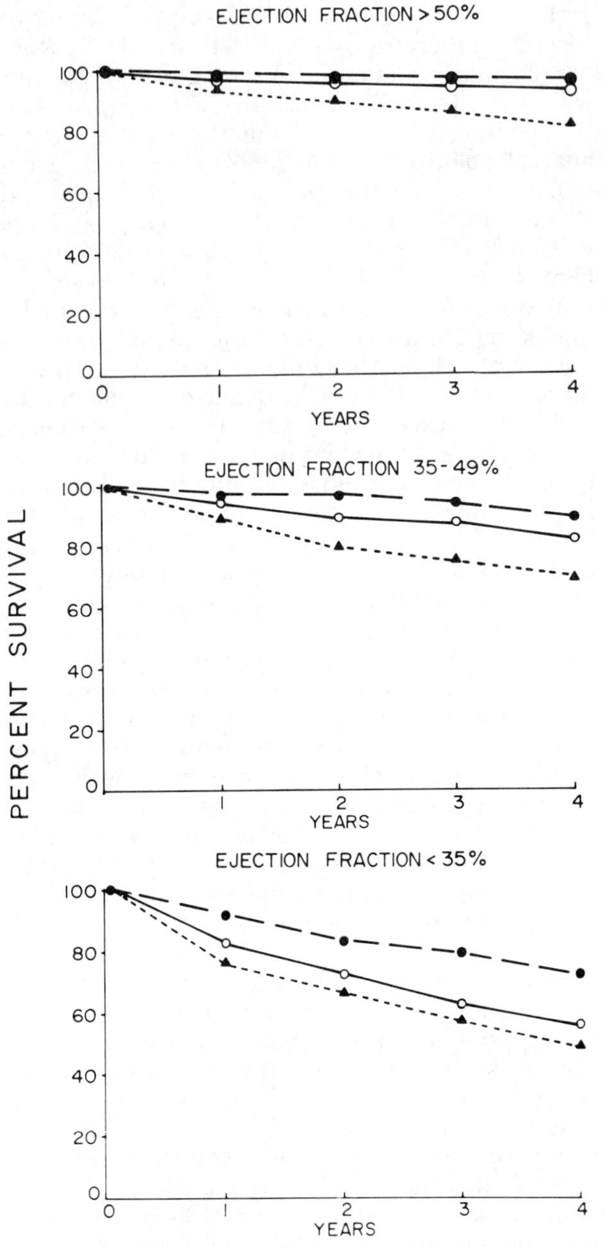

FIGURE 45-4 The 4-year survival in stable patients from the CASS registry: 6791 patients, 73 percent with typical angina pectoris, are included. The importance of left ventricular performance, judged on the basis of ejection fraction, is illustrated. Regional wall motion abnormalities showed a similar trend, i.e., worsening prognosis with increasing wall motion abnormalities for all grades of coronary arteriosclerosis. Single vessel disease = - • -; double vessel disease = - ○ -; triple vessel disease = - ▲ -. *(From M. B. Mock, I. Ringqvist, L. D. Fisher, et al., Survival of Medically Treated Patients in the Coronary Artery Surgery Study (CASS) Registry, Circulation, 66:562, 1982. Redrawn and reproduced with permission from the American Heart Association, Inc., and the author.)*

Fig. 45-4), patients with single-vessel disease with an ejection fraction of less than 35 percent had a survival rate of 72 percent at 4 years, while patients with triple-vessel disease and an ejection fraction greater than 50 percent had a 4-year survival rate of 82 percent. Regional wall motion scores make the same point. Subsets with no wall motion abnormalities and triple-vessel disease had a survival rate of 80 percent at 4 years, while patients with marked regional wall motion abnormalities and single-vessel disease had a survival of 74 percent at 4 years. Of the CASS study patients 73 percent had typical angina, and 48 percent had a history of myocardial infarction (see Fig. 45-4).

The use of angiographic and objective exercise data has improved our ability to utilize noninvasive clinical descriptors in predicting survival. More than 500 patients with stable angina pectoris had angiographic study. Four noninvasive descriptors, resting ST-segment depression on the ECG, history of infarction, history of hypertension, and marked limitation on normal activities (class III to IV using the old classification of the New York Heart Association), divided patients into high- and low-risk groups.[261] In patients in the highest tercile for these noninvasive descriptors, the 6-year mortality rate was high, with a survival rate of 60 percent. In the lowest tercile the 6-year survival rate was much better, 92 percent. The distribution of patients with so-called single-, double-, and triple-vessel disease was the same for each tercile. Patients with left main disease had been excluded. This study again emphasizes the importance of functional capacity and historical factors in addition to extent of coronary arteriosclerosis as major prognostic factors.

The data concerning prognostic implications of angiographic findings in stable reversible myocardial ischemia can be summarized. The patient may have stable angina pectoris; no angina but objective evidence of ischemia; or angina equivalents (dyspnea on exhaustion with effort). The prognosis worsens as the extent of arteriographic abnormality increases. The outlook for so-called single-vessel disease and good ventricular function is good, less than 1 to 2 percent mortality rate each year for the 5 years after presentation. Disease localized to the left anterior descending artery carries a poorer prognosis than a similar degree of disease localized to the right coronary artery. Left main coronary artery lesions carry a very poor prognosis. So-called double- and triple-vessel disease are intermediate. The prognosis of patients with *angina equivalents* may be poor because the complaints are sometimes due to severe disease with global myocardial ischemia. There are, however, inadequate reports on such patients.

Ventriculographic abnormalities are additive and even more powerful in predicting outcome than extent of atherosclerotic lesions.

Radionuclide studies, utilizing tagged red blood cells and ^{201}Tl injections to estimate regional myocardial perfusion, are widely used. There are many reports concerning correlations between the radionuclide studies and angiographic findings, symptoms, and functional capacity. However, there are no systematic studies involving large numbers of well-characterized patients which would let us know if these studies are additive to the information obtained by other techniques in reference to prognosis. A combination of clinical evaluation, determination of ejection fraction by radionuclide ventriculography, and exercise tolerance testing could probably provide the information needed to judge prognosis.

Unstable Subsets

Unstable angina pectoris and prolonged myocardial ischemia without objective evidence of infarction are clinical entities which carry similar connotations in reference to prognosis during the 3 to 6 months following their onset. Retrospective studies emphasize the frequent occurrence of a change in symptoms, in 50 to 75 percent, in patients preceding myocardial infarction.[262–264] Prospective data concerning the frequency of infarction and sudden death in patients who are experiencing the unstable anginal syndromes are fragmentary and will never be refined, since broader definitions and better appreciation of the syndrome ensures its recognition and vigorous treatment, and favorably alters its course. Regardless, it is clear that patients with the unstable angina syndromes experience a significantly higher rate of complication than do patients with stable angina during the 6 months following the onset of the condition.

Gazes[265] studied 140 patients judged to have unstable angina severe enough to require hospitalization and found an 18 percent 1-year mortality rate. The highest mortality rate was in patients who had stable angina prior to the onset of the unstable phase and/or who persisted with frequent episodes of ischemia accompanied by ST-segment elevation after hospitalization. These observations were made prior to availability of current management concepts but serve to emphasize the hazardous nature of the unstable anginal syndromes. In a prospective study, Duncan et al.[266] in Edinburgh studied 251 patients with new or worsening angina who were not hospitalized. These patients were followed for 6 months. In this mildly symptomatic group, 4 percent died, 12 percent developed myocardial infarction, and 31 percent were angina-free.

Other prospectively designed studies have provided useful information, but patient selection, protocol design, and therapy prevent direct comparison of studies and/or accurate estimate of prognosis for broad groups of patients. The cooperative national study[267] provides an enormous amount of descriptive information, but patients with left main coronary atherosclerosis were (understandably) excluded, and there were a large number of "crossovers" from the medical to surgical treatment groups. Protocol design prevented a true assessment of natural history because "crossover" to surgery from the medical treatment group was permitted when symptoms were exacerbated. However, patients assigned to medical therapy had a 10 percent mortality rate, a 19 percent incidence of myocardial infarction, and a 36 percent crossover to surgery for persistent angina during an average follow-up of 30 months after randomization. The incidence of these events was higher in the first few months following randomization.

A more recent prospective study by Gerstenblith et al.[268] has a different experimental design and included patients who had had myocardial infarction in the previous 3 months (35 percent of patients), patients over the age of 70, and those who were not candidates for bypass surgery on the basis of poor distal vessels. The principal reason for the study was an evaluation of drug therapy. However, of 138 patients in the study, 19 percent had sudden death or myocardial infarction and an additional 30 percent (excluding those with left main coronary disease) required bypass surgery in a 4-month follow-up. Although the study demonstrated that nifedipine improved outcome when added to other medical therapy, it emphasized the hazardous nature of the unstable phase. Patients with ST-segment elevation during episodes of pain had a more serious prognosis than those who did not. The incidence of events, sudden cardiac death, myocardial infarction, and symptoms requiring bypass surgery, lessened with time so that 3 to 4 months after the onset of the unstable phase, the number of events was at a very low frequency. These data suggest that the unstable period in such patients may last for 3 or 4 months, an important consideration in reference to therapy and prognosis.

An additional prospective study of unstable angina with a different experimental design yields similar information.[269] In a protocol designed to assess the efficacy of low-dose aspirin 1266 men were studied. Selection criteria excluded patients with recent myocardial infarction (6 weeks) and any clinical factor that might have resulted in an increase in myocardial oxygen consumption (such as paroxysmal tachycardia, anemia, hypoxia, congestive heart failure), and the patients were younger than in the Gerstenblith study. In a 12-week follow-up, 6.7 percent had experienced death or acute myocardial infarction as compared to 10.1 percent in a control placebo group. The death rate in the control group of patients was 3.3 percent during the 3-month study period. These rates, with or without drug, are substantially higher than in patients with stable angina pectoris.

The information available regarding prognosis of patients with the unstable angina syndromes can be summarized. Clinical recognition and *prompt attention* to *evaluation and therapy are of critical importance in patients with new onset or a change in symptoms since the incidence of sudden cardiac death and myocardial infarction in the 3 to 6 months following onset of an unstable anginal syndrome is higher than in stable patients.* Patients exeriencing this presentation of atherosclerotic coronary heart disease represent a broad spectrum. Some will have had stable angina pectoris and/or previous myocardial infarction while others will be experiencing their first manifestation of disease. A higher incidence of left main coronary disease may be present in patients with unstable syndromes. Several studies have reported a 10 to 15 percent incidence of left main coronary artery obstruction which is higher than it is in most reports of stable angina pectoris. Patients who experience ST-segment elevation during episodes or who have episodes persist despite excellent drug therapy or who have had previous symptomatic ischemic heart disease tend to have a worse prognosis than those without such features. Left ventricular function is an important prognostic factor. Finally, the unstable state is a transient phase and judged to persist 3 to 4 months in most patients, following which the patient develops stable angina, and/or becomes asymptomatic. The prognosis then becomes the prognosis of the new clinical subset. A most intriguing area of current research concerns hypotheses which might explain why patients enter the unstable phase of disease.

Prinzmetal's variant angina[32] deserves comment for historical and pathophysiological reasons. A variety of terms have been utilized, but these patients represent an unstable angina subset. These patients have ST-segment elevation during attacks not precipitated by increase in myocardial oxygen demand. These episodes are due to coronary spasm. Coronary spasm is not unique to Prinzmetal's angina and may occur in a variety of other unstable angina states, and also as a prelude to myocardial infarction. Arteriographic study may reveal normal vessels. However, a review of 300 cases of Prinzmetal's angina reported revealed that more than 50 percent of the patients had advanced coronary atherosclerosis. Hence, as is true with any clinical descriptor, the subset of Prinzmetal's variant angina has multiple subsets within it. The first 3 months following the onset of Prinzmetal's angina is a hazardous time. During this period the incidence of sudden death or myocardial infarction is high and has been reported to be 18 percent in 132 patients studied by Waters.[270] The more severe the coronary atherosclerosis, the more disturbed the left ventricular dysfunction, and the less the response to appropriate therapy, the worse the prognosis. The most intriguing aspect of Prinzmetal's variant angina is its cyclic nature. Regardless of the background anatomic features, the disease is often phasic, and when patients are in a period of remission, even ergonovine infusions will not provoke spasm and ST-T changes. Alternatively, many of the episodes while the patients are in the active phase of their disease are asymptomatic since monitoring discloses ST-segment elevation unaccompanied by any symptoms.

An additional large unstable subset of patients comprises those who have isolated, sometimes single, episodes of *prolonged ischemic discomfort* without objective evidence of myocardial infarction. These patients are frequently admitted to coronary care units to "rule out myocardial infarction." Although problems may exist in being confident that these isolated episodes of chest discomfort are of ischemic myocardial origin, if that can be established, the data available indicate that the mortality rate and incidence of myocardial infarction in this group, at 1 to 2 years following the episodes, are very similar to those of patients who are discharged following recovery from a myocardial infarction (discussed in subsequent sections).[271,272]

Coronary Atherosclerosis with Irreversible Myocardial Ischemia and Necrosis

The prognosis in the subsets of irreversible myocardial ischemia and necrosis is best considered by dividing the problem into three phases: very early profound ischemia, evolving infarction, and completed infarction.

Very Early Profound Ischemia

The term *heart attack,* instead of myocardial infarction, is used for the earliest phase since most patients who die in the first few minutes or several hours after the onset of an attack may not have myocardial necrosis demonstrable by current routine techniques. Most die of a catastrophic arrhythmia, primarily ventricular fibrillation, prior to the development of overt necrosis; some die with overwhelming pulmonary edema and shock. Lethal arrhythmias due to ischemia are as much a cause of death as is acute myocardial infarction (necrosis) (see section below on sudden cardiac death and Chap. 32).

In a careful study in Edinburgh, it was determined that of patients destined to die within 30 days subsequent to an acute heart attack, nearly 50 percent will do so in the first 1 to 2 h after onset of the episode, and 70 to 80 percent in the first 24 h. A reasonable statistic is a 30 to 40 percent total mortality rate at 30 days. Hence, as many as 20 of every 100 patients with an acute heart attack die in 1 to 2 h, often before reaching a medical facility.[271,272]

This statistic and the pattern of deaths make it apparent that coronary care unit mortality statistics have little meaning and will vary widely unless the time between the onset of the patient's complaint and arrival at the coronary care unit is known. If admission to the coronary care unit is delayed for some hours, the period of highest mortality is passed, and the mortality in such a coronary care unit will be lower than in a unit whose location and/or admitting arrangements allow arrival of patients very early following the onset of symptoms.

Evolving Myocardial Infarction

The definition of evolving infarction has become very important since thrombolytic therapy has been introduced and surgical intervention (coronary bypass) has been used by a few surgeons. While it is understood that the evolution of an infarction may take place over several days, it is useful to divide the period into the first 4 to 6 h and the subsequent period, because thrombolytic therapy and early surgery should salvage more muscle during the early period of ischemia than later, when more necrosis has developed. The discussion that follows does not take into account the benefit or harm that could occur with the use of thrombolytic therapy or early bypass surgery since more data are needed to determine the influence of these treatments on the prognosis.

The principal determinants of mortality rate after the patient arrives in the emergency room or coronary care unit are shown in Table 45-4. Infarct size and left ventricular function are most important. Past myocardial infarction and older age are also powerful prognostic factors. No clinical technique is available to estimate the extent of infarction precisely, but a combination of clinical and laboratory data which are routinely obtained can help in estimating prognosis. Many studies have utilized clinical observations and simple laboratory tests to estimate prognosis, but these must be considered relatively nonspecific and are of assistance in estimating prognosis only insofar as they indirectly relate to the items in Table 45-4.

The pain and/or discomfort of acute infarction are important in helping to establish the diagnosis, but the ischemic discomfort per se is of no major prognostic significance. *Many patients with extensive and even fatal infarction have little discomfort, sometimes none whatsoever (particularly the elderly).* In addition, other problems during the course of infarction may produce chest discomfort. Such complicating factors include pulmonary embolism, pericarditis, and upper-gastrointestinal disease, especially peptic ulcer problems.

Cardiac arrhythmias are of enormous importance, but there is uncertainty concerning the prognostic implications of arrhythmias. The arrhythmias that occur with advanced left ventricular failure and are associated with other evidence of extensive infarction, including intraventricular conduction defects, do not have independent additional prognostic significance. Similarly, so-called primary ventricular fibrillation, which occurs early in the course of infarction without associated left ventricular dysfunction and responds promptly to defibrillation in the coronary care unit, does not measurably worsen the prognosis. The arguments concerning arrhythmia as an independent prognostic factor in the relationship of arrhythmia to myocardial infarction size have been summarized by Cox.[151] Since most arrhythmias are reasonably easily controlled with currently available therapy and those not readily controlled often have their genesis in a large infarct, usually associated with left ventricular dysfunction, it seems probable that arrhythmias per se are not important prognostic determinants in evolving myocardial infarction. There are occasional spectacular exceptions in patients who otherwise are judged to have a favorable prognosis but experience refractory ventricular arrhythmias and die as a consequence of them.

TABLE 45-4 Prognostic Determinants: Evolving Myocardial Infarction

Infarct size and ventricular function
Clinical manifestations (especially left ventricular dysfunction)
Electrocardiographic changes (especially location of infarct and conduction defects)
Peak enzyme levels
Blood pressure
Previous infarction and scarring
Angina pectoris of more than 3 months' duration
Age
Infarct extension
Heart size (and left ventricular hypertrophy)
Associated diseases
Diabetes
Hypertension
Pulmonary disease

Serial electrocardiographic studies may provide additional insights into infarct size. Transmural infarction denotes larger areas of necrosis than subendocardial infarction. Transmural anterior infarction tends to result in larger infarcts than transmural inferior infarction. The degree of ST-segment elevation and the number of leads with ST-segment elevation in initial tracings give a crude estimate of the infarct size and presage the development of Q waves and eventual scarring. However, past disease, the presence of pericarditis, occasional electrolyte disturbances, and the exact time at which the ECG is recorded all influence the information obtained. Even with complicated techniques and sophisticated analyses, involving extensive mapping using multiple precordial leads, no easily applicable reliable method for clinical use has evolved.

Multiple studies have shown that the peak enzyme level is roughly correlated with infarct size.[155,273] As a clinically useful prognostic feature, a markedly elevated (five or six times normal) value indicates a large infarct and is associated with more frequent complications and higher mortality. On the other hand, a lower value does not necessarily guarantee a favorable prognosis, a matter which would logically follow from considering the items in Table 45-4, which include past infarction and age and infarct extension as important prognostic factors.

Other clinical findings, including a pericardial friction rub, leukocytosis greater than 20,000 per cubic millimeter, and high fever (102° to 103° without complicating cause) are features indicating poor prognosis. Since these features accompany evidence of large transmural infarction and/or congestive heart failure, they are prognostic indicators, but only when considered in light of the total picture.

Increasing age has an important adverse effect on prognosis. Patients over the age of 70 with transmural infarction have a prohibitively high mortality rate, more than 50 percent in a number of series. A variety of disease states, particularly diabetes mellitus (primarily in patients requiring insulin), hypertension, and chronic pulmonary disease, tend to worsen prognosis by producing altered myocardial metabolism or hypoxia, and/or by increasing myocardial oxygen requirements.

Completed Myocardial Infarction[274–277]

Most of the myocardial damage has been done by 6 h after the onset of chest discomfort due to myocardial ischemia. Evolution of the infarct continues but with less shift of ischemia to either normal or necrotic tissue. An infarct is said to be "complete" after 6 h although additional evolutionary changes continue for some days.

The 9 to 12 months following myocardial infarction is a hazardous period. A 6 to 10 percent mortality rate occurs, with most deaths in the first 6 months. In the second and third year following acute myocardial infarction mortality rate is reduced to 3 to 4 percent per year. Extensive investigation of patients 2 to 4 weeks post infarction has clarified the factors which allow a prediction of long-term prognosis.

Treadmill exercise testing in the early postinfarction period is popular and useful. Multiple studies indicate that ST-segment depression and angina during exercise and/or reduced exercise tolerance connote a poor prognosis. A study of 210 patients[103] showed a favorable prognosis if no ST-segment depression was present (2.1 percent mortality rate in the year following infarction) and an extremely high, 27 percent, mortality rate in the 64 patients with ST-segment depression.

Multiple studies have indicated that left ventricular function is a powerful determinant of postmyocardial infarction outcome. The study by a group of Spanish investigators[278] is particularly instructive. The ejection fraction as judged by angiography was the most powerful predictor of 5-year outcome. Patients who had a resting ejection fraction of greater than 50 percent had an extremely low mortality rate while there was increasing mortality as resting ejection fraction reduced. Although the extent of coronary atherosclerotic abnormality was additive, the ejection fraction was a much more powerful discriminator than angiographic abnormality. Figure 45-5 illustrates the point.

In a multicenter study involving 866 patients[279] careful postinfarction assessment disclosed four descriptors that separated patients into widely disparate prognostic groups. Multiple descriptors were studied, but an ejection fraction of less than 40 percent, ventricular premature beats more than 10 per hour, rales in the upper-lung fields during the course of the acute infarction, and New York Heart Association functional class II to IV (old classification) *before* admission were the additive, independent predictive factors. Ejection fraction less than 40 percent was the single most powerful item. One-third of the patients had none of the four factors present, and their mortality rate during the 2 years following the myocardial infarction was less than 3 percent. Figure 45-6 summarizes the data. Although some stud-

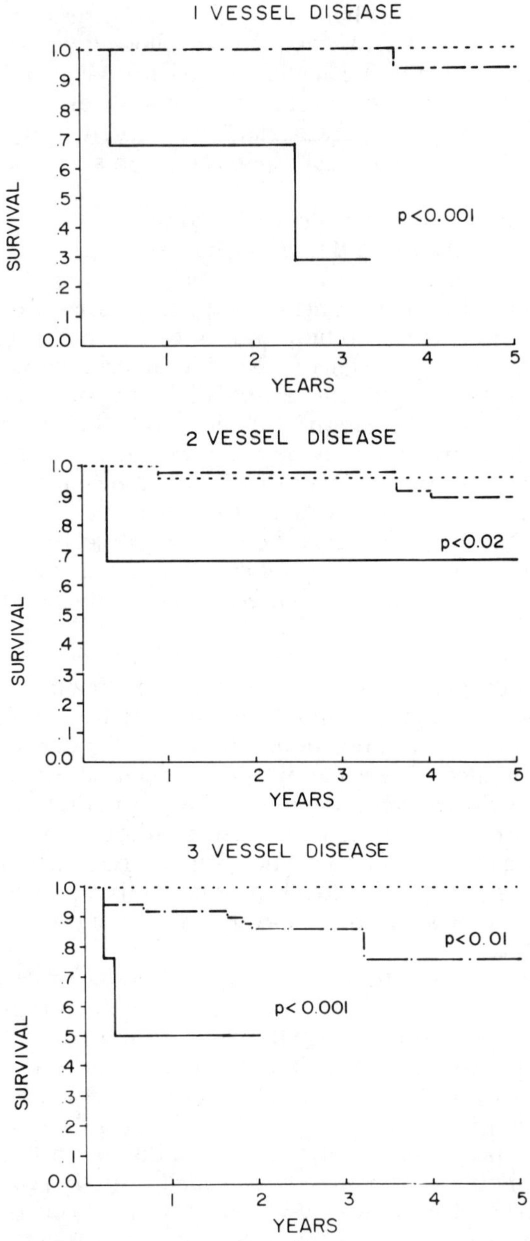

FIGURE 45-5 The relation among coronary atherosclerosis, resting ejection fraction, and 5-year survival in 241 patients evaluated following recovery from acute myocardial infarction. P values represent differences (log-rank test) between the group with an ejection fraction of 50 percent and the other two groups. Ejection fraction > 50 percent = ----; ejection fraction 21–49 percent = • - • -; ejection fraction < 21 percent = ———. *(From G. Sanz, A. Castañer, A. Betriu, et al., Determinants of Prognosis in Survivors of Myocardial Infarction, N. Engl. J. Med., 306:1065, 1982. Abstracted by permission of The New England Journal of Medicine and the author.)*

ies have shown angina pectoris in the early postinfarction period discriminates between those who survive long-term and those who die, this symptom did not differentiate between the groups in this study; perhaps again emphasizing the importance of objective over subjective data.

Further refinement and extension of this risk stratification concept has been attempted utilizing

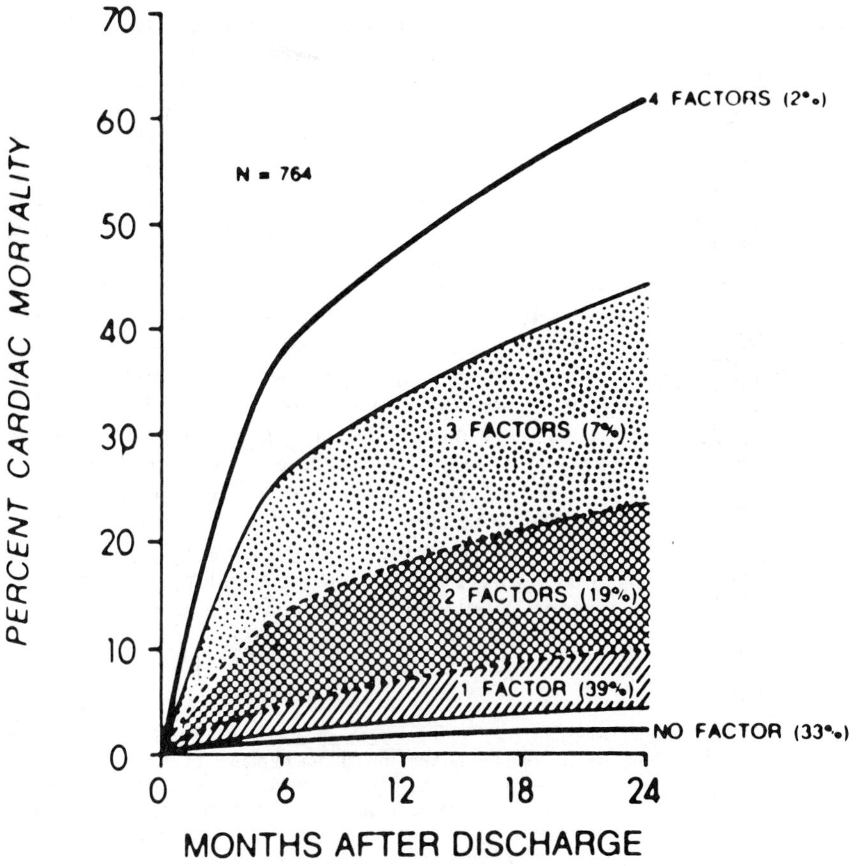

FIGURE 45-6 Risk stratification in 764 (of 866) patients with completed myocardial infarction. Mortality 2 years following myocardial infarction varied from 3 percent, for those with none of the factors, to 60 percent if all four factors were present. The four risk factors were (old) New York Heart Association function class II through IV before admission, pulmonary rales in the upper lung zones during evolving infarction, occurrence of 10 or more ventricular ectopic depolarizations per hour, and a radionuclide ejection fraction below 0.40. The data were obtained during the convalescence period and prior to hospital discharge. The numbers in parentheses denote the percentage of the population with the specified number of factors. (*From Multicenter Postinfarction Research Group, Risk Stratification and Survival after Myocardial Infarction, N. Engl. J. Med., 309:331, 1983. Abstracted by permission of The New England Journal of Medicine and the author.*)

radionuclide techniques.[169,174] Using ^{201}Tl scintigraphy, high-risk postinfarction patients can be identified by the development of more than one discrete defect, redistribution, or increased lung uptake. Using ^{99m}Tc-labeled red blood cells, exercise-induced reduction in ejection fraction and/or an estimate of contractile state have been associated with high risk of events. However, patients have generally been selected, and the numbers of patients involved have been relatively small. The critical item may be an objective estimate of ischemia and ventricular function during exercise rather than the specific technique or endpoint used. The best endpoints are those that are objective and quantitative, and this makes radionuclide studies appealing. There are interpretative problems with these studies. ^{201}Tl studies are more specific than Tc-labeled blood pool studies. Whether data from such studies add independent prognostic information to more simply and less expensively obtained studies seems problematic.

The information concerning prediction of outcome in the completed postinfarction period can be summarized as follows. Left ventricular function and objective evidence of ischemia as judged by exercise testing are the most important determinants. It has been difficult to differentiate the contribution of ventricular ectopy from these two items, but it appears to be an independent additive factor. Preexisting disease, particularly myocardial infarction, and the occurrence of heart failure during the acute infarction are additive factors. When all factors are taken into account, the extent of coronary atherosclerosis on arteriography appears to be a relatively weak contributing factor. Perhaps this is not surprising since a majority, usually 60 to 70 percent, of cases who have suffered myocardial infarction have so-called two- or three-vessel disease, so one would not anticipate this to be a highly discriminatory factor. Refinements in the arteriographic classification of disease would enhance the prognostic value of this factor. Additional items such as age, diabetes, cardiomegaly, and hypertension aid in prognosis.

Complicated Infarction

It is not simple to differentiate uncomplicated myocardial infarction from complicated infarction in many instances. A patient who is pursuing an uncomplicated course may quickly experience an important new event, or some subtle event, not previously appreciated, may become apparent indicating the patient is in a high-risk group. The degree of left ventricular dysfunction may not be easily discernible by bedside examination.

Several investigators have attempted to utilize the multiplicity and complexity of features involved in estimating prognosis in acute infarction by developing a prognostic index which incorporates those factors that have greatest importance and are additive. In such analyses, objective data are given preference over subjective data (e.g., ECG changes in

TABLE 45-5 Discriminant Analysis in a Prognostic Index

Factor	X	Y
Age (yr) (X_1, Y_1):		
<50	0.2	3.9
50–59	0.4	
60–69	0.6	
70–79	0.8	
80–89	1.0	
Position of infarct (X_2, Y_2):		
Anterior transmural	1.0	2.8
Left bundle branch block	1.0	
Posterior transmural	0.7	
Anterior subendocardial	0.3	
Posterior subendocardial	0.3	
Admission systolic blood pressure (mmHg) (X_3, Y_3):		
<55	1.0	10.0
55–64	0.7	
65–74	0.6	
75–84	0.5	
85–94	0.4	
95–104	0.3	
105–114	0.2	
115–125	0.1	
⩾125	0	
Heart size (X_4, Y_4):		
Normal	0	1.5
Doubtfully enlarged	0.5	
Definitely enlarged	1.0	
Lung fields (X_5, Y_5):		
Normal	0	3.3
Venous congestion	0.3	
Interstitial edema	0.6	
Pulmonary edema	1.0	
Previous ischemia (X_6, Y_6):		
No ischemia	0	0.4
Previous angina or infarction	1	

Note: See explanation in text.
Source: R. M. Norris, P. W. T. Brandt, D. E. Caughey, A. J. Lee, and P. J. Scott, A New Coronary Prognostic Index, *Lancet,* 1:274, 1969. Reproduced with permission from the publisher and author.

preference to pain), quantitative information over semiquantitative information (congestion on chest x-ray, or wedge pressure, in preference to rales), and permanent findings over transient features (e.g., the presence of bundle branch block over rhythm disturbances).

The study of Norris and his colleagues[274] illustrates the approach of assessing major prognostic factors by discriminant analysis (Table 45-5 and Fig. 45-7). Six factors obtained on admission to the coronary care unit were selected from several hundred which had been recorded, because they had proved to be additive in establishing prognosis. Sophisticated analysis of the data gives a numerical weighting (X) from 0 (absent) to 1. Each of the six items is further weighted according to the effect it has on mortality (Y). The prognostic index is arrived at by adding the values of the products XY, i.e., $X_1Y_1 \pm \cdots = X_nY_n$ (prognostic index).

To illustrate the use of the index, two patients are described. Consider a 70-year-old man with anterior transmural myocardial infarction, systolic blood pressure of 100 mmHg, enlarged heart, and interstitial edema on x-ray who is known to have had mild angina for 2 years. He has no rales, is free of pain, and clinically looks stable and satisfactory. He is judged to be "much younger" than his stated age. Yet, utilizing the prognostic index, his score is 12.8, and his chances of death are 70 to 80 percent. Alternatively, consider a 40-year-old man without previous angina and with a blood pressure of 110 mmHg, inferior myocardial infarction with complete heart block, and nodal rhythm with rate of 60 who also looks satisfactory. His score is 4.7, and his chances of death are much less than 10 percent.

More recently, schemes to assess left ventricular function, clinically and hemodynamically, have been used to estimate prognosis. These approaches follow directly from the relationship between the extent of left ventricular dysfunction and extent of myocardial necrosis and scarring.

FIGURE 45-7 Numbers of individuals and hospital mortality in six groups of patients with myocardial infarction of increasing severity as assessed by the coronary prognostic index. (*From R. M. Norris, P. W. T. Brandt, D. E. Caughey, A. J. Lee, and P. J. Scott, A New Coronary Prognostic Index,* Lancet, *1:277, 1969. Reproduced with permission from the publisher and author.*)

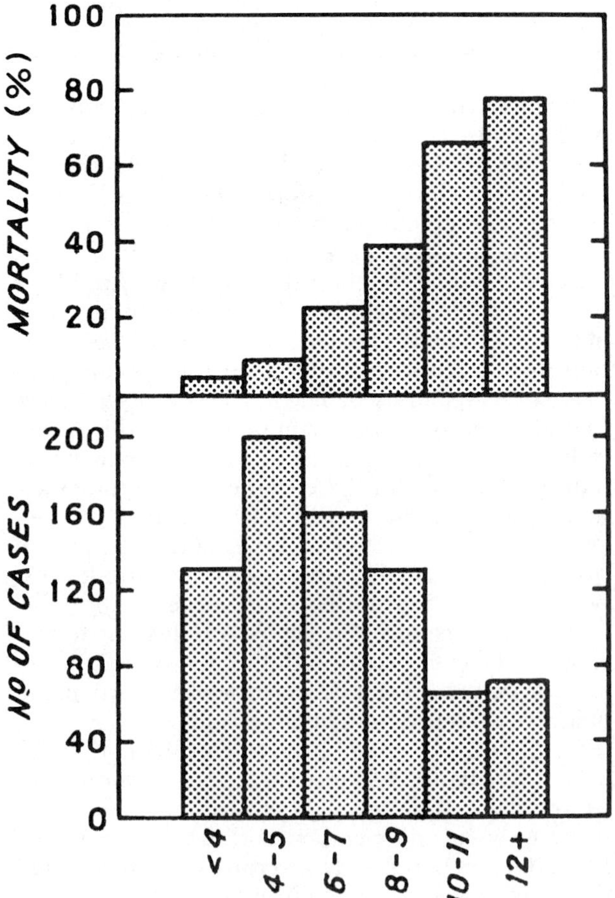

TABLE 45-6 Mortality Rates in Clinical and Hemodynamic Subsets

Subset	Pulmonary Congestion*	Peripheral Hypoperfusion†	% Mortality	
			Clinical	Hemodynamic
I	−	−	1	3
II	+	−	11	9
III	−	+	18	23
IV	+	+	60	51

*Pulmonary-capillary pressure >18 mmHg.
†Cardiac index < 2.2 liters/min/m^2.
Source: J. S. Forrester, G. Diamond, K. Chatterjee, and H. J. C. Swan, Medical Therapy of Acute Myocardial Infarction by Application of Hemodynamic Subsets (First of Two Parts), *N. Engl. J. Med.*, 295(24):1361, 1976. Abstracted by permission of *The New England Journal of Medicine* and the author.

Table 45-6 provides a combination of clinical descriptors and hemodynamic measurements which relate to short-term (30-day) prognosis. Forrester and colleagues[275] collected these data some years ago. It is possible that certain newer approaches and more vigorous drug therapy may have improved prognosis in some groups, but the general trends which are characterized remain correct.

Physicians have long appreciated that a significant proportion of patients with acute myocardial infarction suffer a "recurrent" infarction or "extension" within a few hours or several days. Recent studies utilizing careful serial enzyme and electrocardiographic methods in small numbers of patients indicate that extension is extremely common, possibly affecting 30 to 50 percent of cases in the first week following infarcts.[276,277] This unexpectedly high incidence of infarct extension may be related to case selection. However, it is reasonable to suspect that extension is more common than casual clinical impressions suggest. Diagnosing myocardial extension is not always simple since remodeling of infarct and infarct expansion may occur and be a confounding factor.

Many of the complications that occur in myocardial infarction can be related to the prognostic factors that have already been discussed.[169,174,278,279] However, there are many additional specific complications. The appearance, usually during the first week, of a loud systolic murmur which is associated with the development of acute left ventricular failure in a patient with acute myocardial infarction always arouses a great interest. This is most likely to be a ventricular septal defect, although a rupture of a papillary muscle (or part of it) is an alternative explanation. Probably less than 1 percent of patients have these complications. Both papillary muscle rupture and ventricular septal defect are potentially amenable to surgical therapy, but without surgery, both carry an extremely poor prognosis, with mortality rate in the range of 80 to 90 percent in the several weeks following the event. Interestingly, papillary muscle rupture can occur in a setting of less extensive myocardial infarction than ventricular septal rupture, and the prognosis is better if early surgical intervention is undertaken. The management of ruptured ventricular septum requires considerable judgment and individualization, and is discussed later in this chapter.

Sudden Death

Sudden death is a major consideration when discussing the prognosis of atherosclerotic coronary heart disease since more than half the patients with known ischemic heart disease die suddenly. Of all the patients presenting with ischemic heart disease, sudden death is the initial and final event in nearly one-third. Many definitions for sudden death have been proposed; unexpected cardiac death in a patient with or without preexisting disease within 1 h of having been free of symptoms is a reasonable description. Estimates vary, but it is possible as many as 400,000 sudden cardiac deaths occur in the United States each year. The overwhelming majority are due to atherosclerotic coronary heart disease. The topic is an unusually complex one. In Chap. 32 the matter is considered in detail and the multiple mechanisms and the etiologies involved are discussed.

Most patients with ischemic heart disease who suffer sudden cardiac death have extensive coronary arteriosclerosis, frequently associated with ventricular scarring. Epidemiologic and postmortem studies support this view even when clinical evidence of preexisting atherosclerotic coronary artery disease or prodromal symptoms is absent. Unlike patients who experience myocardial infarction, where a large majority have prodromal symptoms, patients with sudden cardiac death infrequently experience prodromal symptoms. Obviously, these are difficult data to obtain.

The majority of sudden cardiac deaths occur outside the hospital, but valuable information has been provided by an extensive communitywide program of resuscitation in Seattle, Washington. This program demonstrated that the majority of patients who suffer sudden cardiac death outside the hospital do not have myocardial infarction and that there is a high propensity for suffering recurrent sudden cardiac death after the resuscitation if myocardial necrosis is not found. In survivors of out-of-hospital sudden cardiac death, the 1-year mortality rate is 4 percent if acute myocardial infarction occurred compared to 26 percent for the entire group.[280] This interesting statistic might be predicted on the basis of coronary care unit experience, where so-called primary ventricular fibrillation, occurring very early in the course of acute myocardial infarction and unaccompanied by other complications of ventricular dysfunction, does not carry an ominous long-term prognosis when treated promptly. The high incidence of recurrent ventricular fibrillation in the year following resuscitation in noninfarction patients is likely associated with chronic advanced ventricular dysfunction.

Attempts to improve our ability to predict which patients might suffer cardiac death, particularly as the first manifestation of their ischemic heart disease, have resulted in the hypothesis that the risk factors for sudden cardiac death are the same as those for other manifestations of atherosclerotic coronary heart disease. However, because only a minority, probably less than 20 percent, of patients with sudden cardiac death have an acute myocardial infarction at postmortem examination, it seems likely that additional "risk factors" beyond those customarily considered are important in this subset of patients. Epidemiologic studies have not disclosed what they might be, although premature ventricular depolarizations have been intensively studied as discussed below.

The other major subset of patients suffering sudden cardiac death are those who have previously manifested and/or currently experience symptomatic ischemic heart disease. The items listed in Table 45-3 apply to this subset of patients. Multiple studies have demonstrated that left ventricular dysfunction and/or clinical symptoms accompanying left ventricular dysfunction are powerful predictors of sudden cardiac death. In groups of patients with manifest disease and poor ventricular function, the presence of premature ventricular depolarizations, particularly complex forms, is an independent additive feature in most studies. Although it has been complicated to establish premature ventricular depolarization as an independent risk factor, there is now general agreement that such is the case. To date, the important issues concerning the effectiveness of antiarrhythmic drugs in suppressing premature ventricular depolarizations and the influence of such suppression on the incidence of sudden cardiac death have not been resolved and are currently the subject of intense investigation.

Ischemic Cardiomyopathy

The term *ischemic cardiomyopathy* is used in reference to a subset of patients in whom atherosclerotic coronary heart disease is manifested primarily, or exclusively, by myocardial dysfunction and congestive heart failure. It is caused by diffuse fibrosis and/or multiple infarctions.

It is important to differentiate between the subsets of patients with ischemic heart disease and congestive failure and those with ischemic cardiomyopathy. Patients with an important degree of mitral regurgitation, those with discrete aneurysms, and patients who have some degree of myocardial scarring but who manifest an important element of dyspnea accompanying effort angina pectoris must be identified. Such patients benefit from medical therapies, and particularly surgical interventions, which are not appropriate for patients who have ischemic cardiomyopathy.

Some patients with ischemic cardiomyopathy present with congestive heart failure indistinguishable from that of an idiopathic primary cardiomyopathy. This rare presentation is related to patchy fibrosis associated with diffuse severe coronary atherosclerosis in the absence of transmural myocardial infarction. Clinically, it is suspected some such patients may have two conditions, diffuse coronary atherosclerosis and an independent cardiomyopathy.

The more common manifestation of ischemic cardiomyopathy occurs following one, or more frequently multiple, myocardial infarctions with major areas of regional scars. It is possible that this condition is becoming more common in recent years. It is suspected that the use of coronary bypass surgery, which prolongs life in some subsets, may provide an opportunity for developing multiple small myocardial infarctions and areas of fibrosis which eventuate in ischemic cardiomyopathy.

Acknowledging that the term *ischemic cardiomyopathy* encompasses multiple subsets, even after excluding complications not related primarily to left ventricular scarring, the prognosis in these subsets is the poorest of any of the manifestations of atherosclerotic coronary heart disease. Although appreciated for many years, the point has been emphasized since angiographic and functional studies have been systematically carried out during the last 20 years. Studies on relatively large numbers of patients reported in the mid-1970s indicated that conspicuously poor ventricular function, estimated from angiographic studies or left ventricular diastolic pressure, carried extremely high 5-year mortality rates.[252–255] In patients with so-called single-vessel disease, if there was associated marked global left ventricular dysfunction, the 5-year mortality rate was in excess of 50 percent. In one study, 84 percent of the patients were dead 5 years after presentation if clinical congestive heart failure was utilized as the descriptor.[252] In another study, a 31 percent 1-year mortality rate was reported.[281]

A recent series of patients[282] with left ventricular resting ejection fraction less than 36 percent has been reported from the CASS study. In this study 420 patients were followed with medical therapy, approximately one-half for a minimum of 3 years. Analyses of the data are complicated by the fact that slightly more than 50 percent had angina as a primary symptom, and only 20 percent reported congestive heart failure as the principal symptom. In slightly more than 25 percent, the angina was class III or class IV. At a 3-year follow-up, 68 percent of patients who had chest discomfort and severe left ventricular dysfunction survived, while only 55 percent who had principally dyspnea or fatigue (ischemic cardiomyopathy as defined in the above paragraph) survived. Too few patients are reported to allow meaningful survival data beyond 3 years. Despite complexities in interpretation, the extremely poor prognosis is clear. In addition, symptoms are unremitting and progressive when clinical congestive failure is present.

Patients with ischemic cardiomyopathy may die as a consequence of unremitting refractory heart failure or recurrent myocardial infarction, but more suffer sudden cardiac death due to ventricular fibrillation. All patients with ischemic cardiomyopathy have ventricular premature depolarizations, often complex forms, but carefully collected data on the independent importance of this feature have not been obtained.

The data available can be summarized. It is important to be specific in the definition of ischemic cardiomyopathy and to exclude patients who have reversible myocardial ischemia, major mitral regurgitation, or discrete aneurysms. Even with such exclusions, some patients with ischemic cardiomyopathy will have diffuse ventricular dysfunction with small scars and patchy fibrosis, while others will have large scarred areas with regions of well-functioning myocardium, usually with compensatory hypertrophy. It is possible that patients with the well-demarcated scars have a better outlook than those with diffuse dysfunction, but rate of survival is very poor, regardless. Most data would suggest that 40 to 50 percent of patients die within 3 years after presentation, and it is suspected that less than 20 percent survive 5 years. The presence of overt clinical congestive heart failure worsens the prognosis in reference to any objective measurement of left ventricular dysfunction such as end-diastolic pressure, ejection fraction, or wall motion abnormalities.

Recognition, Classification, and Treatment of Patients with Atherosclerotic Coronary Heart Disease

The management of patients with atherosclerotic coronary heart disease includes recognition; classification; and treatment. The latter includes medical treatment, percutaneous transluminal coronary angioplasty, and surgical treatment.

Overriding the therapeutic approach to patients with atherosclerotic heart disease is the recognition of a new goal. It is proper now, with the use of recent diagnostic, prognostic, and therapeutic advances, to establish 10- and 15-year plans for patients with atherosclerotic coronary heart disease. These plans should include the relief of symptoms; improvement of long-term survival; and carefully designed follow-up plans. This is very different to the goal of yesteryear, when efforts were made to relieve symptoms but little was done to improve long-term survival, and follow-up plans were haphazardly designed.

General Considerations

The methods used to identify patients with atherosclerotic coronary heart disease have been discussed earlier in this chapter (see "The Clinical Recognition of Subsets"). The methods used to classify patients are discussed below. The definition of the subsets and sub-subsets of coronary disease is discussed later in this chapter. Certain general considerations regarding the treatment of all patients are discussed below, and specific recommendations for each of the subsets and sub-subsets are given after this section.

Classification (see Chap. 6)

As stated many times in this chapter and in Chap. 6, a system of classification is necessary: for accurate *communication* with others; for *clinical research*; and so that *specific treatment* for the subsets can be implemented. While this is necessary in all of medicine, it is especially applicable to the recognition and treatment of patients with atherosclerotic coronary heart disease. There are three types of classification. They are the New York Heart Association classifications; the American Heart Association classification; and the Canadian Cardiovascular Society classification.

The New York Heart Association (NYHA) classification has been changed. The reader should read the prefaces of the seventh[283] and eighth[284] editions of *Nomenclature and Criteria for the Diagnosis of the Heart and Great Vessels* and compare the contents with the preface of the sixth edition of the same book.[285] The old system (proposed in the first six editions of the book) of classifying heart disease included the establishment of the *etiology*, altered *anatomy*, altered *physiology*, and *functional* and *therapeutic* status of the patient. The Criteria Committee of the New York Heart Association made a rather marked change in the seventh edition[283] of their book. They eliminated the *functional* classification and, in its place, substituted *cardiac status and prognosis*. The *old* functional classification was determined only by the symptoms expressed by a patient. Accordingly, patients with angina pectoris and dyspnea due to heart failure were classified according to their symptoms. The *new* New York Heart Association classification *does not* classify patients according to their *symptoms only*. The reason for the change was stated clearly in the seventh edition[283] of *Criteria and Nomenclature*.

The following excerpts are reprinted below with the permission of the New York Heart Association and its criteria committee and Little, Brown and Company (copyright 1973).

> The Functional and Therapeutic Classification of previous editions required that the physician classify the patient's cardiac status on the basis of symptoms alone, without regard to the etiologic, anatomic, or physiologic diagnoses. Although a consideration of symptomatology is essential for a correct physiologic diagnosis, it is now recognized that a classification of cardiac status based on symptoms alone may be misleading. Symptoms may be absent in the presence of serious anatomic and physiologic abnormalities, and the necessity for medical or surgical intervention may not be appreciated. In addition, symptoms may appear only after serious changes have taken place in the heart and lungs, which can prevent an effective attack upon the underlying defect. Further, some therapies may alter the symptoms and the course of the disease only briefly, whereas others may fundamentally change the course of the disease. Recommendations for therapy can rarely be based on a single diagnostic category; the implications of the other two categories also must be considered.
>
> With these considerations in mind, a new classification, Cardiac Status and Prognosis, is presented. This classification should reflect an accurate assessment of each patient based on the etiologic, anatomic, and physiologic diagnoses and on an understanding of the benefits of present therapies.[283]

The New York Heart Association classification is excellent. It is a generic road map for the practicing physician who is called upon to recognize and treat patients with atherosclerotic coronary heart disease. The physician should insert the specific subset of the disease process into the framework of the NYHA classification. The subsets of atherosclerotic coronary heart disease are depicted in Table 45-1. The recognition and treatment of the subsets will be addressed later in this chapter.

The Canadian Cardiovascular Society classification (Table 6-1) has been accepted by the National Heart, Lung and Blood Institute for use in studies involving coronary bypass surgery. The importance of the Canadian Cardiovascular Society classification was brought into sharp focus by Lucien Campeau of Montreal. His summary is reproduced here with the permission of Dr. Campeau, the American Heart Association, Inc., and the journal *Circulation.*[286] Note the comparison he makes with the New York Heart Association classification and the American Heart Association classification.

> The Canadian Cardiovascular Society proposed in 1972 a grading of effort angina which has since been accepted by the U.S.A. National Heart and Lung Institute for their registry on aortocoronary bypass surgery and for their multi-center randomized study on the long-term results of this surgery. This grading system appears to have some advantages over the classification of the severity of angina proposed by the American Heart Association which appeared in the News Section of *Circulation.*
>
> The Canadian Cardiovascular Society's grading of effort angina is in fact the New York Heart Association functional classification, slightly modified and stated in more precise terms in order to assure reproducibility by independent observers (see Table 6-1). Grade I includes patients in whom angina is provoked by strenuous exertion. It is not clear that Functional Class I of the New York Heart Association includes such patients when one reads its definition: "patients with cardiac disease but without resulting limitations of physical activity." The added statement "ordinary physical activity does not cause undue fatigue, palpitations, dyspnea, or anginal pain" may suggest, however, that severe exertion may provoke pain. The Canadian Cardiovascular Society grades II, III, and IV are detailed descriptions of activities characteristic of the New York Heart Association.
>
> The definition of the New York Heart Association class II is the following: "patients with cardiac disease resulting in slight limitation of physical activity. They are comfortable at rest. Ordinary physical activity results in fatigue, palpitation, dyspnea, or angina pain." The New York Heart Association class III includes: "patients with cardiac disease resulting in marked limitation of physical activity. They are comfortable at rest. Less than ordinary physical activity causes fatigue, palpitation, dyspnea, or anginal pain." "Ordinary physical activity," "slight limitation," and "marked limitation" may lead to different interpretations by independent observers. It was therefore felt necessary to incorporate a detailed description of ordinary activities and the circumstances in which they were carried out. The New York Heart Association class IV includes: "patients with cardiac disease resulting in inability to carry on any physical activity without discomfort. Symptoms of cardiac insufficiency or of the anginal syndrome may be present even at rest." It should be stressed that angina at rest is not mandatory in grade IV effort angina of the Canadian Cardiovascular Society grading nor in the New York Heart Association functional class IV ("the anginal syndrome *may* be present even at rest"). In fact rest angina may be found in patients having grade I to III effort angina, although it is usually observed in more severely disabled patients.
>
> The American Heart Association grading of severity of chest pain differs markedly from the functional class of the New York Heart Association and from the grading of effort angina proposed by the Canadian Cardiovascular Society. The American Heart Association category "mild" is equivalent to the Canadian Cardiovascular Society grade I. The category "moderate" encompasses, however, the Canadian Cardiovascular Society grades II and III. The category "severe" requires that the patient has angina at rest. It seems that this prerequisite may create problems in the classification of patients severely limited in their physical activities but without rest angina. The category "moderate" appears too broad; for instance, it does not separate patients who have angina while walking at a regular pace from patients who experience pain while walking briskly or uphill. Furthermore, "ordinary physical activity which can be considered usual and typical of everyday activity for *that* individual patient" does not allow comparison from patient to patient nor does it permit grouping patients in subsets.

The American Heart Association's classification of severity of chest pain includes emotion as a provocating agent. Since angina produced by exertion and that provoked by emotional stress are not always present to the same degree, the Canadian Cardiovascular Society grading system considers angina of effort separately. It should be noted that emotional stress is not mentioned in the functional classification of the New York Heart Association. It was proposed by the Canadian Cardiovascular Society that nonexertional angina be classified in the following manner: (a) at rest (unprovoked), (b) decubitus (lying down, before sleep), (c) nocturnal (during sleep), and (d) with emotional stress.

We agree with Selzer and Cohn that functional classifications, because of their subjective nature, may lead to bias. They may be meaningless if they are not reproducible by independent observers. A detailed description of the physical activities and of other parameters involved becomes mandatory. We recognize, however, that all functional classifications are subjective in their nature and should be complemented by objective means of evaluation.[286]

The further classification of certain specific subsets into *sub-subsets* will be discussed when the specific subset is discussed. For example, further classification of the subset angina pectoris and the subset myocardial infarction will be discussed later in this chapter.

Many readers will believe that too much space has been allocated to the subject of classification. The subject is so basic and so important to physicians who wish to translate what they "learn" from the literature and lectures to the care of their patients that the use of the allocated textbook space seems justified.

Medical Management (General Discussion)

Certain subjects, discussed in detail in the fifth edition of *The Heart,* will not be dealt with here because the subject matter seems to be accepted. Accordingly, the discussions of ambulatory care; hospital care; posthospital care; equipment and drugs for the office, coronary care unit, and emergency clinic, etc.; personnel; logistics; and education have been deleted from this edition of *The Heart.*

The following items have been chosen for general discussion because they seem timely. The reader is referred to Maurice McGregor's excellent discussion "Myocardial Ischemia—Toward Better Use of the Coronary Care Unit" for additional information on this aspect of medical care.[287]

Physical Rest and Exercise (see Chap. 48)

There is some evidence that persons who are physically active all their lives are less likely to develop coronary atherosclerosis than their sedentary friends. This view has led to jogging clubs and many other group endeavors. The scientific benefit of exercise has not been settled. It is accepted that exercise creates a sense of well-being in the individual who exercises. It improves skeletal muscle strength and permits more physical work to be done with less cardiac work and angina pectoris. Exercise assists in controlling body weight. The pulse rate per minute may be less in the trained individual than in the untrained one. There is evidence that exercise alters the blood lipid levels toward a more favorable pattern. However, it has not been proved that exercise alone prevents coronary atherosclerosis or prolongs life, nor has it been proved that exercise encourages the development of new collateral vessels in the myocardium. Individuals who are engaged in an active "fitness" program often discontinue smoking and obtain a normal body weight. This part of the regimen is obviously useful. Whether or not exercising beyond walking a mile or two each day is useful has not been proved.

Many members of the public have been misled into believing that exercise will *guarantee* they will not have coronary atherosclerosis. This clearly is not true. In addition, deaths have occurred in exercise programs. Regrettably, too, patients with mild heart failure or noncoronary heart disease, such as cardiomyopathy, may unwittingly be placed in exercise programs with disastrous results.

The proper management of the various subsets that make up the full spectrum of coronary atherosclerosis demands the view that there is a time for rest and a time for exercise. Patients with stable angina pectoris should be properly studied, and the need for bypass surgery or angioplasty must be determined before an exercise program is planned for them. Patients with any of the subsets of unstable angina pectoris may require a period of carefully defined rest, coronary arteriography, and possible bypass surgery or coronary angioplasty before unnecessary activity is permitted. The patient with prolonged chest pain due to myocardial ischemia (a condition found in a surprising number of patients with atherosclerosis without objective signs of cardiac muscle necrosis) may require a period of rest, coronary arteriography, and possibly bypass surgery or coronary angioplasty followed by rehabilitation. Patients with evidence of cardiac muscle necrosis require a period of "rest" followed by risk assessment studies before exercise can be permitted. Most patients can be rehabilitated and returned to work without participating in a formal rehabilitation program. Some patients require a properly supervised rehabilitation program in order to encourage them to accept an active life-style including work (see Chap. 48). Patients with complications such as heart failure due to infarction require more rest and less exercise than patients without such complications.

Mental Rest and Patient Psychology (see Chaps. 81 and 82)

The role of emotional tension in the development of coronary atherosclerosis is still debated. There is no debate, however, regarding the effect of emotional tension in the precipitation of angina pectoris. There is also a strong belief that emotional tension can precipitate cardiac arrhythmias and perhaps sudden death in certain susceptible individuals. Patients who are socially isolated and experience considerable emotional stress after myocardial infarction have more than four times the risk of death compared to males without these "risk factors."[288]

The onset of symptoms of atherosclerotic coronary heart disease can produce an emotional crisis in the life of many patients. Some of these individuals may become more disabled than their physical abnormalities justify. The problems of denial, fear, dependence, and depression occur in a surprising number of patients with atherosclerotic coronary heart disease, and these psychological problems may go undetected.

The encouragement of emotional stability and the creation of mental rest require that the physician be aware of the problem; recognize that emotional stability and mental rest are important; try to solve emotional problems without tranquilizers or sedatives; listen to the patient; and possess a willingness to serve as a sophisticated counselor.

The discussion prepared for the Coronary Care Committee of the Council of Clinical Cardiology and the Committee on Medical Education of the American Heart Association should be read by all physicians and coronary care nurses. This excellent discussion was written by Thomas P. Hackett, M.D., and Ned Cassem, M.D. A portion of the discussion is reproduced here with permission of the American Heart Association, Inc., and the authors.[289] Interested readers should refer to refs. 290 to 299.

> The three most common *reasons for psychiatric consultations in the CCU are* anxiety, depression, and management problems. Delirium, which is the scourge of most ICU settings—especially surgical—is rare in the CCU. The pattern of requests for psychiatric consultation follows a different distribution for each problem. Anxiety occurs early in the CCU experience, usually on the first or second day. Depression peaks on the third day and management problems have a bimodal distribution with a higher peak coming on the second day and a lower peak emerging on the fourth day.
>
> Although anxiety is the most common problem for which psychiatric assistance is sought in the CCU, it is by no means as prevalent as might be thought. In a study of 100 patients,[300] half white-collar and half blue-collar workers, 25 were rated as showing no anxiety; only five were found to be severely anxious. Forty were rated as moderate and 30 as mildly anxious. There was no relationship between anxiety and the seriousness of the illness or the patient's socioeconomic background. Anxiety usually stems from one of two sources: the prospect of sudden death, or the appearance of death's heralds—breathlessness, severe chest pain, or complications (arrhythmias, cardioversion, pacemaker insertion).
>
> One less obvious symptom that often evokes anxiety is the sensation of weakness. Particularly when the patient has been robust and hardy, being felled by an MI and feeling weak as a consequence frequently provoke marked anxiety. Patients often regard weakness as proof that their illness is irreversible or that heart damage is permanent. As a result it is wise to anticipate that the patient will feel weak and to explain that this is a normal occurrence after myocardial infarction. Sometimes the sense of weakness is increased by sedatives or tranquilizers. When this is the case, the latter can be reduced or discontinued. In the presence of the subjective complaint of weakness, one should always ask if the patient would prefer no tranquilizer.
>
> We have observed that anxiety is difficult to identify in the CCU because patients consciously or unconsciously deny it. Furthermore, physicians do not have time on rounds to make an adequate judgment of the patient's mental condition. For this reason, we believe that mild-to-moderate anxiety is more common than the outward appearance of patients in the unit might suggest. As a consequence we think it advisable to regard every patient as anxious and to treat him accordingly even though supporting evidence may be lacking. Our suggestion is to order a minor tranquilizer for all patients with the promise that it can be discontinued or decreased. Since the CCU patient is commonly an undercomplainer, unlikely to make routine requests of the nurses, he is less apt to get medication on a p.r.n. basis than if it is regularly ordered. We make it a practice, therefore, to order a standard dose of a benzodiazepine upon entrance into the unit and to inform the patient that if he feels too drowsy for comfort, he should tell the nurse, who will either reduce the dose or withhold the medication. Most patients prefer to be medicated, but there is a small percentage who respond poorly to sedation, and they should be allowed the privilege of having none if they desire. However, it is necessary to emphasize to each patient the importance of mental rest and to assure him that tranquilizers are a standard medication. Too many men equate the need for sedation with weakness, and this kind of thinking should be discouraged.
>
> Depression is the second most common reason for psychiatric consultation in the CCU; it is reactive in nature and rarely assumes psychotic proportions. One would expect a patient with MI to be depressed. He has had a brush with death and has temporarily lost his autonomy and well-being. Loss is invariably followed by grieving which is, after all, a form of depression. The standard signs are a saddened face, disinterest or listlessness, pessimism or hopelessness, slowness of speech or movement, or weeping. Combined with this is the frustration of "Why did it happen to me? Why now? It's the time when I am most needed." In the series of 100 cases mentioned earlier, only six patients were severely depressed whereas 36 were moderately depressed and 33 were mildly depressed. As with anxiety, 25 were rated as not depressed. The depression focuses around damaged self-esteem. Discouraging personal consequences of cardiac damage are foreseen. These include the specter of recurrence, reduced earning power, the inevitable restrictions of activity, sexual incompetence, invalidism, and premature old age.
>
> The treatment of both anxiety and depression involves very simple principles which center chiefly around reassurance based upon explanation and education.[301] Explaining the nature of the infarction and the process of repair may seem a useless waste of the doctor's time,

but such is not the case. We found, for example, that whereas both white-collar and blue-collar patients could define and describe infarction in terms of the damage done to the heart, the white-collar patient was far more aware of the process of repair and how the heart could mend. Some blue-collar patients knew nothing about scar formation and pictured the heart as permanently punctured. Providing information can do more to insure peace of mind than any type of medication.

Much of the depression suffered by the post-coronary patient centers around the fear of not being able to resume work or lead an active life. Most patients have little or no idea of what they will face during convalescence and most are dogged by outmoded stereotypes which equate heart disease with automatic and permanent invalidism. Reminding them that many national and community leaders have sustained heart attacks and yet continue to function normally corrects their thinking. One should then go on to specify individuals known to the patient who have successfully completed convalescence and returned to work. The fact that Presidents Johnson and Eisenhower sustained a coronary without leaving the mainstream of life provides an encouraging framework for the future. The information that eight of the runners who completed a recent Boston Marathon had previously sustained an MI is heartening news for the man in the CCU who is mourning what he regards as the loss of his active life.

Aside from correcting misinformation and educating the patient, the best antidote for depression is, in our opinion, a program of physical conditioning.[302] Some hospitals start patients in such a program on the third CCU day.[303] Most reports to date indicate that both anxiety and depression are less troublesome when the patient is actively engaged in physical conditioning. These programs give the patient a sense of participating in his recovery as well as offering something to fill long stretches of vacant hours. They also restore confidence by demonstrating that activity is possible.

Tranquilizers, particularly the benzodiazepine group (chlordiazepoxide, diazepam, and oxazepam) are important elements in the management of anxiety as well as providing for sleep. If one wants to avoid using barbiturates, doubling the dose of a benzodiazepine will often produce a night of sleep.

Unless the patient is delirious or psychotic, the phenothiazines should not be used for sedation because conduction disturbances and sudden death have been reported in conjunction with their use.[304] The tricyclic antidepressants should be used with caution. Conduction difficulties resulting in cardiac irregularities, including sudden death, have been reported with their use.[305] Since the MAO inhibitors can cause fatal hypertensive crisis unless a tyramine-free diet is adhered to rigidly, they must be used carefully in patients with cardiovascular disease. Depression as mentioned earlier is best treated by starting the patient through inpatient physical conditioning. When programs of early mobilization, as described by Hutter et al.,[306] are more widely practiced, we will probably find less depression as a byproduct.*

Of the two chief management problems, the threat to sign out is the more serious. This usually comes early in the hospital stay when the diagnosis of myocardial infarction is still uncertain. Most of these individuals can be persuaded to stay until the results of the tests have been returned. Should the ECG and enzymes reveal an infarction, it is our experience that most people are willing to remain in the hospital. When such is not the case and the patient is competent, we call in the key figures in his life—wife, children, friends, minister—in an attempt to induce him to stay. Should this fail, we do our best to provide care for him at home, always holding open the option of returning to the hospital.

Another common management problem is the male who makes either sexually provocative comments or physical advances to his nurses. On rare occasions, a man might repeatedly expose himself. The reason for these behavioral aberrations is the sense of threat to virility. Following infarction, men often feel impotent and sexually incompetent. The result is an attempt (often unconsciously motivated) to demonstrate their virility as a means of being reassured of their manhood by the nurses' response. Not infrequently patients do this without realizing the effect it has on the nurses. One patient was appalled when told by the psychiatrist that his "dirty jokes" were offending the nurses. He said, "My God! I thought they enjoyed them even more than I did." Other patients may deny making overtures or comments entirely. When this happens, and the behavior continues even after a psychiatric consultation, the best method of intervention is gentle and compassionate confrontation by individual nurses. On the few occasions we have employed this approach it has succeeded. Even when the individual insists on his innocence, as did one patient, his behavior improves.[289]

Principles of Rehabilitation (see Chap. 48)

The physician must prescribe an activity plan for patients based on *an evaluation of the individual patient.* Many patients with atherosclerotic coronary heart disease do too little physical work and avoid all mental problems, while other patients do too much physical work and take on too many mental problems. The physician must help each individual patient live an active, productive, and safe life within the constraints imposed by the disease process itself. Most of the emphasis has been placed on the rehabilitation of the patient with myocardial infarction (see Chap. 48), but the same goals and principles apply to all patients with atherosclerotic coronary heart disease. Many patients have coronary bypass surgery or coronary angioplasty, and they must be included in our rehabilitation efforts.

The rehabilitation of the patient with myocardial infarction is discussed in Chap. 48. Several points will be emphasized here.

- The use and abuse of bed rest for patients with myocardial infarction and the length of time a patient with myocardial infarction should remain in the hospital will be discussed later in the section dealing with myocardial infarction.
- Proper exercise is important (see Chap. 48). The amount that is helpful and the amount of exercise that is harmful varies with the patient. Rechnetizer

*This paragraph was revised from the original by Dr. Hackett.

et al. have emphasized that no improvement in prognosis occurred in patients who engaged in high-intensity exercise compared to those who engaged in low-intensity exercise. Low-intensity exercise improved fitness.[307]

- The physician should indicate by his or her words and manner that most patients can and should return to and continue to work. This includes most patients who have had coronary bypass surgery or coronary angioplasty. A physician should give considerable thought to the matter before signing disability papers for patients with atherosclerotic coronary heart disease since most patients with the disease are not disabled.
- The act of retirement does not always achieve the goal one believes it will. Many patients become restless and depressed. The mental anguish that is created by retirement may provoke unhappiness and more angina pectoris. Many patients, however, enjoy retirement and manage their disease far better in retirement than they did under stressful employment.
- Friedman and Ulmer emphasize that type A personality is harmful. They also emphasize that type A personality can be changed.[308] This, of course, is an important part of the rehabilitation process of some patients.

Diet and Eating

The dietary recommendations made to the patient are very important. In the past it was believed that *obesity* alone was not a risk factor for the development of coronary atherosclerosis as determined by following patients for a few years. There has always been considerable evidence that individuals who are obese are more likely to have diabetes mellitus, abnormal blood lipid levels, and hypertension, which in turn increase the likelihood for atherosclerosis. Recently Hubert et al.[56] have published the follow-up data on Framingham subjects who were followed for 26 years. They presented data to show that obesity *is* an independent risk factor for coronary disease. This only became evident when patients were followed for a long period of time.

There is little doubt that the health of the citizens of the United States would be vastly improved if each person could achieve normal body weight by limiting caloric intake and, when appropriate, increasing caloric expenditure. The obese patient may have less angina pectoris produced by effort when he or she reduces because less cardiac work is required when there is less weight to move around.

The failure to accomplish weight reduction is often due to the physician's inability to translate the need for weight reduction into effective therapy. The mere giving of a diet form will not accomplish the goal. Instruction and follow-up with a dietician, when available, are the best means of achieving weight reduction. This can be accomplished with due regard to the restriction of total calories, total fat, cholesterol, and carbohydrates (see Chap. 42). Two major deterrents to weight reduction are the use of alcohol and a lack of some form of exercise in conjunction with dietary measures. The patient whose appetite is enhanced because of the omission of smoking poses a special problem requiring more intense treatment for smoking withdrawal and obesity.

In summary, weight reduction is important because it creates an improved body image; enhances a sense of well-being; decreases the likelihood of diabetes mellitus; assists in the control of hypertension and abnormal blood lipid levels; decreases the work of the heart, thereby improving angina pectoris when it is present; and is an independent risk factor for coronary disease worth eliminating.

The patient with angina pectoris may detect the discomfort during or immediately after eating a meal. Some patients note that they can walk less far without angina after eating a meal. Such patients should be advised to eat more slowly, to eat less, not to exercise soon after a meal, and to take nitroglycerin before eating and walking.

The patient with prolonged pain due to myocardial ischemia should not be stressed with a regular diet that requires a moderate amount of chewing. Therefore, it is customary to prescribe a low-calorie, liquid, and soft diet. Iced liquids should be avoided, since cold elevates the blood pressure and precipitates myocardial ischemia in some patients.

The prevention of atherosclerotic coronary heart disease is discussed in Chap. 42.[310–312] The principles set forth in the American Heart Association cookbook should be followed.

Unfortunately, the dietary approach to the treatment of atherosclerotic coronary heart disease is often applied in a most unscientific manner. For example, the obese patient may be obsessed with avoidance of eggs and have no interest in decreasing his or her caloric intake. This, of course, is absurd. It is equally absurd to insist that the patient with extensive coronary atherosclerosis with multiple infarctions and chronic heart failure adhere to a strict diet directed toward lowering the blood lipid levels.

Additional problems may be produced by the prescription of exacting diets. Overzealous family members who constantly insist that the patient follow the "orders" laid down by the physician and who follow the "rules" promulgated by the lay and medical press may unwittingly create much unhappiness.

Sexual Activity

Advice regarding sexual activity is very important. Papadopoulos et al. point out that most studies on sexual activity after myocardial infarction have considered only male patients. They emphasize that female patients need advice and counseling regarding their sexual activity after infarction.[313]

Alcohol[309,314] (see Chap. 74)

Ethyl alcohol is a good tranquilizer, but it must not be abused. It contributes to the obesity. Alcohol may precipitate cardiac arrhythmias, especially atrial fibrillation and flutter, in some patients.[315] It decreases myocardial contractility in experimental animals[316] but does not affect a normal person in an adverse manner. However patients with myocardial dysfunction could experience difficulty. The long-term use of alcohol can cause cardiomyopathy, and lesions can be observed in the myocardial cells of such patients. Alcohol causes vasodilation of the skin vessels due to its action on the central nervous system, but it does not increase coronary blood flow. When ethyl alcohol is given to patients with angina pectoris prior to an exercise test, it may prevent angina from occurring during the test but does not prevent the signs of ischemia from occurring in the ECG.[317] The action of the alcohol seems to be related to its depressing action on the brain.[316] Alcohol, in doses that produce inebriation, does not increase the cerebral circulation. Large doses may increase cerebral blood flow but there is a decrease in cerebral uptake of oxygen.[317] Alcohol may result in elevation of the systemic blood pressure in some patients who use a large amount of it over a long period of time.[318]

Takizawa et al. have presented data suggesting that alcohol can induce attacks of variant angina in some patients.[319]

Shook et al. have reported that the ethanol in an intravenous infusion of nitroglycerin may produce alcohol intoxication and could possibly precipitate arrhythmias and myocardial dysfunction in some patients.[320] Shorey et al. reported a patient in whom the ethanol, used as a diluent for the intravenous preparation of nitroglycerin, precipitated the Wernicke-Korsokoff syndrome.[321]

The idea that alcohol may prevent coronary atherosclerosis is not well founded. Apparently, alcohol increases the concentration of high-density lipoproteins (HDL) and decreases the concentration of low-density lipoproteins (LDL).[317] The undesirable effects of alcohol would prohibit its use for such a purpose.

Coffee[322]

The caffeine in coffee and other beverages may produce cardiac arrhythmias.[323] Although a small dose of a xanthine may decrease the heart rate,[324] larger doses in a sensitive person produce sinus tachycardia; an increase in myocardial contractility; premature ventricular contractions; a decrease in preload;[325] a decrease in peripheral resistance; a transient increase in peripheral blood flow;[324,325] and an increase in cerebral resistance and a decrease in cerebral blood flow and oxygen tension of the brain.[326] It also dilates the coronary arteries, but the increase in coronary blood flow does not reliably keep pace with the oxygen demand of the increased work of the heart muscle.[327]

Thelle et al.[328] studied the effect of coffee drinking on blood lipids. They found it increased the level of cholesterol and triglycerides in men and women and lowered the level of HDL cholesterol in women.

Coffee causes sleepless nights in some people and contributes to esophageal reflux by its ability to lower the tone of the distal esophageal sphincter.

Dobymeyer et al. concluded that caffeine produces tachyarrhythmias in susceptible patients.[329]

Tobacco[330–334] (see Chap. 42)

The inhalation of cigarette smoke not only plays a role in atherogenesis but also increases platelet stickiness and provokes coronary spasm.[333] The latter is extremely important in some patients. Daly et al. have concluded that stopping smoking may still be the most effective action in the treatment of patients with coronary heart disease.[334] Deanfield et al. have recently reported that smoking has a direct and harmful effect on the heart. They further observed that smoking prevented the beneficial action of propranolol, atenolol, and nifedipine.[335] Matsukura et al. have reported on the harmful effects of inhaling tobacco smoke that has been exhaled by others (passive smoking).[336]

While almost all patients should be advised to stop the use of tobacco, it is unreasonable to insist that every elderly patient with severe disease discontinue all the things he or she enjoys.

Drugs Used in the Treatment of Atherosclerotic Coronary Heart Disease and Its Complications

It is not possible to discuss in detail all of the drugs that may be used in patients with coronary disease. The details of the pharmacology of drugs used to alter venous and arterial capacitance are discussed in Chap. 88. The pharmacology of antiarrhythmic drugs is discussed in Chap. 89. The pharmacology of beta blockers and calcium antagonists is discussed in Chaps. 90 and 91. The pharmacology of digitalis and nondigitalis inotropic agents is discussed in Chaps. 92 and 93. The pharmacology of diuretics is discussed in Chap. 94. The pharmacology of streptokinase and other anticoagulants is discussed in Chap. 95. The purpose of the section here is to offer the physician quick access to very practical information regarding certain drugs which are commonly used in patients with coronary disease.

• The administration of *oxygen* is recommended for the patient with chest pain due to myocardial ischemia who is treated in the home, office, or in the street. It is difficult to make continuous and accurate observations during the transfer of a patient from the place where he or she is stricken to the facility where definitive care is to be given, and therefore oxygen is prescribed routinely. When the patient is seen in the coronary care unit, one should make a more accurate assessment regarding the need for oxygen therapy.

The definite indication for oxygen therapy is hypoxia. Patients with cyanosis, tachycardia, heart failure, shock, dyspnea, cough, wheezing, respiratory depression, and an increased respiratory rate should be given oxygen. When these conditions are present, the oxygen should be given at a high rate of flow via a mask or, if the patient has chronic obstructive pulmonary disease, via a Venturi mask. Other modes of oxygen delivery are not as satisfactory. Nasal cannulas irritate the nasal passages and are not satisfactory for "mouth breathers" since they may cause gastric dilation. High flows of oxygen may precipitate respiratory failure in some patients with chronic lung disease.

Opinions differ as to whether oxygen therapy should be given to every patient with prolonged chest discomfort due to myocardial ischemia. There are insufficient data to give a definite answer to the question, but it is unlikely that harm could come from such a practice.

Rawles and Kenmure performed a controlled study involving 203 consecutive patients with myocardial infarction. One group received oxygen and the other group received room air by face masks.[337] There was no significant difference in the number of deaths, mean duration of hospital stay, use of narcotic analgesics, systolic time intervals, and various arrhythmias between the oxygen-treated and room air–treated patients. The mean pulmonary artery pressure, the incidence of sinus tachycardia, and the rise in cardiac enzyme levels were higher in the oxygen-treated group. This suggests that the sicker patients received the oxygen.

Hyperbaric oxygen treatment for prolonged myocardial ischemia has not been found to be consistently useful.[338]

• *Tranquilizers and sedatives* should not be used routinely in all patients with angina pectoris or prolonged myocardial ischemia. Every patient does not require such medication, and many patients receive propranolol, opiates, and other drugs that can dull the thought processes and decrease anxiety. On the other hand, each individual patient with angina or prolonged myocardial ischemia (with or without infarct) should be evaluated for anxiety and a judgment made regarding the need for a tranquilizer.

Tranquilizers and sedatives should not be used indefinitely without careful consideration, since the goal is to rehabilitate the patient (including return to work), and such medical "crutches" do not necessarily encourage emotional rehabilitation. The usual response to the long-term use of sedatives and tranquilizers is that they frequently do not solve the problems for which they are given and an increase in dosage is often requested. As a rule, the new dosage schedule also fails to solve the patient's problems.

Diazepam (Valium) may be given orally in a dose of 2.5 mg four times a day. This drug appears to be as effective and as safe as any other drug although there are few data to indicate its superiority over phenobarbital.

A sedative may be needed to encourage sleep while in the hospital but should not be prescribed for home care unless it seems absolutely necessary. A current favorite is *flurazepam hydrochloride* (Dalmane). The dose is 15 to 25 mg given orally at bedtime.

• *Opiates* are not needed for the relief of chronic angina pectoris. By definition angina pectoris is short-lived, usually lasting 3 to 5 min and occasionally 10 to 15 min. Angina is usually relieved by sublingual nitroglycerin. Opiates are usually required to relieve the pain associated with more prolonged myocardial ischemia, including the pain accompanying acute myocardial infarction. In practice we may use nitroglycerin, a beta blocker, a calcium antagonist, streptokinase, and opiates to relieve the pain of prolonged myocardial ischemia. One must not delay the use of an opiate while waiting and hoping that nitroglycerin and other drugs will relieve the pain. Today, with many drugs available to treat myocardial ischemia, it is unfortunate that the use of opiates is often delayed or never adopted.

Morphine sulfate,[339–344] which is frequently administered for the relief of pain associated with myocardial infarction, can produce respiratory depression; significant changes in the function of the cardiovascular system, including arterial hypotension, especially when the patient is in the upright position; a decrease in cardiac output; and depression of AV conduction, which can occasionally contribute to the production of significant heart block.[339–344] Morphine produces a decrease in arterial resistance and increases dilatation of venous channels in the visceral circulations.[345–347] The decrease in preload and afterload tends to improve ventricular function, but the hypotension that accompanies it may decrease coronary blood flow and produce even more myocardial ischemia.

After the administration of morphine to experimental animals, myocardial contractility slowly increases and reaches its peak in about 30 min.[348] This increased inotropism produced by morphine is the result of a sympathoadrenal discharge, and in experimental animals it is blocked by propranolol or by adrenalectomy.[348] Morphine produces little, if any, myocardial depression in the human being. This is the reason it is used for anesthesia in patients undergoing cardiac surgery (Chap. 79).

The intravenous route of administration of an opiate affords quicker relief with a smaller dosage than the intramuscular injection of the drug. The intramuscular injection of the drug may produce a rise in creatine phosphokinase (CK) which can lead one to falsely diagnose a myocardial infarction. In addition, if respiratory depression occurs secondary to intravenously injected narcotic, it can be promptly recognized and managed, whereas the delayed onset of hypoventilation following intramuscular injection may not be recognized. The drug may be given intramuscularly if the patient has mild pain and the diagnosis has been established.

A dose of 10 mg of morphine sulfate may be diluted in a 10- to 20-ml saline solution and given 2 ml at a time to patients with chest pain due to myocardial infarction. One should pause several minutes between the injection of increments to be certain that respiratory depression does not occur. It is advisable to have a morphine antagonist such as naloxone hydrochloride (Narcan) available. Narcan is the preferred antagonist, because it can reverse the respiratory depression of narcotic overdosage without the risk of augmenting or causing a depression of its own.

Hypoxia is common during the early stages of myocardial infarction, and it may be sharply enhanced by the decreased alveolar ventilation that follows the administration of every opiate at any dosage level regardless of the route of administration. Respiratory depression may be enhanced when opiates are combined with other drugs such as phenothiazine derivatives, and the simultaneous administration of such drugs should be discouraged. It should be emphasized that the amplitude of respiratory excursions may be sufficiently diminished to produce hypoxia even though the respiratory rate remains normal. Pain must be relieved, but we must be aware of the risk of creating hypoxia. In this setting, the hypoxia which occurs can predispose to ventricular fibrillation and cardiac standstill.

Since morphine sulfate is vagotonic, atropine sulfate, 0.5 to 1.0 mg, is advised when morphine produces or contributes to bradycardia, nausea, vomiting, AV block, or nodal rhythm. These complications are especially likely to occur if the myocardial damage is posterior or inferior in location.

Meperidine hydrochloride (Demerol) may be used to relieve the pain of myocardial infarction. It has an atropine-like effect, and on occasion it may increase the ventricular rate in patients with atrial flutter or fibrillation. This drug is preferred when there is inferior myocardial infarction and bradycardia. Meperidine hydrochloride is widely used because it is convenient to administer and is claimed to produce less nausea and respiratory depression than morphine. These advantages are not so apparent to us, and we generally prefer morphine sulfate for patients with anterior myocardial infarction because of its superior ability to relieve pain. The intravenous dose of meperidine hydrochloride (Demerol) is 25 to 50 mg. It should be given slowly and repeated in 15 min if necessary for the relief of pain.

All opiates and their derivatives may produce hypotension and shock by decreasing the peripheral arterial vascular resistance and increasing venous pooling. Potent intravenous diuretics or nitrites may accentuate the hypotension. Opiates must be used with great care in patients with chronic pulmonary disease or myxedema.

Patients may have chest pain due to pericarditis or anxiety following myocardial infarction (see discussion on treatment later, in the section "Complications of Myocardial Infarction" and in Chap. 59). Prednisone is needed to relieve the pain of pericarditis, and opiates should not be used. Furthermore, after determining that the patient's discomfort is not due to ischemia, it is proper to explain to the patient that he or she is not having a "new heart attack."

• *Nitrates* are very useful for the treatment of myocardial ischemia due to obstructive coronary disease and coronary artery spasm.[349–351] The pharmacology of nitrates is discussed in Chap. 88.

There are many preparations of nitrates. Certain forms of the drug can be given by inhalation, sublingually, orally, topically, and intravenously. Table 45-7 was prepared by C. Richard Conti and Robert L. Feldman.[352] It is used with the permission of the publisher and authors. The table shows the generic name, chemical structure, preparation, dose, trade name, and dosing frequency of most of the available preparations.

Nitrates increase the size of the coronary arteries; increase coronary blood flow in some, but not all, patients with coronary obstruction; may decrease coronary blood flow in patients with normal arteries; produce peripheral venous dilatation; decrease right atrial and pulmonary artery pressure; decrease the systemic blood pressure; decrease preload and afterload; increase the heart rate; decrease ventricular wall tension; decrease ventricular end-diastolic volume and pressure; may increase or decrease the cardiac output; and produce relaxation of almost all smooth muscle cells.[352]

The *indications* for the use of nitrates are[352] stable angina pectoris due to obstructive coronary disease; unstable angina pectoris due to obstructive coronary disease (intravenous nitroglycerin may be needed); early infarction; coronary spasm; heart failure (see Chap. 21); and hypertension immediately after bypass surgery.

The *contraindications* to the use of nitrates include a history of undesirable side effects of the drug; hypotension and syncope; hypovolemia; increased intracranial pressure; constrictive pericarditis; and idiopathic hypertrophic cardiomyopathy.

The *adverse reactions* to nitrates are[352] headache; syncope; hypotension; tachycardia; and, rarely, bradycardia; prolongation of the effect of pentobarbital anesthesia; methemoglobinemia, which occurs rarely with large doses of intravenous nitroglycerin; rash from the topical use of the drug; and microwave oven burns which have been reported with certain topical preparations.[353]

Nitrates are excellent drugs for the prevention and treatment of ischemic episodes due to coronary disease. They can be used in combination with beta blockers and calcium antagonists. They may also be used in the treatment of heart failure, where they seem to be most effective when combined with other drugs such as hydralazine (Apresoline).

• *Beta-adrenoceptor blocking drugs* are useful in the treatment of myocardial ischemia, certain arrhyth-

TABLE 45-7 Organic Nitrates Available for Clinical Use

Generic Name	Chemical Structure	Preparation	Dose	Trade Name	Dosing Frequency
Amyl nitrite	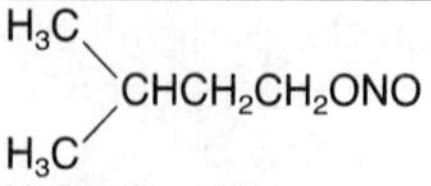	Inhalation	0.18 or 0.3 ml	Vaporale	
Glycerol trinitrate	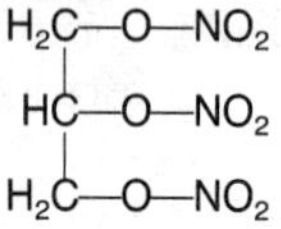	Parenteral	50–100 μg/ml	Nitro-bid IV, Nitroglycerin injection, Nitrostat IV, Tridil	2–4 min (half-life)
		Sublingual	0.15,0.3,0.4,0.6 mg	USP, Nitro-bid, Nitrol, Nitrostat	5–30 min
		Buccal	1,2,5 mg	Susadrin	4–6 h
		Oral	1.3,2.5,6.5,9.0 mg	Nitro-bid, Nitrong, Nitroglycerin capsules, Nitrospan	4–8 h
		Topical	2% over 5,8,10,15,20 cm²	Nitro-bid, Nitrol, and Nitrong ointment, Nitro-disc, Nitro-dur, Transderm-nitro	4–5 h 24–48 h
Isosorbide dinitrate	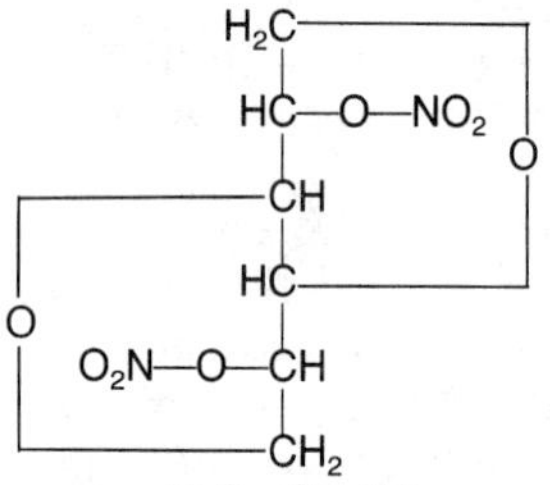	Sublingual	2.5,5 mg	USP, Dilatrate, Iso-bid, Isordil, Laserdil, Sorbide, Sorbitrate	30–60 min
		Chewable	5,10 mg		30–180 min
		Oral	5,10,20,40 mg		2–6 h
Erythrityl tetranitrate	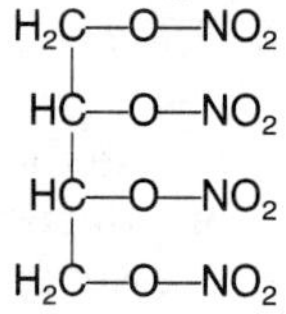	Sublingual	5,10,15 mg	USP, Cardilate	30–60 min
		Oral	10 mg		2–6 h
Pentaerythrityl tetranitrate	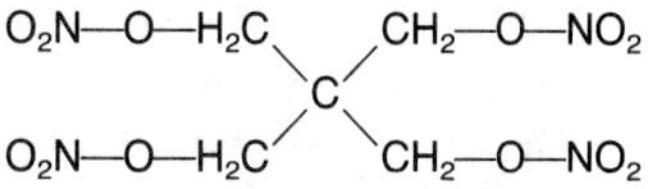	Oral	10,20,30,40,60 mg	USP, Duotrate, Pentritol, Peritrate	4–6 h

Source: C. R. Conti and R. L. Feldman, The Use of Nitrates in the Treatment of Ischemic Heart Disease, in J. W. Hurst (ed.), "Clinical Essays on the Heart," McGraw-Hill Book Company, New York, 1984, vol. 2, p. 4. Reproduced with permission from the publisher and authors.

mias, and hypertension. The pharmacology[354] of beta-adrenoceptor blocking drugs is discussed in Chap. 90.

The names of the drugs, the usual dosage, and the dosing frequency of a few of the drugs are shown in Table 45-8. The table was designed after reading Frishman.[354]

Beta blockers[354] may have a quinidine-like effect or membrane-stabilizing effect on cardiac action potential; may decrease myocardial contractility; decrease the heart rate; decrease the increase in heart rate produced by exercise; may decrease the size of the coronary arteries; may lower the systemic blood pressure; increase atrioventricular conduction time; decrease cardiac output; increase end-diastolic ventricular blood volume and may increase end-diastolic ventricular pressure; and may produce bronchospasm.

The *indications* for the use of beta blockers are:[354] stable and unstable angina pectoris; possibly early in the treatment of myocardial infarction in selected patients (see discussion below); following myocardial infarction; certain forms of hypertension (see Chap. 51); atrial and ventricular arrhythmias (see Chap. 27); hypertrophic cardiomyopathy; and migraine headache.

The *contraindications* to the use of beta blockers are:[354] decrease in myocardial contractility; heart failure; coronary artery spasm; intermittent claudication; bronchospasm; AV block; sick sinus syndrome; hypotension; and a history of adverse reaction to the drugs.

The *adverse reactions* to the drugs are:[354] the precipitation of heart failure, AV block, and the sick sinus node syndrome; coronary spasm; bronchospasm; mental depression; weakness; impotence; and loss of memory; withdrawal of the drugs may precipitate an ischemic event.

The drugs should be used with caution when other drugs such as digitalis or certain calcium antago-

TABLE 45-8 Beta-Adrenergic Blockers Used for the Treatment of Angina Pectoris

Name of Drug	Usual Oral Dose Range	Dosage Frequency*
Atenolol (Tenormin)	50–100 mg	Two times daily
Labetalol (Normodyne, Trandate)	100–400 mg	Three times daily
Metoprolol (Lopressor)	25–100 mg	Four times daily
Nadolol (Corgard)†	40–240 mg	Once daily
Pindolol (Visken)	5–10 mg	Four times daily
Propranolol (Inderal, generic)†	20–80 mg	Four times daily
Propranolol (Inderal-LA)†	40–320 mg	Once daily
Timolol (Blocarden)	5–15 mg	Four times daily

*These are recommended dosing intervals in angina pectoris; however, individual patients may be able to take daily dose less frequently.
†FDA-approved for clinical use in angina pectoris.
Source: Table constructed after reviewing W. H. Frishman, *Clinical Pharmacology of the β-Adrenoceptor Blocking Drugs,* 2d ed., Appleton-Century-Crofts, Norwalk, Connecticut, 1984.

nists, especially verapamil (Calan, Isoptin), are used simultaneously.[354] For example, a certain beta blocker, such as propranolol (Inderal), when used in combination with digitalis and/or verapamil can precipitate AV block; sick sinus syndrome; and hypotension.

Propranolol plus verapamil can produce decreased contractility and precipitate heart failure. On the other hand, propranolol and nitrates or nifedipine (Procardia) when used together have a synergistic effect, and propranolol can blunt the reflex tachycardia produced by nifedipine.

• *Calcium antagonists* may be used for the prevention and treatment of myocardial ischemia due to obstructive coronary disease especially when coronary spasm contributes to the pathophysiology.[355,355a] The drugs may be used in the treatment of hypertension, and one of them, verapamil, can be used to treat atrial arrhythmias and hypertrophic cardiomyopathy.

The pharmacology of the calcium antagonists[355–364] is discussed in Chap. 91.

The calcium antagonists currently available have different actions.[355] Nifedipine, diltiazem (Cardizem), and verapamil increase coronary blood flow by dilating the coronary arteries and improving subendocardial perfusion. All three of the drugs decrease peripheral resistance, but nifedipine is most effective in this regard. In fact, nifedipine may lower the peripheral resistance to the point where there is reflex tachycardia. Verapamil decreases the heart rate more than the other two drugs, and diltiazem decreases the heart rate only slightly. Verapamil decreases myocardial contractility while the other two drugs have little effect on contractility. Verapamil increases AV conduction time and the sinus node rate more than the other two drugs. Diltiazem may do the same but to a lesser degree.

The oral dose of nifedipine is 10 to 40 mg four times a day. The dose of diltiazem is 30 to 90 mg four times a day. The oral dose of verapamil is 80 to 120 mg four times a day (see Table 91-5).

The *indications* for calcium antagonists are:[355] stable[356] and unstable angina pectoris; Prinzmetal's angina;[357] the early phase of infarction; coronary artery spasm; hypertension (nifedipine and diltiazem); atrial flutter and fibrillation (verapamil); idiopathic hypertrophic subaortic stenosis (verapamil).

The *contraindications* are few in number.[355] Verapamil and diltiazem should not be used in patients with the sick sinus syndrome or AV block. Verapamil should be used with great caution or not at all in patients with heart failure.

The *adverse reactions* to the drugs are:[355] edema (nifedipine); mental sluggishness, drowsiness, depression, weakness (all); constipation (verapamil); reflex tachycardia (nifedipine); aggravation of sick sinus syndrome (verapamil and perhaps diltiazem); legs feel "wooden"; constipation (verapamil); and gingival hyperplasia (nifedipine).[365] Diltiazem seems to produce fewer adverse reactions than nifedipine or verapamil.

Schwartz et al. report that the administration of nifedipine does not significantly increase the serum concentration of digoxin as has been reported with verapamil,[356] and Schrager et al. report that diltiazem does not increase digoxin blood levels.[357] Verapamil should be used cautiously with digoxin or a beta blocker since the combination may precipitate the sick sinus syndrome or AV block. Verapamil, by decreasing the renal and extrarenal clearance of digoxin, may increase the serum level of digoxin.

Schanzenbacher et al. report that nifedipine may actually precipitate angina in some patients.[364] When moderate reflex tachycardia develops as the result of the development of slight hypotension, the pressure-rate product may increase, and this may precipitate angina. This response may be blocked with propranolol.

Palatianos et al. reported the hemodynamic basis for sudden cardiovascular collapse early after coronary bypass operation in patients receiving nifedipine. Apparently the peripheral effects of nifedipine last longer than the cardiac effects.[358]

• *Digitalis* remains in the center of controversy (see Chap. 92). Digitalis is useful in the prevention and treatment of certain atrial arrhythmias (see Chap. 27). It is useful in the treatment of heart failure when myocardial cells are capable of responding to its action (see Chap. 21). The question arises, however, whether or not the drug is useful in patients with ischemic heart disease who have congestive heart failure. This, plus the fact that digitalis can cause serious arrhythmias, especially when hypokalemia is present, leads to the arguments surrounding the use of the drug.

The direct effect of digitalis upon the myocardium is to increase the force of myocardial contraction with subsequent increase in oxygen consumption (see Chap. 92). In many patients with angina pectoris, the left ventricular volume and end-diastolic pressure are increased in association with a decrease in the rate of rise of left ventricular pressure. The administration of digitalis to such patients tends to improve these abnormalities. Thus, the net effect of digitalis may be reduction of oxygen consumption and lessening of angina pectoris. On the other hand, digitalis may cause an increased rate of rise of left ventricular pressure which can offset the decreased left ventricular volume and end-diastolic pressure, causing angina at a lower level of exercise.

Ventricular dysfunction is common during angina pectoris, and the pulmonary wedge pressure is often elevated during an attack.[366] Most available studies indicate that digitalis does not prevent angina pectoris, even though there may be improvement of the ventricular performance. Most of the studies, however, have been carried out over a period of 1 to 2 h, using limited amounts of digitalis glycosides intravenously. Optimal use of digitalis over weeks or months has not been evaluated. Clinical impressions of benefit cannot be substantiated, particularly since nitroglycerin, dinitrate isosorbide, and beta-blocking agents may be used in conjunction with digitalis. Theoretically, digitalis may aggravate angina pectoris in patients without left ventricular dilatation, but this is rarely identified in practice.

A trial of digitalis is indicated in patients with chronic ischemic heart disease when any of the following is present: cardiomegaly; large doses of propranolol; significant mitral regurgitation; atrial arrhythmias; S_3 gallop; rales due to pulmonary congestion; or x-ray evidence of interstitial edema.

The use of digitalis in patients with *myocardial infarction* is even more controversial. Morrison et al.[367] studied the effect of digoxin on computer-quantitated ^{201}Tl perfusion scintigrams, left ventricular ejection fraction, and the percentage of abnormally contracting left ventricular regions in 23 patients with myocardial infarction. A correlation was established between MB-CK isoenzyme release and initial radionuclide–gated pool wall estimates of ejection fraction. Digoxin resulted in a minimal but significant improvement in ejection fraction that did not occur at the expense of left ventricular perfusion or regional wall motion.

Marcus points out that several mechanisms may be involved in preventing a digitalis-induced increase in contractility from being translated into an increase in stroke volume and a decrease in left ventricular filling pressure in patients with fresh myocardial infarction.[368] The increase in contractility may increase bulging of the infarcted and ischemic myocardium, thereby dissipating the inotropic effect that it exerts on the remainder of the cardiac muscle. He also emphasizes that the increase in peripheral resistance induced by intravenously administered digitalis produces an increase in afterload and that this effect may oppose the mild inotropic effect of digitalis.

Marcus also points out that different responses are obtained in different patients with infarction who are given digitalis.[368] This occurs because the hemodynamic effects of the drug are the result of the interplay of the direct inotropic effect of the drug on responsive segments of the myocardium, the dissipation of the inotropic action on nonresponsive areas of the myocardium, and the variable effect of the drug on systemic vascular resistance.

The increase in systemic vascular resistance caused by digitalis is partially due to direct arteriolar vasoconstriction. The systemic blood pressure may rise, and pulmonary edema may develop. The increase in rise of systemic vascular resistance may be prevented or diminished by giving digitalis orally or by giving the drug slowly intravenously over a 10-min period, and by using afterload-reducing agents along with the digitalis.

We wish to make the following points regarding the use of digitalis in patients with myocardial infarction:

- Patients with myocardial infarction who exhibit no evidence of heart failure should not receive digitalis because it may increase the ischemia.
- Patients with myocardial infarction who have an S_3 gallop, rales, and/or pulmonary congestion by x-ray should receive digitalis along with a mild diuretic. Some patients should receive drugs to decrease the preload and afterload. Some physicians withhold digitalis and await the results of the diuretic before using digitalis. The value of digitalis in this setting is difficult to prove.
- Digitalis may be used in the treatment of acute pulmonary edema due to myocardial infarction, but it is wise to use it following afterload reduction with a drug such as nitroprusside.
- Digitalis may be given to patients with cardiogenic shock due to myocardial infarction who have normal rhythm, but benefit is rarely apparent.
- Digitalis may be needed to control the ventricular rate of patients with angina or infarction who have atrial fibrillation or flutter. Digitalis not only controls the ventricular rate but may revert the rhythm to normal.
- Digitalis sensitivity is increased in animals with experimentally produced myocardial infarction. We suspect the same is true in patients, but it is un-

common to observe an increase in arrhythmias when proper doses of the drug are used.

Digoxin (Lanoxin) is the current digitalis preparation of choice because its onset of action is sufficiently rapid to use in urgent clinical situations when given intravenously, and its half-life is long enough to ensure a smooth maintenance dose when it is given orally. The initial intravenous loading dose is about 1.0 mg given in divided doses. The maintenance intravenous dose is 0.25 mg daily, assuming normal renal function is present. Less should be used when the creatine is elevated. The initial oral loading dose is 1 mg given in divided doses. This can be followed by 0.5 mg for 2 days and then 0.25 mg daily, assuming renal function is normal. The slow method of giving only 0.125 to 0.25 mg daily without a loading dose is satisfactory when the clinical problem is mild and chronic. The use of digoxin to control atrial fibrillation and flutter requires experience, and one must consider the urgency of the clinical situation, the ventricular rate, the average loading dose, and half-life of the drug. The ventricular rate in patients with atrial fibrillation and flutter should be controlled at 75 to 85 beats per minute after mild exercise. As a rule, more digoxin is needed to prolong conduction in the atrioventricular (AV) node in order to control the ventricular rate in patients with atrial fibrillation and flutter than is needed to increase myocardial contractility. A beta blocker such as propranolol or the calcium antagonist verapamil may be used in conjunction with digoxin for the purpose mentioned above, but such a combination can be harmful if the atrial fibrillation or flutter is a consequence of the sick sinus syndrome.

• The pharmacology of *Coumadin,*[369] *heparin, streptokinase*, and *antiplatelet drugs* is discussed in Chap. 95. The roles of warfarin (*Coumadin*) and *heparin* in the management of atherosclerotic coronary heart disease have not been resolved to everyone's satisfaction.[370–372]

We do not recommend the use of warfarin or heparin for patients with stable angina pectoris. It seems that the use of heparin is gaining favor for the early treatment of coronary events that may be precipitated by coronary thrombosis. Minidose heparin, 5000 units subcutaneously every 8 h, may be used.[373] This applies to patients with unstable angina pectoris or prolonged myocardial ischemia with no objective sign of infarction, and for uncomplicated myocardial infarction. We recommend the use of heparin followed by warfarin in patients with acute myocardial infarction when any of the following conditions is present and when there are no contraindications: (1) cardiac enlargement, (2) suspected or proven ventricular aneurysm, (3) congestive heart failure present prior to acute myocardial infarction, (4) chronic atrial fibrillation, (5) history of infarction, (6) history of thrombophlebitis or embolism, (7) history of a transient ischemic attack, (8) calf tenderness or obvious phlebitis, and (9) obesity or feebleness that prevents ambulation.

We discontinue anticoagulants in patients who develop pericarditis, particularly if the pericardial rub is diffuse or if it persists 24 h. We usually discontinue the drug when the patient is discharged from the hospital. Warfarin should be used cautiously in the presence of renal disease or hepatic disease, or when therapy is required with drugs that interfere with its metabolism. Warfarin should not be used when there is a possibility of dissecting aneurysm or gastrointestinal bleeding. It is discontinued at the end of the period of hospitalization. We rarely use anticoagulants for atherosclerotic coronary heart disease on a long-term basis. Warfarin is started after the baseline prothrombin time has been determined to be normal. A large loading dose of warfarin is no longer recommended. The drug should be given orally 10 mg/day until the therapeutic range is reached, usually in 4 to 5 days. The therapeutic range is considered to be present when the patient's prothrombin time is 2 to 2.5 times the control prothrombin time. Thereafter, the drug dosage is increased or decreased in order to maintain the prothrombin time in this range.

Many drugs interact with warfarin. Drug interaction is a potential problem, especially when warfarin is used over a long period of time and the prothrombin time is measured less frequently. The physician must have ready access to an up-to-date list of drugs that interact with warfarin. The barbiturates, chloral hydrate, chloramphenicol, quinidine, salicylates, clofibrate, etc., are included in the long list. We usually observe no problem with drug interaction when warfarin is not used on a long-term basis and a prothrombin time is done daily while the patient is in the hospital. The problem of drug interaction is a real one when warfarin is used continuously in an effort to prevent pulmonary emboli.

Heparin is used immediately following coronary angioplasty.

The value of potent *fibrinolytic* agents such as *urokinase* and *streptokinase* in the treatment of myocardial infarction has been investigated for several years.[374–377] The pharmacology of these drugs and their use is discussed in Chaps. 95 and 117. The use of intravenous and intracoronary injection of streptokinase in patients with evolving myocardial infarction is currently being investigated[375] since it has become apparent that recent coronary thrombosis seems to play a role in producing the myocardial infarction in most patients. We know now that streptokinase can be injected into a patient with fresh coronary thrombosis with safety to the patient. We know, too, that it will dissolve the clot. We suspect that it will be valuable to some patients but not all patients. We need additional data to determine the indications and value of the intravenous or intracoronary injection of streptokinase. Obviously, other procedures will be needed after the thrombosis is dissolved since the conditions responsible for the thrombus still exist.

"Antiplatelet" drugs have received much attention

in the last few years. The pharmacology of these drugs is discussed in Chap. 95.

Kwaan and Rosen prepared an excellent summary of the antithrombotic effects of aspirin in September 1984.[378] The largest study of the effects of *aspirin* in patients who have recovered from myocardial infarction is the Aspirin Myocardial Infarction Study (AMIS).[379] This is a randomized, double-blind (0.5 g twice a day) study that measured the effects of aspirin versus placebo in 4524 men and women between the ages of 30 and 69 who had a myocardial infarction 8 weeks to 5 years before entry. Over a 3-year observation period, there was no significant difference between the aspirin and placebo groups in total mortality or sudden death rates. On the other hand, the incidence of recurrent, nonfatal myocardial infarction was 22 percent lower in the aspirin group, although this finding was not statistically significant by study criteria. There was also a lower incidence of stroke in the aspirin group; however, this was also not statistically significant. On the basis of AMIS, which is the largest completed and published evaluation of aspirin in the post-myocardial infarction population, the routine prescription of aspirin to all patients who have survived a myocardial infarction is not recommended.

Aspirin is known to inhibit the synthesis of arachidonic acid, cyclic endoperoxides PGH_2, and thromboxane A_2, which aggregate platelets and induce vasospasm. Aspirin also can block the synthesis of prostacyclin (PGI_2), a vasodilator and inhibitor of platelet aggregation produced by the endothelial cells of blood vessels.

In the Boston Collaborative Drug Study, the frequency of prior *aspirin* use among hospitalized patients with a discharge diagnosis of myocardial infarction was compared to the frequency among those with other diagnoses.[380] Markedly lower aspirin use was found in the myocardial infarction group. A prospective, randomized, double-blind trial by Elwood and coworkers compared the effects of 300 mg aspirin a day to those of placebo in men with a recent myocardial infarction.[381] This study showed an overall mortality trend in favor of aspirin, but the results were not statistically significant. The Veterans Administration study reported by Lewis et al. showed that aspirin has a protective effect against myocardial infarction in men with unstable angina. The study also suggested that mortality was decreased in the aspirin-treated group.[382]

The value of *sulfinpyrazone* (Anturane), 200 mg four times a day, has been studied in 1620 patients, starting 25 to 35 days after their acute myocardial infarction.[383,384] This compound inhibits in vivo and in vitro platelet adhesion, aggregation, and the "release reaction" induced by adenosine diphosphate (ADP), collagen, and antigen-antibody complexes. It also inhibits platelet prostaglandin synthesis. Although the initial reports of this study have suggested a significant decrease in sudden death only for the first 6 months after starting the medication, the Federal Drug Administration has withheld approval of this medication following myocardial infarction. Their action has been based upon a number of questions regarding the study design and statistical analysis, particularly patient exclusions, deaths that were not "analyzable," and the criteria used for sudden death. At present, there are insufficient data to recommend the routine administration of sulfinpyrazone to patients following acute myocardial infarction.

In the *Persantine-Aspirin* Reinfarction Study (PARIS-1) study, the effects of combined dipyridamole (Persantine) plus aspirin were compared to the effects of aspirin with placebo in 2026 patients 8 weeks to 5 years after myocardial infarction.[385] The "coronary incidence," or the combination of fatal and nonfatal definite myocardial infarction, was reduced by a statistically significant amount in the combination group for the first 24 months. The reduction in coronary mortality alone was not significantly reduced, though overall total mortality rate was reduced about 17 percent in both of the active treatment groups. The greatest reduction in mortality was seen in the group of patients who entered the study within 6 months after their qualifying myocardial infarction. On the basis of the initial PARIS-1 study, another study is underway with two treatment groups only: the combined Persantine plus aspirin group and the placebo group. The goal is to study 3000 patients equally divided.

Aspirin and dipyridamole are used by some physicians in an effort to decrease the closure rate of vein grafts used in coronary bypass surgery[386] (see later discussion).

Drugs used in the treatment of heart failure are discussed in Chaps. 21, 88, 92 to 94.

The *drugs used in the treatment of shock* are discussed in Chaps. 23 and 88.

The *antiarrhythmic agents* are discussed in Chaps. 27 and 89.

The use of *lipid-lowering drugs* is discussed in Chap. 42.

Drugs such as radioiodine and methimazole (Tapazole) are occasionally used to produce a hypometabolic state in euthyroid patients who have disabling angina despite drug therapy and who are not suitable candidates for coronary bypass surgery or coronary angioplasty.[387] The usual dose of methimazole is 10 mg three times a day.

The Success Rate of Medical Treatment

Fat people tend to remain fat, and the addicted smoker and drinker of alcohol tend to continue their harmful habits, but we in the profession must continue to assist them in their efforts to change.

The new drugs used in the treatment of atherosclerotic heart disease are generally effective. They represent a great advance in the treatment of this disease. Drugs, however, are not always successful in achieving a therapeutic goal, and undesired side effects may prevent their use. Of the patients with class I and II stable angina in the European Coronary Surgery Study, 27 percent were dissatisfied with the relief offered by nitrates and beta blockers (propranolol) and "crossed over" from the medical treatment group to have coronary bypass surgery.[101] Within a 5-year follow-up period 23.5 percent of patients with class I and II stable angina (Canadian classification) in the Coronary Artery Surgery Study (CASS) became dissatisfied with the control of discomfort afforded by nitrates and beta blockers (propranolol) and crossed over from the medical treatment group to have coronary bypass surgery.[78]

No long-term studies are available in which the results of bypass surgery on angina relief and survival are compared with the results of medical treatment which includes nitrates, beta blockers, *and* calcium antagonists.

Opiates, nitrates, beta blockers, and calcium antagonists do not always relieve the pain of acute myocardial infarction.

The drugs used to control cardiac arrhythmias and blood clotting are not always successful in achieving the therapeutic goals established for them.

Some patients cannot take the drugs discussed above because of unwanted side effects.

The cost of medical treatment is considerable when a patient requires nitrates, beta blockers, and calcium antagonists to obtain relief of his or her angina.

Pryor et al. have pointed out that there appears to be an improving prognosis over time in medically treated patients.[388] There is no doubt that the medical treatment of atherosclerotic coronary heart disease has improved enormously, but it is not always successful in preventing the disease, relieving angina pectoris and other complications of decreased coronary blood flow, and prolonging the life of every patient with atherosclerotic coronary heart disease. Accordingly, the intraaortic balloon pump, cardiac pacemakers and cardiac defibrillators, coronary angioplasty, coronary bypass surgery, and surgery for cardiac arrhythmias, ventricular aneurysm, rupture of the interventricular septum, rupture of the papillary muscle, and cardiac transplantation are used.

Percutaneous Transluminal Coronary Angioplasty[389,390] (see Chap. 117)

Gruentzig performed the first coronary angioplasty on a patient in 1978.[51] Since then the technique has been used extensively. The registry, housed at the National Institutes of Health, indicates that by 1983 about 3079 coronary angioplasties had been performed in the United States alone.[391] At the time of this writing, Gruentzig and his colleagues at Emory University Hospital have performed more than 4500 angioplasties.

Gruentzig reported his initial experience with 50 patients in 1979.[52] He was successful in dilating 64 percent of those; however, in the next 50 patients his success rate increased to 86 percent. Of this second group of 50, three had to go directly to surgery because of problems with the dilatation, and one suffered a small myocardial infarction. Gruentzig reported his work again in *Update III: The Heart* in 1979.[53] Gruentzig has worked with his colleagues, King and Douglas, at Emory University since September 1980 and has continued to develop new catheters and improve the technique. The primary success rate is now in the range of 90 percent.

The *indications* for coronary angioplasty have changed during the recent past. Because of a close adherence to a selection protocol, patients who have undergone this procedure at Emory are rather similar. Early in the development of the technique the vast majority of patients had recent-onset angina due to single vessel coronary disease. They were relatively refractory to medical therapy, which made them candidates for coronary bypass surgery. Now, with the development of new catheters, patients with stable angina and unstable angina are believed to be candidates for the procedure. Patients without angina who have objective evidence of ischemia identified by the exercise stress ECG or ^{201}Tl stress test are also occasionally considered for the procedure. Whereas most of these patients would be candidates for bypass surgery, many are not (see later discussion).

The ideal anatomic abnormality determined by arteriography is a noncalcified lesion in the proximal portion of a single coronary artery. If there is a delay in performing the dilatation after subtotal obstruction of an artery has been discovered, there may be total obstruction of the artery when the second arteriogram is performed at the time of the anticipated angioplasty. This progression from subtotal to total obstruction reduces the chance of a successful procedure and indicates that the procedure should be done soon after the initial coronary arteriogram.

About 20 percent of the patients who have had coronary angioplasty at Emory University have had double-vessel coronary disease. About 5 percent of the patients have had triple-vessel disease, and the Emory group believes, based on previous experience, that the procedure is contraindicated in patients with left main coronary artery disease. Others have used the technique in patients with triple-vessel disease.[392,393] We have not recommended the procedure in patients with triple-vessel disease because we believe that randomized trials should be initiated in order to assess the results of coronary angioplasty in patients with multivessel coronary artery obstructions.

The technique of dilatation can be applied to the subtotal occlusion of saphenous vein grafts used in bypass surgery. Occlusion of the distal anastomotic site is the easiest to dilate. Occlusion of the proximal anastomotic site is not as easy to dilate, and midgraft occlusion cannot be dilated.[394]

The *results and goals* of coronary angioplasty are as follows: The primary success rate in the hands of an experienced team is about 90 percent. With experience and the use of new catheters the success rate is about the same in each of the major coronary arteries.

An effort is made to have coronary arteriography performed on every patient 6 months after the procedure. The restenosis rate is about 30 percent. Dilatation is again performed with a 90 percent success rate. The artery tends to remain patent after the second angioplasty.[395]

Angina pectoris and the objective signs of ischemia are usually eliminated following a successful angioplasty. Should angina pectoris or objective signs of ischemia occur before the elective coronary arteriogram is performed, the patient should have prompt coronary arteriography.

We have made no claims that the procedure, done for single-vessel disease, prolongs the life of such patients, and there are no data permitting such a claim for patients with double-vessel or triple-vessel coronary disease. The objective has been twofold:

- To relieve the patient's angina or objective signs of ischemia.
- To prevent as long as possible the development of multivessel coronary disease which places the patient in a high-risk group by using a series of single-vessel dilatations.

The *medical treatment* following coronary angioplasty has changed recently. When successful, the procedure results in an immediate increase in coronary blood flow at rest and during stress testing. The patient is given heparin during the procedure. The patient is given aspirin or aspirin and dipyridamole and a calcium antagonist indefinitely.

The patient is usually discharged from the hospital on the second postangioplasty day. Before leaving the hospital the patient has an exercise stress ECG, exercise ^{201}Tl scan, or radionuclear ventriculogram, and the results are compared to the results of similar tests made prior to the procedure. The cost of angioplasty is, of course, less than the cost of bypass surgery.

The *limitations and complications* of coronary angioplasty are as follows: Years of experience are required for the physician to view a coronary arteriogram and select the proper patients for the procedure. Years of experience are required to achieve the success enjoyed by an experienced team.

As presently applied, the technique is not indicated in patients with chronic total occlusion of the coronary artery; obstruction of the left main coronary artery; lesions that are longer than 1.5 cm; severe multivessel disease, particularly if distal segments are involved; lesions located at or after sharp bends in the artery; or lesions located at the bifurcation of a coronary artery.

The mortality rate of the procedure in experienced hands is about 0.2 percent. Obstructive dissection of the coronary artery occurs in 2.5 percent. About 2.3 percent of the patients will require emergency coronary bypass surgery. There have been no deaths in patients operated on for this reason at Emory. About 1.5 percent of the patients will have a small infarction following coronary angioplasty. Ventricular fibrillation occurs in about 2 percent of the patients, but this has posed no problem for the "operator."

This is a changing field. The recent literature is filled with articles on the subject. It is highly likely, with the improvement of the equipment and increased experience of the "operators," that the technique will be used even more extensively. Perhaps it will be combined with laser treatment, for Gruentzig has taught us that skilled operators can work inside the coronary arteries with safety. Certainly the discussion of coronary angioplasty in the next edition of *The Heart* will be different from the discussion in this edition.

Surgical Treatment—Coronary Bypass Surgery and Other Surgical Techniques

The cardiac surgeons of years past recognized that myocardial ischemia was due to atheromatous obstruction of coronary arteries. They developed many operations in an effort to improve myocardial blood flow in order to relieve angina pectoris and prevent infarction and death. They gradually eliminated a large number of operations that did not help and finally developed coronary bypass surgery[396] (see later discussion). Now it is the most commonly performed surgical procedure at major medical centers in the United States. About 200,000 bypass operations are performed annually in the United States. The total experience of many of the major medical centers is reported in *Clinical Essays on The Heart* (vol. 2).[397]

No operation has been studied as thoroughly as coronary bypass surgery. The operation has captured the interest of many medical investigators and many nonmedical people. The interest in coronary bypass surgery has been great because it represented a "breakthrough" in the treatment of a common, serious disease that defied prevention and satisfactory medical management; it showed the value of modern technology in solving problems; it created controversy; it increased the cost of medical care, which forced our nation to make troublesome value judgments in terms of economic considerations; and it has created a sense of competition—most of which is healthy for the progress of medicine.

Despite the turmoil, coronary bypass surgery has been extremely successful. The procedure, coupled with modern medical therapy, has enormously improved the treatment of patients with atherosclerotic coronary heart disease.

The Importance of Identifying Subsets

Although the importance of identifying subsets of atherosclerotic coronary heart disease has been emphasized throughout this chapter, it is so very important to the care of patients it will be highlighted again.

The term *atherosclerotic coronary heart disease* is a generic term indicating a single disease process. But the disease process produces many different clinical manifestations (see Table 45-1). Patients with similar clinical manifestations are placed in specific categories or subsets. Each subset, then, has its own clinical markers. A subset is not created simply to produce a tidy organizational structure. The identification of a specific subset becomes extremely valuable to the clinician when it is evident that the pathophysiology, clinical characteristics, prognosis, and treatment are rather specific for that particular subset. In addition, there is no way to communicate with colleagues, read the literature, or perform clinical research on patients with atherosclerotic coronary heart disease, or any other disease, without understanding the absolute necessity for identifying subsets—even sub-subsets.

The subset, identified by rather routine clinical skills, can be subdivided into sub-subsets by determining the location of the obstructions in the coronary arteries, the ejection fraction, regional myocardial wall motion (contractility), and myocardial reperfusion.

So the objective in this section is to define the features of the various subsets and sub-subsets that make up the clinical spectrum of coronary disease; to link the sub-subsets with the pathophysiology responsible for them; and to link each of the subsets with specific treatment which is designed to improve the symptoms and prognosis.

Variables To Be Considered

Several variables must be considered when the physician considers the need for coronary bypass surgery. These include the identification of the sub-subset to which the patient belongs (remember the subsets listed in Table 45-1 can be divided into sub-subsets by more refined techniques); the operative mortality rate of the team selected to perform the operation; the morbidity of the procedure; the associated diseases exhibited by the patient; the psychological state of the patient; and the patient's age. *Simply stated, one must consider all aspects of the whole patient in order to make a judgment about the need for coronary bypass surgery.* It is extremely important to realize that the treatment of unstable angina in a 40-year-old male who has no other disease is very different from the treatment prescribed for a 75-year-old male with mild, stable angina who has carotid artery disease and advanced pulmonary emphysema. It is equally important to remember that identification of sub-subsets must be done before a final decision can be made. This may require determination of objective evidence of myocardial ischemia; the extent and location of the obstructing coronary lesions; and the ejection fraction. Finally, and perhaps most importantly, we must remember that it is impossible to predict survival from an analysis of symptoms alone[398] (see later discussion).

Proof That Myocardial Ischemia Is Relieved by Coronary Bypass Surgery

Myocardial ischemia occurs when the pump–coronary artery delivery system fails to deliver an adequate amount of blood to meet myocardial oxygen requirements. When the coronary artery is obstructed, it may not interfere with blood flow to the degree that myocardial ischemia occurs at rest but may prevent adequate myocardial perfusion during exercise. This is referred to as an increase in the *demand* end of the supply-demand system of myocardial perfusion. Myocardial ischemia may occur when coronary artery spasm or coronary thrombosis occurs at the site of coronary artery obstruction. This is referred to as a decrease in the *supply* end of the supply-demand system of myocardial perfusion. This can occur without relationship to an increased demand for an adequate coronary blood flow. Conditions also exist where there is an increase in the demand end of the supply-demand myocardial perfusion system *plus* a decrease in the supply end of the supply-demand system of myocardial perfusion. The latter produces the clinical syndrome that has been called "mixed" angina.

The modern treatment of myocardial ischemia involves either decreasing the *demand* for an increase in coronary blood flow or increasing the *supply* of coronary blood flow. For example, beta blockers decrease the demand for an increase in myocardial perfusion, and coronary bypass surgery improves the supply of coronary blood flow that has been impeded by the obstructing atheroma.

Many studies have demonstrated that myocardial perfusion is in fact improved as a result of bypass surgery. These studies include electromagnetic flow probe measurements made at surgery, xenon flow studies with and without exercise;[399] postoperative exercise electrocardiographic stress testing;[400] atrial pacing studies with measurements of myocardial lactate production;[401] hemodynamic response to exercise;[402] myocardial perfusion scanning with exercise; radionuclear blood pool imaging with exercise showing improvement in ejection fraction postoperatively;[402] and the relation of completeness of revascularization to symptomatic improvement.[403]

Although excellent evidence exists for myocardial perfusion being improved by coronary bypass surgery, the real test of this technique lies in its ability to relieve symptoms and prolong life. Angina relief has been documented in the vast majority of patients who have undergone successful coronary bypass surgery.[79,396,397,404,405] Most centers now report that over 90 percent of the patients who undergo surgery are either free of angina or have their angina significantly improved.[396] Although some of the improvement of angina with surgery is undoubtedly from placebo effect, the relief obtained with coronary bypass surgery is far superior to that obtained with previous operative procedures.

Proof That Life Is Prolonged in Certain Subsets of Patients with Coronary Bypass Surgery[397]

Patients with atherosclerotic coronary heart disease die as a result of cardiac arrhythmias (sudden death), myocardial infarction and shock or pulmonary edema, or chronic heart failure.

When it became apparent that coronary bypass surgery relieved angina pectoris due to myocardial ischemia, it seemed reasonable to believe that the procedure might prolong life by preventing other ischemic events that are known to shorten life. Phrased another way, it seemed unreasonable to believe that coronary bypass surgery could relieve angina pectoris but not be of value in preventing other ischemic events. This led to numerous randomized and nonrandomized studies that were designed to compare the long-term survival of patients assigned to medical treatment with the long-term survival of patients assigned to bypass surgical treatment. Such studies are not easy to implement because, over a 5- and 10-year period during which a study is conducted, both medical treatment (new drugs) and surgical treatment (improved techniques) change. This, plus the "crossover" rates from the medical treatment group to the surgical group because of unacceptable angina, makes it difficult to complete such studies to the satisfaction of all concerned. Despite such difficulties the following data support the concept that bypass surgery prolongs the life of carefully selected patients:

- The Veterans Administration randomized study, reported in 1975, showed the 3-year survival rate of symptomatic patients with left main coronary artery obstruction who had bypass surgery was superior to that of similar patients who were treated medically.[182]
- The results of the European Coronary Surgery Study (1982) also indicated that life is prolonged with bypass surgery in symptomatic patients with left main coronary artery obstruction.[101]
- The Veterans Administration randomized study reported in 1978 showed a trend toward better 5-year survival of symptomatic patients with triple-vessel disease and poor ejection fractions when compared to patients treated medically.[406]
- The *V*eterans *A*dministration *C*oronary *A*rtery *B*y-pass *C*ooperative *S*tudy *G*roup published (1985) their 11-year follow-up of 686 patients who entered the study with stable angina pectoris and who had been randomized to receive either surgical or medical treatment. They found (after 7 years) that patients with triple-vessel disease and impaired left ventricular function who had bypass surgery had superior survival curves compared to similar patients treated medically.[406a]
- The results of the European Coronary Artery Surgery Study indicated the rate of 5-year survival of symptomatic patients with triple-vessel disease who had good ejection fractions was superior to that of similar patients treated medically.[101]
- One of the CASS reports indicated that patients with ischemic symptoms and poor left ventricular function benefit from bypass surgery.[407]
- In 1978 Wynne et al. reported on the value of coronary bypass surgery in patients with multivessel coronary disease who had minimal angina pectoris.[408]
- Kent et al. found that patients who are asymptomatic or mildly symptomatic who have triple-vessel disease and a poor exercise performance on the treadmill have an annual mortality rate of 9 percent.[409] No surgical group has such a high annual mortality rate.
- Hammermeister et al. reported improved survival of patients treated surgically who were asymptomatic or had minimal symptoms with triple-vessel coronary disease and poor left ventricular function[410] compared to similar patients treated medically.
- In 1985 Bonow et al.[410a] reported on a group of patients with triple-vessel coronary disease who were mildly symptomatic but exhibited objective signs of ischemia (ST-segment depression of 1 mm or more) and a decrease in ejection fraction during exercise and who were at high risk during subsequent medical treatment. The survival at 4 years was 71 ± 11 percent. There is no surgically treated group with such a poor 4-year survival.
- The results of the European Coronary Surgery Study showed a trend toward improved survival of symptomatic patients who were treated surgically and who had double-vessel disease when the proximal portion of the left anterior descending artery was obstructed and the ejection fraction was above 0.5.[101] The report of the Coronary Artery Surgery Study published in December 1983 revealed that patients with proximal obstruction of the left anterior descending artery plus obstruction of the right coronary artery had a poorer survival curve than patients with nonproximal obstruction of the left anterior descending artery plus obstruction of the right coronary artery.[410b]
- Leonard Cobb, working with the Seattle Heart Watch, has concluded that patients who experience sudden death but are resuscitated and have coronary bypass surgery live longer than patients who have sudden death but are resuscitated and are treated medically (see Chap. 32).
- There are no data indicating that the 5-year survival rate is improved by bypass surgery in patients when a single coronary artery is obstructed. Concern exists, however, that high-grade obstruction of the proximal portion of the left anterior descending artery is a very serious lesion. Patients with single-vessel disease may die suddenly, have massive infarction, or rupture their papillary muscle. Such patients are not included in clinical trials which require the presence of angina pectoris for entry into the studies.

Clinical Status 10 Years after Coronary Bypass Surgery

Rahmitoola et al. studied the status of patients who had coronary bypass surgery for unstable angina 10 years previously. The 1-month mortality rate was 1.8 percent. The 5-year survival rate was 92 percent, and the 10-year survival rate was 83 percent. Coronary bypass surgery was repeated at a rate of 1 to 2 percent per year; 81 percent of patients were angina-free or only had mild angina.[410c]

Indications for Coronary Bypass Surgery or Coronary Angioplasty To Relieve Myocardial Ischemia

Patients with evidence of myocardial ischemia are often candidates for coronary bypass surgery or coronary angioplasty. The timing of surgery may be determined, in some patients, by the results of the ^{201}Tl scan or nuclear angiogram. Surgery cannot be planned for any patient, however, without careful study of the coronary arteriogram and left ventriculogram. *Obviously, the obstructed coronary arteries must be bypassable, and the ejection fraction must be adequate to consider bypass surgery.*

The Canadian Cardiovascular Society functional classification should be used to grade the angina pectoris (see Table 6-1).

- Patients with class I, II, III, or IV *unstable* angina, or patients with *prolonged myocardial ischemia without objective signs of infarction* who are not suitable candidates for coronary angioplasty are usually candidates for coronary bypass surgery. This includes patients with left main coronary disease, triple-vessel disease, double-vessel disease, and single-vessel disease.[396]
- Patients with class III or IV *stable* angina pectoris who are not suitable candidates for coronary angioplasty should have coronary bypass surgery. Such patients are usually classified as having unacceptable, although stable, angina. This rule applies for patients with left main coronary artery obstruction, triple-vessel obstruction, double-vessel obstruction, and single-vessel obstruction.[78,101]

  Many patients with class III or IV stable angina who have single-vessel disease and a few patients with double-vessel disease are candidates for coronary angioplasty. (Whereas angioplasty is performed by some for patients with double- and triple-vessel disease, we have not used the procedure for patients with triple-vessel disease. We have used it in a small percentage of carefully selected patients with double-vessel disease, but we will await the results of our randomized study before recommending the use of, or the avoidance of, the procedure for multivessel disease).
- Patients with class I or II *stable* angina who have left main coronary artery obstruction; triple-vessel disease with poor exercise performance on the treadmill; or double-vessel disease when one of the obstructions is located in the proximal portion of the left anterior descending artery and a poor exercise performance on the treadmill should have coronary bypass surgery.[101]* Patients with left main equivalent disease, defined as high-grade obstruction of the *proximal* portion of the left anterior descending artery and obstruction of the proximal portion of the circumflex artery, are in this category.

  Many patients with signs or symptoms of myocardial ischemia with single-vessel disease and some patients with double-vessel disease are candidates for coronary angioplasty.
- Patients with class I or II *stable* angina pectoris who have excellent exercise performance on the treadmill (see footnote at bottom of this page), who have single-vessel disease that is not suitable for angioplasty, and who have normal ejection fractions may postpone bypass surgery as long as medication controls the angina to the patient's satisfaction.[78] Fortunately, angioplasty can be used in most of these patients. When angioplasty is not feasible, many physicians would recommend bypass surgery for severe, proximal obstruction of the left anterior descending artery although supportive data for the approach are sparse.

  Patients with class I and II stable angina pectoris and an excellent performance on the treadmill who have double-vessel disease involving the right and circumflex coronary arteries who are not suitable for coronary angioplasty and who have normal ejection fractions can postpone surgery as long as the medication controls the angina to the patient's satisfaction.[78]

  Patients with class I and II stable angina and an excellent exercise performance on the treadmill who have obstruction of the *mid* or *distal* portion

*The CASS[78] did not use the results of exercise stress electrocardiography as a means of matching patients with class I and II stable angina or asymptomatic patients after infarction. The patients assigned to the surgical treatment group or medical treatment group were matched according to vessels involved and ejection fractions. Patients with high-grade obstruction of the left main coronary artery were not included in the study, and most of the patients had excellent ejection fractions. Coplan and Ambrose[102] emphasize the value of the stress test in such patients and believe that the results of the performance of the patients on the treadmill represent an independent prognostic marker.

We agree with this view, and until convinced otherwise by new proof we will continue to be influenced by the exercise electrocardiogram and exercise ^{201}Tl stress tests. This explains why we have inserted the words "who have an excellent performance on the treadmill" in definitions of all subsets of the patients with class I and II stable angina. To bring maximum safety to the patients described in the CASS[78] study we suggest that it is wise to heed the results of the stress electrocardiogram and stress ^{201}Tl test.

The results of the CASS study as reported in November 1983[78] were misinterpreted by many people. The interested reader should review the article written by Gunnar and Loeb,[396a] Lawrie and DeBakey,[396b] and Hurst[396c] since they emphasize an alternative interpretation of the results of the study.

of the left anterior descending artery or one of its branches and obstructions of the right or circumflex coronary artery that are not suitable for coronary angioplasty and who have normal ejection fractions can postpone surgery as long as medication controls the angina to their satisfaction.[78]

The CASS study,[78] in which patients were not matched according to the exercise response, revealed that patients who have class I or II stable angina, or who have no angina after infarction, who have good ejection fractions, but do not have high-grade left main coronary obstruction made up 12.5 percent of a large group of patients who had coronary arteriograms performed because coronary disease was suspected. About 25 percent of the patients treated medically required surgery for unacceptable angina during a 5-year follow-up period.[78] Seven percent of patients with triple-vessel disease who had class I or II stable angina and good ejection fractions required surgery annually.[78]

- Patients *without angina* who have a positive exercise electrocardiogram or positive ^{201}Tl scan indicating reperfusion defect who have single-vessel coronary artery disease and good ejection fractions may be candidates for coronary angioplasty (see earlier discussion). The asymptomatic patient with objective signs of ischemia who has an obstruction in the proximal portion of the left anterior descending coronary artery that is not suitable for angioplasty might be considered for bypass surgery, although few data are available to support this approach.
- Patients who formerly had angina or infarction but currently are *asymptomatic* or have class I or II stable angina should be followed with stress tests (electrocardiographic and radionuclear), and those with positive tests should have coronary arteriograms.

  Patients who are *asymptomatic* or have class I or II stable angina with left main coronary artery obstruction should have bypass surgery.

  Patients who are *asymptomatic* or have class I or II angina due to triple-vessel disease who perform poorly on the treadmill should have bypass surgery.[409] Patients with triple-vessel disease and who have other evidence of left ventricular dysfunction should have surgery. The same applies for asymptomatic patients with double-vessel disease with obstruction of the proximal portion of the left anterior descending artery who have a poor exercise performance on the treadmill.[101]
- *Asymptomatic* patients with left main coronary artery obstruction which is discovered at coronary arteriography performed because of a positive exercise electrocardiogram should have coronary bypass surgery. The same applies for patients with triple-vessel disease and patients with double-vessel disease when one of the obstructions is located in the proximal portion of the left anterior descending coronary artery. The data to support this approach are meager, but a reasonable inference can be made from the data collected on patients with mild angina who have a poor exercise performance and who exhibit the abnormal anatomy described.[101,408–410a]

Other Benefits of Coronary Bypass Surgery[411]

Data regarding the relief of angina pectoris and data regarding improved survival for certain carefully selected subsets of patients with atherosclerotic heart disease are available (see preceding discussion). Data regarding the results of coronary bypass surgery in the prevention of cardiac arrhythmias, myocardial infarction, and heart failure are, however, quite meager. Obviously, bypass surgery that prolongs life prevents or delays disorders that are known to produce death.

- Mason et al. have concluded that coronary bypass surgery decreases the incidence of subsequent infarction in patients with stable angina when compared to the incidence of infarction in similar patients treated medically.[412]
- There are data suggesting that sudden death is diminished in patients who have coronary bypass surgery. Cobbs' data (see later discussion) and data from the European coronary surgery group[101] suggest that sudden death due to a ventricular arrhythmia occurs less often in patients who have had coronary bypass surgery than it does in similar patients who are medically treated. Not all arrhythmias are related to myocardial ischemia, however, and it is not possible to guarantee a patient with atherosclerotic coronary heart disease that bypass surgery will eliminate a troublesome and refractory rhythm disturbance.
- Congestive heart failure may occur less often or may be delayed by coronary bypass surgery. Very few studies have addressed this problem, but one can deduce if the rate of infarctions is delayed that the incidence of heart failure might also be diminished for several years.
- The quality of life is definitely improved in the majority of patients after coronary bypass surgery. The CASS study regarding class I and II stable angina revealed that patients who had surgery had less angina, took fewer drugs, and had less objective evidence of myocardial ischemia than medically treated patients.[78]
- Hamilton et al. have reported that subsequent hospitalization for cardiovascular reasons is significantly diminished in patients who have had bypass surgery compared to those who are treated medically.[413]

What Individual Patients Should Be Told about Coronary Bypass Surgery

The procedure of bypass surgery should be explained carefully to patients who have been selected for the surgery. It is useful to present the patient a diagram of the coronary arteries and to indicate the exact location of the obstructions. Certain individual patients, chosen by their physician, profit by viewing their own coronary arteriogram. The physician should explain that the grafts do not eliminate the obstructions but create detours around them; the procedure does not prevent the disease, which may later appear in other locations and in other coronary arteries; and all grafts do not remain patent indefinitely and an estimate of annual graft closure rate should be given to the patient. The patient in whom surgery is recommended should then be told that all of these considerations, including the operative risk and morbidity of the procedure, have been carefully considered and that surgical intervention seems wise. The physician should explain that angina pectoris is relieved in 90 percent of patients, with complete relief occurring in more than 70 percent. The patient should understand that the angina may return in the years ahead. If the patient for whom surgery is planned is in a subset in which improved rate of survival can be expected from surgical treatment compared to medical treatment, it should be explained.

The physician should not speak for the cardiac surgeon. The physician and surgeon must communicate with each other and coordinate all information and activities, or else the patient may, at times, become confused by what may seem to be, but are not, conflicting statements.

Support of the Family during the Surgical Procedure

There is always apprehension on the part of the families as well as the patient regarding cardiac surgery. The patient's family, as well as the patient, should be oriented to all aspects of the surgical procedures during the preoperative period. This should include a discussion of the relative risks and benefits of the procedure, the time frame involved in the surgical procedure, and the expectations during the immediate recovery phase. Literature for the layman, along with slide and audiocassette programmed instruction on cardiac surgery and the intensive care unit, should be supplied to the family and patient. Trained nursing personnel are invaluable in orienting the patient and family in these matters; however, there is no substitute for time taken by the physician to sit down and answer all remaining questions.

During the operative procedure, a waiting room must be provided and staffed with trained volunteers who receive messages from the operating room and pass them on to the family. At the completion of the operative procedure, the cardiologist and the surgeon should speak with the family members in a realistic and, when possible, in an optimistic tone so that the fears that have been accumulating can be allayed. The physician must have regular daily contact with the family in order to ensure good communication and understanding.

Preoperative Management

Patients with *stable angina* who are selected for surgery are almost always on medical therapy. The challenge in the preoperative period is to avoid changing the program so that the patient becomes unstable while awaiting surgery. Jones et al. found that continuation of the beta blockers until the time of surgery caused no increased risk to the patient at surgery and ensured a smoother course while awaiting the operation.[414] If nitrites and calcium antagonists have been administered, they are continued. Patients are cautioned not to increase their myocardial oxygen requirements during the days preceding surgery but to put off such activities until improved myocardial perfusion is achieved. Antiplatelet drugs should be discontinued, and the bleeding time should be normal. (The use of antiplatelet drugs to improve the patency rate of the saphenous vein grafts is discussed later.)

Patients with *unstable angina*, of course, need more careful observation and preparation prior to surgery. Several studies, including the National Cooperative Study on unstable angina, have emphasized the importance of stabilization of the patient prior to surgical procedure.[415] Although this is not always possible, we feel it is optimal and that vigorous medical therapy should be applied in all patients with unstable angina pectoris. If the pain occurs at rest without provocation, then hospitalization with electrocardiographic monitoring is essential. Beta-blocking drugs and calcium antagonists have been helpful; however, the nitrites, either administered at frequent intervals, or in more serious cases, given by constant intravenous infusion may also be needed to control the angina. A nitroglycerin drip is the most effective means of controlling unstable angina pectoris.[416] The intraaortic balloon pump may be needed when medical treatment fails to relieve the patient.

In patients with *Prinzmetal's angina*, coronary artery spasm often influences the clinical course. If such patients have obstructive coronary disease plus coronary artery spasm and are scheduled for surgery, electrocardiographic monitoring is essential, and a nitroglycerin drip is used to prevent attacks of coronary artery spasm. The calcium antagonists nifedipine and diltiazem are also extremely useful, while verapamil may be contraindicated if AV block occurs at the time of the episode (as it does in some patients with Prinzmetal's angina).

Patients who develop *congestive heart failure and cardiogenic shock* secondary to mechanical derangements such as ventricular septal defect, papillary muscle rupture or dysfunction, or large ventricular aneurysm formation must have vigorous medical therapy applied in order to achieve as much stabilization as possible during preparation for cardiac catheterization and surgery (see later discussion and Chap. 131). Systolic unloading is of course desirable if the blood pressure allows such therapy. Quite often the blood pressure is at shock levels, and systolic unloading can be achieved only by the intraaortic balloon pump. The physician can insert the percutaneous intraaortic balloon pump (see Chap. 129) early in the course of a rupture so that the patient may be stabilized for diagnostic procedures, and thus facilitate a move toward early surgery.

Patients with *severe left main coronary artery stenosis* are a special group and should be managed very aggressively. These patients have a tendency to sudden death[178] and in some cases respond very poorly during and following cardiac catheterization. Many, if not all, patients found at coronary arteriography to have severe left main coronary artery stenosis should be observed in the coronary care unit so the blood pressure and rhythm can be more carefully monitored. Episodes of chest pain should be treated vigorously, and plans for early surgery should be undertaken.[417]

Other high-risk anatomic subsets include those patients with unstable angina who have subtotal occlusion of a major coronary artery, with slow blood flow through the distal segment, preserved wall motion, and absence of Q waves in the ECG. Such patients may be in a precarious position with impending myocardial infarction. The patients should be observed very closely, and careful manipulation of their hemodynamics is necessary in an effort to avoid additional myocardial ischemia. These patients are also potential candidates for very early surgical intervention.

Medical Management during Coronary Bypass Surgery

The cardiac anesthesiologists are highly trained in the use of cardiovascular drugs and in the recognition of myocardial ischemia. This, in large measure, accounts for the safe conduct of most patients through coronary bypass surgery. The major aspects of the anesthetic management are discussed in Chap. 79. Several principles, however, should be reemphasized. Morphine anesthesia has improved the safety of the procedure. Electrocardiographic monitoring from the V_5 lead position has led to early recognition of myocardial ischemia.[418] Hemodynamic monitoring by Swan-Ganz catheters and arterial lines has enabled smooth hemodynamic manipulations throughout the surgical procedure. Principles inherent in induction of anesthesia include the avoidance of an increase in myocardial oxygen requirements and avoidance of hypotension and hypoxia so that myocardial oxygen delivery is maintained. Tachycardia is managed with small intravenous injections of propranolol. Hypertension and ischemic ST segments are corrected with intravenous nitroglycerin.[419] Arrhythmias are identified and managed as they arise. Localized aortic dissection occurs on rare occasion, and surgical repair is usually successful.

Of critical importance during surgery are the techniques that have been developed for myocardial preservation. Most important among these is the hypothermic-potassium cardioplegic arrest now practiced by most cardiovascular teams for coronary bypass surgery (see Chap. 130).

Postoperative Management

Following surgery, the patient is admitted to the intensive care unit, where electrocardiographic and hemodynamic monitoring is achieved. An intraarterial line is continued in order to measure arterial pressure. This also provides a source for frequent arterial blood gas determinations. Central venous pressure, pulmonary artery pressure, and pulmonary capillary wedge pressure are monitored using a Swan-Ganz catheter. The intake and output of fluid, the level of consciousness, and the proper function of the respirator are carefully monitored.[420] Postoperative ECGs are checked for any intraoperative changes, and a baseline postoperative chest x-ray is obtained. In certain patients with a more brittle hemodynamic status, the cardiac output and systemic resistance are determined at frequent intervals.

Mortality

The overall operative mortality rate of coronary bypass surgery at major medical centers is about 1 percent.[397] This low risk has been achieved because of the progress made by a team effort which includes medical cardiologists, cardiac surgeons, cardiac anesthesiologists, excellent intensive care nurses, and excellent floor nurses.

Reoperation is associated with a higher operative mortality. The operative risk is about 2 to 3 percent, and the complications occur more frequently. Laird-Meeter et al. reported that, in their experience, the mortality rate for the first operation was 1.2 percent and for the second operation, 3.8 percent.[420]

Complications and Morbidity

Kuan et al. have recently studied the complications of 365 consecutive patients who had coronary bypass surgery.[421] A summary of their findings is shown in Table 45-9.

Problems that may arise in the *early* preoperative period include myocardial infarction, which occurs in 4 to 6 percent,* excessive bleeding, failure to obtain proper oxygenation, bubble oxygenator-induced immune-compromised syndrome, pneumothorax, hypertension, hypotension, hypervolemia, hypovolemia, arrhythmia, hyperkalemia or hypokalemia, cardiac tamponade, aortic dissection, acidosis, fever, and neurological abnormalities including mental confusion. Stroke, usually due to embolism, occurs in about 1 percent of patients. Coffey et al. reported their experience with patients

*The frequency of myocardial infarction depends upon the adequacy of myocardial preservation during surgery. Coronary artery spasm may also play a role. Most of the perioperative infarcts are small and alter survival curves very little.

TABLE 45-9 Complications of Isolated Coronary Bypass Surgery in 365 Patients

Complications	Short-Term	Long-Term
Minor (total = 54 in 51 patients)		
Atrial fibrillation	25	
Postpericardiotomy syndrome	17	1
Thrombophlebitis, leg	6	
Cellulitis, leg or arm	3	
Phrenic nerve palsy, left	1	
Ileus		
Major (total = 52 in 48 patients)		
Arrhythmias requiring permanent pacer	7	
Mediastinal hemorrhage	5	
With cardiac tamponade	2	
Stroke	5	
Postoperative myocardial infarction	4	
Repeat coronary bypass grafting	2	2
Wound dehiscence	3	
Congestive heart failure	3	
Pneumothorax requiring chest tube	3	
Sternal osteomyelitis	2	1
Pulmonary emboli	2	
Low cardiac output requiring intraaortic balloon pumping	2	
Transient diabetes insipidus	2	
Sternal fracture	1	
Renal failure requiring dialysis	1	
Septic shock	1	
Infective endocarditis	1	
Aortic dissecting aneurysm	1	
Ventricular fibrillation	1	
Leg ulcer requiring amputation		1

Source: P. Kuan, S. B. Bernstein, and M. H. Ellestad, Coronary Artery Bypass Surgery Morbidity, *J. Am. Coll. Cardiol.,* 3(6):1393, 1984. Reproduced with permission from the American College of Cardiology and the author.

who experienced a stroke following coronary bypass grafting in 1983.[422] Corrective measures for excess bleeding include replacement of all deficient clotting factors; if continued bleeding occurs for 2 to 3 h despite such replacement, then surgical reexploration is in order. This is required in about 2 percent of patients, but it does not increase the operative risk. When hypertension is present, intravenous nitroglycerin drip is most effective. When more potent vasodilatation is required, a nitroprusside infusion can be instituted. When diminished cardiac output is present, as evidenced by hypotension, signs of decreased perfusion such as cool cyanotic skin, thirst and diminished urinary output, or a low cardiac output measurement, the next step is to determine the status of the filling pressure of the left ventricle. If the pulmonary capillary wedge pressure is in the low 20s (mmHg), the pressure is increased by fluid loading. If this is ineffective or if the left ventricular filling pressure is already high, then cardiotonic drugs such as isoproterenol, dopamine, epinephrine, or dobutamine hydrochloride are employed. Cardiac tamponade may be responsible for hypotension and poor cardiac output. Emergency surgery may be needed to relieve this serious complication.

The most common arrhythmias seen in the early postoperative period are atrial fibrillation or flutter and ventricular ectopic beats or ventricular tachycardia. Ormerod et al. reported that atrial fibrillation occurred in 27 percent of patients immediately following coronary bypass surgery. The use of propranolol following surgery reduced the incidence of atrial fibrillation to 14.8 percent. Significant ventricular extrasystoles occurred in 3 percent of the patients.[423] Ventricular arrhythmias are usually treated with lidocaine hydrochloride in a bolus of 100 mg followed by a lidocaine drip using 2 to 4 mg/min as needed. Procainamide hydrochloride (Pronestyl) is also used in the early postoperative period. For atrial fibrillation or flutter, it is usually satisfactory to control the rate with digoxin (Lanoxin) and propranolol. Intravenous verapamil may also be useful in controlling atrial tachycardia, atrial fibrillation, and atrial flutter. Defibrillation is used if the cardiac output is inadequate because of an uncontrolled rapid rate despite the drugs just mentioned.

Balloon counterpulsation is rarely needed in the postoperative period unless the patient required balloon pumping preoperatively or when weaned from cardiopulmonary bypass. If the patient comes to the intensive care unit with a balloon pump in place, it is kept operating until the patient is satisfactorily weaned from all medications.

Propranolol, or another beta blocker, is used routinely following surgery by some, but not all, physicians unless there is a contraindication to its use. The value is that it assists in the control of hypertension, decreases the frequency of arrhythmias (see discussion above), and decreases the chances of ischemia by decreasing the pressure-rate product. The drug can be given orally as soon as the patient can swallow. Contraindications to its use are AV block, hypotension, bradycardia, and bronchospasm.

AV conduction disturbances and sinus node dysfunction usually manifest themselves during the operative period. A temporary pacemaker will then be attached to the epicardial surface of the heart prior to returning the patient to the intensive care unit. It is therefore rarely necessary to insert a temporary pacemaker in the intensive care unit. In patients who are unstable, an AV sequential pacemaker is of significant help through the early postoperative period.

The patient is usually moved from the intensive care unit to the postoperative surgical floor within 2 days. The problems that are commonly encountered several days after surgery include the following:

Pericarditis requiring anti-inflammatory therapy with drugs, such as prednisone, occurs in 20 to 30 percent of patients. Atrial arrhythmias usually controlled with digoxin, propranolol, or verapamil may occur. The sick sinus syndrome may appear, in which case a transvenous pacemaker may be needed since the pacemaker placed during surgery has usually been removed by this point. There may be infections, which can range from a superficial surgical wound to the rare, devastating mediastinitis, which may require sternal debridement, mediastinal drainage, and plastic and reconstructive surgery in addition to appropriate antibiotics; pleural effusions, which usually resolve but which may occasionally require thoracentesis; drowsiness and confusion, usually attributed to the postoperative medications. Pulmonary embolism and phlebitis rarely occur. Drug reactions; hypotension; postural hypotension; transient diabetes insipidus;[424] hiccoughs; phrenic nerve paralysis; hoarseness due to vocal chord paralysis; prostatic obstruction and prostatic infarction requiring surgery;[425] unilateral deafness; numbness of the fingers due to unavoidable stretching of the brachial plexus; and depression may also occur.[426] The last problem is an extremely common one, and the reason for it is not entirely understood. Some patients, despite the encouragement of the medical staff, feel an "emotional letdown" following the surgical procedure and undergo a period of significant depression during the first month or so postoperatively.

The postperfusion syndrome, hepatitis, pericarditis, and constrictive pericarditis may occur *following discharge* from the hospital.

The postperfusion syndrome[427] appears in about 2 percent of patients. It begins 3 to 7 weeks following cardiopulmonary bypass and resembles infectious mononucleosis or infectious hepatitis. It is thought to be due to the Ebstein-Barr virus or the cytomegalovirus from transfused blood. The condition is characterized by fever, splenomegaly, lymphadenopathy, a macular papular rash, atypical lymphocytes, and a negative heterophile agglutination reaction. The condition is benign and runs its course without specific treatment.

Hepatitis occurs in about 2 percent of patients. Posttransfusion hepatitis may be due to hepatitis A or hepatitis B virus. The incidence of hepatitis can be decreased if volunteer donors are used and if they are screened for hepatitis. Acquired Immune Deficiency Syndrome (AIDS) has been reported after blood transfusions, but we have not observed it.

Constrictive pericarditis may develop months and years after surgery, and this may lead to pericardiectomy.

Many physicians prescribe no medication at the time the patient is discharged from the hospital. Others recommend the long-term use of beta-blocking drugs, nitrites, and calcium antagonists. The value of such an approach is not known at this time. Long-term antiplatelet therapy is recommended by some physicians (see later discussion). Patients are instructed in the modification of risk factors (see Chap. 42). All smokers are encouraged in the strongest terms to stop, and instructions regarding low-fat, low-cholesterol diets and control of hypertension and diabetes should be given to the patients. Instructions are given for an exercise program of regular walking, and definite plans are made for the patient's return to work. A supervised rehabilitation program is needed for some patients.

The Length of Hospital Stay

The patient is usually discharged on the seventh postoperative day. Some patients go home on the sixth day, and a few remain in the hospital beyond the seventh day.

Accelerated Progression of Atherosclerotic Lesions Proximal to Lesions That Have Been Bypassed

Cashin et al., as well as others, have presented convincing evidence that minimally diseased coronary arteries, defined as showing less than 50 percent internal diameter narrowing, should not be bypassed because the acceleration of the stenosis of the proximal lesions will result.[428]

Graft Patency

Perioperative infarction during or immediately after bypass surgery is usually not due to graft closure. Brindes et al. believe perioperative infarction is usually due to inadequate intraoperative preservation due to severe obstruction of the feeding artery and poor collaterals.[429] Graft closure immediately after surgery can occur, and it is usually due to thrombosis. Graft closure a few months to years after surgery is usually due to fibrosis. Atherosclerosis of the vein graft can occur as a late cause of obstruction.

Grodin et al. performed angiographic studies on 238 patients with saphenous vein grafts and 40 patients with internal mammary grafts at 1 month, 1 year, and at 10 years.[430] The internal mammary artery grafts were more likely to remain patent than the saphenous vein grafts, with 88.5 percent of the internal mammary grafts open at 1 year compared to 76.4 percent of the saphenous vein, and 84.1 percent being open at 10 years compared to 52.8 percent. At 10 years atheromatous changes were more common (43.9 percent) in the saphenous vein grafts than in the internal mammary artery grafts (5.2 percent). Patients who had internal mammary grafts had a better survival rate at 10 years than patients who had saphenous vein grafts.[430] Singh et al.[431] and others[432] have also emphasized that an internal mammary artery graft is more likely to remain patent than a saphenous vein graft.

No other material for grafts has been developed. This is regrettable because the saphenous veins are not perfect in all patients, and arm veins tend to close more often than leg veins.

Some surgeons place a larger number of saphenous vein grafts knowing that some of them are more likely to close than others. Accordingly, subsequent graft closure is not always serious; the seriousness depends on the vessels that are involved.

The Mayo Clinic workers recommend the use of aspirin and dipyridamole in an effort to improve graft patency. They use 100 mg of dipyridamole (Persantine) orally four times a day beginning 2 days before surgery, and on the day of surgery 100 mg is given orally at 6 A.M. and through a nasogastric tube 1 h after surgery. Dipyridamole (75 mg) and aspirin (325 mg) are given by nasogastric tube 7 h after surgery and continued by mouth thereafter.[386]

Brooks et al. have reported on double-blind randomized control trial using aspirin and dipyridamole or a placebo in an effort to improve saphenous vein graft patency. They concluded that there was no significant difference between the treated group and the untreated group of patients.[432a]

Finally, since many saphenous vein grafts are closed at 10 years and since reoperation is associated with a higher operative risk, some investigators have pointed out that patients who have markers indicating a good chance of 5-year survival should delay bypass surgery as long as they are asymptomatic or have mild stable angina pectoris.[78]

Return to Work following Coronary Artery Bypass Graft Surgery

The effect of coronary bypass graft surgery on the patient's work status has been extremely difficult to evaluate. Most investigators have found a discrepancy between the number of patients who are relieved of their symptoms and those who have returned to gainful employment. Several factors, including previous nonemployment status, the patient's desire for retirement, physician and employer recommendation, and economic disincentives to work, account for this discrepancy. At the University of Alabama no overall increase in the working hours are found after surgery.[433] The most important variable was the preoperative work status. Of those patients working preoperatively, 79 percent returned to work postoperatively. The Montreal Heart Institute found the patient's decision to retire after surgery was influenced by the physician's recommendation 60 percent of the time.[434] Some employers also have an unrealistic concern about the patients after coronary artery bypass graft surgery and force them to retire early. This is regrettable because many of these patients are safer risks postoperatively than they were preoperatively. Patients who are highly motivated, especially those who are self-employed, usually return to work. On the other hand, some medical disability plans offer almost the same financial compensation for workers when they are unemployed as when they were fully employed. This disincentive to work is a strong factor in many patients' decision to seek disability status or to "retire" postoperatively.

The importance of the preoperative work status of patients under 65 was evaluated in the Seattle Heart Watch.[435] Of those patients who were working prior to surgery, 82 percent returned to work postoperatively; but only 50 percent of those who were disabled preoperatively returned to work. Of those not working 61 percent stated they were influenced not to work by medical advice.

We surveyed the working status of 2652 patients who underwent coronary artery bypass graft surgery at Emory University Hospital between 1973 and 1979. At a mean follow-up of 20 months, 24 percent of the women and 55 percent of the men were working. These figures are misleading, however, and need further clarification. For example, 16 percent of the men and 48 percent of the women were not employed prior to developing their heart symptoms. Of those who were unemployed at follow-up, only 45 percent of the women and 64 percent of the men said this was because of the heart condition. Of patients who had been employed up until the time of surgery, we found that 81 percent of the women and 89 percent of the men returned to work postoperatively. At the time of the follow-up surgery, 65 percent of the women and 79 percent of the men remained employed. On the other hand, patients who had been disabled prior to surgery were less likely to return to work; 23 percent of the women and 40 percent of the men did so. The age of the patient had a marked effect on the return to work; 77 percent of the men under 40 were working while only 16 percent of the men over 70 were working. The same trend with smaller percentages working also applied to the women. The patients who were not working were asked whether it was because of their heart condition. In general, the young patients gave their heart condition as the reason for not working, but other reasons were mentioned by the older patients who were not working. The patients who had worked up to the time of surgery were the patients most likely to return to work after surgery. Rehabilitation for those who had been disabled prior to surgery was much better for the younger groups.

We surveyed the preoperative variables and related them to the postoperative work status. The most significant factors surveyed were age and preoperative working status. Factors of significance were the preoperative history of congestive heart failure (men), ejection fraction less than 35 percent (men), preoperative myocardial infarctions (men), and abnormal left ventricular contractility (men). The number of women was too small to be significant. In those not working because of their heart condition, the factors related to left ventricular dysfunction were significant; i.e., previous infarction, new Q waves, abnormal contractility, plus completeness of revascularization. Items that were not surveyed but are felt to influence the postoperative work status are the preoperative job (sedentary executive versus manual labor), job satisfaction, and most importantly economic incentive or disincentive to work.[436]

Our approach to younger patients is to explain prior to surgery that continued or resumed employment is an important goal of coronary artery bypass graft surgery. We also try to support the patient in dealing with the employer following surgery. With minor modifications in work status, many of the patients who are not working even because of heart disease could be employed.

Jenkins et al. recently reported the results of their study on the influence of coronary bypass surgery on the physical, psychological, and economic status of a study group which consisted of 318 patients. They found that angina was completely relieved in 69 to 85 percent; disability days were reduced more than 80 percent; 75 percent of employed persons had returned to work; anxiety, depression, fatigue, and sleep problems declined; vigor and well-being improved. They concluded that the great majority of patients are able to resume normal economic and social functioning within 6 months after coronary bypass surgery.[437]

Cost of Medical and Surgical Treatment

Perhaps no item related to medical care has received greater attention than the containment of costs. Certainly medical care had become more and more expensive as high technology has been developed and made available to wide segments of the population. Certain governmental agencies involved in medical planning have also been developed in an effort to control medical costs. Such agencies, of course, are also very expensive.[438]

Coronary bypass surgery, a highly technological and expensive development, has been applied widely. This procedure, more than most others, has received the attention of medical care planners and the public alike. Since coronary bypass surgery is used in patients with atherosclerotic coronary heart disease, the number one health menace in America, we must therefore concern ourselves not only with the cost but also the benefits to be derived, and we must compare surgery with alternative methods of treatment.

Since the course of patients is so variable, the average cost for a patient treated medically for atherosclerotic coronary heart disease cannot be established. The direct cost, of course, includes physician contact, medications, hospitalization, and diagnostic testing as well as treatment for the major complications of atherosclerotic coronary heart disease. More work is needed to establish the cost of this aspect of health care, but it is considerable. If one examines one complication of atherosclerotic coronary heart disease, namely myocardial infarction, which occurs in about 400,000 persons per year and requires an average of about 2 to 3 weeks hospitalization at $300 (plus or minus) per day total cost, then one finds close to 2 billion dollars per year being spent in the treatment of this single complication.

Indirect costs include loss of productivity because of early retirement; days missed from work; decreased ability to perform one's job; fear and anxiety which can be disabling; and death. It is difficult to place a monetary value on these indirect costs to society, but they are great.[438]

Few data exist concerning the comparison of costs between patients treated medically and those treated surgically; however, a few studies have been done.

At Brigham and Women's Hospital, patients undergoing surgery for chronic angina pectoris were evaluated for the number of hospital days in the 2-year period prior to surgery and in the 2 years following surgery.[439] The average duration of hospitalization during the 2 years before surgery was 7.7 days per patient per year, and this was reduced to 1.8 days per patient per year in the period following bypass surgery. The clinicians concluded that the difference (5.9 days per patient per year), based on an average cost of $300 per day, would result in a saving of $1770 per patient per year. The results were more striking when only those patients requiring preoperative hospitalization were analyzed. These had 15.5 days per patient per year preoperatively and only 1.4 days per patient per year postoperatively. At this rate, the cost of surgery would be amortized in less than 2 years assuming that the patient would continue to require 2 weeks/year hospitalization even if surgery had not been done.

Patients with unstable angina pectoris who were part of the national cooperative study group treated at the University of Alabama were evaluated for direct medical cost during the 2 years following randomization.[440] It was found that costs for patients randomized to medical therapy averaged $6226 while those randomized to surgical therapy averaged $10,416. A large percentage of the patients initially randomized to medical treatment later required surgery because of persistent or recurrent symptoms. The cost during the 2-year period for this group (including surgery) averaged $20,059. Certainly one of the most costly medical expenses is the prolonged and repeated hospitalization of patients with intractable or unstable angina pectoris or with complications of myocardial infarction.

Family income decreased less in those patients who were continued on medical therapy without disabling symptoms. This included only 57 percent of those randomized to medical therapy. The other 43 percent had significant symptoms, so surgery was eventually required.[441]

The total cost of medical care appears to be less for patients who have had coronary bypass surgery compared to similar patients who are treated medically.[79,411]

Other Surgical Procedures Used in Patients with Atherosclerotic Coronary Heart Disease

Coronary endarterectomy was popular during the early 1970s.[442] It is currently used frequently by only a few surgeons. Most surgeons believe that it is better to suture the distal end of a saphenous vein graft into a more distal end of the coronary artery when it is severely blocked proximal to the site than to suture it into the artery in an area where the intima has been removed.

Thrombosis is much more likely to follow endarterectomy of the left coronary system (left anterior descending and circumflex arteries) than after endarterectomy of the right coronary artery.

White and Bland used *neurosurgical procedures* to relieve the pain of intractable and disabling angina pectoris.[443] They used cervical sympathectomy and posterior rhizotomy with some success. The patients could still "sense" their angina, but life was more tolerable for them. We rarely use this procedure today.

Partial ileal bypass has been used to lower the blood level of certain lipids.[444,445] The operation consists of a bypass of the distal 200 cm or one-third of the small intestine, whichever value is larger, with restoration of intestinal continuity by an end-to-side anastomosis of the proximal small intestine to the cecum. This operation is not a weight-losing operation and should not be confused with the more extensive 90 percent jejunoileal bypass procedure used to treat obese patients. Partial ileal bypass does not produce malabsorption, except for vitamin B_{12}, which is replaced by supplemental parenteral injection every 2 months. Moore et al.[446] reported the effects of the operation on the plasma lipids and lipoprotein concentrations of 28 male survivors of first infarction. All subjects had a marked reduction in plasma tool cholesterol at 3 months and 1 year after surgery. All but 2 of the 28 subjects had a marked lowering of low-density lipoprotein-cholesterol levels following surgery. Subjects with hypertriglyceridemia prior to surgery had a reduction in triglycerides and low-density lipoprotein-cholesterol levels following surgery, whereas subjects with normal levels of triglycerides prior to surgery had a slight increase in both measurements after surgery. Moore et al.[446] further state that "it remains to be seen whether the use of partial ileal bypass to effect maximal reduction in the atherogenic plasma lipids and lipoproteins will result in a reduction in coronary heart disease risk in man."

Koivisto and Miettinen have recently reported their observations of the long-term effects of ileal bypass on lipoproteins in patients with familial hypercholesterolemia.[447] They state that "most ileal bypass patients were still hypercholesterolemic, and their LDL cholesterol levels, and even more so the LDL apoprotein B levels, were still elevated, indicating that over the long-term ideal bypass could not normalize plasma lipid levels in patients with heterozygous familial hypercholesterolemia and that a combination of surgery with hyperlipidemic drugs may be needed." Illingworth and Connor support such a view with their observation on a patient who had distal ileal bypass but had inadequate lowering of the total and LDL cholesterol until Mevinolin was added to the treatment.[448]

Even if a favorable result can be produced by the procedure, it is unlikely the procedure will ever be used to any degree except in carefully selected patients.

Treatment of Specific Subsets

The preceding discussion highlights, in general terms, the types of treatment that are available for patients with atherosclerotic coronary heart disease.

The subsets of atherosclerotic coronary heart disease discussed below have been identified with the clinician in mind. Each subset represents a category of patients that the clinician must *treat*. The subsets that are listed also take into account current pathophysiological considerations. We have, as Herrick advised,[3] linked specific treatment to specific subsets of the clinical spectrum. This is necessary because the treatment of one specific subset may not be the same as it is for another subset. Clinicians should remember the following points as they approach the patient:

- Stable angina pectoris produced by effort is usually caused by an increase of the demand side of the myocardial oxygen supply-demand system.
- Angina pectoris occurring when the patient is at rest is usually the result of a decrease of the supply side of the myocardial oxygen supply-demand system.
- Angina pectoris and other signs of myocardial ischemia may occur because of a combination of the two abnormal physiological states listed above. This type of angina is referred to as "mixed" angina. There may be an increase in the demand end of the myocardial oxygen-demand system plus a decrease in the supply end of the myocardial oxygen-demand system occurring at the same time.
- Angina pectoris should be considered a direct "signal" of myocardial ischemia. Unfortunately a patient may have a faulty signaling system, and myocardial ischemia may not be recognized until a castastrophic event occurs.[70–76,449–453]
- Angina equivalents produced by effort are often overlooked because the symptoms are commonly due to other conditions and the physician fails to attribute them to myocardial ischemia. There are three types of angina equivalents due to transient left ventricular ischemia. *Dyspnea*, believed to be due to a diminution in left ventricular function and an increase in pulmonary venous pressure and pulmonary edema, may occur. Profound *weakness and fatigue*, associated with a fall in blood pressure of at least 20 mmHg due to poor systolic ventricular function, may occur. *Arrhythmias*, such as ventricular ectopic beats and ventricular tachycardia, produced by effort in patients with atherosclerotic heart disease may be due to myocardial ischemia occurring because of an increase in the demand side of the myocardial oxygen supply-demand system. Similar arrhythmias occurring at rest may be due to myocardial ischemia produced by decreasing the supply side of the myocardial oxygen-demand system. For example, certain subsets of Prinzmetal's angina are characterized by high-grade AV block. The pathophysiology in such cases is

most likely coronary artery spasm plus atheromatous lesions. In fact, as discussed earlier, painless myocardial ischemia is not common. The patient with angina equivalents may have ventricular scarring from previous infarction plus exercise-induced ischemia which produces an additional temporary diminution in myocardial contractility and exercise-induced symptoms. At times painless ischemia dominates the pathophysiological features of the condition.

Angina equivalents may occur with effort and lead one to consider an increase in the demand side of the myocardial oxygen supply-demand system, or they may occur when the patient is at rest, when one should consider a decrease in the supply side of the myocardial oxygen supply-demand system.

- When angina first occurs and when angina occurs at rest, one should consider a decrease in the supply side of the myocardial oxygen supply-demand system. This decrease can be produced by coronary spasm, coronary thrombosis, or the elevation of an atheromatous plaque, or a combination of these.
- Myocardial infarction is usually associated with coronary thrombosis.
- When myocardial ischemia lasts a brief period, as it does with angina produced with effort, the ischemia is reversible, and the heart muscle is not usually damaged. Myocardial ischemia that persists longer than the ischemia responsible for angina pectoris may not cause recognizable permanent myocardial damage. This is called *prolonged myocardial ischemia without objective evidence of necrosis*. When ischemia lasts still longer, or is more intense, there may be, and frequently is, irreversible ischemia and permanent heart muscle damage (*infarction*).

The reason the pathophysiology is discussed here is that we are coming closer now in our efforts to link the clinical features of a patient to the pathophysiology. The altered pathophysiology can then be linked to treatment. For example, angina at rest is more likely to be due to coronary artery spasm than is angina with effort. Accordingly, a calcium antagonist may be more useful in the treatment of angina at rest than a beta blocker.

Coronary Atherosclerosis without Angina or Other Evidence of Ischemia

Definition and Recognition

The individuals give no history of angina or infarction. The exercise stress ECG and radionuclide exercise cardiac scan are normal.

In practice one proves the presence of *nonobstructive* coronary disease when a patient has a coronary arteriogram made for another reason. Nonobstructing atheromatous lesions are defined as being less than 50 percent of the luminal diameter of a coronary artery. Nonobstructing lesions are found in the following way. Most adult patients with valve disease should have a coronary arteriogram prior to valve surgery. Then, too, it is not uncommon for a coronary arteriogram to be made for chest pain that turns out to be noncoronary in origin.

Treatment

The treatment of such patients falls into the realm of preventive medicine (see Chap. 42).

We could *assume* that everyone in the United States is at high risk and is vulnerable atherosclerosis and urge that aggressive preventive measures be used. Regrettably, this would not be a perfect solution to the problem since the method of prevention is imperfect, and the method is not acceptable to everyone. At present we advocate a general prevention program for children, young adults, middle-age persons, and patients after coronary angioplasty or coronary bypass surgery (see Chap. 42). Elderly individuals are different. We use a commonsense approach to elderly patients and would not withhold anything that makes them happy unless it is clearly harmful to them.

We need a simple, inexpensive method of determining the presence and rate of progression of slight coronary atherosclerosis. Should even slight disease be found by such a method, we could then follow the lesions to determine their progression. This concept is important because all lesions do not progress. General preventive measures could be used in the patients who show little or no progression, while aggressive measures, not applicable to everyone, could be instituted in patients whose lesions are progressing. Herein lies the future—the preventive and early detection of disease.*

Patients who have no subjective or objective evidence of myocardial ischemia but have borderline or obstructive lesions discovered by coronary arteriography which has been performed because of valve disease may, at times, have coronary bypass surgery at the time of valve surgery. This special category of patients is discussed later in this chapter and in Chaps. 37 and 38.

Coronary Atherosclerosis with Reversible Myocardial Ischemia—Stable Subsets

Many patients have obstructive coronary atherosclerosis which produces reversible myocardial ischemia and exhibit stable subjective or objective signs of it. Myocardial ischemia develops and subsides in these patients without causing any identifiable permanent myocardial damage. It is important to recognize all of the stable subsets of this category since some of the patients are destined to die suddenly or have a

*It is highly likely that outpatient coronary arteriography, using new catheters and equipment, may become acceptable. Such a procedure would be used initially for research purposes but would later be used routinely in a certain specified population of individuals.

coronary event that will destroy the left ventricle. We must remember that the major goals of treatment are to relieve symptoms, prevent sudden death, and preserve the patient's heart muscle.

Stable Angina Pectoris[454]

Definition and Recognition The patient has noted angina pectoris for at least 60 days. During that time the patient has noted no change in the frequency of angina attacks; precipitating causes; duration of angina; or ease with which it is relieved. The functional status of the patient should be determined by using the guidelines of the Canadian Heart Association (see Table 6-1).

The patient's age, life-style, and coexistent disease should be considered, because they are important items that are needed for the decision-making process in such patients.

About 25 percent of patients suspected as having stable angina pectoris due to atherosclerotic coronary heart disease have normal or minimally diseased coronary arteries.[78] Accordingly, most patients thought to have stable angina pectoris should have a coronary arteriogram and left ventriculogram. Exceptions to this rule are patients whose history has a predictive value less than 90 percent, and who have a negative exercise stress ECG and ^{201}Tl scan; patients who have mild stable angina pectoris and are beyond 75 years of age; and patients who have coexistent disease that would contraindicate bypass surgery. In general, however, patients under 70 years of age who might be candidates for coronary angioplasty or bypass surgery should have a coronary arteriogram and left ventriculogram to confirm the diagnosis, estimate the prognosis, and determine the need for angioplasty or surgery.

Treatment of Stable Angina Pectoris The treatment of stable angina pectoris is determined by many factors.

The treatment of patients with stable angina pectoris who are under the age of 70 depends upon the functional classification; the results of the exercise stress ECG; the results of radionuclide testing; the abnormalities found at coronary arteriography and left ventriculography including the contractility of the myocardium and the ejection fraction; and the existence of other disease.

Patients with class I, II, III, or IV stable angina who have proximal disease of a single coronary artery should be considered for coronary angioplasty (see later discussion).

Patients with class III or IV stable angina who have single-vessel disease and are not ideal candidates for angioplasty should have coronary bypass surgery if their coronary anatomy is suitable.

Patients with class I, II, III, or IV stable angina who have left main coronary artery obstruction should have coronary bypass surgery.

Patients with class I, II, III, or IV stable angina pectoris who have triple-vessel obstruction and a positive exercise ECG or radionuclide scan should have coronary bypass surgery.

Patients with class I, II, III, or IV stable angina pectoris who have high-grade obstruction of the proximal portion of the left anterior descending artery plus obstruction in one other artery and have a poor exercise performance on the treadmill should have coronary bypass surgery.

Patients with class I and II stable angina pectoris who have obstructions of one, two, or three coronary arteries, who have an excellent exercise performance on the treadmill, and who have normal ejection fractions can be treated with nitrates, beta blockers, and calcium antagonists if they are satisfied with their angina control[78] (see footnote on page 949). It should be pointed out that these patients represent a very small subset of patients with stable angina pectoris. Some of the patients are candidates for coronary angioplasty (see later discussion). About 25 percent of these patients will need coronary bypass surgery for unacceptable angina during a 5-year follow-up period.[78]

Nitroglycerin should be used to relieve and prevent anginal episodes in patients with stable angina pectoris. Such patients may need adequate doses of isosorbide dinitrate and a beta blocker such as propranolol or nadolol (Corgard) or timolol (Blocadren) and a calcium antagonist such as diltiazem or nifedipine. Verapamil can be used, but the chance of producing AV block is greater.

The patient must discontinue smoking, attain a normal body weight, and achieve a normal blood pressure. The preventive measures discussed in Chap. 42 should be implemented. Walking is safe exercise for such patients. If more exercise is desired, the patient should enroll in a physician-supervised exercise program.

Positive Electrocardiogram Exercise Test in Asymptomatic Patients

Definition and Recognition The definition and recognition of a positive exercise test in asymptomatic patients are extremely important because sudden death and myocardial infarction are often not preceded by angina pectoris.

The patient may not experience angina pectoris because he or she is inactive. The same patient may, however, have a positive exercise ECG stress test which incudes ST-segment displacement; angina pectoris; dyspnea; extreme exhaustion; and ventricular arrhythmias; or a decrease in systolic blood pressure (usually about 20 mmHg). In a sense the exercise test is an extension of the history because symptoms may occur during the test that have not been noted by the patient during usual daily activities. On the other hand, an ischemic response may appear in the ECG with or without the patient developing symptoms or cardiac arrhythmia during the test.

Painless myocardial ischemia is not rare.[70–76,449–453] There is increasing evidence that painless myocardial ischemia may occur in patients even when the ECG stress test is negative. Ambulatory monitoring may identify these patients. The mechanism of ischemia in such patients may be coronary spasm. Although this is not the subject of the current discussion, these comments are inserted here to emphasize that a negative exercise test does not enable the physician to guarantee all patients that they do not have myocardial ischemia.

Certain asymptomatic patients, especially women, who develop an abnormal ST segment on the treadmill may have their problem clarified with an exercise ^{201}Tl scan, but most male patients with more than 1.5 mm of ST-segment displacement, a fall in blood pressure, and/or symptoms of angina, dyspnea, exhaustion, or ventricular arrhythmia during or just after the treadmill test should have a coronary arteriogram and left ventriculogram. Patients with 2.5 to 3 mm of ST-segment displacement in the ECG during stage I and II of the stress test or who have angina, a fall in blood pressure, dyspnea, exhaustion, or ventricular arrhythmias produced by the treadmill exercise are highly likely to have extensive coronary disease and a poor prognosis. Such patients should have a coronary arteriogram. Patients who only have 1 to 1.5 mm of ST-segment displacement in stage III or IV of the stress test have a better prognosis than the patients described above. Some physicians would have a ^{201}Tl scan performed on these patients, and if the results were negative, they would assume that extensive obstructive coronary disease was not present. If the ^{201}Tl scan result were positive, they would then have coronary arteriography. Other physicians would obtain a coronary arteriogram in such patients and obtain a ^{201}Tl scan only if borderline lesions were found. There are reasons for the different strategies (see concluding section of this chapter).

As usual, a complete examination must be performed in such patients. Remember, a carotid bruit, abdominal aneurysm, and intermittent claudication of the legs due to peripheral atherosclerosis are important markers for the presence of coronary atherosclerosis.

The patient's age, life-style, and coexistent disease should be considered because they are needed for the decision-making process about such patients.

Treatment The treatment of patients who give no history of symptoms but have a positive exercise test usually depends upon the results of the coronary arteriogram and left ventriculogram or radionuclear testing.

There are only a few reports that deal with asymptomatic patients. Accordingly, it is necessary to utilize the data obtained from patients who are mildly symptomatic to determine what should be done regarding patients who have no symptoms.

- Asymptomatic patients with a positive exercise stress test who have high-grade obstruction of the left main coronary artery should have coronary bypass surgery. Such patients have never been studied in a randomized clinical trial, but no one would dare do such a study since all indirect evidence supports the need for urgent surgery.
- Asymptomatic patients with triple-vessel disease who exhibit more than 1.5 mm of ST-segment displacement during the early stages of the exercise ECG; multiple dead areas or multiple areas of reperfusion on the ^{201}Tl scan; or angina, dyspnea, exhaustion, or ventricular arrhythmias during the exercise test; or have a decreased ejection fraction should have coronary bypass surgery.
- Asymptomatic patients with double-vessel disease with one of the obstructions located in the proximal portion of the left anterior descending artery who exhibit greater than 1.5 mm of ST-segment displacement during the early stages of exercise ECG; multiple dead areas or multiple areas of reperfusion on the ^{201}Tl scan; or angina, dyspnea, exhaustion, ventricular arrhythmia, or a fall in blood pressure during the treadmill test should have coronary bypass surgery if coronary angioplasty is not feasible. There are few data to support this view but indirect data do support it.
- Asymptomatic patients with double-vessel disease with the left anterior descending artery not obstructed who exhibit greater than 1.5 mm of ST-segment displacement during the early phase of the exercise electrocardiogram; multiple dead areas or multiple areas of reperfusion on the ^{201}Tl scan; or angina, dyspnea, ventricular arrhythmia, or a fall in blood pressure during the exercise test; or poor ejection fractions should have coronary bypass surgery if coronary angioplasty cannot be performed. There are few data to support this view, but it seems reasonable to approach the problem this way.
- Asymptomatic patients with double-vessel disease in which the left anterior descending artery is spared who exhibit less than 1.5 mm of ST-segment displacement during the exercise stress test; show no more than one dead area or only slight reperfusion in a single area on the ^{201}Tl scan; and do not develop angina, dyspnea, exhaustion, ventricular arrhythmia, or a fall in blood pressure during the exercise test may be treated medically.[78] Such patients must be followed carefully because the obstructive disease may be progressive.
- Asymptomatic patients with single-vessel disease who have a positive exercise electrocardiogram stress test should have coronary angioplasty even if angina, dyspnea, exhaustion, arrhythmias, and a fall in blood pressure do not occur. If the coronary lesion is in the proximal portion of the left anterior descending artery and the stress ECG is markedly positive but angioplasty is not feasible,

then bypass surgery should be performed. There are few data to support the approach, but any experienced physician knows that a high-grade lesion in the proximal portion of the left anterior descending artery is undesirable (see later discussion).

There are few data to indicate the drug therapy that may be indicated in asymptomatic patients who have a proven ischemic response in the exercise ECG. Antiplatelet drugs may be used, but their value is not definitely established. A beta blocker such as nadolol may be used, but the value in the individual patient cannot be evaluated because the patient is asymptomatic. A calcium antagonist may be used if the ST segment is fortuitously discovered to become displaced at times other than during the stress test.

The patient should not smoke, and his or her blood pressure and body weight should be normalized. The American Heart Association diet book should be followed. Walking is acceptable exercise for such patients. If more exercise is desired, the patient should enroll in a supervised exercise program. The preventive measures discussed in Chap. 42 should be implemented.

Angina Equivalents

Definition and Recognition Angina pectoris itself, the most direct patient signal of myocardial ischemia, is not always easy to identify. There are three other complaints, which are indirect signals of myocardial ischemia, that are even more difficult to evaluate. Two of these symptoms, *dyspnea* and *exhaustion*, are due to left ventricular dysfunction which is produced by a more global type of myocardial ischemia. The other disorder, *cardiac arrhythmias*, can be due to transient ischemia of a small area of heart muscle. Ischemia, however, is not always the cause of arrhythmias in patients with coronary disease. These conditions are discussed here because they often represent a reversible subset of myocardial ischemia.

The patient may complain of abrupt *dyspnea*. In extreme form there may actually be pulmonary edema due to left ventricular dysfunction and elevation of pulmonary venous pressure. This condition has been called "left ventricular paralysis." It can also be viewed as transient electrical-mechanical dissociation due to myocardial ischemia. The patient usually complains of new dyspnea produced by effort, but abrupt episodes of severe dyspnea may occur at rest. The physician's dilemma is to exclude hyperventilation, pulmonary embolism, and other types of acute lung disease. The patient may or may not give a history of dyspnea depending on the patient's customary activity. Such patients should not have a stress test without considerable thought and caution. If the test is performed, it will usually reveal ST-segment displacement, an inordinate amount of dyspnea, fatigue, a fall in blood pressure, and occasionally ventricular arrhythmias. The patient may not experience ordinary angina pectoris.

The patient may complain of *chronic fatigue* or have *"episodes" of exhaustion* and weakness which is also due to left ventricular dysfunction and poor left ventricular stroke volume producing a fall in systemic blood pressure. This condition represents a more chronic state of electrical-mechanical dissociation. The complaint may occur while the patient is inactive but is noticed more often in relation to effort. The physician's dilemma is to exclude anxiety and other causes of fatigue such as poor physical fitness. There are, however, few conditions that produce new and abrupt exhaustion with effort. Patients with this complaint should not have an exercise stress test without considerable thought and caution. If the test is performed, it will usually reveal ST-segment displacement, dyspnea, exhaustion, a fall in blood pressure, and occasionally ventricular arrhythmias occurring during the test. The patient may not experience ordinary angina pectoris.

Certain cardiac *arrhythmias* may occur without angina. The patient may have ventricular ectopic beats, ventricular tachycardia, or even ventricular fibrillation produced by effort or occurring at rest. Many of these arrhythmias are due to transient ischemia, but some are not.

Patients suspected of having an angina equivalent should be considered for arteriography. It is accepted, however, that some of the patients with these complaints can be safely exercised by experienced physicians. Accordingly, a radionuclear ventriculogram or a ^{201}Tl scan, when negative, will assist the physician in excluding coronary disease as a cause of these unusual symptoms.

Treatment The treatment of angina equivalents is similar to that of stable angina pectoris or unstable angina pectoris since the equivalents may be stable (present longer than 60 days) or unstable (of recent onset). The results of coronary bypass surgery, if indicated and feasible, are good in patients with dyspnea or exhaustion but unpredictable in patients whose angina equivalent is an arrhythmia.

Coronary Atherosclerosis with Reversible Myocardial Ischemia—Unstable Subsets

Patients with coronary atherosclerosis may have reversible myocardial ischemia and exhibit unstable subjective or objective evidence of it. Myocardial ischemia develops and subsides in such patients without causing any recognizable permanent myocardial damage. It is important to identify all of the unstable subsets since many of the patients are destined to have sudden death or have a coronary event that will destroy the left ventricle. Many patients with unstable ischemic syndromes have an abnormality in the supply end of the myocardial oxygen supply-demand system, and, in general, this is more serious than stable syndromes, when an abnormality of the demand end of the myocardial oxygen-demand system tends to prevail.

Unstable Angina Pectoris

Definition and Recognition *Unstable angina pectoris* is said to be present when angina pectoris first begins; angina pectoris has been present for less than 60 days; angina pectoris is increasing in frequency and duration; angina pectoris is provoked with less than usual stimuli; or angina occurs at rest. Patients with such complaints are considered to be in jeopardy of having a coronary event such as sudden death or myocardial infarction within a few days, weeks, or months.

The physician notes the patient's age, life-style, risk factors, previous infarctions, cardiac status, and extracardiac disease such as pulmonary disease, carotid artery disease, aortic disease, or cerebral disease.

The patient with unstable angina pectoris should be admitted to the hospital for coronary arteriography unless there is some compelling reason not to do so. Advanced age (beyond 75) might be considered to be a relative contraindication to coronary arteriography in patients with unstable angina pectoris. The same applies to the patient who has another serious disease.

Treatment The treatment of unstable angina pectoris is as follows:

- Many patients with uncontrolled unstable angina pectoris should be placed in the coronary care unit.
- Patients with unstable angina pectoris should not, as a rule, have an exercise ECG stress test or an exercise radionuclide stress test.
- Sublingual nitroglycerin should be used to relieve and prevent angina pectoris. Nitroglycerin ointment should be used several times daily, and isosorbide dinitrate should be given orally. An intravenous drip of nitroglycerin is often needed in patients with frequent and recurrent unstable angina pectoris. Diltiazem or nifedipine can be added to the treatment regimen if discomfort continues since the angina is often due to a decrease in the supply end of the myocardial oxygen supply-demand system. A beta blocker such as propranolol or nadolol may also be needed if symptoms continue.
- Coronary artery bypass surgery should be recommended for patients with unstable angina who have left main coronary artery obstruction, triple-vessel coronary artery obstruction, or double-vessel coronary artery obstruction.
- Percutaneous transluminal coronary angioplasty may be recommended for patients with unstable angina who have reachable single-vessel coronary disease.
- Medical management after coronary bypass surgery may include a beta blocker and perhaps an antiplatelet drug. Postangioplasty medical treatment should include antiplatelet drugs and a calcium antagonist.
- Patients with unstable angina who do not have coronary bypass surgery or coronary angioplasty should be treated as if they have a small myocardial infarction. Drug therapy may include long-acting nitrates, a beta blocker, and diltiazem or nifedipine with a beta blocker.
- Patients with unstable angina pectoris should be encouraged to stop smoking, attain a normal body weight, and achieve a normal blood pressure. The principles stated in the American Heart Association cookbook should be the guide for patients under 70 years of age. Exercise is prohibited for patients with unstable angina pectoris until definitive treatment such as angioplasty or bypass surgery has been achieved. After definitive treatment has been completed, a supervised rehabilitation program may be recommended. The preventive measures discussed in Chap. 42 should be implemented.
- Most patients should return to work after bypass surgery or after coronary angioplasty.
- When surgery cannot be performed because of poor distal vessels or myocardial damage and the patient continues to have disabling angina despite nitrates, beta blockers, or calcium antagonists, it may be necessary to use methimazole (Tapazole) or radioactive iodine to reduce the metabolic state. When this form of therapy is needed, it involves a group of patients who may be unable to work.

Postinfarction Angina Pectoris

Definition and Recognition Most patients with myocardial infarction do not have angina pectoris immediately following infarction. Some do, and it is referred to as *immediate* postinfarction angina pectoris. Some patients will have a skip period of weeks before angina appears, and this is referred to as *delayed postinfarction angina pectoris.* These are very serious forms of angina pectoris.

Treatment The patient with fresh infarction who continues to have episodes of myocardial ischemia (*immediate* angina pectoris) is usually receiving a nitroglycerin drip, diltiazem or nifedipine, propranolol, oxygen, etc. Such a patient should have a coronary arteriogram and left ventriculogram to determine the feasibility of coronary bypass surgery. Dead myocardial tissue does not hurt. Therefore, if the coronary anatomy and left ventricular wall motion permit bypass surgery, it should be performed in order to relieve the patient of angina and to salvage the remaining jeopardized myocardium as well.

The patient with *delayed* postinfarction angina should receive vigorous medical therapy but regardless of the results of such therapy should have a coronary arteriogram and left ventriculogram. If conditions are proper, such a patient should have coronary bypass surgery.

Medical management following coronary artery bypass surgery may include a beta blocker and perhaps antiplatelet drugs. The use of a beta blocker depends on the postoperative status of the patient. The patient should not smoke. The diet should incorporate the principles laid down in the American Heart Association cookbook, and the blood pressure should be normalized. Walking is the recommended exercise. If more exercise is desired, the patient should enter a supervised exercise program. The preventive measures discussed in Chap. 42 should be implemented.

Prinzmetal's Angina Pectoris or Variant Angina (see Chap. 46)

Definition and Recognition Patients with Prinzmetal's angina have episodes of myocardial ischemia at rest (see later discussion). The ECG may exhibit transient ST-segment shift that suggests an acute infarction. Prinzmetal described this electrocardiographic abnormality in 1958[32] (Fig. 45-8). On rare occasion transient abnormal Q waves occur during the episode. It is very important to record an ECG during the episode of chest discomfort. Prinzmetal made a brilliant suggestion that the episodes of angina were due to coronary artery spasm in a coronary artery that was already partially occluded with atheroma (see Fig. 45-1). AV block and other arrhythmias may occur during the episodes (see Fig. 45-9). The spasm may occur in otherwise normal coronary arteries, but it more commonly occurs in patients with obstructive coronary disease. Cannon et al. have suggested a syndrome that has similar but not identical pathophysiology. They suggest that the large epicardial coronary arteries may appear normal without spasm, but the small coronary arteries cannot dilate properly when the need arises.[455]

The episodes of variant angina usually occur when the patient is at rest but may rarely occur during treadmill exercise. Smoking tobacco may precipitate angina. Alcohol and cocaine[456] may also precipitate coronary spasm angina.

The physician should note the age of the patient, the "risk factors," and the noncardiac diseases that are present.

Coronary arteriography and left ventriculography should be performed in patients with Prinzmetal's angina pectoris. Special care must be used in the laboratory and plans must be made in advance to use intravenous nitroglycerin and nifedipine if obstinate coronary spasm occurs.

Coronary spasm may be provoked in some patients in whom the diagnosis is not clear by the use of intravenous ergonovine (see Chap. 98). This test should not be used outside the cardiac catheterization laboratory.[188]

Patients with known Prinzmetal's angina do not need an exercise ECG stress test or an exercise radionuclide stress test. Patients who have not been diagnosed as having Prinzmetal's angina but have episodes of chest discomfort at rest in whom the physician suspects angina pectoris should not routinely have a stress test. If the test is performed, it should be done with great caution.

Treatment The treatment of patients with Prinzmetal's angina is as follows:

- Patients who have angina pectoris due to obstructive coronary disease plus coronary spasm or who have coronary spasm with normal coronary arteries may be relieved by nitroglycerin, isosorbide dinitrate, nitroglycerin ointment, or intravenous

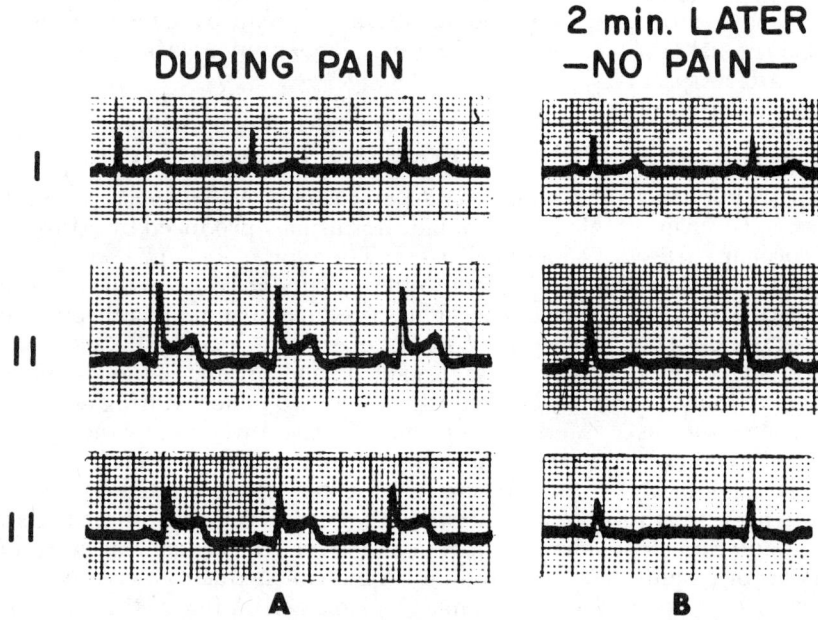

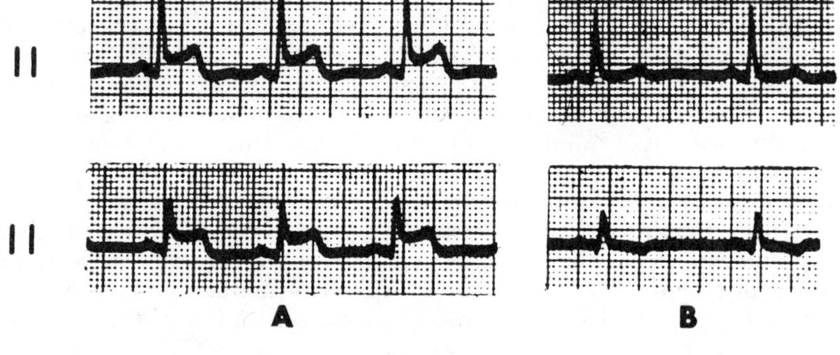

FIGURE 45-8 ECG of variant type of angina pectoris. *A.* During spontaneous pain. Note the ST-segment elevation in leads II and III and slight depression in lead I. *B.* 2 min later. The pain had disappeared and the ECG reverted to normal. (*Legend and illustration from M. Prinzmetal, R. Kennamer, R. Merliss, T. Wada, and N. Bor. Angina Pectoris: I. A Variant Form of Angina Pectoris: Preliminary Report, Am. J. Med., 27:377, 1959. Reproduced with permission from the publisher and author. We wish to thank Dr. Prinzmetal's son for his assistance and kindness in obtaining permission to use this important figure.*)

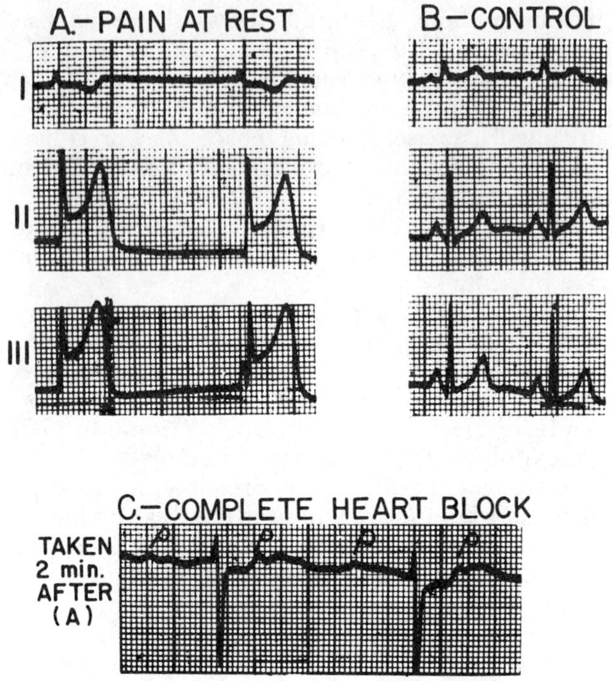

FIGURE 45-9 Transient complete heart block with attacks of pain in the variant form of angina pectoris. *A.* ECG taken during attack of pain in patient at rest. There is marked ST elevation characteristic of the variant form in leads II and III, and reciprocal depression in lead I. Heart block is probably present. (*Courtesy of A. Ekmekci and Z. Kavurt.*) *B.* ECG taken about an hour after the attack of pain. Tracing shows normal sinus rhythm and all symptoms had disappeared. *C.* Transient complete heart block during pain; 10 min after (*C*), patient felt completely well, pain was gone, pulse rate normal. (*Legend and illustration from M. Prinzmetal, R. Kennamer, R. Merliss, T. Wada, and N. Bor. Angina Pectoris: I. A Variant Form of Angina Pectoris. Preliminary Report, Am. J. Med., 27:382, 1959. Reproduced with permission from the publisher and author. We wish to thank Dr. Prinzmetal's son for his assistance and kindness in obtaining permission to use this important figure.*)

nitroglycerin. Nifedipine and diltiazem appear to be the most effective drugs for coronary artery spasm. Verapamil is also useful but may contribute to AV block in patients with Prinzmetal's angina. Some patients with coronary artery spasm are made worse by beta blockers such as propranolol or nadolol.

- Coronary artery surgery is not indicated in patients with coronary artery spasm with normal coronary arteries. Coronary artery bypass surgery is indicated in patients who have coronary artery spasm superimposed upon obstructive coronary disease. This applies to patients with left main coronary artery obstruction, triple-vessel obstruction, double-vessel obstruction, and single-vessel obstruction. Coronary bypass surgery should be used in the majority of such cases, since the disorder is a harbinger of myocardial infarction.
- Percutaneous transluminal coronary angioplasty can be used in carefully selected patients with atheromatous obstruction of the left anterior descending artery, right coronary artery, or circumflex coronary artery. Obviously, great care must be exercised to prevent and manage any superimposed coronary spasm that might develop. In fact, it is likely that coronary spasm will play an important role immediately after coronary angioplasty.
- Medical therapy with nitrates and nifedipine or diltiazem plus antiplatelet drugs should be continued after surgery or coronary angioplasty.
- Patients with coronary spasm with or without obstructive coronary disease due to atheroma should be encouraged to stop smoking (or using tobacco in any form). The patient with obstructive disease should attain normal body weight and normal blood pressure. The dietary principles laid down in the American Heart Association cookbook should be followed except in the elderly. There are no data to support the value of exercise in patients with coronary spasm and normal coronary arteries. Patients with obstructive disease may engage in walking, and if more exercise is desired, the patient should participate in a supervised program. The preventive measures discussed in Chap. 42 should be implemented.
- Patients with Prinzmetal's angina may have spontaneous remissions as emphasized by Waters et al.[457]
- Most patients with obstructive coronary disease plus coronary spasm can return to work after bypass surgery or coronary angioplasty, and after a carefully planned medical regimen has been tested and found to be successful. Patients with coronary artery spasm who have normal coronary arteries and who experience infrequent angina that is controlled with nitrates and nifedipine or diltiazem can continue to work. A few patients are truly disabled.
- When surgery cannot be performed in patients with disabling angina who have spasm and obstructive coronary disease and poor distal vessels or myocardial damage, the patient with disabling angina may benefit from methimazole or radioactive iodine therapy to reduce the metabolic state. Many of these patients cannot work.

Prolonged Myocardial Ischemia without Objective Evidence of Infarction

Definition and Recognition Angina pectoris usually lasts 1 to 5 min. It is usually produced by effort and emotional stress. The type of ischemia we are discussing here often occurs at rest; may awaken the patient at night; lasts 20 to 30 min (it has been called *prolonged angina*); may produce ST-segment depression during an attack; may produce ST-segment elevation (Prinzmetal's phenomenon) during an attack; and may produce T-wave inversion in the electrocardiogram that requires hours or even days to return to normal; but it is not associated with elevations of serum enzyme levels. Most of these patients have progressive obstructive coronary disease, and the symptoms are not solely due to increased myocardial demand for oxygen. A few of these patients have obstructive coronary disease with superimposed coronary artery spasm, and a few have coronary artery spasm with normal coronary arteries. Coronary thrombosis undoubtedly plays a role in some patients.

As usual, the physician takes note of the age of the patient, the "risk factors" that are present, and the other medical problems that are present in the patient.

The patient should be admitted to the hospital. Most of the patients should be admitted to the coronary care unit. Coronary arteriography should be done unless there is evidence of infarction. Advanced age (beyond 75) might be considered to be a relative contraindication to coronary arteriography in patients with this syndrome.

Patients with prolonged chest discomfort due to myocardial ischemia should not routinely have an exercise ECG stress test or an exercise radionuclide stress test performed.

Treatment The management of patients with prolonged myocardial ischemia who exhibit no evidence of infarction is similar to the management of patients with unstable angina pectoris or a small infarction.

- Sublingual nitroglycerin should be used to relieve and prevent the episodes of chest discomfort. Many patients with recurrent episodes of discomfort will require intravenous nitroglycerin to control the pain. Propranolol or nadolol should be given in adequate dosage. Some patients will respond to nitroglycerin ointment and isosorbide dinitrate. Patients with prolonged chest discomfort due to coronary artery spasm superimposed on obstructive coronary disease or coronary artery spasm with otherwise normal coronary arteries may not benefit by the use of propranolol. Such patients should receive adequate doses of nitrates (including intravenous nitroglycerin for recurrent episodes of pain) and a calcium antagonist such as nifedipine or diltiazem.
- Coronary bypass surgery is recommended for those patients whose coronary arteriogram and left ventriculogram reveal the appropriate anatomic finding and acceptable myocardial contractility. As always, advanced age and the presence of additional noncardiac disease should temper the physician's recommendations. Surgery should be recommended for patients who have left main coronary artery obstruction; triple-vessel coronary artery obstruction; and double-vessel coronary artery obstruction. Bypass surgery is not indicated when the syndrome is due to coronary artery spasm without obstructive atheromatous disease (see later discussion).
- Percutaneous transluminal coronary angioplasty may be used in patients with this syndrome who have obstruction of the proximal portion of a single coronary artery.
- Patients who do not have coronary bypass surgery or coronary angioplasty should be treated as if they have a small myocardial infarction.

  There may be a role for the thrombolytic therapy with streptokinase in some of these patients, but the precise role for such treatment has not been delineated (see later discussion in this chapter and Chaps. 95 and 118). Should such therapy be employed, it must be employed as soon as possible following the onset of symptoms.
- Medical therapy may or may not be continued on a long-term basis after coronary bypass surgery. Some physicians would use long-acting nitrates and a beta-blocking drug routinely, while others would use them only if they identify a poor risk group of patients. Nefedipine or diltiazem should be used in the patient with coronary artery spasm superimposed on obstructive coronary disease. Antiplatelet drugs may also be used.
- Calcium antagonists, nitrates, and antiplatelet drugs should be used in patients with coronary artery spasm and otherwise normal coronary arteries.
- Most patients should return to work after coronary bypass surgery or coronary angioplasty and after an appropriate medical regimen has been established.
- The patient should discontinue smoking, attain a normal body weight, and achieve a normal blood pressure. Patients under 70 years of age should follow the principles set forth in the American Heart Association cookbook. An exercise program is contraindicated until a coronary arteriogram is performed and treatment, such as bypass surgery, coronary angioplasty, or medical therapy, has been implemented. A supervised exercise program should not be begun for several weeks following the onset of the event. The preventive measures discussed in Chap. 42 should be implemented.
- When surgery cannot be performed in patients who continue to be disabled with angina due to obstructive coronary disease because of poor distal vessels or myocardial damage, it is occasionally useful to use methimazole or radioactive iodine therapy to reduce the metabolic rate. Regrettably, many patients in this group cannot work, There are no datae to indicate that this approach should be used in patients with coronary spasm and normal coronary arteries (see later discussion).

Coronary Atherosclerosis with Irreversible Myocardial Ischemia and Necrosis

Very Early Profound Ischemia

Definition and Recognition This term—*very early profound ischemia*—is used to designate the patient who has the sudden onset of chest discomfort that is characteristic of myocardial ischemia. The discomfort often occurs when the patient is doing very little and, in fact, may awaken the patient at night. The discomfort usually persists and generally represents the very early phase of myocardial infarction.

The patient, family member, or bystander may call a personal physician, the rescue squad, or ambulance for help. There may be little additional data available. The patient may or may not have had angina or infarction in the past. Obviously, during this phase of very early profound myocardial ischemia the physician is forced to make a decision regarding the cause of the discomfort and its treatment before the ECG is available.

The ECG, when it becomes available, in this setting, may be normal, show T-wave or ST-T wave abnormalities or abnormal Q waves with ST-T abnormalities. The results of the serum enzyme determinations are not available during this early phase and therefore cannot be used in the decision-making process.

Treatment The chest discomfort should be relieved with morphine and meperidine. If the chest discomfort has been present for less than 30 min, an initial trial of sublingual nitroglycerin is appropriate. Oxygen should be administered by mask or nasal prongs. The patient should be examined for physical signs of heart failure, and the blood pressure should be recorded. Surprisingly, the blood pressure may be elevated during the early phase of a "heart attack." The patient's heart rhythm should be monitored continuously since a cardiac arrhythmia and sudden death are the feared complications during this very early phase of potential infarction. Pulmonary edema and shock account for a very small percentage of deaths occurring during this early phase of illness. The earlier death occurs after the onset of irreversible ischemia, the less the likelihood of finding myocardial necrosis at autopsy. One must live a while with myocardial ischemia for the muscle cells to become necrotic.

Paramedics or the physician should give lidocaine during this early period even when the heart rhythm is normal.

The patient should be moved to the coronary care unit as quickly as possible. Initially the patient may be similar to the patient with prolonged myocardial ischemia without objective signs of infarction. As time passes, the patient shifts into the category of patients discussed in the next section, "Early Evolving Myocardial Infarction."

Early Evolving Myocardial Infarction[457a]

Definition and Recognition The former definition of *evolving infarction* implied that all of the abnormalities associated with infarction had evolved through their expected stages of change and had become stable. The patient's chest discomfort had subsided, the ECG had undergone a series of changes beginning with ST-T and T-wave changes followed by the development of abnormal Q waves, and the level of serum cardiac enzymes (MB-CK) had peaked and was declining. This series of changes usually required hours to days.

Now there is a *new definition* for the subset of patients who are seen by the physician within 4 to 6 h after the onset of prolonged chest discomfort. These patients are now referred to as having *early evolving myocardial infarction.* These patients are more likely to have ischemic myocardium that can possibly be salvaged than are patients who are seen 6 and more hours after the onset of myocardial ischemia and chest pain. Appropriate therapy designed to salvage myocardium has a better chance of being successful during this early phase of myocardial injury than it has at a later stage. The patient with *very early profound ischemia* described above becomes the patient described here when the latter survives to be admitted to the coronary care unit without inordinate delay.

Treatment During the past two decades the immediate management of the evolving myocardial infarction has had two major goals: first, to alleviate the patient's discomfort and, second, to transfer the patient to a specialized unit in order to detect and respond to possible complications more expeditiously.[287] In the past 5 years a third, and perhaps overriding goal, has arisen. This goal is the preservation of as much myocardium as possible.

The alleviation or reduction of pain remains an essential element in the care of the patient with an evolving myocardial infarction. The pain and the accompanying anxiety contribute to excessive activity of the autonomic nervous system and to the patient's restlessness. These factors, in turn, increase the metabolic demands of the myocardium. Furthermore, the experience with thrombolytic therapy suggests that pain is the reflection of ongoing ischemia rather than a product of necrotic tissue. Narcotics remain the drugs of choice in the initial attempts to relieve the pain of an evolving myocardial infarction. *Meperidine* or preferably *morphine* should be administered intravenously (see discussion on page 939 for dosage and method of administration). The reduction of pain and anxiety by these drugs will reduce the metabolic demands of the myocardium, which hopefully aids in limiting infarct size.

Measures to relieve pain and limit infarct size may possibly occur simultaneously. The other agent which has become an important element in managing the pain of the evolving myocardial infarction is *intravenous nitroglycerin.* While the predominant antianginal effect of nitroglycerin is due to a reduction in myocardial oxygen demand because of the drug's peripheral hemodynamic effects, the drug does seem to have a direct effect on the coronary circulation. Nitroglycerin appears to act on the coronary circulation primarily by dilating the large epicardial capacitance vessels and the collateral channels. Consequently, in patients with good collateral vessels, nitroglycerin is likely to increase flow into the ischemic regions, which hopefully reduces infarct size.[458,459] Evidence of the beneficial effects of intravenous nitroglycerin when administered in the early hours of a myocardial infarction is preliminary and by no means overwhelming. Nevertheless, data that intravenous nitroglycerin begun within a few hours of the onset of chest pain reduces the likelihood of developing congestive heart failure, infarct extension, or cardiac death with a low prevalence of adverse effects do support its clinical application. Both clinical data[460–462] and studies of animal models suggest that the early administration of nitroglycerin can reduce the predicted extent of myocardial infarction and favorably affect survival.[462]

A reasonable approach would be to begin intravenous nitroglycerin in any patient with discomfort thought to be due to myocardial ischemia that lasts longer than 15 min. The nitroglycerin should be started at a dose of 5 μg/min and increased by 5 μg/min every 10 min until the pain is resolved or the mean arterial pressure is reduced by 10 percent. The adverse effect most frequently encountered is headache, which can usually be controlled with mild analgesics. Sinus tachycardia and hypotension should be avoided by careful titration of the dose because either abnormality has the potential of increasing infarct size. While the potential benefit of intravenous nitroglycerin is open to question, the very low risk of its use when the dosage is carefully controlled gives the drug a favorable risk/benefit ratio. The duration of its use in these circumstances remains unresolved. It is usually given for 24 to 48 h and followed by transdermal administration of nitroglycerin.

The role of *beta blockers* in the treatment of the evolving myocardial infarction is not settled. There is substantial evidence that these pharmacological agents, when administered promptly after coronary occlusion, are successful in limiting the size of experimentally produced infarcts.[140,463–465] Moreover, preliminary clinical results suggest that early intervention with intravenous beta blockers may limit infarct size, especially in patients with evidence of increased sympathetic tone.[466–468] Even more convincing are the data that early intervention with intravenous beta blockers in patients with ongoing myocardial ischemia will reduce the occurrence of an infarction.[466,468] Hjalmarson et al. reported that metoprolol (Lopressor) decreased the 3-month mortality rate of patients with acute infarction compared to a placebo-treated group. They initially gave 15 mg of metoprolol intravenously and then 100 mg orally twice a day.[469,470] While the studies alluding to a beneficial effect of various beta blockers in the early phase of acute myocardial infarction are almost as convincing as those related to intravenous nitroglycerin, the former report a greater prevalence of adverse effects, particularly hypotension and bradyarrhythmias, than do the latter. In other words, the risk/benefit ratio for beta blockers in the evolving myocardial infarction does not seem to be as favorable as it is for nitroglycerin.

Roberts et al. have recently reported that propranolol administered 4 or more h after the onset of symptoms will not limit the size of the infarct.[471] The subset of patients with an evolving myocardial infarction who show evidence of increased sympathetic tone (either with tachycardia or systemic arterial hypertension) should, however, receive intravenous propranolol or metoprolol followed by the oral preparation of propranolol. These drugs may be administered unless there is a contraindication to their use, but we are reluctant to recommend their use routinely. Metoprolol, according to Herlitz et al., does not enhance the development of heart failure.[472]

Thrombolytic therapy[473] is predicated upon the premises that coronary thrombosis is the cause of myocardial infarction and that the most effective means of limiting myocardial necrosis is the early restoration of coronary flow by clot resolution (see Chaps. 95 and 118). There exists a substantial body of data to support each of these premises. Kennedy et al. report a nearly threefold decrease in the 30-day mortality rate of patients with infarction who have been treated with intracoronary streptokinase.[474] While the reported percentage of successful thrombolysis varies between 65 and 95 percent, a reasonable expectation of success with intracoronary administration of presently available lytic agents is 75 percent. The success rate of thrombolysis will vary depending upon the duration of pain prior to the administration of streptokinase or urokinase and upon the artery involved. Lee and associates reported a 75 percent reperfusion rate in patients receiving streptokinase within 5 h of the onset of chest pain versus 50 percent in those treated at 5 to 7 h and 17 percent in those treated beyond 7 h.[475] Rutsch and his associates noted that thrombolysis occurred within 23 min if the thrombus was less than 2 h old and 43 min if the thrombus was older than 4 h.[476] Recanalization of the left anterior descending artery and the right coronary artery requires a briefer infusion time than recanalization of the circumflex coronary artery[476] and is more likely to be successful.

It is imperative that the physician remember that preservation of the myocardium is the goal of thrombolysis and that reestablishing coronary flow is only the means to this end. Studies employing a variety of models and techniques have generally demonstrated that myocardial tissue is available for salvage for at least 2 to 3 h and possibly 6 h after coronary thrombosis.[477–479] Proportionally the greatest loss of muscle will occur in the first hour after occlusion. The time delay inherent in the intracoronary administration of a lytic agent has made the intravenous use of the drug appealing. Furthermore, the intravenous administration is a more widely applicable technique. Some studies suggest that thrombolysis is less often achieved with intravenous administration than with intracoronary administration.[480,481] On the other hand, Ganz et al. have reported success with the intravenous method of therapy, and obviously if future investigation proves the value of the approach, it can be applied to a larger population of patients with infarction.[482] Alderman et al. reported that intracoronary streptokinase had a systemic effect similar to that found with the intravenous use of the drug.[483] The threat of bleeding with systemic administration of the lytic agent would seem to be greater, but the studies reported to date have not substantiated this assumption.[480,484]

The therapeutic benefit, and consequently the exact role of thrombolytic therapy in the evolving myocardial infarction, remains to be absolutely defined. The administration of lytic agents in either manner seems to be appropriate in those patients with ongoing ischemic pain (less than 4 h) who are early in the course of their infarction and who are a part of a clinical trial (see Chap. 118). It is, of course, understood that the patients should have no contraindication to lytic therapy.

Should thrombolytic therapy be successful, it is then necessary to make a decision regarding further treatment, since it is likely the event will occur again. If intravenous streptokinase has been used, it will be necessary to have a coronary arteriogram performed in about 4 days. Further treatment would be dictated by the extent and location of the coronary artery obstructions, the ejection fraction, and ventricular wall motion. If intracoronary streptokinase has been used, the operator has immediate knowledge of the coronary anatomy, ejection fraction, and wall motion. A decision can be made at that time if coronary antioplasty, bypass surgery, or medical therapy is needed. The principles discussed earlier are used to determine the use of angioplasty or surgery in such patients. Surgery, it seems, can be done with relative safety in patients who have had intracoronary streptokinase.

The value, limitations, and harm of thrombolytic therapy are still being evaluated, and no rigid claim of long-term benefit can be stated.

Coronary bypass surgery has been used for patients with early evolving myocardial infarction. Berg et al.[485] have reported success, as determined by the rate of long-term survival, with reasonable operative risk in patients with evolving infarct.

We have used coronary bypass surgery for such patients when the patient was already in the hospital and scheduled for coronary arteriography or bypass surgery and developed persistent chest pain due to myocardial ischemia that was not relieved by intravenous nitroglycerin, beta blockers, calcium antagonists, etc. Occasionally, an intraaortic balloon pump has been used. We simply speed up the timetable for coronary angiography or proceed to coronary bypass surgery. While we are pleased with the results, we have had too few patients to draw conclusions.

Uncomplicated Completed Myocardial Infarction

Definition and Recognition Completed myocardial infarction is said to be present when myocardial necrosis develops in the aftermath of acute myocardial ischemia. The designation *completed* implies that there is little or no ongoing active ischemia.

An infarct is said to be completed by about 6 h after the onset of chest pain that is characteristic of prolonged myocardial ischemia. While it is true that active myocardial ischemia may still be present, the bulk of jeopardized heart muscle has become irreversibly damaged by that point in time. In other words, the modern definition of completed infarct implies that thrombolytic therapy would do little good because most, but not all, of the heart damage has already occurred. Older definitions implied that certain electrocardiographic and enzyme changes had passed through certain specified stages and that no subjective or objective evidence of continued ischemia or necrosis was apparent. In electrocardiographic terms, the patient would have progressed through the stage of ST elevation to the development of pathological Q waves and T-wave inversion. Enzymatic reflection of a completed infarction would be the recording of a consistent decline in the cardiac enzymes from their peak level.

Although complications are not as likely to occur after the fourth day, a completed myocardial infarction should be diagnosed as uncomplicated only at the end of the hospitalization when there has been no evidence of extension of the infarction, recurrent angina pectoris, heart failure, shock, myocardial rupture, dysrhythmia, pericarditis, or systemic embolus. Of course, any myocardial infarction could be termed uncomplicated up to the point one of these events occurred.

Treatment Patients with a myocardial infarction should be admitted to a coronary care unit. Pain should be relieved according to the method described earlier. If the patient is admitted within 1 or 2 h after the onset of symptoms, the patient may be designated as having an evolving infarction. Methods of limiting the size of the infarction including thrombolytic therapy could be considered for such a patient. If the patient is admitted 4 to 6 h after the onset of symptoms, the patient is designated as having a completed infarct, and efforts to limit the size of the infarction are less successful. If, by chance, the patient has not been hospitalized and is first seen within 48 h of the onset of infarction, admission to the coronary care unit is still indicated. Since the major focus of the coronary care unit is the immediate recognition and expeditious treatment of cardiac arrhythmias, the length of stay in this specialized area should be based on the likelihood of a patient manifesting the two arrhythmias of greatest concern, ventricular tachycardia and ventricular fibrillation. The risk of developing primary ventricular fibrillation decreases exponentially with time, with the vast majority of arrhythmic deaths occurring within the first 24 h after myocardial infarction. After the third day following a myocardial infarction, the episodes of life-threatening arrhythmias are fairly evenly distributed over the remainder of the hospitalization.[486] Based upon these data, a patient with an uncomplicated infarction can be transferred from the coronary care unit on the third day.

- Studies pointing out that 31 to 34 percent of in-hospital deaths from acute myocardial infarction occur after discharge from the coronary care unit and that half of these are sudden and unexpected emphasize that certain patients need more prolonged cardiac monitoring.[487,488] Those patients who are prime candidates for late-hospital sudden deaths are those patients who manifest, while in the coronary care unit, one of the following: (1) the arrhythmias of pump failure (sinus tachycardia, atrial flutter, or atrial fibrillation), (2) the arrhythmias of electrical instability (ventricular tachycardia or ventricular fibrillation), (3) acute interventricular conduction disturbances, (4) evidence of circulatory failure (congestive heart failure, pulmonary edema, or significant hypotension), or (5) anterior location of infarction.[487,489] The effectiveness of prolonged monitoring of this select group of patients in an intermediate care unit following coronary care unit discharge is evident in a doubling of the rate of successful resuscitations in patients so treated.[488,490]

  Patients who do not fit into this high-risk subgroup can be discharged from the coronary care unit to a medical floor without continuous monitoring.
- The length of hospitalization following an acute myocardial infarction should likewise depend on the presence or absence of these same complicating factors. If the patient has not manifested the arrhythmias of pump failure, the arrhythmias of electrical instability, evidence of circulatory failure, or advanced AV block during the first 4 days of hospitalization, he or she is very unlikely to do so at any later time.[491] This patient could probably be discharged after 7 days in the hospital.[492,493] A 10- to 14-day hospitalization for the acute uncomplicated myocardial infarction seems more appropriate. The last 3 to 5 days of the hospitalization are generally necessary to resolve the questions pertaining to residual ventricular function, the presence or absence of ventricular ectopy, and the adequacy of the remainder of the coronary circulation. In addition, time is needed for instruction in risk marker modification.
- The *activity* permitted the patient with uncomplicated completed infarction has changed a great deal during the last two decades. In an uncomplicated myocardial infarction, the patient does not need to be confined to bed for longer than 24 h. In fact, the patient may use a bedside commode when needed from the time of admission. The safety and benefits of chair rest were initially elucidated in a publication by Samuel Levine and Bernard Lown in 1951.[494] Beginning with the second day of hospitalization, the patient may sit in a chair twice a day as long as he or she feels comfortable. It should be recognized that allowing patients to sit as long as they are comfortable at each of two sittings is different from allowing them to go from chair to bed ad lib.

  Patients can usually begin to walk in their hospital room on hospital day 5 and walk in the hall at increasing intervals on day 7. The male may shave by day 5, and the patient may take a sit-down bath on day 7.
- The goal of *diagnostic testing* in patients with a completed uncomplicated myocardial infarction is to identify those patients who are at risk of recurrent infarction or sudden death (Chaps. 98 and 109). The fact that the greatest risk of reinfarction and cardiac death is in the first 2 months after hospital discharge[495] is the rationale for completing this evaluation before hospital discharge rather than on a return visit 4 to 8 weeks later.

  Over the past decade, the safety of *submaximal exercise testing* early after an uncomplicated infarction has been established in more than 22 studies involving more than 3300 patients.[496] There were only five major arrhythmias and two deaths reported.[496,497] It must be stressed that these tests were performed on patients manifesting no major complications from their infarction. Furthermore, the patients were exercised to submaximal stress levels.

  Three recent investigations based on correlations between exercise tests and coronary angiography performed prior to hospital discharge revealed that 82 to 90 percent of patients with either exercise-induced angina or ischemic ST-segment responses had multivessel disease while 27 to 55 percent of those patients without angina or ST abnormalities had multivessel disease.[498–500] In other words, the "positive" exercise test was highly predictive of multivessel disease, but the "negative" test did not reliably imply single-vessel disease. The question in these cases is not who has multivessel disease, but who is likely to suffer a future cardiac event. Starling and his associates[501] in an evaluation of 130 survivors of recent uncomplicated infarctions found that only patients with at least one exercise-induced abnormality (ST depression of 1 mm or more, angina, or blunted blood pressure response) had a subsequent fatal cardiac event. Furthermore, patients manifesting at least two of these abnormalities demonstrated a significantly increased risk of death during the following 11 months.[501] The importance of a predischarge evaluation is emphasized by the finding that 10 percent of the patients undergoing a predischarge exercise test could not return for a 6-week reevaluation because of an intercurrent cardiac event. All of these patients were identified by an exercise-related abnormality to be at risk prior to hospital discharge.[502]

Two points are noteworthy in regard to exercise testing following myocardial infarction. First, exercise-induced ventricular arrhythmias provide little prognostic information.[502] This observation perhaps relates to the fact that patients selected for predischarge testing generally have good ventricular function. Second, prior administration of beta blockers does not reduce the accuracy of the test.

Predischarge *exercise ^{201}Tl scintigraphy* seems to have better discriminatory value than the submaximal exercise electrocardiogram test.[503–505] ^{201}Tl defects in more than one discrete coronary vascular region, presence of delayed redistribution, and increased lung uptake of ^{201}Tl were demonstrated to be more sensitive predictors of subsequent cardiac events than ST-segment depression in the electrocardiogram or angina. ^{201}Tl scintigraphy was no better than exercise electrocardiography, however, in predicting a fatal cardiac event.[503] Perhaps the major advantage of ^{201}Tl scintigraphy over routine exercise electrocardiography is that ^{201}Tl scinitigraphy is significantly better at identifying the patient at low risk of a future cardiac event.[503] Again, it is important to emphasize that exercise was submaximal and either symptom-limited or stopped at a heart rate of 120 beats per minute.

Coronary arteriography can be safely performed prior to discharge for hospitalization with an acute myocardial infarction.[503] The arteriographic assessment of the extent of coronary artery disease is an important prognostic indicator in this as well as all other clinical subsets of ischemic heart disease. Coronary arteriography, combined with left ventriculography, is generally thought to be the best method for the assessment of prognosis in coronary artery disease and is, in fact, the gold standard for most studies assessing noninvasive evaluation of the post-myocardial infarction patient.[506] ^{201}Tl scintigraphy prior to discharge suggested that this was superior to coronary arteriography in predicting which patient would experience future cardiac events.[503] An earlier study, however, which coupled the results of coronary arteriography with contrast ventriculography suggested that the information gained from this technique could not be surpassed.[507] A history of previous myocardial infarction coupled with an ejection fraction of less than 40 percent identified all patients who died during a 30-month follow-up. Moreover, none of the patients without a contracting, presumably viable, myocardial segment perfused by a narrowed coronary artery died or had a reinfarction.[507]

The evidence that left ventricular function is the best predictor of survival in the medically treated patient with coronary disease[508] makes *radionuclide ventriculography* a valuable tool to the clinician. Certainly there are many patients with infarction in whom the combination of clinical, electrocardiographic, and enzymatic data is irrefutable evidence that the loss of myocardium and resulting reduction in left ventricular function is small. In contrast, there are other patients, particularly those with previous infarctions or those with enzymatic or electrocardiographic evidence of a large infarction, in whom the level of ventricular function cannot be accurately assessed without ventriculography. Individual patients may have severely depressed left ventricular contractility in the absence of clinical evidence of heart failure. This condition is especially true in the postinfarction patient whose activity in the hospital has been restricted. Radionuclide ventriculography can aid the physician in identifying those patients who are likely to develop heart failure early in the posthospital period.[509] Furthermore, those patients with severely depressed left ventricular function form the cohort in which posthospital sudden death will occur.[510,511] The presence of both poor left ventricular systolic function (less than 40 percent ejection fraction) and complicated ventricular arrhythmia seems to increase significantly the risk of sudden cardiac death in the early posthospital period.[510] While identification of this subset of patients seems appropriate, alteration of the predicted poor chance of survival by therapeutic intervention has not been established.

Gated cardiac blood pool imaging is also a very reliable technique for assessing segmental left ventricular disease. It has been shown to have a 96 percent accuracy in detection of left ventricular aneurysms[512] and has been used successfully in the identification of a false left ventricular aneurysm.[513]

Radionuclide ventriculography has also been demonstrated to be an effective means of identifying patients at the time of hospital discharge who are likely to have a cardiac event during the ensuing 6 months. The test requires the use of supine bicycle ergometry with exercise continued until symptoms develop or a heart rate of 130 is achieved. A fall in left ventricular ejection fraction of at least 5 units, an increase in end-systolic volume of 5 percent, or a failure of the ratio between cuff-determined systolic blood pressure and end-diastolic volume to increase by more than 35 percent reliably identifies the patients who are in a high-risk subset for experiencing a future cardiac event.[514]

Hung et al. have recently reported that exercise radionuclide ventriculography and symptom-limited treadmill testing are superior to ^{201}Tl scintigraphy for prognostic evaluation soon after an uncomplicated myocardial infarction.[515]

Two-dimensional echocardiography can also provide a reliable assessment of left and right ventricular size and function. In fact, a study evaluating noninvasive methods of detecting right ventricular infarction found the echocardiogram to be as accurate as gated photoscintigraphy.[516] Gated radionuclide cardiac imaging is the preferred noninvasive means of assessing ventricular function because of the occasional failure to obtain an adequate echocardiographic image and the ability with photoscintigraphy to reliably quantitate ventricular function.

The major advantage of two-dimensional echocardiography is the capacity to detect mural thrombi. Approximately 17 percent of patients with an acute myocardial infarction have been found to have mural thrombi.[517] The study by Asinger and associates would suggest that all patients with anterior infarction with possible apical involvement should have a two-dimensional echocardiogram.[517] The echocardiogram not only identified those patients with apical akinesis or dyskinesis, which would place them in a high-risk group for developing thrombi, but also detected the thrombus. However, a recommendation to perform echocardiography in all patients with an anterior infarction cannot be made on the basis of this study due to its small number of patients studied and its failure to show therapeutic benefit by medical intervention.

The absence of ventricular ectopy and ventricular tachycardia in the coronary care unit does not exclude their subsequent occurrence in the late hospital phase of a myocardial infarction. Only 16.9 percent of patients have been found to have these ventricular arrhythmias during both phases of their hospitalization.[518] Prolonged *ambulatory electrocardiographic monitoring* is the only reliable means of detecting arrhythmias. Physical examination, symptomatology, and 12-lead electrocardiograms were able to detect only 23 percent of late arrhythmias.[518] Recent studies also indicate that exercise testing is less sensitive than ambulatory electrocardiography in detecting these arrhythmias.[519] While there is consistent evidence that complex ventricular ectopy is an independent contributor to the rates of both overall mortality and sudden death following an infarction,[520,521] the limited efficacy of oral antiarrhythmic agents in abolishing ventricular ectopy[518,522] and the frequent adverse effects of the drugs[522] make it difficult to promote the use of these agents in all such patients. An attempt to abolish complex ventricular ectopy, such as short, unsustained ventricular tachycardia, would appear to be warranted in those patients with poor left ventricular function.

The method used to identify the patient who has had an uncomplicated myocardial infarction and is at high risk for subsequent cardiac events should be selected based on the local availability of and expertise associated with the various methods discussed (exercise electrocardiography, exercise ^{201}Tl scintigraphy, radionuclide ventriculography, echocardiography, and coronary arteriography and left ventriculography).

- *Long-term drug therapy* following uncomplicated completed infarction deserves careful evaluation.

The long-term use of *beta blockers* in patients who have no contraindications to such therapy can be justified. Three large-scale studies of the value of beta-blocker therapy following an acute myocardial infarction have found positive and remarkably similar results.[523] In the timolol (Blocadren) study, there was a reduction of 44.6 percent in the cumulative rate of sudden death over a 17-month follow-up and of 39.3 percent in the total mortality rate with the use of the beta blocker.[524] The total mortality rate during a 25-month follow-up was reduced by 26 percent with the use of propranolol in the Beta-Blocker Heart Attack Trial.[525] The metoprolol-treated group demonstrated a reduction in the death rate of 36 percent over the 90-day follow-up period in the metroprolol study.[469] The duration of such therapy has not been settled. Obviously, as patients grow older contraindication to the use of beta blockers may occur.

Ahumada has recently emphasized that it is possible to identify patients who do not require beta-blocking drugs after myocardial infarction. She reported a review of the literature which revealed that patients who have had only one infarction, who have good ventricular function, no complex ectopy, no angina, and a negative stress test have a mortality rate of 0.6 percent per year. She believes it is unlikely that beta blockers can be proved to prolong the life of such good-risk patients.[526] The editorial written by Griggs et al. on the subject expresses a similar view.[527]

There is no evidence to support the long-term administration of *nitrates* following an uncomplicated myocardial infarction. Certainly, those patients who are demonstrated to have evidence of myocardium in jeopardy of ischemia may benefit from nitrates. On the contrary, there seems to be no rationale for their use in those patients with single-vessel disease and no myocardium in jeopardy of future ischemic events.

Digitalis is not indicated in cases of uncomplicated myocardial infarction. An exception might be those patients found on left ventriculography (either contrast or radionuclide) to have an ejection fraction of less than 40 percent even though they have not yet demonstrated clinical manifestations of heart failure. Digitalis should be used to control the ventricular response to atrial fibrillation and to give inotropic support in those patients with depressed left ventricular contractility.

Antiarrhythmic drugs are not to be use routinely with possibly the exception of the beta blockers. The routine use of lidocaine in the early stages of myocardial infarction can be supported, but its administration should not be continued past 24 h in the uncomplicated patient.

Anticoagulants, such as heparin and coumadin, are not used in the uncomplicated infarction unless there is evidence of a large infarction, a condition preventing rapid ambulation of the patient, a history of previous pulmonary embolus, phlebitis, or transient ischemic attacks. The benefit of placing every patient with an echocardiographically detected mural thrombus on long-term anticoagulation remains to be proved.[528,529]

The first report of the use of *sulfinpyrazone* by the Anturane Reinfarction Trial Research Group demonstrated over an average follow-up of 8.4 months a significant reduction in all cardiac deaths and an even more impressive reduction in sudden death in those patients randomized to the sulfinpyrazone treatment group.[383] The continuation of this study for an average follow-up of 16 months confirmed these earlier findings and established that the reduction in total mortality could be linked to the reduction in numbers of sudden deaths. This protracted study, however, could demonstrate no further therapeutic gain after the initial 6 months.[384] The Anturane Reinfarction Trial has subsequently been challenged because of an imprecise classification scheme and perhaps inappropriate patient exclusion.

An Italian study of similar design using sulfinpyrazone (Anturane) could not demonstrate a reduction in either total mortality or rate of sudden death. This study, however, did demonstrate a reduction in the likelihood of reinfarction or thromboembolic events over 19 months.[530]

The inconsistent results of these studies coupled with the challenges raised to the United States study have eroded the enthusiasm initially shown for sulfinpyrazone. Any future trials with this agent will now have to show an effect which is additive to the effect that is rather consistently reported with beta blockers.

- *Before discharge from the hospital,* the patient should be instructed thoroughly on risk marker modification (see Chap. 42) and given general guidelines as to resuming physical activity. Initially the patient should become fully ambulatory within the home. During the first week at home, the activity level should be restricted to going to the toilet, eating at the family table, and walking in the house. If the weather is pleasant, the patient can begin to take walks outside during the second week at home. These twice-daily walks should be of approximately 5-min duration at a normal pace and can be increased by 5 min/week during the convalescence. The patient may begin to take automobile rides the third week at home and can be allowed to drive brief distances the fourth week at home. Sexual intercourse can be resumed at about the same time.

  Patients can usually return to work at 6 to 8 weeks following hospitalization. Their work day should be cut approximately in half for the first week.

  At the end of their convalescence some patients will benefit from enrollment in a medically supervised exercise program. The benefits of such a program include continued reminders of risk marker modification, improved sense of well-being gained from improved physical conditioning, and self-confidence gained by the patient associating with others having a similar health problem. These programs have not been demonstrated to reduce the incidence of reinfarction or overall mortality[531] or to improve myocardial function.[532]

  The physician must be sensitive to the patient's emotional status since depression is often overlooked. Data have recently been reported indicating that social isolation and severe life stress situations increase the chance of death in the 3 years following infarction by fourfold when compared to controls.[288] Accordingly, the physician should assist in the correction of these conditions whenever possible.

Complicated Completed Myocardial Infarction

Definition and Recognition An infarct is said to be *completed* 6 or more hours after the onset of pain. It is said to be *complicated* when an arrhythmia, persistent and recurrent pain, ventricular dysfunction, reversible hypotensive states, cardiogenic shock, nonarrhythmic cardiac arrest, pericarditis, venous thrombosis and pulmonary embolism, systemic arterial embolism, ventricular septal rupture, papillary muscle dysfunction, papillary muscle rupture, external cardiac rupture, and abnormal emotional responses occur. The complications can be divided into *early complications* and *late complications.*

Early Complications: Cardiac Arrhythmias The reader interested in a detailed discussion of the mechanisms, recognition, and management of *cardiac arrhythmias and conduction abnormalities* may refer to Chaps. 25 to 28. Cardiac arrhythmias complicating transmural or subendocardial myocardial infarction are of similar type and prevalence, and can be discussed together. The clinical distinction between transmural and subendocardial infarction is generally based on the presence or absence of abnormal Q waves in the scalar ECG, although experimental and clinical-pathological studies show that the presence or absence of Q waves does not permit distinction between transmural and subendocardial infarcts.[533] It is, therefore, understandable that the arrhythmia complications are the same.

- *Sinus tachycardia,* sinus rate exceeding 100 beats per minute, complicating myocardial infarction is a nonspecific finding. Pain, anxiety, fever, volume depletion, pericarditis, pulmonary embolus, and cardioaccelerator drugs may produce sinus tachycardia. Persistent sinus tachycardia may be an ominous sign, adumbrating severe left ventricular dysfunction.[534,535] Occasionally, sinus tachycardia may precede other findings of left ventricular dysfunction, such as ventricular gallop or radiographic evidence of pulmonary congestion.

The *treatment* of sinus tachycardia is directed at the underlying cause. Beta-adrenergic blocking drugs may be used to treat patients with evidence of sympathetic nervous system overactivity, sinus tachycardia, or acute systemic arterial hypertension during the first few hours following acute myocardial infarction. Acute or chronic heart failure precludes the use of beta-adrenergic blocking drugs in this setting.

- *Sinus bradycardia*, defined as a sinus rate less than 60 beats per minute, is found in approximately 20 percent of monitored patients. Postulated mechanisms include direct or reflex cholinergic stimulation, sinus node ischemia or infarction, and the release of necrotic tissue products.[536] Iatrogenic causes include morphine sulfate, beta-adrenergic blocking drugs, calcium antagonists, and digitalis. Sinus bradycardia may cause a reduction in cardiac output and contribute to further ischemic injury. Systemic arterial hypotension accompanies sinus bradycardia more commonly in the prehospital phase of myocardial infarction than in the hospital phase.[537] Sinus bradycardia at a rate less than 40 beats per minute usually results in decreased systemic arterial blood flow manifested by cool, clammy skin, hypotension, and light-headedness.[575] The hospital mortality rate is lower in patients with sinus bradycardia, which relates in part to a lower incidence of pump failure.[538]

Experimental and clinical reports present contradictory conclusions concerning the relation of sinus bradycardia to ventricular arrhythmias.[539] In experimental myocardial ischemia, cardiac slowing may induce ventricular tachyarrhythmias by partial recovery of conductivity in a reentry pathway.[540] As a group, patients monitored in a coronary care unit with sinus bradycardia do not experience a greater incidence of ventricular tachycardia or ventricular fibrillation. However, in the first few hours of acute myocardial infarction, ventricular tachyarrhythmias may appear when the heart rate slows, and they may be abolished by increasing the heart rate.[541]

Many patients with sinus bradycardia require no *treatment*, but when decreased peripheral perfusion or heart failure is present, increasing the heart rate may improve both conditions. Some patients with sinus bradycardia have a systolic blood pressure of 90 to 100 mmHg with normal peripheral perfusion and have a benign course without treatment. If frequent premature ventricular depolarizations or more complex ventricular arrhythmias are present, the heart rate should be cautiously increased. Atropine sulfate should be given intravenously in a dose of 0.4 to 0.6 mg.[542] A dose of 0.3 mg or less may cause further sinus node slowing, and a dose of 0.8 mg or more may produce sinus tachycardia. Atropine-induced sinus tachycardia may cause angina pectoris and ventricular arrhythmias. Atropine causes other troublesome side effects, such as urinary retention, increased intraocular tension, psychosis, and visual disturbances. When the pulse rate response to atropine is not satisfactory, atrial or ventricular pacing may be used. Persistent hypotension, despite an increase in heart rate, suggests possible hypovolemia and a need for volume expansion.

- *Sinus node dysfunction* complicates approximately 5 percent of myocardial infarctions and usually occurs in patients with inferior infarction. It has many of the features found in the chronic "sinus node dysfunction" syndrome. The ECG reveals sinus pauses typical of type I or type II second degree sinoatrial block or sinus pauses greater than twice the sinus cycle length. Atrial tachyarrhythmias alternating with bradycardia are seen in one-third of patients. Atrioventricular nodal block may be an accompanying abnormality. Dizziness and syncope are the most common symptoms and result from prolonged sinus pauses associated with subsidiary pacemaker failure. A long pause may follow the termination of an atrial tachyarrhythmia or the spontaneous appearance of advanced sinoatrial block.

Sinus node dysfunction should be *treated* if there is accompanying dizziness, syncope, ventricular arrhythmias, paroxysmal atrial tachyarrhythmias, or hypotension. Potential drug causes of sinus node dysfunction including digitalis, beta-adrenergic blocking drugs, verapamil, class I antiarrhythmic drugs, and morphine sulfate should be eliminated. Atropine will abolish sinus pauses in some patients, particularly if the sinus node dysfunction appears within the first hours of infarction. If atropine fails, temporary intracardiac pacing is required. Patients with the tachycardia-bradycardia syndrome are treated with a temporary pacemaker for control of the bradycardia and antiarrhythmic drugs to suppress the atrial tachyarrhythmias. Sinus node dysfunction is usually short-lived.[543] A permanent pacemaker and antiarrhythmic drugs may be needed if the tachycardia-bradycardia syndrome persists.[544]

- *Atrial premature depolarizations* are found in up to 50 percent of monitored patients with acute myocardial infarction. They are usually not important but may initiate atrial tachyarrhythmias.

Treatment is reserved for atrial premature depolarizations that precipitate an atrial tachyarrhythmia, atrial bigeminy, and beats with coupling intervals less than one-half the sinus P-P interval. The administration of digitalis may not decrease the atrial ectopy but may slow the ventricular rate if atrial fibrillation ensues. Beta-adrenergic blocking drugs or class I antiarrhythmic drugs may be used if digitalis fails.

- *Atrial tachycardia*, defined as three or more consecutive ectopic P waves occurring at a rate greater than 100 beats per minute, is seen in up to 20 percent of patients.[545] However, most episodes are transient and may not require treatment. These brief runs of atrial rhythm appear to be the atrial counterpart of accelerated idioventricular rhythm. Sustained, rapid supraventricular atrial tachycardia is an infrequent arrhythmia following myocardial infarction. Reentry is the most common mechanism for sustained supraventricular tachycardia.

If the tachycardia is rapid and sustained, *treatment* is necessary. The choice of therapy is dictated by the urgency of converting the tachycardia. If the tachycardia is associated with hemodynamic deterioration, synchronous electrical cardioversion should be used. In less urgent situations, medical therapy may be tried. Intravenous verapamil, 5 to 10 mg, terminates most episodes of reentrant supraventricular tachycardia if the reentrant pathway includes the atrioventricular node. Digitalis and propranolol may also be effective. Maneuvers designed to increase vagal tone are commonly used to convert supraventricular tachycardia, but should be used cautiously in patients with acute myocardial infarction. Accordingly, carotid sinus pressure should not be used to revert atrial tachycardia in patients with acute myocardial infarction. Class I antiarrhythmic drugs may be used in combination with digitalis and a beta-adrenergic blocking drug to prevent recurrent episodes. Atrial tachycardia with AV block may be caused by digitalis intoxication, especially if hypokalemia is present.

- *Atrial flutter* is an organized rhythm with the atrial rate ranging between 280 and 320 beats per minute. It is seen in less than 5 percent of patients with myocardial infarction.[546] It is usually associated with a 2:1 atrioventricular conduction ratio; therefore, the ventricular rate will be approximately 150 beats per minute. The rapid ventricular rate will increase myocardial oxygen demand and result in hemodynamic deterioration in many patients. The prompt restoration of a slow ventricular rate is imperative.

  Treatment using synchronized dc cardioversion is generally the preferred therapy for atrial flutter with a rapid ventricular response. Cardioversion will usually terminate atrial flutter and can frequently be achieved with 25 to 50 J. Although digitalis may control the rapid ventricular rate, it may be unsuccessful despite large doses. Verapamil assists in controlling the rapid ventricular rate and may occasionally restore sinus rhythm. The negative inotropic and hypotensive effects of verapamil preclude its use in some patients. Digitalis, verapamil, or beta-adrenergic blocking drugs may slow the ventricular rate if atrial flutter is recurrent and cannot be suppressed. Lidocaine is contraindicated since it may produce 1:1 AV conduction. Occasional patients with inferior infarction develop atrial flutter with a controlled ventricular rate because of ischemic injury to the AV node. Treatment is usually not necessary in these cases.

- *Atrial fibrillation* is the most common atrial tachyarrhythmia complicating myocardial infarction.[546] It may appear de novo, be preceded by atrial premature depolarizations, or follow atrial flutter. Atrial fibrillation is often intermittent and reverts spontaneously to sinus rhythm. Controversy continues regarding the prognostic significance of atrial fibrillation following myocardial infarction. Some investigators find no increase in mortality related to the presence of atrial fibrillation, while other studies show a greater overall early mortality rate in patients with anterior infarction.[546–548] Heart failure is present in most patients with anterior infarction and atrial fibrillation, and the heart failure usually precedes the arrhythmia.

  Atrial fibrillation requires *treatment* because the loss of a synchronized atrial contraction and the rapid irregular ventricular rate may produce further hemodynamic impairment. In contrast to atrial flutter, the rapid ventricular rate is more easily controlled with medical therapy. Digitalis should be administered until satisfactory slowing is achieved. The drug must, of course, be discontinued if digitalis-induced arrhythmias occur. If digitalis fails to slow the ventricular rate, beta-adrenergic drugs or verapamil deserve a trial unless there are contraindications to their use. Prompt electrical cardioversion is necessary when the onset of atrial fibrillation is associated with hypotension, heart failure, or recurrent ischemic chest pain. Occasionally, patients with myocardial infarction have atrial fibrillation related to chronic pulmonary disease, hypoxia, or pulmonary embolism. In these patients, treatment is directed to the underlying medical problem.

- *Accelerated AV junctional rhythm (rate of 60 to 100 beats per minute) and AV junctional tachycardia* result from acceleration of impulse formation in the AV junction. Accelerated junctional rhythms are more frequent in patients with inferior infarction. In general, the rate of the junctional rhythm and the clinical course vary with the site of infarction. With inferior infarction, the junctional rate is only moderately accelerated and the clinical course is usually benign.[549] If the junctional rate exceeds 80 beats per minute, commonly the case in patients with anterior infarction, the hospital mortality rate is high because of accompanying left ventricular dysfunction.[550]

  Accelerated junctional rhythms at rates less than 80 beats per minute rarely require *treatment*. Faster junctional rhythms pose a serious therapeutic problem. Many patients with junctional tachycardia have severe left ventricular dysfunction, and the rapid ventricular rate and loss of atrial kick may further compromise ventricular function. Class I antiarrhythmic drugs deserve a trial, but therapeutic failure is common. Major attention should be directed to treatment of left ventricular dysfunction. Digitalis intoxication should not be overlooked as a cause for accelerated junctional rhythm.

- *Ventricular arrhythmias.* Premature ventricular depolarizations (PVDs) occur in greater than 80 percent of monitored patients with acute infarction. Despite numerous experimental and clinical studies, the pathogenesis of PVDs is incompletely understood, and their treatment remains controversial. Experimental coronary occlusion produces a wide variety of changes in extracellular potassium, pH, P_{O_2}, and P_{CO_2}.[551] The rate and magnitude of these changes are inhomogeneous, both within and at the lateral margin of the ischemic zone. As a result, intraventricular conduction is accelerated in some areas and slowed in others. The nonuniform conduction velocity provides the electrical substrate for reentry.[552] Enhanced automaticity may be an important mechanism for delayed ventricular arrhythmias. For a detailed discussion of the multiple factors involved in the genesis of ventricular arrhythmias, the reader is referred to refs. 553 and 554.

Following myocardial infarction *primary ventricular fibrillation* and *ventricular tachycardia* are not closely related either in appearance time or in inciting mechanisms.[555–557] The incidence of primary ventricular fibrillation is highest in the first 4 h. Primary ventricular fibrillation is precipitated by R-on-T PVDs in the majority of patients, but may follow a late-diastolic PVD or a run of ventricular tachycardia.[556–558] Occasionally, ventricular fibrillation appears without preceding ventricular ectopy. Ventricular tachycardia usually occurs later than 4 h after infarction at a time when frequent, multiformed, and paired PVDs are common.[555] Ventricular tachycardia is rarely induced by R-on-T ventricular ectopic complexes, but is usually initiated by a late-diastolic PVD.[556,557] Degeneration of ventricular tachycardia is the usual cause of ventricular fibrillation that occurs more than 12 h after the onset of infarction.

Although *primary ventricular fibrillation* is commonly incited by an R-on-T premature ventricular depolarization, the R-on-T phenomenon occurs as often in patients without primary ventricular fibrillation and has little predictive value.[557,559] The inadequacy of "warning ventricular ectopy" and the finding that conventional monitoring recognizes less than half the ventricular arrhythmias detected by automated systems prompt some investigators to recommend prophylactic antiarrhythmic therapy for most patients admitted to a coronary care unit.[560]

The *treatment* of ventricular arrhythmias is discussed here and in Chap. 27.

We have *reservations about the routine use of antiarrhythmic prophylaxis.* Since the incidence of primary ventricular fibrillation falls markedly with time following infarction, the most important criterion for prophylactic antiarrhythmic therapy is the patient's time of arrival at the hospital. *When patients reach the hospital within 4 to 6 h of first symptoms, prophylactic antiarrhythmic therapy may be warranted.* Routine lidocaine or procainamide therapy should not be given to patients with hypotension, shock, severe heart failure, bradyarrhythmias, or age greater than 70 years, because of the negative inotropic and chronotropic effects of the drugs. Only one acceptable study demonstrates that prophylactic lidocaine prevents primary ventricular fibrillation.[561] Lidocaine or procainamide are indicated to supress R-on-T PVDs occurring within the first 6 h, and PVDs that are frequent, multiformed, or consecutive in an effort to prevent ventricular tachycardia. Ventricular bigeminy may be treated to improve cardiac output.

A loading dose of 200 mg of lidocaine is given intravenously over 20 min followed by a continuous infusion of 2 to 4 mg/min.[560] The loading dose and infusion rate should be decreased by at least 50 percent in patients with heart failure or primary liver disease, and in patients receiving cimetidine. Confusion, delirium, muscular irritability, slurred speech, and convulsions are important toxic central nervous system effects of lidocaine. Cardiac toxicity is manifested by hypotension, sinus node arrest, or AV block, but these toxic effects are rare. Patients who are sensitive or refractory to lidocaine should receive procainamide, 100 mg intravenously every 5 min, until the arrhythmia is abolished, a dose of 1 g is reached, or untoward drug effects appear. The loading dose is followed by a continuous intravenous infusion of 2 to 4 mg/min or the oral administration of 250 to 500 mg every 3 to 4 h. Hypotension, atrioventricular or intraventricular conduction disturbances, or worsening of the arrhythmia are important side effects seen with acute procainamide administration. Quinidine and beta-adrenergic blocking drugs may be useful in selected patients. Diphenylhydantoin has been tried, but the results are disappointing unless the ventricular ectopy is due to digitalis intoxication. Occasional patients have PVDs that are refractory to antiarrhythmic drugs used singly or in combination. If ventricular tachycardia or ventricular fibrillation does not occur, it may be preferable to accept a certain degree of ectopy rather than risk serious toxicity from large doses of drugs.

A clear distinction between *ventricular tachycardia* and *accelerated idioventricular rhythm* is sometimes impossible because both rhythms may have inconstant cycle lengths and the rate may vary above and below 120 beats per minute. For this discussion, *ventricular tachycardia* is defined as three or more successive ventricular beats at a rate exceeding 120 beats per minute. The usual form of ventricular tachycardia lasts 3 to 12 beats.[556,562] It usually stops spontaneously, but occasionally degenerates into ventricular fibrillation. Ventricular tachycardia lasting no longer than 10 min is infrequent, but has a propensity for evolving into ventricular fibrillation. Shorter-cycle ventricular ectopic beats may interrupt the sustained tachycardia and serve as a warning that fibrillation may be imminent.[563] Taylor et al. find that the corrected

QT interval is frequently prolonged early in acute myocardial infarction, and that prolonged ventricular repolarization predicts complex ventricular tachyarrhythmias within the first 48 h.[564] Our experience suggests that the QT interval does not select patients subject to ventricular tachyarrhythmias unless the QT interval exceeds 0.54 s.

Brief bursts of ventricular tachycardia showing spontaneous termination are treated with lidocaine or procainamide to prevent further episodes. Beta-adrenergic blocking drugs, used in conjunction with other antiarrhythmic drugs, may be useful. Castle, as well as others, recently has emphasized the value of bretylium tosylate in treatment of ventricular tachycardia. The dose is 5 to 10 mg/kg given intravenously over a period of 10 to 20 min.[565] Synchronous cardioversion, 10 to 25 J, is the preferred *treatment for sustained ventricular tachycardia.* Occasionally, ventricular tachycardia may be refractory to all common pharmacological measures. Ideally, an adequate blood level of an antiarrhythmic agent should be demonstrated before a therapeutic failure is declared. A search for any possible contributing factors should be made. Correction of hypokalemia, hypomagnesemia, respiratory acidosis or alkalosis, hypovolemia, digitalis intoxication, and left ventricular dysfunction may control the arrhythmia. When myocardial ischemia is suspected, intensive nitrate and calcium antagonist therapy should be employed. Overdrive cardiac pacing is occasionally successful when other measures fail. If investigational antiarrhythmic drugs are available, various pharmacological trials are warranted. We have observed a favorable reponse to amiodarone in a few patients. In a desperate clinical situation left ventricular infarctectomy with subendocardial resection guided by intraoperative mapping and coronary artery bypass may be tried. The results of this operation are less favorable than in patients with chronic, recurrent ventricular tachycardia.

The incidence of *accelerated idioventricular rhythm* after myocardial infarction varies from 10 to 46 percent.[566] It is defined as three or more consecutive ventricular beats at a rate of 55 to 120 beats per minute. A variable cycle length and intermittent appearance in brief paroxysms are characteristic of accelerated idioventricular rhythm. The paroxysm may begin as an ectopic rhythm beginning in late diastole or may serve as an escape rhythm following sinus node slowing or a postextrasystolic pause. Accelerated idioventricular rhythm frequently stops spontaneously after 3 to 30 beats, or it may be suppressed by acceleration of the dominant cardiac pacemaker. When accelerated idioventricular rhythm persists for several minutes, it is usually associated with 1:1 retrograde ventriculoatrial conduction. Since the atria are controlled by the idioventricular pacemaker, the opportunity for a sinus node capture and suppression of the idioventricular rhythm is lost. Multiform, accelerated idioventricular rhythm is occasionally seen, but it appears as innocuous as the more common uniform variety.[567]

Although patients with accelerated idioventricular rhythm have an increased incidence of ventricular tachycardia, the incidence of ventricular fibrillation and the hospital mortality are not increased.[568] When idioventricular rhythm is associated with ventricular tachycardia, the QRS morphology of the two rhythms is often similar, and the rate of the idioventricular rhythm may be half or some other multiple of that of the ventricular tachycardia.[569] This finding suggests the presence of exit block. The effects of verapamil on this rhythm suggest a possible role of the slow inward current.[567] Accelerated idioventricular rhythm *does not require treatment unless it is associated with rapid ventricular tachycardia or hypotension.* Acceleration of the atrial rate with atropine or atrial pacing may suppress idioventricular rhythm. Lidocaine should not be used unless the sinus rate exceeds 75 beats per minute. Digitalis may cause accelerated idioventricular rhythm and should be omitted.

Resuscitation from *primary ventricular fibrillation,* ventricular fibrillation not associated with shock or heart failure, is quite successful. Approximately 20 percent of patients with primary ventricular fibrillation suffer a recurrence, and the mean time of recurrence is 4 days.[570] When ventricular fibrillation occurs in patients with severe left ventricular dysfunction, the outcome is less favorable. The initial resuscitative efforts are less successful, the recurrence rate is nearly 50 percent, and only 25 percent of patients leave the hospital.[570,571] Approximately 3 percent of patients sustain unexpected ventricular fibrillation after discharge from the coronary care unit. Factors that predispose patients to late ventricular fibrillation include anteroseptal infarction complicated by bundle branch block, persistent heart failure, and recurrent myocardial ischemia.[572] These patients should ideally remain under continuous electrocardiographic monitoring for 2 weeks.

The *treatment for ventricular fibrillation* is immediate cardioversion using a defibrillator storing no more than 400 J. The sooner ventricular fibrillation is reverted, the greater the chances for a successful outcome. Cardioverters should be positioned in a coronary care unit so that emergency defibrillation can be accomplished within 1 min. Following restoration of a supraventricular rhythm, lidocaine or procainamide should be used to help prevent further attacks. Repeated episodes of primary ventricular fibrillation that are refractory to lidocaine or procainamide may be suppressed by intravenous propranolol 1 to 3 mg, or bretylium tosylate 5 to 10 mg/kg intravenously. Bretylium tosylate, an adrenergic blocking agent, raises the ventricular fibrillation threshold in experimental animals. In a randomized blinded clinical trial, bretylium tosylate was compared with lidocaine as initial drug therapy in patients suffering out-of-hospital ventricular fibrillation.[573] Bretylium offered neither significant advantage nor disadvantage when compared with lidocaine.

- The incidence of *AV conduction disturbances* varies between 12 and 25 percent, and the incidence of complete AV block varies from 2 to 10 percent in patients with acute myocardial infarction. AV conduction disturbances following inferior and anterior infarction differ in many respects and will be discussed separately.[574] In some patients, AV block may not conform to such a clear distinction based upon the site of infarction.

AV conduction disturbances occur two to three times more frequently in inferior infarction as compared with anterior infarction. The site of block in most patients with inferior infarction is within the AV node or high in the His bundle.[575] The pathogenesis of AV nodal block following acute infarction is not fully understood, but increased vagal tone and ischemia play a role. Pathological studies show only minor degrees of tissue necrosis, if any, within the AV node and His bundle.

AV block following inferior infarction begins with prolongation of the PR interval, followed by a progression to type I second degree AV block. A further progression to complete heart block may ensue. The QRS morphological characteristics of the junctional escape pacemaker are frequently normal, and its rate is characteristically between 40 and 60 beats per minute. Occasionally, escape pacemakers exhibit a wide QRS complex that may be due to preexisting bundle branch block, bradycardia-dependent bundle branch block, or a ventricular escape rhythm. Electrocardiographic findings of type I AV block or an accelerated AV junctional rhythm may antedate the QRS-complex, ST-segment, and T-wave changes of inferior infarction. When AV block occurs lower in the His bundle, the escape pacemaker rate is usually slower, and the prognosis less favorable. Occasionally, P waves fail to traverse the AV node because of a transient increase in vagal tone. The ECG shows an abrupt increase in the P-wave cycle length and the simultaneous development of AV block.[576] Treatment is rarely required because normal AV conduction returns within a few seconds. These episodes usually occur during the stage of sleep when parasympathetic tone is high and during retching, choking, or straining at stool.

AV block following inferior infarction requires *treatment* only if associated with heart failure, hypotension, syncope, serious ventricular ectopy, or a heart rate less than 40 beats per minute. Atropine is usually effective in improving conduction when AV block appears within hours of infarction, but it is often ineffective when the onset is delayed beyond the first day. Pacemaker therapy is indicated if atropine fails to improve AV conduction.[577] Isoproterenol 0.5 to 2 μg/min may be used if cardiac pacing is not possible. The prognosis for patients with AV block and an escape pacemaker with a narrow QRS complex is quite good. If the AV block is associated with a wide QRS-complex escape pacemaker or severe heart failure, the mortality rate is high. Because AV block following inferior infarction is usually transient, lasting hours or days, permanent pacing is rarely needed.

Heart block complicating anterior infarction results from extensive necrosis involving the bundle branches and surrounding myocardium. Intracardiac electrograms localize the conduction abnormality to the distal His-Purkinje conducting system.[578] AV block following anterior infarction usually develops abruptly, producing many consecutive nonconducted P waves. Occasionally, Mobitz II second degree AV block is seen as an intermediate stage. The idioventricular escape pacemakers are slow and exhibit a wide, bizarre QRS complex, suggesting an origin below the His bundle.

Since the progression to complete heart block is usually sudden, it is important to identify those patients at greatest risk for complete heart block. The conceptual division of the bundle branch system into right bundle branch, anterior division of the left bundle branch, and posterior division of the left bundle branch has produced electrocardiographic criteria for the diagnosis of block of one fascicle or a combination of fascicles. Although this concept is clinically useful, it is an oversimplification of the anatomy of the bundle branches and only approximates the site of intraventricular block.

The *treatment* is not satisfactory. Prophylactic temporary pacemakers should be inserted in patients at high risk of developing complete heart block unless irreparable left ventricular function is present (see Chap. 28).[579] Patients with anterior infarction complicated by new right bundle branch block with either left anterior or left posterior hemiblock, alternating bundle branch block, or preexisting complete left bundle branch block have a significant risk of progressing to complete heart block.[580,581] The problem of selecting patients with newly acquired complete left bundle branch block for pacemaker therapy cannot be resolved without further study. Despite the use of prophylactic pacing, many patients with bundle branch block die in severe pump failure. However, a few patients die as a result of sudden complete heart block; a prophylactic pacemaker would have helped these patients. Patients who survive transient type II AV block or complete heart block need permanent pacemaking to prevent sudden death due to recurrent heart block (see Chap. 28).[580] In the group of patients with bundle branch block or bifascicular block complicating anteroseptal infarction and no transient second degree or complete heart block in the acute stage, permanent pacing is not needed.[582]

Early Complications: Persistent Pain or Recurrent Pain Due to Myocardial Ischemia Pain due to myocardial ischemia requires special attention. Myocardial infarction may not always be an abrupt event. Some patients experience recurrent pain after narcotics during the first 48 h. Creatine kinase isoenzyme curves (MB-CK) and autopsy findings in this setting suggest that progressive myocardial necrosis may be occurring. Progressive myocardial necrosis produces further left ventricular dysfunction and may culminate in cardiogenic shock. Myocardial infarct extension, detected by recurrent elevation of plasma MB-CK, is observed in 14 to 31 percent of patients.[583–585] It occurs more frequently in patients whose electrocardiographic changes of infarction are restricted to the ST-T segment.[585,586] Recurrent chest pain or isolated ST-segment elevation are relatively insensitive indicators of infarct extension, but a combination of pain and ST-segment elevation is highly specific.[583] Infarct extension increases the hospital mortality rate several-fold even in patients without symptomatic heart failure.[583–585]

Persistent or recurrent pain requires prompt *treatment* and adequate relief. The goals of therapy are to increase coronary artery perfusion and to decrease myocardial oxygen demand. As pointed out earlier, intracoronary and intravenous streptokinase are being widely investigated as a means of recanalizing acutely thrombosed coronary arteries.[587,588] Reperfusion in a previously occluded coronary artery usually alleviates persistent chest pain and rapidly decreases ST-segment elevation. In rare patients, reperfusion of an initially obstructed artery and pain relief occur after the sublingual administration of nifedipine.

Patients with anterior infarction may have persistent pain associated with sympathetic nervous system overactivity, despite heavy narcotic administration. Propranolol, given in 1-mg increments, will decrease the heart rate and blood pressure and frequently alleviate the pain. Giving propranolol in this clinical setting is safe if the heart size is normal and overt heart failure is absent. Persistent pain associated with systemic arterial hypertension may respond to intravenous nitroglycerin or sublingual nifedipine. An intravenous infusion of nitroglycerin relieves persistent pain in many normotensive patients.[589] Patients with refractory chest pain or pain associated with hemodynamic instability benefit from hemodynamic monitoring with a Swan-Ganz thermodilution catheter. Hemodynamic monitoring allows for a more precise titration of intravenous nitroglycerin, calcium antagonists, beta-adrenergic blocking drugs, and blood volume expansion. Intraaortic balloon counterpulsation may abolish refractory pain and is especially useful for patients who are hemodynamically unstable. Reduction of myocardial oxygen consumption is the major mechanism by which intraaortic balloon counterpulsation relieves myocardial ischemia.[590] *When chest pain continues despite maximum medical therapy, coronary arteriography and left ventriculography are indicated. The intraaortic balloon pump may be needed prior to cardiac catheterization. Unless there is irreparable left ventricular dysfunction, coronary bypass surgery can be accomplished in these selected patients with a low rate of operative mortality.*[591] Patients requiring mechanical circulatory assistance for adequate peripheral perfusion are usually not surgical candidates, except for correctable mechanical problems such as severe mitral regurgitation or ventricular septal rupture.

Early Complications: Ventricular Dysfunction Ventricular dysfunction is a common complication of infarction. Approximately two-thirds of patients without clinical evidence of heart failure have elevations in left ventricular filling pressure, and one-half have a moderate reduction in resting cardiac output. The extent of acute infarction plus old infarction is the principal factor determining the degree of left ventricular dysfunction. There is a progressive decrease in stroke volume index and ejection fraction and an increase in end-systolic volume with greater degrees of left ventricular impairment.[592,593] The left ventricular end-diastolic volume is not increased substantially except in patients with overt pulmonary edema or cardiogenic shock.[592,593] Contractility in noninfarcted regions is normal or even increased in patients with only moderate hemodynamic impairment, but may be suppressed in patients with severe pump failure, forming an indication for treatment with positive inotropic drugs.

Radionuclide ventriculography provides a means to assess ventricular function serially. The left ventricular ejection fraction offers the best global left ventricular function correlate of regional wall motion abnormality.[593] Abnormal wall motion in the territory supplied by the left anterior descending coronary artery best predicts a reduction in global left ventricular function. A single assessment of left ventricular ejection fraction during the first 24 h following myocardial infarction may not characterize left ventricular performance properly because significant fluctuations may occur in the absence of persistent pain or major therapeutic interventions.[594] A decrease of mean heart rate–blood pressure product, spontaneous thrombolysis, or relief of coronary artery spasm may explain the "spontaneous" improvement observed in some patients. Worsening left ventricular function may occur with acute thinning and dilatation of the infarcted segment. Patients with greatly reduced left ventricular performance continue to show functional abnormality after 4 to 6 weeks. The hemodynamic responses of the right and left ventricles to infarction are distinctly different with anterior and with inferior infarction.[595] Anterior infarction is associated with persistent left ventricular regional dysfunction and transient global right ventricular impairment. The reasons for this temporary right ventricular dysfunction are not apparent. Inferior infarction is associated with minimal to moderate left ventricular impairment and persistent, regional right ventricular abnormality. Right ventricular infarction explains the persistent wall motion abnormality in most patients with inferior infarction. Impaired left ventricular function may improve during convalescence.[596] There is some evidence that stiffening of the infarcted area may improve ventricular performance by preventing bulging and sequestration of blood during systole.[597]

Correlation of physical examination and chest x-ray with hemodynamic measurements shows that the clinical evaluation accurately predicts the hemodynamic state in approximately 80 percent of patients.[598] Clinical evaluation misses a number of patients with a low cardiac output who have normal physical examinations and chest x-rays. This may not be terribly important since patients with a normal physical examination and a normal chest x-ray have a very low rate of hospital mortality. The diagnosis of interstitial pulmonary edema is better made by chest x-ray than by auscultation, since pulmonary rales may be absent with interstitial pulmonary edema and, when present, may be caused by bronchitis or respiratory depression from narcotics.[599] A left ventricular S_3 gallop correlates with left ventricular dysfunction and a pulmonary capillary wedge pressure greater than 12 mmHg. Elevated neck veins do not always indicate elevated pulmonary capillary wedge pressure. For instance, in right ventricular infarction or cor pulmonale the neck veins may be elevated but the wedge pressure may be normal or only minimally elevated. Vigorous diuresis might lower cardiac output in either of these settings. In massive anterior infarction with pulmonary congestion the neck veins may be normal acutely, even though the wedge pressure is very high.

The patient with uncomplicated acute myocardial infarction does not require invasive hemodynamic monitoring. Patients with complications such as heart failure, severe right ventricular infarction, hypotension, persistent pain, or shock benefit from serial hemodynamic measurements.[600,601] Measurements of pulmonary capillary wedge pressure (PCWP) or pulmonary artery end-diastolic pressure (PAEDP) and thermodilution cardiac output are useful in establishing and following treatment. The PAEDP is similar to the left ventricular filling pressure in the absence of mitral valve obstruction or pulmonary vascular disease. Complications due to the intravascular catheter are pulmonary infarction and pulmonary artery rupture. These considerations can be markedly decreased by monitoring the PAEDP and avoiding frequent balloon inflations.

A *treatment* scheme developed by Charles Rackley and his associates is shown in Fig. 45-10. This scheme outlines a therapeutic program based upon the initial hemodynamic measurements. Patients are divided into groups contingent upon the PAEDP and the cardiac index. The reader should also see Chap. 124.

Clinically stable patients with a PAEDP less than 20 mmHg and cardiac index greater than 2.5 liters/min/m^2 may be observed. If ischemic chest pain or systemic arterial hypertension intervene, therapy that reduces myocardial oxygen requirements should be considered. Intravenous nitroglycerin may be used to relieve ischemic pain, but the infusion rate and

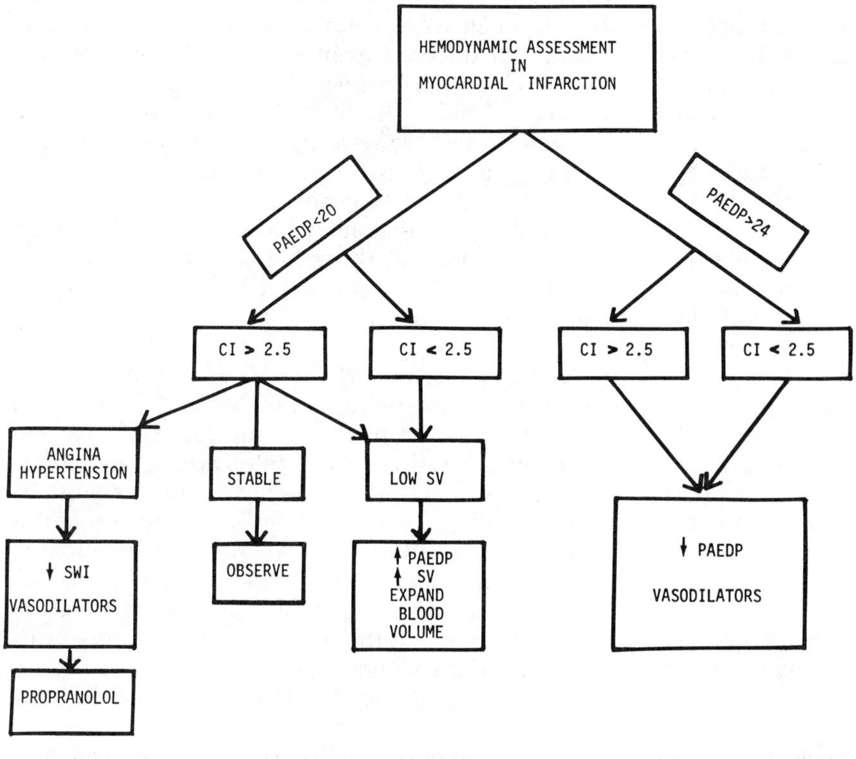

FIGURE 45-10 An approach is illustrated for the management of the patient with acute myocardial infarction based on the hemodynamic measurements and clinical features. PAEDP = pulmonary artery end-diastolic pressure; CI = cardiac index; SWI = stroke work index; SV = stroke volume. (*From C. E. Rackley, R. O. Russell, Jr., J. A. Mantle, and W. J. Rogers. Modern Approach to the Patient with Acute Myocardial Infarction, Curr. Prob. Cardiol. 1(10):1977, p. 40. Reproduced with permission from the publisher and author.*)

PAEDP should be adjusted such that an excessive increase in heart rate or fall in coronary artery perfusion pressure are prevented. Acute hypertension may respond to *sodium nitroprusside,* but nitroprusside should probably be avoided when hypertension is associated with myocardial ischemia.[602] Sublingual nifedipine may decrease blood pressure and myocardial oxygen requirements.[603] Patients with sympathetic overactivity, manifested by sinus tachycardia, hypertension, and a cardiac index above 4.0 liters/min/m^2, are candidates for propranolol.

Volume expansion is the initial treatment when the PAEDP is less than 20 mmHg and the cardiac index is less than 2.5 liters/min/m^2 or is maintained slightly above 2.5 liters/min/m^2 by a sinus tachycardia. Elevating the left ventricular filling pressure may increase the cardiac index and produce a compensatory decrease in heart rate. If the cardiac index remains low despite a PAEDP of 20 to 24 mmHg, the impedence to left ventricular ejection should be reduced by the administration of a vasodilator, such as intravenous nitroglycerin or sodium nitroprusside.

Patients with a PAEDP greater than 24 mmHg will usually have signs or symptoms of interstitial pulmonary edema. The cardiac index may be above or below 2.5 liters/min/m^2. Occasional patients with a first inferior infarction will have pulmonary edema with a global left ventricular ejection fraction greater than 45 percent.[604] *Diuretics and vasodilator drugs* may be used to decrease the left ventricular filling pressure. If a depressed cardiac index persists, positive inotropic agents, digitalis, and catecholamines should be used.

Patients with acute myocardial infarction and left ventricular dysfunction often have a low cardiac output and a high systemic vascular resistance. In the presence of a high left ventricular filling pressure, the administration of sodium nitroprusside or nitroglycerin can substantially reduce this pressure while either maintaining or increasing stroke volume and cardiac output. *Nitroprusside* reduces the mean arterial pressure, PCWP, and left and right ventricular end-diastolic volumes.[602,605] Left ventricular ejection fraction, right ventricular ejection fraction, and stroke volume index generally increase. Improvement in global left ventricular ejection fraction is almost entirely due to improved contraction in the noninfarcted wall segments.[602] Nitroprusside does not affect contraction of infarcted segments, either beneficially or adversely. Animal studies suggest that nitroprusside may have a deleterious effect on blood flow to ischemic areas. Whether this detrimental effect occurs in humans in unknown, but it is prudent to use nitroprusside cautiously in patients with ischemic chest pain and to ensure that an adequate coronary perfusion pressure is maintained. Nitroprusside has beneficial acute hemodynamic effects, but it does not alter hospital mortality.[606,607]

Intravenous nitroglycerin may improve perfusion to ischemic myocardium by increasing collateral blood flow or by reducing left ventricular filling pressure.[608] When nitroglycerin is used for this purpose, careful titration is needed in order to maintain the pressure gradient between aorta and subendocardium. Therefore, the reduction in mean arterial pressure should not exceed the decrease in PCWP. Patients with left ventricular dysfunction benefit from nitroglycerin because it decreases PCWP and systemic vascular resistance and increases cardiac output.[602] Nitroglycerin may cause profound hypotension in patients with right ventricular infarction unless its administration is preceded by adequate volume replacement. Intravenous isosorbide dinitrate enhances cardiac output when the initial systemic vascular resistance is high.[609]

Digitalis may not be needed in mild heart failure but should be given if severe heart failure is present. Digitalis can increase cardiac output and decrease PCWP in some patients with heart failure following myocardial infarction. It produces a small improvement in left ventricular ejection fraction in patients with low resting ejection fractions.[610] The effects of digitalis on ischemic myocardium in human myocardial infarction are unknown. In the canine model ouabain has a salutary effect on ischemic myocardium.[611,612] Ouabain increases blood flow to the ischemic region and improves its mechanical function.

In a series of patients with mild ventricular dysfunction reported by Whitlow et al., a *glucose-insulin-potassium* infusion increased global left ventricular ejection fraction and ejection fraction in the "infarcted zone."[613]

A number of pharmacological interventions may alter acute ischemic injury and infarct size following coronary artery occlusion in experimental animals. It is difficult to extrapolate these data to humans because of differences in collateral blood flow, the extent of coronary artery disease, the mechanism of infarction, and right and left ventricular function. Human studies are seriously limited by the inability to measure the mass of jeopardized ischemic myocardium. Interest has moved away from pharmacological agents that might alter infarct size to interventions such as thrombolytic therapy that may restore perfusion in an occluded artery (see above and Chaps. 95 and 118).

Early Complications: Reversible Hypotensive States

Reversible hypotensive states must be differentiated from shock (see Chaps. 22 and 23). Since cardiogenic shock resulting from extensive loss of cardiac muscle is usually not reversible, emphasis must be placed on the early recognition and treatment of less severe and potentially reparable hypoperfusion states. Although it is not known whether cardiogenic shock can be prevented by aggressive therapy, it is reasonable to assume that the immediate correction of cardiac arrhythmias and abnormalities of blood pressure may lessen the development of cardiogenic shock.[614]

Arterial hypotension is commonly defined as a

systolic arterial blood pressure of less than 100 mmHg, an obviously arbitrary designation. Some patients with chronic systemic arterial hypertension may have decreased peripheral perfusion at a systemic pressure considerably greater than this, while occasional patients at this pressure are normal. Patients in the latter category have a normal or slightly decreased heart rate and a pulse pressure greater than 25 mmHg, and can safely be observed. Arterial hypotension requires treatment if there is peripheral hypoperfusion or if the mean arterial pressure is less than 70 mmHg, a pressure incompatible with adequate myocardial perfusion.

The *bradycardia-hypotension* syndrome is the most frequent correctable cause of peripheral hypoperfusion. Parasympathetic overactivity resulting in bradycardia or hypotension, or both, is noted in approximately one-half of patients seen within 30 min of inferior wall infarction. In experimental animals, the Bezold-Jarisch reflex, an inhibitory reflex characterized by bradycardia and hypotension, is induced by stimulating vagal afferent receptors located primarily in the inferoposterior wall.[615] The precise location of similar receptors in humans is not determined, but the frequent occurrence of bradycardia and hypotension in patients with inferior infarction suggests that the receptors may be in the inferoposterior left ventricular wall. Reperfusion of the right coronary artery, in contrast to the left anterior descending, commonly produced bradycardia and hypotension.[615]

Treatment consists of reversing the bradycardia with atropine, which usually raises the blood pressure. If hypotension persists, central venous blood volume should be increased by leg elevation and volume administration.

Occasional patients with decreased peripheral perfusion have a low cardiac output and a low or normal pulmonary capillary wedge pressure. Volume expansion will increase the cardiac output but may not return it to normal, suggesting that the depressed cardiac output is related to muscle dysfunction as well as hypovolemia. Under these circumstances, additional therapy may include inotropic agents and vasodilators.

Right ventricular infarction deserves special emphasis since it is a potentially reversible cause of cardiogenic shock.[616] Isolated right ventricular infarction is rare, but it accompanies inferoposterior left ventricular infarction in approximately one-third of patients. Postmortem examinations indicate that infarction of the posterior interventricular septum usually accompanies right ventricular free wall infarction. The bedside diagnosis of right ventricular infarction is based upon a constellation of findings of right-sided heart failure with no left-sided signs, including a right ventricular third or fourth heart sound, elevated jugular venous pressure with a large *v* wave and a steep *y* descent, a positive Kussmaul's sign, arterial hypotension, and clear lung fields by x-ray and physical examination.[617] ST-segment elevation equal to or greater than 1 mm in electrocardiographic lead V_4R in the absence of left bundle branch block or other causes of anteriorly directed ST vectors is a fairly sensitive way to diagnose right ventricular injury.[618] The duration of ST-segment elevation in lead V_4R persists for a brief period of time, often disappearing within hours.[619] Radionuclide ventriculography shows right ventricular dilatation, segmental wall motion abnormalities, a decreased right ventricular ejection fraction,[620] and a normal or near normal left ventricular ejection fraction.

The hemodynamic picture is that of acute right ventricular failure with the right-sided filling pressure higher than the left-sided filling pressure. An inspiratory increase in mean right atrial pressure and in right ventricular end-diastolic pressure is commonly found.[617] Systolic pressures in the right ventricle and pulmonary artery are normal, and the left ventricular filling pressure is normal or minimally elevated. Right ventricular infarction may resemble constrictive pericardial disease when there is equilibration of diastolic pressures, a diastolic dip and plateau in both right and left ventricular pressure, and no respiratory decrease in right atrial pressure.[621] These changes result from a decrease in compliance of the right ventricle and possibly the normal pericardium's attempt to restrain a dilating heart. Cor pulmonale may produce a somewhat similar hemodynamic picture but can be distinguished by the elevation of pulmonary artery systolic and diastolic pressures with a normal pulmonary capillary wedge pressure.

The *treatment* is different to that of left ventricular infarction. When severe right ventricular infarction is suspected, blood volume expansion with a colloid solution should be given while preparations are made for hemodynamic monitoring. Volume expansion is continued until hypotension is corrected or the capillary wedge pressure reaches 15 to 20 mmHg. As much as 3 to 6 liters of fluid may be needed during the first 24 h. Treatment with diuretics for a mistaken diagnosis of right-sided cardiac failure is deleterious and is associated with reduced cardiac output and heart failure. Inotropic agents are needed when hypoperfusion persists despite an adequate left ventricular filling pressure. AV block is a common complication of right ventricular infarction and usually requires temporary pacing. AV sequential pacing should be employed in patients with AV block or AV junctional rhythms because a synchronous right atrial contraction may improve right-sided forward flow and help maintain adequate systemic perfusion.[622] Koor et al. reported a patient who had right ventricular infarction associated with severe tricuspid regurgitation.[623] Tricuspid valve replacement produced dramatic improvement.

Right ventricular infarction presents a wide clinical spectrum from a rather benign, uncomplicated disorder to a serious event with AV block and shock. If adequate peripheral perfusion can be maintained until right ventricular function slowly improves, the prognosis is good because left ventricular function is reasonably well preserved. After 2 months, most patients show major improvement in right ventricular ejection fraction. The prognosis is adversely affected by major left ventricular and interventricular septum dysfunction.[624]

Early Complications: Cardiogenic Shock (see Chaps. 22 and 23) Cardiogenic shock complicating acute infarction has two major clinical presentations. A few patients have all the signs of shock on reaching the hospital. Their hemodynamic studies reveal a severely depressed cardiac index and a high pulmonary artery wedge pressure. There is little response to treatment, and death occurs within hours. The irreparable nature of this condition is supported by pathological examination, which reveals acute infarction of greater than 40 percent of the left ventricle. In the usual clinical presentation, shock develops more insidiously. Pathological studies and MB-CK curves suggest that the extensive loss of functioning myocardium occurs in a stepwise fashion.[625] Therapy is designed to interrupt the cycle of progressive myocardial damage. Treatment should be monitored by serial clinical and hemodynamic observations.

An aggressive *treatment* program should be initiated before shock is manifest. Intravenous nitroglycerin may be used to decrease left ventricular filling pressure and to lessen myocardial ischemia. An unacceptably low arterial blood pressure necessitates the addition of a catecholamine. If these measures fail, intraaortic balloon counterpulsation[626] followed by cardiac catheterization and coronary artery bypass grafting should be considered. This treatment must be accomplished expeditiously since the mortality rate increases as the time from infarction lengthens.

Early Complications: Nonarrhythmic Cardiac Arrest[627] Sudden death in patients with acute myocardial infarction is generally assumed to be caused by ventricular fibrillation or asystole. Instantaneous death may also result from sudden electromechanical dissociation without arrhythmias. Electromechanical dissociation is a common cause of unsuccessful cardiac resuscitation in critically ill patients. The unsuccessful resuscitation of these patients is due to myocardial contractile failure rather than absent electrical systole. Adequate electrocardiographic complexes in the absence of audible heart sounds or palpable pulses characterize electromechanical dissociation.[628] This syndrome has many causes. Cardiac rupture with hemopericardium is suggested by the sudden occurrence of electromechanical dissociation, bradycardia, and abrupt distension of neck veins. Since myocardial ischemia results in the rapid disappearance of effective myocardial contractions, ischemia of an extraordinarily large myocardial segment may produce electromechanical dissociation. This has been observed most frequently in patients with coronary artery spasm. Reversal of the syndrome by the administration of sublingual nifedipine or nitroglycerin has been observed. Some investigations suggest that electromechanical dissociation may occasionally be caused by an acute increase in parasympathetic activity or withdrawal of sympathetic activity. The observations that patients with inferior infarction are subject to bradycardia and hypotension, and are less likely to respond to resuscitation attempts by emergency medical personnel, may support this hypothesis. Most commonly, electromechanical dissociation occurs without a detectable inciting event and is fatal.[627] The pathophysiology of electromechanical dissociation is unknown, but the failure of myocardial contractility suggests a depletion of high-energy phosphate bonds.[628]

The *treatment* of electrical-mechanical dissociation is unsatisfactory, and resuscitational efforts are often futile.

Early Complications: Pericarditis (see Chap. 59) A myocardial infarction may extend to the pericardial surface and produce a localized, or occasionally extensive, fibrinous pericardial inflammation. Evidence of pericarditis is usually delayed several days after infarction, with peak incidence within the first week. Occasionally, it may be detected on the day of admission, suggesting that the onset of infarction antedates admission by several days, even when a history of chest discomfort is not obtained. The recognition and prompt treatment of pericarditis is important since the pain may be confused with the pain of myocardial ischemia and cause undue alarm, the chest wall splinting may produce basilar atelectasis, and the accompanying fever may increase the heart rate and myocardial oxygen consumption. While pericarditis may occur without pain, pain is the most common symptom. Characteristically, the pain is aggravated by deep inspiration, change of position, swallowing, or coughing. A pericardial friction rub is not invariably audible. Undoubtedly, a pericardial rub would be heard more often if patients were more frequently examined. Diffuse ST-segment elevation, typical of pericarditis, is usually absent in this setting unless the inflammation is diffuse.

In the setting of myocardial infarction, *treatment* should be instituted for symptomatic pericarditis, whether or not a pericardial friction rub is heard. A single oral dose of 40 mg of methylprednisolone or 8 mg of dexamethasone intravenously will diminish or resolve the pain within hours of administration, and is therefore preferred. Occasionally, a second dose may be needed. Prolonged high-dose corticosteroid therapy should be avoided since corticosteroids retard myocardial healing and might theoretically increase the risk of cardiac rupture. Aspirin and indomethacin are generally effective in relieving the pain though relief may be delayed for 48 h.[629] Anticoagulants are contraindicated in persistent pericarditis because they increase the risk of pericardial bleeding.

The post-myocardial infarction syndrome (Dressler's syndrome) occurs in about 3.3 percent of patients[630] (see Chap. 59). Corticosteroids and nonsteroid anti-inflammatory drugs are useful in its management.

Early Complications: Venous Thrombosis and Pulmonary Embolism The incidence of deep venous thrombosis after myocardial infarction, measured with ^{125}I-labeled fibrinogen scanning, is about 30 percent, with greater risk in patients with varicose veins, previous venous thromboembolism, congestive heart failure, shock, obesity, and age greater than 70 years.[631] In most patients, the venous thrombi are limited to the calf. The risk of clinically detectable pulmonary embolism is negligible unless the venous thrombosis extends more proximally into the popliteal, femoral, or iliac veins. Early ambulation may reduce the incidence of venous thrombosis. Miller et al. found abnormal ^{125}I-labeled fibrinogen scans in only 2 of 21 patients who did leg exercises and sat at the bedside during the initial 3 hospital days.[632] The institution of early ambulation may help explain why pulmonary embolism currently accounts for less than 1 percent of total deaths.

Recognition of pulmonary embolism in patients with recent myocardial infarction may be difficult because episodes of dyspnea, tachypnea, sweating, sinus tachycardia, and atrial tachyarrhythmias, which are suggestive of pulmonary embolism, may also be caused by myocardial ischemia. The diagnostic problem may not be resolved without further studies.

Occasionally, it may be safer to *treat* patients for suspected pulmonary embolus with heparin than to remove them from the coronary care unit for perfusion and ventilation scanning or a pulmonary arteriogram.

Routine prophylactic anticoagulant therapy is not recommended for all patients admitted to the coronary care unit, but should be used for patients at high risk. Both oral anticoagulants and heparin are effective in preventing venous thrombosis if begun soon after myocardial infarction has occurred.[633] Heparin, 5000 units given subcutaneously every 8 to 12 h, decreases the incidence of leg vein thrombosis by two-thirds,[631] without full anticoagulation. The effectiveness of low-dose heparin in preventing pulmonary emboli after myocardial infarction is not known, but the efficacy of low-dose heparin prophylaxis has been demonstrated in patients undergoing elective general surgery, and it is reasonable to assume that it may be useful in patients with acute myocardial infarction.[634] Patients who develop pulmonary emboli should receive intravenous heparin to prolong the partial thromboplastin time to one and one-half to two times control. Heparin should be continued for 7 to 10 days and then supplanted by oral anticoagulants. In addition to bleeding complications, heparin may induce thrombocytopenia.[635]

Early Complications: Systemic Arterial Embolism Systemic arterial emboli originate from left ventricular mural thrombi. Mural thrombi detected by ^{111}In platelet imaging generally occur in akinetic or dyskinetic left ventricular segments. Technically excellent two-dimensional echocardiograms are valuable in detecting left ventricular thrombi.[636] The incidence of systemic embolization has seemingly decreased in recent years for reasons not apparent. Emboli may lodge in visceral arteries and produce infarction of brain, kidney, spleen, or intestine. Sudden coldness, pain, and numbness are the characteristic features of embolization to an extremity. A systemic arterial embolus may be the initial manifestation of an otherwise unsuspected myocardial infarction.

The *treatment* of the embolus depends upon the organ or tissue that it compromises. The treatment of a cerebral embolus is discussed in Chap. 66. Arterial emboli that compromise the blood supply to an extremity may be removed with a balloon catheter. The institution of heparin therapy should follow the surgical procedure. Oral anticoagulation should usually follow heparin administration.

Early Complications: Ventricular Septal Rupture Rupture of the interventricular septum complicates 1 to 3 percent of acute myocardial infarctions and occurs most frequently during the first week after infarction. Ventricular septal rupture most often occurs near the junction of the septum and the anterior or posterior left ventricular free wall. Septal rupture tends to develop in patients experiencing their first transmural infarction in whom collateral flow to the septum is limited.[637] Thinning and dilatation of the acutely infarcted myocardium may be important in the genesis of septal or free wall rupture.[638] Ventricular septal rupture produces an abrupt change in clinical status characterized by cardiogenic shock and/or heart failure. During the period immediately following the rupture, clinical findings of right-sided heart failure are more conspicuous than signs of pulmonary edema. A new holosystolic murmur is heard coincident with the clinical deterioration. The diagnosis is reasonably certain if the new holosystolic murmur is loudest along the lower left sternal border and is accompanied by a thrill. However, the murmur is sometimes loudest at the apex and easily mistaken for a murmur of mitral regurgitation. Bedside right-sided heart catheterization with sequential oximetry makes the differentiation of septal rupture from acute mitral regurgitation relatively straightforward because septal rupture produces an oxygen step-up in the right ventricle. The pulmonary/systemic flow ratio usually exceeds 2:1. Two-dimensional echocardiography with saline contrast provides a reliable means of diagnosing ventricular septal rupture.[639,640]

The clinical course after ventricular septal rupture varies. Rapid hemodynamic deterioration develops in approximately one-half the patients, leading to either early operation or death from cardiogenic shock. Other patients experience slow, progressive deterioration. The remaining patients become hemodynamically stable with medical therapy, but usually have symptomatic heart failure. Perioperative survival is mainly determined by whether cardiogenic shock develops preoperatively.[641] Right ventricular dysfunction may be the major determinant in the development of cardiogenic shock.[641,642] Patients with inferior myocardial infarction and septal rupture usually have extensive right ventricular free wall infarction. Why anterior left ventricular infarction and septal rupture coexist with right ventricular dysfunction is less clear. Conceivably, massive septal infarction with rupture may, in some patients, impair right ventricular function.

Eventual surgical *treatment* (see Chap. 132) of the ventricular septal rupture is generally advisable since the mortality rate with medical management alone exceeds 80 percent. Although the risk is high, early surgical repair should be considered in patients with cardiogenic shock and in patients with progressively increasing or severe heart failure.[641] Intraaortic balloon pumping should be instituted. Balloon counterpulsation may reduce the pulmonary-to-systemic flow rate, and it decreases the risk of preoperative coronary arteriography and left ventriculography. Clinical and hemodynamic improvement resulting from intraaortic balloon pumping is not a reason for deferring surgery, because this improvement is usually temporary. In the few patients whose heart failure is not worsening, vasodilator drugs may produce enough improvement that intraaortic balloon pumping is unnecessary, and angiographic studies and surgery may be delayed for several weeks.

Early Complications: Papillary Muscle Dysfunction Papillary muscle dysfunction develops because of ischemia or infarction of a papillary muscle and the adjacent left ventricular myocardium. The patient's course is determined largely by the extent of ventricular muscle loss, as papillary muscle dysfunction per se is usually not a major factor in determining outcome. The systolic murmur produced by papillary muscle dysfunction may have many different configurations. The murmur is most easily recognized as being due to mitral regurgitation when it is holosystolic or mid to late systolic. Severe mitral regurgitation may be silent when marked left ventricular dysfunction exists. The detection of large *v* waves in the phasic capillary wedge pressure may be the first indication of massive mitral regurgitation.

There are relatively rare situations in which papillary muscle dysfunction may assume major significance. Exceptional patients develop severe mitral regurgitation and pulmonary edema during chest pain episodes. Nitroglycerin may produce a dramatic reversal of the clinical signs of mitral regurgitation and pulmonary edema within minutes. Occasionally, papillary muscle necrosis can lead to fibrosis, shortening, and retraction of one of the mitral leaflets into the body of the left ventricle. The resulting disruption of the normal line of anterior and posterior leaflet closure may cause severe mitral regurgitation. These patients are indistinguishable clinically from patients with papillary muscle rupture, but the two lesions can be differentiated by two-dimensional echocardiography.[640]

Treatment depends upon the severity of the mitral regurgitation and degree of left ventricular dysfunction. Mitral valve replacement may prove beneficial if left ventricular contractility is reasonably well preserved.

Early Complications: Papillary Muscle Rupture[642a] Complete dehiscence of a papillary muscle following myocardial infarction produces massive mitral regurgitation, resulting in pulmonary edema, shock, and death. Partial rupture of a papillary muscle, rupture of one or two of five heads, is not always so catastrophic, thereby allowing time for clinical evaluation and possible surgical correction.[643] Because of a single blood supply, the posteromedial papillary muscle ruptures at least six times more frequently than the anterolateral muscle, which has a dual blood supply from the left anterior descending and left circumflex coronary arteries. Commonly the extent of infarction is small and may be limited to the subendocardium.[643] Half the patients with papillary muscle rupture have single-vessel disease. Theoretically, a small infarction with well-preserved ventricular function may produce greater shearing forces and increase the risk of rupture.

A new systolic murmur may not be heard if the entire papillary muscle is ruptured or the patient is in shock. Patients with partial rupture who survive the acute event usually have a systolic murmur typical of acute mitral regurgitation. Two-dimensional echocardiography is useful in detecting a flail mitral leaflet.[640]

Early surgical *treatment* (see Chap. 132) should be considered in all patients with papillary muscle rupture.[643] Although medical therapy with vasodilator drugs, diuretics, and the intraaortic balloon pump may stabilize the patient's condition, the improvement is often temporary. Urgent surgery is essential in patients with hypotension and pulmonary edema because the prognosis with medical therapy is abysmal. In stable patients, clinical deterioration may be sudden and unpredictable, and thus delay in surgery may be risky.

Early Complications: External Cardiac Rupture External cardiac rupture accounts for 10 to 15 percent of deaths following acute myocardial infarction. It is seldom seen before the sixth decade of life. A transmural infarction with poor collateral circulation to the infarcted area, systemic arterial hypertension during the acute phase of infarction, and dilatation and thinning of the infarct are additional factors that correlate with a higher incidence of rupture.

External cardiac rupture results in hemopericardium with cardiac tamponade, marked neck vein distension, cardiogenic shock, and electromechanical dissociation. Most patients die suddenly without premonitory symptoms. In others, rupture may be suggested by the appearance of chest pain with hypotension and signs of cardiac tamponade. A pericardial friction rub may be heard in a few patients prior to rupture. Pericardial pain that is not improved by the administration of narcotics or corticosteroids may be an indication of impending cardiac rupture. The ECG usually shows the unchanged pattern of myocardial infarction at a time when the blood pressure is unobtainable. Sinus bradycardia followed by a slow AV junctional rhythm commonly develops and may be mediated by vagal stimulation with the afferent limb originating in pericardial stretch receptors.[644]

Treatment is usually not possible because death occurs within a few minutes. An occasional patient may survive long enough to undergo pericardiocentesis, which may temporarily relieve the cardiac tamponade and allow the patient to be moved to the operating room for closure of the defect. Only a few cases of successful repair of the ruptured left ventricle have been reported (see Chap. 132).[645,646]

Early Complications: Emotional Responses Many patients suffering a myocardial infarction pass through states of denial, acceptance, anxiety, and depression before they realistically adapt to their illness (see "Emotional Causes of Chest Discomfort" earlier in this chapter). Physicians must be sensitive to these emotional responses in order to rehabilitate patients physically and mentally. Emotional reactions to myocardial infarction are easily overlooked, especially in patients with serious medical complications. Frequently the nursing staff preempts the physician in recognizing an emotional problem. Some patients relay their fears to the nurse but disguise them from the physician. Nurses play an important role in allaying a patient's fear of electrocardiographic and hemodynamic monitoring equipment by introducing it as a source of protection.

Patients who deny the reality of their illness are easily recognized. They minimize the severity of their condition, appear nonchalant, and complain excessively about the restrictions placed upon them in the coronary care unit. Occasionally, the presentation of denial is less overt. Patients may express an interest in and an understanding of their problem, but their actions belie their words. Denial does not require direct confrontation unless it threatens effective medical care.

Most patients express some anxiety, but it is usually not severe. Anxiety develops from a fear of dying, and the appearance of chest discomfort, weakness, dyspnea, or other symptoms of myocardial infarction.[647] Some degree of depression is found in most patients after myocardial infarction. It is reactive in nature and rarely assumes psychotic proportions.[648] The threat of physical debilitation and loss of self-worth are important contributing factors.

The primary physician should be able to *treat* most emotional problems that arise in patients with myocardial infarction. What is required of the physician is interest, common sense, and time. An explanation of myocardial infarction and its healing is reassuring to most patients. As soon as a patient's short-term course can be predicted with reasonable accuracy, a physical rehabilitation program, including a return to work, should be outlined. Such a discussion may ferret out patients with outmoded ideas of permanent invalidism after myocardial infarction. The need for and expected benefits from a formal cardiac rehabilitation program should be addressed. Minor tranquilizers may be needed for patients with severe anxiety, but the chronic administration of tranquilizers is discouraged. Patients with severe, unrelenting depression require psychiatric consultation.

Late Complications: Angina Pectoris Angina pectoris following myocardial infarction is associated with a poor prognosis. Occasionally, patients who have suffered from angina pectoris lose their pain after a myocardial infarction, but more commonly, angina persists. Some patients develop angina only after recovery from infarction. The presence of an earlier infarction does not alter the management of angina pectoris. However, more extensive left ventricular regional wall motion abnormalities are expected in postinfarction patients.

Intensive medical *treatment* is needed. Postinfarction angina pectoris is usually an indication for coronary arteriography. The decision to intervene with coronary angioplasty or bypass surgery is based upon considerations discussed earlier in this chapter.

Late Complications: Cardiac Arrhythmias Although patients with prior infarction are subject to all types of cardiac arrhythmias, ventricular arrhythmias present the major clinical problem. Myocardial infarction complicated by ventricular aneurysm is a common cause of recurrent, sustained ventricular tachycardia.

Sustained ventricular tachycardia may recur despite empiric *treatment* with multiple antiarrhythmic drugs. The best method for establishing an effective drug regimen in patients with coronary artery disease and refractory ventricular tachycardia remains controversial. Some investigators favor an approach that includes acute testing of multiple drugs during continuous electrocardiographic monitoring and exercise stress testing, and observations during maintenance therapy.[649] If antiarrhythmic drugs abolish salvos of ventricular tachycardia and R-on-T ventricular premature depolarization (PVD), the incidence of sudden death during follow-up is decreased.[649] One disadvantage of this approach is the time required for serial drug testing, which averages 17 hospital days. In addition, the efficacy of this clinical approach needs verification by additional investigators. With programmed ventricular stimulation, an effective drug regimen is found in approximately one-half of the patients in a few days of hospitalization.[650] The incidence of subsequent ventricular tachyarrhythmias is significantly less when effective therapy is found by electrophysiological study.[651,652] Whether this beneficial effect is related to drug action or to selection of patients who are somehow at lower risk remains to be clarified.[651] Most patients who survive out-of-hospital cardiac arrest and who show no objective evidence of myocardial infarction should undergo programmed ventricular stimulation with serial drug testing.[653] Some patients for whom no effective drug can be found are candidates for arrhythmia surgery. Surgery guided by intraoperative mapping frequently eliminates recurrent ventricular tachycardia in patients with a ventricular aneurysm or akinetic segment.[654–656] Patients in whom no drug is predicated to be effective and for whom surgery is contraindicated may be considered for an automatic antitachycardia pacemaker (see Chap. 28) or an automatic implanted defibrillator (see Chap. 106).[657,658]

Cardiac arrest is a major cause of death in survivors of myocardial infarction. Much remains to be learned about how best to identify the patients at risk. We do not recommend routine 24-h ambulatory electrocardiography after acute myocardial infarction. Numerous reports associate complex ventricular ectopy (multiformed, repetitive, begeminal, R-on-T PVDs) with an increased risk of subsequent sudden death.[659,660] However, complex PVDs are found in up to three-fourths of patients monitored for 24 h and are reproducible in only one-half of the patients.[661] The induction of sustained or nonsustained ventricular tachycardia by electrophysiological testing may identify a propensity to subsequent ventricular arrhythmias in some patients, but further studies are needed before this technique can be widely applied.[662]

Monitoring the *treatment* of premature ventricular depolarizations (PVDs) presents a problem. Ambulatory electrocardiographic monitoring has limited value because the day-to-day variation in the number of PVDs is so large that a reduction in the frequency of PVDs cannot be attributed to a therapeutic intervention unless there is an 80 percent or greater reduction in PVDs.[663] The aggravation of ventricular arrhythmias by antiarrhythmic drugs is insufficiently recognized.[664] Detection is easy when a class I antiarrhythmic drug produces marked QT-interval prolongation and torsade de pointes ventricular tachycardia.[665] Unfortunately, the presentation is frequently more subtle and can only be discovered by prolonged electrocardiographic monitoring or ventricular stimulation during periods of drug administration and withdrawal.

Complex PVDs are only one of several factors associated with an increased likelihood of cardiac death. It is frequently difficult to determine whether a higher rate of cardiac mortality is due to complex PVDs or severe left ventricular dysfunction.[651,666,667]

Late Complications: Heart Failure (see Chap. 21) Persistent heart failure after myocardial infarction is a poor prognostic sign. Little spontaneous improvement can be expected after 4 to 6 weeks. Dyspnea associated with physical exertion, emotional stress, or dreaming may be due to severe regional myocardial dysfunction produced by acute ischemia. Preventing myocardial ischemia with medical therapy, coronary angioplasty, or coronary bypass surgery may abolish these episodes of transient "heart failure." Successful therapy may improve the left ventricular ejection fraction during exercise.[668] An important task is to divide patients with heart failure into those with diffuse asynergy and those with a discrete ventricular aneurysm amenable to surgical resection. Radionuclide ventriculography is reasonably accurate in making this distinction.

The *treatment* of heart failure is discussed in Chap. 21. Heart failure due to diffuse hypokinesis may improve with a combination of digitalis, diuretic, and vasodilator therapy. Surgical removal of a ventricular aneurysm with coronary artery bypass grafting is the best treatment for patients with refractory heart failure associated with a discrete aneurysm.

Late Complications: Ventricular Aneurysm A ventricular aneurysm is distinguished by extreme thinning of the cardiac wall with a convex deformity of the external surface. The endocardial surface of the aneurysm tends to show either prominent fibroelastosis or considerable thrombus with little or no fibroelastosis. Patients with ventricular aneurysm and recurrent ventricular tachycardia commonly have extensive fibroelastosis in the aneurysm.[669] Ventricular aneurysms are usually associated with transmural infarction and involve the anterior or apical area in 80 percent of cases. Physical findings that suggest the presence of a ventricular aneurysm include a sustained and broad precordial pulsation at the cardiac apex, a holosystolic precordial pulsation located medially or superiorly to the cardiac apex, and persistent gallop rhythm.

The chest x-ray may disclose a bulge, sharp angulation, or a ledge in the lower left ventricular contour. Calcium is sometimes seen within the aneurysm wall.

Pathological Q waves are recorded on the ECG in most patients. Persistent ST-segment elevation on the resting electrocardiogram is a suggestive but rather insensitive sign. ST-segment elevation may be recorded only during exercise.

Congestive heart failure, ventricular tachyarrhythmias, and arterial embolism are the major complications. Disabling angina pectoris in conjunction with congestive heart failure suggests associated multivessel coronary artery disease. Rupture virtually never occurs unless there is reinfarction at the border of the aneurysm. The prognosis is contingent upon the size of the aneurysm, mechanical function of the remaining myocardium, and the severity of coronary artery disease. The prognosis may be quite good if the aneurysm is small.

Anticoagulant *treatment* is indicated if an arterial embolus or a thrombus is found in the aneurysm on a ventriculogram or two-dimensional echocardiogram. Aneurysmectomy is considered if congestive heart failure, ventricular tachycardia, angina pectoris, or arterial emboli become refractory to medical therapy. Radionuclide ventriculography can identify large aneurysms; however, biplane ventriculograms and a coronary arteriogram are essential prior to surgery. Aneurysmectomy, and when indicated, concomitant coronary revascularization, improve congestive heart failure and angina pectoris in most patients who survive the surgery[670,671] (see Chap. 132). However, standard left ventricular aneurysm resection commonly fails to eliminate ventricular tachyarrhythmias. Surgical procedures guided by endocardial activation sequence mapping achieve greater success because most tissue responsible for generating the arrhythmia can be removed.[655,656]

A *false left ventricular aneurysm* occurs following hemorrhagic dissection into and through an area of transmural infarction. If the parietal pericardium adheres to the epicardium, it may contain the hematoma that has dissected through the left ventricular wall. The confined hematoma stretches and forms a false aneurysm communicating with the left ventricle via a small orifice. A left ventriculogram usually suggests the diagnosis.

Surgical *repair* is generally indicated because a false aneurysm may rupture.

Late Complications: Post-Myocardial Infarction Syndrome (Dressler's Syndrome) (see Chap. 59) The post-myocardial infarction syndrome appears a few weeks or months after myocardial infarction, and is characterized by protracted or recurrent fever, chest pain of the pleuropericardial type, a pericardial friction rub, and left pleural effusion. A pericardial effusion may be detected by echocardiography, but cardiac tamponade is rare. Dressler's syndrome is an uncommon complication of myocardial infarction, and its incidence appears to be decreasing.[672] The etiology of Dressler's syndrome is unknown. Various causes have been proposed, including an autoimmune mechanism, viral infection, and pericardial bleeding produced by anticoagulant therapy. Most patients with Dressler's syndrome also have had early post-myocardial infarction pericarditis.[673]

Treatment with corticosteroids, indomethacin, or aspirin is usually effective. Occasionally patients are subject to recurrent attacks.

Late Complications: Shoulder-Hand Syndrome The shoulder-hand syndrome (periarthritis of the shoulder) was a common complication of myocardial infarction when patients were treated with strict and prolonged best rest. The change from prolonged bed rest to early ambulation has nearly eliminated this problem. Rarely, patients with preexisting disease of the shoulder and medical complications requiring prolonged bed rest develop the shoulder-hand syndrome. It begins from one to several months after infarction with pain, stiffness, and marked limitation of motion of the shoulder joint, shoulder girdle, and arm. If untreated, the skin over the hands and fingers may become tense, shiny, and swollen.

Physiotherapy is the mainstay of *treatment.* Sometimes, intraarticular corticosteroid injection may provide relief.

Late Complications: Emotional Response (see Chap. 82) Emotional distress disproportionate to actual cardiac impairment may prevent complete rehabilitation. Patients who are depressed at their first post-hospital visit are likely to remain so after 6 months.[674] Hypochondriasis, social withdrawal, and invalidism may result.

Ruberman et al. studied 2320 male patients after myocardial infarction. They discovered that the risk of death in a 3-year follow-up period was more than four times greater in males who were socially isolated, had less education, and experienced considerable life stress compared to controls.[288]

This incapacitating state may be prevented in many patients. A *treatment* program of appropriately graded exercise should be instituted soon after infarction. The physical and psychological benefits of a formal cardiovascular rehabilitation program are well-accepted. In some patients with a major depressive disorder, conservative doses of tricyclic antidepressants may be used without adversely affecting ejection fraction or inducing ventricular ectopy.[675] Congestive heart failure, orthostatic hypotension, and intraventricular conduction disturbances are contraindications to tricyclic antidepressants. Recalcitrant depression requires psychiatric consultation.

Sudden Death

Recognition and Definition

When a patient dies within a few minutes or within 2 h, he or she is said to have experienced *sudden death.* There are many causes for such an event, but the most common is myocardial ischemia due to atherosclerotic coronary heart disease (see Chaps. 31, 32, and 43). The abnormal mechanism responsible for death is usually ventricular fibrillation, although cardiac standstill and electrical-mechanical dissociation may be responsible. When such patients are resuscitated, they may, but often do not, give a history of angina pectoris or previous infarction. Such an event is more likely to occur again to these people as compared to patients who have never experienced it.

Treatment
No perfect study has been done which determines the proper treatment of such patients after they have been resuscitated. Leonard Cobb, working with the Seattle Heart Watch, has data to indicate that such patients should have a coronary arteriogram, and when obstructive but operable lesions are found, coronary bypass surgery should be performed. Sudden death may still occur in the operated group, but it is less common than in the group who did not have coronary bypass surgery (see Chap. 32).

After coronary bypass surgery has been performed, other medical measures are indicated. They include Holter monitoring to identify cardiac arrhythmias; variable drug treatment of arrhythmias as determined by long-term monitoring; preventive measures as described in Chap. 42; and carefully supervised rehabilitation.

Syncope (see Chaps. 29 and 30)

Recognition and Definition
Cardiac syncope is defined as transient loss of consciousness due to heart disease. *Near syncope* is the momentary loss of postural tone and a feeling that unconsciousness is pending. The cardiac diseases that may produce syncope are aortic stenosis; idiopathic hypertrophic subaortic stenosis; sick sinus and atrioventricular node syndromes; Lenegre's disease and Lev's disease producing complete heart block; and certain cardiac arrhythmias with or without other disease. Atherosclerotic coronary disease causes myocardial ischemia, which in turn causes cardiac arrhythmias such as ventricular fibrillation and ventricular tachycardia. Such arrhythmias can also occur in patients with atherosclerotic coronary disease when the mechanism of arrhythmia production is not ischemia.

Obviously, ventricular fibrillation will cause syncope if the arrhythmia lasts a short period and sudden death if it persists.

Patients with syncope due to atherosclerotic heart disease may or may not complain of angina pectoris.

Treatment
The treatment obviously depends upon the identification of the type of cardiac arrhythmia. This is done by constantly monitoring the electrocardiogram for a prolonged period of time if the attacks are infrequent. Arrhythmias due to the sick sinus syndrome and fascicular and trifascicular block are usually not due to coronary disease, although it may coexist. Ventricular arrhythmias are more likely to be due to atherosclerotic heart disease. Such patients should have a coronary arteriogram performed, and when operable conditions are found, the patient should have coronary bypass surgery. Following surgery, appropriate antiarrhythmic therapy should be continued. If the arrhythmia continues, then detailed electrophysiological studies should be obtained in an effort to acquire information that would be useful in guiding therapy.

Cardiac Arrhythmias

Recognition and Definition
Cardiac arrhythmias may be associated with atherosclerotic coronary heart disease. This is not to say that reversible myocardial ischemia is always responsible for the arrhythmias. For example, chronic atrial fibrillation and transient atrial fibrillation occur more frequently in patients with known angina pectoris than in patients without angina. This, however, does not prove that the atrial fibrillation is due to reversible ischemia. The rhythm disturbance associated with sick sinus node syndrome is usually not due to ischemia. The cause of this disorder is usually not known. The AV block related to bifascicular block and trifascicular block is usually due to Lenegre's or Lev's disease even in patients with coronary atherosclerosis.

Patients who have a positive response to the exercise stress test and develop ventricular tachycardia or transient ventricular fibrillation usually have reversible myocardial ischemia due to atherosclerotic coronary heart disease.

Some patients with Prinzmetal's syndrome due to obstructive coronary disease plus coronary spasm develop AV block or ventricular arrhythmia during an attack of myocardial ischemia.

These rhythms may be captured on a routine ECG or on a Holter monitor recording when the patient is being studied for palpitation.

Obviously, cardiac arrhythmias due to transient ischemia overlap with the arrhythmias that cause syncope and sudden death.

Treatment
When the exercise test reveals a ventricular arrhythmia with or without an abnormal ST-segment response, the patient should have a coronary arteriogram. When high-grade coronary artery obstruction is found and the distal vessels are adequate, the patient should have coronary bypass surgery. After surgery, if a similar arrhythmia is identified during the treadmill test, the patient should be started on drug therapy such as propranolol or procainamide. If this approach does not solve the problem, then cardiac electrophysiology should be performed.

The patient with Prinzmetal's variant angina who has a cardiac arrhythmia during the episode should have coronary arteriography and coronary bypass surgery if coronary artery obstruction plus coronary spasm is found. Nitrates and calcium antagonists (excluding verapamil) should be used following surgery. If only coronary artery spasm is discovered, surgery is not indicated, and drug therapy with nitrates and calcium antagonists is indicated (excluding verapamil). If episodes of atrioventricular block continue, it may be necessary to insert an artificial pacemaker. If treacherous ventricular arrhythmias continue, it may be necessary to have cardiac electrophysiological studies.

The treatment of ventricular arrhythmias is discussed in Chap. 27. Patients with troublesome and dangerous arrhythmias despite the usual drug therapy may need electrophysiological studies. The patients who have any other clue that coronary disease is present, such as angina or prolonged chest discomfort consistent with myocardial ischemia, a positive exercise electrocardiogram, or a positive radionuclide exercise stress test, should have a coronary arteriogram.

Ischemic Cardiomyopathy

Recognition and Definition
Patients with diffuse myocardial disease due to atherosclerotic coronary heart disease may or may not give a history of angina pectoris or reveal evidence of old myocardial infarction. This condition is commonly seen in diabetic patients. The syndrome is one of cardiac enlargement with chronic heart failure. The disorder must be differentiated from idiopathic congestive cardiomyopathy (see Chap. 58). The identification of hypertrophic cardiomyopathy is less of a problem since the heart is usually not large and heart failure is usually not a prominent feature until late in the course of the disease. The diagnosis of ischemic cardiomyopathy is not always easy since patients with idiopathic congestive cardiomyopathy and hypertrophic cardiomyopathy may have angina pectoris or even prolonged episodes of chest discomfort due to myocardial ischemia and electrocardiographic signs consistent with infarction.

This disorder is discussed here as a subset of irreversible myocardial ischemia because the hearts of some of these patients show diffuse areas of old infarction and dilatation. Chronic myocardial ischemia is undoubtedly present, and reversible myocardial ischemia may be superimposed on the more chronic state. In some patients the latter predominates (see Chap. 43).

The first decision that must be made in a patient with cardiomyopathy is whether or not other diagnostic procedures are indicated.

An exercise stress test should not be done. An echocardiogram can establish the diagnosis of hypertrophic cardiomyopathy. A radionuclide ventriculogram may be used to document the degree of muscle damage and to estimate the ejection fraction in patients with large hearts and heart failure. If the radionuclide ventriculogram suggests that a ventricular aneurysm is present, it is then necessary to obtain a coronary arteriogram and left ventriculogram. Under these circumstances, the etiology can be established. If the radionuclide ventriculogram shows a generalized decrease in contractility, it does not separate a coronary cause from idiopathic cardiomyopathy. A coronary arteriogram will usually reveal little useful information in such patients, since they are rarely candidates for surgery even if coronary disease is found.

Treatment
The treatment of heart failure with digitalis, diuretics, and alteration of the preload and afterload is discussed in Chap. 21.

- Some patients with a ventricular aneurysm may be candidates for cardiac surgery.
- Patients with angina pectoris may respond to nitroglycerin, nitroglycerin ointment, and isosorbide dinitrate.
- Patients with ischemic cardiomyopathy should not use alcohol.
- Patients with ischemic cardiomyopathy should not engage in an exercise program and should restrict their activity to necessary acts. Patients with this disorder frequently become disabled or experience sudden death.
- Cardiac transplantation should be considered in carefully selected patients (see Chap. 136).

Atherosclerotic Coronary Heart Disease in Combination with Other Conditions

The Patient with Chest Pain Who Has Already Had Coronary Bypass Surgery

Definition and Recognition Coronary bypass surgery relieves the symptoms of angina pectoris in 90 percent of patients. Complete relief occurs in 70 to 80 percent of patients. However, patients often have chest pain that is difficult to analyze following coronary bypass surgery. A patient may have pericarditis, chest wall discomfort, the pain of anxiety, or various types of chest pain due to myocardial ischemia. When angina pectoris or prolonged pain due to myocardial ischemia occurs soon after surgery, it is proper to consider thrombosis of the graft, some technical cause of graft closure, or inadequate revascularization at the time of surgery. When the symptoms occur several months after surgery, one should consider obliterative closure of a graft or grafts. When the symptoms occur months to years after surgery, they may be the result of graft closure from fibrosis or atherosclerosis, but they may also be due to progressive coronary disease in the native vessels.

An exercise ECG may show an abnormal ST-segment shift, and the patient may experience angina during the test. Such a test does not solve all problems and a ^{201}Tl scan may be needed. If the patient exhibits a positive response in the stress ECG or if the ^{201}Tl scan is positive, the patient should have a coronary arteriogram (see Chap. 109). This is the only reliable way of determining whether the grafts are patent or whether the coronary atherosclerotic process has progressed in the nongrafted vessels or in areas beyond the graft. Most patients who have a negative exercise electrocardiogram and a negative exercise ^{201}Tl scan can be reassured by the physician that myocardial ischemia is not occurring.

Treatment The management is linked to the diagnosis. If the patient has pericarditis, then treatment with prednisone or indomethacin is indicated. Chest wall pain is usually managed by simple reassurance. Angina pectoris is managed according to the results of the stress ECG, radionuclide test, and coronary arteriographic abnormalities. If the grafts have closed, it is usually necessary to have repeat coronary bypass surgery. Angioplasty can be occasionally used if the artery beyond the graft is narrowed or if stenosis is located in the distal anastomotic site of the vein graft. If the symptoms are due to progressive narrowing in nongrafted vessels, then the feasibility of bypass surgery is determined by the location and extent of obstructing lesions.

The operative mortality rate is increased in patients who have bypass surgery for the second time, and the complication rate is also increased. Medical management must be continued in patients in whom surgery is repeated. Patients who are not candidates for surgery but continue to have unacceptable angina pectoris despite the usual treatment may benefit from drugs that lower the metabolic rate, such as radioactive iodine and methimazole.

The Patient with Coronary Disease and Carotid Artery Disease

Definition and Recognition All patients with evidence of atherosclerotic coronary artery disease must be examined for carotid artery disease, vertebrobasilar arterial disease, abdominal aortic aneurysm, and peripheral vascular disease, and patients with the conditions listed must be examined for atherosclerotic coronary heart disease.

The male patient with an asymptomatic carotid bruit is likely to have evidence of atherosclerotic coronary heart disease within the next several years. A candidate for coronary bypass surgery who also has transient ischemic attacks should have additional studies performed prior to coronary bypass surgery. The patient with transient ischemic attacks should, as a rule, have carotid arteriography. The mortality rate of carotid arteriography is almost zero at Emory University Hospital, but a very small percent of the patients studied for transient ischemic attacks have significant neurological complications as a result of the procedure. This simply implies that the workup and surgical treatment for such patients are very difficult, and much clinical judgment is needed to plan treatment. Patients with asymptomatic carotid bruits who need coronary bypass surgery are also troublesome. Surgeons and anesthesiologists are concerned about such patients since postoperative stroke seems to be more common in them. First of all, one must be certain that the bruit is produced by obstruction in the carotid artery since venous hums occasionally occur in adults, the murmur of aortic stenosis is usually transmitted up the neck, and a relatively unimportant murmur due to stenosis of the origin of the left subclavian artery may be misinterpreted as a carotid bruit. If the carotid bruit is short in duration and noninvasive studies suggest that the vessel is not significantly occluded, an arch aortogram need not be done before coronary bypass surgery is performed. More clinical research is needed on this problem, and for this reason definitive views cannot be expressed.

Treatment The problem is as follows: When should the carotid artery surgery be performed in relation to the coronary bypass surgery? When the patient has transient ischemic attacks from obstructive atherosclerotic disease of the carotid arteries and needs coronary bypass surgery, we have carotid endarterectomy and coronary bypass surgery performed during the same time frame. A vascular surgeon operates on the carotid artery, and, when this is completed, the cardiac surgeon operates on the coronary arteries.

At the present time we do not recommend carotid endarterectomy on a patient who is to have coronary bypass surgery simply because a carotid bruit is heard.

The Patient with Abdominal Aneurysm or Intermittent Claudication Who Needs Coronary Bypass Surgery

Patients with an abdominal aneurysm or disabling intermittent claudication of the legs who need coronary bypass surgery should have the latter operation before surgery is performed for the former conditions. When a patient is unable to perform the usual stress test, it may be necessary to utilize arm exercise testing in order to find objective signs of myocardial ischemia in the ECG or radionuclide stress test. According to Balady, arm exercise testing is less sensitive than leg testing but, he believes, it is a reasonable alternative for patients who are unable to use their lower extremities.[676]

The Patient with Aortic Stenosis and Atherosclerotic Coronary Heart Disease

Definition and Recognition Many patients with valvular aortic stenosis who have angina pectoris or prolonged episodes of myocardial ischemia also have associated obstructive atherosclerotic coronary heart disease. Therefore, a coronary arteriogram should be done at the time of cardiac catheterization to determine whether the angina pectoris is due to aortic stenosis alone or to associated coronary atherosclerosis. It should be recalled that angina pectoris is a definite signal to perform cardiac catheterization, including coronary arteriography, in patients with aortic stenosis.

The patient with aortic stenosis who has no angina pectoris or evidence of prolonged myocardial ischemia should have coronary arteriography performed at the same time cardiac catheterization is performed for aortic stenosis because asymptomatic but severe coronary disease is often present.

Treatment If such patients have high-grade obstructive lesions demonstrated in the coronary arteries, bypass surgery should be performed at the same time that aortic valve surgery is performed, even though the patient has no symptoms of ischemia. There are few data regarding this group of patients, but the plan seems reasonable. Coronary bypass surgery is usually not performed for lesions causing less than 50 percent luminal diameter narrowing although some debate still exists regarding the group of patients. The operative risk in such patients at Emory University Hospital is about 5 percent.

The Patient with Aortic Regurgitation and Atherosclerotic Coronary Heart Disease

Definition and Recognition When angina pectoris or prolonged myocardial ischemia occurs in patients with aortic regurgitation, it is necessary to perform coronary arteriography at the time of cardiac catheterization in order to determine the cause of the ischemic episodes. Obviously, coronary arteriography should also be done in such patients even when there is no history of angina pectoris.

Treatment Coronary bypass surgery should be performed in patients who have high-grade obstructive coronary disease and who have aortic valve replacement performed for aortic regurgitation, whether or not they have angina pectoris. Coronary bypass surgery is usually not performed for lesions causing less than 50 percent luminal diameter narrowing although some debate still exists regarding this group of patients. The operative risk in such patients at Emory University is about 5 percent.

The Patient with Mitral Stenosis and Atherosclerotic Heart Disease

Definition and Recognition Patients with tight mitral stenosis may have chest discomfort due to myocardial ischemia. The angina pectoris may be due to factors other than associated obstructive coronary atherosclerosis, and coronary arteriography is needed to clarify the problem. A coronary arteriogram should be done in most adults who undergo cardiac catheterization for mitral stenosis since it adds little if any risk to the procedure. Young women with tight mitral stenosis and little likelihood of coronary disease may have valve surgery without coronary arteriography.

Treatment Coronary bypass surgery should be performed in patients with high-grade obstructive lesions in the coronary arteries at the same time that surgery for mitral stenosis is performed, even though the patient has no symptoms of ischemia. Coronary bypass surgery is usually not performed for lesions causing less than 50 percent luminal diameter narrowing although some debate still exists regarding this group of patients. The operative risk for patients who are seriously ill with heart failure is, regrettably, 5 to 15 percent depending on the severity of the problem.

The Patient with Mitral Regurgitation with Atherosclerotic Coronary Heart Disease

Definition and Recognition Patients over the age of 35 years who have mitral regurgitation and sufficient signs and symptoms to justify surgery should have coronary arteriography performed when cardiac catheterization is performed. Many patients with mitral regurgitation do have coronary atherosclerosis.

Treatment Coronary bypass surgery should be performed in patients with high-grade obstructive lesions in the coronary arteries at the same time surgery for mitral regurgitation takes place, even though the patient has no symptoms of ischemia. Coronary bypass surgery is usually not performed for lesions causing less than 50 percent luminal diameter narrowing although some debate still exists regarding this group of patients. The operative risk of the combined operation on patients who undergo elective surgery at Emory University Hospital is about 5 percent. When the mitral regurgitation is secondary to coronary heart disease or when the patient is seriously ill with heart failure, the operative risk is about 50 percent.

The Patient with Atherosclerotic Coronary Heart Disease Who Is To Have Surgery for Noncardiac Problems (Abdominal Aneurysm, Gallstones, Prostatic Hypertrophy, etc.)

Many patients with certain subsets of atherosclerotic coronary heart disease who are to undergo surgery for a noncardiac problem should have coronary bypass surgery performed before the elective surgery is performed for noncardiac disease. The usual clinical setting is that of a patient with unacceptable stable angina pectoris or unstable angina with high-grade obstructive lesions in several coronary arteries who also needs gallbladder surgery, prostate surgery, or resection of an abdominal aneurysm, etc.

Reasons for Different Strategies

Years ago little could be done about the prevention, diagnosis, and treatment of coronary disease due to atherosclerosis. People with the disease continued to hurt, they retired, and they died in greater numbers than they do currently. There were arguments regarding the length of time a patient with an infarct should stay in bed and if long-term anticoagulants should, or should not, be given.

Today preventive measures, though far from perfect, are taken more seriously than they were in the past. Opinions still vary about the value of certain aspects of some of the "programs" that the public at large seems to believe should guarantee immortality.

The diagnostic and therapeutic approach may vary from physician to physician and facility to facility. In other words, several different strategies may be utilized in the diagnostic workup and the treatment of similar patients. The purpose of this final note is to offer an explanation for some of the differences in diagnostic methods and treatment that are occurring today.

- All physicians have different views about their own diagnostic accuracy in determining if patients have angina pectoris or do not have angina.
- Diagnostic methods commonly used, in addition to the history, physical examination, and resting ECG are exercise stress electrocardiography; radionuclide stress tests; echocardiography; and coronary arteriography. The equipment, use, and interpretation of the test results and their appropriate usage vary considerably from physician to physician and facility to facility.

  If a facility has poor nuclear cardiology and excellent coronary arteriography, the physician is likely to depend upon coronary arteriography rather than radionuclide tests to assist him or her in decisions about patients. If nuclear cardiology is excellent at the institution, it will be used for decision making more often.
- All physicians do not view predictive values of test results in the same manner. Some physicians and patients will accept a statement that the evidence is 80 percent in favor of no disease, whereas other physicians and patients will not accept such a figure when it is possible, using another technique, to be 95 percent certain there is no disease.
- If a facility has a track record of 5 percent operative mortality for bypass surgery, the physician must be very careful indeed how he or she chooses patients for surgery, since the overall operative risk should be 1 to 2 percent.
- An experienced angioplasty team has fewer complications and more primary success than does an inexperienced team. This profoundly influences the interest a physician has in the procedure.

These are some of the reasons why different diagnostic and therapeutic approaches are used today. In a sense there is no conflict of desire since physicians want the best for their patients. The conflict is not even about the existence of high technology used for diagnosis and treatment. Most physicians realize that modern diagnostic and therapeutic techniques are useful if used properly. The problem is that few places can perform all of the tests or procedures with equal skill. The physician then chooses to work with the elements of the system he or she believes in. This is why the reader will find a slightly different approach (see footnote in legends of figures in Chap. 19) to the recognition and treatment of this disease in Chaps. 19, 32, 43, 45, 98, 108, and 109.

The reader should not interpret the slight differences in the diagnostic and therapeutic approaches depicted in the various chapters as a failure to obtain a perfect "consensus" among authors. The truth is, there *are* different approaches to diagnostic and therapeutic problems. The experience physicians (and authors) have with the disease, their patients, and the diagnostic and therapeutic methods that are available to them determines how they diagnose and treat the disease.

The "bottom line" is, patients with coronary disease have a better future than they had 25 years ago.

References

1. Heberden, W.: Commentaries on the History and Cure of Diseases, in "Angina Pectoris," printed for T. Tayne, Mews-Gate, London, 1802, chap. 70.
2. Heberden, W.: Some Account of a Disorder of the Breast, *Med. Trans. R. Coll. Physicians*, II:59, 1786. (The original mention of angina pectoris was made by Heberden in a lecture before the Royal College of Physicians in London in July 1768.)
3. Herrick, J. B.: Clinical Featuares of Sudden Obstruction of the Coronary Arteries, *JAMA*, 59:2015, 1912.
4. Master, A. M.: Coronary Heart Disease: Angina Pectoris, Acute Coronary Insufficiency and Coronary Occlusion, *Ann. Intern. Med.*, 20:661, 1944.
5. Gillum, R. F., Folsom, A. R., and Blackburn, H.: Decline in Coronary Heart Disease Mortality: Old Questions and New Facts, *Am. J. Med.*, 76(6):1055, 1984.
6. Levy, R. I. (Chairman): The Decline in Coronary Heart Disease Mortality Status and Perspectives on the Role of Cholesterol (joint proceedings of symposiums conducted at the 1984 annual meetings of the American College of Cardiology, Dallas, Texas, and the American College of Physicians, Atlanta, Georgia), *Am. J. Cardiol.*, 54(4):1C, 1984.
7. Benson, R. L.: The Present Status of Coronary Arterial Disease, *Arch. Path. Lab. Med.*, 2:876, 1926.
8. Herrick, J. B.: "A Short History of Cardiology," Charles C Thomas, Springfield, Ill., 1942, pp. 54–62 and 207–229.
9. Proudfit, W. L.: The Fleece Medical Society, *Br. Heart J.*, 46(6):589, 1981.
10. Proudfit, W. L.: Origin of Concept of Ischaemic Heart Disease, *Br. Heart J.*, 50:209, 1983.
11. Home, E.: "A Treatise on the Blood, Inflammation, and Gun Shot Wounds by the Late John Hunter. To Which is Prefixed an Account of the Author's Life by His Brother-in-Law, Everard Home," Thomas Bradford, South Front Street, Philadelphia, 1796. (An earlier edition was published in England in 1794.)
12. Burns, A.: "Observation on Some of the Most Frequent and Important Diseases of the Heart," Hafner Publishing Company, New York, 1964.
13. Osler, W.: "The Principles and Practice of Medicine," 3d ed., D. Appleton & Company, New York, 1899, p. 763.
14. Hurst, J. W.: Obstruction of the Coronary Arteries, *JAMA*, 250(13):1763, 1983.
15. Pruitt, R. D.: Symptoms, Signs, Signals, and Shadows: The Pathophysiology of Angina Pectoris—A Historical Perspective, *Mayo Clin. Proc.*, 58:394, 1983.
16. Howell, J. D.: Early Perceptions of the Electrocardiogram: From Arrhythmia to Infarction, *Bull. Hist. Med.*, 58:83, 1984.
17. Einthoven, W.: The Galvanometric Registration of the

Human Electrocardiogram, Likewise a Review of the Use of the Capillary-Electrometer in Physiology, in F. A. Willius, Cardiac Classics: A Collection of Classic Works on the Heart and Circulation, with Comprehensive Biographic Accounts of the Authors, The C. V. Mosby Company, St. Louis, 1941.
18. Lippmann, G.: Relations entre les Phenomènes Éléctriques et Capillaries, *Ann. Chim. (Phys.), Ser.*, 5:5:494, 1875.
19. Marey, E. J.: Des Variations Éléctriques des Muscles et du Coeur en Particulier, Etudiées au Moyen de l'Electromètre de M. Lippman, *C.R. Acad. Sci. (Paris)*, 82:975, 1876.
20. Ader, C.: Sur un Nouvel Appariel Enregistreur pour Cables Sousmarins, *C.R. Acad. Sci. (Paris)*, 124:1440, 1897.
21. Waller, A. D.: "An Introduction to Human Physiology," 2d ed., Longmans, Green & Co., Ltd., London, 1893.
22. Lewis, T.: "The Mechanism and Graphic Registration of the Heart Beat," 3d ed., Shaw & Sons, London, 1925.
23. Wilson, F. N., MacLeod, A. G., and Barker, P. S.: "The Distribution of the Currents of Action and of Injury Displayed by Heart Muscle and Other Excitable Tissues," University of Michigan Press, Ann Arbor, 1933.
24. Wilson, F. N.: The Distribution of the Potential Differences Produced by the Heart Beat within the Body and at Its Surface, *Am. Heart J.*, 5:599, 1930.
25. Grant, R. P.: "Clinical Electrocardiography: The Spatial Vector Approach," McGraw-Hill Book Company, New York, 1957, p. 255.
26. Bousfield, G.: Angina Pectoris: Changes in Electrocardiogram during Paroxysm, *Lancet*, 2:457, October 5, 1918.
27. Herrick, J. B.: Thrombosis of the Coronary Arteries, *JAMA*, 72:387, 1919.
28. Wood, F. C., and Wolferth, C. C.: Angina Pectoris: The Clinical and Electrocardiographic Phenomenon of the Attack and Their Comparison with the Effects of Experimental Temporary Coronary Occlusion, *Arch. Intern. Med.*, 47:339, 1931.
29. Master, A. M.: Reminiscences of Fifty Years in Cardiology at Mount Sinai with Special Reference to the Two Step Test, *Mt. Sinai J. Med. N.Y.*, 39:486, 1972.
30. Wilson, F.: Foreword, in E. Lepeschkin, "Modern Electrocardiography," The Williams & Wilkins Company, Baltimore, 1951, vol. I, p. 5.
31. Blumgart, H. L., Schlesinger, M. J., and Zoll, P. M.: Angina Pectoris, Coronary Failure and Acute Myocardial Infarction, *JAMA*, 116(2):91, 1941.
32. Prinzmetal, M., Kennamer, R., Merliss, R., Wada, T., and Bor, N.: Angina Pectoris: I., A Variant Form of Angina Pectoris. Preliminary Report, *Am. J. Med.*, 27:374, 1959.
33. LaDue, J. S., Wroblewski, F., and Karmen, A.: Serum Glutamic Oxaloacetic Transaminase Activity in Human Transmural Myocardial Infarction, *Science*, 120:497, 1954.
34. Hurst, J. W.: History of Cardiac Catheterization, in S. B. King, III, and J. S. Douglas, Jr. (eds.), "Coronary Arteriography," McGraw-Hill Book Company, New York, 1985.
35. Forssmann, W.: Die Sondierung des rechten Herzens, *Klin. Wochenschr.*, 8:2085, 1929.
36. Castellanos, A., Pereiras, R., and Lopez, A. Y.: La angiocardiografia, *Rev. de Cien. Med.*, 1:1, 1938.
37. Robb, G. P., and Steinberg, I.: A Practical Method of Visualizing the Heart, the Pulmonary Circulation and the Great Blood Vessels in Man, *J. Clin. Invest.*, 17:507, 1938.
38. White, P. D.: "Heart Disease," 4th ed., The Macmillan Company, New York, 1951.
39. Bland, E. F., and White, P. D.: Coronary Thrombosis (with Myocardial Infarction) Ten Years Later, *JAMA*, 117:1171, 1941.
40. Brunton, T. L.: On the Use of Nitrite of Amyl in Angina Pectoris, *Lancet*, 2:97, 1867.
41. Murrell, W. K.: Nitroglycerine as a Remedy for Angina Pectoris, *Lancet*, 1:80; 151; and 225, 1879.
42. Ahlquist, R. P.: A Study of Adenotropic Receptors, *Am. J. Physiol.*, 53:586, 1948.
43. Fleckenstein, A.: Specific Inhibitors and Promoters of Calcium Action in the Excitation-Contraction Coupling of Heart Muscle and Their Role in Prevention of Production of Myocardial Lesions, in P. Harris and L. Epie (eds.), "Calcium and The Heart," Academic Press, New York, 1971.
44. Tillet, W. S., and Garner, R. L.: The Fibrinolytic Activity of Hemolytic Streptococci, *J. Exp. Med.*, 58:485, 1933.
45. Johnson, A. L., and McCarty, W. R.: The Lysis of Artificially Induced Intravascular Clots in Man by Intravenous Infusions of Streptokinase, *J. Clin. Invest.*, 39:426, 1959.
46. Lawrie, G. M., and Morris, G. C.: The Role of Surgery in the Treatment of Coronary Artery Disease: A Surgical Perspective, Cardiology Series, Baylor College of Medicine, Henry D. McIntosh, M.D. (ed.), vol. 6, no. 4, 1983.
47. Carrel, A.: On the Experimental Surgery of the Thoracic Aorta and Heart, *Am. J. Surg.*, 52:83, 1910.
48. Sabiston, D. C., Jr.: The Coronary Circulation, *Johns Hopkins Med. J.*, 134:320, 1974.
49. Garrett, H. E., Dennis, E. W., and DeBakey, M. E.: Aortocoronary Bypass with Saphenous Vein Grafts: Seven-Year Follow-up, *JAMA*, 223:729, 1973.
50. Dotter, C. T., and Frische, L. H.: Visualization of the Coronary Circulation by Occlusion Aortography: A Practical Method, *Radiology*, 76:502, 1958.
51. Gruentzig, A.: Transluminal Dilatation of Coronary Artery Stenosis, *Lancet*, 1:263, 1978.
52. Gruentzig, A. R., Senning, A., and Siegenthaler, W. E.: Nonoperative Dilatation of Coronary Artery Stenosis: Percutaneous Transluminal Coronary Angioplasty, *N. Engl. J. Med.*, 301:61, 1979.
53. Krayenbuehl, H. P., Gruentzig, A. R., and Siegenthaler, W. E.: Percutaneous Transluminal Coronary Angioplasty, in J. W. Hurst (ed.), "Update III: The Heart," McGraw-Hill Book Company, New York, 1980, p. 35.
54. Stamler, J.: Atherosclerotic Coronary Heart Disease-Etiology and Pathogenesis: The Coronary Risk Factors, in J. Stamler, "Lectures on Preventive Cardiology," Grune & Stratton, New York, 1967, p. 107.
55. Daly, L. D., Mulcahy, R., Graham, I. M., and Hickey, N.: Long-Term Effect on Mortality of Stopping Smoking after Unstable Angina and Myocardial Infarction, *Br. Med. J.*, 287:324, 1983.
56. Hubert, H. B., Feinleib, M., McNamara, P. M., and Castelli, W. P.: Obesity as an Independent Risk Factor for Cardiovascular Disease: A 26-Year Follow-up of Participants in the Framingham Heart Study, *Circulation*, 67(5):968, 1983.
57. Billman, G. E., Schwartz, P. J., and Stone, H. L.: The Effects of Daily Exercise on Susceptibility to Sudden Cardiac Death, *Circulation*, 69(6):1182, 1984.
58. Beard, J. T.: Serum Uric Acid and Coronary Heart Disease, *Am. Heart J.*, 106(2):397, 1983.
59. ten Kate, L. P., Boman, H., Daiger, S. P., and Motulsky, A. G.: Increased Frequency of Coronary Heart Disease in Relatives of Wives of Myocardial Infarct Survivors: Assortative Mating for Lifestyle and Risk Factors?, *Am. J. Cardiol.*, 53(4):399, 1984.
60. Kannel, W. B., Castelli, W. P., Gordon, T., and McNamara, P. M.: Serum Cholesterol, Lipoproteins, and the Risk of Coronary Heart Disease: The Framingham Study, *Am. Intern. Med.*, 74:1, 1971.
61. Hotchkiss, R. S., and Hurst, J. W.: Radiation and the Heart in J. W. Hurst (ed.), "Update V: The Heart," McGraw-Hill Book Company, New York, 1981, p. 205.
62. Schecter, J. P., Jones, S. E., and Jackson, R. A.: Myocardial Infarction in a 27-Year-Old Woman: Possible Complication of Treatment with VP-16-213, Mediastinal Irradiation or Both, *Cancer Chemother. Rep.*, 59:887, 1975.
63. McReynolds, R. A., Gold, G. L., and Roberts, W. C.: Coronary Heart Disease after Myocardial Irradiation for Hodgkin's Disease, *Am. J. Med.*, 60:39, 1976.
64. Stewart, J. R., Cohn, K. E., Fajardo, L. F., Hancock, E. W., and Kaplan, H. S.: Radiation-Induced Heart Disease, *Radiology*, 89:302, 1967.
65. Fajardo, L. F., Stewart, J. R., and Cohn, K. E.: Morphol-

ogy of Radiation-Induced Heart Disease, *Arch. Pathol.*, 86:512, 1968.
66. Stewart, J. R., and Fajardo, L. F.: Dose Response in Human and Experimental Radiation-Induced Heart Disease, *Radiology*, 99:403, 1971.
67. Bagdale, J. D.: Hyperlipidemia and Atherosclerosis in Chronic Dialysis Patients, in W. Drukker, F. M. Parsons, and J. F. Maher (eds.), "Replacement of Renal Function by Dialysis," Martinus Nijhoff, The Hague, 1978, p. 538.
68. Proudfit, W. L.: Variations on a Theme From Heberden: Symptoms in Angina Pectoris, *Cleve. Clin. Q.*, 51:1, 1984.
69. Maouad, J., Fernandez, F., Barrillon, A., Gerbaux, A., and Gay, J.: Diffuse or Segmental Narrowing (Spasm) of the Coronary Arteries During Smoking Demonstrated on Angiography, *Am. J. Cardiol.*, 53(2):354, 1984.
70. Cohn, P. F.: Silent Myocardial Ischemia in Patients with a Defective Anginal Warning System, *Am. J. Cardiol.*, 45:697, 1980.
71. Lindsey, H. E., and Cohn, P. F.: "Silent" Myocardial Ischemia during and after Exercise Testing in Patients with Coronary Artery Disease, *Am. Heart J.*, 95(4):441, 1978.
72. Chierchia, S., Lazzari, M., Freedman, B., Brunelli, C., and Maseri, A.: Impairment of Myocardial Perfusion and Function during Painless Myocardial Ischemia, *J. Am. Coll. Cardiol.*, 1(3):924, 1983.
73. Uretsky, B. F., Farquhar, D. S., Berezin, A. F., and Hood, W. B.: Symptomatic Myocardial Infarction without Chest Pain: Prevalence and Clinical Course, *Am. J. Cardiol.*, 40:498, 1977.
74. Cecchi, A. C., Dovellini, E. V., Marchi, F., Pucci, P., Santoro, G. M., and Fazzini, P. F.: Silent Myocardial Ischemia during Ambulatory Electrocardiographic Monitoring in Patients with Effort Angina, *J. Am. Coll. Cardiol.*, 1(3):934, 1983.
75. Cohn, P. F., Brown, E. J., Wynne, J., Holman, B. L., and Atkins, H. L.: Global and Regional Left Ventricular Ejection Fraction Abnormalities during Exercise in Patients with Silent Myocardial Ischemia, *J. Am. Coll. Cardiol.*, 1(3):931, 1983.
76. Droste, C., and Roskamm, H.: Experimental Pain Measurement in Patients with Asymptomatic Myocardial Ischemia, *J. Am. Coll. Cardiol.*, 1(3):940, 1983.
77. Kannel, W. B., and Abbott, R. D.: Incidence and Prognosis of Unrecognized Myocardial Infarction: An Update on the Framingham Study, *N. Engl. J. Med.*, 311:1144, 1984.
78. CASS Principal Investigators and Their Associates: Coronary Artery Surgery Study (CASS): A Randomized Trial of Coronary Bypass Surgery. Survival Data, *Circulation*, 68(5):939, 1983.
79. CASS Principal Investigators and Their Associates: Coronary Artery Surgery Study (CASS): A Randomized Trial of Coronary Artery Bypass Surgery. Quality of Life in Patients Randomly Assigned to Treatment Groups, *Circulation*, 68(5):951, 1983.
80. Proudfit, W. L., Shirey, E. K., and Sones, F. M., Jr.: Selective Cine Coronary Arteriography: Correlation with Clinical Findings in 1,000 Patients, *Circulation*, 33:901, 1966.
81. Douglas, J. S., Jr., and Hurst, J. W.: Limitations of Symptoms in the Recognition of Coronary Atherosclerotic Heart Disease, in J. W. Hurst (ed.), "Update I: The Heart," McGraw-Hill Book Company, New York, 1979, p. 3.
82. Heyman, A., Wilkinson, W. E., Heyden, S., et al.: Risk of Stroke in Asymptomatic Persons with Cervical Arterial Bruits, *N. Engl. J. Med.*, 302(15):838, 1980.
83. Hurst, J. W., Hopkins, L. C., and Smith, R. B.: Noises in the Neck, *N. Engl. J. Med.*, 302(no. 15):862, 1980.
84. Hammond, E. C., and Garfinkel, L.: Coronary Heart Disease, Stroke and Aortic Aneurysm, *Arch. Environ. Health*, 19:167, 1969.
85. Hertzer, N. R., Beven, E. G., Young, J. R., et al.: Coronary Artery Disease in Peripheral Vascular Patients, *Ann. Surg.*, 199(2):223, 1984.
86. Langou, R. A., Huang, E. K., Kelley, M. J., and Cohen, L. S.: Predictive Accuracy of Coronary Artery Calcification and Abnormal Exercise Test for Coronary Artery Disease in Asymptomatic men, *Circulation*, 62(6):1196, 1980.
87. Haiat, R., Desoutter, P., and Stoltz, J.-P.: Angina Pectoris without ST-T Changes in Patients with Documented Coronary Disease, *Am. Heart J.*, 105(5):883, 1983.
88. Bodenheimer, M. M., Banka, V. S., Trout, R. G., Herman, G. A., Pasdar, H., and Helfant, R. H.: Pathophysiologic Significance of ST and T Wave Abnormalities in Patients with the Intermediate Coronary Syndrome, *Am. J. Cardiol.*, 39:153, 1977.
89. Guthrie, R. B., Vlodaver, Z., Nicoloff, D. M., and Edwards, J. E.: Pathology of Stable and Unstable Angina Pectoris, *Circulation*, 57:105, 1975.
90. Zarling, E. J., Sexton, H., and Milnor, P., Jr.: Failure to Diagnose Acute Myocardial Infarction, *JAMA*, 250(9):1177, 1983.
91. McQueen, M. J., Holder, D., and El-Maraghi, N. R. H.: Assessment of The Accuracy of Serial Electrocardiograms in the Diagnosis of Myocardial Infarction, *Am. Heart J.*, 105(2):258, 1983.
92. Rothfeld, B., Fleg, J. L., and Gottlieb, S. H.: Insensitivity of the Electrocardiogram in Apical Myocardial Infarction, *Am. J. Cardiol.*, 53(6):715, 1984.
93. Movahed, A., and Becker, L. C.: Electrocardiographic Changes of Acute Lateral Wall Myocardial Infarction: A Reappraisal Based on Scintigraphic Localization of the Infarct, *J. Am. Coll. Cardiol.*, 4:660, 1984.
94. Pruitt, R. D.: The Electrocardiogram in Acute Subendocardial Myocardial Infarction, in J. W. Hurst (ed.), "Update IV: The Heart," McGraw-Hill Book Company, New York, 1981, p. 55.
95. Kaplan, B. M. and Berkson, D. M.: Serial Electrocardiograms after Myocardial Infarction, *Ann. Intern Med.*, 60:430, 1964.
96. Horan, L. G., Flowers, N. C., and Johnson, J. C.: Significance of the Diagnostic Q Wave of Myocardial Infarction, *Circulation*, 43:428, 1971.
97. Geft, I. L., Shah, P. K., Rodriquez, L., et al.: ST Elevations in Leads V_1 to V_5 May be Caused by Right Coronary Artery Occlusion and Acute Right Ventricular Infarction, *Am. J. Cardiol.*, 53(8):991, 1984.
98. Helfant, R. H.: Q Wave in Coronary Heart Disease: Newer Understanding of Their Clinical Implications, *Am. J. Cardiol.*, 38:662, 1976.
99. Ferguson, D. W., Pandian, N., Kioschos, J. M., Marcus, M. L., and White, W. W.: Angiographic Evidence That Reciprocal ST-Segment Depression during Acute Myocardial Infarction Does Not Indicate Remote Ischemia: Analysis of 23 Patients, *Am. J. Cardiol.*, 53(1):55, 1984.
100. Mills, R. M., and Greenberg, J. M.: A Clinical Approach to Exercise Tolerance Testing in Coronary Artery Disease, *Clin. Cardiol.*, 6(7):345, 1983.
101. European Coronary Surgery Study Group: Long-Term Results of Prospective Randomised Study of Coronary Artery Bypass Surgery in Stable Angina Pectoris, *Lancet*, 27:1173, 1982.
102. Coplan, N. L., and Ambrose, J. A.: Exercise Stress Tests and the CASS, *J. Am. Coll. Cardiol.*, 4(4):853, 1984.
103. Theroux, P., Waters, D. D., Halphen, C. Debaisieux, J.-C., and Mizgala, H. F.: Prognostic Value of Exercise Testing Soon after Myocardial Infarction, *N. Engl. J. Med.*, 30(7):341, 1979.
104. Philbrick, J. T., Horwitz, R. I., and Feinstein, A. R.: Methodologic Problems of Exercise Testing for Coronary Artery Disease: Groups, Analysis and Bias, *Am. J. Cardiol.*, 46:807, 1980.
105. Fox, K., Selwyn, A., and Shillingford, J.: Precordial Electrocardiographic Mapping after Exercise in the Diagnosis of Coronary Artery Disease, *Am. J. Cardiol.*, 43:541, 1979.
106. Quyyumi, A. A., Raphael, M. J., Wright, C., Bealing, L., and Fox, K. M.: Inability of the ST Segment/Heart Rate Slope to Predict Accurately the Severity of Coronary Artery Disease, *Br. Heart J.*, 51(4):396, 1984.
107. Wohlgemuth, J.: Uber eine neue Methode zur quantia-

tiven Bestimmung des diastatichen Ferments, *Biochem. Ztschr.*, 9:1, 1908.
108. Dreyfus, J. C., Schapira, G., Resnais, J., and Scebat, L.: Le Creatine-kinase Sérique dans le Diagnostic de l'Infarctus Myocardique, *Rev. Fr. Études Clin. Biol.*, 5:386, 1960.
109. Hedworth-Whitty, R. B., Whitfield, J. B., and Richardson, R. W.: Serum γ-glutamyl Transpeptidase Activity in Myocardial Ischaemia, *Br. Heart J.*, 29:432, 1967.
110. Nagai, R., Ueda, S., and Yazaki, Y.: Radioimmunoassay of Cardiac Myosin Light Chain II in the Serum following Experimental Myocardial Infarction, *Biochem. Biophys. Res. Commun.*, 86:683, 1979.
111. Sobel, B. E., and Shell, W. E.: Serum Enzyme Determinations in the Diagnosis and Assessment of Myocardial Infarction, *Circulation*, 45:471, 1972.
112. Cohen, L., Djordjevich, J., and Ormiste, V.: Sereum Lactic Dehydrogenase Isozyme Patterns in Cardiovascular and Other Diseases, with Particular Reference to Acute Myocardial Infarction, *J. Lab. Clin. Med.*, 64:355, 1964.
113. Kjekshus, J. K., and Sobel, B. E.: Depressed Myocardial Creatine Phosphokinase Activity following Experimental Myocardial Infarction in Rabbits, *Circulation Res.*, 27:403, 1970.
114. Shell, W. E., Kjekshus, J. K., and Sobel, B. E.: Quantitative Assessment of the Extent of Myocardial Infarction in the Conscious Dog by Means of Analysis of Serial Changes in Serum Creatine Phosphokinase Activity, *J. Clin. Invest.*, 50:2614, 1971.
115. Sobel, B. E., Roberts, R., and Larson, K. B.: Considerations in the Use of Biochemical Markers of Ischemic Injury, *Circulation Res.*, 38(suppl. I):I-99, 1976.
116. Clark, G. E., Robison, A. K., Gnepp, D. R., Roberto, R., and Sobel, B. E.: Effects of Lymphatic Transport of Enzyme on Plasma Creatine Kinase Time-Activity Curves after Myocardial Infarction in Dogs, *Circulation Res.*, 43:162, 1978.
117. Sobel, B. E., Markham, J., Karlsberg, R. P., and Roberts, R.: The Nature of Disappearance of Creatine Kinase for the Circulation and Its Influence on Enzymatic Estimation of Infarct Size, *Circulation Res.*, 41:836, 1977.
118. Morelli, R. L., Carlson, C. J., Emilson, B., Abendschein, D. R., and Rapaport, E.: Serum Creatine Kinase MM Isoenzyme Sub-bands after Acute Myocardial Infarction in Man, *Circulation*, 67:1238, 1983.
119. Ishikawa, Y., George, S. E., Spaite, D., Hashimoto, H., Sobel, B. E., and Roberts, R.: Distortion of Plasma CK Curves Induced by Reperfusion: Mechanisms and Implications, *Circulation*, 68:III-196, 1983. (Abstract.)
120. Cohen, L., Block, J., and Djordjevich, J.: Sex Related Differences in Isozymes of Serum Lactic Dehydrogenase (LDH), *Proc. Soc. Exp. Biol. Med.*, 126:55, 1967.
121. Rose, L. I., Lowe, S. L., Carroll, D. R., Wolfson, S., and Cooper, K. H.: Serum Lactate Dehydrogenase Isoenzyme Changes after Muscle Exertion, *J. Appl. Physiol.*, 28:279, 1970.
122. Jaffe, A. S., Garfinkel, B. T., Ritter, C. S., and Sobel, B. E.: Elevated Plasma MB Creatine Kinase after Vigorous Exercise in Professional Athletes: A Diagnostic Dilemma, *Am. J. Cardiol.*, 53:856, 1984.
123. Konttinen, A., Hupli, V., Louhija, A., and Hartel, G.: Origin of Elevated Serum Enzyme Activities after Direct-Current Countershock, *N. Engl. J. Med.*, 281:231, 1969.
124. Ehsani, A., Ewy, G. A., and Sobel, B. E.: Effects of Electrical Countershock on Serum Creatine Phosphokinase (CPK) Isoenzyme Activity, *Am. J. Cardiol.*, 37:12, 1976.
125. West, M., Gelb, D., Pilz, C. G., and Zimmerman, H. J.: Serum Enzymes in Disease: Significance of Abnormal Serum Enzyme Levels in Cardiac Failure, *Am. J. Med. Sci.*, 241:350, 1961.
126. Wroblewski, F.: Serum Enzyme and Isoenzyme Alterations in Myocardial Infarction, *Prog. Cardiovasc. Dis.*, 6:63, 1963.
127. Markert, C. L.: Lactate Dehydrogenase Isozymes: Dissociation and Recombination of Subunits, *Science*, 140:1329, 1963.
128. Meltzer, H. Y., Mrozak, S., and Boyer, M.: Effect of Intramuscular Injections on Serum Creatine Phosphokinase Activity, *Am. J. Med. Sci.*, 259:42, 1970.
129. Henry, P. D., Bloor, C. M., and Sobel, B. E.: Increased Serum Creatine Phosphokinase Activity in Experimental Pulmonary Embolism, *Am. J. Cardiol.*, 26:151, 1970.
130. Batsakis, J. G., and Briere, R. O.: Interpretive Enzymology, Charles C Thomas, Springfield, Ill., 1967.
131. Ahumada, G., Roberts, R., and Sobel, B. E.: Evaluation of Myocardial Infarction with Enzymatic Indices, *Prog. Cardiovasc. Dis.*, 18:405, 1976.
132. Varat, M. A., and Mercer, D. W.: Cardiac Specific Creatine Phosphokinase Isoenzyme in the Diagnosis of Acute Myocardial Infarction, *Circulation*, 51:855, 1975.
133. Sobel, B. E., Roberts, R., and Larson, K. B.: Estimation of Infarct Size from Serum MB Creatine Phosphokinase Activity: Applications and Limitations, *Am. J. Cardiol.*, 37:474, 1976.
134. Van Der Veen, K. J., and Willebrands, A. F.: Isoenzymes of Creatine Phosphokinase in Tissue Extracts and in Normal and Pathological Sera, *Clin. Clim. Acta*, 13:312, 1966.
135. Klein, M. S., Shell, W. E., and Sobel, B. E.: Serum Creatine Phosphokinase (CPK) Isoenzymes after Intramuscular Injections, Surgery, and Myocardial Infarction: Experimental and Clinical Studies, *Cardiovasc. Res.*, 7:412, 1973.
136. Konttinen, A., and Somer, H.: Determination of Serum Creatine Kinase Isoenzymes in Myocardial Infarction, *Am. J. Cardiol.*, 29:817, 1972.
137. Roberts, R., and Sobel, B. E.: Isoenzymes of Creatine Phosphokinase and Diagnosis of Myocardial Infarction, *Ann. Intern. Med.*, 79:741, 1973.
138. Roberts, R., Gowda, K. S., Ludbrook, P. A., and Sobel, B. E.: Specificity of Elevated Serum MB Creatine Phosphokinase Activity in the Diagnosis of Acute Myocardial Infarction, *Am. J. Cardiol.*, 36:433, 1975.
139. Ahmed, S. A., Williamson, J. R., Roberts, R., Clark, R. E., and Sobel, B. E.: The Association of Increased Plasma MB CPK Activity and Irreversible Ischemic Myocardial Injury in the Dog, *Circulation*, 54:187, 1976.
140. Maroko, P. R., Kjekshus, J. K., Sobel, B. E., Watanabe, T., Covell, J. W., Ross, J., Jr., and Braunwald, E.: Factors Influencing Infarct Size following Experimental Coronary Artery Occlusions, *Circulation*, 43:67, 1971.
141. Bleifeld, W., Mathey, D., Hanrath, P., Buss, H., and Effert, S.: Infarct Size Estimated from Serial Serum Creatine Phosphokinase in Relation to Left Ventricular Hemodynamics, *Circulation*, 55:303, 1977.
142. Manders, T., Vatner, S., Millard, R., Heyndrickx, G., and Maroko, P. B.: Altered Relationship between Creatine Phosphokinase Release and Infarct Size with Reperfusion in Conscious Dogs, *Circulation*, 52:II-5, 1975.
143. Reimer, K. A., Hackel, D. B., Ideker, R. E., et al.: Comparison of Enzymatic and Anatomic Estimates of Myocardial Infarct Size in Man, *Clin. Res.*, 31:214A, 1983.
144. Shell, W. E., Lavelle, J. F., Covell, J. W., and Sobel, B. E.: Early Estimation of Myocardial Damage in Conscious Dogs and Patients with Evolving Acute Myocardial Infarction, *J. Clin. Invest.*, 52:2579, 1973.
145. Sobel, B. E., Bresnahan, G. F., Shell, W. E., and Yoder, R. D.: Estimation of Infarct Size in Man and Its Relation to Prognosis, *Circulation*, 46:640, 1972.
146. Sobel, B. E., and Shell, W. E.: Diagnostic and Prognostic Value of Serum Enzyme Changes in Patients with Acute Myocardial Infarction, in P. N. Yu and J. F. Goodwin (eds.), "Progress in Cardiology," Lea & Febiger, Philadelphia, 1975, p. 165.
147. Roberts, R., Henry, P. D., and Sobel, B. E.: An Improved Basis for Enzymatic Estimation of Infarct Size, *Circulation*, 52:743, 1975.
148. Thompson, P. L., Fletcher, E. E., and Katavotis, V.: Enzymatic Indices of Myocardial Necrosis: Influence on Short- and Long-Term Prognosis after Myocardial Infarction, *Circulation*, 59:113, 1979.
149. Roberts, R., Ambos, H. D., and Sobel, B. E.: Estimation

of Infarct Size with MB Rather Than Total CK, *Int. J. Cardiol.,* 2:479, 1983.
150. Carter, C. L., and Amundsen, L. R.: Infarct Size and Exercise Capacity after Myocardial Infarction, *J. Appl. Physiol.,* 42:782, 1977.
151. Cox, J. R., Jr., Roberts, R., Ambos, H. D., Oliver, G. C., and Sobel, B. E.: Relations between Enzymatically Estimated Myocardial Infarct Size and Early Ventricular Dysrhythmia, *Circulation,* 53:I-150, 1976.
152. Norris, R. M., Whitlock, R. M. L., Barratt-Boyes, C., and Small, C. W.: Clinical Measurement of Myocardial Infarct Size: Modification of a Method for the Estimation of Total Creatine Phosphokinase Release after Myocardial Infarction, *Circulation,* 51:614, 1975.
153. Roberts, R., Husain, A., Ambos, H. D., Oliver, G. C., Cox, J., Jr., and Sobel, B. E.: Relation between Infarct Size and Ventricular Arrhythmia, *Br. Heart J.,* 37:1169, 1975.
154. Rogers, W. J., McDaniel, H. G., Smith, L. R., Mantle, J. A., Russell, R. O., Jr., and Rackley, C. E.: Correlation of CPK-MB and Angiographic Estimates of Infarct Size in Man, *Circulation,* 54:II-28, 1976.
155. Geltman, E. M., Ehsani, A. A., Campbell, M. K., Schechtman, K., Roberts, R., and Sobel, B. E.: The influence of Location and Extent of Myocardial Infarction on Long-Term Ventricular Dysrhythmia and Mortality, *Circulation,* 60:805, 1979.
156. Gutovitz, A. L., Sobel, B. E., and Roberts, R.: Progressive Nature of Myocardial Injury in Selected Patients with Cardiogenic Shock, *Am. J. Cardiol.,* 41:469, 1978.
157. Tamaki, S., Murakami, T., Kadota, K., et al.: Effects of Coronary Artery Perfusion on Relation between Creatine Kinase-MB Release and Infarct Size Estimated by Myocardial Emission Tomography with Thallium-201 in Man, *J. Am. Coll. Cardiol.,* 2:1031, 1983.
158. Hashimoto, H., Grace, A. M., Billadello, J. J., Gross, R. W., Strauss, A. W., and Sobel, B. E.: Non-denaturing Quantification of Subforms of Canine MM Creatine Kinase Isoenzymes (Isoforms) and Their Interconversion, *J. Lab. Clin. Med.,* 103:470, 1984.
159. Gibson, R. S., and Beller, G. A.: Should Exercise Electrocardiography be Replaced by Radionuclide Methods?, in S. H. Rahimtoola and A. M. Brest (eds.), "Controversies in Coronary Artery Disease," F. A. Davis Company, Philadelphia, 1982, p. 1.
160. Pohost, G. M., Zir, L. M., Moore, R. H., McKusick, K. A., Guiney, T. E., and Beller, G. A.: Differentiation of Transiently Ischemic from Infarcted Myocardium by Serial Imaging after a Single Dose of Thallium-201, *Circulation,* 55:74, 1977.
161. Beller, G. A., Watson, D. D., and Pohost, G. M.: Kinetics of Thallium Distribution and Redistribution: Clinical Applications in Sequential Myocardial Imaging, in H. W. Strauss and B. Pitt (eds.), "Cardiovascular Nuclear Medicine," The C. V. Mosby Company, St. Louis, 1979, p. 225.
162. Beller, G. A.: Radionuclide Techniques in the Evaluation of the Patient with Chest Pain, *Mod. Concepts Cardiovasc. Dis.,* 50:43, 1981.
163. Berger, B. C., Watson, D. D., Taylor, G. J., et al.: Quantitative Thallium-201 Exercise Scintigraphy for Detection of Coronary Artery Disease, *J. Nucl. Med.,* 22:585, 1981.
164. McCarthy, D. M., Blood, D. K., Sciacca, R. R., et al.: Single Dose Myocardial Perfusion Imaging with Thallium-201: Application in Patients with Nondiagnostic Electrocardiographic Stress Tests, *Am. J. Cardiol.,* 43:899, 1979.
165. Botvinick, E. H., Taradash, M. R., Shames, D. M., et al.: Thallium-201 Myocardial Perfusion Scintigraphy for the Clinical Clarification of Normal, Abnormal, and Equivocal Electrocardiographic Stress Tests, *Am. J. Cardiol.,* 41:43, 1978.
166. Guiney, T. E., Pohost, G. M., McKusick, K. A., and Beller, G. A.: Differentiation of False from True Positive Electrocardiographic Responses to Exercise Stress by Thallium-201 Perfusion Imaging, *Chest,* 80:4, 1981.
167. Nygaard, T. W., Gibson, R. S., Ryan, J. M., Gascho, J. A., Watson, D. D., and Beller, G. A.: Prevalence of High Risk Thallium-201 Scintigraphy Findings in Left Main Coronary Artery Stenosis and Comparison to Patients with Multiple- and Single-Vessel Coronary Artery Disease, *Am. J. Cardiol.,* 53:462, 1984.
168. Brown, K. A., Boucher, C. A., Okada, R. D., Newell, J., Strauss, H. W., and Pohost, G. M.: The Prognostic Value of Exercise Thallium-201 Imaging in Patients Presenting for Evaluation of Chest Pain: Comparison to Contrast Angiography, Exercise Electrocardiography and Clinical Data, *Am. J. Cardiol.,* 49:967, 1982.
169. Gibson, R. S., Watson, D. D., Craddock, G. B., et al.: Prediction of Cardiac Events after Uncomplicated Myocardial Infarction: A Prospective Study Comparing Predischarge Exercise Thallium-201 Scintigraphy and Coronary Angiography, *Circulation,* 68(2):321, 1983.
170. Gibson, R. S., Taylor, G. J., Watson, D. D., et al.: Prospective Assessment of Regional Myocardial Perfusion before and after Coronary Revascularization Surgery by Quantitative Thallium-201 Scintigraphy, *J. Am. Coll. Cardiol.,* 1(3):804, 1983.
171. Strauss, H. W., and Boucher, C. A.: Nuclear Cardiology: Radionuclide Angiography, *Am. J. Cardiol.,* 49:1337, 1982.
172. Borer, J. S., Kent, K. M., Bachrach, S. L., et al.: Sensitivity, Specificity and Predictive Accuracy of Radionuclide Cineangiography during Exercise in Patients with Coronary Artery Disease: Comparison with Exercise Electrocardiography, *Circulation,* 60:572, 1979.
173. Jones, R. H., Floyd, R. D., Austin, E. H., and Sabiston, D. C., Jr.: The Role of Radionuclide Angiocardiography in the Preoperative Prediction of Pain Relief and Prolonged Survival following Coronary Artery Bypass Grafting, *Ann. Surg.,* 197(6):743, 1983.
174. Corbett, J. R., Dehmer, G. J., Lewis, S. E., et al.: The Prognostic Value of Submaximal Exercise Testing with Radionuclide Ventriculography before Hospital Discharge in Patients with Recent Myocardial Infarction, *Circulation,* 64:535, 1981.
175. Caldwell, J. H., Hamilton, G. W., Sorensen, S. G., et al.: The Detection of Coronary Artery Disease with Radionuclide Technique: Comparison of Rest-Exercise Thallium Imaging and Ejection Fraction Response, *Circulation,* 61:610, 1980.
176. King, S. B., III, and Douglas, J. S., Jr.: "Coronary Arteriography," McGraw-Hill Book Company, New York, 1985.
177. Adams, D. F., Fraser, D. B., and Abrams, H. L.: The Complications of Coronary Arteriography, *Circulation,* 48:609, 1973.
178. Abrams, H. L., and Adams, D. F.: The Complications of Coronary Arteriography, *Circulation,* 52(suppl. 2):27, 1975.
179. Kennedy, J. W.: Complications Associated with Cardiac Catheterization and Angiography, *Cath. Cardiovasc. Diagnosis,* 8:5, 1982.
180. Cohen, M. V., and Gorlin, R.: Main Left Coronary Occlusive Disease: Clinical Experience from 1964–1974, *Circulation,* 52:275, 1975.
181. King, S. B., III, Douglas, J. S., Jr., and Morris, D. C.: New Angiographic Views for Coronary Arteriography in J. W. Hurst (ed.), "Update IV:The Heart," McGraw-Hill Book Company, New York, 1981, p. 193.
182. Takaro, T., Hultgren, H. N., Lipton, M. J., et al.: The VA Cooperative Randomized Study of Surgery for Coronary Aterial Occlusive Disease: II. Subgroups with Significant Left Main Lesions, *Circulation,* 54(suppl. 3):107, 1975.
183. Jones, E. L., Douglas, J. S., Jr., Craver, J. M., King, S. B., III, et al.: Results of Coronary Revascularization in Patients with Recent Myocardial Infarction, *J. Thorac. Cardiovasc. Surg.,* 76:545, 1978.
184. Welch, C. C., Proudfit, W. L., and Sheldon, W. C.: Coronary Arteriographic Findings in 1000 Women under Age 50, *Am. J. Cardiol.,* 35:211, 1975.
185. Proudfit, W. L., Bruschke, A. V. G., and Sones, F. M., Jr.: Natural History of Obstructive Coronary Artery Disease: Ten Year Study of 601 Non-Surgical Cases, *Prog. Cardiovasc. Dis.,* 21:53, 1978.
186. Curry, R. C., Pepine, C. J., Sabom, E. M., Feldman, R. L.,

Christie, L. G., and Conti, C. R.: Effects of Ergonovine in Patients with and without Coronary Artery Disease, *Circulation,* 56:803, 1977.
187. Muller, J. E., and Gunther, S. J.: Nifedipine Therapy for Prinzmetal's Angina, *Circulation,* 57:137, 1978.
188. Waters, D. D., Theroux, P., Szlachcic, J., et al.: Ergonovine Testing in a Coronary Care Unit, *Am. J. Cardiol.,* 46(6):922, 1980.
189. Hammermeister, K. E., DeRouen, T. A., and Dodge, H. T.: Survival Analyses in Medically and Surgically Treated Patients with Coronary Artery Disease: A Critical Review and Experience in Seattle Heart Watch, a Nonrandomized Series, in J. W. Hurst (ed.), "Update II: The Heart," McGraw-Hill Book Company, New York, 1980, p. 239.
190. Yatteau, R. F., Peter, R. H., Behar, V. S., et al.: Ischemic Cardiomyopathy: The Myopathies of Coronary Artery Disease, *Am. J. Cardiol.,* 34:520, 1974.
191. Trask, N., Califf, R. M., Conley, M. J., et al.: Accuracy and Interobserver Variability of Coronary Cineangiography: A Comparison with Postmortem Evaluation, *J. Am. Coll. Cardiol.,* 3(5):1145, 1984.
192. White, C. W., Wright, C. B., Doty, D. B., et al.: Does Visual Interpretation of the Coronary Arteriogram Predict the Physiologic Importance of a Coronary Stenosis? *N. Engl. J. Med.,* 310(13):819, 1984.
193. Cohen, M. E., White, P. D., and Johnson, R. E.: Neurocirculatory Asthenia, Anxiety Neurosis or the Effort Syndrome, *Arch. Intern. Med.,* 81:260, 1948.
194. Cohen, M. E., and White, P. D.: Life Situations, Emotions, and Neurocirculatory Asthenia (Anxiety Neurosis, Neurasthenia, Effort Syndrome), *Psychosom. Med.,* 13(no. 6):335, 1951.
195. Cohen, M. E., and White, P. D.: Neurocirculatory Asthenia: 1972 Concept, *Milit. Med.,* 137(no. 4):142, 1972.
196. Warren, J. V.: Hyperventilation: A Diagnostic Dilemma, *Primary Cardiol.,* 9(no. 9):127, 1983.
197. Friesinger, G. C., Likas, I., Beirn, R., and Mason, R. E.: Vasoregulatory Asthenia: A Cause for False Positive Electrocardiograms, *Circulation,* 32(suppl. 2):90, 1965. (Abstract.)
198. Marcomichaelakis, J., Donaldson, R., Green, J., et al.: Exercise Testing after Beta-Blockage: Improved Specificity and Predictive Value in Detecting Coronary Heart Disease, *Br. Heart J.,* 43(3):252, 1980.
199. Nordenfelt, O.: Orthostatic ECG Changes and the Adrenergic Beta-Receptor Blocking Agent, Propranolol (Inderal), *Acta Med. Scand.,* 178:393, 1965.
200. Furberg, C.: Adrenergic Beta-Blocking and Electrocardiographical ST-T Changes, *Acta Med. Scand.,* 181:21, 1967.
201. Spodick, D. H.: Pitfalls in the Recognition of Pericarditis, in J. W. Hurst (ed.), "Clinical Essays on the Heart," McGraw-Hill Book Company, New York, vol. 5, 1985, p. 95.
202. Ouzts, H. G., Turner, J. L., Douglas, J. S., Jr., and Hurst, J. W.: Prolonged Chest Pain Suggesting Myocardial Infarction in Patients with Hypertrophic Cardiomyopathy, in J. W. Hurst (ed.), "Update III: The Heart," McGraw-Hill Book Company, New York, 1980, p. 139.
203. Mondor, H.: Tronculité sous-cutanée subaigue de la paroi thoracique antero-laterale, *Mem. Acad. Chir., Paris,* 65:1271, 1939.
204. Long, W. B., and Cohen, S.: The Digestive Tract as a Cause of Chest Pain, *Am. Heart J.,* 100(4):567, 1980.
205. Mellow, M. H.: A Gastroenterologist's View of Chest Pain, *Curr. Prob. Cardiol.,* 7(10):7, 1983.
206. Bernstein, L. M., Fruin, R. C., and Pacini, R.: Differentiation of Esophageal Pain from Angina Pectoris: Role of Esophageal Acid Perfusion, *Medicine,* 41:143, 1962.
207. Castell, D. O.: Achalasia and Diffuse Esophageal Spasm, *Arch. Intern. Med.,* 136:571, 1976.
208. Orlando, R. C., and Bozymski, E. M.: Clinical and Manometric Effects of Nitroglycerin in Diffuse Esophageal Spasm, *N. Engl. J. Med.,* 289:23, 1973.
209. Richter, J. E., and Castell, D. O.: Diffuse Esophageal Spasm: A Reappriasal, *Ann. Intern. Med.,* 100:242, 1984.
210. Gravino, F. N., Perloff, J. K., Yeatman, L. A., and Ippolitti, A. F.: Coronary Arterial Spasm: Response to Ergonovine, *Am. J. Med.,* 70(6):1293, 1981.
211. Koch, K., Calson, G., Long, A., Curry, R. C., and Mathias, J. R.: The Ergonovine Stress Test: A Provocative Test for Diffuse Esophageal Spasm or Variant Angina, *Clin. Res.,* 27:778, 1979. (Abstract.)
212. Dart, A. M., Davies, H. A., Lowndes, R. H., Dalal, J., Ruttley, M., and Henderson, A. H.: Oesophageal Spasm and Angina: Diagnostic Value of Ergometrine (Ergonovine) Provocation, *Eur. Heart J.,* 1:91, 1980.
213. Benjamin, S. B., and Castell, D. O.: Chest Pain of Esophageal Origin: Where Are We, and Where Should We Go?, *Arch Intern. Med.,* 143:772, 1983.
214. Weiser, H. F., Lepsien, G., Golenhofen, K., and Siewert, R.: Clinical and Experimental Studies on the Effect of Nifedipine on Smooth Muscle of the Esophagus and LES, in H. L. Duthie (ed.), "Gastrointestinal Motility in Health and Disease," Lancaster, MTP Press, 1978.
215. Youngs, J., and Nicoloff, D.: Management of Esophageal Perforation, *Surgery,* 65:264, 1969.
216. Hammon, L.: Spontaneous Mediastinal Emphysema, *Bull. Johns Hopkins Hosp.,* 64:1, 1939.
217. Laing, F. C.: Diagnostic Evaluation of Patients with Suspected Cholecystitis, *Surg. Clin. North Am.,* 64(1):3, 1984.
218. Thistle, J. L., and Hofman, A. F.: Efficacy and Specificity of Chenodeoxycholic Acid Therapy for Dissolving Gallstones, *N. Engl. J. Med.,* 289:655, 1973.
219. Schoenfield, L. J., Lachin, J. M., The Steering Committee, and the National Cooperative Gallstone Study Group: Chenodiol (Chenodeoxycholic Acid) for Dissolution of Gallstones: The National Cooperative Gallstone Study: A Controlled Trial of Efficacy and Safety, *Ann. Intern. Med.,* 95(3):257, 1981.
220. Peppercorn, M. A.: Drug Therapy of Peptic Ulcer Disease, *Compr. Therapy,* 9(11):47, 1983.
221. Soergel, K. H.: Acute Pancreatitis, in M. H. Sleisenger and J. S. Fordtran (eds.), "Gastrointestinal Disease," 3d ed., W. B. Saunders Company, Philadelphia, 1983, p. 1462.
222. Moossa, A. R.: Current Concepts: Diagnostic Tests and Procedures in Acute Pancreatitis, *N. Engl. J. Med.,* 311(10):639, 1984.
223. Atlas, D. H.: "Cafe Coronary" from Peanut Butter, *N. Engl. J. Med.,* 296:399, 1977.
224. Heimlich, H. J.: A Life-Saving Maneuver to Prevent Food-Choking, *JAMA,* 234:398, 1975.
225. Lasser, R. B., Bond, J. H., and Levitt, M. D.: The Role of Intestinal Gas in Functional Abdominal Pain, *N. Engl. J. Med.,* 293:524, 1975.
226. Dalen, J. E., and Alpert, J. S.: Natural History of Pulmonary Embolism, *Prog. Cardiovasc. Dis.,* 17(4):259, 1975.
227. Inouye, W. Y., Berggren, R. B., and Johnson, J.: Spontaneous Pneumothorax: Treatment and Mortality, *Dis. Chest,* 51:67, 1967.
228. Dale, W. A., and Lewis, M. R.: Management of Thoracic Outlet Syndrome, *Ann. Surg.,* 181:575, 1975.
229. Lord, J. W., Jr., and Rosati, L. M.: Thoracic-Outlet Syndromes, *Ciba Clin. Symp.,* 23:2, 1971.
230. Roos, D. B.: The Place for Scalenectomy and First-Rib Resection in Thoracic Outlet Syndrome, *Surgery,* 92:1077, 1982.
231. Urschel, H. C., Jr., and Razzuk, M. A.: Management of the Thoracic-Outlet Syndrome, *N. Engl. J. Med.,* 286:1140, 1972.
232. Tietze, A.: Ueber eine eigenartige Haufung von Fallen mit Dystrophie der Rippenknorpel, *Berl. Klin. Wochenschr.,* 58:829, 1921.
233. Karon, E. H., Achor, R. W. P., and Janes, J. M.: Painful Nonsuppurative Swelling of Costochondral Cartilages (Tietze's Syndrome), *Proc. Staff Meet. Mayo Clin.,* 33:45, 1958.
234. Weller, T. H.: Varicella and Herpes Zoster: Changing Concepts of the Natural History, Control, and Importance of a Not-So-Benign Virus (Second of Two Parts), *N. Engl. J. Med.,* 309:1434, 1983.

235. Silverman, M. E., and Hurst, J. W.: Chest Wall Pain: The Great Masquerader, *Chest Pain,* 1:1, 1976.
236. Friesinger, G. C.: Prognosis in Chronic Ischemic Heart Disease, *Trans. Assoc. Am. Physicians,* 91:98, 1981.
237. Friesinger, G. C.: The Reasonable Work-up before Recommending Medical or Surgical Therapy: An Overall Strategy, *Circulation,* 65(suppl. 2):21, 1982.
238. White, N. K., Edwards, J. E., and Dry, T. J.: The Relationship of the Degree of Coronary Atherosclerosis with Age, in Women, *Circulation,* 1:1345, 1950.
239. Ackerman, R. F., Dry, T. J., and Edwards, J. E.: The Relationship of the Degree of Coronary Atherosclerosis with Age, in Men, *Circulation,* 1:645, 1950.
240. Enos, W. F., Holmes, R. H., and Beyer, J. C.: Coronary Disease among United States Soldiers Killed in Action in Korea, *JAMA,* 152:1090, 1953.
241. Erikssen, J., Enge, I., Forfang, K., and Storstein, O.: False Positive Diagnostic Tests and Coronary Angiographic Findings in 105 Presumably Healthy Males, *Circulation,* 54:371, 1976.
242. Cohn, P. F.: Seminar on Asymptomatic Coronary Artery Disease, *J. Am. Coll. Cardiol.,* 1(no. 3):922, 1983.
243. Prospective Randomized Study of Coronary Artery Bypass Surgery in Stable Angina Pectoris: Second Interim Report by the European Coronary Surgery Study Group, *Lancet,* 2:491, 1980.
244. Murphy, M. L., Hultgren, H. N., Detre, K., Thomsen, J., and Takaro, T.: Treatment of Chronic Stable Angina: A Preliminary Report of Survival Data of the Randomized Veterans Administration Cooperative Study, *N. Engl. J. Med.,* 297:621, 1977.
245. Proudfit, W. J., Bruschke, A. V. G., MacMillan, J. P., Williams, G. W., and Sones, F. M., Jr.: Fifteen Year Survival Study of Patients with Obstructive Coronary Artery Disease, *Circulation,* 68:986, 1983.
246. Frank, C. W., Weinblatt, E., and Shapiro, S.: Angina Pectoris in Men: Prognostic Significance of Selected Medical Factors, *Circulation,* 47:509, 1973.
247. Ruberman, W., Weinblatt, E., Goldberg, J. D., Frank, C. W., Shapiro, S., and Chaudhary, B. S.: Ventricular Premature Complexes in Prognosis of Angina, *Circulation,* 61:1172, 1980.
248. McNeer, J. F., Margolis, J. R., Lee, K. L., et al: The Role of the Exercise Test in the Evaluation of Patients for Ischemic Heart Disease, *Circulation,* 57:64, 1978.
249. Dagenais, G. R., Rouleau, J. R., Christen, A., and Fabia, J.: Survival of Patients with a Strongly Positive Exercise Electrocardiogram, *Circulation,* 65:452, 1982.
250. Gohlke, H., Samek, L., Betz, P., and Roskamm, H.: Exercise Testing Provides Additional Prognostic Information in Angiographically Defined Subgroups of Patients with Coronary Artery Disease, *Circulation,* 68:979, 1983.
251. Friesinger, G. C., Page, E. E., and Ross, R. S.: Prognostic Significance of Coronary Arteriography, *Trans. Assoc. Am. Physicians,* 83:78, 1970; also *Circulation,* 49:489, 1974.
252. Bruschke, A. V., Proudfit, W. L., and Sones, F. M., Jr.: Progress Study of 490 Consecutive Nonsurgical Cases of Coronary Disease Followed 5–9 Years: I. Arteriographic Correlations, *Circulation,* 47:1147, 1973; II. Ventriculographic and Other Correlations, *Circulation,* 47:1154, 1973.
253. Burggraf, G. W., and Parker, J. O.: Prognosis in Coronary Artery Disease—Angiographic, Hemodynamic and Clinical Factors, *Circulation,* 51:146:1975.
254. Oberman, A., Jones, W. B., and Riley, C. P.: Natural History of Coronary Artery Disease, *Bull. N.Y. Acad. Med.,* 48:1109, 1972.
255. Killip, T.: National Heart, Lung, and Blood Institute Coronary Artery Surgery Study, *Circulation,* 63(suppl. 1):1, 1981.
256. Mock, M. B., Ringqvist, I., Fisher, L. D., et al.: Survival of Medically Treated Patients in the Coronary Artery Surgery Study (CASS) Registry, *Circulation,* 66:562, 1982.
257. Zir, L. M., Miller, S. W., Dinsmore, R. E., Gilbert, J. P., and Harthorne, J. W.: Interobserver Variability in Coronary Arteriography, *Circulation,* 53:627, 1976.
258. Detre, K. M., Wright, E., Murphy, M. L., and Takaro, T. T.: Observer Agreement in Evaluating Coronary Angiograms, *Circulation,* 52:979, 1975.
259. Bruschke, A. V. G., Proudfit, W. L., and Sones, F. M.: Progress Study of 590 Consecutive Nonsurgical Cases of Coronary Disease Followed 5–9 Years, *Circulation,* 51:1147, 1973.
260. Conley, M. J., Ely, R. L., Kisslo, J., Lee, K. L., McNeer, F., and Rosait, R. A.: The Prognostic Spectrum of Left Main Stenosis, *Circulation,* 57:947, 1978.
261. Detre, K., Peduzzi, P., Murphy, M., et al.: Effect of Bypass Surgery on Survival in Patients in Low- and High-Risk Subgroups Delineated by the Use of Simple Clinical Variables, *Circulation,* 63:1329, 1981.
262. Feil, H.: Premonitory Pain in Coronary Thrombosis, *Am. J. Med. Sci.,* 193:42, 1937.
263. Sampson, J. J., and Eliaser, M.: The Diagnosis of Impending Acute Coronary Artery Occlusion, *Am. Heart J.,* 13:675, 1937.
264. Solomon, H. A., Edwards, A. L., and Killip, T.: Prodromata in Acute Myocardial Infarction, *Circulation,* 40:463, 1969.
265. Gazes, P. C., Mobley, E. M., Faris, M. H., Jr., Duncan, R. C., and Humphries, G. B.: Preinfarctional (Unstable) Angina: A Prospective Study. Ten-Year Follow-up, *Circulation,* 48:331, 1973.
266. Duncan, B., Fulton, M., Morrison, S. L., et al.: Prognosis of New and Worsening Angina Pectoris, *Br. Med. J.,* 1:981, 1976.
267. Unstable Angina Pectoris: National Cooperative Study Group to Compare Medical and Surgical Therapy: I. Report of Protocol—Patient Population, *Am. J. Cardiol.,* 42:839, 1978.
268. Gerstenblith, G., Ouyang, P., Achuff, S. C., et al.: Nifedipine in Unstable Angina: A Double-Blind, Randomized Trial, *N. Engl. J. Med.,* 306:885, 1982.
269. Lewis, H. D., Jr., Davis, J. W., Archibald, D. G., et al.: Protective Effects of Aspirin against Acute Myocardial Infarction and Death in Men with Unstable Angina, *N. Engl. J. Med.,* 309:396, 1983.
270. Waters, D. D., Szlachcic, J., Miller, D., and Theroux, P.: Clinical Characteristics of Patients with Variant Angina Complicated by Myocardial Infarction or Death within 1 Month, *Am. J. Cardiol.,* 49:658, 1982.
271. Armstrong, A., Duncan, B., Oliver, M. F., et al: Natural History of Acute Coronary Heart Attacks: A Community Study, *Br. Heart J.,* 34:67, 1972.
272. Fulton, M., Julian, D. G., and Oliver, M. F.: Sudden Death and Myocardial Infarction, AHA Monograph no. 27, Research in Acute Myocardial Infarction, *Circulation,* 40(suppl. 4):182, 1969.
273. Chapman, B. L.: Correlation of Mortality Rate and Serum Enzymes in Myocardial Infarction: Test of Efficiency of Coronary Care, *Br. Heart J.,* 33:643, 1971.
274. Norris, R. M., Brandt, P. W. T., Caughey, D. E., Lee, A. J., and Scott, P. J.: A New Coronary Prognostic Index, *Lancet,* 1:274, 1969.
275. Forrester, J. S., Diamond, G. A. Charterlee, K., and Swan, H. J. C.: Medical Therapy of Acute Myocardial Infarction by Application of Hemodynamic Subsets. *N. Engl. J. Med.,* 295:1356, 1404, 1976.
276. Reid, P. R., Taylor, D. R., Kelly, D. T., et al.: Myocardial-Infarct Extension Detected by Precordial ST-Segment Mapping, *N. Engl. J. Med.,* 290:123, 1974.
277. Buda, A. J., MacDonald, I. L., Dubbin, J. O., Orr, S. A., and Strauss, H. O.: Myocardial Infarct Extension: Prevalence, Clinical Significance and Problems in Diagnosis, *Am. Heart J.,* 105:744, 1983.
278. Sanz, G., Castaner, A., Betriu, A., et al.: Determinants of Prognosis in Survivors of Myocardial Infarction, *N. Engl. J. Med.,* 306:1065, 1982.
279. The Multicenter Postinfarction Research Group: Risk Stratification and Survival after Myocardial Infarction, *N. Engl. J. Med.,* 309:331, 1983.
280. Cobb, L. A., Hallstrom, A. P., Weaver, D. W., Copass,

M. W., and Haynes, R. E.: Clinical Predictors and Characteristics of the Sudden Cardiac Death Syndrome, in "Proceedings of the First U.S.–U.S.S.R. Symposium on Sudden Death, Yalta, October 3–5, 1977," U.S. Department on Health, Education and Welfare, Public Health Service, National Institutes of Health, D.H.E.W. Publication no. NIH 78-1470, 1978. [See also *N. Engl. J. Med.*, 293:260, 1975 and *Circulation*, 52(III):223, 1975.]
281. Yatteau, R. F., Peter, R. H., Behar, V. S., Bartel, A. G., Rosati, R. A., and Kong, Y.: Ischemic Cardiomyopathy: The Myopathy of Coronary Artery Disease. Natural History and Results of Medical Versus Surgical Treatment, *Am. J. Cardiol.*, 34:520, 1974.
282. Alderman, E. L., Fisher, L. D., Litwin, P., et al.: Results of Coronary Artery Surgery in Patients with Poor Left Ventricular Function (CASS), *Circulation*, 68:785, 1983.
283. New York Heart Association: "Nomenclature and Criteria for Diagnosis of Diseases of the Heart and Great Vessels," 7th ed., Little, Brown and Company, Boston, 1973, p. viii.
284. New York Heart Association: "Nomenclature and Criteria for Diagnosing Diseases of the Heart and Great Vessels," 8th ed., Little, Brown and Company, Boston, 1979.
285. New York Heart Association: "Nomenclature and Criteria for Diagnosing Diseases of the Heart and Great Vessels," 6th ed., Little, Brown and Company, Boston, 1964.
286. Campeau, L.: Letter to the Editor, *Circulation*, 54:522, 1976.
287. McGregor, M.: Myocardial Ischemia: Towards Better Use of the Coronary Care Unit, *Am. J. Med.*, 76:887, 1984.
288. Ruberman, W., Weinblatt, E., Goldberg, J. D., and Chaudhary, B. S.: Psychosocial Influences on Mortality after Myocardial Infarction, *N. Engl. J. Med.*, 311(9):552, 1984.
289. Hackett, T. P., and Cassem, N. H.: "Coronary Care Patient Psychology," American Heart Association, Inc., New York, 1975.
290. Cassem, N. H., Wishnie, H. A., and Hackett, T. P.: How Coronary Patients Respond to Last Rites, *Postgrad. Med.*, 45:147, 1969.
291. Wilson, L. M.: Intensive Care Delirium, *Arch. Intern. Med.*, 130:225, 1972.
292. Browne, I. W., and Hackett, T. P.: Emotional Reactions to the Threat of Impending Death: Study of Patients on Monitor Cardiac Pacemaker, *Ir. J. Med. Sci.*, 6:177, 1967.
293. Hackett, T. P., and Cassem, N. H.: Psychological Effects of Acute Coronary Care, in L. E. Meltzer and A. J. Dunning (eds.), "Textbook of Coronary Care," The Charles Press, Philadelphia, 1972, p. 443.
294. Hackett, T. P., Cassem, N. H., and Wishnie, H. A.: The Coronary Care Unit: An Appraisal of Its Psychological Hazards, *N. Engl. J. Med.*, 279:1365, 1968.
295. Bruhn, J. G., Thurman, A. E., Jr., Chandler, B. C., and Bruce, T. A.: Patients' Reactions to Death in a Coronary Care Unit, *J. Psychosom. Res.*, 14:65, 1970.
296. Druss, R. G., and Kornfeld, D. S.: Survivors of Cardiac Arrest: Psychiatric Study, *JAMA*, 201:291, 1967.
297. Dobson, M., Tattersfield, A. E., Adler, M. M., and McNicol, M. W.: Attitudes and Long-Term Adjustment of Patients Surviving Cardiac Arrest, *Br. Med. J.*, 3:207, 1971.
298. Hackett, T. P.: The Lazarus Complex Revisited, *Ann. Intern. Med.*, 76:135, 1972.
299. Klein, R. F., Kliner, V. A., Zipes, D. P., Troyer, W. G., Jr., and Wallace, A. G.: Transfer from a Coronary Care Unit, *Arch. Intern. Med.*, 122:104, 1968.
300. Hackett, T. P., and Cassem, N. H.: "White- and Blue-Collar Responses to a Heart Attack," paper presented at the American Psychosomatic Society National Meeting, Boston, 1971.
301. Hackett, T. P., and Cassem, N. H.: Detection and Treatment of Anxiety in the Coronary Care Unit, *Am. Heart J.*, 78:727, 1969.
302. Cassem, N. H., and Hackett, T. P.: Psychological Rehabilitation of Myocardial Infarction Patients in the Acute Phase, *Heart and Lung*, 2:382, 1973.
303. Naughton, J. P., and Hellerstein, H. K. (eds.): "Exercise Testing and Exercise Training in Coronary Heart Disease," Academic Press, New York, 1973, p. 311.
304. Lesstma, J. E., and Loenig, K. L.: Sudden Death and Phenothiazines, *Arch. Gen. Psychiatry*, 18:137, 1968.
305. Coull, D. C., Crooks, J., Dingwall-Fordyce, I., Scott, A. M., and Weir, R. D.: Amitriptyline and Cardiac Disease: Risk of Sudden Death Identified by Monitoring System, *Lancet*, 2:590, 1970.
306. Hutter, A. M., Sidel, V. W., Shine, K. I., and DeSanctis, R. W.: Early Hospital Discharge after Myocardial Infarction, *N. Engl. J. Med.*, 288:1141, 1973.
307. Rechnitzer, P. A., Cunningham, D. A., Andrew, G. M., et al.: Relation of Exercise to the Recurrence Rate of Myocardial Infarction in Men: Ontario Exercise-Heart Collaborative Study, *Am. J. Cardiol.*, 51:65, 1983.
308. Friedman, M., and Ulmer, D.: "Treating Type A Behavior and Your Heart," Alfred A. Knopf, New York, 1984.
309. Orlando, J., Aronow, W. S., Cassidy, J., and Prakayh, R.: Effect of Ethanol on Angina Pectoris, *Ann. Intern. Med.*, 84:652, 1976.
310. Gotto, A. M., Jr.: Can the Progression of Atherosclerosis Be Halted?, *Drug Therapy*, 14(5):37, 1984. (Editorial.)
311. Herbert, P. N., and Terpstra, H. M.: Diet and Exercise in the Treatment of Hyperlipoproteinemia, *Drug Therapy*, 14(5):42, 1984.
312. Lees, R. S., and Lees, A. M.: Lipid-Lowering Drugs: Renewed Enthusiasm, *Drug Therapy*, 14(5):57, 1984.
313. Paradopoulos, C., Beaumont, C., Shelley, S. I., and Larrimore, P.: Myocardial Infarction and Sexual Activity of the Female Patient, *Arch. Intern. Med.*, 143(8):1528, 1983.
314. Evans, D. A., Willett, W. C., and Hennekens, C. H.: Alcohol and Coronary Heart Disease, *Am. Heart J.*, 100(4):584, 1980.
315. Engel, T. R., and Luck, J. C.: Effects of Whiskey on Atrial Vulnerability and "Holiday Heart," *J. Am. Coll. Cardiol.*, 1:816, 1983.
316. Wallgren, H., and Barry, H., III: "Actions of Alcohol," American Elsevier Publishing Company, Inc., New York, 1970, vols. I and II.
317. Gilman, A. G., Goodman, L. S., and Gilman, A. (eds.): "Goodman and Gilman: The Pharmacological Basis of Therapeutics," 6th ed., The Macmillan Company, New York, 1980, p. 378.
318. Klatsky, A. L., Friedman, A. D., Sieglaub, A. B., and Gerard, M. J.: Alcohol Consumption and Blood Pressure: Kaiser-Permanente Multiphasic Health Examination Data, *N. Engl. J. Med.*, 296:1194, 1977.
319. Takizawa, A., Yasue, H., Omote, S., et al.: Variant Angina Induced by Alcohol Ingestion, *Am. Heart J.*, 107(1):25, 1984.
320. Shook, T. L., Kirshenbaum, J. M., Hundley, R. F., Shorey, J. M., and Lamas, G. A.: Ethanol Intoxication Complicating Intravenous Nitroglycerin Therapy, *Ann. Intern. Med.*, 101(4):498, 1984.
321. Shorey, J., Bhardwaj, N., and Loscalzo, J.: Acute Wernicke's Encephalopathy after Intravenous Infusion of High-Dose Nitroglycerin, *Ann. Intern. Med.*, 101(4):500, 1984.
322. Goldman, P.: Coffee and Health: What's Brewing?, *N. Engl. J. Med.*, 310(12):783, 1984.
323. Camargo, C. A.: Arrhythmogenic Effects of Caffeine, *N. Engl. J. Med.*, 309(9): 559, 1983. (Letter to the Editor.)
324. Starr, I., Gamble, C. F., Margolies, A., Donal, J. S., Joseph, H., and Engle, E.: A Study of the Action of Commonly Used Drugs on Cardiac Output, Work, and Size, on Respiration, on Metabolic Rate and on the Electrocardiogram, *J. Clin. Invest.*, 16:799, 1937.
325. Ogilvie, R. I., Fernandez, P. G., and Winsberg, F.: Cardiovascular Response to Increasing Theophylline Concentration, *Eur. J. Clin. Pharmacol.*, 12:409, 1977.
326. Moyer, J. H., Miller, S. I., Tashnek, A. B., and Bowman, R.: The Effect of Theophylline with Ethylene Diamine (Aminophylline) on Cerebral Hemodynamics in the Presence of Cardiac Failure with and without Cheyne-Stokes Respiration, *J. Clin. Invest.*, 31:267, 1952.
327. Gilman, A. G., Goodman, L. S., and Gilman, A. (eds.): "Goodman and Gilman: The Pharmacological Basis of Therapeutics, 6th ed., The Macmillan Company, New York, 1980, p. 595.

328. Thelle, D. S., Arnesen, E., and Forde, O. H.: The Tromso Heart Study: Does Coffee Raise Serum Cholesterol?, *N. Engl. J. Med.*, 308(24):1454, 1983.
329. Dobmeyer, J. J., Stine, R. A., Leier, C. V., Greenberg, R., and Schall, S. F.: The Arrhythmogenic Effects of Caffeine in Human Beings, *N. Engl. J. Med.*, 308:814, 1983.
330. "Smoking and Health: A Report of the Surgeon General," U.S. Department of Health, Education and Welfare, Public Health Service, Publ. no. (PHS)79-500066, 1979.
331. Gordon, T., Kannel, W. B., and McGee, D.: Death and Coronary Attacks in Men after Giving Up Cigarette Smoking: A Report from the Framingham Study, *Lancet*, 2:1345, 1974.
332. Kannel, W. B.: Update on the Role of Cigarette Smoking in Coronary Artery Disease, *Am. Heart J.*, 101(3):319, 1981.
333. Klein, L. W., Ambrose, J., Pichard, A., Holt, J., Gorlin, R., and Teichholz, L. E.: Acute Coronary Hemodynamic Response to Cigarette Smoking in Patients with Coronary Artery Disease, *J. Am. Coll. Cardiol.*, 3(4):879, 1984.
334. Daly, L. E., Mulcahy, R., Graham, I. M., and Hickey, N: Long-Term Effect on Mortality of Stopping Smoking after Unstable Angina and Myocardial Infarction, *Br. Med. J.*, 287:324, 1983.
335. Deanfield, J., Wright, C., Krikler, S., Ribeiro, P., and Fox, K.: Cigarette Smoking and the Treatment of Angina with Propranolol, Atenolol, and Nifedipine, *N. Engl. J. Med.*, 310:951, 1984.
336. Matsukura, S., Taminato, T., Kitano, N., et al.: Effects of Environmental Tobacco Smoke on Urinary Cotinine Excretion in Nonsmokers: Evidence for Passive Smoking, *N. Engl. J. Med.*, 311(13):828, 1984.
337. Rawles, J. M., and Kenmure, A. C. F.: Controlled Trial of Oxygen in Uncomplicated Myocardial Infarction, *Br. Med. J.*, 1:1121, 1976.
338. Moon, A. J., Williams, K. G., and Hopkinson, W. I.: A Patient with Coronary Thrombosis Treated with Hyperbaric Oxygen, *Lancet*, 1:18, 1964.
339. Thomas, M., Malmcrona, R., Fillmore, S., and Shillingford, J. J.: Haemodynamic Effects of Morphine in Patients with Acute Myocardial Infarction, *Br. Heart J.*, 27:863, 1965.
340. Vasko, J. S., Henney, R. P., Oldham, H. N., Brawley, R. K., and Morrow, A. G.: Mechanisms of Action of Morphine in the Treatment of Experimental Pulmonary Edema, *Am. J. Cardiol.*, 18:876, 1966.
341. Heney, R. P., Vasko, J. S., Brawley, R. K., Oldham, H. N., and Morrow, A. G.: The Effects of Morphine on the Resistance and Capacitance Vessels of the Peripheral Circulation, *Am. Heart J.*, 72:242, 1966.
342. Pur-Shahriari, A. A., Mills, R. A., Hoppin, F. G., Jr., and Dexter, L.: Comparison of Chronic and Acute Effects of Morphine Sulfate on Cardiovascular Function, *Am. J. Cardiol.*, 20:654, 1967.
343. Hoel, B. L., and Refsum, H. E.: The Effect of Morphine on Arterial Blood Gases in Patients with Acute Myocardial Infarction, *Acta Med. Scand.*, 186:511, 1969.
344. Grendahl, H., and Hansteen, V.: The Effect of Morphine on Blood Pressure and Cardiac Output in Patients with Acute Myocardial Infarction, *Acta Med. Scand.*, 186:515, 1969.
345. Ward, J. M., McGrath, R. L., and Weil, J. V.: Effects of Morphine on the Peripheral Vascular Response to Sympathetic Stimulation, *Am. J. Cardiol.*, 29:659, 1972.
346. Zelis, R., Mansour, E. J., Capone, R. J., and Mason, D. T.: The Cardiovascular Effects of Morphine: The Peripheral Capacitance and Resistance Vessels in Human Subjects, *J. Clin. Invest.*, 54:1247, 1974.
347. Vismara, L. A., Leaman, D. M., and Zelis, R.: The Effects of Morphine on Venous Tone in Patients with Acute Pulmonary Edema, *Circulation*, 54:335, 1976.
348. Vasko, J. S., Henney, R. P., Brawley, R. K., Oldham, H. N., and Morrow, A. G.: The Effects of Morphine on Ventricular Function and Myocardial Contractile Force, *Am. J. Physiol.*, 210:329, 1966.
349. "Second North American Conference on Nitroglycerin Therapy: Perspectives and Mechanisms" (proceedings of a symposium), *Am. J. Med.*, 76(6A):1, 1984.
350. Sonnenblick, E. H.: The Nitrates as Basic Therapy in Coronary Artery Disease, *Cardiovasc. Rev. Rep.*, 5:423, 1984.
351. Whalen, R. E.: Clinical Classification of Angina, *Cardiovasc. Rev. Rep.*, 5:475, 1984.
352. Conti, C. R., and Feldman, R. L.: The Use of Nitrates in the Treatment of Ischemic Heart Disease, in J. W. Hurst (ed.), "Clinical Essays on the Heart," McGraw-Hill Book Company, New York, 1984, vol. 2, p. 3.
353. Murray, K. B.: Hazard of Microwave Ovens to Transdermal Delivery System, *N. Engl. J. Med.*, 310:721, 1984.
354. Frishman, W. H.: Beta-Adrenergic Blockade in the Treatment of Coronary Artery Disease, in J. W. Hurst (ed.), "Clinical Essays on The Heart," McGraw-Hill Book Company, New York, 1984, vol. 2, p. 25.
355. Singh, B. N., Ellrodt, G., and Nademanee, K.: Calcium Antagonists: Cardiocirculatory Effects and Therapeutic Applications, in J. W. Hurst (ed.), "Clinical Essays on The Heart," McGraw-Hill Book Company, New York, 1984, vol. 2, p. 65.
355a. Epstein, S. E. (ed.): Calcium-Channel Blockers: Present Status and Future Directions, *Am. J. Cardiol.*, 55(no. 3):41B–80B, 1985.
356. Schwartz, J. B., Raizner, A., and Akers, S.: The Effect of Nifedipine on Serum Digoxin Concentrations in Patients, *Am. Heart J.*, 107(4):669, 1984.
357. Schrager, B. R., Pina, I., Frangi, M., Applewhite, S., Sequeira, R., and Chahine, R. A.: Diltiazem, Digoxin Interaction?, *Circulation*, 68(suppl. 3):368, 1983.
358. Palatianos, G. M., Mallon, S., and Bolooki, H.: Hemodynamic Basis for Sudden Cardiovascular Collapse after Coronary Bypass Operation in Patients Receiving Nifedipine, *Circulation*, 66(suppl. 3):251, 1983.
359. Stone, P. H., Muller, J. E., Turi, Z. G., Geltman, E., Jaffee, A. S., and Braunwald, E.: Efficacy of Nifedipine Therapy in Patients with Refractory Angina Pectoris: Significance of the Presence of Coronary Vasospasm, *Am. Heart J.*, 106(4):644, 1983.
360. Petru, M. A., Crawford, M. H., Sorensen, S. G., Chaudhuri, T. K., Levine, S., and O'Rourke, R. A.: Short- and Long-Term Efficacy of High-Dose Oral Diltiazem for Angina Due to Coronary Artery Disease: A Placebo-Controlled, Randomized, Double-Blind Crossover Study, *Circulation*, 68(1):139, 1983.
361. Subramanian, V. B.: Comparative Evaluation of Four Calcium Antagonists and Propranolol with Placebo in Patients with Chronic Stable Angina, *Cardiovasc. Rev. Rep.*, 5(1):91, 1984.
362. Hill, J. A., Feldman, R. L., Conti, C. R., Hill, C. K., and Pepine, C. J.: Long-Term Responses to Nifedipine in Patients with Coronary Spasm Who Have an Initial Favorable Response, *Am. J. Cardiol.*, 52(1):27, 1983.
363. Sellers, T. D., Gibson, R. S., Taylor, G. J., et al.: Relation of Therapeutic Response to Nifedipine to Coronary Anatomy and Motion of S-T Segment during Unstable Angina Pectoris, *Am. J. Med.*, 75:57, 1983.
364. Schanzenbacher, P., Deeg, P., Liebau, G., and Kochsiek, K.: Paradoxical Angina after Nifedipine: Angiographic Documentation, *Am. J. Cardiol.*, 53:345, 1984.
365. Ramon, Y., Behar, S., Kishon, Y., and Engelberg, I. S.: Gingival Hyperplasia Caused by Nifedipine—A Preliminary Report, *Int. J. Cardiol.*, 5:195, 1984.
366. Mullar, O., and Rornik, K.: Hemodynamic Consequences of Coronary Heart Disease with Observations during Anginal Pain and on the Effect of Nitroglycerin, *Br. Heart J.*, 20:302, 1958.
367. Morrison, J., Coromilas, J., Robbins, M., et al.: Digitalis and Myocardial Infarction in Man, *Circulation*, 62(1):8, 1980.
368. Marcus, F. I.: Use of Digitalis in Acute Myocardial Infarction, *Circulation*, 62(1):17, 1980. (Editorial.)
369. Wessler, S., and Gitel, S. N.: Warfarin: From Bedside to Bench, *N. Engl. J. Med.*, 311(10):645, 1984.
370. Soffer, A.: Editorial Comment, *Arch. Intern. Med.*, 136:1229, 1976.

371. Rogel, S., and Bassan, M. M.: Anticoagulants in Ischemic Heart Disease, *Arch. Intern. Med.*, 136:1229, 1976.
372. Modan, B., Schor, S. S., and Modan, M.: The Case for Anticoagulants in Acute Myocardial Infarction: How Do You Know You Cannot Do It Better?, *Arch. Intern. Med.*, 136:1231, 1976.
373. Wessler, S.: Prevention of Venous Thromboembolism by Low-Dose Heparin, *Mod. Concepts Cardiovasc. Dis.*, 45:105, 1976.
374. Fratantoni, J. C.: Thrombolytic Therapy, *Am. Heart J.*, 93:271, 1977.
375. Ganz, W., Buchbinder, N., Marcus, H. et al.: Intracoronary Thrombolysis in Evolving Myocardial Infarction, *Am. Heart J.*, 101(1):4, 1981.
376. Laffel, G. L., and Braunwald, E.: Thrombolytic Therapy: A New Strategy for the Treatment of Acute Myocardial Infarction (First of Two Parts), *N. Engl. J. Med.*, 311(11):710, 1984.
377. Laffel, G. L., and Braunwald, E.: Thrombolytic Therapy: A New Strategy for the Treatment of Acute Myocardial Infarction (Second of Two Parts), *N. Engl. J. Med.*, 311(11):770, 1984.
378. Kwaan, H. C., and Rosen, S. T.: Antithrombotic Effects of Aspirin, *Mod. Concepts Cardiovasc. Dis.*, 53(9):47, 1984.
379. Aspirin Myocardial Infarction Study Research Group: A Randomized, Controlled Trial of Aspirin in Persons Recovered from Myocardial Infarction, *JAMA*, 243: 661, 1980.
380. Boston Collaborative Drug Surveillance Group: Regular Aspirin Intake and Acute Myocardial Infarction, *Br. Med. J.*, 1:440, 1974.
381. Elwood, P. C., Cochrane, A. L., Burr, M. L., et al.: A Randomized Controlled Trial of Acetyl Salicylic Acid in the Secondary Prevention of Mortality from Myocardial Infarction, *Br. Med. J.*, 1:436, 1974.
382. Lewis, H. D., Davis, J. W., Archibald, D. G., et al.: Protective Effects of Aspirin against Acute Myocardial Infarction and Death in Men with Unstable Angina, *N. Engl. J. Med.*, 309(7):396, 1983.
383. The Anturane Reinfarction Trial Research Group: Sulfinpyrazone in the Prevention of Cardiac Death after Myocardial Infarction: The Anturane Reinfarction Trial, *N. Engl. J. Med.*, 298:289, 1978.
384. Anturane Reinfarction Trial Research Group: Sulfinpyrazone in the Prevention of Sudden Death after Myocardial Infarction, *N. Engl. J. Med.*, 302:250, 1980.
385. The Persantine-Aspirin Reinfarction Study Research Group: Persantine and Aspirin in Coronary Heart Disease, *Circulation*, 62(3):449, 1980.
386. Chesebro, J. H., Fuster, V., Elveback, L. R., et al.: Effect of Dipyridamole and Aspirin on Late Vein-Graft Patency after Coronary Bypass Operations, *N. Engl. J. Med.*, 310(4):209, 1984.
387. Allee, J. G., and Tedrick, D. L.: Radioiodine Thyroid Ablation for Symptomatic Heart Disease: It Still has A Place, in J. W. Hurst (ed.), "Update V: The Heart," McGraw-Hill Book Company, New York, 1981, p. 237.
388. Pryor, D. B., Harrell, F. E., Jr., Lee, K. L., Califf, R. M., and Rosati, R. A.: An Improving Prognosis over Time in Medically Treated Patients with Coronary Artery Disease, *Am. J. Cardiol.*, 52:444, 1983.
389. Kent, K. M., Mullin, S. M., and Passamani, E. R. (guest eds.): Proceedings of the National Heart, Lung, and Blood Institute Workshop on the Outcome of Percutaneous Transluminal Coronary Angioplasty, *Am. J. Cardiol.*, 53(12):1, 1984.
390. Roberts, A. J., Conti, C. R., and Pepine, C. J.: Symposium: New Techniques in Therapeutic Coronary Catheterization including Intraoperative Angioplasty, *Am. J. Cardiol.*, 107(4):817, 1984.
391. Mullin, S. M., Passamani, E. R., and Mock, M. B.: Historical Background of the National Heart, Lung and Blood Institute Registry for Percutaneous Transluminal Coronary Angioplasty, *Am. J. Cardiol.*, 53(12):3C, 1984.
392. Dorros, G. Stertzer, S. H., Cowley, M., Kent, K., and Williams, D.: Complex Transluminal Coronary Angioplasty: Multivessel Disease and Multiple Dilatations, *Circulation*, 66(suppl. 2):329, 1982. (Abstract.)
393. Hartzler, G. O., Rutherford, B. D., McConahay, D. R., and McCallister, S. H.: Simultaneous Multiple Lesion Coronary Angioplasty—A Preferred Therapy for Patients with Multiple Vessel Disease, *Circulation*, 66(suppl. 2):5, 1982. (Abstract.)
394. Douglas, J. S., Gruentzig, A. R., King, S. B., et al.: Percutaneous Transfemoral Coronary Angioplasty in Patients with Prior Coronary Bypass Surgery, *J. Am. Coll. Cardiol.*, 2:745, 1983.
395. Meier, B., King. S. B., Gruentzig, A. R., et al.: Repeat Coronary Angioplasty, *J. Am. Coll. Cardiol.*, 4:463, 1984.
396. King. S. B., III, and Hurst, J. W.: The Relief of Angina Pectoris by Coronary Bypass Surgery, in J. W. Hurst (ed.), "Update II: The Heart," McGraw-Hill Book Company, New York, 1980, p. 71.
396a. Gunnar, R. M., and Loeb, H. S. C.: An Alternative Interpretation of the Results of the Coronary Artery Surgery Study, *Circulation*, 71(no. 2):193, 1985.
396b. Lawrie, G. M., and DeBakey, M. E.: The Coronary Artery Surgery Study (commentary), *JAMA*, 252(no. 18):2609, 1984.
396c. Hurst, J. W.: Chest Pain: What to Look for in the Work-Up, *Mod. Med.*, 53(4):40, 1985.
397. Hurst, J. W. (ed.): "Clinical Essays on the Heart," McGraw-Hill Book Company, New York, 1984, vol. 2.
398. Lown, B., Podrid, P. J., and Graboys, T. B.: Letter to the Editor, *N. Engl. J. Med.*, 306(11):679, 1982.
399. Lichtlen, P., Mocetti, T., Hlater, J., et al.: Postoperative Evaluation of Myocardial Blood Flow in Aorto-to-Coronary Artery Vein Bypass Grafting Using Xenon-Residue Detection Technique, *Circulation*, 46:445, 1972.
400. Ormond, J., Platt, M., Nels, L., et al.: Thallium 201 Syntography and Exercise Testing in Evaluating Patients Prior to and after Coronary Bypass Surgery, *Circulation*, 56(suppl. 3):131, 1977.
401. Marco, J. D.: Myocardial Perfusion following Bypass Surgery, in J. W. Hurst (ed.), "Update II: The Heart," McGraw-Hill Book Company, 1980, p. 13.
402. Kent, K. M., Borer, J. S., Green, M. V., et al.: Effects of Coronary-Artery Bypass on Global and Regional Left Ventricular Function during Exercise, *N. Engl. J. Med.*, 298:1434, 1978.
403. Tyras, D. H., Admad, N., Kaiser, G. C., et al.: Ventricular Function and the Native Coronary Circulation Five Years after Myocardial Revascularization, *Ann. Thorac. Surg.*, 27:547, 1979.
404. Sheldon, W. C., Rincon, G., Pichard, A. D., Razavi, M., Cheanvechai, C., and Loop, F. D.: Surgical Treatment of Coronary Artery Disease: Pure Graft Operations, with a Study of 741 Patients Followed 3–7 Years, *Prog. Cardiovasc. Dis.*, 18(3):237, 1975.
405. Hurst, J. W.: The "Overshadowed" CASS Report, *Clin. Cardiol.*, 7:193, 1984.
406. Read, R. C., Murphy, M. L., Hulgren, H. N., et al.: Survival of Men Treated for Chronic Stable Angina Pectoris: A Cooperative Randomized Study, *J. Thorac. Cardiovasc. Surg.*, 75:1, 1978.
406a. The Veterans Administration Coronary Artery Bypass Surgery Cooperative Study Group: Eleven-Year Survival in the Veterans Administration Randomized Trial of Coronary Bypass Surgery for Stable Angina Pectoris, *N. Engl. J. Med.*, 311(no. 21):1333, 1984.
407. Alderman, E. L., Fisher, L. D., Litwin, P., et al.: Results of Coronary Artery Surgery in Patients with Poor Left Ventricular Function (CASS), *Circulation*, 68(4):785, 1983.
408. Wynne, J., Cohn, L. H., Collins, J. J., and Cohn, P. F.: Myocardial Revascularization in Patients with Multivessel Coronary Artery Disease and Minimal Angina Pectoris, *Circulation*, 68(suppl. 1):I-92, 1978.
409. Kent, K. M., Rosing, D. R., Ewels, C. J., Lipson, L., Bonow, R., and Epstein, S. E.: Prognosis of Asymptomatic or Mildly Symptomatic Patients with Coronary Artery Disease, *Am. J. Cardiol.*, 49(8):1823, 1982.

410. Hammermeister, K. E., DeRouen, T. A., and Dodge, H. T.: Effect of Coronary Surgery on Survival in Asymptomatic and Minimally Symptomatic Patients, *Circulation,* 62(suppl. 1):I-98, 1980.

410a. Bonow, R. O., Kent, K. M., Rosing, K. K., et al.: Exercise-Induced Ischemia in Mildly Symptomatic Patients with Coronary-Artery Disease and Preserved Left Ventricular Function: Identification of Subgroups at Risk of Death during Medical Therapy, *N. Engl. J. Med.,* 311(no. 21):1339, 1984.

410b. Chaitman, B. R., Davis, K., Fisher, L. D., et al.: A Life Table and Cox Regression Analysis of Patients with Combined Proximal Left Anterior Descending and Proximal Left Circumflex Coronary Artery Disease: Non-left Main Equivalent Lesions (CASS), *Circulation,* 68(no. 6):1163, 1983.

410c. Rahimtoola, S. H., Nunley, D., Grunkemeier, G., Tepley, J., Lambert, L., and Starr, A.: Ten-Year Survival after Coronary Bypass Surgery for Unstable Angina, *N. Engl. J. Med.,* 308:676, 1983.

411. Loop, F. D., Sheldon, W. C., Lytle, B. W., Cosgrove, D. M., and Proudfit, W. L.: The Efficacy of Coronary Artery Surgery, *Am. Heart J.,* 101(1):86, 1981.

412. Mason, D. T., Amsterdam, E. A., DeMaria, A. N., et al.: The Prevention of Myocardial Infarction by Coronary Bypass Surgery, in J. W. Hurst (ed.), "Update II: The Heart," McGraw-Hill Book Company, New York, 1980, p. 103.

413. Hamilton, W. M., Hammermeister, K. E., DeRouen, T. A., Zia, M. S., and Dodge, H. T.: Effect of Coronary Artery Bypass Grafting on Subsequent Hospitalization, *Am. J. Cardiol.,* 51:353, 1983.

414. Jones, E. L., Kaplan, J. A., Dorney, E. R., et al.: Propranolol Therapy in Patients Undergoing Myocardial Revascularization, *Am. J. Cardiol.,* 38:696, 1976.

415. Hutter, A. M., Jr., Russell, R. O., Jr., Resnekov, L., et al.: Unstable Angina Pectoris. National Randomized Study of Surgical vs Medical Therapy: Results in 1, 2 and 3 Vessel Disease, *Circulation,* 55, 56(suppl. 3):60, 1977. (Abstract.)

416. Epstein, S. E., Kent, K. M., Goldstein, R. E., Borer, J. S., and Redwood, D. R.: Reduction of Ischemic Injury by Nitroglycerin during Acute Myocardial Infarction, *N. Engl. J. Med.,* 292:29, 1975.

417. Hurst, J. W.: The Perils of Waiting, in J. W. Hurst (ed.), "Update I: The Heart," McGraw-Hill Book Company, New York, 1980, p. 1137.

418. Kaplan, J. A., and King, S. B.: The Precordial Electrocardiographic Lead (V5) in Patients Who Have Coronary-Artery Disease, *Anesthesiology,* 45(no. 5):570, 1976.

419. Kaplan, J. A., Dunbar, R. W., and Jones, E. L.: Nitroglycerin Infusion during Coronary Artery Surgery, *Anesthesia,* 45:14, 1976.

420. Laird-Meeter, K., van den Brand, M. J. B. M., Serruys, P. W., Penn, O. C. K. M., Haalebos, M. M. P., and Hugenholtz, P. G.: Reoperation after Aortocoronary Bypass Procedure: Results in 53 Patients in a Group of 1041 with Consecutive First Operations, *Br. Heart J.,* 50:157, 1983.

421. Kuan, P., Bernstein, S. B., and Ellestad, M. H.: Coronary Artery Bypass Surgery Morbidity, *J. Am. Coll. Cardiol.,* 3(6):1391, 1984.

422. Coffey, C. E., Massey, E. W., Roberts, K. B., Curtis, S. E., Jones, R. H., and Pryor, D. B.: Occurrence of Stroke following Coronary Artery Bypass Graft Surgery, *Cardiovasc. Rev. Rep.,* 4(11):1455, 1983.

423. Ormerod, O. J. M., McGregor, C. G. A., Stone, D. L., Wisbey, C., and Petch, M. C.: Arrhythmias after Coronary Bypass Surgery, *Br. Heart J.,* 51:618, 1984.

424. Kuan, P., Messenger, J. C., and Ellestad, M. H.: Transient Central Diabetes Insipidus after Aortocoronary Bypass Operations, *Am. J. Cardiol.,* 52:1181, 1983.

425. Taussig, A. S., Hurst, J. W., Ambrose, S. S., and Swell, C. W.: Massive Prostatic Infarction following Aortocoronary Bypass Surgery: A Report of Two Cases, *Clin. Cardiol.,* 7(2):113, 1984.

426. Clements, S. D., Jr., and Hurst, J. W.: Medical Care before, during, and after Coronary Bypass Surgery, in J. W. Hurst (ed.), "Update II: The Heart," McGraw-Hill Book Company, New York, 1980, p. 261.

427. Hodgman, J. R., and Cosgrove, D. M.: Post-Hospital Course and Complications following Coronary Bypass Surgery, *Clev. Clin. Q.,* 43(3):125, 1976.

428. Cashin, W. L., Sanmarco, M. E., Nessim, S. A., and Blankenhorn, D. H.: Accelerated Progression of Atherosclerosis in Coronary Vessels with Minimal Lesions That Are Bypassed, *N. Engl. J. Med.,* 311(13):824, 1984.

429. Brindis, R. G., Brundage, B. H., Ullyot, D. J., McKay, C. W., Lipton, M. J., and Turley, K.: Graft Patency in Patients with Coronary Artery Bypass Operation Complicated by Perioperative Myocardial Infarction, *J. Am. Coll. Cardiol.,* 3(1):55, 1984.

430. Grondin, C. M., Campeau, L., Lesperance, J., Enjalbert, M., and Bourassa, M. G.: Comparison of Late Changes in Internal Mammary Artery and Saphenous Vein Grafts in Two Consecutive Series of Patients 10 Years after Operation, *Circulation,* 70(suppl. 1):I-208, 1984.

431. Singh, R. N., Sosa, J. A., and Green, G. E.: Internal Mammary Artery Versus Saphenous Vein Graft: Comparative Performance in Patients with Combined Revascularization, *Br. Heart J.,* 50:48, 1983.

432. Lytle, B. W., Kramer, J. R., Golding, L. R., et al.: Young Adults with Coronary Atherosclerosis: 10-Year Results of Surgical Myocardial Revascularization, *J. Am. Coll. of Cardiol.,* 4(3):445, 1984.

432a. Brooks, N., Wright, J., Sturridge, M., et al.: Randomised Placebo Controlled Trial of Aspirin and Dipyridamole in the Prevention of Coronary Vein Graft Occlusion, *Br. Heart J.,* 53:201, 1985.

433. Barnes, G. K., Ray, M. J., Oberman, A., and Kouchoukos, N. T.: Changes in Working Status of Patients following Coronary Bypass Surgery, *JAMA,* 238:1259, 1977.

434. David, P.: Contributing Factors Preventing Return to Work of Cardiac Surgery Patients, *Cleve. Clin. Q.,* 45:177, 1978.

435. Hammermeister, K. E., DeRouen, T. A., Curci, H., Blake, B., and Dodge, H. T.: Evidence of Reduction in Rate of Hospitalization for Cardiac Causes as a Result of Coronary Bypass Surgery, *Circulation,* 57,58(suppl. 2):18, 1978.

436. Logue, R. B., King, S. B., and Douglas, J. S.: A Practical Approach to Coronary Artery Disease, with Special Reference to Coronary Bypass Surgery, *Curr. Prob. Cardiol.,* 1(a):1, 1976.

437. Jenkins, C. D., Stanton, B. A., Savageau, J. A., Denlinger, P., and Klein, M. D.: Coronary Artery Bypass Surgery: Physical, Psychological, Social, and Economic Outcomes Six Months Later, *JAMA,* 250:782, 1983.

438. Personal observation by J. Willis Hurst, M.D.

439. Collins, J. J.: The Cost of Coronary Bypass Surgery, in J. W. Hurst (ed.), "Update II: The Heart," McGraw-Hill Book Company, New York, 1980, p. 261.

440. Kronenfeld, J. J., Charles, E. D., Jr., Ween, J. B., et al.: Unstable Angina Pectoris: An Examination of Mode of Therapy and Cost of Therapy, *Circulation,* 6(suppl. 1): 1-16, 1979.

441. Russell, R. O., Wayne, J. B., Kronenfeld, J. J., et al.: Surgical Vs. Medical Therapy for Treatment of Unstable Angina: Changes in Work Status and Family Income, *Am. J. Cardiol.,* 45:34, 1980.

442. Personal communication with Robert Guyton, M.D.

443. White, J. C., and Bland, E. F.: The Surgical Relief of Angina Pectoris, *Medicine,* 27:1, 1948.

444. Buchwald, H.: A Surgical Operation to Lower Circulating Cholesterol, *Circulation,* 28:649, 1980.

445. Buchwald, H., Moore, R. B., and Varco, B. L.: Surgical Treatment of Hyperlipidemia, *Circulation,* 49(suppl. 1):1, 1974.

446. Moore, R. B., Buchwald, H., Varco, R. L., et al.: The Effect of Partial Ileal Bypass on Plasma Lipoproteins, *Circulation,* 62(3):469, 1980.

447. Koivisto, P., and Miettinen, T. A.: Long-Term Effects of Ileal Bypass on Lipoproteins in Patients with Familial Hypercholesterolemia, *Circulation,* 70:290, 1984.

448. Illingworth, D. R., and Connor, W. E.: Hypercholesterolemia Persisting after Distal Ileal Bypass; Response to Mevinolin, *Ann. Intern. Med.,* 100:850, 1984.

449. Clark, L. T., Garfein, O. B., and Dwyer, E. M.: Acute Pulmonary Edema Due to Ischemic Heart Disease without Accompanying Myocardial Infarction: Natural History and Clinical Profile, *Am. J. Med.*, 75:332, 1983.
450. Cohn, J. K., and Cohn, P. F.: Patient Reactions to the Diagnosis of Asymptomatic Coronary Artery Disease—Implications for the Primary Physician and Consultant Cardiologist, *J. Am. Coll. Cardiol.*, 1:956, 1983.
451. Cohn, P. F.: Prognosis and Treatment of Asymptomatic Coronary Artery Disease, *J. Am. Coll. Cardiol.*, 1:959, 1983.
452. Deanfield, J. E., Selwyn, A. P., Chierchia, S., et al.: Myocardial Ischemia during Daily Life in Patients with Stable Angina: Its Relation to Symptoms and Heart Rate Changes, *Lancet*, 2:753, 1983.
453. Maseri, A.: The Changing Face of Angina Pectoris: Practical Implications, *Lancet*, 1:746, 1983.
454. Silverman, K. J., and Grossman, W.: Current Concepts. Angina Pectoris: Natural History and Strategies for Evaluation and Management, *N. Engl. J. Med.*, 310:1712, 1984.
455. Cannon, R. O., Watson, R. M., Rosing, D. R., and Epstein, S. E.: Angina Caused by Reduced Vasodilator Reserve of the Small Coronary Arteries, *J. Am. Coll. Cardiol.*, 1(6):1359, 1983.
456. Schachne, J. S., Roberts, B. H., and Thompson, P. D.: Coronary-Artery Spasm and Myocardial Infarction Associated with Cocaine Use, *N. Engl. J. Med.*, 310:1165, 1984.
457. Waters, D. D., Bourchard, A., and Theroux, P.: Spontaneous Remission Is a Frequent Outcome of Variant Angina, *J. Am. Coll. Cardiol.*, 2(2):195, 1983.
457a. Rackley, C. E. (guest ed.): Symposium on Early Intervention in Acute Myocardial Infarction, *Am. J. Cardiol.*, 54(no. 11):1E, 1984.
458. Mann, T., Cohn, P. F., Holman, L., Green, L. H., Markis, J. E., and Phillips, D. A.: Effect of Nitroprusside on Regional Myocardial Blood Flow in Coronary Artery Disease: Results in 25 Patients and Comparison with Nitroglycerin, *Circulation*, 57:732, 1978.
459. Chiariello, M., Gold, H. K., Leinbach, R. C., Davis, M. A., and Maroko, P. R.: Comparison between the Effects of Nitroprusside and Nitroglycerin on Ischemic Injury during Acute Myocardial Infarction, *Circulation*, 54:766, 1976.
460. Flakerty, J. T., Becker, L. C., Bulkley, B. H., et al.: A Randomized Prospective Trial of Intravenous Nitroglycerin in Patients with Acute Myocardial Infarction, *Circulation*, 68:576, 1983.
461. Bussmann, W. D., Passek, D., Seidel, W., and Kaltenbach, M.: Reduction of CK and CK-MB Indexes of Infarct Size by Intravenous Nitroglycerin, *Circulation*, 63:615, 1981.
462. Jugdutt, B. L., Becker, L. C., Hutchins, G. M., et al.: Effect of Intravenous Nitroglycerin on Collateral Blood Flow and Infarct Size in the Conscious Dog, *Circulation*, 63:17, 1981.
463. Opie, L. H.: Myocardial Infarct Size: II. Comparison of Anti-Infarct Effects of Beta-Blockade, Glucose-Insulin-Potassium, Nitrates, and Hyaluronidase, *Am. Heart J.*, 100(4):531, 1980.
464. Pierce, W. S., Carter, D. R., McGarran, M. H., and Waldhausen, J. A.: Modification of Myocardial Infarct Volume: An Experimental Study in the Dog, *Arch. Surg.*, 107:682, 1973.
465. Miura, M., Thomas, R., Ganz, W., et al.: The Effect of Delay in Propranolol Administration on Reduction of Myocardial Infarct Size after Experimental Coronary Artery Occlusion in Dogs, *Circulation*, 59:1148, 1979.
466. Peter, T., Norris, R. M., Clarke, E. D., et al.: Reduction of Enzyme Levels by Propranolol after Acute Myocardial Infarction, *Circulation*, 57:1091, 1978.
467. Yusuf, S., Peto, R., Bennett, D., Ramsdale, D., Furse, P., Broy, C., and Sleight, P.: Early Intravenous Atenolol Treatment in Suspected Acute Myocardial Infarction, *Lancet*, 2:273, 1980.
468. Herlitz, J., Elmfeldt, D., Hjalmarson, A., Holmberg, S., et al.: Effect of Metoprolol on Indirect Signs of the Size and Severity of Acute Myocardial Infarction, *Am. J. Cardiol.*, 51:1282, 1983.
469. Hjalmarson, A., Herlitz, J., Malek, I., et al.: Effect on Mortality of Metoprolol in Acute Myocardial Infarction, *Lancet*, 8221:823, 1981.
470. Hjalmarson, A., Herlitz, J., Holmberg, S., et al.: The Goteborg Metoprolol Trial—Effects of Mortality and Morbidity in Acute Myocardial Infarction, *Circulation*, 67(suppl. 1):26, 1983.
471. Roberts, R., Croft, C., Gold, H. K., et al.: Effect of Propranolol on Myocardial-Infarct Size in a Randomized Blinded Multicenter Trial, *N. Engl. J. Med.*, 311:218, 1984.
472. Herlitz, J., Hjalmarson, A., Holmberg, S., et al.: Development of Congestive Heart Failure after Treatment with Metoprolol in Acute Myocardial Infarction, *Br. Heart J.*, 51:539, 1984.
473. Little, W. C.: Thrombolytic Therapy of Acute Myocardial Infarction, *Curr. Prob. Cardiol.*, 8(9):7, 1983.
474. Kennedy, J. W., Ritchie, J. L., David, K. B., and Fritz, J. K.: Western Washington Randomized Trial of Intracoronary Streptokinase in Acute Myocardial Infarction, *N. Engl. J. Med.*, 309:1477, 1983.
475. Lee, G., Amsterdam, E. A., Low, R., et al.: Efficacy of Percutaneous Transluminal Coronary Recanalization Utilizing Streptokinase Thrombolysis in Patients with Acute Myocardial Infarction, *Am. Heart J.*, 102:1159, 1981.
476. Rutsch, W., Schartt, M., Mathey, O., et al.: Percutaneous Transluminal Coronary Recanalization: Procedure, Results, and Acute Complications, *Am. Heart J.*, 102:1178, 1981.
477. Reimer, K. A., Lowe, J. E., Rosmussen, M. M., and Jennings, R. B.: The Wavefront Phenomenon of Ischemic Cell Death: 1. Myocardial Infarct Size Vs. Duration of Coronary Occlusion in Dogs, *Circulation*, 56:786, 1977.
478. Maroko, P. R., Libby, P., Ginks, W. R., et al.: Coronary Artery Reperfusion: 1. Early Effects of Local Myocardial Function and the Extent of Myocardial Necrosis, *J. Clin. Invest.*, 51:2710, 1972.
479. Mather, V. S., Guinn, G. A., and Burris, W. H.: Maximal Revascularization (Reperfusion) in Intact Conscious Dogs after 2 to 5 Hours of Coronary Occlusion, *Am. J. Cardiol.*, 36:252, 1975.
480. Schroder, R., Biamino, G., Leitner, E., et al.: Intravenous Short-Term Infusion of Streptokinase in Acute Myocardial Infarction, *Circulation*, 67:536, 1983.
481. Spann, J. F., Sherry, S., Carabello, B. A., et al.: Coronary Thrombolysis by Intravenous Streptokinase in Acute Myocardial Infarction: Acute and Follow-up Studies, *Am. J. Cardiol.*, 53:655, 1984.
482. Ganz, W., Geft, I., Shah, P. K., et al.: Intravenous Streptokinase in Evolving Acute Myocardial Infarction, *Am. J. Cardiol.*, 53:1209, 1984.
483. Alderman, E. L., Jutzy, K. R., Berte, L. E., et al.: Randomized Comparison of Intravenous Versus Intracoronary Streptokinase for Myocardial Infarction, *Am. J. Cardiol.*, 54:14, 1984.
484. Rogers, W. J., Baxley, W. A., Hood, W. P., and Mantle, J. A.: Prospective Randomized Trial of Intravenous Vs. Intracoronary Streptokinase in Myocardial Infarction, *J. Am. Coll. Cardiol.*, 1:629, 1983. (Abstract.)
485. Berg, R., Jr., Selinger, S. L., Leonard, J. J., Grunwald, R. P., and O'Grady, W. P.: Immediate Coronary Artery Bypass for Acute Evolving Myocardial Infarction, *J. Thorac. Cardiovasc. Surg.*, 81:493, 1981.
486. Gable, A. J., Sloman, G., and Robinson, J. S.: Mortality Reduction in a Coronary Care Unit, *Br. Med. J.*, 1:1005, 1966.
487. Graboys, T. B.: In-Hospital Sudden Death after Coronary Care Unit Discharge: A High Risk Profile, *Arch. Intern. Med.*, 135:512, 1975.
488. Grace, W. J., and Yarvote, P. M.: Acute Myocardial Infarction: The Course of the Illness Following Discharge from the Coronary Care Unit: A Description of the Intermediate Coronary Care Unit, *Chest*, 59:15, 1971.
489. Christensen, D., Ford, M., Reading, J., and Castle, C. H.: Sudden Death in the Late Hospital Phase of Acute Myocardial Infarction, *Arch. Intern. Med.*, 137:1675, 1977.

490. Frieden, J., and Cooper, J. A.: The Role of the Intermediate Cardiac Care Unit, *JAMA*, 235:816, 1976.
491. McNeer, J. F., Wallace, A. G., Wagner, G. S., Starmer, C. F., and Rosati, R. A.: The Course of Acute Myocardial Infarction, *Circulation*, 51:410, 1975.
492. McNeer, J. F., Wagner, G. S., Ginsburg, P. B., et al.: Hospital Discharge One Week after Acute Myocardial Infarction, *N. Engl. J. Med.*, 298:229, 1978.
493. Masden, E. B., Hougaard, P., Gilpin, E., and Pedersen, A.: The Length of Hospitalization after Acute Myocardial Infarction Determined by Risk Calculation, *Circulation*, 68:9, 1983.
494. Levine, S. A., and Lown, B.: The "Chair" Treatment of Coronary Thrombosis, *Trans. Assoc. Am. Physicians*, 64:316, 1951.
495. Sloman, J. G., Penington, C., Sutton, L. D., and Hunt, D.: Management of the Late Phase of Acute Myocardial Infarction, *Prog. Cardiol.*, 9:25, 1980.
496. Miller, D. H., and Borer, J. S.: Exercise Testing Early after Myocardial Infarction: Risks and Benefits, *Am. J. Med.*, 72:427, 1982.
497. Gravath, A., Sodermark, T., Winge, T., Volpe, U., and Zetterquist, S.: Early Work Load Tests for Evaluation of Long-Term Prognosis of Acute Myocardial Infarction, *Br. Heart J.*, 39:758, 1977.
498. Dillahunt, P. H., II, and Miller, A. B.: Early Treadmill Testing after Myocardial Infarction: Angiographic and Hemodynamic Correlations, *Chest*, 76:150, 1979.
499. Fuller, C. M., Raizner, A. E., Verani, M. S., et al.: Early Post Myocardial Infarction Treadmill Stress Testing: An Accurate Predictor of Multi-vessel Coronary Disease and Subsequent Cardiac Events, *Ann. Intern. Med.*, 94:734, 1981.
500. Schwartz, K. M., Turner, J. D., Sheffield, L. T., et al.: Limited Exercise Testing Soon after Myocardial Infarction: Correlation with Early Coronary and Left Ventricular Angiography, *Ann. Intern. Med.*, 94:727, 1981.
501. Starling, M. R., Crawford, M. H., Kennedy, G. T., and O'Rourke, R. A.: Exercise Testing Early after Myocardial Infarction: Predictive Value for Subsequent Unstable Angina and Death, *Am. J. Cardiol.*, 46:909, 1980.
502. Starling, M. R., Crawford, M. H., Kennedy, G. T., and O'Rourke, R. A.: Treadmill Exercise Tests Predischarge and Six Weeks Post-Myocardial Infarction to Detect Abnormalities of Known Prognostic Value, *Ann. Intern. Med.*, 94:721, 1981.
503. Gibson, R. S., Watson, D. D., Craddock, G. B., et al.: Prediction of Cardiac Events after Uncomplicated Myocardial Infarction: A Prospective Study Comparing Predischarge Exercise Thallium-201 Scintigraphy and Coronary Angiography, *Circulation*, 68:321, 1983.
504. Dunn, R. F., Freedman, B., Bailey, I. K., Uren, R., and Kelly, D. T.: Non-Invasive Prediction of Multivessel Disease after Myocardial Infarction, *Circulation*, 62:726, 1980.
505. Turner, J. D., Schwartz, K. M., Logic, J. R., et al.: Detection of Residual Jeopardized Myocardial Three Weeks after Myocardial Infarction by Exercise Testing with Thallium-201 Myocardial Scintigraphy, *Circulation*, 61:729, 1980.
506. Turner, J. D., Rogers, W. J., Mantle, J. A., Rackley, C. E., and Russell, R. O.: Coronary Angiography Soon after Myocardial Infarction, *Chest*, 77:58, 1980.
507. Taylor, G. J., Humphries, J. O. P., Mellits, E. D., et al.: Predictors of Clinical Course, Coronary Anatomy and Left Ventricular Function after Recovery for Acute Myocardial Infarction, *Circulation*, 62:960, 1980.
508. Hammermeister, K. E., DeRouen, T. A., and Dodge, H. T.: Variables Predictive of Survival in Patients with Coronary Disease: Selection of Univariate and Multivariate Analyses for the Clinical Electrocardiographic, Exercise, Arteriographic and Quantitative Angiographic Evaluations, *Circulation*, 59:421, 1979.
509. Lyons, K. P., and Olson, H. G.: Correlation between Radionuclide Left Ventricular Ejection Fraction during Acute Myocardial Infarction and Cardiac Death or Congestive Heart Failure, *J. Nucl. Med.*, 21:6, 1980.
510. Schulze, R. A., Strauss, H. W., and Pitt, B.: Sudden Death in the Year following Myocardial Infarction: Relation to Ventricular Premature Contractions in the Late Hospital Phase and Left Ventricular Ejection Fraction, *Am. J. Med.*, 62:192, 1977.
511. Borer, J. S., Rosing, D. R., Miller, R. H., et al.: Natural History of Left Ventricular Function during One Year after Acute Myocardial Infarction: Comparison with Clinical Electrocardiographic and Biochemical Determinations, *Am. J. Cardiol.*, 46:1, 1980.
512. Friedman, M. L., and Castor, R. E.: Reliability of Gated Heart Scintigrams for Detection of Left Ventricular Aneurysm: Concise Communication, *J. Nucl. Med.*, 20:720, 1979.
513. Botvinick, E. H., Shames, D., Hutchinson, J. C., Rose, B., and Fitzpatrick, M.: Non-invasive Diagnosis of a False Left Ventricular Aneurysm with Radioisotope Gated Cardiac Blood Pool Imaging, *Am. J. Cardiol.*, 37:1089, 1976.
514. Corbett, J. R., Dehmer, G. J., Lewis, S. E., et al.: The Prognostic Value of Submaximal Exercise Testing with Radionuclide Ventriculography before Hospital Discharge in Patients with Recent Myocardial Infarction, *Circulation*, 64:535, 1981.
515. Hung, J., Goris, M. L., Nash, E., et al.: Comparative Value of Maximal Treadmill Testing, Exercise Thallium Myocardial Perfusion Scintigraphy, and Exercise Radionuclide Ventriculography for Distinguishing High- and Low-Risk Patients Soon after Acute Myocardial Infarction, *Am. J. Cardiol.*, 53:1221, 1984.
516. Sharpe, D. N., Botvinik, E. H., Shames, D. M., et al.: The Non-Invasive Diagnosis of Right Ventricular Infarction, *Circulation*, 57:483, 1978.
517. Asinger, R. W., Mikell, F. L., Elsperger, J., and Hodges, M.: Incidence of Left Ventricular Thrombosis after Acute Transmural Myocardial Infarction: Serial Evaluation by Two-Dimensional Echocardiography, *N. Engl. J. Med.*, 305:297, 1981.
518. Vismara, L. A., De Maria, A. N., Hughes, J. L., Mason, D. T., and Amsterdam, E. A.: Evaluation of Arrhythmias in the Late Hospital Phase of Acute Myocardial Infarction Compared to Coronary Care Unit Ectopy, *Br. Heart J.*, 37:598, 1975.
519. Ryan, M., Lown, B., and Horn, H.: Comparison of Ventricular Ectopic Activity during 24 Hour Monitoring and Exercise Testing in Patients with Coronary Heart Disease, *N. Engl. J. Med.*, 292:224, 1975.
520. Coronary Drug Research Group: Prognostic Importance of Premature Beats following Myocardial Infarction, *JAMA*, 223:1116, 1973.
521. Ruberman, W., Weinblott, E., Goldberg, J. D., Frank, C. W., and Shapiro, S.: Ventricular Premature Beats and Mortality after Myocardial Infarction, *N. Engl. J. Med.*, 297:750, 1972.
522. Jelinek, M. V., Lohrbauer, L., and Lown, B.: Antiarrhythmic Drug Therapy for Sporadic Ventricular Ectopic Arrhythmias, *Circulation*, 49:659, 1974.
523. Braunwald, E., Muller, J. E., Kloner, R. A., and Maroko, P. R.: Role of Beta-Adrenergic Blockade in the Therapy of Patients with Myocardial Infarction, *Am. J. Med.*, 74:113, 1983.
524. Norwegian Multicenter Study Group: Timolol-Induced Reduction in Mortality and Reinfarction in Patients Surviving Acute Myocardial Infarction, *N. Engl. J. Med.*, 304:801, 1981.
525. Beta-Blocker Heart Attack Trial Research Group: A Randomized Trial of Propranolol in Patients with Acute Myocardial Infarction: I. Mortality Results, *JAMA*, 247:1701, 1982.
526. Ahumada, G. G.: Identification of Patients Who Do Not Require Beta Antagonists after Myocardial Infarction, *Am. J. Med.*, 76:900, 1984.
527. Griggs, T. R., Wagner, G. S., and Gettes, L. S.: Beta-Adrenergic Blocking Agents after Myocardial Infarction: An Undocumented Need in Patients at Lowest Risk, *J. Am. Coll. Cardiol.*, 1:1530, 1983.

528. Meltzer, R. S., Visser, C. A., Kan, G., et al.: Two-Dimensional Echocardiographic Appearance of Left Ventricular Thrombi after Myocardial Infarction, *Am. J. Cardiol.*, 53:1511, 1984.
529. Weinrich, D. J., Burke, J. F., and Pauletto, F. J.: Left Ventricular Mural Thrombi Complicating Acute Myocardial Infarction, *Ann. Intern. Med.*, 100:789, 1984.
530. Sulfinpyrazone in Post-Myocardial Infarction: Report from the Anturane Reinfarction Italian Study, *Lancet*, 1:237, 1982.
531. Palats, L.: Feasibility of Physical Training after Myocardial Infarction and Its Effects on Return to Work for Morbidity and Mortality, *Acta Med. Scand.*, (suppl. 599):7, 1976.
532. Neill, W. A., and Oxendine, J. M.: Exercise Can Promote Coronary Collateral Development without Improving Perfusion of Ischemic Myocardium, *Circulation*, 60:1513, 1979.
533. Phibbs, B.: "Transmural" Versus "Subendocardial" Myocardial Infarction: An Electrocardiographic Myth, *J. Am. Coll. Cardiol.*, 1(2):561, 1983.
534. Norris, R. M., Mercer, C. J., and Yeates, S. E.: Sinus Rate in Acute Myocardial Infarction, *Br. Heart J.*, 34:901, 1972.
535. Crimm, A., Severance, H. W., Jr., Coffey, K., McKinnis, R., Wagner, G. S., and Califf, R. M.: Prognostic Significance of Isolated Sinus Tachycardia during the First Three Days of Acute Myocardial Infarction, *Am. J. Med.*, 76:983, 1984.
536. Rotman, M., Wagner, G. S., and Wallace, A. G. P.: Bradyarrhythmias in Acute Myocardial Infarction, *Circulation*, 45:703, 1972.
537. Pantridge, J. F., Webb, S. W., Adgey, A. A. J., and Geddes, J. S.: The First Hour after the Onset of Acute Myocardial Infarction, in "Progress in Cardiology," Lea & Febiger, Philadelphia, 1974, vol. 3.
538. Wilson, C., and Pantridge, J. F.: ST-Segment Displacement and Early Hospital Discharge in Acute Myocardial Infarction, *Lancet*, 2:1284, 1973.
539. Kent, K. M., Smith, E. R., Redwood, D. R., and Epstein, S. E.: Electrical Stability of Acutely Ischemic Myocardium: Influences of Heart Rate and Vagal Stimulation, *Circulation*, 47:291, 1973.
540. Scherlag, B. J., Kabell, G., Harrison, L., and Lazzara, R.: Mechanisms of Bradycardia-Induced Ventricular Arrhythmias in Myocardial Ischemia and Infarction, *Circulation*, 65:1429, 1982.
541. Adgey, A. A. J., Geddes, J. S., Webb, S. W., Allen, J. P., James, R. G. G., and Zaidi, S. A.: Acute Phase of Myocardial Infarction, *Lancet*, 2:501, 1971.
542. Chadda, K. D., Lichstein, E., Gupta, P. K., and Kourtesis, P.: Effects of Atropine in Patients with Bradyarrhythmia Complicating Myocardial Infarction, *Am. J. Med.*, 63:503, 1977.
543. Hatle, L., Bethen, J., and Tokseth, R.: Sinoatrial Disease in Acute Myocardial Infarction: Long-term Prognosis, *Br. Heart J.*, 38:410, 1976.
544. Parameswara, R., Ohe, T., and Goldberg, H.: Sinus Node Dysfunction in Acute Myocardial Infarction, *Br. Heart J.*, 38:93, 1976.
545. Lesser, L., and Walter, P. F.: Atrial Tachycardia in Acute Myocardial Infarction, *Ann. Intern. Med.*, 86:582, 1977.
546. Liberthson, R. R., Salisbury, K. W., Hutter, A. M., and DeSanctis, R. W.: Atrial Tachyarrhythmias in Acute Myocardial Infarction, *Am. J. Med.*, 60:956, 1976.
547. Julian, D. G., Valentine, P. A., and Miller, G. L.: Disturbances of Rate, Rhythm and Conduction in Acute Myocardial Infarction, *Am. J. Med.*, 37:915, 1964.
548. Cristal, N., Peterburg, I., and Azwarcberg, J.: Atrial Fibrillation Developing in the Acute Phase of Myocardial Infarction: Prognostic Implications, *Chest*, 70:8, 1976.
549. Fishenfeld, J., Desser, K. B., and Benchimol, A.: Nonparoxysmal A-V Junctional Tachycardia Associated with Acute Myocardial Infarction, *Am. Heart J.*, 86:754, 1973.
550. Konecke, L. L., and Knoebel, S. B.: Nonparoxysmal Junctional Tachycardia Complicating Acute Myocardial Infarction, *Circulation*, 45:367, 1972.
551. Gettes, L. S., Hill, J. L., Swito, T., and Kagiyama, Y.: Factors Related to Vulnerability to Arrhythmias in Acute Myocardial Infarction, *Am. Heart J.*, 103:667, 1982.
552. Naito, M., Michelson, E. L., Kaplinsky, E., Dreifus, L. S., David, D., and Blenko, T. M.: Role of Early Cycle Ventricular Extrasystoles in Initiation of Ventricular Tachycardia and Fibrillation: Evaluation of the R-on-T Phenomenon during Acute Ischemia in A Canine Model, *Am. J. Cardiol.*, 49:317, 1982.
553. Lazeara, R., ElSherif, N., Hope, R. R., and Scherlag, B. J.: Ventricular Arrhythmias and Electrophysiological Consequences of Myocardial Ischemia and Infarction, *Circ. Res.*, 42:740, 1978.
554. Wit, A. L., and Bigger, J. T.: Possible Electrophysiological Mechanisms for Lethal Arrhythmias Accompanying Myocardial Ischemia and Infarction, in R. J. Prineas and H. Blackburn (eds.), "Sudden Coronary Death Outside Hospital," *Circulation*, 52(suppl. 3):96, 1975.
555. Campbell, R. W. F., Murray, A., and Julian, D. G.: Ventricular Arrhythmias and Ventricular Fibrillation in Acute Myocardial Infarction, *Am. J. Cardiol.*, 45:462, 1980.
556. Tye, K. H., Samant, A., Desser, K. B., and Benchimol, A.: R on T or R on P Phenomenon? Relation to the Genesis of Ventricular Tachycardia, *Am. J. Cardiol.*, 44:632, 1979.
557. Campbell, R. W. F., Murray, A., and Julian, D. G.: Ventricular Arrhythmias in First 12 Hours of Acute Myocardial Infarction, *Br. Heart J.*, 46:351, 1981.
558. Lie, K. I., Wellens, H. J. J., Downar, E., and Durrer, D.: Observations on Patients with Primary Ventricular Fibrillation Complicating Acute Myocardial Infarction, *Circulation*, 52:755, 1975.
559. El-Sherif, N., Myerburg, R. S., Scherlag, B. J., et al.: Electrocardiographic Antecedents of Primary Ventricular Fibrillation: Value of the R-on-T Phenomenon in Acute Myocardial Infarction, *Br. Heart J.*, 38:415, 1976.
560. Harrison, D. G.: Should Lidocaine be Administered Routinely to All Patients after Acute Myocardial Infarction?, *Circulation*, 58:581, 1978.
561. Lie, K. I., Wellens, H. J., Van Capelle, F. J., and Durrer, D.: Lidocaine in the Prevention of Primary Ventricular Fibrillation, *N. Engl. J. Med.*, 291:1324, 1975.
562. deSoyza, N., Meacham, D., Murphy, M. L., Kane, J. J., Doherty, J. E., and Bissett, J. K.: Evaluation of Warning Arrhythmias before Paroxysmal Ventricular Tachycardia during Acute Myocardial Infarction in Man, *Circulation*, 60:814, 1979.
563. Wellen, H. J. J., Lie, K. I., and Durrer, D.: Further Observations on Ventricular Tachycardia as Studied by Electrical Stimulation on the Heart: Chronic Recurrent Ventricular Tachycardia and Ventricular Tachycardia during Acute Myocardial Infarction, *Circulation*, 49:647, 1974.
564. Taylor, G. J., Crampton, R. S., Gibson, R. S., Stebbins, P. T., Waldman, M. T. G., and Beller, G. A.: Prolonged QT Interval at Onset of Acute Myocardial Infarction in Predicting Early Phase Ventricular Tachycardia, *Am. Heart J.*, 102:16, 1981.
565. Castle, L. (Moderator): Symposium on the Management of Ventricular Dysrhythmias, *Am. J. Cardiol.*, 54(2):1A, 1984.
566. Norris, R. M., and Mercer, C. J.: Significance of Idioventricular Rhythms in Acute Myocardial Infarction, *Prog. Cardiovasc. Dis.*, 16:455, 1974.
567. Sclarovsky, S., Strasberg, B., Fuchs, J., et al.: Multiform Accelerated Idioventricular Rhythm in Acute Myocardial Infarction: Electrocardiographic Characteristics and Response to Verapamil, *Am. J. Cardiol.*, 52:43, 1983.
568. Lichstein, E., Ribas-Meneclier, C., Gupta, P. K., and Chadda, K. D.: Incidence and Description of Accelerated Ventricular Rhythm Complicating Acute Myocardial Infarction, *Am. J. Med.*, 58:192, 1975.
569. deSoyza, N., Bissett, J. K., Kane, J. J., Murphy, M. L., and Doherty, J. E.: Association of Accelerated Idioventricular Rhythm and Paroxysmal Ventricular Tachycardia in Acute Myocardial Infarction, *Am. J. Cardiol.*, 34:667, 1974.
570. Logan, K. R., Mallwaine, W. J., Adgey, A. A. J., and Pan-

tridge, J. F.: Recurrence of Ventricular Fibrillation in Acute Ischemic Heart Disease, *Circulation,* 64:1163, 1981.
571. Conley, M. J., McNeer, J. F., Lee, K. L., Wagner, G. S., and Rosati, R. A.: Cardiac Arrest Complicating Acute Myocardial Infarction: Predictability and Prognosis, *Am. J. Cardiol.,* 39:7, 1977.
572. Lie, K. I., Liem, K. L., Schuilenburg, R. M., David, C. K., and Durrer, D.: Early Identification of Patients Developing Late In-Hospital Ventricular Fibrillation after Discharge from the Coronary Care Unit, *Am. J. Cardiol.,* 41:674, 1978.
573. Haynes, R. E., Chinn, T. L., Copass, M. K., and Cobb, L. A.: Comparison of Bretylium Tosylate and Lidocaine in Management of Out-of-Hospital Ventricular Fibrillation: A Randomized Clinical Trial, *Am. J. Cardiol.,* 48:353, 1981.
574. Scheinman, M. M., Remedios, P., Cheitlin, M. D., et al.: Effects of Antiarrhythmic Drugs on Atrioventricular Conduction in Patients with Acute Myocardial Infarction, *Circulation,* 62(1):20, 1980.
575. Rosen, K. M., Loeb, H. S., Choquimia, R., Sinno, M. Z., Rahimtoola, S. H., and Gunnar, R. M.: Site of Heart Block in Acute Myocardial Infarction, *Circulation,* 42:925, 1970.
576. Massie, B., Scheinman, M. M., Peters, R., Desai, J., Hirschfield, D., and O'Young, J.: Clinical and Electrophysiologic Findings in Patients with Paroxysmal Slowing of the Sinus Rate and Apparent Mobitz Type II Atrioventricular Block, *Circulation,* 58:305, 1978.
577. Tans, A. C., Lie, K. I., and Durrer, D.: Clinical Setting and Prognostic Significance of High Degree Atrioventricular Block in Acute Inferior Myocardial Infarction: A Study of 144 Patients, *Am. Heart J.,* 99:4, 1980.
578. Lie, K. I., Wellens, H. J., Schuilenburg, R. M., Becker, A. E., and Durrer, D.: Factors Influencing Prognosis of Bundle Branch Block Complicating Acute Anteroseptal Infarction: The Value of His Bundle Recordings, *Circulation,* 50:935, 1974.
579. Hindman, M. C., Wagner, G. S., JaRo, M., et al.: The Clinical Significance of Bundle Branch Block Complicating Acute Myocardial Infarction: 1. Clinical Characteristics, Determinants of Mortality, and One-Year Follow-up, *Circulation,* 58:679, 1978.
580. Hindman, M. C., Wagner, G. S., JaRo, M., et al.: The Clinical Significance of Bundle Branch Block Complicating Acute Myocardial Infarction: 2. Indications for Temporary and Permanent Pacemaker Insertion, *Circulation,* 58:589, 1978.
581. Hollander, G., Nadiminti, V., Lichstein, E., Greengart, A., and Sanders, M.: Bundle Branch Block in Acute Myocardial Infarction, *Am. Heart J.,* 105:738, 1983.
582. Haver, R. N. W., Lie, K. I., Liem, K. L., and Durrer, D.: Long-Term Prognosis in Patients with Bundle Branch Block Complicating Acute Anteroseptal Infarction, *Am. J. Cardiol.,* 49:1581, 1982.
583. Buda, A. J., MacDonald, I. L., Dubbin, J. D., Orr, S. A., and Strauss, H. D.: Myocardial Infarction Extension: Prevalence, Clinical Significance, and Problems in Diagnosis, *Am. Heart J.,* 105:744, 1983.
584. Baker, J. T., Bramlet, D. A., Lester, R. M., Harrison, D. G., Roe, C. R., and Cobb, F. R.: Myocardial Infarct Extension: Incidence and Relationship to Survival, *Circulation,* 65:918, 1982.
585. Marmor, A., Geltman, E. M., Schechtman, K., Sobel, B. E., and Roberts, R.: Recurrent Myocardial Infarction: Clinical Predictors and Prognostic Implications, *Circulation,* 66:415, 1982.
586. Forman, R., Cho, S., Factor, S. M., and Kirk, E. S.: Acute Myocardial Infarct Extension into a Previously Preserved Subendocardial Region at Risk in Dogs and Patients, *Circulation,* 67:117, 1983.
587. Rentrop, P., Blanke, H., Karsch, K. R., Kaiser, H., Kostering, H., and Leitz, K.: Selective Intracoronary Thrombolysis in Acute Myocardial Infarction and Unstable Angina Pectoris, *Circulation,* 63:307, 1981.
588. Rogers, W. J., Mantle, J. A., Hood, W. P., Jr., Baxley, W. A., Whitlow, P. L., Reeves, R. C., and Soto, B.: Prospective Randomized Trial of Intravenous and Intracoronary Streptokinase in Acute Myocardial Infarction, *Circulation,* 68:1051, 1983.
589. Curfman, G. D., Heinsimer, J. A., Lozner, E. C., and Fung, H.: Intravenous Nitroglycerin in the Treatment of Spontaneous Angina Pectoris: A Prospective, Randomized Trial, *Circulation,* 67:276, 1983.
590. Williams, D. O., Korr, K. S., Gewirtz, H., and Most, A. S.: The Effect of Intraaortic Balloon Counterpulsation on Regional Myocardial Blood Flow and Oxygen Consumption in the Presence of Coronary Artery Stenosis in Patients with Unstable Angina Pectoris, *Circulation,* 66:593, 1982.
591. Jones, E. L.: Use of the Coronary Bypass Operation in the Treatment of Selected Patients with Myocardial Infarction, in J. W. Hurst (ed.), "Update II: The Heart," McGraw-Hill Book Company, New York, 1980, p. 115.
592. Rigaud, M., Rocha, P., Boschat, J., Farcot, J. C., Bardet, J., and Boudaris, J. P.: Regional Left Ventricular Function Assessed by Contrast Angiography in Acute Myocardial Infarction, *Circulation,* 60:130, 1979.
593. Ohsuzu, F., Boucher, C. A., Newell, J. B., et al.: Relation of Segmental Wall Motion to Global Left Ventricular Function in Acute Myocardial Infarction, *Am. J. Cardiol.,* 51:1275, 1983.
594. Wackers, F. J., Berger, H. J., Weinberg, M. A., and Zaret, R. L.: Spontaneous Changes in Left Ventricular Function Over the First 24 Hours of Acute Myocardial Infarction: Implications for Evaluating Early Therapeutic Interventions, *Circulation,* 66:748, 1982.
595. Marmor, A., Geltman, E. M., Biello, D. R., Sobel, B. E., Siegel, B. A., and Roberts, R.: Functional Response of the Right Ventricle to Myocardial Infarction: Dependence of the Site of Left Ventricular Infarction, *Circulation,* 64:1005, 1981.
596. Kupper, W., Bleifeld, W., Hanrath, P., Mathey, D., and Effert, S.: Left Ventricular Hemodynamics and Function in Acute Myocardial Infarction: Studies during the Acute Phase, Convalescence and Late Recovery, *Am. J. Cardiol.,* 40:900, 1977.
597. Bertrand, M. E., Rosseau, M. F., LaBlanche, J. M., Carre, A. G., and Lekieffre, J. P.: Cineangiographic Assessment of Left Ventricular Function in the Acute Phase of Transmural Infarction, *Am. J. Cardiol.,* 43:472, 1979.
598. Forrester, J. S., Diamond, G. A., and Swan, H. J. C.: Correlative Classification of Clinical and Hemodynamic Function after Acute Myocardial Infarction, *Am. J. Cardiol.,* 39:137, 1977.
599. Leupker, R. V., Caralis, D. G., Voigt, G. C., Burns, R. F., Murphy, L. W., and Warbasse, J. R.: Detection of Pulmonary Edema in Acute Myocardial Infarction, *Am. J. Cardiol.,* 39:146, 1977.
600. Goldenheim, P. D., and Kazemi, H.: Current Concepts: Cardiopulmonary Monitoring of Critically Ill Patients (First of Two Parts), *N. Engl. J. Med.,* 311(11):717, 1984.
601. Goldenheim, P. D., and Kazemi, H.: Current Concepts: Cardiopulmonary Monitoring of Critically Ill Patients (Second of Two Parts), *N. Engl. J. Med.,* 311(11):776, 1984.
602. Swan, H. J. C., Shah, P. K., and Rubin, S.: Role of Vasodilators in the Changing Phase of Acute Myocardial Infarction, *Am. Heart J.,* 103:707, 1982.
603. Ludbrook, P. A., Tietenbrunn, A. J., Reed, F. R., and Sobel, B. E.: Acute Hemodynamic Responses to Sublingual Nifedipine: Dependence on Left Ventricular Function, *Circulation,* 65:489, 1982.
604. Warnowicz, M. A., Parker, H., and Cheitlin, M. D.: Prognosis of Patients with Acute Pulmonary Edema and Normal Ejection Fraction after Acute Myocardial Infarction, *Circulation,* 67:330, 1983.
605. Cohn, J. N.: Vasodilator Therapy: Implications in Acute Myocardial Infarction and Congestive Heart Failure, *Am. Heart J.,* 103:773, 1982.
606. Hockings, B. E. F., Cope, G. D., Clarke, G. M., and Taylor,

R. R.: Randomized Controlled Trial of Vasodilator Therapy after Myocardial Infarction, *Am. J. Cardiol.*, 48:345, 1981.
607. Cohn, J. N., Franciosa, J. A., Francis, G. S., et al.: Effect of Short-Term Infusion of Sodium Nitroprusside on Mortality Rate in Acute Myocardial Infarction Complicated by Left Ventricular Failure, *N. Engl. J. Med.*, 306:1129, 1982.
608. Bussman, W. F., Passek, D., Seidel, W., and Kaltenbach, M.: Reduction of CK and CK-M8 Indexes of Infarct Size by Intravenous Nitroglycerin, *Circulation*, 63:615, 1981.
609. Rabinowitz, B., Tamari, I., Elaza, E., and Neufeld, H. N.: Intravenous Isosorbide Dinitrate in Patients with Refractory Pump Failure and Acute Myocardial Infarction, *Circulation*, 65:771, 1982.
610. Morrison, J., Coromilas, J., Robbins, M., et al.: Digitalis and Myocardial Infarction in Man, *Circulation*, 62:8, 1980.
611. Vatner, S. F., and Baig, H.: Comparison of the Effects of Ouabain and Isoproterenol on Ischemic Myocardium of Conscious Dogs, *Circulation*, 58:654, 1979.
612. Banka, V. S., Yamazaki, H., Agarwal, J. B., Bodenheimer, M. M., and Helfant, R. H.: Effects of Digitalis on Subendocardial and Subepicardial Dysfunction during Acute Ischemia, *Circulation*, 65:1315, 1982.
613. Whitlow, P. L., Rogers, W. J., Smith, L. R., et al.: Enhancement of Left Ventricular Function by Glucose-Insulin-Potassium Infusion in Acute Myocardial Infarction, *Am. J. Cardiol.*, 49:811, 1982.
614. Geddes, J. S., Adgey, A. A. J., and Pantridge, J. F.: Prevention of Cardiogenic Shock, *Am. Heart J.*, 99:243, 1980.
615. Esente, P., Giambartolome, A., Gensini, G., and Dator, C.: Coronary Reperfusion and Bezold-Jarish Reflex (Bradycardia and Hypotension), *Am. J. Cardiol.*, 52:221, 1983.
616. Cohn, J. N.: Right Ventricular Infarction Revisited, *Am. J. Cardiol.*, 43:660, 1979.
617. Cintron, G. B., Hermandez, E., Linares, E., and Aranda, J. M.: Bedside Recognition, Incidence and Clinical Course of Right Ventricular Infarction, *Am. J. Cardiol.*, 47:224, 1981.
618. Klein, H. O., Tordjman, T., Ninio, R., et al.: The Early Recognition of Right Ventricular Infarction: Diagnostic Accuracy of Electrocardiographic V_4R Lead, *Circulation*, 67:558, 1983.
619. Braat, S. H., Brugada, P., DeZwaan, C., Coenegrach, J. M., and Wellers, H. J. J.: Value of Electrocardiogram in Diagnosing Right Ventricular Involvements in Patients with an Acute Inferior Wall Myocardial Infarction, *Br. Heart J.*, 49:368, 1983.
620. Sharpe, D. N., Botvinick, E. H., Shames, D. M., et al.: The Noninvasive Diagnosis of Right Ventricular Infarction, *Circulation*, 57:483, 1978.
621. Lorell, B., Leinbach, R. C., Pohost, G. M., et al.: Right Ventricular Infarction: Clinical Diagnosis and Differentiation from Cardiac Tamponade and Pericardial Constriction, *Am. J. Cardiol.*, 43:465, 1979.
622. Isner, J. M., Fisher, G. P., Del Negro, A. A., and Borer, J. S.: Right Ventricular Infarction with Hemodynamic Decompensation Due to Transient Loss of Active Atrial Augmentation: Successful Treatment with Atrial Pacing, *Am. Heart J.*, 102:792, 1981.
623. Korr, K. S., Levinson, H., Bough, E. W., et al: Tricuspid Valve Replacement for Cardiogenic Shock after Acute Right Ventricular Infarction, *JAMA*, 224(17):1958, 1980.
624. Mikell, F. L., Asinger, R. W., and Hodges, M.: Functional Consequences of Interventricular Septal Involvement in Right Ventricular Infarction: Echocardiographic, Clinical, and Hemodynamic Observations, *Am. Heart J.*, 105:393, 1983.
625. Cutovitz, A. L., Sobel, B. E., and Roberts, R.: Progressive Nature of Myocardial Injury in Selected Patients with Cardiogenic Shock, *Am. J. Cardiol.*, 41:469, 1978.
626. DeWood, M. A., Notske, R. N., Hensler, G. R., et al.: Intra-aortic Balloon Counterpulsation with and without Reperfusion for Myocardial Infarction Shock, *Circulation*, 61:1105, 1980.
627. Raizes, G., Wagner, G. S., and Hackel, D. B.: Instantaneous Nonarrhythmic Cardiac Death in Acute Myocardial Infarction, *Am. J. Cardiol.*, 39:1, 1977.
628. Vincent, J. L., Thijs, L., Weil, M. H., Michaels, S., and Silverberg, R. A.: Clinical and Experimental Studies on Electromechanical Dissociation, *Circulation*, 64:18, 1981.
629. Berman, J., Haffajee, C. I., and Alpert, J. S.: Therapy of Symptomatic Pericarditis after Myocardial Infarction: Retrospective and Prospective Studies of Aspirin, Indomethacin, Prednisone, and Spontaneous Resolution, *Am. Heart J.*, 101:750, 1981.
630. Welin, L., Vedin, A., and Wilhelmsson, C.: Characteristics, Prevalence, and Prognosis of Postmyocardial Infarction Syndrome, *Br. Heart J.*, 50:140, 1983.
631. Emerson, P. A., and Marks, P.: Preventing Thromboembolism after Myocardial Infarction: Effect of Low-Dose Heparin or Smoking, *Br. Med. J.*, 1:18, 1977.
632. Miller, R. R., Lies, J. E., Caretta, R. F., et al.: Prevention of Lower Extremity Venous Thrombosis by Early Mobilization, *Ann. Intern. Med.*, 84:700, 1976.
633. Anticoagulants in Acute Myocardial Infarction: Results of a Cooperative Clinical Trial, *JAMA*, 225:724, 1973.
634. Kakkar, V. V., Corrigan, T. P., and Fossard, D. P.: Prevention of Fatal Postoperative Pulmonary Embolism by Low Doses of Heparin; An International Multicenter Trial, *Lancet*, 2:45, 1975.
635. Bell, W. R., Tomasulo, P. A., Alving, B. M., and Duffy, T. P.: Thrombocytopenia Occurring during the Administration of Heparin: A Prospective Study in 52 Patients, *Ann. Intern. Med.*, 85:155, 1976.
636. Stratton, J. R., Lighty, G. W., Jr., Pearlman, A. S., and Ritchie, J. L.: Detection of Left Ventricular Thrombus by Two-Dimensional Echocardiography: Sensitivity, Specificity, and Causes of Uncertainty, *Circulation*, 66:156, 1981.
637. Hutchins, G. M.: Rupture of the Interventricular Septum Complicating Myocardial Infarction: Pathological Analysis of 10 Patients with Clinically Diagnosed Perforations, *Am. Heart J.*, 97:165, 1979.
638. Schuster, E. H., and Bulkley, B. H.: Expansion of Transmural Infarction: A Pathophysiological Factor in Cardiac Rupture, *Circulation*, 60:1532, 1979.
639. Drobac, M., Gilbert, B., Howard, R., Baigrie, R., and Rakowski, H.: Ventricular Septal Defect after Myocardial Infarction: Diagnosis by Two-Dimensional Contrast Echocardiography, *Circulation*, 67:335, 1983.
640. Mintz, G. S., Victor, M. F., Kotler, M. N., Parry, W. R., and Segal, B. L.: Two-Dimensional Echocardiographic Identification of Surgically Corrective Complications of Acute Myocardial Infarction, *Circulation*, 64:91, 1981.
641. Radford, M. J., Johnson, R. A., Duggett, W. M., Jr., Fallon, J. T., Buckley, M. J., Gold, H. K., and Leinbach, R. C.: Ventricular Septal Rupture: A Review of Clinical and Physiologic Features and an Analysis of Survival, *Circulation*, 64:545, 1981.
642. Grose, R., and Spindola, Franco H.: Right Ventricular Dysfunction in Acute Ventricular Septal Rupture, *Am. Heart J.*, 101:67, 1981.
642a. Clements, S. D., Jr., Story, W. E., Hurst, J. W., Craver, J. M., and Jones, E. L.: Ruptured Papillary Muscle, A Complication of Myocardial Infarction: Clinical Presentation, Diagnosis, and Treatment, *Clin. Cardiol.*, 8(no. 2):93, 1985.
643. Nishimura, R. A., Schaff, H. V., Shub, C., Gersh, B. J., Edwards, W. D., and Tajik, A. M.: Papillary Muscle Rupture Complicating Acute Myocardial Infarction: Analysis of 17 Patients, *Am. J. Cardiol.*, 51:373, 1983.
644. Bates, R. J., Beutler, S., Resnekov, L., and Anagnostopoulos, C. E.: Cardiac Rupture—Challenge in Diagnosis and Management, *Am. J. Cardiol.*, 40:429, 1977.
645. Cobbs, B. W., Jr., Hatcher, C. R., Jr., and Robinson, P. H.: Cardiac Rupture: Three Operations with Two Long-Term Survivals, *JAMA*, 223:532, 1973.
646. Cohn, L. H.: Surgical Management of Acute and Chronic

Cardiac Mechanical Complications Due to Myocardial Infarction, *Am. Heart J.*, 102:1049, 1981.
647. Hackett, T. P., Cassem, N. H., and Wishnie, H. A.: Detection and Treatment of Anxiety in the Coronary Care Unit, *Am. Heart J.*, 78:727, 1969.
648. Hackett, T. P., Cassem, N. H., and Wishnie, H. A.: The Coronary Care Unit: An Appraisal of Its Psychological Hazards, *N. Engl. J. Med.*, 279:1365, 1968.
649. Graboys, T. B., Lown, B., Podrid, P. J., and DeSilva, R.: Long-Term Survival of Patients with Malignant Ventricular Arrhythmia Treated with Antiarrhythmic Drugs, *Am. J. Cardiol.*, 50:437, 1982.
650. Horowitz, L. N., Josephson, M. E., Farshidi, A., Spielman, S. R., Michelson, E. L., and Greenspan, A. M.: Recurrent Sustained Ventricular Tachycardia: 3. Role of the Electrophysiologic Study in Selection of Antiarrhythmic Regimens, *Circulation*, 58:986, 1978.
651. Swerdlow, C. D., Winkle, R. A., and Mason, J. W.: Determinants of Survival in Patients with Ventricular Tachyarrhythmias, *N. Engl. J. Med.*, 308:1436, 1983.
652. Horowitz, L. N., Josephson, M. E., and Kastor, J. A.: Intracardiac Electrophysiologic Studies as a Method for the Optimation of Drug Therapy in Chronic Recurrent Ventricular Arrhythmia, *Prog. Cardiovasc. Dis.*, 23:81, 1980.
653. Ruskin, J. N., DiMarco, J. P., and Garan, H.: Out-of-Hospital Cardiac Arrest: Electrophysiologic Observations and Selection of Long-Term Antiarrhythmic Therapy, *N. Engl. J. Med.*, 303:607, 1980.
654. Klein, H., Karp, R. P., Kouchovkos, N. T., Zorn, G. L., Jr., James, T. N., and Waldo, A. L.: Intraoperative Electrophysiologic Mapping of the Ventricles during Sinus Rhythm in Patients with a Previous Myocardial Infarction, *Circulation*, 66:817, 1982.
655. Horowitz, L. N., Harken, A. H., Kastor, J. A., and Josephson, M. E.: Ventricular Resection Guided by Epicardial and Endocardial Mapping for Treatment of Recurrent Ventricular Tachycardia, *N. Engl. J. Med.*, 302:589, 1980.
656. Mason, J. W., Stinson, E. B., Winkle, R. A., Griffin, J. C., Oyer, P. E., Ross, D. L., and Derby, G.: Surgery for Ventricular Tachycardia: Efficacy of Left Ventricular Aneurysm Resection Compared with Operation Guided by Electrical Activation Mapping, *Circulation*, 65:1148, 1982.
657. Fisher, J. D., Mehra, R., and Furman, S.: Termination of Ventricular Tachycardia with Bursts of Rapid Ventricular Pacing, *Am. J. Cardiol.*, 41:94, 1978.
658. Reid, P. R., Mirowski, M., Mower, M. M., et al.: Clinical Evaluation of the Internal Automatic Cardioverter-Defibrillator in Survivors of Sudden Cardiac Death, *Am. J. Cardiol.*, 51:1608, 1983.
659. Ruberman, W., Weinblatt, E., Goldberg, J. D., Frank, C. W., Chaudhary, B. S., and Shapiro, S.: Ventricular Premature Complexes and Sudden Death after Myocardial Infarction, *Circulation*, 64:297, 1981.
660. Weaver, W. D., Cobb, L. A., and Hallstrom, A. P.: Ambulatory Arrhythmias in Resuscitated Victims of Cardiac Arrest, *Circulation*, 66:212, 1982.
661. Manger, C. V., Lie, K. I., Van Capelle, F. J. L., and Durrer, D.: Limitations of 24 Hour Ambulatory Electrocardiographic Recording in Predicting Coronary Events after Acute Myocardial Infarction, *Am. J. Cardiol.*, 44:1257, 1979.
662. Hamer, A., Vohra, J., Hunt, D., and Stoman, G.: Prediction of Sudden Death by Electrophysiologic Studies in High Risk Patients Surviving Acute Myocardial Infarction, *Am. J. Cardiol.*, 50:223, 1982.
663. Morganroth, J., Michelson, E. L., Horowitz, L. N., Josephson, M. E., Pearlman, A. S., and Dunkman, W. B.: Limitations of Routine Long-Term Electrocardiographic Monitoring to Assess Ventricular Ectopic Frequency, *Circulation*, 58:408, 1978.
664. Velebit, V., Podrid, P., Lown, B., Cohen, B. H., and Graboys, T. B.: Aggravation and Provocation of Ventricular Arrhythmias by Antiarrhythmic Drugs, *Circulation*, 65:886, 1982.
665. Walter, P. F.: Arrhythmias Related to Abnormal Repolarization, in J. W. Hurst (ed.), "Update I: The Heart," McGraw-Hill Book Company, New York, 1979, p. 305.
666. Califf, R. M., Burks, J. M., Behar, V. S., Margolis, J. R., and Wagner, G. S.: Relationships among Ventricular Arrhythmias, Coronary Artery Disease, and Angiographic and Electrocardiographic Indicators of Myocardial Fibrosis, *Circulation*, 57:725, 1978.
667. Kleiger, R. E., Miller, J. P., Thanavaro, S., Province, M. A., Martin, T. F., and Oliver, G. C.: Relationship between Clinical Features of Acute Myocardial Infarction and Ventricular Runs 2 Weeks to 1 year after Infarction, *Circulation*, 63:64, 1981.
668. Battler, A., Ross, J., Jr., Slutsky, R., Pfisterer, M., Ashburn, W., and Froelicher, V.: Improvement of Exercise-Induced Left Ventricular Dysfunction with Oral Propranolol in Patients with Coronary Heart Disease, *Am. J. Cardiol.*, 44:319, 1979.
669. Hockman, J. S., Platia, E. B., and Bulkley, B. H.: Endocardial Abnormalities in Left Ventricular Aneurysms: A Clinicopathologic Study, *Ann. Intern. Med.*, 100:29, 1984.
670. Rogers, W. J., Oberman, A., and Kouchoukos, N. T.: Left Ventricular Aneurysmectomy in Patients with Single Vs. Multivessel Coronary Artery Disease, *Circulation*, 58(suppl. 1):1–50, 1978.
671. Burton, N. A., Stinson, E. B., Oyer, P. E., and Shumway, N. E.: Left Ventricular Aneurysm: Preoperative Risk Factors and Long-Term Postoperative Results, *J. Thorac. Cardiovasc. Surg.*, 77:65, 1979.
672. Lichstein, E. Arsvra, E., Hollander, G., Greengart, A., and Sanders, M.: Current Incidence of Postmyocardial Infarction (Dressler's) Syndrome, *Am. J. Cardiol.*, 50:1269, 1982.
673. Kossowsky, W. A., Lyon, A. F., and Spain, D. M.: Reappraisal of the Postmyocardial Infarction Dressler's Syndrome, *Am. Heart J.*, 102:954, 1981.
674. Stern, M. J., Pascale, L., and Ackerman, A.: Life Adjustment Postmyocardial Infarction, *Arch. Intern. Med.*, 137:1680, 1977.
675. Veith, R. C., Raskind, M. A., Caldwell, J. H., Bornes, R. F., Gumbrecht, G., and Ritchie, J. L.: Cardiovascular Effects of Tricyclic Antidepressants in Depressed Patients with Chronic Heart Disease, *N. Engl. J. Med.*, 306:954, 1982.
676. Balady, G. J., Weiner, D. A., McCabe, C. H., and Ryan, T. J.: Value of Arm Exercise Testing in Detecting Coronary Artery Disease, *Am. J. Cardiol.*, 55(no. 1):37, 1985.

46

Coronary Artery Spasm

D. Gregg Hopkins, M.D.   Donald C. Harrison, M.D.

Approximately 75 years ago William Osler suggested that "spasm or narrowing of a coronary artery, or even of one branch, may so modify the action of a section of the heart that it works with disturbed tension, and there are stretching and strain sufficient to arouse painful sensations."[1] This description, though not the first to mention coronary artery spasm, is representative of early explanations of angina pectoris. However, as pathological studies in the 1930s and 1940s revealed the prevalence of coronary atherosclerosis the concept of arteries as rigid tubes with fixed, obstructive atheromata gained favor, and investigations of myocardial ischemia and angina pectoris focused almost entirely on the myocardial oxygen demand side of the oxygen supply-and-demand equation. In 1959, though, Prinzmetal reported on a group of patients whose angina occurred at rest and was associated with transient, cyclic ST-segment elevation.[2] Termed *variant angina,* this newly appreciated syndrome was thought to be secondary to "temporary occlusion of a large diseased artery with a narrow lumen due to a normal increase in tonus of the vessel wall." Subsequently, this coronary artery spasm has been observed angiographically and shown to reproduce symptoms of angina pectoris and electrocardiographic signs of ischemia in selected patients. A decrement in coronary sinus blood flow corresponding to decreased myocardial oxygen delivery has also been documented during these episodes and precedes any increase in metabolic demand of the myocardium, thus verifying spasm as the primary event.

It is now appreciated that coronary artery spasm plays a much broader role in coronary heart disease than simply an explanation for the relatively uncommon variant angina syndrome. Dynamic coronary tone coupled with varying degrees of fixed atherosclerosis creates a spectrum of clinical manifestations of ischemia.[3] At one extreme of this spectrum is the patient with severe fixed atherosclerotic coronary obstruction, in whom any increase in myocardial oxygen consumption outstrips the supply capability of the coronary artery; vascular tone may become manifest clinically as the appearance of unstable angina. At the other extreme is the syndrome of variant angina with normal coronaries, in which spasm plays a virtually pathognomonic role and can even lead to myocardial infarction and death. Most patients, though, are between these two extremes, having fixed atherosclerotic coronary lesions yet widely varying anginal thresholds. Nonocclusive epicardial coronary spasm may occur to a degree which, though not leading to ischemia at rest, could exhaust the ability of the smaller, autoregulatory "resistance" coronary vessels to respond to increased myocardial oxygen requirements once exertion begins.[4]

Coronary artery spasm can now be recognized as *a reversible focal reduction in coronary artery diameter leading to myocardial ischemia.* This definition excludes "catheter-induced" spasm, which typically occurs in 1 to 2 percent of patients undergoing coronary arteriography and involves the proximal coronary arterial segment adjacent to the catheter tip but generally produces no symptomatic or electrocardiographic evidence of ischemia. It also excludes the diffuse coronary constriction of up to 20 percent of vessel diameter characteristic of the normal response to ergonovine administration.

Physiologic Mechanisms of Coronary Artery Spasm

Vascular Smooth-Muscle Behavior

The cause of coronary artery spasm is not known, but much has been learned in the laboratory about coronary smooth-muscle physiology which is helping to explain some aspects of clinical vasospasm. Most importantly, normal arteries are not immobile conduits. Spontaneous rhythmic activity has been recorded in many isolated arterial samples; human coronary arteries contract at rapid cycle lengths of 60 to 80 ms.[5] Numerous pharmacologic agents that enhance the force of this rhythmic contractility include norepinephrine, acetylcholine, histamine, serotonin, prostaglandins, and ergonovine. Nitroglycerin and calcium channel blockers, on the other hand, inhibit the activity.

This rhythmic motion appears to be related to intracellular calcium concentration (Fig. 46-1). It has long been felt that in vascular smooth muscle, as opposed to cardiac and skeletal muscle, the influx of extracellular calcium plays the major role in excitation. Membrane "channels" which allow this influx of calcium are considered to be opened by two mechanisms: (1) depolarization, with activation of *potential-dependent* channels, and (2) binding of pharmacologic or hormonal agents to receptors. Once the intracellular calcium concentration reaches a critical level the calcium molecule combines with calmodulin, an inactive subunit of the enzyme myosin light chain kinase (MLCK). This calcium-calmodulin complex then binds with MLCK to activate the enzyme for phosphorylation of myosin. The resultant

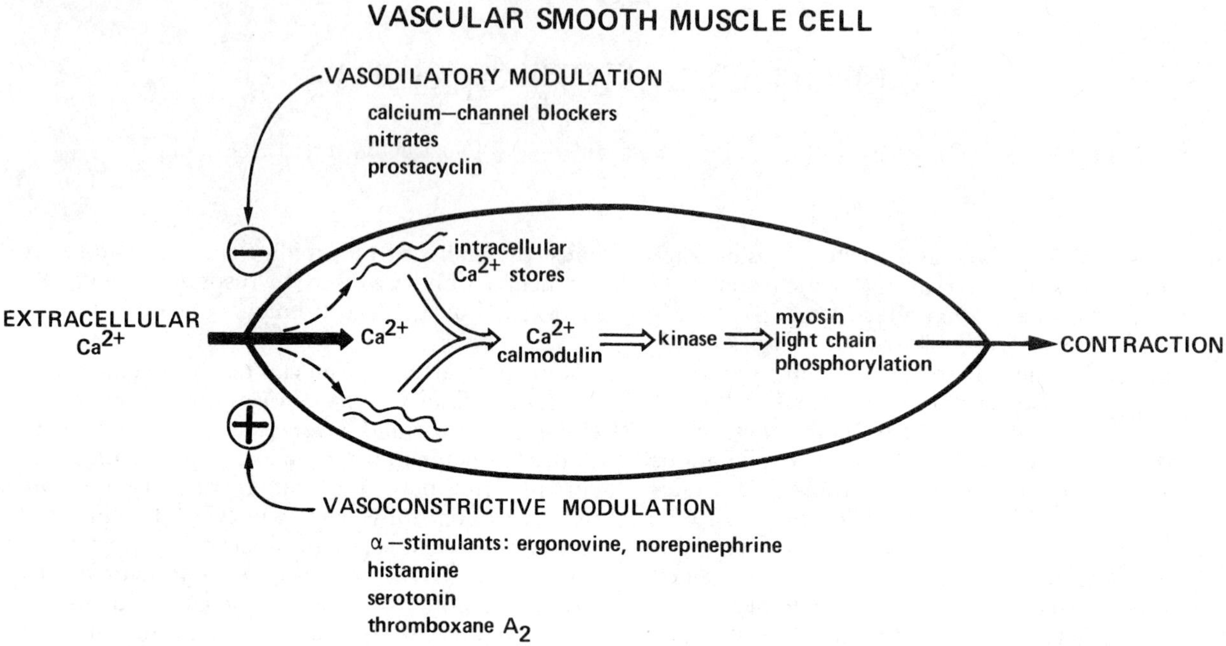

FIGURE 46-1 The role of extracellular and intracellular calcium in vascular smooth-muscle contraction is shown (see text). Agents which directly or indirectly lead to vasodilatation are calcium channel blockers, nitroglycerin, and prostacyclin. Vasoconstrictors include alpha-adrenergic agonists, histamine, serotonin and thromboxane A_2. (*From L. H. Opie, "The Heart: Physiology, Metabolism, Pharmacology, and Therapy," Grune & Stratton, New York, 1984. Reproduced with permission from the publisher and author.*)

interaction with actin initiates contraction of the muscle elements. Work in human coronary artery segments obtained at the time of heart transplantation has revealed a significant role not only for extracellular calcium influx but also for release of intracellular calcium stores with receptor-mediated activation.[6] These intracellular calcium stores are utilized to different degrees by various hormonal and pharmacologic agents. One hypothesis explaining coronary artery spasm is that these intracellular calcium stores are increased in amount at the site of the hypercontractility or are more sensitive to release by extracellular triggering mechanisms.

Causes of Abnormal Vascular Smooth-Muscle Contractility

An association between coronary reactivity and *atherosclerosis* has long been observed. Indeed, clinical spasm of truly normal coronary arteries is uncommon, accounting for only 10 percent of one group of patients with variant angina.[7] In animal studies, a high-cholesterol diet sensitizes vascular smooth muscle to the vasoconstricting effects of ergonovine and increases membrane receptor density to other hormonal agents.[8] Moreover, atherosclerotic segments of human arteries are deficient in prostacyclin production, which could lead to unopposed vasoconstriction and platelet aggregation.[9] Other animal studies indicate that spasm may play a part in the late development of atherosclerosis; a high-cholesterol diet, for example, leads to fixed atherosclerotic lesions only if repeated mechanical constriction is applied or a drug such as vasopressin is administered.[10]

Endogenous *adrenergic influences* play a role in coronary spasm, but probably not a major one. Although alpha-adrenergic blocking agents, such as phentolamine and phenoxybenzamine, can acutely reverse spontaneous or ergonovine-induced coronary spasm, they are not useful in the chronic prevention of such episodes. In addition, normal catecholamine levels have been measured before and during episodes of spasm, with elevated levels appearing only after the onset of ischemia.[11] Furthermore, surgical denervation alone is not effective in preventing coronary spasm, and one patient with spasm occurring in the transplanted heart has been reported. *Parasympathetic agents,* such as methacholine, can also cause coronary vasoconstriction. Their effect is reproducible in vitro but the clinical importance of this mode of coronary spasm is uncertain.

Histamine and *serotonin* are two other agents with pronounced vasoconstricting effects when studied in isolated human coronary artery segments. The highest receptor density for both agents is found in the most proximal portions of the artery segments, where spasm is most commonly observed. Clinically, histamine has produced chest pain and ST-segment elevation in a small number of patients with atypical angina.[12] The serotonin receptor may effect the vasoconstriction seen with ergonovine, for cyproheptadine, an antagonist of the receptor, blocks the action of ergonovine.[13]

The role of *prostaglandins* in the etiology of coronary spasm is not clear. Though episodes of spasm are associated with increased levels of a metabolite of thromboxane A_2 (a prostaglandin which promotes vasoconstriction and platelet aggregation), it is not certain whether this increase precedes ischemia or is secondarily released. In either case, inhibition of prostaglandin synthesis with indomethacin or aspirin can effectively lower thromboxane A_2 metabolites to negligible levels, but ischemic episodes are not prevented.[14]

The well-described circadian patterns of ischemic pain in the variant angina syndrome may be a result of differing metabolic rates throughout the day, resulting in varying *hydrogen ion* concentrations. This could change the degree of calcium channel blockade caused by the hydrogen ion and potentially lead to differences in vasomotor tone in susceptible individuals. Indeed, hyperventilation and TRIS-buffer infusion can produce coronary spasm, presumably through the same mechanism.[15] Though *vasopressin* can cause coronary spasm in pharmacologic doses little is known about its endogenous role.

Clinical Presentations

Variant Angina

As distinguished from classic effort-related angina pectoris, the characteristic feature of variant angina is the occurrence of chest pain at rest, often in a cyclic or predictable pattern, associated with transient ST-segment elevation. Though variant angina is now appreciated to be just one manifestation of coronary spasm, this description is still accurate.

The character of the chest pain—a substernal pressure or tightness which may extend to the jaw, neck, or arm—is identical to that of classic angina. Though it resolves after sublingual nitroglycerin, it may not do so for 20 to 30 min; often more nitrates are required to relieve the pain than are needed with exertional angina.[16] Frequently the anginal episodes are cyclic in nature, recurring at the same time of day, often awakening the patient in the early morning. The disease activity can vary such that multiple daily attacks may occur for a period of time followed by a pain-free interval of several weeks. Often associated with the chest discomfort is dyspnea, probably secondary to the acute rise in left ventricular filling pressure due to the transient ischemia. Syncope, from heart block or tachyarrhythmias, may also be a presenting symptom. Heart block is usually seen with ischemic changes in the inferior leads, whereas ventricular arrhythmias occur in about half of ischemic episodes regardless of the site of spasm.

During an attack of variant angina the electrocardiogram (ECG) usually demonstrates ST-segment elevation similar to the early recordings of an acute myocardial infarction. This is secondary to transmural ischemia caused by transient total occlusion of a large coronary artery (Fig. 46-2). Although ST-segment elevation has long been considered the sine qua non of variant angina, ST-segment depression is just as common.[17] ST-segment depression and elevation may be recorded in the same patient in different anginal attacks or even during the same episode. The ST-segment depression represents subendocardial ischemia and can be secondary to subtotal spasm, involvement of small branch vessels, or the presence of collateral channels from uninvolved arteries. These ST-segment changes may be associated with peaking of T waves or pseudonormalization of inverted T waves. Transient Q waves, an increase in R-wave voltage, and the appearance of inverted U waves in the ischemic region have also been described.[17]

A controversial subject is whether an association exists between coronary artery spasm and systemic disorders characterized by vasospasm. There is evidence that migraine headaches and Raynaud's phenomenon occur with greater frequency in patients with variant angina, but the anginal attacks are generally not temporally related to the headache or digital spasm.[18] Coronary artery spasm has also been implicated in eclampsia and progressive systemic sclerosis, but a precise relation remains to be demonstrated.

Unstable Angina

The term *unstable angina* has long included such manifestations of ischemic heart disease as the new onset of angina and a change in the pattern of a patient's angina. A frequent clinical situation, however, is the patient with repeated episodes of angina at rest associated with ST-segment depression. Although the classical teaching is that these episodes are caused by an increase in myocardial oxygen consumption in the setting of severe coronary artery narrowing, much evidence argues against this view.[19] Hemodynamic and electrocardiographic monitoring in the setting of rest angina has frequently documented a decrement in coronary flow with ST-segment depression as the primary event; heart rate and blood pressure often rise minutes later, generally corresponding with the onset of anginal pain. A transient reduction in coronary blood flow, then, underlies at least this subset of patients with rest pain, though in other patients with unstable angina myocardial oxygen consumption plays the major role.

Effort-Related Angina

Most patients with variant angina have a normal exercise capacity, yet in some, typical chest pain and ST-segment changes can be precipitated by treadmill exercise. Provocation of coronary artery spasm with supine bicycle exercise has also been documented angiographically. The anginal threshold in these patients varies widely and appears to correlate with the baseline activity of the disease process.[20] That is, exercise is more likely to precipitate an anginal episode during a period when frequent spon-

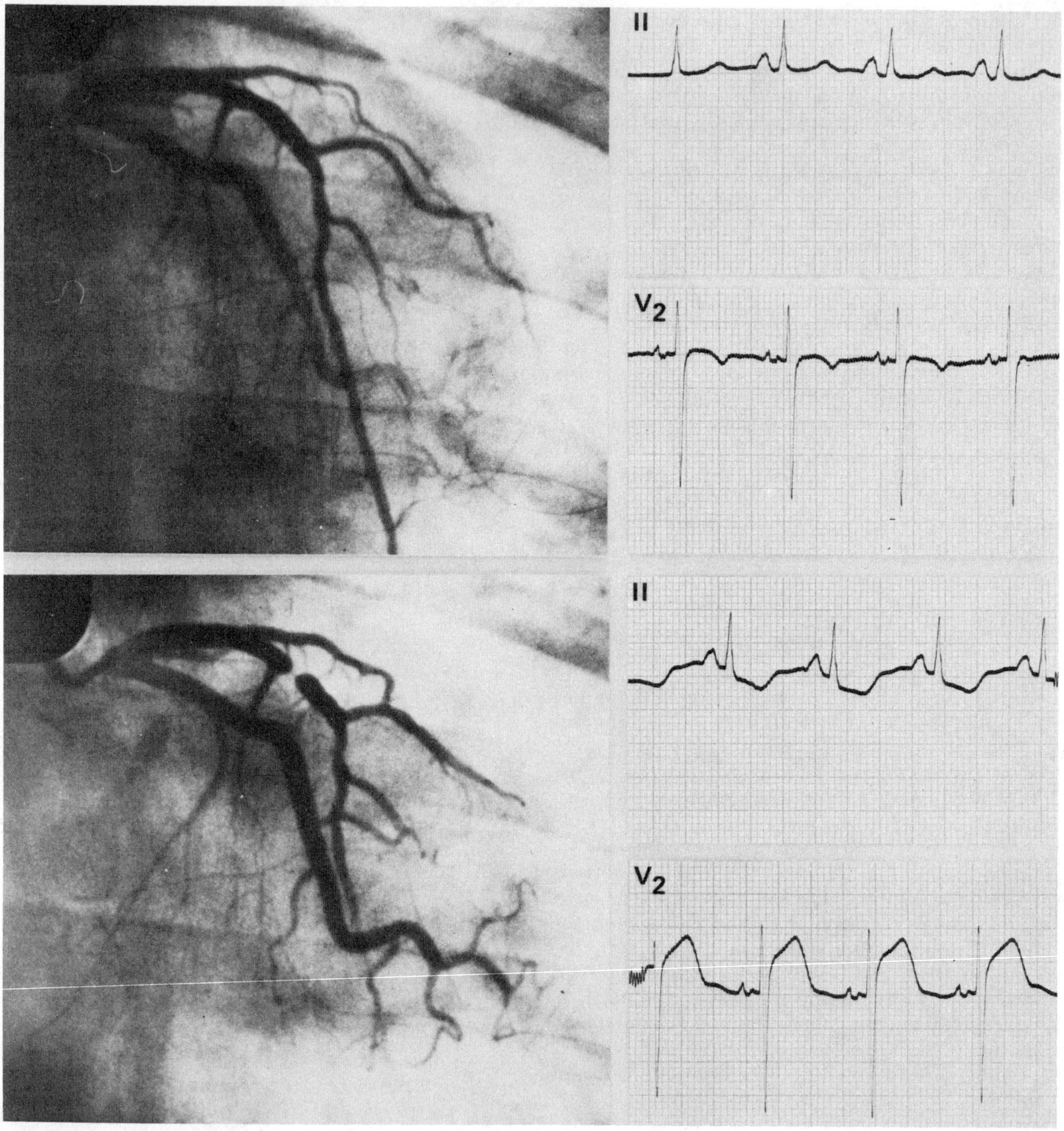

FIGURE 46-2 Coronary artery spasm is demonstrated by left coronary artery contrast medium injection and ECG leads II and V_2 before (*top panel*) and during (*bottom panel*) a spontaneous episode of chest pain. This 40-year-old woman developed frequent episodes of variant angina following an initial episode of chest pain associated with ventricular fibrillation. Therapy with the calcium channel blocker diltiazem resulted in nearly complete prophylaxis of subsequent episodes of variant angina.

taneous attacks of spasm are occurring. There has also been a circadian pattern described, with exercise inducing ST-segment elevation if performed during the morning but not in the afternoon.[21]

In patients with fixed atherosclerotic coronary disease and classic effort-related angina, spasm has also been proposed as an explanation for day-to-day changes in anginal thresholds and "walk-through" phenomena (the early onset of angina during exercise which resolves despite continued exertion).[22] One hypothesis is that minor increments in coronary artery tone could occur which, though not leading to ischemia at rest, significantly alter coronary vascular resistance. Thus, the ischemic threshold during a particular activity would depend not only on the degree of myocardial oxygen consumption but also on changes in the coronary flow response.

Myocardial Infarction

Patients with the variant angina syndrome uncommonly develop myocardial infarction, with those having severe coronary stenoses superimposed on spasm appearing to be most susceptible. Myocardial infarction in the setting of normal coronary arteries is a rare yet recognized finding. Although no definitive evidence of coronary spasm inducing myocardial infarction has been shown, several observations suggest a causative role: (1) infarction has occurred in munitions workers with normal coronary arteries when chronic exposure to nitroglycerin is interrupted,[23] (2) rarely, catheter-induced spasm has led to myocardial damage, and (3) refractory vasospasm in response to ergonovine or vasopressin has been shown to result in myocardial infarction.

The role of spasm in typical myocardial infarction in the setting of atherosclerosis is controversial. Angiographic studies in patients following myocardial infarction have demonstrated that total coronary occlusion is progressively less common the later after infarction the arteriography is performed.[24] Moreover, acute administration of thrombolytic agents shows a high incidence of subtotal stenoses in the vessel supplying the infarcted area once the thrombus has been lysed. This suggests that some process other than obliteration of the coronary lumen with atheroma converts a stenosis to a total occlusion. Circumstantial evidence that this process includes vasoconstriction is the high incidence of observed and inducible coronary spasm both in patients with rest angina who later go on to infarct and in patients immediately after infarction.[25] The vessel in which spasm can be induced is usually the same artery that is involved in the infarction. A likely explanation of myocardial infarction, then, includes not only the interplay of platelet aggregation, thrombus formation, and atheromatous plaque rupture, but also arterial spasm. Yet whether spasm plays a predominantly causative or secondary role in acute infarction needs further study.

Natural History

Although serious complications occur in patients with variant angina, the mortality in most studies remains less than 10 percent.[26] The greatest risk of myocardial infarction and death is in the first month after symptoms begin.[27] This may reflect the impact made by later therapy or be a manifestation of the active stage of the disease. The incidence of myocardial infarction accompanying spasm is clearly highest in those patients with multivessel coronary stenoses. On the other hand, sudden death in patients with the variant angina syndrome is not related to the degree of coronary atherosclerosis. Patients dying suddenly usually, however, have had serious arrhythmias during earlier episodes of spasm, including ventricular fibrillation and tachycardia, high-grade heart block, and asystole.[28] The occurrence of these arrhythmias identifies a subset of patients at particularly high risk of sudden death and should prompt aggressive therapy.

Roughly half of patients with the variant angina syndrome, regardless of the degree of coronary atherosclerosis, experience a spontaneous remission in their disease.[29] This remission frequently occurs within 6 to 12 months after the onset of symptoms and can persist for several years. After a prolonged symptom-free interval, those whose anginal episodes will subside even after withdrawal of medications can be identified by normalization of the ergonovine challenge test. Because the variant angina syndrome is characterized by variations in disease activity, however, careful follow-up is necessary to monitor the duration of this frequently observed clinical remission.

Diagnosis

Spontaneous Episodes of Spasm

A careful history provides the major clues for a diagnosis of variant angina. Documentation of the ECG changes, however, is essential for proper management. On an outpatient basis, the approach will vary depending on the frequency of attacks in the individual patient. If chest pain episodes occur more than once daily, two-lead ambulatory ECG monitoring is useful. Reporting symptoms in a diary or activating the "event marker" on the recording device is important to correlate chest pain with ECG abnormalities. Many brief, asymptomatic ST-segment shifts are recorded in patients with variant angina, suggesting that only prolonged ischemic episodes result in anginal symptoms.

In those with less frequent attacks of pain, transtelephonic ECG monitoring is often helpful.[30] Patients are advised to wear electrodes at all times and simply attach the portable transmitting device during a symptomatic episode. The rhythm strip may then be transmitted to a recording device, using any available telephone, and compared to baseline tracings at a subsequent date. This method extends the monitoring period up to several weeks and facilitates diagnosis in patients with unpredictable and infrequent episodes.

Ergonovine Provocation

Ergonovine maleate, an ergot alkaloid, is a potent smooth-muscle constrictor. It is used to provoke coronary artery spasm when the diagnosis cannot be made during spontaneous episodes of chest pain. Administration of ergonovine is successful at inducing spasm in greater than 90 percent of patients with the true variant angina syndrome. Alternatively, less than 5 percent of patients with atypical chest pain or only effort-related angina have a positive test.[31] Although a small number of patients have been reported with refractory coronary spasm and death following ergonovine administration, this has usually been secondary to the use of excessively high initial or total doses of the drug and delay in using intravenous or intracoronary nitroglycerin to reverse the spasm.[32]

Conti et al.[26] list as contraindications to the test: (1) acute myocardial infarction, (2) uncontrolled chest pain, (3) uncontrolled ventricular arrhythmias, (4) severe hypertension, (5) severe left ventricular dysfunction, (6) severe aortic stenosis, (7) significant left main coronary artery disease, and (8) suspected pregnancy. Stenosis of 90 percent or greater in a major coronary artery is considered a relative contraindication. Ergonovine can safely be given to patients with less severe fixed obstructive disease when the degree of coronary narrowing is insufficient to explain the patient's symptoms.

At Stanford University a positive test requires reproduction of the patient's chest pain, ST-segment elevation or depression, and focal narrowing of a coronary artery of any significant degree (Table 46-1). Diffuse coronary constriction of less than 20 percent luminal diameter occurs in most patients and is not accompanied by chest pain or evidence of myocardial ischemia; this is considered a normal response to ergonovine.[33]

Ergonovine testing can be performed in the coronary care unit in patients with coronary arteries previously documented to be normal, if the clinical history excludes syncope or dizziness suggestive of serious arrhythmias or heart block accompanying the spasm. The same protocol is used, and a positive test is defined as chest pain associated with 1-mm ST-segment elevation or depression. Outpatient testing is as safe and sensitive as testing performed in the catheterization laboratory[34] but should not be done without intravenous nitroglycerin available.

TABLE 46-1 Ergonovine Provocation Protocol

1. No nitrates or calcium channel blockers for at least 12 h prior to test.
2. Prepare ergonovine and nitroglycerin in 10-ml syringes:
   Ergotrate*—mix 2 ampules (0.2 mg each) in 8 ml saline solution for final concentration of 50 μg/ml.
   nitroglycerin—mix 2 tablets (0.4 mg each) in 8 ml saline solution for final concentration of 100 μg/ml. Inject through Millipore† filter.
3. Obtain baseline 12-lead ECG and coronary arteriograms; leave coronary catheter in ostium of coronary artery with suspected involvement, if known.
4. Doses of intravenous Ergotrate:
   First: 1 ml (50 μg)
   ECG after $2\frac{1}{2}$ min
   coronary arteriogram after 3 min
   Second: 2 ml (100 μg)
   ECG after $2\frac{1}{2}$ min
   coronary arteriogram after 3 min
   Third: 5 ml (250 μg)
   ECG after 3 min
   coronary arteriogram after 5 min
   coronary arteriogram of opposite coronary artery
5. Stop test as soon as angina, ST-segment changes, or *focal* coronary spasm occurs. Obtain arteriogram of opposite coronary artery immediately if first coronary arteriogram is negative.
6. Administer sublingual, intravenous, or intracoronary nitroglycerin as soon as spasm is documented.

*Eli Lilly and Co.
†Milex®—GI, Millipore Corp., Bedford, MA.

Treatment

The goals of therapy for coronary artery spasm are to reduce the frequency of anginal attacks and to prevent the serious complications of myocardial infarction and death. The mainstays of treatment, nitrates and calcium channel blockers, rarely fail to accomplish these goals. These two drugs have comparable safety and efficacy, and differ mainly in their dosage, side effects, and suitability to the individual patient. For the 10 percent of patients who do not respond to these agents, beta-adrenergic blockers or a combined medical and surgical approach may be necessary. Surgical treatment in general, however, has shown poor results as compared with the success of bypass grafting for effort-related angina. Little is known about the effects of percutaneous transluminal coronary angioplasty on vasospastic coronary arteries associated with some degree of fixed obstruction, but preliminary results are discouraging.[35]

Nitroglycerin

Sublingual nitroglycerin is successful at terminating most episodes of coronary spasm. In some patients with variant angina, though, relief of pain may take several minutes or higher doses than is the case with exertional angina. Long-acting oral preparations, ointment, and sustained-release patches are also very effective in prophylaxis of chest pain episodes. The major side effects, which can be intolerable to some patients, are headaches and orthostatic hypotension.

When terminating ergonovine-induced coronary spasm, intravenous or intracoronary nitroglycerin is often necessary and should be readily available. Spasm in the immediate postbypass setting, though rare, may also be refractory to all but intravenous or intracoronary administration of nitroglycerin.[36]

Calcium Channel Blockers

These agents are as effective as nitrates at prevention of anginal episodes and may work to prevent myocardial infarction and sudden death as well.[37] The three agents available for use in the United States are nifedipine, verapamil, and diltiazem. These drugs are equivalent in their efficacy and differ mainly in their side effects. For complete elimination of anginal episodes, combined therapy with nitrates and calcium channel blockers is usually necessary.

Nifedipine may be administered orally (30 to 180 mg/day) or sublingually (by puncturing the oral capsule). It is very effective in decreasing the frequency of anginal attacks and is usually better tolerated than nitrates. Nifedipine often causes pedal edema unrelated to heart failure and may also result in reflex tachycardia. This latter effect may require concurrent use of beta-adrenergic blockers in patients with predominantly fixed obstructive coronary disease. No depression of the conduction system or ventricular function occurs with nifedipine.

Verapamil can be given orally (120 to 480 mg/day) or intravenously (in 5-mg increments) and is also effective against coronary artery spasm. A major effect of this drug is suppression of AV node conduction, making it useful in the treatment of AV nodal reentry supraventricular tachycardia and control of the ventricular response to atrial fibrillation and flutter. Beta-adrenergic blockers must be used cautiously in combination with verapamil, as the combined effects on the conduction system and ventricular function can be significant.

Diltiazem is available only as an oral agent (120 to 360 mg/day). It provides excellent protection from episodes of spasm and subsequent cardiac events, and it causes fewer side effects than do most of the other agents. Sinus bradycardia occurs in a small number of patients but may be exacerbated by concurrent use of beta-adrenergic blockers in others.

Beta-Adrenergic Blockers

These agents alone are not effective in the treatment of variant angina. They may actually prolong the duration of ischemic attacks in some patients and possibly increase the frequency of anginal episodes.[38] This is presumably due to unopposed alpha-adrenergic vasoconstrictor tone and blockade of beta-adrenergic vasodilatation. Nonetheless, beta-adrenergic blockers are often useful in patients with rest angina, particularly those with significant associated coronary atherosclerosis. Because the exact, relative contributions of vasospasm and myocardial oxygen consumption to a particular patient's anginal threshold are difficult to gauge, treatment of both processes with a combination of nitrates, calcium channel blockers, and beta-adrenergic blockers is often warranted.

Surgery

Coronary artery bypass grafting alone has not proved successful in the treatment of variant angina. Recurrence of chest pain, higher perioperative mortality, and frequent graft occlusions have been reported. These complications may occur secondary to spasm of nongrafted vessels or spasm at sites distal to or involving the graft anastomosis. Total denervation of the heart has failed to prevent spasm as well. However, studies suggest that coronary artery bypass grafting is safer and more successful in patients with variant angina when combined with sympathetic plexectomy.[39] In small groups of patients with significant coronary atherosclerosis whose attacks of spasm were refractory to medical therapy, this technique prevented recurrence of anginal attacks without the perioperative complications noted in previous reports.

References

1. Osler, W.: Lumleian Lecture on Angina Pectoris, *Lancet*, 1:697, 1910.
2. Prinzmetal, M., Kennamer, R., Merliss, R., Wada, T., and Bor, N.: Angina Pectoris: I. The Variant Form of Angina Pectoris, *Am. J. Med.*, 27:375, 1959.
3. Maseri, A., Pesola, A., Marzilli, M., Severi, S., Parodi, O., L'Abbate, A., Ballestra, A., Maltinti, G., DeNes, D., and Biagini, A.: Coronary Vasospasm in Angina Pectoris, *Lancet*, 2:713, 1977.
4. Epstein, S. E., and Talbot, T. L.: Dynamic Coronary Tone in Precipitation, Exacerbation and Relief of Angina Pectoris, *Am. J. Cardiol.*, 48:797, 1981.
5. Ginsburg, R., Bristow, M. R., Harrison, D. C., and Stinson, E. B.: Studies with Isolated Human Coronary Arteries: Some General Observations, Potential Mediators of Spasm, Role of Calcium Antagonists, *Chest*, 78:180, 1980.
6. Ginsburg, R., Bristow, M. R., Davis, K., Dibiase, A., and Billingham, M. E.: Quantitative Pharmacologic Responses of Normal and Atherosclerotic Isolated Human Epicardial Coronary Arteries, *Circulation*, 69:430, 1984.
7. MacAlpin, R. N.: Relation of Coronary Arterial Spasm to Sites of Organic Stenosis, *Am. J. Cardiol.*, 46:143, 1980.
8. Rinzler, S., Travell, J., Karp, D., and Charleson, D.: Detection of Coronary Atherosclerosis in the Living Rabbit by the Ergonovine Stress Test, *Am. J. Physiol.*, 184:605, 1956.
9. Boullin, D. J., Bunting, S., Blaso, W. P., Hunt, T. M., and Moncada, S.: Responses of Human and Baboon Arteries to Prostaglandin Endoperoxides and Biologically Generated and Synthetic Prostacyclin: Their Relevance to Cerebral Arterial Spasm in Man, *Br. J. Clin. Pharmacol.*, 7:139, 1979.
10. Gutstein, W. H.: Coronary Spasm and Coronary Atherosclerosis, *Am. J. Cardiol.*, 48:389, 1981.
11. Robertson, R. M., Bernard, Y., and Robertson, D.: Arterial and Coronary Sinus Catecholamines in the Course of Spontaneous Coronary Artery Spasm, *Am. Heart J.*, 105:901, 1983.
12. Ginsburg, R., Bristow, M. R., Kantrowitz, N., Baim, D. S., and Harrison, D. C.: Histamine Provocation of Clinical Coronary Artery Spasm: Implications Concerning Pathogenesis of Variant Angina Pectoris, *Am. Heart J.*, 102:819, 1981.
13. Yokoyama, M., Akita, H., Mizutani, T., Fukuzaki, H., and Watanabe, Y.: Hyperreactivity of Coronary Arterial Smooth Muscles in Response to Ergonovine from Rabbits with Hereditary Hyperlipidemia, *Circ. Res.*, 53:63, 1983.
14. Robertson, R. M., Robertson, D., Roberts, L. J., Mass, R. L., FitzGerald, G. A., Friesinger, G. C., and Oates, J. A.: Thromboxane in Vasotonic Angina Pectoris with Evidence from Direct Measurements and Inhibitor Trials, *N. Engl. J. Med.*, 304:998, 1981.
15. Yasue, H., Nagao, M., Omote, S., Takizawa, A., Miwa, K., and Tanaka, S.: Coronary Arterial Spasm and Prinzmetal's Variant Form of Angina Induced by Hyperventilation and Tris-Buffer Infusion, *Circulation*, 58:56, 1978.
16. Ginsburg, R., Schroeder, J. S., and Harrison, D. C.: Coronary Artery Spasm: Pathophysiology, Clinical Presentations, Diagnostic Approaches and Rational Treatment, *West J. Med.*, 136:398, 1982.
17. Maseri, A., and Chierchia, S.: Coronary Artery Spasm: Demonstration, Definition, Diagnosis, and Consequences, *Prog. Cardiovasc. Dis.*, 25:169, 1982.
18. Miller, D., Waters, D. D., Warnica, W., Szlachcic, J., Kreeft, J., and Theroux, P.: Is Variant Angina the Coronary Manifestation of a Generalized Vasospastic Disorder? *N. Engl. J. Med.*, 304:763, 1981.
19. Oliva, P.: Unstable Rest Angina with ST-Segment Depression. Pathophysiologic Considerations and Therapeutic Implications, *Ann. Intern. Med.*, 100:424, 1984.
20. Waters, D. D., Szlachic, J., Bourassa, M. G., Scholl, J.-M., and Theroux, P.: Exercise Testing in Patients with Variant Angina: Results, Correlation with Clinical and Angiographic Features and Prognostic Significance, *Circulation*, 65:265, 1982.
21. Yasue, H., Omote, S., Takizawa, A., Nagao, M., Miwa, K., and Tanaka, S.: Circadian Variation of Exercise Capacity in

Patients with Prinzmetal's Variant Angina: Role of Exercise-Induced Coronary Arterial Spasm, *Circulation*, 59:938, 1979.
22. deServi, S., Specchia, G., Falcone, C., Gavazzi, A., Mussini, A., Angoli, L., Bramucci, E., Ardissino, D., Vaccari, L., Salerno, J., and Bobba, P.: Variable Threshold Exertional Angina in Patients with Transient Vasospastic Myocardial Ischemia. Repeat Exercise Test Results and Therapeutic Implications, *Am. J. Cardiol.*, 51:397, 1983.
23. Lange, R. L., Reid, M. S., Tresch, D. D., Kellan, M. H., Bernhard, V. M., and Coolidge, G.: Nonatheromatous Ischemic Heart Disease following Withdrawal from Chronic Industrial Nitroglycerin Exposure, *Circulation*, 46:666, 1972.
24. DeWood, M. A., Spores, J., Notske, R., Mouser, L. T., Burroughs, R., Golden, M. S., and Lang, H. T.: Prevalence of Total Coronary Occlusion during the Early Hours of Transmural Myocardial Infarction, *N. Engl. J. Med.*, 303:897, 1980.
25. Oliva, P.: What Is the Evidence for and the Significance of Spasm in Acute Myocardial Infarction? *Chest*, 80:730, 1981.
26. Conti, C. R., Pepine, C. J., and Feldman, R. L.: Coronary Artery Spasm, *Baylor Coll. Med. Cardiol. Ser.*, 4:1, 1981.
27. Waters, D. D., Szlachcic, J., Miller, D., and Theroux, P.: Clinical Characteristics of Patients with Variant Angina Complicated by Myocardial Infarction or Death within 1 Month, *Am. J. Cardiol.*, 49:658, 1982.
28. Miller, D. D., Waters, D. D., Szlachcic, J., and Theroux, P.: Clinical Characteristics Associated with Sudden Death in Patients with Variant Angina, *Circulation*, 66:588, 1982.
29. Waters, D. D., Bouchard, A., and Theroux, P.: Spontaneous Remission Is a Frequent Outcome of Variant Angina, *J. Am. Coll. Cardiol.*, 2:195, 1983.
30. Ginsburg, R., Lamb, I. H., Schroeder, J. S., and Harrison, D. C.: Long-Term Transtelephonic Electrocardiographic Monitoring in the Detection and Evaluation of Variant Angina, *Am. Heart J.*, 102:196, 1981.
31. Schroeder, J. S., Bolen, J. L., Quint, R. A., Clark, D. A., Hayden, W. G., Higgins, C. B., and Wexler, L.: Provocation of Coronary Spasm with Ergonovine Maleate. New Test with Results in 57 Patients Undergoing Coronary Arteriography, *Am. J. Cardiol.*, 40:487, 1977.
32. Buxton, A., Goldberg, S., Hirshfeld, J. W., Wilson, J., Mann, T., Williams, D. O., Overlie, P., and Oliva, P.: Refractory Ergonovine-Induced Coronary Vasospasm: Importance of Intracoronary Nitroglycerine, *Am. J. Cardiol.*, 46:329, 1980.
33. Cipriano, P. R., Guthaner, D. F., Orlick, A. E., Ricci, D. R., Wexler, L., and Silverman, J. F.: The Effects of Ergonovine Maleate on Coronary Arterial Size, *Circulation*, 59:82, 1979.
34. Ginsburg, R., Lamb, I. H., Bristow, M. R., Schroeder, J. S., and Harrison, D. C.: Application and Safety of Outpatient Ergonovine Testing in Accurately Detecting Coronary Spasm in Patients with Possible Variant Angina, *Am. Heart J.*, 102:698, 1981.
35. David, P. R., Waters, D. D., Scholl, J.-M., Crepeau, J., Szlachcic, J., Lesperance, J., Hudon, G., and Bourassa, M. G.: Percutaneous Transluminal Coronary Angioplasty in Patients with Variant Angina, *Circulation*, 66:695, 1982.
36. Buxton, A. E., Goldberg, S., Harken, A., Hirshfeld, J., and Kastor, J. A.: Coronary-Artery Spasm Immediately after Myocardial Revascularization. Recognition and Management, *N. Engl. J. Med.*, 304:1249, 1981.
37. Theroux, P., Waters, D. D., and Latour, J.-G.: Clinical Manifestations and Pathophysiology of Myocardial Ischemia with Special Reference to Coronary Artery Spasm and the Role of Slow Channel Calcium Blockers, *Prog. Cardiovasc. Dis.*, 25:157, 1982.
38. Robertson, R. M., Wood, A. J. J., Vaughn, W. K., and Robertson, D.: Exacerbation of Vasotonic Angina Pectoris by Propranolol, *Circulation*, 65:281, 1982.
39. Betriu, A., Pomar, J. L., Bourassa, M. G., and Grondin, C. M.: Influence of Partial Sympathetic Denervation on the Results of Myocardial Revascularization in Variant Angina, *Am. J. Cardiol.*, 51:661, 1983.

47

Nonatherosclerotic Coronary Heart Disease

Donald S. Baim, M.D.
Donald C. Harrison, M.D.

Although myocardial ischemic syndromes (angina pectoris, myocardial infarction, and sudden cardiac death) are nearly always caused by coronary atherosclerosis, they may occasionally result from one of a variety of nonatherosclerotic coronary artery diseases (Table 47-1).[1–3] These relatively uncommon diseases pose several problems to the clinician: (1) they often occur in patients in whom ischemic heart disease is uncommon, unsuspected, or masked by an underlying systemic disease, (2) they may require specialized techniques for diagnosis, and (3) their natural histories and optimal management are incompletely understood. Since specific and potentially lifesaving therapies are often available, the physician should have an overall familiarity with the diagnosis and therapy of these nonatherosclerotic coronary artery diseases.

Congenital Anomalies of the Coronary Circulation

Coronary artery anomalies—variations in the origin, course, or distribution of the coronary arteries—are present in 1 to 2 percent of the population.[4] These anomalies may make angiographic visualization of the coronary circulation more difficult and may increase the risk of coronary artery trauma during cardiac surgery.[3] In addition, certain types of coronary anomalies may cause myocardial ischemia,[5] although most do so in only a fraction of the patients in whom they are present. Evaluation of each patient with a coronary anomaly should therefore include anatomic classification, recognition of the particular anomaly as one capable of producing

TABLE 47-1 Nonatherosclerotic Coronary Artery Disease

1. Congenital anomalies of the coronary circulation
   - *a.* Anomalous origin from the aorta
     - (1) Origin from the contralateral sinus of Valsalva
     - (2) Single coronary artery
     - (3) Atresia of the coronary ostium
   - *b.* Anomalous origin from the pulmonary artery
   - *c.* Coronary artery fistula
   - *d.* Muscle bridge
   - *e.* Coronary artery aneurysm
2. Mechanical insults to the coronary circulation
   - *a.* Coronary artery embolus
   - *b.* Coronary artery dissection
   - *c.* Coronary artery trauma
     - (1) Nonpenetrating trauma
     - (2) Penetrating trauma
     - (3) Trauma during cardiac catheterization or surgery
   - *d.* Coronary thrombosis
3. Progressive nonatherosclerotic coronary occlusive disease
   - *a.* Coronary artery vasculitis
     - (1) Polyarteritis nodosa
     - (2) Systemic lupus erythematosus
     - (3) Wegener's granulomatosis
     - (4) Takayasu's disease
     - (5) Mucocutaneous lymph node syndrome
     - (6) Infection
   - *b.* Intimal proliferation or fibrosis
     - (1) Ionizing radiation
     - (2) Cardiac transplantation
   - *c.* Accumulation of metabolic substances
     - (1) Inborn errors of metabolism
     - (2) Amyloid accumulation
   - *d.* Extrinsic coronary compression

myocardial ischemia, and documentation that ischemia is present. In the symptomatic patient with a coronary anomaly in whom ischemia has been documented by exercise testing, isotopic myocardial perfusion scanning, or transmyocardial metabolic testing, effective corrective surgery is generally possible.

Anomalous Origin from the Aorta

In normal coronary circulation, the right coronary artery originates from a single ostium within the right sinus of Valsalva, and the left coronary artery originates from a single ostium within the left sinus of Valsalva (Fig. 47-1*A*). Abnormally high or low locations of the coronary ostia and the presence within the appropriate sinus of Valsalva of separate ostia for the left anterior descending and circumflex coronary artery branches, or for the right coronary artery and its conus branch, are common minor variations which do not result in myocardial ischemia. Other anomalous patterns of coronary artery origin from the aorta are potential causes of myocardial ischemia even in the absence of atherosclerosis.

Origin from the Contralateral Sinus of Valsalva

When one of the coronary arteries originates from the contralateral sinus of Valsalva, this anomalous vessel must traverse the base of the heart to reach its territory of distribution, passing anterior to, posterior to, or between the aorta and pulmonary artery[6,7] (Fig. 47-1*B*). Acute angulation at the origin of the artery from the aorta may result in anatomic or functional constriction of the proximal portion of the anomalous coronary artery. Anomalous vessels passing between the aorta and pulmonary artery seem to carry an additional risk of ischemia, possibly

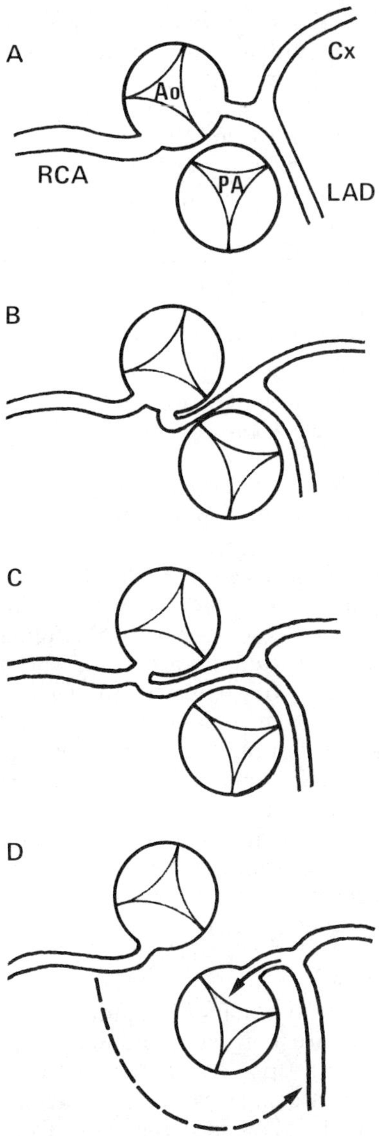

FIGURE 47-1 Representative patterns of anomalous coronary artery origin. *A.* Normal coronary circulation with origin of the right coronary artery (RCA) from the right sinus of Valsalva and origin of the left coronary artery from the left sinus of Valsalva. The aorta (Ao), pulmonary artery (PA), and left anterior descending (LAD) and circumflex (Cx) branches of the left coronary artery are shown. *B.* Anomalous origin of the left coronary artery from the right sinus of Valsalva, with passage of the left main coronary artery between the aorta and pulmonary artery. *C.* Single coronary artery originating from the right sinus of Valsalva, with passage of the left main coronary artery between the aorta and pulmonary artery. *D.* Origin of the left coronary artery from the pulmonary artery, showing the development of collateral flow (dotted arrow) from the right coronary artery and the associated left-to-right shunt into the pulmonary artery (solid arrow).

as a result of being compressed between the great vessels, although this is unlikely at normal pulmonary artery pressure. Abnormal mechanical stresses or flow patterns may enhance the development of coronary atherosclerosis in the anomalous segment.

Origin of the left coronary artery from the right sinus of Valsalva with passage of the proximal left coronary artery between the aorta and pulmonary artery is associated with an increased incidence of exercise-related sudden cardiac death in young patients. In one autopsy study of 33 patients with this anomaly, sudden death occurred in 9 patients (27 percent), generally without prior warning symptoms.[1] Some thus recommend prophylactic coronary artery bypass surgery when this anomaly is detected in young patients.[5,7]

In patients without coronary atherosclerosis, passage of the anomalous left coronary artery either anterior or posterior to both great vessels has been associated with pacing-induced myocardial lactate production and angina pectoris, but does not seem to carry a significant risk of sudden death.[6,8] Angina pectoris has also been reported in patients in whom the right coronary artery originates from the left sinus of Valsalva, but confirmation of myocardial ischemia has been less complete in these patients than in patients with anomalous origin of the left coronary artery.[6] The most common pattern of anomalous aortic origin, origin of the circumflex coronary artery from the right sinus of Valsalva or proximal right coronary artery, does not seem to impose independent ischemic risk.[6]

Single Coronary Artery

Derivation of the entire coronary circulation from a single ostium is a rare coronary anomaly (Fig. 47-1*C*). Approximately 40 percent of patients with this anomaly have an associated congenital cardiac defect, i.e., tetralogy of Fallot, transposition of the great vessels, or improper division of the truncus arteriosis.[9] There is no clear sex predominance for this condition, and the frequency of occurrence of single left and single right coronary arteries is approximately equal.[10] As in the case of anomalous origin from the contralateral sinus of Valsalva, one or more components of the coronary circulation system must cross the base of the heart to reach its territory of distribution, passing anterior to, posterior to, or between the great vessels. These transposed vessels may thereby be exposed to the risks of angulation, compression, and accelerated atherosclerosis. Since the entire myocardium is supplied by way of the single coronary artery, proximal coronary atherosclerosis poses the risk of global myocardial ischemia.

Clinical manifestations of the single coronary artery anomaly depend in part on associated cardiac defects and atherosclerosis, but up to 15 percent of patients with only this anomaly develop severe cardiac complications by age 40.[9] Angina pectoris and myocardial lactate production have been demonstrated in patients with a single coronary artery, in the absence of coronary atherosclerosis or vessel passage between the aorta and pulmonary artery.[10]

Atresia of the Coronary Ostium

Atresia or severe stenosis of one of the coronary ostia, often associated with hypoplasia of the proximal coronary artery, is a rare congenital coronary anomaly, with only seven reported cases.[5,11] The absence of a second coronary ostium may lead to the incorrect diagnosis of a single coronary artery. Because the involved vessel is dependent on collateral flow from the contralateral coronary artery, myocardial ischemia or infarction may develop during infancy. In this sense, patients with ostial atresia bear an angiographic and clinical resemblance to patients with anomalous origin of a coronary artery from the pulmonary artery (see below). Successful coronary artery bypass grafting has been reported in a 10-year-old male with ostial atresia.[11]

Anomalous Origin from the Pulmonary Artery

Origin of a coronary artery from the pulmonary artery rather than from the aorta is a relatively uncommon but severe coronary anomaly. In more than 90 percent of cases, it is the left coronary artery that originates from the pulmonary artery, generally from the left posterior pulmonary sinus[5] (Fig. 47-1*D*). Origin of the right coronary artery, an accessory coronary artery, and both coronary arteries from the pulmonary artery have been described, the last of which is invariably fatal in the neonatal period.[5,12]

As the pulmonary artery pressure falls during the first weeks of life, perfusion of the anomalous coronary artery from the pulmonary artery decreases. Unless adequate collateral flow develops from the contralateral coronary artery, the territory of the anomalous vessel becomes ischemic. Angina pectoris or congestive heart failure with mitral regurgitation may then develop, often accompanied by electrocardiographic manifestation of myocardial ischemia or infarction. This clinical picture, the *infantile syndrome,* develops in approximately 80 percent of affected patients, usually within the first 4 months of life.[5,13] In the absence of surgical correction, this syndrome has an 85 percent first-year mortality, although the mortality is somewhat lower with anomalous origin of the right coronary artery.[12] Those who do not develop the infantile syndrome may present during childhood or adult life with one of the following: asymptomatic murmur, mitral regurgitation, angina pectoris, or sudden death.[13]

Patients surviving infancy tend to have extensive intercoronary collateral flow, with dilatation of both the normal and the anomalous vessels. This collateral flow reverses the direction of blood flow in the anomalous coronary artery, constituting a left-to-right shunt into the pulmonary artery. Despite extensive collateralization, electrocardiographic evidence of ischemia and pathological evidence of subendocardial fibrosis usually persist.

Surgical correction of anomalous coronary artery origin from the pulmonary artery seeks to eliminate the left-to-right shunt and to establish an independent arterial blood supply to the anomalous vessel. Ligation of the anomalous vessel at its origin in combination with saphenous vein aortocoronary bypass grafting has been performed, but it is technically difficult in children under 2 years of age and is associated with a high rate of graft failure.[14] The alternative methods of correction, reimplantation of the anomalous vessel into the aortic root, or end-to-end anastomosis of the anomalous vessel with the subclavian artery, seem more successful in infants. This anomaly is associated with high morbidity and mortality rates, and since suitable techniques are available, early surgical correction appears to be the treatment of choice.

Coronary Artery Fistula

Direct precapillary anastomosis between a major coronary artery and a cardiac chamber or major vessel (superior vena cava, coronary sinus, or pulmonary artery) is the most common hemodynamically significant coronary artery anomaly.[5] Fistulas from the right coronary artery are slightly more common than those from the left coronary artery, and bilateral fistulas are present in 4 to 5 percent of cases[15] (Fig. 47-2). Over 90 percent of the fistulas drain into the venous circulation (right ventricle, 41 percent; right atrium, 26 percent; pulmonary artery, 17 percent; coronary sinus, 7 percent; and superior vena cava, 1 percent). The remaining fistulas drain into the arterial circulation (left atrium, 5 percent; left ventricle, 3 percent).[5] Multiple patterns of anastomosis between the involved coronary artery and the recipient cardiac structure are possible. The involved coronary artery is usually markedly dilated proximal to the fistula, and flow through the fistula may be several times that delivered to the myocardium. When the fistula drains into the venous circulation, a significant left-to-right shunt may be present.[16] Runoff through a fistula may lower intracoronary diastolic pressure and produce myocardial ischemia in some patients by a "coronary steal" phenomenon.[5] Physical examination often reveals a continuous heart murmur, which brings approximately one-half of patients with coronary artery fistulas to medical attention. The chest x-ray is usually normal, but may show evidence of pulmonary overcirculation when a large left-to-right shunt is present, mimicking a patent ductus arteriosus. Electrocardiographic abnormalities are uncommon. Diagnosis is best made by selective coronary angiography, particularly when catheterization to evaluate a continuous murmur has failed to disclose the expected anatomic abnormality. Similar fistulas may result from cardiac trauma.

Since the great majority of patients with coronary fistulas are asymptomatic, the decision regarding surgical correction is complex. Ischemia has been documented in some patients with coronary fistulas and no atherosclerosis,[5] and there is evidence that the majority of patients do become symptomatic with advancing age.[16] In addition to angina and myocardial infarction, congestive heart failure, bacterial endocarditis, and fistula rupture have been described. Since spontaneous fistula closure is rare and since the risk of surgical closure of the fistula is significantly lower in patients under age 20, some authorities have suggested elective fistula ligation in young patients, including those who are asymptomatic.[16] Antibiotic prophylaxis against bacterial endocarditis is recommended.[16]

Muscle Bridge

Intramyocardial segments of the large coronary arteries, particularly the left anterior descending artery, may be subject to systolic compression, or "milking" (Fig. 47-3). While intramyocardial segments of the coronary arteries are present in approximately 20 percent of autopsied hearts,[17] angiographic evidence of systolic compression is

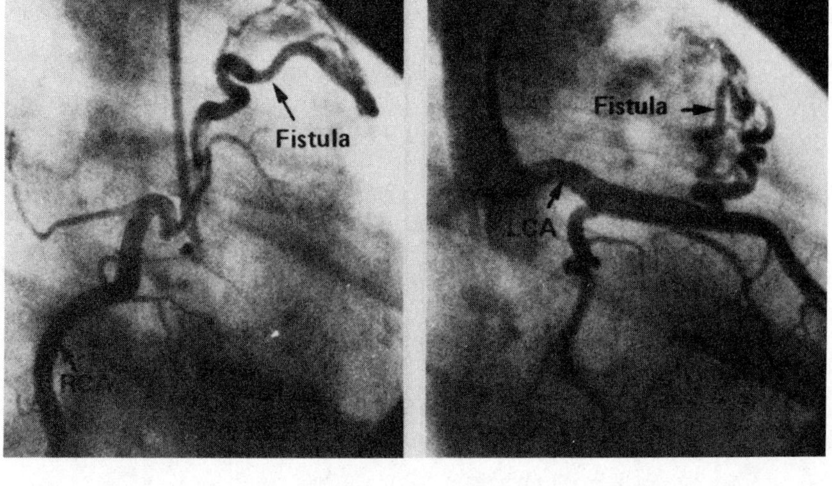

FIGURE 47-2 Bilateral coronary artery to pulmonary artery fistula, originating from the proximal right coronary artery (RCA) and the left anterior descending branch of the left coronary artery (LCA) in an asymptomatic 29-year-old female with a continuous heart murmur. No left-to-right shunt was detected by oximetry.

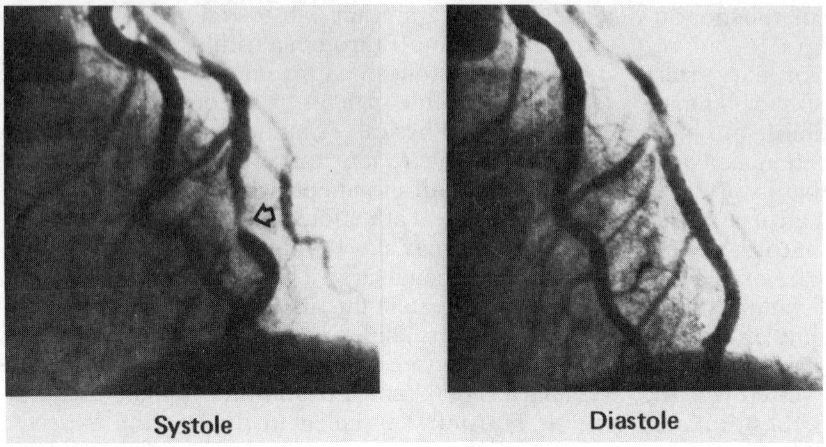

FIGURE 47-3 Systolic compression of the midleft anterior descending coronary artery by a muscle bridge with restoration of the normal coronary artery diameter during diastole in a young male with exercise-induced ventricular tachycardia. Treated with oral propranolol, the patient was free of both arrhythmia and electrocardiographic evidence of myocardial ischemia during maximal treadmill exercise testing. (*Courtesy of Dr. John A. Michal, Santa Barbara, Calif.*)

reported in only 0.5 percent of patients undergoing coronary angiography for chest pain.[18] In most cases angiographic compression is a benign finding, but when a long vessel segment demonstrates systolic compression to less than 25 percent of its diastolic diameter, ischemia may be revealed by exercise, by ^{201}Tl myocardial perfusion scanning, or by coronary sinus pacing—metabolic evaluation, even in the absence of coronary atherosclerosis.[18] Since most coronary flow takes place during diastole, it is not clear how systolic compression alone results in myocardial ischemia. In some symptomatic patients, coronary compression may extend into early diastole, and excessive myocardial oxygen demand may be present as the result of associated left ventricular hypertrophy.[18] Although muscle bridges are a congenital anomaly, symptoms of ischemia may not develop until middle age.

Angina pectoris resulting from systolic coronary artery compression may respond to therapy with beta-adrenergic blocking drugs. When symptoms are refractory to medical therapy and when inducible ischemia has been unequivocally demonstrated, coronary bypass grafting or simple unroofing of the bridged coronary segment has resulted in relief of symptoms and normalization of myocardial perfusion and metabolism.[18,19]

Coronary Artery Aneurysm

Coronary artery aneurysms, localized areas of coronary dilatation relative to adjacent normal arterial segments, occur in approximately 1.5 percent of patients studied by autopsy or coronary angiography.[20] The aneurysms are frequently multiple, may attain a diameter of several centimeters, involve the right coronary artery more frequently than the left,[21] and may be either congenital or acquired. Atherosclerosis, either by stenosis with poststenotic dilatation or by primary destruction of the coronary intima and media, accounts for approximately 50 percent of coronary aneurysms. Atherosclerotic damage may also produce diffuse coronary ectasia rather than focal coronary aneurysm.[2] Other pathological processes which damage the arterial wall, including dissection, trauma, coronary angioplasty, vasculitis, mycotic emboli, syphilis, and mucocutaneous lymph node syndrome, may also lead to aneurysm formation.[20,21] The remainder of coronary aneurysms are felt to be congenital in origin, although many of these may in fact be the residua of prior subclinical vasculitis.

There are no reliable clinical features of coronary artery aneurysm, although a diastolic or continuous heart murmur may occasionally be present.[20] The chest x-ray may show a paracardiac mass or calcification, and while echocardiography may detect the largest and most proximal coronary aneurysms, coronary angiography is required for accurate diagnosis.

The clinical course of patients with coronary artery aneurysms usually depends on the severity of the associated atherosclerotic stenoses. Even in the absence of stenosis, abnormal flow patterns within the aneurysm may lead to thrombus formation with subsequent vessel occlusion, distal thromboembolization, or myocardial infarction.[20] One case has been reported in which a large intramyocardial aneurysm resulted in angina by a coronary steal mechanism. Rupture of a coronary aneurysm is a rare but serious complication.

Surgical therapy of combined stenotic and aneurysmal atherosclerosis consists of ligation of the involved vessel immediately beyond the aneurysm (to eliminate subsequent emboli) and aortocoronary bypass grafting to the distal vessel. Similar surgery has been suggested in patients without stenotic lesions and even in asymptomatic patients with coronary aneurysms.[20] Anticoagulant or antiplatelet therapy may also be of value in this condition.[2] Because aneurysmal changes are frequently present in other vessels, particularly the abdominal aorta, comprehensive arteriographic evaluation is recommended in patients with coronary artery aneurysms.[20,21]

Mechanical Insults to the Coronary Artery Circulation

An acute mechanical insult to a previously normal coronary artery circulation may result in transient myocardial ischemia or myocardial infarction. Circumstantial evidence (recent chest trauma, intercurrent cardiac catheterization, predisposition to arterial embolization) often suggests that an ischemic event is the result of such an insult, but more commonly the clinical picture is indistinguishable from acute atherosclerotic myocardial infarction.

Coronary Artery Embolus

The coronary arteries may be partially protected from embolic events by the acute angulation of the coronary ostia relative to the aortic stream and by their position behind the aortic valve leaflets during systole. When coronary artery emboli do occur, the outcome is dictated by the size of the embolus and its position of impaction in the coronary circulation. Small emboli tend to produce occlusion of a distal branch of one of the coronary arteries (most commonly the left anterior descending artery), resulting in a small area of myocardial necrosis which may not be clinically evident.[22,23] These small emboli appear to be relatively frequent. In one autopsy series they were found in 13 percent of patients with histologically evident myocardial necrosis.[23] Larger coronary artery emboli are relatively less frequent, but generally result in clinically apparent myocardial infarction.

Coronary artery emboli should be considered in the differential diagnosis of acute myocardial ischemia in patients whose clinical condition predisposes them to arterial emboli, including patients with valvular heart disease (endocarditis, noninfected abnormal valve, prosthetic valve), mural thrombus (congestive cardiomyopathy, previous myocardial infarction, atrial fibrillation), left-sided cardiac catheterization, or the anatomic potential for paradoxical embolization.[22,23] Coronary emboli of a variety of materials, including tumor, myocardial or skeletal muscle, and materials used in cardiac surgery, have also been reported. Extracardiac emboli may also be present. In patients sustaining coronary emboli, prompt coronary angiography may show occlusion of the involved vessel, but restudy as soon as 1 month following the acute event may show renewed vessel patency as the result of lysis or recanalization of the embolus.[22]

The role of cardiac surgery in the treatment of acute coronary emboli is yet to be established. When emboli occur during cardiac surgery, embolectomy appears to correct the myocardial ischemia. Embolectomy performed for emboli associated with endocarditis[24] or cardiac catheterization seems to have less influence on the evolution of myocardial infarction.

Coronary Artery Dissection

Hemorrhage into the coronary artery wall, with or without an associated intimal tear, forces the intima into the coronary lumen and may produce distal myocardial ischemia or frank infarction. Coronary artery dissections may occur by extension of aortic root dissection (secondary dissection), or may be limited to the coronary artery (primary dissection). Primary coronary artery dissections may occur as the result of diagnostic coronary angiography, coronary angioplasty, cardiac surgery, or chest trauma (see below), or they may occur spontaneously. Angiographically evident localized coronary dissection occurs in at least 30 percent of patients undergoing coronary angioplasty and may progress to abrupt vessel reclosure in the first hour following the procedure in 2 to 3 percent of patients.[25] In the remaining patients, dissection is not progressive, does not lead to myocardial ischemia, and heals within 2 to 3 months to produce a vessel which appears angiographically normal. Most *spontaneous* dissections occur in women, particularly in the peripartum period.[26,27] Hypertension and coronary atherosclerotic involvement are infrequent, but changes resembling cystic medial necrosis may be present.[26–28] The involved vessel is enlarged and ecchymotic and may rupture. The left anterior descending artery is involved in three-fourths of the cases, usually within 2 cm of its origin.[28]

The diagnosis of coronary artery dissection during life relies on coronary angiography showing extravasation or delayed clearance of contrast, an intimal flap, or the presence of true and false lumina, but dissection may present simply as occlusion of the involved vessel.[27,29]

Coronary Artery Trauma

Nonpenetrating Blunt Trauma

Chest-wall impact, frequently the result of vehicular trauma, may lead to myocardial necrosis by direct myocardial contusion or by occlusive injury to the coronary arteries. This occlusive injury may be the result of coronary artery dissection, thrombosis, or rupture.[30,31] Coronary artery fistulas or aneurysms may develop as late sequelae.[32] The left anterior descending and right coronary arteries are the more frequently involved. The electrocardiogram usually shows a pattern of acute myocardial infarction, but this finding does not distinguish between coronary occlusion and myocardial contusion. This distinction can be made by prompt coronary angiography, but it is of limited clinical utility unless immediate revascularization (bypass surgery, thrombolytic therapy, or angioplasty performed on an emergency basis) is contemplated. Recovery is the rule, although left ventricular aneurysm formation is common.

Penetrating Trauma

Laceration of a coronary artery as in a stab wound or small-caliber gunshot wound may cause acute myocardial ischemia, although the immediate presentation is generally that of acute pericardial tamponade. The left anterior descending and right coronary arteries are most frequently involved. Laceration of small coronary artery branches may be treated with simple ligation without producing significant myocardial ischemia, but ligation of larger vessels often results in a large area of myocardial ischemia (manifested as immediate myocardial discoloration and hypokinesis), necessitating coronary artery bypass grafting.[33] Development of a loud continuous murmur days to months after the original injury may signal the development of a coronary artery fistula. Surgical repair of these fistulas is often only transiently successful, with return of the murmur in the postoperative period; thus surgery should be reserved for patients with evidence of hemodynamic compromise.[32]

Trauma during Cardiac Catheterization or Surgery

Catheterization of the left side of the heart, particularly selective cannulation of the coronary arteries, is associated with a 0.1 to 0.2 percent incidence of myocardial infarction as the result of coronary artery embolization (thrombus, dislodged plaque, air) or coronary artery dissection.[34,35] Coronary artery dissection (particularly that which occurs during percutaneous transluminal angioplasty) and embolization have been reported without ischemic sequelae, but when they result in acute myocardial infarction with hypotension or refractory arrhythmia, urgent coronary artery bypass surgery may be lifesaving.[25] Careful flushing technique and systemic heparinization during coronary angiography have minimized these complications. Laceration of a coronary artery is a potential but rare complication during pericardiocentesis.

Coronary Thrombosis

Coronary thrombosis clearly plays an important role in the evolution of myocardial infarction (see Chaps. 44 and 45). When myocardial infarction develops in the setting of coronary atherosclerosis, superimposed coronary thrombosis is nearly always present. In certain disorders involving thrombocytosis or platelet activation, including polycythemia vera, idiopathic thrombocytosis, thrombotic thrombocytopenia purpura, and multiple myeloma,[36,37] acute myocardial infarction has occurred in the absence of significant underlying atherosclerosis. While this circumstantial evidence points toward primary coronary thrombosis as the cause of infarction, the differentiation between in situ thrombosis and thromboembolus may be difficult.

Progressive Nonatherosclerotic Coronary Occlusive Disease

Progressive nonatherosclerotic coronary occlusion may result from coronary artery vasculitis,[38] intimal proliferation or fibrosis, abnormal accumulation of metabolic substances,[2] or extrinsic coronary artery compression.[39] When the large proximal coronary arteries are involved, angina pectoris or acute myocardial infarction may result, but clinical, angiographic, and even histological differentiation of progressive nonatherosclerotic coronary occlusion from atherosclerosis may be difficult. When the small coronary vessels (0.1 to 1.0 mm in diameter) are involved, as they may be in diabetes mellitus, collagen vascular disease, thrombotic thrombocytopenic purpura, homocystinuria, neuromuscular disorders, or cardiac transplantation, the patient may develop arrhythmias, conduction defects, chest pain, or sudden death despite angiographic normality of the large coronary arteries.[40] The overall prevalence of small-vessel disease and the frequency with which it leads to clinical sequelae are not known.

Coronary Artery Vasculitis

Polyarteritis Nodosa

Polyarteritis nodosa is a systemic necrotizing vasculitis which affects medium and small arteries and is most prevalent in males between the ages of 30 and 60. Some cases appear to be related to hepatitis B antigenemia, allergy, or amphetamine abuse. Approximately two-thirds of affected patients have evidence of coronary artery involvement. In these patients, coronary aneurysm formation or occlusion may lead to myocardial infarction.[38,41]

Systemic Lupus Erythematosus

Systemic lupus erythematosus is a chronic multisystem disease which most commonly affects women between the ages of 20 and 40. Pericarditis and myocarditis are common and may lead to chest pain and electrocardiographic abnormalities. In addition, several young patients with lupus erythematosus have developed acute myocardial infarction despite the absence of conventional coronary atherosclerosis risk factors.[38,42] Pathological examination in these cases showed intimal fibrosis of the coronary arteries, but to what degree this was the result of coronary arteritis rather than atherosclerosis accelerated by the underlying disease or corticosteroid therapy is unclear. In one reported case, however, progressive coronary occlusion was observed on sequential coronary angiograms performed several days apart and was attributed to coronary vasculitis.[43] Coronary vasculitis has also been reported in pathological studies of patients with rheumatoid arthritis and acute rheumatic fever.[38]

Wegener's Granulomatosis
Wegener's granulomatosis is a necrotizing vasculitis which most commonly affects the respiratory tract and kidney. Cardiac involvement is rare, but fibrinoid necrosis of the small- and medium-sized coronary arteries has been described.[38] One case of large-vessel coronary occlusion with myocardial infarction has been reported.[44]

Takayasu's Disease (Pulseless Disease)
Takayasu's disease is predominantly a disease of young Oriental women. Granulomatous panarteritis and fibrosis of the aorta and its large branches lead to stenosis of these vessels, associated with decreased pulse amplitude and vascular bruits. Involvement of the coronary ostia and proximal coronary arteries, which has been described in 16 patients, may lead to angina pectoris or myocardial infarction.[38] This disease is seen with greater frequency in areas such as the west coast with large oriental populations. Successful coronary artery bypass grafting has been performed for this condition.

Mucocutaneous Lymph Node Syndrome (Kawasaki's Disease)
Described by Kawasaki in 1967, this acute febrile illness affects infants and young children. It produces sterile conjunctivitis and oropharyngeal erythema and may lead to a desquamative reaction of the extremities and nonpurulent cervical adenopathy. In approximately 20 percent of patients, intense vasculitis of the coronary vasa vasorum leads to coronary artery aneurysm, thrombosis, or stenotic scarring. Death may result from myocardial ischemia or arrhythmia in 1 to 2 percent of patients, frequently during the recovery phase. Late presentation of myocardial ischemia due to coronary artery aneurysm or stenosis may occur. Coronary artery bypass grafting has been performed successfully on these patients.[38,45,46]

Infection
Syphilis is the most common infectious disease affecting the coronary arteries. Up to one-fourth of patients with tertiary cardiovascular syphilis may have ostial stenosis of one or both coronary arteries, in addition to involvement of the ascending aorta or aortic valve. The right coronary artery is most frequently affected. Angina and myocardial infarction have resulted from syphilitic coronary disease.[47]

Other infections which cause coronary arteritis only rarely include salmonella, tuberculosis, and leprosy.[1] Viral infections have caused abnormalities of the coronary intima in experimental animals and have been proposed as a cause of myocardial infarction in young patients.[48]

Intimal Proliferation or Fibrosis
Fibrous hyperplasia of the coronary arteries may result in myocardial ischemia. This process is most frequently associated with fibromuscular hyperplasia of the renal arteries or the use of methysergide maleate (Sansert).[2] Intimal fibroblastic proliferation and medial calcification is a distinct but idiopathic disease of childhood and may lead to coronary artery obstruction.[3,5] In children with this disorder, other medium-sized arteries may be similarly involved.

Ionizing Radiation
Therapeutic doses of ionizing radiation delivered to the heart may cause pericarditis or myocardial fibrosis. Animal experimentation suggests that cardiac radiation may also injure capillary walls and enhance the development of lesions resembling atherosclerotic plaque in animals fed lipid-rich diets. In a small number of young patients with no conventional risk factors for coronary atherosclerosis, acute myocardial infarction has been reported at varying intervals following therapeutic cardiac radiation.[49] The relation between radiation and coronary atherosclerosis in these patients has not been established.[50]

Cardiac Transplantation
Approximately 20 percent of patients develop significant coronary fibrosis or atherosclerosis within 3 years of cardiac transplantation. Angina pectoris is absent because of cardiac denervation, but myocardial infarction or sudden death may result. This process usually involves the epicardial coronary arteries and is therefore evident on coronary arteriography. Selective fibrosis of the smaller coronary vessels has also been reported. Intimal damage resulting from immunologic rejection is believed to be the initiating injury causing coronary artery disease following cardiac transplantation.[51] In patients who do not experience clinical or biopsy evidence for rejection there is a lesser prevalence of coronary atherosclerosis.

Accumulation of Metabolic Substances
Specific metabolic substances may accumulate in various body tissues as the result of an inborn error of metabolism. Deposition of these substances in the walls of large and small coronary arteries may narrow the vessel lumen and lead to myocardial ischemia. These diseases include the mucopolysaccharidoses (Hunter's and Hurler's diseases),[52] gangliosidoses (Sandhoff's disease and G_{M1}), primary oxalosis, alkaptonuria, and Fabry's disease. Accentuated intimal proliferation of the coronary arteries has been reported in patients with homocystinuria and Friedreich's ataxia.[1–3,5]

In patients with systemic amyloidosis, amyloid may be deposited in the walls of both large and small coronary arteries and may lead to focal myocardial necrosis. The clinical importance of such small areas of necrosis is unclear, but they may contribute to the myocardial dysfunction which results from extensive deposits of amyloid in the myocardium.[53]

Extrinsic Coronary Artery Compression

External compression of the coronary artery may cause progressive narrowing of the vessel lumen. This has been reported in patients with aneurysms of the sinus of Valsalva[39] and in patients with epicardial tumor metastases.[49] Systolic coronary compression by muscle bridges has been discussed previously.

References

1. Cheitlin, M. D., McAllister, H. A., and DeCastro, C. M.: Myocardial Infarction without Atherosclerosis, *JAMA*, 231:951, 1975.
2. Razavi, M.: Unusual Forms of Coronary Artery Disease, *Cardiovasc. Clin.*, 7:25, 1975.
3. Neufeld, H. N., and Blieden, L. C.: Coronary Artery Disease in Children, *Prog. Cardiol.*, 4:119, 1975.
4. Engel, H. J., Torres, C., and Page, H. L., Jr.: Major Variations in Anatomical Origin of the Coronary Arteries: Angiographic Observations in 4,250 Patients without Associated Congenital Heart Disease, *Cathet. Cardiovasc. Diagn.*, 1:157, 1975.
5. Levin, D. C., Fellows, K. E., and Abrams, H. L.: Hemodynamically Significant Primary Anomalies of the Coronary Arteries. Angiographic Aspects, *Circulation*, 58:25, 1978.
6. Kimbiris, D., Iskandrian, A. S., Segal, B. L., and Bemis, C. E.: Anomalous Aortic Origin of Coronary Arteries, *Circulation*, 58:606, 1978.
7. Liberthson, R. R., Dinsmore, R. E., and Fallon, J. T.: Aberrant Coronary Artery Origin from the Aorta. Report of 18 Patients, Review of Literature and Delineation of Natural History and Management, *Circulation*, 59:748, 1979.
8. Chaitman, B. R., Lesperance, J., Saltiel, J., and Bourassa, M. G.: Clinical, Angiographic, and Hemodynamic Findings in Patients with Anomalous Origin of the Coronary Arteries, *Circulation*, 53:122, 1976.
9. Sharbaugh, A. H., and White, R. S.: Single Coronary Artery. Analysis of the Anatomic Variation, Clinical Importance, and Report of Five Cases, *JAMA*, 230:243, 1974.
10. Joswig, B. C., Warren, S. E., Vieweg, W. V., and Hagan, A. D.: Transmural Myocardial Infarction in the Absence of Coronary Arterial Luminal Narrowing in a Young Man with Single Coronary Arterial Anomaly, *Cathet. Cardiovasc. Diagn.*, 4:297, 1978.
11. Byrum, C. J., Blackman, M. S., Schneider, B., Sondheimer, H. M., and Kavey, R. W.: Congenital Atresia of the Left Coronary Ostium and Hypoplasia of the Left Main Coronary Artery, *Am. Heart J.*, 99:354, 1980.
12. Lerberg, D. B., Ogden, J. A., Zuberbuhler, J. R., and Bahnson, H.T.: Anomalous Origin of the Right Coronary Artery from the Pulmonary Artery, *Ann. Thorac. Surg.*, 27:87, 1979.
13. Wesselhoeft, H., Fawcett, J. S., and Johnson, A. L.: Anomalous Origin of the Left Coronary Artery from the Pulmonary Trunk, *Circulation*, 38:403, 1968.
14. Richardson, J. V., and Doty, D. B.: Correction of Anomalous Origin of the Left Coronary Artery, *J. Thorac. Cardiovasc. Surg.*, 77:699, 1979.
15. Baim, D. S., Kline, H., Silverman, J. F.: Bilateral Coronary-Pulmonary Artery Fistulae: Report of Five Cases and Review of the Literature, *Circulation*, 65:810, 1982.
16. Liberthson, R. R., Sagar, K., Berkoben, J. P., Weintraub, R. M., and Levine, F. H.: Congenital Coronary Arteriovenous Fistula. Report of 13 Patients. Review of the Literature and Delineation of the Management, *Circulation*, 59:849, 1979.
17. Geiringer, E.: The Mural Coronary Artery, *Am. Heart J.*, 41:359, 1951.
18. Noble, J., Bourassa, M. G., Petitclerc, R., and Dyrda, I.: Myocardial Bridging and Milking Effect of the Left Anterior Descending Coronary Artery: Normal Variant or Obstruction, *Am. J. Cardiol.*, 37:993, 1976.
19. Grondin, P., Bourassa, M. G., Noble, J., Petitclerc, R., and Dyrda, I.: Successful Course after Supra-Arterial Myotomy for Myocardial Bridging and Milking Effect of the Left Anterior Descending Artery, *Ann. Thorac. Surg.*, 24:422, 1977.
20. Glickel, S. Z., Maggs, P. R., and Ellis, F. H., Jr.: Coronary Artery Aneurysm, *Ann. Thorac. Surg.*, 25:372, 1978.
21. Befeler, B., Aranda, J. M., Embi, A., Mullin, F. L., El-Sherif, N., and Lazzara, R.: Coronary Artery Aneurysms: Study of the Etiology, Clinical Course and Effect on Left Ventricular Function and Prognosis, *Am. J. Med.*, 62:597, 1977.
22. Roberts, W. C.: Coronary Embolism: A Review of Causes, Consequences, and Diagnostic Considerations, *Cardiovasc. Med.*, 3:699, 1978.
23. Prizel, K. R., Hutchins, G. M., and Bulkley, B. H.: Coronary Artery Embolism and Myocardial Infarction, *Ann. Intern. Med.*, 88:155, 1978.
24. Pfeifer, J. F., Lipton, M. J., Oury, J. H., Angell, W. W., and Hultgren, H. N.: Acute Coronary Embolism Complicating Bacterial Endocarditis: Operative Treatment, *Am. J. Cardiol.*, 37:920, 1976.
25. Baim, D. S.: Percutaneous Transluminal Coronary Angioplasty: Analysis of Unsuccessful Procedures as a Guide Toward Improved Results, *Cardiovasc. Intervent. Radiol.*, 5:186, 1982.
26. Claudon, D. G., Claudon, D. B., and Edwards, J. E.: Primary Dissecting Aneurysm of Coronary Artery, *Circulation*, 45:259, 1972.
27. Shaver, P. J., Carrig, T. F., and Baker, W. P.: Postpartum Coronary Artery Dissection, *Br. Heart J.*, 40:83, 1978.
28. Smith, J. C.: Dissecting Aneurysms of Coronary Arteries, *Arch. Pathol.*, 99:117, 1975.
29. Ciraulo, D. A., and Chesne, R. B.: Coronary Arterial Dissection: An Unrecognized Cause of Myocardial Infarction, with Subsequent Coronary Arterial Patency, *Chest*, 73:677, 1978.
30. Allen, R. P., and Liedtke, A. J.: The Role of Coronary Artery Injury and Perfusion in the Development of Cardiac Contusion Secondary to Nonpenetrating Chest Trauma, *J. Trauma*, 19:153, 1979.
31. Cheitlin, M. D.: Cardiovascular Trauma—Key References (Parts I and II), *Circulation*, 65:1529 and 66:244, 1982.
32. Austin, S. M., Applefeld, M. M., Turney, S. Z., and Mech, K. F., Jr.: Traumatic Left Anterior Descending Coronary Artery to Right Ventricle Fistula: Report of Two Cases, *South Med. J.*, 70:581, 1977.
33. Espada, R., Whisennand, H. H., Mattox, K. L., and Beall, A. C., Jr.: Surgical Management of Penetrating Injuries to the Coronary Arteries, *Surgery*, 78:755, 1975.
34. Sethi, G. K., Scott, S. M., and Takaro, T.: Iatrogenic Coronary Artery Stenosis Following Aortic Valve Replacement, *J. Thorac. Cardiovasc. Surg.*, 77:760, 1979.
35. Kennedy, J.: Symposium on Catheterization Complications. Complications Associated with Cardiac Catheterization and Angiography, *Cathet. Cardiovasc. Diagn.*, 8:5, 1982.
36. Virmani, R., Popovsky, M. A., and Roberts, W. C.: Thrombocytosis, Coronary Thrombosis and Acute Myocardial Infarction, *Am. J. Med.*, 67:498, 1979.
37. Ridolfi, R. L., Hutchins, G. M., and Bell, W. R.: The Heart and Cardiac Conduction System in Thrombotic Thrombocytopenia Purpura. A Clinicopathologic Study of 17 Autopsied Patients, *Ann. Intern. Med.*, 91:357, 1979.
38. Parillo, J. E., and Fauci, A. S.: Necrotizing Vasculitis, Coronary Angiitis and the Cardiologist, *Am. Heart J.*, 99:547, 1980.
39. Garcia-Rinaldi, R., Von Koch, L., and Howell, J. F.: Aneurysm of the Sinus of Valsalva Producing Obstruction of the Left Main Coronary Artery, *J. Thorac. Cardiovasc. Surg.*, 72:123, 1976.
40. James, T. N.: Small Arteries of the Heart, *Circulation*, 56:2, 1977.
41. Holsinger, D. R., Osmundson, P. J., and Edwards, J. E.: The Heart in Periarteritis Nodosa, *Circulation*, 25:610, 1962.
42. Meller, J., Conde, C. A., Deppisch, L. M., Donoso, E., and Dack, S.: Myocardial Infarction Due to Coronary Atherosclerosis in Three Young Adults with Systemic Lupus Erythematosus, *Am. J. Cardiol.*, 35:309, 1975.
43. Heibel, R. H., O'Toole, J. D., Curtiss, E. I., Medsger, T. A.,

Jr., Reddy, S. P., and Shaver, J. A.: Coronary Arteritis in Systemic Lupus Erythematosus, *Chest,* 69:700, 1976.
44. Gatenby, P. A., Lytton, D. G., Bulteau, V. G., O'Reilly, B., and Basten, A.: Myocardial Infarction in Wegener's Granulomatosis, *Aust. N. Z. J. Med.,* 6:336, 1976.
45. Onouchi, Z., Shinichiro, S., Kiyosawa, N., et al.: Aneurysms in the Coronary Arteries in Kawasaki Disease—An Angiographic Study of 30 Cases, *Circulation,* 66:6, 1982.
46. Fukushige, J., Nihill, M. R., and McNamara, D. G.: Spectrum of Cardiovascular Lesions in Mucocutaneous Lymph Node Syndrome, *Am. J. Cardiol.,* 45:98, 1980.
47. Holt, S.: Syphilitic Ostial Occlusion, *Br. Heart J.,* 39:469, 1977.
48. Burch, G. E., and Shewey, L. L.: Viral Coronary Arteritis and Myocardial Infarction, *Am. Heart J.,* 92:11, 1976.
49. Kopelson, G., and Herwig, K. J.: The Etiologies of Coronary Artery Disease in Cancer Patients, *Int. J. Radiat. Oncol. Biol. Phys.,* 4:895, 1978.
50. Fajardo, L. F.: Radiation-Induced Coronary Artery Disease, *Chest,* 71:563, 1977. (Editorial.)
51. Mason, J. W., and Strefling, A.: Small Vessel Disease of the Heart Resulting in Myocardial Necrosis and Death Despite Angiographically Normal Coronary Arteries, *Am. J. Cardiol.,* 44:171, 1979.
52. Brosius, F. C., and Roberts, W. C.: Coronary Artery Disease in the Hurler Syndrome, *Am. J. Cardiol.,* 47:649, 1981.
53. Smith, R. R., and Hutchins, G. M.: Ischemic Heart Disease Secondary to Amyloidosis of Intramyocardial Arteries, *Am. J. Cardiol.,* 44:413, 1979.

48

Rehabilitation of the Patient with Atherosclerotic Coronary Heart Disease

Nanette Kass Wenger, M.D.
Gerald F. Fletcher, M.D.

The most important element of all is graded exercise, not on the level but up hills of various grades. The distance walked each day is marked off and is gradually lengthened. In this way the heart is systematically exercised and strengthened.

W. Osler, 1914[1]

Rehabilitative Goals and Categories of Eligible Patients

Rehabilitative management is appropriate for patients with many manifestations of atherosclerotic coronary heart disease. Although patients with myocardial infarction have traditionally been the largest group considered for rehabilitation, this approach is equally important for patients undergoing coronary artery bypass surgery and/or coronary angioplasty, as well as those with stable angina pectoris.

The rehabilitative approach to care is designed to reduce the physical and psychosocial impact of disabling and handicapping conditions by a variety of efforts directed toward the restoration and enhancement of functional status.[2] Rehabilitation ideally begins at the onset of illness and continues during long-term care; the patient's primary physician thus has a pivotal role in initiating and coordinating rehabilitative care. Resources to effect rehabilitation should be available in the local community—in the hospital, in the office of the primary physician, or in a variety of public, governmental, and private community agencies and facilities.

Rehabilitation of the patient with atherosclerotic coronary heart disease involves (1) limitation of the adverse physiological and emotional consequences of the acute illness, (2) identification of patients at increased risk of early reinfarction or sudden cardiac death and the institution of therapy to lessen this risk, (3) control of symptoms by a variety of medical and surgical therapies, with consequent improvement in function, (4) institution of measures designed to retard the progression or induce regression of atherosclerosis, and (5) maintenance and enhancement of residual physiological, psychosocial, and vocational status. The latter involves provision of medical and surgical therapies, as well as education and counseling of the patient and family. The second and third items are addressed in detail in Chapter 45, and the fourth item is reviewed in Chapter 42. The rehabilitative approaches discussed in this chapter include prescriptive physical activity, patient and family education and counseling about coronary disease and its management, psychosocial concerns, and vocational planning.

The current abbreviated hospital stay for patients with an uncomplicated *myocardial infarction*[3] necessitates early and accelerated rehabilitation; a comparable, though modulated, approach is appropriate for patients with complications of myocardial infarction. The 150,000 or more patients who have *coronary artery bypass surgery* each year in the United States now constitute larger components of most rehabilitation programs. Because many of these patients have not sustained a myocardial infarction and have good ventricular function, their rehabilitation potential is great; to date, however, their vocational rehabilitation success has been limited. Functional evaluation helps encourage a prompt return to the prior life-style, including return to work; and intensive risk modification is warranted postoperatively. These considerations are also applicable to the newest group of patients undergoing rehabilitation, those who have had *coronary angioplasty;* however, these patients may require more medication than patients who have had coronary bypass surgery. Patients with *stable angina pectoris,* with or without myocardial infarction, constitute almost one-fourth of the total coronary population. They often have a less structured system of rehabilitative care than do patients after myocardial infarction. Because of their symptoms, they often have more physical limitations and require more medication than other subsets of coronary patients. They often also have greater loss of productivity than patients recovered from myocardial infarction, and their need for comprehensive care may exceed that of patients after uncomplicated infarction. Patients with angina pectoris must be watched closely for changes in the pattern of angina or other markers of myocardial ischemia (exercise-induced ECG abnormalities, arrhythmias, or hypotension) that warrant prompt evaluation and the institution of medical or surgical therapy.

Exercise Testing in Coronary Rehabilitation

A discussion of techniques of exercise testing will be found in Chapter 98.

Predischarge Exercise Testing

Low-intensity exercise testing, preferably prior to discharge from the hospital, may be safely performed at 1 to 3 weeks following myocardial infarction. The level of testing approximates the intensity of physical activity permitted during the last days of the hospitalization. Exercise testing may be conducted to a workload of 3 to $3\frac{1}{2}$ METS (1 MET is equivalent to 3.5 ml O_2 per kilogram of body weight per minute) or that workload evoking a heart rate response below 120 to 130 beats per minute, or 60 percent of age-predicted maximum heart rate. Many laboratories, however, test patients to a sign- or symptom-limited endpoint. Treadmill testing characteristically entails serial 3-min stages of walking at 1.2 miles an hour, initially on the level and then at 3 and 6 percent elevations; other test protocols are available for the treadmill or bicycle ergometer. Arm testing is an alternative for patients with claudication or musculoskeletal problems that render leg testing unfeasible.[4]

Predischarge exercise testing helps identify patients at increased risk for recurrent coronary events[5,6] who may require early angiography—those with a low exercise capacity (below 4 to 6 METs), and those who develop angina, ischemic ST-segment abnormalities, and/or exercise-induced hypotension at low levels of exercise. Attainment of only a low workload,[6a] as well as development of ventricular arrhythmias at low levels of exercise, also suggest an adverse prognosis. Predischarge exercise testing also helps identify patients with a favorable prognosis, and those well-suited for early discharge home, allows definition of safely tolerated activity levels, and often decreases the common fear of post-infarction patients that physical activity may result in recurrent infarction or death. Although most helpful after myocardial infarction, predischarge exercise testing may be of value in selected patients after coronary angioplasty or coronary bypass surgery.

Serial Surveillance with Standard Exercise Testing

Serial exercise testing is indicated at 3- to 6-month intervals, both for patients in supervised exercise regimens and for those exercising individually, to permit revision of the exercise prescription; to define the need for changes in antianginal, antiarrhythmic, or antihypertensive medications; and to indicate the need for further diagnostic studies such as radionuclide imaging or coronary angiography. Serial exercise testing can identify recurrent manifestations of atherosclerosis—progression of the underlying coronary occlusive disease, closure of coronary bypass grafts, or recurrence of obstruction after coronary angioplasty.

Exercise Training

Alterations in Exercise Response of the Coronary Patient[7,8]

Limitation of activity in patients with atherosclerotic coronary disease relates to a discrepancy between myocardial oxygen supply and demand; angina pectoris, left ventricular dysfunction, or electrical instability may all be manifestations of myocardial ischemia. Regional abnormalities of myocardial perfusion, some of which may be evident at rest, often increase with exercise and result in regional alterations of myocardial performance. Stroke volume may decrease, rather than showing the anticipated increase, as the intensity of exercise progresses; if this results in exercise-induced hypotension (inotropic incompetence), the response has poor prognostic significance. Additionally, many patients with atherosclerotic coronary disease do not maintain the linear relationship between increased intensity of workload and increased heart rate response; this chronotropic incompetence also suggests an unfavorable prognosis.

Patients with modest coronary impairment may have a normal cardiac output at rest and at low levels of activity; however, as the intensity of the activity progresses, the restriction of cardiac output, not demonstrated at low workloads, becomes evident. In patients with angina pectoris, the threshold for myocardial ischemia determines the activity intensity at which signs and symptoms of cardiac dysfunction appear. When the increased myocardial oxygen demand of exercise cannot be met by an increase in coronary blood flow (this is usually encountered with coronary obstruction greater than 75 percent of the cross-sectional area), evidence of myocardial dysfunction and electrical instability may appear. This is closely associated with the rate-pressure product, which reflects a well-defined threshold for myocardial ischemia at a given time in a given patient.

Exercise Prescription

Individualized prescriptive physical activity[9–11] is central to rehabilitation. The ultimate goal is long-term, regular exercise of moderate intensity as part of the life-style. The prescriptive components of exercise include its "dosage"—the frequency, duration, and intensity of exercise—as well as the specific type of exercise to be undertaken. Exercise testing is necessary for the accurate and safe prescription of exercise. Age-predicted target heart rates should not be used for coronary patients; the disease, as well as the therapy and the prior state of physical conditioning, may influence the heart rate response to exercise. Exercise test data are used to determine the intensity of exercise appropriate during training; patients should attain a heart rate between 70 and 85 percent of the highest level safely achieved at exercise testing. Coronary patients should never exercise at a level higher than that documented as maintaining an appropriate cardiovascular response during testing. In general the 70 to 75 percent heart rate range for unsupervised exercise and the 80 to 85 percent range for supervised programs have been found to be effective in developing endurance, yet associated with an acceptably low risk of cardiovascular complications.[12] An alternative method for calculating the target heart rate is that of Karvonen; 70 to 85 percent of the difference between the peak exercise test heart rate and the resting heart rate is added to the resting rate. This method may be advantageous for patients whose heart rate is attenuated by beta blockade.

Two or three sessions each week of dynamic exercise, preferably on nonsuccessive days, are generally the minimum frequency recommended to achieve a training effect. Sedentary older patients or deconditioned individuals may improve their physical work capacity with one or two exercise sessions each week. Exercise sessions are generally 45 to 60 min in duration, including warm-up and cool-down periods. Although increased duration and/or frequency of exercise can compensate for decreased intensity, this may be associated with an increase in orthopedic and musculoskeletal injuries and poor adherence to the program.

Dynamic versus Isometric Exercise

The physiological response to *dynamic (isotonic) exercise* is an increase in heart rate that parallels the intensity of the activity, with an associated increase in stroke volume. Systolic blood pressure increases progressively; maintenance of, or slight decrease in, diastolic blood pressure widens the pulse pressure. Increased oxygen extraction, aided by redistribution of blood flow to working muscles, increases the systemic arteriovenous oxygen difference. The volume load on the heart due to dynamic exercise is the basis for its "cardiac conditioning" effect.

The increase in heart rate is modest with *isometric exercise* and is not related to the intensity of the effort. The increase in cardiac output is slight. There is often a precipitous increase in systolic blood pressure, which may provoke angina, left ventricular dysfunction, and/or arrhythmias; this is the basis for limiting isometric activity in patients with recent infarction. Because imposition of a pressure load effects little improvement in cardiovascular function, isolated isometric training has not been a major component of rehabilitative physical activity. Recent data suggest that combined isotonic and isometric training may produce a substantial training effect.[13]

Arm versus Leg Work and Training

Both arm and leg exercise[14] must be included in a training regimen, as their effects are only modestly interchangeable. After leg training, the heart rate and blood pressure responses to leg work decrease, but there is a lesser decrease in responses to arm work. After arm training, the reverse is true. At a comparable oxygen uptake, arm work evokes a higher heart rate and systolic blood pressure response than does leg work. In one study,[15] improvement in exercise performance with the untrained limb was 50 to 75 percent of the change in the trained limb, suggesting that half of the increase in trained limb performance is due to a generalized training effect and the other half is due predominantly to improved oxygen extraction by trained skeletal muscle. Since most occupational and recreational activities entail both arm and leg work, specific arm muscle exercises must be included in rehabilitative training designed to improve performance.

Effect of Cardiovascular Drugs on Exercise Training

Exercise training can be accomplished in patients receiving concomitant drug therapy, and drug therapy may improve the ability to exercise.[16] Nitroglycerin and longer-acting nitrate drugs improve coronary blood flow, decrease venous return, and improve wall motion and thereby increase the ejection fraction; an increased exercise capacity of about 1 MET may occur with the administration of nitrate drugs. Training can also occur in patients receiving calcium-blocking drugs. Despite the decrease in heart rate and blood pressure response with beta-adrenergic blocking drugs, exercise training in patients receiving these agents has been demonstrated to improve physical work capacity. Exercise testing for exercise prescription should be done with patients on the medical regimen planned for their period of training to ensure the proper target rate range recommendation.

The Effect of Training—Appropriate and Inappropriate Expectations

The major beneficial effect of exercise training[10,17] is an improvement in functional capacity. The hemodynamic determinants include an increase in maximal cardiac output and oxygen consumption, a lowering of the heart rate and systolic blood pressure both at rest and at submaximal work levels, and a more rapid return to normal of the exercise heart rate. The decreased myocardial oxygen requirements for submaximal levels of exercise in the trained individual improve the physical work capacity and increase the exercise threshold required to precipitate angina pectoris. A significant amount of "spontaneous" improvement in cardiac function occurs during the early weeks of recovery from myocardial infarction.[17a]

There is no documentation indicating that exercise training alters the coronary lesions demonstrated at arteriography, increases coronary blood flow, or stimulates formation of a coronary collateral circulation in human beings, although studies in experimental animals have demonstrated morphologic adaptations that may be favorable. Radionuclide studies have not delineated a consistent improvement in myocardial perfusion or left ventricular systolic performance in coronary patients after exercise training.[17a–20] The improvement in functional capacity and decrease in symptoms that result from short-term exercise training appear primarily due to peripheral adaptations;[18] there is increased oxygen extraction from the blood, systemic vascular resistance decreases, and skeletal muscle and autonomic nervous system adaptations result in a decreased rate-pressure product.[21] Whether improvement in myocardial performance occurs, even with vigorous exercise, remains controversial,[22] particularly in patients with significant coronary obstruction; protracted, high-intensity exercise training has been described as increasing stroke volume and stroke work, resulting in augmented cardiac function.[21] Neither is there evidence that even prolonged and intense exercise training, as an isolated intervention, favorably alters the natural history of coronary disease,[23–25] although a small multifactorial intervention trial showed a reduction in mortality, particularly in sudden death, during the initial 6 months after infarction, the reduction being associated with exercise training, quality medical care, and patient education.[26] A decrease in fatal reinfarction occurred in exercising patients in the National Exercise and Heart Disease Project, although total reinfarction rate was not altered.[24] Pooling of data from several large controlled exercise trials suggests a 25 to 35 percent survival advantage for exercising subjects, as well as a decrease in recurrent coronary events.[27]

Serum triglyceride levels decrease with exercise. Although changes in total cholesterol levels are not predictable, levels often decrease; the ratio of high-density lipoprotein (HDL) to low-density lipoprotein (LDL) cholesterol also increases in physically active individuals. A beneficial effect of exercise on fibrinolysis and on platelet function has not been substantiated. Even low-intensity short-term exercise seemed adequate to stimulate positive psychosocial, sexual, and vocational changes in patients in the randomized National Exercise and Heart Disease Project.[28]

Not all patients improve their functional capacity with exercise training, often owing to the development of left ventricular dysfunction or cardiac failure at higher levels of exercise. Despite prolonged training, the atherosclerotic coronary obstruction may progress.

Implementation of Rehabilitation

Inpatient or Hospital Phase

The *components* of rehabilitative care for the patient hospitalized for acute myocardial infarction or coronary artery bypass surgery include, in addition to the traditional medical and surgical management, progressive physical activity (often termed *early ambulation*), and patient and family education and counseling.

Progressive Physical Activity (Early Ambulation)
Early ambulation is indicated for most patients after myocardial infarction and coronary bypass surgery to avert or limit the detrimental effects of prolonged bed rest.[29] These include a decrease in physical work capacity due to a decrease in maximal cardiac output; orthostatic intolerance, characterized by orthostatic hypotension and tachycardia due to hypovolemia and a lessened cardiovascular reflex response; increased blood viscosity due to contraction of plasma volume disproportionate to the decrease in red blood cell mass (which, associated with the circulatory stasis of bed rest, predisposes to thromboembolism); and diminution of pulmonary ventilation. Decreases in muscle mass and muscular contractile strength result in inefficient muscular contraction and require more oxygen for comparable work. Deleterious psychological responses to immobilization are discussed subsequently.

Cardiac work is less in the seated than in the supine position. Activity as low-level as sitting in a chair two or three times daily seems sufficient to limit the hypovolemia of immobilization and the resultant orthostatic hypotension; the exposure to gravitational stress, rather than the intensity of the activity, appears to prevent hypovolemia with cardiac underfilling and resultant deterioration of the oxygen transport capacity[30] and effort intolerance.[31]

Similarities in the rehabilitation of patients after myocardial infarction, coronary artery bypass surgery, and angioplasty are more prominent than differences. The patient with an *uncomplicated myocardial infarction* with a favorable prognosis requires accelerated education and progressive physical activity because of the typical early discharge.[3] With *complications of infarction,* particularly left ventricular dysfunction and arrhythmias, a more prolonged hospitalization, a more gradual increase in physical activity, and additional education and counseling may be required. Many such patients will need multiple cardiac drugs and additional diagnostic assessment. Patients after coronary artery bypass surgery, as well as after angioplasty, often have had the opportunity for preoperative education and orientation. Coronary bypass patients usually can be rapidly ambulated and have a short hospital stay, although discomfort at the sternotomy and saphenous vein removal sites may limit mobility. Postoperative pericarditis is common and may result in sinus tachycardia. Postoperative hypovolemia may be manifest by a hypotensive response, often with accompanying tachycardia, to early physical activity.[32] Patients undergoing successful coronary *angioplasty* usually have stable coronary disease with few symptoms and good left ventricular function after the angioplasty. Their hospital stay is brief, and emphasis should be on averting physiological and psychological disability.

Initial guidelines for physical activity in the coronary or surgical intensive care unit are that exercise be low level in intensity (1 to 2 METs), be gradually progressive in work demand, and be supervised to assess whether the patient's response is appropriate. Patients may feed themselves, perform personal care, use a bedside commode, and sit in a bedside chair. Selected arm and leg exercises help maintain muscle tone and increase flexibility and joint mobility. Incentive spirometry is important for the postoperative patient. *Disproportionate responses*[33] to low-level activity include chest discomfort, dyspnea, or palpitations; a heart rate greater than 120 beats or below 50 beats per minute (patients receiving beta-adrenergic blocking drugs should not increase their heart rate by more than 15 to 20 beats per minute above resting level); ST-segment displacement on the ECG or monitor; the appearance of dysrhythmias; or a fall of greater than 10 to 15 mmHg in systolic blood pressure, which usually indicates inadequacy of the cardiac output to meet the activity demand. A systolic blood pressure in excess of 180 mmHg or a diastolic pressure in excess of 110 mmHg suggests the need for antihypertensive therapy. An appropriate response allows the patient to progress to activities of greater intensity; a disproportionate response requires reduction of activity and clinical reassessment, and may indicate otherwise unrecognized cardiac dysfunction.

The goal of physical activity during the remainder of the hospitalization is to help patients achieve a functional level that permits self-care and homebound activities at discharge from the hospital. Household tasks require a work intensity of 2 to 3 METs. Patients continue to perform personal care, sit in a chair for increasing periods of time, and are supervised in selected warm-up dynamic exercises involving the extremities and trunk. The major prescriptive exercise component is walking, with stepwise increases in pace and distance. Elastic stockings are advised during exercise for the postoperative patient to decrease leg pain and edema at the saphenous vein incision sites. The patients who must climb steps at home should practice this in the hospital. Electrocardiographic monitoring or telemetry during early ambulation is required only for selected patients, particularly those with prior serious ventricular ectopy or asymptomatic myocardial ischemia. An early ambulation protocol (Table 48-1), implemented under the supervision of the Emory University School of Medicine, delineates prescribed exercises, in-hospital "daily living" activities, and recreational and educational activities of comparable intensity for a series of steps. The initial two steps are intensive care unit activities; the subsequent five, performed on a general medical or surgical care area, include warm-up exercises and progressive increases in walking.

Early physical activity has not increased the complications of myocardial infarction, and early hospital discharge for appropriately selected patients has not adversely affected short- or long-term morbidity or mortality. Benefits include the prevention of deconditioning, lessened pulmonary atelectasis and thromboembolic complications, and a decrease in anxiety and depression related to the tangible evidence of improvement. Early ambulation makes possible the current shorter hospital stay, savings in medical care costs, and potential improved use of hospital beds. It permits the appropriate performance of predischarge exercise testing. The functional status of patients is improved at hospital discharge; this has been associated with an earlier and more complete return to work.

Patient and Family Education and Counseling

These interventions are designed to provide the information about coronary disease and its management that enables patients and their families to assume some responsibility for their health care on return home. Teaching optimally begins during the acute hospital stay, but, if benefits are to be maintained, medical recommendations must be reinforced after return home and effort must be made to ensure continuity between in-hospital education and counseling and that done on an outpatient basis.

TABLE 48-1 In-Patient Rehabilitation: Seven-Step Myocardial Infarction Program (Revised 1980): Grady Memorial Hospital and the Emory University School of Medicine

Step	Date	M.D. Initials	Nurse/PT Notes	Supervised Exercise	CCU/Ward Activity	Educational-Recreational Activity
CCU						
1	——			Active and passive ROM all extremities, in bed Teach patient ankle plantar and dorsiflexion—repeat hourly when awake	Partial self-care Feed self Dangle legs on side of bed Use bedside commode Sit in chair 15 min 1–2 times/day	Orientation to CCU Personal emergencies, social service aid as needed
2	——			Active ROM all extremities, sitting on side of bed	Sit in chair 15–30 min 2–3 times/day Complete self-care in bed	Orientation to rehabilitation team, program Smoking cessation Educational literature if requested Planning transfer from CCU
Ward						
3	——			Warm-up exercises, 2 METs: Stretching Calisthenics Walk 50 ft and back at slow pace	Sit in chair ad lib To ward class in wheelchair Walk in room	Normal cardiac anatomy and function Development of atherosclerosis What happens with myocardial infarction 1–2 METs craft activity
4	——			ROM and calisthenics, 2.5 METs Walk length of hall (75 ft) and back, average pace Teach pulse counting	OOB as tolerated Walk to bathroom Walk to ward class, with supervision	Coronary risk factors and their control
5	——			ROM and calisthenics, 3 METs Check pulse counting Practice walking few stairsteps Walk 300 ft bid	Walk to waiting room or telephone Walk in ward corridor prn	Diet Energy conservation Work simplification techniques (as needed) 2–3 METs craft activity
6	——			Continue above activities Walk down flight of steps (return by elevator) Walk 500 ft bid Instruct on home exercise	Tepid shower or tub bath, with supervision To OT, cardiac clinic teaching room, with supervision	Heart attack management: Medications Exercise Surgery Response to symptoms Family, community adjustments on return home Craft activity prn
7	——			Continue above activities Walk up flight of steps Walk 500 ft bid Continue home exercise instruction; present information regarding outpatient exercise program	Continue all previous ward activities	Discharge planning: Medications, diet, activity Return appointments Scheduled tests Return to work Community resources Educational literature Medication cards Craft activity prn

In the coronary or surgical intensive care unit (or in the *preprocedure phase* for patients scheduled for angioplasty or coronary bypass surgery), answers to patient's questions should provide reassurance. There should be a brief explanation of the diagnosis, what is to be anticipated, and reasons for regulations, procedures, and equipment. This information helps patients adjust to a life-threatening situation. Emphasis should be placed on the temporary nature of most restrictions and the fact that, as the patient recovers, improvement in cardiac status will result in a decrease in surveillance and intensity of care.

During the remainder of the hospitalization, more detailed education and planning for discharge are appropriate. A brief review of normal cardiac structure and function and of atherosclerotic coronary obstruction is needed. Description of the changes of infarction should emphasize healing. This provides a basis for subsequent recommendations for care, including coronary risk modification and medical or surgical therapy. Angioplasty techniques and coronary bypass surgery should be explained as needed. Many psychosocial outcomes after infarction, angioplasty, or coronary bypass surgery appear related to the patient's perception of health status, which may be favorably altered by education and counseling. Recommendations should be presented for control of associated diseases, particularly hypertension and diabetes, as well as modification of other risk factors, designed to limit subsequent coronary events (see Chap. 42). Because myocardial infarction often has a negative impact on sexuality,[34] resumption of sexual activity should be recommended as appropriate and safe when other daily activities are reinstituted; both partners should be counseled about resumption of sexual intercourse. Patients should be instructed about all medications to be taken at home, the purpose, dosage, desired effects, and potential adverse affects. Many patients have not taken medications prior to the coronary event and may be unfamiliar with problems of taking medications. Patients should be taught the appropriate response to new or recurrent symptoms and how to gain access to emergency medical care. Many hospital centers teach cardiopulmonary resuscitation to families of coronary patients. The role of relaxation techniques and biofeedback training remains to be defined. Although the value of stress management has not been established, the favorable responses in a pilot study are encouraging.[35] Community resources that may be helpful should be identified: counseling and guidance services, home care agencies, vocational rehabilitation facilities and services for job training and placement, services for financial aid, and postcoronary groups or clubs. Family counseling should include life-style adjustments during convalescence, focusing on avoiding unnecessary invalidism of the coronary patient. Because many patients have concern about inadequate or ambiguous information, there should be discussion of tests or procedures planned in subsequent weeks, review of permitted activities and their serial resumption, and preliminary attention to return to work and long-term outlook.

The current shortened duration of hospitalization has altered the provision of education and counseling, limiting the ability to address the patient's and spouse's needs for information and advice and to adequately prepare them for convalescence at home. Although this accelerated care has economic advantages and appears associated with an increased return to work or preillness activity, participation in posthospital community heart clubs or educational groups may further facilitate rehabilitation between discharge from the hospital and return to preillness levels of function, encourage modification of risk-related behaviors, and aid in reinforcing maintenance of these changes. Patients who understand their disease and its management seem to cooperate more effectively in recommendations for care, i.e., the acquisition of knowledge appears to exert a demonstrable effect on behavior.[36]

Outpatient or Ambulatory Phase

Guidelines for exercise for coronary patients in the ambulatory phase are given in Table 48-2.

Therapeutic Exercise Training[9,13,37]

Therapeutic (phase II) exercise training ideally involves medically supervised exercise, at least for the initial weeks after hospital discharge, although economic constraints and logistics often limit the availability of supervised exercise. There is need to assess the role, safety, and effectiveness of unsupervised physical activity. Until data define the safety of unsupervised exercise, interim guidelines suggest that patients with a low maximal functional capacity, severely depressed left ventricular function, complex ventricular arrhythmias, exercise-induced hypotension, or inability to self-monitor the exercise heart rate are at increased risk for adverse events and should be trained in a medically supervised setting.[38] Although unsupervised exercise may be recommended for patients lacking these characteristics, it is preferable that this follow a brief period of observation, instruction, and training in a medically supervised setting. A recent study showed that home and supervised training equally increased the functional capacity of low-risk patients after myocardial infarction; there were no training-related complications.[38a]

The exercise prescription varies with the needs and goals of each patient, age and general health status, current exercise capacity, musculoskeletal competence, prior exercise activity and level of training, planned occupational and recreational activities, and the patient's skills, likes, and dislikes as well as accessibility of exercise equipment. The basic design of the exercise regimen is an initial 5 to 10-minute warm-up period of stretching and range of motion exercises to bring about musculoskeletal and circulatory "readiness" for exercise. A 15- to 45-min endurance component typically initially includes walk-run sequences or exercise on a stationary bicycle or treadmill; these are activities where skill is a minimal component of the intensity of work demand (Table 48-2). Exercise prescription of target heart rate is based on predischarge exercise testing or sign-

TABLE 48-2 Coronary Outpatient Exercise Guidelines: Emory University School of Medicine

Level	Approx. No. of Weeks after Event‡	Calisthenics No. of Repetitions	Medically Supervised: Bicycle Ergometer	Medically Supervised: Arm Ergometer	Medically Supervised: Treadmill or Walk-Jog	Unsupervised: Bicycle Ergometer	Unsupervised: Walk
Phase II (Therapeutic)						(85% of Supervised)	
1	3–4	6	8 min (×2) 35% MET-ET or 50 r/min at 150 KPM	8 min (×2) 30% MET-ET or 100 T at 150 KPM	12 min* 50% MET-ET† or 22-min mile	8 min (×2) 50 r/min at 130 KPM	12 min* 25-min mile
2	3–4	7	8 min (×2) 40% MET-ET or 50 r/min at 225 KPM	8 min (×2) 35% MET-ET or 125 T at 225 KPM	12 min* 60% MET-ET† or 22-min mile	8 min (×2) 50 r/min at 190 KPM	12 min* 25-min mile
3	3–4	8	8 min (×2) 45% MET-ET or 50 r/min at 300 KPM	8 min (×2) 45% MET-ET or 125 T at 300 KPM	12 min* 70% MET-ET† or 20-min mile	8 min (×2) 60 r/min at 225 KPM	12 min* 22-min mile
4	5	10	12 min 45% MET-ET or 60 r/min at 300 KPM	8 min (×2) 45% MET-ET or 150 T at 300 KPM	12 min* 75% MET-ET† or 18-min mile	12 min 60 r/min at 225 KPM	12 min* 20-min mile
5	5	10	15 min 45% MET-ET or 70 r/min at 300 KPM	8 min (×2) 45% MET-ET or 150 T at 300 KPM	12 min* 75% MET-ET† or 18-min mile	15 min 70 r/min at 225 KPM	12 min* 20-min mile
6	5	10	15 min 45% MET-ET or 70 r/min at 300 KPM	8 min (×2) 45% MET-ET or 150 T at 300 KPM	12 min* 75% MET-ET† or 18-min mile	15 min 70 r/min at 255 KPM	12 min* 20-min mile
7‡	6	12	15 min 60 r/min at 300 KPM or 3.7 MET	175 T at 300 KPM or 4.5 MET	1.5 min§ 3.9 MET, 16-min mile walk; or 6.0 MET, 14-min mile walk; or 8.6 MET, 12-min mile jog; or 10.2 MET, 10-min mile jog	15 min 60 r/min at 255 KPM or 3.1 MET	1.5 min 3.9 MET or 16-min mile walk
8‡	7	18	15 min 60 r/min at 450 KPM or 4.9 MET	200 T at 375 KPM or 5.5 MET	2.0 min§ 3.9 MET, 16-min mile walk; or 6.0 MET, 14-min mile walk; or 8.6 MET, 12-min mile jog; or 10.2 MET, 10-min mile jog	15 min 60 r/min at 380 KPM or 4.2 MET	2.0 min 3.9 MET or 16-min mile walk
9‡	9	18	15 min 60 r/min at 450 KPM or 4.9 MET	200 T at 450 KPM or 6.4 MET	2.25 min§ 6.0 MET, 14-min mile walk; or 8.6 MET, 12-min mile jog; or 10.2 MET, 10-min mile jog; or 11.0 MET, 9-min mile jog	15 min 60 r/min at 380 KPM or 4.2 MET	2.25 min 3.9 MET or 16-min mile walk
10‡	11	18	15 min 60 r/min at 600 KPM or 6.1 MET	250 T at 450 KPM or 6.4 MET	2.5 min§ 6.0 MET, 14-min mile walk; or 8.6 MET, 12-min mile jog; or 10.2 MET, 10-min mile jog; or 11.0 MET, 9-min mile jog	15 min 60 r/min at 500 KPM or 5.2 MET	2.5 min 6.0 MET or 14-min mile walk
11‡	12	18	15 min 60 r/min at 600 KPM or 6.1 MET	250 T at 450 KPM or 6.4 MET	2.75 min§ 6.0 MET, 14-min mile walk; or 8.6 MET, 12-min mile jog; or 10.2 MET, 10-min mile jog; or 11.0 MET, 9-min mile jog	15 m 60 r/min at 500 KPM or 5.2 MET	2.75 min 6.0 MET or 14-min mile walk

TABLE 48-2 Coronary Outpatient Exercise Guidelines: Emory University School of Medicine (*continued*)

Level	Approx. No. of Weeks after Event‡	Calisthenics No. of Repetitions	Medically Supervised: Bicycle Ergometer	Medically Supervised: Arm Ergometer	Medically Supervised: Treadmill or Walk-Jog	Unsupervised: Bicycle Ergometer	Unsupervised: Walk
Phase II (Therapeutic) (*continued*)						**(85% of Supervised)**	
12‡	13	18	15 min 60 r/min at 600 KPM or 6.1 MET	250 T at 450 KPM or 6.4 MET	3.00 min§ 6.0 MET, 14-min mile walk; or 8.6 MET, 12-min mile jog; or 10.2 MET, 10-min mile jog; or 11.0 MET, 9-min mile jog	15 min 60 r/min at 500 KPM or 5.2 MET	3.00 min 6.0 MET or 14-min mile walk
Phase III (Maintenance)							
13‡	14 on	18	15 min 60 r/min at 600 KPM or 6.1 MET	250 T at 450 KPM or 6.4 MET	3.00 min 9–12-min mile or 11.0–8.6 MET jog-walk	15 min 60 r/min at 500 KPM or 5.2 MET	3.00 min 6.0 MET or 14-min mile walk

Notes: Levels 1–6, typically accomplished in a 2-week period. Telemetry ECG monitoring may aid in heart rate and rhythm evaluation during this period. Supervised programs, 3 sessions weekly. Unsupervised programs 3–4 sessions weekly. MET-ET = MET level on treadmill test. KPM = bicycle resistance in kilopond meters. T = turns of 60–75 revolutions per minute (r/min).

*Plus an additional 1-min warm-up and 1-min cool-down.

†As designated on exercise treadmill (calibrated).

††Event = myocardial infarction, coronary bypass surgery, or coronary angioplasty.

‡Levels 7–13, rowing machine may be used for 3–5 min, progressing from slight to moderate resistance.

§Select pace on an individual basis considering activity level in previous weeks and patient's cardiovascular status.

Source: G. F. Fletcher and J. D. Cantwell, "Exercise and Coronary Heart Disease," 2d ed., Charles C Thomas, Publisher, Springfield, Ill., 1979, p. 175.

symptom limited testing prior to entering the program. Since these activities primarily train leg muscles, they should be supplemented with arm-training exercises such as selected repetitive calisthenics, use of shoulder wheels, rowing machines, and arm ergometers to provide a variety of training stimuli. With space limitations, "station" training with bicycle ergometry, hand ergometry, rowing machines, and treadmills may be preferable. With more space availability, gymnasium programs can accommodate larger numbers of patients for walk-jog activities; some facilities have indoor or outdoor tracks. Intermittent exercise or alternation of high- and low-intensity activities allows a greater total training workload to be imposed at each exercise session without producing cardiovascular symptoms. The final 5- to 10-min cool-down period entails a gradual decrease in exercise intensity, allowing the heart rate to subside and averting postexercise hypotension. Aerobic games, as an optional recreational component, add variety to an exercise program and improve adherence to the program; they also have the advantage of providing upper-body exercise. Since variations in skills and competitiveness significantly vary the oxygen cost of these activities, they are often limited early in exercise training.

Exercise supervision may not entail an "all-or-none" approach; intermittent supervision at periodic exercise sessions may occur in a community facility, there may be intermittent telephone transmission of the exercise ECG of patients exercising at home,[39] or a combination of these approaches may be used. Periodic transtelephonic ECG transmission has been reported to improve adherence to exercise. Because the risk of exercise-related cardiac complications is not increased in proximity to the acute cardiac event,[40] the appropriate role and duration of ECG surveillance of exercise remain unclear.

Patients in supervised exercise programs without continuous electrocardiographic monitoring should intermittently measure their heart rate response to assure that it remains in the prescribed range and should concomitantly estimate their exercise intensity. Pulse rhythm irregularities require the recording of an ECG rhythm strip; this may be accomplished using the defibrillator paddles as ECG leads. Although complication rates appear lower in exercise programs with continuous ECG monitoring, it is not known whether the ECG monitoring, the closer medical supervision, or differing exercise intensities are the determinants.

Detailed instructions for unsupervised home exercise should be provided in written form. Some initial home exercise regimens involve progressive walking and walk-jog sequences; others serially increase the intensity and duration of use of the stationary bicycle (Table 48-2). As the level of training increases, recreational activities in which skill influences work intensity may add variety to the exercise regimen. Effective endurance activities include rope-jumping, bicycling, skating, swimming, rowing, and aerobic dancing.

The goal of prescriptive exercise is an improvement in cardiovascular function, designated as the *training effect*. Training can increase the maximal oxygen uptake by as much as 20 percent. This appears to be due primarily to peripheral mechanisms, i.e., increased oxygen extraction by trained skeletal muscles as well as redistribution of the cardiac output. These changes lower the heart rate and systolic blood pressure response to submaximal exertion. A benefit that reflects this decrease in the rate-pressure product is that the trained patient experiences less or no angina and fewer or no ischemic electrocardiographic changes at submaximal work levels. Thus, the trained individual functions farther from his or her ischemic threshold in performing usual daily activities and perceives these tasks as requiring less exertion because they require a smaller percentage of the improved physical work capacity.

Exercise training of patients after coronary bypass surgery[41] can increase their activity threshold before the onset of angina, avert deconditioning, optimize musculoskeletal function, and provide psychologic benefits. It often has a favorable effect in modifying coronary risk factors. The magnitude and rate of improvement in work capacity were greater in patients exercising after coronary bypass surgery than in a randomly assigned control group.[42]

Maintenance Exercise Training

Components of the *maintenance* (long-term) phase of rehabilitation include continued medical care, exercise,[43] and education and counseling. (See Table 48-2.)

Because exercise training is designed to maintain adequate physical conditioning, a lifetime pattern of regular activity is necessary. Patients must achieve reasonable independence in exercising, and there should be progressive involvement in exercise that is social, enjoyable, convenient, and appropriate. Most patients who attain a 7- to 8-MET level of performance can progress to an unsupervised or minimally supervised exercise setting; this typically occurs within 3 to 6 months after infarction. Patients leaving supervised exercise programs require counseling about long-term community exercise activities. As with patients in a supervised exercise setting, serial exercise testing is recommended.

Exercise training aids in weight control, favorably affects psychological status, and appears to aid patients in renouncing the sick role and resuming a normal life-style, including return to work.

Special Concerns in Coronary Rehabilitation

The Elderly Patient

Elderly patients currently constitute a progressively larger component of the population with myocardial infarction, coronary artery bypass surgery, and coronary angioplasty.

Myocardial infarction is typically more severe in elderly patients and is associated with increased complications; the prolonged hospitalization may foster additional deconditioning. Elderly patients often become confused in intensive care settings and require concise but repeated explanations, reassurance, and time-and-place orientation. Early mobilization is important to limit functional deterioration, and aged patients tend to be reassured by their ability to perform personal care. Aggressive modification of conventional coronary risk factors has less justification in the elderly, except for advising smoking cessation which appears to be of as much benefit as in younger patients. The emphasis in rehabilitation is a return to the preinfarction life-style. The teaching of energy-conserving techniques of self-care and for performance of household tasks is often needed. Elderly individuals in a posthospital exercise program require a longer time to attain a training effect because of their slower initial adaptation to training and because of the appropriately low intensity of the training stimulus. Warm-up exercises permit more effective training. Because more time is required for the heart rate to return to normal after exercise than for younger patients, longer intervals of rest or low-level activity are necessary between exercise periods. Exercise may modify the decrease in joint mobility that occurs with aging and can enhance neuromuscular coordination. Nevertheless, running and jumping should be limited for elderly patients because these are more likely to cause orthopedic complications. Often simple walking, bicycle ergometry, and/or walking in pools are adequate exercise activities for the elderly. Furthermore, elderly individuals perspire less efficiently so that exercise should be limited in hot and humid environments.[44]

Rehabilitative goals for the elderly patient involve helping the patient to maintain physical capacity, coordination, and mental functional integrity and to readjust to preillness family and community settings.

The Patient with Severe Ventricular Dysfunction

In prior years, patients with severe ventricular dysfunction, typically New York Heart Association classes III and IV,[45] were not considered candidates for rehabilitative physical activity. These patients usually had a more protracted hospital stay and more delayed mobilization. However, as with elderly patients, because low-level physical activity constitutes a large proportion of their physical capacity, even slow walking can provide effective conditioning. An increased duration of activity can compensate for the necessary low intensity and yet produce a training effect. Other important components of rehabilitative care include the teaching of work-simplification techniques, the pacing of activities, working in the sitting position, and taking frequent rest periods.

Recent studies suggest that selected patients with a low exercise capacity, and those with severely impaired left ventricular function, can benefit from exercise training.[46] Low-level physical activity, imposed gradually over a protracted period of time, had no adverse consequences. It may produce a sufficient training effect and improvement in physical work capacity to permit patients to continue independent living. Although there is no improvement in ventricular function, ventricular function does not deteriorate.[46] However, training of these individuals has only been performed in a highly supervised setting with continuous electrocardiographic monitoring; it is not known whether an effective and safe training regimen can occur under other circumstances.

Impaired exercise capacity in patients with congestive heart failure is in part due to inadequate nutritive blood flow to skeletal muscle; factors other than the inability to increase the cardiac output with exercise seem important.[47] The effects of exercise training on skeletal muscle blood flow require investigation.

Psychological Aspects of Rehabilitation

Psychological impairment may limit the recovery of the coronary patient.[48] (See also Chap. 45.) Major psychological problems of coronary patients include anxiety, depression, denial, and dependency. Anxiety and depression contribute to failure to resume sexual function, to engage in social activities, and to make satisfactory life adjustments. Many patients with successful physical recovery after infarction and coronary bypass surgery have residual emotional impairment. Their initial anxiety is realistic, related to fear of dying; "appropriate" denial, characterized by confidence in a favorable outcome, is an effective coping strategy and is associated with an improved prognosis. The characteristic overcompetitive type A patient with a sense of time urgency, whose life-style involves control, adapts poorly to a dependent role in an intensive care unit. These patients also respond poorly to sedation which decreases external perception and augments anxiety. Involving the patient in planning for recovery and teaching self-monitoring of the heart rate response to activity tend to return self-control to the patient and encourage adherence.

Depression is the major emotional problem during convalescence. This may be accentuated by the family's overprotection and often mimics organic illness because of combinations of fatigue, insomnia, memory impairment, headache, and vague chest discomfort. Although depression typically resolves in most individuals, in some it results in long-term invalidism with fear of return to prior life-style, inappropriate early retirement, and withdrawal from social interactions.

The two major intervention strategies which appear to limit psychological complications are education and counseling and physical activity.[28] Rehabilitation involves the behavior and capacities to meet life demands; this coping ability may be enhanced by the acquisition of skills, techniques, and knowledge. Many patients remain psychologically disabled because they inappropriately perceive their excessive severity of infarction and vulnerability to sudden death. The demonstration that modest physical activity can be performed safely provides reassurance and restores self-confidence.

Vocational Aspects of Rehabilitation

About 80 percent of patients with uncomplicated myocardial infarction, if younger than age 65 and employed at the time of infarction, return to work within 2 to 3 months, typically resuming their former jobs.[49] Unfortunately, although the early return to work is high after uncomplicated infarction, the dropout each year is also high. In one group of patients whose return to work by 6 months was 83 percent only 63 percent were gainfully employed at 1 year.[50] Although comparable data are not available for patients with complications of myocardial infarction and residual functional impairment, their estimated return to work rate is 25 to 33 percent.

These data contrast with the data on return to work of patients after coronary bypass surgery; despite their substantial decrease in symptoms, improvement in functional capacity, and reported enhancement of quality of life, the return to work has been limited.[51] The frequency of return to work after angioplasty is comparable to that after coronary bypass surgery, but angioplasty patients return to work earlier.[52]

Analysis of disability after myocardial infarction reveals it to be more dependent on psychological than on physiological problems. Only rarely in the patient with marginal cardiac function does the severity of angina or heart failure preclude or delay return to work. Factors which negatively influence return to work include patients of older age, patients with adequate nonwork income, patients who are anxious or depressed, those who become symptomatic with effort, patients lower on the social class and educational scales, those whose jobs are characterized by high physical activity, and those who perceive their illness as job-related. Patients who do not return to work within 6 months are less likely to ever do so.[51,53] In general, both for patients after infarction and patients after coronary bypass surgery, preoperative work status and the type of occupation (physical effort involved) are predominant factors in the decision to return to work.

A number of patients fail to return to work because of lack of professional assurance that they can safely do so. Exercise testing may permit a more precise assessment of function and help allay the fears of the patient,[54] physician, and employer regarding the capability and safety of a coronary patient's return to work. Exercise testing correlates moderately well with vocational pursuits when consideration is given to differences in temperature, environment, intellectual demands, relation to meals, and emotional stress. Patients who do not develop ischemia or arrhythmia during a symptom-limited dynamic exercise test are typically free of these problems when static and dynamic effort are combined.[55] In addition, since cardiac output, blood pressure, and oxygen uptake do not approach the steady state until about 2 min after the onset of work, occupational myocardial work demand is lower than that of the same level of steady-state exercise. Most occupational work is intermittent, with brief periods of strenuous activity and longer intervals of low-level activity. This explains why individuals with modest cardiac impairment and limitation of cardiac output can tolerate significant workloads of short duration when adequate rest periods are provided. When exercise test results are used to recommend full-time work, a level of about 30 percent of the physical work capacity is appropriate.

A number of nonmedical considerations may influence postoperative work status; they involve the financial, social, disability, and compensation benefits of not returning to work. Appropriate physician and employer attitudes may facilitate reemployment, but the viewpoint of the patient appears to be the major determinant.

Summary

Changes in the pattern of rehabilitative care of coronary patients during the past decade emphasize the current appreciation of the benefits and safety of early activity, as well as long-term exercise training; and an understanding of the prognostic and therapeutic values of exercise testing, angioplasty, coronary bypass surgery, and coronary risk reduction. Current practices are designed to reduce the physical and vocational invalidism and medical care costs associated with coronary disease. The overall consequences should be an improvement in the quality of life and a reduction in the economic burden of disability benefits and premature retirement.

References

1. Osler, W., (ed.): "The Principles and Practice of Medicine," 8th ed., Appleton & Co., New York, 1914, p. 796.
2. Report of the World Health Organization Expert Committee on Disability Prevention and Rehabilitation: Disability Prevention and Rehabilitation, *WHO Tech. Rep. Ser.*, No. 668, Geneva, 1981.
3. Pryor, D. B., Hindman, M. C., Wagner, G. S., Califf, R. M., Rhoads, M. K., and Rosati, R. A.: Early Discharge after Acute Myocardial Infarction, *Ann. Intern. Med.*, 99:528, 1983.
4. Johnston, B. L.: Exercise Testing for Patients after Myocardial Infarction and Coronary Bypass Surgery: Emphasis on Predischarge Phase, *Heart Lung*, 13:8, 1984.
5. Lindvall, K., Erhardt, L. R., Lundman, T., Rehnqvist, N., and Sjogren, A.: Early Mobilization and Discharge of Patients with Acute Myocardial Infarction. A Prospective Study Using Risk Indicators and Early Exercise Tests, *Acta Med. Scand.*, 206:169, 1979.
6. Theroux, P., Waters, D. D., Halphen, C., Debaisieux, J.-C., and Mizgala, H. F.: Prognostic Value of Exercise Testing Soon after Myocardial Infarction, *N. Engl. J. Med.*, 301:341, 1979.
6a. Williams, W. L., Nair, R. C., Higginson, L. A. J., Baird, M. G., Allan, K., and Beanlands, D. S.: Comparison of Clinical and Treadmill Variables for the Prediction of Outcome after Myocardial Infarction, *J. Am. Coll. Cardiol.*, 4:477, 1984.
7. Clausen, J. P.: Circulatory Adjustments to Dynamic Exercise and Effect of Physical Training in Normal Subjects and in Patients with Coronary Artery Disease, *Prog. Cardiovasc. Dis.*, 18:459, 1976.
8. Blomqvist, C. G.: Clinical Exercise Physiology, in N. K. Wenger and H. K. Hellerstein (eds.), "Rehabilitation of the Coronary Patient," 2d ed., John Wiley & Sons, Inc., New York, 1984, p. 179.
9. "The Exercise Standards Book," American Heart Association, 70-041-A, Dallas, 1979.
10. Council on Scientific Affairs: Physician-Supervised Exercise Programs in Rehabilitation of Patients with Coronary Heart Disease, *JAMA*, 245:1463, 1981.
11. American College of Sports Medicine: "Guidelines for Graded Exercise Testing and Exercise Prescription," 2d ed, Lea and Febiger, Philadelphia, 1980.
12. Haskell, W. L.: Cardiovascular Complications during Exercise Training of Cardiac Patients, *Circulation*, 57:920, 1978.
13. Bezucha, G. R., Lenser, M. C., Hanson, P. G., Nagle, F. J.: Comparison of Hemodynamic Responses to Static and Dynamic Exercise, *J. Appl. Physiol.*, 53:1589, 1982.
14. Schwade, J., Blomqvist, C. G., and Shapiro, W.: A Comparison of the Response to Arm and Leg Work in Patients with Ischemic Heart Disease, *Am. Heart J.*, 94:203, 1977.
15. Thompson, P. D., Cullinane, E., Lazarus, B., Carleton, R. A.: Effect of Exercise Training on the Untrained Limb Exercise Performance of Men with Angina Pectoris, *Am. J. Cardiol.*, 48:844, 1981.
16. Wenger, N. K.: Cardiovascular Drugs: Effects on Exercise Testing and Exercise Training of the Coronary Patient, in N. K. Wenger (ed.), "Exercise and the Heart," 2d ed., *Cardiovasc. Clin.*, F. A. Davis Company, Philadelphia, 1985, p. 133.
17. Paterson, D. H., Shephard, R. J., Cunningham, D., Jones, N. L., and Andrew, G.: Effects of Physical Training on Cardiovascular Function following Myocardial Infarction, *J. Appl. Physiol.*, 47:482, 1979.
17a. Hung, J., Gordon, E. P., Houston, N., Haskell, W. L., Goris, M. L., and DeBusk, R. F.: Changes in Rest and Exercise Myocardial Perfusion and Left Ventricular Function 3 to 26 Weeks after Clinically Uncomplicated Acute Myocardial Infarction: Effects of Exercise Training, *Am. J. Cardiol.*, 54:943, 1984.
18. Cobb, F. R., Williams, R. S., McEwan, P., Jones, R. H., Coleman, R. E., and Wallace, A. G.: Effects of Exercise Training on Ventricular Function in Patients with Recent Myocardial Infarction, *Circulation*, 66:100, 1982.
19. Verani, M. S., Hartung, G. H., Hoepfel-Harris, J., Welton, D. E., Pratt, C. M., and Miller, R. R.: Effects of Exercise Training on Left Ventricular Performance and Myocardial Perfusion in Patients with Coronary Artery Disease, *Am. J. Cardiol.*, 47:797, 1981.
20. Scheuer, J.: Effects of Physical Training on Myocardial Vascularity and Perfusion, *Circulation*, 66:491, 1982.
21. Hagberg, J. M., Ehsani, A. A., and Holloszy, J. O.: Effect of 12 Months of Intense Exercise Training on Stroke Volume in Patients with Coronary Artery Disease, *Circulation*, 67:1194, 1983.
22. Ehsani, A. A., Martin, W. H. III, Heath, G. W., and Coyle, E. F.: Cardiac Effects of Prolonged and Intense Exercise Training in Patients with Coronary Artery Disease, *Am. J. Cardiol.*, 50:246, 1982.

23. Wilhelmsen, L., Sanne, H., Elmfeldt, D., Grimby, G., Tibblin, G., and Wedel, H.: A Controlled Trial of Physical Training after Myocardial Infarction. Effects on Risk Factors, Nonfatal Reinfarction, and Death, *Prev. Med.*, 4:491, 1975.
24. Shaw. L. W.: Effects of a Prescribed Supervised Exercise Program on Mortality and Cardiovascular Morbidity in Patients after a Myocardial Infarction. The National Exercise and Heart Disease Project, *Am. J. Cardiol.*, 48:39, 1981.
25. Rechnitzer, P. A., Cunningham, D. A., Andrew, G. M., Buck, C. W., Jones, N. L., Kavanagh, T., Oldridge, N. B., Parker, J. O., Shephard, R. J., Sutton, J. R., and Donner, A. P.: Relation of Exercise to the Recurrence Rate of Myocardial Infarction in Men. Ontario Exercise-Heart Collaborative Study, *Am. J. Cardiol.*, 51:65, 1983.
26. Kallio, V., Hamalainen, H., Hakkila, J., and Luurila, O. J.: Reduction in Sudden Deaths by a Multifactorial Intervention Programme after Acute Myocardial Infarction, *Lancet*, 2:1091, 1979.
27. Shephard, R. J.: The Value of Exercise in Ischemic Heart Disease: A Cumulative Analysis, *J. Cardiac Rehab.*, 3:294, 1983.
28. Stern, M. J., and Cleary, P.: National Exercise and Heart Disease Project. Psychosocial Changes Observed During a Low-Level Exercise Program, *Arch. Intern. Med.*, 141:1463, 1981.
29. Wenger, N. K.: Early Ambulation after Myocardial Infarction: Rationale, Program Components, and Results, in N. K. Wenger and H. K. Hellerstein (eds.), "Rehabilitation of the Coronary Patient," 2d ed., John Wiley & Sons, Inc., New York, 1984, p. 97.
30. Convertino, V., Hung, J., Goldwater, D., and DeBusk, R. F.: Cardiovascular Responses to Exercise in Middle-Aged Men after 10 Days of Bedrest, *Circulation*, 65:134, 1982.
31. Hung, J., Goldwater, D., Convertino, V. A., McKillop, J. H., Goris, M. L., and DeBusk, R. F.: Mechanisms for Decreased Exercise Capacity after Bed Rest in Normal Middle-Aged Men, *Am. J. Cardiol.*, 51:344, 1983.
32. Dion, W. F., Grevenow, P., Pollock, M. L., Squires, R. W., Foster, C., Johnson, W. D., and Schmidt, D. H.: Medical Problems and Physiologic Responses During Supervised Inpatient Cardiac Rehabilitation: The Patient after Coronary Artery Bypass Grafting, *Heart Lung*, 11:248, 1982.
33. Report of Inter-Society Commission for Heart Disease Resources: Optimal Resources for the Care of Patients with Acute Myocardial Infarction and Chronic Coronary Heart Disease, *Circulation*, 65:654B, 1982.
34. Stern, M. J., Pascale, L., and Ackerman, A.: Life Adjustment Postmyocardial Infarction. Determining Predictive Variables, *Arch. Intern. Med.*, 137:1680, 1977.
35. Ornish, D., Scherwitz, L. W., Doody, R. S., Kesten, D., McLanahan, S. M., Brown, S. E., DePuey, E. G., Sonnemaker, R., Haynes, C., Lester, J., McAllister, G. K., Hall, R. J., Burdine, J. A., and Gotto, A. M., Jr.: Effects of Stress Management Training and Dietary Changes in Treating Ischemic Heart Disease, *JAMA*, 249:54, 1983.
36. Hogan, C. A., and Neill, W. A.: Effects of a Teaching Program on Knowledge, Physical Activity, and Socialization in Patients Disabled by Stable Angina Pectoris, *J. Cardiac Rehab.*, 2:379, 1982.
37. Fletcher, G. F.: Exercise in Secondary Prevention and Rehabilitation of Subjects with Coronary Disease, in G. F. Fletcher (ed.), "Exercise in the Practice of Medicine," Futura Publishing Co., Inc., Mt. Kisco, New York, 1982, p. 147.
38. Williams, R. S., Miller, H., Koisch, F. P., Jr., Ribisl, P., and Graden, H.: Guidelines for Unsupervised Exercise in Patients with Ischemic Heart Disease, *J. Cardiac Rehab.*, 1:213, 1981.
38a. Miller, N. H., Haskell, W. L., Berra, K., and DeBusk, R. F.: Home versus Group Exercise. Training for Increasing Functional Capacity after Myocardial Infarction, *Circulation*, 70:645, 1984.
39. Fletcher, G. F., Chiaramida, A. J., LeMay, M. R., Johnston, B. L., Thiel, J. E., and Spratlin, M. C.: Telephonically-Monitored Home Exercise Early after Coronary Artery Bypass Surgery, *Chest*, 86:198, 1984.
40. Hossack, K. F., and Hartwig, R.: Cardiac Arrest Associated with Supervised Cardiac Rehabilitation, *J. Cardiac. Rehab.*, 2:402, 1982.
41. Murray, G. C., and Beller, G. A.: Cardiac Rehabilitation following Coronary Artery Bypass Surgery, *Am. Heart J.*, 105:1009, 1983.
42. Foster, C., Pollock, M. L., Anholm, J. D., Squires, R. W., Ward, A., Dymond, D. S., Rod, J. L., Saichek, R. P., and Schmidt, D. H.: Work Capacity and Left Ventricular Function during Rehabilitation after Myocardial Revascularization Surgery, *Circulation*, 69:748, 1984.
43. Report of the Subcommittee on Exercise/Rehabilitation: Standards for Supervised Cardiovascular Exercise Maintenance Programs, *Circulation*, 62:669A, 1980.
44. Fletcher, G. F.: Influence of Environmental Factors on Exercise Activities in Patient Care, in G. F. Fletcher (ed.), "Exercise in the Practice of Medicine," Futura Publishing Co., Inc., Mt. Kisco, New York, 1982, p. 347.
45. The Criteria Committee of the New York Heart Association: "Diseases of the Heart and Blood Vessels. Nomenclature and Criteria for Diagnosis," 6th ed., Little, Brown and Company, Boston, 1964.
46. Conn, E. H., Williams, R. S., and Wallace, A. G.: Exercise Responses before and after Physical Conditioning in Patients with Severely Depressed Left Ventricular Function, *Am. J. Cardiol.*, 49:296, 1982.
47. Wilson, J. R., Martin, J. L., and Ferraro, N.: Impaired Skeletal Muscle Nutritive Flow during Exercise in Patients with Congestive Heart Failure: Role of Cardiac Pump Dysfunction as Determined by the Effect of Dobutamine, *Am. J. Cardiol.*, 53:1308, 1984.
48. Razin, A. M.: Psychosocial Intervention in Coronary Artery Disease: A Review, *Psychosom. Med.*, 44:363, 1982.
49. Wenger, N. K., Hellertstein, H. K., Blackburn, H., and Castronova, S. J.: Physician Practice in the Management of Patients with Uncomplicated Myocardial Infarction: Changes in the Past Decade, *Circulation*, 65:421, 1982.
50. Stern, M. L., Pascale, L., and McLoone, J. B.: Psychosocial Adaptation following an Acute Myocardial Infarction, *J. Chron. Dis.*, 29:513, 1976.
51. Almeida, D., Bradford, J. M., Wenger, N. K., King, S. B., and Hurst, J. W.: Return to Work after Coronary Bypass Surgery, *Circulation*, 66(suppl. 2):II-205, 1983.
52. Meier, B., and Gruentzig, A. R.: Return to Work after Coronary Artery Bypass Surgery in Comparison to Coronary Angioplasty, International Symposium on Return to Work after Coronary Artery Bypass Surgery, Psychosocial and Economic Aspects, May 10–11, 1984, Rotenburg/Fulda, Federal Republic of Germany. (Abstract.)
53. Smith, H. C., Hammes, L. N., Gupta, S., Vlietstra, R. E., and Elveback, L.: Employment Status after Coronary Artery Bypass Surgery, *Circulation*, 65(suppl. 2):II-120, 1982.
54. Ewart, C. K., Taylor, C. B., Reese, L. B., and DeBusk, R. F.: Effects of Early Postmyocardial Infarction Exercise Testing on Self-Perception and Subsequent Physical Activity, *Am. J. Cardiol.*, 51:1076, 1983.
55. Hung, J., McKillip, J., Savin, W., Magder, S., Kraus, R., Houston, N., Goris, M., Haskell, W., and DeBusk, R.: Comparison of Cardiovascular Response to Combined Static-Dynamic Effort, Postprandial Dynamic Effort and Dynamic Effort Alone in Patients with Chronic Ischemic Heart Disease, *Circulation*, 65:1411, 1982.

Section D

Systemic Arterial Hypertension

49

Pathophysiology of Hypertension

Harriet P. Dustan, M.D.

Determinants of Arterial Pressure

Basic Hemodynamic Principles

Under ordinary circumstances, pressure in the arterial system is maintained within fairly narrow limits in normotensive individuals. The exceptions to this generalization occur during sleep and exercise. During sleep arterial pressure may fall as low as 60/40 mmHg, and during exercise there are marked rises, particularly in systolic pressure.

To understand the hemodynamics of hypertension it may be helpful to review briefly some basic principles of hydrodynamics as they relate to the flow of blood throughout the vascular system. These are well described in texts of cardiovascular physiology.

The flow of liquid in a tube is related to the gradient of pressure along the tube and the resistance the liquid meets as it flows. Resistance (R) cannot be measured directly, so it is expressed as the ratio of the pressure gradient (P) to the flow rate (F):

$$R = \frac{P}{F}$$

Poiseuille's formula describes the relation of flow to the pressure gradient, the radius and length of the tube, and the viscosity of the fluid:

$$F = P\frac{r^4}{lv}\,\mathrm{k}$$

where r = the radius
l = the length of the tube
v = viscosity
k = a constant ($\pi/8$) derived from calculus integration

Combining these two equations we get

$$R = \frac{vl}{r^4} \times \frac{8}{\pi}$$

Within the usual physiological limits of blood viscosity, and since vascular length in an individual does not change abruptly, variations in resistance reflect functional or structural changes in vessel diameter. These equations clearly show the importance of vascular diameter as a determinant of resistance, because radius is raised to the fourth power, which means that small changes in diameter can have a profound effect on flow. This concept is central to an understanding of hypertension.

These fundamental hydrodynamic principles can be translated into clinical terms by the equation:

$$\text{MAP} = \text{CO} \times \text{TPR}$$

where CO (cardiac output) = F
MAP (mean arterial pressure) = P
TPR (total peripheral resistance) = R

MAP is the integrated pressure over one or several cardiac cycles. This integration can be obtained by damping pulsatile pressure or by calculating it as diastolic pressure plus one-third pulse pressure.

TPR is the sum of the resistances in all the vascular beds of the body. These are not necessarily equal, nor do they always change in the same direction. Thus, for example, a fall in TPR does not mean that vasodilation has occurred in each vascular bed; in some it may be unchanged, in others even increased, but enough vasodilation has occurred somewhere to result in an overall decrease.

Volume II

Systems Controlling Arterial Pressure

A General Statement

It is obvious from the above discussion that arterial pressure is determined by flow (cardiac output) and the resistance to flow (TPR). These are direct determinants, and in this grouping is another determinant, aortic impedance, and possibly a fourth, diastolic arterial volume (Table 49-1). *Impedance* is a term used to describe resistance to phasic flow.[1] For the aorta this is particularly apt, because the aorta receives the systolic ejection volume from the left ventricle.

Each time the heart contracts, it ejects a relatively small volume of blood into the arterial system. The arterial system has limited distensibility, is elastic, and is already partly filled (i.e., it contains the volume of blood remaining at the end of diastole). Hence, this ejection creates a pressure pulse. The pulse height is determined not only by the volume ejected and the residual diastolic volume, but also by the elasticity of the aorta. When the aorta is normally elastic, it dampens the pressure of ejection; it dilates, then recoils during diastole, and this recoil provides for diastolic flow. When the elasticity decreases, as with aging or active contraction, the arterial wall does not "give" during ejection and the full force of ejection pressure is expressed. Thus, the condition of the aortic wall is a determinant of arterial pressure.

Diastolic arterial volume is a theoretical function because arterial volume cannot now be measured, nor can the residual volume at the end of diastole. But since flow out of the aorta and large vessels is governed in large measure by the arterioles and precapillary sphincters, it seems logical to consider that diastolic arterial volume is a determinant of pressure. For example, hyperthyroidism is characterized by elevated systolic pressure because of a hyperkinetic heart, and low diastolic pressure because of vasodilation. The latter means a facilitated runoff during diastole and a relatively low diastolic arterial volume.

These direct determinants of arterial pressure are influenced by a variety of systems that basically control arterial pressure. These systems are indirect determinants. As listed in Table 49-1, these are the activity of the central and peripheral autonomic nervous system (primarily the sympathetic component), total body sodium stores and/or the extracellular fluid volume (ECF), the renal pressor system, and salt-active steroids. Although prostaglandins and the kallikrein-kinin system may influence arterial pressure, they will not be discussed here because a clear picture of their roles has not emerged.

TABLE 49-1 Determinants of Arterial Pressure

Direct
Cardiac output
Vascular resistance
Aortic impedance
Diastolic arterial volume
Indirect
Activity of the autonomic nervous system
Body sodium stores and/or extracellular fluid volume
The renal pressor system
Salt-active steroids

These indirect determinants affect cardiac output, vascular resistance, the circulating blood volume, and probably aortic impedance. They are also intimately interrelated. For example, activity of the nervous system influences renin release, which in turn controls aldosterone production, which affects fluid and electrolyte balance; it also has an independent effect on the renal excretion of salt and water. The renal pressor system, through its major polypeptide angiotensin II, besides being potently vasoconstrictive, plays a role in determining the degree of sympathetic nervous activity—both centrally and peripherally—as well as being the major control system for aldosterone release. It also seems to have an effect on salt and water excretion unrelated to aldosterone. It is well recognized that a positive fluid balance suppresses renin production and release and therefore suppresses aldosterone production, while a negative balance has the opposite effect. How salt balance affects activity of the nervous system is still under investigation.

It is these direct and indirect determinants of arterial pressure that are important to any consideration of the pathophysiology of hypertension. In some types of hypertension, their roles have been well defined, while in others we have only a partial picture as to how these various determinants are interrelated.

Systemic Hemodynamics

The formula MAP = CO × TPR indicates the primacy of flow and resistance in the control of arterial pressure. It is obvious from this formula that in the presence of an increased cardiac output, pressure is controlled within the normal range only if vascular resistance falls. The hyperdynamic heart syndrome described by Gorlin[2] dramatizes this because the patients studied were normotensive. In contrast, most of those reported by Frohlich et al.[3] were hypertensive because vascular resistance was either inappropriately normal or slightly elevated.

There are two ways that cardiac output can rise.[4] One is an increase in myocardial contractility with a rise in ejection fraction. This is common in borderline and mild hypertension. The other is an increased "priming of the pump," i.e., an elevated pulmonary blood volume. This has two causes, hypervolemia and a decreased capacity of venous reservoirs that leads to a central translocation of blood, as reflected by an increased ratio of cardiopulmonary volume to total blood volume (CPV/TBV). Hypervolemia occurs rarely in hypertension, but an elevated CPV/TBV ratio is commonly found in mild or borderline hypertension.

Peripheral resistance is controlled by neural, local, and humoral factors. All blood vessels are richly supplied by adrenergic nerves that provide for vasoconstriction. In mild hypertension there is evidence for increased neural tone, while in severe hypertension this does not seem to be the case. Currently, there is much interest in the possibility that an abnormality of the vascular smooth-muscle (VSM) contractile mechanism is the basic fault in hypertension.[5] Work in progress is focused on the control of intracellular Na^+, K^+, and Ca^{2+} because their concentrations determine membrane potential and VSM contractility. Local hormones, such as prostaglandins and kinins, may also play a role in peripheral resistance, but there is no clear evidence as yet that they are important in hypertension.

Neural Mechanisms

The autonomic nervous system, particularly its sympathetic component, plays an important role in circulatory control. Its known importance concerns rapid adjustments to a variety of stimuli, such as changes in posture, intrathoracic pressure, and temperature. In addition, there is a growing body of evidence linking abnormalities of central vasomotor centers to the genesis of experimental hypertension. The spectrum of nervous control abnormalities in clinical hypertensions is not yet known; the most evidence that we have now relates to mild hypertension in which a neural mechanism seems predominant (see below).

The nervous system works to control arterial pressure in two ways. One is through neural reflexes and the other is through an ongoing maintenance of sympathetic vasomotor tone.[6] Reflex control is well demonstrated by the changes that occur when one assumes an upright posture or performs the Valsalva maneuver. Standing causes blood to pool in the distensible veins below heart level, thereby decreasing venous return, lowering central blood volume, and decreasing cardiac output and systolic pressure. The decreased pressure is sensed by mechanoreceptors in the aortic arch and carotid sinus; the mechanoreceptors cease sending inhibitory impulses to the central sympathetic control areas of the brain, resulting in increased sympathetic vasomotor outflow to both venous and arterial sides of the circulation. The resultant venoconstriction stabilizes venous return, cardiac output, and systolic pressure. The arteriolar constriction raises diastolic pressure.

The Valsalva maneuver allows an excellent view of reflex operations. The positive intrathoracic pressure diminishes venous return so that cardiac output and arterial pressure fall. The reflex increase in sympathetic outflow increases heart rate and constricts arterioles. When straining is suddenly stopped, blood rushes into the thorax and the rapidly increasing cardiac output is delivered into a vasoconstricted arterial bed, so pressure rises abruptly. When this happens the mechanoreceptors are stimulated and the resultant central sympathetic inhibition slows heart rate and reduces pressure. Thus, normally, reflex control of the circulation serves to elevate pressure when it falls and reduces it when it rises. Why the mechanism fails in hypertension is not known, but there is evidence for upward resetting of mechanoreceptor sensitivity so that pressure rises are inadequately sensed although pressure decreases are not. What role this plays in hypertension has not been defined.

Ongoing control of sympathetic vasomotor tone is not as easy to demonstrate as reflex mechanisms are. As will be detailed below, there is evidence that this may be elevated in borderline hypertension.

Sympathetic control of the circulation—both reflex and tonic—is carried out through the noradrenergic neuroeffector system.[7] The nerves make and store norepinephrine, which is released from nerve endings by nerve impulses. The beginning of norepinephrine synthesis is with the amino acid tyrosine, which is taken up by brain, peripheral neurons, and chromaffin tissue. In mitochondria, tyrosine is acted upon by tyrosine hydroxylase to form L-dopa, which migrates to the cytoplasm where it is decarboxylated to dopamine. Dopamine, in turn, moves into a specialized compartment, a vesicle, where it is acted upon by dopamine β-oxidase and becomes norephinephrine. Epinephrine derives from the methylation of norepinephrine by action of the enzyme phenylethanolamine-*N*-methyltransferase. The largest amounts of this enzyme are in the adrenal medulla.

Norepinephrine is released from nerve endings in quantities greater than are needed to effect a response. Some escapes into the circulation, some is transformed into normetanephrine by the enzyme catechol *O*-methyltransferase (COMT) and is excreted as such in the urine. Some is deaminated by monamine oxidase and is then methylated by COMT to form vanillylmandelic acid (VMA) and methoxyhydroxyphenylglycol (MHPG), which are excreted in the urine. One final mechanism, reuptake by nerve endings, represents the major pathway whereby the released norepinephrine is disposed of.

Extracellular Fluid Volumes

Extracellular fluid (ECF) and/or body sodium stores are importantly linked with hypertension, but the reasons for their importance have not been determined. ECF is compartmentalized into interstitial fluid and plasma volume. These two compartments are separated by capillary endothelium, through which exchanges of nutrients, gases, electrolytes, and water take place. Sodium is the major cation of the ECF; although most of it is freely exchangeable, bone sodium exchanges slowly. Sodium does get into cells where it has to be extruded by sodium-potassium adenosine triphosphatase (Na-K-ATPase). Intracellular sodium of VSM is currently considered one important factor in the increased vascular resistance that characterizes hypertension.

ECF, particularly its intravascular component plasma volume (PV), plays a significant hemodynamic role.[8] PV and red blood cell mass comprise the total blood volume (TBV), which fills the vascular bed. The venous side of the circulation contains the bulk of the TBV, and the capacity of venous reservoirs below heart level partly determines pulmonary blood volume and is therefore a factor in cardiac output. As will be discussed later, there is substantial evidence for diminished venous capacity in mild or borderline hypertension and in renovascular hypertension, and this, in part, is responsible for the slightly increased cardiac output that is so often found in these types.

PV itself is characteristically diminished in hypertension, the only exception being primary aldosteronism, in which it is often elevated.[9] The mild oligemia probably reflects the effect of high arterial pressure and decreased venous capacity as well, because the veins contain about 75 percent of the TBV, the arteries but 20 percent, and the capillaries 5 percent.[10] PV is determined by sodium balance and arterial pressure. With a negative sodium balance ECF and PV fall, and with a positive sodium balance they increase. The increase in PV is limited in hypertensive people because of pressure natriuresis. Sodium balance is determined not only by sodium intake but also by the ability of the kidney to excrete sodium. It is in the latter regard that the renin-angiotensin-aldosterone system is of importance.

The Renal Pressor System

The kidney produces a proteolytic enzyme, renin, which acts on a plasma protein substrate to split off a 10-amino acid polypeptide, angiotensin I, which in turn is acted upon by converting enzyme to produce an 8-amino acid polypeptide, angiotensin II.[11] This polypeptide is a powerful vasoconstrictor and is the main controlling mechanism for aldosterone release; it increases the activity of the sympathetic nervous system and seems to have a direct inhibiting effect on sodium excretion.

Renin is produced by the juxtaglomerular apparatus. Little is known about renin synthesis, except that it is increased by sodium deprivation and decreased by sodium loading. In contrast, renin release has been extensively defined. It is increased by a fall in renal perfusion pressure (as in hypotension or renal arterial stenosis), by enhanced activity of sympathetic nerves (as in standing), and by oligemia (as in hemorrhage). Also, the amount of sodium (or chloride) transported by the macula densa of the distal tubule is an important factor, since the macula densa and the juxtaglomerular apparatus are in close proximity. When transport of sodium (or chloride) is inhibited by a chlorothiazide diuretic, renin release is increased.

Renin is important in blood pressure control because it is the enzyme that starts the cascade that results in the formation of angiotensin II. Converting enzyme is also important since inhibiting it reduces angiotensin II levels, diminishing the influence of the renal pressor system despite marked increases in levels of angiotensin I and renin.

Although the renal pressor system has received much attention in the past two decades as a prime factor in hypertension, one should realize that it is but one of the systems that control arterial pressure. Increased angiotensin II is the mechanism for renovascular hypertension and the renin-dependent hypertension of end-stage kidney disease, but its primacy has not been determined for the other hypertensions, except that it seems to play no role in primary aldosteronism.

Salt-Active Steroids

Aldosterone is the major salt-active steroid. Its production by the zona glomerulosa of the adrenal cortex is predominantly controlled by angiotensin II.[12] It affects electrolyte homeostasis by increasing sodium reabsorption and facilitating potassium excretion by the distal nephron. Since its production is so strongly influenced by renin release and the formation of angiotensin II, aldosterone levels (in blood or urine) are intimately related to those factors that influence the renal pressor system. Thus, there is a significant positive correlation between plasma renin activity (or angiotensin II levels) and aldosterone levels on the one hand, and a negative correlation between urinary sodium excretion and aldosterone on the other.

Aldosterone is the major steroid influencing potassium homeostasis: Its level increases when potassium intake is large and falls with potassium depletion. In fact, it is now well recognized that the hypokalemia of primary aldosteronism can limit the hyperaldosteronism that characterizes this tumor.

The importance of aldosterone in hypertension is most obvious in primary aldosteronism. In this condition, the increased amounts of the hormone are associated with increases of ECF, PV, and total exchangeable sodium. Aldosterone itself is not pressor, rather it causes a positive sodium balance and a salt-dependent hypertension.[13] Hyperaldosteronism is caused by the hyperreninemia of severe renovascular hypertension and is responsible for the hypokalemia often found. In essential hypertension, there is exaggerated production of aldosterone in response to infusions of angiotensin II and diminished responses to upright posture.[14] However, these abnormalities have not yet been shown to play a role in hypertension.

Definitions of Hypertension

Definition of Hypertension according to Pressure Level

Until very recently there was no unanimity about the definition of hypertension. This disagreement stemmed from two sources: (1) a lack of appreciation of the actuarial statistics that showed a progressively rising mortality beginning with diastolic arterial pressure between 84 to 88 mmHg, and (2) Pickering's demonstration that in any given population arterial pressure is a continuous variable and shows a unimodal, not bimodal, distribution.[15]

The 1984 report of the Third Joint National Committee on the Detection, Evaluation and Treatment of Hypertension (JNC III)[16] has provided a useful categorization of arterial pressure. For diastolic pressure: less than 85 mmHg, normal; 85 to 89 mmHg, high normal; 90 to 104 mmHg, mild hypertension; 105 to 114 mmHg, moderate hypertension; 115 mmHg or over, severe hypertension. People with intermittently elevated pressures are said to have labile hypertension.

Another frequently used classification includes both systolic and diastolic arterial pressure levels. Values of less than 140/90 mmHg are considered normal; 140/90 to 160/95 mmHg, borderline hypertension; more than 160/95, definite hypertension.[17]

The types of hypertension are *isolated diastolic, mixed* (with both diastolic and systolic elevation), and *isolated systolic.*

Isolated diastolic hypertension is extremely rare and is only seen with mild elevations of diastolic pressure (e.g., 120/100 mmHg). It is usually found in children and young adults.

Isolated systolic hypertension is fairly frequent in the elderly and can also accompany aortic coarctation or hyperdynamic circulation in young people. The JNC III report recommends the following classification for systolic pressure when the diastolic is less than 90 mmHg: less than 140 mmHg, normal; 140 to 159 mmHg, borderline isolated systolic hypertension; 160 mmHg or over, isolated systolic hypertension.

The Pathophysiology of Hypertension

Mechanisms of Hypertension—A General Statement

In most people (at least 75 percent of the United States population), arterial pressure is normal and maintained within a relatively narrow range. This means that the control systems regulating arterial pressure are so integrated that when pressure rises it is immediately reduced.

The present perception about the pathogenesis and maintenance of hypertension is that there are abnormalities in the control systems that fail to reduce arterial pressure to normal when it becomes elevated. Thus, this is a "disease of regulation," as first proposed by Page.[18] These abnormalities vary according to the cause of hypertension. Whatever the underlying cause (with the exception of coarctation of the aorta), the basic hemodynamic fault is a failure to control vascular resistance. The hypertension so produced damages the arteries and results in the vascular diseases responsible for premature morbidity and mortality—heart failure, renal failure, strokes, and heart attacks.

The purpose of the following discussion is to delineate what is known of the abnormalities of arterial pressure control systems in various types of hypertension.

Essential Hypertension

Labile, Borderline, and Mild

Labile, borderline, and mild hypertension are combined here because the reported studies have not used the classification of hypertension given above but have included all three types. These types occur frequently. Among the 168,000 people screened for the Hypertension Detection and Follow-Up Program (HDFP), 71.5 percent of the 10,940 hypertensive people had diastolic pressures less than 105 mmHg.[17]

Hemodynamics Hemodynamics has been a topic of considerable interest in the past 20 years, and a fairly clear picture has emerged of the hemodynamic characteristics of these various types of essential hypertension. Widimsky, Fejfarova, and Fejfar[19] and Eich et al.[20] were the first to report a modest increase in cardiac output in young people with slight elevations of diastolic arterial pressure. Since then, extensive investigations have been carried out, and these have been summarized recently by Lund-Johansen[21] and by Julius, Esler, and Randall.[22] It is apparent that a substantial percentage of such patients have elevated cardiac output and normal TPR (Table 49-2). In this case, it would seem that hypertension results because of the increased cardiac output. However, if control mechanisms are normally operational, vascular resistance should be decreased. In support of the conclusion of a peripheral hemodynamic fault is the exercise study of Lund-Johansen.[21] He found that these young hypertensives failed to lower TPR to the same level as normotensive control subjects.

Neural and Volume Factors As shown in Table 49-2, this is a hyperdynamic circulation with an increased heart rate, shortened preinjection period (PEP), diminished preinjection period/left ventricular ejection time ratio (PEP/LVET), and increased mean rate of left ventricular ejection. The reasons for this situation have been extensively investigated, and the evidence obtained points to an increased adrenergic drive to the heart, capacitance vessels, and arterioles. Julius et al.[22] have shown that the increased cardiac output is due to increases in heart rate and stroke volume. The heart rate abnormality is due to increased beta-adrenergic activity and diminished parasympathetic inhibition. The increased stroke volume is not only because of increased myocardial contractility, but also a shunting of blood to the central circulation by diminished capacity of the

TABLE 49-2 Hemodynamic Factors in Various Hypertensions

Group	HR, beats/min	CI, liters/min/m^2	SI, ml/min/m^2	TPR, units/m^2
Normotensive	68	3.05	45	30
Hypertensive				
Labile	75	3.36	46	31
Essential				
No cardiac enlargement	76	2.91	39	45
Cardiac enlargement	74	2.67	36	53
Renovascular	80	3.48	44	37
Renal parenchymal disease	76	3.23	43	41
Primary aldosteronism	83	3.30	41	45

Notes: HR = heart rate; CI = cardiac index; SI = stroke index; TPR = total peripheral resistance.
Source: From data reported in Refs. 25, 36, 37, and 45.

reservoir veins below heart level. Both Tarazi[8] and Safar et al.[23] have demonstrated that such patients have an increased ratio of central blood volume to total blood volume (CBV/TBV) and that this is positively and significantly correlated with stroke volume and/or cardiac output. This increase in cardiac output and CBV is not because of an increased blood volume since this tends to be diminished.

There is also evidence for increased adrenergic stimulation of the peripheral arterial vascular bed. Julius et al.[22] have found that alpha-adrenergic blockade lowered arterial pressure in some patients with hyperdynamic circulation. Earlier, Frohlich et al.[25] used a 50° head-up tilt and the Valsalva maneuver to assess the neurogenic component and demonstrated orthostatic hypertension and an exaggerated overshoot of arterial pressure with the Valsalva maneuver. Such patients were subsequently found to have increased urinary norepinephrine excretion during tilt, yet further evidence for increased noradrenergic activity.

The Renin-Angiotensin-Aldosterone System Since plasma renin activity (PRA) tends to fall with age, it has been difficult to assess the significance of renin levels in young hypertensive patients as opposed to older ones. However, Julius et al.[22] found that those young people with hyperdynamic circulation had higher PRA than those with a normokinetic circulation. Williams et al.[24] have shown that some young, mildly hypertensive patients had abnormal aldosterone responses to acute stimulation.

Moderate and Severe Hypertension

Although established hypertension is important because of increased morbidity and mortality, the prevalence of moderate and severe hypertension is not so great as that of mild hypertension. If the screening performed for the HDFP[15] can be taken as representative of the United States population, only 28.5 percent of the hypertensive subjects were classified as moderate and severe.

When arterial pressure is elevated above the ranges used to designate mild hypertension, the pathophysiology usually changes. Although patients with a hyperdynamic circulation are occasionally encountered, this is unusual.[26] There is little evidence for increased adrenergic activity, and the fault clearly seems to be in the mechanisms controlling vascular resistance.

Hemodynamics The hemodynamic characteristics of established hypertension depend on the height of the arterial pressure, the degree of vasoconstriction, and the presence of cardiac enlargement.[27] In moderate hypertension without evidence of cardiac enlargement, cardiac output is normal and TPR is elevated; left ventricular ejection rate is also normal despite an increase in cardiac work. However, as hypertension becomes more severe and is associated with cardiac enlargement, there is a progressive fall in cardiac output (in the absence of cardiac failure) and a further rise in TPR; the rate of left ventricular ejection is decreased, the PEP becomes prolonged, and the PEP/LVET ratio is increased.

Studies of regional circulations have shown that the elevated resistance is fairly evenly distributed, except in the kidney where it is more intense and in the skeletal muscles where it is slightly less marked.[28] Since the renal vascular bed is particularly vulnerable to damage by extremely high arterial pressure, renal blood flow can be markedly reduced (finally to the point of renal failure) and renal resistance markedly elevated.

Neural and Volume Factors As indicated above, there is little evidence for a prime neural factor in moderate and severe hypertension; in fact, the evidence suggests a diminished neural response to stimuli when hypertension is severe. Frohlich et al.[25] used a head-up tilt and the Valsalva maneuver to study neural participation. In patients with moderate hypertension, both arterial pressure responses to tilt and Valsalva overshoot were normal. Those with severe hypertension had mild orthostatic hypotension and a diminished pressor response to the Valsalva maneuver. Others have shown a decreased baroreceptor reflex sensitivity in patients with established essential hypertension.[29]

Plasma volume is characteristically reduced in patients with moderate and severe hypertension.[10] Since ECF volume is normal, this results in a diminished plasma volume/interstitial fluid volume (PV/IF) ratio. Reasons for this are not apparent, but the reduced PV/IF ratio likely reflects an overall decrease in vascular capacity since treatment with vasodilators and alpha-adrenergic blocking drugs leads to fluid retention and an expanded plasma volume.

Although there is no clear evidence associating increased neural activity with moderate and severe hypertension, three points should be made. One is that adrenergic blocking drugs often reduce supine, as well as standing, arterial pressure, and this effect suggests that there are some patients with a significant neural component. Further, Tarazi and Dustan[30] showed that the fall in arterial pressure produced by the intravenous administration of the ganglion blocker trimethaphan was inversely related to PV: the lower the volume, the greater the decrease in pressure. Finally, Campese et al.[31] have reported that some patients with salt-sensitive hypertension have abnormally elevated plasma catecholamine levels with salt loading. These three observations add a note of caution to the interpretation that neural factors are not abnormal, or may even be relatively unimportant, in moderate and severe hypertension. Since we know so little about the ways in which the central nervous system controls pressure, it is premature to judge the extent of its participation in moderate and severe hypertension.

The Renin-Angiotensin-Aldosterone System There has been much elucidation of this system in moderate and severe hypertension in the past 20 years, but there is still uncertainty as to its primacy as a controlling factor. Brown et al.[32] and Laragh et al.[33] have shown the inverse relation between sodium balance and plasma angiotensin II concentrations with plasma aldosterone and aldosterone excretion rates. There are well-defined, normal relations which serve as a guide to assess the participation of this system in hypertension.

Laragh[34] has emphasized the importance of classifying hypertension according to the PRA into low renin, normal renin, and high renin groups. Excluding renovascular hypertension from consideration, it has been found that PRA is often elevated in patients with severe and/or accelerated hypertension. Further, Brown et al.[35] have shown that in malignant hypertension plasma aldosterone is inappropriately high for the level of angiotensin II, indicating an increased adrenal responsiveness in this state.

Low renin hypertension has been the subject of much research and controversy. The well-established, age-related fall in PRA makes the significance of PRA levels in older hypertensive people difficult to assess; also, PRA is lower in black people than in white. However, it is clear that there are some hypertensive people who have low PRA that is relatively unresponsive to the usual stimuli. The significance of this finding has not yet been revealed.

Renovascular Hypertension

Renovascular hypertension is one of the most common hypertensions of known cause, although its occurrence is numerically small in comparison to the large prevalence of essential hypertension. Depending upon the population studied, its reported incidence has ranged from less than 1 percent to as high as 20 percent. It results from atherosclerotic or fibrous dysplastic stenosis of one or both renal arteries; sometimes fibrous dysplasia affects only branches of the main renal artery. Since the recognition of renovascular hypertension more than 30 years ago, much has been learned about its clinical spectrum and pathophysiology. The hypertension can be borderline, mild, moderate, severe, or accelerated, but whatever the level of pressure, the underlying cause is stimulation of the renal pressor system. There is also indication that the nervous system participates.

Hemodynamics

In renovascular hypertension cardiac output is often modestly elevated even when arterial pressure is high.[36] Peripheral resistance is elevated, in contrast to borderline hypertension with hyperdynamic circulation. Although output and arterial pressure are positively correlated, the modest increase in flow is not the cause of the hypertension, because relief of hypertension by nephrectomy or renal revascularization regularly decreases vascular resistance without necessarily changing cardiac output. Further, in those patients with reduced cardiac output preoperatively, output increases following successful operation.

Neural and Volume Factors

In many patients with renovascular hypertension, evidence of stimulation of the nervous system can be found. There is often an increased rate of left ventricular ejection, the heart rate is slightly elevated, the CBV/TBV ratio is increased, indicating a decreased capacity of venous reservoirs, orthostatic hypertension is frequent, and an exaggerated Valsalva overshoot can often be demonstrated.[37] PV is almost always decreased and correlates negatively with PRA.[38]

The Renin-Angiotensin-Aldosterone System

Regardless of the evidence for increased neural activity in renovascular hypertension, the underlying cause is increased production and release of renin. Hyperreninemia is not a constant finding, but this is because PRA and arterial pressure are positively correlated so that the increased levels of PRA are found only when arterial pressure is moderately to severely elevated.[38] Plasma angiotensin II levels also correlate positively with arterial pressure.[35]

It is not uncommon to find hypokalemia in patients with severe renovascular hypertension. This is a reflection of the angiotensin-induced secondary aldosteronism. Brown et al.[35] have shown that not only were plasma angiotensin II and plasma aldosterone directly related, but that, for any given angiotensin II level, aldosterone concentration was higher than in normal subjects given angiotensin infusions. Thus, such patients have an inappropriate stimulation of aldosterone production.

Hypertension Accompanying Renal Parenchymal Disease

Renal parenchymal disease, either congenital or acquired, is often accompanied by hypertension. It is a common enough cause that screening tests for all hypertensive patients should include a measurement of proteinuria and indexes of renal excretory efficiency (BUN and serum creatinine). It is now known that the hypertension is either renin-dependent or salt-and-water-dependent,[39] or due to both mechanisms. The pathophysiology varies depending on the extent of renal insufficiency and the type of renal disease. The pure renin-dependent hypertension is found most frequently in severe nephrosclerosis, while the pure salt-and-water-dependent type is seen in anephric patients.

Acute Glomerulonephritis

What we know about the pathophysiology of the hypertension of acute glomerulonephritis concerns hemodynamic and volume factors. In two studies, cardiac output was found to be elevated and TPR normal, slightly increased, or slightly decreased.[40,41]

Blood volume has been reported to be normal or increased.[42] Since edema is a characteristic of acute glomerulonephritis, increased PV might be expected. Failure to find this regularly may represent decreased capacity of the vascular bed, an increased capillary permeability, or a decreased fluid reabsorption on the venular limb of the capillary bed because of hypoalbuminemia.

In summary, it seems likely that the hypertension accompanying acute glomerulonephritis results from fluid retention, a hyperdynamic circulation, and failure of the peripheral circulation to respond normally to the increased cardiac output.

Renal Parenchymal Disease without Renal Insufficiency

Again, with renal parenchymal disease without renal insufficiency, understanding of the associated hypertension is primarily concerned with hemodynamic and volume factors.

Frohlich et al.[37] studied a group of hypertensive patients who had pyelonephritis and normal renal function. They were found to have a normal cardiac output and elevated TPR. PV and TBV ranged from reduced to slightly expanded. The striking feature was a positive correlation between pressure and volume in contrast to the negative correlation found in essential and renovascular hypertension. Reasons for this positive relation did not emerge, but because of a similar finding in a patient with chronic renal failure both before and after nephrectomy, the authors suggested that a positive correlation might be the characteristic of volume-dependent hypertension.

Hypertension and Uremia

Renoprival hypertension is the term frequently used for the hypertension of uremia, and it implies a failure of salt-and-water homeostasis. However, as indicated above, some of the hypertension of uremia is renin-dependent.

Hemodynamic and Volume Factors The studies of Onesti et al.[43] have provided a clear picture of the hemodynamics of the hypertension of uremia. In those people with renin-dependent, severe hypertension, cardiac output was found to be decreased, even in the presence of anemia, and vascular resistance extremely high. Nephrectomy produced a marked amelioration of the hypertension, TPR fell, and cardiac output rose.

The patients with salt-and-water-dependent hypertension presented a different hemodynamic pattern. Cardiac output was elevated, but so also was that of the normotensive uremic subjects because the two groups were equally anemic. In the hypertensive subjects vascular resistance was slightly increased, while in the normotensive subjects it was decreased. Thus, the hypertension resulted from an inability to regulate the peripheral circulation.

The importance of salt-and-water balance in the genesis and maintenance of this type of hypertension was shown by a study of anephric patients in whom varying degrees of positive salt-and-water balance occurred during hemodialysis.[43] In the hypertensive patients, diastolic arterial pressure was significantly related to total exchangeable sodium (and, therefore, ECF volume), while in the normotensive patients arterial pressure did not change, regardless of the degree of positive salt-and-water balance.

Neural Factors Since peripheral neuropathy commonly occurs in uremic patients maintained by hemodialysis, the possibility of autonomic neuropathy has been raised as a possible explanation of the changes in arterial pressure—both the hypotension that sometimes occurs with hemodialysis and the hypertension with fluid overload. In the latter regard, this implies a lack of modulation of arterial pressure in response to salt-and-water excess, much like the false tolerance to adrenergic blocking drugs in nonazotemic hypertensions, a tolerance that is known to result from fluid retention. However, there is as yet no evidence that a deficiency of neural control plays any role in this type of hypertension.

The Renin-Angiotensin-Aldosterone System PRA is variable in chronic uremia. As noted before, it is often elevated in nephrosclerosis. As for the other renal diseases,[44] it is usually normal or low in pyelonephritis, polycystic renal disease, and interstitial nephritis. In glomerulonephritis it may be normal or elevated.

Aldosterone does not seem to be a factor controlling hypertension in uremia. Although it is certainly elevated in patients with renin-dependent hypertension, it can have little effect on salt-and-water balance because of the renal insufficiency. Following nephrectomy, when angiotensin II, the major regulator of aldosterone release, is no longer available, aldosterone production becomes dependent upon electrolyte balance.

Primary Aldosteronism

Primary aldosteronism is caused by aldosterone excess resulting from a solitary adenoma of the adrenal gland or from adenomatous hyperplasia. It is not frequent and probably occurs in less than 1 percent of those with hypertension.[12] It is not the only type of steroid hypertension, but it is the most frequent and its pathophysiology has been well described. Other forms include Cushing's syndrome, adrenogenital syndrome, and 17- and 11-hydroxylase deficiencies. The hypertension of primary aldosteronism is salt-and-water-dependent because of the excess aldosterone.[13] The mechanism(s) of the other adrenal cortical types has not been so well worked out.

Hemodynamic and Volume Factors

In primary aldosteronism a broad spectrum of cardiac output and vascular resistance is found.[45] Cardiac output is frequently elevated. It is negatively correlated with arterial pressure, which means that the higher the pressure the less the likelihood of a high output. Intravascular volume plays a singularly direct hemodynamic role in this type of hypertension. PV and TBV are often elevated, and they are positively correlated with cardiac output, but negatively correlated with arterial pressure and TPR. Thus, patients with mild to moderate hypertension are those in whom an elevated cardiac output and blood volume can be expected. These seem to be the hallmarks of primary aldosteronism because Tarazi et al.[45] have shown that it is such patients who can be expected to have solitary adenomas and to achieve normalization of arterial pressure following their removal. The severely hypertensive patients with normal cardiac output and high resistance may either have adenomatous hyperplasia or an aldosteronoma engrafted upon essential hypertension.

Neural Factors

One of the striking features about the high-output type of primary aldosteronism is the hyperdynamic circulation. Cardiac output elevation was found to reflect an increased heart rate, and although stroke volume was not elevated, there was an increased mean rate of left ventricular ejection. These findings suggest increased sympathetic outflow to the heart, but likely reflect the hypervolemia since plasma catecholamine levels have been found to be normal.[13]

The Renin-Angiotensin-Aldosterone System

Autonomous production of aldosterone is the basic cause for the hypertension. Because it is autonomous, angiotensin II no longer functions as a regulator of aldosterone synthesis, and because aldosterone creates a positive fluid balance, plasma renin and angiotensin levels are markedly reduced. Thus, there is no evidence that the renal pressor system plays any role in the hyperaldosteronism or the hypertension.

Pheochromocytoma

Pheochromocytoma is a tumor of chromaffin tissue that releases varying amounts of norepinephrine and epinephrine into the circulation, thus causing hypertension.[46] It can arise from any tissue that contains chromaffin cells. Most tumors occur in the adrenal medulla, while the rest originate in chromaffin cells adjacent to sympathetic ganglia; the latter are usually termed *paragangliomas.*

The bulk of investigations concerning the pathophysiology of pheochromocytoma has concentrated on the excess production of catecholamines and methods to measure them. Thus, we know relatively little about the cardiovascular abnormalities of this type of hypertension.

Because norepinephrine and epinephrine have different effects, the pathophysiological characteristics vary considerably. Hypertension can either be sustained or episodic. Cardiac output has been reported to be normal or elevated.[46,47] Since the increased catecholamine production in a sense substitutes for ongoing neural control of the circulation, it is not surprising that orthostatic hypotension is a common finding. PV is very often reduced, reflecting the generalized vasoconstrictor effect of the catecholamines.[46] PRA has been found to be elevated.[48]

Coarctation of the Thoracic Aorta

Coarctation of the thoracic aorta is a congenital lesion—one of the few developmental defects that cause hypertension and the only one that directly affects the arterial system (see Chap. 36). It is the adult type of coarctation that concerns us here because the infantile variety is so severe and associated with other serious cardiovascular defects that hypertension is only one of the problems to be considered.

This type of hypertension is unique because it results from a localized, not generalized, vascular abnormality—a narrowing or complete obliteration of the thoracic aorta in the region of the ductus. This sharply reduces the volume of the aortic compression chamber so that each stroke volume is delivered into an abnormally small aorta; the result is hypertension above the coarctation and hypotension below. The hypertension is often primarily systolic.

It has long been thought that there is a significant renal pressor component to the hypertension because the kidneys are perfused at an abnormally low pressure. However, increased PRA is not a constant finding.

In reporting a study of systemic and splanchnic hemodynamics in patients with coarctation, Culbertson et al.[49] summarized the previous work as having shown cardiac output to be normal or increased, leg blood flow normal or decreased, arm blood flow normal or increased, and cerebral blood flow increased. In their study of 10 patients, they found cardiac output elevated in six, normal in two, and reduced in two. In only one patient (who also had a reduced output) was TPR raised. Hepatic blood flow was increased, Kirkendall et al.[50] found renal blood flow and glomerular filtration rate to be normal except in patients who had cardiac failure.

Taken as a whole, these findings indicate that coarctation hypertension is characterized by a hyperdynamic circulation with little abnormality of resistance vessels.

References

1. McDonald, D. A.: The Relationship between Pulsatile Pressure and Flow, in "Blood Flow in Arteries," The Williams & Wilkins Company, Baltimore, 1974, p. 118.
2. Gorlin, R.: The Hyperkinetic Heart Syndrome, *JAMA*, 182:823, 1962.
3. Frohlich, E. D., Tarazi, R. C., and Dustan, H. P.: Hyperdynamic Beta-Adrenergic Circulatory State, *Arch. Intern. Med.*, 117:614, 1966.
4. Dustan, H. P., Tarazi, R. C., and Hinshaw, L. B.: Mechanisms Controlling Arterial Pressure, in E. D. Frohlich (ed.), "Pathophysiology: Altered Regulatory Mechanisms in Disease," 2d ed., J. B. Lippincott Company, Philadelphia, 1976.
5. Report of Hypertension Task Force. 9. Vascular Smooth Muscle: Contractile Apparatus, DHEW Publication (NIH) 79-1627.
6. Shepherd, J. T., and Vanhoutte, P. M.: Integrated Responses of the Cardiovascular System to Stress, in "The Human Cardiovascular System, Facts and Concepts," Raven Press, New York, 1979.
7. Wurtman, R. J.: "Catecholamines," Little, Brown and Company, Boston, 1966.
8. Tarazi, R. C.: Hemodynamic Role of Extracellular Fluid, *Circ. Res.*, 38:I-173, 1976.
9. Tarazi, R. C., Dustan, H. P., Frohlich, E.D., Gifford, R. W., and Hoffman, G. C.: Plasma Volume and Chronic Hypertension, *Arch. Intern. Med.*, 125:835, 1970.
10. Rushmer, R. F.: Properties of the Vascular System, in "Cardiovascular Dynamics," W. B. Saunders Company, Philadelphia, 1970.
11. Kaplan, N. M.: The Renin-Angiotensin System, in "Clinical Hypertension," 2d ed., The Williams & Wilkins Company, Baltimore, 1978.
12. Kaplan, N. M.: Primary Aldosteronism, in "Clinical Hypertension," 2d ed., The Williams & Wilkins Company, Baltimore, 1978.
13. Bravo, E. L., Dustan, H. P., and Tarazi, R. C.: Spironolactone as a Nonspecific Treatment for Primary Aldosteronism, *Circulation*, 48:491, 1971.
14. Davies, D. L., Beevers, D. G., Brown, J. J., Cumming,
14. Davies, D. L., Beevers, D. G., Brown, J. J., Cumming,
A. M. M., Fraser, R., Lever, A. F., Mason, P. A., Morton, J. J., Robertson, J. I. S., Titterington, M., and Tree, M.: Aldosterone and Its Stimuli in Normal and Hypertensive Man: Are Essential Hypertension and Primary Hyperaldosteronism without Tumour the Same Condition? *J. Endocrinol.* 81:79P, 1979.
15. Pickering, F.: The Inheritance of Arterial Pressure, in "High Blood Pressure," 2d ed., Grune & Stratton, Inc., New York, 1968, p. 236.
16. The 1984 Report of the Joint National Committee on Detection, Evaluation and Treatment of High Blood Pressure, *Arch. Intern. Med.*, vol. 144, May, 1984.
17. Hypertension Detection and Follow-Up Program Cooperative Group: Five-Year Findings of the Hypertension Detection and Follow-Up Program, *JAMA*, 242:2562, 1979.
18. Page, I. H.: The Mosaic Theory of Hypertension, in K. D. Bock and P. T. Cottier (eds.), "Essential Hypertension," Springer-Verlag, New York, 1960, p. 1.
19. Widimsky, J., Fejfarova, M. H., and Fejfar, Z.: Changes of Cardiac Output in Hypertensive Disease, *Cardiologia*, 31:381, 1957.
20. Eich, R. H., Peters, R. J., Cuddy, R. P., Smulyan, H., and Lyons, R. H.: Hemodynamics in Labile Hypertension, *Am. Heart J.*, 63:188, 1962.
21. Lund-Johansen, P.: Hemodynamics in Essential Hypertension, *Clin. Sci. Mol. Med.*, 59:343, 1980.
22. Julius, S., Esler, M. D., and Randall, O. S.: Role of the Autonomic Nervous System in Mild Human Hypertension, *Clin. Sci. Mol. Med.*, 48:234s, 1975.
23. Safar, M., Weiss, Y. A., London, G. M., Frackowiak, R. F., and Milliez, P. L.: Cardiopulmonary Blood Volume in Borderline Hypertension, *Clin. Sci. Mol. Med.*, 47:153, 1974.
24. Williams, G. H., Rose, L., Dluhy, R. G., et al.: Abnormal Responsiveness of the Renin-Aldosterone System to Acute Stimulation in Patients with Essential Hypertension, *Ann. Intern. Med.*, 72:317, 1970.
25. Frohlich, E. D., Tarazi, R. C., Ulrych, M., Dustan, H. P., and Page, I. H.: Tilt Test for Investigating a Neural Component in Hypertension. Its Correlation with Clinical Characteristics, *Circulation*, 36:387, 1967.
26. Ibrahim, M. M., Tarazi, R. C., Dustan, H. P., Bravo, E. L., and Gifford, R. W., Jr.: Hyperkinetic Heart in Severe Hypertension: A Separate Clinical Hemodynamic Entity, *Am. J. Cardiol.*, 35:667, 1975.
27. Frohlich, E. D., Kozul, V. J., Tarazi, R. C., and Dustan, H. P.: Physiological Comparison of Labile and Essential Hypertension, *Circ. Res.*, 26(suppl. 1):55, 1970.
28. Brod, J., Hejl, Z., Ulrych, M., Fencl, V., and Jirka, J.: General and Regional Hemodynamic Pattern Underlying Essential Hypertension, *Clin. Sci.*, 23:339, 1962.
29. Bristow, J. D., Honour, A. J., Pickering, G. W., Sleight, P., and Smyth, H. S.: Diminished Baroreflex Sensitivity in High Blood Pressure, *Circulation*, 39:48, 1969.
30. Tarazi, R. C., and Dustan, H. P.: Neurogenic Participation in Essential and Renovascular Hypertension, Assessed by Acute Ganglionic Blockade, *Clin. Sci.*, 44:197, 1973.
31. Campese, V. M., Romoff, M. S., Levitan, D., Saglikes, Y., Friedler, R. M., and Massry, S. G.: Abnormal Relationship between Sodium Intake and Sympathetic Nervous System Activity in Salt-Sensitive Patients with Essential Hypertension. *Kidney Int.*, 21:371, 1982.
32. Brown, J. J., Davies, D. L., Lever, A. F., and Robertson, J. I. S.: Variations in Plasma Renin Concentration in Several Physiological and Pathological States, *Can. Med. Assoc. J.*, 90:201, 1964.
33. Laragh, J. H., Sealey, J. E., and Sommers, S. C.: Patterns of Adrenal Secretion and Urinary Excretion of Aldosterone and Plasma Renin Activity in Normal and Hypertensive Subjects, *Circ. Res.*, 19:158, 1966.
34. Laragh, J.: Vasoconstriction—Volume Analysis for Understanding and Treating Hypertension: The Use of Renin and Aldosterone Profiles, *Am. J. Med.*, 55:261, 1973.
35. Brown, J., Casals-Stenzel, J., Cumming, A. M. M., Davies, D. L., Fraser, R., Lever, A., Morton, J., Semple, P. F., Tree,

M., and Robertson, J. I.: Angiotensin II, Aldosterone and Arterial Pressure: A Quantitative Approach, *Hypertension*, 1:159, 1979.
36. Tarazi, R. C., Frolich, E. D., and Dustan, H. P.: Contribution of Cardiac Output to Renovascular Hypertension. Relation to Surgical Treatment, *Am. J. Cardiol.*, 31:600, 1973.
37. Frohlich, E. D., Tarazi, R. C., Dustan, H. P.: Hemodynamic and Functional Mechanisms in Two Renal Hypertensions: Arterial and Pyelonephritis, *Am. J. Med. Sci.*, 261:189, 1971.
38. Dustan, H. P., Tarazi, R. C., and Frohlich, E. D.: Functional Correlates of Plasma Renin Activity in Hypertensive Patients, *Circulation*, 41:555, 1970.
39. Vertes, V., Cangiano, J. L., Berman, L. B., and Gould, A.: Hypertension in End-State Renal Disease, *N. Engl. J. Med.*, 230:978, 1969.
40. DeFazio, V., Cristensen, R. C., Regan, T. J., Baer, L. J., Morita, Y., and Hellems, H. K.: Circulatory Changes in Acute Glomerulonephritis, *Circulation*, 20:190, 1959.
41. Fleisher, D. S., Voci, G., Garfunkel, J., Purugganan, H., Kirkpatrick, J., Wells, C. R., and McElfresh, A. E.: Hemodynamic Findings in Acute Glomerulonephritis, *J. Pediatr.*, 69:1054, 1966.
42. Eisenberg, S.: Blood Volume in Patients with Acute Glomerulonephritis as Determined by Radioactive Chrominum Tagged Red Cells, *Am. J. Med.*, 27:241, 1960.
43. Onesti, G., Kim, K. E., Greco, J. S., Del Guercio, E. T., Fernandes, M., and Swartz, C.: Blood Pressure Regulation in End-State Renal Disease and Anephric Man, *Circ. Res.*, 36/37(suppl. 1):145, 1975.
44. Weidmann, P., and Maxwell, M. H.: The Renin-Angiotensin-Aldosterone System in Terminal Renal Failure, *Kidney Int.*, 8:S–219, 1975.
45. Tarazi, R. C., Ibrahim, M. M., Bravo, E. L., and Dustan, H. P.: Hemodynamic Characteristics of Primary Aldosteronism, *N. Engl. J. Med.*, 289:1330, 1973.
46. Manger, W., and Gifford, R.: "Pheochromocytoma," Springer-Verlag, New York, Heidelberg, Berlin, 1977.
47. Dustan, H. P., Tarazi, R. C., and Bravo, E. L.: Physiologic Characteristics of Hypertension, *Am. J. Med.*, 52:610, 1972.
48. Maebashi, M., Miura, Y., Yoshinaga, K., and Sato, K.: Plasma Renin Activity in Pheochromocytoma, *Jpn. Circ. J.*, 32:1427, 1968.
49. Culbertson, J. W., Eckstein, J. W., Kirkendall, W. M., and Bedel, G. N.: General Hemodynamics and Splanchnic Circulation in Patients with Coarctation of the Aorta, *J. Clin. Invest.*, 36:1537, 1957.
50. Kirkendall, W. M., Culbertson, J. W., Eckstein, J. W.: Renal Hemodynamics in Patients with Coarctation of the Aorta, *J. Lab. Clin. Med.*, 53:6, 1959.

50

Diagnostic Evaluation of the Patient with Hypertension

W. Dallas Hall, M.D.
Gary L. Wollam, M.D.
Elbert P. Tuttle, Jr., M.D.

The utter recklessness with which this condition is overlooked may be compared to that of a man who piles coals upon his engine fire and neglects to take notice of his pressure gauge; anon his boiler bursts, and what cause is there for surprise?
Mahomed, 1879[1]

Proper Measurement of Blood Pressure

Measurement of Blood Pressure

The measurement of blood pressure requires precision as well as the consideration of a number of factors that could result in an erroneous labeling of a normotensive patient as hypertensive.[2] There are a number of possible sources of measurement artifacts. For example, false elevations of auscultatory measurements may be observed when regular-size blood pressure cuffs are used on adult patients whose midarm circumference exceeds 35 cm.[3,4] In addition, auscultatory measurements have also been reported to overestimate intraarterial pressure in some elderly patients, presumably because of "pipestem" arteries in patients with extensive atherosclerosis.[5,6]

The presence of an "auscultatory gap," which is not uncommon in elderly patients with atherosclerosis, can lead to underestimation of systolic pressure, as well as overestimation of diastolic pressure.[7] It occurs more frequently when blood pressure is measured in the sitting or standing positions, and is often observed in elderly patients with high systolic pressures. It can readily be avoided, however, by first estimating systolic pressure by palpation, and continuing to listen over the artery until the mercury falls 20 to 30 mm below the final disappearance of the Korotkoff sounds.

Blood pressure should initially be measured in both arms, and subsequent determinations should be performed in the arm with the highest pressure. In a study of 1000 normal men and women, Amsterdam and Amsterdam found that blood pressure readings in the right arm were generally higher than in the left arm.[8]

The position of the arm during the blood pressure measurement can be a source of variation in blood pressure readings. When blood pressure is measured in the sitting or standing position, lowering the arm from a near-horizontal (i.e., "heart level") position to a near-vertical (i.e., "dependent") position results in an increase in both the systolic and diastolic blood pressure readings. This increase in auscultatory blood pressure measurements with vertical arm displacement has been attributed to changes in hydrostatic pressure.[9,10]

Blood pressure should always be measured in the standing as well as in the supine or sitting position in patients with suspected or established hypertension. This is because the presence of a marked orthostatic decrease in blood pressure, which is especially common in diabetic and elderly patients, can influence the choice of antihypertensive therapy. The normal blood pressure response to assuming the upright position is a slight decrease in systolic and a slight increase in diastolic with little change in mean arterial pressure.[11,12] Standing reductions in systolic pressure of 20 mmHg or more, or mean arterial pressure of 10 percent or more, are often used as criteria for orthostatic hypotension. In general, marked orthostatic decreases in pretreatment blood pressure are more common in hypertensive patients with extensive target organ complications such as cardiomegaly, congestive heart failure, and associated vascular disease,[13] whereas the presence of orthostatic hypertension (i.e., an increase in diastolic pressure exceeding 8 to 10 mmHg upon arising from the supine to the standing position) has been associated with elevated norepinephrine levels and evidence of increased neurogenic tone.[13,14] It may also predict the subsequent response to certain adrenergic blocking drugs such as methyldopa.[15]

Variability of Blood Pressure

In addition to measurement artifacts, there is considerable variation in blood pressure. The variability of blood pressure has been found to increase with age and also with the level of blood pressure; it is more striking with systolic than with diastolic pressure.[16] Some studies have found that the magnitude of variability in systolic pressure and mean arterial pressure is inversely related to baroreceptor sensitivity.[17,18]

Even for normotensive individuals, however, blood pressure varies considerably throughout a 24-h period; isolated intermittent elevations of systolic pressure to levels above 150 mmHg and diastolic pressure to levels of 100 mmHg or greater are not uncommon.[19] In addition, blood pressure follows a circadian rhythm and is generally highest in the late morning and lowest at night.[20] When two or three consecutive blood pressure readings are taken, the first systolic reading is usually 2 to 4 mmHg higher than the second or third readings.[21] Diastolic pressure follows a similar pattern but to a lesser degree.

In addition, Souchek et al. found that the mean of two or three consecutive readings at one visit provided a more accurate prediction of blood pressure status over a subsequent 8-year follow-up period than did a single reading.[22] Furthermore, in the Framingham Study, the mean, maximum, and minimum of three blood pressure measurements obtained during the course of a single hour examination were all equally predictive of the subsequent development of cardiovascular disease.[23] The lowest (i.e., more "basal") of the three blood pressures was no better predictor of cardiovascular disease than the average (or the highest) of the blood pressure measurements.

In addition to variation within a given day, blood pressure exhibits marked variability between days.[24] This variability exceeds that observed within days. Decreases in systolic pressure of 10 to 30 mmHg and diastolic pressure of 5 to 10 mmHg between the first clinic visit, and the second (or third) follow-up visits are common. In the Hypertension Detection and Follow-Up Program, over 30 percent of subjects with average diastolic pressures of 95 mmHg or greater on the initial home screening, had diastolic pressures below 90 mmHg at the time of the second set of measurements approximately one week later.[25] Thus, the time of day, the number of blood pressure measurements taken during the clinic visit, and the variability between visits are all important considerations in the diagnosis of hypertension.[26] In uncomplicated cases with mild or moderate elevations of blood pressure, a minimum of two measurements on each of three different days are recommended to establish a diagnosis of hypertension. However, in patients with labile or borderline elevations of blood pressure, additional visits are frequently required to accurately assess blood pressure status.[27]

Home blood pressure measurement with ambulatory monitoring of daytime pressures by the patient may assist in evaluation of the patient with mild or borderline hypertension.[28] Perloff and associates[29] demonstrated that patients whose ambulatory blood pressures remained high (as compared with the average of three initial office visit pressures) had more target organ complications and experienced an increased number of cardiovascular events over an average follow-up period of 5 years than a group of patients with similar average office pressures but lower average ambulatory pressures. Home blood pressure monitoring may also assist in evaluation of the response to antihypertensive therapy.[30]

Basic Diagnostic Evaluation

The Patient with Mild or Moderate Hypertension

Our recommended evaluation procedures and diagnostic tests for mild to moderate hypertension are summarized in Tables 50-1 and 50-2.[31–33] It is widely

TABLE 50-1 Key Items of the History in Patients with Mild or Moderate Hypertension

Symptoms	
Blurred vision	Impotence
Bronchospasm	Joint pains
Chest pain	Muscle cramps
Claudication	Nocturia
Depression	Palpitations
Dizziness	Polyuria
Dyspnea	Skin rash
Fatigue	Sweating
Flushing	Tingling/cold extremities
Headaches	Unsteadiness
Hematuria	Weakness
	Weight loss or gain

Past Disease History	Diet and Drug History	Family History
Angina	Alcohol	Coronary heart disease
Asthma	Analgesics	Diabetes
Diabetes	BP medications	Hereditary nephritis
Glomerulonephritis	Cigarettes	Hyperlipemia
Gout	Cold remedies	Hyperparathyroidism
Hepatitis	Chewing tobacco	Hypertension
Hypertension	Licorice	Pheochromocytoma
Lupus erythematosus	Nasal sprays	Polycystic kidney disease
Myocardial infarction	Nonsteroidal anti-inflammatory agents	Renal hypoplasia
Peptic ulcer	Oral contraceptives	Thyroid disorders
Pyelonephritis	Potassium (dietary)	
Toxemia	Salt (dietary or tablets)	
Transient ischemic attacks	Tricyclic antidepressants	

held that mild or moderate hypertension is an asymptomatic disease. However, Bulpitt et al.[34] compared the prevalence of clinical symptoms in 99 untreated hypertensive patients with 78 normotensive patients of similar age; they observed that five symptoms (unsteadiness, waking headaches, blurred vision, depression, and nocturia) were significantly more frequent in the group with untreated hypertension. In addition to these five symptoms, the clinician should also ask about each of the other 18 symptoms listed in Table 50-1.

In the initial evaluation, efforts should be made to detect clinical clues to possible causes of secondary hypertension. For example, the presence of coarctation of the aorta is suggested by diminished leg pulses, a delay in the femoral pulse when palpated simultaneously with the radial pulse, a reduced blood pressure in the leg, a coarse systolic murmur at the left sternal border, and rib notching on the chest x-ray. Renovascular hypertension, aldosteronism, renal parenchymal hypertension and pheochromocytoma are discussed in succeeding sections. Acromegaly, hyperthyroidism, hypothyroidism, and Cushing's syndrome should be suspected from the general appearance of the patient.

In the baseline evaluation, the clinician should assess the extent of target organ damage and search for the risk factors of cardiovascular disease. Include a careful history for angina, past myocardial infarction, transient ischemic attacks, stroke, claudication, cigarette smoking, and a family history of cardiovascular events. Listen carefully for bruits over the carotid and femoral arteries as well as the aorta, and grade the amplitude of arterial pulsations in the limbs. Inspect the electrocardiogram for evidence of ischemic heart disease. Measure total and high-density lipoprotein (HDL) cholesterol levels, along with the other recommended routine laboratory tests listed in Table 50-2.

Hypertension is the most common cause of congestive heart failure which, in the Framingham Study, was associated with a 5-year survival of 38 to 57 percent.[35] Hence, the examiner should search for evidence of left ventricular hypertrophy, rales, ventricular gallop, distended neck veins, edema, and other clinical signs of congestive heart failure.

The initial evaluation is also important with regard to the subsequent selection of drug therapy. The therapeutic plan will be modified if there is a past disease history of diabetes, gout, nephrolithiasis, peptic ulcer, breast disease, severe depression, bronchospasm, or various other past illnesses. Also estimate the likelihood of proper adherence to medications and compliance in keeping appointments, because long-term control of hypertension depends on good cooperation by the patient. Choice of dosage schedules and cost of medications also influence effectiveness of therapy.

TABLE 50-2 Key Items of the Physical and Laboratory Examinations in Patients with Mild or Moderate Hypertension

Physical Examination

General	HEENT	Chest	Abdomen	Extremities	Neurological
Appearance	Carotid bruit	Breast	Bruit	Edema	Focal signs
BP (supine or sitting; standing; both arms; one leg)	Fundi	Diastolic murmur	Femoral pulses	Peripheral pulses	Proximal muscle strength
	Neck veins	Rales	Palpable kidneys	Peripheral bruits	
	Ocular bruits	S_3			
Heart rate (supine or sitting; standing)	Temporal arteries	S_4			
		Systolic murmur			
		Wheezes			

Laboratory Examination

General	Kidney	Metabolic	Miscellaneous
Hemoglobin	BUN	Calcium	Chest x-ray
Hematocrit	Creatinine	Cholesterol	Electrocardiogram
White blood count	Urine dipstix	Glucose (fasting)	
	Urine sediment	HDL cholesterol	
		Potassium	
		Uric acid	

The Patient with Severe, Accelerated, or Malignant Hypertension

The major diagnostic criteria for "malignant hypertension" include severe hypertension, generally with diastolic pressure of 125 mmHg or more, in conjunction with target organ damage and altered physiology.[36–38] Diagnostic criteria based on target organ damage include retinal hemorrhages and exudates, papilledema, heart failure, encephalopathy, and renal insufficiency. Diagnostic criteria based on physiologic abnormalities include impaired renal arteriolar perfusion associated with end arteritis, elevated plasma renin and aldosterone levels, increased sympathetic tone, and failure of physiologic negative feedback mechanisms. As a result of differences in the populations defined by these two types of criteria, there is debate over whether "malignant" hypertension ever occurs in association with low-renin states such as primary aldosteronism,[39] diabetic nephropathy,[40] or low-renin essential hypertension;[41] or whether fibrinoid necrosis of renal arterioles is a pathognomonic feature of malignant hypertension[42] and an invariable component of the disease. (See Fig. 50-1 for identification of the categories of findings in malignant hypertension.)

Because of the infrequent occurrence as well as the morbid prognosis associated with severe hypertension, a more aggressive diagnostic approach is indicated. In addition to the items listed in Tables 50-1 and 50-2, plasma renin activity in peripheral or renal venous blood may be helpful in planning therapy. Diagnostic studies for renal artery stenosis (i.e., rapid-sequence intravenous pyelogram, digital subtraction angiography, or renal arteriography) are

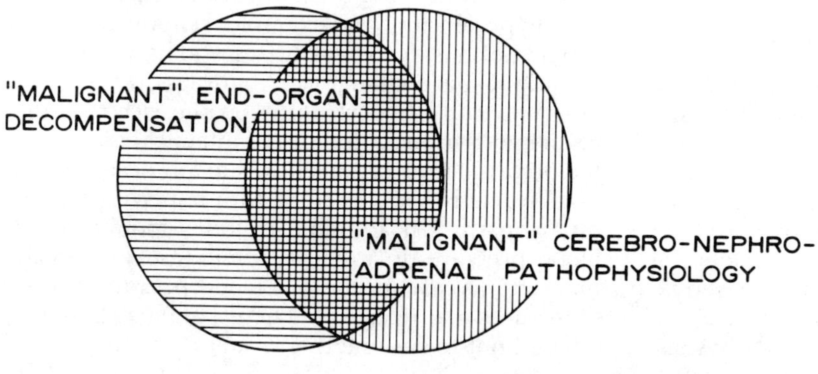

FIGURE 50-1 Venn diagram illustrating how the syndrome of malignant hypertension combines both elements of target organ damage ("malignant" end-organ decompensation) and altered physiology ("malignant" cerebro-nephro-adrenal pathophysiology).

also often indicated in severely hypertensive patients who would be candidates for renal artery angioplasty or surgery. Davis et al.[43] identified renal artery stenosis in 7 percent of black and 42 percent of white patients who presented with diastolic blood pressure of 125 mmHg or over and either flame hemorrhages, cotton-wool exudates, or papilledema. Pheochromocytoma may also present with severe or resistant hypertension, and can usually be excluded by obtaining plasma or urinary tests for catecholamines or their metabolites.

If a patient meets the criteria for "severe" or "malignant" hypertension by any combination of findings listed above, an aggressive search for primary causes of hypertension and a physiologic characterization of his or her blood pressure should be carried out. Qualitative or quantitative estimates of blood volume, cardiac output, peripheral resistance, symmetry of renal perfusion, and kidney size should be considered. In addition, appropriate studies to rule out primary correctable causes of hypertension discussed in later sections of this chapter must be conducted.

The Patient with Labile Hypertension

The examination of patients with labile hypertension should be generally the same as that for mild and moderate hypertension. This is because labile hypertension is associated with an increased risk of cardiovascular disease.[44] Special attention should be given to symptoms suggestive of pheochromocytoma, or to the abuse of alcohol,[45] diet pills,[46] nasal decongestants, or cold remedies containing phenylpropanolamine.[47] Inquire about recent stressful events because emotional stress can be associated with intermittent elevations of the blood pressure.[48] Rapid pulse, dilated pupils, and sweating suggest hyperactivity of the sympathetic nervous system.

There should be no evidence of target organ damage and the biochemical profile and urinalysis should be normal in patients with labile hypertension. The presence of any abnormality should be a cause for concern and may indicate that the seemingly intermittent elevations of blood pressure may actually be more persistent, of longer duration, and/or of greater magnitude than previously appreciated.

The Patient with Isolated Systolic Hypertension

The guidelines for evaluation of mild and moderate hypertension also apply to patients with isolated systolic hypertension. This is because the cardiovascular risks associated with elevated systolic pressure are as great or even greater than those of elevated diastolic pressure.[49,50] Isolated systolic hypertension has been associated with an increased prevalence of diabetes mellitus. Therefore, particular note should be made of symptoms and laboratory values suggestive of glucose intolerance. Elevation of the systolic blood pressure may also be the first clue to the presence of large-vessel atherosclerosis, as well as certain other conditions such as coarctation of the aorta, aortic insufficiency, hyperthyroidism, arteriovenous fistulas, or Paget's disease.

The Athlete with Elevated Blood Pressure

It is not infrequent for athletes to present to the clinician for evaluation of an elevated blood pressure detected on a routine screening or training examination. The usual story is that a physician's clearance and signature are needed before the patient can compete in athletic events. The blood pressure, particularly on the initial office visit, is usually abnormal. The electrocardiogram may show evidence of increased vagal tone (sinus bradycardia, first or second degree atrioventricular block, junctional rhythm) that can revert to normal in the standing position, changes associated with body build (high-amplitude R waves, a semivertical QRS axis), or changes suggestive of ischemia (elevation of the ST segments or inversion of the T waves).[51] An S_3 gallop may be audible[52] and borderline cardiomegaly is often present on the chest x-ray. Isolated systolic hypertension in an unusually tall basketball player may be the first clue to Marfan's syndrome with aortic insufficiency.

Echocardiography frequently reveals increased left ventricular end-diastolic posterior wall and septal wall thickness (and mass index) in highly trained collegiate athletes performing certain types of isometric exercise, such as wrestling, shot-putting, or weight lifting; whereas an elevated left ventricular end-diastolic internal dimension and volume have been reported to be a more characteristic finding in professional athletes participating primarily in isotonic (dynamic) exercise, such as competitive running, swimming, or basketball.[52,53] Almost all these changes can occur in athletes with normal left heart catheterization and widely patent coronary arteries.[54] Great caution, however, must be taken in evaluating such patients because almost 75 percent of reported sudden deaths in young athletes have occurred during major exertion; this risk appears to be accentuated in athletes with hypertrophic cardiomyopathy.[55] Thus, in addition to the usual evaluation, consideration should be given to diagnostic procedures not generally done in the usual asymptomatic patient with hypertension. For example, echocardiography should be considered in athletes who have abnormal ST and T-wave changes (or findings suggestive of left ventricular hypertrophy) on the electrocardiogram and/or clinical findings or a family history (e.g., the occurrence of unexplained sudden death in first-degree relatives) compatible with hypertrophic cardiomyopathy. In addition, cautious monitoring of blood pressure during a treadmill test can reveal a marked increase in diastolic blood pressure, rather than the usual decrease. These patients should be advised not to resume their usual exercise activities until blood pressure is better controlled. Blood pressure monitoring can also be conducted under circumstances that mimic the patient's usual exercise setting (e.g., weight lifting).[56] The blood pressure response to exercise can then be reevaluated following cautious institution of selected antihypertensive therapy.

Diagnosis of Target Organ Damage

Hypertensive Retinopathy

The funduscopic examination helps assess the prognosis as well as the severity of hypertension. Keith, Wagener, and Barker[57] first noted that patients with group I (constriction), II (sclerosis, arteriovenous nicking), III (hemorrhages and exudates), and IV (papilledema) retinopathy had untreated 5-year survivals of 85, 50, 13, and 0 percent, respectively. Arteriovenous nicking and a copper- or silver-wire appearance of the arterioles may be noted in older patients, although these changes indicate arteriosclerosis of any etiology.[58] A large inter- and intraobserver variability limits the value of fine distinctions between the lower grades (i.e., groups I and II) of retinopathy, although most agree that both focal and generalized arteriolar narrowing are retinal vascular signs of hypertension.[59]

Hypertensive Cardiovascular Disease

Two major forms of heart disease occur in the patient with hypertension: coronary heart disease and hypertensive heart disease. Criteria for the diagnosis of coronary heart disease are described elsewhere. The clinical diagnosis of hypertensive heart disease is made by the combined presence of hypertension and left ventricular hypertrophy (LVH) when other causes of LVH are reasonably excluded. Hypertension is the most common cause of LVH.[60] Neither a long duration nor any particular level of severity of blood pressure elevation are necessary prerequisites for LVH because factors other than blood pressure elevation are important for its development. Four noninvasive diagnostic techniques are available currently for clinical assessment of LVH: physical examination, chest x-ray, electrocardiogram (ECG), and echocardiogram (ECHO).

Detection of LVH by physical examination depends on palpation of an enlarged and sustained left ventricular impulse at the apex.[61,62] An enlarged apical impulse is often defined as having a diameter greater than that of a quarter (i.e., more than 2.4 cm); whereas a sustained apical impulse has an outward thrust that lasts one-half to two-thirds or more of the duration of systole. Clinical information is maximized by turning the patient partially on the left side.[63] An apical impulse diameter greater than 3 cm in the left lateral decubitus position is a more sensitive and specific finding of left ventricular enlargement than is the location of the apex impulse 10 cm or more from the midsternal line or lateral to the midclavicular line.[64]

Detection of LVH by chest x-ray is fraught with the problems of defining which portions of the cardiac silhouette belong specifically to the left ventricle. Two methods are used to define cardiomegaly: the cardiothoracic ratio[65] and the cardiac volume.[66,67] The cardiothoracic ratio should not exceed 0.5 in adults, and is usually below 0.45. Normal values for the cardiac volume are 500 ml per M^2 in men and 450 to 490 ml per M^2 in women.

Table 50-3 lists the criteria developed by Romhilt and Estes for an electrocardiographic diagnosis of LVH (five points) or probable LVH (four points).[68] These authors found that LVH is detected by the ECG point-score system in 58 percent of hypertrophied hearts; false-positive results occur in 3 percent. A number of criteria for summed precordial voltage are as sensitive as the point-score system, but are less specific and lead to false-positive readings of LVH in 10 to 15 percent of cases.[69] As defined originally, the "typical" ST segment shift (i.e., "strain pattern") requires both depression of the ST segment (more than 0.5 mm) and inversion of the T wave (0.5 mm or more) in the limb or left precordial leads; the resultant ST segments and T wave vectors must be opposite to the direction of the main QRS vector.[70] Refinements in the Romhilt-Estes point-score system have further improved the specificity of the electrocardiographic diagnosis of LVH.[71]

Electrocardiographic evidence of left atrial abnormality often precedes that of left ventricular abnormality in patients with hypertension. One set of criteria for left atrial abnormality requires two of the following four findings: terminal (negative) atrial forces in $V_1 \geq 0.04$ mm-s, bipeak interval > 0.04 s in deeply notched P waves in any lead, ratio of P

TABLE 50-3 Estes Point-Score System for the Electrocardiographic Diagnosis of Left Ventricular Hypertrophy

	Points*
Amplitude R or S wave in limb lead $\geq$ 20 mm, or S wave in V_1 or $V_2 \geq$ 30 mm, or R wave in V_5 or $V_6 \geq$ 30 mm	3
Terminal negativity of the P wave in V_1 of 1 mm or more in depth and $\geq$ 0.04 s duration	3
ST-T segment vector opposite to QRS vector	3†
QRS axis of $-30°$ or more	2
QRS duration $\geq$ 0.09 s	1
Intrinsicoid deflection (ventricular activation time) $\geq$ 0.05 s in V_5 or V_6	1

*Five or more points equals LVH; four points equals probable LVH.

†Reduced to one point if the patient is receiving digitalis.

Source: Romhilt, D. W., and Estes, E. H., Jr.: A Point-score System for the ECG Diagnosis of Left Ventricular Hypertrophy, *Am. Heart J.*, 75:752, 1968. Adapted and reproduced with permission from the publisher and author.

wave duration to PR segment > 1.6 in lead II, and P wave > 0.3 mv height or > 0.12 s duration in lead II.[72]

Echocardiography has revolutionized the diagnosis of LVH. This is because echocardiographic evidence of LVH is found in many hypertensive patients with normal ECG and chest x-ray. In fact, one study of 234 hypertensive patients revealed cardiomegaly on chest x-ray or LVH on electrocardiography in less than 10 percent of patients who had an echocardiographic increase in left ventricular mass.[73] Four echocardiographic parameters assess left ventricular muscle anatomy: interventricular septal thickness (IVST), posterior wall thickness (PWT), mean myocardial thickness (IVST + PWT/2), and left ventricular mass index (LVMI). In general, two-dimensional echocardiography does not appear to be superior to M-mode echocardiography in assessing left ventricular hypertrophy, provided there are no regional wall motion abnormalities.[74]

Devereax and Reichek[75] correlated the LVMI with the weight of the left ventricle at postmortem examination of 34 adult patients. Eight different echocardiographic estimates of left ventricular mass all correlated strongly with anatomic left ventricular mass. Multiple studies have now documented that the ECHO is both a sensitive and an early indicator of anatomic abnormality of the left ventricle in patients with hypertension.[76–80] Echocardiography is also a useful technique to demonstrate changes in left ventricular anatomy and function following therapy for hypertension.[81–83] The current cost of echocardiography is approximately threefold that of electrocardiography and must be considered in context of the diagnostic and therapeutic yields in individual patients with hypertension.

Hypertensive Cerebrovascular Disease

Cerebrovascular Accidents

Hypertension is the most important risk factor for the development of hemorrhagic or atheroembolic stroke. The incidence of stroke increases with each higher stratum of blood pressure.[84]

Microhemorrhage or occlusion of small vessels may result in small areas of infarction, most frequently in the putamen, thalamus, caudate nucleus, pons, or posterior limb of the internal capsule. These "lacunar" infarcts are often associated with neurological deficits that clear over a period of days to weeks. Four distinct clinical syndromes have been identified: (1) pure motor hemiparesis (weakness of the face, arm, and leg), (2) pure sensory stroke (numbness and sensory loss over the face, arm, trunk, and leg), (3) homolateral ataxia and crural paresis (ataxia of the arm and leg, and weakness of the leg), and (4) dysarthria and clumsy hand (dysarthria, central facial weakness, deviation of the tongue, and weakness and ataxia of the arm).[85] Multiple lacunae may result in pseudobulbar palsy (i.e., the "lacunar state"), characterized by lability of affect, dementia, abnormal gait, dysarthria, incontinence, and bilateral long-tract signs.

Classical cerebrovascular accidents of the hemorrhagic and infarctive types are diagnosed on the basis of the detailed neurological examination. In cerebral infarction, the computerized axial tomography (CT) scan shows a sharply marginated, homogeneous, low-density lesion in a specific vascular territory; whereas in intracerebral hemorrhage the scan usually shows an irregularly shaped, consolidated, high-density mass.[86] The differentiation between a transient ischemic attack (TIA) and a small lacunar infarct is often difficult; although TIAs may recur in a repetitive pattern, lacunar infarcts by definition cannot. Evanescent neurological symptoms or findings in conjunction with a carotid artery bruit justify carotid angiography or ultrasonography in an operable patient, with due attention to potential nephrotoxicity of radiographic contrast material.

Hypertensive Encephalopathy

Hypertensive encephalopathy is a syndrome characterized by acute or subacute alterations in neurological status that occur as the result of elevated arterial pressure, and are reversed by lowering the blood pressure. It usually occurs in the setting of accelerated-malignant hypertension, although severe hypertensive retinopathy may occasionally be absent.[87] This syndrome can occur with almost any variety of hypertension, although it is rare with primary aldosteronism and coarctation of the aorta.

Hypertensive encephalopathy usually presents with severe headache along with confusion, agitation, or lethargy. It is frequently accompanied by nausea, vomiting, and visual disturbances, including scotomata and transient amaurosis. The symptoms generally worsen over 12 to 48 h and seizures, myoclonus, obtundation, and, in some instances, blindness, may develop.

Hypertensive encephalopathy must be distinguished from other disorders that can present with diffuse neurological findings in patients with hypertension.[88,89] Both uremic and hypertensive encephalopathy may present with hypertension, confusion, lethargy, and seizures. However, severe headache and retinal hemorrhages, exudates, or papilledema are more characteristic of hypertensive encephalopathy, whereas uremic encephalopathy is often accompanied by myoclonic jerking in a diffuse asynchronous and asymmetric pattern. Moreover, the symptoms of hypertensive encephalopathy are usually reversed within 12 to 72 h by effective antihypertensive therapy. In malignant hypertension with renal insufficiency, the encephalopathy may well be due to both. Other causes of metabolic encephalopathy (e.g., hyponatremia, hypernatremia, meningitis, encephalitis, drug intoxication, and collagen vascular diseases) should be considered and evaluated as indicated by other signs and symptoms.

Focal seizures and other focal neurologic signs may occur in patients who appear clinically to have hypertensive encephalopathy.[88,89] However, in an autopsy study of patients with the clinical diagnosis of hypertensive encephalopathy, Chester et al.[89] found that focal neurological deficits were almost invariably attributable to gross structural lesions such as cerebral hemorrhage or cerebral infarction. Patients who appear to have hypertensive encephalopathy and exhibit focal neurological signs should undergo further diagnostic evaluation. Computerized axial tomography scanning with or without intravenous contrast medium is the procedure most likely to identify focal areas of intracerebral hemorrhage or infarction, and has largely replaced carotid arteriography in this setting.

Severe hypertension may occur in previously normotensive patients who develop intracranial hemorrhage, or a wide variety of other primary neurological disorders. In these settings, considerable caution must be taken to avoid the erroneous diagnosis of hypertensive encephalopathy. In general, such patients have neither severe hypertensive retinopathy nor LVH.

Nephrosclerosis

The urinalysis, creatinine clearance, kidney size, pyelogram, angiogram, renal scan, and renogram are usually normal in patients with primary hypertension. Sophisticated diagnostic tests, however, often reveal malfunction of the kidney at this stage. These include renal blood flow,[90] filtration fraction,[90] fractional excretion of filtered sodium,[91] change in vascular caliber with vasodilator drugs,[92] and microdetermination of albuminuria.[93]

These special diagnostic tests are not justified in prognostication or in treatment of hypertension when the usual clinical tests of kidney function are within the normal range. If the diagnosis of hypertension can be established when the urinalysis, BUN, and creatinine are normal, the hypertension may be assumed not to be secondary to renal parenchymal disease.

Benign Nephrosclerosis

Abnormalities of standard kidney function tests in patients with long-standing, poorly controlled hypertension, in the absence of intercurrent primary disease of the kidneys, are attributable to benign nephrosclerosis. Under these circumstances low-grade proteinuria (less than 1 g/day) and granular casts may appear, creatinine clearance may fall, and kidneys may shrink slightly. Pyelograms may show poor visualization of the kidneys or excretion of contrast material without distortion of the renal contour or collecting system. Quantitative renal scans and radioactive renograms will provide information on symmetry, size, vascularization, and function of the kidneys at this stage of disease. Although not usually required for the diagnosis of benign nephrosclerosis, renal angiography will show moderately constricted renal blood vessels with increased tortuosity and "cork-screwing" of renal arterioles, but a normal ratio of parenchyma to vascularity of the kidney (Fig. 50-2). Kidney biopsy is not indicated unless hematuria, red blood cell casts, heavy proteinuria, or systemic findings of collagen vascular or neoplastic disease are found.

There is an impression among those who see a large number of end-stage renal disease patients that an appreciable number of patients develop renal failure as a consequence of long-standing, poorly controlled hypertension causing nephrosclerosis. In patients with end-stage renal disease, a credible diagnosis of benign hypertensive nephrosclerosis depends on multiple lines of evidence: that hypertension preceded renal disease by a number of years; that glucose tolerance has been normal prior to renal failure; that microscopic hematuria is absent; that no other intercurrent primary renal disease occurred; that the hypertension was at least moderately severe and poorly controlled; that renal arteriography shows corkscrew arterioles; or that kidney biopsy shows only advanced arteriolar intimal and medial changes with interstitial fibrosis and glomerular atrophy and fibrosis.

Malignant Nephrosclerosis

The renal disease associated with malignant essential hypertension, usually called malignant nephrosclerosis, differs in pathology, physiology, and natural history from the forms of nephrosclerosis described above. As pointed out earlier, the renal failure from malignant hypertension is usually seen in a clinical context of multiple target organ decompensation—retinopathy, encephalopathy, and congestive heart failure. Depending upon definition, it is often or always associated with elevated plasma renin, elevated aldosterone, and increased sympathetic outflow manifested by tachycardia and a hyperdynamic precordium.

The diagnosis of malignant nephrosclerosis can be confirmed by renal arteriography. It is desirable to use less than 10 ml of contrast material per kidney by performing only selective renal arteriograms and thereby avoiding aortograms because large doses of radiographic contrast medium may impair marginally compensated renal function. The "pruning" of the vascular tree with relatively large, poorly perfused kidneys indicates malignant nephrosclerosis (Fig. 50-3).

The urinalysis in malignant nephrosclerosis can range from negative in patients whose lesion is confined to the arterioles, to four-plus proteinuria, hematuria, and red blood cell or pigmented casts in those with associated glomerulitis or interstitial bleeding. Renal biopsy carries extra risk because of the marked elevation of the blood pressure, but may be done successfully following blood pressure control with diazoxide or nitroprusside. One justification for renal biopsy is to evaluate the potential for recovery of function, based on the number of viable glomeruli that can be found.

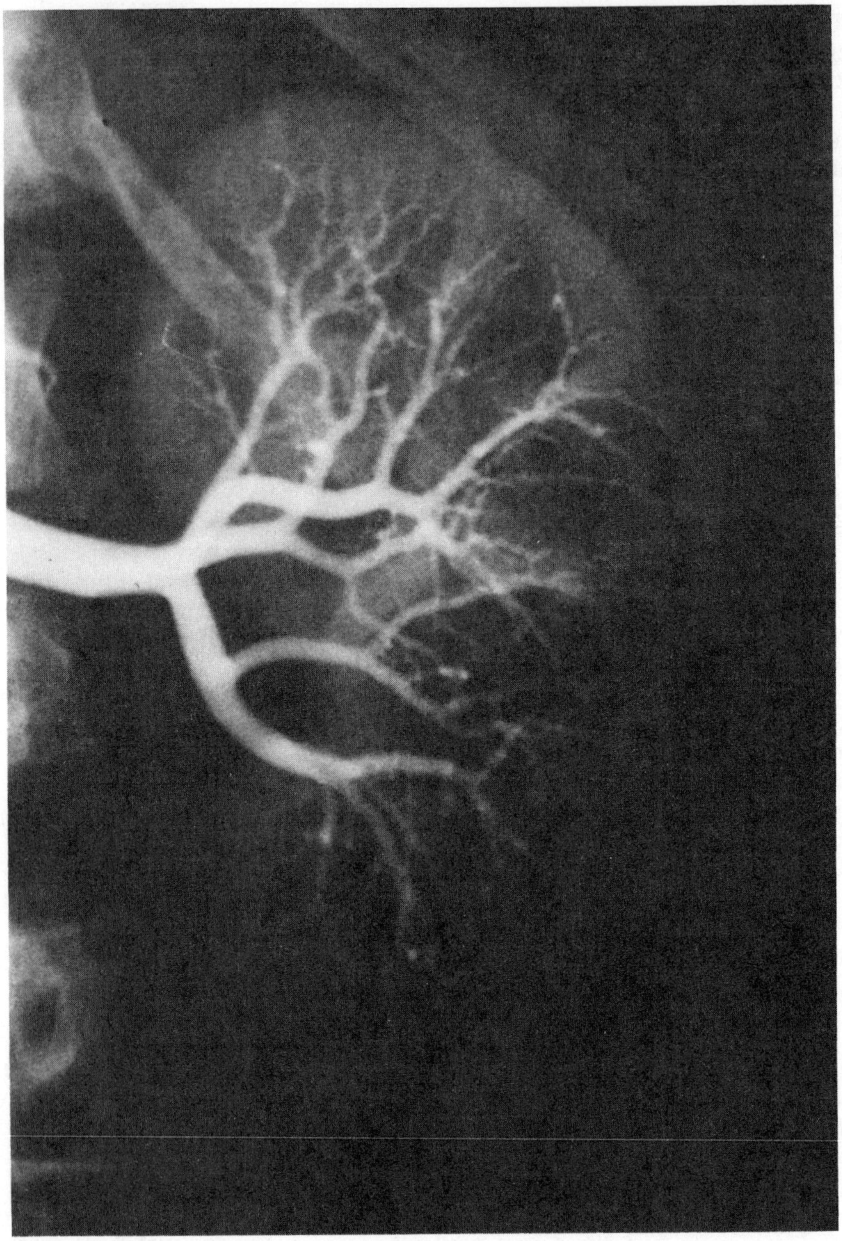

FIGURE 50-2 Tortuosity and corkscrewing of the vessels (represented by white dots in the vascular tree) with preservation of renal mass and good cortical nephrogram in benign nephrosclerosis.

Rapid changes in perfusion pressure secondary to aggressive antihypertensive therapy and evolving vascular pathology make serial creatinine clearance determinations necessary to evaluate short-term changes in renal function.

Quantitation of plasma renin concentration may be desirable in cases of malignant nephrosclerosis with renal failure. It is of clinical value in interpreting the pathologic physiology of the renal failure, in planning for renal transplantation, in choosing drug therapy, and in prescribing for sodium intake and ultrafiltration for hemodialysis. Serum aldosterone concentrations are of physiologic interest, but of minimal diagnostic value in this setting. Serum potassium concentrations are often disproportionately low in the face of oliguric renal failure.

Diagnosis of Secondary Hypertension

The prevalence of causes of secondary hypertension is not known with certainty and estimates have varied from as low as 1 percent or less to as high as 30 percent. The results of several studies are listed in Table 50-4.[94–98] The largest is from the Cleveland Clinic, where the prevalence of secondary hypertension was found to be 11 percent.[94] At present, the best estimate of the prevalence of secondary hypertension in relatively unselected populations would appear to be lower, in the range of 5 to 10 percent. Potentially curable etiologies are even less frequent,[94,99] emphasizing the importance of limiting extensive evaluations to patients in whom the diagnostic yield is likely to be increased.

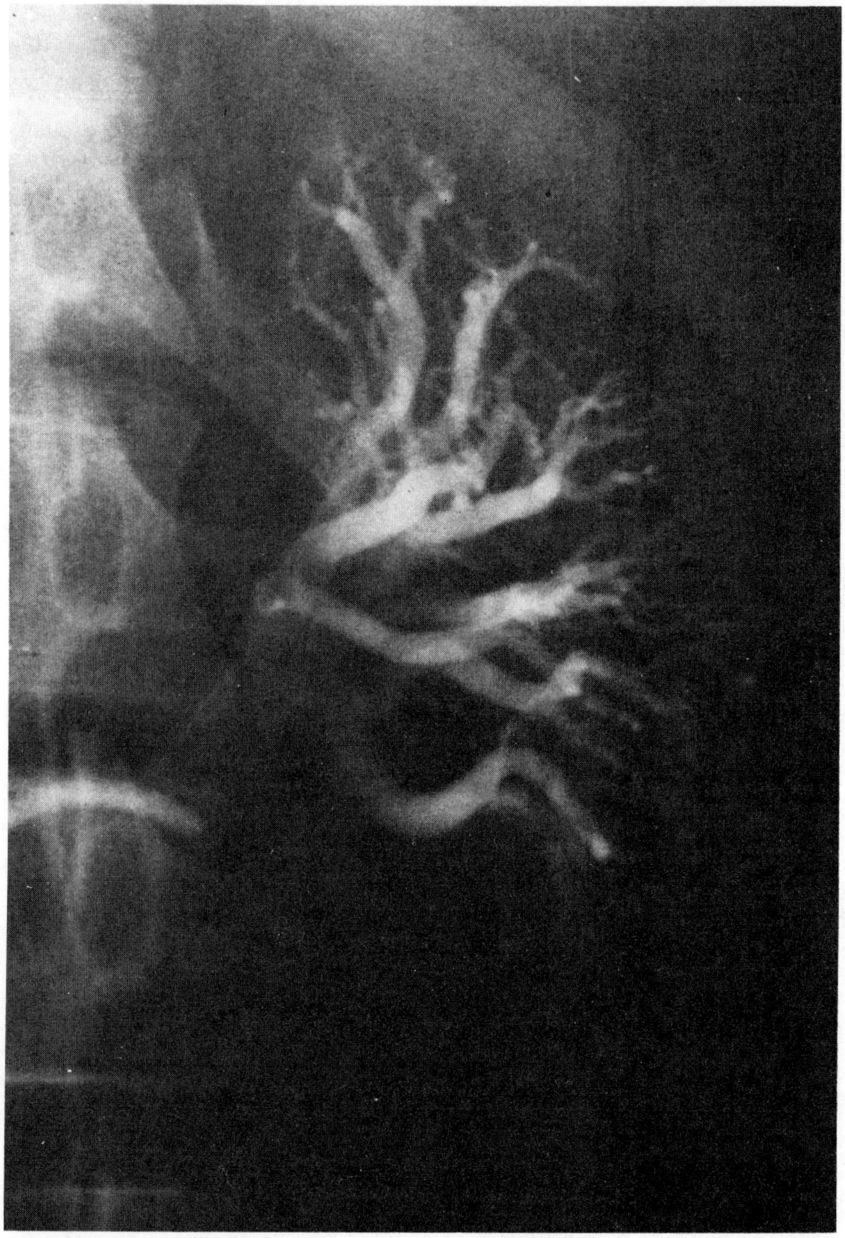

FIGURE 50-3 Distended main branches with "pruning" of small arteries and minimal opacification of the cortical nephrogram despite preservation of renal mass in malignant nephrosclerosis.

TABLE 50-4 Secondary Hypertension in Adults: Results of Five Major Studies

	Reference				
	Gifford[94]	Kennedy[95]	Ferguson[96]	Bech[97]	Berglund[98]
Patient Population	**Partly Referred**	**Partly Referred**	**Partly Referred**	**Partly Referred**	**Randomly Selected***
Number, %	**4939**	**750**	**246**	**482**	**689**
Essential hypertension	89	73	89	79	94
Chronic renal disease	5	17	2	13	4
Renovascular disease	4	6	3	5	0.6
Primary aldosteronism	0.4	0.3	0.4	0.4	0.1
Coarctation	0.6	—	—	0	0.1
Cushing's syndrome	0.2	—	—	—	—
Pheochromocytoma	0.2	0.1	—	0.2	—
Miscellaneous†	—	4	4	3	1

*Randomly selected men between the ages of 47 and 54 years with blood pressure > 175/115.
†Includes oral contraceptive hypertension as well as patients not thoroughly investigated for secondary causes.

Renovascular Hypertension

Prevalence

Renal artery stenosis is the most common potentially curable cause of hypertension. Estimates range from less than 1 percent to as high as 18 percent of the hypertensive population. At the present time, the best estimate of the prevalence of renovascular hypertension in less selected populations of hypertensive patients would appear to be in the range of 3 percent or less (Table 50-4). The prevalence may, in part, depend on the demographic characteristics of the hypertensive population. Below the age of 40, renovascular hypertension may occur more frequently in women than men.[100] Renovascular hypertension is also less common in black hypertensive patients.[101–103]

Clinical Findings (Table 50-5)

The likelihood of renovascular hypertension is increased in several clinical settings, such as the onset of hypertension before age 30 or after age 50. An abdominal bruit is six to nine times more common in renovascular hypertensive patients than in essential hypertensive patients. The presence of severe hypertensive retinopathy (hemorrhages, exudates, or papilledema) also increases the likelihood. The sudden onset of severe hypertension, or the onset of uncontrolled hypertension in a patient whose blood pressure was previously well-controlled, is another clue to renovascular disease. In addition, obesity may be less common among renovascular hypertensive patients than essential hypertensive patients.[103,104]

Pathologic Types of Renal Artery Stenosis

Fibrous dysplasia and atherosclerosis of the renal artery account for the vast majority of cases of renovascular hypertension. Table 50-5 contrasts the clinical features of these two types of renovascular hypertension with those of essential hypertension.

Fibrous Dysplasia With fibrous dysplasia, the onset of hypertension generally occurs before age 35, most prevalently in women. Fibrous dysplasia may involve either or both renal arteries, although the most common presentation is unilateral involvement of the right renal artery.[100] An upper abdominal bruit is detected in approximately 60 percent of patients. Heavy pressure with auscultation deep in the epigastrium enhances detection of abdominal bruits, but an abdominal bruit is by no means a universal finding and is frequently absent or heard intermittently. A bruit originating from a renal artery is generally heard best in the midepigastrium and radiates to one or both upper quadrants. It is usually high-pitched and is occasionally systolic-diastolic or continuous in character. If combined with hypertension of less than 3 years' duration, the presence of a systolic-diastolic bruit is predictive of a favorable response to surgery in patients with fibrous dysplasia.[105]

Atherosclerotic Renovascular Disease Atherosclerotic disease accounts for the largest portion of renovascular hypertensive patients. In contrast to fibromuscular dysplasia, atherosclerotic renovascular disease occurs predominately in men over age 45.

TABLE 50-5 Comparison of the Clinical Characteristics of Essential Hypertension and Renovascular Hypertension (Surgically Cured)

Clinical Characteristics	Essential Hypertension (*N* = 339)	Renovascular Hypertension: Atherosclerosis (*N* = 91)	Renovascular Hypertension: Fibrous Dysplasia (*N* = 84)
History			
Age of onset, years	35	46*	33
Duration, years	3.1	1.9*	2.0*
Sex, % female	40	34	81*
Race, % black	29	7*	10*
Family history of hypertension, %	67	58	41*
Physical			
Obese, %	38	17*	11*
Thin, %	6	13	30*
Systolic BP, mmHg	169	181*	174
Diastolic BP, mmHg	109	108	108
Fundi grade 3 or 4, %	12	26*	10
Abdominal bruit, %	7	41*	57*
Laboratory			
Cardiomegaly (chest x-ray), %	26	26	8*
Serum creatinine > 1.5 mg/dl, %	11	15	2*
Serum potassium < 3.4 meq/l, %	7	14	17*

*Indicates significant difference ($p < 0.05$) when compared with the group with essential hypertension.

Source: Simon, N., Franklin, S.S., Bleifer, K.H. and Maxwell, M.H.: Clinical Characteristics of Renovascular Hypertension, *JAMA*, 220:1209, 1972. Copyright 1972, American Medical Association. Adapted and reproduced with permission from the publisher and author.

In the Cooperative Study of Renovascular Hypertension, approximately 31 percent of patients with atherosclerotic renovascular disease had bilateral lesions; unilateral lesions were more prevalent on the left side.[100] In addition, Shapiro et al.[106] found a high prevalence of diabetes mellitus in patients with atherosclerotic renal artery disease. Abdominal bruits are of less diagnostic value because the atherosclerotic process often involves other arteries.

Special Diagnostic Tests

When renovascular hypertension is suspected, diagnostic evaluation should generally be considered in younger patients (below age 35) who may have fibrous dysplasia of the renal artery. This is particularly true in patients with moderate or severe hypertension of less than 3 years' duration, or when blood pressure is inadequately controlled on three or more antihypertensive drugs. It should also be considered in selected older patients who may have atherosclerotic renovascular disease and are judged to be good candidates for either surgical intervention or angioplasty using the balloon-dilatation technique. Diagnostic testing is not usually indicated in patients with advanced renal failure, and bilateral small kidneys; although improvement in renal function following revascularization has been observed in selected cases with one relatively normal-size kidney.[107]

The evaluation should generally begin with either a rapid-sequence intravenous urogram (IVP) or digital subtraction angiography (DSA). DSA is a relatively new radiologic technique that combines intravenous urography with angiotomography to create subtraction images of the abdominal arteries.[108–111] Rapid injection of a large bolus of contrast material by catheter into the central circulation is required. A technically satisfactory rapid-sequence IVP is abnormal in about 83 percent of patients with renovascular hypertension.[112] Using the newer DSA technique, lesions of the main renal artery may be detected in up to 90 percent or more of cases where adequate visualization is achieved,[108,109] although it is less reliable for detecting segmental renal artery lesions.[110,113] When the index of clinical suspicion is high, or when the risk of complications seems excessive, it may be expedient to proceed directly to renal arteriography. If serum creatinine is greater than 2 mg/dl and especially in diabetics, the total amount of contrast material should be limited to less than 90 ml, and hydration, volume expansion, and diuresis should be ensured.

Once the presence of renal arterial disease has been established, the functional significance of the stenosis must be evaluated to determine if the renal artery lesion is the cause of the hypertension. This is best done by measuring the "renal vein renin ratio": i.e., the ratio of plasma renin activity in blood samples obtained from the venous effluent of each kidney. Blood samples for renal vein renin activity should generally be obtained following sodium depletion (e.g., the administration of oral furosemide, 40 mg bid or tid for 24 to 48 h in conjunction with a low-sodium diet). A reduction of 2 percent or more in baseline body weight is generally considered an adequate diuretic response. The adminstration of a single oral dose of the converting enzyme inhibitor, captopril, 30 to 90 min prior to obtaining renal vein renin studies (in patients not receiving therapy with captopril) may also enhance lateralization in patients with unilateral renal artery disease.[114,115] However, captopril should be used with caution in this setting. This is because acute renal insufficiency (usually reversible following discontinuation of the drug) has been observed in patients with severe bilateral renal artery stenosis, or renal artery stenosis in a solitary kidney, following therapy with converting enzyme inhibitors such as captopril or enalapril.[116,117] A renal vein renin ratio of 1.5 or greater favoring the stenotic side is abnormal, and generally indicates a functionally significant renal artery stenosis.[118] Lateralization may have additional significance when the peripheral plasma renin activity is also elevated and renin secretion from the unaffected kidney is suppressed; i.e., the renal venous renin activity from the unaffected side is approximately equivalent to or less than the renin activity of a sample obtained from the inferior vena cava below the renal veins.[119–122] In general, when renal vein renins reveal a stenotic: nonstenotic ratio of ≥ 1.5, approximately 90 percent of patients will be improved or relieved of hypertension following successful surgical revascularization or nephrectomy. However, up to 50 percent or more of selected patients with nonlateralizing renal vein renin ratios (i.e., < 1.5) may also have a favorable response to surgery.[123] Hence, a lateralizing renal vein renin ratio predicts improvement of hypertension (i.e., "success") with a high degree of accuracy in patients with unilateral renal arterial disease; whereas, a nonlateralizing value does not appear to be a reliable predictor of lack of improvement of hypertension (i.e., "failure") following a technically successful surgical procedure or percutaneous renal angioplasty using the balloon-dilatation technique.[119] The renal vein renin ratio is frequently not reliable for predicting surgical response in patients with bilateral renovascular disease.[120] Peripheral vein renin activity is generally not a useful test for renovascular hypertension because up to 50 percent of patients may have values within the normal range for the particular testing method.[124]

Hypertension Due to Renal Parenchymal Disease

Two types of renal parenchymal hypertension are the acute form associated with glomerulitis in a normal census of nephrons, and the chronic form associated with loss of viable nephron population. In neither of these is plasma renin activity usually very elevated. In contrast to essential hypertension, the urinalysis is typically abnormal in patients with hypertension due to renal parenchymal disease.[125]

Hypertension in Acute Renal Parenchymal Disease

Laboratory evidence of hematuria, especially with red blood cells showing the microrosette evagination of the membrane seen under oil immersion or phase contrast microscopy,[126] red blood cell or hematin-pigmented casts, proteinuria in conjunction with periorbital and/or pedal edema, and elevation of the BUN-to-creatinine ratio to ≥ 15:1 are diagnostic of acute diffuse glomerulitis. The reduction of single nephron urine flow with acute glomerulitis results in a greater reduction of urea clearance (by virtue of its avid reabsorption) than of creatinine clearance. This gives a urea-to-creatinine clearance ratio similar to that which is often called "pre-renal azotemia." A more accurate term for the setting of acute glomerulitis would be *intact nephron azotemia.*

Usually tachycardia and vigorous contractility of the myocardium give the impression of a hyperdynamic circulation unopposed by baroreceptor reflexes. If plasma renin is measured, it is often normal or slightly depressed,[127] but it may be considered elevated relative to the increased blood volume and pressure.

Radiographic examination of the kidneys in hypertensive acute glomerulitis usually shows them to be enlarged or at the upper limit of normal size. Sometimes retrograde pyelography, done because of gross hematuria, reveals large kidneys with a delicate or filigree pattern of the calyces and infundibulum, resulting from intracapsular swelling of the kidney and compression of the collecting system.

Other laboratory tests may confirm the etiologic diagnosis: bacteriologic or serologic evidence of streptococcal infection, antinuclear antibodies, depressed serum complement. If heavy proteinuria is present on qualitative testing, 24-h urine protein and creatinine clearances should be determined to ascertain whether a nephrotic type of protein leak is present. Meltzer and coworkers have pointed out that whereas hypotensive idiopathic nephrotic patients often have high plasma renins, hypertensive nephrotic patients usually have low plasma renins.[128] The nephrotic syndrome has been described in cases of pheochromocytoma[129] and renal artery stenosis.[130]

If the nephrotic syndrome is diagnosed, or if the renal function remains severely depressed after 2 weeks of treatment with appropriate antibiotics, antihypertensive agents, and diuretics, then a kidney biopsy should be performed. Immunologic and ultrastructural classification of the disease will modify diagnosis, prognosis, and therapy. The hypertension of acute glomerulonephritis is usually controlled easily with diuretics and antisympathetic agents.

Hypertension in Chronic Renal Parenchymal Disease

The second major category of renal disease associated with hypertension is that related to loss of nephron population in chronic nephritis. In this type of renal parenchymal hypertension, creatinine clearances and urea clearances are proportionately reduced and the BUN-to-creatinine ratio is normal, approximately 10:1. Urinalysis usually shows moderate proteinuria (0.5 to 2 g/day), moderate numbers of red blood cells, and frequent granular casts with glomerulonephritis, whereas pyuria, white blood cell casts, and bacteriuria are present with pyelonephritis. Pyuria may also be seen with abacterial forms of interstitial nephritis such as analgesic nephropathy.

X-ray studies in chronic nephritis usually show variable degrees of reduction in kidney size. The kidneys are symmetric and smooth in chronic glomerulonephritis, so-called pyelonephritis lenta, and diabetic intercapillary nephrosclerosis. In focal pyelonephritis, they are often irregular in configuration. With advanced uremia, small kidneys indicate irreversibility of the underlying disease. Shrunken kidneys are not good to biopsy because tissue is difficult to obtain from the sclerotic organ and the end-stage histologic pattern is hard to interpret.

When arteriograms are done in advanced parenchymal nephritis, the small kidney shows relatively profuse blood vessels extending almost to the capsule with no cortical tissue remaining (Fig. 50-4). The caliber of the vessels is small, but the number is normal. This angiographic pattern differs considerably from that described for benign or malignant nephrosclerosis.

When chronic renal failure is found in conjunction with diabetes mellitus, the pathologic lesion may be either intercapillary glomerulosclerosis, large- or medium-vessel atherosclerotic disease, or shrunken atrophy with interstitial fibrosis due to deficiency of nutrient blood flow to the kidney. Search for renal artery occlusive disease by radioactive renogram and renal scan allows demonstration of asymmetry of size; renal blood flow helps to identify candidates for vascularization to preserve renal function.

In the hypertension of patients with end-stage renal disease on maintenance hemodialysis, most patients are volume-dependent, but some are renin-mediated. For this reason, as well as to interpret excessive thirst and polydipsia when volume is contracted, plasma renin determinations may be of value. This information is also important if kidney transplantation is planned because posttransplant hypertension is sometimes caused by renin secretion from the native kidneys.

Primary Aldosteronism

Primary aldosteronism (Conn's syndrome) is an uncommon, but potentially curable cause of hypertension. In centers where patients are referred and extensively investigated for primary aldosteronism, this diagnosis has been confirmed in up to 12 percent of patients.[131,132] However, in most studies of the prevalence of known causes of hypertension, pri-

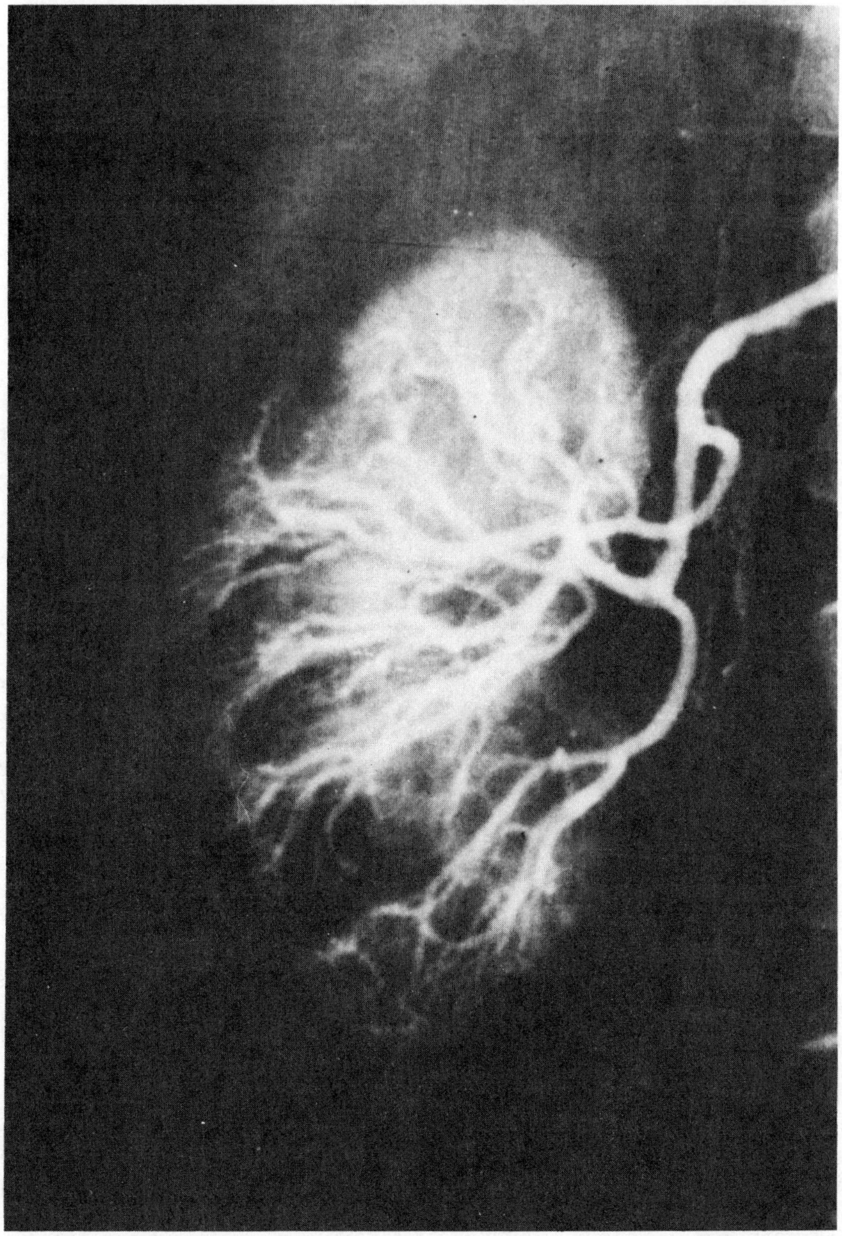

FIGURE 50-4 Disproportionately profuse vasculature of small caliber running out to the capsule of the small kidney with an atrophic cortex in chronic parenchymatous nephritis of various causes.

mary aldosteronism is found in 0.5 percent or less of patients (Table 50-4).

The majority of cases of primary aldosteronism are diagnosed between the ages of 30 and 50 years.[133] The hypertension of primary aldosteronism is usually mild or moderate. Although severe hypertension may be observed,[134] accelerated-malignant hypertension is rare.

Except for hypokalemia, primary aldosteronism does not usually present with clinical manifestations that readily suggest the diagnosis. Occasionally, the presenting feature results from severe potassium depletion (e.g., nocturia, polyuria, polydipsia, proximal muscle weakness, intermittent paralysis, rhabdomyolysis, paresthesias, or tetany).[133] The manifestations of primary aldosteronism may also be temporarily ameliorated during pregnancy.[135,136] This observation has been attributed to the antimineralocorticoid effect of high levels of progesterone.[137]

Hypokalemia

Hypokalemia is the most common manifestation of primary aldosteronism. Typically, hypokalemia is associated with metabolic alkalosis and mild or borderline hypernatremia. Hypomagnesemia may also be observed.[138]

Primary aldosteronism may present with either unprovoked or diuretic-induced hypokalemia. Unprovoked hypokalemia occurs in the absence of diuretics, vomiting, diarrhea, or laxative abuse. It is particularly suggestive of primary aldosteronism because spontaneous hypokalemia is observed in only a small percentage of patients with uncomplicated essential hypertension. The likelihood of diagnosing primary aldosteronism is increased in untreated hypertensive subjects who present with unprovoked hypokalemia.[139,140]

The precipitation of severe hypokalemia by diuretic therapy is frequently the initial clinical manifestation of primary aldosteronism. Mild hypokalemia is observed in up to 40 percent or more of hypertensive patients receiving diuretic therapy, but severe hypokalemia is considerably less common.[141,142] When serum potassium is less than 2.8 to 3.0 meq/liter, the possibility of primary aldosteronism or some other variety of mineralocorticoid hypertension should be considered.

The presence of a normal serum potassium concentration (i.e., "normokalemic primary aldosteronism") in patients who otherwise have the characteristic features of primary aldosteronism has been observed by many.[143] However, when unselected (or partially selected) populations of normokalemic hypertensive subjects have been screened by measuring renin and aldosterone levels, in general, relatively few cases have been found.[139] In addition, most patients with normokalemic primary aldosteronism appear to have bilateral hyperplasia. Of those with adenomas (i.e., the surgically remediable group), relatively few appear to be persistently normokalemic when the serum potassium is checked on multiple occasions.[134]

Other Varieties of Mineralocorticoid Hypertension

Besides primary aldosteronism, there are a number of less frequently encountered varieties of mineralocorticoid hypertension. These are enumerated in Table 50-6. All can cause hypertension and hypokalemia. In most instances, they can be identified by their clinical and laboratory characteristics.[144] For example, the chronic or excessive ingestion of licorice-containing candy and chewing tobacco can cause mineralocorticoid hypertension.[145,146] The elevated blood pressure is caused by an exogenous mineralocorticoid substance, glycyrrhizinic acid, which is a component of licorice extract. Cases of "pseudoaldosteronism" have also been reported following the chronic use of nasal sprays containing 9α-fluoroprednisolone, which are available in some countries in Europe, Africa, and Central and South America.[147]

Confirming the Diagnosis of Primary Aldosteronism

The major criterion for the diagnosis of primary aldosteronism is the demonstration of autonomous overproduction of aldosterone, usually in conjunction with a low plasma renin activity. Typically, plasma renin activity is suppressed to low levels and remains subnormal with volume depletion and upright posture.* Some authorities have advocated use of the plasma renin activity as a screening test for primary aldosteronism. However, approximately 30 percent of essential hypertensive patients (i.e., the subgroup with "low-renin" essential hypertension) also exhibit subnormal plasma renin activity. Furthermore, a random plasma renin activity, obtained without appropriate stimulation, may not be suppressed in up to 10 percent or more of patients with primary aldosteronism,[134,148] and may even be increased in patients receiving spironolactone.

The diagnosis of primary aldosteronism is confirmed by finding plasma or urinary levels of aldosterone that are increased relative to sodium intake and excretion, and that fail to suppress normally with volume expansion. Several methods have been used to test aldosterone suppressibility. These include volume expansion by administration of deoxycorticosterone or fludrocortisone, or by administration of intravenous saline or oral salt loads. The lack of suppression of aldosterone is an important, if not critical, diagnostic feature. This is because considerable overlap exists in the plasma and urinary aldosterone levels of patients with essential hypertension and primary aldosteronism, particularly in circumstances of uncontrolled sodium intake. In patients with primary aldosteronism, plasma aldosterone levels usually fail to suppress below 10 ng/dl following the intravenous administration of 2 liters of normal saline over 4 h.[149]

The ratio of plasma aldosterone to plasma renin activity may also be useful in the diagnosis of primary aldosteronism. Hiramatsu et al.[150] found the ratio of plasma aldosterone concentration (in picograms per deciliter) to plasma renin activity (in nanograms per milliliter per hour) to be less than 200 in patients with essential hypertension, and greater than 400 in patients with aldosterone-secreting adenomas. Lyons et al.[151] reported that the ratio of plasma aldosterone concentration to plasma renin activity in blood samples obtained 2 h following the administration of a single oral dose of captopril, provided better discrimination between essential hypertension and primary aldosteronism than did the baseline (i.e., precaptopril) values. However, further study is warranted to fully establish the validity of this test.

*Several different methods have been used to test renin responsiveness. Most examine the response to 2 to 4 h of upright posture following administration of furosemide (40 to 160 mg over 12 to 24 h). Some methods also employ a low-sodium diet (10 to 15 meq/day for 3 to 5 days) in conjunction with diuretics and upright posture. Under these conditions, a threefold or more increase in baseline plasma renin activity is generally considered normal. Patients with primary aldosteronism usually stimulate minimally or not at all.

TABLE 50-6 Mineralocorticoid Hypertension*

Diagnosis	Age of Onset	Clinical Features	Laboratory Abnormalities
Primary Aldosteronism			
Aldosteronoma	More common between 30 and 50, but can occur at any age	Usually asymptomatic; may present with muscle weakness or periodic paralysis. More common in females.	↑ plasma and urinary aldosterone; ↓ PRA; normal urinary 17-OHCS and 17-KS
Hyperplasia	As above, but tend to be 5 to 10 years older	As above, except male-to-female ratio is approximately 1:1.	As above
Glucocorticoid-suppressible primary aldosteronism	Usually childhood or adolescence	Often familial; clinical and laboratory abnormalities are reversed with dexamethasone.	As above
Indeterminate hyperaldosteronism		Usually associated with mild hypertension; serum potassium frequently normal.	As above; ↑ plasma and urinary aldosterone reported to be suppressed by DOC administration[144]
Cushing's Syndrome	Any age	Cushingoid appearance with or without excessive pigmentation	↑ plasma cortisol; ↑ urinary 17-OHCS, usually not suppressed by low-dose dexamethasone
Congenital Adrenal Hyperplasia			
11-β-hydroxylase deficiency	Usually childhood; occasionally adolescence or early adulthood	Virilization with or without pseudohermaphroditism in females. Precocious puberty in males. Hypokalemia is occasionally observed.	↑ plasma DOC and 11-deoxycortisol, ↑ urinary 17-OHCS and 17-KS (usually suppressed by dexamethasone), ↓ plasma and urinary aldosterone and cortisol, ↓ PRA
17-α-hydroxylase deficiency	Adolescence	Primary amenorrhea and absence of secondary sex characteristics in females. Pseudohermaphroditism in males.	↑ plasma DOC and corticosterone, ↓ urinary 17-OHCS and 17-KS, ↓ plasma and urinary aldosterone and cortisol, ↓ PRA
Exogenous Mineralocorticoids			
Licorice,† carbenoxolone,‡ fludrocortisone, or 9α-fluoroprednisolone	Any age	Excessive licorice ingestion, antacid therapy with carbenoxolone (in use in Great Britain and Canada) or the use of nasal sprays containing 9α-fluoroprednisolone (in use in Europe, Africa, and Central and South America).[147] Fluid retention may occur with all compounds.	↓ plasma and urinary aldosterone, ↓ PRA

17-OHCS = 17-hydroxycorticosteroids; 17-KS = 17-ketosteroids; DOC = 11-deoxycorticosterone; PRA = plasma renin activity.
*All can cause hypertension, hypokalemia, and inappropriate kaliuresis.
†Active ingredient is glycyrrhizinic acid.
‡A derivative of glycyrrhizinic acid.

Differential Diagnosis of Types of Primary Aldosteronism

There are two major pathologic varieties of primary aldosteronism: adrenocortical adenomas (aldosteronomas) and bilateral adrenocortical (zona glomerulosa) hyperplasia. Aldosterone-producing adenomas account for about 80 percent or more of cases. They are almost invariably benign, and women are affected more commonly than men.[133,134] As shown in Table 50-7, aldosteronomas are usually associated with higher levels of aldosterone and more pronounced hypokalemia and hyporeninemia than bilateral hyperplasia.

Bilateral hyperplasia is sometimes referred to as idiopathic hyperaldosteronism or pseudoprimary aldosteronism. In contrast to aldosteronomas, bilateral hyperplasia affects men and women with approximately equal frequency.[134] In addition, some studies have found that patients with hyperplasia, as a group, tend to be older than those with adenoma.[134,148] Other differences have also been described. For example, Gross et al. found that patients with hyperplasia experience a reduction in plasma aldosterone levels following administration of the serotonin antagonist, cyproheptadine; whereas patients with adenomas do not.[152] Moreover, most

TABLE 50-7 Comparison of Findings in Patients with Surgically Proven Adenoma or Hyperplasia

Clinical Findings	Adenoma* (*N* = 38)	Hyperplasia (*N* = 11)
Age, years	42	50
Mean arterial pressure, mmHg	145	144
Serum potassium, meq/liter	2.98	3.44
Serum sodium, meq/liter	143	142
Plasma renin activity (stimulated), ng/ml/3 h	0.45	1.19
Plasma aldosterone (suppressed), ng/dl	35	24
Localization Studies	**Predictive of Adenoma,* % Accuracy**	**Predictive of Hyperplasia, % Accuracy**
Adrenal venography	59	71
Adrenal iodocholesterol scan	46	56
Adrenal venous aldosterone levels	100	62†
Orthostatic fall in plasma aldosterone‡	72	88

*Includes only patients with unilateral adenoma.

†Pertains to the accuracy in identifying unilateral or bilateral disease.

‡Based on a postural decline in plasma aldosterone as predictive of adenoma and the absence of a postural decline as predictive of hyperplasia.

Source: Weinberger, M. H., Grim, C. E., Hollifield, J. W., et al.: Primary Aldosteronism. Diagnosis, Localization, Treatment, *Ann. Intern. Med.*, 90:386, 1979. Adapted and reproduced with permission from the publisher and author.

patients with aldosterone-secreting adenomas exhibit a fall in plasma aldosterone levels after 2 to 4 h of upright posture, whereas those with bilateral hyperplasia usually experience an increase (Table 50-7).[153,154] These findings have led to speculation that bilateral hyperplasia may be due to excessive secretion of some as yet unidentified pituitary hormone.[152,155,156] Investigators from a number of centers have recently reported the isolation of a new aldosterone-stimulating factor from human urine.[157,158]

A number of patients have been described with the typical features of primary aldosteronism, but whose clinical and laboratory abnormalities were reversed with glucocorticoid administration.[159] This variety has been termed *glucocorticoid-suppressible primary aldosteronism.* A specific biochemical defect has not been identified and the etiology is unknown.[155] Bilateral adrenal hyperplasia is the only reported histologic abnormality. Such cases are rare and appear to be familial. Some authors have advocated excluding this possibility by administering a 2-week course of dexamethasone (1 to 2 mg per day) to patients with the presumptive diagnosis of bilateral hyperplasia.[160]

A fourth variety of primary aldosteronism, referred to as "indeterminate hyperaldosteronism," has also been described.[144] In contrast to the other varieties, the increased levels of aldosterone are suppressed by volume expansion following administration of deoxycorticosterone acetate (DOCA). This variety is frequently associated with mild hypertension and a normal serum potassium concentration.

Localization Methods

Once the diagnosis of primary aldosteronism is established, further diagnostic tests are indicated in patients judged to be operative candidates. Evaluation must include efforts to distinguish between adenoma and bilateral hyperplasia, and to localize the side of any tumor-bearing gland.

Adrenal venography is a reasonably accurate method for identifying adenomas larger than 8 to 10 mm in diameter because about 80 percent or more are detected. However, this technique is unreliable for identifying smaller adenomas or for detecting bilateral hyperplasia.

A more sensitive localization method is that of measuring the aldosterone levels of the venous effluent from each adrenal. Regardless of size, aldosteronomas may be localized with about 90 percent accuracy (Table 50-7). The aldosterone levels of venous blood from tumor-bearing glands are often increased up to tenfold or more above those from contralateral uninvolved glands. Bilateral elevation of aldosterone levels is suggestive of bilateral hyperplasia, or the rare circumstance of bilateral adenomas.

Adrenal scintillation scanning with ^{131}I-19-iodocholesterol, or more recently with ^{131}I-6β-iodomethyl-19-norcholesterol (NP-59), is a newer technique based on the uptake of cholesterol by the adrenal gland. Preliminary reports suggest that adenomas are identified with reasonably good accuracy.[161] However, this procedure is not universally available for routine clinical use.

The plasma concentration of 18-hydroxycorticosterone may also distinguish between patients with aldosteronomas and bilateral hyperplasia. The plasma levels of this precursor of aldosterone have, in general, been found to be significantly higher in patients with aldosterone-secreting adenomas than in those with hyperplasia.[162,163] Adenomas larger than 1 cm in diameter may sometimes be identified with the higher resolution CT scanning devices.[161,164]

Pheochromocytoma

The initial clinical suspicion of pheochromocytoma usually occurs because the patient complains of severe headaches (often of the vascular type), inappropriate sweating, or cardiac awareness in the form of palpitations or recurrent arrhythmias.[165] The first hint may occur, however, when the patient has hypertension that is difficult to control; when the patient has inappropriate sinus tachycardia or orthostatic hypotension; when the patient has neurofibromatosis, café-au-lait spots, von Hippel-Lindau disease, Sturge-Weber disease, or tuberous sclerosis; when the patient gives a history of previously catastrophic anesthesia or surgery, especially for cholecystectomy; when he or she gets a pressor response to beta blockers; or when the family history reveals hypertension plus either thyroid carcinoma or hyperparathyroidism.

Urinary Screening Tests

Urinary excretion measurements of total catecholamines, metanephrine, and vanillylmandelic acid are the most commonly used screening tests for pheochromocytoma. Table 50-8 provides data on the sensitivity of these tests in three large series of hypertensive patients.[166–168] All indicate that excretion of metanephrine is the most sensitive urinary screening test. Gitlow et al.[169] reported that a urinary metanephrine (expressed in μg) to creatinine (expressed in mg) ratio above 2.2 identified 90 of 92 patients with pheochromocytoma, but only 2 percent of control subjects without pheochromocytoma. Subsequently, Kaplan et al.[170] documented the usefulness of the metanephrine to creatinine ratio on single-voided urine specimens. The ratio ranged between 0.20 and 0.56 in 10 untreated adult hypertensive patients without pheochromocytoma, whereas the lowest ratio was 2.8 in multiple urine samples from seven adult patients with pheochromocytoma. A ratio above 1 is strongly suggestive of pheochromocytoma in an untreated and otherwise uncomplicated hypertensive patient above 15 years of age.

False-positive urinary metanephrine levels have been noted in patients with coma and increased intracranial pressure,[169] as well as patients with intracranial aneurysms.[171] False-negative urinary metanephrine levels can occur within 24 h following the use of contrast media for angiography or intravenous pyelography.[172]

Plasma Catecholamine Levels

Radioenzymatic measurements of plasma catecholamines, usually both norepinephrine (NE) and epinephrine (E), in the supine and rested state are abnormally elevated in 90 to 96 percent of patients with pheochromocytoma.[173,174] Levels may even be abnormal in occasional patients with normal urinary screening tests or at a time when blood pressure is not elevated. In general, there is minimal overlap between the lowest catecholamine levels of patients with pheochromocytoma and the highest catecholamine levels of either normotensive subjects or patients with essential hypertension. A problem can arise, however, when samples are drawn from patients with essential hypertension who are undergoing acute stress. For example, marked elevations of plasma catecholamines can accompany acute myocardial infarction[175–177] as well as subarachnoid hemorrhage,[178] clonidine withdrawal syndrome,[179] and likely other similarly stressful clinical settings. Less striking but still abnormally elevated plasma catecholamines can also be a consequence of antihypertensive drug therapy, including diuretics,[180,181] hydralazine,[182,183] calcium channel blockers,[182,184] and possibly also prazosin.[185,186]

To reduce the effects of stress or ambulation, most authorities recommend that an indwelling intravenous catheter be placed, and that the patient rest in the supine position for at least 30 min before sampling.

Clonidine Suppression Test

The clonidine suppression test is very useful to differentiate pheochromocytoma from essential hypertension in patients who have been found to have elevated plasma catecholamines.[187] A dose of 0.3 mg of clonidine is given and plasma catecholamine levels are drawn immediately before and 3 h later. Blood pressure and heart rate are reduced similarly in hypertensive pheochromocytoma and nonpheochromocytoma patients. However, plasma norepinephrine (and to a lesser extent epinephrine) is essentially unchanged in patients with pheochromocytoma but reduced markedly in patients with essential hypertension. This is because the central action of clonidine does not block peripheral production of catecholamines. Interestingly, however, the elevated plasma catecholamines that have been observed in some patients with autonomic epilepsy are likewise suppressed by clonidine.[188]

Suppression of plasma norepinephrine in patients with pheochromocytoma (i.e., a false-negative test) has been noted rarely in metastatic, epinephrine-secreting, and otherwise uncomplicated pheochromocytoma.[189,190] For optimal interpretation, the clonidine suppression test should be performed under controlled environmental conditions when the patient is not receiving concomitant antihypertensive therapy.

Anatomic Localization of the Tumor

The intravenous pyelogram with tomography is a relatively insensitive procedure for localization of

TABLE 50-8 Frequency of Positive Urinary Tests in Patients with Pheochromocytoma

	Total Catecholamines	Vanillylmandelic Acid	Metanephrines
Mayo Clinic[166]	47/60 (79%)	37/52 (71%)	50/52 (96%)
Cleveland Clinic[167]	18/27 (67%)	27/33 (82%)	25/25 (100%)
NIH[168]	60/62 (97%)	59/62 (95%)	60/62 (97%)

adrenal pheochromocytomas. Adrenal arteriography will detect 80 to 85 percent of tumors, and adrenal venography will occasionally identify small or hypovascular tumors. Noninvasive computerized axial tomography (CT) scans, however, have replaced angiography as the primary localization procedure, particularly since the vast majority of tumors exceed 3 cm in diameter. The CT scan is effective in localizing intraabdominal pheochromocytomas in 90 percent or more of cases.[191,192] In addition, scintigraphic imaging with ^{131}meta-iodobenzylguanidine (^{131}MIBG), a radiolabeled analogue of guanethidine that is concentrated in adrenergic tissue, has demonstrated pheochromocytoma tumors in several patients in whom the CT scan was negative.[193,194]

References

1. Mahomed, F. A.: On Chronic Bright's Disease, and Its Essential Symptoms, *Lancet,* 1:149, 1879.
2. Kirkendall, W. M., Feinleib, M., Freis, E. D., and Mark, A. L.: Recommendations for Human Blood Pressure Determination by Sphygmomanometers. Subcommittee of the AHA Postgraduate Education Committee, *Hypertension,* 3(4):509A, 1981.
3. Nielsen, P. E., and Janniche, H.: The Accuracy of Auscultatory Measurement of Arm Blood Pressure in Very Obese Subjects, *Acta. Med. Scand.,* 195:403, 1974.
4. Maxwell, M. H., Waks, A. U., Schroth, P. C., Karam, M., and Dornfeld, L. P.: Error in Blood Pressure Measurement Due to Incorrect Cuff Size in Obese Patients, *Lancet,* 2:33, 1982.
5. Taguchi, J. T., and Suwangool, P.: "Pipe-Stem" Brachial Arteries. A Cause of Pseudohypertension, *JAMA,* 228:733, 1974.
6. Spence, J. D., Sibbald, W. J., and Cape, R. D.: Pseudohypertension in the Elderly, *Clin. Sci. Mol. Med.,* 55(suppl. 4):399, 1978.
7. Rodbard, S., and Margolis, J.: The Auscultatory Gap in Arteriosclerotic Heart Disease, *Circulation,* 15:850, 1957.
8. Amsterdam, B., and Amsterdam, A. L.: Disparity in Blood Pressure in Both Arms in Normals and Hypertensives and Its Clinical Significance. A Study of 1,000 Normals and 272 Hypertensives, *N.Y. State J. Med.,* 43:2294, 1943.
9. Mitchell, P. L., Parlin, R. W., and Blackburn, H.: Effect of Vertical Displacement of the Arm on Indirect Blood-Pressure Measurement, *N. Engl. J. Med.,* 271:72, 1964.
10. Kossmann, C. E.: Relative Importance of Certain Variables in the Clinical Determination of Blood Pressure, *Am. J. Med.,* 1:464, 1946.
11. Currens, J. H.: A Comparison of the Blood Pressure in the Lying and Standing Positions: A Study of Five Hundred Men and Five Hundred Women, *Am. Heart J.,* 35:646, 1948.
12. Hall, W. D., Douglas, M. B., and Blumenstein, B. A.: The Standing Blood Pressure in Patients with Hypertension, *Clin. Res.,* 25(3):264, 1977. (Abstract.)
13. Frohlich, E. D., Tarazi, R. C., Ulrych, M., Dustan, H. P., and Page, I. H.: Tilt Test for Investigating a Neural Component in Hypertension. Its Correlation with Clinical Characteristics, *Circulation,* 36:387, 1967.
14. Esler, M. D., and Nestel, P. J.: Sympathetic Responsiveness to Head-Up Tilt in Essential Hypertension, *Clin. Sci.,* 44:213, 1973.
15. Affarah, H. B., Wollam, G. L., Hall, W. D., Wood, M., and Unger, D. J.: The Effect of Therapy with Methyldopa and Hydrochlorothiazide in Black Patients with Essential Hypertension. (Submitted, 1984.)
16. Gordon, T., Sorlie, P., and Kannel, W. B.: Problems in the Assessment of Blood Pressure: The Framingham Study, *Int. J. Epidemiol.,* 5:327, 1976.
17. Watson, R. D. S., Stallard, T. J., Flinn, R. M., and Littler, W. A.: Factors Determining Direct Arterial Pressure and Its Variability in Hypertensive Man, *Hypertension,* 2:333, 1980.
18. Mancia, G., Ferrari, A., Gregorini, L., et al.: Blood Pressure Variability in Man: Its Relation to High Blood Pressure, Age and Baroreflex Sensitivity, *Clin. Sci.,* 59(suppl. 6):401, 1980.
19. Bevan, A. T., Honour, A. J., and Scott, F. H.: Direct Arterial Pressure Recording in Unrestricted Man, *Clin. Sci.,* 36:329, 1969.
20. Drayer, J. I. M., Weber, M. A., DeYoung, J. L., and Wyle, F. A.: Circadian Blood Pressure Patterns in Ambulatory Hypertensive Patients. Effects of Age, *Am. J. Med.,* 73:493, 1982.
21. Armitage, P., Fox, W., Rose, G. A., and Tinker, C. M.: The Variability of Measurements of Casual Blood Pressure. II. Survey Experience, *Clin. Sci.,* 30:337, 1966.
22. Souchek, J., Stamler, J., Dyer, A. R., Paul, O., and Lepper, M. H.: The Value of Two or Three Versus a Single Reading of Blood Pressure at a First Visit, *J. Chronic Dis.,* 32:197, 1979.
23. Kannel, W. B., Sorlie, P., and Gordon, T.: Labile Hypertension: A Faulty Concept? The Framingham Study, *Circulation,* 61:1183, 1980.
24. Glock, C. Y., Vought, R. L., Clark, E. G., and Schweitzer, M. D.: Studies in Hypertension. II. Variability of Daily Blood Pressure Measurements in the Same Individuals Over a Three-Week Period, *J. Chronic Dis.,* 4:469, 1956.
25. Hypertension Detection and Follow-Up Program Cooperative Group: Blood Pressure Studies in 14 Communities. A Two-Stage Screen for Hypertension, *JAMA,* 237:2385, 1977.
26. Rosner, B., and Polk, B. F.: The Implications of Blood Pressure Variability for Clinical and Screening Purposes, *J. Chronic Dis.,* 32:451, 1979.
27. Rosner, B., and Polk, B. F.: Predictive Values of Routine Blood Pressure Measurements in Screening for Hypertension, *Am. J. Epidemiol.,* 117:429, 1983.
28. Julius, S., Ellis, C. N., Pascual, A. V., et al.: Home Blood Pressure Determination. Value in Borderline ("Labile") Hypertension, *JAMA,* 229:663, 1974.
29. Perloff, D., Sokolow, M., and Cowan, R.: The Prognostic Value of Ambulatory Blood Pressures, *JAMA,* 249:2792, 1983.
30. Drayer, J. I. M., Weber, M. A., DeYoung, J. L., and Brewer, D. D.: Long-Term BP Monitoring in the Evaluation of Antihypertensive Therapy, *Arch. Intern. Med.,* 143:898, 1983.
31. Joint National Committee on Detection, Evaluation, and Treatment of High Blood Pressure: The 1984 Report of the Joint National Committee on Detection, Evaluation, and Treatment of High Blood Pressure. *Arch. Intern. Med.,* 144:1045, 1984.
32. Wilber, J. A.: The Minimum Work-Up for Hypertension, *Cardiovasc. Med.,* 2:55, 1977.
33. Bock, K. D.: The Diagnostic Work-Up in Mild Hypertension, in Gross, F. H., and Strasser, T. (eds.): "Mild Hypertension: Natural History and Management," Year Book Medical Publishers, Chicago, 1979, p. 303.
34. Bulpitt, C. J., Dollery, C. T., and Carne, S.: Change in Symptoms of Hypertensive Patients after Referral to Hospital Clinic, *Br. Heart J.,* 38:121, 1976.
35. Kannel, W. B., Castelli, W. P., McNamara, P. M., McKee, P. A., and Feinleib, M.: Role of Blood Pressure in the Development of Congestive Heart Failure, *N. Engl. J. Med.,* 287:781, 1972.
36. Keith, N. M., Wagener, H. P., and Kernohan, J. W.: The Syndrome of Malignant Hypertension, *Arch. Intern Med.,* 41:141, 1928.
37. Schottstaedt, W. E., and Sokolow, M.: The Natural History and Course of Malignant Hypertension with Papilledema, *Am. Heart J.,* 45:331, 1953.
38. Kincaid-Smith, P., McMichael, J., and Murphy, E. A.: The

Clinical Course and Pathology of Hypertension with Papilledema (Malignant Hypertension), *Q. J. Med.*, 105:117, 1958.
39. Kaplan, N. M.: Primary Aldosteronism with Malignant Hypertension, *N. Engl. J. Med.*, 269:1282, 1963.
40. Christlieb, R. A., Kaldany, A., and D'Elia, J. A.: Plasma Renin Activity and Hypertension in Diabetes Mellitus, *Diabetes*, 25(suppl. 2):969, 1976.
41. Ideishi, M., Takii, M., Hiroki, T., and Arakawa, K.: An Accelerated Hypertension with Neither Malignant Nephrosclerosis Nor Elevation of Plasma Renin Activity, *Jpn. Heart J.*, 19:151, 1978.
42. Pitcock, J. A., Johnson, J. G., Share, L., et al.: Malignant Hypertension Due to Musculo-Mucoid Intimal Hyperplasia of Intrarenal Arteries, *Circ. Res.*, 36–37(suppl. 1):133, 1975.
43. Davis, B. A., Crook, J. E., Vestal, R. E., and Oates, J. A.: Prevalence of Renovascular Hypertension in Patients with Grade III or IV Hypertensive Retinopathy, *N. Engl. J. Med.*, 301:1273, 1979.
44. Julius, S., and Schork, N. A.: Borderline Hypertension—A Critical Review, *J. Chronic Dis.*, 23:723, 1971.
45. Klatsky, A. L., Friedman, G. D., Siegelaub, A. B., and Gérard, M. J.: Alcohol Consumption and Blood Pressure. Kaiser-Permanente Multiphasic Health Examination Data, *N. Engl. J. Med.*, 296:1194, 1977.
46. Messerli, F. H., and Frohlich, E. D.: High Blood Pressure. A Side Effect of Drugs, Poisons, and Food, *Arch. Intern. Med.*, 139:682, 1979.
47. Dietz, A. J., Jr.: Amphetamine-Like Reactions to Phenylpropanolamine, *JAMA*, 245:601, 1981.
48. Hall, W. D., and Gunnells, C. T.: Emotional Stress and Hypertension, Workshop Report. National Conference on Emotional Stress and Heart Disease. *J. S.C. Med. Assoc.*, 72(suppl.):82, 1976.
49. Wollam, G. L., and Hall, W. D.: Systolic Hypertension, in Hurst, J. W. (ed.): "Update IV. The Heart," McGraw-Hill Book Company, New York, 1981, p. 135.
50. Hall, W. D., and Wollam, G. L.: Systolic Hypertension, in Harvey, W. P. (ed.): "Current Problems in Cardiology," vol. 7 (no. 6), Year Book Medical Publishers, Inc., Chicago, 1982, p. 1.
51. Lichtman, J., O'Rourke, R. A., Klein, A., and Karliner, J. S.: Electrocardiogram of the Athlete. Alterations Simulating Those of Organic Heart Disease, *Arch. Intern. Med.*, 132:763, 1973.
52. Roeske, W. P., O'Rourke, R. A., Klein, A., Leopold, G., and Karliner, J. S.: Noninvasive Evaluation of Ventricular Hypertrophy in Professional Athletes, *Circulation*, 52:286, 1976.
53. Morganroth, J., Maron, B. J., Henry, W. L., and Epstein, S. E.: Comparative Left Ventricular Dimensions in Trained Athletes, *Ann. Intern. Med.*, 82:521, 1975.
54. Oakley, D. G., and Oakley, C. M.: Significance of Abnormal Electrocardiograms in Highly Trained Athletes, *Am. J. Cardiol.*, 50:985, 1982.
55. Maron, B. T., Roberts, W. C., McAllister, H. A., Rosing, D. R., and Epstein, S. E.: Sudden Death in Young Athletes, *Circulation*, 62:218, 1980.
56. Laird, W. P., and Fixler, D. E.: Acute Blood Pressure Response in Hypertensive Adolescents During Strenuous Weight Lifting, *Clin. Res.*, 26(6):817A, 1978. (Abstract.)
57. Keith, N. M., Wagener, H. P., and Barker, N. D.: Some Different Types of Essential Hypertension: Their Course and Prognosis, *Am. J. Med. Sci.*, 197:332, 1939.
58. van Buchem, F. S. P., Heuvel-Aghina, J. W. M., and Heuvel, J. E. A.: Hypertension and Changes in the Fundus Oculi, *Acta. Med. Scand.*, 176:539, 1964.
59. Kagan, A., Aurell, E., Dobree, J., et al.: A Note on Signs in the Fundus Oculi and Arterial Hypertension: Conventional Assessment and Significance, *Bull. WHO*, 34:955, 1966.
60. Kannel, W. B., Gordon, T., and Offutt, D.: Left Ventricular Hypertrophy by Electrocardiogram. Prevalence, Incidence, and Mortality in the Framingham Study, *Ann. Intern. Med.*, 71:89, 1969.
61. Davie, J. C., Langley, J. O., Dodson, W. H., and Eddleman, E. E., Jr.: Clinical and Kinetocardiographic Studies of Paradoxical Precordial Motion, *Am. Heart J.*, 63:775, 1962.
62. Davids, J. Z.: Apex Impulse, in Walker, H. K., Hall, W. D., and Hurst, J. W. (eds.): "Clinical Methods," 2d ed., Butterworth Publishers, Inc., Boston, 1980, p. 669.
63. Burchell, H. B.: Clinical Recognition of Cardiac Hypertrophy, *Circ. Res.*, 35(suppl. II):116, 1974.
64. Eilen, S. D., Crawford, M. H., and O'Rourke, R. A.: Accuracy of Precordial Palpation for Detecting Increased Left Ventricular Volume, *Ann. Intern. Med.*, 99:628, 1983.
65. Lusted, L. B., and Keats, T. E.: Atlas of Roentgenographic Measurement, ed. 4, Year Book Medical Publishers, Chicago, 1978, p. 225.
66. Keats, T. E., and Enge, I. P.: Cardiac Mensuration by the Cardiac Volume Method, *Radiology*, 85:850, 1965.
67. Glover, L., Baxley, W. A., and Dodge, H. T.: A Quantitative Evaluation of Heart Size Measurements from Chest Roentgenograms, *Circulation*, 47:1289, 1973.
68. Romhilt, D. W., and Estes, E. H., Jr.: A Point-Score System for the ECG Diagnosis of Left Ventricular Hypertrophy, *Am. Heart J.*, 75:752, 1968.
69. Romhilt, D. W., Bove, K. E., Norris, R. J., et al.: A Critical Appraisal of the Electrocardiographic Criteria for the Diagnosis of Left Ventricular Hypertrophy, *Circulation*, 40:185, 1969.
70. Carter, W. A., and Estes, E. H., Jr.: Electrocardiographic Manifestations of Ventricular Hypertrophy; A Computer Study of ECG-Anatomic Correlations in 319 Cases, *Am. Heart J.*, 68:173, 1964.
71. Murphy, M. L., Thernabadu, P. N., Soyza, N. D., et al.: Reevaluation of Electrocardiographic Criteria for Left, Right and Combined Cardiac Ventricular Hypertrophy, *Am. J. Cardiol.*, 53:1140, 1984.
72. Tarazi, R. C., Miller, A., Frohlich, E. D., and Dustan, H. P.: Electrocardiographic Changes Reflecting Left Atrial Abnormality in Hypertension, *Circulation*, 34:818, 1966.
73. Savage, D. D., Drayer, J. I. M., Henry, W. L., et al.: Echocardiographic Assessment of Cardiac Anatomy and Function in Hypertensive Subjects, *Circulation*, 59:623, 1979.
74. Woythaler, J. N., Singer, S. L., Kwan, O. L., et al.: Accuracy of Echocardiography in Detecting Left Ventricular Hypertrophy: Comparison with Postmortem Mass Measurements, *J. Am. Coll. Cardiol.*, 2:305, 1983.
75. Devereax, R. B., and Reichek, N.: Echocardiographic Determination of Left Ventricular Mass in Man. Anatomic Validation of the Method, *Circulation*, 55:613, 1977.
76. Dunn, F. G., Chandraratna, P., de Carvalho, J. G. R., Basta, L. L., and Frohlich, E. D.: Pathophysiologic Assessment of Hypertensive Heart Disease with Echocardiography, *Am. J. Cardiol.*, 39:789, 1977.
77. McFarland, T. M., Alam, M., Goldstein, S., Pickard, S. D., and Stein, P. D.: Echocardiographic Diagnosis of Left Ventricular Hypertrophy, *Circulation*, 57:1140, 1978.
78. Safar, M. E., Lehner, J. P., Vincent, M. I., Plainfosse, M. T., and Simon, A. Ch.: Echocardiographic Dimensions in Borderline and Sustained Hypertension, *Am. J. Cardiol.*, 44:930, 1979.
79. Lehner, J. P., Safar, M. E., Dimitriu, V. M., Simon, A., Carrez, J. P., and Plainfosse, M. T.: Systolic Time Intervals and Echocardiographic Findings in Borderline Hypertension, *Eur. J. Cardiol.*, 9(4):319, 1979.
80. Baker, B. J., Bass, K. M., Scoril, J. A., Kane, J. J., and Murphy, M. L.: M-Mode Echocardiographic Correlates of Left Ventricular Mass: An Anatomic Correlation, *J. Cardiovasc. Ultrasonography*, 1:263, 1982.
81. Schlant, R. C., Felner, J. M., Heymsfield, S. B., et al.: Echocardiographic Studies of Left Ventricular Anatomy and Function in Essential Hypertension, *Cardiovasc. Med.*, 2:477, 1977.
82. Wollam, G. L., Hall, W. D., Porter, V. D., et al.: Time Course of Regression of Left Ventricular Hypertrophy in Treated Hypertensive Patients, *Am. J. Med.*, 75 (suppl. 3A):100, 1983.
83. Drayer, J. I. M., and Weber, M. A.: Echocardiographic Left

Ventricular Hypertrophy in Hypertension, *Chest,* 84:217, 1983.
84. Kannel, W. B., Wolf, P. A., Vertes, J., and McNamara, P. M.: Epidemiologic Assessment of the Role of Blood Pressure in Stroke. The Framingham Study, *JAMA,* 214:301, 1970.
85. Cuneo, R. H., and Caronna, J. J.: The Neurologic Complications of Hypertension, *Med. Clin. North Am.,* 61:565, 1977.
86. Weisberg, L. A.: Computed Tomography in the Diagnosis of Intracranial Disease, *Ann. Intern. Med.,* 91:87, 1979.
87. Gifford, R. W., Jr., and Westbrook, E.: Hypertensive Encephalopathy: Mechanisms, Clinical Features, and Treatment, *Prog. Cardiovasc. Dis.,* 32:115, 1974.
88. Ziegler, D. K., Zosa, A., and Zileli, T.: Hypertensive Encephalopathy, *Arch. Neurol.,* 12:472, 1965.
89. Chester, E. M., Agamanolis, D. P., Banker, B. Q., and Victor, M.: Hypertensive Encephalopathy: A Clinicopathologic Study of 20 Cases, *Neurology (NY),* 28:928, 1978.
90. Goldring, W., Chasis, H., Ranges, H. A., and Smith, H. W.: Effective Renal Blood Flow in Subjects with Essential Hypertension, *J. Clin. Invest.,* 20:637, 1941.
91. Schalekamp, M. A. D. H., Krauss, X. H., Schalekamp-Kuyken, M. P. A., Kolsters, G., and Birkenhäger, W. H.: Studies on the Mechanism of Hypernatriuresis in Essential Hypertension in Relation to Measurements of Plasma Renin Concentration, Body Fluid Compartments, and Renal Function, *Clin. Sci.,* 41:219, 1971.
92. Hollenberg, N. K., Adams, D. F., Solomon, H., Chenitz, W. R., Borger, B. M., and Abrams, H. L.: Renal Vascular Tone in Essential and Secondary Hypertension: Hemodynamic and Angiographic Responses to Vasodilators, *Medicine (Baltimore),* 54:29, 1975.
93. Pedersen, E. B., and Mogensen, C. E.: Effect of Antihypertensive Treatment on Urinary Albumin Excretion, Glomerular Filtration Rate and Renal Plasma Flow in Patients with Essential Hypertension, *Scand. J. Clin. Lab. Invest.,* 36:231, 1976.
94. Gifford, R. W., Jr.: Evaluation of the Hypertensive Patient with Emphasis on Detecting Curable Causes, *Milbank Mem. Fund Q.,* 47:170, 1969.
95. Kennedy, A. C., Luke, R. G., Briggs, J. D., and Stirling, W. B.: Detection of Renovascular Hypertension, *Lancet,* 2:963, 1965.
96. Ferguson, R. K.: Cost and Yield of the Hypertensive Evaluation: Experience of a Community-Based Referral Clinic, *Ann. Intern. Med.,* 82:761, 1975.
97. Bech, K., and Hilden, T.: The Frequency of Secondary Hypertension, *Acta. Med. Scand.,* 197:65, 1975.
98. Berglund, G., Andersson, O., and Wilhelmsen, L.: Prevalence of Primary and Secondary Hypertension: Studies in a Random Population Sample, *Br. Med. J.,* 2:554, 1976.
99. Tucker, R. M., and Labarthe, D. R.: Frequency of Surgical Treatment for Hypertension in Adults at the Mayo Clinic from 1973 through 1975, *Mayo Clin. Proc.,* 52:549, 1977.
100. Maxwell, M. H., Bleifer, K. H., Franklin, S. S., and Varady, P. D.: Cooperative Study of Renovascular Hypertension. Demographic Analysis of the Study, *JAMA,* 220:1195, 1972.
101. Foster, J. H., Oates, J. A., Rhamy, R. K., et al.: Detection and Treatment of Patients with Renovascular Hypertension, *Surgery,* 60:240, 1966.
102. Keith, T. A., III: Renovascular Hypertension in Black Patients, *Hypertension,* 4:438, 1982.
103. Simon, N., Franklin, S. S., Bleifer, K. H., and Maxwell, M. H.: Clinical Characteristics of Renovascular Hypertension, *JAMA,* 220:1209, 1972.
104. Grim, C. E., Luft, F. C., Fineberg, N. S., and Weinberger, M. H.: Responses to Volume Expansion and Contraction in Categorized Hypertensive and Normotensive Man, *Hypertension,* 1:476, 1979.
105. Eipper, D. F., Gifford, R. W., Jr., Stewart, B. H., Alfidi, R. J., McCormack, L. J., and Vidt, D. G.: Abdominal Bruits in Renovascular Hypertension, *Am. J. Cardiol.,* 37:48, 1976.
106. Shapiro, A. P., Perez-Stable, E., and Moutsos, S. E.: Coexistence of Renal Arterial Hypertension and Diabetes Mellitus, *JAMA,* 192:121, 1965.
107. Novick, A. C., Pohl, M. A., Schreiber, M., Gifford, R. W., Jr., and Vidt, D. G.: Revascularization for Preservation of Renal Function in Patients with Atherosclerotic Renovascular Disease, *J. Urol.,* 129:907, 1983.
108. Buonocore, E., Meaney, T. F., Borkowski, G. P., Pavlicek, W., and Gallagher, J.: Digital Subtraction Angiography of the Abdominal Aorta and Renal Arteries. Comparison with Conventional Aortography, *Radiology,* 139:281, 1981.
109. Ingrisch, H., Holzgreve, H., and Frey, K. W.: Visualization of the Renal Arteries During Excretory Urography, *Clin. Sci.,* 59(suppl. 6):419, 1980.
110. Smith, C. W., Winfield, A. C., and Price, R. R., et al.: Evaluation of Digital Venous Angiography for the Diagnosis of Renovascular Hypertension, *Radiology,* 144:51, 1982.
111. Osborne, R. W., Jr., Goldstone, J., Hillman, B. J., Ovitt, T. W., and Malone, J. M.: Digital Video Subtraction Angiography: Screening Technique for Renovascular Hypertension, *Surgery,* 90:932, 1981.
112. Bookstein, J. J., Abrams, H. L., Buenger, R. E., et al.: Radiologic Aspects of Renovascular Hypertension. Part 2. The Role of Urography in Unilateral Renovascular Disease, *JAMA,* 220:1225, 1972.
113. Tucker, W. S., Jr., Smith, C. W., Dean, R. H., Winfield, A. C., and Hollifield, J. W.: Role of Digital Subtraction Angiography (DSA) in the Diagnosis of Renovascular (RV) Hypertension, *Clin. Res.,* 29:834, 1981. (Abstract.)
114. Lyons, D. F., Streck, W. F., Kem, D. C., et al.: Captopril Stimulation of Differential Renins in Renovascular Hypertension, *Hypertension,* 5:615, 1983.
115. Thibonnier, M., Joseph, A., Sassano, P., et al.: Improved Diagnosis of Unilateral Renal Artery Lesions After Captopril Administration, *JAMA,* 251:56, 1984.
116. Hricik, D. E., Browning, P. J., Kopelman, R., Goorno, W. E., Madias, N. E., and Dzau, V. J.: Captopril-Induced Functional Renal Insufficiency in Patients with Bilateral Renal-artery Stenosis or Renal-Artery Stenosis in a Solitary Kidney, *N. Engl. J. Med.,* 308:373, 1983.
117. Fotino, S., and Sporn, P.: Nonoliguric Acute Renal Failure After Captopril Therapy, *Arch. Intern. Med.,* 143:1252, 1983.
118. Strong, C. G., Hunt, J. C., Sheps, S. G., Tucker, R. M., and Bernatz, P. E.: Renal Venous Renin Activity: Enhancement of Sensitivity of Lateralization by Sodium Depletion, *Am. J. Cardiol.,* 27:602, 1971.
119. Maxwell, M. H., Marks, L. S., Lupu, A. N., Cahill, P. J., Franklin, S. S., and Kaufman, J. J.: Predictive Value of Renin Determinations in Renal Artery Stenosis, *JAMA,* 238:2617, 1977.
120. Gunnells, J. C., Jr., McGuffin, W. L., Jr., Johnsrude, I., and Robinson, R. R.: Peripheral and Renal Venous Plasma Renin Activity in Hypertension, *Ann. Intern. Med.,* 71:555, 1969.
121. Stockigt, J. R., Collins, R. D., Noakes, C. A., Schambelan, M., and Biglieri, E. G.: Renal-Vein Renin in Various Forms of Renal Hypertension, *Lancet,* 1:1194, 1972.
122. Vaughan, E. D., Jr., Bühler, F. R., Laragh, J. H., Sealey, J. E., Baer, L., and Bard, R. H.: Renovascular Hypertension: Renin Measurements to Indicate Hypersecretion and Contralateral Suppression, Estimate Renal Plasma Flow, and Score for Surgical Curability, *Am. J. Med.,* 55:402, 1973.
123. Marks, L. S., Maxwell, M. H., Varady, P. D., Lupu, A. N., and Kaufman, J. J.: Renovascular Hypertension: Does the Renal Vein Renin Ratio Predict Operative Results? *J. Urol.,* 115:365, 1976.
124. Grim, C. E., Luft, F. C., Weinberger, M. H., and Grim, C. M.: Sensitivity and Specificity of Screening Tests for Renal Vascular Hypertension, *Ann. Intern. Med.,* 91:617, 1979.
125. Lemann, J., Jr.: Diagnostic Value of Urinalysis in Patients with Hypertension, *Am. J. Surg.,* 107:38, 1964.
126. Fairley, K. F., and Birch, D. F.: Hematuria: A Simple Method for Identifying Glomerular Bleeding, *Kidney Int.,* 21:105, 1982.
127. Birkenhäger, W. H., Schalekamp, M. A. D. H., Schalekamp-Kuyken, M. P. A., Kolsters, G., and Krauss, X. H.:

Interrelations between Arterial Pressure, Fluid-Volumes, and Plasma Renin Concentration in the Course of Acute Glomerulonephritis, *Lancet,* 1:1086, 1970.
128. Meltzer, J. S., Keim, H. J., Laragh, J. H., Sealey, J. E., Jan, K-M., and Chien, S.: Nephrotic Syndrome: Vasoconstriction and Hypervolemic Types Indicated by Renin-Sodium Profiling, *Ann. Intern. Med.,* 91:688, 1979.
129. Rizzuto, V. J., Mazzara, J. T., and Grace, W. J.: Pheochromocytoma with Nephrotic Syndrome, *Am. J. Cardiol.,* 16:432, 1965.
130. Berlyne, G. M., Tavill, A. S., and Baker, S. B.: Renal Artery Stenosis and the Nephrotic Syndrome, *Q. J. Med.,* 33:325, 1964.
131. Grim, C. E., Weinberger, M. H., Higgins, J. T., and Kramer, N. J.: Diagnosis of Secondary Forms of Hypertension. A Comprehensive Protocol, *JAMA,* 237:1331, 1977.
132. Conn, J. W.: Primary Aldosteronism and Primary Reninism, *Hosp. Pract.,* 9:131, October 1974.
133. Conn, J. W., Knopf, R. F., and Nesbit, R. M.: Clinical Characteristics of Primary Aldosteronism from an Analysis of 145 Cases, *Am. J. Surg.,* 107:159, 1964.
134. Ferriss, J. B., Beevers, D. G., and Brown, J. J., et al.: Clinical, Biochemical and Pathological Features of Low-Renin ("Primary") Hyperaldosteronism, *Am. Heart J.,* 95:375, 1978.
135. Biglieri, E. G., and Slaton, P. E., Jr.: Pregnancy and Primary Aldosteronism, *J. Clin. Endocrinol. Metab.,* 27:1628, 1967.
136. Gordon, R. D., and Tunny, T. J.: Aldosterone-Producing-Adenoma (A-P-A): Effect of Pregnancy, *Clin. Exp. Hypertens.,* 4:1685, 1982.
137. Drucker, W. D., Hendrikx, A., Laragh, J. H., Christy, N. P., and Vande Wiele, R. L.: Effect of Administered Aldosterone Upon Electrolyte Excretion During and After Pregnancy in Two Women with Adrenal Cortical Insufficiency, *J. Clin. Endocrinol. Metab.,* 23:1247, 1963.
138. Mader, I. J., and Iseri, L. T.: Spontaneous Hypopotassemia, Hypomagnesemia, Alkalosis and Tetany Due to Hypersecretion of Corticosterone-Like Mineralocorticoid, *Am. J. Med.,* 19:976, 1955.
139. Fishman, L. M., Kuchel, O., Liddle, G. W., Michelakis, A. M., Gordon, R. D., and Chick, W. T.: Incidence of Primary Aldosteronism Uncomplicated "Essential" Hypertension. A Prospective Study with Elevated Aldosterone Secretion and Suppressed Plasma Renin Activity Used as Diagnostic Criteria, *JAMA,* 205:497, 1968.
140. Kaplan, N. M.: Hypokalemia in the Hypertensive Patient: With Observations on the Incidence of Primary Aldosteronism, *Ann. Intern. Med.,* 66:1079, 1967.
141. Veterans Administration Cooperative Study on Antihypertensive Agents: Double Blind Control Study of Antihypertensive Agents: III. Chlorothiazide Alone and in Combination with other Agents; Preliminary Results, *Arch. Intern. Med.,* 110:230, 1962.
142. Morgan, D. B., and Davidson, C.: Hypokalaemia and Diuretics: An Analysis of Publications, *Br. Med. J.,* 2:905, 1980.
143. Conn, J. W., Cohen, E. L., Rovner, D. R., and Nesbit, R. M.: Normokalemic Primary Aldosteronism. A Detectable Cause of Curable "Essential" Hypertension, *JAMA,* 193:100, 1965.
144. Biglieri, E. G., Stockigt, J. R., and Schambelan, M.: Adrenal Mineralocorticoids Causing Hypertension, *Am. J. Med.,* 52:623, 1972.
145. Conn, J. W., Rovner, D. R., and Cohen, E. L.: Licorice-induced Pseudoaldosteronism. Hypertension, Hypokalemia, Aldosteronopenia, and Suppressed Plasma Renin Activity, *JAMA,* 205:80, 1968.
146. Blachley, J. D., and Knochel, J. P.: Tobacco Chewer's Hypokalemia: Licorice Revisited, *N. Engl. J. Med.,* 302:784, 1980.
147. Mantero, F., Armanini, D., Opocher, G., et al.: Mineralocorticoid Hypertension Due to a Nasal Spray Containing 9α-Fluoroprednisolone, *Am. J. Med.,* 71:352, 1981.
148. Weinberger, M. H., Grim, C. E., Hollifield, J. W., et al.: Primary Aldosteronism. Diagnosis, Localization, Treatment, *Ann. Intern. Med.,* 90:386, 1979.
149. Weinberger, M. H.: Primary Aldosteronism: Diagnosis and Differentiation of Subtypes, *Ann. Intern. Med.,* 100:300, 1984.
150. Hiramatsu, K., Yamada, T., Yukimura, Y., et al.: A Screening Test to Identify Aldosterone-Producing Adenoma by Measuring Plasma Renin Activity. Results in Hypertensive Patients, *Arch. Intern. Med.,* 141:1589, 1981.
151. Lyons, D. F., Kem, D. C., Brown, R. D., Hanson, C. S., and Carollo, M. L.: Single Dose Captopril as a Diagnostic Test for Primary Aldosteronism, *J. Clin. Endocrinol. Metab.,* 57:892, 1983.
152. Gross, M. D., Grekin, R. J., Gniadek, T. C., and Villareal, J. Z.: Suppression of Aldosterone by Cyproheptadine in Idiopathic Aldosteronism, *N. Engl. J. Med.,* 305:181, 1981.
153. Ganguly, A., Melada, G. A., Luetscher, J. A., and Dowdy, A. J.: Control of Plasma Aldosterone in Primary Aldosteronism: Distinction between Adenoma and Hyperplasia, *J. Clin. Endocrinol. Metab.,* 37:765, 1973.
154. Biglieri, E. G., Schambelan, M., Brust, N., Chang, B., and Hogan, M.: Plasma Aldosterone Concentration. Further Characterization of Aldosterone-Producing Adenomas, *Circ. Res.,* 34 and 35(suppl. I):183, 1974.
155. Mulrow, P. J.: Glucocorticoid-Suppressible Hyperaldosteronism: A Clue to the Missing Hormone? *N. Engl. J. Med.,* 305:1012, 1981.
156. Franco-Saenz, R., Mulrow, P. J., and Kim, K.: Idiopathic Aldosteronism. A Possible Disease of the Intermediate Lobe of the Pituitary, *JAMA,* 251:2555, 1984.
157. Sen, S., Valenzuela, R., Smeby, R., Bravo, E. L., and Bumpus, F. M.: Localization, Purification, and Biological Activity of a New Aldosterone-Stimulating Factor, *Hypertension,* 3(suppl. I):I–81, 1981.
158. Saito, I., and Saruta, T.: Regulation of Aldosterone Secretion by a New Aldosterone Stimulating Factor, *Jpn. Circ. J.,* 46:523, 1982.
159. Giebink, G. S., Gotlin, R. W., Biglieri, E. G., and Katz, F. H.: A Kindred with Familial Glucocorticoid-Suppressible Aldosteronism, *J. Clin. Endocrinol. Metab.,* 36:715, 1973.
160. Ferriss, J. B., Beevers, D. G., Boddy, K., et al.: The Treatment of Low-Renin ("Primary") Hyperaldosteronism, *Am. Heart J.,* 96:97, 1978.
161. Guerin, C. K., Wahner, H. W., Gorman, C. A., Carpenter, P. C., and Sheedy, P. F., II: Computed Tomographic Scanning Versus Radioisotope Imaging in Adrenocortical Diagnosis, *Am. J. Med.,* 75:653, 1983.
162. Biglieri, E. G., Schambelan, M.: The Significance of Elevated Levels of Plasma 18-Hydroxycorticosterone in Patients with Primary Aldosteronism, *J. Clin. Endocrinol. Metab.,* 49:87, 1979.
163. Bravo, E. L., Tarazi, R. C., Dustan, H. P., et al.: The Changing Clinical Spectrum of Primary Aldosteronism, *Am. J. Med.,* 74:641, 1983.
164. White, E. A., Schambelan, M., Rost, C. R., Biglieri, E. G., Moss, A. A., and Korobkin, M.: Use of Computed Tomography in Diagnosing the Cause of Primary Aldosteronism, *N. Engl. J. Med.,* 303:1503, 1980.
165. Manger, W. M., and Gifford, R. W., Jr.: "Pheochromocytoma," Springer-Verlag, New York, 1977.
166. Remine, W. H., Chong, G. C., van Heerden, J. A., Sheps, S. G., and Harrison, E. G., Jr.: Current Management of Pheochromocytoma, *Ann. Surg.,* 179:740, 1974.
167. DeOreo, G. A., Jr., Stewart, B. H., Tarazi, R. C., and Gifford, R. W., Jr.: Preoperative Blood Transfusion in the Safe Surgical Management of Pheochromocytoma: A Review of 46 Cases, *J. Urol.,* 111:715, 1974.
168. Sjoerdsma, A., Engelman, K., Waldmann, T. A., Cooperman, L. H., and Hammond, W. G.: Pheochromocytoma: Current Concepts of Diagnosis and Treatment, *Ann. Intern. Med.,* 65:1302, 1966.
169. Gitlow, S. E., Mendlowitz, M., and Bertani, L. M.: The Biochemical Techniques for Detecting and Establishing the Presence of a Pheochromocytoma: A Review of Ten Years' Experience, *Am. J. Cardiol.,* 26:270, 1970.
170. Kaplan, N. M., Kramer, N. J., Holland, O. B., Sheps, S. G., and Gomez-Sanchez, C.: Single-Voided Urine Metane-

phrine Assays in Screening for Pheochromocytoma, *Arch. Intern. Med.*, 137:190, 1977.

171. Miller, R., Stark, D. C. C., and Gitlow, S. E.: Paroxysmal Hyperadrenergic State. A Case During Surgery for Intracranial Aneurysm, *Anaesthesia,* 31:743, 1976.
172. Sheps, S., Van Heerden, J., and Sheedy, P., II: Current Approach to the Diagnosis of Pheochromocytoma, in Blaufox, M. D., and Bianchi, C. (eds.): "Secondary Forms of Hypertension. Current Diagnosis and Management," New York, Grune & Stratton, 1981, p. 11.
173. Engelman, K., Portnoy, B., and Sjoerdsma, A.: Plasma Catecholamine Concentrations in Patients with Hypertension, *Circ. Res.,* 27(suppl. 1):141, 1970.
174. Bravo, E. L., Tarazi, R. C., Gifford, R. W., and Stewart, B. H.: Circulating and Urinary Catecholamines in Pheochromocytoma. Diagnostic and Pathophysiologic Implications, *N. Engl. J. Med.,* 301:682, 1979.
175. Videbaek, J., Christensen, N. J., and Sterndorff, B.: Serial Determinations of Plasma Catecholamines in Myocardial Infarction, *Circulation,* 46:846, 1972.
176. Karlsberg, R. P., Cryer, P. E., and Roberts, R.: Serial Plasma Catecholamine Response Early in the Course of Clinical Acute Myocardial Infarction: Relationship to Infarct Extent and Mortality, *Am. Heart J.,* 102:24, 1981.
177. Mueller, H. S., and Ayres, S. M.: Propranolol Decreases Sympathetic Nervous Activity Reflected by Plasma Catecholamines During Evolution of Myocardial Infarction in Man, *J. Clin. Invest.,* 65:338, 1980.
178. Benedict, C. R., and Loach, A. B.: Sympathetic Nervous System Activity in Patients with Subarachnoid Hemorrhage, *Stroke,* 9:237, 1978.
179. Hansson, L., Hunyor, S. N., Julius, S., and Hoobler, S. W.: Blood Pressure Crisis Following Withdrawal of Clonidine (Catapres, Catapresan), with Special Reference to Arterial and Urinary Catecholamine Levels, and Suggestions for Acute Management, *Am. Heart J.,* 85:605, 1973.
180. Lake, C. R., Ziegler, M. G., Coleman, M. D., and Kopin, I. J.: Hydrochlorothiazide-Induced Sympathetic Hyperactivity in Hypertensive Patients, *Clin. Pharmacol. Ther.,* 26:428, 1979.
181. Weidmann, P., Beretta-Piccoli, C., Meier, A., Keusch, G., Glück, Z., and Ziegler, W. H.: Antihypertensive Mechanism of Diuretic Treatment with Chlorthalidone. Complementary Roles of Sympathetic Axis and Sodium, *Kidney Int.,* 23:320, 1983.
182. Murphy, M. B., Scriven, A. J., Brown, M. J., Causon, R., and Dollery, C. T.: The Effects of Nifedipine and Hydralazine Induced Hypotension on Sympathetic Activity, *Eur. J. Clin. Pharmacol.,* 23:479, 1982.
183. Lin, M-S., McNay, J. L., Shepherd, A. M. M., Musgrave, G. E., and Keeton, T. K.: Increased Plasma Norepinephrine Accompanies Persistent Tachycardia After Hydralazine, *Hypertension,* 5:257, 1983.
184. Klein, W., Brandt, D., Vrecko, K., and Härringer, M.: Role of Calcium Antagonists in the Treatment of Essential Hypertension, *Circ. Res.,* 52(suppl. 1):174, 1983.
185. Izzo, J. L., Jr., Horwitz, D., and Keiser, H. R.: Physiologic Mechanisms Opposing the Hemodynamic Effects of Prazosin, *Clin. Pharmacol. Ther.,* 29:7, 1981.
186. Inouye, I., Massie, B., Benowitz, N., Simpson, P., Loge, D., and Topic, N.: Monotherapy in Mild to Moderate Hypertension: Comparison of Hydrochlorothiazide, Propranolol and Prazosin, *Am. J. Cardiol.,* 53:24A, 1984. (Proceedings of a Symposium.)
187. Bravo, E. L., Tarazi, R. C., Fouad, F. M., Vidt, D. G., and Gifford, R. W., Jr.: Clonidine-Suppression Test. A Useful Aid in the Diagnosis of Pheochromocytoma, *N. Engl. J. Med.,* 305:623, 1981.
188. Metz, S. A., Halter, J. B., Porte, D., Jr., and Robertson, R. P.: Autonomic Epilepsy: Clonidine Blockade of Paroxysmal Catecholamine Release and Flushing, *Ann. Intern. Med.,* 88:189, 1978.
189. Halter, J. B., Beard, J. C., Pfeifer, M. A., and Metz, S. A.: Clonidine-suppression Test for Diagnosis of Pheochromocytoma, *N. Engl. J. Med.,* 306:49, 1982. (Letter.)
190. Dupont, A. G., Velkeniers, B., Somers, G., Gerlo, E., and Vanhaelst, L.: Unusual Clonidine-Suppression Test in an Epinephrine-secreting Pheochromocytoma, *N. Engl. J. Med.,* 310:266, 1984. (Letter.)
191. Stewart, B. H., Bravo, E. L., Haaga, J., Meaney, T. F., and Tarazi, R.: Localization of Pheochromocytoma by Computed Tomography, *N. Engl. J. Med.,* 299:460, 1978.
192. Ganguly, A., Henry, D. P., Yune, H. Y., et al.: Diagnosis and Localization of Pheochromocytoma. Detection by Measurement of Urinary Norepinephrine Excretion During Sleep, Plasma Norepinephrine Concentration and Computerized Axial Tomography (CT-Scan), *Am. J. Med.,* 67:21, 1979.
193. Sisson, J. C., Frager, M. S., Valk, T. W., et al.: Scintigraphic Localization of Pheochromocytoma, *N. Engl. J. Med.,* 305:12, 1981.
194. Shapiro, B., Kalff, V., Sisson, J. C., et al.: Intrathoracic Pheochromocytoma a Diagnostic Dilemma Solved by 131-I-Metaiodobenzylguanidine Scintigraphy, *Clin. Res.,* 30(4):722A, 1982. (Abstract.)

51

Treatment of Systemic Hypertension

Gary L. Wollam, M.D.

W. Dallas Hall, M.D.

Until the etiology of essential hypertension is known, its treatment will necessarily be empiric; but with increasing insight into the mechanisms of hypertension and into the clinical pharmacology of the drugs used to treat it, we are emerging from a period of "blind empiricism" into an era of "enlightened empiricism."

R. W. Gifford, Jr., 1975[1,*]

Treatment of Primary (Essential) Hypertension

Pharmacologic Therapy for Mild or Moderate Hypertension

Selection of Initial Therapy (i.e., Step 1) in the Usual Patient

Pharmacologic therapy for hypertension should generally be initiated with low doses of a diuretic, such as the equivalent of 25 mg daily of chlorthalidone or hydrochlorothiazide, or 2 mg daily of trichlormethiazide, (see Table 51-1).[2] If renal function is normal, there is usually no advantage to initiating therapy with a loop diuretic, such as furosemide or bumetanide.

If supine or sitting diastolic blood pressure is not reduced below 90 mmHg after several weeks of diuretic therapy in doses equivalent to 25 to 50 mg daily of hydrochlorothiazide or chlorthalidone, then a beta blocker or a sympatholytic drug such as methyldopa, clonidine, reserpine, guanabenz, or prazosin should be added if there is no contraindication.[2] The dosage should then be increased stepwise until diastolic pressure is reduced below 90 mmHg, or moderate dosage levels are attained in the absence of adverse effects (e.g., the equivalent of 1000 mg daily of methyldopa, 160 mg daily of propranolol, 0.8 mg daily of clonidine, 0.25 mg daily of reserpine). If diastolic pressure remains uncontrolled at these dosage levels, it is often more efficacious to add a vasodilating agent, such as hydralazine, than to proceed immediately to higher doses of the sympatholytic drug. This is because the dose-response relationships of many sympatholytic drugs are such that the greatest therapeutic benefits with the least adverse experiences are usually observed in the low to moderate dosage range. Table 51-2 provides a listing of adverse effects encountered with antihypertensive drugs.

Supplemental Potassium Therapy in Diuretic-Treated Patients

When diuretic therapy is begun in patients with uncomplicated essential hypertension, the serum potassium concentration should be measured prior to treatment, again within 4 weeks after therapy is initiated, and then once or twice a year thereafter. The development of diuretic-induced hypokalemia would appear to be more closely related to the magnitude of the natriuretic response and the increase in aldosterone levels than the particular diuretic agent employed.[3] In general, potassium supplements or a potassium-sparing diuretic should be prescribed when a serum potassium of less than 3.0 to 3.2 meq/liter is confirmed in patients with uncomplicated essential hypertension.[4] In patients with ventricular ectopy and normal renal function, potassium repletion may be desirable with less severe hypokalemia, particularly if there has been a greater than usual postdiuretic decrease in serum potassium (e.g., from 4.8 to 3.8 meq/liter). In patients requiring digitalis preparations, potassium supplementation should generally be prescribed routinely with initial diuretic therapy if the serum potassium is not elevated. When hypokalemia is treated with potassium supplements, doses of at least 40 meq daily are typically required. For example, Licht et al. studied patients with essential hypertension who received therapy with hydrochlorothiazide, 50 mg daily.[5] They found that an average prescribed dose of 37 meq daily of potassium supplements increased the serum potassium level by only 0.2 meq/liter. Morgan and Davidson reported similar findings, although the increase in the mean serum potassium level (i.e., 0.32 meq/liter) was somewhat greater.[6] The use of potassium-sparing diuretics (i.e., amiloride, triamterene, or spironolactone) was associated with somewhat larger increases in the serum potassium concentration.[5,6] In general, potassium supplements should not be used concomitantly with potassium-sparing diuretics because of the risk of hyperkalemia.[7,8]

Sympatholytic Drugs as Initial Therapy

Clinical Settings Associated with Increased Adrenergic Activity There are several clinical settings in which beta blockers or other sympatholytic drugs may be preferable to diuretics as first-line therapy for hypertension. These are enumerated in Table 51-3 and include "high-renin" essential hypertension, the hyperdynamic beta-adrenergic circulatory state, alcohol-withdrawal hypertension, and possibly other settings associated with increased adrenergic tone.

High-renin essential hypertension is more prevalent in patients under age 40.[9] In addition to elevated plasma renin activity, these patients frequently have high plasma norepinephrine levels.[10,11]

*Reproduced with permission from the publisher and author.

TABLE 51-1 Dosage Range for Antihypertensive Drugs

Drugs	Initial Dose (mg/day)	Maximum Dose† (mg/day)
Diuretics		
Thiazide-type		
Bendroflumethiazide	2.5	5
Benzthiazide	25.0	50
Chlorothiazide	250.0	500
Chlorthalidone	25.0	50
Cyclothiazide	1.0	2
Hydrochlorothiazide	25.0	50
Hydroflumethiazide	25.0	50
Indapamide	2.5	5
Methyclothiazide	2.5	5
Metolazone	2.5	5
Polythiazide	2.0	4
Quinethazone	50.0	100
Trichlormethiazide	2.0	4–8
Loop		
Bumetanide‡	1.0	10
Ethacrynic acid‡	50.0	200
Furosemide‡	80.0	480
Potassium-sparing		
Amiloride	5.0	10
Spironolactone‡	50.0	100
Triamterene	50.0	100
Adrenergic Inhibitors		
β-Adrenergic blockers		
Atenolol	25.0	100
Metoprolol‡	50.0	300
Nadolol	20.0	120–320
Oxprenolol‡	160.0	480
Pindolol‡	10.0	60
Propranolol‡	40.0	480
Timolol‡	20.0	60
Central-acting adrenergic inhibitors		
Clonidine‡	0.2	1.2
Guanabenz‡	8.0	32
Methyldopa‡	500.0	2000
Peripheral-acting adrenergic antagonists		
Guanadrel‡	10.0	150
Guanethidine	10.0	100
Reserpine	0.1	0.25
α_1-Adrenergic blocker		
Prazosin‡	1.0	20
Combined α- and β-adrenergic blockers		
Labetalol‡	200.0	1200
Vasodilators		
Hydralazine‡	50.0	300
Minoxidil	5.0	60
Angiotension-converting enzyme inhibitors		
Captopril‡	25.0–37.5	150–300
Enalapril*	10.0	40
Slow channel calcium-entry blocking agents		
Diltiazem§	120.0	240
Nifedipine§	30.0	90–180
Verapamil§	240.0	480

*This drug has not yet been approved by the FDA.
†The maximum suggested dosage may be exceeded in resistant cases.
‡This drug is usually given in divided doses twice daily unless a long-acting formulation is available.
§This drug is usually given in divided doses three times daily.
Source: Adapted in part from The Joint National Committee on Detection, Evaluation, and Treatment of High Blood Pressure: The 1984 Report of the Joint National Committee on Detection, Evaluation, and Treatment of High Blood Pressure, *Arch. Intern. Med.*, 144:1045, 1984. Reproduced with permission of the authors.

TABLE 51-2 Side Effects of Antihypertensive Drugs

Drug	Side Effects
Thiazide-type Diuretics	Dry mouth Weakness Muscle cramps Hyperuricemia/gout Gastrointestinal disturbances Hypomagnesemia Hypokalemia Hyponatremia Hypercalcemia Skin rash Photosensitivity Thrombocytopenia Marrow depression Lithium toxicity Exacerbation of glucose intolerance Hypertriglyceridemia Hypercholesterolemia Sexual dysfunction
Reserpine	Bradycardia Lethargy Lassitude Sexual dysfunction Diarrhea Nasal congestion Depression Peptic ulcer Parkinsonism
Guanethidine or Guanadrel	Bradycardia Orthostatic hypotension Exercise hypotension Diarrhea Weakness Retrograde ejaculation or impotence Interaction with tricyclic antidepressants
Prazosin	Headache Palpitation Drowsiness Dizziness Nausea First-dose syncope Orthostatic hypotension Sexual dysfunction Nightmares Weakness
Hydralazine	Tachycardia* Palpitation* Headache* Flushing* Aggravation of angina* Lupus-like syndrome Drug fever
Captopril or Enalapril†	Occasional hypotension with initial dose Skin rash Angioedema Neutropenia Proteinuria Membranous glomerulopathy Dysgeusia Acute renal failure in bilateral renal artery stenosis (or renal artery stenosis in a solitary kidney)
Methyldopa	Drowsiness Lethargy Sexual dysfunction Positive Coomb's test Hemolytic anemia Abnormal liver tests Hepatitis Drug fever Orthostatic hypotension Depression Myocarditis
Clonidine or Guanabenz	Dry mouth Drowsiness Lethargy Sexual dysfunction Gastrointestinal disturbances Risk of "rebound hypertension" when discontinued abruptly Parotid pain
Beta Blockers or Labetalol	Bradycardia Weakness Lethargy Gastrointestinal disturbances Insomnia Congestive heart failure Prolongation of PR interval Second or third degree heart block Bronchospasm Laryngospasm Aggravation of peripheral arterial insufficiency Nightmares Hallucinations Depression Prolongation of hypoglycemic episode Worsening of diabetes mellitus; hyperosmolar coma Sexual dysfunction Hyperlipemia Positive ANA
Minoxidil	Hypertrichosis Edema (occasionally resulting in anasarca and congestive heart failure) Pericardial effusion Aggravation of coronary insufficiency*
Nifedipine	Headache Hypotension Tachycardia* Edema Erythromelalgia

*Side effects that may sometimes be minimized by the coadministration of a beta blocker or other sympathetic inhibitor (e.g., clonidine).

†This drug has not yet been approved by the FDA.

TABLE 51-3 Clinical Settings Where Beta Blockers or Other Sympatholytic Drugs May Be Appropriate as Initial (i.e., Step 1) Therapy for Hypertension

High-renin essential hypertension (i.e., more prevalent in Caucasians below age 40)
Hyperdynamic beta-adrenergic circulatory state
Alcohol-withdrawal hypertension
Exaggerated orthostatic increase in diastolic pressure (i.e., "orthostatic hypertension")
Hyperlipemia
Postmyocardial infarction/coronary insufficiency
Ventricular ectopy
Selected cases of maturity-onset (i.e., noninsulin-dependent) diabetes mellitus

Blood pressure may be reduced to normotensive levels following treatment with sympatholytic drugs alone.[12,13] High-renin essential hypertension is more common in whites than blacks.[14] Black hypertensive patients as a group have lower plasma renin activity, and tend to be more responsive to diuretic therapy than white hypertensive patients.[15]

Patients with the "hyperkinetic heart syndrome," as described by Gorlin, or the "hyperdynamic beta-adrenergic circulatory state," as described by Frohlich et al., may present with labile or elevated blood pressure in conjunction with symptoms of tachycardia and palpitations.[16,17] Such patients frequently have a hyperdynamic circulation and increased beta-receptor responsiveness. Therapy with a beta blocker such as propranolol is often beneficial.[17,18]

The presence of an exaggerated increase in diastolic pressure upon standing (i.e., orthostatic hypertension) may indicate increased adrenergic tone.[19] Plasma and urinary norepinephrine levels have been found to correlate with the magnitude of the orthostatic increase in diastolic pressure and pulse pressure.[20–22] Preliminary information would suggest that patients with untreated essential hypertension who exhibit exaggerated orthostatic increases in diastolic pressure (i.e., greater than 8 to 10 mmHg upon standing) may have a good initial response to treatment with sympatholytic drugs alone.[23] In addition, Cressman et al. have found that the magnitude of the reduction in blood pressure following 4 weeks of treatment with clonidine correlated with the baseline plasma norepinephrine concentration; the higher the pretreatment norepinephrine level, the greater the reduction in blood pressure with clonidine monotherapy.[24]

In addition to clinical settings associated with increased adrenergic activity, there are a number of other situations in which beta blocker or other sympatholytic drugs may sometimes be appropriate as first-line therapy for hypertension.

Hypertension and Ventricular Ectopy Beta blockers may be preferable to diuretics as initial antihypertensive therapy in patients with ventricular ectopy or in those at increased risk (e.g., postmyocardial infarction, left ventricular hypertrophy) of ventricular arrhythmias.[25] Therapy with the thiazide diuretics has been associated with an increase in ventricular ectopy (including high-grade ventricular arrhythmias) in some cases,[26,27] although not all agree.[28] Ventricular arrhythmias may be, in part, related to the development of hypokalemia,[26,29] although other factors such as hypomagnesemia or stimulation of norepinephrine or epinephrine release may also be involved.[30–32] For further discussion of the use of beta-adrenergic blocking drugs in patients with coronary heart disease and ventricular arrhythmias, see Chap. 90.

Hypertension and Hyperlipemia In patients with coexistent hypertension and hyperlipemia, it may sometimes be appropriate to initiate therapy with certain sympatholytic drugs, such as prazosin or clonidine, which tend to decrease the serum cholesterol concentration.[33,34] For example, Leren et al. performed careful measurements of fasting serum lipid concentrations in 23 hypertensive men who were participants in the Oslo Study.[33] Following 8 weeks of monotherapy with prazosin, an average reduction in the total serum cholesterol concentration of 8.9 percent and a mean decrease in serum triglyceride concentration of 16.2 percent was observed; no significant changes in high-density lipoprotein (HDL) cholesterol occurred. Following 8 weeks of monotherapy with propranolol, the average HDL cholesterol concentration had decreased by 13.0 percent, and the mean serum triglyceride concentration had risen by 24.0 percent; although no significant change in the total serum cholesterol concentration was observed. In a preliminary investigation, Kirkendall et al. reported a reduction in total serum cholesterol concentration following treatment with clonidine,[34] although additional study is warranted to further confirm these findings.

Therapy with thiazide-type diuretics is frequently associated with a mild to moderate increase in the serum cholesterol concentration.[35,36] This is illustrated by the results of the Veterans Administration study on antihypertensive therapy in patients with mild hypertension.[37] In this investigation, careful measurements of fasting serum lipoprotein levels were obtained at baseline and again after 1 year of therapy with chlorthalidone, 50 mg or 100 mg daily, or placebo. The group treated with chlorthalidone experienced an average increase in the total serum cholesterol concentration of 9.9 mg/dl ($p < 0.001$); whereas in the placebo group, no significant change was observed. The serum triglyceride and low-density lipoprotein (LDL) cholesterol concentrations also increased significantly (i.e., 9.8 mg/dl and 12.6 mg/dl, respectively, over placebo) in the group that received treatment with chlorthalidone. Changes in HDL cholesterol concentration were not significant in either group. The rise that occurred in the total serum cholesterol concentration in the chlorthalidone group correlated inversely with the baseline level; i.e., the younger patients with the lowest levels at baseline had the greatest increases. Some investigators have found that the increase in total serum cholesterol following treatment with the thiazide-type diuretics can be ameliorated or prevented with a cholesterol-lowering diet.[36]

In the Multiple Risk Factor Intervention Trial (MRFIT), the use of diuretics markedly attenuated the effects of lipid-lowering diets in reducing the serum cholesterol concentration.[38] For example, of those participants who were randomized to the special intervention group (and who received instruction on dietary weight control and a low saturated fat, low-cholesterol intake), the average reduction in the total serum cholesterol concentration after 24 months of therapy was 6.2 mg/dl in those receiving diuretics as compared with a twofold greater reduction (i.e., 12.7 mg/dl) in those not receiving diuretics. In addition, the average serum triglyceride concentration rose by 10.5 mg/dl in the diuretic group, whereas it fell by 24.0 mg/dl in the group not receiving diuretics.

If worsening of hyperlipemia occurs following therapy with a thiazide-type diuretic, it may be useful to attempt switching to furosemide or spironolactone. Preliminary reports suggest that these diuretics may have less tendency to exacerbate hyperlipemia than the thiazide-type diuretics,[39,40] although some have not found this and further study is warranted.[41]

Hypertension and Glucose Intolerance Hypertensive patients with diabetes mellitus may have increased total body sodium stores.[42] This may explain the clinical observation that diuretic therapy is frequently required to control arterial pressure in such patients.[43] Particularly in patients with evidence of diabetic nephropathy, hypertension appears to be, in part, "volume-dependent";[43] moreover, adequate arterial pressure control is of utmost importance as it may reduce the rate of progression of renal insufficiency.[44,45]

The exacerbation of glucose intolerance that sometimes occurs following the administration of diuretics may, in part, be related to the development of hypokalemia. The mechanism appears to be a suppressive effect of hypokalemia on insulin secretion,[46–48] although other factors may also be involved.[49] The administration of potassium supplements to hypokalemic patients usually leads to improvement of serum glucose levels.[50–52] Some investigators have found that furosemide may have less tendency to exacerbate glucose intolerance than the thiazide-type diuretics.[5,53] In most cases, however, the relative magnitude of this effect would appear to be small, and its clinical significance has not been fully established.

Whenever possible, sympatholytic drugs other than beta blockers should be used to control blood pressure in patients with either insulin-dependent (i.e., type I) or maturity-onset (i.e., type II) diabetes mellitus. This is because beta blockers prolong hypoglycemia following an insulin reaction. They also prevent the development of the tachycardia usually associated with hypoglycemia.[54] However, excessive sweating associated with hypoglycemia does not appear to be prevented and may actually be enhanced by beta blockers.[55,56] The cardioselective drugs appear to have less tendency to prolong hypoglycemia or interfere with the hemodynamic and metabolic responses to hypoglycemia than the nonselective drugs.[55,57,58]

Beta blockers also exacerbate glucose intolerance in some patients with maturity-onset diabetes mellitus.[59] In the Oslo Study, combined therapy with hydrochlorothiazide and propranolol was associated with a significantly greater increase in fasting blood glucose levels than was treatment with hydrochlorothiazide alone or in combination with methyldopa.[60] This effect is presumably due to blockade of $beta_2$-receptor mediated insulin secretion in the pancreas,[61] and there is some evidence that it may be less with the cardioselective beta blockers.[62–64] When therapy with beta blockers is indicated in patients with either maturity-onset or insulin-dependent diabetes mellitus, the cardioselective drugs are better choices.

Hypertension Unresponsive to Diuretic Plus Sympatholytic Therapy

When hypertension does not respond to combined therapy with a diuretic and beta blocker or other sympatholytic drug, then a vasodilator such as hydralazine should be added. The coadministration of hydralazine with a beta blocker antagonizes the reflex tachycardia and increase in cardiac output produced by hydralazine, thus enhancing its therapeutic effect. To a lesser degree, clonidine, methyldopa, reserpine, and guanabenz also blunt the reflex tachycardia of hydralazine. The selective postsynaptic (i.e., $alpha_1$) adrenergic blocking agent, prazosin, can also be substituted in place of the other sympatholytic drugs. However, it appears to be most effective when combined with a beta blocker. In the Veterans Administration Study on antihypertensive agents, the blood-pressure lowering effect of prazosin was comparable to that of hydralazine,[65] although side effects (e.g., orthostatic dizziness, impotence, nightmares) were more frequent with prazosin.

Pharmacologic Therapy for Severe or Resistant Hypertension

In patients with untreated and uncomplicated severe essential hypertension (i.e., in whom a diastolic pressure of 115 mmHg or more is confirmed), it is frequently advisable to initiate therapy concomitantly with a diuretic and a beta blocker or other sympatholytic drug. The patient should be followed closely, however, as marked reductions in arterial pressure (and/or orthostatic hypotension) are sometimes observed, even with relatively low doses of antihypertensive drugs.

Previous studies have indicated that over 90 percent of hypertensive patients who comply with their medications achieve normalization of diastolic pressure with pharmacologic regimens consisting of up to three or more antihypertensive drugs.[66] When blood pressure is uncontrolled on three or more antipressor drugs (i.e., generally consisting of a diuretic, sympatholytic, and vasodilator drug administered in adequate dosages), the term *resistant hypertension* is generally applied.[67] Most cases of bona fide resistant hypertension occur either in the setting of severe essential hypertension complicated by target organ damage (e.g., left ventricular hypertrophy, renal insufficiency, and/or severe hypertensive retinopathy), or in patients with secondary hypertension, particularly renal artery stenosis.

Factors to Consider Prior to Selecting Additional Drug Therapy

Factors that should be considered before additional drug therapy is begun include medication adherence, excessive salt intake, drug interactions, undiagnosed causes of secondary hypertension, and inaccurate measurements of blood pressure.

Lack of adherence to a complex treatment regimen is one of the most frequent causes of uncontrolled hypertension. In many cases, this may be due, at least in part, to patient confusion with regard to the prescribed multidrug regimen. For example, Hulka et al. identified medication errors in 58 percent of a group of predominately middle-class patients.[68] With the exception of the currently available calcium channel blockers, all marketed antihypertensive drugs used in the treatment of hypertension (e.g., diuretic, sympatholytic, vasodilator) can generally be administered on a bid dosage schedule with satisfactory results. In general, patients with uncontrolled hypertension should be asked to bring their medication bottles to each clinic visit, and to briefly review the dosage schedule with the clinician. Finally, in patients who present with unexplained hypertension on a number of occasions during outpatient visits (i.e., particularly when the level of blood pressure control fluctuates markedly between clinic visits for no apparent reason) and noncompliance is suspected, it is sometimes useful to administer the currently prescribed antihypertensive medications (e.g., the P.M. dose of diuretic, sympatholytic, and vasodilator drugs) in the office or clinic, and then recheck blood pressure again after 1 to 3 h. If a marked reduction in blood pressure (i.e., on the order of −35/−20 mmHg) has occurred during this period, then poor medication adherence is implied. This "compliance test" must be administered with caution, however, as marked hypotension can ensue in patients who are taking few, if any, of their prescribed medications.

A 24-h urinary sodium excretion that exceeds 200 meq/day clearly indicates excessive dietary sodium intake, and may explain apparent resistance to diuretic therapy in patients who are receiving multiple antihypertensive drugs.

Nonsteroidal antiinflammatory drugs such as indomethacin have been reported to decrease the natriuretic effect of furosemide and possibly also the thiazide diuretics;[69,70] they may also interfere with the antihypertensive effect of captopril and beta blockers.[71–73] Aspirin may partially interfere with the diuretic effect of spironolactone[74] as well as furosemide.[75] Diphenylhydantoin and other anticonvulsants may also reduce the diuretic potency of furosemide.[76] Tricyclic antidepressants interfere with the antihypertensive effect of guanethidine, clonidine, and possibly methyldopa.[77] How often such drug interactions are actually a cause of resistant hypertension, however, remains to be clarified.

Andersson identified secondary etiologies in 10 percent of patients with refractory hypertension.[78] Diagnostic studies to exclude renal artery stenosis and pheochromocytoma are indicated in most cases. In general, a 24-h urine collection should be obtained on patients with resistant hypertension, and assessed for metanephrine, sodium, and creatinine excretion. This is to exclude the diagnosis of pheochromocytoma and also to assess dietary sodium intake. Other causes of secondary hypertension (e.g., primary aldosteronism, excessive ingestion of licorice-containing candy or chewing tobacco, chronic renal disease, Cushing's syndrome, coarctation of the aorta, collagen vascular diseases) should also be considered (see Chap. 50).

Falsely elevated auscultatory blood pressure measurements are most frequently encountered in obese patients whose midarm circumference exceeds 35 cm, and in elderly patients with extensive atherosclerosis.

Approach to Drug Therapy in Resistant Hypertension

In the approach to drug therapy, it is important to remember that arterial pressure is regulated by volume, neural, and humoral mechanisms; among other factors, these include the plasma and extracellular fluid volumes, the sympathetic nervous system, and the renin-angiotensin system. In some cases, there may be clinical clues to indicate which of these systems may be contributing most to the elevated arterial pressure. For example, patients with exudative or hemorrhagic retinopathy (i.e., related to accelerated or malignant hypertension) or hypertensive encephalopathy usually have elevated plasma renin activity. In this clinical setting, it may be useful to add a converting-enzyme inhibitor, such as captopril or enalapril. Likewise, patients with edema usually need repeated and effective doses of diuretics, and those with persistent tachycardia usually need judicious doses of a beta blocker or other sympatholytic agent as tolerated. In patients with severely impaired left ventricular function, attempts should be made to control hypertension and reflex tachycardia (induced by vasodilator therapy) with sympathetic inhibitors, such as clonidine or guanabenz, which may have less of a depressant effect on myocardial contractility.[79] Beta blockers should generally be avoided for treatment of hypertension in patients with congestive cardiomyopathy. However, in the absence of congestive heart failure, the cautious administration of low doses of pindolol (e.g., 5 mg bid), a beta blocker which possesses substantial intrinsic sympathomimetic activity, has been reported to be useful in selected cases.[80]

When there are no clinical clues, however, it often is useful to select additional drug therapy that acts on each of these systems in succession. For example, when blood pressure remains elevated on adequate doses of a diuretic, beta blocker, and hydralazine (e.g., furosemide 80 mg bid, propranolol 160 mg bid, hydralazine 150 mg bid), it is sometimes useful to add a second sympatholytic drug (e.g., methyldopa, clonidine, or prazosin) that interferes directly with alpha-mediated vasoconstriction.

Following the blockade of sympatholytic reflexes (i.e., generally with a beta blocker combined with a central- or peripheral-acting sympathetic inhibitor), blood pressure is largely "volume dependent" and can generally be lowered by more intensive diuretic therapy.[81] When the response to furosemide is unsatisfactory at a dosage of 160 to 240 mg per day, the cautious addition of a thiazide-type diuretic in low doses (i.e., 25 mg of hydrochlorothiazide or 2.5 mg of metolazone daily or even every other day) is frequently effective in restoring arterial pressure control.[82] However, combined thiazide-furosemide therapy is a potent diuretic regimen, which can result in volume depletion, severe hypokalemia, and an increase in blood urea nitrogen and creatinine concentrations. The risk of hypokalemia is lessened by the concomitant use of converting-enzyme inhibitors, such as captopril and enalapril. These drugs interfere with the formation of angiotensin II, and lessen the secondary aldosteronism and urinary potassium losses that are frequently associated with combined thiazide-furosemide therapy. The addition of captopril can be accomplished by administering a first dose (e.g., usually 12.5 mg) in the office or outpatient clinic, and then assessing the effect on blood pressure after 60 to 90 min. Therapy with captopril can then be initiated at a low but relatively safe dose of 12.5 mg to 25 mg bid, depending on the response to the first dose, which is somewhat predictive of the long-term antihypertensive effect.[83]

In patients with renal insufficiency, the plasma and extracellular fluid volumes tend to be expanded.[84,85] In these settings, hypertension is usually volume-dependent, and more intensified diuretic therapy is often the most effective therapy for establishing arterial pressure control.[86,87]

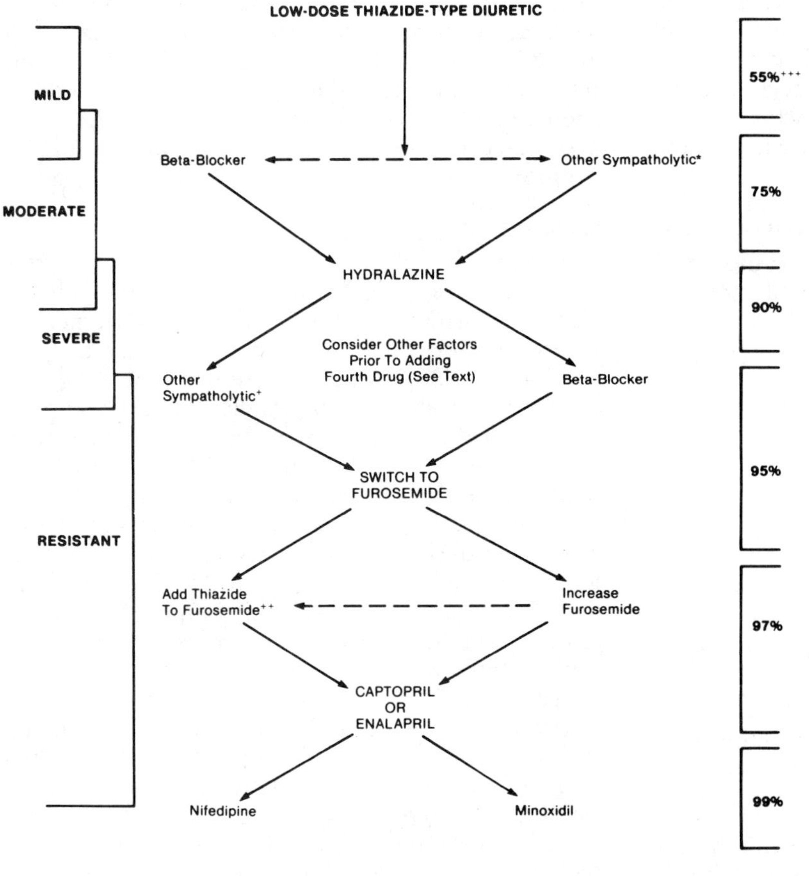

FIGURE 51-1 A typical pharmacologic scheme for the management of progressively severe degrees of essential hypertension. *Methyldopa, clonidine, guanabenz, prazosin, or reserpine. †Such as the addition of either methyldopa, clonidine, or prazosin. ††In patients with accelerated or malignant hypertension, it is often preferable to try converting enzyme inhibitors prior to more vigorous diuresis. †††Estimated percentages of patients usually controlled to diastolic pressures below 90 mmHg if compliant with the prescribed treatment regimen.

Patients with accelerated or malignant hypertension usually have severe hyperreninemia and secondary aldosteronism. In this setting, volume contraction (in the absence of a converting-enzyme inhibitor) can cause further elevation of plasma angiotensin II and aldosterone levels. In such cases, blockade of the renin-angiotensin system with captopril or enalapril should generally be accomplished prior to the institution of more intensified diuretic therapy unless there is evidence of volume overload. However, converting-enzyme inhibitors must be employed with caution in this setting. The likelihood of renovascular hypertension is increased in patients with accelerated or malignant hypertension,[88] and acute renal failure can result from therapy with captopril or enalapril if the patient has bilateral renal artery stenosis or renal artery stenosis in a solitary kidney.[89]

When hypertension remains refractory, then consideration should be given to the use of minoxidil. However, therapy with minoxidil is frequently limited by side effects such as facial hirsutism, serosanguineous pericardial effusions, and marked fluid retention that may be difficult to control. Other treatment modalities include combined alpha-beta blockade with prazosin and propranolol (or labetalol, a combined alpha-beta blocker) or the use of combined central-peripheral alpha-inhibitors (e.g., with methyldopa and prazosin). The latter combination is particularly effective in lowering upright blood pressure (i.e., in patients with severe orthostatic hypertension), but is relatively contraindicated in patients with orthostatic hypotension. The calcium channel blocking agent nifedipine is also a potent antihypertensive drug, which is effective in the management of selected cases of refractory hypertension.[90,91] For further discussion of the calcium channel blocking agents, see Chap. 91.

Fig. 51-1 provides a schematic representation of the previously outlined general approach to pharmacologic therapy in patients with mild or moderate essential hypertension, as well as cases of more severe and resistant hypertension.

Nonpharmacologic Therapy for Selected Cases of Mild Hypertension

Three major nonpharmacologic therapies for elevated blood pressure are dietary salt restriction, weight reduction, and dietary potassium supplementation. These interventions may be used alone or in combination. This is particularly true when diastolic blood pressure is between 90 and 94 mmHg in patients below age 50 who have no other cardiovascular risk factors (e.g., hypercholesterolemia, diabetes mellitus, male sex, black race, family history of cardiovascular disease) or evidence of target organ damage. They are also used as adjunctive measures in patients receiving drug therapy.

Dietary Salt Restriction

Kawasaki and associates[92] have demonstrated that some hypertensive individuals are "salt-sensitive," whereas others are "salt-resistant." Salt-sensitive patients tend to retain sodium, gain weight, and develop a rise in blood pressure on a high-salt diet. In contrast, salt-resistant patients tend to have no change in weight or blood pressure on either a high- or low-salt diet.[93] This individual variability in response to salt helps explain why some persons have excellent blood pressure reduction following dietary salt restriction,[94] whereas in others blood pressure remains unchanged.[95,96]

Extreme degrees of salt restriction are not necessary for improvement of blood pressure. For example, several studies have shown that diets containing 1600 to 2300 mg of sodium per day (i.e., equivalent to 70 to 100 meq of sodium) are associated with average reductions in systolic pressure of −9 to −15 mmHg and decreases in diastolic pressure of −7 to −16 mmHg.[97–100] Salt restriction in the range of 2000 mg sodium daily is thus recommended for the dietary management of most hypertensive patients.

Overnight urine collection is a useful technique to assess compliance to dietary sodium restriction.[101,102] Patients are instructed to empty their bladder at 10:00 P.M., then collect all subsequent urine until 6:00 or 7:00 A.M. the following day. A reasonable intervention goal for most hypertensive patients is reduction of the overnight urinary sodium content by one-third or more. The reduction in salt intake can also be estimated by dipsticks that measure urinary chloride concentrations, although this method would overestimate salt intake in patients taking supplemental potassium chloride. Small group sessions to discuss dietary sodium intake (as reflected by overnight urinary sodium excretion) have been reported to be more effective than the more customary methods of dietary advice or educational programs.[103]

Weight Reduction

Approximately 23 to 36 percent of Americans are overweight, ranging from 19 percent of younger black men to 51 percent of older black women.[104] The prevalence of hypertension is increased by 54 percent to 142 percent in obese patients.

Significant short-term weight loss is usually associated with a reduction in blood pressure. In a review of six controlled studies in hypertensive patients, Hovell[105] calculated an average reduction in blood pressure of −20.7/−12.7 mmHg in patients who accomplished an average weight loss of 11.7 kg. Reisin and associates[106] studied 24 overweight patients with untreated and uncomplicated hypertension and 57 overweight patients who were receiving antihypertensive therapy. After 6 months of an 800- to 1200-calorie diet, the average weight reduction was 10.5 kg, and all but two patients had a meaningful decrease in blood pressure. The reduction in blood pressure correlated with the change in weight. A similar study was conducted by Ramsay et al.[107] on 10 untreated and 39 treated overweight patients with hypertension. A significant correlation between weight change and blood pressure change was found, predicting a fall in blood pressure of −2.5/−1.5 mmHg per kilogram of reduction in body weight. An excellent review of the subject is provided by Langford and Watson.[108]

Dietary Potassium Supplementation
Considerable attention has focused recently on the possible role of a high dietary potassium intake in improving blood pressure in patients with mild hypertension.[109–111] MacGregor and associates[112] studied the effects of oral potassium supplements (60 meq daily for 8 weeks) in 23 hypertensive patients on a normal sodium intake (140 to 169 meq/day). Average blood pressure fell significantly from 154/99 to 148/95 mmHg over an 8-week period.

The blood-pressure lowering effect of supplemental potassium may be greater in patients receiving a high-salt diet. For example, Iimura and colleagues[113] reported a reduction of mean arterial pressure from 114 to 103 mmHg when a high-potassium diet (175 meq daily) was superimposed on a high-salt diet (260 meq daily) in 20 patients with uncomplicated hypertension.

These reductions in mean arterial pressure with supplemental dietary potassium are generally less than those experienced by patients who respond to salt restriction or weight reduction programs. Moreover, the amount of dietary potassium required to demonstrate this effect (i.e., 60 to 175 meq daily) is not obtained easily, and would certainly carry a risk of hyperkalemia if prescribed to patients with undetected renal insufficiency. Hence, supplemental dietary potassium is not currently recommended as primary nonpharmacologic therapy for hypertension, although further study is clearly indicated.

Treatment of Secondary Hypertension

Renovascular Hypertension

Several factors influence the choice between medical or surgical management of renovascular hypertension, or treatment with percutaneous transluminal renal angioplasty (PTRA) using the balloon-dilatation technique. The type of renal artery lesion is of major importance. Patients with fibrous dysplasia are more likely to benefit from surgery or balloon angioplasty than those with atherosclerotic renovascular disease.[114–117]

Grim and Weinberger compared the results of surgery versus balloon angioplasty in the treatment of renovascular hypertension due to fibrous dysplasia and atherosclerosis of the renal artery.[118] In patients with fibrous dysplasia, approximately 90 percent were improved or cured of hypertension, regardless of which procedure was employed, whereas in those with atherosclerosis the improvement rate was substantially higher with surgery than balloon angioplasty.[119] However, some have found balloon angioplasty to be beneficial in the treatment of selected cases of atherosclerotic renovascular disease,[120] although the overall improvement rates for atherosclerotic disease are still substantially below those achieved in patients with fibrous dysplasia.[114,118,119]

In addition to a higher improvement rate, patients with fibrous dysplasia also have a lower operative risk following surgical revascularization than those with atherosclerotic renovascular disease. For example, in the Cooperative Study of Renovascular Hypertension (which involved 15 institutions in the United States), the improvement rate following surgical revascularization or nephrectomy was up to 80 percent in patients with unilateral fibrous dysplasia, whereas the operative mortality was 3 percent.[115,116] This contrasts with the atherosclerotic group, in which the improvement rate was 63 percent and the operative mortality was over 9 percent. The mortality rate associated with balloon angioplasty would appear to be negligible, although complications (e.g., acute renal failure, renal infarction, renal artery dissection) have been reported in up to 16 percent of cases.[114,120,121] Most complications associated with balloon angioplasty are relatively minor (e.g., transient elevations of the serum creatinine), although end-stage renal failure requiring chronic hemodialysis has been reported, mainly in patients with atherosclerotic renovascular disease in a solitary kidney.[118] Restenosis is not an uncommon event, and a substantial number of patients require repeat balloon-dilatation procedures to maintain patency of the renal artery.[118,122]

In general, treatment with balloon angioplasty or surgical revascularization would appear to be preferable to medical treatment in many patients with fibrous dysplasia, particularly when hypertension is of less than three years duration and renal function is not yet impaired. In many cases of atherosclerotic renal artery disease, medical treatment may be preferable to surgery or balloon angioplasty because of the lessened chance of improvement of hypertension. This is particularly true since the advent of converting-enzyme inhibitors such as captopril and enalapril, which interfere with production of angiotensin II. However, converting-enzyme inhibitors must generally be avoided if the renal artery stenosis is severe and bilateral, or if stenosis exists in a solitary kidney. This is because acute deterioration in renal function has been reported to occur in these two settings following the initiation of therapy with captopril or enalapril.[89,123] Surgical intervention or balloon angioplasty may be preferred, however, in selected patients with atherosclerotic renovascular disease;[120,122] this is particularly true in younger patients (i.e., below age 50 or 55) in whom atherosclerosis appears localized to the renal artery and/or when blood pressure cannot be controlled with drug therapy.

In general, hypertension of relatively short duration (i.e., less than 3 years) is more likely to be relieved by surgery than when present for longer periods.[115,124,125] Younger patients are generally better operative candidates because they are more apt to have a shorter duration of hypertension, as well as less target organ damage and associated vascular disease. For example, Lawrie et al. reported on the 5- and 10-year follow-up of 505 hypertensive patients who underwent reconstructive surgery for renovascular disease at Baylor College of Medicine.[126] Age at time of surgery was found to be the most important factor determining long-term blood pressure response; the presence of diffuse atherosclerosis was a less powerful determinant. The factors that correlated best with long-term survival following renal revascularization surgery were age, sex (women fared better than men), and the presence of fibrous dysplasia; persistent severe hypertension and diffuse atherosclerosis exerted important but lesser influences.

Target organ damage (e.g., left ventricular hypertrophy or renal insufficiency) and coronary or cerebral atherosclerosis are also important determinants of operative risk and surgical response. In the Cooperative Study of Renovascular Hypertension, the presence of either angina pectoris, previous myocardial infarction, or renal insufficiency (defined by a serum creatinine of 1.4 mg/dl or greater) was associated with more than a fourfold increase in the mortality rate associated with surgical revascularization or nephrectomy.[116] Elevation of the serum creatinine (in patients with unilateral renal artery stenosis) implies that nephrosclerosis is present in the contralateral kidney and that the chance of a favorable surgical outcome is reduced markedly.[127] However, there are a number of reports (mostly in patients with bilateral atherosclerotic renovascular disease) of improvement of renal function following successful surgical revascularization;[128] the possibility of surgical intervention may warrant consideration in patients with bilateral renal artery stenosis who also have renal insufficiency, more so when one kidney is of relatively normal size.[128]

If the decision has been made to treat renovascular hypertension medically, the clinician must assume responsibility for maintaining arterial pressure control and for periodic assessment of renal size and function. Inadequate control of arterial pressure or further deterioration of renal function may indicate the need for repeat investigations (i.e., renal ultrasound and/or isotopic studies, digital subtraction angiography, renal arteriography, or renal vein renins). This is because the anatomic or functional characteristics of the stenosis may have changed as a result of progression of the disease since the original investigations.

Renoparenchymal Hypertension

Weidmann and Maxwell[129] reported that elevated blood pressure was present in 83 percent of 290 patients with end-stage renal disease presenting to dialysis centers in Australia, Europe, and the United States. The most common types of primary kidney disease associated with hypertension are chronic glomerulonephritis, diabetic nephropathy, polycystic kidney disease, collagen vascular disease, chronic pyelonephritis, and interstitial renal disease, approximately in that order.

Early stages of chronic renal failure associated with hypertension are characterized by a high cardiac output, a relatively normal peripheral resistance, and hypervolemia.[85,130] With the possible exception of patients with accelerated or malignant hypertension, blood pressure correlates better with total body sodium stores than with the level of plasma renin activity.[84] Because of the expanded blood volume and increased body content of sodium, vigorous diuretic therapy is frequently required to control blood pressure.

Diuretics

The hypertension of renal failure is classically responsive to volume depletion. Conversely, inadequate volume contraction is by far the most frequent cause of hypertension that remains uncontrolled, despite seemingly adequate therapy. Thiazide-type diuretics, with the exception of metolazone, are relatively ineffective when the glomerular filtration rate is less than 25 ml/min. Accordingly, loop diuretics such as furosemide, bumetanide, or ethacrynic acid are usually required for patients who have a serum creatinine level above approximately 3 mg/dl. The recommended starting dose for furosemide is 40 mg twice daily, increasing to a maximum total daily dosage of 480 mg as needed. For bumetanide, the recommended initial dosage is 0.5 mg twice daily, increasing to a maximum total daily dosage of 10 mg if necessary. Reduction of body weight is the simplest clinical indicator of diuretic response.

Potassium-sparing diuretics (e.g., spironolactone, triamterene, amiloride) are generally contraindicated in patients with any degree of renal failure because of the risk of hyperkalemia.

Beta Blockers: Propranolol, Metoprolol, and Nadolol

Advanced stages of renal failure are characterized by high cardiac output, increased total peripheral resistance, and expanded plasma and total blood volumes.[131] The elevated blood pressure appears to be mediated primarily by increased total peripheral resistance because red blood cell transfusion corrects the anemia and high cardiac output, but does not improve hypertension.[132] In addition, plasma renin activity is usually higher in hypertensive patients with advanced renal failure than in those with uncomplicated essential hypertension.[133] The increased plasma renin activity, elevated peripheral resistance, and expanded blood volume often require therapy with a sympatholytic drug as well as effective volume contraction in order to achieve adequate control of blood pressure.

Beta blockers are effective antihypertensive drugs in patients with renal failure. As with most other antipressor drugs, however, the reduction in blood pressure may be associated with a modest (i.e., 10 to 20 percent) rise in serum creatinine concentration. Maggiore and associates[134] reported that 160 to 480 mg daily of propranolol was effective in lowering blood pressure in many patients on chronic hemodialysis.

Minimal or no adjustment of the usual dosage of propranolol or metoprolol is required in patients with renal failure even though there is accumulation of the 4-hydroxy and glucuronide metabolites of propranolol[135] and the α-hydroxy metabolite of metoprolol.[136] In contrast, however, nadolol and atenolol are excreted primarily by the kidneys and reduction in dosage is necessary in patients with renal failure. For example, nadolol can be given every other day in patients with creatinine clearances of 10 ml/min or less.[137]

The serum potassium concentration must be monitored closely when beta blockers are used in patients with renal failure. This is because occasional patients manifest more than the usual 0.2 to 0.3 meq/liter rise in serum potassium. Elevation of the serum potassium results mainly from the blockade of beta-receptor-mediated uptake of potassium into muscle.[138]

Vasodilators: Hydralazine and Minoxidil

Hydralazine is effective in lowering total peripheral vascular resistance and reducing blood pressure in patients with renal failure. When blood pressure is lowered with hydralazine, the reflex tachycardia and increased cardiac output tend to preserve renal blood flow. The metabolic degradation of hydralazine is decreased markedly when the glomerular filtration rate is reduced below 40 ml/min. In this setting, the half-life of hydralazine is prolonged twofold or more.[139]

Minoxidil is an extremely potent vasodilator and is generally reserved for patients with resistant hypertension. Like hydralazine, it tends to preserve renal blood flow in patients with chronic renal failure. Volume retention is a prominent side effect of minoxidil, and patients can retain up to 10 lb of edema and develop signs of congestive heart failure during the initial 1 to 2 weeks of therapy if loop diuretics are not used judiciously. Minoxidil can also cause a noninflammatory serosanguineous pericardial effusion that can be confused with uremic pericarditis.

Prazosin

Prazosin is an effective drug in patients with chronic renal failure, although severe orthostatic hypotension can occur.[140,141] Peak plasma levels and the hypotensive effect of prazosin are both increased in patients with chronic renal failure.[142] Unlike propranolol, prazosin does not cause a rise in serum triglyceride levels, or a reduction in the HDL cholesterol concentration in dialysis patients.[143] This "lipid-sparing" effect of prazosin may be particularly advantageous in the subset of dialysis patients who are prone to accelerated atherosclerosis.[144]

Methyldopa

In end-stage renal disease, the half-life of methyldopa is increased approximately twofold and there is an accumulation of the active metabolite, methyldopa-*O*-sulfate. This may account for the orthostatic hypotension sometimes observed following treatment with methyldopa in patients with advanced renal insufficiency.[145] Methyldopa is readily dialyzed and elevation of blood pressure can occur during peritoneal dialysis or hemodialysis.[146]

Clonidine

Clonidine is as effective as either methyldopa or metoprolol in lowering blood pressure in dialysis patients.[147] In end-stage renal disease, the half-life of clonidine is increased approximately twofold, and once daily dosages can usually be employed, starting with 0.1 mg administered at bedtime. The hemodialysance of clonidine is relatively low and postdialysis rebound hypertension is infrequent.[148]

Protein-Binding and Dialysance of Antihypertensive Drugs

Table 51-4 provides a listing of the protein-binding and dialysance of a number of antihypertensive drugs frequently prescribed in patients with renal failure. In general, compounds with a high degree of protein binding are not well dialyzed. The alteration in the plasma half-life of the parent drug or metabolites is indicated for those drugs in which this information is available. Several excellent resources are available for further details.[149–151]

Mineralocorticoid Hypertension

Primary Aldosteronism

The type of adrenal pathology (i.e., adenoma versus hyperplasia) is the most important factor influencing the choice between medical or surgical management of primary aldosteronism. Hypertension is almost always improved or cured by surgery in patients with adenomas. For example, Weinberger et al. reported on the follow-up of 38 patients with primary aldosteronism and unilateral adenoma who underwent surgery;[152] blood pressure was reduced to normotensive levels in 26 cases (or 68 percent). Moreover, hypertension was improved in the remaining 12 cases. Others have reported similar findings, although some have found that only about 50 percent of adenoma cases are cured completely of hypertension.[153,154] In contrast, relatively few patients with bilateral (zona glomerulosa) hyperplasia are surgically cured of hypertension, despite relief of hyperaldosteronism.[152,155] In general, surgical treatment is preferable to medical treatment in patients with aldosteronomas,[152,155,156] whereas medical treatment is almost always preferred in cases of bilateral hyperplasia.[154,157]

Rarely, adrenal, ovarian, and other carcinomas can present with hyperaldosteronism.[158–160] However, the levels of other adrenocortical steroids (e.g., 11-deoxycorticosterone, corticosterone) in addition

TABLE 51-4 Protein-Binding, Dialysance, and Altered Plasma Half-Life of Antihypertensive Drugs Used in Patients with Chronic Renal Failure

			Plasma Half-Life	
Drugs	Serum Protein-Binding, %	Dialysance	Normal, h	End-Stage Renal Disease
Captopril	+ (23–30)	?	4.3	156 h
Clonidine	+ (20–40)	± (27–48 ml/min)	10–17	35–41 h
Methyldopa	+ (< 20)	+ + + (60%)	1.7	3.6 h
Reserpine	+ + (40)	0	46–162	87–323 h
Guanethidine	0	Minimal	120	Unchanged?
Diazoxide	+ + + (85–90)	+ (23–28 ml/min)	17–36	Prolonged > 30 h
Nitroprusside	?	+ + +	0.2	Unchanged
Ethacrynic acid	+ + + (95)	0	1–4	Prolonged > 4 h
Bumetanide	+ + + (85–95)	?	0.8–2	2–3 h
Furosemide	+ + + (90–99)	0	0.5–1.5	2–14 h
Metolazone	+ + + (90–95)	0	6–15	Prolonged > 15 h
Hydralazine	+ + + (85–87)	0	1.7–3	7–16 h
Minoxidil	0	+ (24–43)	4.2	Unchanged?
Metoprolol	+ (12)	+ +	2.5–5	*
Atenolol	0 (< 5)	?	6–9	42 h
Nadolol	+ (20–30)	+ + (46–102 ml/min)	14–24	45 h
Propranolol	+ + + (90–97)	± (18.5 ml/min)	3.5–6	1.1–6.2 h
Pindolol	+ + (57)	?	3–4	Unchanged
Prazosin	+ + + (97)	Minimal	2.5–9	Unchanged
Verapamil	+ + + (90)	Minimal	3–7	?

*The plasma half-life of metoprolol is presumably unchanged, but the half-life of the α-hydroxy metabolite, one-tenth as active as metoprolol, is prolonged from 5 to 60 h.

to aldosterone, are usually elevated.[161] In general, urinary 17-ketosteroid and 17-hydroxycorticosteroid excretion and/or plasma cortisol levels should be measured in patients suspected of having primary aldosteronism to ensure that they are normal. As a precautionary measure, patients who may undergo bilateral exploration and manipulation of the adrenal glands should have glucocorticoids administered during surgery, and then tapered during the postoperative period. Surgical "coverage" with corticosteroids may not always be necessary in patients who undergo unilateral adrenalectomy, provided that the contralateral adrenal gland is unimpaired.[161]

The aldosterone antagonist, spironolactone, is the drug of choice for the treatment of bilateral hyperplasia, as well as for the medical management of patients with adenomas who are unable or unwilling to undergo surgery.[154,162] The usual effective dose of spironolactone ranges between 100 mg and 400 mg per day, and a dose of 200 mg per day or more is frequently required. The addition of a thiazide-type diuretic may further improve blood pressure control, and allow a reduction in the dosage of spironolactone.[163] When patients are unable to tolerate spironolactone because of adverse effects (e.g., gastrointestinal upset, breast tenderness, gynecomastia, menstrual irregularities, impotence), other potassium-sparing diuretics such as triamterene and amiloride can be employed. However, these agents may be less effective than spironolactone in this setting.[154]

In patients with aldosteronomas in whom surgery is planned, spironolactone (or possibly amiloride or triamterene) should be administered preoperatively for a period of 4 to 6 weeks. This allows the attainment of arterial pressure control, as well as normalization of sodium and potassium stores prior to surgery.[154] Some have suggested that preoperative therapy with spironolactone may also reduce the usual period of postoperative hypoaldosteronism following the removal of the adenoma,[164,165] although others have not found this.[166] Postoperative hypoaldosteronism is associated with an increased risk of hyperkalemia,[165] and potassium supplements should not be administered routinely in the postoperative period. Furthermore, the discontinuation of spironolactone therapy several days or more prior to surgery may also reduce the risk of developing hyperkalemia in the postoperative period.[161]

Glucocorticoid-suppressible primary aldosteronism is a rare variety which is often familial (i.e., usually inherited as an autosomal dominant trait). It is associated with the pathologic finding of bilateral adrenocortical hyperplasia. In this subtype of primary aldosteronism, hypertension and hypokalemia are relieved by glucocorticoid replacement therapy (e.g., dexamethasone, 1 to 2 mg daily).[154,167]

Other Varieties of Mineralocorticoid Hypertension

There are a number of other varieties of mineralocorticoid hypertension that are encountered less frequently than primary aldosteronism (see Table 50-6). For example, two varieties of congenital adrenal hyperplasia, the 17-α-hydroxylase and the 11-β-hydroxylase deficiencies, are associated with excessive production of mineralocorticoid hormones and can present with hypertension and hypokalemia.[168–170] The adrenocortical enzymatic defects that characterize these disorders result in deficient production of cortisol and hypersecretion of ACTH. In both of these entities, 11-deoxycorticosterone (DOC) is one of the major mineralocorticoid hormones secreted; plasma renin and aldosterone levels are both generally decreased.[171] Hypertension and hypokalemia are responsive to glucocorticoid-replacement therapy. In the 17-α-hydroxylase deficiency, the enzymatic defect is also present in the ovary and testis, and estrogen or androgen replacement therapy may be indicated.[170,171] Such patients may also be sensitive to low doses of glucocorticoid replacement therapy.[171] For a discussion of Cushing's syndrome, see reference 172.

Pheochromocytoma

Once the diagnosis of pheochromocytoma is established, specific pharmacologic treatment is indicated in preparation for surgery.[173,174] Therapy is selected primarily to reduce the elevated total peripheral resistance that characterizes the hypertension of pheochromocytoma,[175] and to counteract the alpha-mediated vasoconstriction induced by the high levels of norepinephrine. Phentolamine (Regitine), a nonselective alpha blocker, is the recommended initial therapy. Intravenous bolus doses of 1, 2, or 5 mg usually reduce blood pressure promptly, although the effect is transient (i.e., 10 to 20 min), and an intravenous drip is typically required. One hundred mg of phentolamine can be dissolved into 500 ml of dextrose and water, providing a concentration of 200 μg/ml that can be infused initially at a rate of 10 μg/kg/min. Sodium nitroprusside is an effective alternative therapy.[176]

After marked elevations of blood pressure are controlled with parenteral treatment, oral therapy is usually begun with phenoxybenzamine (Dibenzyline), a nonselective alpha blocker. The usual initial dosage in adults is 10 mg twice daily, although total daily doses of 80 to 160 mg are not unusual, and some patients are resistant to even higher doses.[177] Prazosin, a selective blocker of postsynaptic alpha receptors, can be used as alternative therapy,[178,179] although not all patients respond satisfactorily.[180] However, diagnostic tests for pheochromocytoma should be completed prior to instituting therapy with prazosin because it can cause a twofold or more increase in the plasma levels of norepinephrine, as well as a modest rise in urinary vanillylmandelic acid (VMA) excretion.[181]

The usual tachycardia of patients with pheochromocytoma can be exaggerated by the use of either phenoxybenzamine or nitroprusside. Although the tachycardia can be inhibited by beta blockers such as propranolol, these drugs must *not* be used prior to the establishment of adequate alpha blockade. This is because blockade of the $beta_1$ and $beta_2$ receptors, in the setting of continued unopposed stimulation of the alpha receptors, can cause a further rise in blood pressure. Theoretically, this pressor response to beta blockers would be diminished with the use of cardioselective beta blockers such as atenolol or metoprolol, but intravenous preparations of these drugs are not commonly available and clinical experience is thus far limited or absent.

In one case of pheochromocytoma associated with hypertrophic cardiomyopathy, the use of the calcium channel blocker, nifedipine, appeared to interfere with the release of norepinephrine.[182] This contrasts with the usual rise in the level of plasma norepinephrine following the administration of nifedipine to patients with essential hypertension.[183]

As a consequence of the high circulating level of catecholamines,[184] patients with pheochromocytoma often have marked reductions in plasma volume as well as an increased risk of hypotension during anesthesia and surgery. DeOreo and associates[185] demonstrated that transfusion of 2 units of blood within 24 h of surgery was a useful preoperative measure. Vigorous volume repletion prior to surgery has since become a routine procedure for the preoperative management of patients with pheochromocytoma.

The preoperative use of alpha blockers does not completely prevent the marked fluctuations in blood pressure than can occur during anesthesia and surgery in patients with pheochromocytoma.[185] In selected cases, preoperative therapy with alpha blockers may be omitted when difficulty with intraoperative localization of the tumor is anticipated.

The preferred surgical incision is transabdominal, although a flank approach is occasionally used in patients who clearly have unilateral tumors that have been identified by the CT or ^{131}meta-iodobenzylguanidine (^{131}I-MIBG) scan. Adequate surgical removal of a benign tumor is associated with cure of hypertension in 60 to 80 percent of patients, and a 5-year survival of approximately 96 percent.[173] However, 6 to 13 percent of tumors are malignant and the 5-year survival of such cases is only 44 percent. Alpha-methylparatyrosine (Demser), an inhibitor of tyrosine hydroxylase, is used as chemotherapy for malignant tumors that are unresectable or associated with metastases.[186]

Patients with pheochromocytoma, especially those with the familial varieties or with bilateral tumors, should be evaluated routinely for hyperparathyroidism and medullary thyroid carcinoma. Adequate screening includes serum calcium as well as measurements of both parathyroid hormone and calcitonin levels.

Coarctation of the Aorta (see Chap. 36)

Oral Contraceptive Hypertension

Like essential hypertension, a single measurement of elevated blood pressure is insufficient for a diagnosis of hypertension in oral contraceptive users. The diagnosis should be based on elevations of blood pressure that are present on two or more separate occasions.[187]

The treatment of oral contraceptive hypertension consists of discontinuation of the oral contraceptive and substitution of an alternate contraceptive method such as a diaphragm, an intrauterine device, or foam and condoms. Oral contraceptives that contain progestins but no estrogens (i.e., "minipills") may be substituted in selected cases. This is because there is no evidence that the currently marketed type of minipill (i.e., 0.35 mg norethisterone) causes elevation of blood pressure.[188]

In cases where the diagnosis of oral contraceptive-induced hypertension seems well established, no immediate pharmacologic therapy is indicated if the diastolic blood pressure is only mildly elevated (i.e., in the 90 to 104 mmHg range) because blood pressure returns to normal within 3 to 6 months in half to two-thirds of cases.[189] However, when hypertension persists for 6 months or more after discontinuation of the oral contraceptive, the diagnosis of pill-induced hypertension is unlikely and patients should undergo the usual hypertensive diagnostic evaluation and treatment schemes recommended earlier. This is because oral contraceptive use may provoke hypertension in some women who have a predisposition to essential hypertension, or who have an underlying secondary cause of hypertension. For example, the investigation of hypertension in oral contraceptive users has unveiled cases of renal artery stenosis, primary aldosteronism, Cushing's disease, and chronic pyelonephritis.

Furthermore, Woods and associates[190] noted the reappearance of hypertension in seven of 14 women who were followed for periods up to 5 years. In all these cases, blood pressure had normalized initially following discontinuation of the oral contraceptives. Thus, blood pressure should be monitored at regular intervals in all women with hypertension attributed to oral contraceptive use, even if it returns to normal after discontinuation of the pill.

If the diastolic blood pressure is elevated to levels of 105 mmHg or more, the clinician should probably initiate antihypertensive therapy simultaneously with discontinuation of the oral contraceptive. Low-dose diuretic therapy is typically effective in this setting, probably because oral contraceptive hypertension is associated with an increase in blood volume and cardiac output.[191,192] Cases of oral contraceptive hypertension may also respond to blockade of angiotensin II,[193] thus also attesting to a role of renin.[194]

Hypertension may also accompany postmenopausal use of conjugated estrogens such as Premarin.[195] Crane and Harris[196] studied 27 women (average age 54) in whom the onset of hypertension was reported to have occurred after using Premarin (usual dose of 1.25 mg daily) for an average period of 4.7 years. Thirteen of 27 patients (48 percent) became normotensive during an average period of 2½ months following discontinuation of Premarin.

Gestational Hypertension

The two major hypertensive disorders of pregnancy are preeclampsia (toxemia, pregnancy-induced hypertension) and chronic essential hypertension. Together they represent the leading cause of prematurity, fetal death, and maternal death.[197] These risks underscore the importance of early diagnosis and therapy. Following is a summary of the risks and benefits of a variety of antihypertensive drugs used in the pregnant patient.[198–200]

Diuretics

Prophylactic thiazide therapy does not alter the incidence of preeclampsia.[201] Moreover, thiazide therapy for active preeclampsia may be associated with adverse fetal effects including low birth weight,[202] neonatal jaundice, and neonatal thrombocytopenia.[203] The potentially deleterious effects of thiazide diuretics[204] or furosemide[205] on the fetus presumably reflect decreased placental perfusion, as gauged by studies that show impaired conversion of dehydroepiandrosterone sulfate to estradiol.[206] Diuretics are considered relatively contraindicated in patients with preeclampsia, more so since the documentation that these patients have a lower than expected blood volume.[207] In 1977, the FDA summarized the limited utility of diuretics in pregnancy and removed toxemia and hypertension of pregnancy as indications for diuretic therapy.[208] Others disagree and have defended the use of diuretics in hypertensive disorders of pregnancy.[209]

Thiazides and chlorthalidone decrease lactation, but are present in only minimal concentrations in breast milk.[210]

Hydralazine

Marked reductions of blood pressure with hydralazine can be associated with proportional decreases in uterine blood flow[211] or placental function,[205] although hydralazine appears to spare uterine blood flow better than does nitroprusside.[212] Initial oral doses of 25 mg twice daily can be increased to a maximum total daily dose of 300 mg, but the reduction of blood pressure may be limited by reflex sympathetic stimulation, expansion of the blood volume, and hyperreninemia. Hydralazine can also be given intravenously in bolus doses of 5 to 15 mg, or it can be infused as a solution of 25 to 50 mg of hydralazine dissolved into 500 ml of saline solution and given at an initial infusion rate of 0.2 to 0.5 mg/min.

Hydralazine crosses the placenta and appears in breast milk.[213]

Methyldopa

Antihypertensive therapy with methyldopa appears to have particular benefit in reducing the risk of midtrimester abortions when the onset of hypertension is prior to the twentieth week of gestation.[214] In a series of 117 women treated with methyldopa, Redman et al. observed no significant deleterious effects on the fetus.[215] There has been some concern, however, about slight reductions in the head size of neonates born to mothers who have received treatment with methyldopa between the sixteenth and twentieth week of gestation, although head size was reported to return to normal within 6 months following delivery.[216] In addition, methyldopa crosses the placenta and can be associated with slight reductions in neonatal blood pressure during the first 2 days following delivery.[217] Methyldopa may also appear in breast milk, and low plasma levels of the drug have been found in breastfed infants.[210]

Beta Blockers

Propranolol, oxprenolol, metoprolol, atenolol, and the combined alpha-beta blocker, labetalol, have all been used successfully to control hypertension in pregnancy.[218–220] Reductions in blood pressure and fetal outcomes have been as good or better as with the use of either methyldopa or hydralazine. Adverse fetal effects reported following maternal therapy with beta blockers include reduced birth weight, neonatal bradycardia, and neonatal hypoglycemia.

Most beta blockers (e.g., atenolol, metoprolol, nadolol, oxprenolol, pindolol, timolol) are secreted into breast milk in a concentration that is higher than maternal plasma.[210] Propranolol is also secreted into breast milk, but usually in a concentration below that of maternal plasma. Hence, propranolol, at least when prescribed in relatively low doses, may be the preferred drug when a beta blocker is indicated for control of blood pressure in a breastfeeding mother.

Other Antihypertensive Drugs

Reserpine is generally not used in pregnancy because it crosses the placenta, and can cause marked fetal lethargy as well as respiratory distress due to upper airway congestion. Experience with the use of clonidine[221] or prazosin[222] is limited and further study is warranted before any recommendations can be made.

Low doses of diazoxide (i.e., 150 mg or less) given intravenously are effective in reducing blood pressure in patients with severe preeclampsia, but diazoxide abolishes uterine contractility and has also been associated with fetal bradycardias.[223] Sodium nitroprusside is contraindicated in pregnancy because it crosses the placenta and causes fetal cyanide toxicity.[224]

References

1. Gifford, R. W., Jr.: Practical Clinical Pharmacology of Antihypertensive Drugs, in D. G. Vidt (ed.), "Cleveland Clinic Cardiovascular Consultations," Cardiovascular Clinics, vol. 7, F. A. Davis Company, Philadelphia, 1975, p. 143.
2. The Joint National Committee on Detection, Evaluation, and Treatment of High Blood Pressure: The 1984 Report of the Joint National Committee on Detection, Evaluation, and Treatment of High Blood Pressure, *Arch. Intern. Med.*, 144:1045, 1984.
3. Laragh, J. H., Cannon, P. J., Stason, W. B., and Heinemann, H. O.: Physiologic and Clinical Observations on Furosemide and Ethacrynic Acid, *Ann. N.Y. Acad. Sci.*, 139:453, 1966.
4. Kaplan, N. M.: Our Appropriate Concern about Hypokalemia, *Am. J. Med.*, 77:1, 1984. (Editorial.)
5. Licht, J. H., Haley, R. J., Pugh, B., and Lewis, S. B.: Diuretic Regimens in Essential Hypertension. A Comparison of Hypokalemic Effects, BP Control, and Cost, *Arch. Intern. Med.*, 143:1694, 1983.
6. Morgan, D. B., and Davidson, C.: Hypokalaemia and Diuretics: An Analysis of Publications, *Br. Med. J.*, 280:905, 1980.
7. Lawson, D. H.: Adverse Reactions to Potassium Chloride, *Q. J. Med.*, 43:433, 1974.
8. Greenblatt, D. J., and Koch-Weser, J.: Adverse Reactions to Spironolactone. A Report from the Boston Collaborative Drug Surveillance Program, *JAMA*, 225:40, 1973.
9. Morganti, A., Pickering, T. G., Lopez-Ovejero, J. A., and Laragh, J. H.: High and Low Renin Subgroups of Essential Hypertension: Differences and Similarities in Their Renin and Sympathetic Responses to Neural and Nonneural Stimuli, *Am. J. Cardiol.*, 46:306, 1980.
10. Esler, M., Julius, S., Zweifler, A., Randall, O., Harburg, E., Gardiner, H., and DeQuattro, V.: Mild High-Renin Essential Hypertension. Neurogenic Human Hypertension? *N. Engl. J. Med.*, 296:405, 1977.
11. Esler, M., Zweifler, A., Randall, O., and DeQuattro, V.: Pathophysiologic and Pharmacokinetic Determinants of the Antihypertensive Response to Propranolol, *Clin. Pharmacol. Ther.*, 22:299, 1977.
12. Hollifield, J. W., Sherman, K., Zwagg, R. V., and Shand, D. G.: Proposed Mechanisms of Propranolol's Antihypertensive Effect in Essential Hypertension, *N. Engl. J. Med.*, 295:68, 1976.
13. Bühler, F. R., Laragh, J. H., Vaughan, E. D., Jr., Brunner, H. R., Gavras, H., and Baer, L.: Antihypertensive Action of Propranolol. Specific Anti-Renin Responses in High and Normal Renin Forms of Essential, Renal, Renovascular and Malignant Hypertension, *Am. J. Cardiol.*, 32:511, 1973.
14. Freis, E. D., Materson, B. J., and Flamenbaum, W.: Comparison of Propranolol or Hydrochlorothiazide Alone for Treatment of Hypertension. III. Evaluation of the Renin-Angiotensin System, *Am. J. Med.*, 74:1029, 1983.
15. Veterans Administration Cooperative Study Group on Antihypertensive Agents: Comparison of Propranolol and Hydrochlorothiazide for the Initial Treatment of Hypertension. I. Results of Short-Term Titration with Emphasis on Racial Differences in Response, *JAMA*, 248:1996, 1982.
16. Gorlin, R.: The Hyperkinetic Heart Syndrome, *JAMA*, 182:823, 1962.

17. Frohlich, E. D., Tarazi, R. C., and Dustan, H. P.: Hyperdynamic β-Adrenergic Circulatory State. Increased β-Receptor Responsiveness, *Arch. Intern. Med.*, 123:1, 1969.
18. Gillum, R. F., Teichholz, L. E., Herman, M. V., and Gorlin, R.: The Idiopathic Hyperkinetic Heart Syndrome: Clinical Course and Long-Term Prognosis, *Am. Heart J.*, 102:728, 1981.
19. Frohlich, E. D., Tarazi, R. C., Ulrych, M., Dustan, H. P., and Page, I. H.: Tilt Test for Investigating a Neural Component in Hypertension. Its Correlation with Clinical Characteristics, *Circulation*, 36:387, 1967.
20. Eide, I., Campese, V., Stein, D., Eide, K., and DeQuattro, V.: Clinical Assessment of Sympathetic Tone: Orthostatic Blood Pressure Responses in Borderline Primary Hypertension, *Clin. Exp. Hypertens.*, 1:51, 1978.
21. Esler, M. D., and Nestel, P. J.: Renin and Sympathetic Nervous System Responsiveness to Adrenergic Stimuli in Essential Hypertension, *Am. J. Cardiol.*, 32:643, 1973.
22. Esler, M. D., and Nestel, P. J.: Sympathetic Responsiveness to Head-Up Tilt in Essential Hypertension, *Clin. Sci.*, 44:213, 1973.
23. Affarah, H., Wollam, G. L., Hall, W. D., et al.: Unpublished observations, 1984.
24. Cressman, M., Bravo, E. L., and Pohl, M.: Cardiovascular and Neurohumoral Responses to Long-Term Central Sympathetic Inhibition in Essential Hypertension, *Clin. Res.*, 32:329, 1984. (Abstract.)
25. Messerli, F. H., Ventura, H. O., Elizardi, D. J., Dunn, F. G., and Frohlich, E. D.: Hypertension and Sudden Death. Increased Ventricular Ectopic Activity in Left Ventricular Hypertrophy, *Am. J. Med.*, 77:18, 1984.
26. Holland, O. B., Nixon, J. V., and Kuhnert, L.: Diuretic-Induced Ventricular Ectopic Activity, *Am. J. Med.*, 70:762, 1981.
27. Medical Research Council Working Party on Mild to Moderate Hypertension: Ventricular Extrasystoles during Thiazide Treatment: Substudy of MRC Mild Hypertension Trial, *Br. Med. J.*, 287:1249, 1983.
28. Papademetriou, V., Fletcher, R., Khatri, I. M., and Freis, E. D.: Diuretic-Induced Hypokalemia in Uncomplicated Systemic Hypertension: Effect of Plasma Potassium Correction on Cardiac Arrhythmias, *Am. J. Cardiol.*, 52:1017, 1983.
29. Hollifield, J. W., and Slaton, P. E.: Thiazide Diuretics, Hypokalemia and Cardiac Arrhythmias, *Acta. Med. Scand.*, 647(suppl.):67, 1981.
30. Dyckner, T., and Wester, P. O.: Relation between Potassium, Magnesium and Cardiac Arrhythmias, *Acta. Med. Scand.*, 647(suppl.):163, 1981.
31. Hollifield, J. W., and Slaton, P. E.: Cardiac Arrhythmias Associated with Diuretic Induced Hypokalemia and Hypomagnesaemia, in C. Wood and W. Somerville (eds.), "Arrhythmias and Myocardial Infarction: The Role of Potassium," Royal Society of Medicine, London, 1981, p. 17.
32. Struthers, A. D., Whitesmith, R., and Reid, J. L.: Prior Thiazide Diuretic Treatment Increases Adrenaline-Induced Hypokalaemia, *Lancet*, 1:1358, 1983.
33. Leren, P., Foss, P. O., Helgeland, A., Hjermann, I., Holme, I., and Lund-Larsen, P. G.: Effect of Propranolol and Prazosin on Blood Lipids. The Oslo Study, *Lancet*, 2:4, 1980.
34. Kirkendall, W. M., Hammond, J. J., Thomas, J. C., Overturf, M. L., and Zama, A.: Prazosin and Clonidine for Moderately Severe Hypertension, *JAMA*, 240:2553, 1978.
35. Ames, R. P., and Hill, P.: Elevation of Serum Lipid Levels During Diuretic Therapy of Hypertension, *Am. J. Med.*, 61:748, 1976.
36. Grimm, R. H., Jr., Leon, A. S., Hunninghake, D. B., Lenz, K., Hannan, P., and Blackburn, H.: Effects of Thiazide Diuretics on Plasma Lipids and Lipoproteins in Mildly Hypertensive Patients. A Double-Blind Controlled Trial, *Ann. Intern. Med.*, 94:7, 1981.
37. Goldman, A.I., Steele, B. W., Schnaper, H. W., Fitz, A. E., Frohlich, E. D., and Perry, H. M., Jr.: Serum Lipoprotein Levels During Chlorthalidone Therapy. A Veterans Administration–National Heart, Lung, and Blood Institute Cooperative Study on Antihypertensive Therapy: Mild Hypertension, *JAMA*, 244:1691, 1980.
38. Lasser, N. L., Grandits, G., Caggiula, A. W., et al.: Effects of Antihypertensive Therapy on Plasma Lipids and Lipoproteins in the Multiple Risk Factor Intervention Trial, *Am. J. Med.*, 76(suppl. 2A):52, 1984.
39. Ames, R. P., and Hill, P.: Antihypertensive Therapy and the Risk of Coronary Heart Disease, *J. Cardiovasc. Pharmacol.*, 4(suppl. 2):S206, 1982.
40. Ames, R. P., and Peacock, P. B.: Serum Cholesterol During Treatment of Hypertension with Diuretic Drugs, *Arch. Intern. Med.*, 144:710, 1984.
41. Glück, Z., Baumgartner, G., Weidmann, P., et al.: Increased Ratio Between Serum β- and α-Lipoproteins During Diuretic Therapy: An Adverse Effect? *Clin. Sci.*, 55(suppl. 4):325s, 1978.
42. Weidmann, P., Beretta-Piccoli, C., Keusch, G., et al.: Sodium-Volume Factor, Cardiovascular Reactivity and Hypotensive Mechanism of Diuretic Therapy in Mild Hypertension Associated with Diabetes Mellitus, *Am. J. Med.*, 67:779, 1979.
43. Christlieb, A. R.: Diabetes and Hypertension, *Cardiovasc. Rev. Rep.*, 1:609, 1980.
44. Mogensen, C. E.: Long-Term Antihypertensive Treatment Inhibiting Progression of Diabetic Nephropathy, *Br. Med. J.*, 285:685, 1982.
45. Parving, H.-H., Anderson, A. R., Smidt, U. M., Christiansen, J. S., Oxenbøll, B., and Svendsen, P. Aa.: Diabetic Nephropathy and Arterial Hypertension. The Effect of Antihypertensive Treatment, *Diabetes*, 32(suppl. 2):83, 1983.
46. Gorden, P., Sherman, B. M., and Simopoulos, A. P.: Glucose Intolerance with Hypokalemia: An Increased Proportion of Circulating Proinsulin-Like Component, *J. Clin. Endocrinol. Metab.*, 34:235, 1972.
47. Amery, A., Berthaux, P., Bulpitt, C., et al.: Glucose Intolerance during Diuretic Therapy. Results of Trial by the European Working Party on Hypertension in the Elderly, *Lancet*, 1:681, 1978.
48. Helderman, J. H., Elahi, D., Andersen, D. K., et al.: Prevention of the Glucose Intolerance of Thiazide Diuretics by Maintenance of Body Potassium, *Diabetes*, 32:106, 1983.
49. Fajans, S. S., Floyd, J. C., Jr., Knopf, R. F., Rull, J., Guntsche, E. M., and Conn, J. W.: Benzothiadiazine Suppression of Insulin Release from Normal and Abnormal Islet Tissue in Man, *J. Clin. Invest.*, 45:481, 1966.
50. Grunfeld, C., and Chappell, D. A.: Hypokalemia and Diabetes Mellitus, *Am. J. Med.*, 75:553, 1983.
51. McFarland, K. F., and Carr, A. A.: Changes in the Fasting Blood Sugar After Hydrochlorothiazide and Potassium Supplementation, *J. Clin. Pharmacol.*, 17:13, 1977.
52. Rapoport, M. I., and Hurd, H. F.: Thiazide-Induced Glucose Intolerance Treated with Potassium, *Arch. Intern. Med.*, 113:405, 1964.
53. Jackson, W. P. U., and Nellen, M.: Effect of Furosemide on Carbohydrate Metabolism, Blood-Pressure, and other Modalities: A Comparison with Chlorothiazide, *Br. Med. J.*, 2:333, 1966.
54. Abramson, E. A., Arky, R. A., and Woeber, K. A.: Effects of Propranolol on the Hormonal and Metabolic Responses to Insulin-Induced Hypoglycemia, *Lancet*, 2:1386, 1966.
55. Lager, I., Blohmé, G., and Smith, U.: Effect of Cardioselective and Non-Selective β-Blockade on the Hypoglycaemic Response in Insulin-Dependent Diabetics, *Lancet*, 1:458, 1979.
56. Molnar, G. W., and Read, R. C.: Propranolol Enhancement of Hypoglycemic Sweating, *Clin. Pharmacol. Ther.*, 15:490, 1974.
57. Davidson, N. McD., Corrall, R. J. M., Shaw, T. R. D., and French, E. B.: Observations in Man of Hypoglycaemia During Selective and Non-Selective Beta-Blockade, *Scott. Med. J.*, 22:69, 1977.
58. Ostman, J., Arner, P., Haglund, K., Juhlin-Dannfelt, A., Nowak, J., and Wennlund, A.: Effect of Metoprolol and Alprenolol on the Metabolic, Hormonal, and Haemodynamic Response to Insulin-Induced Hypoglycaemia in Hy-

pertensive, Insulin-Dependent Diabetics, *Acta. Med. Scand.*, 211:381, 1982.
59. Podolsky, S., and Pattavina, C. G.: Hyperosmolar Nonketotic Diabetic Coma: A Complication of Propranolol Therapy, *Metabolism*, 22:685, 1973.
60. Helgeland, A., Leren, P., Foss, O. P., Hjermann, I., Holme, I., and Lund-Larsen, P. G.: Serum Glucose Levels during Long-Term Observation of Treated and Untreated Men with Mild Hypertension. The Oslo Study, *Am. J. Med.*, 76:802, 1984.
61. Cerasi, E., Luft, R., and Efendić, S.: Effect of Adrenergic Blocking Agents on Insulin Response to Glucose Infusion in Man, *Acta. Endocrinol.*, 69:335, 1972.
62. Waal-Manning, H. J.: Metabolic Effects of β-Adrenoreceptor Blockers, *Drugs*, 11(suppl. 1):121, 1976.
63. Holm, G., Johansson, S., Vedin, A., Wilhelmsson, C., and Smith, U.: The Effect of Beta-Blockade on Glucose Tolerance and Insulin Release in Adult Diabetes, *Acta. Med. Scand.*, 208:187, 1980.
64. Groop, L., Tötterman, K.-J., Harno, K., and Gordin, A.: Influence of Beta-Blocking Drugs on Glucose Metabolism in Patients with Non-Insulin Dependent Diabetes Mellitus, *Acta. Med. Scand.*, 211:7, 1982.
65. Veterans Administration Cooperative Study Group on Antihypertensive Agents: Comparison of Prazosin with Hydralazine in Patients Receiving Hydrochlorothiazide. A Randomized, Double-Blind Clinical Trial, *Circulation*, 64:772, 1981.
66. Wollam, G. L., and Hall, W. D.: Resistant Hypertension, in M. Fernandes (ed.), "Evolving Concepts in Hypertension," vol. 1, no. 3, Biomedical Information Corporation, New York, 1980, p. 32.
67. Gifford, R. W., Jr., and Tarazi, R. C.: Resistant Hypertension: Diagnosis and Management, *Ann. Intern. Med.*, 88:661, 1978.
68. Hulka, B. S., Cassel, J. C., Kupper, L. L., and Burdette, J. A.: Communication, Compliance, and Concordance between Physicians and Patients with Prescribed Medications, *Am. J. Public Health*, 66:847, 1976.
69. Kramer, H. J., Düsing, R., Stinnesbeck, B., et al.: Interaction of Conventional and Antikaliuretic Diuretics with the Renal Prostaglandin System, *Clin. Sci.*, 59:67, 1980.
70. Patak, R. V., Mookerjee, B. K., Bentzel, C. J., Hysert, P. E., Babej, M., and Lee, J. B.: Antagonism of the Effects of Furosemide by Indomethacin in Normal and Hypertensive Man, *Prostaglandins*, 10:649, 1975.
71. Swartz, S. L., and Williams, G. H.: Angiotensin-Converting Enzyme Inhibition and Prostaglandins, *Am. J. Cardiol.*, 49:1405, 1982.
72. Fujita, T., Yamashita, N., and Yamashita, K.: Effect of Indomethacin on Antihypertensive Action of Captopril in Hypertensive Patients, *Clin. Exp. Hypertens.*, 3:939, 1981.
73. Watkins, J., Abbott, E. C., Hensby, C. N., Webster, J., and Dollery, C. T.: Attenuation of Hypotensive Effect of Propranolol and Thiazide Diuretics by Indomethacin, *Br. Med. J.*, 281:702, 1980.
74. Tweeddale, M. G., and Ogilvie, R. I.: Antagonism of Spironolactone-Induced Natriuresis by Aspirin in Man, *N. Engl. J. Med.*, 289:198, 1973.
75. Planas, R., Arroyo, V., Rimola, A., Pérez-Ayuso, R. M., and Rodés, J.: Acetylsalicylic Acid Suppresses the Renal Hemodynamic Effect and Reduces the Diuretic Action of Furosemide in Cirrhosis with Ascites, *Gastroenterology*, 84:247, 1983.
76. Ahmad, S.: Renal Insensitivity to Furosemide Caused by Chronic Anticonvulsant Therapy, *Br. Med. J.*, 3:657, 1974.
77. Wollam, G. L., Gifford, R. W., Jr., and Tarazi, R. C.: Antihypertensive Drugs: Clinical Pharmacology and Therapeutic Use, in R. N. Brogden and G. S. Avery (eds.), "Antihypertensive Drugs Today," Cardiovascular Drugs, vol. 4, ADIS Press, New York, 1979, p. 1.
78. Andersson, O.: Management of Hypertension. Clinical and Hemodynamic Studies with Special Reference to Patients Refractory to Treatment, *Acta. Med. Scand.*, 617(suppl.):1, 1977.
79. Walker, B. R., Shah, R. S., Ramanathan, K. B., Vanov, S. K., and Helfant, R. H.: Guanabenz and Methyldopa on Hypertension and Cardiac Performance, *Clin. Pharmacol. Ther.*, 22:868, 1977.
80. Plotnick, G. D., Fisher, M. L., Wohl, B., Hamilton, J. H., and Hamilton, B.P.: Improvement in Depressed Cardiac Function in Hypertensive Patients during Pindolol Treatment, *Am. J. Med.*, 76:25, 1984.
81. Dustan, H. P., Tarazi, R. C., and Bravo, E. L.: Dependence of Arterial Pressure on Intravascular Volume in Treated Hypertensive Patients, *N. Engl. J. Med.*, 286:861,1972.
82. Wollam, G. L., Tarazi, R. C., Bravo, E. L., and Dustan, H. P.: Diuretic Potency of Combined Hydrochlorothiazide and Furosemide Therapy in Patients with Azotemia, *Am. J. Med.*, 72:929, 1982.
83. Guillevin, L., Lardoux, M.-D., and Corvol, P.: Effects of Captopril on Blood Pressure, Electrolytes, and Certain Hormones in Hypertension, *Clin. Pharmacol. Ther.*, 29:699, 1981.
84. Beretta-Piccoli, C., Weidmann, P., de Chatêl, R., and Reubi, F.: Hypertension Associated with Early Stage Kidney Disease. Complementary Roles of Circulating Renin, the Body Sodium/Volume State, and Duration of Hypertension, *Am. J. Med.*, 61:739, 1976.
85. Brod, J., Bahlmann, J., Cachovan, M., Hubrich, W., and Pretschner, P. D.: Mechanisms for the Elevation of Blood Pressure in Human Renal Disease. Preliminary Report, *Hypertension*, 4:839, 1982.
86. Dustan, H. P.: Evaluation and Therapy of Hypertension—1976, *Mod. Concepts Cardiovasc. Dis.*, 45:97, 1976.
87. de Planque, B. A., Mulder, E., and Mees, E. J. D.: The Behavior of Blood and Extracellular Volume in Hypertensive Patients with Renal Insufficiency, *Acta. Med. Scand.*, 186:75, 1969.
88. Davis, B. A., Crook, J. E., Vestal, R. E., and Oates, J. A.: Prevalence of Renovascular Hypertension in Patients with Grade III or IV Hypertensive Retinopathy, *N. Engl. J. Med.*, 301:1273, 1979.
89. Hricik, D. E., Browning, P. J., Kopelman, R., Goorno, W. E., Madias, N. E., and Dzau, V. J.: Captopril-Induced Functional Renal Insufficiency in Patients with Bilateral Renal-Artery Stenosis or Renal-Artery Stenosis in a Solitary Kidney, *N. Engl. J. Med.*, 308:373, 1983.
90. Guazzi, M. D., Fiorentini, C., Olivari, M. T., Bartorelli, A., Necchi, G., and Polese, A.: Short- and Long-Term Efficacy of a Calcium-Antagonistic Agent (Nifedipine) Combined with Methyldopa in the Treatment of Severe Hypertension, *Circulation*, 61:913, 1980.
91. Evans, M. G., Jr., Olanoff, L. S., Hurwitz, G., Cowart, T. D., and Conradi, E. C.: Use of Nifedipine as an Adjunct to Current Antihypertensive Therapy, *Arch. Intern. Med.*, 144:985. 1984.
92. Kawasaki, T., Delea, C. S., Bartter, F. C., and Smith, H.: The Effect of High-Sodium and Low-Sodium Intakes on Blood Pressure and Other Related Variables in Human Subjects with Idiopathic Hypertension, *Am. J. Med.*, 64:193, 1978.
93. Fujita, T., Henry, H. L., Bartter, F. C., Lake, C. R., and Delea, C. S.: Factors Influencing Blood Pressure in Salt-Sensitive Patients with Hypertension, *Am. J. Med.*, 69:334, 1980.
94. Luft, F. C., and Weinberger, M. H.: Sodium Intake and Essential Hypertension, *Hypertension*, 4(suppl. III):III–14, 1982.
95. Longworth, D. L., Drayer, J. I. M., Weber, M. A., and Laragh, J. H.: Divergent Blood Pressure Responses during Short-Term Sodium Restriction in Hypertension, *Clin. Pharmacol. Ther.*, 27:544, 1980.
96. Watt, G. C. M., Edwards, C., Hart, J. T., Hart, M., Walton, P., and Foy, C. J. W.: Dietary Sodium Restriction for Mild Hypertension in General Practice, *Br. Med. J.*, 286:432, 1983.
97. Parijs, J., Joosens, J. V., Van der Linden, L., Verstreken, G., and Amery, A. K. P. C.: Moderate Sodium Restriction and Diuretics in the Treatment of Hypertension, *Am. Heart J.*, 85:22, 1973.

98. Carney, S., Morgan, T., Wilson, M., Matthews, G., and Roberts, R.: Sodium Restriction and Thiazide Diuretics in the Treatment of Hypertension, *Med. J. Aust.*, 1:803, 1975.
99. Morgan, T., Adam, W., Gillies, A., Wilson, M., Morgan, G., and Carney, S.: Hypertension Treated by Salt Restriction, *Lancet*, 1:227, 1978.
100. MacGregor, G. A., Markandu, N. D., Best, F. E., Elder, D. M., Cam, J. M., Sagnella, G. A., and Squires, M.: Double-Blind Randomised Crossover Trial of Moderate Sodium Restriction in Essential Hypertension, *Lancet*, 1:351, 1982.
101. Kaplan, N. M., Simmons, M., McPhee, C., Carnegie, A., Stefanu, C., and Cade, S.: Two Techniques to Improve Adherence to Dietary Sodium Restriction in the Treatment of Hypertension, *Arch. Intern. Med.*, 142:1638, 1982.
102. Luft, F. C., Sloan, R. S., Fineberg, N. S., and Free, A. H.: The Utility of Overnight Urine Collections in Assessing Compliance with a Low Sodium Intake Diet, *JAMA*, 249:1764, 1983.
103. Nugent, C. A., Carnahan, J. E., Sheehan, E. T., and Myers, C.: Salt Restriction in Hypertensive Patients. Comparison of Advice, Education, and Group Management, *Arch. Intern. Med.*, 144:1415, 1984.
104. Stamler, R., Stamler, J., Riedlinger, W. F., Algera, G., and Roberts, R. H.: Weight and Blood Pressure. Findings in Hypertension Screening of 1 Million Americans, *JAMA*, 240:1607, 1978.
105. Hovell, M. F.: The Experimental Evidence for Weight-Loss Treatment of Essential Hypertension: A Critical Review, *Am. J. Public Health*, 72:359, 1982.
106. Reisin, E., Abel, R., Modan, M., Silverberg, D. S., Eliahou, H. E., and Modan, B.: Effect of Weight Loss without Salt Restriction on the Reduction of Blood Pressure in Overweight Hypertensive Patients, *N. Engl. J. Med.*, 298:1, 1978.
107. Ramsay, L. E., Ramsay, M. H., Hettiarachchi, J., Davies, D. L., and Winchester, J.: Weight Reduction in a Blood Pressure Clinic, *Br. Med. J.*, 2:244, 1978.
108. Langford, H. G., and Watson, R. L.: Obesity and Hypertension, in P. Sleight and E. D. Freis (eds.), "Cardiology: Hypertension," vol. 1, Butterworth Scientific, London, 1982, p. 340.
109. Heyden, S., Nelius, S. J., and Schneider, K. A.: The Role of Potassium Manipulation in Blood Pressure Control, *Arteriosclerosis*, 3:302, 1983. (Editorial.)
110. Dustan, H. P.: Is Potassium Deficiency a Factor in the Pathogenesis and Maintenance of Hypertension? *Arteriosclerosis*, 3:307, 1983. (Editorial.)
111. Tannen, R. L.: Effects of Potassium on Blood Pressure Control, *Ann. Intern. Med.*, 98:773, 1983.
112. MacGregor, G. A., Smith, S. J., Markandu, N. D., Banks, R. A., and Sagnella, G. A.: Moderate Potassium Supplementation in Essential Hypertension, *Lancet*, 2:567, 1982.
113. Iimura, O., Kijama, T., Kikuchi, K., Miyama, A., Ando, T., Nakao, T., and Takigami, Y.: Studies on the Hypotensive Effect of High Potassium Intake in Patients with Essential Hypertension, *Clin. Sci.*, 61(suppl. 7):77s, 1981.
114. Sos, T. A., Pickering, T. G., Sniderman, K., et al.: Percutaneous Transluminal Renal Angioplasty in Renovascular Hypertension due to Atheroma or Fibromuscular Dysplasia, *N. Engl. J. Med.*, 309:274, 1983.
115. Simon, N., Franklin, S. S., Bleifer, K. H., and Maxwell, M. H.: Clinical Characteristics of Renovascular Hypertension, *JAMA*, 220:1209, 1972.
116. Franklin, S. S., Young, J. D., Jr., Maxwell, M. H., et al.: Operative Morbidity and Mortality in Renovascular Disease, *JAMA*, 231:1148, 1975.
117. Council on Scientific Affairs: Percutaneous Transluminal Angioplasty, *JAMA*, 251:764, 1984.
118. Grim, C. E., and Weinberger, M. H.: Renal Artery Stenosis and Hypertension, *Semin. Nephrol.*, 3:52, 1983.
119. Grim, C. E., Yune, H. Y., Weinberger, M. H., and Donohue, J. P.: Percutaneous Transluminal Dilatation or Surgery in the Management of Renal Vascular Hypertension? *Clin. Sci.*, 61(suppl. 7):485s, 1981.
120. Madias, N. E., Ball, J. T., and Millan, V. G.: Percutaneous Transluminal Renal Angioplasty in the Treatment of Unilateral Atherosclerotic Renovascular Hypertension, *Am. J. Med.*, 70:1078, 1981.
121. Kuhlmann, U., Vetter, W., Gruntzig, A., Schneider, E., Pouliadis, G., Steurer, J., and Siegenthaler, W.: Percutaneous Transluminal Dilatation of Renal Artery Stenosis: 2 Years' Experience, *Clin. Sci.*, 61(suppl. 7):481s, 1981.
122. Levin, D. C.: Percutaneous Transluminal Angioplasty of the Renal Arteries, *JAMA*, 251:759, 1984.
123. Fotino, S., and Sporn, P.: Nonoliguric Acute Renal Failure After Captopril Therapy, *Arch. Intern. Med.*, 143:1252, 1983.
124. Fournier, A., Romeder, J. M., Salmon, D., Meyer, P., and Milliez, P.: Predictive Criteria of Surgical Curability of Renovascular Hypertension. Comparative Assessment Individually and in Combination by Discriminant Analysis, *Acta. Med. Scand.*, 189:391, 1971.
125. Fouad, F. M., Gifford, R. W., Jr., Fighali, S., Mujais, S. K., Novick, A. C., Bravo, E. L., and Tarazi, R. C.: Predictive Value of Angiotensin II Antagonists in Renovascular Hypertension, *JAMA*, 249:368, 1983.
126. Lawrie, G. M., Morris, G. C., Jr., Soussou, I. D., et al.: Late Results of Reconstructive Surgery for Renovascular Disease, *Ann. Surg.*, 191:528, 1980.
127. Vertes, V., Genuth, S., Leb, D. E., and Galvin, J. B.: Unilateral Renal Plasma Flow in the Assessment of Correctable Renovascular Hypertension, *N. Engl. J. Med.*, 273:855, 1965.
128. Novick, A. C., Pohl, M. A., Schreiber, M., Gifford, R. W., Jr., and Vidt, D. G.: Revascularization for Preservation of Renal Function in Patients with Atherosclerotic Renovascular Disease, *J. Urol.*, 129:907, 1983.
129. Weidmann, P., and Maxwell, M. H.: The Renin-Angiotensin-Aldosterone System in Terminal Renal Failure, *Kidney Int.*, 8(suppl. 5):S–219, 1975.
130. Brod, J.: Kidney and Hypertension, in M. D. Blaufox and C. Bianchi (eds.), "Secondary Forms of Hypertension. Current Diagnosis and Management," Grune & Stratton, Inc., New York, 1981, p. 41.
131. Kim, K. E., Onesti, G., Schwartz, A. B., Chinitz, J. L., and Swartz, C.: Hemodynamics of Hypertension in Chronic End-Stage Renal Disease, *Circulation*, 46:456, 1972.
132. Neff, M. S., Kim, K. E., Persoff, M., Onesti, G., and Swartz, C.: Hemodynamics of Uremic Anemia, *Circulation*, 43:876, 1971.
133. del Greco, F., Simon, N. M., Goodman, S., and Rogoska, J.: Plasma Renin Activity in Primary and Secondary Hypertension, *Medicine*, 46:475, 1967.
134. Maggiore, Q., Biagini, M., Zoccali, C., and Misefari, M.: Long-Term Propranolol Treatment of Resistant Arterial Hypertension in Haemodialysed Patients, *Clin. Sci. Mol. Med.*, 48(suppl. 2):73s, 1975.
135. Thompson, F. D., Joekes, A. M., and Foulkes, D. M.: Pharmacodynamics of Propranolol in Renal Failure, *Br. Med. J.*, 2:434, 1972.
136. Hoffmann, K.-J., Regardh, C.-G., Aurell, M., Ervik, M., and Jordö, L.: The Effect of Impaired Renal Function on the Plasma Concentration and Urinary Excretion of Metoprolol Metabolites, *Clin. Pharmacokin.*, 5:181, 1980.
137. Herrera, J., Vukovich, R. A., and Griffith, D. L.: Elimination of Nadolol by Patients with Renal Impairment, *Br. J. Clin. Pharmacol.*, 7(suppl. 2):227s, 1979.
138. Traub, Y. M., Rabinov, M., Rosenfeld, J. B., and Treuherz, S.: Elevation of Serum Potassium During Beta Blockade: Absence of Relationship to the Renin-Aldosterone System, *Clin. Pharmacol. Ther.*, 28:765, 1980.
139. Talseth, T.: Studies on Hydralazine. II. Elimination Rate and Steady-State Concentration in Patients with Impaired Renal Function, *Eur. J. Clin. Pharmacol.*, 10:311, 1976.
140. Curtis, J. R., and Bateman, F. J. A.: Use of Prazosin in Management of Hypertension in Patients with Chronic Renal Failure and in Renal Transplant Recipients, *Br. Med. J.*, 4:432, 1975.
141. Harter, H. R., and Delmez, J. A.: Effects of Prazosin in the Control of Blood Pressure in Hypertensive Dialysis Patients, *J. Cardiovasc. Pharmacol.*, 1(suppl.):S–43, 1979.

142. Stokes, G. S., Monaghan, J. C., Frost, G. W., and MacCarthy, E. P.: Responsiveness to Prazosin in Renal Failure, *Clin. Sci.*, 57(suppl. 5):383s, 1979.
143. Meltzer, V. N., Goldberg, A. P., Tindira, C. A., Naumovich, A. D., and Harter, H. R.: Effects of Prazosin and Propranolol on Blood Pressure and Plasma Lipids in Patients Undergoing Chronic Hemodialysis, *Am. J. Cardiol.*, 53(Proceedings of a Symposium):40A, 1984.
144. Lindner, A., Charra, B., Sherrard, D. J., and Scribner, B. H.: Accelerated Atherosclerosis in Prolonged Maintenance Hemodialysis, *N. Engl. J. Med.*, 290:697, 1974.
145. Myhre, E., Stenbaek, Ö., Brodwall, E. K., and Hansen, T.: Conjugation of Methyldopa in Renal Failure, *Scand. J. Clin. Lab. Invest.*, 29:195, 1972.
146. Yeh, B. K., Dayton, P. G., and Waters, W. C., III: Removal of Alpha-Methyldopa (Aldomet) in Man by Dialysis, *Proc. Soc. Exp. Biol. Med.*, 135:840, 1970.
147. de Fremont, J. F., Coevoet, B., Andrejak, M., et al.: Effects of Antihypertensive Drugs on Dialysis-Resistant Hypertension, Plasma Renin and Dopamine Betahydroxylase Activities, Metabolic Risk Factors and Calcium Phosphate Homeostasis: Comparison of Metoprolol, Alphamethyldopa and Clonidine in a Cross-Over Trial, *Clin. Nephrol.*, 12:198, 1979.
148. Hulter, H. N., Licht, J. H., Ilnicki, L. P., and Singh, S.: Clinical Efficacy and Pharmacokinetics of Clonidine in Hemodialysis and Renal Insufficiency, *J. Lab. Clin. Med.*, 94:223, 1979.
149. Bennett, W. M., Porter, G. A., Bagby, S. P., and McDonald, W. J.: "Drugs and Renal Disease," Churchill Livingstone, New York, 1978.
150. Anderson, R. J., and Schrier, R. W.: "Clinical Use of Drugs in Patients with Kidney and Liver Disease," W. B. Saunders Company, Philadelphia, 1981.
151. Brater, D. C.: "Handbook of Drug Use in Patients with Renal Disease," Improved Therapeutics, Lancaster, Texas, 1982–1983.
152. Weinberger, M. H., Grim, C. E., Hollifield, J. W., et al.: Primary Aldosteronism. Diagnosis, Localization, and Treatment, *Ann. Intern. Med.*, 90:386, 1979.
153. Biglieri, E. G., Schambelan, M., Slaton, P. E., and Stockigt, J. R.: The Intercurrent Hypertension of Primary Aldosteronism, *Circ. Res.*, 26–27(suppl. 1):195, 1970.
154. Ferriss, J. B., Beevers, D. G., Boddy, K., et al.: The Treatment of Low-Renin ("Primary") Hyperaldosteronism, *Am. Heart J.*, 96:97, 1978.
155. Baer, L., Sommers, S. C., Krakoff, L. R., Newton, M. A., and Laragh, J. H.: Pseudo-Primary Aldosteronism. An Entity Distinct from True Primary Aldosteronism, *Circ. Res.*, 26–27(suppl. 1):203, 1970.
156. Conn, J. W.: Primary Aldosteronism and Primary Reninism, *Hosp. Pract.*, 9:131, 1974.
157. Hunt, T. K., Schambelan, M., and Biglieri, E. G.: Selection of Patients and Operative Approach in Primary Aldosteronism, *Ann. Surg.*, 182:353, 1975.
158. Filipecki, S., Feltynowski, T., Poplawska, W., et al.: Carcinoma of the Adrenal Cortex with Hyperaldosteronism, *J. Clin. Endocrinol. Metab.*, 35:225, 1972.
159. Todesco, S., Terribile, V., Borsatti, A., and Mantero, F.: Primary Aldosteronism Due to a Malignant Ovarian Tumor, *J. Clin. Endocrinol. Metab.*, 41:809, 1975.
160. Greathouse, D. J., McDermott, M. T., Kidd, G. S., and Hofeldt, F. D.: Pure Primary Hyperaldosteronism Due to Adrenal Cortical Carcinoma, *Am. J. Med.*, 76:1132, 1984.
161. Weinberger, M. H.: Primary Aldosteronism, in J. Genest, O. Kuchel, P. Hamet and M. Cantin (eds.), "Hypertension. Physiopathology and Treatment," 2d ed., McGraw-Hill Book Company, New York, 1983, p. 922.
162. Gwinup, G., and Steinberg, T.: Differential Response to Thiazides and Spironolactone in Primary Aldosteronism, *Arch. Intern. Med.*, 120:436, 1967.
163. Bravo, E. L., Dustan, H. P., and Tarazi, R. C.: Spironolactone as a Nonspecific Treatment for Primary Aldosteronism, *Circulation*, 48:491, 1973.
164. Kaplan, N. M.: "Clinical Hypertension," 2d ed., The Williams & Wilkins Company, Baltimore, 1978, p. 281.
165. Morimoto, S., Takeda, R., and Murakami, M.: Does Prolonged Pretreatment with Large Doses of Spironolactone Hasten a Recovery from Juxtaglomerular-Adrenal Suppression in Primary Aldosteronism? *J. Clin. Endocrinol. Metab.*, 31:659, 1970.
166. Bravo, E. L., Dustan, H. P., and Tarazi, R. C.: Selective Hypoaldosteronism Despite Prolonged Pre- and Postoperative Hyperreninemia in Primary Aldosteronism, *J. Clin. Endocrinol. Metab.*, 41:611, 1975.
167. Giebink, G. S., Gotlin, R. W., Biglieri, E. G., and Katz, F. H.: A Kindred with Familial Glucocorticoid-Suppressible Aldosteronism, *J. Clin. Endocrinol. Metab.*, 36:715, 1973.
168. Sizonenko, P.-C., Riondel, A.-M., Kohlberg, I. J., and Paunier, L.: 11-β-Hydroxylase Deficiency: Steroid Response to Sodium Restriction and ACTH Stimulation, *J. Clin. Endocrinol. Metabol.*, 35:281, 1972.
169. New, M. I.: Male Pseudohermaphroditism Due to 17α-Hydroxylase Deficiency, *J. Clin. Invest.*, 49:1930, 1970.
170. de Lange, W. E., Weeke, A., Artz, W., Jansen, W., and Doorenbos, H.: Primary Amenorrhea with Hypertension due to 17-Hydroxylase Deficiency. Therapy with Dexamethasone and Ethinyloestradiol, *Acta. Med. Scand.*, 193:565, 1973.
171. Biglieri, E. G., and Kater, C. E.: Adrenal Enzymatic Defects, in J. Genest, O. Kuchel, P. Hamet and M. Cantin (eds.), "Hypertension. Physiopathology and Treatment," 2d ed., McGraw-Hill Book Company, New York, 1983, p. 939.
172. Hamet, P.: Endocrine Hypertension: Cushing's Syndrome, Acromegaly, Hyperparathyroidism, Thyroxicosis, and Hypothyroidism, in J. Genest, O. Kuchel, P. Hamet and M. Cantin (eds.), "Hypertension: Physiopathology and Treatment," 2d ed., McGraw-Hill Book Company, New York, 1983, p. 964.
173. Manger, W. M., and Gifford, R. W., Jr.: "Pheochromocytoma," Springer-Verlag, New York, 1977, p. 304.
174. Manger, W. M., and Gifford, R. W.: Pheochromocytoma, in P. Sleight, and E. D. Freis (eds.), "Cardiology: Hypertension," vol. 1, Butterworth Scientific, London, 1982, p. 153.
175. Levenson, J. A., Safar, M. E., London, G. M., and Simon, A. Ch.: Haemodynamics in Patients with Phaeochromocytoma, *Clin. Sci.*, 58:349, 1980.
176. Lipson, A., Hus, T.-H., Sherwin, B., and Geelhoed, G. W.: Nitroprusside Therapy for a Patient with Pheochromocytoma, *JAMA*, 239:427, 1978.
177. Hauptman, J. B., Modlinger, R. S., and Ertel, N. H.: Pheochromocytoma Resistant to α-Adrenergic Blockade, *Arch. Intern. Med.*, 143:2321, 1983.
178. Wallace, J. M., and Dill, G. P.: Prazosin in the Diagnosis and Treatment of Pheochromocytoma, *JAMA*, 240:2752, 1978.
179. Cubeddu, L. X., Zarate, N. A., Rosales, C. B., and Zschaeck, D. W.: Prazosin and Propranolol in Preoperative Management of Pheochromocytoma, *Clin. Pharmacol. Ther.*, 32:156, 1982.
180. Nicholson, J. P., Jr., Vaughn, E. D., Jr., Pickering, T. G., et al.: Pheochromocytoma and Prazosin, *Ann. Intern. Med.*, 99:477, 1983.
181. Izzo, J. L., Jr., Horwitz, D., and Keiser, H. R.: Physiologic Mechanisms Opposing the Hemodynamic Effects of Prazosin, *Clin. Pharmacol. Ther.*, 29:7, 1981.
182. Serfas, D., Shoback, D. M., and Lorell, B. H.: Phaeochromocytoma and Hypertrophic Cardiomyopathy: Apparent Suppression of Symptoms and Noradrenaline Secretion by Calcium-Channel Blockade, *Lancet*, 2:711, 1983.
183. Corea, L., Miele, N., Bentivoglio, M., Boschetti, E., Agabiti-Rosei, E., and Muiesan, G.: Acute and Chronic Effects of Nifedipine on Plasma Renin Activity and Plasma Adrenaline and Noradrenaline in Controls and Hypertensive Patients, *Clin. Sci.*, 57(suppl. 5):115s, 1979.
184. Cohn, J. N.: Relationship of Plasma Volume Changes to Resistance and Capacitance Vessel Effects of Sympatho-

mimetic Amines and Angiotensin in Man, *Clin. Sci.*, 30:267, 1966.
185. DeOreo, G. A., Jr., Stewart, B. H., Tarazi, R. C., and Gifford, R. W., Jr.: Preoperative Blood Transfusion in the Safe Surgical Management of Pheochromocytoma: A Review of 46 Cases, *J. Urol.*, 111:715, 1974.
186. Engelman, K., and Sjoerdsma, A.: Chronic Medical Therapy for Pheochromocytoma. A Report of Four Cases, *Ann. Intern Med.*, 61:229, 1964.
187. Blumenstein, B. A., Douglas, M. B., and Hall, W. D.: Blood Pressure Changes and Oral Contraceptive Use: A Longitudinal Study of 2676 Black Women in the Southeastern United States, *Am. J. Epidemiol.*, 112:539, 1980.
188. Hall, W. D., Douglas, M. B., Blumenstein, B. A., and Hatcher, R. A.: Blood Pressure and Oral Progestational Agents: A Prospective Study of 119 Black Women, *Am. J. Obstet. Gynecol.*, 136:344, 1980.
189. Kaplan, N. M.: Cardiovascular Complications of Oral Contraceptives, *Annu. Rev. Med.*, 29:31, 1978.
190. Woods, J. W., Algary, W. A., and Stier, F. M.: Oral Contraceptives and Hypertension, *Circulation*, 45–46(suppl. 2):II–82, 1972. (Abstract.)
191. Walters, W. A. W., and Lim, Y. L.: Haemodynamic Changes in Women Taking Oral Contraceptives, *J. Obstet. Gynaecol. Br. Commonw.*, 77:1007, 1970.
192. Lehtovirta, P.: Haemodynamic Effects of Combined Oestrogen/Progestogen Oral Contraceptives, *J. Obstet. Gynaecol. Br. Commonw.*, 81:517, 1974.
193. Streeten, D. H. P., Anderson, G. H., Jr., and Dalakos, T. G.: Angiotensin Blockade: Its Clinical Significance, *Am. J. Med.*, 60:817, 1976.
194. Saruta, T., Saade, G. A., and Kaplan, N. M.: A Possible Mechanism for Hypertension Induced by Oral Contraceptives, *Arch. Intern. Med.*, 126:621, 1970.
195. Pfeffer, R. I.: Estrogen Use, Hypertension and Stroke in Post-Menopausal Women, *J. Chronic Dis.*, 31:389, 1978.
196. Crane, M. G., and Harris, J. J.: Estrogens and Hypertension: Effect of Discontinuing Estrogens on Blood Pressure, Exchangeable Sodium, and the Renin-Aldosterone System, *Am. J. Med. Sci.*, 276:33, 1978.
197. Friedman, E. A., and Neff, R. K.: "Pregnancy Hypertension," PSG Publishing Company, Littleton, Mass., 1977, p. 1.
198. Sullivan, J. M.: Blood Pressure Elevation in Pregnancy, *Prog. Cardiovas. Dis.*, 16:375, 1974.
199. Woods, J. R., Jr., and Brinkman, C. R., III: The Treatment of Gestational Hypertension, *J. Reprod. Med.*, 15:195, 1975.
200. Berkowitz, R. L.: Anti-Hypertensive Drugs in the Pregnant Patient, *Obstet. Gynecol. Surv.*, 35:191, 1980.
201. Kraus, G. W., Marchese, J. R., and Yen, S. S. C.: Prophylactic Use of Hydrochlorothiazide in Pregnancy, *JAMA*, 198:1150, 1966.
202. MacGillivray, I., and Campbell, D. M.: A Prospective Study of Factors Affecting Intrauterine Growth (with an Emphasis on Blood Pressure and Diuretics), in M. D. Lindheimer, A. I. Katz, and F. P. Zuspan (eds.), "Hypertension in Pregnancy," John Wiley & Sons, New York, 1976, p. 23.
203. Rodriguez, S. U., Leikin, S. L., and Hiller, M. C.: Neonatal Thrombocytopenia Associated with Ante-Partum Administration of Thiazide Drugs, *N. Engl. J. Med.*, 270:881, 1964.
204. Gant, N. F., Madden, J. D., Siiteri, P. K., and MacDonald, P. C.: The Metabolic Clearance Rate of Dehydroisoandrosterone Sulfate. III. The Effect of Thiazide Diuretics in Normal and Future Pre-Eclamptic Pregnancies, *Am. J. Obstet. Gynecol.*, 123:159, 1975.
205. Gant, N. F., Madden, J. D., Siiteri, P. K., and MacDonald, P. C.: The Metabolic Clearance Rate of Dehydroisoandrosterone Sulfate. IV. Acute Effects of Induced Hypertension, Hypotension, and Naturesis in Normal and Hypertensive Pregnancies, *Am. J. Obstet. Gynecol.*, 124:143, 1976.
206. Gant, N. F., and Worley, R. J.: "Hypertension in Pregnancy. Concepts and Management," Appleton-Century-Crofts, New York, 1980, p. 61.
207. Assali, N. S., and Vaughn, D. L.: Blood Volume in Pre-Eclampsia: Fantasy and Reality, *Am. J. Obstet. Gynecol.*, 129:355, 1977.
208. Kennedy, D., Whitehorn, W. V., and Martin, E. W.: Limited Usefulness of Diuretics in Pregnancy, *FDA Drug Bull.*, 7:7, 1977.
209. Burrow, G. N., and Ferris, T. F.: "Medical Complications During Pregnancy," 2d ed., W. B. Saunders Company, Philadelphia, 1982, p. 22.
210. White, W. B.: Management of Hypertension During Lactation, *Hypertension*, 6:297, 1984.
211. Ladner, C. N., Weston, P. V., Brinkman, C. R., III, and Assali, N. S.: Effects of Hydralazine on Uteroplacental and Fetal Circulations, *Am. J. Obstet. Gynecol.*, 108:375, 1970.
212. Ring, G., Krames, E., Shnider, S. M., Wallis, K. L., and Levinson, G.: Comparison of Nitroprusside and Hydralazine in Hypertensive Pregnant Ewes, *Obstet. Gynecol.*, 50:598, 1977.
213. Liedholm, H., Wählin-Ball, E., Hanson, A., Ingemarsson, I., and Melander, A.: Transplacental Passage and Breast Milk Concentrations of Hydralazine, *Eur. J. Clin. Pharmacol.*, 21:417, 1982.
214. Leather, H. M., Hymphreys, D. M., Baker, P., and Chadd, M. A.: A Controlled Trial of Hypotensive Agents in Hypertension in Pregnancy, *Lancet*, 2:488, 1968.
215. Redman, C. W. G., Beilin, L. J., Bonnar, J., and Ounsted, M. K.: Fetal Outcome in Trial of Antihypertensive Treatment in Pregnancy, *Lancet*, 2:753, 1976.
216. Moar, V. A., Jeffires, M. A., Mutch, L. M. M., and Redman, C. W. E.: Neonatal Head Circumference and the Treatment of Maternal Hypertension, *Br. J. Obstet. Gynaeco.*, 85:933, 1978.
217. Whitelaw, A.: Maternal Methyldopa Treatment and Neonatal Blood Pressure, *Br. Med. J.*, 283:471, 1981.
218. Rubin, P. C.: Beta-Blockers in Pregnancy, *N. Engl. J. Med.*, 305:1323, 1981.
219. Thorley, K. J., McAinsh, J., and Cruickshank, J. M.: Atenolol in the Treatment of Pregnancy-Induced Hypertension, *Br. J. Clin. Pharmacol.*, 12:725, 1981.
220. Lamming, G. D., Pipkin, F. B., and Symonds, E. M.: Comparison of the Alpha and Beta Blocking Drug, Labetalol, and Methyl Dopa in the Treatment of Moderate and Severe Pregnancy-Induced Hypertension, *Clin. Exp. Hypertens.*, 2:865, 1980.
221. Johnston, C. I., and Aickin, D. R.: The Control of High Blood Pressure During Labour with Clonidine ("Catapres"), *Med. J. Aust.*, 2:132, 1971.
222. Davey, D. A., and Dommisse, J.: The Management of Hypertension in Pregnancy, *S. Afr. Med. J.*, 58:551, 1980.
223. Pennington, J. C., and Picker, R. H.: Diazoxide and the Treatment of the Acute Hypertensive Emergency in Obstetrics, *Med. J. Aust.*, 2:1051, 1972.
224. Lewis, P. E., Cefalo, R. C., Naulty, J. S., and Rodkey, F. L.: Placental Transfer and Fetal Toxicity of Sodium Nitroprusside, *Gynecol. Obstet. Invest.*, 8:46, 1977. (Abstract.)

Section E

Pulmonary Hypertension and Pulmonary Heart Disease

52

Pulmonary Hypertension: Mechanism and Recognition

Hiroshi Kuida, M.D.

Pulmonary hypertension may be defined as a pathophysiologic condition in which the blood pressure in the pulmonary circulation is elevated above the normal range for a given situation. It is not a disease. Nominally, this term refers to elevated pressure in the pulmonary arterial system, but there are conditions in which pressures in the pulmonary capillaries and veins also may be elevated. As in the case of systemic hypertension, there are many causes of pulmonary hypertension.[1] The situations in which pulmonary pressures are measured are relevant to the definition of pulmonary hypertension because pulmonary vascular pressures are dynamic phenomena; they change depending on physiologic circumstances. In this regard, pulmonary vascular pressures are somewhat different than systemic vascular pressures, wherein arterial blood pressure is regulated within a physiologic range by an intricate mechanoreceptor neural reflex control system and wherein increase in systemic venous pressure has little direct effect on arterial blood pressure. It is appropriate, therefore, to consider relevant features of the normal pulmonary circulation as a preamble to considering the subject of pulmonary hypertension.

Normal Pulmonary Circulation

Human pulmonary circulation serves many functions, but its raison d'être is that of providing the blood phase of respiratory gas exchange. Lungs provide a large oxygen consumption capacity (utilized during exercise) that is achieved by the matching of a very large alveolar ventilatory with an equally generous pulmonary blood flow capacity. Normally these linked functions are accomplished at relatively low energy expenditure because the two pumps involved, the diaphragm and chest wall in the case of breathing and the right ventricle in the case of pulmonary circulation, move their tidal and stroke volumes, respectively, under low pressures.

Pulmonary Vascular Pressures

The pressure in the pulmonary venous system plays an important role in determining pulmonary artery pressure. Left atrial pressure normally is determined by pressure in the left ventricle during diastole. The latter, so-called left ventricular filling pressure, is determined by the relationship between the distensibility (or compliance) of the left ventricle and its filling or end-diastolic volume (Chap. 3). At rest, this pressure averages approximately 5 ± 5 mmHg and may reach values up to 15 to 20 mmHg during heavy exercise. Pressures of this magnitude, albeit low, comprise a significant fraction of the corresponding pulmonary artery pressures, on the order of a third to as much as half. The pressures in the pulmonary capillaries and veins can be estimated by measuring the so-called pulmonary artery wedge pressure by catheterization of the right side of the heart. This pressure is very nearly the same as those in the left atrium and in the left ventricle during diastole, 5 to 12 mmHg at rest.

The left ventricular diastolic or left atrial pressure, therefore, represents the "floor," so to speak, below which pulmonary venous, capillary, and arterial pressure upstream cannot be. Any situation or condition which causes this venous effluent pressure to rise will produce at the very least a comparable (pari passu) increase in pulmonary capillary and arterial pressure, assuming no other effects are elicited (as we shall see later, this assumption is not necessarily valid).

The teleologic value and importance of a low pulmonary capillary venous pressure are readily discernible. The osmotic pressure of plasma, owing to the plasma proteins, principally albumin, constitutes a reabsorptive force for fluid transport across the capillary endothelium. In the systemic capillaries, this inward pressure of roughly 25 to 30 mmHg is offset by the opposing (i.e., filtration) capillary hydrostatic pressure of essentially equivalent magnitude. Thus, the net pressure gradient for bulk fluid transport across the capillary membrane is neutral. In the pulmonary capillaries the same plasma osmotic pressure is not offset because of the low capillary blood pressure. The resulting imbalance favors reabsorption rather than filtration of fluid, a desirable situation conducive to gas- instead of water-filled alveolar spaces. This consideration is particularly important in dependent (that is, below heart level) lung segments (such as the lung bases in the erect posture), where the effect of gravity raises the capillary venous pressure above that in the left atrium by as much as 5 to 8 mmHg.[2]

The normally low pulmonary capillary venous pressure combined with equally high arterial conductance (see below) confers the advantage of permitting a low pulmonary arterial pressure. The normal value of roughly 15 mmHg mean pulmonary artery pressure in healthy resting subjects at sea level testifies to this benefit, which is that pressure development by the right ventricular pump is kept low. This feature is what makes for an efficient blood flow component of respiratory gas exchange: it is accomplished at a low cardiac energy expenditure even when the demand for such gas exchange is high. The architecture of the normal right ventricle mirrors this hemodynamic situation in being relatively thin-walled compared with that of the left ventricle.

Pulmonary Vascular Conductance

Pulmonary vascular conductance by the Poiseuille relationship (Chaps. 3, 49) is the relation of blood flow to the longitudinal driving pressure gradient between the pulmonary artery and left atrium. (Some prefer the reciprocal relationship, pressure difference to blood flow, which yields vascular resistance.) Conductance or resistance represents a calculated abstraction which reflects the conducting or resisting properties of inaccessible tube systems:[1]

$$G = \frac{\overline{\mathrm{CO}}}{\overline{\mathrm{PAP}} - \overline{\mathrm{LAP}}} \quad \text{or} \quad R = \frac{\overline{\mathrm{PAP}} - \overline{\mathrm{LAP}}}{\overline{\mathrm{CO}}}$$

where
G = pulmonary vascular conductance
R = pulmonary vascular resistance
$\overline{\mathrm{CO}}$ = cardiac output
$\overline{\mathrm{PAP}}$ = mean pulmonary artery pressure
$\overline{\mathrm{LAP}}$ = mean left atrial pressure

Since the normal pulmonary circulation conducts the entire cardiac output under all conditions, it is clear that resting pulmonary blood flow is only a fraction, perhaps a fourth to a fifth, of that during vigorous exercise when cardiac output increases to as much as 20 to 25 liters/min in healthy, conditioned persons. Thus, what the pulmonary artery pressure is during exercise is more significant than what it is at rest when the flow is a mere 4 to 6 liters/min. It is remarkable that the high pulmonary blood flows during exercise, especially in the upright posture, are associated with only a modestly higher mean pulmonary artery pressure than those at rest. Thus, the mean pulmonary artery pressure may double during heavy exertion. It is obvious that since cardiac output, which is relatively high in mammals, is conducted through the pulmonary vessels at a low driving pressure gradient, vascular conductance is high and resistance low. It is also clear that, during exercise, since the proportional increase in blood flow normally is greater (four times) than the increase in pressure difference (two times), vascular conductance becomes even greater. This effect can be illustrated with representative conductance values:

Rest:
$\overline{\mathrm{CO}}$ = 5 liters/min
$\overline{\mathrm{PAP}}$ = 15 mmHg
$\overline{\mathrm{LAP}}$ = 5 mmHg

$$G = \frac{5}{15 - 5} = 0.5 \text{ liter/min/mmHg}$$

Exercise:
$\overline{\mathrm{CO}}$ = 20 liters/min
$\overline{\mathrm{PAP}}$ = 25 mmHg
$\overline{\mathrm{LAP}}$ = 10 mmHg

$$G = \frac{20}{25 - 10} = 1.3 \text{ liters/min/mmHg}$$

There are probably two major reasons for increased vascular conductance during exercise. The first is the passive effect of higher intravascular pressures on distensible blood vessels causing their dilation. The second, and perhaps more important, is the probable recruitment of more blood vessels, especially in apical lung segments, not only because of augmented pressures but also because of larger fluctuations in lung volume associated with greater ventilatory effort. It is also possible that sympathetic beta-adrenoreceptor stimulation causes pulmonary vascular as well as bronchial smooth-muscle relaxation leading to active vasodilation.

Other examples of the adaptability of pulmonary vascular conductance are provided by occlusion experiments and by augmented pulmonary blood flow associated with large left-to-right intracardiac shunts in patients with congenital atrial septal defect (Chap. 36). In the latter it is not unusual for measured pulmonary blood flows to exceed 20 liters/min even though pulmonary artery pressure remains normal or only minimally elevated. This gives conductance values in the same range as those during exercise in the absence of ventilatory or neural mechanisms augmenting conductance. Balloon occlusion of one of the branches of the main pulmonary artery has been shown to divert the entire cardiac output through the contralateral unoccluded lung with only a small increase (a few millimeters of mercury) in pulmonary artery pressure, thus increasing conductance in the unoccluded lung significantly. These examples, which represent the opposite of pulmonary hypertension, dramatize what a drastic derangement even mild pulmonary hypertension (at rest) represents in reflecting a loss of this adaptive capacity.

Definition of Pulmonary Hypertension

Lest it be misconstrued from the foregoing that pulmonary vessels are totally passive under normal circumstances, two conditions are worth mentioning that are relevant to the definition of pulmonary hypertension. The first is fetal pulmonary circulation (Chap. 36). The second is the effect of alveolar hypoxia (high-altitude dwelling or exposure) on pulmonary vessels (Chap. 84).

Because pulmonary circulation in the fetus serves no respiratory function, pulmonary blood flow is virtually nonexistent. Flow is kept low by the combined effects of the patent foramen ovale and ductus arteriosus through which potential pulmonary flow is shunted to the systemic circulation and by the high vascular resistance afforded by constricted muscular pulmonary arterioles and the unexpanded lungs. Since pulmonary arterial and aortic pressures are virtually equal in the fetus, pulmonary hypertension is the normal condition antepartum. Dramatic changes occur at birth with the onset of breathing.[3] Lung expansion itself, due to elastic forces and the high oxygen concentration, suddenly opens lung vessels and increases pulmonary vascular conductance. This allows rapid increase in pulmonary blood flow and lowers pulmonary artery pressure. Involution of vascular smooth muscle hypertrophy and ductus closure take several hours to days. Thus, the normal low-resistance, low-pressure pulmonary circulation is a situation that evolves postpartum from one that is initially quite the opposite.[4] Occasionally the regression of abundant pulmonary vascular smooth muscle fails to take place, and in some types of congenital heart disease (see below) persistence of the fetal pattern is essential for survival (Chap. 36). These situations result in persisting pulmonary hypertension with its attendant consequences.

It is firmly established that natural or experimental alveolar hypoxia elicits constriction of precapillary pulmonary arterioles in a number and variety of mammalian species, including humans (Chap. 84). The magnitude of this effect is variable both within as well as among species. It is the fact that humans live or choose to climb at high terrestrial elevations, to fly airplanes or to ride balloons to high altitudes, that makes this consideration relevant. The question arises whether there is a level of hypoxic pulmonary artery pressure elevation relative to the degree of hypoxic exposure that can be considered "normal," responses above which can be considered "true" pulmonary hypertension.[5] Regrettably, there is no universally accepted answer to this question.

Peñaloza et al.[6] carried out hemodynamic studies in 38 healthy, lifelong native residents of Morococha in the Peruvian Andes. At this elevation of roughly 14,000 ft above sea level, where ambient oxygen partial pressure is only about 80 mmHg (compared with 159 mmHg at sea level), resting pulmonary artery pressure averaged 28 mmHg compared with 12 mmHg in 25 residents of Lima, Peru (sea level). At comparable levels of exercise, the mean pulmonary artery pressure increased to 60 mmHg in the altitude dwellers and to only 18 mmHg in those living at sea level.[7] Other variables such as cardiac output and pulmonary artery wedge pressure were normal. Therefore, calculated pulmonary vascular conductance was only a third of normal at rest and failed to increase during exercise in the hypoxic environment.

From the sea-level perspective it is easy to conclude that altitude dwellers suffer pulmonary hypertension due to pulmonary vascular obstruction (i.e., vasoconstriction) secondary to alveolar hypoxia. But to those who live generation after generation at elevations above 5000 ft without untoward consequences, by and large, the pathophysiologic label has no more consequence than that of relative polycythemia, hypocapnia, increased red blood cell 2,3-DPG, or compensated respiratory alkalosis, all normal chronic acclimation responses to altitude dwelling (Chap. 84).

Although pulmonary hypertension can be quantified by the pulmonary artery pressure level, the rationale for this practice does not apply to the pulmonary circulation as it does in systemic hypertension. In systemic hypertension the assumption that resting cardiac output is not a variable (i.e., it is "normal") is valid in the vast majority of cases. Thus, the blood pressure level by itself correctly estimates the magnitude of vascular obstruction by the Poiseuille relation.

In pulmonary hypertension the cardiac output is unpredictable. Usually it is decreased compared to normal if pulmonary hypertension is severe, but this is variable. It would be distinctly unusual for pulmonary blood flow to be so depressed that an obstruction would not be associated with an increase in pressure upstream of the impediment, but it happens. On the other hand, pulmonary hypertension may exist in the presence of increased blood flow in congenital heart disease. Thus, accurate quantitation of obstructions in the pulmonary circulation optimally requires measurement of conductance (or resistance) flow in relation to pressure gradient.

Mechanisms (Pathophysiology) and Syndromes of Pulmonary Hypertension

The level of cardiac output is determined by systemic tissue needs and by physiologic control mechanisms involving the systemic circulation. The baroreceptor reflex mechanism is but one of the latter. Thus, in the absence of disease the right ventricle is not a primary determinant of cardiac output since it pumps along what it receives in the way of systemic venous return. When obstructions develop in the pulmonary circulation, it is on the right ventricle that the extra load impinges to maintain output to meet demand. To the extent that the right ventricle succeeds in maintaining output, it is inevitable that pressure will rise upstream of the obstructing lesion. If, faced with the added load of generating a higher systolic pressure, the right ventricle fails to maintain cardiac output at the appropriate normal level, then the right ventricle becomes a primary determinant of cardiac output and the left ventricle passively pumps along what it receives. In these situations, whether they occur only during exercise or are present at rest as well, the right ventricle has failed.

Syndromes of Obstruction to Pulmonary Blood Flow

Obstructions in the pulmonary circulation extend from the main pulmonary artery to the left ventricle. In general, the hemodynamic effect of an obstruction is a rise in pressure proximal to or upstream from the obstruction, a lowering of blood flow (cardiac output), or a combination of these two. The farther downstream the obstruction occurs, the greater the vascular segments involved in elevated pressure. The location of obstructive lesions determines clinical and physiologic consequences. It is clinically useful and physiologically rational to separate obstructions proximal to the capillary bed from those that occur downstream to it.

Postcapillary Obstruction

Postcapillary obstructions in the pulmonary veins (venocclusive disease), left atrium (myxoma), mitral valve (stenosis), or left ventricle (hypertrophy or failure) cause capillary blood pressure to increase. Capillary hypertension has a pathophysiologic or symptom-limited ceiling determined by plasma osmotic pressure. Reaching or exceeding this pressure produces congestion of the pulmonary parenchyma at the very least, and frank alveolar edema at worst.

Elevation of pulmonary capillary pressure obligatorily raises pulmonary arterial pressure by a comparable amount. In fact, typically the pulmonary artery diastolic pressure is virtually identical to increased downstream mean capillary venous (i.e., pulmonary artery wedge) pressure. This finding is indicative of the absence of significant precapillary obstruction. In some patients, however, chronic elevation of capillary pressure is accompanied by increased precapillary resistance. This phenomenon is characterized by a disproportionate increase in pulmonary artery (including diastolic) pressure compared with pulmonary artery wedge pressure. This was first described and is most common in patients with mitral stenosis,[8] the prototypical lesion causing capillary venous hypertension. The syndrome, termed *secondary pulmonary vascular disease,* also occurs, although to a lesser extent, in patients with chronic left-sided heart failure due to any cause. The mechanism by which postcapillary obstruction elicits this precapillary response is unknown, but it tends to be progressive and is believed to reflect arteriolar vasoconstriction since, in patients with mitral stenosis, it usually remits, albeit incompletely, when valve obstruction is surgically relieved. There is clinical evidence which suggests that the phenomenon affords protection against pulmonary capillary congestion and edema in some patients.

The sine qua non for diagnosing postcapillary obstruction is an elevated pulmonary artery wedge pressure. If this occurs in the absence of an elevated left ventricular diastolic pressure, the obstruction lies between the pulmonary veins and mitral valve. Echocardiography, which permits specific evaluation of mitral valve stenosis, left atrial size, and presence or absence of a left atrial tumor, has dramatically improved our ability to assess the specific location and consequences of postcapillary obstruction (Chap. 39). Patients with pulmonary hypertension associated with postcapillary obstruction are not included in the classification of cor pulmonale (see below), despite the fact that many of these patients have severe pulmonary hypertension and chronic right-sided heart failure. It is worth recalling that Paul White pointed out in 1936 that the most common cause of right-sided heart hypertrophy and failure was chronic left-sided heart failure.[9]

Congenital Heart Disease and Pulmonary Hypertension

Congenital heart diseases constitute a major category of disorders associated with pulmonary hypertension. The diversity of congenital lesions results in a variety of mechanisms for pulmonary hypertension (see Chap. 36). In congenital mitral and aortic valve stenosis, for example, postcapillary obstruction (increased left ventricular filling resistance in the case of severe aortic stenosis) causes pulmonary hypertension presumably by the same mechanism as in adult acquired diseases of the same name.

Precapillary Obstruction
It was indicated previously that there are congenital heart lesions in which precapillary pulmonary vascular obstruction and consequent pulmonary hypertension are essential for life (see Chap. 36). The lesions are characterized by a large defect connecting the ventricles[10] (single ventricle or ventricular septal defect) or the aortic and pulmonary arterial roots (large patent ductus arteriosus or aortopulmonary window).[11] A large communication precludes a systolic pressure difference between the connected chambers (or vessels) both before and after birth. In this circumstance, pulmonary hypertension is obligatory and survival depends on precapillary pulmonary vascular resistance being sufficiently increased to prevent elevation of pulmonary capillary pressure and excessive left-to-right shunting, and to allow an adequate systemic blood flow. In ventricular septal defect (so-called Eisenmenger's disease or syndrome) the aortic and pulmonary systolic pressures are obligatorily equal but diastolic (and mean) pressures usually are different, aortic being higher. In aortic–pulmonary artery defects, both systolic and diastolic pressures are equal. Since in these lesions systolic pressures in the pulmonary and systemic circuits are equal, the vascular conductances of the systemic and pulmonary systems are directly proportional to the blood flow rates. As long as pulmonary conductance exceeds systemic, pulmonary blood flow will exceed systemic and the shunt will be in the left-to-right direction. Quantitatively the shunt may be large or small. The usual situation, however, is that the pulmonary conductance progressively diminishes over time (i.e., obstruction increases). Thus, the magnitude of left-to-right shunting gradually decreases and eventually results in a reversal of shunt and cyanosis later in life.

Since survival after birth in these cases depends on a persisting elevated precapillary pulmonary vascular resistance, it is easy to conceive that it is mechanistically accounted for by persistence of the fetal medial (i.e., vascular smooth muscle) hypertrophy pattern.[1] Pathologic findings are consistent with this interpretation.[12] The mechanism of progression of vascular obstruction in these cases is unknown, but may share some of the mechanisms that have been speculated upon in other congenital lesions characterized by increased pulmonary flow due to left-to-right shunting, such as atrial septal defect.[13]

It is well established that any congenital defect characterized by a left-to-right shunt regardless of the anatomic "level" of the shunt (atria, ventricles, or large vessels) or its magnitude, may be accompanied early or late in the course by secondary pulmonary hypertension due to precapillary vascular obstruction (i.e., secondary pulmonary vascular disease) (Chap. 36). Shunts at the ventricular and large vessel levels are more apt to elicit this response than those at the atrial level, and it seems to occur more frequently in altitude dwellers than in similar patients living at sea level presumably because one mechanism for pulmonary vasoconstriction (hypoxia) is added to another. Indications for surgical closure of such defects hinge on the magnitude of the vascular obstruction. In successful surgical cases pulmonary hypertension is significantly relieved, largely because of reduction in flow but in some cases also because of relief of vasospasm.

Cor Pulmonale

In the presently accepted classification all other forms of pulmonary hypertension, that is, those excluding postcapillary obstruction syndromes and congenital heart disease, fall into the generic category of cor pulmonale, right-sided heart disease (i.e., hypertrophy or failure) associated with chronic or acute lung disease (Chaps. 54, 55). The lung disease may involve virtually any aspect of the respiratory mechanism including the respiratory centers in the medulla, respiratory neurons, the chest cage (including spine), diaphragm, airways, pleura, lung parenchyma, and pulmonary vessels.

The central pathophysiologic theme of cor pulmonale is pulmonary arterial hypertension secondary to precapillary obstruction. The precapillary locus and mechanism of obstruction are quite variable in the many types of cor pulmonale.[1] Most are acquired lesions that tend to occur late in life. It is pulmonary hypertension that connects these various obstructive lesions to the right side of the heart. Since the diagnostic term and its classification antedated the presently available means for detecting as well as quantifying pulmonary hypertension, it is not difficult to perceive why the cardiac component (right ventricular hypertrophy and/or failure) had to be evident before the diagnosis could be made. In systemic hypertension, it is the ease and specificity of detecting hypertension itself that make it possible to identify the disease long before and even exclusive of the advent of left ventricular hypertrophy or failure. The list of specific entities that fall into this category of pulmonary hypertension is so long that a classification scheme based on mechanism of obstruction may have merit. However, multiple mechanisms may be involved rather than just one.

Hypoxemia-Induced Pulmonary Hypertension
Hypoxemia-induced pulmonary hypertension is a significant category of cor pulmonale because of the number of people who reside at high terrestrial elevations around the world such as the Peruvian Andes,

the Bolivian Altiplano, the American Rockies, the Himalayas, Mexico City, and elsewhere. Mountaineers, of course, now climb everything, including Mount Everest (over 29,000 ft), without using oxygen tanks! At this highest terrestrial elevation the oxygen partial pressure is only a third of that at sea level (159 mmHg). Perhaps a more important reason for the importance of this category is the high worldwide incidence of disorders of the respiratory apparatus in which significant chronic hypoxemia occurs. Chronic alveolar hypoventilation from any of a large number of disparate causes[14] leads to hypoxic pulmonary vasoconstriction and pulmonary hypertension even though the lung parenchyma and pulmonary vessels may have been structurally normal initially. Therapeutic relief of chronic alveolar hypoventilation or hypoxemia by ventilatory assist or oxygen usually is accompanied by a demonstrable fall in pulmonary artery pressure and calculated vascular resistance, but often is incomplete.

Perhaps the most dramatic examples of hypoxia-induced pulmonary hypertension are demonstrated by two different altitude-related illnesses. The first is Monge's disease, or chronic mountain sickness, pulmonary hypertension, hypoxemia, and polycythemia described in Peruvian native Indians living at elevations above 12,000 ft. The second is known as high-altitude pulmonary edema (HAPE).[15] In contrast with lifelong altitude residence (Monge's disease), HAPE, also an uncommon disorder, occurs most commonly in children returning to their high-altitude communities after a sojourn at sea level[16] or in newcomers to altitude, often mountaineers,[17] skiers,[16] or soldiers (1965 border war between India and China).[18] Typically, physical activity within a few days of arrival at altitude (usually over 8000 to 10,000 ft) causes progressive dyspnea, headache, cyanosis, and lassitude. If untreated, the subject goes on to develop frank pulmonary edema. Deaths have occurred. Treatment is simple and effective: either 100% oxygen inhalation or descent to a lower elevation (the latter is effective in Monge's disease as well). Typical (composite) hemodynamic findings during the acute phase include hypoxemia, moderate pulmonary arterial hypertension, normal pulmonary artery wedge and left-sided heart filling pressures, normal ventilation, and normal cardiac output. Chest roentgenograms show findings of patchy, predominantly perihilar pulmonary edema. Hultgren proposed a possible, and what may be the only plausible, mechanism to explain the consistent findings of pulmonary edema and pulmonary arterial hypertension in the absence of an elevated pulmonary artery wedge pressure.[15] The hypothesis is that patchy, but widespread, hypoxic pulmonary arteriolar vasoconstriction occurs sufficiently to cause pulmonary artery pressure to increase; this shunts blood flow to unconstricted lung vascular segments wherein capillary pressure is increased and causes lung edema.

Mechanical Obstruction

Mechanical obstruction represents another large category of cor pulmonale (Chap. 54), mainly because of the commonness of pulmonary thromboembolism. Of course, many other substances besides blood clots can impact in pulmonary arteries and block them. Air, amniotic fluid, fat (from fractured long bones), tumor cells, ova of parasites, and endocarditic vegetations in the right side of the heart are examples. In some, the obstructive effect is purely mechanical; that is, it causes reduction in vascular cross section. In others (perhaps a majority?), primary or aggravative pulmonary vasoconstriction occurs. A number and variety of vasoactive intermediaries have been implicated as causes of this secondary effect, prominently various prostaglandins, amines, and polypeptides.

The abrupt onset of vascular obstruction in some of these cases renders it the only category of acute cor pulmonale. In fact, if the occlusion is massive, the clinical presentation is that of shock or even sudden death rather than that of cor pulmonale. At the opposite extreme are cases of recurrent emboli that are individually so small as to have no clinical or physiologic effect, but in the aggregate, over a prolonged period, produce miliary embolization and insidiously progressive cor pulmonale. Clinically, such patients are indistinguishable from those with so-called primary pulmonary hypertension (Chap. 53) in whom, by definition, no etiologic factor can be identified.

Among the causes of mechanical obstruction of the pulmonary circulation besides thromboembolism is a disparate group of disorders characterized by structural (i.e., anatomical) obliteration of the pulmonary vascular cross section in association with pathologic processes involving the lung parenchyma. The mechanism of vascular obstruction is not only highly variable in these disorders; in many, multiple mechanisms are involved. Most of these disorders involve parenchymal (including vascular) disease produced by physical, chemical, or infectious agents. In others the mechanism of obstruction either is unknown (emphysema in a nonsmoker, for example), or is speculative (autoimmunity in rheumatoid pulmonary angiitis, for example). Most of these are slowly progressive chronic disorders, but occasionally, such as in the adult respiratory distress syndrome (ARDS), the presentation is dramatically precipitous (i.e., shock lung).

Because different respiratory components may be involved such as terminal airways, alveoli, alveolar macrophages, and alveolar surface active material, in many of these diseases the ventilatory derangement tends to dominate both the clinical presentation and pathophysiology in comparison with that of vascular obstruction. In addition, respiratory abnormalities also may lead to localized or diffuse alveolar hypoxia and inflammatory processes may be associated with release of vasoactive intermediaries.

These, acting alone or in concert, tend to superimpose vasoconstrictive obstruction on vascular obliteration, thus compounding pulmonary hypertension.

This category of cor pulmonale is large and clinically significant both because of the different mechanisms by which the pulmonary vascular cross section is compromised and also because some of the individual disorders are so common. Pulmonary emphysema and chronic obstructive lung disease alone account for a significant population worldwide. The pneumoconioses, of course, have a strong occupational relationship.

Whether the disorder is common or rare or of known or unknown etiology, an important feature, as far as classification is concerned, is that the underlying disorder responsible or presumed to be responsible for pulmonary vascular obstruction be identifiable. These diseases, along with those associated with hypoxic vasoconstriction and thromboembolism, constitute the category of secondary pulmonary hypertension in cor pulmonale.

The Right Ventricle in Pulmonary Hypertension

The right ventricular response to pulmonary hypertension varies depending on a number and variety of variables, including (1) congenital versus acquired vascular obstruction and, in the latter, whether it appears early in life or later; (2) rapidity of progression of pulmonary hypertension; (3) severity of vascular obstruction; and (4) activity status of the patient. These variables have an impact on the development and magnitude of compensatory right ventricular hypertrophy and on right ventricular failure.

The capacity of the right ventricle to hypertrophy in response to increased load is greater in utero and in infancy and early childhood than later in life. Accordingly, the right ventricle in congenital heart lesions, such as pulmonic stenosis, obligatory pulmonary hypertension associated with large defects (see above), and failure of involution of fetal vascular medial hypertrophy pattern (with or without shunts), demonstrates striking degrees of hypertrophy. Such hypertrophy is sufficiently compensatory that high, even systemic level, right ventricular systolic pressure is sustained for many years, even decades, before overt right ventricular failure ensues. Hypoxic vasoconstrictive pulmonary hypertension present from birth, such as in high-altitude natives, also elicits compensatory right ventricular hypertrophy that permits persons to enjoy a normal life-style with full activity. For any degree of obstruction, the more active the person, the higher the cardiac output and the more severe the degree of exercise-induced pulmonary hypertension.

At the opposite extreme are disorders that abruptly obstruct the pulmonary circulation, such as pulmonary thromboembolism and acute mountain sickness. A suddenly increased pressure load on the right ventricle is poorly tolerated because of the inability of the normally thin-walled right ventricle to develop and sustain high wall tension and stress. Acute dilatation in this setting produces a vicious circle of escalating wall tension (i.e., both components of the Laplace equation, $T = Pr$, increase). Dilatation thins the right ventricular free wall, leading to increased wall stress. Acute right ventricular failure characterized by reduced cardiac output and elevated filling pressure occur if the magnitude of obstruction is sufficiently great.

Between these extremes of chronic hypertrophy and acute failure is a spectrum of pathophysiologic circumstances wherein both the rate of development and progression as well as the magnitude of vascular obstruction vary. In general, the earlier in life and more slowly progressive obstruction develops and the milder its degree, the more compensatory hypertrophy is likely to be, with avoidance of right ventricular failure. However, if pulmonary hypertension is progressive and reaches high levels, eventual failure is almost inescapable.

Clinical Recognition of Pulmonary Hypertension

Pulmonary hypertension produces stereotypical clinical manifestations whose pathophysiologic basis is reasonably straightforward. These relate to the effects of pulmonary hypertension per se, to right ventricular hypertrophy resulting therefrom, or to right ventricular failure. The manifestations appear in their "purest" form in so-called primary pulmonary hypertension because they are "uncontaminated" by manifestations of underlying (i.e., causative) disease processes as in cases of secondary pulmonary hypertension. Variability in clinical manifestations relates to the rate of progression of pulmonary vascular obstruction, the severity of hypertension, and to the activity status of the patient.

Symptoms

Dyspnea and easy fatigue are virtually universally present when pulmonary hypertension is severe. However, they are absent in mild cases and only irregularly present when pulmonary hypertension is moderate and depend on patients' activity status. Dyspnea is thought to result from diminished lung compliance and fatigue from a low cardiac output.

Syncope is another nonspecific symptom associated with severe pulmonary hypertension. It is far less common than dyspnea but it may be dramatic in its frequency in some cases, especially in primary pulmonary hypertension. Transient cerebral ischemia due to reduced cerebral blood flow is the most likely mechanism since it tends to be associated with exertion or orthostasis when there is failure of the right ventricle to maintain cardiac output to meet demand.

Severe pulmonary hypertension also may be associated with chest pain. The term *hypercyanotic angina* was used earlier to describe chest pain in patients with congenital heart disease and pulmonary hypertension. Regardless of etiology or pathophysiologic mechanism, some patients with pulmonary hypertension have typical angina pectoris in the absence of obstructive coronary artery disease. In such patients it is presumed that right ventricular myocardial ischemia results from the combined effects of severe hypertrophy and reduced coronary blood flow. In other patients, chest pain is nondescript. The mechanism of these syndromes is even less certain but aneurysmal dilatation of the main and main branch pulmonary arteries may be involved in some.

An important, even critical, point to be emphasized here is that the symptoms described above occur only when pulmonary hypertension is severe and of long standing. In and of itself, mild to moderate pulmonary hypertension usually is clinically "silent" with regard to symptomatology. Thus, clinical recognition of pulmonary hypertension in its earlier stages relies on more sensitive criteria.

Physical Examination

The physical findings attributable to pulmonary hypertension also relate to hypertension per se, right ventricular hypertrophy, and right ventricular failure. Hypertension is reflected in an accentuated pulmonic component of the second heart sound and a palpable systolic pulsation in the second left parasternal intercostal space. Dilatation of the main pulmonary artery and valve annulus often results in a systolic ejection click and/or a descrescendo diastolic murmur along the left sternal border of pulmonic valve regurgitation. Right ventricular hypertrophy produces a palpable left parasternal thrust or heave and, if present from infancy or childhood, may cause an asymmetric bulge of the left anterior hemithorax. Hypertrophy also may be associated with a third heart sound (S_4, or atrial gallop rhythm). A corollary of this phenomenon is a prominent *a* or presystolic wave in the jugular veins. The signs of right ventricular failure consist of an early diastolic third heart sound (S_3), evidence of systemic venous hypertension, and tissue congestion. A dilated right ventricle and tricuspid valve annulus may cause functional tricuspid regurgitation (holosystolic murmur that may be accentuated by inspiration) and prominent venous *v* waves.

Laboratory Examination

Laboratory data also reflect effects of pulmonary hypertension, right ventricular hypertrophy, and right ventricular failure. The ECG is not very sensitive, but in severe pulmonary hypertension typically shows tall, peaked P waves in leads II, III, and aV_F characteristic of right atrial enlargement (so-called P pulmonale), right axis deviation (mean QRS axis $> +110°$), predominant R deflection of QRS in lead V_1 (right ventricular hypertrophy), and T-wave inversion with ST-segment depression in precordial leads V_1 to V_3.

Routine roentgen films of the chest usually reveal enlargement of the main pulmonary artery and its major branches with attenuated terminal (i.e., distal or peripheral one-third) radicles in the absence of intracardiac shunt. The right atrium and ventricle are enlarged in appropriate projections.

The echocardiogram is probably more sensitive than either the electrocardiogram or chest roentgenograms in revealing enlargement of cardiac chambers and blood vessels. Unfortunately echocardiography is a significantly more costly procedure and itself lacks sensitivity as well as specificity in detecting mild or moderate pulmonary hypertension.[19]

Cardiac catheterization of the right side of the heart continues to be the definitive diagnostic procedure in patients with pulmonary hypertension. However, not all patients need to be subjected to this invasive procedure. It is impossible to specify universally applicable criteria for selecting patients who should be studied. Virtually all patients with suspected congenital heart disease should be studied to determine operability and prognosis. On the other hand, most other patients with secondary pulmonary hypertension, with the exception of those with mitral stenosis, probably do not require catheterization unless precise quantification of pulmonary hypertension is important or vasodilator therapy is to be undertaken. Patients in whom a clinical diagnosis of primary pulmonary hypertension is arrived at by exclusion should be studied to exclude remediable disorders and to quantify vascular obstruction. Patients with severe pulmonary hypertension tend to be hemodynamically fragile; thus, catheterization carries a higher risk.[20]

Radionuclide perfusion lung scanning and pulmonary angiography have the same diagnostic applicability to patients with suspected or established pulmonary hypertension as to those without—that is, to determine the presence of discrete thromboembolic lesions. Resolution of these techniques, however, is compromised to some extent by alterations accompanying vascular obstruction associated with pulmonary hypertension independent of thromboembolism. In general, they are not widely applicable, and angiography carries a higher risk when pulmonary hypertension is severe.[21]

References

1. Harris, P., and Heath, D.: "The Human Pulmonary Circulation," Churchill Livingstone, New York, 1977.

2. West, J. B.: "Respiratory Physiology," The Williams & Wilkins Company, Baltimore, 1974.
3. Dawes, G. S.: Changes in the Circulation at Birth, *Br. Med. Bull.*, 17:148, 1961.
4. Emmanouilides, G. C., Moss, A. J., Dreffie, E. R., Jr., and Adams, F. H.: Pulmonary Arterial Pressure Changes in Human Newborn Infants from Birth to Three Days of Age, *J. Pediatr.*, 65:327, 1964.
5. Vogel, J. H. K., Weaver, W. F., Rose, R. L., Blount, S. G., Jr., and Grover, R. F.: Pulmonary Hypertension on Exertion in Normal Man Living at 10,500 Feet (Leadville, Colorado), *Med. Thorac.*, 19:269, 1962.
6. Peñaloza, D., Sime, F., Banchero, N., Gamboa, R., Cruz, J., and Marticorena, E.: Pulmonary Hypertension in Healthy Men Born and Living at High Altitude, *Am. J. Cardiol.*, 11:150, 1963.
7. Peñaloza, D., Sime, F., Banchero, N., and Gamboa, R.: Pulmonary Hypertension in Healthy Men Born and Living at High Altitude, *Med. Thorac.*, 19:257, 1962.
8. Lewis, B. M., Gorlin, R., Houssay, H. E. J., and Dexter, L.: Clinical and Physiological Correlations in Patients with Mitral Stenosis, *Am. Heart J.*, 43:2, 1952.
9. Thompson, W. P., and White, P. D.: The Commonest Cause of Hypertrophy of the Right Ventricle—Left Ventricular Strain and Failure, *Am. Heart J.*, 12:641, 1936.
10. Tikoff, G., Schmidt, A. M., Thorne, J. L., and Kuida, H.: Clinical and Physiologic Sequelae of Large Ventricular Septal Defects, *Am. J. Med.*, 42:497, 1967.
11. Tikoff, G., Echegaray, H. M., Schmidt, A. M., and Kuida, H.: Patent Ductus Arteriosus Complicated by Heart Failure, *Am. J. Med.*, 46:43, 1969.
12. Wagenvoort, C. A.: The Pulmonary Arteries in Infants with Ventricular Septal Defect, *Med. Thorac.*, 19:162, 1962.
13. Dalen, J. E., Haynes, F. W., and Dexter, L.: Life Expectancy with Atrial Septal Defect: Influence of Complicating Pulmonary Vascular Disease, *JAMA*, 200:422, 1967.
14. Fishman, A. P., Turino, G. M., and Bergofsky, E. H.: The Syndrome of Alveolar Hypoventilation, *Am. J. Med.*, 23:333, 1957.
15. Hultgren, H. N., Lopez, C. E., Lundberg, E., and Miller, H.: Physiologic Studies of Pulmonary Edema of High Altitude, *Circulation*, 29:393, 1964.
16. Fred, H. L., Schmidt, A. M., Bates, T., and Hecht, H. H.: Acute Pulmonary Edema of Altitude: Clinical and Physiologic Observations, *Circulation*, 25:929, 1962.
17. Houston, C. S.: Acute Pulmonary Edema of High Altitude, *New Engl. J Med.*, 263:478, 1960.
18. Singh, I., Kapila, C. C., Khanna, P. K., Nanda, R. B., and Rao, B. D.: High-Altitude Pulmonary Edema, *Lancet*, 1:229, 1965.
19. Algeo, S., Morrison, D., Ovitt, T., and Goldman, S.: Noninvasive Detection of Pulmonary Hypertension, *Clin. Cardiol.*, 7:148, 1984.
20. Caldini, P., Gensini, C. G., and Hoffman, M. S.: Primary Pulmonary Hypertension with Death during Right Heart Catheterization: A Case Report and a Survey of Reported Fatalities, *Am. J. Cardiol.*, 4:519, 1959.
21. Primary Pulmonary Hypertension: A Fatality during Pulmonary Angiography. Clinical Conference from Boston University School of Medicine (G. Snider, moderator), *Chest*, 64:628, 1973.

53

Primary Pulmonary Hypertension

Hiroshi Kuida, M.D.

It is of high importance that students of medicine should learn more clearly than they do to distinguish between factual knowledge and conception. Diagnosis is a system of more or less accurate guessing, in which the end-point achieved is a name. These names applied to disease come to assume the importance of specific entities, whereas they are for the most part no more than insecure and therefore temporary conceptions.

Sir Thomas Lewis, M.D., 1944[1]

The overwhelming majority of cases of pulmonary hypertension are ascribable to an identifiable underlying disease process which provides a pathophysiologic basis for pulmonary vascular obstruction.[2] The general categories of these, as outlined in Chap. 52, include (1) elevated capillary pressure, especially when chronic; (2) congenital heart defects with left-to-right shunting; (3) cor pulmonale of acute or chronic variety with subcategories of (*a*) hypoxic pulmonary vasoconstriction, (*b*) mechanical obstruction due either to thromboembolism or to obliteration of vasculature associated with pulmonary parenchymal diseases, (*c*) vasoconstriction by vasoactive intermediaries, and (*d*) combinations of the above. While no universally valid statistics are available as documentation, the above categories of secondary pulmonary hypertension should account for at least 99 percent of cases of pulmonary hypertension.[3] The main reason that the incidence of pulmonary hypertension in the general population cannot be adequately documented is because definitive detection continues to require venous (right side of the heart) cardiac catheterization. There are no widely applicable and reliable noninvasive techniques for diagnosing pulmonary hypertension, especially when it is mild in degree.[3a]

When a meticulous and ongoing search is made for all the underlying causes of pulmonary hypertension and none is found, then it is appropriate to entertain the presumptive diagnosis of primary pulmonary hypertension, that is, documented pulmonary hypertension in the demonstrated absence of clinically detectable cause. The terms *presumptive* and *detectable* are important here because, as will be discussed below, not all pathologically demonstrable causes of secondary pulmonary hypertension are necessarily clinically detectable. Thus, primary pulmonary hypertension is a rare disorder, comprising less than 1 percent of cases of pulmonary hypertension from all causes documented by cardiac catheterization. Not only is it rare, it continues to be an enigma, as Paul Wood claimed.[4]

Nomenclature and Classification

While *primary pulmonary hypertension* is the term most commonly used,[3] other designations of this disorder include idiopathic,[5,6] essential,[7] solitary,[8] and unexplained[9] pulmonary hypertension. Nomenclature and classification of this condition have been complicated in recent years with the introduction of new diagnostic concepts and terminology.

Before the advent of cardiac catheterization, primary pulmonary hypertension was primarily of pathologic interest.[10] Dresdale et al. correlated clinical and hemodynamic findings with autopsy data and were first to suggest a distinctive clinical presentation.[11] The widespread application of cardiac catheterization has resulted in documentation of severe hemodynamic obstruction and confirmed the stereotypical clinical presentation.[5–9,12–17] However, autopsy-diagnosed thromboembolic pulmonary hypertension in which the clinical and hemodynamic findings were indistinguishable from those in primary pulmonary hypertension has been reported.[18–21] This experience led to the speculation that perhaps some, if not all, cases of primary pulmonary hypertension represented recurrent, clinically silent pulmonary thromboembolism. On the other hand, autopsy examination of certain clinically and hemodynamically similar cases failed to reveal characteristic vascular lesions. McGuire et al.[22] proposed that only these extremely rare cases represented the true, presumably vasospastic, functional obstructive disease that deserved the designation *primary pulmonary hypertension,* thus preserving the analogy with essential systemic hypertension.

More recently the Wagenvoorts[23] proposed the concept that pathologic discrimination between the clinically silent form of recurrent pulmonary thromboembolism and primary pulmonary hypertension could be made and that it was possible to distinguish yet a third pathologic entity, pulmonary venocclusive disease,[24–28] which also could be misconstrued as primary pulmonary hypertension. These workers reviewed pathologic material in 156 cases of supposedly autopsy-confirmed primary pulmonary hypertension submitted to them from 51 medical centers around the world. Surprisingly, in nearly a third of the cases, the original diagnosis was judged erroneous. In 31 cases, the correct diagnosis was considered to be chronic thromboembolism. Of interest in the submitted material were three previously reported cases that had no pulmonary vascular lesions. In all three, "distinct vascular alterations were present although only one case, in our opinion, belonged to the group of cases of vasoconstrictive primary pulmonary hypertension."[23] They also commented that "cases without distinct vascular lesions did not occur in our material." Subsequently, Harris and Heath[29] and Edwards and Edwards[30] concurred with the conclusion that thromboembolic pulmonary hypertension and primary pulmonary hypertension, along with pulmonary venocclusive disease, are pathologically distinct, although potentially clinically uniform, entities. Harris and Heath use the term *unexplained pulmonary hypertension,* and Edwards and Edwards use the term *clinical primary pulmonary hypertension* for antemortem clinical diagnoses of such cases to avoid using primary pulmonary hypertension for cases that potentially have pathologically identifiable causes. The concept of three pathologically distinct entities was adopted at the World Health Organization Conference on Primary Pulmonary Hypertension held in Geneva, Switzerland, in 1973, but the terms *unexplained pulmonary hypertension* and *primary pulmonary hypertension* are considered synonymous in the report of the meeting.[3] Thus, diagnosis of primary pulmonary hypertension as originally conceived, that is, all known causes excluded, theoretically cannot be made without pathologic confirmation. When so confirmed, the term *classical* or *vasoconstrictive primary pulmonary hypertension* is used to distinguish this particular form of unexplained pulmonary hypertension.[23]

The confusion in diagnosis and classification is highlighted by the discrepancy between researchers: Paul Wood, who was never proved wrong in his ability to diagnose primary pulmonary hypertension clinically,[6] and the Wagenvoorts, who found that even pathologic diagnosis may be erroneous. While clinicians undoubtedly will continue to make the diagnosis of primary pulmonary hypertension on the basis of clinical and hemodynamic criteria, Paul Wood notwithstanding, they should be prepared to be proved wrong if and when their patients are autopsied. It is doubtful, however, that pathologic classification represents the final word on this disorder.

Etiology and Pathogenesis

The etiology of primary pulmonary hypertension is, of course, unknown. Most agree, however, that it is, with rare exception, an acquired condition.[23] There are certain clinical aspects of the disease that have stimulated speculation about etiologic or pathogenetic mechanisms:

- Women's predisposition to the disease, female/male sex-incidence ratios averaging greater than 3:1.[23]
- The relationship of pregnancy to disease onset or aggravation, raising the possibility that amniotic fluid or thromboplastin-induced fibrin embolism might be initiating or perpetuating factors.[5,31]

- The common occurrence of Raynaud's phenomenon in association with primary pulmonary hypertension raising the possibility that primary pulmonary hypertension might represent a form of autoimmune or collagen vascular disease.[23,32–34]
- Reports of familial aggregation of cases, raising the issue of a genetic basis or predisposition to primary pulmonary hypertension.[32,35,36] In one particular family, abnormal fibrinolysis was demonstrated.[36]
- The occurrence in a few central European countries of outbursts of the disease that seemed circumstantially to be related to the anorexigenic compound aminorex.[3,37–39]
- The demonstration over the years of several unequivocal pulmonary vasoconstrictive mediators such as hypoxia, serotonin, and prostaglandin $F_2\alpha$.
- The occurrence of primary pulmonary hypertension in children, an age group in which thromboembolism is rare, in roughly equal sex distribution.

In reviewing these as well as other possible etiologic factors, a compelling case could not be made for any single factor causing the vasoconstriction believed to be the root cause of vascular obstruction.[23] Recent reports[40] linking pulmonary hypertension with use of oral contraceptive drugs are ominous, but to date there have been no large-scale outbreaks as in the case of aminorex. An alternative interpretation of this wide array of associative factors is that, not unlike essential hypertension, primary pulmonary hypertension is a complex, multifactorial syndrome of diverse contributory etiologies and that its terminal course is uniform.

Pathophysiology

The physiologic determinants of pulmonary artery pressure can be gleaned from the Poiseuille relationship:

$$\text{PAP} = k\frac{\text{CO}}{r^4} + \text{PCP}$$

where PAP = pulmonary artery pressure
CO = cardiac output
r = radius or bore of flow-limiting vessels
PCP = pulmonary capillary pressure
k = a proportionality constant

In primary pulmonary hypertension, pulmonary artery pressure is elevated, pulmonary capillary pressure is normal, and cardiac output normal or decreased; hence r is diminished. It is, therefore, an example of vascular obstruction, i.e., diminished vascular conductance or increased resistance. What is far from obvious is the mechanism of the initiation of vasoconstriction and the perpetuation, or progression, of the obstruction.

Pathology

There is no specific pulmonary vascular lesion in primary pulmonary hypertension. Indeed, the arteriopathy of primary pulmonary hypertension is virtually identical, in every respect, to that seen more commonly associated with congenital cardiovascular defects accompanied by shunting and severe pulmonary hypertension.[41] Particular types of lesions (discussed below) also have been described in diseases other than congenital heart disease. For example, plexiform lesions have been found in pulmonary hypertension secondary to cirrhosis or portal vein thrombosis,[42] and other types of dilatation lesions are seen in pulmonary hypertension associated with schistosomiasis.[23] Fibrinoid medial necrosis-arteritis is considered to be a nonspecific response to severe and/or rapid pressure elevation of whatever cause.[41] Fishman has proposed that this may also be true for plexiform lesions.[43] However, when other causes of pulmonary hypertension are carefully excluded using evidence other than pulmonary vasculopathy, the pathologic findings in primary pulmonary hypertension are considered to be distinctive.

Pathologic lesions in primary pulmonary hypertension in approximate ascending order of relative diagnostic specificity are as follows: (1) typical atherosclerotic plaques in the large, elastic pulmonary arteries; (2) medial hypertrophy of small muscular arteries; (3) so-called dilatation lesions, including medial degeneration and atrophy with dilatation, angiomatous and plexiform lesions, and veinlike branches of hypertrophied, usually occluded, muscular arteries; and (4) intimal fibrosis and fibroelastosis in typical onionskin, laminated proliferation. In the aggregate these lesions constitute so-called plexogenic pulmonary arteriopathy, and they supposedly represent the pathologic substrate of "classical" primary pulmonary hypertension.[24]

The pathology of these lesions has been detailed by Wagenvoort, Heath, and Edwards.[41] The vasculopathy in primary pulmonary hypertension is characterized by considerable variability and patchy distribution of focal lesions. Indeed, the majority of vessels remain normal-looking or show only varying degrees of medial hypertrophy. Medial hypertrophy may be the only finding in children, and there are isolated reports of catheterization-documented cases of severe pulmonary hypertension in adults in whom no lesions or, at most, only mild medial hypertrophy was found. Apparently the presence, number, type, or combination of lesions found does not necessarily correlate with clinical or hemodynamic features. However, this may only reflect the fact that by the time most patients come to postmortem examination, the process is sufficiently far advanced that a wide pathologic spectrum is not being evaluated.

The pathology of the two entities besides plexogenic pulmonary arteriopathy that may give rise to clinical and hemodynamic findings indistinguishable from those of primary pulmonary hypertension deserves comment. The first is recurrent (or chronic) pulmonary thromboembolism. Pathologic diagnosis of this entity hinges on identification of thromboembolic lesions in various stages of organization in muscular pulmonary arteries and arterioles.[23] Intimal fibrosis and thickening are common but usually eccentrically located in the form of pads rather than concentric and laminated rings as in the case of onionskin lesions. Recanalized and septate thrombi are considered to be different from, but may mimic, plexiform and angiomatous lesions, which are absent. Necrotizing arteritis also is absent, but medial hypertrophy and pulmonary atherosclerosis may be present. The other pathologic entity, pulmonary venocclusive disease, is distinctive in showing what are considered to represent postthrombotic occlusion of pulmonary veins with patchy capillary engorgement and nonspecific secondary arteriopathy.[23]

Clinical Diagnosis

The typical or classic case of primary pulmonary hypertension is not difficult to diagnose if it is accepted that clinical distinction of cases of pulmonary hypertension secondary to clinically silent recurrent pulmonary embolism cannot be made. While the symptoms outlined in Chap. 52 are nonspecific,[44] their occurrence in a young woman with unequivocal physical and laboratory manifestations of pulmonary hypertension and right ventricular hypertrophy constitute a dramatic presentation.[13] Usually, cardiac catheterization is performed to exclude the remote possibilities of occult congenital heart disease or mitral valve stenosis.

The real challenge of this disorder is making the diagnosis before pulmonary hypertension of sufficient severity or duration has existed to produce easily detectable manifestations of pulmonary hypertension and right ventricular hypertrophy. This is especially pertinent now that vasodilator drug therapy looms as an efficacious possibility and in consideration of the concept that treatment will be more likely to be successful if instituted before fixed obstructive lesions develop. In practical terms, this means exercising a high index of suspicion and surveillance of the diagnosis of primary pulmonary hypertension in any patient who has unexplained effort dyspnea or episodes of light-headedness, or who manifests equivocal findings of right ventricular hypertrophy.

Treatment

The treatment objective in primary pulmonary hypertension is clear enough; it is to relieve vascular obstruction, but achieving it has been difficult and often frustrating. Pharmacologic therapy is based on the notion that pathophysiologic vasospasm is an important contributor to or the cause of vascular obstruction. To this end, a number and variety of vasoactive drugs have been tested for therapeutic efficacy by many investigators for over two decades. The results of these tests can be fairly characterized as covering the spectrum from tantalizing successes to dismal failures (i.e., deaths). Beneficial effects have been reported even in patients with thromboembolism.[45]

It is not difficult to specify characteristics of the ideal drug; i.e., one that (1) is effective orally and intravenously without tachyphylaxis, (2) reduces or blocks pulmonary vasoconstriction exclusively without other pharmacologic effects (such as on systemic vessels or on cardiac output), and (3) has no undesirable side effects. Drug efficacy research in primary pulmonary hypertension is made difficult by several considerations, including (1) rarity of the disorder, (2) the requirement for invasive studies (also lack of noninvasive monitoring of chronic therapy), and, perhaps most importantly, (3) potential lack of uniformity, both qualitatively and quantitatively, of cases. The recent availability of a number and variety of effective vasodilator drugs for the treatment of systemic hypertension has resulted in their trial in primary pulmonary hypertension. The rationale for such trials is based on earlier observations of vasodilatory effects of such parenteral agents as acetylcholine and tolazoline.[46,47] The "newer" drugs include isoproterenol,[48–51] diazoxide,[52–54] continuous O_2,[55] hydralazine,[56–59] phentolamine,[59,60] calcium channel blockers,[61–66] and nitroglycerin.[67]

The interesting result of these trials is the lack of consistency both among and within studies. Of course, it has not been possible to conduct randomized placebo-blinded studies nor to systematically control for stage or severity of disease process, much less for possible differences in etiology. Yet another problem is the definition of a beneficial effect. The optimal vasodilatory effect of lowering pulmonary artery pressure without increasing resting cardiac output unduly is the exception rather than the rule. Reduction in calculated pulmonary vascular resistance is commonly reported, but in many of these cases increase in cardiac output exceeds the fall, if any, in pulmonary artery pressure. Thus, while pulmonary resistance falls, right ventricular minute work changes little or, in fact, may increase. The latter is hardly a desirable effect in a disease where right ventricular failure is the most common cause of disability and death.

Since long-standing, severe pulmonary hypertension predisposes to fixed pulmonary vascular lesions such as "onionskin" fibrosis or plexiform lesions, or may provoke arteritis, it is reasonable that cases diagnosed earlier in the overall course of the disorder and/or when pulmonary hypertension was milder in severity stand to achieve greater benefit from vasodilator therapy. Thus, early diagnosis is an important therapeutic goal. Selection of the therapeutic agent can be made rationally only by hemodynamic trial-and-error testing of drugs available for oral administration or topical application. The available literature on such trials, characterized by conflicting or unpredictable results, does not permit a preference priority. Undoubtedly, newer agents will become available as the search for the ideal drug for the treatment of systemic hypertension continues. The commercial imperative to develop "pure" pulmonary vasodilator drugs is not nearly so pressing, unfortunately. The national registry of cases of primary pulmonary hypertension, undertaken by the NHLBI, is a valuable first step in the systematic study of this disorder and, hopefully, will be followed by multicenter, long-term, drug-efficacy trials.

The issue of anticoagulation therapy also is a vexing problem. The rationale is to curtail thromboembolic episodes in those patients who have this form of unexplained pulmonary hypertension. Anticoagulation therapy would not be expected to have a beneficial effect on patients with classic or plexogenic primary pulmonary hypertension, although these patients are by no means immune to thromboembolism. The occasional patient who exhibits hemoptysis, presumably from rupture of dilatation lesions, could be made worse. No general recommendation concerning anticoagulation therapy is therefore possible. However, it may be reasonable to initiate anticoagulation therapy at the slightest provocation.

Chronic, especially nocturnal, oxygen therapy may be worth trying under certain circumstances, such as (1) in patients residing at higher elevations to preclude aggravative hypoxic pulmonary vasoconstriction, (2) in patients who exhibit significant arterial blood oxyhemoglobin desaturation, and (3) in patients who respond to acute oxygen inhalation by a drop in pulmonary artery pressure during hemodynamic study.

References

1. Lewis, T.: Reflections upon Reform in Medical Education, *Lancet,* 1:619, 1944.
2. Blount, S. G., Jr., and Grover, R. F.: Pulmonary Hypertension, in J. W. Hurst, (ed.), "The Heart," 4th ed., McGraw-Hill Book Company, New York, 1978, p. 1456.
3. Hatano, S., and Strasser, T. (eds.): "Report on a WHO Meeting on Primary Pulmonary Hypertension in October 1973," World Health Organization, Geneva, 1975.
3a. Algeo, S, Morrison, D., Ovitt, T., and Goldman, S.: Noninvasive Detection of Pulmonary Hypertension, *Clin. Cardiol.,* 7:148, 1984.
4. Wood, P.: Primary Pulmonary Hypertension, in: "Diseases of the Heart and Circulation," 2d ed., Eyre & Spottiswoode, Ltd., London, 1956, p. 83.
5. Shepherd, J. T., Edwards, J. E., Burchell, J. B., Swan, H. J. C., and Wood, E. H.: Clinical Physiological and Pathological Consideration in Patients with Idiopathic Pulmonary Hypertension, *Br. Heart J.,* 19:70, 1957.
6. Heath, D., Whittaker, W., and Brown, J.: Idiopathic Pulmonary Hypertension, *Br. Heart J.,* 19:83, 1957.
7. Schafer, H., Blain, J. M., Ceballos, R., and Bing, R. J.: Essential Pulmonary Hypertension: A Report of Clinical-Physiologic Studies in 3 Patients with Death Following Catheterization of the Heart, *Ann. Intern. Med.,* 44:505, 1956.
8. Evans, W., Short, D. S., and Bedford, D. E.: Solitary Pulmonary Hypertension, *Br. Heart J.,* 19:93, 1957.
9. Wade, G., and Ball, J.: Unexplained Pulmonary Hypertension, *Q. J. Med.,* 26:83, 1957.
10. Brenner, O.: Pathology of the Vessels of the Pulmonary Circulation, *Arch. Intern. Med.,* 56:211, 1935.
11. Dresdale, D. T., Schultz, M., and Michtom, R. J.: Primary Pulmonary Hypertension, *Am. J. Med.,* 11:686, 1951.
12. Chapman, D. W., Abbott, J. P., and Latson, J.: Primary Pulmonary Hypertension: Review of the Literature and Results of Cardiac Catheterization in Ten Patients, *Circulation,* 15:35, 1957.
13. Kuida, H., Dammin, G. J., Haynes, F. W., Rapaport, E., and Dexter, L.: Primary Pulmonary Hypertension, *Am. J. Med.,* 23:166, 1957.
14. Yu, P. N.: Primary Pulmonary Hypertension: Report of Six Cases and Review of Literature, *Ann. Intern. Med.,* 49:1138, 1958.
15. Sleeper, J. C., Orgain, E. S., and McIntosh, H. D.: Primary Pulmonary Hypertension: Review of Clinical Features and Pathologic Physiology with a Report of Pulmonary Hemodynamics Derived from Repeated Catheterization, *Circulation,* 26:1358, 1962.
16. Farrar, J. F.: Idiopathic Pulmonary Hypertension, *Am. Heart J.,* 66:128, 1963.
17. Shane, S. J., Aterman, K., Roy, D. L., and Chandler, B. M.: Primary Pulmonary Hypertension: A Review and Report of Five Cases. *Can. Med. Assoc. J.,* 91:145, 1964.
18. Fowler, N. O., Black-Schaffer, B., Scott, R. C., and Gueron, M.: Idiopathic and Thromboembolic Pulmonary Hypertension, *Am. J. Med.,* 40:331, 1966.
19. Castleman, B., and Bland, E. F.: Organized Emboli of Tertiary Pulmonary Arteries, *Arch. Pathol.,* 42:581, 1946.
20. Owen, R. W., Thomas W. A., Castleman, B., and Bland, E. F.: Unrecognized Emboli to the Lungs with Subsequent Cor Pulmonale, *N. Engl. J. Med.,* 249:919, 1953.
21. Goodwin, J. F., Harrison, C. V., and Wilcken, D. E. L.: Obliterative Pulmonary Hypertension and Thromboembolism, *Br. Med. J.,* 1:701, 1963.
22. McGuire, J., Scott, R. C., Helm, R. A., Kaplan, S., Gall, E. A., and Diehl, J. P.: Is There an Entity Primary Pulmonary Hypertension? *A.M.A. Arch. Intern. Med.,* 99:917, 1957.
23. Wagenvoort, C. A., and Wagenvoort, N.: Primary Pulmonary Hypertension: A Pathologic Study of the Lung Vessels in 156 Clinically Diagnosed Cases, *Circulation,* 42:1163, 1970.
24. Brown, C. H., and Harrison, C. V.: Pulmonary Veno-Occlusive Disease, *Lancet,* 2:61, 1966.
25. Heath, D., Segel, M. B., and Bishop, J.: Pulmonary-Veno-Occlusive Disease, *Circulation,* 34:242, 1966.
26. Weisser, K., Wyler, F., and Gloor, F.: Pulmonary Veno-Occlusive Disease, *Arch. Dis. Child.,* 42:322, 1967.
27. Heath, D., Scott, O., and Lynch, J.: Pulmonary Veno-Occlusive Disease, *Thorax,* 26:663, 1971.
28. Rosenthal, A., Vawter, G., and Wagenvoort, C. A.: Intrapulmonary Veno-Occlusive Disease, *Am. J. Cardiol.,* 1:78, 1973.
29. Harris, P., and Heath D.: Unexplained Pulmonary Hypertension, in "The Human Pulmonary Circulation," 2d ed., Churchill Livingstone, Edinburgh, 1977, p. 418.
30. Edwards, W. D., and Edwards J. E.: Clinical Primary Pulmonary Hypertension, Three Pathologic Types, *Circulation,* 56:884, 1977.
31. Olley, P. M., and Whitaker, W.: Postpartum Pulmonary Hypertension, *Obstet, Gynecol.,* 29:369, 1967.
32. Walcott, B., Burchell, H. B., and Brown, A. L.: Primary Pulmonary Hypertension, *Am. J. Med.,* 49:70, 1970.
33. Celoria, G. C., Fierdell, G. H., and Sommer, S. C.: Raynaud's Disease and Primary Pulmonary Hypertension, *Circulation,* 22:1055, 1960.

34. Winters, W. L., Jr., Joseph, R. R., and Learner, N.: "Primary" Pulmonary Hypertension and Raynaud's Phenomenon, Case Report and Review of the Literature, *Arch. Intern. Med.*, 114:821, 1964.
35. Hendrix, G. H.: Familial Primary Pulmonary Hypertension, *South Med. J.*, 67:981, 1974.
36. Inglesby, T. V., Singer, J. W., and Gordon, D. S.: Abnormal Fribrinolysis in Familial Pulmonary Hypertension, *Am. J. Med.*, 55:5, 1973.
37. Gurtner, H. P., Gertsch, M., Salzmann, C., Scherrer, M., Stucki, P., and Wyss, F.: Haufen sich die primar Vascularen formen des Chronischen Cor Pulmonale? *Schweiz. Med. Wochenschr.*, 98:1579, 1968.
38. Schwingshackl, H., Armor, H., and Dienstl, F.: "Primare" Pulmonale hypertonie bei sieben jungeren Frauen, *Dtsch. Med. Wochenschr.*, 94:639, 1969.
39. Lang, E., Haupt, E. J., Kohler, J. A., and Schmidt, J.: Cor Pulmonale durch Appetitizugler?, *Munch. Med. Wochenschr.*, 111:405, 1969.
40. Kleiger, R. E., Boxer, M., Ingham, R. E., and Harrison, D. E.: Pulmonary Hypertension in Patients Using Oral Contraceptives: A Report of Six Cases, *Chest*, 69:143, 1976.
41. Wagenvoort, C. A., Heath, D., and Edwards, J. E.: "The Pathology of the Pulmonary Vasculature," Charles C Thomas, Publisher, Springfield, Ill., 1964.
42. Naeye, R. L.: "Primary" Pulmonary Hypertension with Coexisting Portal Hypertension, *Circulation*, 22:376, 1969.
43. Fishman, A. P.: Plexiform Lesions, *Pathol. Microbiol. Basel*, 43:242, 1975.
44. Trell, E., and Lindstrom, C.: Primary and Chronic Thromboembolic Pulmonary Hypertension: Clinical and Pathoanatomic Observations, *Acta Med. Scand. (Suppl.)*, 534:1, 1972.
45. Dantzker, D. R., and Bower, J. S.: Partial Reversibility of Chronic Pulmonary Hypertension Caused by Pulmonary Thromboembolic Disease, *Am. Rev. Resp. Dis.*, 124:129, 1981.
46. Dresdale, D. T., Michtom, R. J., and Schultz, M.: Recent Studies in Primary Pulmonary Hypertension Including Pharmacodynamic Observations on Pulmonary Vascular Resistance, *Bull N.Y. Acad. Med.*, 30:195, 1954.
47. Grover, R. F., Reeves, J. T., and Blount, S. G.: Tolazoline Hydrochloride (Priscoline), an Effective Pulmonary Vasodilator, *Am. Heart J.*, 61:5, 1961.
48. Shettigar, U. R., Hultgren, H. N., Specter, M., Martin, R., and Davies, H. D.: Primary Pulmonary Hypertension, Favorable Effect of Isoproterenol, *N. Engl. J. Med.*, 295:1414, 1976.
49. Daoud, F. S., Reeves, J. T., and Kelly, D. B.: Isoproterenol as a Potential Pulmonary Vasodilator in Primary Pulmonary Hypertension, *Am. J. Cardiol.*, 42:817, 1978.
50. Belman, M. J., Tiep, B. L., and Westinghouse, W. D.: Isoproterenol in Pulmonary Hypertension, *N. Engl. J. Med.*, 298:51, 1978.
51. Elkayam, U., Freshman, W. H., Yoran, C., Strom, J., Sonnenblick, E. H., and Cohen, M.: Unfavorable Hemodynamic and Clinical Effects of Isoproterenol Therapy in Primary Pulmonary Hypertension, *Cardiovasc. Med.*, 3:1177, 1978.
52. Wang, S. W. S., Pohl, J. E. F., Rowlands, D. J., and Wade, E. G.: Diazoxide in Treatment of Primary Pulmonary Hypertension, *Br. Heart J.*, 40:572, 1978.
53. Klinke, W. P., and Gilbert, J. A. L.: Diazoxide in Primary Pulmonary Hypertension, *N. Engl. J. Med.*, 302:91, 1980.
54. Rubino, J. M., and Schroeder, J. S.: Diazoxide in Treatment of Primary Pulmonary Hypertension (Correspondence), *Br. Heart J.*, 42:362, 1979.
55. Nagasaka, Y., Akutsu, H., Lee, Y. S., Fujimoto, S., and Chikamori, J.: Long-Term Favorable Effect of Oxygen Administration on a Patient with Primary Pulmonary Hypertension, *Chest*, 74:299, 1978.
56. Rubin, L. J., and Peter, H. R.: Oral Hydralazine Therapy for Primary Pulmonary Hypertension, *N. Engl. J. Med.*, 302:69, 1980.
57. Lupi-Herrera, E., Sandoval, J., Sloane, M., and Bialostozky, D.: The Role of Hydralazine Therapy for Pulmonary Arterial Hypertension of Unknown Cause, *Circulation*, 65:645, 1982.
58. Kronzon, I., Cohen, M., and Wener, H. E.: Adverse Effect of Hydralazine in Patients with Primary Pulmonary Hypertension, *JAMA*, 247:3112, 1982.
59. Ruskin, J. N., and Hutter, A. M.: Primary Pulmonary Hypertension Treated with Oral Phentolamine, *Ann. Intern. Med.*, 90:772, 1979.
60. Cohen, M. L., and Kronzon, I.: Adverse Hemodynamic Effects of Phentolamine in Primary Pulmonary Hypertension, *Ann. Intern. Med.*, 95:591, 1981.
61. Landmark, K., Refsum, A. M., Simonsen, S., and Storstein, O.: Verapamil and Pulmonary Hypertension, *Acta Med. Scand.*, 204:299, 1978.
62. Camerini, F., Alberti, E., Klugman, S., and Salvi, A.: Primary Pulmonary Hypertension: Effects of Nifedipine, *Br. Heart J.*, 44:352, 1980.
63. Kambara, H., Fujimoto, K., Wakabayashi, A., and Kawai, C.: Primary Pulmonary Hypertension: Beneficial Therapy with Diltiazem, *Am. Heart J.*, 101:230, 1981.
64. Berkenboom, G., Sobolski, J., and Stoupel, E.: Failure of Nifedipine Treatment in Primary Pulmonary Hypertension (Correspondence), *Br. Heart J.*, 47:511, 1982.
65. Crevey, B. J., Dantzker, D. R., Bower, J. S., Popat, K. D., and Walker, S. D.: Hemodynamic and Gas Exchange Effects of Intravenous Diltiazem in Patients with Pulmonary Hypertension, *Am. J. Cardiol.*, 49:578, 1982.
66. Melot, C., Naeije, R., Mols., P., Vandenbossche, J., and Denolin, H.: Effects of Nifedipine on Ventilation Perfusion Matching in Primary Pulmonary Hypertension, *Chest*, 8:203, 1983.
67. Pearl, R. G., Rosenthal, M. H., Schroeder, J. S., and Ashton, J. P. A.: Acute Hemodynamic Effects of Nitroglycerine in Pulmonary Hypertension, *Ann. Intern. Med.*, 99:9, 1983.

54

Pulmonary Embolism

James E. Dalen, M.D.   Joseph S. Alpert, M.D.

That, therefore, which according to the ordinary nomenclature is called suppurative phlebitis, is neither suppurative, nor yet phlebitis, but a process which begins with a coagulation, with the formation of a thrombus in the blood, and afterwards presents a stage in which the thrombi soften, so that the whole history of the process is contained in the history of the thrombus.

Rudolf Virchow, 1858[1]

Pulmonary Embolism

Each year there are approximately 200,000 deaths in the United States due to pulmonary embolism. In half the cases, it is the major cause of death; in the other half it is a significant contributing cause in patients who have other major diseases. The majority of deaths occur in patients who are not treated because the diagnosis is not established.[2] The mortality of untreated pulmonary embolism is 20 to 30 percent. If the diagnosis is established and appropriate treatment instituted, mortality is less than 10 percent.[3]

In nearly all cases pulmonary embolism originates as deep venous thrombosis (DVT) in the proximal deep venous system in the lower legs. The factors that predispose to deep venous thrombosis are shown in Table 54-1. The optimal strategy for preventing fatal pulmonary embolism is to recognize those patients who are at increased risk of DVT, and then to institute appropriate prophylactic treatment to prevent DVT and pulmonary embolism.

Prevention of Deep Venous Thrombosis

There are multiple techniques to prevent DVT, as shown in Table 54-2. In medical patients without contraindications, low-dose heparin, 5000 units subcutaneously every 12 h is very effective in preventing DVT.[4,5] In patients at particular risk, e.g., in those undergoing hip replacement, in hip fractures, and in men undergoing urological procedures, low-dose heparin does not provide adequate protection. In these circumstances intravenous dextran or the combination of dihydroergotamine and low-dose heparin are appropriate forms of prophylaxis.[6,7] In patients at increased risk of bleeding such as those undergoing neurosurgical procedures, external compression devices have been shown to be effective.[8,9] It should be noted that in patients undergoing elective surgery these prophylactic therapies should begin prior to the induction of anesthesia. Deep venous thrombosis begins to occur while patients are anesthetized in the operating room.

Diagnosis of Deep Venous Thrombosis

If the prophylactic therapies listed above are instituted, the risk of DVT and its potentially lethal complication, pulmonary embolism, is greatly diminished.

If prophylactic treatment is not utilized or if it fails, the clinician must be prepared to recognize DVT when it first occurs, in order to institute treatment to prevent pulmonary embolism. The classic sign of DVT, unilateral leg swelling, occurs in the minority of cases; most episodes of DVT are clinically silent. Therefore, the detection of DVT requires the clinician to be vigilant, and to perform venography or noninvasive tests whenever DVT is suspected.

The most sensitive and specific test for the recognition of DVT is venography.[10,11] A disadvantage of venography is that it is invasive and somewhat uncomfortable, and therefore is rarely performed more than once on a given patient.

Scanning the legs after the injection of fibrinogen

TABLE 54-1 Risk Factors for Deep Venous Thrombosis

Prior history of venous thrombosis
Surgical procedures
Trauma to lower extremities
Bed rest, immobility
Congestive heart failure
Malignancy (including occult malignancy)
Pregnancy
Oral contraceptive agents
Obesity
Advanced age

TABLE 54-2 Prevention of Deep Venous Thrombosis

Anticoagulation
Low-dose subcutaneous heparin
Warfarin
Platelet active agents
Aspirin
Dextran
Other agents
Dihydroergotamine
Prevention of venous stasis
Graded compression stockings
Intermittent pneumatic compression

labeled with ^{125}I is very sensitive in the diagnosis of DVT.[12] The disadvantage of this test is that the ^{125}I must be injected prior to the development of DVT. This test can be used preoperatively in patients who are at risk of intra- or postoperative DVT.

The Doppler technique is another noninvasive test for the diagnosis of DVT. The value of the Doppler technique is compromised by the fact that its accuracy is highly dependent upon the expertise of the operators. The sensitivity and specificity of this technique in detecting DVT vary widely in different medical centers.

The impedance plethysmography (IPG) technique is extremely useful in evaluating patients with suspected DVT.[13] This noninvasive technique can be performed at the bedside in 15 to 20 min. It takes advantage of the fact that the electrical impedance in the lower extremities is easily measured, and is directly related to venous volume in the legs. The baseline electrical impedance in the legs is measured and then a blood pressure cuff is inflated above venous pressure in the proximal thigh. The change in electrical impedance as venous volume increases is recorded with a strip chart. The cuff is then released. If the deep venous system is patent and free of occlusive thrombus, there is a prompt venous outflow and electrical impedance returns to baseline over a period of seconds. If the deep venous system is obstructed, the return of electrical impedance to baseline is delayed. Correlation between a unilaterally positive IPG and venography exceeds 90 percent. A bilaterally normal IPG nearly excludes proximal (above the knee) DVT. The test is less sensitive to DVT confined to the distal leg (below the knee). If the IPG is positive in both legs, venography should be performed because DVT may or may not be present. The IPG is extremely useful in detecting DVT at the bedside.[12,14]

If proximal DVT is detected, treatment with intravenous heparin for 10 days, followed by oral warfarin therapy should be given to prevent pulmonary embolism. Without treatment, pulmonary embolism occurs in 50 percent of patients with proximal DVT. The probability of pulmonary embolism in patients with DVT limited to the distal lower extremity is less than 10 percent. Therefore, in an asymptomatic patient, many physicians would not institute heparin treatment in this circumstance. Repeat IPG to make certain that there has not been extension to the proximal venous circulation is indicated if DVT limited to the distal lower extremity is not treated.

Some have advocated fibrinolytic treatment with urokinase or streptokinase in patients with symptomatic proximal DVT to prevent the postphlebitic syndrome. However, incidence of the postphlebitic syndrome in patients treated with heparin is uncertain. Direct evidence that fibrinolytic therapy prevents the postphlebitic syndrome in patients with DVT has not been presented.

Diagnosis of Acute Pulmonary Embolus

One of the reasons that the diagnosis of acute pulmonary embolism is frequently missed is that a given episode of acute pulmonary embolism may present as one of three different clinical syndromes: acute cor pulmonale, pulmonary infarction or hemorrhage, or acute "unexplained" dyspnea.[15] The pathophysiology, signs, and symptoms of these three syndromes are quite different. The differential diagnosis and the appropriate diagnostic workup also are different. In order to detect acute pulmonary embolism, the clinician must be prepared to recognize each of these three syndromes of acute pulmonary embolism.

Pulmonary Infarction or Hemorrhage

This is the commonest way that pulmonary embolism presents. More than 50 percent of all patients in whom pulmonary embolism is diagnosed have signs or symptoms of pulmonary infarction. The classic symptom of pulmonary infarction is the abrupt onset of pleuritic chest pain, with or without dyspnea. Hemoptysis occurs in a minority of patients. Pleuritic pain in patients with pulmonary infarction is caused by intraalveolar hemorrhage due to the influx of blood from the bronchial collateral circulation into obstructed portions of the distal pulmonary circulation.[16] Pulmonary angiography in these patients demonstrates submassive embolism with obstruction of distal branches of the pulmonary circulation.

Pulmonary hemorrhage due to bronchial arterial collateral flow usually causes a pulmonary infiltrate as detected by chest x-ray. The other chest x-ray abnormalities in patients with pulmonary infarction include an elevated diaphragm due to splinting of respiration, or a small pleural effusion which is usually unilateral and may or may not be bloody. One or more of these three chest x-ray abnormalities is present in more than two-thirds of patients with pulmonary infarction.[17]

On physical examination, tachypnea as evidenced by a respiratory rate greater than 20 per min is nearly always present. Signs of right ventricular failure are absent. Examination of the lungs usually reveals rales, wheezes, or evidence of a pleural effusion. A pleural friction rub may be present. Evidence of deep venous thrombosis is present in a minority of cases.

The principal differential diagnosis in patients presenting with pulmonary infarction is viral or bacterial pneumonitis. A history of a viral prodrome, or of a shaking chill with fever or purulent sputum points to pneumonitis.

The most useful laboratory tests in patients with suspected pulmonary infarction include the chest x-ray, white blood cell count (WBC) and differential, gram stain of sputum if available, and arterial blood gases. The WBC, differential, and sputum examination help to diagnose bacterial pneumonia. The arterial blood gases in patients with pulmonary infarction will nearly always demonstrate hypocapnia and respiratory alkalosis secondary to tachypnea. However, since pulmonary infarction usually occurs in patients with submassive pulmonary embolism, the arterial P_{O_2} may be in the normal range in patients without prior lung disease.

The most useful screening test for pulmonary embolism is the perfusion ventilation lung scan.[17] The most specific finding for acute pulmonary embolism is the presence of large segmental perfusion defects that ventilate normally.[18] The IPG is also useful in patients suspected of acute pulmonary embolism, in that it is positive in the vast majority of patients with acute pulmonary embolism.[14,19] If the diagnosis remains uncertain after evaluation of the clinical findings, IPG, and ventilation/perfusion (V/Q) lung scan, pulmonary angiography may be indicated for definitive diagnosis.

Acute Cor Pulmonale

Acute cor pulmonale, the most dramatic presentation of acute pulmonary embolism, occurs when pulmonary embolism has been sufficiently massive to obstruct more than 60 to 75 percent of the pulmonary circulation.

The body's normal response to acute pulmonary embolism is to increase cardiac output and to increase right ventricular systolic pressure to overcome the increased afterload in the pulmonary circulation. The normal right ventricle can acutely increase its systolic pressure to about 50 to 60 mmHg. Acute increases in right ventricular systolic pressure beyond this level lead to acute right ventricular dilatation and increased filling pressures. As the right ventricle dilates and fails, its stroke volume decreases, leading to decreased cardiac output, hypotension, and possible cardiac arrest.[20]

In addition to acute dyspnea, patients with acute cor pulmonale may present with signs of an acute decrease in cardiac output: hypotension, syncope,[21] or cardiac arrest. On physical examination the vital signs reveal tachypnea and tachycardia, and possible hypotension. Signs of acute right ventricular failure—distended neck veins, right-sided S_3 gallop, and a parasternal heave—are usually present. The lungs are clear; signs of DVT may be present. Dependent upon the clinical setting, the differential diagnosis includes acute myocardial infarction, hypovolemia, or sepsis.

The most useful diagnostic tests in patients with suspected acute cor pulmonale are the ECG, measurement of central venous pressure, and arterial blood gas analysis.

The ECG in patients with acute cor pulmonale will usually show a new S_1 Q_3 T_3 pattern,[22] incomplete right bundle branch block,[17] or other signs of right ventricular ischemia.[23] The ECG helps to exclude acute myocardial infarction.

Measurement of central venous pressure may be critical in establishing the diagnosis of acute cor pulmonale in patients who present with hypotension or cardiovascular collapse. If hypotension is present and is due to acute cor pulmonale, right atrial and central venous pressure will be elevated.[20] If central venous pressure is normal or low, it suggests that the hypotension may be due to hypovolemia or acute (left ventricular) infarction.

Arterial blood gases in patients with acute cor pulmonale will show significant hypoxemia as well as hypocapnia. The chest x-ray is not helpful in the diagnosis of acute cor pulmonale.

Once the diagnosis of acute cor pulmonale has been suspected, it should be confirmed by V/Q lung scan or pulmonary angiography. In unstable patients in whom surgical therapy may be indicated, it may be appropriate to proceed directly to pulmonary angiography for definitive diagnosis.

Acute, Unexplained Dyspnea

The diagnosis of pulmonary embolism is most difficult in patients with submassive pulmonary embolism who do not sustain pulmonary infarction. As noted, if pulmonary embolism obstructs less than 60 percent of the pulmonary circulation acute cor pulmonale does not occur; the ECG remains normal and there are no signs of right ventricular failure on physical examination. If pulmonary infarction does not occur, pleuritic pain is absent and there are no abnormalities on chest x-ray. In this circumstance, the primary symptom of acute pulmonary embolism is the sudden onset of dyspnea. The only abnormalities on physical examination are tachypnea, possible tachycardia, and anxiety. The lungs are clear, there are no signs of acute right ventricular failure. Signs of DVT may be present. The ECG and chest x-ray are normal.

The principal differential diagnoses in patients with acute dyspnea due to pulmonary embolism are left ventricular failure, pneumonia, and the hyperventilation syndrome. Left ventricular failure and pneumonia can be excluded by further history, physical examination, and chest x-ray. The remaining alternative diagnosis, the hyperventilation syndrome, can be excluded by arterial blood gas analysis. Patients presenting with dyspnea due to acute pulmonary embolism nearly by definition can be expected to have significant hypoxemia. Measurement of arterial blood gases while the patient breathes room air may be the only way to distinguish between potentially lethal pulmonary embolism and benign hyperventilation.

As with the other syndromes of acute pulmonary embolism, IPG examination is very helpful. The diagnosis should be confirmed by V/Q lung scan or pulmonary angiography.

Laboratory Tests in Diagnosing Pulmonary Embolism

Chest X-Ray

The chest x-ray is most useful in evaluating patients with pleuritic pain who are suspected of having pulmonary infarction. Most patients with pulmonary infarction have an infiltrate, elevated hemidiaphragm due to splinting, or a pleural effusion which is usually small, unilateral, and which may or may not be bloody.[17] In patients with acute cor pulmonale or acute unexplained dyspnea without pulmonary infarction, the chest x-ray is usually normal or may show subtle, nonspecific findings.

ECG

The ECG is most helpful in evaluating patients with massive pulmonary embolism complicated by acute cor pulmonale. In these patients the ECG helps to exclude myocardial infarction and will usually demonstrate ECG correlates of acute cor pulmonale: new $S_1\,Q_3\,T_3$ pattern, new incomplete right bundle branch block, or other signs of right ventricular ischemia.[17,22,23] These ECG findings are transient and resolve as right ventricular failure resolves. In patients with submassive pulmonary embolism, the ECG is not helpful. It may show nonspecific ST changes or sinus tachycardia.

Arterial Blood Gases

The vast majority of patients with acute pulmonary embolism have tachypnea, therefore the arterial blood gases will demonstrate hypocapnia and respiratory alkalosis.[17] The Pa_{O_2} (breathing room air) will be decreased in patients with massive embolism and in patients presenting with dyspnea due to pulmonary embolism. In patients with pulmonary infarction who have submassive pulmonary embolism, the Pa_{O_2} may be "normal" or near normal if there is no prior pulmonary disease. The arterial blood gases should be measured while the patient is breathing room air. In patients receiving supplemental oxygen, who do not have overt, significant, coexistent pulmonary disease, it is only necessary to discontinue supplemental oxygen for 5 to 10 min to assess baseline values.[24]

Ventilation/Perfusion Lung Scans (V/Q Scans)

Perfusion lung scans are extremely sensitive in detecting pulmonary embolism; a normal multiple-view perfusion scan excludes acute pulmonary embolism.[17,25] Unfortunately, perfusion defects are not specific for pulmonary embolism, but can be due to a wide variety of other pulmonary abnormalities. The specificity of lung scans is increased by the use of ventilation as well as perfusion scans (see Chap. 113).

The abnormality most consistent with acute pulmonary embolism is the presence of multiple large segmental defects by perfusion scan that ventilate normally.[18,26] The probability of pulmonary embolism with this set of findings exceeds 90 percent.

Unfortunately, the findings by V/Q scan very frequently are nonspecific. The perfusion scan may show defects that are nonsegmental. The ventilation scan may show that the perfusion defects ventilate normally. In this circumstance, the diagnosis of acute pulmonary embolism is neither excluded nor confirmed.[26] The clinician must evaluate the total clinical findings. If a nonspecific lung scan is coupled with a strong clinical picture of pulmonary embolism, and there is no other viable explanation of the patient's symptoms, it may be appropriate to proceed to pulmonary angiography and/or to treat for acute pulmonary embolism. The same nonspecific lung scan findings coupled with a weak clinical story for pulmonary embolism may be sufficient to dismiss the diagnosis of pulmonary embolism. The IPG is especially helpful when the lung scan is nonspecific. If the IPG is negative, it is usually appropriate to conclude that the patient does not have pulmonary embolism. If the IPG is unilaterally positive, the diagnosis of pulmonary embolism should be pursued by performing pulmonary angiography or venography.

It is important to recognize that the diagnosis of acute pulmonary embolism is not made by the results of the lung scan alone. The clinician must evaluate the clinical findings and the results of IPG and arterial blood gases as well as the results of the lung scan.

Pulmonary Angiography

Pulmonary angiography is clearly the most accurate test for the diagnosis of acute pulmonary embolism.[27] Unfortunately, pulmonary angiography is not available at all hospitals, and it has the disadvantage of being an invasive test. The mortality of pulmonary angiography when performed by an experienced team is very low.[28] However, the morbidity of pulmonary angiography is substantial. It is an uncomfortable procedure that few patients wish to have repeated. For these reasons, we do not recommend that pulmonary angiography be performed in all patients in whom pulmonary embolism is suspected. Rather, we would reserve the use of pulmonary angiography for those patients having the specific indications noted in Table 54-3 (see Chap. 113).

The primary contraindication of pulmonary angiography is a history of severe, systemic reactions to contrast media. Relative contraindications include the presence of significant ventricular ectopic activity, left bundle branch block, and coexistent life-threatening disease.[28] Pulmonary angiography should be performed with great caution in patients with suspected primary pulmonary hypertension. If angiography is performed in such patients, main-

TABLE 54-3 Indications for Pulmonary Angiography

1. When examination of clinical findings, V/Q scan, and IPG are inconclusive
2. Relative contraindication to anticoagulation
3. When surgical therapy may be indicated
4. Recurrent pulmonary embolism, despite therapy
5. Young patient with uncertain predisposition to DVT

stream injections into the central pulmonary artery must not be performed. Rather, injections of small amounts of contrast media should be made selectively into distal portions of the pulmonary circulation that have been noted to have perfusion defects by lung scan.

Pulmonary angiography should only be performed by physicians experienced in cardiac catheterization. The complications of pulmonary angiography include those due to right-sided heart catheterization (arrhythmias, cardiac perforation) and reactions to contrast media. The electrocardiogram and systemic blood pressure should be monitored continuously. Right-sided heart pressures should be measured and recorded.

In patients with submassive pulmonary embolism, it is not necessary to perform mainstream injections to visualize the entire pulmonary circulation. Rather, selective or subselective injections should be made into areas shown to have perfusion defects by lung scan. We find hand injections of contrast through a balloon-tipped catheter to be ideal.[29] The artery is occluded with the balloon and the injection is made distal to the occlusion, utilizing cineangiography. The diagnostic finding of acute pulmonary embolism is the visualization of intraluminal clot.[27]

In patients with acute cor pulmonale due to massive pulmonary embolism, in whom pulmonary embolectomy may be indicated, mainstream injection into the main pulmonary artery with the use of cut film or cineangiography is appropriate. In this circumstance, the total pulmonary circulation, including the main and proximal right and left pulmonary arteries, must be visualized.

Venography

Venography, which is more widely available than pulmonary angiography, is a useful test in several circumstances (see Chap. 114).[10,11] In patients with nonspecific findings by lung scan who have a positive IPG, venography is ideal. If the venogram demonstrates deep venous thrombosis, the treatment is the same as if acute pulmonary embolism had been documented.

Occult Cancer in Patients with Pulmonary Embolism

It has long been recognized that patients with clinically evident cancer are at increased risk of venous thromboembolism. It is also well recognized that an unusual form of venous thrombosis, thrombophlebitis migrans, may be a clue to the presence of occult cancer. Thrombophlebitis migrans involves superficial veins, often at atypical sites such as the arms, may be migratory, and may be resistant to anticoagulant therapy.[30,31]

Data have indicated that the far more common form of venous thrombosis, deep venous thrombus, and its complication, pulmonary embolism, may also be a clue to the presence of occult cancer, especially in young patients.[32] A wide variety of malignancies may be present, including gastrointestinal tract, lung, breast, uterus, and prostate.

Given this association, the evaluation of the patient with venous thrombosis or pulmonary embolism should obviously include a complete history and physical examination, including breast and pelvic examination in women and examination of the prostate in men. Further diagnostic evaluation will be guided by the results of the history and physical examination.

In the follow-up of patients with pulmonary embolism, in addition to the concern for recurrent pulmonary embolism, the clinician should be alert to signs or symptoms of early cancer.

Paradoxical Embolism

Paradoxical embolism of the systemic circulation is a rare complication of deep venous thrombosis that may occur in patients who have an intracardiac defect (ASD, VSD, PDA, or pulmonary AV fistula) or who have a patent foramen ovale. The vast majority of reported cases of paradoxical embolism have occurred in patients with a patent foramen ovale,[33] which is present in 27 percent of the adult population.[34]

In normal circumstances, left atrial pressure exceeds right atrial pressure, thereby compressing a flap across the foramen ovale in the left atrium. In order for a venous thrombus to cross a patent foramen ovale, the pressure in the right atrium must be greater than in the left atrium. The commonest acute cause of right atrial pressure exceeding left atrial pressure is acute cor pulmonale secondary to acute massive pulmonary embolism.[33]

The usual clinical profile of a patient with paradoxical embolism is that of massive pulmonary embolism causing acute cor pulmonale in a patient without prior heart disease who has an asymptomatic patent foramen ovale. The increased right atrial pressure causes a right-to-left shunt across the foramen ovale. If another venous thrombus is dislodged from the deep venous system, it may cross the foramen to enter and embolize the systemic circulation. The commonest site of systemic embolism is the brain. Additional sites include the extremities and the coronary arteries.

Paradoxical embolism should be considered whenever systemic embolism occurs without the usual predisposing causes: atrial fibrillation, mitral valve disease, myocardial infarction, prosthetic heart valves, or cardiomyopathy. In this circumstance, the presence of pulmonary embolism should be sought. If there is evidence of acute pulmonary embolism in addition to unexplained systemic embolism, the presence of a right-to-left intracardiac shunt should be sought by means of indicator dilation curves,[35] angiography, or echocardiography.[36]

Paradoxical embolism tends to recur, and is usually fatal. If the diagnosis is confirmed during life, recurrent episodes can be prevented by means of interruption of the inferior vena cava.

It should be noted that paradoxical embolism may occur without acute pulmonary embolism, in patients with intracardiac defects complicated by right-to-left shunts, and in patients with chronic cor pulmonale with right ventricular failure.[33]

Treatment of Acute Pulmonary Embolism

The therapeutic modalities available for patients with acute pulmonary embolism can be divided into two groups: prophylactic and definitive therapy. Prophylactic therapy is based on the concept that the body's intrinsic fibrinolytic system can dissolve essentially all thromboembolic material that finds its way into the pulmonary vascular bed. Such dissolution usually leads to resolution of the pathophysiologic changes associated with acute pulmonary embolism over a period of 7 to 14 days.[20] Thus, prophylactic therapy aims at preventing further embolic episodes, thereby allowing the body's fibrinolytic defenses to resolve thromboembolic material that has already reached the lungs. Examples of prophylactic therapy include anticoagulation with heparin and warfarin, and venous interruption. Prophylactic therapy with anticoagulants is initiated as soon as the clinician has a high index of suspicion for the diagnosis of pulmonary embolism. If further diagnostic evaluation fails to confirm the diagnosis, anticoagulation is discontinued.

Definitive therapy focuses its impact on thromboemboli that already exist in the pulmonary vascular bed. Definitive therapy attempts to remove or dissolve such emboli in order to effect a more rapid resolution of the pathophysiologic sequelae of pulmonary embolism. Examples of a definitive treatment for pulmonary embolism include exogenously administered fibrinolytic agents and pulmonary embolectomy. Supportive measures, e.g., fluid and pressor administration, often precede or accompany definitive therapy and are terminated once the patient's hemodynamic status is stable.

Prophylactic Therapy: Anticoagulation[37–41] (see Chap. 95)

Intravenous heparin is the initial prophylactic treatment of choice for acute pulmonary embolism. Heparin in a dosage higher than that required to block thrombin-fibrinogen interaction can relieve bronchoconstriction; heparin may also decrease the high pulmonary vascular resistance associated with acute pulmonary embolism. Several investigators have reported striking success using high-dose intravenous heparin in patients with massive pulmonary embolism, in whom the prognosis was guarded. Table 54-4 represents a recommended dosage schedule for heparin tailored to the severity of the thromboembolic process.

The incidence of bleeding during heparin therapy is determined not by the dose of heparin, but by a defect in the wall of a blood vessel. Therefore, contraindications to anticoagulants include patients who are potential bleeders, e.g., those with active peptic ulcer disease, esophageal varices, any hemorrhagic diathesis, severe liver or kidney disease, severe hypertension, intracranial disease, and recent surgery on brain, spinal cord, joints, or genitourinary tract.

As noted in Table 54-4, heparin is continued for 7 to 10 days and overlaps oral warfarin therapy until a prothrombin time of 1.2 to 1.6 times control is achieved. Warfarin is usually started at a dose of 5 mg per day for the first 3 days of therapy. Thereafter, warfarin dosage is adjusted up or down, according to the results of the prothrombin time. At that point, heparin is discontinued and final regulation of the prothrombin time is achieved by altering the dosage of warfarin. Oral anticoagulants

TABLE 54-4 Prophylactic Therapy for Treatment of Thrombophlebitis and Pulmonary Embolism

Diagnosis	Heparin Dosage
Deep venous thrombosis without pulmonary embolism or with minor pulmonary embolism	5000 U IV loading dose followed by 1000–1500 U IV per hour (24,000 U/24 h); check partial thromboplastin time (PTT) 4 h after initiating infusion and adjust heparin dose to prolong PTT to $1\frac{1}{2}$ to 2 times control. Warfarin is started on approximately day 2–3 with changeover from heparin occurring approximately on day 7–10.
Major pulmonary embolism with or without right ventricular failure and hypotension	10,000–15,000 U IV loading dose followed by 1500–2000 U IV per hour (36,000 U/24 h); check PTT 4 h after initiating infusion and adjust heparin dose to prolong PTT to $1\frac{1}{2}$ to 2 times control (employ smaller loading and infusion dosage for smaller individuals or patients with hepatic and/or renal insufficiency). Warfarin is started on approximately day 5–6 (if patient is stable) with changeover from heparin occurring approximately on day 8–12.

should be continued for as long as the patient continues to have an underlying predisposition to thromboembolism, e.g., bed rest. In the patient with a fracture, this period of time should be for 2 months after the cast or traction is removed and the individual is ambulatory. If predisposition to thromboembolism is transitory, patients who have suffered an episode of acute pulmonary embolism should receive oral anticoagulation for 3 to 6 months.

In the cardiac patient or other individual with permanent predisposition to thromboembolism, anticoagulation should be lifelong. An alternative to daily oral warfarin is injection of subcutaneous heparin every 8 to 12 h for a minimum of 12 weeks. Subcutaneous heparin dosage is adjusted to maintain the activated partial thromboplastin time (APTT) to one-and-one-half times the control value.[42]

Anticoagulant dosage schedules have advised prolongation of the APTT or prothrombin time to as much as two-and-one-half times control. However, recent experience favors more modest prolongation of clotting parameters without any resultant loss of therapeutic efficacy and with a decreased risk for hemorrhagic complications.[43] Heparin plasma activity is significantly shortened in some patients with acute pulmonary embolism, presumably as a result of active intravascular coagulation on the surface of pulmonary thromboemboli in the pulmonary vascular bed.[44] Heparin administered as a continuous infusion results in fewer hemorrhagic complications than delivering this drug by intermittent bolus technique.[45] Hemorrhagic complications of heparin are more common in elderly females than in any other patient group.[46]

Heparin can cause an immunologically mediated thrombocytopenia. Such decreases in platelet counts may occur in as many as 5 to 33 percent of patients receiving intravenous heparin. Onset of heparin-associated thrombocytopenia usually occurs 6 to 12 days after initiation of therapy. Occasionally, heparin-associated thrombocytopenia develops together with arterial thrombosis that may be life-threatening.[47,48]

Other medical therapy is often required in patients with acute pulmonary embolism regardless of whether prophylactic or definitive treatment is elected. For example, apprehension, pain, and respiratory distress usually respond to intravenous morphine sulfate as required. Oxygen is administered by nasal cannulae or mask. Hypotension or shock usually requires intravenous infusion of isoproterenol, 1 mg diluted in 500 ml of 5% dextrose in water, or the more potent l-norepinephrine bitartrate (Levophed), 2 ml of 0.2% Levophed in 500 ml of 5% dextrose in water. The rate of infusion is determined by the response of the blood pressure.

Prophylactic Therapy: Venous Interruption[49,50]

Venous interruption is also a form of prophylactic therapy in that it is performed to prevent further episodes of venous thromboembolism from reaching the pulmonary vascular bed. The first form of venous interruption to be performed was bilateral common femoral vein ligation. This type of venous interruption is simple to perform and entails minimal risk in the patient without heart disease since local anesthesia is employed. However, further embolism occurs in 5 to 10 percent of cases, usually because clot is present above the tie at the time of surgery. Surgical interruption of the vena cava just below the renal veins carries a risk of 2 to 5 percent in patients without heart disease. If the patient is in left-sided heart failure, the in-hospital mortality is approximately 20 percent; if left-and right-sided heart failure are present, the risk is 50 percent.[49] Essentially the same risk exists for femoral vein ligation in patients with heart failure, secondary to the high mortality rate of recurrent thromboembolism in patients with prior heart failure. If a pelvic source of embolism exists, the left ovarian vein must also be ligated. This latter procedure does not result in interruption of pregnancy or prevent future pregnancies.

Interruption of the vena cava is highly effective in preventing further episodes of thromboembolism. Interruption of the inferior vena cava is indicated (1) when embolism occurs in patients receiving anticoagulants; (2) when anticoagulants are contraindicated; (3) when diseases predisposing to venous thrombosis and pulmonary embolism are prominent and persistent; (4) when septic embolism occurs; and (5) in some patients with massive embolism in whom a further episode of embolism would be fatal.

At present, the commonest form of venous interruption is not surgical, but rather the insertion of a Mobin-Uddin inferior vena caval filter. Schlosser reviewed the experience with more than 5000 patients who had undergone insertion of a Mobin-Uddin filter.[51] In these patients, nonfatal recurrent emboli occurred in 1.8 percent and fatal recurrent embolism developed in 0.5 percent. When the more recently developed 28-mm filter was employed in 2500 patients, nonfatal embolic recurrences occurred in only 0.5 percent of patients while fatal recurrences were noted in 0.1 percent.[51] Filter migration is also said to be reduced with the 28-mm device.

Morbidity following vena caval clipping or filter insertion is largely the result of subsequent total occlusion of the vena cava below the site of the clip or filter. Such occlusion is said to occur in 50 percent or more of patients who undergo these procedures. Morbid events secondary to total occlusion of the vena cava include postphlebitic limb syndrome, unilateral or bilateral leg swelling, and mild venous claudication.[52,53] It has been suggested that administration of anticoagulants following clip or umbrella insertion markedly reduces the incidence of vena caval occlusion and the attendant morbid events.[53]

Another form of inferior vena caval filter that has recently gained popularity is the Kim-Ray Greenfield stainless-steel wire filter.[54] This device is inserted in a manner similar to that employed for the Mobin-Uddin filter, i.e., via a venous cutdown on the common femoral or internal jugular vein. Both of these approaches utilize local anesthesia, thereby avoiding the risks associated with the general anesthesia necessary for inferior vena caval clip or filter insertion. Some surgeons feel that long-term inferior vena caval patency rate is higher with the Kim-Ray Greenfield filter than with the Mobin-Uddin device.[54]

Follow-Up of Patients Treated with Prophylactic Therapy[55,56]

The excellent prognosis of patients with pulmonary embolism in whom the diagnosis is suspected, confirmed, and prophylactic treatment initiated has been documented.[3,55] Indeed, death secondary to pulmonary embolism is almost invariably the result of massive obstruction of the pulmonary vascular bed by thromboembolism.[3] Such patients usually die within minutes to hours following the acute episode, often before diagnosis and therapy are even considered. However, if the diagnosis is made and appropriate prophylactic therapy initiated, the outlook is excellent, even in patients with massive embolism complicated by right ventricular failure but in the absence of hypotension.[3] Patients with massive embolism, right ventricular failure, and systemic arterial hypotension represent that subgroup of patients with pulmonary embolism who have the highest mortality.[3,56] As noted below, it is only this subgroup of patients who are potential candidates for definitive therapy since prognosis is excellent for all other patient subgroups treated with less morbid therapy, i.e., prophylactic therapy.

The overall hospital mortality of all patients treated for acute pulmonary embolism is 8 percent.[3] Individuals with massive pulmonary embolism obstructing 50 percent or more of the pulmonary vascular bed have a hospital mortality of 16 percent. As noted earlier, most of the deaths in these latter patients occur in individuals with right ventricular failure and systemic hypotension.[3] Preexisting heart disease also worsens the prognosis in patients with acute pulmonary embolism by predisposing the patient to the development of right ventricular failure and hypotension with the embolic insult.

Resolution of pulmonary embolism occurs by two mechanisms: in vivo fibrinolysis and mechanical changes in the location of clots within the pulmonary vascular bed. Embolic obstruction resolves by approximately 10 to 20 percent during the first 24 h after acute pulmonary embolism.[2] Complete resolution can occur as soon as 14 days after the acute event, but remains incomplete in some patients until weeks after embolism.[20] The hemodynamic abnormalities associated with pulmonary embolism, i.e., pulmonary hypertension and right ventricular failure in patients with massive embolism, resolve as the pulmonary emboli resolve.[20,57]

Thus, the late prognosis of the patient with acute pulmonary embolism depends on two factors: (1) whether the diagnosis of pulmonary embolism is made and appropriate therapy is initiated, and (2) the presence of associated medical illness, e.g., heart disease. Further modest resolution of pulmonary embolism occurs for 3 to 4 months following discharge from the hospital. Thereafter, little if any further resolution occurs. Approximately two-thirds of patients with acute pulmonary embolism have complete resolution of their embolism. The remainder have partial resolution of much of the thromboembolic material. Most individuals with partial resolution of embolism do not develop chronic cor pulmonale. It is only the rare patient with recurrent untreated or inadequately treated pulmonary embolism who develops chronic cor pulmonale.[2,55] Recurrences of pulmonary embolism are rare in patients who are adequately treated and in whom appropriate prophylactic measures are undertaken against further episodes of thromboembolism.

Definitive Therapy: Rationale

As noted earlier, most patients with pulmonary embolism have an excellent prognosis as long as the diagnosis is suspected and confirmed, and treatment initiated. Individuals with massive embolism, right ventricular failure, and hypotension represent a subgroup of patients with acute pulmonary embolism who have a high hospital mortality (32 percent).[3] It is in this subgroup of patients that one would expect benefits to accrue from a direct, definitive attack on the thromboemboli present in the pulmonary vascular bed. This subgroup represents a small minority of the total population of patients with acute pulmonary embolism. This small subgroup might benefit from definitive therapy, i.e., embolectomy or fibrinolytic dissolution of thromboemboli. To date, unequivocal proof is lacking that definitive therapy in comparison with prophylactic therapy leads to decreased mortality in this group of patients.

Definitive Therapy: Embolectomy[56,58]

Pulmonary embolectomy (Trendelenburg's operation) was introduced at the turn of the century, but met with only occasional success. The introduction of cardiopulmonary bypass made the performance of embolectomy feasible. However, surgical mortality associated with embolectomy remains high, approximately 30 to 50 percent, since the operation is usually performed on patients who are in profound shock. Most individuals who require embolectomy die before it can be performed. Conversely, many patients who survive embolectomy might have survived with less vigorous therapy.[56]

The primary indication for embolectomy is the presence of right ventricular failure and systemic arterial hypotension requiring vasopressors in a patient with bilateral central pulmonary emboli documented by pulmonary angiography. In this setting, embolectomy may be lifesaving. In the absence of hypotension, pulmonary embolectomy is not indicated even if massive pulmonary embolism is documented by angiography. Such patients survive without embolectomy if further embolism is prevented by administering prophylactic therapy.[56]

Contraindications to pulmonary embolectomy include recurrent pulmonary embolism without angiographic evidence of occluded central pulmonary arteries, pulmonary arterial systolic pressure in excess of 70 mmHg, severe underlying heart disease complicated by heart failure, and marked pulmonary insufficiency secondary to severe pulmonary disease, i.e., chronic obstructive lung disease.

An alternative to operative pulmonary embolectomy which requires a thoracotomy is percutaneous pulmonary embolectomy employing a special catheter.[59,60] This technique involves percutaneous, transvenous introduction of a steerable suction catheter into the pulmonary artery under fluoroscopic guidance. Emboli are aspirated via the catheter, thereby removing them from the pulmonary vascular bed. Multiple retrievals of embolic material by the catheter are usually required before an improvement occurs in the abnormal hemodynamic pattern engendered in the pulmonary vascular bed by the emboli. A vena caval filter is usually inserted at the end of this procedure.[60] Experience with this technique is currently modest. Further work is required in order to define the applicability and success rate of catheter pulmonary embolectomy.

Elective pulmonary embolectomy for chronic, unresolved pulmonary thromboembolism is considerably more successful than is the emergency operation. Daily et al. reviewed their experience with four such patients, three of whom survived the operation and were markedly improved.[61] Moser et al. reviewed their experience with 15 such patients, 13 of whom survived and were improved following surgery.[62] Benotti et al. reviewed their own experience and that of the English literature with respect to this syndrome.[63] These latter authors identified 30 patients in whom extensive clinical and hemodynamic data were available. The mean age of these individuals was 45 years; most complained of dyspnea. Roentgenographic, arterial blood gas, and electrocardiographic findings were nonspecific; perfusion lung scans were invariably abnormal. Most patients had mild to moderate pulmonary hypertension at rest. Operative mortality was 20 percent in the 20 patients who underwent elective pulmonary embolectomy, and operative results ranged from good to excellent.[63] It seems evident that operative pulmonary embolectomy is best suited to patients with chronic, unresolved pulmonary thromboembolism. Only an occasional individual benefits from emergency pulmonary embolectomy.

Definitive Therapy: Fibrinolytic Therapy (see Chap. 118)

The search for an agent to dissolve thromboemboli in human beings has been long and complex. The two agents that have been most extensively studied are streptokinase and urokinase. The efficacy of urokinase in the treatment of acute pulmonary embolism in human beings was assessed in a national cooperative trial sponsored by the National Heart and Lung Institute.

In this multicenter trial, one-half of the patients were treated with a 12-h infusion of urokinase, while the remainder received a 12-h infusion of heparin.[64] After completion of the 12-h infusions, therapy was the same in both groups: intravenous heparin followed by oral warfarin. Pulmonary angiography and right heart catheterization were repeated after the initial infusion of heparin or urokinase; multiple follow-up lung scans were obtained over a period of 2 weeks.

Repeat pulmonary angiography demonstrated greater, albeit modest, resolution of embolism in the group treated with urokinase. However, 5 days after the initial treatment, resolution of embolism as determined by lung scanning was the same in both groups. Hospital mortality was the same for both groups.

Hemorrhagic complications were significant: moderate or severe bleeding occurred in 27 percent of the heparin-treated group and in 45 percent of the urokinase-treated patients.[64] Although these early results were somewhat encouraging, the modest degree of resolution of embolism and the major bleeding complications indicated that urokinase therapy was far from ideal for all patients with acute pulmonary embolism.

A second NIH-sponsored trial compared a 24-h infusion of urokinase with that of streptokinase in 167 patients with angiographically documented pulmonary embolism. Urokinase and streptokinase were equally effective.[65] There was no significant benefit derived from 24 h of thrombolytic infusion as compared with 12 h. Significant bleeding occurred in more than one-third of patients treated with urokinase or streptokinase; bleeding was sufficiently severe in 14 percent of patients to require transfusion.[65]

The 1980 NIH Consensus Conference on Thrombolytic Therapy and Thrombosis recommended that this form of treatment be widely applied to patients with documented pulmonary embolism with associated hemodynamic abnormalities.[65] However, it is important to note that thrombolytic therapy did not alter mortality secondary to pulmonary embolism in either of these two trials. Patients with massive embolism fared just as well as with heparin (prophylactic) therapy as with thrombolytic (definitive) therapy. With respect to morbidity, only one study purports to demonstrate reduced morbidity with thrombolytic therapy as compared with routine anticoagulation.[66] These authors observed that two indexes of pulmonary function, pulmonary capillary blood volume and pulmonary diffusing capacity, were significantly better in pulmonary embolism patients treated with thrombolytic therapy as compared with individuals who received routine anticoagulation.[66] The clinical significance of these observations is unknown.

Major concern persists among clinicians concerning the incidence of bleeding complications in patients treated with thrombolytic therapy. Estimates of this incidence range from 5 to 45 percent.[67–70] Since estimates of bleeding complications with thrombolytic therapy vary, contraindications to this form of therapy are noted to be variable depending on the individual investigator's perception of the risk of hemorrhage. Thus, firm indications for the use of thrombolytic agents in patients with acute pulmonary embolism are lacking at present. We agree with Genton who recommends that thrombolytic therapy is potentially most useful in that small group of patients with documented massive pulmonary embolism with severe hemodynamic abnormalities, especially if these individuals manifest cardiac or pulmonary decompensation.[71]

The dosage of urokinase for patients with acute pulmonary embolism is an initial intravenous infusion of 4400 IU per kilogram of body weight dissolved in 15 ml of sterile water given over 10 min. Maintenance therapy is then initiated: 4400 IU per kilogram of body weight per hour for a total of 12 h. Each hour's dosage of urokinase is dissolved in 15 ml of sterile water. Streptokinase is given as an initial loading dose of 250,000 IU dissolved in normal saline solution or 5% dextrose in water and administered over 30 min. Maintenance therapy consists of 100,000 IU per hour for 24 h.[68] Bell and Meek recommend determination of thrombin time, prothrombin time, partial thromboplastin time, and platelet count before initiating thrombolytic therapy in order to screen for preexisting coagulation disorders. During thrombolytic therapy, these investigators advise that thrombin times be measured every 4 to 8 h.[68] The thrombin time should be prolonged to between two and five times the normal control value in seconds to confirm that adequate fibrinolysis has been achieved.[68]

Pulmonary Embolism in Pregnancy[72]

Pulmonary embolism during pregnancy represents a difficult diagnostic and therapeutic problem. Lung scanning and pulmonary angiography involve ionizing radiation exposure for both mother and fetus. Consequently, the diagnosis often remains tentative. Therapy is also problematic since warfarin crosses the placenta and reaches the fetal circulation. With respect to diagnosis, it is usually our policy to pursue the diagnostic evaluation of pulmonary embolism aggressively, even in pregnancy, since untreated pulmonary embolism carries a 30 percent mortality.[3]

The treatment of pulmonary embolism during pregnancy is hazardous.[72] Prophylactic therapy must continue throughout pregnancy and the puerperium. Heparin does not cross the placental barrier and so represents no hazard to the fetus, but it is difficult to administer for more than 2 weeks. Warfarin derivatives do cross the placenta and can result in significant fetal mortality. Interruption of the pregnancy to avert further embolism is usually not appropriate. Ligation of the femoral veins does not protect against emboli arising from pelvic and gluteal veins. Interruption of the inferior vena cava and left ovarian vein is a highly effective preventive procedure. However, this operation entails a surgical risk of about 2 percent in experienced hands; there is little risk of miscarriage after the first trimester, and no interference with future pregnancies.[49] When pulmonary embolism occurs in the first trimester, the appropriate treatment is a 10-day course of heparin, followed by subcutaneous heparin (5000 units bid), administered by the patient at home. Heparin is used after delivery until the patient is fully ambulatory. In selected cases, inferior vena caval interruption is appropriate.

Hall et al. reviewed the complications associated with anticoagulant therapy during pregnancy.[73] Heparin therapy was associated with hemorrhage (10 percent), spontaneous abortion (2 percent), stillbirths (13 percent), early infant mortality (7 percent), and chronic complications in 1 percent of surviving children. Warfarin therapy was complicated by fetal developmental abnormalities (nasal hypoplasia, mental retardation) in 7 percent of infants, spontaneous abortion (9 percent), and stillbirths (8 percent). Consequently, these authors recommend avoidance or termination of pregnancy in patients who require anticoagulant therapy.[73] It is thus evident that pulmonary embolism during pregnancy represents a severe challenge to the clinician.

Special Types of Pulmonary Embolism

Robert C. Schlant, M.D.*

Fat Embolism[74–97]

In 1861 Zenker[98] described the postmortem findings of fat emboli in the lungs, and in 1873 Bergmann[99] described the classic triad for the fat embolism syndrome (FES) of dyspnea (respiratory insufficiency), confusion (neurologic dysfunction), and petechiae.

The entrance of free globules of fat into systemic veins most often occurs after fractures of long bones, especially of the tibia and femur after automobile accidents. Fat may also enter following direct injury to subcutaneous fat tissue by contusion, concussion, or burns; childbirth or poisoning; the use of a pump oxygenator; or simulated high-altitude flights. Some less common causes include alcoholism, fatty metamorphosis of the liver, decompression sickness, sickle cell crisis, multiple blood transfusions, sternal-splitting incisions for cardiac surgery, and external cardiac massage.

*The remainder of this chapter was kindly written by Robert C. Schlant, M.D.

The exact pathophysiology of the fat embolism syndrome (FES) is unknown and probably is different in different patients. At least some of the fatty emboli are caused by mechanical obstruction in the pulmonary circulation produced by the release of depot fat from traumatized bone since myeloid tissue can occasionally be identified in the pulmonary vessels.[74,82,85] There is also evidence that physiobiochemical alterations in the natural emulsion of circulating fats can result in the production of macroglobules of fat that can also act as emboli. Other physiobiochemical mechanisms that have been suggested as contributing to the syndrome include the following: the release of thromboplastin substances from the traumatized tissues with platelet aggregation; excess free fatty acidemia from the superimposition of fat on platelet aggregations; the liberation of toxic free fatty acids in the lungs by enzymatic hydrolysis of embolic fat, and the subsequent pulmonary capillary leak syndrome and curtailment of lung surfactant activity;[84] the release of vasoactive and bronchoactive substances such as bradykinin, histamine, or serotonin from pulmonary microthrombi; traumatic shock; and defects in the coagulation system.[79,81] The often sudden drop in hematocrit is usually related to blood losses in fractured extremities, to extensive pulmonary hemorrhages, or, less frequently, to associated disseminated intravascular coagulation (DIC). Thrombocytopenia frequently develops in individuals with fat embolism, probably as a result of platelet adhesion and sequestration to fat droplets in the lung.[78]

The fat droplets vary in size and may obstruct smaller branches of the pulmonary artery, including arterioles and capillaries. The fat globules may also traverse the pulmonary circulation and block arterioles and capillaries of the brain, skin, kidney, heart, and other organs.

Patients may develop an acute respiratory distress syndrome (ARDS) with extensive intrapulmonary hemorrhage and damage to the pulmonary vascular endothelium and parenchyma. In fact, it is frequently difficult to distinguish between the FES and ARDS.

Clinically, patients usually have a lucid interval of 6 h to several days (classically, 24 to 40 h) following trauma before the first symptoms or signs of fat embolism are recognized. Most features of the syndrome result from fat emboli either to the lungs or brain. Cardiorespiratory manifestations of pulmonary fat emboli include tachypnea, dyspnea, tachycardia up to 140 beats per minute, hypoxemia, and pyrexia to 39.4°C (103°F). Individuals with severe respiratory distress may become cyanotic. Patients with fat embolism syndrome often have copious bronchial secretions, which may be hemorrhagic. The cerebral symptoms, which may occur simultaneously with or after the pulmonary symptoms, include headache, increasing irritability, disturbances of consciousness, disorientation, delirium, confusion, restlessness, convulsions, apathy, stupor, and coma. As noted above, patients with fat embolism may present with or develop the full clinical picture of adult respiratory distress syndrome.[92] Oliguria and even anuria may develop.

The signs of systemic fat embolism include petechiae, especially on the anterior chest, axillary folds, neck, fundi, and conjunctivae. Rarely, fat emboli are seen in the retinal vessels. In some patients the petechiae, whether spontaneous or induced, may be related to the associated thrombocytopenia although small fat emboli may be found in biopsy of cutaneous capillaries adjacent to the petechiae.[100] The prothrombin time and partial thromboplastin time may be increased whereas the plasma concentration of fibrinogen may be reduced. Serum calcium may be decreased, presumably because of the interaction between the increased fatty acids and calcium, but serum lipase and tributyrinase concentrations are usually elevated. A frozen section of clotted blood examined for fat may be of some diagnostic value early in the course of the fat embolism syndrome, particularly in patients with a Pa_{O_2} less than 60 mmHg.[87,91] The findings of fat droplets in sputum or urine are also suggestive but not diagnostic of fat embolism.[77] Arterial hypoxemia is one of the earliest and most important laboratory findings. The chest roentgenogram usually shows extensive fluffy infiltrates or, occasionally, only hazy, fine stippling throughout both lungs. The chest x-ray may also be compatible with pulmonary edema.[93]

There is no specific therapy for fat embolism, and the most important principle is the maintenance of pulmonary oxygenation and function. It is important to correct the arterial hypoxemia that is almost always present and, occasionally, quite marked. This therapy usually requires supplemental inspiratory oxygen and occasionally assisted ventilation, at times with positive end-expiratory pressure (PEEP). Although 100% inspiratory oxygen may be necessary initially, this should later be reduced to 40% to avoid oxygen toxicity. Frequent determinations of arterial blood gas concentrations are necessary. It has been suggested that massive doses of corticosteroids, which may decrease alveolar damage, are useful and possibly lifesaving, although there are still no really adequate clinical trials.[75,76,83,86,88,90,95,97] Doses are usually hydrocortisone, 1 to 2 g/day, or methylprednisolone, 13 mg/kg/day, for 3 to 5 days. Low doses of heparin were formerly recommended to decrease platelet adhesiveness. Theoretically, however, the stimulatory effect of heparin upon lipase activity in the lung might be detrimental by increasing the amount of toxic fatty acids in the lungs. Other former therapies no longer used include low-molecular-weight dextran,[80] intravenous ethyl alcohol, hypothermia, or various detergents.[78]

Air Embolism[101–106]

Air may enter the circulation in the course of intravenous infusions, pneumoperitoneum, knee-chest position in the puerperium, uterine douches, surgical procedures on the neck or brain, retroperitoneal air injection, irrigation of nasal sinuses, tubal or vaginal insufflation, orogenital sex,[106] or rapid pressure decompression or heart-lung bypass. The lethal dose varies with the age, condition, and position of the patient and the rapidity of air entry. It varies between 5 and 15 ml/kg. Death results either from an "air lock" in the right ventricle or from air embolism to the lungs with resultant pulmonary vascular obstruction and secondary reflex pulmonary vasoconstriction.[101,102] It is likely that only very minute (if any) volumes of air traverse the pulmonary capillaries. Clinically, air embolism is associated with the sudden onset of dyspnea, shock, and cyanosis. Frequently, there is a loud, continuous churning or "millhouse" murmur or noise over the precordium produced by the air and blood in the right ventricle. Venous air embolism can also result in diffuse pulmonary injury with subsequent development of the adult respiratory distress syndrome.[103] Marked ventilation-perfusion abnormalities develop as a result of air in the pulmonary vascular bed.[104] Air bubbles in cardiac chambers can be detected by echocardiography.[107]

Treatment consists of turning the patient on the left side with the head in a dependent position in an effort to displace the air bolus from the right ventricular outflow tract to the right ventricular apex or right atrium, and to trap the air in the superior portion of the right atrium; aspiration of air through a needle or catheter inserted into the right ventricle; and support of respiration with 100% oxygen.[105] Closed-chest cardiac massage has also been used successfully, particularly when air embolism occurs during a neurosurgical or neck operation.[108]

Amniotic Fluid Embolism[109–116]

Amniotic fluid embolism as a cause of maternal mortality was first described in 1926 by Meyer[109] and was more firmly established as a clinical syndrome in 1941 by Steiner and Luschbaugh.[110] The incidence has been variably stated from 1 in 8000 to 1 in 80,000 live births. It remains one of the more common causes of maternal death during legal abortion, labor, delivery, and the immediate postpartum period. Predisposing factors are increased age and parity, premature placental separation, intrauterine fetal death, oversized baby, prolonged and vigorous labor with tumultuous uterine contractions, uterine rupture, large doses of oxytocin, meconium contamination of amniotic fluid, and abortion induced by intraamniotic injection of saline or glucose.[114]

The amniotic fluid, containing meconium, epithelial squamae, mucin, amorphous debris, lipids, bile pigments, or lanugo, enters the maternal circulation either through the venous sinuses of the uteroplacental site or through the endocervical veins. The pulmonary embolic manifestations are primarily due to the solid contents of the amniotic fluid, since most experiments have indicated that filtered amniotic fluid produces minimal pulmonary vascular response. Occasionally, amniotic fluid material can be detected in the vessels of the lungs, heart, kidneys, and brain.[111]

Disseminated intravascular coagulation (DIC) develops in a significant number of patients who survive the initial pulmonary embolic event. It is produced by the entry into the circulation of a large amount of thromboplastic substances in the amniotic fluid. The coagulation process is initiated, leading to the consumption of factors V and VIII, prothrombin, and fibrinogen. If consumption proceeds more rapidly than repletion, deficiencies of these factors can develop. The fibrinolytic enzyme system is activated as a compensatory mechanism, resulting in the production of large amounts of fibrin degradation products, which act as inhibitors of thrombin, interfere with normal fibrin polymerization, and impair platelet function. This process may result in severe vaginal hemorrhage. Fibrin deposition throughout the microvasculature aggravates the pulmonary embolic manifestations and may produce hypoperfusion with profound alteration in function of almost every organ in the body.

Clinically, most episodes occur near the end of the first stage of labor and are manifested by the abrupt onset of severe dyspnea, hypotension and shock, tachypnea, tachycardia, cyanosis, evidence of acute cor pulmonale and of pulmonary edema, and apprehension. The latter may rapidly progress to semicoma or coma. Generalized convulsions, cardiac arrest, and death may occur suddenly. Chest pain is relatively unusual. About 25 to 50 percent of patients die within the first hour, and the survivors are still at great risk of life from either irreversible shock or the subsequent development of profuse vaginal bleeding. There may be bleeding from venipuncture sites and all body orifices or into skin and mucosa. Acute renal failure may develop secondary to hypotension. The mortality in patients with the full amniotic fluid embolism syndrome exceeds 80 percent.[114]

Laboratory findings usually reflect deficiencies of all coagulation factors, especially low fibrinogen levels and a low platelet count.

Treatment [110,111,113,115,116] consists of (1) general supportive measures for thromboembolism with hypotension and/or respiratory distress; (2) immediate evacuation of the uterus to remove the basic cause of the diffuse intravascular coagulation process; (3) for hemorrhage, administration of fresh frozen plasma, platelets as necessary, and packed red blood cells as needed for anemia; and (4) if bleeding persists and especially if fibrinogen and factor VIII are low, the administration of cryoprecipitate, which contains fibrinogen and factor VIII.[115,116] There has been some controversy regarding the use of fibrinogen, which promotes clotting and hemostasis, since it theoretically might produce more deposition of fibrin. The management of amniotic fluid embolism is greatly assisted by monitoring intraarterial blood pressure, central venous pressure, pulmonary artery pressure with a Swan-Ganz catheter, and urinary output.

Tumor Embolism[117–120]

In addition to pulmonary metastases resulting from the dissemination of malignant tumors, acute and subacute cor pulmonale may be produced by emboli of malignant tissue cells to the pulmonary arteries and capillaries. These emboli may originate from the primary site of the tumor or from other sites such as the liver or inferior vena cava, to which the tumor has spread. Tumor emboli occur with virtually any type of malignancy, and their frequency is surely higher than the rarity of reported cases would indicate. Tumor emboli are relatively more common in patients with renal carcinoma, primary hepatic carcinoma, gastric carcinoma, and trophoblastic tumors (chorioepithelioma).

Since trophoblastic tumors, even with extensive pulmonary metastases, may respond well to chemotherapy,[118,119] it is imperative to consider this diagnosis whenever a female patient has symptoms of acute dyspnea, pleurisy, cough, or hemoptysis, or unexplained signs of pulmonary hypertension following a hydatidiform mole, abortion, or normal pregnancy. Occasionally, trophoblastic pulmonary emboli may not occur until several years after the initiating pregnancy, and the patient may be asymptomatic in the interval, although there is usually amenorrhea, excessive menstrual bleeding or discharge, or other disturbances of menses. Since uterine curettage is often negative, diagnosis is best established by measurement of urinary gonadotropin excretion. Radiological changes in the lungs resulting from metastasis of trophoblastic tumors may take one or more of the following forms: (1) discrete, usually well-defined, and rounded opacities; (2) "snowstorm" patterns with multiple, small, less well defined opacities; and (3) changes resulting from embolic occlusion of the pulmonary arteries without invasion of the lung parenchyma. Of interest is the study of 50 asymptomatic puerperal patients, 13 of whom had pulmonary scan defects thought to be due to asymptomatic trophoblastic emboli.[120]

Cor pulmonale, i.e., right-sided heart failure, occasionally results from hematogenous or lymphogenous spread of tumor. It can be subacute, occurring over the course of a week or 10 days, or appear more slowly with a clinical picture of chronic right-sided heart failure.[117]

Rare Causes of Embolism

Among the many very rare forms of pulmonary embolism are those due to cotton fiber, talc or other particulate matter in contaminated heroin, hair, barium sulfate crystals after barium enema, vegetable material, bullets, shotgun shot, cardiac catheters, indwelling venous catheters, bone marrow, brain tissue, parasites, cardiac vegetations, foam cells from rupture of atheromata of an enlarged pulmonary artery, liver cells, and bile thromboembolism.[121,122]

References

1. Virchow, R. I. K.: "Cellular Pathology as Based upon Physiological and Pathohistology," 7th Am. ed., translated by Frank Chance, Robert M. DeWitt, New York, 1860, p. 236.
2. Dalen, J. E., and Alpert, J. S.: Natural History of Pulmonary Embolism, *Prog. Cardiovasc. Dis.*, 17(4):259, 1975.
3. Alpert, J. S., Smith, R., Carlson, J., Ockene, I. S., Dexter, L., and Dalen, J. E.: Mortality in Patients Treated for Pulmonary Embolism, *JAMA*, 236:1477, 1976.
4. Kakkar, V. V.: The Logistic Problems Encountered in the Multicenter Trial of Low-Dose Heparin Prophylaxis, *Thromb. Haemost.*, 41:105, 1979.
5. Halkin, H., Goldberg, J., Modan, M., and Modan, B.: Reduction of Mortality in General Medical In-Patients by Low-Dose Heparin Prophylaxis, *Ann. Intern. Med.*, 96:561, 1982.
6. Kakkar, V. V., Stamatakis, J. D., Bentley, P. G., et al.: Prophylaxis for Postoperative Deep-Vein Thrombosis, Synergistic Effect of Heparin and Dihydroergotamine, *JAMA*, 241:39, 1979.
7. Pedersen, B., and Christiansen, J.: Thromboembolic Prophylaxis with Dihydroergotamine-Heparin in Abdominal Surgery, *Am. J. Surg.*, 145:788, 1983.
8. Moser, G., Krahenbuhl, B., Barroussel, R., Bene, J. J., Donath, A., and Rohner, A.: Mechanical Versus Pharmacologic Prevention of Deep Venous Thrombosis, *Surg. Gynecol. Obstet.*, 152:448, 1981.
9. Coe, N. P., Collins, R. E. C., Klein, L. A., et al.: Prevention of Deep Vein Thrombosis in Urological Patients: A Controlled, Randomized Trial of Low-Dose Heparin and External Pneumatic Compression Boots, *Surgery*, 83:230, 1978.
10. Rabinov, K., and Paulin, S.: Roentgen Diagnosis of Venous Thrombosis in the Leg, *Arch. Surg.*, 104:134, 1972.
11. Hull, R., Hirsh, J., Sackett, D. L., et al.: Clinical Validity of a Negative Venogram in Patients with Clinically Suspected Venous Thrombosis, *Circulation*, 64:622, 1981.
12. Hull, R., Hirsh, J., Sackett, D. L., and Stoddart, G.: Cost Effectiveness of Clinical Diagnosis, Venography, and Noninvasive Testing in Patients with Symptomatic Deep-Vein Thrombosis, *N. Engl. J. Med.*, 304:1561, 1981.
13. Wheeler, H. B., O'Donnell, J. A., Anderson, F. A., Jr., and Benedict, K., Jr.: Occlusive Impedance Phlebography: A Diagnostic Procedure for Venous Thrombosis and Pulmonary Embolism, *Prog. Cardiovasc. Dis.*, 17(3):199, 1974.
14. Moser, K. M., and LeMoine, J. R.: Is Embolic Risk Conditioned by Location of Deep Venous Thrombosis? *Ann. Intern. Med.*, 94:439, 1981.
15. Dalen, J. E., and Dexter, L.: Pulmonary Embolism, *JAMA*, 207:1505, 1969.
16. Dalen, J. E., Haffajee, C. I., Alpert, J. S., Howe, J. P., III, Ockene, I. S., and Paraskos, J. A.: Pulmonary Embolism, Pulmonary Hemorrhage and Pulmonary Infarction, *N. Engl. J. Med.*, 296:1431, 1977.
17. Szucs, M. M., Jr., Brooks, H. L., Grossman, W., et al.: Diagnostic Sensitivity of Laboratory Findings in Acute Pulmonary Embolism, *Ann. Intern. Med.*, 74:161, 1971.
18. Hull, R. D., Hirsh, J., Carter, C. J., et al.: Pulmonary Angiography, Ventilation Lung Scanning, and Venography for Clinically Suspected Pulmonary Embolism with Abnormal Perfusion Lung Scan, *Ann. Intern. Med.*, 98:891, 1983.
19. Sasahara, A. A., Sharma, G. V. R. K., and Parisi, A. F.: New Developments in the Detection and Prevention of Venous Thromboembolism, *Am. J. Cardiol.*, 43:1214, 1979.
20. Dalen, J. E., Banas, J., Jr., Brooks, H., Evans, G., Paraskos,

J., and Dexter, L.: Resolution Rate of Acute Pulmonary Embolism in Man, *N. Engl. J. Med.*, 280:1194, 1969.
21. Thames, M. D., Alpert, J. S., and Dalen, J. E.: Syncope in Patients with Pulmonary Embolism, *JAMA*, 238:2509, 1977.
22. McGinn, S., and White, P. D.: Acute Cor Pulmonale Resulting from Pulmonary Embolism, *JAMA*, 104:1473, 1935.
23. Stein, P. D., Dalen, J. E., McIntyre, K. M., Sasahara, A. A., Wenger, N. K., and Willis, P. W., III: The Electrocardiogram in Acute Pulmonary Embolism, *Prog. Cardiovasc. Dis.*, 17:247, 1975.
24. Howe, J. P., III, Alpert, J. S., Rickman, F. D., Spackman, D. G., Dexter, L., and Dalen, J. E.: Return of Arterial P_{O_2} Values to Baseline after Supplemental Oxygen in Patients with Cardiac Disease, *Chest*, 67:256, 1975.
25. Kipper, M. S., Moser, K. M., Kortman, K. E., and Ashburn, W. L.: Longterm Follow-Up of Patients with Suspected Pulmonary Embolism and a Normal Lung Scan, *Chest*, 82:411, 1982.
26. Cheely, R., McCartney, W. H., Perry, J. R., et al.: The Role of Noninvasive Tests Versus Pulmonary Angiography in the Diagnosis of Pulmonary Embolism, *Am. J. Med.*, 70:17, 1981.
27. Stein, P. D., O'Connor, J. F., Dalen, J. E., et al.: The Angiographic Diagnosis of Acute Pulmonary Embolism: Evaluation of Criteria, *Am. Heart J.*, 73:730, 1967.
28. Dalen, J. E., Brooks, H. L., Johnson, L. W., Meister, S. G., Szucs, M. M., Jr., and Dexter, L.: Pulmonary Angiography in Acute Pulmonary Embolism: Indications, Techniques, and Results in 367 Patients, *Am. Heart J.*, 81:175, 1971.
29. Benotti, J. R., Alpert, J. S., and Dalen, J. E.: Superiority of Balloon-Occlusion Pulmonary Cineangiography in the Diagnosis of Pulmonary Embolism, *Chest*, 84:341, 1983. (Abstract.)
30. Greenberg, E., Divertie, M. B., Woolner, L. B.: A Review of Unusual Systemic Manifestations Associated with Carcinoma, *Am. J. Med.*, 36:106, 1964.
31. Lieberman, J. S., Borrero, J., Urdaneta, E., and Wright, I. S.: Thrombophlebitis and Cancer, *JAMA*, 177:542, 1961.
32. Gore, J. M., Appelbaum, J. S., Green, H. L., Dexter, L., and Dalen, J. E.: Occult Cancer in Patients with Acute Pulmonary Embolism, *Ann. Intern. Med.*, 96:556, 1982.
33. Meister, S. G., Grossman, W., Dexter, L., and Dalen, J. E.: Paradoxical Embolism. Diagnosis During Life, *Am. J. Med.*, 53:292, 1972.
34. Hagen, P. T., Scholz, D. G., and Edwards, W. D.: Incidence and Size of Patent Foramen Ovale During the First 10 Decades of Life: An Autopsy Study of 965 Normal Hearts, *Mayo Clin. Proc.*, 59:17, 1984.
35. Banas, J., Jr., Meister, S. G., Gazzaniga, A. B., O'Connor, N., Haynes, F. W., and Dalen, J. E.: A Simple Technique for Detecting Small Defects of the Atrial Septum, *Am. J. Cardiol.*, 28:467, 1971.
36. Higgins, J. R., Strunk, B. L., and Schiller, N. B.: Diagnosis of Paradoxical Embolism with Contrast Echocardiography, *Am. Heart J.*, 107:375, 1984.
37. Clagett, G. P., and Saltzman, E. W.: Prevention of Venous Thromboembolism, *Prog. Cardiovasc. Dis.*, 17(5):345, 1975.
38. Genton, E., and Hirsh, J.: Observations in Anticoagulant and Thrombolytic Therapy in Pulmonary Embolism, *Prog. Cardiovasc. Dis.*, 17(5):335, 1975.
39. Barritt, D. W., and Jordan, S. C.: Anticoagulant Drugs in the Treatment of Pulmonary Embolism. A Controlled Trial, *Lancet*, 1:1309, 1960.
40. Kernahan, R. J., and Todd, C.: Heparin Therapy in Thromboembolic Disease, *Lancet*, 1:621, 1966.
41. Colman, R. W.: Prophylaxis and Treatment of Thromboembolism Based on Pathophysiology of Clotting Mechanisms, in A. P. Fishman (ed), "Pulmonary Diseases and Disorders," New York, McGraw-Hill Book Co., 1980, p. 827.
42. Hull, R., Delmore, T., Carter, C., et al.: Adjusted Subcutaneous Heparin Versus Warfarin Sodium in the Long-Term Treatment of Venous Thrombosis, *N. Engl. J. Med.*, 306:189, 1982.
43. Hull, R., Hirsh, J., Jay, R., et al.: Different Intensities of Oral Anticoagulant Therapy in the Treatment of Proximal Vein Thrombosis, *N. Engl. J. Med.*, 307:1676, 1982.
44. Hirsh, J., VanAken, W., Gallus, A. S., Dollery, C. T., Cade, J. F., and Yung, W. L.: Heparin Kinetics in Venous Thrombosis and Pulmonary Embolism, *Circulation*, 53:691, 1976.
45. Salzman, E. W., Deykin, D., Shapiro, R. M., and Rosenberg, R.: Management of Heparin Therapy—Controlled Prospective Trial, *N. Engl. J. Med.*, 292:1046, 1975.
46. Jick, H., Sloane, D., Borda, I. T., and Shapiro, S.: Efficacy and Toxicity of Heparin in Relation to Age and Sex, *N. Engl. J. Med.*, 279:284, 1968.
47. Bell, W. R., Tomasulo, P. A., Alving, B. M., and Duffy, T. P.: Thrombocytopenia Occurring During the Administration of Heparin—A Prospective Study in 52 Patients, *Ann. Intern. Med.*, 85:155, 1976.
48. King, D. J., and Kelton, J. G.: Heparin-Associated Thrombocytopenia, *Ann. Intern. Med.*, 100:535, 1984.
49. Crane, C.: Venous Interruption for Pulmonary Embolism: Present Status, *Prog. Cardiovasc. Dis.*, 17(5):329, 1975.
50. Bomalaski, J. S., Martin, G. J., Hughes, R. L., and Yao, J. S. T.: Inferior Vena Cava Interruption in the Management of Pulmonary Embolism, *Chest*, 82:767, 1982.
51. Schlosser, V.: Umbrella Filter Implantation as Prophylaxis Against Pulmonary Embolism, *Eur. Soc. Cardiovasc. Radiol.*, 23:329, 1979.
52. Askew, A. R., and Gardner, A. M.: Long-Term Follow-Up of Partial Caval Occlusion by Clip, *Am. J. Surg.*, 140:441, 1980.
53. Adelson, J., Steer, M. L., Glotzer, D. J., et al.: Thromboembolism after Insertion of the Mobin-Uddin Caval Filter, *Surgery*, 87:184, 1980.
54. Greenfield, L. J.: Technical Considerations for Insertion of Vena Caval Filters, *Surg. Gynecol. Obstet.*, 148:422, 1979.
55. Paraskos, J. A., Adelstein, S. J., Smith, R. E., et al.: Late Prognosis of Acute Pulmonary Embolism, *N. Engl. J. Med.*, 289:55, 1973.
56. Alpert, J. S., Smith, R. E., Ockene, I. S., et al.: Treatment of Massive Pulmonary Embolism: The Role of Pulmonary Embolectomy, *Am. Heart J.*, 89:413, 1975.
57. McIntyre, K. M., and Sasahara, A. A.: Hemodynamic and Ventricular Responses to Pulmonary Embolism, *Prog. Cardiovasc. Dis.*, 17(3)175, 1974.
58. Sautter, R. D., Myers, W. O., Ray, J. F., III, and Wenzel, F. J.: Pulmonary Embolectomy: Review and Current Status, *Prog. Cardiovasc. Dis.*, 17(5):371, 1975.
59. Hietala, S. O., and Greenfield, L. J.: Percutaneous Pulmonary Embolectomy by the Transvenous Route, *Eur. Soc. Cardiovasc. Radiol.*, 23:325, 1979.
60. Greenfield, L. J., and Zocco, J. J.: Intraluminal Management of Acute Massive Pulmonary Thromboembolism, *J. Thorac. Cardiovasc. Surg.*, 77:402, 1979.
61. Daily, P. O., Johnston, G. G., Simmons, C. J., et al.: Surgical Management of Chronic Pulmonary Embolism, *J. Thorac. Cardiovasc. Surg.*, 79:523, 1980.
62. Moser, K. M., Spragg, R. G., Utley, J., and Daily, P. O.: Chronic Thrombotic Obstruction of Major Pulmonary Arteries: Results of Thromboendarterectomy in 15 Patients, *Ann. Intern. Med.*, 99:299, 1983.
63. Benotti, J. R., Ockene, I. S., Alpert, J. S., and Dalen, J. E.: The Clinical Profile of Unresolved Pulmonary Embolism, *Chest*, 84:669, 1983.
64. Urokinase Pulmonary Embolism Study Group: The Urokinase Pulmonary Embolism Trial, *Circulation*, 47(suppl. II):1, 1973.
65. Consensus Development Conference Report: Thrombolytic Therapy in Thrombosis: A National Institutes of Health Consensus Development Conference, *Ann. Intern. Med.*, 93:141, 1980.
66. Sharma, G. V. R. K., Burleston, V. A., and Sasahara, A. A.: Effect of Thrombolytic Therapy on Pulmonary-Capillary Blood Volume in Patients with Pulmonary Embolism, *N. Engl. J. Med.*, 303:842, 1980.
67. Marder, V. J.: Are We Using Fibrinolytic Agents Often Enough? *Ann. Intern. Med.*, 93:136, 1980.

68. Bell, W. R., and Meek, A. G.: Guidelines for the Use of Thrombolytic Agents, *N. Engl. J. Med.*, 301:1266, 1979.
69. Dalen, J. E.: The Case Against Fibrinolytic Therapy, *J. Cardiovasc. Med.*, 5:798, 1980.
70. Sasahara, A. A.: The Case for Fibrinolytic Therapy, *J. Cardiovasc. Med.*, 5:794, 1980.
71. Genton, E.: Thrombolytic Therapy of Pulmonary Thromboembolism, *Prog. Cardiovasc. Dis.*, 21:333, 1979.
72. Evans, G., Dalen, J. E., and Dexter, L.: Pulmonary Embolism During Pregnancy, *JAMA*, 206:320, 1968.
73. Hall, J. G., Pauli, R. M., and Wilson, K. M.: Maternal and Fetal Sequelae of Anticoagulation During Pregnancy, *Am. J. Med.*, 68:122, 1980.
74. Gauss, H.: The Pathology of Fat Embolism, *Arch. Surg.*, 9:593, 1924.
75. Ashbaugh, D. G., and Petty, T. L.: The Use of Corticosteroids in the Treatment of Respiratory Failure Associated with Massive Fat Embolism, *Surg. Gynecol. Obstet.*, 123:493, 1966.
76. Liljedahl, S., and Westermark, L.: Aetiology and Treatment of Fat Embolism: Report of Five Cases, *Acta Anaesthesiol. Scand.*, 11:177, 1967.
77. Tederschi, C. G., Castelli, W., Kropp, G., and Tedeschi, L. G.: Fat Macroglobulinemia and Fat Embolism, *Surg. Gynecol. Obstet.*, 126:83, 1968.
78. Oh, W. H., and Mital, M. A.: Fat Embolism: Current Concepts of Pathogenesis, Diagnosis and Treatment. *Orthop. Clin. North Am.*, 9:769, 1968.
79. Bradford, D. S., and Dick, H. M.: Fat Embolism: Report of a Case and Discussion of Current Concepts of Pathogenesis and Treatment. *Clin. Orthop.*, 65:218, 1969.
80. Rokkanen, P., Lahdensuu, M., Kataja, J., and Julkunen, H.: The Syndrome of Fat Embolism: Analysis of Thirty Consecutive Cases Compared to Trauma Patients with Similar Injuries, *J. Trauma.*, 10:299, 1971.
81. Bradford, D. S., Foster, R. R., and Nossel, H. L.: Coagulation Alterations, Hypoxemia, and Fat Embolism in Fracture Patients. *J. Trauma*, 10:307, 1971.
82. Peltier, L. F.: The Diagnosis and Treatment of Fat Embolism, *J. Trauma*, 11:661, 1971.
83. Herndon, J. H., Riseborough, E. J., and Fischer, J. E.: Fat Embolism: A Review of Current Concepts, *J. Trauma*, 11:673, 1971.
84. Fonte, D. A., and Hausberger, F. X.: Pulmonary Free Acids in Experimental Fat Embolism, *J. Trauma*, 11:668, 1971.
85. Kerstell, J.: Pathogenesis of Post-Traumatic Fat Embolism, *Am. J. Surg.*, 121:712, 1971.
86. Fischer, J. E., Turner, R. H., Herndon, J. H., and Riseborough, E. J.: Massive Steroid Therapy in Severe Fat Embolism, *Surg. Gynecol. Obstet.*, 132:667, 1971.
87. Dines, D. E., Linscheid, R. L., and Didier, E. P.: Fat Embolism Syndrome, *Mayo Clin. Proc.*, 47:237, 1972.
88. Rokkanen, P., Alho, A., Avikainen, V., et al.: The Efficacy of Corticosteroids in Severe Trauma, *Surg. Gynecol. Obstet.*, 138:69, 1974.
89. Moylan, J. A. and Evenson, M. A.: Diagnosis and Treatment of Fat Embolism, *Annu. Rev. Med.*, 28:85, 1977.
90. Alho, A., Saikku, K., Eerola, P., et al.: Corticosteroids in Patients with a High Risk of Fat Embolism Syndrome, *Surg. Gynecol. Obstet.*, 147:358, 1978.
91. Renne, J., Wuthier, R., House, E., et al.: Fat Macroglobulinemia Caused by Fractures or Total Hip Replacement, *J. Bone Joint Surg.*, 60A:613, 1978.
92. Oh, W. H., and Mital, M. A.: Fat Embolism: Current Concepts of Pathogenesis, Diagnosis, and Treatment, *Orthop. Clin. North Am.*, 9:769, 1978.
93. Curtis, A. M., Knowles, G. D., Putman, C. E., et al.: The Three Syndromes of Fat Embolism: Pulmonary Manifestations, *Yale J. Biol. Med.*, 52:149, 1979.
94. Gossling, H. R., and Donohue, T. A.: The Fat Embolism Syndrome. *JAMA*, 241:2740, 1979.
95. Guenter, C. A., and Braun, T. E.: Fat Embolism Syndrome. Changing Prognosis, *Chest*, 79:143, 1981.
96. Gossling, H. R., and Pellegrini, V. D., Jr.: Fat Embolism Syndrome: A Review of the Pathophysiology and Physiological Basis of Treatment. *Clin. Orthop.*, 165:68, 1982.
97. Schonfeld, S. A., Ploysongsang, Y., DiLisio, R., et al.: Fat Embolism Prophylaxis with Corticosteroids. A Prospective Study in High-Risk Patients, *Ann. Intern. Med.*, 99:438, 1983.
98. Zenker, F. A.: "Beitrage zur Anatomie und Physiologie der Lunge," Braunsdorf, Dresden, 1861.
99. Bergmann, E. B.: Ein Fall todlicher Fettembolie, *Berl. Klin. Wochenschr.*, 10:385, 1873.
100. Whitaker, A. C.: Traumatic Fat Embolism. Report of Two Cases with Recovery, *Arch. Surg.*, 38:182, 1939.
101. Berglund, E., and Josephson, S.: Pulmonary Air Embolization in the Dog. I. Hemodynamic Changes in Repeated Embolizations, *Scand. J. Clin. Lab. Invest.*, 26:97, 1970.
102. Josephson, S.: Pulmonary Air Embolization in the Dog: II. Evidence and Location of Pulmonary Vasoconstriction. *Scand. J. Clin. Lab. Invest.*, 26:113, 1970.
103. Ence, T. J., and Gong, H., Jr.: Adult Respiratory Distress Syndrome after Venous Air Embolism, *Am. Rev. Resp. Dis.*, 119:1033, 1979.
104. Hlastala, M. P., Robertson, H. T., and Ross, B. K.: Gas Exchange Abnormalities Produced by Venous Gas Emboli, *Respir. Physiol.*, 36:1, 1979.
105. Yee, E. S., Verrier, E. D., and Thomas, A. N.: Management of Air Embolism in Blunt and Penetrating Thoracic Trauma, *J. Thorac. Cardiovasc. Surg.*, 85:661, 1983.
106. Bray, P., Myers, R. A., and Cowley, R. A.: Orogenital Sex as a Cause of Nonfatal Air Embolism in Pregnancy, *Obstet. Gynecol.*, 61:653, 1983.
107. Rodigas, P. C., Meyer, F. J., Haasler, G. B., et al.: Intraoperative 2-Dimensional Echocardiography: Ejection of Microbubbles from the Left Ventricle after Cardiac Surgery, *Am. J. Cardiol.*, 50:1130, 1982.
108. Ericsson, J. A., Gottlieb, J. D., and Sweet, R. B.: Closed-Chest Cardiac Massage in the Treatment of Venous Air Embolism, *N. Engl. J. Med.*, 270:1353, 1964.
109. Meyer, J. R.: Embolia Pulmonar Amino-Caseosa. *Brasil Med.*, 2:301, 1926.
110. Steiner, P. E., and Luschbaugh, C. C.: Maternal Pulmonary Embolism by Amniotic Fluid as a Cause of Obstetric Shock and Unexpected Deaths in Obstetrics, *JAMA*, 117:1245, 1941.
111. Liban, E., and Raz, S.: A Clinicopathologic Study of Fourteen Cases of Amniotic Fluid Embolism, *Am. J. Clin. Pathol.*, 51:477, 1969.
112. Peterson, E. P., and Taylor, H. B.: Amniotic Fluid Embolism: An Analysis of 40 Cases, *Obstet. Gynecol.*, 35:787, 1970.
113. Jewett, J. F.: Amniotic-Fluid Infusion, *N. Engl. J. Med.*, 292:973, 1975.
114. Morgan, M.: Amniotic Fluid Embolism, *Anaesthesia*, 34:20, 1979.
115. Sterner, S., Campbell, B., and Davies, S.: Amniotic Fluid Embolism, *Ann. Emerg. Med.*, 13:343, 1984.
116. Rogers, G. P., and Heymach, G. J., III: Cryoprecipitate Therapy in Amniotic Fluid Embolization, *Am. J. Med.*, 76:916, 1984.
117. Durhan, J. R., Ashley, P. F., and Dorenclamp, D.: Cor Pulmonale Due to Tumor Emboli: Review of Literature and Report of a Case, *JAMA*, 175:757, 1961.
118. Bagshawe, K. D., and Noble, M. I. M.: Cardiorespiratory Aspects of Trophoblastic Tumors, *Q. J. Med.*, 35:39, 1966.
119. Li, M. C.: Trophoblastic Disease: Natural History, Diagnosis and Treatment, *Ann., Intern. Med.*, 74:102, 1971.
120. Ross, M., Nowicki, K., and Rangarajan, N. S.: Asymptomatic Pulmonary Embolism during Pregnancy, *Obstet. Gynecol.*, 37:131, 1971.
121. Mehta, S., and Rubenstone, A. I.: Pulmonary Bile Thromboemboli: A Report of Two Cases, *Am. J. Clin. Pathol.*, 47:490, 1967.
122. Dimmick, J. E., Bove, K. E., McAdams, A. J., and Benzing, G., III: Fiber Embolization—Hazard of Cardiac Surgery and Catheterization, *N. Engl. J. Med.*, 292:685, 1975.

55

Chronic Cor Pulmonale

Joseph C. Ross, M.D.

John H. Newman, M.D.

So it appears that whereas one ventricle, the left, suffices for distributing the blood to the body, and drawing it from the vena cava, as is the case in all animals lacking lungs, nature was compelled, when she wished to filter blood through the lungs, to add the right ventricle. . . . Thus the right ventricle may be said to be made for the sake of transmitting blood through the lungs, not for nourishing them.

William Harvey, 1628[1]

Definition

Cor pulmonale is a term which signifies the effect of lung dysfunction in the right side of the heart. Thus, cor pulmonale is a secondary form of heart disease. There are many conditions which can lead to cor pulmonale, but the common thread in each case is pulmonary hypertension, leading to dilatation with or without hypertrophy of the right ventricle. The systemic consequences of cor pulmonale relate to alterations in cardiac output, salt and water homeostasis, and, in many cases, gas exchange in the lung. Right-sided heart disease arising from dysfunction of the left side of the heart or from congenital heart disease is excluded in the definition of cor pulmonale.[2] Pulmonary venous obstruction may or may not be considered within the definition of cor pulmonale. As a concept, cor pulmonale was introduced over 200 years ago but the exact origin of the term is uncertain.[3] Osler commented in the first edition of his textbook that "hypertrophy of the right ventricle . . . results from increased resistance in the pulmonary circulation, as in cirrhosis of the lung and emphysema."[4] McGinn and White apparently were the first to use the term *acute cor pulmonale* in the discussion of a case of massive thromboembolism in 1935.[5] William Harvey's discussion of the relationship of the right side of the heart and lung in *De Motu Cordis*[1] showed remarkable insight into the limitations of that muscular structure.

Incidence and Etiologies

Emphysema and chronic bronchitis cause over 50 percent of cases of cor pulmonale in this country. The prevalence of cor pulmonale is difficult to determine because not all cases of chronic lung disease develop cor pulmonale and because routine physical examination and laboratory tests are relatively insensitive to the presence of pulmonary hypertension. It has been estimated that cor pulmonale accounts for 5 to 10 percent of organic heart disease, and cor pulmonale was present in 20 to 30 percent of admissions for heart failure in one study.[6]

Approximately 30,000 persons per year die of chronic obstructive lung diseases in this country, and it is likely that cor pulmonale is a complication in a high percentage of cases. Gazes found that of cases of heart disease which came to autopsy, 9.2 percent had cor pulmonale.[6] Chronic cor pulmonale occurs most frequently in male smokers, 50 to 60 years old, although the incidence in women is increasing as heavy smoking in females becomes more prevelant. A list of all diseases which may lead to cor pulmonale would be extensive and is not included in this chapter, but the major types of disease processes are listed in Table 55-1. Because cor pulmonale denotes the response of the right side of the heart to pulmonary hypertension, it is more useful to understand the pathophysiology of pulmonary hypertension and to categorize diseases by mechanism.

Pathophysiology

Common factors in all cases of cor pulmonale are increased pulmonary vascular resistance and pulmonary hypertension. Mechanisms causing and po-

TABLE 55-1 Etiologies of Chronic Cor Pulmonale by Mechanism of Pulmonary Hypertension

1. Hypoxic vasoconstriction
   a. Chronic bronchitis and emphysema, cystic fibrosis
   b. Chronic hypoventilation
      (1) Obesity
      (2) Sleep apnea
      (3) Neuromuscular disease
      (4) Chest wall dysfunction
   c. High-altitude dwelling and chronic mountain sickness
2. Occlusion of the pulmonary vascular bed
   a. Pulmonary thromboembolism, parasitic ova, tumor emboli
   b. Primary pulmonary hypertension
   c. Venocclusive disease
   d. Pulmonary angiitis from systemic disease
      (1) Collagen vascular disease
      (2) Drug-induced lung disease
3. Parenchymal disease with destruction of vascular surface area
   a. Chronic bronchitis and emphysema
   b. Bronchiectasis, cystic fibrosis
   c. Diffuse interstitial disease
      (1) Pneumoconioses
      (2) Sarcoid, idiopathic pulmonary fibrosis, histiocytosis x
      (3) Tuberculosis, chronic fungal infection
      (4) Acute respiratory distress syndrome
      (5) Collagen vascular disease

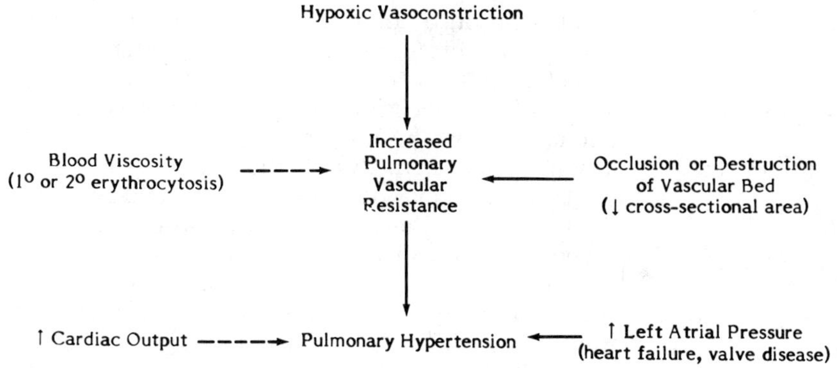

FIGURE 55-1 Mechanisms of the production of pulmonary hypertension. Dashed arrows represent mechanisms that increase pulmonary artery pressure but are not sufficient alone to cause pulmonary hypertension. Left-sided heart failure causes pulmonary hypertension but not increased pulmonary vascular resistance unless the process is chronic and vascular damage occurs. Cor pulmonale is the result of lung disease involving constriction, occlusion, or destruction of the vascular bed.

tentiating pulmonary hypertension are shown in Fig. 55-1. Fortunately, most pulmonary diseases or disorders do not produce enough pulmonary hypertension to cause cor pulmonale.

Normal Pulmonary Circulation

The primary function of the unique low-pressure, low-resistance pulmonary circulation is to provide blood for gas exchange, and it is ideally suited to optimize that function. It receives and transmits the entire cardiac output with a low-pressure head primarily because of three characteristics: (1) pulmonary arteries are thin-walled with little resting muscular tone; (2) there is negligible vasomotor control by the autonomic nervous system in the adult; (3) many small arterioles and capillaries are nonperfused at rest, but can be recruited when needed to expand the pulmonary vascular bed, resulting in a decreased pulmonary vascular resistance. Normal mean pulmonary artery pressure (PAP) is about 12 to 17 mmHg; PAP $>$ 20 mmHg signifies pulmonary hypertension. Flow of blood through pulmonary capillaries is accompanied by a pressure drop of only 5 to 9 mmHg (pulmonary artery to left atrial pressure) compared with an arterial to venous gradient of 90 mmHg in the systemic circuit. Thus normal pulmonary vascular resistance is 10 to 20-fold less than systemic vascular resistance.

Pulmonary Hypertension

The effective cross-sectional area of the pulmonary vascular bed must be reduced by more than 50 percent before any change in pulmonary artery pressure can be detected at rest, but exercise will cause increased pressure at lower levels of increased blood flow. Obliterative vascular diseases increase pulmonary vascular resistance by vascular occlusion, while diffuse interstitial diseases act primarily by compression and obliteration of small vessels. It is now well established, however, that arteriolar constriction is the predominant cause of pulmonary hypertension.

Pulmonary Arteriolar Constriction

The most important cause of pulmonary vasoconstriction is alveolar hypoxia. The mechanism of this effect is not clear. It is thought to be due to mediator release from some unknown effector cell or a direct action of hypoxia on pulmonary vascular smooth muscle.[7] The degree of hypoxic vasoconstriction is dependent primarily on the alveolar oxygen tension (Pa_{O_2}) and, when Pa_{O_2} is about 55 torr (7.3 kPa), pulmonary artery pressure rises sharply (Fig. 55-2).

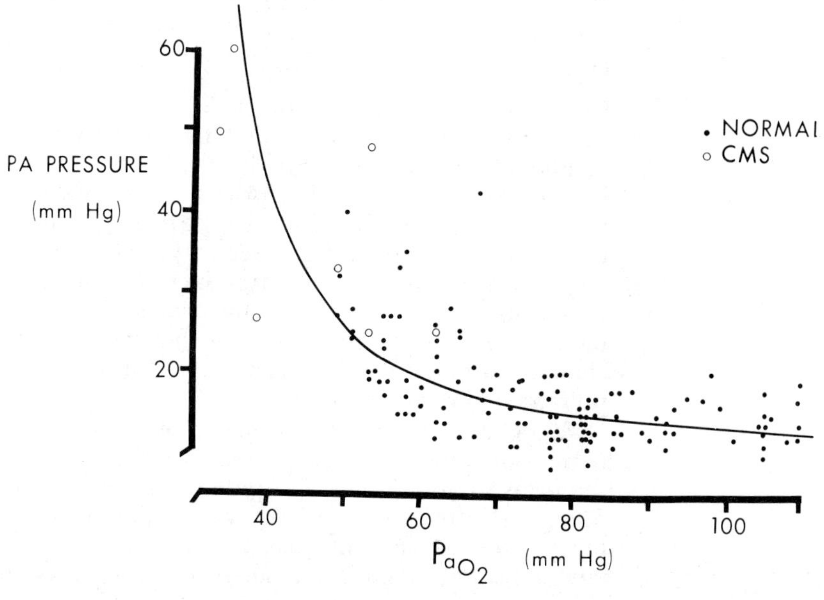

FIGURE 55-2 Pulmonary artery pressure as a function of Pa_{O_2} in normal residents of cities of different altitudes, and patients with chronic mountain sickness (CMS). Pulmonary artery pressure rises steeply as Pa_{O_2} decreases below 55 torr. (*From J. T. Reeves and R. F. Grover, High Altitude Pulmonary Hypertension and Pulmonary Edema, Prog. Cardiol., 4:105, 1975. Reproduced with permission from the publisher and authors.*)

TABLE 55-2 Pulmonary Vasomotor Tone

Dilator	Constrictor
Beta-adrenergic agonists	Alpha-adrenergic agonists
Histamine H_2	Histamine H_1
Prostacyclin (PGI_2)	PGE_2, $PGF_{1\alpha}$, thromboxane A_2
Acetylcholine	Serotonin
O_2	Hypoxia
Bradykinin	Angiotensin II

When the pulmonary artery pressure is greater than 40 mmHg, arterial oxygen saturation is very likely less than 75 percent.[8] There is large individual variability in the hypoxic pressor response, and hypoxic vasoconstriction is enhanced by acidosis and blunted by alkalosis. Acidosis also has a mild direct pressor effect on the pulmonary circulation.[9] Extensive investigations into the mechanism of hypoxic vasoconstriction have shown that local and circulating mediators of pulmonary vascular tone are capable of modulating the hypoxic pressor response, but that no single mediator yet discovered is responsible (Table 55-2). Hypoxic vasoconstriction in a region of lung where ventilation is diminished probably serves to maximize net arterial oxygenation by diverting blood from the hypoxic region to better ventilated areas. Because the pulmonary vascular bed is capable of large recruitment, localized hypoxic vasoconstriction does not cause pulmonary hypertension. Generalized hypoxia causes generalized hypoxic vasoconstriction and the development of pulmonary hypertension (Fig. 55-3). Obliteration of blood vessels was once thought to be the primary cause of hypertension in chronic obstructive pulmonary disease (COPD), but it is clearly of secondary importance. In COPD, the first episodes of alveolar hypoxia may occur during sleep, and gradually become worse thereafter.[10] Any cause of alveolar hypoventilation (Table 55-1) can result in chronic cor pulmonale through the mechanism of hypoxic pulmonary vasoconstriction, even from entities as different as diffuse obstructive lung disease and kyphoscoliosis.[11]

FIGURE 55-3 Hypoxic pulmonary vasoconstruction maximizes arterial oxygenation by diverting blood away from areas of regional hypoxia toward better-ventilated zones. Generalized hypoxia causes generalized hypoxic vasoconstriction and results in pulmonary hypertension. [*From J. H. Newman, Pulmonary Vascular Reactivity in Primary Pulmonary Edema, Semin. Resp. Med., 4(4):299, 1983. Reproduced with permission from the publisher and author, and courtesy of J. V. Weil.*]

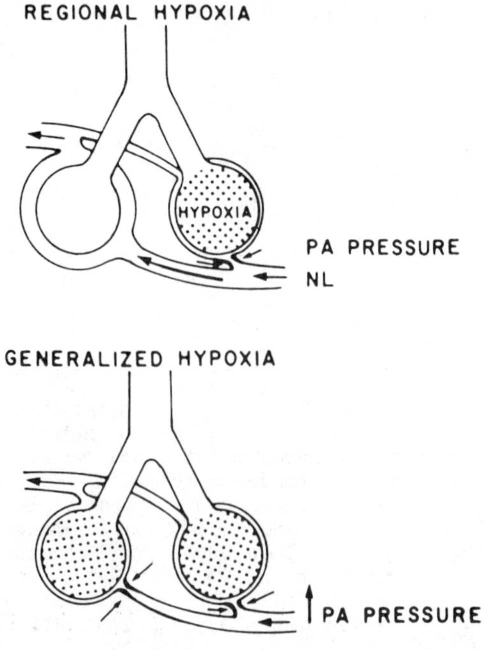

Other Factors Which Increase Pulmonary Hypertension

After the cross-sectional area of the pulmonary vascular bed has become reduced, increases in cardiac output, heart rate, and blood volume, or direct effects of acidosis and/or hypoxia on the myocardium, may contribute to pulmonary hypertension. Increased blood flow (i.e., exercise) will require the generation of a higher pulmonary artery pressure and, in such a situation, the effects of hypoxia and acidosis will also be exaggerated.[8] Sustained hypoxemia causes secondary erythrocytosis. Blood viscosity increases rapidly after the hematocrit exceeds about 55 percent, raising pulmonary vascular resistance and also decreasing cerebral function. If left ventricular failure is superimposed on an already reduced pulmonary vascular bed, a higher pulmonary artery pressure will occur in response to a stimulus. Once established, pulmonary hypertension may be self-perpetuating. Enson et al.[12] found that a sustained increase in pulmonary vascular resistance in patients with diffuse lung disease caused anatomic changes in the walls of small arteries, further increasing pulmonary vascular resistance. Chronic hypoxia alone results in muscularization of pulmonary arterioles and exaggerated increases in pulmonary artery pressure with stimuli.[13]

Right Ventricular Response to Pulmonary Hypertension

The right ventricle is thin-walled and better able to handle an increase in volume load than to meet an increased pressure load. The primary cause of right ventricular failure, therefore, is a chronic pressure load (afterload). Small increases in pulmonary artery pressure may result in large increases in right ventricular work. Pulmonary hypertension at rest indicates advanced disease and, at that stage, small changes in blood flow will cause large increases in pulmonary artery pressure.

Response of the right ventricle to pulmonary hypertension depends on the acuteness and severity of the pressure load. Acute cor pulmonale (see Chap. 54) occurs after a sudden and severe stimulus (i.e., massive pulmonary embolus), with ventricular dilatation and failure but no hypertrophy. Chronic cor pulmonale, however, is associated with a more slowly evolving and slowly progressive hypertension,[14] and the responses may include increased protein synthesis and right ventricular hypertrophy.[15] The severity of the hypertension, the rapidity with which it becomes severe, and the possible eventual onset of right ventricular failure are influenced by factors which intercede intermittently, such as (1) *alterations in ventilatory function,* causing alveolar pressure changes with effects on chamber function; (2) *alterations in gas exchange* with more or less severe hypoxemia, hypercapnia, and acidosis; (3) *alterations in volume load* as influenced by exercise, heart rate, polycythemia, or renal retention of salt and water associated with cor pulmonale. At some stage, the myocardium is unable to function at the high-pressure load, dilates, and fails. That may occur relatively early in patients with chronic bronchitis because of sustained hypoxemia, but occurs later in patients with diffuse lung disease because the degree of right ventricular hypertrophy helps to maintain blood flow, even when the pulmonary artery pressure is high.[12]

Left Ventricular Function in Cor Pulmonale

Dysfunction of the left ventricle occurs in patients with cor pulmonale, but the evidence available now indicates that cor pulmonale per se does not cause disease of the left side of the heart. The likelihood, in most cases, is that left-sided heart dysfunction coexisting with cor pulmonale results from other known causes such as coronary ischemia or systemic hypertension. Certainly left ventricular failure is a serious complication in cor pulmonale because the increase in lung water further impairs lung function, increases the work of breathing, increases pulmonary artery pressure, impairs gas exchange, and may induce respiratory failure. When underlying disease of the left ventricle is also present, the direct effects of hypoxia, hypercapnia, and acidosis arising from primary lung disease may precipitate left ventricular failure.[16,17]

Several lines of evidence point to direct effects of lung dysfunction and right ventricular hypertrophy on performance of the left ventricle.[18] Wide swings in transpulmonary pressure in obstructive lung disease can reduce left ventricular filling and increase left ventricular afterload.[19] Hypertrophy and elevated end-diastolic pressure of the right ventricle in cor pulmonale can reduce left ventricular compliance and impair left ventricular filling through effects on the shared ventricular septum.[20] Despite these effects, most patients with chronic cor pulmonale demonstrate normal resting cardiac output, pulmonary artery wedge pressure, and normal resting left ventricular ejection fraction. The majority of patients with abnormal left ventricular ejection fraction in either compensated or decompensated chronic lung disease probably have demonstrable coronary artery disease.[21]

Edema Formation and Cor Pulmonale

Systemic edema occurs in some cases of chronic cor pulmonale. The mechanism is poorly understood but is probably related to increased systemic venous pressure, hypercarbia, and hypoxemia.[22] The presence of pulmonary hypertension per se does not appear to be sufficient to cause fluid retention unless pressures are excessively high as in primary pulmonary hypertension. Decreased clearance of aldosterone from the passively congested liver contributes to salt retention, but is likely not an initiating event. Plasma volume is, however, increased in chronic cor pulmonale.[23]

Hypercarbia stimulates plasma renin activity, and hypercarbic, edematous patients with chronic obstructive lung disease have increased plasma levels of aldosterone and antidiuretic hormone.[24] This pattern occurs despite oxygen therapy in these patients.[24] Thus not only increased salt retention but also impaired water excretion contributes to edema in chronic hypercapnia. The renal effects of moderate hypoxia are less pronounced, unless the Pa_{O_2} is in the 30 to 45 torr (4 to 6 kPa) range, where decrease in urine formation occurs. Other mechanisms of edema formation are increased systemic capillary hydrostatic pressure, related to increased venous pressure and blood volume, and perhaps a direct effect of hypoxia on peripheral tissue.

Many mechanisms appear to be operating to produce edema in chronic cor pulmonale, several of which are related to the primary pulmonary dysfunction. The exact pattern and sequence of events leading to edema are difficult to determine in any specific case. Pulmonary edema and pleural effusion are not seen as a consequence of cor pulmonale.

Diseases Causing Cor Pulmonale

Complete discussion of all causes of cor pulmonale is not within the scope of this chapter, but features of some diseases (Table 55-1) will be described.

Chronic Obstructive Pulmonary Disease

Chronic obstructive lung diseases cause cor pulmonale through several interrelated mechanisms, including hypoventilation, hypoxemia from ventilation/perfusion ($\dot{V}/\dot{Q}$) mismatch, and destruction of perfused surface area. When chronic bronchitis predominates, cough productive of sputum is the common symptom, and the striking $\dot{V}/\dot{Q}$ inequality leads to hypoxemia, hypercarbia, erythrocytosis, and early onset of cor pulmonale ("blue bloaters").[25] When emphysema predominates, dyspnea on exertion is the most prominent symptom, and these patients ("pink puffers")[25] have less $\dot{V}/\dot{Q}$ inequality and less hypoxemia at rest, and, therefore, develop cor pulmonale later. Some of the differences between blue bloaters and pink puffers may relate to ventilatory drives; patients with low drives may be more likely to fit the blue bloater category, whereas pink puffers strive to maintain normal arterial pH and gas tension.[26] *Physical examination* shows an increase in the thoracic diameter, low diaphragm, hyperresonance to percussion, decreased breath sounds with expiratory wheezes, distant heart sounds, distended neck veins during expiration, and a palpable (but not enlarged) liver. *Chest roentgenogram* may show characteristic changes of emphysema such as hyperlucent lungs, bullae, increased anteroposterior (AP) diameter, and flattened diaphragm. On the other hand, it may not show these characteristic findings nor be indicative of the severity of the physiological impairment. *Pulmonary function tests* show large residual volume and total lung capacity, decreased forced vital capacity, and decreased expiratory flow rates (FEV_1, MMEF). *Arterial blood* studies at rest are often normal when disease is mild but, in severe disease, show decreased P_{O_2}, increased P_{CO_2}, and decreased pH. With cor pulmonale, Pa_{O_2} is likely to be less than 55 torr (7.3 kPa). Desaturation increases with exercise and frequently during sleep. $\dot{V}/\dot{Q}$ inequality and hypoventilation both contribute to the hypoxemia. Pa_{CO_2} more than 45 torr (6 kPa) indicates either *net* or *general* alveolar hypoventilation. Asthma is a form of chronic obstructive pulmonary disease, but it rarely, if ever, leads to chronic cor pulmonale.[27]

Diffuse Interstitial Lung Disease

Patients with diffuse interstitial lung disease have dyspnea, tachypnea, exercise intolerance, and frequently clubbing of the digits. The chest roentgenogram shows diffuse reticular, reticulonodular, or fibrotic lesions, but the appearance does not always correlate well with physiological impairment. A lung biopsy is usually required to identify the basic pathologic process, and, even then, the exact etiology may not always be determined. Pulmonary function tests show a restrictive process with reduced lung volumes, decreased compliance, and decreased diffusing capacity, without airways obstruction. At first, Pa_{O_2} decreases during exercise but is kept at normal levels at rest by hyperventilation while Pa_{CO_2} is normal or low. As the disease becomes more severe, Pa_{CO_2} is low at rest. The course and prognosis of interstitial lung disease depend on the specific disease, and there is wide variation among and within diseases.[28,29] The presence of cor pulmonale in interstitial lung disease implies extensive, severe lung dysfunction.

Hypoventilation Syndromes

Some disorders (i.e., kyphoscoliosis) may impair or restrict mechanics of ventilation so that it is inadequate to maintain gas exchange, causing *general* alveolar hypoventilation. Extreme obesity may be associated with hypoventilation, cyanosis, polycythemia, and somnolence (without lung disease), often called the Pickwickian syndrome.[30] Patients with daytime somnolence, morning headaches, and personality disturbances have been found to have periodic apnea during sleep associated with sleep deprivation, loud snoring, hypoxemia, and hypercapnia caused by upper airway obstruction (i.e., tongue, enlarged tonsils, or collapse of pharyngeal walls).[31] Brainstem abnormalities may cause respiratory center depression and primary hypoventilation. Diagnosis of hypoventilation is confirmed by a depressed ventilatory response to inhaled CO_2, tests of voluntary hyperventilation, or sleep studies. It has become apparent recently that disordered ventilation during sleep is a major component of many hypoventilation syndromes.[32]

Pulmonary Vascular Diseases

Chronic cor pulmonale is a consequence of several diseases that are limited to the pulmonary vessels. Primary pulmonary hypertension and recurrent pulmonary emboli are two of the most important causes of cor pulmonale and are described in detail in Chaps. 52 and 53. Sickle cell disease, from SS or SC hemoglobinopathy, can cause cor pulmonale after multiple episodes of pulmonary infarction from focal pulmonary sickling or from thromboembolism.[33] Venocclusive disease is a rare disease of the veins which presents with pulmonary hypertension and pulmonary edema. There is one report of a beneficial response to immunosuppressive therapy in that disease.[34] Cirrhosis of the liver is usually associated with pulmonary vasodilatation, but occasionally a disorder seemingly identical to primary pulmonary hypertension emerges.[35,36] Collagen vascular diseases can cause cor pulmonale by primary vasculitis as well as by diffuse interstitial fibrosis. Systemic sclerosis, systemic lupus erythematosis (SLE), and rheumatoid arthritis (RA) are the collagen vascular syndromes which most commonly cause pulmonary arteritis. Patients with SLE and RA frequently present with primary interstitial lung disease. Occasionally, the appearance is that of cor pulmonale, without prominent interstitial disease but with primary pulmonary arteritis.[37]

Cor Pulmonale: Clinical Manifestations

Clinical manifestations of cor pulmonale are often obscured by the signs and symptoms of underlying disease and are, therefore, closely related to the pulmonary disease or disorder. It is absolutely necessary first to recognize the type of underlying disease and then look for cor pulmonale.

History

When left ventricular failure occurs, the immediate effect on the pulmonary vascular bed and on lung function produces symptoms and is an early indicator. No such situation exists with cor pulmonale. The symptoms are mainly those related to progression of the underlying disease or disorder. Heart failure occurs insidiously, causing further impairment of lung function, but frequently is misinterpreted as worsening of the underlying disease. The diagnosis is often not made until significant right ventricular hypertrophy or overt right ventricular failure is present, but cor pulmonale should be considered in any patient with pulmonary hypertension and, particularly, with chronic hypoxemia. There is no history which is specific for cor pulmonale. Episodes of leg edema, atypical chest pain, dyspnea on exertion, exercise-induced peripheral cyanosis, prior respiratory failure, and excessive daytime somnolence are all historical clues suggesting the presence of cor pulmonale.

Physical Examination

The signs are easiest to detect when cor pulmonale is associated with long-standing pulmonary hypertension. The earliest sign of pulmonary hypertension is an accentuated pulmonic component of S_2, which may also be palpable in the pulmonic area, and right ventricular lift of the sternum may be seen. With very high pulmonary artery pressure, characteristic diastolic and systolic murmurs of pulmonary valvular and tricuspid valvular insufficiency are heard along with a systolic ejection sound and right ventricular S_3 gallop. In overt right ventricular failure, cardiac enlargement, distended neck veins, hepatomegaly, and peripheral edema are present. Right ventricular failure is frequently accompanied by hypoxemia and cyanosis. Symptoms and signs suggestive of heart failure, such as dyspnea, orthopnea, peripheral edema, palpable liver, and distended neck veins, however, can be observed in patients with COPD without right ventricular failure. When neck veins are distended during inspiration as well as expiration, however, right ventricular failure is more likely present. Hyperinflated lungs alter the position of the heart and frequently make the examination difficult. The apical impulse and the right ventricular lift are often not palpable and the right ventricular S_3 gallop is heard in the epigastrium along the sternum. Heart sounds may be best heard below the xyphoid. Right ventricular failure is usually precipitated by some acute episode (i.e., respiratory infection) and associated with cyanosis and significant hypoxemia, hypercapnia, and acidosis. Extremities may be warm owing to peripheral vasodilatation caused by hypercapnia.

Chest Roentgenogram

The radiographic findings of pulmonary hypertension in patients with normal lung parenchyma (such as early mitral stenosis) are well described.[38] Most diseases that cause cor pulmonale produce grossly abnormal chest roentgenograms, and the radiologic diagnosis of pulmonary hypertension in these diseases is more difficult. Right ventricular enlargement may be difficult to detect in the vertical heart of emphysema, and comparison with previous films may be helpful. In the most obvious cases of cor pulmonale, there is right ventricle and pulmonary artery enlargement, but pulmonary hypertension precedes right ventricular dilatation. The most sensitive indicator of pulmonary hypertension is measurement of the dimensions of the right and left pulmonary arteries. Enlargement is considered to exist if the diameter of the right descending pulmonary artery is greater than 16 mm[39] and the left descending pulmonary artery is greater than 18 mm.[40] These findings occurred in 43 of 46 patients with known pulmonary hypertension,[40] but the true sensitivity and specificity of these measurements are not known.

Electrocardiogram

ECG patterns are influenced by many factors such as pulmonary artery pressure, pulmonary vascular resistance, rotation and displacement of the heart by hyperinflated lungs, arterial blood gases, myocardial ischemia, and metabolic disturbances. The value of the ECG in diagnosis of cor pulmonale, therefore, is dependent on the underlying disease and complicating conditions. Absence of changes indicating right ventricular disease does not rule out cor pulmonale since the ECG may be normal in advanced cor pulmonale. The classic right ventricular hypertrophy pattern is seen more often when there is anatomic restriction of the pulmonary vascular bed. An example of right ventricular hypertrophy is shown in Fig. 55-4. Fishman[2] noted that standard

FIGURE 55-4 Electrocardiogram in a patient with cor pulmonale. The mean QRS axis was +120°. The tall, peaked P waves indicate right atrial enlargement. The tall R waves in leads V_1 to V_3 and deep S wave in V_6 and the associated T-wave changes indicate right ventricular hypertrophy. (*From N. F. Voelkel and J. T. Reeves, Primary Pulmonary Hypertension, in "Pulmonary Vascular Diseases," Marcel Dekker, Inc., New York, p. 612. Reproduced with permission from the authors, and by courtesy of J. Ray Pryor and Marcel Dekker, Inc.*)

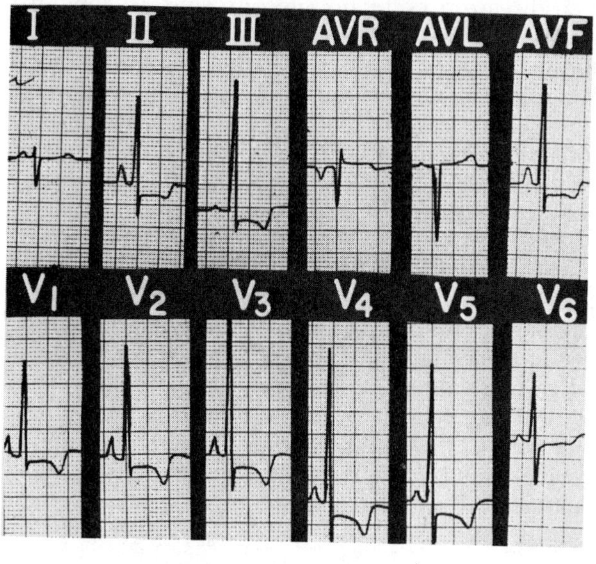

criteria for right ventricular enlargement were absent in two-thirds of patients with COPD who had right ventricular hypertrophy on postmortem examination. It has been suggested that, when classic right ventricular hypertrophy changes are absent, diagnosis be based on the combination of rS in V_5 to V_6; right axis deviation (RAD), qR in aV_R; and "P pulmonale."[41] Tall peaked P waves in leads II, III, and aV_F may reflect positional changes rather than right atrial enlargement. Right bundle branch block occurs in about 15 percent of patients.[41] Arrhythmias are infrequent in uncomplicated cor pulmonale but when present are mostly supraventricular and may reflect blood gas abnormalities, hypokalemia, or excess of drugs such as digitalis, theophylline, and beta agonists. Ventricular arrhythmias, when they occur, are associated with a high mortality rate. Serial ECGs are usually helpful, particularly in patients with COPD.

Special Laboratory Studies

The echocardiogram is not reliable in determining right ventricular size, but investigations are being done regarding the use of ultrasound for noninvasive measurement of pulmonary artery pressure. Quantitative first pass radionuclide angiocardiography is a useful technique for noninvasive assessment of right ventricular function and shows an abnormal right ventricular ejection fraction in patients with cor pulmonale.[42] Thallium 201 myocardial imaging has shown right ventricular free wall thickening in patients with pulmonary hypertension, even when right ventricular hypertrophy is not detected by ECG.[43]

Right-Sided Heart Catheterization

Right-sided heart catheterization is the only technique available for the direct measurement of pulmonary artery pressure and pulmonary artery wedge pressure. It is occasionally important in differentiating cor pulmonale from left ventricular failure when disease presentation is confusing. In cor pulmonale, pulmonary artery diastolic pressure is significantly higher than wedge pressure, unlike left ventricular failure or mitral stenosis where the diastolic-wedge pressure gradient is smaller. Mean pulmonary artery pressure is very high in obliterative vascular diseases, but only moderately high in interstitial lung diseases until arterial hypoxemia is present.[44] In COPD, pulmonary artery pressure is related to the level of hypoxemia and usually will be decreased by O_2 administration.[45] About 50 percent of patients with COPD will have pulmonary hypertension at rest although, in those patients with normal resting values, pulmonary artery pressure may rise with exercise.[46] Serial catheterizations in patients with COPD and pulmonary hypertension have revealed remarkable stability of pulmonary hemodynamics.[46]

Management

The primary lung disease is the focus of therapy since the right ventricular pressure work load must be reduced. If right ventricular failure has not appeared, a goal is to prevent its onset. When it appears, it should be treated, but the response will be poor unless cardiac work is reduced by control of pulmonary hypertension.

Treatment to Decrease Pulmonary Hypertension

Relief of hypoxia is of prime importance in reducing pulmonary hypertension, either to prevent or to treat cor pulmonale. That may be done in two ways: (1) treatment of the underlying disease, and (2) O_2 administration. Neither will lower pulmonary artery pressure in all patients since hypertension is often intractable in those with an anatomic restriction of the vascular bed. With the onset of right ventricular failure, however, most patients with chronic cor pulmonale do have some hypoxic pulmonary vasoconstriction, and all should be treated with oxygen in amounts adequate to restore arterial O_2 tension to greater than 60 torr (8 kPa). Corticosteroids may be helpful in some patients with interstitial lung disease and patients with a bronchospastic component of COPD. Measures should be instituted to treat the systemic disease with which obliterative vascular disease is associated or to prevent further emboli, if that is the problem.

In COPD, the primary focus is relief of hypoxemia by restoration of effective ventilation or by O_2 administration. Net alveolar ventilation may be improved by therapy, including bronchodilators for bronchospasm, antibiotics to prevent or treat acute exacerbations of bronchitis, bronchial toilet for removal of secretions, and avoidance of airway irritants such as tobacco smoke. Tranquilizers, sedatives, and narcotics must be avoided in unstable patients and in patients with hypoventilation. Correction of hypoxia and acidosis may produce a striking reduction in pulmonary artery pressure. In diseases which alter lung function but not structure, effective alveolar ventilation must be restored by treatment of the underlying disease or by use of mechanical ventilation. Ventilatory stimulants may be useful in some cases of decreased ventilatory drives.[47]

Adequate oxygenation may well prevent the onset of heart failure, both acutely and over a long period of time. Any patient with cor pulmonale and right ventricular failure should be given O_2 if it is required to restore Pa_{O_2} to levels greater than 60 torr (8 kPa), but cautiously when Pa_{CO_2} is high and the threat of respiratory acidosis is present. When low-flow nasal O_2 causes significant increases in Pa_{CO_2}, mechanical ventilation may be required to relieve hypoxia. Studies[48] have also shown that home oxygen therapy, nocturnal or continuous, is beneficial in keeping patients with severe COPD functioning better for longer periods of time and may be effective both in treating cor pulmonale and in postponing its onset.

Treatment of Heart Failure

Cor pulmonale is heart disease, and, while treatment of the lung disease and relief of hypoxia are necessary to reduce cardiac work, general principles also apply. Digitalis, diuretics, and phlebotomy are appropriate measures for treatment of right ventricular failure.

Beneficial effects of digitalis are not as obvious with right ventricular failure as with left ventricular failure, and arrhythmias caused by digitalis may occur at relatively low serum levels in patients with hypoxia and acidosis. Susceptibility to digitalis intoxication is enhanced in pulmonary disease.[49] Its use in cor pulmonale, therefore, has been controversial. Nevertheless, studies[50] have shown that digitalis improves right ventricular function in cor pulmonale, and it is an appropriate drug for treatment of right ventricular failure when given cautiously and in carefully controlled dosage levels. It should not be used during the acute phases of respiratory insufficiency when there are large fluctuations in levels of hypoxemia and acidosis, but reserved for the time when hypoxemia is stabilized. Heart rate cannot be used as a guide to the dosage level required for digitalization. It is also reasonable to question whether patients with cor pulmonale who continue to have overt right ventricular failure, after relief of hypoxemia and intensive therapy for the underlying lung disease, will benefit from the use of digitalis.

Vasodilator therapy to reduce right ventricular afterload has been recognized as a potential treatment strategy for years. Vasodilator therapy has the disadvantage of being secondary therapy, not aimed at the primary lung dysfunction. Evidence exists that it may well be beneficial in some cases.[51]

Diuretics are effective in the treatment of right ventricular failure, and indications for their use are the same as in other forms of heart disease. Pulmonary function is improved by diuretics in patients with COPD who have hypervolemia.[52] The effects of diuretics should be carefully monitored by measurement of Pa_{O_2}, Pa_{CO_2}, and pH, since acid-base abnormalities are often present in cor pulmonale. Contraction alkalosis can be a problem in hypercarbic patients with a large buffer base who have had vigorous diuresis.

Phlebotomy, when the hematocrit is more than 55 to 60 percent, may reduce pulmonary artery pressure and pulmonary vascular resistance and, possibly, improve right ventricular function.[53] The phlebotomy should be done cautiously, taking only small volumes (200 to 300 ml).

Natural History and Prognosis

Prognosis depends on control of pulmonary hypertension, but prognoses for cor pulmonale and the underlying lung disease are not necessarily the same. Patients with COPD have hypoxic pulmonary hypertension which is, to a great extent, reversible, and right ventricular failure can be improved with appropriate therapy. Even with repeated episodes of right ventricular failure, some patients have long survival times.[25,54] The pink puffers live longer than the blue bloaters.[25]

With anatomic restriction of the vascular bed, pulmonary artery pressure may at first be elevated only during exercise but, after further restriction, hypertension becomes sustained at rest and intensified during exercise. Once right ventricular failure occurs, prognosis is poor, but even though right ventricular failure occurs most often in the terminal phase of illness, there are reports of 7- to 8-year survival rates after the diagnosis of cor pulmonale.[55]

In patients with alveolar hypoventilation but no alteration in lung structure, the natural history is one of progressive worsening of pulmonary hypertension due to sustained hypoxemia, hypercapnia, and, eventually, cor pulmonale and right ventricular failure. If alveolar ventilation is improved prior to the development of nonreversible changes in vessel walls, prognosis is good.

Even with modern techniques for diagnosis and management, prognosis for the underlying disease has not been greatly improved. The prognosis for cor pulmonale, however, is much better because of newer techniques for early recognition of the problem, better understanding of the role of hypoxia, and the early application in many patients of measures to prevent or relieve pulmonary hypertension.

References

1. Harvey, W.: "Exercitatio de Motu Cordis et Sanguinis in Animalibus," Francofurti Guilielem Fitzeri, 1628, C. D. Leake (trans.), Charles C Thomas, Springfield, Ill., 1928.
2. Fishman, A. P.: State of the Art: Chronic Cor Pulmonale, *Am. Rev. Resp. Dis.,* 14:755, 1976.
3. Richards, D. W.: The Right Heart and the Lung with Some Observations on Teleology (The J. Burns Amberson Lecture), *Am. Rev. Resp. Dis.,* 94:691, 1966.
4. Osler, W.: "The Principles and Practice of Medicine," D. Appleton & Company, Inc., New York, 1892, p. 632.
5. McGinn, S., and White, P. D.: Acute Cor Pulmonale Resulting from Pulmonary Embolism, Its Clinical Recognition, *JAMA,* 104:1473, 1935.
6. Gazes, P. C.: "Clinical Cardiology: A Bedside Approach," Year Book Medical Publishers, Inc., Chicago, 1975, p. 171.
7. Bohr, D. F.: The Pulmonary Hypoxic Response: State of the Field, *Chest,* 71:244, 1977.
8. Burrows, B.: Arterial Oxygenation and Pulmonary Hemodynamics in Patients with Chronic Airways Obstruction, *Am. Rev. Resp. Dis.,* 110(suppl.):64, 1974.
9. Enson, Y., Giuntini, C., Lewis, M. L., Morris, T. Q., Ferrer,

M. I., and Harvey, R. M.: The Influence of Hydrogen Ion Concentration and Hypoxia on the Pulmonary Circulation, *J. Clin. Invest.*, 43:1146, 1964.
10. Boysen, P. G., Block, A. J., Wynne, J. W., Hunt, L. A., and Flick, M. R.: Nocturnal Pulmonary Hypertension in Patients with Chronic Obstructive Pulmonary Disease, *Chest*, 76:536, 1979.
11. Bergofsky, E. N.: Respiratory Failure in Disorders of the Thoracic Cage, *Am. Rev. Resp. Dis.*, 119:643, 1979.
12. Enson, Y., Thomas, H. M. III, Bosken, C. H., et al.: Pulmonary Hypertension in Interstitial Lung Disease: Relation of Vascular Resistance to Abnormal Lung Structure, *Trans. Assoc. Am. Phys.*, 88:248, 1975.
13. Fried, R., Meyrick, B., Rabinovetch, M., and Reid, L.: Polycythemia and the Acute Hypoxic Response in Awake Rats Following Chronic Hypoxia, *J. Appl. Physiol.*, 55(4):1167, 1983.
14. Enson, Y.: Pulmonary Heart Disease: Relation of Pulmonary Hypertension to Abnormal Lung Structure and Function, *Bull. N.Y. Acad. Med.*, 53:551, 1977.
15. Morkin, F.: Activation of Synthetic Processes in Cardiac Hypertrophy, *Circ. Res.*, 35(suppl. 2):37, 1974.
16. Fishman, A. P.: The Left Ventricle in "Chronic Bronchitis and Emphysema," *N. Engl. J. Med.*, 285:402, 1971.
17. Murphy, M. L., Adamson, J., and Hutcheson, F.: Left Ventricular Hypertrophy in Patients with Chronic Bronchitis and Emphysema, *Ann. Intern. Med.*, 81:307, 1974.
18. Matthay, R. A., and Berger, H. O.: Cardiovascular Function in Cor Pulmonale, in "Clinics in Chest Medicine," W. B. Saunders Company, Philadelphia, 4(2):269, 1983.
19. Buda, A.J., Pinsky, M. R., Ingels, N. B., Daughters, G. T., Stinson, E. B., and Alderman, E. L.: Effect of Intrathoracic Pressure on Left Ventricular Performance, *N. Engl. J. Med.*, 301:453, 1979.
20. Bermis, C. E., Sehur, J. R., Borkenhagen, D., Sonnenblick, E. H., and Vrachel, C. W.: Influence of Right Ventricular Filling Pressure on Left Ventricular Pressure and Dimension, *Circ. Res.*, 34:498, 1974.
21. Steele, P. S., Ellis, J. H., VanDyke, D., Sutton, F., Creagh, E., and Davies, H.: Left Ventricular Ejection Fraction in Severe Chronic Obstructive Airways Disease, *Am. J. Med.*, 59:21, 1975.
22. Berns, A. S., and Schrier, R. S.: The Kidney in Heart Failure, in W. N. Suki and G. Eknoyan (eds.), "The Kidney in Systemic Disease," John Wiley & Sons, Inc., New York, 1981, p. 569.
23. Harvey, R. M., Ferrer, M. I., Richards, D. W., and Cournand, A.: Influence of Chronic Pulmonary Disease on the Heart and Circulation, *Am. J. Med.*, 10:719, 1951.
24. Farber, M. D., Roberts, L. R., Weinberger, M. H., Robertson, G. L., Fineberg, M. S., and Manfredi, F.: Abnormalities of Sodium and H_2O Handling in Chronic Obstructive Lung Disease, *Arch. Intern. Med.*, 142:1326, 1982.
25. Filley, G. F., Beckwitt, H. J., Reeves, J. T., and Mitchell, R. S.: Chronic Obstructive Bronchopulmonary Disease: II. Oxygen Transport in Two Clinical Types, *Am. J. Med.*, 44:26, 1968.
26. Mountain, R., Zwillich, C., and Weil, J.: Hypoventilation in Obstructive Lung Disease, *N. Engl. J. Med.*, 298:521, 1978.
27. Thurlbeck, W. M., Henderson, J. A., Fraser, R. G., and Bates, D. V.: Chronic Obstructive Lung Disease: A Comparison between Clinical, Roentgenologic, Functional and Morphological Criteria in Chronic Bronchitis, Emphysema, Asthma and Bronchiectasis, *Medicine*, 48:81, 1970.
28. Winterbauer, R. H., Hammer, S. P., Hallman, K. O., et al.: Diffuse Interstitial Pneumonitis, Clinicopathological Correlations in 20 Patients Treated with Prednisone/Azathioprine, *Am. J. Med.*, 65:661, 1978.
29. Crystal, R. G., Bitterman, P. B., Rennard, S. I., Nance, A. J., and Keogh, B. A.: Interstitial Lung Diseases of Unknown Cause (2 parts), *N. Engl. J. Med.*, 310:54 and 310:235, 1984.
30. Burwell, C. S., Robin, E. D., Whaley, R. D., and Bickleman, A. G.: Extreme Obesity Associated with Alveolar Hypoventilation—A Pickwickian Syndrome, *Am. J. Med.*, 21:811, 1956.
31. Sackner, M. A., Landa, J., Forrest, T., and Gruneltch, D.: Periodic Sleep Apnea: Chronic Sleep Deprivation Related to Intermittent Upper Airway Obstruction and Central Nervous System Disturbance, *Chest*, 67:164, 1975.
32. Guilleminault, C., and Dement, W. C.: "Sleep Apnea Syndromes," Allen R. Liss, Inc., New York, 1978.
33. Gerry, J. L., Buckley, B. H., and Hutchins, G. M.: Clinicopathologic Analysis of Cardiac Dysfunction in 52 Patients with Sickle Cell Anemia, *Am. J. Cardiol.*, 42:211, 1978.
34. Wagenvoort, C. A.: Pulmonary Veno-Occlusive Disease, Entity or Syndrome? *Chest*, 69:82, 1976.
35. Fritts, W. H.: Systemic Circulatory Adjustments in Hepatic Disease, *Med. Clin. North Am.*, 47:563, 1963.
36. Segel, N., Kay, J. M., Bayley, T. J., and Paton, A.: Pulmonary Hypertension with Hepatic Cirrhosis, *Br. Heart J.*, 30:575, 1968.
37. Perez, D., and Kramer, N.: Pulmonary Hypertension in Systemic Lupus Erythematosis: Report of Four Cases and Review of the Literature, *Semin. Arthritis Rheum.*, 11:177, 1981.
38. Moore, C. B., Kraus, W. L., and Dork, D. S.: The Relationship Between Pulmonary Arterial Pressure and Roentgenographic Appearance in Mitral Stenosis, *Am. Heart J.*, 58:576, 1959.
39. Chang, C. H.: The Normal Roentgenographic Measurement of the Right Descending Pulmonary Artery in 1,085 Cases, *Am. J. Roentgenol.*, 87:929, 1962.
40. Matthay, R. A., Schwarz, M. I., and Ellis, J. H.: Pulmonary Artery Hypertension in Chronic Obstructive Pulmonary Disease: Chest Radiographic Assessment, *Invest. Radiol.*, 16:95, 1981.
41. Padmavati, S., and Raizada, V.: Electrocardiogram in Chronic Cor Pulmonale, *Br. Heart J.*, 34:648, 1975.
42. Berger, H. J., Matthay, R. A., Loke, J., Marshall, R. C., Gottschalk, A., and Zaret, B.: Assessment of Cardiac Performance with Quantitative Radionuclide Angiocardiography: Right Ventricular Ejection Fraction with Reference to Findings in Chronic Obstructive Pulmonary Disease, *Am. J. Cardiol.*, 41:897, 1978.
43. Cohen, H. A., Baird, M. G., Rouleau, J. R., et al.: Thallium 201 Myocardial Imaging in Patients with Pulmonary Hypertension, *Circulation*, 54:790, 1976.
44. Bishop, J. M., and Cross, K. W.: Use of Other Physiological Variables to Predict Pulmonary Arterial Pressure in Patients with Chronic Respiratory Disease: Multi Center Study, *Eur. Heart J.*, 2:509, 1981.
45. Stark, R. D., Finnegan, P., and Bishop, J. M.: Longterm Domiciliary Oxygen in Chronic Bronchitis with Pulmonary Hypertension, *Br. Med. J.*, 3:467, 1973.
46. Schrijen, F., Uffholtz, H., Polu, J. M., and Poincelot, F.: Pulmonary and Systemic Hemodynamic Evolution in Chronic Bronchitis, *Am. Rev. Resp. Dis.*, 117:25, 1978.
47. Morgan, E. J., and Zwillich, C. W.: The Obesity-Hypoventilation Syndrome, *West. J. Med.*, 129:387, 1978.
48. Nocturnal Oxygen Therapy Trial Group: Continuous or Nocturnal Oxygen Therapy in Hypoxemic Chronic Obstructive Lung Disease: A Clinical Trial, *Ann. Intern. Med.*, 93:391, 1980.
49. Green, L. H., and Smith, T. W.: The Use of Digitalis in Patients with Pulmonary Disease, *Ann. Intern. Med.*, 87:459, 1977.
50. Smith, D. E., Bissett, J. K., Phillips, J. R., Doherty, J. E., and Murphy, M. L.: Improved Right Ventricular Systolic Time Intervals after Digitalis in Patients with Cor Pulmonale and Chronic Obstructive Pulmonary Disease, *Am. J. Cardiol.*, 41:1299, 1978.
51. Rubin, L. J.: Cardiovascular Effects of Vasodilator Therapy for Pulmonary Arterial Hypertension, in R. Matthay (ed.), "Cardiovascular-Pulmonary Interactions in Normal and Diseased Lungs," W. B. Saunders Company, Philadelphia, 1983, p. 309.
52. Gertz, I., Hedenstierna, G., and Wester, P. O.: Improvement

in Pulmonary Function with Diuretic Therapy in the Hypervolemic and Polycythemic Patient with Chronic Obstructive Pulmonary Disease, *Chest,* 75:146, 1979.
53. Weisse, A. B., Moschos, C. B., Frank, M. J., Levinson, G. E., Cannella, J. E., and Regen, T. J.: Hemodynamic Effects of Staged Hematocrit Reduction in Patients with Stable Cor Pulmonale and Severely Elevated Hematocrit Levels, *Am. J. Med.,* 58:92, 1975.
54. Weitzenblum, E., Loiseau, A., Hirth, C., Mirholm, R., and Rasaholinjanohary, J.: Course of Pulmonary Hemodynamics in Patients with Chronic Obstructive Pulmonary Disease, *Chest,* 75:656, 1979.
55. Ferrer, M. I.: Cor Pulmonale (Pulmonary Heart Disease): Present-Day Status, *Am. Heart J.,* 89:657, 1975.

Section F

Endocarditis

56

Infective and Noninfective Endocarditis

David T. Durack, M.B., D.Phil.

Definitions and Terminology

Infective endocarditis is the disease caused by microbial infection of the endothelial lining of the heart. Its characteristic lesion is a *vegetation,* which usually develops on a heart valve but occasionally appears elsewhere on the endocardium or on the lining of a large artery. This last case, more accurately termed *infective endarteritis,* produces a clinical syndrome closely resembling infective endocarditis. Among the many acronyms and abbreviations to be found in the literature, these few are convenient and useful enough to deserve perpetuation:

SBE: Subacute bacterial endocarditis
ABE: Acute bacterial endocarditis
NVE: Native valve endocarditis
PVE: Prosthetic valve endocarditis
NBTE: Nonbacterial thrombotic endocarditis

The terms *subacute* and *acute bacterial endocarditis* (SBE and ABE) remain in common use, and have descriptive value. SBE evolves over several weeks or months; it is usually caused by organisms of low virulence, such as viridans streptococci, which possess limited ability to infect other tissues.[1–4] In contrast, ABE evolves over days to weeks; the progress is hectic, complications develop earlier, and the diagnosis is usually made in less than 2 weeks.[4–7] ABE is most often caused by primary pathogens such as *Staphylococcus aureus* which are capable of causing invasive infection at other sites in the body.

Infection engrafted upon a heart valve that was either previously normal or damaged by congenital or acquired disease is termed *native valve endocarditis* (NVE). Infection of an artificial valve is termed *prosthetic valve endocarditis* (PVE). This is arbitrarily defined as *early* PVE when it occurs within the first 2 months after surgery, and as *late* PVE thereafter.[8–10]

The term *noninfective endocarditis* refers to sterile vegetations within the heart. Endocard*itis* is a partial misnomer in this context, because the lesions are thrombotic rather than inflammatory in nature. The central importance of thrombosis in this condition is emphasized appropriately by the term *nonbacterial thrombotic endocarditis* (NBTE), which is broadly defined here to describe any sterile vegetation. This includes a spectrum of lesions ranging from microscopic aggregates of platelets to the large vegetations of marantic endocarditis, which typically affects some patients with terminal malignancy.[11–13]

Infective endocarditis is designated best by naming the infecting organism, e.g., *Staph. aureus* endocarditis or *Aspergillus* PVE. This terminology is both specific and informative in that it allows useful inferences on natural history, prognosis, and treatment of the case in question.

Historical Note

Riviere, in 1646, Lancisi, in 1706, and Morgagni, in 1761, described patients who died with endocarditis in the seventeenth and eighteenth centuries.[14] Jean-Baptiste Bouillaud introduced the terms *endocardium* and *endocarditis* between 1824 and 1835. Virchow was familiar with the necropsy appearance of valvular vegetations by 1846, but the microbial etiology of infective endocarditis was not fully appreciated until Virchow, Winge, and Heiberg independently demonstrated bacteria in vegetations between 1869 and 1872.[14]

Sir William Osler studied the disease extensively.[15] He chose infective endocarditis as the subject for his Goulstonian lectures of 1885, in which he summarized the current state of knowledge as follows: "We may assume that the etiological, clinical, and anatomical characters of the disease have been fairly well ascertained, and that we have got about as far towards a full knowledge of the affection as the ordinary means at our disposal will permit. The inquiry now enters upon another stage, and it remains for experimental investigation to determine, if possible, the relation of the endocarditis to those diseases with which it is most frequently associated."[16]

Further major contributions to knowledge of natural history, pathogenesis, and pathology of the disease were made by Lenharz, Harbitz, and Schottmuller[14] in Germany, by Horder[17] in England, and by Blumer,[1] Thayer,[2] Allen,[18] Libman and Friedberg,[19] and Beeson[20] in the United States. In 1955, Kerr published a classic monograph summarizing the state of knowledge on subacute bacterial endocarditis to that date.[3]

The history of early attempts to treat endocarditis is closely linked to the story of penicillin. The first patient to receive parenteral penicillin was a young man with streptococcal endocarditis who was treated by Dawson in October, 1940, at Columbia University in New York.[21] Although the patient received far too little penicillin to effect a cure, his treatment antedated the first administration of penicillin to a patient by Florey's team in Oxford[22] by several months.[23] After initial failures, by 1944 it had been established that penicillin,[24] unlike sulfonamides,[25] could cure most cases of streptococcal endocarditis. Subsequently, Bloomfield,[26] Hunter,[27] Finland,[28] Geraci,[29] Weinstein,[30] and their colleagues contributed important early studies on antibiotic treatment of endocarditis.

Epidemiology

The Evolution of Endocarditis

Infective endocarditis today is a different disease from that seen in the preantibiotic era, when its salient clinical features were exhaustively described.[1–3] During the past 20 years, treatises on the "changing face" of "modern endocarditis"[31–39] have identified the following trends:

- The median age of patients has increased.
- The ratio of males to females has risen.
- The proportion of acute cases has risen.
- Fewer patients develop the classic physical signs of advanced SBE such as Osler's nodes, finger clubbing, or Roth's spots.
- The proportion of cases due to streptococci has fallen slightly.
- The proportion of cases caused by gram-negative bacilli, fungi, and miscellaneous unusual microbes has increased.

These striking changes in the clinical features and epidemiology of infective endocarditis cannot be explained by alterations in the virulence of the infecting microorganisms. Rather, they are due to changes in the susceptible population, to earlier treatment of patients with subacute disease before advanced manifestations develop, and to the impact of antibiotic therapy.[35,36]

The Susceptible Host

Changes in the population at risk are the most important factors responsible for evolution of the clinical spectrum of endocarditis.[36] The prevalence of rheumatic valvular disease, formerly the most common substrate for endocarditis, has steadily decreased in developed countries; meanwhile, the number of children with congenital heart disease surviving due to palliative or corrective surgery has increased. The proportion of elderly people in the population of developed countries has increased, and endocarditis in the elderly has become more common, even though degenerative valvular disease seems to present a relatively low risk for infection.[40] The median age of patients with endocarditis has risen steadily for three decades, from about 30 to about 50 years of age. At present, approximately one-fourth of all patients are over 60 years of age. Over the same period the proportion of males with endocarditis has increased. Male patients now outnumber females by approximately 2:1 overall, and by as much as 5:1 among patients over 60 years of age.[35–42]

Preexisting Heart Disease

Some patients develop endocarditis even though they have no known heart disease. This is most common in cases of ABE, especially in children less than 2 years of age[43–45] and in narcotic addicts.[46–49] Approximate figures for the frequency of the main predisposing factors in children, adults, and addicts are given in Table 56-1.

The relative propensity of various cardiac lesions to become infected can be estimated by noting their frequency in published series of cases of infective endocarditis, even though there is wide variation among individual studies. Cardiac abnormalities have been ranked according to the risk that they seem to carry for development of infective endocarditis in Table 56-2.

Mitral valve prolapse (MVP) occupies an interesting position in the spectrum of heart lesions that can predispose to endocarditis.[52–56] This common condition increases an individual's risk for infective endocarditis by five- to eightfold.[53,54] MVP is now known to underlie a significant proportion of cases of infective endocarditis.[53–56] In the past many such cases must have been wrongly attributed to mild rheumatic mitral valve damage. Although MVP is common, infective endocarditis is rare, so the risk that any individual with MVP will develop infective

TABLE 56-1 Approximate Frequency of the Major Preexisting Cardiac Lesions in Patients with Infective Endocarditis

	Children under 2 Years Old, %	Children 2–15 Years Old, %	Adults 15–50 Years Old, %	Adults > 50 Years Old, %	Adults Who Are IV Drug Abusers, %
No known heart disease	50–70	10–15	10–20	10	50–60
Congenital heart disease	30–50	70–80	20–30	10–20	10
Rheumatic heart disease	Rare	10–20	30–40	20–30	10
Degenerative heart disease	0	0	Rare	10–20	Rare
Previous cardiac surgery	5	10–15	10–20	10–20	10–20
Previous endocarditis	Rare	5	5	5–10	10–20

Source: Adapted from Refs. 33–51.

TABLE 56-2 Estimates of the Relative Risk for Infective Endocarditis Posed by Various Cardiac Lesions

Relatively High Risk	Intermediate Risk	Very Low or Negligible Risk
Prosthetic heart valves	Mitral valve prolapse	Atrial septal defects
Aortic valve disease	Pure mitral stenosis	Arteriosclerotic plaques
Mitral insufficiency	Tricuspid valve disease	Coronary artery disease
Patent ductus arteriosus	Pulmonary valve disease	Syphilitic aortitis
Ventricular septal defect	Previous infective endocarditis	Cardiac pacemakers
Coarctation of the aorta	Asymmetrical septal hypertrophy	Surgically corrected cardiac lesions (without prosthetic implants, more than 6 months after operation)
Marfan's syndrome	Calcific aortic sclerosis	
	Hyperalimentation or pressure-monitoring lines that reach the right atrium	
	Nonvalvular intracardiac prosthetic implants	

Source: Adapted from Refs. 33, 41, 50–57.

endocarditis during his or her lifetime remains low.[53,54]

Endocarditis in Parenteral Drug Abusers

Intravenous drug abusers are at high risk for infective endocarditis.[46–49] Bacteremias related to parenteral drug abuse are common, either from direct intravenous injection of bacteria or arising secondarily from local infections at injection sites (cellulitis, abscesses, or suppurative thrombophlebitis). Narcotic addicts seldom use sterile injection technique, sometimes even taking water from toilet bowls to dissolve their drugs. Nevertheless, the organisms that cause drug-related endocarditis are more often derived from the addict's normal surface flora than from the drug itself or its solvent.[58] Strains of *Staph. aureus* cause more cases of endocarditis among parenteral drug abusers than any other species (about 50 percent of all cases), but infections with gram-negative bacilli, especially *Pseudomonas* species[59,60] (15 percent) or fungi[61] (5 percent) are notably more common than in nonaddicts (Table 56-3). *Candida parapsilosis* and other *Candida* species are the most common fungi causing drug-related endocarditis, but occasional infections with a wide range of other fungal species have been recorded.[61] Polymicrobial and culture-negative infections each occur in about 5 percent of addicts with endocarditis.[46,47]

The disease in addicts frequently follows an acute course,[5,46–49] reflecting the high frequency of *Staph. aureus* infection. This partly explains the overall modest increase in the proportion of acute to subacute cases that has been observed over the past 25 years.[36]

The incidence of right-sided valvular infection is much higher among parenteral drug abusers (especially those infected by *Staph. aureus*) than among any other group of patients with endocarditis. In various series of patients, the tricuspid valve has been involved in 40 to 70 percent, and the aortic and/or mitral valve in 30 to 48 percent.[46–49] Tricuspid vegetations commonly embolize to the lungs, causing multiple small radiological opacities due to septic pulmonary infarcts. This is a highly characteristic finding in addicts with acute right-sided infection.[5,46–49] Nevertheless, it should be remembered that infection will be limited to the left side in about half of addicts with endocarditis.[47] More than one valve, on either side, may be infected simultaneously. Pulmonary valve infection is unusual even among narcotic addicts, occurring in only some 2 percent of cases.

Endocarditis after Cardiac Surgery

Cardiac surgery has created a new population of patients at high risk for infective endocarditis. The

TABLE 56-3 Frequency of Various Organisms Causing Infective Endocarditis*

	NVE, %	IV Drug Abusers, %	Early PVE, %	Late PVE, %
Streptococci	65	15	10	35
Viridans, alpha-hemolytic	35	5	<5	25
Strep. bovis (group D)	15	<5	<5	<5
Strep. fecalis (group D)	10	8	<5	<5
Other streptococci	<5	<5	<5	<5
Staphylococci	25	50	50	30
Coagulase-positive	23	50	20	10
Coagulase-negative	<5	<5	30	20
Gram-negative aerobic bacilli	<5	5	20	15
Fungi	<5	5	10	5
Miscellaneous bacteria	<5	5	5	5
Diphtheroids, propionibacteria	<1	<5	5	<5
Other anaerobes	<1	<1	<1	<1
Rickettsia	<1	<1	<1	<1
Chlamydia	<1	<1	<1	<1
Polymicrobial infection	<1	5	5	5
Culture-negative endocarditis	5–10	5	<5	<5

*These are representative figures collated from the literature; wide local variations in frequency are to be expected. *Source:* Adapted from Refs. 33, 35, 41, 46–51, 61–64. NVE = native valve endocarditis; PVE = prosthetic valve endocarditis.

number and variety of cases of postcardiotomy endocarditis has increased steadily since the 1950s, when surgeons first noted that *Staphylococcus epidermidis* endocarditis occurred fairly frequently after operations to split stenotic mitral valves.[65] It is probable that these organisms were sometimes inoculated directly onto the endocardium through minor rents in the surgeon's glove, made during palpation of rough, calcified valves. Subsequently, *Staph. epidermidis,* which rarely infects native valves, has become a leading cause of both early and late PVE (Table 56-3).[8–10,66,67] Contamination of blood circulating through the pump oxygenator with *Staph. epidermidis* can initiate infection at the time of operation, resulting in early PVE.[68] In late PVE, the source of bacteremia causing infection is usually unknown, but is presumed to be the normal flora of the skin or gastrointestinal tract.

Gram-negative bacilli and fungi also infect prosthetic valves much more frequently than native valves, especially in early postoperative cases.[67] The spectrum of organisms causing late PVE more nearly resembles that of subacute native valve infection (Table 56-3).

The incidence of postcardiotomy endocarditis has decreased over the past 20 years, due to improving techniques and possibly to use of prophylactic antibiotics, although this is unproven. Figure 56-1 shows the curve for incidence of PVE per month after valve replacement. The peak time of onset is about 5 weeks after operation; the patient's risk quickly falls to a much lower level thereafter.[10] This important curve emphasizes the fact that *Staph. epidermidis* and certain other organisms are often inoculated during or immediately after surgery, while streptococci infect the prosthesis during bacteremias that may occur at any time. Review of the literature indicates that in recent years a rate of about 1 percent for early PVE is representative, although this varies quite widely between hospitals.[8–10,67] Clearly, an incidence of early PVE that is *persistently* 3 percent or higher is unacceptable, and should lead to review of surgical and infection-control techniques in that unit.

Reported experience with late PVE has gradually increased,[8–10,69] reflecting longer follow-up of patients who escape early PVE but remain at higher risk for infective endocarditis each year thereafter than people with native valves. Late PVE occurs at a rate of about 1 percent per year.[67,70] Aortic valve prostheses are two to five times more likely to be infected than mitral prostheses (1 to 2 percent per year versus 0.4 percent).[9,57] Interestingly, these fig-

FIGURE 56-1 Incidence of prosthetic valve endocarditis (PVE) over 24 months after valve replacement. The hazard function has been stratified according to the infecting organisms. *(From T. S. A. Ivert, W. E. Dismukes, C. G. Cobbs, et al.: Prosthetic Valve Endocarditis, Circulation, 69:223, 1984. Reproduced by permission of the American Heart Association, Inc., and the author.)*

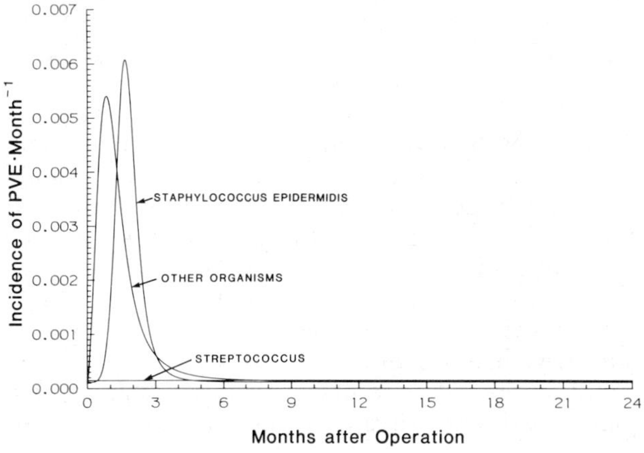

ures suggest that the annual risk for late infection of a mitral valve prosthesis may be no higher than that for chronic rheumatic disease affecting a native mitral valve.

Fortunately, coronary artery bypass grafting, which is the most common operation performed today in the United States, carries a negligible risk for infective endocarditis because the endocardium is not breached.

Endocarditis in Children

Infective endocarditis occurs at all ages, but is relatively uncommon during childhood and rare during infancy.[43–45,71] Reviews of clinical experience indicate that endocardial infection in infants and very young children most often develops in association with obvious infection elsewhere. Thus, infective endocarditis should be considered as a rare complication of septicemia caused by staphylococci or group B streptococci, or of pneumonia, other respiratory tract infections, osteomyelitis, and severe burns.[43,44] Endocarditis in these settings is likely to be caused by invasive pathogens, therefore following an acute course. In older children, subacute disease without an obvious portal of entry for the organisms is more common. *Haemophilus influenzae* type b endocarditis is very rare, even though this organism is the most common cause of bacteremia in children.

The leading underlying cardiac lesions are the tetralogy of Fallot and other forms of cyanotic congenital heart disease, aortic stenosis, patent ductus arteriosus, ventricular septal defect, pulmonary stenosis, and coarctation of the aorta.[43,44,51] In most series, preexisting rheumatic heart disease is much less common than congenital disease. No underlying cardiac disease is found in about 15 percent of children with endocarditis, but the proportion is much higher in those less than 2 years of age (Table 56-1). Atrial septal defects of the ostium secundum type very rarely become infected.

Diagnosis of infective endocarditis is more difficult in children, especially infants. The physician's attention is frequently focused on a serious primary bacteremic infection, so that endocarditis may be an unexpected finding at necropsy. The clinical manifestations of acute rheumatic fever may mimic endocarditis (and vice versa), but fortunately the two conditions rarely coexist. The choice of antibiotic treatment for children should be governed by the same principles as for adults, with appropriate dose adjustment for age. As in adults, valve replacement or other potentially curative surgical treatment should not be delayed "until the infection is eradicated" if the child has heart failure that does not respond well to medical therapy.

Endocarditis in Gynecologic and Obstetric Patients

When endocarditis occurs as a complication of pregnancy, it is most likely to develop at the time of delivery, or in the puerperium.[73] Normal delivery presents a low risk for endocarditis, even in the presence of preexisting valvular disease,[74] but bacteremias associated with perinatal infective complications such as endometritis, parametritis, septic thrombophlebitis in pelvic veins, or urinary tract infection can seed the endocardium.[73] Septic abortion or pelvic infection related to intrauterine contraceptive devices can also provide the portal of entry for bacteremia resulting in endocarditis.[75] The organisms most often involved are *Streptococcus fecalis,* group B streptococci, *Staph. aureus,* and occasionally *Bacteroides* or gram-negative enteric bacilli.

Nosocomial Endocarditis

Hospital-acquired infective endocarditis has become more common.[50,76] Pelletier and Petersdorf[50] found no less than 35 examples of probable nosocomial endocarditis among 125 cases (28 percent). This is not surprising, because intensive medical care can predispose to endocarditis in many ways. Iatrogenic endocardial damage can be produced by surgery, by intracardiac pressure-monitoring catheters, by ventriculoatrial shunts, and by hyperalimentation lines if they reach into the right atrium. Portals of entry for microorganisms are provided by wounds, biopsy sites, pacemakers, intravenous and arterial catheters, urinary catheters, and intratracheal airways. Nosocomial bacteremias arising from local infections are common in seriously ill patients, while infected solutions are sometimes accidentally infused intravenously.

All these factors may coexist in severely burned patients. Ehrie and his colleagues[77] found either NBTE or infective endocarditis at autopsy in all of six burned patients who sustained repeated episodes of bacteremia while a pressure-monitoring catheter was maintained in the right side of the heart. This important observation has been confirmed in another necropsy study of patients with flow-directed pulmonary artery catheters.[77a] Of 55 patients, 29 had one or more right-sided endocardial lesions, including 13 with thrombi and 4 with infective endocarditis.[77a] On the other hand, catheterization of the right side of the heart for brief periods in patients without bacteremia, as in a coronary care unit, presents a very low risk of causing infective endocarditis.

The leading organisms causing nosocomial endocarditis are staphylococci, *Candida* species, and gram-negative bacilli. *Staph. aureus* is especially associated with wound infections, cellulitis, and cannula infections; *Staph. epidermidis* with ventriculoatrial shunts; and *Candida albicans* with parenteral alimentation.

Nosocomial endocarditis can involve native or prosthetic valves. Prognosis for nosocomial native valve endocarditis is worse than for other forms of native valve infection. These patients usually have serious underlying diseases which may delay diagnosis of endocarditis by obscuring the symptoms and signs, while the organisms most commonly involved are more difficult to eradicate than streptococci.

Hemodialysis and Endocarditis
Creation of an arteriovenous shunt for hemodialysis predisposes to infective endocarditis in two ways: by providing a ready portal of entry for bacteremia, and by increasing cardiac output. Lillehei[78] showed that dogs with surgically created arteriovenous fistulas were predisposed to develop not only infective *endarteritis* at the site of the shunt, but *endocarditis* as well. Therefore, it is not surprising that endocarditis has been reported in 2 to 6 percent of patients on long-term hemodialysis via either arteriovenous fistulas or cannulas. In a review of 35 cases, *Staph. aureus* was the most common etiologic organism, followed by viridans streptococci and *Strep. fecalis.*[79] The diagnosis of endocarditis was difficult to make in this group of patients, partly because coexisting intravascular infection at the shunt site often confused the clinical picture. Mortality was high (53 percent). Early recognition and aggressive treatment of both shunt infections and endocarditis in dialysis patients are necessary to improve this figure.[79]

Infective Endarteritis
Intravascular infection outside the heart itself can mimic most of the clinical manifestations of endocarditis, including vascular and immunologic phenomena. In the past, about one-quarter of all patients with an uncorrected patent ductus arteriosus developed bacterial endarteritis.[3] Infections located at coarctations of the aorta, while well known, were less frequent; endocarditis of an associated bicuspid aortic valve was three times more common than endarteritis on the coarctation. Endarteritis occasionally complicates traumatic arteriovenous fistulas, but arteriosclerotic aneurysms rarely become infected. When bacterial endarteritis does occur within an aneurysm, the organisms usually grow in a multilayered thrombus in the lumen of the aneurysm rather than in vegetations.

The spectrum of organisms causing infective endarteritis is similar to that found in endocarditis except for a higher frequency of gram-negative bacillary infection (especially *Salmonella*) in arteriosclerotic aneurysms. The pattern of embolization observed will differ according to the site of infection; thus petechiae may occur on the skin of the lower extremities in a patient with an infected abdominal aneurysm, and infarctions occur in the lungs of a patient with an infected dialysis fistula in the forearm.

Because many of the congenital or acquired vascular lesions that predispose to endarteritis can be corrected by modern surgery, endarteritis is seldom seen today in developed countries, except in arteriovenous shunts constructed for hemodialysis (see "Nosocomial Endocarditis" above).

The Etiologic Organisms

The range of microbial species that can cause infective endocarditis is extraordinarily wide, yet only a few species account for the great majority of infections. On native valves, streptococci and staphylococci together cause more than 80 percent of infections.[33,41,50] Native valve infections caused by *Staph. epidermidis,* enteric bacilli, and fungi are uncommon. Among intravenous drug abusers and patients with prosthetic valves, however, the incidence of infection due to these organisms is much higher. Table 56-3 offers representative figures culled from the literature for the relative frequency of the major etiologic organisms on native valves, in drug addicts, and on prosthetic valves. It should be emphasized that local experience differs widely between medical centers.

Streptococci cause more cases of endocarditis than any other group of organisms.[41,50,51,80] Alpha-hemolytic or viridans streptococci account for the majority of these cases. The viridans streptococci are ubiquitous (although outnumbered by anaerobes) in the oropharyngeal and gastrointestinal flora. They are low-grade pathogens, often recovered from clinical specimens in mixed culture with other organisms, but seldom themselves causing disease. Their strong association with SBE is therefore determined by the frequency with which they enter the bloodstream and by their ability to adhere to endocardium, rather than by their virulence. In order of frequency, these species cause SBE most often: *Streptococcus sanguis, Streptococcus mutans, Streptococcus intermedius,* and *Streptococcus mitis.*[80–83] A few cases are caused by nutritionally dependent strains that require media supplemented with L-cysteine or pyridoxine for growth.[91–93] These strains are harder to isolate from blood[94] and harder to eradicate with antibiotic treatment than the other viridans streptococci.

Group D streptococci are next in frequency among the streptococci as the cause of endocarditis.[84–86] The nonenterococcal group D species, *Streptococcus bovis,* accounts for about one-fifth of streptococcal cases. Gastrointestinal lesions, especially cancers of the colon, are commonly present in patients who develop *Strep. bovis* bacteremia and/or endocarditis.[87–89] Hence, recovery of this species from blood cultures should prompt an early investigation for colonic disease, whether or not the patient has gastrointestinal symptoms. Strains of *Strep. fecalis* (enterococci) cause about 10 percent of streptococcal cases. It is said that this species causes endocarditis "in young women and old men," because it is found in association with infections of the genital and urinary tract in women of childbearing age, and of the urinary tract in men with prostatic enlargement.[85,87]

Streptococcus pneumoniae endocarditis has become uncommon since the advent of penicillin. This species causes acute endocarditis.[90] In debilitated alcoholics, coexisting pneumococcal pneumonia and pneumococcal meningitis may be present. This triad, known as Austrian's syndrome, carries an extremely poor prognosis.[90]

Many other species and strains of streptococci occasionally cause endocarditis, but they are rare compared with the viridans and group D organisms.

Staph. aureus is the leading cause of acute bacterial endocarditis. It is the predominant etiologic organism in narcotic addicts with endocarditis[38–40] and frequently causes PVE.[55] Because it is an invasive primary pathogen, patients with staphylococcal ABE often develop disseminated disease with metastatic infections in bone, joints, eye, or brain.[75,76]

Staph. epidermidis, which is an uncommon cause of NVE, gives rise to an indolent, subacute, or chronic infection on native valves.[77] In striking contrast, it is a common cause of PVE, which may follow either an acute or subacute clinical course.[53,55]

Although most of the species of gram-negative bacilli that colonize and/or infect humans have been reported to cause endocarditis in at least a few cases, they account for a very small proportion of cases of native valve endocarditis. For example, cases of endocarditis caused by *Escherichia coli* and *Klebsiella* are rare,[60] even though these two species are by far the most frequent cause of gram-negative bacteremias. The reasons for this striking disparity are probably multiple, including low adhesiveness of gram-negative enteric bacilli to heart valves[98,99] and fibrin.[100,101] Despite these factors, two special populations are at increased risk of gram-negative endocarditis: drug addicts and patients with prosthetic valves. Gram-negative bacilli account for 13 to 20 percent of endocarditis in intravenous drug abusers.[46–49] *Pseudomonas* species, *Serratia,* and *Enterobacter* species predominate. Gram-negative bacilli cause 20 to 30 percent of early PVE and 10 to 20 percent of late PVE.[66,67]

Interesting but unusual cases caused by species of *Salmonella, Brucella, Acinetobacter,* and other gram-negative bacilli have been reviewed by Cohen et al.[60] Endocarditis caused by anaerobic bacteria is rare (1 percent or less of cases,[63] perhaps because the oxygen tension in heart blood is too high to favor growth of these species on the endocardium.

Among the less common forms of infective endocarditis, a significant number of cases are caused by the "HACEK" group of organisms (*Haemophilus, Actinobacillus, Cardiobacterium, Eikenella,* and *Kingella*).[102,103] Cases caused by *Haemophilus* predominate in this group. Endocarditis caused by this genus is usually due to *Haemophilus aphrophilus, Haemophilus paraphrophilus,* or *Haemophilus parainfluenzae,*[102–104] and very rarely to *Haemophilus influenzae,* even though *Haemophilus influenzae* is more virulent and more frequently found in the blood than the other species.

Neisseria gonorrhoeae causes an acute form of the disease,[2] often involving the right side of the heart. Like the pneumococcus, *N. gonorrhoeae* has become uncommon as a cause of endocarditis since introduction of penicillin.[41,102]

Although many species of *fungi* can infect the endocardium, only two genera account for the great majority: *Candida* and *Aspergillus.*[61,105,106] *Candida* causes native valve infections in narcotic addicts and in patients receiving parenteral alimentation, while *Aspergillus* often involves prosthetic valves. Fungal infection of native valves in nonaddicts is rare (Table 56-3).

Culture-Negative Endocarditis

Culture-negative endocarditis is the term used when a patient has infective endocarditis but *blood* cultures are persistently negative.[107–109] In these cases, a working diagnosis based on clinical manifestations can sometimes be confirmed by the progress of the disease and response to empirical treatment. If blood cultures remain negative, an etiologic diagnosis can be made only by detecting organisms in an infected embolus, or in vegetations excised during surgery or at necropsy.

The reported incidence of culture-negative endocarditis varies widely. Among large unselected series of cases collected from several different hospitals, 15 to 20 percent of cases may be culture-negative.[41,107–109] Smaller series of patients studied by a single clinical and laboratory team that is highly experienced in evaluation of endocarditis usually show only 5 percent or fewer culture-negative cases.[76] This low figure carries an important clinical implication: *diagnoses other than endocarditis should be meticulously excluded before a diagnosis of culture-negative endocarditis is accepted.*

Negative blood cultures should be expected from about one-third of patients with *Candida* NVE or PVE,[61] and from most patients with *Aspergillus* endocarditis.[106] The incidence of negative blood cultures is slightly higher in SBE of long duration. Recent antibiotic therapy may transiently render blood cultures negative without achieving cure, but in most cases organisms will reappear in the blood within a few days of discontinuing antibiotics. The blood of a few patients with active bacterial endocarditis remains persistently culture-negative after receiving a short course of antibiotics.[50]

Rare causes of infective endocarditis with negative blood cultures include mycobacteria,[110] Q fever,[111–113] and chlamydia.[114,115] Q fever endocarditis is a chronic, febrile systemic illness with prominent hepatic as well as cardiac valvular involvement.[111–113] Chlamydial endocarditis is even more rare; a few cases have been reported in bird fanciers.[114,115] In such cases the etiologic diagnosis can only be established by specialized culture techniques, serology, or examination of vegetations using immunofluorescent antibodies.

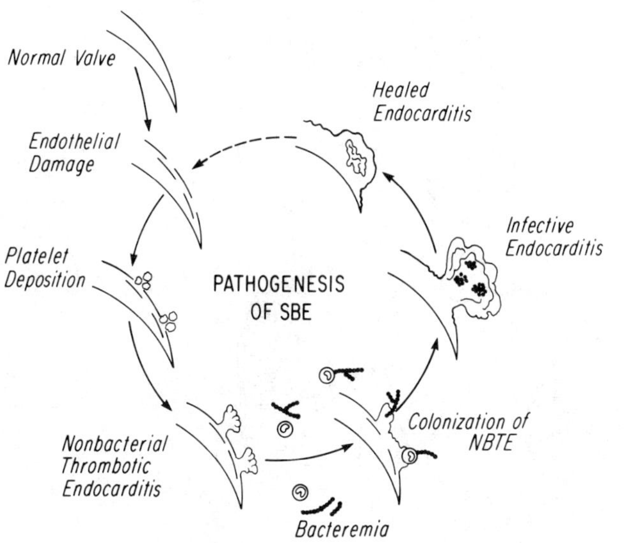

FIGURE 56-2 A diagram illustrating the main events in pathogenesis of subacute bacterial endocarditis (SBE).

The Influence of Antibiotics

Although the advent of antibiotics revolutionized treatment of endocarditis, the overall incidence of the disease has neither fallen nor risen strikingly during the antibiotic era. It is true that availability of rapidly effective treatments for pneumococcal pneumonia and gonorrhea was probably responsible for the striking decrease in incidence of endocarditis caused by *Strep. pneumoniae* and *N. gonorrhoeae* since 1944, and that the incidence of endocarditis caused by miscellaneous unusual antibiotic-resistant organisms has increased slightly during the antibiotic era.[35,41,42] Apart from these special cases, the widespread use of antimicrobial agents seems to have exerted considerably less influence than alterations in the populations at risk (described above) on the changing epidemiology of endocarditis.[36] Prophylactic use of antibiotics before medical procedures that cause bacteremia has not reduced the incidence of endocarditis significantly; this is not surprising because only a small proportion of all cases can be attributed to such procedures.[37,116]

Pathogenesis and Pathology

A general concept of the pathogenesis of NBTE and SBE is presented in Fig. 56-2.

Noninfective Endocarditis

Sterile thrombotic lesions (NBTE) may develop on heart valves in a wide variety of clinical conditions.[117] Small aggregates of platelets have been found occasionally on normal valves, but they occur frequently on the surfaces of valves damaged by congenital or rheumatic disease,[118] or by infective endocarditis. Marantic endocarditis occurs most often in patients with advanced malignancy,[11–13] but may also complicate other chronic wasting diseases or uremia. Sterile vegetations (termed *Libman-Sacks endocarditis,* see Chap. 73) sometimes develop in patients with systemic lupus erythematosus.

The common factor leading to platelet deposition is endothelial damage. This exposes subendothelial connective tissue containing collagen fibers, which in turn causes platelets to aggregate at the site. These microscopic platelet thrombi may embolize away harmlessly, or they may be stabilized by fibrin to form larger vegetations of NBTE. This process can be duplicated experimentally by passing a catheter into the heart of an animal; NBTE forms at sites of endothelial damage.[119] In humans, intracardiac pressure-monitoring catheters produce identical lesions.[77] Both experimental[120] and human[77a,117] NBTE can be colonized by circulating bacteria, resulting in infective endocarditis.

The vegetations of NBTE are friable white or tan masses, usually situated along the lines of valve closure. These vary greatly in size, being sometimes microscopic but frequently rather large and exuberant, with a corresponding tendency to cause extensive infarctions when they break off and are carried to the myocardium, spleen, kidney, brain, mesentery, or extremities. There is little inflammatory reaction at the site of attachment, so that fresh vegetations can often be picked off easily with forceps, leaving a valve surface that looks normal to the naked eye.[117] It is not surprising that such easily dislodged vegetations frequently embolize (Plate 7A).

Histologically, the vegetations of NBTE consist of degenerating platelets interwoven with strands of fibrin forming a bland, eosinophilic mass, featureless except for occasional trapped leukocytes.[117,119]

Infective Endocarditis

The essential event leading to development of infective endocarditis is attachment of microorganisms circulating in the bloodstream onto an endocardial surface. If the microbes persist and multiply there, infective endocarditis results. In the case of SBE, which usually develops on previously abnormal valves, the circulating bacteria probably colonize preexisting NBTE.[117] It is not known whether ABE, which often affects apparently normal valves, develops in like manner by colonization of microscopic sterile vegetations, or by direct invasion of normal endothelium. In the case of intravenous drug abuse, particulate matter injected intravenously may damage valvular endothelium and thus cause formation of minute platelet thrombi.

Once lodged upon NBTE, bacteria multiply rapidly, soon reaching high numbers and then entering

TABLE 56-4 Approximate Frequency of Anatomic Location of Vegetations in SBE, ABE, and Endocarditis Associated with IV Drug Abuse

	SBE, %	ABE, %	Endocarditis in IV Drug Abusers, %
Left-sided valves	85	65	40
Aortic	15–26	18–25	25–30
Mitral	38–45	30–35	15–20
Aortic and mitral	23–30	15–20	13–20
Right-sided valves	5	20	50
Tricuspid	1–5	15	45–55
Pulmonary	1	Rare	2
Tricuspid and pulmonary	Rare	Rare	3
Left- and right-sided sites	Rare	5–10	5–10
Other sites (patent ductus, VSD, coarctation, jet lesions)	10	5	5

Source: Adapted from Refs. 41, 46–51, 95, and 122.

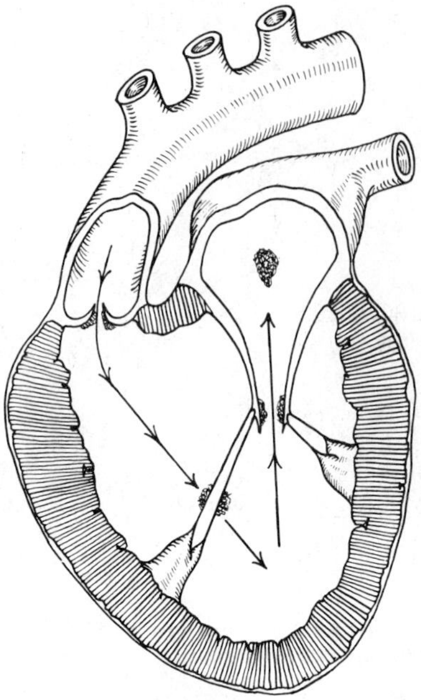

FIGURE 56-3 A diagram to illustrate the sites where endocarditis occurs in aortic and mitral insufficiency. The arrows at left indicate a high-velocity regurgitant stream passing through the orifice of an incompetent aortic valve into a low-pressure sink (left ventricle in diastole). Vegetations appear on the ventricular surface of the aortic valve. The regurgitant stream may cause a jet lesion on the chordae tendineae of the anterior leaflet of the mitral valve. Arrow at right shows regurgitation from the high-pressure source of the left ventricle during systole into the left atrium, with vegetations developing on the atrial surface of the mitral valve. Vegetations also can occur on the jet lesion where the regurgitant stream through the mitral valve strikes the atrial endocardium—MacCallum's patch. *(From S. Rodbard, Blood Velocity and Endocarditis, Circulation, 27:18, 1963. Reproduced by permission of the American Heart Association, Inc., and the author.)*

a resting phase.[120] The vegetation provides an ideal supporting stroma for bacteria colonies, into which essential nutrients can diffuse from the blood. The presence of bacteria is a powerful stimulus for further thrombosis, possibly mediated by thromboplastin generated by leukocytes when they are exposed to fibrin.[121] New layers of fibrin are deposited around growing bacteria, causing the vegetations to enlarge.[119]

Knowledge of the usual location of vegetations is important to both understanding and management of endocarditis. Approximate figures for the incidence with which vegetations are found at various sites are given in Table 56-4.

The frequency of involvement of each valve is directly proportional to the mean blood pressure upon it;[122] thus, the left side of the heart is involved much more often than the right. This rule is reliable for SBE, but does not hold true for acute endocarditis in drug abusers. In that group, tricuspid infection predominates, due to invasion of the valve by primary pathogens, especially *Staph. aureus* (Table 56-4).

Vegetations are usually located on the downstream side of anatomic abnormalities in the heart or great vessels. This observation is explained by the work of Rodbard, who developed the unifying concept that endocarditis usually occurs where blood flows from a high-pressure source (e.g., left ventricle) through a narrow orifice (e.g., stenotic aortic valve) into a low-pressure sink (e.g., aorta).[123] Illustrative examples from human disease include aortic stenosis, ventricular septal defect (VSD), coarctation, and mitral regurgitation. Experimentally, Rodbard showed that bacteria carried in an aerosol flowing through a constricted tube into an area of low pressure were deposited upon the walls of the tube immediately beyond the constriction, due to Venturi pressure effects and turbulence.[123] These observations fit well with the actual location of vegetations found at necropsy in cases of endocarditis (Fig. 56-3). Vegetations also may develop on *jet lesions,* which are areas of endothelial roughening and reactive fibrosis at sites where a swift, turbulent regurgitant stream of blood strikes the endothelium.[124] MacCallum's patch on the wall of the left atrium in some patients with mitral regurgitation is an example of a jet lesion; an infected vegetation occasionally develops at this site (Fig. 56-3).

The vegetations of infective endocarditis vary greatly in morphology, from small, warty nodules to large, cauliflower-like polypoid masses (Plate 7B). Their color also varies widely, from white to tan to greenish-gray.[125,126] In general, the vegetations found in ABE and in fungal endocarditis are larger than those of SBE. Histologically, colonies of microorganisms are found embedded in a fibrin-platelet matrix.[119,120,126] Although the inflammatory reaction at the site of attachment may be extensive, even progressing to form a frank abscess, the vegetations themselves characteristically contain relatively few leukocytes. Those few phagocytes present are prevented from reaching bacteria by layers of fibrin,

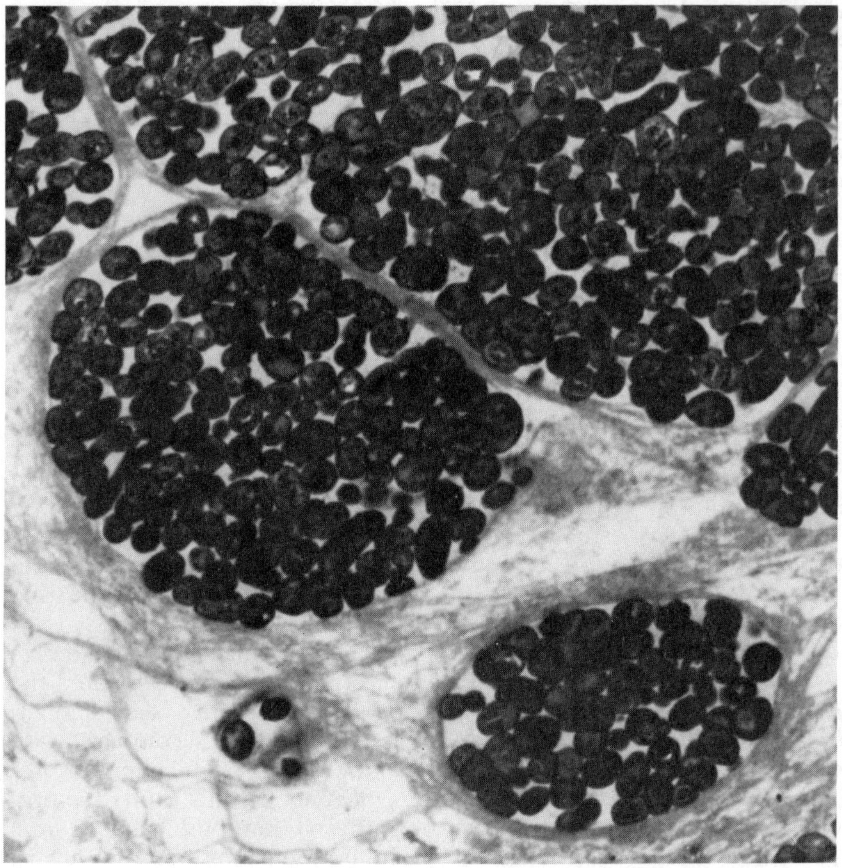

FIGURE 56-4 Electron micrograph of a vegetation of experimental streptococcal endocarditis (× 7800). Note the very large number of cocci, the protective layers of fibrin, and the absence of leukocytes—all factors that influence the results of therapy. *(From D. T. Durack, Experimental Bacterial Endocarditis: IV. Structure and Evolution of Very Early Lesions, J. Pathol., 115:81, 1975. Copyright 1975, John Wiley & Sons, Ltd. Reproduced with permission from John Wiley & Sons, Ltd. and author.)*

which form protective barriers around colonies (Fig. 56-4).

Formation of an abscess is one of the most important complications of valvular infection.[125,126] Abscesses often develop by direct extension of valvular infection into the fibrous cardiac skeleton, that is, the ring of supporting connective tissue around the valves. From here, abscesses can extend further into the adjacent myocardium. Hematogenous spread occasionally leads to development of abscesses elsewhere in the myocardium.

Abscesses develop more often during the course of ABE because this form of endocarditis is caused by primary pathogens capable of direct invasion of tissues. They are rare in SBE, unless a valvular prosthesis is present. Abscesses are found in the great majority of patients who die with active prosthetic valve infection, often spreading around the sewing ring of the prosthesis and causing partial dehiscence of the prosthetic valve.[126] Because these valve ring abscesses are located close to the conduction system, conduction disturbances and arrhythmias are common clinical manifestations.

The Role of Immunity in Endocarditis

Presence of bacteria in endocardial vegetations stimulates the humoral immune system to produce nonspecific antibodies. This can result in a polyclonal increase in gamma globulins, positive rheumatoid factor, and occasional false-positive serological tests for syphilis.[127] Rheumatoid factor develops in about half of patients with SBE, and can provide a useful diagnostic clue in culture-negative cases; it reverts to negative after eradication of the organisms.[128–130] Antiendocardial and antisarcolemmal antibodies have been detected in 60 to 100 percent of cases;[131] they are more commonly found in SBE than ABE.

Specific antibodies to many of the commensal organisms that cause SBE may be present in low titer before infection. Titers rise during active infection[3] and fall after treatment. Obviously, specific antibody prevents neither infection nor reinfection of the endocardium because reinfections with the same species have been reported. It has been claimed that preexisting humoral immunity actually *predisposes* to endocarditis,[3,132] and that "a high titer of agglutinating antibody for the infecting organism" is a prime factor in pathogenesis.[132] However, this hypothesis is based only upon theoretical considerations and uncontrolled observations in animals.[133,134] It is most unlikely that high titers of agglutinating antibody could exist for all the myriad organisms that may cause endocarditis, while controlled animal experiments suggest that high titers of specific antistreptococcal antibodies actually *protect* against streptococcal endocarditis.[135] Thus, the reality of the humoral *response* to endocardial infection is undisputed, but the evidence that preexisting antibody promotes development of endocarditis remains unconvincing.[136]

Hemolytic complement levels are low in about 30 percent of patients early in the course of endocarditis, rising later, and returning to normal after treatment.[137,138] The lowest levels are found in patients with immune complex glomerulonephritis.

Circulating immune complexes have been detected in 82 to 97 percent of patients with either ABE or SBE.[137–140] Higher concentrations correlated with presence of extracardiac manifestations such as arthritis, splenomegaly, and glomerulonephritis, with longer duration of illness, and with hypocomplementemia. Several studies confirm that glomerulonephritis in patients with endocarditis is mediated by immune complexes.[141–143] It seems likely that arthritis and tenosynovitis, and possibly pericarditis, Osler's nodes, and Roth spots,[137,139,140] also may represent inflammatory responses involving immune complexes, but this has not been proved.

Antibodies to teichoic acids were found in the serum of 14 of 15 patients with *Staph. aureus* endocarditis.[144] Because these antibodies were seldom found in patients who did not have staphylococcal endocarditis, their detection may be useful in diagnosis of occasional uncertain cases.[144,145] This test is unnecessary in diagnosis and management of most cases of endocarditis.

Healed Endocarditis

Even in active, untreated endocarditis, evidence of healing can be found.[126,136] Histiocytes slowly advance into the base of vegetations, while endothelium begins to cover the surface from the periphery. This attempt at healing fails in untreated cases, but progresses to completion during and after successful treatment. Macrophages ingest bacterial debris and fibrin, while fibroblasts organize the lesions by laying down collagen fibers. Endocardium gradually covers the surface of the shrinking vegetations. Calcium is often deposited at the site of old bacterial colonies. Dead, but still recognizable, gram-positive cocci can sometimes be found in sections of valves resected at operation or necropsy, months after infection has been eradicated by antibiotic treatment. The healed valve is often scarred, and thickened by new collagen; it may be perforated or ruptured, and the supporting structures may be damaged. Therefore, residual functional valvular abnormalities, varying from insignificant to severe, are common. Valvular function often continues to deteriorate at an unpredictable rate after infection is eradicated, due to mechanical stresses. Whether or not adequate hemodynamic function is preserved, the scarred valve surface remains susceptible to reinfection.

Experimental Endocarditis

Because the primary cardiac lesions are inaccessible to direct study in living patients, investigators long ago turned to animal models.[136,146] Bacterial infections of the endocardium in laboratory animals were successfully produced as early as the 1880s. Subsequent studies have contributed significantly to our understanding of the disease; for example, the crucial importance of endothelial damage in pathogenesis was established in animals before 1890, at a time when human investigations were limited to clinical case studies.[136]

Later studies in animals demonstrated that arteriovenous fistulas and other high-output states predispose to endocarditis,[78] confirmed the hypothesis (derived from human necropsy observations) that the lesion of NBTE is a receptive nidus upon which circulating bacteria readily lodge,[120] and allowed studies of the earliest stages of growth of vegetations.[119] Experiments showing that most bacteria in vegetations are in a metabolically inactive, resting phase helped to explain why antibiotic treatment must be continued longer than for other infections to cure endocarditis. Other experiments demonstrated the reduced propensity of gram-negative bacilli and anaerobes to colonize vegetations when compared with gram-positive cocci, the role of complement in protecting against *E. coli* endocarditis, and the protective effect of humoral immunity against oral streptococci. The immune response to endocardial infection, including demonstration of immune complexes in serum, healing, effect of anticoagulants, and the comparative efficacy of preventive and therapeutic antibiotics have all been examined in animals with endocarditis.[136,146,147]

For obvious reasons, most of these studies could not have been performed in human beings. Thus, an appreciation of the contribution of experimental studies is essential for a full understanding of this protean disease.

Clinical Manifestations

The clinical and laboratory manifestations of infective endocarditis can be conveniently grouped under three headings (Table 56-5):

- Evidence of a systemic infection
- Evidence of an intravascular lesion
- Evidence of an immunologic reaction to infection

History

The symptoms of subacute endocarditis develop insidiously and with great variability.[3,33,41,50,148] Fevers, chills, rigors, and night sweats provide evidence of systemic infection. General malaise with anorexia, fatigue, and weakness is typical. The patient often loses weight. Headaches and musculoskeletal complaints including myalgias, arthralgias,

TABLE 56-5 Summary of the Major Clinical Manifestations of Infective Endocarditis

	History	Examination	Investigations
Manifestations of systemic infection	Fever, chills, rigors, sweats, malaise, weakness, lethargy, delirium, headache, anorexia, weight loss, backache, arthralgia, myalgia Portal of entry: Oropharynx, skin Urinary tract Drug addiction Nosocomial bacteremia	Fever Pallor Weight loss Asthenia Splenomegaly	Anemia Leukocytosis (variable) Raised ESR Blood cultures positive Abnormal CSF
Manifestations of intravascular lesion	Dyspnea, chest pain, focal weakness, stroke, abdominal pain, cold and painful extremities	Murmurs Signs of cardiac failure Petechiae—skin, eye, mucosae Roth spots, Osler's nodes Janeway lesions Splinter hemorrhages Stroke Mycotic aneurysm Ischemia or infarction of viscera or extremities	Blood in urine Chest roentgenogram Echocardiography Arteriography Liver-spleen scan Lung scan, brain scan, CT scan Histology, culture of emboli
Manifestations of immunologic reactions	Arthralgia, myalgia, tenosynovitis	Arthritis Signs of uremia Vascular phenomena Finger clubbing	Proteinuria, hematuria, casts, uremia, acidosis Polyclonal increases in gamma globulins Rheumatoid factor, decreased complement, and immune complexes in serum Antistaphylococcal teichoic acid antibodies

Source: Adapted from Refs. 33, 41, 50, and 148.

and back pains are fairly common.[149] This symptom complex is often described by the patient or physician as "a flulike illness."

Evidence of an intravascular lesion is provided by symptoms of left- or right-sided heart failure and by manifestations of embolization such as focal neurological injury, chest pain, flank pain, left upper quadrant pain, hematuria, or ischemia of an extremity. Symptoms usually persist and worsen intermittently over 4 to 8 weeks before the diagnosis is made.[150]

In the acute form of infective endocarditis, the symptoms are both accelerated and accentuated in severity. Patients experience hectic fevers, rigors, and prostration, usually leading to admission to hospital within a few days.[5,95,96]

Symptoms of cardiac failure may develop or worsen suddenly in either acute or subacute disease, due to mechanical complications such as perforation of a valve leaflet, rupture of one of the chordae tendineae, or development of functional stenosis from obstruction of blood flow by large vegetations. Alternatively, heart failure may develop insidiously or preexisting chronic heart failure may worsen due to progressive damage to the valves or associated structures. Myocarditis, or myocardial infarction due to coronary artery embolism, may contribute to heart failure.

Physical Examination

General Appearance

Patients with endocarditis may appear acutely or chronically ill. Evidence of systemic infection is provided by chills, rigors, and sweating. Asthenia and recent weight loss often are notable. Anemia, mild or severe, is common in all forms of endocarditis, so that many patients are pallid. The skin of some with long-standing SBE will show the sallow hue of uremia.[3]

Vascular Phenomena

Patients with endocarditis may show a variety of striking physical findings arising from vascular abnormalities. If present, these are diagnostically useful, even though all have been found at times in conditions other than endocarditis. *Petechiae* are common in both SBE and ABE, and rare in NBTE. In a few cases the petechiae possess a pale central spot. Most are due to microembolization to small vessels in the skin or mucous membranes. Capillary fragility, evidenced by a positive tourniquet test, accounts for the petechiae in some cases, while patients with ABE caused by a virulent bacterial pathogen may develop petechiae due to disseminated intravascular coagulation.

Splinter Hemorrhages
Linear subungual hemorrhages, resembling tiny splinters of wood under the nail but not reaching the nail margin, are found in about 10 percent of patients with SBE. Because splinter hemorrhages are found in some 5 to 8 percent of patients admitted to hospital who do not have endocarditis, they are of limited diagnostic value.[151] They are probably caused by microembolization to linear capillaries under the nail.

Osler's Nodes
Osler's nodes occur in 10 to 20 percent of patients with SBE, and in less than 10 percent of patients with ABE.[152] They are painful, tender erythematous nodules in the skin of the extremities, most usually in the pulp of the fingers. Occasionally the center of these pea-sized, red lesions is pale, but necrosis does not occur. They are probably caused by inflammation around the site of lodgment of small, infected emboli in distal arterioles, because the etiologic organism can be recovered from the lesions, at least in acute cases.[153] Possibly some of these lesions are caused by inflammation at the site of an immunologic reaction, especially in subacute cases.[140]

Janeway Lesions
These are flat, nontender red spots, small in size (less than 5 mm) and irregular in outline, found on the palms and soles of a few patients with SBE and ABE. Unlike petechiae, they are not hemorrhagic and therefore will blanch on pressure.[3,34]

Eye Lesions
Conjunctival petechiae show up as small, bright-red hemorrhages that are easily seen if the upper and lower eyelids are everted. These are not specific for endocarditis, being found after cardiac surgery and occasionally in septicemia (Plate 7C). Nevertheless, discovery of conjunctival hemorrhages in a patient with fever and heart murmur makes the diagnosis of endocarditis highly likely.

Retinal hemorrhages are found in 10 to 25 percent of cases of both SBE and ABE. They are quite variable in appearance. Some simply represent petechiae in the retina; their round or flame-shaped outline is determined by the layer of the retina in which they develop. Those with a white or yellow center surrounded by a bright-red, irregular halo are known as Roth spots (Plate 6C).[3,4,34] They probably represent cytoid bodies and associated hemorrhage caused by microinfarction of retinal vessels.

Loss of vision during the course of endocarditis can occur from embolization to the brain or to the retinal artery, from optic neuritis, or from ophthalmitis. *Endophthalmitis* may occur in patients with *Candida* endocarditis and fungemia. The typical retinal lesions are rounded, white, cotton-like exudates with extension into the vitreous and overlying vitreous haze.[154] *Panophthalmitis* occurs in some patients with ABE due to hematogenous spread of virulent pathogens. This occurs most often in narcotic addicts infected with *Staph. aureus, Pseudomonas,* and fungi.

Clubbing of the Fingers
Previously common in SBE, finger clubbing is now found in less than 10 percent of cases. The pathogenesis of this reaction, which usually resolves after eradication of the infecting organism, is not understood.

Embolization
Decreased or absent arterial pulses in an extremity may signal occlusion of a large artery by a fragment of vegetation. Focal neurological signs may develop transiently or progress to a completed stroke due to embolization of a cerebral artery (see "Complications" below). Infarctions of the spleen, kidney, or bowel can present with pain and tenderness on palpation of the abdomen, mimicking an acute abdominal event such as bowel obstruction or peritonitis. Myocardial infarction due to obstruction of a coronary artery can cause heart failure or death, and is sometimes an unexpected finding at necropsy in patients who die with active disease. These complications are illustrated in Plates 7D to H.

Splenomegaly
Development of moderate splenomegaly is still common, occurring in about one-third of patients with ABE and one-half of those with SBE. The spleen is usually soft and only slightly tender except in the case of recent embolic infarction, when palpation may be very painful. Radionuclide scanning may reveal infarction, or occasionally a splenic abscess.

Cardiac Examination
The pulse is often rapid due to fever or congestive failure. Irregularities of rhythm may indicate presence of an abscess near the conducting system. Underlying or newly developed aortic incompetence associated with infective endocarditis may result in a collapsing pulse. Peripheral arteries should be palpated for evidence of occlusion by emboli or for the pulsatile swelling of a mycotic aneurysm.

One or more *murmurs* are present in virtually all patients at some stage of the disease. Even though some of the classic findings of infective endocarditis are less often seen today than formerly, the classic triad of *fever, anemia, murmur* should still suggest this disease, providing one remembers that these manifestations are nonspecific. They may be absent initially. Up to 15 percent of patients do not have a murmur when first seen. These are more likely to be patients with right-sided or acute endocarditis than patients with left-sided SBE. The murmurs most often found in association with endocarditis are those of mitral and aortic regurgitation. Pure mitral stenosis is complicated by SBE much less often than mitral incompetence with or without associated stenosis. Development of a new aortic insufficiency murmur during a febrile illness strongly suggests the diagnosis of endocarditis, because this finding is seldom associated nonspecifically with increased blood flow due to fever and anemia.

"Changing murmurs" are not a common finding in SBE, despite a persistent misconception to the contrary. This error is partly based upon misreading of Osler's words in which he pointed out that murmurs usually do *not* change much during SBE: "a very slight change in the character of the heart murmur in spite of the . . . most extensive vegetations and alterations in the valve."[155] It is true that appearance of *new* murmurs is not rare in SBE. New murmurs and changing murmurs may be found in patients with ABE.

Complications

Heart Failure

Heart failure is the single most important complication of infective endocarditis.[41,50,156] No other factor exerts such a critical influence on prognosis. Cates and Christie[157] in 1950 reported a death rate of 37 percent among 314 patients with SBE who had no heart failure, and 85 percent in 94 who had moderate or severe failure. In a more recent series,[156] congestive failure occurred in 55 percent, but was much more common in patients with aortic valve disease (75 percent) than with mitral (50 percent) or tricuspid disease (19 percent).

Sudden onset or worsening of left ventricular failure is common during the course of ABE due to perforation or destruction of a valve leaflet or rupture of chordae tendineae, but also occurs in some patients with SBE for the same reasons. Occasionally, bulky vegetations occlude the valve orifice causing functional stenosis; this is most likely to occur in fungal infection of prosthetic valves.

Embolization

This complication is recognized in 12 to 35 percent of patients with SBE and 50 to 60 percent with ABE, but necropsy findings indicate that many arterial emboli go undetected. Pelletier and Petersdorf[50] reported a 50 percent incidence of major arterial emboli in 125 cases, affecting brain (25 cases), lung (17), coronary artery (8), spleen (8), extremities (8), gut (4), and eye (3).

Neurological Manifestations

Involvement of the nervous system during the course of endocarditis is both common and clinically important.[158–160] Jones[158] found neurological abnormalities in 110 of 385 patients (29 percent); Ziment[159] reviewed 21 studies and concluded that the nervous system was involved in 40 to 50 percent of patients with endocarditis. A wide range of syndromes occurs, including toxic confusional states, psychiatric symptoms, minor or major strokes (Plate 71), meningoencephalitis, and cranial or peripheral nerve lesions. It is important to know that the presenting complaint involves the nervous system in 10 to 15 percent of patients with endocarditis.

Of 55 patients with cerebrovascular complications of endocarditis, four-fifths suffered infarction and one-fifth hemorrhage.[158] Infarction is usually due to embolism, most often to the middle cerebral arteries, while hemorrhage can be a complication of either emboli or mycotic aneurysms.[50,158–160]

A *meningeal reaction* occurs in 7 to 15 percent of patients, especially those with staphylococcal ABE.[33,158–160] This may be mistakenly diagnosed as due to acute bacterial meningitis because the cerebrospinal fluid (CSF) contains polymorphonuclear leukocytes and slightly raised protein concentration. However, the glucose is usually normal and CSF culture is usually negative; the other abnormalities will resolve during treatment of the underlying disease. True bacterial meningitis occurs in some patients with pneumococcal endocarditis[90] and occasionally in staphylococcal ABE.

Cerebritis may develop in brain tissue surrounding small infected emboli lodged in cerebral vessels in both SBE and ABE, often with associated meningoencephalitis. Computerized tomography often reveals multiple areas of cerebritis, especially in acute staphylococcal endocarditis. In patients with ABE this inflammatory reaction in the brain may progress to form a brain abscess, but more often cerebritis will resolve uneventfully during antibiotic treatment of the underlying disease. Brain abscesses are distinctly uncommon in patients with SBE.

Mycotic Aneurysm

This complication develops in only 3 to 15 percent of patients with infective endocarditis, but the local consequences of expansion and rupture can be very serious, especially in the brain (Plate 71). In order of frequency, the sites most often involved are the proximal aorta, including the sinuses of Valsalva (25 percent of cases), arteries to the viscera (24 percent), to the extremities (22 percent), and to the brain (15 percent).[161] Unfortunately, intracerebral aneurysms are often multiple.

Mycotic aneurysms develop when the wall of an artery is damaged by the inflammatory response to microbes.[136] These reach the arterial wall via microemboli to vasa vasorum, or by impaction of a larger infected embolus in the lumen. The arterial wall is apparently a poor culture medium for bacteria when compared with a valvular vegetation, because the organisms responsible for weakening the vessel often die out spontaneously, even if untreated. The mycotic aneurysm may continue to enlarge even when living organisms are no longer present, due to the physical effects of arterial blood pressure (Plate 71).

Differential Diagnosis

Because the clinical manifestations of endocarditis are numerous and often nonspecific, the differential diagnosis of this disease is very wide.[3,33,41,50,148] Of the many conditions that may be considered, only a few leading examples will be listed here.

ABE shares many clinical features with nonendocarditic septicemias due to *Staph. aureus, Neisseria,* pneumococci, and gram-negative bacilli. Pneumonia, meningitis, brain abscess, stroke, malaria, acute pericarditis, vasculitis, and disseminated intravascular coagulation may cause diagnostic confusion.

SBE must be considered in the workup of every patient with fever of unknown origin. Its manifestations can mimic those of rheumatic fever, osteomyelitis, tuberculosis, meningitis, intraabdominal infections, salmonellosis, brucellosis, glomerulonephritis, myocardial infarction, stroke, endocardial thrombi, atrial myxoma, connective tissue diseases, vasculitis, occult malignancy (especially lymphomas), chronic cardiac failure, pericarditis, and even psychoneurosis.

Investigations

Routine Laboratory Tests

Anemia is usual in SBE and fairly common in ABE. This is most often of the hypoproliferative type, with a normochromic, normocytic smear, but may be hemolytic in ABE. Chronic low-grade hemolysis due to a prosthetic valve may confuse the blood picture.

Leukocytosis is an unreliable manifestation of SBE. A low-grade, variable elevation of the leukocyte count with some immature forms is characteristic, but in many cases the leukocyte count is normal. A high granulocyte count with an increase in band forms is commonly found in patients with ABE. These neutrophils may show toxic granulation, and in a few cases of ABE staphylococci can be identified inside them on examination of a Gram-stained smear of the buffy coat of the peripheral blood.[162] Abnormal histiocytes may be found in smears of peripheral blood in one-third of patients with SBE.[163]

The erythrocyte sedimentation rate is almost always elevated. A fall of greater than 50 mm/h is common in SBE, while the rate of fall is variable in ABE.

Urinalysis shows microscopic hematuria and/or slight proteinuria in about 50 percent of cases, even in the absence of specific renal complications.[3,41,148] Red blood cell casts and heavy proteinuria are found in those patients who develop immune complex glomerulonephritis, often in association with decreased total serum complement.[141] Gross hematuria suggests that renal infarction has occurred. A positive test for rheumatoid factor is found in 40 to 50 percent of cases of SBE,[128–130] but rarely in ABE. A polyclonal increase in gamma globulins is characteristic. Occasional false-positive serological tests for syphilis occur.[127]

Blood Cultures

Isolation of an organism from the blood is the most important step in diagnosis of endocarditis. Blood cultures should be drawn from *all patients with fever and heart murmur,* unless their illness is clearly due to another disease or the fever resolves within a few days without treatment. Cultures should also be taken from susceptible patients with other nonspecific symptoms or signs consistent with endocarditis, to help rule out that diagnosis.

Beeson, Brannon, and Warren showed that bacteremia in SBE is usually continuous.[20] The number of organisms per milliliter of blood varies widely, but is usually between 1 and 100 organisms per milliliter in subacute cases. Therefore, most blood samples will be positive, and it is usually not necessary to take a large number of cultures.[93,164] Pelletier and Petersdorf[50] found that *all* blood cultures taken were positive in 68 percent of 125 patients. Similarly, Werner noted that the etiologic organism was recovered from cultures taken on the first day of admission in 93 percent of patients with culture-positive endocarditis.[165]

Katsu found that arterial cultures were positive slightly more often than venous cultures (72 percent versus 64 percent of 313 cases), and reported 40 cases in which arterial but not venous cultures were positive.[166] Although this difference was significant, it seems too small to justify obtaining arterial cultures in every case. The following practical approach is suggested: for SBE, draw three separate venous blood cultures on the first day. If these cultures show no growth by the second day, draw two more venous cultures. If all are negative on the third day *but the diagnosis of endocarditis still seems likely,* draw two more venous cultures and one arterial blood culture. If the patient had received prior antibiotic therapy, three more venous samples may be taken over the following week, looking for a late recrudescence of bacteremia after partial treatment. For ABE, draw three venous blood cultures and begin empirical antibiotic therapy, because treatment should not be delayed until culture results are available in acute endocarditis.

Because *Staph. epidermidis*[62] and diphtheroids[167] can cause endocarditis, special care must be taken during venipuncture to avoid contamination of the specimen with these common skin organisms, which would result in diagnostic confusion. For each cul-

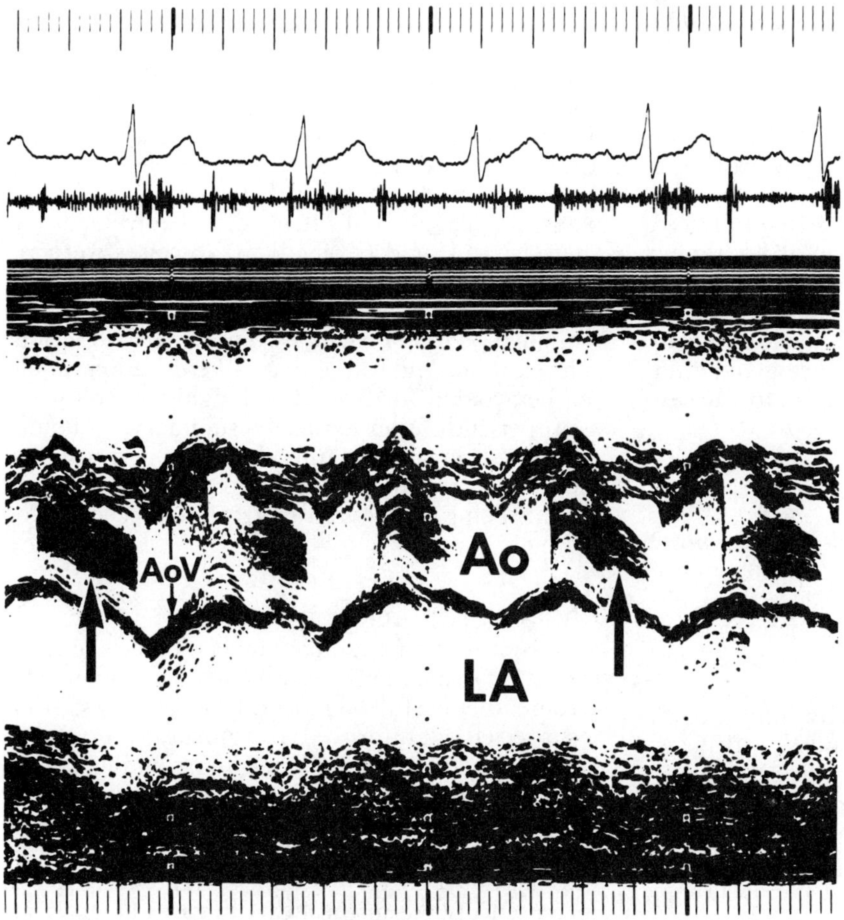

FIGURE 56-5 The echocardiogram shows dense, fuzzy echoes on the diastolic portion of the aortic valve (arrows) that are virtually diagnostic of valvular vegetations. Ao = aortic; AoV = aortic valve; LA = left atrium. *(Courtesy of Dr. Joel Felner.)*

ture, 10 to 20 ml of blood should be drawn and divided equally between one unvented anaerobic bottle of medium and one vented bottle. Media should be adequately supplemented to allow growth of fastidious, nutritionally variant bacteria.[91–93] Cultures should be incubated for at least 3 weeks, and Gram stains made at intervals even if no growth is apparent on inspection. Pour plates can help to distinguish contaminants from true positive cultures.

Electrocardiography

Electrocardiography should be performed upon admission to hospital and repeated at intervals according to progress during treatment. This may reveal evidence of otherwise silent myocardial infarction due to embolization of a vegetation to a coronary artery. A disturbance of conduction that develops during the course of endocarditis suggests extension of infection into the myocardium. This may be due to focal myocarditis or to an abscess located close to the conduction system.[69]

Echocardiography

The detection of valvular vegetations or abnormal echoes consistent with vegetations by echocardiography can be vitally important in diagnosis of endocarditis, but enthusiasm for this technique must be tempered by knowledge of its limitations (Fig. 56-5).[168,169] *A negative study does not rule out endocarditis.* The sensitivity of M-mode echocardiography for detection of vegetations in proven cases of endocarditis is 40 to 50 percent, while two-dimensional sector scanning is somewhat more sensitive.[168] Vegetations less than 3 to 4 mm in size cannot be detected, and all the leaflets of the tricuspid, pulmonary, and aortic valves cannot be visualized in every case. Thus, false-negative echocardiograms are common with either technique, particularly when the tricuspid valve is infected. For example, Andy and colleagues found echocardiographic indications of endocarditis in all of three patients with aortic valve infections, and in only 12 of 20 with tricuspid infection.[170] Echocardiography is more likely to detect the larger vegetations typical of acute infection in narcotic addicts and of fungal endocarditis than the smaller lesions often found in SBE. Vegetations on prosthetic valves are difficult to demonstrate. Complications of endocarditis such as rupture of a valve leaflet, chordal rupture, aortic root abscess, or myocardial abscess can be demonstrated in some cases.

The specificity of echocardiography is limited by occasional false-positive readings for "vegetations" that do not exist. These are particularly common in patients with myxomatous degeneration of the mitral valve.[169]

Sequential echocardiograms performed during treatment can assist materially in making decisions on the necessity and timing for surgery by providing objective assessments of cardiac function. For example, premature mitral valve closure due to raised end-diastolic pressure is a useful echocardiographic sign indicating severe aortic regurgitation, usually requiring valve replacement.[171] However, sequential echocardiographic studies intended to document disappearance of vegetations during and after treatment are not reliable as the criterion for success or failure of antibiotic therapy.[172]

Roentgenography

The most important contribution of the chest x-ray in assessment of endocarditis is to provide evidence of early congestive heart failure, because this complication carries such important implications for both prognosis and management (see "Complications" above).

Presence of multiple small patchy infiltrates in the lungs of an intravenous drug abuser with fever strongly suggests the diagnosis of septic emboli arising from right-sided infective endocarditis.[46–49] Valvular calcification may identify a previously abnormal valve, thus aiding the localization of presumed intravascular infection. Widening of the aorta may be caused by a mycotic aneurysm.

Fluoroscopy can demonstrate abnormal motion of a prosthetic valve, indicating presence of a vegetation or partial dehiscence of the valve from the aortic root. This information often helps to decide whether valve replacement is needed during management of PVE.

Computerized axial tomography can be helpful in defining the cause of focal neurological lesions in patients with endocarditis, especially infarction, hemorrhage from a mycotic aneurysm, or brain abscess. Angiography may be necessary to demonstrate mycotic aneurysms in the brain or elsewhere.

Cardiac Catheterization and Cineangiography

This investigation is usually not necessary for patients who respond well to antimicrobial therapy without developing cardiac failure. When treatment seems to be failing and/or operation is considered, cardiac catheterization and cineangiography can provide vital information. Anatomic abnormalities such as valvular lesions, congenital defects, coronary artery disease, or asymmetrical septal hypertrophy, coarctation of the aorta, or mycotic aneurysm can be defined. Occasionally, a previously unsuspected diagnosis such as presence of a sinus of Valsalva aneurysm will be made. Physiological measurements including cardiac output, pressures on the left and right sides of the heart, and the degree of aortic regurgitation may help to decide whether valve replacement is indicated, and influence the timing of operation. Welton and colleagues reviewed 35 patients who underwent cardiac catheterization during active endocarditis.[173] The clinical assessment was materially modified by catheterization in 23 patients, the diagnosis of site of valve involvement was altered in 14, and 6 valve ring abscesses were revealed. Surgery was postponed or cancelled in 6 patients when catheterization revealed only mild hemodynamic abnormalities. There were no serious complications, indicating that catheterization should not be avoided for fear of dislodging emboli when a proper indication exists. In summary, catheterization and cineangiography should be performed in most patients with infective endocarditis when operation is being considered or treatment seems to be failing.

Radionuclide Imaging

Liver-spleen imaging may reveal defects due to splenic infarction, thus confirming embolization. This is sometimes useful diagnostically when endocarditis is suspected but unproved. In animals, experimental vegetations have been located by scanning for radiolabeled platelets deposited from the bloodstream onto a growing endocardial lesion.[174] The potential value of this test for diagnosis of human endocarditis has not yet been proved. Ga^{67} scans have shown increased uptake in the heart in cases of endocarditis, but this technique is presently of little value because of the high incidence of false positives.[175]

Natural History and Prognosis

Infective endocarditis is one of the very few infectious diseases that is almost universally fatal if untreated. Spontaneous recovery did occur occasionally in the preantibiotic era,[3] but most cases reported to have "recovered" probably had illnesses other than infective endocarditis. The interval between onset of symptoms and death in patients with untreated subacute disease varied widely, with a median time to death of about 6 months.[3] Almost all patients with acute infective endocarditis died in less than 4 weeks.

Heart failure is by far the most adverse prognostic factor.[156,157] Others include renal failure, culture-negative disease, gram-negative or fungal infection, prosthetic valve infection, and development of abscesses in the valve ring or myocardium. Favorable prognostic factors include youth, early diagnosis and treatment, and penicillin-sensitive streptococcal infection. Prognosis is good for many young drug addicts with *Staph. aureus* infection of the tricuspid valve.[5,176]

Eradication of the etiologic organisms ("microbiological cure") can be achieved in a high proportion of all patients with bacterial endocarditis. How-

TABLE 56-6 An Estimate of Bacteriologic Cure Rates for Various Forms of Endocarditis*

Native Valve Endocarditis	Antimicrobial Therapy Alone		Antimicrobial Therapy Plus Surgery	
Viridans streptococci, group A streptococci, *Strep. bovis,* pneumococci, gonococci	98		98	
Strep. fecalis	90		90	
Staph. aureus (in young drug addicts)	90		>90	
Staph. aureus (in elderly patients with chronic underlying diseases)	50		70	
Gram-negative aerobic bacilli†	40		65	
Fungi	<5		50	
Prosthetic Valve Endocarditis	**Early PVE**	**Late PVE**	**Early PVE**	**Late PVE**
Viridans streptococci, group A streptococci, *Strep. bovis,* pneumococci, gonococci	‡	80	‡	90
Strep. fecalis	‡	60	‡	75
Staph. aureus	25	40	50	60
Staph. epidermidis	20	40	60	70
Gram-negative aerobic bacilli†	<10	20	40	50
Fungi	<1	<1	30	40

*Morbidity and mortality will be significantly greater than these figures for *bacteriologic* cure indicate.
†Excluding *Haemophilus* species.
‡Insufficient data to estimate rate.
Source: Adapted from Refs. 10, 29, 30, 35, 50, 51, 69, 178, 179, 192–195.

ever, both early and long-term mortality rates remain significant because of preexisting disease and damage already caused before infection is eradicated. Survival curves after admission with infective endocarditis show a significant number of late deaths despite "cure."[10,178] Analysis of experience over the past 20 years allows a reasonably accurate formulation of the prognosis for microbiologic cure among the various subgroups of patients with infective endocarditis. Approximate figures are listed in Table 56-6.

Recurrent Endocarditis

Recurrent endocarditis is a general term that includes both *relapses* and *reinfections.* The frequency of relapse after treatment for each of the different forms of infective endocarditis can be predicted from published experience (Table 56-6). Because occasional relapses occur even after an optimal treatment regimen has been used, follow-up clinical evaluation including blood cultures should be meticulously performed during the first 2 months after treatment. Most relapses occur within a few weeks of ending treatment, but living organisms can persist in seemingly healed vegetations for many months, and may cause occasional late relapse.

The term *reinfection* refers to a new episode of endocarditis occurring after cure of a previous episode.[178] Usually a different etiologic organism is involved, but if it appears identical to the previous organism, one cannot be certain whether an episode of recurrent endocarditis represents a true reinfection or a relapse.

Patients remain permanently at risk of reinfection after cure of infective endocarditis because of residual valve scarring (Fig. 56-1). Second episodes are fairly common, being recorded in from 2 to 31 percent of cases.[3,35,178] This wide variation in reported incidence is partly due to variable duration of follow-up. Intravenous drug abusers and patients with severe periodontitis are at highest risk for reinfection. Occasional patients have suffered three or more separate episodes of infective endocarditis.[178] Patients who have previously had native-valve endocarditis are at higher risk for prosthetic valve infection (often with a different organism) for reasons that are not yet understood.[10]

Treatment of Infective Endocarditis

General Principles

The principal aims of management are to eradicate the infecting organism as soon as possible, to operate with correct timing if surgical intervention should be required, and to treat complications. Because infective endocarditis carries significant risk of death even when well managed, it is important that treatment be continued long enough to ensure that relapse will not occur. On the other hand, patients with the most favorable forms of endocarditis should not be subjected to unnecessarily long and expensive treatment in hospital. This can happen when physicians exercise excessive caution based on outdated rules of thumb such as "all cases of endocarditis should be treated for at least 6 weeks." In fact, some patients with endocarditis require treatment for much longer than 6 weeks, while many can be cured in only 2 weeks.

Antimicrobial Therapy

Microbiological Tests

To choose and regulate antibiotic therapy correctly, certain basic microbiologic information on the infecting organism is required.[93] For group A streptococcal and pneumococcal endocarditis, nothing more than positive identification of the organism is necessary because these organisms are still sensitive to low concentrations of penicillin, with very rare exceptions. For other species of streptococci, for staphylococci, and for most other bacteria, both the minimal inhibitory concentration (MIC) and minimal bactericidal concentration (MBC) of relevant antibiotics should be determined. Some of these organisms will be resistant to intermediate or high concentrations of penicillin,[179,180] while others may be tolerant, that is, inhibited but not killed by antibiotic levels achievable in serum.[181,182]

The serum bactericidal titer (SBT or Schlichter test) is frequently used to monitor treatment of endocarditis.[30,64,93] In this test, the infecting organism is exposed in vitro to the patient's serum, which is drawn while the patient is receiving antibiotic treatment, to determine the maximal dilution of serum that will inhibit and kill the organism. Based upon empirical clinical experience, it is often said that the SBT should be 1:8 or higher at intervals during each day of treatment. However, the interpretation and clinical relevance of this test remain controversial.[183] Proof that the patient's serum is actually capable of killing the infecting organism reassures the clinician, but for streptococcal and staphylococcal endocarditis this can usually be achieved without difficulty, and SBTs are often very high (e.g., 1:128 to 1:1024). Therefore, SBTs need not be measured repeatedly during management of most patients with endocarditis. Measurement of the SBT is most likely to be clinically helpful when treating unusual organisms, when using unusual antibiotics, when using unusual regimens (such as oral treatment), or when treatment appears to be failing.

Intermittent dosage regimens that result in widely fluctuating SBTs are traditionally employed for treatment of endocarditis and are usually effective. Whether maintenance of continuous high SBTs would offer any therapeutic benefit over intermittent dosing regimens is not known; perhaps continuous infusion of antibiotic would be desirable for treatment of gram-negative organisms, which regrow more rapidly than gram-positive organisms when antibiotic levels fall below the minimal inhibitory concentration.

Choice of Antibiotic

Bactericidal antibiotics should be chosen for treatment of endocarditis whenever possible.[30,64] Although cases have occasionally been cured with bacteriostatic drugs such as tetracycline and chloramphenicol, results of treatment with these agents are usually poor.[184] This is because host defense mechanisms are inadequate in the vegetation. Relatively few phagocytes are present, and even these are hampered by protective layers of fibrin around the colonies of bacteria (Fig. 56-3). To effect cure, antibiotic therapy must eradicate organisms completely, without the help of phagocytes to eliminate the subpopulation of microbes that are relatively resistant to antibiotics because they are in the resting phase. In this important respect infective endocarditis differs strikingly from bacterial pneumonia, where phagocytes are plentiful and bacteriostatic antibiotics are usually effective. Nevertheless, it may occasionally be necessary when treating unusual organisms to use a bacteriostatic antibiotic in combination with other drugs to achieve optimal antibacterial effect. When treatment with unusual combinations of antibiotics is needed, in vitro laboratory tests should be performed to find out whether synergism, indifference, or antagonism exists between them.

For the common forms of bacterial endocarditis caused by gram-positive organisms, published experience is so extensive that specific therapeutic regimens can be recommended with confidence.[176,185] Standard regimens for streptococcal and staphylococcal endocarditis are listed in Table 56-7.

Staph. epidermidis PVE is difficult to eradicate with antibiotics alone.[97] These staphylococci are frequently resistant to semisynthetic penicillins and other antibiotics. A regimen combining vancomycin, rifampin, and an aminoglycoside chosen according to sensitivity tests is most likely to succeed, but results are unpredictable. The organism may develop resistance to rifampin during treatment.

Treatment for endocarditis due to less common organisms must be chosen on the basis of more limited published experience,[60,103,186] together with the results of tests performed upon the infecting organism in the microbiology laboratory. Treatment often must be individualized. In general, one of the betalactam antibiotics should be included in the regimen whenever possible. Combinations of two or more antibiotics are often employed. The list of potentially useful regimens for these rarer forms of infective endocarditis is too long to detail here.

Empirical Therapy

When the etiologic organism is not known, the choice of empirical therapy should depend upon whether the patient has acute or subacute disease. ABE requires broad-spectrum therapy that will cover *Staph. aureus* as well as many species of streptococci and gram-negative bacilli. SBE requires a regimen that will treat most streptococci including *Strep. fecalis.*

TABLE 56-7 Treatment Regimens for Infective Endocarditis Caused by Gram-Positive Cocci

Organism	Regimen	Duration, weeks	Comments
Alphahemolytic (viridans) streptococci; *Strep. bovis*	1. Penicillin G 2 million units IV every 6 h *plus* streptomycin 7.5 mg/kg every 12 h IM,* *or*	2	Standard regimen, for patients less than 65 years old without renal failure, eighth-nerve defects, or serious complications
	2. Penicillin G 4 million units IV every 6 h *plus* streptomycin 7.5 mg/kg every 12 h IM (for first 2 weeks only)* *or*	4	For patients with complicated disease, e.g., CNS involvement, shock, moderately penicillin-resistant streptococci, failed previous treatment
	3. Penicillin G 4 million units every 6 h IV, *or*	4	For patients more than 65 years old, with renal failure or eighth-nerve defects
	4. Cefazolin 2 g IV every 8 h, *or*	4	For patients allergic to penicillins
	5. Vancomycin 15 mg/kg IV every 12 h	4	For patients allergic to penicillins and cephalosporins
Group A streptococci, *Strep. pneumoniae*	1. Penicillin G 2 million units IV every 6 h, *or*	2–4	These organisms are usually highly sensitive to penicillin; 2 weeks should be adequate for many patients
	2. Cefazolin 1 g IV every 8 h	2–4	
Strep. fecalis (streptomycin sensitive) and other penicillin-resistant streptococci	1. Penicillin G 3 million units IV q 4 h *plus* streptomycin 7.5 mg/kg q 12 h IM* *or*	4–6	4 weeks should be adequate for most cases with symptoms present for less than 3 months
	2. Vancomycin 15 mg/kg IV every 12 h *plus* gentamicin 1.0 mg/kg IV every 12 h	4–6	For patients allergic to penicillin; 4 weeks should be adequate for most cases
Strep. fecalis (streptomycin-resistant) and other penicillin-resistant streptococci	1. Ampicillin 2 g IV every 4 h *plus* gentamicin 1.0 mg/kg IV every 8 h, *or*	4–6	4 weeks should be adequate for most cases with symptoms present for less than 3 months
	2. Vancomycin 15 mg/kg IV every 12 h IV *plus* gentamicin 1.0 mg/kg IV every 12 h	4–6	For patients allergic to penicillin; 4 weeks should be adequate for most cases
Staph. aureus	1. Nafcillin 2 g IV every 4 h, *or*	4 or longer	Standard regimen
	2. Nafcillin as above, *plus* gentamicin 1.5 mg/kg IV every 8 h for the first 3–5 days only, *or*	4 or longer	For patients with severe disseminated staphylococcal disease, synergy may be advantageous during early stages of treatment
	3. Cefazolin 2 g IV every 8 hr, *or*	4 or longer	For patients allergic to penicillins
	4. Vancomycin 15 mg/kg IV every 12 h	4 or longer	For patients allergic to penicillins and cephalosporins; for methicillin resistant strains

*Gentamicin 1.0 mg/kg intravenously every 12 h for 2 weeks may be substituted for streptomycin, if desired, to avoid intramuscular injections. The dose of streptomycin should not exceed 500 mg per dose in any regimen employing streptomycin.

Source: Adapted with slight modification from D.T. Durack: Infectious Endocarditis, in J.B. Wyngaarden and L.H. Smith (eds.), "Cecil Textbook of Medicine," 17th ed., W. B. Saunders Company, Philadelphia, 1985, p. 1540. Reproduced with permission from the publisher and author.

To meet these requirements, the following suggestions are offered:

For ABE: Nafcillin 2.0 g IV every 4 h
plus
ampicillin 2.0 g IV every 4 h
plus
gentamicin 1.5 mg/kg IV every 8 h

For SBE: Ampicillin 2.0 g IV every 4 h
plus
gentamicin 1.5 mg/kg IV every 8 h

Treatment should be adjusted if and when the etiologic organism is identified. In those few cases where empirical therapy is administered as a therapeutic trial to help confirm a diagnosis, treatment should be continued without interruption or unnecessary changes for at least 2 weeks; otherwise no useful diagnostic information will be gained.

Duration of Therapy

Extensive experience with treatment of the common forms of endocarditis provides sufficient grounds for recommendations on adequate duration of therapy (Table 56-7). An exception to this is *Staph. aureus* endocarditis. The natural history of this disease is highly variable; some patients recover swiftly without complications,[5] but others remain febrile for several weeks, often with extracardiac manifestations of disseminated staphylococcal disease such as osteomyelitis. While 4 weeks of therapy will be adequate for most cases, this must not be regarded as a rigid rule because some patients require treatment for 6 weeks, 8 weeks, or even longer to achieve cure. For *Strep. fecalis* endocarditis, 4 weeks' treatment will usually be adequate. However, the relapse rate seems to be higher in patients with mitral valve infection and in those who have had symptoms for more than 3 months.[86] These patients should be treated for 6 weeks.

In general, the less extensive the published experience with a particular infective agent, the more one should lean toward prolonging treatment in order to provide a reasonable margin of safety. Guidelines for duration of treatment for gram-positive organisms are listed in Table 56-7, but not for other organisms, because the duration required for these varies greatly according to individual circumstances in each patient.

Anticoagulant Therapy and Endocarditis

Can anticoagulant therapy be started or continued safely during treatment of endocarditis? This is a common and vexing question. Even though the infected vegetation is essentially a thrombotic lesion, there is no evidence that anticoagulation has any useful therapeutic effect in endocarditis. On the contrary, early experience showed that simultaneous treatment with penicillin plus heparin carried a higher risk of fatal intracerebral hemorrhage from mycotic aneurysm or infarction than treatment with penicillin alone.[189] For this reason anticoagulation was considered to be strongly contraindicated in patients with endocarditis, until more recent experience showed that warfarin could be given safely during treatment of patients with prosthetic valve infections.[190,191] Presently available information suggests the following simple guidelines for patients with infective endocarditis:

- Avoid use of heparin entirely (except for immediate treatment of massive pulmonary embolism).
- Discontinue or avoid anticoagulation if possible.
- Anticoagulate with warfarin if there is a clear-cut indication, taking extra care not to allow the prothrombin time to rise above 1.5 times normal values.
- Choose an antibiotic treatment regimen that does not require intramuscular injections, if anticoagulation is instituted.

Role of Surgery

Optimal management requires operative intervention during treatment of certain patients with endocarditis.[72,192,195] This most often involves replacement of a valve to reverse cardiac failure due to newly developed or worsening valvular lesions. Because prosthetic valve infection is more difficult to eradicate with antibiotics than native valve infection, replacement of an infected prosthesis is often necessary for cure. Repeated major emboli constitute a relative indication for valve replacement (see "Management of Complications" below). Occasionally, a patient remains "septic" despite antibiotic therapy; operation may then be required to control infection itself, rather than its hemodynamic consequences. Operation to close a patent ductus arteriosus or septal defect, to excise a coarctation of the aorta, or to relieve asymmetrical septal hypertrophy may be required as part of treatment of endocarditis engrafted upon these lesions. Other indications for surgery will be considered under "Management of Complications" below.

Correct timing is the essence of good surgical management of endocarditis.[72,190,194] If operation is undertaken too soon, the risks of operative death and the early and late morbidity associated with valve replacement may be inflicted upon the patient unnecessarily, because some patients will respond to medical therapy so well that operation can be postponed indefinitely. If operation can be delayed safely, antibiotic therapy should eradicate or at least greatly reduce the population of organisms of the valve, thus increasing the chance that an artificial valve can be inserted if necessary without itself becoming infected. If time is available for effective treatment of complications such as septicemia, renal failure, pneumonia, myocarditis, and conduction defects before operation, ventricular function will improve and operative risk will be correspondingly lower. On the other hand, if surgery is too long delayed, patients may die suddenly, or their hemodynamic status may deteriorate so seriously that operation is no longer feasible. This is a tragic error because many such patients could have been saved by earlier operation.[192–196] Thus, both the decision to operate and the timing of operation are of critical importance.

Careful, frequent reexamination of the patient, together with echocardiography and sometimes cardiac catheterization to confirm the clinical findings, is indicated in every case where operation may be needed. The decision to operate should be influenced also by knowledge of the natural history of the type of endocarditis being treated. For example, penicillin-sensitive streptococcal endocarditis can almost always be cured bacteriologically (Table 56-6), and the immediate prognosis is good providing cardiac failure does not supervene. Thus, operation should usually be considered only for those patients with cardiac failure that does not respond well to medical treatment. Similarly, youthful narcotic addicts with acute staphylococcal endocarditis have a good prognosis,[5,176] so operation usually should be reserved for those who develop serious heart failure. At the other end of the spectrum, the likelihood that fungal prosthetic valve endocarditis can be eradicated with antifungal drugs alone is negligible, even in the absence of heart failure (Table 56-6). Such patients usually should undergo valve replacement early, without waiting to test the remote possibility that antifungal treatment could eradicate the infection. Other examples of patients who are highly likely to require operation are those with gram-negative infection of prosthetic valves and patients with valve ring abscesses. Aortic valve involvement, staphylococcal infection in a non-drug addict, and gram-negative or fungal etiology should be regarded as other relative indications favoring early valve replacement.[69,72,195]

Because of the possible need for surgery during the course of any case of endocarditis, it is desirable that patients be managed in consultation with a thoracic surgical unit. Such consultation should be obtained early, so that an operation can be performed without delay if it becomes necessary during the course of treatment. Sudden onset of aortic or mitral valvular incompetence with consequent acute left ventricular failure can occur without warning, even in the most favorable forms of endocarditis.

Management of Complications

Heart Failure

Development of moderate or severe cardiac failure due to structural valvular damage indicates the need for immediate surgery in most patients with endocarditis, even if the intracardiac infection is still active.[69,72,193–196] In patients with milder heart failure the decision should be individualized, always remembering that lives may be lost unnecessarily if cardiac function suddenly worsens to the extent that operation is either very hazardous or no longer possible.

Emboli

Occurrence of one or more significant arterial emboli during treatment of endocarditis is a relative indication for surgery. However, the predictable early and long-term mortality and morbidity rates of valve replacement must be weighed against the fact that the likelihood of further emboli is highly unpredictable. For this reason, embolization is much less satisfactory as an indication for valve replacement than is cardiac failure.[196] In the author's opinion, operative intervention during antibiotic treatment should seldom be undertaken solely "to prevent further emboli," unless the patient has suffered more than one or two proven major emboli.

Renal Failure

Patients who died with SBE before 1955 frequently had developed chronic renal failure.[3] Subsequently, both the incidence of renal failure and its importance as a cause of death have greatly diminished. Earlier diagnosis and antibiotic treatment have forestalled the development of immune complex glomerulonephritis in many patients. In those few (about 5 percent) who still develop this complication of SBE, timely dialysis will maintain the patient until antibiotic treatment removes the bacterial antigen that triggered immune complex nephritis. Renal function usually normalizes smoothly once infection has been controlled, but recovery may take weeks or months. In a few cases creatinine clearance worsens for a time despite effective antibacterial treatment, perhaps reflecting persistence of bacterial antigen in vegetations after bacteriologic cure. Some patients with septicemia, shock, or disseminated intravascular coagulation associated with ABE develop acute renal failure and require dialysis as part of their intensive care.

Mycotic Aneurysm

This complication is diagnosed in only about 5 percent of patients with infective endocarditis, but the local consequences of expansion and rupture can be very serious, especially in the brain.

Small aneurysms sometimes will resolve spontaneously after antibiotic therapy. Once they grow larger than 1 or 2 cm in diameter, resolution is unlikely; the aneurysm will enlarge and eventually rupture despite eradication of the etiologic bacteria. Surgery is indicated for accessible aneurysms before this can occur.

Intracerebral aneurysms pose a much more difficult therapeutic dilemma because they are often multiple and relatively inaccessible. Large aneurysms or aneurysms that have bled intracranially should be clipped if possible. An individualized decision must be made on whether or not to operate on smaller aneurysms that have not leaked or ruptured.

The Problem of Prophylaxis

Because bacteremias occur during dental or other surgical procedures,[197–199] prophylactic antibiotics are frequently given to susceptible patients in an attempt to prevent bacterial endocarditis. Although prevention of such a serious infection is obviously desirable, many relevant questions remain unanswered. These include:

- Is antibiotic prophylaxis effective?
- What is the risk of developing bacterial endocarditis after an episode of bacteremia?
- Which operations and diagnostic procedures should be covered?
- Which patients should receive antibiotics?
- What antibiotic regimens will be most effective?

Although the risk of infection has not been quantitated, it is sufficiently low that most of these questions probably cannot be answered by clinical trials; the number of susceptible patients required to provide significant results would be far too large.[95,172]

Less than one in five cases of SBE and even fewer cases of ABE follow identifiable medical procedures that cause transient bacteremias;[37,197,198] therefore the proportion of cases that is potentially preventable by antibiotics is small. However, because endocarditis causes serious morbidity and mortality, prevention of even a few cases would be worthwhile.

For this reason, presently accepted standards of practice require that an antibiotic regimen be administered before certain dental and surgical procedures to patients with known heart lesions which pose a significant risk for endocarditis.

Several hundred cases of streptococcal endocarditis following dental and genitourinary tract procedures have been recorded, so that the causative role of these procedures may be regarded as fairly well established.[197,198] A rather short "incubation period" for endocarditis is typical, in that most of these patients noticed symptoms within 2 weeks of the procedure.[150] However, it should be emphasized that the link between a case of endocarditis and a recent procedure causing bacteremia cannot be proved, because asymptomatic, low-grade bacteremias occur very commonly related to everyday events such as chewing and cleaning the teeth.[197]

In the absence of specific information, empirical recommendations[200,201] for prophylaxis of bacterial endocarditis must be made on the basis of indirect information. This includes the reported frequency of bacteremia after various procedures (Table 56-8), the relative risk posed by the patient's cardiac lesion (Table 56-2), case reports of prophylaxis failures,[55] in vitro susceptibility studies on the relevant organisms, especially streptococci, and experimental studies in laboratory animals.[147]

For the individual patient, the decision to give prophylaxis should be made by assessing two main factors: the risk posed by the preexisting cardiac lesion and the risk posed by the procedure that might cause bacteremia. For example, if a patient with a prosthetic valve undergoes prostatic resection, antibiotic prophylaxis should be given because both factors present significant risk for endocarditis. On the other hand, if a patient with mitral valve prolapse is scheduled for gastroscopy, prophylaxis is not necessary because the risk for endocarditis in this setting is very low.[199] Obviously, such risk assessments may be inaccurate; in many situations uncertainties inevitably will remain. To meet a reasonable standard of care, the health-care professional should (1) know of the patient's cardiac lesion, (2) inform the patient that a small risk of endocarditis exists, (3) then make a reasoned decision as to whether to give prophylaxis along the lines described above. Patient and physician preferences may influence the final decision.

Attempted prophylaxis does not always succeed. Of 52 recently recorded cases of apparent prophylaxis failure, 42 involved patients with heart disease who received oral penicillin or erythromycin, usually to cover dental procedures.[55]

Common errors in attempted prevention of endocarditis are starting antibiotics too early, continuing too long, using low doses, covering tooth extractions but not lesser dental procedures, and confusing prevention of rheumatic fever (long-term, low-dose) with prevention of endocarditis (short-term, high-dose).[116]

Based on present information prophylaxis is probably *not* necessary for minor dental procedures that do not involve the gums, such as simple fillings above the gum line and adjustment of orthodontic appliances. When a dentist cleans and scales the teeth, however, the gums are always involved and susceptible patients should receive a prophylactic antibiotic regimen.[200]

In the absence of pelvic infection, prophylaxis for endocarditis in patients with heart lesions is probably not required to cover normal delivery, therapeutic abortion, dilation and curettage, and insertion or removal of intrauterine contraceptive devices. Similarly, antibiotics need not be given before many common procedures such as cardiac catheterization, insertion of temporary pacemakers, endotracheal intubation, bronchoscopy, endoscopy, or radiographic contrast studies of the upper and lower gastrointestinal tract. However, some physicians choose to cover even these low-risk procedures in patients with prosthetic valves because they are at higher risk for endocarditis than patients with native valves. Specific regimens suggested for prophylaxis of endocarditis are listed in Table 56-9.

Cardiac surgeons presently administer antibiotics to virtually all patients undergoing intracardiac surgery, attempting to prevent both wound infections and endocarditis. This practice is rational and traditional, but as with prophylaxis of endocarditis in other settings, its efficacy has not been conclusively proved.[202–204] Current recommendations call for parenteral administration of an antistaphylococcal antibiotic just prior to operation, then continued for 1 or 2 further doses (Table 56-9). The regimen may be modified if local experience shows that cases of early PVE caused by *Staph. epidermidis* or gram-negative bacilli have occurred with significant frequency (Table 56-9).

TABLE 56-8 Incidence of Transient Bacteremia after Various Dental, Surgical, or Diagnostic Procedures

Extraction of one or more teeth	82%
Periodontal surgery	88%
Brushing teeth	40%
Tonsillectomy	38%
Esophageal dilatation	45%
Catheter removal after urologic surgery	50%
Prostatectomy (sterile urine)	11%
Prostatectomy (infected urine)	57%
Normal delivery	4–11%
Diagnostic procedures:	
Bronchoscopy	0–15%
Barium enema	10%
Liver biopsy	10%
Upper GI endoscopy	4%
Sigmoidoscopy	0–5%
Colonoscopy	5%

Source: Adapted from Refs. 197–199 and from D. T. Durack, Prophylaxis of Infective Endocarditis, in G. L. Mandell, R. G. Douglas, and J. E. Bennett (eds.), "Principles and Practice of Infectious Diseases," John Wiley & Sons, New York, 1979, p. 701. Copyright 1979, John Wiley & Sons. Reproduced with permission from John Wiley & Sons, editor, and author.

TABLE 56-9 Suggested Regimens for Prophylaxis of Infective Endocarditis*

Standard Regimen	
For dental procedures and oral or upper respiratory tract surgery	Penicillin V 2.0 g orally 1 h before, then 1.0 g 6 h later†
Special Regimens	
Parenteral regimen for high-risk patients; also for gastrointestinal (GI) or genitourinary (GU) tract procedures	Ampicillin 2.0 g IM or IV *plus* gentamicin 1.5 mg/kg IM or IV, 0.5 h before†
Parenteral regimen for penicillin-allergic patients	Vancomycin 1.0 g IV *slowly* over 1 h, starting 1 h before; *add* gentamicin 1.5 mg/kg IM or IV if GI or GU tract involved†
Oral regimen for penicillin-allergic patients (oral and respiratory tract only)	Erythromycin 1.0 g orally 1 h before, then 0.5 g 6 h later†
Oral regimen for minor GI or GU tract procedures	Amoxicillin 3.0 g orally 1 h before, then 1.5 g 6 h later†
Parenteral regimen for cardiac surgery including valve replacement	Cefazolin 2.0 g IV on induction of anesthesia, repeated 8 and 16 h later‡ *or* Vancomycin 1.0 g IV *slowly* over 1 h starting on induction of anesthesia, then 0.5 g IV 8 and 16 h later‡

*Note that (1) these regimens are empirical suggestions; no regimen has been proved effective for prevention of endocarditis, and prevention failures may occur with any regimen, (2) these regimens are not intended to cover all clinical situations; the practitioner should use his or her own judgment on safety and cost-benefit issues in each individual case, (3) one or two additional doses may be given if the period of risk for bacteremia is prolonged.

†Pediatric dosages: ampicillin 50 mg/kg; erythromycin 20 mg/kg for first dose, then 10 mg/kg; gentamicin 2 mg/kg; penicillin V and amoxicillin; for children who weigh more than 60 lb, use same as for adults; for children less than 60 lb, use one-half the adult dose; vancomycin 20 mg/kg.

‡Vancomycin is preferred if *Staph. epidermidis* is an important cause of postoperative infection in that hospital. Gentamicin 1.5 mg/kg IV or IM may be added to each dose, only if postoperative gram-negative infections have occurred with significant frequency.

Source: D.T. Durack, Nine Controversies in the Management of Infective Endocarditis, in R.G. Petersdorf et al. (eds.), "Update V: Harrison's Principles of Internal Medicine," McGraw-Hill Book Company, New York, 1984, p. 35. Adapted and reproduced with permission of the publisher and author.

References

1. Blumer, G.: Subacute Bacterial Endocarditis, *Medicine* 2:105, 1923.
2. Thayer, W. S. T.: Studies on Bacterial (Infective) Endocarditis, *Johns Hopkins Hosp. Rep.*, 22:1, 1926.
3. Kerr, A. J., Jr.: "Subacute Bacterial Endocarditis," Charles C Thomas, Springfield, Ill., 1955.
4. Hermans, P. E.: The Clinical Manifestations of Infective Endocarditis, *Mayo Clin. Proc.*, 57:15, 1982.
5. Chambers, H. F., Korzeniowski, O. M., and Sande, M. A., with the National Collaborative Endocarditis Study Group: *Staphylococcus aureus* Endocarditis: Clinical Manifestations in Addicts and Nonaddicts, *Medicine*, 62:170, 1983.
6. Arnett, E. N., and Roberts, W. C.: Pathology of Active Infective Endocarditis: A Necropsy Analysis of 192 Patients, *Thorac. Cardiovasc. Surgeon*, 30:327, 1982.
7. Weinstein, L.: Infective Endocarditis, in E. Braunwald (ed.), "Heart Disease: A Textbook of Cardiovascular Medicine," W. B. Saunders Company, Philadelphia, 1984, p. 1136.
8. Baumgartner, W. A., Miller, D. C., Reitz, B. A., Oyer, P. E., Jamieson, S. W., Stinson, E. B., and Shumway, N. E.: Surgical Treatment of Prosthetic Valve Endocarditis, *Ann. Thorac. Surg.*, 35:87, 1983.
9. Wilson, W. R., Danielson, G. K., Guiliani, E. R., and Geraci, J. E.: Prosthetic Valve Endocarditis, *Mayo Clin. Proc.*, 57:155, 1982.
10. Ivert, T. S. A., Dismukes, W. E., Cobbs, C. G., Blackstone, E. H., Kirklin, J. W., and Bergdahl, L. A. L.: Prosthetic Valve Endocarditis, *Circulation*, 69:223, 1984.
11. MacDonald, R. A., and Robbins, S. L.: The Significance of Nonbacterial Thrombotic Endocarditis: An Autopsy and Clinical Study of 78 Cases, *Ann. Intern. Med.*, 46:255, 1957.
12. Barry, W. E., and Scarpelli, D.: Nonbacterial Thrombotic Endocarditis, *Arch. Intern. Med.*, 109:151, 1962.
13. Bryan, C. S.: Nonbacterial Thrombotic Endocarditis in Patients with Malignant Tumors, *Am. J. Med.*, 46:787, 1969.
14. Major, R. H.: Notes on the History of Endocarditis, *Bull. Hist. Med.*, 17:351, 1945.
15. Pruitt, R. D.: William Osler and his Goulstonian Lectures on Malignant Endocarditis, *Mayo Clin. Proc.*, 57:4, 1982.
16. Osler, W.: The Goulstonian Lectures on Malignant Endocarditis, *Br. Med. J.*, 1:467, 522, 577, 1885.
17. Horder, T.: Infective Endocarditis, with an Analysis of 150 Cases and with Special Reference to the Chronic Form of the Disease, *Q. J. Med.*, 2:229, 1909.
18. Allen, A.: Nature of Vegetations of Bacterial Endocarditis, *Arch. Pathol.*, 27:661, 1939.
19. Libman, E., and Friedberg, C. K.: "Subacute Bacterial Endocarditis," Oxford University Press, Oxford, New York, 1941.
20. Beeson, P. B., Brannon, E. S., and Warren, J. V.: Observations on the Site of Removal of Bacteria from the Blood in Patients with Bacterial Endocarditis, *J. Exp. Med.*, 81:9, 1945.
21. Dawson, M. H., and Hunter, T. H.: The Treatment of Subacute Bacterial Endocarditis with Penicillin, *JAMA*, 127:129, 1945.
22. Abraham, E. P., Chain, E., Fletcher, C. M., Florey, H. W., Gardner, D., Heatley, N. G., and Jennings, M. A.: Further Observations on Penicillin, *Lancet*, 2:177, 1941.
23. Durack, D. T.: Review of Early Experience in Treatment of Bacterial Endocarditis, 1940–1955, in A. L. Bisno (ed.), "Infective Endocarditis," Grune & Stratton, New York, 1981.
24. Loewe, L., Rosenblatt, P., Greene, H., and Russell, M.: Combined Penicillin and Heparin Therapy of Subacute Bacterial Endocarditis: Report of Seven Consecutive Successfully Treated Patients, *JAMA*, 124:144, 1944.
25. Galbreath, W. R., and Hull, E.: Sulfonamide Therapy of Bacterial Endocarditis, *Ann. Intern. Med.*, 18:201, 1943.
26. Bloomfield, A. L., Armstrong, C. D., and Kirby, W. M. M.: The Treatment of Subacute Bacterial Endocarditis with Penicillin, *J. Clin. Invest.*, 24:251, 1945.
27. Hunter, T. H.: The Treatment of Some Bacterial Infections of the Heart and Pericardium, *Bull. N. Y. Acad. Med.*, 28:213, 1952.
28. Finland, M.: Treatment of Bacterial Endocarditis, *N. Engl. J. Med.*, 250:372, 1954.

29. Geraci, J. E.: The Antibiotic Therapy of Bacterial Endocarditis: Therapeutic Data on 172 Patients Seen from 1951 through 1957; Additional Observations on Short-Term Therapy (Two Weeks) for Penicillin-Sensitive Streptococcal Endocarditis, *Med. Clin. North Am.*, 42:1101, 1958.
30. Weinstein, L., and Schlesinger, J.: Treatment of Infective Endocarditis, *Prog. Cardiovasc. Dis.*, 16:275, 1973.
31. Kaye, D., McCormack, R. C., and Hook, E. W.: Bacterial Endocarditis: The Changing Pattern since Introduction of Penicillin Therapy. *Antimicrob. Agents Chemother.*, 1961, p. 37.
32. Uwaydah, M. M., and Weinberg, A. N.: Bacterial Endocarditis—A Changing Pattern, *N. Engl. J. Med.*, 273:1231, 1965.
33. Lerner, P. I., and Weinstein, L.: Medical Progress: Infective Endocarditis in the Antibiotic Era, *N. Engl. J. Med.*, 274:199, 1966.
34. Finland, M., and Barnes, N. W.: Changing Etiology of Bacterial Endocarditis in the Antibacterial Era: Experiences at Boston City Hospital, *Ann. Intern. Med.*, 72:341, 1970.
35. Garvey, G. J., and Neu, H. C.: Infective Endocarditis—An Evolving Disease: A Review of Endocarditis at the Columbia-Presbyterian Medical Center, 1968–1973, *Medicine*, 57:105, 1978.
36. Durack, D. T., and Petersdorf, R. G.: Changes in the Epidemiology of Endocarditis: In E. L. Kaplan and A. V. Taranta (eds.), "Infective Endocarditis," American Heart Association, AHA Monograph no. 52, 1977, p. 3.
37. Bayliss, R., Clarke, C., Oakley, C., Somerville, W., and Whitfield, A. G. W.: The Teeth and Infective Endocarditis, *Br. Heart J.*, 50:506, 1983.
38. Bayliss, R., Clarke, C., Oakley, C. M., Somerville, W., Whitfield, A. G. W., and Young, S. E. J.: The Microbiology and Pathogenesis of Infective Endocarditis, *Br. Heart J.*, 50:513, 1983.
39. Bayliss, R., Clarke, C., Oakley, C., Somerville, W., Whitfield, A. G. W., and Young, S. E. J.: The Bowel, the Genitourinary Tract and Infective Endocarditis, *Br. Heart J.*, 51:339, 1983.
40. Ries, K.: Endocarditis in the Elderly, in D. Kaye (ed.), "Infective Endocarditis," University Park Press, Baltimore, 1977, p. 143.
41. Weinstein, L., and Rubin, R. H.: Infective Endocarditis—1973, *Prog. Cardiovasc. Dis.*, 16:239, 1973.
42. Kaye, D.: Definitions and Demographic Characteristics, in D. Kaye (ed.), "Infective Endocarditis," University Park Press, Baltimore, 1977, p. 1.
43. Johnson, D. H., Rosenthal, A., and Nadas, A. S.: A Forty Year Review of Bacterial Endocarditis in Infancy and Childhood, *Circulation*, 51:581, 1975.
44. Rosenthal, A., and Nadas, A. S.: Infective Endocarditis in Infancy and Childhood, in S. H. Rahimtoola, (ed.), "Infective Endocarditis," Grune & Stratton, New York, 1978, p. 149.
45. Johnson, C. M., and Rhodes, K. H.: Pediatric Endocarditis, *Mayo Clin. Proc.*, 57:86, 1982.
46. El-Khatib, M. R., Wilson, F. M., and Lerner, A. M.: Characteristics of Bacterial Endocarditis in Heroin Addicts in Detroit, *Am. J. Med. Sci.*, 271:147, 1976.
47. Stimmel, B., and Dack, S.: Infective Endocarditis in Narcotic Addicts, in S. H. Rahimtoola (ed.), "Infective Endocarditis," Grune & Stratton, New York, 1978, p. 195.
48. Reisberg, B. E.: Infective Endocarditis in the Narcotic Addict, *Prog. Cardiovasc. Dis.*, 22:193, 1979.
49. Cannon, N. J., and Cobbs, C. G.: Infective Endocarditis in Drug Addicts, in D. Kaye (ed.), "Infective Endocarditis," University Park Press, Baltimore, 1977, p. 111.
50. Pelletier, L. L., and Petersdorf, R. G.: Infective Endocarditis: A Review of 125 Cases from the University of Washington Hospitals, 1963–72, *Medicine*, 56:287, 1977.
51. Kaplan, E. L., Rich, H., Gersony, W., and Manning, J.: A Collaborative Study of Infective Endocarditis in the 1970's: Emphasis on Patients Who Have Undergone Cardiovascular Surgery, *Circulation*, 59:327, 1979.
52. Corrigall, D., Bolen, J., Hancock, E. W., and Popp, R. L.: Mitral Valve Prolapse and Infective Endocarditis, *Am. J. Med.*, 63:215, 1977.
53. Clemens, J. D., Horwitz, R. I., Jaffe, C. C., Feinstein, A. R., and Stanton, B. F.: A Controlled Evaluation of the Risk of Bacterial Endocarditis in Persons with Mitral-Valve Prolapse, *N. Engl. J. Med.*, 307:776, 1982.
54. Beton, D. C., Brear, S. G., Edwards, J. D., and Leonard, J. C.: Mitral Valve Prolapse: An Assessment of Clinical Features, Associated Conditions and Prognosis, *Q. J. Med.*, 52:150, 1983.
55. Durack, D. T., Kaplan, E. L., and Bisno, A. L.: Apparent Failure of Endocarditis Prophylaxis: Analysis of 52 Cases Submitted to a National Registry, *JAMA*, 250:2318, 1983.
56. Clemens, J. D., and Ransohoff, D. F.: A Quantitative Assessment of Pre-dental Antibiotic Prophylaxis for Patients with Mitral-Valve Prolapse, *J. Chronic Dis.*, 37:531, 1984.
57. Wang, K., Gobel, F. L., and Gleason, D. F.: Bacterial Endocarditis in Idiopathic Hypertrophic Subaortic Stenosis, *Am. Heart J.*, 89:359, 1975.
58. Tuazon, C. U., and Sheagren, J. N.: Increased Staphylococcal Carrier Rate among Narcotic Addicts, *J. Infect. Dis.*, 129:725, 1974.
59. Reyes, M. P., and Lerner, A. M.: Current Problems in the Treatment of Infective Endocarditis Due to *Pseudomonas aeruginosa*, *Rev. Infect. Dis.*, 5:314, 1983.
60. Cohen, P. S., Maguire, H. J., and Weinstein, L.: Infective Endocarditis Caused by Gram-Negative Bacteria: A Review of the Literature, 1945–1977, *Prog. Cardiovasc. Dis.*, 22:205, 1980.
61. McLeod, R., and Remington, J. S.: Fungal Endocarditis, in S. H. Rahimtoola (ed.), "Infective Endocarditis," Grune & Stratton, New York, 1978, p. 211.
62. Keys, T. F., and Hewitt, W. L.: Endocarditis Due to Micrococci and *Staphylococcus epidermidis*, *Arch. Intern. Med.*, 132:216, 1973.
63. Felner, J. M., and Dowell, V. R.: Anaerobic Bacterial Endocarditis, *N. Engl. J. Med.*, 283:1189, 1970.
64. Scheld, W. M., and Sande, M. A.: Endocarditis and Intravascular Infections, in G. L. Mandell, R. G. Douglas, and J. E. Bennett (eds.), "Principles and Practice of Infectious Diseases," 2nd ed., John Wiley & Sons, New York, 1984.
65. Resnekov, L.: Staphylococcal Endocarditis following Mitral Valvotomy, with Special References to Coagulase-Negative *Staphylococcus albus*, *Lancet*, 2:587, 1959.
66. Kloster, F. E.: Infective Prosthetic Valve Endocarditis, in S. H. Rahimtoola (ed.), "Infective Endocarditis," Grune & Stratton, New York, 1978, p. 291.
67. Watanakunakorn, C.: Prosthetic Valve Infective Endocarditis, *Prog. Cardiovasc. Dis.*, 22:181, 1979.
68. Frater, R. W. M., and Santos, G. H.: Sources of Infection in Open Heart Surgery, *N.Y. State J. Med.*, 74:2386, 1974.
69. Karchmer, A. W., Dismukes, W. E., Buckley, M. J., and Austen, W. G.: Late Prosthetic Valve Endocarditis: Clinical Features Influencing Therapy, *Am. J. Med.*, 64:199, 1978.
70. Rossiter, S. J., Stinson, E. B., Oyer, P. E., Miller, D. C., Schapira, J. N., Martin, R. P., and Shumway, N. E.: Prosthetic Valve Endocarditis: Comparison of Heterograft Tissue Valves and Mechanical Valves, *J. Thorac. Cardiovasc. Surg.*, 76:795, 1978.
71. Mendelsohn, G., and Hutchins, G. M.: Infective Endocarditis during the First Decade of Life, *Am. J. Dis. Child.*, 133:619, 1979.
72. Stinson, E. B.: Surgical Treatment of Infective Endocarditis, *Prog. Cardiovasc. Dis.*, 22:145, 1979.
73. Lein, J., and Stander, R. W.: Subacute Bacterial Endocarditis following Obstetric and Gynecologic Procedures, *Obstet. Gynecol.*, 13:568, 1959.
74. Sugrue, D., Blake, S., Troy, P., and MacDonald, D.: Antibiotic Prophylaxis against Infective Endocarditis after Normal Delivery—Is It Necessary?, *Br. Heart J.*, 44:499, 1980.
75. Cobbs, C. G.: IUD and Endocarditis, *Ann. Intern. Med.*, 78:451, 1973.

76. von Reyn, C. F., Levy, B. S., Arbeit, R. D., Friedland, G., and Crumpacker, C. S.: Infective Endocarditis: An Analysis Based on Strict Case Definitions, *Ann. Intern. Med.*, 94:505, 1981.
77. Ehrie, M., Morgan, A. P., Moore, F. D., and O'Connor, N. E.: Endocarditis with Indwelling Balloon-Tipped Pulmonary Artery Catheter in Burn Patients, *J. Trauma*, 18:664, 1978.
77a. Rowley, K. M., Clubb, K. S., Walker Smith, G. J., and Cabin, H. S.: Right-Sided Infective Endocarditis as a Consequence of Flow-Directed Pulmonary-Artery Catheterization. A Clinicopathologic Study of 55 Autopsied Patients, *N. Engl. J. Med.*, 311:1152, 1984.
78. Lillehei, C. W., Bobb, J. R. R., and Visscher, M. B.: The Occurrence of Endocarditis with Valvular Deformities in Dogs with Arteriovenous Fistulas, *Ann. Surg.*, 132:577, 1950.
79. Cross, A. S., and Steigbigel, R. T.: Infective Endocarditis and Access Site Infections in Patients on Hemodialysis, *Medicine*, 55:453, 1976.
80. Brennan, R. O., and Durack, D. T.: The Viridans Streptococci in Perspective, in J. S. Remington and M. N. Swartz (eds.), "Current Clinical Topics in Infectious Diseases," McGraw-Hill Book Company, New York, 1984, vol. 5, p. 253.
81. Facklam, R. R.: Physiological Differentiation of Viridans Streptococci, *J. Clin. Microbiol.*, 5:184, 1977.
82. Harder, E. J., Wilkowske, C. J., Washington, J. A., III, and Geraci, J. E.: *Streptococcus mutans* Endocarditis, *Ann. Intern. Med.*, 80:364, 1974.
83. Malacoff, R. F., Frank, E., and Andriole, V. T.: Streptococcal Endocarditis (Nonenterococcal, non-Group A), *JAMA*, 241:1807, 1979.
84. Moellering, R. C., Jr., Watson, B. K., and Kunz, L. J.: Endocarditis Due to Group D Streptococci: Comparison of Disease Caused by *Streptococcus bovis* with that Produced by Enterococci, *Am. J. Med.*, 57:239, 1974.
85. Mandell, G. L.: Enterococcal Endocarditis, in D. Kaye (ed.), "Infective Endocarditis," University Park Press, Baltimore, 1977, p. 101.
86. Wilson, W. R., Wilkowski, C. J., Wright, A. J., Sande, M. A., and Geraci, J. E.: Treatment of Streptomycin-Susceptible and Streptomycin-Resistant Enterococcal Endocarditis, *Ann. Intern. Med.*, 100:816, 1984.
87. Levy, B. S., von Reyn, C. F., Arbeit, R. D., Friedland, G., and Crumpacker, C.: More on *S. bovis* and Bowel Carcinoma, *N. Engl. J. Med.*, 298:572, 1978.
88. Murray, H. W., and Roberts, R. B.: *Streptococcus bovis* Bacteremia and Underlying Gastrointestinal Disease, *Arch. Intern. Med.*, 138:1097, 1978.
89. Klein, R. S., Catalano, M. T., Edberg, S. C., Casey, J. I., and Steigbigel, N. H.: *Streptococcus bovis* Septicemia and Carcinoma of the Colon, *Ann. Intern. Med.*, 91:560, 1979.
90. Strauss, A. L., and Hamburger, M.: Pneumococcal Endocarditis in the Penicillin Era, *Arch. Intern. Med.*, 118:190, 1966.
91. Carey, R. B., Gross, K. C., and Roberts, R. B.: Vitamin B^6-Dependent *Streptococcus mitior* (*mitis*) Isolated from Patients with Systemic Infections, *J. Infect. Dis.*, 131:722, 1975.
92. Ellner, J. J., Rosenthal, M. S., Lerner, P. I., and McHenry, M. C.: Infective Endocarditis Caused by Slow-Growing, Fastidious, Gram-Negative Bacteria, *Medicine*, 58:145, 1979.
93. Washington, J. A., II: The Role of the Microbiology Laboratory in the Diagnosis and Antimicrobial Treatment of Infective Endocarditis, *Mayo Clin. Proc.*, 57:22, 1982.
94. Roberts, W. C.: Characteristics and Consequences of Infective Endocarditis (Active or Healed or Both) Learned from Morphologic Studies, in S. H. Rahimtoola (ed.), "Infective Endocarditis," Grune & Stratton, New York, 1978, p. 55.
95. Pankey, G. A.: Acute Bacterial Endocarditis at the University of Minnesota Hospitals, 1939–1959, *Am. Heart J.*, 64:583, 1962.
96. Watanakunakorn, C., Tan, J. S., and Phair, J. P.: Some Salient Features of *Staphylococcus aureus* Endocarditis, *Am. J. Med.*, 54:473, 1973.
97. Karchmer, A. W., Archer, G. L., and Dismukes, W. E.: *Staphylococcus epidermidis* Causing Prosthetic Valve Endocarditis: Microbiologic and Clinical Observations as Guides to Therapy, *Ann. Intern. Med.*, 98:447, 1984.
98. Gould, K., Ramirez-Ronda, C. H., Holmes, R. K., and Sanford, J. P.: Adherence of Bacteria to Heart Valves *in vitro*, *J. Clin. Invest.*, 56:1364, 1975.
99. Holmes, R. K., and Ramirez-Ronda, C. H.: Adherence of Bacteria to the Endothelium of Heart Valves, in "Infective Endocarditis," an American Heart Association Symposium, AHA Monograph no. 52, 1977, p. 12.
100. Scheld, W. M., Valone, J. A., and Sande, M. A.: Bacterial Adherence in the Pathogenesis of Endocarditis: Interaction of Bacterial Dextran, Platelets and Fibrin, *J. Clin. Invest.*, 61:1394, 1978.
101. Durack, D. T., and Beeson, P. B.: Protective Role of Complement in Experimental *E. coli* Endocarditis, *Infect. Immun.*, 16:213, 1977.
102. Kaye, D.: Infecting Microorganisms, in D. Kaye (ed.), "Infective Endocarditis," University Park Press, Baltimore, 1977, p. 43.
103. Geraci, J. E., and Wilson, W. R.: Endocarditis Due to Gram-Negative Bacteria, *Mayo Clin. Proc.*, 57:145, 1982.
104. Jemsek, J. G., Greenberg, S. B., Gentry, L. O., Welton, D. E., and Mattox, K. L.: *Haemophilus parainfluenzae* Endocarditis; Two Cases and Review of the Literature in the Past Decade, *Am. J. Med.*, 66:51, 1979.
105. Rubinstein, E., Noriega, E. R., Simberkoff, M. S., Holzman, R., and Rahal, J. L., Jr.: Fungal Endocarditis: Analysis of 24 Cases and Review of the Literature, *Medicine*, 54:331, 1975.
106. Kammer, R. B., and Utz, J. P.: *Aspergillus* Species Endocarditis: The New Face of a Not So Rare Disease, *Am. J. Med.*, 56:506, 1974.
107. Cannady, P. B., Jr., and Sanford, J. P.: Negative Blood Cultures in Infective Endocarditis: A Review, *South. Med. J.*, 69:1420, 1976.
108. Pesanti, E. L., and Smith, I. M.: Infective Endocarditis with Negative Blood Cultures; An Analysis of 52 Cases, *Am. J. Med.*, 66:43, 1979.
109. Van Scoy, R. E.: Culture-Negative Endocarditis, *Mayo Clin. Proc.*, 57:149, 1982.
110. Wainwright, J.: Tuberculous Endocarditis: A Report of 2 Cases, *South African Med. J.*, 56:731, 1979.
111. Turck, W. P. G., Howitt, G., Turnberg, L. A., Fox, H., Longson, M., Matthews, M. B., and Das Gupta, R.: Chronic Q Fever, *Q. J. Med.*, 45:193, 1976.
112. Wilson, H. G., Neilson, G. H., Galea, E. G., Stafford, G., and O'Brien, M. F.: Q Fever Endocarditis in Queensland, *Circulation*, 53:680, 1976.
113. Kimbrough, R. C., Ormsbee, R. A., Peacock, M., Rogers, W. R., Bennetts, R. W., Raaf, J., Krause, A., and Gardner, C.: Q Fever Endocarditis in the United States, *Ann. Intern. Med.*, 91:400, 1979.
114. Ward, C., and Ward, A. M.: Acquired Valvular Heart Disease in Patients Who Kept Pet Birds, *Lancet*, 2:734, 1974.
115. Van der Bel-Kahn, J. M., Watanakunakorn, C., Menefee, N. G., Long, H. D., and Dieter, R.: *Chlamydia trachomatis* Endocarditis, *Am. Heart J.*, 95:627, 1978.
116. Durack, D. T.: Prophylaxis of Infective Endocarditis, in G. L. Mandell, R. G. Douglas, and J. E. Bennett (eds.), "Principles and Practice of Infectious Diseases," 2nd ed., John Wiley & Sons, New York, 1984.
117. Angrist, A., Oka, M., and Nakao, K.: Vegetative Endocarditis, *Pathol. Ann.*, 2:155, 1967.
118. Grant, R. T., Wood, J. E., Jr., and Jones, T. D.: Heart Valve Irregularities in Relation to Subacute Bacterial Endocarditis, *Heart*, 14:247, 1927.
119. Durack, D. T.: Experimental Bacterial Endocarditis: IV. Structure and Evolution of Very Early Lesions, *J. Pathol.*, 115:81, 1975.
120. Durack, D. T., and Beeson, P. B.: Experimental Bacterial Endocarditis: I. Colonization of a Sterile Vegetation, *Br. J. Exp. Pathol.*, 53:44, 1972.

121. Van Ginkel, C. J. W., Thorig, L., Thompson, J., Oh, J. I. H., and Van Aken, W. G.: Enhancement of Generation of Monocyte Tissue Thromboplastin by Bacterial Phagocytosis: Possible Pathway for Fibrin Formation on Infected Vegetations in Bacterial Endocarditis, *Infect. Immun.*, 5:388, 1979.
122. Lepeschkin, E.: On the Relation between the Site of Valvular Involvement in Endocarditis and the Blood Pressure Resting on the Valve, *Am. J. Med. Sci.*, 224:318, 1952.
123. Rodbard, S.: Blood Velocity and Endocarditis, *Circulation*, 27:18, 1963.
124. Edwards, J. E., Jr., and Burchell, H. B.: Endocardial and Intimal Lesions (Jet Impact) as Possible Sites of Origin of Murmurs, *Circulation*, 18:946, 1958.
125. Buchbinder, N. A., and Roberts, W. C.: Left-Sided Valvular Active Infective Endocarditis: A Study of Forty-Five Necropsy Patients, *Am. J. Med.*, 53:20, 1972.
126. Roberts, W. C.: Characteristics and Consequences of Infective Endocarditis (Active or Healed or Both) Learned from Morphologic Studies, in S. H. Rahimtoola (ed.), "Infective Endocarditis," Grune & Stratton, New York, 1978, p. 55.
127. Phair, J. P., and Clarke, J.: Immunology of Infective Endocarditis, *Prog. Cardiovasc. Dis.*, 22:137, 1977.
128. Williams, R. C., and Kunkel, H. G.: Rheumatoid Factor, Complement and Conglutinin Aberrations in Patients with Subacute Bacterial Endocarditis, *J. Clin. Invest.*, 41:666, 1962.
129. Messner, R. P., Laxdal, T., Quie, P. G., and Williams, R. C.: Rheumatoid Factor in Subacute Bacterial Endocarditis—Bacterium, Duration of Disease or Genetic Predisposition, *Ann. Intern. Med.*, 68:746, 1968.
130. Sheagren, J. N., Tuazon, C. U., Griffin, C., and Padmore, N.: Rheumatoid Factor in Acute Bacterial Endocarditis, *Arthritis Rheum.*, 19:877, 1976.
131. Maisch, B., Eichstadt, H., and Kochsiek, K.: Immune Reactions in Infective Endocarditis: I. Clinical Data and Diagnostic Relevance of Antimyocardial Antibodies, *Am. Heart J.*, 106:329, 1984.
132. Weinstein, L., and Schlesinger, J. J.: Pathoanatomic, Pathophysiologic, and Clinical Correlations in Endocarditis, *N. Engl. J. Med.*, 291:832, 1974.
133. Wadsworth, A. B.: A Study of the Endocardial Lesions Developing during Pneumococcus Infection in Horses, *J. Med. Res.*, 34:279, 1919.
134. Mair, W.: Pneumococcal Endocarditis in Rabbits, *J. Pathol. Bacteriol.*, 26:426, 1923.
135. Durack, D. T., Gilliland, B. G., and Petersdorf, R. G.: Effect of Immunization on Susceptibility to Experimental *Streptococcus mutans* and *Streptococcus sanguis* Endocarditis, *Infect. Immun.*, 22:52, 1978.
136. Durack, D. T., and Beeson, P. B.: Pathogenesis of Infective Endocarditis, in S. H. Rahimtoola (ed.), "Infective Endocarditis," Grune & Stratton, New York, 1978, p. 1.
137. Bayer, A. S., Theofilopoulos, A. N., Eisenberg, R., Dixon, F. J., and Guze, L. B.: Circulating Immune Complexes in Infective Endocarditis, *N. Engl. J. Med.*, 295:1500, 1976.
138. Bayer, A. S., Theofilopoulos, A. N., Tillman, D. B., Dixon, F. J., and Guze, L. B.: Use of Circulating Immune Complex Levels in the Serodifferentiation of Endocarditis and Nonendocarditis Septicemias, *Am. J. Med.*, 66:58, 1979.
139. Maisch, B., Mayer, E., Schubert, U., Berg, P. A., and Kochsiek, K.: Immune Reactions in Infective Endocarditis: II. Relevance of Circulating Immune Complexes, Serum Factors, and Cytotoxicity in Endocarditis, *Am. Heart J.*, 106:338, 1984.
140. Cabane, J., Godeau, P., Hereeman, A., Acar, J., Digeon, M., and Bach, J. F.: Fate of Circulating Immune Complexes in Infective Endocarditis, *Am. J. Med.*, 66:277, 1979.
141. Gutman, R. A., Striker, G. E., Gilliland, B. C., and Cutler, R. E.: The Immune Complex Glomerulonephritis of Bacterial Endocarditis, *Medicine*, 51:1, 1972.
142. Levy, R. L., and Hong, R.: The Immune Nature of Subacute Bacterial Endocarditis (SBE) Nephritis, *Am. J. Med.*, 64:645, 1973.
143. Wilson, J. W., Houghton, D. C., Bennett, W. M., and Porter, G. A.: The Kidney in Infective Endocarditis, in S. H. Rahimtoola (ed.), "Infective Endocarditis," Grune & Stratton, New York, 1978, p. 179.
144. Crowder, J. G., and White, A.: Teichoic Acid Antibodies in Staphylococcal and Nonstaphylococcal Endocarditis, *Ann. Intern. Med.*, 77:87, 1972.
145. Nagel, J. G., Tuazon, C. U., and Cardella, T. A.: Teichoic Acid Serologic Diagnosis of Staphylococcal Endocarditis: Use of Gel Diffusion and Counter-Immunoelectrophoretic Methods, *Ann. Intern. Med.*, 82:13, 1975.
146. Freedman, L. R., and Valone, J., Jr.: Experimental Endocarditis, *Prog. Cardiovasc. Dis.*, 22:169.
147. Durack, D. T.: Experience with Prophylaxis of Experimental Endocarditis, in E. L. Kaplan and A. V. Taranta (eds.), "Infective Endocarditis," American Heart Association, AHA Monograph no. 52, 1977, p. 28.
148. McAnulty, J. H., Rahimtoola, S. H., Demots, H., and Griswold, H. E.: Clinical Features of Infective Endocarditis, in S. H. Rahimtoola (ed.), "Infective Endocarditis," Grune & Stratton, New York, 1978, p. 125.
149. Churchill, M. A., Geraci, J. E., and Hunder, G. G.: Musculoskeletal Manifestations of Bacterial Endocarditis, *Ann. Intern. Med.*, 87:754, 1977.
150. Starkebaum, M., Durack, D., and Beeson, P.: The "Incubation Period" of Subacute Bacterial Endocarditis, *Yale J. Biol. Med.*, 50:49, 1977.
151. Kilpatrick, Z. M., Greenberg, P. A., and Sanford, J. P.: Splinter Hemorrhages—Their Clinical Significance, *Arch. Intern. Med.*, 115:730, 965.
152. Howard, E. J.: Osler's Nodes, *Am. Heart J.*, 59:633, 1960.
153. Alpert, J. S., Krous, H. F., Dalen, J. E., O'Rourke, R. A., and Bloor, C. M.: Pathogenesis of Osler's Nodes, *Ann. Intern. Med.*, 85:471, 1976.
154. Edwards, J. E., Jr., Foos, R. Y., Montgomerie, J. Z., and Guze, L. B.: Ocular Manifestations of *Candida* Septicemia: Review of Seventy-six Cases of Hematogenous *Candida* Endophthalmitis, *Medicine*, 53:47, 1974.
155. Osler, W.: Chronic Infective Endocarditis, *Q. J. Med.*, 2:219, 1909.
156. Mills, J., Utley, J., and Abbott, J.: Heart Failure in Infective Endocarditis: Predisposing Factors, Course and Treatment, *Chest*, 66:151, 1974.
157. Cates, J. E., and Christie, R. V.: Subacute Bacterial Endocarditis: A Review of 442 Patients Treated in 14 Centres Appointed by the Penicillin Trials Committee of the Medical Research Council, *Q. J. Med.*, 20:93, 1951.
158. Jones, H. R., Siekert, R. G., and Geraci, J. E.: Neurologic Manifestations of Bacterial Endocarditis, *Ann. Intern. Med.*, 71:21, 1969.
159. Ziment, I.: Nervous System Complications in Bacterial Endocarditis, *Am. J. Med.*, 47:593, 1968.
160. Pruitt, A. A., Rubin, R. H., Karchmer, A. W., and Duncan, G. W.: Neurologic Complications of Bacterial Endocarditis, *Medicine*, 57:329, 1978.
161. Stengel, A., and Wolferth, C. C.: Mycotic (Bacterial) Aneurysms of Intravascular Origin, *Arch. Intern. Med.*, 31:527, 1923.
162. Powers, D. L., and Mandell, G. L.: Intraleukocytic Bacteria in Endocarditis Patients, *JAMA*, 227:313, 1974.
163. Engle, R. L., and Koprowska, I.: The Appearance of Histiocytes in the Blood in Subacute Bacterial Endocarditis, *Am. J. Med.*, 26:965, 1959.
164. Belli, J., and Waisbren, B. A.: The Number of Blood Cultures Necessary to Diagnose Most Cases of Bacterial Endocarditis, *Am. J. Med. Sci.*, 232:284, 1956.
165. Werner, A. S., Cobbs, C. G., Kaye, D., and Hook, E. W.: Studies on the Bacteremia of Bacterial Endocarditis, *JAMA*, 202:199, 1967.
166. Katsu, M.: "Spectrum of Endocarditis in Japan and Current Treatment" (proceedings, 8th World Congress of Cardiology, Tokyo, 1978), p. 536.
167. Gerry, J. L., and Greenough, W. B.: Diphtheroid Endocarditis: Report of Nine Cases and Review of the Literature, *Johns Hopkins Med. J.*, 139:61, 1976.

168. Mintz, G. S., Morris, M. D., and Kotler, N.: Clinical Value and Limitations of Echocardiography, *Arch. Intern. Med.*, 140:1022, 1980.
169. Chandraratna, P. A. N., and Langevin, D. O.: Limitations of the Echocardiogram in Diagnosing Valvular Vegetations in Patients with Mitral Valve Prolapse, *Circulation*, 56:436, 1978.
170. Andy, J. J., Sheikh, M. M., Nayab, A., Barores, B. O., Fox, L. M., Curry, C. L., and Roberts, W. C.: Echocardiographic Observations in Opiate Addicts with Active Infective Endocarditis, *Am. J. Cardiol.*, 40:17, 1977.
171. DeMaria, A. N., King, J. F., Salel, A. E., Caudill, C. C., Miller, R. R., and Mason, R. P.: Echography and Phonography of Acute Aortic Regurgitation in Bacterial Endocarditis, *Ann. Intern. Med.*, 82:329, 1975.
172. Stewart, J. A., Silimperi, D., Harris, P., Wise, N. K., Franker, T. D., and Kisslo, J.: Echocardiographic Documentation of Vegetative Lesions in Infective Endocarditis: Clinical Implications, *Circulation*, 61:374, 1980.
173. Welton, D. E., Young, J. B., Raizner, A. E., Ishimori, T., Adyanthaya, A., Mattox, K. L., Chahine, R. A., and Miller, R. R.: Value and Safety of Cardiac Catheterization during Active Infective Endocarditis, *Am. J. Cardiol.*, 44:1306, 1979.
174. Riba, A. L., Takur, M. L., Gottschalk, A., Andriole, V. T., and Zaret, B. L.: Imaging Experimental Infective Endocarditis with Indium 111–Labeled Blood Cellular Components, *Circulation*, 59:336, 1979.
175. Miller, M. H., and Casey, J. I.: Infective Endocarditis: New Diagnostic Techniques, *Am. Heart J.*, 96:123, 1978.
176. Korzeniowski, O., Sande, M. A., and the National Collaborative Endocarditis Study Group: Combination Antimicrobial Therapy for *Staphylococcus aureus* Endocarditis in Patients Addicted to Parenteral Drugs and in Nonaddicts: A Prospective Study, *Ann. Intern. Med.*, 97:496, 1982.
177. Durack, D. T.: Nine Controversies in the Management of Infective Endocarditis, in R. G. Petersdorf, et al. (eds.), "Update V: Harrison's Principles of Internal Medicine," McGraw-Hill Book Company, New York, 1984, p. 35.
178. Ormiston, J. A., Neutze, J. M., Agnew, T., Lowe, J. B., and Kerr, A. R.: Infective Endocarditis: A Lethal Disease, *Aust. N.Z. J. Med.*, 11:620, 1981.
179. Kaye, D.: Cure Rates and Long Term Prognosis, in D. Kaye (ed.), "Infective Endocarditis," University Park Press, Baltimore, 1977, p. 201.
180. Welton, D. E., Young, J. B., Gentry, W. O., Raizner, A. E., Alexander, J. K., Chahine, R. A., and Miller, R. R.: Recurrent Infective Endocarditis: Analysis of Predisposing Factors and Clinical Features, *Am. J. Med.*, 66:932, 1979.
181. Blount, J. G.: Bacterial Endocarditis, *Am. J. Med.*, 38:909, 1965.
182. Pulliam, L., and Hadley, W. K.: Resistance of Viridans Streptococci to Penicillin, *N. Engl. J. Med.*, 300:1442, 1979.
183. Denny, A. E., Peterson, L. R., Gerding, D. N., and Hall, W. H.: Serious Staphylococcal Infections with Strains Tolerant to Bactericidal Antibiotics, *Arch Intern. Med.*, 139:1026, 1979.
184. Brennan, R. O., and Durack, D. T.: Therapeutic Significance of Penicillin Tolerance in Experimental Streptococcal Endocarditis, *Antimicrob. Agents Chemother.*, 23:273, 1983.
185. Reller, L. B., and Stratton, C. W.: Serum Dilution Test for Bactericidal Activity: II. Standardization and Correlation with Antimicrobial Assays and Susceptibility Tests, *J. Infect. Dis.*, 136:196, 1977.
186. Kane, L. W., and Finn, J. J., Jr.: The Treatment of Subacute Bacterial Endocarditis with Aureomycin and Chloromycetin, *N. Engl. J. Med.*, 244:623, 1951.
187. Bisno, A. L., Dismukes, W. E., Durack, D. T., et al.: AHA Committee Report: Treatment of Infective Endocarditis Due to Viridans Streptococci, *Circulation*, 63:730A, 1981.
188. Watanakunakorn, C.: Antimicrobial Therapy of Endocarditis Due to Less Common Bacteria, in A. L. Bisno (ed.), "Treatment of Infective Endocarditis," Grune & Stratton, New York, 1981.
189. Katz, L. N., and Elek, S. R.: Combined Heparin and Chemotherapy in Subacute Bacterial Endocarditis, *JAMA*, 124:149, 1944.
190. Kanis, J. A.: The Use of Anticoagulants in Bacterial Endocarditis, *Postgrad. Med. J.*, 50:312, 1974.
191. Wilson, W. R., Geraci, J. E., Danielson, G. K., Thompson, R. L., Spittell, J. A., Jr., Washington, J. A., II, and Giuliani, E. R.: Anticoagulant Therapy and Central Nervous System Complications in Patients with Prosthetic Valve Endocarditis, *Circulation*, 57:1004, 1978.
192. McAnulty, J. H., and Rahimtoola, S. H.: Surgery for Infective Endocarditis, *JAMA*, 242:77, 1979.
193. Jung, J. Y., Saab, S. B., and Almond, C. H.: The Case for Early Surgical Treatment of Left-Sided Primary Infective Endocarditis: A Collective Review, *J. Thorac. Cardiovasc. Surg.*, 70:509, 1975.
194. Wilson, W. R., Danielson, G. K., Giuliani, E. R., Washington, J. A., II, Jaumin, P. I., and Geraci, J. E.: Valve Replacement in Patients with Active Infective Endocarditis, *Circulation*, 58:585, 1978.
195. Richardson, J. V., Karp, R. B., Kirklin, J. W., and Dismukes, W. E.: Treatment of Infective Endocarditis: A 10-Year Comparative Analysis, *Circulation*, 58:589, 1978.
196. Durack, D. T.: Nine Controversies in the Management of Endocarditis, in R. G. Petersdorf (ed.), "Update V: Harrison's Principles of Internal Medicine," McGraw-Hill Book Company, New York, 1984, p. 35.
197. Everett, E. D., and Hirschmann, J. V.: Transient Bacteremia and Endocarditis Prophylaxis: A Review, *Medicine*, 56:61, 1977.
198. Sullivan, N. M., Sutter, V. L., Mims, M. M., Marsh, V. H., and Finegold, S. M.: Clinical Aspects of Bacteremia after Manipulation of the Genitourinary Tract, *J. Infect. Dis.*, 127:49, 1973.
199. Shorvon, P. J., Eykyn, S. J., and Cotton, P. B.: Gastrointestinal Instrumentation, Bacteraemia and Endocarditis, *Gut*, 24:1078, 1983.
200. American Heart Association Committee on Prevention of Bacterial Endocarditis: Prevention of Bacterial Endocarditis, *Circulation*, 70:1123A, 1984.
201. Prevention of Bacterial Endocarditis, *The Medical Letter*, 26:4, 1984.
202. Goodman, J. S., Schaffner, W., Collins, H. A., Battersky, E. J., and Koenig, M. G.: Infection after Cardiovascular Surgery: Clinical Study including Examination of Antimicrobial Prophylaxis, *N. Engl. J. Med.*, 278:117, 1968.
203. Schaffner, W.: Antibiotic Prophylaxis in Valvular Replacement Surgery, in R. J. Duma (ed.), "Infections of Prosthetic Heart Valves and Vascular Grafts," University Park Press, Baltimore, 1977, p. 313.
204. Myerowitz, P. D., Caswell, K., Lindsay, W. G., and Demetre, M. N.: Antibiotic Prophylaxis for Open Heart Surgery, *J. Thorac. Cardiovasc. Surg.*, 73:625, 1977.

Section G

Myocardial Disease

57

Myocarditis

Nanette Kass Wenger, M.D.
Walter H. Abelmann, M.D.
William C. Roberts, M.D.

Hence this inflammation almost always terminates fatally; but the death which it usually occasions may happen instantly or somewhat slowly. Thus carditis *has been known to become fatal in a very few days; while in other instances, when the disease has attained to its highest degree, the most alarming symptoms partially disappear, and a sort of convalescence is established; sometimes even the patient is restored to apparent health; he then flatters himself with a near and perfect cure; but the most intelligent physician perceives only a transformation, or degeneration of the disease into another affection slower, but not less severe, as a* chronic organic *disease is then established, mortal in all cases.*

Jean Nicolas Corvisart, 1806[1]

Etiology

This chapter addresses only myocarditis of infectious etiology. Myocarditis, an inflammatory process involving the myocardial wall, may result from virtually any bacterial, viral,[2] rickettsial, mycotic,[3] and parasitic[4] organism. It affects persons of all ages and in all areas of the world. The frequency of specific etiologic agents for infectious myocarditis varies with the age of the patients surveyed; with the geographic location; with the endemic or epidemic occurrence of infectious diseases; with the sophistication of public health measures, especially immunization and sanitation programs; with the availability of effective medication; and with a specific patient's associated disease and/or therapy. The immune-deficient host is at special risk.

In the United States and western Europe, most cases of acute myocarditis appear to be caused by viruses. Because it is often difficult to prove the viral etiology of cases of myocarditis that occur sporadically, such cases are often referred to as *idiopathic myocarditis.* The Coxsackie B enterovirus is especially cardiotropic in humans; it is the most common cause of viral heart disease, although Coxsackie pericarditis occurs more commonly than myocarditis.[5] Not infrequently, myocarditis and pericarditis occur together; one then speaks of *myopericarditis.* Coxsackievirus infections commonly occur in epidemics, particularly in the summer and early fall, and about 5 percent of infections involve the heart. Coxsackie B 1–5 and A 4, 16 are the strains most commonly implicated. The echovirus group of enterovirus also may cause acute myopericarditis, especially types 9, 11, and 22.[6,7]

In an endemic area for *Trypanosoma cruzi,* the patient with acquired cardiomyopathy, arrhythmia, and a right bundle branch block electrocardiographic pattern probably has *chronic Chagas' disease.*[8,9] Indeed, chronic Chagas' disease is the most common form of heart disease in some areas of South America, affecting an estimated 7 million persons.[10] The highest frequency is in the third and fourth decades of life, affecting primarily males from rural areas.

Trichinosis is the most prevalent helminthic infestation in humans; myocarditis is the most frequent and serious complication, accounting for the preponderance of trichinosis fatalities.

Cardiac *echinococcosis* is most frequently encountered in sheep-raising areas such as Uruguay, Australia, New Zealand, and the Mediterranean countries. This feature of the history often helps make the diagnosis. The heart is involved in about 1 percent of patients with hydatidosis, a predominantly hepatic-pulmonary disease. Men in the second to fifth decade of life are most commonly affected.[11]

The specific etiologic diagnosis of infectious myocarditis is often based on the extracardiac manifestations of the disease, as the clinical cardiovascular syndromes and myocardial morphologic alterations are similar for many different etiologic agents. Most commonly, the cardiovascular manifestations are but a minor presentation of a systemic infection in which noncardiac symptoms predominate. Even when a causative organism is isolated, it is often not known whether direct invasion and tissue damage by the infectious agent or a toxic, allergic, or hypersensitivity response to this agent is responsible for the clinical, electrocardiographic, and morphologic manifestations.

Pathology (Morphologic Features)

If myocarditis is defined as the *presence of extravasated leukocytes in the myocardial interstitium,* most patients diagnosed during life as having myocarditis do not have this process confirmed morphologically because death during the acute episode is rare; conversely, most patients with "myocarditis" observed at necropsy have not had this diagnosis made or suspected during life. If one adheres to the above definition, by far the most common cause of acute myocarditis is acute myocardial infarction secondary to coronary arterial narrowing from severe atherosclerosis, because this process is characterized at one stage by the presence of numerous inflammatory cells in the left ventricular wall. Indeed, acute myocardial infarction in the latter portion of the nineteenth century and during the first decades of the twentieth century was called *acute myocarditis* at necropsy; today, the myocardial necrosis resulting from coronary atherosclerotic narrowing is no longer placed in the "myocarditis" category. Nevertheless, myocardial inflammation in the absence of associated stainable microorganisms probably should not be considered myocarditis unless the lumens of the major epicardial coronary arteries are relatively free of atherosclerotic plaques. The degenerative myocardial morphologic changes in the patient with established myocarditis may be variably influenced by concomitant hypoxia, hypotension, electrolyte derangements, nutritional deficiencies, drug therapy, etc.; administration of corticosteroid hormones or other immunosuppressive agents may modify the interstitial inflammatory process.

The most common cause of acute myocarditis in humans is believed to be a virus, particularly the Coxsackie B enterovirus. Fortunately, viral myocarditis, with rare exceptions, is a benign condition and therefore confirmation of the presence of extravasated leukocytes in the myocardial interstitium is rare. Furthermore, viruses have never been unequivocally identified in human myocardium by electron microscopic studies, although a number of viruses have been isolated from human hearts. Experimental myocarditis has been produced with a number of viruses associated with human myocarditis, and viral replication in myocardial tissue has been repeatedly demonstrated in association with varying degrees of cellular infiltration and myocytolysis. When a viral illness clinically is associated with signs or symptoms of cardiac dysfunction and the patient dies, death generally occurs several weeks, months, or even years after the acute illness; examination of the myocardium at this late stage typically discloses only increased amounts of fibrous tissue in the myocardial interstitium and no extravasated inflammatory cells. Such was the case in a patient with acute mumps who died several months after the acute illness from progressive congestive cardiac failure[12] (Fig. 57-1).

Today, the most common circumstance in which "myocarditis" is observed at necropsy is in patients with suppressed immunologic responses because of treatment with corticosteroid or other immunosuppressive drugs, chemotherapeutic agents, or both. Although foci of inflammatory cells are fairly commonly observed in the myocardial walls of these immunosuppressed patients, "myocarditis" is rarely diagnosed or suspected during life, presumably because signs and symptoms from dysfunction of one or more noncardiac body organs dominate the clinical presentation or at least overshadow signs or symptoms of cardiac dysfunction. Among 420 necropsy patients with acute leukemia,[13] 29 (7 percent) had acute myocarditis at necropsy, caused by a variety of organisms (Table 57-1); but only a few of these 29 patients had a diagnosis of "acute myocarditis" made during life (Figs. 57-2 to 57-4; Plate 8-A). The myocarditis consisted primarily of focal myocardial abscesses, and the myocardial walls between the abscesses appeared normal or nearly normal.

Among patients dying of diphtheria, myocarditis is found at necropsy in about 70 percent.[14] The principal myocardial findings among those dying during the first 2 weeks of illness consist of a focal mononuclear cell infiltrate, mainly cardiac histiocytes, plasma cells, and lymphocytes, associated with degeneration of adjacent myocardial fibers. During the third week of illness, fibrous tissue replaces the degenerated monocytes. The potent exotoxin of diphtheria has been identified as being responsible for the degeneration or necrosis of the myocardial fibers; myocardial lesions are characterized by the prevalence of fatty changes, triglyceride deposition, and depletion of carnitine.

Certain infections have a fairly predictable effect on the heart. Chagas' disease, which infrequently is fatal during the acute illness, leads to generalized cardiomegaly, with right-sided cardiac dilatation more severe than the left-sided dilatation (Fig. 57-5). Additionally, the myocardial walls at the apices of each cardiac ventricle appear to be preferentially involved, so that this portion of the wall becomes thin and scarred and bulges. The right bundle branch of the conduction system also appears to be preferentially affected since complete right bundle branch

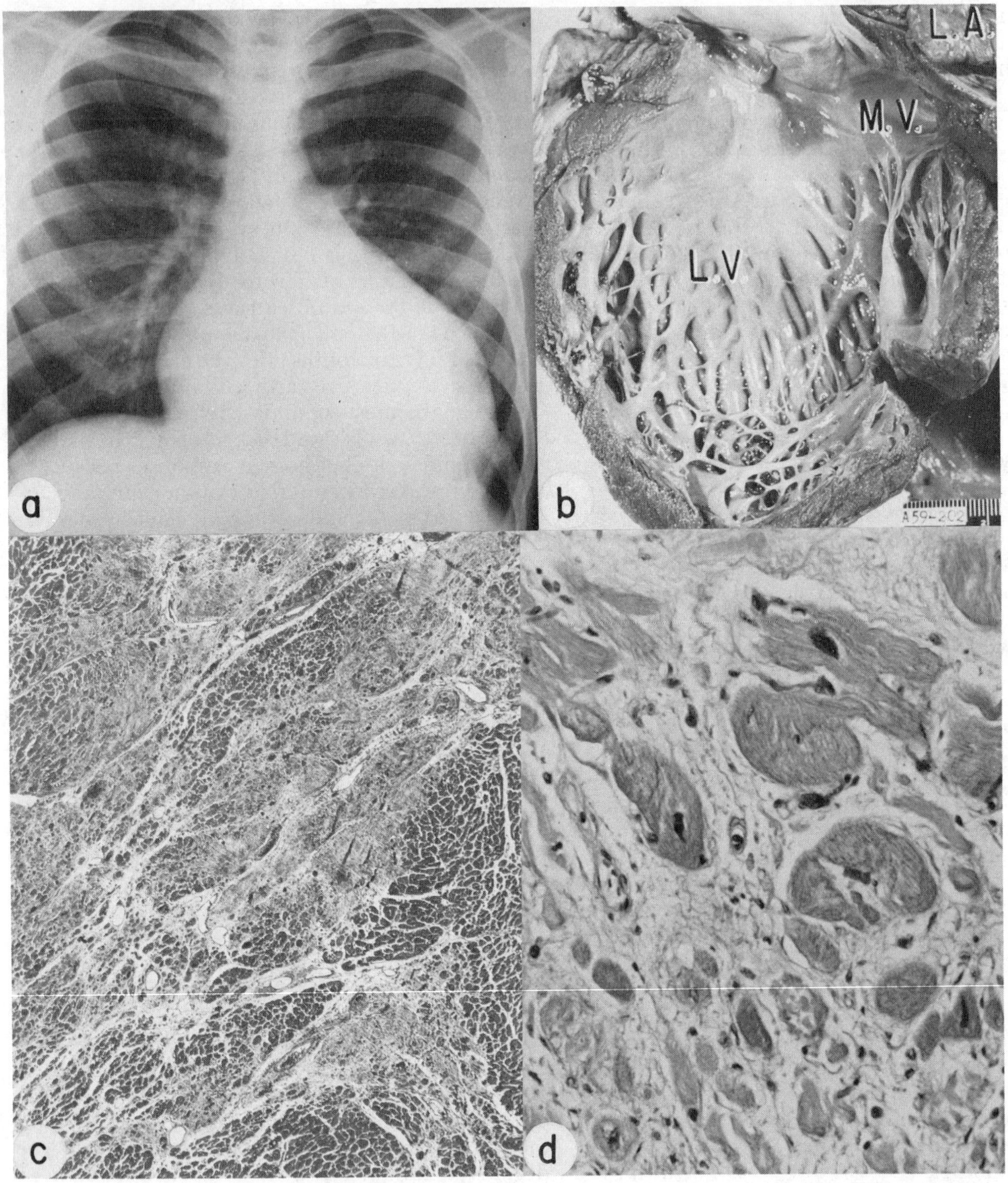

FIGURE 57-1 The heart of a patient with mumps myocarditis. This 17-year-old boy died 8 months after the onset of well-documented mumps. At the time of the acute illness, tachycardia was noted; it persisted, the heart progressively enlarged, and congestive heart failure appeared. He died of the latter. *a.* Chest radiograph showing cardiomegaly. *b.* Opened left ventricle (LV), aortic valve, and aorta. The chamber is dilated and the endocardium is mildly but diffusely thickened. MV = anterior mitral leaflet; LA = left atrial appendage. The heart weighed 550 g. Thrombi are present in the apex. *c.* Photomicrograph of portion of left ventricular wall showing replacement fibrosis (Masson stain; ×35). *d.* Close-up view of another area showing degeneration of myocardial fibers and loose interstitial fibrosis (Hematoxylin and eosin stain; ×235). (*From W. C. Roberts and S. M. Fox III, Mumps of the Heart. Clinical and Pathological Features, Circulation, 32:342, 1965. Reproduced by permission of the American Heart Association, Inc., and the authors.*)

block is extremely common. Inflammatory cells are nearly always absent in patients with chronic Chagas' disease.

Trichinosis, although usually benign, has been fatal during the acute illness; when observed at this stage, it is characterized by inflammatory cells, mainly eosinophils, within the myocardial interstitium[15] (Plate 8-B). The specific diagnosis, however, is based on an appropriate history and the finding of trichina cysts within the diaphragm or tongue or both. Ventricular endocardial damage with superimposed thrombosis appears related to the associated eosinophilia (Plate 8-B).

Echinococcosis is acquired by humans by ingestion of the hexacanth embryo of the tapeworm *Echinococcus granulosus,* which penetrates the intes-

TABLE 57-1 Focal Myocarditis in Acute Leukemia[13]

Staphylococcus aureus	6
Pseudomonas sp.	7
Clostridium perfringens	2
Escherichia coli	1
Candida albicans	5
Mucor	2
Aspergillus sp.	2
Aspergillus sp. + *Candida* sp.	1
Cytomegalic inclusion disease	1
Toxoplasma gondii	2
Total	29 of 420 (7%)

tinal wall and enters the portal system. The hydatid cysts form most often in the liver (about 70 percent), next in the lung (about 20 percent), and rarely in the heart (about 1 percent). The left ventricular wall is the most frequent site in the heart, with epicardium next, right ventricle next, and atrial wall least commonly involved.[4] After invading the heart, the parasite grows rapidly; the resulting unilocular cyst compresses adjacent myocardium, causing atrophy or necrosis. Eventually the cyst dies, its wall becomes fibrotic with or without calcific deposits, and, unless strategically situated or large enough to cause mechanical difficulties, it produces no symptoms of cardiac dysfunction. The cysts vary in size from pinhead to grapefruit. Although they originate within the myocardial wall, cysts may project into a cardiac chamber or into the pericardial space; occasionally they may rupture into either. A foreign-body reaction consisting of multinucleated giant cells, macrophages, and eosinophils is frequently found in the adventitial wall of the cardiac cyst.

Many patients with fatal active infective endocarditis have foci of inflammation (microabscesses) associated with stainable organisms within the left ventricular myocardial wall[16] (Figure 57-6). These inflammatory foci appear to be embolic in origin, the result of dislodgment of a portion of a valvular vegetation with embolization to one or more small intramural coronary arteries. With rare exceptions, however, these inflammatory foci do not appear numerous enough or large enough to cause myocardial dysfunction.

Certain organisms tend to invade the walls of small arteries, specifically the intramural (intramyocardial) coronary arteries; after burrowing through the vascular walls, they produce an inflammatory reaction in the perivascular myocardium. Such organisms include *Pseudomonas;* certain fungi, particularly *Mucor* and *Aspergillus,* and occasionally *Candida* (Plate 8-C); and *Rickettsia rickettsii* (Rocky Mountain spotted fever).[13,17] A few organisms attack the myocardial cell itself, stimulating an adjacent inflammatory response. These organisms in-

FIGURE 57-2 Location of *Candida albicans* abscesses (dots) in a young man who died of leukemia. Clinically, evidence of myocardial dysfunction was not apparent. RA = right atrium; RV = right ventricle; LA = left atrium; LV = left ventricle.

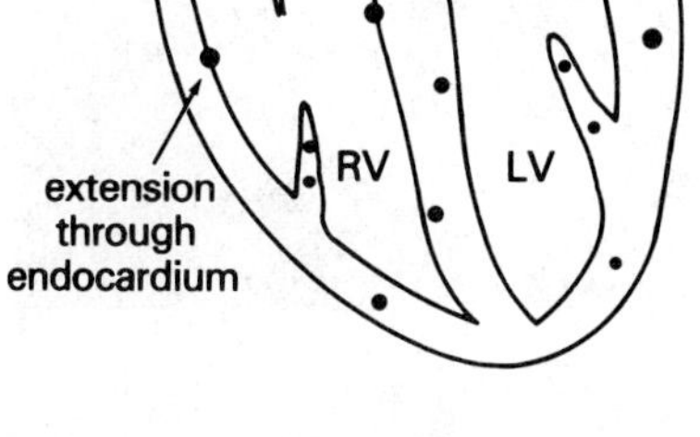

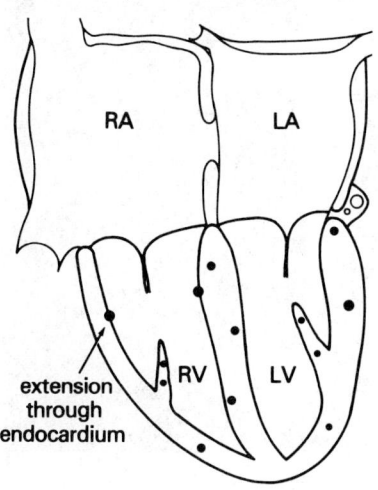

FIGURE 57-3 Serial ECGs from a 27-year-old man with acute lymphocytic leukemia and toxoplasmosis of the heart. His illness was characterized by paroxysmal arrhythmias (atrial fibrillation and atrial tachycardia). He died with ventricular fibrillation; *Toxoplasma gondii* organisms were found in myocardial cells. (*From W. C. Roberts, G. P. Bodey, and P. T. Wertlake, The Heart in Acute Leukemia. A Study of 420 Autopsy Cases, Am. J. Cardiol., 21:388, 1968. Reproduced with permission from the publisher and authors.*)

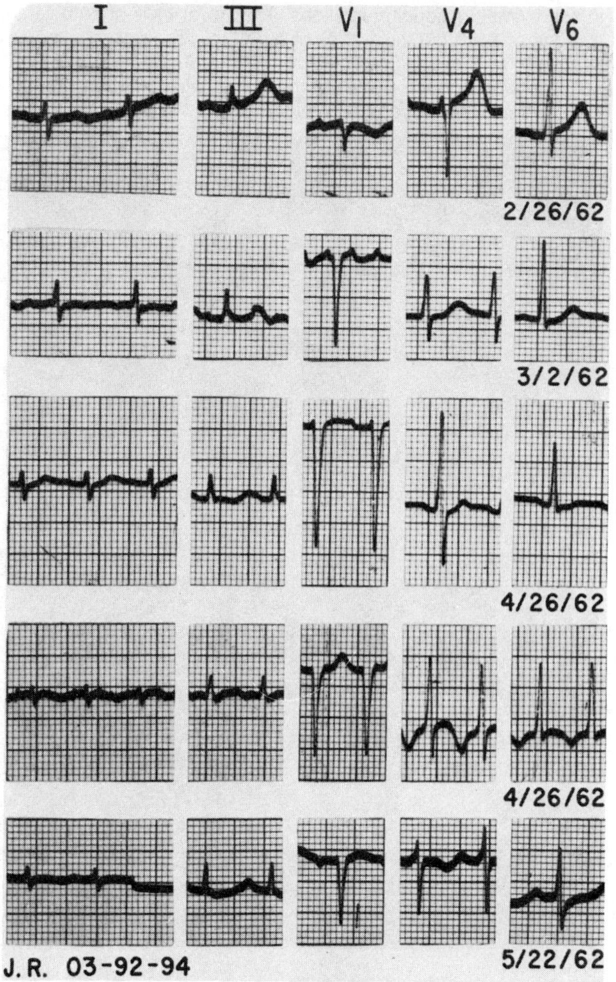

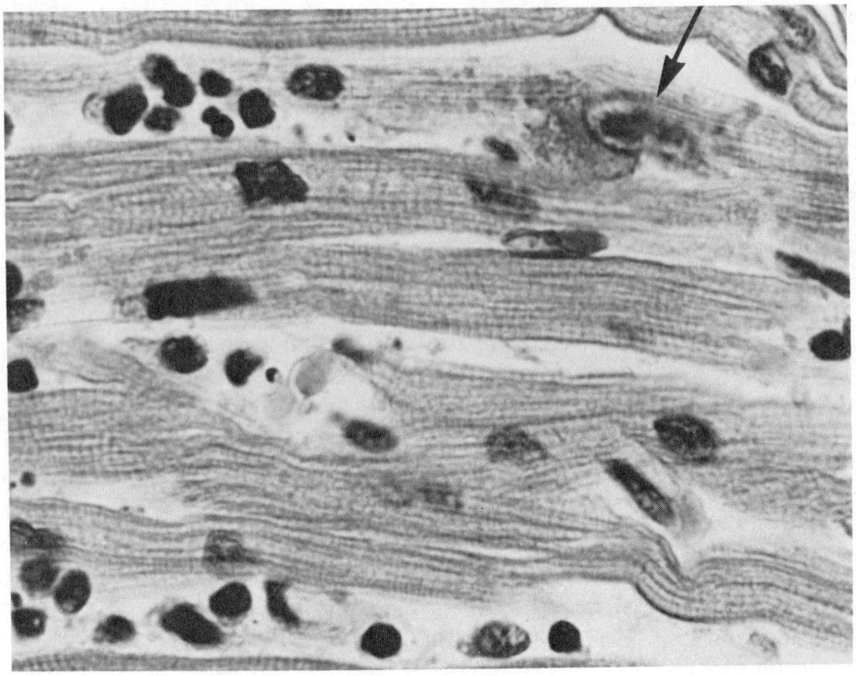

FIGURE 57-4 Cytomegalic inclusion disease of the heart. This 8-year-old girl with acute lymphocytic leukemia of 8 months duration had clear lung fields by chest roentgenogram 7 days before death. During the last 4 days of life she gained 3 kg in weight; and fever [to 41°C (105.2°F)], tachypnea (to 80 breaths per minute), pulmonary rales, and finally hypotension developed. ECG 24 h before death showed left bundle branch block; chest roentgenogram 30 min before death showed changes consistent with acute pulmonary edema. At necropsy, cytomegalic inclusion bodies were found in numerous organs, including the heart. Section of myocardium showing cytomegalic inclusion body (arrow) and surrounding acute inflammatory cells. (Hematoxylin and eosin; ×900 reduced by 14 percent.) (*From W. C. Roberts, G. P. Bodey, and P. T. Wertlake: The Heart in Acute Leukemia. A Study of 420 Autopsy Cases, Am. J. Cardiol., 21:388, 1968. Reproduced with permission from the publisher and authors.*)

FIGURE 57-5 Hearts of 2 patients who died from Chagas' disease. The anterior half of each specimen has been removed showing the four walls and cavities. *a.* The right side of the heart is more dilated than the left. Although there is scarring of the apical portions of each ventricle, no intracavitary thrombi, ventricular thrombi, or ventricular aneurysms are present. Weight is 350 g. *b.* Both ventricles are dilated to approximately equal proportions. The apical walls of both ventricles are extremely thinned and thrombi are present above the thinned portions of each ventricle. Weight is 560 g. [Specimens submitted to one of us (WCR) by Dr. Joao B. M. Janini, Chief of Pathology, University of Brasilia, Brasilia, Brazil. We are indebted to him for allowing us to study these patients.] (*From W. C. Roberts and V. J. Ferrans, Morphologic Observations in the Cardiomyopathies, in N. O. Fowler (ed.), Myocardial Disease, Grune & Stratton, Inc., New York, 1973. Reproduced by permission from the publisher and author.*)

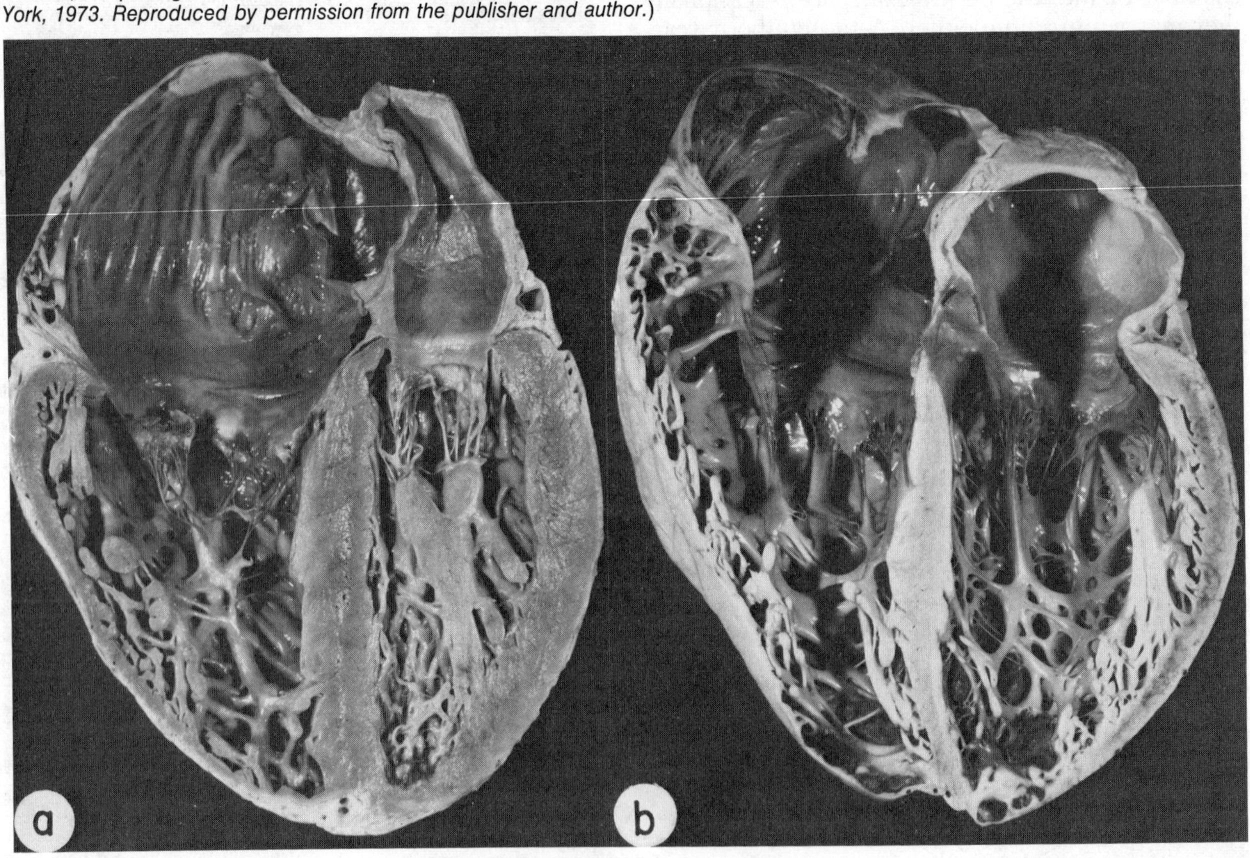

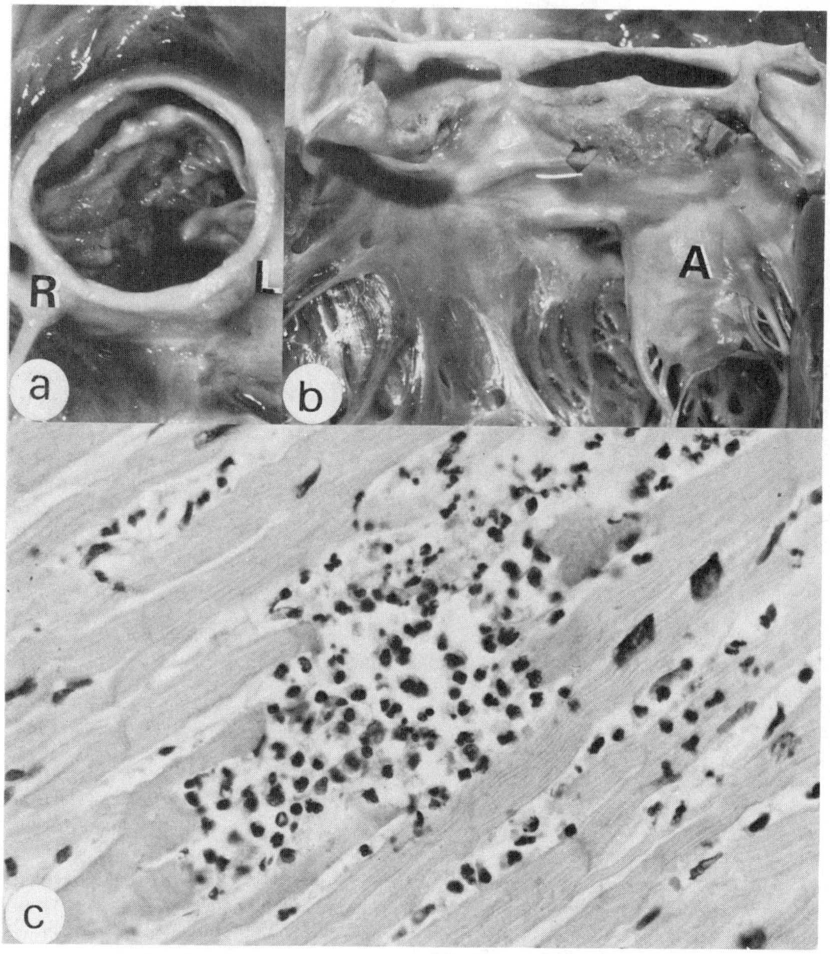

FIGURE 57-6 *Staphylococcus aureus* endocarditis involving a congenitally bicuspid aortic valve in a 55-year-old woman. She had never had symptoms of cardiac disease; chills, fever, and mental confusion appeared $4\frac{1}{2}$ months before death. Blood cultures were positive for *S. aureus*; penicillin, 40 million units per day intravenously for 4 weeks, followed by 24 million units per day intramuscularly for 2 weeks, was given. A grade 4/6 early diastolic blowing basal murmur appeared, and the diastolic blood pressure fell to 20 mmHg. Six days after penicillin was stopped she had a shaking chill and blood cultures were again positive for *S. aureus*. Over the next 3 months she was treated with various combinations of penicillin, methicillin, cephalothin, and vancomycin; each time antibiotics were withdrawn, blood cultures again grew *S. aureus*. Signs of congestive cardiac failure increased progressively, the diastolic blood pressure rose to 60 mmHg, and the aortic regurgitant murmur became almost inaudible several days before death. *a*. Bicuspid aortic valve viewed from above. Both the right (R) and left (L) coronary arteries arise from the anterior sinus. *b*. Opened aortic valve and left ventricle. Perforations are present in both cusps. A = anterior mitral leaflet. *c*. Histologic section showing microabscess in left ventricular wall. (Hematoxylin-eosin stain; ×400.) (*From W. C. Roberts, Characteristics and Consequence of Infective Endocarditis (Active or Healed or Both) Learned from Morphologic Studies, in S. H. Rahimtoola (ed.), "Infective Endocarditis," Grune & Stratton, Inc., New York, 1978, p. 55. Reproduced by permission from the publisher and author.*)

clude *Toxoplasma gondii* (Plate 8-A) and cytomegalic inclusion disease (Fig. 57-4).[13]

Gas gangrene (*Clostridium perfringens*) may involve cardiac striated muscle just as it does peripheral striated muscle. Gas bubbles, bordered by microorganisms without inflammatory response, replace large portions of the myocardial wall (Fig. 57-7). Many granulomatous diseases affect the myocardium, and all are associated with inflammatory cells (myocarditis). The most common is sarcoidosis; this condition is discussed in Chapter 58.

Sudden death occurred in a child who had no precordial murmur and who at autopsy had numerous mononuclear cells throughout the myocardial walls. In addition, small fibrin deposits and Anitschkow myocytes were observed on or in the mitral leaflets, and Aschoff bodies were present in the left atrial endocardium. Thus, acute rheumatic fever may be present with fulminating myocarditis, and the valvular involvement may be clinically silent.[18] Rheumatic myocarditis is discussed in Chapter 62.

Although rare, acute myocarditis may produce sudden death as the initial manifestation of an illness; such was the case in a 33-year-old man recently studied at necropsy (Fig. 57-8).

Pathophysiology

Virus replication in the heart may result in a temporary or permanent change in myocardial structure and function.[19] In viral myocarditis, the characteristic latent period between the acute systemic infection and the onset of clinical myocarditis strongly implicates activation of an autoimmune mechanism, possibly related to alteration of the myocardial cell by virus replication.[20]

Alternative explanations for viral myocarditis include direct cellular destruction by the virus or viral alteration of cellular energy systems. "Conditioning factors" such as hypoxemia, malnutrition, pregnancy, bacterial infection, ethanol intake, corticosteroid or immunosuppressive therapy, ionizing radiation, intensive exercise, and heat or cold stress, may facilitate the initial viral infection and/or activate latent or dormant viruses.[21]

Alteration of pulmonary or systemic vascular resistance during viral infections may compromise cardiac function; viral infections commonly also cause pericarditis, and less often valvulitis.

Some specific forms of myocarditis have characteristic pathophysiologic alterations. The diphtheria

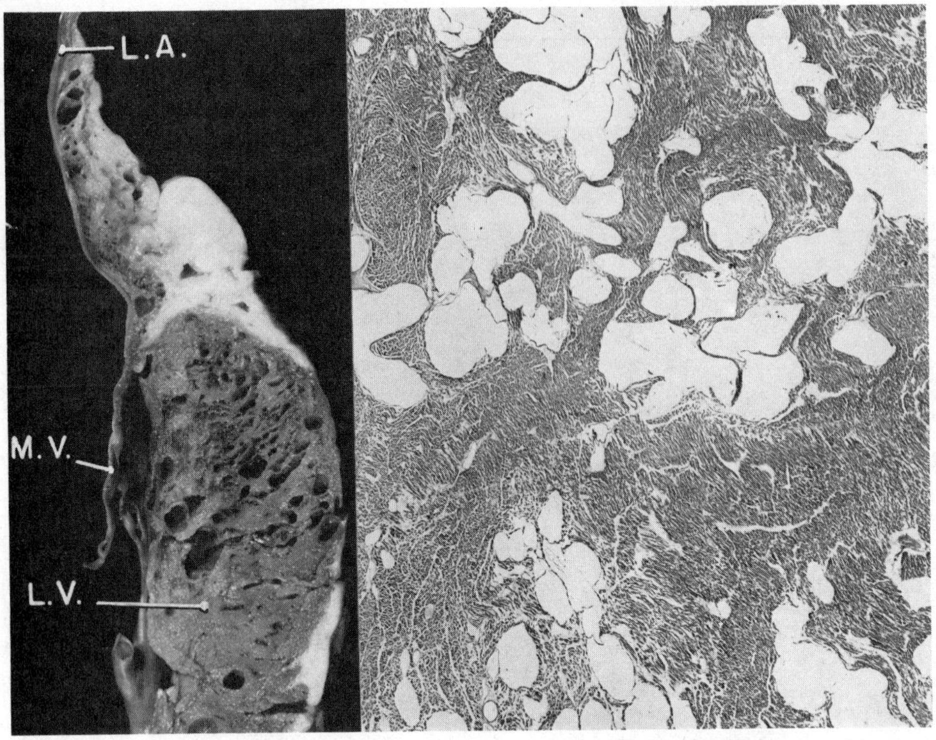

FIGURE 57-7 Gas gangrene of the myocardial wall in a 54-year-old man who had hemochromatosis and terminal *Clostridium perfringens* septicemia. *Left:* A cut section of the left atrium (LA), atrioventricular sulcus, posterior leaflet of mitral valve (MV), and left ventricle (LV). Numerous gas cysts are present in the myocardial walls of both atria and ventricles as well as in the adipose tissue of the atrioventricular sulcus. *Right:* Photomicrograph of section of left ventricular myocardium demonstrating the numerous gas cysts. (Hematoxylin and eosin stain; ×14.) (*From W. C. Roberts and C. W. Berard, Gas Gangrene of the Heart in Clostridial Septicemia, Am. Heart J., 74:482, 1967. Reproduced with permission from the publisher and authors.*)

FIGURE 57-8 Photomicrographs of portions of left ventricular myocardium from a 33-year-old man who suddenly died at home. He had been healthy until 3 weeks before death when he had an upper respiratory infection but continued his usual activities. At necropsy, the heart was of normal size but numerous inflammatory cells, mainly mononuclear and unassociated with microorganisms, were present in all sections of the myocardial wall. [Hematoxylin and eosin stains; ×220 (*left*), ×500 (*right*).]

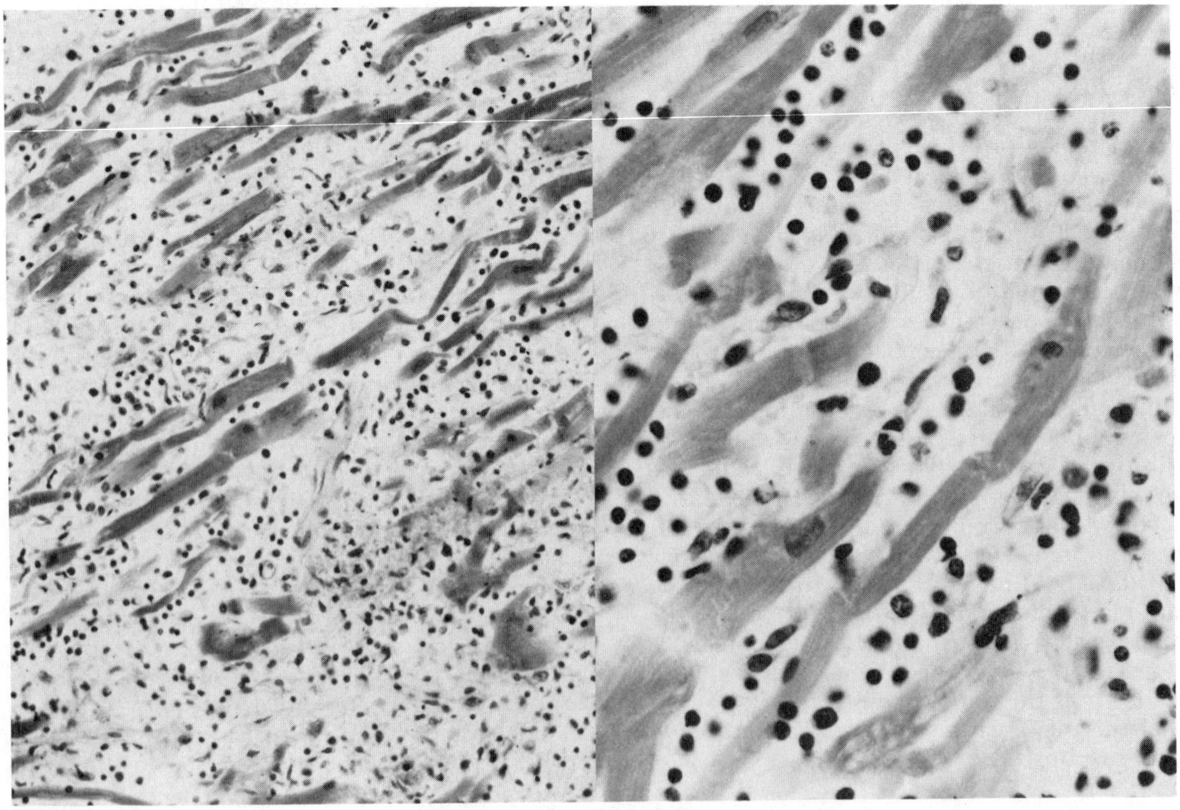

circulating endotoxin produces a disturbance of cellular respiration, apparently acting as a competitive analogue once the host's cytochrome b is depleted; thus, organs with high-energy requirements (heart, nerves, etc.) are first affected.[22] These alterations of cellular metabolism may result in electrocardiographic depolarization abnormalities, even without irreversible myocardial cell necrosis. Diphtheria toxin has a special affinity for the conduction system, and damage to this system is a prominent feature of diphtheritic myocarditis.

Because myocarditis generally involves both ventricles, the manifestations of right ventricular failure may predominate. Elevated ventricular diastolic pressures and volumes are often necessary to maintain even a low stroke volume when impairment of myocardial function is present. Any tachy- or bradyarrhythmia may compromise the stroke volume and further reduce cardiac output.

In acute Chagas' myocarditis, the triatome-transmitted trypanosomes multiply within the myofiber; myofiber rupture occasions the inflammatory response (Plate 8-D). The neurotoxic properties of *T. cruzi* are evident in the chronic myocarditis where the severe autonomic ganglion, cardiac nerve, and conduction system inflammation and degeneration contrasts with the mild muscle damage. This is the basis for the frequent conduction disturbances, tachyarrhythmias, and heart block; as well as impairment of autonomic control.[23]

In trichinosis, since the *Trichinella spiralis* larvae never encyst in the myocardium, the myocarditis has been postulated to be a nonspecific inflammatory manifestation of the larval invasion of the myocardium, a reaction to the death of the parasite, or a hypersensitivity or toxic response to *T. spiralis.*

Taenia echinococcus hexacanth embryos invade the myocardium via the coronary and/or lymphatic circulation. The pea-size to grapefruit-size pseudocyst which forms in the myocardium may produce surrounding muscle ischemia from compression, may interfere with heart valve function, or may impair conduction. Myocardial density, particularly in the ventricles, limits cyst growth and favors formation of daughter cysts. The cyst may rupture into a cardiac chamber or into the pericardium, depending on its location and the direction of least resistance. Cyst rupture is often evident as anaphylaxis, due to sensitization to hydatid protein.

Clinical Manifestations: General Considerations

Clinical manifestations are variable and probably depend on the extent and location of the myocardial inflammatory process, as well as the associated systemic illness. Patients may be asymptomatic, may have minimal to extreme manifestations of congestive heart failure, may have arrhythmias or conduction disturbances or both, or may have sudden death as their initial manifestation of the illness.[24,25]

The manifestations of the underlying systemic infection may overshadow cardiac symptoms and signs. On the other hand, increased preload and/or afterload secondary to the systemic disease may increase cardiac work and precipitate heart failure. Similarly, preexistent heart disease may lower the threshold for acute cardiac manifestations.

History

The typical clinical picture of myocarditis consists of fatigue, dyspnea, palpitations, and occasionally precordial discomfort. Although the chest pain is typically pleuropericardial, often reflecting the associated pericarditis, the combination of precordial discomfort and electrocardiographic abnormalities may be misinterpreted as myocardial infarction. Dizziness or syncope may be manifestations of arrhythmia. Recently, considerable emphasis has been placed on myalgia and peripheral muscle tenderness as presaging cardiac involvement in viral infections.[26] These early nonspecific symptoms occur during the first few weeks of a systemic infection. Symptoms of the systemic manifestations of the illness—nausea, vomiting, diarrhea, malaise, arthralgias, skin rash, upper respiratory tract symptoms, etc.—often mask the features of myocarditis, which may become evident only in early convalescence.

Physical Examination

The patient may or may not appear ill. There may be persistent fever, but the tachycardia is disproportionate to the degree of fever. This excessive tachycardia, both at rest and with effort, should alert the clinician to the diagnosis of myocarditis. Subsidence of the tachycardia or its responsiveness to digitalis therapy is clinical evidence of improvement of the myocarditis. Rarely, unexplained but profound bradycardia occurs.

In patients with viral infection who have dyspnea and pulmonary congestion, these symptoms are often attributed to viral pneumonia. Some of these patients have viral myocarditis, often manifesting biventricular failure. In the symptomatic patient with myocarditis, the heart is usually enlarged, hypotension is frequent with a narrow pulse pressure, and the murmurs of mitral and/or tricuspid insufficiency may be present; other findings include a faint first heart sound, distension of the neck veins, often loud atrial and ventricular gallop sounds, pulsus alternans, hepatomegaly, and peripheral edema.[27] Oliguria may be further evidence of the low cardiac output state. Pericardial or pleuropericardial rubs are common; when they occur in association with heart failure, myocarditis should be seriously considered. Supraventricular or ventricular arrhythmias are typical, and pulmonary or systemic embolization may be evident. Disturbances of conduction are frequent. Less commonly, the presentation in the patient with fulminant disease is one of circulatory collapse, progressing to clinical shock. Evidence of preexisting heart disease may make the diagnosis of superimposed myocarditis difficult.

The more diagnostic clinical manifestations of myocarditis rarely occur at the height of the infectious illness, but rather become evident during convalescence as the signs and symptoms of the systemic infection are subsiding. Not infrequently, the constitutional manifestations of the acute infectious disease overshadow the myocardial involvement, so that it may remain undetected or be recognized only by a late complication. Conversely, especially in viral infections, the systemic infection may be subclinical without abnormal physical findings and the myocarditis manifest as isolated arrhythmia, conduction disturbance, or heart failure, easily misdiagnosed as ischemic heart disease. In these latter patients, evidence of a systemic illness—fever, lymphadenopathy, cutaneous eruptions, pneumonitis, pleural effusion, muscle tenderness, or splenomegaly—may suggest the etiologic diagnosis.

Chest Roentgenogram

The chest roentgenogram is frequently abnormal. The cardiac silhouette may be enlarged from ventricular cavity dilatation or pericardial effusion or both. Evidence of interstitial pulmonary edema and/or prominence of the superior vena cava or azygos vein may be present with more severe myocardial involvement. This enlarged cardiac silhouette must be differentiated from pericardial effusion (see Chaps. 15 and 59).

Electrocardiogram

There are frequent but nonspecific electrocardiographic alterations: sinus tachycardia, atrial and ventricular rhythm disturbances, atrioventricular and ventricular conduction defects, low voltage, and ST-T abnormalities. Serious ventricular arrhythmias or cardiac arrest in a previously healthy young adult warrants evaluation for myocarditis.

Special Laboratory Tests

Routine Blood Tests

Mild to moderate leukocytosis may be present, with a variable preponderance of polymorphonuclear leukocytes or lymphocytes; the percentage of eosinophils may increase with recovery. Eosinophilia may indicate a parasitic infection. The erythrocyte sedimentation rate is typically elevated, and serial determinations help assess the clinical course and response to therapy. However, in some patients with marked hepatic congestion, the sedimentation rate may not be elevated. Elevation of cardiac serum enzymes—CK (creatine kinase), LDH (lactic dehydrogenase), and SGOT (glutamic oxaloacetic transaminase)—will vary with the extent of myocardial necrosis. Serial determinations of enzymes and isoenzymes may help assess progression or subsidence of the myocarditis.

Other Tests for Infective Agents

Laboratory tests to define the etiologic agent are recommended for all patients, although a specific etiologic agent is not often found. Blood cultures, aerobic and anaerobic, can identify many bacterial pathogens. Acute and convalescent serum titers can identify *Mycoplasma pneumoniae* and antistreptolysin titer can indicate a streptococcal infection.

Infectious mononucleosis (Monospot test and Epstein-Barr viral antibody titers), hepatitis (surface antigen), etc., can be identified by appropriate studies. Urine and serum tests can establish cytomegalovirus infection. Acute and convalescent (2 to 6 weeks after illness) serum samples can define recent viral infection by a fourfold or greater rise in virus-neutralizing antibody, complement-fixing antibody, and hemagglutination-inhibiting antibody titers to specific viruses; however, this only suggests that viral infection is the etiology of the myocarditis.

Throat washings, feces, and urine should be cultured for viruses, as should pericardial or pleural fluid if obtained. The routine availability of diagnostic viral laboratory tests should enable identification of specific forms of viral myocarditis; however, virus recovery is usually possible only during the initial phase of the illness. This is a prerequisite for the development of special viral vaccines (as for rubella), of viricidal drugs, of interferon-inducers, etc.[21]

Skin Tests

Skin testing is valuable to identify tuberculosis as a potential etiology of the myocarditis, particularly the development of a positive skin test.

Echocardiography

This simple noninvasive procedure is most valuable to help evaluate chamber size and left ventricular function, initially and serially (Fig. 57-9). It may reveal significant chamber enlargement, notwithstanding a normal roentgenographic silhouette. It allows identification of pericardial effusion, and can readily be performed at the bedside of an acutely ill patient. It may also help exclude other forms of heart disease, particularly preexisting valvular heart disease. However, transient regional wall motion abnormalities may simulate myocardial infarction. A recent report described correlation of the wall motion abnormalities with the severity of the disease and electrocardiographic T-wave abnormalities.[27a] Serial echocardiograms may help guide the subsequent management of the patient.

Nuclear Imaging of the Heart

Radionuclide ventriculography can also assess ventricular function and wall motion, features that can be followed serially to document the impact of the

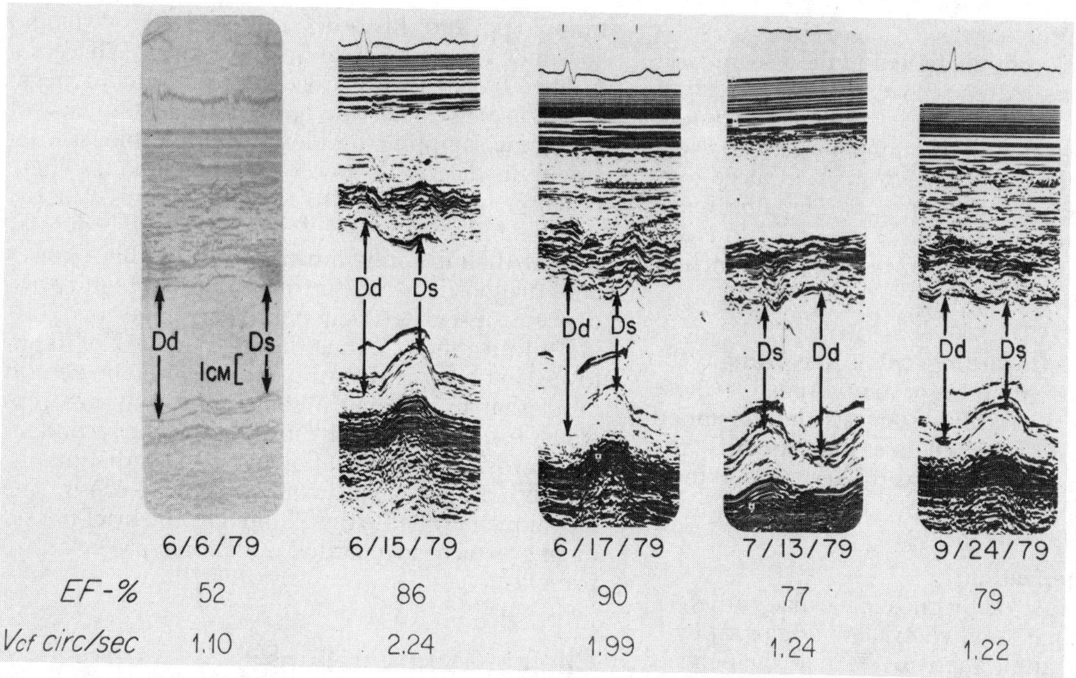

FIGURE 57-9 Serial M-mode echocardiograms from a 34-year-old male with acute viral myocarditis who presented with cardiogenic shock. The first study shows hypokinesis of the posterior wall of the left ventricle. Nine days later, movement of the posterior wall is normal. Dd = left ventricular end-diastolic diameter; Ds = left ventricular end-systolic diameter; EF = ejection fraction (normal, 55 percent); Vcf = mean velocity of circumferential fiber shortening (normal, 1.29 ± 0.23 circ/sec).

infection upon ventricular function (Fig. 57-10). It is increasingly recognized that acute myocarditis may not only present with classical biventricular global dysfunction, but may manifest regional hypokinesis or dyskinesis, especially at the apex. Furthermore, involvement may favor only one ventricle. Myocardial imaging with ^{99m}Tc pyrophosphate or gallium may reveal uptake in some patients with myocarditis as evidence of diffuse or focal myocardial necrosis or inflammation; whereas a positive test appears of diagnostic value, a negative one is not; the sensitivity and specificity of a positive test require validation.[27b]

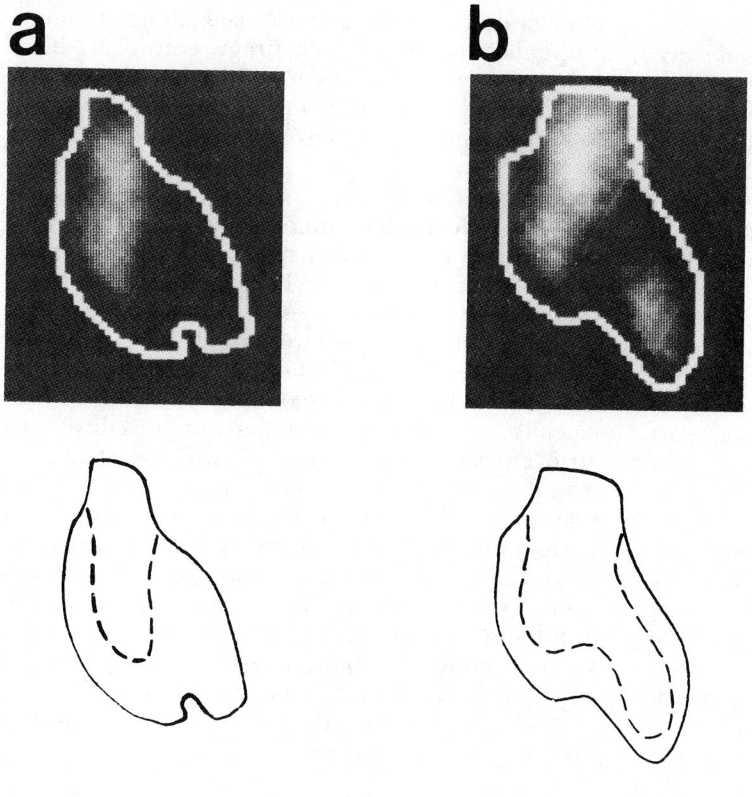

FIGURE 57-10 Modified left anterior oblique view of two radionuclide ventriculograms from a 20-year-old male who presented with acute viral pericarditis and developed congestive heart failure 1 month later. *a.* The normal study (ejection fraction 60 percent) was done when the patient developed pericarditis. *b.* A study done at the time of congestive heart failure shows a dilated left ventricle with an ejection fraction of 20 percent and apical, lateral, and inferior wall akinesis. There is also systolic bulging of the apex. The broken lines in the drawings refer to end systole. The solid lines refer to end diastole.

Exercise Testing
This procedure is contraindicated in the patient with acute myocarditis. After recovery, however, serial exercise testing can document residual functional impairment, help define recommended activity levels, and may identify treatable exercise-induced dysrhythmia. Some patients with apparent subsidence of myocarditis may have chest pain, rhythm disturbances, and evidence of myocardial dysfunction for many months.

Continuous Electrocardiographic Recording
In patients with symptoms of arrhythmia or whose etiology of the myocarditis suggests the likelihood of arrhythmia, this procedure may identify the rhythm disturbance and assess the response to therapy.

Cardiac Catheterization
The principal role of diagnostic cardiac catheterization and coronary and ventricular angiography—other than the application to the management of severe heart failure and cardiogenic shock—lies in the differential diagnosis of remediable pericardial, congenital, coronary, or valvular heart disease. Hemodynamically, myocarditis is usually characterized by biventricular pump failure, with low cardiac output, elevated filling pressures, increased ventricular volumes, and decreased ejection fraction. However, in the presence of fever, anemia, or tachycardia, cardiac output and ejection fraction may be normal or even increased. Furthermore, there may be evidence of impaired diastolic function.

Endomyocardial Biopsy (See Chap. 108)
More than 20 years have elapsed since Sakakibara and Konno[28] introduced the bioptome for transvenous biopsy of the right ventricular endomyocardium. This method has become well established as the safest approach to cardiac biopsy and can be used also transarterially for biopsy of the left ventricle. This technique has been applied increasingly to aid in the diagnosis of myocarditis, especially in patients who present with congestive heart failure or serious ventricular arrhythmias of recent onset, without evidence of coronary or valvular heart disease.[29,30] To date the sensitivity and specificity of this diagnostic technique have not been established.

Histopathologic evidence of inflammatory heart muscle disease has been reported in 1 to 25 percent of patients with dilated, congestive cardiomyopathy so studied.[29–34] Comparable abnormal biopsies have, however, also been obtained from patients who presented with arrhythmias and conduction disturbances rather than heart failure. Thus far, examination of biopsy tissue has generally been limited to histopathology and electron microscopy. Viruses are cultured only rarely from biopsy specimens, in part because biopsy is likely to be performed after the short period of viral replication in heart muscle. Immunologic and histochemical analyses of biopsy specimens remain research procedures. Whereas a positive biopsy is of great diagnostic value, a negative biopsy does not rule out myocarditis, in view of the great sampling problem. Multiple biopsies increase the diagnostic power of this technique. There remains uncertainty as to what constitutes a biopsy positive for myocarditis.[34a] Whereas some consider greater than five inflammatory cells per high-power field diagnostic of myocarditis,[33] others require evidence of associated degenerative changes or "fraying" of myofibers.[32] In addition to the lack of definitive criteria for myocarditis, it must also be kept in mind that myocardial inflammation may not represent infectious myocarditis, but may be secondary to necrosis of other etiology, e.g., radiation, ischemia, collagen vascular disease, or sarcoidosis. The technique may be further limited by the brief period during which myocardial inflammatory cells are present.

Clinical Manifestations: Specific Forms of Myocarditis

Diphtheria

Myocarditis, which occurs in 10 to 25 percent of patients with diphtheria, is the major cause of death from this infection.

Clinical Manifestations
The earliest cardiovascular symptoms are not related to myocarditis but to toxemia and respiratory obstruction; hypoxia is due to membrane formation and edema in the oropharynx. The early findings of myocarditis include tachycardia, faint heart sounds, and gallop rhythm, which progress to overt heart failure and circulatory collapse. Complete heart block may develop. The circulatory collapse is due both to the vasomotor paralysis and the myocarditis.

Laboratory Examination
Electrocardiographic abnormalities and elevated serum levels of cardiac enzymes may be the earliest evidence of myocarditis. ST-T electrocardiographic changes, the first evidence of acute myocarditis, usually appear in the second week of illness; conduction abnormalities, especially bundle branch block, follow (Fig. 57-11). The development of bundle branch block is associated with a 50 percent mortality.[35] An atrioventricular conduction disturbance, characteristically complete heart block, is an ominous sign that warns of incipient congestive heart failure and peripheral circulatory failure; an 80 to 100 percent mortality rate is reported among patients who develop complete heart block. Most electrocardiographic abnormalities regress in survivors within several months, although occasionally partial to complete heart block may persist. Marked elevation of the serum transaminase levels likewise signals a poor prognosis.

Coxsackie B Myocarditis

Viral infection of the heart is not infrequent and Coxsackievirus is the most common etiologic agent.

Clinical Manifestations

In infancy, Coxsackie B myocarditis, often fatal in nursery epidemics, is an acute fulminating illness with fever, respiratory distress, cyanosis, extreme tachycardia or arrhythmia, cardiac dilatation, congestive heart failure, and circulatory collapse. Gallop rhythm is common, and murmurs are rare.

Typically, acute Coxsackie myopericarditis is a benign disease in the adult. On the other hand, severe Coxsackie B myopericarditis, often with pleurodynia, is reported with increasing frequency; fever, arrhythmias, severe congestive heart failure, and pericarditis with effusion are common. Heart block, shock, and/or sudden death may occur. The disease occurs more commonly in men; the pain and electrocardiographic abnormalities may mimic myocardial infarction.[36]

Laboratory Examination

Viral involvement of the AV node has been implicated as the cause of the arrhythmias and electrocardiographic abnormalities. ST-segment displacement occurs frequently, and T-wave abnormalities and low voltage may also be present.

Cardiac enzyme levels may be elevated, and there is often cardiac enlargement on the chest x-ray. Echocardiography best demonstrates the contribution of a pericardial effusion to the cardiac enlargement; it also may reveal chamber enlargement not evident roentgenographically and permits detection and quantification of left ventricular dysfunction. Radionuclide ventriculography may also be valuable. Viral confirmation is best done by isolation from blood or urine, or from throat or rectal swabs; antibody titer determinations require acute and convalescent sera.[5]

Echovirus Myocarditis

Clinical Manifestations

In the adult, symptomless myocarditis is characteristically associated with myalgia, and an electrocardiogram is recommended for patients with this symptom.[26] Nursery infections are typically more severe. In the symptomatic patient, tachycardia and tachypnea may progress to arrhythmias, evidence of pericarditis, heart failure, and occasional cardiovascular collapse.

Laboratory Examination

Variable conduction abnormalities, arrhythmias, and abnormalities mimicking myocardial infarction may be noted in the electrocardiogram (Fig. 57-12); cardiac enlargement may be evident on chest x-ray, with echocardiography differentiating this from pericardial effusion. The virus may be isolated from urine, throat, or stool. A fourfold increase in serum antibody neutralizing titers is diagnostic.

Acute Chagas' Disease (South American Trypanosomiasis)[23]

Clinical Manifestations

Acute Chagas' disease, most common in early childhood, is characteristically asymptomatic and unrecognized. Patients with chronic Chagas' disease often deny a prior acute illness. A chagoma, or swelling at the site of entry of the parasite, may suggest the diagnosis, as may characteristic unilateral palpebral edema (Romana's sign) on the side of the facial lesion. Fever, sweating, muscular pain, diarrhea, and vomiting occur. Some patients also develop tachycardia, cardiomegaly, congestive heart failure, or nonspecific electrocardiographic changes, but arrhythmias are notably absent.

Laboratory Examination

The diagnosis can be confirmed by a positive blood smear or the more sensitive xenodiagnostic study; xenodiagnosis consists of allowing laboratory-bred, parasite-free triatomes to feed upon the patient's forearm and ingest and concentrate the parasites in their feces, where they are identified. Complement-fixation tests are usually positive after 6 weeks.

Chronic Chagas' Disease[23]

Clinical Manifestations

The clinical presentation of chronic Chagas' myocarditis is one of insidious, progressive cardiac enlargement, initially asymptomatic, but eventually resulting in protracted congestive heart failure. Associated fever, tachycardia, frequent arrhythmias, anemia, hypertension, or preexisting heart disease may lower the threshold for heart failure. Mitral and tricuspid insufficiency usually become evident and pulmonary embolization is common. An abnormal left ventricular impulse may reflect the frequent apical aneurysm formation.[37] Precordial pain may be present. Fixed splitting of the second heart sound, due to right bundle branch block, is frequent. Complete heart block, high-grade ventricular ectopy, and atrial fibrillation have a grave prognostic significance, both aggravating the congestive heart failure and predisposing to sudden cardiac death.

Laboratory Examination

Confirmatory laboratory evidence includes a positive Machado-Guerreiro complement-fixation reaction and a positive xenodiagnostic study. A circulating antibody (EVI), which appears to have high clinical specificity, can be demonstrated by immunofluorescent techniques to react with endocardium, vascular structures, and interstitium of striated muscle in 95 percent of patients with Chagas' heart

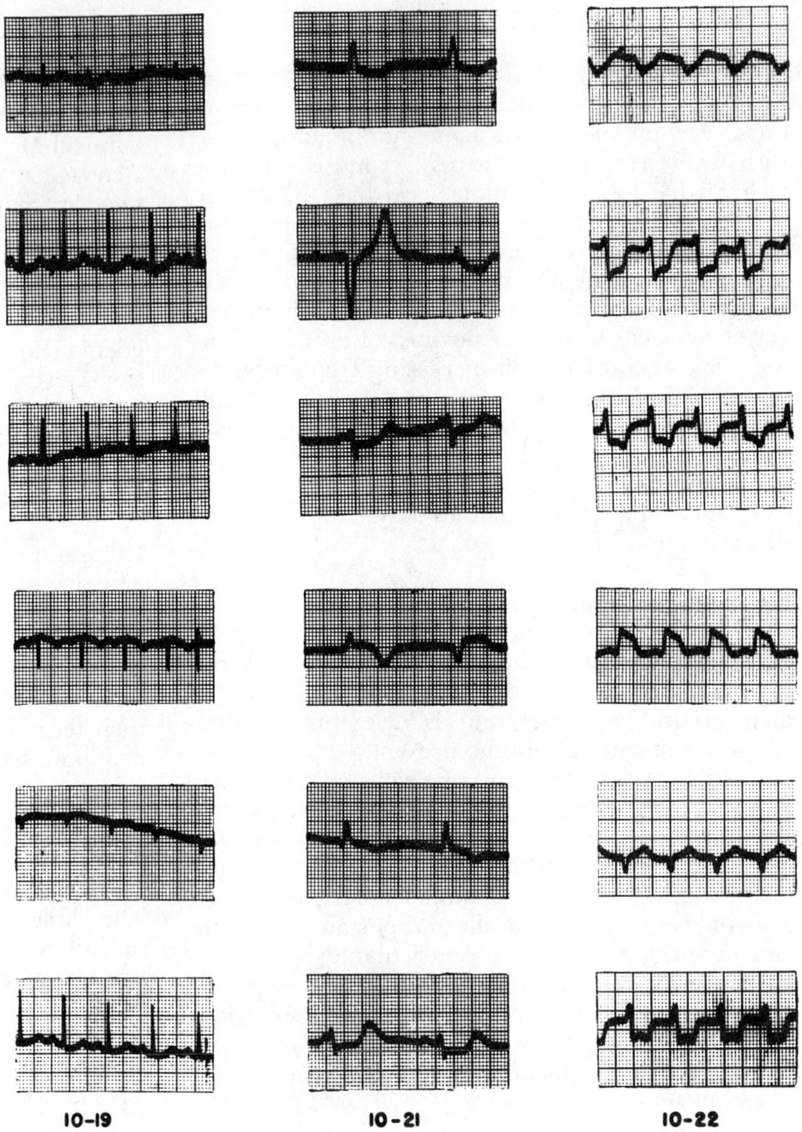

FIGURE 57-11 Fatal diphtheritic myocarditis in an 8-year-old girl. 10-19, sinus tachycardia; 10-21, complete heart block, multiple ectopic ventricular beats, marked ST-T changes; 10-22, no P waves seen, rapid tachycardia with marked alteration in QRS contour, and profound ST-T changes. *A.* Extremity leads. *B.* Precordial leads (*facing page*).

A

disease and in 45 percent of asymptomatic individuals with *Trypanosoma cruzi* infection.[38]

Electrocardiographic abnormalities occur in 87 percent of patients with chronic Chagas' disease and are often the initial manifestation of illness. Right bundle branch block with a superiorly oriented QRS axis is the most common electrocardiographic abnormality, encountered in over 50 percent of patients. Arrhythmias, atrioventricular block, conduction defects, and abnormalities of the P and T waves are common. Conduction system dysfunction is evident early in the course of the disease, even before patients become symptomatic.

Arrhythmias, especially ventricular extrasystoles, may be provoked by effort; the appearance of ventricular premature beats on the exercise electrocardiogram in Chagas' myocarditis has a diagnostic value similar to ST segment displacement in coronary atherosclerotic heart disease. Chronotropic incompetence is also described, even in asymptomatic patients, and may reflect the autonomic dysfunction of Chagas' disease.[38a]

Characteristic abnormalities of left ventricular wall motion, seen at ventriculography, reflect anteroapical aneurysm formation;[39] apical aneurysm and dyskinesis can also be detected by two-dimensional echocardiography.[40]

Trichinosis

Clinical Manifestations

The diagnosis of trichinosis should be considered in any patient with periorbital edema and marked muscle tenderness, even without a history of pork

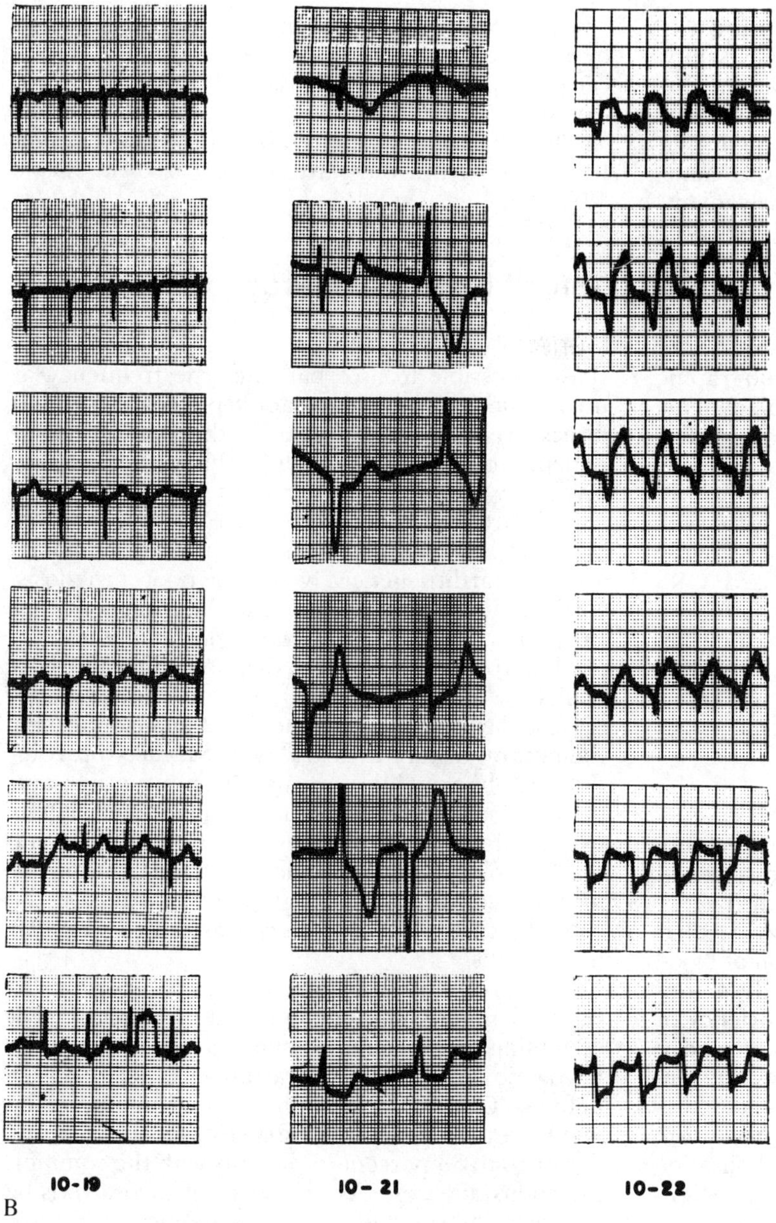

B

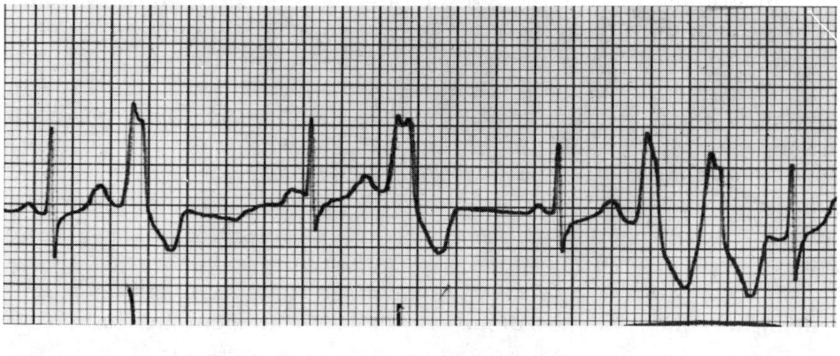

FIGURE 57-12 Lead II rhythm strip from a 16-year-old male, taken 3 months after Echovirus 11 viral myocarditis, showing persistent frequent premature ventricular beats with occasional couplets.

ingestion. Cardiac complications appear in the second or third week of illness, as systemic symptoms are abating.[41] Dyspnea, cardiac enlargement, substernal pain, tachycardia, arrhythmia, and congestive heart failure may, at times, mimic the presentation of myocardial infarction. Cardiac manifestations, concomitant with cerebral involvement, become maximal in the fourth to eighth week of illness and subsequently subside.

Laboratory Examination
Eosinophilia is characteristic. Skeletal muscle biopsy may be diagnostic. Transient electrocardiographic abnormalities occur in about one-third of patients with trichinosis, often in the absence of cardiac symptoms. They parallel other evidence of myocarditis, appearing in the second or third week of illness, being most pronounced at about the sixth week and gradually disappearing. Nonspecific T-wave changes are most frequent, with decreased QRS voltage, ventricular premature beats, and conduction abnormalities also observed. The electrocardiogram may mimic that of myocardial infarction.[42]

Echinococcosis

Clinical Manifestations
In an endemic area, the diagnosis of cardiac echinococcosis should be suggested by the presence of echinococcus cysts elsewhere in the body, the history of an anaphylactic shock syndrome, and a peculiar cardiac murmur probably due to obstruction of blood flow by a large cyst.[43] Other cardiac manifestations include chest pain due to coronary insufficiency or pericarditis, tachycardia, palpitations, congestive heart failure, and Stokes-Adams syncope due to atrioventricular conduction abnormalities.

The first symptoms of intracardiac cyst rupture may be due to pulmonary or cerebral embolization of the daughter cysts; either of these complications may result in sudden death. Cyst rupture may result in acute pericarditis with tamponade,[44] with the late complication of constrictive disease.

Laboratory Examination
Eosinophilia is common, as is a positive intradermal (Casoni) reaction and a complement-fixation titer. A bizarre and often calcified cardiac shadow is present on the chest roentgenogram. Electrocardiographic ST-T ischemic changes (due to cyst compression of surrounding heart muscle) are particularly evident in the precordial leads and may localize an echinococcal cyst prior to surgery. Occasional P-wave changes have been reported with atrial cysts, and atrioventricular block has been documented with septal cysts. Arrhythmias and conduction abnormalities are not unusual. Electrocardiographic abnormalities may be reversible following excision of a cardiac echinococcal cyst.

Angiocardiographic examination delineates the cyst and confirms the diagnosis;[11] coronary arteriography may further aid in cyst localization. Echocardiography may also identify a hydatid cyst by location and appearance.[45]

Clinical features and therapy for the less common forms of myocarditis are summarized in Table 57-2.

Natural History and Prognosis

General Considerations

It is impossible to ascertain the true frequency of myocarditis, because most adult patients with mild disease recover spontaneously; the percentage of patients that blend into "idiopathic dilated cardiomyopathy" is not known. Patients who present with large hearts and heart failure have an unpredictable but generally poor prognosis. Diphtheritic and Chagas' myocarditis generally have a poor prognosis. Myocarditis in infancy and childhood and during pregnancy is often a fulminant and fatal illness.

Myocarditis is difficult to diagnose clinically, particularly when mild and without impairment of cardiovascular function; thus neither the incidence nor the natural history is clearly defined. Electrocardiographic abnormalities are usually nonspecific, and the bacteriologic, biochemical, and immunologic tests used to identify the causative organisms are of value only when positive. As previously stated, it is uncommon to identify the etiology of myocarditis in the sporadic case, and such cases are termed *idiopathic* myocarditis.

Myocarditis, as diagnosed by areas of focal or diffuse inflammation, is encountered in 1 to 5 percent of routine postmortem examinations; however, even histologic criteria for myocarditis are not precisely defined. Electrocardiographic abnormalities, in the absence of other clinical evidence of myocarditis, occur in 10 to 33 percent of patients with the common infectious diseases. The diagnosis of myocarditis by this criterion depends on the frequency of electrocardiographic recordings, particularly during convalescence. Infectious myocarditis, as diagnosed by electrocardiogram, other noninvasive studies, or histologic abnormalities[46] is encountered during a systemic infection in many patients who present trivial or no clinical evidence of cardiovascular involvement.

Although the outlook is generally favorable and most patients recover rapidly, a significant number have recurrent or chronic myocarditis, and some patients succumb to a fulminant acute illness. Indeed, acute myocarditis is not an unusual cause of sudden death in young adults (Fig. 57-8).[24,25] Prior acute myocarditis[46] or chronic recurrent infectious myocarditis is a possible cause of chronic cardiomyopathy[47–49] and has also been implicated as a cause of postinfectious asthenia. Some patients with apparent idiopathic dilated cardiomyopathy have evidence of myocardial viral antigens by fluorescent

TABLE 57-2 Rarer Forms of Myocarditis

Etiology	Distinctive Features: Physical Examination	Distinctive Features: Laboratory	Distinctive Features: Morphological Manifestations	Specific Therapy*	Reference
Bacterial					
Diphtheria	See text	See text	See text	See text	—
Tuberculosis	Arrhythmias	Arrhythmias	Tubercles with caseation	Isoniazid, plus rifampin, plus ethambutol or streptomycin	Claiborne, *Am. J. Cardiol.*, 33:920, 1974
Typhoid fever (*Salmonella*)	Early: peripheral circulatory collapse; ? endotoxin effect Late: congestive heart failure	—	Coronary arteritis Abscesses	Chloramphenicol Vasopressor drugs	Diem, *Am. J. Trop. Med. Hyg.*, 23:218, 1974
Scarlet fever Rheumatic fever	—	—	Valve lesions Aschoff bodies	Penicillin G Salicylates Corticosteroid hormones	Ewy, *Am. Heart J.*, 78:259, 1969
Meningococcemia	Circulatory collapse	Disseminated intravascular coagulation	Petechiae	Penicillin Isoproterenol	Denmark, *Arch. Intern. Med.*, 127:238, 1971
Infective endocarditis	—	—	Valve vegetations Microabscesses	Depends on specific etiology	Roberts, *Cardiovasc. Med.*, 3:699, 1978
Staphylococcal Pneumococcal Gonococcal infection	—	—	Abscesses Valve vegetations	Antistaphylococcal penicillin (staph) Penicillin G (pneumo) Penicillin G (gono)	—
Clostridial infection	—	—	Air cysts with organisms in wall	Penicillin G	Roberts, *Am. Heart J.*, 74:482, 1967
Psittacosis (*Chlamydia psittaci*)	—	—	Psittacosis inclusion bodies in plasma cells	Tetracycline	Sutton, *Am. Heart J.*, 81:597, 1971
Chlamydia trachomatis	Heart failure	—	—	Tetracycline, erythromycin	Grayston, *JAMA*, 246:2823, 1981
Brucellosis	—	—	—	Tetracycline plus streptomycin	Buczynska-Hencner, *Pol. Tyg. Lek.*, 20:761, 1966
Actinomycosis	—	—	Abscesses with actinomycotic granules	Penicillin G or tetracycline	Edwards, *Am. J. Dis. Child.*, 41:1419, 1931
Tetanus	—	—	Nerve cell degeneration	Penicillin G Tetanus antitoxin Propranolol	Murphy, *Med. J. Aust.*, 2:542, 1970
Tularemia	—	—	—	Streptomycin	—
Meliodosis	Mimic AMI	Mimic AMI	Abscesses	Tetracycline plus streptomycin	Baumann, *Ann. Intern. Med.*, 67:836, 1967
Legionnaires' disease	Heart failure	—	—	Erythromycin	Gross, *Chest*, 79:232, 1981
Spirochetal					
Syphilis	Arrhythmias, heart block Conduction abnormalities		Gumma	Penicillin G	Boss, *Ann. Intern. Med.*, 55:824, 1961
Leptospirosis	Valve "pseudostenosis" Arrhythmias	Arrhythmias	Focal hemorrhage Edema Necrosis	Penicillin G Tetracycline	Nusynowitz, *Hawaii Med. J.*, 23:41, 1963

*With appreciation to Dr. Jonas A. Shulman, Professor of Medicine (Infectious Diseases), Emory University School of Medicine, for review of drug therapy.

Notes: (—) indicates no distinctive physical findings, laboratory data, or morphologic manifestations other than heart failure and nonspecific cardiac enlargement; or no specific therapy. References for diseases discussed in text cited at end of chapter.

TABLE 57-2 Rarer Forms of Myocarditis (*continued*)

	Distinctive Features				
Etiology	**Physical Examination**	**Laboratory**	**Morphological Manifestations**	**Specific Therapy***	**Reference**
Spirochetal (*continued*)					
Relapsing fever	Vasoconstriction Hypotension Heart failure Conduction abnormalities, arrhythmias	Conduction abnormalities, arrhythmias	—	Tetracycline Penicillin	Judge, *Arch. Pathol.*, 97:136, 1974
Lyme disease	—	Conduction abnormalities Complete heart block	—	Penicillin Tetracycline ± Prednisone	Steere, *Ann. Intern. Med.*, 93:8, 1980
Rickettsial					
Typhus	—	—	Vasculitis	Tetracycline or chloramphenicol	Woodward, *Ann. Intern. Med.*, 53:1130, 1960
Rocky Mountain spotted fever	Hypovolemia, hypotension Peripheral vascular collapse	—	Vasculitis	Colloid Tetracycline or chloramphenicol	Walker, *Arch. Pathol. Lab. Med.*, 104:171, 1980
Q fever	—	—	—	Tetracycline	Barraclough, *Br. Med. J.*, 2:423, 1975
Viral					
Coxsackie B	See text	See text	See text	See text	—
Echovirus	See text	See text	See text	See text	—
Poliomyelitis	Pulmonary edema Vascular collapse	—	—	Tracheostomy Oxygen Vasopressor drugs	Trimbos, *Folia Med. Neerl.*, 1963, p. 49
Influenza	Peripheral circulatory failure Arrhythmias, complete heart block	Arrhythmias, complete heart block	Myofiber necrosis	Pacemaker ? Amantadine for influenza A	Verel, *Am. Heart J.*, 92:290, 1976
Mumps	—	Complete heart block	—	—	Arita, *Br. Heart J.*, 46:342, 1981
Infectious mononucleosis (virus Epstein-Barr)	—	—	Abnormal perivascular lymphocytes	Corticosteroid hormones	Hudgins, *JAMA*, 235:2626, 1976
Viral hepatitis	—	—	—	—	Bell, *JAMA*, 218:387, 1971
Rubella	Congestive heart failure	ECG: mimic AMI	Extensive myocardial vacuolation necrosis	—	Ainger, *Cardiol. Dig.*, 2:21, 1967
Rubeola	Pericarditis Arrhythmias	—	—	—	Guistra, *AMA J. Dis. Child.*, 79:487, 1950
Rabies	—	—	—	Vaccine	Roux, *Coeur Med. Intern.*, 15:37, 1976
Varicella	—	Bundle branch block Arrhythmia	Eosinophilic intranuclear inclusion bodies	—	Fiddler, *Br. Heart J.*, 39:1150, 1977
Mycoplasma pneumoniae	Myalgia	ECG: mimic AMI Arrhythmias	—	Erythromycin	Ponka, *Acta. Med. Scand.*, 206:77, 1979
Lymphocytic choriomeningitis	—	—	—	—	Thiede, *Arch. Intern. Med.*, 109:104, 1962
Viral encephalitis	—	—	—	—	Ungar, *Am. J. Clin. Pathol.*, 18:48, 1948
Herpes simplex	—	—	—	? Adenine arabinoside	Bell, *Am. Heart J.*, 74:309, 1967
Cytomegalovirus	—	—	Intranuclear inclusion bodies	—	Wilson, *Br. Heart J.*, 34:865, 1972

TABLE 57-2 Rarer Forms of Myocarditis (*continued*)

	Distinctive Features				
Etiology	**Physical Examination**	**Laboratory**	**Morphological Manifestations**	**Specific Therapy***	**Reference**
Viral (*continued*)					
Variola	—	—	—	—	—
Herpes zoster	—	—	—	? Acyclovir	—
Adenovirus infection	—	—	—	—	Henson, *Am. J. Dis. Child.*, 121:334, 1971
Arbovirus infection	Arrhythmias Heart failure	Arrhythmias	—	—	Obeyesekere, *Am. Heart J.*, 85:186, 1973
Respiratory syncytial virus	—	—	—	—	Giles: *JAMA*, 236:1128, 1976
Viral hemorrhagic fever	Shock	—	Myocardial hemorrhage	—	Milei, *Am. Heart J.*, 104:1385, 1982
Mycotic					
Blastomycosis	—	—	Tubercle with caseation and giant cells	Amphotericin B	Baker, *Am. J. Pathol.*, 13:139, 1937
Candidiasis	Debilitated or immunosuppressed host	ECG: Bundle branch block, AV block, mimic AMI	Multiple abscesses with pseudohyphae, yeast forms	Amphotericin B	Franklin, *Am. J. Cardiol.*, 38:924, 1976
Aspergillosis	Debilitated or immunosuppressed host	—	Granulomas or microabscesses; mycelial and filamentous forms	Amphotericin B	Williams, *Am. J. Clin. Pathol.*, 61:247, 1974
Histoplasmosis	—	—	Granulomas *H. capsulatum* in phagocytes	Amphotericin B	Owen, *Am. J. Med.*, 32:552, 1962
Sporotrichosis	—	—	—	Amphotericin B Potassium iodide	Collins, *Arch. Dermatol.*, 56:523, 1947
Coccidioidomycosis	—	—	Miliary granulomas with *C. immitis* spherules	Amphotericin B	Reingold, *Am. J. Clin. Pathol.*, 20:1044, 1950
Cryptococcosis	—	—	*C. neoformans* in granulomas	Amphotericin B plus 5-fluorocytosine	Jones, *Br. Heart J.*, 27:462, 1965
Mucormycosis	Debilitated or immunosuppressed host	—	Septic thromboses	Amphotericin B	Virmani, *Am. J. Clin. Path.*, 78:42, 1982
Protozoal					
Chagas' disease	See text	See text	See text	See text	—
Sleeping sickness (trypanosomiasis)	—	Frequent ECG abnormalities and arrhythmias	—	Early infection: *T. gambiense*—Pentamidine *T. rhodesiense*—Suramin Late infection: Melarsoprol	Poltera, *Br. Heart J.*, 38:827, 1976
Toxoplasmosis	—	Arrhythmias	Parasitized myofiber → rupture	Pyrimethamine plus trisulfapyrimidines	Leak, *Am. J. Cardiol.*, 43:841, 1979
Malaria	Peripheral circulatory collapse Angina	—	Parasitized RBC Myocardial vascular occlusion	Chloroquine unless resistant falciparum—then quinine, pyrimethamine and sulfonamides	Herrera, *Arch. Inst. Cardiol. Mex.*, 30:26, 1960
Leishmaniasis	—	—	Clasmatocytes with Leishman-Donovan bodies	Stibogluconate	Benhamou, *Arch. Mal. Coeur*, 31:81, 1938

TABLE 57-2 Rarer Forms of Myocarditis (*continued*)

	Distinctive Features				
Etiology	**Physical Examination**	**Laboratory**	**Morphological Manifestations**	**Specific Therapy***	**Reference**
Protozoal (*continued*)					
Balantidiasis	—	—	—	Tetracycline	Sidorov, *Ann. Anat. Pathol.*, 12:711, 1935
Sarcosporidiosis	—	—	Sarcocysts in myofiber with basophilic bodies	—	Arai, *J. Mt. Sinai Hosp.*, 15:367, 1949
Amebiasis	—	—	Microabscesses	Metronidazole	Markowitz, *Am. J. Clin. Pathol.*, 62:619, 1974
Helminthic					
Trichinosis	See text	See text	See text	See text	—
Echinococcosis	See text	See text	See text	See text	—
Schistosomiasis	Cor pulmonale	—	Microscopic pseudotubercle or granuloma	*S. japonicum:* Praziquantel *S. haematobium* and *S. Mansoni:* Niridazole, Praziquantel	Lima, *Rev. Inst. Med. Trop. São Paulo*, 11:290, 1969
Ascariasis	—	—	—	Mebendazole Pyrantel pamoate	Ferreira, *Rev. Med. Aeroaut.*, 15:35, 1963
Heterophydiasis	—	—	—	Tetrachloroethylene	Africa, *Acta. Med. Philippina*, Monograph Series, no. 1, 118, 1940
Filariasis	Congestive heart failure	Eosinophilia	Pericardial effusion Restrictive endocarditis	Corticosteroid hormones Diethylcarbamazine	Tatibouet, *Semaine Hop., Paris*, 37:3418, 1961
Paragonimiasis	—	—	—	Bithional Praziquantel	Kean, "Parasites of the Human Heart," Grune & Stratton, New York, 1964, p. 104
Strongyloidiasis	—	—	—	Thiabendazole	Kyle, *Ann. Intern. Med.*, 29:1014, 1948
Cysticerocosis	—	—	Myocardial scolex-containing cysts	—	Ibarra-Perez, *South. Med. J.*, 65:484, 1972
Visceral larva migrans	—	—	Allergic granulomatosis	Corticosteroid hormones Thiabendazole	Becroft, *N.Z. Med. J.*, 63:729, 1964

antibody and other techniques.[50] Cellular damage by the virus is postulated to trigger immunologic responses; their relationship to collagen formation, defective suppressor T-cell function, etc., is unknown.[32]

Although infectious myocarditis is thought to be acute, benign, and self-limiting in most instances, among patients who come to the attention of cardiologists a disproportionate number have significant heart failure, arrhythmias, conduction disturbances, or a combination of these, and the prognosis is more guarded. Subacute and chronic forms of myocarditis have long been recognized, and a chronic and progressive form has been described in detail by Kline and Saphir.[51] Recently, Fenoglio and associates,[31] on the basis of study of 34 patients with congestive heart failure and biopsy evidence of myocarditis, distinguished three forms of the disease: acute myocarditis, characterized by diffuse interstitial inflammation and extensive acute cellular damage; rapidly progressive myocarditis, presenting with focal acute and healing cell damage and extensive fibrosis; and chronic myocarditis, characterized by focal inflammation and cell damage. The prognosis of the first two forms was quite poor, with a rapid downhill course; and that of the chronic form better, with a less malignant course. No data regarding etiology were provided. Other investigators, however, dispute the prognostic value of endomyocardial biopsy.

Specific Forms of Myocarditis

In diphtheria, the early onset of myocarditis and the presence of severe electrocardiographic abnormalities indicate a grave prognosis. Regression of electrocardiographic abnormalities parallels the recovery from myocarditis.[22] The patient who recovers from diphtheritic myocarditis may have persistent atrioventricular conduction abnormalities for months or years, but this is generally the sole evidence of residual heart disease.

In patients with Coxsackie myocarditis, complete recovery is characteristic, but residual electrocardiographic abnormalities, cardiac enlargement, and constrictive pericarditis have been reported,[52] as has recurrence of illness.[53] Persistent, symptomatic complete heart block has necessitated pacemaker implantation.[54] Echovirus myocarditis is generally characterized by recovery.

Recovery from acute Chagas' myocarditis, with subsidence of cardiac manifestations, usually occurs within a few months, and the patient appears well for the ensuing 10 to 20 years. Some fatalities, however, occur with acute Chagas' disease from heart failure and/or meningoencephalitis. By contrast, chronic Chagas' myocarditis is characterized by progressive, unrelenting congestive heart failure. The almost invariable arrhythmias make syncope and sudden death common, in patients both with and without congestive heart failure.

Recovery is the rule in trichinosis myocarditis, and residual chronic disease is unusual.

When cardiac echinococcosis is diagnosed in the uncomplicated stage of the disease, prior to cyst rupture, surgical excision is curative. After cyst rupture, the prognosis varies with the site of the metastatic daughter cysts.

Treatment

General Considerations

All patients with suspected acute myocarditis should be admitted to the hospital for observation. Patients with pericardial effusion, cardiac rhythm abnormalities, congestive heart failure, evidence of myocardial ischemia, hypotension, or shock should be placed in an intensive care facility for closer surveillance of electrocardiographic and hemodynamic changes.

Medical management of the patient with infectious myocarditis includes (1) specific therapy for the underlying infection; (2) general measures, designed primarily to decrease cardiac work; and (3) control of the complications of myocarditis: congestive heart failure, cardiogenic shock, heart block,[54] arrhythmias, and thromboembolism.

Restriction of physical activity reduces the work of the heart and is designed to decrease residual myocardial damage and promote healing. Clinical and noninvasive assessment of myocardial function by physical examination, continuous ECG recording, echocardiography, and radionuclide ventriculography should determine the duration of convalescence recommended after an acute infectious illness in an attempt to minimize myocardial damage. This is the only measure directed specifically at the myocarditis, as the value of drugs that suppress inflammation and/or autoimmune responses remains controversial.[55]

Corticosteroid hormones appear relatively contraindicated in early infectious myocarditis, particularly myocarditis of viral etiology,[19] as inhibition of interferon synthesis and suppression of systemic defense mechanisms may increase viral replication and virulence and permit dissemination of the infection. In general, the use of corticosteroid hormones appears justified only in carefully selected patients with intractable heart failure, severe life-threatening arrhythmias, or severe systemic toxicity; steroids should be reduced in dosage and then stopped as soon as feasible. However, immunosuppressive therapy with corticosteroid hormones and azathioprine has been described as clinically, hemodynamically, and histologically effective in small numbers of patients followed with serial endomyocardial biopsy studies;[31,55–57] patients with inflammatory infiltrates, but not those with fibrosis, are described to respond to therapy. Because immunosuppressive therapy is potentially harmful, and adverse effects have been described both in animal models of myocarditis and in humans, clinical trial assessment of the role of immunosuppression appears warranted.

Antipyretic agents are usually indicated, both for the comfort of the patient and because fever and its hemodynamic consequences increase myocardial work. Aspirin is contraindicated in the patient receiving oral anticoagulation or in the patient who may have hemorrhagic pericarditis.

A regimen of modified bed rest is of the utmost importance, with the caloric requirements of a particular physical activity guiding its permission or restriction. For example, the use of a bedside commode requires less work than the use of a bedpan; and sitting in a chair may require less cardiac work than being recumbent in bed. Furthermore, the patient with considerable dyspnea may be more comfortable sitting in a chair than recumbent in bed. A passive or mild, active, supervised physical activity program of low-level caloric expenditure will help prevent atrophy of the muscle mass and help decrease venous stasis and the propensity to thromboembolism. Alcohol use and undernutrition should be avoided, as should cigarette smoking. Small, frequent meals may decrease cardiac work in the severely impaired patient.

Routine supplemental oxygen is indicated for hypoxemic patients, as well as those with tachycardia or low cardiac output. Experimental data suggest that hypoxemia may potentiate viral infection; a low-cardiac-output state with a widened arteriovenous oxygen difference will decrease the partial pressure of oxygen at the tissue (myocardial) level. Hypoxemia occurs commonly in patients with influenza and poliomyelitis myocarditis. Correction of anemia will also improve oxygen delivery to tissues. The use of hyperbaric oxygen acutely or on a long-term basis remains experimental. Similarly, the rationale for, and the results of, the administration of polarizing solutions (glucose, insulin, and potassium) are debatable. Therapy with interferon and other antiviral agents remains experimental.

Control of congestive heart failure involves the reduction of systemic tissue oxygen requirements by restriction of activity, control of fever, management of tachyarrhythmias, the augmentation of myocardial contractility by the administration of digitalis, and the diminution of fluid retention by sodium restriction and the use of diuretic agents. Some patients with myocarditis may have sinus tachycardia as rapid as 140 to 160 beats per minute. Propranolol in small doses may be of value in slowing the heart rate, in hope that this benefit will outweigh the decrease in myocardial contractility. Other tachyarrhythmias may also be treated with propranolol with the same concern. With diuretic use, serum potassium levels must be determined serially, as hypokalemia may cause arrhythmias and myocardial abnormalities. Excessive diuresis must be avoided, as a decreased circulating blood volume may produce hypotension or clinical shock. Preload and afterload reducing agents may considerably improve cardiac compensation.

Digitalis in doses somewhat greater than the average recommended amount may be necessary to control the congestive heart failure, particularly in patients with atrial fibrillation; patients receiving such dosages should be observed carefully for digitalis toxicity. Some patients with acute myocarditis seem unusually sensitive to the usual doses of digitalis. Variables determining digitalis dosages include electrolyte levels, cardiac rhythm, the severity of any associated hepatic and/or renal diseases, and possibly the adequacy of myocardial oxygenation; serum digitalis levels may help guide therapy. At times, digitalis cannot completely reverse the myocardial failure in patients with acute myocarditis, particularly in the presence of very severe disease, associated anemia, arrhythmias, or pulmonary embolization. Specific therapy to combat the infection may be required before the congestive heart failure can be controlled. The role of other positive inotropic agents is as yet unknown.[58]

Patients with a low-cardiac-output state, commonly associated with severe congestive heart failure, require serial monitoring of cardiac filling pressures via a flow-directed pulmonary artery catheter (Swan-Ganz), with capabilities to measure cardiac output. Dobutamine appears particularly valuable because of its predominant inotropic activity with limited vasoconstrictor and arrhythmogenic effects; it may be combined with a parenteral vasodilator drug, e.g., nitroprusside. The patient with severe heart failure whose blood pressure is maintained may respond to combinations of preload and afterload reducing agents, e.g., nitrate drugs, hydralazine, prazosin, or captopril. If the response to drugs that alter preload, afterload, and contractility is unsatisfactory, temporary circulatory assistance with intraaortic balloon counterpulsation may prove beneficial. An occasional patient with cardiogenic shock, in whom dehydration and hypovolemia related to the underlying acute infection may play a role, will respond to colloid or fluid administration.

Intractable congestive cardiac failure, shock, or both in a patient with acute myocarditis may in time prove an indication for temporary partial or total cardiopulmonary bypass.

In those varieties of acute myocarditis characterized by frequent arrhythmias, continuous monitoring for disturbances of cardiac rhythm is recommended. An intensive care unit, where personnel and equipment for cardiac resuscitation, defibrillation, and pacing are readily available, provides optimal care. Arrhythmias should be detected and treated early, before cardiac disturbances become life-threatening. The antiarrhythmic drugs—quinidine, procainamide, propranolol, disopyramide, etc.—concomitantly depress myocardial contractility and must be used with caution in the patient with myocarditis. Temporary or permanent cardiac pacing is often lifesaving for patients with bradyarrhythmias.

Prophylactic heparin administration in therapeutic doses may prevent thromboembolic complications in the patient with severe congestive cardiac failure in whom no specific contraindications to anticoagulation are present. Anticoagulant therapy, initially with heparin and subsequently with a warfarin derivative, is indicated in patients with systemic or pulmonary embolism; but may present a problem with hemopericardium if pericarditis is a prominent feature. All patients with evidence of pericarditis or pericardial effusion require careful surveillance for the development of pericardial tamponade.

Early diagnosis of infectious diseases and institution of appropriate chemotherapy may decrease the frequency of infectious myocarditis; the preventive role of vaccination and immunization against infectious disease is obvious. Thus, vaccination against diphtheria and poliomyelitis has eliminated the myocarditis due to these viruses. Vaccines against the influenza viruses and against pneumococcus clearly have preventive value.

Specific Forms of Myocarditis

In the patient with diphtheritic myocarditis, intubation with positive pressure ventilation may be necessary; erythromycin and diphtheria antitoxin should be administered. Digitalis must be used cautiously because of the high incidence of complete heart block. Electrocardiographic monitoring is requisite for all patients with abnormal electrocardiograms. The patient should be kept at bed rest as long as electrocardiographic abnormalities or undue tachycardia on exertion are present; these may persist for 6 to 8 weeks after the onset of diphtheria. Temporary[59] or permanent implanted cardiac pacemakers[60] and mechanically assisted circulation may markedly reduce fatalities from diphtheritic myocarditis. Nevertheless, primary prevention by immunization against diphtheria is the approach of choice.

There is minimal experience with specific antiviral agents such as amantadine and idoxuridine in patients with Coxsackie and other viral myocarditis.

A patient with laboratory-acquired acute Chagas' disease was seen by one of us (NKW). Although she recovered from the acute illness before diagnosis and without therapy, a course of treatment with the investigational drug Bayer 2502 was given; this drug, an S-nitrofuran known as nifurtimox, available widely in South America as Lampit, is effective in the acute stages of the disease, but some strains of *T. cruzi* are resistant, and the effectiveness of the drug against tissue forms in the chronic disease is limited in tolerable doses.[61] In chronic Chagas' disease propranolol or other antiarrhythmic agents in combination with ventricular demand pacing appear beneficial for the many patients who have both life-threatening ventricular tachyarrhythmias and episodes of high-degree atrioventricular block. The high risk of death from thromboembolism warrants anticoagulation.[62] There is no known specific therapy; preventive measures involve vector control.

Corticosteroid hormone therapy diminishes the myocardial inflammatory response in trichinosis myocarditis and produces striking clinical improvement. Thiabendazole is effective therapy.[63] Proper cooking of pork and pork products can virtually eliminate human trichinosis.

Surgical excision of a cardiac echinococcal cyst is ideally performed before the cyst ruptures into the pericardial cavity or a cardiac chamber; this permits curative surgery.

Summary

Acute myocarditis may be caused by almost any infectious agent, is probably much more prevalent then generally recognized, and affects primarily the young. Although generally benign in its course, it may be accompanied by significant arrhythmias, conduction disturbances, heart failure, cardiogenic shock, and sudden unexpected death. Late sequelae may include recurrent arrhythmias, abnormalities of conduction, and congestive cardiomyopathy. Newer noninvasive techniques may facilitate earlier recognition and therapy. The role of endomyocardial biopsy requires validation, and the effect of immunosuppressive therapy has yet to be determined. It is believed that prompt recognition may prevent early or late complications and reduce deaths, but data from controlled studies are not available. Vaccination against infections potentially associated with acute myocarditis is of preventive value.

References

1. Corvisart, J. N.: Essai sur les Maladies et les Lesions Organiques du Coeur, Paris, 1806, English translation by Jacob Gates, MMSS, 1812, pp. 182–189 and 299–303.
2. Lansdown, A. B. G.: Viral Infections and Diseases of the Heart, *Prog. Med. Virol.*, 24:70, 1978.
3. Walsh, T. J., Hutchins, G. M., Bulkley, B. H., and Mendelsohn, G.: Fungal Infections of the Heart: Analysis of 51 Autopsy Cases, *Am. J. Cardiol.*, 45:357, 1980.
4. Kean, B. H., and Breslau, R. C.: "Parasites of the Human Heart," Grune & Stratton, New York, 1964.
5. Hirschman, S. Z., and Hammer, G. S.: Coxsackie Virus Myopericarditis. A Microbiological and Clinical Review, *Am. J. Cardiol.*, 34:224, 1974.
6. Bell, E. J., and Grist, N. R.: Echo Viruses, Carditis, and Acute Pleurodynia, *Am. Heart J.*, 82:133, 1971.
7. Lewes, D., Rainford, D. J., and Lane, W. F.: Symptomless Myocarditis and Myalgia in Viral and *Mycoplasma pneumoniae* Infections, *Br. Heart J.*, 36:924, 1974.
8. Santos-Buch, C. A.: American Trypanosomiasis: Chagas' Disease, *Internat. Rev. Exper. Pathol.*, 19:63, 1979.
9. Rosenbaum, M. B.: Chagasic Myocardiopathy, *Prog. Cardiovasc. Dis.*, 7:199, 1964.
10. Puigbo, J. J., Rhode, J. R. N., Barrios, H. G., Suarez, J. A., and Yepez, C. G.: Clinical and Epidemiological Study of Chronic Heart Involvement in Chagas' Disease, *Bull. WHO,* 34:655, 1966.
11. Murphy, T. E., Kean, B. H., Venturini, A., and Lillehei, C. W.: Echinococcus Cyst of the Left Ventricle: Report of a Case with Review of the Pertinent Literature, *J. Thorac. Cardiovasc. Surg.*, 61:443, 1971.
12. Roberts, W. C., and Fox, S. M. III: Mumps of the Heart. Clinical and Pathologic Features, *Circulation,* 32:342, 1965.
13. Roberts, W. C., Bodey, G. P., and Wertlake, P. T.: The Heart in Acute Leukemia. A Study of 420 Autopsy Cases, *Am. J. Cardiol.*, 21:388, 1968.
14. Gore, I., and Saphir, O.: Myocarditis Associated with Acute Nasopharyngitis and Acute Tonsillitis, *Am. Heart J.*, 34:831, 1947.
15. Andy, J. J., O'Connell, J. P., Daddario, R. C., and Roberts, W. C.: Trichinosis Causing Extensive Ventricular Mural Endocarditis with Superimposed Thrombosis. Evidence that Severe Eosinophilia Damages Endocardium, *Am. J. Med.*, 63:824, 1977.
16. Roberts, W. C.: Characteristics and Consequences of Infective Endocarditis (Active or Healed or Both) Learned from Morphologic Studies, in S. H. Rahimtoola (ed): "Infective Endocarditis," Grune & Stratton, New York, 1977, p. 55.
17. Ihde, D. C., Roberts, W. C., Marr, K. C., Brereton, H. D., McGuire, W. P., Levine, A. S., and Young, R. C.: Cardiac Candidiasis in Cancer Patients, *Cancer,* 41:2364, 1978.
18. Ewy, G. A., Lotz, M., Geraghty, M., Marcus, F. I., and Roberts, W. C.: Clinical Pathologic Conference, *Am. Heart J.*, 78:259, 1969.
19. Lerner, A. M., Wilson, F. M., and Reyes, M. P.: Enteroviruses and the Heart (with Special Emphasis on the Probable Role of Coxsackie Viruses, Group B, Types 1–5), I. Epidemiological and Experimental Studies, II. Observations in Humans, *Mod. Concepts Cardiovasc. Dis.*, 44:7, 11, 1975.
20. Woodruff, J. F.: Viral Myocarditis. A Review, *Am. J. Pathol.*, 101:427, 1980.
21. Burch, G. E., and Giles, T. D.: The Role of Viruses in the Production of Heart Disease, *Am. J. Cardiol.*, 29:231, 1972.
22. Ledbetter, M. K., Cannon, A. B., II, and Costa, A. F.: The Electrocardiogram in Diphtheritic Myocarditis, *Am. Heart J.*, 68:599, 1964.
23. Amorim, D. S.: Chagas' Disease, in P. N. Yu and J. F. Goodwin (eds): "Progress in Cardiology," vol. 8, Lea & Febiger, Philadelphia, 1979, p. 235.
24. Wentworth, P., Jentz, L. A., and Croal, A. E.: Analysis of Sudden Unexpected Death in Southern Ontario, with Emphasis on Myocarditis, *Can. Med. Assoc. J.*, 120:676, 1979.
25. Lambert, E. C., Menon, V. A., Wagner, H. R., and Vlad, P.: Sudden Unexpected Death from Cardiovascular Disease in Children. A Cooperative International Study, *Am. J. Cardiol.*, 34:89, 1974.
26. Lewes, D.: Viral Myocarditis, *Practitioner,* 216:281, 1976.
27. Woodward, T. E., Togo, Y., Lee, Y.-C., and Hornick, R. B.: Specific Microbial Infections of the Myocardium and Pericardium. A Study of 82 Patients, *Arch. Intern. Med.*, 120:270, 1967.
27a. Nieminen, M. S., Heikkila, J., and Karjalainen, J.: Echocardiography in Acute Infectious Myocarditis: Relation to

Clinical and Electrocardiographic Findings, *Am. J. Cardiol.*, 53:1331, 1984.

27b. O'Connell, J. B., Henkin, R. E., Robinson, J. A., Subramanian, R., Scanlon, P. J., and Gunnar, R. M.: Gallium-67 Imaging in Patients with Dilated Cardiomyopathy and Biopsy-proven Myocarditis, *Circulation*, 70:58, 1984.

28. Sakakibara, S., and Konno, S.: Endomyocardial Biopsy, *Jpn. Heart J.*, 3:537, 1962.

29. Fowles, R. E., and Mason, J. W.: Endomyocardial Biopsy, *Ann. Intern. Med.*, 97:885, 1982.

30. Nippoldt, T. B., Edwards, W. D., Holmes, D. R., Jr., Reeder, G. S., Hartzler, G. O., and Smith, H. C.: Right Ventricular Endomyocardial Biopsy: Clinicopathologic Correlates in 100 Consecutive Patients, *Mayo Clin. Proc.*, 57:407, 1982.

31. Fenoglio, J. J., Jr., Ursell, P. C., Kellogg, C. F., Drusin, R. E., and Weiss, M. B.: Diagnosis and Classification of Myocarditis by Endomyocardial Biopsy, *N. Engl. J. Med.*, 308:12, 1983.

32. Olsen, E. G. J.: Myocarditis—A Case of Mistaken Identity? *Br. Heart J.*, 50:303, 1983.

33. Edwards, W. D., Holmes, D. R., Jr., and Reeder, G. S.: Diagnosis of Active Lymphocytic Myocarditis by Endomyocardial Biopsy: Quantitative Criteria for Light Microscopy, *Mayo Clin. Proc.*, 57:419, 1982.

34. Parrillo, J. E., Aretz, H. T., Palacios, I., Fallon, J. T., and Block, P. C.: The Results of Transvenous Endomyocardial Biopsy can Frequently Be Used to Diagnose Myocardial Diseases in Patients with Idiopathic Heart Failure. Endomyocardial Biopsies in 100 Consecutive Patients Revealed a Substantial Incidence of Myocarditis, *Circulation*, 69:93, 1984.

34a. Kereiakes, D. J., and Parmley, W. W.: Myocarditis and Cardiomyopathy, *Am. Heart J.*, 108:1318, 1984.

35. Harris, L. C., and Nghiem, Q. X.: Cardiomyopathies in Infants and Children, *Prog. Cardiovasc. Dis.*, 15:255, 1972.

36. Saffitz, J. E., Schwartz, D. J., Southworth, W., Murphree, S., Rodriguez, E. R., Ferrans, V. J., and Roberts, W. C.: Coxsackie Viral Myocarditis Causing Transmural Right and Left Ventricular Infarction without Coronary Narrowing, *Am. J. Cardiol.*, 52:644, 1983.

37. Aldama-Luebbert, A., Nasrallah, A. T., Garcia, E., and Hall, R. J.: Ventricular Aneurysm in Chagas' Myocardiopathy: Clinical, Epidemiologic, Angiographic Features, *Texas Med.*, 72:55, 1976.

38. Cossio, P. M., Laguens, R. P., Diez, C., Szarfman, A., Segal, A., and Arana, R. M.: Chagasic Cardiopathy. Antibodies Reacting with Plasma Membrane of Striated Muscle and Endothelial Cells, *Circulation*, 50:1252, 1974.

38a. Pereira, M. H. B., Brito, F. S., Ambrose, J. A., Pereira, C. B., Levi, G. C., Neto, V. A., and Martinez, E. E.: Exercise Testing in the Latent Phase of Chagas' Disease, *Clin. Cardiol.*, 7:261, 1984.

39. Hammermeister, K. E., Caeiro, T., Crespo, E., Palmero, H., and Gibson, D. G.: Left Ventricular Wall Motion in Patients with Chagas's Disease, *Br. Heart J.*, 51:70, 1984.

40. Acquatella, H., Schiller, N. B., Puigbo, J. J., Giordano, H., Suarez, J. A., Casal, H., Arreaza, N., Valecillos, R., and Hirschhaut, E.: M-mode and Two-dimensional Echocardiography in Chronic Chagas' Heart Disease. A Clinical and Pathologic Study, *Circulation*, 62:787, 1980.

41. Gray, D. F., Morse, B. S., and Phillips, W. F.: Trichinosis with Neurologic and Cardiac Involvement: Review of the Literature and Report of Three Cases. *Ann. Intern. Med.*, 57:230, 1962.

42. Kirschberg, G. J.: Trichinosis Presenting as Acute Myocardial Infarction, *Can. Med. Assoc. J.*, 106:898, 1972.

43. de los Arcos, E., Madurga, M. P., Leon, J. P., Martinez, J. L., and Urquia, M.: Hydatid Cyst of Interventricular Septum Causing Left Anterior Hemiblock, *Br. Heart J.*, 33:623, 1971.

44. Perez-Gomez, F., Duran, H., Tamames, S., Perrote, J. L., and Blanes, A.: Cardiac Echinococcosis: Clinical Picture and Complications, *Br. Heart J.*, 35:1326, 1973.

45. Limacher, M. C., McEntee, C. W., Attar, M., Nelson, J. G., DeBakey, M. E., and Quinones, M. A.: Cardiac Echinococcal Cyst: Diagnosis by Two-dimensional Echocardiography, *JACC*, 2:574, 1983.

46. Pankey, G. A.: Effect of Viruses on the Cardiovascular System, *Am. J. Med. Sci.*, 250:103, 1965.

47. Kawai, C., Matsumori, A., Kitaura, Y., and Takatsu, T.: Viruses and the Heart: Viral Myocarditis and Cardiomyopathy, in P. N. Yu and J. F. Goodwin (eds.), "Progress in Cardiology," vol. 7, Lea & Febiger, Philadelphia, 1978, p. 141.

48. Abelmann, W. H.: Viral Myocarditis and its Sequelae, *Am. Rev. Med.*, 24:145, 1973.

49. O'Connell, J. B.: Evidence Linking Viral Myocarditis to Dilated Cardiomyopathy in Humans, in Robinson, J. A., and O'Connell, J. B. (eds): "Myocarditis: Precursor of Cardiomyopathy," D. C. Heath and Co., Lexington, Mass., 1983, p. 93.

50. Cambridge, G., MacArthur, C. G. C., Waterson, A. P., Goodwin, J. F., and Oakley, C. M.: Antibodies to Coxsackie B Viruses in Congestive Cardiomyopathy, *Br. Heart J.*, 41:692, 1979.

51. Kline, I. K., and Saphir, O.: Chronic Pernicious Myocarditis, *Am. Heart J.*, 59:681, 1960.

52. Smith, W. G.: Coxsackie B Myopericarditis in Adults, *Am. Heart J.*, 80:34, 1970.

53. Sainani, G. S., Krompotic, E., and Slodki, S. J.: Adult Heart Disease Due to the Coxsackie Virus B Infection, *Medicine*, 47:133, 1968.

54. Schieken, R. M., and Myers, M. G.: Complete Heart Block in Viral Myocarditis, *J. Pediatr.*, 87:831, 1975.

55. Mason, J. W., Billingham, M. E., and Ricci, D. R.: Treatment of Acute Inflammatory Myocarditis Assisted by Endomyocardial Biopsy, *Am. J. Cardiol.*, 45:1037, 1980.

56. Daly, K., Richardson, P. J., Olsen, E. G. J., Morgan-Capner, P., McSorley, C., Jackson, G., and Jewitt, D. E.: Acute Myocarditis. Role of Histological and Virological Examination in the Diagnosis and Assessment of Immunosuppressive Treatment, *Br. Heart J.*, 51:30, 1984.

57. Melvin, K. R., Richardson, P. J., Olsen, E. C. J., Daly, K., and Jackson, G.: Peripartum Cardiomyopathy due to Myocarditis, *N. Engl. J. Med.*, 307:731, 1982.

58. Baim, D. S., McDowell, A. V., Cherniles, J., Monrad, E. S., Parker, J. A., Edelson, J., Braunwald, E., and Grossman, W.: Evaluation of a New Bipyridine Inotropic Agent—Milrinone—in Patients with Severe Congestive Heart Failure, *N. Engl. J. Med.*, 309:748, 1983.

59. Matisonn, R. E., Mitha, A. S., and Chesler, E.: Successful Electrical Pacing for Complete Heart Block Complicating Diphtheritic Myocarditis, *Br. Heart J.*, 38:423, 1976.

60. Gallez, A., and Bernard, R.: La Myocardite Diphterique: Utilisation de L'entrainement Electrosystolique Temporaire dans un Cas Compliqué de Bloc Auriculo-ventriculaire Complet, *Acta. Cardiol.*, 26:88, 1971.

61. Gutteridge, W. E.: Chemotherapy of Chagas's Disease: The Present Situation, *Trop. Dis. Bull.*, 73:699, 1976.

62. Oliveira, J. S. M., de Araujo, R. R. C., Navarro, M. A., and Muccillo, G.: Cardiac Thromboses and Thromboembolism in Chronic Chagas' Heart Disease, *Am. J. Cardiol.*, 52:147, 1983.

63. Stone, O. J., Stone, C. T., Jr., and Mullins, J. F.: Thiabendazole—Probable Cure for Trichinosis, *JAMA*, 187:536, 1964.

58

Cardiomyopathy and Myocardial Involvement in Systemic Disease

Nanette Kass Wenger, M.D.
John F. Goodwin, M.D.
William C. Roberts, M.D.

The heart is a kind of center where all disorders converge. All the ills of the rest of the body reflect on this organ. As soon as some part is irritated or inflamed, the heart may partake of its suffering.

J.-B. de Senac, 1749[1]

Definitions and Classification

The term *cardiomyopathy* connotes any structural and/or functional abnormality of ventricular myocardium. Because practically all cardiac diseases affect the structure or function of the myocardium, in this chapter *cardiomyopathy* is used to designate a condition affecting primarily the myocardium, unassociated with significant narrowing of the extramural coronary arteries, systemic hypertension, anatomic valvular heart disease, congenital malformation of the heart and vessels, or intrinsic pulmonary parenchymal or vascular disease. We have chosen to classify cardiomyopathy etiologically as "heart muscle disease of unknown cause"[2] as distinct from "myocardial involvement in systemic disease"[3] (rare specific heart muscle disease[2]). No causative or associated condition can be identified in most patients with cardiomyopathy. Cardiomyopathies are now considered in three major groups[4,5] based on abnormalities of structure and function: *dilated, hypertrophic,* and *restrictive/obliterative.* The major characteristics of each are presented in Fig. 58-1 and Table 58-1 (see also Chap. 17). The World Health Organization (ISFC Task Force on the Definition and Classification of Cardiomyopathies) adopted basically the same classification: dilated, hypertrophic, and restrictive.[6]

Dilatation of the ventricles is the predominant feature of the dilated type, and the descriptive term *dilated cardiomyopathy* (DC) is therefore applied. Myocardial mass also is increased. The cardinal feature of the *hypertrophic* type is the absence of cavity dilatation, associated with a considerable increase in myocardial mass (hypertrophy); cavity size may be normal or decreased. *Restrictive/obliterative cardiomyopathy* denotes restriction of filling of the ventricles by endocardial or myocardial disease or both, producing hemodynamic and clinical responses similar to constrictive pericarditis; the cavity size is decreased. The hallmark is thus an abnormality of diastolic function. *Obliterative* cardiomyopathy may be viewed as a more severe form of the restrictive type in which endocardial disease is usually paramount; it is therefore considered as a stage in progression. Heart muscle disease of unknown cause will be discussed in these three categories, although the features may merge in the sequential clinical course of an individual patient.

Familial cardiomyopathy[7] has been used to denote heart muscle disease occurring in more than one family member; it most frequently is applicable to hypertrophic cardiomyopathy, but a familial tendency is occasionally noted in dilated cardiomyopathy. We do not use this nonspecific designation in classification.

The term *ischemic cardiomyopathy* has been used to describe patients with occlusive atherosclerotic coronary artery disease who develop progressive heart failure as the predominant manifestation. The term tends to be misleading, although it distinguishes these patients from those with dilated cardiomyopathy who have insignificant coronary narrowing. Ischemic cardiomyopathy is not a true "cardiomyopathy" because the heart muscle disease is secondary to coronary arterial narrowing.

In certain patients presenting with cardiac dysrhythmias, this may be the initial manifestation of cardiac and skeletal myopathies.[8] In one study, most patients with ventricular tachycardia and normal cardiac mechanical function had abnormal myocardium, challenging the concept of idiopathic ventricular tachycardia.[8a]

Dilated Cardiomyopathy

Etiology

Dilated cardiomyopathy (DC) is the most common of the cardiomyopathies. The striking features are cardiomegaly with dilatation of both ventricles, impairment of systolic function, and increased myocardial mass. The dilatation is more impressive than the hypertrophy, and the disease characteristically affects both ventricles. Rarely a right ventricular type, notable for ventricular arrhythmias, is seen, known as arrhythmogenic right ventricular dysplasia.[9]

Etiologic Features, Potentiating Conditions, Causal Relations, and Risk Factors

A number of conditions appear to be related to or identified with dilated cardiomyopathy. These in-

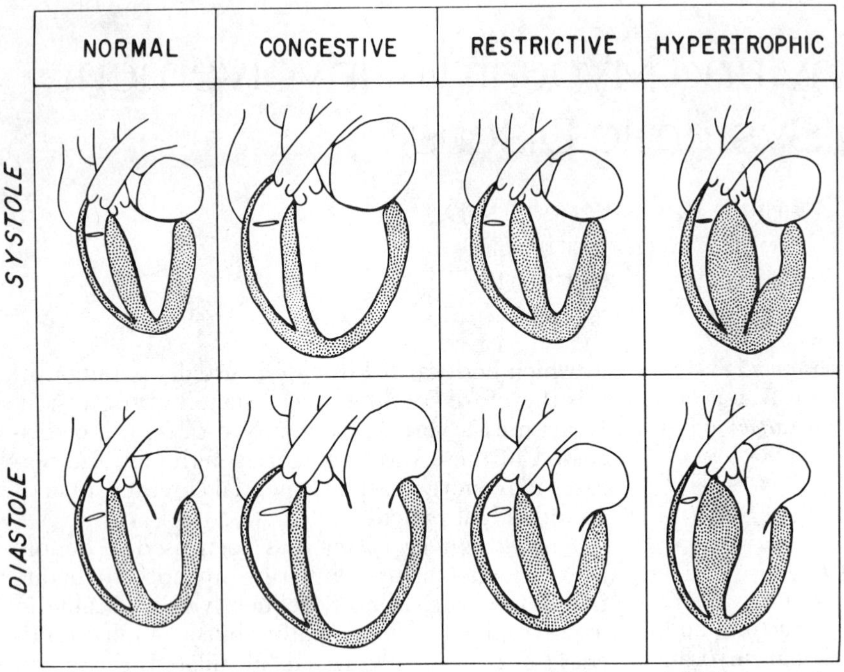

FIGURE 58-1 Diagram of the 50° left anterior oblique view of the heart in the different types of cardiomyopathy at end systole and end diastole. (*From M. R. Goldman and C. A. Boucher, Value of Radionuclide Imaging Techniques in Possessing Cardiomyopathy, Am. J. Cardiol., 46:1232, 1980. Reproduced with permission from the publisher and author.*)

clude alcohol abuse, systemic arterial hypertension, pregnancy and the puerperium, immunologic disorders, viral infections,[5] and a number of chemical and physical agents that produce toxic effects on the myocardium.

Alcohol Abuse

Consumption of large quantities of alcohol over long periods of time (see Chap. 74) may be followed by ventricular dilatation, cardiomegaly, poor left ventricular contractile function, and heart failure (alcoholic heart disease). A direct causal relation between alcohol ingestion and heart disease is well-supported. The features are indistinguishable from those of dilated cardiomyopathy except that the heart failure often remits if alcohol is abandoned and recurs if consumption is resumed. Eventually permanent cardiac damage occurs, and progressive deterioration sets in despite abstinence. The quantity of alcohol required to damage myocardium is difficult to assess, and the way(s) in which alcohol may affect the heart are uncertain. Individual variation and the duration of alcohol abuse are important variables. There is little evidence to suggest that alcohol plays an important etiologic role in dilated cardiomyopathy except as a potentiating or conditioning factor in patients who already have, or are susceptible to, cardiac damage for other reasons: associated nutritional deficiencies, particularly of thiamine, may

TABLE 58-1 Characteristics of the Three Main Types of Cardiomyopathy

Characteristics	Dilated	Hypertrophic	Restrictive/ Obliterative
Myocardial mass	↑→↑↑	↑↑↑	nl→↑
Ventricular cavity size	↑↑→↑↑↑↑	↓↓→nl	↓
Dilated atrial cavities	+	+	+
Endocardial thickening	0→+	+*	+ + +
Myocardial infiltration	0	0	0→+†
Asymmetric septal hypertrophy	0	+	0
Myocardial fiber disorientation	0	+	0
Abnormal intramural coronary arteries	0	+	0
Endocardial plaque, LV outflow tract	0	+	0
Contractile function	↓↓↓	↑↑→↓	nl→↓
Ventricular inflow resistance	0	+ +	+
Ventricular outflow "obstruction"	0	0⇄+	0
LV filling pressure	↑↑	nl	↑
Mitral regurgitation	+	+	+
Thickened mitral valve	0	+	±
Intracardiac thrombi	+	0	+

*Limited to mural endocardium of outflow tract in apposition to anterior mitral leaflet.
†Only with amyloid; none with EMF.

contribute to the heart failure, as may the arrhythmias and systemic hypertension that are concomitants of alcohol abuse.

Systemic Arterial Hypertension
High blood pressure is not infrequently associated with dilated cardiomyopathy in the early stages, and differentiation of dilated cardiomyopathy from hypertensive heart disease early on may be difficult (see Chaps. 49 to 51). Although hypertension may cause congestive cardiomyopathy in some patients,[10,11] it is uncertain how frequently it is a major factor.

Pregnancy and the Puerperium
The etiology of peripartal cardiomyopathy (cardiac failure occurring during the latter part of pregnancy or in the puerperium without other evidence of heart disease) remains obscure. The features are those of dilated cardiomyopathy, and it has been suggested that the occurrence of pregnancy is fortuitous. However, the absence of heart disease before pregnancy and the tendency to recur with subsequent pregnancies suggest that it is a specific condition (see Chap. 69).

Genetic Predisposition
Stressful events, such as physical restraint and exposure to cold, precipitated heart failure in asymptomatic but genetically cardiomyopathic hamsters; this did not occur in genetically normal hamsters. Extrapolation to cardiomyopathy in human beings is premature (see Chap. 35).

Microvascular Spasm
Microvascular spasm with myocytolysis and cell loss, followed by reactive hypertrophy and progressively reduced contractility owing to both of these features, has been described in animal models. Because pretreatment with verapamil prevented the cardiomyopathy, as well as the microvascular spasm, increased calcium flux across the sarcolemma has been postulated to cause the cell hypercontraction, mitochondrial calcification, and myocyte necrosis.[12]

Infective and Immunologic Aspects
The association between acute viral infection and dilated cardiomyopathy is also obscure. In both animals and human beings, apparent dilated cardiomyopathy has developed after an acute Coxsackie or arbovirus myocarditis. Although virus has not been isolated from the myocardium of human beings with dilated cardiomyopathy, viral antigens can be demonstrated in biopsy specimens. Patients with a brief history of dilated cardiomyopathy may have very high titers to Coxsackie B, but endomyocardial biopsy has not shown virus infection or myocarditis.[13] Four possibilities include (1) chance association between prior virus infection and dilated cardiomyopathy, (2) opportunistic virus infection of an already damaged heart, (3) direct infection of the myocardium, and (4) virus infection that precipitates an immunologic reaction that damages myocardium (see also Chap. 57).

The last seems most likely and deserves further study, especially since disordered cellular immunity is found in patients with dilated cardiomyopathy, including some undergoing cardiac transplantation.[14,15] It is important to differentiate cardiomyopathy resulting from viral myocarditis with necrosis and fibrosis from the cardiomyopathy that occurs after apparent complete recovery from the acute viral illness. It has been theorized that viruses may modify the antigenic properties of the hosts' myocardial cells so as to initiate production of autoantibodies that subsequently impair myocardial function. The presence of heart reactive antibodies, immunoglobulins, antinuclear factors, and bound gamma globulin in the myocardium of some patients further suggests an immunologic process. Suppressor lymphocytes may play a role in preventing or ameliorating myocardial damage.[15] An abnormality in cellular immunity may result in progressive myocardial damage leading to dilated cardiomyopathy. Conversely, another study reports no consistent disorder of humoral immunity.[16] Alternatively, certain individuals may have a preexisting, possibly inherited, disorder of cellular immunity that renders them more vulnerable to the effects of viral infection. Evidence is accumulating that viral disease may progress to dilated cardiomyopathy.[17–19]

Allied Conditions and Experimental Studies
Clues to the causation of dilated cardiomyopathy may be obtained from a similar morphological and functional abnormality of known toxic cause. *Daunorubicin* produces direct myocardial toxicity by specific effects on enzyme function that cause progressive myocardial damage, pump failure, and death.[20] The mechanism of cardiac toxicity of this antineoplastic agent is likely related to binding of the drug to DNA in nuclei and mitochondria; once bound, the drug is only very slowly liberated from the cell. Cardiac muscle cells cannot reproduce; hence, inhibition of protein synthesis resulting from alteration in the DNA end plates persists; cumulative interference with normal protein regeneration, replenishment, and growth could explain the delayed onset of toxicity and the fact that adults appear more vulnerable than children, and the elderly most vulnerable of all.

Cardiomyopathy due to small quantities of *cobalt,*[21] used as a frothing agent in beer, presents as dilated cardiomyopathy. The condition can be produced experimentally when conditioning factors, particularly protein deficiency, necessary for reproduction of the human type of the disease, are present. Cobalt cardiomyopathy seems to have disappeared with removal of the cobalt additive from beer.

Selenium deficiency has been regarded as a cause of heart muscle disease, indistinguishable from dilated cardiomyopathy, in the People's Republic of

China (Keshan disease). It is not clear whether selenium deficiency alone is responsible, because other deficiencies have been described in association; selenium deprivation increases the incidence of fatal Coxsackie myocarditis in young mice. Selenium deficiency may increase platelet aggregation due to impaired glutathione peroxidase activity.[22]

Catecholamines and Autonomic Function

The administration of large quantities of catecholamines to human beings may produce subendocardial necrosis, and pheochromocytoma may rarely present as a cardiomyopathy.[23] Some animal experiments show that catecholamines increase the rate of protein synthesis and induce hypertrophy without preceding decompensation. However, a defect in the adrenergic receptor–adenyl cyclase system has been demonstrated in the rat; this may contribute to attenuation of the inotropic adrenergic response to stress.[24] High sympathetic tone in human beings with cardiomyopathy may potentially induce increased protein synthesis, hypertrophy, necrosis, and deterioration in cardiac function; however, sympathetic tone does not seem unduly high in patients with dilated congestive cardiomyopathy.

Heart rate responses to isometric exercise and phenylephrine are depressed in patients with dilated cardiomyopathy, both with and without heart failure.[25] Furthermore, histological studies have shown a significant reduction in the number of parasympathetic neurons in the right atrial wall.[26] These results suggest that parasympathetic function is impaired even at an early stage.[27] This may possibly be a predisposing factor for arrhythmia and sudden death. In a myocardial biopsy study from Japan,[28] some patients with dilated cardiomyopathy had lower levels of myocardial norepinephrine (myocardial catecholamine depletion) than consistent with the degree of hypertrophy, interstitial fibrosis, and severity of the heart failure, but mean plasma epinephrine and norepinephrine levels were significantly elevated in these patients with dilated cardiomyopathy.

Thyroid Hormone

In response to a pressure load, the immature rate has an elevated level of thyroid hormone and altered composition of ventricular isomyosin; cardiac enlargement occurs without depression of myocardial function. Thyroid status and isomyosin composition do not change in the mature rat, increased myofiber efficiency does not occur, and hemodynamic function deteriorates (see Chap. 72).

Epidemiology

Idiopathic dilated cardiomyopathy occurs worldwide in persons of all ages and races, but more commonly in men than in women. A genetic predisposition is unusual, but occurs occasionally,[29] perhaps as a result of an inherited immunologic deficiency.

Pathology

The major morphological feature of DC is dilatation of both ventricular cavities (Fig. 58-2). Although the degree of dilatation of both cavities is usually similar, occasionally one ventricle is more dilated than the other. Although the left is usually more severely affected, right ventricular dilated cardiomyopathy with evidence during life of preserved left ventricular function is described.[30] The ventricular dilatation is associated with poor ventricular contractility, which in turn results in a low ejection fraction and high end-systolic volume. The latter appears to limit atrial emptying, which in turn leads to a high atrial end-diastolic volume with resulting atrial dilatation.

The large end-systolic ventricular volume causes relative stasis of blood in the apical portions of the ventricular cavities and this often results in intracavitary thrombosis (Fig. 58-3). Thrombi also are frequent in one or both atrial appendages, presumably also the consequence of poor atrial emptying and relative stasis of blood in the appendages. The most frequent locations of thrombi in patients with DC are left ventricle, right ventricle, right atrial appendage, and, lastly, left atrial appendage. About 75 percent of patients have left ventricular thrombi at necropsy. Thrombus occurs rarely in the atria or right ventricle without thrombi also being present in the left ventricle. In addition to fibrin thrombi, focal endocardial thickenings often are present, probably representing "healed" or organized thrombi. The intracardiac thrombi may give rise to pulmonary and systemic emboli.

The heart is always increased in weight; the average is just under 600 g. Despite the increased weight, the maximal thickness of the left ventricular free wall and the ventricular septum is often less than 1.5 cm.

Although interstitial myocardial fibrosis of varying degree usually is present by histological examination, left ventricular free wall scarring is evident by gross inspection in only about 25 percent of patients. Even when scarring is observed grossly, it is usually limited to the papillary muscle and subendocardium (inner one-half of wall). Thus, the poor myocardial contractility cannot be explained by ventricular scarring.

The leaflets of the four cardiac valves are usually normal, but occasionally the margins of the mitral and tricuspid valve leaflets are focally thickened by fibrous tissue. The latter is most frequent in patients with atrioventricular (AV) valvular regurgitation for long periods of time. These valvular thickenings appear to be secondary to the regurgitation, and do not themselves cause valvular regurgitation. The cause of valvular regurgitation in these patients is generally considered to be papillary muscle dysfunction, because the tricuspid and mitral valvular annuli are usually only mildly dilated (< 25 percent above normal); however, a recent echocardiographic study suggests that mitral annular enlargement is the chief determinant.[31]

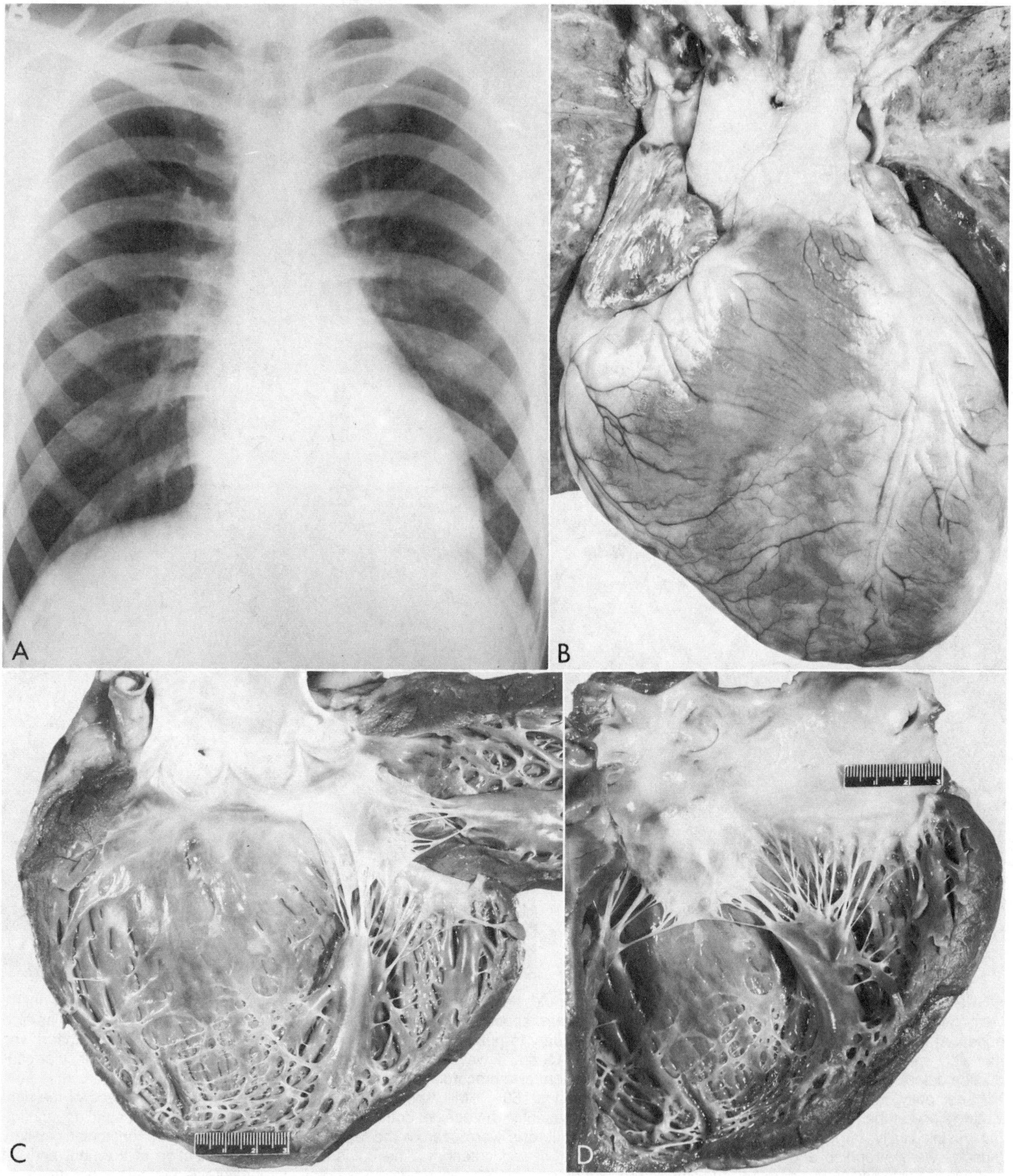

FIGURE 58-2 Idiopathic dilated cardiomegaly in a 22-year-old white man (A61-56) who had been well until 5 years before death when he had the onset of pleuritic-type pain followed by congestive cardiac failure. Electrocardiogram showed nonspecific T-wave changes. After a 4-month hospitalization, he was entirely well until 2 months before death, when an upper respiratory infection precipitated overt congestive heart failure. Thereafter, the heart failure progressively worsened and the heart enlarged. A grade 2/6 apical systolic murmur appeared.

At necropsy, the heart weighed 570 g, and both ventricles were very dilated (*A* to *D*). The valves and coronary arteries were normal. Histological sections of left ventricular wall showed only mild interstitial fibrosis. *A.* Chest roentgenogram during last week of life. *B.* Anterior aspect of heart. The pericardial sac contained 50 ml of serous fluid. *C.* Opened left ventricle, aortic valve, and aorta. Small, focal endocardial thickenings are present. *D.* Opened left atrium, mitral valve, and left ventricle. The mitral annulus is not dilated.

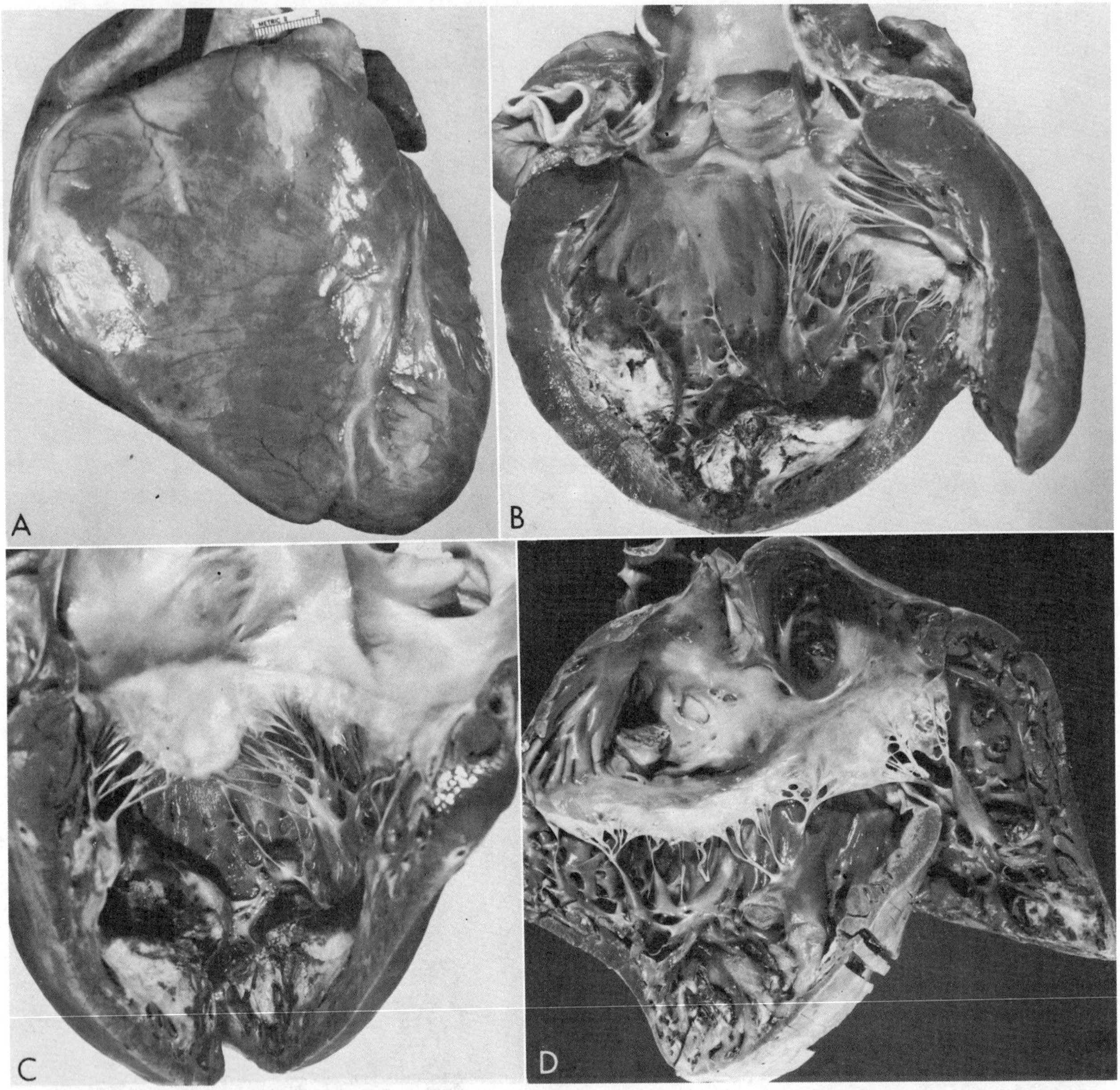

FIGURE 58-3 Idiopathic dilated cardiomegaly in a 36-year-old black man (A69-199), a habitual alcoholic, who had been well until 2 years before death when evidence of congestive cardiac failure appeared. The latter gradually worsened, and various arrhythmias also appeared. Finally, pulmonary infiltrates, proved to be secondary to pulmonary emboli, precipitated death. By radiograph the heart was markedly enlarged. Electrocardiogram showed low voltage. Q- and T-wave changes suggesting old infarction, and intraventricular conduction defect. The patient never had chest pain, hypertension, or a precordial murmur.

At necropsy, the heart plus the intracardiac thrombi weighed 750 g. "Milk spots" were present over the anterior surface of the right ventricle and at the left ventricular apex (*A*). Thrombi were present in the apex of both ventricles (*B* to *D*) and in the right atrial appendage (*D*). Histologically, large foci of replacement and interstitial fibrosis were seen in the left ventricular wall. Both left ventricular papillary muscles were atrophied and severely scarred. *A.* Heart as viewed anteriorly. The notch present at the junction of the right and left ventricular apices was considered at one time to be diagnostic of the African condition, endomyocardial fibrosis, but this is not the case, as shown by this patient. *B.* Opened left ventricle, aortic valve, and aorta showing the large apical thrombus. *C.* Opened left atrium, mitral valve, and left ventricle. The mitral annulus is not dilated. *D.* Opened right atrium, tricuspid valve, and right ventricle showing a thrombus at the apex of the ventricle.

Histological studies of the myocardial walls disclose nonspecific changes. Many myocardial cells appear hypertrophied; others, atrophied. The amount of fibrous tissue between myocardial cells usually is increased. Inflammatory cells are absent. The intramural coronary arteries are normal. Electron microscopy has confirmed these histological observations and demonstrated other nonspecific changes including cellular edema; increased numbers of lipid droplets, lysosomes, and lipofuscin granules; dilatation of the tubules of the sarcoplasmic reticulum and the T system; mild myofibrillar damage, and various mitochondrial alterations. The mitochondria vary in size; many are smaller than normal. No virus particles have been observed in the myocardium of patients with fatal cardiomyopathy. The changes in the myocardium of patients with histories of habitual alcoholism are indistinguishable from those of patients without such histories. In general, the extent of the degenerative changes in the myocardial cells correlates with the duration and severity of cardiac dysfunction.

Although it is well-recognized that DC may be confused clinically with atherosclerotic coronary heart disease, separation of the two at necropsy may present problems if one adheres rigidly to a definition that includes "absence of coronary arterial disease." How much coronary arterial narrowing is permissible to allow the diagnosis of DC? Because fatal atherosclerotic coronary heart disease is commonly associated with cross-sectional area luminal narrowing of greater than 75 percent, a 75 percent cutoff point appears reasonable. Furthermore, there is apparently no reduction in flow through a tube (coronary artery) until more than 75 percent of the cross-sectional area of the lumen is obliterated. Obviously, the associated coronary atherosclerosis usually presents no problem in the younger patients, but it might in the older ones. In dilated cardiomyopathy, the degree of myocardial disorder is grossly out of proportion to any coronary arterial disease that is present. In so-called ischemic cardiomyopathy, the coronary artery disease is severe and widespread and consistent with the degree of myocardial disorder.

Abnormal Physiology (see also Chap. 20)

Hemodynamic changes are those of failure of the heart as a pump (Fig. 58-4). In the early stages, a reduced stroke volume may be compensated for by tachycardia, which maintains the cardiac output. The minute volume, however, does not rise normally with exercise; this causes an increase in end-diastolic pressure of the left ventricle and produces dyspnea. In the late stages, both minute volume and stroke volume are reduced. However, for a long time period the ventricles may be dilated and the patient asymptomatic. Exercise capacity, in other words, relates poorly to the functional status of the ventricle. Stimulation of an increased force of contraction due to increased end-diastolic fiber length by the Frank-Starling mechanism achieves the same stroke volume with less myocardial fiber shortening; eventually, however, the disadvantage of dilatation greatly outweighs the advantages. According to Laplace's law, dilatation is accompanied by greater wall tension and pressure, which invoke a greater metabolic need and oxygen demand. There is, in addition, a decreased rate of fiber shortening, diminished maximal rate of rise of pressure (max dP/dt), and diminished velocity of ejection. It is likely that the increased myocardial mass is at least in part compensatory and tends to maintain overall cardiac function. The greater the hypertrophy, the better the compensation and the prognosis.[4] The reduced ejection fraction is inversely related to left ventricular end-diastolic pressure;[11] systolic and diastolic ventricular volumes are increased.

Reduced oxygen saturation of the mixed venous blood occurs in most patients and results in a high arteriovenous oxygen difference. Increased pulmonary venous pressure causes symptoms of pulmonary venous congestion. Pulmonary artery pressure and pulmonary vascular resistance are often modestly increased as a result of left ventricular failure, but severe pulmonary hypertension is unusual; chronic elevation of pulmonary arterial pressure may ultimately precipitate right-sided heart failure.

Decreased renal perfusion, owing to a low cardiac output, stimulation of the renin-angiotensin-aldosterone system, and enhanced sympathetic activity all participate in increasing the intracardiac volume, but may increase the peripheral vascular resistance as well; the latter initiates a vicious cycle, causing further reduction of the cardiac output.

Chest pain in the presence of normal coronary arteries appears, at least in part, to be due to increased extravascular coronary resistance. The exercise-induced increase in left ventricular end-diastolic volume and pressure, as well as the decreased ejection fraction, may limit the dilatory capacity of the coronary arteries with resultant subendocardial ischemia.[32]

Clinical Manifestations

History

The insidious onset of left ventricular failure is manifest by dyspnea, initially on exertion and then

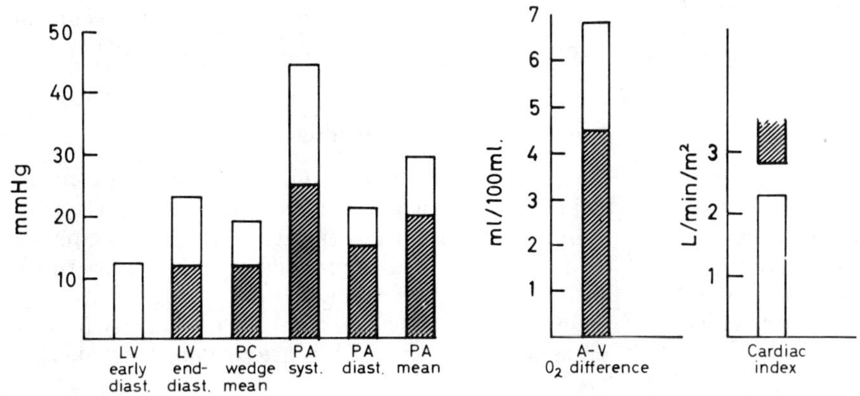

FIGURE 58-4 Results of hemodynamic study in congestive cardiomyopathy (30 catheterizations of the right side of the heart and 14 catheterizations of the left side of the heart). Average values. Shaded area, normal values. (*From A. Kristinsson, "Diagnosis, Natural History and Treatment of Congestive Cardiomyopathy," Ph.D. thesis, University of London, 1969. Reproduced with permission from the publisher and author.*)

at rest, a nocturnal dry cough, and at times pulmonary edema followed by symptoms of right-sided congestive heart failure. In many patients there may be symptoms mimicking an upper respiratory tract infection before heart failure develops. Chest pain may occur, particularly with exertion.

Physical Examination
The abnormal physical signs are those resulting from congestive heart failure. The patient may be breathless on slight exertion or even at rest; the skin is cool, pale, and slightly cyanosed. The peripheral veins are constricted, and the arterial pulse is small in volume. Pulsus alternans is evident in advanced disease. Tachycardia at rest is common. The jugular venous pressure is elevated, sometimes substantially. When there is sinus rhythm, a prominent *a* wave is usually followed by a poor *x* descent and a prominent systolic wave due to tricuspid regurgitation. With atrial fibrillation, the *a* wave is absent and is replaced by a single wave due to a combination of right atrial filling and tricuspid regurgitation. The left ventricular impulse is located outside the midclavicular line and is usually of poor quality, but may be forceful. A presystolic impulse also may be evident. Pulsation to the left of the lower sternum may be due to right ventricular dilatation.

Systolic murmurs of mitral and tricuspid regurgitation are common, rarely loud, and often diminish in intensity with treatment. Gallop rhythm is almost invariable; a third heart sound, due to rapid filling, is common, indicating a dilated, poorly functioning left ventricle. A fourth sound, resulting from the high left ventricular diastolic pressure, is frequently present but may be poorly audible due to its low frequency. When the heart rate exceeds 100 to 110 beats per minute, the third and fourth heart sounds may produce a single sound in middiastole, a summation gallop. The second heart sound shows reversed splitting if there is left bundle branch block. Pulmonary valve closure is accentuated when pulmonary arterial hypertension is present.

The blood pressure often is normal, despite a reduced pulse pressure due to poor cardiac output. At times peripheral vasoconstriction may increase the blood pressure. Pericardial effusion may be present. Examination of the lungs reveals basal rales and frequently pleural effusions. When right-sided failure is severe, there often is hepatomegaly. The liver may pulsate, a reflection of severe tricuspid regurgitation. Peripheral edema is common. Ascites also may occur.

Chest Roentgenogram
There is considerable cardiomegaly due mainly to dilatation of both ventricles. The left and right atria may be enlarged, the right atrium more than the left, as a result of tricuspid regurgitation (Fig. 58-5). The pulmonary vascular pattern is that of pulmonary venous hypertension, reflecting redistribution of flow to the upper-lobe vessels. Interstitial

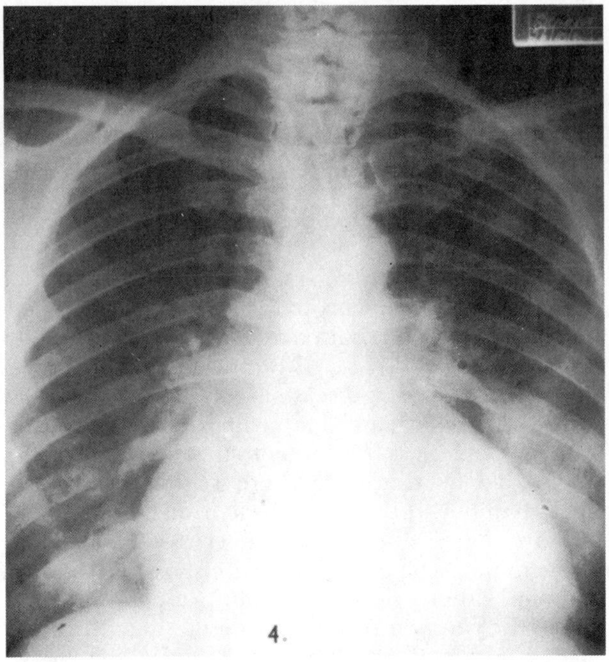

FIGURE 58-5 Posteroanterior chest radiograph of a patient with dilated cardiomyopathy. The heart is greatly enlarged, including the pulmonary arteries and right atrium. The superior vena cava is prominent due to right-sided heart failure. Incipient pulmonary edema is present due to left-sided heart failure.

costophrenic lines are common. The main pulmonary arteries are slightly enlarged; pleural effusions may be present, as may be pulmonary infarction. The heart has a water-bottle shape when there is a pericardial effusion.

Electrocardiogram
The electrocardiogram is characteristically abnormal, but the changes are usually nonspecific, with flat or inverted T waves. Sinus tachycardia is frequent. There is often an atrial abnormality and evidence of modest left ventricular hypertrophy, which is occasionally severe with disease of long standing. QRS complexes are usually of low voltage. The frontal plane axis is abnormal in 40 percent of patients; atrial fibrillation occurs in 25 percent; and atrial flutter, junctional rhythm, supraventricular tachycardia, first degree and complete heart block, and ventricular tachycardia have all been noted. Left bundle branch block occurs in about 20 percent of patients. Q waves may be present in the precordial leads, mimicking myocardial infarction.[33] (Fig. 58-6)

Special Laboratory Studies

Blood and Urine Tests The red and white blood cell counts are usually normal; the erythrocyte sedimentation rate is often elevated. Serum proteins are usually normal, but abnormal globulins may result from hepatic insufficiency due to heart failure. Occasionally, abnormal cardiac enzyme activity may be present. Serum iron levels are usually normal. Lev-

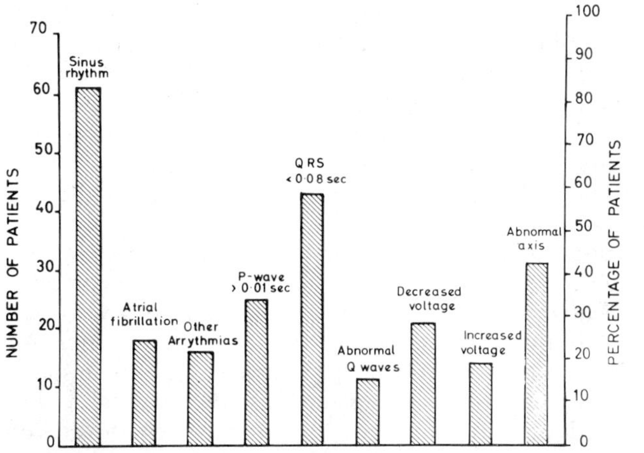

FIGURE 58-6 Electrocardiographic abnormalities in a series of 74 patients with congestive cardiomyopathy. (*From A. Kristinsson, "Diagnosis, Natural History and Treatment of Congestive Cardiomyopathy," Ph.D. thesis, University of London, 1969. Reproduced with permission from the publisher and author.*)

els of vanillylmandelic acid in the urine are usually normal.[11]

Phonocardiogram Phonocardiogram confirms the gallop sounds and systolic murmurs of mitral and tricuspid regurgitation.

Echocardiogram (Fig. 58-7) Increased cavity size of both ventricles and poor movement of the posterior (free) wall of the left ventricle, with paradoxical movement of the septum, is common; septal and free wall thicknesses are normal or nearly so. The mitral valve apparatus is located close to the posterior wall, and the distance from the anterior mitral leaflet to the septum is increased. The amplitude of separation of the mitral valve leaflets is usually decreased, and the rate of circumferential shortening of the myocardial wall is markedly reduced. A pericardial effusion may be evident. Two-dimensional echocardiography may identify left ventricular mural thrombi.[34] Usually there is global hypokinesia of the ventricle, but regional dyskinesia occurs, probably as a result of regional scarring. Segmental wall motion abnormalities cannot be used to differentiate ischemic from nonischemic cardiomyopathy; prognosis is often better than with diffuse wall motion abnormalities.[34a] Echocardiography is valuable to define the extent of dysfunction and dilatation of the left ventricle, but is of no value in indicating the cause. Pulsed Doppler echocardiography may aid in the quantitative assessment of left ventricular systolic function.[35]

Ambulatory Electrocardiogram Identification of frequent pairs of ventricular ectopic beats or episodes of ventricular tachycardia on a 24-h ambulatory electrocardiogram identified patients with dilated cardiomyopathy and a reduced ejection fraction who were at high risk of dying suddenly.[36]

Radionuclide Imaging Techniques Blood pool imaging confirms the biventricular dilatation and global decrease in contractility. The left ventricle is usually more involved than the right. The ejection fraction may be as low as 10 to 15 percent. Serial radionuclide examinations can help assess the course of the disease and the response to therapy.[37] Perfusion defects on thallium scanning occur in patients with dilated cardiomyopathy, so this test cannot reliably distinguish between cardiomyopathy and coronary artery disease.[38]

FIGURE 58-7 Echocardiogram illustrating congestive cardiomyopathy. Echocardiographic sweep from the aorta and left atrium (left) to the apex of the left ventricle (right). The aorta is slightly increased in size and the wall motion is decreased, consistent with diminished left ventricular stroke output. The left atrium is increased in size. The left ventricular cavity is markedly dilated, with decreased septal and posterior wall motion. The mitral valve has a "double diamond" configuration, with decreased leaflet excursion and a marked increase in the distance between the anterior leaflet and the ventricular septum, characteristic of a decreased left ventricular ejection fraction. The left ventricular cavity, rather than tapering normally at the apex, remains dilated. These findings are consistent with congestive cardiomyopathy. Ao = aorta; LA = left atrium; MV = mitral valve; RV = right ventricle; LV = left ventricle. (*Courtesy of Dr. Joel Felner, Emory University School of Medicine.*)

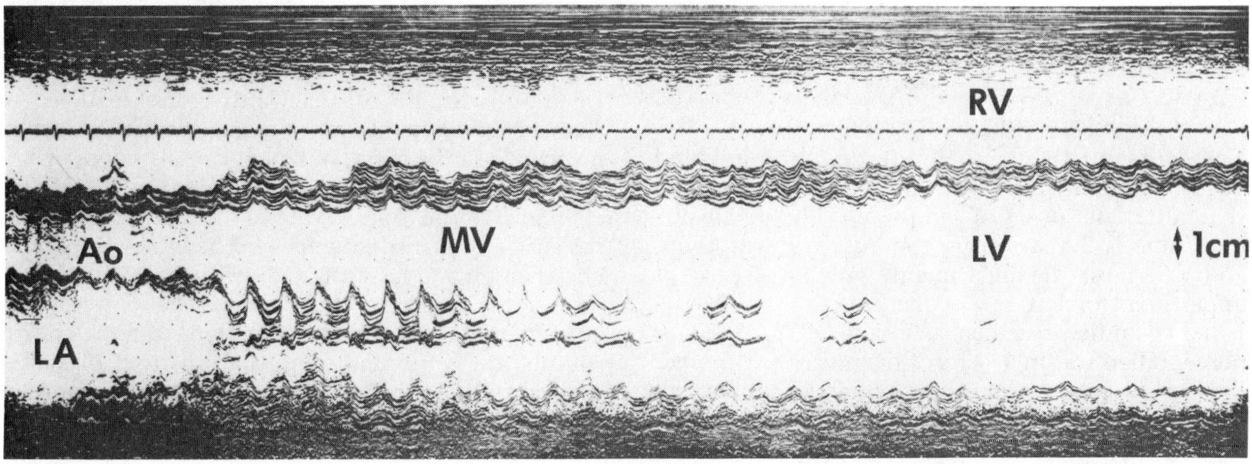

Systolic Time Intervals The ratio of pre-ejection period (PEP) to left ventricular ejection time (LVET) is abnormal. The PEP/LVET ratio varies inversely with the ejection fraction, and ratios greatly above normal (0.43) are common.

Angiocardiogram This reveals a diffusely enlarged left ventricle with generalized hypokinesis and poor contraction. The normal pear-shaped contour of the left ventricle is replaced by diffuse globular enlargement. Regional dyskinesis, when occasionally present, may make differentiation from coronary heart disease with myocardial infarction impossible unless coronary arteriography is performed. Filling defects of the left ventricle due to intracavitary thrombus are seen on occasion. The left atrium is usually slightly, but seldom greatly, enlarged; mitral regurgitation is usually only slight or moderate. Coronary arteriography characteristically shows widely patent vessels.

Endomyocardial Biopsy Endomyocardial biopsy is a useful investigative technique. Studies of enzymes in the various subcellular organelles have shown reduced levels of mitochondrial dehydrogenases and myofibrillar ATPase and increased lactic dehydrogenase, suggesting that impaired myocardial contractility may be associated with impairment of mitochondrial energy production and consequent enhanced anaerobic glycolysis.[39] No specific biopsy changes have been found to indicate a cause for the condition. As a method of diagnosis in an individual patient, endomyocardial biopsy is unlikely to be rewarding and is not recommended as a routine procedure, as the findings are usually nonspecific.[40] An exception is the young patient with a brief history of heart failure who may respond to corticosteroid or immunosuppressive therapy.[41] In such patients, biopsy is indicated to differentiate dilated cardiomyopathy from myocarditis. Also, when specific heart muscle disease is suspected, biopsy may be helpful. It is also valuable for the diagnosis of acute rejection of the transplanted heart and may be of value in the evaluation of cardiotoxicity from anthracycline chemotherapy. The role of endomyocardial biopsy in monitoring the treatment of patients with dilated cardiomyopathy remains uncertain, with little value demonstrated to date.

Natural History and Prognosis

The course of DC is usually steadily downhill, and death commonly ensues within 6 months to several years after the onset of symptoms. The mean survival time is 3 years from the onset of symptoms, and prognosis depends mainly on the severity of impairment of left ventricular function.[41a] Of 104 patients studied between 1960 and 1973, about 70 percent died within 2 years of diagnosis.[42] Although the overall prognosis is not good, about 20 percent of patients may do well.

The main complications of dilated cardiomyopathy are manifestations of severe heart failure. Atrial fibrillation increases the risk of embolism, but embolism commonly occurs with sinus rhythm from thrombus in the dilated, poorly contractile left ventricle. However, systemic emboli were not more frequent in patients with left ventricular thrombus demonstrated by two-dimensional echochardiography than in those without evidence of thrombi. Pulmonary embolism is common, arising from both the peripheral veins and the right side of the heart. Repeated small pulmonary emboli may progressively obliterate the pulmonary vascular bed and increase right-sided heart failure. Repeated pulmonary embolism also may be evident as unexplained tachycardia, disturbances of consciousness, fever, or dyspnea. There may be clinical evidence of increasing pulmonary hypertension and central venous pressure; hemoptysis and icterus may occur particularly when pulmonary infarction develops. Ventricular arrhythmias may be as frequent as in hypertrophic cardiomyopathy and are an important potential cause of sudden death, but may go undetected unless regular ECG monitoring is carried out. The severity of left ventricular dysfunction, however, may better predict the risk of sudden death than the results of ambulatory electrocardiography.[43]

When heart failure develops, energetic treatment commonly produces a remission; the patient improves for months, and occasionally the disease remains indolent for years. Relapse then occurs, recurring episodes of heart failure become increasingly difficult to control, and finally the patient is in a state of intractable congestive cardiac failure which proves fatal. Death can occur suddenly from ventricular fibrillation or occasionally from embolism.

Differential Diagnosis[44]

The differential diagnosis includes causes of congestive heart failure. Organic valvular or congenital heart diseases can usually be readily differentiated; principal differentials include atherosclerotic coronary heart disease, hypertensive heart disease, and heart muscle disease secondary to specific systemic disorders.

Atherosclerotic Coronary Heart Disease

In atherosclerotic coronary heart disease there is characteristically a history of angina pectoris or acute myocardial infarction, but such can also occur with dilated cardiomyopathy. On the other hand, ischemic cardiomyopathy due to coronary atherosclerosis may occur in patients who have never experienced angina. Many patients with coronary heart disease do not have abnormalities on physical examination of the heart, although third or fourth heart sounds are common. Abnormal, diffuse, or paradoxical pulsation of the left ventricle, superior and internal to the apex impulse, suggests a ventricular aneurysm, but these abnormalities can occur with dilated cardiomyopathy. The electrocardiogram can show evidence of previous infarction but can be misleading because Q waves may be present in some patients with dilated congestive cardiomyopathy and normal coronary arteries. Conduction defects may occur in both disorders, but the left bundle branch block is far more common in cardiomyopathy. Segmental asynergy (by two-dimensional echocardiography or radionuclide angiography) suggests coronary artery disease, as do large circumferential perfusion defects with ^{201}Tl-myocardial imaging.[37] Absolute proof is dependent on demonstration of coronary artery narrowing by arteriography; however, in most patients, dilated cardiomyopathy can be diagnosed with accuracy by clinical methods. (See Chap. 45.)

Hypertensive Heart Disease
Patients with established hypertensive heart disease usually have marked left ventricular enlargement and evidence of long-standing hypertensive vascular disease elsewhere in the body, particularly the optic fundi, before heart failure develops (see Chaps. 49 to 51). Moreover, episodes of left ventricular failure are usually related to substantial increases in systemic blood pressure. Difficulty may arise in differential diagnosis when heart failure persists despite only moderate hypertension. Differential diagnosis then may include hypertensive heart disease, atherosclerotic coronary heart disease, and dilated cardiomyopathy, with the presence of cardiac pain favoring coronary heart disease.

Myocardial Involvement in Systemic Disease
These disorders (see Chaps. 72 to 76) constitute an important group because accurate diagnosis is essential for specific treatment. Clinical examination, by revealing evidence of systemic disease, can often identify many disorders. Examples of cardiac features useful in differential diagnosis are a tendency to arrhythmias and heart block in both sarcoidosis and the peripheral myopathies, and a pericardial friction rub in polyarteritis, systemic lupus erythematosus, and viral infection.

Hypertrophic Cardiomyopathy
Occasionally when outflow tract gradients are absent in hypertrophic cardiomyopathy (HC), the condition may resemble dilated cardiomyopathy, particularly when atrial fibrillation and congestive heart failure are present (see later discussion). A history of chest pain is far more common in hypertrophic than in dilated congestive cardiomyopathy, as is a history of syncope. The jerky, ill-sustained arterial pulse of hypertrophic cardiomyopathy, while not as striking in patients without, as in those with, gradients, may still be retained and contrasts with the small-volume pulse of dilated cardiomyopathy. If sinus rhythm is present, the palpable presystolic left ventricular impulse is an important sign of hypertrophic cardiomyopathy. Systolic murmurs can be present in both dilated and hypertrophic cardiomyopathy; in dilated cardiomyopathy they are due to mitral and tricuspid atrioventricular regurgitation secondary to ventricular dilatation, and in hypertrophic cardiomyopathy to an aortic outflow tract gradient and mitral regurgitation. The murmur in hypertrophic cardiomyopathy is of late onset, spindle-shaped, and heard at the left sternal edge and apex; the systolic murmurs of dilated cardiomyopathy, while they may be spindle-shaped, are usually pansystolic, start earlier, and are usually best heard at the lower left sternal border and the cardiac apex. The electrocardiogram in hypertrophic cardiomyopathy shows considerably greater QRS voltage and more marked ST-T wave abnormalities than those in dilated cardiomyopathy. The echocardiogram is valuable in diagnosis, mainly when attention is directed to the dimensions of the left ventricle; these are reduced in hypertrophic cardiomyopathy and increased in dilated cardiomyopathy. Observing the position of the mitral valve is also useful; it is displaced toward the septum in hypertrophic cardiomyopathy and toward the posterior wall of the left ventricle in dilated cardiomyopathy. The movement of the posterior (free) wall of the left ventricle tends to be poor in dilated cardiomyopathy and normal or greater than normal in hypertrophic cardiomyopathy. In occasional patients, angiography is required to differentiate these conditions.

In patients with heart failure, the question What is the heart failure due to? must always be asked. Common causes of heart failure, or apparent heart failure, that are not always appreciated include recurrent pulmonary embolism, infective endocarditis, severe anemia, thyrotoxicosis, and pericardial effusion with tamponade. Rare causes are atrial myxoma, tricuspid stenosis, and obliterative pulmonary hypertension. Occasionally, severe aortic stenosis with heart failure and a low cardiac output may present without an obvious murmur and simulate dilated congestive cardiomyopathy; calcification of the aortic valve is a useful diagnostic feature. Usually when the heart failure improves and cardiac output increases, the murmur becomes obvious.

Heart failure is not always due to impairment of systolic contractile function; it may be due to impairment of filling of the left ventricle or both ventricles, which in turn leads to a reduction in effective cardiac output. Diastolic heart failure is seen in hypertrophic cardiomyopathy, endomyocardial fibrosis, amyloid heart disease, and constrictive pericarditis. These conditions are termed *diastolic heart disease.*

Treatment

Medical treatment of dilated cardiomyopathy remains unsatisfactory. Control of heart failure by the usual means is essential,[45] with specific care taken to avoid digitalis toxicity. It is advisable to withdraw alcohol completely. There is no evidence that smoking is deleterious to patients with dilated cardiomyopathy, but its adverse effects on the lungs, heart, and circulation make it unwise. A nutritious diet with vitamin supplementation is recommended. Prolonged bed rest or at least prolonged reduction of activity may be useful and may delay the onset of relapse into heart failure in some patients. However, the possibility that graded exercise might diminish the risk of arrhythmia and improve prognosis should be explored. Possibly the increase in parasympathetic tone and decrease in sympathetic tone of effort, noted in an experiment in dogs, might explain the protective effect of exercise.[46] Activity should be restricted for about a year after the first episode of heart failure. Pregnancy is inadvisable.

The use of corticosteroid hormones is controversial. They have little or no value in established dilated cardiomyopathy, but may help patients with heart failure due to a specific heart muscle disease with evidence of an autoimmune disorder and patients with subacute myocarditis.[41] Young patients with a brief history of heart failure may obtain benefit from corticosteroid hormone (and possibly immunosuppressive drug) treatment, but evidence for myocarditis should be sought from endomyocardial biopsy.[41]

Reduction of the resistance to left ventricular ejection, with a resultant improvement in cardiac performance is the basis for vasodilator therapy. Vasodilator therapy appears of benefit symptomatically, at times dramatically so, but does not improve the rate of survival. Hydralazine (50 to 300 mg/day) reduces systemic vascular resistance, increases cardiac output, and causes a fall in left ventricular end-diastolic pressure. Tachycardia does not occur because of blunted chronotropic reflexes.[47] Common side effects include headache, nausea, facial flushing, and fever; occasionally a lupus erythematosus-like syndrome may develop. Side effects are usually confined to patients who are slow acetylators. Prazosin, another peripheral vasodilator, has a similar effect to hydralazine but with fewer complications; a disadvantage is a tendency to tachyphylaxis. Captopril, an angiotensin-converting enzyme inhibitor, may improve cardiocirculatory function by selective arteriolar dilatation.[48] Nitrates may also be used to reduce left ventricular preload and afterload. Isosorbide dinitrate in a dose of 10 to 20 mg four times daily can be used alone or in conjunction with other vasodilator agents. The effect of the combination of nitrate drugs and hydralazine appears synergistic. Vasodilators are contraindicated when the systemic blood pressure is low, i.e., at or below 100 mmHg systolic, and in patients in cardiogenic shock.

Salbutamol, a primarily beta$_2$-adrenergic stimulant, has a peripheral vasodilator and possibly a positive inotropic action with larger doses; given acutely by continuous intravenous infusion at a rate of 2 to 8 μg/min, it produced clinical improvement, with an increase in cardiac output and stroke volume, a decrease in left ventricular end-diastolic pressure, and a slight decrease in systemic blood pressure.[49] Tachycardia, hyperglycemia, and hypokalemia are disadvantages.

The use of positive inotropic agents such as dobutamine and dopamine is becoming more promising, as is the combination of positive inotropic agents and vasodilator drugs, which may exert a synergistic benefit. The combination of intravenous infusion of dobutamine with a vasodilator appears of benefit. A number of new drugs that can be given orally, such as prenalterol, pirbuterol, amrinone, and milrinone, have a positive inotropic action.[50–53] It is not always easy to determine whether beneficial effects are due to the direct positive inotropy or to the vasodilator effects of these drugs. Some of these drugs have undesirable side effects such as thrombocytopenia and impaired liver function. The mechanism of action of amrinone and milrinone is not known, although an increase in intracellular calcium is postulated as a cause of increased inotropy. The role of these newer inotropic agents in the management of patients with dilated cardiomyopathy and their effects on prognosis are as yet uncertain; they appear to improve exercise capacity and quality of life, despite progression of the underlying disease. The use of two vasodilator agents, one of which acts on preload as well as afterload, and the other on afterload alone, such as nitrites or nitroprusside in combination with hydralazine, has been found advantageous. Some agents improve hemodynamics and metabolism,[50] others mainly affect symptoms and effort tolerance. With all, the effects usually wear off; whether this is due to tachyphylaxis or a worsening of the disease is not known. Claim has been made that vasodilator therapy, in addition to improving cardiac function, may improve myocardial cellular morphology and reduce hypertrophy.[54] Since calcium transport into the sarcoplasmic reticulum is related to heart muscle relaxation, modification of the effects of the calcium-calmodulin–dependent protein kinases that regulate this function may be an alternate approach to the treatment of heart failure. Details of the pharmacological treatment of congestive heart failure are found in Chap. 21. There is no drug specific for the heart failure of dilated cardiomyopathy. If viral infection proves to be an important cause, the goal to strive for will be early detection and effective viral chemotherapy, before immunologic faults have become irreversible.

Although ventricular arrhythmias are associated with an unfavorable prognosis, the role of antiarrhythmic therapy remains to be defined; pacemakers may be lifesaving.

The use of selective beta-adrenergic blockade has been advocated, beginning with small doses and gradually increasing unless there is deterioration. Dramatic effects have been reported, especially in patients with high resting heart rates.[55] Improvement in both myocardial function and in rate of survival is described.[55] The rationale of this treatment is not fully understood, although slowing of the heart rate as occurs with bed rest and limitation of excessive catecholamine stimulation of the failing heart have been suggested. Few randomized trials are available,[56] some show no improvement,[57] and while some patients may benefit, caution is advised until the results of the multicenter trial that is planned are available.

Anticoagulant drugs are important to prevent the frequent systemic and pulmonary embolism, particularly in patients with atrial fibrillation, those who require prolonged immobilization, who have extensive edema, and a low cardiac output; substantial benefit has recently been documented even for patients with sinus rhythm.[42] The dose of oral anticoagulant required may be less than usual because of depressed hepatic function due to the severe heart failure.

The only *surgical treatment* of dilated cardiomyopathy is that of cardiac transplantation; it should be considered in young patients in the terminal phases of the disease, and may improve prognosis.[58] A substantial improvement in survival of cardiac transplantation recipients is evident in recent years (see Chap. 36).

Occasionally improvement may occur with mitral valve replacement in patients with considerable mitral regurgitation. It is often uncertain, however, whether such patients have dilated congestive cardiomyopathy or primary mitral valve disease with secondary ventricular involvement. If left ventricular function is severely damaged, mitral valve replacement is very unlikely to help and may be fatal.

Hypertrophic Cardiomyopathy

Nomenclature

This condition has been described by many names, the two most frequently initially used being *idiopathic hypertrophic subaortic stenosis*[59] in North America and *hypertrophic obstructive cardiomyopathy* in Europe. These terms overemphasize the "obstructive" element or phase of the disease. HC is the current name of choice, emphasizing the predominant increase in ventricular muscle mass. In many cases a familial incidence has been noted. The inheritance is not sex-linked and is dominant, but because of the great variability in the extent and severity of the disease, many familial cases are probably not detected, so that all patients may, in fact, inherit the disease. It is likely that the disorder is genetically transmitted, a concept reenforced by the association with specific leukocyte antigen phenotypes[60,61] and the frequent echocardiographic abnormalities in asymptomatic family members. Immunogenetic factors linked to HLA seem to play a role in the "obstructive" but not the "nonobstructive" aspects of hypertrophic cardiomyopathy.[61] The genetic basis has been reviewed recently.[62]

Etiology

There are only speculations as to etiology. The resemblance of the disorganized myofibrillar lesions to those in a primitive heart, such as the salamander's; the presence of the abnormality at birth; and the familial occurrence all suggest a disorder of myocardial development in utero.[63] The direction of the mechanical forces of contraction normally determine the pattern of orientation of muscle fibers.[64] The arrangement and orientation of myofibrils into parallel lines in the embryonic heart may be altered by abnormally oriented forces.[63] The myofibrillar arrangement in hypertrophic cardiomyopathy suggests a cell type less well differentiated than that of the fully developed myocardium.

The reason for abnormal orientation of myofibrils in hypertrophic cardiomyopathy[5,65] may be a genetically determined *aberration of catecholamine function* in the embryo heart. Although there is no direct proof, circumstantial evidence, both clinical and experimental, supports this theory. Clinically, a number of conditions with catecholamine dysfunction occur in association with hypertrophic cardiomyopathy: systemic arterial hypertension, pheochromocytoma, neurofibromatosis, lentiginosis, and Friedreich's ataxia; indeed, Friedreich's ataxia is the most commonly associated condition. The responses to beta-adrenergic stimulation and beta blockade in acute observation of systolic and diastolic function of the left ventricle, respectively, are also persuasive. The increase in outflow tract gradient and ventricular stiffness produced by isoproterenol and the decrease in gradient and reduction in stiffness produced by beta-adrenergic blocking agents suggest that catecholamine function is abnormal.

Experimentally, subhypertensive infusions of norepinephrine can produce ventricular hypertrophy in the dog, with hemodynamic and angiographic changes similar to hypertrophic cardiomyopathy.[66] Nerve growth factor, the glycoprotein which enhances sympathetic nerve growth and cardiac adrenergic innervation, produces a left ventricular pressure gradient, increased septal thickness, and myocardial fibrillar disarray when given to newborn puppies.[67] More recently, further studies in dogs have suggested that the ventricular septum may be susceptible to cyclic adenosine monophosphate (AMP) depletion, leading to hypertrophy similar to that seen in HC.[68] A study of patients with HC might show increased adrenergic activity and decreased stores of cyclic AMP and adenosine triphosphate (ATP). Other hormones may be implicated. For example, reversible echocardiographic features of hypertrophic cardiomyopathy have been described in infants of diabetic mothers.[69] Administration of large doses of triac to pregnant rats produced myofibrillar disarray in the offspring,[70] and an association in human beings between thyrotoxicosis and hypertrophic cardiomyopathy has been suggested.

Hypertrophic cardiomyopathy may therefore result from an inherited abnormality of handling catecholamines by the developing myocardium. It is unlikely to be due to a direct effect of excessive catecholamine action, but myofibrillar disarray may prevent the orderly arrangement of the myofibrils, stimulate further hypertrophy, and impair both contraction and relaxation. It has been suggested that faulty interaction between norepinephrine and the myocardial adrenergic receptor sites may cause failure of regression of myocardial disarray and disproportionate septal thickness in animal fetal hearts.[71]

Pathology

At necropsy, the heart in hypertrophic cardiomyopathy (HC) has a constellation of certain predictable, characteristic, although not absolutely specific, features (Figs. 58-8 and 58-9): (1) greater thickening of the ventricular septum than the left ventricular free wall (95 percent); (2) small or normal-sized left and right ventricular cavities (95 percent); (3) mural endocardial plaque, left ventricular outflow tract (75 percent; mainly adults); (4) thickened mitral valve (75 percent; mainly adults); (5) dilated atria (100 percent; adults); (6) abnormal intramural coronary arteries (50 percent; see Fig. 58-10); and (7) disorganization of myocardial fibers in the ventricular septum (95 percent; see Fig. 58-11).[72]

The chief morphological abnormality in HC resides in the ventricular septum. As pointed out by Teare in his initial description of this condition,[73] the ventricular septum nearly always is thicker than the left ventricular free wall. Among adult necropsy patients, the maximal thickness of ventricular septum averages 3.0 cm, and the maximal thickness of left ventricular free wall 1.8 cm.[74] The thickest portion of the septum is located about midway between the aortic valve and left ventricular apex; this level corresponds approximately to the apex of right ventricle. Although the ventricular septum is thicker than normal, the left ventricular free wall is usually, but not always, thicker than normal.

Although ventricular asymmetry, i.e., a signifi-

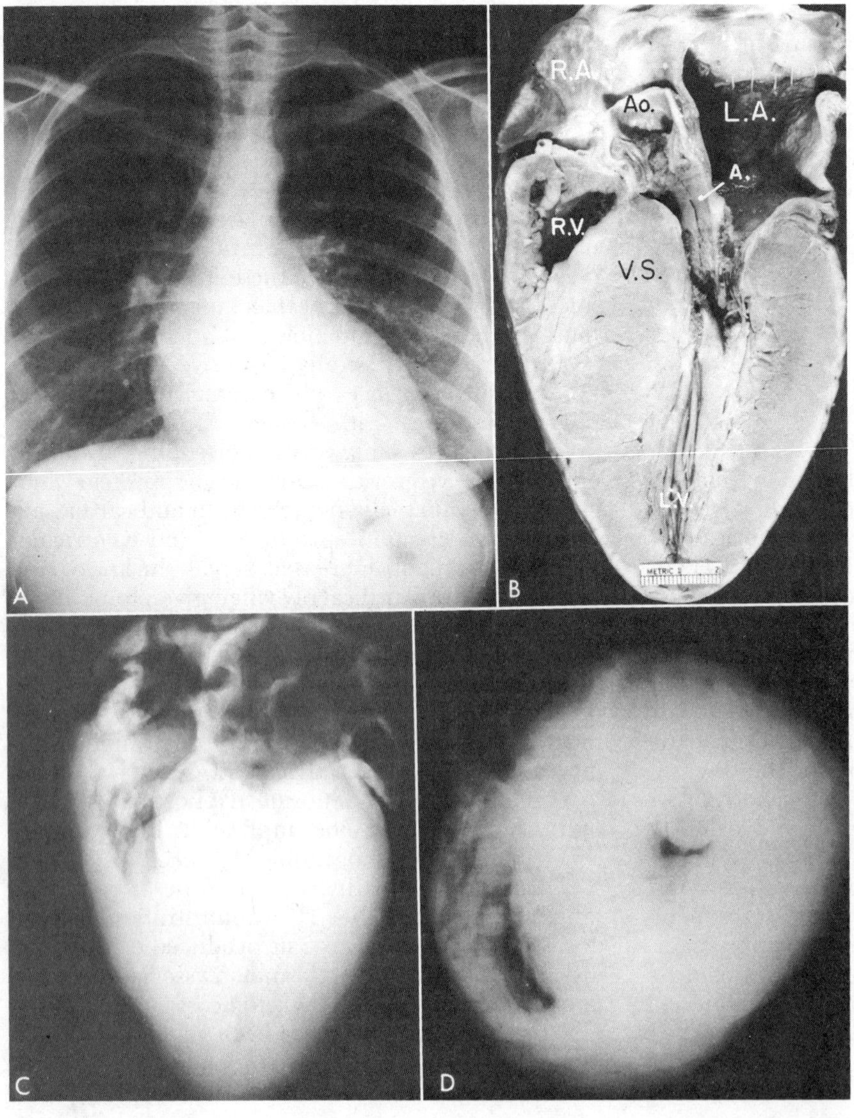

FIGURE 58-8 Hypertrophic cardiomyopathy of the obstructive type. This 36-year-old woman (A67-121) developed congestive cardiac failure during her second pregnancy at age 32. When studied at age 34, she had a grade 3/6 precordial systolic murmur, loudest over the apex, and audible third and fourth heart sounds. Electrocardiogram showed bilateral bundle branch block with left axis deviation and prolongation (0.23 s) of the PR interval. Catheterization disclosed a 75-mmHg peak systolic pressure gradient at rest between left ventricle (160/18) and femoral artery (85/50), and a 125-mmHg gradient with provocation (Valsalva). The premature ventricular contraction response was positive for hypertrophic cardiomyopathy (HC). She died during an episode of rapid heart action. She was known to have multiple premature ventricular contractions on occasions.

At necropsy, the heart was enlarged (*A*), weighing 450 g; the left ventricular cavity was small (*B* to *D*), and the ventricular septum (V.S.) was much thicker than the left ventricular (L.V.) free wall. There was little room in the left ventricular cavity for the mitral leaflets, and contact lesions (fibromas) were present on the ventricular aspect of the anterior (*A*) mitral leaflet and on the adjacent left ventricular mural endocardium (*B*). Ao. = aorta; R.V. = right ventricle. This is the typical "muscle-bound" heart in which the ventricular cavities are minute in comparison to the mass of ventricular muscle. Both right (R.A.) and left (L.A.) atria are dilated.

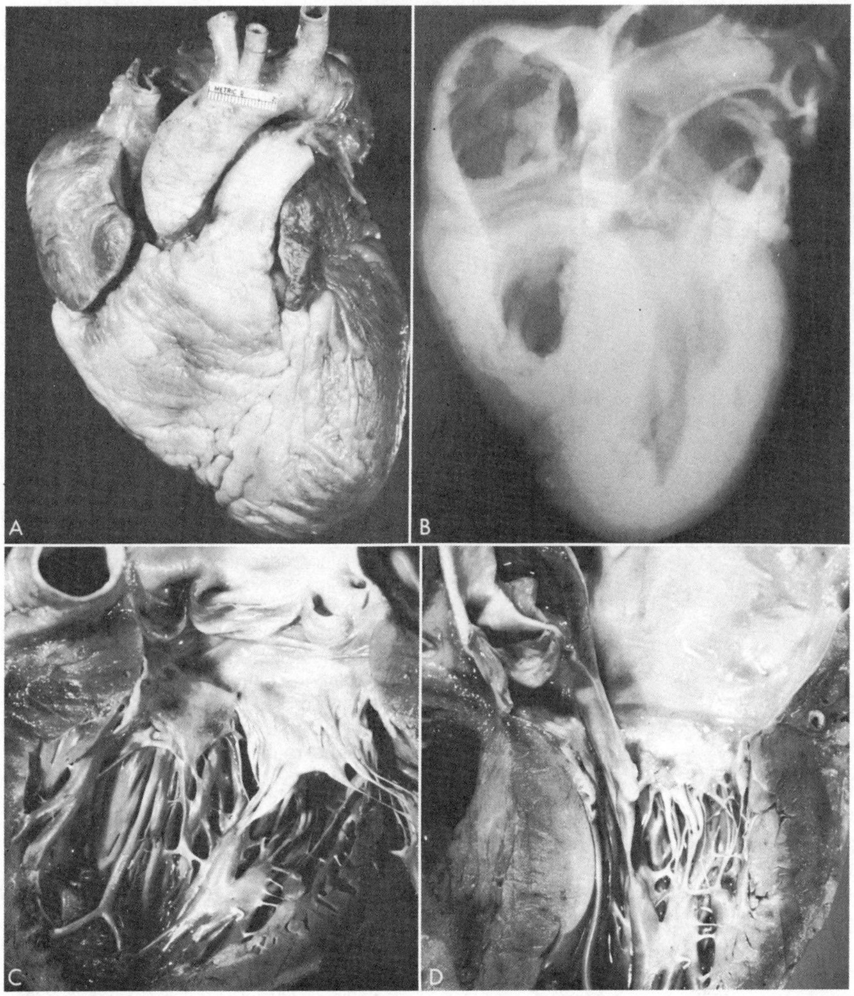

FIGURE 58-9 Hypertrophic cardiomyopathy. This 33-year-old man (A68-185) had no systolic pressure gradient at rest between left ventricle and brachial artery, but a 33-mmHg gradient was provoked by isoproterenol. He died of sudden unilateral hemiparesis which appeared 6 days after the catheterization. He had been asymptomatic when examined at age 26 when a grade 2 to 3/6 precordial systolic murmur, loudest at the apex, was heard. Catheterization at that time showed a 30-mmHg peak systolic gradient at rest between left ventricle and brachial artery, and it rose to 85 mmHg with ouabain provocation. He became symptomatic (exertional and nocturnal dyspnea) 6 months before death, when atrial fibrillation appeared. The precordial murmur then was only intermittently audible.

At necropsy, the heart weighed 450 g; both atria were dilated, but neither ventricle was dilated (*A*). The ventricular septum was thicker than the left ventricular free wall (*B*). A mural endocardial plaque was present in the left ventricular outflow tract, and the corresponding anterior mitral leaflet was thickened (*C* and *D*). The longitudinal cut of the heart in *D* clearly shows that the ventricular septum is thicker than the left ventricular free wall.

cant difference in maximal thickness of ventricular septum and left ventricular free wall, is a characteristic morphological feature of HC, about 5 percent of patients at necropsy have ventricular symmetry, i.e., equal maximal thickness of the ventricular septum and left ventricular free wall.[75] Thus, although asymmetric septal hypertrophy (ASH) is a highly sensitive marker for HC, it is not specific for this condition.[75] Ventricular septa thicker than left ventricular free walls have been reported in conditions causing thinning of the left ventricular free wall relative to the septum and in conditions causing thickening of the septum relative to the free wall. The most common cause of preferential septal thickening is right ventricular systolic hypertension from any of a variety of conditions. Disproportionate septal thickening usually occurs early in the intrauterine development of the heart.

Among patients with HC, the thickness of the ventricular septum is not dependent on the presence of a left ventricular outflow tract gradient at rest, and, indeed, the thickness of the septum is similar in patients with and without outflow gradients at rest. Although examination of the septum is not helpful in separating patients with from those without left ventricular outflow gradients at rest, examination of the basal portion of the left ventricular free wall (posterior or posterolateral portion) permits delineation between these two groups.[76] In patients with the "obstructive" type of HC, this posterobasal portion of the left ventricular free wall represents the thickest portion of free wall, whereas in patients with the nonobstructive type of HC (Fig. 58-12), this posterobasal portion is thinner than normal and is often pointed like a bird's bill. In the patients with gradients at rest, the thickest portion of left ventricular free wall is about midway between the base of the posterior mitral leaflet and the apex of the left ventricle.

Another abnormality in the ventricular septum in patients with HC is focal myocardial fiber disarray or disorganization. This abnormality, also described by Teare,[73] occurs in about 95 percent of patients, depending on how "septal disorganization" is defined.[77] Small foci of groups of myocardial fibers not parallel to one another in the ventricular septum are common in normal developing and adult hearts. When the definition of "septal disorganization" is rigid and quantitation of the amount of disorganization is introduced, about 90 percent of patients

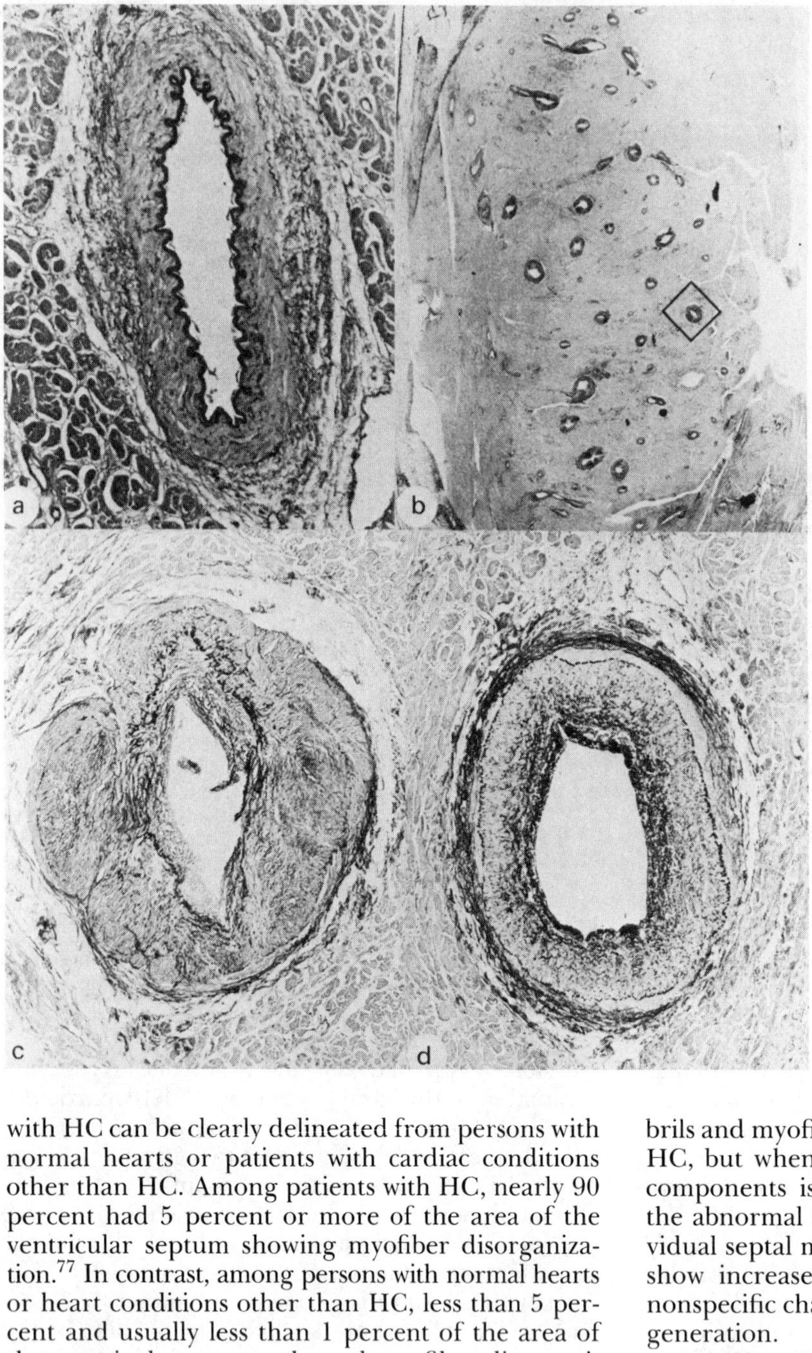

FIGURE 58-10 Intramural coronary arteries in ventricular septum in HC in three different patients. *a.* A normal artery (in a patient with HC), ×140. *b.* Low-power (×4) photomicrograph of portion of ventricular septum showing marked prominence of the intramural coronary arteries in another patient. The arteries appear to be increased in number, size, and wall thickness. *c.* The artery enclosed by the box in *b* is shown here, ×90. *d.* This artery, from another patient, has marked intimal thickening by fibroelastic proliferation, in contrast to the artery shown in *c*, which shows no delineation between intima and media. Elastic van Gieson stains; reduced 18 percent. [*From W. C. Roberts, Congenital Cardiovascular Abnormalities Usually "Silent" until Adulthood: Morphologic Features of the Floppy Mitral Valve, Valvular Aortic Stenosis, Discrete Subvalvular Aortic Stenosis, Hypertrophic Cardiomyopathy, Sinus of Valsalva Aneurysm, and the Marfan Syndrome, in W. C. Roberts (ed.), "Congenital Heart Disease in Adults," Cardiovasc. Clin., Philadelphia, F. A. Davis Company, 1979, p. 407. Reproduced with permission from the publisher and author.*]

with HC can be clearly delineated from persons with normal hearts or patients with cardiac conditions other than HC. Among patients with HC, nearly 90 percent had 5 percent or more of the area of the ventricular septum showing myofiber disorganization.[77] In contrast, among persons with normal hearts or heart conditions other than HC, less than 5 percent and usually less than 1 percent of the area of the ventricular septum showed myofiber disorganization.[78]

Although "septal disorganization" of greater than 5 percent of the ventricular septum occurs in about 90 percent of patients with HC, about 10 percent of patients have less than 5 percent of the area of the septum showing disarray, and a few of them have absolutely no disarray.[76] Thus, like ventricular asymmetry, "septal disorganization" of greater than 5 percent of the septum occurs in most patients with HC, but this abnormality may involve a smaller area of the septum, or, rarely, may be entirely absent.

Not only does disorganization of myocardial fibers occur, but ultrastructural studies have shown disarray of myofibrils and myofilaments within individual cells.[63] Again, the abnormalities of myofibrils and myofilaments are not absolutely specific for HC, but when disorganization of these subcellular components is found in other cardiac conditions, the abnormal cells are in small numbers. The individual septal myocardial cells in HC also frequently show increased amounts of Z-band material and nonspecific changes of cellular hypertrophy and degeneration.

Myofiber disarray in the left and right ventricular free walls is more difficult to determine by light microscopy than that in the ventricular septum. Ultrastructural examination of the left and right ventricular free walls, however, has disclosed many bizarrely shaped, disorganized cells in the ventricular free walls of patients without obstruction, whereas the bizarrely shaped and disorganized myocardial fibers are virtually absent from the ventricular free walls in patients with obstruction.[76] Thus, the disorientation of groups of myocardial cells and the disarray of myofibrils and myofilaments within individual myocardial cells is not the result of left ventricular outflow obstruction or high intraventricular systolic pressures.

The functional or clinical significance of "septal

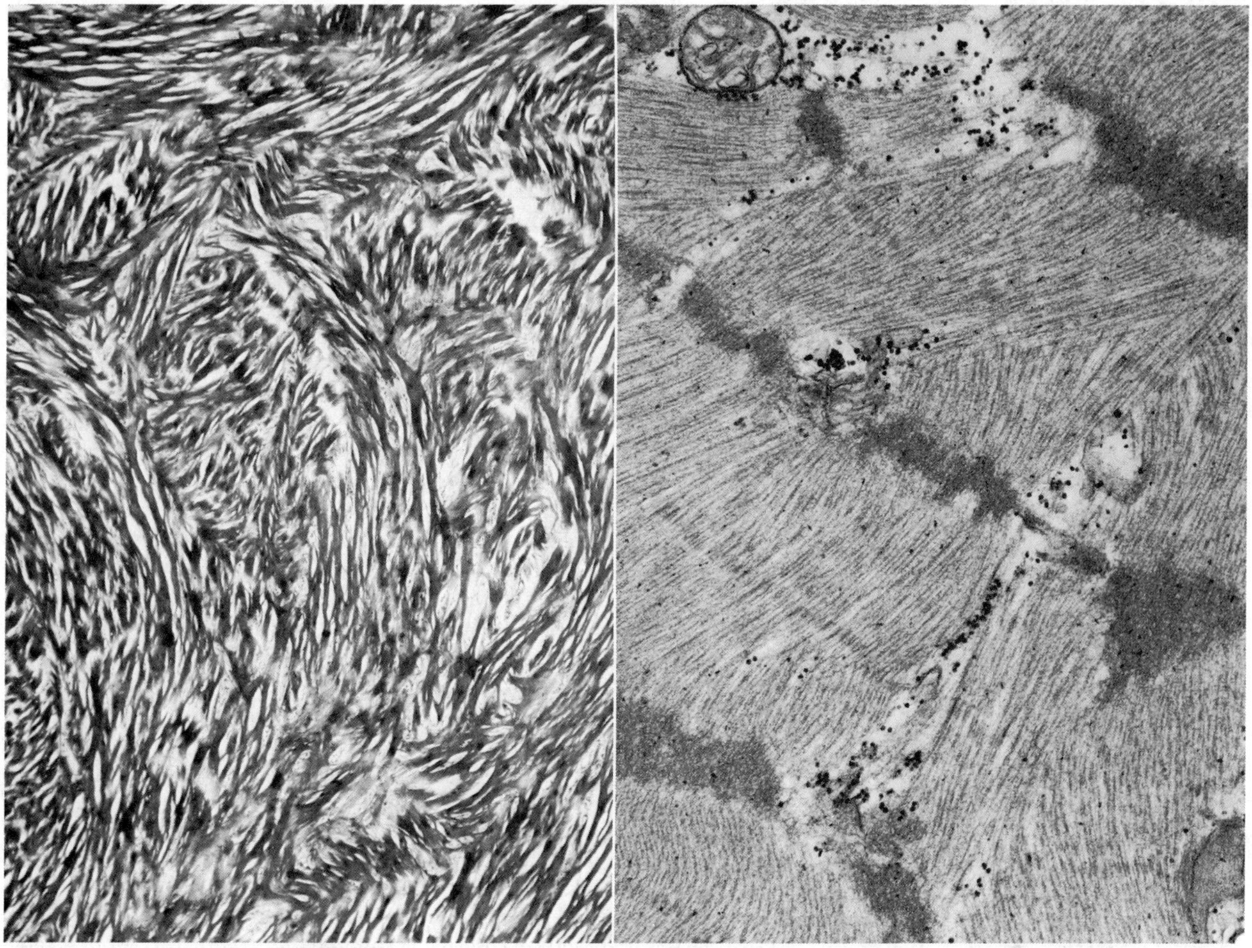

FIGURE 58-11 Histological (*left*) and ultrastructural (*right*) features of ventricular septum of hypertrophic cardiomyopathy. *Left,* from a 19-year-old man with the obstructive type. There is marked disorganization of muscle bundles and bizarre arrangement of muscle cells. Masson's trichrome stain, ×60. *Right,* from a 39-year-old woman with the obstructive type. There is markedly abnormal orientation of the myofibrils and widening of the Z bands, ×47,000.

disorganization" is not entirely clear. Among the patients studied at necropsy,[75] those with high percentages of the septum showing disorganization were younger, had a higher frequency of premature deaths involving more than one member of the same family, and had thicker ventricular septa than those with low percentages of area of the septum involved. Comparisons of the presence or degree of left ventricular outflow obstruction, length of symptoms of cardiac dysfunction, mode of death, arrhythmias, etc., were not significantly different in patients with high as opposed to low percentages of septal area involved by disorganization.

A further abnormality of the ventricular septum in patients with HC is the presence of abnormal intramural coronary arteries in about one-half of patients.[72] The abnormalities in the intramural coronary arteries are striking, and consist of increased number and size of arteries with thickened walls and narrowed lumens. The thickening results from proliferation of smooth muscle cells and collagen in both the media and the intima. Also, mucoid deposits (acid mucopolysaccharide material) are increased. Like disproportional septal thickening (causing ventricular asymmetry) and septal disorganization, abnormality of the intramural coronary arteries is not specific for HC, but is more striking in HC than in most other conditions. Similar abnormality of the intramural coronary arteries is observed in patients and in Newfoundland dogs with discrete subaortic stenosis, in patients with tunnel subaortic stenosis, in normal human fetuses, and in newborns with aortic valve atresia.[72]

The significance of the changes in the intramural coronary arteries in patients with HC is unknown. Their presence or absence does not correlate with any analyzed clinical parameter, including presence of or degree of left ventricular outflow tract "obstruction," age, sex, presence of cardiac dysfunction, chest pain, or length of symptoms of cardiac dysfunction. The cause of the striking abnormalities of the intramural coronary arteries also is uncertain. In each of the four conditions in which this degree of abnormality has been observed (namely HC, discrete and tunnel subaortic stenosis, and aortic valve atresia) the septum is extremely thick, and movement of the septum during life as shown by M-mode echocardiography appears to be extremely limited.

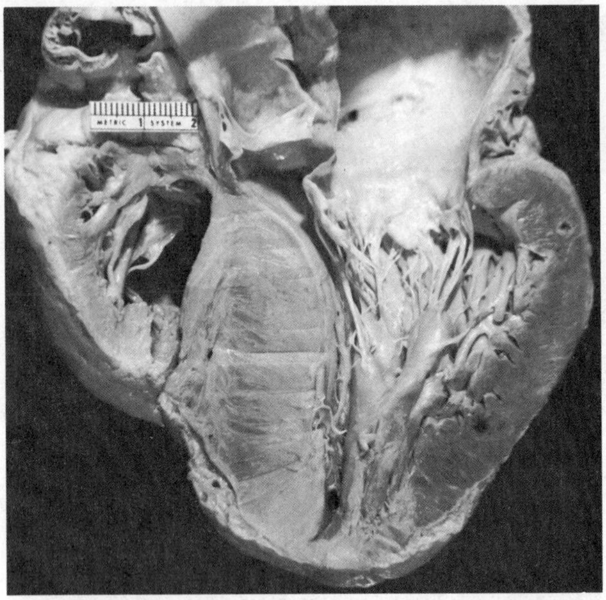

FIGURE 58-12 Hypertrophic cardiomyopathy of the nonobstructive type. This 33-year-old woman (A67-70) became mildly symptomatic when 15 years of age. She had three pregnancies without difficulty, but during the fourth she had overt congestive cardiac failure. When evaluated at age 28, she had exertional dyspnea, chest pain, and occasional episodes of dizziness. Several other family members also had HC. A grade 2/6 precordial systolic murmur, loudest at the apex, and a fourth heart sound were audible. Electrocardiogram showed left bundle branch block and premature ventricular contractions. The cardiac silhouette was enlarged by radiograph. No systolic gradient was present between left ventricle (108/34 mmHg) and brachial artery (114/64 mmHg) at rest. By age 30, the angina, dyspnea, and dizziness were worse and more frequent; syncope had occurred once. On repeat catheterization, still no systolic gradient was present between left ventricle (97/30 mmHg) and femoral artery (102/58) at rest, but a 9-mmHg gradient was provoked by isoproterenol. The premature ventricular contraction response was normal. Repeat catheterization 2 years later showed virtually identical findings. The left ventricular angiocardiogram was interpreted as showing "cavity obliteration." She was found dead in bed at home 4 months later.

At necropsy, the heart weighed 430 g. The ventricular septum was much thicker than the left ventricular free wall, which was of normal thickness. The mitral leaflets were only slightly thickened, and no endocardial mural plaque was present in the left ventricular outflow tract. Both atria were dilated.

This case is typical of the nonobstructive variety of hypertrophic cardiomyopathy and is characterized by normal thickness of at least the basal portion of the left ventricular free wall.

In a study of 26 patients, impaired or paradoxical septal motion was directly related to ventricular tachycardia.[80] It is possible that the severe septal thickening prevents adequate expansion of these vessels during ventricular diastole so that flow through them during this phase of the cardiac cycle is greatly reduced. The fibrous-smooth muscle cell response, in turn, may serve to obliterate the unused lumen. This does not explain the large size of these arteries. It is possible that proliferation of smooth muscle cells in the walls of these arteries represents a response to the same stimulus which causes severe hypertrophy and abnormal configuration of many striated myocardial cells. The major extramural coronary arteries are of unusually wide bore and smooth.

A fourth abnormality of the ventricular septum in adults with HC is the occurrence of a fibrous plaque on the mural endocardium of the outflow portion of the septum.[74] This fibrous thickening is in direct apposition to the ventricular aspect of the anterior mitral leaflet and is the result of contact between the valvular and mural endocardium. The mural plaque, in other words, is the anatomic equivalent of the "systolic anterior motion (SAM)" of the anterior mitral leaflet observed on echocardiogram in HC and occasionally in other conditions. The obstruction in HC, when present, almost certainly begins at a level corresponding to the distal margin of the anterior mitral leaflet and with the caudal margin of the septal endocardial plaque. The mural endocardial septal plaque is present more frequently and is thicker in patients with "obstruction" at rest compared to those without outflow obstruction at rest.

It appears that HC is primarily a disease of the ventricular septum and that the morphological abnormalities in it are apparent at the gross, microscopic, and ultrastructural levels. Other portions of the heart, however, are also affected in HC. These other abnormalities include decreased ventricular cavity size, especially in systole, lack of ventricular cavity dilatation, increased atrial cavity size, varying degrees of interstitial myocardial fibrosis (particularly in the ventricular septum), thickening of the posterior as well as the anterior mitral leaflet, and, in older patients, calcification of the mitral annulus.[74]

The cause of the relatively small sizes of the ventricular cavities is unclear. The septum, on the average about twice normal thickness, occupies space normally represented by cavity. Furthermore, the ventricular free walls, on the average about one-third thicker than normal, also probably compromise slightly the intracavitary space. The cavity is described as slitlike and angulated in its midportion. Additionally, the greater thickness of the septum makes this structure relatively noncompliant. Although the left ventricular free wall in HC (by echocardiography) usually contracts vigorously (in contrast to the septum), it appears to have little capacity to distend outward. Whatever the explanation, ventricular cavity size is rarely enlarged. The rare patients with dilated ventricular cavities have either nonscarred left and/or right ventricular free walls of normal thickness or scarred ventricular free walls of less than normal thickness.[78] Dilatation may occur after massive myocardial necrosis, severe mitral regurgitation, or very widespread myofibrillar disarray. Dilatation may also occur after operative septotomy-septectomy in HC.

The impression of ventricular cavity size as observed at necropsy may be misleading because the cavity at necropsy represents the size at the end of ventricular systole. This information was derived by comparing the left ventricular free wall thickness at necropsy to that measured by echocardiogram during life. The thickness at necropsy corresponds to the thickness during ventricular systole, not diastole.

In contrast to the ventricular cavities, the atrial cavities, at least in adults, are always dilated. The dilatation appears to be a response to difficulty in filling the relatively small and stiff ventricular cavities.

Not only is the anterior mitral leaflet thickened, but often (more frequently in patients with obstruction) the posterior mitral leaflet is as well. The thickening of both mitral leaflets is probably the consequence of the turbulence of blood flow and of the small left ventricular cavity. The position of the mitral valve in the small left ventricle causes abnormal contact of the leaflets with themselves, and also causes apposition of the anterior leaflet to the septum. The mitral valve is thus crumpled within the left ventricle. In patients without gradients, the basal portion of the left ventricular cavity is larger than in patients with gradients because of the thinning of the basal portion of free wall posteriorly and laterally. The focal fibrous thickening of the posterior mitral leaflet probably results from abnormal contact during ventricular systole because there is not enough room in the ventricular cavity to easily accommodate the leaflets and chordae. The ventricle and mitral leaflets in this respect may be regarded as similar to an accordion. The mitral leaflet thickening in HC is somewhat analogous to that which occurs normally as a consequence of aging. With aging, the left ventricular cavity becomes smaller, presumably in response to the lowered cardiac output; the mitral leaflets thicken; the left ventricular muscle becomes less compliant; and the left atrium dilates in response to increased work required to fill the small left ventricle. Similar mechanisms appear to be accelerated in HC.

Most patients with HC have some degree of mitral regurgitation. It is not related to annular dilatation because the mitral annulus is not dilated. Furthermore, the leaflet thickening, in and of itself, is not extensive enough to cause valvular regurgitation. The most likely explanation appears to be abnormal bending of the papillary muscles, particularly the anterolateral one. These structures may be bent abnormally by the bulging ventricular septum with resulting excessive tension on the chordae tendineae preventing closure of the mitral orifice. Although focal scars are usually present in the papillary muscles, they cannot account for the regurgitation. Although usually mild in HC, mitral regurgitation may be the predominant clinical feature of this condition. It may be severe enough to threaten life, and then mitral valve replacement may be not only advisable but lifesaving. Despite its advocacy by some investigators, mitral valve replacement in HC is hazardous and unwarranted for a number of reasons,[79] unless there is major mitral regurgitation. There is no indication to remove a mitral valve that is working well.

Abnormal Physiology[59]

The predominant feature of the abnormal physiology in hypertrophic cardiomyopathy is decreased ventricular compliance with impedance to diastolic filling. Abnormalities of both systolic and diastolic function are due to the chaotic architecture of the myofibrils which, by their abnormal alignment, disturb effective contraction and relaxation. When some myofibrils contract at abnormal angles to each other, they create abnormal tensions; while some cells contract, others may relax, producing incoordination of contraction and relaxation.

Complex abnormalities of diastolic function are both global and regional and are due to the abnormal architecture, the increased stiffness of the left ventricle, and the fibrosis, which may be extensive. Filling of the left ventricle may be slower than normal. Most patients have a greatly prolonged isovolumic relaxation period, the interval from aortic valve closure to the opening of the mitral valve; this results from delay in the opening of the mitral valve, reflecting the reduced rate of fall of left ventricular pressure. The rapid filling period of the left ventricle is prolonged in many patients.[81] The diastolic transverse dimension of the ventricle is normal, but the end-systolic dimension is reduced, making the peak rate of change of dimension during filling greater than normal. In general, the peak filling rate is normal, but the filling pattern is disturbed because of impaired relaxation and the abnormal shape of the cavity.[82] The abnormalities of diastolic function can be aggravated by beta-adrenergic stimulation and diminished by beta-adrenergic blockade.[83] Although many patients have a prolonged isovolumic relaxation period, some have a shortened period; this may impair myocardial oxygenation. Reduction in the isovolumic relaxation period decreases coronary flow, 30 percent of which normally occurs during this period. The disorders of diastolic function have yet to be fully evaluated; their net effect is to impair filling of the left ventricle and thus compromise cardiac function.

Abnormalities of systolic function were recognized before those of diastolic function. The main feature that led to the recognition of the disease was the peak systolic pressure differential across the outflow tract of the left ventricle, below the aortic valve. The lability of the gradient from time to time in the same patient and its provocation by an ectopic beat, by inotropic stimulation, by a reduction in left ventricular cavity size, or by lowered aortic diastolic pressure all suggest a dynamic process. The massively hypertrophied left ventricle causes a powerful contraction which is abnormally coordinated, presumably the result, at least in part, of the disturbed architecture of the myocardium. Initial contraction is rapid, with the major content of the left ventricle expelled in the first half of systole; end-systolic volume is below normal. A pressure gradient develops after the initial contraction. The left ventricular cavity is small and the mitral valve is displaced toward the hypertrophied septum, which leaves little room for the outflow tract (Fig. 58-13). Powerful contraction can produce an intracavity gradient even in a normal heart;[84] this is accentuated in hypertrophic

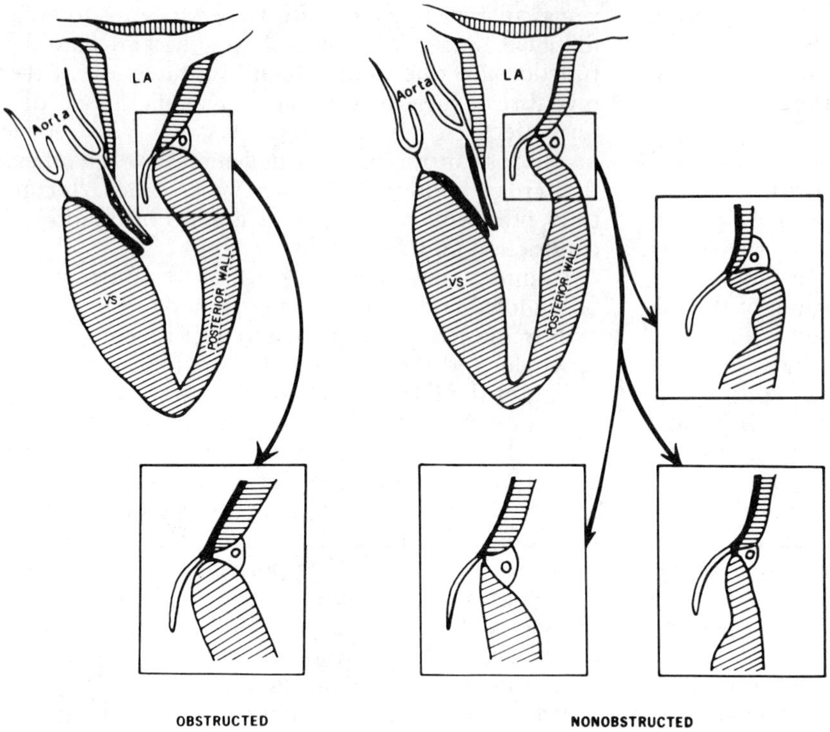

FIGURE 58-13 Diagram illustrating the major differences between the obstructed and nonobstructed types of hypertrophic cardiomyopathy. In the obstructed type, the most basal portion of posterior and lateral left ventricular free walls is rounded and thick. In the nonobstructed type, the left ventricular free wall beneath the posterior mitral leaflet is thinned and pointed.

cardiomyopathy, especially when left ventricular size is further reduced by diminution of afterload or reduction in the circulating blood volume. The question remains as to whether true *obstruction* occurs, or whether *elimination* of the ventricular cavity by the factors mentioned is an important cause of gradients and the reduction in effective cardiac output. Since there is no correlation between left ventricular outflow pressure differential and symptoms or prognosis, it is questionable whether it is an important basic feature. The importance of a gradient should not be neglected because (1) in patients with substantial gradients the administration of inotropic drugs such as digitalis[85] or the volume-depleting effects of diuretic drugs may intensify the pressure differential with castatrophic results; (2) in very symptomatic patients with a substantial gradient, partial incision or excision or both of portions of the hypertrophied septum can produce remarkable symptomatic improvement; and (3) a persistent gradient should raise suspicion of an additional fixed outflow tract obstruction such as aortic valvular or discrete subvalvular stenosis. In a small proportion of patients, there is apparent spontaneous increase or decrease of the outflow gradient, but this is most often associated with clinical deterioration.[86]

Many factors are involved in the production of a systolic gradient in the left ventricle: powerful contraction; apposition of the mitral valve apparatus to the hypertrophied septum; large papillary muscles; abnormal shape and reduced systolic cavity size; and possibly a Venturi effect. Although its importance should not be minimized, a systolic gradient should not be assumed to indicate true obstruction to outflow.[87]

Clinical Manifestations[59,85,88]

The wide clinical spectrum of hypertrophic cardiomyopathy depends on the extent and the severity of the disease, its rate of progression, the presence or absence of a gradient, the degree of familial involvement, and the age of the patient.

History

The main symptoms are dyspnea and chest pain. Dyspnea is due to the increased pulmonary venous pressure occasioned by the high left ventricular end-diastolic pressure. Tachycardia from any cause limits the time available for filling the ventricle and tends to increase dyspnea. Angina may be due to relative ischemia of the greatly hypertrophied myocardium, probably related to diminished diastolic blood flow to the subendocardium caused by impairment of relaxation, especially in patients with a prolonged isovolumic relaxation period. It is likely that narrowing of the intramyocardial coronary arteries results from abnormal relaxation of the greatly hypertrophied muscle. Palpitations, dizziness, and syncope all suggest arrhythmias, but syncope can also be due to sudden reduction in filling of the left ventricle or sudden elimination of the left ventricular cavity in systole. These symptoms are not related to the presence or magnitude of the resting outflow tract pressure gradient. Older patients tend to be more symptomatic.

Physical Examination

The physical habitus of the patient is usually normal. They are often active, athletic people. About 15 percent have moderate systemic arterial hypertension. The physical signs depend to some extent on the presence of a systolic pressure gradient within the left ventricle, found in approximately 40 percent of patients. When a gradient is present, there are three dominant physical signs:[88]

- A *systolic murmur* (Fig. 58-14) of late onset with a clear interval following the first sound; it is spindle-shaped and ends at aortic valve closure. It is heard at the left sternal border and the apex and may radiate to the axilla, but is not well-heard in the aortic area and occasionally radiates to the neck. The murmur reflects the late onset of the gradient and the mitral regurgitation that always accompanies it. It is intensified by standing and the Valsalva maneuver and lessened with squatting and handgrip. Postextrasystolic potentiation is also characteristic. An associated thrill may be palpated between the lower left sternal border and the cardiac apex. A systolic murmur can be heard in the absence of a gradient. Possible explanations include a gradient in the outflow tract of the *right* ventricle; turbulence set up by the powerfully contracting, abnormally shaped left ventricle; or mitral regurgitation due to secondary changes in the mitral valve.
- The *arterial pulse* is characteristically of normal volume but abrupt, ill-sustained, and jerky in quality. The abrupt nature is due to the powerful initial contraction of the left ventricle, with collapse resulting from development of a gradient. The peak pressure is the percussion wave, and a tidal wave on the downstroke is often prominent, resulting in the bifid or bisferiens configuration (see Chap. 9). Atrial fibrillation is present in approximately 10 percent of patients.
- The *cardiac apical impulse* is formed by the left ventricle which produces a powerful but ill-sustained pulsation. Interruption of systolic ejection by the outflow gradient may produce a bifid systolic impulse. This ventricular impulse is preceded by a forceful atrial one, sometimes giving a "triple" character to the apex impulse. The presystolic impulse is due to the powerful atrial contraction needed to fill the poorly compliant left ventricle, and is a prominent feature in many patients; a triple impulse is uncommon.

An accentuated *a* wave in the jugular venous pulse and third and fourth heart sounds, the latter of such low pitch that it may be difficult to hear, may be present. A low-pitched mitral diastolic murmur due to abnormal filling of the stiff ventricle and encroachment on the inflow tract of the left ventricle by the hypertrophied septum may be heard, giving a false impression of mitral valve stenosis. Aortic valve closure is usually normal in intensity. Sometimes pulmonary valve closure is accentuated due to reactive or passive pulmonary hypertension.

When there is no gradient, the clinical signs are far less easy to assess. Often there is no murmur and there may be no gallop sounds. The arterial pulse, although often abrupt and ill-sustained, is usually not impressive. The most important detectable sign is the palpable left atrial impulse, best elicited with the patient turned onto the left side.

With a right ventricular outflow gradient, there is an increase in the *a* wave of the jugular venous pulse and a delay in pulmonary valve closure.

Chest Roentgenogram

This is the least helpful of all the noninvasive studies, because the cardiac silhouette is often normal. Features suggesting increased left atrial pressure may be present, such as prominence of the left atrial appendage, interstitial pulmonary edema, and enlargement of the pulmonary arteries. In patients with severe disease, the cardiac silhouette is increased in size, and there may be a bulge on the left cardiac border due to hypertrophy of the free wall of the left ventricle. Since dilatation of the left ventricular cavity is unusual, an increase in the cardiac silhouette suggests massive, generalized ventricular wall thickening and atrial dilatation.

Electrocardiogram

The characteristic features include the increased QRS voltage and T-wave inversion of left ventricular hypertrophy; left anterior hemiblock; Q waves in the

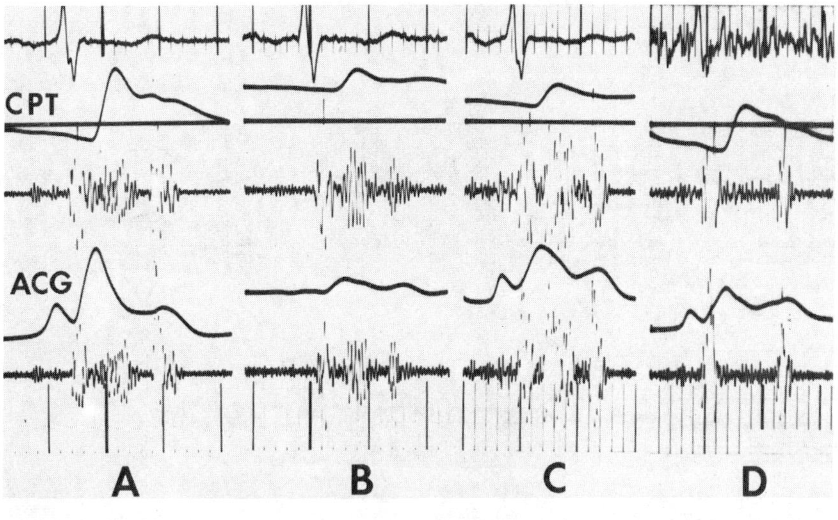

FIGURE 58-14 Phonocardiogram, carotid pulse tracing (CPT), and apexcardiogram (ACG) of a patient with hypertrophic cardiomyopathy. *A.* Control record. The CPT has a rapid upstroke and spike-and-dome pattern; the ACG has a large *a* wave and a bifid systolic impulse (the so-called triple impulse); and phonocardiograms from the second left intercostal space (*top*) and cardiac apex (*bottom*) show a midsystolic murmur. *B.* Taken during squatting. Shows a decrease in the systolic murmur. *C.* Taken during standing. Shows an increase in the systolic murmur. *D.* Taken during isometric handgrip. Shows a marked diminution in the systolic murmur. (*Courtesy of Dr. Joel Felner, Emory University School of Medicine.*)

inferior and left precordial leads; left atrial abnormality; and a short PR interval (Fig. 58-15). Occasionally a delta wave of preexcitation is present. Q waves usually represent massive septal hypertrophy and fibrosis but may occasionally be the result of transmural infarction. Evidence of right ventricular hypertrophy, in addition to left, may occur. In occasional patients the electrocardiogram may show no abnormality, and in others merely the changes of left ventricular hypertrophy. Progression of T-wave changes has been noted with time, but its significance is uncertain. Abnormal ST-segment shift is common. The tracing may simulate the electrocardiogram of myocardial infarction. Reduction in precordial QRS voltage may indicate progression of hypertrophy or fibrosis.[89] "Giant" inverted T waves and high precordial QRS voltage are described with apical HC.[89a] Asymptomatic ventricular arrhythmias are common, are often not seen on the routine ECG, but are detected with ambulatory monitoring.[90]

Special Laboratory Studies

Echocardiogram (see Fig. 58-16 and Chap. 120) This is the main noninvasive investigative technique for diagnosis; it can also serve to assess the results of therapy. Many of the individual features described are not specific for hypertrophic cardiomyopathy, and caution should be exercised in echocardiographic diagnosis unless all features are present[91]: (1) disproportionate thickness of the ventricular septum with a ratio of septum to posterior left ventricular wall of more than 1.5; (2) apparently poor septal contraction but vigorous movement of the free wall of the left ventricle; (3) reduced systolic dimension of the cavity; (4) anterior displacement of the mitral valve toward the septum; (5) reduced rate of closure of the mitral valve, and (in patients with a gradient) systolic anterior motion of the mitral valve and midsystolic closure of the aortic valve. Asymmetric septal hypertrophy (ASH) is not synonymous with hypertrophic cardiomyopathy and may be found in other conditions. Its occurrence in families, however, suggests that it may indicate hypertrophic cardiomyopathy. Prominent systolic anterior motion (SAM) of the anterior mitral leaflet, midsystolic aortic valve closure (MSCAV), and increased left atrial size on M-mode echocardiography suggest outflow obstruction at rest in contrast to latent or absent outflow obstruction.[92] SAM and/or MSCAV, in one series, were found in 82 percent of patients with and 35 percent of patients without gradients; neither SAM nor MSCAV was seen in hypertension.[93]

Based on a disproportionate increase in septal thickness and/or systolic anterior motion of the mitral leaflet by M-mode echocardiography, study of the Framingham cohort and offspring showed that HC was not rare in a free-living population-based sample, especially in the elderly, was occasionally familial, was often associated with other cardiovascular disorders, and often masqueraded as other cardiac disorders.[94]

While M-mode echocardiography is valuable in assisting in diagnosis and in following the disease, two-dimensional techniques appear superior in revealing nonuniform hypertrophy of parts of the septum and in characterizing mitral apparatus ab-

FIGURE 58-15 Electrocardiogram (at one-half standardization) of a patient with hypertrophic cardiomyopathy. There is left ventricular hypertrophy, with increased voltage, ST-segment and T-wave changes, and a left atrial abnormality. (*Courtesy of Dr. Joel Felner, Emory University School of Medicine.*)

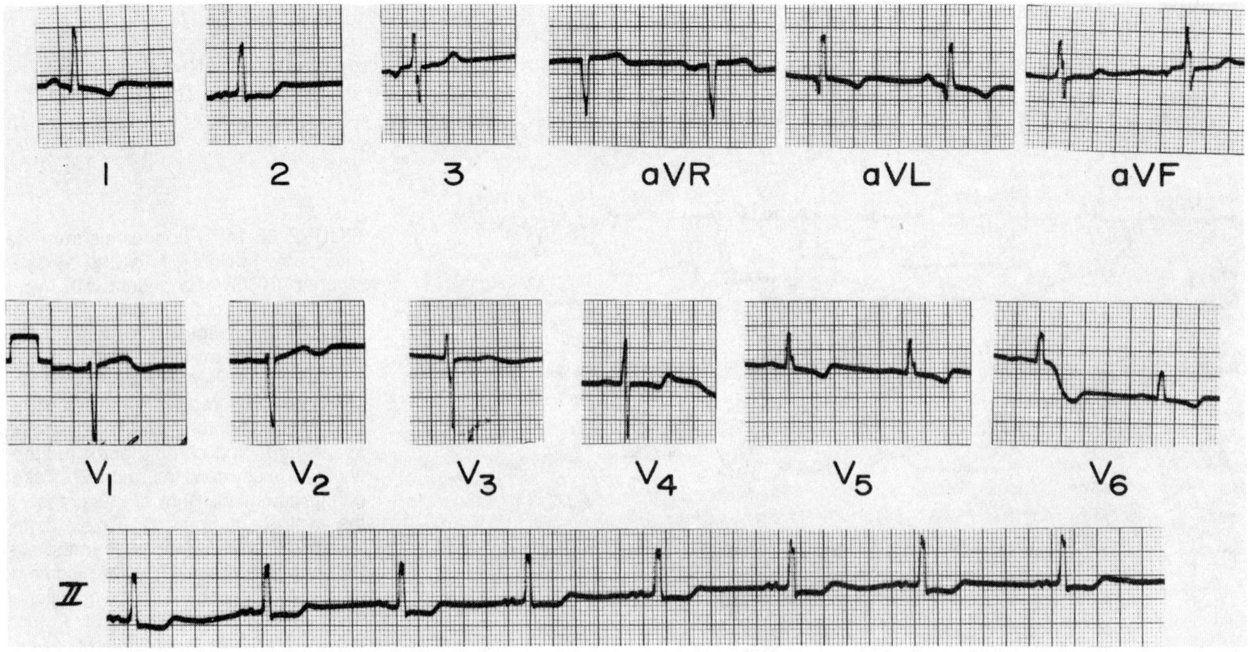

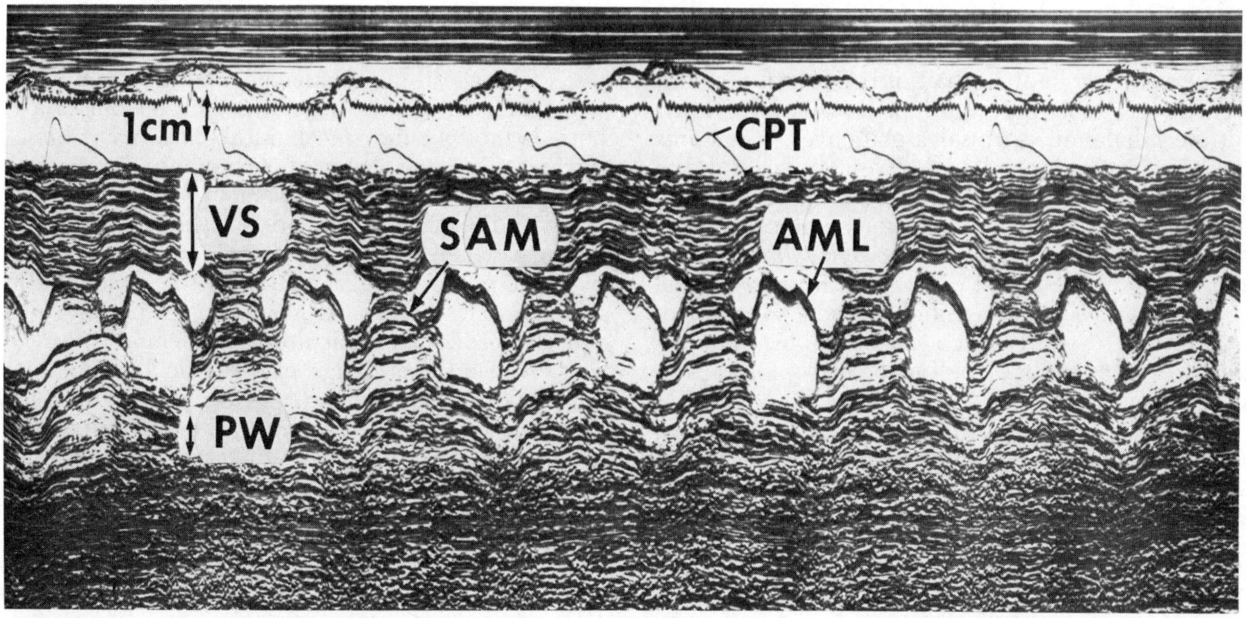

FIGURE 58-16 Echocardiogram of the left ventricle at the level of the mitral valve and a carotid pulse tracing from a patient with proven hypertrophic cardiomyopathy. The CPT shows a rapid upstroke and a spike-and-dome pattern. The echocardiogram shows a small left ventricular cavity with asymmetric septal hypertrophy; the ventricular septum to posterior wall ratio is 1:9. The mitral valve demonstrates systolic anterior motion and in diastole almost touches the septum. CPT = carotid pulse tracing; VS = ventricular septum; PW = posterior wall; SAM = systolic anterior motion; AML = anterior mitral leaflet. (*Courtesy of Dr. Joel Felner, Emory University School of Medicine.*)

normalities not always detectable by the limited access of the M-mode technique.[34] These data may enable improved classification of patients with this disorder, with possible therapeutic and prognostic implications. Hypertrophy is not always asymmetric; in a two-dimensional echocardiographic study from the Royal Postgraduate Medical School, hypertrophy was symmetrical in 31 percent, asymmetric septal in 55 percent, and distal ventricular in 14 percent of patients.[95]

Radionuclide Imaging Techniques (see Chap. 109) Tc-labeling of the blood pool confirms the decreased ventricular systolic volume and can document myocardial contractility, mitral valve function, obstruction when present, and septal and cavity configuration; serial evaluations help characterize the course of the disorder and response to therapy. Myocardial imaging with ^{201}Tl defines the increased myocardial mass and configuration.[37]

Experience at the Royal Postgraduate Medical School with gated blood pool scanning showed a high ejection fraction (80 to 90 percent) in many patients with HC. The percentage of stroke volume ejected in the initial 30 percent, the initial 50 percent, and the first 80 percent of systole was significantly greater than normal, and did not differ whether or not there was an outflow tract gradient, supporting the interpretation that true obstruction does not occur.[96]

Gated blood pool scanning with ^{99m}Tc also showed that both systolic and diastolic function tended to be abnormal in those patients at risk of sudden death. Digitization of left ventricular cineangiograms revealed that hyperdynamic systolic function and impaired filling were markers of an increased risk of sudden death.

Phonocardiogram, Systolic Time Intervals, and Apex Cardiogram Phonocardiography confirms the clinical analysis of the murmurs and may sometimes reveal a fourth heart sound that is not audible. Study of the systolic time intervals documents prolongation of the isovolumic relaxation period in most patients and an increased left ventricular ejection time and pre-ejection period. Apex cardiography shows a large *a* wave due to powerful atrial contraction.

Cardiac Catheterization and Angiocardiogram (see Chap. 108)[85] Angiocardiography is an important diagnostic test and is often definitive. It is indicated when surgery is considered. In diastole, the ventricle is angulated, the shape resembling a banana; end-diastolic volume is normal. In systole, the cavity in about half the patients is slitlike and the end-systolic volume is reduced. Increase in systolic and diastolic volumes is unusual, occurring in less than 5 percent of patients, and is associated with severe heart failure, severe secondary mitral regurgitation, or massive transmural infarction of the left ventricle. The apex of the left ventricle may be isolated from the outflow portion by apposition of the lateral wall and septum, or the cavity may be virtually eliminated. Papillary muscles are enlarged and project into the cavity, and contrast medium may be seen in the interstices of the trabeculae carneae in the shape of a star. In patients with a gradient, mitral regurgitation at least of slight degree is invariable. Coronary arteriograms are usually normal.

Withdrawal tracings from the apex and left ventricle to the aorta show a gradient within the body of the ventricle in about half of patients at rest and a further 15 to 20 percent on provocation with amyl nitrate inhalation, a Valsalva maneuver, an ectopic beat or isoproterenol. The left ventricular end-diastolic pressure is usually elevated. Gradients tend to occur in the mid rather than in the apical part of the left ventricle and are associated with forward movement of the mitral valve apparatus toward the septum. This sign is significant when seen angiographically, though its echocardiographic counterpart (SAM) is not specific for hypertrophic cardiomyopathy.

Endomyocardial Biopsy This technique, while possibly useful for research purposes, should not be part of routine diagnostic study. Reading disorganization on a biopsy specimen is unreliable,[40] for the disease is patchy and the disordered geometry of the septum may render investigation hazardous.

Natural History and Prognosis[59]

The natural history is extremely variable, ranging from long life with few or no symptoms[97] to rapidly progressive disease, fatal in a few years or less. The disease has been noted in infancy. Most patients pursue a stable course over a period of about 10 years, some deteriorating and a few even improving. With a younger age of onset, there is often biventricular involvement and an increased occurrence of severe obstruction, congestive heart failure, and sudden death. Half of the patients with hypertrophic cardiomyopathy die suddenly.[98,99] The prediction of sudden death is difficult, but clues include diagnosis in childhood, syncope at diagnosis, family history of sudden death, symptoms, and, in older patients, impairment of systolic and diastolic function.[100] Prolonged peak filling rate and high ejection fraction are hemodynamic clues. Evidence of serious ventricular arrhythmias on ambulatory ECG monitoring is the best predictor of prognosis, but presentation in childhood alone carries a similar hazard. There is no relation between outflow tract gradient and symptoms or prognosis. The development or increase of the intensity of the murmur usually suggests progression of the disease, but disappearance of the murmur does not indicate improvement; in fact, the reverse. As systolic function becomes impaired, the gradient diminishes or disappears, with disappearance of the murmur.[97] The development of atrial fibrillation usually causes severe clinical deterioration because of loss of the atrial kick and adversely affects prognosis. Many patients develop congestive heart failure at this time and systemic embolism may occasionally occur. Gross mitral regurgitation may also result in heart failure. Ventricular dilatation most often results from transmural infarction, typically silent and usually in the absence of significant narrowing of the epicardial coronary arteries.[78]

Sudden Death

Sudden death is the commonest form of termination of life, is often unexpected, and may be the initial manifestation of the disease.[98] The causes are both hemodynamic (mechanical) and arrhythmic. Arrhythmia is probably the commonest cause of sudden death.[101] Gradients may be produced by positive inotropic stimulation such as exercise, tachycardia, emotion, or positive inotropic drugs, all of which can cause elimination of the cavity of the left ventricle. Sudden decrease of ventricular volume, as produced by acute hypovolemia, hypotension, or vasodilator drugs, may augment the outflow tract gradient and add to the hazard. Sudden increase of resistance to inflow to the left ventricle is an important factor and tends to be aggravated by tachycardia, which shortens the time available for filling. In one patient monitored during a syncopal episode the blood pressure became unrecordable and the left ventricular outflow tract murmur disappeared. No arrythmia was recorded, suggesting a hemodynamic mechanism such as acute reduction in ventricular volume due to cavity elimination in systole and impairment of filling of the left ventricle in diastole; the patient recovered.[102]

Arrhythmia

While atrial fibrillation is well-recognized, until recently other arrhythmias were not thought important in hypertrophic cardiomyopathy. Contemporary studies using ambulatory electrocardiography have shown frequent supraventricular arrhythmias; ventricular premature contractions and short runs of ventricular tachycardia are common, and the risk of sudden death appears higher in patients with ventricular arrhythmias.[103] Exercise testing appears less sensitive than ambulatory ECG monitoring in detecting arrhythmias. The mechanisms of arrhythmia are complex. Preexcitation of the ventricle due to bypass tracts has been reported,[104] and delta waves with a short PR interval are sometimes seen. If atrial fibrillation occurs in a patient with preexcitation, rapid irregular impulses may be conducted to the ventricle, simulating ventricular fibrillation. Ventricular arrhythmias are likely to be due to local preexcitation or automaticity related to patchy fibrosis and myofibrillar disarray in the ventricles in the region of the conduction tissue. A high incidence of sustained ventricular tachycardia or ventricular fibrillation was evident with programmed electrical stimulation.[105]

Congestive Heart Failure

Congestive heart failure occurs in a few patients, often related to the onset of atrial fibrillation[97] or to extensive myocardial necrosis.[78] The factors leading to congestive heart failure include atrial fibrillation with loss of the atrial kick, increased resistance to ventricular inflow, tachycardia, and impairment of systolic function. The most important factor may be the systolic pump failure which adds to the severe diastolic disorder already present. Verapamil has been described to increase the early rapid left ventricular diastolic filling, thereby decreasing dependence on the filling contribution of atrial systole; this may reduce the risk of life-threatening hemodynamic decompensation with the onset of atrial fibrillation or other tachyarrhythmias.[106] Usually the systolic volume of the left ventricle remains small, and the characteristic appearance at end systole on angiography is preserved. Occasionally, the left ventricle may dilate, usually the result of myocardial necrosis; it may also occur after septal resection. Dilatation of the left ventricle does not exclude the diagnosis, as the other angiographic and necropsy features remain, especially the fibrous thickening of the anterior mitral valve leaflet and the impingement plaque on the septum. The diagnosis of hypertrophic cardiomyopathy with congestive heart failure can be extremely difficult, although echocardiography and angiocardiography can provide important evidence.

Systemic Embolism, Infective Endocarditis, and Severe Mitral Regurgitation

Systemic embolism, infective endocarditis, and severe mitral regurgitation are additional hazards. Systemic embolism is uncommon, occurring in only about 10 percent of patients, but is more likely when atrial fibrillation has developed. Embolism may also result from infective endocarditis, which is by no means uncommon and usually occurs on the mitral valve. Severe mitral regurgitation occurs in less than 5 percent of patients and may be the result of previous infection, damage to the valve by turbulence, or mitral annular calcification.

Pregnancy

Pregnancy is well-tolerated. Oakley and associates documented no perinatal death of mother or infant in the outcome of 54 pregnancies in 23 patients.[107] The genetic hazards of pregnancy are probably not great. In view of the variability and severity of the disease and the good prognosis in many patients, it does not seem reasonable to advise against pregnancy if only one parent has the disease. If both parents have the disease, or if there is a strong history on one side of the family, the matter should be reconsidered, and the situation explained to the prospective parents.

Differential Diagnosis

Hypertrophic cardiomyopathy can mimic a large number of cardiovascular disorders and may coexist with some. In patients with outflow tract gradients, the differential diagnosis lies between valvular aortic stenosis, discrete subaortic stenosis, pulmonary stenosis, ventricular septal defect, and mitral regurgitation of other types.

In *mitral regurgitation and ventricular septal defect,* the arterial pulse is not sustained due to the increased volume load and "runoff" from the left ventricle, but neither mitral regurgitation nor ventricular septal defect is associated with a pronounced presystolic impulse, and the murmur is usually holosystolic. In subvalvular mitral regurgitation, the murmur may be spindle-shaped, and difficulty can be experienced in differentiating this from hypertrophic cardiomyopathy (which should be considered as a diagnostic possibility in any patient with mitral regurgitation).

In *valvular aortic stenosis,* the pulse is anacrotic and often slowly rising and of small amplitude; the murmur is longer and starts earlier than in hypertrophic cardiomyopathy. It is heard at the base and radiates to the neck. In *congenital valvular aortic stenosis,* an ejection click is the rule, often heard best at the apex. In *discrete subaortic stenosis,* the pulse may be similar to that of hypertrophic cardiomyopathy, but aortic valve closure is soft or absent and an aortic diastolic murmur is common.

Difficulties arise when valvular aortic stenosis is mild, the murmur is short, and the pulse nonspecific in character. Difficulty may also be experienced in discrete subaortic stenosis if aortic valve closure is audible and there is no early diastolic murmur. Particular difficulty may arise when more than one lesion is present, such as a bicuspid aortic valve or valvular aortic stenosis in association with hypertrophic cardiomyopathy. Exact diagnosis may not be possible clinically, but bizarre electrocardiographic changes with deeply inverted T waves, inferior and precordial Q waves, and a short PR interval should suggest hypertrophic cardiomyopathy. The possibility of multiple lesions must always be kept in mind; in such cases, although echocardiography may be valuable, cardiac catheterization and angiocardiography are essential.

Patients should be examined for aortic valve calcium. If present, it indicates valvular aortic stenosis and virtually excludes *coexistence* of hypertrophic cardiomyopathy. However, mitral annular calcium is common in older patients with hypertrophic cardiomyopathy.

Other types of mitral valve disease may be difficult to differentiate from hypertrophic cardiomyopathy, particularly when atrial fibrillation and mitral valve calcium are present. Echocardiography is helpful in showing the characteristic features of hypertrophic cardiomyopathy, but angiocardiography may be essential for differentiation. If there is a family history or the findings are unusual in a patient with mitral regurgitation thought to be of rheumatic origin, hypertrophic cardiomyopathy should be considered. Mitral stenosis may be simulated in patients with a middiastolic murmur at the apex. In some patients, relative stenosis may occur from bulging of the septum into the outflow tract of the left ventricle. The presence of a presystolic impulse is useful when the patient is in sinus rhythm. Careful auscultation, phonocardiography, and echocardiography will usually differentiate the early diastolic third sound of hypertrophic cardiomyopathy from the opening snap of mitral stenosis. The characteristic thickening of the mitral valve and forward diastolic movement of the posterior leaflet in mitral stenosis on the echocardiogram are not present in hypertrophic cardiomyopathy.

When the systolic murmur is soft or absent, the following conditions must be considered: *primary pulmonary hypertension; prolapsing mitral valve; left atrial myxoma; atherosclerotic coronary heart disease;* and *angina with normal coronary arteries.* When the left ventricular end-diastolic pressure is high and both passive and reactive pulmonary hypertension occur, the signs may be similar to those of primary pulmonary hypertension. Prolapse of the mitral valve may be difficult to distinguish from hypertrophic cardiomyopathy, because of its midsystolic murmur and sometimes jerky pulse. There is often a midsystolic click, and the presystolic impulse is not felt. However, prolapse may coexist with hypertrophic cardiomyopathy.

In patients with hypertrophic cardiomyopathy with right ventricular outflow obstruction, the findings may mimic pulmonary stenosis. Evidence of septal or left ventricular hypertrophy on the electrocardiogram may be a useful differentiating clue.

Left atrial myxoma is an uncommon diagnosis which should be considered in any patient with unusual mitral murmurs, especially if systemic embolism has occurred or there are features suggesting infective endocarditis. Both of the latter can also occur in hypertrophic cardiomyopathy. Echocardiography usually resolves the problem, but angiocardiography may be needed.

Atherosclerotic coronary heart disease may be suggested when angina is prominent, there are no physical findings of hypertrophic cardiomyopathy, and the electrocardiographic abnormalities suggest infarction or are nonspecific. Diagnosis may not always be possible without coronary arteriography and left ventricular angiography, but important clinical clues may be found. If the history of angina is long and begins in childhood, hypertrophic cardiomyopathy is more likely. If the electrocardiogram shows severe left ventricular hypertrophy, septal hypertrophy, bizarre T-wave changes, and septal Q waves without obvious findings or history of recent myocardial infarction, the diagnosis is likely to be hypertrophic cardiomyopathy. Careful search for a presystolic apical impulse can be rewarding, and echocardiography may reveal the diagnosis. In hypertrophic cardiomyopathy, the coronary arteries are typically large and smooth. In 10 to 15 percent of patients, hypertrophic cardiomyopathy and atherosclerotic coronary artery disease may coexist.

When congestive heart failure develops, the diagnosis usually suggested is dilated cardiomyopathy or ischemic heart disease with heart failure, but without preceding angina or infarction. With sinus rhythm, a presystolic impulse is a useful clue to hypertrophic cardiomyopathy; when atrial fibrillation has developed, differentiation from dilated cardiomyopathy may be impossible, although the left ventricular impulse is usually more powerful and thrusting in hypertrophic than in dilated cardiomyopathy.

Treatment

Prevention

There is no known method of preventing the disease, and the best that can be done is to try to minimize the consequences. The most important hazard is sudden death; this predominates among younger patients. Any circumstance that favors the development of a gradient or increases resistance to filling of the left ventricle should be avoided. Violent exercise, tachycardia, sudden fall in blood pressure or blood volume, and fainting increase vulnerability, as do positive inotropic and vasodilator drugs, which should be avoided.

It had been hoped that propranolol would reduce sudden death because of its effect on ventricular function in acute observations and because of its antiarrhythmic action.[83] Unfortunately this expectation has not been achieved, except perhaps for very large doses.[108] Because of the association between ventricular arrhythmias and sudden death,[109] antiarrhythmic therapy appears indicated. The drugs that have been specifically investigated are calcium-blocking agents, notably verapamil,[110] and the antiarrhythmic agent amiodarone. Theoretically, verapamil should be useful because of its action on the slow calcium channel, but ambulatory electrocardiographic studies show no diminution of ventricular arrhythmias in patients treated with verapamil.[111] There is thus far no evidence that verapamil prevents sudden death, though it appears to improve hemodynamics and exercise capacity[112,113] and perhaps diminish myocardial hypertrophy; diastolic function appears improved.[110] However, asystolic sudden death has occurred with verapamil therapy;[114] abnormalities of atrioventricular conduction due to verapamil may necessitate pacemaker implantation. Amiodarone has diminished the frequency of ventricular arrhythmias on ambulatory electrocardiography and may be the drug of choice. Amiodarone improves prognosis by preventing ventricular tachycardia. It is not known whether it will influence cardiac pain or dyspnea, but it was originally introduced to treat angina and has a weak beta-adrenergic blocking effect. Prevention of sudden death may depend upon prophylaxis of arrhythmias (amiodarone) and improvement in compliance and filling of the left ventricle (beta-blocking or calcium-blocking agents), together with restriction of inappropriate tachycardia. Because of the danger of heart block, amiodarone and verapamil should not be given together.

Antibiotic prophylaxis is indicated to avert infective endocarditis.

Medical Treatment

The treatment of hypertrophic cardiomyopathy is at the crossroads. Current knowledge does not permit exact recommendations, although new information that is rapidly being gathered may resolve this problem. (See also Chap. 21.)

Angina and dyspnea respond to large does of beta-adrenergic blocking agents in about 70 percent of patients. Agents with a cardioselective action are not as satisfactory as those without[115] because their effect on outflow tract gradient is less. The drug of choice is propranolol, which should be given in maximum tolerated doses to produce as complete beta-adrenergic blockade as possible. Early studies with beta-blocking agents suggested improvement in diastolic function,[83] and subsequent investigation using diastolic time intervals suggested improved left ventricular filling in some, but not all, patients,[116] presumably because of the very complex, variable, and regional disorder of diastolic function. All patients should have an ambulatory ECG study for at least 24 to 48 h; if this shows multiple episodes of ventricular arrhythmia, antiarrhythmic treatment is indicated; amiodarone is the most effective drug and appears to improve prognosis.[109,111,117,117a] Combinations of drugs require further investigation for safety and effectiveness.

Patients with mild disease who are asymptomatic, without a distinctly abnormal resting ECG or marked septal thickening, and who have no obvious family history or ventricular arrhythmia on ambulatory ECG recording probably do not need specific therapy but should be kept under observation. Those with a definite family history should receive treatment with either propranolol or verapamil in hope of retarding progression of the disease.

Calcium-Blocking Agents The action of verapamil is uncertain and somewhat confusing. Both sudden death and acute pulmonary edema have been attributed to it,[118] and great care is necessary in its administration. It should always be started in the hospital, beginning with the lowest effective dose and slowly increasing, watching carefully for signs of pulmonary congestion or conduction defects. Verapamil should not be given to patients with pulmonary venous pressures of 20 mmHg or more or with conduction defects.[118] Moreover, it is uncertain which patients should receive verapamil and on what basis. A sensible approach would be to reserve it for patients in whom symptoms persist despite beta-adrenergic blocking treatment and in whom there are no specific contraindications.

Nifedipine appears more promising than verapamil because of its effect on improving ventricular filling.[119,120] Vasodilation, as with verapamil,[118] may cause adverse effects by producing hypotension and reducing the volume of the left ventricle, although it has been suggested that systemic vasodilation and ventricular unloading might actually help improve diastolic function.[120] The exact indications for the use of nifedipine in hypertrophic cardiomyopathy are not yet clear.

Verapamil and beta-adrenergic blocking agents should probably not be administered concomitantly, though nifedipine has been given with beta-blocking drugs to patients with coronary heart disease without apparent hazard.

Diltiazem appears to improve left ventricular relaxation and diastolic filling without altering left ventricular systolic function.[120a]

Amiodarone (see Chap. 27) Amiodarone is indicated to reduce the risk of sudden death due to arrhythmia, but it should not be given if there is evidence of atrioventricular block; its action does not occur for 5 to 10 days after administration, and cumulative effects may result. It does not appear to depress left ventricular function at rest.[120b] Since it contains iodine which may unmask subclinical thyroid disorders, thyroid function must be watched. Side effects are dose-related.[121] After a loading dose, the maintenance dose should be 200 to 400 mg/day for 5 or 6 days of the week. It commonly causes corneal deposits which, apart from slightly tinting vision, do not appear to affect visual acuity or damage the eye. Other side effects include photosensitivity, impaired liver function, and pulmonary fibrosis. Nausea may occur for a few days after oral treatment is begun. Amiodarone may be combined with a beta-blocking agent. As an alternative, sotalol, which has both antiarrhythmic amiodarone-like action and a beta-blocking effect, may be used. The combination of amiodarone and nifedipine awaits evaluation.

Congestive Heart Failure When congestive heart failure develops, treatment becomes difficult. There is little risk of provoking a gradient, so diuretics may be used as in other forms of congestive heart failure. Digitalis is not absolutely contraindicated, but its benefits are uncertain. Amiodarone is more satisfactory for stabilizing atrial fibrillation or converting it to sinus rhythm. Propranolol is unlikely to be of benefit and may be contraindicated, although small doses may help control atrial fibrillation. Although most patients who develop congestive heart failure lose the outflow tract gradient, this is not always so, and such patients present a uniquely difficult problem. If medical treatment is unavailing, surgical treatment by septal resection must be considered; but the risk is high in the presence of heart failure. If heart failure is the result of severe mitral regurgitation, mitral valve replacement may produce dramatic improvement.

Atrial fibrillation should be regarded as a medical emergency. Electrical defibrillation should be attempted at once after heparin administration. If successful, attempt should be made to maintain sinus rhythm with amiodarone. If reversion to sinus rhythm is not possible or if relapse into atrial fibrillation occurs, continued anticoagulant therapy is necessary. Atrial fibrillation is generally a poor prognostic sign.

When systemic arterial hypertension is associated with hypertrophic cardiomyopathy, vasodilator and diuretic drugs should be avoided if there is a systolic gradient in the absence of congestive heart failure.

There is a limited role for pacemaker therapy. The indications are complete heart block with an unacceptably slow heart rate or Stokes-Adams syncope; atrial tachyarrhythmias alternating with the bradycardia; and symptoms which respond to propranolol but which cannot be relieved without unacceptable bradycardia. Pacing the right ventricle may, by premature contraction of the ventricle, relieve the outflow tract gradient, but the value of this maneuver is uncertain. Physiological pacemakers which maintain atrial function may be of value in the future.

Surgical Treatment

Partial septal resection is advised for selected patients. Operation always consists of an incision into the ventricular septum, with or without resection of part of the septum. Generally, symptoms are relieved, gradients are nearly always abolished, and mitral regurgitation almost always disappears.[122] Reduction or addition of the gradient appears due primarily to surgical enlargement of the left ventricular outflow tract area.[122a] The indication is symptoms unrelieved by intensive medical treatment in a patient with a ventricular outflow gradient of at least 50 mmHg at rest or with provocation and evidence of a very thick ventricular septum. Surgical treatment should not be undertaken unless there is a gradient and/or appreciable mitral regurgitation. Septal resection affords symptomatic relief, but there is no certainty that it prolongs life. The operative mortality and late postoperative mortality rates each approximate 8 percent. Congestive cardiac failure may occur long after operation. Mitral valve replacement is rarely justified except for the patient with severe intractable mitral regurgitation, usually secondary to leaflet or chordal damage from infective endocarditis. Analysis of published results[123] have not encouraged the widespread use of septal resection because of relatively high mortality rates, no definite benefit to prognosis, and uncertainty as to the rationale or mode of action of surgery. Nevertheless, one recent series describes a 77 percent 10-year survival rate and prominent symptomatic improvement,[124] and another no operative death among 36 patients and a 1.6 percent annual mortality rate.[125]

Laser myoplasty may be an alternative to myotomy or myectomy.[126]

Restrictive/Obliterative Cardiomyopathy

Restrictive cardiomyopathy (RC) is present when diastolic ventricular volume and stretch are impaired by morphological endocardial, subendocardial, or myocardial lesions; the hemodynamic abnormality is a limitation of ventricular filling, leading to a decreased cardiac output. Good systolic function is usually present, especially in the earlier stages of the disease.[127] The most common cause worldwide is probably endomyocardial fibrosis, with or without eosinophilia. When this process becomes extensive, the ventricular cavity may become reduced in size, i.e., the "obliterative" phase.[65]

In the western world, the restrictive form is the least prevalent of the cardiomyopathies and is due to Loeffler's endomyocardial fibrosis with eosinophilia; amyloid disease may produce a similar but not identical hemodynamic effect. On rare occasions, other infiltrative processes such as hemochromatosis/hemosiderosis may produce a restrictive picture; at times, no specific infiltrative disorder is evident.[127a]

Tropical Endomyocardial Fibrosis and Loeffler's Endomyocardial Disease (Eosinophilic Endomyocardial Disease[6])

Until recently, tropical endomyocardial fibrosis (EMF) and Loeffler's disease were considered separate entities. Newer evidence suggests that they are basically the same disease,[128,129] though possibly produced by different endomyocardial irritants and with some different features due to environmental conditions. They will be considered as one entity in the following discussion.

Tropical cases are found in humid zones in the equatorial belt throughout the world—southern India; parts of Latin America; central east, and west Africa. Endomyocardial fibrosis is by no means the commonest heart disease in the tropics. For example, in equatorial Africa, it accounts for only approximately 10 percent of cardiac disease. It mainly affects older children and young adults of both sexes. Endomyocardial fibrosis is commonest in the rain forest districts, and there is apparently a seasonal incidence, with new cases appearing most frequently during the rainy season.[130]

Etiology

The cause of tropical endomyocardial fibrosis is unknown, but seems related to the tropical environment. The episodes of fever and irregular exacerbations of the disease suggest an infective origin. Many prior theories of etiology, primarily dietary, have not proved tenable. The similarity to the pathology of the endomyocardial fibrosis in Loeffler's hypereosinophilic disease suggests that some disorder of the eosinophil may be common to both tropical and nontropical cases. Although slight eosinophilia is common in tropical endomyocardial fibrosis, profuse eosinophilia is seldom if ever seen; minor degrees of eosinophilia are common in tribal African areas as a result of helminthic infestation. Immunologic studies suggest that the inhabitants prone to develop EMF differ in their immunologic makeup from those who are less susceptible. The immunologic pattern is characterized by high levels of malarial antibody immunoglobin and IgM circulating autoantibodies to thyroid and gastric parietal cell mucosa; however, these immunologic patterns may be the result of infection and may not be etiologically important.

The Eosinophil and Endomyocardial Fibrosis

The term *hypereosinophilic syndrome*[131] has been coined to describe persistent marked blood eosinophilia combined with diffuse eosinophilic infiltration of organs, associated with significant cardiac and immunologic abnormalities. The association between blood eosinophilia and severe endomyocardial disease has been documented, although questions remain about the morphological and clinical characteristics of the cardiac damage and the preferred approach to diagnosis and management. In a recent review,[132] 84 percent of patients with the hypereosinophilic syndrome had some evidence of cardiac disease, the most frequent finding being biventricular heart failure. Precordial murmurs were common, mostly arising from the mitral valve. Most patients had a total white blood cell count above 100,000 per cubic millimeter with eosinophilia from 30 to 75 percent. The eosinophils appeared morphologically abnormal. The known causes of the eosinophilia include parasitic[133] and other infections, leukemia and other malignancies, and collagen and other diseases characterized by vasculitis; often no cause for the eosinophilia can be ascertained. A number of noncardiovascular findings characterize the patient with idiopathic hypereosinophilia with an increased risk of developing endomyocardial fibrosis: male sex, positive HLA-Bw44, splenomegaly, thrombocytopenia, elevated serum vitamin B_{12} level, hypogranular or vacuolated eosinophils, and abnormal early myeloid precursors in the blood.[134]

Special studies[132] of the eosinophils in EMF show that they are frequently immunologically abnormal. The vacuolated and degranulated eosinophils appear to produce an abnormal substance that may damage the myocardium and endocardium; raised serum concentrations of eosinophilic granule cationic proteins are described, and these granules have been shown to be thrombogenic. These characteristics are only found when the eosinophil count is substantially increased. It seems likely that Loeffler's endomyocardial disease is due to an immunologic disorder of peculiar clones of eosinophils, for all eosinophils in a patient with the disease do not behave in the same way.

Pathology

In both eosinophilic endomyocardial disease and eosinophilic leukemia there is endocardial fibrosis of one or both ventricles and severe eosinophilia (Fig. 58-17). Death is usually the result of congestive cardiac failure. From examination of previous reports and of necropsy patients, the clinical and some morphological features of eosinophilic leukemia and Loeffler's endocarditis appear similar. Certain similarities also exist between African EMF (Fig. 58-18) and EMF with eosinophilia, described by others as Loeffler's endocarditis or eosinophilic leukemia. The mural endocardial thickening in the ventricles is seen in both conditions, and blood eosinophilia may occur in EMF.

That Loeffler's fibroplastic parietal endocarditis and tropical EMF of the African are basically the same disease at different stages of development is an attractive hypothesis[74,128,129,135] (Fig. 58-19). Patients with eosinophilia associated with a transient, benign, febrile illness, such as tropical eosinophilia or Loeffler's pneumonia, may represent one end of the spectrum. Patients with severe EMF and no blood eosinophilia may represent the other end. Between these two extremes there may be patients who still have eosinophilia but less extensive endocardial scarring. The latter process is still active, and thus eosinophilia is still present, but as the inflammatory process dies down, cardiac scar tissue remains and eosinophilia disappears. The large epicardial coronary arteries are patent.

Endomyocardial biopsy examination has documented an acute necrotic stage,[135a] a thrombotic stage, and a late fibrotic stage. In the acute stage there is marked inflammatory infiltration with eosinophils, periarterial infiltration, and myocytolysis. In the thrombotic stage, extensive superimposition of

FIGURE 58-17 Patient with cardiomegaly, congestive cardiac failure, and blood eosinophilia. *a.* Opened right atrium (RA), tricuspid valve, and right ventricle (RV). *b.* Opened left atrium (LA), mitral valve (AML = anterior mitral leaflet; PML = posterior mitral leaflet), and left ventricle (LV). The endocardium of both ventricles is extensively thickened and antemortem thrombus is present in both apices. Both left ventricular papillary muscles (A = anterolateral and P = posteromedial) are severely scarred, and both extra- and intramural coronary arteries were normal. Both atria and ventricles are dilated. (*From W. C. Roberts, L. M. Buja, and V. J. Ferrans, Löffler's Fibroplastic Parietal Endocarditis, Eosinophilic Leukemia, and Davies' Endomyocardial Fibrosis: The Same Disease at Different Stages? Pathol. Microbiol., 35:90, 1970. Reproduced with permission from S. Karger AG, Basel, and author.*)

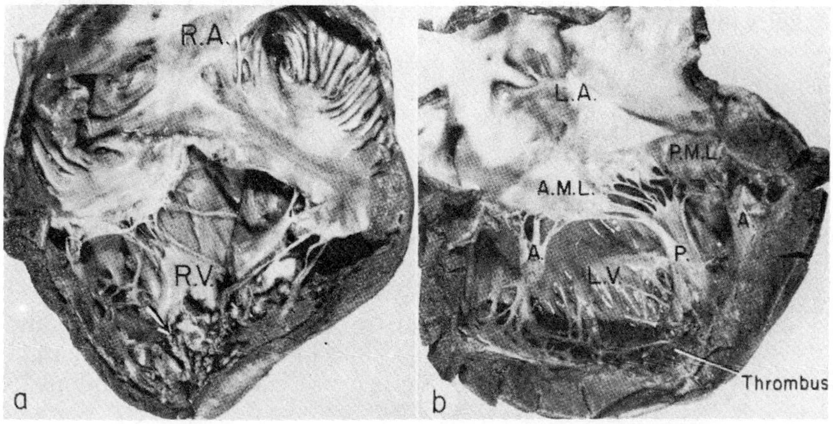

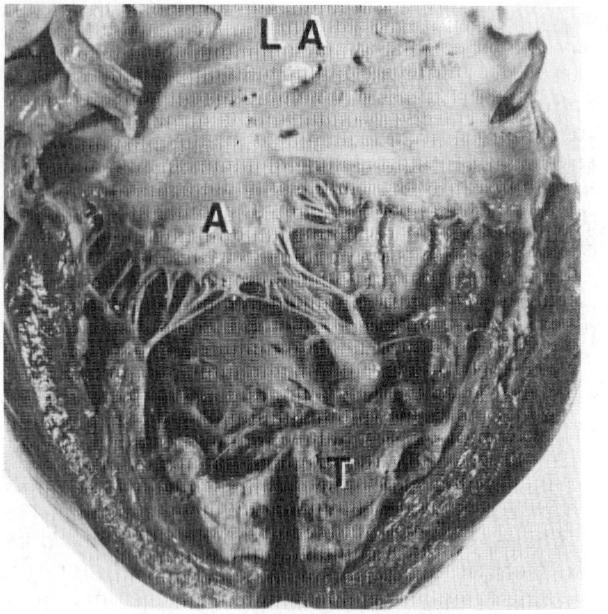

FIGURE 58-18 Davies' endomyocardial fibrosis of the African. Opened left atrium (LA), mitral valve, and left ventricle. A large thrombus (T) is present at the left ventricular apex, and the posterior mitral leaflet is adherent to the underlying mural endocardium. Process involves the endocardium of the entire inflow portion of the left ventricle. The presence of the large thrombus and the absence of dense endocardial fibrous tissue probably indicates that the process in this patient was of relatively recent onset. A = anterior mitral leaflet. (Photograph given to W. C. Roberts by Gregory T. O'Connor, who spent 2 years in Kampala, Uganda.) (*From B. J. Maron, and W. C. Roberts, Cardiovasc. Clin., 11:35, 1980. Reproduced with permission from the publisher and author.*)

thrombus on a thickened endocardium is the main feature. Some fibrosis is present, and the fibrotic stage takes up to 2 years to develop. In the fibrotic stage the eosinophils tend to disappear, and dense fibrosis occurs in the endocardium and myocardium.[129] Although fibrosis is maximal at the ventricular apex, involvement of the papillary muscles and chordae tendineae results in valvular regurgitation, the fibrosis may extend into the ventricular outflow tract, and there is progressive encroachment on the ventricular chamber.

Endocardial mural fibrin deposition in the right ventricle, containing altered eosinophils, caused intractable heart failure in a patient with eosinophilic leukemia; surgical removal and tricuspid valve replacement provided palliation.[136]

Abnormal Physiology

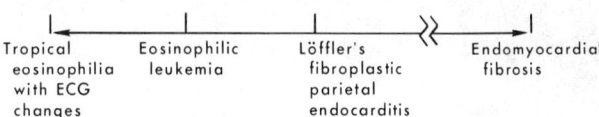

The most important abnormality in tropical EMF is a restriction of ventricular filling, produced initially by the endocardial fibrosis and later by progressive obliteration of the ventricle by masses of fibrous tissue and thrombus, with contraction and scarring of the ventricular wall (see Chap. 20). The distortion of the ventricular cavity and the involvement of the papillary muscles and chordae tendineae produce considerable mitral and tricuspid regurgitation. Rapid ventricular filling occurs in early diastole, with the noncompliant ventricle limiting late diastolic filling. The restrictive element is evidenced by the steep x and y descents of the jugular venous pulse and by the high mean pressure of the right atrium. The obliterative process in the right ventricle produces a pattern similar to that of constrictive pericarditis, with a "dip-and-plateau" contour; there is a sharp early diastolic dip with a high end-diastolic plateau. Peak pressures in the right atrium and right ventricle in ventricular systole may be identical. Inspiration increases the venous pressure and diminishes the arterial pressure, although these changes are less impressive than in constrictive pericarditis. Partial obliteration of the ventricular cavity reduces the stroke volume so that compensatory tachycardia is needed to maintain the cardiac output. The involvement of the myocardium secondary to the endocardial process eventually impairs systolic function. With severe right ventricular involvement, the right atrium may assume an enormous size. Pulmonary hypertension is common when there is predominant involvement of the left ventricle with mitral regurgitation.

FIGURE 58-19 Diagram illustrating spectrum of endomyocardial disease with and without eosinophilia.

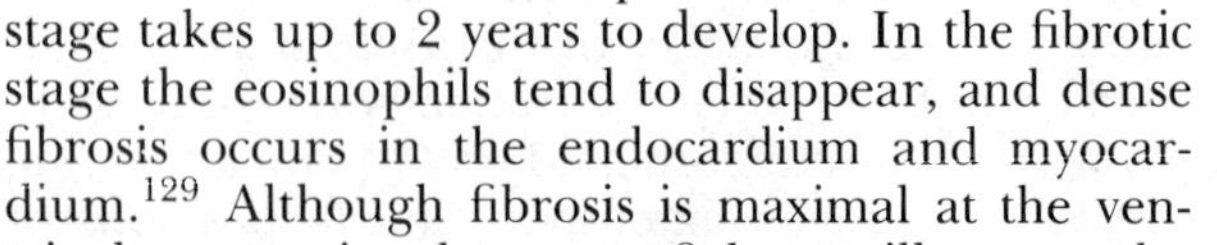

Before obliteration of the right ventricular cavity occurs, while the process is still in the restrictive phase, distinction from constrictive pericarditis may be difficult. Important differential features are the similarity of the diastolic pressures in both ventricles in constrictive pericarditis but not in restrictive cardiomyopathy, and the frequency of pulmonary hypertension in restrictive cardiomyopathy but not in constrictive pericarditis (see also Chap. 59).

The features of Loeffler's disease and tropical EMF are closely similar, but there are some differences.

Clinical Manifestations of Eosinophilic Endomyocardial Disease

The acute initial illness in EMF is characterized by edema, breathlessness, and fever. These symptoms commonly remit, and the individual may remain well for an interval. Following the initial illness, there may also be progressive tiredness and general ill health with prolonged fever. Development of hepatomegaly with ascites and dyspnea with cough may reflect right and left ventricular failure, respectively. Sinus tachycardia is common, and episodes of atrial fibrillation may occur. In the established disease, the clinical picture is usually of severe right-sided heart failure, in many respects resembling constrictive pericarditis. Massive pericardial effusion may occasionally cause tamponade. If the left ventricle is also involved, dyspnea, rales in the lungs, and often mitral regurgitation are present. Tropical endomyocardial fibrosis has a *right ventricular form,* a *left ventricular form,* and a *mixed form* with involvement of both ventricles. When right and left ventricular disease coexist, the right ventricular signs usually predominate; most patients appear to have disease of both ventricles.

Left Ventricular EMF The *history* in left ventricular endomyocardial fibrosis is of predominant dyspnea and cough, but symptoms of right-sided heart failure are also commonly present. The presence of dyspnea strongly suggests left ventricular EMF. *Physical examination* reveals evidence of a low cardiac output, mitral regurgitation, and pulmonary hypertension. Mitral regurgitation, however, is not invariable. The murmur of mitral regurgitation may be maximal at onset and diminuendo at termination, when the relatively unaffected anterior mitral valve apparatus can prevent mitral regurgitation at end systole. The jugular venous pulse shows a distinct *a* wave, and the arterial pulse is of small volume. Sinus rhythm is usual, but atrial fibrillation can occur. There is usually a third heart sound at the apex. Embolic phenomena are relatively common, particularly when there is atrial fibrillation. Left ventricular involvement appears associated with a poorer prognosis.

The *chest roentgenogram* shows moderate cardiac enlargement with evidence of an elevated left atrial pressure and pulmonary venous congestion. Enlargement of the left atrium can be substantial when mitral regurgitation is severe. A linear calcific deposit may be seen in the region of the obliterated apex of the left ventricle. Small pleural effusions are present. The *electrocardiogram* shows left ventricular hypertrophy and a left atrial abnormality, often with associated right ventricular hypertrophy as a result of pulmonary hypertension. QRS voltage is diminished.

Right Ventricular EMF Isolated right ventricular EMF is less common, even in patients with predominant right-sided findings. On *physical examination,* in the right ventricular form, there is substantial ascites but no peripheral edema. The liver is enlarged, the face may be puffy, and there is occasional exophthalmos. The jugular venous pressure is greatly elevated, with a large systolic wave and sharp *y* descent. The venous pressure rises with inspiration. Ventricular pulsation is not impressive, as the right atrium occupies most of the area usually taken up by the right ventricle. There can be a holosystolic murmur of tricuspid regurgitation, and a right ventricular third heart sound is prominent. The heart sounds are often soft, due to pericardial effusion. The arterial pulse is small and decreases with inspiration. There is tachycardia, and central cyanosis is often present, probably due to uneven ventilation-perfusion. Areas of lung which are perfused but not ventilated serve as intrapulmonary shunts, allowing systemic venous blood to reach the pulmonary veins. Angiographic studies have shown that the azygos vein fills from the right atrium, suggesting blood flow through the azygos system to the pulmonary veins, bypassing the right side of the heart.[130]

The clinical features of 15 patients with the hypereosinophilic syndrome were recently described.[137]

On *chest roentgenogram,* the cardiac silhouette is massive, due mainly to the enormous right atrium and the pericardial effusion. The lung fields may appear underfilled. Occasionally calcific deposits are present in the thickened endocardial fibrous tissue at the right ventricular apex. Small pleural effusions are not infrequent. The *electrocardiogram* shows low-voltage QRS complexes and flat or inverted T waves. The P waves are usually large, indicating a right atrial abnormality. Right axis deviation may be present.

Special Laboratory Studies There are no consistent biochemical abnormalities of *blood tests.* Disordered liver function in advanced cases is probably secondary to the elevated venous pressure and low cardiac output. There is usually anemia and mild or moderate eosinophilia.

M-mode *echocardiography* (Fig. 58-20) may show increased bright echoes in the endocardium but is often unrewarding, except to demonstrate pericardial effusion and to define the functional consequences of the disease.[138] Two-dimensional echocardiography is of value in demonstrating the obliteration of the apices of the ventricles and the presence of thrombus, especially in the apical four-chamber view; bright, patchy echoes at the cavity surface suggest calcification, and there is evidence of involvement of the papillary muscles and posterior atrioventricular valve. Preserved ventricular contractility and atrial dilatation are prominent.[139] Color-coded, amplitude-processed cross-sectional echocardiography can provide information about the extent and severity of the disease and be used to confirm a clinical diagnosis.[138]

Gated blood pool scanning (*radionuclide imaging*) aids in differentiation from dilated cardiomyopathy by defining the normal to diminished ventricular cavity size.[37]

Angiocardiography characteristically shows reduction in the size of the ventricles and thickening of the endocardium. The apices of both ventricles tend to be blunted, smooth, and sometimes truncated as if amputated; the left ventricular shape may resemble a boxing glove. Contractile function remains good until the late stages. Distortion of the ventricular cavity and reduction in cavity size are important differential features from constrictive pericarditis. The presence of a pericardial effusion is confirmed by a gap between the contrast medium in the right atrium and the outer border of the right cardiac silhouette. Severe mitral and tricuspid regurgitation are common. Selective coronary cineangiography, revealing a vascular blush, lends support to the presence of

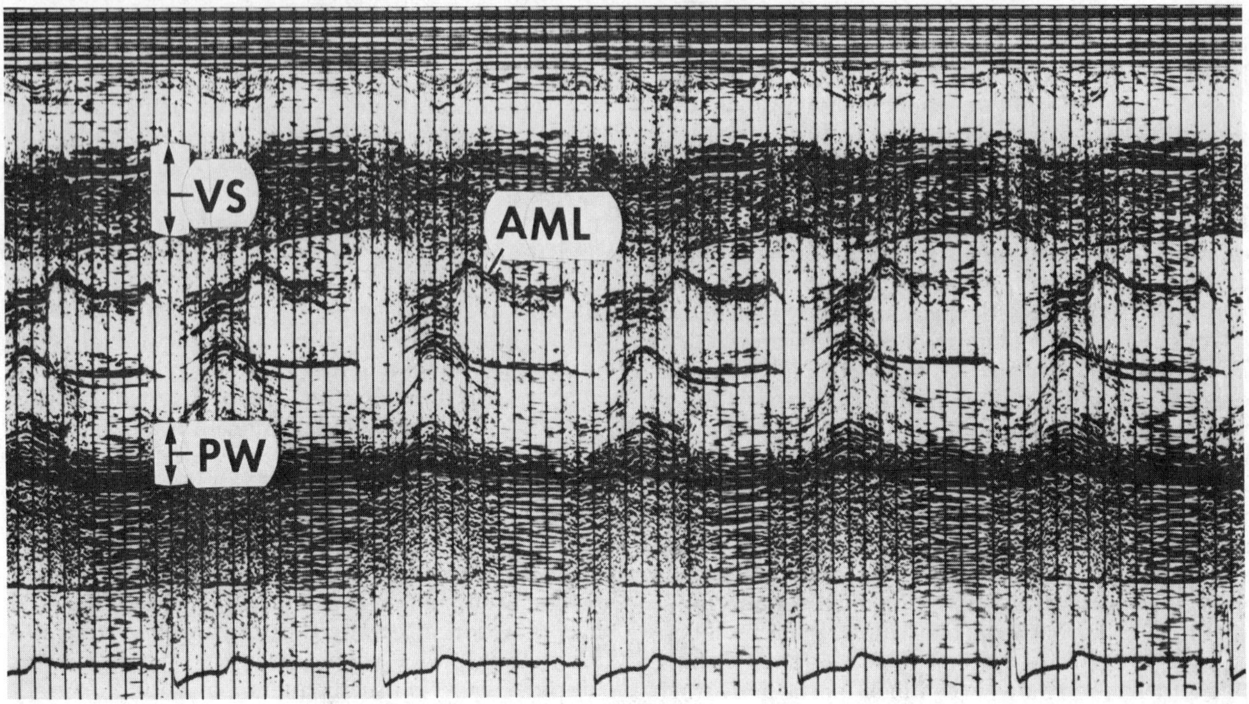

FIGURE 58-20 Echogram of the left ventricle at the level of the mitral valve from a patient with hemochromatosis. The septum and posterior wall are symmetrically hypertrophied, each measuring 2.1 cm. The excursion and systolic thickening of the septum, however, are reduced; posterior wall motion is normal. The left ventricular cavity size is at the lower limit of normal, but the fractional shortening or ΔD is normal. The anterior mitral leaflet shows a decreased diastolic slope, consistent with decreased left ventricular compliance. VS = ventricular septum; PW = posterior wall; AML = anterior mitral leaflet. (*From J. M. Felner, and R. C. Schlant, "Echocardiography: A Teaching Atlas," Grune & Stratton, Inc., New York, 1976. Reproduced with permission from the publisher and author.*)

the mural thrombus in the evolutionary patterns of the disease.[140]

Although the diagnosis often can be confirmed by echocardiography, *endomyocardial biopsy* is helpful in delineating the stage of the disease and thus guiding treatment.[141] With skill, the risk of embolism is small.

Differential Diagnosis

In right-sided tropical endomyocardial fibrosis when the heart is of moderate size, differentiation must be made from *constrictive pericarditis,* an important distinction being the absence of pericardial calcification in EMF. However, calcification can occur within the ventricles and may simulate calcium in the pericardium. When pericardial effusion is present, the differential diagnosis includes tuberculous or pyogenic infection. Distinction must be made also from other conditions producing a very large right atrium, such as severe *Ebstein's anomaly.* The characteristic auscultatory features and the right bundle branch block of Ebstein's anomaly are absent in tropical EMF. Echocardiography, angiocardiography, and at times intracardiac electrography should clarify the diagnosis. Important to differentiate from right ventricular endomyocardial fibrosis is right atrial myxoma, which can also mimic constrictive pericarditis. Echocardiography can be diagnostic, but angiocardiography is sometimes needed.

Treatment

Medical Treatment The medical treatment of eosinophilic endomyocardial disease is unrewarding because the cause is unknown. Treatment concentrates on the usual measures for heart failure (see Chap. 21) and on anticoagulant drugs to prevent systemic embolism. Digitalis may be of little value because the tachycardia is a compensatory one necessary to maintain an adequate cardiac output, but when rapid atrial fibrillation is present, digitalis is required to slow the ventricular rate. Ascites may be tapped when abdominal distension is extreme, but paracentesis should be avoided except when essential because of the protein loss entailed. Fluids should be rigidly restricted and diuretics used carefully. Pericardioperitoneal shunts have been beneficial with massive recurrent pericardial effusion.[142]

If eosinophilia is present, additional management is warranted. With clear evidence of eosinophilic leukemia, antimetabolic treatment may be helpful, but in most cases eosinophilic leukemia is not the cause. Corticosteroid and immunosuppressive drugs have been used with little success; the effect on the abnormal eosinophils tends to be transient. Corticosteroid hormones are often helpful in the short term; the usual treatment for heart failure, including anticoagulant drugs to prevent embolism, is necessary.

A recent prospective study of 26 patients with the hypereosinophilic syndrome suggested that prednisone and/or hydroxyurea therapy could stabilize or reverse the symptomatic and echocardiographic abnormalities.[143] Prednisolone has been described as useful in treating episodes of heart failure, and vincristine and hydroxyurea have been helpful in treating the hypereosinophilic syndrome.[137,141] Plasma exchange caused a fall in eosinophilic counts in filariasis.[137] There are no reports of bone marrow transplantation.

Recently *surgical treatment* of EMF has had considerable success, at least in the short term.[144] It consists of resection of the thickened and obliterating endocardial tissue (endomyocardiectomy) with repair or replacement of the regurgitant mitral and tricuspid valves if required.[141] With predominant right ventricular disease, placement of a Glenn shunt between the superior vena cava and pulmonary artery can augment pulmonary blood flow.[144] It is uncertain whether surgical treatment will be effective in the long term, because it is unlikely to affect the progress of the underlying disease.

Amyloid Disease of the Heart[145,146]

Classification

Amyloid disease of the heart may occur with or without manifestations in other organs and can be considered either as a cardiomyopathy or as myocardial involvement in systemic disease (specific heart muscle disease). Because prominent manifestations of restrictive cardiomyopathy without symptomatic involvement of other organ systems are common, it is discussed here. Amyloid deposits in the heart extensive enough to cause cardiac dysfunction are seldom isolated to the heart. Cardiac amyloidosis causing dysfunction is thus usually part of a systemic disorder. It occurs more commonly in men of at least middle age.

Elderly patients with minute amyloid deposits in the heart may have isolated cardiac involvement, but these deposits are not of sufficient size to cause cardiac dysfunction.

Amyloidosis is a rare disease, characterized by the accumulation of a protein polysaccharide complex which contains specific binding sites for anti-gamma globulin antiserum as well as other serum proteins such as fibrinogen, albumin, and complement. Amyloid deposition may rarely occur on a familial basis.

Pathology

Amyloid may be deposited in any portion of the heart (Fig. 58-21), and the deposits may be large (grossly visible) or small (microscopic-sized).[147] When cardiac dysfunction results from cardiac amyloidosis, the heart weight is increased, and amyloid deposits are grossly visible and diffusely distributed throughout the ventricular walls, which have a firm, rubbery consistency.[148] Histologically, most ventricular myocardial cells are surrounded by amyloid fibrils. Thus, not only is ventricular motion restricted but most myofibers are constricted by the amyloid deposits. In addition to being in the myocardial interstitium, amyloid is deposited in the walls and in the lumina of the intramural coronary arteries, in the mural endocardium, particularly in the atria, in valvular endocardium, in the epicardium, and in both conduction tissue and cardiac nerves. The endocardial deposits usually are not large enough to produce valvular dysfunction. The deposits in the lumina of the small coronary arteries, however, may lead to focal myocardial ischemia with resulting necrosis and fibrosis.[149] Despite the frequent arrhythmias and conduction abnormalities, the amount of amyloid deposition in the conducting myocardium is minimal in comparison to that present in contracting myocardium. Nevertheless, conduction and rhythm disturbances are more common in these patients than in those of similar age and sex without cardiac amyloidosis. Amyloid may be viewed as an "acellular cancer" in that the deposits infiltrate within and between normal tissues but no cells are present in the proliferating material. Massive infiltration of the heart is characteristic of patients with symptomatic cardiac disease.

Although the ventricular walls are made rigid by heavy amyloid deposits, the ventricular cavities are not dilated unless another cardiac condition also is present. Thus, cardiac amyloidosis joins hypertrophic cardiomyopathy and constrictive pericarditis as a cause of diastolic heart disease, where congestive heart failure may occur in the absence of ventricular cavity dilatation. The atria, in contrast, usually are dilated. The enlargement of the cardiac silhouette on roentgenogram in this condition may well be related to the atrial dilatation, although pericardial effusion may be present. Petechiae may be present on the heart surface. Diagnosis of clinically significant cardiac amyloidosis should be questioned in the absence of congestive cardiac failure and electrocardiographic low voltage.[146]

Abnormal Physiology

In patients with restrictive cardiomyopathy, hemodynamic studies reveal elevation of both right and left ventricular systolic pressures; both early and late diastolic pressures in the left ventricle are also substantially elevated. The cardiac index is low and the ejection fraction significantly reduced. The syndrome differs hemodynamically from constrictive pericarditis and restrictive cardiomyopathy due to endomyocardial disease in that the speed of filling of the ventricle is reduced throughout diastole, there is no initial rapid filling, and no left ventricular third heart sound is heard.[150]

The diastolic fault in amyloid disease, while differing from HC in a number of ways, may produce a clinical presentation that is not dissimilar. The amyloid diastolic faults are very different. The left ventricle in early or mild amyloid disease contracts well, but systolic function is diminished later. Amy-

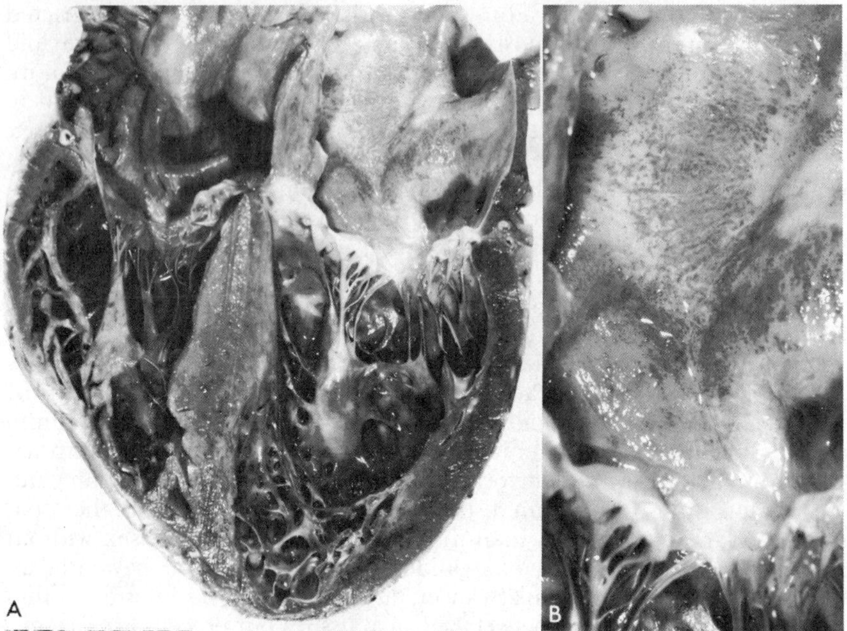

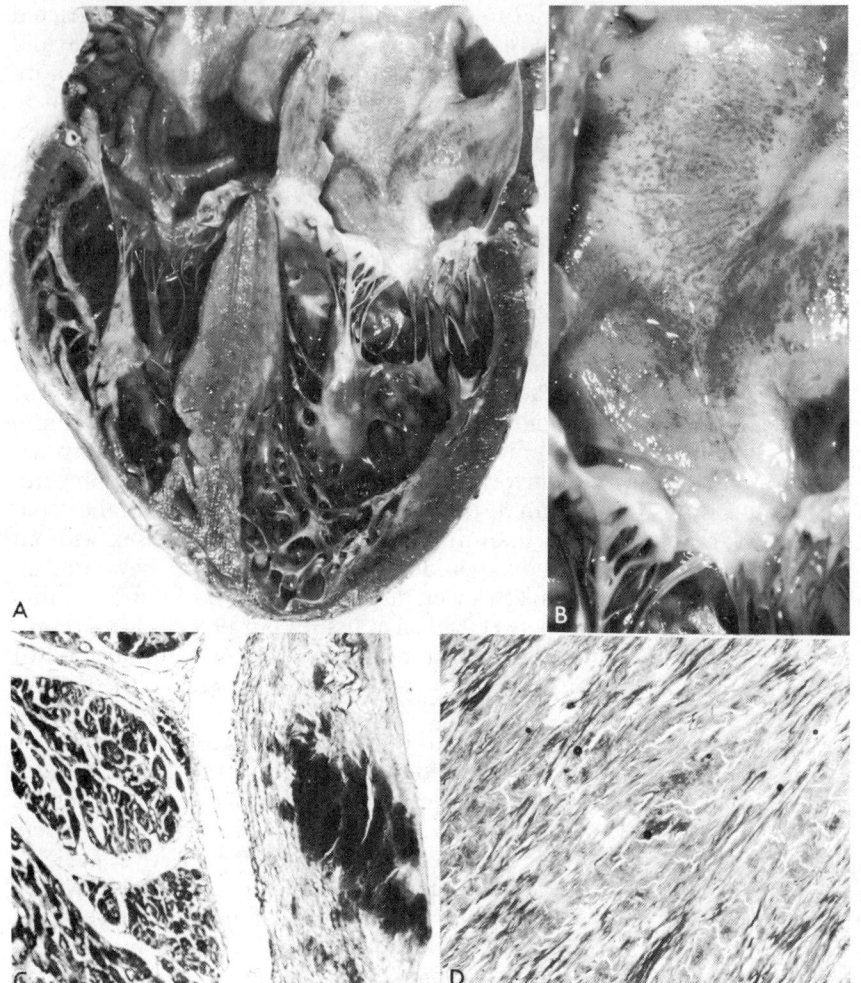

FIGURE 58-21 Cardiac amyloidosis. *A.* Posterior half of the heart in an 86-year-old man (A68-18) who had angina pectoris and healed myocardial infarction as well as large amyloid deposits. *B.* A close-up of left atrial endocardium. The waxy lesions on this endocardium represent amyloid deposits and are indicative of extensive ventricular amyloid deposits. *C.* Photomicrograph of left atrial endocardial amyloid deposit, ×107. *D.* Amyloid has infiltrated extensively a left ventricular papillary muscle, ×32. Crystal violet stain (*C* and *D*).

loid disease does not show the distortion of the ventricles found in endomyocardial fibrosis.

Clinical Manifestations

History The earliest cardiac finding is exertional dyspnea,[151] progressing to paroxysmal nocturnal dyspnea and heart failure. A history of chest pain is common, and fatigue and edema are noted.

Physical Examination In addition to lesions of tongue and mucous membranes, there may be petechiae, purpura, or peripheral neuropathy. Cutaneous circumorbital bruising has been described. Orthostatic hypotension may reflect autonomic nerve infiltration. Kussmaul's sign (inspiratory increase in neck vein distension) may be evident, with prominent *x* and *y* descents of the jugular venous pulse. Abnormal signs, however, may be confined to the heart. When the heart is stiff, inelastic, and resistant to filling, it manifests some features of restrictive cardiomyopathy and may resemble constrictive pericarditis. When amyloid deposits are extensive, however, left ventricular systolic function becomes impaired, and a syndrome of dilated cardiomyopathy emerges. Murmurs of atrioventricular valvular regurgitation are characteristic. Patients tend to be severely ill, with marked cardiac failure and a low cardiac output manifest by a low systolic blood pressure and narrow pulse pressure. A pericardial effusion may be present. Arrhythmias and conduction disturbances are frequent and often result in sudden death. Bradycardia is common, with both persistent atrial standstill and the sick sinus syndrome described. Amyloid infiltration may damage the sinoatrial (SA) node so that sinus rhythm does not resume after defibrillation of an arrhythmia.

Electrocardiogram The electrocardiogram characteristically shows low-voltage complexes but no specific repolarization changes. Arrhythmias and conduction defects are common; there may be atrioventricular block. Q waves, predominantly inferior, may simulate myocardial infarction. The distinctive combination of low electrocardiographic voltage and an increase in left ventricular mass on the echocardiogram, both compatible with increased amyloid infiltration, is valuable in diagnosis and appears to indicate the severity of the disease.[152]

Chest Roentgenogram There is cardiomegaly on the chest roentgenogram, often with pulmonary congestion. Cardiac pulsations are diminished at fluoroscopy. Pericardial effusion may cause an enlarged cardiac silhouette.

Special Laboratory Studies M-mode *echocardiogram* study demonstrates normal left ventricular dimensions in diastole, but reduced amplitude of pulsation of the septum and posterior (free) wall, and an increased systolic dimension. Pericardial effusion may be detected. There is an increase in left ventricular mass. On occasion the septum may be thicker than the left ventricular free wall, simulating hypertrophic cardiomyopathy; and right ventricular wall thickness may be increased. The rate of outward movement of the posterior wall of the left ventricle and the slope are gentler than normal, indicating slow ventricular filling. Two-dimensional echocardiography may aid in differentiation from hypertrophic cardiomyopathy and may better define right ventricular and atrial involvement;[34] a "granular sparkling" appearance of the thickened myocardium, particularly in the endocardial layer, has been described as virtually diagnostic of cardiac amyloidosis,[153,153a] but is also found in myocarditis with severe fibrosis and is quite common in HC. Color-coded two-dimensional studies show a characteristic uniform pattern of the myocardium. Asymmetric hypertrophy of the septum due to amyloid deposition has been reported.[154] Conversely, amyloid deposition involving primarily the small coronary vessels may not cause abnormal myocardial wall thickening. Early aortic valve closure may reflect the decreased cardiac output.

Using radionuclide imaging techniques ^{201}Tl-imaging may aid in differentiation from constrictive pericarditis by identifying the increased wall thickness of an infiltrative cardiomyopathy. It has been claimed that diagnosis may be assisted by increased diffuse uptake of ^{99m}Tc-pyrophosphate in areas of increased left ventricular wall thickness determined by echocardiography,[154,155] particularly when combined with noninvasive tests of ventricular function; two-dimensional echocardiography seems superior in detecting cardiac amyloidosis.[155a] Computed tomographic (CT) imaging of the chest may identify a thickened pericardium, differentiating constrictive pericarditis from restrictive cardiomyopathy.[37,156]

Angiocardiogram reveals coarse trabeculation of the left ventricle and impressive papillary muscle indentation. *Ambulatory electrocardiography* shows frequent complex ventricular ectopic activity, as well as supraventricular arrhythmias; the former correlated well with the presence of heart failure and even more strongly with an abnormal echocardiogram in a recent report. All four patients who died suddenly had abnormal echocardiograms and complex ventricular arrhythmias.[157]

Endomyocardial biopsy is diagnostic.

Treatment

Treatment of amyloid heart disease is highly unsatisfactory; most patients have progressive deterioration and die within a year or so after the onset of heart failure. Sensitivity to digitalis limits its use, and excessive diuresis may cause cardiovascular collapse. AV conduction defects may necessitate pacemaker placement, and success in pacing is variable. Arrhythmias are often refractory to therapy. No current method can remove amyloid from tissue, though plasma exchange has been tried.

Carcinoid Heart Disease

This problem is discussed in Chap. 61. Although valvular lesions predominate, metastatic carcinoid lesions may be found in the myocardium (Fig. 58-22), and endocardial thickening is described.[158] The acellular hyalinized collagenous material on the atrial and/or ventricular endocardium may restrict filling.[159]

Endocardial Fibroelastosis (see Chap. 36)

Classification

Endocardial fibroelastosis (EFE) does not fit into the classification of cardiomyopathy. It involves the left ventricle of infants and children, often on a familial basis.

Severe EFE is commonly described in two forms: the primary or idiopathic form in which other heart disease is absent, and the secondary form in which there is left-sided congenital heart disease such as coarctation of the aorta, aortic stenosis, mitral stenosis, or atresia.

Pathology

See Fig. 58-23.

Clinical Manifestations

The disease is notable for the early development of severe heart failure, often unresponsive to medical treatment. The clinical picture is of dilated cardiomyopathy, but the left ventricle appears peculiarly spherical and immobile, with the cavity smooth and

FIGURE 58-22 Carcinoid, metastatic to the myocardium. Nests of small, regular cells are arranged in an organoid pattern. × 150. (*Courtesy of the Department of Pathology, Emory University School of Medicine.*)

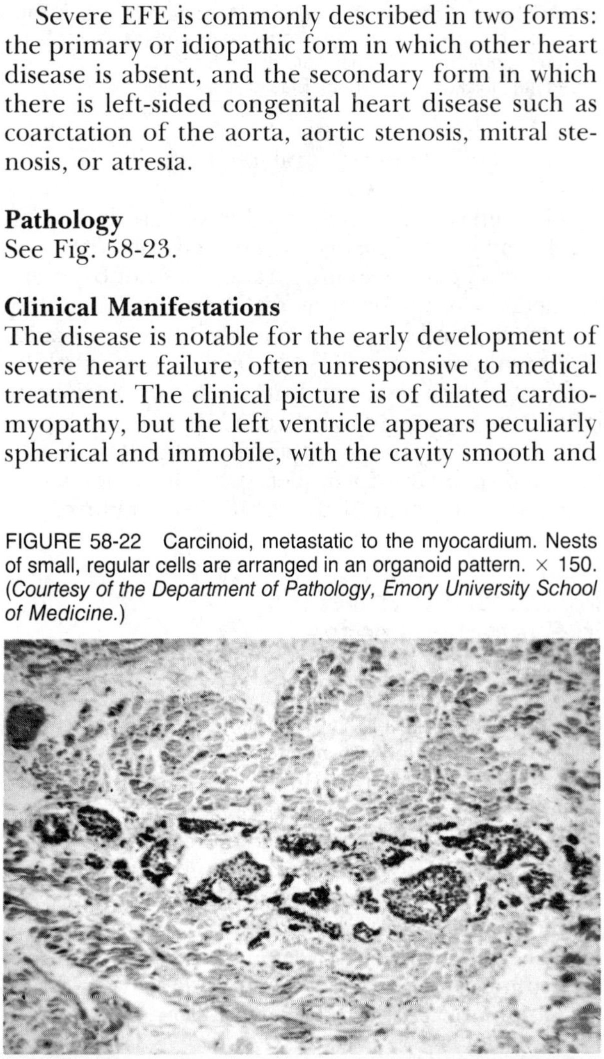

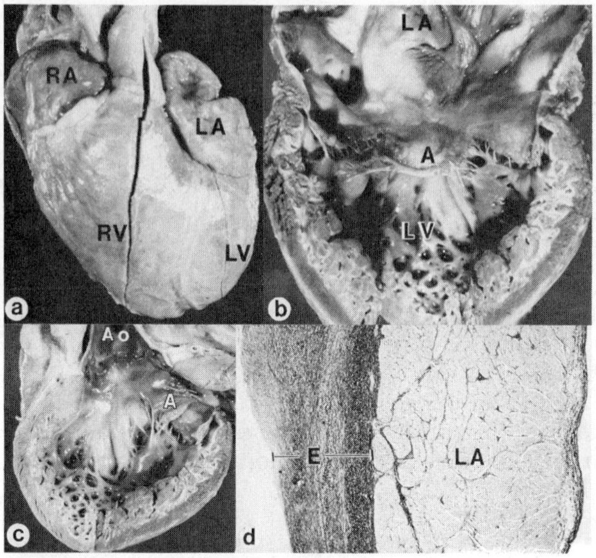

FIGURE 58-23 Heart of a 6-month-old boy (A66-220) with congenital endocardial fibroelastosis. The child had evidence of congestive heart failure throughout life. The final event was acute pneumonia. The heart at necropsy showed typical morphological features of this condition. *a.* Exterior of heart. All four chambers are dilated, the right ventricle (RV) slightly more than the left ventricle (LV). RA = right atrium; LA = left atrium. *b.* Opened left atrium, mitral valve, and left ventricle showing diffuse endocardial fibrosis of both chambers. The anterior (A) mitral leaflet is slightly thickened. *c.* Opened aorta (Ao), aortic valve, and left ventricle. *d.* Photomicrograph of left atrial wall. Its endocardium (E) is about three times thicker than normal. Elastic tissue stain.

not indented. Severe mitral regurgitation is common.

The clinical and angiographic picture is one of severe myocardial disease without characteristics of endocardial disease. This paradox has not been explained, possibly because differentiation between myocarditis and endocardial fibroelastosis in infants is difficult or impossible. Indeed, endocardial fibroelastosis as a separate entity has been questioned; it has been suggested to be secondary to severe heart failure resulting from congenital cardiac lesions, the so-called primary form being a misnomer. The management is that of congestive heart failure.

Myocardial Involvement in Systemic Disease

Myocardial structural and functional abnormalities are an integral part of a wide variety of systemic diseases. Systemic manifestations often overshadow the myocardial abnormalities, but the latter occasionally dominate the clinical presentation.

The myocardial lesions may be diffuse or localized. When the myocardium is *diffusely* involved, the clinical picture may resemble that of myocarditis or cardiomyopathy (see also Chap. 57) with cardiac enlargement and progressive congestive heart failure; arrhythmias, embolic phenomena, and sudden death are common. On the other hand, a myocardial abnormality may be recognized only by an abnormal electrocardiogram, or identified as an incidental finding at postmortem examination. When the myocardial involvement is *localized,* it may produce arrhythmias, obstruction to blood flow, or electrocardiographic abnormalities, or it may be an incidental finding at autopsy. Both diffuse and localized myocardial lesions may be associated with valvular (endocardial) and/or pericardial disease.[160]

The diagnostic problem in myocardial disease is complex because similar clinical syndromes may result from widely differing histological abnormalities; in addition, related etiologic factors may produce different histological patterns. The specific etiologic diagnosis of the myocardial disease often depends on extracardiac manifestations of the disease; these may remove it from the designation of cardiomyopathy (idiopathic myocardial disease).[2]

Systemic diseases with myocardial involvement will be considered in the following categories:

- infectious disease
- sarcoidosis
- nutritional disorders
- metabolic disorders
- endocrine disorders
- hematologic diseases
- neurological and neuromuscular diseases
- collagen vascular diseases
- neoplastic diseases
- chemical and drug effects (toxicity and hypersensitivity)
- physical causes
- miscellaneous systemic syndromes

Infectious Diseases

See Chap. 57.

Sarcoidosis

Sarcoidosis is a multisystem granulomatous disorder which cannot be classified etiologically. It is discussed as a separate entity because of the frequency of cardiac manifestations. Myocardial sarcoid occurs equally among whites and blacks, despite the marked predominance of systemic sarcoidosis in blacks. There is an equal sex incidence.[161]

Pathology

In cardiac sarcoidosis (Figs. 58-24 and 58-25), portions of myocardial wall are replaced by sarcoid granulomas;[162] hard granulomas are found in the heart in about 20 percent of patients with sarcoidosis studied at necropsy. Although sarcoid lesions are never limited to the heart, most patients with cardiac sarcoidosis have prominent symptoms of cardiac dysfunction. In other words, a patient with sarcoidosis either has dominant cardiac involvement or the heart is spared. The cardiac deposits preferentially involve the cephalad portion of the ventricular septum, producing severe conduction disturb-

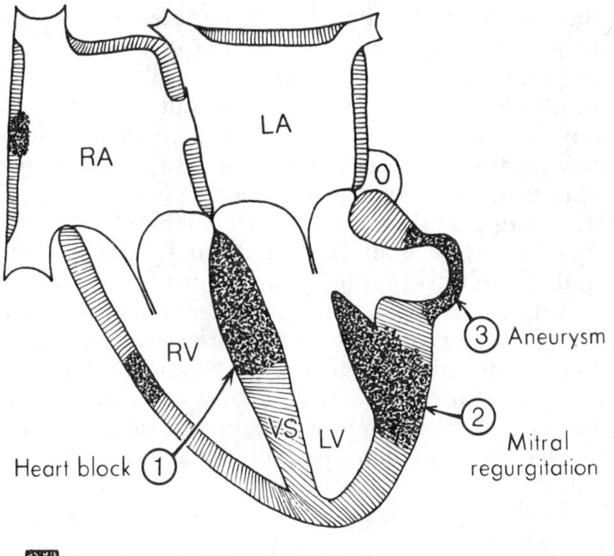

FIGURE 58-24 Cardiac sarcoidosis. Diagram showing the more frequent locations of sarcoid granulomas in the heart and their more frequent functional consequences.

ances,[163] particularly complete heart block; or the left ventricular papillary muscles and the adjacent free walls, producing papillary muscle dysfunction with resultant mitral regurgitation; or right or left ventricular free walls, which, after corticosteroid therapy, may scar (explaining the electrocardiographic pattern of "myocardial infarction") and lead to ventricular aneurysm. Ventricular arrhythmias, particularly tachycardias, are a frequent consequence. Sudden death is common and may be the initial manifestation of sarcoidosis.[164] Pericardial involvement is uncommon, but tamponade and constriction have been described.

Clinical Manifestations

History Myocardial involvement occurs in the second and third decades of life. Dyspnea and palpitations are frequent. Occasionally, atypical chest pain or Stokes-Adams syncope occur. Although about 20 percent of patients with sarcoid have autopsy evidence of cardiac involvement, only about 5 percent have cardiovascular symptoms.[165,166]

Physical Examination Sarcoid heart disease should be suspected in a patient with systemic sarcoidosis who develops unexplained cardiac arrhythmias or conduction abnormalities; cardiac murmurs, particularly of severe mitral regurgitation; or progressive congestive heart failure. Complete heart block without apparent cause in a young adult should suggest myocardial sarcoidosis.[167]

FIGURE 58-25 Cardiac sarcoidosis. Shown here is a longitudinal section through anterolateral (*A*) papillary muscle in a 26-year-old woman (PGGH #A-70-541) who had been asymptomatic until 10 days before her death, when dyspnea appeared. The dyspnea rapidly worsened, and when hospitalized on the day of death, she was in acute pulmonary edema. The blood pressure was 80/70 mmHg, heart rate 160 beats per minute, and a grade 3 to 4/6 pansystolic blowing murmur, which radiated to the axilla, was audible. Chest roentgenogram showed congested lungs, cardiomegaly, and prominent hilar adenopathy. Electrocardiogram showed nonspecific ST-T wave changes and atrial hypertrophy. She developed complete heart block and died shortly thereafter.

At necropsy, large, firm white deposits were present in the walls of all four cardiac chambers and completely replaced both left ventricular papillary muscles (*A*). On histological section, the firm white areas represented hard granulomas typical of sarcoidosis (*B*). H&E; ×400. Similar hard granulomas were present in lymph nodes, liver, spleen, and lung. Stains for acid-fast organisms, other bacteria, and fungi were negative.

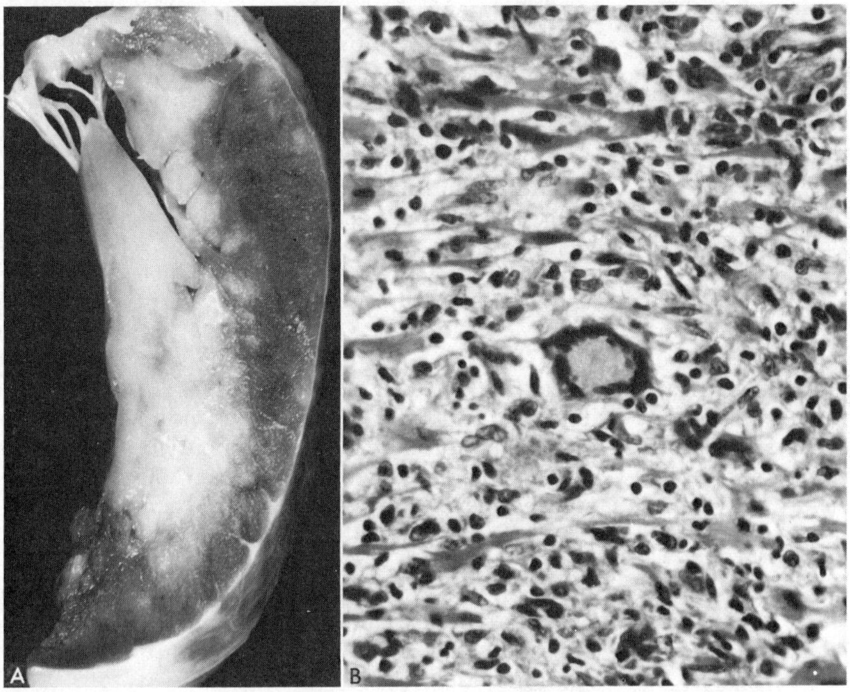

Atrioventricular conduction disturbances, particularly complete heart block with Stokes-Adams syncope, are common. Ventricular arrhythmias, often difficult to control, occur next most commonly and may result in sudden death. Congestive heart failure is common with cor pulmonale, but is less frequent in myocardial sarcoid. On occasion, with extensive myocardial sarcoid infiltration, a component of restrictive cardiomyopathy may be evident. Clinical evidence of pericardial involvement is rare; constrictive pericarditis is unusual, but pericardial effusion is reported.[168] Valve involvement is uncommon, except for mitral annular calcification possibly secondary to the chronic hypercalcemia.[162]

Electrocardiogram As many as 50 percent of patients demonstrate an electrocardiographic abnormality. Abnormalities of rhythm, conduction, and repolarization occur commonly in the absence of cardiovascular symptoms. Arrhythmias are often paroxysmal, and serial electrocardiograms show varying conduction abnormalities. The electrocardiogram may mimic myocardial infarction. Exercise testing and ambulatory ECG recording are recommended to identify ventricular dysrhythmias.[169]

Chest Roentgenogram Sarcoid is usually suspected because of hilar lymphadenopathy or pulmonary nodular reticulation. Radiological findings vary with the extent of myocardial involvment, cor pulmonale, and pericardial effusion.

Special Laboratory Studies A positive Kveim test supports the diagnosis, as does a positive lymph node, scalene node, or liver biopsy. Transbronchial lung biopsy should be considered. Myocardial radionuclide imaging may identify areas of decreased or absent perfusion, compatible with sarcoid infiltration,[170] helping to differentiate myocardial sarcoidosis from cardiac dysfunction secondary to pulmonary sarcoidosis and to detect myocardial sarcoidosis in patients without clinical evidence of heart disease. Endomyocardial biopsy is valuable when positive[171] and may permit initiation of therapy, but the patchy distribution of myocardial sarcoid limits interpretation of a negative biopsy.

Natural History and Prognosis

Patients with cardiac dysfunction due to cardiac sarcoidosis rarely have other organ dysfunction.[164] Two-thirds of patients die suddenly, either from heart block or ventricular arrhythmias,[161] and these tend to be the patients with extensive grossly evident myocardial sarcoid. The clinical course of symptomatic cardiac sarcoidosis tends to be short, with three-fourths of patients dying within 2 years of the onset of cardiac symptoms.[166]

Treatment

Myocardial involvement appears to be an indication for corticosteroid hormone therapy, regardless of the severity of the systemic disease. Ventricular performance may improve.[171] Q waves, arrhythmias, and atrioventricular and intraventricular blocks have resolved both with[168,172] and without steroid therapy. The arrhythmias are often refractory to digitalis and many antiarrhythmic agents; these drugs may potentiate the atrioventricular block.[165] Beta-adrenergic blocking agents may decrease the severity of arrhythmias and sudden death. Quinidine, with and without propranolol, has also been effective.[169]

Implantation of a permanent demand pacemaker may be useful with high-degree atrioventricular block to prevent sudden death. In one young patient with a ventricular aneurysm due to sarcoid, multiform ventricular beats and refractory ventricular tachycardia responded dramatically to aneurysm resection.[173]

Nutritional Disorders (see Chap. 74)

Beriberi

Oriental (Shoshin) beriberi, usually caused by malnutrition, is characterized by high-output cardiac failure, often associated with syncope, shock, and rapid death. In the western hemisphere, it has occasionally been associated with excessive beer drinking.[174] Occidental beriberi, most common in alcoholic men, presents both right and left ventricular failure, often without evidence of a hyperkinetic circulation; it is often misdiagnosed as atherosclerotic coronary heart disease or alcoholic or other cardiomyopathy. (See also Chap. 24.)

The cardiac manifestations are probably due to a potentially reversible derangement of carbohydrate metabolism, with effects similar to those of hypoxemia. Inability of the myocardium to utilize oxygen and the decreased metabolic demand for oxygen may decrease coronary flow. Myocardial energy production is impaired by lack of cocarboxylase; thus, fats rather than carbohydrates must provide the major source of energy. High-output cardiac failure, with decreased myocardial oxygen extraction[174a] and consumption, imposes an additional workload on a heart already handicapped by this metabolic defect.[175]

The heart failure is responsive, at least in part, to thiamine administration.

Pellagra

The cardiovascular disturbances and electrocardiographic abnormalities have been attributed to both nicotinic acid deficiency and the frequently associated beriberi. Exertional dyspnea, tachycardia, palpitations, and edema are described, but all may not be due to heart disease. The regression of electrocardiographic changes in 40 percent of patients with pellagra parallels clinical improvement. Niacin therapy is specific, but multivitamin therapy is generally recommended.[176]

Scurvy

Sudden death may occur in patients with severe scurvy and appears due to myocardial involvement.[177] The myocardium may show fatty degeneration. Severe scurvy should be considered as a medical emergency requiring immediate intravenous ascorbic acid; this frequently reverses the abnormal electrocardiogram.[178]

Hypervitaminosis D

Gross and microscopic deposits of calcium in the heart, particularly in individual necrotic myofibers (dystrophic calcification), occur in patients with hypervitaminosis D.[179] The electrocardiographic abnormalities of hypercalcemia may be present. The ST-T alterations may reflect myocardial damage (see "Supravalvular Aortic Stenosis," Chap. 36).

Kwashiorkor

This disease is most common in Africa, affecting primarily persons on a high-carbohydrate, low-protein diet. There is striking atrophy and disintegration of the conduction system, which may be the basis for the atrioventricular conduction disturbances and unexplained sudden death.[180] Other cardiac lesions include biventricular dilatation and hypertrophy, myofiber atrophy, and endocardial mural thrombosis. The patients demonstrate tachycardia, low-output cardiac failure, and extreme edema. Pulmonary and peripheral emboli are common, as is sudden death, the latter often in the first week of recovery.

Nonspecific ST-T abnormalities are the most frequent electrocardiographic alterations.[181] Potassium therapy reverses the electrocardiographic abnormalities;[175] and the electrocardiogram also becomes normal with clinical improvement. The heart is small on roentgenologic examination.

The patients respond to bed rest and adequate diet in all but the latter stages of the disease, but characteristically relapse with return to physical activity and an inadequate diet.

Metabolic Disorders

Amyloidosis

See p. 1213.

Pheochromocytoma

Predominantly epinephrine-secreting pheochromocytomas (see Chaps. 50 and 72) may mimic a cardiomyopathy.[182] The catecholamine-induced myocardial damage is due to inability of the coronary circulation to meet the increased metabolic demands of the myocardium; catecholamines probably also cause constriction of small coronary arteries.

The clinical findings are those of congestive heart failure, tachycardia, and arrhythmias. Associated hypertrophic cardiomyopathy has been reported. Adrenergic blocking agents commonly reverse the electrocardiographic abnormalities, and preoperative therapy with phenoxybenzamine and propranolol may reduce the surgical risk in patients with pheochromocytoma with cardiomyopathy. Tumor removal is associated with hemodynamic, electrocardiographic, and clinical improvement of the cardiomyopathy.

Cardiac Glycogenosis

Cardiac glycogenosis (glycogen storage disease of the heart, Pompe's disease, glycogenosis type II) is an autosomal recessive disorder of carbohydrate metabolism, due to a deficiency of acid maltase, occurring equally in both sexes. Excessive normal glycogen accumulates in cardiac and skeletal muscle and in other tissues.[183] Energy deprivation contributes to the cardiomyopathy. The specific metabolic defect is absence of the enzyme alpha-glucosidase. McPhie delineated five categories of glycogenosis; cardiac involvement is prominent only in type II. Electrocardiographic abnormalities have been described in patients with glycogenosis other than type II;[184] and myocardial involvement was recorded with type III (Cori's disease).[185] Biochemical analysis of an endomyocardial biopsy speciman enabled the diagnosis of type III disease in a young adult.[186]

Pathology The ventricles are massive with thick walls and normal chambers (Fig. 58-26); the atria are normal. The myocardial fibers are enlarged, with diffuse and extensive vacuolation, producing a lacework pattern.[183]

Clinical Manifestations The age of onset of symptoms is a diagnostic clue, as heart failure usually occurs between 2 and 6 months, and always before

FIGURE 58-26 Glycogen storage disease of the heart. Massive thickening of the left ventricular wall and thickening of the left ventricular endocardium. (*Courtesy of the Department of Pathology, Emory University School of Medicine.*)

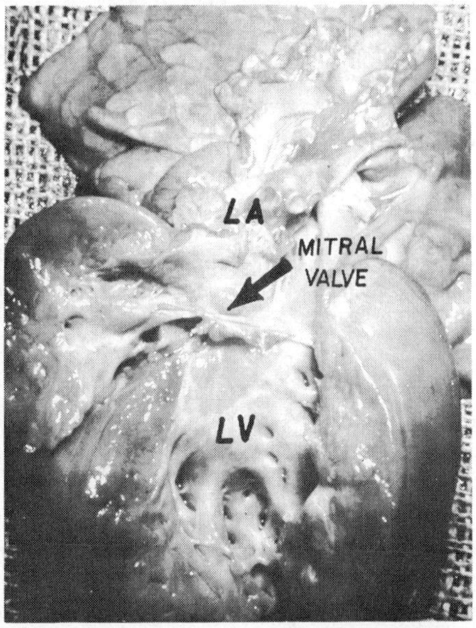

18 months. The presentation includes feeding difficulty, cyanosis, dyspnea, sweating, tachycardia, massive cardiac enlargement, susceptibility to respiratory infection, and terminal congestive heart failure. Generalized muscle weakness and hypotonia, large tongue, hyporeflexia, and other neurological deficits are also present, and a similar disorder is often described in a sibling.

Glycogen storage disease with massive left ventricular hypertrophy may also present as hypertrophic cardiomyopathy, as a massively hypertrophied ventricular septum may encroach upon both right and left ventricular outflow tracts. Digitalis may be harmful with muscular outflow tract obstruction. Sudden death is common in the first year of life, presumably due to arrhythmia. Death in infancy or early childhood is the rule, usually related to heart failure or respiratory infection.

Increased glycogen in a skeletal muscle biopsy confirms the diagnosis, as does absence of alpha-glucosidase activity in skeletal muscle, liver biopsy tissue, or blood leukocytes. Periodic acid Schiff staining of peripheral blood lymphocytes demonstrates glycogen granules; and decreased lymphocyte acid maltase activity further confirms the diagnosis. The blood sugar, glucose, and galactose tolerance are normal, as is response to glucagon and epinephrine; these distinguish between Pompe's disease and other types of glycogen storage disease.

The electrocardiogram shows left ventricular hypertrophy, with strikingly increased QRS voltage and a short PQ interval[187] (Fig. 58-27). These findings[183] distinguish this abnormality from other causes of left ventricular hypertrophy in infancy. Preexcitation and right ventricular hypertrophy may occur. Massive generalized cardiac enlargement and pulmonary congestion are characteristic roentgenographic findings (Fig. 58-28).

The echocardiogram demonstrates an enormously thickened ventricular septum and ventricular walls. Systolic anterior motion of the mitral valve and outflow tract obstruction have been described.[188] Angiocardiography demonstrates a massive, thick-walled left ventricle, often with an outflow tract gradient. Right ventricular obstruction may also occur (Fig. 58-28).

FIGURE 58-27 Glycogen storage disease of the heart in a 3-month-old infant. There is biventricular hypertrophy with massively increased QRS voltage and Wolff-Parkinson-White conduction. (*Courtesy of the Electrocardiographic Laboratory, Grady Memorial Hospital.*)

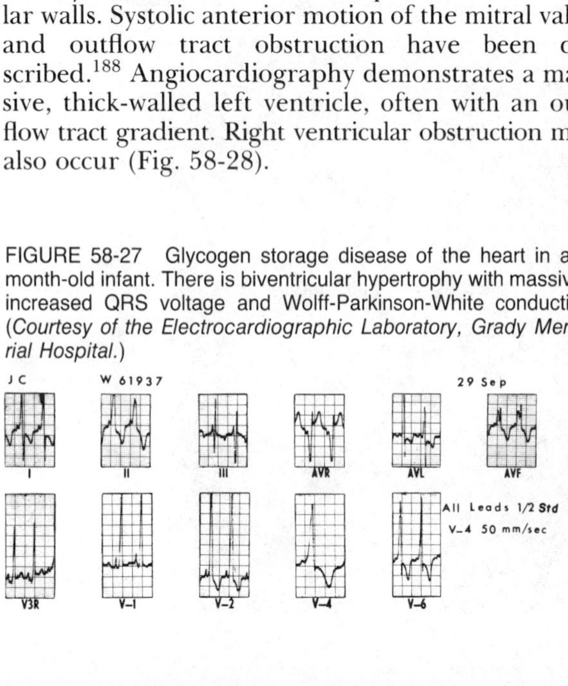

This condition must be differentiated from other causes of severe heart failure in infancy: endocardial fibroelastosis, anomalous left coronary artery, coronary sclerosis of infancy, and acute myocarditis.

Treatment No specific therapy exists. Surgical resection of the hypertrophied ventricular septum has been unrewarding, as has administration of acid maltase. Digitalis must be administered with caution because of problems with preexcitation and arrhythmias.

Other Glycogen Abnormalities of the Myocardium

Congenital Nodular Glycogenic Infiltration Infiltration of the myocardium with glycogen, previously known as *rhabdomyoma,* is the most common cardiac "tumor" in the pediatric age group and is associated with tuberous sclerosis in approximately 50 percent of cases. These solitary or multiple "tumors" are not encapsulated but merge with surrounding myocardium. The gray-purple nodules are usually incidental findings at autopsy, but may cause arrhythmias and AV block with sudden death. Fatality was 52 percent in the first year of life, and 86 percent before puberty in one series of patients. Symptomatic "tumors" are potentially amenable to surgery.[189]

Glycogen in Familial Cardiomyopathy Increased myocardial glycogen has also been reported with familial cardiomyopathy, with normal function of all enzymes absent in known forms of glycogenosis.[190]

McArdle's Syndrome

In this metabolic myopathy, deficient glycogen breakdown in muscle is due to lack of muscle phosphorylase. There is autosomal recessive inheritance. Profound skeletal muscle weakness is evident, with pain and stiffness on exercise. Clinical cardiovascular disease is unusual, although PR prolongation and intraventricular conduction defects[191] have been described.

Systemic Carnitine Deficiency

Familial cardiomyopathy, with endocardial fibroelastosis demonstrated at autopsy, has been associated with severe plasma and tissue carnitine deficiency. Treatment with oral L-carnitine improved myocardial function. This may be a treatable cause of familial cardiomyopathy.[192]

Polysaccharide Storage Disease

The precise metabolic abnormality is not defined. Nonmetachromatic neutral polysaccharide is deposited in the myocardium, and cellular vacuolation and abnormal glycogen deposition have been described.[184]

Dyspnea, palpitations, and syncope may occur. Cardiac enlargement and systolic murmurs are described. Electrocardiographic abnormalities include

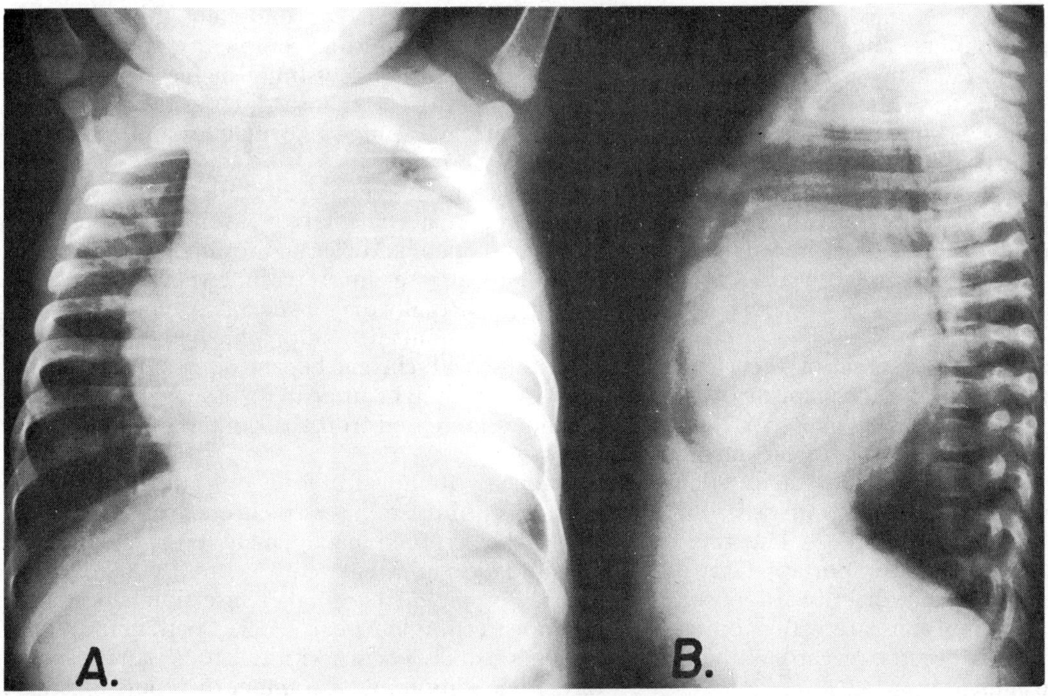

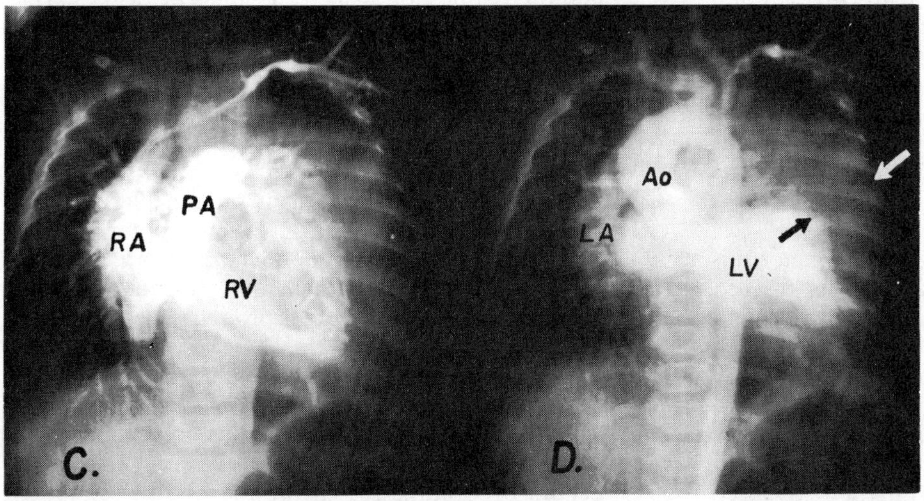

FIGURE 58-28 Glycogen storage disease of the heart. *A* and *B*. Massive generalized cardiomegaly with pulmonary congestion. Cardiac pulsations were normal at fluoroscopy. *C* and *D*. Venous angiocardiogram demonstrating distortion of the right ventricular outflow tract secondary to hypertrophy of the interventricular septum and left ventricle (between arrows). (*Courtesy of the Cardiac Catheterization Laboratory, Grady Memorial Hospital.*)

biventricular and left ventricular hypertrophy and conduction abnormalities.

Hemochromatosis

Hemochromatosis must be considered in males with cardiomyopathy without apparent cause, since this is a potentially remediable cause of myocardial damage. The metabolic disorder is characterized by excessive tissue iron deposition. Since the use of insulin as therapy for diabetes, cardiac failure rather than diabetes and its complications is the leading cause of death in hemochromatosis. Fifteen percent of patients present with cardiac symptoms, and cardiac disease occurs in the absence of bronze skin pigmentation and diabetes. Cardiac involvement is characteristic in patients with hemochromatosis developing in childhood or early adult life.[193]

Pathology (Fig. 58-29) For years it was debated whether or not iron deposition in the heart could cause cardiac dysfunction. Just as with amyloid, cardiac dysfunction will occur if the cardiac iron deposits are large enough;[194] cardiac dysfunction does not occur in patients with only microscopically visible iron deposits and usually occurs when the deposits are grossly visible. In contrast to amyloid deposits which are between myocardial cells, the iron deposits are within myofibers. The iron deposits are most extensive in ventricular myocardium, particularly in the epicardium, less in atrial myocardium, and least in conducting as contrasted to contracting myocardium. Most patients with large cardiac iron deposits have arrhythmias, conduction disturbances, and congestive cardiac failure. In contrast to amyloid, the ventricular cavities typically are dilated. Thus, the rusty brown iron-infiltrated heart is a weak heart, not a strong one.

Abnormal Physiology The genesis of the cardiac damage is unknown, as is the mechanism of iron entry into myocardial cells. There is no correlation between the accumulation of iron in the myocardium, the interstitial fibrosis, and cardiac functional impairment. However, patients with grossly visible cardiac iron all have heart failure.[195] The rate of iron deposition may be more important than the absolute quantity of iron. Cardiac iron deposition occurs only after other organs are saturated with iron; iron deposition is greater in cardiac than in skeletal or smooth muscle.

The hemodynamic pattern is often of dilated cardiomyopathy;[193] however, a pattern resembling restrictive cardiomyopathy with impairment of myocardial relaxation as well as contraction suggests a mechanical cause of the cardiac failure, such as myocardial or endocardial fibrosis. Intracellular disruption by iron deposition—resulting in decreased mitochondria and myofibrils—suggests that it can cause myocardial dysfunction.[196]

Clinical Manifestations Hemochromatosis is recognizable by the classic tetrad of liver disease, diabetes mellitus, heart disease, and skin pigmentation. The dominant cardiac abnormalities are heart failure and arrhythmias. The patient is dyspneic, with cardiomegaly, stasis cyanosis, edema, and ascites. Arrhythmias, AV block, and rapidly progressive biventricular congestive heart failure respond poorly to digitalis and diuretic therapy. Unexplained precordial pain is described. Paroxysmal atrial tachycardia and atrial fibrillation are the most frequent arrhythmias; they relate to atrial rather than conduction system iron deposition; iron is rarely deposited in conduction tissue. Ventricular arrhythmias are less common, despite ventricular iron deposition.

The *electrocardiogram* shows diminished QRS voltage, conduction disturbances, and nonspecific repolarization changes. Electrocardiographic abnormalities may be the earliest evidence of cardiac involvement. A large globular heart with feeble pulsations and biventricular hypertrophy is seen at *roentgenographic* examination (Fig. 58-29); it may mimic pericardial effusion, constrictive pericarditis, beriberi, or myxedema heart disease. *Echocardiography* or *radionuclide angiography* in the early stages shows a nondilated, concentrically thickened left ventricle with diminished compliance; late in the illness, the picture is indistinguishable from dilated cardiomyopathy.[196] Echocardiographic and radionuclide angiographic abnormalities may antedate clinical disease.[196a]

Confirmatory evidence includes excessive iron deposits in a sternal marrow aspirate and/or liver biopsy specimen, and elevated serum iron and serum ferritin levels; serum ferritin levels in excess of 1 g/ml are virtually diagnostic. HLA typing may differentiate patients with idiopathic hemochromatosis from those with chronic hepatic disease; patients with HLA-A3 and -B14 appear to have genetically determined increased iron absorption.

Treatment Removal of iron by repeated venesection, except in patients with chronic refractory anemia, is the accepted management to reverse the iron accumulation and may require 1 to 2 years of treatment. Permanent pacemaker insertion can control syncope in complete heart block. Death in untreated patients usually occurs within 1 to 2 years of onset of cardiac symptoms. A number of reports describe patients who have had regression of symptoms, hemodynamic abnormalities, and cardiac enlargement with repeated venesection;[193,195,196a,197,198] the iron content of liver biopsy specimens can guide the duration of therapy. The role of chelation remains controversial.

Acquired Hemochromatosis
Acquired hemochromatosis is seen in patients with refractory anemias requiring multiple transfusions.[199] The anatomic abnormalities are indistinguishable from idiopathic hemochromatosis. Chelating agents to remove excess iron may be of value.[196]

Fabry's Disease (Angiokeratoma Corporis Diffusum Universale)
Cardiac failure is a common cause of death in this inherited abnormality of glycolipid metabolism, which occurs predominantly in the male. This sex-linked disorder is variably and incompletely recessive, with severest manifestations in the homozygous male.[200] Abnormal glycolipid deposition in blood vessel walls and myocardium is due to deficiency of the enzyme ceramide trihexosidase.

Pathology Myofibers are fragmented, with striking vacuolation due to glycolipid deposition; ceramide trihexoside may also be deposited in the coronary arteries (contributing to myocardial infarction), conduction system, and heart valves.[184,201]

Clinical Manifestations Angiokeratosis and corneal opacities are common. Crises are characterized by fever and burning pain in the extremities. Cardiovascular manifestations include left ventricular hypertrophy and cardiac failure. Hypertension is com-

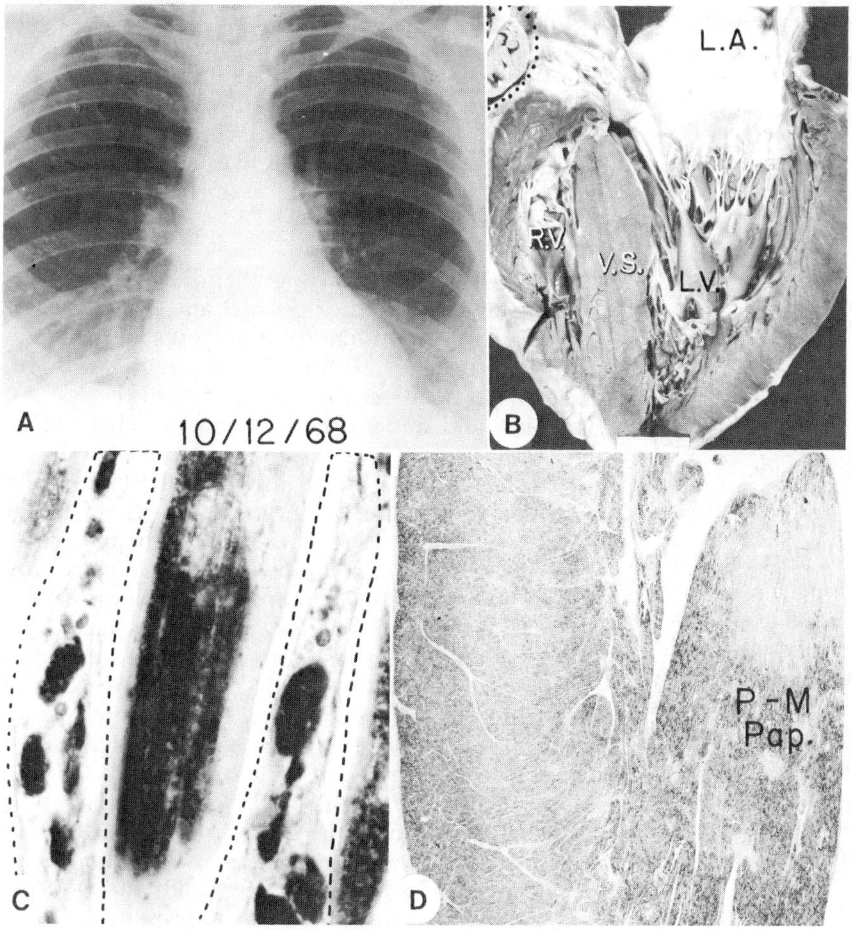

FIGURE 58-29 Cardiac hemosiderosis in a 42-year-old woman (68-327) with sickle cell anemia. She had received 260 units of blood when congestive cardiac failure developed 6 years before death. Chest roentgenogram (*A*) showed cardiomegaly. By the time of death she had received 359 units of blood (90 g iron). At necropsy, the walls of the right and left ventricles and left atrium were rusty brown due to extensive iron deposits (*B*). The right atrial wall in contrast was tan (*B*) and only minute particles of iron were present in it by histological examination. *C.* Photomicrograph of several myocardial cells showing huge deposits of iron in them. Despite large deposits of iron in working myocardium, no iron deposits were observed in conducting myocardium. Longitudinal section of left ventricular wall including posteromedial (P-M) papillary muscle is shown in *D.* Foci of necrosis and fibrosis are present. The necrotic and fibrotic areas probably are anatomic indicators of chronic myocardial hypoxemia, a result of the chronic anemia. Prussian blue iron stains; ×628 (*C*), ×3 (*D*).

mon, generally due to renal failure; angina pectoris and myocardial infarction may occur. Cardiac murmurs may be heard.

The *electrocardiogram* may show changes of left ventricular hypertrophy or myocardial infarction. Sinoatrial block, pre-excitation, atrial fibrillation, and right bundle branch block have been recorded. Cardiac enlargement is evident on *chest roentgenogram,* and pulmonary vascular congestion may be present. Increased left ventricular wall thickness on *echocardiography* probably reflects myocardial glycosphingolipid deposition.[202]

There is no effective therapy, although enzyme replacement may be feasible.[202]

Tay-Sachs Disease

This neurodegenerative autosomal recessive trait, prominent in Jewish families, is due to hexosaminidase A deficiency. Gangliosides are important constituents of cell membranes; deposition of abnormal gangliosides in the myocardium may explain the electrocardiographic derangements.[184]

Cardiovascular symptoms are unusual in these children with mental retardation, decerebrate rigidity, and a cherry-red macula, who die in early childhood. Electrocardiographic abnormalities include a wide QRS-T angle, QT prolongation, and abnormal T waves.

Sandhoff's Disease

This autosomal recessive disorder of glycosphingolipid metabolism, due to hexosaminidase A and B deficiency, resembles Tay-Sachs disease. Morphological abnormalities include endocardial fibroelastosis; redundancy and hooding of the mitral valve, with abnormal myxoid valve tissue; and coronary luminal narrowing due to fibroblastic proliferation.[184] Congestive heart failure and mitral regurgitant murmurs are present.

Electrocardiographic changes include T-wave abnormalities and left ventricular hypertrophy. Diagnosis is made by finding globoside in the urinary sediment or by measuring plasma globoside or hexosamine activity.

G_{MI} Gangliosidosis

Galactosidase deficiency is characteristic of this autosomal recessive trait. Foamy histiocytes with vacuolation are seen, with thickening of the mitral and tricuspid valves.[184] One-third of patients have cardiovascular involvement.

Progressive psychomotor retardation, hepatosplenomegaly, and skeletal abnormalities are present. Cardiovascular symptoms are unusual, and electrocardiographic abnormalities are nonspecific.

Niemann-Pick Disease

This autosomal recessive disorder is characterized by excessive tissue sphingomyelin with foam cells in the myocardium. Clinical cardiac dysfunction is rare.

Gaucher's Disease

Hereditary beta-glucosidase deficiency allows accumulation of glycosyl ceramide in body tissues. Myofiber infiltration, when symptomatic, presents as dilated cardiomyopathy,[203] although on occasion a restrictive component results from excessive cerebroside deposition. Diagnosis has been made by right ventricular endomyocardial biopsy.[204]

Isolated Cardiac Lipidosis

Isolated myofiber lipid accumulation has been reported in a few infants. Lipid accumulates in myocardial cells, producing myofibril degeneration. The lipid is primarily triglyceride with some free fatty acids. The infants, who often have central nervous system symptoms, develop cardiac enlargement and heart failure. Arrhythmias are common, and they and/or the heart failure are the cause of death.[205] Conduction disturbances and biventricular hypertrophy are seen on the electrocardiogram.

Porphyria

Despite an absence of cardiac symptoms and cardiovascular abnormalities in porphyria, pigment deposition and myocardial fiber disintegration are frequent.

Electrocardiographic abnormalities of diminished QRS voltage, left axis deviation, and repolarization changes during an attack of acute porphyria occurred in a patient with a normal electrocardiogram between attacks.[206] Completely normal electrocardiograms have also been reported in patients with porphyria, even during an acute attack.

Mucopolysaccharidosis[207]

Genetically determined disturbances of mucopolysaccharide metabolism are distinguished biochemically by the mucopolysaccharides deposited in tissues and/or excreted in the urine (see also Chap. 47). Enzymatic defects have not been identified.

Hurler's Syndrome (Gargoylism, Mucopolysaccharidosis I) Clinical cardiovascular disease is present in more than 70 percent of patients with Hurler's syndrome (gargoylism). There is deposition of a complex macromolecular glycoprotein in the parenchymal cells and supporting connective tissue of most organ systems. It is inherited both as an autosomal and as a sex-linked recessive trait.

Morphological examination reveals that the myocardial and connective tissue cells are swollen, hypertrophied, and vacuolated. Myocardial involvement is most prominent adjacent to blood vessels; large cells filled with storage material interfere with myocardial contractility. There are biventricular cardiac hypertrophy; nodulation and thickening of the heart valves, especially the mitral valve; endocardial sclerosis; and intimal proliferation of the coronary and pulmonary arteries.[208]

Clinical Manifestations Signs and symptoms usually appear between the ages of 1 and 2 years, when glycoprotein accumulation interferes with tissue growth, structure, and function. Mental retardation, skeletal deformities with dwarfed growth, corneal opacities, and hepatosplenomegaly are characteristic.

Cardiomegaly and murmurs of valve deformity, particularly mitral regurgitation,[209] with resultant congestive heart failure, comprise the major cardiac abnormalities. Clinical coronary insufficiency is rare, despite the usually severe coronary narrowing. Thoracic deformities, pulmonary disease, hypertension, hypoproteinemia, and anemia contribute to the cardiovascular symptoms. Cardiac failure is the cause of death in two-thirds of patients with Hurler's syndrome, with death occurring at an average age of 11 years.

At *roentgenographic* examination, there is generalized cardiomegaly (Fig. 58-30) and calcification of the mitral valve ring; this is the most common cause of mitral annulus calcification in childhood. No specific *electrocardiographic* pattern is present. *Echocardiography* may help identify valvular abnormalities and calcific deposits, as well as myocardial abnormalities[210] (Fig. 58-31).

FIGURE 58-30 Generalized cardiac enlargement and prominent bronchovascular markings in a child with Hurler's syndrome. (*Courtesy of the Department of Radiology, Emory University School of Medicine.*)

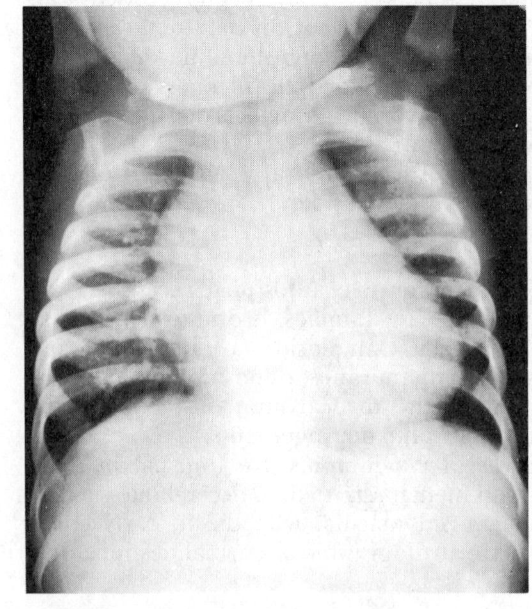

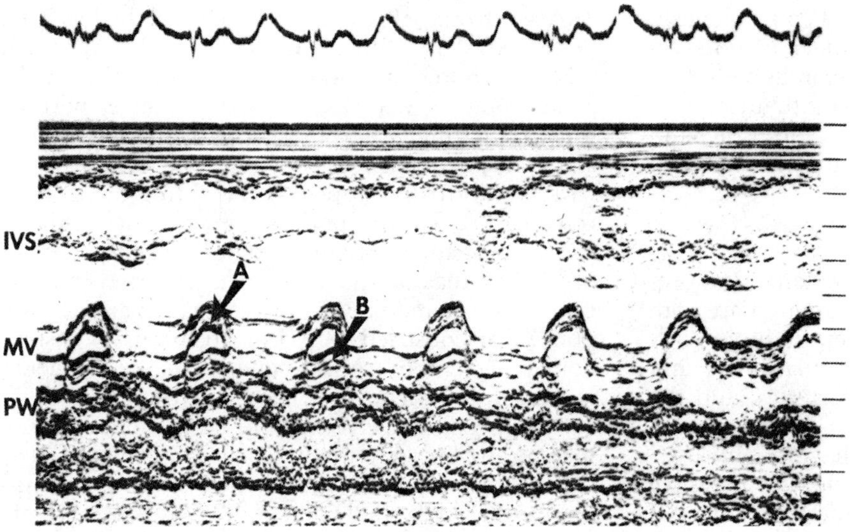

FIGURE 58-31 Hurler's syndrome. Thickening of the anterior (*A*) and posterior (*B*) leaflets of the mitral valve on an echocardiogram. (*Courtesy of Dr. Dorothy Brinsfield, Emory University School of Medicine.*)

Excessive dermatan sulfate and heparitin sulfate are excreted in the urine.

Treatment is nonspecific and unsatisfactory.

Other Mucopolysaccharidoses[184] Patients with other forms of mucopolysaccharidosis have few cardiac manifestations except valvular lesions.

Fucosidosis Fucose accumulation in tissues, with predominant progressive cerebral degeneration, produces dementia, loss of muscle strength, spasticity, and decerebrate rigidity. Cardiac enlargement and arrhythmias occur.[184] Electrocardiographic abnormalities are nonspecific; premature ventricular beats are common.

Refsum's Syndrome (Heredopathia Atactica Polyneuritiformis)

This autosomal recessive disorder of lipid metabolism is characterized by phytanic acid accumulation due to impaired oxidative degeneration.[211] Cardiovascular involvement occurs in most patients. The myocardium shows atrophic cells and fibrosis; the autonomic nerves, sinus node, and His bundle are abnormally prominent due to phytanic acid accumulation, mainly in the myelin sheath.

Chronic polyneuropathy, cerebellar ataxia, and retinitis pigmentosa are seen. More severe cardiac involvement is associated with the presence of ophthalmoplegia, ptosis, and facial weakness. Stokes-Adams syncope and sudden death are described. Electrocardiographic conduction and repolarization abnormalities; arrhythmias, especially complete heart block; and QT prolongation are encountered.

A diet low in phytanic acid and standard antiarrhythmic therapy are recommended.

Primary Xanthomatosis

Patients with familial hypercholesterolemic xanthomatosis (type II hyperlipoproteinemia) have premature atherosclerotic coronary artery disease (see also Chap. 45). Cardiovascular symptoms are due to coronary disease with myocardial infarction and xanthomatous infiltration of the myocardium. Focal lipid deposits and fibrosis involve the myocardium. Acquired aortic stenosis, with foamy macrophages and cholesterol clefts in the aortic valve, has been described.

In addition to the presentation as coronary disease or rarely, aortic stenosis, hereditary normocholesterolemic xanthomatosis may present as dilated cardiomyopathy with congestive heart failure, arrhythmias, and conduction abnormalities. Treatment is discussed in Chap. 45.

Hand-Schüller-Christian Disease

Lipid accumulation may be secondary to a reticuloendothelial cell abnormality, as no disturbance of lipid metabolism has been demonstrated.[212] Xanthomatous deposits, mainly cholesterol and neutral fat, occur in many organs and organ systems including the myocardium. The classic triad includes exophthalmos, diabetes insipidus, and bony defects of the calvarium. There is little correlation between cardiovascular infiltrates and symptoms. The clinical course is slowly progressive. There is no specific therapy.

Gout

Urate deposits in the heart may involve the intima of the coronary arteries; the valvular endocardium, usually of the mitral valve; the pericardium; and the myocardium. In a patient with gout, a mitral valve tophus extended through the myocardium into the epicardium, compressing the left circumflex coronary artery, causing myocardial infarction.

Arrhythmias, including atrioventricular block, are the major manifestations. Hypertension is secondary to renal disease. Pericarditis has been described. Bigeminal rhythm in a patient with gout was unresponsive to quinidine and procainamide but subsided, on several occasions, after probenecid; the arrhythmia was presumed due to a gouty deposit. Complete heart block during an attack of gout resolved to a Wenckebach phenomenon and then to first degree atrioventricular block with uricosuric therapy, decrease in uric acid concentration, and disappearance of clinical gout; urate deposition in the conduction system was implicated.[213]

Oxalosis

Primary oxalosis, a rare hereditary defect (autosomal recessive), and secondary hyperoxaluria are both characterized by calcium oxalate deposition in body tissues. Crystals are seen in myocardial fibers and interstitial tissue, in the coronary arteries, and the conduction system.[214,215]

Patients with primary oxalosis have nephrolithiasis, nephrocalcinosis, and renal failure. Congestive heart failure may occur. Cardiac arrhythmias and conduction abnormalities have been described, with complete heart block presenting as a medical emergency.[133] Hemorrhagic pericardial effusion has been seen.[184] In patients with renal insufficiency, secondary oxalosis may also cause heart failure and conduction abnormalities, including complete heart block.[216]

There is no known therapy. Pacemaker implantation may be indicated. In patients with uremia and secondary oxalosis, hemodialysis may decrease calcium oxalate deposition.[216]

Ochronosis (Alkaptonuria)

This disorder is due to a deficiency of homogentisic oxidase. Areas of gray-blue to purple-black pigmentation occur in the myocardium and coronary arteries; ochronotic pigment granules are deposited preferentially in collagen and fibrous tissue but do not evoke an inflammatory cell response.[217] Atheromata in coronary arteries have a blue-black pigmentation.

There is only modest cardiovascular disease compared with the striking anatomic lesions. Aortic and mitral valve disease with calcification may produce murmurs; aortic and left ventricular aneurysms usually produce few symptoms. Homogentisic acid is present in the urine, producing dark urine. A diet low in phenylalanine is recommended.

Hypokalemia

See Chaps. 72 and 77.

Uremia

The frequent cardiovascular manifestations include congestive heart failure, arrhythmias, pericarditis, and left ventricular hypertrophy, and may be due to hypertensive cardiovascular disease, electrolyte imbalance, fluid overload, anemia, atherosclerotic coronary artery disease, the arteriovenous fistula used for hemodialysis, and/or metastatic myocardial calcification. (See also Chap. 76.) Whether a true uremic cardiomyopathy exists remains controversial. Calcium deposition in small myocardial arteries evokes intimal proliferation and fibrosis with luminal narrowing and ischemic myocardial damage.

A syndrome of uremic cardiomyopathy has been described[218] in patients treated for chronic renal failure by a low-protein diet: massive cardiomegaly, gallop sounds, decreased blood pressure, pericarditis, arrhythmias, and marked sensitivity to cardiac glycosides.

The pericarditis appears related to the degree of renal failure. Uremic pericarditis is characteristically serosanguineous to hemorrhagic, hence the danger of fatal cardiac tamponade when heparin is administered for hemodialysis. Occasionally cardiac tamponade or constrictive pericarditis occurs; constriction appears more frequent in hemodialyzed patients, in part due to heparin-related bleeding.

Nonspecific electrocardiographic abnormalities may be attributed to the hypertension, anemia, electrolyte abnormalities, and pericarditis. In patients on chronic renal dialysis, conduction defects, complete heart block, and even sudden death appear related to metastatic calcification of the conduction system.[219] Patients on a high-fat, low-protein renal failure diet for many years may also have increased atherosclerotic coronary heart disease which may produce electrocardiographic abnormalities. Constrictive pericarditis should be suspected when the cardiac silhouette decreases in size with persistent or increased congestive heart failure.

All abnormalities of uremic cardiomyopathy improve or disappear after hemodialysis. The role of the protein-restricted diet in the development of cardiomyopathy is uncertain. Pericarditis and pericardial effusion can usually be controlled by dialysis, indomethacin therapy, and/or pericardiocentesis. Constriction may require pericardiectomy.

Endocrine Diseases

See Chap. 72.

Hematologic Diseases

Leukemia

See Chap. 61.

Myeloma

Cardiac disease with myeloma is unusual since myeloma nodules rarely involve the myocardium and pericardium. Characteristically, patients have no cardiovascular symptoms. Cardiac tamponade and digitalis-resistant atrial fibrillation, the latter due to SA node myeloma infiltration, have been described.[220] The diagnosis of myeloma should suggest the high frequency of association with amyloid.

Sickle Cell Anemia

Cardiovascular manifestations are due to chronic anemia; pulmonary arterial thromboses, leading to cor pulmonale; and myocardial disease caused by thrombosis of small intracardiac blood vessels.[221] Biventricular dilatation and hypertrophy, myofiber hypertrophy, arteritis with proliferation and thrombosis, and myocardial degeneration, necrosis, and fibrosis are noted. There is no consensus as to whether this is, indeed, a cardiomyopathy.

Cardiomegaly is present in most patients, usually associated with exertional dyspnea and systolic murmurs. Congestive heart failure is a late manifestation. The frequent pulmonary and mitral murmurs, coupled with the joint symptoms of sickle cell disease, often lead to the misdiagnosis of rheumatic fever and rheumatic heart disease. Although dyspnea is the predominant symptom, symptoms and electrocardiographic changes of myocardial ischemia occurred in a 22-year-old man during a sickle cell crisis; the electrocardiogram reverted to normal after the crisis, and myocardial infarction was not demonstrated at subsequent postmortem examination. There is no specific electrocardiographic pattern.[222] Decreased exercise performance is due primarily to the decreased oxygen-carrying capacity of the blood; this may result in an exercise-induced decrease in pump function and in myocardial ischemia.[223]

There is no satisfactory specific therapy.

Sickle Cell Trait Cardiomyopathy

A cardiomyopathy has been described in sickle cell trait without anemia; congestive heart failure, pulmonary thromboembolism, and sudden death were the major manifestations. Chronic alcohol ingestion seemed an important determinant, either acting directly as a myocardial toxin or facilitating sickling from resulting systemic acidosis.[224]

Anaphylactoid Purpura

Clinical and electrocardiographic evidence of myocardial damage occur at the onset of anaphylactoid (Henoch-Schönlein) purpura. The changes appear immunologically mediated, probably reflecting arteriolar and capillary vasculitis. Endomyocardial biopsy has demonstrated IgA and C3 in intramyocardial vessel walls.[225] Symptoms are usually mild, and cardiac involvement may be overlooked. Heart failure, retrosternal pain, and arrhythmias, particularly atrial fibrillation, nodal rhythm, heart block, and conduction disturbances may develop. Electrocardiographic abnormalities vary from nonspecific ST-T alterations to those of myocardial infarction.

Immunosuppressive therapy is recommended.

Thrombotic Thrombocytopenic Purpura

Thrombotic thrombocytopenic purpura is characterized by thrombocytopenic purpura, a microangiopathic hemolytic anemia, fever, and renal and neurological involvement. The thrombotic microcirculatory lesions with hemorrhage and necrosis in the myocardium and conduction system may explain the heart failure, arrhythmias, and occasional cardiac arrest. Anemia may augment the cardiac dysfunction.[226]

Hereditary Hemorrhagic Telangiectasia

A typical telangiectatic lesion was demonstrated in the ventricle by histological examination and postmortem coronary angiography in a patient with chest pain, syncope, left bundle branch block, and arrhythmias.[227]

Neurological and Neuromuscular Disease[228]

Progressive (Duchenne's) Muscular Dystrophy[229]

Cardiac involvement occurs in more than half the patients with this sex-linked, recessively inherited disorder which almost exclusively severely affects the male. There is no correlation between the extent of skeletal muscle disease and the severity of cardiac symptoms or electrocardiographic abnormalities. Cardiac manifestations may antedate the neuromuscular disease; one report describes predominant cardiomyopathy.

Pathology Fatty and fibrous replacement of the myocardium occurs, with selective scarring of the posterobasal left ventricle and posteromedial papillary muscle; this unusual location is not explained. The lesion correlates well with the electrocardiographic and vectorcardiographic[230] abnormalities. However, comparable electrocardiographic abnormalities occur in asymptomatic female carriers. Myocardial cells are atrophic, with loss of striation, vacuolation, fragmentation, and nuclear degeneration. Multifocal dystrophic involvement of the conduction system suggests an anatomic basis for the frequent arrhythmias and conduction abnormalities.[231,232]

James[233] noted generalized noninflammatory degenerative changes in small myocardial arteries, including those supplying the sinus and AV nodes, and suggested this as a basis for the arrhythmias; the epicardial coronary arteries are characteristically normal. Sinoatrial node artery occlusion was demonstrated angiographically in Duchenne's muscular dystrophy; postmortem examination showed that this was due to noninflammatory degeneration. Myocardial artery abnormalities correlate poorly with the localization of myocardial scarring.

Mitral valve prolapse is often described.

Clinical Manifestations The neuromuscular disease is diagnosed by the triad of peculiar waddling gate, large calves, and the "climbing up the legs" phenomenon, characteristically beginning in childhood. Tachycardia is the earliest sign of cardiac involvement; this characteristic finding persists during sleep, is often associated with arrhythmia and cardiac enlargement (Fig. 58-32), and may reflect sympathetic hyperactivity. Although gallop rhythm is frequent, symptoms of congestive heart failure are generally absent because of prolonged inactivity or bed rest. Arrhythmia or infection precipitates overt cardiac failure. Mitral regurgitant murmurs may be due to papillary muscle dysfunction. Chest pain is probably musculoskeletal in origin.[234] Death is usual in the second decade, often from respiratory infection; sudden death is not uncommon.

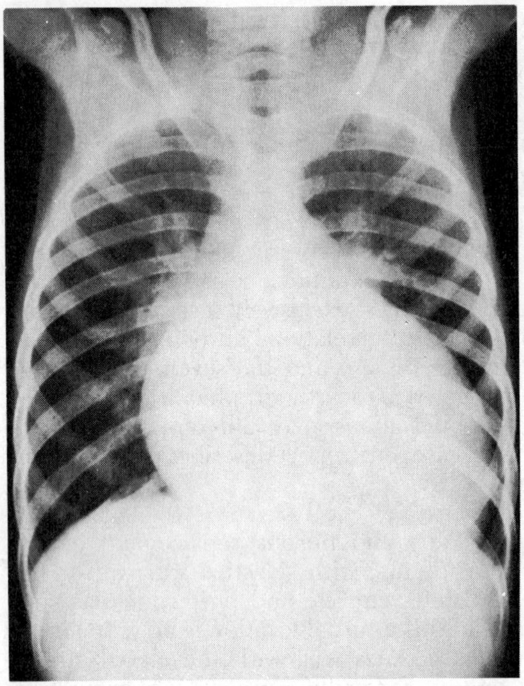

FIGURE 58-32 Generalized cardiac enlargement and pulmonary venous congestion in a 10-year-old boy with muscular dystrophy. (*Courtesy of Crippled Children's Division, Georgia Department of Public Health.*)

The *electrocardiogram* is the earliest and most sensitive indication of cardiac involvement and is abnormal in 40 to 90 percent of patients.[234] The distinctive changes include tall R waves in the right precordial leads and deep Q waves in the inferior limb leads and left precordial leads;[235] identical electrocardiographic abnormalities may be present in affected family members and asymptomatic female carriers with serum abnormalities.[236] The mechanism of these ECG changes is not known, but a genetic determinant has been postulated. However, muscle weakness, predominantly pelvic girdle, documented in some female carriers, raises the possibility of a latent cardiomyopathy. Tachycardia is characteristic; arrhythmias and P-wave abnormalities are common; conduction defects, a short PQ interval, and nonspecific T-wave changes are seen (Fig. 58-33).

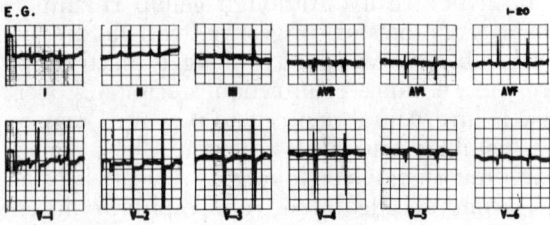

Determination of cardiac size and configuration on *chest roentgenogram* may be complicated by thoracic deformities and elevated diaphragms, due to diaphragmatic dystrophy. Serum creatine kinase (CK) levels are elevated. *Echocardiogram* shows a relaxation abnormality (decreased diastolic endocardial velocity) of the posterior left ventricular wall, which may be more specific than the electrocardiogram in identifying early cardiac involvement.[237] A decrease in left ventricular wall thickness with progression of the disease probably reflects myofibril loss and fibrosis.

FIGURE 58-33 Muscular dystrophy in a 10-year-old boy. The electrocardiogram mimics posterolateral wall myocardial infarction. (*Courtesy of Crippled Children's Division, Georgia Department of Public Health.*)

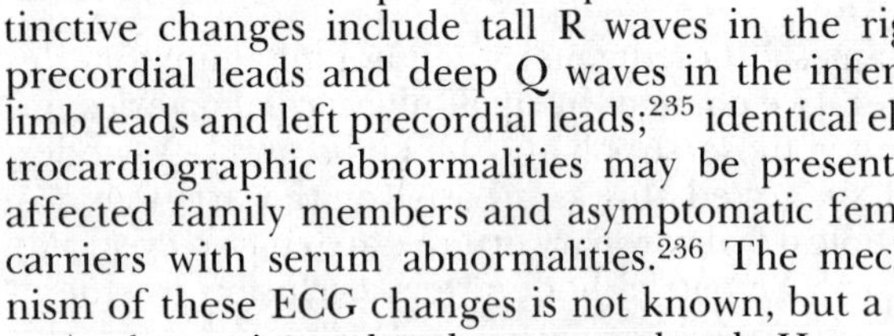

Treatment There is no specific therapy. Heart failure responds to usual management. Because the neuromuscular transmission-excitation-contraction mechanism in skeletal muscle is compromised, antiarrhythmic drugs with neuromuscular effects may cause adverse responses; procainamide may induce muscle weakness, and verapamil has been described to precipitate respiratory failure.[238] The role of prophylactic pacemaker insertion in patients with conduction disturbances requires evaluation.

Cardiomyopathy in Other Forms of Nonmyotonic Muscular Dystrophy

Cardiomyopathy occurs in the limb-girdle type (Erb's), the fascioscapulohumeral type (Landouzy-Dejerine), and the limb-girdle–pseudohypertrophic type of nonmyotonic muscular dystrophy, but manifestations are less prominent and specific than in the Duchenne type, and the prognosis is much better.[229] Gallop sounds, cardiac enlargement, and minor electrocardiographic abnormalities occur.[234] Heart failure is unusual. Rhythm and conduction disturbances are seen. Fascioscapulohumeral dystrophy has been associated with persistent atrial standstill.[239]

X-Linked Humeroperoneal Neuromuscular Disease

Mild muscular disability but life-threatening cardiovascular complications occur; sudden death is common in young adult life. The distal leg and proximal arm weakness and contractures begin in the first decade, progress slowly, and stabilize in the second decade. Palpitations, awareness of a slow pulse, and syncope are the only cardiac symptoms. Bradycardia is prominent, often with a diffuse and displaced apex impulse, and nonspecific murmurs. Heart failure is notably absent.

Atrial abnormalities are universal—P-wave abnormalities, atrial arrhythmias, varying atrioventricular block, and permanent atrial paralysis with junctional bradycardia.[240] Sinus arrest with infranodal junctional rhythm is described. Both neuropathy and myopathy of the peripheral musculature are suggested by electromyograms and muscle biopsy. Ventricular function is normal.

Permanent pacing is recommended, irrespective of atrial activity, with ventricular rates below 50 because of the high incidence of sudden cardiac death.[240]

Friedreich's Ataxia

The original description of heritable progressive spinocerebellar degeneration noted cardiac involvement—arrhythmia, cardiac enlargement, and congestive failure—in five of six patients. Cardiovascular disease occurs in one-third to one-half of patients, with cardiac symptoms often the initial manifestation. No relation is documented between the severity of the neurological disease, the family history of ataxia, and the severity of the heart disease.

Etiology of the Cardiomyopathy The cardiac disease has been attributed to scoliosis or chest deformity causing cor pulmonale, coronary artery narrowing or occlusion, neurogenic or toxic causes, rheumatic or congenital factors, etc. The association of Friedreich's ataxia and hypertrophic cardiomyopathy has received attention; both diseases are familial, both affect the myocardium, both have similar electrocardiographic abnormalities, and both become symptomatic in the same age group; an etiologic link is questioned,[241] possibly an abnormality of catecholamine function. Other studies dispute this relationship.[242]

Pathology Cardiac involvement is virtually universal: cardiac hypertrophy and dilatation, fatty degeneration, interstitial fibrosis, and eosinophilic and lymphocytic infiltrates. Collagen replaces degenerating myofibers, and compensatory hypertrophy of remaining muscle cells occurs. Mural thrombosis occurs. Coronary arteries vary from normal to diffusely involved with atheromatous lesions. Infiltration of the Purkinje fibers of the AV node and conducting system by fibrous tissue disrupts normal excitation and may explain the arrhythmias. The cardiomyopathy has also been attributed[243] to extensive medial degeneration and intimal hyperplasia of the small intramural coronary arteries; arrhythmias, most commonly atrial fibrillation and paroxysmal supraventricular tachycardia, may also be due to involvement of the SA and AV node arteries.

Clinical Manifestations[244] There is onset in adolescence of progressive skeletal deformities, ataxia, and a dysarthric scanning speech; death due to congestive heart failure or intercurrent infection usually occurs within 20 years after onset of symptoms. Palpitations due to arrhythmia and exertional dyspnea are common; angina is rare. The classic findings include inappropriate sinus tachycardia, arrhythmias, cardiac enlargement, nonspecific murmurs, and congestive heart failure. Congestive heart failure is rare before age 10 and is due to myocardial disease, with or without cor pulmonale. Hypertrophic cardiomyopathy may also occur, with outflow gradients and murmurs disappearing as the disease becomes more extensive. The loss of atrial systole with the onset of atrial fibrillation may precipitate heart failure. Occasional peripheral emboli result from the mural thrombi.

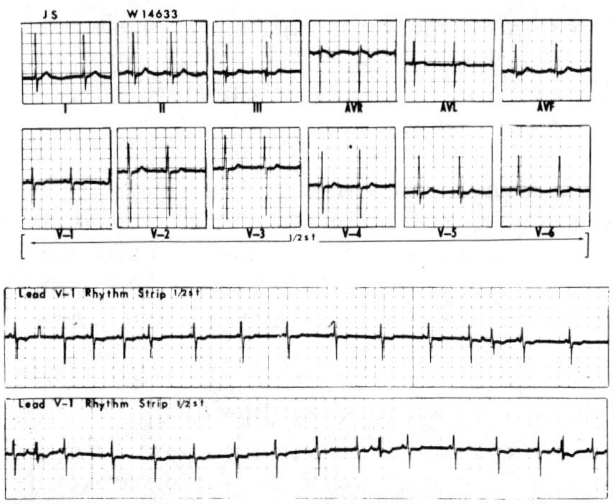

FIGURE 58-34 Twenty-one-year-old man with Friedreich's ataxia, a congestive heart failure, and recurrent arrhythmias. There is electrocardiographic evidence of biventricular hypertrophy and nonspecific ST-T abnormalities. A wandering supraventricular pacemaker is demonstrated on the rhythm strips. *(Courtesy of Electrocardiographic Laboratory, Grady Memorial Hospital.)*

The *electrocardiogram* is abnormal (Fig. 58-34) in about 90 percent of patients.[229] ST-T changes suggestive of left ventricular ischemia are an almost constant abnormality. AV block and bundle branch block are frequent. Atrial fibrillation is also seen. Right and left ventricular hypertrophy are described. Electrocardiographic abnormalities may appear rapidly and are sometimes reversible.[229] Electrocardiographic abnormalities are unrelated to age, sex, or disease duration but are more common with severe neurological disease. Affected members of the same family tend to show the same electrocardiographic patterns. The electrocardiographic abnormalities and cardiac morphological changes correlate poorly.

The *vectorcardiogram* may show earlier evidence of cardiac involvement than the electrocardiogram and more closely parallel the neurological involvement.[245] Generalized cardiac enlargement, pulmonary vascular congestion, and marked thoracic bony deformities are present on *chest roentgenogram*; the severe scoliosis renders heart size difficult to evaluate. At *cardiac catheterization* there is an increased filling pressure in both ventricles, with a small stroke volume.[246] Serial *echocardiographic* examinations have been described to reliably evaluate the development of hypertrophic cardiomyopathy;[241] however, concentric left ventricular wall thickening is described as characteristic.[242]

Treatment There is no specific therapy. Standard management of heart failure and arrhythmias is appropriate.

Roussy-Lévy Hereditary Polyneuropathy

This disorder is characterized by manifestations of both peroneal muscular atrophy and Friedreich's ataxia, with abnormalities occurring relatively independently within a family; there is an autosomal dominant inheritance. The cardiomyopathy resembles Friedreich's ataxia.[247]

Myotonia Atrophica (Steinert's Disease)
This slowly progressive illness is inherited as an autosomal dominant; clinical manifestations become evident in the third and fourth decades. The pathogenesis of the cardiac abnormalities remains obscure.

Cardiac involvement usually occurs late, but occasionally may antedate recognition of the disease. There is no correlation between the severity of the muscular disease and cardiac disease or electrocardiographic abnormalities, but cardiac involvement is present in two-thirds of patients and is considered responsible for sudden death.

The infranodal conduction system seems selectively involved, with lesser abnormality of the sinus node and myocardium; heart failure is less common than are rhythm disturbances.[247a]

Pathology Autopsy and endomyocardial biopsy studies disclose diffuse myocardial fibrosis with fatty infiltration. Conduction system fibrosis is described. Electron microscopy shows vacuolation of the sarcoplasmic reticulum and mitochondrial abnormalities; damage to the sarcoplasmic reticulum may explain the conduction abnormalities.[229] Some reports describe electrocardiographic conduction and rhythm abnormalities as the only cardiovascular manifestations and suggest that the cardiac disturbances may be metabolic.

Clinical Manifestations Delayed muscle relaxation, atrophy, increased skeletal muscle tone, expressionless face, cataracts, premature frontal baldness, gastrointestinal muscular disorders, and gonadal atrophy are evident.

Dyspnea and palpitations are common. Findings include sinus bradycardia with a weak pulse; split S_1 and an S_4, producing a triple rhythm; and hypotension. Heart failure, which occurs in less than 10 percent of patients, is a late manifestation.[229] The sinus bradycardia of myotonia contrasts with the sinus tachycardia of Duchenne's dystrophy and Friedreich's ataxia. Atrial flutter or fibrillation, when present, rarely requires digitalis because high-degree atrioventricular block is characteristic.[229]

Murmurs, chest pain, or other evidence of heart disease is rare; an increased frequency of mitral valve prolapse is described.[248] Syncope may be due to ventricular fibrillation, complete heart block, or extreme bradycardia. Sudden death has been described. Alveolar hypoventilation results in hypercapnea, hypoxemia, pulmonary hypertension, and right ventricular failure.

The *electrocardiogram* is the earliest and most sensitive index of cardiac involvement and is abnormal in 60 to 85 percent of patients.[248] Electrocardiographic abnormalities are common in the absence

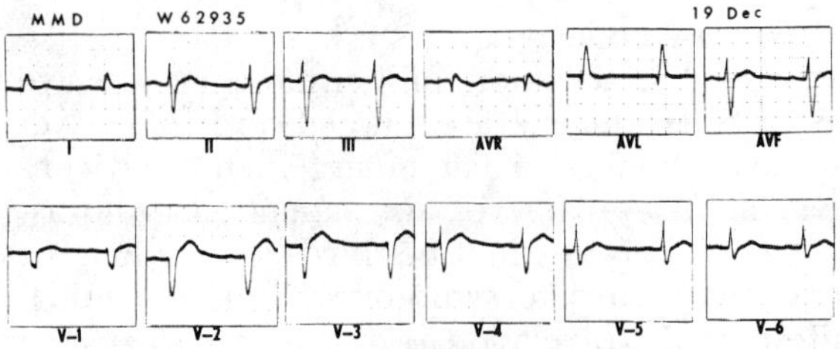

FIGURE 58-35 Electrocardiogram mimicking anterior myocardial infarction. This patient with myotonia atrophica has no symptoms referable to the cardiovascular system. (*Courtesy of Electrocardiographic Laboratory, Grady Memorial Hospital.*)

of clinical heart disease.[249] Atrioventricular and intraventricular conduction defects are frequent; serial studies may show gradual progression. Abnormalities may mimic myocardial infarction (Fig. 58-35). Conduction defects and changes in ventricular activation on the vectorcardiogram occurred in 60 percent of patients with myotonia atrophica, consistent with autopsy reports of myocardial involvement. Electrocardiographic abnormalities are comparable in older and younger patients, suggesting little influence of coronary atherosclerosis. *His bundle electrocardiography* with atrial pacing has documented marked impairment of His-Purkinje conduction.[249,250] However, since electrophysiological studies cannot predict progression of conduction system disease, they are recommended only for symptomatic patients.[250] External His bundle recording can serially assess the distal conduction abnormality.[248] *Chest roentgenogram* is typically unremarkable, and *echocardiography* shows normal ventricular function.[248]

Treatment Stokes-Adams syncope is treated with an implanted cardiac pacemaker.[251] Mitral valve prolapse necessitates prophylaxis against infective endocarditis.

Myasthenia Gravis
Myofiber necrosis with acute and chronic inflammatory infiltrates is noted, particularly associated with thymoma. This may represent a progressive "autoimmune" myocardial disorder and explain the occurrence of arrhythmias, heart failure, and electrocardiographic abnormalities.[252] Alternatively, myocardial changes may be due to hypokalemia or bronchopneumonia.

Variable generalized weakness follows use of voluntary muscles; heart failure is unusual. Tachycardia, arrhythmia, dyspnea, and precordial oppression occur in some patients. Nonspecific electrocardiographic ST-T abnormalities were reported to disappear with neostigmine therapy; transitory electrocardiographic changes of acute infarction were described during a myasthenic crisis. Terminal QRS notching may represent myocardial involvement; this abnormality did not regress with anticholinesterase therapy or thymectomy.[252] There is no specific abnormality on chest roentgenogram.

Drugs used to treat cardiovascular problems may adversely affect myasthenia. Quinidine may aggravate the myasthenia, and procainamide and lidocaine may interfere with neuromuscular transmission; cardioversion is preferable for arrhythmia management. Morphine may be dangerous, as vagotonic drugs have an increased effect in myasthenic patients and since morphine is potentiated by neostigmine.[253]

Tuberous Sclerosis

Pale-gray myocardial tumor masses, composed of fat tissue, have been described in patients with tuberous sclerosis;[254] the relation between these lipomas of the heart and the cerebral tubers is unknown.

Chronic Progressive External Ophthalmoplegia (Kearns' Syndrome)

Patients with chronic progressive external ophthalmoplegia (CPEO) also have pigmentary degeneration of the retina, ataxia, facial and limb weakness, and cardiac abnormalities. It is not known whether this represents a primary myopathy, a denervation atrophy, or a metabolic defect. Ultrastructural demonstration of increased glycogen and abnormal mitochondria suggests a cardiomyopathy, although there is no clinically manifest myocardial disease.[255] Familial occurrence has been noted.

Dizziness and syncope may occur. Conduction disturbances, particularly right bundle branch block and left axis deviation, are noted. Atrioventricular block tends to be progressive, and complete heart block may occur. Abnormalities of AV conduction are demonstrated in the His bundle electrogram. Ventricular function is normal at cardiac catheterization.

Prophylactic demand pacemaker insertion is recommended because sudden death is common.[256]

Amyotrophic Chorea with Acanthocytosis

Congestive cardiomyopathy has been described with this hereditary syndrome, which includes limb wasting, choreiform movements, and areflexia, in association with normolipoproteinemic acanthocytes.[257] Abnormal lipoprotein metabolism is implicated.

Familial Centronuclear Myopathy

This slowly progressive, familial, wasting skeletal muscle disease begins at birth and is associated with ptosis, hyporeflexia, and cardiomyopathy. Fibrosis and myofiber hypertrophy occur.[258] Congestive heart failure is prominent. Electrocardiographic and electromyographic abnormalities are nonspecific. Creatine kinase levels are elevated. Standard management for heart failure is recommended.

Kugelberg-Welander Syndrome (Juvenile Progressive Spinal Muscular Atrophy)

This syndrome is characterized by onset in childhood of proximal, followed by distal, limb muscle atrophy and weakness. This non-sex-linked, recessively inherited disorder has a slowly progressive course.[259] There is fibrosis of the atria, ventricles, and conduction system. Atrial arrhythmias and atrioventricular conduction abnormalities occur, with cardiac enlargement and heart failure. Elevation of cardiac serum enzyme levels is described. Pacemaker therapy may be required.

Collagen Vascular Disease

See Chap. 73.

Neoplastic Diseases

See Chap. 61.

Chemical and Drug Effects (Toxicity and Hypersensitivity) (see also Chap. 78)

Toxicity

The fundamental mechanisms underlying the toxic effects of chemicals and drugs on the myocardium are largely unknown. Cell injury has been postulated to be mediated by microvascular spasm, the formation of highly reactive oxygen radicals, calcium ion excess, nutritional or metabolic abnormalities, a variety of vasoactive hormones, and abnormalities in cellular hormone receptors, occurring alone or in combinations.

Ethyl Alcohol See Chap. 74.

Cobalt (Beer-Drinkers') Cardiomyopathy See Chap. 74.

Emetine and Chloroquine Cardiovascular toxicity occurs in most patients receiving emetine for amebiasis and schistosomiasis because of the small therapeutic/toxic ratio. Similar, but milder, abnormalities occur with chloroquine, but toxicity of combined therapy appears additive.

Myocardial degeneration (Fig. 58-36) occurs without an inflammatory response. Selective mito-

FIGURE 58-36 Emetine toxicity. Focal myocytolysis of the myocardium with interstitial and focal perivascular infiltration of lymphocytes. (*Courtesy of the Departments of Pathology, Emory University School of Medicine and the Atlanta Veterans Administration Medical Center.*)

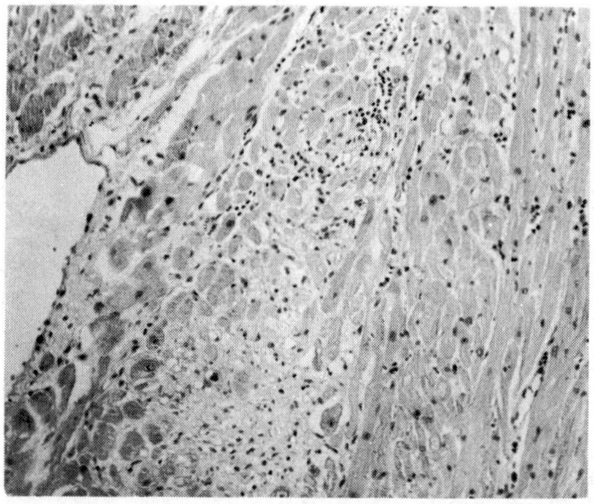

chondrial damage appears reversible with cessation of therapy. Electrocardiographic abnormalities may be functional, since they can be prevented or reversed by potassium administration; disturbance of potassium metabolism can be implicated in both the electrocardiographic changes and the neuromuscular toxicity. Emetine inhibits mitochondrial oxidative phosphorylation; this may partially account for the cardiotoxicity.[260]

Dyspnea and precordial pain occur; the mechanism is not known. With dehydroemetine, parenteral therapy causes more toxicity than oral, and adults have more toxicity than children.[261] As with quinidine, chloroquine idiosyncrasy presents as a cardiovascular emergency. Adrenalin is an effective antidote. Arrhythmias, hypotension, tachycardia, and sudden death are risks of emetine therapy. Dehydroemetine toxicity is manifest as tachycardia and gallop sounds. Chloroquine toxicity causes decreased cardiac output and bradycardia.

Almost invariable electrocardiographic T-wave abnormalities and QT prolongation occur after the first week of emetine therapy (Fig. 58-37);[261] because of the prolonged duration of action, electrocardiographic alterations may appear only after completion of therapy. Repolarization changes and conduction disturbances are described; terminal ventricular fibrillation was recorded. Electrocardiographic abnormalities persist or progress during emetine therapy but characteristically regress within a month or two after drug cessation. The initial abnormality—precordial T-wave inversion—is usually the last to disappear. Electrocardiographic abnormalities with dehydroemetine are less marked and of shorter duration than those due to emetine.[261] Conduction abnormalities and arrhythmias occur with chloroquine toxicity.

The chest roentgenogram is usually normal. Cardiac serum enzyme elevations, myocardial in origin, are encountered.

Bed rest is advocated during emetine and chloroquine therapy, with frequent clinical and electrocardiographic evaluation; emetine appears contraindicated in patients with heart disease. Occurrence of cardiovascular abnormalities is an indication for immediate cessation of emetine, even in the absence of electrocardiographic alterations; this appears prudent, as the mechanism of emetine toxicity is poorly understood. Clinical and electrocardiographic abnormalities regress with cessation of therapy.

FIGURE 58-37 Emetine toxicity. Sinus tachycardia, QT-interval prolongation, and nonspecific ST-T abnormalities are present. *(Courtesy of Electrocardiographic Laboratory, Atlanta Veterans Administration Medical Center.)*

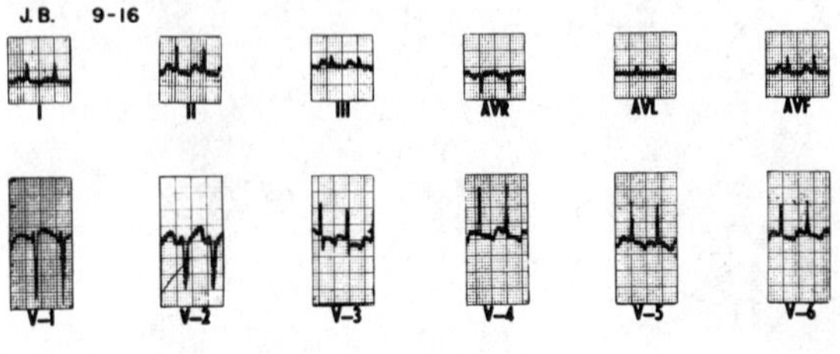

Phenothiazine Drugs (Chlorpromazine, Thioridazine) (see also Chap. 78) Arrhythmias and electrocardiographic abnormalities are common with phenothiazines; thus, these psychotropic drugs are relatively contraindicated in patients with cardiovascular disease, particularly atherosclerotic coronary heart disease. Potentially hazardous cardiac arrhythmias also occur in patients without heart disease receiving customary therapeutic doses,[262] despite the antiarrhythmic effect of these drugs in experimental animals.

Focal interstitial myocardial necrosis is reported in individual patients. Acid mucopolysaccharide deposition around intramyocardial arterioles, in the conduction system, subendocardium, and papillary muscles was seen in patients who died suddenly. Phenothiazine drugs alter myocardial catecholamines; increased circulating norepinephrine may predispose to arrhythmias, cardiac catecholamine depletion may depress myocardial contractility, or both mechanisms may obtain. Hypotension is the most common cardiovascular side effect, due to inhibition of centrally mediated pressor reflexes or to alpha-adrenergic blockade.

Electrocardiographic ST-T changes occur in about half of patients, apparently dose- and duration-related; PR and QT prolongation are common. T-wave amplitude decreases, and prominent U waves are seen. Intraventricular conduction disturbances occur, particularly with higher doses. The electrocardiogram returns to normal when phenothiazines are discontinued (Fig. 58-38).

Quinidine and procainamide are not recommended to treat the arrhythmias, as they may further decrease conduction velocity and reinforce the arrhythmia. Psychotropic therapy should be discontinued and lidocaine, which enhances conduction velocity, should be used.[262] Pacing may be used for overdrive suppression and to treat an underlying bradycardia after tachyarrhythmia reversion.[263]

Tricyclic Antidepressant Drugs[262,264] See Chap. 78.

Lithium[265,266] See Chap. 78.

Methysergide[267] ***(see also Chap. 78)*** The major adverse effect of methysergide (Sansert) is retroperitoneal and pleuropulmonary fibrosis; endocardial fibroelastosis similar to that of the carcinoid syndrome also occurs. Methysergide is chemically similar to serotonin, which may explain the similarity of these cardiac lesions. However, carcinoid lesions are predominantly right-sided whereas methysergide affects the left side of the heart for the most part. Coronary ostial stenosis is described.

Cyclophosphamide Massive doses of this antineoplastic agent can produce myocardial necrosis and

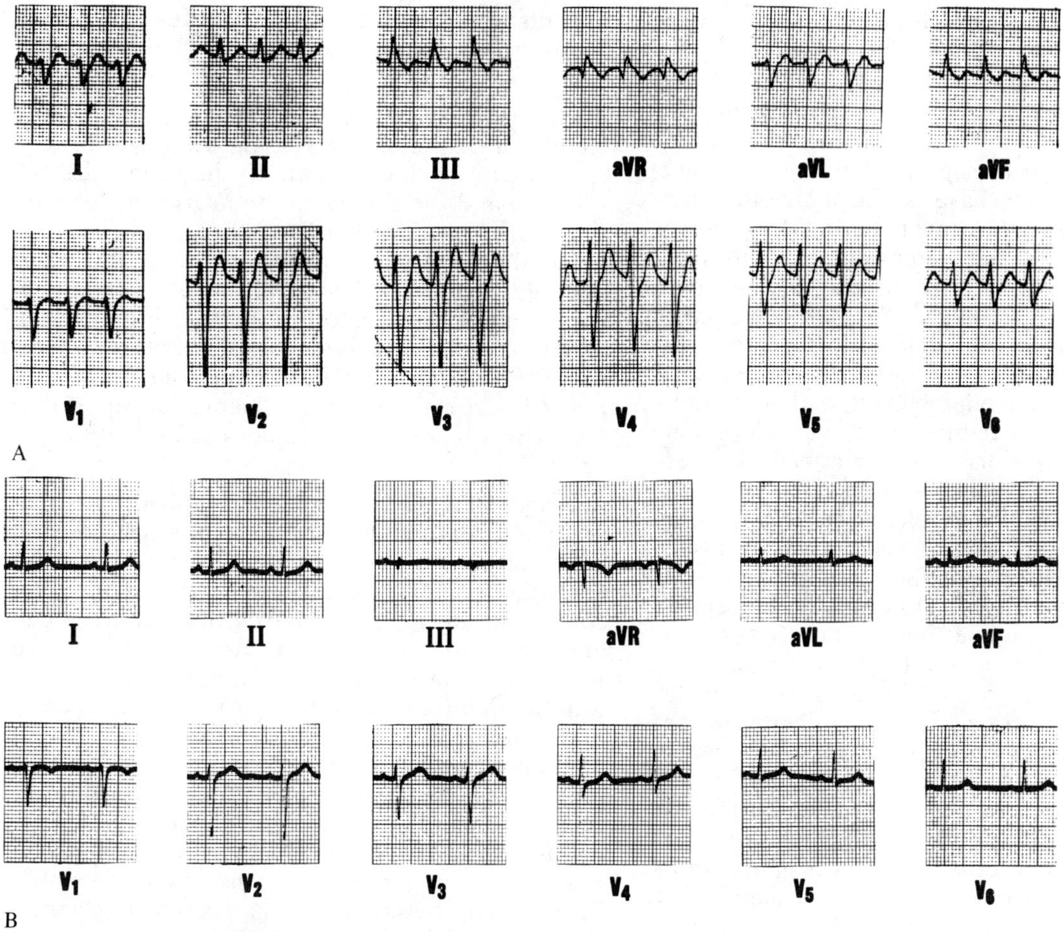

FIGURE 58-38 *A.* Thioridazine (Mellaril) poisoning. Normal serum electrolyte levels. *B.* Normal ECG after recovery. (*Courtesy of Electrocardiographic Laboratory, Grady Memorial Hospital.*)

hemorrhagic myocarditis with capillary microthrombosis and fibrin deposition in the interstitium and in myofibers.[268] Heart failure and/or pulmonary edema are acute in onset and unresponsive to therapy. Elevated serum enzyme levels indicate myocardial damage; and decreased voltage, ST-T wave changes, and QT prolongation appear on the electrocardiogram. Intensive cyclophosphamide dose regimens are not justified. Cardiac function should be monitored clinically and by serum enzyme levels and electrocardiographic changes during therapy.

Daunorubicin See p. 1183.

Adriamycin (Doxorubicin) (see also Chap. 78) Adriamycin is an effective antineoplastic agent used to treat lymphoma, leukemia, and solid tumors. Cardiac toxicity is the major factor limiting its use; the precise mechanism is not known, but free radical generation and peroxidation of subcellar membranes may be involved. A single rapid infusion of 60 to 75 mg/m^2 is usually given at 21-day intervals. Adriamycin binds to tissue (including heart) DNA and inhibits nucleic acid synthesis. There is decreased beta-adrenergic receptor density in the failing heart. Cardiac enlargement and mural thrombi occur. There is myocardial interstitial fibrosis with cellular loss. Electron microscopy shows loss of contractile substance with mitochondrial swelling and distortion.[270]

The cardiotoxic effects may be acute, subacute, or chronic. Transient electrocardiographic abnormalities—ST-T changes, premature ventricular beats, supraventricular tachycardia—occur in 5 to 30 percent of patients during the first few days of drug administration; these changes are unrelated to subsequent cardiomyopathy and are not dose-dependent. A toxic myocarditis and occasionally pericarditis may occur within days or weeks, often related to a single high dose. Rapidly progressive biventricular failure appears 1 to 6 months after completion of chemotherapy. Cardiomyopathy is unrelated to prior heart disease. A conspicuous decrease in QRS voltage occurs with the onset of clinical cardiomyopathy, but the electrocardiogram is insensitive in detecting early myocardial dysfunction. There is rapid cardiac dilatation and pulmonary vascular congestion on chest roentgenogram. Depression of ventricular function is more profound and recovery time longer as the cumulative dose of adriamycin increases. In severe toxicity, there is profound, intractable biventricular failure, with death commonly occurring within weeks.

Although heart failure was less common below a total dose of 550 mg/m^2 of adriamycin, cardiotoxicity did occur, and often higher antineoplastic doses were needed. Echocardiographic and systolic time interval abnormalities have not been able to detect early cardiomyopathy in time to permit dose restriction. However, newer noninvasive, load-independent indexes of left ventricular systolic performance appear promising.[270] Radionuclide ejection fractions appear helpful, but endomyocardial biopsy was reported by some to be a more sensitive technique.[271] In patients requiring additional doxorubicin who have a reduced ejection fraction, endomyocardial biopsy has been described as determining the safety of additional anthracycline therapy, with some patients able to tolerate up to a cumulative dose of 1000 mg/m^2.[271] Alteration of the dosing schedule may also permit increased therapy with lessened cardiotoxicity.[272] However, other reports suggest that serial radionuclide ejection fraction determinations can more safely guide doxorubicin therapy, even in patients with a moderately depressed ejection fraction.[273] Although endomyocardial biopsy seems the most specific method to assess myocardial toxicity, serial exercise radionuclide left ventricular ejection fraction determinations may be more cost-effective in identifying high-risk patients.[274] The role of proton nuclear magnetic resonance (NMR) techniques is being investigated.[275] A synergistic effect is evident between x-irradiation and other antitumor antibiotics and adriamycin in producing cardiotoxicity;[271] advanced age and underlying heart disease also increase risk. The heart failure is relatively unresponsive to inotropic drugs and mechanical ventricular assistance. Combined therapy with digitalis, diuretics, and peripheral vasodilators occasionally is of benefit.

Chronic Arsenic Poisoning Acute interstitial myocarditis may occur during arsenical therapy of syphilis, usually associated with dermatitis. An allergic cause is postulated. Interstitial myocarditis, endocardial thickening, and mural thrombus formation occur. Dyspnea, cardiac enlargement, and progressive congestive heart failure are associated with nonspecific T-wave changes and QT prolongation on the electrocardiogram.[276] There is no specific therapy.

Acute Arsenic Poisoning Acute arsenic poisoning is the most common acute heavy metal poisoning. Arsenic interferes with respiratory enzyme systems and may produce myocardial hypoxemia. Multiple focal subepicardial hemorrhages occur within the first few hours. There are no cardiac symptoms, and no cardiovascular disease is evident in patients who recover. Electrocardiographic changes are of myocardial ischemia and QT prolongation; electrocardiographic abnormalities disappear more rapidly in patients receiving BAL (British antilewisite, dimercaprol) than in untreated patients.[276]

Acute Arsine Gas Poisoning Arsine gas causes red blood cell hemolysis, decreasing the oxygen-carrying capacity of the blood. Both the myocardial hypoxemia and the arsenic in the heart muscle at autopsy may produce cardiac lesions: subepicardial hemorrhage, myocardial degeneration, and interstitial edema.[277] The severity of the illness relates to the extent of toxic exposure. Poisoning may terminate fatally due to acute myocardial failure. Abnormal T waves appear on the electrocardiogram. There is red blood cell hemolysis. Therapy is supportive; BAL (British antilewisite) is not useful.

Antimony Fuadin, tartar emetic, Astiban, and other antimony compounds used to treat schistosomiasis frequently produce myocardial damage. Myocardial disturbances may occur early in therapy or after completion of treatment. Cardiovascular symptoms are uncommon, but sudden death from arrhythmias is not unusual. Almost invariable electrocardiographic abnormalities appear by the end of a course of antimony.

Nonspecific ST-T changes and a prolonged QT interval are frequent;[278] arrhythmias and conduction abnormalities have an ominous prognosis. Electrocardiographic abnormalities increase as the duration of therapy increases and usually regress after drug cessation. Arrhythmias and conduction abnormalities require termination of therapy.

l-Norepinephrine, Epinephrine, and Isoproterenol Lesions similar to those seen with pheochromocytoma may occur following therapy with l-norepinephrine. This is also described with epinephrine, isoproterenol, and angiotensin infusion. Focal myocardial necrosis, an inflammatory infiltrate, edema, and epicardial hemorrhages are present. Epinephrine platelet-aggregating effects may produce myocardial necrosis; pretreatment of animals with anti-platelet agents decreases epinephrine-induced myocardial necrosis.[279] Chest pain has been reported. Electrocardiographic changes are of myocardial injury and ischemia. Ischemic electrocardiographic changes may also be due to hypertension, increased myocardial oxygen demand, coronary endothelial damage, hypokalemia, etc.

These changes may also represent a toxic myocarditis. The role of antiplatelet agents remains controversial.

Dextroamphetamine Long-term use of high-dose dextroamphetamine was associated with clinical findings of cardiomyopathy and myocardial morphological changes similar to those of pheochromocytoma. Catecholamine toxicity is postulated.[280] Acute cardiomyopathy is also described with intravenous amphetamine abuse.[281]

Phenylpropanolamine Catecholamine toxicity is also postulated as the mechanism of myocardial injury after ingestion of the sympathomimetic amine phenylpropanolamine, used in decongestant and appetite suppressant formulations.[282]

Carbon Monoxide[283,284] ***(see Chaps. 78 and 87)*** Acute and chronic carbon monoxide poisoning may cause myocardial infarction or injury. Cardiac damage is due both to hypoxemia, as carbon monoxide diminishes oxygen transport capacity, and to a direct toxic effect on myocardial mitochondria. Carbon monoxide replaces the oxygen in oxyhemoglobin and decreases tissue oxyhemoglobin dissociation. Hemorrhagic and necrotic lesions, probably hypoxemic, have a predilection for the papillary muscles and subendocardial left ventricle. Endocardial injury may be associated with mural thrombosis. Rupture of the heart has occurred.

Cobalt (see also p. 1183) Fatal cobalt cardiomyopathy occurred in an industrial exposure.[285] There was excessive cobalt accumulation in the myocardium, and the histological abnormalities were like those of beer-drinkers' cardiomyopathy. The patient demonstrated heart failure, chest pain, cyanosis, electrocardiographic abnormalities, and shock.

Hydrocarbons (Fluorinated)[286,287] ***(see Chaps. 78 and 87)*** Aerosol inhalation toxicity is due to fluorocarbon compounds used as aerosol propellants. Morphological abnormalities include myofiber fragmentation and loss of cross-striations.

Phosphorus Death in the first 12 to 24 h after phosphorus poisoning is usually cardiovascular in origin. Later deaths are due to hepatic failure. Phosphorus inhibits amino acid incorporation into myocardial proteins, with resultant cardiac dysfunction. A direct toxic effect of phosphorus on the myocardium and peripheral blood vessels depresses myocardial contractility and lowers systemic vascular resistance; there is unresponsiveness to adrenergic agents.[288] The myocardial lesion is fatty degeneration with myofiber necrosis.

Ventricular fibrillation or peripheral vascular collapse indicates a grave prognosis. Electrocardiographic abnormalities occur in over 50 percent of patients; changes appear related to the amount of phosphorus ingested. Nonspecific ST-T abnormalities[289] and QT interval prolongation regress with clinical improvement. Nevertheless, sudden death due to malignant ventricular arrhythmias may occur after improvement of the respiratory and neurological complications, typically due to the torsade de pointes ventricular tachycardia associated with QT prolongation. Electrical pacing is recommended to shorten the QT interval and eliminate the arrhythmia.[290] Isoproterenol may also be used. ECG monitoring is indicated until the QT interval has returned to normal.

Fluoride Excessive fluoride exerts a direct toxic action on cardiac muscle. Additional cardiovascular abnormalities may result from the hypocalcemia due to the calcium-binding effect of fluoride.[291] Cardiac arrhythmias may be fatal.

Mercury ST-segment and T-wave abnormalities, QT prolongation, and arrhythmias occurred[292] with mercury poisoning; a mercury-containing fungicide had been inadvertently ingested.

Lead Clinical and electrocardiographic assessment of myocardial damage should be part of the management of chronic lead poisoning. Lead poisoning from lead-contaminated stills may exacerbate the alcoholic cardiomyopathy of moonshine whiskey drinkers; cardiac function improved in one group of such patients after chelation of the lead with calcium EDTA (ethylenediaminetetraacetic acid). The myocardial dysfunction may be due to the hypertension of lead nephropathy and/or a direct toxic effect on the myocardium.[293] Interstitial fibrosis, inflammatory cells, and a serous exudate has been described in patients dying of chronic lead poisoning.

Frequent cardiomyopathy, heart failure, and chest pain occurred in young patients with chronic occupational lead poisoning. Electrocardiographic sinus bradycardia, shortened PQ interval, premature ventricular beats, and nonspecific ST-T changes subsided after therapy with EDTA. EDTA and supportive management are indicated.

Scorpion Venom[294] ***(see also Chap. 78)*** Scorpion sting myocardial toxicity is more common than neurotoxicity, and often is the cause of death. Scorpion venom is a potent sympathetic stimulator; cardiovascular manifestations and myocardial morphological abnormalities are due to the elevated circulating catecholamines. The papillary muscles and subendocardium are prominently involved; these hypoxemic lesions are probably related to the inotropic effect of catecholamines.

Myocarditis has been reported due to the sting of a scorpion, *Tityus trinitatis*. Heart rate and rhythm disturbances were frequent; transient murmurs were heard. Reversible tachycardia, pulmonary edema, and peripheral circulatory failure have been described secondary to *Buthus tamulus* scorpion bites. The sting of the yellow scorpion, *Buthus quinquestriatus*, frequently results in hypertension, anxiety, profuse perspiration, and pulmonary edema.[294] Circulatory collapse may follow.

Electrocardiographic conduction changes, ST-T abnormalities, or QT prolongation occurred in 76 percent of patients with *Tityus trinitatis* sting. Changes mimicking myocardial infarction occurred from *Buthus tamulus* bites, and abnormal Q and T waves persisted in one patient. Myocardial serum enzyme levels may be elevated. Adrenergic blocking agents appear of value in treatment and in prevention of cardiomyopathy.[294]

Black Widow Spider Venom In addition to the common neurotoxicity accompanying black widow (*Lactrodectus m. tredecimguttatus*) spider bites, atrial fibrillation and blood pressure lability are described. Urinary catecholamine levels were elevated; beta blockade therapy was beneficial.[295]

Snake Venom[296] See Chap. 78.

Wasp Venom[297] See Chap. 78.

Tick Paralysis Cardiac enlargement and cardiac failure occurred after regression of neurological changes in a child with tick paralysis. [298] Nonspecific electrocardiographic abnormalities were also transient.

Hypersentivity

This discussion of drug hypersensitivity considers direct damage to myocardium. Drug-induced cardiomyopathies[299] which result from interference with cellular metabolic activity have been discussed in the preceding section; drugs which damage myocardium through an allergic mechanism are next considered. Drug-induced electrocardiographic abnormalities generally reflect a direct or indirect effect on the electrical activity of the heart; occasionally drug effect is directly on the myofiber; most electrocardiographic abnormalities are reversible as the drug is metabolized or eliminated.[300]

Anaphylaxis Even in patients without heart disease, sensitization by exogenous agents may result in acute anaphylaxis with primarily cardiovascular manifestations. Anaphylactic reactions produce profound hypotension and can precipitate myocardial infarction in patients with coronary atherosclerosis. Dyspnea, cyanosis, chest pain, syncope, and recurrent arrhythmias may also mimic myocardial infarction with shock. Electrocardiographic nonspecific ST-T changes and abnormalities of impulse formation and conduction are recorded; possible explanations include myocardial antigen-antibody reactions, a pharmacological effect of the mediator subtances of anaphylaxis, effects of the drugs (e.g., epinephrine) used to treat the anaphylaxis, myocardial hypoxemia, etc. Antihistamine therapy is generally effective.[301]

Serum Sickness Serum sickness is characterized anatomically by a generalized vasculitis and necrotizing arteritis; coronary, myocardial, and pericardial artery involvement explain the clinical presentations.[302] There may be tachycardia, arrhythmia, hypotension, the pain and friction rub of pericarditis, and the pain of myocardial infarction. Electrocardiographic transient ST-T and conduction abnormalities are common; changes may mimic myocardial infarction. Corticosteroid hormone therapy is recommended.

Sulfonamide Interstitial mononuclear and eosinophilic perivascular infiltrates can occur in patients who receive sulfonamide drugs. With severe sulfonamide hypersensitivity, granulomatous myocardial lesions, myofiber necrosis, and petechial hemorrhages were noted at autopsy. A similar picture has been due to sulfonylurea antidiabetic therapy.[303] One group of patients with these abnormalities at autopsy had no cardiac symptoms, and only 50 percent had clinical sulfonamide hypersensitivity. Severe heart failure has also been described; electrocardiographic abnormalities are nonspecific. Sulfonamide cardiomyopathy has been reported to subside after digitalis and corticosteroid hormone therapy.[304]

Penicillin Granulomatous and diffuse interstitial myocardial abnormalities occur in penicillin hypersensitivity reactions, with and without clinical cardiac symptoms and electrocardiographic abnormalities. Classic granulomatous lesions predominated in the papillary muscles; myofiber necrosis and eosinophilic and inflammatory cellular exudates were present. Bradycardia and transient ST-T electrocardiographic changes probably represent myocardial involvement. Pericarditis with effusion has been described.[305] Dilated cardiomyopathy, unrelated to an acute allergic reaction, was presumed secondary to oxacillin, as cardiac function returned to normal after discontinuation of the drug.[306]

Phenylbutazone Profound interstitial myocardial changes, indistinguishable from other drug-hypersensitivity lesions, may occur with phenylbutazone. Abnormalities include focal perivascular granulomas, muscle necrosis, eosinophilic and acute inflammatory cellular reaction, and fibrinoid degeneration.[307] Chest pain, tachycardia, hypotension, and heart failure have been reported during and after phenylbutazone therapy in recommended doses.[307] Pericarditis has also been described. Electrocardiographic changes are compatible with myocardial ischemia.

Smallpox Vaccine "Myocarditis" and "pericarditis," presumed due to an antigen-antibody reaction, have been described 1 to 2 weeks after smallpox vaccination. The time lag suggests that viremia is not implicated. Cardiovascular complications are less common than neurological or dermatologic reactions. Since 1972 smallpox vaccination is not required in the United States because the potential complications were considered more serious than the risk of smallpox infection. Fatal smallpox reactions are characterized by acute myocardial degeneration, particularly of the left ventricle. The illness is generally mild, with spontaneous recovery, although chest pain, dyspnea, and rapid heart rate have been described. Severe heart failure may occur.[309] Death has also occurred without premonitory cardiac symptoms. The ST-T changes on the electrocardiogram and occasional arrhythmias disappear in patients who survive. Corticosteroid hormone therapy and routine heart failure management are indicated.

Cholera Vaccine Cardiovascular complications of cholera vaccine administration (as with tetanus and smallpox) suggest an allergic myocardial reaction. One patient had arrhythmia, syncope,[309] eosinophilia, and an elevated antimyocardial antibody titer suggesting an allergic picture. The electrocardiogram may show arrhythmias and/or changes of myocardial ischemia. Arrhythmia management is indicated.

Aureomycin (Chlortetracycline) In Aureomycin hypersensitivity,[310] fibrinoid necrosis and a diffuse infiltrate of eosinophils, lymphocytes, and Anitschkow myocytes were seen in the myocardium.

Methyldopa An inflammatory myocarditis, consistent with hypersensitivity, was encountered in five patients who died suddenly circumstantially associated with methyldopa therapy; four had hypersensitivity hepatitis.[311]

Antituberculous Drugs With *streptomycin,* widespread myofiber necrosis, eosinophilic and inflammatory cell infiltrates, and petechial myocardial hemorrhages occurred in a patient who died suddenly during chemotherapy for tuberculosis; it was presumed due to streptomycin allergy.[311] Chest discomfort was the only cardiac abnormality.

In another fatal case during antituberculous chemotherapy with *para-amino-salicylic acid,* the myofibers were fragmented, multinucleate giant cells were present, there was an inflammatory cell infiltrate, and IgG appeared localized along the myofiber sarcolemma. Heart failure, pericardial effusion, hypotension, and ventricular irritability occurred. Death was attributed to amino-salicylic acid hypersensitivity, known to cause cardiac dilatation and transient arrhythmias.[313]

Phenindione Fatal "myocarditis" was described[314] due to sensitivity to phenindione (Danilone) anticoagulation.

Acetaminophen (Paracetamol) Myocardial necrosis and electrocardiographic abnormalities are seen with large doses of paracetamol.[315] It is not certain whether this represents a toxic or hypersensitivity response.

Reserpine, Guanethidine Biochemical and structural myocardial lesions occur in experimental animals after prolonged reserpine and guanethidine therapy, apparently not related to catecholamine depletion. Focal inflammatory necrosis, deranged lipid and glycogen metabolism, and depression of mitochondrial oxidative enzymes [316] may be a toxic or hypersensitivity effect or may be related to catecholamine depletion.

Physical Causes

Radiation

High-dose therapeutic radiation (see also Chap. 78) to the thorax may damage the heart and pericardium. Radiation may predispose to or accelerate coronary atherosclerosis. Pericardial fibrosis is most common; myocardium is among the most radiation-resistant tissues, but patchy fibrosis and necrosis may occur. The coronary arteries become thickened and hyalinized; the narrowed lumen may result in myocardial infarction. Endocardial fibrosis and fibroelastosis may produce cardiac murmurs by valve distortion. Fibrosis of the conduction system produces complete heart block. Electron microscopy shows disorganization of the mitochondria, myofibrils, nucleus, and sarcolemma, differing from abnormalities of ischemic myocardial disease.[317]

The diagnosis should be considered in patients who have received extensive radiation to the chest who present unusual clinical or electrocardiographic evidence of heart disease.[318]

Electric Shock[319]

See Chap. 78.

Trauma

Isolated focal myocardial disease has been documented among pilots killed in aircraft accidents, but not in the nonpilot air crew killed in the same accidents. Since there was no evidence that trauma caused the myocardial damage, sudden cardiac death may have been due to focal myocardial disease.[320]

Posttraumatic myocardial ossification has been described.[321] Ventricular aneurysm has resulted from blunt trauma.[322] (See also Chap. 60.)

Heatstroke

The myofiber degeneration, petechial hemorrhages, and interstitial edema may be due to direct tissue injury, hypoxemia, metabolic abnormalities, and so forth.[323] Myocardial damage due to heatstroke is evidenced by electrocardiographic ST-T wave changes and conduction abnormalities which appear reversible in survivors. Serum LDH isoenzyme elevation compatible with cardiac damage is seen.

Hypothermia

Myocardial hemorrhage and infarction may be due to the profound hypotension; hemoconcentration and sludging of blood in the capillaries are associated with ventricular dilatation.[324]

Miscellaneous Systemic Syndromes

Rejection Cardiomyopathy[325]

Morphological alterations of allograft rejection include necrotizing arteritis and vascular fibrinoid necrosis, myocytolysis, edema, and a mononuclear cell reaction.

Cardiac function deterioration is evident as decreased exercise tolerance and heart failure. Temperature, heart rate, and sedimentation rate rise. About three-fourths of patients remain asymptomatic. Decreased electrocardiographic voltage is the most reliable sign of late acute rejection. Arrhythmias and conduction abnormalities also occur. Enlargement of the cardiac silhouette due to cardiac dilatation and/or pericardial effusion is encountered. Endomyocardial (percutaneous transcatheter) biopsy provides early identification.

Immunosuppressive therapy and corticosteroid hormones may reverse the process and permit good long-term cardiac function in most patients. Early identification by endomyocardial biopsy permits augmentation of immunosuppressive therapy and has increased recipient survival.[326,327]

Cardiomyopathy of Aging

It is doubtful whether there is a true cardiomyopathy of aging (see also Chap. 71). Many factors probably contribute to heart failure in the elderly apart from hypertension, atherosclerotic coronary artery disease, valvular disease, and pulmonary heart disease. Degenerative calcification of the mitral and aortic valve rings and cusps, which may be complicated by infective endocarditis; and fibrosis of the cardiac skeleton may cause cardiac illness in the elderly; and senile cardiac amyloidosis may be contributory.

Rheumatoid Disease and Ankylosing Spondylitis

See Chap. 73.

Reiter's Disease

Pericardial, myocardial, and valvular involvement are associated with the arthritis, urethritis, and conjunctivitis of Reiter's disease, particularly after recurrent attacks. The aortic valve cusps are thickened; the edges are rolled and cordlike, and the valve ring is dilated, with collagen replacement of muscle and elastica. Acute pericarditis is diagnosed by a friction rub, often associated with pain; gallop sounds and apical systolic murmurs also occur. Aortic regurgitation is a late complication of severe recurrent disease. Rarely, cardiac involvement may be the sole manifestation.[328] Electrocardiographic abnormalities include PQ prolongation which may progress to complete heart block,[329] QRS widening, and nonspecific ST-T changes. Pacemaker implantation may be necessitated by the complete heart block. Corticosteroid therapy may transiently reverse the conduction abnormalities.

Of interest is that patients with HLA-B27, even without evidence of Reiter's disease or ankylosing spondylitis, appear to have a genetic predisposition to develop complete heart block.[330]

Cogan's Syndrome

About one-third of patients with Cogan's syndrome (nonsyphilitic interstitial keratitis and bilateral deafness) have cardiovascular manifestations.[331] Fibrinoid necrosis of the aortic valve may produce aortic regurgitation. Angiitis of myocardial arteries may result in myocardial ischemia and necrosis. Cardiac enlargement; heart murmurs, particularly aortic regurgitation; and congestive failure are prominent.

Behçet's Disease

Recurrent oral and genital ulceration with relapsing iritis of unknown cause constitute Behçet's disease. Vasculitis is a prominent component of this multisystem disorder. Cardiac manifestations include myocarditis with cardiac enlargement, gallop sounds, pericardial friction rub, conduction disturbances, and arrhythmias. Thrombophlebitis is common. Aneurysms of large arteries may occur, as may valvular disease and myocardial infarction; one patient had myocardial infarction and resultant ventricular aneurysm due to vasculitic coronary occlusion.[332] Circulating immune complexes have been demonstrated.[333] Corticosteroid therapy is often effective.

Noonan's Syndrome

Noonan's syndrome (see also Chap. 36) has a phenotype similar to Turner's syndrome but has no chromosomal abnormalities. Congenital heart disease, particularly valvular pulmonary stenosis, is common. Left ventricular cardiomyopathy, with and without symptoms, both of the obstructive and nonobstructive variety, is also a feature. Rapidly progressive obstructive cardiomyopathy refractory to therapy, has been described.[334]

Pseudoxanthoma Elasticum (Groenblad-Strandberg Syndrome)

Primary cardiac abnormalities have not often been reported in this heritable connective tissue disorder, but may occasionally be the mode of presentation or the cause of death. Cardiovascular morphologic abnormalities are present in most patients. A pearly white endocardial thickening may involve the valves; collagen and elastic fibers may encase the conduction system.[335] Calcification and fragmentation of the myocardial artery elastica are seen. Characteristic crêpelike cutaneous lesions and retinal angioid streaks are present. Cardiac enlargement, heart failure, arrhythmias, and murmurs of valve deformity from the endocardial thickening are present. Angina pectoris and Stokes-Adams syncope have occurred. Premature advanced arterial disease may occur in the myocardium and peripheral vessels. There is no specific therapy.

Weber-Christian Disease (Relapsing Febrile Nodular Nonsuppurative Panniculitis)

There is little morphological cardiac involvement except for focal necrosis of epicardial fat. Periarteritis and endarteritis of myocardial and pericardial blood vessels with vascular occlusion could explain the clinical abnormalities. In a recent case, there were granulomatous foci with central necrosis and surrounding histiocytes, lymphocytes, and eosinophils identical to those in the skin.[336] The disease is most common in women in the second to fourth decade and is characterized by painful subcutaneous nodules. Cardiac enlargement and heart failure may occur. There are nonspecific electrocardiographic abnormalities. There is no specific therapy.

Juvenile Xanthogranuloma (Neuroxanthoendothelioma)
This generally self-limiting skin disease of infants and children is amenable to radiation therapy. There is occasional visceral involvement, including cardiac, with xanthogranulomas. Xanthogranulomatous "tumors" of the epicardium were reported to produce symptomatic hemopericardium.[337]

Scleredema of Buschke
This generally self-limiting skin infiltration with acid mucopolysaccharides often follows a respiratory infection and occasionally has associated systemic manifestations. There is firm, nonpitting edema of the face and thorax. Pericardial effusion and heart failure resolve as the skin infiltrate clears; hence, this cardiomyopathy has a good prognosis.[338] ST-T electrocardiographic changes and decreased QRS voltage also resolve as the skin infiltrate clears. Skin biopsy is diagnostic. There is no specific therapy, but corticosteroid hormone administration has been associated with recovery.[339]

Wegener's Granulomatosis
The classic triad of nonhealing midline granuloma of the nose, pulmonary infiltrate, and renal disease may progress to systemic involvement, presumably with an allergic panarteritis. Myocardial abnormalities include focal necrotizing vasculitis, granulomatous lesions, fibrinoid degeneration, myofiber necrosis, and an inflammatory cell infiltrate, at times with giant cells. Cardiac enlargement, congestive heart failure, and pericarditis with effusion occur; the association with mitral stenosis appears fortuitous, related to anatomic study of the left atrial appendage removed at surgery.[340] Cytotoxic drugs, with or without corticosteroid hormones, appear of value.

Reye's Syndrome
This rapidly fatal disease of young children is characterized by encephalopathy and fatty degeneration of the viscera. The cause is unknown, but there appears to be association with aspirin administration during the febrile phase of influenza or chickenpox viral illness. Cardiac involvement may contribute to the fatal outcome. In one study, intramyocardial fat droplets were universal in the atria and present to a lesser extent in the ventricles. Extensive fat was described in the bundle of His, bundle branches, and Purkinje fibers. Electron microscopy revealed mitochondrial swelling with fragmentation of the cristae; fat droplets were present between clusters of mitochondria.[341] Fatty accumulation in the Purkinje system suggests that bundle branch block and complete heart block may be important clinical problems. Cardiovascular symptoms or signs are unusual. No specific cardiovascular management appears warranted.

Lentiginosis
All patients with lentiginosis should be evaluated for cardiomyopathy. The relation to previously described familial pigmented spots with cardiac murmurs and electrocardiographic abnormalities is uncertain. An association with atrial myxoma is suggested. Skin melanin and myocardial norepinephrine are chemically related, and an enzyme defect or precursor abnormality has been suggested.[342] Cardiac enlargement and/or systolic murmurs should suggest cardiomyopathy in patients with prominent widespread lentigines. There is progressive massive atrioventricular septal hypertrophy with bilateral outflow tract obstruction.

The disease is often mild at onset, but increases in severity; at times progression of the cardiomyopathy is associated with increase in lentiform moles. Electrocardiographic abnormalities are variable and nondiagnostic. Surgical septectomy has had variable success, and propranolol is suggested.

Mulibrey Nanism
This autosomal recessive disorder is characterized by prenatal-onset growth failure, muscular hypotonia, enlarged cerebral ventricles and cisternae, and ocular fundal changes. The name indicates involvement of *mu*scle, *li*ver, *br*ain, and *ey*e. The major cardiac abnormality is constrictive pericarditis.[343] Patchy collagenous myocardial fibrosis occurs beneath a thickened pericardium which often has flecks of calcium. Symptoms and signs of cardiac failure vary in severity. Nonspecific P- and T-wave abnormalities are present; arrhythmias may occur. Cardiac enlargement with diminished pulsation is evident at fluoroscopy. Echocardiography confirms pericardial thickening. The cardiac catheterization findings are those of constrictive pericarditis. Pericardiectomy has effected marked clinical and hemodynamic improvement in sicker patients; conservative management is recommended in milder cases.

Ulcerative Colitis
Recurring myopericarditis has been described during relapses of chronic ulcerative colitis.[344] Retrosternal discomfort, pleuritic chest pain, and a pericardial friction rub may be present. Nonspecific ST-T electrocardiographic abnormalities resolve with corticosteroid hormones.

Whipple's Disease (Intestinal Lipodystrophy)
Clinical cardiac findings and gross cardiac lesions occur in the majority of patients with intestinal lipodystrophy; however, the extent of cardiac involvement appears unrelated to the severity and duration of Whipple's disease. Large macrophages

with PAS-positive granules, identical to those in the intestine, occur in the pericardium, myocardium, and heart valves. Adhesive pericarditis, focal myocardial fibrosis, and valvular fibrosis with deformity are present.[345] Rod-shaped bodies, possibly bacteria, are evident in the heart valves and myocardium. Cardiac murmurs, particularly mitral; pericardial friction rubs; and congestive heart failure are encountered. Electrocardiographic abnormalities are common but nonspecific. There is often a favorable response to antibiotic therapy.

References

1. de Senac J.-B.: "Traité de la Structure du Coeur, de son Action et de ses Maladies," Jacques Vincent, Paris, Preface, vol. 1, 1749, p. XI.
2. Goodwin, J. F., and Oakley, C. M.: The Cardiomyopathies, *Br. Heart J.*, 34:545, 1972.
3. Wenger, N. K.: Myocardial Involvement in Systemic Disease, in J. W. Hurst (ed.), "The Heart," 4th ed., McGraw-Hill Book Company, New York, 1978, p. 1590.
4. Goodwin, J. F.: Congestive and Hypertrophic Cardiomyopathies: A Decade of Study, *Lancet,* 1:731, 1970.
5. Goodwin, J. F.: Prospects and Predictions for the Cardiomyopathies, *Circulation,* 50:210, 1974.
6. Report of the WHO/ISFC Task Force on the Definition and Classification of Cardiomyopathies, *Br. Heart J.*, 44:672, 1980.
7. O'Connell, J. B., Fowles, R. E., Robinson, J. A., Subramanian, R., Henkin, R. E., and Gunnar, R. M.: Clinical and Pathological Findings of Myocarditis in Two Families with Dilated Cardiomyopathy, *Am. Heart J.*, 107:127, 1983.
8. Dunnigan, A., Pierpont, M. E., Smith, S. A., Breningstall, G., Benditt, D. G., and Benson, D. W., Jr.: Cardiac and Skeletal Myopathy Associated with Cardiac Dysrhythmias, *Am. J. Cardiol.*, 53:731, 1984.
8a. Sugrue, D. D., Holmes, D. R., Jr., Gersh, B. J., et al.: Cardiac Histologic Findings in Patients with Life-Threatening Ventricular Arrhythmias of Unknown Origin, *J. Am. Coll. Cardiol.*, 4:952, 1984.
9. Pietras, R. J., Lam, W., Bauernfiend, R., Sheikh, A., Palileo, E., Strasberg, B., Swiryn, S., and Rosen, K. M.: Chronic Recurrent Right Ventricular Tachycardia in a Patient without Ischemic Heart Disease: Clinical, Hemodynamic, and Angiographic Findings, *Am. Heart J.*, 105:357, 1983.
10. Brockington, I. F., and Edington, G. M.: Adult Heart Disease in Western Nigeria: A Clinicopathological Synopsis, *Am. Heart J.*, 83:27, 1972.
11. Kristinsson, A.: "Diagnosis, Natural History and Treatment of Congestive Cardiomyopathy, Ph.D. Thesis, University of London, Royal Postgraduate Medical School of London, 1969.
12. Factor, S. M., Minase, T., Cho, S., Dominitz, R., and Sonnenblick, E. H.: Microvascular Spasm in the Cardiomyopathic Syrian Hamster: A Preventable Cause of Focal Myocardial Necrosis, *Circulation,* 66:342, 1982.
13. Cambridge, G., MacArthur, C. G. C., Waterson, A. P., Goodwin, J. F., and Oakley, C. M.: Antibodies to Coxsackie B Viruses in Congestive Cardiomyopathy, *Br. Heart J.*, 41:692, 1979.
14. Anderson, J. L., Fowles, R. E., Bieber, C. P., and Stinson, E. B.: Idiopathic Cardiomyopathy, Age and Suppressor-Cell Dysfunction as Risk Determinants of Lymphoma after Cardiac Transplantation, *Lancet,* 2:1174, 1978.
15. Fowles, R. E., Bieber, C. P., and Stinson, E. B.: Defective In Vitro Suppressor Cell Function in Idiopathic Congestive Cardiomyopathy, *Circulation,* 59:483, 1979.
16. Lowry, P. J., Thompson, R. A., and Littler, W. A.: Humoral Immunity in Cardiomyopathy, *Br. Heart J.*, 50:390, 1983.
17. Goodwin, J. F.: Future Trends in Cardiomyopathy: Part I. Prediction for the Cardiomyopathies, in P. N. Yu and J. F. Goodwin (eds.), "Progress in Cardiology," Lea & Febiger, Philadelphia, 1981, vol. 10, p. 175.
18. Daly, K., Richardson, P.-J., Olsen, E. G. J., Pattison, J., Jackson, G., and Jewitt, D. E.: Immunosuppressive Therapy in Acute Inflammatory Myocarditis, *Circulation,* 63–64:IV–27, 1981.
19. Shapiro, L. M., Rozkovec, A., Cambridge, G., Hallidie-Smith, K. A., and Goodwin, J. F.: Myocarditis in Siblings Leading to Chronic Heart Failure, *Eur. Heart J.*, 4:742, 1983.
20. Editorial: Daunorubicin and the Heart, *Br. Med. J.*, 4:431, 1974.
21. Rona, G., and Chappel, C. I.: Pathogenesis and Pathology of Cobalt Cardiomyopathy, in Z. E. Bajusz and G. Rona (eds.), "Cardiomyopathies. Recent Advances in Studies on Cardiac Structure and Metabolism," vol. 2, University Park Press, Baltimore, 1973, p. 407.
22. Selenium Perspective, *Lancet,* 1:685, 1983. (Editorial.)
23. Schaffer, M. S., Zuberbuhler, P., Wilson, G., Rose, V., Duncan, W. J., and Rowe, R. D.: Catecholamine Cardiomyopathy: An Unusual Presentation of Pheochromocytoma in Children, *J. Pediatr.*, 99:276, 1981.
24. Corder, D. W., Heyliger, C. E., Beamish, R. E., and Dhalla, N. S.: Defect in the Adrenergic Receptor–Adenylate Cyclase System during Development of Catecholamine-Induced Cardiomyopathy, *Am. Heart J.*, 107:537, 1984.
25. Amorim, D. S., Dargie, H. J., Heer, K., et al.: Is There Autonomic Impairment in Congestive (Dilated) Cardiomyopathy?, *Lancet,* 1:525, 1981.
26. Amorim, D. S., and Olsen, E. G. J.: Assessment of Heart Neurons in Dilated (Congestive) Cardiomyopathy, *Br. Heart J.*, 47:11, 1982.
27. Dargie, H. J., and Goodwin, J. F.: Catecholamines, Cardiomyopathies and Cardiac Function, in P. N. Yu and J. F. Goodwin (eds.), "Progress in Cardiology," Lea & Febiger, Philadelphia, 1982, vol. 11, p. 93.
28. Kawai, C., Yui, Y., Hoshino, T., Sasayama, S., and Matsumori, A.: Myocardial Catecholamines in Hypertrophic and Dilated (Congestive) Cardiomyopathy: A Biopsy Study, *J. Am. Coll. Cardiol.*, 2:834, 1983.
29. Emanuel, R., Withers, R., and O'Brien, K.: Dominant and Recessive Modes of Inheritance of Idiopathic Cardiomyopathy, *Lancet,* 2:1065, 1971.
30. Fitchett, D. H., Sugrue, D. D., MacArthur, C. G., and Oakley, C. M.: Right Ventricular Dilated Cardiomyopathy, *Br. Heart J.*, 51:25, 1984.
31. Boltwood, C. M., Tei, C., Wong, M., and Shah, P. M.: Quantitative Echocardiography of the Mitral Complex in Dilated Cardiomyopathy: The Mechanism of Functional Mitral Regurgitation, *Circulation,* 68:498, 1983.
32. Opherk, D., Schwarz, F., Mall, G., Manthey, J., Baller, D., and Kubler, W.: Coronary Dilatory Capacity in Idiopathic Dilated Cardiomyopathy: Analysis of 16 Patients, *Am. J. Cardiol.*, 51:1657, 1983.
33. Gau, G. T., Goodwin, J. F., Oakley, C. M., Olsen, E. G. J., Rahimtoola, S. H., Raphael, M. J., and Steiner, R. E.: Q Waves and Coronary Arteriography in Cardiomyopathy, *Br. Heart J.*, 34:1034, 1972.
34. DeMaria, A. N., Bommer, W., Lee, G., and Mason, D. T.: Value and Limitations of Two-Dimensional Echocardiography in Assessment of Cardiomyopathy, *Am. J. Cardiol.*, 46:1224, 1980.
34a. Wallis, D. E., O'Connell, J. B., Henkin, R. E., Costanzo-Norden, M. R., and Scanlon, P. J.: Segmental Wall Motion Abnormalities in Dilated Cardiomyopathy: A Common Finding and a Good Prognostic Sign, *J. Am. Coll. Cardiol.*, 4:674, 1984.
35. Gardin, J. M.,Iseri, L. T., Elkayam, U., Tobis, J., Childs, W., Burn, C. S., and Henry, W. L.: Evaluation of Dilated Cardiomyopathy by Pulsed Doppler Echocardiography, *Am. Heart J.*, 106:1057, 1983.
36. Meinertz, T., Hofmann, T., Kasper, W., Treese, N., Bechtold, H., Stienen, U., Pop, T., Leitner, E. V., Andre-

sen, D., and Meyer, J.: Significance of Ventricular Arrhythmias in Idiopathic Dilated Cardiomyopathy, *Am. J. Cardiol.,* 53:902, 1984.

37. Goldman, M. R., and Boucher, C. A.: Value of Radionuclide Imaging Techniques in Assessing Cardiomyopathy, *Am. J. Cardiol.,* 46:1232, 1980.
38. Dunn, R. F., Uren, R. F., Sadick, N., Bautovich, G., McLaughlin, A., Hiroe, M., and Kelley, D. T.: Comparison of Thallium-201 Scanning in Idiopathic Dilated Cardiomyopathy and Severe Coronary Artery Disease, *Circulation,* 66:804, 1982.
39. Peters, T. J., Wells, C., Oakley, C. M., Brooksby, I. A. B., Webb-Peploe, M., and Coltart, D. J.: Enzyme Studies on Myocardial Biopsies in Congestive Cardiomyopathy, *Br. Heart J.,* 37:780, 1975.
40. Ferrans, V. J., and Roberts, W. C.: Myocardial Biopsy: A Useful Diagnostic Procedure or Only a Research Tool? *Am. J. Cardiol.,* 41:965, 1978.
41. Mason, J. W., Billingham, M. E., and Ricci, D. R.: Treatment of Acute Inflammatory Myocarditis Assisted by Endomyocardial Biopsy, *Am. J. Cardiol.,* 45:1037, 1980.

41a. Schwarz, F., Mall, G., Zebe, H., Schmitzer, E., Manthey, J., Scheurlen, H., and Kübler, W.: Determinants of Survival in Patients with Congestive Cardiomyopathy: Quantitative Morphologic Findings and Left Ventricular Hemodynamics, *Circulation,* 70:923, 1984.

42. Fuster, V., Gersh, B. J., Giuliani, E. R., Tajik, A. J., Brandenburg, R. O., and Frye, R. L.: The Natural History of Idiopathic Dilated Cardiomyopathy, *Am. J. Cardiol.,* 47:525, 1981.
43. von Olshausen, K., Schafer, A., Mehmel, H. C., Schwarz, F., Senges, J., and Kubler, W.: Ventricular Arrhythmias in Idiopathic Dilated Cardiomyopathy, *Br. Heart J.,* 51:195, 1984.
44. Johnson, R. A., and Palacios, I.: Dilated Cardiomyopathies of the Adult, *N. Engl. J. Med.,* 307:1051, 1119, 1982.
45. Chatterjee, K.: Digitalis Versus Newer Inotropic Agents: Which to Use, *Drug Therapy,* 12:83, 1982.
46. Billman, G. E., Schwartz, P. J., and Stone, H. L.: The Effects of Daily Exercise in Susceptibility to Sudden Cardiac Death, *Circulation,* 69:1182, 1984.
47. Fitchett, D. H., Marin Neto, J. A., Oakley, C. M., and Goodwin, J. F.: Hydralazine in the Management of Left Ventricular Failure, *Am. J. Cardiol.,* 44:303, 1979.
48. Faxon, D. P., Halperin, J. L., Creager, M. A., Gavras, H., Schick, E. C., and Ryan, T. J.: Angiotensin Inhibition in Severe Heart Failure: Acute Central and Limb Hemodynamic Effects of Captopril with Observations on Sustained Oral Therapy, *Am. Heart J.,* 101:548, 1981.
49. Sharma, B., and Goodwin, J. F.: Beneficial Effect on Salbutamol on Cardiac Function in Severe Congestive Cardiomyopathy: Effect on Systolic and Diastolic Function of the Left Ventricle, *Circulation,* 58:449, 1978.
50. Kupper, W., Schutt, M., Hamm, C. W., Kuck, K. H., Hanrath, P., and Bleifeld, W.: Hemodynamic and Cardiac Metabolic Effects of the New β_1 Agonist Prenalterol in Patients with Cardiac Failure, *Eur. Heart J.,* 4:573, 1983.
51. Packer, M.: Vasodilator and Inotropic Therapy for Severe Chronic Heart Failure: Passion and Skepticism, *J. Am. Coll. Cardiol.,* 2:841, 1983.
52. Beta-agonists and Heart Failure. *Lancet,* 2:1063, 1983. (Editorial.)
53. Baim, D. S., McDowell, A. V., Cherniles, J., Monrad, E. S., Parker, J. A., Edelson, J., Braunwald, E., and Grossman, W.: Evaluation of a New Bipyridine Inotropic Agent—Milrinone—in Patients with Severe Congestive Heart Failure, *N. Engl. J. Med.,* 309:748, 1983.
54. Unverferth, D. V., Mehegan, J. P., Magorien, R. D., Unverferth, B. J., and Leier, C. V.: Regression of Myocardial Cellular Hypertrophy with Vasodilator Therapy in Chronic Congestive Heart Failure Associated with Idiopathic Dilated Cardiomyopathy, *Am. J. Cardiol.,* 51:1392, 1983.
55. Waagstein, F., Hjalmarson, Å., Swedberg, K., and Wallentin, I.: Beta-Blockers in Dilated Cardiomyopathies: They Work, *Eur. Heart J.,* 4(suppl. A):173, 1983.
56. Ikram, H., and Fitzpatrick, M. A.: Beta Blockade for Dilated Cardiomyopathy: The Evidence against Therapeutic Benefit, *Eur. Heart J.,* 4(suppl. A):179, 1983.
57. Currie, P. J., Kelly, M. J., McKenzie, A., Harper, R. W., Lim, J. L., Federman, J., Anderson, S. T., and Pitt, A.: Oral Beta-Adrenergic Blockade with Metoprolol in Chronic Severe Dilated Cardiomyopathy, *J. Am. Coll. Cardiol.,* 3:203, 1984.
58. Hassell, L. A, Fowles, R. E., and Stinson, E. B.: Patients with Congestive Cardiomyopathy as Cardiac Transplant Recipients: Indications for and Results of Cardiac Transplantation and Comparison with Patients with Coronary Artery Disease, *Am. J. Cardiol.,* 47:1205, 1981.
59. Braunwald, E., Lambrew, C. T., Morrow, A. G., Pierce, G. E., Rockoff, S. D., and Ross, J. Jr.: Idiopathic Hypertrophic Subaortic Stenosis, *Circulation,* 29/30 (suppl. IV):1, 1964.
60. Matsumori, A., Hirose, K., Wakabayashi, A., Kawai, C., Nabeya, N., Sakurami, T., and Tsuji, K.: HL-A and Hypertrophic Cardiomyopathy, *Am. Heart J.,* 97:428, 1979.
61. Kishimoto, C., Kaburagi, T., Takayama, S., Yokoyama, S., Hanyu, I., Takatsu, Y., and Tomimoto, K.: Two Forms of Hypertrophic Cardiomyopathy Distinguished by Inheritance of HLA Haplotypes and Left Ventricular Outflow Tract Obstruction, *Am. Heart J.,* 105:988, 1983.
62. Emanuel, R., and Withers, R.: Genetics of the Cardiomyopathies, in P. N. Yu and J. F. Goodwin (eds.), "Progress in Cardiology," Lea & Febiger, Philadelphia, 1983, vol. 12, p. 211.
63. Ferrans, V. J., Morrow, A. G., and Roberts, W. C.: Myocardial Ultrastructure in Idiopathic Hypertrophic Subaortic Stenosis; A Study of Operatively Excised Left Ventricular Outflow Tract Muscle in 14 patients, *Circulation,* 45:769, 1972.
64. Manasek, F. J.: Histogenesis of the Embryonic Myocardium, *Am. J. Cardiol.,* 25:149, 1970.
65. Goodwin, J. F.: Cardiomyopathy: An Interface between Fundamental and Clinical Cardiology, in S. Hayase and S. Murao (eds.), "Cardiology" (Proceedings VIII World Congress of Cardiology, Tokyo, 1978), Excerpta Medica, Amsterdam, 1979, p. 103.
66. Blaufuss, A. H., Laks, M. M., Garner, D., Ishimoto, B. M., and Criley, J. M.: Production of Ventricular Hypertrophy Simulating "Idiopathic Hypertrophic Subaortic Stenosis" (IHSS) by Subhypertensive Infusion of Norepinephrine (NE) in the Conscious Dog, *Clin. Res.,* 23:77A, 1975.
67. Witzke, D. J., and Kaye, M. P.: Hypertrophic Cardiomyopathy Induced by Administration of Nerve Growth Factor, *Circulation,* 53/54 (suppl. 2):II–88, 1976.
68. Raum, W. J., Laks, M. M., Garner, D., and Swerdloff, R. S.: β-Adrenergic Receptor and Cyclic AMP Alterations in the Canine Ventricular Septum during Long-Term Norepinephrine Infusion: Implications for Hypertrophic Cardiomyopathy, *Circulation,* 68:693, 1983.
69. Way, G. L., Ruttenberg, H. D., Eshaghpour, E., Nora, J. J., and Wolfe, R. R.: Hypertrophic Obstructive Cardiomyopathy in Infants of Diabetic Mothers, *Circulation,* 53/54(suppl. 2):II–105, 1976.
70. Olsen, E. G. J., Symons, C., and Hawkey, C.: Effect of Triac on the Developing Heart, *Lancet,* 2:221, 1977.
71. Perloff, J. K.: Pathogenesis of Hypertrophic Cardiomyopathy: Hypotheses and Speculations, *Am. Heart J.,* 101:219, 1981.
72. Roberts, W. C.: Congenital Cardiovascular Abnormalities Usually "Silent" until Adulthood: Morphologic Features of the Floppy Mitral Valve, Valvular Aortic Stenosis, Discrete Subvalvular Aortic Stenosis, Hypertrophic Cardiomyopathy, Sinus of Valsalva Aneurysm, and the Marfan Syndrome, in W. C. Roberts (ed.), "Congenital Heart Disease in Adults," *Cardiovasc. Clin.,* F. A. Davis Company., Philadelphia, 1979, p. 407.
73. Teare, D.: Asymmetrical Hypertrophy of the Heart in Young Adults, *Br. Heart J.,* 20:1, 1958.
74. Roberts, W. C., and Ferrans, V. J.: Pathologic Anatomy of the Cardiomyopathies: Idiopathic Dilated and Hyper-

trophic Types, Infiltrative Types, and Endomyocardial Disease with and without Eosinophilia, *Hum. Pathol.*, 6:287, 1975.
75. Maron, B. J., and Epstein, S. E.: Hypertrophic Cardiomyopathy. Recent Observations Regarding the Specificity of Three Hallmarks of the Disease: Asymmetric Septal Hypertrophy, Septal Disorganization and Systolic Anterior Motion of the Anterior Mitral Leaflet, *Am. J. Cardiol.*, 45:141, 1980.
76. Henry, W. L., Clark, C. E., Roberts, W. C., Morrow, A. G., and Epstein, S. E.: Differences in Distribution of Myocardial Abnormalities in Patients with Obstructive and Nonobstructive Asymmetric Septal Hypertrophy (ASH): Echocardiographic and Gross Anatomic Findings, *Circulation*, 50:447, 1974.
77. Maron, B. J., and Roberts, W. C.: Quantitative Analysis of Cardiac Muscle Cell Disorganization in the Ventricular Septum of Patients with Hypertrophic Cardiomyopathy, *Circulation*, 59:689, 1979.
78. Maron, B. J., Epstein, S. E., and Roberts, W. C.: Hypertrophic Cardiomyopathy and Transmural Myocardial Infarction without Significant Atherosclerosis of the Extramural Coronary Arteries, *Am. J. Cardiol.*, 43:1086, 1979.
79. Roberts, W. C.: Operative Treatment of Hypertrophic Obstructive Cardiomyopathy: The Case against Mitral Valve Replacement, *Am. J. Cardiol.*, 32:377, 1973.
80. Doi, Y. L., McKenna, W. J., Chetty, S., Oakley, C. M., and Goodwin, J. F.: Prediction of Mortality and Serious Ventricular Arrhythmia in Hypertrophic Cardiomyopathy: An Echocardiographic Study, *Br. Heart J.*, 44:150, 1980.
81. Alvares, R. F., Shaver, J. A., Gamble, W. H., and Goodwin, J. F.: Isovolumic Relaxation Period in Hypertrophic Cardiomyopathy, *J. Am. Coll. Cardiol.*, 3:71, 1984.
82. Sanderson, J. E., Gibson, D. G., Brown, D. J., and Goodwin, J. F.: Left Ventricular Filling in Hypertrophic Cardiomyopathy: An Angiographic Study, *Br. Heart J.*, 39:661, 1977.
83. Webb-Peploe, M. M., Croxson, R. S., Oakley, C. M., and Goodwin, J. F.: Cardioselective Beta-Adrenergic Blockade in Hypertrophic Obstructive Cardiomyopathy, *Postgrad. Med. J.* (*Suppl.*), 47:93, 1971.
84. Grose, R., Maskin, C., Spindola-Franco, H., and Yipintsoi, T.: Production of Left Ventricular Cavitary Obliteration in Normal Man, *Circulation*, 64:448, 1981.
85. Braunwald, E., Morrow, A. G., Cornell, W. P., Aygen, M. M., and Hilbish, T. F.: Idiopathic Hypertrophic Subaortic Stenosis: Clinical, Hemodynamic and Angiographic Manifestations, *Am. J. Med.*, 29:924, 1960.
86. Ciró, E., Maron, B. J., Bonow, R. O., Cannon, R. O., and Epstein, S. E.: Relation between Marked Changes in Left Ventricular Outflow Tract Gradient and Disease Progression in Hypertrophic Cardiomyopathy, *Am. J. Cardiol.*, 53:1103, 1984.
87. Murgo, J. P.: Does Outflow Obstruction Exist in Hypertrophic Cardiomyopathy? *N. Engl. J. Med.*, 307:1008, 1982.
88. Goodwin, J. F.: The Frontiers of Cardiomyopathy, *Br. Heart J.*, 48:1, 1982.
89. McKenna, W. J., Borggrefe, M., England, D., Deanfield, J., Oakley, C. M., and Goodwin, J. F.: The Natural History of Left Ventricular Hypertrophy in Hypertrophic Cardiomyopathy: An Electrocardiographic Study, *Circulation*, 66:1233, 1982.
89a. Vacek, J. L., Davis, W. R., Bellinger, R. L., and McKiernan, T. L.: Apical Hypertrophic Cardiomyopathy in American Patients, *Am. Heart J.*, 108:1501, 1984.
90. Frank, M. J., Watkins, L. O., Prisant, M., Stefadouros, M. A., and Abdulla, A. M.: Potentially Lethal Arrhythmias and Their Management in Hypertrophic Cardiomyopathy, *Am. J. Cardiol.*, 53:1608, 1984.
91. Doi, Y. L., McKenna, W. J., Gehrke, J., Oakley, C. M., and Goodwin, J. F.: M Mode Echocardiography in Hypertrophic Cardiomyopathy: Diagnostic Criteria and Prediction of Obstruction, *Am. J. Cardiol.*, 45:6, 1980.
92. Gilbert, B. W., Pollick, C., Adelman, A. G., and Wigle, E. D.: Hypertrophic Cardiomyopathy: Subclassification by M-Mode Echocardiography, *Am. J. Cardiol.*, 45:861, 1980.
93. Doi, Y. L., Deanfield, J. E., McKenna, W. J., Dargie, H. J., Oakley, C. M., and Goodwin, J. F.: Echocardiographic Differentiation of Hypertensive Heart Disease and Hypertrophic Cardiomyopathy, *Br. Heart J.*, 44:395, 1980.
94. Savage, D. D., Castelli, W. P., Abbott, R. D., Garrison, R. J., Anderson, S. J., Kannel, W. B., and Feinleib, M.: Hypertrophic Cardiomyopathy and Its Markers in the General Population: The Great Masquerader Revisited: The Framingham Study, *J. Cardiovasc. Ultrasonography*, 2:41, 1983.
95. Shapiro, L. M., and McKenna, W. J.: Distribution of Left Ventricular Hypertrophy in Hypertrophic Cardiomyopathy: A Two-Dimensional Echocardiographic Study, *J. Am. Coll. Cardiol.*, 2:437, 1983.
96. Sugrue, D. D., McKenna, W. J., Dickie, S., Myers, M. J., Lavender, J. P., Oakley, C. M., and Goodwin, J. F.: Relation between Left Ventricular Gradient and Relative Stroke Volume Ejected in Early and Late Systole in Hypertrophic Cardiomyopathy. Assessment with Radionuclide Cineangiography, *Br. Heart J.*, 52:602, 1984.
97. Swan, D. A., Bell, B., Oakley, C. M., and Goodwin, J. F.: Analysis of Symptomatic Course and Prognosis and Treatment of Hypertrophic Obstructive Cardiomyopathy, *Br. Heart J.*, 33:671, 1971.
98. Hardarson, T., de la Calzada, C. S., Curiel, R., and Goodwin, J. F.: Prognosis and Mortality of Hypertrophic Obstructive Cardiomyopathy, *Lancet*, 2:1462, 1973.
99. Shah, P. M., Adelman, A. G., Wigle, E. D., Gobel, F. L., Burchell, H. B., Hardarson, T., Curiel, R., de la Calzada, C., Oakley, C. M., Goodwin, J. F., and Yu, P. N.: The Natural (and Unnatural) Course of Hypertrophic Obstructive Cardiomyopathy—A Multicenter Study, *Circulation*, 47/48(suppl. 4):IV–5, 1973.
100. McKenna, W., Deanfield, J., Faruqui, A., England, D., Oakley, C., and Goodwin, J.: Prognosis in Hypertrophic Cardiomyopathy: Role of Age and Clinical, Electrocardiographic and Hemodynamic Features, *Am. J. Cardiol.*, 47:532, 1981.
101. Goodwin, J. F., and Krikler, D. M.: Arrhythmia as a Cause of Sudden Death in Hypertrophic Cardiomyopathy, *Lancet*, 2:937, 1976.
102. McKenna, W., Harris, L., and Deanfield, J.: Syncope in Hypertrophic Cardiomyopathy, *Br. Heart J.*, 47:177, 1982.
103. McKenna, W.: The Significance and Treatment of Arrhythmias in Hypertrophic Cardiomyopathy, "Proceedings of the VIII Asian Pacific Congress of Cardiology," A 163, p. 43.
104. Krikler, D. M., Davies, M. J., Rowland, E., Goodwin, J. F., Evans, R. C., and Shaw, D. B.: Sudden Death in Hypertrophic Cardiomyopathy: Associated Accessory Atrioventricular Pathways, *Br. Heart J.*, 43:245, 1980.
105. Anderson, K. P., Stinson, E. B., Derby, G. C., Oyer, P. E., and Mason, J. W.: Vulnerability of Patients with Obstructive Hypertrophic Cardiomyopathy to Ventricular Arrhythmia Induction in the Operating Room: Analysis of 17 Patients, *Am. J. Cardiol.*, 51:811, 1983.
106. Bonow, R. O., Frederick, T. M., Bacharach, S. L., Green, M. V., Goose, P. W., Maron, B. J., and Rosing, D. R.: Atrial Systole and Left Ventricular Filling in Hypertrophic Cardiomyopathy: Effect of Verapamil, *Am. J. Cardiol.*, 51:1386, 1983.
107. Oakley, G. D. G., McGarry, K., Limb, D. G., and Oakley, C. M.: Management of Pregnancy in Patients with Hypertrophic Cardiomyopathy, *Br. Med J.*, 1:1749, 1979.
108. Frank, M. J., Stefadouros, M. A., Watkins, L. O., Prisant, L. M., and Abdulla, A. M.: Rhythm Disturbances in Hypertrophic Cardiomyopathies: Relationship to Symptoms and the Effect of 'Complete' β Blockade, *Eur. Heart J.*, 4(suppl. F):235, 1983.
109. McKenna, W. J., England, D., Doi, Y. L., Deanfield, J. E., Oakley, C., and Goodwin, J. F.: Arrhythmia in Hypertrophic Cardiomyopathy: I. Influence on Prognosis, *Br. Heart J.*, 46:168, 1981.

110. Chatterjee, K., Raff, G., Anderson, D., and Parmley, W. W.: Hypertrophic Cardiomyopathy—Therapy with Slow Channel Inhibiting Agents, *Prog. Cardiovasc. Dis.*, 25:193, 1982.
111. McKenna, W. J., Harris, L., Perez, A., Krikler, D. M., Oakley, C., and Goodwin, J. F.: Arrhythmia in Hypertrophic Cardiomyopathy: II. Comparison of Amiodarone and Verapamil in Treatment, *Br. Heart J.*, 46:173, 1981.
112. Rosing, D. R., Kent, K. M., Borer, J. S., Seides, S. F., Maron, B. J., and Epstein, S. E.: Verapamil Therapy: A New Approach to the Pharmacologic Treatment of Hypertrophic Cardiomyopathy: (I) Hemodynamic Effects, *Circulation*, 60:1201, 1979; (II) Effects on Exercise Capacity and Symptomatic Status, *Circulation*, 60:1208, 1979.
113. Hanrath, P., Schluter, M., Sonntag, F., Diemert, J., and Bleifeld, W.: Influence of Verapamil Therapy on Left Ventricular Performance at Rest and during Exercise in Hypertrophic Cardiomyopathy, *Am. J. Cardiol.*, 52:544, 1983.
114. Perrot, B., Danchin, N., and de la Chaise, A. T.: Verapamil: A Cause of Sudden Death in a Patient with Hypertrophic Cardiomyopathy, *Br. Heart J.*, 51:352, 1984.
115. Hubner, P. J. B, Ziady, G. M., Lane, G. K., Hardarson, T., Scales, B., Oakley, C. M., and Goodwin, J. F.: Double-Blind Trial of Propranolol and Practolol in Hypertrophic Cardiomyopathy, *Br. Heart J.*, 35:1116, 1973.
116. Alvares, R. F., and Goodwin, J. F.: Non-invasive Assessment of Diastolic Function in Hypertrophic Cardiomyopathy on and off Beta Adrenergic Blocking Drugs, *Br. Heart J.*, 48:204, 1982.
117. McKenna, W. J., Oakley, C. M., and Goodwin, J. F.: The Influence of Amiodarone on Survival in Hypertrophic Cardiomyopathy, *Circulation*, 68(suppl. 3):III–161, 1983.
117a. McKenna, W. J., Harris, L., Rowland, E., Kleinebenne, A., Krikler, D. M., Oakley, C. M., and Goodwin, J. F.: Amiodarine for Long-Term Management of Patients with Hypertrophic Cardiomyopathy, *Am. J. Cardiol.*, 54:802, 1984.
118. Epstein, S. E., and Rosing, D. R.: Verapamil: Its Potential for Causing Serious Complications in Patients with Hypertrophic Cardiomyopathy, *Circulation*, 64:437, 1981.
119. Lorell, B. H., Paulus, W. J., Grossman, W., Wynne, J., and Cohn, P. F.: Modification of Abnormal Left Ventricular Diastolic Properties by Nifedipine in Patients with Hypertrophic Cardiomyopathy, *Circulation*, 65:499, 1982.
120. Paulus, W. J., Lorrell, B. H., Craig, W. E., Wynne, J., Murgo, J. P., and Grossman, W.: Comparison of the Effects of Nitroprusside and Nifedipine on Diastolic Properties in Patients with Hypertrophic Cardiomyopathy: Altered Left Ventricular Loading or Improved Muscle Inactivation? *J. Am. Coll. Cardiol.*, 2:879, 1983.
120a. Suwa, M., Hirota, Y., and Kawamura, K.: Improvement in Left Ventricular Diastolic Function During Intravenous and Oral Diltiazem Therapy in Patients with Hypertrophic Cardiomyopathy: An Echocardiographic Study, *Am. J. Cardiol.*, 54:1047, 1984.
120b. Sugrue, D. D., Dickie, S., Myers, M. J., Lavender, J. P., and McKenna, W. J.: Effect of Amiodarine on Left Ventricular Ejection and Filling in Hypertrophic Cardiomyopathy as Assessed by Radionuclide Angiography, *Am. J. Cardiol.*, 54:1054, 1984.
121. McKenna, W. J., Rowland, E., and Krikler, D. M.: Amiodarone: The Experience of the Past Decade, *Br. Med. J.*, 287:1654, 1983.
122. Maron, B. J., Koch, J.-P., Kent, K. M., Epstein, S. E., and Morrow, A. G.: Results of Surgery for Idiopathic Hypertrophic Subaortic Stenosis, *J. Cardiovasc. Med.*, 5:145, 1980.
122a. Spirito, P., Maron, B. J., and Rosing, D. R.: Morphologic Determinants of Hemodynamic State after Ventricular Septal Myotomy-Myectomy in Patients with Obstructive Hypertrophic Cardiomyopathy: M Mode and Two-Dimensional Echocardiographic Assessment, *Circulation*, 70:984, 1984.
123. McKenna, W. J., and Goodwin, J. F.: The Natural History of Hypertrophic Cardiomyopathy, in W. P. Harvey (ed), *Current Problems in Cardiology*, Year Book Medical Publishers, Chicago, 1981, vol. 6, p. 1.
124. Beahrs, M. M., Tajik, A. J., Seward, J. B., Giuliani, E. R., and McGoon, D. C.: Hypertrophic Obstructive Cardiomyopathy: Ten- to 21-Year Follow-up after Partial Septal Myectomy, *Am. J. Cardiol.*, 51:1160, 1983.
125. Fighali, S., Krajcer, Z., and Leachman, R. D.: Septal Myomectomy and Mitral Valve Replacement for Idiopathic Hypertrophic Subaortic Stenosis: Short- and Long-term Follow-up, *J. Am. Coll. Cardiol.*, 3:1127, 1984.
126. Isner, J. M., Clarke, R. H., Pandian, N. G., et al.: Laser Myoplasty for Hypertrophic Cardiomyopathy: In vitro Experience in Human Postmortem Hearts and in vivo Experience in a Canine Model (Transarterial) and Human Patient (Intraoperative), *Am. J. Cardiol.*, 53:1620, 1984.
127. Chew, C. Y. C., Ziady, G. M., Raphael, M. J., Nellen, M., and Oakley, C. M.: Primary Restrictive Cardiomyopathy: Non-tropical Endomyocardial Fibrosis and Hypereosinophilic Heart Disease, *Br. Heart J.*, 39:399, 1977.
127a. Siegel, R. J., Shah, P. K., and Fishbein, M. C.: Idiopathic Restrictive Cardiomyopathy, *Circulation*, 70:165, 1984.
128. Roberts, W. C., Buja, L. M., and Ferrans, V. J.: Löffler's Fibroplastic Parietal Endocarditis, Eosinophilic Leukemia, and Davies' Endomyocardial Fibrosis: The Same Disease at Different Stages?, *Pathol. Microbiol.*, 35:90, 1970.
129. Olsen, E. G. J., and Spry, C. J. F.: The Pathogenesis of Löffler's Endomyocardial Disease, and Its Relationship to Endomyocardial Fibrosis, in P. N. Yu and J. E. Goodwin (eds.), "Progress in Cardiology," Lea & Febiger, Philadelphia, 1979, vol. 8, p. 281.
130. Parry, E. H. O.: Endomyocardial Fibrosis, in G. Wolstenholme and M. O'Connor (eds.), "Cardiomyopathies," Ciba Foundation Symposium, Churchill, London, 1964, p. 322.
131. Chusid, M. J., Dale, D. C., West, B. C., and Wolff, S. M.: The Hypereosinophilic Syndrome. Analysis of Fourteen Cases with Review of the Literature, *Medicine*, 54:1, 1975.
132. Spry, C. J. F., and Tai, P. C.: Studies on Blood Eosinophils. II. Patients with Löffler's Cardiomyopathy, *Clin. Exp. Immunol.*, 24:423, 1976.
133. Andy, J. J., Bishara, F. F., and Soyinka, O. O.: Relation of Severe Eosinophilia and Microfilariasis to Chronic African Endomyocardial Fibrosis, *Br. Heart J.*, 45:672, 1981.
134. Harley, J. B., Fauci, A. S., and Gralnick, H. R.: Noncardiovascular Findings Associated with Heart Disease in the Idiopathic Hypereosinophilic Syndrome, *Am. J. Cardiol.*, 52:321, 1983.
135. Roberts, W. C., Liegler, D. G., and Carbone, P. P.: Endomyocardial Disease and Eosinophilia: A Clinical and Pathologic Spectrum, *Am. J. Med.*, 46:28, 1969.
135a. Herzog, C. A., Snover, D. C., and Staley, N. A.: Acute Necrotising Eosinophilic Myocarditis, *Br. Heart J.*, 52:343, 1984.
136. Fournial, G., Schlanger, R., Berthoumieu, F., Pris, J., Marco, J., and Echapasse, H.: Surgery for Cardiac Complications Caused by Endocardial Mural Fibrin Deposits in a Hypereosinophilic Syndrome, *Circulation*, 65:1010, 1982.
137. Spry, C. J. F., Davies, J., Tai, P. C., Olsen, E. G. J., Oakley, C. M., and Goodwin, J. F.: Clinical Features of Fifteen Patients with the Hypereosinophilic Syndrome, *Q. J. Med.*, 52:1, 1983.
138. Vijayaraghavan, G., Davies, J., Sadanandan, S., Spry, C. J. F., Gibson, D. G., and Goodwin, J. F.: Echocardiographic Features of Tropical Endomyocardial Disease in South India, *Br. Heart J.*, 50:450, 1983.
139. Acquatella, H., Schiller, N. B., Puigbó, J. J., Gómez- Mancebo, J. R., and Suarez, C.: Value of Two-Dimensional Echocardiography in Endomyocardial Disease with and without Eosinophilia: A Clinical and Pathologic Study, *Circulation*, 67:1219, 1983.
140. Balakrishnan, K. G., Sasidharan, K., Venkitachalam, C. G., and Sapru, R. P.: Coronary Angiographic Features in Endomyocardial Fibrosis, *Cardiology*, 70:121, 1983.
141. Davies, J., Spry, C. J. F., Sapsford, R., Olsen, E. G. J., de Perez, G., Oakley, C. M., and Goodwin, J. F.: Cardiovas-

cular Features of 11 Patients with Eosinophilic Endomyocardial Disease, *Q. J. Med.*, 52:23, 1983.
142. Adebonojo, S. A., and Jaiyesimi, F.: Pericardioperitoneal Shunt for Massive Recurrent Pericardial Effusion in Patients with Endomyocardial Fibrosis, *Int. Surg.*, 62:349, 1977.
143. Parrillo, J. E., Borer, J. S., Henry, W. L., Wolff, S. M., and Fauci, A. S.: The Cardiovascular Manifestations of the Hypereosinophilic Syndrome: Prospective Study of 26 Patients, with Review of the Literature, *Am. J. Med.*, 67:572, 1979.
144. Cherian, G., Vijayaraghavan, G., Krishnaswami, S., Sukumar, I. P., John, S., Jairaj, P. S., and Bhaktaviziam, A.: Endomyocardial Fibrosis: Report on the Hemodynamic Data in 29 Patients and Review of the Results of Surgery, *Am. Heart J.*, 105:659, 1983.
145. James, T. N.: Pathology of the Cardiac Conduction System in Amyloidosis, *Ann. Intern. Med.*, 65:28, 1966.
146. Case Records of the Massachusetts General Hospital, *N. Engl. J. Med.*, 290:1474, 1974.
147. Buja, L. M., Khoi, N. B., and Roberts, W. C.: Clinically Significant Cardiac Amyloidosis: Clinicopathologic Findings in 15 Patients, *Am. J. Cardiol.*, 26:394, 1970.
148. Roberts, W. C., and Waller, B. F.: Cardiac Amyloidosis Causing Cardiac Dysfunction: Analysis of 54 Necropsy Patients, *Am. J. Cardiol.*, 52:137, 1983.
149. Smith, R. R. L., and Hutchins, G. M.: Ischemic Heart Disease Secondary to Amyloidosis of Intramyocardial Arteries, *Am. J. Cardiol.*, 44:413, 1979.
150. Chew, C., Ziady, G. M., Raphael, M. J., and Oakley, C. M.: The Functional Defect in Amyloid Heart Disease: The "Stiff Heart" Syndrome, *Am. J. Cardiol.*, 36:438, 1975.
151. Przybojewski, J. Z., Daniels, A. R., and Van der Walt, J. J.: Primary Cardiac Amyloidosis: A Review of the Literature, *S. Afr. Med. J.*, 57:831, 1980.
152. Carroll, J. D., Gaasch, W. H., and McAdam, K. P. W. J.: Amyloid Cardiomyopathy: Characterization by a Distinctive Voltage/Mass Relation, *Am. J. Cardiol.*, 49:9, 1982.
153. Siqueira-Filho, A. G., Cunha, C. L. P., Tajik, A. J., Seward, J. B., Schattenberg, T. T., and Giuliani, E. R.: M-Mode and Two-Dimensional Echocardiographic Features in Cardiac Amyloidosis, *Circulation*, 63:188, 1981.
153a. Nicolosi, G. L., Pavan, D., Lestuzzi, C., Burelli, C., Zardo, F., and Zanuttini, D.: Prospective Identification of Patients with Amyloid Heart Disease by Two-Dimensional Echocardiography, *Circulation*, 70:432, 1984.
154. Falk, R. H., Lee, V. W., Rubinow, A., Hood, W. B., Jr., and Cohen, A. S.: Sensitivity of Technetium-99m-Pyrophosphate Scintigraphy in Diagnosing Cardiac Amyloidosis, *Am. J. Cardiol.*, 51:826, 1983.
155. Wizenberg, T. A., Muz, J., Sohn, Y. H., Samlowski, W., and Weissler, A. M.: Value of Positive Myocardial Technetium-99m–Pyrophosphate Scintigraphy in the Noninvasive Diagnosis of Cardiac Amyloidosis, *Am. Heart J.*, 103, 468, 1982.
155a. Eriksson, P., Backman, C., Bjerle, P., Eriksson, A., Holm, S., and Olofsson, B.-O.: Noninvasive Assessment of the Presence and Severity of Cardiac Amyloidosis. A Study in Familial Amyloidosis with Polyneuropathy by Cross Sectional Echocardiography and Technetium-99m Pyrophosphate Scintigraphy, *Br. Heart J.*, 52:321, 1984.
156. Isner, J. M., Carter, B. L., Bankoff, M. S., Pastore, J. O., Ramaswamy, K., McAdam, K. P. W. J., and Salem, D. N.: Differentiation of Constrictive Pericarditis from Restrictive Cardiomyopathy by Computed Tomographic Imaging, *Am. Heart J.*, 105:1019, 1983.
157. Falk, R. H., Rubinow, A., and Cohen, A. S.: Cardiac Arrhythmias in Systemic Amyloidosis: Correlation with Echocardiographic Abnormalities, *J. Am. Coll. Cardiol.*, 3:107, 1984.
158. Grahame-Smith, D. G.: The Carcinoid Syndrome, *Am. J. Cardiol.*, 21:376, 1968.
159. Roberts, W. C., and Sjoerdsma, A.: The Cardiac Disease Associated with the Carcinoid Syndrome (Carcinoid Heart Disease), *Am. J. Med.*, 36:5, 1964.
160. Perloff, J. K., Lindgren, K. M., and Groves, B. M.: Uncommon or Commonly Unrecognized Causes of Heart Failure, *Prog. Cardiovasc. Dis.*, 12:409, 1970.
161. Porter, G. H.: Sarcoid Heart Disease, *N. Engl. J. Med.*, 263:1350, 1960.
162. Roberts, W. C., McAllister, H. A., Jr., and Ferrans, V. J.: Sarcoidosis of the Heart: A Clinicopathologic Study of 35 Necropsy Patients (Group I) and Review of 78 Previously Described Necropsy Patients (Group II), *Am. J. Med.*, 63:86, 1977.
163. Fawcett, F. J., and Goldberg, M. J.: Heart Block Resulting from Myocardial Sarcoidosis, *Br. Heart J.*, 36:220, 1974.
164. Virmani, R., Bures, J. C., and Roberts, W. C.: Cardiac Sarcoidosis: A Major Cause of Sudden Death in Young Individuals, *Chest*, 77:423, 1980.
165. Wheeler, R. C., and Abelmann, W. H.: Cardiomyopathy Associated with Systemic Diseases, *Cardiovasc. Clin.*, 4:283, 1972.
166. Matsui, Y., Iwai, K., Tachibana, T., Fruie, T., Shigematsu, N., Izumi, T., Homma, A. H., Mikami, R., Hongo, O., Hiraga, Y., and Yamamoto, M.: Clinicopathological Study on Fatal Myocardial Sarcoidosis, *Ann. N.Y. Acad. Sci.*, 278:455, 1976.
167. Fleming, H. A.: Sarcoid Heart Disease, in C. Symons, T. Evans, and A. G. Mitchell (eds.), "Specific Heart Muscle Disease," Wright, Bristol, 1983, p. 90.
168. Gozo, E. G., Jr., Cosnow, I., Cohen, H. C., and Okun, L.: The Heart in Sarcoidosis, *Chest*, 60:379, 1971.
169. Stein, E., Stimmel, B., and Siltzbach, L. E.: Clinical Course of Cardiac Sarcoidosis, *Ann. N.Y. Acad. Sci.*, 278:470, 1976.
170. Kinney, E. L., Jackson, G. L., Reeves, W. C., and Zelis, R.: Thallium-Scan Myocardial Defects and Echocardiographic Abnormalities in Patients with Sarcoidosis without Clinical Cardiac Dysfunction: An Analysis of 44 Patients, *Am. J. Med.*, 68:497, 1980.
171. Lorell, B., Alderman, E. L., and Mason, J. W.: Cardiac Sarcoidosis: Diagnosis with Endomyocardial Biopsy and Treatment with Corticosteroids, *Am. J. Cardiol.*, 42:143, 1978.
172. Friedman, H. S., Parikh, N. K., Chander, N., and Calderon, J.: Sarcoidosis with Incomplete Bilateral Bundle Branch Block Pattern Disappearing following Steroid Therapy: An Electrophysiological Study, *Eur. J. Cardiol.*, 4:141, 1976.
173. Lull, R. J., Dunn, B. E., Gregoratos, G., Cox, W. A., and Fisher, G. W.: Ventricular Aneurysm Due to Cardiac Sarcoidosis with Surgical Cure of Refractory Ventricular Tachycardia, *Am. J. Cardiol.*, 30:282, 1972.
174. Stefadouros, M. A., El Shahawy, M., and Witham A. C.: Shoshin in Georgia: A Case of Acute Fulminant Cardiac Beriberi, *J. Med. Assoc. Ga.*, 65:149, 1976.
174a. Pereira, V. G., Masuda, Z., Katz, A., and Tronchini, V., Jr.: Shoshin Beriberi: Report of Two Successfully Treated Patients with Hemodynamic Documentation. *Am. J. Cardiol.*, 53:1467, 1984.
175. Alexander, C. S.: Nutritional Heart Disease, *Cardiovasc. Clin.*, 4:221, 1972.
176. Rachmilewitz, M., and Braun, K.: Electrocardiographic Changes and the Effect of Niacin Therapy in Pellagra, *Br. Heart J.*, 7:72, 1945.
177. Sament, S.: Cardiac Disorders in Scurvy, *N. Engl. J. Med.*, 282:282, 1970.
178. Shafar, J.: Rapid Reversion of Electrocardiographic Abnormalities after Treatment in Two Cases of Scurvy, *Lancet*, 2:176, 1967.
179. Bauer, J. M., and Freyberg, R. H.: Vitamin D Intoxication with Metastatic Calcification, *JAMA*, 130:1208, 1946.
180. Sims, B. A.: Conducting Tissue of the Heart in Kwashiokor, *Br. Heart J.*, 34:828, 1972.
181. Swanepoel, A., Smythe, P. M., and Campbell, J. A. H.: The Heart in Kwashiokor, *Am. Heart J.*, 67:1, 1964.
182. Garcia, R., and Jennings, J. M.: Pheochromocytoma Masquerading as a Cardiomyopathy, *Am. J. Cardiol.*, 29:568, 1972.
183. Ehlers, K. H., Hagstrom, J. W. C., Lukas, D. S., Redo, S. F., and Engle, M. A.: Glycogen-Storage Disease of the Myo-

cardium with Obstruction to Left Ventricular Outflow, *Circulation,* 25:96, 1962.
184. Blieden, L. C., and Moller, J. H.: Cardiac Involvement in Inherited Disorders of Metabolism, *Prog. Cardiovasc. Dis.,* 16:615, 1974.
185. Miller, C. G., Alleyne, G. A., and Brooks, S. E. H.: Gross Cardiac Involvement in Glycogen Storage Disease Type III, *Br. Heart J.,* 34:862, 1972.
186. Olson, L. J., Reeder, G. S., Noller, K. L., Edwards, W. D., Howell, R. R., and Michels, V. V.: Cardiac Involvement in Glycogen Storage Disease: III. Morphologic and Biochemical Characterization with Endomyocardial Biopsy, *Am. J. Cardiol.,* 53:980, 1984.
187. Ruttenberg, H. D., Steidl, R. M., Carey, L. S., and Edwards, J. E.: Glycogen-Storage Disease of the Heart: Hemodynamic and Angiocardiographic Features in 2 Cases, *Am. Heart J.,* 67:469, 1964.
188. Rees, A., Elbl, F., Minhas, K., and Solinger, R.: Echocardiographic Evidence of Outflow Tract Obstruction in Pompe's Disease (Glycogen Storage Disease of the Heart), *Am. J. Cardiol.,* 37:1103, 1976.
189. Fenoglio, J. J., Jr., McAllister, H. A., Jr., and Ferrans, V. J.: Cardiac Rhabdomyoma: A Clinicopathologic and Electron Microscopic Study, *Am. J. Cardiol.,* 38:241, 1976.
190. Öckerman, P. A., and Berlin, S.-O.: Biochemical Studies in Familial Cardiomyopathy: With Special Reference to the Differential Diagnosis from Known Types of Glycogen Storage Disease, *Acta Med. Scand.,* 176:277, 1964.
191. Ratinov, G., Baker, W. P., and Swaiman, K. F.: McArdle's Syndrome with Previously Unreported Electrocardiographic and Serum Enzyme Abnormalities, *Ann. Intern. Med.,* 62:328, 1965.
192. Tripp, M. E., Katcher, M. L., Peters, H. A., Gilbert, E. F., Arya, S., Hodach, R. J., and Shug, A. L.: Systemic Carnitine Deficiency Presenting as Familial Endocardial Fibroelastosis: A Treatable Cardiomyopathy, *N. Engl. J. Med.,* 305:385, 1981.
193. Short, E. M., Winkle, R. A., and Billingham, M. E.: Myocardial Involvement in Idiopathic Hemochromatosis. Morphologic and Clinical Improvement Following Venesection, *Am. J. Med.,* 70:1275, 1981.
194. Buja, L. M., and Roberts, W. C.: Iron in the Heart: Etiology and Clinical Significance, *Am. J. Med.,* 51:209, 1971.
195. Easley, R. M., Jr., Schreiner, B. F., Jr., and Yu, P.N.: Reversible Cardiomyopathy Associated with Hemochromatosis, *N. Engl. J. Med.,* 287:866, 1972.
196. Arnett, E. N., Nienhuis, A. W., Henry, W. L., Ferrans, V. J., Redwood, D. R., and Roberts, W. C.: Massive Myocardial Hemosiderosis: A Structure-Function Conference at the National Heart and Lung Institute, *Am. Heart J.,* 90:777, 1975.
196a. Dabestani, A., Child, J. S., Henze, E., et al.: Primary Hemochromatosis: Anatomic and Physiologic Characteristics of the Cardiac Ventricles and Their Response to Phlebotomy, *Am. J. Cardiol.,* 54:153, 1984.
197. Bomford, A., and Williams, R.: Long Term Results of Venesection Therapy in Idiopathic Haemochromatosis, *Q. J. Med.,* 45:611, 1976.
198. Candell-Riera, J., Lu, L., Serés, L., Gonzáles, J. B., Batlle, J., Permanyer-Miralda, G., García-del-Castillo, H., and Soler-Soler, J.: Cardiac Hemochromatosis: Beneficial Effects of Iron Removal Therapy: An Echocardiographic Study, *Am. J. Cardiol.,* 52:824, 1983.
199. Engle, M. A., Erlandson, M., and Smith, C. H.: Late Cardiac Complications of Chronic, Severe, Refractory Anemia with Hemochromatosis, *Circulation,* 30:698, 1964.
200. Ferrans, V. J., Hibbs, R. G., and Burda, C. D.: The Heart in Fabry's Disease: A Histochemical and Electron Microscopic Study, *Am. J. Cardiol.,* 24:95, 1969.
201. Desnick, R. J., Blieden, L. C., Sharp, H. L., Hofschire, P. J., and Moller, J. H.: Cardiac Valvular Anomalies in Fabry Disease. Clinical, Morphologic, and Biochemical Studies, *Circulation,* 54:818, 1976.
202. Bass, J. L., Shrivastava, S., Grabowski, G. A., Desnick, R. J., and Moller, J. H.: The M-Mode Echocardiogram in Fabry's Disease, *Am. Heart J.,* 100:807, 1980.
203. Smith, R. R. L., Hutchins, G. M., Sack, G. H., Jr., and Ridolfi, R. L.: Unusual Cardiac, Renal and Pulmonary Involvement in Gaucher's Disease: Interstitial Glucocerebroside Accumulation, Pulmonary Hypertension and Fatal Bone Marrow Embolization, *Am. J. Med.,* 65:352, 1978.
204. Edwards, W. D., Hurdey, H. P., III, and Partin, J. R.: Cardiac Involvement by Gaucher's Disease Documented by Right Ventricular Endomyocardial Biopsy, *Am. J. Cardiol.,* 52:654, 1983.
205. Deacon, J. S. R., Gilbert, E. F., Viseskul, C., Herrmann, J., Angevine, J. M., Opitz, J. M., and Albert, A. E.: Familial Cardiac Lipidosis, *Birth Defects,* 10:181, 1974.
206. Eilenberg, M. D., and Scobie, B. A.: Prolonged Neuropsychiatric Disability and Cardiomyopathy in Acute Intermittent Porphyria, *Br. Med. J.,* 1:858, 1960.
207. McKusick, V. A., Neufeld, E. F., and Kelly, T. E.: The Mucopolysaccharide Storage Diseases, in J. B. Stanbury, J. B. Wyngaarden, and D. S. Frederickson (eds.), *"The Metabolic Basis of Inherited Disease,"* 4th ed., McGraw-Hill Book Company, New York, 1978, p. 1282.
208. Renteria, V. G., Ferrans, V. J. and Roberts, W. C.: The Heart in the Hurler Syndrome. Gross, Histologic, and Ultrastructural Observations in Five Necropsy Cases, *Am. J. Cardiol.,* 38:487, 1976.
209. Krovetz, L. J., Lorincz, A. E., and Schiebler, G. L.: Cardiovascular Manifestations of the Hurler Syndrome: Hemodynamic and Angiocardiographic Observations in 15 Patients, *Circulation,* 31:132, 1965.
210. Schieken, R. M., Kerber, R. E., Ionasescu, V. V., and Zellweger, H.: Cardiac Manifestations of the Mucopolysaccharidoses, *Circulation,* 52:700, 1975.
211. Campbell, A. M. G., and Williams, E. R.: Natural History of Refsum's Syndrome in a Gloucestershire Family, *Br. Med. J.,* 3:777, 1967.
212. Miller, A. A., and Ramsden, F.: Neural and Visceral Xanthomatosis in Adults, *J. Clin. Pathol.,* 18:622, 1965.
213. Virtanen, K. S. I., and Halonen, P. I.: Total Heart Block as a Complication of Gout, *Cardiologia,* 54:359, 1969.
214. Pikula, B., Plamenac, P., Ćurčić, B., and Nikulin, A.: Myocarditis Caused by Primary Oxalosis in a 4-Year-Old Child, *Virchows Arch (Pathol. Anat.),* 358:99, 1973.
215. Massie, B. M., Bharati, S., Scheinman, M. M., Lev, M., Desai, J., Rubeson, E., and Schmidt, W.: Primary Oxalosis with Pan-Conduction Cardiac Disease: Electrophysiologic and Anatomic Correlation, *Circulation,* 64:845, 1981.
216. Salyer, W. R., and Hutchins, G. M.: Cardiac Lesions in Secondary Oxalosis, *Arch. Intern. Med.,* 134:250, 1974.
217. Lichtenstein, L., and Kaplan, L.: Hereditary Ochronosis: Pathologic Changes Observed in Two Necropsied Cases, *Am. J. Pathol.,* 30:99, 1954.
218. Bailey, G. L., Hampers, C. L., and Merrill, J. P.: Reversible Cardiomyopathy in Uremia, *Trans. Am. Soc. Artif. Intern. Organs,* 13:263, 1967.
219. Arora, K. K., Lacy, J. P., Schacht, R. A., Martin, D. G., and Gutch, C. F.: Calcific Cardiomyopathy in Advanced Renal Failure, *Arch. Intern. Med.,* 135:603, 1975.
220. Atkinson, K., McElwain, T. J., and Mackay, A. M.: Myeloma of the Heart, *Br. Heart J.,* 36:309, 1974.
221. Oliveira, E., and Gómez-Patiño, N.: Falcemic Cardiopathy: Report of a Case, *Am. J. Cardiol.,* 11:686, 1963.
222. Uzsoy, N. K.: Cardiovascular Findings in Patients with Sickle Cell Anemia, *Am. J. Cardiol.,* 13:320, 1964.
223. Hellenbrand, W., Brown, J., Covitz, W., Gallagher, D., Geer, M., Leff, S., and Talner, N.: Cardiovascular Performance in Sickle Cell Disease, *Circulation,* 68(suppl. 3):III-163, 1983.
224. Fleischer, R. A., and Rubler, S.: Primary Cardiomyopathy in Nonanemic Patients: Association with Sickle Cell Trait, *Am J. Cardiol.,* 22:532, 1968.
225. Kereiakes, D. J., Ports, T. A., and Finkbeiner, W.: Endomyocardial Biopsy in Henoch-Schönlein Purpura, *Am. Heart J.,* 107:382, 1984.
226. Ridolfi, R. L., Hutchins, G. M., and Bell, W. R.: The Heart

and Cardiac Conduction System in Thrombotic Thrombocytopenic Purpura. A Clinicopathologic Study of 17 Autopsied Patients, *Ann. Intern. Med.*, 91:357, 1979.
227. Miller, C. L., and Murphy, M. L.: Hereditary Hemorrhagic Telangiectasia: Demonstration of a Myocardial Lesion by Postmortem Coronary Angiography, *J. Arkansas Med. Soc.*, 73:64, 1976.
228. James, T. N.: Primary and Secondary Cardioneuropathies and their Functional Significance, *J. Am. Coll. Cardiol.*, 2:983, 1983.
229. Perloff, J. K.: Cardiac Involvement in Heredofamilial Neuromyopathic Diseases, *Cardiovasc. Clin.*, 4:333, 1972.
230. Ronan, J. A., Jr., Perloff, J. K., Bowen, P. J., and Mann, O.: The Vectorcardiogram in Duchenne's Progressive Muscular Dystrophy, *Am. Heart J.*, 84:588, 1972.
231. Sanyal, S. H., and Johnson, W. W.: Cardiac Conduction Abnormalities in Children with Duchenne's Progressive Muscular Dystrophy: Electrocardiographic Features and Morphologic Correlates, *Circulation*, 66:853, 1982.
232. Perloff, J. K.: Cardiac Rhythm and Conduction in Duchenne's Muscular Dystrophy: A Prospective Study of 20 Patients, *J. Am. Coll. Cardiol.*, 3:1263, 1984.
233. James, T. N.: Observations on the Cardiovascular Involvement, Including the Cardiac Conduction System, in Progressive Muscular Dystrophy, *Am. Heart J.*, 63:48, 1962.
234. Perloff, J. K., deLeon, A. C., Jr., and O'Doherty, D.: The Cardiomyopathy of Progressive Muscular Dystrophy, *Circulation*, 33:625, 1966.
235. Perloff, J. K., Roberts, W. C., de Leon, A. C., Jr., and O'Doherty, D.: The Distinctive Electrocardiogram of Duchenne's Progressive Muscular Dystrophy: An Electrocardiographic-Pathologic Correlative Study, *Am. J. Med.*, 42:179, 1967.
236. Mann, O., de Leon, A. C., Jr., Perloff, J. K., Simanis, J., and Horrigan, F. D.: Duchenne's Muscular Dystrophy: The Electrocardiogram in Female Relatives, *Am. J. Med. Sci.*, 255:376, 1968.
237. Heymsfield, S. B., McNish, T., Perkins, J. V., and Felner, J. M.: Sequence of Cardiac Changes in Duchenne Muscular Dystrophy, *Am. Heart J.*, 95:283, 1978.
238. Zalman, F., Perloff, J. K., Durant, N. N., and Campion, D. S.: Acute Respiratory Failure Following Intravenous Verapamil in Duchenne's Muscular Dystrophy, *Am. Heart J.*, 105:510, 1983.
239. Baldwin, B. J., Talley, R. C., Johnson, C., and Nutter, D. O.: Permanent Paralysis of the Atrium in a Patient with Facioscapulohumeral Muscular Dystrophy, *Am. J. Cardiol.*, 31:649, 1973.
240. Waters, D. D., Nutter, D. O., Hopkins, L. C., and Dorney, E. R.: Cardiac Features of an Unusual X-Linked Humeroperoneal Neuromuscular Disease, *N. Engl. J. Med.*, 293:1017, 1975.
241. Van der Hauwaert, L. G., and Dumoulin, M.: Hypertrophic Cardiomyopathy in Friedreich's Ataxia, *Br. Heart J.*, 38:1291, 1976.
242. Gottdiener, J. S., Hawley, R. J., Maron, B. J., Bertorini, T. F., and Engel, W. K.: Characteristics of the Cardiac Hypertrophy in Friedreich's Ataxia, *Am. Heart J.*, 103:525, 1982.
243. James, T. N., and Fisch, C.: Observations on the Cardiovascular Involvement in Friedreich's Ataxia, *Am. Heart J.*, 66:164, 1963.
244. Cote, M., Davignon, A., Pecko-Drouin, K., Solignac, A., Geoffroy, G., Lemieux, B., and Barbeau, A.: Cardiological Signs and Symptoms in Friedreich's Ataxia, *Can. J. Neurol. Sci.*, 3:319, 1976.
245. Gregorini, L., Valentini, R., and Libretti, A.: The Vectorcardiogram in Friedreich's Ataxia, *Am. Heart J.*, 87:158, 1974.
246. Cote, M., Davignon, A., Elias, G., Solignac, A., Geoffroy, G., Lemieux, B., and Barbeau, A.: Hemodynamic Findings in Friedreich's Ataxia, *Can. J. Neurol. Sci.*, 3:333, 1976.
247. Lascelles, R. G., Baker, I. A., and Thomas, P. K.: Hereditary Polyneuropathy of Roussy-Lévy Type with Associated Cardiomyopathy, *Guys. Hosp. Rep.*, 119:253, 1970.
247a. Perloff, J. K., Stevenson, W. G., Roberts, N. K., Cabeen, W., and Weiss, J.: Cardiac Involvement in Myotonic Muscular Dystrophy (Steinert's Disease): A Prospective Study of 25 Patients, *Am. J. Cardiol.*, 54:1074, 1984.
248. Gottdiener, J. S., Hawley, R. J., Gay, J. A., DiBianco, R., Fletcher, R. D., and Engel, W. K.: Left Ventricular Relaxation, Mitral Valve Prolapse, and Intracardiac Conduction in Myotonia Atrophica: Assessment by Digitized Echocardiography and Noninvasive His Bundle Recording, *Am. Heart J.*, 104:77, 1982.
249. Josephson, M. E., Caracta, A. R., Gallagher, J. J., and Damato, A. N.: Site of Conduction Disturbances in a Family with Myotonic Dystrophy, *Am. J. Cardiol.*, 32:114, 1973.
250. Prystowsky, E. N., Pritchett, E. L. C., Roses, A. D., and Gallagher, J.: The Natural History of Conduction System Disease in Myotonic Muscular Dystrophy as Determined by Serial Electrophysiological Studies, *Circulation*, 60:1360, 1979.
251. Clements, S. D., Jr., Colmers, R. A., and Hurst, J. W.: Myotonia Dystrophica: Ventricular Arrhythmias, Intraventricular Conduction Abnormalities, Atrioventricular Block and Stokes-Adams Attacks Successfully Treated with Permanent Transvenous Pacemaker, *Am. J. Cardiol.*, 37:933, 1976.
252. Luomanmäki, K., Hokkanen, E., and Heikkilä, J.: Electrocardiogram in Myasthenia Gravis: Analysis of a Series of 97 Patients, *Ann. Clin. Res.*, 1:236, 1969.
253. Gibson, T. C.: The Heart in Myasthenia Gravis, *Am. Heart J.*, 90:389, 1975.
254. Pomerleau, O. F., and Schwarz, H. J.: Tuberous Sclerosis with Unusual Findings: A Case Report, *J. Maine Med. Assoc.*, 60:137, 1969.
255. Charles, R., Holt, S., Kay, J. M., Epstein, E. J., and Rees, J. R.: Myocardial Ultrastructure and the Development of Atrioventricular Block in Kearns-Sayre Syndrome, *Circulation*, 63:214, 1981.
256. McCormish, M., Compston, A., and Jewitt, D.: Cardiac Abnormalities in Chronic Progressive External Ophthalmoplegia, *Br. Heart J.*, 38:526, 1976.
257. Faillace, R. T., Kingston, W. J., Nanda, N. C., and Griggs, R. C.: Cardiomyopathy Associated with the Syndrome of Amyotrophic Chorea and Acanthocytosis, *Ann. Intern. Med.*, 96:616, 1982.
258. Verhiest, W., Brucher, J. M., Goddeeris, P., Lauweryns, J., and DeGeest, H.: Familial Centronuclear Myopathy Associated with "Cardiomyopathy," *Br. Heart J.*, 38:504, 1976.
259. Tanaka, H., Uemura, N., Toyama, Y., Kudo, A., Ohkatsu, Y., and Kanehisa, T.: Cardiac Involvement in the Kugelberg-Welander Syndrome, *Am. J. Cardiol.*, 38:528, 1976.
260. Murphy, M. L., Bulloch, R. T., and Pearce, M. B.: The Correlation of Metabolic and Ultrastructural Changes in Emetine Myocardial Toxicity, *Am. Heart J.*, 87:105, 1974.
261. Dempsey, J. J., and Salem, H. H.: An Enzymatic Electrocardiographic Study on Toxicity of Dehydroemetine, *Br. Heart J.*, 28:505, 1966.
262. Fowler, N. O., McCall, D., Chou, T.-C., Holmes, J. C., and Hanenson, I. B.: Electrocardiographic Changes and Cardiac Arrhythmias in Patients Receiving Psychotropic Drugs, *Am. J. Cardiol.*, 37:223, 1976.
263. Stimmel, B.: "Cardiovascular Effects of Mood-Altering Drugs," Raven Press, New York, 1979.
264. Jefferson, J. W.: A Review of the Cardiovascular Effects and Toxicity of Tricyclic Antidepressants, *Psychosom. Med.*, 37:160, 1975.
265. Palileo, E. V., Coelho, A., Westveer, D., Dhingra, R., and Rosen, K. M.: Persistent Sinus Node Dysfunction Secondary to Lithium Therapy, *Am. Heart J.*, 106:1443, 1983.
266. Tilkian, A. G., Schroeder, J. S., Kao, J., and Hultgren, H.: Effect of Lithium on Cardiovascular Performance: Report on Extended Ambulatory Monitoring and Exercise Testing before and during Lithium Therapy, *Am. J. Cardiol.*, 38:701, 1976.
267. Bana, D. S., MacNeal, P. S., LeCompte, P. M., Shah, Y., and Graham, J. R.: Cardiac Murmurs and Endocardial

Fibrosis Associated with Methysergide Therapy, *Am. Heart J.*, 88:640, 1974.
268. Mills, B. A., and Roberts, R. W.: Cyclophosphamide-Induced Cardiomyopathy: A Report of Two Cases and Review of the English Literature, *Cancer*, 43:2223, 1979.
269. Buja, L. M., Ferrans, V. J., and Roberts, W. C.: Drug-Induced Cardiomyopathies, *Adv. Cardiol.*, 13:330, 1974.
270. Borow, K. M., Henderson, I. C., Neuman, A., Colan, S., Grady, S., Papish, S., and Goorin, A.: Assessment of Left Ventricular Contractility in Patients Receiving Doxorubicin, *Ann. Intern. Med.*, 99:750, 1983.
271. Bristow, M. R., Mason, J. W., Billingham, M. E., and Daniels, J. R.: Dose-Effect and Structure-Function Relationships in Doxorubicin Cardiomyopathy, *Am. Heart J.*, 102:709, 1981.
272. Torti, F. M., Bristow, M. R., Howes, A. E., Aston, D., Stockdale, F. E., Carter, S. K., Kohler, M., Brown, B. W., Jr., and Billingham, M. E.: Reduced Cardiotoxicity of Doxorubicin Delivered on a Weekly Schedule: Assessment by Endomyocardial Biopsy, *Ann. Intern. Med.*, 99:745, 1983.
273. Choi, W. B., Berger, H. J., Schwartz, P. E., Alexander, J., Wackers, F. J. T., Gottschalk, A., and Zaret, B. L.: Serial Radionuclide Assessment of Doxorubicin Cardiotoxicity in Cancer Patients with Abnormal Baseline Resting Left Ventricular Performance, *Am. Heart J.*, 106:638, 1983.
274. McKillop, J. H., Bristow, M. R., Goris, M. L., Billingham, M. E., and Bockemuehl, K.: Sensitivity and Specificity of Radionuclide Ejection Fractions in Doxorubicin Cardiotoxicity, *Am. Heart J.*, 106:1048, 1983.
275. Thompson, R. C., Lojeski, E. W., Ratner, A. V., Fallon, J. T., and Pohost, G. M.: Detection of Adriamycin Cardiotoxicity using Proton NMR Techniques, *Circulation*, 68:III–387, 1983.
276. Glazener, G. S., Ellis, J. G., and Johnson, P. K.: Electrocardiographic Findings with Arsenic Poisoning, *Calif. Med.*, 109:158, 1968.
277. McKinstry, W. J., and Hickes, J. M.: Emergency—Arsine Poisoning, *Arch. Intern. Med.*, 100:34, 1957.
278. Somers, K., and Rosanelli, J. D.: Electrocardiographic Effects of Antimony Dimercaptosuccinate ("Astiban"), *Br. Heart J.*, 24:187, 1962.
279. Haft, J. I., Gershengorn, K., Kranz, P. D., and Oestreicher, R.: Protection against Epinephrine-Induced Myocardial Necrosis by Drugs that Inhibit Platelet Aggregation, *Am. J. Cardiol.*, 30:838, 1972.
280. Smith, H. J., Roche, A. H. G., Jagusch, M. F., and Herdson, P. B.: Cardiomyopathy Associated with Amphetamine Administration, *Am. Heart J.*, 91:792, 1976.
281. Call, T. D., Hartneck, J., Dickinson, W. A., Hartman, C. W., and Bartel, A. G.: Acute Cardiomyopathy Secondary to Intravenous Amphetamine Abuse, *Ann. Intern. Med.*, 97:559, 1982.
282. Pentel, P. R., Mikell, F. L., and Zavoral, J. H.: Myocardial Injury after Phenylpropanolamine Ingestion, *Br. Heart J.*, 47:51, 1982.
283. Anderson, R. F., Allensworth, D. C., and deGroot, W. J.: Myocardial Toxicity from Carbon Monoxide Poisoning, *Ann. Intern. Med.*, 67:1172, 1967.
284. Corya, B. C., Black, M. J., and McHenry, P. L.: Echocardiographic Findings after Acute Carbon Monoxide Poisoning, *Br. Heart J.*, 38:712, 1976.
285. Barborik, M., and Dusek, J.: Cardiomyopathy Accompanying Industrial Cobalt Exposure, *Br. Heart J.*, 34:113, 1972.
286. James, F. W., Kaplan, S., and Benzing, G., III: Cardiac Complications following Hydrocarbon Ingestion, *Am. J. Dis. Child.*, 121:431, 1971.
287. Harris, W. S.: Toxic Effects of Aerosol Propellants on the Heart, *Arch. Intern. Med.*, 131:162, 1973.
288. Talley, R. C., Linhart, J. W., Trevino, A. J., Moore, L., and Beller, B. M.: Acute Elemental Phosphorus Poisoning in Man: Cardiovascular Toxicity, *Am. Heart J.*, 84:139, 1972.
289. Rao, S., and Brown, R. H.: Acute Yellow Phosphorus Rat Poisoning, *Ill. Med. J.*, 145:128, 1974.
290. Ludomirsky, A., Klein, H. O., Sarelli, P., Becker, B., Hoffman, S., Taitelman, U., Barzilai, J., Lang, R., David, D., DiSegni, E., and Kaplinsky, E: Q-T Prolongation and Polymorphous ("Torsade de Pointes") Ventricular Arrhythmias Associated with Organophosphorus Insecticide Poisoning, *Am. J. Cardiol.*, 49:1654, 1982.
291. Goodman, L. S., and Gilman, A.: "The Pharmacologic Basis of Therapeutics," 3d ed, The Macmillan Company, New York, 1965, p. 816.
292. Dahhan, S. S., and Orfaly, H.: Electrocardiographic Changes in Mercury Poisoning, *Am. J. Cardiol.*, 14:178, 1964.
293. Freeman, R.: Reversible Myocarditis Due to Chronic Lead Poisoning in Childhood, *Arch. Dis. Child.*, 40:389, 1965.
294. Gueron, M., and Yarom, R.: Cardiovascular Manifestations of Severe Scorpion Sting: Clinicopathologic Correlations, *Chest*, 57:156, 1970.
295. Weitzman, A., Margulis, G., and Lehmann, E.: Uncommon Cardiovascular Manifestations and High Catecholamine Levels Due to "Black Widow" Bite, *Am. Heart J.*, 93:89, 1977.
296. Chadha, J. S., Ashby, D. W., and Brown, J. O.: Abnormal Electrocardiogram after Adder Bite, *Br. Heart J.*, 30:138, 1968.
297. Levine, H. D.: Acute Myocardial Infarction following Wasp Sting: Report of Two Cases and Critical Survey of the Literature, *Am. Heart J.*, 91:365, 1976.
298. Pearn, J. H.: A Case of Tick Paralysis with Myocarditis, *Med J. Australia*, 1:629, 1966.
299. Wenzel, D. G.: Drug-Induced Cardiomyopathies, *J. Pharmacol. Sci.*, 56:1209, 1967.
300. Surawicz, B., and Lasseter, K. C.: Effect of Drugs on the Electrocardiogram, *Prog. Cardiovasc. Dis.*, 13:26,1970.
301. Harkavy, J.: Cardiac Manifestations Due to Hypersensitivity, *Ann. Allerg.*, 28:242, 1970.
302. Langsjoen, P. H., and Stinson, J. C.: Acute Fatal Allergic Myocarditis: Report of a Case, *Dis. Chest*, 48:440, 1965.
303. Field, J. B., and Federman, D. D.: Sudden Death in a Diabetic Subject during Treatment with BZ-55 (Carbutamide), *Diabetes*, 6:67, 1957.
304. MacSearraigh, E. T. M., and Patel, K. M.: Cardiomyopathy as a Complication of Sulphonamide Therapy, *Br. Med. J.*, 3:33, 1968.
305. Schoenwetter, A. H., and Silber, E. N.: Penicillin Hypersensitivity, Acute Pericarditis, and Eosinophilia, *JAMA*, 191:136, 1965.
306. Fighali, S., Strickman, N. E., and Hall, R. J.: Congestive Cardiomyopathy Presumably Secondary to Oxacillin, *Tex. Heart Inst. J.*, 10:421, 1983.
307. Hodge, P. R., and Lawrence, J. R.: Two Cases of Myocarditis Associated with Phenylbutazone Therapy, *Med. J. Australia*, 1:640, 1957.
308. Matthews, A. W., and Griffiths, I. D.: Post-vaccinial Pericarditis and Myocarditis, *Br. Heart J.*, 36:1043, 1974.
309. Gavrilesco, S., Streian, C., and Constantinesco, L.: Tachycardie Ventriculaire et Fibrillation Auriculaire, Associées, Après Vaccination Anticholérique, *Acta Cardiol.*, 28:89, 1973.
310. Kline, I. K., Kline, T. S., and Saphir, O.: Myocarditis in Senescence, *Am. Heart J.*, 65:446, 1963.
311. Mullick, F. G., and McAllister, H. A.: Myocarditis Associated with Methyldopa Therapy, *JAMA*, 237:1699, 1977.
312. Chatterjee, S. S., and Thakre, M. W.: Fiedler's Myocarditis: Report of a Fatal Case following Intramuscular Injection of Streptomycin, *Tubercle*, 39:240, 1958.
313. Barrett, D. A., II, Dalldorf, F. G., Barnwell, W. H., II, and Hudson, R. P.: Allergic Giant Cell Myocarditis Complicating Tuberculosis Chemotherapy, *Arch. Pathol.*, 21:201, 1971.
314. Kerwin, A. J.: Fatal Myocarditis Due to Sensitivity to Phenindione, *Can. Med. Assoc. J.*, 90:1418, 1964.
315. Sanerkin, N. G.: Acute Myocardial Necrosis in Paracetamol Poisoning, *Br. Med. J.*, 3:478, 1971.
316. Sun, S.-C., Sohal, R. S., Colcolough, H. L., and Burch, G. E.: Histochemical and Electron Microscopic Studies of

the Effects of Reserpine on the Heart Muscle of Mice, *J. Pharmacol. Exp. Ther.*, 161:210, 1968.

317. Burch, G. E., Sohal, R. S., Sun, S.-C., Miller, G. C., and Colcolough, H. L.: Effects of Radiation on the Human Heart: An Electron Microscopic Study, *Arch. Intern. Med.*, 121:230, 1968.
318. Biran, S., Hochmann, A., and Stern, S.: Therapeutic Irradiation of the Chest and Electrocardiographic Changes, *Clin. Radiol.*, 20:433, 1969.
319. Elmino, O., and Rossi, A.: Alterazioni Cardiovascolari in Alcuni Casi di Trauma Elettrico, *Folia Med.*, 48:164, 1965.
320. Stevens, P. J., and Ground, K. E. U.: Occurrence and Significance of Myocarditis in Trauma, *Aerosp. Med.*, 41:776, 1970.
321. Grossman, C. M.: Posttraumatic Ossification of the Myocardium, *J. Trauma,* 14:85, 1974.
322. Berkoff, H. A., Rowe, G. G., Crummy, A. B., and Kahn, D. R.: Asymptomatic Left Ventricular Aneurysm: A Sequela of Blunt Chest Trauma, *Circulation,* 55:545, 1977.
323. Kew, M. C., Tucker, R. B. K., Bersohn, I., and Seftel, H. C.: The Heart in Heatstroke, *Am. Heart J.*, 77:324, 1969.
324. Duguid, H., Simpson, R. G., and Stowers, J. M.: Accidental Hypothermia, *Lancet,* 2:1213, 1961.
325. Hastillo, A., Willis, H. E., and Hess, M. L.: The Heart as a Target Organ of Immune Injury, in W. P. Harvey (ed.), "Current Problems in Cardiology," vol. 6, Year Book Medical Publishers, Chicago, 1982.
326. Mason, J. W., and Billingham, M. E.: Myocardial Biopsy, in P. N. Yu and J. F. Goodwin (eds.), "Progress in Cardiology," Lea & Febiger, Philadelphia, 1980, vol. 9, p. 113.
327. Brooksby, I. A. B., Coltart, D. J., and Webb-Peploe, M. M.: Progress in Endomyocardial Biopsy, *Mod. Concepts Cardiovasc. Dis.*, 44:65, 1975.
328. Collins, P.: Aortic Incompetence and Active Myocarditis in Reiter's Disease, *Br. J. Vener. Dis.*, 48:300, 1972.
329. Bottiger, L. E., and Edhag, O.: Heart Block in Ankylosing Spondylitis and Uropolyarthritis, *Br. Heart J.*, 34:487, 1972.
330. Bergfeldt, L., Vallin, H., and Edhag, O.: Complete Heart Block in HLA B27 Associated Disease: Electrophysiological and Clinical Characteristics, *Br. Heart J.*, 51:184, 1984.
331. Eisenstein, B., and Taubenhaus, M.: Nonsyphilitic Interstitial Keratitis and Bilateral Deafness (Cogan's Syndrome) Associated with Cardiovascular Disease, *N. Engl. J. Med.*, 258:1074, 1958.
332. Schiff, S., Moffatt, R., Mandel, W. J., and Rubin, S. A.: Acute Myocardial Infarction and Recurrent Ventricular Arrhythmias in Behçet's Syndrome, *Am. Heart J.*, 103:438, 1982.
333. James, D. G., and Thomson, A.: Recognition of the Diverse Cardiovascular Manifestations in Behçet's Disease, *Am. Heart J.*, 103:457, 1982.
334. Hirsch, H. D., Gelband, H., Garcia, O., Gottlieb, S., and Tamer, D. M.: Rapidly Progressive Obstructive Cardiomyopathy in Infants with Noonan's Syndrome: Report of Two Cases, *Circulation,* 52:1161, 1975.
335. Huang, S., Kumar, G., Steele, H. D., and Parker, J. O.: Cardiac Involvement in Pseudoxanthoma Elasticum: Report of a Case, *Am. Heart J.*, 74:680, 1967.
336. Wilkinson, P. J., Harman, R. R. M., and Tribe, C. R.: Systemic Nodular Panniculitis with Cardiac Involvement, *J. Clin. Pathol.*, 27:808, 1974.
337. Eller, J. L.: Roentgen Therapy for Visceral Juvenile Xanthogranuloma, Including a Case with Involvement of the Heart, *Am. J. Roentgenol.*, 95:52, 1965.
338. Johnson, M. L., and Ikram, H.: Scleroedema of Buschke: An Uncommon Cause of Cardiomyopathy, *Br. Heart J.*, 32:720, 1970.
339. Erlichman, M., and Glaser, J.: Buschke's Scleredema with Right-Sided Heart Failure: Echocardiographic and Clinical Observations, *Cardiology,* 70:344, 1983.
340. Saheta, N. P.: Cardiomyopathy and Mitral Stenosis Associated with Wegener's Granulomatosis, *Indian Heart J.*, 19:144, 1967.
341. Morales, A. R., Bourgeois, C. H., and Chulacharit, E.: Pathology of the Heart in Reye's Syndrome (Encephalopathy and Fatty Degeneration of the Viscera), *Am. J. Cardiol.*, 27:314, 1971.
342. Somerville, J., and Bonham-Carter, R. E.: The Heart in Lentiginosis, *Br. Heart J.*, 34:58, 1972.
343. Tuuteri, L., Perheentupa, J., and Rapola, J.: The Cardiopathy of Mulibrey Nanism, A New Inherited Syndrome, *Chest,* 65:628, 1974.
344. Mowat, N. A. G., Bennett, P. N., Finlayson, J. K., Brunt, P. W., and Lancaster, W. M.: Myopericarditis Complicating Ulcerative Colitis, *Br. Heart J.*, 36:724, 1974.
345. McAllister, H. A., Jr., and Fenoglio, J. J., Jr.: Cardiac Involvement in Whipple's Disease, *Circulation,* 52:152, 1975.

Section H

The Pericardium and Its Diseases

59

Diseases of the Pericardium

Ralph Shabetai, M.D.

I think it to have been made by nature to prevent the heart from becoming completely dry. So the wounds of Christ exuded water along with blood.

William Harvey[1]

This statement appears in the Prelectiones of the great William Harvey in reference to Chapter 19, verse 34, of the gospel of St. John in which we read that when Christ's side was pierced on the Cross by the centurion's lance "came thereout blood and water."

Anatomy of the Pericardium

The pericardium consists of a tough, fibrous outer coat with discrete attachments to the sternum, great vessels, and diaphragm, and an inner membranous coat. The fibrous coat is lined by a serosal layer of cuboidal cells one layer thick. Together, the fibrous pericardium and its serosal membrane comprise the parietal pericardium. The serosal membrane is reflected over the epicardial surface of the heart, together with which it forms the visceral pericardium. The pericardial cavity is enclosed between these two serosal layers and normally contains from 15 to 50 ml of clear fluid,[2] which is an ultrafiltrate of blood plasma.[3] The pericardium has a number of recesses, the most important of which is the oblique sinus. The left atrium lies anterior to the oblique sinus and is, strictly speaking, largely an extrapericardial chamber. This relationship explains why pericardial effusion behind the posterior wall of the left ventricle is usually not seen also behind the left atrium.

The phrenic nerves are embedded in the parietal pericardium, explaining diaphragmatic paralysis when the phrenic nerves are injured when opening the pericardium.

The superior and inferior pericardiosternal ligaments attach the pericardium to the sternum. Ligaments also attach the pericardium firmly to the diaphragm. The connective tissue of the pericardium becomes contiguous with the adventitia of the great vessels to provide the superior tether. These attachments maintain the heart in its normal position and are so arranged that external forces exerted on the pericardium by respiration or changes in body posture tend to cancel each other and maintain the heart position constant.[4]

Histology

The major constituent of the parietal pericardium is the fibrosa, the chief ingredient of which is compactly arranged collagen fibers disposed in three layers oriented approximately at equal angles to each other.[4] The collagen bundles have an accordion-like appearance. The elastin fibers are much less numerous, do not occur in dense bundles, and tend to be oriented at right angles to adjacent collagen fibers. The predominance of collagen and its anatomical configuration are important in the viscoelastic properties of pericardium.

Ultrastructure

Scanning electron micrographs disclose that the pericardium is far from being an inert mass of connective tissue, but rather is highly organized with microvilli and cilia for production and absorption of fluid and facilitation of movement of the serosal surfaces over each other.[5]

Mechanical (Viscoelastic) Properties of the Pericardium

The pressure-volume curve of the pericardium is characterized by an initial flat portion during which volume is increased with little or no change in pressure, followed by a "knee" leading to the final portion, during which pressure rapidly increases with little or no increase in volume[6] (Fig. 59-1). Normal pericardial pressure is subatmospheric and thus several millimeters of mercury lower than the pressure in the atria and the ventricular diastolic pressures, indicating that although the pericardium appears to fit the heart quite snugly, the heart is not normally engaged by the pericardium. There is appreciable day-to-day and moment-to-moment variation in cardiac volume, but the pericardial volume exceeds cardiac volume by perhaps 10 to 20 percent, the difference constituting the pericardial reserve volume that allows physiological changes in cardiac volume to occur without restriction by the pericardium.

The pericardium limits or prevents acute pathological distension of the heart once the pericardial reserve volume has been used up and the pericardium is stretched. The pericardium has then reached the steep portion of its pressure-volume relation and the wavy bundles of pericardium have straightened out and become inextensible. The stress-strain curve of excised pericardium is similar to the pressure-volume curve of the whole pericardium.[7] Most observers consider the pericardium anisotropic, a finding that can be explained by the directionality of the collagen bundles. The pericardium stretches more in the short than the long axis of the heart and this anisotropy persists after the pericardial attachments are cut.

When the pericardium is subjected to constant stretch over a period of time the tension in it drops (creep). Creep allows for slight relief of pericardial pressure in acute cardiac tamponade. It has been suggested that with growth of the heart, the collagen fibers are rearranged within the intracellular substance, allowing the pericardium to creep and so adapt to the increased cardiac size,[8] but the magnitude of creep is unlikely to be sufficient to account for this adaptation. Instead, in response to chronic cardiac enlargement, the pericardium undergoes hypertrophy and becomes more compliant.[9]

Normal Pericardial Fluid: Amount and Turnover

As little as 15 ml of pericardial fluid can be detected by echocardiography.[10] On the other hand, the average amount of pericardial fluid found routinely at autopsy of patients free from pericardial and cardiac disease averages 50 ml.[1]

There are no published data on the turnover of normal human pericardial fluid, but in patients with pericardial effusion, it was noted that losses of albumin from the pericardial cavity averaged 1.86 g/day. The albumin disappeared from the pericardial cavity exponentially and accumulated in corresponding concentration in the blood.[11] The membrane characteristics of the pericardium favor removal over accumulation of fluid.[12] Erythrocytes labeled with a radiopharmaceutical can be detected in the peripheral blood within a few hours but it may take several days for all the cells to be absorbed.

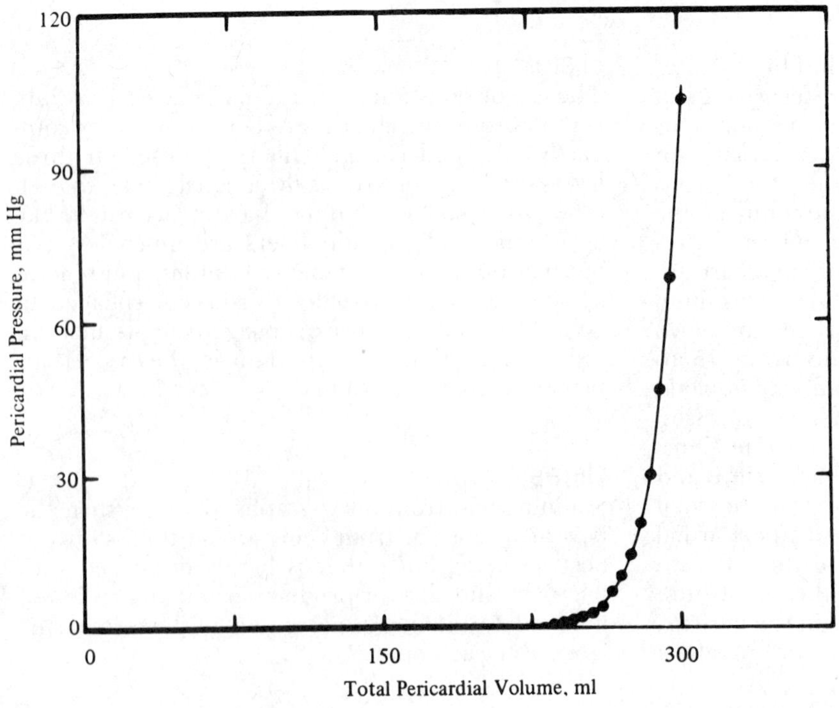

FIGURE 59-1 Pericardial pressure-volume curve (canine). (*From J. P. Holt: The Normal Pericardium, Am. J. Cardiol., 26:455, 1970. Reproduced with permission from the publisher and author.*)

Pericardial Pressure

Pericardial pressure measured by a catheter in the pericardial cavity is subatmospheric and essentially equal to pleural pressure throughout the respiratory cycle.[13] Superimposed on the large respiratory fluctuations of pericardial pressure are smaller fluctuations related to the events of the cardiac cycle, pericardial pressure being lowest during ventricular ejection. Liquid pressure within the pericardial cavity is lower than pericardial surface pressure measured by an intrapericardial balloon which may give a more accurate estimate of pericardial restraint on the heart.[14]

Functions of the Pericardium

Numerous experiments have demonstrated that the pericardium restrains cardiac volume, yet no adverse consequences follow congenital absence or surgical removal of the pericardium. The thin-walled right ventricle and atrium are more subject to the influence of the pericardium than the more resistant thick-walled left ventricle.[15] Interactions among the cardiac chambers, especially in diastole, but also in systole, are more pronounced with the pericardium intact.[16]

The pericardium exerts a powerful restraining effect on the size of the heart in situations of acute volume overload, particularly those that involve all four cardiac chambers, but the role of the pericardium in normal physiology and in chronic cardiac enlargement remains controversial. Conventional *liquid* pressure within the pericardium suggests that pericardial influence on the heart in these circumstances is small,[17] but pericardial *surface* pressure measured by an intrapericardial balloon, suggests that pericardial restraint may be important in chronic heart failure in which right atrial pressure may closely approximate intrapericardial pressure.[14] However, the few attempts to treat congestive heart failure by pericardiectomy have not met with resounding success.

Pericardial pressure is strongly influenced by the intrathoracic pressure, which must be kept normal or be measured when measuring ventricular diastolic compliance.

Other Pericardial Functions

The pericardium maintains the heart in a relatively fixed position and functionally optimal shape within the mediastinum. The thin layer of pericardial fluid reduces friction on the epicardium and equalizes gravitational forces over the surface of the heart; transmural cardiac pressures, therefore, do not change during acceleration or differ regionally within cardiac chambers.[18] Negative pressure in the pericardium augments atrial filling during ventricular systole. The pericardium acts as a barrier to inflammation from contiguous structures, and may buttress the thinner portions of the myocardium.

Acute Viral and Idiopathic Pericarditis

Like the squeak of leather on a new saddle under a rider, or grating in the knee joint on moving the patella over the femoral condyles.

V. Collin[19]

Acute fibrinous or dry pericarditis is a syndrome associated with characteristic chest pain, pericardial friction rub, and specific ECG changes. A great variety of conditions are associated with acute pericarditis (Table 59-1). The following description refers to viral and idiopathic pericarditis without significant effusion. Viral infection is often presumed rather than proven, many cases being classified as idiopathic. Common viral infections causing acute pericarditis are those due to echovirus and coxsackievirus.

Pathology

The acute fibrinous deposits give rise to the characteristic bread-and-butter appearance of the pericardium described by Laennec: "the knobbed appearance of this exudation is very like what would result from the sudden separation of two pieces of slab joined by a pretty thick layer of butter." In addition to fibrin deposition the usual changes of acute inflammation are found.[20]

History

There may be a prodromal phase characterized by fever and myalgia. The characteristic symptom is chest pain, the nature of which varies appreciably among patients, and perhaps with etiology. In some cases the pain is indistinguishable from that of myocardial infarction; in others it strongly simulates pleurisy. Often the pain of acute pericarditis lies between the extremes, being retrosternal without radiation to the arms but exacerbated by respiration. Characteristically, pericardial pain is relieved by sitting up, and a typical, although not common, radiation is to the trapezius ridge.

Physical Examination

The characteristic physical finding of acute pericarditis is the pericardial friction rub which is superficial, scratchy, or creaky, and heard anywhere or everywhere over the precordium, but most commonly between the lower left sternal edge and the cardiac apex. Pericardial friction rubs are usually best appreciated with the diaphragm of the stethoscope applied firmly and with respiration suspended. In some patients they are best heard in the sitting position. Most pericardial friction rubs are independent of the respiratory cycle, but on occasion they are louder during inspiration. The classic

TABLE 59-1 Etiology of Pericarditis*

I. Trauma
- *A.* Pericardiotomy
- *B.* Indirect trauma to chest
- *C.* Transeptal catheterization
- *D.* Pressure injection of contrast media
- *E.* Perforation of right ventricle by indwelling catheter
- *F.* Implantation of epicardial pacemaker
- *G.* Blow to chest
- *H.* Perforation of right ventricle with catheter for parenteral nutrition

II. Viral infections
- *A.* Coxsackie B5, B6
- *B.* Echovirus
- *C.* Adenovirus
- *D.* Infectious mononucleosis
- *E.* Influenza
- *F.* Lymphogranuloma venereum
- *G.* Chickenpox
- *H.* *Mycoplasma pneumoniae*

III. Bacterial infections
- *A.* *Staphylococcus*
- *B.* Pneumococcus
- *C.* Meningococcus
- *D.* *Streptococcus*
- *E.* *Haemophilus influenzae*
- *F.* Psittacosis
- *G.* *Salmonella*
- *H.* Tuberculosis

IV. Amebiasis

V. Echinococcus cysts

VI. Fungus infections—histoplasmosis, aspergillosis, blastomycosis, coccidioidomycosis

VII. *Rickettsia*

VIII. Radiation

IX. Amyloidosis

X. Tumors
- *A.* Primary
  - 1. Mesothelioma
    - *a.* Rhabdomyosarcoma
    - *b.* Teratoma
    - *c.* Fibroma
    - *d.* Leiomyofibroma
    - *e.* Lipoma
    - *f.* Angioma
  - 2. Metastatic
    - *a.* Bronchogenic carcinoma
    - *b.* Carcinoma of breast
    - *c.* Lymphoma
    - *d.* Leukemia
    - *e.* Melanoma
- *B.* Sarcoid
  - 1. Collagen disease
    - *a.* Rheumatic fever
    - *b.* Lupus erythematosus
    - *c.* Rheumatoid arthritis
    - *d.* Vasculitis
    - *e.* Polyarteritis nodosa
    - *f.* Scleroderma
    - *g.* Dermatomyositis

XI. Anticoagulants
- *A.* Heparin
- *B.* Coumadin

XII. Myocardial infarction—post-myocardial infarction pericarditis (Dressler's syndrome)

XIII. Idiopathic thrombocytopenic purpura

XIV. Drugs
- *A.* Procainamide
- *B.* Cromolyn sodium
- *C.* Hydralazine
- *D.* Dantrolene
- *E.* Methysergide

XV. Dissecting aneurysm

XVI. Infective endocarditis (SBE) with valve ring abscess

XVII. Thymic cyst

*Principal causes of pericardial disease and pericardial heart disease. Most can cause pericardial effusion, cardiac tamponade, and/or constrictive pericarditis. The commoner causes of these syndromes are mentioned under the syndromes and under specific disorders.

pericardial friction rub is triphasic with components in atrial systole, ventricular systole, and ventricular diastole,[21] but frequently the rub is biphasic, and occasionally there is only a single component. Pericardial friction, especially when of uremic origin, may be palpable. The triphasic pericardial friction rub is virtually unmistakable, but biphasic rubs must be distinguished from the to-and-fro murmur of aortic valve disease, and monophasic rubs are often mistaken for systolic murmurs. In the differential diagnosis one must consider, in addition to cardiac murmurs, mediastinal crunch and artifacts produced by rubbing of the skin against the stethoscope.

Pericardial friction rubs vary in intensity from hour to hour and day to day, sometimes transiently disappearing altogether. Pericardial fluid does not prevent the rub.

Depending upon etiology, there may be fever and other signs of inflammation or systemic illness. Atrial arrhythmias, perhaps owing to the subepicardial location of the sinus node,[22] may be observed but are rare in the absence of concomitant heart disease.[23]

Electrocardiogram

Electrocardiographic changes of acute pericarditis evolve through four stages.[24] In the first, which occurs within hours or days of the onset of pericarditis, there is widespread ST-segment elevation, commonly involving all three standard limb leads and most of the precordial leads. Reciprocal depression is usually found in leads aV_R and V_1. ST-segment elevation seldom reaches 5 mm and monophasic patterns are not seen. In some cases the PR segment is depressed[25] (Fig. 59-2), a useful sign in

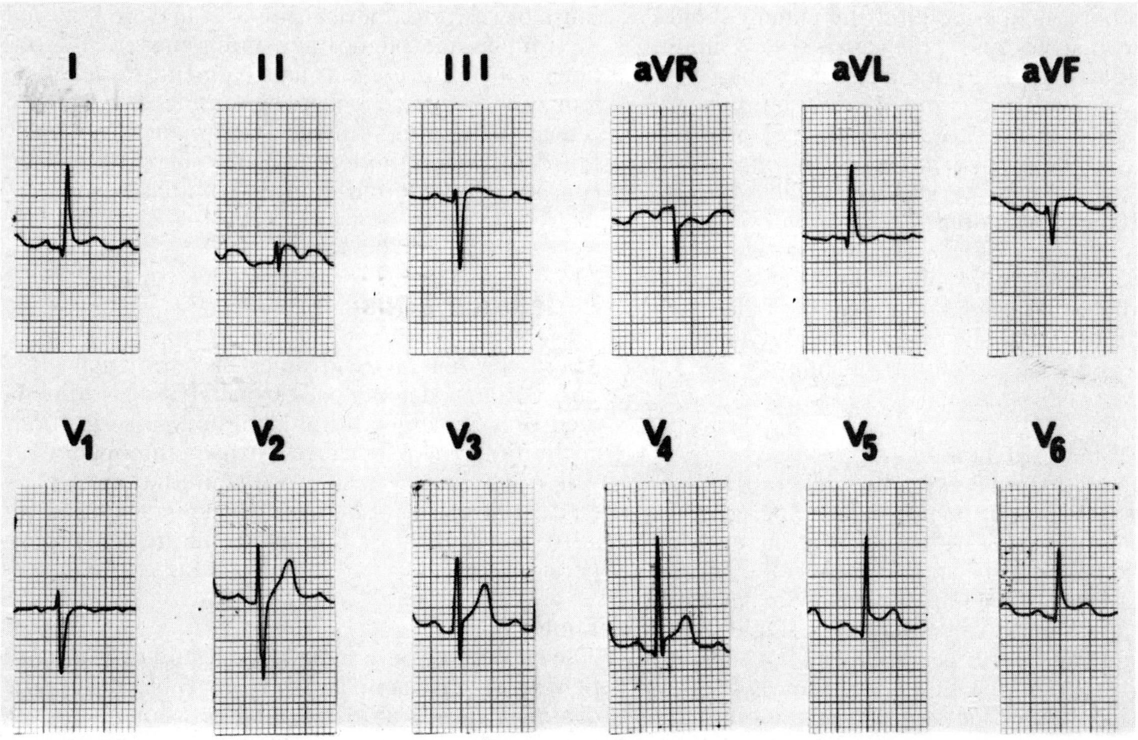

FIGURE 59-2 Electrocardiogram in acute pericarditis showing PR-segment depression and ST-segment elevation. (*From R. Shabetai, "The Pericardium," Grune & Stratton, New York, p. 359, 1981. Reproduced with permission from the publisher and author.*)

differentiating acute pericarditis from early repolarization variants.[26] During the succeeding several days the ST and PR segments return toward isoelectric and the electrocardiogram becomes normal (stage 2). There may be no further progression, but the T waves may become inverted (stage 3). Abnormal T waves may be permanent, or the electrocardiogram may revert to normal for a second time (stage 4).

ST-segment elevation in acute pericarditis can usually be distinguished from that of acute myocardial infarction by the absence of Q waves, the upwardly concave ST segments, and the absence of associated T-wave inversion. During evolution, the electrocardiogram of acute myocardial infarction does not pass through a normal pattern before T-wave inversion occurs. The acute ST-segment elevation of Prinzmetal's variant of angina is more transitory and is associated with transient ischemic pain. The early repolarization variant which is common in young individuals, especially blacks and athletes, and among patients in psychiatric institutions, may simulate the ECG of acute pericarditis. In these cases PR-segment depression is not seen and the ECG pattern does not evolve in a manner consistent with pericarditis.

Other Laboratory Findings

The erythrocyte sedimentation rate is almost always elevated. Leukocytosis is present early but, depending on etiology, may give way to lymphocytosis. Cardiac enzymes are usually normal, but may be elevated when there is extensive epicarditis. The results of pyrophosphate and gallium scintigrams may be positive when there is associated myocarditis.[27]

ECG changes in acute pericarditis imply inflammation of the epicardium. The epicardium is frequently spared in uremic pericarditis in which fibrin deposition may be extensive while inflammatory changes are minimal. In these cases ECG signs of pericarditis do not occur. The occurrence of first degree heart block or bundle branch block suggests more widespread myocarditis.

In the absence of pericardial effusion or severe myocarditis the echocardiogram and the chest radiograph remain normal. Computerized tomography is seldom resorted to, but in difficult cases can be relied upon to demonstrate the thickened and inflamed pericardium.[28]

Differential Diagnosis

The early stages of acute pericarditis may be confused with acute myocardial infarction. In cases of doubt the issue is clarified over the subsequent 24 to 36 h by the clinical course and serial changes in the ECG and the plasma level of cardiac enzymes. Dissecting hematoma of the aorta may be misdiagnosed as pericarditis, or may cause pericarditis.

Treatment

When acute pericarditis is of known etiology it may respond to treatment of the underlying cause. For viral and idiopathic pericarditis, the patient should be given an analgesic and if the pain is severe should be confined to bed. The patient should be observed for pericardial effusion and cardiac tamponade. Usually aspirin suffices for the control of pain but it may have to be given every 3 or 4 h for the first 48 h. The pain of acute pericarditis usually responds to 25 to 100 mg of indomethacin given every 4 h. Ibuprofen (Motrin), 400 mg four times a day, is also effective. Corticosteroids should not be given unless it is clear that nonsteroidal treatment has failed, and when resorted to must be tapered and discontinued as rapidly as the clinical course will allow.

Recurrent Pericarditis

One of the most troublesome disorders of the pericardium is relapsing or recurrent acute pericarditis. This may occur with or without pericardial effusion and occasionally is associated with pleural effusions or parenchymal pulmonary lesions. Why in some instances acute pericarditis may be a single illness and in others may recur is not known, but this phenomenon suggests that in some instances at least, acute pericarditis is, or sets up, an autoimmune process.

The course may extend over many years[30] with numerous recurrences which may be spontaneous, but more commonly are associated with discontinuing or reducing the dose of anti-inflammatory agents. When associated with pericardial effusion, relapsing pericarditis can cause cardiac tamponade.

Treatment

Recurrences are usually so severe that treatment must be given; quite commonly chest discomfort, fever, or dyspnea are not controlled by large doses of nonsteroidal drugs, but yield only to steroids. Once steroids are administered there is real danger of dependency and development of steroid-induced abnormalities.[29] When the physician is forced to use steroids every effort must be made to establish the minimal dose that will control pericarditis. In very ill patients, predisone is begun at a high dose such as 60 mg/day, but within a few days of clinical resolution, rapid tapering must be begun. Tapering may be easier when steroids are combined with nonsteroidal agents and when they are given on alternate days. In the most difficult cases relapses occur every time the dose of predisone is reduced below 5 to 10 mg/day. When this occurs the patient should be maintained for several weeks on the lowest suppressive dose. Occasionally, steroid-resistant cases respond to immunosuppressive treatment, but this too is undesirable and should be avoided except as a last resort. When treatment with steroids and perhaps azathioprine has failed after several years to produce permanent remission (there are no reports of cyclosporine treatment) pericardiectomy may be considered. It must, however, be recognized that pericardiectomy may abbreviate rather than end the cause of relapsing pericarditis and may be followed by troublesome pleural and pulmonary manifestations that require vigorous treatment. Pericardiectomy is therefore a resort to be considered only when repeated attempts at medical treatment have clearly failed and when there is evidence or well-grounded concern about steroid-induced complications.

Pericardial Effusion

There are several syndromes of pericardial effusion. At one extreme, pericardial effusion is discovered only during routine laboratory investigation; at the other, it may cause cardiac tamponade. Effusion may be the principal manifestation of pericardial disease or may be an incidental finding in acute pericarditis, or it may complicate constrictive pericarditis.

Etiology

The etiology of pericardial disease and by inference pericardial effusion, is given in Table 59-1. The common causes of pericardial effusion are acute pericarditis (viral or idiopathic), neoplastic (usually bronchogenic, mammary, or lymphoma), postradiation, and posttraumatic. Somewhat less common are pericardial effusions induced by drugs and occurring with collagen vascular diseases, particularly rheumatoid arthritis and lupus erythematosus. Pericardial effusion is an important component of the postpericardiotomy syndrome and many cases of Dressler's syndrome.

Diagnosis

There are no specific symptoms. Likewise, clinical signs such as a quiet precordium, an increased area of cardiac dullness, and cardiac dullness percussable beyond the apex beat are so nonspecific and so rarely employed that the diagnosis of pericardial effusion has become a matter of knowing when to suspect it and confirm its presence by echocardiography. On occasion, pericardial effusion is found by chance on the chest radiograph, a radionucleotide ventriculogram, an echocardiogram, or during cardiac catheterization.

Pericardial effusion must be kept in mind whenever a patient with a disorder that may affect the pericardium is encountered, and it should be strongly suspected in such patients when there is evidence of pericardial involvement. Particularly suspect are patients with cancer of the lung or breast, patients undergoing hemodialysis, patients with unexplained enlargement of the cardiopericardial silhouette and patients with unexplained increased venous pressure.

The most specific and sensitive test is echocardiography,[31] which should be performed whenever there is a reasonable suspicion of a pericardial effusion. Pericardial liquid appears on the M-mode echocardiogram as an echo-free space. In smaller effusions the echo-free space is behind the left ventricle, but larger effusions are associated with an additional space in front of the right ventricle (Fig. 59-3). Two-dimensional echocardiography serves to further quantify the amount and distribution of pericardial effusion,[32] and also may demonstrate fibrinous adhesions.[33] Echocardiography may also indicate whether the pericardium is thickened. When analyzing the echocardiogram of a patient with pericardial effusion one can estimate, by determining the dimensions of the cardiac chambers, whether apparent enlargement of the heart can be entirely accounted for by pericardial effusion, or whether there is underlying enlargement of the heart itself. By assessing wall motion one can determine whether there is underlying heart failure.

Silent Pericardial Effusion

Routine echocardiography[34] has shown that silent pericardial effusions are common,[35] especially in hemodialysis patients. Similarly, echocardiography reveals pericardial effusion in a significant proportion of patients with clinically dry pericarditis.

It is possible to estimate the size of a pericardial effusion by echocardiography,[36] but for clinical purposes it is only necessary to separate small, moderate, and large effusions. Small effusions are detected by an echo-free space confined to the area behind the left ventricle, and are not associated with an anterior clear space or enlargement of the cardiac silhouette. Moderate effusions are characterized by a posterior echo-free space larger than a centimeter and with an anterior space, especially during systole. Cardiac enlargement may not be apparent with chest radiography unless earlier films are available for comparison. Massive effusions are associated with great enlargement of the cardiopericardial silhouette and large echo-free spaces around the heart throughout the cardiac cycle.

Technique

To identify pericardial effusion by M mode, the controls are adjusted to damp out all cardiac structures except the pericardium and are then adjusted to display in addition the epicardium, myocardium, and endocardium.[37] Normal structures and spaces may mimic pericardial effusion;[38,39] these include the space between vertebrae and myocardium, the gap between papillary muscle and free wall, pleural effusion,[40] cyst, hematoma (especially postoperative), giant left atrium,[40] calcified mitral valve annulus,[41] and tumors.[42] Two-dimensional echocardiography allows better identification of normal and abnormal structures with corresponding reduction of false-positive diagnosis.[43]

Chest radiography is not specific. There is overall enlargement of the cardiac silhouette and the lung fields are less congested than in cardiac failure. However, this combination is difficult to distinguish from four-chamber cardiac enlargement with tricuspid regurgitation. Rarely, the pericardium and

FIGURE 59-3 M-mode echocardiogram showing moderate pericardial effusion. Pericardial fluid is present anteriorly (PE) and posteriorly (PPE). RVW = right ventricular wall; IVS = interventricular septum; endo = endocardium; epi = epicardium; MV = mitral valve, LA = left atrium. (*From R. Shabetai, "The Pericardium," Grune & Stratton, New York, 1981. Reproduced with permission from the publisher and author.*)

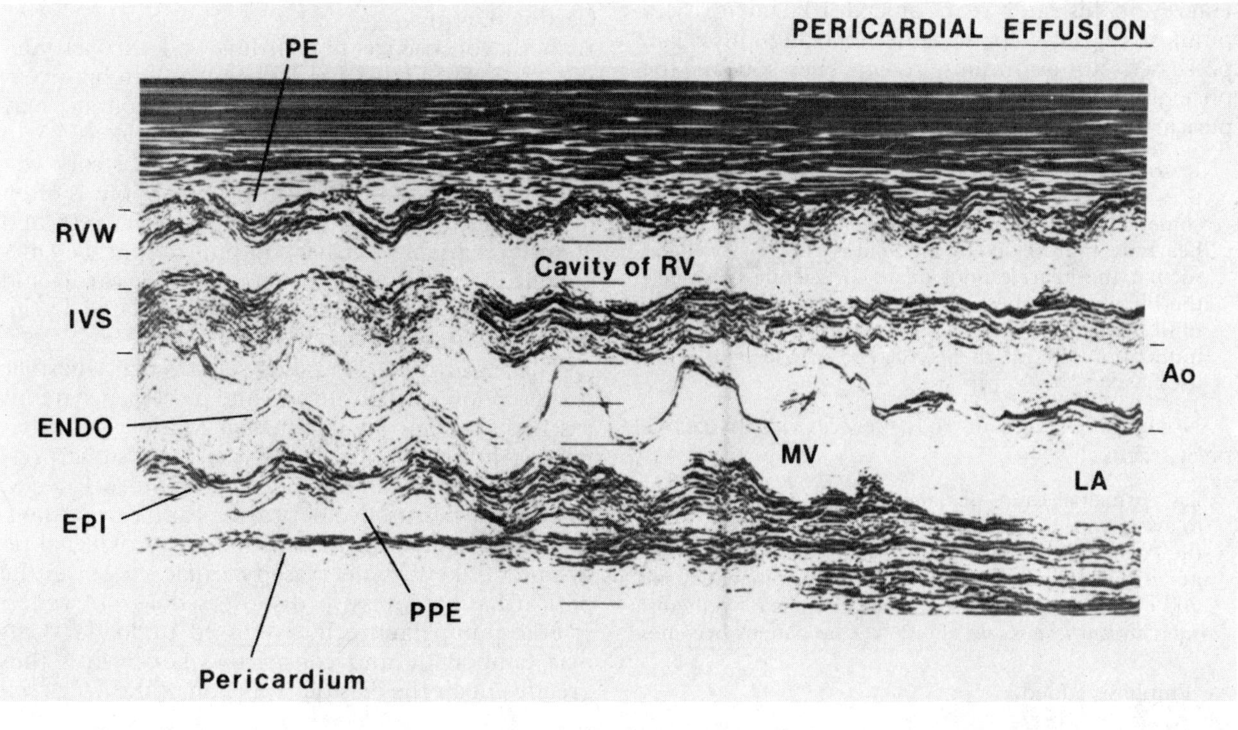

cardiac edge can be distinguished as separate shadows along the left heart border.[44]

Nature of the Fluid

In certain situations it is mandatory to determine the nature of the pericardial fluid. In patients with neoplastic disease it is necessary to determine whether pericardial effusion indicates invasion of the pericardium or a postradiation phenomenon. In cases of bacterial or other nonviral infections it becomes necessary to discover whether the pericardial effusion is an exudate and to culture pericardial fluid; suspected tuberculous pericarditis is a case in point. The presence of blood in pericardial fluid is less ominous than in pleural or peritoneal fluid, since it may be found in pericardial effusions of almost any etiology, including viral and idiopathic pericarditis.

There are clinical situations in which it is unnecessary to obtain pericardial fluid for analysis; for example, when pericardial effusion is found in a patient with typical viral or idiopathic pericarditis, pericardiocentesis should not be considered unless the effusion fails to respond to anti-inflammatory treatment or cardiac tamponade develops. Likewise, when a patient undergoing chronic hemodialysis develops pericardial effusion, pericardial fluid need be obtained only when the clinical course suggests a different etiology or when there is suspicion of hemodynamic embarrassment.

The Pericardial Compressive Syndromes

Richard Lower (1631–1691), a colleague of William Harvey in his later years at Oxford University, a pulmonary physiologist and practicing physician, possessed an astonishing comprehension of the physiology of cardiac tamponade and constrictive pericarditis. In 1669, he wrote:

> It sometimes happens that a profuse effusion oppresses and inundates the heart. The envelope becomes filled in hydrops of the heart; the walls of the heart are compressed by the fluid circling everywhere, so that the heart cannot dilate sufficiently to receive the blood; then the pulse becomes exceedingly small, until finally it becomes utterly suppressed by the great inundation of fluid, thence succeed syncope and death itself.[45]

Norman Chevers in 1842 described constrictive pericarditis:

> The principal cause of dangerous symptoms appears to arise from the occurrence of gradual contraction in the layers of adhesive matter which have been deposited around the heart, compressing its muscular tissue and embarrassing its systolic and diastolic movements, *but more particularly the latter** . . . the patient becomes incapable of continued muscular exertion and always liable to suffer from dropsy and other serous effusions.[46]

*Emphasis added.

Pathophysiology of Compression of the Heart by the Pericardium

Constrictive pericarditis, cardiac tamponade, and restrictive cardiomyopathy are three conditions which restrict diastolic filling. Impaired cardiac filling is manifested by reduced ventricular volumes, elevated ventricular diastolic pressure, and reduced diastolic compliance. Secondarily, cardiac output is reduced.[47]

In both cardiac tamponade and constrictive pericarditis, the heart is surrounded by either pericardial fluid under increased pressure or by a noncompliant scar which prevents the heart from attaining its normal diastolic dimensions. The generalized nature of compression by constrictive pericarditis or cardiac tamponade equilibrates the filling pressures of the two sides of the heart. In both conditions left ventricular and right ventricular diastolic pressures are equal to each other and to the pressure in both atria. Cardiac compression rarely induces reactive pulmonary hypertension, therefore the pulmonary arterial diastolic pressure is the same as the common ventricular filling pressure.

Central Venous Pressure

When the filling pressure of the right ventricle is increased by pericardial fluid or constrictive pericarditis, the central venous pressure must increase if circulation is to be maintained. The diagnosis of significant constriction or tamponade is not tenable when the central venous pressure is normal.

Cardiac Output

In both constrictive pericarditis and cardiac tamponade cardiac output is reduced, and in both conditions left ventricular end-diastolic volume may be diminished,[7,48] sometimes to as little as 25 to 30 ml/M^2, which is less than the normal stroke volume. Compensatory tachycardia ensues but is often insufficient to maintain cardiac output at rest, and almost invariably cardiac output cannot be adequately increased during exercise. Tachycardia and elevated vascular resistance[49] are mediated by increased sympathetic tone.[50]

The syndrome of raised ventricular diastolic pressure, low cardiac output, and increased systemic vascular resistance mimic cardiac failure. In cardiac failure, however, raised ventricular diastolic pressure is a manifestation of myocardial insufficiency, whereas in constrictive pericarditis and cardiac tamponade it is an expression of increased external restraint.[47] Likewise, decreased cardiac output in the pericardial compressive disorders does not reflect systolic pump failure but reduced preload.[47] Cardiac tamponade and constrictive pericarditis thus greatly impair the diastolic function of the heart, but impairment of systolic performance, when it occurs, is a late manifestation.

The Differing Pathophysiology of Constrictive Pericarditis and Cardiac Tamponade

The similarities between constrictive pericarditis and cardiac tamponade are fundamental to understanding compressive disorders of the heart, but distinction between their pathophysiologies is crucial in understanding their respective clinical and laboratory findings.

In cardiac tamponade intrapericardial pressure is elevated and can be reliably measured. The elevated intrapericardial pressure is exerted on the heart throughout the cardiac cycle with slight momentary relief during ventricular ejection, when intrapericardial pressure falls a little as cardiac volume diminishes. In severe cardiac tamponade venous return is halted in diastole when cardiac volume and intrapericardial pressure are maximal (Fig. 59-4).

Normal cardiac filling is bimodal. A surge of venous return occurs at the onset of ventricular ejection marked by the *x* descent of venous pressure and a small drop in intrapericardial pressure; a second surge occurs in diastole when the tricuspid valve opens and the *y* descent is inscribed.[51] The venous return in cardiac tamponade is unimodal, confined to ventricular systole, and corresponds with the *x* descent of venous pressure[52] (Fig. 59-5).

The waveform of venous pressure in constrictive pericarditis differs from that of cardiac tamponade. In constrictive pericarditis, cardiac volume is set by the pericardial scar and under no circumstances can the heart exceed this set volume, which is attained near the end of the first third of diastole (Fig. 59-4). During ejection there is little impediment to venous return, and therefore the normal systolic surge of venous return and *x* descent of venous pressure are preserved. Cardiac compression is still insignificant at end systole, so that when the tricuspid valve opens, blood rushes into the ventricles at a supranormal rate, registering a precipitous *y* descent of venous pressure. Thus, as in normal physiology, in constrictive pericarditis venous return is bimodal, but the diastolic surge and *y* descent are equal to or greater than the *x* descent and the systolic surge[52] (Fig. 59-4).

Respiratory Variation and Central Venous Pressure

In cardiac tamponade, the inspiratory fall in intrathoracic pressure is transmitted to the pericardial space. Thus, although intrapericardial pressure is elevated, it falls during inspiration almost as much as the pleural pressure, increasing transmural pericardial pressure (pericardial minus pleural pressure) only 1 or 2 mmHg.[53] The inspiratory drop in pericardial pressure is transmitted into the right heart chambers, so that despite the elevated intrapericardial pressure the normal inspiratory increase in systemic venous return is preserved.[53] In constrictive

FIGURE 59-4 Diagram illustrating differences between constrictive pericarditis and cardiac tamponade. In constrictive pericarditis the heart is not restricted at end systole, so the heart fills rapidly during early diastole, creating the dip of ventricular pressure and the *y* descent of atrial pressure. When cardiac volume reaches the limit set by the diseased pericardium, further filling cannot take place, creating the late plateau of ventricular diastolic pressure. Atrial filling is bimodal, so atrial pressure displays sharp *x* and *y* descents. In cardiac tamponade the heart is compressed throughout the cardiac cycle by the pressure of pericardial fluid. Pulsus paradoxus occurs, and the early diastolic dip of ventricular pressure and the *y* descent of atrial pressure are absent. In constrictive pericarditis early diastolic filling is abnormally rapid, but no filling occurs in mid- and late diastole.

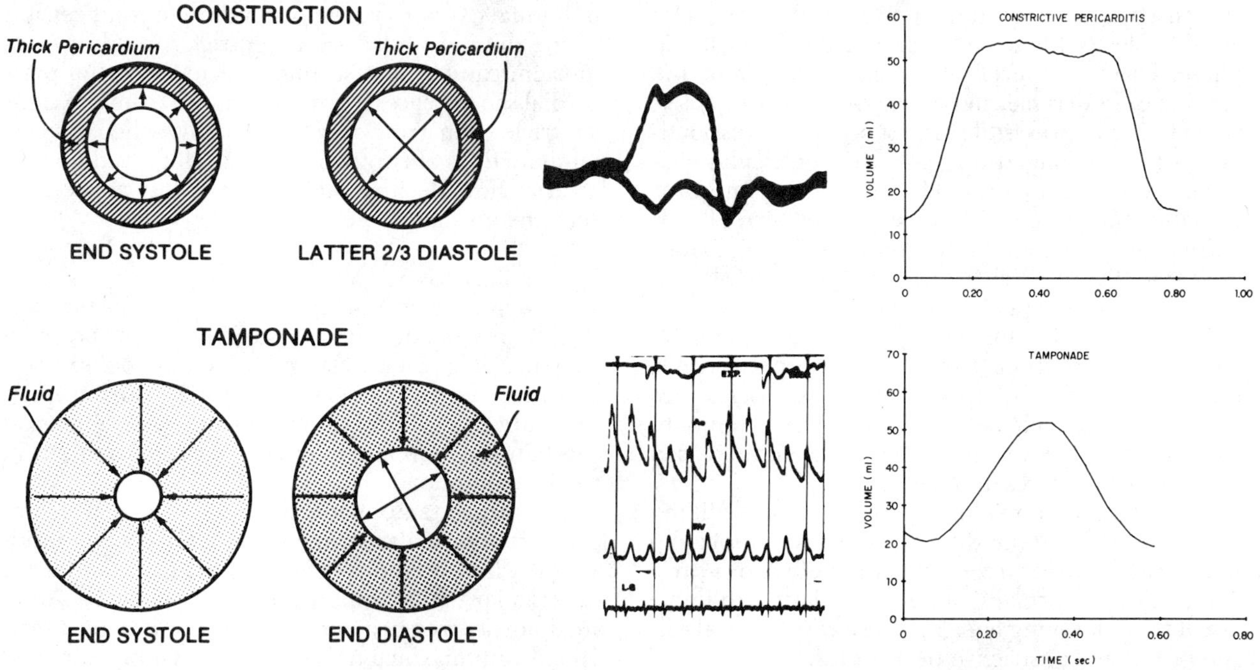

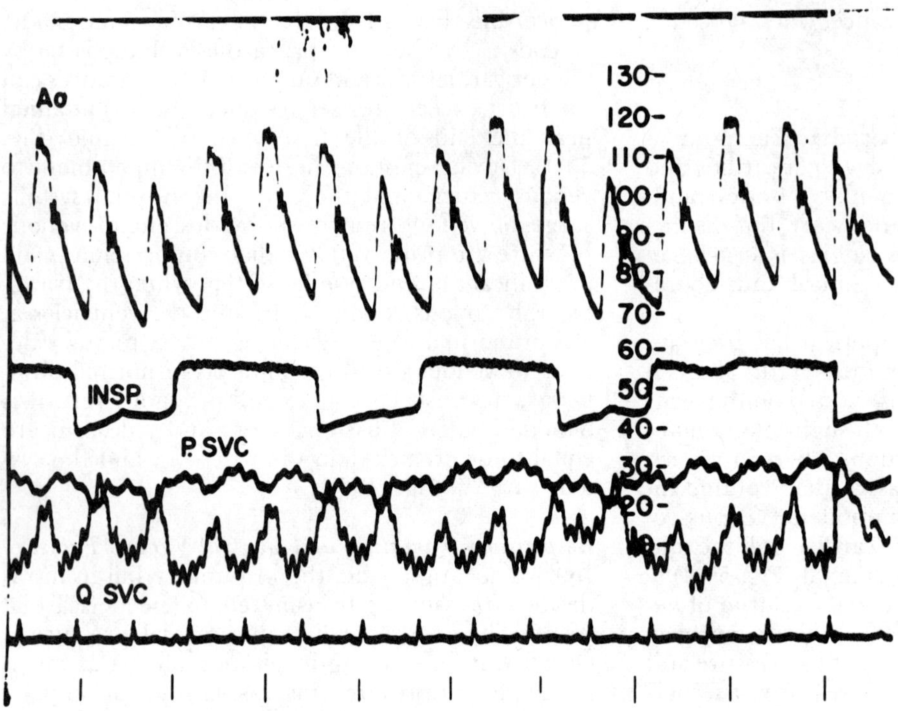

FIGURE 59-5 Cardiac catheterization of a patient with tamponade. From above, aortic pressure showing pulsus paradoxus, respiration, superior vena caval (SVC) pressure, and blood flow velocity. During inspiration (insp.) pressure declines and flow increases in the SVC. The SVC pressure shows a sharp *x* but no *y* descent. The SVC flow is monophasic, peaking at the *x* descent. SVC pressure (and pericardial pressure not shown) were 27 mmHg.

pericarditis, however, the intrapericardial space is obliterated; decreased intrathoracic pressure during inspiration is not transmitted to the heart, therefore venous pressure does not fall and systemic venous pressure fails to rise.

In constrictive pericarditis early diastolic filling is faster than normal; consequently the ventricular diastolic pressure is characterized by a dip in early diastole.[54] In normal physiology, the early diastolic filling period is followed by diastasis and a second period of rapid filling associated with atrial systole. In constrictive pericarditis, however, the ventricles are completely filled by the end of the rapid filling phase. Diastasis therefore persists throughout the remainder of diastole, and except in the mildest cases, rapid filling in presystole cannot occur. Corresponding to the prolonged diastasis, the ventricular diastolic pressure remains unchanged but elevated for the latter two-thirds of diastole. The pattern of ventricular diastolic pressure in constrictive pericarditis is frequently referred to as the "dip and plateau pattern" or the "square-root sign."

Small ventricles and impeded venous return favor filling by suction.[55] In constrictive pericarditis, the end-systolic volumes of the ventricles are reduced[52] and their recoil is rapid. The prominent early diastolic pressure dip may indicate increased suction during early diastole.

In cardiac tamponade, ventricular diastolic filling is reduced throughout diastole; an early diastolic dip in ventricular pressure, the *y* descent of venous pressure,[56] and abnormally rapid early diastolic filling[52] are absent, denoting a major pathophysiological difference from constrictive pericarditis.

Mechanism of Reduced Left Ventricular Volume in Cardiac Tamponade

The thick-walled left ventricle resists reduction of its volume by direct compression.[57] Several experimental observations support this idea. In dogs, when systemic venous return is diverted and returned by a pump at a slow rate to the right atrium, pericardial pressure can be raised to 20 mmHg without inducing pulmonary congestion or arterial hypotension.[53] This suggests that a major cause of reduced left ventricular volume in cardiac tamponade is decreased pulmonary venous return secondary to compression of the thinner-walled right ventricle. In fresh postmortem canine hearts, fluid injected into the pericardial sac displaces a greater volume from the right ventricle than from the left. Finally, when cardiac tamponade is abruptly induced in dogs, pulmonary arterial flow declines immediately, but aortic flow remains normal for several cardiac cycles.[57]

Pulsus Paradoxus

Pulsus paradoxus is an abnormally large inspiratory decline in systemic arterial systolic pressure and pulse pressure (Fig. 59-4). Normally, systolic blood pressure declines up to about 10 mmHg during quiet inspiration. A number of normal and abnormal mechanisms combine to create pulsus paradoxus in cardiac tamponade.

In cardiac tamponade systemic arterial pressure and left ventricular stroke volume fall during inspiration when pulmonary arterial pressure and right ventricular stroke volume increase.[58] However, minimal aortic pressure and flow do not exactly correspond with maximal pulmonary arterial pressure and flow. Rather, maximal pulmonary arterial pressure and flow precede maximal aortic pressure and flow by one to three beats.[59] This observation is not compatible with the hypothesis that competition between the two sides of the heart for fixed pericardial space is the sole cause of pulsus paradoxus in cardiac tamponade.[53] In normal dogs intrapleural and intrapericardial pressures fall equally during inspiration. However, in tamponade transmural pericardial pressure rises slightly with inspiration.[53] Inspiratory augmentation of systemic venous return in cardiac tamponade increases the volume of the right side of the heart at the expense of the left side. The volume of the left side of the heart may be decreased in part by bulging of the intraventricular septum from right to left[60] and in part by increased transmural pericardial pressure.

The hemodynamic effect of inspiration has been simulated by rapidly adding a small volume of blood to the venous return of dogs studied during apnea while the right side of the heart was supported by a constant flow pump.[53] When intrapericardial pressure was normal the addition of blood to the venous return caused an immediate increase in pulmonary arterial pressure, no immediate change in aortic pressure, but a later increase. Pericardial pressure did not increase. When the experiment was repeated in the presence of cardiac tamponade the sudden increase in systemic venous return was again followed by an early increase in pulmonary arterial pressure, but now there was a simultaneous increase in intrapericardial pressure and a drop in aortic pressure. Aortic pressure rose two or three beats later. This experiment confirms the importance of inspiratory expansion of the volume of the right side of the heart in the genesis of pulsus paradoxus when pericardial pressure is elevated.

In cardiac tamponade, pulsus paradoxus appears when both ventricles fill against a common resistance. Therefore, when left ventricular diastolic pressure is elevated by coexisting left ventricular disease, pulsus paradoxus does not develop in cardiac tamponade.[61] Atrial septal defect prevents reciprocal inspiratory changes in the filling of the two sides of the heart, and therefore in this condition too, cardiac tamponade can occur without pulsus paradoxus.[62] In patients with aortic incompetence cardiac tamponade may occur without pulsus paradoxus.

The increased volume of the right side of the heart in inspiration occurring when the pericardium is overstretched causes the ventricular septum to bulge to the left. This decreases left ventricular compliance at the same time that transmural pericardial pressure is increased. Pulmonary venous return is diminished and negative thoracic pressure is transmitted to the aorta, increasing left ventricular afterload. Two or three cardiac cycles following the inspiratory augmentation of right ventricular stroke volume, the augmented volume appears in the aorta, but by this time the respiratory phase has shifted to expiration. Finally, left ventricular stroke volume falls more sharply than normal in response to decreased ventricular filling in cardiac tamponade because the small ventricle is operating on the steep ascending limb of the Starling curve.[63] Additional factors including inspiratory traction by the diaphragm on the already taut pericardium,[64] reflex changes in vascular resistances and cardiac contractility,[65] and increased respiratory effort owing to pulmonary congestion modify the already complex effect of inspiration on aortic pressure in cardiac tamponade.

Pulsus paradoxus is much less common in constrictive pericarditis than in cardiac tamponade. This may be because in the former, inspiratory increase in venous return[53] and the volume of the right side of the heart seldom occur. When pulsus paradoxus does occur in constrictive pericarditis it may be because there is pericardial effusion in addition[66] or that its mechanism differs, inasmuch as the intrapericardial space is obliterated and the position of the ventricular septum relative to the two ventricles is not altered by respiration.[67]

Ventricular Function and Coronary Blood Flow

In constrictive pericarditis and cardiac tamponade systolic function usually is unimpaired.[47] Longstanding calcific constrictive pericarditis may invade the myocardium and coronary vessels, leading to conduction disturbances and impaired ventricular function.[68]

In cardiac tamponade ventricular function remains normal and is often supranormal. Unrelieved extreme tamponade is fatal because circulation ceases when venous pressure cannot increase to equal the pericardial pressure. Diminution of myocardial perfusion in these cases is aggravated by direct compression of the major coronary arteries[69] and abnormal transmyocardial distribution.[70]

Clinical Features of Cardiac Tamponade

Etiology

Virtually any disease that can affect the pericardium may cause pericardial effusion, and tamponade may complicate virtually any pericardial effusion. However, the common causes are few.

Acute tamponade is usually caused by trauma, which may be iatrogenic, or by rupture of the heart or aorta. The trauma may be penetrating or blunt. Rupture of the heart may occur during acute myocardial infarction, and rupture of the aorta may complicate aneurysm or dissecting hematoma. Iatrogenic injuries include perforation during cardiac catheterization or pacing, cardiac laceration during attempted pericardiocentesis, and contusion during resuscitation. Subacute cardiac tamponade occurs in a variety of conditions, of which the most common are idiopathic or viral pericarditis and neoplastic and dialysis-related pericardial disease.

Cardiac Tamponade Syndromes

Acute Cardiac Tamponade

Tamponade may be so sudden that symptoms are not complained of. In less drastic circumstances victims of chest trauma with cardiac tamponade may complain of severe shortness of breath accompanied by chest tightness. Occasionally, there is pericardial pain, but its characteristics are usually obscured by the pain of other injuries.

The venous pressure is greatly elevated and the systemic arterial pressure severely depressed. Pulsus paradoxus can be appreciated except when hypotension is extreme. When pulsus paradoxus is not obvious in the radial pulse, it may be detected in larger vessels. In striking contrast to these abnormalities of venous and arterial pressure, the precordium is quiet, cardiac activity often being impalpable (Beck's triad).[70] In the most severe cases, consciousness may be impaired; but for the raised venous pressure, such patients appear to be in shock.

When cardiac tamponade complicates a diagnostic procedure, the patient complains of discomfort, generalized uneasiness, and precordial pain. Systemic arterial pressure falls, pulsus paradoxus appears, venous pressure rises, and severe tissue hypoperfusion appears. Fluoroscopy shows that the cardiac silhouette has increased and that its pulsations have diminished or disappeared.

Cardiac tamponade should be suspected in any likely victim of recent chest trauma who appears in apparent shock. The suspicion is increased when venous pressure is high and pulsus paradoxus is present. When circumstances are at their most pressing an immediate therapeutic trial of rapid infusion of fluid and diagnostic pericardiocentesis should be carried out. If the threat of death is more remote, pericardiocentesis should be delayed until the presence of pericardial fluid can be demonstrated by prompt echocardiography, but when tamponade occurs in the diagnostic laboratory where pressures are being monitored and fluoroscopy is on hand, the diagnosis can be safely established without waiting for echocardiography.

Another cause of acute cardiac tamponade is cardiac rupture complicating acute myocardial infarction. This catastrophe must be differentiated from cardiogenic shock (see "Specific Pericardial Disorders").

Subacute Cardiac Tamponade

A disconcertingly large number of diseases can cause cardiac tamponade. The common ones, however, are idiopathic or viral pericarditis, neoplastic invasion of the pericardium, and nephrogenic pericardial disease.

Symptoms Symptoms may be divided into three categories: those of the underlying illness, those of the accompanying pericardial disease, and those of cardiac compression. Many patients with inflammatory pericarditis give a history of prodromal fever, myalgia, and arthralgia. Patients with neoplastic disease may have symptoms associated with the neoplasm itself and its treatment. In some patients there is pericardial pain similar to that of acute pericarditis, but this more often is absent. The symptoms of cardiac compression include rapidly progressive dyspnea accompanied by fullness or tightness in the chest, occasionally with dysphagia. The course may be less rapid, allowing time for increase in weight and abdominal girth, and the rapid onset and progression of edema.

Physical Examination The examination shows raised venous pressure and lowered systemic arterial pressure with pulsus paradoxus.[71] When there is underlying cardiac disease, the precordium may not be unusually quiet, the apex beat may be palpated, and even cardiac enlargement is not uncommon.[72]

The abnormalities of venous pressure described under "Pathophysiology of Compression of the Heart by the Pericardium" can often be recognized at the bedside. The mean pressure is elevated. When the patient's thorax and neck are placed at the elevation that maximizes the jugular venous pulsations, inspiratory decline in the height of pulsations can be appreciated. The *x* descent is recognized as an inward pulsation of the internal jugular pulse coincident with the carotid pulse. These abnormalities, together with equal diastolic pressures on the two sides of the heart and reduced ventricular volumes, can also be demonstrated by cardiac catheterization (Fig. 59-5). Catheterization, at least of the right side of the heart, with comparisons of right atrial and pulmonary wedge pressures should be carried out if there is doubt about the diagnosis, or if underlying heart disease is suspected. In the latter instance a full cardiac catheterization and angiographic procedure is required.[71]

Severe pulsus paradoxus is recognized as disappearance of the pulse at the height of inspiration. Less severe pulsus paradoxus is felt as a decrease in pulse amplitude during inspiration. Pulsus paradoxus is difficult to evaluate or may be absent when there is shock[73] and is confounded by labored rapid breathing, atrial fibrillation, and frequent extrasystoles. The severity of pulsus paradoxus can be estimated with the sphygmomanometer. The cuff must be deflated evenly and slowly while the patient's respirations are observed. In pulsus paradoxus, the Korotkov sound is initially heard only during expiration. As the cuff pressure falls, this sound becomes audible throughout the respiratory cycle. The difference in systolic pressure between these events is an estimate of pulsus paradoxus.

In some cases it is necessary to document venous and arterial pressure by intravenous recordings and this procedure should precede and accompany pericardiocentesis whenever possible. The inspiratory drop in systemic arterial systolic and pulse pressure can then be accurately quantified, and the *x* descent of venous pressure can be identified as coinciding with the QRS complex. The tracing verifies inspiratory decline in venous or right atrial pressure and absence or severe attenuation of the *y* descent.

Echocardiogram in Cardiac Tamponade The diagnosis of cardiac tamponade is seldom secure without echocardiographic demonstration of pericardial effusion. Only under exceptional circumstances should pericardial drainage be undertaken without prior echocardiography to document the effusion, and perhaps corroborate tamponade. Two-dimensional echocardiography has proven the value of compression of the right atrium[74] and diastolic collapse of the right ventricle[75] as evidence of cardiac tamponade. Less specific signs include exaggerated respiratory variation in ventricular dimensions[60] and the E-F slope of mitral valve closure[76] and pseudoprolapse of the mitral valve. More specific but less common is pendular swinging of the heart within the pericardial fluid.[77] This phenomenon can be recognized by M-mode studies, but is dramatically demonstrated by two-dimensional echocardiography and is frequently associated with electrical alternans.[78]

Electrocardiogram in Cardiac Tamponade Frequently, there are no diagnostic electrocardiographic findings. Electrical alternans of the P wave, QRS complex, and T wave is virtually specific for cardiac tamponade, but is uncommon. Alternation of the QRS complex alone is more common but less specific.[79] Pericardial fluid tends to lower QRS voltage and there may be associated abnormalities of the T waves[80] (Fig. 59-6).

Less Common Syndromes of Cardiac Tamponade

Low-Pressure Cardiac Tamponade Cardiac tamponade may develop when pericardial pressure is but modestly increased.[80a] The clinical picture is subtle. The venous pressure is increased only a few centimeters of water above normal, although inspection reveals absence or diminution of the *x* descent. The blood pressure is normal and pulsus paradoxus is not striking and may be absent. There may be no symptoms. Causes include severe dehydration, overly vigorous diuresis, and massive extrapericardial blood loss.

The diagnosis is made by keeping in mind the possibility of pericardial effusion in diseases which may reasonably involve the pericardium. Echocardiography can then confirm the effusion, and sometimes tamponade, and leads to examination of the neck veins. The diagnosis is established when catheterization of the right atrium and pericardial sac shows equal pressures, and hemodynamic improvement follows removal of pericardial fluid (Fig. 59-7).

Effusive Constrictive Pericarditis When the pericardium is scarred but also contains fluid under pressure, cardiac tamponade results. When the fluid is aspirated the features of constrictive pericarditis are unmasked.[66] This syndrome may occur in tuberculous pericarditis and in patients undergoing hemodialysis (see "Constrictive Pericarditis").

Cardiac Tamponade and Preexisting Heart Disease A commonly encountered example of cardiac tamponade modified by preexisting cardiac abnormalities is furnished by the hemodialysis population, in whom hypertrophy, fibrosis, and decreased compliance of the left ventricle are common.[81] The venous pressure may be affected by abnormalities unrelated to the pericardium; hypertension is common and cardiac output may be elevated by anemia and the access shunt. A third or fourth heart sound, cardiac murmurs, cardiac enlargement, and a left ventricular heave may be found in spite of cardiac tamponade. The electrocardiogram frequently shows ischemic or hypertensive myocardial disease which obscures the findings of pericardial disease. The echocardiogram discloses enlargement and impaired function of the cardiac chambers in addition to the pericardial effusion. Furthermore, pulsus

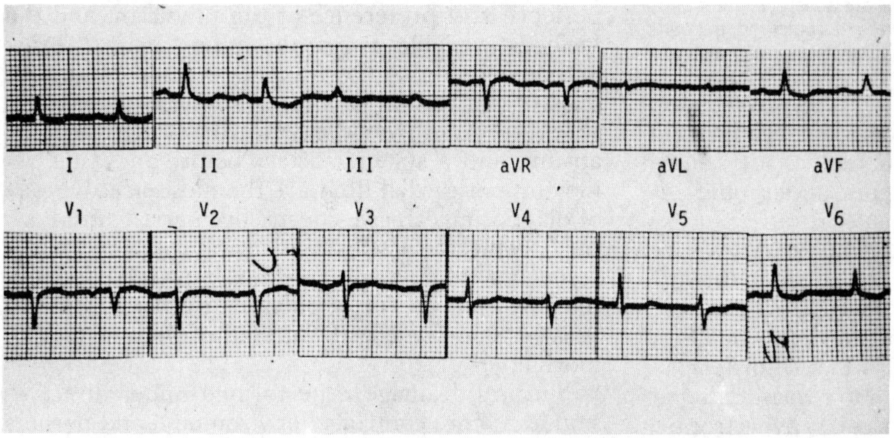

FIGURE 59-6 Alternans of QRS in cardiac tamponade. (*From R. Shabetai, "The Pericardium," Grune & Stratton, New York, 1981. Reproduced with permission from the publisher and author.*)

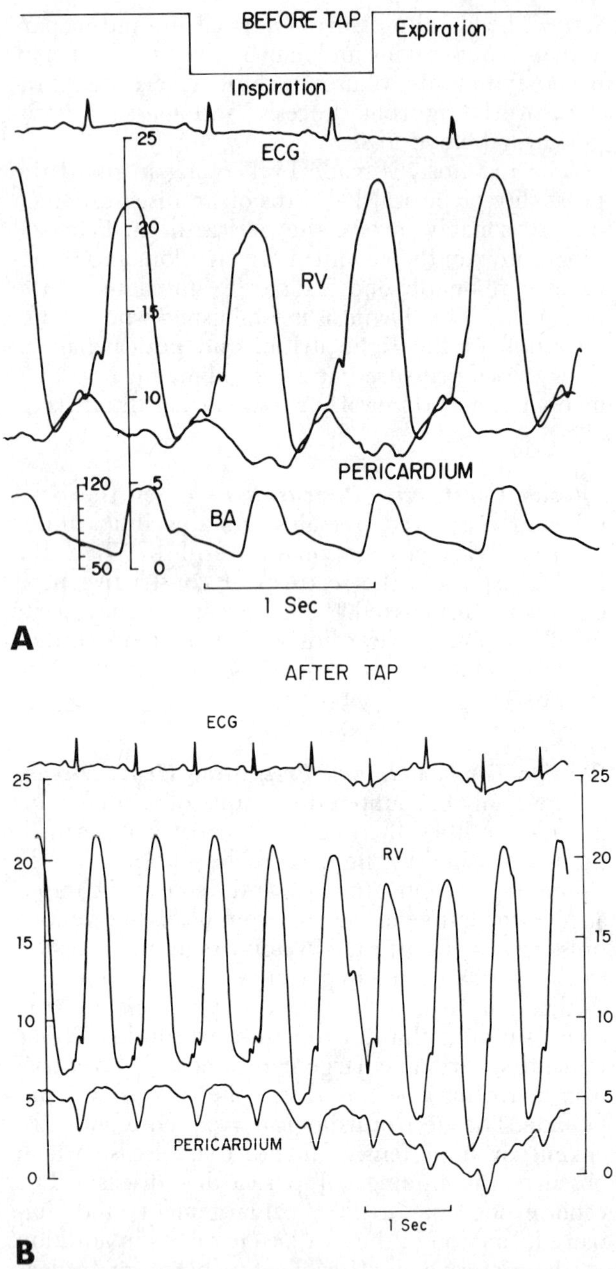

FIGURE 59-7 *A.* Low-pressure cardiac tamponade; tracing obtained during cardiac catheterization. Right ventricular diastolic pressure is only slightly elevated, but is equal to pericardial pressure. Hypotension and pulsus paradoxus are absent. *B.* After pericardiocentesis: Little hemodynamic change has occurred, but pericardial pressure is consistently lower than ventricular diastolic pressure. RV = right ventricle.

paradoxus is absent.[61] One must not require the classical presentation of cardiac tamponade before making the diagnosis in patients undergoing dialysis. Rather, any rise in venous pressure not explained by fluid overload, or a fall in blood pressure not explained by overdialysis, should lead to the suspicion of cardiac tamponade, especially when there is unexplained enlargement of the heart by chest radiography (see "Specific Pericardial Disorders").

Cardiac tamponade is difficult to recognize in patients with severe right ventricular hypertrophy. Specific criteria have not been published, but diastolic collapse of the right side of the heart is prevented.[75]

Atypical Cardiac Tamponade Fluid in the pericardial space or mediastinum may be localized, compressing one side of the heart or one cardiac chamber.[82] Selective compression of the right side is more common; but localized left-sided compression has been reported.[83] Localized cardiac tamponade from blood clots occurs after surgical operations on the heart.[84] Recognition may be difficult, and echocardiography may be inconclusive. In cases of clinical doubt, surgical exploration is fully justified, and when it confirms the diagnosis produces dramatic relief.

Differential Diagnosis of Cardiac Tamponade

The differential diagnosis depends to a great extent on associated abnormalities. Many cases are confused with cardiac failure, having in common raised venous pressure, low cardiac output, and apparent cardiac enlargement. Abnormalities of jugular venous pressure in such cases may be attributed to cardiac failure and tricuspid regurgitation. The correct diagnosis can be arrived at by echocardiography and analysis of the jugular pulsations. Many cases are confused with shock, particularly after acute myocardial infarction; indeed, both may be present. The superior vena caval syndrome may be mistaken for cardiac tamponade especially when the obstructing mass is mistaken for pericardial effusion, but in this case, although venous pressure is increased, pulsations are absent.

Treatment of Cardiac Tamponade

Pericardiocentesis versus Open Drainage

Most often, the only effective treatment is to drain the fluid. Early cardiac tamponade complicating idiopathic or viral pericarditis may remit with anti-inflammatory treatment. The pericardium may be drained via pericardiocentesis, or by limited pericardiectomy. The choice depends upon the cause of effusion, the general health of the patient, the experience and preference of the physician, and the facilities available. Pericardiocentesis permits exact hemodynamic diagnosis and evaluation of the effects of pericardial drainage.[85] Simultaneous pressure recordings from the pericardial space, the right atrium, and a systemic artery before and after removing pericardial fluid are the most effective way of diagnosing effusive-constrictive pericarditis. Pericardiocentesis is less expensive and consumes fewer resources than surgical drainage procedures. On the other hand, even in good hands, pericardiocentesis is associated with morbidity and occasional mortality.[86]

Surgical drainage is performed under direct vision in a more controlled environment and permits pericardial biopsy. If done from the subxiphoid route, local anesthesia may suffice. If a more extensive procedure is needed the incision can be extended cephalad for pericardiectomy. Intraoperative hemodynamic measurements are seldom satisfactory, although when fluid spurts from a pericardiotomy, cardiac tamponade is a reasonable supposition.

The need for repeated pericardiocentesis is an indication for open drainage. In effusive-constrictive pericarditis, fluid drainage alone does not suffice but must be followed by pericardiectomy.

Pharmacological Interventions

Experimental studies[49] to the contrary notwithstanding, pharmacological treatment of cardiac tamponade should not be thought of other than as a temporizing measure. The most important step is to expand the intravascular volume with blood, plasma, dextran, or even saline solution. Agents such as isoproterenol may be given to sustain venous and arterial pressures, and a vasodilator such as nitroprusside can be given to overcome the intense arterial vasoconstriction.[49]

Constrictive Pericarditis

Etiology

Constrictive pericarditis may follow almost any pericardial reaction and should be suspected should any patient who has had pericardial disease develop increased central venous pressure. Again, a few causes account for the vast majority. Many are idiopathic and some are posttraumatic. There is a small but definite incidence of constrictive pericarditis complicating operations on the heart and pericardium.[87] Neoplasia may invade the pericardium and is an important cause of constrictive pericarditis, effusive-constrictive pericarditis, and cardiac tamponade. Constrictive pericarditis may appear months to years after mediastinal radiation.[88] In the United States, tuberculosis is progressively less important in the etiology of constrictive pericarditis,[89] but cases following tuberculosis and other infections of the pericardium are still encountered.

Symptoms

The usual symptoms are indistinguishable from those of congestive heart failure, but there may have been prior pericarditis. Dyspnea and fatigue[87] are common, and in longstanding cases, weight gain, edema, and ascites make their appearance.

Physical Examination

Signs suggesting congestive heart failure in patients who lack an appropriate etiology and in whom evidence for cardiac abnormalities is not forthcoming should be suspected of constrictive pericarditis. This suspicion is heightened by evidence of preexisting pericardial disease or disorders that affect the pericardium. The venous pressure is almost invariably elevated and is characterized by the preservation of both *x* and *y* descents. Frequently the *y* descent, an inward jugular pulsation asynchronous with the carotid pulse, is dominant. Peripheral edema is common, the liver is enlarged, and ascites may be disproportionate.

In some cases the apex beat is impalpable, in others systolic retraction of the chest wall may be present. As there may be preexisting cardiac enlargement, displacement of the apex beat must not be taken as evidence against constrictive pericarditis. Likewise, systolic murmurs are common, and the pericardial knock may be difficult to distinguish from a third heart sound.

In chronic cases, the pericardium may be calcified,[88] but may not be in subacute pericarditis, which is increasingly replacing chronic pericarditis in the spectrum of pericardial disease.[89] P mitrale is common as long as sinus rhythm is maintained, but in chronic cases atrial fibrillation is the rule.[90] Nonspecific repolarization changes consist for the most part of widespread T-wave inversion.[24] When the scar involves the myocardium or coronary arteries, depolarization changes, such as bundle branch block, and conduction delay between atrium and ventricle may be found.[91] Liver function tests are often abnormal, sometimes grossly so.

Cardiac Catheterization

Catheterization and angiography are done to assess the severity of constriction, determine cardiac function, discover underlying heart disease, and to exclude restrictive cardiomyopathy. The findings (Fig. 59-8) are those discussed under pathophysiology.

FIGURE 59-8 Cardiac catheterization tracings from a patient with constrictive pericarditis. *A.* Pressures recorded simultaneously from both ventricles. *B.* Simultaneous right atrial and ventricular pressures showing early diastolic dip and *x* and *y* descents. *C.* Simultaneous pulmonary wedged and superior vena caval (SVC) pressures. *D.* Simultaneous pulmonary arterial and SVC pressures. [*From R. Shabetai and W. Grossman, Profiles in Constrictive Pericarditis, Restrictive Cardiomyopathy and Cardiac Tamponade, in W. Grossman (ed.), "Cardiac Catheterization and Angiography," 2d ed., Lea & Febiger, Philadelphia, 1980, p. 360. Reproduced with permission from the publisher, editor, and author.*]

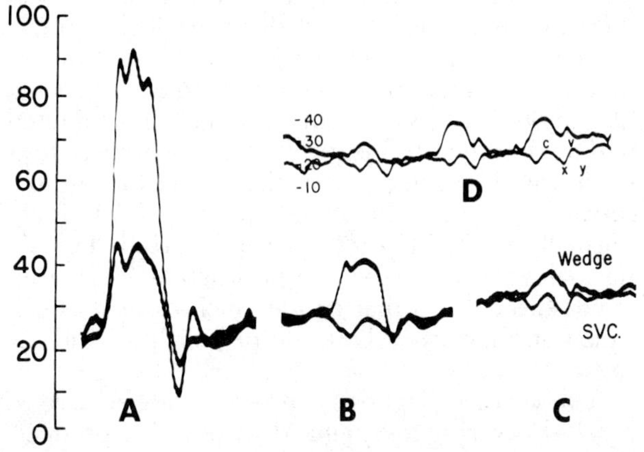

Differential Diagnosis
The most commonly encountered erroneous diagnosis is cirrhosis of the liver. However, in cirrhosis the central venous pressure is not increased. Differentiation from right-sided heart failure with tricuspid regurgitation can be difficult; systemic congestion characterizes both disorders, and both are characterized by a prominent *y* descent of venous pressure. Furthermore, severe tricuspid regurgitation can be present without a loud murmur, and the *v* wave may not be impressive. Tricuspid regurgitation mitigates pulmonary congestion leading to further confusion with constrictive pericarditis. In right-sided heart failure, the etiology is usually apparent and there is right ventricular hypertrophy and enlargement. The electrocardiogram may show P pulmonale, right axis deviation, and right ventricular hypertrophy. Imaging studies show enlargement and dysfunction of the right side of the heart.

Right ventricular infarction may produce a hemodynamic picture indistinguishable from constrictive pericarditis, with prominent *y* descent and absent respiratory variation in central venous pressure, early diastolic dip of ventricular pressure and equal diastolic pressures on the two sides of the heart.[91a] This differential diagnosis is particularly difficult when it arises in patients who have undergone saphenous vein bypass grafting operations because they are at risk for both postoperative constrictive pericarditis and right ventricular infarction. Severe lesions of arteries supplying the right ventricle, and evidence by imaging techniques of right ventricular dysfunction are good clues to right ventricular infarction.

Restrictive cardiomyopathy may also reproduce the hemodynamic picture of constrictive pericarditis. Restrictive cardiomyopathy is not common, but may characterize some cases of amyloid heart disease,[92] idiopathic myocardial disease, and other storage diseases.[93] When left ventricular diastolic pressure greatly exceeds right ventricular diastolic pressure, the diagnosis usually is not in doubt,[90] but exceptional cases of localized constrictive pericarditis occur.[94] It is when restrictive cardiomyopathy with equal left and right ventricular diastolic pressures must be distinguished from constrictive pericarditis without pericardial calcification that the real difficulty arises. Exercise,[95] pharmacological interventions,[96] and fluid challenge may be used to try to induce separation between left and right ventricular diastolic pressures, but experience is so limited that neither the specificity or sensitivity of these tests is known. The same reservation applies to the observation that the rate of early diastolic filling is abnormally rapid in constrictive pericarditis but abnormally slow in restrictive pericarditis.[97] Another major difficulty is that entities such as mediastinal radiation may affect both the pericardium and the myocardium.

The correct diagnosis can sometimes be arrived at by discovering a systemic disease with a predilection either for the myocardium (amyloidosis) or the pericardium (tuberculosis). Major conduction disturbances and depolarization abnormalities, while possible in constrictive pericarditis,[91] favor cardiomyopathy.

The thickened parietal pericardium may be visualized by echocardiography[98] or by computerized tomography.[99] The analogue of the hemodynamic early diastolic dip of pericardial pressure may be recognized echocardiographically by rapid expansion of ventricular dimensions in early diastole followed by a long period during which there is little or no change. This abnormality is present in both restrictive cardiomyopathy and constrictive pericarditis, but preservation of motion of the interventricular septum and notching of the motion of the septum in patients with P mitrale[67] favor constrictive pericarditis.

Attention to the preceding points usually serves to distinguish constrictive pericarditis from restrictive cardiomyopathy. When doubt remains, endomyocardial biopsy may disclose myocardial disease.[100] When an experienced cardiologist remains in doubt following full investigation, exploratory thoracotomy with a view to possible pericardiectomy is fully justified, though fortunately seldom required.

Syndromes of Constrictive Pericarditis

Chronic Calcific Constrictive Pericarditis This is the classical constrictive pericarditis that is now becoming less common. The clinical picture is striking, with severe cachexia, anasarca, massively increased venous pressure, and atrial fibrillation. Calcium frequently surrounds the whole pericardium and is best seen in lateral or oblique projections of the chest radiograph. Liver dysfunction is severe, amounting to failure, with spider angiomata, bilirubin retention, and even altered states of consciousness.

Subacute Constrictive Pericarditis This form of constrictive pericarditis is becoming more common at the expense of chronic constrictive pericarditis. Frequently, the pericardium is not calcified and the course may be over a matter of weeks or months to 2 or 3 years. Subacute constrictive pericarditis may follow upon rheumatoid arthritis[101] and *H. influenzae* infections, especially in children. Diagnosis depends upon careful evaluation of venous pressure in patients with systemic diseases that may involve the pericardium.

Postoperative Constrictive Pericarditis Considering the number of intrapericardial surgical operations, it is surprising that the incidence of postoperative constrictive pericarditis does not exceed the 0.2 percent reported in a careful retrospective study.[102] In these operations the pericardium is subject to cellular injury and is exposed to blood, foreign materials, and local hypothermia, all of which might induce inflammation. There is considerable variation in whether and how the pericardium is closed after cardiac operations and in the techniques employed for myocardial preservation, yet no specific factors, save possibly the use of iodine solutions,[103] have been implicated as an etiologic factor.

Occult Constrictive Pericarditis This is defined as constrictive pericarditis so mild that it is not detectable without fluid challenge.[104] In the first series reported the patients complained of nondescript chest pain for which they underwent cardiac catheterization and coronary arteriography. Many reported previous acute pericarditis. Hemodynamic studies revealed normal atrial and ventricular pressures, but following the infusion of approximately a liter of saline solution in roughly 10 min, the right atrial pressure waveform assumed the characteristics of constrictive pericarditis, and the diastolic pressures in the two ventricles became equal. At subsequent operation, the pericardium was thickened and fibrosed, findings that were confirmed by histological examination.

This form of constrictive pericarditis must be rare, and its existence, though frequently sought, is seldom found. Caution is advised in applying rapid, large fluid challenges to patients undergoing cardiac catheterization; furthermore, the induction of hemodynamic changes suggesting constrictive pericarditis by this technique should seldom if ever be taken alone as an indication for pericardiectomy.[105]

Effusive Constrictive Pericarditis This condition results from combined cardiac tamponade and constrictive pericarditis[66] and may occur in tuberculous pericarditis, nephrogenic pericardial disease, and in neoplastic or postradiation pericardiopathy. The clinical and hemodynamic presentation is that of cardiac tamponade. Pericardiocentesis, however, reveals persistence of raised venous pressure, absent respiratory variation of the venous pulse which shows a prominent *y* descent that was not present before pericardiocentesis, and a prominent *y* descent (Fig. 59-9).

Localized Constrictive Pericarditis Localized constrictive pericarditis is rare, but occasionally a localized band constricts the inflow or outflow region of one or more of the cardiac chambers. The clinical picture then simulates valve disease or venous obstruction[105a] (Fig. 59-10).

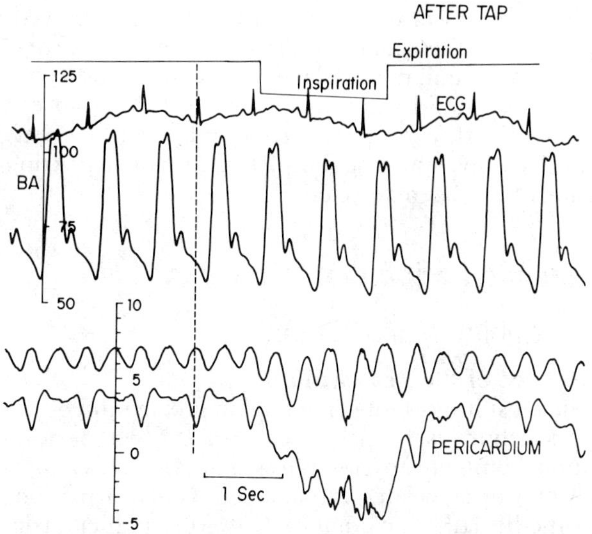

FIGURE 59-9 Recording made during cardiac catheterization of a patient with effusive-constrictive pericarditis due to bronchogenic carcinoma. The tracings were obtained during pericardiocentesis which has lowered pericardial pressure; however, right atrial pressure elevation persists and the tracing shows prominent *x* and *y* descents and absent respiratory variation. (*From R. Shabetai, "The Pericardium," Grune & Stratton, New York, 1981, p. 273. Reproduced with permission from the publisher and author.*)

Treatment

The treatment of constrictive pericarditis is usually surgical pericardiectomy. The mildest cases can be followed without surgical treatment, but when jugular venous pressure is consistently raised beyond 7 or 8 mmHg, or requires medical treatment for its control, pericardiectomy should be carried out. In the most extreme cases of severe longstanding constrictive pericarditis with profound cachexia and liver dysfunction, it has been argued that treatment with a diuretic and digitalis should suffice,[105] but many surgeons disagree.

Pericardiectomy is commonly carried out via a median sternotomy, although some surgeons prefer thoracotomy. The risk has declined but is still in the range of 5 percent.[106] The risk is increased by heavy calcification, especially involving the epicardium, and

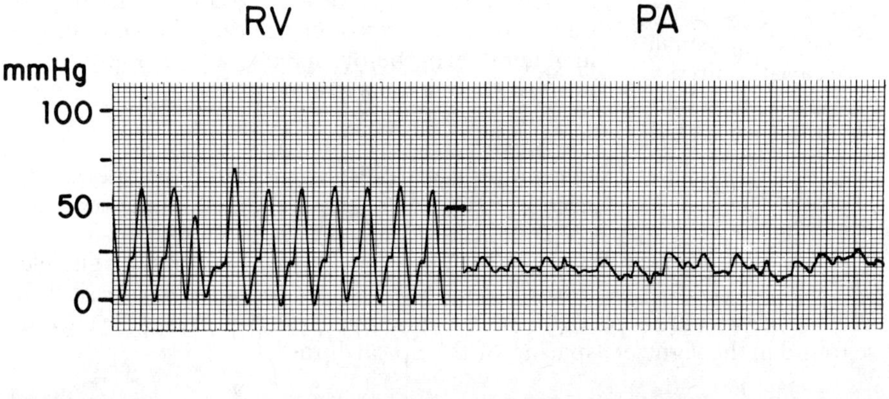

FIGURE 59-10 Pressure tracing from the pulmonary artery (PA) and right ventricle (RV) of a patient with extrinsic pulmonary stenosis caused by a localized band of pericardial constriction which developed after rupture of the esophagus. (*From R. Shabetai, "The Pericardium," Grune & Stratton, New York, 1981, p. 208. Reproduced with permission from the publisher and author.*)

when the visceral pericardium must be removed. Recovery of normal venous pressure and cardiac performance may be delayed weeks or months, but it is more rapid when the operation is carried out before the disease is too chronic and when the pericardiectomy is almost complete and all constricting bands have been resected.[107]

Specific Pericardial Disorders

Congenital Malformations

Absence of the Pericardium

The most important congenital malformation of the pericardium is partial absence of the left pericardium; complete absence is less common. This anomaly may be associated with congenital malformations of the heart,[108] including patent arterial duct, atrial septal defect, mitral stenosis, tetralogy of Fallot, tricuspid regurgitation, and Eisenmenger physiology. Association with mitral valve prolapse has also been reported.

Diagnosis Most cases come to attention because of an abnormality on the chest roentgenogram. The heart tends to be shifted to the left, and its left border is elongated, showing prominent separation between the aorta and pulmonary artery. Lucencies caused by interposition of lung may be seen between the pulmonary artery segment and the aortic knob, and between the left hemidiaphragm and the base of the heart.

Most patients are symptomless, but chest pain is reported by a significant proportion, perhaps related to torsion of the great vessels. Recurrent pulmonary infections may be a significant feature. Physical findings are not often helpful, but a conspicuous left ventricular heave in the anterior or midaxillary line may be found when the deficiency is substantial. A systolic murmur may be present, and on occasion diastolic murmurs have been described.

Laboratory Findings The electrocardiogram in complete absence of the left side of the pericardium usually shows incomplete right bundle branch block. In the presence of induced or spontaneous pneumothorax air enters the pericardial space and outlines the pericardium.

Clinical Course and Treatment Total and very small deficiencies are not associated with pathophysiological changes. Medium-size defects may allow herniation of the left atrium, which may then strangulate and require surgical closure or enlargement of the defect to reduce the herniation and prevent recurrence.

Pericardial Cysts

Pericardial cysts vary greatly in size, are smooth and rounded, and most commonly are found in the right cardiophrenic angle. They are benign and produce no local or general symptoms. Their importance lies in differentiation from neoplasm. The roentgenographic appearance of pericardial cysts is highly characteristic and the nature of the lesion can be confirmed by computerized tomography.

Dialysis-Related and Uremic Pericardial Disease

Etiology

The association of pericardial disease with renal failure has been widely recognized since its description by Richard Bright.[109] Bright's report referred to end-stage renal disease in which pericarditis still occurs, but of greater importance is pericarditis complicating chronic dialysis. The mechanism, in spite of considerable investigation and speculation, remains unknown. The theory that uremic pericarditis is a chemical reaction to retained products of metabolism fails to account for the lack of relationship between the level of blood urea nitrogen or other nitrogenous metabolites and the frequency of pericarditis. Pericarditis is less common in patients undergoing peritoneal as compared with hemodialysis, suggesting a possible role for "middle molecules." The hemorrhagic diathesis, an important component of the uremic syndrome, may predispose to pericarditis, a predisposition which may be aggravated by even regional heparinization. Nephrogenic pericarditis is highly vascular, consequently uremia or dialysis-related pericardial effusion is usually bloody. The clinical manifestation may be acute fibrinous pericarditis, pericardial effusion, or cardiac tamponade. Classical constrictive pericarditis is a rare sequel, but effusive constrictive pericarditis is an important complication in the dialysis population.

The etiology in dialyzed patients may be different from that in end-stage renal failure. It is possible that some cases are caused by living agents introduced into the bloodstream during hemodialysis, or that pericarditis is an immune response to a component of the hemodialysis equipment or fluid.[110] Renal insufficiency is associated with increased susceptibility to infection; therefore the possibility of viral, tuberculous, or even bacterial pericarditis must not be neglected. Since neoplasia, ischemic heart disease, and thyroid disease occur in this population, it is wise to consider the differential diagnosis in general terms before making a presumptive diagnosis of dialysis-related pericarditis.

Diagnosis

Fibrinous pericarditis is manifested by a pericardial friction rub, which may be coarse, and sometimes palpable. Chest pain occurs in about two-thirds of patients and fever in the vast majority.[110] The electrocardiogram is of little value since the classical ST-segment elevation may not be present, reflecting sparing of the epicardium.[111]

Pericardial effusion should be suspected whenever there is a sudden unexplained increase in the apparent size of the heart, but differentiation from fluid overload or congestive heart failure is important. Unexplained cardiac enlargement or hemodynamic deterioration suggest either cardiac tamponade, fluid imbalance, or heart failure. Physicians caring for patients undergoing hemodialysis must be constantly on the alert for cardiac tamponade, especially as the clinical manifestations may be atypical, and are difficult to distinguish from cardiac and cardiovascular deterioration. Recognition and good treatment are essential as cardiac tamponade remains one of the principal causes of hemodialysis-associated morbidity, and in 20 percent of cases terminates fatally.[112]

Treatment
Acute pericarditis without hemodynamic manifestations is treated by intensified dialysis.[81] Nonsteroidal anti-inflammatory agents may accelerate resolution, but may aggravate bleeding. Pericardial effusions without associated changes in venous or arterial pressure are usually treated the same way; a salutory response may be anticipated.

Considerable controversy exists regarding the optimal management of large, persistent, or recurrent pericardial effusion, and especially of cardiac tamponade. A conservative approach to early cardiac tamponade is intensification of hemodialysis combined with either nonsteroidal agents or prednisone. More severe tamponade is an indication for pericardial drainage. The instillation of nonabsorbable steroids directly into the pericardial space has been advocated,[113] but experience with this technique is small.

The Pericardium and Myocardial Infarction

Pericardial Friction Rub in Acute Myocardial Infarction
A pericardial friction rub occurs in approximately 10 percent of patients with acute myocardial infarction[114] and perhaps more commonly since it is often transitory. Shaggy fibrinous pericarditis may be found overlying Q-wave infarctions. However, pericarditis can occur in non-Q-wave infarctions, and sometimes pericardial friction rubs are audible in patients with inferior wall myocardial infarction, suggesting that pericarditis may sometimes be an immune reaction to myocardial damage.

The pain is difficult or impossible to distinguish from angina, extension of infarction, or pulmonary embolism. Similarly, it is often impossible to recognize pericarditis on the electrocardiogram during evolution of an acute myocardial infarction. Echocardiography has demonstrated that silent pericardial effusion may accompany myocardial infarction.

The most practical aspect of acute pericarditis in myocardial infarction is to what extent it contraindicates or modifies treatment with anticoagulants. A pericardial friction rub occurring in the first 2 or 3 days and not accompanied by pericardial effusion or evidence suggesting cardiac tamponade need not modify standard practice, which in any case is variable. Pericarditis occurring later in the course, or accompanied by pericardial effusion or tamponade is a contraindication. Thrombolytic therapy is almost always begun before pericarditis develops. Acute pericarditis does not of itself alter the prognosis, but tends to be associated with larger infarctions and hence with a higher incidence of arrhythmia and a higher mortality.[115]

Dressler's Syndrome
Dressler described a syndrome comprising chest pain, pleurisy, pericardial friction rub, fever, and leukocytosis, sometimes associated with pulmonary infiltrate.[116] This complication, described almost in its entirety in the title of the original description[116] usually occurs weeks or months after the causative infarction, but may occur while the patient is still in the hospital. Most authorities consider it a separate entity from acute pericarditis occurring within the first 48 h,[117] but pericarditis associated with myocardial infarction may be an immune reaction to myocardial damage.[118] The postmyocardial infarction syndrome may be caused by a combination of viral activation and myocardial antibodies,[119] bringing it into line with the clinically similar postpericardiotomy syndrome, for which there is strong evidence supporting this dual etiology.[120]

Diagnosis is scarcely tenable without a pericardial friction rub, and is strengthened by the presence of pericardial effusion. When Dressler's syndrome occurs soon after infarction the differential diagnosis must include extension of the infarction, or pulmonary embolism. Later cases must be distinguished from a second infarction and unstable angina. Symptoms and signs usually subside rapidly with treatment with nonsteroidal anti-inflammatory drugs, but more resistant cases need steroids. Over succeeding months or years there may be several recurrences that require treatment.

The postmyocardial infarction syndrome appears to be decreasing in prevalence,[119] possibly reflecting the decreased use of Coumadin in acute myocardial infarction.

Postpericardiotomy Syndrome

This is a syndrome with features indistinguishable from acute idiopathic pericarditis or Dressler's syndrome, occurring after operations in which the pericardium is opened. The syndrome occurs in children and adults and is not more common in those undergoing operation for rheumatic heart disease. Epidemiological studies have shown high levels of both antiheart antibody and viral titers.[120] Differential diagnosis is from overt postoperative complications associated with pleurisy, pleural effusion, pericardial effusion, chest pain, and fever.

Treatment
Treatment is with corticosteroids or nonsteroidal anti-inflammatory agents. Recurrences may require reinitiation of treatment.

Posttraumatic Pericardial Syndrome

A virtually indistinguishable syndrome may follow blunt and sharp chest trauma. Common to all these conditions is injury to the pericardial mesothelium, myocardial injury, and blood in the pericardial space.

Treatment is with anti-inflammatory drugs.

Neoplastic Pericardial Disease

A number of primary and secondary neoplasms may involve the myocardium and pericardium. Secondary neoplasia of the pericardium is more common than primary, the leading offenders being carcinoma of the breast and lung, lymphoma, and leukemia. Mesothelioma is the commonest primary pericardial neoplasm and may respond to treatment with doxorubicin and cyclophosphamide.[121] Melanoma may involve the myocardium extensively, yet seldom produces clinical findings except when the pericardium is involved.

Uncommon Neoplasms
Rare metatastic neoplasms of the pericardium include carcinoma of the colon, esophagus, kidney, ovary, prostate, and stomach, and sarcoma.[122] Rare primary neoplasms include lymphangioma, hemangioma,[123] and teratoma.[124]

Clinical Features The most common manifestation is pericardial effusion; indeed, the commonest cause of cardiac tamponade observed on medical wards is neoplasm. Occasionally, tamponade is the initial finding, but more commonly patients are already known to have cancer. The differential diagnosis of the combination of a proven pericardial effusion and an intrathoracic mass lies between cardiac tamponade and the superior vena caval syndrome. In the former the characteristic pulsations of the jugular veins can be observed, whereas in the latter the distended neck veins do not pulsate. Respiratory distress, pulsus alternans, and tachycardia may obscure pulsus paradoxus, which otherwise occurs in cardiac tamponade but not in the superior vena caval syndrome. A pericardial friction rub may be present, but electrocardiographic signs of pericarditis usually are lacking. The pericardial fluid is almost always bloody.

The pericardium itself is frequently normal in gross appearance but may be thickened, sometimes sufficiently to encase the heart. Uncommonly, effusive-constrictive pericarditis is found. Neoplastic cells can be recovered from the pericardial fluid in the majority of cases, especially when the services of a skilled exfoliative cytologist are available. Rarely, sympathetic pericardial effusion occurs in thoracic neoplasms that do not involve the pericardium.

Treatment Metastatic pericardial effusion almost invariably indicates an inoperable lesion. Treatment is therefore palliative, with the goals being to ameliorate symptoms and prevent death from cardiac tamponade, except in otherwise terminal individuals. Procedures should be as limited as possible and yet meet these goals. There is considerable controversy over the relative merits of pericardiocentesis and open drainage with biopsy. In the latter, the less extensive subxiphoid incision should be used whenever possible. The need for frequently repeated pericardiocenteses can be reduced by draining the fluid via an intrapericardial catheter for several hours. The ultimate choice depends upon the extent of neoplasia, the general condition of the patient, and local preferences. The decision is best made jointly by the patient's physician, an oncologist, and a cardiologist or cardiac surgeon. Tetracycline can be instilled via an intrapericardial catheter and may succeed in preventing recurrences of pericardial effusion or cardiac tamponade.[125] This is usually followed by transient pain and fever, but surprisingly, not by constrictive pericarditis. Few controlled trials of instilling chemotherapeutic agents are available because of the infrequency, varied clinical presentation, and frequent need for emergency treatment.

Radiation-Induced Pericardial Disease

Exposure of the mediastinum to radiation involves the risk of pericardial and myocardial damage. By far the greatest experience has been in patients treated for Hodgkin's disease. The acute reaction of the pericardium to radiation is fibrinous inflammation, often accompanied by effusion. The less common chronic response usually takes the form of constrictive pericarditis, sometimes effusive-constrictive pericarditis. The latency between exposure and constriction is often remarkably long. In one series of seven patients the lesion developed between 51 and 268 months after radiotherapy.[126]

The pathophysiology is unknown. The acute lesion has been studied mainly in experimental animals[127] but only occasionally in humans.[128] The myocardial, and by inference the pericardial, microcirculation is extensively damaged, resulting in ischemic injury to the tissue. The common opinion that the chronic lesion occurs only after 4000 rad has been delivered is not backed by statistical evidence. The incidence increases when anteriorly weighted thoracic mantle field techniques are employed. It has been suggested that reactivation of a latent virus in the pericardium[127] may occur, and that radiation may damage the pericardial lymphatics.[127] The lesion appears to be more common in patients who have also received adjunctive chemotherapy.[127]

The acute lesion usually subsides within 2 years without sequel. The chronic lesion produces the typical picture of constrictive pericarditis, or effusive-constrictive pericarditis. In the effusive stage the differential diagnosis is recurrence of the neoplasm. Examination of pericardial fluid is then helpful, as the fluid is positive in about 30 percent of cases.[129] Cytological examination of pericardial fluid is reliable in breast and lung cancer, but less so in lymphoma and leukemia in which pericardial biopsy may be needed.[130] Acute radiation-induced pericarditis can be managed symptomatically along the same lines as acute idiopathic pericarditis; the response is usually gratifying. Pericardial effusions when not causing tamponade can also be managed conservatively. Constrictive pericarditis requires pericardiectomy unless there is prohibitive associated endomyocardial fibrosis. Significant impairment of left ventricular systolic function indicates severe myocardial damage, but frequently systolic function is preserved in spite of extensive myocardial fibrosis. In case of doubt, endomyocardial biopsy may be helpful, but good results may accrue from pericardiectomy when the biopsy shows mild endomyocardial fibrosis.[130]

Hypersensitivity and Collagen-Vascular Pericardial Disease

Rheumatoid Arthritis

Necropsy studies yield an overall incidence of pericardial disease associated with rheumatoid disease of about 30 percent,[131] a prevalance that was known to Charcot.[132] The clinical incidence is appreciably lower except when echocardiograms are performed on patients with rheumatoid arthritis who have no symptoms of pericardial disease.[133] Rheumatoid pericardial disease is usually self-limiting, but may lead to acute or chronic pericardial effusion, subacute or chronic constrictive pericarditis, or cardiac tamponade.

Rheumatoid pericardial disease appears to be more common in middle-aged males in whom the arthritis was of acute onset. Serological tests for rheumatoid disease are usually positive, and typical rheumatoid nodules are common.

Associated cardiac abnormalities, including mitral valve involvement[123] and heart block,[134] are important but less common.

Constrictive pericarditis is usually subacute and seldom calcified. Pericardiectomy may be required within months of the first diagnosis of acute pericarditis[135] and almost always within 5 years.

Systemic Lupus Erythematosus

Pericardial disease develops in nearly all patients when life is prolonged by steroid treatment. The usual lesion is fibrinous pericarditis, but large pericardial effusions may develop.[136] Both cardiac tamponade[137] and constrictive pericarditis[138] have been described. Rarely, pericarditis is the initial manifestation. The pericardial fluid usually has a high content of protein and a normal or slightly reduced glucose content. As in rheumatoid arthritis, the complement level is low and LE cells may be found.

Other Connective Tissue Diseases

Pericardial involvement may be found in systemic sclerosis (scleroderma) when it is often associated with cardiomyopathy. The pericardial fluid does not contain antibodies, immune complexes, or low levels of complement. There may be associated cardiac disease, and in some of the cases pericardial involvement is secondary to uremia.[139]

Drug-Induced Pericardial Disease

Pericardial abnormalities may develop in response to a number of drugs, of which the more important are hydralazine, procainamide, and daunorubicin.[140] Pericardial abnormalities have also been reported with psycofuranine, isonicotinic acid, and isoniazid. Pericarditis induced by penicillin presumably is a hypersensitivity reaction. Cardiac tamponade has been reported after administration of cromolyn sodium[141] and physergide.[142] In patients with lupus nephritis treated with hydralazine it may be difficult to know whether pericarditis is drug-induced or is a manifestation of the disease. Minoxidil may cause pericardial effusion.[143]

Infectious (Nonviral) Pericarditis

Tuberculous Pericarditis

The pericardium is infected via lymphatic spread; frequently no other, and especially no pulmonary lesion is detectable. Tuberculosis of the pericardium is now rare in the western hemisphere. In a series of 72 pericardiectomies performed between 1974 and 1980, none was for tuberculous constrictive pericarditis.[144] Likewise, in two reviews of pericardiocentesis tuberculosis was proven in only three of 173[85] and four of 52.[86]

Most of the detailed descriptions antedate chemotherapy. Furthermore, the features emphasized in those years of plentiful clinical material, such as insidious onset, lack of constitutional symptoms, thick pericardium by air contrast, and bloody pericardial effusion, are not sufficiently specific to be of use to the modern clinician.[145] On the other hand, when untreated, tamponade, effusive-constrictive pericarditis, and chronic calcific constriction are common sequels. Consequently, in spite of its rarity, the possibility of tuberculosis must be considered in virtually every case of acute pericarditis, pericardial effusion, cardiac tamponade, or constrictive pericarditis.

The dire consequences of missing the diagnosis has led to the practice of presumptive diagnosis based on such indirect evidence as contacts, skin tests, chronicity, and therapeutic trial. It is now quite impossible to tell either from personal experience or literature review how many patients treated for tuberculous pericarditis really had the disease, or what would have been the consequences of withholding treatment until Koch's postulates were fulfilled. Tubercle bacilli may fail to grow from the pericardial fluid of patients subsequently proven to have had tuberculous pericarditis[146] and even pericardial biopsy can be negative in such patients.[147]

Treatment A potent triple drug regimen, such as rifampin 600 mg, isoniazid 300 mg, and ethambutol 15 mg/kg should be prescribed. After several months isoniazid should be discontinued, but the other two drugs are given for 18 months after activity has subsided. Concurrent treatment with corticosteroids has been proposed[148] but its role remains unsettled.

Histoplasmosis

Most cases of histoplasmosis of the pericardium occur in the Ohio and Mississippi Valleys and western Appalachia.[149] Rarely, *Histoplasma* can be recovered from pericardial fluid,[150] but more commonly diagnosis depends upon serology, which must be tested before it is modified by intradermal injections of histoplasmin. A titer exceeding 1:32 favors recent or active infection. Distinction from tuberculosis can be difficult using clinical criteria and because neither organism is easy to culture, but adenopathy favors histoplasmosis. Calcific constrictive pericarditis is a documented outcome.[151]

Treatment

Proven active disease, especially with tamponade, should be treated with a total course of 35 to 40 mg/kg of amphotericin B.[152]

Tuberculosis may occur in association with histoplasmosis[153] and when disseminated these diseases may cause adrenal insufficiency.[154]

Other Organisms

The pericardium may also be infected by *Blastomyces,* and *Candida albicans,* the latter usually after immunosuppressive or broad-spectrum antibiotic treatment. *Actinomyces israeli* and *Nocardia asteroides* may also affect the pericardium and can cause constriction.[155] Purulent pericarditis may complicate pulmonary aspergillosis. Sporotrichosis and mucormycosis were not included in a review,[156] to which the reader is referred for references regarding specific fungal pericarditides.

Treatment

Unlike histoplasmosis, these infections do not remit spontaneously, therefore pericardiectomy should be carried out whenever possible.

Bacterial and Other Pyogenic Infections of the Pericardium

Purulent pericarditis has decreased in frequency because of effective antibiotics, but when it occurs it is serious, carrying a high risk of mortality. The combination of pericarditis and septicemia demands a relentless search for the causative organism. It is most important to obtain at least four blood cultures, which should be tested on a wide range of media so that fastidious organisms as well as the more common pyrogens will grow. Immunological studies for tuberculosis, *Hemophilus influenzae, Streptococcus, Toxoplasma,* and *Entameba histolytica* should be done.

The antibiotic control of common infections has led to a change in the spectrum of bacterial pericarditis. The previously common pneumococcal pericarditis, a direct consequence of pneumococcal pneumonia, and streptococcal pericarditis, has given way to infections caused by resistant *Staphylococcus,* anaerobes, fungi, and commensal organisms. Consequently, the population at risk has shifted to the extremes of age, the debilitated, and the immunosuppressed.[157]

Treatment

Infections due to penicillin-sensitive organisms can be brought under control by large doses of penicillin, which achieve therapeutic concentration in the pericardial fluid.[158]

The definitive treatment of purulent pericarditis is surgical drainage. Meningococcal pericarditis is a metastatic infection, usually from the nasopharynx. Meningococcal pericarditis may occur in the absence of meningitis[159] and frequently the purulent serosanguineous pericardial exudate is sterile because of previous antibiotic treatment, but in some cases sterile pericardial effusion is thought to be an immune reaction.[160] The disease should yield to penicillin, but surgical drainage is often required, and constrictive pericarditis needing pericardiectomy may occur acutely.[161]

Staphylococcal pericarditis is an extremely serious illness and frequently fatal, especially when it is a complication of cardiac surgery or staphylococcal endocarditis. Systemic illness is profound and the pericardial exudate tenacious and loculated. Vigorous and aggressive treatment must be directed at every aspect of the disease, including control of the primary infection, removal of infected venous and arterial catheters, administration of appropriate antibiotics, and surgical drainage. Pericardiocentesis never suffices but surgical decompression must be carried out.[162]

Gram-negative organisms such as *Pseudomonas aeruginosa, Klebsiella pneumoniae,* and *Escherichia coli* produce pericarditis by hematogenous spread in the gravely debilitated.[163] Antibiotic treatment is beset with difficulties in selection and toxicity, and surgical drainage may be required. Pericarditis may result from hematogenous spread or by direct extension of anaerobic infections.[164] Treatment must include drainage of both the primary focus and the pericardium.

Purulent pericarditis in children carries a high mortality and may lead rapidly to constrictive pericarditis.[164] *Hemophilus influenzae* and meningococci are the most common offenders, but pneumococcal pericarditis still occurs in infants and children. Prognosis remains poor despite modern treatment.

Miscellaneous Diseases of the Pericardium

Myxedema Pericardial Disease

Pericardial effusion occurs in about one-third of patients with myxedema. There is no correlation between pericardial effusion and the level of thyroid activity. Cardiomegaly is often the first clue, but may be due to coexisting heart disease. The pericardial effusion rarely causes symptoms, although tamponade has been reported.[165] The pericardial fluid is usually clear, but may be myxomatous, and is high in cholesterol until restoration of the euthyroid state.

Cholesterol Pericarditis

Cholesterol pericarditis may be idiopathic, but more commonly is found in myxedema, tuberculosis, or rheumatoid disease. The effusions are often large, but because they develop slowly, tamponade is uncommon. The associated inflammation may provoke constrictive pericarditis.[166] The cholesterol may be liberated from injured pericardial cells, or lysed from red corpuscles, or develop as a consequence of lymphatic obstruction.[167]

Chylopericardium

Chylopericardium is usually idiopathic, but may be associated with surgical or traumatic injury of the thoracic duct, or neoplastic obstruction of the lymphatic drainage. The diagnosis is established by examination of the pericardial fluid, which is milky-white when allowed to stand, and contains fat globules and increased levels of cholesterol and triglycerides. The milky appearance clears promptly after the addition of ether. Treatment is by drainage, and if the thoracic duct is injured, it must be ligated. Lymphopericardium is less common than chylopericardium and is usually secondary to lymphangioma. Pericardial involvement has also been reported in echinococcosis,[168] Degos' disease,[169] and pseudomyxoma peritoneae.[170]

Uncommon Causes

There are a number of syndromes associated with pericardial effusion, although the mechanism is unclear. These include Reiter's syndrome,[171] ulcerative colitis,[172] Whipple's disease,[173] thalassemia,[174] atrial septal defect,[175] and Sipple's syndrome.[176] Pericardiopathy may also occur as part of mechanical disorders such as the chylous reflux syndrome,[177] inversion of the diaphragm,[178] pancreatic fistula,[179] and in diabetic ketoacidosis.[180]

Constrictive pericarditis is a component of mulibrey nanism. *Mulibrey* is an acronym for *mu*scle-*li*ver-*br*ain-*ey*e, the organs principally affected by this autosomal recessive disorder found mainly in Finland.[181] Other features include yellow dots on the ocular fundi, fibrous dysplasia of the long bones, and an abnormally shaped skull, and sella turcica.

A patient with Behçet's syndrome with pericardial effusion and mixed cryoglobulinemia who responded to treatment with indomethacin has been reported.[182] There is also a report of pericardial perforation of a gastric ulcer into the pericardium secondary to a phytobezoar in an oligophrenic man.[183]

References

1. Whitteridge, G.: The Anatomical Lectures of William Harvey, Prelectiones Anatomie Universalis De Musculis, Livingstone, 1964, Edinburgh, p. 249.
2. Roberts, W. C., and Spray, T. L.: Pericardial Heart Disease: A Study of its Causes, Consequences, and Morphologic Features, in D. H. Spodick (ed.), "Pericardial Diseases," F. A. Davis, Philadelphia, 1976, p. 17.
3. Gibson, A. T., and Segal, M. B.: A Study of the Composition of Pericardial Fluid with Special Reference to the Probable Mechanism of Fluid Formation, *J. Physiol. (Lond.)*, 277:635, 1940.
4. Elias, H., and Boyd, L. J.: Notes on the Anatomy, Embryology and Histology of the Pericardium, *J. New York Med. Coll.*, 2:50, 1960.
5. Ishihara, T., Ferrans, V. J., Jones, M., Boyce, S. W., Kawanamni, O., and Roberts, W. C.: Histologic and Ultrastructural Features of the Normal Human Parietal Pericardium, *Am. J. Cardiol.*, 46:746, 1980.
6. Holt, J. P.: The Normal Pericardium, *Am. J. Cardiol.*, 26:455, 1970.
7. Rabkin, S. W., and Ping, H. H.: Mathematical and Mechanical Modeling of Stress-Strain Relationship of Pericardium, *Am. J. Physiol.*, 229:896, 1975.
8. Lee, J. M. and Boughner, D. R.: Mechanics of Canine Pericardium in Different Test Environments, *Circ. Res.*, 49:533, 1981.
9. Freeman, G. L., and LeWinter, M. M.: Pericardial Adaptations during Cardiac Dilatation in Dogs, *Circ. Res.*, 54:29, 1984.
10. Horowitz, M. S., Schultz, C. S., Stinson, E. B., Harrison, D. C., and Popp, R. L.: Sensitivity and Specificity of Echocardiographic Diagnosis of Pericardial Effusion, *Circulation*, 50:239, 1974.
11. Hollenberg, M., and Dougherty, J.: Lymph Flow and ^{131}I Albumin Resorption from Pericardial Effusions in Man, *Am. J. Cardiol.*, 24:514, 1969.
12. Pegram, B. L., and Bishop, V. S.: An Evaluation of the Pericardial Sac as a Safety Factor during Cardiac Tamponade, *Cardiovasc. Res.*, 9:715, 1975.
13. Morgan, B. C., Guntheroth, W. C., and Dillard, D. H.: The Relationship of Pericardial to Pleural Pressure during Quiet Respiration and Cardiac Tamponade, *Circ. Res.*, 16:493, 1965.
14. Smiseth, O. A., Refsum, H., Junemann, M., et al.: Ventricular Diastolic Pressure-Volume Shifts during Acute Ischemic Left Ventricular Failure in Dogs, *J. Am. Coll. Cardiol.*, 3:966, 1984.
15. Ditchey, R., Engler, R. L., LeWinter, M. M., et al.: The Role of the Right Heart in Acute Cardiac Tamponade in Dogs, *Circ. Res.*, 48:701, 1981.
16. Janicki, J. S., and Weber, K. T.: The Pericardium and Ventricular Interaction Distensibility and Function, *Am. J. Physiol.*, 238:H494, 1980.
17. Tyson, G. S., Maier, G. W., Olsen, C. O., David, J. W., and Rankin, J. S.: Pericardial Influences on Ventricular Filling in the Conscious Dog. An Analysis Based on Pericardial Pressure, *Circ. Res.*, 54:173, 1984.
18. Banchero, N., Rutihauser, W. J., Tsakiris, A. G., and Wood,

E. H.: Pericardial Pressure during Transverse Acceleration in Dogs without Thoracotomy, *Circ. Res.*, 20:65, 1967.
19. Collin, V.: Quoted in L. J. Boyd and H. Elias, Contributions to Diseases of the Heart and Pericardium. I. Historical Introduction, *Bull. N.Y. Med. Coll.*, 18:1, 1955.
20. Laennec, R. T. H.: "A Treatise on Diseases of the Chest," translated from the French by John Forbes, T and G Underwood, London, 1821, p. 264.
21. Spodick, D. H.: Acoustic Phenomena in Pericardial Disease, *Am. Heart J.*, 81:114, 1971.
22. James, T. N.: Pericarditis and the Sinus Node, *Arch. Intern. Med.*, 110:305, 1962.
23. Spodick, D. H.: Frequency of Arrhythmias in Acute Pericarditis Determined by Holter Monitoring, *Am. J. Cardiol.*, 53:842, 1984.
24. Surawicz, B., and Lasseter, K. C.: Electrocardiogram in Pericarditis, *Am. J. Cardiol.*, 26:671, 1970.
25. Spodick, D. H.: Diagnostic Electrocardiographic Sequences in Acute Pericarditis: Significance of PR Segment and PR Vector Changes, *Circulation*, 48:575, 1973.
26. Wanner, W. R., Schaal, S. F., Bashore, T. M., Norton, V. J., Lewis, R. P., and Fullerson, R. P.: Repolarization Variant versus Acute Pericarditis: A Prospective Electrocardiographic and Echocardiographic Evaluation, *Chest*, 83:180, 1983.
27. O'Connell, J. B., Robinson, J. A., Henkin, R. E., and Gunnar, R. M.: Gallium-67 Citrate Scanning for Noninvasive Detection of Inflammation in Pericardial Diseases, *Am. J. Cardiol.*, 46:879, 1980.
28. Hackney, D., Slutsky, R., Mattrey, R., et al.: Experimental Pericardial Effusion Evaluated by Computerized Tomography, *Radiology*, 151:145, 1984.
29. Connoly, D. C., and Burchell, H. B.: Pericarditis: A Ten Year Survey, *Am. J. Cardiol.*, 7:7, 1961.
30. Burchell, H. B.: Problems in the Recognition and Treatment of Pericarditis, *Lancet*, 74:465, 1954.
31. Teicholz, L. E.: Echocardiographic Evaluation of Pericardial Diseases, *Prog. Cardiovasc. Dis.*, 21:133, 1978.
32. Haaz, W. S., Mintz, G. S., Kotler, M. N., Parry, W., and Segal, B. L.: Two Dimensional Echocardiographic Recognition of the Descending Thoracic Aorta: Value in Differentiating Pericardial from Pleural Effusion, *Am. J. Cardiol.*, 46:739, 1980.
33. Martin, R. P., Bowden, R., Filly, K., and Popp, R. L.: Intrapericardial Abnormalities in Patients with Pericardial Effusion. Findings by Two Dimensional Echocardiography, *Circulation*, 61:568, 1980.
34. Riba, A. L., and Morganroth, J.: Unsuspected Substantial Pericardial Effusions Detected by Echocardiography, *JAMA*, 236:2623, 1976.
35. Goldstein, D. H., Nagar, C., Srivastava, N., Schacht, R. A., Ferris, F. Z., and Flowers, N. C.: Clinically Silent Pericardial Effusions in Patients on Long Term Hemodialysis, *Chest*, 72:744, 1977.
36. Horowitz, M. S., Schultz, C. S., Stinson, E. B., Harrison, D. C., and Popp, R. L.: Sensitivity and Specificity of Echocardiographic Diagnosis of Pericardial Effusion, *Circulation*, 50:239, 1974.
37. Feigenbaum, H.: Echocardiographic Diagnosis of Pericardial Effusion, *Am. J. Cardiol.*, 26:475, 1970.
38. Hagan, A. D.: Evaluation of Pericardial Diseases by M Mode and Two Dimensional Echocardiography, in D. T. Mason (ed.), "Advances in Heart Disease," vol. 3, New York, Grune & Stratton, 1980, pp. 699–702.
39. Come, P. C., Riley, M. F., and Fortuin, N. J.: Echocardiographic Mimicry of Pericardial Effusion, *Am. J. Cardiol.*, 39:112, 1977.
40. Shah, P.: Echocardiography in Pericardial Disease, in P. S. Reddy, D. F. Leon, and J. A. Shaver (eds.), "Pericardial Disease," New York, Raven Press, 1981, p. 130.
41. Hirschfield, D. S., and Emilson, B. B.: Echocardiogram in Calcified Mitral Valve Annulus, *Am. J. Cardiol.*, 36:354, 1975.
42. Foote, W. C., Jefferson, C. M., and Price, H. L.: False Positive Echocardiographic Diagnosis of Pericardial Effusion: Result of Tumor Encasement of the Heart Simulating Constrictive Pericarditis, *Chest*, 71:546, 1976.
43. Martin, R. P., Rakowski, H., French, J., and Popp, R. L.: Localization of Pericardial Effusion with Wide Angle Phased Array Echocardiography, *Am. J. Cardiol.*, 42:904, 1978.
44. Tehranzadeh, J., and Kelley, M. J.: The Differential Density Sign of Pericardial Effusion, *Radiology*, 133:23, 1979.
45. Lower, R.: "Tactatus de Corde, Item de Motu et Colare Sanguinis et Chyli in Sum Transiti," London, J. Allestry, 1969.
46. Chevers, N.: Observations of Diseases of the Orifice and Valves of the Aorta, *Guy's Hosp. Rep.*, 7:387, 1842.
47. Gaasch, W. H., Peterson, K. L., and Shabetai, R.: Left Ventricular Function in Chronic Constrictive Pericarditis, *Am. J. Cardiol.*, 34:107, 1974.
48. Craig, R. J., Whalen, R. E., Behar, V. S., and McIntosh, H. D.: Pressure and Volume Changes in Acute Pericardial Tamponade, *Am. J. Cardiol.*, 22:65, 1968.
49. Fowler, N. O., Gabel, M., and Holmes, J. C.: Hemodynamic Effects of Nitroprusside and Hydralazine in Experimental Cardiac Tamponade, *Circulation*, 57:563, 1978.
50. Pegram, B. L., Kardon, M. B., and Bishop, V. S.: Changes in Left Ventricular Internal Diameter with Increasing Pericardial Pressure, *Cardiovasc. Res.*, 9:707, 1975.
51. Brecher, G. A.: "Venous Return," New York, Grune & Stratton, 1956, p. 111.
52. Shabetai, R., Fowler, N. O., and Guntheroth, W. G.: The Hemodynamics of Cardiac Tamponade and Constrictive Pericarditis, *Am. J. Cardiol.*, 26:480, 1970.
53. Shabetai, R., Fowler, N. O., Fenton, J. C., and Masangkay, M.: Pulsus Paradoxus, *J. Clin. Invest.*, 44:1882, 1965.
54. Hansen, A. T., Eskildsen, P., and Gotzsche, H.: Pressure Curves from the Right Auricle and the Right Ventricle in Chronic Constrictive Pericarditis, *Circulation*, 3:881, 1951.
55. Brecher, G. A.: Critical Review of Recent Work on Ventricular Diastolic Suction, *Circ. Res.*, 6:554, 1958.
56. DeCristofaro, D., and Liv, C. K.: The Hemodynamics of Cardiac Tamponade and Blood Volume Overload in Dogs, *Cardiovasc. Res.*, 3:298, 1968.
57. Ditchey, R., Engler, R. L., LeWinter, M. M., et al.: The Role of the Right Heart in Acute Cardiac Tamponade in Dogs, *Circ. Res.*, 48:701, 1981.
58. Shabetai, R., Fowler, N. O., and Gueron, M.: The Effects of Respiration on Aortic Pressure and Flow, *Am. Heart J.*, 65:525, 1963.
59. Shabetai, R., Fowler, N. O., and Bruanstein, J. R.: Transmural Ventricular Pressures and Pulsus Paradoxus in Experimental Cardiac Tamponade, *Dis. Chest.*, 39:557, 1961.
60. Settle, H. P., Adolph, R. J., Fowler, N. O., Engel, P., Agruss, N. S., and Levenson, N. I.: Echocardiographic Study of Cardiac Tamponade, *Circulation*, 56:951, 1977.
61. Reddy, P. S., Curtiss, E. L., O'Toole, J. D., and Shaver, J. A.: Cardiac Tamponade: Hemodynamic Observations in Man, *Circulation*, 58:265, 1978.
62. Kronzon, I., and Winer, H. E.: Absence of Paradoxical Pulse in Patients with Atrial Septal Defect and Cardiac Tamponade, *Am. J. Cardiol.*, 41:446, 1978. (Abstract.)
63. Friedman, H. S., Sakurai, H., Choe, S.-S., Lajam, F., and Celis, A.: Pulsus Paradoxus: A Manifestation of Marked Reduction of Left Ventricular End Diastole Volume in Cardiac Tamponade, *J. Thorac. Cardiovasc. Surg.*, 79:74, 1980.
64. Dock, W.: Inspiratory Traction on the Pericardium, *Arch. Intern. Med.*, 108:837, 1961.
65. Friedman, H. S., Lajam, F., Saman, O., et al.: Effect of Autonomic Blockade on the Hemodynamic Findings of Acute Cardiac Tamponade, *Am. J. Physiol.*, 232:H5, 1977.
66. Hancock, E. W.: Subacute Effusive-Constrictive Pericarditis, *Circulation*, 43:183, 1971.
67. Tei, C., Child, J. S., Tanaka, H., and Shan, P. M.: Atrial Systolic Notch on the Interventricular Septal Echogram: An Echocardiographic Sign of Constrictive Pericarditis, *J. Am. Coll. Cardiol.*, 1:907, 1983.
68. Jarmakani, J. M. M., McHale, P. A., and Greenfield, J. C.:

The Effect of Cardiac Tamponade on Coronary Hemodynamics in the Awake Dog, *Cardiovasc. Res.*, 9:112, 1975.
69. Wechsler, A. S., Auerbach, B. J., Graham, T. C., and Sabiston, D. C.: Distribution of Intramyocardial Blood Flow during Pericardial Tamponade: Correlation with Microscopic Anatomy and Intrinsic Myocardial Contractility, *J. Thorac. Cardiovasc. Surg.*, 68:867, 1974.
70. Beck, C. S.: Two Cardiac Compression Triads, *JAMA*, 104:714, 1935.
71. Katz, L. N., and Gauchat, H. W.: Observations on Pulsus Paradoxus (with Special Reference to Pericardial Effusions), *Arch. Intern. Med.*, 33:371, 1924.
71a. Shabetai, R., Mangiardi, L., Bhargava, V., Ross, J., Jr., and Higgins, C. B.: The Pericardium and Cardiac Function, *Prog. Cardiovasc. Dis.*, 22:107, 1979.
72. Guberman, B. A., Fowler, N. O., Engel, P. J., Gueron, M., and Allen, J. M.: Cardiac Tamponade in Medical Patients, *Circulation*, 64:633, 1981.
73. Cohn, J. N., Pinkerson, A. L., and Tristani, F. E.: Mechanism of Pulsus Paradoxus in Clinical Shock, *J. Clin. Invest.*, 46:1744, 1967.
74. Gillam, L. D., Guyer, D. E., Gibson, T. C., King, M. E., Marshall, J. E., and Weyman, A. E.: Hemodynamic Compression of the Right Atrium, a New Echocardiographic Sign of Cardiac Tamponade, *Circulation*, 68:294, 1983.
75. Leimgruber, P. P., Klopfenstein, H. S., Wann, L. S., and Brooks, H. L.: The Hemodynamic Derangement Associated with Right Ventricular Diastolic Collapse in Cardiac Tamponade: an Experimental Echocardiographic Study, *Circulation*, 68:612, 1983.
76. D'Cruz, I. A., Cohen, H. C., Parbhu, R., and Glick, G.: Diagnosis of Cardiac Tamponade by Echocardiography. Changes in Mitral Valve Motion and Ventricular Dimensions, with Special Reference to Paradoxical Pulse, *Circulation*, 52:460, 1975.
77. Feigenbaum, H., Zaky, A., and Grabhorn, L. L.: Cardiac Motion in Patients with Pericardial Effusion: A Study Using Reflected Ultrasound, *Circulation*, 34:611, 1966.
78. Price, E. C., and Dennis, E. W.: Electrical Alternans, Its Mechanism Demonstrated, *Circulation*, 39(suppl. III):165, 1969.
79. Littman, D., and Spodick, D. H.: Total Electrical Alternation in Pericardial Disease, *Circulation*, 27:912, 1958.
80. Toney, J. C., and Kolmen, S. N.: Cardiac Tamponade: Fluid and Pressure Effects on Electrocardiographic Changes, *Proc. Soc. Exp. Biol. Med.*, 121:642, 1966.
80a. Antman, E. M., Gargill, V., and Grossman, W.: Low Pressure Cardiac Tamponade, *Ann. Intern. Med.*, 91:403, 1979.
81. Shabetai, R., and Rostand, S. G.: Nephrogenic Pericardial Disease. Contemporary Issues in Nephrology, 13, in R. A. O'Rourke, B. M. Brenner, and J. H. Stein (eds.), "The Heart and Renal Disease," Churchill Livingstone, New York, 1984.
82. Hardesty, R. L.: Delayed Postoperative Cardiac Tamponade: Diagnosis and Management, in P. S. Reddy, D. F. Leon, and J. S. Shaver (eds.), "Pericardial Disease," New York, Raven Press, 1981, p. 341.
83. Yacoub, M. H., Cleland, W. P., and Deal, C. W.: Left Atrial Tamponade, *Thorax*, 21:306, 1966.
84. Engleman, R. M., Spencer, F. C., Reed, G. E., and Tice, D. A.: Cardiac Tamponade following Open Heart Surgery, *Circulation*, 41(suppl. 2):11–165, 1970.
85. Krikorian, J. G., and Hancock, E. W.: Pericardiocentesis, *Am. J. Med.*, 65:808, 1978.
86. Wong, B., Murphy, J., Chang, C. J., and Hassenein, K.: The Risk of Pericardiocentesis, *Am. J. Cardiol.*, 44:1110, 1979.
87. Paul, O., Castleman, B., and White, P. D.: Chronic Constrictive Pericarditis: A Study of 53 Cases, *Am. J. Med. Sci.*, 216:361, 1948.
88. Andrews, G. W. S., Pickering, G. W., and Sellors, T. H.: The Aetiology of Constrictive Pericarditis with Special Reference to Tuberculosis Pericarditis, Together with a Note on Polyserositis, *Q. J. Med.*, 17:291, 1948.
89. Shabetai, R.: The Pericardium: An Essay on Some Recent Developments, *Am. J. Cardiol.*, 42:1036, 1978.
90. Wood, P.: Chronic Constrictive Pericarditis, *Am. J. Cardiol.*, 7:48, 1961.
91. Levine, H. D.: Myocardial Fibrosis in Constrictive Pericarditis: Electrocardiographic and Pathologic Observations, *Circulation*, 48:1268, 1973.
91a. Lorrel, B., Leinback, R. C., Pohost, G. M., et al.: Right Ventricular Infarction. Clinical Diagnosis and Differential Diagnosis from Cardiac Tamponade and Pericardial Constriction, *Am. J. Cardiol.*, 43:465, 1979.
92. Meany, E., Shabetai, R., Bhargava, V., et al.: Cardiac Amyloidosis, Constrictive Pericarditis and Restrictive Cardiomyopathy, *Am. J. Cardiol.*, 38:547, 1976.
93. Goodwin, J. F., and Oakley, C. M.: The Cardiomyopathies, *Br. Heart J.*, 34:345, 1972.
94. Schire, V., Gostman, M. S., and Beck, W.: Unusual Diastolic Murmurs in Constrictive Pericarditis and Constrictive Endocarditis, *Am. Heart J.*, 76:4, 1968.
95. McHenry, M. M., Ord, J. W., Johnson, R. R., et al.: Exercise Performance and Stroke Volume Changes in Two Patients with Constrictive Pericarditis, *Am. Heart J.*, 70:180, 1965.
96. Nakhjavan, F. K., and Goldberg, H.: Hemodynamic Effect of Catecholamine Stimulation in Constrictive Pericarditis, *Circulation*, 42:487, 1970.
97. Tyberg, T. I., Goodyear, A. V. N., Hurt, V. W., Alexander, J., and Langou, R. A.: Left Ventricular Filling in Differentiating Restrictive Cardiac Amyloid Cardiomyopathy and Constrictive Pericarditis, *Am. J. Cardiol.*, 47:791, 1981.
98. Candell- Riera, J., del Castillo, G., Permanyer-Miralda, G., and Soler-Soler, J.: Echocardiographic Features of the Interventricular Septum in Chronic Constrictive Pericarditis, *Circulation*, 57:1154, 1978.
99. Doppman, J. L., Rienmuller, R., Lissner, L., et al.: Computer Tomography in Constrictive Pericardial Disease, *J. Comput. Assist. Tomogr.*, 5:1, 1981.
100. Swanton, R. H., Brooksby, I. A. B., Davies, M. J., Coltart, D. J., Jenkins, B. S., and Webb-Peploe, M. M.: Systolic and Diastolic Ventricular Function in Cardiac Amyloidosis, *Am. J. Cardiol.*, 39:658, 1977.
101. Keith, T. A.: Chronic Constrictive Pericarditis in Association with a Rheumatoid Disease, *Circulation*, 25:477, 1962.
102. Kutcher, M. A., King, S. B., III, Alimurung, B. N., Craver, J. M., and Logue, R. B.: Constrictive Pericarditis as a Complication of Cardiac Surgery: Recognition of an Entity, *Am. J. Cardiol.*, 50:742, 1982.
103. Marsa, R., Mehta, S., Willis, W., and Balley, L.: Constrictive Pericarditis after Myocardial Revascularization, *Am. J. Cardiol.*, 44:117, 1979.
104. Bush, C. A., Stang, J. M., Wooley, C. F., and Kilman, J. W.: Occult Constrictive Pericardial Disease. Diagnosis by Rapid Volume Expansion and Correction by Pericardiectomy, *Circulation*, 56:924, 1977.
105. Fowler, N. O.: Constrictive Pericarditis: New Aspects, *Am. J. Cardiol.*, 50:1014, 1982.
105a. Shabetai, R.: "The Pericardium," Grune & Stratton, New York, 1981, pp. 206–208.
106. Culliford, A. T., Lipton, M., and Spencer, F. C.: Operation for Chronic Constrictive Pericarditis: Do the Surgical Approach and Degree of Pericardial Resection Influence the Outcome Significantly? *Ann. Thorac. Surg.*, 29:146, 1980.
107. Sommerville, W.: Constrictive Pericarditis with Special Reference to the Change in Natural History Brought About by Surgical Intervention, *Circulation*, (suppl. V):V–102, 1968.
108. Nasser, W. K.: Congenital Absence of the Left Pericardium, *Am. J. Cardiol.*, 26:470, 1970.
109. Bright, R.: Tabular View of the Morbid Appearances in a Hundred Cases Connected with Albuminous Urine, *Guy's Hosp. Rep.*, 1:380, 1836.
110. Compty, C. M., Cohen, S. L., and Shapiro, F. L.: Pericarditis in Chronic Uremia and Its Sequels, *Ann. Intern. Med.*, 75:173, 1971.

111. Beaudry, G., Nakamoto, S., and Kolff, W. J.: Uremic Pericarditis and Tamponade in Chronic Renal Failure, *Ann. Intern. Med.,* 64:990, 1966.
112. Compty, C. M., Wathen, R. L., and Shapiro, F.L.: Uremic Pericarditis, in D. H. Spodick (ed.), "Uremic Pericarditis," F. A. Davis, Philadelphia, 1976, p. 220.
113. Buselmeir, T. J., Simmons, R. L., Najarian, J. S., Mauer, S. M., Matas, A. J., and Kjellstrand, C. M.: Uremic Pericardial Effusion, *Nephron,* 16:371, 1976.
114. Parkinson, J., and Bedford, D. E.: Cardiac Infarction and Coronary Thrombosis, *Lancet,* 1–214:4, 1928.
115. Kahn, A. H.: Pericarditis of Myocardial Infarction: Review of the Literature with Case Presentation, *Am. Heart J.,* 90:788, 1975.
116. Dressler, W.: A Post Myocardial Infarction Syndrome. Preliminary Report of a Complication Resembling Idiopathic Benign Pericarditis, *JAMA,* 160:1379, 1956.
117. Lichstein, E., Arsura, E., Hollander, G., Greengart, A., and Sanders, M.: Current Incidence of Post Myocardial Infarction (Dressler's) Syndrome, *Am. J. Cardiol.,* 50:1269, 1982.
118. Kossowsky, W. A., Lyon, A. F., and Spain, D. M.: Reappraisal of the Post Myocardial Dressler's Syndrome, *Am. Heart J.,* 102:954, 1981.
119. Burch, G. E., and Colcolough, H. L.: Postcardiotomy and Postinfarction Syndromes—a Theory, *Am. Heart J.,* 80:290, 1970.
120. Engle, M. A., Zabriskie, J. B., Senterfit, L. B., Gay, W. A., Jr., O'Loughlin, J. E., Jr., and Ehlers, K. H.: Viral Illness and the Post Pericardiotomy Syndrome. A Prospective Study in Children, *Circulation,* 62:1151, 1980.
121. Artman, K.: Current Concepts: Malignant Mesothelioma, *N. Engl. J. Med.,* 303:200, 1980.
122. Applefeld, M. M., and Pollock, S. H.: Cardiac Disease in Patients Who Have Malignancies, *Curr. Probl. Cardiol.,* 4:6, 1980.
123. Syed, S., and Jung, R. T.: Cardiac Tamponade Caused by Metastasising Hemangio-Endothelial Sarcoma of the Liver, *Br. Heart J.,* 40:697, 1978.
124. Arciniegas, E., Hakimi, M., Forooki, Z. Q., and Green, E. W.: Intrapericardial Teratoma in Infancy, *J. Thorac. Cardiovasc. Surg.,* 79:306, 1980.
125. Davis, S., Sharma, S. M., Blumberg, E. D., and Kim, C. S.: Intrapericardial Tetracycline for the Management of Cardiac Tamponade Secondary to Malignant Pericardial Effusion, *N. Engl. J. Med.,* 299:1113, 1978.
126. Applefeld, M. M., Slawson, R. G., Hall-Craigs, M., Green, D. C., Singleton, R. T., and Wiernik, P. H.: Delayed Pericardial Disease after Radiotherapy, *Am. J. Cardiol.,* 47:210, 1981.
127. Ruckdeschel, J. C., Chang, P., Martin, R., et al.: Radiation Related Pericardial Effusions in Patients with Hodgkin's Disease, *Medicine,* 54:245, 1975.
128. Schneider, J. S., and Edwards, J. E.: Irradiation Induced Pericarditis, *Chest,* 75:560, 1979.
129. King, D. T., and Nieberg, R. K.: The Use of Cytology to Evaluate Pericardial Effusion, *Am. Clin. Lab. Sci.,* 9:18, 1979.
130. Hancock, E. W.: Pericardial Disease in Patients with Neoplasm, in P. S. Reddy, D. F. Leon, and J. A. Shaver (eds.), "Pericardial Disease," Raven Press, New York, 1981, p. 327.
131. Bywaters, E. G. L.: The Relation between Heart and Joint Disease "Rheumatoid Heart Disease" and Chronic Post-rheumatic Arthritis (Type Jaccoud), *Br. Heart J.,* 12:101, 1950.
132. Charcot, J. M.: "Clinical Lectures on Senile and Chronic Diseases," New Sydenham Soc., London, 95, 1881, pp. 172–175. (Translated by N. S. Tuke.)
133. Prakash, R., Atassi, A., Poske, R., and Rosen, K. M.: Prevalence of Pericardial Effusion and Mitral Valve Involvement in Patients with Rheumatoid Arthritis without Cardiac Symptoms. An Echocardiographic Evaluation, *N. Engl. J. Med.,* 289:597, 1973.
134. Gelson, A., Sanderson, J. M., and Carson, P.: Rheumatoid Pericardial Effusion with Heart Block Treated by Pericardiectomy and Implantation of Permanent Pacemaker, *Br. Heart J.,* 39:113, 1977.
135. Burney, D. P., Martin, C. E., Thomas, C. S., Fisher, R. D., and Bender, H. W.: Rheumatoid Pericarditis, *J. Thorac. Cardiovasc. Surg.,* 77:511, 1979.
136. Brigden, W., Bywaters, E. G. L., Lessof, M. H., and Ross, I. P.: The Heart in Systemic Lupus Erythematosus, *Br. Heart J.,* 22:1, 1960.
137. Bergen, S. S., Jr.: Pericardial Effusion, a Manifestation of Systemic Lupus Erythematosus, *Circulation,* 22:144, 1960.
138. Bulkley, B. H., and Roberts, W. C.: The Heart in Systemic Lupus Erythematosus and the Changes Induced in It by Corticosteroid Therapy. A Study of 36 Necropsy Patients, *Am. J. Med.,* 58:243, 1975.
139. Sackner, M. A., Heinz, R., and Steinberg, A.: The Heart in Scleroderma, *Am. J. Cardiol.,* 17:542, 1966.
140. Fowler, N. O.: "Cardiac Diagnosis and Treatment," 3d ed., Harper & Row, Hagerstown, 1980, p. 978.
141. Slater, E. E.: Cardiac Tamponade and Peripheral Eosinophilia in a Patient Receiving Cromolyn Sodium, *Chest,* 73:878, 1978.
142. Orlando, R. C., Moye, P., and Barnett, T. B.: Methysergide Therapy and Constrictive Pericarditis, *Ann. Intern Med.,* 88:213, 1978.
143. Houston, M. C., McChesney, J. A., and Chatergee, K.: Pericardial Effusion Associated with Minoxidil Therapy, *Arch. Intern. Med.,* 91:511, 1971.
144. Logue, R. B.: Etiology, Recognition and Management of Pericardial Disease, in J. W. Hurst (ed.), "The Heart," 5th ed., McGraw-Hill, New York, 1982, p. 1383.
145. Gleckman, R. A.: Nonviral Infectious Pericarditis, in D. H. Spodick (ed.), "Pericardial Diseases," F. A. Davis, Philadelphia, 1976.
146. Suzman, S.: Tuberculous Pericarditis, *Br. Heart J.,* 5:19, 1943.
147. Cheitlin, M. D., Serfas, L. J., Sebar, S. S., et al.: Tuberculous Pericarditis: Is Limited Pericardial Biopsy Sufficient for Diagnosis? *Am. Rev. Respir. Dis.,* 98:287, 1968.
148. Lyons, H. A., Rooney, J. J., and Crocco, J. A.: Tuberculous Pericarditis, *Ann. Intern. Med.,* 68:1175, 1968.
149. Kirchner, S. G., Heller, R. M., Sell, S. H., and Altemeier, W. A.: The Radiological Features of *Histoplasma* Pericarditis. *Pediatr. Radiol.,* 7:7, 1978.
150. Young, E. J., Vainrub, B., and Musher, D. M.: Pericarditis due to Histoplasmosis, *JAMA,* 240:1750, 1978.
151. Wooley, C. F., and Hosier, D. M.: Constrictive Pericarditis due to *Histoplasma capsulatum, N. Engl. J. Med.,* 264:1230, 1961.
152. Bennett, J. E.: Chemotherapy of Systemic Mycoses, *N. Engl. J. Med.,* 290:30, 1974.
153. Goodwin, R. A., Jr., Snell, J. D., Jr., Hubbard, W. N., et al.: Relationship in Combined Pulmonary Infections with *Histoplasma capsulatum* and *Mycobacterium tuberculosis, Am. Rev. Respir. Dis.,* 96:990, 1967.
154. Sarosi, G. A., Voth, D. W., Dahl, B. A., et al.: Disseminated Histoplasmosis: Results of Long Term Follow-Up, *Ann. Intern. Med.,* 75:511, 1971.
155. Chavez, C. M., and Conn, J. H.: Constrictive Pericarditis due to Infection with *Nocardia asteroides, Chest,* 61:79, 1972.
156. Fowler, N. O.: Infectious Pericarditis, *Prog. Cardiovasc. Dis.,* 16:23, 1973.
157. Klacsman, P. G., Bulkley, B. H., and Hutchins, G. M.: The Changed Spectrum of Purulent Pericarditis: An 86 Year Autopsy Experience in 200 Patients, *Am. J. Med.,* 63:666, 1977.
158. Tan, J. S., Holmes, J. C., Manitas, G. T., and Fowler, N. O.: Antibiotic Level in Pericardial Fluid, *J. Clin. Invest.,* 53:7, 1974.
159. Miller, H. I.: Acute Pericarditis as a Presenting Feature of Meningococcal Septicemia, *Am. J. Med. Sci.,* 9:1570, 1973.
160. Pierce, H. I., and Cooper, E. B.: Meningococcal Pericarditis, *Arch. Intern. Med.,* 129:918, 1972.
161. Scott, L. P., Knot, D., Perury, L. W., and Pineros-Torres,

F. J.: Meningococcal Pericarditis. Report of 2 Cases Complicated by Acute Constrictive Pericarditis, *Am. J. Cardiol.*, 29:104, 1972.
162. Symbar, P. N., Ware, R. E., and DiOrio, D. A.: Purulent Pericarditis. A Review of Diagnostic and Surgical Principles, *South. Med. J.*, 67:46, 1974.
163. Gould, K., Barnett, J. A., and Sanford, J. P.: Purulent Pericarditis in the Antibiotic Era, *Arch. Intern. Med.*, 134:923, 1974.
164. Caird, R., Conway, N., and McMillan, I. K. R.: Purulent Pericarditis Followed by Early Constriction in Young Children, *Br. Heart J.*, 35:201, 1973.
165. Smolar, E. N., Rubin, J. E., Avramides, A., and Carter, A. C.: Cardiac Tamponade in Primary Myxedema and Review of the Literature, *Am. J. Med. Sci.*, 272:345, 1976.
166. Stanley, R. J., Subramanian, R., and Lie, J. T.: Cholesterol Pericarditis Terminating as Constrictive Calcific Pericarditis, *Am. J. Cardiol.*, 46:511, 1980.
167. Brawley, R. K., Vesco, J. S., and Morrow, A. G.: Cholesterol Pericarditis. Considerations of its Pathogenesis and Treatment, *Am. J. Med.*, 41:235, 1966.
168. Shojaee, S., and Hutchins, G. M.: Echinococcosis Complicated by Purulent Pericarditis, *Chest*, 73:79, 1978.
169. Pierce, R. N., and Walker Smith, G. J.: Intrathoracic Manifestations of Dego's Disease (Malignant Atrophic Papulosis), *Chest*, 73:79, 1978.
170. Mets, T., Van Hove, W., and Louis, H.: Pseudomyxoma Peritonei: Report of a Case with Extraperitoneal Metastasis and Invasion of the Spleen, *Chest*, 72:792, 1977.
171. Gsonka, G. W., and Oates, J. K.: Pericarditis and Electrocardiographic Changes in Reiter's Syndrome, *Br. Med. J.*, 1:866, 1957.
172. Mihass, A. A., and Dasher, C. A.: Pericarditis Associated with Granulomatous Colitis, *Am. J. Gastroenterol.*, 68:494, 1977.
173. Vliestra, R. E., Lie, J. T., Kuhl, W. E., Danielso, G. K., and Roberts, M. K.: Whipple's Disease Involving the Pericardium. Pathological Confirmation during Life, *Aust. N.Z. J. Med.*, 8:649, 1978.
174. Engle, M. A.: Cardiac Involvement in Cooley's Anemia, *Ann. N.Y. Acad. Sci.*, 119:694, 1964.
175. Just, H., and Mattingly, T. W.: Interatrial Septal Defect and Pericardial Disease, *Am. Heart J.*, 76:157, 1968.
176. Westfried, M., Mandel, D., Alderate, M. N., Groopman, J., and Minkowitz, S.: Sipple's Syndrome with a Malignant Pheochromocytoma Presenting as Pericardial Effusion, *Cardiology*, 63:305, 1978.
177. Toltzis, R. J., Rosenthal, A., Fellows, K., Castenada, A. R., and Nadas, A. S.: Chylous Reflux Syndrome Involving the Pericardium and Lung, *Chest*, 74:457, 1978.
178. Rogers, C. I., and Meridith, H. C.: Osler Revisited: An Unusual Cause of Inversion of the Diaphragm, *Radiology*, 125:596, 1977.
179. Davidson, E. D., Horney, J. T., and Salter, P. P., III: Internal Pancreatic Fistula to the Pericardium and Pleura, *Surgery*, 85:478, 1979.
180. McNicholl, B., Murray, J. P., Egan, B., and McHugh, P.: Pneumomediastinum and Diabetic Hyperpnoea, *Br. Med. J.*, 4:493, 1968.
181. Cumming, G. R., Kerr, R., and Ferguson, C. C.: Constrictive Pericarditis with Dwarfism in Two Siblings (Mulibrey Nanism), *J. Pediatr.*, 88:569, 1976.
182. Scarlett, J. A., Kistner, M. L., and Yang, L. C.: Behçet's Syndrome. Report of a Case Associated with Pericardial Effusion and Cryoglobulinemia Treated with Indomethacin, *Am. J. Med.*, 66:146, 1979.
183. Bianchi, C., DiBonito, L., Fonda, F., and Sauli, G.: Pericardial Perforation of a Gastric Ulcer Secondary to a Phytobezoar, *Panminerva Med.*, 19:353, 1977.

Section I

Traumatic Heart Disease

60

Traumatic Heart Disease

Panagiotis N. Symbas, M.D. Daniel Arensberg, M.D.

One of the leading causes of death and morbidity in our society is traumatic injuries. A significant number of these injuries are due to trauma to the heart and great vessels. With the improvement of emergency transportation networks an increasing number of patients with traumatic injuries to the heart and great vessels now reach the hospital alive.

Injury to the heart and great vessels may be due to penetrating and nonpenetrating trauma. A penetrating injury requires a vector for the physical force, such as an instrument inflicting a stab wound, or a missile that penetrates the heart or great vessels, or rarely by a needle that migrates through the wall of an adjacent organ such as the esophagus, or, very rarely, by a missile embolus reaching the heart through the venous system. Nonpenetrating injuries, on the other hand, are cardiovascular lesions resulting from physical forces acting externally upon the body. These forces can act through any one or a combination of several of the following mechanisms: (1) unidirectional force against the chest; (2) bidirectional or compressive force against the thorax; (3) indirect forces, i.e., compression of the abdomen and lower extremities resulting in a marked increase of intravascular pressure; (4) decelerative forces; and (5) concussive forces. The last is a category indicating a jarring force that interferes with cardiac rhythm, but which is not of sufficient magnitude to produce a significant anatomic lesion. All of these mechanisms may occur with or without actual fracture of bony structures of the chest wall.[1,2]

As the diagnostic and therapeutic modalities for the management of heart diseases have become more complex and more invasive, another group of mechanical injuries has become increasingly important. This group consists of iatrogenic trauma, comprising the complications of cardiopulmonary resuscitation, diagnostic cardiac catheterization, and regional angiocardiography.[3,4] These techniques have resulted in nonpenetrating contusive injuries to the pericardium and the myocardium, and penetrating cardiac injuries. The increasing use of invasive catheters and electrode pacemakers has also led to a corresponding increase of penetrating cardiac lesions, nonbacterial thrombotic endocarditis, and bacterial endocarditis, as well as an increasing incidence in the migration of therapeutic and intravenous catheters to the heart or pulmonary vascular beds.[5–10]

Two additional categories of heart trauma not due to mechanical injury are sufficiently distinctive to warrant separate classification. The first category encompasses cardiac injuries due to ionizing radiation, which predominantly causes pericarditis but may also result in myocardial injury.[11,12] The second includes the group of cardiac injuries due to electric current, which most often produces either atrial or ventricular dysrhythmias but may also cause burns of the heart and great vessels.

A few penetrating injuries and many nonpenetrating injuries of the heart are well tolerated, as clinical experience and experimental studies have indicated. Consequently, the majority of these lesions are infrequently diagnosed, since their initial clinical manifestation may be relatively minimal, and the lesion may be overlooked unless specific studies are obtained.[1,2,13,14] Frequently these cardiac injuries are overshadowed by the more overt manifestations of cerebral, abdominal, or musculoskeletal trauma. For these reasons and because only the more severe injuries are reflected in autopsy studies, the actual incidence of traumatic heart disease remains obscure.

Injury of the Heart, the Aorta, and the Great Vessels from Penetrating Trauma

The chest wall offers very little protection to the heart from stab and projectile wounds. These wounds may produce a variety of cardiac lesions including (1) penetrating wound of the pericardium; (2) penetrating wound of the cardiac wall; (3) penetrating wound of the interventricular septum; (4) perforating or lacerating wound of the cardiac valves, chordae tendineae, or papillary muscle; and (5) lacerating or perforating wound of the coronary vessels.

Penetrating or lacerating wounds of the heart are caused by knives, sharp objects, bullets, or other projectiles, and less commonly by the inward displacement of a rib or sternal fragment. These wounds are most frequently associated with penetrating wounds of the precordium, although they may also occur in patients with penetrating wounds of the chest, neck, and upper abdomen. The area of exposure to the anterior chest wall of each cardiac chamber and the intrapericardial great vessels differs markedly: 55 percent of the anterior surface is right ventricle, 20 percent left ventricle, 10 percent right atrium, 10 percent great vessels, and 5 percent vena cava.[1] The relative incidence of penetrating wounds to each of these structures coincides with their percentage of exposure to the anterior chest wall. Although this is true for both stab and projectile wounds, the latter frequently produce injury to the heart at more than one site.[14–17]

Almost half of the individuals who have incurred stab wounds of the heart may be expected to survive for a sufficient time to reach medical treatment.[18] Gunshot or other projectile injuries carry a more serious outlook, and perhaps only 10 to 20 percent of these individuals will fall into a salvageable category. The multiplicity of heart and great-vessel lesions that may be produced by penetrating wounds is indicated in Table 60-1. The pathophysiological consequences of penetrating wounds of the heart and great vessels depend upon the mode, sight, and size of the injury, and especially the state of the pericardial wound.[18,19] Lacerating or penetrating wounds frequently result in immediate hemorrhage of varying magnitude. The severity of the hemorrhage and whether it is intra- or extrapericardial determine the clinical picture and dictate the requirement of therapy. Where there is intrapericardial hemorrhage with a sealed pericardial wound, cardiac tamponade is the major threat;[20] whereas when the pericardial wound is open and bleeding occurs freely into the pleural space, loss of circulating blood volume is the major danger. The management of penetrating wounds should be based primarily on the prompt diagnosis and the clinical manifestations, with appropriate emergency resuscitative procedures and surgical treatment as indicated. The treatment of these lesions, when they are manifested with massive and/or continuous intrapleural hemorrhage, is immediate surgical repair. When the presenting clinical picture is that of cardiac tamponade, the treatment should consist of palliative pericardiocentesis, followed by immediate thoracotomy and cardiorrhaphy.[21–29] Immediate surgical repair appears to be the treatment of choice for all penetrating cardiac wounds, and pericardiocentesis should be used in patients with cardiac tamponade only to provide time for a safe operation. The unpredictable course of patients with a favorable response to pericardiocentesis, the propensity of these wounds to rebleed, and the possibility of coronary artery injury coupled with the advances in cardiac anesthesia and cardiac surgery greatly favor the immediate surgical treatment of penetrating cardiac wounds.

There are many residual or delayed sequelae of penetrating wounds of the heart, including structural defects such as (1) a ventricular or atrial septal defect; (2) aorta or coronary artery to cardiac chamber fistula; (3) aorta to pulmonary artery communications; (4) atrioventricular defects; (5) laceration of valve leaflets, cusps, or chordae tendineae; and (6) ventricular aneurysms.[19] The complications of infection, pericarditis, embolization, and dysrhythmias may also occur. These sequelae should always be suspected in patients who have sustained penetrating wounds of the heart or the chest. When symptoms and signs of a structural defect are detected, cardiac catheterization should be performed

TABLE 60-1 Penetrating Wounds of the Heart

1. Pericardial damage
   a. Laceration or perforation
   b. Hemopericardium with or without cardiac tamponade
   c. Serofibrinous or suppurative pericarditis
   d. Pneumopericardium
   e. Constrictive pericarditis
2. Myocardial damage
   a. Laceration
   b. Penetration or perforation
   c. Retained foreign body
   d. Structural defects
      (1) Aneurysm formation
      (2) Septal defects
      (3) Aorticocardiac fistula
3. Valvular injury
   a. Leaflet or cusp injury
   b. Papillary muscle or chordae tendineae laceration
4. Coronary artery injury
   a. Laceration or thrombosis with or without myocardial infarction
   b. Arteriovenous fistula
   c. Aneurysm
5. Embolism
   a. Foreign body
   b. Thrombus (septic or sterile)
6. Infective endocarditis
7. Rhythm or conduction disturbances

Note: We wish to thank Loren F. Parmley, M.D., and Thomas W. Mattingly, M.D., for permission to modify the table they prepared for the first edition (1966) of *The Heart.*

to define the lesion and its hemodynamic significance. Once evaluated, the proper mode of therapy should be determined by collaboration of the cardiologist and thoracic surgery team.[19,30]

Recurrent posttraumatic pericarditis, a phenomenon complicating approximately 20 percent of all cases of penetrating heart wounds, has been noted and is similar to the postcardiotomy syndrome seen after cardiac surgery. Symptomatic management is the treatment of choice for this syndrome unless cardiac tamponade or other sequelae, such as purulent or constrictive pericarditis, require surgical intervention.

Coronary artery injuries, depending upon the size of the injured vessel, can result in cardiac tamponade and varying degrees of myocardial ischemia or myocardial infarction. In these patients, survival is dependent upon the proper restoration of the coronary artery blood flow by repair or bypass of the injured major branches of the coronary arterial system, or the ligation of smaller terminal vessels.[31] Coronary artery aneurysms and arteriovenous fistulas are rare sequelae of injury, and treatment should be individualized.[18,32]

Penetrating wounds may result in the retention of a projectile within the heart. Embolization of such a foreign body, or of the thrombus associated with it, has occurred.[33] The possibility of bacterial endocarditis is also present if the projectile is not completely embedded in the myocardium. In addition, several patients with intracardiac projectiles have developed cardiac neurosis with an almost maniacal desire for removal of the foreign body. These possible complications suggest that after precise angiographic localization, elective extraction may be the preferred management of such projectiles in the heart. If a projectile enters one of the large venous channels, embolization to the heart or pulmonary arteries may occur. Embolization of a foreign body from the left side of the heart to the systemic arterial system may be a serious consequence of such a retained object.[34] A potentially embolic foreign body in the heart or, similarly, a foreign body which has embolized to the systemic circulation should be surgically removed without delay unless it has resulted in a significant neurological deficit. Projectiles adjacent to or embedded within the wall of one of the great arteries should be extracted to prevent subsequent erosion and bleeding.

The pathophysiology of penetrating wounds to the great vessels is quite similar to that of penetrating wounds to the heart. In addition to the obvious results of either immediate or delayed hemorrhage, a penetrating wound of the great vessels may result in the formation of a false aneurysm, with possible subsequent rupture, or of an arteriovenous fistula, producing either immediate or latent signs and symptoms of congestive heart failure.[35,36] Traumatic arteriovenous fistulas are occasionally complicated by the development of bacterial endarteritis and endocarditis.[37] These traumatic vascular lesions should be detected and repaired as soon as possible.

Injury of the Heart, the Aorta, and the Great Vessels from Blunt Trauma

The forces that produce nonpenetrating lesions of the heart and great vessels are of such a nature that external evidence of chest injury may be meager or nondetectable in almost one-third of the traumatized patients. This lack of evidence of chest wall injury along with the frequent presence of other more obvious injuries to the body may, in many cases, cause failure or prevent the early diagnosis of cardiovascular lesions of this type.

The wide variety of injuries produced by nonpenetrating trauma is summarized in Table 60-2. The pathological lesions of myocardial contusion may vary considerably in extent and character, ranging from small areas of petechiae or ecchymosis, which may be either subepicardial or subendocardial, to contusion of the full thickness of the myocardial wall and, finally, to actual rupture of the heart.[2] Although minor insignificant myocardial contusion of the right ventricle is the most frequently occurring lesion, the most fatal lesion is that of myocardial rupture, as has been demonstrated by necropsy study. Myocardial rupture is extremely difficult to treat because of the rapid demise of the patient, and very often, when traumatic cardiac rupture has occurred,

TABLE 60-2 Nonpenetrating Trauma of the Heart

1. Pericardial injury
   a. Hemopericardium
   b. Rupture or laceration
   c. Serofibrinous pericarditis
   d. Constrictive pericarditis
2. Myocardial injury
   a. Contusion
   b. Rupture of free cardiac wall, early or delayed
   c. Rupture of septum
   d. Aneurysm
   e. Laceration
3. Disturbances of rhythm or conduction
4. Valve injury
   a. Rupture of valve leaflets, cusp, or chordae tendineae
   b. Contusion of papillary muscle
5. Coronary artery injury
   a. Thrombosis with or without myocardial infarction
   b. Arteriovenous fistula
   c. Laceration with or without myocardial infarction
6. Great-vessel injury
   a. Rupture
   b. Aneurysm formation
   c. Aorta–cardiac chamber fistula
   d. Thrombotic occlusion

Note: We wish to thank Loren F. Parmley, M.D., and Thomas W. Mattingly, M.D., for permission to modify the table they prepared for the first edition (1966) of *The Heart*.

it is only one of many severe body injuries that could have resulted in death. Although cardiac rupture is, in most instances, not amenable to therapy, there have been reports of successful surgical repair.[38] Rupture of the atrium or the interventricular septum may not be rapidly fatal, and successful surgical repair is often possible. In the case of interventricular septal rupture, surgical repair is accomplished optimally after medical therapy has allowed for the hemodynamic stabilization of the patient.[30–41]

Patients with myocardial contusion may be asymptomatic or may complain of pain that is identical in character, location, and radiation to the pain of myocardial ischemia and/or myocardial infarction. In severe cardiac injuries, all the clinical features of a well-developed myocardial infarction may be present. The patient may complain of typical chest pain starting immediately after or within several hours following the trauma.[42] An angina-like syndrome may also be initiated by the contusion, but it is usually transient unless there is concomitant coronary artery injury or, more likely, the antecedent presence of occult coronary atherosclerotic heart disease.[43] Coronary thrombosis may result from nonpenetrating trauma, but this is a rare event and is usually associated with existing coronary atherosclerotic heart disease.[44] The rarity of this lesion is demonstrated by the fact that in a series of 546 necropsy cases of nonpenetrating cardiac trauma, not a single instance of coronary thrombosis was found. Electrocardiographic evidence compatible with myocardial infarction may follow myocardial contusion, yet coronary arteriography may fail to demonstrate a coronary occlusion.[45] Coronary arteriography has also been used to demonstrate coronary occlusion presumably on a traumatic basis in the absence of electrocardiographic evidence of myocardial injury.[46] Laceration of a coronary artery from nonpenetrating injury may occur, producing cardiac tamponade or, on very rare occasions, a coronary artery fistula.[47]

Dyspnea and hypotension may also be presenting symptoms. In mild or moderate myocardial contusion, any of these signs may be transient in nature, or frequently absent. Cardiac failure is relatively rare, and, when present, the possibility of an associated cardiac injury, such as ventricular septal rupture or rupture of one of the cardiac valve leaflets, is very great. Hemopericardium, with or without signs and symptoms of cardiac tamponade, may be associated with myocardial contusion.

Although myocardial contusion is primarily manifested pathologically by hemorrhage within the myocardium, varying degrees of necrosis do occur. Ususally this is minimal and healing is complete, with little or no obvious scar or impairment of myocardial function. Large contusions, however, may cause a decrease in cardiac output, and extensive necrosis may lead to either rupture or, rarely, to congestive heart failure and formation of a true or false aneurysm.[48–51] Rupture of a true aneurysm is rare, whereas a false aneurysm is subject to this complication. Other complications from cardiac aneurysms include dysrhythmia, congestive heart failure, and mural thrombosis with embolism.[52] Because of these complications, surgical repair is advisable. Posttraumatic ventricular aneurysms, as well as septal defects, can be successfully repaired.[1] Localized areas of necrosis or hemorrhage involving the cardiac conduction system may produce varying degrees of atrioventricular block or any of the different types of intraventricular conduction defects.[2]

Electrocardiographic studies may be the only clinical clue that myocardial contusion has occurred.[53–57] Changes consistent with acute pericarditis may be seen. When there is more extensive contusion, the electrocardiographic abnormalities may be similar to those produced by a myocardial infarction. Atrial and ventricular dysrhythmias of all types may also occur and, undoubtedly, ventricular tachycardia and ventricular fibrillation may be the cause of death in some contusive injuries.

Elevated serum enzyme levels may be suggestive of myocardial injury, but these may be elevated as a result of other body trauma. Isoenzyme determinations, however, such as the MB creatine kinase (MB-CK) level and the cardiac-specific lactic dehydrogenase (LDH) level, may be of value in differentiating cardiac contusion from other tissue injuries.[58]

Radiocardiography may provide an additional means of detecting myocardial injury. Myocardial radioisotope scanning in dogs with experimentally induced contusion of the heart has shown that the areas of injury can be identified.[48,59] The clinical application of gated blood pool studies for the detection of impaired ventricular performance following myocardial contusion appears very promising. Further refinement of these techniques can be expected to allow earlier and more accurate diagnosis of myocardial injury.

More recently, two-dimensional echocardiography has been shown to be of value in the early diagnosis of a number of functional and intracardiac abnormalities associated with cardiac contusions.[60,61]

The treatment of myocardial contusion, like that of myocardial infarction, is symptomatic. A 1- to 3-week period of bed rest, gradual ambulation, and the prevention and early treatment of dysrhythmias are the most important therapeutic measures. The increased irritability of the heart must also be considered when one is deciding what drugs to use in the recently traumatized patient. For this reason, general anesthesia should be delayed when feasible. If surgical treatment for some other injury is necessary, the knowledge and the presence of a myocardial contusion should guide the anesthetist in the management and selection of any anesthetic and other supporting agent.

Anticoagulants should not be administered because they may precipitate bleeding within the myocardium or pericardial space. Digitalis should be used in the presence of congestive cardiac failure. Conventional antiarrhythmic agents can be given for control of any ectopic rhythms in the presence of a contused ventricular myocardium. If the myocardial contusion is severe, support with inotropic drugs and balloon counterpulsation may be necessary.

Valvular laceration, primarily involving the atrioventricular valves, is an infrequent result of nonpenetrating cardiac injury. This injury usually occurs in the presence of severe cardiac trauma resulting in death.[2] The aortic valve is most commonly involved in the surviving patient, characteristically leading to the rapid development of congestive heart failure secondary to aortic regurgitation.[62] It should be noted, however, that the onset of aortic regurgitation may be delayed for some time.[63] Mitral valvular laceration may have somewhat similar hemodynamic consequences, but this lesion is seldom encountered clinically. In contrast, tricuspid valve injury may be tolerated for years before surgical correction is required.[64] In addition to the more common complications of congestive heart failure and dysrhythmias, endocarditis occasionally may also develop.[65]

Papillary muscle or chordae tendineae rupture and laceration occur more frequently than valvular lacerations. Myocardial contusion may also result in papillary muscle dysfunction with secondary mitral or tricuspid regurgitation.[66] The clinical outcome depends on whether the structures involved are on the right side of the heart, where the lesion may be well tolerated, or on the left side of the heart, where the high-pressure system can lead to more serious hemodynamic sequelae. The murmurs produced by these lesions are generally typical of valvular regurgitation, but unusual high-pitched systolic and diastolic murmurs of variable intensity may also result. Traumatic tricuspid regurgitation may be present despite the absence of any detectable murmur.[67] Prompt and correct diagnosis by appropriate hemodynamic, echocardiographic, and angiographic studies is important. Operative techniques employing extracorporeal circulation and the use of valve prostheses or bioprostheses for the surgical correction of these lesions are readily available.

Pericardial lesions are often overlooked and heal without incident. Hemopericardium, however, may occur and, if hemorrhage is severe, cardiac tamponade will rapidly occur. When hemopericardium is suspected, echocardiography is an effective tool for confirming the diagnosis. If there is slow oozing of blood into the pericardium, often evoking a pericardial reaction, tremendous dilatation of the pericardial sac may develop over an extended period of time. Symptoms and signs of traumatic pericarditis are similar to those of pericarditis produced by a wide variety of causes. The syndrome of recurrent pericarditis, similar to the post-myocardial infarction syndrome, may develop, but this occurs less frequently with blunt than with penetrating cardiac injuries. Pericardial laceration is usually well tolerated, but herniation of the heart may occur, rarely leading to more serious consequences and death.[68,69]

Rupture of the aorta is the most common blunt injury of the great vessels. Rupture or avulsion of the great arteries (brachiocephalic, common carotid, and left subclavian) and venae cavae have been also observed. Because of the variety of mechanical forces produced by blunt trauma (Fig. 60-1) combined with anatomic factors,[1] the most frequent sites of rupture of the aorta in blunt injuries are the descending aorta just distal to the origin of the left subclavian artery (aortic isthmus), and the ascending aorta just proximal to the origin of the brachiocephalic artery.[70,71] Because of the high association of ascending aortic rupture with severe cardiac injury, the overwhelming majority of patients surviving aortic rupture for a sufficient period of time to receive definitive surgical correction are those who sustained rupture of the aortic isthmus.[70] Other sites of rupture of the thoracic aorta and the rupture of the abdominal aorta are much less common. The initial survival of the patient with aortic rupture is about 20 percent and is due to the formation of a false aneurysm, the wall of which consists of adventitia, the parietal pleura, and other mediastinal structures. The intactness of these structures maintains continuity of the circulation.

The common manifestations of traumatic rupture of the aorta are severe chest and midscapular pain, a new murmur, dyspnea, increased pulse amplitude, and hypertension of the upper extremities.[72] Some patients, however, are surprisingly free of any major symptoms or signs. Hoarseness, evidence of a superior vena cava syndrome, paraplegia, and anuria are less frequent manifestations. Although occasionally there are no obvious signs of

FIGURE 60-1 Diagrammatic illustration of the forces acting upon the aortic wall during rupture of the aorta from blunt trauma. (*From P. N. Symbas, "Traumatic Injuries of the Heart and Great Vessels," Charles C Thomas, Publisher, Springfield, Ill. 1971, p. 153. Reproduced with permission from the author. Courtesy of Charles C Thomas, Publisher, Springfield, Ill.*)

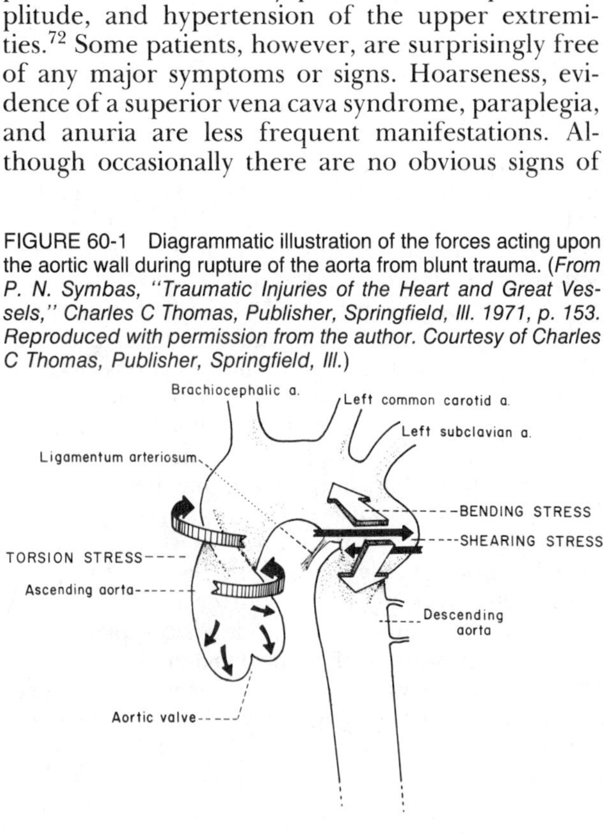

external injury, patients with rupture of the aorta usually have associated injuries of the skeleton, abdominal viscera, or central nervous system. The coexisting injuries may mask the signs of aortic rupture. For this reason any patient who has sustained severe blunt trauma or who has been exposed to major deceleration forces should be suspected of having aortic rupture, particularly if an increased pulse pressure and upper-extremity hypertension are present. Chest roentgenography is of great diagnostic value in patients with aortic rupture. Widening of the superior mediastinal shadow, disappearance of the aortic knob shadow, depression of the left main bronchus, and displacement of the trachea to the right are common roentgenographic abnormalities associated with this injury (Fig. 60-2). The only definite way, however, to establish the diagnosis of aortic rupture is by aortography. This should be performed immediately in all patients whose history, physical examination, or routine chest roentgenogram suggests the possibility of this injury. Surgical treatment should then be immediately undertaken with particular attention to provisions for perfusion of the kidney and spinal cord.

A chronic false aortic aneurysm may be discovered months or years after blunt trauma to the great vessels. Rupture of the aneurysm may occur at any time after its formation. Rarely, the complications of peripheral embolization from the thrombus contained within the aneurysm or the development of bacterial endoaortitis or chronic pseudocoarctation may occur.[73–75] Because of the relative instability of these aneurysms and the potential complications, surgical correction is the treatment of choice.

FIGURE 60-2 *A.* Chest roentgenogram of a young male who shortly before admission was involved in automobile accident. Note the mediastinal widening. *B.* Aortogram the same day showing a false aneurysm distal to the origin of the left subclavian artery and two filling defects, one proximal and one distal to the aneurysm.

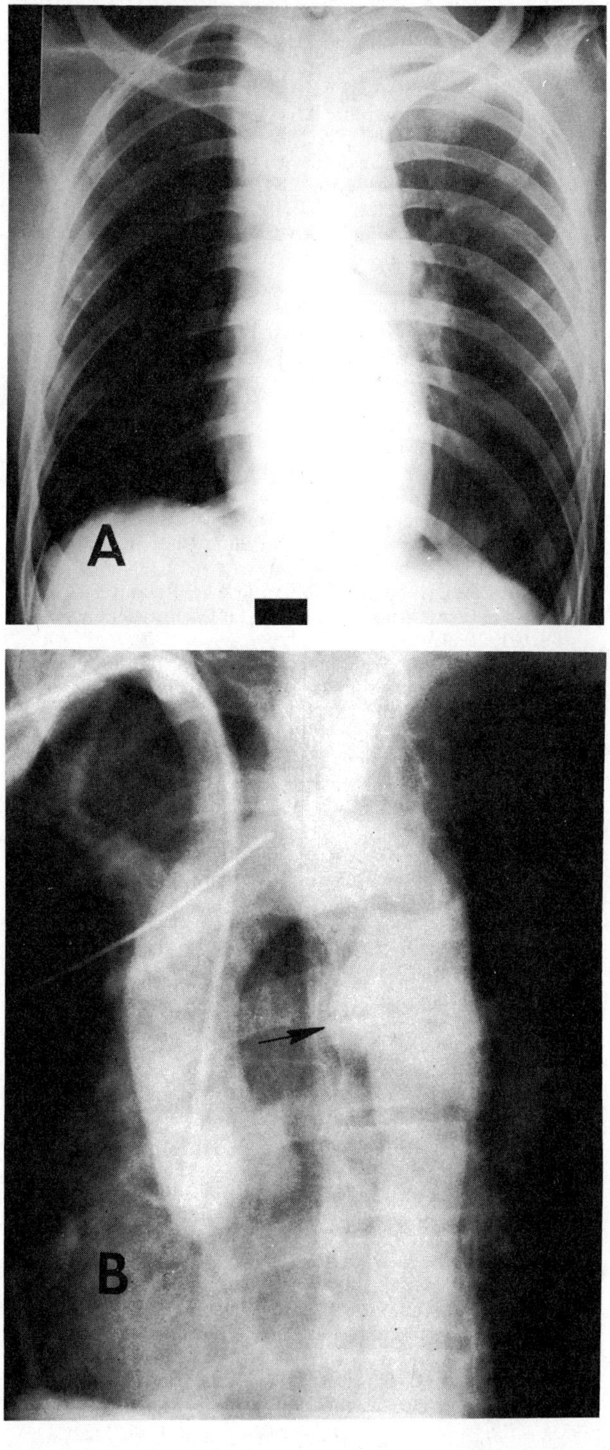

References

1. Symbas P. N.: "Trauma to the Heart and Great Vessels," Grune & Stratton, Inc., New York, 1978, p. 2.
2. Parmley, L. F., Manion, W. C., and Mattingly, T. W.: Nonpenetrating Traumatic Injury of the Heart, *Circulation,* 18:371, 1958.
3. Baldwin, J. J., and Edwards, J. E.: Rupture of Right Ventricle Complicating Closed Chest Cardiac Massage, *Circulation,* 53:562, 1976.
4. Gorlin, R.: Perforations and Other Cardiac Complications: A Cooperative Study on Cardiac Catheterization Performed and Other Cardiac Complications, *Circulation,* 37(suppl. 3):36, 1968.
5. Peters, R. W., Scheinman, M. M., Raskin, S., and Thomas, A. N.: Unusual Complications of Epicardial Pacemakers, *Am. J. Cardiol,* 45:1088, 1980.
6. Meyer, J. A., and Millar, K.: Perforation of the Right Ventricle by Electrode Catheters: A Review and Report of Nine Cases, *Ann. Surg.,* 168:1048, 1968.
7. Fitts, C. T., Barnett, T., Webb, C. M., Sexton, J., and Yarbrough, D. R., III: Perforating Wounds of the Heart Caused by Central Venous Catheters, *J. Trauma,* 10:764, 1970.
8. Pace, N. L., and Horton, W.: Indwelling Pulmonary Artery Catheters—Their Relationship to Aseptic Endocardial Vegetation, *JAMA,* 233:893, 1975.
9. Greene, J. J., Fitzwater, J. E., and Clemmer, T. P.: Septic Endocarditis and Indwelling Pulmonary Artery Catheters, 233:891, 1975.
10. Bloomfield, B. A.: Techniques of Nonsurgical Retrieval of Iatrogenic Foreign Bodies of the Heart, *Am. J. Cardiol.,* 27:538, 1971.
11. Cohn, K. E., Stewart, R. J., Fajardo, L. F., and Hancock, E. W.: Heart Disease Following Radiation, *Medicine,* 46:281, 1967.
12. Morton, D. L., Glancy, D. L., Joseph, W. L., and Adkins, P. C.: Management of Patients with Radiation-Induced Peri-

carditis with Effusions: A Note on the Development of Aortic Regurgitation in Two of Them, *Chest,* 64:291, 1973.
13. Moritz, A. R., and Atkins, J. P.: Cardiac Contusions: An Experimental and Pathologic Study, *Arch. Pathol.,* 25:445, 1938.
14. Samson, P. C.: Battle Wounds and Injuries of the Heart and Pericardium: Experiences in Forward Hospitals, *Ann. Surg.,* 127:1127, 1948.
15. Elkin, D. C.: The Diagnosis and Treatment of Wounds of the Heart, *JAMA,* 70:398, 1955.
16. Valle, A. R.: War Injuries of the Heart and Mediastinum, *Arch. Surg.,* 70:398, 1955.
17. Warshaw, L. J.: "The Heart in Industry," Hoeber Medical Division, Harper & Row, Publishers, Inc., New York, 1960, chap. 15.
18. Parmley, L. F., Mattingly, T. W., and Manion, W. C.: Penetrating Wounds of the Heart and Aorta, *Circulation,* 17:953, 1958.
19. Symbas, P. N., DiOrio, D. A., Tyras, D. H., Ware, R. E., and Hatcher, C. R., Jr.: Penetrating Cardiac Wounds. Significant Residual and Delayed Sequelae, *J. Thorac. Cardiovasc. Surg.,* 66:526, 1973.
20. Isaacs, J. P.: Sixty Penetrating Wounds of the Heart, *Surgery,* 45:696, 1959.
21. Decker, H. R.: Foreign Bodies in the Heart and Pericardium—Should They Be Removed?, *J. Thorac. Surg.,* 9:62, 1939.
22. Schechter, D. C., and L. Gilbert: Injuries of the Heart and Great Vessels Due to Pins and Needles, *Thorax,* 24:246, 1969.
23. Sugg, W. L., Rea, W. J., Ecker, R. R., Webb, W. R., Rose, E. F., and Shaw, R. R.: Penetrating Wounds of the Heart: An Analysis of 459 Cases, *J. Thorac. Cardiovasc. Surg.,* 56:531, 1968.
24. Ransdell, H. T., Jr., and Glass, H., Jr.: Gunshot Wounds of the Heart: Review of 20 Cases, *Am. J. Surg.,* 99:788, 1960.
25. Wilkinson, A. H., Jr., Buttram, T. L., Reid, W. A., and Howard, J. M.: Cardiac Injuries: An Evaluation of Immediate and Long-Range Results of Treatment, *Ann. Surg.,* 147:347, 1958.
26. Cooley, D. A., Dunn, J. R., Brockman, H. LeR., and DeBakey, M. E.: Treatment of Penetrating Wounds of the Heart: Experimental and Clinical Observations, *Surgery,* 37:882, 1955.
27. Symbas, P. N., Harlaftis, N., and Waldo, W. J.: Penetrating Cardiac Wounds: A Comparison of Different Therapeutic Methods, *Ann. Surg.,* 183:377, 1976.
28. Trinkle, H. H., Toon, R. S., Franz, J. L., Arom, K. V., and Graves, F. L.: Affairs of the Wounded Heart: Penetrating Cardiac Wounds, *J. Trauma,* 19:467, 1979.
29. Breaux, E. P., Dupont, J. B., Albert, H. M., Bryant, L. R., and Schechter, F. G.: Cardiac Tamponade Following Penetrating Mediastinal Injuries: Improved Survival with Early Pericardiocentesis, *J. Trauma,* 19:461, 1979.
30. Whisennard, H. H., Van Pelt, S. A., Beall, A. C., Jr., Mattox, K. L., and Espada, R.: Surgical Management of Traumatic Intracardiac Injuries, *Ann. Thorac. Surg.,* 28:530, 1979.
31. Heitzman, E. J., and Heitzman, G. C.: Myocardial Infarction Following Penetrating Wounds of the Heart, *Am. J. Cardiol.,* 7:283, 1961.
32. Konecke, L. L., Spitzer, S., Mason, D., Kasparian, H., and James, P. M., Jr.: Traumatic Aneurysm of the Left Coronary Artery, *Am. J. Cardiol.,* 27:221, 1971.
33. Bland, E. F., and Beebe, G. W.: Missiles in the Heart: A 20-Year Follow-Up Report of World War Cases, *N. Engl. J. Med.,* 274:1039, 1966.
34. Symbas, P. N., and Harlartis, N.: Bullet Emboli in the Pulmonary and Systemic Arteries, *Ann. Surg.,* 185:318, 1977.
35. Symbas, P. N., Schlant, R. C., Logan, W. D., Jr., Lindsay, J., MacCannell, K. L., and Zakaryia, M.: Traumatic Aorticopulmonary Fistula Complicated by Postoperative Low Cardiac Output Treated with Dopamine, *Ann. Surg.,* 165:614, 1967.
36. Smith, V. M., Hughes, C. W., Sapp, O., Joy, R. J. T., and Mattingly, T. W.: High-Output Circulatory Failure Due to Arteriovenous Fistula, *Arch. Intern. Med.,* 100:883, 1957.
37. Parmley, L. F., Orbison, J. A., Hughes, C. W., and Mattingly, T. W.: Acquired Arteriovenous Fistulas Complicated by Endarteritis and Endocarditis Lenta Due to *Streptococcus faecalis, N. Engl. J. Med.,* 250:305, 1954.
38. Trueblood, H. W., Wuerflein, R. D., and Angell, W. W.: Blunt Trauma Rupture of the Heart, *Ann. Surg.,* 177:66, 1973.
39. Cary, F. H., Hurst, J. W., and Arentzen, W. R.: Acquired Interventricular Defect Secondary to Trauma: Report of Four Cases, *N. Engl. J. Med.,* 258:355, 1958.
40. Stephenson, L. W., MacVaugh, H., and Kastor, J. A.: Tricuspid Valvular Incompetence and Rupture of the Ventricular Septum Caused by Nonpenetrating Trauma, *J. Thorac. Cardiovasc. Surg.,* 77:768, 1979.
41. Rotman, J., Peter, R. H., Sealy, W. C., and Morris, J. J., Jr.: Traumatic Ventricular Septal Defect Secondary to Nonpenetrating Chest Trauma, *Am. J. Med.,* 48:127, 1970.
42. Kissane, R. W.: Traumatic Heart Disease: Nonpenetrating Injuries, *Circulation,* 6:421, 1952.
43. Stern, T., Wolf, R. Y., Reichart, B., Harrington, O. B., and Crosby, V. G.: Coronary Artery Occlusion Resulting from Blunt Trauma, *JAMA,* 230:1308, 1974.
44. Levy, H.: Traumatic Coronary Thrombosis with Myocardial Infarction, *Arch. Intern. Med.,* 84:261, 1949.
45. Hawthorne, J. W., Kantrowitz, P. A., Dinsmore, R. E., and Sanders, C. A.: Traumatic Myocardial Infarction: Report of a Case with Normal Coronary Angiogram, *Ann. Intern. Med.,* 66:341, 1967.
46. DeMuth, W. E., Jr., and Zinsser, H. F.: Myocardial Contusion, *Arch Intern. Med.,* 115:434, 1965.
47. Forker, A. D., and Morgan, J. R.: Acquired Coronary Artery Fistula from Nonpenetrating Chest Injury, *JAMA,* 215:289, 1971.
48. Doty, D. B., Anderson, A. E., Rose, E. F., Raymundo, J. G., Chiu, C. L., and Ehrenhaft, J. L.: Cardiac Trauma: Clinical and Experimental Correlations of Myocardial Contusion, *Ann. Surg.,* 180:452, 1974.
49. Silver, G. M., Stampinato, N., Favaloro, R. G., and Groves, L. K.: Ventricular Aneurysm and Blunt Chest Trauma, *Chest,* 63:628, 1973.
50. Killen, D. A., Gobbel, W. G., Jr., France, R., and Vix, V. A.: Post-Traumatic Aneurysm of the Left Ventricle, *Circulation,* 39:101, 1969.
51. Singh, R., Nolan, S. P., and Schrank, J. P.: Traumatic Left Ventricular Aneurysm: Two Cases with Normal Coronary Angiograms, *JAMA,* 234:412, 1975.
52. Basta, L. L., Takeshita, A., Theilen, E. O., and Ehrenhaft, J. L.: Aneurysmectomy in Treatment of Ventricular and Supraventricular Tachyarrhythmias in Patients with Postinfarction and Traumatic Ventricular Aneurysms, *Am. J. Cardiol.,* 32:693, 1973.
53. Kissane, R. W., Fidler, R. S., and Koons, R. A.: Electrocardiographic Changes Following External Chest Injury to Dogs, *Ann. Intern. Med.,* 11:907, 1937.
54. Louhimo, I.: Heart Injury after Blunt Trauma, *Acta Chir. Scand.,* vol. 1 (suppl. 380), 1965.
55. Dolara, A., Morando, P., and Pampaloni, M.: Electrocardiographic Findings in 98 Consecutive Nonpenetrating Chest Injuries, *Dis. Chest,* 52:50, 1967.
56. Jones, F. L., Jr.: Transmural Myocardial Necrosis after Nonpenetrating Cardiac Trauma, *Am. J. Cardiol.,* 26:419, 1970.
57. DeMuth, W. E., Jr., Baue, A. E., and Odom, J. A., Jr.: Contusions of the Heart, *J. Trauma,* 7:443, 1967.
58. Tonkin, A. M., Lester, R. M., Guthrow, C. E., Roe, C. R., Hackel, D. B., and Wagner, G. S.: Persistence of MB Isoenzyme of Creatine Phosphokinase in Serum after Minor Iatrogenic Cardiac Trauma, *Circulation,* 51:627, 1975.
59. Martin, L. G., Larose, J. H., Sybers, R. G., Tyras, D. H., and Symbas, P. N.: Myocardial Perfusion Imaging with ^{99m}Tc-Albumin Microspheres, *Radiology,* 107:367, 1973.
60. Miller, F. H., Jr., Seward, J. B., Gersh, B. J., Tajik, A. J., and Mucha, P., Jr.: Findings in Cardiac Trauma, *Am. J. Cardiol.,* 50:1022, 1982.
61. Pandian, N. G., Skorton, D. J., Doty, D. B., and Kerber, R. E.: Immediate Diagnosis of Acute Myocardial Contusion

by Two-Dimensional Echocardiography: Studies in a Canine Model of Blunt Chest Trauma, *J. Am. Coll. Cardiol.,* 2:488, 1983.
62. Payne, D. D., DeWeese, J. A., Mahoney, E. B., and Murphy, G. W.: Surgical Treatment of Traumatic Rupture of the Normal Aortic Valve, *Ann. Thorac. Surg.,* 17:223, 1974.
63. Case Records of the Massachusetts General Hospital, Case 3-1976, *N. Engl. J. Med.,* 294:152, 1976.
64. Liu, S., Sako, Y., and Alexander, C. S.: Traumatic Tricuspid Insufficiency, *Am. J. Cardiol.,* 26:200, 1970.
65. Morgan, M. G., Glasser, S. P., and Sanusi, I. D.: Bacterial Endocarditis Occurrence on a Traumatically Ruptured Aortic Valve, *JAMA,* 233:810, 1975.
66. Schroeder, J. S., Stinson, E. B., Bieber, C. P., Wexler, L., Shumway, N. E., and Harrison, D. C.: Papillary Muscle Dysfunction Due to Nonpenetrating Chest Trauma, Recognition in a Potential Cardiac Donor, *Br. Heart J.,* 34:645, 1972.
67. Marvin, R. F., Schrank, J. P., and Nolan, S. P.: Traumatic Tricuspid Insufficiency, *Am. J. Cardiol.,* 32:723, 1973.
68. Munchow, O. B. G., Carter, R., Vannix, R. S., and Anderson, F. S.: Cardiac Arrest Due to Ventricular Herniation: Report of a Case of Two Successful Cardiac Resuscitations, *JAMA,* 173:1350, 1960.
69. Anderson, M., Fredens, M., and Olesson, K. H.: Traumatic Rupture of the Pericardium, *Am. J. Cardiol.,* 27:566, 1971.
70. Parmley, L. F., Mattingly, T. W., Manion, W. C., and Jahnke, E. J., Jr.: Nonpenetrating Traumatic Injury of the Aorta, *Circulation,* 17:1086, 1958.
71. Symbas, P. N., Tyras, D. H., Ware, R. E., and DiOrio, D. A.: Traumatic Rupture of the Aorta, *Ann. Surg.,* 178:6, 1973.
72. Symbas, P. N., Tyras, D. H., Ware, R. E., and Hatcher, C. R., Jr.: Rupture of the Aorta: A Diagnostic Triad, *Ann. Thorac. Surg.,* 15:405, 1973.
73. Gulkin, T. A., and Ashbury, A. K.: Fragment of Great-Vessel Wall Causing Cerebral Embolism, *N. Engl. J. Med.,* 277:751, 1967.
74. Stryker, W. A.: Traumatic Saccular Aneurysms of the Thoracic Aorta, *Am. J. Clin. Pathol.,* 18:152, 1948.
75. Kinley, C. E., and Chandler, B. M.: Traumatic Aneurysm of Thoracic Aorta: A Case Presenting as a Coarctation, *Can. Med. Assoc. J.,* 96:279, 1967.

Section J

Neoplastic Disease of the Heart

61

Neoplastic Heart Disease

Robert J. Hall, M.D. Denton A. Cooley, M.D.

The heart is too noble an organ to be attacked by a primary tumor.

Jean-Baptiste de Senac[1]

Tumors of the heart, while uncommon, present in protean ways and challenge the acumen of the physician. Although they have been observed since the seventeenth century,[2] antemortem diagnosis was rare before 1950. The first diagnosis, aided by angiography, and attempted surgical removal of an intracardiac myxoma were reported in 1952.[3] The first successful removal using cardiopulmonary bypass was performed in 1955.[2] Subsequently, increased clinical awareness coupled with angiographic and noninvasive diagnostic techniques has led to more frequently correct diagnoses.[4–6]

The heart may be the site of a primary tumor or be invaded secondarily by malignancies that arise in adjacent or remote organs. Whether involving primary or secondary tumors, neoplastic heart disease can be expressed in only a limited variety of ways (Table 61–1). In the presence of neoplastic disease, the occurrence of pericardial pain, effusion, tamponade, constriction, rapid increase in heart size, new heart murmurs, electrocardiographic changes, atrial or ventricular arrhythmias, atrioventricular block, or unexplained heart failure are suggestive of secondary invasion of the heart. The triad of obstruction, embolization, and constitutional manifestations characterizes intracavitary tumors, especially myxomas.

Primary Tumors of the Heart

While less common than secondary tumors, primary tumors of the heart are far more challenging to both the physician and the surgeon. They usually present as intracavitary lesions, and most—over 75 percent—are benign.[7] Current surgical techniques permit removal and potential "cure" in a considerable number of patients with primary tumors, necessitating an awareness of the clinical and hemodynamic presentation of these tumors.

Primary tumors of the heart and pericardium are rare, occurring with a frequency of 0.001 to 0.28 percent in reported or collected postmortem series.[7] Myxomas are the most common of the primary tumors and constitute nearly 50 percent of all histologically benign tumors of the heart. The frequency and classification of 533 primary tumors and cysts of the heart and pericardium collected by the Armed Forces Institute of Pathology can be seen in Table 61-2.[8]

Cardiac Myxomas

Intracardiac myxoma is the most frequent benign tumor of the heart. While most (75 percent) are located in the left atrium, myxomas are also found in the right atrium (18 percent), right ventricle (4 percent), and left ventricle (4 percent).[8] Atrial myxomas usually originate from the region of the fossa ovalis but may arise from a variety of locations within the atria, mitral annulus,[5] mitral valve itself,[9] or the inferior vena cava.[10]

Pathology

Attached to the endocardium by a broad base, myxomas are usually pedunculated, polypoid, and friable, although some may have a smooth surface and be rounded (Fig. 61-1). Sessile myxomas are uncommon.[5] Myxomas appear as a soft, gelatinous, mucoid, usually gray-white mass, often with areas of hemorrhage or thrombosis. They vary from 1 to 15 cm in diameter with most measuring 5 to 6 cm.[8]

TABLE 61-1 General Manifestations of Neoplastic Heart Disease

Pericardial Involvement
Pericarditis, pain
Pericardial effusion
Radiographic enlargement
Arrhythmia, predominantly atrial
Tamponade
Constriction
Myocardial Involvement
Arrhythmias, ventricular and atrial
Electrocardiographic changes
Radiographic enlargement:
Generalized
Localized
Conduction disturbances and heart block
Congestive heart failure
Coronary involvement:
Angina, infarction
Intracavitary Tumor
Cavity obliteration
Valve obstruction and valve damage
Embolic phenomena; systemic, neurological, coronary
Constitutional manifestations

On microscopic examination the myxoma is comprised of an acid mucopolysaccharid myxoid matrix in which are embedded polygonal cells (*lepidic cells*) and occasional blood vessels. Channels, often filled with red blood cells, communicate from the surface to deep within the tumor and are lined by endothelial-like cells resembling multipurpose mesenchymal cells from which the tumor is purported to arise. Similar endothelial cells line the surface of the tumor; however, fibrin, erythrocytes, and organized thrombi also may be present on the surface. Cystic areas, focal or gross hemorrhage, calcification, rarely bone formation, and even hematopoietic tissue comprise the multiple although uncommon variations that may be present.[8]

A neoplastic rather than a thrombotic origin of myxomas[11] is supported by the ultrastructural characteristics of the tumor,[12–15] the results of biochemical analyses,[16] and the cultural properties of the tumor cell.[8,17] While myxomas can recur because of their incomplete removal,[18–20] and distant growth of embolic myxomatous material has been observed,[18,21,22] the existence of a true malignant cardiac myxoma remains doubtful.[7] The occurrence of multiple tumors within the left atrium,[19] bilaterally in each atrium,[23,24] or simultaneously in the atrium and ventricle[25] raises the possibility of multicentric origin rather than recurrence of the tumor.

Age, Sex, and Familial Occurrence

Most patients with myxomas are from 30 to 60 years of age,[4] although myxomas have been discovered in children[26] and infants,[27] neonates,[28] and the elderly.[29] Children have a higher incidence of ventricular myxomas than adults.[26,30] A higher incidence in females has characterized most series.[4,5] Familial occurrence has been reported,[31,32] and in these examples males predominate, tumors are divided equally on both sides of the heart, and opposite atria are usually involved in afflicted members. In one report, three of four involved members had multiple myxomas.[32]

General or Constitutional Manifestations

While asymptomatic patients with myxoma (Fig. 61-1*C*) have been reported,[25,33] most present with one or more effects of a triad of constitutional, embolic, or obstructive manifestations.[4,5] Cardiac myxomas provoke systemic illness in 90 percent of the patients, characterized by weight loss, fatigue, fever, anemia (often hemolytic), elevated sedimentation rate, and elevated serum immunoglobulin concentration formed in response to either tumor embolization, degenerative changes within the tumor itself, or changes in the normal cardiac muscle. The globulin fraction most frequently elevated is

TABLE 61-2 Tumors and Cysts of the Heart and Pericardium

Type	Number	Percent
Benign		
Myxoma	130	24.4
Lipoma	45	8.4
Papillary fibroelastoma	42	7.9
Rhabdomyoma	36	6.8
Fibroma	17	3.2
Hemangioma	15	2.8
Teratoma	14	2.6
Mesothelioma of the AV node	12	2.3
Granular cell tumor	3	
Neurofibroma	3	
Lymphangioma	2	
Subtotal	319	59.8
Pericardial cyst	82	15.4
Brochogenic cyst	7	1.3
Subtotal	89	16.7
Malignant		
Angiosarcoma	39	7.3
Rhabdomyosarcoma	26	4.9
Mesothelioma	19	3.6
Fibrosarcoma	14	2.6
Malignant lymphoma	7	1.3
Extraskeletal osteosarcoma	5	
Neurogenic sarcoma	4	
Malignant teratoma	4	
Thymoma	4	
Leiomyosarcoma	1	
Liposarcoma	1	
Synovial sarcoma	1	
Subtotal	125	23.5
Total	533	100.00

Source: H. A. McAllister, Jr., and J. J. Fenoglio, Jr., "Tumors of the Cardiovascular System," Armed Forces Institute of Pathology, Washington, D.C., 1978. Reproduced with permission of the author.

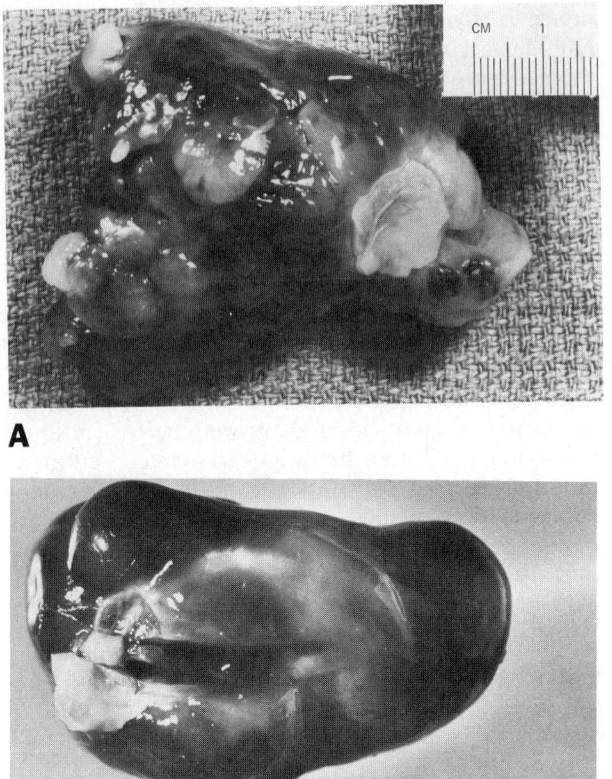

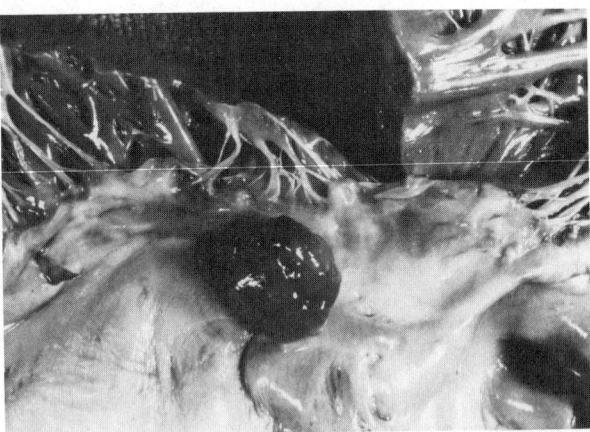

FIGURE 61-1 Left atrial myxomas. *A.* More polypoid and irregular. *B.* Smooth-surfaced and rounded. Attachment to and portion of the atrial septum are seen on each tumor. *C.* An asymptomatic sessile myxoma attached above the posterior leaflet of the mitral valve was found coincidentally at necropsy.

IgG and, only rarely, IgA.[4,17] Continuous immunologic stimulation by products from an atrial tumor can result in malignant transformation of immunocytes with resulting IgG multiple myeloma.[34] Less common findings are leukocytosis, thrombocytopenia, clubbing, Raynaud's phenomenon, and breast fibroadenomas.[4] Polycythemia may result from tumor erythropoietin production.[35]

Patients with hemolytic anemia have features of intravascular mechanical destruction which may be accompanied by pancytopenia. Hemolytic anemia is more likely to occur in patients with calcified myxomas,[33] occurring more commonly in the right atrium. Multiple pigmented lesions occasionally have been reported in patients with atrial myxoma.[36] A myxoma embolus to the skin has been confirmed by biopsy.[37] The protracted multisystemic symptoms produced by myxomas may mimic connective tissue disease.[38]

Infected Myxoma

An intracavitary myxoma rarely becomes infected, and blood cultures have demonstrated a variety of organisms.[31–42] Most patients present with major neurological embolic events. Surgical resection should be carried out promptly before catastrophic embolic complications occur.[31,43]

Embolization

Systemic tumor embolization occurs in 40 to 50 percent of patients with left atrial myxoma,[4] with tumor fragments or surface clots most commonly embolizing to arteries in the brain, kidneys, extremities, and aortic bifurcation.[44] Rarely does a complete left atrial myxoma become detached and lodge in the aortic bifurcation.[42] Histologic examination of emboli recovered at operation from a peripheral artery can aid in diagnosing an otherwise unsuspected intracardiac myxoma.[7,37,42,45,46] Systemic embolization, especially in a young patient with normal sinus rhythm, should arouse suspicion of a myxoma, once bacterial endocarditis has been ruled out.

Central Nervous System Tumor embolization of the central nervous system constitutes about one-half of all embolic events caused by left atrial myxomas,[46] may represent the first symptomatic manifestation,[17,21,46,47] and is more common in the left hemisphere.[48] Embolization may be to the extracranial or intracranial cerebral vessels, with the former being amenable to surgical removal.[21,47] Onset of the neurological deficit may be gradual or sudden.

Sudden alterations in consciousness may be caused by prolapse of a pedunculated tumor with resulting valvular obstruction and marked reduced output. Such episodes of syncope can be mistaken for seizure activity and thus delay recognition of the true cardiac cause.[46]

Intracranial Aneurysms Intracranial mycotic aneurysms secondary to myxomatous emboli have been demonstrated angiographically. They have caused symptoms years after surgical removal of the intracardiac myxoma and histologically have been the site of invasion and proliferation of myxomatous tissue replacing the vessel wall. Late rupture with intracranial hemorrhage has been reported.[21] Care must be taken during surgical removal of an intracardiac myxoma to avoid embolization, not only because of the immediate consequences of an embolic phenomena, but because viable metastatic foci may cause symptoms years later.[21] As a consequence, the patient who has sustained cerebral emboli is not necessarily "cured" even after the primary tumor has been removed surgically.[48]

Retinal Artery Embolism Tumor embolization to the retinal artery can occur with transient[46] or permanent[49] visual impairment, confirmed by ophthalmoscopic[46] and histopathologic[49] evidence of particulate embolic matter in the retinal artery. The left eye is involved twice as frequently as the right eye, presumably the consequence of the more direct takeoff of the left internal carotid artery from the aorta.[49] Only rarely has occlusion of the retinal artery occurred in the absence of multifocal neurological manifestations, usually in the distribution of the ipsilateral middle cerebral artery.

Coronary Artery Embolism The occurrence of acute myocardial infarction at an unusually young age should cause one to suspect nonatherosclerotic and embolic causes. Myxomatous embolic occlusion of the coronary artery has been documented by both angiography in living patients and histology at postmortem study.[7,50] Myocardial infarction occasionally is the first manifestation of a myxoma.[50,51]

Left Atrial Myxoma

General Features Constitutional manifestations and embolic potential are common, to varying degrees, in patients with myxoma in any intracavitary location. The cardiac manifestations, symptoms, and physical findings are the consequence of the intracavitary mass and are unique to the particular location of the tumor. Myxomas of the left atrium may obstruct either the mitral or pulmonary venous orifices and produce symptoms and manifestations of pulmonary venous hypertension, secondary pulmonary hypertension, and right-sided heart failure. The clinical symptoms include dyspnea on exertion, orthopnea, paroxysmal nocturnal dyspnea, acute pulmonary edema, cough, and hemoptysis, along with palpitations, chest pain, fatigue, and peripheral edema. Episodes of syncope or dizziness are frequent, and sudden death may occur. A marked effect on the severity of any symptom caused by a change in position of the patient, especially if recumbency relieves dyspnea,[4,52] is suggestive of myxoma, but this occurs infrequently.

Physical Examination On physical examination the first heart sound is loud and frequently split, with the second component corresponding to the tumor expulsion from the mitral orifice. The pulmonic component of the second sound is accentuated, and an early diastolic sound, the "tumor plop," is usually heard 80 to 120 ms after the aortic closure sound,[4,53] resembling, but not as sharp as and of lower frequency than, an opening snap. The tumor plop may be confused with either an opening snap of the mitral valve or a third heart sound, and follows the aortic closure sound at an interval which is intermediate between these events. Suspicion of a left atrial myxoma should be raised when one hears what is considered to be an inordinately early "third heart sound" associated with auscultatory features suggestive of mitral regurgitation, or an unusually late low-pitched "opening snap" accompanying features consistent with severe mitral stenosis (Fig. 61-2).

An apical diastolic or apical systolic murmur, or both, are present in many patients. The auscultatory findings may vary from time to time or with a change in position of the patient.[4,52–54] Features of pulmonary hypertension are frequent. A shorter clinical history and the persistence of sinus rhythm are in contrast to features of rheumatic mitral valvular disease. Rarely, there may be a murmur of aortic regurgitation, the origin of which is unclear, although damage to the valve by the mobile tumor has been suggested as the cause.[55]

Electrocardiogram and Chest X-Ray Results of electrocardiography are nonspecific, reflecting hemo-

FIGURE 61-2 Recordings of a patient with a cystic left atrial myxoma including (*top*) the electrocardiogram; (*middle*) phonocardiograms from the pulmonic area (PA) at high frequency, and from the apex (AP) at medium frequency; and (*bottom*) the echocardiogram at the level of the mitral valve. Time lines equal 0.01-s intervals. The right ventricle (RV), septum (IVS), and posterior wall of the left ventricle (PW) are identified. The loud component of the first sound (M_1) is delayed (Q to M_1 = 0.09 s). The pulmonic second sound (P_2) is accentuated. Multiple linear tumor echoes (TE) are seen behind the anterior leaflet to the mitral valve (ALMV), first appearing at the mitral level 0.04 s after onset of mitral opening and completing the forward movement 0.09 s after onset of mitral opening, at which point the tumor plop (TP) is recorded. The A_2-TP interval measures 0.10 s.

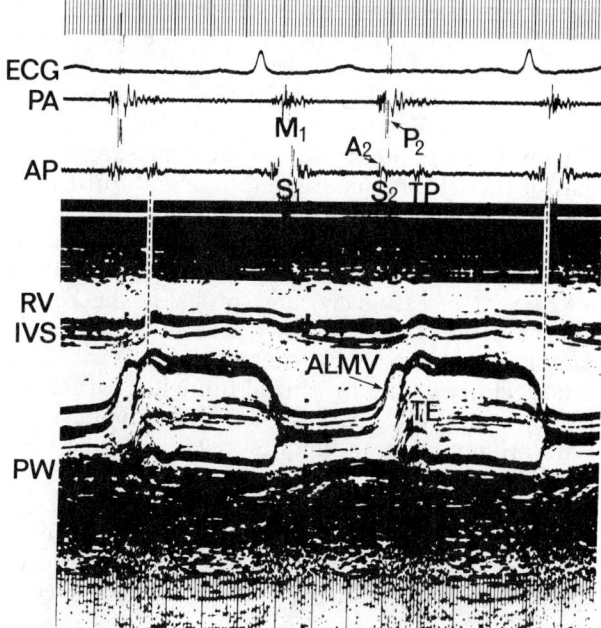

dynamic alterations similar to those of mitral valvular disease; however, sinus rhythm is generally the rule. The chest roentgenogram reveals left atrial enlargement and the characteristic changes of pulmonary venous congestion and pulmonary hypertension. Absence of mitral valve calcification, and a left atrium smaller than might be expected in a patient with severe rheumatic mitral disease, are helpful differentiating clues. Calcification may be evident in the tumor even on routine chest x-ray,[56] but it is better visualized and the motion is better appreciated at fluoroscopic examination.

The "wrecking-ball" effect of a calcified mobile myxoma may cause destruction of the mitral valve or rupture of chordae tendineae and may produce severe mitral regurgitation.[52,57]

Apexcardiogram The apexcardiogram may demonstrate a prominent notching of the early systolic rise which coincides with the loud, delayed component of the first heart sound resulting from sudden expulsion of the tumor from the left ventricle into the left atrium.[58,59] This notch also has been noted in some normal subjects and in an occasional patient with rheumatic mitral stenosis.[60]

Echocardiography Since Shattenberg[58] first reported the characteristic echocardiographic recordings of a left atrial myxoma, the value of ultrasound in the noninvasive diagnosis of intracavitary tumors[4–6,17,59,61] has been well documented. M-mode echocardiographic studies in patients with a prolapsing left atrial myxoma typically demonstrate a diminished EF slope of the anterior leaflet of the mitral valve,[61] behind which a dense array of wavy tumor echoes is seen. These tumor echoes typically appear a short interval following the opening movement of the mitral leaflets, due to the inertial lag in movement of the tumor after onset of diastole and opening of the mitral leaflets. The tumor plop coincides with the completion of this anterior movement of tumor echoes (Fig. 61-2). A similar array of tumor echoes may be seen in the left atrial chamber during ventricular systole. False-positive and false-negative studies occur,[62] and nonprolapsing myxomas of the left atrium are detected, with difficulty, by M-mode echocardiography.[61] Fluttering of the anterior leaflet of the mitral valve has been reported in association with a nonprolapsing left atrial myxoma.[33] Occasionally, and probably the consequence of its acoustic density, even a large mobile tumor may not produce the classic array of wavy echoes either within the mitral funnel or within the left atrium (Fig. 61-2).[58,62–65] Two-dimensional echocardiographic techniques readily clarify such cases.[66,67]

Two-Dimensional Echocardiography Two-dimensional echocardiography enhances visualization of the tumor—its size, shape, position, ultrasonic echo pattern, attachment, and motion characteristics (Fig. 61-3).[61,68,69] It is sufficiently reliable in many patients to permit immediate operative intervention without additional invasive studies.[69,70] A nonprolapsing left atrial myxoma more likely will be detected by two-dimensional echocardiography,[61,63] as will a prolapsing myxoma from which M-mode imaging yields atypical findings because of its acoustic density.[58,63,65–67] False-negative two-dimensional echographic studies, however, also have been reported.[71] The ability afforded by two-dimensional echocardiography to visualize all four chambers simultaneously permits recognition of multiple tumors[72] or tumors in less common locations.[37,73] Continuous-wave Doppler ultrasound has shown characteristic deflections that coincide with tumor motion.[74] The diagnosis of ball thrombus in the left atrium, difficult with M-mode echocardiography, may be facilitated by two-dimensional echocardiography.[75,76]

Gated Radionuclide Cardiac Imaging Gated radionuclide imaging of the isotopically tagged blood pool also has resulted in detection of left atrial myxomas. An abnormal area of diminished activity was detected, and the size and motion of the tumor defined.[77] This technique has also helped define intracavitary tumors in other chambers[78,79] and biatrial tumors.[23]

Catheterization Cardiac catheterization invariably demonstrates significant pulmonary capillary wedge and pulmonary arterial hypertension.[4] A notch on the ascending limb of the left ventricular pressure curve, comparable to that seen on the apexcardiogram, results from expulsion of the myxoma from the left ventricle, which decreases left ventricular volume suddenly. When a large left atrial tumor or a left atrial ball thrombus obstructs the mitral orifice but does not prolapse into the left ventricular cavity, this notch is absent.[75,80,81] Similarly, a rapid y descent of the pulmonary wedge or left atrial pressure curve is the consequence of sudden decrease of left atrial volume when the tumor prolapses into the left ventricle.[81,82] The notch, or "hold," on the rapid y descent appears to be caused by the slightly delayed tumor prolapse through the mitral orifice.[83] The large v wave, at times as great as 75 mmHg, even in the absence of significant mitral regurgitation, reflects the space-occupying effect of the tumor within the left atrium. When the clinical picture is that of mitral stenosis, these findings are highly suggestive of a space-filling defect in the atrium.[82] Large left atrial myxomas that obstruct the mitral orifice without prolapsing into the left ventricle demonstrate a slow y descent.[81] Abnormal diastolic anterior motion of a catheter passed retrogradely in the left ventricle, caused by displacement due to a prolapsing left atrial myxoma, has been observed fluoroscopically.[84] Rarely is a left atrial myxoma associated with a congenital

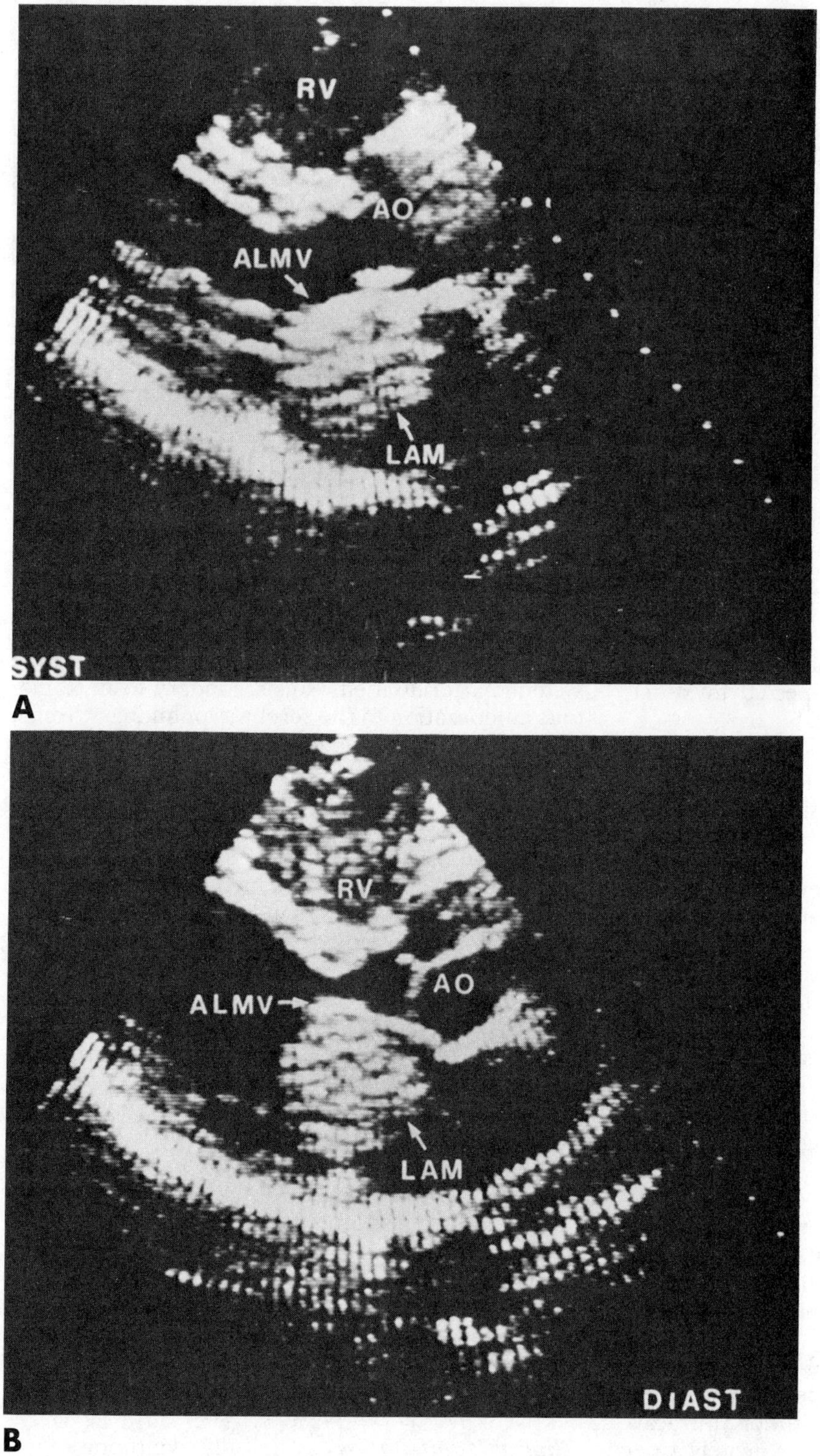

FIGURE 61-3 Two-dimensional echocardiograms, long axis parasternal view, (*A*) in systole and (*B*) in diastole, from a 56-year-old woman. A large left atrial myxoma (LAM) is seen in the left atrium behind the anterior leaflet of the mitral valve (ALMV). The myxoma prolapses and fills the mitral orifice during diastole. The right ventricle (RV) and aorta (AO) are identified. This tumor was attached to the posterior leaflet of the mitral valve and adjacent posterior wall of the left atrium.

atrial septal defect with an accompanying left-to-right shunt.[85]

Angiography Angiography characterizes the size, location, and mobility of the tumor (Fig. 61-4).[4] Left ventricular injection of opaque medium may fail to delineate the tumor,[4,9,86] although there is usually sufficient regurgitation of opaque medium through the mitral valve, or deep enough penetration of the prolapsing myxoma into the left ventricle, to permit recognition of the tumor mass.[63,87] Injection of contrast medium into the pulmonary artery, with attention to the levophase of the angiogram, is diagnostic in all patients except those with small tumors. In a patient with an unsuspected left atrial myxoma, systemic embolization of tumor fragments to the cen-

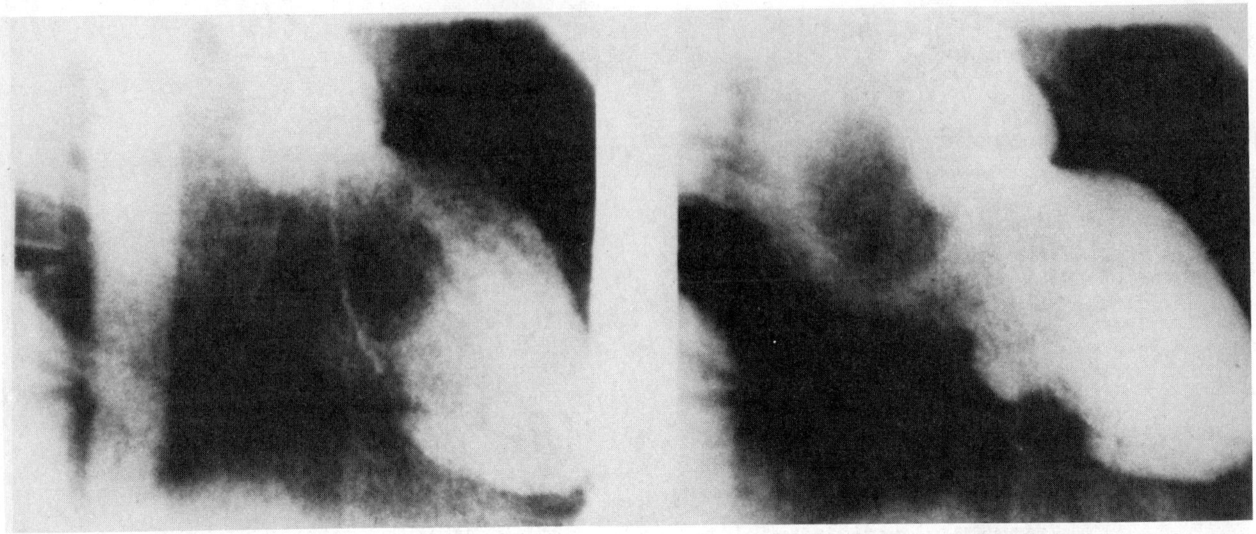

FIGURE 61-4 Left ventriculogram in the right anterior oblique view. A mobile left atrial myxoma is seen as a space-filling defect within the mitral valve in diastole (*left*), and sufficient mitral regurgitation is present to delineate the myxoma in the left atrium in systole (*right*).

tral nervous system may complicate transseptal approach to the left atrium and left atrial angiography.[88] The frequency, however, of unsuspected myxoma is reduced greatly by echo imaging.

Coronary Angiography Coronary angiography may demonstrate a vascular blush in the tumor from branches of both the right and left coronary arteries; and both left and right atrial myxomas and a right ventricular myxoma have been demonstrated in this manner.[87,89,90] Occasionally, an atrial myxoma in a patient with false-negative echocardiographic findings will be discovered in this fashion.[65] Neovascularization of a left atrial thrombus accompanying mitral stenosis may produce an appearance similar to a tumor blush.[91] Aneurysms or occlusion of the coronary artery caused by tumor emboli have also been demonstrated by coronary angiography.[51,65] Results of noninvasive imaging such as two-dimensional echocardiography have proved sufficiently reliable and accurate in the diagnosis of left atrial myxoma that cardiac catheterization appears to be indicated primarily for patients with additional heart disease and for those over 40 years of age to rule out concomitant coronary artery disease.[87,92]

Differential Diagnosis Left atrial myxomas most often present as, and must be differentiated from, mitral valvular disease. At our institution, intracavitary myxomas were present in approximately 1 per 100 patients requiring mitral valve surgery.[4] Characteristically, the clinical course is relatively recent in origin, distinguishing myxoma from rheumatic mitral valvular disease, although occasionally the course may span many years. Rarely both conditions may coexist.[90] Fever, constitutional symptoms, and embolic phenomena mimic infective endocarditis, and on rare occasions the myxoma itself may be infected. Muscle pain, skin rash, and Raynaud's phenomenon may simulate peripheral vasculitis, and myxomatous emboli may be found on muscle biopsy.[30] Multiple systemic arterial aneurysms secondary to myxomatous embolization to the cerebral, pulmonary, renal, and muscular arteries have mimicked polyarteritis nodosa.[24,39,93] Similarly, coronary artery aneurysmal dilatation and myocardial infarction have been attributed to coronary myxoma embolization.[65,94] The clinical picture at times has been suggestive of acute rheumatic fever[95] and acute myocarditis.[96] The correct diagnosis will be suspected if the physician maintains a high index of clinical suspicion in patients with diverse and protean features—especially when cardiac, embolic, and constitutional manifestations coexist. The advent of echocardiographic imaging of the heart has greatly facilitated the recognition of intracavitary tumors.

Right Atrial Myxoma

Myxomas in the right atrial cavity constitute about one-fifth of all myxomas and tend to be more solid, have a wider attachment, and involve a greater amount of the atrial wall or septum than those in the left atrium.[37] They originate from a variety of locations within the right atrium, including the inferior margin of the foramen ovale,[5,97] and characteristically produce tricuspid valve obstruction. They rarely arise from the inferior vena cava.[10]

Clinical Manifestations Clinically, symptoms of low cardiac output and manifestations of systemic venous hypertension are present with a prominent jugular venous *a* wave, hepatomegaly, ascites, edema, and cyanosis, which may be episodic and vary with the position of the patient. Persistence of normal sinus rhythm is common; however, sinus rhythm is also frequent in patients with rheumatic tricuspid stenosis. Intermittent episodes of syncope and abrupt onset of dyspnea, features never seen with rheumatic tricuspid stenosis,[52] are reported in one-third of these patients.[79,80] The pendular action of a prolapsing right atrial myxoma, especially when it is calcified, may damage or destroy the tricuspid valve and produce severe tricuspid insufficiency.[52,98]

Pulmonary Emboli While embolic tumor phenomena are reputed to occur less frequently with right than with left atrial myxomas, pulmonary emboli have been reported,[97] at times are extensive,[98,99] and may produce irreversible pulmonary hypertension.[100] Wide dissemination of myxomatous embolization to the pulmonary arteries has been reported with active infiltration of the media[18] and formation of aneurysms.[24] Paradoxical embolization may occur if an interatrial communication exists.[31]

Systemic Manifestations Constitutional symptoms are less frequent in patients with a right atrial myxoma.[73] Anemia, polycythemia,[100,101] and cyanosis have been reported. Polycythemia and cyanosis may be caused by right-to-left shunting through a patent foramen ovale or atrial septal defect,[31,102] low cardiac output and hypoxemic stimulation of the bone marrow, or intravascular hemoconcentration,[101] or may result from erythropoietin production by the tumor.[35]

Auscultation On auscultation a loud early systolic sound may be heard. This sound occurs as late as 80 ms after the mitral component of the first sound[103] and results from expulsion of the tumor from the right ventricle. A crescendo murmur with inspiratory augmentation preceding this loud tumor expulsion sound is probably caused by early systolic tricuspid regurgitation while the valve is still held open by the tumor.[103] There may be a long diastolic murmur or, more commonly, only a late diastolic rumble, augmented by inspiration, accompanying atrial systole. If major injury to the tricuspid valve occurs, the murmur of tricuspid regurgitation will be present and large *v* waves will be seen in the jugular venous column. An early diastolic sound may be heard but is less constant than the tumor plop accompanying a left atrial myxoma. The changing quality of the sound and murmurs, their closeness to the ear, and their friction-like quality may mimic a pericardial rub.[73]

Electrocardiogram and Chest X-Ray Results of electrocardiography are often normal, although right atrial enlargement frequently is suggested.[97] Low-voltage right axis deviation and varying degrees of right bundle branch block are reported.[79] The chest roentgenogram may reveal some prominence or enlargement of the right atrial shadow and, occasionally, of the right ventricle. An important radiologic feature is the mild or moderate degree of cardiomegaly, considering the severe clinical state of the patients.[103] Calcification in the tumor may be recognized on plain film or at fluoroscopy and is more common in patients with myxomas in the right atrium (Fig. 61-5).

Echocardiography M-mode imaging may demonstrate a dense cluster of echoes behind the tricuspid valve or in the right ventricle during diastole.[14,23,79,104] It was not until the advent of two-dimensional imaging, however, that the presence of masses within the right atrium could be evaluated reliably.[68,69,105,106]

Catheterization and Angiography Cardiac catheterization demonstrates elevated right atrial pressure, prominence of the *a* wave, and a diastolic gradient between the right atrium and right ventricle. Notching of the upstroke of the right ventricular pressure curve has been noted[59,97] and is similar to that seen in patients with prolapsing left atrial myxomas. Similarly, a collapsing *y* descent has been described with marked inspiratory augmentation.[97] Angiography is diagnostic of right atrial myxoma, and contrast medium should be injected into either the superior or inferior vena cava to avoid dislodging any portion of the tumor.

FIGURE 61-5 Lateral chest roentgenogram showing dense calcification of a right atrial myxoma.

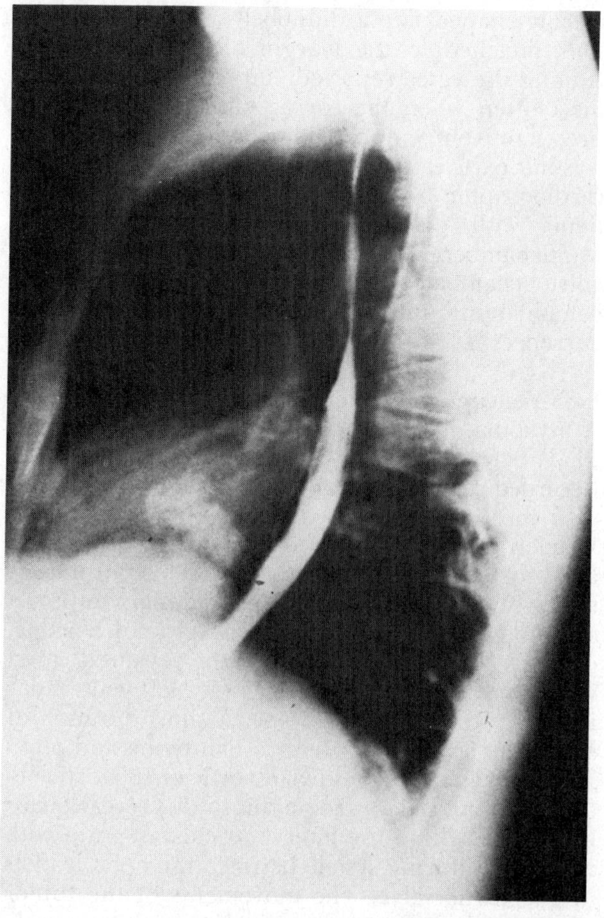

Differential Diagnoses The clinical features of right atrial myxoma resemble rheumatic tricuspid valvular disease, although the latter is always accompanied by significant mitral[103] and, frequently, aortic valve disease. There are many similarities to the manifestations of constrictive pericarditis and Ebstein's anomaly of the tricuspid valve. Episodic dyspnea, sudden syncope, and variability of symptoms and findings with position of the patient may serve as helpful clues. Changing murmurs, along with fever and anemia, can be suggestive of infective endocarditis. Tricuspid stenosis and insufficiency are prominent in patients with carcinoid syndrome, but involvement of the pulmonary valve and other features of a carcinoid tumor will usually serve to distinguish it from a right atrial myxoma. Obstruction of the right ventricular outflow tract may be the dominant finding in some examples of familial obstructive myopathy and may resemble a right atrial tumor.[103] Pulmonary embolization of other diverse etiologies, with secondary thromboembolic pulmonary hypertension and right-sided heart failure, may be mimicked by right atrial myxoma. An awareness of the protean manifestations along with evidence from echocardiographic or radionuclide imaging usually will facilitate a correct diagnosis.

Bilateral Atrial Myxoma
An atrial myxoma may pass through the foramen ovale and be present in both atria. The tumor is usually shaped like a dumbbell with the common stalk attached to the margin of the fossa ovalis. Among the cases reported, surgery was successful most often when the correct diagnosis was made preoperatively, emphasizing the importance of ultrasonic exploration of all chambers.[23] Similar echocardiographic findings have been reported in patients with discrete tumors in each atrium.[72] Multichambered cardiac myxomas occasionally involve chambers other than the usual biatrial combination[51] and are more frequent in familial occurrences.[31]

Left Ventricular Myxoma
A myxoma originates from the left ventricle in 2.5 to 4 percent of reported cases of myxoma.[7,73] Recorded cases are found in the younger age groups, with most patients being under 30 years of age. Women are involved three times more often than men. Systemic emboli, mostly cerebral, occur in two-thirds of the patients, and constitutional symptoms are almost conspicuously absent. Attacks of syncope, occurring in nearly one-half of the reviewed cases, were more frequent in patients with left ventricular myxomas than any other type. A short duration of symptoms is also characteristic. Symptoms and physical findings are suggestive of aortic or subaortic obstruction, and echocardiographic studies reveal a mass of echoes behind the interventricular septum with movement during systole between the open leaflets of the aortic valve. The movements of the tumor mass are demonstrated particularly well by two-dimensional echocardiography.[73,107] Echoes from the intracavitary left ventricular mass must be differentiated from left ventricular thrombi, which are usually apical but occasionally are pedunculated, and from ventricular septal rhabdomyomas.[108]

Right Ventricular Myxoma
Myxomas of the right ventricle are as infrequent as are those occurring in the left ventricle. The patient will have symptoms and manifestations of right-sided heart failure, syncope, unexplained fever, and a murmur consistent with pulmonary stenosis. An "ejection sound" has been reported as well as delayed closure of the pulmonary valve. A right-sided tumor plop may be heard in diastole.[109] Calcium in the tumor may be recognized on roentgenogram. A gradient across the right ventricular outlet is characteristic,[109] and the tumor can be visualized angiographically.[110] Pulmonary emboli may occur.[111] Two-dimensional echocardiography is superior to M-mode studies of right ventricular intracavitary masses,[112] yet cannot distinguish tumor from thrombus.[113] Other tumors, producing similar outflow tract obstruction, occur rarely within the right ventricle.[114]

Surgery for Intracavitary Myxoma
Surgical resection of a myxoma is the only acceptable therapy and, in view of the dangers of embolization and sudden death, should be performed promptly.[37] For complete removal of left atrial myxoma, we use a biatrial approach, excising a full thickness of interatrial septum if the tumor is attached to the region of the fossa ovalis (Fig. 61-6).[19,115,116] Right atrial myxomas are commonly attached to the fossa ovalis, and a full thickness of atrial septum also should be resected with right-sided tumors. Since fragmentation and embolization of the tumor are an ever-present threat, vigorous palpation and other manipulations of the heart should be avoided until cardiopulmonary bypass is initiated.[21,37] We usually induce ventricular fibrillation to reduce the possibility of fragmentation of the gelatinous tumor. Left atrial myxomas have been removed successfully during pregnancy, utilizing cardiopulmonary bypass, with subsequent uncomplicated completion of a full-term pregnancy.[70,117,118] Surgical removal of a right ventricular myxoma in a neonate has been reported.[28]

By its movement within the heart, the tumor may traumatize either atrioventricular valve, which may require replacement or repair by annuloplasty.[4] Arrhythmias and conduction disturbances may follow surgical removal of left atrial myxomas.[119] Recurrence of atrial myxomas are rare and usually occur within a 48-month period.[19,20]

Other Benign Primary Cardiac Tumors

Rhabdomyoma
The most frequent cardiac tumor in infants and children[7,120] is a rhabdomyoma and is probably a hamartoma rather than a true neoplasm.[121] They

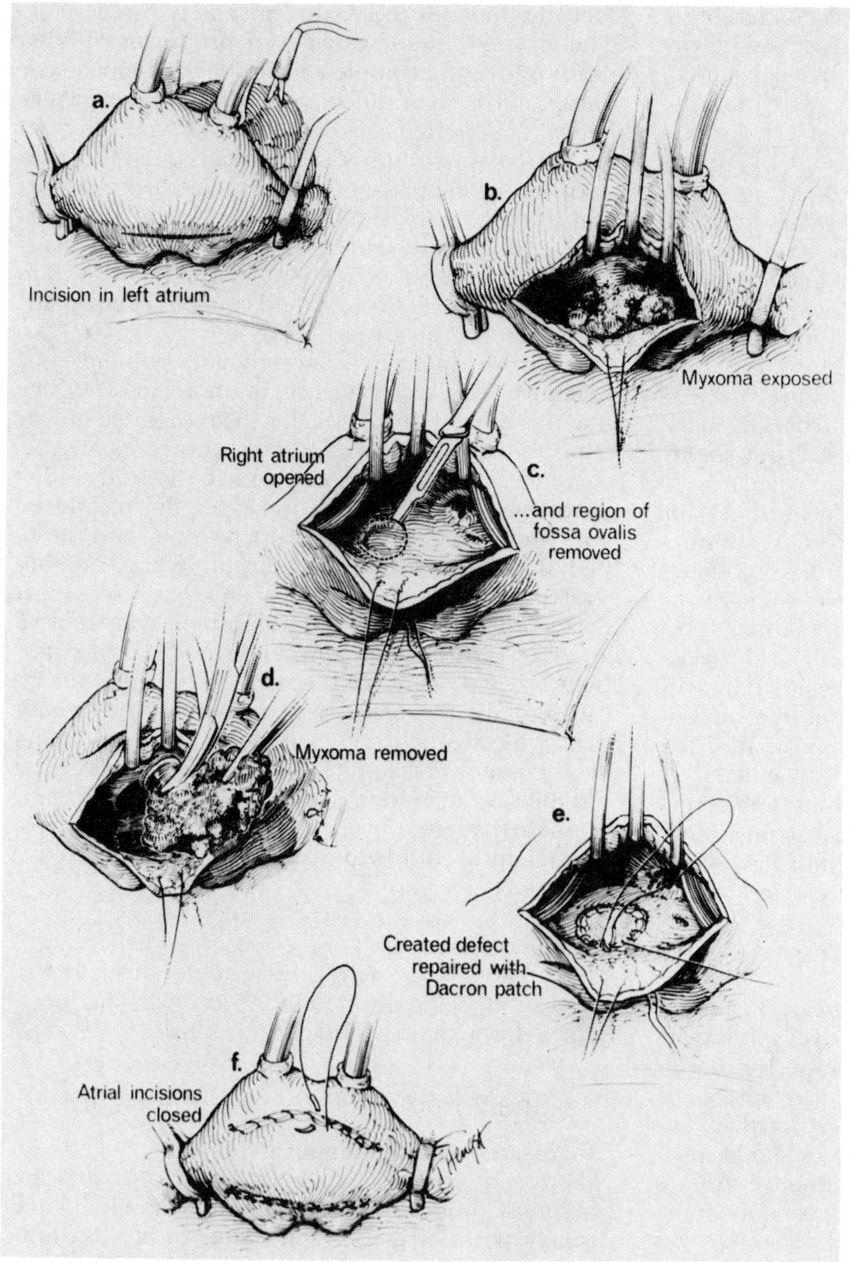

FIGURE 61-6 Drawing illustrating resection of a typical left atrial myxoma with a broad attachment to the interatrial septum near the fossa ovalis. The ascending aorta is cross-clamped and the left atrium is opened near the interatrial groove (*a*). After the pedicle of the tumor is located (*b*), a separate incision is made in the right atrium (*c*). The interatrial septum is opened near the fossa ovalis and a portion of the interatrial septum is excised. The tumor is removed through the left atriotomy (*d*). The resultant atrial defect is closed with a knitted Dacron patch (*e*). The atrial chambers and atrioventricular valve areas should be thoroughly inspected for additional tumor implants or fragments before the atriotomy incisions are closed (*f*). (*From D. A. Cooley and J. C. Norman, "Techniques in Cardiac Surgery," Texas Medical Press, Houston, 1975, p. 211. Reproduced with permission from the publisher and authors.*)

are usually multiple and most often involve the ventricular myocardium. Associated tuberous sclerosis is present in one-third of the patients. Presenting symptoms may be caused by cardiac obstructive phenomena, arrhythmias, atrioventricular block, pericardial effusion, or even sudden death.[122,123] At times these tumors mimic pulmonary stenosis and can produce hypoxic spells like those seen with tetralogy of Fallot.[120] Ventricular outlet gradients, angiographic abnormalities, and, more recently, echocardiographic[120,124–127] and radionuclide angiographic[128] demonstrations of the tumor can lead to successful surgical resection of the tumor, which may be pedunculated and freely movable or project from the ventricular or septal wall.[120,125,129] Multiplicity of tumors does not contraindicate surgery, as these tumors appear to have little capacity for further growth. Pedunculated rhabdomyomas that arise from the left atrium and cause mitral stenosis have been reported.[122]

Fibroma

Fibromas are usually ventricular and intramural and, although reported cases have occurred in the age range from newborn to 65 years, most occur in infants and children.[7,130,131] Calcification is common. Sudden death has been reported in nearly one-third of the patients, presumably due to involvement of the conduction system, production of arrhythmias, or obstruction of the outflow tract of the left ventricle.[131–133] Two-dimensional echocardiography accurately delineates intramural ventricular tumors.[134] Left axis deviation may occur as an interesting electrocardiographic feature. Total or partial resection of the tumor to relieve obstruction has been reported,[94] with excellent probability of long-term survival.[133] Cardiac transplantation has been used in the management of a young adult with a nonresectable (1030 g) left ventricular fibroma.[135]

Papillary Fibroelastoma

Also referred to as *papillomas* or *papillary fibromas,* papillary fibroelastomas arise from the cardiac valves or occasionally from the ventricular endocardium, are most commonly seen in patients over 50 years of age, and are usually a coincidental finding at surgery or postmortem examination. There is a predilection for involvement of the aortic valve,[13] where angina and sudden death may result from coronary ostial occlusion caused by the fronds of the villous tumor.[7,13] Obstruction of the right ventricular outflow tract has been reported in patients with a papillary tumor of the tricuspid valve.[136] The tumor is histologically different from Lambl's excrescences, which are degenerative in origin and usually situated on the ventricular aspect of the semilunar valve along the line of closure.[7,137,138] Papillary fibroelastomas are also incorrectly confused with polypoid myxomatous valvular lesions in children, which probably represent incomplete differentiation of the valve and may involve any valve with equal frequency.[7] Two-dimensional echocardiographic recognition of papillary fibroelastomas arising from cardiac valves and mural endocardium have been reported,[139,140] and successful surgical excision has followed clinical recognition.[140–143]

Lipoma

Lipomas may occur throughout the heart, including the pericardium. They may be massive; the largest reported cardiac tumor was an intrapericardial lipoma.[144] Intrapericardial lipomas may cause pericardial effusion, be mistaken for a pericardial cyst, or present as asymptomatic cardiac or mediastinal enlargement.[145,146] Intramyocardial lipomas are encapsulated and usually small.[7] An occasional lipoma arising from the mitral or tricuspid valve may resemble an atrial myxoma on echocardiographic examination[147] and must also be differentiated from a cyst[12,101,148] or lymphangioma of the mitral valve.[100]

Lipomatous hypertrophy of the atrial septum is a nonencapsulated hyperplasia of adipose tissue and may not represent a true tumor. Varying in size from 2 to 8 cm, the tumescence may bulge into the atrial cavity and become a factor in the differential diagnosis of intracavitary masses. Although at times found coincidentally at postmortem study, lipomatous hypertrophy of the atrial septum can be associated with sudden death,[149] unexplained supraventricular rhythm and conduction disturbances, and recurrent pericardial effusion.[150] This association has been considered fortuitous by some observers.[7] The two-dimensional echocardiographic features, especially from the subcostal approach, are distinctive and reveal sparing of the area of the fossa ovalis.[151]

Mesothelioma of the Atrioventricular Node

The smallest tumor capable of producing sudden death by causing complete heart block or ventricular fibrillation is mesothelioma of the atrioventricular node.[7,152] Reported ages of patients have ranged from the newborn period to the ninth decade of life, with a strong female preponderance. While the exact origin of these cystic tumors has been disputed, most believe they arise from arrests in development,[152] and other terms have been applied to them, such as lymphangioepithelioma[152] and congenital polycystic tumor of the atrioventricular node.[153,154] In vivo recognition remains unreported, although the cystic structure may exceed 3 cm or more in size. The tumor is usually large enough to be recognized grossly at postmortem examination and, despite its rare occurrence, should be suspected in all cases of sudden death without apparent cause, especially in children and young adults.[7,155,156] Most patients with mesothelioma of the atrioventricular node have demonstrated complete heart block and have recurrent Stokes-Adams attacks. Even with complete heart block a narrow QRS is common, and these patients may pursue a stable course for years. Electrophysiological study discloses a block proximal to the His bundle.[155] Electronic pacing should aid in maintaining an adequate cardiac rate; yet examples of electrical instability and sudden death reflect a special hazard in these patients, even during diagnostic electrophysiological studies and after initiation of effective ventricular pacing.[7,154]

Hemangiomas

Hemangiomas are rare cardiac tumors usually discovered at postmortem study. Coronary angiography yields a characteristic tumor blush.[157–160]

Malignant Primary Tumors of the Heart

Angiosarcoma (Hemangiosarcoma)

Almost all primary malignant cardiac tumors are sarcomas, most frequently an angiosarcoma,[161] and usually originate in the right atrium or pericardium. Intense vascularity may produce a continuous murmur.[162] One-fourth of all angiosarcomas will, in part, be intracavitary with valvular obstruction, and characteristically will manifest right-sided heart failure and pericardial tamponade with hemorrhagic fluid.[163] Echocardiography and angiography are helpful in the diagnosis.[164,165] Coronary angiography may demonstrate angiomatous vessels over the tumor area.[166] The course is rapid, and widespread metastases make surgery impractical.[165] Radiation and chemotherapy may offer some relief of symptoms.[7,162,166,167]

Rhabdomyosarcoma

A rhabdomyosarcoma is the second most frequent primary sarcoma of the heart and, like an angiosarcoma, is prevalent in males. There is no single chamber predilection; multiple sites are common, and significant obstruction of at least one valve is present in one-half of the patients.[168,169] Excision of the main tumor mass combined with radiation and chemotherapy has been advocated as the treatment for patients with primary malignant tumor of the heart, but in general the prognosis is poor and survival short.[7,170–173]

Other Malignant Primary Tumors
Fibrosarcoma, liposarcoma,[174] primary malignant lymphoma, and occasional sarcomas of other basic cell types constitute the remaining but infrequent primary malignant cardiac tumors.[7,175,176] These tumors may also obstruct cardiac chambers or valves[177–182] and have been resected surgically, allowing some favorable palliation.[174,176,182,183]

Tumors of the Pericardium

Pericardial Cysts
Pericardial, or mesothelial, cysts are the most frequent benign "tumors" of the pericardium. They are usually found coincidentally on routine radiographic examination of the chest; however, 25 to 30 percent of the patients will have chest pain, dyspnea, cough, or paroxysmal tachycardia. Pericardial cysts occur most frequently in the third or fourth decade of life and equally among men and women. The right costophrenic location is the most common. Only rarely will the cyst connect with the pericardial cavity. Clinically and radiographically, they resemble other tumors of the pericardium such as hemangioma, lymphangioma, or lipoma, as well as retrosternal hernia, a pericardial fat pad, or eventration of the diaphragm. Two-dimensional echocardiography[184] and computed tomography are most helpful in the differential diagnosis. Surgical excision completely relieves symptoms and confirms the diagnosis.[7,13]

Teratoma
Most teratomas are extracardiac, yet intrapericardial, and arise and receive their blood supply from the root of the aorta or pulmonary artery through the vasa vasorum. Most are found in infants and children, with a strong female preponderance.[7] One case has been diagnosed in utero by aid of fetal echocardiography.[185] Recurrent, nonbloody pericardial effusion is common in children with this tumor, and intrapericardial teratoma is the most likely diagnosis in this setting.[186] Embarrassment of cardiac function results from expansion of the tumor to considerable proportions, at times up to 15 cm in diameter. Surgical excision is the only effective therapy[7] and is curative since the tumor is rarely malignant.[187] In fact, the first successful operation for any type of cardiac tumor was done in 1938 when Beck removed an intrapericardial teratoma.[186] A teratoma is rarely intracardiac, arises from the interventricular septum, and can be excised successfully.[188]

Mesothelioma
Mesothelioma ranks third in frequency among malignant tumors of the heart and pericardium.[8,189,190] Clinical manifestations resemble pericarditis, constrictive pericardial disease, or vena caval obstruction. Aspiration and histologic examination of the usually bloody pericardial fluid may be diagnostic. Among those affected, males outnumber females by a ratio of 2:1, with peak incidence in the third to fifth decades. The prognosis is poor, surgical excision is usually impossible, and treatment with irradiation and chemotherapy generally produces only temporary improvement.

Intrapericardial Pheochromocytoma
Pheochromocytoma may rarely be localized within the pericardium. Diagnosis by ^{131}I scintigraphy and by computed tomography has been described.[191]

Secondary Tumors of the Heart

General Considerations

Metastatic tumors invade the heart, pericardium, or both from a primary origin in some other organ 20 to 40 times more frequently than primary tumors of the heart.[192,193] Tumors of other organs gain access to the heart by direct contiguous growth from an adjacent structure, hematogenous spread, lymphatic portals, or direct growth along the vena cava or pulmonary veins.[192,194,195] Development of otherwise unexplained cardiac symptoms or manifestations, cardiac enlargement, tachycardia, arrhythmias, or heart failure in the presence of neoplastic disease should be suggestive of cardiac metastases.

Frequency and Origin of Secondary Tumors
In 4375 autopsies of patients who died of cancers recorded by the Harvard Cancer Commission, myocardial metastases were present in 146 patients (3.4 percent).[192] In a series of 2547 consecutive autopsies performed at Walter Reed General Hospital, a total of 980 cases of malignant disease were observed. The heart was the site of metastatic tumor in 5.7 percent of the cases and the heart, including the pericardium, in 13.9 percent.[193] In other series cardiac metastases have been present in a range as wide as 1.5 to 21 percent of patients with malignant tumors.[196] An increased prevalence of secondary cardiac neoplasms in recent years is possibly related to more vigorous surgical and radiation treatment of patients with primary neoplasms.[197] The relative infrequency of cardiac metastases has been attributed to the strong kneading action of the heart, the metabolic peculiarities of striated muscle, rapid coronary blood flow, and lymphatic connections which drain afferently from the heart.[192]

Cardiac metastases occur with all types of primary tumors: carcinomas, sarcomas, leukemias, lymphomas,[198] Kaposi's sarcoma, myeloma,[199] etc.

No malignant tumor tends particularly to metastasize to the heart, with the possible exception of malignant melanoma, which involves the myocardium in over 50 percent of cases.[196] Cardiac metastases occur most frequently from bronchogenic carcinoma and carcinoma of the breast, being found in one-third of the cases. Cardiac infiltration, often macroscopic, is seen in one-half of cases of leukemia and in one-sixth of cases of lymphoma, particularly reticulum cell sarcoma.[200]

Metastatic cardiac tumors are 16[201] to 40[175] times more common than primary cardiac tumors, and carcinomatous invasion is more frequent than sarcomatous invasion. Cardiac metastases occur most frequently in patients over age 50, with an equal sex incidence.[202] Metastatic tumor of the heart has been described in 0.1 to 6.4 percent of selected autopsies and in 1.5 to 20.6 percent of patients dying of malignant tumors.[201,202]

Cardiac metastases are encountered with widespread systemic tumor dissemination; only rarely is metastatic tumor limited to the heart or pericardium. Carcinomatous metastases are generally grossly visible, multiple, discrete, small, white, firm nodules; microscopically they resemble the primary tumor and the metastases in other organs. Diffuse infiltration is characteristic of sarcomatous metastases. Necrosis is uncommon.[202]

Metastatic tumors are classically thought to reach the heart by embolic hematogenous spread, by lymphatic spread, or by direct invasion, in descending order of frequency.[202] Recently, cardiac lymphatics have been reported to be the chief pathway of tumor metastases to the heart; lymphatic obstruction by tumor results in myocardial interstitial edema, and the secondary pressure on the myofibers may contribute to the eventual cardiac decompensation,[203] particularly in the patient with underlying coronary atherosclerotic heart disease.

Lymphatic spread of tumors is particularly frequent with carcinoma of the bronchus and the breast; the proximity of the heart to major mediastinal lymphatic channels seems to explain the high incidence of cardiac metastases from mediastinal tumors.[202]

Manifestations

Secondary involvement of the heart may be recognized as a pathologic finding without clinical manifestations. More often, however, such involvement is symptomatic and on rare occasions may be the first or only[204] expression of a remote primary tumor. Recognition of neoplastic heart disease is dependent upon the physician's awareness of the probability of occurrence and diverse manners of presentation. At times, as with rapidly developing tamponade, recognition and appropriate therapy must be undertaken promptly. Secondary tumors of the heart may involve the pericardium, myocardium, endocardium, valves, and coronary arteries. Direct invasion of the heart through the venae cavae or pulmonary veins,[205] or an expanding myocardial implant, can produce an intracavitary tumor mass and result in obstruction to flow or cause valvular obstruction.[206] Depending on the character and location of the cardiac lesion, a variety of manifestations may serve to identify cardiac involvement, especially in a patient known to have a malignancy.[52,207]

Pericardial Involvement

Pericardial involvement is often first manifested by chest pain aggravated by inspiration and pericardial friction rub. Increased fluid accumulation, often but not always bloody, may result in progressive cardiac enlargement on roentgenogram, with symptoms and signs of cardiac tamponade. Reduced electrocardiographic QRS voltage can be expected. Electrical alternans, generally seen in patients with large effusions and serious tamponade,[208] usually necessitates prompt pericardiocentesis. The echocardiogram will demonstrate pericardial effusion and may also demonstrate changes suggestive of cardiac tamponade. The association of large quantities of pericardial fluid with tumor encasing the heart frequently results in persistent cardiac constriction, even after the fluid is withdrawn by pericardiocentesis.[209] Two-dimensional echocardiography and computed tomography (CT) are both useful for detecting pericardial metastases (Fig. 61-7).[210,211]

Myocardial Involvement

Atrial arrhythmias are common, probably because the atrium has less mobility and hence is invaded more often. Atrial flutter and fibrillation are frequent, and the patient with either may be unusually resistant to conventional therapy. Ventricular extrasystoles and even serious ventricular arrhythmias may accompany invasion of a tumor into the myocardium. Conduction disturbances and complete heart block have been reported.[212,213] Widespread muscle involvement by tumor invasion or obstruction of the cardiac lymphatic drainage system may cause congestive failure. Myocardial damage and heart failure also may result from some of the chemotherapeutic agents used in the treatment of patients with neoplastic diseases, and combined radiotherapy and chemotherapy may synergistically increase cardiac damage.[214] (See Chap. 58.) The most frequent electrocardiographic abnormalities seen in patients with neoplastic heart disease are nonspecific changes of the ST segment and the T wave due to myocardial or pericardial involvement by the tumor. Pronounced and prolonged ST-segment elevation, in the absence of myocardial infarction, may occur with tumor invasion of the heart.[215]

Coronary Artery Involvement

In patients with a malignant tumor, angina or myocardial infarction may result from concomitant atherosclerosis,[214] coronary occlusion by tumor embolization,[216] or external coronary compression by the

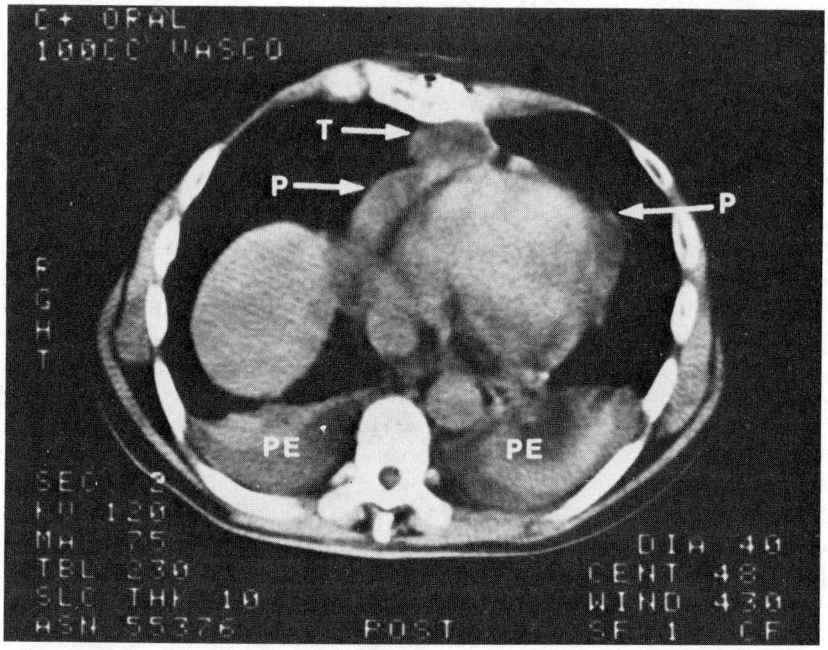

FIGURE 61-7 Computerized axial tomographic section of the chest at the cardiac level, of a patient with metastatic renal cell carcinoma to the anterior mediastinum (T) and the pericardium. Extensive pericardial involvement (P) by the tumor is evident. Bilateral pleural effusions (PE) are also evident. (*Courtesy of Dr. F. Parker Gregg, Department of Radiology, St. Luke's Episcopal Hospital, Houston, Texas.*)

tumor,[217] as well as from coronary fibrosis or accelerated atherogenesis in patients who have received irradiation to the mediastinum.[214] The electrocardiographic pattern of myocardial infarction also can result from massive invasion of the myocardium by a tumor[214,218] or from a large pericardial effusion.[193,219]

Intracavitary Tumor

Extensions of tumors such as renal cell carcinoma,[185] hepatocellular carcinoma,[220] and uterine leiomyosarcoma[221] along the inferior vena cava and into the right atrium can present as an intracavitary obstructive mass. Intracavitary metastases or an expanding myocardial tumor may progressively obliterate a cardiac chamber or result in a valvular obstruction[222–225] and, rarely, produce fever of unknown origin.[204] Successful surgical resection has been reported.[226,227] Right atrial and tricuspid obstruction by an intracavitary mass can mimic pericardial constriction[226] either from tumor invasion or from previous intensive radiotherapy to the mediastinum.[228] Systemic or pulmonary emboli, so common with primary tumors of the heart, are uncommon with secondary tumors.

Diagnostic Studies

Echocardiography, especially two-dimensional,[210,229] radionuclide imaging of the cardiac and pulmonary blood pool,[230] and radiographic CT scanning[231] facilitate identification of pericardial effusion and intracavitary and pericardial masses.[210,231–233] Pericardiocentesis not only affords prompt symptomatic relief from pericardial tamponade but often provides a definitive cytologic diagnosis.[234,235] Angiocardiography provides diagnostic information on filling defects and chamber displacement, as well as evidence of pericardial effusion or thickening. Results of endomyocardial biopsy may contribute to the diagnosis in some cases.[236] Bone formation in metastatic osteogenic sarcoma occasionally may be visible radiographically.[237]

Treatment

Malignant pericardial effusion usually recurs rapidly following pericardiocentesis. Depending upon the cytologic type and radiosensitivity of the tumor, radiation to the cardiac area,[238,239] with or without systemic chemotherapy, is the treatment of choice. The heart can tolerate 2000 to 4000 rad, beyond which the risk of radiation-induced pericardial, myocardial, and valvular[240] damage is increased. Patients with malignant pericardial effusions have responded to systemic chemotherapy[241] and to intrapericardial administration of fluorouracil, Au, mechlorethamine hydrochloride,[207,242] and tetracycline.[243] Persistent reaccumulation of fluid may require surgical creation of a pericardial "window."[244–246] Patients with myocardial infiltration by tumor also respond to radiation therapy and systemic chemotherapy.[207] Heart block is treated with temporary or permanent electronic pacing as conditions dictate. Surgical removal of intracavity obstructing secondary tumors may ameliorate symptoms and prolong survival,[223,231,247–249] as may chemotherapy in the occasional patient.[228]

Special Considerations

Leukemia

Leukemic infiltration of the heart is usually found at postmortem study and generally is not suspected before death.[250–252] Cardiac infiltrates were found in 69 percent of the postmortem studies of patients with acute leukemia, with most having pericardial involvement.[252] Cardiac symptoms were unusual. Chronic lymphocytic leukemia reportedly has caused myocardial infiltration in some patients,[253] as well as mitral valve dysfunction[254] and congestive heart failure.[255] Myocardial rupture has been reported as an early manifestation of acute myeloblastic leukemia.[256] Massive pericardial effusion, often hemorrhagic,[257] and pericardial tamponade[258] have been reported, although overt pericardial effusion is not common. Management consists of pericardiocentesis and chemotherapy; and, occasionally, surgical decompression of the pericardium is necessitated by recurrent tamponade.[258] Infective endocarditis, commonly fungal, may complicate acute leukemia. Because of advances in treatment and improved long-term remission in patients with acute lymphoblastic leukemia, complicating infective endocarditis has been managed by valve replacement.[259]

Carcinoid Heart Disease

While carcinoid tumors are never primary in the heart, and only rarely metastasize to the heart and pericardium, products of the tumor produce a distinctive endocardial and valvular pathologic pattern.[260] Carcinoid tumors originally were described by Oberndorfer in 1907.[260a] Tumors producing the carcinoid syndrome most commonly arise in the gastrointestinal tract, although they may arise in the bronchus, biliary tract, pancreas, and testis (Strickman et al.).[260] Primary ovarian carcinoid tumors associated with the carcinoid syndrome have been seen.[261] Appendiceal carcinoids, while common, rarely metastasize or produce the carcinoid syndrome. Ileal carcinoids, containing cytoplasmic granules which take up and reduce silver salts (argentaffinity), frequently metastasize to the liver and produce the carcinoid syndrome. These carcinoids contain a high concentration of 5-hydroxytryptamine (5-HT), excreted mainly as 5-hydroxyindoleacetic acid (5-HIAA) in the urine. Bronchial, pancreatic, and gastric carcinoid tumors differ morphologically and histochemically, carry a worse prognosis, and metastasize more widely than ileal tumors. They also produce 5-HT and excrete 5-HIAA in the urine; however, the clinical picture may be atypical. Carcinoid tumors of the rectum have a negative argentaffin reaction and are not associated with abnormalities of 5-HT synthesis or the carcinoid syndrome. While they bear no morphological or histochemical relation to the more typical carcinoid tumor, occasionally carcinomas of the bronchus, pancreas, or thyroid may secrete humoral substances that produce the carcinoid syndrome. In gastrointestinal carcinoid disease, the fact that the production of the syndrome depends upon secretion of tumor products into the systemic circulation unfortunately delays its occurrence until after liver metastases have occurred. The carcinoid syndrome, resulting from the systemic effect of circulating vasoactive amines, consists of cutaneous flushing, intestinal hypermobility, bronchial constriction, edema, and cardiac lesions.

Cardiac Lesions

The right side of the heart is involved more commonly than the left (Fig. 61-8). Left-sided involvement occurs with bronchial tumors, in the presence of an intraatrial communication, or, in the absence of such a communication, when there is extensive right-sided heart involvement. Grossly visible, glistening white-yellow deposits are found on the pulmonary and tricuspid valves and, to varying degrees, on the right atrial and ventricular endocardium. Contraction of these deposits leads predominantly to pulmonary stenosis and tricuspid insufficiency and occasionally may produce a restrictive type of myopathy.[260] Mitral valve involvement may result in both stenosis and insufficiency. On microscopic examination the endocardial lesions consist of superficial deposits of fibrous tissue beneath a normal endothelium. Metastatic lesions may be found in the myocardium. Both 5-HT and bradykinin have been implicated in the pathogenesis of the cardiac lesions.[260]

Clinical Manifestations

Carcinoid heart disease cannot be recognized clinically until cardiac murmurs and signs of right-sided heart failure develop—especially elevated jugular venous pressure with inspiratory augmentation of the *v* wave, which is characteristic of tricuspid regurgitation. A harsh pansystolic lower sternal border murmur with inspiratory accentuation is common, frequently followed by an early diastolic filling

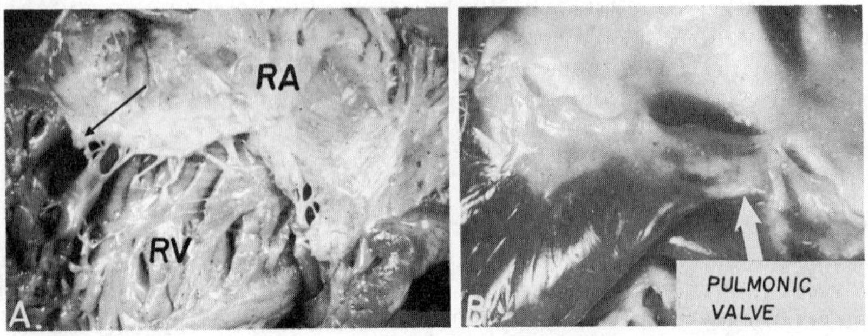

FIGURE 61-8 Valvular changes in carcinoid heart disease. *A.* The tricuspid valve shows nodular thickening along the valve margin (arrow), with scarring and retraction of the valve and the chordae tendineae. *B.* The pulmonic valve shows thickening and retraction of all leaflets. RV = right ventricle; RA = right atrium.

sound and diastolic rumble. A separate left upper sternal systolic ejection murmur of pulmonary stenosis may or may not be identified separately. Murmurs of concomitant valvular involvement are rarely identified. There may be a parasternal heave and systolic pulsation of the liver, although enlargement and multinodular irregularity of the liver, ascites, and edema may be features of hepatic metastases per se.

On roentgenogram of the chest the lung fluids are clear; the pulmonary trunk is normal in size; and the size of the heart may be normal or show evidence of right ventricular and atrial enlargement. The electrocardiogram may show evidence of right atrial enlargement, but right ventricular hypertrophy is rare. Echo imaging reveals right ventricular volume overload and abnormal right-sided valves. The tricuspid valve is typically thickened, retracted, and fixed in a semiopen position. Saline contrast studies document tricuspid valve regurgitation. The echographic changes are distinctive of carcinoid heart disease, are useful in following its progression, and may detect subclinical involvement.[262]

Cardiac catheterization usually reveals predominant tricuspid regurgitation with a large right atrial systolic wave as well as some degree of tricuspid diastolic gradient. Angiography demonstrates thickening and doming of both the pulmonary and tricuspid valves. Injection of contrast medium into the pulmonary artery provides evidence of pulmonary regurgitation which is rarely appreciated clinically, on the basis of auscultation of a separate diastolic murmur. A large transpulmonary valve gradient and marked elevation of right ventricular pressure are unusual. A low cardiac output with wide arteriovenous oxygen difference usually dominates the picture by the time cardiac catheterization is performed.

Diagnosis of carcinoid heart disease depends upon clinical recognition of the characteristic right-sided heart findings in the setting of systemic features of the carcinoid syndrome. Rarely, the diagnosis is made postoperatively after tricuspid valve replacement.[263] In cases of ileal carcinoid disease, clinical recognition of multinodular deformity, along with radionuclide or CT imaging of the enlarged liver, serves to identify the prerequisite metastases to this organ.[260,264] Carcinoid tumors that originate in the location that can release metabolic products outside the portal circulation will not share these latter characteristics. Urinary excretion of 5-HIAA is markedly elevated, and heavy diversion of tryptophan to this metabolic pathway may result in profound hypoproteinemia and nicotinamide deficiency (pellagra).

Treatment

Current chemotherapeutic programs are at least partially effective in some patients with extensive liver metastases. When hepatic metastases are present, removing the primary ileal lesion is indicated only if it is large and is producing mechanical obstruction. Occasionally large hepatic metastases are few in number, and resection may afford symptomatic relief. Newer techniques of catheter embolization may permit segmental hepatic ablation in selected patients. In contrast, removal of an extraportal primary tumor can result in rapid resolution of cardiac failure.[261] Some of the manifestations of the carcinoid syndrome may be blocked by alpha-adrenergic blockers and serotonin antagonists.[260,265]

Valve Replacement

Since heart failure is a frequent cause of disability and death when carcinoid heart disease complicates the carcinoid syndrome, tricuspid valve replacement and pulmonary valvotomy, with outflow tract enlargement if necessary, have been recommended when hemodynamically indicated.[260,261,264,266,267] Only a small number of patients have had valve surgery; however, selected patients have experienced clinical improvement even in the presence of extensive hepatic metastases, reflecting the slow progression and potential for long-term survival with this tumor.[260,264] Carcinoid plaque extending onto bioprosthetic valves as early as 8 months after surgery has been reported.[268] Since the mechanism of valvular fibrosis in this entity is unknown, implantation of a bioprosthetic valve is not recommended,[264] although use of tissue valves has been reported by several groups.[260] Anesthetic considerations require an understanding of the effects of release of humoral substances. However, with proper care and planning, general anesthesia can be conducted with minimal risk.[260,269]

References

1. Primary Cardiac Tumors, *Scott Med. J.*, 20:103, 1975.
2. Newman, H. A., Cardell, A. R., and Pritchard, R. W.: Intracardiac Myxomas Literature Review and Report of Six Cases, One Successfully Treated, *Am. Surg.*, 33:219, 1966.
3. Goldberg, H. P., Glenn F., Dotter, C. T., and Steinberg, I.: Myxoma of the Left Atrium: Diagnosis Made during Life with Operative and Post Mortem Findings, *Circulation*, 6:762, 1952.
4. Peters, M. N., Hall, R. J., Cooley, D. A., Leachman, R. D., and Garcia E.: The Clinical Syndrome of Atrial Myxoma, *JAMA*, 230:694, 1974.
5. St. John Sutton, M. G., Mercier, L. A., Giuliani, E. R., and Lie, J. T.: Atrial Myxomas: A Review of Clinical Experience in 40 Patients, *Mayo Clin. Proc.*, 55:371, 1980.
6. Bulkley, B. H., and Weiss, J. L.: Atrial Myxomas: Triumph of Machine over Man, *Chest*, 75:537, 1979.
7. McAllister, H. A., Jr.: Primary Tumors and Cysts of the Heart and Pericardium, in W. P. Harvey (ed.), "Current Problems in Cardiology," Year Book Medical Publishers, Inc., Chicago, May 1979, vol. IV, no. 2.
8. McAllister, H. A., Jr., and Fenoglio, J. J., Jr.: "Tumors of the Cardiovascular System," Armed Forces Institute of Pathology, Washington, D.C., 1978.
9. Sandrasagra, F. A., Oliver, W. A., and English, T. A. H.: Myxoma of the Mitral Valve, *Br. Heart J.*, 42:221, 1979.

10. Devig, P. M., Clark, T. A., and Aaron, B. L.: Cardiac Myxoma Arising from the Inferior Vena Cava, *Chest,* 78:784, 1980.
11. Salyer, W. R., Page, D. L., and Hutchins, G. M.: The Development of Cardiac Myxomas and Papillary Endocardial Lesions from Mural Thrombus, *Am. Heart J.,* 89:4, 1975.
12. Feldman, P. S., Horvath, E., and Kovacs, K.: An Ultrastructural Study of Seven Cardiac Myxomas, *Cancer,* 40:2216, 1977.
13. Fine, G.: Primary Tumors of the Pericardium and Heart, *Cardiovasc. Clin.,* 5:207, 1973.
14. Frishman, W., Factor, S., Jordan, A., Hellman, C., Elkayam, U., Lejemtel, T., Strom, J., Unschuld, H., and Becker, R.: Right Atrial Myxoma: Unusual Clinical Presentation and Atypical Glandular Histology, *Circulation,* 59:1070, 1979.
15. Wold, L. E., and Lie, J. T.: Scanning Electron Microscopy of Intracardiac Myxoma, *Mayo Clin. Proc.,* 56:198, 1981.
16. Bashey, R. I., and Nochumson, S.: Cardiac Myxoma: Biochemical Analyses and Evidence for Its Neoplastic Nature, *N.Y. State J. Med.,* 79:29, 1979.
17. Glasser, S. P., Bedynek, J. L., Hall, R. J., Hopeman, A. R., Treasure, R. L., McAllister, H. A., Jr., Esterly, J. A., Manion, W. C., and Sanford, H. S.: Left Atrial Myxoma: Report of a Case Including Hemodynamic, Surgical, Histologic and Histochemical Characteristics, *Am. J. Med.,* 50:113, 1971.
18. Read, R. C., White, H. J., Murphy, M. L., Williams, D., Sun, C. N., and Flanagan, W. H.: The Malignant Potentiality of Left Atrial Myxoma, *J. Thorac. Cardiovasc. Surg.,* 68:857, 1974.
19. Jugdutt, B. I., Rosall, R. E., and Sterns, L. P.: An Unusual Case of Recurrent Left Atrial Myxoma, *Can. Med. Assoc. J.,* 112:1099, 1975.
20. Cleveland, D. C., Westaby, S., and Karp, R. B.: Treatment of Intra-Atrial Cardiac Tumors, *JAMA,* 249:2799, 1983.
21. Desousa, A. L., Muller, J., Campbell, R., Batnitzky, S., and Rankin, L.: Atrial Myxoma: A Review of the Neurological Complications, Metastases, and Recurrences, *J. Neurol. Neurosurg. Psych.,* 41:1119, 1978.
22. Pastakia, B.: Malignant Atrial Myxoma Presenting as Intercranial Mass, *Chest,* 75:531, 1979.
23. Dashkoff, N., Boersma, R. B., Nanda, N. C., Gramiak, R., Anderson, M. N., and Subramanian, S.: Bilateral Atrial Myxomas: Echocardiographic Considerations, *Am. J. Med.,* 65:361, 1978.
24. Leonhardt, E. T., and Kullenberg, K. P.: Bilateral Atrial Myxomas with Multiple Arterial Aneurysms—A Syndrome Mimicking Polyarteritis Nodosa, *Am. J. Med.,* 62:792, 1977.
25. Morgan, D. L., Palazola, J., Reed, W., Bell, H. H., Kindred, L. H., and Beauchamp, G. D.: Left Heart Myxomas, *Am. J. Cardiol.,* 40:611, 1977.
26. Steinke, W. E., Perry, L. W., Gold, H. R., McClenathan, J. E., and Scott, L. P.: Left Atrial Myxoma in a Child, *Pediatrics,* 49:580, 1972.
27. Nakata, K., Onouchi, Z., Tomisawa, M., and Gotto, M.: Right Ventricular Myxoma in Infancy, *Jpn. Circ. J.,* 40:1183, 1976.
28. Balsara, R. K., and Pelias, A. J.: Myxoma of Right Ventricle Presenting as Pulmonic Stenosis in a Neonate, *Chest,* 83:145, 1983.
29. Guillet, P., Baconnet, C., Labrousse, A., Aigueperse, I., André, A., Grosgogeat, Y, Laurenceau, J. L., Temkina, J., and Vanetti, A.: Left Atrial Myxoma in the Elderly: Diagnosis by M-Mode and Bidimensional Echocardiography, *J. Am. Geriatr. Soc.,* 29:453, 1981.
30. Burech, D. L., Teska, D. W., and Haynes, R. E.: Right Atrial Myxoma in a Child, *Am. J. Dis. Child.,* 131:750, 1977.
31. Powers, J. C., Falkoff, M., Heinle, R. A., Nanda, N. C., Ong, L. S., Weiner, R. S., and Barold, S. S.: Familial Cardiac Myxoma: Emphasis on Unusual Clinical Manifestations, *J. Thorac. Cardiovasc. Surg.,* 77:782, 1979.
32. Crawford, F. A., Jr., Selby, J. H., Jr., Watson, D., and Joransen, J.: Unusual Aspects of Atrial Myxoma, *Ann. Surg.,* 188:240, 1978.
33. Ciraulo, D. A.: Mitral Valve Fluttering: An Echocardiographic Feature of Left Atrial Myxoma, *Chest,* 76:95, 1979.
34. Graham, S. L., and Sellers, A. L.: Atrial Myxoma with Multiple Myeloma, *Arch. Intern. Med.,* 139:116, 1979.
35. Burns, E. R., Schulman, I. C., and Murphy, M. J., Jr.: Hematologic Manifestations and Etiology of Atrial Myxoma, *Am. J. Med. Sci.,* 284:17, 1982.
36. Atherton, D. J., Pitcher, D. W., Wells, R. S., and MacDonald, D. M.: A Syndrome of Various Cutaneous Pigmented Lesions, Myxoid Neurofibromata and Atrial Myxoma: The NAME Syndrome, *Br. Assoc. Dermatol.,* 103:421, 1980.
37. O'Neil, M. B., Jr., Grehl, T. M., and Hurley, E. H.: Cardial Myxomas: A Clinical Diagnostic Challenge, *Am. J. Surg.,* 138:68, 1979.
38. Kaminsky, M. E., Ehlers, K., Engle, M. E., Klein, A. A., Levin, B. R., and Subramanian, V. A.: Atrial Myxoma Mimicking a Collagen Disorder, *Chest,* 75:93, 1979.
39. Thomas, M. H.: Myxoma Masquerading as Polyarteritis Nodosa, *J. Rheumatol.,* 8:133, 1981.
40. Rajpal, R. S., Leibsohn, J. A., Leikweg, W. G., Gross, C. M., Olinger, G. N., Rose, H. D., and Bamrah, V. S.: Infected Left Atrial Myxoma with Bacteremia Simulating Infective Endocarditis, *Arch. Intern. Med.,* 139:1176, 1979.
41. Joseph, P., Himmelstein, D. V., Mahowald, J. M., and Stullman, W. S.: Atrial Myxoma Infected with Candida: First Survival, *Chest,* 78:340, 1980.
42. Sweiger, M. J., Hafer, J. G., Jr., Brown, R., and Gianelly, R. E.: Spontaneous Cure of Infected Left Atrial Myxoma Following Embolization, *Am. Heart J.,* 99:630, 1980.
43. Flynn, W., Garcia-Rinaldi, R., Roehm, J. O., Jr., and Crawford, E. S.: Surgical Treatment of Infected Right Atrial Myxoma, *Ann. Thorac. Surg.,* 27:242, 1979.
44. Bradham, R. R., Gregorie, H. B., Jr., Howell, J. S., Jr., Ribers, C. F., Jr., and Barnwell, W. H.: Aortic Obstruction from Embolizing Cardiac Myxoma, *J. S. C. Med. Assoc.,* 75:7, 1979.
45. Chadda, K. D., Pochaczevsky, R., Gupta, P. K., Lichstein, E., and Schwartz, I. S.: Nonprolapsing Atrial Myxoma; Clinical, Echocardiographic, and Angiographic Correlations, *Angiology,* 29:179, 1978.
46. Tipton, B. K., Robertson, J. T., and Robertson, J. H.: Embolism to the Central Nervous System from Cardiac Myxoma: Report of Two Cases, *J. Neurosurg.,* 47:937, 1977.
47. Thompson, J. R., and Simmons, C. R.: Arterial Embolus: Manifestations of Unsuspected Myxoma, *JAMA,* 228:864, 1974.
48. Roeltgen, D. P., Weimer, G. R., and Patterson, L. F.: Delayed Neurologic Complications of Left Atrial Myxoma, *Neurology,* 31:8, 1981.
49. Cogan, D. G., and Wray, S. H.: Vascular Occlusions in the Eye from Cardiac Myxomas, *Am. J. Ophthalmol.,* 80(3):396, 1975, pt. 1.
50. Tanabe, J., Williams R. L., and Diethrich, E. B.: Left Atrial Myxoma: Association with Acute Coronary Embolization in an 11-Year-Old Boy, *Pediatrics,* 63:778, 1979.
51. Balk, A. H. M., Wagenaar, S. S., and Bruschke, A. V. G.: Bilateral Cardiac Myxomas and Peripheral Myxomas in a Patient with Recent Myocardial Infarction, *Am. J. Cardiol.,* 44:767, 1979.
52. Harvey, W. P.: Clinical Aspects of Cardiac Tumors, *Am. J. Cardiol.,* 21:328, 1968.
53. Martinez-Lopez, J. I.: Sounds of the Heart in Diastole, *Am. J. Cardiol.,* 34:594, 1974.
54. Goodwin, J. F.: The Spectrum of Cardiac Tumors, *Am. J. Cardiol.,* 21:307, 1968.
55. Rose, M. R., Fox, A. C., Glassman, E., and Reed, G. E.: Left Atrial Myxoma and Aortic Regurgitation: Case Report, *J. Thorac. Cardiovasc. Surg.,* 68:797, 1974.
56. Sharratt, G. P., Grover, M. L., and Monro, J. L.: Calcified Left Atrial Myxoma with Floppy Mitral Valve, *Br. Heart J.,* 42:608, 1979.

57. Case Records of the Massachusetts General Hospital, Weekly Clinicopathological Exercises: Case 42-1973, *N. Engl. J. Med.*, 289:853, 1973.
58. Giuliani, E. R., Lemire, F., and Schattenberg, T. T.: Unusual Echocardiographic Findings in a Patient with Left Atrial Myxoma, *Mayo Clin. Proc.*, 53:469, 1978.
59. Nasser, W. K., Davis, R. H., Dillon, J. C., Tavel, M. E., Helmen, C. H., Feigenbaum, H., and Fisch, C.: Atrial Myxoma: II. Phonocardiographic, Echocardiographic, Hemodynamic, and Angiographic Features in Nine Cases, *Am. Heart J.*, 83:810, 1972.
60. Becker, L. C., Klaus, A. P., and Humphries, J. O.: Early Systolic Notch in the Apexcardiogram in Mitral Stenosis, *Am. Heart J.*, 86:582, 1973.
61. Salcedo, E. E., Adams, K. V., Lever, H. M., Gill, C. C., and Lombardo, H.: Echocardiographic Findings in 25 Patients with Left Atrial Myxoma, *J. Am. Coll. Cardiol.*, 1:1162, 1983.
62. Kotler, M. N., Segal, B. L., and Parry, W. R.: Role of Echocardiography in the Diagnosis of Bacterial Endocarditis, Cardiac Tumors, Wolff-Parkinson-White Syndrome, Mitral Annular Calcification, Aortic Root Dissection, and Marfan's Syndrome, *Cardiovasc. Clin.*, 9:167, 1978.
63. Vozzi, C. R., Pechacek, L. W., Garcia, E., Mathur, V. S., de Castro, C. M., and Hall, R. J.: Two-Dimensional Echocardiography in the Diagnosis of Unusual Left Atrial Myxomas, *Cardiovasc Dis. Bull. Tex. Heart Institute*, 7:246, 1980.
64. DeMaria, A. N., Vismara, L. A., Miller, R. R., Neumann, A., and Mason, D. T.: Unusual Echographic Manifestations of Right and Left Heart Myxomas, *Am. J. Med.*, 59:713, 1975.
65. Stewart, J. A., Warnica, J. W., Kirk, M. E., and Winsberg, F.: Left Atrial Myxoma: False Negative Echocardiographic Findings in a Tumor Demonstrated by Coronary Arteriography, *Am. Heart J.*, 98:228, 1979.
66. Moses, H. W., and Nanda, N. C.: Real Time Two-Dimensional Echocardiography in the Diagnosis of Left Atrial Myxoma, *Chest*, 78:788, 1980.
67. Rahilly, G. T., and Nanda, N. C.: Two-Dimensional Echocardiographic Identification of Tumor Hemorrhages in Atrial Myxomas, *Am. Heart J.*, 101:237, 1981.
68. DePace, N. L., Soulen, R. L., Kotler, M. N., and Mintz, G. S.: Two Dimensional Echocardiographic Detection of Intraatrial Masses, *Am. J. Cardiol.*, 48:954, 1981.
69. Liu, H. Y., Panidis, I., Soffer, J., and Dreifus, L. S.: Echocardiographic Diagnosis of Intracardiac Myxomas, *Chest*, 84:63, 1984.
70. Donahoo, J. S., Weiss, J. L., Gardner, T. J., Fortuin, N. J., and Brawley, R. K.: Current Management of Atrial Myxoma with Emphasis on a New Diagnostic Technique, *Ann. Surg.*, 189:763, 1979.
71. Come, P. C., Rileyl, M. F., Markis, J. E., and Malagold, M.: Limitations of Echocardiographic Techniques in Evaluation of Left Atrial Masses, *Am. J. Cardiol.*, 48:947, 1981.
72. Fitteret, J. D., Spicer, M. J., and Nelson, W. P.: Echocardiographic Demonstration of Bilateral Atrial Myxomas, *Chest*, 70:282, 1976.
73. Meller, J., Teichholz, L. E., Pichard, A. D., Matta, R., Litwak, R., Herman, M. V., and Massie, K. F.: Left Ventricular Myxoma: Echocardiographic Diagnosis and Review of the Literature, *Am. J. Med.*, 63:816, 1977.
74. Boughner, D. R., and Persaud, J. A.: Transcutaneous Continuous Wave Doppler Ultrasound in the Diagnosis of Left Atrial Myxoma, *Chest*, 79:322, 1981.
75. Sunagawa, K., Orita, Y., Tanaka, S., Kikuchi, Y., Nakamura, M., and Hirata, T.: Left Atrial Ball Thrombus Diagnosed by Two-Dimensional Echocardiography, *Am. Heart J.*, 100:89, 1980.
76. LeJemtel, T., Strom, J., Jordan, A., Becker, R., and Aronson, R. S.: Left Atrial Thrombus Occluding the Mitral Orifice, *Cardiovasc. Rev. Rep.*, 2:56, 1981.
77. Pohost, G. M., Pastore, J. O., McKusick, K. A., Chiotellis, P. N., Kapellakis, G. Z., Myers, G. S., Dinsmore, R. E., and Block, P. C.: Detection of Left Atrial Myxoma by Gated Radionuclide Cardiac Imaging, *Circulation*, 55:88, 1977.
78. Meyers, S. N., Shapiro, S. E., Barresi, V., DeBoer, A. A., Pavel, D. I., Gracey, D. R., Suhre, D. E., and Buehler, J. H.: Right Atrial Myxoma with Right to Left Shunting and Mitral Valve Prolapse, *Am. J. Med.*, 62:208, 1977.
79. Case Records of the Massachusetts General Hospital, Weekly Clinicopathological Exercises: Case 14-1978, *N. Engl. J. Med.*, 298:834, 1978.
80. Willey, R. F., Matthews, M. B., and Walbaum, P. R.: An Unusual Case of Large Right Atrial Myxoma, *Br. Heart J.*, 44:108, 1980.
81. Sung, R. J., Ghahramani, A. R., Mallon, S. M., Richter, S. E., Sommers, L. S., Gottlieb, S., and Meyerburg, R. J.: Hemodynamic Features of Prolapsing and Nonprolapsing Left Atrial Myxoma, *Circulation*, 51:342, 1975.
82. Pitt, A., Pitt, B., Schaeffer, J., and Criley, J. M.: Myxomas of the Left Atrium: Hemodynamic and Phonocardiographic Consequences of Sudden Tumor Movement, *Circulation*, 36:408, 1967.
83. Ognibene, A. J., and Nelson, W. P.: Atrial Myxoma: Comments on Hemodynamic Alterations—Report of a Case, *Dis. Chest*, 52:699, 1967.
84. Rausch, J. M., Reinke, R. T., Peterson, K. L., and Higgins, C. B.: Abnormal Left Ventricular Catheter Motion: An Ancillary Angiographic Sign of Left Atrial Myxoma, *Am. J. Roentgenol.*, 126:1155, 1976.
85. Hamer, J. P. M., Nieveen, J., Bergstra, A., Blickman, J. R., and Homan van der Heide, J. N.: Left Atrial Myxoma Moving from Right to Left Ventricle, *Acta Med. Scand.*, 205:527, 1979.
86. Martinez, E. C., Giles, T. D., and Burch, G. E.: Echocardiographic Diagnosis of Left Atrial Myxoma, *Am. J. Cardiol.*, 33:281, 1974.
87. Shapiro, J. M., Kronzon, I., and Winer, H. E.: Diagnosis of Left Atrial Tumors by Coronary Angiography and Left Ventriculography, *Cathet. Cardiovasc. Diagn.*, 5:41, 1979.
88. Pindyck, F., Peirce, E. C., II, Baron, M. G., and Lukban, S. B.: Embolization of Left Atrial Myxoma after Transseptal Cardiac Catheterization, *Am. J. Cardiol.*, 30:569, 1972.
89. Stroobandt, R., Peiessens, J., and DeGeest, H.: Arterial Blood Supply to a Left Atrial Myxoma Diagnosed by Coronary Arteriography: Report of a Case, *Eur. J. Cardiol.*, 5:477, 1977.
90. Shapiro, M. R., Cohen, M. V., Gross R., and Spindola-Franco, H.: Diagnosis of Left Atrial Myxoma by Coronary Angiography Eight Years Following Open Mitral Commissurotomy, *Am. Heart J.*, 105:325, 1983.
91. Bochna, A. J., and Falicov, R. E.: Diagnosis of Intracardiac Thrombi in Mitral Stenosis and Left Ventricular Dysfunction: Use of Selective Coronary Arteriography, *Arch. Intern. Med.*, 140:759, 1980.
92. Ennker, J., Daniel, W., Doehring, W., and Oelert, H.: Surgical Experience with Left Atrial Myxomas, *Herz*, 8:227, 1983.
93. Huston, K. A., Combs, J. J., Jr., Lie, J. T., and Giuliani, E. R.: Left Atrial Myxoma Simulating Peripheral Vasculitis, *Mayo Clin. Proc.*, 53:752, 1978.
94. Tanabe, J., Williams, R. L., and Diethrich, E.B.: Left Atrial Myxoma: Association with Acute Coronary Embolization in an 11-Year-Old Boy, *Pediatrics*, 63:778, 1979.
95. Lortscher, R. H., Toews, W. H., Nora, J. J., Wolfe, R. R., and Spangler, R. D.: Left Atrial Myxoma Presenting as Rheumatic Fever, *Chest*, 66:302, 1974.
96. Neches, W. H., Park, S. C., Lenox, C. C., Zuberbuhler, J. R., and Siewers, R. D.: Left Atrial Myxoma: Clinical Presentation Suggesting Acute Myocarditis, *JAMA*, 229:1906, 1974.
97. Roguin, N., Amikam, S., and Riss, E.: Prolapsing Right Atrial Myxoma: Clinical and Haemodynamic Considerations, *Br. Heart J.*, 39:577, 1977.
98. Hickie, J. B., Gibson, H., and Windsor, H. M.: "The Wrecking Ball": Right Atrial Myxoma, *Med. J. Aust.*, 2:82, 1970.

99. Muroff, L. R., and Johnson, P. M.: Right Atrial Myxoma Presenting as Nonresolving Pulmonary Emboli: Case Report, *J. Nucl. Med.*, 17:890, 1976.
100. Vidne, B., Atsmon, A., Aygen, M., and Levy, M. J.: Right Atrial Myxoma: Case Report and Review of the Literature, *Isr. J. Med. Sci.*, 7:1196, 1971.
101. Siggillino, J. J., Crawley, C. J., Clauss, R. H., Reed, G. E., and Tice, D. A.: Myxoma of the Right Atrium with Polycythemia, *Arch. Intern. Med.*, 3:178, 1963.
102. Natarajan, P., Vijayanagar, R. R., Eckstein, P. F., Bognolo, D. A., Toole, J. C.: Right Atrial Myxoma with Atrial Septal Defect: A Case Report and Review of the Literature, *Cathet. Cardiovasc. Diagn.*, 8:267, 1982.
103. Barlow, J., Fuller, D., and Denny, M.: Case Report: A Case of Right Atrial Myxoma with Special Reference to an Unusual Phonocardiographic Finding, *Br. Heart J.*, 24:120, 1962.
104. Pernod, J., Piwnica, A., and Duret, J. C.: Right Atrial Myxoma: An Echocardiographic Study, *Br. Heart J.*, 40:201, 1978.
105. Riggs, T., Paul, M. H., DeLeon, S., and Ilbawi, M.: Two Dimensional Echocardiography in Evaluation of Right Atrial Masses: Five Cases in Pediatric Patients, *Am. J. Cardiol.*, 48:961, 1981.
106. Oldershaw, P. J., and Coll, L.: Echocardiographic Appearances of Right Atrial Thrombus, *Clin. Cardiol.*, 5:544, 1982.
107. Mazer, M. S., and Harrigan, P. R.: Left Ventricular Myxoma: M-Mode and Two-Dimensional Echocardiographic Features, *Am. Heart J.*, 104:875, 1982.
108. DeJoseph, R. L., Shiroff, R. A., Levenson, L. W., Martin, C. E., and Zelis, R. F.: Echocardiographic Diagnosis of Intraventricular Clot, *Chest*, 71:417, 1977.
109. Hada, Y., Wolfe, C., Murray, G. F., and Craige, E.: Right Ventricular Myxoma: Case Report and Review of Phonocardiographic and Auscultatory Manifestations, *Am. Heart J.*, 100:871, 1980.
110. Yakirevich, V., Glazer, Y., Ilie, B., and Vidne, M.: Myxoma of the Pulmonary Valve Causing Severe Pulmonic Stenosis in Infancy (letter), *J. Thorac. Cardiovasc. Surg.*, 83:936, 1982.
111. Gonzalez, A., Altieri, P. I., Marquez, E., Cox, R. A., and Castillo, M.: Massive Pulmonary Embolism Associated with a Right Ventricular Mxyoma, *Am. J. Med.*, 69:795, 1980.
112. Stern, M. J., Cohen, M. V., Fish, B., and Rosenthal, R.: Clinical Presentation and Non-Invasive Diagnosis of Right Heart Masses, *Br. Heart J.*, 46:552, 1981.
113. Van Osdol, K. D., Hall, R. J., Warda, M., Massumi, A., and Klima, T.: Right Ventricular Thrombus: Clinical and Diagnostic Features, *Tex. Heart Inst. J.*, 10:359, 1983.
114. Betancourt, B., Defendini, E. A., Johnson, C., DeJesus, M., Pavia-Villamil, A., Cruz, A. D., and Medina, J. C.: Severe Right Ventricular Outflow Tract Obstruction Caused by an Intracavitary Cardiac Neurilemoma, *Chest*, 75:522, 1979.
115. Cooley, D. A., and Norman, J. C.: "Techniques in Cardiac Surgery," Texas Medical Press, Inc., Houston, Tex., 1975, p. 211.
116. Kabbani, S. S., and Cooley, D. A.: Atrial Myxoma: Surgical Considerations, *J. Thorac. Cardiovasc. Surg.*, 65:731, 1973.
117. Gasarotto, D., Bortolotti, U., Russo, R., Betti, D., Schivazappa, L., and Thiene, G.: Surgical Removal of a Left Atrial Myxoma during Pregnancy, *Chest*, 75:390, 1979.
118. Trimakas, A. P., Maxwell, K. D., Berkay, S., Gardner, T. J., and Achuff, S. C.: Fetal Monitoring during Cardiopulmonary Bypass for Removal of a Left Atrial Myxoma during Pregnancy, *Johns Hopkins Med. J.*, 144:156, 1979.
119. Bateman, T. M., Gray, R. J., Raymond, M. J., Chaux, A., Czer, L. S. C., and Matloff, J. M.: Arrhythmias and Conduction Disturbances Following Cardiac Operation for the Removal of Left Atrial Myxomas, *J. Thorac. Cardiovasc. Surg.*, 86:601, 1983.
120. Mahoney, L., Schieken, R. M., and Doty, D.: Cardiac Rhabdomyomas Simulating Pulmonic Stenosis, *Cathet. Cardiovasc. Diagn.*, 5:385, 1979.
121. Fengolio, J. J., Jr., McAllister, H. A., Jr., and Ferrans, V. J.: Cardiac Rhabdomyoma: A Clinicopathologic and Electron Microscopic Study, *Am. J. Cardiol.*, 38:241, 1976.
122. Kuehl, K. S., Perry, L. W., Chandra, R., and Scott, L. P., III: Left Ventricular Rhabdomyoma: A Rare Cause of Subaortic Stenosis in the Newborn Infant, *Pediatrics*, 46:464, 1970.
123. Violette, E. J., Hardin, N. J., and McQuillen, E. N.: Sudden Unexpected Death Due to Asymptomatic Cardiac Rhabdomyoma, *J. Forensic Sci.*, 26:599, 1981.
124. Milner, S., Abramowitz, J. A., and Levin, S. E.: Rhabdomyoma of the Heart in a Newborn Infant: Diagnosis by Echocardiography, *Br. Heart J.*, 44:224, 1980.
125. Spooner, E. W., Farina, M. A., Shaher, R. M., and Foster, E. D.: Left Ventricular Rhabdomyoma Causing Subaortic Stenosis—The Two-Dimensional Echocardiographic Appearance, *Pediatr. Cardiol.*, 2:67, 1982.
126. Duncan, W. J., Rowe, R. D., Freedom, R. M., Izukawa, T., and Olly, P. M.: Space-Occupying Lesions of the Myocardium: Role of Two-Dimensional Echocardiography in Detection of Cardiac Tumors in Children, *Am. Heart J.*, 104:780, 1982.
127. Marx, G. R., Bierman, F. Z., Matthews, E., and Williams, R.: Two-Dimensional Echocardiographic Diagnosis of Intracardiac Masses in Infancy, *J. Am. Coll. Cardiol.*, 3:827, 1984.
128. Starshak, R. J., and Sty, J. R.: Radionuclide Angiocardiography: Use in the Detection of Myocardial Rhabdomyoma, *Clin. Nucl. Med.*, 3:106, 1978.
129. Gutierrez De Loma, J., Villagra, F., De Leon, J. P., Casanova, M., Collando, R., and Brito, J. M.: Rhabdomyoma of the Heart, *J. Cardiovasc. Surg.*, 23:149, 1982.
130. Hoen, A. G., and Ellis, E. J.: Intramural Fibroma of the Heart, *Am. J. Cardiol.*, 17:579, 1966.
131. Reul, G. J., Jr., Howell, J. F., Rubio, P. A., and Peterson, P. A.: Successful Partial Excision of an Intramural Fibroma of the Left Ventricle, *Am. J. Cardiol.*, 36:262, 1975.
132. Oliva, P. B., Breckinridge, J. C., Johnson, M. L., Brantigan, C. P., and O'Meara, O. P.: Left Ventricular Outflow Obstruction Produced by a Pedunculated Fibroma in a Newborn: Clinical, Angiographic, Echocardiographic and Surgical Observations, *Chest*, 74:590, 1978.
133. Williams, D. B., Danielson, G. K., McGoon, D. C., Feldt, R., H., and Edwards, W. D.: Cardiac Fibroma: Long-Term Survival After Excision, *J. Thorac. Cardiovasc. Surg.*, 84:230, 1982.
134. Biancaniello, T. M., Meyer, R. A., Gaum, W. E., and Kaplan, S.: Primary Benign Intramural Ventricular Tumors in Children: Pre- and Postoperative Electrocardiographic, Echocardiographic, and Angiocardiographic Evaluations, *Am. Heart J.*, 103:852, 1982.
135. Jamieson, S. W., Gaudiani, V. A., Reitz, B. A., Oyer, P. E., Stinson, E. B., and Shumway, N. E.: Operative Treatment of Unresectable Tumor of the Left Ventricle, *J. Thorac. Cardiovasc. Surg.*, 81:797, 1981.
136. Anderson, K. R., Fiddler, G. I., and Lie, J. T.: Congenital Papillary Tumor of the Tricuspid Valve: An Unusual Cause of Right Ventricular Outflow Obstruction in a Neonate with Trisomy E., *Mayo Clin. Proc.*, 52:665, 1977.
137. Cha, S. D., Incarvito, J., Chang, K. S., and Maranhao, V.: Giant Lambl's Excrescences of Papillary Muscle and Aortic Valve Echocardiographic, Angiographic, and Pathologic Findings, *Clin. Cardiol.*, 4:51, 1981.
138. Fitzgerald, D., Gaffney, P., Dervan, P., Doyle, C. T., Horgan, J., and Nelligan, M.: Giant Lambl's Excrescence Presenting as a Peripheral Embolus, *Chest*, 81:516, 1982.
139. Almagro, U. A., Perry, L. S., Choi, H., and Pintar, K.: Papillary Fibroelastoma of the Heart: Report of Six Cases. *Arch. Pathol. Lab. Med.*, 106:318, 1982.
140. Shub, C., Tajik, A. J., Seward, J. B., Edwards, W. D., Pruitt, R. D., Orszulak, T. A., and Pluth, J. R.: Cardiac Papillary Fibroelastomas: Two-Dimensional Echocardiographic Recognition, *Mayo Clin. Proc.*, 56:629, 1981.
141. Ong, L. S., Nanda, N. C., and Barold, S. S.: Two-Dimen-

sional Echocardiographic Detection and Diagnostic Features of Left Ventricular Papillary Fibroelastoma, *Am. Heart J.*, 103:917, 1982.
142. Marvasti, M. A., Obeid, A. E., Cohen, P. S., Giambertolomei, A., and Parker, F. B.: Successful Removal of Papillary Endocardial Fibroma, *Thorac. Cardiovasc. Surgeon*, 31:254, 1983.
143. Frumin, H., O'Donnell, L., Kerin, N. Z., Levine, F., Nathan, L. E., Jr., and Klein, S. P.: Two-Dimensional Echocardiographic Detection and Diagnostic Features of Tricuspid Papillary Fibroelastoma, *J. Am. Coll. Cardiol.*, 2:1016, 1983.
144. Moulton, A. L., Jaretzki, A., III, Bowman, F. O., Jr., Silverstein, E. F., and Bregman, D.: Massive Lipoma of Heart, *N.Y. State J. Med.*, 76:1820, 1976.
145. Shumacker, H. B., Jr., and Leshnower, A. C.: Extracavitary Lipoma of the Heart: Operative Resection, *Ann. Thorac. Surg.*, 18:411, 1974.
146. Reyes, L. H., Rubio, P. A., Korompai, F. L., and Guinn, G. A.: Lipoma of the Heart, *Intern. Surg.*, 61:179, 1976.
147. Barberger-Gateau, P., Paquet, M., Desaulniers, D., and Chenard, J.: Fibrolipoma of the Mitral Valve in a Child: Clinical and Echocardiographic Features, *Circulation*, 58:955, 1978.
148. Leatherman, L., Leachman, R. D., Hallman, G. L., and Cooley, D. A.: Cyst of the Mitral Valve, *Am. J. Cardiol.*, 21:428, 1968.
149. Voigt, J., and Agdal, N.: Lipomatous Infiltration of the Heart: An Uncommon Cause of Sudden, Unexpected Death in a Young Man, *Arch. Pathol. Lab. Med.*, 106:497, 1982.
150. Tschirkov, A., and Stegaru, B.: Lipomatous Hypertrophy of Interatrial Septum Presenting as Recurring Pericardial Effusion and Mistaken for Constrictive Pericarditis, *Thorac. Cardiovasc. Surgeon*, 27:400, 1979.
151. Fyke, F. E., III, Tajik, A. J., Edwards, W. D., and Seward, J. B.: Diagnosis of Lipomatous Hypertrophy of the Atrial Septum by Two-Dimensional Echocardiography, *J. Am. Coll. Cardiol.*, 1:1352, 1983.
152. Manion, W. C., Nelson, W. P., Hall, R. J., and Brierty, R. E.: Benign Tumor of the Heart Causing Complete Heart Block, *Am. Heart J.*, 83:535, 1972.
153. Paulson, S. M., and Kristensen, I. B.: So-Called Mesothelioma of the Atrioventricular Node, *Submicrosc. Cytol.*, 13:667, 1981.
154. James, T. N., and Galakhov, I.: De Subitaneis Mortibus: XXVI. Fatal Electrical Instability of the Heart Associated with Benign Congenital Polycystic Tumor of the Atrioventricular Node, *Circulation*, 56:667, 1977.
155. Hellemans, I. M., van Hemel, N. M., and Kooyman, C. A.: Atrioventricular Block in Childhood Caused by Mesothelioma, *PACE*, 4:216, 1981.
156. Travers, H.: Congenital Polycystic Tumor of the Atrioventricular Node: Possible Familial Occurrence and Critical Review of Reported Cases with Special Emphasis on Histogenesis, *Hum. Pathol.*, 13:25, 1982.
157. Raabe, D. S., Fischer, J. C., and Brandt, R. L.: Cavernous Hemangioma of the Right Atrium: Presumptive Diagnosis by Coronary Angiography, *Cathet. Cardiovasc. Diagn.*, 2:389, 1976.
158. Tabry, I. F., Nassar, V. H., Risk, G., Touma, A., and Dagher, I. K.: Cavernous Hemangioma of the Heart: Case Report and Review of the Literature, *J. Thorac. Cardiovasc. Surg.*, 69:415, 1975.
159. Stoupel, E., Primo, G., Kahn, R. J., le Clerc, J. L., de Wilde, P., Deuvaert, F., and Toussaint, C.: Cardiac Tamponade with Renal Failure due to Hemangioma of the Heart, *Acta Cardiol.*, 34:345, 1979.
160. Boden, W. E., Funk, E. J., Carleton, R. A., Benham, I., Khan, A. H., Lasser, A., and McEnany, M. T.: Left Ventricular Hemangioma Masquerading as Mycoplasma Pericarditis, *Am. Heart J.*, 106:771, 1983.
161. Panella, J. S., Paige, M. L., Victor, T. A., Sermerdjian, R. A., and Heuter, D. C.: Angiosarcoma of the Heart, Diagnosis by Echocardiography, *Chest*, 76:21, 1979.
162. Bjerregaard, P., and Baandrup, U.: Haemangioendotheliosarcoma of the Heart: Diagnosis and Treatment, *Br. Heart J.*, 42:734, 1979.
163. Strohl, K. P.: Angiosarcoma of the Heart: A Case Study, *Arch. Intern. Med.*, 136:928, 1976.
164. Shackell, M., Mito, A., Williams, P. L., and Sutton, G. C.: Angiosarcoma of the Heart, *Br. Heart J.*, 41:498, 1979.
165. Marni, E., Pedroni, E., Magrini, U., Mariani, P., Richichi, I., and Vigan'o, M.: Angiosarcoma of the Heart: Report of a Case in a 9-Year-Old Boy, *Med. Pediatr. Oncol.*, 11:336, 1983.
166. Ugarte, M., Alonso-Pulpon, L., Gonzalez-Villa, J., De Artaza, M., and Martin-Judez, V.: Coronary Arteriographic Findings in a Case of Primary Angiosarcoma of the Heart, *Eur. Heart J.*, 3:577, 1982.
167. Glancy, D. L., Morales, J. B., Jr., and Roberts, W. C.: Angiosarcoma of the Heart, *Am. J. Cardiol.*, 21:413, 1968.
168. Van Bruggen, H. W., and de Koning, J.: Pulmonic Stenosis Caused by a Malignant Tumor of the Heart, *Am. Heart J.*, 76: 526, 1968.
169. Schmaltz, A. A., and Apitz, J.: Primary Rhabdomyosarcoma of the Heart, *Pediatr. Cardiol.*, 2:73, 1982.
170. Coe, G. C.: Primary Rhabdomyosarcoma of the Heart, *Am. Heart J.*, 52:1124, 1960.
171. Schwartz, J. E., Schwartz, G. P., Judson, P. L., Siebel, J. E., and Trumbull, H. R.: Complete Resection of a Primary Cardiac Rhabdomyosarcoma: Case Report, Review of the Literature, and Management Recommendations, *Cardiovasc. Dis. Bull. Tex. Heart Inst.*, 6:413, 1979.
172. Baldelli, P., De Angeli, D., Dolora, A., Diligenti, L. M., Marchi, F., and Salvatore, L.: Primary Fibrosarcoma of the Heart, *Chest*, 62:234, 1972.
173. Gough, J. C., Connolly, C. E., and Kennedy, J. D.: Primary Sarcoma of the Heart: A Light and Electron Microscopic Study of Two Cases, *J. Clin. Pathol.*, 32:601, 1979.
174. Murtra, M., Mestres, C. A., Igual, A., Cubells, J., Espinosa, M., Benasco, C., and Ballestra, F.: Primary Liposarcoma of the Right Ventricle and Pulmonary Artery: Surgical Excision and Replacement of the Pulmonic Valve by a Björk-Shiley Tilting Disc Valve, *Thorac. Cardiovasc. Surgeon*, 31:172, 1983.
175. Bearman, R. M.: Primary Leiomyosarcoma of the Heart, *Arch. Pathol.*, 98:62, 1974.
176. Yashar, J., Witoszka, M., Savage, D. D., Klie, J., Dyckman, J., Yashar, J. H., Reddick, R. L., Watson, D. C., and McIntosh, C. L.: Primary Osteogenic Sarcoma of the Heart, *Ann. Thorac. Surg.*, 28:594, 1979.
177. Case Records of the Massachusetts General Hospital, Weekly Clinicopathological Exercises: Case 43-1971, *N. Engl. J. Med.*, 285:1016, 1971.
178. Frandsen, N. E., Anderson, G., and Nielsen, J. R.: Malignant Mesenchymoma of the Heart Presenting as Mitral Stenosis, *Acta Med. Scand.*, 209:235, 1981.
179. Donovan, V. M., Summer, W., Hutchins, G. M.: Left Atrial Lieomyosarcoma: Manifestation as Unexplained Pulmonary Vascular Disease, *Arch. Intern. Med.*, 142:1923, 1982.
180. Terashima, K., Aoyama, K., Nihei, K., Nito, T., Imai, Y., Takahashi, K., and Daidoji, S.: Malignant Fibrous Histiocytoma of the Heart, *Cancer*, 52:1919, 1983.
181. Ceretto, W. J., Miller, M. L., Shea, P. M., Gregory, C. W., and Vieweg, W. V.: Malignant Mesenchymoma Obstructing the Right Ventricular Outflow Tract, *Am. Heart J.*, 101:114, 1981.
182. Magovern, G. J., Yusuf, M. F., Liebler, G. A., Pugh, R. P., and Joyner, C. R.: The Surgical Resection and Chemotherapy of Metastatic Osteogenic Sarcoma of the Right Ventricle, *Ann. Thorac. Surg.*, 29:76, 1980.
183. Mori, K., Itoh, H., Kanaya, H., Onoe, T., Ohka, T, Lin, S., Matsubara, F., Ohmura, K., Magara, T., Tsuchiya, K., and Iwa, T.: Malignant Fibrous Histiocytoma of the Heart, *Jpn. Circ. J.*, 47:188, 1983.
184. Pezzano, A., Belloni, A., Faletra, F., Binaghi, G., Colli, A., and Rovelli, F.: Value of Two-Dimensional Echocardiog-

raphy in the Diagnosis of Pericardial Cysts, *Eur. Heart J.*, 4:238, 1983.
185. De Geeter, B., Kretz, J. G., Nisand, I., Eisenmann, B., Kieny, M. T., and Kieny, R.: Intraperiocardial Teratoma in a Newborn Infant: Use of Fetal Echocardiography, *Ann. Thorac. Surg.*, 35:664, 1983.
186. Reynolds, J. L., Donahue, J. K., and Pearce, C. W.: Intrapericardial Teratoma: A Cause of Acute Pericardial Effusion in Infancy, *Pediatrics*, 43:71, 1969.
187. MacDonald, S., Fay, J. E., and Lynn, R. M.: Intrapericardial Teratoma: A Continuing Challenge, *Can. J. Surg.*, 26:81, 1983.
188. Maeta, H., Hiyama, T., Okamura, K., Iriyama, T., Yamaguchi, T., Tamura, T., Mitsui, T., and Hori, M.: Successful Excision of Intracardiac Teratoma, *J. Thorac. Cardiovasc. Surg.*, 83:909, 1982.
189. Sytman, A. L., and MacAlpin, R. N.: Primary Pericardial Mesothelioma: Report of Two Cases and Review of the Literature, *Am. Heart J.*, 81:760, 1971.
190. Yilling, F. P., Schlant, R. C., Hertzler, G. L., and Krzyaniak, R.: Pericardial Mesothelioma, *Chest*, 81:520, 1982.
191. Saad, M. F., Frazier, O. H., Hickey, R. C., and Samaan, N. A.: Intrapericardial Pheochromocytoma, *Am. J. Med.*, 75:371, 1983.
192. Prichard, R. W.: Tumors of the Heart: Review of the Subject and Report of One Hundred and Fifty Cases, *Arch. Pathol.*, 51:98, 1951.
193. DeLoach, J. F., and Haynes, J. W.: Secondary Tumors of Heart and Pericardium: Review of the Subject and Report of One Hundred Thirty-Seven Cases, *Arch. Intern. Med.*, 92:224, 1953.
194. Timmis, A. D., Smallpeice, C., Davies, A. C., MacArthur, A. M., Grishen, P., and Jackson, G.: Intracardiac Spread of Intravenous Leiomatosis with Successful Surgical Excision, *N. Engl. J. Med.*, 303:1043, 1980.
195. Kadir, S., and Coulam, C. M.: Intracaval Extension of Renal Cell Carcinoma, *Cardiovasc. Int. Radiol.*, 3:180, 1980.
196. Glancy, D. L., and Roberts, W. C.: The Heart in Malignant Melanoma: A Study of 70 Autopsy Cases, *Am. J. Cardiol.*, 21:555, 1968.
197. Lockwood, W. B., and Broghamer, W. L., Jr.: The Changing Prevalence of Secondary Cardiac Neoplasms as Related to Cancer Therapy, *Cancer*, 45:2659, 1980.
198. McDonnell, P. J., Mann, R. B., and Bulkley, B. H.: Involvement of the Heart by Malignant Lymphoma: A Clinicopathologic Study, *Cancer*, 4:944, 1982.
199. Atkinson, K., McElwain, T. J., and Mackay, A. M.: Myeloma of the Heart, *Br. Heart J.*, 36:309, 1974.
200. Roberts, W. C., Glancy, D. L., and De Vita, V. T., Jr.: Heart in Malignant Lymphoma (Hodgkin's Disease, Lymphosarcoma, Reticulum Cell Sarcoma and Mycosis Fungoides): A Study of 196 Autopsy Cases, *Am. J. Cardiol.*, 22:82, 1968.
201. Griffiths, G. C.: A Review of Primary Tumors of the Heart, *Prog. Cardiovasc. Dis.*, 7:465, 1965.
202. Hanfling, S. M.: Metastatic Cancer to the Heart: Review of the Literature and Report of 127 Cases, *Circulation*, 22:474, 1960.
203. Kline, I. K.: Cardiac Lymphatic Involvement by Metastatic Tumor, *Cancer*, 29:799, 1972.
204. Hood, R. P., Geraci, J. E., Broadbent, J. C., and Titus, J. L.: Metastatic Squamous Cell Carcinoma of the Heart Presenting as Fever of Unknown Origin, *Mayo Clin. Proc.*, 62:556, 1967.
205. Onuigbo, W. I.: Direct Extension of Cancer Between Pulmonary Veins and the Left Atrium, *Chest*, 62:444, 1972.
206. Johnson, I., and Popple, A. W.: Right Ventricular Outflow Tract Obstruction Secondary for Small Intestinal Lymphoma, *Br. Heart J.*, 43:593, 1980.
207. Smith, L. H.: Secondary Tumors of the Heart, *Rev. Surg.*, 33:223, 1976.
208. Hernandez-Lopez, E., and Chahine, R. A.: Simultaneous Electrical and Mechanical Alternans in Pericardial Effusion, *Arch. Intern. Med.*, 140:840, 1980.
209. Mann, T., Brodie, B. R., Grossman, W., and McLaurin, L.: Effusive-Constrictive Hemodynamic Pattern Due to Neoplastic Involvement of the Pericardium, *Am. J. Cardiol.*, 41:781, 1978.
210. Moncada, R., Baker, M., Salinas, M., Demos, T. C., Churchill, R., and Love, L.: Diagnostic Role of Computed Tomography in Pericardial Heart Disease: Congenital Defects, Thickening, Neoplasms, and Effusions, *Am. Heart J.*, 103:163, 1982.
211. Chandraratna, P. A. N., and Arnow, W. S.: Detection of Pericardial Metastasis by Cross-Sectional Echocardiography, *Circulation*, 63:197, 1981.
212. Redwine, D. B.: Complete Heart Block Caused by Secondary Tumors of the Heart: Case Report and Review of Literature, *Tex. Med.*, 70:59, 1974.
213. Kubac, G., Doris, I., Ondra, M., and Davey, P. W.: Malignant Granular Cell Myoblastoma with Metastatic Cardiac Involvement: Case Report and Echocardiogram, *Am. Heart J.*, 100:227, 1980.
214. Kopelson, G., and Herwig, K. J.: The Etiologies of Coronary Artery Disease in Cancer Patients, *Int. J. Rad. Oncol. Biol. Phys.*, 4:895, 1978.
215. Hartman, R. B., Clarke, P. I., and Schulman, P.: Pronounced and Prolonged ST Segment Elevation: Pathognomonic Sign of Tumor Invasion of the Heart, *Arch. Intern. Med.*, 142:1917, 1982.
216. Vermani, R., Khedekar, R., Robinowitz, M., and McAllister, H.: Tumor Embolization in Coronary Artery Causing Myocardial Infarction, *Arch. Pathol. Lab. Med.*, 107:243, 1983.
217. Franciosa, J. A., and Lawrinson, W.: Coronary Artery Occlusion Due to Neoplasm: A Rare Cause of Acute Myocardial Infarction, *Arch. Intern. Med.*, 128:797, 1971.
218. Lubell, D. L., and Goldfarb, C. R.: Metastatic Cardiac Tumor Demonstrated by ^{201}Thallium Scan, *Chest*, 78:98, 1980.
219. Salem, B. I., Schnee, M., Leatherman, L. L., de Castro, C. M., and Benrey, J.: Electrocardiographic Pseudo-Infarction Pattern: Appearance with a Large Posterior Pericardial Effusion after Cardiac Surgery, *Am. J. Cardiol.*, 42:681, 1978.
220. Kato, Y., Tanaka, N., Kobayashi, K., Ideda, T., Hattori, N., and Nonomura, A.: Growth of Hepatocellular Carcinoma into the Right Atrium: Report of Five Cases, *Ann. Intern. Med.*, 99:472, 1983.
221. Maurer, G., and Nanda, N. C.: Two-Dimensional Echocardiographic Identification of Intracardiac Leiomyomatosis, *Am. Heart J.*, 103:915, 1982.
222. Birmingham, C. L., and Peretz, D. I.: Metastatic Carcinoma Presenting as Obstruction to the Right Ventricular Outflow Tract: Report of a Case Review of the Literature, *Am. Heart J.*, 97:229, 1979.
223. Stark, R. M., Perloff, J. H., Glick, H. J., Hirshfield, J. W., Jr., and Devereaux, R. B.: Clinical Recognition and Management of Cardiac Metastatic Disease: Observations in a Unique Case of Alveolar Soft-Part Sarcoma, *Am. J. Med.*, 63:653, 1977.
224. Steffens, T. G., Mayer, H. S., and Das, S. K.: Echocardiographic Diagnosis of a Right Ventricular Metastatic Tumor, *Arch. Intern. Med.*, 140:122, 1980.
225. Hurst, J. W., and Cooper, H. R.: Neoplastic Disease of the Heart, *Am. Heart J.*, 50(5):782, 1955.
226. Kaku, K., Kawashima, Y., Kitamura, S., Nakano, S., Mori, T., Beppu, S. U., Kozuka, T., Sakurai, M., Katayama, S., Tanizawa, O., and Sonoda, T.: Resection of Lieomyosarcoma Originating in Internal Iliac Vein and Extending into Heart via Inferior Vena Cava, *Surgery*, 89:604, 1981.
227. Luck, S. R., DeLeon, S., Shkolnik, A., Morgan, E., and Labotka, R.: Intracardiac Wilms' Tumor: Diagnosis and Management, *J. Pediatr. Surg.*, 17:551, 1982.
228. Garfein, O. B.: Lymphosarcoma of the Right Atrium: Angiographic and Hemodynamic Documentation of Response to Chemotherapy, *Arch. Intern. Med.*, 135:325, 1975.
229. Johnson, M. H., and Soulen, R. L.: Echocardiography of Cardiac Metastases, *AJR*, 141:677, 1983.

230. Avila Ramirez, E., and Martinez Guerra, G.: Radionuclide Angiography: As Diagnostic Method for Wilms' Tumor with Direct Extension into the Heart, *Pediatr. Radiol.,* 12:301, 1982.
231. Watts, F. B., Jr., Zingas, A. P., Das, L., and Cushing, B. A.: Computed Tomographic Diagnosis of an Intracardiac Metastasis from Osteosarcoma, *CT,* 7:271, 1983.
232. Wolverson, M. K., Grider, R. D., Sundaram, M., Heiberg, E., and Johnson, F.: Demonstration of Unsuspected Malignant Disease of the Pericardium by Computed Tomography, *CT,* 4:330, 1980.
233. Gross, B. H., Glazer, G. M., and Francis, I. R.: CT of Intracardiac and Intrapericardial Masses, *AJR,* 140:903, 1983.
234. Reyes, C. V., Strinden, C., and Banerji, M.: The Role of Cytology in Neoplastic Cardiac Tamponade, *Acta Cytol.,* 26:299, 1982 (Baltimore). (Abstract.)
235. Posner, M. R., Cohen, G. I., and Skarin, A. T.: Pericardial Disease in Patients with Cancer: The Differentiation of Malignant from Idiopathic and Radiation-Induced Pericarditis, *Am. J. Med.,* 71:407, 1981.
236. Hanley, P. C., Shub, C., Seward, J. B., and Wold, L. E.: Intracavitary Cardiac Melanoma Diagnosed by Endomyocardial Left Ventricular Biopsy, *Chest,* 84:195, 1983.
237. Seibert, K. A., Rettenmier, C. W., Waller, B. F., Battle, W. E., and Levine, A. S.: Osteogenic Sarcoma Metastatic to the Heart, *Am. J. Med.,* 73:136, 1982.
238. Charm, W. C., Freiman, A. H., Carstens, P. H. B., and Chu, F. C. H.: Radiation Therapy of Cardiac and Pericardial Metastases, *Radiology,* 114:701, 1975.
239. Quraishi, M. A., Costanzi, J. J., and Hokanson, J.: The Natural History of Lung Cancer with Pericardial Metastases, *Cancer,* 51:740, 1983.
240. Warda, M., Khan, A., Massumi, A., Mathur, V., Klima, T., and Hall, R. J.: Radiation-Induced Valvular Dysfunction, *J. Am. Coll. Cardiol.,* 2:180, 1983.
241. Primrose, W. R., Clee, M.D., and Johnston, R. N.: Malignant Pericardial Effusion Managed with Vinblastine, *Clin. Oncol.,* 9:67, 1983.
242. Lokich, J. J.: The Management of Malignant Pericardial Effusions, *JAMA,* 224:1401, 1973.
243. Davis, S., Sharma, S. M., Blumberg, E. D., and Kim, C. S.: Intrapericardial Tetracycline for the Management of Cardiac Tamponade Secondary to Malignant Pericardial Effusion, *Med. Intell.,* 229:1113, 1975.
244. Applequist, P., Maamies, T., and Gröhn, P.: Emergency Pericardiotomy as Primary Diagnostic and Therapeutic Procedure in Malignant Pericardial Tamponade: Report of Three Cases and Review of the Literature, *J. Surg. Oncol.,* 21:18, 1982.
245. Hankins, J. R., Satterfield, J. R., Aisner, J., Wiernik, P. H., and McLaughlin, J. S.: Pericardial Window for Malignant Pericardial Effusion, *Ann. Thorac. Surg.,* 30:465, 1980.
246. Prague, R. L., Wilson, C. H., and Bender, H. W., Jr.: The Subxiphoid Approach to Pericardial Disease, *Ann. Thorac. Surg.,* 34:6, 1982.
247. Ravikumar, T. S., Topulos, G. P., Anderson, R. W., and Grage, T. B.: Surgical Resection for Isolated Cardiac Metastases, *Arch. Surg.,* 118:117, 1983.
248. Melvin, K. N., Howard, R. J., Rakowski, H., Goldman, B. S., and El-Maraghi, N. R.: Embryonal Carcinoma of the Testis with Metastases to the Right Atrium, *Can. J. Surg.,* 26:86, 1983.
249. Poole, G. V., Jr., Meredith, J. W., Breyer, R. H., and Mills, S. A.: Surgical Implications in Malignant Cardiac Disease, *Ann. Thorac. Surg.,* 36:484, 1983.
250. Bierman, H. R., Perkins, E. K., Orega, P.: Pericarditis in Patients with Leukemia, *Am. Heart J.,* 43:413, 1952.
251. Terry, L. N., and Kligerman, M. M.: Pericardial and Myocardial Involvement by Lymphomas and Leukemias, *Cancer,* 25:1003, 1970.
252. Roberts, W. C., Bodey, G. C., and Wertlake, P. T.: The Heart in Acute Leukemia: A Study of 420 Autopsy Cases, *Am. J. Cardiol.,* 21:388, 1968.
253. Schwartz, J. B., and Shamsuddin, A. M.: The Effects of Leukemic Infiltrates in Various Organs in Chronic Lymphocytic Leukemia, *Hum. Pathol.,* 12:432, 1981.
254. Meltzer, V., Korompai, F. L., Mathur, V. S., and Guinn, G. A.: Surgical Treatment of Leukemic Involvement of the Mitral Valve, *Chest,* 67:119, 1975.
255. Applefeld, M. M., Milner, S. D., Vigorito, R. D., and Shamsuddin, A. K. M.: Congestive Heart Failure and Endocardial Fibroelastosis Caused by Chronic Lymphocytic Leukemia, *Cancer,* 46:1479, 1980.
256. Björkholm, M., Ost, A., and Biberfeld, P.: Myocardial Rupture with Cardiac Tamponade as a Lethal Early Manifestation of Acute Myeloblastic Leukemia, *Cancer,* 50:1967, 1982.
257. Cassis, N., Jr., and Porterfield, J.: Massive Hemopericardium as the Initial Manifestation of Chronic Myelogenous Leukemia, *Arch. Intern. Med.,* 142:2193, 1982.
258. Liepman, M. K., and Goodlerner, S.: Surgical Management of Pericardial Tamponade as a Presenting Manifestation of Acute Leukemia, *J. Surg. Oncol.,* 17:183, 1981.
259. Crofts, M. A., Morgan-Capner, P., Sharp, J. C., McLeod, A. A., and Keates, J. R.: Fungal Endocarditis in a Patient with Acute Leukaemia Treated by Valve Replacement, *Br. Med. J.,* 284:574, 1982.
260. Strickman, N. E., Rossi, P. A., Massumkhani, G. A., and Hall, R. J.: Carcinoid Heart Disease: A Clinical Pathologic, and Therapeutic Update, *Curr. Probl. Cardiol.,* 6:1, 1982.
260a. Oberndorfer, S.: Karzenoid tumoren des dunndarms. *Frankfurt Ztschr. Pathol.,* 1:426, 1907.
261. Sworn, M. J., Edlin, G. P., McGill, D. A., and Mousley, J. S.: Tricuspid Valve Replacement in Carcinoid Syndrome Due to Ovarian Primary, *Br. Med. J.,* 280:85, 1980.
262. Howard, R. J., Drobac, M., Rider, W. D., Keane, T. J., Finlayson, J., Silver, M. D., Wigle, E. D., and Rakowski, H.: Carcinoid Heart Disease: Diagnosis by Two-Dimensional Echocardiography, *Circulation,* 66:1059, 1982.
263. Kessler, M. R.: Carcinoid Heart Disease: A Unique Case of Postvalvotomy Diagnosis, *Arch. Intern. Med.,* 143:1615, 1983.
264. Hendel, N., Leckie, B., and Richards, J.: Carcinoid Heart Disease: Eight-Year Survival Following Tricuspid Valve Replacement and Pulmonary Valvotomy, *Ann. Thorac. Surg.,* 30:391, 1980.
265. Grahame-Smith, D. G.: The Carcinoid Syndrome, in P. K. Body and L. E. Rosenberg (eds.), "Metabolic Control and Disease," 9th ed., W. B. Saunders Company, Philadelphia, 1980, p. 1703.
266. Gutierrez, F. R., McKnight, R. C., Jaffe, A. S., Ludbrook, P. A., Biello, D., and Weldon, C. S.: Double Porcine Valve Replacement in Carcinoid Heart Disease, *Chest,* 81:101, 1982.
267. Miller, B. R., Vohr, F. H., Christian, F. V., and Singh, A. K.: Cardiac Valvular Replacement in Carcinoid Heart Disease, *Am. J. Med.,* 75:896, 1983.
268. Schoen, F. J., Hausner, R. J., Howell, J. F., Beazley, H. L., and Titus, J. L.: Porcine Heterograft Valve Replacement in Carcinoid Heart Disease, *J. Thorac. Cardiovasc. Surg.,* 81:100, 1981.
269. Hurst, J. W., Whitworth, H. B., O'Donoghue, S., et al.: Heart Disease due to Ovarian Carcinoid: Successful Replacement of the Pulmonary and Tricuspid Valves with Porcine Heterografts and Removal of the Tumor, in J. W. Hurst (ed.), "Clinical Essays on the Heart," vol. 5, McGraw-Hill Book Co., New York, 1985, p. 177.

Section K

Rheumatic Fever

62

Acute Rheumatic Fever and Its Management*

Gene H. Stollerman, M.D.

Definition

Rheumatic fever is a diffuse inflammatory disease which is a delayed nonsuppurative sequel of pharyngeal infection with group A streptococci. In its typical form, the disease is an acute febrile illness characterized by inflammation of the joints, heart, skin, and nervous system. The clinical manifestations usually include migratory polyarthritis, pancarditis, Sydenham's chorea, erythema marginatum, and subcutaneous nodules in varying combinations. Although the name *acute rheumatic fever* emphasizes involvement of the joints, the disease owes its major importance to the involvement of the heart, which can be fatal during the acute attack or can lead to rheumatic heart disease, a chronic condition due to scarring and deformity of the heart valves. Patients who have suffered an initial attack of rheumatic fever are at high risk of developing recurrences following group A streptococcal pharyngeal infections.

Etiology and Pathogenesis

Etiology

Several lines of evidence have established the etiologic relationship between group A streptococcal infection and rheumatic fever.[1,2] Outbreaks of acute rheumatic fever tend to accompany epidemics of streptococcal sore throat. In long-term prospective follow-up studies, rheumatic fever has been shown to recur only as a result of intercurrent streptococcal infections. Both primary and secondary attacks of the disease can be prevented by prompt treatment or prevention of streptococcal infections by antimicrobial therapy.[1,3]

Pathogenesis

To initiate the rheumatic process group A streptococci must infect the pharynx. Streptococcal infections of the skin or other extrapharyngeal sites will not cause the disease.[4,5] Furthermore, throat infections with some group A strains appear to produce rheumatic fever rarely or not at all.[6] A relatively small percentage of patients who sustain a streptococcal infection subsequently develop acute rheumatic fever. The organism cannot be found in the lesions when rheumatic fever appears after a latent period of several days or weeks after the acute streptococcal infection. No streptococcal product has been identified as a cause of the rheumatic lesions, nor has it been shown that the lesions are due to a direct effect of a tissue toxin or an immunologic process. Purified proteins from streptococcal cell membranes have been shown to be immunologically cross-reactive with sarcolemmal tissue,[7] and patients with rheumatic fever (with or without carditis) often have circulating antibodies to heart tissue.[8] Experimentally, tissue cultures of embryonic guinea pig heart can be damaged by lymphocytes sensitized to group A streptococci.[9] These findings have suggested that the myocardial lesions of rheumatic fever are the result of autoimmunity induced by streptococcal antigens, but the cytopathic nature of the immunologic reactions has not been verified.

*Portions of this chapter appeared in Chapter 257 of Petersdorf et al.: *Harrison's Principles of Internal Medicine*, 10th ed.

Incidence and Epidemiology

Acute rheumatic fever appears most frequently between the ages of 5 and 15 when streptococcal pharyngitis is most intense. It is extremely rare in infancy but may appear at any age. The geographic distribution, incidence, and severity of rheumatic fever are closely correlated with the frequency and severity of streptococcal disease in a given population. In epidemics of severe exudative streptococcal pharyngitis, the attack rate of rheumatic fever averages approximately 3 percent in untreated patients.[10] The attack rate, however, appears to be much lower when streptococcal pharyngitis is sporadic and mild and due to strains of lesser rheumatic potential.[11,12] Eradication of the infection by penicillin can reduce the attack rate of rheumatic fever when treatment is begun up to 10 days after the onset of pharyngitis.

Secondary rheumatic attack rates (those following streptococcal infections in patients who have had previous attacks of rheumatic fever) are increased to as high as 5 to 50 per 100 streptococcal infections and are related to the virulence of reactivating infections.[13] Moreover, the frequency of secondary attacks of rheumatic fever is much greater in subjects with rheumatic heart disease than in those who had acute rheumatic fever but not rheumatic carditis during the prior rheumatic attack. With the passage of years, the tendency for subjects to suffer recurrences of rheumatic fever following streptococcal infections declines but remains higher than the attack rate in the general population even after more than a decade.

A family history of rheumatic fever is commonly elicited; yet the concordance of the disease in identical twins is approximately 20 percent,[14] a figure which does not exceed that of poliomyelitis or tuberculosis, suggesting only a limited genetic predisposition to rheumatic fever. Although it has been vigorously investigated, the association of acute rheumatic fever with specific histocompatibility antigens has not yet been established.

The incidence of acute rheumatic fever, and the associated mortality rate, like those of septic streptococcal sore throat and scarlet fever, have been decreasing for several years in countries where housing and economic conditions have been steadily improving. The rate of decline has probably been accelerated by the wide use of antimicrobial therapy. The decrease may also be due to a change in the prevalence of rheumatogenic streptococcal strains. Despite its dramatic decline in relatively affluent countries, acute rheumatic fever is a major cause of death and disability from heart disease wherever poor economic conditions, overcrowding, and substandard housing are common. Thus, rheumatic fever and rheumatic heart disease remain an important priority of public health programs in the poorest countries and populations in the world and particularly in such regions as South Africa, India, the Middle East, China, southeast Asia, Micronesia, and many parts of South America.

Pathology

The pathology of rheumatic fever is characterized by diffuse proliferative and exudative inflammatory lesions in the connective tissues, particularly around small blood vessels.

Cardiovascular Lesions

The disease is distinct, pathologically because of its unique lesions of the heart and because of its tendency to spare other organs from serious damage. All the layers of the heart—endocardium, myocardium, and pericardium—may be involved, giving rise to the term *rheumatic pancarditis*. The most distinctive and specific pattern of rheumatic inflammation is found in the myocardial *Aschoff body*. This lesion, a submiliary granuloma, when present in its classic form, is considered to be pathognomonic of rheumatic fever. The origin of these Aschoff cells, or Anitschkow "myocytes," has been the subject of some controversy; it is unclear whether they are myocytes or of interstitial origin.[15] Aschoff bodies with more productive and less exudative changes may persist for many years after clinical evidence of carditis has subsided and remain as the lingering traces of chronic rheumatic inflammation in patients with rheumatic heart disease, particularly those who go on to develop mitral stenosis.[16]

Rheumatic endocarditis is characterized by a verrucous valvulitis which causes swelling, edema, and deformity of the valves, and leads to the most serious permanent cardiac damage once the risk of heart failure from the "toxic," exudative phase of myocarditis is over. Healing of the valvulitis may occur with fibrous thickening and adhesion of the valve commissures and chordae tendineae, leading to variable degrees of regurgitation and stenosis. Valvular deformity occurs most commonly in the mitral and aortic valves, less frequently in the tricuspid valves, and almost never in the pulmonary valves.

Rheumatic pericarditis consists of a serofibrinous effusion, causing "shaggy" elements of fibrin to be deposited on the heart's surface. Despite such heavy fibrinous and sometimes sanguineous effusions, pericardial constriction does not occur although the pericardium may become calcified.

Clinical Features

The major clinical manifestations of rheumatic fever are polyarthritis, carditis, chorea, erythema marginatum, and subcutaneous nodules. These major manifestations may occur singly or in various combinations following a latent period of 1 to 5 weeks (mean of 18 days) after streptococcal infection (usually much later in the case of chorea; see below). Surprisingly, as many as one-third of patients with acute rheumatic fever cannot recall the antecedent streptococcal sore throat.

Arthritis

The classic attack of rheumatic fever presents as an acute migratory polyarthritis associated with the usual signs and symptoms of an acute febrile illness, and cannot be distinguished from many other forms of acute infectious polyarthritis when joint involvement is the only major manifestation of the disease. The large joints of the extremities are most frequently affected, but any joint may be involved. Permanent scarring of the joints does not occur. As pain and swelling subside in one joint, others tend to become involved in "migratory" fashion, although such migration is not invariable and several large joints may become inflamed simultaneously. For polyarthritis to be acceptable as a criterion for the diagnosis of rheumatic fever, it should involve at least two joints, should be associated with at least two minor manifestations such as fever or elevation of erythrocytes in the sedimentation rate, and, most importantly, should be associated with a high titer of one or more streptococcal antibodies.[17]

Acute Rheumatic Carditis

Carditis, if it is to occur, usually appears within the first 3 weeks of the attack.[18] It first manifests itself by the appearance of the heart murmurs of either mitral or aortic regurgitation or both (the former more frequently). When acute polyarthritis is the presenting symptom, attention of the physician should be drawn to the heart, and carditis can usually be detected by the presence of the murmurs early in the attack. If isolated carditis is the initial manifestation, however, the onset may be insidious or even subclinical. In its most severe form, carditis causes death from acute myocardial failure. The fulminating form of rheumatic carditis has now become relatively rare, however. In contrast to the seriousness of the prognosis, rheumatic carditis most often causes no symptoms of its own. It is often diagnosed only because arthritis or chorea directs the patient to a physician, unless isolated carditis is associated with the pain of pericarditis or is severe enough to cause symptoms of heart failure or fever and constitutional symptoms such as weakness, fatigue, and anorexia. For this reason, patients whose rheumatic fever is manifested only by carditis are frequently not diagnosed, and in later life it may be discovered that they have rheumatic heart disease without a definite history of rheumatic fever.

Carditis occurs in 40 to 50 percent of first attacks of acute rheumatic fever although the incidence of various rheumatic manifestations varies with age. Carditis is most frequent during an initial rheumatic attack in the youngest age groups and is relatively rare in adult cases. Moreover, there tends to be an inverse relationship between the severity of arthritis and the severity of carditis.

The hallmarks of clinically active rheumatic carditis are (1) organic heart murmurs not previously present or a distinct change in the character of a preexisting heart murmur, (2) cardiac enlargement, (3) congestive heart failure, and (4) pericardial friction rubs or signs of effusion. In actuality, rheumatic carditis is almost always associated with one or more characteristic murmurs. The diagnosis must be suspect in the absence of such murmurs unless they are obscured by a loud pericardial friction rub or severe tachycardia. Of those patients who develop carditis in their first rheumatic attack, the murmurs are present in 75 percent during the first week of the illness and in 85 percent by the third week.[18] Virtually all murmurs appear within 3 months except perhaps in those patients with slight degrees of aortic or mitral regurgitation which may be heard for the first time some months later after maximal exercise or effort is permitted. The three murmurs of rheumatic carditis are apical systolic, apical middiastolic, and basal diastolic.

The apical middiastolic murmur, also known as the Carey Coombs murmur, begins immediately following the third heart sound and ends prior to the first heart sound. It is low-pitched and does not radiate widely. The murmur can also be heard in other situations characterized by rapid flow across the mitral valve (e.g., established mitral regurgitation in chronic rheumatic heart disease, other forms of carditis with marked cardiac dilatation, thyrotoxicosis, anemia).

The basal diastolic murmur of aortic regurgitation begins immediately following the second heart sound. The aortic regurgitation murmur may be heard only intermittently. Occasionally there is a transient cooing or high-pitched crying ("seagull") quality to the murmur during the active stage of rheumatic valvulitis of either mitral or aortic origin.

In addition to murmurs, cardiomegaly, frank congestive heart failure, and pericarditis, other manifestations of carditis in acute rheumatic fever include tachycardia which persists during sleep and gallop rhythms of S_3, S_4, or summation types. Abnormalities of atrioventricular conduction are quite common. The most common of these is first degree heart block. Second degree block, complete heart block, and atrioventricular dissociation may also be observed. Atrial fibrillation, on the other hand, is usually a feature of chronic rather than acute rheumatic heart disease. Prolongation of the PR interval and other changes in the ECG are very common but do not in themselves indicate acute carditis, and their presence or absence is unrelated to the subsequent development of chronic rheumatic heart disease.[19]

Chronic Rheumatic Carditis

The presenting picture in chronic rheumatic carditis is one of chronic heart failure in a patient with a markedly dilated heart and with physical, electrocardiographic, and x-ray findings of mitral regurgitaton. Differentiating this syndrome from other forms of chronic myocarditis may be difficult, if not impossible, when the other associated extracardiac features of rheumatic fever are absent. Although rheumatic fever does not produce *isolated* myocarditis but rather is almost invariably associated with pancarditis, the pericardial inflammation may not be evident and the mitral valvulitis might not be distinguishable from other causes of mitral regurgitation that are due to dilatation of the mitral ring. In such cases one must search diligently for clues such as evanescent pericardial rubs, pericardial effusion, transient aortic regurgitation, subcutaneous nodules, erythema marginatum, and subtle signs of chorea.

Chronic rheumatic myocarditis may run a fatal course over a period of months or even several years. Often, however, the patient improves, sometimes rather suddenly, and may even recover cardiac reserve dramatically in association with the disappearance of systemic manifestations of the chronic inflammatory process. The heart may remain large or may decrease somewhat in size. In occasional instances it may even return to normal size, but with varying degrees of valvular insufficiency. Such a course signals the termination of the "toxic" phase of the rheumatic process, and thereafter the course of rheumatic heart disease depends on the variables in healing cited below.

Chorea

Chorea is a disorder of the central nervous system characterized by sudden, aimless, irregular movements and is often accompanied by emotional instability. Chorea may appear after a long latent period, as long as several months after the antecedent streptococcal infection, and at a time when all other manifestations of rheumatic fever have abated and antistreptococcal antibodies have returned to normal. When no previous rheumatic manifestations are present, the syndrome is called *pure chorea.* More often chorea begins 1 to 3 months after the antecedent streptococcal infection but always later than polyarthritis.[20] When the former is absent, chorea may first direct the physician's attention to the presence of active carditis and other manifestations of the acute rheumatic attack.

The duration of chorea in hospitalized patients is usually between 2 and 4 months, but this neurological manifestation of acute rheumatic fever may last for only a week or may persist for several years. It leaves no permanent CNS sequelae. Chorea is the only manifestation of acute rheumatic fever which shows a striking difference in sex incidence. Before puberty the incidence is the same in boys and girls, but as the male matures sexually, chorea becomes rare; it is not found in the fully mature adult male. On the other hand, female hormones tend to aggravate chorea and the disease may be exacerbated by pregnancy.

Subcutaneous Nodules

Subcutaneous nodules are usually small, painless, firm, discrete, and freely movable swellings ranging in size from a few millimeters to 2 cm and found over bony prominences and along extensor tendons. They are frequently unnoticed by the patient and need to be sought for carefully in the physical examination. They are often evanescent and are easily overlooked. These nodules are most often observed in patients with protracted carditis and are seldom observed in mild rheumatic fever.

Erythema Marginatum

Erythema marginatum is a nonpruritic, pink, erythematous rash occurring on the trunk and proximal extremities—never on the face or hands. It begins as pink or red macules which fade centrally and extend peripherally in the pattern of enlarging circles. The erythema blanches completely and may change before ones eyes. Erythema marginatum appears to be a vasomotor phenomenon and anatomic lesions are not found. The process may go on intermittently for weeks or months. Erythema marginatum may appear early in the attack but sometimes is seen only during convalescence, and its course seems to be uninfluenced by anti-inflammatory therapy nor is its persistence necessarily an adverse prognostic sign.

Minor Clinical Criteria

Certain clinical features occur quite regularly in rheumatic fever but are also common to many other inflammatory diseases and are, therefore, of minor diagnostic value except as they support the major manifestations as diagnostic criteria. They include fever, arthralgia, abdominal pain, tachycardia, and epistaxis.

Laboratory Findings

No laboratory test in itself is diagnostic of rheumatic fever. The appraisal of rheumatic activity by laboratory findings is, however, of value since various tests are useful to indicate the persistence of rheumatic inflammation when clinical manifestations subside.

Streptococcal Antibody Tests for Preceding Streptococcal Infection

Because of the latent period between streptococcal sore throat and the onset of the early manifestations of rheumatic fever, streptococcal antibody levels will always be increased except when rheumatic fever is not discovered until many months after the pharyngeal infection, such as may happen in the case of pure chorea or chronic rheumatic carditis.[20] The antibodies may already be declining, or low, if the interval between the acute streptococcal infection and the detection of rheumatic fever has been longer than 2 months. Except in these instances, one should be reluctant to make the diagnosis of acute rheumatic fever in the absence of serological evidence of a recent streptococcal infection. The most widely used and best standardized test is the antistreptolysin O titer (ASO). In general, single titers of at least 250 Todd units in adults and at least 333 units/ml in children over 5 years of age are considered to be increased. A varying percentage of the normal population may show titers of this magnitude depending upon the general prevalence and intensity of streptococcal infections. In the early stages of rheumatic fever, about 20 percent of patients may have a low or borderline ASO titer; in such cases it is advisable to obtain another streptococcal antibody test such as the antideoxyribonucleotidase B (anti-DNase B) or antihyaluronidase titers. The antistreptozyme test (ASTZ) is a hemagglutination reaction test to a concentrate of extracellular streptococcal antigens adsorbed to red blood cells. It is a very sensitive indicator of streptococcal infection in that virtually all patients with acute rheumatic fever have titers in excess of 200 units/ml.[21] The actual value of all streptococcal antibody tests is in ruling out rheumatic fever in cases of isolated polyarthritis when no antibody rise can be detected. Rheumatic polyarthritis invariably occurs within 4 to 5 weeks of streptococcal infection at a time when streptococcal antibody responses are maximal.

Increased streptococcal antibodies, however, do not reflect rheumatic activity per se, and their rate of decline is independent of the course of the rheumatic attack.[2]

Isolation of Group A Streptococci

Throat cultures are less satisfactory than antibody tests as supporting evidence of recent streptococcal infection. Throat cultures usually fail to reveal group A streptococci when the rheumatic attack begins, or such organisms are present in very small numbers and are difficult to find. In addition, a significant number of normal individuals, especially children, carry group A streptococci in their throats intermittently, and positive cultures may be difficult to interpret.

Acute Phase Reactants

The erythrocyte sedimentation rate (ESR) and the test for C-reactive protein (CRP) in serum are useful although nonspecific detectors of the presence of an inflammatory process. Unless the patient has received corticosteroids, salicylates, or other aspirin-like compounds, these reactions are almost invariably abnormal in patients presenting with arthritis or carditis, whereas they are often normal in patients with the delayed onset of chorea. Prolongation of the PR interval of the electrocardiogram is frequent in acute rheumatic fever (about 25 percent of all cases with and without carditis), and other ECG changes are common but nondiagnostic. Anemia occurs commonly due to the suppression of erythropoiesis such as is found in many inflammatory diseases.

Course and Prognosis

The course of rheumatic fever cannot be predicted at the onset of the disease, but despite its variability in any given case, generalizations can be made on a statistical basis. Thus, 75 percent of acute rheumatic attacks abate within 6 weeks and 90 percent within 12 weeks, and less than 5 percent persist for more than 6 months. The persistent forms of the disease are the stubborn prolonged bouts of chronic rheumatic carditis described above or prolonged attacks of Sydenham's chorea. Once all evidence of rheumatic inflammation has abated, however, and more than 2 months has elapsed after withdrawal of all antirheumatic suppressive therapy with adrenal corticosteroids or aspirin-like compounds, rheumatic fever does not recur in the absence of new streptococcal infections. The frequency of recurrence is then dependent upon the frequency and severity of streptococcal infections, and is further influenced by the presence or absence of rheumatic heart disease and the duration of freedom from the last attack.[13]

Rheumatic Carditis and the Course of Rheumatic Heart Disease

The long-term prognosis of acute rheumatic fever is correlated most closely with the severity of carditis during the acute attack. Approximately 95 percent of patients who escape rheumatic carditis during their initial attack and are kept free of recurrences by careful prophylactic therapy (see below) will have no stigmata of rheumatic heart disease when examined a decade later.[22] Patients who show evidence of mild acute carditis (i.e., apical systolic murmur of mild mitral regurgitation without heart failure or pericarditis) have a fairly good prognosis in that only 30 percent will have organic heart murmurs after 10 years of observation. Approximately 40 percent of subjects with basal or apical *diastolic* murmurs and

70 percent of those with heart failure and/or pericarditis during their acute attack will have residual heart disease. Prognosis is the worst for those who have rheumatic heart disease and suffer recurrent rheumatic attacks.

In the longest *prospective* study of acute rheumatic fever, two forms of mitral stenosis could be distinguished: (1) the early appearance of a severely deformed valve within 5 years of the acute attack which occurred with equal distribution in both sexes and often carried a fatal prognosis owing to the hemodynamics of severe valvular dysfunction; and (2) the insidious development of mitral stenosis, primarily in women and in those who had experienced mild mitral valvulitis and who had no recurrent attacks to explain the progression of the disease.[23]

In order to help clarify the diagnosis of rheumatic fever and to avoid overdiagnosis, the American Heart Association has published a modification of the Jones criteria (Table 62-1). They are not meant to substitute for sound medical judgment but are recommended as a guide for the diagnosis of questionable cases. The finding of two major, or of one major and two minor, criteria indicates a high probability of the presence of rheumatic fever if supported by evidence of preceding streptococcal infection. The absence of the latter should always make the diagnosis suspect except when rheumatic manifestations are discovered long after the antecedent infection as in chorea or low-grade carditis. Because the prognosis may vary greatly according to the major manifestations, for recording purposes the diagnosis of acute rheumatic fever should be followed by a list of the major manifestations present, e.g., rheumatic fever manifested by polyarthritis and carditis. An indication of the severity of carditis (cardiac enlargement, congestive heart failure) is also advisable for future reference.

TABLE 62-1 Jones Criteria (Revised)

Major Manifestations	Minor Manifestations
Carditis	Fever
Polyarthritis	Arthralgia
Chorea	Previous rheumatic fever or rheumatic heart disease
Erythema marginatum	Elevated ESR or positive CRP
Subcutaneous nodules	Prolonged PR interval

Plus, supporting evidence of preceding streptococcal infection: history of recent scarlet fever; positive throat culture for group A streptococcus; increased ASO titer or other streptococcal antibodies.

Source: G. H. Stollerman, M. Markowitz, A. Taranta, and L. W. Wannamaker, Jones Criteria (Revised) for Guidance in the Diagnosis of Rheumatic Fever, *Circulation,* 32:664, 1965. Reproduced with permission from the American Heart Association, Inc., and the authors.

Treatment

No measures are known which will cure rheumatic fever or change the course of the attack. Good supportive therapy, however, may reduce its morbidity and mortality rates.

Antibiotic Therapy

As soon as acute rheumatic fever is diagnosed, a course of penicillin should be given to ensure the elimination of group A streptococci from the throat, even when throat cultures are negative. An effective course is either a single injection of 1.2 million units of benzathine penicillin G intramuscularly (IM) or 600,000 units of procaine penicillin IM daily for 10 days. Penicillin, even in large doses, will not reduce ultimate heart damage, nor will it influence the course of the attack, but once initiated it should be given continuously, as prophylaxis against intercurrent streptococcal infection, with one of the regimens described below.

Suppressive Therapy

Acute arthritis can be relieved with codeine or with salicylates or other nonsteroidal anti-inflammatory drugs. Although codeine will relieve pain but not inflammation, the rheumatic attack will be briefer in duration with this drug than when agents are used to suppress inflammation. Nonetheless, the effectiveness with which aspirin and aspirin-like compounds suppress the arthritis of acute rheumatic fever makes it difficult to deny patients the symptomatic benefits of these drugs. For patients without carditis, corticosteroids are unnecessary. When aspirin is used in the therapy of acute rheumatic fever, starting daily doses of 100 to 150 mg/kg in children and 6 to 8 g in adults given in five to six divided doses are recommended as a full therapeutic test. Indomethacin or other aspirin-like compounds effective in lower doses may be employed.

It is preferable, therefore, to begin treatment of patients with carditis with salicylates or compounds with similar pharmacologic action.[23] If these drugs fail to reduce fever and to relieve heart failure, corticosteroid therapy may be promptly substituted. Prednisone, the corticosteroid most commonly employed, is administered in initial doses of 60 to 120 mg or higher when necessary in four divided doses daily. After the signs and symptoms of rheumatic inflammation have been brought under control by anti-inflammatory agents, treatment should be continued until the sedimentation rate approaches near normal values and the test for C-reactive protein is negative. Treatment should be maintained for several weeks thereafter before tapering the dose. Poststeroid "rebounds" can often be avoided by an overlapping course of salicylate therapy when steroids are slowly withdrawn over a 2-week period. Salicylates may then be continued for an additional

2 to 3 weeks. Rheumatic rebounds that are mild are best allowed to abate spontaneously without resuming anti-inflammatory treatment so as to avoid further prolongation of the attack. About 5 percent of rheumatic attacks persist for more than 6 months. These chronic attacks are most likely to occur in patients with severe carditis and in those who have had previous episodes. The healing process should be followed with weekly tests for C-reactive protein and erythrocyte sedimentation rate.

Prevention of Recurrence

Recurrences are preventable by continuous chemoprophylaxis against recurrent streptococcal sore throat. The most efficient and effective regimen for this purpose is a monthly injection of 1.2 million units of benzathine penicillin G.[24] The discomfort and disadvantages of this regimen have to be weighed against the probability of recurrence in each individual case. Those with recent rheumatic fever, rheumatic heart disease, and multiple previous attacks, and particularly those who are exposed to an environment in which the risk of streptococcal pharyngitis is great, deserve the most effective form of protection. A second choice is an oral regimen of either 1 g sulfadiazine daily in a single dose or 200,000 units of penicillin G given twice daily on an empty stomach. The decision to continue prophylaxis beyond 5 years should be conditioned by the following variables: the presence of rheumatic heart disease (which greatly increases the risk and seriousness of recurrences), previous bouts of carditis, exposure to epidemiologic settings with a high incidence of streptococcal disease, and particularly exposure to populations in which acute rheumatic fever is prevalent. Such variables should be carefully considered before prophylaxis is terminated.

Prevention of Initial Rheumatic Attacks

First attacks of rheumatic fever may be prevented if group A streptococcal pharyngitis is treated promptly and adequately.[3] In communities where group A streptococcal pharyngitis is diagnosed early and treated well and where socioeconomic standards are high, streptococcal pharyngitis occurs with diminished frequency. In these communities, the group A streptococci found in schoolchildren's throats may be of relatively low virulence and may cause rheumatic fever far less frequently, or not at all, when transmitted to others.[1,5,6,25–29]

Streptococcal pharyngitis is adequately treated by a single intramuscular injection of 600,000 units of benzathine penicillin G in very young children or 1.2 million units in patients age 10 or older. Alternate plans of parenteral therapy or combined parenteral and oral therapy should produce consistent penicillinemia over a period of at least 10 days. If oral penicillin is employed, at least 200,000 units four times daily is recommended. Erythromycin in daily doses of 1 g for 10 days may be substituted in penicillin-sensitive individuals, although erythromycin resistance is a growing problem in some populations[26,27] wherein this antibiotic is used extensively for upper respiratory infections. Tetracycline is no longer recommended because of increasing worldwide frequency of strains of group A streptococci resistant to this antibiotic. So far, all group A streptococci have remained extremely sensitive to penicillin G. With the marked decline in streptococccal pharyngitis and rheumatic fever in many populations, the need for treatment of simple pharyngitis with the regimens recommended above has been questioned.[27,28] Some authorities therefore recommend not treating common simple pharyngitis in populations wherein rheumatic fever has disappeared but rather making a selective throat culture for beta-hemolytic streptococci. A negative culture's high predictive value in such circumstances may make antibiotic therapy of simple sore throat unnecessary more than 90 to 95 percent of the time.[29]

References

1. Stollerman, G. H.: "Rheumatic Fever and Streptococcal Infection," Grune & Stratton, Inc., New York, 1975.
2. Stollerman, G. H., Lewis, A. J., Schultz, I., and Taranta, A.: Relationship of Immune Response to Group A Streptococci to the Course of Acute, Chronic and Recurrent Rheumatic Fever, *Am. J. Med.*, 20:163, 1956.
3. Denny, F. W., Wannamaker, L. W., Brink, W. R., Rammelkamp, C. H., Jr., and Custer, E. A.: Prevention of Rheumatic Fever: Treatment of the Preceding Streptococcal Infection, *JAMA*, 143:151, 1950.
4. Wannamaker, L. W.: The Chain That Links the Heart to the Throat, *Circulation*, 48:9, 1973.
5. Stollerman, G. H.: Nephritogenic and Rheumatogenic Group A Streptococci, *J. Infect. Dis.*, 120:258, 1969.
6. Bisno, A. L.: The Concept of Rheumatogenic and Nonrheumatogenic Group S Streptococci, in S. E. Read and J. B. Zabriskie (eds.), "Streptococcal Diseases and the Immune Response," Academic Press, New York, 1980, p. 789.
7. Van deRijn, I., Zabriskie, J. B., and McCarty, M.: Group A Streptococcal Antigens Cross-Reactive with Myocardium: Purification of Heart-Reactive Antibody and Isolation and Characterization of the Streptococcal Antigen, *J. Exp. Med.*, 146:579, 1977.
8. Kaplan, M. H., and Svec, K. H.: Immunologic Relation of Streptococcal and Tissue Antigens: II. Presence in Human Sera of Streptococcal Antibody Cross-Reactive with Heart Tissue: Association with Streptococcal Infection, Rheumatic Fever, and Glomerulonephritis, *J. Exp. Med.*, 119:651, 1964.
9. Yang, L. C., Soprey, P. R., Wittner, M. K., and Fox, E. N.: Streptococcal-Induced Cell-Mediated Immune Destruction of Cardiac Myofibers in Vitro, *J. Exp. Med.*, 146:344, 1977.
10. Rammelkamp, C. H., Denny, F. W., and Wannamaker, L. W.: Studies on the Epidemiology of Rheumatic Fever in the Armed Services, in L. Thomas (ed.), "Rheumatic Fever." University of Minnesota Press, Minneapolis, 1952.
11. Stollerman, G. H.: The Relative Rheumatogenicity of Strains of Group A Streptococci, *Mod. Concepts Cardiovasc. Dis.*, 64:35, 1975.
12. Bisno, A. L., Pearce, I. A., Wall, H. P., Moody, M. D., and

Stollerman, G. H.: Contrasting Epidemiology of Acute Rheumatic Fever and Acute Glomerulonephritis: Nature of the Antecedent Streptococcal Infection, *N. Engl. J. Med.*, 283:561, 1970.

13. Taranta, A., Kleinberg, E., Feinstein, A. R., Wood, H. F., Tursky, E., and Simpson, R.: Rheumatic Fever in Children and Adolescents: A Long-Term Epidemiologic Study of Subsequent Prophylaxis, Streptococcal Infections, and Clinical Sequelae: V. Relation of the Rheumatic Fever Recurrence Rate per Streptococcal Infection to Preexisting Clinical Features of the Patients, *Ann. Internal. Med.*, 60(suppl. 5):58, 1964.
14. Taranta, A., Metrakos, J. D., and Uchida, I.: Rheumatic Fever in Monozygotic and Dizygotic Twin, *Circulation*, 20:778, 1959. (Abstract.)
15. Becker, C. G., and Murphy, G. E.: On the Pathology of Rheumatic Heart Disease, in S. E. Read and J. B. Zabriskie (eds.): "Streptococcal Diseases and the Immune Response," Academic Press, New York, 1980, p. 23.
16. Virmani, R., and Roberts, W. C.: Aschoff Bodies in Operatively Excised Atrial Appendages and in Papillary Muscles: Frequency and Clinical Significance, *Circulation*, 55:559, 1977.
17. Stollerman, G. H., Markowitz, M., Taranta, A., and Wannamaker, L. W.: Jones Criteria (Revised) for Guidance in the Diagnosis of Rheumatic Fever, *Circulation*, 32:664, 1965.
18. Massell, B. F., Fyler, D. C., and Roy, S. B.: The Clinical Picture of Rheumatic Fever: Diagnosis, Immediate Prognosis, Course and Therapeutic Implications, *Am. J. Cardiol.*, 1:436, 1958.
19. Feinstein, A. R., Wood, H. F., Spagnuolo, M., et al.: Rheumatic Fever in Children and Adolescents: VII. Cardiac Changes and Sequelae, *Ann. Intern. Med.*, 60(suppl. 5):87, 1964.
20. Taranta, A., and Stollerman, G. H.: The Relationship of Sydenham's Chorea to Infection with Group A Streptococci, *Am. J. Med.*, 20:170, 1956.
21. Bisno, A. L., and Ofek, I.: Serologic Diagnosis of Streptococcal Infection: Comparison of a Rapid Hemagglutination Technique with Conventional Antibody Tests, *Am. J. Dis. Child.*, 127:676, 1974.
22. United Kingdom and United States Joint Report: The Natural History of Rheumatic Fever and Rheumatic Heart Disease: Ten-Year Report of a Cooperative Clinical Trial of ACTH, Cortisone and Aspirin, *Circulation*, 32:457, 1965.
23. Combined Rheumatic Fever Study Group: A Comparison of the Effect of Prednisone and Acetylsalicylic Acid on the Incidence of Residual Rheumatic Heart Disease, *N. Engl. J. Med.*, 262:895, 1960.
24. Wood, H. F., Feinstein, A. R., Taranta, A., Epstein, J. A., and Simpson, R.: Rheumatic Fever in Children and Adolescents: A Long-Term Epidemiologic Study of Subsequent Prophylaxis, Streptococcal Infections, and Clinical Sequelae: III. Comparative Effectiveness of Three Prophylaxis Regimens in Preventing Streptococcal Infection and Rheumatic Recurrences, *Ann. Intern. Med.*, 60(suppl. 5):31, 1964.
25. Siegel, A. C., Johnson, E. E., and Stollerman, G. H.: Controlled Studies of Streptococcal Pharyngitis in a Pediatric Population: I. Factors Related to the Attack of Rheumatic Fever, *N. Engl. J. Med.*, 265:559, 1961.
26. Maruyama, S., Yoshioka, H., Fujita, K., Takimoto, M., and Satake, Y.: Sensitivity of Group A Streptococci to Antibiotics; Prevalence of Resistance to Erythromycin in Japan, *Am. J. Dis. Child.*, 133:1143, 1979 (November).
27. Stollerman, G. H.: Global Changes in Group A Streptococcal Diseases and Strategies for Their Prevention, in G. H. Stollerman (ed.). "Advances in Internal Medicine," Year Book Medical Publishers, Inc., Chicago, 1982, pp. 373–406.
28. Stollerman, G. H.: Pharyngitis: Management in an Era of Declining Rheumatic Fever, in S. T. Shulman (ed.), Praeger, New York, 1983, p. 47.
29. Stollerman, G. H.: Global Strategies for the Control of Rheumatic Fever, *JAMA* 249:931, 1983. (Editorial.)

Section L

Syphilis and the Cardiovascular System

63

Syphilis and the Cardiovascular System

J. O'Neal Humphries, M.D.   Bernadine Healy Bulkley, M.D.

For one pleasure, a thousand pains.
From an engraving by Jacques Laniet (1659–1663)

Aortitis is the primary cardiovascular manifestation of syphilis and results most commonly in aortic regurgitation, aortic aneurysm, and coronary artery ostial obstruction. Less commonly myocarditis, myocardial gumma formation, and peripheral arterial obstruction may occur. Though the relation of the venereal disease syphilis to aortitis was considered for several centuries, it was not until the beginning of the twentieth century that this relation was established and widely accepted. The number of years between the primary venereal infection and the symptomatic presentation of aortitis no doubt contributed to the lack of recognition of the relation.

Syphilis is sometimes referred to as *lues,* which literally means "pestilential disease." Many present-day authors will use the terms *syphilis* and *lues* or *syphilitic* and *luetic* interchangeably, though in the distant past *lues* often meant "plague."

Infectious Process and Natural History

Soon after the primary infection the *Treponema pallidum* spirochetes invade the body and spread by vascular transmission to all parts of the body. For some unclear reason these organisms are likely to cause an inflammatory process in the small vasa vasorum vessels in the intimal layer of the aorta. The involved arteries become narrowed or obstructed and surrounded by lymphocytes, plasma cells, and occasionally giant cells, as evidenced by the granulomatous or gummatous reaction. These processes lead to patchy but extensive necrosis of the muscular and elastic elements of the media, followed by replacement with fibrous tissue, which may eventually become calcified. This necrosis and scarring of the media cause gross changes of the intima, characterized by deep furrowing between elevated patches or plaques, which are shiny or glistening. These changes of the intima produce the distinctive "tree-bark" appearance of syphilitic aortitis. Although this pattern is distinctive, it is not diagnostic of syphilis since it may also be seen in aortitis of other etiology, such as ankylosing spondylitis.

The process is most intense just above the sinuses of Valsalva, becomes less intense after the origin of the brachiocephalic artery, even less intense beyond the left subclavian, and is very rarely of any consequence below the renal arteries.

The damage to the media may lead to extreme thinning, which allows for bulging or aneurysm formation of the aortic wall. This usually develops in one portion of the wall. The bulge or aneurysm has a saccular appearance, but diffuse or fusiform dilatation may occur. Since the media is densely scarred, dissection is exceedingly unlikely to develop as a consequence of syphilis.

Syphilitic aortitis proximal to the sinuses of Valsalva may involve the ostia of the coronary arteries, but the process does not extend distally along the coronary arteries beyond 1 cm.

Syphilis also causes extensive damage to the fibrous ring of the aortic valve and results in marked dilatation of the ring. This dilatation of the ring and accompanying separation of leaflets causes the aortic valve regurgitation; the valve leaflets themselves are not significantly involved by the syphilitic process.

The change in the size of the ring produces enormous stress in the individual leaflet, and this may result in some thickening or stiffening of the leaflets and eventually rolling or frank collapse of the free margin, which increases the severity of the aortic regurgitation. Obstruction to left ventricular outflow with aortic stenosis is not produced by syphilis.

Infection in the wall of the aorta and aortic valve ring develops during the secondary or bacteremic phase of syphilis. However, the resulting inflammatory process is extremely low-grade, so that significant damage leading to the pathological pictures described above, the tertiary stage, may not develop for 5 to 50 years; the period from the initial infection to the clinical presentation as an aneurysm or aortic regurgitation is termed the *latent period.* Latent periods as short as 1 to 2 years have been reported but are extremely rare, and 5 to 15 years represents the more usual latent period. There is some evidence that the activity of the process in untreated cases does not continue beyond 20 years; i.e., all damage occurs within the first 20 years.[1] On the other hand, the results of the damage may be progressive even after adequate treatment. Thus the size of an aortic aneurysm will continue to increase, and left ventricular failure due to severe aortic valve regurgitation will progress despite the absence of active disease.

Syphilitic involvement of the aorta may occur and not cause any symptoms or difficulty for many years, and in approximately one-third of cases may never cause symptoms or become clinically apparent. Nevertheless, if asymptomatic cardiovascular syphilis is recognized, appropriate antibiotic treatment is indicated.

Clinical Manifestations

Aortic Regurgitation

Aortic regurgitation due to syphilis ranges in severity from trivial, manifest only by a faint decrescendo diastolic murmur along the left sternal border and perhaps an accentuated aortic second sound, to severe with great left ventricular enlargement and congestive heart failure. This complication of syphilis, as well as the other cardiovascular manifestations of syphilis, usually presents in the late or tertiary stage of the disease; the usual patient is a male between 40 and 55 years of age.

Mild Aortic Regurgitation

Trivial aortic regurgitation caused by syphilis may not have specific features to distinguish this process from other etiologies of mild pure aortic regurgitation. An aortic second sound which is increased in intensity and has a ringing or tambour-like quality introducing the decrescendo diastolic murmur would favor a syphilitic origin (Fig. 63-1), although chronic systemic hypertension may have similar auscultatory findings. An ejection click may be present in syphilitic aortic valve or bicuspid aortic valve. Signs of significant aortic stenosis and mild aortic regurgitation would exclude a syphilitic origin of aortic valve disease. Also, clear evidence of mitral valve

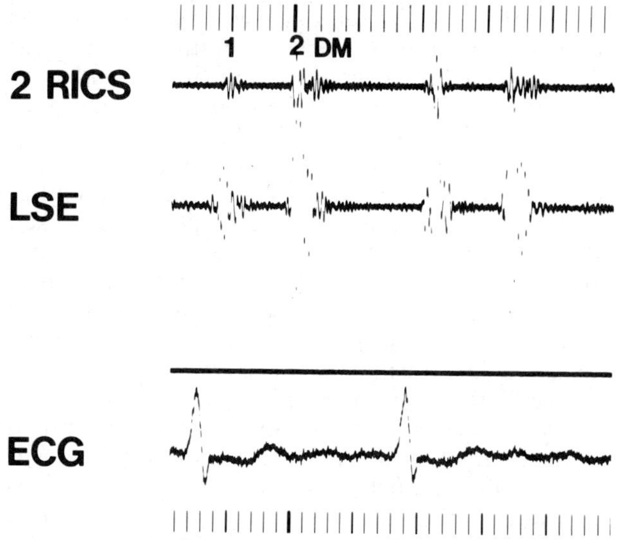

FIGURE 63-1 Phonocardiogram of a patient with cardiovascular syphilis with mild aortic regurgitation. Note the loud second sound; the ring or tambour-like quality is noted by the multiple, regular vibrations of the sound.

disease on physical or laboratory examination would be strong evidence against a syphilitic origin of the valve disease. Care must be taken not to attribute an Austin Flint murmur to evidence of mitral valve disease. This murmur is not encountered in the presence of only trivial or mild aortic regurgitation.

The importance of recognizing syphilis as the cause of trivial aortic regurgitation is related more to instituting proper antibiotic therapy than it is to the management of the hemodynamic consequences of the mild valvular regurgitation. However, mild aortic regurgitation usually progresses to severe aortic regurgitation in a matter of years, even though the infectious aspect of the disease has been treated by adequate antibiotic therapy.

Moderate or Severe Aortic Regurgitation

The peripheral signs of significant aortic regurgitation are seen in their classic form in more severe degrees of syphilitic aortic regurgitation. In fact, most of the peripheral signs of aortic regurgitation were probably initially described in patients with syphilis, including de Musset's head bobbing, Quincke's capillary pulses, Duroziez's sign, Traube's pistol shots, and Corrigan's collapsing pulses. These signs are often seen in the same patient, since they represent the consequences of the same hemodynamic phenomenon, namely, a large stroke volume and significant collapse of the vascular system due to aortic regurgitation and peripheral vasodilatation. The systolic blood pressure is high and the diastolic blood pressure is low, often approaching zero. The skin is warm and moist and the patient complains of excessive perspiration with little or no effort. The left ventricle is enlarged and there may or may not be signs of pulmonary and systemic congestion.

Again, the second sound may have a ringing or tambouric quality but may be diminished or absent. The high-pitched diastolic murmur is loud and long; this murmur may be heard best along the right lower sternal border and is often louder there than along the left lower sternal border. This murmur location of syphilitic aortic regurgitation is shared with other causes of aortic regurgitation associated with marked dilatation of the root of the aorta including Marfan's syndrome, myxomatous degeneration of the valve, osteogenesis imperfecta, and relapsing polychondritis.[2] A loud, harsh systolic murmur is usually present; this murmur may even be associated with a thrill at the right upper sternal border and in the suprasternal notch. Though the systolic murmur is loud, it is not long and does not represent true aortic stenosis or obstruction to left ventricular outflow, but rather reflects the turbulence created by the large stroke volume crossing stiffened, irregular aortic valve cusps into a large, dilated aortic root.

The diastolic murmur may have a musical or even "honking" quality caused by regular vibrations of the margin of a leaflet, especially the noncoronary leaflet (Fig. 63-2). The quality and intensity of the murmur are such that it is widely transmitted and may even be heard without a stethoscope at a distance from the chest. This musical diastolic murmur is especially likely to develop with syphilitic aortic regurgitation, since the free margins of the leaflets are stretched and poorly supported by the dilated aortic valve ring. In this setting the free margin of the leaflet may roll back or evert and thus allow the tense margin to be set into regular vibration during regurgitant flow.[3]

An Austin Flint murmur is often heard in patients with moderate or severe aortic regurgitation of any cause (see Chaps. 11 and 37). The mitral diastolic rumble of Austin Flint may simulate the rumble of mitral stenosis. Mitral valve calcification as detected on the chest x-ray indicates a rheumatic etiology, and echocardiography reliably identifies mitral stenosis and is thus of great assistance in distinguishing an Austin Flint rumble from a mitral stenosis rumble.

The most frequent consequence of severe aortic regurgitation is left ventricular failure and pulmonary congestion, though other symptoms such as angina pectoris or syncope may precede or accompany the symptoms of heart failure. The left ventricle is usually markedly dilated and hypertrophied by the time syphilitic aortic regurgitation has produced left ventricular failure. The clinical course is one of progressive disability despite the introduction of a medical program including appropriate antibiotics, restriction of activities, digitalis, diuretics, and arterial and venous dilators. A large experience with the use of arterial and venous dilators in syphilitic aortic regurgitation is not available. Within a year of the onset of heart failure nearly one-half of the patients will have died and the majority will have died within 5 years.[4] Aortic valve replacement offers definite improvement in clinical status and in the prognosis. However, the beneficial effects of aortic valve surgery for syphilitic aortic regurgitation are not as good as for aortic regurgitation of other etiologies, because the left ventricle is usually so enormously enlarged and dilated and because of syphilitic involvement of other portions of the vascular system.[5] Overall prognosis is also poor because of involvement of other organ systems, especially the central nervous system.

Aortic Aneurysm

Aneurysms of the aorta are a direct result of syphilitic aortitis. Most commonly they develop in the thoracic aorta, especially the ascending portion, and are saccular or fusiform and never dissecting in nature. They produce symptoms by encroaching on surrounding structures or by leakage. The latter can

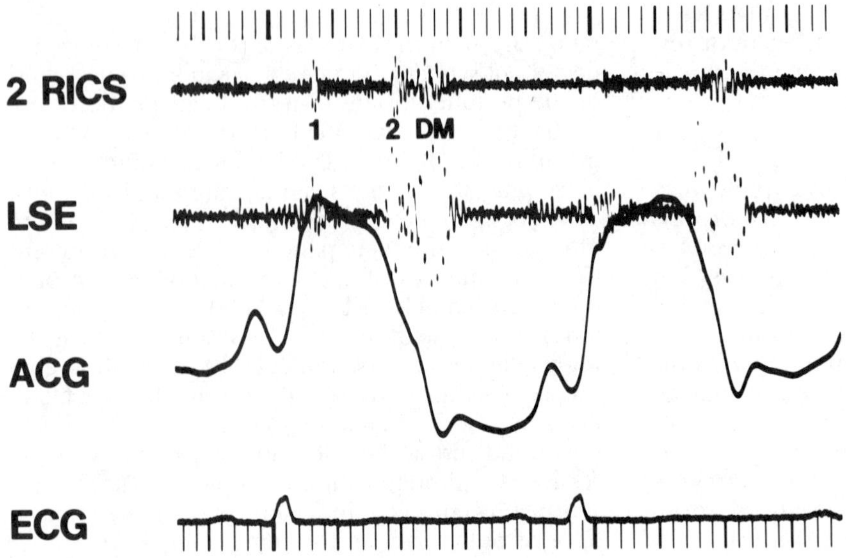

FIGURE 63-2 Phonocardiogram of a patient with moderate syphilitic aortic regurgitation. The diastolic murmur (DM) is very loud and musical with a "honking" quality.

be abrupt (termed *rupture*) and cause rapid collapse and death; the rupture can be the initial manifestation of the illness, but it is usually preceded by a period of time during which other symptoms, especially pain, are present. Rupture may occur into various parts of the thoracic cavity, including the pleura, bronchus, esophagus, or pulmonary artery, or may actually appear externally through the skin. Rarely, the aneurysm may be below the diaphragm, but it will be above the renal arteries. This contrasts with atherosclerotic abdominal aortic aneurysms of the elderly, which develop at the level of the renal arteries or below. With syphilitic abdominal aneurysm, rupture occurs into the retroperitoneal space.

Though rupture may be the initial presentation, far more often prolonged periods of pain and evidence of pressure on surrounding structures precede the rupture. The pain is usually constant and boring but later may become excruciating and pulsatile. The location of the pain depends on the location of the aneurysm, but it may be parasternal; high, mid, or low back; or epigastric.[6] Other symptoms are related to the compression of surrounding structures, such as hoarseness related to pressure on the recurrent laryngeal nerve, an irritating nonproductive cough due to pressure on the bronchi, and dysphagia due to pressure on the esophagus.

Abnormal physical findings develop only very late in the course when the aneurysm has become quite large. A pulsatile mass may be present high to the right of the sternum or in the back along the course of the aorta. Adhesions around the aneurysm may attach it to the trachea and a tracheal tug may be present; this is detected by grasping the thyroid cartilage between the thumb and the index finger and lifting gently to either side. If the trachea and aorta are adherent, a downward tug will be felt with each heartbeat. Increased retrosternal dullness to percussion, especially if it is high, may suggest aneurysm of the ascending aorta or another anterior mediastinal mass.

Syphilitic aortic regurgitation is present in about one-half of the patients with the aneurysm, in which case the signs of aortic regurgitation will also be present.

The x-ray of the chest may be normal even in the presence of a large aneurysm, but the x-ray may demonstrate a high anterior mediastinal mass, which may or may not be pulsatile on fluoroscopy (Fig. 63-3). Linear calcification reflecting severe intimal atherosclerosis overlying the segment of the aorta involved by syphilis is rather typical of this condition; delineation of this calcium on chest x-ray or fluoroscopy may help in determining the location and extent of the aneurysm. With huge aneurysms, erosion of the sternum, ribs, or spine may be seen. Displacement of the esophagus by some aneurysms may be seen on radiography after a barium swallow.

Contrast angiography is the most accurate method to demonstrate the presence of an aneurysm and to precisely determine its location, size, and the involvement of branch arteries (Fig. 63-4). Improvement in radioisotope angiography, sonography, and computerized axial tomography may allow these techniques or other noninvasive methods of visualizing thoracic contents to play an increasing role in the evaluation of aortic aneurysms.

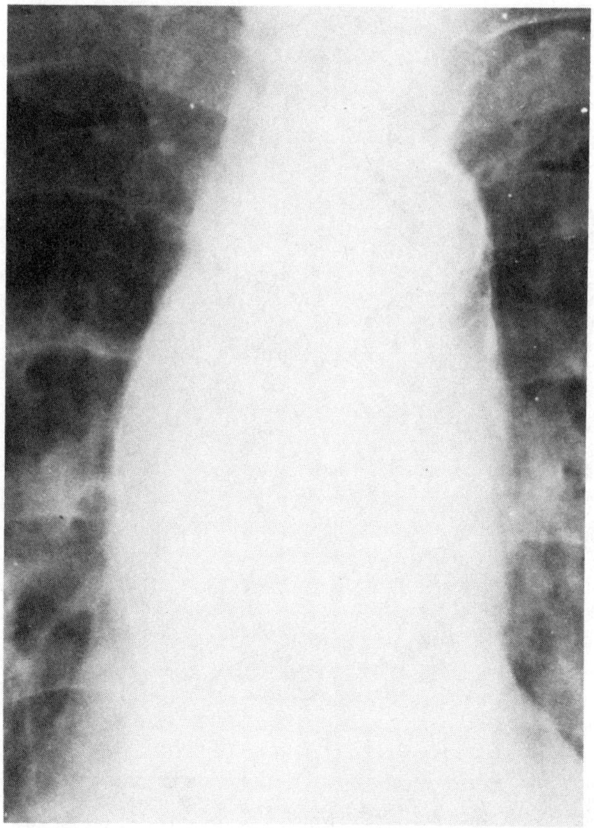

FIGURE 63-3 Chest x-ray of a patient with a syphilitic aneurysm of the ascending aorta noted as a prominence of the high right mediastinal shadow. Note the calcification in the wall of the aorta in the edge of the right mediastinal shadow. (*Courtesy of David B. Propert, M. D., Department of Medicine, University of South Carolina School of Medicine, Columbia, S.C.*)

Giant cell aortitis may produce aortic regurgitation, and the chest x-ray may show linear calcification of the aortic wall. This condition is differentiated from syphilitic aortitis by appropriate serological testing.[7]

Coronary Ostial Disease

As noted, syphilis typically causes a proximal aortitis, and this process may extend so far proximally that the orifices of the coronary arteries become partially or even totally obstructed by the intimal syphilitic changes. This may lead to typical angina pectoris or sudden cardiac death. Angina due to syphilitic ostial disease is usually associated with other evidence of syphilitic cardiovascular disease such as aortic regurgitation or aortic aneurysm, but occasionally this may be the only symptom caused by the involvement of the vascular system. Rarely, coronary ostial disease may cause impaired left ventric-

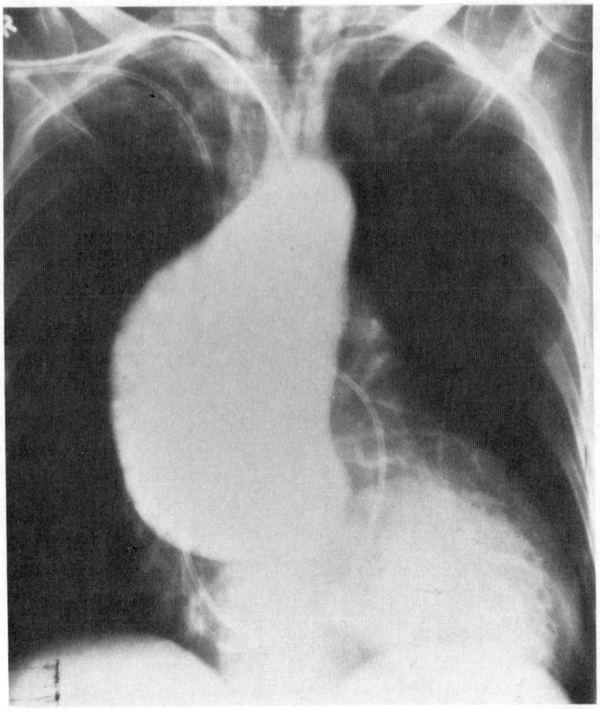

A

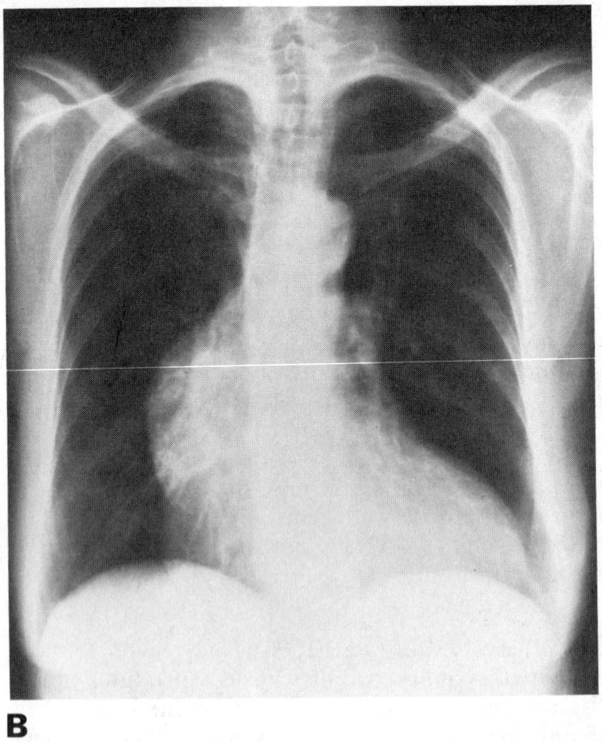

B

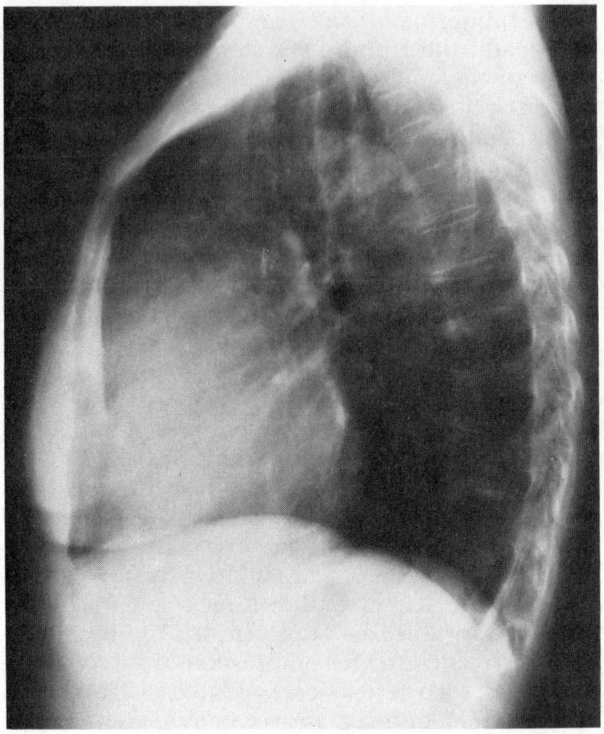

C

FIGURE 63-4 *A.* Aortogram of a patient with a syphilitic aneurysm of the ascending aorta and associated aortic regurgitation. The absence of dilatation of the sinuses of Valsalva in the presence of an aneurysm of the ascending aorta favors the diagnosis of syphilis rather than cystic medical necrosis. *B.* and *C.* Faint calcification in the wall of the aneurysm seen on the PA and lateral chest x-ray of this patient favors a syphilitic etiology. (*Courtesy of Robert I. White, Jr., M.D., Department of Radiology, Johns Hopkins School of Medicine and Hospital, Baltimore, Md.*)

ular dysfunction without angina or aortic regurgitation,[8] but myocardial infarction is very rare.

Angina in the patient with severe syphilitic aortic regurgitation may occur in the absence of any obstructive coronary disease, or may be due to coronary artery obstruction caused by either syphilitic ostial disease or associated atherosclerotic disease. Coronary arteriography is usually necessary to be certain which of these possibilities explains the angina in any particular patient. The presence of calcium in the wall of the ascending aorta and/or the absence of recognized atherosclerotic risk factors favor but do not establish syphilitic ostial disease.[9]

Less Common Presentations

Acute myocarditis is reported during the early, bacteremic phase of syphilis, but is usually mild and runs a self-limited course even without antibiotic therapy of the infectious process. The same process that involves the wall of the aorta may involve other systemic arteries and lead to cerebral or ocular vascular insufficiency.[10] Gumma may infiltrate the myocardium and involve portions of the conducting system of the heart causing conduction defects, including complete heart block, or provoke ectopic beats or tachyarrhythmias.[11]

Diagnosis and Treatment

As the screening tests for syphilis are simple, safe, and inexpensive, and the treatment both safe and effective, the tests should be performed on anyone who might possibly have the disease. This is especially true for the early stages of syphilis at the time of the primary skin or mucous membrane infection, or soon thereafter during the secondary hematogenous dissemination.

The serological tests for syphilis are of two basic types and both depend on the fact that systemic infection by the *T. pallidum* spirochete induces the development of a number of antibodies. Some of these are nonspecific and react with components of normal animal tissue (e.g., beef heart cardiolipin). Others specifically react with pathogenic treponemes.

The nonspecific tests (e.g., VDRL and Wassermann) are inexpensive and easily and quickly performed and thus are used primarily as screening tests. They are very sensitive during the early stages of syphilis but are often only weakly positive or even negative in tertiary syphilis. Cardiovascular syphilis falls into the latter category, and thus a negative screening test does not exclude syphilis as the etiology of a particular cardiovascular lesion. Also, the screening tests may be positive, usually only weakly and transiently, in diseases other than syphilis, e.g., systemic lupus erythematosus and infectious mononucleosis.

The specific tests are highly sensitive (close to 100 percent) and specific (also close to 100 percent) but are relatively expensive. If the patient has or has had tertiary syphilis, the high sensitivity and specificity remain even after proper antibiotic treatment. The most widely used is the fluorescent treponemal antibody absorption test (FTA-ABS). After absorption of the serum with extracts of nonpathogenic treponemes, the presence of antibodies capable of reacting with killed *T. pallidum* are detected by fluorescent technique. Other specific tests include the *T. pallidum* immobilization (TPI) test and Reiter protein complement-fixation (RTCF) test. In a patient suspected of having cardiovascular syphilis, one of the specific tests should be obtained. A positive test will prove that the patient has or has had syphilis. Even this does not prove that any particular cardiovascular lesion is due to syphilis, but it certainly adds valuable information to the total clinical evaluation.

In a patient with a weakly positive nonspecific test for syphilis without an obvious clinical picture of syphilis, one of the specific tests should be obtained. If the specific test is positive the patient should be treated for syphilis, but if it is negative a search for one of the other illnesses which cause false-positive nonspecific tests should be instituted.

Once the diagnosis of cardiovascular syphilis is established the patient should be given 2.4 million units of benzathene penicillin three times at weekly intervals. The cerebrospinal fluid should be tested for evidence of neurovascular syphilis, which, if present, should be treated with larger doses of penicillin for a longer period of time. Whether even large doses of penicillin eradicate all treponemes is debated, but proper treatment may prevent or at least retard further tissue damage by continued active low-grade infection and inflammation. In patients who are allergic to penicillin, tetracycline or erythromycin can be used.

Treatment of the specific cardiovascular lesions of syphilis requires the consideration of surgery. Valve replacement is necessary to correct severe syphilitic aortic regurgitation. (See Chap. 37.) The hemodynamic indications for valve replacement and the surgical technique, risks, and results are not that different than for other causes of aortic regurgitation. If the aortic regurgitation is of long standing and the left ventricle greatly dilated, the benefits of surgery will be limited.[4] Also, the risk of surgery will be considerably increased if there is associated aneurysm formation or coronary ostial obstruction.

Any aneurysm causing symptoms should be resected. (See Chap. 132.) An aneurysm large enough to be seen on chest x-ray probably should be resected. It is likely to continue increasing in size and the threat of rupture is great enough to justify the surgical risk except in unusual circumstances such as complicating illnesses and very advanced age.

When an aortic aneurysm is asymptomatic, but suspected because of a positive serological test for syphilis and/or the finding of a large aorta or calcification in the wall of the ascending aorta, the diagnosis should be confirmed by aortography. If the aneurysm is present and is larger than 7 to 8 cm in width, then serious consideration for surgical replacement of the aneurysm by a graft is appropriate.

Syphilitic obstruction of the coronary ostia can be relieved by endarterectomy in most instances, but occasionally one or more vein bypass grafts may be necessary and should be successful in providing adequate coronary artery flow in the absence of extensive atherosclerosis of the same vessels.

Conclusions

The rarity of syphilis in the United States in the 1980s makes the challenge of recognizing and properly treating a cardiovascular disorder due to this infection greater than ever.[12] A physician must be familiar with the clinical presentations of this process, including the totally asymptomatic presentation, and must have an organized plan of evaluation to establish or exclude the presence of cardiovascular syphilis. Once the diagnosis of cardiovascular syphilis is established, the patient should be treated with antibiotics, and the consequences of the disorder, both present and potential, should be considered before deciding whether to recommend surgical intervention.

References

1. Kampmeier, R. H.: Final Report on the "Tuskegee Syphilis Study," *South. Med. J.*, 67:1349, 1974.
2. Harvey, W. P., Corrado, M., and Perloff, J. K.: Right-Sided

Murmur of Aortic Insufficiency, *Am. J. Med. Sci.*, 245:533, 1963.
3. McKusick, V. A.: "Cardiovascular Sound in Health and Disease," The Williams & Wilkins Company, Baltimore, 1958.
4. Webster, B., Rich, C., Jr., Dense, P., Moore, J. E., Nicol, C. S., and Padget, P.: Studies in Cardiovascular Syphilis: III. The Natural History of Syphilitic Aortic Insufficiency, *Am. Heart J.*, 46:117, 1953.
5. Grabau, W., Emanuel, R., Ross, D., Parker, J., and Hegde, M.: Syphilitic Aortic Regurgitation: An Appraisal of Surgical Treatment, *Br. J. Vener. Dis.*, 52:366, 1976.
6. Leung, J. S. M., Mok, C. K., Leong, J. C. Y., and Chan, W. C.: Syphilitic Aortic Aneurysm with Spinal Erosion, *J. Bone Joint Surg.*, 59:89, 1977.
7. Klein, R. G., Hunder, G. G., Stanson, A. W., and Shepps, S. G.: Large Artery Involvement in Giant Cell (Temporal) Arteritis, *Ann. Intern. Med.*, 83:806, 1975.
8. Holt, S.: Syphilitic Ostial Occlusion, *Br. Heart J.*, 39:469, 1977.
9. Higgins, C. B., and Reinke, R. T.: Nonsyphilitic Etiology of Linear Calcification of the Ascending Aorta, *Diagn. Rad.*, 113:609, 1974.
10. Appen, R. E., Wray, S. H., and Cogan, D. G.: Central Retinal Artery Occlusion, *Am. J. Ophthal.*, 79:374, 1975.
11. Lev, M., and Bharati, S.: Atrioventricular and Intraventricular Conduction Disease, *Arch. Intern. Med.*, 135:405, 1975.
12. Burch, G. E.: Trends in the Incidence of Disease in the United States, *Am. Heart J.*, 88:807, 1974.

Section M

Diseases of the Blood Vessels

64

Diseases of the Aorta

Joseph Lindsay, Jr., M.D.
Michael E. DeBakey, M.D.
Arthur C. Beall, Jr., M.D.

The aorta, structurally and functionally uncomplicated, manifests disease in a limited number of ways. Disease may weaken its wall, and such weakness may result in aneurysm, dissection, or rupture. Its lumen may be occluded, but occlusion of the main trunk is less frequently a manifestation of aortic disease than is occlusion of the origin of one of its major branches.

A considerable variety of disease processes affect the aorta. Most involve other tissues as well, but certain congenital anomalies affect the aorta exclusively.

We propose first to review the various diseases which affect the aorta together with their pathogenetic mechanism and the characteristic pathological features of the aortic involvement. In the second portion of this chapter we will review the major clinical problems that result from aortic disease and will suggest diagnostic and therapeutic approaches to them.

Etiologic and Pathogenetic Considerations in Aortic Disease

Atherosclerosis

Some degree of atherosclerosis of the aorta inevitably accompanies aging. Intimal depositions of lipid, *fatty streaks,* appear before age 10 and may constitute the initial manifestation. Elevated gray-yellow intimal plaques containing soft, yellow, lipid-rich material make their appearance in young adulthood. As the years pass, hemorrhage into these plaques, calcification, ulceration, and superimposed thrombus complete the typical lesion. While atherosclerosis is initially an intimal process, the media underlying segments of severe involvement is weakened and aneurysm formation begins. Progression of intimal disease and further buildup of thrombus may occlude the lumen of the aorta or, more often, the origin of a major branch vessel.[1] The severity of the process varies from individual to individual. Diabetes, hypercholesterolemia, smoking, and hypertension are among the factors that appear to accelerate the process.

Atherosclerosis is characteristically most severe in the abdominal aorta and tends to spare the ascending segment. Atherosclerotic plaqueing is severe in the proximal portion only in a few special situations, for example, in patients with diabetes mellitus. In these individuals atherosclerosis is characteristically of great severity throughout the aorta. Individuals with type II hyperlipemia are another exception to the rule that the ascending aorta is spared. Roberts found severe atherosclerotic changes in the ascending segment in patients with both homozygous and heterozygous forms of the disorder.[2] Luetic aortitis provides another example of severe atherosclerotic change in the ascending aorta. Since syphilis affects the ascending segment with great frequency, atherosclerosis can be of greatest severity in that area since it tends to overlie regions of aortitis.[1,2]

Careful radiographic examination of asymptomatic individuals provides insight into the frequency of this process and supports necropsy evidence for its predilection for the abdominal aorta. In one epidemiologic study, lateral abdominal radiographs demonstrated calcification of this segment in 10 percent of men aged 40 and in 65 percent of men aged 64. Moreover, nearly 4 percent of those 60 to 64 years of age could be said to have an abdominal aortic aneurysm.[3]

As might be expected from the above information, aortic atherosclerosis is manifested clinically most often as either aneurysm or occlusion of the abdominal aorta.

Medial Degeneration

Changes of Aging

With advancing age the aorta becomes dilated, elongated, and less elastic. These changes result from degeneration of the elastic and smooth muscle fibers of the media. Collagen fibers increase in number, and the amount of mucoid ground substance (acid mucopolysaccharide) increases.[1,4] Clinical problems do not result but tortuosity and ectasia of the aorta are commonly observed in chest radiographs of elderly individuals.

Unusually severe and premature degeneration has been reported in certain patients for half a century. It has been thought to be important in the pathogenesis of aortic dissection. Gsell applied the term *medionecrosis* and Erdhiem coined the still popular name *cystic medial necrosis.* Investigators now suggest that this latter term is not appropriate.[1,4] Necrosis of tissue is not observed, and "cystic" areas of mucoid ground substance are probably the result of dropout of degenerated elastic fibers or smooth muscle cells.

Marfan's Syndrome and Idiopathic Cystic Medial Degeneration

Massive degeneration of elastic fibers in the aortic media is the characteristic cardiovascular abnormality in patients with Marfan's syndrome.[1,5–7] Similar lesions, severe enough to result in clinical aortic disease, are encountered in individuals with none of the other features of that disorder. Such patients are said to have *idiopathic cystic medial degeneration* or *anuloaortic ectasia.*[8,9]

McKusick has termed Marfan's syndrome a "heritable disorder of connective tissue."[5] In its most complete presentation, skeletal, ocular, and cardiovascular anomalies are present. Long extremities, particularly long, thin hands and feet (*arachnodactyly*), a high-arched palate, deformities of the thoracic cage, lax ligaments, and sparse muscle mass are outstanding musculoskeletal aberrations. Subluxated or frankly dislocated lenses attributable to lax supporting ligaments are characteristic. In the cardiovascular system, in addition to the aortic changes, myxomatous transformation of the aortic and mitral valves may produce valvular incompetence.[5,6] Neither the biochemical defect nor the specific component of connective tissue affected has been identified.[6,7] Moreover, there is disagreement as to whether or not those individuals who have none of the skeletal or ocular anomalies but whose aortic lesion is identical with that of patients with Marfan's syndrome represent a forme fruste of the syndrome or are examples of another disorder.[7–9]

Medial degeneration is most severe at the aortic root. Consequently, aneurysm of the proximal aorta, including the sinuses of Valsalva, is the most frequent clinical consequence. Rupture of such aneurysms or the hemodynamic effects of aortic regurgitation result in premature death in many of these individuals. Aortic dissection is somewhat less frequent if one excludes the intimal tears and associated limited medial disruption commonly encountered within the aneurysm.[10,11] One should be careful not to conclude that the presence of a typical, extensive aortic dissection confirms the diagnosis of Marfan's syndrome in patients who have less-than-convincing skeletal and ocular manifestations.

Exceptionally, medial degeneration severe enough to result in aneurysm, rupture, or dissection is found in the main pulmonary arteries or in the aorta distal to the ascending segment.[5]

Aortitis

Bacterial Aortitis and Mycotic Aneurysm[12–14]

Bacteria may involve the aortic wall directly from contiguous tissue, but more frequently invading organisms are blood-borne, entering the aortic wall from the lumen or from vasa vasorum. Since the intact endothelium is quite resistant to bacterial invasion, a previously damaged area almost always provides the site for infection. For this reason, secondarily infected aneurysms are more common than aneurysms resulting solely from bacterial infection.

Aneurysms resulting from damage to the aortic wall by bacterial infection are termed *mycotic aneurysms.* Although infective endocarditis is the background against which mycotic aneurysms most often appear, they may result from septicemia unassociated with endocarditis. In this setting, the *Salmonella* group of organisms is particularly noteworthy. Mycotic aneurysms occasionally are found when no bacteremia can be demonstrated.

Direct invasion of the wall of the aorta adjacent to an aortic valve involved with bacterial endocarditis may result in valve ring abscess or in rupture of a sinus of Valsalva.

Spread of tuberculous infection from adjacent lymph nodes may cause caseous necrosis of the aortic wall, producing aneurysm, rupture, or both.

Syphilitic Aortitis

Syphilitic involvement of the cardiovascular system, including the aorta, is discussed in Chap. 63.

Nonspecific Aortitis[15]

Stenosis or obstruction of the aorta and its branches, dilatation and aneurysm formation, or aortic regurgitation may be produced by aortitis. This lesion may be a lone abnormality, or it may appear in association with rheumatic fever or rheumatoid arthritis, and in such diverse conditions as scleroderma and Hodgkin's disease.

A great variety of names have been applied to those instances in which there is no associated disease, but at the moment, any differences seem a matter of geographic distribution and sex incidence, since distinct etiologic, pathogenetic, and histological differences are not readily apparent. Much of what will follow by way of description of the clinical and pathological features of Takayasu's arteritis can be applied to these instances of aortopathy.

Takayasu's Disease

This inflammatory disorder of the aorta, of its major branches, and of the pulmonary artery is named for the Japanese ophthalmologist who first called attention to the funduscopic findings of the disease. Because of the frequency with which the brachiocephalic vessels are occluded, it has been labeled *pulseless disease* and *aortic arch syndrome.*[15]

Etiology The cause is unknown. Clinical and serological data suggest an "autoimmune" process. Recently a genetic predisposition has been suggested because of clustering of the disorder in certain families and because of the frequency of certain human leukocyte antigen (HLA) types in these kindreds.[16]

Pathology On histological examination a panarteritis is found during active stages of the disease; in late stages fibrous scarring, intimal proliferation and thrombosis result in occlusion of the affected vessel.

The origins of the brachiocephalic vessels typically are involved, resulting in the loss of radial and carotid pulses. The abdominal branches of the aorta may be affected as well. Aneurysms or acquired coarctation may result from lesions in the aorta itself. The pulmonary artery is often found to be involved, and the pulmonary hypertension may be found at catheterization.[17]

Clinical Manifestations[17–19] Only in the Orient have large series of Takayasu's disease been collected; however, the disorder is found worldwide. The disease develops during the second or third decade in 70 to 80 percent of cases; but it has been reported in childhood and middle life. Females predominate 8:1 to 9:1 over males.

Constitutional symptoms occur during the early or "prepulseless" period of the disease. Fever, night sweats, malaise, weight loss, arthralgia, anemia, nausea, and vomiting are frequently reported. An elevated erythrocyte sedimentation rate, anemia, and serum protein abnormalities are often present, as are splenomegaly, skin rash, Raynaud's phenomenon, and occasionally positive serological tests for lupus erythematosus or rheumatoid arthritis. It will be recognized that many features of this disorder reflect altered immune mechanisms.

Cardiac manifestations may result from aortic regurgitation or coronary occlusion. Angina pectoris, heart failure, and myocardial infarction are reported. Pericarditis has been occasionally observed clinically, but more commonly, healed pericarditis is noted at autopsy. Aortic regurgitation may result from a deformed aortic valve or may be due to dilatation of the aortic root in response to inflammation of the wall.

Ischemia of the nervous system is commonly encountered. Syncope, formerly attributed to enhanced carotid sinus sensitivity, more probably reflects cerebral ischemia due to the obstruction of the brachiocephalic vessels.

The wreathlike anastomoses about the optic disks to which Takayasu first directed attention are believed to result from ischemia of the retina. Ocular ischemia may also be manifested by transient loss of vision, cataracts, corneal opacity, and iridal atrophy.

Occlusion of the abdominal branches of the aorta has resulted in bowel infarction and in renovascular hypertension; however, intermittent claudication due to aortoiliofemoral obstruction is rather unusual.

Recently attention has been directed toward an understanding of the special problems which may arise during pregnancy in patients with this disorder. Hypertension is a frequent and troublesome problem, but outcome for mother and child are acceptable when meticulous obstetrical care is provided.[20,21]

Natural History and Prognosis Two phases are recognized: an active phase during which arterial inflammation is ongoing and a chronic phase dominated by evidence of arterial occlusion. Unless a life-threatening complication of the latter is present, a protracted course is to be expected.

Management An assessment of the results of therapy is difficult since the disease typically runs a chronic course. Adrenocorticosteroids appear to be effective in suppressing the inflammation of the active phase. Anticoagulation and immunosuppressive therapy have also been utilized. Sporadic reports of surgical therapy of the chronic occlusions have appeared.

Giant Cell Arteritis[22]

Giant cell arteritis (temporal arteritis, polymyalgia rheumatica) may involve the aorta. The histological picture of the disorder and its peak incidence in late life seem to set it apart from other varieties of aortitis. Like them it may produce occlusion of aortic arch vessels, aneurysm of the ascending aorta, aortic regurgitation, and aortic dissection.

Aortitis Due to Ankylosing Spondylitis and to Reiter's Syndrome[22,23]

Etiology The etiology of ankylosing spondylitis is unknown. Reiter's syndrome usually follows nongonorrheal urethritis or, less commonly, infectious dysentery. Recently, it has been learned that more than 90 percent of individuals afflicted with one of these disorders have HLA-B27, an antigen quite infrequent in the general population. This observation may be a clue to a common pathogenetic mechanism.[24]

Pathology The aortitis found in these disorders is remarkably similar to that of syphilis, and as in syphilis severe aortic regurgitation may result. Unlike syphilis, adventitial thickening extends below the aortic valve to involve the membranous ventricular septum and the base of the mitral valve. When histological examination is carried out, focal destruction of elastic tissue of the media is seen, but that layer is not thickened as are the intima and adventitia. An obliterative endarteritis of the vasa vasorum may be observed. The aortic root is dilated. The valve cusps are thickened and retracted, and their edges are rolled.

Such aortitis is more frequent in patients with spondylitis of long duration, in those with peripheral joint complaints in addition to spondylitis, and in patients who have the iritis which accompanies this disorder.

Clinical Manifestations Aortic regurgitation is the most frequent clinical manifestation of these forms of aortitis. It may be severe and life-threatening.

Congenital Anomalies of the Aorta

Patent ductus arteriosus, coarctation of the aortic isthmus, aortopulmonary window, aneurysm of the aortic sinuses, and anomalies of the aortic arch are considered in the section of this text dealing with congenital heart disease (see Chap. 36).

Aortic aneurysm is at times found in patients with congenital aortic stenosis, patent ductus arteriosus, and congenital coarctation. In fact, aortic dissection or spontaneous rupture is fatal in a significant number of patients with coarctation.[25,26] Furthermore, bacterial infection of the aortic wall distal to the coarcted segment may produce mycotic aneurysm and rupture.[26]

Congenital kinking, so-called pseudocoarctation of the aorta, may present as a mediastinal mass or as a systolic murmur. It may produce an appreciable reduction or delay in the femoral pulses. True coarctation may be ruled out only by angiography and the demonstration that no pressure difference exists between the upper and lower aortic segments. The abnormality is a sharp downward angulation of the aorta at the attachment of the ligamentum arteriosum.[27,28]

Coarctation of the descending thoracic aorta or of the abdominal aorta is rare. It can be attributed to healed aortitis in some instances, but more often it is thought to be congenital. Such coarctations, either congenital or acquired, may take the form of localized narrowing or of elongated hypoplastic segments.[29]

The clinical features of the abdominal or thoracoabdominal coarctation are similar to those of the more common variety in that upper-extremity hypertension is present while feeble pulses and hypotension are found in the legs. Attention may be directed to the unusual location of the stenosis by a bruit in the lumbar or umbilical area. Intermittent claudication is more frequent in patients with coarctation of the abdominal aorta than in those patients with the more classic site of narrowing. This is particularly true when the obstruction is distal to the renal arteries. Visceral arteries arising at the site of the constriction may be stenosed, hypoplastic, or thrombosed. Severe hypertension may result from renal ischemia.[29]

Life expectancy in patients with the more distal sites of aortic coarctation is reduced to the same degree as in patients with stenosis of the aortic isthmus. For this reason, surgical correction is considered in most instances.[29]

Clinical Manifestations of Aortic Disease

Aneurysm

Aneurysms develop at sites of medial weakness. Susceptible points may be congenital or acquired. Hypertension, frequently present in patients with aneurysm, exposes weakness that might not otherwise be manifested and may accelerate degeneration of the aortic wall. Once begun, aneurysm formation is promoted by physical laws, particularly that of Laplace. Expansion and rupture frequently result.

Fusiform and *saccular* aneurysms are described. In the former, circumferential dilatation, a result of a diffuse area of weakness, produces a spindle-shaped deformity. In the latter, balloon-like dilatation occurs, beginning at a narrow neck. Many aneurysms are not pure examples of either. By the time the aortic wall has been stretched to aneurysmal size, little or no recognizable aortic tissue is present. The wall is composed entirely of fibrous tissue.

Whether fusiform or saccular, the lumen of the aneurysm characteristically contains laminated clot. Roberts believes that rupture would be more frequent were it not for additional wall strength provided by the thrombus.[1] Often a saccular aneurysm is filled with clot, and the circumference of a fusiform aneurysm is nearly covered with laminated thrombus. Because the aneurysm contains a clot, angiographic opacification of the aortic lumen may not clearly delineate the size or extent of the aneurysm.

Thoracic Aneurysm

Etiology As has been noted, atherosclerosis is by far the most frequent cause of aortic disease and, thus, of aneurysm. Syphilitic aneurysms, frequently encountered in the past, are now uncommon. Cystic medial degeneration and chronic aortic dissection now produce thoracic aneurysms more often than does syphilis.[30–34] Aneurysms of the aorta rarely may result from bacterial or tuberculous aortitis or from noninfectious aortitis such as giant cell arteritis or Takayasu's disease.[34]

Pathology Since atherosclerosis tends to spare the ascending aorta, aneurysms attributable to this process are characteristically located in the arch and descending segments. They tend to be fusiform and to extend over a considerable length. Some extend into the abdomen. An associated abdominal aneurysm is frequent and should be sought.[30–34]

Syphilis and cystic medial degeneration have a predilection for the ascending aorta. Cystic medial degeneration tends to be most severe at the aortic root. The dilatation characteristically involves all three aortic sinuses. The diameter of the aorta tapers to normal before the takeoff of the arch vessels. Angiographically, the appearance has been called "Florence flask aorta." This characteristic pattern is seen in Marfan's syndrome as well as in instances of idiopathic cystic medial degeneration.[1,10,11,32] Syphilitic aneurysms typically begin at the sinotubular junction and are most severe in the ascending aorta. They often include the arch and proximal descending aorta and, more often than atherosclerotic aneurysms, are saccular in configuration. One or more aortic sinuses is occasionally involved.[32]

Clinical Manifestations Many, perhaps most, thoracic aneurysms are asymptomatic and are detected incidentally as a result of a chest radiograph. Aortic regurgitation may be the sole manifestation when only the intrapericardial aorta is affected as with cystic medial degeneration. In such cases marked dilatation of the aortic root may be discovered during echocardiographic, angiographic, or scintigraphic examination directed toward investigation of the aortic incompetence.

Chest pain, described as deep and aching or throbbing, has been the most frequent symptom reported in patients with thoracic aneurysm.[31,33] Pain may be associated with erosion of ribs or vertebrae but more often is not. The appearance of pain clearly related to a thoracic aneurysm may signal expansion and threatened rupture.

Because the aortic arch and proximal descending aorta are fixed by the brachiocephalic arteries and lie across the mediastinum, aneurysms of these segments produce symptoms by compression of adjacent structures more frequently than do those in the ascending or distal descending aorta. Compression of the tracheobronchial tree may be attended by cough or dyspnea. Tracheal deviation or "tug" may be detected on physical examination. Pressure on the esophagus may result in dysphagia, rarely quite severe. Hoarseness may result from the compression of the recurrent laryngeal nerve. Adjacent vascular structures may be compressed, resulting in pulmonary arterial stenosis or superior vena caval syndrome.[30,32]

Rupture can be the initial manifestation of a thoracic aneurysm. Exsanguination into the mediastinum, pleural space, tracheobronchial tree, or the esophagus may be the fatal consequence. Hemoptysis preceding fatal hemorrhage by several weeks is a little known complication of descending thoracic aneurysms that become adherent to the adjacent lung. Aortovenous fistula can be produced from rupture of an aneurysm into one of the great veins or into the pulmonary artery. Since the pericardium envelops the ascending aorta, rupture at this site produces hemopericardium and cardiac tamponade.[32]

Diagnostic Studies The chest radiograph is the most useful screening examination for the detection of thoracic aneurysm. Examination in several projections, fluoroscopy, or tomography may be useful. In instances in which only the proximal ascending aorta is dilated, none of these techniques may detect the aneurysm since that segment of the aorta lies within the cardiac silhouette. Echocardiography is valuable for screening for dilatation of the aortic root. Aortography may be essential to verify the presence of an aneurysm or to assess its extent.

Computer-assisted radiographic techniques (computerized tomography and digital subtraction angiography) are gaining wide acceptance. There seems little doubt that such techniques will soon obviate the need for invasive aortography in many circumstances.

Natural History and Prognosis Most of the data concerning the natural history of thoracic aortic aneurysm come from retrospective analyses of hospital experience,[31,33] but some come from an epidemiologic study in a community.[34] If aortic dissection is excluded, the vast majority of the cases studied have been examples of atherosclerotic aneurysm, and these predominantly involve the descending aortic segment. Joyce's study suggested a 50 percent 5-year and a 70 percent 10-year mortality rate for patients found to have thoracic aneurysm.[31] More recent studies have suggested that the 5-year mortality rate may approach 75 percent.[33,34] One-third to one-half of deaths result from rupture of the aneurysm.[31,33,34] The location of the aneurysm did not influence the mortality rate figures, but advanced age, an aneurysm more than 6 cm in size, the presence of hypertension, and the association of other cardiovascular disease all increased the risk of death. The presence of symptoms reflecting large aneurysms or impending rupture also was associated with reduced rate of survival.

The outlook for patients with ascending aortic aneurysm attributable to cystic medial degeneration may be even more grim. McKusick's group reported that 52 of 56 patients with Marfan's syndrome died as a consequence of aortic disease (i.e., rupture of an aneurysm, dissection, or congestive heart failure attributable to severe aortic regurgitation).[35]

Management Operative repair presently constitutes the only effective therapy for thoracic aneurysms. It is most urgently indicated for patients with large aneurysms, especially in the presence of symptoms suggesting expansion or compression of an adjacent structure. Cardiac failure from aortic regurgitation or aortocameral fistula may also necessitate operative repair. Resection is less urgent in small, asymptomatic lesions.

A consideration of the severity of any associated disease is also important in selection of patients for operation. As compared to an individual without other disease, the patient with coronary or cerebrovascular disease has greater operative risk and a smaller risk of dying of rupture of the aneurysm before succumbing to the associated vascular disease.

Surgical therapy consists in replacing the resected aneurysmal segment with a Dacron graft attached to relatively normal aorta proximally and distally. Specific surgical procedures vary with the site of the aneurysm and the need for maintaining circulation to distal parts of the body during the necessary period of aortic occlusion (Fig. 64-1). Accordingly, thoracic aneurysms are divided into those involving[36] the ascending aorta, those involving the transverse arch of the aorta containing origins of the brachiocephalic vessels, and those involving the descending thoracic aorta distal to the left common carotid artery.

For aneurysms of the ascending aorta, total cardiopulmonary bypass is required.[30,38] The myocardium is protected by coronary arterial perfusion or cold cardioplegia during the period that the coronary ostia are exposed. The aneurysm is opened, and a woven Dacron graft is sutured in place from within the aneurysm with continuous sutures. Finally, the aneurysmal sac is trimmed and sutured around the graft. If the aneurysm has distorted the aortic valve and made it incompetent, the leaflets are excised and a prosthetic valve is sutured in place with interrupted sutures before completion of the proximal aortic anastomosis.

For aneurysms of the transverse arch of the aorta, total cardiopulmonary bypass is also required. Additionally, extracorporeal perfusion of the brachiocephalic vessels or profound hypothermia is necessary to protect the brain. A woven Dacron graft is sutured to relatively normal aorta proximally and distally from within the aneurysm, after which aortic circulation is reestablished. The innominate, left common carotid, and left subclavian vessels are then attached individually to the aortic graft with woven Dacron grafts of approximate size. The walls of the aneurysm are trimmed and sutured together around the grafts.

Aneurysms arising distal to the left common carotid artery do not require extracorporeal circulation.[37,38] Although we previously recommended left atrial to femoral artery bypass during the period of aortic occlusion and others have recommended temporary shunts around the aneurysm, in recent years we have not used these adjuncts because they have been found not to prevent certain complications, including particularly spinal cord ischemia, which occurs in about 3 to 4 percent of the cases, and they have been associated with a number of complications. The aorta is clamped proximally and distally to the aneurysm while the blood pressure is controlled proximally by the intravenous administration of nitroprusside, and the aneurysm is opened. Bleeding from the orifices of the intercostal arteries is controlled within the aneurysm by figure-of-eight sutures, and a woven Dacron graft is sutured to relatively normal aorta proximal and distal to the aneurysm. Finally, the walls of the aneurysm are trimmed and sutured around the graft.

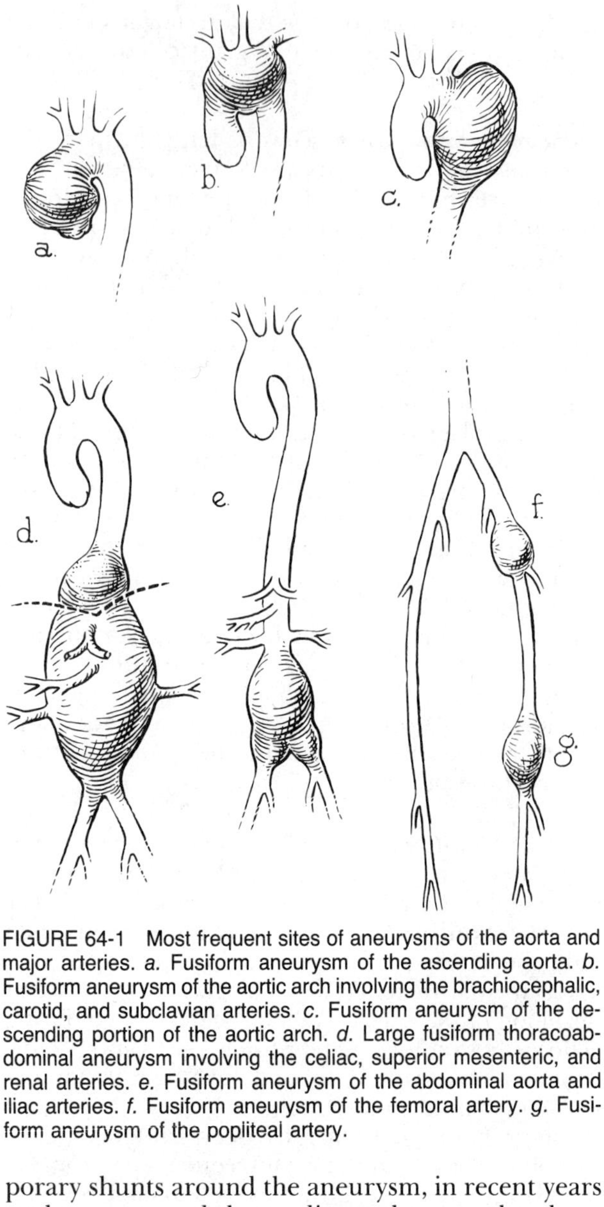

FIGURE 64-1 Most frequent sites of aneurysms of the aorta and major arteries. *a.* Fusiform aneurysm of the ascending aorta. *b.* Fusiform aneurysm of the aortic arch involving the brachiocephalic, carotid, and subclavian arteries. *c.* Fusiform aneurysm of the descending portion of the aortic arch. *d.* Large fusiform thoracoabdominal aneurysm involving the celiac, superior mesenteric, and renal arteries. *e.* Fusiform aneurysm of the abdominal aorta and iliac arteries. *f.* Fusiform aneurysm of the femoral artery. *g.* Fusiform aneurysm of the popliteal artery.

Results of these methods of surgical treatment at Baylor College of Medicine have been most encouraging. Overall surgical mortality rate for aneurysms of the ascending or descending thoracic aorta is around 15 percent, although it is somewhat higher for those affecting the transverse arch and origins of the brachiocephalic vessels. Follow-up studies on these patients for more than 30 years provide evidence of maintenance of good results with long-term survival.[38] Deaths during this period have usually been due to associated diseases or other causes, although aneurysms occasionally develop in later years in other parts of the aorta and require surgical treatment.

Abdominal Aneurysm

Etiology Virtually all abdominal aneurysms are atherosclerotic. Rare examples of traumatic, congenital, and mycotic origin have been reported.[1,39]

Pathology These aneurysms are, as a rule, fusiform but may be saccular. They occur almost exclusively distal to the renal arteries, extend to the aortic bifurcation, and often involve the iliac arteries. Rarely, extension above the renal arteries and involvement of the thoracoabdominal aorta is encountered. These unusual lesions, unlike the more distal aneurysms that involve only the origin of the inferior mesenteric artery, threaten the origins of major visceral arteries.[39,40]

Clinical Manifestations Abdominal aortic aneurysm is uncommon before age 50. The typical patient is a man in his seventh or eighth decade.

Most cases are asymptomatic and are first detected in the course of an examination for an unrelated, or dubiously related, abdominal symptom. Occasionally, the patient reports for care because he has detected an abdominal mass.

When pain can definitely be attributed to the aneurysm, especially if it is of recent onset, it is likely to herald rupture.[41] Constant midabdominal, lumbar, or pelvic pain, which may be severe and may have a boring quality, found in a patient with a palpable expansile abdominal mass should suggest to the physician the likelihood of expanding abdominal aneurysm and impending rupture.

Unless the patient is obese, physical examination will almost always disclose an abdominal mass in the periumbilical area and slightly to the left of the midline. If definite expansile movement can be detected, the diagnosis of abdominal aneurysm is reasonably secure. Bruits may be audible, and femoral pulses are reduced in some patients.[39]

Since most abdominal aneurysms are clinically silent, a life-threatening complication may be the initial manifestation. The most frequent of these is rupture. Rapid exsanguination may result from rupture of the aneurysm into the peritoneal cavity. Fortunately, more often the rupture is into the retroperitoneal space, where hemorrhage may be retarded. Symptoms of abdominal pain and findings of hemorrhagic shock may persist for hours or days, allowing the patient to come under medical attention. Rarely, the rupture is locally confined for a prolonged period. In such instances, the patient may present a diagnostic problem of abdominal pain, fever, and evidence of slight to moderate blood loss. Secondary rupture probably always ensues, although there can be a delay of several weeks.[39,40]

In rare cases abdominal aneurysms rupture into adjacent, retroperitoneal structures. An aortovenous fistula with a continuous murmur, a high-output state, and congestive heart failure follow rupture of the aneurysm into the inferior vena cava.[42] Rupture into the duodenum results in gastrointestinal bleeding,[43] but such aortoduodenal fistulas are more common following graft replacement of the terminal aorta.

An unruptured aneurysm may have other serious complications. Acute thrombosis of aneurysms occurs rarely, mimicking saddle embolism.[44] Furthermore, it has been shown that embolization of thrombus or atherosclerotic debris from abdominal aneurysms to the lower extremities is relatively frequent.[45] Intestinal obstruction from duodenal compression and peripheral edema from inferior vena cava blockade have rarely been reported, since the mobility of these retroperitoneal structures allows their displacement rather than compression by the aneurysm.

Rarely, secondary bacterial infection of an aortic aneurysm will give rise to fever, leukocytosis, and abdominal pain.[13,14] It would appear that infection leads to rupture of the aneurysm.

Diagnostic Studies When characteristic eggshell calcification partially outlines the mass, the diagnosis of abdominal aneurysm can be confirmed by anteroposterior and lateral radiographs of the abdomen. In some instances, aortography provides confirmation or additional information regarding the extent of the aneurysm and the presence or absence of involvement of branch vessels.[46] It may be misleading, however, since the lumen of the aneurysm is characteristically filled with laminated thrombus.

Recently, ultrasound has proved quite valuable. Not only can the diagnosis be confirmed or denied, but ultrasound may also be valuable in following patients with aneurysms in whom expectant therapy is initially elected. Progressive enlargement of the aneurysm can readily be detected by serial examination.[47]

The recent introduction of computerized axial tomography provides an additional accurate means for the diagnosis and follow-up of these lesions. Together with ultrasound, this technique may obviate the need for aortography in many instances.[48]

Natural History Rupture is a major threat to the lives of patients with an abdominal aneurysm. The risk of dying from this complication seems roughly 1 in 3.[39] It is greater when the aneurysm exceeds 6 cm in diameter. As is the case with thoracic aneurysms, individuals with associated coronary or cerebrovascular disease are less apt to die of rupture because of the lethality of their "organ-fixed atherosclerotic" disease.

Management Since operative repair of abdominal aneurysms can now be accomplished with a mortality rate well under 5 percent,[39] operative repair can be recommended for almost all patients, excepting only those with advanced associated disease.

Symptomatic aneurysms require urgent operative treatment since early rupture can be confidently predicted. A ruptured abdominal aneurysm constitutes a surgical emergency. Prompt operative therapy can salvage a majority of these individuals. Death is otherwise virtually inevitable.

Operation for an abdominal aortic aneurysm does not require maintenance of the distal circulation.[49,50] The aorta is clamped proximally between the aneurysm and the renal arteries, and the iliac arteries are clamped distally. The aneurysm is opened, and bleeding from the orifices of the lumbar arteries is controlled from within the aneurysm by figure-of-eight sutures. If the aortic bifurcation is not affected by the aneurysm, a Dacron tube graft may be used to restore circulation. If the bifurcation and the proximal iliac arteries are affected, a Dacron bifurcation graft is required. From within the aneurysm the graft is sutured proximally to relatively normal aorta and distally to the aortic bifurcation or to the iliac arteries individually. Finally, the aneurysmal walls are trimmed and sutured over the graft.

We have used this method of treatment in more than 10,000 patients for more than 30 years. Risk of operation depends primarily on the presence or absence of rupture, associated heart disease or hypertension, and the patient's age. Our experience has shown that the 5- to 10-year survival rate for patients operated on for aneurysms of the abdominal aorta closely parallels that for comparable age groups in the normal population. Surgical treatment is therefore recommended for all patients with aneurysms of the abdominal aorta unless a surgical contraindication exists.

Aortic Dissection

Pathology[51–53]

Longitudinal cleavage of the aortic media by a dissecting hematoma is the cardinal feature of aortic dissection (Fig. 64-2). The separation of medial fibers usually does not completely encircle the lumen, but the entire length of the vessel is often involved. The plane of dissection tends to follow the lateral margin of the ascending aorta and the superior aspect (the greater curvature) of the arch. In the descending aorta it is most often lateral but may be medial or may spiral "barber pole" fashion.

An intimal tear connects the true aortic lumen with the cleavage plane, or false lumen, near the proximal limit of the dissection in almost all instances (Fig. 64-3). These tears are most often single and transverse in orientation, but exceptions are frequent. "Secondary" or "reentry" tears, located more distally along the false channel, are also common.

It is important to recognize the distinct nature of this lesion. The term *dissecting aneurysm* is often applied but leads to confusion with an entirely separate problem—expanding or leaking aneurysm of atherosclerotic or luetic origin. *Aortic dissection* is a much more suitable label, particularly since aneurysm formation is not a feature of the acute phase.

The ascending aorta is involved in about two-thirds of all aortic dissections. The intimal ("entry") tear typically is located a few centimeters above the aortic valve. Medial dissection may be confined to the as-

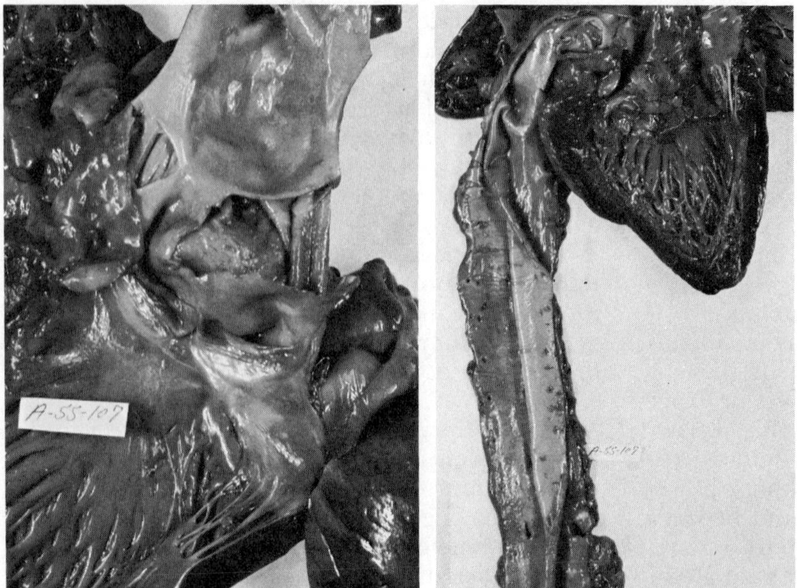

A B

FIGURE 64-2 Dissecting aortic aneurysm. *A.* The large intimal rent may be seen a few centimeters above the aortic cusps. *B.* The false channel created by the dissecting hematoma is shown. Notice the cleanly sheared layers of aortic media.

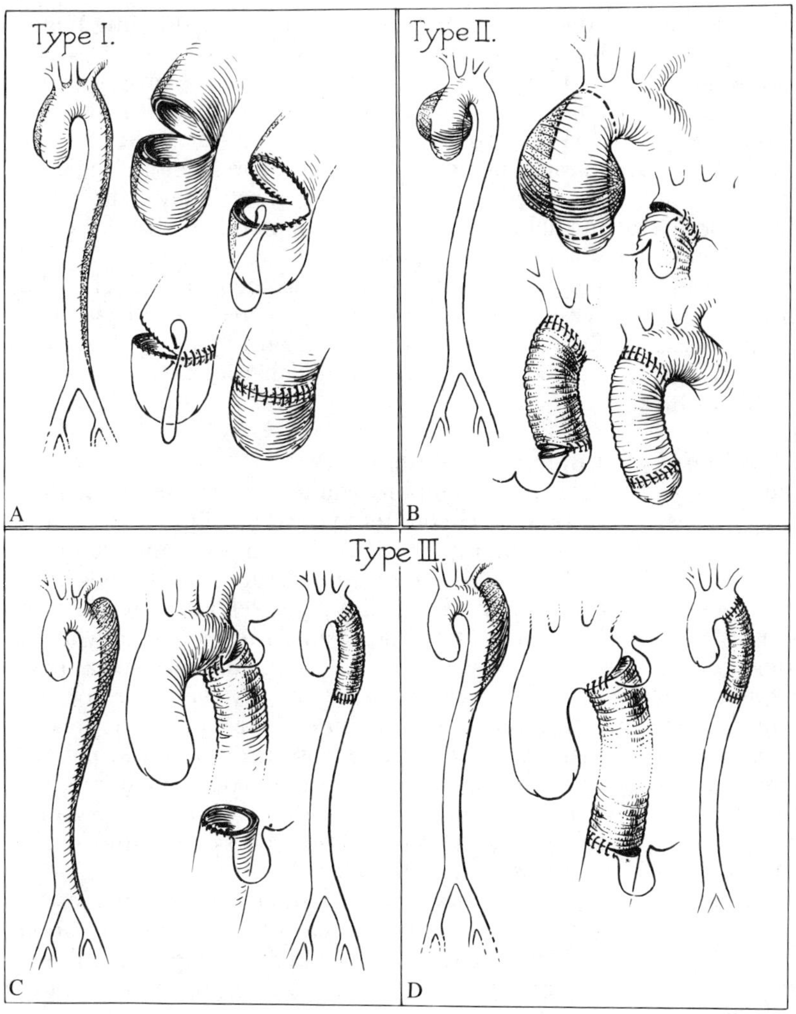

FIGURE 64-3 Surgical classification of dissecting aneurysms of the aorta based on anatomic and pathological patterns of the lesions and their respective methods of surgical treatment.

cending aorta, but far more frequently it extends beyond the arch, often to the aortic bifurcation. Dissections limited to the descending aorta constitute about one-quarter of all cases and are the second most frequent anatomic type. In such cases, the proximal limit of the medial hematoma is near the left subclavian artery, and the cleavage plane extends down the aorta for varying distances. As in ascending dissection, an entry tear is characteristically located near its proximal limit. These two most common types of aortic dissection may be conveniently referred to as proximal and distal dissection, depending on the presence or absence of involvement of the ascending aorta.

A small number of cases do not follow these two patterns. In some, the medial cleavage is short and limited to the aortic arch or to the ascending or descending segments. A few lack an intimal tear. In one rather frequently encountered variation, an entry tear is located just beyond the left subclavian artery as in the distal type, but the dissection extends into the ascending aorta, as in the proximal variety.

The most widely applied nomenclature is that of DeBakey (Fig. 64-3). In his classification, proximal dissection is type I and distal dissection is type III. Type II includes dissection limited to the ascending aorta, a small, heterogeneous group. Apart from length, some are indistinguishable from type I, but some have distinctive characteristics. These include chronic dilatation of the ascending aorta and the aortic sinuses, multiple intimal tears, and limited medial dissection. Cystic medial degeneration of the proximal aorta is present. Some, but not all, of these patients have musculoskeletal or ocular manifestations of Marfan's syndrome.

External rupture, by far the most common cause of death from aortic dissection, tends to occur at the site of the entrance tear. Rupture of a proximal dissection therefore produces hemopericardium and cardiac tamponade. Hemorrhage into the mediastinum or either pleural space may also occur. Rupture of distal dissection characteristically takes place into the left pleural space. Death from external rupture may be abrupt, but in a substantial number of individuals temporary cessation of hemorrhage results from falling aortic pressure and increasing tension in the periaortic tissue.

In approximately half of patients with proximal dissection, medial hematoma undermines the aortic valve, rendering it incompetent. Fortunately, it is unusual for very serious hemodynamic consequences to appear during the acute phase.

Occlusion of a branch vessel of the aorta by aortic dissection occurs in about half of patients with proximal dissection and commonly, but less frequently, with the distal type. The results may be catastrophic, particularly in proximal dissection, since the blood supply to the brain and heart is jeopardized. Occlusion of renal or splanchnic arteries may produce life-threatening complications in either type. Severe hypertension and acute renal failure may attend renal artery occlusion. The iliac arteries are the vessels most frequently compromised. While not life-threatening, their obstruction may be dramatic and painful.

The aortic wall that has been weakened by aortic dissection is often the site of saccular aneurysm formation. Rupture of these aneurysms is a major cause of late death.

Pathogenesis[51–56]

Arterial hypertension seems clearly to be a factor in the genesis of aortic dissection. Hypertension, or evidence of its existence, can be found in 80 percent of patients. The mechanism by which hypertension promotes medial dissection is uncertain, since it has been difficult to duplicate the process in experimental animals, even at arterial pressures far in excess of those seen clinically. Increased arterial pressure may certainly expose existing medial weakness. Furthermore, it may accelerate the usual degenerative processes of aging and thereby weaken the aortic wall.[4]

Histological evidences of medial degeneration in the aorta of patients with this disorder have been noted since the description by Gsell and by Erdheim 50 years ago of what has been called *cystic medial necrosis*. The presence of such abnormalities has led to the belief that weakening of the aortic media is of great importance in the pathogenesis of this process. The frequency with which dissecting hematoma is noted in Marfan's syndrome and in experimental lathyrism supports this notion. The recent work of Schlatmann and Becker[4,55] suggests that cystic medial degeneration is a nonspecific response to injury, for example, long-standing hypertension, and is not a specific entity.

The role of the intimal tear in the production of aortic dissection is debated. Some investigators feel that the proximal tear is quite important in allowing luminal blood to split the aortic media. Others advocate a more traditional view. They believe that medial weakness leads to hemorrhage from the vasa vasorum and, consequently, formation of an intramural hematoma which splits the medial layers. They reason that the intimal tears are secondary, citing the approximately 10 percent of cases without intimal tear as evidence for their thesis.

Clinical Manifestations[51–53,58,59]

The most common fatal aortic disease, medial dissection, is encountered several times each year in large general hospitals. It is most common in the fifth through the seventh decades of life, but it has been reported in children as well as in the very old. It is at least twice as common in men as in women.

Certain congenital lesions of the aorta (e.g., coarctation and bicuspid aortic valve) are associated with increased frequency of dissection. A greater-than-expected incidence is encountered in patients with aortic stenosis. The same is true of patients with Marfan's syndrome and those with exactly similar aortic lesions, but without the skeletal and ocular features of that disorder.[56,57]

Iatrogenic vascular trauma may produce extensive aortic dissection. It may rarely complicate cardiac catheterization, coronary bypass surgery, cardiopulmonary bypass, or interaortic balloon counterpulsation.

It has been said that most instances of dissection of the aorta in young women have occurred during pregnancy, and that pregnancy, either because of its effects on the aortic wall or because of attendant hemodynamic stress, predisposes to medial dissection. Only about 60 instances of the concurrence of pregnancy and dissection have been reported, most in the form of single case reports.[60] Thus, selective reporting may account for this apparent relationship.

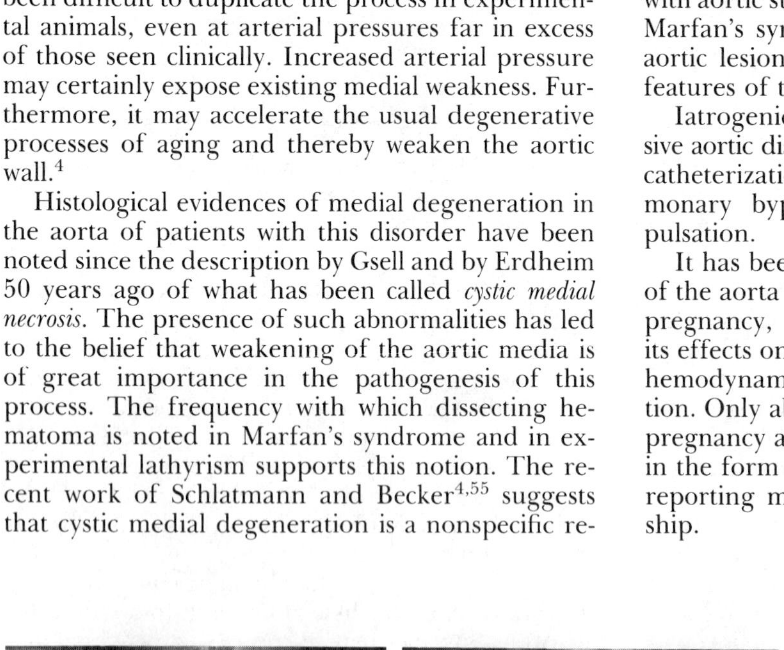

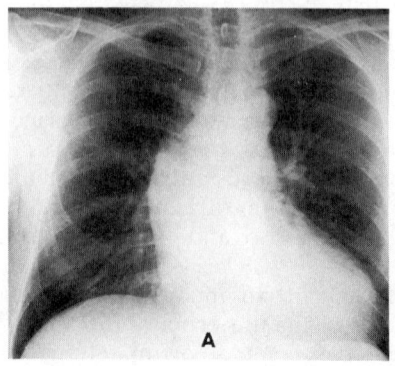

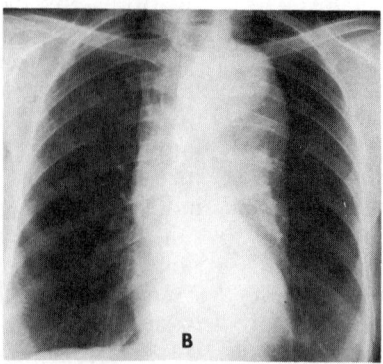

FIGURE 64-4 *A.* Type I aortic dissection. Characteristic appearance on chest roentgenogram. Note the marked dilatation of the ascending aorta. The aorta may appear normal on the roentgenogram early in the course of aortic dissection. *B.* Type III aortic dissection. In contrast to type I, marked distortion of the aortic arch and dilatation of the descending portions are typical, as seen in this radiograph of a patient with dissection beginning distal to the arch vessels.

History Pain in the midline of the trunk is the presenting complaint in the vast majority of instances of aortic dissection. It may seem to the patient that the pain is centered in the anterior chest, interscapular area, abdomen, or lumbar area. Thus, myocardial infarction, pancreatitis, cholecystitis, perforated peptic ulcer, and back strain are among the conditions that may be simulated. There are certain features of the discomfort which should alert the examiner. The pain of aortic dissection is typically quite severe—the worst ever experienced. It may be "cutting," "ripping," or "tearing" in quality. Classically, it is at its most intense from inception, rather than gradually building in intensity. These features, while typical, are often not present. The tendency for the pain of dissection to locate in more than one of the four cited areas of the trunk, either simultaneously or sequentially, is helpful. Suspicion should be aroused particularly by pain occurring both above and below the diaphragm.

Aortic dissection is painless when abrupt appearance of a neurological defect renders the patient unable to perceive or to describe pain. This situation may result from occlusion of an aortic branch to the brain. Furthermore, syncope, a common initial manifestation, may alter consciousness and may distract both the patient and the examiner from any concomitant discomfort. Syncope has proved to be an ominous sign; frequently, it has been associated with rupture into the pericardial space.

When pain is not prominent, occlusion by the dissection of the femoral or the subclavian artery may be the major clinical feature. Arterial embolism may be simulated.

Rarely, the acute episode is clinically silent or nearly so. In such instances, chronic dissection is detected during study of patients with aortic regurgitation, aortic aneurysm, or occlusion of an arterial branch of the aorta.

Physical Examination In the great majority of patients in whom the ascending aorta is involved, careful physical examination will disclose an altered arterial pulse or the murmur of the aortic regurgitation. In distal dissection, aortic regurgitation is rarely seen, and alteration in an arterial pulse is less common. Thus, in the proper setting, the presence of one of these findings greatly increases the suspicion of aortic dissection, but their absence does not deny the diagnosis. Indeed many, perhaps most, patients with distal dissection have neither of these cardinal findings.

Other physical findings may be helpful, but unfortunately they are infrequently found. The sternoclavicular joint on either side may be pulsatile. A gently lifting sensation in the area of this articulation indicates aortic dilatation. Systolic cardiac murmurs and arterial bruits over the thorax or abdomen can be present and useful in drawing attention to a vascular problem, but they are nonspecific. A palpable abdominal mass, consisting of a dilated aorta or a related hematoma, is a valuable but infrequent sign.

Most patients will be found to have hypertension. In some, it will be very severe. Extreme elevations in blood pressure are encountered particularly in patients with distal dissection. Diastolic pressures as high as 160 mmHg are known and may reflect humoral consequences of renal ischemia.

On the other hand, hypotension is detected in perhaps a fifth of patients with proximal dissection. This finding indicates aortic rupture and results from hypovolemia or from cardiac tamponade.

Laboratory Studies At this writing, only radiological examination is of much value in establishing the proper diagnosis. Sonography or computerized tomography may be helpful, but neither is as readily obtained as a chest x-ray nor as valuable as an aortogram.

The aortic shadow is abnormal on routine chest radiography in 80 to 90 percent of cases.[59] Thus, while a normal aortic silhouette on a good-quality film does not completely exclude the diagnosis, it is strong evidence against it. Dilatation of the ascending aorta, indicated by protrusion of its shadow from the right side of the mediastinum, is a characteristic finding in proximal dissection. Dilatation of the aortic knob and descending thoracic aorta is typical of distal disease (Fig. 64-4). These findings are nonspecific, but certain other changes are more diagnostic. Progressive widening of the aortic silhouette on serial films, a lobulated or serrated margin of the aortic shadow, and a "double-lumen" effect created by a less radiopaque false channel are more specific, but less common. The same can be said for detection of intimal calcification more than 6 mm inside the margin of the aorta.[61]

Aortography is presently the most definitive diagnostic tool. In experienced hands, it is safe and almost always conclusive. Two aortic channels can usually be identified because of the variation in intensity and timing of their opacification. It is often possible to identify a linear lucency representing the aortic intima and media separating the two channels (Figs. 64-5 and 64-6). At times, the false channel is not opacified because of thrombosis. In such cases, the true lumen will appear to be compressed and to lie at a distance from one of the margins of the aortic shadow. The resulting appearance of a thickened aortic wall can be produced by thrombosis within an aneurysm, aortitis, and mediastinal hematoma or tumor, but the aortic lumen is not significantly compressed in these disorders, and, therefore, they can usually be differentiated.[61]

Less invasive imaging techniques have been investigated for their utility in this disorder. Of these, greatest experience has been attained with computed tomography (CT) after intravenous administration of contrast agents. Initial reports suggest that this may be as valuable as aortography for the detection of aortic dissection.[62] Digital subtraction

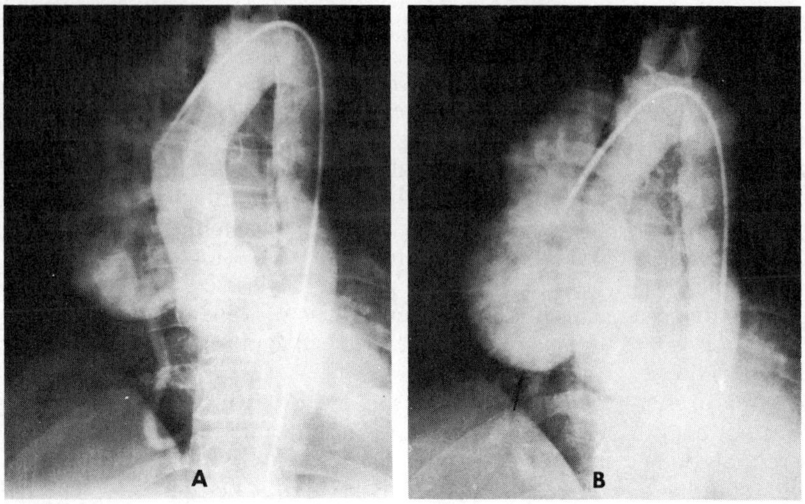

FIGURE 64-5 Serial frames from an aortogram of a patient with type I aortic dissection. Contrast material is seen to fill a tremendously dilated false channel. This accounts for the dilatation of the ascending aorta noted in Fig. 64-4.

angiography and echocardiography also offer promise.

Natural History and Prognosis[51–53,58,59]

A precise estimate of the prognosis of the patient with aortic dissection is not possible. Virtually all reports since the late 1960s have been concerned with aggressive pharmacological therapy or with surgical intervention. We must therefore look to older reports for insights. From these, it may be estimated that 38 percent of patients dies in the initial 24 h and that the mortality rate continues to be high during the first and second weeks. Fifty percent have succumbed by 48 h, 70 percent by 1 week, and 80 percent by 2 weeks.

FIGURE 64-6 Aortic dissection, type III. A typical aortogram of a patient with aortic dissection beginning distal to the arch vessels. The narrowed true lumen is filled with contrast material and does not occupy the entire aortic shadow. Contrast material can be seen entering the false channel just beyond the left subclavian artery.

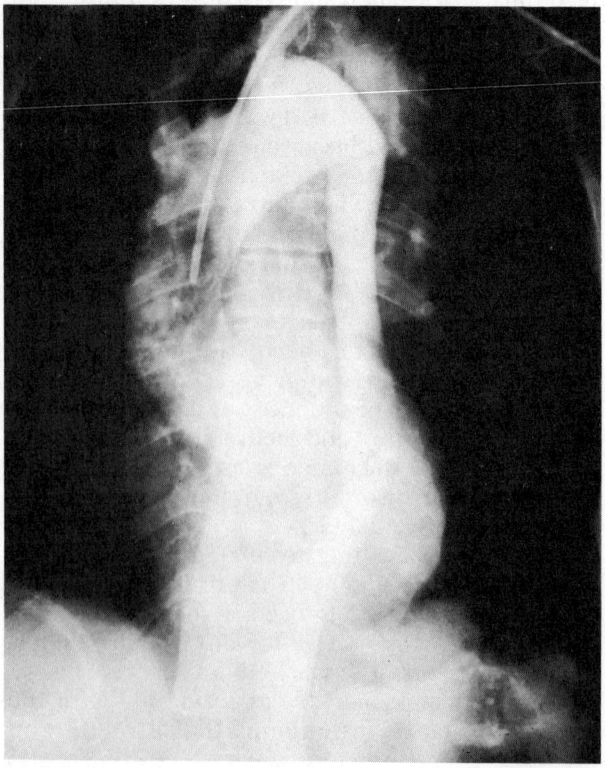

Certain subgroups are identifiable. Hypotension (blood pressure, less than 100 mmHg) usually indicates aortic rupture and a very serious immediate prognosis. Almost all such patients have proximal dissection. They constitute about one-quarter of all patients with ascending aortic dissection. On the other hand, the survival of patients whose dissection is located distal to the arch vessels appears more favorable, at least during the initial 2 weeks, considered to constitute the acute phase. In the classic study of Hirst et al.,[51] only 50 of 239 (21 percent) patients with an intimal tear located in the arch or ascending aorta lived for more than 2 weeks, whereas 47 of 104 (45 percent) of patients with an intimal tear located at the aortic isthmus or beyond survived for that time. Thus, the mortality rate in patients who have acute dissection involving the proximal aorta and have blood pressure of 100 mmHg or less approaches 100 percent in the absence of definitive therapy. Those with distal dissection experience about a 50 percent mortality rate in the first 2 weeks. The mortality rate of normotensive or hypertensive patients with ascending aortic dissection is probably intermediate.

Patients who survive the first 2 weeks continue to experience a high mortality rate in the first year. About half of the survivors die within 3 months and an additional 10 percent within a year of the onset of their illness. The lucky few who pass the first anniversary apparently may expect reasonable longevity. Late deaths may be due to cerebrovascular complications of hypertension, heart failure from severe aortic regurgitation, rupture of a saccular aneurysm complicating aortic dissection, or as a direct or indirect result of neurological injury sustained during the dissection.

Management[52,53]

The patient with acute aortic dissection is managed most effectively in a critical care unit in which close surveillance of cardiac rhythm, hemodynamic parameters, and neurological signs can be maintained.

Control of pain may be difficult, even with large doses of narcotics. The pain will often subside, however, following appropriate blood pressure reduction.

Drug therapy that appears to arrest, at least temporarily, the progression of the medial dissection and to avoid thereby fatal complications was first described by Wheat, Palmer, and their associates. They reasoned that reduction of hydraulic stress on the aortic wall, by both lowering aortic pressure and diminishing the vigor of contraction of the left ventricle (and thereby the rate of rise of aortic pressure), would be beneficial. They successfully employed a regimen consisting of intravenous trimethaphan camsylate for acute pressure reduction, and reserpine and guanethidine for subacute and chronic management. Other workers have employed methyldopa, propranolol, and sodium nitroprusside. Hydralazine and diazoxide are probably contraindicated since they produce reflex inotropic stimulation of the left ventricle. Sodium nitroprusside may also have this fault; however, it has been employed successfully and offers definite advantages over trimethaphan insofar as ease of utilization is concerned. Propranolol should be used with nitroprusside, in addition to a diuretic such as furosemide.

Not all patients with acute aortic dissection have an increased blood pressure. As has been mentioned, hypotension reflecting rupture of the aorta is present in about 20 percent of cases. Furthermore, some patients are found to have blood pressure only slightly greater than the 100 to 120 mmHg that is the target for drug treatment. The authors believe that pharmacological therapy is of dubious value in such patients, although propranolol may be tried as a means of reducing the rate of rise of aortic pressure.

The role of drug therapy vis-à-vis operative treatment has been a matter of considerable debate during the past 15 years. Presently, fairly general agreement exists regarding the choice for most patients.[63] Certain individuals are inoperable because of advanced age, severe associated disease, or severe neurological injury consequent to the dissection. Supportive care is given for such patients, and pharmacological therapy is added for those who are hypertensive. Hypotensive patients, obviously not candidates for drug therapy, usually have aortic leak and require immediate surgery. For the remainder, a choice exists between "medical" and "surgical" treatment.

Experience in the past decade has suggested that patients with distal dissection can be managed successfully through the acute phase by means of drug therapy. Unlike the situation in patients with proximal dissection, complications which dictate immediate operation occur in a minority.

On the other hand, severe aortic regurgitation, occlusion of a major branch artery, and threatened rupture are common in patients with proximal dissection. Surgery may be mandatory. Furthermore, experience has shown that even in uncomplicated patients with dissection involving the ascending aorta, rate of survival is improved by early operative intervention.

Because it appears that rate of long-term survival is better after opertive therapy than after drug therapy alone, it would seem wise to recommend surgery for selected "good-risk" patients who have survived the acute phase. Risk of rupture of a saccular aneurysm at the site of the dissection and of progressive aortic regurgitation (the major late fatal complications) is eliminated.

Surgical techniques for aortic dissection are based on the origin of the dissecting process and its extent.[64–66] Surgical treatment for type I aneurysms consists in transection of the ascending aorta with use of cardiopulmonary bypass, obliteration of the false lumen by approximation of the inner and outer walls of the dissecting process with a continuous suture proximally and distally, and end-to-end anastomosis of the transected aorta. In patients in whom this method of direct repair is not applicable, it may be necessary to resect the proximal segment and restore vascular continuity by means of a Dacron patch or tube graft. Many patients have aortic valvular incompetence, secondary to loss of commissural support of the valve leaflets. This condition is usually corrected by suture approximation of the inner and outer layers of the dissecting process, with resultant resuspension of the valve, although some patients may require prosthetic valvular replacement.

Surgical treatment for type II aneurysms consists essentially in resection and graft replacement of the entire ascending aorta with use of cardiopulmonary bypass. Aortic valvular incompetence is more common in this type than in type I and is less often amenable to reparative techniques because of the usually more chronic nature of the dissecting process. Under such circumstances prosthetic replacement of the aortic valve usually is performed concomitantly with graft replacement of the ascending aorta.

Surgical treatment for type III aneurysms consists in resection of the descending thoracic aorta above the level of the origin of the dissecting process (usually at, or just below, the origin of the left subclavian artery), obliteration of the distal false passage by suture closure of the inner and outer layers, and replacement of the excised segment with an aortic graft.

Analysis of experience with more than 600 patients treated by these surgical methods at Baylor College of Medicine indicates gratifying results, with an operative mortality rate of about 20 percent. Follow-up observations extending over more than 30 years show maintenance of good functional activity.[66]

Acquired Occlusive Disease of the Aorta and Its Major Branches

Chronic Occlusive Disease of the Arch Vessels[67]

Etiology Atherosclerosis accounts for more than 90 percent of instances of occlusion of the innominate, carotid, or subclavian arteries. Takayasu's arteritis, luetic aortitis, neoplastic obstruction, and trauma account for almost all the remainder.

Pathology Atherosclerotic lesions tend to be located at arterial bifurcations and are therefore characteristically found at the origin of the arch vessels, at the bifurcation of the common carotid arteries. The proximal left subclavian artery is the most common site of an obstructing lesion.

Clinical Manifestations Occlusion at the origin of one of the arch vessels often does not produce symptoms because of the many possibilities for collateral connections. Upper-extremity ischemia is particularly unusual. The occurrence of symptoms of cerebral ischemia suggests that more than one lesion is present, that there are lesions in more distal arteries, that collateral circulation is compromised, or that a *steal syndrome* is present. Details of the clinical manifestations of cerebrovascular disease are discussed in Chap. 66.

The steal syndromes are of particular interest. In its classic presentation, *subclavian steal* is triggered by vigorous motion of the arm on the side of severe proximal subclavian arterial occlusion. Symptoms of cerebral ischemia result. Because of the subclavian occlusion, blood flow to the arm cannot be increased sufficiently to maintain arterial pressure in the face of exercise-induced vasodilatation, and blood is "stolen" from the cerebral circulation. That is, blood delivered to the brain through the carotid arteries is diverted via the circle of Willis and proceeds in a direction opposite from that of normal flow through the ipsilateral vertebral artery to the exercising arm. In innominate artery steal, a much more unusual problem, retrograde flow through the ipsilateral carotid artery may be an additional hazard.

Meticulous assessment of the carotid, temporal, and upper-extremity pulses, measurement of the blood pressure in both arms, and careful auscultation for bruits in the neck and supraclavicular areas usually will detect brachiocephalic occlusive disease. These observations should be part of the physical examination not only of patients with neurological or upper-extremity symptoms but also of asymptomatic patients as well, since even asymptomatic patients with carotid bruits have an increased risk of subsequent stroke or transient ischemic attack.

Laboratory Studies Noninvasive techniques have been developed to aid in the assessment of the severity of arterial obstruction in this area. These techniques are particularly pertinent to the evaluation of a patient with a carotid bruit. The pressure within the arterial system distal to the carotid obstruction may be assessed by ophthalmodynamometry or, more recently, by ocular pneumoplethysmography, techniques by which the pressure in the ophthalmic artery is estimated. Ultrasound techniques employing the Doppler principle may provide useful information regarding blood flow in the obstructed artery and may demonstrate reversal of flow in steal syndromes. Definitive identification of the severity and location of the occlusion depends upon arteriography. This may be accomplished via the transfemoral catheter approach, but intravenous arteriography employing digital subtraction imaging is now obviating the need for this examination in many instances.

Management Occlusive diseases of the vessels arising from the aortic arch lend themselves to surgical treatment when patent segments are present distally in the neck. These diseases are best considered as proximal and distal occlusions, although both may occur in the same patient. Distal occlusions usually affect the carotid bifurcations or origins of the vertebral arteries and are discussed in Chap. 66. Proximal occlusions usually occur in the vessels at or near their origins from the aortic arch and are best corrected by use of the bypass principle.

The proximal end of a graft is attached to the side of the ascending aorta, and the distal end (or ends) of the graft is attached to patent arterial segments in the neck or supraclavicular region distal to the occlusion. The ascending aorta is exposed through a second or third right anterior intercostal incision. Using a partial occlusion clamp and end-to-side anastomosis, the surgeon attaches the proximal end of the graft to the aorta. The patent distal arterial segments are exposed through separate incisions in the neck and supraclavicular regions. The distal end of the graft is drawn retrosternally through a tunnel made by blunt dissection and is attached to the side of the patent distal segment. In the presence of multiple occlusions, the appropriate limbs are attached to the sides of the other patent arterial segments. Knitted Dacron velour tubes 6 to 8 mm in diameter are used for this purpose.

Results of this form of treatment have been most gratifying. In virtually all patients with only proximal occlusion of vessels arising from the aortic arch, normal circulation has been restored. In patients with combined proximal and distal occlusions, the success rate varies with the ability to correct the distal occlusion.

Abdominal Angina

The etiology, pathology, clinical manifestations, and diagnosis of occlusive disease of the mesenteric vessels are discussed in Chap. 67. Patients with abdominal angina may be treated by endarterectomy, excision and graft replacement, or bypass graft, the last procedure being preferable for most patients.[68] The abdominal aorta is exposed between the renal and common iliac arteries. The proximal end of the graft is attached to the side of the abdominal aorta in this region, and the other end of the graft is carried behind the transverse mesocolon and stomach and sutured to the side of the normal hepatic or splenic artery. Since the occlusive process usually does not affect the trifurcation of the celiac artery, attachment of the graft to the hepatic or splenic arteries provides complete revascularization of the celiac distribution. One end of a second tube is sutured to the side of the graft, and the other end is carried through a tunnel in the small-intestinal mesentery under the duodenum and is attached to the side of the superior mesenteric artery distal to the site of occlusion. Knitted Dacron velour tubes 8 mm in diameter are used in most patients.

Renovascular Hypertension

In Chaps. 49 and 50 renal arterial occlusive disease is discussed as a cause of hypertension. Surgical treatment for renovascular hypertension is directed toward correction of renal ischemia.[69] Patients with well-localized disease may be treated by endarterectomy and patch graft angioplasty. For more extensive segmental occlusion, the end-to-side bypass principle is preferred. The proximal end of an 8-mm Dacron velour graft is attached to the abdominal aorta below the origin of the renal arteries, and the distal end of the graft is attached to the side of the renal artery distal to the obstruction. Bifurcation grafts are, of course, required in the treatment of bilateral disease when this method is used. The bypass graft method has been particularly effective in restoring normal circulation to both the kidneys and the lower limbs in patients with combined occlusive disease of the aorta, iliac arteries, and renal arteries.[70] The proximal end of the renal arterial graft is attached to the side of the aortic segment of the aortoiliac bypass graft in these patients. In a small number of patients, reconstructive operation is impossible because of the site and extent of the disease. In these, nephrectomy or partial nephrectomy may be required.

The use of renal artery angioplasty is discussed in Chap. 117.

Chronic Aortoiliac Obstruction[71]

Etiology-Pathology In 1923, Leriche called attention to the symptoms produced by slowly progressive occlusion of the terminal aorta and iliac vessels. Atherosclerotic occlusion of the area of the aortic bifurcation with superimposed thrombosis of the stenotic area is usually found when obstruction is complete. Unlike saddle embolus or sudden thrombosis, the manifestations of ischemia are typically present for months or years before the sufferer seeks medical attention.

Most individuals with atherosclerotic occlusion of the terminal aorta also have atherosclerotic disease elsewhere. Associated occlusive disease in the femoral or popliteal arteries and in the coronary or cerebral circulation is often found.

Clinical Manifestations Men are affected with far greater frequency than women, the highest prevalence being in the fifth, sixth, and seventh decades. Some investigators have felt that, as a group, patients with aortoiliac occlusion are younger than those with arteriosclerosis obliterans of the femoropopliteal arteries.

Pain in the low back, buttocks, or thighs produced by exercise and relieved by brief periods of rest is virtually pathognomonic of aortoiliac occlusion. Claudication may occur in the calf or foot in association with the more proximal distress and may be the sole complaint. Patients commonly report inability to maintain a penile erection if inquiry is made in this regard.

Absence of or marked reduction in the femoral pulses is characteristic. More distal lower-extremity pulses are reduced or absent, and bruits are commonly audible over the femoral arteries and in the midline of the abdomen near the umbilicus. Low skin temperature, diminished hair growth, atrophy of the skin and subcutaneous tissue, and diminished muscle bulk in the lower extremities are common but not universal findings. Frank gangrene is not frequently encountered, and amputation for ischemia is seldom required.

Differentiation of this disorder from congenital coarctation of the aorta and from aortitis is usually possible on clinical grounds. However, aortography will be needed to define the pathological anatomy precisely.

Natural History and Prognosis A protracted course is usual. Typically, symptoms are slowly progressive, but about half of these individuals experience periods of accelerated progression of their symptoms. Such periods have been attributed to extension of the aortoiliac thrombosis or to occlusion of collateral vessels.

Chances of survival for persons with Leriche syndrome appear to be less favorable than for those in a control population matched for age and sex, but death rarely results from the aortoiliac disease. Death may occasionally be due to occlusion of the renal arteries by proximal extension of the thrombotic process. Coronary heart disease and cerebrovascular disease are largely responsible for the accelerated death rate in these patients.

Treatment Chronic aortoiliac occlusion may be partial or complete and may occur alone or in association with femoropopliteal occlusive disease as discussed in Chap. 65. For aortoiliac occlusion, the end-to-side bypass with a flexible, knitted, Dacron bifurcation graft is the preferable method of treatment.[72] One end of the graft is attached to the side of the uninvolved abdominal aorta above the obstruction, and the other ends are drawn through tunnels made behind the peritoneum and attached to the side of distal patent segments, either in the external iliac arteries or in the common femoral arteries opposite the origins of the deep femoral arteries in the groins.

In the absence of femoropopliteal occlusive disease, this method has been successful in restoring normal distal circulation in about 98 percent of patients. Even in patients with combined aortoiliac and femoropopliteal disease, bypass of the aortoiliac occlusion alone with revascularization of the deep femoral arterial system may be adequate to relieve symptoms. When this is not the case, extension of the bypass to the popliteal region can be considered. Follow-up observations in these patients for more than 30 years have provided evidence of maintenance of good long-term results with a relatively low recurrence rate of about 5 percent if only the aortoiliac region is involved.[73]

Recently the technique of percutaneous transluminal angioplasty devised by Grüntzig[74,75] has been applied in several centers in the treatment of iliac and femoropopliteal obstructive atherosclerotic disease. The early success rate appears to be satisfactory, but the long-term patency rate remains to be determined. This technique is applicable in highly selected cases in which the stenotic occlusive lesion is well-localized and involves a relatively short segment.

Acute Aortoiliac Occlusion[76–78]

Etiology The terminal aorta and its branches, the iliac arteries, may be acutely occluded by a large embolus (*saddle embolus*), in the course of aortic dissection, as a result of trauma, or by spontaneous thrombosis. None of these events is common; however, Deterling estimates that the aortic bifurcation is the site of 25 percent of the emboli which threaten the viability of the lower extremities.[79]

The underlying cause is usually recognizable from the clinical picture. This is particularly true in the case of trauma and of aortic dissection. The great majority of emboli large enough to occlude the terminal aorta are thrown off from the heart. Thus, embolus must be considered in patients with mitral stenosis, atrial fibrillation, or myocardial infarction. Rarely, a saddle embolus may originate in a severely atherosclerotic aorta or in a vegetation resulting from infective endocarditis. Acute thrombosis superimposed on aortic atherosclerosis may occur when there is considerable reduction in blood flow through these vessels, as may be the case in shock or severe congestive failure.[80]

Clinical Manifestations The victim almost always complains of moderate or severe pain in the legs and, less often, in the abdomen, lumbosacral area, and perineum. Numbness is commonly reported in the ischemic areas. The pulses typically are absent in the legs, although at times faint femoral pulsations may be detected. The legs are cold and pale. Sensory function and motor power are reduced, and total paralysis of both legs is not unusual. Massive muscle ischemia may produce myoglobinemia and severe, acute renal failure.

The mortality rate is high not only because of the severity of the vascular insult, but also because serious underlying heart disease is usually present.

Management In contrast to chronic aortoiliac occlusion, acute obstruction to flow does not allow for the formation of collateral circulation. Immediate operative intervention is necessary for patient survival. The procedure employed will depend upon the etiology of the occlusion.

Treatment for aortic dissection has been discussed previously. Acute aortoiliac occlusion due to trauma with an intimal tear producing dissection may be corrected by the bypass graft technique described for chronic aortoiliac occlusion. In patients with acute aortoiliac occlusion due to a saddle embolus, consideration also must be given to treatment of the underlying disease, such as concomitant open mitral commissurotomy at the time of embolectomy, in order to prevent recurrent embolization to such vital organs as the brain.

Although aortoiliac embolectomy may be performed directly through an incision in the distal aorta or proximal iliac arteries, this approach requires laparotomy in a severely ill patient, and it does not provide the means for removing the more distally lodged embolic material which frequently is present in these patients. The preferable approach is to expose both common femoral arteries in the groins and, through transverse arteriotomies, to remove both proximally and distally lodged embolic material by the use of balloon-tipped Fogarty catheters. Care must be taken to prevent further embolization in the opposite leg while these catheters are passed proximally, but even large amounts of embolic material contained in the distal aorta itself can be safely removed in this manner, even with use of a local anesthetic when the general condition of the patient contraindicates general anesthesia.

Results of such procedures usually are good as far as restoring circulation. Subsequent mortality rates, however, remain high because of the underlying disease that caused the saddle embolus in many of these patients, particularly those with myocardial infarction and a mural thrombus. Nevertheless, by the use of a local anesthetic and Fogarty catheters operation is possible in virtually all patients.

References

1. Roberts, W. C.: The Aorta: Its Acquired Diseases and Their Consequences as Viewed from a Morphologic Perspective, in J. Lindsay, Jr., and J. W. Hurst (eds.), "The Aorta," Grune & Stratton, New York, 1979, p. 51.
2. Roberts, W. C., Ferrans, V. J., Levy, R. I., and Fredrickson, D. S.: Cardiovascular Pathology in Hyperlipoproteinemia, *Am. J. Cardiol.*, 31:557,1973.
3. Schilling, F. J., Christakis, G., Hempel, H. H., and Orbach, A.: The Natural History of Abdominal Aortic and Iliac Ath-

erosclerosis as Detected by Lateral Abdominal Roentgenograms in 2663 Males, *J. Chron. Dis.*, 27:37, 1974.
4. Schlatmann, T. J. M., and Becker, A. E.: Histologic Changes in the Normal Aging Aorta, *Am. J. Cardiol.*, 39:13, 1977.
5. McKusick, V. A.: "Heritable Disorders of Connective Tissue," 4th ed., C. V. Mosby, St. Louis, 1972, p. 61.
6. Pyeritz, R. E., and McKusick, V.A.: The Marfan Syndrome: Diagnosis and Management, *N. Engl. J. Med.*, 300:772, 1979.
7. Pyeritz, R. E., and McKusick, V. A.: Basic Defects in the Marfan Syndrome, *N. Engl. J. Med.*, 305:1011, 1981.
8. Emanuel, R., Ng, R. A. L., Marcomichelakis, J., Moores, E. C., Jefferson, K. E., MacFaul, P. A., and Withers, R.: Formes Frustes of Marfan's Syndrome Presenting with Severe Aortic Regurgitation, *Brit. Heart J.*, 39:190, 1977.
9. Lemon, D. K., and White, C. K.: Anuloaortic Ectasia: Angiographic, Hemodynamic and Clinical Comparison with Aortic Valve Insufficiency, *Am. J. Cardiol.*, 41:482, 1978.
10. Roberts, W. C., and Honig, H. S.: The Spectrum of Cardiovascular Disease in the Marfan Syndrome, *Am. Heart J.*, 104:115, 1982.
11. Crawford, E. S.: Marfan's Syndrome, *Ann. Surg.*, 198:487, 1983.
12. Bennett, D. E.: Primary Mycotic Aneurysms of the Aorta, *Arch. Surg.*, 94:758, 1967.
13. Bennett, D. E., and Cherry, J. K.: Bacterial Infection of Aortic Aneurysms: A Clinico-Pathologic Study, *Am. J. Surg.*, 113:321, 1967.
14. Jarrett, F., Darling, R. C., Mundth, E. D., and Austin, W. G.: Experience with Infected Aneurysms of the Abdominal Aorta, *Arch. Surg.*, 110:1281, 1975.
15. Landle, A., and Berkmen, Y. M.: Aortitis—Pathologic Clinical, and Arteriographic Review, *Radiol. Clin. North Am.*, 14:219, 1976.
16. Isohisa, I., Numano, F., Maezawa, H., and Sasazuki, T.: Hereditary Factors in Takayasu's Disease, *Angiology*, 33:98, 1982.
17. Ishikawa, K.: Natural History and Classification of Occlusive Thromboaortopathy (Takayasu's Disease), *Circulation*, 57:27, 1978.
18. Ishikawa, K: Survival and Morbidity after Diagnosis of Occlusive Thromboaortopathy (Takayasu's Disease), *Am. J. Cardiol.*, 47:1026, 1981.
19. Morooka, S., Saito, Y., Nonaka, Y., Gyotoku, Y., and Sugimoto, T.: Clinical Features and Course of Aortitis Syndrome in Japanese Women Older than 40 Years, *Am. J. Cardiol.*, 53:859, 1984.
20. Ishikawa, K., and Matsura, S.: Occlusive Thromboaortopathy (Takayasu's Disease) and Pregnancy, *Am. J. Cardiol.*, 50:1293, 1982.
21. Wong, V. C. W., and Wang, R. Y. C.: Pregnancy and Takayasu's Arteritis, *Am. J. Med.*, 75:597, 1983.
22. Bulkley, B. H., and Roberts, W. C.: Ankylosing Spondylitis and Aortic Regurgitation, *Circulation*, 43:1014, 1973.
23. Good, A. E.: Reiter's Disease: A Review with Special Attention to Cardiovascular and Neurologic Sequelae, *Semin. Arthritis Rheum.* 3:253, 1974.
24. Bluestone, R., and Pearson, C. M.: Ankylosing Spondylitis and Reiter's Syndrome: Their Interrelationship and Association with HLA B27, *Adv. Intern. Med.*, 22:1, 1977.
25. Nikaidoh, H., Idriss, F. S., and Riker, W. L.: Aortic Rupture in Children as a Complication of Coarctation of the Aorta, *Arch. Surg.*, 107:838, 1973.
26. Edwards, J. E.: Aneurysms of the Thoracic Aorta Complicating Coarctation, *Circulation*, 48:195, 1973.
27. Hoeffel, J. C., Henry, M., Mentre, B., Louis, J. P., and Pernot, C.: Pseudocoarctation or Congenital Kinking of the Aorta, *Am. Heart J.*, 89:428, 1975.
28. Smyth, P. T., and Edwards, J. E.: Pseudocoarctation, Kinking, or Buckling of the Aorta, *Circulation*, 46:1027, 1972.
29. Ben-Shoshan, M., Rossi, N. P., and Korns, M. E.: Coarctation of the Abdominal Aorta, *Arch Pathol.*, 95:221, 1973.
30. DeBakey, M. E., and Noon, G. P.: Aneurysms of the Thoracic Aorta, *Mod. Concepts Cardiovasc. Dis.*, 44:53, 1975.
31. Joyce, J. W., Fairbairn, J. F., II, Kincaid, O. W., and Juergens, J. L.: Aneurysms of the Thoracic Aorta, *Circulation*, 29:176, 1964.
32. Lindsay, J. Jr.: Thoracic Aneurysms, in J. Lindsay, Jr., and J. W. Hurst, (eds.), "The Aorta," Grune & Stratton, New York, 1979, p. 121.
33. Pressler, V., and McNamara, J. J.: Thoracic Aortic Aneurysm: Natural History and Treatment, *J. Thorac. Cardiovasc. Surg.*, 79:489, 1980.
34. Bickerstaff, L. K., Pairolero, P. C., Hollier, L. H., et al.: Thoracic Aortic Aneurysms: A Population-Based Study, *Surgery*, 92:1103, 1982.
35. Murdock, J. L., Walker, B. A., Halpern, B. L., Kuzma, J. W., and McKusick, V. A.: Life Expectancy and Causes of Death in the Marfan Syndrome, *N. Engl. J. Med.*, 286:804, 1972.
36. DeBakey, M. E., and Noon, G. P.: Aneurysms of the Sinuses of Valsalva, in D. C. Sabiston and F. C. Spencer (eds.), "Gibbon's Surgery of the Chest," 3d ed. W. B. Saunders Company, Philadelphia, 1976, p. 903.
37. Crawford, E. S., and Rubio, P. A. Reappraisal of Adjuncts to Avoid Ischemia in the Treatment of Aneurysms of the Descending Thoracic Aorta, *J. Thorac. Cardiovasc. Surg.*, 66:693, 1973.
38. DeBakey, M. E., McCollum, C. H., and Graham, J. M.: Surgical Treatment of Aneurysms of the Descending Thoracic Aorta: Long-Term Results in 500 Patients, *J. Cardiovasc. Surg.*, 19:571, 1978.
39. Weintraub, A. M., and Gomes, M. N.: Clinical Manifestations of Abdominal Aortic Aneurysm, in J. Lindsay, Jr., and J. W. Hurst (eds.), "The Aorta," Grune & Stratton, New York, 1979.
40. Gore, I., and Hirst, A. E., Jr.: Arteriosclerotic Aneurysms of the Abdominal Aorta: A Review, *Prog. Cardiovasc. Dis.*, 16:113, 1973.
41. Dodenhoff, T., and Cos, E. F.: The Acutely Symptomatic Aneurysm: A Surgical Emergency, *Am. Surg.*, 35:691, 1969.
42. Gourdin, F. W., Salam, A. A., Smith, R. B., III, and Perdue, G. D.: Aortovenous Fistulas Due to Ruptured Infrarenal Aortic Aneurysms, *South. Med. J.*, 75:913, 1982.
43. Pfeiffer, R. B.: Successful Repair of Three Primary Aortoduodenal Fistulae, *Arch. Surg.*, 117:1098, 1982.
44. Johnson, J. M., Gaspar, M. R., Morris, H. J., and Rosental, J. J.: Sudden and Complete Thrombosis of Aortic and Iliac Aneurysms, *Arch. Surg.*, 108:792, 1974.
45. Williams, G. M., Harrington, D., Burdick, J., and White, R. F.: Mural Thrombus of the Aorta, *Ann. Surg.*, 194:737, 1981.
46. Brewster, D. C., Retana, A., Waltman, A. C., and Darling, R. C.: Angiography in the Management of Aneurysms of the Abdominal Aorta, *N. Engl. J. Med.*, 292:822, 1975.
47. Hardy, D. C., Lee, J. K. T., Weyman, P. G., and Melson, G. L.: Measurement of the Abdominal Aortic Aneurysms, *Radiology*, 141:821, 1981.
48. Eriksson, I., Forsberg, J. O., Hemmingsson, A., and Lindgren, P. G.: Preoperative Evaluation of Abdominal Aortic Aneurysms: Is There a Need for Aortography? *Acta Chir. Scand.*, 147:533, 1981.
49. DeBakey, M. E., Crawford, E. S., Cooley, D. A., Morris, G. C., Jr., Royster, T. S., and Abbott, W. P.: Aneurysms of the Abdominal Aorta: Analysis of Graft Replacement Therapy One to Eleven Years after Operation, *Ann. Surg.*, 160:622, 1964.
50. DeBakey, M. E.: Aneurysmectomy of the Abdominal Aorta, *Surg. Tech. Illus.*, 1:5, 1976.
51. Hirst, A. E., Jr., Johns, V. J., and Kime, S. W.: Dissecting Aneurysms of the Aorta: A Review of 505 Cases, *Medicine* (Baltimore), 37:217, 1958.
52. Lindsay, J., Jr.: Aortic Dissection, in J. Lindsay, Jr., and J. W. Hurst (eds.), "The Aorta," Grune & Stratton, New York, 1979, p. 239.
53. Wheat, M. W., Jr.: Acute Dissecting Aneurysm of the Aorta: Diagnosis and Treatment—1979, *Am. Heart J.*, 99:373, 1980.
54. Roberts, W. C.: Aortic Dissection: Anatomy, Consequences, and Causes, *Am. Heart J.*, 101:195, 1981.
55. Schlatmann, T. J. M., and Becker, A. F.: Pathogenesis of Dissecting Aneurysms of the Aorta, *Am. J. Cardiol.*, 39:21, 1977.
56. Wilson, S. K., and Hutchins, G. M.: Aortic Dissecting Aneu-

rysms: Causative Factors in 204 Subjects, *Arch. Pathol. Lab. Med.*, 106:175, 1982.
57. Larson, E. W., and Edwards, W. D.: Risk Factors for Aortic Dissection: A Necropsy Study of 161 Cases, *Am. J. Cardiol.*, 53:849, 1984.
58. Lindsay, J., Jr., and Hurst, J. W.: Clinical Features and Prognosis in Dissecting Aneurysm of the Aorta, *Circulation*, 35:880, 1967.
59. Slater, E. E., and DeSanctis, R. W.: The Clinical Recognition of Dissecting Aortic Aneurysm, *Am. J. Med.*, 60:625, 1976.
60. Konishi, Y., Tatsuta, N., Kumada, K., et al.: Dissecting Aneurysm during Pregnancy and the Puerperium, *Jap. Circulation*, 44:726, 1980.
61. Jang, G. C., Brody, W. R., and Dinsmore, R. E.: Radiologic Diagnosis in Aortic Disease, in J. Lindsay, Jr., and J. W. Hurst (eds.), "The Aorta," Grune & Stratton, New York, 1979, p. 296.
62. Thorsen, M. K., San Dretto, M. A., Lawson, T. L., Foley, W. D., Smith, D. F., and Berland, L. L.: Dissecting Aortic Aneurysms: Accuracy of Computed Tomographic Diagnosis, *Radiology*, 148:773, 1983.
63. Doroghazi, R. M., Slater, E. E., De Sanctis, R. W., Buckley, M. J., Austin, W. G., and Rosenthal, S.: Long-Term Survival of Patients with Treated Aortic Dissection, *J. Am. Coll. Cardiovasc.*, 3:1026, 1984.
64. DeBakey, M. E., Beal, A. C., Jr., Cooley, D. A., Crawford, E. S., Morris, G. C., Jr., Garret, H. E., and Howell, J. F.: Dissecting Aneurysms of the Aorta, *Surg. Clin. North Am.*, 46:1045, 1966.
65. DeBakey, M. E.: The Development of Vascular Surgery, *Am. J. Surg.*, 137:697, 1979.
66. DeBakey, M. E., McCollum, C. H., Crawford, E. S., et al.: Dissection and Dissecting Aneurysms of the Aorta: Twenty-Year Follow-Up of Five Hundred Twenty-Seven Patients Treated Surgically, *Surgery*, 92:1118, 1982.
67. Smith, R. B., III, and Perdue, G. D., Jr.: Aortic Arch Syndromes, in J. Lindsay, Jr., and J. W. Hurst (eds.), "The Aorta," Grune & Stratton, New York, 1979, p. 225.
68. McCollum, C. H., Graham, J. M., and DeBakey, M. E.: Chronic Mesenteric Arterial Insufficiency: Results of Revascularization in 33 Cases, *South. Med., J.*, 69:1266, 1976.
69. Lawrie, G. M., Morris, G. C., Jr., Soussou, I. D., Starr, D. S., Silvers, A., Glasser, D. H., and DeBakey, M. E.: Late Results of Reconstructive Surgery for Renovascular Disease, *Ann. Surg.*, 191:528, 1980.
70. Lawrie, G. M., Morris, G. C., Jr., and DeBakey, M. E.: Long-Term Results of Treatment of the Totally Occluded Renal Artery in 40 Patients with Renovascular Hypertension, *Surgery*, 88:753, 1980.
71. Perdue, G. D., Jr. and Smith, R. B., III: Chronic Aortoiliac Occlusion, in Lindsay, Jr., and J. W. Hurst (eds.), "The Aorta," Grune & Stratton, New York, 1979, p. 189.
72. Liddicoat, J. E., Bekassy, S. M., Dang, M. H., and DeBakey, M. E.: Complete Occlusion of the Infrarenal Abdominal Aorta: Management and Results in 64 Patients, *Surgery*, 77:467, 1975.
73. DeBakey, M. E.: Patterns of Atherosclerosis and Rates of Progression, in R. Paoletti and A. M. Gotto, Jr., (eds.), *Atherosclerosis Reviews*, Raven Press, New York, 1978, vol. 3, p. 1.
74. Grüntzig, A., and Hopff, H.: Perkutane Rekanalisation chronischer arterieller Verschlusse mit einem neuen Dilatationskatheter, *Dtsch. Med. Wochenshr.*, 99:2502, 1974.
75. Grüntzig, A.: Perkutane Dilatation von Kronarstenosen. Beschreibung eines neuen Kathetersystems. *Klin. Wochenshr.*, 54:543, 1976.
76. Perdue, G. D., Jr., and Smith, R. B., III: Acute Aortoiliac Occlusion, in J. Lindsay, Jr., and J. W. Hurst (eds.), "The Aorta," Grune & Stratton, New York, 1979, p. 169.
77. Schatz, I. J., and Stanley, J. C.: Saddle Embolus of the Aorta, *JAMA*, 235:1262, 1976.
78. Busuttil, R. W., Keehn, G., Milliken, J., et al.: Aortic Saddle Embolus, *Ann. Surg.*, 197:698, 1983.
79. Deterling, R. A.: Acute Arterial Occlusion, *Surg. Clin. North Am.*, 46:587, 1966.
80. Danto, L. A., Fry, W. J., and Kraft, R. O.: Acute Aortic Thrombosis, *Arch. Surg.*, 104:569, 1972.

65

Diseases of the Peripheral Arteries

Jess R. Young, M.D.

I never looked upon the Heart as the maker of the blood, but only as an Engine that caused the blood to circulate, driving it forcibly in to the Arteries, and by its opening, giving way for the blood to come in again out of the Veins.

Anton van Leeuwenhock, 1632–1723[1]

Chronic Occlusive Arterial Diseases

The term *chronic occlusive arterial disease* refers to those disorders, usually due to atherosclerosis, that as a result of occlusion of large- and medium-sized arteries, cause various degrees of chronic ischemia of a number of organs, organ systems, and peripheral tissues. These include the brain, heart, kidneys, and other visceral organs, and the upper and lower extremities. Chronic ischemia in each of these arterial beds tends to assume characteristic anatomic, pathological, and clinical patterns. In this section those diseases that produce chronic ischemia of the aorta and peripheral arteries will be discussed. The term *peripheral vascular disease* relates to a variety of diseases affecting the arteries, veins, and lymphatics and should not be used as a synonym for chronic occlusive arterial disease. Other sections in this chapter will be devoted to conditions which produce ischemia caused by acute arterial occlusion and arterial spasm.

Arteriosclerosis Obliterans

The term *arteriosclerosis obliterans* refers to chronic occlusive disease of the aorta and its branches to the extremities as a result of atherosclerosis. *Arteriosclerosis* is the accepted diagnostic term by common usage. Occasionally terms such as *atherosclerotic occlusive disease, chronic occlusive arterial disease, obliterative arteriosclerosis,* and *peripheral arterial disease* are also used.

Arteriosclerosis obliterans is by far the most common disease causing chronic ischemia of the lower extremities, accounting for about 95 percent of cases.[2] The disease affects the elderly, most often persons older than age 50. Men are affected more often than women in ratios of about 5:1 to 10:1.[2] The incidence of diabetes mellitus among patients with arteriosclerosis obliterans ranges from 20 to 33 percent. Approximately 90 percent of patients with peripheral disease have atherosclerosis elsewhere.[3]

Etiology

There is a close association between smoking and arteriosclerosis obliterans. When first examined, approximately 90 percent of patients with arteriosclerosis obliterans are smokers, and the incidence of progression of the disease and the failure of arterial grafts is much higher in patients who continue to smoke. Results of the Framingham study showed that intermittent claudication occurred about twice as often among cigarette smokers as among nonsmokers, and the risk tended to increase with the intensity of the habit.[4] Other risk factors in arteriosclerosis obliterans are diabetes mellitus, hyperlipidemia, hypertension, obesity, and atherosclerosis elsewhere, particularly in the coronary arteries.[3]

Pathology

The atherosclerotic lesion in the large- and medium-sized arteries supplying the extremities is similar pathologically to that occurring elsewhere in the body, and characteristically patients with arteriosclerosis obliterans have a high incidence of atherosclerosis affecting the coronary arteries and the arteries supplying the brain.[3] In addition to the atherosclerotic lesions in the larger arteries of the extremities, arteriolar and capillary lesions in diabetic patients consist of endothelial proliferation and thickening of the basement membrane.

Pathophysiology

The basic pathophysiological alteration produced by chronic occlusive arterial disease, regardless of its underlying cause, is ischemia of tissues supplied by the obstructed arteries. The severity of the ischemia is dependent upon the site and extent of the arterial disease and upon the adequacy of the collateral circulation. A hemodynamically significant arterial obstruction will usually result in compensatory collateral circulation that bypasses the obstructed segment.[5] The stimulus for development of collaterals may be the abnormal pressure gradient across the collateral bed or the increased flow velocity through the collateral vessels. The resistance of the collateral pathway is always greater than the resistance in the original unobstructed artery. Thus, even with the development of prominent collateral vessels, the flow through the collateral bed will never be equal to the flow through the unobstructed artery.

Clinical Manifestations

As with atherosclerosis elsewhere, arteriosclerosis obliterans develops slowly and insidiously over a period of years. At first the disease will be mild, and since only a minimal pressure gradient across the lesion will be present, the patient will have no symptoms. With time the disease progresses; a collateral circulation will develop, and its ultimate capacity to carry blood will determine the severity of the symptoms and signs. Early in the course of the disease the flow through the collateral arteries is usually adequate to maintain the viability of the affected extremity but is not sufficient to prevent symptoms during exercise, and the typical symptoms of intermittent claudication will appear. If the disease progresses, the collateral vessels may become occluded, causing more ischemia. The patient may experience pain when at rest, and ultimately ulceration and gangrene may ensue.

Occasionally acute thrombosis on an atherosclerotic plaque will occur as a primary event in a patient without previous symptoms of arterial insufficiency, but, more often, it occurs as a secondary event superimposed on preexisting disease. In such a situation, an adequate collateral circulation does not have time to develop, resulting in marked acute ischemia which, if not surgically corrected promptly, may progress to gangrene and necessitate amputation.

Intermittent Claudication The characteristic symptom of occlusive arterial disease affecting the extremities is intermittent claudication. It is a symptom related to muscle ischemia. When a muscle is exercised to the point that the blood supply cannot meet the demand of the exercising muscle, discomfort occurs. This may be aching, cramping, severe fatigue, or occasionally numbness brought on by walking a certain distance and quickly relieved by rest. The distance required to bring on the symptom may vary from a few steps to several blocks, or it may occur only when walking rapidly uphill. The patient need not sit down to obtain relief, which usually will come within 1 to 3 min. When the distress is relieved, the patient can walk the same distance again. The distance will decrease if the disease progresses and increase if a good collateral circulation forms. Intermittent claudication most often occurs in the muscles of the calf, because these are most active during walking and their blood supply is affected by occlusive disease in any artery proximal to them. Intermittent claudication may also occur in other regions such as the buttocks, hips, thighs, and feet. There is close correlation between the site of the claudication and the arterial segment affected by the occlusive disease.

Rest Pain If the disease progresses, more extensive segments of the arteries become involved, the collateral vessels may become occluded, and resting blood flow is greatly reduced, despite maximal reduction in peripheral vascular resistance. The tissues become ischemic and painful at rest (rest pain) and necrosis may ensue. Rest pain is different from intermittent claudication in that it always occurs in the foot, usually in the forefoot and toes. There are often associated complaints of coldness and numbness. The pain is severe and relentless; it is worse at night when the patient is in bed. Relief is obtained by sitting up and hanging the leg over the side of the bed or spending the night in a chair with the legs dependent. Such prolonged dependency may cause edema, which further compromises blood flow because of the increased extravascular pressure.

Vascular Physical Examination

Similar to the history, the physical findings in arteriosclerosis obliterans are typical, logical, and readily apparent to the eyes and hands. In most instances, a thorough history and an adequate vascular physical examination result in an accurate diagnosis of occlusive arterial disease.

Palpation of Pulses Careful palpation of pulses at all locations in the lower extremities is an important part of every complete physical examination. A diagnosis of chronic occlusive arterial disease is not possible when the arterial pulses are unequivocally normal. However, in the presence of partial or complete occlusion with a rich collateral circulation in a sedentary person, it is possible to have mild chronic occlusive arterial disease without any symptoms of

FIGURE 65-1 Radial compression test of Allen, which may be employed to test for patency of the ulnar and radial arteries and the palmar arterial arch. *A.* While the examiner occludes the radial artery, the patient squeezes the blood out of the hand by making a tight fist. *B.* While radial compression is maintained by the examiner, the patient opens the hand. If color does not return to the hand within 3 s, occlusion of the ulnar artery or the ulnar side of the palmar arch is usually present. By compressing the ulnar artery and repeating the maneuver, it is possible to test for patency of the radial artery and the radial side of the palmar arch. Compression tests are more difficult to perform on the foot and give less satisfactory results.

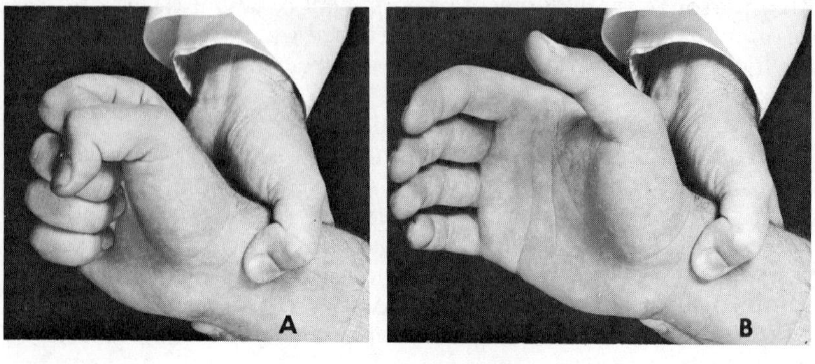

intermittent claudication. In such instances the distal pulses, although present, are definitely reduced. Occasionally a patient will complain of intermittent claudication, usually in the hips or buttocks due to aortoiliac disease, but on examination the peripheral pulses seem adequate. In this situation the pulses may disappear when the patient walks to the point of discomfort. This occurs because muscle hypoxia causes maximal dilatation of the distal muscular bed at the time of the claudication. This lowers the peripheral resistance and drops the arterial pressure, and the pulses disappear. The phenomenon can be demonstrated well by noninvasive instrumentation.

Arterial pulsations may be unimpaired at the wrist or ankle when the occlusive disease is confined to the palmar or plantar arches or the digital arteries themselves. In situations such as this, compression tests, such as Allen's test (Fig. 65-1), are useful in making the clinical diagnosis.

Systolic bruits heard over the abdominal aorta, particularly at the level of the umbilicus and over the femoral arteries in the groin, are common in older persons. These bruits indicate some intimal disease but are not closely related to the degree of occlusion present. However, in the absence of an arterial venous communication, bruits with both systolic and diastolic components usually indicate definite occlusive arterial disease. Bruits in the lower extremities may be misleading, so final evaluation is best made by observing other aspects of the vascular examination, particularly the palpation of the peripheral pulses and by noninvasive laboratory tests.

Postural Color Changes Postural color changes that occur in the feet with elevation of the legs, followed by dependency, provide important additional information concerning the degree of ischemia present in arteriosclerosis obliterans. When ischemia is moderate or severe, pallor of the involved foot will occur during elevation. The leg should be elevated at about 60° or more until the maximum amount of pallor develops, usually within 1 min. During elevation, the hypoxia of the tissues of the foot occurs so that upon dependency, immediately following the period of elevation, rubor of the foot develops. This is caused by maximal dilatation of the arterioles and capillaries of the foot (reactive hyperemia), the compensatory mechanism to correct the hypoxia.

Trophic Changes When arterial insufficiency is mild, such as in the patient with stenosis or occlusion with a good collateral circulation, the nutrition of the foot is good; the skin is warm and pink, and hair and nail growth is good. However, with chronic severe ischemia, trophic changes occur, and the foot becomes cold, with loss of hair, poor nail growth, and dry, scaly skin. Ischemic ulcers usually occur on the toes, the most distal part of the arterial bed, but they may occur in the heel, ankle, or leg after trauma (Fig. 65-2). Ischemic ulcers are necrotic, crusted, or gangrenous with poorly defined, often cyanotic, borders.[6] They are associated with severe unrelenting pain. Infection is usually absent, or superficial, because of the poor blood supply.

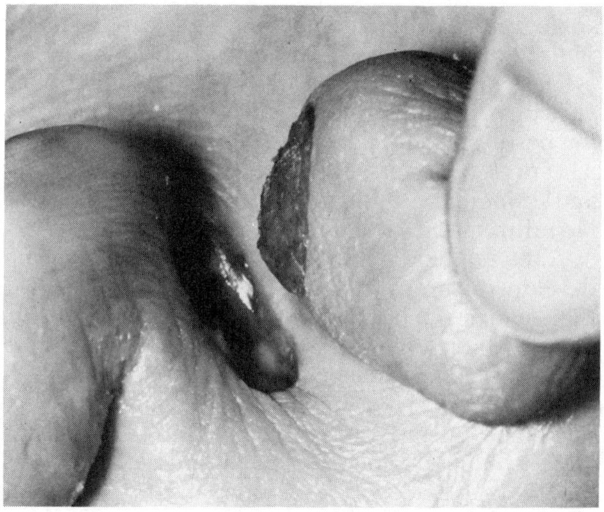

A

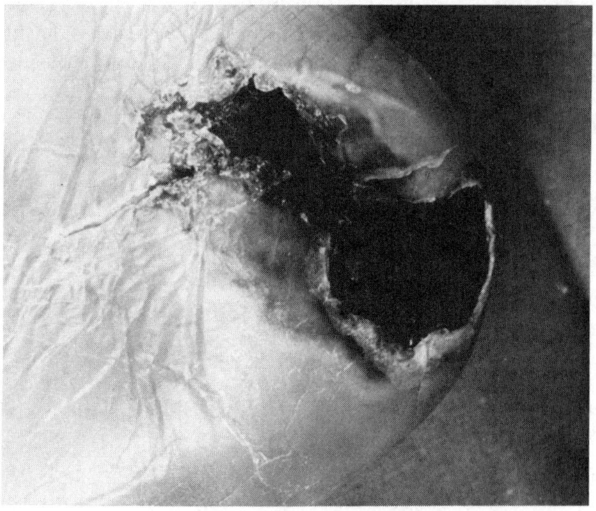

B

FIGURE 65-2 Characteristic ulcers in arteriosclerosis obliterans. *A.* Ischemic ulcers on abutting surfaces of two toes ("kissing ulcers"). *B.* Gangrenous heel ulcer.

Further progression of the occlusive disease results in gangrene, the end-stage lesion. It usually begins on a toe or the heel, often in and around an area of ulceration, and spreads proximally to larger areas of the foot. Rapid development of large areas of gangrene is caused by trauma, acute arterial occlusion, or an overwhelming infection in a diabetic foot.

Diagnosis

Noninvasive Diagnostic Techniques[7] The advent of noninvasive instrumentation in the diagnosis of occlusive arterial disease has provided a valuable intermediate step between the clinical examination and angiography. Although the diagnosis can be made clinically in most cases, the examination is limited by the experience of the observer, who may have difficulty palpating pulses or may be unfamiliar with the postural color changes that occur with ischemia. The present noninvasive instruments are practical and economical, and yield accurate and reproducible information.

Although new instruments and methods are being developed, the most practical and well proven for the diagnosis of occlusive arterial disease are (1) the Doppler ultrasonic velocity detector, which is simple to use, relatively inexpensive, and accurate for diagnosing occlusive arterial disease; and (2) the segmental plethysmograph, which measures changes in blood volume during systole and diastole in the segment of the extremity being measured.

The degree of arterial insufficiency is measured by comparing the Doppler ankle systolic pressure with the brachial systolic pressure. With a blood pressure cuff around the ankle, the Doppler systolic pressure is taken over the posterior tibial or dorsalis pedis artery and compared to the brachial systolic pressure. The ankle systolic pressure normally is equal to or greater than the brachial systolic pressure. The severity of the arterial insufficiency is determined by the ratio of ankle to brachial pressure as follows:

No arterial insufficiency—0.9 to 1.0 or greater
Mild arterial insufficiency—0.7 to 0.9
Moderate arterial insufficiency—0.5 to 0.7
Severe arterial insufficiency—less than 0.5

More extensive studies can be performed in the vascular laboratory. During measurement of arterial flow in various segments of the lower extremities, the location of the lesions and the severity of the disease can be assessed. This makes possible a rational decision as to the need for angiography and possible revascularization. Furthermore, follow-up can be done during the course of medical treatment or following surgery. The data obtained are objective and can be recorded in the patient's record.

Angiography[8] Adequate angiography will demonstrate the arterial supply to the lower extremities from the level of the renal arteries to the feet and to the upper extremities from the origin of the subclavian arteries to the hands. This study will complement the physical and noninvasive examinations. Angiograms are indicated for every patient who requires revascularization and for patients in whom clinical and noninvasive examinations do not provide sufficient information for adequate evaluation.

Differential Diagnosis

Usually the diagnosis of chronic occlusive arterial disease presents less difficulty than the establishment of the specific cause of the arterial obstruction. Trauma, arterial embolism, and acute arterial thrombosis usually can be ruled out on the basis of the history. Acute occlusions are characterized by the sudden onset of severe ischemia with findings of the five P's: pain, pallor, paresthesia, paralysis, and pulselessness. In such cases, there is usually a history of intermittent claudication or atherosclerotic or rheumatic heart disease.

Takayasu's disease occurs in young women and affects branches of the aorta, usually the arch, but occasionally the visceral, renal, and extremity arteries. Fever, malaise, weight loss, and an elevated sedimentation rate may be characteristics of the onset of the disease. Diagnosis is made by angiography of the aorta and its branches. Rarely, fibromuscular hyperplasia occurs in the peripheral arteries, and isolated cases of involvement of the external iliac, brachial, and femoral arteries have been reported. The diagnosis can be made only by angiography.

Arteritis associated with collagen disease is a multisystem disease manifested by general and diverse symptoms. It may cause cutaneous infarcts, ischemic purpura, and digital gangrene with normal arterial pulses because usually only the small arteries are affected.

Atheromatous or fibrin emboli, which arise in ulcerated plaques or aneurysms in the aorta and arteries of the lower extremities, cause small scattered ischemic lesions in the toes, feet, or legs. Occasionally the small emboli lodge in the visceral and renal arteries. Usually the peripheral pulses are normal or reduced. This condition occurs in older persons with evidence of atherosclerosis elsewhere.

Buerger's disease (thromboangiitis obliterans) is described in the next section of this chapter. It is a chronic, progressive, inflammatory disease that causes occlusion of the small arteries of the feet and hands, and progresses proximally. The disease usually occurs in men younger than age 40 who smoke. Superficial phlebitis occurs in 40 percent of these patients.

The cauda equina syndrome is caused by narrowing of the lumbar canal by spondylosis, disease of the intervertebral disks, or spinal cord tumor. It is characterized by a symptom complex which mimics intermittent claudication. Burning, tingling, numbness, weakness, and occasionally pain in the hips, thighs, and calves are brought on by walking and standing. Most often the patient obtains relief only by sitting or lying recumbent. The differential diagnosis is often difficult because these patients are older and arteriosclerosis obliterans may coexist. The diagnosis is confirmed by roentgenograms of the lumbosacral spine, computed tomographic scanning of the lumbosacral spine, noninvasive testing in the vascular laboratory before and after exercise, and, if necessary, angiography and myelography.[9]

In the diabetic with arterial insufficiency and diabetic neuropathy, it is often difficult to distinguish between rest pain due to ischemia or pain due to the neuropathy. Ischemic rest pain is chronic and severe, and is relieved by dependency or walking. The distress of neuropathy is usually a numb, burning sensation, or a dysesthesia which is worse at night and is not relieved by dependency or walking. The foot is often warm, and although the pulses may be diminished or absent, the signs of ischemia may not be advanced. Noninvasive studies in the vascular laboratory will often distinguish between these two conditions.

The popliteal artery entrapment syndrome causes intermittent claudication in the calf of young persons. It is caused by entrapment of the popliteal artery by the gastrocnemius muscle as the result of an anomaly in which the popliteal artery passes medial to or through the fibers of the medial head of the gastrocnemius.[10] During walking the popliteal artery is compressed by the muscle, cutting off arterial flow. On examination at rest the peripheral pulses are normal. This condition can be highly suspected after examination in the vascular laboratory before and after exercise, but angiography is diagnostic and shows medial deviation of the popliteal artery at the knee.

There are several distressing and often disabling functional conditions of the lower extremities that are unfamiliar to the practicing physician and are often misdiagnosed as vascular disorders. These are muscular pain (fibrositis, tension myalgia), a common condition manifested by aching legs and tight, tender hamstring and calf muscles; the disuse phenomenon; reflex sympathetic dystrophy; and the restless leg syndrome. The patient's bitter complaints alarm the physician, and, in the absence of an obvious musculoskeletal disorder, the complaints are often attributed to the area with which the physician is least knowledgeable, the peripheral vascular system. Occasionally the symptoms are attributed to poor arterial circulation, especially if there is sympathetic nerve overactivity, but most often the diagnosis of thrombophlebitis is made on the basis of aching, tender legs. A careful physical examination and noninvasive studies in the vascular laboratory can confirm the absence of vascular disease and thus reassure the patient.

Homocystinuria should be suspected when occlusive arterial disease occurs in children or young adults who also have one or more of the following: congenital skeletal anomalies similar to those in Marfan's syndrome, thrombophlebitis, osteoporosis, mental retardation, ectopia lentis, cutaneous flushing, and evidence of coronary disease, cerebrovascular disease, or both.

Prognosis

Arteriosclerosis obliterans is not invariably a progressive disease. Generally speaking, 75 percent of the patients remain the same or improve and 25 percent become worse. In a study of 104 patients with intermittent claudication studied by angiography, 82 remained stable and 22 became worse during a follow-up period from 6 months to 8 years, with a mean of 2.5 years.[11] Of the 22 patients who became worse, only 6 required amputation because of gangrene. In the Framingham experience the amputation rate was 5 percent in a cohort of 125 patients with intermittent claudication over a period of 18 years.[12] The remainder had only worsening of the claudication. Progression occurs more frequently in superficial femoral arteries than in other vessels, and in the extremities of patients 50 years or older and in the extremities of manifest diabetics. Progression occurs more frequently in arterial segments immediately proximal to occlusions than in the distal segments.

It has been well established that the risk factors of hypertension, hyperlipemia, smoking, left ventricular hypertrophy on the electrocardiogram, and glucose intolerance are precursors common to all three major atherosclerotic disorders: stroke, coronary artery disease, and arteriosclerosis obliterans.[4] The life expectancy of patients with arteriosclerosis obliterans is compromised because of the high frequency of concomitant atherosclerotic complications in the brain and heart.[3] The occlusive disease in the extremities contributes little to the increased mortality rate.

Medical Treatment

All patients with arteriosclerosis obliterans should be instructed in a medical treatment program. Although some patients require surgery because of the severity of the disease, this only relieves symptoms or accomplishes limb salvage and has no beneficial effect on atherogenesis, either locally or in other arterial beds. The goals of medical treatment are as follows:

- To increase the blood supply to the limb by stimulating the development of a collateral circulation
- To protect the leg and foot from injury
- To relieve ischemic pain
- To treat ischemic ulcers
- To control associated diseases, such as heart disease, hypertension, diabetes mellitus, hyperlipemia, and obesity

In order to prevent progression of the disease and avoid complications, the following should be the cornerstones of medical therapy:

- Abstinence from smoking
- Exercise in the form of walking
- Careful care of the feet
- Diet

Smoking Although there is no evidence to substantiate it, the prevalence of cigarette smoking in arteriosclerosis obliterans is suggestive of an etiologic relationship. Therefore, the patient should stop smoking completely and permanently. It is well known that tobacco causes peripheral vasoconstriction and probably inhibits the development of collateral circulation. Since the patient has complete control over this risk factor that is so important in the progression of the disease, it is important to explain the reasons for stopping smoking in simple, understandable terms.

Exercise Much convincing evidence has accumulated which indicates that the most effective treatment for intermittent claudication is physical exercise, particularly walking. Maximum walking distance can be at least doubled and often increased severalfold.[13] The patient should exercise from 30 to 60 min daily, walking to the point of distress and then continuing to walk as far as pain tolerance will permit. The patient should then stop and allow the discomfort to disappear, and then walk again as far as can be tolerated, repeating this exercise for the prescribed period. The exact mechanism by which the walking distance is increased is not clear, and although there is some evidence that exercise increases the collateral circulation, the results of other studies suggest that better coordination of muscles, and perhaps some sort of beneficial metabolic change are the mechanisms responsible. The maximum benefit from the exercise program requires at least 3 months, but the program should be continued indefinitely.

Foot Care In most patients who undergo amputation, the initiating factor that leads to gangrene is some avoidable injury. Therefore, as a preventive measure, all patients with chronic occlusive arterial disease, regardless of the cause, should be given careful and detailed instructions in the care and hygiene of ischemic extremities. Instructions in foot care and the avoidance of thermal, chemical, and mechanical trauma are available from the American Heart Association. The feet should be kept clean by bathing them in lukewarm water [35 to 37.7°C (95 to 100°F)] with a mild soap, rinsing them in clear, tepid water, and then gently drying them with a soft towel, being particularly careful to dry between the toes. Nonmedicated talc should be dusted on lightly, and if the skin is scaly or dry, a small amount of lanolin should be rubbed in gently. The patient should wear clean socks daily and comfortable shoes that do not bind or rub. New shoes should be broken in gradually. Advice should be given regarding care of the nails, avoidance of the extremes of hot and cold temperature, and the proper treatment of dermatophytosis. Ingrown toenails, corns, and calluses should be treated by a physician or a podiatrist who is aware that the patient has arterial insufficiency.

Diet Despite the current preoccupation with diets and drugs to lower cholesterol and triglyceride levels, there is still no clear-cut evidence that such measures are of *significant* benefit to most patients with symptomatic atherosclerosis of the peripheral arteries. Such factors as the expense, safety, convenience, and side effects of drugs must be balanced against the possibility of future benefit. Until more decisive evidence is available, decisions regarding diet and lipid-lowering agents will continue to be difficult to make and even more difficult to vindicate. Younger patients, however, would more likely benefit from a reduction in serum lipid values than older patients (see Chap. 42).

Drug Therapy Over the years a variety of drugs have been advocated for the treatment of arteriosclerosis obliterans, particularly so-called vasodilating drugs. Experience has shown that none of these agents is capable of selectively dilating main arteries or collateral vessels supplying an ischemic extremity.[14] When these agents are prescribed in amounts sufficient to cause vasodilatation, the effect is generalized, causing the well-known and predictable physiological reaction of hypotension, tachycardia, syncope, and even shock. Such a reaction is intolerable and harmful to the patient and of no benefit to an ischemic limb. For these reasons, drugs advocated for vasodilation have no place in the treatment of chronic occlusive disease.

Since beta-adrenergic blocking agents can worsen intermittent claudication, their use should be avoided, if possible, in patients with arterial insufficiency.

Treatment of Pain The management of ischemic rest pain, ischemic ulcers, and gangrene can be one of the most difficult problems in the treatment of arteriosclerosis obliterans. Elevation of the head of the bed 4 to 6 in can increase blood flow to the limb and can help relieve nocturnal rest pain. Mild ischemic pain can usually be controlled by the judicious use of salicylates or propoxyphene hydrochloride (Darvon); not infrequently it is necessary to administer narcotics such as morphine sulfate or levorphanol tartrate (Levo-Dromoran). The latter in dosages of 2 mg every 4 to 6 h, with or without chlorpromazine hydrochloride (Thorazine), is particularly helpful, with less risk of addiction. Along with the analgesic a tranquilizer may be helpful in alleviating the anxiety often associated with severe pain and may potentiate the effect of the analgesics.

Treatment of Ischemic Ulcers and Gangrene Ischemic ulcers and gangrene signify advanced disease and are the most feared complications of arteriosclerosis obliterans. Important in the management of these complications are bed rest with elevation of the head of the bed, relief of pain, eradication of infection, and improvement of the arterial blood supply, if possible. In this situation arterial reconstruction can be a limb-saving procedure. To help eradicate or prevent infection and to effect cleanliness, the affected part may be soaked in a lukewarm solution of 3% boric acid, physiological saline, or mild soap (such as Ivory Snow) for 20 min, once or twice daily. The basic principle is to use a bland, nonirritating, nonsensitizing solution. A 1:10,000 solution of potassium permanganate may be used as a foot soak when active dermatophytosis is present, which is usually the case when an ulcer is between the toes.

After soaking, the lesion should be rinsed with clear, lukewarm water, patted dry with a soft towel, and dressed with a clear, dry dressing. To protect the foot while the patient is in bed, pressure on the heel or malleoli can be prevented by the use of protective pads, bulky bandages, or foam rubber boots.

Because severe ischemia does not encourage deep or spreading infections, systemic antibiotics are usually not necessary unless the ischemic ulcerations are associated with obvious cellulitis or lymphangitis, or unless there is evidence of systemic infection with chills and fever.

Surgery and Other Modes of Treatment

Before any revascularization procedure is considered, every patient with arteriosclerosis obliterans who has symptoms limited to intermittent claudication should first be treated with the medical program described previously. If the symptoms do not improve after 2 or 3 months on this program and the patient is economically incapacitated (unable to work) or if the symptoms progress, surgical therapy should be considered. If the patient has severe ischemia with rest pain, ulceration, or gangrene, revascularization is indicated, if possible, in an attempt to salvage the limb.

The decision is dependent not only upon the symptoms but also upon the angiographic findings and on the patient's general condition. In view of the high incidence of atherosclerosis elsewhere, especially in the coronary arteries,[3] the patient should be carefully evaluated as a surgical risk. Careful selection of patients minimizes the operative risk and often will make possible the choice of a less extensive procedure, such as a femorofemoral graft or a femoral profundoplasty, for poor-risk patients.

Arteriosclerosis obliterans causes chronic occlusive disease in four general areas: (1) aortoiliac, (2) femoropopliteal, (3) both aortoiliac and femoropopliteal (combined disease), and (4) popliteal-tibial. Since the indications for surgical treatment, the operative techniques, and the results differ depending upon the arterial segment affected, each segment will be discussed separately. Complete arteriography from the abdominal aorta to the distal tibial arteries is indispensable for proper evaluation in all cases.

Aortoiliac Disease Patients with occlusive disease affecting the aortoiliac area, with patent femoropopliteal segments, complain only of intermittent claudication. Since the collateral circulation around the aortoiliac segment is rich, perfusion of the lower extremities seldom, if ever, becomes critically reduced so as to threaten viability. Therefore, many patients can accept the nuisance of the claudication and do well on a medical program of treatment. Surgical correction should be considered for those patients with economically disabling intermittent claudication or rapidly progressive disease.

Since by definition these patients have adequate inflow from the proximal abdominal aorta and good outflow in the femoropopliteal segment, they are operable from a technical standpoint. The surgical technique most commonly employed entails the use of an aortofemoral bypass graft with a suitable prosthesis and, less commonly, an aortoiliac graft, providing the external iliac arteries are normal. An endarterectomy may be performed in those cases in which the occluded segment is short and well localized. The results following aortofemoral bypass procedures and endarterectomy are gratifying since the early and late patency rate is 90 percent. If one iliac segment is occluded and the other is widely patent, femorofemoral bypass grafting can be done as an elective procedure and for patients who are poor risks for the more extensive abdominal procedure. The results of this technique are acceptable but not quite as good as aortoiliac or aortofemoral procedures.

Aortoiliac and Femoropopliteal Disease (Combined Disease) Patients with combined disease may have presenting symptoms of claudication at a short distance or of severe ischemia in the form of rest pain or early gangrene. The criteria for revascularization are less strict than in the aortoiliac group since frequently the surgery is performed for limb salvage rather than for relief of intermittent claudication. The reconstructive procedure of choice consists of aortofemoral bypass grafting. Localized endarterectomies of the common femoral and profunda femoris arteries, with or without profundoplasty, are frequently necessary to ensure good runoff. It is usually not necessary to correct associated occlusions of the superficial femoral arteries since most patients (85 percent) obtain relief of rest pain, and claudication is frequently entirely relieved or greatly improved after only the proximal obstruction is corrected. When necessary, femoropopliteal reconstruction can be performed at a later date.

Patients who are considered poor surgical risks because of serious associated disease may be successfully treated with the use of the less traumatic extraanatomic bypasses (axillofemoral and femorofemoral), since surgical dissection is minimal and the procedures can be performed under local anesthesia. The results almost approach those observed with the standard aortofemoral bypass.

Femoropopliteal Disease Segmental occlusion of the superficial femoral arteries seldom results in severe ischemia; therefore, surgical treatment is rarely needed. The claudication frequently improves with a walking program. It is only when the occlusive disease includes the popliteal or tibial arteries that severe ischemia occurs.

When operation is necessary, the recommended procedure is femoropopliteal bypass grafting utilizing a reversed or in situ autogenous saphenous vein. The success rate of this procedure is 60 to 80 percent at 1 year and 50 to 70 percent at 5 years.[15] If a saphenous vein is not available, polytetrafluoroethylene (PTFE, Gore-Tex) or human umbilical vein, which have patency rates almost comparable to those of the saphenous vein, can be used.

Popliteal-Tibial Disease Distal disease of this type commonly occurs in the patient with diabetes mellitus. Occasionally a bypass procedure to a distal tibial or peroneal artery is possible, but in most cases the disease is diffuse and the runoff is poor. In such cases, lumbar sympathectomy may be helpful, but frequently amputation is inevitable.

Transluminal Angioplasty

The role of percutaneous transluminal dilatation of atherosclerotic lesions of the peripheral arteries is presently still being defined. The clinical indications for its use in arteriosclerosis obliterans are the same as for reconstructive surgery: economically incapacitating intermittent claudication, rest pain, ulceration, and minor gangrene. It may have particular value for patients who are poor risks for surgery or for patients with severe inoperable disease who are facing amputations. The angiographic indications are short, isolated segments of stenosis or occlusion in the iliac, superficial femoral, and popliteal arteries. The procedure may be used to dilate proximal arteries, such as the iliac, during the course of distal surgery.

Morphological changes caused by the procedure are desquamation of endothelial cells, intimal disruption, splitting of the atheromatous plaque, and subsequent deposition of platelets and fibrin.[16] The long-term pathophysiological changes are unknown.

For dilation of iliac artery stenoses, immediate success rates range from 79 to 93 percent, and 70 to 80 percent of the treated vessels may be patent after 2 to 3 years.[15] In the treatment of femoral artery stenoses, primary success rates range from 73 to 84 percent, and the patency rates after 2 years range from 57 to 75 percent.[17] Complications are infrequent and include acute occlusion due to thrombosis or embolism and arterial wall perforation. These may require immediate surgical correction; therefore, when transluminal angioplasty is done, the vascular surgical team should be available.

The advantages of this procedure are its nonsurgical nature, the use of local anesthesia, early ambulation, and reduced hospital stay. In addition, in dilation of the iliac arteries the risk of severing autonomic nerves is avoided.

Thrombolytic Therapy

The role of thrombolytic therapy in arterial occlusive disease is still evolving. Streptokinase and urokinase seem to be equally effective in acute arterial occlusions. Marked improvement has been achieved in the majority of patients whose thrombosis has been present for less than 10 days.[18] Although standard systemic doses have been employed in most patients, a low dose of lytic agents infused through arterial catheters adjacent to the thrombus has also been effective, and seems to be more effective in lysing chronic occlusions.[19] Thrombolytic agents appear to be most useful in patients with arterial or graft thrombosis at the time of an acute episode or after failure of reconstructive surgery. Some of these patients may require a secondary procedure such as transluminal angioplasty or bypass grafting to maintain patency.

Sympathectomy

Lumbar sympathectomy is indicated when the signs and symptoms of ischemia progress, despite adequate medical treatment, and revascularization procedures are infeasible or inadvisable. Lumbar sympathectomy does not increase blood flow to the muscles and, therefore, does not relieve intermittent claudication. Perfusion to the skin may increase and rest pain may be relieved, and minor ulcerations may heal in approximately 50 percent of patients.

Amputation

When the blood supply to an extremity is reduced to a degree insufficient to support tissue viability, resulting in irreversible gangrene, nonhealing ulcers, or intractable pain, and when reconstructive surgery is not possible, or fails, amputation is indicated. The lowest possible level of amputation should be done. Transmetatarsal amputations are frequently possible in the diabetic patient with distal disease. On the other hand, higher levels of amputation are usually necessary in patients with arteriosclerosis obliterans. Preservation of the knee, whenever possible, is of great importance in rehabilitation of the amputee. This is especially true in the older patient who is debilitated and weak and has poor balance, poor vision, and multiple-system disease. The vascular laboratory may offer helpful guidelines, but the level of amputation can be quickly decided once the incision for the below-knee amputation is made. If free bleeding occurs, the below-knee amputation will most likely heal well.

Optimum results following amputation are obtained when a team trained in amputations—a surgeon, prosthetist, psychiatrist, and family physician—works with the patient.

Thromboangiitis Obliterans (Buerger's Disease)

After arteriosclerosis obliterans, thromboangiitis obliterans (Buerger's disease), though relatively rare, is the next most common cause of chronic, occlusive arterial disease of the extremities.

Etiology

The cause of thromboangiitis obliterans is not definitely known, but the direct relationship to cigarette smoking appears to be indisputable. The angiitis most likely represents a poorly understood sensitivity reaction to tobacco. The disease occurs only in smokers; cessation of smoking will arrest the disease and persistence in smoking will cause occlusion of the more proximal arteries and result in amputation. A cellular sensitivity to collagen has also been demonstrated in patients with thromboangiitis obliterans,[20] suggesting that this may be an etiologic factor and raising the possibility of diagnosing the disease by immunologic means.

Pathology and Pathophysiology

The pathological findings in thromboangiitis obliterans, as described by Buerger in his classic article published in 1908,[21] are usually distinctly different from those of arteriosclerosis obliterans, except in the late stages when old, occluding, organized thrombi may be seen to fill the lumina of arteries that demonstrate considerable perivascular fibrosis.

In the acute and subacute stages, thromboangiitis obliterans is characterized by an intense inflammatory reaction that, unlike atherosclerosis, involves the veins as well as the arteries. Thromboangiitis obliterans characteristically affects medium-sized and small arteries initially; atherosclerosis usually involves arteries of large caliber. The visceral arteries rarely are affected by thromboangiitis obliterans, but they are commonly the sites of atherosclerosis. Thromboangiitis obliterans is a true panarteritis (or panphlebitis), as all coats of the vessel are affected and the process often extends into the perivascular tissues, leading to fibrosis and scarring that firmly bind together the artery, vein, and nerve. Characteristically, the involvement is segmental, with normal segments interspersed between segments of inflammation. Proliferation of the endothelium and invasion of all three coats by lymphocytes and fibroblasts are common characteristics of this disease. Polymorphonuclear leukocytes are present in the acute stage and for this reason are more likely to be seen in veins because biopsies can be obtained more easily than in the arteries, which are not usually obtained for microscopic study until the disease has reached the chronic stage. Giant cells may be found both in arteries and in veins during the acute stage. The arterial lumen is compromised by proliferation of the endothelium and invasion of the intima by lymphocytes, but final occlusion is usually the result of thrombus, which characteristically is intensely cellular and becomes organized rapidly. Necrosis of the arterial wall does not occur; the internal elastic lamina is preserved, and aneurysm formation as the result of thromboangiitis obliterans is extremely rare.

As in arteriosclerosis obliterans, the pathophysiological abnormality in thromboangiitis obliterans is ischemia, initially of the fingers and toes as the result of obstruction of the small arteries. Since small, often end, arteries are involved, the collateral circulation is meager and often absent, accounting for the early onset of tissue necrosis.

Clinical Manifestations

Thromboangiitis obliterans affects young men and women, usually before age 40. The incidence of the disease in women appears to be increasing, probably because of the large number who now smoke, and women constitute approximately 5 to 10 percent of cases. The disease seems to have a more severe onset and more rapid course than arteriosclerosis obliterans.

The initial symptom may be intermittent claudication, which is described in detail in the previous section on arteriosclerosis obliterans. In thromboangiitis obliterans intermittent claudication most often affects the foot, usually the arch, and is characteristic enough to be considered a useful guide in the diagnosis of this disease. Claudication may also occur in the calf as well as the foot, but when it does, the disease is further advanced, and rest pain, ulceration, and gangrene are usually also present. Intermittent claudication in Buerger's disease does not occur in the thigh or hip and rarely in the hand.

Symptoms at rest in both the upper and lower extremities are early manifestations of this disease. These consist of coldness, sweating, and pain of a digit, hand, or foot. The pain is usually worse at night, causing the patient to hang the extremity down or spend the night sleeping in a chair. Ulcerations and gangrene usually start at the tip of a toe or finger (Fig. 65-3), frequently involving the nail. The pain is severe and persistent, often interfering with eating and sleeping.

Diagnosis

The history of a young man who smokes and has intermittent claudication or painful ulcers of the digits and who, on physical examination, has arterial insufficiency in the small vessels of the hands or feet usually will have the diagnosis of thromboangiitis obliterans.

Angiography will reveal normal arteries proximal

FIGURE 65-3 Ischemic ulcer on fingertip of patient with thromboangiitis obliterans.

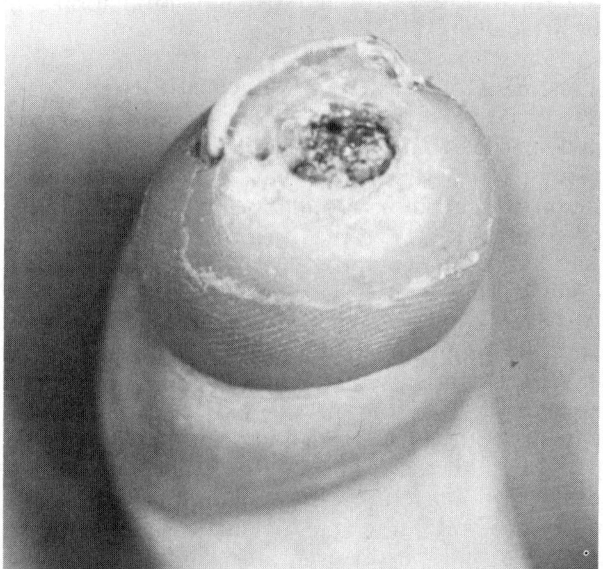

to the ankle and wrist. Early in the course of the disease segmental occlusions will be seen in the digital arteries of the toes or fingers. Between these occlusions the arteries appear normal ("skip areas"). As the disease progresses, the medium-sized arteries may become involved and are identified on the arteriogram as abrupt occlusions of an artery in the plantar or palmar arches, a tibial artery at the ankle, or radial or ulnar artery at the wrist. The collateral arteries are small, often have a corkscrew appearance, and connect the skip areas in the digits, feet, and hands. In contrast, in arteriosclerosis obliterans the arteriographic findings are usually more proximal, and with atherosclerosis the arteries are irregular with obvious diffuse involvement.

Differential Diagnosis

The disease can usually be easily differentiated from arteriosclerosis obliterans because of the typical clinical picture described previously. Not only is the patient younger, but diabetes mellitus, hyperlipemia, and atherosclerosis elsewhere are usually not present. Carotid, abdominal, and femoral bruits are not present on physical examination. When the upper extremities are involved, Raynaud's phenomenon is rarely present, and scleroderma, rheumatoid arthritis, and other collagen disease are absent on physical examination.

Acute arterial occlusion has a sudden onset in a patient with heart disease or preexisting arteriosclerosis obliterans. Emboli from atherosclerotic plaques or aneurysms occur in older persons with obvious generalized atherosclerosis or palpable aneurysms.

Prognosis

Thromboangiitis obliterans is a greater threat to limb survival than is arteriosclerosis obliterans. It presents no threat to life expectancy. The amputation rate for thromboangiitis obliterans in patients who will not stop smoking is high. If the patient stops smoking, the disease will be arrested and amputation can be avoided.

Treatment

Treatment of thromboangiitis obliterans is simple and specific; the patient should stop smoking completely and permanently. This should include cessation of cigar smoking and pipe smoking. Upon the cessation of smoking, the disease will become quiescent and no longer progress. The damage already done will not be reversed, but as the collateral circulation develops, ischemic ulcers will heal and rest pain will disappear. Depending upon the amount of arterial insufficiency, intermittent claudication of the arch of the foot may persist. Unfortunately, some patients with thromboangiitis obliterans appear to be more addicted to smoking than normal patients or those with arteriosclerosis obliterans; and despite every method known to persuade them to stop smoking, they persist even after multiple amputations (Fig. 65-4).

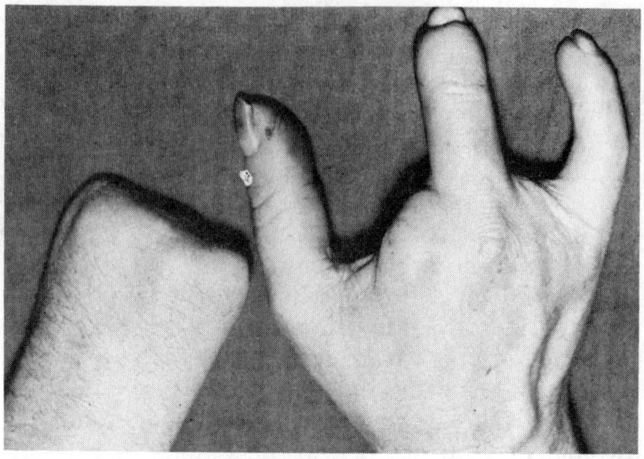

FIGURE 65-4 Upper extremities of patient with thromboangiitis obliterans who refused to stop smoking.

Patients with ischemic ulcers or gangrene should be hospitalized and placed on bed rest with the head of the bed elevated. The ulcers should be treated as described in the section on arteriosclerosis obliterans. Adequate analgesics should be prescribed because the ischemic lesions of thromboangiitis obliterans are extremely painful. Oral vasodilators are of no use. Since overactivity of the sympathetic nervous system, manifested by coldness, sweating, and cyanosis, is a prominent feature of thromboangiitis obliterans, lumbar or dorsal sympathetic blocks will relieve pain and cause warming of the extremity and are useful adjuncts to medical treatment. Sympathectomy may dramatically help the patient with severe disease who has stopped smoking permanently.

Amputation is indicated for irreversible gangrene but should be deferred, if possible, until the patient has stopped smoking, conservative measures have been instituted, and the gangrene has become well demarcated. In many cases, if the patient responds to conservative treatment, a gangrenous digit may slough spontaneously. Most often, amputations are limited to the toes, transmetatarsal segments of the foot, or fingers. In advanced cases higher amputation is necessary. In the lower extremity it should always be possible to limit the amputation to below the knee level.

Acute Arterial Occlusion of the Extremities

When a major artery to an extremity suddenly becomes occluded, survival of the patient as well as of the limb often depends on prompt and intelligent management.

Etiology

The two most common causes of sudden occlusion of a peripheral artery are embolization and thrombosis in situ. Emboli originate within the cardiac chambers in approximately 80 to 90 percent of reported cases. Rheumatic mitral valvulitis with subsequent enlargement of the left atrium, acute myocardial infarction, and chronic congestive heart failure from any cause predispose to the formation of mural thrombi within the left ventricle or left atrium, which may become detached and lodge as emboli in peripheral arteries. The presence of atrial fibrillation enhances the likelihood of formation of mural thrombus but is not an essential prerequisite. Cardiac surgical procedures, such as excision of ventricular aneurysm, valve replacement, and occasionally coronary bypass surgery, may be complicated by systemic embolism. Peripheral embolism arising from a valve or the left atrium may occur as a late complication of prosthetic valve replacement. The incidence of embolic phenomena has dropped sharply in recent years as the result of the introduction of less thrombogenic valves and the use of anticoagulants. Intriguing but rare is the paradoxical embolus, which arises from a venous thrombus and is transported to the peripheral arterial circulation through a septal defect with a right-to-left shunt. Usually one or more previous pulmonary emboli have set the stage for the paradoxical embolus by increasing the blood pressure in the pulmonary circuit and right side of the heart, thereby creating a right-to-left shunt through an otherwise asymptomatic atrial septal defect. The most common peripheral site for an embolus to lodge is the bifurcation of the common femoral artery (45 percent), followed by an iliac artery (19 percent), a popliteal artery (14 percent), the aorta (9 percent), and the axillary and brachial arteries (6 percent).[22] Unusual types of embolism sporadically reported are those of bullets, catheters, and other foreign bodies. Atheromatous debris from a diseased aorta may be responsible for the sudden appearance of small areas of cutaneous gangrene on the feet and toes.

Sudden local thrombosis in an artery usually occurs at the site of an atherosclerotic plaque. Sometimes sudden arterial thrombosis is the first clinical manifestation of peripheral atherosclerosis, but more often it occurs as an unexpected complication of symptomatic arteriosclerosis obliterans. Acute arterial thrombosis occurs occasionally as a complication of thromboangiitis obliterans, polyarteritis nodosa, polycythemia vera, lupus erythematosus, and scleroderma. Thrombosis may occur suddenly in arteries with no intimal disease, presumably because of a hypercoagulable state of the blood, resulting from such abnormal physiological states as dehydration, anemia, hypotension, stress, or stasis. This type of primary or simple arterial thrombosis may complicate acute infectious diseases, carcinomatosis, chronic ulcerative colitis, congestive heart failure, or any chronic debilitating disease.

Dissecting aneurysm of the thoracic aorta occasionally has presenting symptoms of acute arterial occlusion of one or both of the lower extremities. The rare syndrome of entrapment of the popliteal artery by the medial head of the gastrocnemius muscle, a developmental anomaly of young men, may result in popliteal artery thrombosis.[10] The anterior tibial compartment syndrome or extensive soft tissue injury to any fascial compartment can result in compression and thrombosis of the arteries contained within the compartment as the result of hemorrhage or edema.[23]

Pathology

Sudden interruption of blood flow through a major artery to an extremity results in acute ischemia of the tissues supplied by the diseased artery. If adequate collateral circulation is present, recovery without permanent residual effect is possible. In the absence of collateral circulation, however, ischemia may progress to necrosis and gangrene, with loss of a portion of the extremity.

Clinical Manifestations

Diagnosis of sudden arterial occlusion is usually correctly made in the presence of the typical clinical picture characterized by acute onset of pain, coldness, numbness, and hypesthesia of the involved extremity. In half the cases of sudden arterial occlusion, however, the onset is gradual and pain is not the initial symptom. In 25 percent of cases, pain is entirely absent and the only symptoms may be numbness and coldness. The most important physical sign in establishing the diagnosis of sudden arterial occlusion is the absence of severe impairment of pulsations in arteries that were known, or were assumed, to have had palpable pulses. The acutely ischemic extremity appears pale or cyanotic, is cold and hypesthetic, and the superficial veins are collapsed. In the latter stages muscular weakness can sometimes be demonstrated.

Once the diagnosis of sudden arterial occlusion is confirmed, it is important to determine the level of the occlusion and to differentiate, if possible, between embolus and thrombosis in situ. Emboli usually lodge at bifurcations where the caliber of the artery is suddenly reduced. The site of the occlusion is peripheral to the most distal point at which normal pulsations are noted and proximal to the line at which the temperature of the skin changes from low to normal and to the zone of hypesthesia. When sudden arterial occlusion occurs in the presence of overt heart disease, especially if atrial fibrillation is present, it is most likely due to embolization. Recent myocardial infarction should be considered in every patient with acute arterial occlusion; therefore, a careful history and an electrocardiogram should be obtained. When arterial occlusion occurs in the course of chronic occlusive arterial diseases and in the absence of overt heart disease, it can usually be attributed to thrombosis in situ. When both these predisposing factors are present or when both are absent, an exact etiological diagnosis may not be possible. Fortunately, medical therapy for the ischemic limb is the same, regardless of whether thrombosis or embolism has caused the ischemia.

Natural History and Prognosis

Without treatment acute arterial occlusion (embolism and thrombosis) results in gangrene in about 50 percent of cases.[24] Approximately 40 percent of patients with untreated sudden arterial occlusion die, because most of them are elderly and have serious cardiovascular disease.

There seems to be little doubt that since the discovery of anticoagulants and their use on a long-term basis, the prognosis is better for survival of both life and limb because recurrent thromboembolism is prevented. The introduction by Fogarty and Cranley[25] of the balloon catheter for extraction of thrombi and emboli was a revolutionary advance in surgery for acute arterial occlusion. This relatively simple procedure, which can be done under local anesthesia if necessary, has greatly increased the limb salvage rate and somewhat lowered the mortality rate, although this remains high in all current reported series.

Although prognosis for limb survival is somewhat worse when sudden arterial occlusion is caused by thrombosis than when it is caused by embolism, the site of the occlusion has an even greater bearing on the outcome. Prognosis for survival of an upper extremity is far better than that for a lower extremity,[26] and the prognosis for survival of a lower limb is worst when the aorta or common iliac artery is occluded; the prognosis becomes more favorable as the site of occlusion becomes more distal.

Treatment

Embolectomy, thromboendarterectomy, or bypass grafting is the treatment of choice if the site of occlusion is at or proximal to the popliteal artery, if the ischemia is severe, if irreversible ischemic changes have not already taken place, and if the condition of the patient is good enough to make the risks acceptable. Unfortunately, most patients with embolic arterial occlusion have serious heart disease, and the risk associated with embolectomy, even under local anesthesia, is considerable. Surgical treatment for sudden arterial occlusion may be successful even after many hours have elapsed.[26] (See Chap. 135.)

As soon as sudden arterial occlusion has been diagnosed, heparin sodium should be administered intravenously without delay, unless its use is strongly contraindicated. Even though surgical treatment is being considered, it is advisable to maintain anticoagulation therapy until shortly before the operation. If the coagulation time is unduly prolonged, the effect of heparin can be neutralized immediately before operation with protamine sulfate. For prompt anticoagulant effect, aqueous heparin should be administered intravenously (100 units per kilogram of body weight), either by intermittent injection or by continuous drip; this dose may be repeated every 4 h. It should be emphasized that anticoagulant therapy is contraindicated if sudden arterial occlusion is caused by dissecting aneurysm or by atheromatous embolization.

In addition to anticoagulation, relief of pain and of arterial spasm is an urgent consideration in the management of sudden arterial occlusion. Adequate doses of narcotics should be given as often as necessary to relieve pain. A warm environmental temperature is one of the best measures to relieve arterial spasm, so the patient should be assigned to a room where the temperature can be maintained between 26.4 and 29.4°C (80 and 85°F). In addition, it is often advisable to wrap the involved extremity loosely in cotton to preserve body heat and to protect it from trauma.

The blocking of appropriate sympathetic ganglia has been advocated in the treatment of sudden arterial occlusion. This should be done before heparin is administered and should not be repeated while effective anticoagulation therapy is being maintained because of the danger of bleeding at the sites of injection. Anticoagulation therapy is more important than regional sympathetic blocks in the management of sudden arterial occlusion, so anticoagulant drugs should not be withheld for any significant period of time.

The head of the bed should be elevated on 8- or 10-in-high blocks, so that the feet are in a dependent position and the effect of gravity will increase the flow of blood into the ischemic extremity.

Various vasodilator drugs administered intravenously or directly into the affected artery proximal to the occlusion have been advocated, but there is no evidence that they produce any lasting benefit.

The efficacy of streptokinase and urokinase in the treatment of sudden arterial occlusion is actively being studied and is most promising.[18] If these agents are to be used, they should be added to conventional anticoagulation therapy, not used instead of it. The roles of hyperbaric oxygen and of low-molecular-weight dextran (Rheomacrodex) in the management of sudden arterial occlusion have not been definitively evaluated, but it would appear that the latter holds more promise in the treatment of acute arterial occlusion than in the treatment of chronic occlusive arterial disease.

In patients with systemic arterial emboli the source should be determined because recurrence is common. Mitral stenosis and ventricular and arterial aneurysms can be surgically corrected. An attempt can be made to convert atrial fibrillation to normal sinus rhythm. When the source of embolism cannot be eliminated, the patient should receive long-term oral anticoagulation therapy in an attempt to prevent future emboli.

Peripheral and Visceral Arterial Aneurysms

Arterial aneurysms may be classified as true aneurysms, false aneurysms, and dissecting aneurysms (dissecting hematomas). Aneurysms of the thoracic and abdominal aorta and dissecting aneurysms are discussed in Chap. 64.

True Aneurysms

True aneurysms are localized dilatations of arteries that result from atrophy of the media; they may be fusiform or saccular.

Etiology

Most arterial aneurysms are arteriosclerotic. Syphilitic aneurysms have seldom been encountered since the advent of penicillin. When they do occur, they are almost always located in the ascending portion or the arch of the thoracic aorta. Mycotic aneurysms are also rare. Trauma sometimes results in true aneurysmal formation, especially in the thoracic aorta, but usually trauma causes false aneurysms rather than true aneurysms.

Clinical Manifestations

Arteriosclerotic aneurysms occur mainly in men, usually older than age 50. They are frequently multiple, so that discovery of one aneurysm should stimulate the search for others.

The most common site for peripheral aneurysms is the popliteal artery. Popliteal aneurysms produce symptoms of acute arterial occlusion if mural thrombus abruptly propagates to occlude the artery or if it gives rise to emboli distally. When popliteal aneurysms become large enough to exert pressure on the medial popliteal nerve, they also may cause pain in the popliteal region, and they will cause edema and venous distension if the popliteal vein is compressed. The diagnosis usually is made easily by palpating a pulsating, expansile mass in the popliteal space. When thrombosis of the aneurysm has occurred, a firm, nonpulsatile mass may be felt. In doubtful cases, femoral arteriography or ultrasound scanning may be helpful. Most aneurysms of the femoral artery are easily palpable just above or below the inguinal ligament. Like aneurysms of the popliteal artery, they can suddenly cause signs and symptoms of ischemia in the lower extremity because of acute thrombosis within the aneurysms or embolization of mural thrombi. Aneurysms of the iliac artery usually cause no symptoms until they rupture. Diagnosis can be made by palpating an expansile, pulsatile mass in the abdomen above the inguinal ligament. Aneurysms may also occur in the brachiocephalic (innominate), subclavian, femoral, radial, and ulnar arteries. The appearance of pulsatile masses in these regions is a clue to diagnosis.

Visceral aneurysms are rare and are usually asymptomatic until they rupture. Hypertension associated with aneurysms of the renal artery is usually mild unless there is associated occlusive disease of the renal arteries. Hematuria is sometimes the only clue to a renal artery aneurysm. The diagnosis of visceral aneurysm may be suggested by plain roentgenograms of the abdomen that show circular areas of calcification. Visceral aneurysms not containing calcium will cast no shadows on plain roentgenograms. Aortography has led to greater awareness of visceral aneurysms that sometimes are found incidentally when this procedure is done for other diagnostic purposes. Splenic and renal aneurysms are the exception to the rule that aneurysms occur predominantly in men. Trastek and his coworkers[27] reported that 87 percent of their patients with splenic artery aneurysms were women. In another study 60 percent of patients with aneurysms of the renal artery were women.[28] Microaneurysms are a consistent pathological feature of medial fibroplasia of the renal artery, which sometimes causes hypertension in young women. The triad of abdominal pain, gastrointestinal hemorrhage, and jaundice should be suggestive of the diagnosis of aneurysms of the hepatic artery. Epigastric pain (sometimes radiating to the back), nausea, and vomiting are symptoms caused by celiac artery aneurysms. The diagnosis of visceral artery aneurysms is confirmed by angiography, which is a safe procedure and should be employed whenever abdominal symptoms cannot be explained satisfactorily.

Treatment

Surgical extirpation with appropriate arterial reconstruction is the treatment of choice for most aneurysms of peripheral arteries if the patient's condition is good enough to permit operation. Splenic and renal aneurysms are particularly likely to rupture during the third trimester of pregnancy; therefore routine resection is recommended only in women of childbearing age. In others, aneurysmectomy should be considered if the aneurysm is symptomatic, if it is more than 1.5 cm in diameter, or if it is enlarging. There is insufficient knowledge of the natural history of aneurysms of the celiac and hepatic arteries to justify any statement regarding the necessity for resection of these lesions. In general, the onset of symptoms heralds the rupture of an aneurysm, and the indication for operation becomes accordingly urgent. Surgical treatment of aneurysms is discussed in Chap. 64.

False Aneurysms

False aneurysms result from rupture of true aneurysms, from penetrating trauma to an artery, or from a disruption of an arterial graft at the suture line. The clinical manifestations are similar to those of true aneurysms, consisting of an expansile, pulsatile mass. On the basis of clinical history it may be possible to suspect that an aneurysm is false rather than true, but only a pathological diagnosis can distinguish between the two. The distinguishing feature of the false aneurysm is the break in continuity of all three coats of the arterial wall, permitting the extravascular accumulation of blood in adjacent tissues. The wall of the false aneurysmal sac is therefore composed of a mixture of organized blood clot and dense connective tissue. Clinically, the diagnosis and management of false aneurysms are the same as those already described for true aneurysms.

Arteriospastic Diseases

Acrocyanosis, livedo reticularis, and Raynaud's phenomenon result from spasm of small arteries and arterioles in the skin and subcutaneous tissues without actual organic occlusion. Although they usually occur separately, two of these conditions and sometimes all three may occur concomitantly.

Etiology

The cause of arteriospasm, which is the common denominator of these three conditions, is unknown.

Clinical Manifestations

Typically, the arteriospastic disorders affect young women. The clinical manifestations are localized to the skin of the extremities and are characterized by changes in color and temperature. The location, appearance, and duration of the color changes are important in making a differential diagnosis of the arteriospastic disorders. In addition to the typical color changes of the skin, the hands and feet may be chronically cold and often tend to perspire excessively.

Acrocyanosis is the rarest and most innocuous of the arteriospastic disorders. The arteriospasm is persistent and confined to the hands or feet, or both; as a result they are chronically cyanotic. The cyanosis tends to be less severe in a warm environment, but it usually does not disappear entirely and is a source of embarrassment to the patients, who are usually young women. Major arterial pulsations are always palpable, although at times it is necessary for the patient to be in a warm environment to demonstrate them. The absence of clubbing and cyanosis elsewhere and the lack of heart murmurs and other signs of heart disease serve to distinguish this benign condition from cyanotic heart disease. The prognosis is excellent, inasmuch as gangrene and other complications of ischemia never occur.

Livedo reticularis, a common condition, is characterized by mottled or reticulated cyanotic discoloration of the skin (Fig. 65-5). Livedo reticularis not only involves the hands and feet but may extend onto the arms and legs, and, in some cases, is apparent on the buttocks and the trunk. The reticulated, or fishnet, pattern of cyanosis is more notable when the patients are in a cold environment or are emotionally upset, but it usually can be demonstrated to some degree at all times. Livedo reticularis may be primary, in which case it exists in the absence of any underlying or causative disease, or it may be secondary to such conditions as systemic lupus erythematosus, polyarteritis nodosa, cryoglobulinemia, or cholesterol embolization from an abdominal aortic aneurysm or an atherosclerotic abdominal aorta. Primary, or idiopathic, livedo reticularis infrequently leads to complications and is usually only cosmetically objectionable to the patient. Secondary, or symptomatic, livedo reticularis sometimes results in ischemic ulcerations at the tips of the digits or in the malleolar areas. The ischemic ulcerations resulting from livedo reticularis may be difficult to heal, but amputation is seldom if ever necessary.

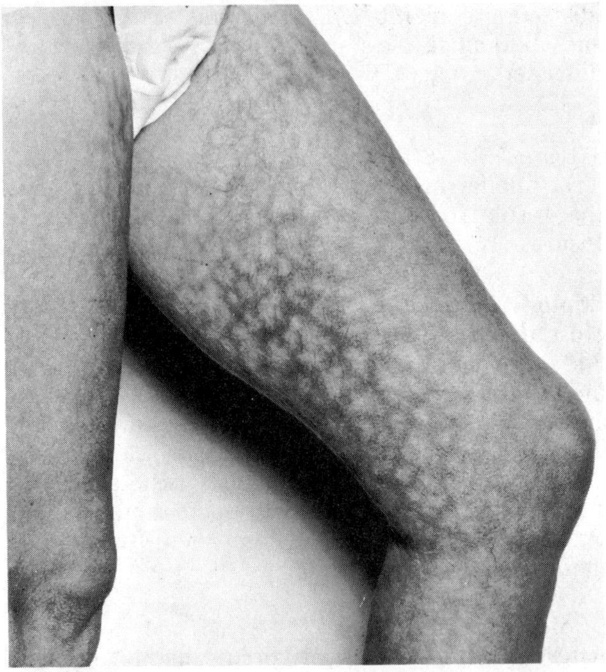

FIGURE 65-5 Mottled, reticulated cyanosis of livedo reticularis involving the thigh and to a lesser extent the leg. *(From R. W. Gifford, Jr., Arteriospastic Disorders of the Extremities, Circulation, 27:970, 1963. Reproduced with permission from the American Heart Association, Inc., and the author.)*

Raynaud's phenomenon is characterized by intermittent changes in color of the skin of the fingers or toes or both (Fig. 65-6). The change in color persists for only a few minutes at a time. Rarely is the entire hand or foot affected, and often only one or two digits at a time are involved. Typically the affected digits turn dead white (pallor phase), after which they become cyanotic (cyanotic phase). Before normal color returns to the affected parts, they may become excessively hyperemic (rubor phase) because of reactive vasodilation. Raynaud's phenomenon can occur without the rubor phase, but pallor or cyanosis or both must be present before the diagnosis of Raynaud's phenomenon is tenable. The color changes of Raynaud's phenomenon are usually induced by exposure of the affected extremity or the entire body to a cool or cold environment. The typical color changes occasionally occur when the patient is emotionally upset, and sometimes they occur for no obvious reason.

Raynaud's phenomenon is often secondary to some disease or condition that may not be clinically obvious at the time when the vasospastic phenomena

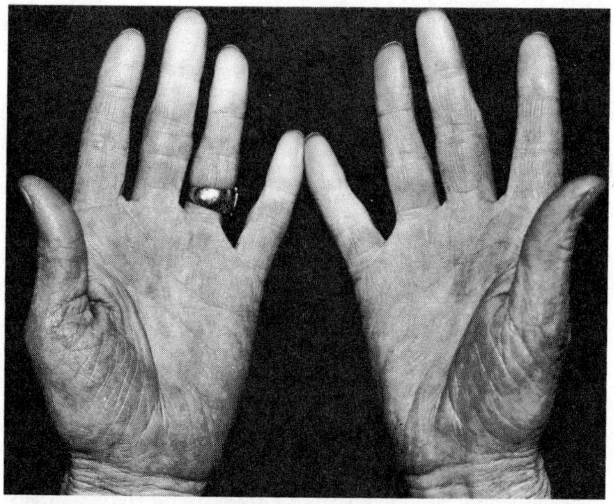

FIGURE 65-6 Pallor phase of Raynaud's phenomenon involving the fingers. (*From R. W. Gifford, Jr., Arteriospastic Disorders of the Extremities, Circulation, 27:970, 1963. Reproduced with permission from the American Heart Association, Inc., and the author.*)

first appear. Among the most common causes of secondary Raynaud's phenomenon are rheumatoid arthritis, systemic lupus erythematosus, systemic scleroderma, and the use of beta-adrenergic blocking drugs or ergotamine preparations. Other less common causes of Raynaud's phenomenon are the chronic use of grinding or vibrating tools, the late results of cold injury, thoracic outlet syndrome, arteriosclerosis obliterans, thromboangiitis obliterans, lead and arsenic intoxication, and blood abnormalities such as cryoglobulins, cold agglutinins, and macroglobulins. Indications that Raynaud's phenomenon may be secondary to some underlying disease include onset after age 50, especially in men; unilateral Raynaud's phenomenon, especially when confined to one or two digits; rapid progression to ulceration shortly after onset of symptoms; extensive ulceration or gangrene; and presence of fever, systemic symptoms, anemia, and elevated sedimentation rate.

The diagnosis of primary Raynaud's phenomenon, or *Raynaud's disease,* cannot be made until the diseases and conditions mentioned above have been excluded, and at least 2 years have elapsed since the onset of symptoms to permit any underlying disease to become manifest.

Extensive gangrene does not occur as a complication of Raynaud's disease, and major amputations are never necessary. The chief complications are sclerodactylia, which refers to sclerodermatous changes that remain confined to the skin of the digits (in contradistinction to progressive involvement of systemic scleroderma), and trophic changes, such as ulceration, superficial necrosis, scarring, and fissuring of the tips of the digits, or chronic paronychia.

The prognosis for patients with secondary Raynaud's phenomenon depends on the underlying disease and may be dismal in regard to survival and cutaneous necrosis.

Treatment

Most patients with acrocyanosis, livedo reticularis, or Raynaud's disease require no specific treatment other than reassurance that the condition is benign and will not lead to major amputation, as so many of them fear. They should be advised to avoid unnecessary exposure to cold and to wear warm clothing as well as gloves whenever they go out in cool or cold weather. Patients with Raynaud's disease should avoid mechanical and chemical trauma as much as possible. Repeated exposure of the hands to water and detergents leads to drying and fissuring of the skin. Patients with Raynaud's disease should be advised to apply am emollient such as lanolin to the fingers at least twice daily, more often if the hands are exposed to water and detergents. These precautions are not so necessary for patients with acrocyanosis and livedo reticularis, since dryness and fissuring of the skin are less likely to occur in these conditions.

Vasodilating drugs are not necessary in the routine management of any of these diseases. If symptoms are unusually severe or bothersome, nifedipine (Procardia) in doses of 10 to 20 mg three or four times daily may be helpful. Other vasodilating drugs are neither as well tolerated nor as effective as nifedipine.

Sympathectomy may be beneficial in all these conditions. Since acrocyanosis is primarily a cosmetic defect that never leads to complications, sympathectomy is seldom if ever advisable. When livedo reticularis is complicated by ischemic ulcerations, sympathectomy may be helpful in healing them and keeping them healed. Sympathectomy should be advised for patients with Raynaud's disease when conservative measures fail to prevent or to control ischemic ulcerations at the tips of the digits.

Treatment of ischemic ulcerations secondary to livedo reticularis or Raynaud's disease is similar to that already discussed for ulcerations secondary to chronic occlusive arterial disease.

References

1. Willius, F. A., and Keys, T. E.: "Cardiac Classics," The C. V. Mosby Company, St. Louis, 1941, p. 118.
2. Juergens, J. L., Spittell, J. A., Jr., and Fairbairn, J. F. II: "Allen-Barker-Hines Peripheral Vascular Diseases," 5th ed., W. B. Saunders Company, Philadelphia, 1980.
3. Hertzer, N. R., Beven, E. G., Young, J. R., et al.: Coronary Artery Disease in Peripheral Vascular Patients: A Classification of 1000 Coronary Angiograms and Results of Surgical Management, *Ann. Surg.*, 199:223, 1984.
4. Kannel, W. B., and Shurtleff, D.: The Framingham Study: Cigarettes and the Development of Intermittent Claudication, *Geriatrics*, 28:61, 1973.
5. Barnes, R. W.: Hemodynamics for the Vascular Surgeon, *Arch. Surg.*, 115:216, 1980.

6. Roenigk, H. H., and Young, J. R.: "Leg Ulcers," Harper & Row, Publishers, Inc., Hagerstown, Md., 1975, p. 265.
7. Kempczinski, R. F., and Rutherford, R. B.: Current Status of the Vascular Diagnostic Laboratory, *Adv. Surg.*, 12:1, 1978.
8. Wendt, A. J., Jr.: Peripheral Arteriography—An Overview of Its Origins and Present Status, *CRC Crit. Rev. Clin. Radiol. Nucl. Med.*, 6:369, 1975.
9. Goudreau, J. J., Creasy, J. K., Flanigan, D. P., et al.: Rational Approach to the Differentiation of Vascular and Neurogenic Claudication, *Surgery*, 84:749, 1978.
10. Iawi, T., Susumu, K., Kyoichi, S., et al.: Diagnostic and Pathological Considerations in the Popliteal Artery Entrapment Syndrome, *J. Cardiovasc. Surg.*, 24:243, 1983.
11. Imparato, A. M., Kim, G., Davidson, T., and Crowley, J. G.: Intermittent Claudication: Its Natural Course, *Surgery*, 78:795, 1975.
12. Kannel, W. B., and Shurtleff, D.: The Natural History of Arteriosclerosis Obliterans, *Cardiovasc. Clin.*, 3:37, 1971.
13. Schersten, T.: Indications and Methods of Exercise Training of Patients with Intermittent Claudication, *Pract. Cardiol.*, 8:45, 1982.
14. Coffman, J. D.: Vasodilator Drugs in Peripheral Vascular Disease, *N. Engl. J. Med.*, 300:713, 1979.
15. Bergan, J. J., Flinn, W. R., and Yao, J. S. T.: Operative Therapy of Peripheral Vascular Disease, *Prog. Cardiovasc. Dis.*, 26:273, 1984.
16. Block, P. C., Myler, R. K., Stertzer, S., and Fallon, J. T.: Morphology after Transluminal Angioplasty in Human Beings, *N. Engl. J. Med.*, 305:382, 1981.
17. Beljan, J. R., Cooper, T., Dolan, W. D., et al.: Percutaneous Transluminal Angioplasty: Council on Scientific Affairs Report, *JAMA*, 251:764, 1984.
18. Sharma, G. V. R. K., Cella, G., Parisi, A. F., and Sasahara, A. A.: Thrombolytic Therapy, *N. Engl. J. Med.*, 306:1268, 1982.
19. Risius, B., Zelch, M. C., Graor, R. A., Geisinger, M. A., Smith, J. A. M., and Piraino, D. W.: Catheter-Directed Low Dose Streptokinase Infusion: A Preliminary Experience, *Radiology*, 150:349, 1984.
20. Adar, R., Papa, M. Z., Halpern, Z., et al.: Cellular Sensitivity to Collagen in Thromboangiitis Obliterans, *N. Engl. J. Med.*, 308:1113, 1983.
21. Buerger, L.: Thromboangiitis Obliterans: A Study of the Vascular Lesions Leading to Presenile Spontaneous Gangrene, *Am. J. Med. Sci.*, 135:567, 1908.
22. Thompson, J. E., Sider, L., Raub, P. S., Austin, D. I., and Patman, R. D.: Arterial Embolectomy: A 20 Year Experience with 163 Cases, *Surgery*, 67:212, 1970.
23. Hyde, G. L., Peck, D., and Powell, D. C.: Compartment Syndromes: Early Diagnosis and a Bedside Operation, *Am. Surg.*, 49:563, 1983.
24. McKechnie, R. E., and Allen, E. V.: Sudden Occlusion of Arteries of the Extremities: A Study of 100 Cases of Embolism and Thrombosis, *Surg. Gynecol. Obstet.*, 63:231, 1936.
25. Fogarty, T. J., and Cranley, J. J.: Catheter Technic for Embolectomy, *Ann. Surg.*, 161:325, 1965.
26. Sheiner, M. S., Zelter, J., and MacIntosh, E.: Arterial Embolectomy in the Modern Era, *Can. J. Surg.*, 25:373, 1982.
27. Trastek, V. F., Pairolero, P. C., Joyce, J. W., Hollier, L. H., and Bernatz, P. E.: Splenic Artery Aneurysms, *Surgery*, 91:694, 1982.
28. Soussou, I. D., Starr, D. S., Lawrie, G. M., and Morris, Jr., G. C.: Renal Artery Aneurysm: Long-Term Relief of Renovascular Hypertension by in Situ Operative Correction, *Arch. Surg.*, 114:1410, 1979.

66

Cerebrovascular Disease and Neurological Manifestations of Heart Disease

Gary R. Kilgo, M.D.
James F. Toole, M.D.
Terence B. McGhee, M.D.

Apoplexy is a paralysis of the whole body, of sensation, of understanding and motion; wherefore to get rid of a strong attack of apoplexy is impossible, and of a weak not easy.

Aretaeus[1]

Stroke may be a devastating or even fatal event. The prognosis varies, but if the patient survives, he or she is often left with a significant deficit. Thus the emphasis of management is on stroke prevention. Controversy exists, however, as to how prevention can best be accomplished. Extensive clinical studies have elucidated the risk factors for stroke and the warning signs and symptoms of impending stroke. Modern technology has provided a variety of means by which to investigate the cardiovascular system. Still, many questions remain unanswered and often management is ultimately highly individualized.

The neurological manifestations of vascular and cardiac disease may be reflected by either focal or diffuse lesions. The ability to localize the areas of involvement in the nervous system is an important factor in diagnosis as well as in following disease progression. A knowledge of neuroanatomy and cerebrovascular anatomy in particular is indispensable in this regard. Detailed discussion of each neurovascular syndrome is beyond the scope of this chapter and the reader is referred to the various standard textbooks on the subject.

Atherosclerosis

Atherosclerosis produces neurological signs and symptoms through involvement of the arterial tree anywhere from the aorta to the intracranial vessels. In the aortocervical vessels, sites of predilection are the origins of the aortic arch vessels, the vertebral origins from the subclavian vessels, and the carotid bifurcations. Intracranially the carotid siphon, the circle of Willis, and proximal portions of the anterior, middle, and posterior cerebral arteries, along with the vertebrobasilar system, are involved most frequently and severely. Turbulence arising in bifurcations, angulations, dilatations, and tortuosities may result in injury to the intimal lining and predispose to atheromatous deposition. Cerebral symptoms may be caused by atherothrombotic occlusion of the vessel or by artery-to-artery emboli.

Neurological Manifestations

Asymptomatic Bruit

Bruits in the cervical region may be clues to the presence of atherosclerosis. They may, however, represent other processes such as turbulent flow through carotid tortuosities or referred cardiac murmurs. Furthermore, the absence of a bruit does not exclude atherosclerosis. A bruit may also reflect increased flow through one carotid system in an effort to compensate for stenosis in the opposite system. It follows that an asymptomatic bruit is a rather nonspecific finding, although not one that should be ignored. Soft, high-frequency bruits at the angle of the mandible that persist into diastole correlate with the greater degrees of stenosis.[2] With disease progression, however, the bruit may become inaudible as flows decrease.

The prevalence of asymptomatic carotid bruits is about 4 percent overall and increases with age; bruits are more common in women.[3,4] The risk of subsequent infarction compared with that in populations without bruits is increased. The location of the infarction, however, does not correlate with the location of the bruit.[5] Thus, asymptomatic bruits, when attributable to atherosclerosis, should be regarded as reflecting generalized rather than isolated vascular disease.

Transient Ischemic Attack

Transient ischemic attacks (TIAs) are episodes of focal neurological dysfunction resulting from reversible interruption of the cerebral blood flow. These attacks usually last only a few minutes; by definition they do not last more than 24 h. Symptoms produced are, of course, dependent on the part of the vascular system involved.

Prospective studies suggest that the overall incidence of stroke after TIA varies from 6 to 30 percent within a year, with the majority occurring during the first month. Carotid system TIAs are more likely to be followed by infarction than are vertebrobasilar system TIAs.

The pathogenesis of TIAs is debated. Postulated causes include (1) thromboembolism from arterial or cardiac sources, (2) intermittent local thrombosis in arteries stenosed by atherosclerosis, (3) abnormalities of blood constituents, (4) alteration of systemic blood pressure, and (5) cardiac dysrhythmias.

Intuitively it would seem that emboli should be randomly distributed with no two causing identical symptoms. This is not always the case, however, even though repeated stereotypical events probably more often represent critical local stenosis with temporary reduction of flow by either thrombosis or hemodynamic changes. The clinical distinction between embolic events and insufficiency attacks is often difficult.

Thromboembolic Cerebral Infarction

The most important precursor to atherosclerotic cerebral infarction is hypertension, and the incidence of infarction rises in proportion to blood pressure.[6] Other contributing factors include increasing age, diabetes mellitus, hyperlipidemia, hypercoagulable states, and cigarette smoking. Thrombosis is suggested clinically by stepwise progression of symptoms which build to a maximum neurological deficit. Often this occurs during the night and the patient awakens with a deficit. On the other hand, an embolism from an arterial plaque is more likely to occur when the patient is active, producing maximal effects at the onset.

Diagnostic Evaluation

Noninvasive Studies

There has been a rapid increase in the technology available for use in investigating the integrity of the cerebrovasculature. Much emphasis has been placed on being less invasive. B-mode ultrasonic scanners provide a real-time two-dimensional view of the extracranial carotid system. Image resolution may reach 0.5 to 1.0 mm.[7] Although capable of outlining even small atheromatous deposits and ulcerations with clarity, B-mode scanners are generally unable to distinguish tight stenoses from occlusions. Doppler scanning is more appropriate in this regard. Thus these two methods complement each other. These tests are often done along with phonoangiography, which provides a visual record of any bruits. All these tests give information about disease locally in the extracranial portion of the cerebral vessels. Several indirect noninvasive tests are likewise available to assess intracranial portions. Periorbital Doppler examination assesses an important anastomotic link between the external and internal carotid systems. Normally flow is out of the orbit. With significant internal carotid stenosis, flow is reversed. Likewise, ophthalmodynamometry and oculoplethysmography are indirect tests of the internal carotid system.

Computed Cranial Tomography

In TIA, computed cranial tomography (CCT) scan shows no abnormality related to the acute event. In such cases, as is true early in infarction, the CCT scan is done mostly to exclude processes which can mimic ischemic events. With infarction, the CCT scan may become positive within 48 h with the earliest signs being decreased parenchymal density and variable mass effect on adjacent structures. Over several weeks or months, the picture changes and may ultimately show focal cerebral atrophy.

Angiography

In order to demonstrate both intra- and extracranial vessels, an arteriographic study must be done. Digital subtraction angiography (DSA) by the intravenous technique is a safe, relatively noninvasive procedure which may be done on an outpatient basis. Spatial resolution is, however, inferior to that of conventional angiography. The DSA technique may also be applied intraarterially, in which case resolution is improved with the advantage of requiring a smaller load of contrast material. The best spatial resolution, however, is obtained with conventional angiography. There is risk associated with the better imaging, however; Faught and associates found a 12.2 percent complication rate using the retrofemoral approach, but most report a lower complication rate.[8] Risk factors included the number of TIAs, the number of arteries injected, and the presence of diabetes. Females had more complications than males. Not surprisingly, the greater the stenosis of a given artery the more likely it was to undergo a complication.

Nuclear Magnetic Resonance Tomography

Nuclear magnetic resonance (NMR) tomography makes use of the natural properties of charged particles to align themselves in a magnetic field and to be perturbed by radio-frequency energy pulses. Following the pulse of energy, the particles realign themselves and emit radio signals which can be reconstructed by computers to create a two-dimensional tomographic image of the brain. Advantages of NMR over CCT are the absence of x-ray exposure and improved contrast between structures. Although current clinical applications are based on proton analyses, the potential ability to study phosphate in vivo may allow one to follow metabolic changes in ischemic and infarcted brains and thus assess response to therapeutic maneuvers.

Management

Asymptomatic Atherosclerosis

Because the natural history and risk of stroke in asymptomatic bruit are unknown, there is a wide range of approaches to its management. One approach is observation. Another begins with the use of the noninvasive studies and intravenous DSA to define the vascular anatomy. For stenoses which exceed 70 percent of the cross-sectional area of the artery, hemispheric perfusion may be in jeopardy and carotid endarterectomy should be considered. The same is true for bilateral stenosis of greater than 50 percent. Stenoses of lesser degree and asymptomatic occlusions are managed medically as outlined below. Although some physicians may recommend surgery for ulcerated plaques, it may be just as reasonable to treat the asymptomatic patient with antiplatelet agents or anticoagulants and periodically repeat the noninvasive studies to see if the lesions reendothelialize with time.

If surgical intervention is planned, the intracranial portion of the cerebral vessels must be imaged to rule out tandem stenoses; if DSA is insufficient, then conventional angiography should be used. The same risk factors for endarterectomy as outlined below for TIA should be considered in the decision-making process.

Symptomatic Atherosclerosis

Transient Ischemic Attack All patients who suffer TIAs must be evaluated for hypertension, diabetes mellitus, cardiac disease, clotting abnormalities, hyperlipidemia, and erythrocytosis. Patients with definite carotid system TIAs who are surgical candidates should undergo cerebral angiography in an attempt to define the lesion responsible for the symptoms. Patients with less well-defined TIAs should be evaluated initially by noninvasive studies, and possibly DSA. A decision regarding angiography can then be made on the basis of the clinical and laboratory studies. Patients with vertebrobasilar insufficiency should undergo arteriography only when surgical intervention is anticipated or when the diagnosis is still in question.

Patients with angiographically demonstrated stenosis of greater than 70 percent or with ulcerated plaques should be considered for endarterectomy. There is no clear evidence that endarterectomy decreases the risk of stroke but it may diminish the frequency of TIAs. The most benefit is to be anticipated in patients who have a good life expectancy, who have carotid bifurcation stenosis or ulcerated plaques on the symptomatic side, and who have little disease intracranially or in the opposite carotid system.

Mortality and morbidity rates for carotid endarterectomy vary from center to center. Sundt has grouped patients according to risk factors for complications of endarterectomy.[9] Neurologically and medically stable patients have a mortality and serious morbidity rate of 1 to 2 percent when endarterectomy is performed by an experienced surgeon. Patients with major medical risks, including angina pectoris, myocardial infarction less than 6 months previously, congestive heart failure, chronic obstructive pulmonary disease, blood pressure greater than 180/110, severe obesity, or age greater than 70 years have a 7 percent risk of serious complication, primarily in the form of myocardial infarction. Patients who are unstable neurologically at the time of surgery have a 10 percent risk of subsequent morbidity, primarily in the form of cerebral infarction. Ennix found that patients with symptomatic coronary artery disease have a 22 percent mortality during endarterectomy, but when coronary artery bypass is performed before or in conjunction with endarterectomy the incidence is reduced to 3 percent.[10]

Patients who do not have surgically amenable lesions, or who have significant operative risk factors or posterior circulation TIAs, should be considered for anticoagulation therapy, provided that hypertension or other contraindications are not present. However, the evidence that anticoagulants decrease the incidence of TIAs is equivocal; this therapy neither increases survival chances nor reduces the incidence of subsequent cerebral infarction, and bleeding complications may be severe.[11]

In those patients who require long-term therapy, and for whom operation or anticoagulation therapy is contraindicated, antiplatelet therapy is indicated. Aspirin has been shown to decrease the risk of death and cerebral infarction in men, though not in women.[12] Efforts to define the dosage of aspirin which maximally reduces the platelet aggregator thromboxane without also decreasing the platelet inhibitor prostacycline are underway. Some studies suggest such a dose may be as low as 40 mg every other day.[13] Dipyridamole is commonly added to the aspirin regimen although it has not been shown conclusively to be beneficial.

Thromboembolic Infarction Treatment of cerebral infarction is mainly supportive and includes good nursing care, early ambulation, nutritional support, and prevention of complications such as aspiration, phlebitis, and decubitus ulcers. Blood pressure control is important but acutely the diastolic pressure should not be lowered below 100 mmHg for fear of increasing infarct size. Most evidence suggests that corticosteroids are not of benefit in ischemic cerebral infarction, though occasionally patients with large infarcts and signs of edema by CCT appear to improve with their use.[14] Anticoagulants are of no benefit in completed infarction but are indicated when neurological signs are fluctuating or evolving, providing hemorrhage has not occurred. The CCT is particularly effective in delineating hemorrhage. Physical and rehabilitative therapy is begun once the patient is stabilized. Life-style changes, including the institution of a low-cholesterol diet and cessation of cigarette smoking, may be helpful. Depending on the degree of deficit and general medical condition, the patient may still be a candidate for surgical intervention.

Hypertensive Cerebrovascular Disease

Hypertension is a major risk factor in cerebral vascular disease; complications include lacunar infarction, parenchymal hemorrhage, hypertensive encephalopathy, and acceleration of atherosclerosis.

Lacunar Infarction

Lacunar infarctions result from occlusions of vessels 100 to 400 μm in diameter which are the small penetrating branches of the large cerebral arteries; they are for the most part due to microatheromata and lipohyalinosis.[15] Lacunar syndromes are characterized by the relative purity of the clinical deficits they produce. At least 20 clinical syndromes have been described, but the most common are pure motor and pure sensory deficits.

Lacunar infarctions are diagnosed clinically. Because of the size of the vessel involved and lesions produced, arteriography and CCT may not be able to document their presence. NMR may be more successful than CCT.

Patients with lacunar infarctions most often improve spontaneously. Adequate blood pressure control is the mainstay of treatment. Antiplatelet agents may slow microatheromatous deposition but this is unproved.

Intracerebral Hemorrhage

The pathogenesis of hypertensive hemorrhage is related to the development of degenerative changes in the perforating arteries, notably the formation of Charcot-Bouchard microaneurysms. Certain locations are favored, most commonly the basal ganglia. In these patients there is an abrupt onset of hemiplegia, often with headache, nausea, and vomiting, with deviation of the eyes toward the side of the hemorrhage. There is often a rapid deterioration of consciousness. Second most commonly involved is the thalamus, with a similar clinical picture, except sensory components may be more prominent and the eyes may be deviated downward and toward the nose. Pontine hemorrhage constricts the pupils and the patient quickly becomes comatose. Cerebellar hemorrhage presents a variety of clinical manifestations, including severe ataxia, nausea, vomiting, and occasionally nystagmus.

CCT easily makes the diagnosis of intracranial hemorrhage. Lumbar puncture may confirm the extension into the subarachnoid space but is hazardous when intracranial pressure is elevated.

Treatment of intracranial hemorrhage consists of immediate lowering of blood pressure, mannitol and steroids to reduce edema, and surgical evacuation of accessible clots. The overall prognosis for survival is poor, but is related to the size of the hemorrhage.

Hypertensive Encephalopathy

The term *hypertensive encephalopathy* should be reserved for a specific entity seen in patients with severe hypertension who have the subacute onset of headache, convulsions, and altered mental status. The syndrome may be associated with severe hypertensive retinopathy, papilledema, and renal insufficiency. Focal neurological signs are not uncommon. These signs and symptoms probably result from widespread vascular spasm, which, in combination with fibrinoid degeneration of small arteries, lead to microinfarction and brain edema.

Lumbar puncture is hazardous in patients with hypertensive encephalopathy. Although these patients may have cerebral edema on CCT scan and diffuse slowing on EEG, hypertensive encephalopathy is more often a clinical diagnosis.

Intravenous sodium nitroprusside is often the initial drug of choice in hypertensive encephalopathy, but its use requires close monitoring.[16] The neurological deficits generally improve as blood pressure is lowered.

Other Occlusive Vascular Disorders

Vasculitis

The aortocervical vasculature can be involved in a variety of disease states which may produce neurological deficits. Takayasu's disease is an idiopathic inflammatory process causing stenosis and obstruction of the great vessels arising from the aortic arch. It occurs primarily in young females. In older individuals, temporal arteritis causes segmental narrowing of medium-sized and large arteries, and patients present with headache and visual loss. Other types of arteritis, including granulomatous arteritis, polyarteritis nodosa, and lupus arteritis may involve smaller intracranial vessels.

Mechanical Obstruction

Mechanical alteration, including coils and kinks of the internal carotid artery, can harbor thrombotic material generated by turbulent blood flow. Removal of these abnormal areas may alleviate symptoms in patients with recurrent TIAs.

Fibromuscular Dysplasia

Fibromuscular dysplasia, a nonatherosclerotic, noninflammatory idiopathic process, causes stenosis and aneurysmal dilatation of the large arteries in the neck. The entity is characteristically seen in young women who present clinically with symptoms and signs of internal carotid ischemia. Diagnosis is made arteriographically by demonstrating alternating areas of stenosis and dilatation, causing a "string-of-beads" appearance. Saphenous vein grafting and bougie recanalization of the artery can be useful.

Dissection

Neurological symptoms may be caused by spontaneous or traumatic dissections of the great vessels supplying the brain. Sometimes the preceding trauma is quite trivial. The pathological mechanism is often not clear, and even children may be affected. Arteriography reveals the classic "string sign."

Venous Occlusion

Aseptic thrombosis of a cerebral vein or sinus most often occurs postoperatively or during the postpartum period. It may follow local infection as well. There may be an associated increase in intercranial pressure, headache, localized weakness, and seizures. In general, anticoagulation therapy is not recommended.

Cerebral Embolism

Clinical Manifestations

Most studies suggest that 15 to 20 percent of all cerebral infarctions are embolic. The most common source is the heart, followed by emboli from atherothrombotic plaques in the arterial system, as discussed above. In contrast to thrombotic infarction, embolic events are abrupt in onset and tend to improve rapidly. Other clues are seizures during the acute event, multiple areas of involvement, and the demonstration of a potential embolic source. Eighty percent of emboli occur in the carotid territory, while 20 percent occur in the vertebrobasilar circulation.[17]

Causes

Valvular Heart Disease

Rheumatic Heart Disease Rheumatic heart disease most often affects the mitral and aortic valves. Mitral valve involvement correlates best with thromboembolism. Mitral stenosis alone or combined with insufficiency leads to systemic embolization in up to 20 percent of patients. Pure mitral insufficiency causes embolization in 3 percent. Associated aortic valve involvement does not affect the embolization rate.[18] Emboli tend to be more common in patients over 40 with moderate to severe valve involvement, left atrial enlargement, and atrial fibrillation. Atrial fibrillation in rheumatic heart disease increased 17-fold the risk of stroke, according to data from the Framingham Study.[19]

Mitral Valve Prolapse Mitral valve prolapse is so common that it is practically considered to be a normal variant. However, in a large series from the Mayo Clinic, 3.5 percent of these patients had histories of a prior cerebrovascular ischemic event.[20] This places the risk of stroke in this population four times that above normal subjects. Thromboembolism is postulated to be the basis for these events. Autopsied cases have confirmed thrombotic material overlying myxomatous valves, at the site of attachment of the valves to the atrial wall.

Bicuspid Aortic Valve Bicuspid aortic valve represents another common anomaly. By predisposing to endocarditis, this valvular anomaly may lead to cerebral embolism. It is also postulated that thrombotic deposits embolize in a manner similar to that occurring in mitral valve prolapse.[21]

Ischemic Heart Disease
Cerebral infarction occurs after acute myocardial infarction in about 2 percent of patients, and temporal relations suggest that the cause is embolism arising from mural thrombi adherent to infarcted endocardium. Peak incidence occurs during the first month. Patients at increased risk are those with congestive heart failure, atrial fibrillation, extremely high serum creatine kinases, and elevated plasma fibrinogen.[22,23]

In healed myocardial infarction, the relation to embolic events is less well established. In this group cerebral atherosclerosis is probably a more important cause of stroke. Ventricular aneurysm formation, however, may serve as a source for systemic embolization.[24]

Dysrhythmias
The Framingham Study has shown that chronic atrial fibrillation even without associated valvular disease increased the risk of embolic stroke almost sixfold.[19] Furthermore, in men it was found that stroke often preceded the development of chronic atrial fibrillation, suggesting that transient but undetected atrial fibrillation was present beforehand.[25] Systemic embolization may be more likely when the atrial rhythm is changing either spontaneously or through electrical or drug-induced cardioversion.

Prosthetic Valves
Prosthetic valves are important causes of embolic cerebral infarction. Turbulent flow, stasis, and injury to blood components all contribute to thrombosis, most often at the junction of the prosthesis to normal tissue. Neither the site of the new valve nor the presence of atrial fibrillation affects the incidence of thromboembolic disease; however, cloth-covered prostheses decrease the frequency of emboli, and porcine valves appear to be the least emboligenic.

Infective Endocarditis
Infective endocarditis carries a 15 to 30 percent risk of embolism.[26] Emboli are septic and can cause a variety of manifestations, the most common of which is a hemiplegic stroke. Meningitis may occur either as a septic process or as a sterile reaction to hemorrhage or parenchymal infection. Mycotic aneurysms involving the distal arterial branches may develop and ultimately bleed. Generalized vasculitis and brain abscess may occur and predispose to hemorrhage. Up to 50 percent of patients may experience confusion or even psychosis. It is unclear whether this is due to multiple cerebral emboli or to toxemia alone. Transient ischemic attacks due to microembolism are uncommon but do occur.[27]

Nonbacterial Thrombotic Endocarditis
Sterile vegetations occurring on the heart valves of patients with carcinoma result in a condition known as nonbacterial thrombotic endocarditis (NBTE). This is a recognized source of potential emboli. The most commonly associated neoplasms are lung, breast, and pancreas. The incidence of cerebral infarction is reported to be as high as 50 percent.[28] The mitral valve is most frequently involved and the middle cerebral arteries are the most often embolized. In many of these patients infarction is the cause of death. Vegetations are usually small, do not interfere with cardiac function, and, in general, do not cause cardiac murmurs. Antecedent valve disease predisposes to the development of NBTE.

Atrial Myxoma
Up to one-third of patients with left atrial myxoma will present with symptoms or signs of cerebral embolization. This may involve thrombotic material or more often tumor fragments. Cerebral embolization gives rise to a variety of clinical pictures.[29] Acute occlusion of a vessel causes cerebral infarction. Metastasis of tumor with vessel wall invasion causes either gradual vascular occlusion, aneurysm formation, or intracerebral mass lesion. Constitutional symptoms, anemia, and an elevated sedimentation rate are common.

Paradoxical Emboli
Unexplained cerebral embolism in patients with deep-vein thrombosis, particularly if temporally related to pulmonary embolism, should raise the suspicion of paradoxical embolization. Atrial and ventricular septal defects, patent ductus arteriosus, cyanotic congenital heart disease, and patent foramen ovale are possible underlying lesions.

Other Causes of Cardiogenic Emboli
Cardiac decompensation of any kind can cause pulmonary venostasis with subsequent thromboemboli which may occlude cerebral arteries. Severe cardiomyopathy may give rise to cerebral emboli when poor cardiac contractility causes stasis and intracardiac thrombosis. Cerebral emboli have been reported with Libman-Sacks endocarditis in patients with lupus erythematosis.[30]

Diagnosis
The extent to which the stroke patient is investigated for embolic disease depends on the clinical setting. Every patient should be screened for risk factors through a thorough history and physical examination, chest x-ray, and electrocardiogram. The CCT scan may suggest emboli by showing single or multiple lucencies which may be intermixed at times with areas of hemorrhage. Epileptiform discharges on electroencephalogram also suggest an embolic rather than thrombotic event. Analysis of cerebrospinal fluid in infarction due to embolism in general

is normal. In the case of septic emboli harboring highly virulent organisms, the formula is most commonly purulent and the cultures positive.[31] An aseptic or normal formula may accompany less virulent organisms. Echocardiography should be done if mitral valve disease, mural or atrial thrombi, ventricular aneurysm, or atrial myxoma is suspected. Cerebral angiography may reveal multiple filling defects, and in the case of bacterial endocarditis or atrial myxoma, peripheral aneurysm formation may be seen. Cardiac catheterization may be necessary to document an intracardiac communication. Continuous ambulatory electrocardiographic monitoring is indicated to demonstrate intermittent atrial fibrillation.

Management

In general, anticoagulation therapy with heparin should be undertaken once a probable cardiac source is demonstrated to accompany an embolic event because of the high reembolization rate during the first few weeks.[32] Heparin is withheld, however, in hemorrhagic infarction as detected by CCT or cerebrospinal fluid (CSF) analysis, native valve endocarditis, and mitral valve prolapse. Also, in patients with uncontrolled hypertension and large infarcts with massive edema, anticoagulation therapy is either not used or at least postponed. Anticoagulation therapy is not without risk but may be considered for patients with prosthetic valve endocarditis who embolize.[33] Warfarin is used for long-term anticoagulation therapy. The duration of therapy depends on the clinical setting. For example, the risk of further embolization is low 3 months after myocardial infarction, and anticoagulants may be discontinued. In chronic atrial fibrillation, however, the risk continues and, therefore, so should the anticoagulation therapy.

Treatment of endocarditis is generally medical and consists of appropriate antibiotic therapy, with care to select those drugs which achieve effective concentrations in CSF and brain tissue.[26] Multiple emboli have been suggested as an indication for surgical interventions in active endocarditis.[34] Antiplatelet agents are recommended as the initial treatment for patients with mitral valve prolapse and cerebral symptoms. Full anticoagulation therapy can be considered if symptoms persist.

The management of asymptomatic individuals who are at risk for embolization is often more controversial. It may range from attempts to prevent risk factor progression as with antimicrobial prophylaxis for rheumatic heart disease to the more directly antiembolic intervention of full anticoagulation therapy. The goal naturally is to prevent even the initial embolus without causing side effects from therapy. With myocardial infarction, anticoagulation therapy has been shown to reduce the incidence of stroke.[35] It is recommended that the patient with a large myocardial infarct, congestive heart failure, aneurysm formation, or clot on echocardiogram should undergo anticoagulation therapy. Likewise the patient with severe rheumatic heart disease with obvious mitral stenosis, enlarged left atrium, heart failure, atrial fibrillation, or atrial thrombi on echocardiogram should be treated with anticoagulants. Mild rheumatic heart disease may not warrant anticoagulants. Anticoagulation therapy also significantly lowers the embolization rate in patients with prosthetic valves.[36,37] The addition of dipyridamole to warfarin therapy may have an additional benefit.[24] Embolization rates from prosthetic valves of course depend on valve type; in general porcine valves do not require anticoagulation therapy. The risk of embolization during elective cardioversion is 1 to 2 percent and may be reduced by anticoagulation therapy for several weeks prior to the procedure. If atrial fibrillation is refractory and there are no contraindications, indefinite prophylactic anticoagulation therapy is recommended by some.

Cerebral Hypoperfusion

Manifestations

Cerebral hypoperfusion resulting from cardiac disease leads to a variety of neurological symptoms and signs. The nature of these depends on the specific cardiac impairment, duration of hypoperfusion, and presence of coexisting cerebrovascular disease. Such cerebral manifestations may be focal, diffuse, transient, or permanent. They may range from simple syncope with full recovery to anoxic encephalopathy and death.

Causes

Dysrhythmias

Investigations by Corday and Irving suggest that most cardiac dysrhythmias cause a reduction in cerebral blood flow.[38] Ventricular tachycardia causes the greatest impairment. Supraventricular tachycardia can likewise impair output with higher rates of ventricular response. Bradyarrhythmias with rates above 40 beats per minute generally cause symptoms when the patient is erect but not supine. Premature ventricular or atrial contractions, depending on their timing, are associated with smaller stroke volumes and thus if frequent may impair cardiac output. Cessation of perfusion leads to prompt symptoms; asystole causes loss of consciousness within 5 s.

Patients with arrhythmias may have symptoms of generalized cerebral insufficiency, most notably light-headedness and syncope. Sudden loss of consciousness associated with cardiac dysrhythmias is referred to as the Stokes-Adams attack. Transient focal deficits are rare in cardiac dysrhythmia; Reed and coworkers noted only four such episodes in 290 patients.[39] When focal symptoms do occur they may be secondary to a stenotic artery with relative ischemia in the area supplied by it. Serious prolonged arrhythmias may lead to hypoxic-ischemic encephalopathy and death.

Myocardial Dysfunction

Myocardial dysfunction produces cerebral manifestations by impairing contractility. In moderate cardiac decompensation, cerebral blood flow and metabolism are maintained at the expense of the systemic circulation. Nevertheless, in extreme degrees of failure, compensatory mechanisms fail and cerebral symptoms are more likely.

Valvular and Mechanical Dysfunction

Some cardiac disorders may interfere mechanically with cardiac output and secondarily decrease cerebral blood flow. Syncopal attacks and seizures are described in the course of aortic stenosis, and have been attributed to diminished cardiac output, carotid sinus hypersensitivity, or cardiac rhythm disturbance.[40] Increased peripheral blood flow during exertion in the face of a fixed cardiac output may result in decreased flow to the brain and cause symptoms. Similar cerebral symptoms, particularly syncope, are seen in other cardiac diseases with relatively fixed output, most notably idiopathic hypertrophic subaortic stenosis.

Left atrial myxoma can cause cerebral symptoms by intermittent mitral valve obstruction. Patients may present with syncope or seizures. In a similar fashion, left atrial thrombi interfere with venous return and reduce cardiac output with resulting cerebral hypoperfusion.

Other Causes of Hypoperfusion

Effort-induced syncope can be a significant diagnostic feature in primary pulmonary hypertension.[41] The exact etiology is unknown but the syncope may be due to a vasovagal reaction originating in the wall of the pulmonary artery. Syncope may also accompany pulmonary embolus, perhaps through a similar mechanism. Similarly, reflex slowing of the heart rate through a hypersensitive carotid sinus or in response to severe pain may also lead to momentary loss of consciousness. Impairment of venous return, as during the Valsalva maneuver with coughing, has on rare occasion caused syncope.

Diagnosis

The diagnostic evaluation begins with a thorough history and physical examination. Syncope due to dysrhythmia is generally sudden in onset and brief. In contradistinction to seizure disorders, there is no aura or postictal drowsiness or confusion. At times a few clonic movements of the limbs and even a generalized tonic-clonic seizure may be caused by cerebral hypoperfusion and complicate the diagnostic workup. In those patients with repeated transient symptoms, ambulatory ECG monitoring over 24 h has been shown to be of diagnostic value.[42] Certain maneuvers such as cardiac sinus massage may be undertaken in an effort to reproduce the patients' symptoms.

Focal cerebral deficits in association with hypoperfusion should lead to simultaneous investigation of the cerebral vasculature. Border territories between major vascular beds, even in absence of focal vascular disease, are subject to infarction during periods of hypoperfusion. These are known as *watershed infarctions.*

Management and Prognosis

Patients with dysrhythmias causing cerebral symptoms will benefit from either antiarrhythmic agents or a pacemaker. If the precise correlation between rhythm disturbances and symptoms cannot be made, a diagnostic-therapeutic trial of antiarrhythmic medication may be useful. Mechanical, valvular, and contractile impairments are managed according to the specifics of the clinical situation. Fixed neurological deficits are managed as outlined above for completed cerebral infarction. In general, hypoxic-ischemic encephalopathy has a dismal prognosis. Of 210 patients in one series, only 10 percent of those who presented in coma had a good recovery.[43]

Complications of Cardiac Catheterization and Surgery

Cardiac Catheterization

Central nervous system complications of cardiac catheterization for the purpose of arteriography are rare. In a large prospective study involving over 7500 patients, only 2 had cerebral events.[44] Postulated causes include embolization from thrombotic deposits on the catheter surface or on catheter-traumatized endothelium, and in situ cerebral venous thrombosis from dehydration; hypotension during the procedure has also been implicated. In the review of Dawson and Fischer only 10 cases with central nervous system complications were found, and of the embolic events, 50 percent involved the posterior circulation.[45]

Cardiac Surgery

In a review of 1669 survivors of coronary artery bypass surgery, 64 (over 3.8 percent) suffered cerebral complications which included altered mental status, stroke, and seizures.[46] Those with altered mental status consisted of a large group with self-limited delirium and a smaller group with hypoxic-metabolic encephalopathy. The latter usually was reflective of hypotension, hypoxia, stroke, aortic dissection, or air embolus intraoperatively or metabolic dysfunction postoperatively. Embolic materials generated during surgery and extracorporeal circulation include muscle, calcium, cholesterol, fibrin-platelet aggregates, silicon, and fat. Although small-pore filters have reduced most particulate emboli, fat globules still manage to pass through and embolize.

Postoperative stroke is often of unclear etiology but proposed mechanisms include embolization from vein graft anastomosis, mural thrombosis secondary to myocardial infarction, arrhythmias, and postoperative hypercoagulability.

Similar factors are present for open heart procedures. In mitral valvulotomy procedures, Geldof et al. found the incidence of cerebral embolism in patients with thrombi in the left atrium and with mitral valve calcifications to be 19 percent.[47] Without thrombi or calcified valves, the incidence of embolism is only about 2 percent. In autopsy studies of patients dying after open heart surgery, Brierly found localized cerebral disease in the majority of cases, while diffuse changes typical of cerebral anoxia were rare.[48] Resection of postinfarction ventricular aneurysm is also associated with thrombotic embolism.

Intracranial hemorrhages have been reported following cardiac surgery, usually in the form of subarachnoid bleeding or small scattered lesions. Humphreys et al. reported 16 patients with surface intracranial hematomas, and postulated that intraoperative anticoagulants, positioning of the patient's head on the table, and alterations in blood osmolality may be responsible.[49]

Cardiac transplantation is associated with many of the same complications that occur with other cardiac surgery. In addition, however, are the delayed complications, which for the most part involve infection of the nervous system with opportunistic organisms as a result of immunosuppression therapy.

Prevention of the above complications is obviously the most important form of treatment. Meticulous attention to prevention of air embolism, prompt correction of hypotension, and the addition of small-pore filters to the extracorporeal circulation can significantly reduce the incidence of complications. Cerebral function monitoring using a modified electroencephalogram is an effective means of identifying most cortical disturbances during the operative period. Once a cerebral deficit has occurred, hypothermia, sedation, and diuretic agents may prolong survival.

Congenital Heart Disease

Neurological complications occur in about 25 percent of patients with congenital heart disease.[50] In cyanotic heart disease, probably the most common symptom is episodic loss of consciousness or convulsion due to hypoxia, where rapid changes in the amount of venous blood reaching the systemic circulation are encountered. Exertion increases cyanosis and dyspnea and is followed by loss of consciousness, although it is rare that no preceding signs are noted. Convulsions are particularly common in patients with tetralogy of Fallot.

Cerebral abscess occurs if venous blood bypasses the lungs and flows directly into the systemic circulation, indicating a possible protective role of the pulmonary capillary bed in removing bacteria from the blood. Cerebral abscess is uncommon in children below 2 years of age.

Cerebral infarction, usually presenting as acute hemiplegia, is more common with transposition of the great vessels and tricuspid atresia, usually during the first year of life. In cyanotic congenital heart disease the most common cause of infarction is cerebral venous thrombosis, and many such cases occur before the age of 4.[51] Theoretical causes include hyperviscosity with polycythemia, altered red blood cell morphology, and dilatation and stagnation of cerebral vessels. In some instances probably all these factors contribute. The superior sagittal sinus is involved in the majority of cases, followed by the lateral and sigmoid sinuses. Arterial thrombus is less common, and intracardiac thrombosis does not occur.

Treatment consists of correction of hyperviscous blood by phlebotomy and volume replacement, but this provides only temporary relief. Heparin and other anticoagulants do not seem to prevent central nervous system vessel thrombotic occlusions in congenital heart disease and may be contraindicated because many venous thrombi are hemorrhagic.

References

1. McHenry, L. C., Jr.: "Garrison's History of Neurology," Charles C Thomas, Publisher, Springfield, Ill., 1969, p. 374.
2. Hurst, J. W., Hopkins, L. C., and Smith, R. B., Jr.: Noises in the Neck, *N. Engl. J. Med.*, 302:862, 1980.
3. Sandok, B. A., Whisnant, J. P., Furlan, A. J., and Mickell, J. L.: Carotid Artery Bruits: Prevalence Survey and Differential Diagnosis, *Mayo Clin. Proc.*, 57:227, 1982.
4. Wolf, P. A., Kannel, W. B., Sorlie, P., and McNamara, P.: Asymptomatic Carotid Bruit and Risk of Stroke, *JAMA*, 245:1442, 1981.
5. Heyman, A., Wilkinson, W. E., Heyden, S., et al.: Risk of Stroke in Asymptomatic Persons with Cervical Arterial Bruits, *N. Engl. J. Med.*, 302:838, 1980.
6. Wolf, P. A., Kannel, W. B., and Verter, J.: Current Status of Risk Factors for Stroke, *Neurol. Clin.*, 1:317, 1983.
7. Cebul, R. D., and Ginsberg, M. D.: Non-invasive Neurovascular Tests for Carotid Artery Disease, *Ann. Intern. Med.*, 97:867, 1982.
8. Faught, E., Trader, S. D., and Hanna, G. R.: Cerebral Complications of Angiography for Transient Ischemia and Stroke: Prediction of Risk, *Neurology*, 29:4, 1979.
9. Sundt, T. M., Jr., Sandok, B. A., and Whisnant, J. P.: Carotid Endarterectomy: Complications and Preoperative Assessment of Risk, *Mayo Clin. Proc.*, 50:301, 1975.
10. Ennix, C. L., Jr., Lawrie, G. M., Morris, G. C., et al.: Improved Results of Carotid Endarterectomy in Patients with Symptomatic Coronary Disease: An Analysis of 1546 Consecutive Carotid Operations, *Stroke*, 10:112, 1979.
11. Genton, E., Barnett, H. J. M., Fields, W. S., Gent, M., and Hoak, J. C.: Cerebral Ischemia: The Role of Thrombosis and of Antithrombotic Therapy, *Stroke*, 8:150, 1977.
12. The Canadian Cooperative Stroke Study Group: A Randomized Trial of Aspirin and Sulfinpyrazone in Threatened Stroke, *N. Engl. J. Med.*, 299:53, 1978.

13. Hanley, S. P., Bevan, J., Cockbill, S. R., and Heptinstall, S.: A Regimen For Low-Dose Aspirin?, *Br. Med J.*, 285:1299, 1982.
14. Anderson, D. C. and Crawford, R. E.: Corticosteroids in Ischemic Stroke, *Stroke*, 10:68, 1979.
15. Mohr, J. P.: Lacunes, *Stroke*, 13:3, 1982.
16. Dinsdale, H. B.: Hypertensive Encephalopathy, *Stroke*, 13:717, 1982.
17. Calkins, R. A.: Cerebral Embolism, *Arch. Intern. Med.*, 130:430, 1972.
18. Neilson, G. H., Calea, E. G., and Hassock, K. F.: Thromboembolic Complications of Mitral Valve Disease, *Aust. N.Z. J. Med.*, 8:372, 1978.
19. Wolf, P. A., Dowber, T. R., Thomas, H. E., and Kannel, W. B.: Epidemiologic Assessment of Chronic Atrial Fibrillation and Risk of Stroke: The Framingham Study, *Neurology*, 28:973, 1978.
20. Sandok, B. A., and Giuliani, E. R.: Cerebral Ischemic Events in Patients with Mitral Valve Prolapse, *Stroke*, 13:448, 1982.
21. Pleet, A. B., Massey, E. W., and Vengrow, M. E.: TIA, Stroke, and the Bicuspid Aortic Valve, *Neurology*, 31:1540, 1981.
22. Thompson, P. L., and Robinson, J. S.: Stroke After Acute Myocardial Infarction: Relation to Infarct Size, *Br. Med. J.*, 2:457, 1978.
23. Fulton, R. M., and Duckett, K.: Plasma Fibrinogen and Thromboemboli after Myocardial Infarction, *Lancet*, 2:1161, 1976.
24. Reeder, G. S., Lengyel, M., Tajik, A. J., Seward, J. B., Smith, H. C., and Danielson, G. K.: Mural Thrombus in Left Ventricular Aneurysm, *Mayo Clin. Proc.*, 56:77, 1981.
25. Kannel, W. B., Abbott, R. D., Savage, D. D., and McNamara, P. M.: Epidemiologic Features of Chronic Atrial Fibrillation: The Framingham Study, *N. Engl. J. Med.*, 306:1018, 1982.
26. Greenlee, J. E., and Mandell, G. L.: Neurologic Manifestations of Infective Endocarditis: A Review, *Stroke*, 4:958, 1973.
27. Siekert, R. G., and Jones, H. R., Jr.: Transient Cerebral Ischemic Attacks Associated with Subacute Bacterial Endocarditis, *Stroke*, 1:178, 1970.
28. Kooiker, J. C., MacLean, J. M., and Sumi, S. M.: Cerebral Embolism, Marantic Endocarditis and Cancer, *Arch. Neurol.*, 33:260, 1976.
29. Desousa, A. L., Muller, J., Campbell, R. L., Batnitsky, S., and Rankin, L.: Atrial Myxoma: A Review of the Neurological Complications, Metastases, and Recurrences, *J. Neurol. Neurosurg. Psych.*, 41:1119, 1978.
30. Fox, I. S., Spence, A. M., Wheelis, R. F., and Healey, L. A.: Cerebral Embolism in Libman-Sacks Endocarditis, *Neurology*, 30:487, 1980.
31. Pruitt, A. A., Rubin, R. H., Karchmer, A. W., and Duncan, G. W.: Neurologic Complications of Bacterial Endocarditis, *Medicine*, 57:329, 1978.
32. Easton, J. D., and Sherman, D. G.: Management of Cerebral Embolism of Cardiac Origin, *Stroke*, 11:433, 1980.
33. Wilson, W. R., Geraci, J. E., Danielson, G. K., et al.: Anticoagulation Therapy and Central Nervous System Complications in Patients with Prosthetic Valve Endocarditis, *Circulation*, 57:1004, 1978.
34. Dinubile, M. J.: Surgery in Active Endocarditis, *Ann. Intern. Med.*, 96:650, 1982.
35. Cooperative Clinical Trial: Anticoagulants in Acute Myocardial Infarction, *JAMA*, 225:724, 1973.
36. Moggio, R. A., Hammond, G. L., Stansel, H. C., and Glenn, W. W. L.: Incidence of Emboli with Cloth-Covered Starr Edwards Valve without Anticoagulation and with Varying Forms of Anticoagulation, *J. Thorac. Cardiovasc. Surg.*, 72:296, 1978.
37. Sullivan, J. M., Hanken, D. E., and Gorlin, R.: Pharmacologic Control of Thromboembolic Complications of Cardiac-Valve Replacement, *N. Engl. J. Med.*, 284:1391, 1971.
38. Corday, E., and Irving, D. W.: Effect of Cardiac Arrhythmias on the Cerebral Circulation, *Am. J. Cardiol.*, 6:803, 1960.
39. Reed, R. L., Siekert, R. G., and Meredith, J.: Rarity of Transient Focal Cerebral Ischemia in Cardiac Dysrhythmia, *JAMA*, 223:893, 1973.
40. Anderson, M. W., Kelsey, J. R., Jr., and Edwards, J. E.: Clinical and Pathological Considerations in Cases of Calcific Aortic Stenosis, *JAMA*, 149:9, 1952.
41. Dressler, W.: Effort Syncope as an Early Manifestation of Primary Pulmonary Hypertension, *Am. J. Med. Sci.*, 223:131, 1952.
42. Jonas, S., Klein, I., and Dimant, J.: Importance of Holter Monitoring in Patients with Periodic Cerebral Symptoms, *Ann. Neurol.*, 1:470, 1977.
43. Levy, D. E., Bates, D., Coronna, J. J., et al.: Prognosis in Nontraumatic Coma, *Ann. Intern. Med.*, 94:293, 1981.
44. Davis, K., Kennedy, J. W., Kemp, H. G., Jr., Judkins, M. P., Gosselin, A. J., and Killip, T.: Complications of Coronary Arteriography from the Collaborative Study of Coronary Artery Surgery, *Circulation*, 59:1105, 1979.
45. Dawson, D. M., and Fischer, E. G.: Neurologic Complications of Cardiac Catheterization, *Neurology*, 27:496, 1977.
46. Coffey, C. E., Massey, E. W., Roberts, K. B., Curtis, S., Jones, R. H., and Pryor, D. B.: Natural History of Cerebral Complications of Coronary Artery Bypass Graft Surgery, *Neurology*, 33:1416, 1983.
47. Geldof, Ch.P., Roos, J. P., and Brom, A. G.: Embolism Following Mitral Valvotomy, *Acta Cardiol. Brux*, 26:392, 1971.
48. Brierly, J. B.: Neuropathological Findings in Patients Dying after Open Heart Surgery, *Thorax*, 18:291, 1963.
49. Humphreys, R. P., Hoffman, H. J., Mustard, W. T., and Trusler, G. A.: Cerebral Hemorrhage Following Heart Surgery, *J. Neurosurg.*, 43:671, 1975.
50. Tyler, H. R., and Clark, D. B.: Cerebrovascular Accidents in Patients with Congenital Heart Disease, *Arch. Neurol. Psych.*, 77:483, 1957.
51. Cottrill, C. M., and Kaplan, S.: Cerebral Vascular Accidents in Cyanotic Congenital Heart Disease, *Am. J. Dis. Child.*, 125:484, 1973.

67

Vascular Disease of the Digestive System

W. Scott Brooks, Jr., M.D.

As occlusion of the mesenteric vessels is usually associated with heart disease or atheromatous arteries or cirrhosis of the liver, we must not expect much from operative treatment. Nevertheless, patients with symptoms of intestinal obstruction cannot be left unrelieved. We have yet much to learn about thrombosis, and there are on record a few cases in which the origin of the process could not be satisfactorily explained, and in which there was no serious complication which would make an operation unfavorable. Pilliet's theory that a bacterial inflammation in the intestine may start a thrombus in the veins is the most encouraging suggestion we have met. Possibly more cases will appear with purely local lesions. If so, this condition seems to me to offer a chance for an occasional surgical success.

J. W. Elliot, 1895[1]

More often than not, vascular disease in the digestive system presents as an emergency to an unsuspecting physician who thinks first of digestive disorders and second, if at all, of intestinal ischemia. Although occlusive mesenteric vascular disease is increasing in frequency as medical progress prolongs survival rates, intestinal ischemia still remains one of the less common disorders of the digestive system. Awareness of several clinical features should direct the physician to the timely selection of correct diagnostic studies.

Vascular diseases of the intestine may be grouped into six categories: (1) acute occlusion of a major splanchnic artery or vein, resulting in intestinal infarction; (2) nonocclusive mesenteric ischemia, often leading to infarction; (3) transient intestinal ischemic attack; (4) recurrent mesenteric ischemia due to gradual narrowing and occlusion of splanchnic arteries; (5) systemic vascular disease affecting the splanchnic vessels, which may simulate the symptoms of recurrent mesenteric ischemia; and (6) other types of vascular lesions.

Acute Occlusion of a Major Splanchnic Vessel

Superior Mesenteric Artery Occlusion

Etiology

Acute occlusion of the superior mesenteric artery is a sudden, catastrophic, usually fatal event resulting in extensive ischemia and gangrene of the intestine. The etiology of superior mesenteric artery ischemia is either thrombotic, in association with atheromatous disease of the vessel, or embolic, in association with heart failure or arrhythmia, recent arterial manipulation by catheter, or surgery. Atheromatous disease most commonly affects the origin of the superior mesenteric artery, and, for this reason, thrombosis tends to occur at this point. Arterial emboli more often lodge farther down the superior mesenteric artery as the artery narrows. Collateral circulation is available to the superior mesenteric artery through the inferior mesenteric artery or through the celiac artery. With gradual occlusion of the superior mesenteric artery, these collaterals are often able to maintain adequate blood flow to the intestine. With acute occlusion, however, these collaterals prove to be inadequate to provide blood to the extensive area supplied by the superior mesenteric artery. In addition, with thrombic disease, vessels other than the superior mesenteric artery are often involved as well. For these reasons, acute occlusion of the superior mesenteric artery by thrombosis usually results in extensive infarction of the small bowel and colon (Fig. 67-1). Ischemia secondary to embolism is also abrupt. The embolus often lodges at the level of the ileocolic artery or below, and a less extensive infarction occasionally results. Embolism has been reported following cardiac catheterization, mitral valve commissurotomy, and aortic surgery.[2] (See Fig. 67-2.)

Abnormal Physiology

Whether acute intestinal ischemia is caused by embolus or by sudden thrombosis, the lesion precipitates an extremely complex alteration of the normal physiology. Mucosal ischemia occurs initially, producing mucosal edema and hemorrhage. Later the muscularis is affected and, lastly, the peritoneal surface. Massive plasma volume depletion occurs with loss into the intestinal tract. Severe metabolic acidosis and bacterial invasion of the bowel, peritoneum, and bloodstream occur. These catastrophic events are usually seen in patients with existing serious cardiovascular disease. It is not surprising, therefore, that the survival figures have not improved significantly during the last two decades.

Clinical Manifestations

The clinical manifestations of bowel ischemia are multiple, but the presence of pain is universal. The characteristic picture is that of a restless patient in obvious distress from severe abdominal pain but with a paradoxically normal abdominal examination. This reference is found repeatedly throughout the literature and reflects the fact that mucosal ischemia precedes serosal ischemia, that is, that the pain from

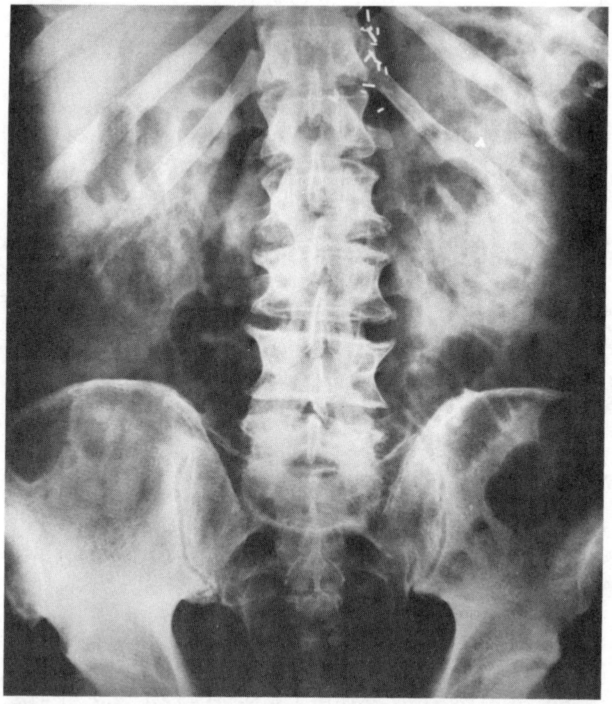

A

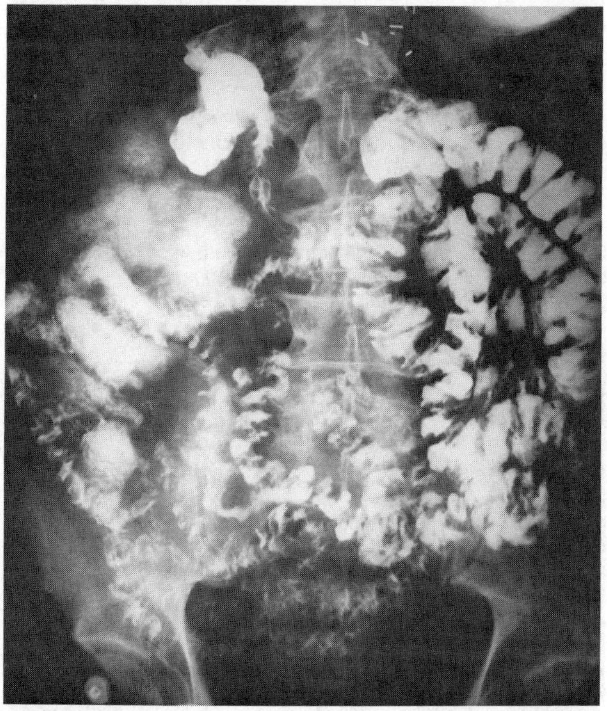

B

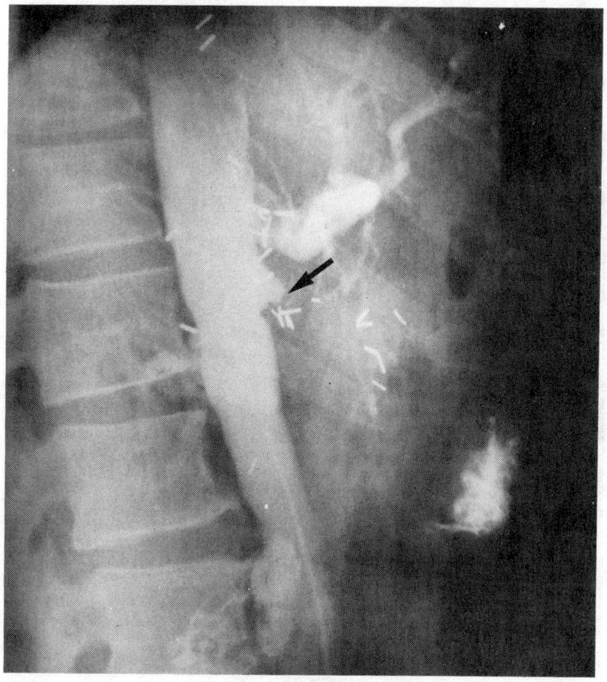

C

FIGURE 67-1 Thrombosis of superior mesenteric artery. *A.* Initial abdominal film showing multiple air-filled small bowel loops with separation of loops and thickened mucosa. *B.* Small bowel follow-through showing marked mucosal abnormality with more prominent thickening of folds, separation of bowel loops, and dilution of barium. *C.* Lateral aortogram showing acute occlusion at the ostea of the superior mesenteric arteries (arrow).

ischemia precedes clinical signs of infarction. This is a relatively unusual clinical finding and should alert the physician to the possibility of an acute vascular event in the abdomen. With other abdominal diseases, guarding, rebound, or at least abdominal tenderness are present. Surprisingly, these may all be absent in the patient with acute mesenteric ischemia. The location of the pain, however, is variable, although usually midabdominal. Occult blood may be present in the stool or in the gastric contents. Leukocytosis is usually present, as is evidence of hemoconcentration. The serum amylase is often twice normal but may not be elevated at all.

Special Laboratory Studies

Mesenteric arteriography should be utilized when a diagnosis is uncertain or if embolus is suspected. Often this will expedite the operative approach. Whether all patients with suspected occlusion should have angiography is unresolved, but most vascular surgeons feel that their approach is improved with this anatomic information available.

Management

The nonoperative management of acute occlusion of a major splanchnic vessel is uniformly fatal. Exploration is done for resection of nonviable intestine and for revascularization. The mortality rate in patients with acute mesenteric vascular occlusion from all causes is approximately 85 percent. For patients with occlusion secondary to embolus, the mortality rate is lower although only slightly. Boley and coworkers have adapted an aggressive approach to early diagnosis and treatment using intraarterial papaverine in conjunction with surgery, reducing the mortality rate to 55 percent.[3] Occasionally surgery

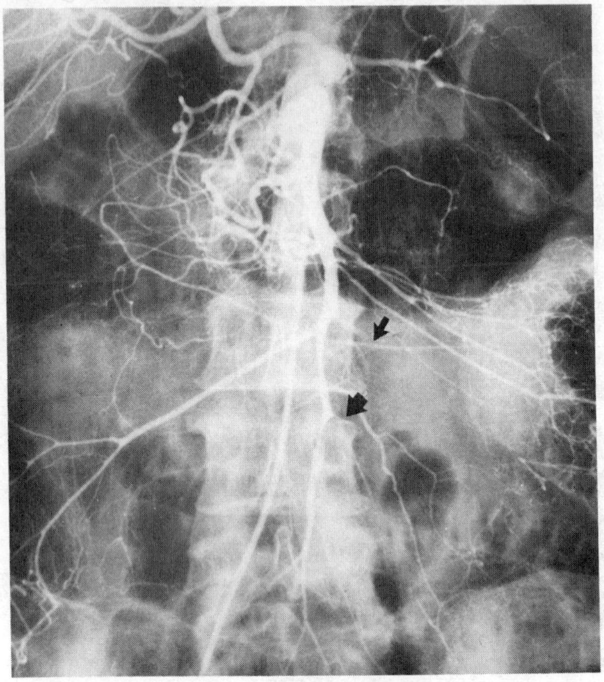

FIGURE 67-2 Embolism to the superior mesenteric artery following cardiac catheterization. This patient developed acute abdominal pain shortly after cardiac catheterization by the femoral approach. Superior mesenteric arteriogram demonstrates two areas of vascular cutoff in the distribution of the superior mesenteric artery. This patient had resection of infarcted bowel and did well postoperatively.

is not advised because of a patient's moribund condition and because the results from surgery, even in the best of circumstances, are poor.

Embolic occlusion of the celiac axis is rare. Because of efficient collateral circulation through the marginal artery, embolus to the inferior mesenteric artery usually does not result in bowel necrosis if the superior mesenteric artery is patent.

Atheromatous embolism to the smaller branches of the splanchnic arteries often causes gastrointestinal ulcerations and bleeding but may cause no significant bowel ischemia unless progressive thrombosis involves the arterial arcades, where the usually rich anastomoses exist.

Mesenteric Venous Occlusion

Mesenteric venous occlusion[4–6] may present with a clinical picture similar to that of a major arterial occlusion, with acute abdominal pain progressing to intestinal infarction. Etiologic factors include liver disease with cirrhosis and portal hypertension, polycythemia vera, migratory thrombophlebitis, antithrombin III deficiency, thrombosis secondary to intraabdominal sepsis or previous surgical procedures, thrombosis associated with oral contraceptives, and spontaneous occlusion of the superior mesenteric vein.

The abdominal pain associated with mesenteric venous occlusion tends to occur over several days, becoming progressively more severe. The distinction from arterial thrombosis must be made by angiographic criteria, indicating the absence of arterial occlusion with arterial spasm and prolongation of the arterial phase. A characteristic small bowel pattern of edematous submucosa with long transitional zones at either end has been described in venous obstruction (Fig. 67-3). Mesenteric venous thrombosis causes hemorrhagic necrosis of the intestine unless the rate of occlusion is slow enough to allow the development of adequate collaterals. Early diagnosis and resection of necrotic bowel are essential for survival in the acute case. Postoperative anticoagulation therapy is recommended.[5]

Portal Vein Occlusion

Thrombosis of the portal vein may present with acute intestinal infarction; more often thrombosis causes no acute problem but presents later as portal hypertension. Surgical ligation of the portal vein is feasible and results in transient engorgement of the intestines. The catastrophic events which may follow the sudden thrombosis of the portal vein are likely to be due to the simultaneous thrombosis of the mesenteric veins. More gradual occlusion of the portal vein results in portal hypertension alone.

Hepatic Vein Occlusion

Hepatic vein occlusion may involve either the major or the small hepatic veins. This occlusion is usually secondary to oral contraceptive agents, polycy-

FIGURE 67-3 Mesenteric venous occlusion. Abdominal film demonstrating marked separation of bowel loops with thickening of folds and haziness indicating the presence of peritoneal fluid.

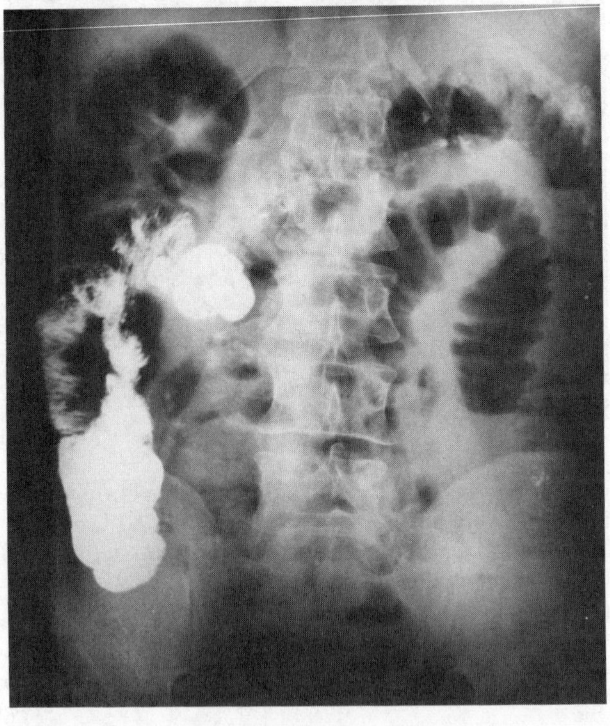

themia, infection, or tumor, but may occur spontaneously. Shock, for whatever reason, may result in massive hemorrhagic necrosis of the liver along the distribution of the efferent (central) veins.

Congestive heart failure with pressures elevated secondarily in the hepatic vein may cause jaundice. Although heart failure is associated occasionally with hepatic anoxia and centrilobular necrosis, cardiac cirrhosis is uncommon, seen only in cases of longstanding heart failure.

Nonocclusive Infarction

Intestinal infarction without recognizable vascular occlusion usually occurs as a result of hypoperfusion, particularly in the setting of acute myocardial infarction, severe congestive heart failure, or cardiac arrhythmias.[7] Digitalis, known to be a potent vasoconstrictor in the mesenteric circulation, may be an additional precipitating factor in these circumstances.

Nonocclusive mesenteric ischemia is felt to represent approximately one-third of the cases of acute intestinal infarction. Hypoperfusion initiates a number of physiological events similar to those outlined above. Bacteria invade the ischemic mucosa, resulting in a progression of the ischemic injury and a release of endotoxin. Further hypotension may result from sequestration of fluid in the intestine. Bleeding and ulceration follow the initial mucosal ischemia, but if circulation is restored recovery may be complete. Strictures may result from ischemia progressing to involve the muscular areas of the intestine.

The clinical picture of nonocclusive infarction is similar to that described above for patients with acute vascular occlusion, with pain being the predominant feature. This syndrome should be suspected in all elderly patients with congestive heart failure in whom abdominal pain appears during or after severe stress such as cardiac decompensation, myocardial or pulmonary infarction, or infection; or in debilitated patients during postoperative convalescence. If bloody diarrhea and shock develop in such a clinical setting, the diagnosis of nonocclusive ischemia must always be considered. Specific diagnosis depends on selective mesenteric angiography demonstrating the patency of both the splanchnic arteries and mesenteric veins in association with other evidence of ischemia such as radiographic changes of "thumb printing" resulting from mucosal edema.

Management of these patients is difficult because they are often poor operative risks. If peritoneal signs are present, infarction is likely. Ideally, nonocclusive ischemia should be recognized prior to this event. An attempt should be made to restore perfusion with vasodilators such as papaverine or phenoxybenzamine, or with splanchnic block in addition to correction of any existing hypovolemia. Because of the danger of circulatory overload, the left ventricular filling pressure should be constantly monitored by a Swan-Ganz catheter. Antibiotic therapy for the control of septicemia from the invading microorganisms has been recommended. In general, the nonoperative treatment is similar to that of gram-negative sepsis. If the patient is a reasonable operative risk, early laparotomy should be done with resection of gangreneous segments. Often a second-look approach is utilized to confirm viable bowel in a patient with a limited resection and questionable areas at the time of the initial operation. The mortality rate is high for this poor-risk patient group.

Transient Intestinal Ischemic Attack

Ischemic Colon Syndrome

Occlusion of branches of the *inferior mesenteric artery* results in transient ischemia of a portion of the colon (ischemic colitis). The collateral circulation usually remains adequate to maintain viability of the bowel wall, but reduction of the blood flow causes ischemic changes in the mucosa. Since the colon is rich in bacteria, such areas of mucosal ischemia are rapidly converted to areas of inflammation, necrosis, and ulceration. Ischemic colitis may be seen following inadvertent inferior mesenteric artery ligation, as a complication of a colonic obstruction secondary to carcinoma, or following aortic aneurysm surgery; it also may be seen occurring spontaneously.[8] Since changes in luminal pressure in the colon may affect colonic blood flow, minor arteriosclerotic changes in the colon vessels in association with some alteration in colonic pressure may be a precipitating factor in the ischemic event.

Typically, ischemic colitis occurs in patients over 50 years of age. The onset of symptoms is usually acute. Abdominal pain may be constant or cramping, generally localized in the lower part of the abdomen or in the left side of the abdomen. The onset of pain may be accompanied by an urge to defecate. The patient may have nausea and vomiting; often there is occult blood in the stool, or bright red blood and blood clots are passed rectally. Fever and leukocytosis are common. The splenic flexure–descending colon area is the most frequently involved portion of the colon. This portion represents the marginal area for the superior mesenteric and inferior mesenteric systems and constitutes the region most affected by systemic hypotension.

Barium enema may show a mass lesion or mucosal edema manifested by a pseudotumor or thumb printing. As the lesion progresses, it may become indistinguishable from idiopathic ulcerative colitis. Healing may lead to stricture formation.

Occlusion of the inferior mesenteric artery or one of its branches commonly occurs without intestinal infarction. Resection of the ischemic intestine may be required if signs of peritoneal inflammation develop indicating infarction. More often, the lesion is self-limited and will heal without a permanent defect; consequently immediate surgery is not required. Angiography is probably not necessary in the typical clinical setting.

Superior Mesenteric Artery Ischemia

Occasionally, superior mesenteric artery branches are involved in a transient ischemic attack and may produce a pseudotumor appearance as described above. Both embolic and thrombotic occlusions of a small branch of the mesenteric artery have been associated with ulceration of the small intestinal mucosa and subsequent stricture formation. The lesions may heal without perforation or necrosis or they may progress to stricture. It is possible that these vascular lesions are responsible for the small intestinal strictures usually attributed to enteric coated potassium chloride, for these strictures are sometimes found independent of potassium ingestion.

Recurrent Mesenteric Ischemia

The term *abdominal angina* is one well known to most physicians and readily conjures up the image of a patient with ischemic abdominal pain in response to the digestive stress of eating. The common use of this term is somewhat unfortunate (and incorrect) because angina refers to "strangling" and denotes pressure or tightness, while mesenteric ischemia often induces sharp, cramping pain. Use of nitroglycerine may be harmful. Thus, the term *recurrent mesenteric ischemia* is preferred.

Etiology

The etiology of recurrent mesenteric ischemia is commonly secondary to atheromatous disease involving the proximal superior mesenteric artery. Occasionally, tumor, particularly carcinoid tumor, can produce this syndrome.

Clinical Manifestations

The classic symptom of recurrent mesenteric ischemia is postprandial abdominal pain. This may begin soon after the completion of a meal or may be delayed as long as an hour or two. Generally the pain is poorly localized, often periumbilical, and may radiate to the back. The pain is usually intense; it may be constant and gnawing, but usually it is colicky. Some patients may also develop abdominal distension, bloating, and nausea. The pain may subside gradually within 30 to 60 min, but, more often, it lasts for several hours. There is no medication which can consistently prevent or ameliorate the pain of recurrent mesenteric ischemia. Specifically, nitroglycerine is of no therapeutic value; indeed, by reducing aortic pressure, it may be expected to decrease splanchnic perfusion even further and may accentuate bowel ischemia.

Some patients are able to control their pain by eating small amounts at a time. In most patients, however, the size of the meal is not related to the severity of their symptoms. Any solid or liquid food can precipitate pain. The food-pain sequence eventually conditions the patient to avoid eating. Consequently weight loss may become a dominant problem. It should be emphasized that the symptoms of recurrent mesenteric ischemia are not specific and vary considerably from patient to patient.

Physical examination usually shows nonspecific abdominal tenderness. The most significant diagnostic finding is a bruit heard in the epigastrium or midabdomen. The patient should be turned during auscultation because the bruit may change as the mesentery shifts. A bruit has been described in from 50 to 90 percent of the patients. It should be stressed that a bruit in the abdomen may arise from sources other than narrowing of the splanchnic arteries, or, in the case of vascular narrowing, the patient's symptoms may be due to some other cause.

Special Laboratory Studies

Measurable malabsorption may be present in 30 percent of cases and undoubtedly contributes to weight loss. This is presumably due to damage of the intestinal mucosal function and structure due to recurrent ischemia. The patient usually will not have a history of steatorrhea because the food intake is too small to permit development of this symptom. Unwillingness to eat fatty foods because of fear of pain makes the chemical determination of fecal fat excretion difficult to interpret.

Occult blood in the stool is a frequent finding. The source of gastrointestinal bleeding is not known. Conventional barium x-rays of the intestine as a rule are unremarkable.

Recurrent mesenteric ischemia is suspected on the basis of clinical findings, but the diagnosis must be correlated and the extent of the arterial disease must be defined by angiography. Aortography with lateral exposures is of aid in identifying lesions at the orifice of the vessels (see Fig. 67-4). The occlusive lesion commonly involved the ostium or the proximal 2 cm of the main arterial trunk. It may involve a proximal segment of the artery without including the orifice. When narrowing involves a longer, more distal segment, elective angiography of the suspected vessels may give superior diagnostic information. During operation, decreased or absent pulsations of the involved vessels and their branches may be easily overlooked and the correct diagnosis missed unless these arteries are deliberately palpated.

Angiographic findings should be interpreted with caution. Postprandial abdominal pain in an older patient may not be due to mesenteric ischemia, even though the angiogram shows atherosclerotic narrowing of the splenic vessels. The patient should have a complete workup to rule out the many digestive disorders which might result in postprandial abdominal pain. Significant atheromatous narrowing

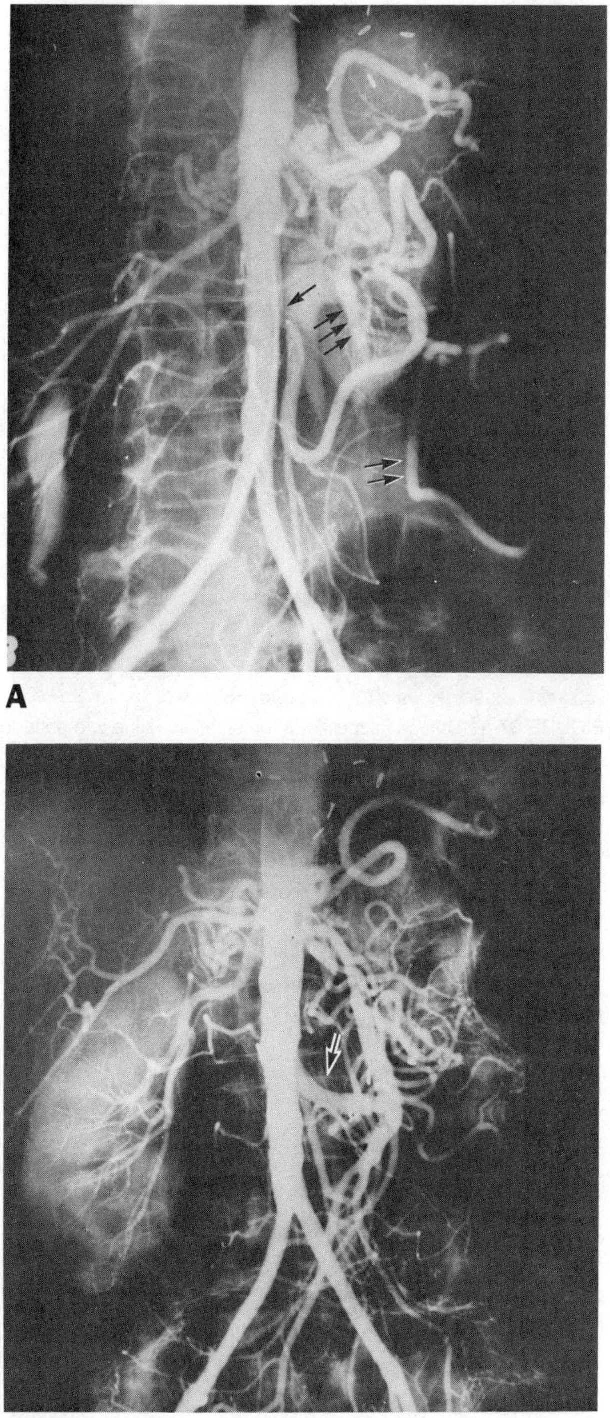

FIGURE 67-4 Recurrent mesenteric ischemia. *A.* Lateral aortogram demonstrating no flow to the liver, narrowed and more prominent inferior mesenteric artery (arrow), prominent marginal artery of Drummond (double arrow), late retrograde filling of the superior mesenteric artery through collaterals (triple arrow). *B.* Follow-up study 2 years later showing bypass graft (arrow) with good filling of the superior mesenteric artery on the initial injection and improved filling of the hepatic artery.

of the superior mesenteric artery has been reported to occur in 37 to 40 percent of unselected patients in two series of autopsies, yet the clinical syndrome of recurrent mesenteric ischemic attacks is quite uncommon. Dick and coworkers found that a reduction of the total cross-sectional area of the celiac and the superior and inferior mesenteric arteries to less than two-thirds of normal was required before symptoms of ischemia appeared.[9]

Recurrent mesenteric ischemia is usually characterized by involvement of the superior mesenteric artery with gradual occlusion. A potentially extensive collateral circulation exists between the branches of the celiac axis and the superior and inferior mesenteric arteries. Collateral circulation between these three major branches usually becomes adequate to compensate for the narrowing or occlusion of one or two of the splanchnic arteries. The potential of adequate collateral circulation is so great that both the inferior mesenteric and the celiac arteries have been ligated without incident. Therefore, narrowing or occlusion of at least two of the three major visceral vessels of the abdominal aorta is required to produce clinically significant bowel ischemia. Of interest is the patient described by Chiene in 1869, who was found at autopsy to have complete occlusion of the celiac and the superior and inferior mesenteric arteries.[10] This patient had no symptoms of mesenteric ischemia during life.

Management

Recurrent mesenteric ischemia attacks necessitate mesenteric revascularization as soon as possible, for many patients with this syndrome will experience complete mesenteric artery thrombosis and extensive infarction. Hollier and associates have emphasized the importance of complete revascularization where multiple vessels are involved, as a safeguard against future ischemia should one vessel fail again.[11] Percutaneous transabdominal angioplasty of the mesenteric arteries is also feasible for relief of mesenteric artery obstruction. Golden has reported successful angioplasty of the superior mesenteric artery in six of seven cases, but only short-term follow-up studies are available.[12]

Single Vessel Stenosis

While prevailing opinion indicates the involvement of two vessels, Bircher and coworkers reported arteriosclerotic involvement of the superior mesenteric artery alone in four patients who were successfully operated upon for recurrent mesenteric ischemia.[13]

Compression of the celiac axis by a fibrous band has been claimed to be the cause of recurrent mesenteric ischemia in numerous reports. This opinion remains controversial, however. Drapanas saw such a lesion demonstrated by angiography in 90 of 692 patients (13 percent) for a period of 4 years.[14] All these patients had causes of their symptoms other than celiac artery compression. Evans, in reviewing the follow-up of 59 patients with celiac compression syndrome, urged a skeptical and cautious approach to these patients, as long-term follow-up did not bear out the initial good results noted.[15]

One must interpret with great caution vague and unexplained abdominal symptoms associated with celiac artery stenosis. When the narrowing of the celiac axis is demonstrated by selective celiac angiography rather than lateral aortography, the appearance may be due to artifact. In addition, while the finding of an epigastric bruit often represents celiac compression, the majority of these lesions are asymptomatic.[16]

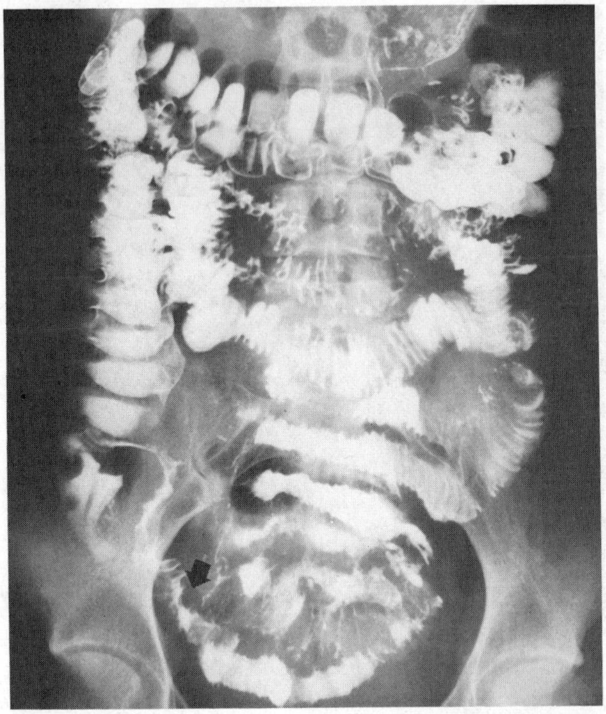

FIGURE 67-5 Diffuse vasculitis of the small intestine in a patient with lupus erythematosus. The small bowel series shows quite well the separation of bowel loops throughout the length of the small intestine, indicating thickening of the small bowel due to edema. Mucosal folds are prominent as well with thumb printing in the distal ileum (arrow).

Systemic Vascular Disease Affecting the Digestive System

The symptoms of recurrent mesenteric ischemia may be caused by involvement of the splanchnic arteries in a generalized vascular disease. The symptoms are indistinguishable from those caused by atheromatous occlusion.

Thromboangiitis Obliterans

Visceral involvement with thromboangiitis obliterans has been well documented, although this lesion may be difficult to differentiate from arteriosclerosis. The small inflammatory reaction in the ileum caused by this vascular lesion may be confused with early regional enteritis.

Periarteritis Nodosa

Periarteritis nodosa involves the gastrointestinal tract in about half the patients with this disease. The most common manifestation is abdominal pain. Indeed the splanchnic arteries may be the only ones so affected. The segmental destruction of the arteriolar wall associated with small aneurysmal dilatation and ischemia may result in focal ulcerations or, at times, perforation of the viscera. Gastrointestinal bleeding may occur, but it is rarely severe. Although involvement of branches of the hepatic or cystic artery is common, only an occasional patient develops clinical manifestations of liver disease before the terminal episode. Periarteritis may produce hepatic infarctions. In some patients with periarteritis nodosa, the hepatic lesions dominate the clinical picture; such patients are usually suspected to have primary liver disease.

Lupus Erythematosus

In patients with lupus erythematosus, small vessel involvement of the abdominal viscera may be associated with vasculitis in the bowel or in the pancreas. The peritoneum may be involved with polyserositis (Fig. 67-5).

Hypertension

Ulceration of the intestine due to necrotizing arteritis has been described in malignant hypertension.

Congenital Angiomas

The gastrointestinal tract may be involved with angiomas in either of two forms: hereditary hemorrhagic telangiectasia, with or without cutaneous or nasopharyngeal involvement, or angiomas associated with hypertrophy of one or both limbs. Osler in 1901 noted liver involvement when he first described hemorrhagic telangiectasia.[17] In some cases arteriovenous shunting may cause epigastric bruit and hepatic coma. Angiomas may be the source of occult gastrointestinal bleeding which may be severe and is often recurrent. Twenty patients who had hemorrhagic hereditary telangiectasia were evaluated by angiography. All but two had marked arteriovenous shunting within the liver; multiple arteriovenous anastomoses were demonstrated in the pancreas, spleen, small bowel, and the visceral vessels of the mesentery.[18] It seems that angiodysplasia within the abdominal viscera is a consistent and integral part of hemorrhagic hereditary telangiectasia.

Pseudoxanthoma Elasticum

Pseudoxanthoma elasticum is commonly associated with vascular lesions. These lesions occur both in the mesentery and in the pancreas and may be associated with massive gastrointestinal hemorrhage.

Amyloidosis

Vascular involvement of the abdominal viscera is more conspicuous in primary than in secondary amyloidosis. In an extensive review of primary amyloidosis, vascular involvement of the gastrointestinal tract was found in 70 percent of cases, with the liver being involved in 35 percent of the cases.[19]

Isolated Vascular Lesions

Postoperative Mesenteric Arteritis

Some patients develop necrotizing splanchnic arteritis after successful operative correction of coarctation of the aorta.[20] This process usually affects the branches of the superior mesenteric artery. In its full-blown form, arteritis leads to bowel ischemia, ulceration, and gangrene. This lesion developed most commonly in children between 8 and 12 years of age. The symptoms usually begin between the third and tenth postoperative days; if left untreated, the condition progresses rapidly to gangrene of the intestine, peritonitis, and death. This syndrome should be suspected in patients whose blood pressure begins to rise instead of decreasing to normal after surgery. The increase of diastolic pressure exceeds that of the systolic pressure, resulting in a narrowed pulse pressure. These patients have increasingly severe abdominal pain and leukocytosis. The development of the full-blown syndrome can be prevented by prompt and effective parenteral antihypertensive therapy such as intravenous sodium nitroprusside.

Angiodysplasia of the Colon

No discussion of vascular disease of the digestive system would be complete without mention of angiodysplasia. Angiodysplasia is characterized by arteriovenous lesions that develop in the elderly and may cause repeated gastrointestinal bleeding. Often it is very difficult to demonstrate these lesions with standard diagnostic techniques. These lesions have been described by a number of names in the literature, including angiomas, hemangiomas, arteriovenous malformations, and vascular ectasias. There has been good evidence to suggest that these lesions are often associated with the presence of aortic stenosis in the elderly. One such study looked at patients coming to surgery for either mitral or aortic valve disease. Patients with aortic valve disease were found more often to have a history of gastrointestinal bleeding than the patients with mitral valve disease. In addition, in 20 percent of the patients with aortic disease the source of the bleeding could not be identified.

Careful vascular inspection of resected colons by Boley et al.[22] has demonstrated vascular ectasias of the colon in 8 of 15 colons resected for carcinoma in patients over 60 years of age. This study indicates that the ectasia is a result of intermittent low-grade obstruction of the submucosal veins, apparently due to muscular contraction and distension of the cecum and right colon over the years. As a result of this obstruction, degenerative changes ultimately occur, producing ectasias. Boley et al. believe that the physiological effects of aortic stenosis do not contribute to the development of these ectasias. They suggest though, that because of low perfusion pressure and low pulse pressure, ischemic necrosis of the single layer of endothelium between the ectasia and the colon lumen may occur, accounting for the bleeding that is seen more commonly in these patients.

The majority of these lesions are located on the right side of the colon and usually present with significant hemorrhage of dark red blood. Barium studies are usually normal in this group. These lesions may be missed by colonoscopy. Arteriography remains the best single study for identification of these lesions. Occasionally transillumination of the colon may reveal these otherwise obscure lesions. Surgical resection of the involved area is indicated once these lesions are identified, as recurrent bleeding is the rule rather than the exception.

References

1. Elliot, J. W.: The Operative Relief of Gangrene of the Intestine Due to Occlusion of the Mesenteric Vessels, *Ann. Surg.*, 21:9, 1895.
2. Ottinger, L. W.: The Surgical Management of Acute Occlusion of the Superior Mesenteric Artery, *Ann. Surg.*, 188:721, 1978.
3. Boley, S. J., Feinstein, F. R., Sammartano, R., Brandt, L. J., and Sprayregen, S.: New Concepts in the Management of Emboli of the Superior Mesenteric Artery, *Surg. Gynecol. Obstet.*, 153:561, 1981.
4. Clemmett, A. R., and Chang, J.: The Radiologic Diagnosis of Spontaneous Mesenteric Venous Thrombosis, *Am. J. Dig. Dis.*, 63:209, 1975.
5. Grendall, J. H., and Ockner, R. K.: Mesenteric Venous Thrombosis, *Gastroenterology*, 82:358, 1982.
6. Skinner, D. B., Zarins, C. K., and Moossa, A. R.: Mesenteric Vascular Disease, *Am. J. Surg.*, 128:835, 1974.
7. Ottinger, L. W.: Nonocclusive Mesenteric Infarction, *Surg. Clin. North Am.*, 54:689, 1974.
8. Williams, L. F., and Wittenberg, J.: Ischemic Colitis: A Useful Clinical Diagnosis, But Is It Ischemic?, *Ann. Surg.*, 182:439, 1975.
9. Dick, A. P., Graff, R., Gregg, D. M., Peters, N., and Sarner, M.: An Arteriographic Study of Mesenteric Arterial Disease, *Gut*, 8:206, 1967.
10. Chiene, J.: Complete Obliteration of Coeliac and Mesenteric Arteries, *J. Anat. Physiol.*, 3:65, 1869.
11. Hollier, L. H., Bernatz, P. E., Pairolero, P. C., Payne, W. S., and Osmundson, P. J.: Surgical Management of Chronic Intestinal Ischemia: A Reappraisal, *Surgery*, 90:940, 1981.
12. Golden, D. A., Ring, E. J., McLean, G. K., and Freiman, D. B.: Percutaneous Transabdominal Angioplasty in Treatment of Abdominal Angina, *Am. J. Roentgenol.*, 139:247, 1982.
13. Bircher, J., Bartholomew, L. G., Cain, J. C., and Adson, M. A.: Syndrome of Intestinal Arterial Insufficiency ("Abdominal Angina"), *Arch. Intern. Med.*, 117:362, 1966.
14. Drapanas, T.: Quoted in S. A. Marable, M. F. Kaplan, F. M. Beman, and W. Molnar, Celiac Compression Syndrome, *Am. J. Surg.*, 115:101, 1968.
15. Evans, W. E.: Long-Term Evaluation of the Celiac Band Syndrome, *Surgery*, 76:867, 1974.

16. Ottinger, L. W.: Mesenteric Ischemia, *N. Engl. J. Med.*, 307:535, 1982.
17. Osler, W.: On Multiple Hemorrhagic Telangiectases with Recurring Hemorrhages, *Q. J. Med.*, 1:53, 1901.
18. Bean, W. B.: "Vascular Spiders and Related Lesions of the Skin," Charles C Thomas, Publisher, Springfield, Ill., 1958, p. 132.
19. Levine, R. A.: Amyloid Disease of the Liver, *Am. J. Med.*, 33:349, 1962.
20. Benson, W. R., and Sealy, W. C.: Arterial Necrosis Following Resection of Coarctation of Aorta, *Lab. Invest.*, 5:359, 1956.
21. McNamara, J. J., and Austen, G. G.: Gastrointestinal Bleeding Occurring in Patients with Acquired Valvular Diseases, *Arch. Surg.*, 97:538, 1968.
22. Boley, S. J., Sammartano, R., Adams, A., DiBiase, A., Kleinhaus, S., and Sprayregen, S.: On the Nature and Etiology of Vascular Ectasias of the Colon: Degenerative Lesions of Aging, *Gastroenterology*, 72:650, 1977.

68

Diseases of the Peripheral Veins and the Venae Cavae

Garland D. Perdue, Jr., M.D.   Robert B. Smith III, M.D.

Ulceration is not a direct consequence of varicosity, but of other conditions of the venous system with which varicosity is not infrequently a complication.

John Gay, 1867[1]

Descriptive knowledge of diseases of the venous side of the circulation dates at least to the time of Hippocrates. Understanding of these diseases is overshadowed by the more dramatic advances in knowledge of diseases of the heart and arteries, and the victim of venous disease benefits less from medical care than might otherwise be the case. Knowledge is available, however, to understand, recognize, and treat diseases of the veins with consistent benefit.

Anatomy

Superficial veins lie in the subcutaneous fat and receive tributaries from the dermal plexus, which coalesce to form the branches and main subcutaneous trunks. Deep veins receive tributaries from the muscle, form the paired conduits accompanying the intermediate arteries, and ultimately flow together to form larger veins which, in turn, are the tributaries of the venae cavae. The two sets of conduits in the extremities intercommunicate through connecting channels called perforators. Semilunar valves in extremity veins are profuse and function as check valves to interrupt the long hydrostatic column of blood and prevent reflux as blood is moved toward the heart. Valves are not present in veins of the trunk.

Physiology

Veins are thin-walled, collapsible, and under low pressure. Systemic veins, apart from the splanchnic system, have little sympathetic innervation and little vasomotor reactivity, though cutaneous veins do expand and contract as a part of the thermoregulatory mechanism. Inflow to systemic veins is regulated by cardiac output and, more importantly, by dilatation or contraction of the precapillary arterioles.

Venous pressure is the result of the rapidity of filling and the pressure transmitted from the arterial side. Owing to the upright posture, venous return to the heart is against gravity, but right ventricular contraction and the thoracic bellows allow a pressure gradient to exist. Veins from the muscular areas are squeezed during exercise with more rapid emptying and refilling.

Abnormal states of the systemic veins usually combine pathological and anatomical changes with disturbance of the normal venous drainage of the affected part.

Inflammatory Diseases

Severe inflammation involving vein walls is usually confined to superficial veins. Localized and often migratory areas of thrombophlebitis are occasionally seen in patients with connective tissue diseases and other causes of vasculitis, and in patients with advanced cancer. Thrombophlebitis is rarely the presenting manifestation of any of these disorders, and reflects an advanced disease state.

Perivascular inflammation may be initiated by cellulitis and lymphangitis when trauma, disruption of skin with fungal infections, or other sources of bacterial invasion are present. Secondary thrombosis within the vein may follow. Most instances of vein thrombosis have an inflammatory reaction that is sterile. Thrombosis may be initiated by external trauma or may occur spontaneously in patients with varicose veins, where stasis of blood flow contributes to the development of intravascular thrombus. Inflammation may be severe and associated with high temperature. While this causes an acute and significant illness, the thrombus and inflammatory reaction usually remain confined to the superficial vein. Noteworthy exceptions occur when the proximity of the thrombus and inflammatory reaction to the saphenofemoral junction, the saphenopopliteal junction, or to a major perforator (usually present in the thigh along Hunter's canal) may result in extension of the thrombus to the deep venous system. Spontaneous superficial thrombophlebitis occurs most often in veins about the knee level or in the calf; therefore, extension to the deep venous system is a marked exception rather than the rule.

The most frequently observed inciting trauma is the cannulation of veins for the administration of fluids and medication. Needle penetration of the vein wall and the use of indwelling catheters is less injurious than the use of thrombogenic solutions and medications infused into the vein. Septic thrombosis may occur with bacterial contamination. The longer the vein is used, the greater the incidence of thrombophlebitis. Pulmonary embolism is rare, but is more likely to occur when a catheter has been placed into a larger vein of the trunk (Fig. 68-1).

Treatment consists of removal of the cannula or catheter if present, with rest and elevation of the affected part. Application of warm compresses is felt to be symptomatically helpful by many patients. Spontaneous resolution is often slow, with persistent local induration in some patients for many weeks.

When superficial thrombophlebitis is confined to the calf or lower thigh, the patient may remain ambulatory as discomfort permits, provided external elastic support is used. Hospitalization and anticoagulant drugs are not required unless there is progressive propagation of thrombus, or occurrence in proximity to major communications with the deep venous system. The usefulness of anti-inflammatory drugs is questionable. Surgical excision of varicosities containing thrombus may be chosen in occasional instances to accomplish treatment of varicose veins and simultaneously hasten healing of the inflammatory mass. Excision may also be used, together with appropriate antibiotic therapy, to hasten resolution of septic thrombophlebitis in accessible veins.

Deep Venous Thrombosis

Intravascular thrombosis in deep veins is a serious illness which may cause death due to pulmonary embolism. It is less widely appreciated that it often produces lingering chronic disability and multiple late complications. Prevention of fatal pulmonary embolism and late disability requires understanding of causes, evolution of the disease, preventive measures, and proper treatment. Virchow's triad of stasis of blood flow, injury to vein wall, and hypercoagulability of blood remains the basis for evaluation of potential causes. It is more likely to occur in those patients whose blood is made hypercoagulable by various disease states such as dehydration, extensive soft tissue injury, and polycythemia vera. Throm-

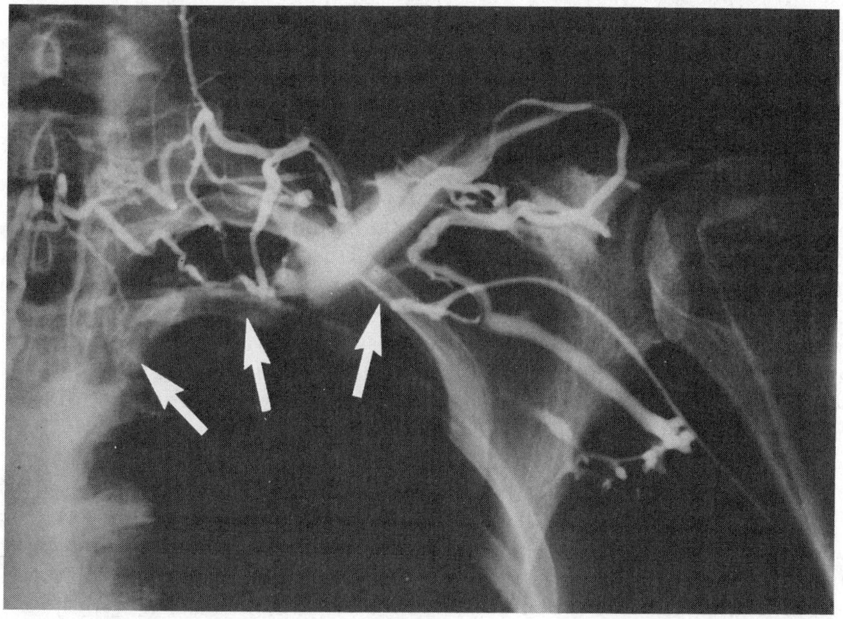

FIGURE 68-1 Catheter-induced thrombosis of left subclavian and brachiocephalic vein. Arrows indicate totally occluded venous segment. An extensive collateral network is evident in the cervical and superior mediastinal regions.

bosis may occur in the presence of extrinsic pressure on large veins and in the presence of venous anomalies. There is a definite increase in the frequency of intravenous thrombosis, thrombophlebitis, and pulmonary embolus in women taking oral contraceptives that contain estrogen.[2] The increase in frequency is about four to six times the expected frequency in the most satisfactory large studies. Since spontaneous intravenous thrombosis can occur in normal individuals not taking oral contraceptives, however, it may be difficult to prove that oral contraceptives are responsible in an individual patient.

The most frequently observed common denominator appears to be impedance to and stasis of venous drainage toward the heart. Owing to absence of valves in the veins of the trunk, hydrostatic pressure is transmitted to the veins of the lower extremity when the lower half of the body is in a dependent position. Increased pressure and diminished drainage from the lower extremity cause relative stasis in individuals immobilized from injury, surgery, or illness and may even be seen after prolonged sitting during extended travel. Because there are multiple potential causes and no single dominant cause, it is necessary to search for the most probable etiology in individual patients.[3]

Development of the thrombus tends to be insidious, and pulmonary embolism may be the first and only presenting symptom. Embolism is more likely to occur early than after the clot is well established and becomes adherent to the vein wall. (Pulmonary embolism is discussed more extensively in Chap. 54.) When the thrombus occurs in the iliac or upper femoral vein, it is often marked by sudden swelling of the entire limb because of massive outflow occlusion (Fig. 68-2). Thrombosis in any sizable vein causes venous hypertension, the development of passive congestion, and accompanying limb swelling and tenderness. As the thrombus matures, it becomes more adherent to the vein wall, but through clot retraction and lysis recanalization may follow. A tail of thrombus may propagate into the eddies of the moving bloodstream, serving as the source for pulmonary embolism, even while the thrombus undergoes organization (Fig. 68-3).

Diagnosis of deep-vein thrombosis by clinical methods is notoriously inaccurate and should not be relied upon except as a means of increasing suspicion when physical findings are positive.[4] The signs are the result of chronic passive congestion caused by the venous occlusion. Perivascular hemorrhage may occur with some inflammatory response, and muscle tissues are swollen with edema. Tenderness to direct palpation over any portion of the deep vein or to inflation of a blood pressure cuff over the calf or thigh (Lowenberg's cuff sign) are frequently present. Pain upon stretching the gastrocnemius muscle (Homan's sign) is a nonspecific finding which is sometimes present. Asymmetrical ankle edema and increase in calf or thigh circumference are the most reliable physical signs. Dilatation of superficial veins, altered skin temperature, and mottling or cyanosis of skin may be seen. Diagnosis should never be dependent on presence or absence of any of these signs; accurate diagnosis requires further assessment by noninvasive methods or phlebography.

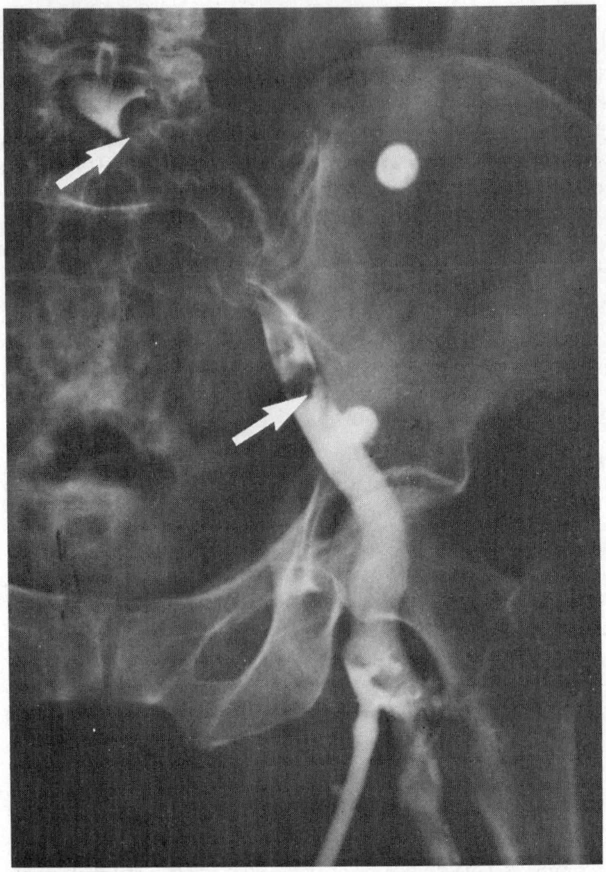

FIGURE 68-2 Left iliac vein thrombosis. Note mural filling defect (between the arrows) causing almost complete obstruction of the vein. There is also an absence of collateral drainage resulting in severe venous outflow impairment of the limb.

Doppler ultrasound may be used to demonstrate flow over the larger veins. The audible venous flow is augmented by distal compression and diminished by performance of the Valsalva maneuver, and varies with respiration. Absence of flow strongly suggests obstruction due to thrombus in one of the large veins being tested, but a mural thrombus producing incomplete obstruction may not be detected. The flow, as heard with Doppler ultrasound, may be recorded, and more sophisticated instrumentation for measurement of segmental plethysmography and calculation of venous output is available in most vascular laboratories. The combination of use of Doppler ultrasound and a segmental plethysmograph is highly accurate in indicating the presence of thrombus in larger veins.[5] Small thrombi in calf veins are less readily detected (and less likely to cause major pulmonary embolism).[6]

^{125}I-labeled human serum fibrinogen is incorporated into fresh thrombus, and a demonstrable focus of radioactivity after administration of radioac-

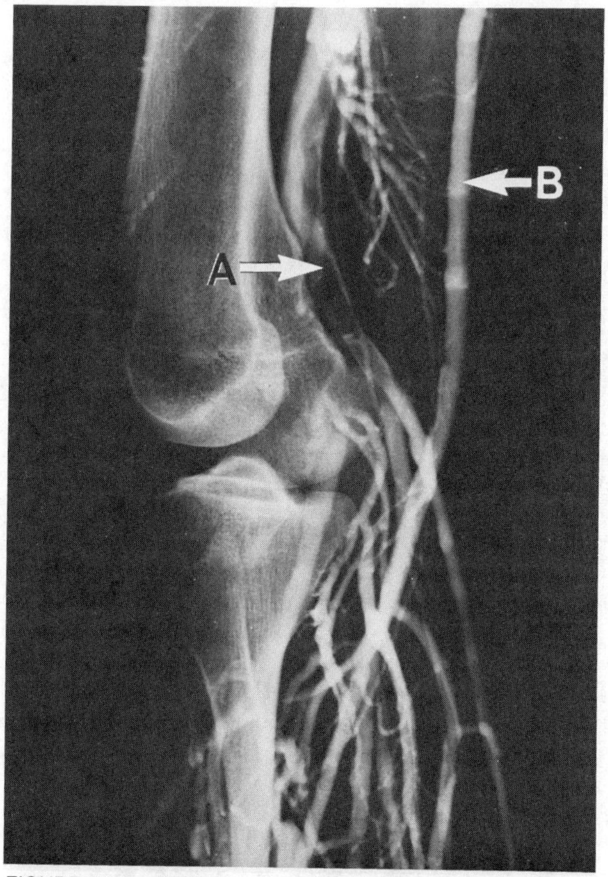

FIGURE 68-3 Occlusion of popliteal vein and propagation of a "tail of thrombus," proximally. There is an intraluminal filling defect (*A*) in popliteal vein. Note patent greater saphenous vein (*B*).

tive fibrinogen may be used to detect developing thrombi.[7] This is a useful research tool, but has little place in clinical practice. The examination is accurate over the calf and lower thigh, but less accurate over the upper thigh and trunk. Many of the thrombi detected are clinically insignificant, and, finally, the method is expensive and not practical because of the special training and experience required to implement it.

Phlebography should be done for accurate diagnosis of deep venous thrombosis when clinical suspicion is strong, screening test with Doppler ultrasound is positive, or segmental plethysmography is equivocal.[8] Complete filling of the leg and pelvic veins by percutaneous injection of contrast material into veins of the feet can be obtained. A tourniquet at the ankle should partially occlude distal superficial veins to divert contrast material into the deep venous system. Compression over the femoral vein, or a second tourniquet at the knee, can be left in position until exposure of x-ray film over the calf and, after release, x-ray films over the femoral vein can be exposed as the contrast material flows proximally. Reflux into the deep femoral and internal iliac veins, as far as the first competent valve, can be achieved if the patient performs a Valsalva maneuver. Intermittent firm pressure on the calf may improve the flow of contrast material when proximal exposure is being obtained. Occasionally it is necessary to do percutaneous puncture of femoral veins for filling of the iliac veins and venae cavae. Good visualization of the deep venous system will reveal filling defects, mural thrombi, and segments of complete occlusion. Incorrect interpretation may follow inadequate injection of contrast material or visualization of old areas of obstruction in patients with previous episodes of deep venous thrombosis. Patients who are not candidates for standard phlebography because of contrast allergy can safely undergo radioisotopic phlebography to establish the diagnosis.

When diagnosis is confirmed by phlebography, the patient should be placed on bed rest with the foot of the bed elevated approximately 30° to provide maximal gravity drainage of the lower extremities.[9] This position should be maintained until the patient is free of edema and all tenderness has subsided. At that point, limited ambulation with effective external elastic support can be begun and increased as the patient remains free of edema and tenderness. Effective external support consists of a heavyweight elastic stocking applied evenly to avoid wrinkles in areas of compression. Calf compression is probably sufficient, since attempts to compress the thigh do little to divert venous flow into the deep venous system and are often accompanied by wrinkling or rolling of the stocking, which creates a tourniquet and defeats the purpose. Several commercial stockings are available that provide a pressure of approximately 40 mmHg at the ankle level with a gradient of decreasing pressure up to the knee level.

Anticoagulant drugs are used in order to prevent additional thrombus formation or propagation of existing thrombus. Continuous intravenous infusion of heparin to maintain activated partial thromboplastin time at twice normal levels is most effective. Careful regulation of the infusion to avoid excessive anticoagulant effect diminishes hemorrhagic complications. Intermittent intravenous infusion is favored by many but is subject to inaccuracy in maintaining anticoagulant effect. Heparin therapy is best maintained until the patient is ambulatory without evidence of recurrent thrombus formation. The value of subsequent oral anticoagulation therapy with warfarin is controversial.[10] Strict laboratory control of dosage is required to maintain effective anticoagulation, and excessive variations in drug effect probably do harm. If initiated, oral anticoagulants may be used for periods up to 3 months. There is little justification for more prolonged use with inaccurate dosage control.

Streptokinase and urokinase are powerful activators for the conversion of plasminogen to plasmin, which catalyzes fibrin breakdown. The value of these drugs in enhancing natural dissolution is limited by side effects and by the fact that older thrombi become increasingly resistant to lysis.

Surgical thrombectomy is rarely needed, though

instances of impending venous gangrene caused by massive outflow occlusion may be reversed by thrombectomy.[11] Interruption of venous channels from the lower extremity may be done for prevention of pulmonary embolism. This is best reserved for those infrequent instances of recurrent pulmonary embolism occurring in spite of normal treatment measures and effective heparin therapy. Venous interruption, when required, is best accomplished by partial occlusion of the inferior vena cava. An external clip which narrows the vena cava but allows blood flow while preventing passage of thrombi can be applied. Alternatively, the placement of an intraluminal device, such as the Mobin-Uddin umbrella or the Greenfield filter, is favored by many.[12]

Partial interruption of the vena cava by any method avoids the problem of sudden decrease in venous return to the heart associated with complete ligature. Complications of operation or placement of intraluminal devices are frequent enough so that these procedures are reserved for patients in whom treatment by other methods has failed. It is particularly important to note that partial interruption by any method may be converted to complete interruption by thrombosis in situ or by migration of distal thrombi impinging on the obstructing device. Obstruction of the vena cava adds to the consequences of deep venous thrombosis in producing chronic venous hypertension.

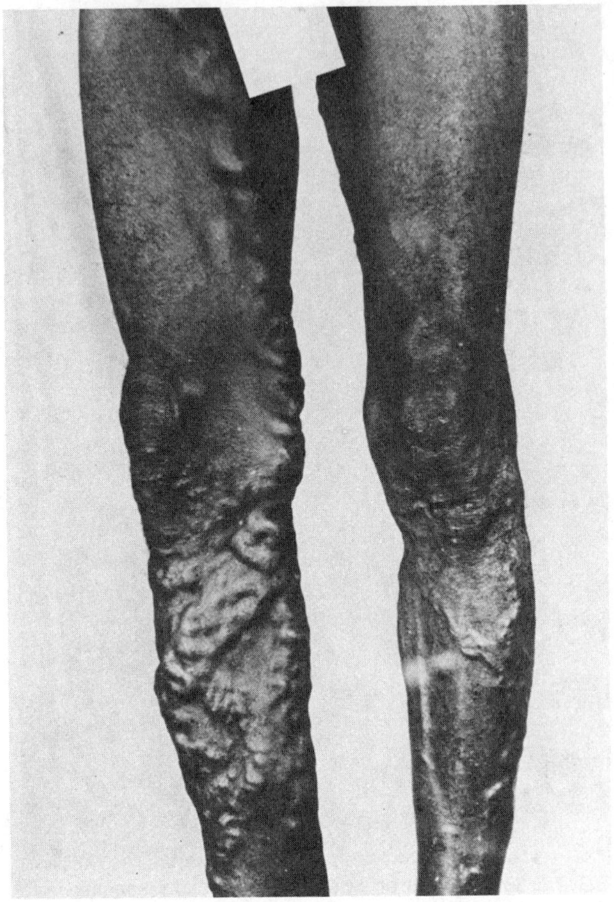

FIGURE 68-4 Severe varicose veins.

Chronic Venous Hypertension

Varicose Veins

Varicose veins are superficial veins that have become dilated and tortuous (Fig. 68-4). They contrast with the normal hypertrophy of veins seen in athletic individuals. Primary varicose veins are caused by incompetent valves in the saphenous system or in perforators connecting the saphenous and deep venous system. Secondary varicose veins are associated with incompetent valves in the deep venous system as well.

The cause of primary varicose veins is incompetence or ineffectiveness of valves at the saphenofemoral or saphenopopliteal junction and, less frequently, in one of the large perforating veins found in Hunter's canal or just above the ankle over the posterior tibial vein. Approximately two-thirds of patients give a family history that reveals varicose veins in a close relative. The hereditary defect is not known, but the common factor may be a congenital absence of one or more valves or, alternatively, primary connective tissue deficiency in which a lower collagen and elastin content is present with a corresponding increase in distensibility of the vein wall.[13] Acquired valvular incompetence may follow direct injury to the vein or local inflammatory thrombosis with fibrosis as healing occurs. Given the conditions of ineffective valves and distensibility of the vein wall, the assumption of prolonged upright posture and increases in intraabdominal and intrathoracic pressure contribute to further development. Varicose veins in women often begin during the first pregnancy. Branches of the saphenous system have less muscular tissue than the saphenous trunks; therefore, enlargement and tortuosity of dilated veins are often more apparent in primary branches than in the saphenous trunk itself.

Symptoms of varicose veins include cosmetic disfigurement, aching pain in the leg noted especially with prolonged dependency, and sometimes such paresthetic sensations as stinging, burning, or crawling localized to a particular varix. Many patients are asymptomatic, and severe pain is almost invariably the result of another cause.

Postcapillary venous dilatation is a type of intradermal varix marked by a flare or starburst radiation of branch veins from a central point in the skin. The condition is harmless, though distressing because of paresthesia and cosmetic disfigurement.

Varicose veins are usually visible and diagnosis is straightforward. Dilated veins are readily emptied by palpation and "stripping" the vein toward the heart, or by elevation of the limb above the heart. Rapid reflux filling is demonstrated when the emptied vein is replaced in the dependent position. The point of origin of reflux is usually at the orifice of the long or short saphenous trunk, but occasionally over a perforating vein in Hunter's canal or in the lower third of the leg. Ballottement of the proximal part of the vein causes a palpable or audible thrust over the distal vein. The short saphenous vein is subfascial through much of its course, and valvular incompetence is less readily demonstrated by inspection and palpation. The Doppler instrument is useful in demonstrating reflux in this instance. Branch veins of the long or short saphenous trunk are frequently those most readily visible, but it is important to recognize that these are almost invariably associated with an incompetent proximal valve present in the saphenous trunk itself.

Complications of varicose veins are infrequent. Spontaneous external hemorrhage is rare, but may occur in long-standing varices covered by thin, atrophic skin. More often, small hemorrhages or ecchymoses may occur in the subcutaneous tissues. Superficial thrombosis can occur with varying degrees of inflammatory reaction, and occasionally a type of dermatitis characterized by dry, scaly, itching skin over cuticular and subcuticular venules is seen. Excessive use of medicated creams and ointments may cause superimposed, atopic dermatitis. Intractable ulceration is rare, unless associated with deep venous hypertension as well.

Lightweight external elastic support may give some relief of symptoms and cover up cosmetic disfigurement. The most effective treatment is stripping of the involved saphenous trunk and major dilated tributaries.[14] After stripping, residual branch veins are effectively obliterated by injection of a sclerosing agent.[15] Results of surgical treatment are generally quite satisfactory, though some patients require additional ligations or periodic sclerotherapy for optimum cosmetic results. Intradermal varices are not readily eliminated by any method. Large, conspicuous ones may be made somewhat less conspicuous by injection of sclerosing solutions or electrodesiccation.

Deep Venous Hypertension

In many instances of deep venous thrombosis, clot retraction and fibrinolysis allow recanalization and complete dissolution of the thrombus. Residual thrombus becomes adherent to the vein wall and organizes with healing by fibrosis. Recanalization is rarely complete, and persistent areas of segmental occlusion are often present. Moreover, fibrosis of the vein wall is often adjacent to or involves a venous valve. Incompetence of a valve is functionally more important in causing venous hypertension than segmental occlusion, since increased hydrostatic pressure impedes venous flow more severely than diminution of the caliber of the venous outflow tract. Impairment of venous drainage of the dependent limb and resulting venous hypertension cause insidious development of late disability, which may become severe only after years of patient or physician inattention.

Ideal management of deep venous thrombosis requires elimination of edema during early treatment and continuing efforts to prevent recurrence thereafter. Edema is the visible symptom and physical finding indicating inadequate control of venous hypertension. Treatment begins with prophylaxis. Patients having had deep venous thrombosis should be carefully educated as to the nature and importance of their problem and the means of control. A way of life which stresses avoidance of venous stasis and the patient's role in prevention of edema should be carefully explained.

The consequences of uncontrolled deep venous hypertension include chronic venous engorgement, often visible in the cuticular capillary network in the region of the ankle. This is accompanied by lymphedema, which worsens during the hours of limb dependency and improves during rest with the limb in the horizontal or elevated position. Venous engorgement may cause petechial hemorrhages in the dermis or subcutaneous fat. An inflammatory reaction follows that often includes subcutaneous fat necrosis. As healing occurs, fibrosis in the subcutaneous fat and dermis causes thickening of skin, fixation to underlying fatty tissues, loss of skin appendages in the affected area, and development of pigmentation from hemosiderin (Fig. 68-5). The scarring results in impaired nutrition of the skin by impedance of flow in the dermal arterioles. Minor trauma or spontaneous disruption of skin continuity may lead to spreading tissue necrosis and a chronic venous ulcer (Fig. 68-6). The sites of predilection for venous ulcers are those areas where perforating veins are present, especially above the medial malleolus where perforating communications between the posterior tibial and superficial veins are especially prominent. Sustained deep venous hypertension causes valves in the perforating veins to become incompetent, with reversal of flow and extreme venous engorgement. The calf muscle pump becomes ineffective, owing to "leakage" of blood by reflux out of these perforating veins.

Clinical diagnosis is based on the presence of chronic lymphedema and characteristic skin changes of pigmentation, induration, and loss of skin appendages in the affected area. A history of lymphedema for several years following an episode of probable thrombophlebitis is usually given. Incompetent perforators are often palpable, and reflux may be detected with Doppler ultrasound. Similarly, loss of valves in the deep veins is demonstrated by audible reflux. Secondary varicose veins may be present, but they are often absent. Segmental plethysmography may demonstrate impairment of venous output from an extremity, and phlebography outlines the anatomical characteristics.

When there is appropriate treatment from the beginning of postphlebitic care, most complications can be avoided in all but rare exceptions. All too

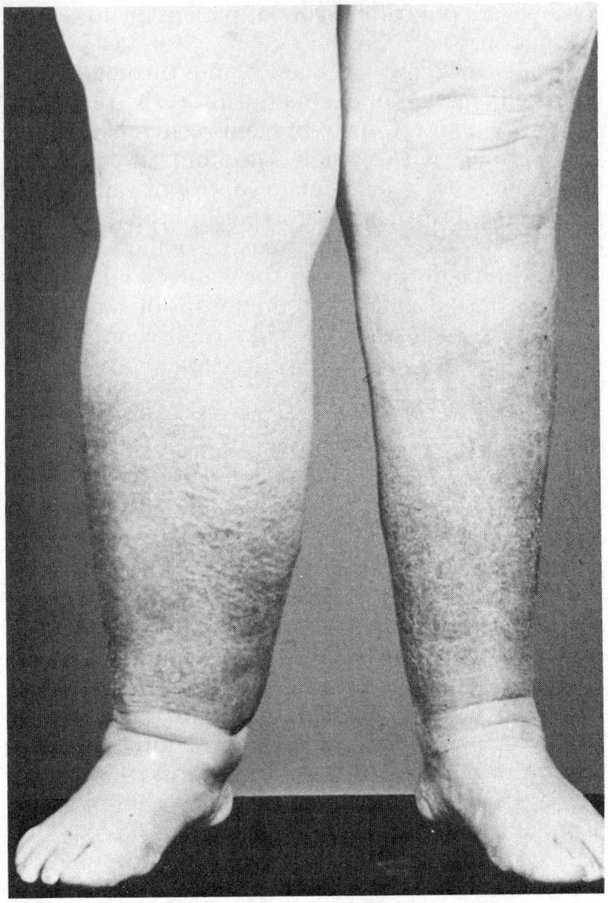

FIGURE 68-5 Edema, hyperpigmentation, and scaling dermatitis in a patient having bilateral deep venous hypertension due to previous iliofemoral thromboses.

often an intervening period of inattention to the problem of lymphedema occurs, and the patient is seen with advanced changes that are not reversible. In many instances, venous ulceration is already present.[16] Both prophylaxis and therapy, however, require inclusion of the following methods. Patients having lymphedema should sleep with the foot of the bed elevated approximately 30° to accomplish nocturnal gravity drainage. Frequent interruption of prolonged periods of limb dependency should be stressed, and sufficient periods of gravity drainage during the day should be identified to minimize lymphedema. Effective external elastic support should be prescribed. A pressure of at least 40 mmHg at the ankle impedes reflux through perforators. Longer-length stockings are difficult to fit properly, patient acceptance is poor, and the extra length serves little useful purpose, since the area of maximum venous pressure and reflux through incompetent perforators is confined to the calf and ankle in most patients. Replacement stockings are required every 3 to 4 months because of loss of fit. It should be stressed to the patient that the aim is the avoidance of lymphedema or, failing this, its minimization so that daytime lymphedema is reversed during the hours of rest.

FIGURE 68-6 Chronic venous ulcers complicating deep venous hypertension. Note signs of long-standing venous insufficiency in the surrounding skin.

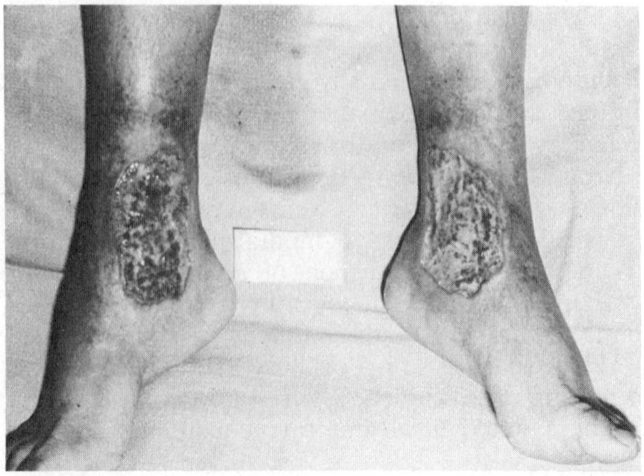

Small venous ulcers may heal with institution of appropriate gravity drainage and external support. Local care of the ulcer per se usually requires only mechanical cleansing. A myriad of topical preparations exist, but indications for their use in venous ulcers are the exception rather than the rule. Large, resistant ulcers may require excision and split-thickness skin grafting. Interruption of incompetent perforators is mandatory to prevent prompt recurrence. Disconnection operations for subfascial interruption of incompetent perforators stop reflux from deep veins; occasionally, reflux in superficial veins makes their interruption also desirable. Reconstruction of vein valves and ingenious bypasses for areas of segmental venous obstruction are procedures applicable to a minority of patients. The therapeutic value of the latter procedures is not firmly established, but several methods appear promising in selected patients. No method of therapy is curative, and both patient and physician should be reconciled to continuing care of a chronic condition.

Diseases of the Venae Cavae

Superior Vena Caval Obstruction

Obstruction of the superior vena cava is often dramatic with severe consequences, but sometimes it occurs gradually and symptoms are mild if sufficient venous collateral flow develops concomitantly. Edema of the face, neck, and upper extremities, strutted neck veins, prominent superficial venous collaterals over the upper chest, and plethoric cyanosis of the skin of the brachiocephalic region may be apparent. A marked increase in symptoms occurs if the patient bends forward or lies flat. Cerebral edema may develop with associated headache, lethargy, visual blurring, and seizures. Edema of the laryngeal structures can produce hoarseness or respiratory distress. Causes of superior vena caval obstruction include (1) compression or invasion by neoplasms (bronchogenic carcinoma, lymphoma, or metastatic tumors), (2) thrombosis induced by indwelling venous catheters, (3) involvement by mediastinal inflammatory disease, or (4) progressive constriction caused by idiopathic fibrosing mediastinitis.[17] Aortic arch aneurysms, external trauma, and surgical procedures are less frequent causes of superior vena caval obstruction. Confirmation and localization of the level of obstruction can be obtained by phlebography; more precise identification of etiology requires diagnostic procedures used to detect intrathoracic or mediastinal lesions.

Treatment depends upon the cause of obstruction. Malignant lesions are almost certainly nonresectable; palliative treatment can be attempted with radiation therapy, chemotherapy, and diuretics. If the condition is due to thrombosis induced by a central venous catheter, the venous line should be removed and the patient treated with heparin anticoagulation. Symptoms of venous hypertension frequently improve as the vena cava is recanalized or as collateral circulation develops. Successful surgical interventions have been reported in a few patients with benign disease by the creation of collateral runoff through the azygous venous system or by direct replacement of the occluded venous segment.[18] Prosthetic or autogenous tissue bypass grafts often become occluded because of low pressure and volume of flow.

Inferior Vena Caval Obstruction

Acute obstruction of the infrarenal inferior vena cava produces massive edema and plethoric cyanosis of the lower torso and legs, and distended superficial veins over the trunk. If the vena caval obstruction occurs above the renal vein orifices, or if intracaval thrombus extends cephalad to that level, the patient may have hematuria, nephrotic syndrome, and renal failure, and death occurs in a significant number. Inferior vena caval obstruction is most often caused by propagation of thrombus from the iliac veins but can also result from surgical manipulation and from compression or invasion by primary or metastatic tumors. Intracaval extensions of renal cell carcinoma are relatively common, but primary venous tumors are rare. Retroperitoneal fibrosis causes gradual compression of the inferior vena cava in occasional instances.

The treatment for thrombotic occlusion of the infrarenal vena cava is the same as for deep venous thrombosis of the lower extremities. If the process extends above and occludes both renal veins, direct surgical thrombectomy may be warranted. Likewise, operative intervention may be justified to remove an obstructing intracaval tumor in conjunction with nephrectomy for renal cancer. Efforts to resect a segment of the inferior vena cava and to reconstruct that vessel by the use of prosthetic grafts are usually unsuccessful, and carry a significant risk of pulmonary embolism.

Budd-Chiari Syndrome

This uncommon but frequently fatal disorder is characterized by occlusion of the hepatic vein ostia by progressive endophlebitis with resultant hepatic outflow obstruction (Fig. 68-7). This causes portal hypertension and centrilobular necrosis of the liver. Approximately one-third of patients with Budd-Chiari syndrome have associated obstruction of the retrohepatic inferior vena cava as a result either of compression by the massively engorged liver or from propagation of thrombus into the vena caval lumen. Patients with significant vena caval obstruction in addition to hepatic outflow occlusion have leg edema as well as tense ascites, jaundice, hepatomegaly, and abdominal pain. Differential diagnosis includes intraabdominal neoplasms, constrictive pericarditis, tuberculous peritonitis, pancreatic ascites, and severe right-sided heart failure. Accurate diagnosis depends upon appropriate contrast roentgenography and pressure measurements in the inferior vena cava and hepatic veins. Treatment of Budd-Chiari syndrome with caval obstruction is much different from the therapy offered to patients without associated caval obstruction, wherein a side-to-side portasystemic vein shunt offers good palliation. Such a shunt is contraindicated in the presence of retrohepatic vena caval obstruction, since portal decompression will not succeed if the gradient between the portal system and the systemic vein is negligible. Instead, one must rely on more conserv-

FIGURE 68-7 Mural thrombus in (*A*) retrohepatic inferior vena cava of a patient with Budd-Chiari syndrome. "Coning" (*B*) or narrowing of the interior vena cava (IVC) is produced by compression from the enlarged, congested liver. Note patent left renal vein (*C*).

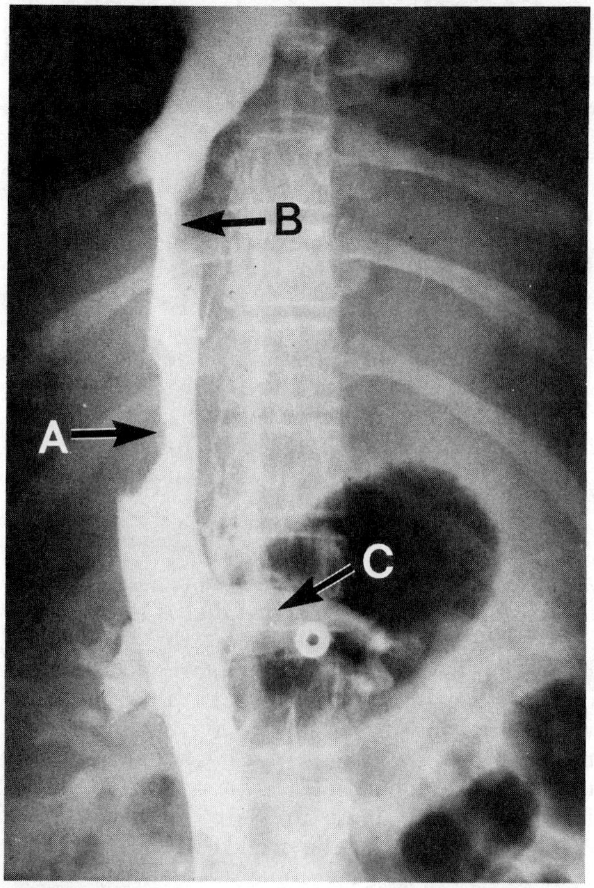

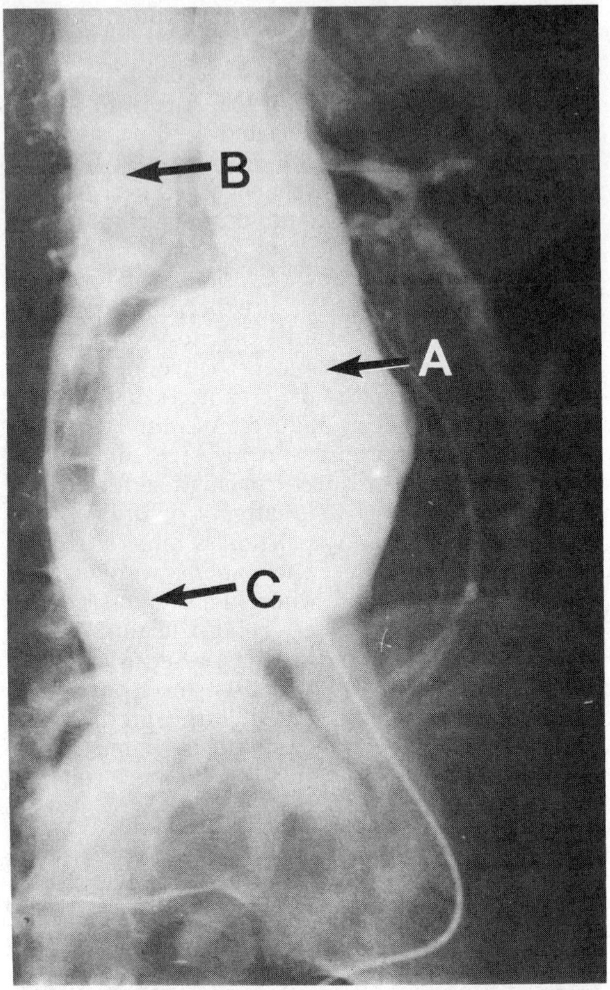

FIGURE 68-8 Aortic aneurysm with aortocaval fistula. Arrow *A* indicates the aneurysm, *B* shows the inferior vena cava opacified immediately via the arteriovenous connection, and *C* points out the site of rupture of the aneurysm into adjacent inferior vena cava.

ative therapy (fibrinolytic agents, anticoagulants, diuretics, and, possibly, a peritoneovenous shunt) or on the performance of a formidable surgical procedure, such as the insertion of a prosthetic graft from the portal system across the diaphragm into the right atrium or pulmonary artery.[19] A small number of reports have appeared describing successful surgical disobliteration of the involved vessels in conjunction with a hepatic tumor resection or the direct operative removal of obstructing venous webs.

Aortocaval Fistula

Acquired aortocaval fistulas are unusual and result most often from rupture of an atherosclerotic aneurysm of the abdominal aorta into the adjacent inferior vena cava or one of its tributaries. Penetrating trauma can cause this condition, but the majority of victims probably do not survive to reach medical attention. The classic signs of arteriovenous connection at this location include refractory congestive heart failure, widened pulse pressure, tachycardia, leg edema, and a loud machinery-like murmur over the abdomen, flank, or back. Renal insufficiency and hematuria are seen in some patients. Confirmation of the diagnosis is readily obtained by an aortogram, which demonstrates rapid venous filling via the fistula (Fig. 68-8). Appropriate therapy is urgent repair of the aortic aneurysm with suture closure of the caval opening from within the aneurysm sac.[20] Accurate diagnosis and prompt surgical intervention should result in survival of the majority of patients with this life-threatening variety of arteriovenous fistula.

References

1. Gay, J.: On Varicose veins of the Lower Extremities, in "The Lettsomian Lecture of 1867," Churchill and Sons, London, 1868, 171 pp.
2. Kaplan, N. M.: Cardiovascular Complications of Oral Contraceptives, *Ann. Rev. Med.,* 29:31, *u.* 1978.
3. Kakkar, V. V., Howe, C. T., Nicolaides, A. N., Renney, J. T. G., and Clarke, M. B.: Deep Vein Thrombosis of the Leg; Is There a "High Risk" Group?, *Am. J. Surg.,* 120:527, 1970.
4. Cranley, J. J., Canos, A. J., and Sull, W. J.: The Diagnosis of Deep Venous Thrombosis; Fallibility of Clinical Symptoms and Signs, *Arch. Surg.,* 111:34, 1976.
5. Barnes, R. W., Russell, H. E., Wu, K. K., and Hoak, J. C.: Accuracy of Doppler Ultrasound in Clinically Suspected Venous Thrombosis of the Calf, *Surg. Gynecol. Obstet.,* 143:425, 1976.
6. Kakkar, V. V., Corrigan, T. P., and Fossard, D. P.: Prevention of Fatal Postoperative Pulmonary Embolism by Low Doses of Heparin; An International Multicentre Trial, *Lancet,* 2:45, 1975.
7. Hirsh, J., and Gallus, A. S.: ^{125}I-Labeled Fibrinogen Scanning; Use in the Diagnosis of Venous Thrombosis. *JAMA,* 223:970, 1975.
8. Rabinov, K., and Paulin, S.: Roentgen Diagnosis of Venous Thrombosis in the Leg, *Arch. Surg.,* 104:134, 1972.
9. Adar, R., and Salzman, E. W.: Treatment of Thrombosis of Veins of the Lower Extremities, *N. Engl. J. Med.,* 292:348, 1975.
10. Clagett, G. P., and Salzman, E. W.: Prevention of Venous Thromboembolism in Surgical Patients, *N. Engl. J. Med.,* 290:93, 1974.
11. Lansing, A. M., Davis, W. M.: Five-Year Follow-Up Study of Iliofemoral Venous Thrombectomy, *Ann. Surg.,* 168:620, 1968.
12. Greenfield, L. J., Stewart, J. R., and Crute, S.: Improved Technique for Insertion of Greenfield Vena Caval Filter, *Surg. Gynecol. Obstet.,* 156:217, 1983.
13. Dodd, H., and Cockett, F. B.: "The Pathology and Surgery of the Veins of the Lower Limb," Churchill Livingstone, Edinburgh, 1976, p. 59.
14. Lofgren, E. P., and Lofgren, K. A.: Recurrence of Varicose Veins after the Stripping Operation, *Arch. Surg.,* 102:111, 1971.
15. Hobbs, J. T.: Compression Sclerotherapy of Varicose Veins, in J. J. Bergan and J. S. T. Yao (eds.), "Venous Problems," Year Book Medical Publishers, Inc., Chicago, 1978, p. 89.
16. Dale, W. A.: The Swollen Leg, in "Current Problems in Surgery," Year Book Medical Publishers, Inc., Chicago, 1973, p. 26.
17. Fairbairn, J. F. II, Juergens, J. L., and Spittell, J. A., Jr. (eds.), "Peripheral Vascular Diseases," 4th ed., W. B. Saunders Company, Philadelphia, 1972, p. 552.
18. Cooley, D. A., and Wukasch, D. C.: "Techniques in Vascular Surgery," W. B. Saunders Company, Philadelphia, 1979, p. 226.
19. Cameron, J. L., and Maddrey, W. C.: Mesoatrial Shunt. A New Treatment for the Budd-Chiari Syndrome, *Ann. Surg.,* 187:402, 1978.
20. Baker, W. H.: Arteriovenous Fistulas of the Aorta and Its Major Branches, in R. B. Rutherford (ed.), "Vascular Surgery," W. B. Saunders Company, Philadelphia, 1977, p. 807.

PART VI

The Heart and Other Medical Problems

Part V of this book is devoted to a discussion of the disease processes that affect the heart and blood vessels (see introduction to Part V). For the most part, the diseases described in Part V begin in the heart and blood vessels themselves. These might be termed *primary diseases* of the heart and blood vessels. However, a large number of diseases and conditions affecting the heart and blood vessels actually originate in other organs. Under these circumstances, the involvement of the heart may be termed *secondary heart disease.* These diseases and conditions are discussed in this part of the book. In addition, there are a number of other issues that are important to patients with heart disease. These diverse topics are also discussed in Part VI.

Section A

The Heart and Certain Physiological Conditions

69

Heart Disease and Pregnancy

John H. McAnulty, M.D.
James Metcalfe, M.D.
Kent Ueland, M.D.

If disease during pregnancy is to be well managed, the physiological changes of pregnancy must first be known.
C. Sidney Burwell, M.D., 1958[1]

Heart disease in a pregnant woman affects the health of two individuals; the well-being of both the mother and the fetus must be considered in managing the disease. Potential dangers to the mother fall into several categories. First, by imposing a hemodynamic burden, pregnancy may result in her disability or death. On the basis of recorded experience, pregnancy is particularly dangerous to women with some specific cardiac abnormalities; these include Eisenmenger's syndrome,[2,3] primary pulmonary hypertension,[4] Marfan's syndrome,[5] and significant mitral stenosis.[6]

Second, pregnancy may aggravate preexisting maternal heart disease. Pregnant women with some forms of heart disease are at risk of developing bacterial endocarditis, particularly at the time of labor and delivery, and this can turn a previously tolerable cardiac abnormality into one that requires immediate attention. It has been suggested that rheumatic fever is also more likely to recur during pregnancy, sometimes resulting in severe symptoms and compromising pregnancy.[6–9]

Third, in rare instances, pregnancy may cause heart disease. During labor and delivery bacteremia may occur and bacterial endocarditis can develop. In addition, a peripartum cardiomyopathy may develop in individuals with previously normal hearts.[10–12]

In women with heart disease, fetal health may be jeopardized for a number of reasons. The fetus depends upon an adequate and continuous supply of well-oxygenated maternal blood to the uterus and is at risk of abnormal organogenesis or death should this supply be compromised. When maternal heart disease is severe, this risk is significant; fetal wastage exceeds 50 percent in women with severe congenital heart disease.[1,4,13–16]

In addition, if the mother has congenital heart disease, the fetus has an increased likelihood of being born with heart disease. Congenital heart disease is recognized in 0.8 percent of all live births in the United States.[17–19] If one of the parents has congenital heart disease, the offspring has up to a 15 percent chance of having a similar abnormality.[15–19] This increases to 50 percent when the abnormality is an autosomal dominant trait, as is the case with idiopathic hypertrophic subaortic stenosis or with Marfan's syndrome. Finally, even if the mother and fetus survive pregnancy, the child has an increased chance of losing its mother because of the mortality rate associated with heart disease.

Cardiovascular Adjustments at Various Stages of Pregnancy

Changes in the cardiovascular system during a normal pregnancy are remarkable, so it is not surprising that certain maternal cardiac abnormalities are

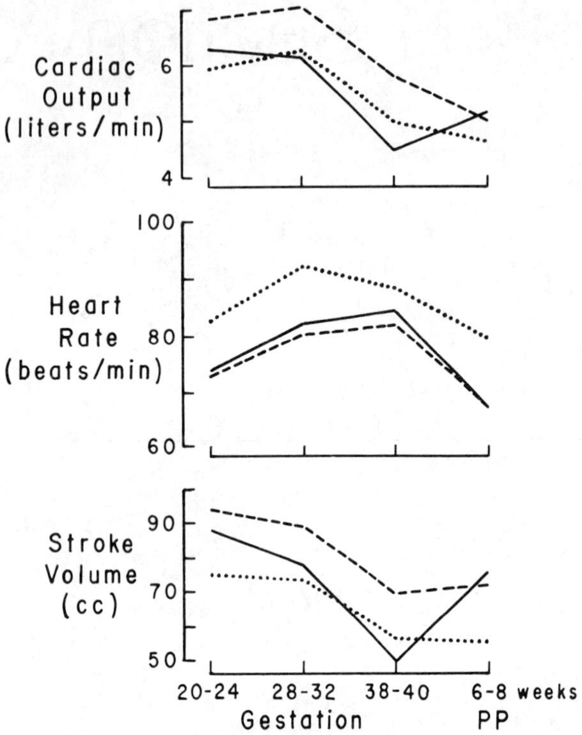

FIGURE 69-1 The effects of time in gestation and of maternal position upon the cardiovascular system of the mother. Data were obtained at three periods during gestation and once postpartum. Solid line = supine; broken line = side; dotted line = sitting.

not well tolerated (Fig. 69-1). Even in the woman without heart disease, the hemodynamic adjustments can result in symptoms and signs which are sometimes difficult to distinguish from those associated with cardiac abnormalities.

Sodium and water retention occur. Plasma volume begins to increase as early as 6 weeks after conception, approaches its maximum in the second trimester,[20] and approximates $1\frac{1}{2}$ times normal by the time of delivery.[21] Total body water increases steadily throughout pregnancy by 6 to 8 liters; most is extracellular.[22] Sodium retention results in an excess accumulation of 500 to 900 meq by the time of delivery. Although these changes contribute to the hemodynamic alterations of pregnancy, they do not adequately explain all of them.

The most significant hemodynamic change occurring in the maternal circulation during pregnancy is an increase in resting cardiac output. As shown in Fig. 69-2, this begins in the first trimester and reaches levels of 30 to 50 percent above values in nonpregnant individuals by the middle trimester. The cardiac output may remain elevated to this degree throughout the rest of the pregnancy, but it is sensitive to changes in position, which affect venous return to the heart.[21,23,24] Early in pregnancy the increase in resting cardiac output is due mainly to an increase in stroke volume, a variable which falls later in pregnancy coincident with the progressive elevation in heart rate.[21] Initially the increased cardiac output is associated with a decreased arteriovenous oxygen difference, but this gradually widens as resting oxygen consumption increases progressively and at term reaches a level 20 percent above that of the nonpregnant state.[21]

As shown in Fig. 69-1, when measurements are made in the supine position, the resting cardiac output of the woman near term in pregnancy is, on the average, lower than that of the postpartum woman. This decrement is attributed to compression of the inferior vena cava by the enlarged uterus, which results in a decreased venous return and a fall in cardiac output, even in women with adequate venous collaterals. In a few women, presumably those whose collaterals are not well developed, maintenance of the supine position may result in alarming hypotension and bradycardia, a vasovagal syndrome which has been called the "supine hypotensive syndrome of pregnancy."[25–27] During labor, cardiac output increases with each uterine contraction (compared with the time between contractions), but the magnitude of the increase varies depending on the anesthesia used and on body position.

Immediately after vaginal delivery, cardiac output may increase by as much as 60 to 80 percent. With a cesarean section there may be a transient fall in output and blood pressure.[28] In the postpartum period relative bradycardia is common, and resting cardiac output falls progressively to normal levels over the course of a few weeks. It is possible that these postpartum changes are affected by lactation, but the effects of lactation on maternal hemodynamics have not been studied in humans.

The increase in cardiac output is accompanied by a fall in systemic vascular resistance. This occurs early in pregnancy and is associated with a slight fall in mean arterial blood pressure,[21,29] which returns to the level of the nonpregnant state before delivery.[30] The changes in cardiac output and total systemic vascular resistance do not accurately reflect changes in the resistance of specific vascular beds, which regulate the distribution of the increased maternal cardiac output. A schematic summary of the distribution of cardiac output in a resting woman at several stages of pregnancy is shown in Fig. 69-2. This is a composite, using data from a variety of studies, but the general outlines are probably correct. By the end of the first trimester, uterine flow has increased by only 50 to 100 ml/min over that of the nonpregnant state; it increases to 200 ml/min by 28 weeks of pregnancy and reaches 1200 ml/min above the baseline at term.[31–33] In twin pregnancies uterine flow is even higher. This progressive expansion of uterine blood flow is out of phase with the total rise in resting maternal cardiac output, which reaches its peak in the middle trimester.

When redistribution of flow is required in order to serve the mother, uterine blood flow falls.[34,35] Excitement, heat, exercise, or a decrease in venous return have all been shown to result in decreased uterine blood flow. Though exercise may temporarily

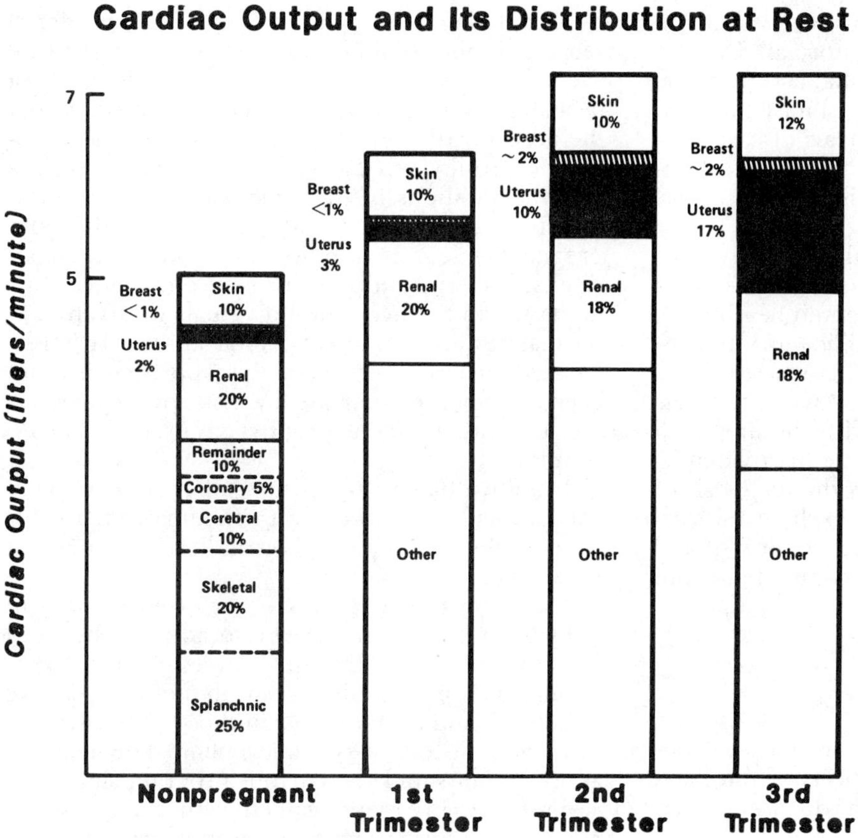

FIGURE 69-2 The distribution of increased cardiac output in association with human pregnancy. The data are fragmentary, especially early in pregnancy, and are nonexistent in the postpartum period. The change in flow to each region is labeled.

divert blood flow away from the pregnant uterus, it is not apparent that this transient diversion has any detrimental effect on the fetus. This question has become more important with the increasing enthusiasm for exercise in this country. There is not enough evidence available to suggest that the healthy pregnant woman should avoid recreational exercise.

The hemodynamic responses of a pregnant woman to exercise are somewhat different from those of nonpregnant women. For a given level of exercise in the sitting position there is a greater increase in oxygen consumption compared to that of the nonpregnant state.[36,37] This is associated with a relatively smaller rise in arteriovenous oxygen difference than that produced by the same exercise in nonpregnant women.

The mechanisms evoking the hemodynamic changes of pregnancy are not clear. Recognizing the similarity between the hemodynamic changes of human pregnancy and those found in patients with an arteriovenous fistula, Burwell et al. suggested that the low-resistance shunt created by the placental vascular bed might be the basis for the hemodynamic change.[38] It is now recognized that maternal cardiac output increases long before there is any significant change in uterine blood flow, so Burwell's explanation is not adequate for the observed changes in resting cardiac output. At the present time it seems most likely that changes in the levels of steroid hormones are the most significant contributors to the hemodynamic changes of pregnancy, possibly by altering compliances throughout the maternal vascular system and in the heart.[39–41]

Clinical Evaluation of the Pregnant Woman

Effects of Hemodynamic Changes

The recognition and definition of heart disease is difficult at any time, and this is particularly true during pregnancy. Easy fatigability, dyspnea, chest pain, palpitations, and syncope are symptoms of heart disease, but all are common in normal pregnant women. Examination may be equally misleading. Peripheral edema occurs in as many as 80 percent of normal pregnant women, and pulmonary rales, visible neck vein pulsations, a third heart sound, and systolic murmurs are not uncommon.

Although it is difficult to differentiate evidence of heart disease from the normal cardiovascular changes of pregnancy, there are symptom complexes and physical findings that should cause concern about associated heart disease. Dyspnea severe enough to limit activity and true orthopnea or paroxysmal nocturnal dyspnea are not normal during pregnancy and should lead to further evaluation. Hemoptysis cannot be considered normal. Syncope occurring with exertion is not normal and warrants evaluation. If chest discomfort limits activity, worsens, or is typical of ischemic heart disease, further evaluation may be warranted because occasionally a pregnant woman has ischemic cardiac events.[42–47]

Physical findings can also signal the presence of heart disease. Cyanosis may be due to causes other than heart disease, but its cause should be defined. The same is true of clubbing. Systolic murmurs are common in pregnancy, but one of grade 3/6 intensity or greater deserves evaluation. Atrioventricular valve flow murmurs may occur with the increased cardiac output of pregnancy,[48] but a diastolic murmur is so unusual that it warrants the diagnosis of heart disease if care is taken to exclude internal mammary flow sounds (the mammary souffle) and a venous hum which has a diastolic component; both are common in normal pregnancy.

General Considerations

Each patient and each cardiac lesion must be considered individually, but some aspects of the diagnosis and management of heart disease during pregnancy apply in all cases.

Health Priorities

Fetal well-being should be considered as part of each diagnostic and management consideration, but the highest priority should be given to maternal health. If there are alternatives to drug intervention, such as appropriate manipulation of the environment or maternal activity, these measures are preferable. But if drugs, diagnostic studies, or surgery are required for the maximum security of the mother, they should be used.

Management

Preconceptual counseling is always appropriate. Each woman should be advised about the risks of the pregnancy to herself and to a child, and she should be told of the long-term significance of her heart disease, particularly if it could be potentially limiting or may shorten her life span.

In the woman with heart disease it is appropriate to minimize stress on the heart when this does not inappropriately limit her day-to-day functioning. Measures should be taken to avoid anxiety and systemic illnesses such as anemia and infection. In addition to its adverse effects in the woman, cigarette smoking is associated with a handicap to fetal growth and development and should be discouraged.[49] Immunization against rubella, measles, mumps, polio, tetanus, and influenza is appropriate in the years prior to pregnancy.[50–52] Once pregnancy has begun, vaccination with live organisms is inadvisable.

Each lesion is unique and must be considered separately, but certain issues must be considered with every cardiac lesion. The hemodynamic status must be assessed with each visit and a decision made about the need for diagnostic studies or intervention. Antibiotic prophylaxis against endocarditis using the recommendations of the American Heart Association is as applicable to pregnancy as to the nonpregnant state.[53] In addition, antibiotic prophylaxis against bacterial endocarditis is recommended during labor and delivery in individuals with valve abnormalities and some congenital lesions. It is recognized that the benefit of this approach has not been documented, but the low risk and expense associated with antibiotic prophylaxis make its use appropriate.

In individuals with a history of rheumatic fever and particularly in those with rheumatic heart disease, antibiotic prophylaxis is indicated to prevent recurrences.[54]

Thromboembolic events occur often enough in individuals with heart disease to address the need for anticoagulation therapy. Anticoagulants are a requirement in all individuals with mechanical valve prostheses and are desirable in those with valve disease and a history of systemic emboli. The need for anticoagulants and the current program should be reviewed in pregnant women with valve disease, however, because warfarin derivatives cross the placental barrier and put the fetus at increased risk of abnormal development and hemorrhage (see the section "Anticoagulants" below). Whenever possible, alternatives to warfarin therapy should be used in the woman who is pregnant.

Cardiovascular Disease in Pregnancy

Each of the abnormalities discussed in the remainder of this chapter is covered in detail in other sections of this book. We will relate them to pregnancy and will consider (1) the potential problems during pregnancy, emphasizing the effects of the normal hemodynamic changes on each lesion (Table 69-1), (2) the demonstrated risk to the mother and fetus, and (3) the management of mother and fetus during pregnancy.

Rheumatic Fever

Clinically recognized rheumatic fever is disappearing in the United States.[55,56] However, it is still the most common cause of heart disease seen in pregnant women, and it remains a problem throughout much of the world.[56,57] In addition, it has been suggested that rheumatic fever is more likely to occur during pregnancy,[6–9] a reason for the more aggressive use of antibiotic prophylaxis against rheumatic fever in pregnant women and in women capable of pregnancy. Myocarditis occurring during pregnancy may be due to other causes, but its occurrence

TABLE 69-1 Effects of Pregnancy on Heart Disease

Cardiac Lesion	Relevant Hemodynamic Change in Pregnancy	Result	Time of Greatest Risk	Demonstrated Risks	Management
Myocardial Disease					
Rheumatic fever; myocarditis; cardiomyopathy	↑ Blood volume ↑ Cardiac output	↑ Pulmonary capillary pressure ↓ Cardiac output	>12 weeks	Uncommon: ↑ Maternal morbidity	Treat pulmonary congestion Avoid pregnancy if left ventricular failure is present
Valve Deformities					
Mitral stenosis	↑ Cardiac output ↑ Heart rate ↑ Blood volume ↓ Pulmonary vascular resistance	↑ Pulmonary capillary pressure	> 12 weeks (when hemodynamic changes become significant)	↑ Maternal morbidity and mortality from pulmonary congestion and pulmonary edema ↓ Fetal growth and ↑ fetal loss	Limit demands for cardiac output, based on symptoms Avoid tachycardia Treat tachyarrhythmia
	Obstruction of inferior vena cava by uterus Blood loss at delivery	↓ Venous return ↓ LA filling ↓ LV filling ↓ Cardiac output	Late in pregnancy when supine (labor, delivery, surgery) and postpartum	Possible explanation of some maternal deaths	Maintain venous return, especially if symptoms of ↓ cardiac output occur
Mitral regurgitation (includes mitral prolapse when complicated by important mitral regurgitation)	↑ Blood volume	↑ Pulmonary capillary pressure	> 12 weeks	Uncommon: pregnancy is usually uneventful	Rx of pulmonary congestion if it occurs (restrict sodium intake, diuretics)
Aortic stenosis	Obstruction of inferior vena cava by uterus Blood loss at delivery	↓ Venous return ↓ LV filling ↓ Cardiac output	Late in pregnancy when supine (labor, delivery, surgery) and postpartum	↑ Maternal mortality uncommon because aortic stenosis is rare in pregnancy	Maintain venous return Strict limitation of activity, and if symptoms persist, proceed to valve surgery or interruption of pregnancy
Aortic regurgitation	↑ Blood volume	↑ Pulmonary capillary pressure	> 12 weeks	Uncommon: pregnancy is usually uneventful	Rx of pulmonary congestion if it occurs (restrict sodium intake, diuretics)
Pulmonary stenosis	Obstruction of inferior vena cava by uterus Blood loss at delivery	↓ Venous return ↓ LV filling ↓ Cardiac output	Late in pregnancy when supine (labor, delivery, surgery) and postpartum	Uncommon: pregnancy is usually uneventful	Maintain venous return
Congenital Lesions					
Shunts:					
Left-to-right (septal defect, patent ductus)	↑ Cardiac output ↑ Blood volume ↓ Pulmonary vascular resistance	↑ Pulmonary capillary pressure	> 12 weeks	Uncommon: pregnancy is usually uneventful	Rx of pulmonary congestion if it occurs (restrict sodium intake, diuretics)
Right-to-left (Eisenmenger's syndrome, tetralogy of Fallot)	↓ Peripheral vascular resistance Obstruction of inferior vena cava by uterus Blood loss at delivery	↑ Shunting and ↓ venous return ↓ Pulmonary blood flow	Late in pregnancy when supine (labor, delivery, surgery) and postpartum	↑ Maternal mortality due to sudden death ↓ Fetal growth and ↑ fetal loss	Avoid pregnancy Maintain venous return

TABLE 69-1 Effects of Pregnancy on Heart Disease (*Continued*)

Cardiac Lesion	Relevant Hemodynamic Change in Pregnancy	Result	Time of Greatest Risk	Demonstrated Risks	Management
Coarctation of the aorta	Obstruction of inferior vena cava by uterus	↓ Venous return ↓ LV filling ↓ Cardiac output	Late in pregnancy when supine (labor, delivery, surgery) and postpartum	Uncommon: pregnancy is usually uneventful	Maintain venous return
	↑ Blood volume ↑ Pulse pressure ↑ Steroid hormones ? Tendency to ↑ hypertension	Distension of aortic root	> 12 weeks	Aortic rupture Dissection of aorta Rupture of intracranial aneurysm	Delay pregnancy until Rx optimal Treat hypertension and minimize ↑ pulse pressure
Pulmonary Hypertension					
Any cause	Obstruction of inferior vena cava by uterus Blood loss at delivery	↓ Venous return ↓ LV filling ↓ Cardiac output	Late in pregnancy when supine (labor, delivery, surgery) and postpartum	↑ Maternal mortality due to sudden death	Avoid pregnancy Maintain venous return Try to lower pulmonary vascular resistance
Developmental Abnormalities					
Idiopathic hypertrophic subaortic stenosis	Obstruction of inferior vena cava by uterus ↑ Heart rate Blood loss at delivery	↓ Venous return ↓ LV filling ↑ LV obstruction ↓ Cardiac output		↑ Maternal morbidity during pregnancy	Maintain venous return β-adrenergic blockade to ↓ LV outflow obstruction
	↑ Blood volume	↑ Pulmonary capillary pressure	> 12 weeks	↑ Maternal morbidity during pregnancy	Rx of pulmonary congestion, especially diuretics
Marfan's syndrome	↑ Blood volume ↑ Pulse pressure ↑ Steroid hormones	Distension of aortic root	> 12 weeks	↑ Maternal mortality from aortic dissection or rupture	Avoid pregnancy Minimize ↑ pulse pressure

Note: This table summarizes the theoretical basis for concern about specific heart lesions in relation to the cardiovascular changes which normally occur during pregnancy. Under "Management" we list specific recommendations for each lesion, omitting consideration of general recommendations for prophylaxis against rheumatic fever and bacterial endocarditis, maintenance of general health, and precautions against anemia, infections, anxiety, and fatigue. The statement *Avoid pregnancy* means that the lesion has a documented high risk during pregnancy. Accordingly, in our opinion, pregnancy is inadvisable, and if it occurs, an early interruption is advised.

should raise the consideration of rheumatic fever, particularly in women with a previous episode. When congestive heart failure develops, it should be treated with standard therapy.

Valve Disease

Mitral Valve Disease

Significant heart disease in women usually involves the mitral valve and is rheumatic in origin.

Mitral Stenosis The increased cardiac output, tachycardia, and fluid and sodium retention of pregnancy may cause hemodynamic deterioration in the patient with mitral stenosis. Symptoms attributable to an increase in left atrial pressure with associated pulmonary vascular congestion and bronchial vein distension occur in up to 25 percent of patients with mitral stenosis during pregnancy.[4,6] They usually become apparent by the twentieth week and may be aggravated still further at the time of labor and delivery with the associated increases in heart rate and cardiac output. Maternal death from pulmonary edema may occur but is rare when there is careful attention to the management of congestive heart failure.[1,4,6] Although potentially at risk from the elevated left atrial pressure, the patient with significant mitral stenosis also depends upon this pressure to fill the left ventricle adequately and thus to maintain cardiac output. The pregnant woman is liable to sudden shifts in the distribution of blood volume and is, therefore, at increased risk of a sudden decline in left atrial pressure and a consequent dramatic fall in cardiac output. This may also increase maternal and fetal morbidity and may be the explanation for the death of women with mitral stenosis who had no previous congestive heart failure.[6]

Management of the patient with mitral stenosis should include rheumatic fever prophylaxis[54] and prophylaxis against endocarditis.[53] When severe mitral stenosis is identified prior to pregnancy, mitral commissurotomy should be undertaken before conception. When a woman with mitral stenosis becomes pregnant, no definitive treatment is needed unless symptoms develop, but restriction of activity to minimize symptoms is appropriate. If symptoms of pulmonary congestion develop, attempts should be made to control them with further restriction of activity and sodium intake. If an arrhythmia develops or pulmonary congestion persists, standard medical therapy is required. Should these symptoms be unremitting despite medical therapy, mitral commissurotomy can be performed during pregnancy,[58,59] however, the use of surgery is diminishing, even among its advocates. If necessary, open heart surgery with valve replacement can be performed, but fetal loss may be as high as 33 percent.[58] If thromboembolic complications develop, anticoagulation therapy is required, but again, warfarin derivatives should be avoided if possible because of the danger to the fetus.[60–62]

Mitral Regurgitation Mitral regurgitation from any cause is generally well tolerated during pregnancy. Unlike mitral stenosis, it may be due to a variety of causes, and it is of value to understand its etiology in considering the management during pregnancy. When it is caused by rheumatic fever, antibiotic prophylaxis against streptococcal infection is indicated. The presence of mitral regurgitation necessitates the need for prophylaxis against endocarditis at the time of labor and delivery. Occasionally, the hemodynamic alterations of a normal pregnancy can overwhelm the capabilities of the heart with a regurgitant mitral lesion and result in symptoms of congestive heart failure. These should be treated in the routine manner. In our experience surgery for mitral regurgitation has not been necessary during pregnancy.

Mitral Valve Prolapse The mitral valve prolapse syndrome warrants discussion not because it is dangerous but because it is so common. It occurs in 5 to 10 percent of young adults.[63–66] There is some familial tendency toward the development of the syndrome; but there is no clear genetic pattern of inheritance.[63,67,68] Pregnancy, with its changes in vascular resistance and blood volume, may alter the physical findings in the syndrome, either enhancing or diminishing them.[69] It is not clear that the occasional problems associated with the syndrome (endocarditis, arrhythmia, cerebral emboli, or mitral regurgitation) are more likely to occur during pregnancy, and no treatment is recommended except the use of prophylactic antibiotics at the time of labor and delivery.

Aortic Valve Disease

Aortic Stenosis Usually a congenital abnormality,[70] aortic stenosis is more common in males than in females, and so is infrequently encountered during pregnancy. It is so rare that we may have underestimated its danger in the past. A woman with aortic stenosis may very rarely get into difficulty during pregnancy with volume overload and associated congestive heart failure, but it is hypovolemia that puts these patients at greatest potential risk. Any significant fall in venous return can result in a dramatic fall in cardiac output with resulting cerebral or cardiac ischemia. In addition, with this fall in cardiac output, uterine blood flow may be compromised. With aortic stenosis maternal mortality rates up to 17 percent have been reported during pregnancy.[71] Mortality seems to be most likely to occur when the patient is predisposed to hypovolemia, for example, at the time of interruption of pregnancy, at which time the mortality rate approaches 40 percent. A fetal mortality rate of 32 percent has also been noted in these women.[71]

If a woman is found to have severe aortic stenosis prior to pregnancy, surgical correction before conception is advisable. This not only offers protection to the mother and fetus, but also decreases the incidence of congenital heart disease in the infant.[15] In most women of this age a commissurotomy will suffice. If a valve must be inserted prior to pregnancy, the issue of long-term anticoagulation therapy should be considered a relative indication for use of a heterograft rather than a mechanical prosthesis. In the patient with aortic stenosis who is already pregnant, measures to avoid hypovolemia and to restrict activity are appropriate. If symptoms develop, activity should be limited still further. If symptoms are progressive and cannot be controlled, interruption of pregnancy or aortic valve surgery should be performed.

Aortic Insufficiency Like aortic stenosis, aortic insufficiency is not common in young women, and like the other major regurgitant lesion, mitral insufficiency, it is usually well tolerated during pregnancy. Should heart failure develop, standard treatment is appropriate. Antibiotic prophylaxis at the time of labor and delivery is indicated. If aortic insufficiency develops in a patient with endocarditis and if the infection is not rapidly controlled or if hemodynamic deterioration occurs, early surgery should be considered despite the pregnancy. The mortality rate associated with medical therapy alone is high in such patients.[72–74]

Pulmonary Valve Disease

Hemodynamically significant pulmonary valve lesions are uncommon in pregnancy. As the use and abuse of intravenous drugs increase, the frequency of pulmonary valve damage may rise. When the diagnosis of pulmonary valve disease is made, prophylactic antibiotics against endocarditis are appropriate.

Tricuspid Valve Disease

Also uncommon, tricuspid valve disease, particularly tricuspid insufficiency, may be increasing because of the use of intravenous drugs and resultant endocarditis. Tricuspid valve disease is well tolerated during pregnancy, and no special considerations are in order other than prophylaxis against bacterial endocarditis.

Congenital Heart Disease

An increasing number of women with congenital heart disease are reaching childbearing age and many are capable of conception. Each abnormality has its unique relation to pregnancy but some considerations applicable in all cases were discussed in the introduction to this chapter.

Pulmonary Hypertension

It is recognized that pulmonary hypertension may not be simply the result of congenital heart disease and that it is frequently related to some of the abnormalities discussed below, but its danger warrants emphasis here. *Pulmonary hypertension is a contraindication to pregnancy.* Whether primary (with no recognizable cause) or secondary (due to prolonged left-to-right shunting, drug abuse, or recurrent pulmonary emboli), the risks to the lives of the mother and the child are significant. The maternal mortality rate approaches 50 percent in those with primary pulmonary hypertension,[75,76] and when the hypertension is due to Eisenmenger's syndrome, the maternal mortality rate ranges from 30 to 70 percent.[1,77,78] Death may occur during gestation or in the postdelivery period.[1,78] The fetal mortality rate exceeds 40 percent even when the mother survives. If pregnancy occurs in a woman with pulmonary hypertension, interruption should be recommended. If this recommendation is not accepted, aggressive attempts to avoid hypovolemia are essential, especially during and after delivery. A sudden fall of venous return limits the ability of the right ventricle to pump blood through the fixed pulmonary vascular resistance, often resulting in a cascading hemodynamic and metabolic deterioration with subsequent death.

Congenital Heart Disease without Associated Cyanosis

Left-to-Right Shunts Some women with left-to-right shunts reach adulthood and become pregnant, occasionally with no previous recognition of the cardiac abnormality. Others will have undergone surgical correction prior to pregnancy, but residual defects may remain. Although left-to-right shunting increases the chance of pulmonary hypertension, right ventricular failure, arrhythmias, emboli, and congestive heart failure, it is not clear that these complications are made more likely by pregnancy. The degree of shunting is affected by the relative resistances in the systemic and pulmonary vascular circuits; both fall during pregnancy and the changes are normally similar, so there is no significant alteration in the degree of shunting during pregnancy.[21] Those with shunts also have right ventricular volume overload. As with other volume overload conditions, pregnancy is reasonably well tolerated.

Pregnancy is well tolerated by patients with an uncomplicated atrial secundum defect and no specific treatment is indicated. The same is true for ostium primum defects, but they are more often associated with other cardiac and congenital abnormalities which may increase the risks associated with pregnancy. Endocarditis is rare with uncomplicated atrial septal defects; antibiotic prophylaxis is not required.

Ventricular septal defects and patency of the ductus arteriosus are more likely to be recognized and thus corrected early in life, prior to pregnancy. If present, however, they too are well tolerated during pregnancy. Endocarditis can occur and antibiotic prophylaxis is appropriate.

With any left-to-right shunting there is a risk of thrombosis and emboli but routine anticoagulation therapy is not appropriate. Should congestive heart failure develop from a left-to-right shunt, standard therapy is indicated.

Obstructive Lesions Obstructive lesions of the left side of the heart include the previously discussed aortic valve stenosis, and also supra- as well as subaortic valve stenosis. In general, surgical correction prior to pregnancy for any of these lesions may protect the mother during pregnancy and, of interest, may significantly reduce the incidence of congenital heart disease in the offspring.[15] This suggests that the hemodynamic effects of left ventricular obstructive lesions affect fetal development, presumably by affecting uterine perfusion.

Although there are a variety of left ventricular obstructive disease processes, two syndromes warrant some discussion: coarctation of the aorta and hypertrophic obstructive cardiomyopathy.

Coarctation of the Aorta. Although coarctation usually affects males, it may occur in women and may be associated with a bicuspid aortic valve. Coarctation and its associated lesions shorten life span, but affected individuals often reach childbearing age and may conceive. These individuals are at risk of aortic root dissection and of cerebral hemorrhage due to rupture of associated intracranial aneurysms and from complications of prolonged hypertension. The risk of these events is even higher during pregnancy, with an overall maternal mortality rate in these patients of approximately 3 percent.[4,79] Cardiac complications are common in those who survive.[79–81] Should pregnancy occur in a patient with a coarctation, treatment of hypertension is indicated. Care should be taken to avoid major swings in blood pressure, and prophylactic antibiotics against endocarditis are appropriate.

Hypertrophic Obstructive Cardiomyopathy. Recognized with increasing frequency, hypertrophic obstructive cardiomyopathy is usually inherited as an autosomal dominant condition. Because its dynamic characteristics are affected by changes in ventricular volume and vascular resistance, it might be expected that pregnancy would not be well tolerated. The normal fall in peripheral vascular resistance during pregnancy and the tendency to hypotension due to obstructed venous return or to blood loss at the time of delivery both tend to increase the outflow tract obstruction, an undesirable consequence. In addition, the emotional variations and the intermittent discomfort of pregnancy, labor, and delivery are likely to be associated with increased catecholamine levels, which might also increase outflow obstruction. An increase in both the number and severity of symptoms has been noted in women with obstructive cardiomyopathy during pregnancy, but death of a pregnant woman with this problem has not been reported.[82–85]

Management of patients with hypertrophic obstructive cardiomyopathy should include avoidance of hypovolemia. Beta-adrenergic blocking agents have been used at the time of labor and delivery,[82] but it is not clear that their use is necessary on a prophylactic basis.[85] If the patient develops angina or tachyarrhythmia, these drugs may be instituted during pregnancy, though the potential effects of beta-adrenergic blockade on the fetus should be considered. Prophylactic antibiotics are needed at the time of labor and delivery as these women are at risk of developing endocarditis on their mitral valve.

Obstructions to right ventricular outflow are also preferably corrected prior to pregnancy. This will decrease not only maternal morbidity but, as with correction of left-sided obstruction lesions, may decrease the incidence of congenital heart disease in the offspring.[15] If pregnancy occurs prior to correction however, a safe pregnancy results in most cases. Treatment should be directed at avoiding intervascular volume depletion. The dangers of right ventricular obstruction due to increased pulmonary vascular resistance were emphasized in the discussion of pulmonary hypertension.

Cyanotic Congenital Heart Disease

Congenital cardiac lesions resulting in cyanosis are frequently complex and deserve individual consideration. An increasing number of women with cyanotic congenital heart disease are living 3 to 4 decades and are becoming pregnant.

Women with tetralogy of Fallot may accomplish a full-term pregnancy, but they and their fetuses are at increased risk of morbidity and mortality.[13,14] In addition, as with any form of cyanotic heart disease, the children are likely to be small at birth and fetal wastage is high. Alterations in pulmonary or peripheral vascular resistance and in venous return may cause sudden changes in pulmonary or peripheral blood flow, which may result in symptoms or death. Surgical correction of the cardiac lesion prior to pregnancy should decrease the maternal and fetal risk although the baby continues to have an increased chance of having congenital heart disease.[15]

Even women with transposition of the great arteries (some with single ventricles) may become pregnant. Maternal risk is difficult to evaluate because "therapeutic interruption" is carried out in many series, but the majority of women will survive pregnancy.[15] Fetal loss, however, approaches 50 percent. Partial or complete surgical correction of the lesion prior to pregnancy will decrease the spontaneous abortion rate.

Marfan's Syndrome

Marfan's syndrome is easily recognizable when classic, but otherwise the diagnosis is often difficult to establish. It has been recommended that evidence of subluxated ocular lenses and of aortic root disease be required in order to make a definitive diagnosis of the syndrome.[5,86] Pregnancy is particularly dangerous for patients with this syndrome. First, half the offspring will inherit the problem. Second, the life span of a parent with Marfan's syndrome is reduced to half of normal, which must be considered when contemplating the future of the child. Third, and perhaps most important, the risk of death from aortic rupture or dissection is high during pregnancy.[87] This may be particularly true if the aortic root is enlarged ($>$ 40 mm by echocardiogram has been used as one criteria).[88] For all these reasons, women with Marfan's syndrome should be advised to avoid pregnancy. If the diagnosis of Marfan's syndrome is definite, the risks of pregnancy are so high that interruption should be recommended. Should the parents elect to continue with the pregnancy, the mother's activity should be restricted and hypertension should be prevented. Beta blockade has never been proved to be of value when used on a prophylactic basis, but its use in pregnant patients with Marfan's syndrome seems reasonable. Prophylactic antibiotics against endocarditis should be used with labor and delivery because there is a high incidence of mitral valve prolapse and of aortic valve regurgitation with the syndrome.[89]

Congestive (Dilated) Cardiomyopathies

A congestive cardiomyopathy preceding pregnancy is uncommon. If an affected woman is symptomatic or has cardiomegaly, pregnancy should be avoided because it tends to aggravate the symptoms and because the associated risk of fetal and maternal mortality is increased. If pregnancy occurs, treatment should include limitation of activity. If heart failure occurs and persists despite standard treatment, interruption of pregnancy must be considered.

A cardiomyopathy can occur in association with pregnancy, during the peripartum period.[10–12] The etiology of this cardiomyopathy is uncertain, but its pathological changes are similar to those of other types of congestive cardiomyopathies. Endomyocardial biopsy studies have suggested the presence of inflammation early in the course of the disease.[90] In the United States, peripartum cardiomyopathy occurs most commonly in black women, especially in those who are multiparous, older, pregnant (or postpartum) with twins, and those whose pregnancy is complicated by hypertension. Prognosis of the cardiomyopathies is poor if heart size does not return to normal within 6 months after pregnancy. Although a previous history of postpartum cardiomyopathy is not an absolute contraindication to another pregnancy, it is a relative contraindication.[12] The infant mortality rate in pregnant patients with congestive heart failure approaches 10 percent and can reach 30 percent. These statistics are cited to emphasize the point that congestive heart failure is exceptionally hazardous and should be treated aggressively.

Coronary Artery Disease

Myocardial infarction and angina pectoris during pregnancy have been reported.[42–47] The causes of the coronary obstruction have been thromboemboli, dissection, and presumed spasm, as well as atherosclerosis. Standard medical therapy is most appropriate but coronary artery bypass surgery has been utilized.[47]

Cardiac Arrhythmias

Pregnant women frequently experience dizziness, palpitations, and syncope—symptoms which may be attributed to cardiac arrhythmias. It has been suggested that tachyarrhythmias, particularly atrial tachyarrhythmias, occur more frequently in pregnant women,[91–93] but this has never been demonstrated. However, arrhythmias are not uncommon during pregnancy. As in the nonpregnant state, management should be undertaken with deliberate effort to avoid drug treatment. Attempts to manipulate the environment in terms of eliminating stimulants, fatigue, and anxiety are always appropriate. When medical treatment is required, standard medications should be used. If cardioversion is necessary, it appears to be tolerated without problems to the mother and child.[94] As in the nonpregnant state, drug treatment of asymptomatic atrial or ventricular premature beats is not justified.

Bradyarrhythmias may also occur during pregnancy.[91,95] They generally do not require treatment unless they result in symptoms or in clear compromise of maternal hemodynamics. Even complete heart block, which in this age group is most likely to be congenital in origin, is consistent with successful pregnancy.[96]

Pregnancy and Cardiac Surgery

Valve Surgery

Individuals who have undergone commissurotomy or surgical repair of a valve almost always have a residual deformity. They should be managed in the same way as other patients with valve disease. The use of antibiotics at the time of labor and delivery is advised, and those with rheumatic valve disease should take antibiotics chronically to prevent recurrences of rheumatic fever. Patients who are symptomatic from the valve disease despite surgery require careful evaluation, and consideration of further surgery before pregnancy is undertaken. Some will not have sufficient relief from surgery to permit a safe pregnancy.

Prosthetic Valves

Pregnancy in patients with prosthetic valves is associated with increased risks, though in most it can be carried to completion without complications.[97] All patients with *mechanical* prosthetic heart valves require full anticoagulation therapy. Because of the risks to the fetus from the warfarin derivatives, women with mechanical prostheses should be instructed in the use of heparin therapy when contemplating pregnancy or when pregnant.[60,61]

Prophylactic antibiotics must be used at the time of dental and surgical procedures and at the time of labor and delivery. If endocarditis develops in a pregnant woman with a prosthetic valve, aggressive antibiotic therapy must be instituted. If the infection is not immediately controlled, replacement of the prosthesis is required.[73,74,98]

Patients with heterograft prostheses, like those with mechanical prostheses, are at increased risk of developing bacterial endocarditis and require antibiotic prophylaxis. The single advantage of heterografts over mechanical prostheses is their lower susceptibility to thrombosis and thromboembolic events. For this reason, it is an advantage for a young woman planning pregnancy to have a tissue valve, recognizing that replacement may eventually be required. If an individual with a heterograft valve has an embolic event, anticoagulants (heparin during pregnancy) should be instituted.

Pregnancy after Surgery for Congenital Lesions

The risks of pregnancy in this group of patients depend upon the residual lesions and the type of surgery. Surgical correction, even if not complete, increases maternal safety, fetal viability, and decreases the chance of congenital heart disease in the infant.[15] Patients with persistent pulmonary hypertension are at high risk of maternal and fetal mortality. If residual defects are present, or if a patch, conduit, or artificial valve has been inserted, antibiotics should be used with dental and surgical procedures and with labor and delivery.

The Use of Cardiovascular Drugs in Pregnancy

It is best to avoid medications during pregnancy when possible. However, if the cardiovascular function of the mother indicates the need for a drug, it should not be withheld.

Diuretics

Diuretics should be reserved for women with congestive heart failure uncontrolled by sodium restriction. Although it was once advised that they be used in an uncomplicated pregnancy to prevent preeclampsia, this is now discouraged. The relative advantages and risks of the available diuretics are not altered by pregnancy.

Inotropic Agents

Indications for the use of digitalis are not changed by pregnancy.[99] Both digoxin and digitoxin cross the placental barrier, and fetal serum levels approximate those in the mother.[100] The same dose of digoxin will, in general, yield lower maternal serum levels during pregnancy than in the nonpregnant state, so measurement of blood levels may be required if the desired clinical effect is not achieved.[100] Digitalis may shorten the duration of gestation and labor, possibly because of an effect on the myometrium similar to the inotropic effect of digitalis on the myocardium.[101]

When intravenous inotropic or vasopressor agents are required, the standard agents (dopamine, norepinephrine, dobutamine) may be used, but the fetus is jeopardized because all the available preparations result in decreased uterine blood flow and may stimulate uterine contractions.

Adrenergic Receptor Blockade

It is not uncommon for women of childbearing age to be taking beta-blocking agents, most often for treatment of hypertension or tachyarrhythmias.[99] All the relative contraindications to the use of beta blockade exist during pregnancy. Beta blockade has been used to treat gestational hyperthyroidism with its associated tachycardia and tremor without adverse effects,[102] but there is evidence from animal studies that propranolol lowers umbilical blood flow.[103] In addition, beta blockers have the potential of initiating premature labor.[104] The potential for a chronic increase in uterine tone induced by these drugs could result in a small and infarcted placenta, and potentially in a low-birth-weight infant.[105] All the available beta-blocking agents cross the placenta, are present in human breast milk, and can reach significant clinical levels in the fetus or the newborn. If these agents are used during pregnancy it is appropriate to monitor fetal heart rate carefully, as well as the infant's heart rate, blood sugar, and respiratory status after delivery.[82,106–109]

Adrenergic blockade with phentolamine or phenoxybenzamine is rarely required in pregnancy. Occasionally—for example, in a patient with a pheochromocytoma—an appropriate drug effect has been achieved with no threat to maternal or fetal survival.[110]

Antiarrhythmic Agents

Information on the use of quinidine, procainamide, or disopyramide in pregnancy is sparse. Of these, quinidine has been used most frequently without clear adverse effects unique to pregnancy.[111] Little has been written about the use of procainamide or disopyramide, but an occasional problem has been encountered for each.[112–114] If a patient with a dangerous arrhythmia requires urgent treatment, the intravenous use of these agents is justified. Lidocaine is the preferred parenteral agent when applicable. Bretylium tosylate is a distant second as it may adversely affect uterine perfusion.

Calcium Channel Blocking Agents

Nifedipine, verapamil, and diltiazem have not been demonstrated to adversely affect pregnancy. Each, however, is a peripheral vasodilator and could lower blood pressure sufficiently to decrease uterine blood flow. Each crosses the placenta and is found in breast milk, but adverse effects on the fetus or infant have not been reported. Verapamil is as effective in managing supraventricular arrhythmias during pregnancy as at other times.[114]

Vasodilator Agents

While none of the vasodilators are contraindicated, the preload and afterload reducers have the potential for adversely affecting uterine perfusion.[112] Many also cross the placenta and fetal effects have not been well defined. Hydralazine and the nitrate preparations have been most frequently used with good fetal tolerance. There is little information available on the effects of captopril on the fetus although animal studies suggest impaired fetal viability. Nitroprusside use may result in fetal accumulation of thiocyanate and cyanide, but its use is justified in life-threatening situations.[115]

Anticoagulants

Concerns about the use of anticoagulants in pregnancy have already been expressed. The warfarin derivatives pose the usual significant risks to the mother: a 1 to 5 percent chance per year of a significant bleeding episode and up to a 10 percent chance per year of a minor hemorrhage. The fetus is at an even higher risk because warfarin derivatives cross the placenta. Fetal exposure during the first 2 months results in a 15 to 25 percent incidence of malformations from the so-called warfarin embryopathy syndrome (facial abnormalities, optic atrophy, digital abnormalities, epithelial changes, and mental impairment).[60,116–119] Although organogenesis is reasonably complete by the end of the first trimester, fetal risk continues: warfarin increases the chance of fetal bleeding or maternal intrauterine bleeding and may cause mental or visual impairment in the fetus. Safety from this drug is not granted in the third trimester either, as the risk of hemorrhage persists, particularly at the time of labor and delivery. Although pregnancy has been well tolerated and successfully accomplished in patients on long-term anticoagulant therapy,[97,119] it is best to avoid warfarin derivatives whenever possible. One alternative is to use no anticoagulants, but in some patients, particularly in those with prosthetic heart valves or those with recurrent embolic episodes, this is not acceptable. The preferred alternative is the use of heparin, which does not cross the placental barrier. Although the mother continues to be at risk of bleeding, fetal development is not endangered. Women can be instructed in the outpatient use of heparin, and its use is preferable to warfarin. This is particularly important at the time of conception and in the first trimester.

Antiplatelet agents increase the chance of maternal bleeding and cross the placenta. The most commonly used of them, aspirin, is associated with an increased incidence of abortion and fetal growth retardation.[120] Its inhibition of prostaglandin synthesis may also result in closure of the ductus arteriosus during fetal life.[121]

Obstetric Drugs and Their Cardiac Effects

Drugs Used to Stimulate the Uterus

Significant hemodynamic changes may be associated with attempts to induce or suppress labor. The injection of hypertonic solutions into the uterus to produce abortion may result in hypervolemia and, if saline is used, hypernatremia. Prostaglandins E_2 and $F_{2\alpha}$ are employed as agents for inducing labor, both at term and for therapeutic abortion. Hemodynamic alterations are not observed in the low doses generally recommended.

Drugs Used to Quiet the Uterus

Ethyl alcohol administered intravenously in hypertonic concentrations is sometimes used to avert premature labor. Alcohol itself has important effects on the myocardium, especially in patients with heart disease.[122] In addition, substantial alterations in fluid balance may occur, especially when prolonged infusion is necessary to maintain uterine quiescence. Ritodrine, isoxsuprine hydrochloride, terbutaline, and other beta-sympathomimetic amines are sometimes used to stop premature labor. All cause an increase in heart rate and contractility and should not be used when diabetes, hypertension, or heart disease complicate pregnancy. The use of ritodrine and terbutaline at term has been associated with pulmonary edema.[123–125] Evidence up to this point indicates that the pulmonary edema is not due to left ventricular failure. It responds promptly to cessation of the beta-sympathomimetic amine and administration of diuretics.

Drugs Used at Delivery

Adequate analgesia for pain minimizes the hemodynamic burden of labor and reduces the danger of pulmonary edema precipitated by tachycardia. The anesthetic technique employed for delivery should depend on the training and competence of the anesthesiologist. Subarachnoid block, epidural block using an anesthetic solution containing epinephrine, or balanced general anesthesia (thiopental sodium, nitrous oxide, oxygen, and succinylcholine) are all associated with major, although transient, hemodynamic changes.[29] Epidural anesthesia without epinephrine in the anesthetic solution is the most effective of the techniques explored so far in maintaining hemodynamic stability.[28] Scopolamine is contraindicated because of the restlessness and tachycardia it evokes, and atropine should be used in minimal doses and with caution. A term delivery in a well-managed patient offers the best hope of a successful outcome for both mother and child. Although term cesarean section has historically been associated with a high maternal mortality rate in patients with mitral stenosis, with modern techniques and in skilled hands, surgical delivery may be preferable to labor for the rare patient in or on the verge of pulmonary edema at term.[126]

Diagnostic Procedures for Heart Disease during Pregnancy

The use of diagnostic procedures should be considered especially carefully during pregnancy because of potential risks to the mother and the child. Unless the normal changes of pregnancy are recognized, the findings may be misinterpreted. An electrocardiogram, though safe, should be obtained only when indicated to help deal with specific clinical problems. Nonspecific ST-T abnormalities have been reported during pregnancy, but their significance is not clear. There has also been a suggestion that a shift in the electrical axis on the electrocardiogram occurs during pregnancy, but these findings have not been universally accepted.[127]

All x-ray procedures should be avoided, particularly in early pregnancy. There is the risk of abnormal fetal organogenesis or of increasing the incidence of malignancy, particularly leukemia.[128] The American College of Radiology has stated that interruption of pregnancy is not justified in pregnant women who have had chest x-ray evaluation.[129]

A cardiac ultrasound evaluation is of no known risk to the mother or to the fetus, but it should be performed only when clinically indicated.

Cardiac catheterization should be avoided because of the dangers of fluoroscopic exposure and because of the potentially adverse effects of introducing foreign material into the cardiovascular system of a pregnant woman. However, if the woman is at particular risk from her heart disease, the procedure should be performed. It is important to emphasize that any woman who is about to undergo x-ray examination or cardiac catheterization should be questioned about the possibility of being pregnant.

References

1. Burwell, C. S., and Metcalfe, J.: "Heart Disease and Pregnancy: Physiology and Management," Little, Brown and Company, Boston. 1958.
2. Jones, A. M., and Howitt, G.: Eisenmenger Syndrome in Pregnancy, *Br. Med. J.*, 1:1627, 1965.
3. Loffer, F. D.: Eisenmenger's Complex and Pregnancy, *Obstet. Gynecol.*, 29:235, 1967.
4. Szekely, P., and Snaith, L.: "Heart Disease and Pregnancy," Churchill and Livingstone, Edinburgh, London, 1974, p. 171.
5. Pyeritz, R. E., and McKusick, V. A.: The Marfan's Syndrome: Diagnosis and Management, *N. Engl. J. Med.*, 300:772, 1979.
6. Szekely, P., Turner, R., and Snaith, L.: Pregnancy and the Changing Pattern of Rheumatic Heart Disease, *Br. Heart J.*, 35:1293, 1973.
7. Clinch, J.: Chorea Gravidarum, *Hosp. Med.*, 2:317, 1967.
8. Lewis, B. V., and Parsons, M.: Chorea Gravidarum, *Lancet*, 1:284, 1966.
9. Ueland, K., and Metcalfe, J.: Acute Rheumatic Fever in Pregnancy, *Am. J. Obstet. Gynecol.*, 95:586, 1966.
10. Demakis, J. G., and Rahimtoola, S. H.: Peripartum Cardiomyopathy, *Circulation*, 44:964, 1971.
11. Demakis, J. G., Rahimtoola, S. H., Sutton, G. C., Meadows, W. R., Szanto, P. B., Tobin, J. R. and Gunnar, R. M.: Natural Course of Peripartum Cardiomyopathy, *Circulation*, 44:1053, 1971.
12. Burch, G. E.: Heart Disease and Pregnancy, *Am. Heart J.*, 93:104, 1977.
13. Mever, E. C., Tulsky, A. S., Sigmann, P., and Silver, E. N.: Pregnancy in the Presence of Tetralogy of Fallot: Observations on Two Patients, *Am. J. Cardiol.*, 14:874, 1964.
14. Jacoby, W., Jr.: Pregnancy with Tetralogy and Pentalogy of Fallot, *Am. J. Cardiol.*, 14:866, 1964.
15. Whittemore, R., Hobbins, J. C., and Engle, M. A.: Pregnancy and Its Outcome in Women with and without Surgical Treatment of Congenital Heart Disease, *Am. J. Cardiol.*, 50:641, 1982.
16. Whittemore, R.: Congenital Heart Disease: Its Impact on Pregnancy, *Hosp. Prac.*, 18:65, December 1983.
17. Mitchell, S. C., Korones, S. B., and Berendes, H. W.: Congenital Heart Disease in 56,109 Births: Incidence and Natural History, *Circulation*, 43:323, 1971.
18. Nora, J. J., and Nora, A. H.: The Evolution of Specific Genetic and Environmental Counseling in Congenital Heart Diseases, *Circulation*, 57:205, 1978.
19. Roberts, N.: A Predictive Study of Congenital Heart Disease and Need for Care, *West. J. Med.*, 129:19, 1978.
20. Chesley, L. C.: Plasma and Red Cell Volumes during Pregnancy, *Am. J. Obstet. Gynecol.*, 112:440, 1972.
21. Metcalfe, J., and Ueland, K.: Maternal Cardiovascular Adjustments to Pregnancy, *Prog. Cardiovasc. Dis.*, 16:363, 1974.
22. Lindheimer, M. D., and Katz, A. I.: Sodium and Diuretics in Pregnancy, *N. Engl. J. Med.*, 288:891, 1973.
23. Lees, M. M., Taylor, S. H., Scott, D. B., and Kerr, M. G.: A Study of Cardiac Output at Rest throughout Pregnancy, *J. Obstet. Gynaecol. Br. Commonw.*, 74:319, 1967.
24. Rubler, S., Damani, P. M., and Pinto, E. R.: Cardiac Size and Performance during Pregnancy Estimated with Echocardiography, *Am. J. Cardiol.*, 40:534, 1977.
25. Katz, R., Karliner, J. S., and Resnick, R.: Effects of a Natural Volume Overload State (Pregnancy) on Left Ventricular Performance in Normal Human Subjects, *Circulation*, 58:434, 1978.
26. Kerr, M. G.: The Mechanical Effects of the Gravid Uterus in Late Pregnancy, *J. Obstet. Gynaecol. Br. Commonw.*, 72:513, 1965.
27. Kerr, M. G., Scott, D. B., and Samuel E.: Studies of the Inferior Vena Cava in Late Pregnancy, *Br. Med. J.*, 1:532, 1964.
28. Ueland, K., Akamatsu, T. J., Eng, M., Bonica, J. J., and Hansen, J. M.: Maternal Cardiovascular Dynamics: VI. Cesarean Section under Epidural Anesthesia without Epinephrine, *Am. J. Obstet. Gynecol.*, 114:775, 1972.
29. Christianson, R. E.: Studies on Blood Pressure during Pregnancy: I. Influence of Parity and Age, *Am. J. Obstet. Gynecol.*, 125:509, 1976.
30. Gallery, E. D. M., Hunyo, S. N., Ross, M., and (Hunyor) Györy, A. Z.: Predicting the Development of Pregnancy-Associated Hypertension: The Place of Standardized Blood-Pressure Measurement, *Lancet*, 1:1273, 1977.
31. Assali, N. S., Rauramo, L., and Peltonen, T.: Measurement of Uterine Blood Flow and Uterine Metabolism: VIII. Uterine and Fetal Blood Flow and Oxygen Consumption in Early Human Pregnancy, *Am. J. Obstet. Gynecol.*, 79:86, 1960.
32. Metcalfe, J., Romney, S. L., Ramsey, L. H., Reid, D. E., and Burwell, C. S.: Estimation of Uterine Blood Flow in Normal Human Pregnancy at Term. *J. Clin. Invest.*, 34:1632, 1955.
33. Greenberg, B. H., Schutz, R., Grunkemeier, G. L., and Griswold, H. E.: Acute Effects of Alcohol in Patients with Congestive Heart Failure, *Ann. Intern. Med.*, 97:171, 1982.
34. Roman-Ponce, H., Thatcher, W. W., Caton, D., Barron, D. H., and Wilcox, C. J.: Effects of Thermal Stress and Epinephrine on Uterine Blood Flow in Ewes. *J. Anim. Sci.*, 46:167, 1978.
35. Morris, M., Osborn, S. B., and Wright, H. P.: Effective Uterine Blood-Flow during Exercise in Normal and Preeclamptic Pregnancies, *Lancet*, 2:481, 1956.
36. Ueland, K., Novy, M. J., and Metcalfe, J.: Cardiorespiratory Responses to Pregnancy and Exercise in Normal Women and Patients with Heart Disease, *Am. J. Obstet. Gynecol.*, 115:4, 1973.
37. Guzman, C. A., and Caplan, R.: Cardiorespiratory Response to Exercise during Pregnancy, *Am. J. Obstet. Gynecol.*, 108:600, 1970.
38. Burwell, C. S., Strayhorn, W. D., Flickinger, D., Corlette, M. B., Bowerman, E. P., and Kennedy, J. A.: Circulation during Pregnancy, *Arch. Intern. Med.*, 62:979, 1938.
39. Hoversland, A. S., Parer, J. T., and Metcalfe, J.: Hemodynamic Adjustments in the Pygmy Goat during Pregnancy and Early Postpartum, *Biol. Reprod.*, 10:578, 1974.
40. Dhindsa, D. S., Metcalfe, J., and Hummels, D. H.: Responses to Exercise in the Pregnant Pygmy Goat, *Respir. Physiol.*, 32:299, 1978.
41. Hosenpud, J. D., Hart, M. V., Morton, M. J., and Hohimer, A. R.: Chronic Estrogen Administration Increases Left Ventricular Size and Stroke Volume, *Clin. Res.*, 31:192A, 1983. (Abstract.)
42. Beary, J. F., Summer, W. R., and Bulkley, B. H.: Postpartum Acute Myocardial Infarction: A Rare Occurrence of Uncertain Etiology, *Am. J. Cardiol.*, 43:158, 1979.
43. Shaver, P. J., Carrig, T. F., and Baker, W. P.: Postpartum Coronary Artery Dissection, *Br. Heart J.*, 40:83, 1978.
44. Ahronheim, J. H.: Isolated Coronary Periarteritis: Report of a Case of Unexpected Death in a Young Pregnant Woman, *Am. J. Cardiol.*, 40:287, 1977.
45. Jewett, J. F.: Two Dissecting Coronary-Artery Aneurysms Post Partum, *N. Engl. J. Med.*, 298:1255, 1978.
46. Ciraulo, D. A., and Markovitz, A.: Myocardial Infarction in Pregnancy Associated with a Coronary Artery Thrombus, *Arch. Intern, Med.*, 139:1046, 1979.
47. Majdan, J. F., Walinśky, P., Cowchock, S. F., Wapner, R. J., and Plzak, L., Jr.: Coronary Artery Bypass Surgery during Pregnancy, *Am. J. Cardiol.*, 52:1145, 1983.
48. Cutforth, R., and MacDonald, C. B.: Heart Sounds and Murmurs in Pregnancy. *Am. Heart J.*, 71:741, 1966.
49. Abel, E. L.: Smoking during Pregnancy: A Review of Effects on Growth and Development of Offspring, *Hum. Biol.*, 52:593, 1980.
50. Rao, P. S.: Prevention of Heart Disease in Infants and Children, *Curr. Probl. Pediatr.*, 7:1, 1977.
51. Rubella Vaccine: Recommendation of the Public Health Service Advisory Committee on Immunization Practices, Center for Disease Control, DHEW, Atlanta, Ga., *Ann. Intern. Med.*, 88:543, 1978.
52. Rimland, D., McGowan, J. E., and Shulman, J. A.: Immu-

nization for the Internist, *Ann. Intern. Med.*, 85:622, 1976.
53. Kaplan, E. L., Anthony, B. F., Bisno, A., Durack, D., Houser, H., Millard, H. D., Sanford, J., Shulman, S. T., Stillerman, M., Taranta, A., and Wenger, N.: Prevention of Bacterial Endocarditis, *Circulation,* 56:139A, 1977.
54. Kaplan, E. L., Bisno, A., Derrick, W., Facklam, R., Gordis, L., E. Houser, H. B., Jackson, W. H., Millard, H. D., Shulman, S. T., Taranta, A. V., and Wanamaker, L. W.: Prevention of Rheumatic Fever, *Circulation,* 55:1, 1977.
55. Bland, E. F.: Declining Severity of Rheumatic Fever: A Comparative Study of the Past Four Decades, *N. Engl. J. Med.*, 262:597, 1960.
56. Krause, R. M.: The Influence of Infection on the Geography of Heart Disease, *Circulation,* 60:972, 1979.
57. Padmaviti, S.: Rheumatic Fever and Rheumatic Heart Disease in Developing Countries, *Bull. World Health Org.*, 56:543, 1978.
58. Snaith, L., and Szekely, P.: Cardiovascular Surgery in Relation to Pregnancy, in S. L. Marcus and C. C. Marcus (eds.), "Advances in Obstetrics and Gynecology," The Williams & Wilkins Company, Baltimore, 1967, p. 220.
59. Commerford, P. J., Hastie, T., and Beck, W.: Closed Mitral Valvotomy: Actuarial Analysis of Results in 654 Patients over 12 Years and Analysis of Preoperative Predictors of Long-Term Survival, *Ann. Thorac. Surg.*, 33:473, 1982.
60. Stevenson, R. E., Burton, M., Ferlauto, G. J., and Taylor, H. A.: Hazards of Oral Anticoagulants during Pregnancy, *JAMA,* 243:1549, 1980.
61. Hall, J. G., Pauli, R. M., and Wilson, K. M.: Maternal and Fetal Sequelae of Anticoagulation during Pregnancy, *Am. J. Med.*, 68:122, 1980.
62. Merrill, L. K., and VerBurg, D. J.: The Choice of Long-Term Anticoagulants for the Pregnant Patient, *Obstet. Gynecol.*, 47:711, 1976.
63. Devereux, R. B., Perloff, J. K., Reichek, N., and Josephson, M. E.: Mitral Valve Prolapse, *Circulation,* 54:3, 1976.
64. Barlow, J. B., and Pocock, W. A.: The Problem of Nonejection Systolic Clicks and Associated Mitral Systolic Murmurs: Emphasis on the Billowing Mitral Leaflet Syndrome, *Am. Heart J.*, 90:636, 1976.
65. Markiewicz, W., Stoner, J., London, E., Hunt, S. A., and Popp, R. L.: Mitral Valve Prolapse in One Hundred Presumably Healthy Young Females, *Circulation,* 53:464, 1976.
66. Procacci, P. M., Savran, S. V., Schreiter, S. L., and Bryson, A. L.: Prevalence of Clinical Mitral-Valve Prolapse in 1,169 Young Women, *N. Engl. J. Med.*, 294:1086, 1976.
67. Shell, W. E., Walton, J. A., Clifford, M. E., and Willis, P. W. III: The Familial Occurrence of the Syndrome of Mid-Late Systolic Click and Late Systolic Murmur, *Circulation,* 39:327, 1969.
68. Rizzon, P., Biasco, G., Brindicci, G., and Mauro, F.: Familial Syndrome of Midsystolic Click and Late Systolic Murmur, *Br. Heart J.*, 35:245, 1973.
69. Haas, J. M.: The Effect of Pregnancy on the Midsystolic Click and Murmurs of the Prolapsing Posterior Leaflet of the Mitral Valve, *Am. Heart J.*, 92:407, 1976.
70. Roberts, W. C.: The Congenitally Bicuspid Aortic Valve. A Study of 85 Autopsy Cases, *Am. J. Cardiol.*, 26:72, 1970.
71. Arias, F., and Pineda, J.: Aortic Stenosis in Pregnancy, *J. Reprod. Med.*, 20:229, 1970.
72. McAnulty, J. H., and Rahimtoola, S. H.: Surgery for Infective Endocarditis, *JAMA,* 242:77, 1979.
73. Wilson, W. R., Danielson, G. K., Giulani, E. R., Washington, J. A. II, Jaumin, P. M., and Geraci, J. E.: Valve Replacement in Patients with Active Infective Endocarditis, *Circulation,* 58:585, 1978.
74. Pelletier, L. L., Jr., and Petersdorf, R. G.: Infective Endocarditis: A Review of 125 Cases from the University of Washington Hospitals, 1963–1972, *Medicine,* 56:287, 1977.
75. Nielsen, N. C., and Fabricius, J.: Primary Pulmonary Hypertension with Special Reference to Prognosis, *Acta. Med. Scand.*, 170:731, 1961.
76. McCaffrey, R. N., and Dunn, L. J.: Primary Pulmonary Hypertension in Pregnancy, *Obstet. Gynecol. Survey,* 19:567, 1964.
77. Neilson, G., Galea, E. G., and Blunt, A.: Eisenmenger's Syndrome and Pregnancy, *Med. J. Aust.*, 1:431, 1971.
78. Cutforth, R., Catchlove, B., Knight, L. W., and Dudgeon, G.: The Eisenmenger Syndrome and Pregnancy, *Aust. N. Z. J. Obstet. Gynaecol.*, 8:202, 1968.
79. Deal, K., and Wooley, C. F.: Coarctation of the Aorta and Pregnancy, *Ann. Intern. Med.*, 78:706, 1973.
80. Barash, P. G., Hobbins, J. C., Hook, R., Stansel, H. C., Jr., Whittmore, R., and Hehre, F. W.: Management of Coarctation of the Aorta during Pregnancy, *J. Thorac. Cardiovasc. Surg.*, 69:781, 1975.
81. Mortensen, J. D., and Ellsworth, H. S.: Coarctation of the Aorta in Pregnancy: Obstetric and Cardiovascular Complications before and after Surgical Correction. *JAMA,* 191:596, 1965.
82. Kolibash, A. J., Ruiz, D. E., and Lewis, R. P.: Idiopathic Hypertrophic Subaortic Stenosis in Pregnancy, *Ann. Intern. Med.*, 82:791, 1975.
83. Brown, A. K., Doukas, N., Riding, W. D., and Jones, E. W.: Cardiomyopathy and Pregnancy, *Br. Heart J.*, 29:387, 1967.
84. Turner, G. M., Oakley, C. M., and Dixon, H. G.: Management of Pregnancy Complicated by Hypertrophic Obstructive Cardiomyopathy, *Br. Med. J.*, 4:281, 1968.
85. Oakley, G. D. G., McGarry, K., Limb, D. G., and Oakley, C. M.: Management of Pregnancy in Patients with Hypertrophic Cardiomyopathy, *Br. Med. J.*, 1:1749, 1979.
86. McKusick, V. A.: "Hereditable Disorders of Connective Tissue," 4th ed., The C. V. Mosby Company, St. Louis, 1972, p. 61.
87. Murdoch, J. L., Walker, B. A., Halpern, B. L., Kuzma, J. W. and McKusick, V. A.: Life Expectancy and Causes of Death in the Marfan Syndrome, *N. Engl. J. Med.*, 286:804, 1972.
88. Pyeritz, R. E.: Maternal and Fetal Complications of Pregnancy in the Marfan Syndrome, *Am. J. Med.*, 71:784, 1981.
89. Brown, O. R., DeMots, H., Kloster, F. E., Roberts, A., Menashe, V. D., and Beals, R. K.: Aortic Root Dilatation and Mitral Valve Prolapse in Marfan's Syndrome: An Echocardiographic Study, *Circulation,* 52:651, 1975.
90. Melvin, K. R., Richardson, P. J., Olsen, E. G., Daly, K., and Jackson, G.: Peripartum Cardiomyopathy Due to Myocarditis, *N. Engl. J. Med.*, 307:731, 1982.
91. Mendelson, C. L.: Disorders of the Heartbeat during Pregnancy, *Am. J. Obstet. Gynecol.*, 72:1268, 1956.
92. Szekely, P., and Snaith, L.: Paroxysmal Tachycardia in Pregnancy, *Br. Heart J.*, 15:195, 1953.
93. Bellet, S.: "Essentials of Cardiac Arrhythmias. Diagnosis and Management," W. B. Saunders Company, Philadelphia, 1972, p. 257.
94. Schroeder, J. S., and Harrison, D. C.: Repeated Cardioversion during Pregnancy: Treatment of Refractory Paroxysmal Atrial Tachycardia during 3 Successive Pregnancies, *Am. J. Cardiol.*, 27:445, 1971.
95. Copeland, G. D., and Stern, T. N.: Wenckebach Periods in Pregnancy and Puerperium, *Am. Heart J.*, 56:291, 1958.
96. Kenmore, A. C. F., and Cameron, A. J. V.: Congenital Complete Heart Block in Pregnancy, *Br. Heart J.*, 29:910, 1967.
97. Casanegra, P., Avilés, G., Maturana, G., and Dubernet, J.: Cardiovascular Management of Pregnant Women with a Heart Valve Prosthesis, *Am. J. Cardiol.*, 36:802, 1975.
98. Kloster, F. E.: Infective Prosthetic Valve Endocarditis, in S. H. Rahimtoola (ed.) "Infective Endocarditis," Grune & Stratton, Inc., New York, 1978, p. 291.
99. Brinkman, C. R. III, and Woods, J. R., Jr.: Effects of Cardiovascular Drugs during Pregnancy, *Cardiovasc. Med.*, 1:231, 1976.
100. Rogers, M. C., Willerson, J. T., Goldblatt, A., and Smith, T. W.: Serum Digoxin Concentrations in Human Fetus, Neonate and Infant, *N. Engl. J. Med.*, 287:1010, 1972.
101. Weaver, J. B., and Pearson, J. F.: Influence of Digitalis on Time of Onset and Duration of Labor in Women with Cardiac Disease, *Br. Med. J.*, 3:519, 1973.
102. Bullock, J. L., Harris, R. E., and Young, R.: Treatment of

Thyrotoxicosis during Pregnancy with Propranolol, *Am. J. Obstet. Gynecol.*, 121:242, 1975.
103. Chez, R. A., Ehrenkranz, R. A., Oakes, G. K., Walker, A. M., Hamilton, L. A., Jr., Brennan, S. C., and McLaughlin, M. K.: Effects of Adrenergic Agents on Ovine Umbilical and Uterine Blood Flows, in L. D. Longo and D. D. Reneau (eds.), "Fetal and Newborn Cardiovascular Physiology," vol. 2: "Fetal and Newborn Circulation," Garland STPM Press, New York and London, 1978, p. 1.
104. Barden, T. P., and Stander, R. W.: Myometrial and Cardiovascular Effects of an Adrenergic Blocking Drug in Human Pregnancy, *Am. J. Obstet. Gynecol.*, 101:91, 1968.
105. Sabom, M. B., Curry, R. C., Jr., and Wise, D. E.: Propranolol Therapy during Pregnancy in a Patient with Idiopathic Hypertrophic Subaortic Stenosis: Is It Safe?, *South. Med. J.*, 71:328, 1978.
106. Tunstall, M. E.: The Effect of Propranolol on the Onset of Breathing at Birth. *Br. J. Anesth.*, 41:792, 1969.
107. Datta, S., Kitzmiller, J. L., Ostheimer, G. W., and Schoenbaum, S. C.: Propranolol and Parturition, *Obstet. Gynecol.*, 51:577, 1978.
108. Habib, A., and McCarthy, J. S.: Effects on the Neonate of Propranolol Administered during Pregnancy, *J. Pediatr.*, 91:808, 1977.
109. Pruyn, C. S., Phelan, J. P., and Buchanan, G. C.: Long-Term Propranolol Therapy in Pregnancy: Maternal and Fetal Outcome, *Am. J. Obstet. Gynecol.*, 135:485, 1979.
110. Schenker, J. G., and Chowers, I.: Pheochromocytoma and Pregnancy: Review of 89 Cases, *Obstet. Gynecol. Survey*, 26:739, 1971.
111. Hill, L. M., and Malkasian, G. D., Jr.: The Use of Quinidine Sulfate throughout Pregnancy, *Obstet. Gynecol.*, 54:366, 1979.
112. Tamari, I., Eldar, M., Rabinowitz, M., and Newfeld, H. N.: Medical Treatment of Cardiovascular Disorders during Pregnancy, *Am. Heart J.*, 104:1357, 1982.
113. Leonard, R. F., Braun, T. E., and Levy, A. M.: Initiation of Uterine Contractions by Disopyramide during Pregnancy, *N. Engl. J. Med.*, 299:84, 1978.
114. Rotmensch, H. H., Elkayam, U., and Frishman, W.: Antiarrhythmic Drug Therapy during Pregnancy, *Ann. Intern. Med.*, 98:487, 1983.
115. Stempel, J. E., O'Grady, J. P., Morton, M. J., and Johnson, K. A.: Use of Sodium Nitroprusside in Complications of Gestational Hypertension, *Obstet. Gynecol.*, 60:533, 1982.
116. Pauli, R. M., Madden, J. D., Kranzler, K. J., Culpepper, W., and Port, R.: Warfarin Therapy Initiated during Pregnancy and Phenotypic Chondrodysplasia Punctata, *J. Pediatr.*, 88:506, 1976.
117. Raivio, K. O., Ikonen, E., and Saarikoski, S.: Fetal Risks Due to Warfarin Therapy during Pregnancy, *Acta Paediatr. Scand.*, 66:735, 1977.
118. Sherman, S., and Hall, B. D.: Warfarin and Fetal Abnormality, *Lancet*, 1:692, 1976.
119. Fillmore, S. J., and McDevitt, E.: Effects of Coumarin Compounds on the Fetus, *Ann. Intern. Med.*, 73:731, 1970.
120. Corby, D. G.: Aspirin in Pregnancy and Fetal Effects, *Pediatrics*, 62:930, 1978.
121. Rudolph, A. M.: Effects of Aspirin and Acetaminophen in Pregnancy and in the Newborn, *Arch. Intern Med.*, 141:358, 1981.
122. Lunnell, N. O., Nylund, N. E., Lewander, R., and Sarby, B.: Uteroplacental Blood Flow in Pre-Eclampsia Measurements with Indium-113m and a Computer-Linked Gamma Camera. *Clin. Exp. Hypertens. B*, 1:105, 1982.
123. Stubblefield, P. G.: Pulmonary Edema Occurring after Therapy with Dexamethasone and Terbutaline for Premature Labor: A Case Report. *Am. J. Obstet. Gynecol.*, 132:341, 1979.
124. Elliott, H. R., Abdulla, U., and Haves, P. J.: Pulmonary Oedema Associated with Ritodrine Infusion and Betamethasone Administration in Premature Labour, *Br. Med. J.*, 2:799, 1978.
125. Hosenpud, J. D., Morton, M. J., and O'Grady, J. P.: Cardiac Stimulation during Ritodrine Hydrochloride Tocolytic Therapy, *Obstet. Gynecol.*, 62:52, 1983.
126. Ferraris, G., and Gambotto, C.: Cesarean Section as the Method of Choice for Patients with Cardiac Decompensation, *Minerva Ginec.*, 14:198, 1962.
127. Schwartz, D. B., and Schamroth, L.: The Effect of Pregnancy on the Frontal Plane QRS Axis, *J. Electrocardiog.*, 12:279, 1979.
128. Bonebrake, C. R., Noller, K. L., Loehnen, C. P., Muhm, J. R., and Fish, C. R.: Routine Chest Roentgenography in Pregnancy, *JAMA*, 240:2747, 1978.
129. United States Food and Drug Administration, Bureau of Radiological Health: Chest X-Ray as a Screening Procedure for Cardiopulmonary Disease, A Policy Statement, DHEW Publication 73-8036, 1973.

70

The Heart in Athletes

Andrew G. Wallace, M.D.

Speaking generally, all parts of the body which have a function, if used in moderation and exercised in labours to which each is accoustomed, become thereby healthy and well developed, and age slowly; but if unused and left idle, they become liable to disease, defective in growth, and age quickly.
Hippocrates[1]

The relation between athletic performance and the heart can be approached from several points of view. Maximal performance in many forms of athletic activity is determined by the heart and circulation because of their dominant role in oxygen transport. Performance, oxygen transport, and peak cardiac capacity are all increased by training. Protagonists of physical fitness adhere to the view that health and longevity can be enhanced through exercise. Others note that exercise is the most severe stress to which the cardiovascular system is subjected and that such stress may be harmful or even fatal in subjects with underlying heart disease. Historically, many physicians felt that prolonged exercise caused heart disease. This chapter reviews the cardiovascular responses to acute exercise, the cardiac changes that accompany training, the athlete's heart, sudden death during athletic activities, and, finally, the office examination of the athlete.

Physiological Response to Acute Exercise

Circulatory adjustments to dynamic exercise involve local changes in muscle, blood pressure, and cardiac output; the need to eliminate efficiently the energy not utilized for mechanical work; and the role of the nervous system in helping to mediate these adjustments.[1,2,3]

The earliest component of the circulatory response to exercise is a large reduction in the resistance offered by nutrient blood vessels in working muscle (Fig. 70-1). Blood flow to resting muscle averages 4 to 7 ml per 100 g of tissue. This flow rate may increase to 50 to 75 ml per 100 g during maximal activity. The increase in blood flow to muscle is mediated largely by the opening of capillary beds that are not open at rest; it occurs despite the fact that during activity blood flow decreases with each contraction as a result of the extravascular compressive forces exerted by contracting muscles.[4] Current data indicate that the fall in vascular resistance during exercise is caused by the drop in tissue P_{O_2} and perhaps by the release of vasodilator agents including potassium, adenosine, lactic acid, and carbon dioxide.

During near maximal sustained dynamic exercise, skeletal muscle metabolism is principally aerobic. The large increase in adenosine triphosphate (ATP) generation is met by a correspondingly increased uptake of oxygen. Since the need for oxygen is only partially fulfilled by the increase in local flow, extraction of oxygen also increases from approximately 5 to 15 ml per 100 ml of nutrient flow.

Investigators have reported a nearly linear relation between oxygen uptake and cardiac output during exercise.[5] The mechanisms that enable a heart to pump five or more times its resting cardiac output during exercise are dominated by the increase in heart rate, which is most closely related to the increase in flow (Fig. 70-2). During maximal effort, however, changes in heart rate alone cannot account for the increased output of the heart. Dimensional studies in animals and humans[6] have shown that stroke volume is also augmented and this augmentation is caused by increased systolic emptying of the ventricle from the same or a slightly increased left ventricular end-diastolic volume. Thus, while heart

FIGURE 70-1 Schematic representation of the cardiopulmonary system of a human being in the resting state (*left panel*) and during peak upright exercise (*right panel*). Blood flow in milliliters per minute to each organ, representative of those observed at rest and during maximal exercise, is noted. (*From J. H. Mitchell and G. Blomqvist, Maximal Oxygen Uptake, N. Engl. J. Med., 284:1018, 1971. Reprinted by permission of The New England Journal of Medicine and the author.*)

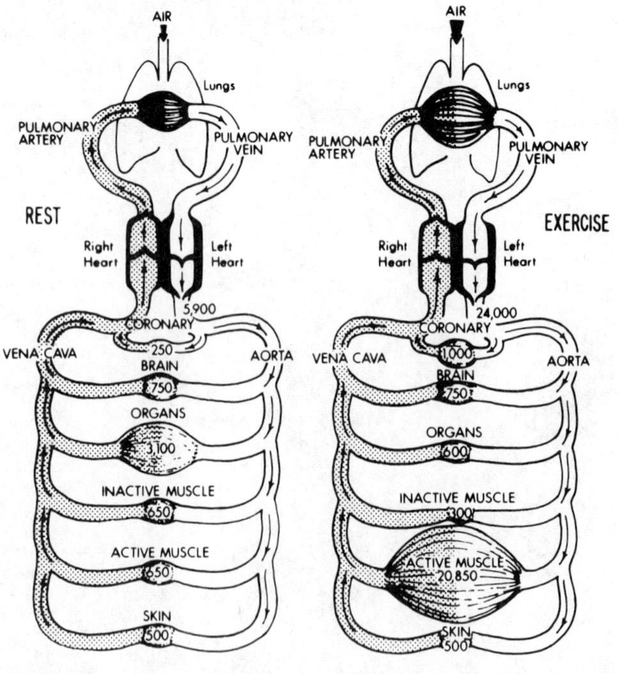

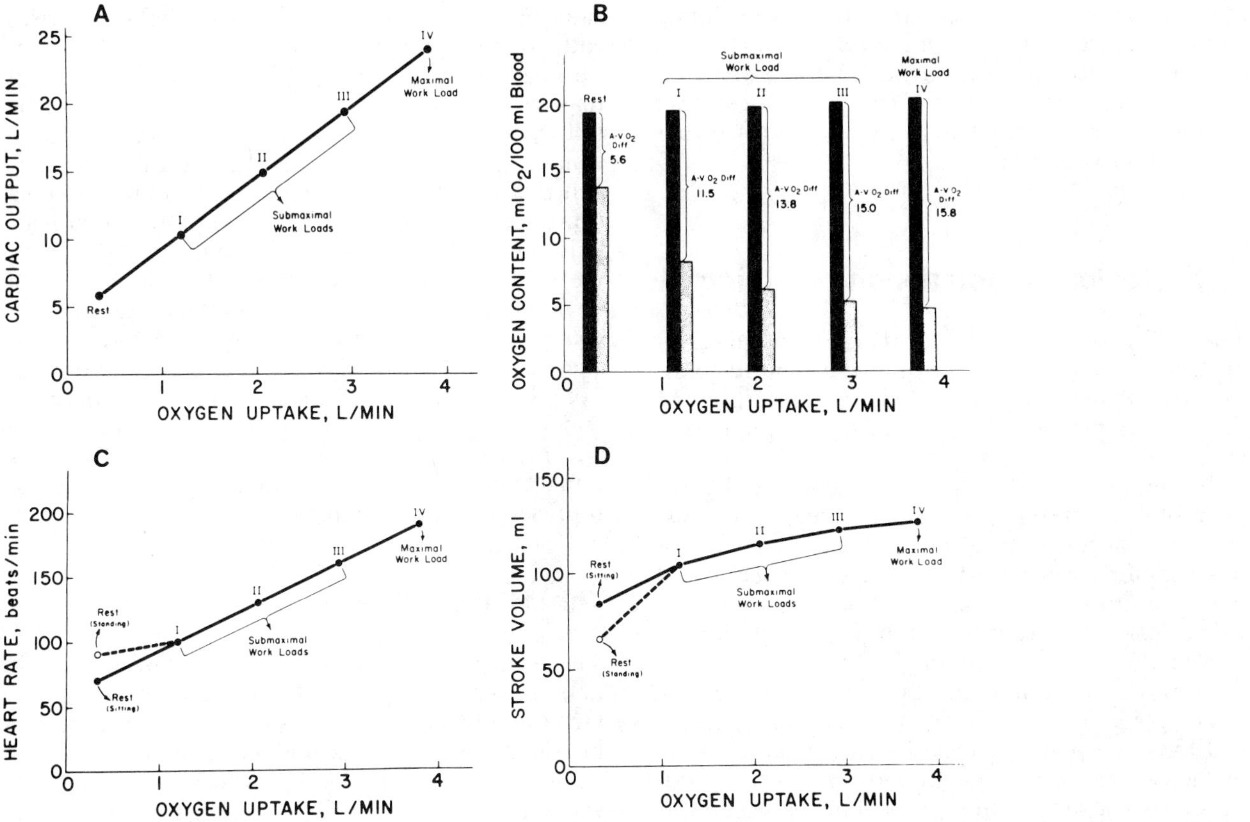

FIGURE 70-2 Hemodynamic responses to upright exercise. In each panel workload is shown as oxygen uptake on the horizontal axis. *A.* Changes in cardiac output. *B.* Changes in arteriovenous oxygen difference. *C.* Changes in heart rate. *D.* Changes in stroke volume. Roman numerals I to IV represent work states on treadmill. (*From J. H. Mitchell and G. Blomqvist: Maximal Oxygen Uptake, N. Engl. J. Med., 284:1018, 1971. Reprinted by permission of The New England Journal of Medicine and the author.*)

rate increases per se play the predominant role in augmentation of flow in response to exercise, the inotropic effects of increased sympathetic nervous activity and, to a lesser extent, Starling forces also play a role. The importance of sympathetic augmentation of heart rate and contractility with exercise is evidenced by the fact that endurance and cardiac output at maximal effort are attenuated by approximately 20 to 40 percent after pharmacological blockage of cardiac beta-adrenergic receptors.

Other features of the cardiovascular response to dynamic exercise include a prominent increase in systolic blood pressure, a modest increase in mean arterial pressure, and little change or a slight decrease in diastolic pressure. The increase in mean systemic arterial pressure at a time when cardiac output is four to five times normal reflects a significant drop in total peripheral vascular resistance, largely as a consequence of marked vasodilatation in exercising muscles. Exercise is accompanied by an increase of sympathetic nerve activity. Sympathetically mediated vasoconstriction of resistance vessels occurs in nearly all areas except those vascular beds supplying the exercising muscle.[7] Thus, during exercise there is vasoconstriction in the kidney, in the splanchnic vascular bed, and in skeletal muscle that is not doing work.

An additional feature of the integrated circulatory response to exercise is a sympathetically mediated increase in the tone of large veins in both exercising and nonexercising parts.[8] This increased tone of capacitance vessels allows the venous system to regulate cardiac output more efficiently. The net effect of venoconstriction is to enhance venous return at any given right atrial pressure and to assure that cardiac output will not be limited by an inadequate return of blood.

During exercise, body temperature increases gradually because of the tremendous heat load generated by exercising muscle. Heat loss occurs almost entirely through the skin. The mechanisms of this heat transfer include radiation, conduction, convection, and evaporation.[2] The most important factor in the control of body temperature during exercise, however, is the ability of the circulation to carry heat from its source (exercising muscle) to its site of dissipation (skin). Furthermore, as the heat load that must be dissipated increases, cutaneous vasodilatation leads to an increase of blood volume contained within the skin. With exercise of moderate to high intensity and of long duration, the requirements for cutaneous vasodilatation become prominent, and a circulatory adjustment referred to as *drift* develops. Drift is characterized by a further increase in heart rate, a drop in venous pressure and stroke volume, and a decrease in arterial pressure. These changes appear to be accounted for in large part by the drop in cutaneous vascular resistance and venous tone, minimizing the increase in body temperature that would otherwise occur.

Physiological Adaptations to Training

The ability to enhance performance through training is well known. In recent years the scientific basis for this fact has been elucidated and the interest of the cardiologist has been addressed to the phenomenon.

In the broadest sense, training involves enhancement of skill, strength, and endurance. It is the last of these that concerns us here. An earlier section of this chapter dealt with the changes in peripheral muscle and cardiovascular function when an individual makes the transition from rest to either submaximal or maximal sustained effort.

Endurance training increases maximal aerobic capacity, i.e., maximal oxygen uptake. Since maximal oxygen uptake defines the functional capacity of the cardiovascular system and reflects the product of cardiac output and arteriovenous oxygen difference, it follows that a change in $V_{O_2\ max}$ must reflect a corresponding change in maximal cardiac output or maximal extraction of oxygen by the periphery or both. The amount that $V_{O_2\ max}$ increases with training is inversely proportional to the preconditioning V_{O_2} and to age. For any given increase in $V_{O_2\ max}$ due to conditioning, about half of the effect is attributable to a peripheral component, i.e., increased capacity to extract oxygen from arterial blood, and about half of the effect is due to increased perfusion. The peripheral component of this effect involves changes in skeletal muscle structure and metabolism. Numerous studies have shown that training increases the size and number of mitochondria per gram of muscle; the level of mitochondrial enzyme activity per gram of mitochondrial protein; the capacity of muscle to oxidize fat, carbohydrate, and ketones; myoglobin levels; and the capacity to generate ATP.[9–11]

The central component of the training effect is characterized by a reduction in heart rate and blood pressure and an increase in stroke volume at any given submaximal workload.[12] With maximal effort peak heart rate is unaltered by training, stroke volume is enhanced, and maximal arteriovenous oxygen difference is enhanced. The increased oxygen uptake is attributable almost equally to a widened arteriovenous oxygen difference and an increase in cardiac output. In world-class athletes maximal oxygen uptake is 65 to 85 ml/kg, and maximal cardiac output averages about 30 to 33 liters/min.

The hemodynamic and metabolic effects of training are accompanied by changes in cardiac dimensions and ultrastructure.[13–15] Cardiac size increases with training whether estimated by x-ray, by echocardiogram, or by angiography. Cardiac volume and mass increase. These are changes that can also be induced in experimental animals subjected to a training program. In one series the estimated left ventricular volume of distance runners was 60 percent greater than that of sedentary normal individuals. The left ventricular volume of distance swimmers was 80 percent greater than that of the control subjects. In experimental animals the ultrastructural changes that accompany hypertrophy induced by exercise have been analyzed carefully. The dimensions and volume of the myocyte appear to increase, and there is a proportional increase in myofibrils and mitochondria per cell. In summary, the structural changes appear to be physiological and are best represented as an extension of normal growth.

The Athlete's Heart

The term *athlete's heart* was used to describe deviations from normal on the physical exam, chest x-ray, and ECG in individuals who have participated in competitive athletics and have undergone prolonged physical training.[16,17] Before 1940, these deviations from normal were often regarded as a form of heart disease caused by excessive physical exercise. However, studies in Great Britain in the 1930s suggested that heart disease was rarely, if ever, caused by exercise. Rather, the cardiovascular changes observed in athletes appear to be a part of a normal physiological adaptation to training, and most of the changes are reversible when training is discontinued.

The pulse rate of a well-trained athlete is typically slow (40 to 60 beats per minute), and the normal respiratory variation in pulse rate may be exaggerated. Blood pressure is normal and the jugular venous pressure and pulse are normal. Evidence of cardiac enlargement is usually absent by physical exam, although x-ray and echocardiography[15] frequently demonstrate an enlarged heart.

In 1929 Herxheimer reported on chest radiography in Olympic athletes and noted evidence of cardiac enlargement.[17a] The heart of an athlete has a globular shape and the cardiothoracic ratio is frequently 0.50 or greater. Heart volumes estimated from biplane chest x-rays have been shown to correlate with maximal oxygen uptake, cardiac output, and stroke volume. All chambers participate equally in the cardiac enlargement of conditioning.

A third heart sound (S_3) is heard in a majority of trained athletes, and a fourth sound (S_4) is audible in about half. These sounds are usually maximal when the athlete is in the supine position and diminish with standing. They are of no known clinical significance. A systolic heart murmur is heard in about 40 percent of endurance athletes; it is best heard over the pulmonic or aortic area, is ejection in quality, and is short in duration. The carotid pulse is normal and the murmur does not produce a thrill. Diastolic murmurs are rarely, if ever, caused by exercise training and warrant appropriate further study.

Many electrocardiographic changes have been observed in athletes and have ultimately been ascribed to the consequences of training.[18,19] These changes can be divided into three major categories: (1) changes of rhythm and conduction, (2) changes of the P wave and QRS complex, and (3) alterations of repolarization leading to changes of the ST-T wave. Among rhythm and conduction changes, sinus bradycardia with or without sinus arrhythmia is common. Frequently, sinus slowing is sufficient to lead to a wandering atrial rhythm and junctional or ventricular escape beats. The PR interval is prolonged in about 25 percent of athletes when the pulse rate is below 50 beats per minute, and occasional periods of Wenckebach second degree AV block are observed. All these changes in rate and rhythm are normal after exercise or atropine administration. Changes in the P wave compatible with right or left atrial enlargement or both are common. An increase in QRS amplitude (but without prolongation) is seen in over 40 percent of athletes and may suggest right or left ventricular hypertrophy. Axis deviation and a strain pattern are absent, however. The ST-T wave changes are of two types. First, an elevated and early takeoff of the T wave (early repolarization) is common. Less frequent, but particularly common in blacks, is the "juvenile T pattern," with inverted T waves in the anterior precordial leads.

There are many reports of echocardiograms in athletes.[15] When the echocardiogram demonstrates an enlarged left ventricle, the diastolic dimensions of the atrial chambers and the right ventricle are also usually increased. Left ventricular thickness is increased in endurance athletes and in weight lifters. In lifters this increased mass is proportional to the increase in body weight (i.e., heart mass/lean body mass ratio is normal). In runners, on the other hand, the increase in left ventricular dimensions with training appears to revert to normal when training is discontinued.

The athlete's heart does not represent a disease state. Rather, it consists of findings on physical exam, x-ray, ECG, and echocardiogram that reflect the known physiological adaptations to training, one of which is physiological hypertrophy of the heart.

Sudden Death in Athletes

Cardiovascular deaths during exercise or competitive sports attract attention, but are fortunately uncommon. The annual incidence of sudden death in individuals between the ages of 1 and 30 ranges from 2 to 7 per 100,000, and of these about 8 percent are related to exercise. After the age of 30 the incidence of sudden death rises sharply to 50 to 60 per 100,000. However, with increasing age the percent of cases of sudden death related to exercise decreases to about 2 percent. Rose reviewed 44 deaths that occurred during sports activities between 1961 and 1969.[20] In individuals 15 to 19 years of age, in whom heat stroke as a cause of death could be eliminated, 38 deaths occurred. Autopsy data showed congenital heart disease in 6, myocarditis in 2, coronary artery disease in 2, rheumatic heart disease in 2, and myocardial contusion in 2. In the remainder a cause could not be determined. In 1978 Maron[21] reported on autopsy studies findings in 21 sports-related deaths in a group ranging from 14 to 30 years of age. Hypertrophic cardiomyopathy was noted in 7, concentric left ventricular hypertrophy in 5, congenital coronary artery anomalies in 4, atherosclerotic coronary artery disease in 2, Marfan's syndrome with aortic rupture in 2, and no identifiable cause in 1. Subsequent reports[22,23] support the view that in individuals under age 30 hypertrophic cardiomyopathies and congenital coronary lesions dominate as causes of sports-related sudden death. In those over age 30, atherosclerotic coronary artery disease dominates.[24]

Office Examination of the Athlete

The AMA Committee on Medical Aspects of Sports recommends that all students taking part in vigorous competitive athletics have a physical examination before participating. Most agencies that sponsor athletics from high school to professional levels now require all athletes to have a medically supervised examination annually. These examinations seek (1) to define the general state of health, (2) to disclose any defects that might contraindicate participation, and (3) to identify and correct any condition that might predispose the athlete to injury.

The extent of such health examinations varies widely and is not regulated by law. The AMA recommends that high school athletes be examined by their family physician. College and professional athletes are examined in a more structured way, usually by a team physician. At the professional level, the medicolegal implications assume greater proportion, and examinations tend to be more thorough and more frequent. However, even in professional sports, how extensive the exam should be is still unresolved.

Many of the conditions that constitute special problems for the athlete fall within the orthopedic sphere and will not be dealt with here. Others are of concern to the general internist and include (1) absence of paired organs, of which the eye and kidney are of greatest concern, (2) bleeding disease such as idiopathic thrombocytopenic purpura (ITP), (3) sickle cell anemia and trait, (4) epilepsy, (5) uncontrolled insulin-dependent diabetes, (6) asthma, and (7) malignancies. Of these, sickle cell anemia, a single eye, and bleeding diseases are regarded by most doctors as absolute contraindications to competitive contact sports. The cardiovascular conditions of special concern include congenital heart disease, hypertension, and arrhythmias.

Among the causes of sudden death in athletes below the age of 30, hypertrophic cardiomyopathy, congenital coronary artery abnormalities, and arrhythmias are the most frequent. Paroxysmal atrial tachycardia or fibrillation is most likely to be detected from the history, while premature ventricular beats or complete atrioventricular (AV) block will be noted most often on physical exam. Any such signs should be further examined by ECG. Paroxysmal atrial tachycardia (PAT) or paroxysmal atrial fibrillation (PAF), arrhythmias related to the Wolff-Parkinson-White (WPW) syndrome, and complete AV block are commonly regarded as contraindications to athletic participation. Isolated premature ventricular beats are innocuous unless associated with the long-QT-interval syndrome.

Congenital coronary artery lesions may cause symptoms or death in infants, but they are usually asymptomatic in teens and young adults. They are detected only when a murmur is heard (mitral regurgitation or a continuous murmur), which leads to an ECG. The fact that congenital coronary lesions and hypertrophic cardiomyopathy usually present in teenage or early adult life as asymptomatic murmurs emphasizes the importance of a careful physical exam. Either is an absolute contraindication to athletic participation. Patients with congenital heart disease and left-to-right shunts have a diminished maximal cardiac output, but if the shunt is small, exercise within the individual's physiological limitations poses no known risk. Cyanotic heart disease and congenital or acquired outflow obstruction, i.e., aortic or pulmonic stenosis or coarctation of the aorta, preclude athletics. Except in cases with coarctation, hypertension is not associated with any known risk and does not contraindicate athletics unless the blood pressure is at severely elevated levels and is unresponsive to treatment. Other conditions that prevent athletic performance include active myocarditis (rheumatic or viral), active pericarditis, and heart failure of any cause.

Among college and professional athletes, especially basketball players, the physician should be alert to stigmata of Marfan's syndrome or to an aortic diastolic murmur that might suggest cystic medial necrosis of the aorta and enhanced risk of dissection or rupture.

The evaluation of athletes with symptoms or a family history of early coronary heart disease should include an exercise stress test. An increasing number of professional teams are including the stress test in their routine preparticipatory exam, although in many cases it is being used primarily to assess fitness and not as a diagnostic test. Since males in the second and third decade of life are afflicted with coronary disease and since few occupations place greater physical demand on the heart than professional athletics, physiological testing of athletes under conditions of stress designed to stimulate their professional activities seems prudent. However, it should be noted that among athletes with physiological hypertrophy of the heart from training, the incidence of false-positive treadmill exercise tests approaches 10 percent, or nearly three times higher than the incidence of false-positive tests among unconditioned control subjects of the same age.[25]

References

1. "Hippocrates": English translation by E. T. Withington, Putnam, New York, vol. 3, 1927, p. 339.
2. Rowell, L. B.: Human Cardiovascular Adjustments to Exercise and Thermal Stress, *Physiol. Rev.*, 54:75, 1974.
3. Scheuer, J., and Tipton, C. M.: Cardiovascular Adaptations to Physical Training, *Annu. Rev. Physiol.*, 30:221, 1977.
4. Zierler, K. L., Masseri, A., Kalssen, G., Rabinowitz, D., and Burgess, J.: Muscle Metabolism during Exercise, *Trans. Assoc. Am. Phys.*, 81:266, 1968.
5. Chapman, C. B.: The Physiology of Muscular Exercise: A Symposium, *Circ. Res.*, 20(suppl. 1):1, 1967.
6. Rerych, S. K., Scholz, P. M., Sabiston, D. C., and Jones, R. H.: Effects of Training on the Left Ventricular Function in Normal Subjects, *Am. J. Cardiol.*, 43:1067, 1979.
7. Smith, E. E., Guyton, A. C., Manning, R. D., and White, R. J.: Integrated Mechanisms of Cardiovascular Response and Control during Exercise in the Normal Human, *Prog. Cardiovasc. Dis.*, 18:421, 1976.
8. Clement, D. L., and Shepherd, J. T.: Regulation of the Peripheral Circulation during Muscular Exercise, *Prog. Cardiovasc. Dis.*, 19:23, 1976.
9. Gollnick, P. D., Ianuzzo, C. D., and King, D. W.: Ultrastructure and Enzyme Changes in Muscle with Exercise, in "Advances in Experimental Medicine and Biology," Plenum Press, New York, 1971, vol. II, p. 69.
10. Holloszy, J. O.: Adaptations of Muscular Tissue to Training, *Prog. Cardiovasc. Dis.*, 18:445, 1976.
11. Havel, R. J.: Influence of Intensity and Duration of Exercise on Supply and Use of Fuels, in "Advances in Experimental Medicine and Biology," Plenum Press, New York, 1971, vol. II, p. 315.
12. Clausen, J. P.: Effects of Physical Training on Cardiovascular Adjustments to Exercise in Man, *Physiol. Rev.*, 57:779, 1977.
13. Gilbert, C., Nutter, S., Meymsfield, S., Perkins, J., and Schlant, R.: The Endurance Athlete: Cardiac Structure and Function. *Circulation*, 51(suppl. 2):115, 1975.
14. Ehsani, A. A., Hagbery, J. M., and Hickson, R. C.: Rapid Changes in Left Ventricular Dimensions and Mass in Response to Physical Conditioning and Deconditioning, *Am. J. Cardiol.*, 42:52, 1978.
15. Gilbert, C. A., Nutter, D. O., and Felner, J. M.: Echocardiographic Study of Cardiac Dimensions and Function in the Endurance Trained Athlete, *Am. J. Cardiol.*, 40:528, 1977.
16. Gott, P. H., Roselle, H. A., and Crampton, R. S.: The Athletic Heart Syndrome, *Arch. Intern. Med.*, 122:340, 1968.
17. Raskoff, W. J., Goldman, S., and Cohn, K.: The Athletic Heart, *JAMA*, 236:158, 1976.
17a. Herxheimer, H.: Die Herzgrosse der Amsterdamer Olympia Teilnehmer. *Klin. Wochenschr.*, 8:402, 1929.
18. Smith, W. G., Cullen, K. J., and Thorburn, I. D.: Electrocardiograms of Marathon Runners in the 1962 Commonwealth Games, *Br. Heart J.*, 26:469, 1964.
19. Schamroth, L., and Jokl, E.: Market Sinus and AV Nodal Bradycardia with Interference-Dissociation in an Athlete, *J. Sports Phys. Fitness*, 9:128, 1969.
20. Rose, K. D.: The Potential for Cardiovascular Accidents in Athletes with a Heart Problem, *Med. Sci. Sports*, 1:144, 1969.
21. Maron, B. J., Roberts, W. C., McCallister, H. A., Rosing, D. R., and Epstein, S. E.: Etiology of Sudden Death in Athletes, *Circulation*, 57(suppl. 2):236, 1978.

22. Kennedy, H. L., Whitlock, J. A., and Buckingham, T. A.: Cardiovascular Sudden Death in Young Persons, *J. Am. Coll. Cardiol.*, 3:485, 1984.
23. Waller, B. F., Newhouse, P., Pless, J., Foster, L., and Wills, E.: Exercise Related Sudden Death in 27 Conditioned Subjects Aged Less Than 30 and Greater Than 30 Years: Coronary Abnormalities Are the Culprit, *J. Am. Coll. Cardiol.*, 3:621, 1984.
24. Thompson, P. D., Stern, M. P., Williams, P., Duncan, K., Haskell, W. L., and Wood, P. D.: Death during Jogging or Running, *JAMA*, 242:1265, 1979.
25. Spirito, P., Maron, B. J., Bonow, R. O., and Epstein, S. E.: Prevalence of and Significance of Abnormal ST Segment Responses to Exercise in a Young Athletic Population, *Am. J. Cardiol.*, 51:166, 1983.

71

Cardiovascular Aging and Adaptation to Disease

Myron L. Weisfeldt, M.D.   Gary Gerstenblith, M.D.

Time has laid his hand upon my heart, gently, not smiting it, but as a harper lays his open palm upon his harp to deaden its vibrations.

Longfellow[1]

Introduction

Difficulties in the Study of Aging

All of us have a preconception that cardiovascular function as well as many other bodily functions decreases substantially during the latter portion of the life span of an individual. Part of this bias is certainly related to the fact that cardiovascular disease is prevalent in our population and its prevalence and severity increase with age.[5] Frequently when cardiovascular function is objectively decreased in an older individual and there is no apparent etiology, the changes are ascribed to aging. As discussed in detail in this chapter, this bias is for the most part unfounded and in fact is not substantiated if one examines a *disease-free* older population.

In order to understand the magnitude and mechanisms of age changes in cardiovascular function we must be clear as to certain definitions and limitations of available information. First, it is important to be clear as to the use, in this context, of the term *aging*. Although aging occurs during all phases of life, including the early phase of growth and development, these early changes are not the subject of this discussion. The cardiovascular changes referred to in this discussion are those that occur during *adulthood*. Second, one must acknowledge that it is often extremely difficult to dissociate aging from disease. For example, for many years it has been controversial as to what level of blood pressure represents a normal age-associated increase in blood pressure and what level indicates the presence of a disease, systemic hypertension. This debate continues, and there are advocates of the notion that it is impossible in this circumstance to dissociate disease from aging. There are others who believe that a clear-cut disease can be defined.

In attempting to decipher true age changes from those of disease, there are several important factors to remember. For the human species the prevalence of autopsy evidence of ischemic heart disease in those over 60 years of age dying of other causes is approximately 50 percent. Thus, only studies in which significant efforts are made to eliminate subjects with ischemic heart disease can appropriately be viewed as an examination of aging separate from disease. It is reassuring that many of the observations that have been made recently with regard to those aspects of cardiovascular function which do and do not change with aging are predictable from studies in experimental animals of a number of species. In most of these species, ischemic heart disease is not common. In addition, it is possible to eliminate those animals with disease.

Third, many factors will affect cardiovascular function over the life span of the animal which may or may not be looked upon as aging-induced changes. These factors include environmental factors such as temperature and toxins to which the person may be exposed. Life-style is another factor which varies over the life span of an individual and influences cardiovascular function and includes the degree of nutrition and cardiovascular fitness or conditioning. Also there may be age-associated alterations in the function of other organ systems, such as the thyroid gland, which secondarily affect the heart and its structure, function, and response to other hormones. Although the broad stroke outline of age-associated changes in cardiovascular function can now be formulated from available data in human beings and experimental animals, many of these issues of secondary determination of age-associated alterations in cardiovascular function remain to be investigated.

Finally, it should be recognized that not only is there difficulty in dissociating disease from aging but also the manifestations of cardiovascular disease in any given individual may in part be age-determined. Aging may increase or decrease the rate of disease progression. In addition, the severity of the disease-induced functional decline likely depends on the aging substrate upon which the disease is superimposed. The response to treatment in the individual with cardiovascular disease may also be determined in part by aging. For example, there is some evidence of a decrease in the potency of the inotropic response to digitalis glycosides and catecholamines with aging.[4,9,10,17,22,23] Such an age-associated decrease in response to agents which are used pharmacologically may well affect the response to treatment in any given older individual with severe heart disease. These issues are complex, and current knowledge does not even allow a clear definition of all of the relevant issues.

Normal Aging

Cardiovascular Aging as a Selective Process

Cardiovascular age changes appear in a selective rather than an overall fashion.[28] Again, the general bias is that all aspects of bodily function decrease similarly with aging. For the cardiovascular system this does not appear to be the case. The ability of the cardiac muscle to develop tension is well-maintained.[6] Also the inotropic response of the cardiac muscle to direct inotropic stimulation of the myofibrils with calcium is well-maintained[9] as are global aspects of left ventricular function at rest.[14,15] In contrast, there is a striking decrease in the response to stimulation of beta-sympathetic receptors of cardiovascular tissues.[4,12,17] This decrease in beta-sympathetic response is manifest in terms of a decreased inotropic response of cardiac muscle to catecholamine or sympathetic stimulation, a decrease in arterial vasodilating response as well as a decrease in the heart rate or chronotropic response. With exercise and other forms of left ventricular loading in human beings there is enhanced use of the Frank-Starling mechanism to compensate for the increased workload and lower inotropic state due to the decreased response to catecholamines.[14,21]

The Function of the Cardiac Muscle

Isolated cardiac muscle from rats, guinea pigs, and other species show a remarkable maintenance of ability to develop tension when studied in vitro. As shown in Fig. 71-1, the rate of rise in tension and the maximum tension achieved under isometric conditions is unchanged with age. This lack of any age change in tension development or the rate of tension rise is true over the entire resting length-tension curve of isolated cardiac muscle.[6]

There appears to be a small decrease in the velocity of shortening in cardiac muscle at similar loads in muscles from senescent animals. The decrease has been ascribed to a decrease in adenosine triphosphatase (ATPase) activity of the myofibrils, but this finding remains controversial, and studies show no major age change in myosin ATPase activity.[20,27] This decrease in shortening velocity may result from increased stiffness during contraction, which also appears to be characteristic of cardiac muscles of senescent animals.[17]

The most striking and consistent change in mechanical performance of isolated cardiac muscle from senescent animals is prolonged duration of contraction and relaxation (Fig. 71-1).[16] There are a number of studies in human beings using noninvasive estimates of relaxation rate and duration that suggest a similar prolongation of duration of contraction and a slower relaxation phase of the cardiac cycle.[18] This age-associated prolongation of relaxation has been attributed to a decrease in myocardial sarcoplasmic reticulum calcium sequestration with increased age and prolonged duration of action potential.[17,19] Contraction duration and relaxation are thought to be determined in part by the sarcoplasmic reticulum as well as by the duration of calcium entry during depolarization and repolarization. Aging is associated with a measurable decrease in the velocity of calcium uptake by sarcoplasmic reticulum. In younger animals a similar prolongation of relaxation and decreased velocity of calcium uptake by sarcoplasmic reticulum is seen following hypertrophy due to pressure overload. There is a small amount of hypertrophy present in animals and human beings with aging. This hypertrophy may be secondary to the increased impedance to left ventricular ejection as a result of stiffer arteries.[25] In experimental animals the age-associated prolongation of relaxation can be decreased by intense exercise.[26] A hastening of the course of contraction and enhancement of relaxation is seen with exercise conditioning in experimental animals of all ages. Thus, it is possible that the age-associated prolongation of duration of contraction is both a reflection

FIGURE 71-1 Typical isometric twitch in a young adult (------) and in aged (———) isolated cardiac muscle. Note that the rate of rise in tension and maximum tension achieved do not differ with age but that the duration of contraction is prolonged, primarily due to slowed and delayed relaxation.

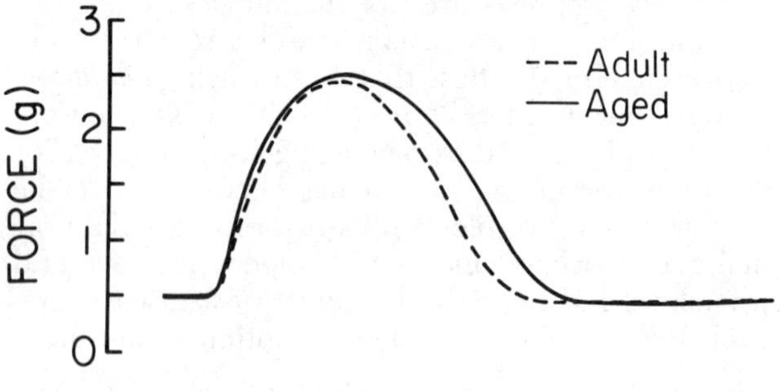

of the age-associated mild hypertrophy of cardiac muscle and deconditioning due to a lower overall level of physical activity with aging.

The broad conclusion of studies of isolated cardiac muscle function with age is that the ability to develop tension and the rate of tension development are normal and that there is some prolongation of the duration of contraction due to a delayed and decreased rate of relaxation. The velocity of shortening, particularly at low loads, is also decreased.

Left Ventricular Function in Human Beings at Rest

Paralleling these features of the function of isolated cardiac muscle in experimental animals are studies of left ventricular function in human beings with age.[12,13,28] Studies utilizing both echocardiographic and radionuclide scintigraphy for assessment of left ventricular volumes have shown that left ventricular function is well-maintained with age.[14,15,21] At rest cardiac volumes and output are not age-related. Even following pharmacological beta-adrenergic blockade, echocardiographically determined left ventricular dimension is unchanged at end diastole and end systole in normal individuals, even into the ninth decade of life.

With beta-adrenergic blockade and an increase in left ventricular afterload induced by raising blood pressure via alpha-sympathetic vasoconstriction there is some evidence of diminished intrinsic left ventricular function.[21] The magnitude of this decrease in function, however, is small. In older subjects there is a small increase in the left ventricular end-diastolic dimension with the increase in afterload following beta blockade. Since end-systolic dimension is unchanged, the increased end-diastolic dimension indicates use of the Frank-Starling mechanism. Thus, to meet the afterload stress there is use of the enhanced function of cardiac muscle resulting from an increase in muscle length or greater ventricular volume in older individuals. Young individuals could meet this afterload stress without enlargement of the left ventricle during diastole or apparent use of the Frank-Starling mechanism. It is important to note that this age difference in ability to deal with afterload stress was not present unless the stress was preceded by beta-adrenergic blockade.

In contrast, a number of studies have shown alterations of aspects of left ventricular function which are likely consequent to a delayed time course of left ventricular pressure fall reflecting slow relaxation. There is, with age, an increase in the interval between aortic closure and mitral valve opening.[18] Second, there is an age-associated decrease in the velocity of left ventricular filling during the rapid early diastolic filling phase of the cardiac cycle.[15] This decrease in the velocity of left ventricular filling in the early phase of the cardiac cycle is probably a reflection of a slowing of left ventricular relaxation.

In summary, in a normal person at rest, there is no major age-associated change in left ventricular function. However, evidence of the prolonged relaxation which is characteristic of aging cardiac muscle can be easily identified in human beings at rest in terms of a prolonged isovolumic phase of diastole and slowed early diastolic left ventricular filling.

Prolonged relaxation may influence overall cardiac function of the older individual, particularly in the presence of disease. As discussed below, these alterations in relaxation are not of sufficient magnitude to have any major impact on the cardiovascular response to exercise when disease is not present. But, in the presence of ischemic heart disease, for example, one would predict that delayed and prolonged relaxation would tend to compromise subendocardial blood flow. This may be particularly true in the presence of a tachycardia since prolonged relaxation would accentuate the detrimental effect of an abbreviated diastole. If relaxation is prolonged, then left ventricular diastolic pressure is higher for a longer period and particularly at rapid heart rates may profoundly compromise subendocardial blood flow. Should the heart rate be sufficiently rapid, as with ventricular tachycardia, and relaxation sufficiently long, left ventricular end-diastolic pressure will be elevated and filling of the left ventricle restricted as a result of inadequate time for relaxation during diastole or incomplete relaxation between beats.

Inotropic Response of Cardiac Muscle

Studies of the isolated cardiac muscle show a striking decrease in the response of tissue from older animals to certain inotropic factors. There is a decrease with age in the inotropic response to catecholamines and digitalis glycosides.[9,10,17] It is important to note that in terms of both the response of cardiac muscle to calcium and the response of myofibrils upon direct exposure to calcium following chemical removal of the cell membrane, the inotropic response to calcium is well sustained. This fact and the maintained intrinsic cardiac muscle function with increasing age indicate that myofibrillar contractile function is selectively well maintained with aging. In contrast, the striking decrease in the inotropic response to catecholamines suggests an important alteration in the response to these specific agents along the cascade of biochemical events that lead from receptor stimulation to increased myofibrillar contractile activity.

Studies of Guarnieri and associates suggest that the age-associated decrease in the inotropic response to catecholamines is *not* receptor-mediated.[23] Receptor number and affinity in rat cardiac muscle appears unchanged. Also, the response to dibutryl cyclic adenosine monophosphate (AMP), an agent which results in a catecholamine-like inotropic response without involving the cell membrane receptor, also shows an age-associated decrease similar in magnitude to that seen with catecholamines. The

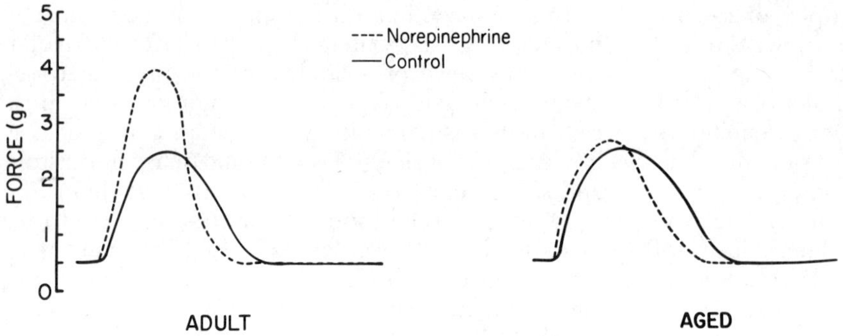

FIGURE 71-2 Typical isometric twitch in a young adult and in aged isolated cardiac muscle before (———) and after (------) exposure to norepinephrine. There is no significant increase in maximum tension or rate of tension development in the aged muscle although the enhanced relaxation effect due to the catecholamines is relatively unaffected by age.

ability of catecholamines to enhance relaxation is less severely impaired than is the inotropic response to catecholamines.

Thus, in senescent myocardium, the duration of contraction is shortened by catecholamines in the face of a markedly diminished inotropic state, and this results in a significantly lower peak tension developed by isolated cardiac muscle of the senescent animals relative to the adult animals in the presence of beta-sympathetic stimulation (Fig. 71-2).

The inotropic response to postextrasystolic potentiation in cardiac muscle from senescent animals is well-maintained and similar to the calcium response. The response to digitalis glycosides in experimental animals is also markedly decreased with age. This decreased response to digitalis glycosides is present in both rats and dogs. In the dog the toxic effects of the digitalis in terms of producing ventricular tachycardia are unchanged with age so that the therapeutic-to-toxic ratio is much less favorable in the senescent dog than it is in the younger adult dog.[10] It is unclear whether these observations in experimental animals are applicable in human beings. There have been no major studies of this relation in normal people.

Peripheral Vasculature

In terms of the load which the central vasculature presents to the left ventricle, there are several age-associated alterations of importance. The arterial wall itself, as with most cardiac and noncardiac tissues, shows increased intrinsic stiffness with age. This is almost certainly a reflection of an increase in the amount and a change in the character of the connective tissue components with age. An increase in stiffness of the aorta alone would tend to increase the vascular load on the ventricle since the heart would eject into a stiffer, more resistant structure. This increase in load is lessened somewhat by the age-associated dilation of the aorta. Dilation results in the ejection of blood into a larger structure which thus needs to change its inner dimension less to accommodate the stroke volume. The increase in the aorta size does increase the impedance to ejection due to the increase in the mass of arterial blood within the aorta, but the extent to which this inertial mass contributes to left ventricular load is not clear. The increase in arterial stiffness which occurs with age almost certainly is the major factor contributing to the documented increase in pulse wave velocity in human beings with age, and is likely an important contributor to the age-associated increase in systolic blood pressure which is observed even in healthy individuals.

In passing, it is important to note that the increase in systolic blood pressure with age *at rest* is relatively modest when efforts are made to examine subjects without evidence of atherosclerotic disease. In most studies, the mean for the population increases no more than 10 to 20 mmHg at rest. Systolic blood pressure increases markedly with exercise, and the differential between adult and aged individuals with regard to systolic blood pressure is much greater with exercise than at rest. As discussed below, this may result from less arterial vasodilation during exercise in the elderly. It is possible that the increase in the vascular load at rest in the aged individual contributes to left ventricular load and is a factor which accounts for the age-associated increase in left ventricular mass or hypertrophy with age. However, it is important to emphasize that this hypertrophy with aging is modest.

The most striking age change in the arterial vasculature parallels directly the age change in cardiac muscle: that is, a decrease in the response to beta-sympathetic stimulation.[4,24] There is a distinct age-associated decrease in the vasodilating response to beta-sympathetic stimulation. That this is a specific decrease in the response to beta-sympathetic stimulation is shown by the fact that the vasodilator response to other vasodilating agents such as nitrates or nitrites is relatively well maintained with age compared to the decrease in response to beta stimulation.

From this observation in isolated aorta, one can speculate that during exercise a major factor in augmenting the load on the left ventricle during ejection is decreased arterial vasodilation. With exercise, cardiac output rises markedly. Systolic blood pressure reflects the net effect of the increased filling of all arterial structures as a result of augmented cardiac output and arterial vasodilatation through beta-sympathetic stimulation. Systolic blood pressure and therefore left ventricular systolic load rises to a higher level in older than in younger adult humans. Strong support for this notion has been obtained during exercise in beagle dogs that have chronically been equipped with measuring devices. These studies show that dynamic impedance to left ventricular ejection is much greater during exercise in 10- to 14-year-old dogs compared to 1- to 4-year-old dogs.[25] The increased impedance with age is not present at rest. The age difference in impedance during exercise can be entirely eliminated by beta-sympathetic blockade. That is to say, the load on the left ventricle during ejection is the same in adult and senescent animals following beta blockade whereas before beta blockade the load is much greater in the older dogs. These observations, therefore, support the concept that in the young adult sympathetic arterial vasodilation limits left ventricular load. In the aged dog this response to beta stimulation is lost, and systolic pressure and ventricular load are much greater. Beta blockade eliminates the ability of the young adult animal to vasodilate and converts the hemodynamic response of the younger adult dog to one which is very similar to that of the aged dog.

One of the major unanswered questions in terms of the peripheral vascular physiological response of the older individual is the influence of age on the ability of exercising skeletal muscle to effect vasodilatation and augment blood flow. Less diversion of blood from the splanchnic and renal beds to actual exercising skeletal muscle may also be an important contributor to the age-associated alteration in exercise response and exercise ability.

Other Aspects of the Intrinsic Cardiovascular Response

In addition to the altered inotropic and vasodilator response to beta-sympathetic stimulation there is a clear age-associated decrease in the chronotropic response to catecholamines. The maximum heart rate response to beta-sympathetic stimulation has been shown to be diminished in the senescent beagle dog both before and after vagal blockade.[22]

Although the studies to date are not extensive, there appears to be no major age-associated alteration in the coronary vasculature with age. There are some anatomic data suggesting an age-associated decrease in the capillary density, but in part this decrease in capillary density is accounted for by the mild hypertrophy discussed above. The few studies that have been performed to assess vasodilating ability of the coronary vasculature show no major age-associated alteration. For many years it was thought that there was a marked age-associated decrease in overall left ventricular function which was ascribable to altered coronary flow due to diminished capillarity or altered oxygen delivery on the basis of increased resistance to oxygen diffusion. Studies in the rat in recent years have not supported these conclusions, and in fact, this particular theory of cardiovascular aging has fallen from favor. Such a mechanism of cardiovascular aging would, of course, conflict directly with the evidence for the selectivity and the maintenance of intrinsic cardiac muscle function with age as well as for the normal inotropic response of cardiac muscle and the left ventricle to certain types of inotropic stimulation such as calcium and postextrasystolic potentiation.

Cardiovascular Response to Exercise in Human Beings

The age-associated decrease in the ability to exercise and in the maximum ability to consume oxygen during exercise with age has long been a subject of scientific investigation.[12,28] On the basis of early studies which claimed a marked decrease in resting cardiac function in normal aging people, it had long been held that the major factor contributing to the decrease in exercise ability with age was a diminished ability to augment cardiac output with exercise in aged individuals.

Although no study to date clearly identifies the factors which limit ability to exercise in normal human beings, the age-associated reduction in exercise ability is not due to a straightforward limitation of the ability to increase cardiac output as a result of a marked reduction of overall cardiac function. Among the possible mechanisms of the decrease are any or all of the following:

- Increased work of breathing or overall pulmonary function
- Decreased blood flow to skeletal muscle
- Alterations in metabolism in skeletal muscle and/or sensation of fatigue
- Psychological factors
- An indirect mechanism whereby the physiological alterations that occur in cardiac function with age lead to an increased sense of fatigue or increased respiratory demands

Although clearly we cannot answer the question as to what factor or factors limit exercise ability with age, we can in a descriptive way examine rather carefully the age-associated alterations in cardiovascular response to exercise that occur at each achievable level of exercise of work performance up to the maximal level for an individual.

Figure 71-3 lists those factors which contribute to maximal cardiac output during exercise or any other form of stress. There are four factors which contribute to maximal output capacity of the left ventricle. They are maximal heart rate, the maximal cardiac inotropic state, the minimal impedance to left ventricular ejection, and the maximal use of the Frank-Starling mechanism. That is to say, if the other three factors are held constant and there is a change in any one of the factors in the direction indicated, there would be an augmentation of cardiac output. In contrast, a change in any of these factors in the opposite direction would contribute to a limitation

CONTRIBUTE TO EXERCISE CARDIAC OUTPUT	AGED	AGED AT SAME WORKLOAD
HEART RATE INCREASE	LESS	LOWER HEART RATE
AFTERLOAD DECREASE	LESS	LARGER END-
INOTROPY INCREASE	LESS	SYSTOLIC VOLUME
FRANK-STARLING USE	MORE	LARGER END-DIASTOLIC AND STROKE VOLUMES

FIGURE 71-3 Factors that contribute to increased cardiac output during stress and the influence of age on the response of these factors to exercise stress.

of maximal cardiac output. This assumes that there is no limitation in venous return. Thus, if heart rate does not increase to the same degree in the elderly compared to the adult individual, this would contribute to lowering cardiac output capacity. Similarly, if contractility does not increase as much, maximum cardiac output capacity would be limited. Also, if impedance to left ventricular ejection did not decrease as much in the elderly as in the adult, this would tend to limit maximum cardiac output capacity. Finally, if there were limitations in the use of the Frank-Starling mechanism, this would lead to limitation of maximum cardiac output capacity. On the other hand, if the Frank-Starling mechanism and increased fiber length could be easily utilized, this reserve mechanism for augmenting cardiac function could compensate for alterations in the other three variables which might limit exercise capacity. It is, in fact, this pattern of response which has been shown to be present in normal aging human beings with exercise. There is a clear decrease in the maximum heart rate response with exercise in the elderly. There is also evidence of a decrease in cardiac inotropic response and an increase in impedance to ejection during exercise in the elderly. These three age-associated alterations in cardiovascular function serve to diminish maximum cardiac output capacity. There appears to be, though, a readily available and effective use of the Frank-Starling reserve which compensates to a very significant degree in normal elderly individuals, and maintains cardiac output even at rather high workload levels.

These specific conclusions are based on an extensive study of 61 normal individuals from the Baltimore Longitudinal Study on Aging.[14] The Baltimore Longitudinal Study population is a group of individuals who have been volunteer research subjects for up to 25 years. These individuals have appeared for general medical evaluation, including a detailed description of cardiovascular status, on a biannual basis. Thus, within this population, subjects could be screened so as to eliminate with some confidence those with manifest cardiovascular disease. Only those subjects who had no evidence of cardiovascular disease on physical examination or stress testing participated in this study. In these individuals bicycle exercise was performed while gated cardiac blood pool scans (see Chap. 109) were obtained during each level of exercise up to the maximum. Absolute left ventricular volumes and cardiac output were measured.

In these subjects at rest there was a slightly higher systolic blood pressure with age but no change in left ventricular end-diastolic volume, left ventricular end-systolic volume, or ejection fraction.

With exercise, there were three major age-associated alterations in the measured cardiovascular variables. First, as expected, there was a lower heart rate response to exercise at each workload level. This is likely related to the decreased chronotropic sympathetic response associated with aging. Second, in the younger individuals, the end-systolic volume diminished with exercise, reflecting enhanced inotropic state and effective vasodilation of the arterial vasculature related to the normal beta-sympathetic response to exercise. In the elderly individuals end-systolic volume did not decrease with exercise. This almost certainly reflects both the decreased cardiac inotropic response and a decreased aortic vasodilator response or increased impedance to ejection as suggested by the animal studies discussed above. Third, there was a striking increase in the end-diastolic volume with exercise in the elderly individuals. In the normal younger individuals there was a minimal increase in end-diastolic volume at any level of exercise. That is to say, the younger individuals did not utilize the Frank-Starling mechanism to augment stroke volume and cardiac output and relied completely and successfully on an augmented heart rate, inotropic state of the ventricle, and a decrease in impedance to ejection. In the elderly individuals, with each stepwise increase in exercise there was a stepwise increase in end-diastolic volume, indicating a reliance on and effective utilization of the Frank-Starling mechanism. The increase in end-diastolic volume was quantitatively greater than the increase in end-systolic volume, thus leading to a considerable augmentation in stroke volume. Thus, there was an age-associated increase in stroke volume during any level of exercise which was ascribable to enhanced use of the Frank-Starling mechanism. This greater increase in stroke volume in the elderly compensated for the lower heart rate response to exercise, and resulted in maintenance of the cardiac output at all levels of exercise. Cardiac output was the same in elderly and younger individuals at any specific exercise workload.

Summarizing from another perspective, cardiac output response to exercise is unchanged at any given level of workload in normal human beings from age 20 to 80 years. There is a marked difference, though, in the mechanisms used to maintain cardiac output in the elderly. The increase in heart rate, the inotropic response, and the reduction of impedance to left ventricular ejection were less in the elderly. This is compensated for by an increased use of the Frank-

Starling mechanism reflected by a progressive step-by-step increase in end-diastolic volume as exercise workload increases.

There is extensive clinical utility and use of the ejection fraction at rest and at exercise in identification of heart disease and in assessing severity and prognosis. Age changes in ejection fraction are important to understand so that no error is made in the elderly in terms of ascribing what is normal to disease or of ascribing to disease what is normal aging. As noted above, ejection fraction is unchanged at rest with age, reflecting the unchanged end-diastolic and end-systolic volumes. During exercise in elderly individuals, the ejection fraction tends to increase less than the increase that is present in younger individuals. The increase in ejection fraction in younger individuals reflects the decrease in end-systolic volume with maintenance of end-diastolic volume, and thus reflects the inotropic stimulation of the left ventricle and the vasodilating response of the central vasculature of the adult during exercise. In the elderly individual, the ejection fraction increases with exercise, but the increase is less than in the younger individuals. This is because the increase in end-diastolic volume is relatively greater with advanced age than is the increase in end-systolic volume during exercise. Thus, a decrease in ejection fraction from rest to exercise would likely reflect the presence of disease and not be due to aging alone.

Cardiovascular Disease in Aging

Hypertension

It is well established that a marked elevation of diastolic blood pressure at any age constitutes a disease which is identifiable and warrants treatment. There is a modest, normal increase in diastolic pressure during the early portion of adulthood but beyond midlife, in general, a consistent blood pressure above 90 mmHg diastolic is considered abnormal, indicating the presence of disease.

Abnormal systolic blood pressure is probably an indication of the presence of disease and indication for treatment as well.[2,3] Although aging is associated with an increase in arterial stiffness and a decrease in sympathetic arterial vasodilating response, systolic blood pressure at rest shows very little age-associated increase when the subjects under study are well selected for no evidence of disease. It is very important to recognize that with exercise older individuals without evidence of cardiovascular disease do have a greater increase in systolic pressure than younger individuals. Therefore, it is important in assessing systolic blood pressure in the elderly to be certain that measurements are obtained under basal conditions. Elevated systolic blood pressure at rest is increasingly recognized as a risk factor associated with subsequent cardiovascular disease. In the middle-aged group it is clear that drugs which lower systolic blood pressure are useful in lowering subsequent cardiovascular risk of patients with clearly elevated systolic blood pressure. There are ongoing studies which suggest that therapy in the older segment of the population is valuable as well.[29]

It is unclear whether etiological factors that are associated with hypertension in the young are the same as those in the older segment of the population. There is some evidence to suggest that sympathetic hyperfunction is more often associated with hypertension in the young than in the elderly.[30] Also since aging per se is associated with a decrease in sympathetic responsiveness, it is not surprising that there is an increasing emphasis in considering the age of the patient when selecting antihypertensive therapy. For example, in younger individuals beta blockade is considered first- or second-line treatment of hypertension, whereas in the elderly beta-adrenergic blockade is not emphasized. This may reflect, in part, the age-associated decrease in overall beta-sympathetic responsiveness. Vasodilator drugs are increasingly viewed as the first line of treatment in older individuals.

Ischemic Heart Disease

Although age is the most important risk factor for manifest ischemic heart disease, the potency of other specific risk factors is so significant that the disease can be manifest in severe form at any age. Since, in general, age is associated with more severe, diffuse atherosclerosis and more damage to the left ventricle, almost all clinical manifestations of ischemic heart disease have a higher mortality rate and a worse outcome in an older population. Thus, mortality rates in acute myocardial infarction, unstable angina, heart failure, and arrhythmias are all increased in the elderly. It is not surprising that evidence of functioning collateral vessels is greater in older individuals, who likely have had a longer duration of disease, than in younger individuals at the same stage in ischemic heart disease. The presence of these collaterals likely indicates not only some protection against acute occlusive episodes but also increased overall severity of disease with each of the vessels having more severe atherosclerosis. In general, therapy of ischemic heart disease is unrelated to the age of the individual patient. There are social, psychological, and other factors which make surgery seem less desirable as a form of treatment of ischemic heart disease in older individuals, and yet where appropriate, the results of surgical therapy of ischemic heart disease in older individuals are rewarding. Age adds relatively little to surgical risk over and above other factors which, of course, correlate with more severe disease and thereby correlate with age.[31]

Congestive Heart Failure

Congestive heart failure due to aging alone is a hypothesis which has, by and large, been refuted by appropriate clinical investigation and careful observation.[7] Although amyloid accumulates with age in cardiac tissues, this accumulation alone is not correlated with the presence of abnormal function except in the presence of very extensive infiltration and deposition which occur with amyloid heart disease. Congestive heart failure thus is primarily due to coronary and hypertensive heart disease occurring in conjunction with factors relating to aging and likely influencing the course of the illness and the response to therapy.

The factors which are associated with aging and which may affect the severity of the clinical manifestations of heart failure include increased impedance to left ventricular ejection particularly with exercise or stress. This would tend to aggravate congestive failure. Also the age-associated decrease in sympathetic responsiveness may decrease the ability of the older person to augment heart rate and cardiac function under the stress of heart disease particularly in the setting of acute depression of left ventricular function. Finally, the prolonged duration of contraction and delayed relaxation may lead to a reduction in subendocardial myocardial blood flow due to shortened diastole both in ischemic heart disease and other disease states in which subendocardial perfusion may be limited, e.g., left ventricular hypertrophy in association with aortic valvular stenosis.

The treatment of congestive heart failure in the elderly is complicated by an age-associated decrease in renal function. This results in decreased excretion of such important drugs as digitalis glycosides, whose toxic effects may be induced by relatively little increases in circulating drug levels.[8] As discussed above, animal studies suggest that the toxicity of digitalis in terms of inducing arrhythmias in the elderly individual is similar to that in the young or middle-aged adult, but the increase in inotropy associated with the administration of digitalis glycosides seems to be diminished in both isolated heart muscle and the intact left ventricle of the aged animal. Extrapolation of these data to human beings is risky, but certainly there is some possibility that digitalis glycosides may be less beneficial and potentially are more likely to be toxic.

There is some possibility that vasodilator therapy of heart failure is more appropriate in an elderly individual. Clearly, the risk of this therapy might be increased in the presence of cerebrovascular disease, but vasodilator therapy might be useful in the setting of increased impedance to ejection and likely decreased inotropic responsiveness to other agents.

Electrophysiology

Loss of pacemaker and conducting cells in otherwise normal hearts has been identified in the elderly.[11] Thus, there appears to be some age-associated predisposition in the elderly to sinus node dysfunction as well as to abnormalities of conduction in the atrioventricular (AV) node and the His-Purkinje system, including the bundle branches.

Supraventricular and ventricular arrhythmias also increase in frequency with aging. This is broadly the case and seems unassociated at this point with specific evidence of cardiovascular disease. It would appear that arrhythmias in the elderly are to be approached in the same fashion as in younger individuals. In general, arrhythmias which are asymptomatic or unassociated with evidence of distinct cardiac disease can be viewed as less serious than ectopic ventricular activity associated with evidence of overtly manifest cardiac disease. In the latter case it is generally thought, in the elderly as in the young, that it is useful to attempt to eliminate ventricular ectopic activity with antiarrhythmic drugs. Again, age-associated alterations in renal and hepatic function as well as perhaps increasing severity of disease makes toxicity with antiarrhythmic drugs more likely to occur in elderly individuals than in young individuals.

Valvular Heart Disease

The frequent valvular heart disease in the elderly is calcific aortic stenosis. In the sixth to seventh decade this condition is most frequently due to congenitally bicuspid aortic valve whereas in more elderly patients calcific aortic stenosis is most likely due to primary aortic degenerative changes. The appearance of clinically significant aortic stenosis may be very rapid in this age group, as calcification and severe scarring occur rather abruptly. Within 6 to 18 months the disease in some patients may progress from mild aortic stenosis to very severe obstruction. Clinical recognition of valvular aortic stenosis is difficult in the elderly. Systolic murmurs are common from a number of etiologies, and the murmur of significant aortic stenosis may be difficult to recognize. The association of left ventricular hypertrophy helps to identify clinically the severity of the condition. By far the most helpful study one can perform in screening an elderly subject for significant aortic stenosis is an echocardiogram looking for severe aortic valve calcification and decreased mobility. Signs of left ventricular hypertrophy are also helpful in suggesting aortic stenosis. It should be noted, however, that primary hypertrophy of the left ventricle in association with symptoms of heart failure and other symptoms similar to aortic stenosis including angina and arrhythmias is not uncommon and is at times a source of confusion. Aortic regurgitation also results from degenerative changes within the proximal aorta and valve although symptomatic aortic regurgitation is unlikely. It should be remembered that there is some increase in susceptibility for patients with degenerative aortic valve disease to bacterial endocarditis. Often instructions with regard to antibiotic prophylaxis are not as vigorously imparted to elderly subjects with evidence of valvular disease as it is to younger individuals.

With regard to the mitral valve, symptomatic mitral regurgitation in the elderly is most often related to ischemic heart disease and papillary muscle dysfunction. Myxomatous degeneration of the mitral valve rather than rheumatic heart disease is probably the next leading cause of mitral regurgitation.

References

1. Longfellow, H. W.: "The Golden Legend," part IV, "The Cloisters," 1872.
2. Kannel, W. B.: Blood Pressure and the Development of Cardiovascular Disease in the Aged, in F. I. Caird, J. L. C. Dall, and R. D. Kennedy, (eds.), "Cardiology in Old Age," Plenum Press, New York and London, 1976, p. 143.
3. Kennedy, R. D. L.: High Blood Pressure and Its Management, in F. I. Caird, J. L. C. Dall, and R. D. Kennedy (eds.), "Cardiology in Old Age," Plenum Press, New York and London, 1976, p. 181.
4. Fleish, J. H.: Further Studies of the Effect of Aging on Beta-Adrenoreceptor Activity of Rat Aorta, *Br. J. Pharmacol.*, 42:311, 1971.
5. White, N. K., Edwards, J. E., and Dry, T. J.: The Relationship of the Degree of Coronary Atherosclerosis with Age in Men, *Circulation,* 1:645, 1950.
6. Weisfeldt, M. L., Loeven, W. A., and Shock, N. W.: Resting and Active Mechanical Properties of Carneae from Aged Male Rats, *Am. J. Physiol.*, 220:1921, 1977.
7. Pomerance, A.: Pathology of the Heart with and without Cardiac Failure in the Aged, *Br. Heart J.*, 27:697, 1965.
8. Ewy, G. A., Kapadia, G. G., Yao, L., Lullin, M., and Marcus, F. I.: Digoxin Metabolism in the Elderly, *Circulation,* 39:449, 1969.
9. Gerstenblith, G., Spurgeon, H. A., Froehlich, J. P., Weisfeldt, M. L., and Lakatta, E. G.: Diminished Inotropic Responsiveness to Ouabain in Aged Rat Myocardium, *Circ. Res.*, 44:517, 1979.
10. Guarnieri, T., Spurgeon, H. A., Froehlich, J. P., Weisfeldt, M. L., and Lakatta, E. G.: Diminished Inotropic Response but Unaltered Toxicity to Acetylstrophanthidin in the Senescent Beagle, *Circulation,* 60:1548, 1979.
11. Lev, M.: The Pathology of Complete Atrioventricular Block, *Prog. Cardiovasc. Dis.*, 6:317, 1964.
12. Gerstenblith, G., Lakatta, E. G., and Weisfeldt, M. L.: Age Changes in Myocardial Function and Exercise Response, *Prog. Cardiovasc. Dis.*, 19:1, 1976.
13. Brandfonbrenner, M., Landowne, M., and Shock, N. W.: Changes in Cardiac Output with Age, *Circulation,* 12:557, 1955.
14. Rodeheffer, R. J., Gerstenblith, G., Becker, L. C., Fleg, J. L., Weisfeldt, M. L., and Lakatta, E. G.: Exercise Cardiac Output Is Maintained with Advancing Age in Healthy Human Subjects: Cardiac Dilation and Increased Stroke Volume Compensate for a Diminished Heart Rate, *Circulation,* 69:203, 1984.
15. Gerstenblith, G., Frederiksen, J., Yin, F. C. P., Fortuin, N. J., Lakatta, E. G., and Weisfeldt, M. L.: Echocardiographic Assessment of a Normal Adult Aging Population, *Circulation,* 56:273, 1977.
16. Lakatta, E. G., Gerstenblith, G., Angell, C. S., Shock, N. W., and Weisfeldt, M. L.: Prolonged Contraction Duration in Aged Myocardium, *J. Clin. Invest.*, 55:61, 1975.
17. Lakatta, E. G., and Yin, F. C. P.: Myocardial Aging: Functional Alterations and Related Cellular Mechanisms, *Am. J. Physiol.*, 242 (*Heart Circ. Physiol.*, 11):H927, 1982.
18. Harrison, T. R., et al.: The Relation of Age to the Duration of Contraction, Ejection, and Relaxation of the Normal Human Heart, *Am. Heart J.*, 67:189, 1964.
19. Froehlich, J. P., Lakatta, E. G., Beard, E., Spurgeon, H. A., Weisfeldt, M. L., and Gerstenblith, G.: Studies of Sarcoplasmic Reticulum Function and Contraction Duration in Young Adult and Aged Rat Myocardium, *J. Mol. Cell. Cardiol.*, 10:427, 1978.
20. Alpert, N. R., Gale, H. H., and Taylor, N.: The Effect of Age on Contractile Protein ATPase Activity and the Velocity of Shortening, in R. D. Tanz, F. Kalaler, and J. Kobentz (eds.), "Factors Influencing Myocardial Contractility," Academic Press, New York, 1967, p. 127.
21. Yin, F. C. P., Raizes, G. S., Guarnieri, T., et al.: Age-Associated Decrease in Ventricular Response to Hemodynamic Stress during Beta-Adrenergic Blockade, *Br. Heart J.*, 40:1349, 1978.
22. Yin, F. C. P., Spurgeon, H. A., Greene, H. L., Lakatta, E. G., and Weisfeldt, M. L.: Age-Associated Decrease in Heart Rate Response to Isoproterenol in Dogs, *Mech. Ageing Dev.*, 10:17, 1979.
23. Guarnieri, T., Filburn, C. R., Zitnik, G., Roth, G. S., and Lakatta, E. G.: Contractile and Biochemical Correlates of Beta-Adrenergic Stimulation of the Aged Heart, *Am. J. Physiol.*, 239 (*Heart Circ. Physiol.*, 8):H501, 1980.
24. Fleisch, J. H., and Hooker, C. S.: The Relationship between Age and Relaxation of Vascular Smooth Muscle in the Rabbit and Rat, *Circ. Res.*, 38:243, 1976.
25. Yin, F. C. P., Weisfeldt, M. L., and Milnor, W. R.: The Role of Aortic Input Impedance in the Decreased Cardiovascular Response to Exercise with Aging in the Dog, *J. Clin. Invest.*, 68:28, 1981.
26. Spurgeon, H. A., Steinback, M. F., and Lakatta, E. G.: Prolonged Contraction Duration in Senescent Myocardium Is Prevented bv Exercise, *Am. J. Physiol.* (In press.)
27. Bhatnager, G. M., Walford, G. D., Beard, E., and Lakatta, E. G.: Dissociation of Time to Peak Force (TPF) and Myofibrillar ATPase Activity (MF-ATPase) with Aging of the Myocardium, *J. Mol. Cell Cardiol.*, 16:203, 1984.
28. Weisfeldt, M. L. (ed.): "The Aging Heart: Its Function and Response to Stress," Raven Press, New York, 1980.
29. Hypertension Detection and Follow-Up Program Cooperative Group: Five-Year Findings of the Hypertension Detection and Follow-Up Program: II. Mortality by Race, Sex and Age, *JAMA,* 242:2572, 1979.
30. Messerli, F. H., Frohlich, E. D., Suarez, D. H., et al.: Borderline Hypertension: Relationship between Age, Hemodynamics, and Circulating Catecholamines, *Circulation,* 64:760, 1981.
31. Gersh, B. J., Kronmal, R. A., Frye, R. L., et al.: Coronary Arteriography and Coronary Artery Bypass Surgery: Morbidity and Mortality in Patients aged 65 Years or Older: A Report from the Coronary Artery Surgery Study, *Circulation,* 67:483, 1983.

Section B

Cardiac Involvement in Systemic Disease

72

The Heart and Endocrine Diseases

John R. K. Preedy, M.D.
Stephen D. Clements, Jr., M.D.
Harry K. Delcher, M.D.

Whilst the nourishment of a part is indispensible to its existence; the influence which it exerts upon the circulating fluids may be more or less needful for healthful subsistence of the entire body.

Thomas Wilkinson King, 1836[1]

Thyroid Disease and the Heart

Hyperthyroidism

Hyperthyroidism can be defined as increased thyroid hormone activity, virtually always due to increased thyroid hormone concentration in extracellular fluid. (The terms *hyperthyroidism* and *thyrotoxicosis* are used interchangeably.)

Criteria for Diagnosis

The minimum requirement for the diagnosis consists of an elevation of the plasma total thyroxine (T_4) and/or plasma total triiodothyronine (T_3), together with an increased radioactive T_3 uptake (rT_3U) test. The latter is an inverse measurement of plasma protein binding of thyroid hormones, and should not be confused with plasma T_3. Plasma T_4 (and to a lesser extent plasma T_3) can be increased or decreased solely by an increase or a decrease in plasma protein binding. Thus, an estimate of binding is essential. In general, concordant results (all tests increased or all tests decreased) indicate thyroid dysfunction, whereas discordant results (plasma T_4 and T_3 increased, rT_3U decreased; or plasma T_4 and T_3 decreased, rT_3U increased) indicate an increase or a decrease in protein binding, respectively. Theoretically, determining the level of plasma "free" (unbound) T_4, which is independent of protein binding, should be an accurate test for hyperthyroidism, and is so used. However, the level of plasma free T_4 is most often calculated from an equation involving the levels of plasma T_4 and plasma rT_3U, not by separate testing. As a correction for abnormal protein binding, this procedure is not very accurate. In addition, one might wish to document any abnormalities of protein binding. Causes of abnormalities of protein binding are given in Table 72-1.

Thyrotoxicosis with elevations of plasma T_3 only, or accompanied by a minimal elevation of plasma T_4, is occasionally seen and is known as "T_3 toxicosis."[2] Plasma T_3 is often suppressed in old age, or in patients severely ill from any nonthyroidal cause.[3] In such cases the plasma T_4 only may be elevated.

In mild or borderline cases, the thyrotropin-releasing hormone–thyroid-stimulating hormone (TRH-TSH) test is useful.[4] In the normal, there is a substantial elevation of plasma TSH after intravenous TRH, whereas in hyperthyroidism the TSH rise is markedly blunted, or does not occur.

TABLE 72-1 Protein Binding of Thyroid Hormones

Increased	Decreased
Pregnancy	Nephrotic syndrome
Estrogen administration (including oral contraceptives)	Hepatic cirrhosis
	Malnutrition
	Testosterone administration

Cause of Hyperthyroidism

Having established the presence of hyperthyroidism, one must proceed to establish the cause (see Table 72-2). The treatment differs, depending on the disease entity. Causes can conveniently be divided into those with low plasma TSH levels (some of which are quite common) and those with raised TSH levels (all of which are quite rare).

Differentiation of the various causes may present some difficulty. The presence of exophthalmos and/or the rare pretibial myxedema makes the diagnosis of Graves' disease, but these features may not be present. Toxic thyroid nodule is diagnosed by demonstrating the nodule at physical examination, and by radioactive iodine scan. In subacute thyroiditis, the thyroid is quite painful and tender, the only cause where this is so. In Hashimoto's disease, the antithyroglobulin and antimicrosomal antithyroid antibodies are markedly increased in 90 percent of cases. Silent thyroiditis, a recently described self-limiting form of hyperthyroidism, is accompanied by low radioactive iodine uptake in a nontender enlarged thyroid.[5] The condition may occur in the postpartum period. Excess thyroid hormone ingestion may be diagnosed by history, but in many cases the history is concealed. Diagnosis is made by finding no thyroid enlargement and a low thyroid radioactive iodine uptake, signs shared only with the extremely rare struma ovarii.

The conditions causing thyrotoxicosis with raised plasma TSH or TSH-like material are usually diagnosed prior to the detection of the hyperthyroidism, and will not be further discussed here.

TABLE 72-2 Causes of Hyperthyroidism

Low or Low Normal TSH	Raised TSH*
Graves' disease	Choriocarcinoma
Toxic thyroid nodule (single or multinodular)	Testicular cancer
Subacute thyroiditis	Struma ovarii
Hashimoto's disease	TSH-producing pituitary tumors
Silent thyroiditis	
Excess thyroid hormone ingestion	

*Or TSH-like material.

Clinical Features

Symptoms Nervousness, irritability, agitation, and anxiety are the principal features. These are common to a number of conditions, and thus the recognition of mild hyperthyroidism may be delayed. Emotional lability is part of this picture, the patient bursting into tears for no good reason. Depression is common. There is often weakness, which may be nonspecific, but may also be due to easily demonstrated generalized muscular weakness or weakness of specific muscle groups. Heat intolerance is a frequent complaint. The patient is comfortably warm when others are complaining of the cold. Edema of the legs may occur. Dyspnea may worry some patients. There is often a family history of thyroid diseases, with or without hyperthyroidism.

Secondary amenorrhea is common. A variety of mental disturbances may be seen, in addition to those mentioned above, including psychotic symptoms, and these may in fact be the presenting feature.[6]

Abnormal Physical Signs Thyroid enlargement is usually, but not always present (see list of causes in Table 72-2). When the thyroid is palpated from behind, a constellation of physical signs is often detected at the same time, namely, thyroid enlargement, warm, moist skin, tremor of the whole body, rapid heart rate, atrial fibrillation, and pounding carotid arterial pulses.

There is a stare, with or without true exophthalmos. The exophthalmometer, an inexpensive but neglected instrument, is of diagnostic value in determining the presence of mild degrees of exophthalmos. Exophthalmos may be bilateral, unilateral, or asymmetrical. The deep tendon reflexes are typically brisk, sometimes excessive, and muscle atrophy, general or regional, may be apparent.

Special Clinical Presentations In addition to the usual or classical presentation described above, there are two modes of presentation where the diagnosis may be difficult. The first is mild hyperthyroidism, in which the condition itself is in a mild form and the clinical features therefore are minimal. The second is apathetic hyperthyroidism,[7] in which although the disease is present to a moderate or even severe degree, the clinical features are masked. The importance of these presentations is that the presence of hyperthyroidism may easily be missed, with potentially serious consequences.

In mild thyrotoxicosis, plasma T_4, plasma T_3, and rT_3U are measured several times at intervals of a few days. If all levels are consistently above normal, this is in favor of hyperthyroidism. The TRH-TSH test is particularly useful here. Even in mild thyrotoxicosis, the thyroid is enlarged (except in excessive thyroid hormone ingestion and, rarely, in apathetic hyperthyroidism). This is quite helpful diagnostically.

In apathetic hyperthyroidism, the condition may be severe, but the clinical features are minimal or easily missed, as mentioned above. The condition usually occurs in older women, accompanied by loss of weight. The patient is apathetic rather than agitated. The thyroid is only slightly enlarged, and may even be impalpable. There may be a rapid regular pulse, or atrial fibrillation. Unless the hyperthyroidism is recognized, the patient may be scheduled for surgery for an unrelated condition, with a high risk of thyroid storm. Thyroid storm may also follow an infection. Once apathetic hyperthyroidism is suspected, it is easily diagnosed: plasma T_4, T_3, and rT_3U are markedly elevated.

Cardiovascular Features
The cardiovascular features of hyperthyroidism are often impressive. Symptoms include palpitations, increased cardiac awareness with sensations of pulsations in the abdomen, extremities, and head due to wide pulse pressure. If arrhythmias are present, they may be sensed as irregularities of the pulse. Exertional dyspnea and easy fatigability may also be present.

The signs found in hyperthyroidism include sinus tachycardia, bounding peripheral pulses, increased systolic pressure with wide pulse pressure. The peripheral blood flow is increased, producing warm skin and plethora with visible capillary pulsations in the nailbeds and palpable pulsations in the fingertips.[8] The cardiac apex is forceful, the first heart sound is loud, and the pulmonary component of the second is often accentuated. Third heart sounds are common; fourth heart sounds are rare. A venous hum may be present. Many of these features reflect high cardiac output and low peripheral resistance.[8]

A scratchy sound is sometimes heard at the second left intercostal space that is similar to a friction rub. This is the so-called Means-Lerman scratch and is most notable in full expiration. It may be caused by a bounding pulmonary artery expanding in the pericardial sac or against the adjacent pleura. Very rarely diastolic murmurs are heard at the apex and simply reflect high diastolic flow rates over the atrioventricular (AV) valves.

Mitral valve prolapse with various auscultatory manifestations has been noted by Channick et al. to be more frequent in hyperthyroidism:[9] 40 consecutive patients were studied along with 40 controls. The incidence of mitral valve prolapse in the hyperthyroid group was 43 percent compared to the 18 percent in the control group. The prevalence of prolapse did not seem related to the activity of the hyperthyroidism, in that findings of mitral valve prolapse persisted after the hyperthyroid state had been adequately treated.[9]

Sinus tachycardia is the most commonly found rhythm in thyrotoxicosis; however, various other arrhythmias are well known. Atrial fibrillation is a frequent arrhythmia in thyrotoxicosis and may be associated with a rapid ventricular response. The ventricular rate is, on the average, faster than it is when atrial fibrillation occurs in euthyroid patients. In addition, digitalis medication does not easily control the ventricular rate. Treatment of the hyperthyroid state results in reversion to normal sinus rhythm in the majority of cases. In one study of 163 patients with thyrotoxic atrial fibrillation, 101 reverted to sinus rhythm after the euthyroid state was reached.[10] Spontaneous reversion was noted to be highly unlikely if the duration of atrial fibrillation exceeded 13 months or was still present 4 months after the euthyroid state was reached. Therefore, cardioversion should be considered if the atrial fibrillation persists for 4 months after the euthyroid state has been reached. As usual, anticoagulation is indicated prior to cardioversion to decrease the incidence of systemic embolism.

In addition to atrial arrhythmias, various ventricular arrhythmias may occur. Ventricular ectopic beats and other ventricular arrhythmias may be found but are uncommon. An occasional patient in the hyperthyroid state has been noted to have a prolonged PR interval, second degree AV block or even complete heart block.[11] A small percentage of hyperthyroid individuals will have the Wolff-Parkinson-White syndrome.[12]

Angina pectoris is a frequent phenomenon in individuals with thyrotoxicosis. Myocardial infarction is less common. Several mechanisms may be responsible for ischemic discomfort. In the presence of fixed obstructive disease in the coronary arteries, the oxygen demands are higher than usual, and ischemia can occur. Embolization to the coronary circulation also may occur if atrial fibrillation is present. Thrombosis of a coronary artery is occasionally seen, and coronary spasm has been documented.

The possibility of direct myocardial damage from the thyrotoxic state has been mentioned as has small vessel coronary disease. The cardiomegaly that is sometimes seen in thyrotoxicosis with heart failure usually reverses with treatment of the thyrotoxicosis.

Angina pectoris in individuals with thyrotoxicosis sometimes has different characteristics. It may occur at rest, may progress rapidly, and improves with treatment of the thyrotoxicosis. Coronary spasm has been implicated and documented in the right coronary artery at the time of arteriography.[13] The mechanism of the spasm is unclear, but some type of autonomic imbalance may be present allowing activation of alpha receptors. Ergonovine-induced spasm also has been documented in an individual whose angina pectoris disappeared with treatment of thyrotoxicosis and returned with thyroid hormone replacement therapy.[14] Transmural myocardial infarction has even been documented to occur in an individual with thyrotoxicosis without obvious obstructive lesions on arteriogram.

Thyroid Hormone and the Heart At the bedside of an individual with thyrotoxicosis, one gets the impression that there is much overactivity of the sympathetic nervous system. Rapid pulse, warm skin, active precordium, and wide pulse pressure all suggest that catecholamine activity is high. The similarity between the hyperthyroid state and that of catecholamine excess has been noted by many observers.

In recent years, however, it has been shown that it is not primarily the action of the sympathetic nervous system that accounts for the dynamic state of the circulation in hyperthyroidism but rather the direct action of thyroid hormone on the cardiovascular system. The following paragraphs deal with the effects of thyroid hormone on the cardiovascular system and the interaction of thyroid hormone with the autonomic nervous system.

The effect of thyroid hormone on the heart and in turn on the myocardial cell has been investigated in some detail. However, the mechanisms involved are not yet entirely apparent.

Markowitz and Yater reported in 1932 that 2-day-old chick embryo heart cells beat more rapidly when exposed to thyroid hormone.[15] At this age, neural elements have not developed, suggesting a direct effect of thyroid hormone on the cells. Buccino studied the force-velocity curves in papillary muscles from hyperthyroid cats and demonstrated augmented contractility.[16] The fact that sympathetic blockade or depletion of catecholamine stores with reserpine does not entirely block these effects also offers evidence that there is a direct effect of thyroid hormone on cardiac tissues.

Protein synthesis is augmented by thyroid hormone, and the effect of thyroid on the heart may be mediated via this mechanism.[17,18] Increases in the number of functional enzyme complexes and the synthesis of myocin and myocin adenosine triphosphatase (ATPase) all take part in this effect. Thyroid hormone may also regulate the expression of the genes coding for the alpha and beta heavy chains of myocin isoenzymes.[19]

The tachycardia and arrhythmias seen in hyperthyroidism have also been investigated. Arnsdorf and Childers demonstrated in rabbit atria that thyroxine induces sinus tachycardia and a shortening of the effective refractory period.[20] These changes were shown to be direct and not mediated by catecholamines or acetylcholine. Johnson et al. studied sinoatrial node and muscle cells in the atria of euthyroid, hypothyroid, and hyperthyroid rabbits and found that thyrotoxic atria had a higher heart rate, increased rate of diastolic depolarization, and decreased duration of the action potential in the sinoatrial node cells.[21] Hypothyroid tissue demonstrated an opposite effect. It was postulated that membrane conductance of potassium may be selectively and directly influenced by thyroid hormone. These factors certainly play roles in the sinus tachycardia and the development of atrial fibrillation seen in hyperthyroidism.

The Thyroid and the Autonomic Nervous System[22,23]

Early observations of the hyperdynamic circulation seen in hyperthyroidism led to conclusions that the autonomic nervous system was responsible. Indeed the high cardiac output, increased systolic blood pressure, tachycardia, and arrhythmias resemble states of sympathetic excess.

Quantitation of plasma levels of noradrenaline (as norepinephrine was previously called) suggested that the autonomic nervous system was not responsible for the hyperdynamic state. Christensen et al. demonstrated lower noradrenaline levels in hyperthyroid subjects.[24] In normal individuals the levels of noradrenaline paralleled the normal increases in pulse rate. In hypothyroid subjects plasma noradrenaline levels were generally three times as high as baseline levels in normal subjects. Additional studies focused on the enzyme, dopamine-β-hydroxylase (DBH), which is responsible for catalyzing the conversion of dopamine to norepinephrine. DBH is present in presynaptic vesicles of the sympathetic nervous system and in chromaffin granules of the adrenal medulla and is released simultaneously with stimulation of these tissues. Noth measured low DBH levels in hyperthyroidism that rose to normal levels with treatment.[25] Even in thyroid storm DBH levels are low and increase with treatment.

The mechanism of the interaction between the autonomic nervous system and thyroid hormone is still not entirely clear. Hyperthyroid subjects have been tested with infusions of norepinephrine and show no increased responses when compared to normal subjects.[26,27] This suggests that there is no increased sensitivity to catecholamines in the hyperthyroid state. Another interesting study by Williams et al. measured an increase in the number of cardiac beta receptors and suggested that the reversal of symptoms in hyperthyroidism is secondary to blockage of excessive adrenergic receptors.[28] Other evidence, however, has made it clear that additional factors are present in hyperthyroidism.

In 1979, Rutherford et al. demonstrated that with induction of hyperthyroidism in the conscious dog there are substantial increases in left ventricular contractility resulting from a direct effect of thyroid hormone and also increased beta-adrenergic activity.[29] The contractile responses to exogenous norepinephrine and isoproterenol were not augmented. Propranolol reduced myocardial contractility more in hyperthyroid than in the euthyroid state. Therefore, some enhancement of beta activity is present, but this is in addition to the direct effect of thyroid hormone.

Practical Considerations

Practical considerations center around two cardiovascular abnormalities.

- Hyperthyroidism should be considered in any patient with *atrial fibrillation.* This is especially true when the ventricular rate is faster than usual (i.e., 180 to 190 beats per minute) and when digitalis does not control the rate.
- *Congestive heart failure* may be precipitated or aggravated by hyperthyroidism in a patient with heart disease. This is due, as a rule, to uncontrolled atrial fibrillation but may possibly be related to superimposed hyperthyroid cardiomyopathy. On rare occasion heart failure may be due to thyrotoxicosis alone, and because of this the evidence for thyrotoxic cardiomyopathy must be considered. Forfar et al. have presented evidence in favor of cardiomyopathy due to hyperthyroidism. They used

exercise radionuclide ventriculography to measure the left ventricular ejection fraction at rest and after exercise and concluded that there was a reversible functional cardiomyopathy that is due to excess circulating thyroid hormone.[30]

Treatment

This, of course, depends on the cause of the hyperthyroidism (see Table 72-2). A toxic thyroid nodule is easily and satisfactorily treated by removal at surgery (after suitable preparation, see below). The hyperthyroidism of subacute thyroiditis is self-limiting to a few weeks, and is usually mild. It seldom requires treatment. The same is true of lymphocytic thyroiditis. Occasionally, treatment with the beta blocker propranolol, 20 to 40 mg twice a day, may be useful. Excess thyroid hormone ingestion is treated by discontinuation or reduction of the dose into the therapeutic range if treatment with thyroid hormone is indicated.

The hyperthyroidism of Hashimoto's disease used to be considered mild and self-limiting. However, either the disease has altered its characteristics or the well-known overlap with Graves' disease has become more pronounced, with the result that moderate or severe hyperthyroidism of long duration is now seen in Hashimoto's disease quite commonly. Thus, the treatment is now similar to that for Graves' disease (see below).

As with several of the conditions mentioned above, the hyperthyroidism of Graves' disease is eventually self-limiting, but the duration of the hyperthyroidism may vary from 6 months to 20 years or more, and the duration in the individual case cannot be predicted. Although mild hyperthyroidism in the young subject does little harm, and could be followed for a few months looking for an early remission, in practice all patients with hyperthyroid Graves' disease need treatment for the hyperthyroidism.

The treatment options are threefold, namely, antithyroid drugs, radioactive iodine, and subtotal thyroidectomy. All three treatments are generally comparable in their therapeutic value, and in many cases the decision may involve the personal preference of the patient.

Antithyroid Drugs The drugs currently used are the antithyroid substances propylthiouracil and methimazole, and the beta blocker propranolol. Occasionally, stable iodine may be used, especially in the preparation of the patient for surgery. Propylthiouracil and methimazole are quite similar, and there is little to choose between them. One may be substituted for the other, if minor toxic effects, such as skin rash, appear. An appropriate regime for a newly diagnosed patient might be propranolol 20 mg three times a day, and propylthiouracil 250 mg three times a day.

The thrice-daily dosage of propylthiouracil is reduced to 200 mg after about 2 weeks, then gradually reduced to 100 mg after about 8 weeks. The maintenance thrice-daily dosage could be 50 mg or less.

The dosage of propylthiouracil must be monitored by the plasma T_4 and T_3, since patients respond differently. The time taken for the plasma T_4 and T_3 to return to normal (the therapeutic endpoint) is quite variable, usually 6 to 10 weeks. It is easy to undertreat and to overtreat, particularly the latter, the patient appearing with hypothyroidism 2 to 3 months after the start of treatment.

When treatment with propylthiouracil is well-advanced, propranolol may be discontinued. The advantage of using propranolol lies in the relatively rapid effect (about 24 h) as compared with the slow effect of propylthiouracil.

Propranolol is substantially free of significant side effects in the small dosage recommended. Side effects with propylthiouracil treatment are usually absent, or quite minor, such as skin rash. Very rarely cholestatic jaundice and vasculitis have been reported. A rare but quite serious complication is agranulocytosis. This usually occurs within the first 3 months of therapy. Patients should be warned to stop the drug if they get a sore throat or fever, and immediately report to the physician. The agranulocytosis usually responds to discontinuation of the drug. False alarms are common, especially in the winter months, but this has to be accepted.

The main action of propylthiouracil is to reduce thyroidal synthesis of T_4 and T_3. The effect is reversible on discontinuation of the drug. Therefore, the patient will relapse unless there has been spontaneous remission of the Graves' disease in the meanwhile. There is presently no reliable way of telling when the Graves' disease is in remission while the patient is still under treatment with propylthiouracil. The drug has to be discontinued, and the plasma T_4 and T_3 followed. If the hormone levels rise, the Graves' disease is not in remission. The drug is then started again, or another form of treatment considered. This procedure is cumbersome and is a disadvantage of drug treatment. However, long-term treatment with antithyroid drugs remains a useful therapeutic regime.

In severe hyperthyroidism or thyroid storm the antithyroid drugs propylthiouracil and methimazole are of little use because of their slow action, although it has been suggested that propylthiouracil may be helpful due to its effect in depressing the peripheral conversion of T_4 to T_3.[30] Propranolol is given in larger doses, such as 40 mg every 4 h. Propranolol acts peripherally to reduce the effects of circulating thyroid hormone, and is therefore of particular value. Iodide may also be given as saturated solution of potassium iodide, 5 drops every 4 h, although the dosage is by no means critical. Iodide is thought to act principally by reducing the release of preformed thyroid hormone from the gland, and thus may have a beneficial effect. However, if iodide is given, it is essential to give propylthiouracil (or methimazole) at the same time, to avoid the rare but serious Jod Basedow effect.[31] The thyroid is usually depleted of iodide in severe hyperthyroid Graves' disease. If iodide is given, the thyroid uses this raw material to make increased quantities of thyroid hormone, the opposite of the effect required. Propylthiouracil blocks this increased synthesis.

Radioactive Iodine The logistics of this treatment are extremely simple, that is, the administration of radioactive iodine (^{131}I) in one dose by mouth. However, calculation of the dose for each patient remains quite unsatisfactory. Underdosage occurs and overdosage is common. Overdosage has a cumulative effect, and it is likely that 50 percent of the patients treated will eventually become hypothyroid. Apart from this, there are virtually no side effects. The risk of increased cancer of the thyroid can now almost be excluded. Radioactive iodine is not given to pregnant women on general grounds, nor to children under 14 years of age. Many clinics do not give radioactive iodine to patients under 25, but this seems unnecessarily cautious. Radioactive iodine is particularly valuable in the older population, say over 50, where there may be objections to long-term drug treatment and to surgery. There is also less time remaining to become hypothyroid.

Radioactive iodine acts slowly, as would be expected, the effect becoming apparent in about 3 months. It is not necessary to give any preliminary drug treatment before radioactive iodine, but in cases where it is desirable to get the hyperthyroidism under control as soon as possible, as in an older person with a compromised cardiovascular system, then propranolol and propylthiouracil may be given as described above for 3 months or so. Propranolol does not affect radioactive iodine treatment. However, propylthiouracil must be discontinued 3 days before radioactive iodine treatment, and for a week afterwards. A convenient schedule would be to start propranolol, give the radioactive iodine, and start propylthiouracil 1 week later, discontinuing all the drugs after 3 months or so.

After radioactive iodine, the patient should be followed with T_4 and TSH determinations every month or two, to detect early evidence for undertreatment (T_4 remains high), or overtreatment (TSH rises to above-normal levels and T_4 falls to low normal levels or below). If after 1 year the patient is euthyroid, then the patient should be followed with plasma TSH determination at 6-monthly intervals for the rest of his or her life. The first sign of hypothyroidism will be a slowly increasing plasma TSH. Treatment can then be started before symptoms supervene (see under "Hypothyroidism").

Subtotal Thyroidectomy This form of treatment has been available for 50 years or more. Its value was somewhat eclipsed as the newer treatments described above were introduced, but more recently the advantages of surgery have again been recognized.[32] These advantages consist principally of speed (the patient is hopefully cured immediately following the operation) and a shorter follow-up. A follow-up period (for continued hyperthyroidism or hypothyroidism) of longer than 6 or 12 months is usually not necessary. These features are particularly attractive to the younger adult, and surgery can confidently be recommended in this group.

An overriding consideration is the availability of a surgeon experienced specifically in thyroid surgery. If this specific experience is not available, surgery should not be considered.

The patient must be rendered euthyroid before operation, using a drug regime such as described above (propranolol and propylthiouracil). The endpoint is a normal level of plasma T_4 and plasma T_3. When this is achieved, iodide in the dose described above should be added to the regime for 2 to 3 weeks before surgery. Propylthiouracil should be discontinued 3 days before surgery. The addition of iodide and discontinuation of propylthiouracil is necessary to decrease the vascularity and friability of the gland.

In the hands of an experienced thyroid surgeon, the incidence of serious complications, such as section of the recurrent laryngeal nerve or hypoparathyroidism, is negligible. The principal untoward results are continued or recurrent hyperthyroidism, and hypothyroidism. The incidence of these two side effects is relatively low, in comparison with the other treatments. If they do occur, then antithyroid drugs, radioactive iodine, or thyroid hormone treatment, as appropriate, remain available.

Subtotal thyroidectomy would, of course, not be recommended in older patients, or where there was some general contraindication to surgery, such as coexistent heart disease.

Cardiovascular Aspects of Treatment for Hyperthyroidism Treatment of the patient with thyrotoxicosis and cardiovascular involvement involves acute treatment with digitalis, diuretics, and beta blockers and ultimately decreasing the production of thyroid hormone. Atrial fibrillation with a rapid ventricular response associated with congestive heart failure is a distressing combination. Beta blockers and digoxin will slow the ventricular response to some degree.

Propranolol can be given as a 1-mg dose intravenously and repeated in increments of 1 mg every 10 to 15 min up to 5 mg until the ventricular rate is slowed. Intravenous digoxin can also be given initially, followed by oral administration. If pulmonary congestion is present, intravenous furosemide (Lasix) is helpful. Hours to days of intensive care is required to obtain a satisfactory state. After intravenous therapy is started, oral therapy should follow with digoxin, propranolol, and antithyroid therapy. Beta blockers are especially helpful in calming the peripheral effects in thyrotoxicosis.

When using beta-blocking agents in thyrotoxicosis, some care must be exercised. There is no doubt that improvement in the peripheral symptoms occurs with beta blockade.[34] Anxiety, agitation, hyperreflexia, palpitations, and hyperkinesis are improved. The exact mechanism of this improvement is yet unclear. Propranolol has some nerve depressant effect in addition to its beta-adrenergic blocking properties. Peripheral oxygen consumption and demands remain excessive in hyperthyroidism, and if beta blockade is accomplished to the degree of compromising oxygen delivery, damage could be done to peripheral tissues. One therefore should exercise caution with beta blockers in treatment of thyrotoxicosis in the presence of heart failure.[27]

Hypothyroidism

Hypothyroidism can be defined as decreased thyroid hormone activity due to a decreased concentration of thyroid hormone(s) in extracellular fluid, and also, in rare cases, to resistance to thyroid hormone(s) at the cellular level. Resistance syndromes will not be further discussed here. The terms *hypothyroidism* and *myxedema* are used interchangeably, although some reserve the term myxedema for more severe hypothyroidism.

Criteria for Diagnosis

The minimum requirement for the diagnosis of hypothyroidism depends on the cause. In primary hypothyroidism (see Table 72-3) the minimum is a decrease in plasma thyroxine (T_4) below the normal concentration with a marked increase in plasma TSH. In secondary hypothyroidism (Table 72-3), the concentrations of plasma T_4 and plasma TSH are both low. The rT_3U should also be estimated to exclude decreased T_4 binding by plasma proteins as a cause for the low plasma T_4 level (see Table 72-1). (Secondary hypothyroidism is more difficult to diagnose than the primary form, and additional information is usually needed.) Plasma triiodothyronine (T_3) is not a sensitive indicator of hypothyroidism. A low plasma T_3 is regularly seen in severe nonthyroidal illness.

Causes of Hypothyroidism

Having made the diagnosis of hypothyroidism, it is necessary to establish the cause. As with hyperthyroidism, the treatment differs with the disease process.

As mentioned above, hypothyroidism can be divided into primary and secondary causes, the primary resulting from intrinsic disease of the thyroid, and the secondary resulting from TSH deficiency. TSH is, of course, secreted by the adenohypophysis, which is in turn under hypothalamic control. The principal causes of hypothyroidism are given under each heading in Table 72-3. Additionally, the causes of primary hypothyroidism are divided into those with goiter and those without. (*Goiter* is simply an enlargement of the thyroid.)

Identification of the Various Causes Athyreotic cretinism is usually diagnosed in the first week of life, following the use of screening tests at birth, e.g., plasma T_4, plasma TSH, or both. Occasionally the diagnosis is missed at birth, and the patient is seen in childhood or even early adult life.

Juvenile myxedema is seen between the ages of approximately 8 and 16.[35] These cases may remain undiagnosed for long periods. The onset is quite insidious. A falling-off of academic achievement, with unexplained low grades, is often the first symptom. Forgetfulness, loss of interest, cessation of growth, and gain in weight are later features. When eventually diagnosed, the internist is often surprised at the extent to which the thyroid tests are compromised.

Hashimoto's disease (late stage) is diagnosed by markedly raised antithyroid antibody levels, as described under "Hyperthyroidism."

There are about six biosynthetic defects.[36] Some of these are not particularly rare (e.g., the organification defect). The detailed diagnosis of individual defects is beyond the range of this chapter. However, the presence of a soft, symmetrical thyroid enlargement, low-normal or low plasma T_4, high plasma

TABLE 72-3 Causes of Primary and Secondary Hypothyroidism

Primary Hypothyroidism		Secondary Hypothyroidism (TSH deficiency)
No Goiter	**Goiter**	
Athyreotic cretinism	Hashimoto's disease (late stage)	Destructive lesions in and around the adenohypophysis and hypothalamus
Juvenile myxedema		Isolated TSH deficiency
Adult idiopathic myxedema	Biosynthetic defects	
Destruction of thyroid	Goitrogens	
Thyroidectomy*†	Food	
	Drugs	
Radioactive iodine therapy*†	Subacute thyroiditis	
External radiation	Ectopic thyroid	
	Iodide deficiency	

*Some remaining nodular thyroid tissue is often palpable.
†Hypothyroidism may be temporary, occurring shortly after treatment.

TSH, high radioactive iodine uptake, and a family history of goiter is strongly suggestive of a biosynthetic defect.

Goitrogen ingestion can be diagnosed by history.[37] Rarely, an excess of certain vegetables may cause mild goitrogen-induced hypothyroidism. A variety of drugs can cause hypothyroidism (in addition to the antithyroid drugs mentioned in the previous section). Examples of such drugs are iodide, lithium, sulfonylureas, *p*-aminosalicylic acid, and phenylbutazone. The hypothyroidism is seldom severe, unless previous intrinsic thyroid disease is present.

Hypothyroidism as a rare result of subacute thyroiditis is diagnosed by a history of a tender enlarged thyroid within the last year or so.

An ectopic thyroid can be felt in the neck or seen under the tongue. It is usually first diagnosed in childhood.

Clinical Features

The clinical features depend upon the severity and type of hypothyroidism, and the age of the patient. Thus, the mild hypothyroidism often seen in biosynthetic defects will be clinically different from the severe hypothyroidism seen in adult idiopathic myxedema. The presentation of juvenile myxedema is somewhat different from that of adult idiopathic myxedema (see above). The clinical features of secondary hypothyroidism are generally less pronounced than those of primary hypothyroidism.

In the majority of instances (thyroidectomy would be an exception), the onset of clinical features is quite insidious. For instance, it is estimated that in the average case of adult idiopathic myxedema symptoms and signs are present for 6 months before the disease is recognized. This is in part due to the slowly progressive failure of the thyroid, and in part due to the similarity between the clinical features of hypothyroidism and those of the aging process. Adult idiopathic myxedema occurs principally in older women, and the patient's complaints are often attributed to increasing years.

What follows is a description of the symptoms and signs in typical cases of adult idiopathic myxedema.

Symptoms Intellectual functions are impaired. In particular, there is poor memory. Mental disturbance, including psychotic behavior, may occur, and this may be a presenting feature. Patients will complain of sleepiness, and there will be diminished mental, as well as physical, activity. Cold intolerance is common, and the patient feels worse in the winter. Weight gain occurs, but this is not usually very marked. Constipation can be severe. There are complaints of brittleness and thinning of the hair, including the eyebrows. Nails may also be brittle. If the onset is before the menopause, menorrhagia may occur. Galactorrhea is rarely seen, which is surprising since plasma TRH tends to be elevated, and TRH is a potent stimulator of prolactin secretion by the adenohypophysis.[38] There is often a family history of thyroid disease, with or without hypothyroidism.

Abnormal Physical Signs The thyroid is not palpable in adult idiopathic myxedema. The facial appearance may be striking. The upper and lower eyelids are puffy, the face is rounded and loses its contours. There is pallor, often but not always due to anemia. The skin is thickened, dry, and scaly, and may feel cold to the touch. The voice is coarse and deepened. On obtaining deep tendon reflexes, a delayed relaxation phase is regularly seen. The patient is seen to be abnormally still, the face is expressionless, and normal spontaneous limb movements are diminished.

A rare presentation is that of "myxedema coma" or severe myxedema.[39] This is often precipitated by exposure to cold or infection. The patient has a subnormal body temperature. The condition has a high mortality rate.

The clinical cardiovascular features of hypothyroidism are described later.

The Heart and Hypothyroidism

Zondek in 1918 introduced the term *myxedema heart* and characterized the heart as being dilated both on left and right sides, slow in action, with normal blood pressure. He went on to describe "lowering of the auricular wave and the T-wave" on electrocardiogram.[40] Early reports emphasized the lack of response to digitalis, and reversible radiographic findings in response to thyroid hormone therapy. It was also pointed out that the cardiac findings were part of the overall myxedematous state and not a separate cardiac entity. Even at that time the microscopic findings of interstitial edema with some degree of fibrosis in the hearts of myxedematous individuals was recognized.[41]

It is understandable that in the past cardiac function in hypothyroidism has been of particular interest. Individuals with extreme edema, bradycardia, and complaints of dyspnea, fatigue, and at times chest pain are, of course, suspected of having some primary cardiac disease. The following paragraphs deal with the status of the heart in hypothyroid subjects.

Myocardial function in the hypothyroid state has been evaluated experimentally. Early thoughts concerning the sensitivity of myocardial adrenergic receptors to catecholamines were clarified by information in human beings that plasma catecholamine levels were low in hyperthyroid subjects and as much as three times normal in hypothyroid patients.[24]

In 1967, Buccino demonstrated that papillary muscles from cats made hypothyroid had decreased velocity of shortening, decreased rate of tension development, and a prolonged duration of activity.[16] The isometric tensions developed in hypothyroid states in this study were only slightly decreased. The inotropic response to norepinephrine and strophanthidin in the hypothyroid state was much more than in the hyperthyroid state, again suggesting a separate effect of thyroid hormone on the myocardium.

Cardiac output in hypothyroid individuals is reduced.[42] This is a result of decreased heart rate and decreased stroke volume. With exercise, cardiac output increases by increasing heart rate and stroke volume. Systemic vascular resistance is increased and arteriovenous oxygen differences are not much different, at rest or with exercise, in hypothyroid individuals versus normal subjects. Metabolic demands are generally decreased, and circulation times are longer than normal. The overall circulation is slowed down in hypothyroidism but increases appropriately with exercise. Circulation times are measurably slowed in hypothyroidism.[43] Central venous pressures are normal[44] unless cardiac tamponade is present.

Clinical Cardiovascular Features of Hypothyroidism

The cardiovascular features of hypothyroidism parallel the systemic features when the condition is advanced. Generalized edema due to increased capillary permeability is a prominent finding in hypothyroidism.[45] Other complaints include fatigue, dyspnea, and sometimes angina pectoris. Paroxysmal nocturnal dyspnea is uncommon. Bradycardia is common, contributing to the low cardiac output. Jugular venous pressure may be normal unless significant pericardial effusion and cardiac compression is present.

The *cardiac shadow at x-ray is commonly enlarged* in hypothyroidism, often secondary to *pericardial effusion*. Large effusions of greater than 2 liters have been noted. The fluid accumulates slowly, and the pericardial sac is usually very distensible, making cardiac tamponade usually very distensible, making cardiac tamponade unlikely although it has been reported to occur.[46] Repeated pericardiocentesis followed by thyroid hormone supplements usually is adequate for treatment of tamponade; however, occasionally surgical treatment is required.[47,48] Elevated cholesterol content (normal < 70 mg/dl[49]) is sometimes found in the pericardial fluid of hypothyroid individuals. Rarely the fluid may demonstrate a scintillating, shimmering state described in 1919 by Alexander as "gold paint" appearance.[50] Cholesterol accumulates in the pericardial fluid for a number of reasons including impaired transport and breakdown of lipoproteins.[51]

The *electrocardiogram* shows *bradycardia* and nonspecific T-wave abnormalities. *Low voltage of P waves and QRS complexes* may be present, especially if a large pericardial effusion is present.[41] Complete heart block has been noted in a patient with myxedema that disappeared with treatment with thyroid hormone.[52] Also, complete heart block has been reported in a newborn hypothyroid child who did not respond to replacement therapy.[53] Two patients have been reported with the torsade de pointes type of repeated ventricular fibrillation who were documented to be hypothyroid, and whose QT prolongation and ventricular arrhythmias disappeared with treatment with thyroid hormone.[54]

The *echocardiogram* is a sensitive indicator of *pericardial effusion*. Kerber and Sherman reported a 30 percent incidence of pericardial effusion detected by echocardiogram in a group of patients with hypothyroidism. Furthermore, cardiomegaly on chest x-ray and low voltage on electrocardiogram could not be reliably used to detect the effusion.[55]

Another interesting finding is the suggestion by echocardiographic study that a *reversible form* of *cardiomyopathy* sometimes occurs in hypothyroidism. Santos et al. described a series of patients with dyspnea on exertion, dizziness, syncope, and angina-like pericardial pain.[56] These individuals had a high incidence of *asymmetrical septal hypertrophy*, while some had abnormal septal excursion and abnormalities of the anterior mitral valve leaflet. These abnormalities resolved with thyroid hormone treatment. In those patients whose angina pectoris disappears with thyroid replacement (a paradoxical response), asymmetrical hypertrophy may be present. Drugs such as digitalis, diuretics, and vasodilators should be avoided in this group of patients.

The angina-like chest pain that disappears in this group of patients may explain this rather paradoxical response to thyroid replacement in hypothyroid patients in general. Individuals who get worse with thyroid therapy may have fixed obstructive lesions in their coronary arteries.

The question of accelerated atherosclerosis in hypothyroidism has been investigated for years. Hyperlipoproteinemia (type III) is common in myxedema. Hypertension, aggregation and sludging of red blood cells, and platelet fibrin particles may be contributing factors. Autopsy studies have suggested a higher frequency of severe atherosclerosis in hypothyroidism, compared with a control group of similar age.[57] On the other hand, we have restudied two patients at 2 and 5 years after they were made hypothyroid for treatment of angina pectoris, and no significant progression of disease was noted.[58] Although arteriograms were not available in the series of patients treated with radioactive iodine by Blumgart, the same impression, that is, no apparent progression of atherosclerotic lesions, was obtained.[59] Thus, despite postmortem studies and lipid abnormalities increased progression of atherosclerosis in individuals with myxedema remains in question.

Treatment

In primary hypothyroidism treatment is principally directed toward the hypothyroidism itself. There is no specific treatment for any of the conditions causing primary hypothyroidism (with the exception of goitrogenic foods and goitrogenic drugs, which should be discontinued, if possible). In secondary hypothyroidism the causative lesion frequently requires treatment, e.g., a tumor in the pituitary area.

In both primary and secondary hypothyroidism the treatment of the hypothyroidism is the administration of thyroid hormone by mouth. In secondary hypothyroidism, tests should be carried out to determine whether adrenal failure is also present, in which case it is obligatory to add a glucocorticoid (e.g., cortisol acetate) to the regimen. In such circumstances it is dangerous to treat with thyroid hormone alone, since an acute adrenal crisis may be precipitated.

The treatment of hypothyroidism is one of the most satisfactory in medicine. It is simple, cheap, virtually 100 percent effective, and is free of side effects in the uncomplicated case. The treatment usually does not need monitoring.

A number of preparations are available, but only one is free from objection, namely, sodium *l*-thyroxine (T_4). The old-fashioned dessicated thyroid extract, which stood us in excellent stead for so many years, is not well-standardized, and contains variable amounts of T_3. Preparations of triiodothyronine (T_3), or preparations containing T_3, are contraindicated because of the rapid absorption and consequent peaking of T_3 in the bloodstream at levels which are above normal.[60] This is felt to be deleterious, especially in the older patient with heart involvement. This effect does not occur with sodium *l*-thyroxine.

The therapeutic dosage of sodium *l*-thyroxine falls in the range of 0.1 to 0.2 mg/day by mouth. The dose can be taken all at once. Divided doses are not necessary. The actual maintenance dose (within the range given) is determined arbitrarily, taking into account the size of the patient. A small, frail, elderly woman, for instance, would be given 0.1 mg/day, and a large, middle-aged man would be given 0.2 mg/day. The dose range is now lower than that previously recommended.[61] It is not necessary to vary the dosage, once decided. Provided the patient continues to take the dose prescribed, follow-up is rarely necessary. This, of course, assumes that the thyroxine content of the tablets is, and remains, as stated on the label.

It has been suggested that the dose of T_4 for any individual patient should be titrated using plasma TSH as the endpoint, the object being to keep plasma TSH within the normal range. Although theoretically attractive, there are practical problems. Plasma TSH is often undetectable in the normal, so that the difference between adequate or excessive dosage with T_4 frequently cannot be determined. The TSH assay is unreliable in the lower concentration range. Attempts to use plasma TSH in this way have resulted in excessively high T_4 dosage (above the dose range given above).[62] It should be noted that recommended replacement treatment is with T_4 only. The thyroid secretes T_4 and some T_3. This may affect the interpretation of "normal" levels of plasma TSH. The appropriate timing of plasma TSH determination in relation to changes in T_4 dosage is uncertain. T_4 has a long half-life of 8 days. Additionally, the body may adjust the dose to its particular requirements by altering the metabolism (and possibly the absorption) of T_4.[63] In conclusion, the monitoring of T_4 dosage with plasma TSH appears difficult to do, unnecessary, and not cost-effective.

Note also that plasma T_4 and plasma T_3 cannot be used for this purpose. With replacement of T_4 only (as recommended), the plasma T_4 tends to run at a high-normal level, or even slightly above normal, especially with the 0.2 mg/day dose. This should not be taken as an indication to reduce the dose. (Plasma TSH and plasma T_4 determinations are, of course, useful in cases of suspected noncompliance.)

The initial dosage schedule is an important consideration. In partial or recent hypothyroidism, the full replacement dose may be given immediately. In younger subjects where the hypothyroidism is apparently of long standing, the initial T_4 dose can be 0.05 mg/day for a month or so. Then the dosage can be increased slowly every month to a maintenance level. A more cautious schedule is necessary in older patients or where there is coexistent cardiovascular disease. It is generally believed that an initial high (full replacement) or rapidly increasing dose may precipitate angina of effort, myocardial infarction, arrhythmias, heart failure, etc.[64] Although the few cases reported have mostly involved T_3 administration, with its rapid peaking effect already referred to,[60] caution should also be observed with T_4. An initial daily dose of 0.025 mg/day should be given for 4 to 6 weeks, increasing by 0.025 mg daily every 4 weeks, until the maintenance dosage range is reached. In the unusual case, angina may appear. This is an indication to return to the previous dose for a further period.

Cardiovascular Aspects of Treatment Treatment of individuals with hypothyroidism and heart disease requires caution,[64] as mentioned above. If significant coronary obstruction is present, symptoms of angina pectoris may become manifest as thyroid replacement therapy is begun, as already mentioned. Nitroglycerin may result in hypotension and even syncope if total blood and plasma volume is reduced, as is sometimes seen in myxedema.[65] Propranolol is helpful in treatment of angina pectoris, but profound bradycardia can result. As mentioned in earlier sections, the effect of thyroid hormone on the myocardium is somewhat independent of the adrenergic nervous system, and the inotropic and chemotrophic effects of supplemental thyroid hormone may not be significantly blocked by propranolol. This may allow angina pectoris to occur.

Coronary bypass surgery offers significant relief of angina pectoris in individuals with hypothyroidism and coronary atherosclerotic heart disease. We have, for a long period, used radioactive iodine to treat incapacitating angina pectoris, and in that group have in recent years done coronary arteriography and coronary bypass surgery. Finlayson reported eight of these patients who had had thyroid ablation previously, and also five other patients with profound hypothyroidism who had either coronary bypass surgery or valve surgery (one patient).[58] All of these patients survived surgery, and some interesting observations were made. Our patients did not have profound alterations of mental status postoperatively or problems with thermoregulation or respiratory control. Enhancement or prolongation of the effect of drugs such as morphine was not apparent.

In most of our patients thyroid supplements were withheld for 2 weeks prior to operation and generally administered at the time revascularization was complete or as tolerated in the intensive care units. Hypertension did develop occasionally, as did ventricular ectopy that seemed related to thyroid hormone treatment and caused doses to be withheld or delayed. Aggressive monitoring, digoxin, and corticosteroids in addition to thyroxine permits these individuals to have a reasonably normal postoperative period despite being profoundly hypothyroid preoperatively. Neither in our series nor that of Paine did hyponatremia due to inappropriate water retention pose a significant problem.[65]

Although individuals with hypothyroidism can be successfully managed through cardiac surgery, all situations involving drug administration must be approached cautiously. Digitalis may reach abnormally high levels because of altered metabolism. Sedatives, analgesics, and tranquilizers may have prolonged effects. One must use medications cautiously and test out the response to each dose, watching for cumulative effects.

Parathyroid Disease and the Heart

Primary Hyperparathyroidism

The diagnosis of primary hyperparathyroidism[66] is usually made by discovering an elevated serum calcium level and elevated parathyroid hormone levels.

Hypercalcemia due to hyperparathyroidism may cause cardiac arrhythmias and cardiac arrest. This complication does not usually occur, however, unless the serum level is about 16 mg/dl or greater. Digitalis toxicity (arrhythmias) may occur in patients with hypercalcemia, and an intravenous injection of a calcium-containing solution may be dangerous to a patient who is receiving digitalis.

The effect of hypercalcemia on the electrocardiogram is discussed in Chap. 77.

The reader is referred to standard textbooks of endocrinology for a discussion of the treatment for hyperparathyroidism.

Hypoparathyroidism

Hypocalcemia due to hypoparathyroidism may prolong the QT interval in the electrocardiogram (see Chap. 77). Myocardial contractility may improve when hypocalcemia is corrected. This usually makes little difference but can in patients with heart failure and diminished contractility.

The reader is referred to standard textbooks of endocrinology for a discussion of the recognition and treatment of hypoparathyroidism.

Pituitary Disease and the Heart

Acromegaly and the Heart[66]

Acromegaly was described as a separate clinical entity by Marie[67] in 1886, and cardiomegaly as an associated finding was noted by Huchard[68] in 1895 and Fournier[69] in 1896. Since then, cardiovascular abnormalities have been well documented to accompany acromegaly; but their exact relation to this condition remains to be clarified.

Acromegaly is due to an increase in the production growth hormone by a pituitary gland tumor. The serum level of growth hormone is usually greater than 10 ng/ml.

Cardiomegaly, congestive heart failure, cardiac arrhythmias, systemic arterial hypertension, and atherosclerosis all contribute to the cardiovascular morbidity in individuals with acromegaly and are largely responsible for decreased life expectancy.

Cardiovascular Manifestations Associated with Acromegaly

The *cardiomegaly* associated with acromegaly has been investigated since the days of Huchard in 1895.[68] One would expect some degree of enlargement of the heart proportional to the enlargement of other organs. However, disproportionate cardiac enlargement occurs in one-third to one-quarter of patients with acromegaly, but seldom exceeds 200 percent of normal.[70] One might also expect some cardiac enlargement from the increased peripheral demands of organomegaly; however, this is not the entire explanation since a significant number of individuals with acromegaly have hearts larger than expected for the degree of organomegaly present, and also symptomatic heart disease is more common than expected. McGuffin noted that of 57 patients with acromegaly 9 had symptomatic heart disease, and 7 of the 9 had symptoms of congestive heart failure.[71]

Hypertension plays a role in contributing to cardiomegaly. In McGuffin's series of 57 patients, 13 had clearly defined hypertension that was described as mild, uncomplicated, and responsive to medical therapy.[71] Balzer demonstrated a 34 percent incidence of significant hypertension in another series.[72] Although some individuals may tolerate the elevated pressure well, it has been reported to be poorly tolerated and leads to cardiomegaly.[72] Low plasma renin activity has been documented in some individuals with acromegaly.[73]

Although *arrhythmias* are not frequent, ventricular premature beats and intraventricular conduction defects have been noted. Frequent arrhythmias suggests that hyperthyroidism should be investigated.[71]

Coronary atherosclerotic heart disease is present in some patients with acromegaly. Although accelerated atherosclerosis is frequently mentioned, only 2 of 57 patients in McGuffin's series were said to have had coronary atherosclerotic heart disease.[71] In the series of 27 patients from the Mayo Clinic reported by Lie, significant coronary disease was present in only 11 percent. There is no doubt that hypertension and diabetes act as risk factors in acromegaly, but the incidence of documented coronary atherosclerotic heart disease in the above series is lower than expected, if indeed atherosclerosis is accelerated. Growth hormone affects carbohydrate and lipid metabolism. It is clear that up to one-half of patients with acromegaly have some disturbance of glucose metabolism, and 10 to 15 percent have definable diabetes.[70,71,74] Cholesterol elevations are not common and hyperlipoproteinemia is exceptional.[71,74] Aloia found only 2 of 25 patients to have hyperlipoproteinemia and postulated that in the absence of diabetes, the individual with acromegaly was generally not at unusual risk for atherosclerosis.[74]

The *heart at postmortem* examination in those individuals with acromegaly has been of considerable interest. Lie reported cardiomegaly in 22 of 27 patients (81 percent) with acromegaly who had postmortem examination.[70] The cardiomegaly occurred in those who had a history of hypertension and also in those who were normotensive. In this group of 27 patients, only 15 percent had diabetes and only 11 percent had definable coronary disease. Myocardial hypertrophy was common, as was fibrosis. A lymphomonocellular infiltrate or focal myocarditis was present in 59 percent. Another interesting finding was thickening of the walls of intramural vessels unrelated to scar tissue in 22 percent of patients. Four of the patients with small-vessel disease had hypertension, and one had diabetes. Another study of muscle tissue in individuals with acromegaly suggested that there is a 10 percent increase in collagen tissue per gram of muscle.[75] This, too, could account for left ventricular dysfunction. Lie's series noted a 19 percent incidence of focal myocardial disarray. It is unknown whether this was related to any findings of asymmetrical septal hypertrophy or hypertrophic cardiomyopathy.

Discussion

Available information suggests that the heart enlarges and left ventricular dysfunction does occur in acromegaly. There are isolated reports of patients with congestive heart failure, cardiomegaly, and no definable underlying cause such as coronary disease, hypertension, or diabetes. One such case had worsening problems with congestive heart failure that improved after hypophysectomy.[76]

Another interesting series of reports in groups of patients with acromegaly employs the echocardiogram for detection of cardiac abnormalities. Smallridge found that 6 of 27 patients who were followed clinically had symmetrical septal hypertrophy, 8 of 27 had concentric hypertrophy, and 13 of 27 were normal. Initial growth hormone levels were greater in those with asymmetrical septal hypertrophy and concentric hypertrophy than in normal people.[77] Savage found 80 percent of a group of 25 individuals with acromegaly had abnormal echocardiograms, including 13 without other signs of symptoms of cardiac involvement.[78] Most commonly, left ventricular mass was increased (64 percent). In this series, the degree of hypertrophy showed no relation to growth hormone levels pre or post treatment, or with the known duration of the acromegaly. All patients in this group with hypertension had increased left ventricular mass or wall thickness.

Many factors contribute to cardiac abnormalities in acromegaly. At this point, no specific cardiomyopathy has been defined, but with more follow-up and the further use of echocardiography, additional support for this possibility may be forthcoming.

Treatment

The treatment of acromegaly is surgical removal of the pituitary adenoma, and if this is not feasible, the use of radiation therapy. This may not, however, alter the course of the cardiovascular disease.

Pituitary Insufficiency

There is little direct effect of anterior pituitary insufficiency on the heart and circulation. The effect that does occur is related to thyroid insufficiency and adrenal insufficiency.

Adrenal Disease and the Heart

Cushing's Disease

The reader is referred to the chapter by P. Hamet in J. Genest, O. Juchel, P. Hamet, and M. Cantin's "Hypertension: Physiopathology and Treatment," 2d ed., McGraw-Hill Book Company, New York, 1983, p. 964, for an excellent discussion of Cushing's disease.

Primary Hyperaldosteronism

The reader is referred to Chaps. 49 to 51 for a discussion of hyperaldosteronism.

Other Varieties of Mineralocorticoid Hypertension

The reader is referred to Chaps. 49 to 51 for a discussion of these disorders.

Primary Adrenal Insufficiency (Addison's Disease)[22]

In addition to the classic findings of weakness and hyperpigmentation of the skin there may be hypotension, postural hypotension, and a small heart.

The reader is referred to standard textbooks of endocrinology for information on the recognition and treatment of Addison's disease.

Pheochromocytoma

The reader is referred to Chaps. 49 to 51 for a discussion of pheochromocytoma.

Oral Contraceptives and Menopausal Estrogen Therapy

Estrogens are naturally occurring hormonal steroids, usually regarded as the "female sex hormones," although in fact they are also secreted by the male in substantial amounts. The steroid hormone progesterone could also be regarded as a female sex hormone. Estrogens are responsible for the development of the genitalia and secondary sexual characteristics in the female. They are also responsible (with other hormones) for the inception and maintenance of the menstrual cycle, and (again with other hormones) for the inception and maintenance of pregnancy. The principal naturally occurring estrogens are estradiol-17β, estrone, estriol, and estrone sulfate.

Estrogens are secreted by the ovary, testicle, and placenta. There is also substantial extraglandular conversion of circulating androgens ("male sex hormones") to estrogens.

Therapy with estrogens can be divided into physiological and pharmacological. In ovarian failure, the normal secretion of estrogen by the ovary would be replaced by administered estrogens in physiological amounts at the appropriate time. This is an important, but somewhat rare, use of estrogens. Far more common is the pharmacological use of estrogens in the form of oral contraceptive agents, or in the treatment of complications of the menopause and of other conditions (Table 72-1).

A practical difficulty in therapy with estrogens is that the principal naturally occurring estrogens are not active when given by mouth. (Estrone sulfate is an exception.) In response to this difficulty, a number of synthetic estrogens have been developed over the years. Oral preparations currently in use are ethinyl estradiol-17β and mestranol, both derivatives of estradiol-17β. These substances are the principal estrogen constituents of oral contraceptives. Stilbestrol is less frequently used. The naturally occurring preparation conjugated equine estrogens, containing principally estrone sulfate, is in general use.

Therapeutic Uses of Estrogens

These are numerous. If oral contraceptives are included, then estrogen administration is one of the most widespread treatments in use today. A list of current therapeutic uses is given in Table 72-4. In the past, estrogens have been used for other conditions, but these uses have been substantially discontinued. The conditions treated include acne, hirsutism, atherosclerosis (prevention), threatened abortion, and premenstrual tension. Estrogens were also used in a pregnancy test. There may be some indication for estrogens in the treatment of endometriosis, and in height control in tall pubertal girls.

TABLE 72-4 Therapeutic Uses of Estrogens

Oral contraceptives	Mammary carcinoma with metastases
Menopausal symptoms Suppression of lactation	Prostatic carcinoma with metastases
Senile vaginitis Dysfunctional uterine bleeding Dysmenorrhea	Osteoporosis

Complications of Estrogen Therapy

In view of the widespread use of estrogens throughout the world, particularly in forms of oral contraceptives, an appraisal of the side effects or complications of estrogen therapy is essential (See Table 72-5).

Where estrogens are given with another hormone or hormones, it is necessary to know which hormone is producing a particular side effect. Oral contraceptive agents contain an estrogen (see above) and a progestogen. It is generally agreed that most of the complications noted in the use of oral contraceptives are due to the estrogen component. It is further agreed that the presence of the progestogen is protective against one of the major complications of estrogen therapy, namely, increased risk of endometrial carcinoma.[79] For this reason, estrogens should now be given only in combination with a progestogen, if the uterus is present. Sequential administration, that is, an estrogen followed by the addition of a progestogen, has been discontinued.

TABLE 72-5 Complications of Estrogen Therapy*

Mild, Occasionally Serious	
Breakthrough vaginal bleeding	Urinary tract infections
Nausea and vomiting	Abnormal glucose tolerance
Fluid retention	Post-oral contraceptive amenorrhea
Pigmentation of the skin	Hyperprolactinemia
Migraine headaches	Cholestatic jaundice
Hyperlipoproteinemia	*Arterial hypertension*
	Increased risk of gallstones
Serious, May Be Life-Threatening	
Peripheral vein thrombosis	
Pulmonary embolism	
Cerebral thrombosis and embolism	
Coronary artery thrombosis	
Benign liver tumors; hemorrhage	
Carcinoma of endometrium (but see discussion in text)	

*The cardiovascular complications are shown in italics.

Nevertheless, estrogens have in fact been given alone up to the present time for menopausal symptoms, and for osteoporosis. Some of our information regarding the complications of estrogen therapy refers to such treatment, as well as to the use of oral contraceptives.[81] The data regarding endometrial cancer provide an example.

The complications of estrogen therapy can be divided into two categories (1) mild, occasionally serious and (2) serious, potentially life-threatening, as shown in Table 72-5.

It is of interest that oral contraceptives probably have a protective effect against benign breast tumors, ovarian cysts, ovarian tumors, and possibly against carcinoma of the breast.

Perusal of the above lists of complications indicates several which are of particular interest to the cardiologist, and therefore need special comment. Fluid retention is not usually marked, and can often be ignored, except in patients already predisposed to fluid retention, such as mild heart failure. In these cases, estrogen therapy should be avoided. Hyperlipoproteinemia[82] is seen in a substantial portion of subjects taking oral contraceptives. This is not usually serious and is reversible on discontinuation of the contraceptives. But oral contraceptives should be avoided in patients with evidence of preexisting symptomatic atheroma, when this can be determined, and preexisting hyperlipoproteinemia.

A diabetic glucose tolerance test is used in some subjects taking oral contraceptives. This effect is also mild and reversible, and can possibly be ignored in the majority of patients. It may be a mild complication in the management of a diabetic subject. There is some question regarding increased incidence of arterial hypertension in oral contraceptive users. This subject is dealt with at length elsewhere (see Chap. 50).

In the serious category, increased incidence of carcinoma of the endometrium is a concern. The incidence in subjects treated with estrogen alone for menopausal symptoms rises from 35 cases per 100,000 population to 245 cases, according to one estimate, an increase of 700 percent.[83] However, the overall incidence remains low, and the administration of a progestogen with the estrogen, as is now recommended, substantially avoids this increased risk (see above). Benign liver tumors are serious only because of the potential for hemorrhage. They usually disappear on discontinuation of the oral contraceptive.

The principal concern for the cardiologist is the increase in thromboembolic disease, with the life-threatening potential (Table 72-6). In these conditions, there is apparently no protective effect from the administration of progestogen concurrently. The subject has been extensively reviewed.[80,84–87] The increased incidence of these complications in oral contraceptive users is illustrated in Table 72-6. The figures were obtained from several publications.

TABLE 72-6 Thromboembolic Disease*

	Controls	Users	Increase, %
Superficial vein thrombosis	200	300	50
Deep vein thrombosis and pulmonary thrombosis	20	110	550
Cerebrovascular thrombosis	10	40	400
Coronary artery thrombosis			
Age 30–39 years	2	6	300
Age 40–44 years	10	57	600

*Increased incidence in oral contraceptive users (cases per 100,000 population).

Source: The figures shown above were obtained from several publications: Johansson et al.,[80] Sartwell and Stolley,[84] Stadel,[85] Vessey and Mann,[86] and Kaplan.[87]

Although these figures indicate an increased incidence of the various thrombotic manifestations in oral contraceptive users, the overall incidence remains quite low, except perhaps in superficial vein thrombosis, which is the least harmful.

Recommendations regarding Treatment with Estrogens

Such recommendations involve the usual consideration of cost/benefit ratio. Some aspects have already been discussed. On general grounds, estrogens should be given in the lowest dose and for the shortest period feasible. This general principle has a somewhat limited value since several applications (e.g., contraception, osteoporosis) clearly require administration over long periods of time. However, the principle does apply to the treatment of menopausal symptoms. Estrogens should only be given for those specific complications where they are known to be beneficial (e.g., hot flashes, vaginitis), and only for as long as is strictly necessary.

Preexisting conditions that may predispose to any of the complications, particularly the serious complications, should be documented clearly and assessed. Usually, the presence of such conditions is a contraindication to the use of estrogens in any form. These conditions include most forms of heart disease, preexisting fluid retention, especially in early heart failure, urinary tract infections, hyperlipoproteinemia, gallstones, depression, and possibly diabetes mellitus. It is of particular importance to avoid estrogens in subjects with a history of thromboembolic episodes or any condition predisposing to such episodes, such as prosthetic heart valves.

In spite of the above logical restrictions on the use of estrogens, estrogen-progestogen mixtures, usually in the form of one of the oral contraceptives, remain an effective method for the treatment of a number of conditions, and are, of course, particularly effective as contraceptives. Careful observation of the restrictions enhances their value.

Osteoporosis (premenopausal, menopausal, or postmenopausal) falls into a particular category.[88] Estrogen treatment has been used intermittently for several decades, without any clear indication of its benefit. More recently, however, substantial evidence has come to hand indicating that estrogens are useful in decreasing the rate of bone loss, provided they are started at the menopause, or no later than 2 years following the menopause.[89] At present, categories of persons in whom treatment is recommended are (1) those in whom evidence of osteoporosis is already present at or within 3 years following the menopause and (2) those in a high-risk category for osteoporosis,[90] namely, patients with short stature, fair hair, nulliparity, early menopause, or a family history of osteoporosis.

Pancreatic Disease and the Heart

Hyperinsulinism[22]

An excess of insulin, due to the secretion of an islet cell adenoma or from an excess of administered insulin, may produce acute hypoglycemia. This in turn produces hypokalemia and catecholamine release, which can alter the electrocardiogram (see Chap. 77). This effect can be partially blocked with beta-blocking drugs.

Hypoglycemia may precipitate angina pectoris in patients with coronary disease. Patients with angina who are receiving beta-blocking drugs who become hypoglycemic may develop hypertension during the episode.

Diabetes Mellitus

Diabetes mellitus can be defined as an elevated plasma glucose level due to insufficient insulin effect. In children there is virtually always a decrease in the number of pancreatic beta cells and the output of insulin. When diabetes begins as an adult, obesity is usually present. Circulating insulin levels are higher than in the lean nondiabetic but not as high as would be expected for an obese nondiabetic individual with a similar level of plasma glucose. The criteria for the diagnosis of glucose intolerance are shown in Table 72-7.[92]

TABLE 72-7 Criteria for Diagnosis of Glucose Intolerance

1. Glucose intolerance in the nonpregnant adult (diabetes mellitus):
   a. Fasting blood sugar (FBS) greater than 140 mg/dl × 2, or
   b. Decompensated diabetes mellitus, or
   c. A glucose tolerance test (GTT)* in a properly prepared individual with 2-h glucose > 200 mg/dl, *and* one other glucose ($\frac{1}{2}$-h, 1-h, $1\frac{1}{2}$-h, or 3-h) > 200 mg/dl.
2. Gestational diabetes (GDM):
   a. Screen at 24–28 weeks' gestation. Give 50 g of glucose orally any time of day and regardless of nutritional status. Measure the plasma glucose 1 h later:
      (1) If the glucose is > 190 mg/dl, diagnose GDM.
      (2) If the glucose is 140 to 190 mg/dl, proceed to full GTT.
   b. Oral GTT with 100 g glucose: Diagnose GDM if two or more glucoses ≥ FBS, 105 mg/dl; 1-h, 190 mg/dl; 2-h, 165 mg/dl; 3-h, 145 mg/dl.
3. Impaired glucose tolerance (IGT): A GTT in a properly prepared individual, with 2-h glucose > 140 mg/dl but < 200 mg/dl *and* one other glucose ($\frac{1}{2}$-h, 1-h, $1\frac{1}{2}$-h, or 3-h) > 200 mg/dl.

*Proper preparation for GTT includes being ambulatory, off diabetogenic drugs, on 3 days of at least 300 g/day of carbohydrate, fasting 8–12 h, and 75 g of glucose.

Heart Disease in Patients with Diabetes

The importance of heart disease in the individual with diabetes did not become apparent until the risk of death from diabetic coma decreased. This was elegantly demonstrated by Elliot P. Joslin's review of 18,055 deaths compiled by the Statistics Bureau of the Metropolitan Life Insurance Company. Eras of diabetes care from 1895 to 1957 were noted and the cases separated into cause of death with coma and without coma. Death from coma decreased from 63.8 percent to 1.1 percent and death from a primary cardiac cause increased from 6.1 percent to 50.2 percent.[91] Most cardiac deaths are secondary to coronary atherosclerotic heart disease. Additional cardiac dysfunction may be secondary to autonomic neuropathy, microangiopathy, and/or myopathy. Heart disease in a young individual with insulin-dependent diabetes is likely to be due to multiple etiologies, while heart disease in an individual with gestational diabetes may be a pure reversible cardiomyopathy. Impaired glucose tolerance only leads to an increased risk of developing coronary atherosclerotic heart disease. Table 72-8 lists the current nomenclature for classifying diabetes together with the heart abnormalities associated with each type.[92]

The symptoms associated with diabetic autonomic neuropathy, myopathy, and coronary athero-

TABLE 72-8 Cardiovascular Abnormalities Associated with the Different Types of Diabetes

Classification of Diabetes	Principal Cardiovascular Abnormalities at Increased Risk
Diabetes mellitus*	
Type I (IDDM)	Cardiomyopathy, ASCVD,† autonomic neuropathy
Type II (NIDDM)	ASCVD†
Gestational diabetes mellitus	Cardiomyopathy, fetal hypertrophic subaortic stenosis
Impaired glucose control	ASCVD†

*IDDM = insulin-dependent diabetes mellitus; NIDDM = non-insulin-dependent diabetes mellitus.
†Atherosclerotic cardiovascular disease.

sclerotic heart disease overlap. Decreased exercise tolerance is common to all. The individual with longstanding diabetes can have spells of sweating, anxiety, or shortness of breath while sleeping, at rest, or with exercise, and feel better sitting and/or drinking orange juice. Measurement of pulse, blood pressure, and glucose when symptomatic or during an exercise test can help separate the contribution of diabetic control and of autonomic neuropathy to the symptoms.

Decreased vibratory perception in the distal limb is an early indicator of diabetic peripheral neuropathy. Peripheral neuropathy is the earliest and most common chronic complication of diabetes. Vibratory perception also decreases with aging. Normally a 128-cycle tuning fork struck maximally can be felt for over 25 s on the toe. Less than 15 s in the person under 40 or less than 10 s in the person over 40 suggests a significant peripheral neuropathy and an increased risk of autonomic neuropathy.[93] Autonomic neuropathy has a grave prognosis.[94] The most sensitive and specific indicator of cardiac autonomic neuropathy is a fixed heart rate as defined by lack of R-R variation on electrocardiogram monitoring while the subject breathes deeply 6 times per minute.[97] Postural hypotension is another common cardiovascular autonomic neuropathy.

The presence of retinopathy also increases the risk of cardiac disease.[95] Individuals with diabetic renal failure may also have significant coronary artery disease. Of 21 patients assessed angiographically with no clinical or electrocardiographic evidence of coronary atherosclerotic heart disease 9 had significant abnormalities angiographically; 8 of the 9 with coronary artery disease were asymptomatic.[96]

A recently described abnormal physical finding that may correlate with cardiac disease is contractures of the hands. When holding the fingers juxtaposed (as in a prayer) the fourth and fifth fingers should completely come together in the normal person. This is not attained in diabetes. The finding occurs particularly in growing children with diabetes.[98] It will be interesting to see if this stiffness in the hands has a similar histopathology to the stiffness in the heart. A vectorcardiogram change, "bites," has been reported to be more frequent in two studies of diabetics.[99,100]

The Relation between the Heart and Diabetic Complications

Diabetic Neuropathies Diabetic neuropathy presents both as an acute complication, mononeuropathy, and as a chronic complication, symmetrical diffuse polyneuropathy of sensory, motor, and autonomic nerves.[101] Young women, middle-aged men, and the elderly seem particularly at risk with these complications. There is decreased perception of pain, paresthesias that are sometimes incapacitating, and functional abnormalities of viscera, proximal muscle, and the heart.

Alterations in heart rate, orthostatic hypotension, and insulin edema are relatively common as clinical problems.

Computer programs are available utilizing standard electrocardiograms that allow calculation of the loss of R-R variation with deep breathing.[102] In one prospective study 56 percent of diabetic patients with autonomic neuropathy died within the next 5 years.[94] Hilstead performed resting and exercise studies on three groups of insulin-dependent diabetes mellitus (IDDM, see classification of diabetes) patients: those with no neuropathy, mild neuropathy, and severe neuropathy. Severe neuropathy was associated with resting tachycardia, systolic hypertension, and decreased R-R variation with deep breathing. The pulse pressure narrowed and the pulse rate failed to increase as much with exercise in individuals with severe neuropathy as in those without neuropathy. Exercise tolerance was also significantly reduced. Individuals with even mild neuropathy had less marked but similar and significant differences in cardiac performance when compared to normal people.[103]

Postural hypotension in diabetics is most commonly seen after bed rest, diuretics, or antihypertensive medications. The blood pressure can fall with exercise and at the peak time of action of insulin in some patients with neuropathy.[104] These symptoms are easily mistaken for insulin reactions.

The treatment for the postural symptoms is elevation of the head of the bed, increased salt intake, reduction of diuretics, leg binders, instruction to the patient to sit on the bed 5 min before standing, and occasionally fludrocortisone or indomethocin (see Chap. 30).[105] In the presence of autonomic neuropathy insulin increases the tendency to pool fluid in the visceral space. Some patients develop diffuse swelling of face and hands, knee effusions, and ankle edema as they recover from diabetic ketoacidosis. This is probably due to the effect of insulin in increasing vascular permeability, particularly in patients with neuropathy.[106,107] Diuretics must be used cautiously.

Diabetic neuropathy is less improved when the glucose is controlled to an average blood glucose of 150 mg/dl or less.[108] Improved glucose control will also increase R-R variation (reflecting improvement in an autonomic neuropathy).[102] Investigational drugs that block the conversion of glucose to sorbitol appear to prevent nerve damage from high blood glucose levels and may have a place in therapy in the future.[109]

Chest pain secondary to mononeuropathy is rare. This pain can be almost as severe as herpes zoster and can be misinterpreted as cardiac in origin. It will start suddenly and is usually continuous. Mapping a dermatome with a pin confirms the neural etiology, and relief of pain with a nerve block can help the patient understand that the pain is due to a nerve, not to the heart.

Silent (painless) myocardial infarction is a bothersome problem that occurs in diabetic individuals not infrequently. Neuropathy was demonstrated in the heart in five cases of painless infarction, leading to the theory that there is a lesion of the afferent nerves that conduct pain.[110] In the Framingham study 7 of 18 diabetics (39 percent) had silent or unrecognized myocardial infarctions, while 53 of 241 nondiabetics (22 percent) had silent myocardial infarctions.[111] Likewise myocardial ischemia may be painless. Decreased exercise tolerance and breathlessness may be the only symptoms of infarction or angina.

Sympathetic neuropathy particularly involves the lower extremity. There is evidence that chronic neuropathic foot ulcers are in fact due to sympathetic neuropathy. There are interesting reports of increased cardiac output and increased blood flow to the foot with arteriovenous shunts, venous dilation, poor tissue perfusion, and intractable edema.[112,113] Ephedrin, a sympathomimetic, helped reduce lower-extremity edema in a few patients with severe autonomic neuropathy and intractable edema.[114] This drug obviously should be used cautiously in a patient with possible coronary atherosclerotic heart disease.

Microangiopathy and Cardiomyopathy

At autopsy, typical microaneurysms were found in the diabetic hearts of three out of six persons with long-standing diabetes. The microaneurysms were not localized to any one layer of the left ventricular myocardium. Extensive interstitial fibrosis and myocardial degeneration was noted in all six patients both in areas of microaneurysms and in areas without. Fusiform dilations were also present in isolated segments of vessels.[115]

Quadriceps and myocardial biopsy specimens were obtained from 24 patients undergoing coronary artery bypass surgery. There were 8 patients with a normal glucose tolerance test (nondiabetic), 8 patients with a fasting plasma glucose less than 130 mg/dl but an elevated 2-h glucose (chemically diabetic), and 8 patients on insulin (overtly diabetic). There was significant laminar thickening of the capillaries from the overtly diabetic patients and early thickening of the chemically diabetic. Pericapillary edema was documented with irregular laminar thickening of the myocardial capillaries in the overtly diabetic.[116] *Chronic microvascular changes of diabetes clearly occur in the heart.*

In the rat, hyperglycemia for over a month results in a depression in calcium-stimulated ATPase activity in cardiac sarcoplasmic reticulum. This defect, along with a decrease in the force of contraction by the heart, is reversible with insulin.[123,124] A number of human studies show decreased myocardial performance in the diabetic and in some cases reversibility with insulin.

Shapiro studied ventricular function by computer analysis of echocardiograms from 142 diabetics. The presence of microvascular complications was coded as 0 = no retinopathy, no proteinuria, and no neuropathy; 1 = mild retinopathy (less than 10 red dots per eye) or mild proteinuria (1 or 2 +) or mild neuropathy (absent ankle jerks and vibratory sense in the feet); 2 = severe retinopathy, 3 or 4 + proteinuria, or peripheral neuropathy and autonomic neuropathy. The 12 young diabetic subjects with no complications had normal diastolic variables of left ventricular function. All other groups of diabetics had significantly delayed mitral valve opening. Forty-four diabetics with severe microvascular complications had abnormalities in all variables of diastolic functions measured compared to normal. These abnormalities were unlike those found in 16 control subjects with coronary artery disease. *The diabetic myocardium, while not hypertrophied, had similar properties to those of myocardial hypertrophy with abnormal compliance.*[117] Preclinical echocardiographic changes of probable preclinical cardiomyopathy were also found in younger (under age 25) diabetics.[118]

Valk et al. studied six under-30-year-old patients with insulin-dependent diabetes of less than 3 years' duration. None had evidence of retinopathy or nephropathy, but all had an elevated glycosylated hemoglobin as evidence of recent hyperglycemia. They were studied initially and after 7 to 10 days of good glucose control. The plasma volume increased 12 percent; the hematocrit decreased 9 percent; the plasma norepinephrine and epinephrine after peak exercise decreased; the resting and postexercise heart rates decreased, as did diastolic volumes and ejection fraction. They concluded that early insulin-dependent diabetes is associated with a reversible hyperdynamic cardiac state.[119]

Fein has written an excellent review on heart disease in diabetes.[120] *A reversible cardiac dysfunction* has also been reported in new-onset type 2 non-insulin-dependent diabetes. After 3 to 8 months of intense diet treatment the mean glucose decreased from 200 to 140 mg/dl; the heart rate–corrected preejection period decreased from 139 to 135 ms; and the heart rate–corrected left ventricular ejection time increased from 400 to 410 ms. When the patients were grouped according to those whose glucose level improved by more than 54 mg/dl and those whose glucose level did not, a significant cardiac change was noted only in those with the significant glucose change.[121] It is of interest that women with diabetes only during gestation had a prolonged ejection period and a shorter left ventricular ejection time. This disappeared after glucose tolerance normalized 5 weeks post delivery.[122]

The Framingham study reported an increased incidence of congestive heart failure in diabetics not accounted for by accompanying atherogenic traits. This suggests the clinical importance of diabetic cardiomyopathy.[123]

Macrovascular Disease (Atherosclerosis) and Diabetes Mellitus

The relative risk for cardiovascular disease (Framingham study 20-year follow-up) for men was 2.1 and women 2.7. The association of diabetes with other risk factors markedly increased the probability of subsequent cardiovascular disease.[111] Average shortening of life expectancy was 8 years.[126] The increased risk of female diabetics could be partially explained by the increased number of accompanying risk factors.[111,126–128]

While diabetics had more coronary atherosclerotic heart disease and more diffuseness of coronary atherosclerotic heart disease, the prognosis appears unrelated to the duration or the severity of the diabetes mellitus.[129] Jarrett reviewed the evidence that impaired glucose tolerance is associated with the same increase in risk of coronary atherosclerotic heart disease as diabetes mellitus. He questioned whether diabetes develops in individuals who possess characteristics which increase the risk of atherosclerotic coronary artery disease in addition to the risk of developing diabetes.[130] Families of diabetics had increased rates of coronary atherosclerotic disease. The one exception was families of insulin-dependent diabetics (patients who were never taken off insulin).[131] This is of interest since in this one group of patients the etiology of the diabetes is thought to be totally related to the beta cell while in the other types of diabetes there are periods of high insulin levels before diabetes develops.

Another explanation for the association of macrovascular disease and mild abnormalities of carbohydrate tolerance is that the atherosclerosis is related to lipid levels or insulin. Pietri et al. compared two intensive diabetes treatment regimes: multiple injections and home glucose monitoring versus continued insulin infusion by pump. The plasma glucose and triglyceride levels improved in both programs. With pump therapy the final average glucose was 108 mg/dl versus 134 mg/dl with multiple insulin injections. The total cholesterol and low-density lipoprotein (LDL) cholesterol levels improved only in the pump patients with the lower glucose. They concluded that it required almost perfect metabolic control to affect plasma cholesterol and LDL cholesterol.[132] Camerini-Davalos et al. demonstrated increased capillary basement membrane thickening in muscle biopsies in 41 asymptomatic individuals with only minimal abnormalities of glucose tolerance.[133] They also showed prospectively over a period of approximately 3 years that the glucose tolerance and the capillary basement membrane thickening improved in 23 individuals treated with an oral hypoglycemic agent but not in 18 individuals on placebo. They concluded that microangiopathy may be present in a considerable number of patients with asymptomatic diabetes and that the changes can be improved if the glucose tolerance is improved.[133]

High peripheral levels of insulin may have a deleterious effect. Insulin has been shown to have a salt-retaining action. Treatments that result in lower insulin levels may improve blood pressure.[134] Patients on over 50 units of insulin a day are more at risk for cardiovascular disease than patients on less than 50 units. In 7246 nondiabetic working men followed for an average of 63 months the fasting plasma insulin level and the fasting insulin glucose ratio were positively associated with nonfatal myocardial infarction and coronary-related deaths.[135] It will take many more years to prove if a diet and/or exercise program that helped lower the insulin levels to normal affected prognosis.

One of the most controversial studies on cardiovascular events and treatment of diabetes is that of the University Group Diabetes Program. The patients treated with increasing doses of insulin averaged a plasma glucose 50 mg/dl lower than the tolbutamide or placebo-treated group but had no improvement in the risk of myocardial infarction.[136] Tolbutamide was associated with a slightly increased risk of myocardial infarction. The risk factors were more significant in the tolbutamide group.[136] In a dog model tolbutamide improved the plasma glucose but still was associated with further reduction of left ventricular function and altered morphology of myocardium.[137] Based on today's data the judgment to use insulin or oral hypoglycemic agents in type II non-insulin-dependent diabetes cannot be based on the goal to increase the life expectancy from coronary artery disease.

When a diabetic patient complains of fatigue, autonomic neuropathy, cardiomyopathy, or coronary atherosclerotic heart disease may be present. Fatigue may be an anginal equivalent. Twelve asymptomatic diabetic males had exercise testing with scintigraphy. Their average age was 48.7 years, and the average duration of diabetes was 7.8 years. Seven (58.3 percent) had an abnormal exercise electrocardiogram or a myocardial perfusion defect on scintigraphy. Only 1 of 12 normal volunteers of average age 48.9 years had an abnormality.[119] Of 21 insulin-dependent diabetes with renal failure 9 had significant coronary artery disease on angiography.[98] Thus, coronary atherosclerotic heart disease is increased and should be suspected in diabetic patients with retinopathy, nephropathy, or symptoms of fatigue on exertion.

Cardiomyopathy in the Fetus

As discussed earlier, there appears to be a type of diabetic cardiomyopathy in patients with diabetes. A different type of cardiomyopathy is observed in the fetus of the poorly controlled diabetic mother (see discussion below). The reader is referred to Fein's excellent review of this subject.[120]

Pregnancy and the Newborn

The diabetic mother is at increased cardiovascular risk, primarily if there is clinical evidence of coronary atherosclerotic heart disease.[138] As mentioned earlier, gestational diabetes results in changes in cardiac performance of the mother, reversible after delivery. If the diabetes is poorly controlled during the pregnancy, then the fetus is at risk for an unusual form of *hypertrophic cardiomyopathy*. In a prospective study of 23 pregnancies in the year 1977, three infants had septal hypertrophy and two had right ventricular wall hypertrophy.[139] The fetus produces increased amounts of insulin in response to the maternal hyperglycemia. This results in macrosomia, which includes glycogen, fat, and muscle buildup. Good blood glucose control in the mother prevents the congenital anomalies, respiratory distress, and macrosomia.[138] The cardiac findings and treatment in the infants is *similar to those of adults with idiopathic hypertrophic subaortic stenosis.*[140] Digitalis should be avoided. One fetus developed tachycardia. The mother was successfully treated with 160 mg of propranolol daily with a reduction of fetal heart rate to 120 to 160 beats per minute.[141] The functional stenosis usually disappears in 4 to 7 days.[140] This is one of the few reversible forms of hypertrophic cardiomyopathy.

Treatment of Heart Disease in the Patient with Diabetes Mellitus

As mentioned, heart disease in a person with diabetes is usually not a single entity but a combination of disorders. The dominant cardiac problems are coronary atherosclerotic heart disease, congestive heart failure, sinus tachycardia, decreased exercise tolerance, fluid retention, particularly after insulin treatment for diabetes out of control, postural hypotension worsened by exercise and insulin, and difficulty with wound healing and in tolerating stress. The relative clinical significance of a cardiomyopathy is still unclear, but it may be more common and significant than previously thought.

Acute Myocardial Infarction Making the diagnosis if a patient is in diabetic ketoacidosis can be difficult due to the electrocardiographic effects of hyper- and hypokalemia.[142] It is important to think of possible myocardial infarction in diabetic patients with atypical complaints. In one series 42 percent of diabetics presented with no chest pain, versus 6 percent of nondiabetics.[143]

Once the diagnosis is made, management will be similar (Chap. 45) to that of nondiabetics. The stress of the infarction raises the plasma glucose. The initial plasma glucose in 26 diabetic patients who had a medium time of 5 h from infarction was used with the rate of insulin dropping from 3.4 to 2.1 units/h by the twelfth hour of infusion.[144] Since diet is erratic, a continuous insulin infusion is a reasonable choice. Hypoglycemia is certainly to be avoided, since in animal studies of hypoglycemia after infarction there is an increase in myocardial damage.[145]

Insulin is an anabolic hormone and may have a therapeutic place even in the nondiabetic who has had a myocardial infarction. A "polarizing" infusion of glucose, potassium, and insulin results in an elevated blood glucose and potassium and a lowering of blood urea nitrogen and free fatty acids.[99,146] Ventricular arrhythmias may decrease. The ejection fraction was noted to increase and the pulmonary arterial end-diastolic pressure and end-diastolic and end-systolic volumes to decrease.[147] High-dose insulin and glucose are also sometimes used after cardiac surgery. The glucose and insulin patients had an increase in cardiac output and dopamine-stimulated cardiac output when compared with 10 similar patients receiving only sorbitol.[148] The use of glucose potassium and insulin after myocardial infarction in nondiabetics is still controversial. Despite the earlier evidence on the value of good glucose control this procedure elevates the glucose. It is of note that hyperglycemia in animals must persist for over 10 days before any deleterious effect on cardiac performance is noted, and current use of these polarizing solutions has been limited to a few days.

Angina Pectoris Due to Coronary Atherosclerosis Nonselective beta-adrenergic blocking drugs like propranolol used in angina pectoris can mask the symptoms of hypoglycemia with unopposed alpha stimulation and an increase in blood pressure. The cautious use of beta-blocking drugs in the IDDM patient would require monitoring of blood glucose to detect hypoglycemia. Gluconeogenesis by the liver is also reduced, so that recovery from hypoglycemia is slower. With patients not on insulin beta blockers result in less endogenous insulin release, with the result that glucose tolerance can deteriorate. These side effects are lessened with a cardioselective blocker like metoprolol.[149] Calcium channel blockers offer a mode of therapy that does not interfere with diabetes management. Nitrites and beta blockers can increase the risk of postural hypotension, particularly if autonomic neuropathy is present.

Hypertension Postural hypotension may occur during the use of any antihypertensive. This is most common in the patient with autonomic neuropathy. Hyporeninemic hypoaldosteronism, which occurs in diabetes, may increase the risk of hyperkalemia. Potassium-sparing diuretics should be used very cautiously and potassium should not be routinely replaced in diabetic patients on thiazide or loop diuretics. The reflex tachycardia of hydralazine can be avoided with prazosin. Because of unusually powerful hypotensive effects of the first dose, prazosin should always be started at bedtime.

Congestive Heart Failure Diabetic patients are at increased risk for congestive heart failure due to hypertension, coronary atherosclerotic heart disease, or cardiomyopathy. Sometimes the heart may not dilate, and a restrictive type of cardiomyopathy may be present.[150] If hyperglycemia is also present and treated, fluid moves with the glucose and failure may improve. Improvement in plasma glucose as mentioned earlier also improves cardiac performance. Edema appearing after poor control has been corrected may be "insulin edema" and not congestive heart failure. Intravascular volume may be decreased and diuretics can result in hypotension. The edema secondary to insulin usually clears spontaneously over 4 to 6 days. Otherwise management of the diabetic patient with congestive heart failure is similar to that of the nondiabetic (Chap. 21).

Surgery in Diabetics

Kahn et al. reported cardiac disease in 63 percent of a series of 100 diabetic patients undergoing lower-limb amputation. There was a 9 percent mortality rate with 6 of the 9 deaths being due to myocardial infarction.[151] Femoropopliteal vein grafts have poorer results in diabetics than in nondiabetics; the 45 percent 5-year graft patency compared with 72 percent at 5 years for nondiabetics.[152] Coronary bypass surgery is offered to diabetics as well as nondiabetics. In one study there was slightly more operative risk but similar quality to the coronary vessels and a similar outcome.[153]

Three explanations have been given for the glucose intolerance which occurs with anesthesia:[154] (1) because of decreased sensitivity of the cell membrane to the action of insulin, tissues exposed to anesthesia require more insulin for the same effect when compared with tissues not exposed to anesthesia, (2) less insulin is released in relation to the same plasma glucose level with anesthesia than without anesthesia, and (3) there is direct stimulation of glycogenolysis by anesthesia. In cardiac bypass procedures where blood glucose levels have become high in individuals with borderline diabetes, there have been reports of rapid spontaneous lowering of plasma glucose and potassium, with subsequent arrhythmias, presumably secondary to recovery from the above effects after anesthesia. The use of glucose monitoring during surgery allows high glucose levels to be detected and to be treated sooner.

There are many ways to manage diabetic patients undergoing general or cardiac surgery. The most common is to administer 1 to 2 units of regular insulin per hour intravenously as a continuous infusion and monitor the glucose every 1 to 2 h.[155] The following program can be helpful after cardiac bypass when stress factors are changing rapidly. The unit must be capable of measuring the glucose hourly.

- Piggyback an insulin drip starting at a rate per hour about three-quarters the usual hourly insulin dosage and change the insulin drip based on the hourly glucose determination. A formula such as

  $$(\text{Blood glucose} - 60)0.03 = \text{units of regular insulin per hour}$$

  can be used to adjust the insulin. Hold drip for 1 h when the glucose first goes under 150 mg/dl. Example: Glucose = 280 mg/dl; (280 − 60) = 220 × .03 = 6.6 units/h. For patients who are likely to be insulin-resistant or sensitive to lower insulin levels you can change the multiplier to 0.04 or 0.02, respectively.

Wound Healing and Diabetes

Wound healing is unquestionably slow in the person with long-standing diabetes.[156–159] This may, at times, increase the risk of infection following coronary bypass surgery.

Overview of Diabetes[160–172]

Diabetes mellitus is a common disease and directly and indirectly causes heart disease. The treatment of the disease has changed greatly in the last 10 years.

The reader is referred to a standard textbook of endocrinology for details regarding treatment.

References

1. King, Thomas Wilkinson: Observations on the Thyroid, *Guys Hosp. Rep.*, 1:441, 1836.
2. Hollander, C. S., Nihel, N., Burday, S. Z., Mitsuma, T., Schenkman, L., and Blum, M.: Clinical and Laboratory Observations in Cases of Triiodothyronine Toxicosis Confirmed by Radioimmunoassay, *Lancet,* 1:609, 1972.
3. Bermudez, F., Surks, M. I., and Oppenheimer, J. H.: High Incidence of Decreased Serum Triiodothyronine Concentration in Patients with Nonthyroidal Disease, *J. Clin. Endocrinol. Metab.*, 41:27, 1975.
4. Ormston, B. J., Garry, R., Cryer, R. J., and Besser, G. M.: Thyrotropin Releasing Hormone as a Thyroid Function Test, *Lancet,* 2:10, 1971.
5. Woolf, P. D.: Transient Painless Thyroiditis with Hyperthyroidism: A Variant of Lymphocytic Thyroiditis?, *Endocrine Rev.*, 1:411, 1980.
6. Eayrs, J. T.: Influence of the Thyroid on the Central Nervous System, *Br. Med. Bull.*, 16:122, 1960.
7. Apathetic Thyrotoxicosis, *Lancet,* 2:809, 1970. (Editorial.)
8. Stewart, H. J., and Evans, W. F.: The Peripheral Blood Flow in Hyperthyroidism, *Am. Heart J.*, 20:715, 1940.
9. Channick, B. J., Adlin, E. V., Marks, A. D., Denenberg, B. S., McDonough, M. T., Chakko, C. S., and Spann, J. F.: Hyperthyroidism and Mitral Valve Prolapse, *N. Engl. J. Med.*, 305:497, 1981.
10. Nakazawa, H. K., Sakurai, K., Hamada, N., Momotani, N., and Ito, K.: Management of Atrial Fibrillation in the Post-Thyrotoxic State, *Am. J. Med.*, 72:903, 1982.
11. Eraker, S. A., Wickamasekaran, R., and Goldman, S.: Complete Heart Block with Hyperthyroidism, *JAMA*, 239:1644, 1978.
12. Skanghir, I. M., and Benerjee, J.: Wolff-Parkinson-White Syndrome Associated with Thyrotoxicosis, *Am. J. Cardiol.*, 8:431, 1961.
13. Wei, J. Y., Senecin, A., Green, H. L., and Achaff, S. C.: Coronary Spasm with Ventricular Fibrillation during Thyrotoxicosis: Response to Attaining Euthyroid State, *Am. J. Cardiol.*, 43:335, 1979.
14. Featherstone, H. J., and Steward, D. K.: Angina in Thyrotoxicosis, Thyroid-Related Coronary Artery Spasm, *Arch. Intern. Med.*, 143(3):554, 1983.
15. Markowitz, C., and Yater, W. M.: Response of Explanted Cardiac Muscle to Thyroxine, *Am. J. Physiol.*, 100:162, 1932.
16. Buccino, R. A., Spann, J. F., Pool, P. E., and Braunwald, F.: Influence of the Thyroid State on the Intrinsic Contractile Properties and the Energy Stores of the Myocardium, *J. Clin. Invest.*, 46:1669, 1967.
17. Morkin, E., Flink, I. L., and Goldman, S.: Biochemical and Physiologic Effects of Thyroid Hormone on Cardiac Performance, *Prog. Cardiovasc. Dis.*, 25:435, 1983.

18. Banerjee, S. K.: Computer Studies of Atrial and Ventricular Myocin from Normal, Thyrotoxic and Thyroidectomized Rabbits, *Circ. Res.*, 52:131, 1983.
19. Mahdavi, V., and Nadal-Ginard, B.: The Genetics of Myocin Regulation, *Cardiology*, 1(6):21, 1984.
20. Arnsdorf, M. F., and Childers, R. W.: A Trial Electrophysiology in Experimental Hyperthyroidism in Rabbits, *Circ. Res.*, 26:575, 1970.
21. Johnson, P. N., Freedberg, A. S., and Marshall, J. M.: Action of Thyroid Hormone on the Transmembrane Potentials from Sinoatrial Cells and Actual Muscle Cells in Isolated Atria of Rabbits, *Cardiology*, 58:273, 1973.
22. Christy, J. H., and Clements, S. D.: The Heart and Endocrine Disease, in J. W. Hurst (ed.), "The Heart," 5th ed., McGraw-Hill Book Company, New York, 1982, p. 1548.
23. Williams, G. H., and Braunwald, E.: Endocrine and Nutritional Disorders and Heart Disease, in E. Braunwald (ed.), "Heart Disease," W. B. Saunders Company, Philadelphia, 1984, p. 726.
24. Christensen, N. J.: Increased Levels of Plasma Noradrenaline in Hypothyroidism, *J. Clin. Endocrinol. Metab.*, 36:587, 1973.
25. Noth, R. H., and Spaulding, S. W.: Decreased Serum Dopamine-Beta-Hydroxylase in Hyperthyroidism, *J. Clin. Endocrinol. Metab.*, 39:614, 1974.
26. Aoki, V. S., Wilson, W. R., and Theilen, E. O.: Studies of the Reputed Augmentation of the Cardiovascular Effects of Catecholamines in Patients with Spontaneous Hyperthyroidism, *J. Pharmacol. Exp. Ther.*, 181:362, 1967.
27. Van der Shoot, J. B., and Moran, N. C.: An Experimental Evaluation of the Reputed Influence of Thyroxin on the Cardiovascular Effects of Catecholamines, *J. Pharmacol. Exp. Ther.*, 149:336, 1965.
28. Williams, L. T., Lefkowitz, R. J., Watanabe, A. M., Hathaway, D. R., and Besch, H. R.: Thyroid Hormone Regulation of Beta-Adrenergic Receptor Number, *J. Biol. Chem.*, 252:2787, 1977.
29. Rutherford, J. D., Vatner, S. F., and Braunwald, E.: Adrenergic Control of Myocardial Contractility in Conscious Hyperthyroid Dogs, *Am. J. Physiol.*, 237:590, 1979.
30. Forfar, J. C., Muir, A. L., Sawers, S. A., and Toft, A. D.: Abnormal Left Ventricular Function in Hyperthyroidism: Evidence for a Possible Reversible Cardiomyopathy, *N. Engl. J. Med.*, 307:1165, 1982.
31. Geffner, D. L., Azukizawa, M., and Hershman, J. M.: Propylthiouracil Blocks Extrathyroidal Conversion of Thyroxine to Triiodothyronine, *J. Clin. Invest.*, 55:224, 1975.
32. Iodide-Induced Thyrotoxicosis, *Lancet*, 2:1072, 1972. (Editorial.)
33. Bradley, E. L., and Liechty, R. D.: Modified Subtotal Thyroidectomy for Graves' Disease: A Two-Institution Study, *Surgery*, 94:955, 1983.
34. Grossman, W., Robin, N. I., Johnson, L. W., Brooks, H., Selenkow, H. A., and Dexter, L.: Effects of Beta Blockade on the Peripheral Manifestation of Thyrotoxicosis, *Ann. Intern. Med.*, 70:963, 1969.
35. DeGroot, L. J., and Stanbury, J. B.: "The Thyroid and Its Diseases," John Wiley and Sons, New York, 1975, p. 489.
36. Lever, E. G., Medeiros-Neto, G. A., and DeGroot, L. J.: Inherited Disorders of Thyroid Metabolism, *Endocrine Rev.*, 4:213, 1983.
37. Clements, F. V.: Naturally Occurring Goitrogens, *Br. Med. Bull.*, 16:133, 1960.
38. Onishi, T., Miyai, K., Aono, T., Shioji, T., Yamamoto, T., Okada, Y., and Kumahara, Y.: Primary Hypothyroidism and Galactorrhea, *Am. J. Med.*, 63:373, 1977.
39. Blum, M.: Myxedema Coma, *Am. J. Med. Sci.*, 264:432, 1972.
40. Zondek, H.: Das Myxodemem Herz, *Munch. Med. Wochenschr.*, 65:1180, 1918.
41. Lerman, J., Clark, R. J., and Means, J. H.: The Heart in Myxedema, *Ann. Intern. Med.*, 6:1251, 1933.
42. Graettinger, J. S., Muenster, J. J., Selverston, L. A., and Campbell, J. A.: A Correlation of Clinical and Hemodynamic Studies in Patients with and without Heart Failure, *J. Clin. Invest.*, 38:1316, 1959.
43. Stewart, H. J., and Evans, W. F.: The Peripheral Blood Flow in Myxedema as Compared with that in Hyperthyroidism, *Am. Heart J.*, 23:175, 1942.
44. Golden, J. S., and Brams, W. A.: Venous Pressure in Thyroid Dysfunction, *Am. Heart J.*, 9:802, 1933–34.
45. Lang, K.: Capillary Permeability in Myxedema, *Am. J. Med. Sci.*, 208:5, 1944.
46. Martin, J., and Spathis, G. S.: Case of Myxedema with a Huge Pericardial Effusion and Cardiac Tamponade, *Br. Med. J.*, 2:83, 1965.
47. Smolar, E. N., Rubin, J. E., Avramides, A., and Carter, A. C.: Cardiac Tamponade in Primary Myxedema and Review of the Literature, *Am. J. Med. Sci.*, 272:345, 1976.
48. Silverstone, F. A.: Recurrent Heart Failure with Tamponade Due to Pericardial Effusion: Improvement following Pleural-Pericardial Fenestration, *Ann. Intern. Med.*, 42:937, 1955.
49. Pericardial Disease and Cholesterol Resorption, *JAMA*, 198:480, 1966. (Editorial.)
50. Alexander, J. S.: A Pericardial Effusion of "Gold Paint" Appearance Due to the Presence of Cholesterin, *Br. Med. J.*, 2:463, 1919.
51. Davis, P. J., and Jacobson, S.: Myxedema with Cardiac Tamponade and Pericardial Effusion of "Gold Paint" Appearance, *Arch. Intern. Med.*, 120:615, 1967.
52. Lee, J. K., and Leurs, J. A.: Myxedema with Complete AV Block and Adams-Stokes Disease Abolished with Thyroid Medication, *Br. Heart J.*, 24:253, 1962.
53. Syed, A. A.: Congenital Heart Block and Hypothyroidism, *Arch. Dis. Child.*, 53:256, 1978.
54. Fredlund, B. O., and Olsson, S. B.: Long QT Interval and Ventricular Tachycardia of "Torsade de Pointe" Type in Hypothyroidism, *Acta Med. Scand.*, 213:231, 1983.
55. Kerber, R. E., and Sherman, B.: Echocardiographic Evaluation of Pericardial Effusion in Myxedema; Evidence and Biochemical and Clinical Correlations, *Circulation*, 52:823, 1975.
56. Santos, A. D., Miller, R. P., Pathenpurakal, K. M., Wallace, W. A., Cave, W. T., and Himajora, L.: Echocardiographic Characterization of the Reversible Cardiomyopathy of Hypothyroidism, *Am. J. Med.*, 68:675, 1980.
57. Steinberg, A. D.: Myxedema and Coronary Artery Disease—A Comparative Autopsy Study, *Ann. Intern. Med.*, 68:338, 1968.
58. Finlayson, D. C., and Kaplan, J. A.: Myxedema and Open Heart Surgery: Anaesthesia and Intensive Care Unit Experience, *Can. Anaesth. Soc. J.* 29:543, 1982.
59. Blumgart, H. L., Freedberg, A. S., and Kurland, G. S.: Treatment of Incapacitated Euthyroid Cardiac Patients with Radioactive Iodine: Summary of Results in Treatment of 1070 Patients with Angina Pectoris or Congestion Failure, *JAMA*, 157:1, 1955.
60. Surks, M. I., Schadlow, A. R., and Oppenhelmer, J. H.: A New Radioimmunoassay for Plasma L-Triiodothyronine: Measurements in Thyroid Disease and in Patients Maintained on Hormonal Replacement, *J. Clin. Invest.*, 51:3104, 1972.
61. Hoffman, D. P., Surks, M. I., Oppenhelmer, J. H., and Weitzman, E. D.: Response to Thyrotropin Releasing Hormone: An Objective Criterion for the Adequacy of Thyrotropin Suppression Therapy, *J. Clin. Endocrinol.*, 44:892, 1977.
62. Bratkovich, I. E., Mashiter, K., Joplin, G. F., and Cassar, J.: Serum T_4, T_3, and TSH Levels in Primary Hypothyroidism during Replacement Therapy with Thyroxine, *Metabolism*, 32:745, 1983.
63. Braverman, L. E., Vagenakis, A. G., Downs, P., Foster, A. E., Sterning, K., and Ingbar, S. H.: Effects of Replacement Doses of Sodium *l*-Thyroxine on the Peripheral Metabolism of Thyroxine and Triiodothyronine in Man, *J. Clin. Invest.*, 52:1010, 1973.
64. Levine, H. D.: Compromise Therapy in the Patient with Angina Pectoris and Hypothyroidism: A Clinical Assessment, *Am. J. Med.*, 69:411, 1980.
65. Paine, T. D., Rogers, W. J., Baxley, W. A., and Russell,

R. D.: Coronary Arterial Surgery in Patients with Incapacitating Angina Pectoris and Myxedema, *Am. J. Cardiol.*, 40:226, 1977.

66. Christy, J. H., and Clements, S. D., Jr.: The Heart and Endocrine Disease, in J. W. Hurst, (ed.), "The Heart," 5th ed., McGraw-Hill Book Company, New York, 1982, p. 1560.
67. Marie, P.: Sur Deux Cas d'Acromegalie; Hypertrophie Singulière non Congénitale des Extremités Supérieures, Inferieures et Céphalique, *Rev. Med. Paris*, 6:297, 1886.
68. Huchard, H.: Anatomie Pathologique, Lesions et Trombles Cardiovasculaires de l'Acromegalie, *J. Praticiens*, 9:249, 1895.
69. Fournier, J. B. C.: Acromegalie et Trombles Cardiovasculares," thesis, Paris, 1896, no. 3.
70. Lie, J. T., and Grossman, S. J.: Pathology of the Heart in Acromegaly: Anatomic Findings in 27 Atrophied Patients, *Ann. Heart J.*, 100:41, 1980.
71. McGuffin, W. L., Sherinan, B. M., Roth, J., Gorden, P., Kahn, R., Roberts, W. C., and Frommer, P. L.: Acromegaly and Cardiovascular Disorders: A Prospective Study. *Ann. Intern. Med.*, 81:11, 1974.
72. Balzer, R., and McCullagh, E. P.: Hypertension in Acromegaly, *Am. J. Med. Sci.*, 237:449, 1959.
73. Cain, J. P., Williams, G. P., and Pluky, R. G.: Plasma Renin Activity and Altosterone Secretion in Patients with Acromegaly, *J. Clin. Endocrinol. Metab.*, 34:73, 1972.
74. Aloia, J. F., Roginsky, M. S., and Field, R. A.: Absence of Hyperlipidemia in Acromegaly, *J. Clin. Endocrinol. Metab.*, 35:92, 1972.
75. Kellgren, J. H., Ball, J., and Tuthen, G. K.: The Articular and Other Limb Changes in Acromegaly, *Q. J. Med.*, 21:405, 1952.
76. Pepine, C. J., and Aloia, J.: Heart Muscle Disease in Acromegaly, *Am. J. Med.*, 48:530, 1970.
77. Smallridge, R. C., Rajfer, S., Davra, J., and Schaaj, M.: Acromegaly and the Heart, an Echocardiographic Study, *Am. J. Med.*, 66:22, 1979.
78. Savage, D. D., Henry, W. L., Eastman, R. L., Bour, J. S., and Gorden, P.: Echocardiographic Assessment of Cardiac Anatomy and Function in Acromegalic Patients, *Am. J. Med.*, 67:823, 1979.
79. Kaufman, D. W., Shapiro, S., Slone, D., Rosenberg, L., Meittinen, O. S., Stolley, P. D., Knapp, R. C., Leavitt, T., Jr., Watring, W. G., Rosenschein, N. B., Lewitt, J. L., Jr., Schottenfield, D., and Engle, R. L., Jr.: Decreased Risks of Endometrial Cancer among Contraceptive Users, *N. Engl. J. Med.*, 303:1045, 1980.
80. Johansson, S., Vedin, A., and Wilhelmsson, C.: Myocardial Infarction in Women, *Epidemiol. Rev.*, 5:67, 1983.
81. Rosenfield, A.: The Pill: An Evaluation of Recent Studies, *Johns Hopkins Med. J.*, 150:177, 1982.
82. Wallace, R. B., Hoover, J., Barrett-Connor, E., Rigkind, B. M., Hunninghake, D. B., Macuenthon, A., and Heiss, G.: Altered Plasma Lipid and Lipoprotein Levels Associated with Oral Contraceptive and Estrogen Use, *Lancet*, 2:111, 1979.
83. Antunes, C. M. F., Stonny, P. D., Rosenshein, N. B., Davies, J. L., Tonascia, J. A., Brown, C., Burnett, L., Ruthedge, A., Pokempner, M., and Garcia, R.: Endometrial Cancer and Estrogen Use: Report of a Large Case Control Study, *N. Engl. J. Med.*, 300:9, 1979.
84. Sartwell, P. E., and Stolley, P. D.: Oral Contraception and Vascular Disease, *Epidemiol. Rev.*, 4:95, 1982.
85. Stadel, B. V.: Oral Contraceptives and Cardiovascular Disease, *N. Engl. J. Med.*, 305:612 (part 1) and 672 (part 2), 1981.
86. Vessey, M. P., and Mann, J. I.: Female Sex Hormones and Thrombosis: Epidemiological Aspects, *Br. Med. Bull.*, 34:157, 1978.
87. Kaplan, N. M.: Cardiovascular Complications of Oral Contraceptions, *Ann. Rev. Med.*, 29:31, 1978.
88. Heath, H., III: Progress Against Osteoporosis, *Ann. Intern. Med.*, 98:1011, 1983.
89. Lindsay R., Hart, D. M., Aitken, J. M., MacDonald, E. B., Anderson, J. G., and Clark, A. C.: Long-Term Prevention of Postmenopausal Osteoporosis by Estrogen, *Lancet*, 1:1038, 1976.
90. Heaney, R. P.: In L. V. Avioli (ed.), "The Osteoporotic Syndrome," Grune & Stratton, New York, 1983. p. 123.
91. Joslin, E. P., Root, H. F., White, P., and Marble, A.: "The Treatment of Diabetes Mellitus," 10th ed. Lea & Febiger, Philadelphia, 1959, p. 188.
92. National Diabetes Data Group: Classification and Diagnosis of Diabetes Mellitus and Other Categories of Glucose Intolerance, Appendix II, *Diabetes*, 28:64, 1979.
93. Sundkvist, G.: Autonomic Nervous Function in Asymptomatic Diabetic Patients with Signs of Peripheral Neuropathy, *Diabetes Care*, 4:529, 1981.
94. Ewing, D. J., Campbell, I. W., Clarke, B. F., Edinburgh, M. B.: Assessment of Cardiovascular Effects in Diabetic Autonomic Neuropathy and Prognostic Implications, *Ann. Intern. Med.*, 92:308, 1980.
95. Smith, S. E., Smith, S. A., and Brown, P. M.: Cardiac Autonomic Dysfunction in Patients with Diabetic Retinopathy, *Diabetologia*, 21:525,1981.
96. Weinrauch, L., D'Elia, J. A., Healy, R. W., Gleason, R. E., Christlieb, A. R., and Leland, O. S., Jr.: Asymptomatic Coronary Artery Disease: Angiographic Assessment of Diabetics Evaluated for Renal Transplantation, *Circulation*, 58:1184, 1978.
97. Mackay, J. D., Page, M. McB., Cambridge, J., and Watkins, P. J.: Diabetic Autonomic Neuropathy, The Diagnostic Value of Heart Rate Monitoring, *Diabetologia*, 18:441, 1980.
98. Rosenbloom, A. L., Silverstien, J. H., Riley, W. J., and Maclaren, N. K.: Limited Joint Mobility in Childhood Diabetes: Family Studies, *Diabetes Care*, 6:370, 1983.
99. Zoneraich, S., (ed.): "Diabetes and the Heart," Charles C Thomas, Publisher, Springfield, Ill., 1978, p. 207.
100. Giampietro, O., Santoro, G., Rossi, M., Luche, A. D., Giusti, C., and Navalesi, R.: Vectocardiographic "Bites" as Possible Early Findings of Cardiac Involvement in Diabetic Patients without Clinical Evidence of Heart Disease, *Angiology—J. Vasc. Dis.*, 33:668, 1982.
101. Brown, M. J., and Asbury, A. K.: Diabetic Neuropathy, *Ann. Neurol.*, 15:2, 1984.
102. Chipps, D. R., Kraegen, E. W., Zelenka, G. S., McNamara, M. E., and Chisholm, D. J.: Cardiac Beat to Beat Variation: Age Related Changes in the Normal Population and Abnormalities in Diabetics, *Aust. N. Z. J. Med.*, 11:614, 1981.
103. Hilstead, J.: Pathophysiology in Diabetic Autonomic Neuropathy: Cardiovascular, Hormonal, and Metabolic Studies, *Diabetes*, 31:730, 1982.
104. Page, M. McB., and Watkins, P. J.: Provocation of Postural Hypotension by Insulin in Diabetic Autonomic Neuropathy, *Diabetes*, 25:90, 1976.
105. Watt, S. J., Tooke, J. E., Perkins, C. M., and Lee, M. R.: The Treatment of Idiopathic Orthostatic Hypotension: A Combined Fludrocortisone and Flurbiprofen Regime, *Q. J. Med.*, 50:205, 1981.
106. Saudek, C. D., Boulter, P. R., Knopp, R. H., and Arky, R. A.: Sodium Retention Accompanying Insulin Treatment of Diabetes Mellitus, *Diabetes*, 23:240, 1974.
107. Gundersen, H. J. G., and Christensen, N. J.: Intravenous Insulin Causing Loss of Intravascular Water and Albumin and Increased Adrenergic Nervous Activity in Diabetics, *Diabetes*, 26:551, 1977.
108. Pirart, J.: Diabetes Mellitus and Its Degenerative Complications: A Prospective Study of 4,400 Patients Observed between 1947 and 1973, *Diabetes Care*, 1:168, 1978.
109. Judzewitsch, R. G., Jaspan, J. B., Polonsky, K. S., et al.: Aldose Reductase Inhibition Improves Nerve Conduction Velocity in Diabetic Patients, *N. Engl. J. Med.*, 308:119, 1983.
110. Faerman, I., Faccio, E., Milei, J., Nunez, R., Jadzinsky, M., Fox, D., and Rapaport, M.: Autonomic Neuropathy and Painless Myocardial Infarction in Diabetic Patients, *Diabetes*, 26:1147, 1977.
111. Kannel, W. B., and McGhee, D. L.: Diabetes and Cardiovascular Risk Factors: The Framingham Study, *Circulation*, 59(1):8, 1979.
112. Ward, J. W.: The Diabetic Leg, *Diabetologia*, 22:141, 1982.

113. Deanfield, J. E., Daggett, P. R., and Harrison, M. J. G.: The Role of Autonomic Neuropathy in Diabetic Foot Ulceration, *J. Neurol. Sci.*, 47:203, 1980.
114. Edmonds, M. E., Archer, A. G., and Watkins, P. J.: Ephedrine: A New Treatment for Diabetic Neuropathic Oedema, *Lancet*, 1:548, 1983.
115. Factor, S. M., Okun, E. M., and Minase, T.: Capillary Microaneurysms in the Human Diabetic Heart, *N. Engl. J. Med.*, 320:384, 1980.
116. Fischer, V. W., Barner, H. B., and LaRose, L. S.: Quadriceps and Myocardial Capillary Basal Laminae, Their Comparison in Diabetic Patients, *Arch. Pathol. Lab. Med.*, 106:336, 1982.
117. Shapiro, L. M.: Echocardiographic Features of Impaired Ventricular Function in Diabetes Mellitus, *Br. Heart J.*, 47:439, 1982.
118. Lababidi, Z. A., and Goldstein, D. E.: High Prevalence of Echocardiographic Abnormalities in Diabetic Youths, *Diabetes Care*, 6:18, 1983.
119. Valk, T. W., Shapiro, B., Frager, M. S., Kalff, V., Gross, M. D., Arastu, M., Savage, P. J., and Thrall, J. H.: Cardiac Function in Uncomplicated Insulin-Dependent Diabetes Mellitus: Alterations Reversed by Improved Glucose Control, *Nucl. Med. Communications*, 3:238, 1982.
120. Fein, F. S.: Heart Disease in Diabetes, *Cardiovasc. Rev. Rep.*, 3(6):877, 1982.
121. Uusitupa, M., Siitonen, O., Aro, A., Korhonen, T., and Pyorala, K.: Effect of Correction of Hyperglycemia on Left Ventricular Function in Non-Insulin-Dependent (Type 2) Diabetics, *Acta Med. Scand.*, 213:363, 1983.
122. Cellina, G., Lo Cicero, G., Brina, A., and Zanchetti, A.: Reversible Alteration of Myocardial Function in Gestational Diabetes, *Eur. Heart J.*, 4:59, 1983.
123. Kannel, W. B., Hjortland, M., and Costelli, W. P.: Role of Diabetes in Congestive Heart Failure: The Framingham Study, *Am. J. Cardiol.*, 34:29, 1974.
124. Ganguly, P. K., Pierce, G. N., Dhalla, K. S., and Dhalla, N. S.: "Defective Sarcoplasmic Reticular Calcium Transport in Diabetic Cardiomyopathy," The American Physiology Society, New York, 1983, E528.
125. Schaible, T. F., Malhotra, A., Bauman, W. A., and Scheuer, J.: Left Ventricular Function after Chronic Insulin Treatment in Diabetic and Normal Rats, *J. Mol. Cell. Cardiol.*, 15:445, 1983.
126. Bale, C. S., and Entmacher, P. S.: Estimated Life Expectancy of Diabetics, *Diabetes*, 26:434, 1977.
127. Heyden, S., Heiss, G., Bartel, A. G., and Hames, C. G.: Sex Differences in Coronary Mortality among Diabetics in Evans County, Georgia, *Chron. Dis.*, 33:265, 1980.
128. Wingard, D. L., Barrett-Conner, E., Criqui, M. H., and Suarez, L.: Clustering of Heart Disease Risk Factors in Diabetic Compared to Nondiabetic Adults, *Am. J. Epidemiol.*, 117:19, 1983.
129. Vigorita, V. J., Moore, G. W., and Hutchins, G. M.: Absence of Correlation between Coronary Arterial Atherosclerosis and Severity or Duration of Diabetes Mellitus of Adult Onset, *Am. J. Cardiol.*, 46:535, 1980.
130. Jarrett, R. L.: Type 2 (Non-Insulin-Dependent) Diabetes Mellitus and Coronary Heart Disease—Chicken, Egg or Neither?, *Diabetologia*, 26:99, 1984.
131. Krolewski, A. S., Czyzyk, A., Kopczynski, J., and Rywik, S.: Prevalence of Diabetes Mellitus, Coronary Heart Disease and Hypertension in the Families of Insulin Dependent and Insulin Independent Diabetics, *Diabetologia*, 21:520, 1981.
132. Pietri, A., Dunn, F. L., and Raskin, P.: The Effect of Improved Diabetic Control on Plasma Lipid and Lipoprotein Levels: A Comparison of Conventional Therapy and Continuous Subcutaneous Insulin Infusion, *Diabetes*, 29:1001, 1980.
133. Camerini-Davalos, R. A., Velasco, C., Glasser, M., and Bloodworth, J. M. B., Jr.: Drug-Induced Reversal of Early Diabetic Microangiopathy, *N. Engl. J. Med.*, 309:1551, 1983.
134. DeFronzo, R. A.: The Effect of Insulin on Renal Sodium Metabolism, *Diabetologia*, 21:165, 1981.
135. Ducimetiere, P., Exchwege, E., Papoz, L., Richard, J. L., Claude, J. R., and Rosselin, G.: Relationship of Plasma Insulin Levels to the Incidence of Myocardial Infarction and Coronary Heart Disease Mortality in a Middle-aged Population, *Diabetologia*, 19:205, 1980.
136. The University Group Diabetes Program: Effects of Hypoglycemic Agents on Vascular Complications in Patients with Adult-Onset Diabetes: VIII. Evaluation of Insulin Therapy: Final Report, *Diabetes*, 31(suppl. 5):1, 1982.
137. Wu, C. F., Haider, B., Ahmed, S. S., Oldewurtel, H. A., Lyons, M. M., and Regan, T. J.: The Effects of Tolbutamide on the Myocardium in Experimental Diabetes, *Circulation*, 55:200, 1977.
138. Mintz, D. H., Skyler, J. S., and Chez, R. A.: Diabetes Mellitus and Pregnancy, *Diabetes Care*, 1:49, 1978.
139. Gutgesell, H. P., Speer, M. E., and Rosenberg, H. S.: Characterization of the Cardiomyopathy in Infants of Diabetic Mothers, *Circulation*, 61:441, 1980.
140. Halliday, H. L.: Hypertrophic Cardiomyopathy in Infants of Poorly-Controlled Diabetic Mothers, *Arch. Dis. Child.*, 56:258, 1981.
141. Teuscher, A., Bossi, E., Imhof, P., Erb, E., Stocker, F. P., and Weber, J. W.: Effect of Propranolol on Fetal Tachycardia in Diabetic Pregnancy, *Am. J. Cardiol.*, 42:304, 1978.
142. Fuller, P. J., Colman, P. G., Harper, R. W., and Stockigt, J. R.: Transient Anterior Electrocardiographic Changes Simulating Acute Anterior Myocardial Infarction in Diabetic Ketoacidosis, *Diabetes Care*, 5:118, 1982.
143. Bradley, R. F., and Schonfeld, A.: Diminished Pain in Diabetic Patients with Acute Myocardial Infarction, *Geriatrics*, 17:322, 1962.
144. Gwilt, D. J., Nattrass, M., and Pentecost, B. L.: Use of Low-Dose Insulin Infusions in Diabetics after Myocardial Infarction, *Br. Med. J.*, 285:1402, 1982.
145. Libby, P., Maroko, P. R., and Braunwald, E.: The Effect of Hypoglycemia on Myocardial Ischemic Injury during Acute Experimental Coronary Artery Occlusion, *Circulation*, 51:621, 1975.
146. Rogers, W. J., Segall, P. H., McDaniel, H. G., Mantle, J. A., Russell, R. O., and Rackley, C. E.: Prospective Randomized Trial of Glucose-Insulin-Potassium in Acute Myocardial Infarction: Effects on Myocardial Hemodynamics, Substrates and Rhythm, *Am. J. Cardiol.*, 43:801, 1979.
147. Whitlow, P. L., Rogers, W. J., Smith, L. R., McDaniel, H. G., Papapietro, S. E., Mantle, J. A., Logic, J. R., Russell, R. O., and Rackley, C. E.: Enhancement of Left Ventricular Function by Glucose-Insulin-Potassium Infusion in Acute Myocardial Infarction, *Am. J. Cardiol.*, 49:811, 1982.
148. Haider, W., Coraim, F., Duma, L., et al.: Effect of Insulin on Cardiac Output after Open Heart Surgery (Wirksamkeit Hoher Insulindosen Auf Die Pumplestung Des Herzens Nach Offenen Herzoperationer), *Anaethesist (Berl.)*, 30:305, 1981.
149. Smith, J. W.: Therapy of Heart Disease in the Patient with Diabetes Mellitus, in G. A. Eur and R. Bressler (eds), "Cardiovascular Drugs and the Management of Heart Disease," p. 719, Raven Press, New York, 1982.
150. Dodek, A., Kassebaum, D. G., and Bristow, J. D.: Pulmonary Edema in Coronary Artery Disease without Cardiomegaly, *N. Engl. J. Med.*, 286:1347, 1972.
151. Kahn, O., Wagner, W., and Bersman, A. N.: Mortality of Diabetic Patients Treated Surgically for Lower Limb Infection and/or Gangrene, *Diabetes*, 23:287, 1974.
152. LoGerfo, F. W., Corgon, J. D., and Mannick, J. A.: Improved Results with Femoropopliteal Vein Grafts for Limb Salvage, *Arch. Surg.*, 112:567, 1977.
153. Verska, J. J., and Walker, W. J.: Aortocoronary Bypass in the Diabetic Patient, *Am. J. Cardiol.*, 35:774, 1975.
154. Delcher, H. K.: Surgery in the Patient with Endocrine Disorders, in M. F. Lubin, H. K. Walker, and R. B. Smith (eds.), "Medical Management of the Surgical Patient," Butterworth Publishers, Woburn, Mass., 1982, p. 461.
155. George, K., Alberti, M. M., Gill, G. V., and Elliott, M. J.: Insulin Delivery during Surgery in the Diabetic Patient, *Diabetes Care*, 5:65, 1982.

156. Artis, W. M., Fountain, J. A., Delcher, H. K., and Jones, H. E.: A Mechanism of Susceptibility to Mucormycosis in Diabetic Ketoacidosis: Transferrin and Iron Availability, *Diabetes,* 31:1109, 1982.
157. Bagdale, J. D., Stewart, M., and Walters, E.: Impaired Granulocyte Adherence: A Reversible Defect in Host Defense in Patients with Poorly Controlled Diabetes, *Diabetes,* 27:677, 1978.
158. Kennedy, L., and Baynes, J. W.: Non-enzymatic Glucosylation and the Chronic Complications of Diabetes: An Overview, *Diabetologia,* 26:93, 1984.
159. Rubinstein, A., Pierce, C. E., and Bloomgarden, Z.: Rapid Healing of Diabetic Foot Ulcers with Continuous Subcutaneous Insulin Infusion, *Am. J. Med.,* 75:161, 1983.
160. Cahill, G. F., Jr., and McDevitt, H. O.: Insulin-Dependent Diabetes Mellitus: The Initial Lesson, *N. Engl. J. Med.,* 304:1454, 1981.
161. Wolf, E., Spencer, K. M., and Cudworth, A. G.: The Genetic Susceptibility of Type 1 (Insulin-Dependent) Diabetes: Analysis of the HLA-DR Association, *Diabetologia,* 24:224, 1983.
162. Rubinstein, P., Fedun, W. B., Witt, M. E., Cooper, L. Z., and Ginsberg-Fellner, F.: The HLA System in Congenital Rubella Patients with and without Diabetes, *Diabetes,* 31:1088, 1982.
163. Srikanta, S., Ganda, O. P., Eisenbarth, G. S., and Soeldner, J. S.: Islet-Cell Antibodies and Beta-Cell Function in Monozygotic Triplets and Twins Initially Discordant for Type I Diabetes Mellitus, *N. Engl. J. Med.,* 308:322, 1983.
164. Ganda, O. P., Srikanta, S., Brink, S. J., et al.: Differential Sensitivity to B-Cell Secretagogues in "Early," Type 1 Diabetes Mellitus, *Diabetes,* 33:516, 1984.
165. Schmidt, M. I., Hadji-Georgopoulos, A., Rendell, M., Margolis, S., and Kowarski, A.: The Dawn Phenomenon, an Early Morning Glucose Rise: Implications for Diabetic Intraday Blood Glucose Variation, *Diabetes Care,* 4:579, 1981.
166. Mirouze, J.: Insulin Treatment: A Non-Stop Revolution, *Diabetologia,* 25:209, 1983.
167. Nuttall, F. Q.: Diet and the Diabetic Patient, *Diabetes Care,* 6:197, 1983.
168. West, K. M.: "Epidemiology of Diabetes and Its Vascular Lesions," Elsevier-North Holland, New York, 1978.
169. Zimmet, P.: Type 2 (Non-Insulin-Dependent) Diabetes—An Epidemiological Overview, *Diabetologia,* 22:399, 1982.
170. Genuth, S. M.: Plasma Insulin and Glucose Profiles in Normal, Obese, and Diabetic Persons, *Ann. Intern. Med.,* 79:812, 1973.
171. Logothetopoulos, J.: Islet Cell Regeneration and Neogenesis, in N. Freinkel and D. F. Steiner, (eds.), "Handbook of Physiology," vol. 1, "Endocrinology," Waverly Press, Baltimore, 1972, p. 67.
172. UK Prospective Study of Therapies of Maturity-Onset Diabetes: I. Effect of Diet, Sulphonylurea, Insulin or Biguanide Therapy on Fasting Plasma Glucose and Body Weight over One Year: Multi-centre Study, *Diabetologia,* 24:404, 1983.

73

The Heart and Collagen Vascular Disease

Bernadine Healy Bulkley, M.D.   J. O'Neal Humphries, M.D.

The collagen vascular diseases represent a subset of the arthritides and rheumatic disorders. These collagen vascular diseases are systemic in nature, commonly linked by a diffuse abnormality of vasculature, and characterized by diffuse idiopathic, inflammatory lesions. Notably affected are joints, muscles, and connective tissue linings such as pleura and pericardium, and their inflammation accounts for the major symptoms. Serious morbidity and mortality, however, are most often linked to involvement of the kidneys, brain, and the heart. Specific collagen vascular–type diseases which may have major cardiac involvement include systemic lupus erythematosus, polyarteritis nodosa, rheumatoid arthritis, ankylosing spondylitis, and progressive systemic sclerosis (Table 73-1). The etiology of these assorted disorders remains uncertain, however, and as their pathogenesis is unveiled, it is likely that different causes may become apparent, making their association under the umbrella of "collagen vascular disease" less appropriate.

Systemic Lupus Erythematosus

Systemic lupus erythematosus (SLE) is one of the more common of the collagen vascular diseases; it tends to affect women more than men, and although all ages are susceptible, it occurs most frequently in the second and third decades of life. A genetic predisposition to SLE has been suggested. A disease of unknown etiology, SLE appears to be a form of hypersensitivity or autoimmune disorder. The sterile inflammatory process of SLE involves multiple organ systems and in particular skin, joints, kidneys, brain, heart, and virtually all serous membranes. Systemic lupus erythematosus may present clinically in a variety of forms reflecting the target organ involved. Fevers, arthritis and arthralgias, skin rashes, and pleuritis are among the most common early signs of this condition. The immunologic abnormalities of SLE, which have now been well-characterized, enable the underlying systemic disorder to be recognized despite the multiplicity and fre-

TABLE 73-1 Primary Cardiac Manifestations of the Collagen Vascular Diseases*

Disease	Pericardium	Myocardium	Endocardium (Valves)	Coronary Arteries
Systemic lupus erythematosis	++	+	++	+/−
Progressive systemic sclerosis	+	++	0	++
Polyarteritis nodosa	+/−	+	0	++
Ankylosing spondylitis	0	+/−	++	0
Rheumatoid arthritis	++	+	+	0

*++ = major site of involvement; + = may be involved, but less frequently; +/− = rarely involved; 0 = not involved.

quent complexity of clinical presentation. Elevated serum gamma globulin concentrations and cryoproteins are common findings. The majority of patients have at some point in the course of their illness positive lupus erythematosus (LE) cell preparations. Less specific are the antinuclear and anticytoplasmic antibodies and rheumatoid factor which are frequently identified. Serum complement is decreased in the majority of patients with SLE, and insofar as serum complement is usually normal or elevated in other collagen vascular–type disorders, such as rheumatoid arthritis, polyarteritis nodosa, scleroderma, and disseminated infections, this serologic test may be useful in diagnosis of SLE.[1,2]

Lupus may run an acute, fulminating course, but most often is characterized by a chronic course marked with exacerbations and remissions, and the 10-year survival rate is reported in excess of 80 percent. When patients die of SLE, it is most often in the setting of acute renal failure, central nervous system disease, or associated infection. Primary cardiac involvement is less commonly a cause of significant morbidity or death.

Primary Cardiac Involvement in SLE

Pericarditis of SLE

Systemic lupus erythematosus may cause a pancarditis with abnormalities of pericardium, endocardium, myocardium, and the coronary arteries. Pericardial involvement is the most frequent of these, as observed clinically and also at autopsy.[3,4] Clinical studies have described pericardial effusions at some point in the clinical course of over half of patients with active SLE, and an "idiopathic" benign pericarditis may antecede the other clinical signs of lupus in up to 4 percent of patients.[3] In the majority of SLE patients, the pericardial involvement is clinically silent, and if manifest, runs a benign course. On rare occasion lupus pericarditis may lead to pericardial constriction[3,5] and acute cardiac tamponade.[6] Serological studies of pericardial fluid may be useful in diagnosis of lupus pericardial effusions, although in most instances the size of the pericardial effusion is not sufficiently large to allow aspiration.

A diffuse fibrofibrinous pericarditis is most typically associated with SLE. The pericardial fluid contains some mononuclear white cells, and occasionally LE cells. In patients with long-standing lupus who have been successfully treated with anti-inflammatory agents, pericarditis appears to occur with the same frequency, but at autopsy, the lesion is less extensive and more apt to be a healed fibrous, as opposed to a more active fibrinous, pericarditis.[4] Lupus erythematosus patients with pericarditis, particularly those who are debilitated by their systemic disease and renal failure and additionally are immunosuppressed, are at greater risk for purulent pericarditis.[7] This last secondary complication of lupus erythematosus pericarditis is likely the most malignant and life-threatening consequence of the pericardial lesion.

Endocarditis of SLE

The cardiovascular lesion of systemic lupus erythematosus that has received the most attention is the "atypical veruccous endocarditis" first described by Libman and Sacks in 1924,[8] long before lupus was recognized as a systemic disease. The lesions, as they were first described and subsequently attributed to systemic lupus erythematosus,[9] are fibrofibrinous, sterile vegetations which may develop on both surfaces of any of the four cardiac valves, but with a preponderance for the left-sided valves, particularly the undersurface of the mitral valve (Fig. 73-1). These "verrucae" are similar to those of nonbacterial thrombotic endocarditis (NBTE) or "marantic" endocarditis, the valve lesion which may occur in patients with debilitating illness or malignancies, particularly of the stomach or pancreas. The Libman-Sacks lesions may differ from marantic endocarditis in that focal necrosis of valve leaflets, and mononuclear infiltrates may also occur. At times, hematoxylin bodies, which are believed to be a histological counterpart to the LE cells, may be identified within the lesions. Although the endocarditis of SLE is usually unassociated with valve dysfunction and is most often clinically silent, it may be observed at autopsy in up to 40 percent of patients with SLE. The end stage, or healed form, of the verrucous endocarditis of SLE is a fibrous plaque. In some instances if the thrombotic lesions are extensive enough, their healing may be accompanied by focal scarring and deformity of the underlying valve tissue. It is likely that this healed, end-stage form of SLE endocarditis is most apt to lead to val-

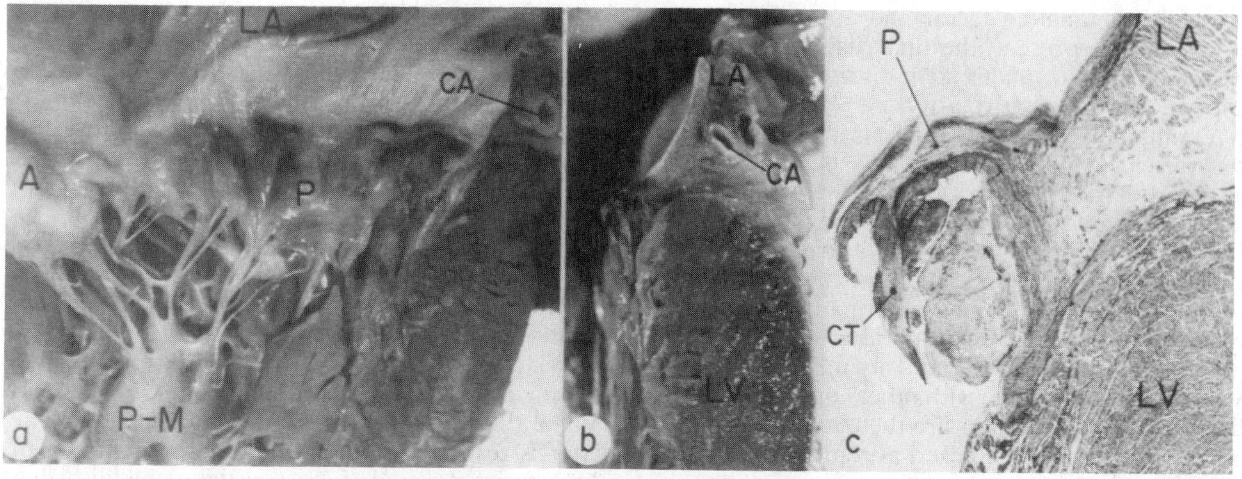

FIGURE 73-1 Systemic lupus erythematosus. Shown here is an example of the endocarditis that may occur in systemic lupus erythematosus. The left atrium (LA) and left ventricle (LV) are open. Fibrofibrinous "verrucae" which are present on the undersurface of the posterior leaflet (P) of the mitral valve, as shown here, not surprisingly are often clinically silent. A = anterior leaflet of mitral valve; CA = left circumflex coronary artery; P-M = papillary muscle. H&E, ×8. *(From B. H. Bulkley and W. C. Roberts, The Heart in Systemic Lupus Erythematosus and the Changes Induced in It by Corticosteroid Therapy, Am. J. Med., 58:243, 1975. Reproduced with permission from the publisher and author.)*

vular dysfunction, and in particular mitral or aortic insufficiency.[10–12] As with the pericardial disease, the verrucous endocardial lesions of SLE pose an increased risk of infective endocarditis, particularly in the immunosuppressed patient.

Myocarditis
Myocarditis is an uncommon cardiac manifestation of systemic lupus erythematosus. Focal interstitial and perivascular mononuclear cell infiltrates associated with small areas of cell necrosis and replacement fibrosis may be observed at autopsy. Although a flagrant myocarditis with ventricular arrhythmias, heart block, and heart failure may occur, this is distinctly uncommon.

Coronary Artery Disease
Coronary artery involvement may occur in systemic lupus erythematosus, but it is an infrequent cardiac manifestation of SLE. Abnormalities of the small intramural vessels of the heart include focal fibrinoid necrosis and thromboembolic occlusion, but are rarely associated with myocardial necrosis or fibrosis. Arteritis of the sinus node artery in association with scarring of both sinus and atrioventricular nodes has been reported[13] and may account for some of the rhythm and conduction disturbances seen in these patients.

Secondary Effects of Systemic Lupus Erythematosus upon the Heart

Many, if not most, of the clinically significant cardiac problems occurring in patients with SLE are secondary occurrences. Systemic hypertension, which is common in patients with SLE, particularly those with renal disease and long-standing steroid therapy, is the major cause of cardiac enlargement and heart failure. Uremic pericarditis may occur in those with severe renal failure and be difficult to distinguish clinically from lupus erythematosus pericarditis. There is some evidence that coronary atherosclerosis may be more prevalent in the relatively young patient population with systemic lupus erythematosus who have been subject to the added risk factors of hypertension, renal failure, and longstanding corticosteroid therapy.[4]

Therapy

Therapy of cardiovascular lupus erythematosus is the therapy of the underlying disease, namely corticosteroids with or without added cytotoxic agents such as azathioprine and cyclophosphamide. In addition, systemic hypertension, congestive heart failure, and arrhythmias should be treated with standard therapeutic measures. Rarely pericardial effusions have mandated pericardiocentesis, and lupus erythematosus valvulitis has required valve replacement.[11,12]

Polyarteritis Nodosa

Polyarteritis nodosa is another disease entity of unknown cause that falls within the "collagen vascular" spectrum. It is characterized by segmental necrotizing inflammation of the medium- to small-sized arteries throughout the body, resulting in disease and dysfunction of multiple organ systems. Commonly involved by polyarteritis are the skin, kidneys, gastrointestinal tract, spleen and lymph nodes, central nervous and musculoskeletal systems, and the heart. Although the sedimentation rate and serum gamma globulins may be elevated in polyarteritis, and occasionally rheumatoid factor and antinuclear antibodies may be present, the final diagnosis rests on the combination of multisystem disease clinically and biopsy evidence of active arteritis.[14,15]

As inflammatory necrotizing arteritis may occur in a variety of disorders generally believed to fall outside the disease category of polyarteritis nodosa, other causes and types of arteritis are generally excluded before the diagnosis of polyarteritis nodosa is made. Specifically excluded and classed as separate entities are granulomatous or giant cell arteritis, hypersensitivity angiitis, temporal arteritis, and arteritis involving the aorta and its major branches. Also, arteritis associated with other connective tissue disorders, when the latter are the major clinical disease form, are not recognized as representing polyarteritis nodosa.[15]

Cardiac Involvement in Polyarteritis Nodosa

The heart, and specifically the coronary arteries, is a frequent target of polyarteritis nodosa. Seen most commonly is a vasculitis of the distal extramural and subepicardial coronary arteries just as they penetrate the myocardium (Fig. 73-2). The lesions are characterized by inflammatory infiltration of media and adventitia. More advanced lesions show necrosis and inflammation of the full thickness of the vessel wall including the intima, with prominent involvement of the surrounding perivascular connective tissue (Fig. 73-2). More advanced lesions are frequently associated with thrombosis and focal aneurysmal dilatation due to the vascular necrosis. The latter is responsible for the nodular appearance of the arteries deemed characteristic of this disorder.

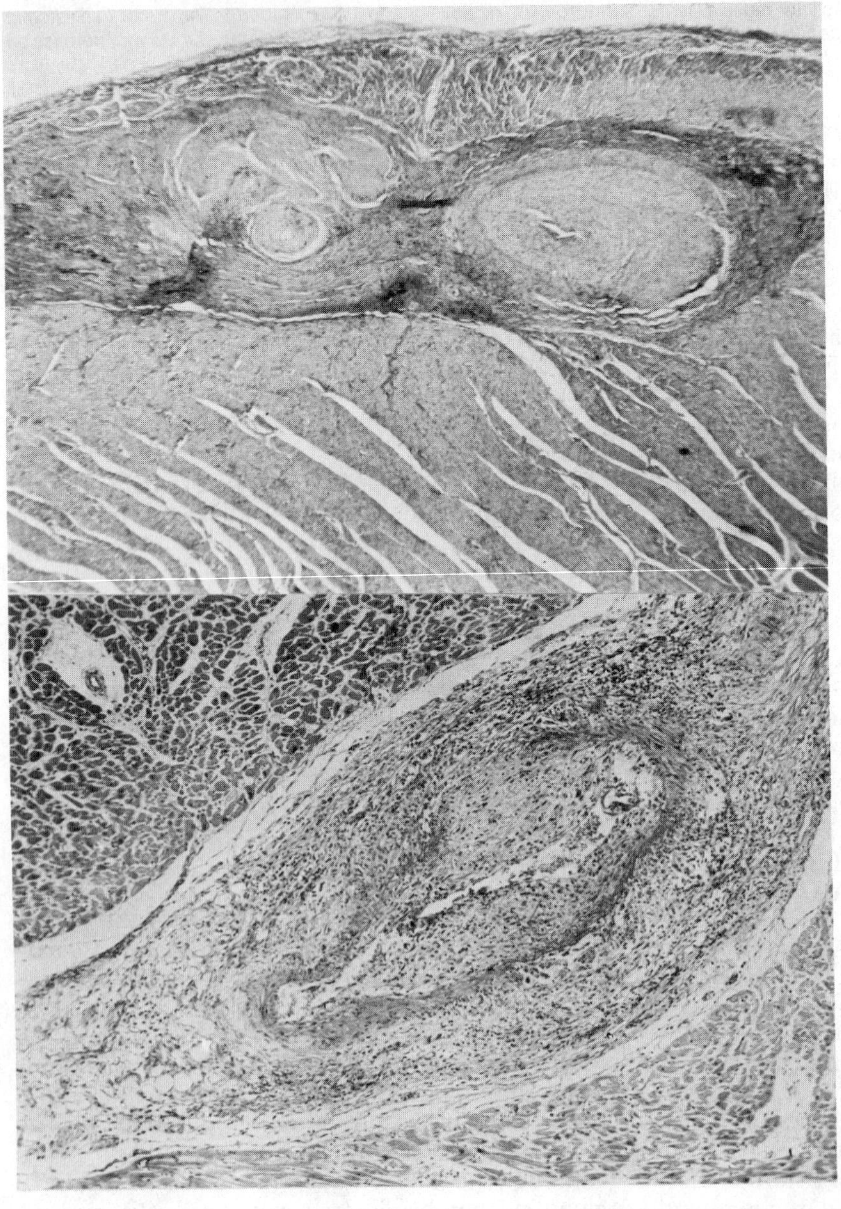

FIGURE 73-2 Polyarteritis nodosa. Shown are examples of the necrotizing vasculitis affecting the extramural (*top*) and intramural (*bottom*) coronary arteries in polyarteritis. The intramural artery shows a necrotizing arteritis with inflammation involving the full thickness of the vessel. H&E, *top*, ×7; *bottom*, ×22.

A later stage of the vasculitic process is evident as the lesions heal, first showing the formation of granulation tissue and subsequently fibrous tissue replacement of the original components of the artery. In this healing phase, intimal proliferation leading to coronary artery luminal narrowing is evident.[16,17]

The coronary arterial disease of polyarteritis nodosa not surprisingly may lead to myocardial infarction. In keeping with the predominantly distal and intramural coronary involvement, the myocardial necrosis and subsequent replacement fibrosis tend to be focal and patchy throughout the left ventricle. This is in contrast to the large areas of grossly visible, regional, subendocardial or transmural necrosis typically seen in the myocardial infarction caused by coronary atherosclerosis.

Conduction system abnormalities have been identified in the hearts of patients with polyarteritis nodosa.[18,19] James[18] has pointed out that the size and location of the sinoatrial (SA) node and atrioventricular (AV) node arteries make them prime targets for polyarteritis. The perivascular inflammation of these vessels is more apt to lead to myocardial dysfunction, as the AV and SA node tissue closely surrounds these vessels and is included in the perivascular inflammatory reaction. Atrial and ventricular conduction disturbances may be a primary manifestation of polyarteritis, despite minimal involvement of vessels elsewhere in the heart.

Other cardiac abnormalities that may be seen in patients with polyarteritis nodosa are those which are likely secondary to the underlying systemic hypertension and renal disease. Cardiomegaly and left ventricular hypertrophy most often represent secondary cardiac manifestations of this disease. Similarly, pericarditis may develop in a patient with polyarteritis, but mostly in association with renal disease.

Clinical Manifestations of Cardiac Disease in Polyarteritis

Despite the dramatic involvement of coronary arteries that may accompany polyarteritis nodosa, the most frequent cardiovascular abnormalities seen in patients with this disease are unrelated to the coronary arteries per se. Systemic hypertension occurs in approximately 90 percent of patients, and this in combination with chronic renal failure is the most likely cause of the congestive heart failure which may develop in up to 60 percent of patients with this disease.[14,15] Patients with polyarteritis nodosa may also develop acute myocardial infarction, posing the diagnostic uncertainty as to whether the myocardial injury is due to coronary arteritis with secondary thrombosis or to atherosclerosis, in a population which is typically middle-aged, male, steroid-treated, and susceptible to atherosclerotic coronary disease, as well.

Therapy

Treatment of the heart disease in polyarteritis nodosa is directed at the specific cardiac dysfunction, and corticosteroid and other anti-inflammatory agents as administered for the underlying disease.[20]

Rheumatoid Arthritis

Rheumatoid arthritis is characterized by its deforming erosion of the joints resulting from chronic synovial inflammation and proliferation. The most common of the collagen vascular diseases, it tends to affect women twice as often as men, and may run in families. Joint symptoms dominate its course, and symmetrical involvement of the hands and wrists is most common. Other joints of the upper and lower extremities and the temporomandibular and sternoclavicular joints may also be affected. More common systemic manifestations of rheumatoid arthritis include fevers, weight loss, anemia, subcutaneous rheumatoid nodules, and lymphadenopathy. Less frequently, pleuritis and a diffuse, necrotizing vasculitis may occur.

Pericardial Involvement in Rheumatoid Arthritis

Cardiac involvement is most uncommon in rheumatoid arthritis, but when it occurs, it may take a variety of forms. A diffuse, nonspecific fibrofibrinous pericarditis has been described in roughly 30 percent of patients with rheumatoid arthritis.[21] The pericarditis may be clinically silent in the majority of these patients, overshadowed by pleuritis or joint pain. Its clinical course tends to be benign but as in most instances of pericardial inflammation, sizable effusions may require pericardiocentesis, and pericardial constriction may necessitate pericardiectomy.[22] Chronic, symptomatic pericarditis in and of itself may require a course of corticosteroid therapy.

Myocardial and Endocardial Involvement in Rheumatoid Arthritis

Rarely rheumatoid nodules may focally infiltrate the heart, including the myocardium and the four cardiac valves (Fig. 73-3).[23] These nodules may lead to no symptoms, but if extensive enough, or strategically located, they may produce cardiac compromise. Rheumatoid nodules developing within the valve leaflets may result in mild valvular insufficiency; if the nodule becomes necrotic, perforation of the leaflet may occur and lead to severe valvular insufficiency.[24] The incidence of such valvular infiltration has been estimated at 1 to 2 percent from autopsy studies. Although distinctly uncommon, arrhythmias and conduction disturbances and congestive heart failure may also result from rheumatoid myocarditis.

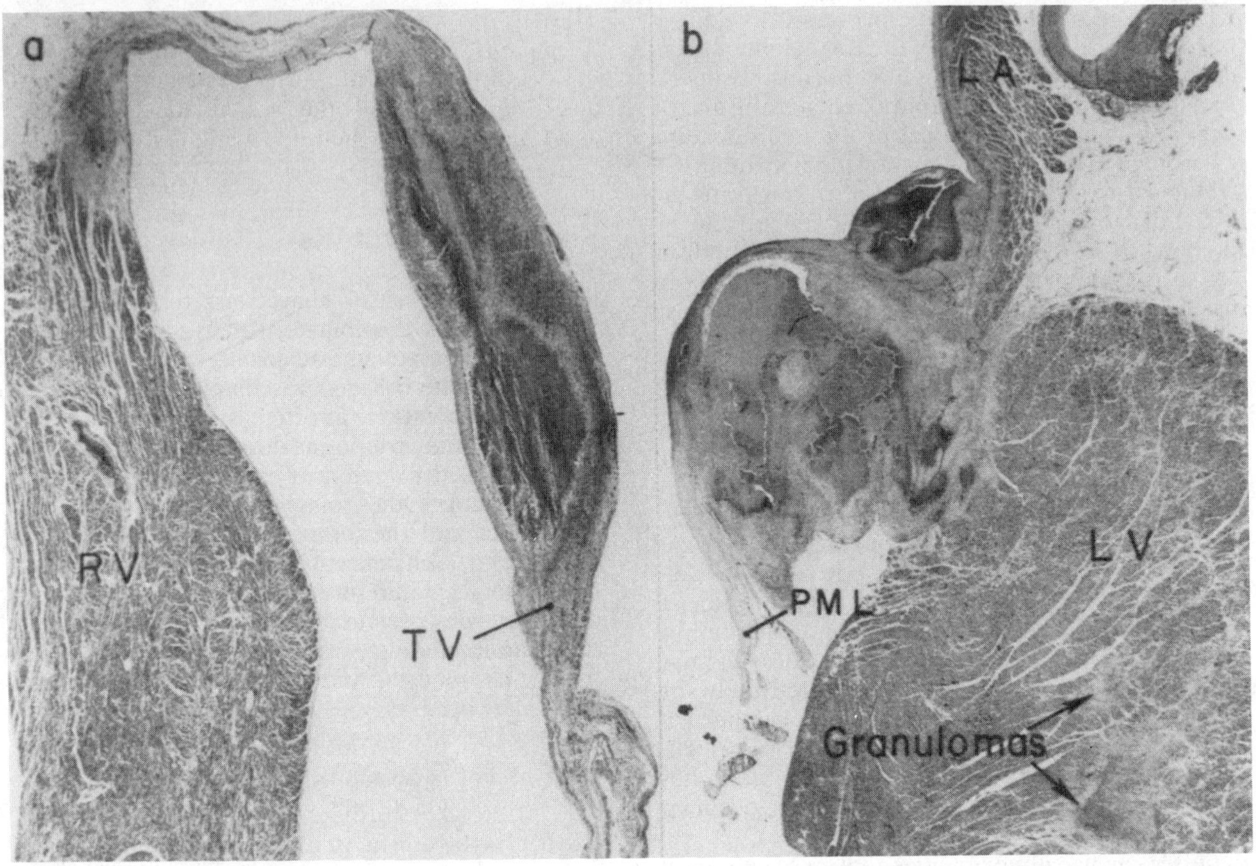

FIGURE 73-3 Rheumatoid arthritis. Shown in *a* is a tricuspid valve (TV), and in *b* a mitral valve infiltrated by rheumatoid nodules. In addition granulomas are present within the left ventricular (LV) wall. LA = left atrium; PML = posterior mitral leaflet; RV = right ventricle. H&E, × 12 (*a*); ×6.5 (*b*). (*From W. C. Roberts, J. C. Dangel, and B. H. Bulkley, Nonrheumatic Valvular Cardiac Disease: A Clinicopathologic Survey of 27 Different Conditions Causing Valvular Dysfunction, Cardiovasc. Clin., 5:333, 1973. Reproduced with permission from the publisher and author.*)

Therapy

As most of the cardiac lesions of rheumatoid arthritis are clinically silent, it is not known whether the specific therapies used in rheumatoid arthritis, including salicylates, indomethacin, penicillamine, and corticosteroids, are effective therapy for treating cardiac involvement. Conventional treatment of pericarditis, arrhythmias, and conduction disturbances which may occur in patients with rheumatic arthritis is utilized when these disorders produce clinical symptoms.

Ankylosing Spondylitis

Ankylosing spondylitis, also called rheumatoid spondylitis, is now recognized as an entity related to, but distinct from, rheumatoid arthritis. Ankylosing spondylitis is characterized by a progressive inflammatory lesion of the spine, leading to chronic back pain, deforming dorsal kyphosis, and in its advanced stage, fusion of the costovertebral and sacroiliac joints with immobilization of the spine. This condition affects mainly men, generally first occurring early in life, but with a chronic progressive course of 20 to 30 years.[25,26] Identification of the HLA-B27 histocompatibility antigen in nearly all patients with ankylosing spondylitis has confirmed its genetic occurrence and also its relationship to other collagen vascular states with a high prevalence of this antigen, such as Reiter's syndrome and juvenile arthritis.

The Heart in Ankylosing Spondylitis

Cardiovascular disease in ankylosing spondylitis takes the form of a sclerosing inflammatory lesion generally limited to the aortic root area. The inflammatory process, which extends immediately above and below the aortic valve, typically causes aortic insufficiency.[27] As the inflammatory process extends below the aortic valve, it may infiltrate the basal portion of mitral valve which is in continuity with the aortic valve and cause mitral insufficiency.[28] Extension of the inflammatory lesion into the top of the ventricular septum, immediately below the aortic valve, accounts for the associated conduction disturbances which may occur (Fig. 73-4).

The major clinical manifestation of ankylosing spondylitis is aortic regurgitation, which may occur

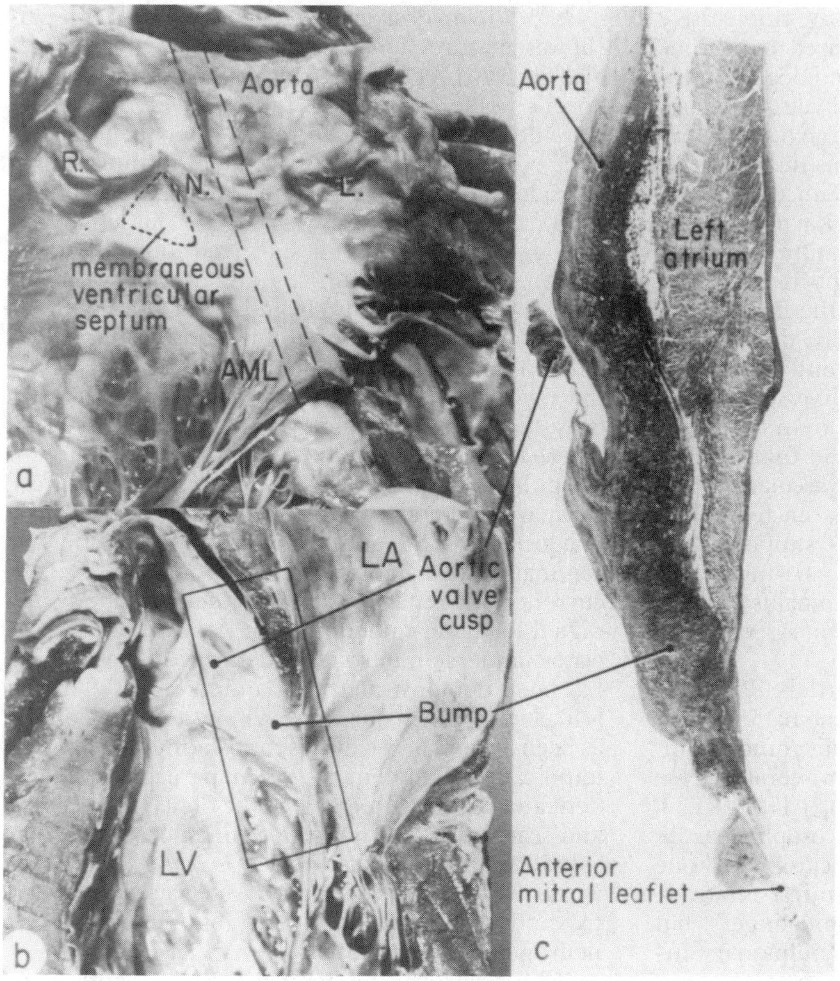

FIGURE 73-4 Ankylosing spondylitis. Aortic insufficiency, in this condition, results from the thickening of the aortic root immediately above and below the aortic valve (*a*) leading to a subvalvular bump, and thickening of the base of aortic valve and anterior leaflet of mitral valve (*b,c*). Shown in (*a*) is the opened left ventricle (LV) with the right (R), noncoronary (N), and left (L) aortic valve cusps grossly thickened. The region of the membranous ventricular septum lying beneath the valve is the site of AV nodal conduction tissue. Phosphotungstic acid-hematoxylin stain, ×3. (*From B. H. Bulkley and W. C. Roberts, Ankylosing Spondylitis and Aortic Regurgitation: Description of the Characteristic Cardiovascular Lesion from Study of Eight Necropsy Patients, Circulation, 48:1014, 1973. Reproduced with permission from the American Heart Association, Inc., and the author.*)

in up to 10 percent of patients with this condition, but mostly becomes manifest in the later years of the illness. For example, among patients with signs of spondylitis for 10 years, only 2 percent have clinical evidence of aortic insufficiency; by 30 years that number increases fivefold.[25,27]

Conditions which may be related to ankylosing spondylitis, including Reiter's syndrome and psoriatic arthropathy, can also develop an aortic root inflammatory lesion similar to ankylosing spondylitis.[29]

Therapy

Drug therapy for ankylosing spondylitis is primarily directed at relief of the pain and discomfort of back pain by salicylate or other anti-inflammatory agents such as indomethacin and phenylbutazone. Corticosteroids are generally not used in this condition except when iritis occurs. The inflammatory lesion of the heart generally runs a clinically silent course until aortic insufficiency develops, and by that time an inflammatory component to the condition is not prominent. Accordingly, clinical evidence of cardiac involvement of ankylosing spondylitis is not an indication for corticosteroid therapy. Heart failure and conduction disturbances are managed conventionally. Not infrequently, however, the aortic insufficiency of ankylosing spondylitis may become severe enough to warrant aortic valve replacement,[27] and patients with aortic insufficiency should be monitored closely.

Progressive Systemic Sclerosis

Progressive systemic sclerosis (PSS) was first identified over 2 centuries ago, and characterized by virtue of its striking skin manifestations; hence the name *scleroderma.* The systemic nature of this disease, and in particular its ability to affect the heart, has only been apparent in recent years. In 1943, Soma Weiss[30] described a pattern to the cardiac dysfunction of nine patients with scleroderma, and correlated these charges with abnormalities in the heart at autopsy in two of them. Moreover, he recognized that the cardiac disease was a manifestation of an underlying primary vascular disorder, or collagen vascular disease.

As we recognize scleroderma today, progressive systemic sclerosis (PSS) is characterized by fibrous thickening of the skin, and fibrous and degenerative alterations of the fingers, and of certain target organs, particularly esophagus, small and large bowels, kidneys, lung, and heart. Central to this degenerative process are diffuse vascular lesions. Functionally the vascular disorder is characterized by Raynaud's phenomenon, which is a prominent feature of scleroderma; Raynaud's disease of the digits is present in almost all patients with PSS, and is the first clinical symptom in the majority. Structurally, the vascular lesions show intimal proliferation and adventitial scarring of small and medium-sized vessels including arterioles. The underlying pathophysiology of scleroderma which links structure and function is a Raynaud's phenomenon of visceral vasculature that leads to focal vascular lesions and parenchymal necrosis and fibrosis. This concept is supported by findings in the heart, as well as in the lungs and kidneys.[31–33] The etiology of PSS remains elusive, however, and the role of the immune system in its pathophysiology is unclear.

Like most collagen vascular disorders, PSS may have variable clinical expression. Some patients may have predominantly skin involvement; others minimal skin abnormalities but severe visceral disease which may therefore evade diagnosis.[34] The CREST (calcinosis, Raynaud's phenomenon, esophageal abnormality, sclerodactylia, telangiectasia) is one scleroderma variant which can manifest relatively mild skin changes limited to face and fingers, but severe lung disease with a primary pulmonary hypertension picture.[35] "Overlap syndromes" are seen when a patient with typical features of PSS also demonstrates features of systemic lupus erythematosus or rheumatoid arthritis. Although scleroderma may run a long and benign course, malignant renal, lung, or cardiac disease may occur with rapid deterioration and death at a young age.

The Cardiovascular System and PSS

Cardiovascular disease in patients with PSS, as with most other collagen vascular disorders, may be due either to a primary involvement of the heart with the sclerosing disease or secondary to disease of the kidney or the lungs. In approaching PSS patients with cardiovascular disease, one must first make this distinction.

Primary PSS of the Heart

When the heart is involved directly by scleroderma, a myocardial fibrosis occurs which bears no direct relationship to large- or small-vessel occlusions or anatomic abnormalities. The fibrosis tends to be patchy, involving all levels of the myocardium unpredictably, and the right ventricle as often as the left. Focal patchy myocardial cell necrosis may also be evident, and at autopsy over three-quarters of patients with myocardial PSS had foci of necrosis.[32,36] The myocardial necrosis associated with patent vasculature suggests strongly that the myocardial fibrosis of PSS does not occur de novo, like a fibrous tissue cancer, but rather develops as most scars do, as the end-stage repair after tissue necrosis.[32,37] The type of necrosis evident in the heart of scleroderma patients is myofibrillar degeneration, or contraction band necrosis (Fig. 73-5). This lesion may develop if myocardium is subjected to transient occlusion with reperfusion—as would occur with vascular spasm. (It may also be induced experimentally by exposing myocardium to high doses of catecholamine.) Thus, the morphological characteristics of the myocardial lesion of primary cardiac PSS are consistent with a Raynaud's phenomenon of the heart. There is evidence that a Raynaud's phenomenon of the pulmonary arterioles may be responsible for the "primary" pulmonary hypertension–type lesion which may occur in PSS, and also that the kidneys in PSS can manifest Raynaud's type phenomena. The concurrence of renal Raynaud's phenomenon when digital Raynaud's phenomenon was induced by cold water immersion in some patients with scleroderma has been demonstrated by Cannon et al.[33] Thus, it is likely that the major visceral manifestations of PSS as seen in the heart, lungs, and kidney have as an important component the vascular reactivity so evident and readily detectable in the digits; the necrosis and scarring of the fingertips which occurs as a result of the reactivity also develops in the viscera similarly afflicted. Why the small vessels are hyperreactive and in spasm is not known, but almost surely a neurogenic factor is operative.

With regard to the heart per se the cause of the myocardial necrosis and fibrosis which develops in the setting of patent extramural and intramural vessels is not yet fully established. That the myocardial disease relates in part to immunologic abnormalities or to primary and unrestrained fibrous tissue proliferation remains a possibility. The growing body of evidence to date, however, suggests that the vascular system—and particularly the smaller arteries and arterioles—is the primary target organ of progressive systemic sclerosis, and the cardiac sclerosis of scleroderma may be a consequence of focal intermittent and progressive ischemic injury.

As mentioned above, morphological study suggested a myocardial Raynaud's phenomenon because of the structural nature of the myocardial cell injury. Subsequently, several functional studies have suggested that microvascular spasm is occurring in patients with cardiac scleroderma. Transient perfusion defects identified by ^{201}Tl-radionuclide imaging in the setting of patent coronary arteries have been identified in patients with progressive systemic sclerosis and symptomatic cardiac disease, for example.[38] Other investigators have demonstrated cold-induced perfusion defects in patients with scleroderma.[39] Decreased coronary reserve has also been reported in patients with widely patent coronary arteries.

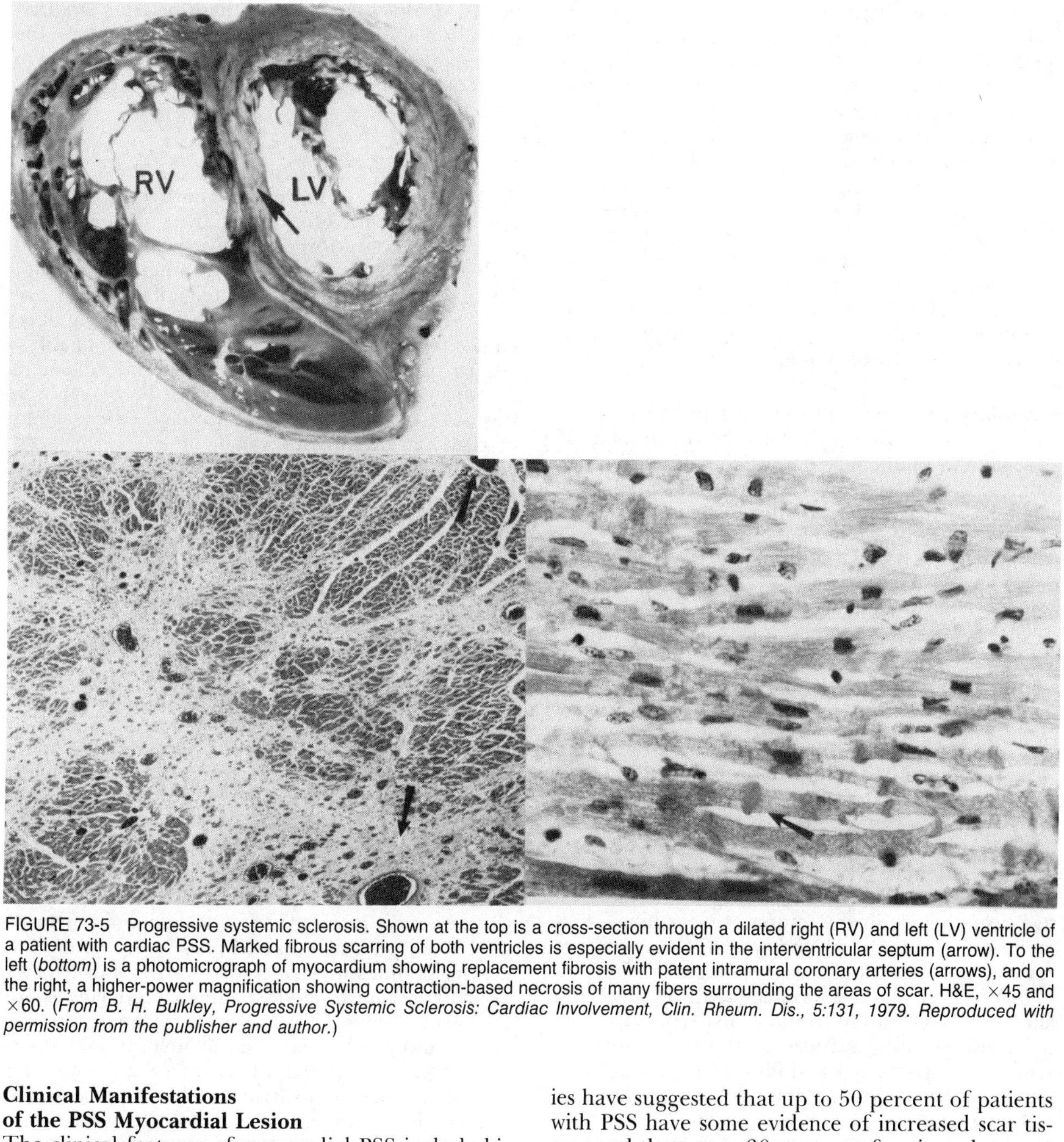

FIGURE 73-5 Progressive systemic sclerosis. Shown at the top is a cross-section through a dilated right (RV) and left (LV) ventricle of a patient with cardiac PSS. Marked fibrous scarring of both ventricles is especially evident in the interventricular septum (arrow). To the left (*bottom*) is a photomicrograph of myocardium showing replacement fibrosis with patent intramural coronary arteries (arrows), and on the right, a higher-power magnification showing contraction-based necrosis of many fibers surrounding the areas of scar. H&E, ×45 and ×60. (*From B. H. Bulkley, Progressive Systemic Sclerosis: Cardiac Involvement, Clin. Rheum. Dis., 5:131, 1979. Reproduced with permission from the publisher and author.*)

Clinical Manifestations of the PSS Myocardial Lesion

The clinical features of myocardial PSS include biventricular congestive heart failure, atrial and ventricular arrhythmias, myocardial infarction, angina pectoris, and sudden cardiac death.[37] These clinical manifestations reflect the underlying conditions of myocardial necrosis and fibrosis, and may at times mimic ischemic heart disease due to coronary atherosclerosis. If the myocardial injury is extensive enough, leading to dilated hypodynamic ventricles, a congestive cardiomyopathy picture may be simulated.

The true incidence of the primary myocardial lesion of PSS is not known, and the extent to which clinical cardiac dysfunction reflects the typical myocardial lesion is not always apparent. Autopsy studies have suggested that up to 50 percent of patients with PSS have some evidence of increased scar tissue, and that up to 30 percent of patients have extensive lesions in their hearts.[37,40,41] Some clinical cardiac abnormality, including symptoms of heart failure or abnormal rhythm with conduction disturbances, may occur in 30 to 40 percent of patients with PSS, and in roughly one-half of them the cardiac disorder is due to primary myocardial scleroderma. Among those patients with severe myocardial involvement morphologically, clinically manifest cardiac disease is evident in close to 90 percent.[37]

Pericardial and Endocardial Disease

Pericarditis may occur in 20 percent or more of patients with PSS.[40] Although in as many as two-thirds of patients with pericarditis, the pericarditis is due to renal failure, there are some who develop a fibrofibrinous or fibrous pericarditis for which no other apparent cause is evident. Exudative pericardial effusions may accompany scleroderma pericarditis, and have been reported to be as large as 1000 ml.[30] Although rare, constrictive pericarditis may result from the pericardial sclerosis.

Scleroderma is virtually unique among the collagen vascular–type diseases in that it rarely, if ever, affects cardiac valves. Mild, focal, nonspecific thickening of valve tissue has been described in hearts from patients with PSS,[40] but no characteristic or consistent valve lesion has been recognized. Clinically evident valvular dysfunction due to scleroderma per se is virtually nonexistent.

Secondary Cardiovascular Disease in PSS

Since scleroderma most frequently manifests itself as renal and pulmonary parenchymal disease, with pulmonary and systemic hypertension, cardiovascular disease secondary to these is common. Left ventricular hypertrophy and congestive heart failure may be associated with long-standing systemic hypertension and renal disease. Uremic pericarditis may occur. Cor pulmonale with marked right ventricular hypertrophy and right-sided heart failure may result from long-standing severe pulmonary scleroderma.

Pulmonary Hypertensive Disease of PSS

Although the pulmonary fibrosis of scleroderma has been known for years, the recognition of a "primary" pulmonary hypertensive lesion independent of parenchymal disease came later. Patients with this primary pulmonary vascular lesion tend to develop rapidly progressive dyspnea and right-sided congestive heart failure in the setting of clear lungs. Pulmonary pressures reach the systemic level and are refractory to treatment. Morphologically the pulmonary arterial lesions show the range of advanced alterations (medial and intimal hyperplasia, plexiform lesions, and necrotizing arteritis) seen in Eisenmenger syndromes and idiopathic primary pulmonary hypertension. Arterial vasospasm is believed to be a major component of "primary" pulmonary hypertension, and the association is supported by angiographic studies. On occasion vasodilators such as tolazoline may induce partial lowering of pressure, but the fixed pulmonary lesions and focal thrombotic occlusions which virtually always accompany the advanced stages of this condition make restoration of normal pressures unlikely. It is of interest that Raynaud's phenomenon of the digits accompanies idiopathic primary pulmonary hypertension in about one-third of patients,[42] suggesting that vascular hyperreactivity may be a common link between this idiopathic lung disease and scleroderma.

Although severe pulmonary hypertension is a less common manifestation of scleroderma, it is one which carries the gravest of prognoses. Sudden unexpected death is common in these patients, and hypotension and death may occur precipitously in the setting of what would appear to be relatively benign procedures such as pericardiocentesis or cardiac catheterization.

Treatment of PSS Cardiovascular Disease

At the present time there is no known effective therapy.[43] Treatment of the cardiovascular disease is standard therapy for congestive heart failure and arrhythmias as they present. Although vasodilator therapy would appear indicated, there is no evidence that nitrates are effective for treating Raynaud's phenomenon, or the other systemic manifestations of PSS. Whether the newer, more potent vasodilators currently available will be of value in this disease has yet to be determined. Other agents of potential therapeutic value for PSS cardiac disease include D-penicillamine and corticosteroids, but none have proven efficacy either for the systemic disease or its cardiac manifestations.

Summary: The Collagen Vascular Diseases and the Heart

The term *collagen vascular diseases* encompasses a broad spectrum of diseases and dysfunctions. Their cardiac afflictions tend to be characteristic and in many cases serve to distinguish the disorders from each other (Table 73-1). In ankylosing spondylitis and related conditions such as Reiter's syndrome, the aortic root is involved primarily; secondarily there are aortic valve and conduction system dysfunctions. Systemic lupus erythematosus leads to a pancarditis; when endocarditis is present, it is the mitral valve which is most often affected. Rheumatoid arthritis affects the pericardium and only rarely do inflammatory nodules involve cardiac valves and myocardium. Polyarteritis nodosa and scleroderma spare the cardiac valves, but affect the coronary arteries mainly and produce secondarily myocardial lesions. The cardiac manifestations of the collagen vascular disease may be the overriding clinical presentation in many instances, and must be distinguished from the similar presentations of other conditions such as infective endocarditis, idiopathic cardiomyopathy, and benign recurrent pericarditis.

References

1. Harvey, A. M., Shulman, L. E., Tumulty, P. A., Conley, C. L., and Schoenrich, E. A.: Systemic Lupus Erythematosus: A Review of the Literature and Clinical Analysis of 138 Cases, *Medicine,* 33:291, 1954.
2. Dubois, E. L.: "Lupus Erythematosus: A Review of the Current Status of Discoid and Systemic Lupus Erythematosus and their Variants," 2d ed., McGraw-Hill Book Company, New York, 1974.
3. Hejtmancik, M. R., Wright, J. C., Quint, R., and Jennings,

F. L.: The Cardiovascular Manifestations of Systemic Lupus Erythematosus, *Am. Heart J.*, 68:119, 1964.
4. Bulkley, B. H., and Roberts, W. C.: The Heart in Systemic Lupus Erythematosus and the Changes Induced in It by Corticosteroid Therapy. A Study of 36 Necropsy Patients, *Am. J. Med.*, 58:243, 1975.
5. Yurchak, P. M., Levine, S. A., and Gorlin, R.: Constrictive Pericarditis Complicating Disseminated Lupus Erythematosus, *Circulation*, 31:113, 1965.
6. Bergen, S. S., Jr.: Pericardial Effusion, A Manifestation of Systemic Lupus Erythematosus, *Circulation*, 22:144, 1960.
7. Klacsmann, P. G., Bulkley, B. H., and Hutchins, G. M.: The Changed Spectrum of Purulent Pericarditis: An 86 Year Autopsy Experience in 200 Patients, *Am. J. Med.*, 63:666, 1977.
8. Libman, E., and Sacks, B.: A Hitherto Undescribed Form of Valvular and Mural Endocarditis, *Arch. Intern. Med.*, 33:701, 1924.
9. Gross, L.: The Cardiac Lesion in Libman-Sacks Disease with a Consideration of Its Relationship to Acute Diffuse Lupus Erythematosus, *Am. J. Pathol.*, 16:375, 1940.
10. Bulkley, B. H., and Roberts, W. C.: Systemic Lupus Erythematosus as a Cause of Severe Mitral Regurgitation: A New Problem in an Old Disease, *Am. J. Cardiol.*, 35:305, 1975.
11. Paget, S. A., Bulkley, B. H., Grauer, L. E., and Seningen, R.: Mitral Valve Disease of Systemic Lupus Erythematosus: A Cause of Severe Congestive Heart Failure Reversed by Valve Replacement, *Am. J. Med.*, 59:134, 1975.
12. Seningen, R. P., Borer, J. S., Redwood, D. R., Bulkley, B. H., and Paget, S. A.: Libman-Sacks Endocardoma: Diagnosis during Life with Radiographic, Fluoroscopic and Angiocardiographic Findings, *Radiology*, 113:597, 1974.
13. James, T. N., Rupe, C. E., and Monto, R. W.: Pathology of the Cardiac Conduction System in Systemic Lupus Erythematosus, *Ann. Intern. Med.*, 63:402, 1965.
14. Zeek, P. M.: Periarteritis Nodosa and Other Forms of Necrotizing Angiitis, *N. Engl. J. Med.*, 248:764, 1953.
15. Alarcon-Segovia, D.: The Necrotizing Vasculitides: A New Pathogenetic Classification, *Sym. Rheum. Dis.*, 61:241, 1977.
16. Holsinger, D. R., Osmundson, P. J., and Edwards, J. E.: The Heart in Periarteritis Nodosa, *Circulation*, 25:610, 1962.
17. Schrader, M. L., and Bulkley, B. H.: The Heart in Polyarteritis Nodosa: A Clinicopathologic Study of 36 Patients, *Am. J. Cardiol.* 45:395, 1980. (Abstract.)
18. James, T. N., and Birk, R. E.: Pathology of the Cardiac Conduction System in Polyarteritis Nodosa, *Arch. Intern. Med.*, 117:561, 1966.
19. Thiene, G., Valente, M., and Rossi, L.: Involvement of the Cardiac Conducting System in Panarteritis Nodosa, *Am. Heart J.*, 95:716, 1978.
20. Fauci, A. S., Haynes, B. F., and Katz, P.: The Spectrum of Vasculitis: Clinical, Pathologic, Immunologic and Therapeutic Considerations, *Ann. Intern. Med.*, 89:660, 1978.
21. Bacon, P. A., and Gibson, D. G.: Cardiac Involvement in Rheumatoid Arthritis: An Echocardiographic Study, *Ann. Rheum. Dis.*, 33:20, 1974.
22. Liss, J. P., and Bachmann, W. T.: Rheumatoid Constrictive Pericarditis Treated by Pericardiectomy: Report of a Case and Review of the Literature, *Arthritis Rheum.*, 13:869, 1970.
23. Weintraub, A. M., and Zwaifler, N. J.: The Occurrence of Valvular and Myocardial Disease in Patients with Chronic Joint Deformity: A Spectrum, *Am. J. Med.*, 35:145, 1963.
24. Roberts, W. C., Dangel, J. C., and Bulkley, B. H.: Nonrheumatic Valvular Cardiac Disease: A Clinicopathologic Survey of 27 Different Conditions Causing Valvular Dysfunction, *Cardiovasc. Clin.*, 5:333, 1973.
25. Graham, D. C., and Smythe, H. A.: The Carditis and Aortitis of Ankylosing Spondylitis, *Bull. Rheum. Dis.*, 9:171, 1958.
26. Julkunen, H.: Rheumatoid Spondylitis—Clinical and Laboratory Study of 149 Cases Compared with 182 Cases of Rheumatoid Arthritis, *Acta Rheum. Scand.* 172 (suppl. 4):24, 1962.
27. Bulkley, B. H., and Roberts, W. C.: Ankylosing Spondylitis and Aortic Regurgitation: Description of the Characteristic Cardiovascular Lesion from Study of Eight Necropsy Patients, *Circulation*, 48:1014, 1973.
28. Roberts, W. C., Hollingsworth, J. F., Bulkley, B. H., Jaffe, R. B., Epstein, S. E., and Stinson, E. B.: Combined Mitral and Aortic Regurgitation in Ankylosing Spondylitis: Angiographic and Anatomic Features, *Am. J. Med.*, 56:237, 1974.
29. Paulus, H. E., Pearson, C. M., and Pitts, W.: Aortic Insufficiency in 5 Patients with Reiter's Syndrome, *Am. J. Med.*, 53:464, 1972.
30. Weiss, S., Stead, E. A., Warren, J. V., and Bailey, O. T.: Scleroderma Heart Disease: With a Consideration of Certain Other Visceral Manifestations of Scleroderma, *Arch. Intern. Med.*, 71:749, 1943.
31. Sackner, A. M., Akgun, N., Kimbel, P., and Lewis, D. H.: The Pathophysiology of Scleroderma Involving the Heart and Respiratory System, *Ann. Intern. Med.*, 60:611, 1964.
32. Bulkley, B. H., Ridolfi, R. L., Salyer, W. R., and Hutchins, G. M.: Myocardial Lesions of Progressive Systemic Sclerosis: A Cause of Cardiac Dysfunction, *Circulation*, 53:483, 1976.
33. Cannon, P. J., Hassar, M., Case, D. B., Casarella, W. J., Sommers, S. C., and LeRoy, E. C.: The Relationship of Hypertension and Renal Failure in Scleroderma (Progressive Systemic Sclerosis) to Structural and Functional Abnormalities of the Renal Cortical Circulation, *Medicine*, 53:1, 1974.
34. Bulkley, B. H., Klacsmann, P. G., and Hutchins, G. M.: Angina Pectoris, Myocardial Infarction and Sudden Death with Normal Coronary Arteries: A Clinicopathologic Study of 9 Patients with Progressive Systemic Sclerosis, *Am. Heart J.*, 95:563, 1978.
35. Salerni, R., Rodnan, G. P., Leon, D. F., and Shaver, J. A.: Pulmonary Hypertension in the CREST Syndrome Variant of Progressive Systemic Sclerosis (Scleroderma), *Ann. Intern. Med.*, 86:394, 1977.
36. Leinwand, I., Duryee, A. W., and Richter, M. N.: Scleroderma (based on a study of over 150 cases), *Ann. Intern. Med.*, 42:1003, 1954.
37. Bulkley, B. H.: Progressive Systemic Sclerosis: Cardiac Involvement, *Clin. Rheum. Dis.*, 5:131, 1979.
38. Follansbee, W. P., Curtiss, E. I., Medsger, T. A., Jr., et al.: Physiologic Abnormalities of Cardiac Function in Progressive Systemic Sclerosis with Diffuse Scleroderma, *N. Engl. J. Med.*, 310:142, 1984.
39. Alexander, E. L., Firestein, G. S., Leitl, G., et al.: Scleroderma Heart Disease: Evidence for Cold-Induced Abnormalities of Myocardial Function and Perfusion, *Arthritis Rheum.*, 24:558, 1981. (Abstract.)
40. Sackner, A. M., Heinz, E. R., and Steinberg, A. J.: The Heart in Scleroderma, *Am. J. Cardiol.*, 17:542, 1966.
41. D'Angelo, W. A., Fries, J. F., Masi, A. T., and Shulman, L. E.: Pathologic Observations in Systemic Sclerosis (Scleroderma): A Study of Fifty-eight Autopsy Cases and Fifty-eight Matched Controls, *Am. J. Med.*, 46:428, 1969.
42. Walcott, G., Burchell, H. B., and Brown, A. L.: Primary Pulmonary Hypertension, *Am. J. Med.*, 71:749, 1970.
43. D'Angelo, W. A.: Progressive Systemic Sclerosis: Management, *Clin. Rheum. Dis.*, 5:263, 1979.

74

The Heart, Alcoholism, and Nutritional Disease

Timothy J. Regan, M.D.

Alcohol is capable of producing a subacute myocarditis, often misdiagnosed because of the slowness of its evolution, and the coexistence in the terminal period of cardiac murmurs and albuminuria.

H. Vaquez, 1921[1]

Heart Disease in Alcoholism

A cardiovascular response directly related to alcohol use was earlier suggested by Paul D. White, who observed paroxysmal arrhythmias, precipitation of congestive failure in cardiac patients, and increase in angina pectoris.[2] That cardiac abnormalities can be produced in the absence of other causes of heart disease has been suggested more recently by several clinical studies.[3,4] With the advent of technology enabling noninvasive as well as invasive evaluation of heart function, it has become possible to consider the question of cardiac involvement in subjects who abuse alcohol but have not yet developed clinical abnormalities.

Increments of left ventricular end-diastolic pressure and diminished stroke volume responses during the stress of exercise or increased afterload have been elicited in noncardiac subjects.[5,6] The type of beverage does not appear to be a determinant since these abnormalities have been observed in individuals using wine exclusively[7] or those who used spirits predominantly.[8,9] A more advanced form of this subclinical disease has been observed in which up to 50 percent of the asymptomatic alcoholic subjects had modest left ventricular hypertrophy as determined by M-mode echocardiographic criteria.[10] Invasive testing has demonstrated reduced indexes of contractility.[6] The subclinical state has been further defined; we now recognize a presumably early stage with increased wall thickness but normal diastolic internal diameter and a later stage in which internal diameter is increased without an abnormality in wall dimension.[11]

Heart Failure

As cardiac dysfunction progresses to low cardiac output failure in alcoholics, pulmonary congestion may lead to dyspnea on exertion or during sleep. Cardiomegaly may be moderate in extent during an initial episode of decompensation in the absence of mitral regurgitation due to papillary muscle insufficiency. After correction of heart failure, heart size may approximate normal. Electrocardiographic changes usually exhibit the range of changes seen in other causes of heart failure. Occasionally a peripheral arterial or pulmonary embolism is the initial manifestation. No consistent pattern of alcohol abuse is associated with the onset of heart failure. A period of intensified drinking may be reported, but recurrent illness can apparently occur after a period of abstinence in some patients. Clinical evidence of peripheral neuropathy or hepatic cirrhosis is usually not associated with alcoholic cardiomyopathy.

Diagnosis of this form of cardiomyopathy may be obscured when the patient presents with elevated arterial blood pressure. Although seen with other causes of cardiomyopathy, hypertensive episodes may be more frequent with this disease entity. This response has been reported in noncardiac alcoholics during the late intoxication–early withdrawal period in up to one-half of patients observed in an outpatient setting, usually without the development of a classical withdrawal illness.[12]

Arterial pressure may be moderately elevated for several days with spontaneous decline thereafter to a normal level.[13] Substantial elevations may require up to a week for spontaneous normalization and are usually associated with sinus tachycardia. After a short period of abstinence arterial pressures in noncardiac alcoholics do not appear to differ from those of a control group.[8,14] In periods up to a year, the normotensive state was found to persist when the patient remained abstinent.[11] Whether transient blood pressure elevation is an important factor in the pathogenesis of the cardiac syndromes associated with alcoholism is an unsettled question.

Except for alcohol abuse, precipitating factors that can be readily associated with the episode of heart failure are usually not present. However, two decades ago, cobalt was suggested as a contributory etiological factor in beer drinkers, in that heart failure seemed to appear after cobalt salts were added to the beer and disappeared when the use of cobalt was discontinued.[15] The course of the disease in these patients differed from that in the usual alcoholic cardiomyopathic patient in that they went rapidly downhill, and marked myocytolysis was present on morphological examination. In moonshine drinkers, lead has also been implicated as a factor that promotes the development of cardiomyopathy.[16]

The course of alcoholic cardiomyopathy is variable depending to a large degree on the extent of cardiac involvement. The outlook is relatively poor in those who continue to ingest ethanol in substantial amounts. This is illustrated in a series of 108 patients admitted to hospital with a diagnosis of congestive cardiomyopathy of multiple etiologies.[17]

Two-thirds of the alcoholic group was dead within 3 years, while one-third of the nonalcoholic group succumbed. An earlier series of 64 alcoholic patients was followed over a 4-year period.[18] Fully one-third remained abstinent, and the mortality rate in this group was 9 percent, although only a minority exhibited clinical improvement. In those who remained actively alcoholic more than one-half had succumbed. Presumably, at certain stages of the disease the pathogenetic mechanisms may continue unabated despite traditional pharmacological management and abstinence from alcohol. The encouraging results of abstinence in this study may well have been exaggerated since this group of individuals seemed to have less severe cardiac disease on entrance into the study. In a smaller series 10 patients from Japan who remained abstinent for a decade were found to have all survived.[19] These responses to abstinence support the view that the major etiological element in this disease is ethyl alcohol.

Pharmacological therapy for cardiac decompensation depends on the state of cardiac disease when the patient is first seen. The use of Antabuse for alcoholism in cardiac patients may be associated with complications. Dopamine-beta-hydroxylase, which is involved in the synthesis of norepinephrine, is inhibited by this agent,[20] and this may limit the sympathetic system's compensatory response in the myocardium. During the first episode of heart failure if the patient has had symptoms for a relatively short time and has only modest cardiomegaly and pulmonary congestion, the patient may be managed initially by diuretics to diminish the volume overload. As the disease progresses, there is presumably a role for preload and afterload reducing agents, but long-term efficacy has not been reported. Digitalis can contribute to the management of congestive heart failure in the advanced stages of the disease and is most useful in the control of atrial fibrillation or sinus tachycardia. Although confinement to bed rest for many months has been suggested as aiding in management,[21] the enforced abstinence from alcohol was presumably the most important feature.

Arrhythmias

Heart disease related to alcoholism may have an arrhythmia as the initial manifestation. Cardiac arrhythmias developing in these circumstances probably are often considered idiopathic in origin, since little or no clinical evidence of heart disease may remain after resolution of the dysrhythmia, and the extent of alcohol use may not be realized.

To elucidate this problem a group of subjects without overt cardiomyopathy or enlarged heart was selected on the basis of alcoholism and acute intoxication with the presence of arrhythmias.[14] Supraventricular arrhythmias predominated, and atrial fibrillation was the most common arrhythmia. Cardioversion or pharmacological intervention was frequently required, but sinus rhythm was restored spontaneously in some. Plasma electrolytes on admission were usually normal. The same arrhythmia as during the original episode was present during subsequent recurrence. Some days after restoration of normal sinus rhythm, these patients were assessed by high-speed electrocardiogram. The observed moderate delays in conduction were considered the background for the genesis of the acute arrhythmias.[14] This entity has been termed the "holiday heart" syndrome because of frequent presentation over holidays or weekends. The acute cardiac rhythm disturbance occurs in association with heavy ethanol consumption in a person who chronically abuses ethanol without other clinical evidence of heart disease. It should be noted that in an urban hospital setting, alcoholism was reported to be the commonest cause of new onset atrial fibrillation in patients under 50 years of age.[22]

An accurate estimate of the incidence of arrhythmias in the population addicted to alcohol is not available. However, evaluation of patients with a Holter monitor during intoxication and early withdrawal stages has revealed several points of interest.[23] Subjects were excluded if arrhythmias or evidence of cardiac ischemia were present on the admission ECG. Of the 60 patients monitored during the initial 12 or 24 h, 12 had high composite arrhythmia scores. This was due to the presence of ventricular premature contractions. On biochemical assays of the serum, high concentrations of plasma catecholamine were found. After baseline observations, interventions with the beta-adrenergic receptor inhibitor propanolol reduced the incidence of arrhythmia. This response supports the view that the sympathetic system has an important role in the genesis of these arrhythmias.

Magnesium deficiency is fairly common with chronic alcohol abuse, particularly in patients with severe withdrawal reactions. There is no clear evidence that deficits of this cation give rise to arrhythmias. However, some cardiomyopathic alcoholics with arrhythmias secondary to digitalis excess may respond to therapeutic doses of magnesium.[24] Another variable pertinent to the question of arrhythmogenesis is sleep apnea and the attendant oxygen desaturation. This has been described in asymptomatic individuals at blood ethanol levels above 80 mg/dl,[25] but there are no data relating to the syndrome associated with alcohol abuse.

Sudden unexpected death has been reported in alcoholics. This phenomenon has been attributed to cardiac arrest which is supported by the observation of a reduced ventricular fibrillation threshold in an animal model of chronic alcoholism.[26] In a medical examiner's report from Baltimore without morphological examination of the heart[27] fatty liver was the principal evidence of alcohol abuse. A similar phenomenon was subsequently observed in a predominantly rural population with characteristics that mirrored those of the general alcoholic population.[28] There were 411 sudden deaths over a 4-year period in subjects with fatty liver, a majority of whom had detectable blood levels of ethanol. In a series of 50 autopsies in which 30 individuals died suddenly, the histories indicated that all had been alcoholics for years.[29] Of the 30, 17 had alcoholemia when they succumbed. The sudden death group had greater degrees of myocardial hypertrophy, foci of fibrosis, and necrosis with mononuclear cell infiltration.

Determinants of Alcoholic Heart Disease

The evidence that ethanol and/or its metabolites are the etiologic basis for alcoholic cardiomyopathy is circumstantial. The major positive supportive feature is the history of ethanol ingestion in intoxicating amounts for many years, frequently marked by periods of spree drinking.

Animal models have been shown to develop functional, biochemical, and morphological abnormalities, but congestive heart failure and significant arrhythmias have not been reported, in part related to the duration of ethanol exposure. However, the reduced mortality rate in patients who become abstinent supports the view that ethanol is the major factor in development of the disease.[18,19,21]

In an epidemiological survey of a working population the risk of cardiovascular death was increased when chronic alcohol consumption exceeded five drinks a day.[30] In terms of variables, in addition to ethanol abuse that may affect the development of cardiomyopathy, several factors have been considered to be potentially important. Cigarette use is common in the person addicted to alcohol and may be a contributory factor. In contrast to alcoholic cirrhosis, clinically evident malnutrition is usually not present in the cardiac patient.[3,4] In females, the disease is rare prior to the age of menopause.[9] A genetic predisposition evaluated in the terms of the HLA antigens has not yet been demonstrated.

Pathophysiology

As concerns mechanism there is presumably some direct effect of ethanol or its metabolites as well as a neurohumoral influence upon the heart over the long term which may interact with adaptive processes that tend to reduce pathological effects. While the pathogenesis of collagen accumulation in terms of synthesis and degradation has not been defined, the early decrease of diastolic compliance of the left ventricle seen experimentally is most likely related to this alteration of interstitium.[31] After several years left ventricular contractility may be impaired.[31,32] There was an associated accumulation of water and Na^+ in cardiac cells without a reduction of K^+, perhaps related to the altered membrane phospholipid composition. In view of the dilatation of sarcoplasmic reticulum observed by electron microscopy,[31] it was postulated that dysfunction of the tubular membranes might limit the rate of Ca^{2+} availability to contractile protein, and thus diminish contractile performance, without a change in total Ca^{2+}.[32] Although high-energy phosphate levels are not altered, an inhibitory effect of long-term ethanol use on myosin ATPase and Ca^{2+}-activated myofibrillar ATPase have been demonstrated.[32]

Protein synthesis in the cardiac cell might be anticipated to be adversely affected by chronic ethanol exposure. However, in experiments to determine the ability of chronic ethanol feeding to affect the process of myocardial hypertrophy during chronic aortic pressure overload[33] the hypertrophic response was unimpaired. Moreover, ribonucleic acid, a determinant of protein synthesis, was not found to be diminished in the alcoholic animals over a period of 14 weeks.[33] Data on the activity of lysosomal enzymes in this experimental cardiomyopathy are not yet available.

When the disease is clinically evident, there appears to be some degree of impaired synthesis or accelerated degradation of contractile protein, inasmuch as lysis of myofibrils is frequently observed on morphological study of advanced cardiomyopathy, which may antecede the appearance of rapid clinical deterioration. An immunological basis for the progression of alcoholic cardiomyopathy has been considered.[34] However, circulating heart antibodies assessed by immunofluorescent methods were rarely present in patients with alcoholic cardiomyopathy, in contrast to the recognized immunological entities such as Dressler's syndrome.

In examination of biopsy specimens from patients or autopsy tissue preparations, no distinctive features have been revealed in the patients with alcoholic heart disease as compared to other causes of congestive cardiomyopathy.[35] Quite early in the prefailure stage there would appear to be dilatation of the sarcoplasmic reticulum and the undifferentiated portion of the intercalated disk, but these changes are apparently obscured at later stages of disease, when considerable myocytolysis may be seen. An increase of fibrous tissue is a usual finding and may take the form of an increase in the interstitial collagen component or replacement of myocardial fibers. Small vessels are usually normal, but in the areas of fibrous tissue accumulation vessels may occasionally show wall thickening. It was thought that these vascular abnormalities were secondary in nature.[35]

Vitamins

Beriberi

While not readily reproduced in animals, the key features of thiamine deficiency include a high cardiac output associated with arteriolar vasodilatation. Although it has been the classic view that right ventricular failure is dominant when symptoms develop, several studies have documented a significant elevation of left ventricular end-diastolic and pulmonary capillary wedge pressures.[36]

Depression of left ventricular function during the acute phase of beriberi heart disease has been described. In addition, the persistence of a chronic cardiac abnormality after treatment with thiamine suggests that alcoholism, usually present in subjects with beriberi on the North American continent, may be responsible. The frequently reversible nature of the cardiac abnormalities in subjects who were apparently not alcoholic has been indicated in American prisoners of war in World War II.[37]

Other Vitamins

Unequivocal direct effects of deficiencies of vitamin A and niacin on heart muscle in humans have not been established. Scurvy, however, can be associated with sudden death.[38] Human volunteers on a vitamin C–deficient diet have reported dyspnea and chest pain associated with PR prolongation and ST-segment abnormalities,[38] and ECG abnormalities can be reversed rapidly with parenteral vitamin C. In experimental vitamin B_6 deficiency, cardiomyopathic changes at postmortem were present in the rat,[39] but the human counterpart has yet to be described. Excess doses of vitamin D in human beings have been associated with deposits of calcium as well as the shortened QT interval of hypercalcemia.[40] Mild excesses of vitamin D_3 have recently been shown to intensify atherosclerosis in nonhuman primates.[41]

Vitamin E and Selenium

In recent years a cardiomyopathy has been described in China affecting infants and children.[42] The pathology is characterized by local myocardial necrosis, fibrosis, and hypercontraction bands. The disease has a regional distribution in agricultural areas invariably poor in the selenium content of the staple grains and soil. Supplementation of the diet with selenium was found to be effective as a preventive. In view of a seasonal variation, other factors have been considered of importance in pathogenesis. Although isolated selenium deficiency that produces cardiomyopathy has not been described in experimental animal models, a combination of selenium and vitamin E deficiencies has been shown to produce diffuse patchy necrosis of the myocardium in young swine.[43] An abnormality of cell lipid peroxidation was thought to affect membrane lipids with resultant disturbance of intracellular electrolyte and water composition as well as energy production.

Cachexia

Severe weight loss in individuals who have relatively normal initial body weights may have important cardiovascular consequences, particularly in infants and children.

The nutritional deficiency that characterizes protein-calorie undernutrition has been studied by a number of investigators. In human adult volunteers on a semistarvation regimen, a significant reduction of heart rate, stroke volume, cardiac output, and heart size was observed during the development of cachexia.[44] Cardiac output, however, did not appear to fall out of proportion to the diminished metabolic requirements. In addition, a recent study of patients with undernutrition secondary to a variety of chronic disease states found by echocardiography that the reduced cardiac output was associated with a diminished left ventricular end-diastolic diameter and mass.[45] When adjusted for body weight, the cardiac index was higher than that of normal controls. Additional observations in a group of individuals with anorexia nervosa showed that the systolic ejection phase indexes of left ventricular function were normal.[46] These patients responded to exercise in a normal fashion. The patients in this study were considered to have an adult marasmus type of syndrome which did not significantly affect cardiac function. In an analysis of 93 malnourished children studied at autopsy in Costa Rica, there were 14 cases considered to have primary congestive heart failure resulting from either marasmus or kwashiorkor.[47] On histological examination, interstitial edema was frequently observed. Substantial degrees of vacuolization within myocardial fibers with apparent disorganization of myofibrillar structure were observed.

In primary protein-calorie undernutrition, the weight of the evidence indicates that the adult heart, though atrophied, will usually function normally prior to refeeding. Studies of young children, supported by some experimental data, suggest that substantial histological abnormality of the myocardium may occur. In some of the children, heart failure may be attributable to the undernutrition. A potential for arrhythmias and sudden death has been postulated but not established.

Hyperalimentation

Therapeutic feeding by the enteric or parenteral route has assumed increasing importance in a variety of acutely ill patients. Although the initial hemodynamic changes during such therapy have not been delineated, the acute responses to oral feeding in the normally nourished are of interest in terms of the cardiovascular changes that occur.

During oral feeding in human beings, diets with mixed caloric composition induce an increase of cardiac output associated with a decline in systemic vascular resistance within 20 min after completion of the meal.[48] The cardiac output rise is essentially due to an increase of stroke volume without a change in left ventricular filling pressure, implying an increase in contractility. In patients who have postprandial angina pectoris at rest, stroke volume is diminished while pulmonary wedge pressure is elevated, suggesting cardiac decompensation.[48] Coronary vasoconstriction secondary to a reflex from the gastrointestinal tract has been suggested as a mechanism. In subjects who develop postprandial lipemia after a high-fat meal, the onset of pain is later, after an interval of 3 to 4 h.[49] The hemodynamic responses during postprandial lipemia in normal persons differ from mixed caloric administration in that stroke output and pulmonary wedge pressures are unaltered.[50] A mild decrease of coronary blood flow in normal persons[50] may be sufficiently exaggerated in the presence of coronary atherosclerosis to precipitate angina.

Patients with chronic cardiac disease may suffer forms of malnutrition similar to those described for the general hospital population.[51] An extreme form, the syndrome of cardiac cachexia, is attributable to anorexia, decreased intestinal absorption of food, and perhaps a change in the distribution of substrates absorbed into the circulatory system. Patients with cardiac cachexia appear to have increased morbidity and mortality rates when compared to noncachectic patients similar in age, sex, and severity of heart disease. In a prospective study of cardiac patients undergoing surgery, the effects of short-term force feeding up to 1500 calories were evaluated.[52] The lack of effect on morbidity and mortality rates was perhaps related to the fact that feeding was begun just prior to operation and continued for approximately 5 days. The effects of longer-term preparation of patients before surgery require investigation.

Adults with chronic undernutrition without underlying heart disease may develop heart failure during hyperalimentation.[45] Under the conditions of rapid repletion, a state resembling congestive heart failure may develop, characterized by hypermetabolism, ventricular gallop, augmented cardiac output, and normal ejection fraction. Rapid resolution follows diuretic therapy, a slower rate of hyperalimentation, and a reduction in the daily intake of sodium.

During hyperalimentation some patients may develop hypophosphatemia. As in other circumstances producing this anion deficit, significant cardiac effects may ensue. In such patients this may take the form of diminished left ventricular function which is improved during phosphate administration.[53] In patients without mechanical defects by echocardiogram, a significant increase in the incidence of arrhythmias was observed without reduction in the plasma concentrations of other electrolytes.[54] Those who exhibited nonsustained ventricular tachycardia were each improved by normalizing plasma phosphate levels with oral supplements.

The child recovering from protein-calorie undernutrition appears to be at high risk for developing cardiac abnormalities during the repletion process, including sudden death.[55] Hypervolemia in the presence of an atrophic heart is a probable basis for congestive heart failure. Fever, sepsis, pneumonia, and electrolyte imbalance may all contribute to or aggravate the circulatory abnormalities.

References

1. Vaquez, H.: "Maladies du Coeur," Baillière et Fils, Paris, France, 1921, p. 308.
2. White, P. D.: "Heart Disease," The Macmillan Company, New York, 1951, p. 597.
3. Brigden, W., and Robinson, J.: Alcoholic Heart Disease, *Br. Med. J.*, 2:1283, 1964.
4. Burch, G. E., and Walsh, J. J.: Cardiac Insufficiency in Chronic Alcoholism, *Am. J. Cardiol.*, 6:864, 1960.
5. Gould, L., Shariff, M., and Lilieto, M.: Cardiac Hemodynamics in Alcoholic Patients with Chronic Liver Disease and Presystolic Gallop, *J. Clin. Invest.*, 48:860, 1969.
6. Regan, T. J., Levinson, G. E., Oldewurtel, H. A., Frank, M. J., Weisse, A. B., and Moschos, C. B.: Ventricular Function in Noncardiacs with Alcoholic Fatty Liver: Role of Ethanol in the Production of Cardiomyopathy, *J. Clin. Invest.*, 48:397, 1969.
7. Levi, G. F., Quadri, A., Ratti, S., et al.: Preclinical Abnormality of Left Ventricular Function in Chronic Alcoholics, *Br. Heart J.*, 39:35, 1977.
8. Spodick, D. H., Pigott, W. M., and Chirife, R.: Preclinical Cardiac Malfunction in Chronic Alcoholism: Comparison with Matched Normal Controls and with Alcohol Cardiomyopathy, *N. Engl. J. Med.*, 287:677, 1972.
9. Wu, C. F., Sudhakar, M., and Jaferi, G., et al.: Preclinical Cardiomyopathy in Chronic Alcoholics: A Sex Difference, *Am. Heart J.*, 91:281, 1976.
10. Askanas, A., Udoshi, M., and Sadjadi, S. A.: The Heart in Chronic Alcoholism: A Noninvasive Study, *Am. Heart J.*, 88:9, 1980.
11. Matthews, E. C., Jr., Gardin, J. M., and Henry, W. L., et al.: Echocardiographic Abnormalities in Chronic Alcoholics with and without Overt Congestive Heart Failure, *Am. J. Cardiol.*, 47:570, 1981.
12. Saunders, J. B., Beevers, D. G., and Paton, A.: Alcohol-Induced Hypertension, *Lancet*, 2:654, 1981, Sept 26.
13. Whitfield, C. L., Thompson, G., Lamb, A., et al.: Detoxification of 1024 Alcohol Patients without Psychoactive Drugs, *JAMA*, 239:1409, 1978.
14. Ettinger, P. O., Wu, C. F., De La Cruz, C., Jr., et al.: Arrhythmias and the "Holiday Heart": Alcohol-Associated Cardiac Rhythm Disorders, *Am. Heart J.*, 95:555, 1978.
15. Morin, Y., and Daniel, P.: Quebec Beer-Drinkers Cardiomyopathy: Etiological Consideration, *Can. Med. Assoc. J.*, 97:926, 1967.
16. Asokan, S. K., and Witham, A. G.: Myocardial Malfunction of Unknown Cause, *Cardiovasc. Clin.*, 4:113, 1972.
17. Bory, M., Mancini, J., Djiane, P., et al.: Les Myocardiomyopathies Ethyliques, *Nouv. Presse Med.*, 6:3295, 1977.
18. Demakis, J. G., Proskey, A., Rahimtoola, S. H., et al.: The Natural Course of Alcoholic Cardiomyopathy, *Ann. Intern. Med.*, 80:293, 1974.
19. Koide, T., Kato, A., Takabatake, Y., et al.: Variable Prognosis in Congestive Cardiomyopathy: Role of Left Ventricular Function, Alcoholism, and Pulmonary Thrombosis, *Jap. Heart J.*, 21:451, 1980.
20. Mussacchio, J., Kopin, I. J., and Snyder, S.: Effect of Disulfiram on Tissue Norepinephrine Content and Subcellular Distribution of Dopamine, Tyramine, and Their β-hydroxylated Metabolites, *Life Sci.*, 3:769, 1964.
21. McDonald, C. D., Burch, G. E., and Walsh, J. J.: Alcoholic Cardiomyopathy Managed with Prolonged Bed Rest, *Ann. Intern. Med.*, 74:681, 1971.
22. Lowenstein, S. R., Gabow, P. A., Cramer, J., Oliva, P. B., and Ratner, K.: The Role of Alcohol in New-Onset Atrial Fibrillation, *Arch. Intern. Med.*, 143:1882, 1983.
23. Zilm, D. H., Jacob, M. S., MaCleod, S. M., et al.: Propranolol

and Chlordiazepoxide Effects on Cardiac Arrhythmias during Alcohol Withdrawal, *Alcoholism: Clin. Exp. Res.,* 4:400, 1980.
24. Iseri, L. T., Freed, J., and Bures, A. R.: Magnesium Deficiency and Cardiac Disorders, *Am. J. Med.,* 58:837, 1975.
25. Taasan, V. C., Block, A. J., Boysen, P. G., et al.: Alcohol Increases Sleep Apnea and Oxygen Desaturation in Asymptomatic Men, *Am. J. Med.,* 71:240, 1981.
26. De La Cruz, C. L., Jr., Haider, B., Oldewurtel, H. A., et al.: The Effect of Ethanol on Ventricular Electrical Stability in the Chronic Alcoholic Animal, in S. Zoneracih (ed.), "Diabetes and the Heart," Charles C Thomas, Publisher, Springfield, Ill., p. 123.
27. Kramer, K., Kuller, L., and Fisher, R.: The Increasing Mortality Attributed to Cirrhosis and Fatty Liver, in Baltimore (1957–1966), *Ann. Intern. Med.,* 69:272, 1968.
28. Randall, B.: Sudden Death and Hepatic Fatty Metamorphosis: A North Carolina Survey, *JAMA,* 243:1723, 1980.
29. Velisheva, L. D., Goldina, B. G., and Boguslavsky,, V. I.: "Proceedings: U.S.A.-U.S.S.R. First Joint Symposium on Sudden Death" (DHEW Publication no. NIH-78-1470), U.S. Government Printing Office, Washington, D.C., 1977, p. 377.
30. Dyer, A. R., Stamler, J., Paul, O., et al.: Alcohol Consumption, Cardiovascular Risk Factors, and Mortality in Two Chicago Epidemiologic Studies, *Circulation,* 56:1067, 1977.
31. Thomas, G., Haider, B., Oldewurtel, H. A., et al.: Progression of Myocardial Abnormalities in Experimental Alcoholism, *Am. J. Cardiol.,* 46:233, 1980.
32. Sarma, J. S. M., Shigeaki, I., Fischer, R., et al.: Biochemical and Contractile Properties of Heart Muscle after Prolonged Alcohol Administration, *J. Mol. Cell. Cardiol.,* 8:951, 1976.
33. Whitman, V., Schuler, H. G., and Musselman, J.: Effects of Chronic Ethanol Consumption on the Myocardial Hypertrophic Response to a Pressure Overload in the Rat, *J. Mol. Cell. Cardiol.,* 12:519, 1980.
34. Trueman, T., Thompson, R. A., Cummins, P., et al.: Heart Antibodies in Cardiomyopathies, *Br. Heart J.,* 46:296, 1981.
35. Olsen, E. G. J.: The Pathology of Cardiomyopathies: A Critical Analysis, *Am. Heart J.,* 98:385, 1979.
36. Wagner, P. I.: Beriberi Heart Disease: Physiologic Data and Difficulties in Diagnosis, *Am. Heart J.,* 69:200, 1965.
37. Allemn, R. J., and Stollerman, G. H.: The Course of Beriberi Heart Disease in American Prisoners-of-War in Japan, *Ann. Intern. Med.,* 28:949, 1948.
38. Sament, S.: Cardiac Disorders in Scurvy, *N. Engl. J. Med.,* 282:282, 1970.
39. Mulvaney, D. A., and Seronde, J., Jr.: Electrocardiographic Changes in Vitamin B_6 Deficient Rats, *Cardiovasc. Res.,* 13:506, 1979.
40. Bauer, J. M., and Freyberg, R. H.: Vitamin D Intoxication with Metastatic Calcification, *JAMA,* 130:1208, 1946.
41. Taylor, C. B., Peng, S. K., Tham, P., and Mikkelson, B.: Influence of Mild Excesses of Vitamin D_3 on Arterial Wall and Its Role in Arteriosclerosis, *Arterial Wall,* 4:229, 1978.
42. Keshan Disease Research Group of the Chinese Academy of Medical Sciences, Beijing: Epidemiologic Studies on the Etiological Relationship of Selenium and Keshan Disease, *Chinese Med. J.,* 92:477, 1979.
43. Van Vleet, J. F., Ferrans, V. J., and Ruth, G. R.: Ultrastructural Alterations in Nutritional Cardiomyopathy of Selenium–Vitamin E Deficient Swine: I. Fiber Lesions, *Lab. Invest.,* 37:188, 1977.
44. Keys, A., Brozek, J., Henschel, A., Mikelsen, O., and Taylor, H.: "The Biology of Human Starvation," University of Minnesota Press, Minneapolis, 1950, p. 607.
45. Heymsfield, S. B., Bethel, R. A., Ansley, J. D., Gibbs, D. M., Felner, J. M., and Nutter, D. O.: Cardiac Abnormalities in Cachectic Patients before and during Nutritional Repletion, *Am. Heart J.,* 95:584, 1978.
46. Gottdiener, J. S., Gross, H. A., Henry, W. L., Borer, J. S., and Ebert, M. H.: Effects of Self-Induced Starvation on Cardiac Size and Function in Anorexia Nervosa, *Circulation,* 58:425, 1978.
47. Piza, J., Troper, L., Cespedes, R., Miller, J. H., and Berenson, G. S.: Myocardial Lesions and Heart Failure in Infantile Malnutrition, *Am. J. Trop. Med. Hyg.,* 20:343, 1971.
48. Figueras, J., Singh, B. N., Ganz, W., and Swan, H. J. C.: Hemodynamic and Electrocardiographic Accompaniments of Resting Postprandial Angina, *Br. Heart J.,* 42:402, 1979.
49. Kuo, P. T., and Joyner, C. R., Jr.: Angina Pectoris Induced by Fat Ingestion in Patients with Coronary Artery Disease: Ballistocardiographic and Electrocardiographic Findings, *JAMA,* 153:1008, 1955.
50. Regan, T. J., Binak, K., Gordon, S., DeFazio, V., and Hellems, H. K.: Myocardial Blood Flow and Oxygen Consumption during Postprandial Lipemia and Heparin-Induced Lipolysis, *Circulation,* 23:55, 1961.
51. Bistrian, B. R., Blackburn, G. L., Vitale, J., Cochran, D., and Naylor, J.: Prevalence of Malnutrition in General Medical Patients, *JAMA,* 235:1567, 1976.
52. Abel, R. M., Fischer, J. E., Buckley, M. J., Barnett, G. O., and Austen, W. G.: Malnutrition in Cardiac Surgical Patients: Results of a Prospective Randomized Evaluation of Early Postoperative Parenteral Nutrition, *Arch. Surg.,* 111:45, 1976.
53. O'Connor, L. R., Wheeler, W. A. S., and Bethune, J. E.: Effect of Hypophosphatemia on Myocardial Performance in Man, *N. Engl. J. Med.,* 297:901, 1977.
54. Venditti, F., Panezai, F., Marotta, C., et al.: Hypophosphatemia and Cardiac Arrhythmias, *Clin. Res.,* 31:223A, 1983. (Abstract.)
55. Wharton, B. A., Balmer, S. E., Somers, K., and Templeton, A. C.: The Myocardium in Kwashiorkor, *Q. J. Med.,* 38:107, 1969.

75

The Heart and Obesity

James K. Alexander, M.D.

Sudden death is more common in those who are naturally fat than in the lean.

Hippocrates[1]

Although a predisposition to circulatory disorders with obesity has long been recognized, it is noteworthy that the mechanisms underlying this relationship are at best only partially defined. In this chapter, potential linkages between obesity and hypertension, coronary heart disease, cardiomyopathy, and cor pulmonale are reviewed, with some background information on adipose tissue circulation and observations on therapy.

Adipose Tissue Circulation

Although adipose tissue is an active metabolic organ, oxygen delivery under resting conditions in human beings necessitates a blood flow of only 2 to 3 ml/min per 100 g as indicated by inert gas washout techniques, or less than one-twentieth that of the brain.[2]

Nonetheless, of considerable importance is the degree to which adipose tissue serves as a blood volume reservoir and to which lipocyte metabolism is flow-dependent. With hemorrhage-induced hypotension in dogs, the decrement in adipose tissue blood volume and flow is much greater than that in other organs, and adipose tissue oxygen uptake falls concomitantly.[3] In addition to metabolic demands and circulating blood volume, a variety of factors may produce profound hemodynamic alterations in the adipose tissue vascular bed, including sympathetic nervous influences, humoral agents, blood and tissue oxygen tension, blood pH, temperature, exercise, and mechanical compression.[4] Since adipose tissue blood flow is a function of both cell number and size,[5] increments in adipose depot volume secondary to either cellular hyperplasia or hypertrophy are accompanied by augmented flow. In extremely obese subjects, for example, in whom both hyperplasia and hypertrophy exist, adipose tissue flow may approximate one-half the total cardiac output at rest.[6] Weight loss involves reduction in adipocyte cell size but not number in obese subjects. Thus cardiac output falls as regression of adipocyte hypertrophy lowers total adipose tissue weight and flow,[7] while flow per kilogram adipose tissue actually increases due to increased adipocyte number.[8]

Obesity and Hypertension

The association of hypertension with obesity has long been established. In a survey of more than 1 million persons screened by the Community Hypertension Evaluation Clinic program across the United States from 1973 to 1975, a significantly increased prevalence of hypertension with overweight was found in all age groups, for men and women, whites and blacks, independent of family history.[9] The prevalence rate of hypertension in overweight subjects averaged 100 percent above that for underweight or normal weight subjects 20 to 30 years old, and 50 percent above that for the age group 40 to 64. A correlation between body bulk, skin fold thickness, or calculated body fat and blood pressure is demonstrable in obese young adults.[10,11] However, this correlation tends to disappear after middle age, while change in weight, that is, weight gain over the long term, assumes the predominant role in the development of sustained hypertension associated with obesity.[12] Despite this association, surveys of large numbers of hypertensive patients indicate that the impact of obesity as a risk factor for hypertension is modest.[13,14]

That the mechanism(s) of obesity hypertension differs from those of essential or renovascular hypertension is suggested by the observations that (1) measurements of blood volume and renin levels in obese subjects do not correlate with the presence or absence of hypertension,[15,16] (2) systemic vascular resistance is less in obese than in lean hypertensives,[15,16] (3) weight loss effects a reduction in blood pressure of obese hypertensives despite unrestricted dietary salt intake in the normal range.[17] Currently the etiopathogenesis of obesity hypertension is unknown. For several hypotheses advanced, involving elevated aldosterone levels, altered response to pressor agents, mechanical capillary compression in adipose depots, and elevated blood insulin levels, there is no firm supporting evidence.[18,19] In addition, some explanation must be found for the fact that most obese people are not hypertensive, and even with extreme obesity one-third are normotensive.[10,15]

Direct intraarterial pressure measurements indicate that hypertension is not artifactual in obese subjects.[20,21] Although large arm circumference usually results in overestimation of systolic and diastolic blood pressures by the indirect cuff method, in obese subjects there is no correlation between measurements obtained by the direct intraarterial and indirect cuff methods based solely on arm circumference.[20] Furthermore, in any sizable series, significant discrepancies of both and over- and underestimation are found, unpredictable on the basis of arm circumference or blood pressure level. Nevertheless, a reasonable approximation of blood pressure level may be obtained when the degree of obesity is not extreme, utilizing a cuff containing a bladder 42 cm in length. In very obese individuals with unusual arm configuration, difficulty in wearing the cuff, or inconsistent readings, direct intraarterial measurement is recommended before prolonged antihypertensive therapy is initiated.[20,21]

Although weight reduction does not always bring about normotension in obese hypertensives, a favorable effect may be expected in about one-half such cases regardless of age or relative weight.[22] Modest weight loss is often associated with significantly reduced blood pressure.[23] Maintenance of lowered weight makes for a stable reduction in pressure, whereas regain of weight is frequently accompanied by return of hypertension.[24] There appears to be no information regarding the effect of weight reduction on the incidence of cardiovascular complications in obese hypertensives. Long-term follow-up studies indicate that the mortality among obese hypertensives is significantly lower than among nonobese hypertensives.[25,26]

Obesity and Coronary Heart Disease

Excess mortality rate associated with overweight more than 30 to 40 percent above the norm (largely due to various manifestations of cardiovascular disease) is well documented.[27,28] However, a great preponderance of evidence based on epidemiologic, pathological, and angiographic studies indicates that obesity (increased adipose tissue), as distinct from overweight, is not an independent risk factor for coronary heart disease. Utilizing the ^{3}H-dilution method to quantitate body fat, and correlating coronary heart disease and its various associated risk factors to obesity, the contribution of obesity per se to coronary disease is small or nonexistent, whereas serum cholesterol and systolic blood pressure are potent risk factors.[29] Large-scale epidemiologic studies with long-term follow-up using skin fold thickness or other indexes of obesity have supported the same conclusions.[30,31] Autopsy studies on the incidence and severity of coronary atherosclerosis in persons dying of accidental cause in different ethnic and geographic groups show no effect of obesity on the extent of atherosclerosis,[32] and coronary angiographic investigations of the extent of disease versus relative body weight are confirmatory.[33,34] Of interest is the observation that in extremely obese subjects virtually no coronary atheroma is found at postmortem examination.[35] Although numerous possibilities have been explored, it appears at present that the principal link between coronary disease and marked obesity is the extent to which the latter predisposes to hypertension.[36]

In men, no effect of obesity (relative weight greater than 20 percent of "ideal") can be demonstrated in early or late mortality rates after myocardial infarction,[37,38] but obese women appear to be at greater risk for early recurrence.[39] A recent large-scale survey has indicated a significantly elevated in-hospital postinfarction mortality rate of 43 percent in obese diabetic women, associated with frequent congestive heart failure.[40] Obesity does not emerge as a risk factor for sudden death due to coronary disease.[41] As regards stable angina pectoris in obese subjects, decrements in body weight greater than 20 percent may be required for symptomatic improvement.[42] In obese persons with coronary disease subject to sleep apnea, serious arrhythmias may occur, disappearing on reversal of the apneic syndrome with weight loss.[43,44]

The Cardiomyopathy of Obesity

It is now well-established that in morbidly obese individuals there may develop a syndrome of chronic circulatory congestion associated with diastolic and sometimes systolic left ventricular dysfunction.[36] Its pathological, physiological, and clinical features appear sufficiently distinctive to warrant its characterization as *obesity cardiomyopathy*.

In the first systematic effort to evaluate cardiac anatomy at necropsy, Smith and Willius in 1933 reported four cases of congestive heart failure in markedly obese subjects without evidence of hypertension or other cardiovascular disease.[45] These authors found a roughly linear increment in heart weight with increasing body weight, so that in a series of 135 overweight patients the average heart weight of the men was 444 g, 150 g greater than the predicted weight at comparable height, and for women 345 g, 95 g more than the predicted. Subsequent postmortem studies have demonstrated that the increased heart weight of obese subjects is largely due to left ventricular hypertrophy, sometimes with right ventricular hypertrophy as well, and that congestive heart failure is a frequent finding with extreme obesity at autopsy.[35,46] Although not specific for obesity, and usually without significant functional consequence, fatty infiltration of the myocardium (usually the right ventricle) may develop in some obese subjects, occasionally with involvement of the conduction system.[47–49]

Appraisal of circulatory dynamics in morbidly obese patients indicates that abnormal hemodynamic patterns antedate the development of frank congestive failure for many years. Plasma and circulating blood volumes in very obese subjects are both increased as compared to volumes in subjects at ideal weight. Hematocrit tends to be normal or slightly increased. The increment in blood volume is correlated with the amount of excess body weight, reflecting an increase in the size of the vascular bed. When the body weight is 100 kg in excess of the ideal, for example, the blood volume is 10 liters, or about twice that predicted for the ideal weight.[6] Augmentation of blood volume is paralleled by an increment in cardiac output, also correlated with the amount of excess body weight.[6] Since resting heart rate is normal or only slightly increased, high cardiac output is effected by a large stroke volume. Systemic arteriovenous difference is only modestly widened. Therefore, cardiac output increases largely in proportion to body oxygen consumption, which in turn increases in proportion to body weight.[50] In the absence of frank congestive failure, increases in cardiac output with exercise in very obese subjects are comparable to those in subjects at ideal weight.[51]

Studies on the regional distribution of blood flow in the high-cardiac-output state of obesity indicate that cerebral blood flow per unit brain weight is normal. Since no change in brain weight occurs with obesity, total cerebral flow is also in the normal range.[6] Renal blood flow is normal or slightly reduced in obese subjects when compared to predicted flow at ideal body weight.[6] By contrast, splanchnic flow in obesity is high compared with that at predicted ideal weight. However, the increases in splanchnic flow, ranging up to 800 ml/min in very obese subjects, are by no means sufficient to account for the increments in cardiac output in these same individuals, which reach levels as high as 5 liters/min.[6] The absence of significant changes in organ blood flow suggests that the increment in resting cardiac output with extreme obesity is largely distributed to fat tissue depots.

Heart catheterization studies indicate that there is a high incidence of hemodynamic alterations in extremely obese persons. About 75 percent of these subjects have pulmonary hypertension at rest or during exercise, with elevated systemic pressure in the majority of cases.[7,15] Left ventricular end-diastolic pressure is elevated at rest or during exercise, resulting in pulmonary hypertension usually without a transpulmonary diastolic pressure gradient.[7,52]

Further insight into the pathogenesis of congestive failure in morbidly obese patients is provided by recent echocardiographic studies.[53] In concordance with pathological studies, eccentric hypertrophy of varying degree is demonstrable involving the left ventricular septum and free wall. Indexes of left ventricular systolic performance such as ejection fraction and velocity of circumferential fiber shortening may be normal or depressed. Further analysis of the data demonstrates that the ratio of diastolic cavity radius to wall thickness is increased in patients with compromised ventricular systolic function, indicating an elevated ventricular wall tension. However, in those subjects with preserved left ventricular systolic performance, the ratio of diastolic cavity radius to wall thickness is normal, consistent with normal wall tension. Characteristically, failure of the left ventricle occurs in the presence of elevated wall tension, thought to be secondary to "inadequate" hypertrophy.[54] Thus, as long as myocardial hypertrophy parallels pressure and volume changes in the ventricle, systolic performance will be well maintained; but when hypertrophy is not adequate to maintain a normal wall tension, this signals depressed function. Whether left ventricular systolic dysfunction develops or not, these patients have left ventricular diastolic dysfunction caused by left ventricular hypertrophy and diminished diastolic chamber compliance.[53,55] Thus, exercise or any state tending to increase venous return to the heart will tend to make for elevated left ventricular filling pressure and will predispose to pulmonary congestion. A central congestive state in very obese patients is indicated by a decreasing ratio of central blood volume to left ventricular diastolic pressure (an index of distensibility) as total blood volume increases.[52]

Therefore, two mechanisms appear to operate in the pathogenesis of recurrent bouts of circulatory congestion in patients with chronic severe exogenous obesity. In one group of patients, pulmonary and systemic vascular congestion develop as a consequence of chronic volume overload superimposed upon the effect of diminished diastolic ventricular compliance caused by ventricular hypertrophy. Left ventricular systolic performance is preserved in this group, and the symptoms and signs of pulmonary and systemic congestion are secondary to diastolic dysfunction alone. In the other group, chronic volume overload and high cardiac output with or without accompanying hypertension result in myocardial hypertrophy which is inadequate, such that the wall thickness/cavity radius ratio is reduced, ventricular wall stress is elevated, and left ventricular systolic dysfunction is superimposed. The prognosis for those with normal left ventricular systolic performance appears to be better than for those with disordered systolic function. Indeed, it is not unusual for patients with preserved left ventricular systolic performance to present with recurrent bouts of pulmonary and systemic congestion for many years (Fig. 75-1). Since the clinical presentation in these two groups may be essentially the same, differentiation will usually require appraisal of left ventricular systolic function by echocardiographic, radionuclide, or angiographic techniques.

Limited observations suggest that the prevalence of congestive heart failure in extremely obese subjects is about 10 percent.[56] However, in a longitudinal sense it may be much more commonly encountered, since it appears to be present at autopsy more often than not.[35] Body weight is usually twice the predicted norm or more, and rapid weight gain may precipitate or exacerbate congestive symptoms. Progressively increasing dyspnea and orthopnea are characteristic, whereas acute pulmonary edema is uncommon. The terminal phase is sometimes char-

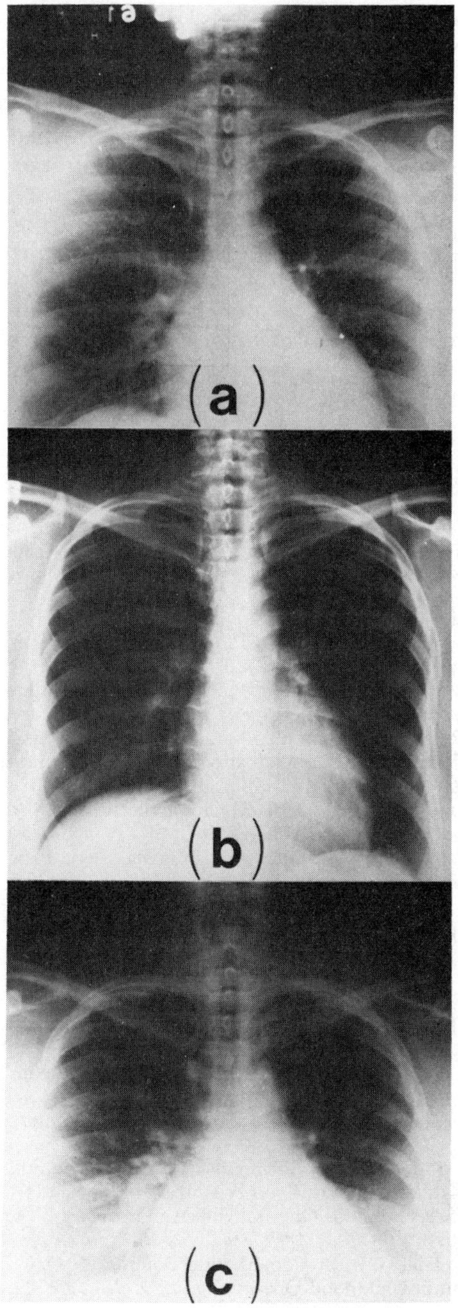

FIGURE 75-1 Chest films of a woman first presenting with severe pulmonary and systemic congestion at age 29, weight 184 kg (*a*). At age 31, weight reduction to 157 kg was associated with decrements in heart size and pulmonary congestion (*b*). Recurrence of cardiomegaly and pulmonary congestion attended regain of weight at age 37 (*c*). At age 43, weight 195 kg, echocardiogram demonstrated normal left ventricular systolic performance, with ejection fraction 64 percent, mean velocity of circumferential fiber shortening 1.36 circ/s. Left ventricular septal and posterior wall thicknesses were increased to 1.7 and 2.0 cm, respectively, and EF slope was reduced to 30 mm/s, suggesting reduced left ventricular compliance. Left atrial dimension was enlarged to 5.2 cm. By age 48 atrial fibrillation had developed. [*From J. K. Alexander, The Cardiomyopathy of Obesity, Prog. Cardiovasc. Dis., 27(5):325, 1985. Reproduced with permission from Grune & Stratton, Inc., and the author.*]

acterized by rapid weight gain due to fluid retention, with increasing somnolence, mental confusion, and coma.[35] Frequent occurrence of sudden death is well documented by case reports.[57] Hypertension may or may not be present. Presystolic gallop rhythm may be heard, but cardiac murmurs are usually absent. Frequent electrocardiographic findings include left deviation of the QRS axis in the frontal plane,[58] or low-voltage, right axis deviation and P pulmonale.[59] Despite gross anatomic involvement, electrocardiographic evidences of left ventricular hypertrophy are absent.[36] Recurrent bouts of congestion predispose to the development of atrial fibrillation or flutter,[60] in association with left atrial enlargement[61] (Fig. 75-1). Conduction defects secondary to fatty infiltration of the conduction system are probably implicated in the predisposition to sudden death.[48,49]

Sleep Apnea and Obesity Hypoventilation Syndrome

Although sleep apnea occurs in a variety of clinical settings, somewhat more than 50 percent of patients so afflicted are obese.[62,63] They are usually men, 40 to 60 years of age, with degrees of obesity varying from moderate to extreme. Daytime hypersomnia is frequent. Significant increases in systemic and pulmonary artery pressures occur cyclically during apnea, and with a rapid succession of apneic spells there may be a progressive rise in both.[64] Apnea may be accompanied by decrements in arterial O_2 tension to 50 mmHg or less, with moderate increases in CO_2 tension. Cardiac arrhythmias are frequent during apnea, involving sinus arrest, asystole up to 6 s, heart block, and ventricular tachycardia.[65] Thus, the potential for sudden death in these patients is clear.[43] All of the hemodynamic and arrhythmic effects induced by sleep apnea may be reversed in some cases by tracheostomy, and when hypertension coexists, blood pressure may fall to or toward normal.[64,65]

A syndrome of hypoventilation, cyanosis, and somnolence, with resultant chronic hypoxemia, hypercapnia, respiratory acidosis, and polycythemia occurs in about 5 percent of extremely obese persons.[56,57] The sequence of physiological events leading to the obesity hypoventilation syndrome is initiated by the development of sleep apnea.[66] Transient bouts of hypoxia with apnea eventually cause blunting of the hypoxic ventilatory drive, and in conjunction with diminished chest wall compliance and increased respiratory work, a reduced ventilatory response to CO_2 as well. Chronic hypoxemia and hypercapnia stimulate pulmonary vasoconstriction, so that the effects of augmented pulmonary vascular resistance are superimposed upon the underlying hemodynamic derangements of severe obesity, namely, increased pulmonary blood volume and flow, with left atrial hypertension. Thus, a transpulmonary diastolic pressure gradient may exist in conjunction with elevated pulmonary venous pressure.[52] As a consequence, biventricular hypertrophy with pulmonary and systemic congestion characterizes the clinical and postmortem picture,[36] though occasionally right-sided involvement may predominate. Hypoventilation is reversible with weight reduction, and the attendant improvement in arterial blood gases is associated with a fall in pulmonary artery pressure and reduction or elimination of the transpulmonary diastolic pressure gradient.[52] Several case reports document the disappearance of P pulmonale, T-wave inversion in leads V_1 to V_3, and right axis deviation after weight reduction in the electrocardiograms of obese subjects with hypoventilation syndrome.[59,60,67]

Therapeutic Considerations and Weight Reduction

Diuretic therapy is the most urgently indicated measure in the management of the obesity congestive state, together with judicious use of oxygen. Though cardioversion may be considered in an emergency setting, rapid ventricular rate in the presence of atrial fibrillation or flutter is usually controlled satisfactorily with digitalis administration. Early appraisal of left ventricular function by echocardiogram or radionuclide study may be helpful with regard to determining the need for an inotropic agent, as well as the potential for use of beta blockade or calcium antagonists to control arrhythmia. Since there is no evidence of altered Na-K-ATPase (adenosine triphosphatase) activity with obesity,[68] and serum levels relate to lean body mass rather than total-body weight,[69] higher digoxin dosage based on body weight may result in toxicity. Vasodilator therapy is indicated for control of severe hypertension and may be useful in the setting of left ventricular systolic dysfunction with elevated blood pressure or pulmonary hypertension. Although there are no studies specifically examining its efficacy in very obese congested subjects, considering the relatively high incidence of venous thrombophlebitis and pulmonary embolism, use of low-dose heparin prophylaxis would seem reasonable.

Low-calorie sodium-restricted regimens appear to be just as effective as fasting for weight reduction, and less hazardous. Ventricular fibrillation may result from potassium depletion with fasting, sometimes preceded by QT prolongation, lactic acidosis, or ventricular dysfunction.[70–73] Experimental and clinical studies indicate that marked dietary caloric restriction or fasting leads to diminished sympathetic nervous system activity, which, together with natriuresis and contraction of plasma volume, may provoke postural hypotension, dizziness, and syncope.[74–77]

The hemodynamic alterations accompanying obesity are largely reversible with weight reduction. Decrements in body oxygen consumption, blood volume, and cardiac output are proportional to the amount of weight loss. Blood volume and cardiac output fall approximately 30 ml and 30 ml/min per kilogram weight loss, respectively.[7] Oxygen consumption, cardiac output, and stroke volume during exercise are less for the same workload after weight reduction.[78]

However, persistent elevation of left ventricular filling pressure with exercise suggests that myocardial hypertrophy may not regress over periods as long as 3 years following weight reduction.[7]

References

1. Chadwick, J., and Mann, W. N.: "The Medical Works of Hippocrates," Aphorisms, sect. II, 44, Charles C Thomas, Springfield, Ill., 1950, p. 154.
2. Nielsen, S. L.: Measurement of Blood Flow in Adipose Tissue from the Washout of Xenon-133 after Atraumatic Labelling, *Acta Physiol. Scand.*, 84:187, 1972.
3. Kovach, A. G., Rossell, S., Sandar, P., Koltay, E., Kovach, E., and Tomka, N.: Blood Flow, Oxygen Consumption and Free Fatty Acid Release in Subcutaneous Adipose Tissue during Hemorrhagic Shock in Control and Phenoxybenzamine-Treated Dogs, *Circ. Res.*, 25/26(suppl. 6):733, 1970.
4. Rossell, S., and Belfrage, E.: Blood Circulation in Adipose Tissue, *Physiol. Rev.*, 59(4):1078, 1979.
5. DiGirolamo, M., and Eposito, J.: Adipose Tissue Blood Flow and Cellularity in the Growing Rabbit, *Am. J. Physiol.*, 299:107, 1975.
6. Alexander, J. K., Dennis, E. W., Smith, W. G., Amad, K. H., Duncan, W. C., and Austin, R. C.: Blood Volume, Cardiac Output and Distribution of Systemic Blood Flow in Extreme Obesity, *Cardiovasc. Res. Cent. Bull.*, 1:39, 1962.
7. Alexander, J. D., and Peterson, K. L.: Cardiovascular Effects of Weight Reduction, *Circulation*, 45:310, 1972.
8. Nielsen, S. L., and Larsen, O.: Relationship of Subcutaneous Adipose Tissue Blood Flow to Thickness of Subcutaneous Tissue and Total Body Fat Mass, *Scand. J. Clin. Lab. Invest.*, 31:383, 1973.
9. Stamler, R., Stamler, J., Riedlinger, W. F., Algera, G., and Roberts, R. H.: Weight and Blood Pressure: Findings in Hypertension Screening of One Million Americans, *JAMA*, 240:1607, 1978.
10. Court, J. M., Hill, G. J., Dunlop, M., and Boulton, T. O. C.: Hypertension in Childhood Obesity, *Am. J. Cardiol.*, 35:523, 1975.
11. Evans, J. G., and Rose, G.: Hypertension, *Br. Med. Bull.*, 27:73, 1971.
12. Abraham, S., Collins, G., and Nordsieck, M.: Relationship of Childhood Weight Status to Morbidity in Adults, *Health Services and Mental Health Administration Health Rep.*, 86:273, 1971.
13. Kannel, W., Brand, N., Skinner, J., Dawber, T., and McNamara, P.: Relation of Adiposity to Blood Pressure and Development of Hypertension: The Framingham Study, *Ann. Intern. Med.*, 67:48, 1967.
14. Keys, A.: Coronary Heart Disease in Seven Countries, *Circulation*, 4(4)(suppl. 1), 1970.
15. Alexander, J. K.: Obesity and the Circulation, *Mod. Concepts Cardiovasc. Dis.*, 32:799, 1963.
16. Messerli, F. H., Christie, B., DeCarvalho, J. G. R., Aristimuno, G. G., Suraz, D. H., Dreslinski, G. R., and Frohlich, E. D.: Obesity and Essential Hypertension: Hemodynamics, Intravascular Volume, Sodium Excretion, and Plasma Renin Activity, *Arch. Intern. Med.*, 141:81, 1981.
17. Reisin, E., Able, R., Modal, M., et al.: Effect of Weight Loss

without Salt Restriction of the Reduction of Blood Pressure in Overweight Hypertensive Patients, *N. Engl. J. Med.*, 198:1, 1979.
18. Sims, E. A. H., Phiney, S. D., and Waswani, A.: The Management of Hypertension Associated with Obesity, *Int. J. Obesity*, 3:215, 1978.
19. Simmons, V. P.: Circulatory Pathophysiology: I. The Role of Capillary Compression in the Etiology of Essential (Idiopathic) Hypertension, *J. Insurance Med.*, 12(2):2, 1981.
20. Kvols, L. K., Rohlfing, B. M., and Alexander, J. K.: A Comparison of Intraarterial and Cuff Blood Pressure Measurements in Very Obese Subjects, *Cardiovasc. Res. Cent. Bull.*, 7:118, 1969.
21. Nielsen, P. E., and Janniche, H.: The Accuracy of Auscultatory Measurement of Arm Blood Pressure in Very Obese Subjects, *Acta Med. Scand.*, 195:403, 1974.
22. Ashley, F. W., Jr., and Kannel, W. B.: Relation of Weight Change to Changes in Atherogenic Traits: The Framingham Study, *J. Chronic Dis.*, 27:103, 1974.
23. Greminger, P., Studer, A., Luscher, T., Mutter, B., Grimm, J., Siegenthaler, W., and Vetter, W.: Gewichstreduktion und Blutdruck, *Schweiz. Med. Wocheuschr.*, 112:120, 1982.
24. Adlersberg, D., Coler, H., and Laval, J.: Effect of Weight Reduction on Course of Arterial Hypertension, *J. Mt. Sinai Hosp.*, 12:984, 1946.
25. Frant, R., and Groen, J.: Prognosis of Vascular Hypertension: A Nine-Year Follow-Up Study of Four Hundred and Eighteen Cases, *Arch. Intern. Med.*, 85:727, 1950.
26. Sokolow, M., and Perloff, D.: The Prognosis of Essential Hypertension Treated Conservatively, *Circulation*, 23:697, 1961.
27. Keys, A.: Overweight, Obesity, Coronary Heart Disease and Mortality, *Nutr. Rev.*, 38:197, 1980.
28. Sorlie, P., Gordon, T., and Kannel, W. B.: Body Build and Mortality: The Framingham Study, *JAMA*, 243:1828, 1980.
29. Weinsier, R. L., Fuchs, R. J., Kay, T. D., Triebwasser, J. H., and Lancaster, M. C.: Body Fat: Its Relationship to Coronary Heart Disease, Blood Pressure, Lipids and Other Risk Factors Measured in a Large Male Population, *Am. J. Med.*, 61(6):815, 1976.
30. Kannel, W. B., and Gordon, T.: Physiological and Medical Concomitants of Obesity and the Framingham Study, in G. A. Bray (ed.),"Obesity in America," NIH Publication no. 79-359:135, 1979.
31. Keys, A.: "Seven Countries: A Multivariate Analysis of Death and Coronary Heart Disease," Harvard University Press, Cambridge, 1980.
32. Montenegro, M. R., and Solberg, L. A.: Obesity, Body Weight, Body Length and Artherosclerosis, *Lab. Invest.*, 18:594, 1968.
33. Cramer, K., Paulin, S., and Werko, L.: Coronary Angiographic Findings in Correlation with Age, Body Weight, Blood Pressure, Serum Lipids and Smoking Habits, *Circ. Res.*, 33:888, 1966.
34. Anderson, A. J., Barboriak, J. J., and Rimm, A. A.: Risk Factors and Angiographically Determined Coronary Occlusion, *Am. J. Epidemiol.*, 107(1):8, 1978.
35. Alexander, J. K., and Pettigrove, J. R.: Obesity and Congestive Heart Failure, *Geriatrics*, 22:101, 1967.
36. Alexander, J. K.: Obesity and the Heart, *Curr. Prob. Cardiol.*, 5(3), 1980.
37. Pell, S., and D'Alonso, C.: A Three-Year Study of Myocardial Infarction in a Large Employed Population, *JAMA*, 175:463, 1961.
38. Frank, C. W., Weinblatt, E., Shapiro, S., and Sager, R. V.: Physical Inactivity as a Lethal Factor in Myocardial Infarction among Men, *Circulation*, 34:1022, 1966.
39. Marmor, A., Sobel, B. E., and Roberts, R.: Factors Presaging Early Recurrent Myocardial Infarction ("Extension"), *Am. J. Cardiol.*, 48:603, 1981.
40. Tansey, M. J., Opie, L. H., and Kennally, B. M.: High Mortality in Obese Women Diabetics with Acute Myocardial Infarction, *Br. Med. J.*, 1:1624, 1977.
41. Romo, M., and Ruosteeuoja, R.: Sudden Coronary Death: Incidence and Common Risk Factors, *Adv. Cardiol.*, 25:1, 1978.
42. Sharma, B., Thadami, U., and Taylor, S. H.: Cardiovascular Effects of Weight Reduction in Obese Patients with Angina Pectoris, *Br. Heart J.*, 74:36, 1974.
43. Kryger, M., Quesney, L. P., Holder, D., Gloor, P., and Macleod, P.: The Sleep Deprivation Syndrome of the Obese Patient, *Am. J. Med.*, 56:531, 1974.
44. Shaw, T. R. D., Carroll, R. J. M., and Craib, I. A.: Cardiac and Respiratory Standstill during Sleep, *Br. Heart J.*, 40:1055, 1978.
45. Smith, H. L., and Willius, F. A.: Adiposity of the Heart, *Arch. Intern. Med.*, 52:911, 1933.
46. Amad, R. H., Brennan, J. C., and Alexander, J. K.: The Cardiac Pathology of Chronic Exogenous Obesity, *Circulation*, 32:740, 1965.
47. Spain, D. M., and Cathcart, R. T.: Heart Block Caused by Fat Infiltration of the Interventricular Septum ("Cor Adiposum"), *Am. Heart J.*, 32:659, 1946.
48. Balsaver, A. M., Morales, A. R., and Whitehouse, F. W.: Fat Infiltration of Myocardium as a Cause of Cardiac Conduction Defect, *Am. J. Cardiol.*, 19:216, 1967.
49. James, T. N., Frame, B., and Coates, E. O.: De Subitaneis Mortibus: III. Pickwickian Syndrome, *Circulation*, 48:1311, 1973.
50. White, R. I., and Alexander, J. K.: Body Oxygen Consumption and Pulmonary Ventilation in Obese Subjects, *J. Appl. Physiol.*, 20:197, 1965.
51. Alexander, J. K.: Obesity and Cardiac Performance, *Am. J. Cardiol.*, 14:860, 1964.
52. Kaltman, A. J., and Goldring, R. M.: Role of Circulatory Congestion in the Cardiorespiratory Failure of Obesity, *Am. J. Med.*, 60:645, 1976.
53. Alexander, J. K., Woodard, C. B., Quinones, M. A., and Gaasch, W. H.: Heart Failure from Obesity, in M. Mancini, B. Lewis, and F. Cantaldo (eds.), "Medical Complications of Obesity," Academic Press, London, 1978.
54. Ford, L. E.: Heart Size, *Circ. Res.*, 39:297, 1976.
55. Wilcken, D. E.: Left Ventricular Volume in Man: The Relation to Heart Rate and to End-Diastolic Pressure, *Aust. Ann. Med.*, 17(suppl. 3):195, 1968.
56. Alexander, J. K., Amad, K., and Cole, V. W.: Observations on Some Clinical Features of Extreme Obesity with Particular Reference to Cardiorespiratory Effects, *Am. J. Med.*, 32:512, 1962.
57. MacGregor, M. I., Block, A. J., and Ball, W. C., Jr.: Serious Complications and Sudden Death in the Pickwickian Syndrome, *Johns Hopkins Med. J.*, 126:279, 1970.
58. Axelrad, M. A., and Alexander, J. K.: The Electrocardiogram and Cardiac Anatomy in Obesity, *Clin. Res.*, 13:25, 1965.
59. Lillington, G. A., Anderson, M. A., and Brandenburg, R. O.: The Cardio-Respiratory Syndrome of Obesity, *Dis. Chest*, 32:1, 1957.
60. Estes, E. H., Jr., Sieker, H. O., McIntosh, H. D., and Kelser, G. A.: Reversible Cardiopulmonary Syndrome with Extreme Obesity, *Circulation*, 16:179, 1957.
61. Cueto Garcia, L., Laredo, C., Arriaga, J., and Gonzalez Barranco, J.: Echocardiographic Findings in Obesity, *Rev. Invest. Clin. (Mex.)*, 34:235, 1982.
62. Guilleminault, C., Tilkian, A., and Dement, W. C.: The Sleep Apnea Syndromes, *Ann. Rev. Med.*, 27:465, 1976.
63. Weitzman, E. D.: The Syndrome of Hypersomnia and Sleep-Induced Apnea, *Chest*, 75:414, 1979.
64. Schroeder, J. S., Motta, J., and Guilleminault, C.: Hemodynamic Studies in Sleep Apnea, in C. Guilleminault and W. C. Dement (eds.), "Sleep Syndromes," Alan R. Liss, New York, 1978.
65. Tilkian, A., Motta, J., and Guilleminault, C.: Cardiac Arrhythmias in Sleep Apnea Syndromes," Alan R. Liss, New York, 1978.
66. Sharp, J. T., Barrocas, M., and Chokroverty, S.: The Cardiorespiratory Effects of Obesity, *Clin. Chest Med.*, 1:103, 1980.
67. Cayler, G. G., Mays, J., and Riley, H. D., Jr.: Cardiorespiratory Syndrome of Obesity (Pickwickian Syndrome) in Children, *Pediatrics*, 27:237, 1961.
68. Beutler, E., Kuhl, W., and Sacks, P.: Sodium-Potassium-

ATPase Activity Is Influenced by Ethnic Origin and Not by Obesity, *N. Engl. J. Med.*, 309:756, 1983.
69. Ewy, G. A., Groves, B. M., Ball, M. F., Mimmo, L., Jackson, B., and Marcus, F.: Digoxin Metabolism in Obesity, *Circulation*, 33:810, 1971.
70. Cubberly, P. T., Polster, S. A., and Schulman, C. L.: Lactic Acidosis and Death after Treatment of Obesity by Fasting, *N. Engl. J. Med.*, 272:628, 1965.
71. Spencer, I. O. B.: Death during Therapeutic Starvation for Obesity, *Lancet*, 1:1288, 1968.
72. Garnett, E. S., Barnard, D. L., Ford, J., Goodbody, R. A., and Woodehouse, J. A.: Gross Fragmentation of Cardiac Myofibrils after Therapeutic Starvation for Obesity, *Lancet*, 1:914, 1969.
73. Sandhofer, F., Dienstl, F., Bolzano, K., and Schwingshackl, H.: Severe Cardiovascular Complication Associated with Prolonged Starvation, *Br. Med J.*, 1:462, 1973.
74. Sigler, M. H.: The Mechanism of the Natriuresis of Fasting, *J. Clin. Invest.*, 55:377, 1975.
75. Landsberg, L., and Young, J. B.: Fasting, Feeding, and Regulation of the Sympathetic Nervous System, *N. Engl. J. Med.*, 298:1295, 1978.
76. Jung, R. T., Shetty, P. S., Barrand, M., Callingham, B. A., and James, W. P. T.: Role of Catecholamines in Hypotensive Response to Dieting, *Br. Med. J.*, 1:12, 1979.
77. DeHaven, J., Sherwin, R., Hendler, R., and Felig, P.: Nitrogen and Sodium Balance and Sympathetic-Nervous System Activity in Obese Subjects Treated With a Low Calorie Protein or Mixed Diet, *N. Engl. J. Med.*, 302:477, 1980.
78. Backman, L., Freyschuss, U., Hallberg, D., and Melcher, A.: Reversibility of Cardiovascular Changes in Extreme Obesity, *Acta. Med. Scand.*, 205:367, 1979.

76

The Heart and Chronic Renal Failure

Susan K. Fellner, M.D.

Control of extracellular fluid volume; regulation of serum osmolality through urinary dilution and concentration; reabsorption and secretion of electrolytes; participation in acid-base balance; and secretion of hormones such as renin, erythropoietin, and 1,25-dihydroxycholecalciferol are important functions of the normal kidney. When these functions are perturbed, there may be profound effects upon the cardiovascular system. In recent years, clearer understanding of the pathophysiology of renal failure coupled with new techniques of therapy have greatly prolonged the survival of patients with advanced kidney disease managed either conservatively or with some form of chronic dialysis. This enlarging and increasingly elderly population of patients provides a challenge to physicians for meticulous medical management.

Physiological Consequences of Renal Failure

Sodium

Even patients with severe impairment of renal function are able to preserve sodium balance to a remarkable degree by varying the fractional reabsorption of filtered sodium. Whereas normal individuals may excrete less than 1 percent of filtered sodium while ingesting a 4-g sodium diet, those with severe renal insufficiency (glomerular filtration rate of only 10 percent of normal) may excrete 10 percent of filtered sodium. Nonetheless, we modern human beings, with our nearly universal intake of salt greater than our needs, are likely to overwhelm the capacity of our kidneys when renal insufficiency develops. We then put ourselves at risk for the development of circulatory congestion, hypertension, and congestive heart failure. The cornerstone of therapy is dietary control of salt intake, not always an easy undertaking without considerable patient education. When diuretics are required, a long-acting thiazide plus a "loop" diuretic given twice daily will usually produce a diuresis. The thiazide-like drug metolazone appears to be efficacious even in advanced renal insufficiency, possibly because of a dual action in the proximal tubule and the cortical diluting segment of the ascending limb.[1] Patients with advanced renal failure may lose lean body weight. Therefore, it is necessary to reassess periodically not only current renal function, but lean body mass as well.

Occasionally patients with chronic renal disease may become sodium-depleted as a consequence of overly enthusiastic dietary salt restriction or therapy with diuretics. Furthermore, patients whose renal disease is characterized by destruction of medullary and interstitial architecture may be liable to urinary salt wasting. The resulting reduction in effective arterial volume can impair renal perfusion, thereby worsening existing renal insufficiency. Likewise, overly vigorous therapy with antihypertensive drugs or afterload-reducing agents can reduce renal plasma flow and glomerular filtration.

During the course of progressive renal failure, a

single patient may have problems with both sodium overload and sodium depletion. Because of anorexia and nausea, some patients may lose lean body mass and become volume-overloaded at a weight at which they were previously isovolemic. Declining renal function will change the dietary limitations for salt and responsiveness to a given diuretic regimen. Periodic reevaluation of lean body weight, sodium balance, and intravascular volume is a necessary and important facet of the long-term management of such patients.

Potassium

The effects of hyperkalemia upon the heart and the acute treatment of hyperkalemia with bicarbonate, insulin and glucose, calcium, and ion-exchange resins are well known and will not be discussed here.

The chronically diseased kidney is able to increase the secretion of potassium sufficiently to keep the level of serum potassium below 6 meq/liter until the terminal stages of renal failure with oliguria are reached or unless other circumstances modify excretion or load. If sodium intake is rigidly restricted, insufficient sodium is delivered to the distal tubule for active reabsorption and creation of luminal electronegativity necessary for potassium secretion. Severe heart failure will limit distal exchange because of avid proximal sodium reabsorption. In this setting, diuretics are helpful in preventing hyperkalemia by increasing distal delivery of sodium and increasing urine flow. Worsening of acidosis will increase extracellular potassium levels when cellular potassium is released as hydrogen ions enter. Potassium is also released into the plasma in those circumstances associated with cellular destruction such as pneumonia, gastrointestinal bleeding, and shock.

Despite the fact that chronic renal failure may be associated with reduced total-body stores of potassium,[2] hypokalemia is rarely seen, even in those conditions in which secondary hyperaldosteronism or distal tubular potassium wasting is a prominent feature of the earlier stage of the disease. Patients undergoing chronic hemodialysis provide an important exception. Dialysate potassium in most centers is about 2.5 meq/liter. These patients are therefore subject to wide swings of serum potassium during dialysis at which time problems with spontaneous arrhythmias or digitalis intoxication may occur. Consequently, some patients may require adjustment of dietary potassium or dialysis with a higher potassium bath. Patients undergoing continuous ambulatory peritoneal dialysis (CAPD) often develop hypokalemia because their peritoneal dialysis solution is potassium-free. An increase in dietary intake of potassium-rich foods will generally suffice.

Calcium

Ionized calcium is usually reduced in chronic renal failure.[3] Diminished synthesis of 1,25-dihydroxycholecalciferol by the diseased kidney, particularly in the setting of high levels of intracellular phosphate, impairs gut absorption of calcium. Skeletal resistance to the action of parathyroid hormone in advanced renal failure also occurs. When hyperphosphatemia is present, complexing of calcium by phosphate further reduces the amount of ionized calcium available for metabolic work. Serum phosphate is maintained at nearly normal levels because of stimulation of parathyroid hormone secretion until the glomerular filtration rate falls to about 25 ml/min, at which point the increased secretion of parathyroid hormone is no longer able to prevent phosphate retention by inhibiting tubular reabsorption of phosphate because filtration of phosphate is so low. Restriction of dietary phosphate and the use of phosphate-binding gels with meals are therefore an important part of the management of patients with renal insufficiency.

Disorders of calcium and phosphorus metabolism in chronic renal disease have a variety of effects upon the cardiovascular system, including vascular calcifications, myocardial calcification, and hypotension. Arterial samples from patients with chronic renal failure show calcification of the internal elastic lamina, medial ground substance, and medial elastic fibers. Lipid deposition, on the other hand, is scanty. The severity of the vascular changes correlates with the duration of uremia and hypertension.[4] When the product of serum calcium and phosphorus concentration expressed in milligrams per deciliter exceeds 70 to 80, metastatic calcifications are likely to occur in the cornea of the eye, the interstitial tissues, the lung, renal tubules, and the media of small and medium-sized arteries. Such arterial calcifications can result in coronary occlusion or peripheral vascular ischemia to the point of gangrene.[5]

An unusual and potentially fatal variety of metastatic calcification involves the atrioventricular node and conducting system of the heart, resulting in atrioventricular block.[6] In addition, some patients with persistently elevated calcium-phosphorus product may develop a calcific cardiomyopathy characterized by intractable heart failure and atrioventricular block, and pathologically by metastatic calcification, degeneration, and fibrosis of the myocardium.[7]

Some undialyzed patients with uremia and hypocalcemia demonstrate relative hypotension and evidence of low cardiac output, which may be reversible following the infusion of calcium. Shackney and Hasson[8] have reviewed the cardiovascular effects of hypocalcemia, suggesting several possible mechanisms for hypocalcemic hypotension: (1) myocardial contractility is reduced in the presence of low concentrations of ionized calcium; (2) the magnitude of the contractile response of vascular smooth muscle varies directly, within limits, with calcium concentration; and (3) the release of norepinephrine from the adrenal medulla and from sympathetic postganglionic fibers varies directly with the concentration of calcium. When faced with the clinical problem of hypotension and/or low cardiac output in an uremic patient, one should consider the possibility of low levels of ionized calcium as a contributing factor. Care must be taken not to precipitate digitalis intoxication with rapid infusions of calcium. Patients with chronic renal failure may be treated with oral calcium carbonate and vitamin D analogues. It is imperative, however, that phosphorus be reduced toward normal levels first in order to prevent creation of a dangerously high calcium-phosphorus product.

Acidosis

Metabolic acidosis resulting from the titration of total-body buffer stores by unexcreted hydrogen ions is an invariable concomitant of chronic renal failure. Patients with chronic renal failure develop heart failure from a variety of causes: volume overload, hypertension, and anemia, to name but a few. Severe metabolic acidosis may convert a state of marginal myocardial compensation to one of failure with pulmonary edema because of the effect of acidosis in reducing left ventricular contractility, decreasing myocardial responsiveness to catecholamines, and constricting the venous system.[9]

In oliguric patients, dialysis may offer the only solution to relieving congestive overload and acidosis. Nonoliguric patients with chronic renal failure may respond to therapy with oral sodium bicarbonate or other alkaline salts.

Anemia

The pathogenesis of the anemia of renal insufficiency is complex.[10] Depending on the nature of the renal disease and the amount of renal parenchyma remaining, there is a relative or absolute deficiency of erythropoietin. Inhibitors of hematopoiesis are present in uremic serum. Red blood cell survival is shortened. Occult blood loss from the hemodialysis machine or from the gastrointestinal tract is common. When it is felt that anemia per se is contributing to disturbed cardiovascular function, restoration of the hematocrit to 20 to 25 percent with the cautious transfusion of packed red blood cells may be beneficial. Therapy with oral or parenteral iron, androgenic steroids, and dialysis improves the anemia of many patients with end-stage renal disease. Patients undergoing CAPD appear to increase red blood cell mass more than those on hemodialysis.

Azotemia

As glomerular filtration rate falls, urea and other specific products of nitrogen metabolism accumulate in the blood. These compounds may well be responsible for many of the symptoms of the uremic syndrome. Whether such nitrogenous compounds directly affect the heart remains a subject of controversy. The myocardial effects of urea, creatinine, guanidinosuccinic acid, and methylguanidine have been studied in experimental animals, with variable results.[11,12] Recent work in human subjects[13] suggests that the beneficial effect of isovolemic hemodialysis on myocardial contractility derives from changes in ionized calcium rather than from removal of uremic toxins.

Specific Complications of Chronic Renal Failure

Bacterial Endocarditis in Dialysis Patients

Reports of bacterial endocarditis in hemodialysis patients began to appear in the medical literature in 1966. Review of these studies[14] shows that *Staphylococcus aureus* was the infecting organism in the majority of cases. The aortic valve was more commonly involved than the mitral valve; several examples of tricuspid valve infection were cited.

Hemodialysis vascular access infection is the predisposing factor in the vast majority of dialysis patients who develop bacterial endocarditis. External Silastic arteriovenous cannulas (Quinton-Scribner), now rarely used except for patients with acute renal failure, have a high rate of infection and thrombosis. Subcutaneous arteriovenous fistulas (Brescia) uncommonly become infected, whereas fistulas created with synthetic material or bovine heterografts are more prone to thrombosis, infection, and aneurysm formation. A high (62 percent) rate of *Staphylococcus aureus* colonization of the nose, throat, or skin in patients receiving long-term hemodialysis is an additional risk factor.[15] Impaired resistance to infection is characteristic of end-stage renal failure and may therefore further enhance a dialysis patient's susceptibility to infection.

Bacterial endocarditis has been considered a rare complication of acquired arteriovenous fistulas in human beings.[16] Lillehei and associates[17] were able to produce bacterial endocarditis without deliberate introduction of bacteria in normal dogs in which they had created very large arteriovenous fistulas. They concluded that the greatly increased cardiac workload was sufficient to predispose these animals to the development of bacterial endocarditis.

Bacterial endocarditis in hemodialysis patients has become uncommon in recent years. Aggressive management of all infections, prompt removal of infected vascular access, and use of native subcutaneous fistulas whenever possible have helped to prevent this complication in dialysis patients. Antibiotic prophylaxis is used with dental manipulations. While vancomycin is a popular antibiotic for gram-positive infections because of its long half-life in patients with renal failure, it cannot be used once every 5 to 7 days as has been recommended by some. Patient-to-patient variability is wide, and therefore one must follow serum levels to perform therapy properly.

Pericarditis

Nearly 150 years have elapsed since Richard Bright first described pericarditis in patients dying of renal failure.[18] Regular dialysis for patients with end-stage renal disease came into being about 20 years ago. It is only in the past decade, however, that we have recognized the distinction between true uremic pericarditis and the pericarditis that afflicts patients undergoing chronic hemodialysis. The reader is referred to several excellent recent reviews.[19–21]

The incidence of true *uremic pericarditis,* that is, pericarditis occurring in previously undialyzed patients or in patients whose dialysis has been interrupted, is difficult to assess. Because uremic pericarditis is often asymptomatic, its presence may be missed unless evidence is specifically sought. Yoshida[22] in a study of 150 uremic patients detected pericardial effusion by echocardiography in 62 percent. Only 7 percent of these patients were symptomatic. Earlier and more aggressive treatment of patients with renal failure over the past several years has probably prevented the development of uremic pericarditis that was heretofore more prevalent.

Typical symptoms of pericarditis occur in uremic patients, but they are less severe than those with dialysis-associated pericarditis.[19] Chest pain occurs in 32 to 83 percent; rubs in 57 to 100 percent. Fever, leukocytosis, hemodynamic compromise, and tamponade occur far less frequently than with dialysis-associated pericarditis. Effusions are serous or serosanguineous. The pathological findings of uremic and dialysis-associated pericarditis are similar. Baldwin and Edwards have reviewed the findings in the former.[23] Both the visceral and parietal pericardium show fibrinous exudate with fibrinous adhesions almost invariably present; organizing perivascular tissue is seen; mononuclear inflammatory cells are common. Concomitant myocarditis may be present.

The etiology of uremic pericarditis has classically been ascribed to azotemia, largely because of the prompt response to intensive dialysis. Young et al.[24] in a prospective study over 8 months in new dialysis patients found a disappearance of the pericardial effusion in only one-third. They feel that volume overload may contribute to the presence of pericardial effusion in uremia. Intensive dialysis for a period of 10 to 14 days is recommended therapy. Although there is no proof that anticoagulation can produce hemorrhagic effusions, hemodialysis is performed with the lowest possible doses of heparin. Corticosteroids and indomethacin have not been shown to alter the course of pericarditis, except to decrease fever[25] and possibly to improve pain.

The occurrence of pericarditis in regularly dialyzed patients is usually called *dialysis-associated pericarditis.* This does not imply, however, that the dialysis procedure is in any way implicated in the etiology of the disorder. Precisely how many chronic dialysis patients have or develop pericardial effusion is difficult to assess on clinical grounds alone. Echocardiography may detect pericardial effusion in as many as 28 percent of asymptomatic dialysis patients.[19] Symptomatic or clinically apparent pericarditis occurs in far fewer dialysis patients.

Symptoms of dialysis-associated pericarditis include chest pain, which may be pleuritic in nature, malaise, dyspnea, cough. Fever and a pericardial friction rub occur in over 90 percent of patients. Leukocytosis is somewhat less common. Unlike uremic pericarditis, dialysis-associated pericarditis effusions are often hemorrhagic and the risk of tamponade is high. Tamponade is unusual in asymptomatic patients with dialysis-associated pericarditis but may complicate the course of as many as 20 percent of symptomatic patients. Hypotension in the absence of volume depletion occurring during the course of a hemodialysis treatment is often the earliest warning of impending tamponade. Paradoxical pulse and strutted neck veins are later signs, and their absence should not delay the institution of diagnostic procedures. While the electrocardiogram is abnormal in most patients, only in about one-third are the classic findings of pericarditis seen.

The etiology of dialysis-associated pericarditis is likely multifactorial. In one study,[26] bacterial infection (in shunts, surgical wounds, respiratory tract, or blood) preceded pericarditis in 14 of 25 patients. Tissue catabolism from infection may perturb biochemical balance sufficiently to put one at risk for pericarditis. Some, but not all, investigators have noted an increase in pericarditis following surgery. Rising titers of influenza and Coxsackie B virus antibody were found in four of five patients with pericarditis by Osanloo.[27] A viral-like prodrome has been noted by other investigators in a minority of patients. Ayus and colleagues[21] believe that dialysis-associated pericarditis may represent unresolved uremic pericarditis that becomes manifest after the institution of dialysis. Thus, although bacterial and viral infection, surgery, stress, and reduction in biochemical control have all been implicated in the predisposition for pericarditis, there still remain a few patients undergoing chronic dialysis for whom we have no ready explanation for the development or emergence of symptomatic pericarditis.

The treatment of dialysis-associated pericarditis with augmented dialysis meets with success in only about half of patients so treated. Renfrew et al.[19] has recommended the instillation of poorly absorbable steroids into the pericardial sac. Fuller et al.[28] have reported that five of five patients with intractable pericarditis recovered after percutaneous drainage and instillation of triamcinolone hexacetonide. Others find this procedure too hazardous. Because of the presence of fibrinous adhesions between the visceral and parietal pericardium, pericardiocentesis may be difficult as well as dangerous.

Those patients who are unresponsive to conservative management or who have tamponade require surgery. Ribot and colleagues[29] recommend subxiphoid pericardiostomy with creation of a 7-cm window (with drain) as a safe and effective procedure. However, because the pericardial window has been associated with closure requiring exploration or with the development of late constriction, other groups recommend wide pericardiectomy.[20,30] Pericardial window was associated with a 33 percent recurrence rate of tamponade in the experience of Dean et al.,[30] who reserve creation of a window for emergencies. They performed wide anterior pericardiectomy in 22 uremic patients, of whom 20 survived. The result was felt to be excellent in 19.

Myocardial Dysfunction

The existence of a specific uremic cardiomyopathy has been a subject of debate since it was first proposed by Bailey, Hampers, and Merrill in 1967.[31] They described five patients who had global cardiomegaly, atrial and ventricular arrhythmias, typical electrocardiographic changes, sensitivity to digitalis, and reversal of the syndrome following dialysis. Whether dialysis simply improved volume overload, hypertension, anemia, or calcium-phosphorus abnormalities or removed a cardiotoxic factor or factors is not known. In support of the existence of an intrinsic uremic cardiomyopathy, Prosser and Parsons[32] cite the following data: (1) In isolated rat heart preparations, perfusates containing combinations of urea, creatinine, guanidinosuccinic acid, and methylguanidine had a cardiac depressant effect. (2) The elevated intracellular sodium content characteristic of uremic cells might result in impaired myocardial function. (3) Vitamin D is necessary for the proper function and structure of sarcoplasmic endoreticulum in muscle cells. Possibly the deficiency of 1,25-dihydroxycholecalciferol in chronic renal failure leads to functional impairment of myocardial cells. In contrast, most students of the subject of myocardial dysfunction in uremia feel that when one excludes the contributions of preexisting heart disease, anemia, increased preload and afterload, workload from arteriovenous fistulas, acidosis, and reduced ionized calcium, a specific cardiomyopathy is rare or absent.[21,33] Nonetheless, myocardial dysfunction is common in patients with chronic renal failure. Ayus, Frommer, and Young[21] have reviewed several studies which examined the echocardiographic abnormalities of undialyzed patients with chronic renal failure. Left ventricular hypertrophy was present in 30 to 78 percent; left ventricular dilatation in 15 to 28 percent. Evidence of left ventricular systolic dysfunction ranged from 25 to 39 percent.

Of primary importance in the evaluation of a renal failure patient with heart disease is the exclusion of other myocardial disorders. Long-standing hypertension, invariably associated with hypertensive heart disease, is an important cause of end-stage renal failure in the United States. Diabetes mellitus, amyloidosis, systemic sclerosis, and vasculitis may affect the heart as well as the kidneys. Cardiomyopathy occurring in an uremic patient is not necessarily uremic cardiomyopathy.

Of equal importance in the assessment of cardiac dysfunction in uremic patients is the contribution to workload made by anemia, peripheral arteriovenous fistula, pressure-volume overload, and hypoxemia. It is the exceptional patient with chronic renal failure who does not have *anemia.* A significant inverse correlation exists between hematocrit and cardiac index in hemodialyzed patients. Capelli and Kasparian[34] studied the relation between cardiac index and level of hematocrit in nine patients, with their arteriovenous fistulas or shunts both occluded and nonoccluded. Cardiac index fell from about 6 liters/min/m^2 at a hematocrit of 20 to about 2 liters/min/m^2 at a hematocrit of nearly 40. They also noted a direct correlation between peripheral resistance and hematocrit, with a range of peripheral resistance between about 900 to 3400 dyn·s/cm^{-5} as hematocrit varied between 20 and nearly 40. In the same group of patients cardiac output was measured before (7.4 liters/min) and after (6.3 liters/min) occlusion of dialysis arteriovenous fistula.

The *arteriovenous fistulas* of hemodialysis patients usually carry a flow of between 250 and 750 ml/min, although flows as high as 10 liters/min have been reported. In and of itself, the fistula is not likely to produce heart failure, but it may well pose an additional hemodynamic load to an already burdened heart. Anderson and coworkers[35] have described six patients and reviewed nine from the literature with high-output cardiac failure from forearm arteriovenous fistulas created for dialysis. Following compression of the fistula, cardiac output decreases from 0.3 to 11.0 liters/min (mean 2.9 liters/min). Improvement in cardiac failure following surgical intervention occurred in 13 of 14 patients. Patients who have exhausted forearm vessels may have brachial or even femoral fistulas created for dialysis. They would have a somewhat greater myocardial workload because of the greater flow through these vessels.

Hypoxemia is yet another burden for the hearts of some patients with chronic renal failure. Pulmonary vascular congestion from extracellular fluid volume overload is common in patients approaching the need for dialysis and in dialyzed patients immediately before their next hemodialysis treatment. Hypoxemia may occur during the dialysis procedure itself. Implicated in causing hypoxemia have been complement activation and pulmonary vascular leukostasis from blood contact on the cellophane membrane of the hemodialyzer;[36] hypoventilation in response to reduced blood carbon dioxide content, occurring particularly during dialysis with large-surface-area dialyzers;[37] and dialysis with acetate-containing dialysate.

Plasma *volume overload* is prevalent in undialyzed patients and those on chronic hemodialysis in the interdialytic period. Weight gains of 1 kg daily are average; noncompliant patients may gain 7 to 8 kg of fluid in a 3-day period. The consequences of such an increase in preload are obvious. What is less obvious are the hemodynamic effects of hemodialysis in patients with normal or abnormal left ventricular function, and the effect of hemodialysis on myocardial function independent of a reduction in extracellular volume. Hung and coworkers[38] have measured left ventricular ejection fraction before and after hemodialysis in 20 uremic patients. Ejection fraction and contraction were normal in 15 (6 of whom had congestive heart failure) and did not change with dialysis. In the five patients with abnormal contractility and ejection fraction, long-term hemodialysis resulted in improvement in these functions in three. Their study, while demonstrating the beneficial effect of long-term dialysis in some patients with the physiology of congestive cardiomyopathy, does not answer the question of whether this was improvement in "uremic cardiomyopathy" or the effect of improvement in control of plasma volume overload and hypertension.

Nixon et al.[39] have studied hemodialysis patients undergoing hemodialysis with volume loss, with ultrafiltration only, and with hemodialysis without volume loss. Pure ultrafiltration resulted in a reduction in end-diastolic volume and stroke volume without significant change in end-systolic volume or mean velocity of circumferential fiber shortening. In contrast, hemodialysis produced a decrease in end-systolic volume and an increase in stroke volume, without a change in end-diastolic volume. Velocity of circumferential fiber shortening doubled. They concluded that pure volume loss produced a Frank-Starling effect, while dialysis shifted the ventricular function curve because of an increase in left ventricular contractility. In a subsequent study, these investigators[13] attempted to assess the independent effects of removing uremic toxins, increasing plasma bicarbonate, or increasing *ionized calcium* on myocardial contractility during hemodialysis. They suggest that an increase in blood ionized calcium that occurs during the dialysis procedure is of key importance in the observed improvement in myocardial contractility.

Parathyroid hormone (PTH) has been proposed as a possible myocardial toxin in patients with chronic renal failure.[40] Studies in heart cells in tissue culture[41] and in isolated guinea pig auricles[42] lend support to this theory. Improvement in left ventricular function in 22 patients with secondary hyperparathyroidism following parathyroidectomy was noted by Drueke et al.[43] The possible role of changes in levels of ionized calcium or *1,25-dihydroxycholecalciferol (1,25-D_3)* in this study is unknown. It is quite likely that the deficiency of 1,25-D_3 characteristic of patients with chronic renal failure plays a role in myocardial dysfunction. Calcium transport in the sarcoplasmic reticulum of skeletal muscle in rabbits with experimental uremia is impaired; the defect was improved with the administration of 1,25-D_3.[44] Depressed calcium transport in fragmented sarcoplasmic reticulum from the hearts of uremic rats had also been noted.[45]

Pulmonary Edema

Pulmonary edema in patients with chronic renal failure is usually the result of cardiac failure, congestive overload, or both. However, a pattern of pulmonary edema extending from the hilum in a sharply defined butterfly configuration can be seen in uremias in the absence of obvious pulmonary vascular congestion. Whether or not this pattern is specific for uremia has been a subject of debate. The peripheral clear areas seen on chest x-ray may be the consequence of hyperventilation in response to uremic acidosis. The alveolar fluid, which is rich in protein and fibrin, might result from increased capillary permeability, possibly caused by "uremic toxins."[46] Rackow and associates[47] have performed hemodynamic studies and pulmonary edema fluid analysis in two uremic patients with acute pulmonary edema but without evidence of cardiac dysfunction. From their studies they conclude that uremic pulmonary edema results from (1) alterations of the intravascular Starling forces such that the plasma colloid osmotic pressure–pulmonary artery wedge pressure gradient is reduced, thereby permitting increased ultrafiltration of fluid into the lung, and (2) the efflux of protein-rich fluid into the lung because of a marked increase in pulmonary capillary membrane permeability.

Atherosclerotic Heart Disease

Older studies of patients undergoing chronic maintenance hemodialysis have suggested that such patients have an accelerated rate of atherosclerosis and an increased mortality rate from cardiovascular disease.[48,49] More recent work refutes the assertion that chronic dialysis is associated with accelerated atherosclerosis.[50,51] A major problem in early studies was the failure to exclude patients with established coronary atherosclerotic heart disease prior to the institution of dialysis. Rostand and coworkers[51] studied the incidence of ischemic heart disease in 382 patients over a 6-year period. Of 101 patients with ischemic heart disease, only 39 (20 percent) developed evidence of disease *after* institution of dialysis, and more than one-half of these were within the first year. They suggest that the incidence of ischemic heart disease is not different in dialysis patients compared to matched controls; that coronary atherosclerosis affected long-term survival rate only in patients with preexisting disease; and that autopsy studies did not show accelerated atherosclerosis. More recently, these same investigators have studied the relationship of coronary risk factors to ischemic heart disease in patients undergoing maintenance hemodialysis.[52] Using regression analysis, they found that increased age, white race, and diastolic hypertension were significantly correlated with ischemic heart disease.

Both Haire[53] and Vincenti[54] consider that a predominant risk factor for the development of atherosclerosis in patients with end-stage renal disease is sustained hypertension prior to the initiation of dialytic therapy. Since prolonged hypertension before dialysis is instituted and poor control of hypertension despite dialysis are such important risk factors for the development of atherosclerosis and ischemic heart disease, it is crucial that a major ef-

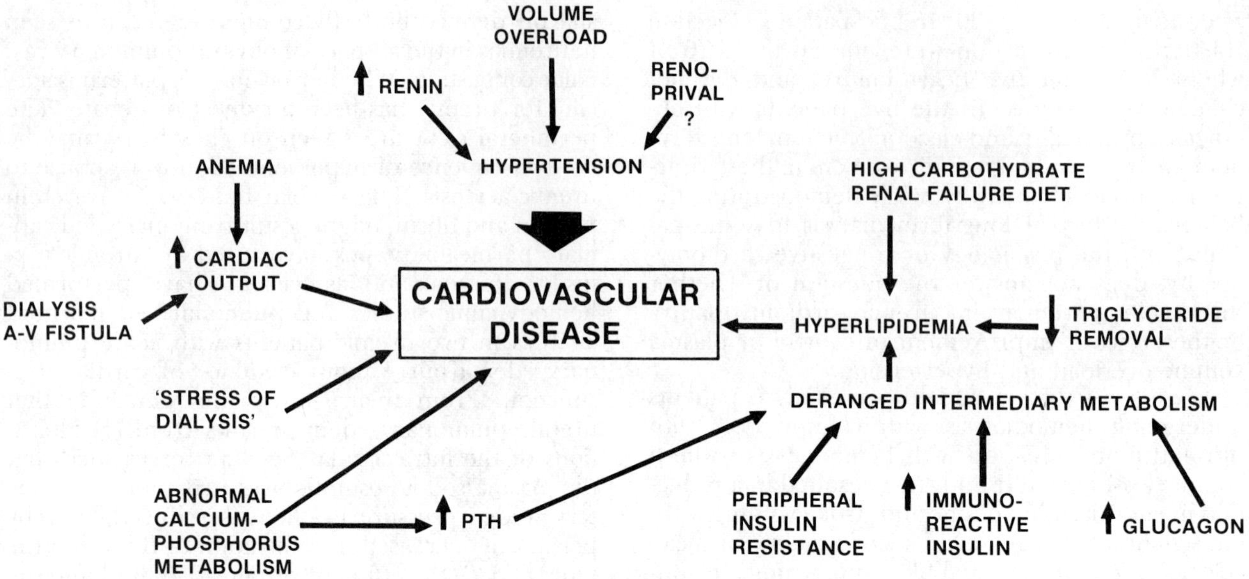

FIGURE 76-1 Possible etiologic factors in the development of cardiovascular disease in dialysis patients.

fort be made on the part of physicians to normalize blood pressure.

A variety of physiological and biochemical abnormalities characteristic of uremia have been implicated in the pathogenesis of cardiovascular disease in patients with chronic renal failure. These are shown in Fig. 76-1. Except for the possibility of hyperlipidemia, none of these has been conclusively shown to accelerate atherogenesis in patients with renal failure. Rapoport[55] suggests that elevated levels of triglycerides and defective high-density lipoprotein composition in patients on chronic hemodialysis may be a mechanism for accelerated atherosclerosis. In contrast Rostand[52] was unable to identify hypertriglyceridemia as a coronary risk factor in 320 dialysis patients.

References

1. Puschett, J. B.: Physiologic Basis for the Use of New and Older Diuretics in CHF, *Cardiovasc. Med.,* 2:119, 1977.
2. Bilbrey, G. L., Carter, N. W., White, M. G., Schilling, J. F., and Knochel, J. D.: Potassium Deficiency in Chronic Renal Failure, *Kidney Int.,* 4:423, 1973.
3. Massry, S. G.: Divalent Ion Metabolism in Renal Osteodystrophy, in S. G. Massry and R. J. Glassrock (eds.), "Textbook of Nephrology," The Williams and Wilkins Company, Baltimore, 1983.
4. Ibels, L. S., Alfrey, A. C., Huffer, W. E., Craswell, P. W., Anderson, J. T., and Weil, R.: Arterial Calcifications and Pathology in Uremic Patients Undergoing Dialysis, *Am. J. Med.,* 66:790, 1979.
5. Friedman, S. A., Novack, S., and Thomason, G. E.: Arterial Calcifications and Gangrene in Uremia, *N. Engl. J. Med.,* 280:1392, 1969.
6. Henderson, R. R., Santiago, L. M., Spring, D. A., and Harringtonn, A. R.: Metastatic Myocardial Calcification in Chronic Renal Failure, *N. Engl. J. Med.,* 284:1252, 1971.
7. Arora, K. K., Lacy, J. P., Schact, R. A., Martin, D. G., and Gutch, L. F.: Calcific Cardiomyopathy in Advanced Renal Failure, *Arch Intern. Med.,* 135:603, 1975.
8. Shackney, S., and Hasson, J.: Precipitous Fall in Serum Calcium, Hypotension and Acute Renal Failure after Intravenous Phosphate Therapy for Hypercalcemia, *Ann. Intern. Med.,* 66:906, 1967.
9. Mitchell, J. H., Wildenthal, K., and Johnson, R. L.: The Effects of Acid-Base Disturbances on Cardiovascular and Pulmonary Function, *Kidney Int.,* 1:375, 1972.
10. Fisher, J. W.: Mechanism of the Anemia Chronic Renal Failure, *Nephron,* 25:106, 1980.
11. Scheuer, J., and Stezoski, S. W.: The Effect of Uremic Compounds on Cardiac Function and Metabolism, *J. Mol. Cell. Cardiol.,* 5:287, 1973.
12. Kersting, F., Brass, H., and Heintz, R.: Uremic Cardiomyopathy: Studies on Cardiac Function in the Guinea Pig, *Clin. Nephrol.,* 10:109, 1978.
13. Henrich, W. L., Hunt, J. M., and Nixon, J. V.: Increased Ionized Calcium and Left Ventricular Contractility during Hemodialysis, *N. Engl. J. Med.,* 310:19, 1984.
14. Cross, A. S., and Steigbigel, R. T.: Infective Endocarditis in Patients on Hemodialysis, *Medicine,* 55:453, 1976.
15. Kirmani, N., Tuazon, D. K., Munoy, H. W., Panish, A. E., and Sheagren, J. W.: *Staphylococcus aureus* Carriage Rate of Patients Receiving Long-Term Hemodialysis, *Arch. Intern. Med.,* 138:1657, 1978.
16. Hook, W., Wainer, H., McGee, T., and Sellers, T., Jr.: Acquired Arteriovenous Fistula with Bacterial Endarteritis and Endocarditis, *JAMA,* 164:1450, 1957.
17. Lillehei, C. W., Bobb, J. R. R., and Visscher, M. P.: Occurrence of Endocarditis with Valvular Deformities in Dogs with Arteriovenous Fistulas, *Ann. Surg.,* 132:577, 1950.
18. Bright, R.: Tabular View of the Morbid Appearances in 100 Cases Connected with Albuminous Urine: With Observations, *Guys Hosp. Rep.,* 1:338, 1836.
19. Renfrew, R., Buselmeier, T. J., and Kjellstrand, C. M.: Pericarditis and Renal Failure, *Ann. Rev. Med.,* 31:345, 1980.
20. Marini, P. V., and Hull, A. R.: Uremic Pericarditis: A Review of Incidence and Management, *Kidney Int.,* 7(suppl. 2):S163, 1975.
21. Ayus, J. C., Frommer, J. P., and Young, J. B.: Cardiac and Circulatory Abnormalities in Chronic Renal Failure, *Semin. Nephrol.,* 1:112, 1981.
22. Yoshida, K., Shiina, A., Asano, Y., and Hosoda, S.: Uremic Pericardial Effusion: Detection and Evaluation of Uremic Pericardial Effusion by Echocardiography, *Clin. Nephrol.,* 13:260, 1980.
23. Baldwin, J. J., and Edwards, J. E.: Uremic Pericarditis as a Cause of Cardiac Tamponade, *Circulation,* 53:896, 1976.
24. Young, J. B., Frommer, P., Ayus, J. C., et al.: Effect of Di-

alysis on Pericardial Effusion: A Prospective Echocardiographic Study in End-Stage Renal Failure Patients, *Circulation,* 62(4)(suppl. 2):111, 1980.
25. Spector, D., Alfred, H., Siedlecki, M., and Briefel, G.: A Controlled Study of the Effect of Indomethadin in Uremic Pericarditis, *Kidney Int.,* 24:663, 1983.
26. Comty, C. M., Cohen, S. L., and Shapiro, F. L.: Pericarditis in Uremia and Its Sequels, *Ann. Intern. Med.,* 75:173, 1971.
27. Osanloo, E., Shalhoub, R. J., Cioffi, R. F., and Parker, R. H.: Viral Pericarditis in Patients Receiving Hemodialysis, *Arch. Intern. Med.,* 139:301, 1979.
28. Fuller, T. J., Knochel, J. P., Brennan, J. P., Fetner, C. D., and White, M. G.: Reversal of Intractable Uremic Pericarditis by Triamcinolone Hexacetonide, *Arch. Intern. Med.,* 137:979, 1976.
29. Ribot, S., Frankel, H. J., Gielchinsky, I., and Gilbert, L.: Treatment of Uremic Pericarditis, *Clin. Nephrol.,* 2:127, 1974.
30. Dean, R. H., Killen, D. A., Daniel, R. A., and Collins, H. A.: Experience with Pericardiectomy, *Ann. Thorac. Surg.,* 15:378, 1973.
31. Bailey, G. L., Hampers, C. L., and Merrill, J. P.: Reversible Cardiomyopathy in Uremia, *Trans. Am. Soc. Artif. Intern. Organs,* 13:263, 1967.
32. Prosser, D., and Parsons, V.: The Case for a Specific Uraemic Cardiomyopathy, *Nephron,* 15:4, 1975.
33. Gueron, M., Berlyne, G. M., Nord, E., and Ben Ari, J.: The Case against a Specific Uraemic Cardiomyopathy, *Nephron,* 15:2, 1975.
34. Capelli, J. P., and Kasparian, H.: Cardiac Work Demands and Left Ventricular Function in End-Stage Renal Disease, *Ann. Intern. Med.,* 86:261, 1967.
35. Anderson, C. B., Codd, J. R., Graff, R. A., Groce, M. A., Harter, H. R., and Newton, W. T.: Cardiac Failure and Upper Extremity Arteriovenous Fistulas, *Arch. Intern. Med.,* 136:292, 1976.
36. Ivanovich, P., Cheuweth, D. E., Schmidt, R., et al.: Symptoms and Activation of Granulocytes and Complement with Two Dialysis Membranes, *Kidney Int.,* 24:758, 1983.
37. Tolchin, W., Roberts, J. L., and Lewis, E. J.: Respiratory Gas Exchange by High-Efficiency Hemodialyzers, *Nephron,* 21:137, 1978.
38. Hung, J., Harris, P. J., Uren, R. F., Tiller, D. J., and Kelly, D. T.: Uremic Cardiomyopathy—Effect of Hemodialysis on Left Ventricular Function in End-Stage Disease, *N. Engl. J. Med.,* 302:546, 1980.
39. Nixon, J. V., Mitchell, J. H., McPhaul, J. J., and Henrich, W. L.: Effect of Hemodialysis on Left Ventricular Function, *J. Clin. Invest.,* 71:377, 1983.
40. Massry, S. G.: The Toxic Effects of Parathyroid Hormone in Uremia, *Semin. Nephrol.,* 3:306, 1983.
41. Bogin, E., Massry, S. G., and Harary, I.: Effect of Parathyroid Hormone on Rat Heart Cells, *J. Clin. Invest.,* 67:1215, 1981.
42. Lhoste, F., Drueke, T., Laino, S., and Boissier, J. R.: Cardiac Interaction between Parathyroid Hormone, β-Adrenoreceptor and Verapamil in the Guinea Pig in Vitro, *Clin. Exp. Pharmacol. Physiol.,* 7:119, 1980.
43. Drueke, T., Fleury, J., Touri, Y., et al.: Effect of Parathyroidectomy on Left Ventricular Function in Hemodialysis Patients, *Lancet,* 1:112, 1980.
44. Matthews, C., Heimberg, K. W., Ritz, E., et al.: Effect of 1,25-Dihydroxycholecalciferol on Impaired Calcium Transport by the Sarcoplasmic Reticulum in Experimental Uremia, *Kidney Int.,* 11:227, 1977.
45. Penpargkue, S., Bhan, A. K., and Scheuer, J.: Studies of Subcellular Control Factors in Hearts of Uremic Rats, *J. Lab. Clin. Med.,* 88:563, 1976.
46. Schwartz, E. E., and Onesti, G.: The Cardiopulmonary Manifestations of Uremia and Renal Transplantation, *Radiol. Clin. North Am.,* 10:569, 1972.
47. Rackow, W. C., Fein, I. A., Sprung, C., and Grodmand, R. S.: Uremic Pulmonary Edema, *Am. J. Med.,* 64:1084, 1978.
48. Lindner, A., Charra, B., Shenard, D. J., and Scriber, B. H.: Accelerated Atherosclerosis in Prolonged Maintenance Hemodialysis, *N. Engl. J. Med.,* 290:697, 1974.
49. Bryan, F.: "National Dialysis Registry," *Proceedings of the 6th Annual Contractors' Conferences of the Artificial Kidney Program of the National Institute of Arthritis, Metabolism and Digestive Disease,* Bethesda, Maryland, 1973, p. 201.
50. Burke, J. F., Frances, G. C., Moore, L. L., et al.: Acceluate Atherosclerosis in Chronic-Dialysis Patients—Another Look, *Nephron,* 21:181, 1978.
51. Rostand, S. G., Gretes, J. C., Kirk, K. A., Rutsky, E. A., and Andreoli, T. E.: Ischemic Heart Disease in Patients with Uremic Undergoing Maintenance Hemodialysis, *Kidney Int.,* 16:600, 1979.
52. Rostand, S. G., Kirk, K. A., and Rutsky, E. A.: Relationship of Coronary Risk Factors to Hemodialysis-Associated Ischemic Heart Disease, *Kidney Int.,* 22:301, 1982.
53. Haire, H. M., Shenard, D. J., Scardapane, D., Curtis, F. K., and Brunzell, J. D.: Smoking, Hypertension and Mortality in a Maintenance Dialysis Population, *Cardiovasc. Med.,* 3:1163, 1978.
54. Vincenti, F., Amend, W. J., Abele, J., Feduska, N. J., and Salvatierra, O., Jr.: The Role of Hypertension in Hemodialysis-Associated Atherosclerosis, *Am. J. Med.,* 68:363, 1980.
55. Rapoport, J., Aviram, M., Chaimovitz, C., and Brooks, J. G.: Defective High-Density Lipoprotein Composition in Patients on Chronic Hemodialysis, *N. Engl. J. Med.,* 299:1326, 1978.

77

Electrolytes and the Heart

Charles Fisch, M.D.

After the publication of a paper in the Journal of Physiology, Vol. III., No. 5, entitled "Concerning the influence exerted by each of the Constituents of the Blood on the Contraction of the Ventricle," I discovered, that the saline solution which I had used had not been prepared with distilled water, but with pipe water supplied by the New River Water Company. As this water contains minute traces of various inorganic substances, I at once tested the action of saline solution made with distilled water and I found that I did not get the effects described in the paper referred to. It is obvious therefore that the effects I had obtained are due to some of the inorganic constituents of the pipe water.

Sydney Ringer, 1883[1]

The reason for the use of tap water was that Ringer, himself busy, trusted the preparation of his solutions to his laboratory technician, Fiedler, who could not see the point of spending all that time distilling water for Dr. Ringer, who would not notice any difference if the salt solution was made up with tap water.[2] Ringer soon realized, however, that the vigorous activity of the frog heart exposed to tap water was due to Ca and that Ca was essential for normal contraction of the frog heart.[1] He also became aware of the importance of K for normal cardiac function,[3] and of the antagonism between K and Na and between Na and Ca.[1,4] These early observations have been confirmed and detailed by a number of investigators.[5]

K, Na, and Ca are the major ions responsible for normal electrical activity of the heart. In addition, Ca is the messenger that initiates excitation-contraction coupling and, along with Mg and P, is involved in the steps leading to myocardial contraction.

While K, Ca, Na, Mg, and P all influence the electrical and mechanical properties of the heart, the clinically recognizable abnormalities of electrolyte disturbances are largely due to changing K and Ca concentration.[6]

The Transmembrane Action Potential

In order to understand the effect of changing electrolyte concentration on the electrical and mechanical behavior of the heart, it is useful to review the sequence of transmembrane voltage changes resulting in transmembrane action potential (TAP) and the electrolyte fluxes generally responsible for such changes.

During diastole (phase 4 of the TAP) the membrane is largely permeable to K with a net loss of intracellular K. Due to this selective permeability to K, the magnitude of the transmembrane resting potential (TRP) is dependent largely on the transmembrane concentration gradient of K. In the ventricular myocardial cell this gradient is approximately −90 mV. The relation of TRP to K is expressed in the Nernst equation, which predicts that an increase in extracellular K decreases the TRP (becomes less negative), while a lowering of the extracellular K results in hyperpolarization, or an increase in TRP (becomes more negative).[7,8]

A greater-than-threshold stimulus produces a rapid inward shift of Na so that the interior ultimately becomes positively charged. Following onset of the rapid inward Na-carried current, and at a point when the transmembrane potential (TMP) is reduced to about −40 mV, a second, slow inward current carried by Ca through specific "slow channels" is activated. This slow current is responsible for the terminal portion of phase 0 and for the plateau, or phase 2, of the TAP (Fig. 77-1).

The slow Ca current is characterized by a low transmembrane resting potential (TRP), low amplitude of TAP, slow rate of depolarization as compared with rapid Na-dependent voltage change, very slow propagation velocity, graded response to applied stimuli, refractoriness exceeding duration of TAP, and a low safety factor for propagation.[9]

The rate of rise of phase 0, a significant determinant of the speed of conduction, is to a great extent dependent on the magnitude of the TRP. The greater (more negative) the TRP at the onset of phase 0, the greater the rate of rise of phase 0 and greater the speed of conduction. At any given point in time, the relationship of the rate of change of phase 0 to the TRP expresses membrane responsiveness. Since an increase in extracellular K lowers the TRP, the rate of rise of phase 0 will be reduced and conduction depressed[10] (Fig. 77-2).

It should be noted that reduction of the TRP will bring the TRP closer to the threshold potential (TP), and the strength of a stimulus needed to reduce the TRP to TP (excitability) will be decreased. Consequently, conduction depression due to reduction of TRP may, within narrow ranges of hyperkalemia, be preceded by an increase in excitability and conduction.[11] As a result, conduction alteration due to changing K concentration may reflect the altered rate of rise of phase 0 as well as changing excitability.

The slow depolarization during phase 4, which characterizes the automatic cells, is most likely due to a gradual influx of Na at a time when K efflux is diminished or completely inhibited.[12]

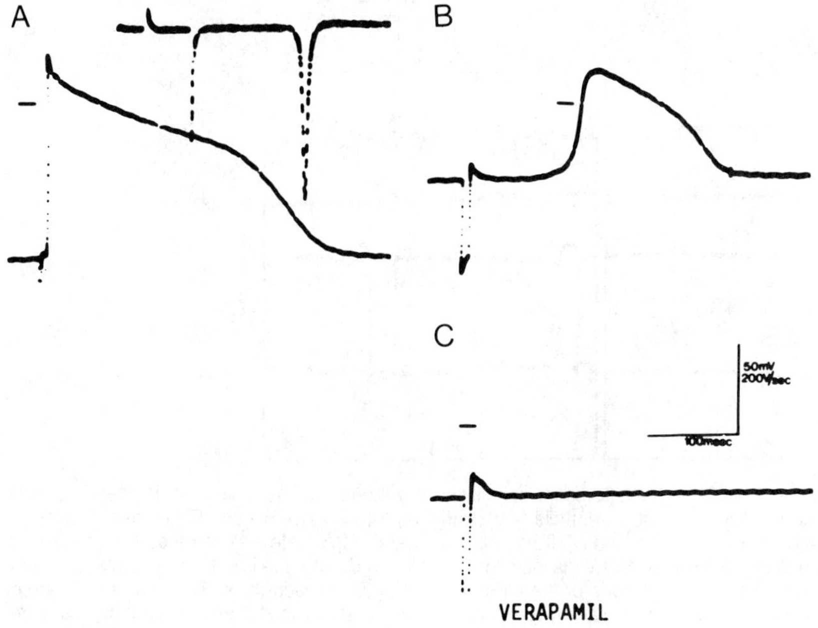

FIGURE 77-1 This figure illustrates slow Ca-dependent transmembrane current. In *A* the TAP is normal. Following superfusion with K and reduction of TMP, a TAP due to slow Ca-carried current is recorded (*B*). The characteristics of the Ca-dependent TAP are described in the test. Administration of verapamil, a Ca blocker, eliminates the Ca-dependent TAP (*C*).

Potassium

Hyperkalemia and Conduction

In 1911, Mathison, while infusing K and observing the sequence of atrioventricular (AV) contraction in a cat heart, noted that the cation induced AV block.[13]

Largely because of the fact that the specialized conduction tissue is most often more resistant to K than the myocardium, AV block due to K, other than simple prolongation of PR, was assumed rare or unlikely. It was not until some 50 years after Mathison that a systematic study of the effect of K in AV conduction clearly indicated that experimental AV block can be induced with relative ease. These studies also demonstrated the dual effect on AV conduction, namely an initial acceleration followed by depression.[14,15]

At plasma levels of 6.0 and 6.5 meq/liter, AV conduction is accelerated, and at levels of about 7.5 meq/liter or higher, conduction is depressed.[15,16] In a clinical setting the accelerating effect of mild hyperkalemia may improve AV conduction,[17,18] and similarly an increase in excitability may restore responsiveness to external stimulation. However, because it is difficult to maintain the plasma K levels within the narrow therapeutic range, K is rarely, if ever, used to enhance AV conduction or restore responsiveness to stimulation. In the intact animal, the antivagal effect of K contributes to enhancement of AV conduction.[19,20]

In dogs, an increase of plasma K concentration to an average of 8.4 meq/liter results, almost uniformly, in a variety of AV conduction abnormalities.[21] At times, complete AV block is induced when both P and QRS waves are still present, indicating that under certain conditions the AV conduction system is less resistant to the depressing effects on K than either the atrial or ventricular tissue[10,21] (Fig.

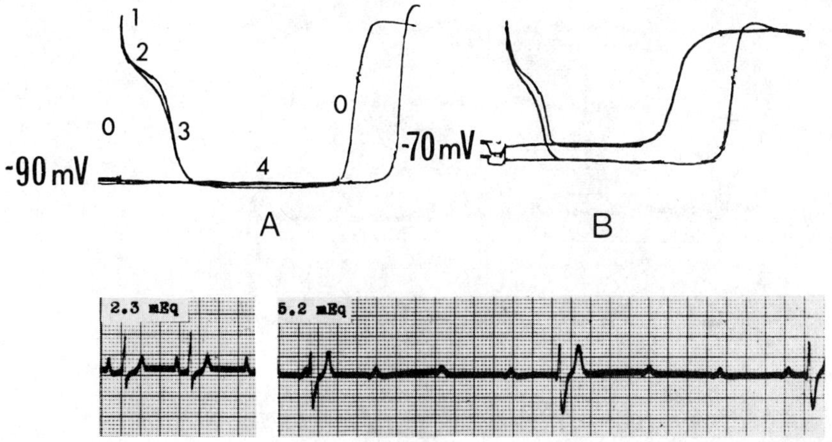

FIGURE 77-2 This figure illustrates the electrophysiological basis for AV block due to K. *A*. Two TAPs are recorded about 1 mm apart, with a rapid sweep seen to the right. The latter shows the rapid upstroke of phase 0 and the delay of conduction between the two microelectrodes. *B*. The TRP is reduced to −70 mV by administration of K. This resulted in slowing of the upstroke of phase 0 and a prolongation of conduction time between the two microelectrodes. *C*. K-induced AV block in a digitalized animal. (*From C. Fisch, Relation of Electrolyte Disturbances to Cardiac Arrhythmias, Circulation, 47:408, 1973. Reproduced with permission from the American Heart Association, Inc., and the author.)*

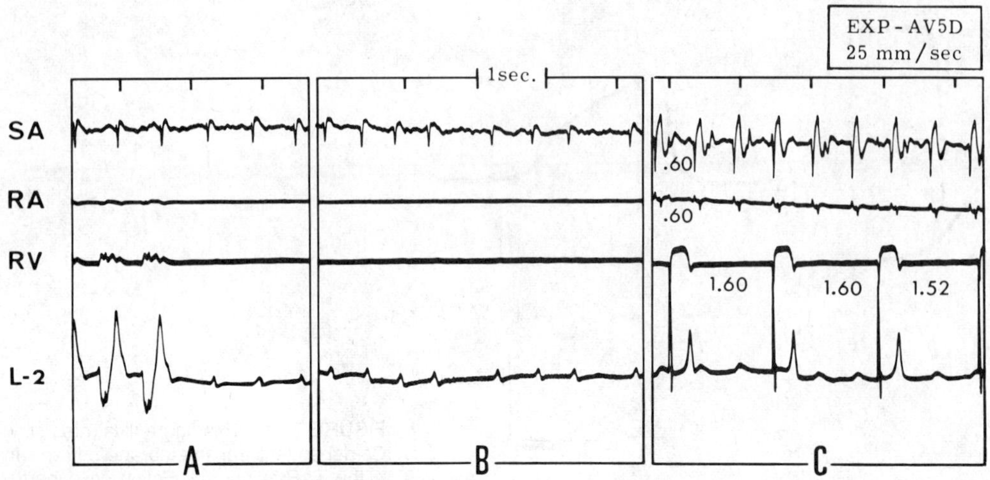

FIGURE 77-3 This figure illustrates K-induced AV block and a differential sensitivity of various cardiac tissues to K. Records were obtained from the region of the SA node (SA), right atrium (RA), right ventricle (RV), and lead II (L-2). The RA and RV leads fail to record electrical activity at a time when P waves are still present in L-2 (*A* and *B*). This indicates that the SA node and some parts of the atrium are less sensitive to K than the ventricular myocardium. The complete AV dissociation recorded in *C*, after the K infusion was discontinued, indicates that the junction is less resistant to K than either the SA node or the atrial and ventricular myocardium. The normal duration of the QRS in presence of prolonged P wave indicates that the ventricular myocardium is more resistant to K than the atrial myocardium. (*From C. Fisch, K. Greenspan, and R. R. Edmands, Complete Atrioventricular Block due to Potassium, Circ. Res., 19:373, 1966. Reproduced with permission from the American Heart Association, Inc., and the author.*)

77-3). His bundle studies localize the initial AV delay or block above the bundle of His, followed by block below the bundle of His. However, with rapid infusion, K preferentially depresses conduction below the bundle of His.[22]

The uniformity with which one can produce AV block in the dog is in striking contrast to the paucity of such observations in clinical hyperkalemia. In fact, in spontaneous clinical hyperkalemia, AV block greater than a simple prolongation of the PR is yet to be reported. However, high-degree AV block has been documented in humans following administration of large doses of K for treatment of arrhythmias,[13,23] or in the course of clinical investigation of the effects of K (Figs. 77-4 and 77-5). The discrepancy between the incidence of AV block in experi-

FIGURE 77-4 This figure demonstrates the effects in human beings of rapidly administered K. The control (*A*) illustrates sinus rhythm with PVC, some followed by retrograde atrial activation. With rapid infusion of K (*B*), the PVCs are promptly eliminated. Further infusion depresses the SA node and is followed by an idioventricular escape rhythm with ventricular bigeminy. It is possible that suppression is that of the atrial myocardium with sinoatrial block, rather than depression of sinus node activity. After K infusion is discontinued, the rhythm returns to control (*C*). (*From C. Fisch, E. F. Steinmetz, and R. B. Chevalier, Transient Effect of Intravenous Potassium on A-V Conduction and Ventricular Ectopic Beats, Am. Heart J., 60:220, 1960. Reproduced with permission from the publisher and author.*)

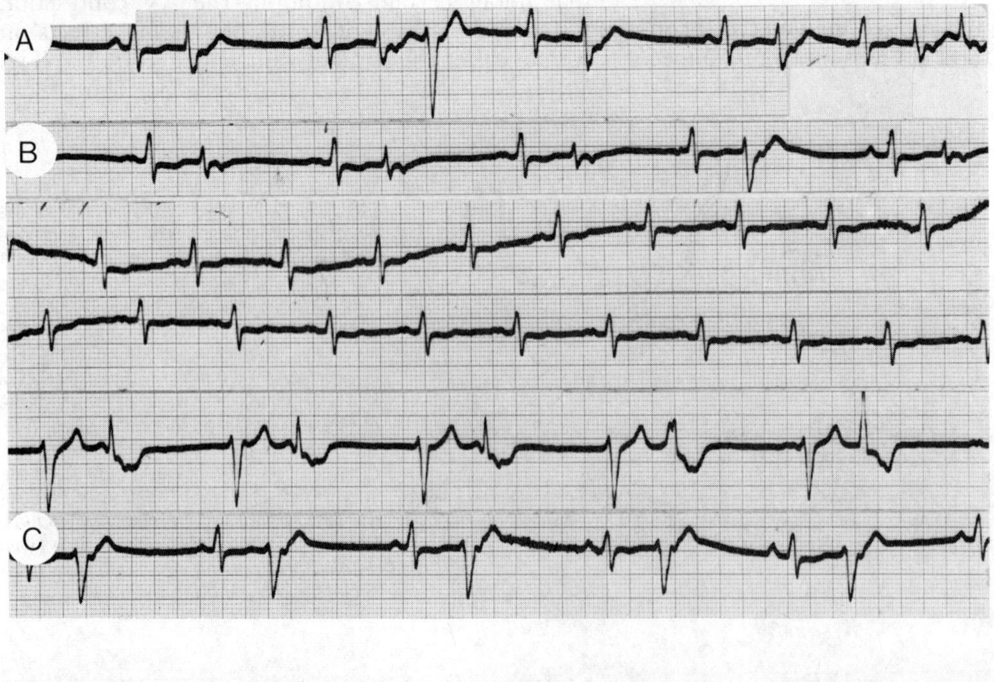

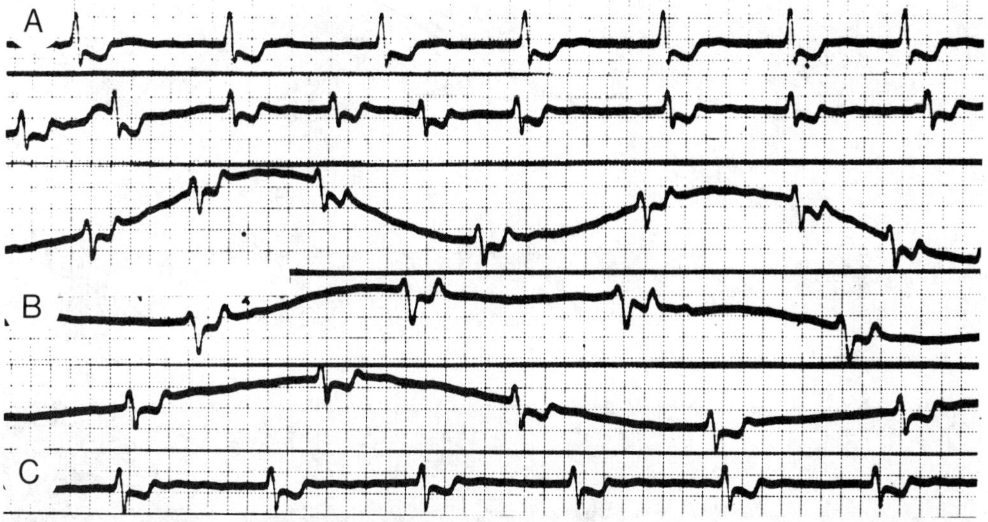

FIGURE 77-5 Effect of rapid administration of K to a patient with atrial fibrillation. *A*. Recorded at a plasma K of 4.5 meq/liter. Illustrates atrial fibrillation with normal intraventricular conduction. With rapid infusion of K, complete AV dissociation and intraventricular conduction appeared at a plasma K of 6.2 meq/liter (*B*). Control rhythm resumed after the infusion was discontinued (*C*).

mental and clinical hyperkalemia may be explained by the fact that experimental hyperkalemia is most likely an expression of pure K effect, while clinical hyperkalemia is ordinarily accompanied by disturbances of acid-base balance and electrolyte concentration other than K. Furthermore, the rate of rise of K differs, being more rapid in the experimental setting and much slower in diseased states. However, regardless of the metabolic variables affecting the ECG in clinical hyperkalemia, the effect is predominantly that of K because the ECG changes are not too dissimilar from those seen when serum K is elevated experimentally. In slowly developing hyperkalemia, the mechanism of death is cardiac standstill due to diffuse depression of intraventricular conduction,[24] and only occasionally due to ventricular fibrillation.

In the intact, lightly anesthetized dog with a slow heart rate and sinus arrhythmia, elevation of plasma K levels to about 6.5 meq/liter results in sinus tachycardia followed by a gradual slowing of the sinus rate as plasma K levels rise to a level of 7.5 to 8.0 meq/liter.

In addition to the depolarizing effect of K, the cation-induced vagal potentiation has been shown to contribute to depression of conduction.[25]

Hypokalemia and Conduction

In the experimental animal, hypokalemia may cause delay of AV conduction and block,[13,15] with depression of intraventricular conduction less common. The exact mechanism of conduction delay is not clear, but it may be related to hyperpolarization of the myocardial cell, with a stronger stimulus required to bring the TRP to TP. It may also be related to excitation of the cell before the latter repolarizes completely; at such a time the takeoff potential is reduced, which results in depression of conduction.[26] In contrast to experimental hypokalemia, in clinical hypokalemia prolongation of PR and QRS is rare.[13]

Potassium-Induced Arrhythmias

Rapid administration of K induces junctional[27] or ventricular ectopic rhythms and, terminally, ventricular fibrillation.[24] The fact that the ectopy is accompanied by K-induced depression of conduction suggests that the predominant mechanism of the arrhythmia may be reentry rather than automaticity. Ectopic rhythms other than junctional are relatively rare in clinical hyperkalemia, except as a terminal event.

Both experimental and clinical hypokalemia are accompanied by ectopic rhythms. A wide spectrum of atrial, junctional, and ventricular arrhythmias is encountered in humans. The arrhythmias may result from enhanced automaticity of latent pacemaker fibers due to decreased K conductance and efflux of K in face of an influx of Na.[28,29] In addition, it has been shown that duration of recovery of TAP may exceed the duration of the refractory period. As a result, a propagated impulse can be elicited before complete recovery of TAP takes place, and when the TRP is reduced and closer to TP, thus requiring a weaker stimulus for excitation.[26] Slowing of conduction by hypokalemia may contribute to reentrant arrhythmias.

Effect of Potassium on Preexisting Arrhythmias

K suppresses ectopic arrhythmias and is very effective for prompt control of life-threatening arrhythmias, particularly when they are due to digitalis tox-

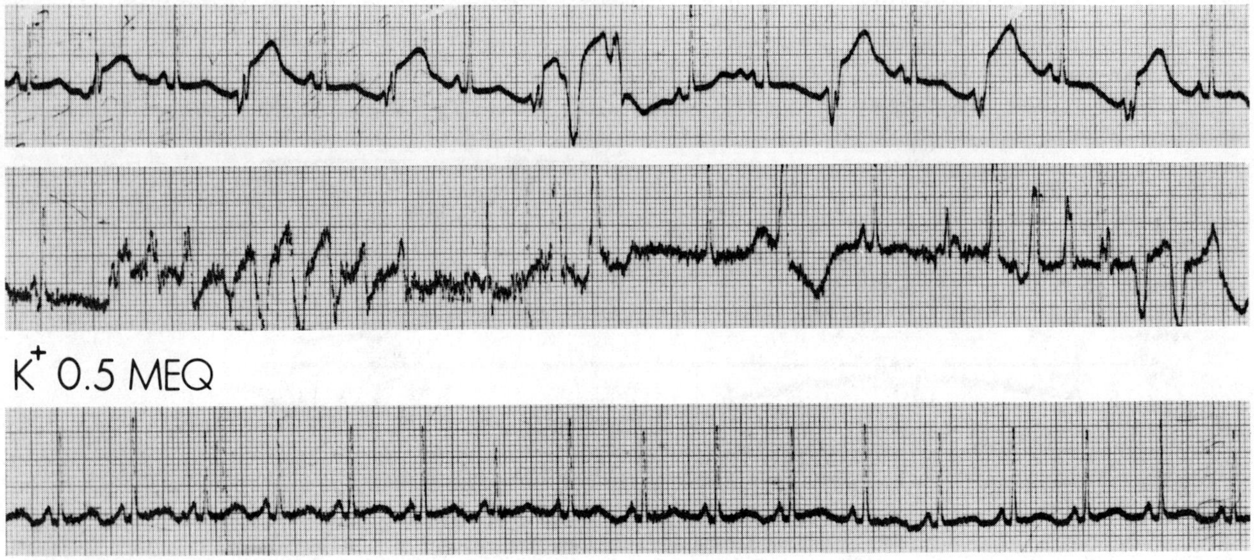

FIGURE 77-6 This figure illustrates the antiarrhythmic properties of K in a digitalis-intoxicated patient. The plasma K is 4.0 meq/liter. The upper two strips represent the chaotic ventricular arrhythmia, which responded promptly to a 0.5-meq bolus of K. It is not advisable to administer K rapidly.

icity (Fig. 77-6). The suppression of arrhythmias is in large measure independent of the control plasma K level or the mechanism of the arrhythmia. The fact that K influences both automaticity and conduction probably explains the striking efficacy of K as an antiarrhythmic agent.

The inhibition of diastolic depolarization hyperkalemia is thought to be due to an increase in membrane conductance and efflux of K, resulting in a more negative TRP.[28,29]

Potassium and Differential Sensitivity of Cardiac Tissue

Ordinarily, the ventricular myocardium is less sensitive to K than the atrial myocardium, and the specialized fibers of the sinoatrial (SA) node and the bundle of His are least sensitive.[7] In addition, the internodal atrial tracts may exhibit a selective resistance to K and perhaps play a role in preferential sinoventricular conduction.[30,31] Some of the factors which may modify the sensitivity of the cardiac tissue to K include other electrolytes, pH, O_2 saturation, the rate of change of plasma K level, and the etiology and severity of the underlying heart disease. All these and perhaps other factors need to be considered in evaluation of the relative sensitivity of cardiac tissues to K.

Occasionally the rate of change of K level, and not only the absolute level, may determine the effect of K on impulse formation and conduction. For example, a rapid increase in K concentration from hypokalemic to normal levels may result in bradycardia, cardiac arrest, or depression of conduction.[32] Such unexpected events are attributed to a sudden increase in negativity of the TRP secondary to increased K conductance in response to a rise of extracellular K concentration.

Potassium and Digitalis

The interrelation of digitalis and K is clinically important, because the effects of digitalis are modified by K. This interrelation may be manifested by (1) depression of digitalis ectopia by K, (2) emergence of digitalis ectopia during hypokalemia,[32–34] and (3) enhancement of digitalis-induced depression of conduction by K.

As early as 1918, Loewi found that in the experimental animal K suppresses digitalis-induced ectopic rhythms.[35] This observation was subsequently confirmed in humans.[36] The mechanism of suppression of the automatic arrhythmias is probably related to activation of the ATPase pump by the K, with an increase of K conductance, and efflux resulting in depression of phase 4 depolarization. In case of reentry, it is likely that K interrupts the reentrant pathway by altering conduction.

The observation that hyperkalemia, particularly if induced rapidly, enhances the depression of conduction by digitalis is expected. Both drugs are known to depress conduction and, furthermore, by blocking K transport, digitalis allows for a more rapid rise of the plasma K level.[33] An inappropriately rapid rate of administration of K to humans or animals intoxicated with digitalis results in depression of SA, intraatrial, AV, and intraventricular conduction.[15,36,37]

Because of the different sensitivities of the Purkinje and AV junctional tissues to K, there is a significantly wide margin of safety between the antiectopic and AV depression effects of K.[38] This margin of safety permits judicious administration of K for control of life-threatening digitalis-induced arrhythmias, even in the presence of simple AV conduction delay.

Hyperkalemia and the ECG

Hyperkalemia, either experimental or spontaneous, such as complicates renal failure, results in altered depolarization and repolarization. The former is manifest by prolongation of the P and QRS waves and the PR interval, while the latter is manifest by changing amplitude and configuration of the T wave. The correlation of the ECG changes and plasma K concentration differs depending on whether hyperkalemia is induced experimentally or results from clinical disorders such as renal failure. The electrocardiographic changes tend to parallel the plasma levels when K is infused in animals[39] or in course of clinical studies in human beings. In human beings exhibiting spontaneous clinical hyperkalemia, the ECG changes occur at much lower plasma level, and the correlation with the electrocardiogram is not as good as it is when hyperkalemia is induced by infusion. This difference has been ascribed to the fact that during clinical hyperkalemia disturbances of other electrolytes and changing acid-base balance play an important role. Such changes play a minor role during rapid infusion of K. The so-called tented T wave with a narrow base is usually the earliest change noted during infusion and is seen at a plasma level of approximately 5.7 meq/liter. The QRS widens uniformly at a plasma K level of 9 to 11 meq/liter and may at times be associated with a current of injury simulating pericarditis or myocardial infarction.[40] At a plasma level of 7 meq/liter the P wave is altered, becoming lower and prolonged due to depression of intraatrial conduction, and the PR interval lengthens. Not infrequently the prolongation of the PR interval progresses to second degree AV block. The P wave becomes unrecognizable at plasma levels over 8.5 meq/liter, and if the infusion is continued, ventricular fibrillation or cardiac arrest results at a K level of approximately 12 meq/liter.

Hyperkalemia depresses the perinodal tissue conduction and may result in SA exit block, either type I or type II.[37,38] The exit block is ascribed to the fact that the SA fibers are more resistant to the depressing action of K than is the atrial myocardium. In other words, the SA impulse is generated but fails to propagate because of the depression of intraatrial conduction. Occasionally junctional rhythms are also recorded.

As in the animal, the earliest ECG abnormality in human beings is a tall T wave which is characteristically peaked, its ascending and descending limbs symmetrical, and the base narrow.[41–43] This is the previously referred to tented T wave seen in approximately 20 percent of patients with hyperkalemia.[44–46] Because of proximity effect the T-wave changes are best noted in leads V_2 to V_4. With gradually increasing plasma level the P wave ultimately disappears and the PR interval is prolonged. Because of disappearance of the P wave, recognition of arrhythmias is often impossible (Fig. 77-7). The R-wave amplitude decreases, a deep S wave appears, and the QRS shows progressive widening terminating in a sine wave. On rare occasions, a current of injury resembling that of myocardial infarction or pericarditis may appear[40] (Fig. 77-8). The elevated K depresses intraventricular conduction, and the widened QRS may resemble all known forms of intraventricular conduction defects. These may include, from time to time, right bundle branch block, left bundle branch block, anterior or posterior fascicular block, or a combination of the above. The intraventricular conduction defects can be differentiated from the classic bundle branch blocks because hyperkalemia induces uniform depression of conduction resulting in aberration of both the initial and the terminal portion of the QRS (Fig. 77-8 and 77-9). As in the experimental animal, hyperkalemia can induce SA block either type I or type II and passive or accelerated escape junctional or ventricular rhythms. Because of the hyperkalemia-induced aberration, it may be difficult or impossible to differentiate junctional from ventricular ectopy.

It has been shown that administration of K to patients with inverted T waves, the inversion a result of physiological influences, will alter the T-wave vector, the latter becoming normal. However, the K has no effect on inverted T wave due to organic disease such as may be present in ischemic heart disease or as a result of administration of drugs.[47–49]

Hypokalemia and the ECG

In 1937, Bellet and Dyer noted that patients treated for diabetic coma exhibited prolongation of QT interval, depression of ST segment, and T-wave changes.[50] This was shown to be due to hypokalemia associated with diabetic acidosis.[51]

In the isolated heart hypokalemia may result in AV and intraventricular conduction delays, prolongation of the ST segment, and alteration of the T wave.[52]

In clinical hypokalemia the characteristic change is an exaggerated U wave but without any significant change in QT duration.[53] It is frequently difficult to separate the ST segment from the U wave because of a gradual fusion of the two. On rare occasions hypokalemia is associated with inversion of the T wave and loss of amplitude of the QRS (Fig. 77-10). Specific criteria for recognition of hypokalemia have been suggested.[54,55]

A diagnosis of hypokalemia can be made with a reasonable degree of accuracy when the plasma K concentration is lower than 2.3 meq/liter.[56] It should be remembered, however, that the electrocardiac pattern of hypokalemia is not specific for that disorder because it can be seen following adminis-

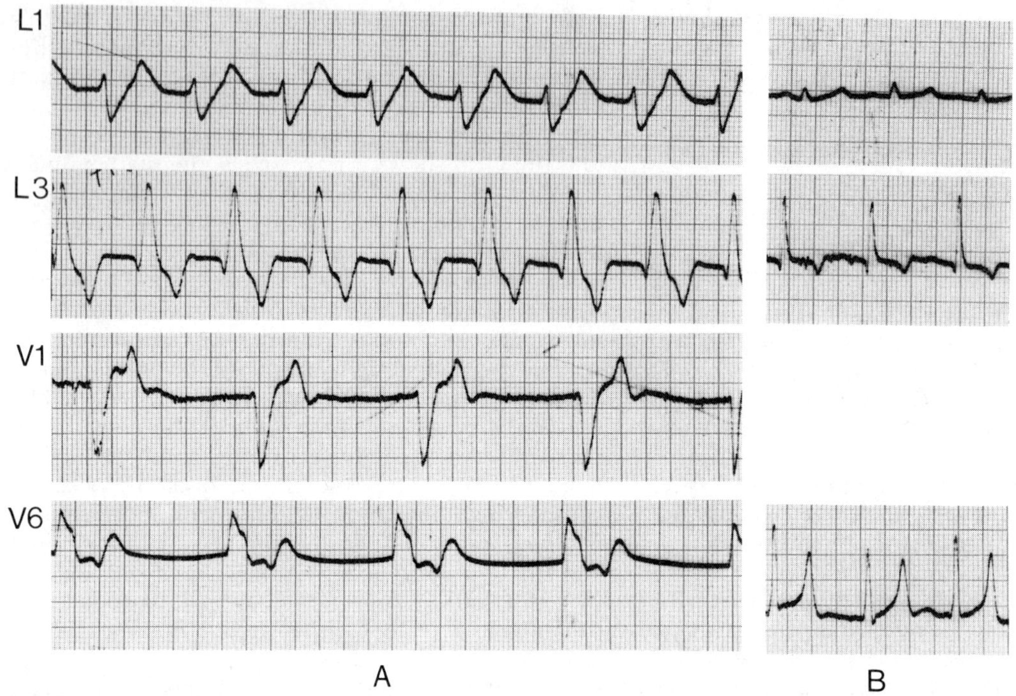

FIGURE 77-7 This figure illustrates the difficulties encountered in analysis of the rhythm in presence of hyperkalemia. *A.* This ECG was recorded at a plasma K level of 9.1 meq/liter with a blood urea nitrogen of 270 mg/dl and CO_2 of 10 meq/liter. P waves are absent, making a definitive diagnosis of the rhythm difficult, if not impossible. The possible atrial rhythms include (1) SA rhythm without identifiable P waves with a 2:1 SA block in leads V_1 and V_6; (2) SA rhythm with 1:1 AV conduction in leads I and III with 2:1 conduction in V_1 and V_6; (3) sinus slowing in V_1 and V_6; (4) SA arrest or atrial fibrillation with a junctional tachycardia with 1:1 exit in leads I and III and 2:1 exit in leads V_1 and V_6. The QRS is prolonged to 0.20 s with prolongation of both the initial and terminal portions, best seen in leads III and V_6, respectively. *B.* Recorded after treatment of the hyperkalemia. (*From C. Fisch, Relation of Electrolyte Disturbances to Cardiac Arrhythmias, Circulation, 47:408, 1973. Reproduced with permission from the American Heart Association, Inc., and the author.*)

FIGURE 77-8 This figure illustrates the current of injury occasionally seen in hyperkalemia. The plasma K at 7:00 p.m. was 9.1 meq/liter and illustrates, in addition to prolongation of the PR and diffuse intraventricular conduction delay, a current of injury simulating acute myocardial infarction. The ST-segment elevation is best seen in leads III, V_1, and V_2. Following treatment of the hyperkalemia (10:30 p.m.), the tracing, with exception of an abnormal T in lead I, is normal.

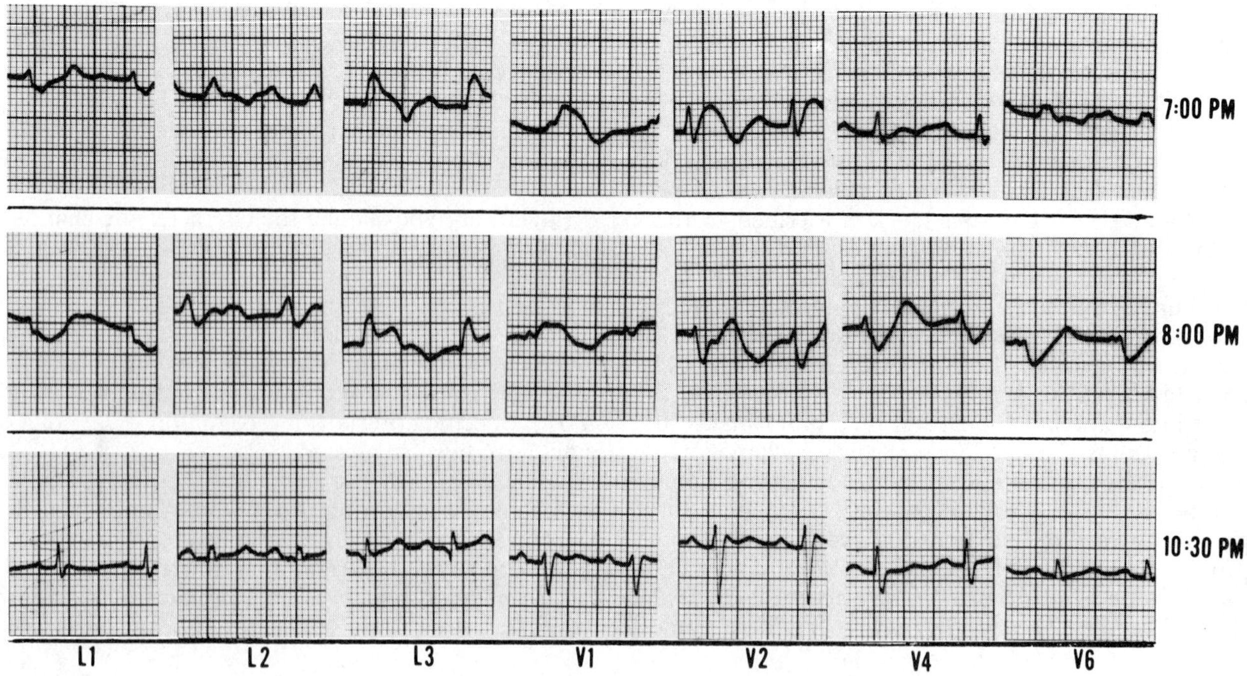

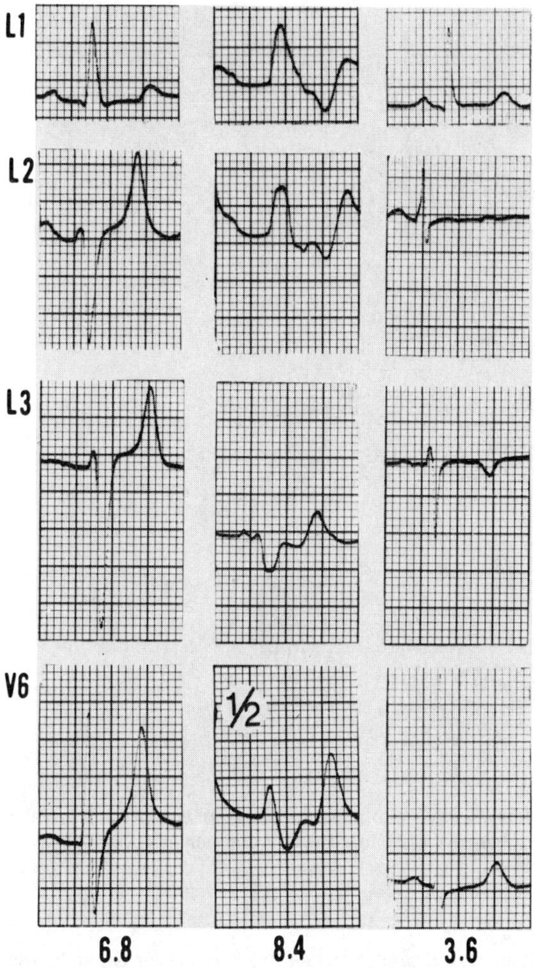

FIGURE 77-9 K and the ECG. After treatment and at a level of 3.6 meq/liter, the PR, QRS, and T waves are normal. At 6.8 meq/liter, the PR and QRS are prolonged, with a shift of the QRS axis to the left, and the T waves are symmetrical, narrow-based, and tall—the so-called tented T waves. At a K level of 8.4 meq/liter there is further prolongation of PR, the P wave becoming difficult to identify, the QRS axis shifted to the right, and the QRS prolonged to 0.20 s. The characteristic prolongation of both the initial and terminal portions of the QRS is best illustrated in V_6.

tration of drugs, particularly digitalis and antiarrhythmic agents in the presence of ventricular hypertrophy and bradycardia.[57,58]

Potassium and Contractility

Although Ca is the primary and most important electrolyte involved in the process of contraction, changes in K level may alter contractility.[59] The effect of changing K level on contractility has been studied only in the animal. The experimental animal manifests a positive inotropic effect in response to hypokalemia, which may be secondary to changes in Ca and Na. The latter is suggested by the observation that a decrease in extracellular K concentration makes the frog heart more sensitive to inotropic effect of Ca, an effect attributed to a demonstrable increase in Ca uptake.[60] In the dog, within K levels of 1.6 and 15 meq/liter intracardiac pressure, cardiac output, and force of left ventricular contraction are normal.[61] However, rapid administration of K causes a decrease in ventricular contractile force.

Calcium

Calcium and Transmembrane Action Potential

Changing Ca level alters the plateau, or phase 2, of the TAP. Hypocalcemia prolongs phase 2 and the duration of the action potential, and hypercalcemia decreases the duration of phase 2 and the duration of action potential. At levels from 1.2 to 20.9 meq/liter, the effect on phase 3 and TRP is minimal.[62–64] Only at levels which are mostly likely incompatible with life does hypocalcemia reduce the TRP and increase the slope of phase 4 depolarization. Thus, within clinically encountered levels of Ca concentration, the ion is without any significant effect on either the magnitude of the TRP or slope of phase 4 depolarization, the two variables important in the genesis of arrhythmias.

The slow inward Ca-carried slow current contributes to the terminal portion of phase 0 and the plateau, or phase 2. Although the exact role of this current in the clinical setting is not yet fully understood, some of the characteristics of these slow potentials, especially the slow depolarization with slow propagation and longer refractory period, could result in arrhythmias by providing the essential link for reentrant arrhythmias, namely very slow conduction. This low-amplitude, Ca-dependent action potential has been shown, under some circumstances, to exhibit properties of automaticity.[65] In the normal heart the sinus and AV nodal TAP resemble the slow Ca action potential and may well depend on the slow Ca current. This assumption is strengthened by the fact that the spontaneous rate of SA discharge is reduced, AV nodal-cell activity depressed, and AV conduction prolonged or blocked by Ca current-blocking agents such as verapamil. It is possible that during acute myocardial infarction, partial depolarization by the increased extracellular K concentration may result in slow depolarization arrhythmias.[66–68] This possibility remains to be proved.

By altering the membrane permeability to Na or K or both, Ca may be involved in the genesis of late and perhaps early afterdepolarizations. It is postulated that a release of intracellular Ca, independent of the Ca-carried current, alters the Na and K permeability, and this in turn results in afterdepolarizations[69] (Fig. 77-11). Preliminary evidence suggests that diastolic afterpotentials may be responsible for some forms of clinical arrhythmias.[70,71]

It has also been suggested that the increased influx of Ca during rapid stimulation, by increasing membrane conductance to K, and hyperpolarization

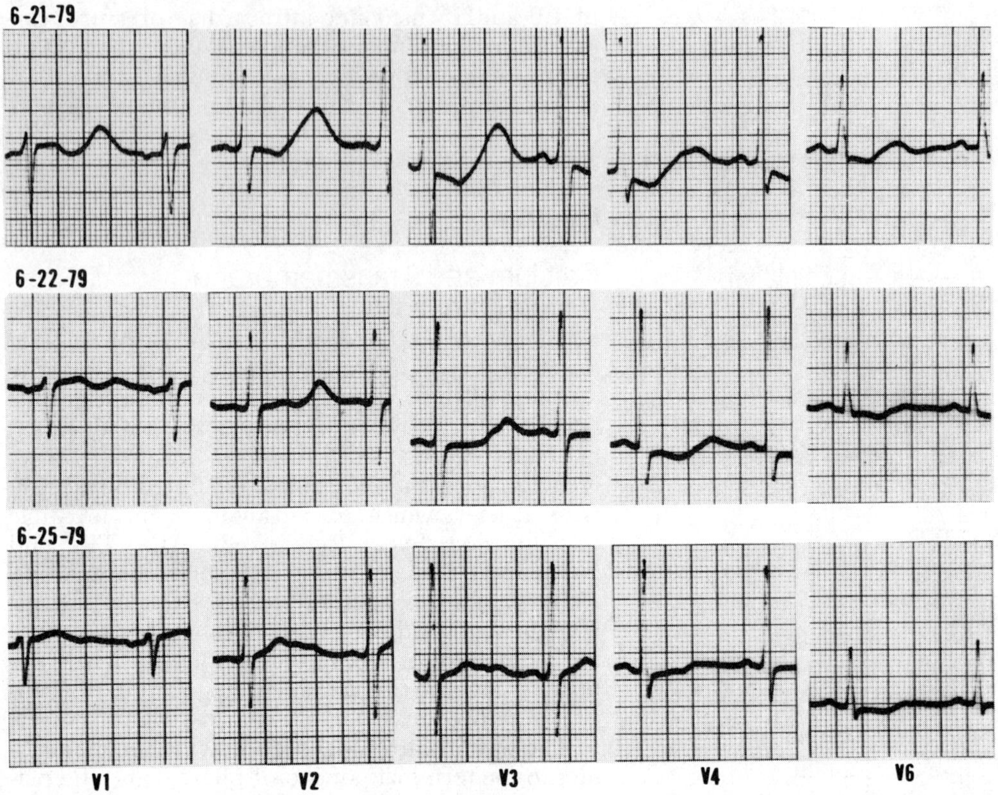

FIGURE 77-10 This figure illustrates the ECG changes of hypokalemia. A striking U wave with a marked prolongation of QU interval is recorded on June 21, 1979. The K level at that time was 1.3 meq/liter. With replacement of K, there was a gradual improvement with a normal QT and U wave recorded on June 25, 1979, at a plasma K of 3.9 meq/liter.

FIGURE 77-11 This figure illustrates diastolic afterpotentials (triggered automaticity) very likely related to intracellular Ca shift. The Purkinje fiber is superfused with $2 \times 10^{-7}M$ acetylstrophanthidin. The basic driving cycle length is gradually shortened from 500 (*A*) to 300 ms (*F*). At a cycle length of 500 ms, 28 min after onset of superfusion, cessation of pacing is followed by a nonpropagated diastolic afterpotential. Similar nonpropagated potential is noted in *C, D, E,* and *F.* The afterpotential results in a full action potential with repetitive responses noted in *F,* paralleling the duration of superfusion with acetylstrophanthidin and the rate of stimulation.

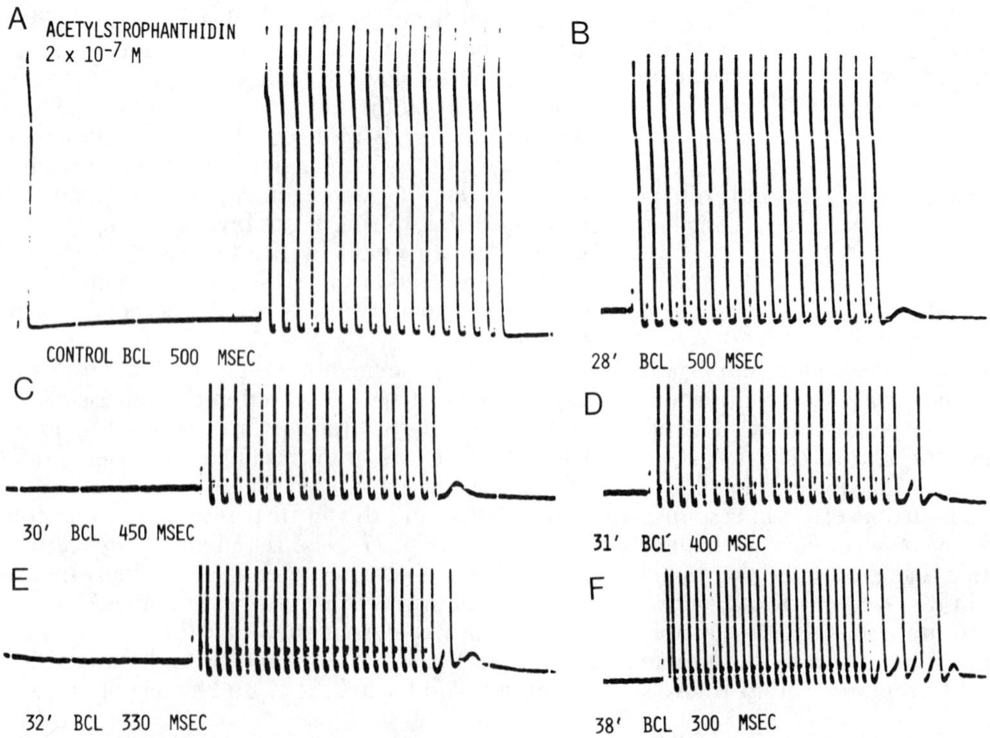

of the cell may be the mechanism responsible for the overdrive suppression of pacemakers.[72]

In the intact experimental animal, marked elevation of the plasma Ca level may depress intraventricular conduction and induce ventricular premature systoles and fibrillation.[62] In patients with extreme elevation of Ca concentration, prolongation of PR, or higher degrees of AV block and prolongation of the QRS have been reported.[6] As a rule, however, arrhythmias do not complicate clinical hypercalcemia.

By reducing the Ca to one-twentieth of its normal concentration, a situation not seen in clinical medicine, arrhythmias can be induced in animals. An interesting and potentially clinically useful relationship exists between K and Ca. K-induced depression of conduction and ectopia can be reversed by administration of Ca. This reversal is probably related to an increase of the TRP by Ca.

The suggestion that elevation of Ca level enhances digitalis arrhythmias needs confirmation. The fact that lowering Ca level with ethylenediaminetetracetic acid (EDTA) can reverse arrhythmias supports such a relationship. However, this intervention affects both the arrhythmias due to digitalis and those not related to digitalis.[63,64]

Calcium and the Surface ECG

The relation between Ca level and the ECG was noted by Carter and Andrus in 1922.[73] The changes in plasma level of Ca are reflected in the ECG by altered duration of the ST segment and QT interval. Hypocalcemia prolongs phase 2 of the TAP, and this is mirrored in the ECG by prolongation of the ST segment and the QT interval. The QaT (Q to apex of T) and the QT intervals are prolonged. However, the corrected QT (QT_c) rarely exceeds 140 percent of the normal. If the QT exceeds that number, the U wave is likely to be included in the measurement. Neither phase 3 of the TAP nor the T wave of the ECG is altered by the hypocalcemia[53] (Fig. 77-12*B*). Hypocalcemia combines with hyperkalemia to produce an easily recognizable pattern and is most often seen in patients with chronic renal disease. This pattern is characterized by prolongation of the ST segment and appearance of a tented T wave (Fig. 77-12*C*). Similarly, hypocalcemia in association with hypokalemia may exhibit a prolonged ST segment with prominent terminal wave consisting of both the T and U waves. While the ST is prolonged, the total QU remains normal.[53]

Elevation of Ca level in an electrophysiological preparation or in human beings results in foreshortening of phase 2 of the TAP and of the electrocardiographic ST segment (Fig. 77-12*A*).

There is a lack of correlation between the corrected QT (QT_c) and the serum Ca concentration, because the QT is affected by a variety of physiological and pharmacological interventions. Of the different components of the QT, the interval from

FIGURE 77-12 *A.* Recorded at a Ca level of 17.0 Mg/dl. Illustrates the short ST segment characteristic of hypercalcemia. *B.* Recorded at a Ca level of 5.9 mg/dl. Shows the prolongation of the ST of hypocalcemia. *C.* Recorded at a K level of 6.2 meq/liter, Ca of 5.3 mg/dl, and P of 12.2 mg/dl. The prolongation of QT due to hypocalcemia, terminated by the tented T of hyperkalemia, is characteristic of both hypocalcemia and hyperkalemia seen in chronic renal disease.

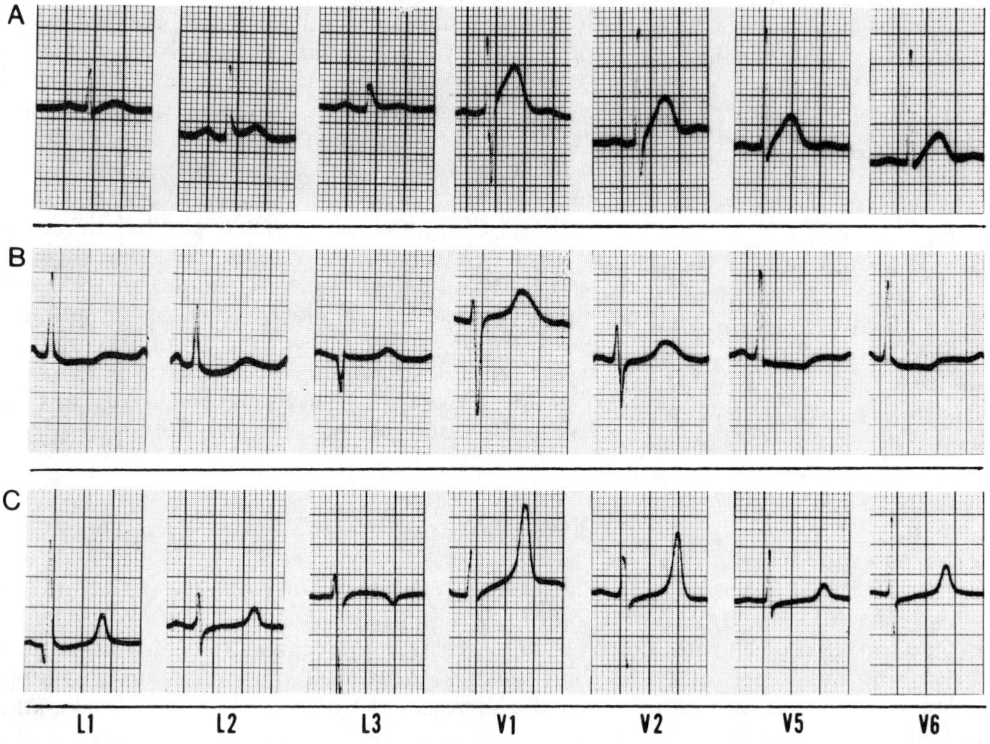

the Q to the apex of the T (QaT) can be measured most precisely and shows the best correlation with Ca level.[74] Given a state of pure hypocalcemia, such as can be induced by EDTA, there is a reasonable correlation between the Ca concentration and the duration of the ST segment.[75]

Calcium and Contractility

The need of Ca for proper mechanical function of cardiac tissue was clearly demonstrated by Ringer.[1] A large body of evidence supports the concept that Ca provides the essential link for excitation-contraction coupling. Ca in the extracellular space couples excitation to contraction by two mechanisms. First, by providing the ionic current carried through the slow channel and, second, by releasing intracellularly stored Ca from the longitudinal system into the sarcoplasm. The Ca released from intracellular stores combines with the Ca which entered the cell as part of the slow-channel current, resulting in a significant increase of free intracellular Ca. The free Ca diffuses into the myofibrils; combines with troponin, which in its Ca-free state inhibits the myosinactin interaction; and releases this inhibition. Actin combines with myosin, and adenosine triphosphate (ATP) is split by the Ca-dependent ATPase. The released energy is transformed into mechanical work with the actin filaments sliding over the myosin filaments, and shortening of the myofibrils results.[75–78]

Despite the fundamental importance of Ca in the process of contraction, chronic hypocalcemia has not been shown to result in heart failure. Occasionally, acutely induced hypocalcemia may be associated with depression of ventricular function.[79] However, with the advent and increasing use of Ca channel-blocking agents, interference with the function of Ca in excitation-contraction coupling and modulation of contractility may become clinically important.

Magnesium

Mg is involved in the function of enzymes which utilize ATP as a substrate, including the Na-K-ATPase, the source of energy for the "sodium pump." Consequently, intracellular Mg deficiency may be associated with an increase in intracellular Na and Ca, and a loss of K. Similarly, an increase of Mg theoretically can result in an intracellular decrease of Na and Ca, and an increase in K.[80,81] This interdependence of the electrophysiological effects of Mg, Ca, Na, and K makes ECG recognition of Mg alteration difficult, if not impossible.

Abnormalities of Mg concentration encountered in clinical situations affect the TAP only in the presence of hypocalcemia.[82] The effect of high Mg concentration on phase 0 is similar to that of K, with a decrease in upstroke velocity, which may explain the antiarrhythmic effect of Mg.[55] The effect on phase 2 resembles that of Ca, with low Mg concentrations prolonging, and high Mg concentrations shortening the plateau, or phase 2. Very significant prolongation of phase 2 can be induced by low concentrations of Ca and Mg.

In the experimental animal, early ECG signs of hypomagnesemia are those of a slight widening of QRS, peaked T, and ST depression. As the deficiency becomes more severe, QRS widens further, and conduction disturbances and arrhythmias may appear.[81,83] These changes may be a manifestation of relative extracellular hyperkalemia due to loss of intracellular K.[84]

Elevation of extracellular Mg to a level of 6 to 10 meq/liter depresses AV and intraventricular conduction.[61,85,86] This may be due to slowing of the upstroke velocity of phase 0, a mechanism similar or identical to that induced by hyperkalemia. SA and AV block occur at about 15 meq/liter, and cardiac arrest may be expected at levels 15 to 22 meq/liter.[85] However, neuromuscular and respiratory paralysis usually precede the cardiac arrest.

Whether or not alteration of Mg concentration within clinical ranges induces arrhythmias is unclear. To date there is very little evidence that clinical hypomagnesemia gives rise to arrhythmias. Study of children with protein-calorie malnutrition and depressed levels of Mg failed to disclose any arrhythmias except for sinus tachycardia, and this was not felt to be due to low Mg levels.[87]

As a rule, abnormalities of the ST segment due to changing Mg concentration cannot be identified in the surface ECG because these are dominated by Ca.[56] However, administration of Mg may result in a statistically significant shortening of QT.[80]

The relationship of low Mg level to digitalis-induced arrhythmias in animals is of potential interest. Lowering the Mg level by dialyzing with an Mg-free solution reduces the amount of acetylstrophanthidin necessary to induce arrhythmia. The arrhythmia is promptly abolished in most, but not all, of the animals by administration of magnesium sulfate solution.[88] Because of the severe and rapid reduction of Mg, it is questionable whether these results can be extrapolated to clinical situations. Digitalis toxicity accompanied by hypomagnesemia can be suppressed with Mg.[88] The question of the specificity of Mg as an antiarrhythmic agent for digitalis arrhythmias needs further study, for, as in the case of K, Mg suppresses arrhythmias due to digitalis, as well as those not due to the glycoside.

Phosphorus

Phosphorus is essential for production and utilization of high-energy phosphate compounds such as ATP and creatine phosphate. It is also important for the function of ATP-dependent cation pump activity, such as Ca-ATPase. Thus, the uptake and intracellular distribution of Ca within myocardial cells depend upon adequate stores of phosphate. It seems reasonable, therefore, that hypophosphatemia and P depletion, by affecting either the energy production cycle or Ca transport mechanisms, could have a deleterious effect on myocardial function.[89] Preliminary reports suggest that this might be the case. Animals with dietary-induced P depletion may exhibit evidence of depression of myocardial function, which is reversed with P repletion. The impairment of myocardial function associated with P depletion is independent of the left ventricular volume, resistance to ventricular ejection, or ventricular rate.[90]

Isolated clinical observations indicate that in certain conditions, such as infusion of large doses of insulin[91] or in critically ill patients, hypophosphatemia may occur and be associated with myocardial depression, which is reversed following phosphate repletion.[89,92] Such observations suggest the possibility that reversible congestive cardiomyopathy may be associated with, or due to, hypophosphatemia.[89] However, the observations relating hypophosphatemia to clinical myocardial disorder must be considered preliminary.

Lithium

Although not a naturally occurring electrolyte, lithium (Li) has assumed an importance in cardiac electrophysiology because of its wide use in the management of depressive states.

Although reversible T-wave changes are the most common ECG abnormality due to Li,[93,94] dysfunction of the SA node has emerged as the characteristic and clinically significant complication of Li therapy. Disordered sinus node function may be manifested by sinus bradycardia, SA arrest, or exit block, either type I (Wenckebach) or type II (Mobitz II). These side effects occur most often with Li within the therapeutic levels. The effect on the SA node appear to be selective, as suggested by a normal PR, QRS, and, in the His electrogram,[95,96] a normal AH with only a slightly prolonged HV interval.

References

1. Ringer, S.: A Further Contribution Regarding the Influence of the Different Constituents of Blood on the Contraction of the Heart, *J. Physiol.,* 4:29, 1883.
2. Dale, H.: Accident and Opportunism in Medical Research, *Br. Med. J.,* 2:451, 1948.
3. Ringer, S.: Concerning the Influence Exerted by Each of the Constituents of Blood on Contraction of the Ventricle, *J. Physiol.,* 3:380, 1882.
4. Ringer, S.: On the Mutual Antagonism between Lime and Potash Salts in Toxic Doses, *J. Physiol.,* 5:247, 1884.
5. Scherf, D., and Schott, A.: "Extrasystoles and Allied Arrhythmias," Wm. Heineman Medical Books Ltd., Bath, Great Britain, 1973, pp. 763, 777, 784.
6. Fisch, C.: Relation of Electrolyte Disturbances to Cardiac Arrhythmias, *Circulation,* 47:408, 1973.
7. Hoffman, B. F., and Cranefield, P. F.: "Electrophysiology of the Heart," McGraw-Hill Book Company, New York, 1960.
8. Hecht, H. H.: Some Observations and Theories Concerning the Electrical Behavior of Heart Muscle, *Am. J. Med.,* 30:720, 1961.
9. Bailey, C. J., Elharrar, V., and Zipes, D. P.: Slow Channel Depolarization and Control of Arrhythmias, *Ann. Rev. Med.* 29:417, 1978.
10. Fisch, C., Greenspan, K., and Edmands, R. R.: Complete Atrioventricular Block Due to Potassium, *Circ. Res.,* 19:373, 1966.
11. Mendez, C., Erlij, D., and Moe, G. K.: Indirect Action of Epinephrine on Intraventricular Conduction Time, *Circ. Res.,* 14:318, 1964.
12. Vassalle, M.: Automaticity and Automatic Rhythms, *Am. J. Cardiol.,* 28:245, 1971.
13. Mathison, G. C.: The Effect of Potassium Salts upon the Circulation and Their Action on Plain Muscle, *J. Physiol. (Lond.),* 42:471, 1911.
14. Fisch, C.: Effect of K on A-V Conduction, *Circulation,* 41:575, 1970 (editorial).
15. Fisch, C., Knoebel, S. B., Feigenbaum, H., and Greenspan, K.: Potassium and Monophasic Action Potential, Electrocardiogram, Conduction and Arrhythmias, *Progr. Cardiovasc. Dis.,* 8:387, 1966.
16. Carvalho, A. P. De, and Langan, W. B.: Influence of Extracellular Potassium Levels on Atrioventricular Transmission, *Am. J. Physiol.,* 205:375, 1963.
17. Bettinger, J. C., Surawicz, B., Bryfogle, J. W., Anderson, B. N., and Bellet, S.: The Effect of Intravenous Administration of Potassium Chloride on Ectopic Rhythms, Ectopic Beats, and Disturbances of A-V Conduction, *Am. J. Med.,* 21:521, 1956.
18. Fisch, C., Steinmetz, E. F., and Chevalier, R. B.: Transient Effect of Intravenous Potassium on A-V Conduction and Ventricular Ectopic Beats, *Am. Heart J.,* 60:220, 1960.
19. Feigenbaum, H., Wunsch, C., and Fisch, C.: Effect of Intracoronary Infusion of Potassium on the Vagal Action on A-V Transmission, *J. Clin. Invest.,* 44:399, 1965.
20. Fisch, C., Feigenbaum, H., and Bowers, J. A.: The Inhibition of Acetylcholine Induced A-V Block by Potassium, *J. Clin. Invest.,* 42:563, 1963.
21. Fisch, C., Feigenbaum, H., and Bowers, J. A.: The Effect of Potassium on Atrioventricular Conduction of Normal Dogs, *Am. J. Cardiol.,* 11:487, 1963.
22. Cohen, H. C., Gozo, E. G., and Pick, A.: The Nature and Type of Arrhythmias in Acute Experimental Hyperkalemia in the Intact Dog, *Am. Heart J.,* 82:777, 1971.
23. Brown, H., Tanner, G. L., and Hecht, H. H.: The Effects of Potassium Salts in Subjects with Heart Disease, *J. Lab. Clin. Med.,* 37:506, 1951.
24. Nahum, L. H., and Hoff, H. E.: Observations on Potassium Fibrillation, *J. Pharmacol. Exp. Ther.,* 65:322, 1939.
25. Howell, W. H.: Vagus Inhibition of the Heart and Its Relation to the Inorganic Salts of the Blood, *Am. J. Physiol.,* 15:280, 1906.
26. Gettes, L. S., Surawicz, B., and Shiue, J. C.: Effect of High K, Low K, and Quinidine on QRS Duration and Ventricular Action Potential, *Am. J. Physiol.* 203:1135, 1962.
27. Fisch, C., Feigenbaum, H., and Bowers, J. A.: Nonparoxysmal A-V Nodal Tachycardia Due to Potassium, *Am. J. Cardiol.,* 14:357, 1964.
28. Gettes, L., and Surawicz, B.: Effects of Low and High Concentrations of Potassium on the Simultaneously Recorded Purkinje and Ventricular Action Potentials of the Perfused Pig Moderator Band, *Circ. Res.,* 23:717, 1968.
29. Vassalle, M.: Cardiac Pacemaker Potentials at Different Extra- and Intracellular K Concentrations, *Am. J. Physiol.,* 208:770, 1965.
30. Vassalle, M., and Hoffman, B. F.: The Spread of Sinus Activation during Potassium Administration, *Circ. Res.,* 17:285, 1965.
31. Hoffman, B. F., and Cranefield, P. F.: The Physiological Basis of Cardiac Arrhythmias, *Am. J. Med.,* 37:670, 1964.

32. Surawicz, B., and Gettes, L. S.: Two Mechanisms of Cardiac Arrest Produced by Potassium, *Circ. Res.*, 12:415, 1963.
33. Fisch, C., Greenspan, K., Knoebel, S. B., and Feigenbaum, H.: Effect of Digitalis on Conduction of the Heart, *Progr. Cardiovasc. Dis.*, 6:343, 1964.
34. Lown, B., Weller, J. M., Wyatt, N., Hoigne, R., and Merrill, J. P.: Effects of Alterations of Body Potassium and Digitalis Toxicity, *J. Clin. Invest.*, 31:648, 1952. (Abstract.)
35. Loewi, O.: Uber den Zusammenhang zwischen Digitalis und Kalziumwirkung, *Arch. Exp. Pathol. Pharmacol.*, 82:366, 1918a.
36. Sampson, J. J., Alberton, E. C., and Kondo, B.: The Effects on Man of Potassium Administration in Relation to Digitalis Glycosides with Special Reference to Blood Serum Potassium, the Electrocardiogram and Ectopic Beats, *Am. Heart J.*, 26:164, 1943.
37. Fisch, C., Martz, B. C., and Priebe, F. H.: Enhancement of Potassium-Induced Atrioventricular Block by Basic Doses of Digitalis Drugs, *J. Clin. Invest.*, 39:1885, 1960.
38. Fisch, C., Steinmetz, E. F., Fasola, A. F., and Martz, B. L.: Effect of Potassium and "Toxic" Doses of Digitalis on the Myocardium, *Circ. Res.*, 7:424, 1959.
39. Winkler, A. W., Hoff, H. E., and Smith, P. K.: Electrocardiographic Changes and Concentration of Potassium in Serum following Intravenous Injection of Potassium Chloride, *Am. J. Physiol.*, 124:478, 1938.
40. Levine, H. D., Wanzer, S. H., and Merrill, J. P.: Dialyzable Currents of Injury in Potassium Intoxication Resembling Acute Myocardial Infarction of Pericarditis, *Circulation*, 13:29, 1956.
41. Thomson, W. A. R.: Potassium and the T Wave of the Electrocardiogram, *Lancet*, 1:808, 1939.
42. Keith, N. M., Burchell, H. B., and Baggenstoss, A. H.: Electrocardiographic Changes in Uremia Associated with a High Concentration of Serum Potassium: A Report of Three Cases, *Am. Heart J.*, 27:817, 1944.
43. Nadler, C. S., Bellet, S., and Lanning, M.: Influence of the Serum Potassium and Other Electrolytes on the Electrocardiogram in Diabetic Acidosis, *Am. J. Med.*, 5:838, 1948.
44. Levine, H. D., Vazifdar, J. P., Lown, B., and Merrill, J. P.: "Tent-Shaped" T Waves of Normal Amplitude in Potassium Intoxication, *Am. Heart J.*, 43:437, 1952.
45. Braun, H. A., Surawicz, B., and Bellet, S.: T Waves in Hyperpotassemia, *Am. J. Med. Sci.*, 230:147, 1955.
46. Merrill, J. P., Levine, H. D., Somerville, W., Smith, S., III: Clinical Recognition and Treatment of Acute Potassium Intoxication, *Ann. Intern. Med.*, 33:797, 1950.
47. Goldberger, E., Pokress, M. J., and Stein, R.: Effect of Potassium on Downward T Waves of Precordial Leads of Normal Children, *Am. Heart J.*, 37:418, 1949.
48. Sharpey-Schafer, E. P.: Potassium Effects on T Wave Inversion in Myocardial Infarction and Preponderance of a Ventricle, *Br. Heart J.*, 5:80, 1943.
49. Wasserburger, R. H., and Corliss, R. J.: Value of Oral Potassium Salts in Differentiation of Functional and Organic T Wave Changes, *Am. J. Cardiol.*, 10:673, 1962.
50. Bellet, S., and Dyer, W. W.: The Electrocardiogram during and after Emergence from Diabetic Coma, *Am. Heart, J.*, 13:72, 1937.
51. Holler, J. W.: Potassium Deficiency Occurring during the Treatment of Diabetic Acidosis, *JAMA*, 131:1186, 1946.
52. Butcher, W. A., Wakim, K. G., Essex, H. E., Pruitt, R. D., and Burchell, H. B.: The Effect of Changes in Concentration of Cations on the Electrocardiogram of the Isolated Perfused Heart, *Am. Heart J.*, 43:801, 1952.
53. Surawicz, B., and Lepeschkin, E.: The Electrocardiographic Pattern of Hypopotassemia with and without Hypocalcemia, *Circulation*, 8:801, 1953.
54. Surawicz, B., Braun, H. A., Crum, W. B., Kemp, R. L., Wagner, S., and Bellet, S.: Quantitative Analysis of the Electrocardiographic Pattern of Hypopotassemia, *Circulation*, 16:750, 1957.
55. Weaver, W. F., and Burchell, H. B.: Serum Potassium and the Electrocardiogram in Hypokalemia, *Circulation*, 21:505, 1960.
56. Surawicz, B.: Relationship between Electrocardiogram and Electrolytes, *Am. Heart J.*, 73:814, 1967.
57. Van Buchem, F. S. P.: The Electrocardiogram and Potassium Metabolism: Electrocardiographic Abnormalities in Primary Aldosteronism and Familial Periodic Paralysis, *Am J. Med.*, 23:376, 1957.
58. Schwartz, W. B., Levine, H. D., and Relman, A. S.: The Electrocardiogram in Potassium Depletion: Its Relation to the Total Potassium Deficit and the Serum Concentration, *Am J. Med.*, 16:395, 1954.
59. Leonard, E., and Hajdu, I.: Action of Electrolytes on the Contractile Mechanism of the Cardiac Muscle Cell, in "Handbook of Physiology," sec. 2: "Circulation," vol. 1, American Physiology Society, Washington, D.C., 1962, p. 151.
60. Thomas, L. J., Jr.: Increase of Labeled Calcium Uptake in Heart Muscle during Potassium Lack Contracture, *J. Gen. Physiol.*, 43:1193, 1960.
61. Surawicz, B., Chlebus, H., and Massellemi, A.: Hemodynamic and Electrocardiographic Effects of Hyperpotassemia: Differences in Response to Slow and Rapid Increases in Concentration of Plasma K, *Am. Heart J.*, 73:647, 1967.
62. Surawicz, B., and Gettes, L. S.: Effect of Electrolyte Abnormalities on the Heart and Circulation, in H. L. Conn, Jr., and O. Horwitz (eds.), "Cardiac and Vascular Disease," Lea & Febiger, Philadelphia, 1971, p. 539.
63. Weidman, S.: Effects of Calcium Ions and Local Anaesthetics on Electrical Properties of Purkinje Fibres, *J. Physiol.*, 129:568, 1955.
64. Temte, J. V., and Davis, L. D.: Effect of Calcium Concentration on the Transmembrane Potentials of Purkinje Fibers, *Circ. Res.*, 20:32, 1967.
65. Aronson, R. S., and Cranefield, P. F.: The Effect of Resting Potential on the Electrical Activity of Canine Cardiac Purkinje Fibers Exposed to Na-Free Solution or Ouabain, *Pfluegers Arch.*, 347:101, 1974.
66. Zipes, D. P., Besch, H. R., Jr., and Watanabe, A. M.: Role of the Slow Current in Cardiac Electrophysiology, *Circulation*, 51:761, 1971.
67. Wit, A. L., and Friedman, P. L.: Basis for Ventricular Arrhythmias Accompanying Myocardial Infarction, *Arch. Intern. Med.*, 135:459, 1975.
68. Cranefield, P. F.: "The Conduction of Cardiac Impulse," Futura Publishing Company, Mount Kisco, New York, 1975, p. 308.
69. Cranefield, P. F.: Action Potentials, Afterpotentials and Arrhythmias, *Circ. Res.*, 41:415, 1977.
70. Knoebel, S. B., and Fisch, C.: Accelerated Junctional Escape, *Circulation*, 50:151, 1974.
71. Rosen, M. R., Fisch, C., Hoffman, F. F., Danilo, P., Jr., and Knoebel, S. B.: Can Accelerated A-V Junctional Escape Rhythms Be Explained by Delayed After-Depolarization? *Am. J. Cardiol.*, 45:1272, 1980.
72. Vassalle, M.: The Relationship among Pacemakers: Overdrive Suppression, *Am. Heart Assoc. Monogr.*, 62:47, 1978.
73. Carter, E. P., and Andrus, E. C.: Q-T Interval in Human Electrocardiogram in Absence of Cardiac Disease, *JAMA*, 78:1922, 1922.
74. Nierenberg, D. W., and Ransil, B. J.: QaTc Interval as a Clinical Indicator of Hypercalcemia, *Am. J. Cardiol.*, 44:243, 1979.
75. Surawicz, B., MacDonald, M. G., Kaljot, V., and Bettinger, J. C.: Treatment of Cardiac Arrhythmias with Salts of Ethylenediaminetetraacetic Acid (EDTA), *Am. Heart J.*, 58:493, 1959.
76. Olson, R. E.: Introduction, in P. Harris and L. Opie (eds.), "Calcium and the Heart," Academic Press, New York, 1971, p. 1.
77. Fleckenstein, A.: Specific Pharmacology of Calcium in Myocardium, Cardiac Pacemakers and Vascular Smooth Muscle, *Ann. Rev. Pharmacol. Toxicol.*, 17:149, 1977.
78. Winegrad, S.: Electromechanical Coupling in Heart Muscle, "Handbook of Physiology," sec. 2: "The Cardiovascular System," vol. 1, American Physiological Society, Bethesda, Md., 1979, p. 393.

79. Layzer, R. B., and Rowland, L. P.: Cramps, *N. Engl. J. Med.*, 285:31, 1971.
80. Kleeman, C., and Singh, B. N.: Serum Electrolytes and the Heart, in M. H. Maxwell and C. R. Kleeman (eds.), "Clinical Disorders of Fluid and Electrolyte Metabolism," McGraw-Hill Book Company, New York, 1979, p. 166.
81. Davis, W. H., Ziady, F.: The Effect of Oral Magnesium Chloride Therapy on the QT_c and QU_c Intervals of the Electrocardiogram, *S. Afr. Med. J.*, 53:591, 1978.
82. Dyckner, T., and Wester, P. O.: Ventricular Extrasystoles and Intracellular Electrolytes before and after Potassium and Magnesium Infusing in Patients on Diuretic Treatment, *Am. Heart J.*, 97:12, 1979.
83. Surawicz, B., Lepeschkin, E., and Herrlich, H. C.: Low and High Magnesium Concentrations at Various Calcium Levels; Effect on the Monophasic Action Potential, Electrocardiogram, and Contractility of Isolated Rabbit Hearts, *Circ. Res.*, 9:811, 1961.
84. Krasner, B. S.: Cardiac Effects of Magnesium with Special Reference to Anaesthesia: A Review, *Can. Anaesth. Soc. J.*, 26:181, 1979.
85. Seta, K., Kleiger, R., Hellerstein, E. F., Lown, B., and Vitale, J. J.: Effect of Potassium and Magnesium Deficiency on the Electrocardiogram and Plasma Electrolytes of Pure Bred Beagles, *Am. J. Cardiol.*, 17:516, 1966.
86. Smith, P. K., Winkler, A. W., and Hoff, H. E.: Electrocardiographic Changes and Concentration of Magnesium in Serum following Intravenous Rejection of Magnesium Salts, *Am. J. Physiol.*, 126:720, 1939.
87. Singh, R. B., Singh, V. P., Jha, V. K., and Katiyar, B. C.: Magnesium and the Heart, *Acta Cardiol.*, 31:401, 1976.
88. Rosen, E. U.: The Controversial Role of Magnesium in Protein-Calorie Malnutrition, *Am. Heart J.*, 82:1, 1971.
89. Seller, R. H., Cangiano, J., Kim, K. E., Mendelssohn, S., Brest, A. N., and Swartz, C.: Digitalis Toxicity and Hypomagnesemia, *Am. Heart J.*, 79:57, 1970.
90. O'Connor, L. R., Wheeler, W. S., and Bethune, J. E.: Effect of Hypophosphatemia on Myocardial Performance in Man, *N. Engl. J. Med.*, 297:901, 1977.
91. Fuller, T. J., Nichols, W. W., Brenner, B. J., and Peterson, J. C.: Reversible Depression in Myocardial Performance in Dogs with Experimental Phosphorus Deficiency, *J. Clin. Invest.*, 62:1194, 1978.
92. Swaminathan, R., Morgan, D. B., Ionescu, M., and Hill, G. L.: Hypophosphatemia and Its Consequences in Patients following Open Heart Surgery, *Anaesthesia*, 33:601, 1978.
93. Rector, W. G., Jr., Jarzobski, J. A., and Levin, H. S.: Sinus Node Dysfunction Associated with Lithium Therapy: Report of a Case and a Review of the Literature, *Neb. Med. J.*, 64:193, 1979.
94. Tilkian, A. G., Schroeder, J. S., Kao, J., and Hultgren, H.: Effect of Lithium on Cardiovascular Performance: Report on Extended Ambulatory Monitoring and Exercise Testing before and during Lithium Therapy, *Am. J. Cardiol.*, 38:701, 1976.
95. Wellens, H. J., Cats, V. M., and Duren, D. R.: Symptomatic Sinus Node Abnormalities following Lithium Carbonate Therapy, *Am. J. Med.*, 59:285, 1974.
96. Carmeliet, E. E.: Influence of Lithium Ions on the Transmembrane Potential and Cation Content of Cardiac Cells, *J. Gen. Physiol.*, 47:501, 1964.

78

Effect of Noncardiac Drugs, Radiation, Electricity, and Poisons on the Heart

I. Sylvia Crawley, M.D.

This chapter deals with a number of deleterious side effects of treatments[1] and environmental agents on the heart. Man-made illnesses are not uncommonly the result of man-made inventions and treatments, possibly cures, for other illnesses. Environmental factors are not necessarily under the control of human beings, but when they are, we must take the responsibility of their potential effects on our health.

Noncardiac Drugs

Psychotropic Agents

The major cardiac effects of psychotropic agents will be discussed. The reader is referred to several recent reviews for more detailed discussion including potential drug interactions, and literature citations.[2–4]

Tricyclic Antidepressants

Tricyclic antidepressants, including the tertiary (amitriptyline, doxepin, imipramine, trimipramine) and secondary (desipramine, nortriptyline, protriptyline) agents, have potentially serious cardiovascular effects. These dangers have been overemphasized, and with appropriate patient selection and monitoring, they can be used safely even in patients with cardiovascular disease.[2–5] The major effects include an increase in heart rate, orthostatic hypotension, electrocardiographic changes, and depression of ventricular function.

A slight increase in heart rate is common and may persist for days to months after discontinuing therapy.[4,6] The rate rarely exceeds 100 beats per minute. This effect is more common with the tertiary amines, especially amitriptyline.[4] Orthostatic hypotension occurs in up to 20 percent of patients and is more troublesome in patients with some degree of orthostasis prior to treatment.[2,4] This side effect is less with nortriptyline and possibly with doxepin.[2]

The most common electrocardiographic changes include nonspecific ST and T-wave changes and slight prolongation of QT interval, PR interval, and QRS duration.[3] PR prolongation is the result of prolonged HV conduction.[7] The tricyclics have a quinidine-like property and may exert both antiarrhythmic and arrhythmogenic effects. The effectiveness of imipramine as an antiarrhythmic agent has been demonstrated.[3,8]

Depression of left ventricular function is usually minimal with therapeutic doses. Severe preexisting left ventricular dysfunction is an important consideration, although patients with moderate dysfunction may be treated safely.[3,9]

Although the tricyclic antidepressants have potentially serious cardiac effects, they may be used safely in many patients with cardiovascular disease with appropriate considerations of their effects and drug interactions.

Tricyclic overdose frequently presents a special cardiac management problem.[3] Electrocardiographic changes frequently include sinus tachycardia, prolongation of PR, QRS and QT, ST and T-wave changes, and bundle branch block. Torsade de pointes ventricular tachycardia may require temporary pacing. Hemodynamic monitoring may be necessary to provide appropriate therapy for hypotension. Continuous cardiac monitoring is indicated for the duration of electrocardiographic changes[10] including QT prolongation.

Other Antidepressants

Newer generation antidepressants may have fewer cardiovascular effects.[2,3] Amoxapine and maprotiline do have the potential for effects similar to the tertiary and secondary tricyclic agents, especially with overdose.[10a] Maprotiline is considered to have fewer cardiac effects including less orthostatic hypotension, but it has recently been reported to cause torsade de pointes ventricular tachycardia.[11] Trazodone has almost no anticholinergic effects and is less likely to cause tachycardia. Orthostatic hypotension is less frequent, and based on animal studies it is unlikely to cause problems with intracardiac conduction.[3] Overdose would be expected to be less complicated by cardiac effects.[3] A recent report of ventricular arrhythmias possibly aggravated by trazodone in two patients with heart disease is disturbing and demands further evaluation.[12]

Mianserin, buproprion, nomifensine, and fluvoxamine may promise to have significantly fewer cardiac effects both with therapeutic doses and overdose.[13] Although not yet released in the United States, several studies of buproprion have demonstrated few cardiovascular effects with little orthostatic hypotension, no effects on intracardiac conduction by electrocardiogram, and no cardiac complications of overdose.[14–16]

Monoamine Oxidase Inhibitors

Monoamine oxidase (MAO) inhibitors do not produce tachycardia and have little direct cardiac effects.[2–4] QT prolongation and atrial arrhythmias have been reported.[4] They do frequently produce orthostatic hypotension, and for this reason they are usually avoided in patients with cardiac and cerebrovascular disease.

The potential interaction of MAO inhibitors with other drugs and tyramine-containing substances resulting in a hypertensive crisis limit the use of MAO inhibitors in many patients. This interaction may persist for at least 2 weeks after discontinuing the drug.[3]

A new short-acting reversible MAO inhibitor is being evaluated which may prove to cause minimal orthostatic hypotension.[17]

Lithium

Lithium, as the citrate or carbonate salt, has infrequent cardiac effects in therapeutic doses, even in patients with heart disease.[3] Suppression of automaticity, especially of the sinus node, is the most common significant effect. Sinus node suppression with a slow escape rhythm may occur even with therapeutic doses and is probably more common in patients with preexisting sinus node disease or in patients taking other medications having a similar effect.[3] Permanent pacing has been used to allow continuation of lithium therapy.[3]

Electrocardiographic changes are common and simulate hypokalemia. A decrease in amplitude or inversion of the T waves and U waves are frequent.[3,4] QT prolongation may occur. Although rare, PR prolongation, bundle branch block, and complete heart block are reported. Despite isolated reports of ventricular arrhythmias, lithium may have antiarrhythmic properties.[3]

There are no data to confirm the concern that lithium suppresses left ventricular function, although the long-term effects, especially in patients with pretreatment myocardial dysfunction, have not been studied.

Bradyarrhythmias are the most frequent cardiac effect of overdose and may require temporary transvenous pacing.[3]

Phenothiazine Antipsychotic Agents

Phenothiazine antipsychotic agents, particularly those of low potency, chlorpromazine and thioridazine, have significant cardiac effects.[3,18] An increase in heart rate occurs frequently, even to 100 beats per minute. Orthostatic hypotension is more frequent with parenteral than oral administration. T-wave changes in the electrocardiogram are common and occur variably in any patient and are influenced by drugs and the fasting state.[3] They may persist for 2 weeks after discontinuing therapy.[3] QT prolongation may occur. Bundle branch block, complete heart block, and atrial and ventricular arrhythmias have been reported but are not common with therapeutic doses.[3]

Sudden death has occurred in patients receiving phenothiazines, but no risk factor can be identified. The mechanism of death is thought to be cardiac arrhythmia, either ventricular tachycardia or complete heart block.[3]

Overdose with the phenothiazines produces serious cardiovascular effects similar to those of the tricyclic agents including electrocardiographic changes, hypotension, and arrhythmias. Torsade de pointes ventricular tachycardia also occurs.[3]

Chemotherapeutic Agents

Doxorubicin

Electrocardiographic changes during the course of therapy are common. They are not usually clinically important, regress in weeks to months, and generally do not predict subsequent cardiomyopathy. The most common are ST-T-wave changes, but QRS changes may also occur, and, less frequently, atrial or ventricular arrhythmias.[19] A reduction in QRS voltage has been used as a predictor of cardiomyopathy but is unreliable.[20,21]

Cardiomyopathy is the most serious cardiotoxic effect. The overall incidence of clinically apparent heart failure is reported in up to 9 percent of patients.[19] Subclinical left ventricular dysfunction is probably more frequent. In one series, 14 percent of 101 patients receiving 430 or more mg/m^2 developed clinical congestive heart failure while 21 percent of the asymptomatic patients also had abnormal resting left ventricular ejection fractions.[22]

A total dose of over 550 mg/m^2 is associated with a much higher incidence of cardiomyopathy of up to 30 percent.[19] Other factors which may increase the chance of cardiomyopathy even with doses below 550 mg/m^2 include prior radiation therapy,[20,23] the schedule of administration,[24] preexisting heart disease, uncontrolled hypertension,[20] and possibly the associated use of other chemotherapeutic agents.[19,20] A higher incidence is also reported in young children and older adults.[19,23] Serial assessment of left ventricular function may aid in the safe administration to selected patients with prior left ventricular dysfunction.[25] A study utilizing endomyocardial biopsy as a measure of myocardial damage failed to demonstrate an association with use of other chemotherapeutic agents, hypertension, age, or history of cardiac disease.[24] Although this study supports the value of a weekly schedule of administration, the conclusions are based on endomyocardial biopsies and not clinical follow-up.

The clinical presentation of doxorubicin cardiomyopathy is that of a congestive cardiomyopathy which usually occurs within days to a few months and mostly within the first year after therapy, but occasionally much later.[19,26] The clinical course is variable from an acute, fulminating heart failure and cardiogenic shock to a gradually progressive deterioration.[27] A few patients improve and appear to regress with medical therapy, but the overall mortality rate is reported to be as high as 61 percent.[19,28] The older patient, over age 45 years, is more likely to progress than the younger patient.[22]

A number of noninvasive methods have been utilized in an attempt to detect early evidence of left ventricular dysfunction in order to terminate therapy at a safer dosage or to provide greater antineoplastic effectiveness with higher doses without added risk to the myocardium. Systolic time intervals and echocardiography have not proved to produce adequate sensitivity or specificity.[29] Noninvasive assessment of end-systolic left ventricular function may provide better sensitivity and specificity, but further studies are needed.[30] The value of radionuclide determination of left ventricular ejection fraction, both at rest and with exercise, has been reported.[25] One recent study suggests that with assessment of both resting and exercise determinations, few false-negative results will be obtained. However, a few patients will have false-positive results (41 percent specificity), and invasive testing may be necessary to assess the safety of further therapy.[29]

Endomyocardial biopsy and histopathological assessment of the degree of myocardial damage are thought to be the most reliable measure of myocardial toxicity.[29,31] Its clinical usefulness is limited since it is invasive and requires special expertise. The validity of the histopathology in determining a safe dose is challenged. The histopathology is not specific for doxorubicin toxicity, and the myocellular damage seen on endomyocardial biopsy may not accurately reflect the extent of changes throughout the myocardium.[23] Coupled, however, with right-sided heart catheterization with resting and exercise hemodynamics it remains the most definitive method of evaluating dosage safety.[29,31a]

Daunorubicin

The cardiac toxicity of daunorubicin is similar to that of doxorubicin. The electrocardiographic changes are similar. They are not related to dosage, are usually transient, and do not predict subsequent cardiomyopathy.[19,32] The overall incidence of cardiomyopathy seems to be slightly less than with doxorubicin. There are limited studies assessing relative risk. Total dosage less than 600 mg/m^2 is associated with an incidence of 1.5 percent while the incidence increases to 12 percent with a dosage over 1000 mg/m^2. Children seem to be at greater risk.[33] The onset of symptoms may be a little later than with doxorubicin, but there are some instances of myocarditis-pericarditis developing during treatment.[27,34] The literature also suggests that daunorubicin cardiomyopathy is less likely to respond to therapy. Available noninvasive studies for early detection are limited.[19]

Other Chemotherapeutic Agents

5-Fluorouracil may rarely cause myocardial ischemia or myocardial infarction.[19]

Vincristine and vindesine, both vinca alkaloids, have been reported to cause myocardial infarction.[19,35] Vindesine has also been reported to cause angina pectoris.[36] Orthostatic hypotension occurs in approximately 8 percent of patients receiving vincristine.[37]

Cyclophosphamide may cause myocardial necrosis when used in large doses, especially when combined with other agents.[19]

Mitoxantrone has been reported to cause congestive heart failure, impairment of left ventricular function, and histological changes in some patients.[38,39] The potential risk of cardiotoxicity remains to be determined.

Amsacrine (AMSA) may cause ventricular arrhythmias especially in the presence of hypokalemia.[40] Congestive heart failure is reported, and noninvasive measures of left ventricular function suggest a relationship to dose and to prior anthracycline therapy.[41,42] Mitomycin, busulfan, cisplatinum, and methotrexate rarely cause cardiac toxicity.[19]

Oral Contraceptive Agents

Soon after the introduction of oral contraceptive agents in 1960, the potential risks of cardiovascular disease became apparent.[43] Numerous studies since that time have addressed the question of incidence, risk factors, and pathogenesis. Most investigators agree that there is an increased incidence of hypertension, myocardial infarction, cerebrovascular accidents, and thromboembolic disease in users of oral contraceptives. Some reviews provide summaries of these observations.[43–45] The use of oral contraceptive agents not only increases these risks but also in the presence of other risk factors multiplies the chances of certain cardiovascular complications.[44]

Myocardial Infarction

The incidence of myocardial infarction in premenopausal women is rare, but this risk is three to four times greater in oral contraceptive users in general.[46] However, in certain subsets, this risk is even more striking. Users who also smoke have a 7 to 39 times greater risk of myocardial infarction compared to those who neither smoke nor use the pill.[47,48] The greatest risk with this combination is in the older age group.[47] The risk of myocardial infarction is also significantly increased with other risk factors for coronary atherosclerotic heart disease, and in the age group over 35 years.[48] A study suggests that although the cardiovascular risk decreases after discontinuing use, some residual risk remains especially in those who were users for 5 years or longer.[46]

The mechanism of myocardial infarction is unclear. A significant percentage of women under age 50 who have a myocardial infarction are oral contraceptive users, and many of these will not have angiographic evidence of atherosclerotic disease. Most often there is a single-vessel discrete lesion or normal vessels.[45,49,50] Conversely, the occurrence of coronary atherosclerotic heart disease or myocardial infarction with normal coronary arteries in nonusers under age 50 is also recognized. The oral contraceptives are known to affect lipid metabolism, decrease glucose tolerance, cause hypertension, and adversely effect hemostasis (hypercoagulability), and these factors may contribute to coronary artery disease and/or thrombosis.[44] In addition, coronary spasm has also been implicated.[51]

Hypertension

The majority of users will have a mild elevation, and 4 to 5 percent will have significant rise in blood pressure, representing an incidence two to three times that of nonusers.[44,45] In most cases the hypertension is mild to moderate and reversible after discontinuing use. A few instances of malignant hypertension have been reported.[52] One study of black women followed for 6 to 24 months did not demonstrate any significant effect on blood pressure.[53] Hypertension is more likely in users who are older or who have a past history or family history of hypertension.[45] The duration of use and the amount of estrogen in the preparation may also contribute.

The effects of these agents on the renin-angiotensin system and sodium metabolism have been investigated as possible mechanisms of the hypertension.[54]

Thromboembolism

The relative risk of superficial or deep lag vein thrombosis or pulmonary embolism in oral contraceptive users is 4 to 10 times that of nonusers, representing a significant morbidity rate but rare death.[43,45] Factors which predispose to this complication are past history of thromboembolic disease, medical or surgical trauma, and the amount of estrogen in the agent.[45] This risk is resolved within 1 month after nonuse. Smoking has not been implicated as an additional risk factor for this complication.[43,45]

This effect is thought to result from a decrease in venous tone and an increase in coagulability caused by these agents.[43,45]

Cerebrovascular Accidents

The relative risk of cerebrovascular events in oral contraceptive users may be as great as nine times that of nonusers.[45] Factors which increase the chances of this complication include hypertension, smoking, migraine headaches, and hypercholesterolemia. Residual risk, especially for subarachnoid hemorrhage, after discontinuing use has been reported.[45]

As with myocardial infarction, cerebrovascular accidents seem to be related to more than atherosclerosis. Intimal hyperplasia and the hypercoagulable state may contribute to the pathogenesis.[45]

Use of Oral Contraceptive Agents

The use of these agents should be avoided in women over age 35 or of any age when there is preexisting risk for hypertension, coronary atherosclerosis, or thromboembolic disease. The combination of smoking and oral contraceptive use is especially risky. The lowest effective dose should be used and blood pressure monitored regularly for the duration of use. Consideration should be given to temporarily discontinuing use during any surgery or trauma.[45]

Miscellaneous Agents

Caffeine

Caffeine has a sympathomimetic amine effect on the cardiovascular system. Hemodynamic responses of acute administration include an increase in blood pressure and heart rate.[55] These effects are blunted with chronic use but are greater in the older individual.[56] Blood pressure elevation is even greater during exercise.[57] The influence of caffeine consumption on therapy of hypertension has been emphasized.[57]

Caffeine is thought to have an arrhythmogenic effect on the heart.[56,57] Electrophysiological studies are limited. One study has demonstrated no change in conduction times, a shortened refractory period of the right atrium, atrioventricular node, and right ventricle, and an increased frequency of sustained tachycardia induced by the extrastimulus technique. This latter effect was especially frequent in patients with a prior history of arrhythmias.[58] Animal studies have also demonstrated the arrhythmogenic potential of caffeine.[59]

The mechanism of action of caffeine on the heart is not known.[56,58] Although elevations of catecholamines may occur with acute administration, this effect is less frequent with chronic use.[55,59a] The role of caffeine as a risk factor for coronary artery disease is not well established.[56]

Caffeine toxicity causes marked catecholamine release and may be associated with tachyarrhythmias, hypotension, metabolic acidosis, hyperglycemia, and hypokalemia.[60] Fatalities are rare.[61]

Theophylline

Theophylline has both chronotropic and ionotropic effects on the heart.[62] The most common cardiac effect with therapeutic doses is a slight increase in heart rate with minimal effects on blood pressure. Patients with severe obstructive lung disease or heart disease are subject to atrial and ventricular arrhythmias.[62] A significant positive ionotropic effect by both oral and intravenous (aminophylline) administration has been demonstrated in human beings. This effect may be due to its direct effect on the heart, the release of catecholamines, or a reduction in peripheral resistance.[63] This ionotropic effect may be attenuated in the presence of beta-adrenergic blockade.[64]

Toxicity is associated with sinus tachycardia, atrial and ventricular arrhythmias, and hypotension. Hypokalemia may occur. Dialysis may be helpful in patients with refractory arrhythmias or hypotension.[65]

Terbutaline

Terbutaline is a selective beta$_2$-adrenergic agonist. It causes a slight increase in heart rate and pulse pressure without an increase in mean arterial pressure. Nonspecific T-wave changes (decreased amplitude) and J-point ST depression have been observed.[66–68] Similar to theophylline, atrial and ventricular arrhythmias may occur, especially in patients with preexisting heart disease or other precipitating factors. hypokalemia may occur.[69,70]

Terbutaline has been demonstrated to have a beneficial hemodynamic effect in patients with congestive heart failure and cardiogenic shock.[69,71–74]

The use of terbutaline in the treatment of premature labor may have significant cardiac complications.[75]

Albuterol

Albuterol, marketed as Salbutamol in Europe, is a highly selective beta$_2$-adrenergic agonist used as a bronchodilator and in the treatment of premature labor. It appears to have few cardiovascular effects, similar to terbutaline.[76] Similarly, hypokalemia may occur.[77] Aerosol therapy, since it produces effective bronchodilation with little systemic effects, has few cardiac effects.[78]

Overdose has fewer serious cardiac effects compared to theophylline.[79] Hypokalemia and sinus tachycardia occur, but serious cardiac arrhythmias are uncommon.[79]

Ergotamine

Ergotamine causes constriction of smooth muscles. There is constriction of peripheral vessels and an increase in blood pressure and peripheral vascular resistance.[80] Cardiac output may increase in patients with orthostatic hypotension.[80] The lower extremities are most commonly involved by peripheral vasoconstriction.[81] An aortic arch syndrome has recently been reported.[81] Intravenous sodium nitroprusside is useful in the therapy of prolonged vasoconstriction.[82]

The use of ergonovine maleate in the diagnosis of coronary artery spasm is recognized. Ergotamine is frequently used in the treatment of migraine headaches. Myocardial infarction is a known complication of this therapy.[83]

Levodopa

Levodopa has few cardiac affects in patients without heart disease. It does cause an increase in the amount of circulating dopamine which may beneficially increase cardiac output in patients with heart failure.[84] Orthostatic hypotension is common, especially early in therapy, and is usually transient but may persist.[85] Due to the cardiac-stimulating effects of dopamine, arrhythmias, including sinus tachycardia and atrial and ventricular arrhythmias, may occur.[86] Levodopa may increase atrioventricular conduction.[86] These effects are more likely early in therapy or in patients with ischemic heart disease.[87] They are less likely with concomitant beta-adrenergic blockade.[86,87] Symptomatic postural hypotension may be treated with fludrocortisone.[85]

Methysergide
Methysergide can cause retroperitoneal, pulmonary, and cardiac fibrosis. Cardiac involvement may effect the endocardium, myocardium, valves, and rarely the aorta.[88,89] The mitral and aortic valves are most commonly involved, but effects on the tricuspid and pulmonary valves have been reported.[88] Lesions are more frequently regurgitant than stenotic.[89] The mechanism is unknown, but the pathology is similar to that seen in carcinoid heart disease. Periodic interruption of therapy with methysergide is recommended and thought to significantly reduce the incidence of cardiac involvement.[89] Patients should be monitored frequently for the development of murmurs during therapy. Methysergide should be discontinued when new murmurs are detected. Regression of the valvular lesion may occur although valve replacement is required in some cases.[89] Patients with known valvular disease should not be given this drug.[88]

Liquid Protein Diets
Liquid protein diets and therapeutic starvation are both reported to be associated with sudden death.[90] Electrocardiographic changes are not uncommon. Atrial and ventricular arrhythmias may occur. QT prolongation and torsade de pointes ventricular tachycardia are responsible for some reported cases of sudden death.[91,92] Potassium and magnesium deficiency and perhaps changes in the autonomic nervous system are possible mechanisms of this complication.[90]

Cimetidine
Cimetidine infrequently causes any cardiac effects.[93,94] Although electrophysiological studies have not demonstrated any effect on sinus node function,[95,96] instances of severe bradycardia have been reported with oral and intravenous administration.[93,94] Hypotension, asystole, and atrial and ventricular arrhythmias have also been reported with intravenous use.[97] These complications appear more likely with larger doses, when given rapidly through a central venous line, or in patients with cardiac or renal disease.[93,94] The antagonist effect on histamine H_2 receptors in the heart has been postulated as the mechanism of these effects.[98]

Ranitidine, a recently released H_2-receptor antagonist, has also been reported to cause bradycardia.[99]

Radiation

The proximity of the radiation field in the treatment of thoracic neoplasms necessitates radiation exposure to cardiac structures. Although initially the heart was thought to be radioresistant, it is apparent that cardiac effects are common and that the pericardium is most commonly involved.[100,101,101a] Some degree of myocardial fibrosis is frequently seen microscopically and occasionally produces significant left ventricular dysfunction. Coronary artery disease, conduction system defects, and valvular lesions have also been described.[101] Although these complications should not preclude the use of radiation therapy for a potential cure, the recognition of these problems allows for appropriate therapy.[102]

Heart disease due to radiation therapy is usually considered to occur within 1 to 2 years after therapy. Delayed cardiac disease is being recognized more frequently.[102–105]

Pericardial Effects

Clinical Recognition
The spectrum of pericardial disease is no different than that from causes other than radiation and includes acute pericarditis, asymptomatic effusion, tamponade, constriction, and effusive constrictive pericarditis.[101] The reported incidence of pericardial involvement varies from 2 to 40 percent.[106–110] This wide variation is due in part to variable risk factors and limitations of retrospective studies. Most early studies reported a 6 to 9 percent incidence. Studies utilizing an increase in the size of the cardiac silhouette as diagnostic for pericardial effusion report a higher incidence of 20 to 30 percent.[106,107] Asymptomatic effusion is probably the most common manifestation and frequently occurs within the first year after radiation therapy.[101,106]

Acute Pericarditis Acute pericarditis may cause typical chest pain, pericardial rub, and electrocardiographic changes. It usually occurs several months after treatment, but it may appear years later. Transient symptoms and/or signs may occur during treatment.[109]

Pericardial Effusion Pericardial effusion is frequently asymptomatic and can persist without hemodynamic alteration for months to years.[101] Progression to tamponade or constriction occurs. In the evaluation of the size of the cardiac silhouette during therapy it is important to appreciate that a decrease in size may occur early during therapy, presumably due to weight loss and a reduction in intravascular volume.[107] The pericardial effusion is usually exudative and may be loculated over the anterior and inferior surfaces of the heart.[106]

Cardiac Tamponade Cardiac tamponade can occur early after therapy or late. It is preceded by brief or long-standing pericardial effusion. Tamponade may also complicate constrictive pericarditis and cause effusive constrictive physiology.[101]

Constrictive Pericarditis Constrictive pericarditis can develop during the first year or two after therapy but may also present several to many years later and may be effusive-constrictive.[101,103] Dyspnea is a common symptom and can be mistaken for radiation lung disease.[103]

Management

Medical Therapy Medical therapy with nonsteroidal anti-inflammatory agents is indicated in symptomatic acute pericarditis. Steroids are especially useful for patients when symptoms are refractory to nonsteroidal agents or when tamponade physiology is present.[101]

Pericardiocentesis Pericardiocentesis is indicated for relief of tamponade. Hemodynamic monitoring during this procedure can be helpful in recognizing effusive constrictive physiology and the need for pericardioectomy.[101] Loculation of fluid may preclude effective pericardiocentesis in some patients. The fluid has a high protein content, and the diagnostic usefulness for involvement with Hodgkin's disease is limited.[101] Other malignancies may manifest positive cytology. The development of pericardial effusion in a patient who has received radiation therapy should not be presumed to be due to malignant involvement since aggressive medical and surgical therapy is appropriate when radiation is the cause.

Surgery Surgery is indicated in patients with moderately severe constriction or tamponade, and possibly when an asymptomatic pericardial effusion persists beyond 6 months.[111,112] In selected patients surgical morbidity is low and the results generally good.[111] Patients who have concomitant and significant myocardial fibrosis may not benefit from pericardiectomy.[113]

Myocardial Effects

Clinical Recognition and Management

Some degree of myocardial fibrosis is commonly seen on microscopic examination especially in the right ventricle and the anterior portion of the left ventricle. Noninvasive tests may demonstrate some degree of right and left ventricular dysfunction even in the asymptomatic patient.[102,104,105] Significant dysfunction, however, seems most common in association with severe pericardial disease. A congestive cardiomyopathy may result, and the medical management is dictated by this physiology.

Coronary Artery Effects

Clinical Recognition and Management

Angina pectoris or myocardial infarction may occur in patients following radiation therapy to the chest. Although the evidence is circumstantial in some cases, pathological findings support an etiologic relationship which is especially suspected in young patients.[109] This complication tends to occur some years after radiation therapy. The incidence is unknown. The process may involve a single or all three major coronary arteries. Management should include not only the indicated medical therapy but also coronary angiography and consideration of coronary artery bypass surgery.[114] Prior radiation therapy is no contraindication as long as the prognosis for the underlying disease is good.[114] Usual surgical techniques are hindered only by mild to moderate pericardial fibrosis not unlike that seen in patients with previous coronary artery bypass surgery.[114]

Valvular and Conduction System Effects

Clinical Syndromes and Management

Valvular regurgitant lesions have been described in only a few cases and include aortic and mitral regurgitation.[101] They do not appear to be of any hemodynamic importance.

Conduction system abnormalities including bundle branch blocks and complete heart block should be kept in mind during long-term follow-up of these patients for appropriate recognition and therapy with a permanent pacemaker.[101,115,116]

Risk Factors

The frequency of heart disease following radiation exposure is related in part to a number of identified variables.[101,110] Since pericardial involvement is the most frequent, this problem is the subject of most studies. A total dose exceeding 4000 rad increases the incidence of pericardial disease. With few exceptions the radiation source is not thought to be an important variable.[113] Radiation therapy that utilizes an anterior port only or an anterior and posterior port but with greater than 60 percent of the total dose by the anterior port may cause more problems.[107] Retreatment increases the chances of pericardial disease, from 6 to 40 percent in one series.[110] The volume of the heart included in the radiation field is important. Staging of therapy may help reduce the incidence since port size can be reduced as the tumor regresses in size.[108]

A greater extent of mediastinal involvement in Hodgkin's disease may contribute to more frequent pericarditis.[107] Concomitant chemotherapy has not been demonstrated to influence the incidence of pericarditis. Certain chemotherapeutic agents do affect the myocardium and may add to the radiation effects. Steroid withdrawal may precipitate acute pericarditis.[117] Hypothyroidism as a result of radiation exposure must be considered as a possible cause of pericardial effusion.[108] A high incidence of thyroid function abnormalities, low thyroxine, and elevated thyroid-stimulating hormone has been reported although clinically apparent hypothyroidism is uncommon.[118] The incidence may be increased by the use of lymphangiography just prior to radiation therapy.[118]

The extent of myocardial involvement is greater in those patients with the most severe pericardial damage and is also presumed to be related to similar risk factors. Other important variables which may be responsible for the development of coronary artery disease have not been identified. Animal studies have demonstrated that a high-cholesterol diet increases the incidence of coronary artery disease due to radiation exposure.[101]

Pathogenesis

Although there are numerous observations of the late effects of radiation on the heart in human beings, information regarding the acute effects is limited.[101] Animal studies have provided a model from which the pathogenesis in human beings is reasonably extrapolated. These studies have demonstrated an *acute* exudative phase (6 to 48 h) involving the pericardium, myocardium, endocardium, and vessels, a *latent* phase (2 to 70 days) during which electron microscopy reveals capillary damage, and a *late* phase of progressive pericardial exudation, fibrosis, and effusion, and myocardial fibrosis.[109]

Pericardial damage,[101] initially cellular with possibly an autoimmune response, initiates the resulting fibrosis. Obstruction to lymphatic drainage of the pericardium by this fibrotic process and possibly damage to mediastinal lymphatics by radiation and or neoplastic involvement further contribute to the development of pericardial effusion. The degree and rapidity of accumulation of fluid and the severity of the fibrosis in the visceral and parietal pericardium determine the subsequent hemodynamic alterations.

Myocardial fibrosis is the result of ischemia.[119] Initial damage to the capillary endothelium results in rupture and/or thrombosis of those vessels. This decrease in capillary bed causes myocardial ischemia and fibrosis. The involvement is more obvious in the anterior part of the heart including the right ventricle and the anterior portion of the left ventricle.[115] The extent of involvement is variable, as is the degree of ventricular dysfunction which may be apparent only by noninvasive or invasive testing. It may be responsible for persistent heart failure after pericardiectomy for constrictive pericarditis,[120] since it is usually most severe in association with severe pericardial involvement.

Coronary artery pathology is thought to be slightly different from the typical atherosclerotic process. Endothelial damage to the coronary arteries, formation of endothelial plaques, and adventitial fibrosis do occur. Unlike the typical atherosclerotic process there is a greater loss of smooth muscle cells and more frequent adventitial fibrosis.[115] The process is most prominent in the proximal segments of the coronary arteries.

Conduction system involvement is thought to result from vascular damage, subsequent ischemia, and fibrosis of the conduction system.[121]

Valvular lesions and endocardial thickening result from the endothelial cellular damage, exudation, and fibrosis.

Electricity

This section will deal with the cardiovascular effects of electrical injuries related to live wires and the electricity of nature—lightning. Iatrogenic problems related to electroconvulsive therapy will also be reviewed. Exposure to electrical fields has been implicated as a cause of adverse cardiac effects, but recent reviews have not revealed any clear-cut cause and effect.[122]

Environmental Accidents

Accidental contact with electricity may occur in the home, where children are particularly vulnerable,[123] or on the job, especially to electrical workers, but also on any job in which electrical equipment is used. The hospital environment has become increasingly hazardous. There are approximately 1200 deaths related to electrical accidents per year.[124] Lightning injury also causes death to at least 100 people per year, representing a 30 percent mortality rate in reported cases.[125,126] People who are involved in outdoor activities, i.e., golfers, hikers, farmers, are especially vulnerable.

Electrophysiology

The degree of total-body injury from electricity is determined by many factors: the amount of electrical energy delivered, the duration of the current, the resistance of the skin, the path of the current through the body, and the tissue damage along the way.[127] Alternating current, even of relatively low voltage is of greater hazard than direct current since tetanic muscle contractions prevent the "let-go" phenomenon. Exposure to a current over the "let-go," but less than the ventricular fibrillation, threshold can cause respiratory arrest and death without direct cardiac effects.[126,128,129] Although burn injury is considered to be a common complication of electrical accidents, only about one-half of deaths due to contact with low voltage (less than 1000 V) are associated with burns.[129] High-tension wires (1000 V or greater) produce greater internal burn injuries, more like a crush injury, in addition to cardiovascular and central nervous system effects.[130] Lightning is of extremely high voltage, but is brief in duration, and is a direct current.[125] Although deep burns do occur, they are less frequent, and a characteristic superficial burn is common.[131,132] A lightning strike may be direct, a side flash, or a stride potential (see below), and to some extent this determines the extent and severity of injury.[133]

The path of the electrical current through the body, entry-to-exit sites, also determines the cardiac and central nervous system effects. A current path from arm to arm or arm to leg is more likely to cause direct cardiac effects. A stride potential, leg-to-leg entry-to-exit sites, is infrequently associated with direct cardiac effects. A current path involving the head or a large current path from arm to arm may cause direct respiratory depression by its effect on the respiratory center.[126]

Cardiovascular Effects

A person struck by lightning may be comatose and without pulses or respirations. The immediate cardiac effect may be a direct result of the electrical current on the heart, causing asystole or ventricular fibrillation, or an indirect result of apnea and hypoxia, causing cardiac arrest.[132,134] Pulseless extremities may persist after normal cardiac activity resumes due to severe peripheral vasoconstriction.

During the hours following injury other cardiac effects may be observed.[135–138] Sinus tachycardia and nonspecific ST and T-wave changes are probably the most common. Arrhythmias may also occur, including ventricular ectopic beats, ventricular tachycardia, atrial ectopic beats, atrial tachycardia, and sinus bradycardia. Conduction abnormalities including bundle branch block and, rarely, complete heart block are also reported. Acute myocardial infarction is rare but can occur and not become manifest for several hours after the injury.[133] This effect may be complicated by significant left ventricular dysfunction including pulmonary edema.[135,137,139] The ST and T-wave changes, including prolongation of the QT interval, may be due to direct effects on the myocardium or may be secondary to electrical injury to the central nervous system. Intense catecholamine release may occur after injury and cause severe hypertension and tachycardia. One case of cardiac rupture has been reported.[140] These late cardiac effects may occur without initial cardiopulmonary arrest.

Victims of electrical accidents are subject to similar cardiac effects. Up to 36 percent of victims of electrical injury who seek medical care are found to have electrocardiographic changes, including cardiac arrhythmias or evidence of myocardial damage.[130,141] When electrical injury causes extensive burns and tissue necrosis, there may be additional secondary cardiac effects due to hypovolemia, electrolyte abnormalities, and infection.

Management and Prognosis

Immediate cardiopulmonary resuscitation should be instituted and continued for a prolonged period.[127,132,142] Spontaneous respirations may not occur for 30 min or more. Nonreactive pupils may be the result of transient central nervous system effects and are no contraindication to resuscitation attempts.[143] Based on reports of successful recovery after prolonged unconsciousness, it has been suggested that basal metabolism is significantly reduced after a lightning strike. In a lightning accident involving a number of victims, attention should be immediately directed to victims who are "apparently dead."[125,144] In such instances, death is rare when cardiopulmonary arrest does not occur.[125] In any electrical injury the victim may have complete cardiopulmonary arrest, respiratory arrest only, or only transient paralysis of extremities or muscles of respiration.

Since cardiac effects may not be immediately apparent, victims should be observed for development of arrhythmias or myocardial infarction.[137] Hypertension and tachycardia secondary to the catecholamine release may be managed with an intravenous beta-adrenergic blocking agent.[143]

Recovery from the cardiac effects of electrical injury is usually good with electrocardiographic abnormalities resolving within a few weeks.[133,135] A number of patients who developed significant left ventricular dysfunction have been observed to return to near-normal myocardial function.[135,136,139]

Electroconvulsive Therapy

Electroconvulsive therapy (ECT) has been utilized in the treatment of various psychiatric illnesses since the late 1930s.[145] Morbidity during its early use was related to musculoskeletal injury as well as cardiopulmonary complications.[146] Present-day use is modified with pharmacological agents which provide greater safety, although the major complications continue to be cardiovascular.[145]

The cardiac effects relate to the electroshock as well as to medications used to modify the response.[145] After the administration of atropine or scopolamine, general anesthesia is accomplished with a short-acting agent; muscle paralysis is achieved with succinylcholine. The grand mal seizure is most commonly produced with an alternating current of 70 to 170 V for 0.1 to 1.0 s, applied either bilaterally or unilaterally to the head.[145] The onset of the seizure is associated with immediate vagal stimulation which would produce a profound bradycardia without prior anticholinergic blockade. This is followed by a sympathetic stimulus with tachycardia and hypertension.[147] During the first few minutes after the seizure, cardiac arrhythmias may develop including ventricular and atrial ectopic rhythms and brady- or tachyarrhythmias.[148] Additional electrocardiographic changes during this time may include ST and T-wave changes, QRS changes, and QT prolongation.[148,149] The T-wave changes may simulate acute subendocardial infarction or hyperkalemia.[150,151] Although some electrocardiographic change is common, the changes are usually of short duration and of no clinical importance.[148,149] Acute pulmonary edema after ECT is reported, but it is unclear whether it is neurogenic or cardiac in origin.[152] Sudden death after ECT has been reported rarely.

Pathogenesis of Cardiovascular Effects

The stimulus of the electric shock to the central nervous system including the autonomic nervous system is responsible for many of the changes in heart rate and blood pressure, which are independent of any motor activity related to the seizure.[147] A significant transient elevation of catecholamines has been demonstrated and may contribute to the tachycardia and hypertension.[153] In addition, the repolarization changes in the electrocardiogram are similar to those described with other problems of the central nervous system.

The anesthetic agent may also contribute to the electrocardiographic changes. Fewer abnormalities have been noted with methohexital than with thiopental.[148] Hypoxia and/or respiratory acidosis may develop during the period of apnea immediately following the induction of general anesthesia and increase the chances of arrhythmias.[148] An increase in serum potassium may be seen due to both the effects of succinylcholine and the electroconvulsive therapy. This increase, however, is small and rarely of clinical significance.[154] Preexisting heart disease or medications, especially cardiac or psychotropic agents, may also increase the risk of cardiovascular complications.

Recognition and Management

Preanesthetic assessment should be directed at identifying those patients with the greatest potential risk of major complications from ECT.[148] Uncontrolled hypertension, recent myocardial infarction, unstable angina pectoris, congestive heart failure, and arrhythmias may increase the risk of cardiovascular complications. Electrolyte abnormalities should be corrected prior to therapy, and the appropriateness of medications, especially cardiac and psychotropic agents, should be assessed. Preexisting pulmonary disease may also increase the chances of hypoxia and respiratory acidosis.

Attention to the anesthesia procedure regarding agents chosen, amount given, and ancillary respiratory support is also critical to the cardiopulmonary safety of the procedure. Cardiac monitoring should be done in all patients during and following the procedure until their full recovery from anesthesia.

Additional drug modification has been employed in selected patients. The use of small doses of a beta-adrenergic blocking agent given intravenously may blunt the tachycardia and hypotension and reduce the frequency of ventricular ectopic beats.[145,153] This can be especially useful in patients who are at risk of cardiac complications due to these effects. Pretreatment with lidocaine is reported to raise the seizure threshold to the shock stimulus, necessitating higher energy levels to effect a seizure.[155] A similar effect has been reported with clonidine.[156] Nitroprusside, begun intravenously just prior to the procedure, has also been used to blunt the hypertensive response.[157] There is one report of asystole associated with the administration of 1 mg of propranolol intravenously prior to ECT. This patient had electrocardiographic evidence of old myocardial infarction and was not given an anticholinergic agent prior to ECT.[158]

Patients who are on chronic anticoagulation with coumarin derivatives may be managed during ECT by the temporary use of intravenous heparin, which can be discontinued 6 to 8 h prior to and resumed shortly after the procedure.[159] Patients with permanent pacemakers also require special consideration. Currently used pacemakers are probably not affected by the ECT current.[160] Conversion to the fixed-rate mode with an external magnet over the generator may afford additional safety.[161]

Determinations of serum creatine phosphokinase activity have demonstrated a mild elevation of total levels in a few patients following ECT due to an increase in skeletal muscle fraction without elevations of the MB fraction.[162]

Although ECT frequently does cause transient electrocardiographic and hemodynamic changes, it continues to be a safe mode of therapy for selected psychiatric illnesses. Attention to patient selection and the details of the procedure is an important determinant of its safety.

Poisons

This section will deal with a number of environmental contacts which demonstrate the ubiquitous nature of agents which can cause cardiac toxicity. The possible cardiac effects of these agents will be reviewed. The reader is referred to other sources for their overall toxicology.

Plants

Cardiac Glycoside–Like Effects

The oleander plant (*Nerium oleander*) contains oleandroside, oleandrin, and nerioside.[163,164] The lily of the valley plant (*Convallaria majalis*) contains convallarin, convallamarin, and convallatoxin.[163] The Jerusalem cherry contains solanocapsine (leaves) and solanine (berry), and the unripe berries of the jessamine (*Cestrum diurnum* and *nocturnum*) contain solanine.[163,164] Both the potato plant and the green tubers also contain solanine.[165] Other plants known to contain substances with cardiac glycoside-like effects include milkweed (*Asclepias species*), *Hollarrhena* species of Asia, pheasant's eye (*Adonis vernalis*), green hellebore (*Helleborus viridis*), Christmas rose (*Helleborus niger*), and the wall flower (*Cheirina cheiri*).[164,166]

The cardiac effects of poisoning with these plants are similar to those of digitalis toxicity.[163,166,167]

Other Cardiotoxic Effects

The larkspur (*Delphinium*), both the plant and the seed, contains delphinine, a substance similar to aconitine, which causes myocardial depression, cardiac arrhythmias, and hypotension.[163,167] The Jimson weed (*Datura stramonium*) contains a belladonna alkaloid, and the mature berries of the day-blooming or night-blooming jessamine contain a tropane-related alkaloid. Both have anticholinergic effects. The castor bean (*Ricinus communis*) contains ricin, a toxalbumin, which in severe cases causes hypotension and circulatory collapse.[163] Mistletoe (*Phorandendron serotinum*), both the plant and berries, contains beta-phenethylamine and tyramine and can cause severe hypertension.[163] The Carolina jessamine (*Gelsemium sempervirens*) has mostly central nervous system effects, but the alkaloids gelsemine and gelsemicine have cardiac depressant effects.[163,167]

Snakes and Scorpions

There are approximately 250 species of venomous snakes.[168] In the United States there are 19.[169] Rattlesnakes, copperheads, and cottonmouths, all of the Crotalidae family, are responsible for the majority of bites. The coral snake, of the Elapidae family, is less frequently the cause.[170] Snake venom, in general, contains substances which affect the coagulation system, cellular components of the blood, endothelium of vessels, the nervous system, including the cardiorespiratory centers and myoneural junction, and the heart.[169] The effects of a specific snake venom, however, may have more effects on one system than another.[168] The cardiotoxins also are variable in any snake venom and are thought to have variable mechanisms of action and cardiac effects.[171] Animal studies have demonstrated that these cardiotoxins may augment myocardial contraction to systolic arrest or may have a negative ionotropic effect. They may also cause cardiac arrhythmias.[171]

Animal studies demonstrate that certain *Crotalus* venoms cause a severe decrease in systemic arterial pressure and an increase in pulmonary artery pressure. The exact mechanism of these effects is unclear. A decrease in circulating blood volume due to venous pooling, especially in the lungs, and thromboembolism in the pulmonary vascular bed have been observed.[168] Clinically, there may be severe hypotension which can be due to the negative ionotropic effect of the venom on the myocardium, but importantly, to loss of intravascular volume due to increased permeability of blood vessels with plasma and blood loss in the tissues. Multiple pulmonary emboli are also seen in patients who survive 12 or more hours.[168]

Scorpion (order Scorpionida) venom can cause hypertension and electrocardiographic changes of myocardial infarction. Pulmonary edema may occur.[172] Arrhythmias, conduction disturbances, and myocarditis have been described.[173] Animal studies suggest that the scorpion toxin acts indirectly on the heart via the release of acetylcholine and catecholamines.[171]

Arthropods

Direct cardiac effects of the venom of bees, yellow jackets, hornets, and wasps (Hymenoptera order) are difficult to establish. Electrocardiographic changes of myocardial ischemia or infarction, chest pain, and pulmonary edema are reported.[174] These problems are usually in association with anaphylaxis and its treatment. Cardiac arrhythmias also occur in association with anaphylaxis or systemic symptoms. One case has been described in which arrhythmias occurred in the absence of systemic symptoms.[175]

Animal studies of bee venom have demonstrated major electrocardiographic changes, suggesting a direct cardiotoxic effect.[171]

Halogenated Hydrocarbons

Halogenated hydrocarbon exposure may occur in the home or in industrial environments. These substances are used in fire extinguishers as propellants, solvents, and refrigerants.[176] They are used in the manufacture of pesticides and plastics.[177] Cardiac effects include arrhythmias and sudden death.[178] These compounds depress myocardial contractility and sensitize the heart to the arrhythmogenic effects of epinephrine.[176] Cardiac effects may also result indirectly from hypoxia or the effects of these compounds on the central nervous system. Sudden death, presumably due to arrhythmias, may occur, or cardiopulmonary effects including pulmonary edema may occur hours after exposure.[177,179]

Carbon Monoxide

For many people, exposure to carbon monoxide is a potential environmental hazard of daily life. The industrial environment provides an even greater potential for poisoning.

Carbon monoxide has an affinity for hemoglobin that is much greater than that of oxygen. The cardiac effects are the result of hypoxia. These effects are determined by the degree of carbon monoxide exposure, the hemoglobin concentration, and the presence or absence of coronary or myocardial disease. A decrease in exercise performance occurs even in normal individuals with low-level exposure. Patients with angina pectoris have a greater reduction in exercise tolerance.[180]

Carbon monoxide poisoning causes myocardial ischemia most commonly manifest as ST and T-wave changes on the electrocardiogram, and atrial and ventricular arrhythmias. Severe exposure can cause extensive myocardial necrosis and cardiomyopathy. Myocardial infarction may occur as a result of myocardial necrosis or coronary occlusion. These cardiac effects may not become apparent for days after exposure.[181]

References

1. Gilman, A. G., and Goodman, L. S. (eds.): "The Pharmacological Basis of Therapeutics," The Macmillan Company, New York, 1980.
2. Jefferson, J. W.: Treating Affective Disorders in the Pres-

ence of Cardiovascular Disease, *Psychiatr. Clin. North Am.*, 6:141, 1983.
3. Crawley, I. S., and Kolodner, R. M.: The Effects of Psychotropic Drugs on the Heart, in J. W. Hurst (ed.), "Clinical Essays on the Heart," McGraw-Hill Book Company, New York, 1983, p. 285.
4. Cassem, N.: Cardiovascular Effects of Antidepressants, *J. Clin. Psychiatry*, 43:22, 1982.
5. Raskind, M., Veith, R., Barnes, R., and Gumbrecht, G.: Cardiovascular and Antidepressant Effects of Imipramine in the Treatment of Secondary Depression in Patients with Ischemic Heart Disease, *Am. J. Psychiatry*, 139:1114, 1982.
6. Taylor, D. J. E., and Braithwaite, R. A.: Cardiac Effects of Tricyclic Antidepressant Medication: A Preliminary Study of Nortriptyline, *Br. Heart J.*, 40:1005, 1978.
7. Vohra, J., Burrows, G., Hunt, D., and Sloman, G.: The Effect of Toxic and Therapeutic Doses of Tricyclic Antidepressant Drugs on Intracardiac Conduction, *Eur. J. Cardiol.*, 3:219, 1975.
8. Connolly, S. J., Mitchell, B., Swerdlow, C. D., Mason, J. W., and Winkle, R. A.: Clinical Efficacy and Electrophysiology of Imipramine for Ventricular Tachycardia, *Am. J. Cardiology*, 53:516, 1984.
9. Veith, R. C., Raskind, M. A., Caldwell, J. H., Barnes, R. F., Gumbrecht, G., and Ritchie, J. L.: Cardiovascular Effects of Tricyclic Antidepressants in Depressed Patients with Chronic Heart Disease, *N. Engl. J. Med.*, 306:954, 1982.
10. Hulten, B.-A., and Heath, A.: Clinical Aspects of Tricyclic Antidepressant Poisoning, *Acta. Med. Scand.*, 213:275, 1983.
10a. Parker, J., and Lahmeyer, H.: Maprotiline Poisoning: A Case of Cardiotoxicity and Myoclonic Seizures, *J. Clin. Psychiatry*, 45:312, 1984.
11. Herrmann, H. C., Kaplan, L. M., and Bierer, B. E.: Q-T Prolongation and Torsades de Pointes Ventricular Tachycardia Produced by the Tetracyclic Antidepressant Agent Maprotiline, *Am. J. Cardiol.*, 51:904, 1983.
12. Janowsky, D., Curtis, G., Zisook, S., Kuhn, K., Resovsky, K., and LeWinter, M.: Ventricular Arrhythmias Possibly Aggravated by Trazodone, *Am. J. Psychiatry*, 140:796, 1983.
13. Roos, J. C.: Cardiac Effects of Antidepressant Drugs: A Comparison of the Tricyclic Antidepressants and Fluvoxamine, *Br. J. Clin. Pharmacol.*, 15:439S, 1983.
14. Wenger, T. L., and Stern, W. C.: The Cardiovascular Profile of Bupropion, *J. Clin. Psychiatry*, 44:176, 1983.
15. Farid, F. F., Wenger, T. L., Tsai, S. Y., Singh, B. N., and Stern, W. C.: Use of Bupropion in Patients Who Exhibit Orthostatic Hypotension on Tricyclic Antidepressants, *J. Clin. Psychiatry*, 44:170, 1983.
16. Wenger, T. L., Cohn, J. B., and Bustrack, J.: Comparison of the Effects of Bupropion and Amitriptyline on Cardiac Conduction in Depressed Patients, *J. Clin. Psychiatry*, 44:174, 1983.
17. Gasic, S., Korn, A., Eichler, H. G., Oberhummer, I., and Zapotoczy, H. G.: Cardiocirculatory Effects of Moclobemide (RO 11-1163), A New Reversible, a Short-Acting MAO-Inhibitor with Preferential Type A Inhibition in Healthy Volunteers and Depressive Patients, *Eur. J. Clin. Pharmacol.*, 25:173, 1983.
18. Risch, S. C., Groom, G. P., and Janowsky, D. S.: Interfaces of Psychopharmacology and Cardiology, Part 2, *J. Clin. Psychiatry*, 42:47, 1981.
19. Von Hoff, D. D., Rozencweig, M., and Piccart, M.: The Cardiotoxicity of Anticancer Agents, *Semin. Oncol.*, 9:23, 1982.
20. Minow, R. A., Benjamin, R. S., Lee, E. T., and Gottlieb, J. A.: Adriamycin Cardiomyopathy—Risk Factors, *Cancer*, 39:1397, 1977.
21. Ali, M. K., Soto, A., Maroongroge, D., et al.: Electrocardiographic Changes after Adriamycin Chemotherapy, *Cancer*, 43:465, 1979.
22. Dresdale, A., Bonow, R. O., Wesley, T., et al.: Prospective Evaluation of Doxorubicin-Induced Cardiomyopathy Resulting from Postsurgical Adjuvant Treatment of Patients with Soft Tissue Sarcomas, *Cancer*, 52:51, 1983.
23. Isner, J. M., Ferrans, V. J., Cohen, S. R., et al.: Clinical and Morphologic Cardiac Findings after Anthracycline Chemotherapy: Analysis of 64 Patients Studied at Necropsy, *Am. J. Cardiol.*, 51:1167, 1983.
24. Torti, F. M., Bristow, M. R., Howes, A. E., et al.: Reduced Cardiotoxicity of Doxorubicin Delivered on a Weekly Schedule, *Ann. Intern. Med.*, 99:745, 1983.
25. Choi, B. W., Berger, H. J., Schwartz, B. E., et al.: Serial Radionuclide Assessment of Doxorubicin Cardiotoxicity in Cancer Patients with Abnormal Baseline Resting Left Ventricular Performance, *Am. Heart J.*, 106:638, 1983.
26. Gottlieb, S. L., Edmiston, W. A., Jr., and Haywood, L. J.: Late, Late Doxorubicin Cardiotoxicity, *Chest*, 78:880, 1980.
27. Bristow, M. R., Thompson, P. D., Martin, R. P., Mason, J. W., Billingham, M. E., and Harrison, D. C.: Early Anthracycline Cardiotoxicity, *Am. J. Med.*, 65:823, 1978.
28. Cohen, M., Kronzon, I., and Lebowitz, A.: Reversible Doxorubicin-Induced Congestive Heart Failure, *Arch. Intern. Med.*, 142:1570, 1982.
29. McKillop, J. H., Bristow, M. R., Goris, M. L., Billingham, M. E., and Bockemuehl, K.: Sensitivity and Specificity of Radionuclide Ejection Fractions in Doxorubicin Cardiotoxicity, *Am. Heart J.*, 106:1048, 1983.
30. Borow, K. M., Henderson, I. C., Neuman, A., et al.: Assessment of Left Ventricular Contractility in Patients Receiving Doxorubicin, *Ann. Intern. Med.*, 99:750, 1983.
31. Mason, J. W., Bristow, M. R., Billigham, M. E., and Daniels, J. R.: Invasive and Noninvasive Methods of Assessing Adriamycin Cardiotoxic Effects in Man: Superiority of Histopathologic Assessment Using Endomyocardial Biopsy, *Cancer Treat. Rep.*, 62:857, 1978.
31a. Kantrowitz, N. E., and Bristow, M. R.: Cardiotoxicity of Antitumor Agents, *Prog. Cardiovasc. Dis.*, 27:195, 1984.
32. Von Hoff, D. D., Rozencweig, M., Layard, M., Slavik, M., and Muggia, F. M.: Daunomycin-Induced Cardiotoxicity in Children and Adults: A Review of 110 Cases, *Am. J. Med.*, 62:200, 1977.
33. Von Hoff, D. D., and Layard, M.: Risk Factors for Development of Daunorubicin Cardiotoxicity, *Cancer Treat. Rep.*, 65(suppl. 4):19, 1981.
34. Harrison, D. T., and Sanders, L. A.: Pericarditis in a Case of Early Daunorubicin Cardiomyopathy, *Ann. Intern. Med.*, 85:339, 1976.
35. Somers, G., Abramow, M., Wittek, M., and Naets, J. P.: Myocardial Infarction: A Complication of Vincristine Treatment?, *Lancet*, 2:690, 1976.
36. Yancey, R. S., and Talpaz, M.: Vindesine-Associated Angina and ECG Changes, *Cancer Treat. Rep.*, 66:587, 1982.
37. DiBella, N. J.: Vincristine-Induced Orthostatic Hypotension: A Prospective Clinical Study, *Cancer Treat. Rep.*, 64:359, 1980.
38. Unverferth, D. V., Unverferth, B. J., Balcerzak, S. P., Bashore, T. A., and Neidhart, J. A.: Cardiac Evaluation of Mitoxantrone, *Cancer Treat. Rep.*, 67:343, 1983.
39. Schell, F. C., Yap, H-Y., Blumenschein, G., Valdivieso, M., and Bodey, G.: Potential Cardiotoxicity with Mitoxantrone, *Cancer Treat. Rep.*, 66:1641, 1982.
40. McLaughlin, P., Salvador, P. G., Cabanillas, F., and Legha, S. S.: Ventricular Fibrillation following AMSA, *Cancer*, 52:557, 1983.
41. Vorobiof, D. A., Iturralde, M., and Falkson, G.: Amsacrine Cardiotoxicity: Assessment of Ventricular Function by Radionuclide Angiography, *Cancer Treat. Rep.*, 67:1115, 1983.
42. Steinherz, L. J., Steinherz, P. G., Mangiacasale, D., Tan, C., and Miller, D. R.: Cardiac Abnormalities after AMSA Administration, *Cancer Treat. Rep.*, 66:483, 1982.
43. Stadel, B. V.: Oral Contraceptives and Cardiovascular Disease (First of Two Parts), *N. Engl. J. Med.*, 305:612, 1981.
44. Stadel, B. V.: Oral Contraceptives and Cardiovascular Disease (Second of Two Parts), *N. Engl. J. Med.*, 305:672, 1981.
45. Dalen, J. E., and Hickler, R. B.: Oral Contraceptives and Cardiovascular Disease, *Am. Heart J.*, 101:626, 1981.
46. Slone, D., Shapiro, S., Kaufman, D. W., Rosenberg, L., Miettinen, O. S., and Stalley, P. D.: Risk of Myocardial Infarction in Relation to Current and Discontinued Use of Oral Contraceptives, *N. Engl. J. Med.*, 305:420, 1981.
47. Salonen, J. T.: Oral Contraceptives, Smoking and Risk of

Myocardial Infarction in Young Women, *Acta. Med. Scand.*, 212:141, 1982.

48. Rosenfield, A.: The Pill: An Evaluation of Recent Studies, *Johns Hopkins Med. J.*, 150:177, 1982.
49. Engle, H.-J., and Lichtlen, P. R.: Coronary Atherosclerosis and Myocardial Infarction in Young Women—Role of Oral Contraceptives, *Eur. Heart J.*, 4:1, 1983.
50. Morris, D. C., Hurst, J. W., and Logue, R. B.: Myocardial Infarction in Young Women, *Am. J. Cardiol.*, 38:299, 1976.
51. Jugdutt, B. I., Stevens, G. F., Zacks, D. J., Lee, S. J. K., and Taylor, R. F.: Myocardial Infarction, Oral Contraception, Cigarette Smoking, and Coronary Artery Spasm in Young Women, *Am. Heart J.*, 106:757, 1983.
52. Hodsman, G. P., Robertson, J. I. S., Semple, P. F., and Mackay, A.: Malignant Hypertension and Oral Contraceptives: Four Cases, with Two Due to the 30 μg Oestrogen Pill, *Eur. Heart J.*, 3:255, 1982.
53. Blumenstein, B. A., Douglas, M. B., and Hall, W. D.: Blood Pressure Changes and Oral Contraceptive Use: A Study of 2676 Black Women in the Southeastern United States, *Am. J. Epidemiol.*, 112:539, 1980.
54. McAreavey, D., Cumming, A. M. M., Boddy, K., et al.: The Renin-Angiotensin System and Total Body Sodium and Potassium in Hypertensive Women Taking Oestrogen-Progestagen Oral Contraceptives, *Clin. Endocrinol.*, 18:111, 1983.
55. Curatolo, P. W., and Robertson, D.: The Health Consequences of Caffeine, *Ann. Intern. Med.*, 98:641, 1983.
56. Izzo, J. L. Jr., Chosal, A., Kwong, T., Freeman, R. B., and Jaenike, J. R.: Age and Prior Caffeine Use Alter the Cardiovascular and Adrenomedullary Response to Oral Caffeine, *Am. J. Cardiol.*, 52:769, 1983.
57. Lane, J. D.: Caffeine and Cardiovascular Responses to Stress, *Psychosom. Med.*, 45:447, 1983.
58. Dobmeyer, D. J., Stine, R. A., Leier, C. V., Greenberg, R., and Schaal, S. F.: The Arrhythmogenic Effects of Caffeine in Human Beings, *N. Engl. J. Med.*, 308:814, 1983.
59. Paspa, P., and Vassalle, M.: Mechanism of Caffeine-Induced Arrhythmias in Canine Cardiac Purkinje Fibers, *Am. J. Cardiol.*, 53:313, 1984.

59a. Robertson, D., Hollister, A. S., Kincaid, D., et al.: Caffeine and Hypertension, *Am. J. Med.*, 77:54, 1984.

60. Benowitz, N. L., Osterloh, J., Goldschlager, N., Kaysen, G., Pond, S., and Forham, S.: Massive Catecholamine Release from Caffeine Poisoning, *JAMA*, 248:1097, 1982.
61. McGee, M. B.: Caffeine Poisoning in a 19-Year-Old Female, *J. Forensic Sci. Soc.*, 25:29, 1980.
62. Van Dellen, R. G.: Theophylline: Practical Application of New Knowledge, *Mayo Clin. Proc.*, 54:733, 1979.
63. Matthay, R. A., Berger, H. J., Davies, R., Loke, J., Gottschalk, A., and Zaret, B. L.: Improvement in Cardiac Performance by Oral Long-Acting Theophylline in Chronic Obstructive Pulmonary Disease, *Am. Heart J.*, 104:1022, 1982.
64. Conrad, K. A., and Prosnitz, E. H.: Cardiovascular Effects of Theophylline: Partial Attenuation by Beta-Blockade, *Eur. J. Pharmacol.*, 21:109, 1981.
65. Greenberg, A., Piraino, B. H., Kroboth, P. D., and Weiss, J.: Severe Theophylline Toxicity: Role of Conservative Measures, Antiarrhythmic Agents, and Charcoal Hemoperfusion, *Am. J. Med.*, 76:854, 1984.
66. Greefhorst, A. P. M., and van Herwaarden, C. L. A.: Ventilatory and Haemodynamic Effects of Terbutaline Infusion during $Beta_1$-Selective Blockade with Metoprolol and Acebutolol in Asthmatic Patients, *Eur. J. Pharmacol.*, 23:203, 1982.
67. Whitsett, T. L., Manion, C. V., and Wilson, M. F.: Cardiac, Pulmonary and Neuromuscular Effects of Clenbuterol and Terbutaline Compared with Placebo, *Br. J. Clin. Pharmacol.*, 12:195, 1981.
68. Greefhorst, A. P. M., and van Herwaarden, C. L. A.: Ventilatory and Haemodynamic Effects of Prenalterol and Terbutaline in Asthmatic Patients, *Eur. J. Clin. Pharmacol.*, 24:173, 1983.
69. Wang, R. Y. C, Lee, P. K., Yu, D. Y. C., Tse, T. F., and Chow, M. S. S.: Terbutaline Infusion in Cardiogenic Shock: Acute Hemodynamic Effects and Clinical Responses, *J. Clin. Pharmacol.*, 23:355, 1983.
70. Gross, T. L., and Sokol, R. J.: Severe Hypokalemia and Acidosis: A Potential Complication of Beta-Adrenergic Treatment, *Am. J. Obstet. Gynecol.*, 138:1225, 1980.
71. Wang, R. Y. C, Lee, P. K., Yu, D. Y. C, Tse, T. F., and Chow, M. S. S.: Myocardial Metabolic Effects of Intravenous Terbutaline in Patients with Severe Heart Failure Due to Coronary Artery Disease, *J. Clin. Pharmacol.*, 23:362, 1983.
72. Slutsky, R.: Hemodynamic Effects of Inhaled Terbutaline in Congestive Heart Failure Patients without Lung Disease: Beneficial Cardiotonic and Vasodilator Beta-Agonist Properties Evaluated by Ventricular Catheterization and Radionuclide Angiography, *Am. Heart J.*, 101:556, 1981.
73. Wang, R. Y. C, Tse, T. F., Yu, D. Y. C., Lee, P. K., and Chow, M. S. S.: Beneficial Hemodynamic Effects of Intravenous Terbutaline in Patients with Severe Heart Failure, *Am. Heart J.*, 104:1016, 1982.
74. Hooper, W. W., Slutsky, R. A., Kocienski, D. E., et al.: Right and Left Ventricular Response to Subcutaneous Terbutaline in Patients with Chronic Obstructive Pulmonary Disease: Radionuclide Angiographic Assessment of Cardiac Size and Function, *Am. Heart J.*, 104:1027, 1982.
75. Katz, M., Robertson, P. A., and Creasy, R. K.: Cardiovascular Complications Associated with Terbutaline Treatment for Preterm Labor, *Am. J. Obstet. Gynecol.*, 139:605, 1981.
76. Legge, J. S., Gaddie, J., and Palmer, K. N. V.: Comparison of Two Oral Selective $Beta_2$-Adrenergic Stimulant Drugs in Bronchial Asthma, *Br. Med. J.*, 1:637, 1971.
77. Phillips, P. J., Vedig, A. E., Jones, P. L., et al.: Metabolic and Cardiovascular Side Effects of the $Beta_2$-Adrenoceptor Agonists Salbutamol and Rimiterol, *Br. J. Clin. Pharmacol.*, 9:483, 1980.
78. Lee, H., Izquierdo, R., and Evans, H. E.: Cardiac Response to Oral and Aerosol Administration of Beta Agonists, *J. Pediatr.*, 103:655, 1983.
79. Prior, J. G., and Cochrane, G. M.: Self-Poisoning with Oral Salbutamol, *Br. Med. J.*, 282:1932, 1981.
80. Tfelt-Hansen, P., Kanstrup, I.-L., Christensen, N. J., and Winkler, K.: General and Regional Haemodynamic Effects of Intravenous Ergotamine in Man, *Clin. Sci.*, 65:599, 1983.
81. Feneley, M. P., Morgan, J. J., McGrath, M. A., and Egan, J. D.: Transient Aortic Arch Syndrome with Dysphagia Due to Ergotism, *Stroke*, 14:811, 1983.
82. Carr, P.: Self-Induced Myocardial Infarction, *Postgrad. Med. J.*, 57:654, 1981.
83. Klein, L. S., Simpson, R. J., Jr., Stern, R., Hayward, J. C., and Foster, J. R.: Myocardial Infarction following Administration of Sublingual Ergotamine, *Chest*, 82:375, 1982.
84. Rajfer, S. I., Anton, A. H., Rossen, J. D., and Goldberg, L. I.: Beneficial Hemodynamic Effects of Oral Levodopa in Heart Failure, *N. Engl. J. Med.*, 310:1357, 1984.
85. Hoehn, M. M.: Levodopa-Induced Postural Hypotension: Treatment with Fludrocortisone, *Arch. Neurol.*, 32:50, 1975.
86. Goldberg, L. I., and Whitsett, T. L.: Cardiovascular Effects of Levodopa, *Clin. Pharmacol. Ther.*, 12:376, 1971.
87. Koch-Weser, J.: Drug Therapy of Parkinsonism, *N. Engl. J. Med.*, 295:814, 1976.
88. Mason, J. W., Billingham, M. E., and Friedman, J. P.: Methysergide-Induced Heart Disease: A Case of Multivalvular and Myocardial Fibrosis, *Circulation*, 56;889, 1977.
89. Bana, D. S., MacNeal, P. S., LeCompte, P. M., Shay, Y., and Graham, J. R.: Cardiac Murmurs and Endocardial Fibrosis Associated with Methysergide Therapy, *Am. Heart J.*, 88:640, 1974.
90. Pringle, T. H., Scorbie, I. N., Murray, R. G., Kesson, C. M., and Maccuish, A. C.: Prolongation of the QT Interval during Therapeutic Starvation: A Substrate for Malignant Arrhythmias, *Int. J. Obes.*, 7:253, 1983.
91. Michiel, R. R., Sneider, J. S., Dickstein, R. A., Hayman, H., and Eich, R. H.: Sudden Death in a Patient on a Liquid Protein Diet, *N. Engl. J. Med.*, 298:1005, 1978.
92. Singh, B. N., Gaarder, T. D., Kanegae, T., Goldstein, M.,

Montgomerie, J. Z., and Mills, H.: Liquid Protein Diets and *Torsade de Pointes*, *JAMA*, 240:115, 1978.
93. Boyce, M. J.: Cimetidine and the Cardiovascular System, in J. H. Baron (ed.), "Cimetidine in the 80's," Churchill Livingstone, Edinburgh, 1981, p. 227.
94. Freston, J. W.: Cimetidine: II. Adverse Reactions and Patterns of Use, *Ann. Intern. Med.*, 97:728, 1982.
95. Gould, L., Reddy, C. V. R., Singh, B. K., and Zen, B.: Electrophysiologic Properties of Cimetidine in Man, *PACE*, 4:3, 1981.
96. Engel, T. R., and Luck, J. C.: Histamine$_2$ Receptor Antagonism by Cimetidine and Sinus-Node Function, *N. Engl. J. Med.*, 301:591, 1979.
97. MacMahon, B., Bakshi, M., and Walsh, M. J.: Cardiac Arrhythmias after Intravenous Cimetidine, *N. Engl. J. Med.*, 305:832, 1981.
98. Cardiovascular Histamine H$_2$ Receptors, *Lancet*, 2:421, 1982. (Editorial.)
99. Koch-Weser, J.: Ranitidine: A New H$_2$-Receptor Antagonist, *N. Engl. J. Med.*, 309:1368, 1983.
100. Selwyn, A. P.: The Cardiovascular System and Radiation, *Lancet*, 2:152, 1983.
101. Hotchkiss, R. S., and Hurst, J. W.: Radiation and the Heart, in J. W. Hurst (ed.), "Update V: The Heart," McGraw-Hill Book Company, New York, 1981, p. 205.
101a. Stewart, J. R. and Fajardo, L. F.: Radiation-Induced Heart Disease: An Update, *Prog. Cardiovasc. Dis.*, 27:173, 1984.
102. Applefeld, M. M., and Wiernik, P. H.: Cardiac Disease after Radiation Therapy for Hodgkins Disease: Analysis of 48 Patients, *Am. J. Cardiol.*, 51:1697, 1983.
103. Applefeld, M. M., Cole, J. F., Pollock, S. H., et al.: The Late Appearance of Chronic Pericardial Disease in Patients Treated by Radiotherapy for Hodgkins Disease, *Ann. Intern. Med.*, 94:338, 1981.
104. Gottdiener, J. S., Katin, M. J., Borer, J. S., Bacharoch, S. L., and Green, M. V.: Late Cardiac Effects of Therapeutic Mediastinal Irradiation, *N. Engl. J. Med.*, 308:569, 1983.
105. Burns, R. J., Bar-Shlomo, B.-Z., Druck, M. N., et al.: Detection of Radiation Cardiomyopathy by Gated Radionuclide Angiography, *Am. J. Med.*, 74:297, 1983.
106. Martin, R. G., Ruckdeschell, J. C., Chang, P., Byhardt, R., Bouchard, R. J., and Wiernik, P. H.: Radiation-Related Pericarditis, *Am. J. Cardiol.*, 35:216, 1975.
107. Pierce, R. H., Hafermann, M. D., and Kagen, A. R.: Changes in the Transverse Cardiac Diameter following Mediastinal Irradiation for Hodgkin's Disease, *Radiology*, 93:619, 1969.
108. Poussin-Rosillo, H., Nisce, L. Z., and Lee, B. J.: Complications of Total Nodal Irradiation of Hodgkin's Disease Stages III and IV, *Cancer*, 42:437, 1978.
109. Stewart, J. R., and Fajardo, L. F.: Radiation-Induced Heart Disease: Clinical and Experimental Aspects, *Radiol. Clin. North Am.*, 9:511, 1971.
110. Stewart, J. R., and Fajardo, L. F.: Dose Response in Human and Experimental Radiation-Induced Heart Disease, *Radiology*, 99:403, 1971.
111. Morton, D. L., Glancy, D. L., Joseph, W. L., and Adkins, P. C.: Management of Patients with Radiation-Induced Pericarditis with Effusion: A Note on the Development of Aortic Regurgitation in Two of Them, *Chest*, 64:291, 1973.
112. Kagen, A. R., Hafermann, M., Hamilton, M., Pierce, R., Morton, D., and Johnson, R.: Etiology, Diagnosis and Management of Pericardial Effusion after Irradiation, *Radiol. Clin. Biol.*, 41:171, 1971.
113. Greenwood, R. D., Rosenthal, A., Cassady, R., Jaffe, N., and Nadas, A. S.: Constrictive Pericarditis in Childhood Due to Mediastinal Irradiation, *Circulation*, 50:1033, 1974.
114. Annest, L. S., Anderson, R. P., Li, W., and Hafermann, M. D.: Coronary Artery Disease following Mediastinal Radiation Therapy, *J. Thorac. Cardiovasc. Surg.*, 85:257, 1983.
115. Brosius, F. C., Waller, B. F., and Roberts, W. C.: Radiation Heart Disease: Analysis of 16 Young (Aged 15 to 33 Years) Necropsy Patients Who Received Over 3,500 Rads to the Heart, *Am. J. Med.*, 70:519, 1981.
116. Kereiakes, D. J., Morady, F., and Ports, T. A.: High-Degree Atrioventricular Block after Radiation Therapy, *Am. J. Cardiol.*, 51:1233, 1983.
117. Castellino, R. A., Glatstein, E., Turbow, M. M., Rosenberg, S., and Kaplan, H. S.: Latent Radiation Injury of Lungs and Heart Activated by Steroid Withdrawal, *Ann. Intern. Med.*, 80:593, 1974.
118. Schimpff, S. C., Diggs, C. H., Wiswell, J. G., Salvatore, P. C., and Wiernik, P. H.: Radiation-Related Thyroid Dysfunction: Implications for the Treatment of Hodgkin's Disease, *Ann. Intern. Med.*, 92:91, 1980.
119. Fajardo, L. F., and Stewart, J. R.: Pathogenesis of Radiation-Induced Myocardial Fibrosis, *Lab. Invest.*, 29:244, 1973.
120. Westerhof, P. W., and van der Putte, S. C. J.: Radiation Pericarditis and Myocardial Fibrosis, *Eur. J. Cardiol.*, 4:213, 1976.
121. Cohen, S. I., Bharati, S., Glass, J., and Lev, M.: Radiotherapy as a Cause of Complete Atrioventricular Block in Hodgkin's Disease, *Arch. Intern. Med.*, 141:676, 1981.
122. Bonnell, J. A.: Effects of Electric Fields Near Power-Transmission Plant, *J. R. Soc. Med.*, 75:933, 1982.
123. Thompson, J. C., and Ashwal, S.: Electrical Injuries in Children, *Am. J. Dis. Child.*, 137:231, 1983.
124. Hughes, J. H.: Electrical Injury, *Ariz. Med.*, 37:760, 1980.
125. Cooper, M. A.: Lightning Injuries: Prognostic Signs for Death, *Ann. Emerg. Med.*, 9:134, 1980.
126. Bernstein, T.: Effects of Electricity and Lightning on Man and Animals, *J. Forensic Sci.*, 18:3, 1973.
127. Dixon, G. F.: The Evaluation and Management of Electrical Injuries, *Crit. Care Med.*, 11:384, 1983.
128. Sances, A., Jr., Larson, S. J., Myklebust, J., and Cusick, J. F.: Electrical Injuries, *Surg. Gynecol. Obstet.*, 149:97, 1979.
129. Wright, R. K., and Davis, J. H.: The Investigation of Electrical Deaths: A Report of 220 Fatalities, *J. Forensic Sci.*, 25:514, 1980.
130. Butler, E. D., and Gant, T. D.: Electrical Injuries, with Special Reference to the Upper Extremities: A Review of 182 Cases, *Am. J. Surg.*, 134:95, 1977.
131. Kleinot, S., Klachko, D. M., and Keeley, K. J.: The Cardiac Effects of Lightning Injury, *S. Afr. Med. J.*, 40:1141, 1966.
132. Apfelberg, D. B., Masters, F. W., and Robinson, D. W.: Pathophysiology and Treatment of Lightning Injuries, *J. Trauma*, 14:453, 1974.
133. Myers, G. J., Colgan, M. T., and Van Dyke, D. H.: Lightning-Strike Disaster among Children, *JAMA*, 238:1045, 1977.
134. Strasser, E. J., Davis, R. M., and Menchey, M. J.: Lightning Injuries, *J. Trauma*, 17:315, 1977.
135. Lewin, R. F., Arditti, A., and Sclarovsky, S.: Non-Invasive Evaluation of Electrical Cardiac Injury, *Br. Heart J.*, 49:190, 1983.
136. Jackson, S. H. D., and Parry, D. J.: Lightning and the Heart, *Br. Heart J.*, 43:454, 1980.
137. Kleiner, J. P., and Wilkin, J. H.: Cardiac Effects of Lightning Stroke, *JAMA*, 240:2757, 1978.
138. Burda, C. D.: Electrocardiographic Changes in Lightning Stroke, *Am. Heart J.*, 72:521, 1966.
139. Chia, B. L.: Electrocardiographic Abnormalities and Congestive Cardiac Failure Due to Lightning Stroke, *Cardiology*, 68:49, 1981.
140. Kirchmer, J. T., Larson, D. L., and Tyson, K. R. T.: Cardiac Rupture following Electrical Injury, *J. Trauma*, 17:389, 1977.
141. Solem, L., Fischer, R. P., and Strate, R. G.: The Natural History of Electrical Injury, *J. Trauma*, 17:487, 1977.
142. Kobernick, M.: Electrical Injuries: Pathophysiology and Emergency Management, *Ann. Emerg. Med.*, 11:633, 1982.
143. Hanson, G. C., and McIlwraith, G. R.: Lightning Injury: Two Case Histories and a Review of Management, *Br. Med. J.*, 4:271, 1973.
144. Taussig, H. B.: "Death" from Lightning—and the Possibility of Living Again, *Ann. Intern. Med.*, 68:1345, 1968.
145. Weiner, R. D.: The Psychiatric Use of Electrically Induced Seizures, *Am. J. Psychiatry*, 136:1507, 1979.
146. Hurwitz, T. D.: Electroconvulsive Therapy: A Review, *Compr. Psychiatry*, 15:303, 1974.
147. Brown, M. L., Huston, P. E., Hines, H. M., and Brown,

G. W.: Cardiovascular Changes Associated with Electroconvulsive Therapy in Man, *AMA Arch. Neurol. Psychiatry,* 69:601, 1953.
148. Gerring, J. P., and Shields, H. M.: The Identification and Management of Patients with a High Risk for Cardiac Arrhythmias during Modified ECT, *J. Clin. Psychiatry,* 43:140, 1982.
149. Woodruff, R. A., Pitts, F. N., and McClure, J. N.: The Drug Modification of ECT: I. Methohexital, Thiopental, and Preoxygenation, *Arch. Gen. Psychiatry,* 18:605, 1968.
150. Gould, L., Gopalaswamy, C., Chandy, F., and Kim, B.: Electroconvulsive Therapy-Induced ECG Changes Simulating a Myocardial Infarction, *Arch. Intern. Med.,* 143:1786, 1983.
151. Graybar, G., Goethe, J., Levy, T., Phillips, J., Youngberg, J., and Smith, D.: Transient Large Upright T-Wave on the Electrocardiogram during Multiple Monitored Electroconvulsive Therapy, *Anesthesiology,* 59:467, 1983.
152. Buisseret, D.: Acute Pulmonary Edema following Grand Mal Epilepsy and as a Complication of Electric Shock Therapy, *Br. J. Dis. Chest,* 76:194, 1982.
153. Jones, R. M., and Knight, P. R.: Cardiovascular and Hormonal Responses to Electroconvulsive Therapy, *Anaesthesia,* 36:795, 1981.
154. Bali, I. M.: The Effect of Modified Electroconvulsive Therapy on Plasma Potassium Concentration, *Br. J. Anaesth.,* 47:398, 1975.
155. Hood, D. D., and Mecca, R. S.: Failure to Initiate Electroconvulsive Seizures in a Patient Pretreated with Lidocaine, *Anesthesiology,* 58:379, 1983.
156. Elliott, R. L.: Case Report of a Potential Interaction between Clonidine and Electroconvulsive Therapy, *Am. J. Psychiatry,* 140:1238, 1983.
157. Giraulo, D., Lind, L., Salzman, C., Pilon, R., and Elkins, R.: Sodium Nitroprusside Treatment of ECT-Induced Blood Pressure Elevations, *Am. J. Psychiatry,* 135:1105, 1978.
158. Decina, P., Malitz, S., Sackeim, H. A., Holzer, J., and Yudofsky, S.: Cardiac Arrest during ECT Modified by Beta-Adrenergic Blockade, *Am. J. Psychiatry,* 141:298, 1984.
159. Alexopoulos, G. S., Nasr, H., Young, R. C., Wilkstrom, T. R., and Holzman, S. R.: Electroconvulsive Therapy in Patients on Anticoagulants, *Can. J. Psychiatry,* 27:46, 1982.
160. Blitt, C. D.: Electroconvulsive Therapy with a Cardiac Pacemaker, *Anesthesiology,* 45:580, 1976.
161. Abiuso, P., Dunkelman, R., and Proper, M.: Electroconvulsive Therapy in Patients with Pacemakers, *JAMA,* 240:2459, 1978.
162. Taylor, P. J., Von Witt, R. J., and Fry, A. H.: Serum Creatinine Phosphokinase Activity in Psychiatric Patients Receiving Electroconvulsive Therapy, *J. Clin. Psychiatry,* 42:103, 1981.
163. Ellis, M. D.: Poisonous Plants, in M. D. Ellis (ed.), "Dangerous Plants, Snakes, Arthropods, and Marine Life," Hamilton Press, Hamilton, Ill., 1975, p. 3.
164. Van Stee, E. W.: Cardiovascular Toxicology: Foundations and Scope, in E. W. Van Stee (ed.), "Cardiovascular Toxicology," Raven Press, New York, 1982, p. 1.
165. Polson, C. J., Green, M. A., and Lee, M. R.: "Clinical Toxicology," 3d ed., J. B. Lippincott Company, Philadelphia, 1983, p. 401.
166. Moeschlin, S.: "Poisoning, Diagnosis and Treatment," Grune & Stratton, New York, 1965, p. 543.
167. Akera, T., and Brown, B. S.: Cardiovascular Toxicology of Cardiotonic Drugs and Chemicals, in E. W. Van Stee (ed.), "Cardiovascular Toxicology," Raven Press, New York, 1982, p. 109.
168. Russell, F. E.: Pharmacology of Animal Venoms, *Clin. Pharmacol. Ther.,* 8:849, 1967.
169. Arena, J. M.: "Poisoning, Toxicology, Symptoms, Treatment," 4th ed., Charles C Thomas, Publisher, Springfield, Ill., 1979, p. 558.
170. Huang, T. T., Lewis, S. R., and Lucas, B. S., III: Venomous Snakes, in M. D. Ellis (ed.), "Dangerous Plants, Snakes, Arthropods, and Marine Life," Hamilton Press, Hamilton, Ill., 1975, p. 123.
171. Lefer, A. M., and Curtis, M. T.: Cardiotoxicity of Naturally Occurring Animal Peptides, in E. W. Van Stee (ed.), "Cardiovascular Toxicology," Raven Press, New York, 1982, p. 221.
172. Horen, W. P.: Insect and Scorpion Sting, *JAMA,* 221:894, 1972.
173. Alagesan, R., Srinivasaraghavan, J., Balambal, R., Haranath, K., Subramanyam, N., and Thiruvengadam, K. V.: Transient Complete Right Bundle Branch Block following Scorpion Sting, *J. Indian Med. Assoc.,* 69:113, 1977.
174. Levine, H. D.: Acute Myocardial Infarction following Wasp Sting: Report of Two Cases and Critical Survey of the Literature, *Am. Heart J.,* 91:365, 1976.
175. Rowe, S. F., Greer, K. E., and Hodge, R. H. Jr.: Electrocardiographic Changes Associated with Multiple Yellow Jacket Stings, *South. Med. J.,* 72:483, 1979.
176. Zakhari, S., and Aviado, D. M.: Cardiovascular Toxicology of Aerosol Propellants, Refrigerants, and Related Solvents, in E. W. Van Stee (ed.), "Cardiovascular Toxicology," Raven Press, New York, 1982, p. 281.
177. Polson, C. J., Green, M. A., and Lee, M. R.: "Clinical Toxicology," 3d ed., J. B. Lippincott Company, Philadelphia, 1983, p. 138.
178. Weill, H.: Cardiorespiratory Effects of Inhalant Occupational Exposures, *Circulation,* 63:250A, 1981.
179. Garriott, J., and Petty, C. S.: Death from Inhalant Abuse: Toxicological and Pathological Evaluation of 34 Cases, *Clin. Toxicol.,* 16:305, 1980.
180. Turino, G. M.: Effect of Carbon Monoxide on the Cardiorespiratory System. Carbon Monoxide Toxicity: Physiology and Biochemistry, *Circulation,* 63:253A, 1981.
181. Moeschlin, S.: "Poisoning, Diagnosis and Treatment," Grune & Stratton, New York, 1965, p. 225.

Section C

The Heart and Anesthesia

79

Anesthesia and the Patient with Cardiovascular Disease

Carl C. Hug, Jr., M.D., Ph.D.

The anesthesiologist faces a unique set of problems in the anesthetic management and life support of the patient with cardiovascular disease. On top of the basic disease processes are superimposed (1) the effects of anesthetic drugs on the cardiovascular, autonomic, endocrine, and other organ systems; (2) manipulation of vital functions influencing hemodynamics (e.g., ventilation, fluid and electrolyte balance); and (3) the stresses of the surgical operation, including noxious stimulation, abnormal positioning of the patient, trauma to vital organs, blood and fluid losses, alterations of body temperature, sudden changes in regional perfusion (tourniquet or vascular clamping, extracorporeal circulation), and activation of reflexes (carotid body compression during endarterectomy, airway stimulation during laryngoscopy and bronchoscopy).

In meeting these challenges, the anesthesiologist depends on the cooperation of the surgeons, physician consultants, nurses, technicians, and all the other members of the patient care team. High-fidelity communication and good working relationships are essential to the best possible outcome in patient care. It takes effort to develop an understanding of the other person's viewpoints, and this chapter is intended to convey the viewpoint of one anesthesiologist who enjoys the benefits and responsibilities of being a member of a very good team caring for a large number of patients with cardiovascular disease undergoing anesthesia and intensive care for cardiac and noncardiovascular surgery.

The details of anesthetic techniques and perioperative life support are readily available in recently published textbooks.[1–4] These details will be considered here only to the extent necessary to bridge gaps in our understanding of what is needed for good patient care.

Modern Precepts of Anesthesiology

Anesthesia Is Essential for Patient Well-Being

Historically, anesthesia has been considered as a reversible, controlled degree of coma that kept the patient comfortable and unmoving. These objectives are still important and their implications for good patient care have been broadened considerably.

Patient comfort goes beyond the absence of pain. It includes the lack of awareness of frightening circumstances that otherwise would engender stress responses and leave the patient with unpleasant recollections and perhaps contribute to the evolution of postoperative psychosis.[5] Even in the absence of pain the patient may be uncomfortable because of the loss of control of and inability to escape from the threatening circumstances. The requirement to maintain a constant, perhaps uncomfortable, and unusual body position, the perception of pressure, movement, sounds, and other sensations, and the intimidating appearance of masks, needles, tubes, equipment, and instrumentation all contribute to apprehension and initiate physiological stress responses. Such responses are inappropriate for the circumstances since the patient does not wish to fight or to flee the operation, which is needed and wanted.

Other nonpsychological sources of physiological stress responses include trauma to tissues, noxious stimulation of the nervous system, blood loss and shifts of body fluids, anesthetic side effects and toxicity, and alterations in the functions of vital organs.

Physiological stress responses are not only unneeded, but they can be detrimental if they increase metabolic work and place greater demands on cardiovascular and pulmonary systems at a time when their ability to respond is limited.

The Anesthesiologist Facilitates the Operation

Obviously some procedures require conditions that even the most cooperative patient could not tolerate emotionally, reflexly, or otherwise. Beyond rendering the patient compliant, the anesthesiologist can facilitate exposure and manipulation of the operative site (e.g., through muscular relaxation, one-lung ventilation), decrease blood loss (e.g., through creation of deliberate hypotension, hemodilution, replacement of coagulation factors), determine integrity and viability of organ systems (e.g., through evoked responses, electroencephalogram activity), and prevent accidents (e.g., by monitoring of body position, grounding of electrical instrumentation).

By vigilant monitoring of the patient's vital functions and prompt correction of abnormalities, the anesthesiologist allows the operators to focus on accomplishment of the procedure to the best of their abilities. In situations in which the operative procedure itself impairs vital organ function, the anesthesiologist can assist the surgeon by giving warning of dangerous levels of impairment and by treating the patient so as to minimize the impact of such physiological trespass.

The Anesthesiologist's Objectives

The classic triad of anesthetic objectives includes (1) analgesia, (2) unconsciousness (or relief of anxiety with regional anesthesia), and (3) muscular relaxation. The modern list of objectives includes these three plus (4) suppression of undesirable autonomic and endocrine responses to stress, (5) maintenance of hemodynamic stability, and (6) support of vital organ function. Thus, the anesthesiologist deals with both anesthesia and life support.

Anesthetic Drugs and Techniques

The anesthesiologist now has available a rather large number of anesthetic drugs and techniques. For purposes of understanding and communication, it is useful to classify them (Table 79-1) and to make some generalizations about them, but the reader will have to refer to anesthesia textbooks and journals for important details.

General anesthetics in sufficient dosage can achieve unconsciousness, muscular relaxation, and obtundation of reflexes. Although halothane, enflurane, and isoflurane qualify as general anesthetics, their side effects, especially on the cardiovascular system, limit the dose that will be tolerated safely by any patient, particularly one with cardiovascular disease.[8] Thus, these general anesthetics are rarely used alone. Usually they are combined with other drugs to achieve a satisfactory anesthetic state with a relatively low dose. Since most of the side effects and toxicities of the individual drugs are dose-dependent, these can often be minimized by using combinations of drugs. The combination of individual drugs selected for their specific effects allows the anesthesiologist to meet the anesthetic objectives more effectively and safely than is possible with a single general anesthetic drug.

In fact, an inhalational anesthetic is more often used today as a supplement to other drugs than as the primary anesthetic in a patient with cardiovascular disease. As a supplement it can contribute to unconsciousness and to the control of sympathetic and hemodynamic responses to noxious stimulation. The ability of halothane (and perhaps enflurane and isoflurane as well) to reduce myocardial oxygen demand may be beneficial in the patient with ischemic heart disease, but the merits of this indication for its use are still being debated, especially since it has potentially contravening effects (i.e., systemic hypotension, dysrhythmias).[9–11]

The predominant practice among anesthesiologists is to select individual drugs for specific objectives related to both anesthesia and life support. Some

TABLE 79-1 Anesthetic Drugs and Techniques in Current Use

- I. General anesthesia
  - A. Inhalation anesthetics (see Table 79-2)
  - B. Intravenous anesthetics (see Table 79-2)
  - C. Muscle relaxants (see Table 79-3)
- II. Regional anesthesia and analgesia[6]
  - A. Spinal
    - 1. Drugs
      - a. Local anesthetics
      - b. Narcotic analgesics (analgesia only)[7]
    - 2. Techniques
      - a. Intrathecal (subarachnoid)
      - b. Epidural
      - c. Caudal
  - B. Nerve conduction block
    - 1. Local anesthetics
    - 2. Examples of sites
      - a. Brachial plexus
      - b. Intercostal nerves
      - c. Femoral-sciatic nerves
  - C. Intravenous regional anesthesia (Bier's block):[6] local anesthetic injected into venous system of a limb isolated by a tourniquet from the central circulation
  - D. Local anesthetic infiltration: intradermal, subcutaneous, submucosal
  - E. Topical anesthesia: application of local anesthetic to mucous membranes
  - F. Autonomic ganglia and plexus block: local anesthetic injected to block reflex activity

TABLE 79-2 Indications for Use and Limiting Features of Drugs Commonly Employed in General Anesthesia

Class and Drugs	Principal Anesthetic Effects	Cardiovascular Indications for Use	Side Effects Limiting Dose
Inhalation anesthetics:[8] Halothane (Fluothane) Enflurane (Ethrane) Isoflurane (Forane)	Unconsciousness Muscular relaxation Somatic reflex suppression Autonomic reflex suppression	To control hypertension and tachycardia	Hypotension Cardiac depression Dysrhythmias
Nitrous oxide	Analgesia Sleep Amnesia Unconsciousness (high concentrations)	Can deepen or lighten anesthesia rapidly in relation to changing intensity of noxious stimulation	Hypoxemia Cardiac depression Diffusion into air-filled spaces Decreased vitamin B_{12} activity[12]
Narcotic analgesics:[8,13] Morphine Fentanyl (Sublimaze) Sufentanil (Sufenta)	Analgesia Sleep Unconsciousness (high doses) Antitussive (↑ toleration of endotracheal tube) Apnea (facilitates controlled ventilation) Suppression of sympathetic and endocrine stress responses[14]	To avoid myocardial depression To avoid tachycardia and hypertension	Prolonged ventilatory depression Vasodilation Morphine: histamine release, edema
Ketamine[8,15]	Analgesia Unconsciousness	To maintain (increase) sympathetic tone (e.g., sick sinus syndrome, cardiac tamponade, hypovolemia)	Tachycardia and hypertension Postoperative dysphoria, psychosis
Benzodiazepines:[8,16] Diazepam (Valium) Lorazepam (Ativan) Midazolam	Anxiolytic Sleep Amnesia Anticonvulsant	To avoid myocardial depression	Interactions with narcotic analgesics to produce hypotension (↓ systemic vascular resistance) and to prolong recovery (coma, ventilatory depression)
Barbiturates:[8,16] Thiopental (Pentothal) Methohexital (Brevital)	Sleep Unconsciousness	To induce anesthesia To deepen anesthesia rapidly	Hypotension Cardiac depression
Etomidate[17–19] (Amidate)	Sleep Unconsciousness	To induce and to maintain unconsciousness To deepen anesthesia rapidly	Adrenal cortical suppression[20] Interaction with narcotic analgesics to prolong recovery
Tranquilizers:[8] Chlorpromazine (Thorazine) Droperidol (Inapsine)	Enhanced narcotic analgesic effects Antiemetic	To control hypertension and sympathetic responses to noxious stimulation	Hypotension Vasodilation Dysphoria

of the properties of the drugs commonly used in anesthesia are listed in Tables 79-2 and 79-3 for the purpose of illustrating their contributions to a general anesthetic plan. Not infrequently, an anesthetic drug is chosen because of its effects on the cardiovascular and autonomic nervous systems (e.g., ketamine to maintain and enhance sympathetic tone in the patient with cardiac tamponade).[24]

Combinations of anesthetic drugs and techniques are often useful. For example, spinal anesthesia for an operation on the lower portions of the body provides analgesia, muscular relaxation, and obtundation of reflexes to the noxious stimulation of surgery. It also can improve perfusion of the lower body by reducing sympathetically mediated arteriolar constriction.[25] The addition of diazepam and nitrous oxide can provide sleep and amnesia or unconsciousness, and in the event of an unexpectedly long operation, the nitrous oxide will provide analgesia as the level of spinal anesthesia recedes.

Cardiovascular drugs are often included in the anesthesia and life-support plans of the anesthesiologist. For example, a small intravenous dose of propranolol injected just prior to laryngoscopy and tracheal intubation will obtund the tachycardia and hypertension that are often produced by these procedures.[26] An intravenous bolus dose of nitroprusside (0.2 to 1 μg/kg) can quickly and transiently lower arterial blood pressure to facilitate cannulation and decannulation of the aorta during cardiac oper-

TABLE 79-3 Indications for Use of Muscle Relaxants

Type of Drug	Autonomic and Cardiovascular Effects	Indications for Use
Depolarizing:		
Succinylcholine (Anectine)	Vagal activation Bradycardia	Rapid-onset paralysis of short duration To avoid sympathetic and cardiovascular stimulation To avoid sympathetic depression and hypotension
Nondepolarizing:		
d-Tubocurarine Metocurine (Metubine)	Histamine release Ganglionic blockade Hypotension	To minimize hypertensive episodes
Atracurium (Tracrium)[22]	Histamine release (with rapid injection)	Paralysis of short duration To avoid autonomic changes
Pancuronium (Pavulon) Gallamine (Flaxedil)	Vagal blockade Inhibition of catecholamine uptake by nerve terminal Tachycardia Hypertension	To maintain sympathetic tone To avoid cardiovascular depression To counteract vagal-mediated bradycardia (e.g., induced by narcotic anesthetics)
Vecuronium (Norcuron)[23]	None	To avoid autonomic and cardiovascular changes

Source: Miller and Morris,[21] Basta et al.,[22] and Fehey et al.[23]

ations. These drugs are especially useful for the control of hemodynamic responses to very transient noxious stimulation.

The contributions of preanesthetic medication to the production and maintenance of anesthesia should not be overlooked. Morphine not only reduces the patient's anxiety and discomfort related to preanesthetic procedures (e.g., percutaneous vascular cannulation) but it also reduces the dosage of halothane and other anesthetic drugs required to achieve a satisfactory depth of general anesthesia.[27] Continuation of chronic antihypertensive therapy and beta-adrenergic receptor blockade up to the time of anesthesia and surgery not only continues to benefit the patient in the preoperative period but also frequently facilitates the control of blood pressure intraoperatively and in the immediate postoperative period.[28,29] Of course, the anesthesiologist needs to be mindful of the potential interactions of premedicant and anesthetic drugs.[30,31]

The Anesthesiologist's Challenge

Monitoring[32]

Anesthesia is not therapeutic and the anesthesiologist keeps in mind the admonition "First, do no harm!" The goal is to return the anesthetized patient to the same (or better) mental and physical status that existed preoperatively. Given the physiological trespasses of anesthesia and surgery, it is apparent that the anesthesiologist has to detect adverse trends and changes in the patient's condition as early as possible, especially in patients with reduced physiological reserves as a result of their disease(s). Such changes tend to happen suddenly and to develop rapidly. Hence, it is essential for the anesthesiologist to be knowledgeable and skillful in monitoring techniques that range from simple to sophisticated. The seal of the American Society of Anesthesiologists contains the word *vigilance* above a lighthouse tower (Fig. 79-1). A summary of monitoring techniques used intra- and postoperatively in the management of patients with cardiovascular disease is shown in Table 79-4.

The emphasis on monitoring is clearly justified by the risks to which the patient may be exposed and by the goal of having the patient recover as rapidly and completely as possible.

Other considerations that support the rather liberal intraoperative use of sophisticated and direct hemodynamic monitoring are the following:

- The purposes of monitoring include (1) identification of the problem, (2) assessment of its severity, and (3) evaluation of its treatment. In the perioperative period, especially in the operating suite, problems arise suddenly, and their ultimate impact on the patient's well-being is determined by how rapidly and effectively they are corrected or controlled. It seems eminently logical that adverse trends and ominous signs be detected as early as possible and that the anesthesiologist should use the most efficient techniques available for the monitoring of those organ systems in which prob-

TABLE 79-4 Monitoring Techniques for the Patient with Cardiovascular Disease

I. Routine (for all patients undergoing general and regional anesthesia)
  A. Inspection
    1. Depth of anesthesia
      a. Somatic responses to command, noxious stimulation (e.g., eye opening, movement, coughing)
      b. Sympathetic responses (e.g., sweating, tearing, mydriasis) to noxious stimulation
    2. Adequacy of ventilation
      a. Inspiration, expiration
      b. Color of skin, mucous membranes, operative site
    3. Body position
      a. Physiological effects (ventilation, hemodynamics, intracranial pressure, etc.)
      b. Patient safety (skin, nerves, vasculature, joints, eyes, etc.)
  B. Palpation
    1. Skin
      a. Temperature
      b. Perfusion (capillary refill)
    2. Pulses
      a. Rate and rhythm
      b. Fullness
    3. Muscle tone
  C. Auscultation (precordial and esophageal stethescopes)
    1. Ventilation
    2. Heart sounds
    3. Blood pressure (sphygmomanometry)
  D. Devices
    1. Electrocardiograph
    2. Temperature probe
    3. Oxygen analyser (inspired gas)
    4. Ventilator–patient disconnection alarm
    5. Peripheral nerve stimulator (muscle relaxant effect)
    6. Electrical safety alarms (e.g., electrocautery grounding)
II. Additional routine monitoring for major surgical operations
  A. Central venous pressure
  B. Arterial blood gases, acid-base balance, potassium concentration (An indwelling arterial cannula permits rapid, convenient sampling and direct arterial blood pressure monitoring; see III, B below.)
  C. Urine
    1. Volume and concentration (specific gravity)
    2. Composition (e.g., protein, hemoglobin)
  D. Specialized monitoring for particular operations, e.g., *neurosurgical*
    1. Electroencephalogram
    2. Evoked potentials (spinal cord integrity)
    3. Intracranial pressure
    4. Cerebral blood flow
    5. Air embolism (sitting position)
      a. Precordial Doppler
      b. Pulmonary artery catheter
      c. End-tidal gas analysis (CO_2 analyser, mass spectrometer)
III. Advanced cardiovascular monitoring for the patient with cardiac disease undergoing noncardiac surgery
  A. Multiple electrocardiographic leads[33]
    1. Dysrhythmia detection facilitated by prominent P wave
      a. Standard limb lead II
      b. MCL_1
      c. Esophageal stethoscope lead[34]
      d. Pacing leads of pulmonary artery catheter (atrial and ventricular electrograms)[35]
    2. Ischemia detection
      a. Precordial lead V_5 or V_6 (anterolateral)
      b. Limb lead II (inferior)
      c. Precordial lead V_1 or V_{-4} (posterolateral)
  B. Intraarterial cannula
    1. Direct systemic arterial pressure measurement
      a. Mean blood pressure monitoring, essential with the following:
        1. Unstable hemodynamics
        2. Deliberate hypotension
        3. Extracorporeal circulation
        4. Ventricular assist device
      b. Estimation of left ventricular contractility (upstroke indicative of dP/dt)
      c. Moment-to-moment correlation with factors affecting hemodynamics (e.g., body position, surgical manipulation, ventilatory cycle)
      d. Detection of changes in pulse waveform (e.g., for assessment of dysrhythmias, vascular resistance, cardiac output, timing of intraaortic balloon pump)
      e. Monitoring rate and rhythm in pacemaker-dependent patient during periods of ECG interference by electrocautery
    2. Rapid, convenient sampling of arterial blood for estimation of the following:
      a. Respiratory gases
      b. pH and acid-base balance
      c. Hematocrit, hemoglobin concentration and oxygen saturation
      d. Blood coagulation status
      e. Serum electrolyte concentrations
      f. Serum glucose, lactate
      g. Serum protein concentrations and oncotic pressure
      h. Serum enzymes
      i. Serum creatinine and blood urea nitrogen
  C. Ventricular performance analysis[36–39]
    1. Preload
      a. Right ventricle
        1. Central venous pressure
        2. Right atrial pressure
      b. Left ventricle
        1. Pulmonary arterial occlusion pressure
        2. Pulmonary arterial diastolic pressure
        3. Left atrial pressure
    2. Cardiac output
      a. Thermodilution
      b. Dye dilution
    3. Vascular resistance calculation
      a. Systemic
      b. Pulmonary
    4. Other indexes of cardiac performance
      a. Stroke volume
      b. Stroke work
      c. Estimation of compliance (elastance)
    5. Experimental techniques for intraoperative detection of impaired ventricular contraction
      a. Cardiokymograph[40]
      b. Esophageal echocardiography[41,42]
  D. Assessment of tissue perfusion
    1. Overall systemic perfusion
      a. Metabolic acid-base balance
      b. Mixed venous blood[43]
        1. Oxygen partial pressure
        2. Hemoglobin saturation
      c. Calculation of oxygen consumption and carbon dioxide production
    2. Central nervous system global perfusion
      a. Electroencephalogram[44]
      b. Cerebral blood flow measurements[45]
    3. Cardiac global perfusion
      a. Systemic blood pressure vs. ventricular end-diastolic pressure
      b. Coronary sinus blood lactate concentration
    4. Pulmonary perfusion
      a. Shunt
      b. Dead space
IV. Monitoring for cardiac surgery with extracorporeal circulation: All of the above plus
  A. Coagulation-anticoagulation tests[46]
    1. Activated clotting time
    2. Heparin-protamine titration
    3. Central laboratory coagulation profile, platelet count, and special tests (specific coagulation factors, fibrinogen concentration, etc.)
  B. Multiple sites of body temperature measurement
    1. Pharyngeal
    2. Rectal or urinary bladder
    3. Surface (e.g., toe)
    4. Pulmonary arterial blood (thermodilution catheter)
    5. Intramyocardial
  C. Serum potassium, calcium
  D. Special tests
    1. Oncotic pressure
    2. Serum glucose
V. Monitoring specific disease states, e.g., *diabetes mellitus*
  A. Serum glucose
  B. Ketoacidosis

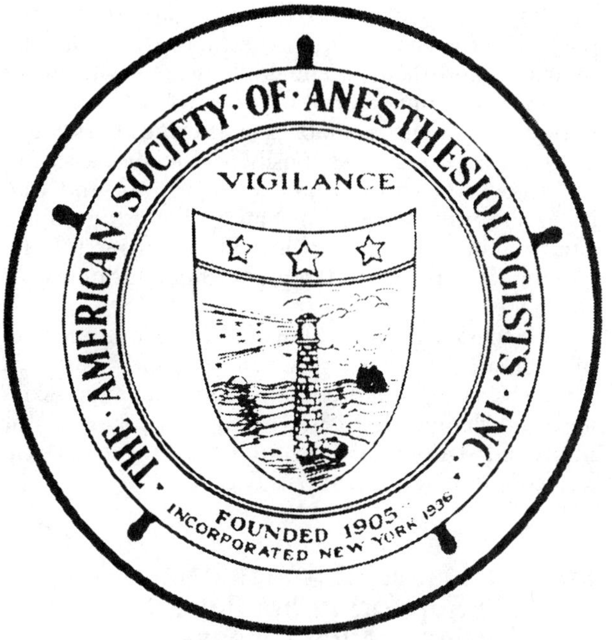

FIGURE 79-1 The seal of the American Society of Anesthesiologists.

lems are most likely to occur. Rapid and direct assessment of hemodynamics is likely to benefit the patient with cardiovascular disease.[47]

- The benefits of hemodynamic monitoring in patients undergoing cardiac surgery have been realized in amazingly low mortality and morbidity rates.[48] These same benefits can be realized in the patient with cardiovascular disease and undergoing noncardiac surgery. It is likely that the benefits will be greater in the noncardiac surgical patient because (1) the surgery does not correct or directly improve cardiovascular function, and (2) the surgeon and anesthesiologist do not have the benefit of diagnostic clues evident when the heart is directly accessible to inspection and palpation as it is during cardiac surgery.
- The traditional signs of cardiovascular dysfunction are often modified and obscured by anesthesia and surgery. Whereas brain, heart, lung, and kidney function can be assessed in the awake patient for indications of the adequacy of their perfusion, the situation is quite different in anesthetized patients in whom the brain is variably depressed by anesthetic drugs; cardiovascular function is altered by anesthetic drugs and changes in body position, circulating blood volume, etc.; pulmonary ventilation and perfusion are affected by mechanical ventilation, the composition of the inspired gas mixture, and changes in cardiac output and pulmonary vascular resistance; and urine volume and concentration reflect translocation of body fluids and endocrine alterations induced by anesthesia and surgery. Even skin perfusion is an unreliable indicator of the adequacy of overall cardiovascular function because of the multiple factors that lead to cutaneous vasodilation and vasoconstriction during anesthesia and surgery. Moreover, the patient with cardiovascular disease often has or develops concurrent impairment of several organ systems, and it is not possible to distinguish the contributions of inadequate perfusion from intrinsic pathophysiological processes.
- The patient with cardiovascular disease encounters cardiovascular stress in the perioperative period that is unpredictable in timing, intensity, and duration. Physicians caring for the patient have to make a rapid assessment of the situation and of its response to their treatment. The patient's exposure to stressful events continues into the postoperative period as does the need for immediate direct assessment of cardiovascular function. In fact, most perioperative myocardial infarctions occur 2 or more days after noncardiac surgery, and many suspect this reflects decreasing diagnostic vigilance and delayed treatment of hemodynamic abnormalities.[49,50]

Little-Known, Important Facts and Circumstances of Anesthesia and Surgery

The depth of anesthesia represents the balance between noxious stimulation and drug depression of the central and autonomic nervous systems. It is an everyday observation that a dose of anesthetic drug producing anesthesia and cardiovascular depression in the *unstimulated* patient proves to be inadequate to maintain unconsciousness and to prevent tachycardia and hypertension in response to skin incision and electrocauterization of subcutaneous tissues. Often the most intense stimulation is so brief that the anesthesiologist is faced with the dilemma of giving a large dose of an anesthetic in anticipation of the stimulation and with the risk of excessive and undesirably prolonged side effects or of maintaining a relatively light level of anesthesia and treating the responses to intense stimulation with other drugs (e.g., short-acting alpha- or beta-adrenergic receptor blockers). The latter are often preferable because it is difficult to predict which patients will exhibit undesirable responses to transient noxious stimuli, and because these drugs have a rapid onset and act directly on the organ or tissue responding to the stimulation.

Minor operations of brief duration not infrequently require a major anesthetic and life-support plan. When the procedure compromises vital functions, no matter how briefly this compromising situation is likely to exist, the stage is set for catastrophe if the physicians and others caring for the patient are not prepared to act promptly and effectively. In some situations, prevention is the only satisfactory answer. Thus, the trachea must be intubated when the anesthetist is denied access to and control of the airway. Tracheal intubation usually requires a general anesthetic to provide both patient comfort and control of the patient's somatic and autonomic reflex responses.

The use of local or regional anesthesia does not preclude major risks to the patient, especially in the presence of cardiovascular disease. As noted above, stressful conditions place these patients at considerable risk of untoward cardiovascular responses. Local anesthesia does not control other causes of patient discomfort (e.g., body position), and it does not prevent anxiety, apprehension, and the associated responses of the autonomic nervous system. The dose of sedative drugs required to control these psychological and autonomic responses may be so large as to compromise protective airway reflexes, ventilation, and other vital functions. In such cases, direct control of the airway and ventilation under general anesthesia may be considerably safer than local or regional anesthesia alone. And the risks of local anesthetic side effects and toxicity cannot be ignored. Toxicity may be manifest as CNS stimulation and/or depression and as cardiac depression.[51] Neither is a desirable side effect of local anesthesia in any patient, especially one with cardiovascular disease.

If the surgical operation is technically successful and yet the patient does not do well in the perioperative period, there is a tendency to attribute problems to the effects of anesthetic drugs and to inadequacies of anesthetic and life-support care. Of course, faulty anesthetic and life-support management contributes to postoperative morbidity and death, but our understanding of physiology, pharmacology, and other medical sciences is imperfect and incomplete, and there are effects and events for which the cause and explanation are unknown, or at best uncertain.[52,53] *Coincidence in time is not proof of a cause-effect relation.*

Anesthesiologists have been focusing on clinical investigations in the operating and postanesthetic recovery rooms. There is a great need for them to extend their efforts further into the postoperative period and to evaluate the impact of anesthetic and life-support procedures on the ultimate outcomes for their patients.[54] A few longer-term studies are beginning to be reported in the anesthesiology literature, but the larger medical community remains unaware of them. There needs to be a much broader interaction of anesthesiologists with their peers in other medical specialties. Sharing of experiences and cross-fertilization of ideas can only be beneficial to patient care. The anesthesiologist is experienced in acute and intensive care of patients and, because of the nature of modern anesthesia, has developed extraordinary knowledge and experience in the management of problems related to the nervous, pulmonary, and cardiovascular systems.[55] In the case of each individual patient, the anesthesiologist gains unique, firsthand experience in the operating room that can be useful in the postoperative period. This is especially true in terms of pulmonary and cardiovascular function and the patient's responses to drugs and other interventions. Moreover, the anesthesiologist is the expert in recovery from anesthesia, the potential effects of residual anesthetic drugs on vital functions, and their potential interactions with drugs that may be administered in the early postoperative period. It is only reasonable that the anesthesiologist assume the primary responsibility for the patient in the recovery room or intensive care unit and that he or she convey the information that has accumulated to the physicians who will be caring for the patient after recovery from anesthetic influences is complete.

Anesthesiologists are subspecializing along the lines of their surgical colleagues. With common interests, similar working schedules, and complementary skills and knowledge, there is tremendous potential for improved patient care through teaching, research, and cooperative clinical practice.

Specific Issues of Anesthesia and Life Support in the Patient with Cardiovascular Disease

The specific details of designing an anesthetic and life-support plan for a patient with a particular type of cardiovascular disease are well-described elsewhere.[1–4, 56–58] What follows is a more general consideration of what the anesthesiologist takes into consideration in designing and implementing such plans. The focus is on two types of cardiac disease in adults: coronary artery disease and acquired valvular heart disease. The reader is referred elsewhere for discussions related to congenital and other acquired forms of heart disease.[1,3,4,58]

Preoperative Assessment of the Patient with Heart Disease

In addition to the information pertinent to the anesthetic management of any patient (outcome of previous anesthetics, drug allergy, airway anatomy, hepatorenal function, etc.), the anesthesiologist caring for the patient with cardiac disease focuses on some key points of cardiopulmonary function. Some of this information can only be obtained with the cooperation of the cardiologist-internist.

Coronary Artery Disease

The anesthesiologist will be caring for the patient in both the awake and the anesthetized states with varying degrees of noxious stimulation. Information about factors precipitating angina pectoris and the ranges of heart rate and systemic blood pressure at rest and during exercise-induced angina pectoris (i.e., stress test) are especially useful in setting the upper and lower limits of these variables that will be considered to be acceptable during anesthesia and surgery. With knowledge of the location of significant coronary artery lesions and of the ECG leads in which changes indicative of ischemia were evident in the past, the anesthesiologist can arrange a limited number of ECG leads to the greatest potential advantage intraoperatively. The patient's responses to chronic prophylactic therapy as well as to acute treatment of angina pectoris provide guidelines for intraoperative therapy of myocardial ischemia (e.g., sublingual nifedipine for the patient prone to coronary artery spasm).[59]

An assessment of ventricular function is helpful in making choices of monitoring techniques and anesthetic drugs. Particularly useful information includes an estimate of exercise tolerance, details about any recent episode of cardiac failure and the responses to therapy, and the results of a very recent radiographic examination of the chest. If the patient has undergone laboratory studies (ventriculography, echocardiography, nuclear scanning), information about ventricular ejection fraction, end-diastolic pressures, wall motion abnormalities, and valvular function can be very helpful to the anesthesiologist.[60] It should be noted, however, that we frequently find disparity between preoperative assessments of ventricular function and the measurements made in the operating room prior to the induction of anesthesia. Of course, time has passed, the patient's condition may have changed, and the circumstances are quite different in the perioperative period. For these reasons, advanced hemodynamic monitoring is indicated in all patients with symptomatic coronary artery disease except those judged to be physically fit, without trace of ventricular impairment, and facing minimal risks of cardiac injury during and after the operation.

Valvular Heart Disease

Estimates of cardiac function at rest and of cardiac reserve in the face of increases in the demand for cardiac work are obviously helpful to the anesthesiologist designing plans for anesthesia, monitoring, and life support of the patient with valvular heart disease. Given the potential for rapidly developing and sometimes extreme degrees of stress imposed on cardiac function during the intra- and postoperative periods, it is better to err on the side of more-than-needed rather than less-than-necessary sophistication of hemodynamic monitoring and therapeutic preparedness; and it should be remembered that valvular heart disease often involves impairment of other organ systems, especially the lungs, and that these systems are stressed in the perioperative period, and further compromise of their function can lead to a vicious cycle of deterioration.

In the case of valvular heart disease the anesthesiologist is especially concerned about ventricular function (as discussed above) and also about circulating blood volume, fluid and electrolyte balance, diuretic therapy, fluid and dietary restrictions, heart rate and dysrhythmias and their response to therapy, relative degrees of valvular stenosis and insufficiency for purposes of afterload and preload manipulation, condition of the coronary circulation, and pulmonary and hepatorenal function. In the case of elective surgery, the anesthesiologist wants to be sure that the patient is in the best possible condition to withstand the circumstances of anesthesia, surgery, and the postoperative period. The postoperative period is most important since the intensity of monitoring and the readiness to respond to adverse changes will be less than in the operating room, even if the patient is in an intensive care unit. It has been said that with modern anesthetic techniques it is relatively easy to take a very sick patient through the anesthetic and operation compared to the difficult struggle of bringing that same patient through the periods of recovery and early convalescence successfully.

The Influence of Preoperative Medications[2,31,61]

Both the continuation of chronic drug therapy and preanesthetic analgesia and sedation should be ordered by the anesthesiologist for the night before and day of operation. Not only is the anesthesiologist responsible for the patient's care during the period of most of the actions of these drugs, but an anesthetic and life-support plan based on their presence or absence must be designed. For example, the requirements of a narcotic anesthetic (narcotic dose, anesthetic and cardiovascular drug supplements) are considerably different in the presence of a therapeutic level of an adrenergic beta-receptor blocking drug than in its absence.[62,63]

Preoperative medications especially useful to the anesthesiologist caring for patients with cardiac disease are listed in Table 79-5.

TABLE 79-5 Preoperative Medications for the Patient with Cardiovascular Disease

The following chronic medications are generally continued up to the time of surgery, often with a dose administered orally on the morning of surgery:
- Adrenergic beta-receptor blocking drugs
- Antihypertensives
- Bronchodilators
- Calcium-channel-blocking drugs
- Corticosteroids
- Potassium

The following drugs may or may not be given on the morning of surgery:
- Antidysrhythmic drugs
- Digitalis glycosides
- Long-acting insulin preparations (usually substituted by regular insulin)

For elective surgery, the following drugs are usually discontinued 1 or more days prior to surgery:
- Antidepressants:
  - MAO inhibitors (discontinued 2 to 3 weeks)
  - Tricyclics
- Diuretics

Assessment of Risks of Perioperative Morbidity and Death in the Patient with Cardiovascular Disease

Hypertension

Preoperative systolic blood pressure is a predictor of postoperative morbidity.[64] In the long-term management of hypertension, the focus has been on the diastolic blood pressure. Unfortunately, existing studies of perioperative morbidity fail to answer the questions: (1) Does the level of diastolic blood pressure correlate with perioperative morbidity and mortality rates? There is a strong tendency to believe that diastolic blood pressures sustained at 120 mmHg or above increase risks and should be treated before undertaking elective surgery.[65] (2) Does preoperative therapeutic control of hypertension reduce perioperative risks? The answer is probably "yes" according to the following reasoning: Hemodynamic fluctuations are less in treated compared to untreated hypertensive people.[65,66] Major deviations of intraoperative arterial blood pressure from preoperative levels have been correlated with myocardial ischemia.[61,65–67] The prevalent view among anesthesiologists is that it is preferable to have hypertension well-controlled preoperatively, to continue chronic antihypertensive therapy up to the time of anesthesia and surgery, and to be prepared to deal with potential drug interactions[31,61] in the perioperative period. Most importantly, the anesthesiologist and other physicians caring for the hypertensive patient should have a therapeutic plan in mind for the control of hypertensive episodes intra- and postoperatively when the effects of chronic therapy are declining and the patient is not able to take oral medications.

Cardiac Disease

Numerous studies and literature reviews have focused on the relationships of various factors to the outcome of anesthesia and surgery (both cardiac and noncardiac) in patients with known cardiac disease. The increased risks of perioperative myocardial reinfarction and death in patients with a recent (less than 6 months old) infarction compared to patients without a recent infarction have been documented by several groups of investigators.[49,50,68] Multiple contributing factors have been identified and shown to be interactive in their apparent effects on outcome (Table 79-6; also see Table 80-1).[68,69] Some of these factors (e.g., age) are immutable; others can be ameliorated preoperatively (e.g., correction of arrhythmias, treatment of congestive heart failure) or controlled in the perioperative period. It seems that the experience gained in the management of patients undergoing coronary artery surgery can be applied to the management of similar patients for noncardiac surgery with a resulting reduction of morbidity and mortality. Advanced hemodynamic monitoring and prompt correction of abnormalities are given most of the credit for the improved outcome.[47]

The practical implications of these findings are that there is no cut-and-dried answer to the question of whether a patient with cardiovascular disease should or should not undergo a particular elective surgical procedure. As noted above, the problems of intraoperative management of even the sickest patient are usually less than those associated with complications arising postoperatively. In our experience it seems that some of the latter can be addressed successfully by continuation of intensive monitoring and therapy, but the difficult dilemmas of costs versus benefits have to be faced.

In the case of the patient with angina pectoris, there is a basic question to be answered before proceeding with elective noncardiac surgery: Should the patient undergo diagnostic evaluation of coronary artery disease? Certainly if the patient is a candidate for such studies without regard to an elective noncardiac surgical problem, the tests should be done, and if definite treatment (e.g., medical, angioplasty, surgical) of coronary artery disease is indicated, this should be accomplished prior to, or perhaps concurrently with, the elective surgical operation.[70] Although admittedly limited, the existing data suggest that prior coronary artery bypass grafting reduces the risk of complications of major noncardiac surgery in patients with a significant history of coronary artery disease.[71]

If, on the other hand, the patient has a history of stable angina pectoris, is in generally good physical condition, and does not have other cardiac risk factors (see Table 80-1),[68] then it seems satisfactory to proceed with anesthesia and elective surgery using appropriate monitoring to detect myocardial is-

TABLE 79-6 Reasons to Postpone Noncurative Surgical Operations*

High-grade fever
High-output heart failure (e.g., thyroid storm)
Congestive heart failure
Cardiogenic shock
Acute myocardial infarction
Critical coronary artery stenosis
Unstable angina pectoris
Hemodynamically significant dysrhythmia
Severe hypokalemia
Shock or uncontrolled hypotension (anaphylaxis, sepsis)
Hypovolemia, low blood volume
Clinically significant anemia
Severe renal failure
Severe hepatic failure
Inability to secure airway
Aspiration pneumonitis
Clinically significant, uncontrolled bronchospasm
Pneumonia
Adult respiratory distress syndrome
Pneumothorax

*Condition should be corrected or controlled therapeutically prior to the induction of anesthesia.

chemia and being prepared to treat such episodes promptly. There is no clear-cut basis for choosing one particular type of anesthetic drug or technique, but the anesthesiologist should be mindful of the anesthetic drugs' effects in relation to the pathophysiology of coronary artery disease and with regard for the effects of the anesthetic technique on the detectability of ischemic episodes.[11,72,73]

There are a number of classifications of heart disease, cardiac function, angina pectoris (see elsewhere in this book), and general physical status (American Society of Anesthesiologists[74]) that serve to describe and to classify patients for various purposes (e.g., research, professional fees). These can be used to identify high-risk patients, but they have limited ability to predict the outcomes of anesthesia and surgery, either cardiac or noncardiac, in any individual patient; witness the low morbidity and mortality rates in high-risk patients undergoing myocardial revascularization.[48]

Reasons to Postpone Elective Surgery

Anesthesiologists join their physician colleagues in striving for the best possible outcome for patients under their care. Their concerns for patient well-being extend beyond the intraoperative period. They should be reluctant to deny or to delay the benefits of a surgical operation to a patient, but they must be certain that the patient is as well prepared as possible for the stresses of anesthesia, surgery, and recovery. These concerns must be weighed against the urgency of the operation.

Except for hemorrhage that cannot be controlled without direct surgical intervention, there are few occasions in which it is necessary and prudent to abridge safe anesthetic practices in hurrying to begin an operation. And there are some definite reasons to delay or to postpone a surgical operation (Table 79-6). These reasons are all-the-more important in the patient with cardiovascular disease and limited reserves with which to withstand physiological trespass.

In most instances the decision to delay or to proceed can be made by discussion of the relative merits and risks of the various alternatives. The conditions listed in Table 79-6 are intended to draw attention to particularly risky circumstances that need to be balanced against the benefits of immediately proceeding with the operation.

Design of a Plan for Anesthesia and Life Support

Four essential considerations enter into the design of a plan for anesthesia and life support:

- The patient's informed consent
- The patient's mental and physical conditions
- The surgeon's objectives and procedures
- Provisions for postoperative care

It is the anesthesiologist's responsibility to recommend a general course of action, along with an appropriate explanation of its potential benefits and risks, to the patient based on the above considerations, but the patient must give consent to that general plan. To the extent that the patient witholds consent, the anesthesiologist may be limited in options (e.g., general versus regional anesthesia). If the anesthesiologist finds these limitations too restrictive for the patient's safety and well-being, and the patient holds to the restrictions, the anesthesiologist like any other physician is best advised to decline to care for the patient for an elective procedure. Fortunately, such situations are very rare in cases of patients with cardiac disease, but all must remember the patient's rights and the physicians' responsibilities.

The anesthesiologist and surgeon must have an understanding of each other's objectives. In selecting anesthetic drugs, monitoring techniques, an approach to airway management, etc., it is essential that the anesthesiologist be aware of the surgeon's needs (e.g., positioning of the patient, muscular relaxation, drugs to be injected by the surgeon into the operative site, special techniques such as deliberate hypotension). In turn, the surgeon should be cognizant of the conditions produced by the anesthesiologist's technique (e.g., potential for awareness of the patient, degree of muscular relaxation, expected benefits and potential complications of the anesthetic drugs).

In the event of complications, high degrees of mutual understanding, respect, and cooperation are essential to rapid correction of the problem and a satisfactory outcome. Subsequently, it is the anesthesiologist's responsibility to inform the patient and family members about complications related to anesthesia and intraoperative life-support management. The discussion of the problems is ideally done in the presence of the surgeon so that the patient and family members are presented with an appropriately complete, precise, and consistent account. In any event, the surgeon should *not* undertake this responsibility.

The anesthesiologist, surgeon, and in some cases, the internist-cardiologist must understand and be in agreement about the plans for postoperative care of the patient. Does the patient go from the operating room to an intensive care unit? Should the patient's ventilation be supported mechanically? What criteria will be used to judge the patient's readiness for extubation? What monitoring techniques are possible given the facilities of the hospital and which are appropriate for the patient? Who will coordinate the patient's postoperative care including the control of pain and anxiety, therapy of cardiovascular dysfunction, fluid and blood replacement, etc.?

There are some aspects of patient care management by the anesthesiologist that are not known or understood by colleagues in other specialties. Some of these are presented briefly because they are important in postoperative care of the patient, especially when responsibility for this care is transferred from the anesthesiologist to another physician.

Drug Administration

There is no justification for administering a water-soluble or water-compatible drug by any route other than intravenously in the perioperative period when the patient has an indwelling intravenous cannula. First of all, there are a number of advantages to intravenous drug administration:

- The onset of drug action is more rapid and predictable because the delay and variability of absorption are avoided.
- The titration of drug dosage to patient response is facilitated by the rapid onset and early occurrence of the peak effect.
- Prompt detection of drug overdose is favored by the earlier occurrence of its peak effect, often while the physician or nurse is still in the vicinity and attentive toward the patient. The chances of toxicity developing later are reduced by the progressive decline of drug concentrations following an intravenous injection.[75]
- Drug action can be maintained by a continuous intravenous infusion.[76]
- Pain and local tissue reactions associated with nonintravenous parenteral injections are avoided. Phlebitis from intravenous injection of an irritant drug preparation can be minimized by injecting it into a rapidly flowing stream of intravenous fluids.

Second, there are disadvantages of using other than an intravenous route in the perioperative period:

- Blood flow to sites of absorption is highly variable as a result of anesthesia, stress responses, hypothermia, and changes in blood volume. Delayed absorption can lead to unexpected, later-occurring drug effects and toxicity.
- Delay in relief of pain actually increases analgesic dose requirements, and the patient's anxiety increases as well.[77,78]

And third, the notion of greater safety and lesser risks of side effects for nonintravenous drug administration is false. Although transiently higher blood levels of the drug occur after intravenous injection compared to other routes of administration, these are usually inconsequential. If an excessive drug effect occurs, it will be soon after drug injection when doctors and nurses are most alert to the possibility of overdose, and the peak effect will be of shorter duration. Variability in absorption and the correspondingly reduced ability to titrate drug dose to intensity of response make nonintravenous routes more hazardous in the vast majority of cases. The important exceptions are drugs that produce severe cardiovascular effects when injected rapidly, but even in these cases, a slow intravenous infusion may prevent hemodynamic changes and still allow the benefits of intravenous administration.

Recovery from Anesthetic Drugs

Recovery from anesthetic drugs, both inhalational and intravenous agents, usually is biphasic. The initial phase of recovery proceeds rapidly as the inhalational drug is exhaled and is redistributed from the central nervous system to other tissues (e.g., skeletal muscle, fat).[79] Intravenous drugs undergo a similar redistribution from brain to nonnervous tissues.[80,81] So there is the tendency for the patient to become responsive shortly (within minutes) after discontinuing administration of the anesthetic. However, complete recovery is typically a slow and prolonged process reflecting the gradual elimination of drug that has accumulated in tissues that serve as a reservoir to maintain low drug concentrations in blood and brain for hours to days. Ultimate recovery depends on the continued excretion of inhalational agents by the lung and also on their metabolism in the liver.[79] Intravenous agents are metabolized primarily in the liver and also are excreted by the kidney.[80,81] There are several important implications of these facts.

(1) Although consciousness may be regained fairly soon after anesthetic administration has ceased, the patient may remain depressed (i.e., lethargic, sleeping, hypoventilating) for many hours. During this slow phase of recovery the patient may be quite sensitive to even very small doses of analgesics and other CNS depressants. In fact, the mere lack of noxious stimulation may allow the patient to manifest the ventilatory and other depressant effects of the residual anesthetic drugs. Most cases of recurrent coma and ventilatory depression are due to either a lack of stimulation and/or the administration of another depressant drug.[82]

(2) Recovery will be more prolonged if factors interfering with anesthetic elimination are encountered. In some cases, the surgical procedure itself alters anesthetic elimination.[83,84]

(3) Although there may be antagonists able to counteract the actions of residual anesthetic drugs, the antagonists should be used cautiously because of their undesirable and sometimes dangerous side effects, especially in patients unable to tolerate cardiovascular stress. For example, the administration of naloxone can virtually eliminate the coma and ventilatory depression produced by morphine-like drugs. However, naloxone antagonism of narcotic analgesics can lead to the unmasking of pain, initiation of nausea and retching, and sympathetic nervous system stimulation which often is associated with hypertension, tachycardia, and dysrhythmias.[85] Serious complications including pulmonary edema, ventricular fibrillation, aneurysmal rupture, and death have been attributed to the injection of naloxone in the postoperative period following the intraoperative use of narcotic analgesics as part of the anesthetic plan.[86]

Antagonists such as the anticholinesterases for skeletal muscle relaxants and benzodiazepine hypnotics and analeptic drugs such as doxapram also have undesirable side effects. None of the narcotic or other type of antagonists have pharmacokinetic characteristics matching those of residual anesthetic drugs. Consequently it is impractical to attempt to maintain a precise degree of antagonism so that desirable degrees of analgesia and sedation are retained. Moreover there is the risk of recurrent depression as the antagonist is eliminated in the face of a more persistent anesthetic drug.

In the critically ill and hemodynamically unstable patient, these risks of using antagonists usually make it desirable to continue ventilatory support while the residual anesthetic drugs are eliminated. In such cases, the persistence of analgesia and sedation may be desirable and the patient may actually benefit from mechanical ventilation (see below).

Fluid and Blood Replacement

The type and quantities of intravenous fluids administered intraoperatively by anesthesiologists are often puzzling to the internist. The following points are pertinent to controversies that arise.

The surgical patient's fluid requirements exceed the quantity usually described as "maintenance" (i.e., replacement of urinary and insensible losses). The greater-than-normal requirements are related to preoperative fluid restriction [nothing-by-mouth (NPO) status of 6 to 24 h], blood loss, evaporation from surgically exposed tissue surfaces, and the translocation of fluid from blood and extracellular space into cells or other inaccessible "third spaces."[87] Although the mechanisms of this translocation are not certain, it is clear that the functional extracellular fluid volume decreases during major surgery. Even though the fluid is not lost from the body, it must be replaced in order to maintain a normal blood volume and to preserve normal cardiovascular and renal function. As a consequence, it is not uncommon for patients to gain considerable body weight associated with fluid accumulation during major intrathoracic and abdominal surgery. If done precisely this fluid replacement does *not* predispose the patient to the development of congestive heart failure and pulmonary edema.[87–89] Usually the excess body weight is shed by a spontaneous diuresis that commences during the second or third postoperative day as the third space fluid begins to be mobilized. Rarely is it necessary to administer a diuretic to initiate the mobilization in the patient with normal cardiovascular function. Patients with impaired cardiac function may benefit from diuretic therapy to facilitate renal function as the third-space fluid begins to reenter and expand the circulating blood volume.

Because of the relentless translocation of extracellular fluid to inaccessible third spaces, a functional hypovolemia can develop in the face of signs indicative of fluid volume overload (e.g., weight gain, edematous tissues). Even urine volume and concentration may give misleading information because of the effects of stress-related endocrine changes and the administration of drugs affecting renal perfusion and tubular function. Thus, the perioperative need for intravenous fluids is most precisely determined by measuring central venous and pulmonary artery occlusion pressures and the cardiovascular responses to a fluid challenge (i.e., cardiac performance curves, see below). This approach is especially important in the patient with cardiac disease in which optimal cardiovascular function is achieved in a rather narrow range of ventricular preload. Careful and reliable monitoring seems to be even more important when one recognizes that fluid shifts to the third space may total several liters during a major cardiac or abdominal operation.[55,87]

Since the major perioperative reductions in circulating blood volume are related to blood loss and the translocation of extracellular fluid, the anesthesiologist replaces these losses with fluids of a composition resembling extracellular fluid, such as lactated Ringer's solution. Although the debate about the replacement of such losses with purely crystalloid solutions or colloids continues, it should be remembered that albumin and other proteins distribute across capillary membranes and increase oncotic pressure of both plasma and interstitial fluid. Thus, the lung parenchyma is not protected against edema formation, and may actually be at greater risk because of the slow removal of protein by the pulmonary lymphatic system.[90,91] The rate of protein diffusion into the lung interstitium obviously is faster when pulmonary capillary permeability is increased (e.g., after the extracorporeal circulation of blood, with sepsis). The transient and limited benefit and the possibility of deleterious changes argue against the routine use of expensive protein solutions for replacement of intraoperative losses of extracellular fluids.

Although the patient's NPO status in the preoperative period may indicate the inclusion of glucose (dextrose) in intravenous fluids, it should be noted that the patient typically becomes glucose-intolerant and insulin-resistant during major surgical operations.[92] A reasonable compromise is to include 50 g of glucose in the first liter of intravenous fluid (5% dextrose) and to omit glucose from intravenous fluids thereafter. These recommendations may be modified for the patient with diabetes mellitus, in which case frequent measurements of serum glucose should guide the administration of both insulin and glucose.[93]

Hemodynamic Problems

In addition to the usual manifestations and complications of particular cardiovascular diseases, the anesthesiologist encounters other hemodynamic variables unique to, or at least more frequent in, the perioperative period. Changes in blood volume, hematocrit (oxygen-carrying capacity, blood viscosity), vascular tone (histamine release, alterations of the endocrine and sympathetic nervous systems), cardiac rate, rhythm and contractility (anesthetic drugs, ventilatory changes) are not uncommon in the intraoperative period (Table 79-7). There is the necessity of having a set of therapeutic priorities and a rational approach to the management of these complex and interrelated variables. Sometimes the approach to particular problems differs when they develop acutely in the intraoperative setting from that likely to be followed traditionally by the internist dealing with a similar problem on a more chronic basis. Limitations of space and unnecessary duplication of what has already been published elsewhere are reasons for not detailing the apparent and the real differences here. But a few things learned by the cardiac anesthesiologist have broad applications in noncardiac surgery, intensive care, and perhaps in other settings.

The pulmonary artery catheter with a thermocouple for cardiac output measurements by thermodilution has increased the accuracy of diagnosis and revolutionized the therapy of hypotension and low-cardiac-output states. While the debate about its use frequently focuses on the usefulness and validity of pulmonary artery occlusion pressure, the major advantages of this device are overlooked. The ability to measure cardiac output, to calculate systemic and pulmonary vascular resistances, and to relate these variables to central venous and pulmonary artery occlusion pressures provides all of the essential information for constructing ventricular performance curves (mentally or on paper).[94,95] Such curves tell the real story of cardiac function and of its responses to various therapeutic measures (Fig. 79-2).

TABLE 79-7 Causes of Hypotension and Low Cardiac Output in the Perioperative Period

- ↓ Preload:
  - Hypovolemia
  - Venodilation (drugs, histamine)
  - Anaphylactoid reaction
  - Severe tachycardia
  - Atrioventricular dissociation
  - Tamponade
  - Right ventricular (RV) failure [↓ left ventricular (LV) preload]
  - Pulmonary arterial embolism (↓ LV preload)
- Bradycardia:
  - Drug side effect or toxicity
  - Sick sinus syndrome
- ↓ Contractility:
  - Anesthetics and other drugs
  - Ischemia
  - Infarction
  - Dysrhythmias
  - Acid-base imbalance
  - Cardiomyopathy and ventricular dysfunction
- Cardiac surgery:
  - Inadequate myocardial preservation intraoperatively
  - Coronary artery embolism (air, particulate matter)
  - Persistent cardiac pathology
  - Operative trauma
- ↑ Afterload
  - ↑ Sympathetic nervous system activity
  - ↑ Renin-angiotensin and other endocrine vasopressors
  - Side effect of sympathomimetic inotropic drugs
  - Thromboembolism—systemic (LV) or pulmonary (RV) arterial systems
- ↓ Afterload (Hypotension)
  - Anaphylactoid reaction
  - Fever
  - Septic shock
  - Hypercarbia (direct effect of CO_2 on vasculature)
  - Drug side effect or toxicity

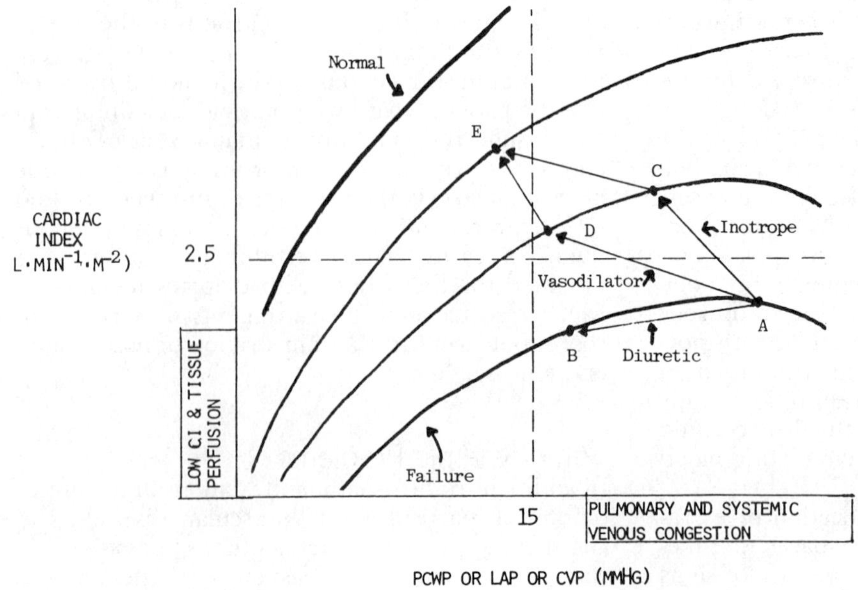

FIGURE 79-2 Ventricular performance curves and their modification by drug therapy. (Point A) Low perfusion and venous congestion. (Point B) Diuretic reduces ventricular filling pressures but does not increase, and may decrease, systemic perfusion. (Point C) Inotrope increases systemic perfusion and partially reduces excessively high ventricular end-diastolic pressures. The addition of a diuretic or vasodilator can reduce the latter (Point E). (Point D) Vasodilator reduces ventricular filling pressures and vascular resistance. If the latter effect is relatively greater than the former, cardiac output increases. An increased cardiac output is accomplished by the addition of an inotrope (Point E).

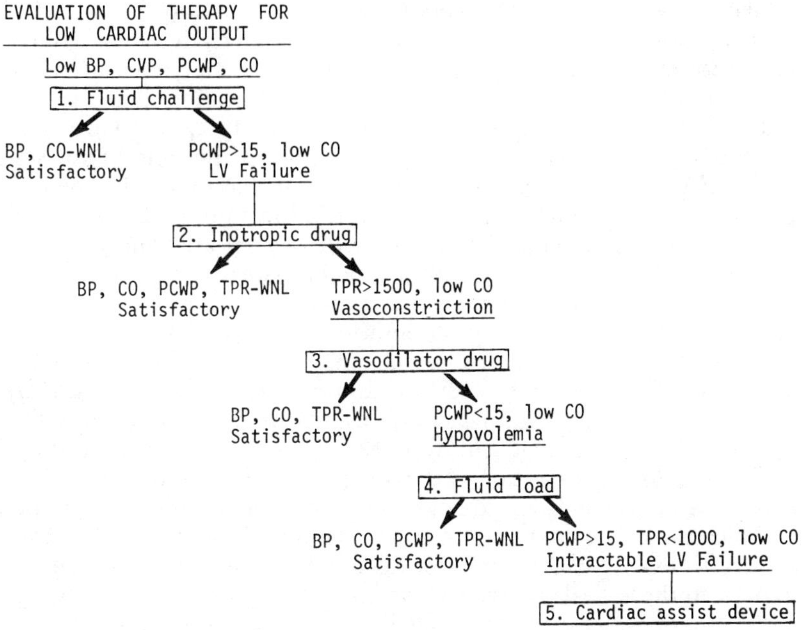

FIGURE 79-3 Algorithm of therapeutic steps in treating low cardiac output syndrome. BP = systemic blood pressure, mmHg; CO = cardiac output, 1 per minute; CVP = central venous pressure, mmHg; PCWP = pulmonary capillary wedge pressure (or pulmonary artery occlusion pressure), mmHg; TPR = total peripheral resistance (or systemic vascular resistance), dyn · s^{-1} · cm^{-5}; and WNL = within normal limits. (*From C. C. Hug, Jr., Anesthesia for Cardiac Surgery, in R. D. Miller (ed.), "Anesthesiology," Churchill Livingstone, New York, 1981, p. 1019. Copyright 1981 by Churchill Livingstone Inc., New York. Reproduced with permission from the publisher and author.*)

The maneuverability of the operating table provides an easy and practical means of varying ventricular filling pressures rapidly and safely.

Combining such diagnostic assessments with a knowledge of pharmacology, the anesthesiologist is in a position to select an appropriate combination of drugs and other therapeutic modalities (Figs. 79-3 and 79-4) and to quickly determine how effective they are in remedying hemodynamic problems. In these life-supporting maneuvers, the anesthesiologist and "intensivist" (see below) need to be mindful of a series of priorities for cardiovascular function and patient survival (Table 79-8).

FIGURE 79-4 Cardiac performance characterized by the relation of cardiac index to pulmonary artery occlusion pressure. (*Adapted from J. S. Forrester and D. D. Waters, Hospital Treatment of Congestive Heart Failure: Management According to Hemodynamic Profile, Am. J. Med., 65:173, 1978. Reproduced with permission from the publisher and authors.*)

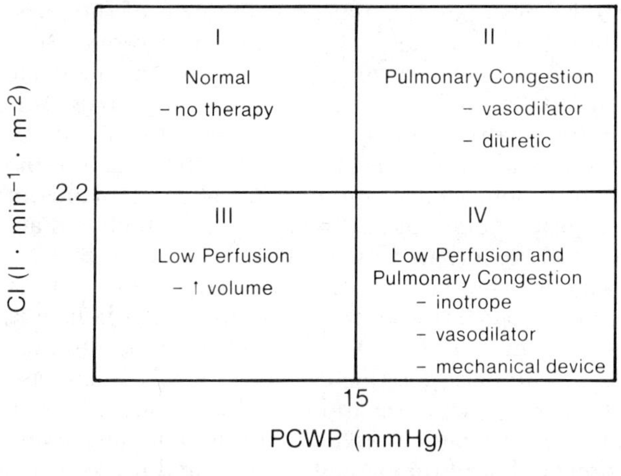

Ventilation in the Postoperative Period

The primary indication for mechanical support of ventilation is hypercarbia. In the absence of pulmonary disease, hypercarbia develops (1) if the response of the brainstem respiratory centers to the partial pressure of carbon dioxide (Pa_{CO_2}) is depressed, (2) if the mechanics of ventilation are impaired, or (3) if the rate of body metabolism increases beyond the capacity of the lungs to excrete carbon dioxide (e.g., in malignant hyperthermia).

TABLE 79-8 Therapeutic Priorities for Cardiovascular Function and Patient Survival

1. Systemic blood pressure must be sufficient to perfuse the heart and brain.
2. Heart rate should be appropriate to maintain cardiac output and to minimize myocardial oxygen demand.
3. Cardiac output (CO) should be adequate to support organ function and to provide for oxygen demands throughout the body.
4. Systemic vascular resistance should be adjusted to provide an adequate cardiac output and to facilitate the perfusion of splanchnic and peripheral tissues.
5. Pulmonary artery occlusion (PAOP) and central venous pressures should be adjusted to the levels required for optimal ventricular performance without producing pulmonary and venous congestion.
   a. If CO and PAOP are low, increase PAOP.
   b. If CO is satisfactory and PAOP is high, decrease PAOP.
   c. If CO is satisfactory and PAOP is low, merely observe.
6. Relieve systemic edema once otherwise satisfactory hemodynamic function has been stabilized for a period of time (hours to days).

Source: C. C. Hug, Jr., Hemodynamic Instability: A Rationale for Therapy, in "1983 Annual Refresher Course Lectures," American Society for Anesthesiologists, Atlanta, Georgia, lecture 137, p. 1.

All anesthetic drugs depress the ventilatory responses to Pa_{CO_2}, and as long as these drugs persist in the body, they have the potential to produce hypercarbia.[96] The potential for ventilatory depression is greater in the absence of stimulation, when the patient is asleep, and when several CNS depressants are combined, especially narcotic analgesics with hypnotics or residual anesthetic drugs. As noted elsewhere, recovery from these drugs can be a prolonged process when it depends on the relatively slow elimination phase ($t\frac{1}{2}$ β).

Muscle relaxants impair the mechanics of ventilation as do a number of other factors present in surgical patients (e.g., pain-limiting ventilatory effort, restrictive surgical dressings, certain body positions).[97]

Unless the physician is willing and prepared to correct the basic cause of hypercarbia (e.g., by administering antagonist or analeptic drugs which have side effects, see above), it may be necessary to extend the mechanical support of ventilation into the postoperative period.

Besides preventing hypercarbia, mechanical ventilation has some potentially useful advantages. Along with oxygen supplementation of the inspired gas mixture, various modes of mechanical ventilation have been used to improve oxygenation and to lessen the work of breathing, which can represent as much as 25 percent of the body's oxygen utilization in the postoperative period.[98]

Criteria for using mechanical ventilation postoperatively include a reduced vital capacity (< 15 ml/kg) and impairment of inspiratory force (< -20 cmH_2O); hypercarbia in excess of 50 mmHg, especially if a trend toward recovery is not apparent; a significant pulmonary arteriovenous shunt (Pa_{O_2} < 300 mmHg with $FI_{O_2} = 1$), and a large pulmonary dead space ($VD/VT > 0.6$).[99]

Criteria for discontinuing mechanical ventilation reflect the patient's recovered ability to meet these minimum levels of spontaneous ventilatory function, and in addition, usually include (1) significant improvement in any acute pulmonary parenchymal disease, (2) hemodynamic stability and the ability to sustain the work of spontaneous ventilation, and (3) a favorable assessment of the patient's general condition with signs pointing toward progressive improvement.

In some patients, especially those with cardiovascular disease, there may be some difficult decisions to make. Do the benefits of continuing artificial ventilation outweigh the side effects and risks? The presence of an endotracheal tube can be a source of discomfort and stress, impairs the patient's ability to cough and to clear secretions, and presents the risk of tracheal and laryngeal damage.[100] The use of a ventilator interferes with ambulation and nutrition, and alters the normal pattern of intrathoracic pressure changes. In the short term these side effects and risks are minimal, but their importance increases with the passing of time. Moreover, artificial ventilation is expensive.

The Intensivist

Critically ill patients require relatively long term continuation of the life-supporting measures initiated before or during the operation. Patients with cardiovascular disease are especially prone to experience impaired function in multiple organ systems because of the central role played by the cardiovascular system in the function of all tissues and organs. The delivery of oxygen and nutrients and the removal of metabolic wastes are fundamental to organ survival and function.

In the postoperative intensive care, as in the intraoperative management, of such patients it is important to remain continuously vigilant to suddenly developing adverse events and ominous trends. The ultimate survival of the patient depends on prompt correction of detrimental changes. Although the intensive care nurse is a capable monitor of the patient's progress with the aid of more or less sophisticated monitoring devices, the nurse's abilities to take corrective actions are limited by a number of factors (e.g., legal, educational). It is impossible for the physician to write orders in advance to cover every eventuality, and therefore it is essential that a physician familiar with the patient and experienced in the management of complex acute medical problems be continuously available to direct the necessary corrective actions. In order to meet this need on a broad scale and to allow other specialists to pursue their other important activities (e.g., the internist holding office hours, the surgeon operating in the same or another hospital), a new specialist has developed, the *intensivist*.[55]

The American Board of Medical Specialties has approved critical care medicine as a subspecialty of anesthesiology, internal medicine, pediatrics, and surgery. Members of the Society of Critical Care Medicine have been instrumental in developing training programs that in time may lead to subspecialty certification. These programs are aimed at persons who are already certified in anesthesiology, internal medicine, pediatrics, or surgery. Among their goals in education, research, and clinical practice is the development of physicians able to diagnose and treat acutely developing problems in one or more vital organ systems.[101] In many ways, the intensivist in the postoperative period is the twin of the anesthesiologist in the surgical operating room. Both employ the basic principles of acute care medicine and utilize sophisticated monitoring and diagnostic techniques to guide intravenous drug use and other therapeutic modalities to support life while the patient is subjected to the extraordinary demands of surgical operations and recovery from them. In addition, the intensivist may be called upon to care for patients who have experienced extensive trauma or who are suffering multiple organ system failure as a concomitant of a severe and widespread disease.

In the perioperative care of critically ill patients it makes good sense, and is probably most efficient, for the anesthesiologist and intensivist to have a very similar view of the patient so that the things learned in the operating room can be put to advantage in the immediate and even longer term periods of postoperative care. It seems eminently logical for those diagnostic and therapeutic measures found to be effective intraoperatively to be continued without interruption as the patient is transferred from one room (operating room) to another (recovery room, intensive care unit). Similarly, the retrial of ineffective measures seems pointless when the condition of the patient remains essentially unchanged.

References

1. Kaplan, J. A. (ed.): "Cardiac Anesthesia," Grune & Stratton, New York, 1979.
2. Kaplan, J. A. (ed.): "Cardiac Anesthesia," vol. 2, "Cardiovascular Pharmacology," Grune & Stratton, New York, 1983.
3. Ream, A. K., and Fogdall, R. P. (eds.): "Acute Cardiovascular Management: Anesthesia and Intensive Care," J. B. Lippincott Company, Philadelphia, 1982.
4. Tarhan, S. (ed.): "Cardiovascular Anesthesia and Postoperative Care," Year Book Medical Publishers, Chicago, 1982.
5. Becker, R., Katz, J., Polonius, M. J., and Speidel, H. (eds.): "Psychopathological and Neurological Dysfunctions following Open-Heart Surgery," Springer-Verlag, Berlin-Heidelberg, 1982.
6. Cousins, M. J., and Bridenbaugh, P. O. (eds.): "Neural Blockade in Clinical Anesthesia and Management of Pain," J. B. Lippincott Company, Philadelphia, 1980.
7. Cousins, M. J., and Mather, L. E.: Intrathecal and Epidural Administration of Opioids Analgesics, *Anesthesiology,* 61:276, 1984.
8. Hug, C. C., Jr.: Anesthetic Agents and the Patient with Cardiovascular Disease, in A. K. Ream and R. P. Fogdall (eds.), "Acute Cardiovascular Management: Anesthesia and Intensive Care," J. B. Lippincott Company, Philadelphia, 1982, p. 247.
9. Smith, G.: Beneficial Effects of Halothane on Myocardial Ischemia, *Anesthesiology,* 55:479, 1981.
10. Kissin, I., Stanbridge, R., Bishop, S. P., et al.: Effect of Halothane on Myocardial Infarct Size in Rats, *Can. Anaesth. Soc. J.,* 28:239, 1981.
11. Wilkinson, P. L., Hamilton, W. K., Moyers, J. R., et al.: Halothane and Morphine–Nitrous Oxide Anesthesia in Patients undergoing Coronary Artery Bypass Operation—Patterns of Intraoperative Ischemia, *J. Thorac. Cardiovasc. Surg.,* 82:372, 1981.
12. Sharer, N. M., Nunn, J. F., Royston, J. P., and Chanarin, I.: Effects of Chronic Exposure to Nitrous Oxide on Methionine Synthetase Activity, *Br. J. Anaesth.,* 55:693, 1983.
13. Moldenhauer, C. C., and Hug, C. C., Jr.: Use of Narcotic Analgesics as Anaesthetics, *Clin. Anesth.,* 2:107, 1984.
14. Hall, G. M.: Fentanyl and the Metabolic Response to Surgery, *Br. J. Anaesth.,* 52:561, 1980. (Editorial).
15. White, R. F.: Ketamine—Its Use as an Intravenous Anaesthetic, *Clin. Anesth.,* 2:43, 1984.
16. Reves, J. G., and Kissin, I.: Pharmacology of Anesthetic Drugs: Intravenous Anesthetics, in J. A. Kaplan (ed.). "Cardiac Anesthesia," vol. 2, "Cardiovascular Pharmacology," Grune & Stratton, New York, 1983, p. 3.
17. Etomidate for Induction of Anesthesia, *Med. Lett. Drugs Ther.,* 25:71, 1983.
18. Criado, A., Maseda, J., Navarro, E., et al.: Induction of Anesthesia with Etomidate: Hemodynamic Study of 36 Patients, *Br. J. Anaesth.,* 52:803, 1980.
19. Gooding, J. M., Weng, J.-T., Smith, R. A., et al.: Cardiovascular and Pulmonary Responses following Etomidate Induction of Anesthesia in Patients with Demonstrated Cardiac Disease, *Anesth. Analg.,* 58:40, 1979.
20. Wagner, R. L., White, P. F., Kan, P. B., et al.: Inhibition of Adrenal Steroidogenesis by the Anesthetic Etomidate, *N. Engl. J. Med.,* 310:1415, 1984.
21. Miller, R. D., and Morris, R. B.: Muscle Relaxants, in J. A. Kaplan (ed.), "Cardiac Anesthesia," vol. 2, "Cardiovascular Pharmacology," Grune & Stratton, New York, 1983, p. 79.
22. Basta, S. J., Ali, H. H., Saverese, J. J., et al.: Clinical Pharmacology of Atracurium Besylate (BW33A): A New Nondepolarizing Muscle Relaxant, *Anesth. Analg.,* 61:723, 1982.
23. Fahey, M. R., Morris, R. B., Miller, R. D., et al.: Clinical Pharmacology of ORG NC45 (Norcuron TM): A New Nondepolarizing Muscle Relaxant, *Anesthesiology,* 55:6, 1981.
24. Ebert, J., Patel, K., Gelman, S., and McElvein, R. B.: The Hemodynamic Response to Ketamine in Patients with Pericardial Tamponade, *Anesthesiology,* 57:A28, 1982.
25. Greene, N. M.: "Physiology of Spinal Anesthesia," Williams & Wilkins Company, Baltimore, 1969.
26. Prys-Roberts, C., Foëx, P., Biro, G. P., and Roberts, J. G.: Studies of Anaesthesia in Relation to Hypertension V: Adrenergic Beta-Receptor Blockade, *Br. J. Anaesth.,* 45:671, 1973.
27. Saidman, L. J., and Eger, E. I., II: Effect of Nitrous Oxide and of Narcotic Premedication on the Alveolar Concentration of Halothane Required for Anesthesia, *Anesthesiology,* 25:302, 1964.
28. Goodloe, S. L.: Essential Hypertension, in R. K. Stoelting and S. F. Dierdorf (eds.), "Anesthesia and Co-Existing Disease," Churchill Livingstone, New York, 1983, p. 99.
29. Slogoff, S., Keats, A. S., and Ott, E.: Preoperative Propranolol Therapy and Aortocoronary Bypass Operations, *JAMA,* 240:1487, 1978.
30. Slogoff, S.: Beta-Adrenergic Blockers, in J. A. Kaplan (ed.), "Cardiac Anesthesia," vol. 2, "Cardiovascular Pharmacology," Grune & Stratton, New York, 1983, p. 181.
31. Smith, N. T., Miller, R. D., and Corbascio, A. N. (eds.): "Drug Interactions in Anesthesia," Lea & Febiger, Philadelphia, 1981.
32. Hug, C. C., Jr.: Monitoring, in R. D. Miller (ed.), "Anesthesia," Churchill Livingstone, New York, 1981, p. 157.
33. Kaplan, J. A., and Wells, P. H.: Electrocardiographic Monitoring, in A. K. Ream and R. P. Fogdall (eds.), "Acute Cardiovascular Management: Anesthesia and Intensive Care," J. B. Lippincott Company, Philadelphia, 1982, p. 163.
34. Kates, R. A., Zaidan, J. R., and Kaplan, J. A.: Esophageal Lead for Intraoperative Electrocardiographic Monitoring, *Anesth. Analg.,* 61:781, 1982.
35. Zaidan, J. R., and Curling, P. E.: Cardiac Dysrhythmias—Recognition and Management, in R. K. Stoelting, P. G. Barash, and T. J. Gallagher (eds.), "Advances in Anesthesia," vol. 2, Year Book Medical Publishers, Chicago, 1985.
36. Barash, P. G., Chen, Y., Kitahata, L. M., et al.: The Hemodynamic Tracking System: A Method of Data Management and Guide for Cardiovascular Therapy, *Anesth. Analg.,* 59:169, 1980.
37. Forrester, J. S., and Waters, D. D.: Hospital Treatment of Congestive Heart Failure: Management According to Hemodynamic Profile, *Am. J. Med.,* 65:173, 1978.
38. Mason, D. T., Awan, N. A., Joye, J. A., et al.: Treatment of Acute and Chronic Congestive Heart Failure by Vasodilator-Afterload Reduction, *Arch. Intern. Med.,* 140:1577, 1980.
39. Meretoja, O. A., and Laaksonen, V. O.: Hemodynamic Effects of Preload and Sodium Nitroprusside in Patients Subjected to Coronary Bypass Surgery, *Circulation,* 58:815, 1978.
40. Bellows, W. H., Bode, R. H., Levy, J. H., et al.: Noninvasive Detection of Periinduction Ischemic Ventricular Dysfunction by Cardiokymography in Humans, *Anesthesiology,* 60:155, 1984.
41. Cahalan, M. K., Kremer, P. F., Beaupre, P. N., et al.: Consistency and Reproducibility of Transesophageal Two-Dimensional Echocardiography, *Anesth. Analg.,* 63:194, 1984.
42. Cahalan, M. K., Kremer, P. F., Beaupre, P. N., et al.: Intraoperative Myocardial Ischemia Detected by Transesophageal 2-Dimensional Echocardiography, *Anesthesiology,* 59:A164, 1983.

43. Waller, J. L., Kaplan, J. A., Bauman, D. I., and Craver, J. M.: Clinical Evaluation of a New Fiberoptic Catheter Oximeter during Cardiac Surgery, *Anesth. Analg.*, 61:676, 1982.
44. Levy, W. J., Grundy, B. L., and Smith, N. T.: Monitoring the Electroencephalogram and Evoked Potentials during Anesthesia, in L. J. Saidman and N. T. Smith (eds.), "Monitoring in Anesthesia," 2d ed., Butterworth & Company (Publishers), Boston, 1984, p. 227.
45. Sundt, T. M., Sharbrough, F. D., Piepgras, D. G., et al.: Correlation of Cerebral Blood Flow and Electroencephalographic Changes during Carotid Endarterectomy, *Mayo Clin. Proc.*, 56:533, 1981.
46. Glass, D. D.: Management of Blood and Coagulation, in J. A. Kaplan (ed.), "Cardiac Anesthesia," vol. 2. "Cardiovascular Pharmacology," Grune & Stratton, New York, 1983, p. 441.
47. Rao, T. L. K., Jacobs, K. H., and El-Etr, A. A.: Reinfarction following Anesthesia in Patients with Myocardial Infarction, *Anesthesiology*, 59:499, 1983.
48. Jones, E. L., Hurst, J. W., King, S. B., and Hatcher, C. R., Jr.: Clinical Factors Influencing Survival and Adequacy of Revascularization after Coronary Bypass Operation, *Int. J. Cardiol.*, 2:109, 1982.
49. Steen, P. A., Tinker, J. H., and Tarhan. S.: Myocardial Reinfarction after Anesthesia and Surgery, *JAMA*, 239:2566, 1978.
50. Eerola, M., Eerola, R., Kaukinen, S., and Kaukinen, L.: Risk Factors in Surgical Patients with Verified Preoperative Myocardial Infarction, *Acta Anaesthesiol. Scand.*, 24:219, 1980.
51. Covino, B. G., and Vassallo, H. G.: "Local Anesthetics: Mechanisms of Action and Clinical Use," Grune & Stratton, New York, 1976.
52. Keats, A. S.: What Do We Know about Anesthetic Mortality?, *Anesthesiology*, 50:387, 1979.
53. Hamilton, W. K.: Unexpected Deaths during Anesthesia: Wherein Lies the Cause?, *Anesthesiology*, 50:381, 1979.
54. Keats, A. S.: The Rovenstine Lecture, 1983: Cardiovascular Anesthesia: Perceptions and Perspectives, *Anesthesiology*, 60:467, 1984.
55. Kirby, R. R., and Smith, R. A.: The Anesthesiologist and Intensive Care, in R. D. Miller (ed.), "Anesthesia," Churchill Livingstone, New York, 1981, p. 1435.
56. Prys-Roberts, C. (ed.): Hypertension, Ischemic Heart Disease, and Anesthesia, *Int. Anesthesiol. Clin.*, 18(4), 1980.
57. Philbin, D. M. (ed.): Anesthetic Management of the Patient with Cardiovascular Disease, *Int. Anesthesiol. Clin.* 17(1), 1979.
58. Radnay, P. A., and Nagashima, H. (eds.): Anesthetic Considerations for Pediatric Cardiac Surgery, *Int. Anesthesiol. Clin.*, 18(1), 1980.
59. Nussmeier, N. A., Curling, P. E., Murphy, D. A., et al.: Nifedipine: Cardiovascular Effects after Sublingual Administration during Fentanyl-Pancuronium Anesthesia in Man, *Anesthesiology*, 59:A34, 1983.
60. Mangano, D. T.: Preoperative Assessment of Cardiac Catheterization Data: Which Parameters Are Most Important?, *Anesthesiology*, 53:s106, 1980.
61. Roizen, M. F.: Preoperative Evaluation of Patients with Diseases That Require Special Preoperative Evaluation and Intraoperative Management, in R. D. Miller (ed.), "Anesthesia," Churchill Livingstone, New York, 1981, p. 21.
62. Sill, J. C., Nugent, M., Moyer, T. P., et al.: Influence of Propranolol Plasma Levels on Hemodynamics during Coronary Artery Bypass Surgery, *Anesthesiology*, 60:455, 1984.
63. Stanley, T. H., De Lange, S., Boscoe, M. J., and De Bruijn, N.: The Influence of Chronic Propranolol Therapy on Cardiovascular Dynamics and Narcotic Requirements during Operation in Patients with Coronary Artery Disease, *Can. Anaesth. Soc. J.*, 29:319, 1982.
64. Schneider, A. J. L., Knoke, J. D., Zollinger, R. M., Jr., et al.: Morbidity Prediction using Pre- and Intraoperative Data, *Anesthesiology*, 51:4, 1979.
65. Prys-Roberts, C., Meloche, R., and Foëx, P.: Studies of Anaesthesia in Relation to Hypertension: I. Cardiovascular Responses of Treated and Untreated Patients, *Br. J. Anaesth.*, 43:122, 1971.
66. Goldman, L., and Caldera, D. L.: Risks of General Anesthesia and Elective Operation in the Hypertensive Patient, *Anesthesiology*, 50:285, 1979.
67. Mauney, F. M., Jr., Ebert, P. A., and Sabiston, D. C., Jr.: Postoperative Myocardial Infarction: A Study of Predisposing Factors, Diagnosis and Mortality in a High Risk Group of Surgical Patients, *Ann. Surg.*, 172:497, 1970.
68. Goldman, L., Caldera, D. L., Nussbaum, S. R., et al.: Multifactorial Index of Cardiac Risk in Noncardiac Surgical Procedures, *N. Engl. J. Med.*, 297:845, 1977.
69. Goldman, L. L.: Cardiac Risks and Complications of Noncardiac Surgery, *Ann. Surg.*, 198:780, 1983.
70. Jones, E. L., Craver, J. M., Michalik, R. A., et al.: Combined Carotid and Coronary Operations: When Are They Necessary?, *J. Thorac. Cardiovasc. Surg.*, 87:7, 1984.
71. Cruchley, P. M., Kaplan, J. A., Hug, C. C., Jr., et al.: Noncardiac Surgery in Patients with Prior Myocardial Revascularization, *Can. Anaesth. Soc. J.*, 30:629, 1983.
72. Kistner, J. R., Miller, E. D., Jr., Lake, C. L., et al.: Indices of Myocardial Oxygenation during Coronary Artery Revascularization in Man with Morphine Versus Halothane Anesthesia, *Anesthesiology*, 50:324, 1979.
73. Merin, R. G., Verdouw, P. D., and de Jong, J. W.: Myocardial Function and Metabolic Responses to Ischemia in Swine during Halothane and Fentanyl Anesthesia, *Anesthesiology*, 56:84, 1982.
74. American Society of Anesthesiologists: New Classification of Physical Status, *Anesthesiology*, 24:111, 1963.
75. Hug, C. C., Jr.: Pharmacokinetics of Drugs Administered Intravenously, *Anesth. Analg.*, 57:704, 1978.
76. Wagner, J. D.: A Safe Method for Rapidly Achieving Plasma Concentration Plateaus, *Clin. Pharmacol. Ther.*, 16:691, 1974.
77. Hug, C. C., Jr.: Improving Analgesic Therapy, *Anesthesiology*, 53:441, 1980.
78. Tamsen, A., Hartvig, P., Fagerlund, C., and Dahlstrom, B.: Patient-Controlled Analgesic Therapy, Part II: Individual Analgesic Demand and Analgesic Plasma Concentrations of Pethidine in Postoperative Pain, *Clin. Pharmacokinetics*, 7:164, 1982.
79. Eger, E. I., II: "Anesthetic Uptake and Action," Williams & Wilkins Company, Baltimore, 1974.
80. Prys-Roberts, C., and Hug, C. C., Jr. (eds.): "Pharmacokinetics of Anesthesia," Blackwell Scientific Publications, Oxford, 1984.
81. Stanski, D. E., and Watkins, W. D.: "Drug Disposition in Anesthesia," Grune & Stratton, New York, 1982.
82. Hug, C. C., Jr.: Pharmacokinetics and Dynamics of Narcotic Analgesics, in C. Prys-Roberts and C. C. Hug, Jr. (eds.), "Pharmacokinetics of Anaesthesia," Blackwell Scientific Publications, Oxford, 1984.
83. Elfstrom, J.: Drug Pharmacokinetics in the Postoperative Period, *Clin. Pharmacokinetics*, 4:16, 1979.
84. Holley, F. O., Ponganis, K. U., and Stanski, D. R.: Effect of Cardiopulmonary Bypass on the Pharmacokinetics of Drugs, *Clin. Pharmacokinetics*, 7:234, 1982.
85. Hug, C. C., Jr.: New Narcotic Agonists and Antagonists in Anaesthesia, *Can. Anaesth. Soc. J.*, 31:s5, 1984.
86. Andree, R. A.: Sudden Death following Naloxone Administration, *Anesth. Analg.*, 59:782, 1980.
87. Giesecke, A. H., Jr.: Perioperative Fluid Therapy—Crystalloids, in R. D. Miller (ed.) "Anesthesia," Churchill Livingstone, New York, 1981, p. 865.
88. Lowe, R. J., Moss, G. S., Jilek, J., et al.: Crystalloid Versus Colloid in the Etiology of Pulmonary Failure after Trauma, A Randomized Trial in Man, *Crit. Care Med.*, 7:107, 1979.
89. Virgilio, R. W., Rice, C. L., Smith, D. E., et al.: Crystalloid Vs Colloid Resuscitation: Is One Better? A Randomized Clinical Study, *Surgery*, 85:129, 1979.
90. Strum, J. A., Carpenter, M. A., Sewis, F. R., Jr., et al.: Water and Protein Movement in the Sheep Lung after Septic Shock: Effect of Colloid Versus Crystalloid Resuscitation, *J. Surg. Res.*, 26:233, 1979.
91. Holcroft, J. W., Trunkey, D. D., and Carpenter, M. A.: Extravasation of Albumin in Tissues of Normal and Septic Baboons and Sheep, *J. Surg. Res.*, 26:341, 1979.

92. Palumbo, P. J.: Blood Glucose Control during Surgery, *Anesthesiology*, 55:94, 1981.
93. Elliott, M. J., Gill, G. V., Home, P. D., et al.: A Comparison of Two Regimens for the Management of Diabetes during Open-Heart Surgery, *Anesthesiology*, 60:364, 1984.
94. Hug, C. C., Jr.: Hemodynamic Instability: A Rationale for Therapy, in "1983 Annual Refresher Course Lectures," American Society of Anesthesiologists, Atlanta, Georgia, lecture 137, p. 1.
95. Mangano, D. T., Van Dyke, D. C., and Ellis, R. J.: The Effect of Increasing Preload or Ventricular Output and Ejection in Man: Limitations of the Frank-Starling Mechanism, *Circulation*, 62:535, 1980.
96. McClain, D. M., and Hug, C. C., Jr.: Pharmacokinetics and Dynamics of Opiates, *Int. Anesthesiol. Clin.*, 22, (4):75, 1984.
97. Jones, J. G. (ed.): Effects of Anesthesia and Surgery on Pulmonary Mechanisms and Gas Exchange, *Int. Anesthesiol. Clin.*, 22(4), 1984.
98. Wilson, R. S., Sullivan, S. F., Malm, J. R., et al.: The Oxygen Cost of Breathing following Anesthesia and Cardiac Surgery, *Anesthesiology*, 39:387, 1973.
99. Smith, R. A.: Respiratory Care, in R. D. Miller (ed.), "Anesthesia," Churchill Livingstone, New York, 1981, p. 1379.
100. Bishop, M. J., Weymuller, E. A., and Fink, B. R.: Laryngeal Effects of Prolonged Intubation, *Anesth. Analg.*, 63:335, 1984.
101. Shoemaker, W. C., Thompson, E. L., and Holbrook, P. R. (eds.): "Textbook of Critical Care," W.B. Saunders Company, Philadelphia, 1984.

80

Evaluation and Management of Patients with Heart Disease Who Undergo Noncardiac Surgery*

R. Bruce Logue, M.D.

The patient with heart disease who undergoes noncardiac surgery is subject to many alterations in homeostasis without the possibility of improvement of pump function or blood supply that occurs with cardiac surgery.

Risks (General Considerations)[1]

With any given type of heart disease, the risks of noncardiac surgery may increase in the older age group, during emergency surgery, with surgery in the chest or the upper part of the abdomen, and in the presence of functional class III and class IV disease (old New York Heart Association classification), and in the presence of other significant systemic disease. A useful preoperative index of risks encountered during anesthesia and surgery has been formulated by Goldman et al. after a review of 1001 cases (Table 80-1).[2] The authors found the risk to be minimal with 0 to 5 points (as assigned in Table 80-1) and increased to the range of 5 percent with 6 to 12 points. With class III, 13 to 25 points, the risk of nonfatal cardiac complications increased to

*The content of this chapter is similar to, but not identical with, the text published in *Current Problems in Cardiology*.[4] This summary is presented with the permission of Year Book Medical Publishers and the authors.

TABLE 80-1 Risk Index

Factor	Points
1. S_3 gallop or jugular venous distension	11
2. Transmural or subendocardial infarction within 6 months	10
3. More than 5 premature ventricular contractions per minute at any time	7
4. Abnormal rhythm or frequent atrial premature contractions in preoperative ECG	7
5. Age over 70 years	5
6. Emergency operation	4
7. Intrathoracic, intraperitoneal, or aortic site surgery	3
8. Important aortic stenosis	3
9. Poor general medical condition*	
a. $P_{O_2} < 60$ or $P_{CO_2} > 50$ mmHg	
b. $K < 3.0$ or $HCO_3 < 20$ meq/liter	
c. BUN > 50 or Cr > 3.0 mg/dl	
d. Abnormal SGOT, signs of chronic liver disease, or patient bedridden from noncardiac causes	
Class I† = 0–5 total points	
Class II† = 6–12 total points	
Class III† = 13–25 total points	
Class IV† = 26 or more points	

*BUN = blood urea nitrogen; Cr = creatinine; SGOT = serum glutamic oxaloacetic transaminase.
†Old New York Heart Association functional classification.
Source: L. Goldman, Cardiac Risks and Complications of Noncardiac Surgery, *Ann. Intern. Med.*, 98:504, 1984. This table has been modified with the permission of the publisher and author.

the range of 22 percent, and with class IV (26 or more points) 22 percent of patients studied had nonfatal cardiac complications, and in addition there was a 56 percent mortality rate due to cardiac causes.

It is well-recognized that there may be left-sided heart failure with interstitial edema in the x-ray in the presence of a normal pulse rate, no S_3 gallop, and no rales.[3] The experienced physician knows that an S_3 gallop is an important auscultatory sign but may occur relatively late in the course of pump dysfunction and failure. There may be significant wall motion abnormality with reduced ejection fraction determined by angiography, echocardiography, or radioisotope scan in the absence of clinical symptoms or abnormal physical findings. Jugular venous distension is more often due to left-sided heart failure with elevated wedge and pulmonary artery pressure of some duration.

Preoperative Evaluation

Excellent evaluation can be obtained with a thorough history, physical examination, ECG, and x-ray of the chest. Important elements in assessment are as follows:[4]

- Is there a history of angina pectoris? Is it stable or unstable?
- Is there a history of ECG evidence of previous myocardial infarction? Was the infarction remote or did it occur within 3 to 6 months?
- Has the patient had prior or is there present congestive heart failure?
- Is there dyspnea on exertion or paroxysmal nocturnal dyspnea?
- Is there significant hypertension? Has it been appropriately treated? What is the current drug regimen?
- Are there significant murmurs indicating valvular or congenital heart disease, mitral valve prolapse, cardiomyopathy, or idiopathic hypertrophic subaortic stenosis (IHSS)? Does the patient have a prosthetic valve?
- Is there cardiomegaly by physical examination and x-ray?
- Is there any disturbance of cardiac rhythm? If arrhythmia is present, what medication is being given? Is there a history of symptoms due to heart block? Does the patient have a pacemaker?
- Any history of transient ischemic attacks (TIAs) or prior stroke?
- Is the patient a cigarette smoker and are there symptoms of chronic obstructive lung disease? What is the patient's exercise tolerance?
- Any history of renal disease, diabetes, or hepatic disease?
- Is there significant extracardiac systemic disease?
- Has there been previous anesthetic experience? Any untoward effects?
- Any intolerance to drugs?
- Has the patient received steroid therapy within 6 months?
- Is patient taking antiplatelet drugs or Coumadin?
- Is there important anemia that may require packed red blood cell transfusion?
- Is there history of previous phlebitis or pulmonary embolism?
- What is the functional classification of heart disease?

The Place of the Electrocardiogram

A baseline tracing allows comparison of changes developing during surgery and the postoperative period. Ischemic ST depression or elevation gives immediate evidence of impairment of myocardial oxygen demand or delivery. This commonly occurs during induction or at times when there are no symptoms or other signs of disturbed physiology. Such changes may aid in the identification of coronary spasm.

The importance of an abnormal preoperative ECG was highlighted by a study of 365 tracings by Mauney et al.,[5] showing old infarction, left ventricular hypertrophy, left bundle branch block, or abnormal ST-T. Perioperative infarction developed in 8.2 percent of the patients, with a 53.3 percent mortality rate; 301 patients showed no change, but 9 died of myocardial infarction; 30 with symptoms suggesting infarction had changes confined to the ST-T interval, and 34 without symptoms had ST-T changes compatible with subendocardial infarction.

Special Procedures

Treadmill exercise tests may identify myocardial ischemia in the asymptomatic patient or may indicate ischemia of varying severity in the symptomatic patient and in the patient who has had previous bypass surgery. The predictability and sensitivity of the test are good in individuals at high risk and in the presence of known coronary disease, but there may be false positives and negatives. Thallium exercise tests are sensitive and have higher predictability but are not 100 percent reliable. A reduced exercise ejection fraction with exercise MUGA scan suggests coronary disease in the absence of other disorders, but this test is not as helpful as Tl-exercise scans. Postoperatively, isotope scans may aid in the identification of myocardial infarction, and may be particularly helpful in the recognition and management of dominant right ventricular myocardial infarction. MUGA scans afford evidence of pump dysfunction in patients with valvular heart disease and diffuse myocardial disease and give some data on the severity of disease and attendant risks as well as the need for hemodynamic monitoring or possible surgery. In selected instances, coronary angiography may be indicated if there has been infarction within 6 months or in the presence of unstable angina. Such patients may require coronary bypass prior to elective surgery. Current experience indicates the value of this approach.[6–8]

Coronary Disease

The widespread prevalence of coronary atherosclerosis makes this disorder the most common cardiac problem faced with anesthesia and surgery. It is often associated with other disease, i.e., hypertension, valvular heart disease, cardiomyopathy, cerebral vascular disease, abdominal aortic aneurysm, and peripheral vascular disease. Recognition of coronary disease remains a major problem. Approximately one-half of acute myocardial infarctions occur without prior angina; thus, there is a large asymptomatic population, so that perioperative infarction may surprise the anesthesiologist and clinician. Currently the most cost-efficient test for identifying such patients is the treadmill exercise test, but it is not routinely indicated in young individuals; it may be worthwhile in the middle-aged male, particularly in the presence of multiple risk factors. Tl-exercise tests have increased predictability and specificity. However, the fourfold increase in cost makes it impractical as a routine screening procedure. It is helpful in selected instances, where the routine treadmill test gives equivocal results or in the patient with history of previous infarction, angina, or coronary bypass. MUGA scans showing reduced ejection fraction in response to exercise in the absence of other causes of heart disease may suggest coronary atherosclerosis in the asymptomatic patient. All tests require that the patient be able to exercise to an appropriate heart rate sufficient to bring out ischemia. Echocardiography may indicate regional wall motion abnormalities as a clue to coronary disease.

The electrocardiogram is normal in about 60 percent of patients with angina pectoris and may have returned to normal after myocardial infarction. Because of this, approximately 50 percent of patients with old infarctions at autopsy may not have shown diagnostic ECG changes. Furthermore, even acute myocardial infarction may be missed due to lack of diagnostic ECG changes and alterations of cardiac enzymes. Thus, 46 percent of 100 acute infarcts at autopsy were undiagnosed during life.[9] The lack of Q waves of 0.04-s duration and rise in enzymes do not rule out acute myocardial infarction. The most common error is excluding acute myocardial infarction with a compatible history and changes confined to the ST-T interval. Subendocardial infarction may demonstrate such changes or no changes. When changes are present, they may identify previous infarction unknown to the patient (one-quarter in the Framingham series).[10]

With a history of intermittent episodes of angina and angina during sleep with no reproducible relation to effort, one must consider Prinzmetal variant angina with spasm of normal or obstructed arteries. Direct current Holter monitoring may demonstrate ST elevation occurring with or without associated symptoms and may confirm the diagnosis. Less often ST elevation in the ECG during distress may point to the diagnosis. Ergonovine provocative testing studied in 1000 patients with coronary disease indicated spasm in 64 percent of patients with obstructive lesions, in 20 percent of patients within 6 weeks following acute myocardial infarction, in 5 percent of those with stable angina, and in 15 percent of patients with unstable angina.[11] Identification of spasm suggests the use of calcium blockers along with nitrates.

Risks in Patients with Coronary Disease

The important assessment of surgical risk is determined largely by whether angina is stable or unstable (unstable angina being associated with higher reinfarction and mortality rates). The risk of infarction in such patients increases fivefold, and the mortality rate is three to four times greater than for infarction unrelated to surgery. The higher risk reflects the fact that those with severe ischemia following recovery from a heart attack have a higher mortality within 6 months, leaving a more favorable group for possible surgery. The incidence of perioperative infarction is about 0.2 to 0.6 percent in those with no prior history of infarction and about 6 percent in those with a prior history of a heart attack (see Tables 80-2 and 80-3). The risk of infarction is increased in the presence of cardiomegaly, significant hypertension, and ischemic ST depression in the resting ECG, and with intraoperative hypotension (Table 80-4).[12] Wells and Kaplan,[17] using intraarterial blood pressure monitoring, ECG monitoring at V_5, intravenous nitroglycerin, and Swan-Ganz catheter monitoring, reported no infarctions in 48 patients operated on within 3 months of acute myocardial infarction. Rao and El-Etr[18] using similar techniques reported reinfarction in only 7.8 percent of 38 patients operated on within 3 months of infarction, with a 5.3 percent mortality rate. Thirty-nine patients operated on within 3 to 6 months after an acute myocardial infarction suffered reinfarction in 3.5 percent of cases with no deaths. For the first time reduced reinfarction and mortality rates have been reported; more studies are needed to substantiate the value of newer techniques.

TABLE 80-2 Risk of Myocardial Infarction with No History of Prior Infarct

Source	Sample Size	Incidence, %	Mortality, %
Topkins and Artusio[14]	12,054	0.66	26
Tarhan et al.[12]	32,033	0.13	42

TABLE 80-3 Risk of Myocardial Infarction with History of Prior Infarction

Source	Size of Sample	Incidence, %	Mortality, %
Knapp et al.[13]	427	6	58
Topkins and Artusio[14]	658	6.5	70
Tarhan et al.[12]	422	6.6	53
Steen et al.[15]	587	6.1	69

TABLE 80-4 Coronary Patients at Increased Risk

1. Unstable angina
2. Acute myocardial infarction within 3–6 months
3. Congestive heart failure
4. Refractory ventricular arrhythmia
5. Where available
   a. Ejection fraction (EF) < 35
   b. Impaired EF with exercise on MUGA scan
   c. Main left coronary disease
6. Cardiomegaly
7. ST depression in resting ECG
8. Moderate or severe hypertension
9. Systolic blood pressure greater than 180 mmHg
10. Emergency operation
11. Intrathoracic or upper abdominal surgery
12. Prior transient ischemic attack (TIA) or stroke
13. Hypotension during surgery

Beta blockers reduce the incidence of reinfarction in addition to having an antiarrhythmic effect and by decreasing renin-angiotensin reducing blood pressure. Our current practice is to treat all patients known to have coronary disease with beta blockers or calcium blockers. If beta blockers are used, they should be continued up to the time of surgery. Intravenous increments may be needed during the intraoperative period, and the drugs should be resumed as soon as possible in the postoperative period. Cessation of therapy may induce hyptertension, tachycardia, ischemia, or infarction, particularly if weaning over a period of days or weeks is not carried out. Substitution of calcium blockers does not prevent the "withdrawal syndrome" but may enhance symptoms such as flushing and tachycardia due to vasodilatation produced. Patients with angina who currently may be preferentially treated by calcium blockers include those with (1) intolerance to beta blockers, (2) bradycardia, (3) Raynaud's syndrome, (4) vasospastic angina, and (5) symptomatic peripheral vascular disease. Diltiazem seems better tolerated than nifedipine or verapamil, but nifedipine is preferred if bradycardia or block is present or results from the other drugs. Nitrate therapy should be adjusted.[19] Nitroglycerin paste may be applied 1 h prior to surgery, provided there is no postural hypotension. Intravenous nitroglycerin is helpful in reducing the incidence of ischemia during surgery.[16] The dose can be rapidly titrated according to the indications given by hemodynamic monitoring. It should be continued in the postoperative period for 48 h or longer if myocardial ischemia or infarction occurs and should be weaned slowly over a period of 6 h. Adequate preanesthetic sedation may prevent ischemia due to anxiety.

Digitalis

Digitalization is recommended for patients with congestive heart failure, cardiomegaly, atrial tachycardia, atrial fibrillation, or atrial flutter, and for those with severely depressed ejection fractions determined by MUGA scan or angiography. Those with S_3 gallop or interstitial edema in the x-ray receive digitalis. Additional indications are nocturnal angina, congenital heart disease with left-to-right shunts, and lobectomy or pneumonectomy in patients over 40. The latter recommendation is controversial but is made because of the approximately 15 percent incidence of supraventricular arrhythmias, even though there is no evidence of reduction of the incidence. Patients with chronic obstructive lung disease are more susceptible to digitalis intoxication, which is in part related to futile attempts to slow the ventricular rate in the presence of hypoxia, hypercarbia, and respiratory acidosis. Multifocal atrial tachycardia seen with pulmonary disease does not respond to digitalis but may respond to verapamil.

Digitalization should be completed 1 to 2 days before surgery when possible. If necessary, digoxin can be given intravenously, 0.25 mg with additional 0.25-mg doses at 4-h intervals for a total dose of 0.75 mg. Maintenance doses are adjusted for elderly patients or those with renal insufficiency. Concurrent use of quinidine may raise the serum digoxin level and predispose to toxicity.[20]

Digitalis toxicity is determined by the presence of such symptoms as loss of taste for cigarettes or food, anorexia, nausea, vomiting, visual disturbances, or symptoms of cerebral dysfunction. More importantly, disturbances of rhythm such as multifocal premature ventricular contractions (PVCs), short runs of ventricular tachycardia, atrioventricular (AV) dissociation, sinus bradycardia, or AV block may occur. The clinical signs and symptoms and the electrocardiogram identify possible toxicity, but confirmation is resolution of these indications within 24 to 48 h after omission of the drug. Serum digoxin levels do not indicate toxicity; the level may be in the normal range in the presence of toxicity and in the abnormal range without toxicity. It is axiomatic that the serum potassium be maintained at normal levels. Magnesium deficiency is less commonly associated with toxicity than is hypokalemia.

Arrhythmias and Heart Block

Patients with atrial tachyarrhythmias should be digitalized prior to surgery. The presence of frequent premature ventricular contractions (PVCs) does not require treatment, although some recommend treatment if there are more than five PVCs per minute.[1] Multifocal PVCs, R-on-T phenomenon, and runs of ventricular tachycardia should probably be treated by appropriate drugs, provided digitalis intoxication, hypokalemia, ischemia, or clinical pump dysfunction do not require correction. Patients who have had ventricular fibrillation not related to the early hours or days of myocardial infarction should receive antiarrhythmic drugs. Procainamide and beta blockers are commonly used. Disopyramide is useful but has negative inotropic effects and may occasionally precipitate congestive heart failure or ventricular tachycardia of varying types, including torsades de pointes, particularly in the presence of a prolonged QT interval and hypokalemia. Quinidine and procainamide may have similar effects. Patients on large doses of the above drugs that develop unexplained syncope are suspect for torsades de pointes, and the drugs should be omitted.

During anesthesia if drugs are required for treatment of ventricular tachyarrhythmias, lidocaine is conventionally used with due care to avoid cerebral and myocardial depression that can be noted in association with anesthetic agents. Amiodarone is an effective antiarrhythmic agent with significant side effects but may be the preferred treatment of arrhythmias associated with bypass tracts and hypertrophic cardiomyopathy. Temporary pacing may be rarely required for the sick sinus syndrome or for refractory ventricular tachycardia.

Most patients with complete heart block will have had permanent pacemakers. For the rare individual who is in complete heart block requiring emergency surgery, a temporary pacemaker is indicated with later insertion of a permanent pacemaker. Pacing is not required for first degree AV block but is indicated for Mobitz type II AV block with wide QRS. The presence of bifascicular block in the asymptomatic individual does not require pacing since complete heart block is extremely rare: 98 patients with bifascicular block including 25 with AV block did not develop complete heart block during surgery. Another study of 44 patients with right bundle branch block and left axis deviation showed a single instance of complete heart block.[22] The asymptomatic patient with bradycardia of 40 to 50 beats per minute does not require pacing, but with complaints of dizziness, near syncope or syncope, and/or paroxysmal atrial fibrillation pacing is indicated. Such patients are prone to atrial standstill.

Pacemaker function should be checked in those with permanent pacemakers to determine whether there is regular capture and whether the rate is within 4 beats of the set rate. Holter monitoring is indicated in the symptomatic patient who at observation has normal pacing. Replacement of the battery component is indicated in the presence of malfunction. The use of electrocautery during surgery is safe, provided the grounding pad is well removed from the pacemaker generator. If electrocautery is required within 18 in, the pacemaker should be converted to the fixed mode by the appropriate sterile magnet available from the manufacturer of the unit.

Hypertension[23,24]

Most patients with hypertension can undergo anesthesia and surgery without complications provided there is not significant atherosclerotic disease of the coronary and cerebral arteries and renal function is normal or near normal and the heart is compensated. Asymptomatic carotid artery stenosis carries a risk of stroke in the range of 1 to 3 percent. This is increased if there has been prior transient ischemic attack (TIA) or stroke. Noninvasive studies can identify those with significant stenosis. Critical to management is maintenance of blood pressure within limits of normal for the particular patient with avoidance of postural hypotension as well as hypertensive crises, not only during surgery but also in the postoperative period. Two-thirds of the strokes in the presence of carotid bruits are due to other causes such as embolism, hemorrhage, or thrombosis.[25]

The blood pressure should be adequately controlled without postural hypotension or hypokalemia, and treatment should be continued until surgery. Hypotension due to overtreatment may induce myocardial infarction or stroke. It is particularly important to continue beta blockers throughout surgery and the postoperative period. Surgery may be successfully carried out with intraoperative control of the blood pressure in the patient without prior treatment, so that it is not necessary to delay elective surgery unless the diastolic blood pressure is above the range of 110 mmHg.[1]

Hypertensive patients may develop myocardial ischemia or infarction with normal coronary arteries. Pressure-dependent areas of the subendocardium may become ischemic with either abrupt rise in blood pressure or fall in blood pressure. Where diuretic therapy has been administered preoperatively, there may be some contraction of blood volume, subjecting the patient to hypotension during surgery.

In addition to myocardial depression and vasodilatation from anesthetic agents, there may be pronounced swings in blood pressure due to stimulation of the sympathetic nervous system. This response is accentuated in the hypertensive patient. Intraarterial monitoring of blood pressure in addition to constant monitoring of ECG lead V_5 provides essential information in management. Activation of receptors in the larynx and trachea at intubation may produce severe hypertension and tachycardia. Beta blockers, sodium nitroprusside, and sodium pentothal or diazepam may counteract this response in conjunction with increasing the depth of anesthesia. Sternal splitting, rib retraction, skin incisions, hypocapnia due to excessive ventilation, volume loading, and cross-clamping of the aorta may induce a rise in blood pressure from catechol stimulation. While hypertensive crises from clonidine withdrawal are rare, they may be managed by propranolol and phentolamine. Drugs that are helpful when given intravenously include nitroglycerin 50 to 200 μg/min, sodium nitroprusside 24 to 400 μg/min, phentolamine 1 to 3 mg, hydralazine 10 to 20 mg, and alpha methyldopa 125 to 500 mg.[4] Renal vasoconstriction with decreased blood flow may produce oliguria. Cerebral blood flow may be reduced by varying mechanisms that are not well understood at this time. If a hypertensive crisis produces pulmonary edema, phlebotomy, sodium nitroprusside, and furosemide are effective with due care to avoid overdiuresis. Arrhythmias incident to catechol stimulation generally respond to measures that control the blood pressure and only occasionally require antiarrhythmic medication. Hypotension may be counteracted by reduction of anesthetic agents, fluid loading, calcium, dopamine, dobutamine, phenylephrine, or ephedrine. Epinephrine and norepinephrine should be avoided in the hypertensive patient.

Abrupt decreases of blood pressure to levels ordinarily considered normal may in the hypertensive patient produce ischemia in vascular beds. Clinical shock may rarely occur in the setting of blood pressure plunging to levels that would ordinarily be normal. A decrease of 30 percent in the systolic blood pressure has been associated with an increased frequency of myocardial ischemia and infarction,[12] and similar decrease in systolic pressure may induce TIAs in the susceptible patient.[26]

Postoperatively, blood pressure elevation may be induced by anxiety and inadequate control of pain by opiates and sedatives, fluid overload, excessive sodium intake, and failure to resume beta blockers or other antihypertensive medication. Medication for control of blood pressure should be resumed orally or through nasogastric tube as soon as possible. Using beta blockers, sodium nitroprusside, nitroglycerin, apresoline, alpha methyldopa, and diuretics, interim medication can be given by vein. Sublingual nifedipine or nitroglycerin may be effective when used for sudden rises in blood pressure. Uncontrolled hypertension in the postoperative period may produce myocardial infarction and has been cited as a factor in the occurrence of neurological deficits after carotid artery surgery.[27]

Systolic Hypertension

Systolic hypertension is more common in the elderly and is associated with an increased incidence of coronary and cerebral vascular disease. Like abdominal aortic aneurysm, it indicates arteriosclerosis in one vascular bed and the likelihood of vascular disease in other organs. There remains unanswered the question of what degree of control is needed and whether overzealous attempts to lower pressure may carry more hazard than benefit. Postural hypotension may occur in some without treatment but is commonly accentuated by therapy with occasional production of stroke. Many would withhold treatment of blood pressure less than 170/90, and if treatment is given, it is essential to avoid postural hypotension. Particular care is needed if there has been previous TIA in the basilar-vertebral artery distribution.

Valvular Heart Disease

The major valve disease in older patients is calcific aortic stenosis. The presence of angina, syncope, or congestive heart failure with aortic stenosis indicates the need for valve replacement prior to major elective surgery. Bedside clues to significant gradients are a slow-rising carotid impulse of small volume, broad, sustained apex impulse, and left ventricular hypertrophy in the ECG. While the blood pressure and pulse pressure are often low, major stenosis can be present even in the face of a systolic blood pressure of 150 mmHg.

Today, significant aortic insufficiency is more often due to annuloaortic ectasia than to previous rheumatic fever. The heart is often large in the absence of symptoms. Echocardiographic demonstration of an end-systolic volume of greater than 55 mm and exercise ejection fraction reduced to a level of 35 percent or less indicates severe disease.

Mitral stenosis is the common valve problem in females and males under 40. Mitral insufficiency may be rheumatic or due to myxomatous changes and prolapse of the mitral leaflets with or without chordal rupture. This is the most common cause of isolated severe regurgitation requiring valve replacement in some hospitals.[28]

Exercise isotope scans and/or cardiac catheterization may be needed in selected instances of valvular heart disease, including aortic stenosis, to determine severity, attendant risks, and possible need for valve replacement.

Congenital Heart Disease

Patients with left-to-right shunts, including patent ductus arteriosus, secundum atrial septal defect, and ventricular septal defect, with no evidence of heart failure, can undergo anesthesia and surgery with minimal risks. The same is true for valvular pulmonary stenosis and for mild aortic valvular stenosis. Patients with primary pulmonary hypertension, critical aortic stenosis, tetralogy of Fallot, or other types of cyanotic heart disease are at increased risk. The presence of congestive heart failure is associated with greater rates of morbidity and mortality. Tetralogy of Fallot is sensitive to decreased peripheral vascular resistance, which may increase right-to-left shunting with increased hypoxia, further myocardial depression, and metabolic acidosis. Catecholamine stimulation, pulmonary vasoconstriction, and infundibular spasm have been involved as factors in right-to-left shunting. Severe pulmonary hypertension requires an adequate filling pressure, and patients with this condition are more susceptible to ventricular fibrillation with overdiuresis.

Mitral Valve Prolapse; Idiopathic Hypertrophic Subaortic Stenosis

Prolapse of the mitral valve without significant mitral regurgitation entails no surgical risk, albeit prophylaxis for bacterial endocarditis is indicated. Severe mitral regurgitation increases the susceptibility to congestive failure.

Hypertrophic subaortic stenosis is associated with 10 to 15 percent risk of sudden death. Postural hypotension may occur spontaneously but also with alarming symptoms of angina and dyspnea after diuresis. The onset of atrial fibrillation requires prompt fluid loading and conversion to sinus rhythm. Nitrates and digitalis may increase the obstructive gradient while beta blockers and calcium antagonists improve pump function.

Prosthetic Valves

Thromboembolism, hemorrhage due to anticoagulants, and bacterial endocarditis occur with increased frequency with prosthetic valves. Those on anticoagulants require that these be stopped preoperatively. Two regimens are used:

1. Coumadin is discontinued 2 to 3 days prior to surgery and resumed 5 mg daily postoperatively until a therapeutic range is obtained.
2. Some advocate reversing the effect of Coumadin 24 h before surgery followed by heparin in the postoperative period for several days while prothrombin time is brought within range by Coumadin.

In a study of 44 patients undergoing noncardiac surgery, 5 had anticoagulants continued until surgery and 3 had perioperative hemorrhage. Two fatal instances of thromboembolism occurred postoperatively in 13 patients in whom anticoagulants were stopped 3 to 5 days before surgery.[29] Tinker et al.[30] felt that there was minimal risk of thromboembolism when anticoagulants were stopped 1 to 2 days preoperatively in 180 operations on 159 patients. There was 13 percent bleeding in those with prolonged prothrombin times at the time of surgery.

Antibiotic Prophylaxis for Endocarditis

Prophylaxis is recommended for patients with any type of valvular heart disease, prolapse of the mitral valve, hypertrophic subaortic stenosis, or calcified aortic valve or mitral annulus. Unfortunately, bacterial endocarditis may occur in the absence of known congenital or valvular heart disease and may be particularly overlooked in the elderly: in 42 patients over age 60, infection was suspected in only 40 percent of the total group and in only 9 percent of those having no murmur.[31] In some series one-quarter to one-half of fatal cases of endocarditis occur on normal valves.[32] Continued infection has been reported in the presence of abdominal abscess and prolonged use of Swan-Ganz catheters.[33] For antibiotic regimens, see Chap. 56.

Chronic Obstructive Lung Disease

Smoking should be omitted days to weeks prior to surgery. If a patient can walk up one flight of steps comfortably, any lung disease present poses no risk with surgery. Those with symptomatic disease may benefit from bronchodilators, expectorants, hydration, chest physiotherapy, and, in selected instances, antibiotics. Higher risks may be identified by a maximum breathing capacity less than 50 percent and an FEV_1 of less than 2 liters or 50 percent of predicted value and a Pa_{CO_2} greater than 45 mmHg. The functional residual capacity decreases up to 25 percent in the first 24 h with surgery in the upper part of the abdomen associated with decreased diaphragmatic excursion.[34] Atelectasis, pneumothorax, and pulmonary infection are not uncommon. Those with severe disease may require mechanical ventilation for several days.

Congestive Heart Failure

Congestive heart failure should be controlled by appropriate medication without the development of hypokalemia or postural hypotension. Clinical signs and symptoms and the x-ray are used to determine adequacy of treatment. It is important to avoid overdiuresis and having the patient at "dry weight," which predisposes to hypotension during anesthesia. The status of digitalization should be reviewed so that there is no toxicity. Renal insufficiency may dictate a maintenance dose of digoxin of 0.125 mg daily or every other day. Of crucial importance is that the serum potassium be maintained at a level of approximately 4 meq/liter. If atrial fibrillation is present, the ventricular rate should be controlled to a rate of 60 to 80 beats per minute by digitalis with increments of Inderal as needed. In the presence of AV block, the ventricular rate may remain slow, unrelated to the dose of digitalis. The "sick sinus node syndrome" may require less digitalis and avoidance of other drugs such as beta blockers, diltiazem, verapamil, quinidine, and procainamide. Corrective surgery for congenital or valvular heart lesions may be needed in some patients prior to major elective operations.

Postoperative Problems

Low Cardiac Output

The most common cause of a low cardiac output is decreased filling pressure due to a contracted blood volume. Leakage of fluid at the site of surgery and in other vascular beds produces sequestration of some of the circulating blood volume. The plasma volume may be reduced as much as 50 percent for as long as a week with major abdominal surgery.[35] Thus, the common problem faced is hypovolemia, and this can be aggravated by fever, sweating, blood loss, vomiting, ileus, nasogastric suction, diuretics, anaphylaxis, hyperglycemia, and prolonged administration of inotropes. If monitoring catheters are present, the wedge pressure will be low, in the range of 10 to 12 mmHg. Postural hypotension is a helpful clue to the need for fluid. Sinus tachycardia, oliguria, constricted veins on the dorsum of the hand, dry, pale tongue, and when advanced, cool, clammy skin and blotchy "blueness of knees" are common findings. Cerebral symptoms of confusion, restlessness, agitation, or insomnia may be present. The circulating blood volume may be reduced even though the patient has gained weight from accumulation of fluid in the extravascular space. One should avoid the common error of giving diuretics to the cardiac patient when oliguria occurs in the absence of pulmonary congestion in the x-ray. Fluid administration with 0.5 *N* saline is usually adequate, but plasma expanders may be needed. Other causes of a low cardiac output are myocardial ischemia or necrosis, arrhythmia, onset of congestive heart failure due to fluid overload or reabsorption, onset of heart block, or pulmonary embolism. Rarely, there may be pulmonary capillary leakage with elevated pulmonary artery pressures but with normal wedge pressure. This noncardiac cause of pulmonary edema can be due to hypersensitivity to blood or plasma, sepsis, shock, oxygen toxicity, aspiration of gastric contents, or drugs. Fluid loading, monitored by pulmonary pressures, and mechanical ventilation with positive end expiratory pressure (PEEP) is needed.

Congestive heart failure may occur at the termination of surgery when positive pressure ventilation is stopped with consequent increased venous return and raised filling pressure. Those susceptible to failure may develop it several days later when third-space fluid is mobilized.[36]

Shock not responding to volume loading or inotropic drugs may be improved with intraaortic balloon assist, accepting the 10 percent failure rate and 10 percent incidence of limb ischemia.[37].

Arrhythmias

Arrhythmias require identification and correction of disturbed physiology such as anemia, hypoxemia, hypercarbia, hypovolemia, or myocardial ischemia. Appropriate antiarrhythmic drugs are used concomitantly while precipitating factors are managed. Ventricular premature beats and tachycardia may be due to the presence of a Swan-Ganz catheter, and simple removal of the catheter may stop arrhythmia. Lidocaine is the first-line treatment of ventricular arrhythmia or tachycardia. The sudden onset of a regular rate of 150 is commonly due to atrial flutter with 2:1 block. If aberrancy is present and the QRS widened, the rhythm should not be confused with ventricular tachycardia. Therapy for the latter with lidocaine would be appropriate but might be hazardous for the former. Lidocaine may produce 1:1 conduction, then ventricular tachycardia and ventricular fibrillation. Paroxysmal atrial flutter or fibrillation may respond to 0.25 mg digoxin given intravenously (IV) to the digitalized patient. Verapamil may be used as initial treatment, and 15 percent may return to normal sinus rhythm. In others the ventricular rate may slow, and conversion can be obtained by intravenous procainamide or intramuscular quinidine. If the ventricular rate does not slow adequately, 1-mg increments of Inderal at 5-min intervals may effect slowing and/or conversion. Monotherapy is always preferred, but practically, one often requires the use of multiple antiarrhythmic agents with "layering technique" to obtain a normal sinus rhythm. Prompt dc cardioversion is used in the presence of shock or pulmonary edema.

Coronary Disease

Acute myocardial infarction probably occurs during surgery in most instances, even though ECG and enzyme evidence may be delayed several days. This is also suggested by the fact that pain is present in only approximately one-half of cases. Any complaints of chest, arm, shoulder, or interscapular discomfort should be viewed with suspicion. Hypotension occurring during surgery or the postoperative period, onset of interstitial or alveolar pulmonary edema, arrhythmia, or dyspnea demand evaluation. An electrocardiogram and chest x-ray should be routinely obtained postoperatively and several days later.

Infections

Fever and infections increase the metabolic demands of the heart and may produce tachycardia and hypotension. Infections should be promptly controlled by removal of venous and arterial lines, incision and drainage of abscesses, and appropriate antibiotics. Urinary catheters should be removed as soon as possible, and single straight catheterization should be used whenever possible. Venous catheters may be a source of septicemia and are often associated with signs of local phlebitis.[38] Where such is suspected, one should obtain cultures from the catheter tip at the time of removal. If Swan-Ganz catheters remain in place over a long period of time, they may be a source of sepsis and bacterial endocarditis.[33] Septic shock due to gram-negative organisms or staphylococcus is catastrophic, with a high mortality rate. When suspected, blood cultures should be obtained and antibiotics promptly given using a cephalosporin and aminoglycoside and vancomycin in addition, if staphylococcus is a possibility. Large volumes of fluid are required with Swan-Ganz monitoring. Some use 3 mg/kg dexamethasone with a repeat dose in 4 h. Antibiotics are adjusted when cultures and sensitivities of organisms are obtained.

References

1. Goldman, L.: Cardiac Risks and Complications of Noncardiac Surgery, *Ann. Intern. Med.*, 98:504, 1983.
2. Goldman, L., Caldera, D. L., Nussbaum, S. R., et al.: Multifactorial Index of Cardiac Risk in Non-Cardiac Surgery, *N. Engl. J. Med.*, 297:845, 1977.
3. Logue, R. B., Rogers, J. V., and Gay, B. B.: Subtle Roentgenographic Signs of Left Heart Failure, *Am. Heart J.*, 65:464, 1963.
4. Logue, R. B., and Kaplan, J.: The Cardiac and Non-Cardiac Surgery, *Curr. Probl. Cardiol.*, 7(2), 1982.
5. Mauney, F. M., Jr., Ebert, P. A., and Sabiston, D. C., Jr.: Postoperative Myocardial Infarctions, *Ann. Surg.*, 172:497, 1970.
6. Mahar, L. J., Steen, P. A., Tinker, J. H., Vliestra, R. E., Smith, H. C., and Pluth, J. R.: Perioperative Infarction in Patients with and without Bypass Grafts, *J. Thorac. Surg.*, 76:533, 1978.
7. McCullom, C. H., Garcia-Rinaldi, R., Graham, J. M., DeBakey, M. E.: Myocardial Revascularization Prior to Subsequent Major Surgery in Patients with Coronary Artery Disease, *Surgery*, 81:302, 1977.
8. Crawford, E. S., Morris, G. S., Howell, J. F., Flynn, W. F., and Moorhead, D. T.: Operative Risk in Patients with Previous Coronary Bypass, *Ann. Thorac. Surg.*, 26:215, 1978.
9. Zarling, E. J., Sexton, H., and Milnor, P.: Failure to Diagnose Acute Myocardial Infarction: The Clinicopathologic Experience at a Large Community Hospital, *JAMA*, 250:1177, 1983.
10. Kannel, W. B., Feinleib, M., Dawber, T. R., and McNamara, P. M.: Clinical Features of Unrecognized Myocardial Infarction: Silent and Symptomatic—18 Year Follow-up, *Am. J. Cardiol.*, 32:127, 1973.
11. Bertrand, M. E., LaBlanche, J. M., Filmant, P. V., et al.: Frequency of Provoked Coronary Arterial Spasm in 1089 Consecutive Patients Undergoing Coronary Arteriography, *Circulation*, 65:1299, 1982.
12. Tarhan, S., Moffitt, J. H., Taylor, W. F., and Gioliana, E. R.: Myocardial Infarction after General Anesthesia, *JAMA*, 220:2566, 1972.
13. Knapp, R. B., Topkins, M. J., and Artusio, J. F., Jr.: The Cerebrovascular Accident and Coronary Occlusion in Anesthesia, *JAMA*, 182:337, 1962.
14. Topkins, M. J., and Artusio, J. F.: Myocardial Infarction and Surgery, *Anesth. Analg.*, 43:716, 1964.
15. Steen, P. A., Tinker, J. H., and Tarhan, S.: Myocardial Reinfarction after Anesthesia and Surgery, *JAMA*, 239:2566, 1978.
16. Kaplan, J. A., Dunbar, R. W., and Jones, E. L.: Nitroglycerin Infusions during Coronary Artery Surgery, *Anesthesiology*, 45:14, 1976.
17. Wells, P. H., and Kaplan, J. A.: Optimal Management of Patients with Ischemic Heart Disease for Noncardiac Surgery by Complementary Anesthesiologist and Cardiologist Interaction, *Am. Heart J.*, 102:1029, 1981.
18. Rao, T. I. K., and El-Etr, H. A.: Myocardial Infarction following Anesthesia in Patients with Recent Infarction, *Anesth. Analg.*, 60:271, 1981. (Abstract.)
19. Glasser, S. P.: Non-Cardiac Surgery in the Cardiac Patient, *Cardiology Series, Baylor College of Medicine*, 6(3):10, 1983.
20. Leahey, E. B., Reiffel, J. A., Giardina, E. V., and Bigger, T.: The Effect of Quinidine and Oral Antiarrhythmic Drugs on Serum Digoxin: A Prospective Study, *Ann. Intern. Med.*, 92:605, 1980.
21. Belloci, F., Santarelli, P., di Gennaro, M., et al.: The Risk of Cardiac Complications in Surgical Patients with Bifascicular Block: A Clinical and Electrophysiologic Study of 98 Patients, *Chest*, 77:3, 1980.
22. Pastore, J. O., Yurchak, P. M., Janis, K. M., Murphy, J. D., and Zior, L. M.: The Risk of Advanced Heart Block in Surgical Patients with Right Bundle Branch Block and Left Axis Deviation, *Circulation*, 57:677, 1978.
23. Goldman, L., and Caldera, D.: Risks of General Anesthesia and Elective Operation in the Hypertensive Patient, *Anesthesiology*, 50:293, 1978.
24. Pickering, T. G.: Anesthesia and Surgery for the Hypertensive Patient, *Cardiovasc. Rev. Rep.*, 4(12):1569, 1983.
25. Wolf, P. A., Kannel, W. B., Sorlie, P., et al.: Asymptomatic Carotid Bruit and Risk of Stroke: The Framingham Study, *JAMA*, 245:1442, 1981.
26. Ruff, R.L.: Transient Ischemic Attack Associated with Hypotension in Hypertensive Patients with Carotid Artery Stenosis, *Stroke*, 12:353, 1981.
27. White, J. S., Sirinek, K. B., and Root, H. D.: Morbidity and Mortality of Carotid Endarterectomy: Rates of Occurrence in Asymptomatic and Symptomatic Patients, *Arch. Surg.*, 116:409, 1981.
28. Waller, B. F., Morrow, A. G., Maron, A. A., et al.: Etiology of Clinically Isolated Severe, Chronic, Pure Mitral Regurgitation: Analysis of 97 Patients over 30 Years of Age Having Mitral Valve Replacement, *Am. Heart J.*, 104:276, 1982.
29. Katholi, R. E., Nolan, L. P., and McGuire, L. B.: Living with Prosthetic Valves: Subsequent Noncardiac Operations and the Risk of Thromboembolism or Hemorrhage, *Am. Heart J.*, 92:162, 1976.
30. Tinker, J. H., and Tarhan, S.: Discontinuing Anticoagulant Therapy in Surgical Patients with Cardiac Valve Prostheses: Observations in 180 Operations, *JAMA*, 239:738, 1978.
31. Thell, R., Martin, F. H., and Edwards, O. E.: Bacterial Endocarditis in Subjects 60 Years or Older, *Circulation*, 51:174, 1975.
32. Roberts, W. C., and Bucklinder, N. A.: Healed Left-sided Infective Endocarditis: A Clinicopathologic Study of 59 Patients, *Am. J. Cardiol.*, 40:876, 1977.
33. Powell, D. C., Bevins, B. A., Bell, R. M., et al.: Bacterial Endocarditis in the Critically Ill Surgical Patient, *Arch. Surg.*, 116:311, 1981.
34. Epstein, P. E.: Preoperative Evaluation of the Patient with Pulmonary Disease, in "Pulmonary Diseases and Disorders," 2d ed., McGraw-Hill Book Company, New York, 1980.
35. Hoye, R. C., Bennett, S. H., Glenn, G. W., et al.: Fluid Volume and Albumin Kinetics Occurring with Major Surgery, *JAMA*, 222:1255, 1972.
36. Cooperman, L. H., and Price, H. L.: Pulmonary Edema in the Postoperative Period: A Review of 40 Cases, *Ann. Surg.*, 172:883, 1970.
37. Goldman, B., and Hill, T. A.: Comparative Analysis of Percutaneous Balloon Pump Catheter Insertions, *Cardiac Assists*, 1(4):1, 1984.
38. Bentley, D. W., and Lepper, M. H.: Septicemia Related to Indwelling Venous Catheters, *JAMA*, 206(8):1749, 1968.

Section D

Emotional Stress, Psychiatric Conditions, and the Heart

81

The Heart and Emotional Stress

James C. Buell, M.D.   Robert S. Eliot, M.D.

My life is in the hands of any scoundrel who chooses to put me in a passion.

John Hunter, 1776[1]

Psychological Stress

The concept that people's circumstances and emotions importantly influence their circulation was long ago accepted by observant students of humanity. Few folklore notions have enjoyed as widespread and persistent popularity as those that ascribe sudden death to emotional shock; and throughout history, anecdotes appear in which people die suddenly in the throes of fear, rage, grief, humiliation, or joy. Scientific scrutiny now provides insight into potential mechanisms and pathways linking stress to cardiovascular disease.

A contemporary definition offered by the First National Conference on Emotional Stress and Heart Disease describes stress as "an obviously painful or adverse force which induces distress or strain upon both the emotional and physical makeup." Appley and Trumbull[2] point out that as a psychological concept, stress has been used not only to refer to extreme environmental or psychosocial conditions but also as a substitute for what one might call anxiety, conflict, ego threat, frustration, or threat to security. Lazarus[3] has suggested that we view psychological stress more broadly, including not only stimulus and response but also the intervening psychological experimental factors which ultimately determine stimulus-response relations.

Thus, in discussions of psychological stress, it is apparent that the term *stress* affords little understanding. It means stimulus to some, response to some, interaction to others, and complex combinations of conditions to still others. Nevertheless, definition of the term *psychological stress* should reflect the idea that behavior and emotion occur at the interface between the environment and the individual and are highly colored by perception. Given these considerations, adherence to terms of stimulus-and-response parameters that are operationally sound and descriptive seems the most acceptable course to take in a discussion of stress.

Psychophysiology: The Physiological Concomitants of Emotional Perception

Although animal models are less cognitively complex than their human counterparts, there is little doubt that emotional stress can induce changes in cardiovascular physiology and promote pathophysiological mechanisms. Work summarized by Mason[4] has clearly demonstrated that psychosocial stimuli in animals can elicit at least two distinct neuroendocrine responses. One pathway involves arousal of the pituitary adrenal cortical system and the other that of the sympathetic adrenal medullary system. Such arousals occur during confrontations between various members of the social group as they seek food, territory, and mates. Social interactions leading to downward displacement in the hierarchy lead to stimulation of the pituitary adrenocortical system, accompanied by mental depression, decreased gonadotropin levels, enhanced vagal activity, gluconeogenesis, and pepsin production (vigilance or playing-dead reaction). The sympathetic adrenal medullary system is called into play as competitive behavior is invoked in an attempt to maintain status and to prevent threatened loss of esteem or related objects of attachment (alarm reaction). When of sufficient magnitude and duration, either response can elicit pathophysiological consequences.

The strongest evidence for implicating psychosocial and behavioral factors in pathophysiological processes derives from manipulations of the social hierarchy of a designated animal species. Henry[5] has demonstrated that socially deprived mice, when introduced into an established colony with an established hierarchy, develop a significant incidence of hypertension, myocardial hypertrophy, progressive arteriosclerosis, myocardial fibrosis, and renal failure. The physiological consequences of such psychosocial provocations are engrafted upon a foundation of cultural and genetic predisposition. Aggressive and submissive behavior are attended by distinct urinary excretion patterns of, respectively, catecholamine or corticosteroid precursors and metabolites until social roles are firmly established. Once roles are established and accepted within the social hierarchy, excessive neuroendocrine activity ceases.

When subordinate male tree shrews protected by a wire-mesh partition are continuously exposed to confrontation by a dominant and aggressive male of the same species, the subordinates fall into coma and die of uremia within 2 to 16 days, manifesting a sustained state of sympathetic arousal.[6]

The dominant hamadryas male baboon develops an intense attachment to his mate. When separated from her but able to witness the introduction of a new consort, the male will manifest chronic agitation, and some develop hypertension, coronary insufficiency, or acute myocardial infarction.[7] Investigators have separated swine from their littermates after primary social bonds were formed and subsequently demonstrated that the separated and isolated animals had a significantly greater incidence, extent, and severity of coronary atherosclerosis. During life, isolated swine manifest obviously depressed behavior.[8] New Zealand rabbits housed singly and then crowded develop early death with severe myocardial necrosis and later deaths with foci of myocardial fibrosis and compensatory myocardial hypertrophy, suggesting the development of a catecholamine-induced cardiomyopathy.[9]

Following Pavlovian conditioning some animals exhibiting neurotic behavior develop marked cardiovascular responses and alterations of diurnal physiological patterns outside the testing chamber.[10]

Using avoidance conditioning investigators have demonstrated alterations in cardiac electrophysiological properties. Dogs have been trained to diminish coronary blood flow without altering systemic hemodynamics, demonstrating that coronary circulation can be independently controlled by the central nervous system during stressful behavioral contingencies.[11] In avoidance yoke procedures, both animals receive the same number and temporal pattern of shocks, but only the avoidance animal has control over whether the shock will occur. Yoked helpless monkeys tend to develop physical deterioration with severe bradycardia and ventricular arrest (playing-dead reaction) whereas the avoidance monkey develops ECG abnormalities and myocardial degenerative lesions (alarm reaction).[12] Here it appears that the key difference leading to divergent pathologies is the perceived element of control.[12]

Thus, animal experimentation indicates that environmental manipulators and circumstances can elicit physiological responses and that such responses are mediated through perception of the social environment rather than resulting from direct actions of the social stimuli on the individual. If emotional arousal is avoided, physical stressors such as fasting fail to elicit notable neuroendocrine responses.[13] For instance, fasted monkeys exposed to the sights and sounds of feeding by their cohorts develop marked increases in urinary cortisol excretion, whereas isolated monkeys provided nonnourishing fruit-flavored pellets show no increased cortisol excretion at all.[13] Thus, personal assessment of the social environment arouses emotions which produce physiological responses. A stimulus inhibited at higher levels by interaction with coping patterns will be perceived as irrelevant; if perceived as relevant, however, arousal is triggered, and further responses are initiated.

The fact that the same experimental design may produce different results in different species or, by altering time frames or options, produce different results in the same species indicates that the impact and countenance of psychological stress is highly individual. Whether an event is stressful depends upon a complex amalgam of variables, including genetic predisposition, early social experience, and a lifelong process of conditioning and cultural factors. The resultant perceptions constitute the psychological prism through which daily events are uniquely and individually refracted (sociocultural brain). Considering the disproportionate size of neocortical structures in humans, and the nearly limitless variety of human perspectives and behaviors, it is hardly surprising that clinical investigations of psychosocial stress and cardiovascular disease have produced less consistent results than animal experimentation.

Nevertheless, it is interesting that the prevalence of coronary heart disease and hypertension generally parallels the increasing complexity, instability, and ambiguity of perceived social roles and hierarchies, whether we speak of animals or human beings.

Epidemiology of Stress-Related Cardiovascular Disease

Regarding socioeconomic factors, the highest coronary disease rates appear to be found in Finland and the United States, with the lowest rates in Greece,

Yugoslavia, and Japan. Occupation and marital status inconsistently correlate with coronary disease. However, the associated way of life for an occupation appears to contribute to coronary risk above and beyond the physical labor involved in the job itself. Within the multiple types of medical practices, the prejudged "high-stress" areas of general practice and anesthesiology have higher coronary rates than the "low-stress" areas of pathology and dermatology.[14] When comparing age groups of 40 to 69 years, the prevalence of coronary disease in dermatologists is 3.2 percent as compared with 11.9 percent in general practitioners. A greater vulnerability has been noted among English general physicians, who have about twice as high an incidence of coronary disease as other members of the medical profession between the ages of 40 and 64 years.[15]

Social mobility and status incongruity may be valid predictors only in certain places or at certain times, only for certain presentations of disease, or only when other variables are present. A major limitation of such demographic approaches is that they deal almost exclusively with the environment, ignoring coping and behavior. If stress represents the interaction between the *perceived* environment and the coping energies of an organism, there is apt to be great variability in correlations obtained from studies concerned exclusively with the environment. If, on the other hand, the broad array of published articles dealing with psychological and social variables and their relation to atherosclerosis and coronary heart disease are viewed together, a very clear pattern emerges. Those psychosocial factors most closely expected to involve intense, sustained overstimulation of the central nervous system have the most consistently positive associations with the risk of coronary heart disease. Conversely, those variables most removed from central nervous system involvement have the weakest associations.

Thus, there is considerable evidence suggesting that coronary disease is strongly associated with anxiety, depression, psychophysiological complaints, sleep disturbances, fatigue, and emotional drain.[16–19] While investigations regarding sleep disturbances are limited, associations with cardiovascular disease are a highly consistent finding. Having somewhat less strength and consistency as predictors of coronary risk are such variables as work overload, life dissatisfactions, and chronic conflict situations. Finally, such social and structural variables as social mobility, migration, educational level, and number of life-change events are less certain to be uniformly a cause for intense central nervous system arousal or distress, and therefore less consistently and strongly associated with risk of coronary disease.

Arrhythmias and Sudden Death

Far back in recorded history, people are described as dying during emotional upheaval. Almost 2000 years ago, Celsus[20] described how emotional states could influence the heart. In more recent times, such influences have been causally implied by, for instance, Hunter's[1] prediction of the circumstances of his death and Cannon's[21] observations on voodoo death.

A large number of experimental animal studies have strongly implicated psychological stress in the precipitation of arrhythmias and sudden death. Human studies and clinical reports have also demonstrated that psychological stress can precipitate significant rhythm disturbances.[22–25] Several reports have recently appeared in the literature documenting the effects of psychological stress in lowering the threshold for ventricular fibrillation and sudden death both in animals and in human beings.[16,26,27]

Corbalan[28] and his coworkers have demonstrated that before coronary arterial obstruction, psychological stress lowered the vulnerable period threshold for repetitive ventricular responses by 82 percent. After myocardial infarction, presentation of stressful stimuli provoked adverse ventricular arrhythmias, including ventricular tachycardia and early extrasystoles with T-wave interruption.[28] Since liberation of catecholamines appears to be a common phenomenon in stress situations, the administration of catecholamines has been utilized to duplicate the effects of stress seen in experimental animals.

The administration of catecholamines to dogs results in histopathological features of myocardial necrosis which are similar, if not identical, to those observed in cases of sudden cardiac death in human beings.[29] This type of myocardial necrosis, termed *coagulative myocytolysis,* is associated with sudden cardiac death and is characterized by the presence of anomalous contraction bands visible under ordinary staining techniques. Metabolic studies demonstrate a remarkable reduction of total high-energy phosphates in all layers of the myocardium with preferential depletion in the subendocardial region.[30] Impaired metabolic energy production is also indicated by the elevation of myocardial lactate following isoproterenol infusion. Such histological and metabolic responses can be largely abated by administration of beta-blocking agents.[30]

Many years ago, Raab[31] demonstrated that corticosteroid administration potentiated and augmented the myocardial degenerative influences of catecholamines administered to animals. Such experimentation strongly suggests that the combination of heightened sympathetic arousal following a complete sense of hopelessness and helplessness is a particularly lethal combination for the development of sudden death.[26] The ability of psychological stress to elicit such responses has also been documented in a variety of studies. Although sudden cardiac death may occur with or without coronary atherosclerosis, it is most usually found in the presence of coronary atherosclerosis. Psychological stress can precipitate malignant rhythm disturbances, and exaggerated sympathetic influences can reproduce the histological lesions most commonly seen in sudden death. There is evidence that psychological stress also plays another role in the pathogenesis of coronary heart disease.

Coronary Atherosclerosis

There is little doubt that emotional stress can aggravate established coronary heart disease, as manifested by Hunter's[1] prediction of the circumstances surrounding his death. In addition, the physiological concomitants of emotional arousal, including tachycardia, enhanced velocity of myocardial fiber shortening, increased systemic vascular resistance, and a lowered threshold to ventricular fibrillation induced by catecholamines, may all logically be suspected to aggravate established angina pectoris or heart failure. What is less well appreciated is the likelihood that emotional stress participates in the pathogenesis of coronary atherosclerosis and myocardial infarction.

In animal experimentation, major environmental factors have been identified and controlled far more readily and more completely than is possible with corresponding factors in human society. It has been shown that hypercholesterolemia and aortic atherosclerosis in cholesterol-fed rabbits may be either augmented or reduced by drugs which stimulate or depress the central nervous system.[32] Nerem[33] has reported a marked decrease in aortic plaques in cholesterol-fed rabbits when the animals were petted and fondled as compared to standard handling and care of cholesterol-fed animals. There was no difference in serum cholesterol levels between animals receiving "tender loving care" and the standard animal prototype. Greater degrees of hypercholesterolemia and coronary atherosclerosis have also been evoked in rats fed an atherogenic diet and exposed to a particular form of stress than in their unstressed controls.[34]

Similarly, although intimal changes are rare in the coronary arteries of wild immature monkeys, changes in the intima observed in immature caged rhesus monkeys are common after $1\frac{1}{2}$ to 3 months of captivity and have been interpreted as a response to emotional stress.[35] Andrus[36] published one attempt to induce atherosclerosis in chimpanzees through high-fat, high-cholesterol feeding. In that study, it was interesting that although there were more aortic fatty streaks in the experimental animals than in controls, this difference was less pronounced in the epicardial coronary arteries, and there was no difference in the cerebral arteries. Stout and Bohorquez[37] found epicardial and cerebral atherosclerosis in two of their chimpanzees which was significantly advanced over that found in the other members of the cohort. The diets of all the chimpanzees contained 10 percent of total calories as fat. Both animals manifesting predominant coronary and cerebral atherosclerosis had adjusted poorly to captivity, showing neurotic traits such as stereotyped posturing, hoarding of food and other objects, and poor socialization with peer animals in the colony.

Steinberg and Shafrir[38] and others have demonstrated in animals that cortisol enhances the ability of epinephrine to trigger sharp blood lipid increases under the influence of psychic stress. They observed a marked and almost immediate rise in the nonesterified fatty acids followed by a slower but definite rise in serum cholesterol. According to Sabin,[39] free fatty acids are irritating, and an excess may cause subendocardial hemorrhage and small mural thrombi. Raab and Humphreys[40] have shown that catecholamines also diminish myocardial efficiency by wasting oxygen in a disproportionate fashion. Through this action, the hormones are capable not only of increasing myocardial vulnerability in the presence of coronary atherosclerosis but of inducing severe potentially necrotizing myocardial hypoxia in animals with perfectly normal coronary vessels. Indeed, Raab[41] and his associates have produced myocardial necrosis in rats solely by subjecting these animals to sensory and emotional stresses.

Groover et al.[42] have also reported myocardial infarction without demonstrable atherosclerosis in baboons subjected to the emotional storm induced by trapping and caging. Still and Heiffer[43] observed sharp increases in viscosity mediated through the action of the sympathetic nervous system as the result of emotional stimuli in animals. Similarly, Haft[44] has demonstrated that microvascular platelet aggregation, often associated with necrosis, may occur in the hearts of animals receiving prolonged epinephrine infusion. These and other animal experiments demonstrate that certain pathological processes can be created in the face of neuroendocrine excesses. These neuroendocrine responses are apparently invoked through the limbic system mediated by cognitive perception.

Whereas the role of metabolic risk factors in the development of coronary heart disease is well documented, the role of psychosocial factors is rather more fiercely disputed. Nevertheless, few today would entirely dismiss the influence of psychosocial factors on the development of coronary heart disease, and recognition of their role is perhaps epitomized by the acceptance of type A behavior as a statistically validated risk factor.[45] Studies linking psychosocial factors with coronary heart disease have been large in quantity but variable in quality, and this latter attribute must bear much responsibility for the delayed recognition in associating behavior, personality, stress, and coronary heart disease.

The validity of all accepted risk factors is based upon postulated mechanisms in the atherosclerotic process, including endothelial trauma, lipid availability and deposition, smooth muscle cell proliferation, vasospasm, and thrombosis. The neuroendocrine responses precipitated by emotion include those of excess catecholamine production and/or corticosteroid production. Among the known physiological effects of catecholamines are those of enhanced lipid mobilization; increased platelet adhesiveness and aggregation; lowered threshold to generation of arrhythmia; increased secretion of glucagon, thyroxine, calcitonin, parathyroid hormone, renin, erythropoietin, and gastrin; and diminished insulin secretion. Glucocorticoids convert protein into carbohydrate and fat, have a minor antagonistic effect on insulin, promote the development of diabetes, foster hyperlipemia and hypercholesterolemia, enhance water diuresis, diminish circulating lymphocytes, reduce leukocytosis and polycythemia, increase platelet counts, lower the electrical excitation threshold of the brain, increase gastric acidity and pepsin production, block growth hormone secretion, decrease calcium absorption, enhance angiotensinogen production, sensitize arterioles to the pressor effect of catecholamines, and decrease the inflammatory response. There is extensive evidence that cortisol could play a role in atherogenesis. Cortisol has been shown to increase the activity of catecholamines and synthesizing enzymes in the adrenal medulla as well as to inhibit the activity of enzymes which break down catecholamines.[46] Henry[47] has reviewed an extensive literature documenting the following effects of glucocorticoids: (1) increased serum lipids; (2) increased atherosclerosis in dogs fed an atherogenic diet; and (3) increased number of dead or injured cells in arterial endothelium. It has been shown by Schmidt, Ekstein, and Debug, in 1966, that corticosteroids potentiate alpha-adrenergic vascular responses to catecholamines, an effect which is likely mediated by inhibition of extraneuronal clearance pathways for catecholamines by corticosteroids.[48] Hydrocortisone administration to human beings has been shown to acutely reduce beta receptor density in lymphocytes and increase beta receptor density in granulocytes; however, the long-term effect is to increase beta receptor density in both types of cells.[49]

The administration of corticosteroids has been associated with acceleration of atherosclerosis in patients with rheumatoid arthritis.[50] Most directly implicating corticosteroids and atherogenesis is the observation of increased morning cortisol levels among patients with more severe coronary atherosclerosis compared to patients with minimal or no disease.[51] In viewing the consequences of naturally occurring excesses, accelerated atherosclerosis, hypertension, and suicide constitute the main causes of death in Cushing's syndrome, whereas the sequelae of pheochromocytoma include hypertensive crises, myocardial infarction with or without coronary disease, arrhythmias, and catecholamine myocarditis.

Type A and Coronary-Prone Behavior

Even though Sir William Osler,[52] as early as 1920, described an apparent relation between arteriosclerosis and a high-pressure life, the issue of psychosocial factors in coronary heart disease has had a contentious history. Although others subsequently had commented on the association between high-pressure living and coronary proneness, it was Friedman and Rosenman[53] who popularized the term *type A* and statistically validated its significance through the prospective Western Collaborative Group Study.[54] The fully developed type A behavior pattern connotes speed, impatience, hostility, competitive drive, and a sense of an effort-oriented person caught up in a joyless struggle. The diagnosis is made using a structured interview with the subjects' responses graded for mannerisms and verbal styles of loud, explosive, rapid, and accelerated speech, short response latency, hostility, and a tendency to verbal competition.

The mechanisms through which type A behavior operate are conjectural; however, the prevalence of certain biochemical and physiological phenomena appear highly associated with fully developed type A behavior. These include elevated serum cholesterol levels, elevated pre- and postprandial serum triglycerides; enhanced platelet aggregation; faster clotting time, higher excretion of norepinephrine, particularly when provoked by emotional challenge; a higher average serum level of corticotropin; a greater insulinemic response to glucose; a decreased growth hormone response to arginine; and greater lability and magnitude of blood pressure response under reward-contingent time-demand tasks.[54]

Glass's[55] observations that the type A personality is vulnerable to depression are in accord with a study by Thomas, Ross, and Duszynski[56] of physicians with myocardial infarctions who readily became depressed even as students. Likewise Bruhn[57] and colleagues found coronary-prone individuals to be effort-oriented people whose achievements gave them little satisfaction. A lack of contentment appears to correlate with a higher incidence of angina pectoris, and conversely, the study of Medalie and Goldbourt[58] suggests that a spouse's love and support is an ameliorating factor when all other risk factors are comparable. These investigators found that anxiety, all severe psychosocial problems, and especially family problems showed a strong association with the subsequent development of angina pectoris.

It is therefore important to make a distinction between the well-defined and statistically validated risk factor of global type A behavior pattern, and the ill-defined but constantly evolving total concept of coronary-prone behaviors. For example, cultural determinants are likely to be important modifiers. The cross-cultural study of Cohen et al. of the relation between type A behavior and coronary heart disease among Japanese Americans living in Hawaii demonstrated that men who were culturally mobile and type A had a two to three times greater risk of coronary disease than men with either characteristic alone.[59] Whether one speaks of the type A pattern of behavior or a disruption of social roots, the way one behaves in terms of adaptation to life carries with it certain health consequences.

Vaillent[60] has published a 40-year prospective study of 93 healthy young men which looks at modes of adaptation. Even with the contributions of smoking, suicide, alcohol use, obesity, and age at death of parents and grandparents controlled for, correlations between the mode of psychological defense and physical health remain significant. The most mature defense mechanisms include humor, altruism, sublimation, and suppression and are associated with persistent health through middle age in 80 percent of men who deploy these defense mechanisms. In contrast, only one-third of men characteristically deploying immature defense mechanisms were still in excellent health at age 55. Perhaps mature defenses while defending against stress are more realistic adaptive behaviors and more socially acceptable, thus binding people together in social support, which in and of itself appears to confer protection. Henry and Stevens[61] have written about an effective cultural canon being protective against cardiovascular disease. Another type of behavior apparently linked to risk for cardiovascular disease is that of physiological response to psychological stress.

Psychophysiological Response Pattern

If by behavior one means the actions or reactions of human beings or animals under specified circumstances, then measuring physiological changes to psychological stress provides one promising avenue for categorizing individuals having enhanced vulnerability to psychological stress.[62] As an example, studies by Rose, Jenkins, and Hurst[63] on air traffic controllers indicate that those normotensive controllers subsequently developing hypertension showed greater reactivity and larger blood pressure responses on the job than their peers who remained normotensive throughout this 3-year study. The 23-year study of Keys found that blood pressure reactivity to the cold pressor test was the single best predictor of coronary disease.[64] Theorell[65] and colleagues had the opportunity to examine twin pairs discordant for coronary heart disease and found that hyperkinetic circulatory responses during stressful interview were seen in the less healthy twin as reflected by ballistocardiography. Thus, whereas neurophysiological and neuroendocrine activation patterns have significant genetic components, behavioral factors also appear to be important in orchestrating the timetable for development of disease.

Falkner et al. over a follow-up period of 41 months compared adolescents with borderline blood pressure elevations to a normotensive, family history-negative control population.[66] Of borderline hypertensive adolescents 56 percent developed fixed essential hypertension. At the time of initial evaluation, they had a strong family history of essential hypertension, higher resting heart rate and blood pressure, and a greater cardiovascular response to mental stress compared to the normotensive, family history-negative, control population. Time series analysis of the stress phase also demonstrated a rhythmic cardiovascular response in the normotensive group not present in the hypertensive group. The results indicate that adolescents with borderline hypertension displaying hyperphysiological responses to mental stress had a greater risk of essential hypertension than previously reported.

Panin and Sokolov[67] studied psychophysiological and biochemical factors in Soviet polar regions and also found that subjects suffering from coronary heart disease tended to show elevated serum 11-hydroxycorticosteroid levels. Hypertensive subjects showed higher free fatty acid levels, which they interpreted to imply activation of the sympathoadrenal medullary system. Our group has studied the cardiovascular response to emotional stress during a stressful interview in post-myocardial infarction patients and in matched control subjects.[68] Cardiovascular hyperreactivity (so-called hot-reacting) was more common in reinfarction patients than in those without coronary heart disease. Extreme cardiovascular reactivity was comparable to type A behavior pattern and better than hypertension or level of physical activity in predicting future coronary events. These results suggest that psychophysiological stress testing may be a useful adjunctive procedure for detecting the potential victim of early reinfarction.[69]

Thus, the individual's physiological response to mental provocation appears to have discriminating and predictive value.[70] It is our opinion that detection of untoward physiological responses to psychological provocation identifies those individuals particularly vulnerable to the cardiovascular effects of psychological stress. Much as exercise stress testing has added an extra dimension to the diagnostic capacity of the electrocardiogram, monitoring of physiological responses to nonphysical stress may provide additionally useful information in the detection, diagnosis, and management of cardiovascular disorders.

Hypertension

Hypertension affects more than 30 million working Americans and can be traced to an identifiable cause in less than 10 percent of the cases. The role of adverse psychosocial situations in the pathogenesis of hypertension has been referred to earlier in the work of Henry.[5] While the strength of evidence in the clinical area is less than that in objective, controlled animal experiments, psychosocial factors such as socioeconomic level, crime rate, residential change, and overcrowding have been linked with hypertension.

Harburg and colleagues[71] have shown that blacks living in areas of Detroit with a low-stress environment had less hypertension than their counterparts living in high-stress areas. Gampel and coworkers[72] have reported that there was less hypertension among rural than urban Zulus, and, of the latter, more of those who clung to traditional cultural practices and seemed unable to successfully adapt to the demands of urban living were hypertensive. One can reasonably assume that change in diet and sodium intake probably attends such migrations. However, in general, a remarkable contrast can be found between industrialized and primitive societies that demonstrates the relative absence of hypertension in the latter. In reality, the agonistic society of Henry's[21] animal experiments is similar to the society of urbanized, industrialized human beings.[73] Different genetic strains of the same rodent species manifest different temperaments and potential for developing hypertension, and it is likely that similar modifiers are operative in the clinical setting. The mosaic theory of pathophysiology proposed by Page[74] seems appropriate in reviewing the socioenvironmental link with hypertension seen in a variety of epidemiologic studies.

Beyond considerations of environmental provocation, psychological and behavioral aspects are also worthy of note. Work by Alexander[75] suggests that the hypertensive personality may be described as an individual who frequently manifests inhibited and poorly expressed rage and anger. It has been proposed that this inhibited rage or anger turned inward results in stimulation of the automatic nervous system, which causes the release of significant amounts of norepinephrine leading to acute and eventually chronic hypertension. Elser[76] has reported that in psychometric testing, patients with high-renin hypertension exhibited suppressed hostility linked to increased sympathetic activity. In these patients, the hypertension was concluded to be neurogenic and possibly psychosomatic in origin. Such individuals are described as withdrawn, not easily communicative, and tending to avoid confrontation with people even when rage is justified.

Studies have indicated that 25 to 40 percent of patients with essential hypertension are characterized by higher basal circulating catecholamine levels and by higher sympathetic activity in response to postural changes.[77] The identification of these patients as a separate entity is desirable, since it is possible that the evolution of the hypertensive disease and response to therapy may differ in this group.

Light et al. have found that competitive mental tasks significantly reduced the urinary sodium and fluid excretion by young men with one or two hypertensive parents or with borderline hypertension.[78] In this high-risk group, the degree of retention was exactly related to the magnitude of heart rate increase during stress, suggesting common mediation by way of the sympathetic nervous system. Thus, psychological stress appears to induce changes in renal excretory functions in the genetically predisposed subject that may play an important role in the long-term regulation of blood pressure.

Whether observations linking personality, behavior, and neuroendocrine mechanisms with hypertension constitute valid clues to the pathogenesis of essential hypertension or a protective response to genetic vulnerability or even a functional defect as a consequence of the disease process remains to be elucidated. However, a wide variety of experimental and clinical observations implicate psychosocial and behavioral factors in the phenomena of essential hypertension. The interaction between mind and environment engrafted upon a genetic substrate is a complex topic for study. Yet the concept that essential hypertension represents specific disturbances or shifts in the bias of physiological regulatory mechanisms is consistent with observed epidemiologic, experimental, and clinical data. Since either adrenal medullary or adrenal cortical systems can lead to hypertension and are known to be activated by psychosocial stimuli, it is not too difficult to see that repeated exposure to such stimuli can lead to structural vascular thickening and mechanically increased resistance. Whereas initially the imbalance is probably reversible, chronically repeated and sustained arousals are hypothesized to result in a permanent disregulatory state and, perhaps, fixed hypertension. While one cannot underestimate the importance of psychosocial and neuroendocrine facilitation early, it is likely that these become less significant in the later stages of hypertension.

Anxiety Neurosis

The term *anxiety neurosis* refers to a syndrome in which cardiovascular, respiratory, and nervous symptoms are prominent features in the absence of an explanatory medical diagnosis. The syndrome referred to in 1864 by Hartshorne[79] as "cardiac muscular exhaustion" and in 1871 by DaCosta[80] as "irritable heart syndrome" has undergone many name changes. This psychophysiological syndrome is also known as cardiac neurosis, disordered action of the heart, soldier's heart, effort syndrome, Holmgren's vasoregulatory asthenia,[81] Gorlin's hyperkinetic heart syndrome,[82] Frohlich's hyperdynamic beta-adrenergic circulatory state,[83] and neurocirculatory asthenia.

Patients with anxiety neurosis have complaints of a moderate to severe degree of dyspnea, palpitations, chest pain, nervousness, anxiousness, or fatigue. Among the most commonly reported aggravating factors are emotion-provoking situations, illness, hard physical labor, pregnancy, and military service.[84,85] Dyspnea is one of the most common and characteristic symptoms, and Christie has termed these cases with marked respiratory complaints *respiratory neurosis*.[86] Generally, the patient feels respiratory distress both at rest and with exertion, but the degree of effort necessary to produce dyspnea varies extraordinarily according to emotional state. Sighing respirations are quite characteristic and are a helpful diagnostic sign. Precordial nonanginal pain is suffered by most patients and may be characterized either as fleeting sticks and stabs and/or dull and aching left thoracic pain of prolonged duration.[85] The patient may relate the pain to exertion, but it usually occurs after exertion and is associated with fatigue rather than effort. Tachycardia and epigastric complaints in the solar plexus are commonly reported.

A large number of clinical and experimental laboratory studies have been made of patients with this disorder, but they have not added much to the clinical picture for arriving at a diagnosis. Standard blood chemistry findings are unremarkable. In various research studies, abnormalities have been found in fingernail capillaries, oxygen consumption, blood lactate, palmar sweat, during psychological testing, during muscular work, and with painful stimuli.[84,85] Exercise tends to cause an abnormal rise in blood lactate level,[84] and administration of lactate to such patients could induce anxiety attacks in the vast majority.[87] Diminished work capacity is reflected by a lower maximal oxygen consumption than normal and a narrow arteriovenous oxygen difference.[81]

Electrocardiographic repolarization abnormalities have been reported by some authors, but there is no characteristic ECG pattern for the syndrome.[88] The ECG changes, referred to as *sympathicotonic*, can also appear in controls.[89] Most clinicians feel that arrhythmias related exclusively to anxiety neurosis are not especially frequent.[90] Friedman,[91] however, has noted various arrhythmias, including extrasystoles, paroxysmal tachycardia, and atrial fibrillation, occurring at the time of onset of sharp precordial pain. He believes the arrhythmias coincide with episodic neurogenic discharges in more than half the patients with anxiety neurosis.

Anxiety neurosis is considered to be a psychiatric disorder, although constitutional and hereditary factors may play a role in its development. The discussions concerning the relation of mitral valve prolapse to psychiatric issues and older literature concerning anxiety neurosis attest to the complexity of factors involved.[92,93] Sympathetic hyperactivity has been reported in both anxiety neurosis and mitral valve prolapse, but the etiologic relations remain obscure for these disorders.[83,93] The fact that some of the patient's symptoms can be aggravated or reproduced by administration of isoproterenol and blocked by propranolol[83,94–96] has led to speculation that increased beta-adrenergic receptor responsiveness or catecholamine production may be an important mechanism in the syndrome.[97] While beta-adrenergic blocking drugs decrease the patient's awareness of heart action, it is not certain that they reduce other symptoms of the disorder.

This condition tends to persist for years with periods of exacerbation and remission. A small number of patients may recover entirely, and some will show improvement.[98] The outlook for disappearance of symptoms is poor when there is a serious psychiatric background and a long history of symptoms, and when the syndrome of anxiety neurosis appears after relatively brief and minor strain.[99] On the other hand, a good symptomatic result may be anticipated if the syndrome appears acutely, after a prolonged and very intense emotional and physical strain in a person without previous significant psychomotor or personality derangement. Thus, if a single precipitating cause can be discovered and eliminated, the prognosis is better than if there is a lifelong global pattern of neurotic behavior in an individual.

Winning and retaining the patient's confidence and providing reassurance are the most important measures in the management of most patients with this syndrome. This is usually accomplished by a careful, detailed history and physical examination, and the demonstration of a complete understanding of and interest in the patient's symptoms. Reassurance should not stop with the exclusion of organic heart disease but should include an emphasis on the good prognosis for life expectancy and the low incidence of disability.[85] Precipitating factors should be identified, explained, and dealt with in terms of the total life situation of the patient and his or her attitudes and emotional reactions. Intensive psychotherapy or psychoanalysis appears no better than simple reassurance, appropriate drug therapy for acute episodes, and advice about aggravating factors.[98] Drug therapy consists of tranquilizers or antidepressants in circumstances of acute stress symptoms, but these drugs do not appear to be helpful in the long-term management of the disorder. Beta-adrenergic blocking agents may be used to reduce tachycardia and some of the hyperkinetic circulatory manifestations.

Comment

Although the etiologic relation between emotional stress and heart disease remains complex and controversial, the ability of the human mind to influence physiological functions is acknowledged. When taken together, studies of animals and humans that relate psychosocial and behavioral factors to cardiovascular disease provide justification for the conclusion that such factors are potentially quite important.

Evaluation of the interaction of psychosocial and biological factors both in laboratory studies of pathogenesis and clinical studies of management will clarify important relations. Key factors to be considered are individual perceptions of events, assessment of coping and other supportive counterbalancing forces, and utilization of more precise and accurate testing systems. It is our belief that better understanding of the relationship between complex emotions and the heart will open the gateway to practical clinical advances in the prevention and rehabilitation of cardiovascular disease.

References

1. Home, E.: A Short Account of the Author's Life, in J. Hunter (ed.), "A Treatise on the Blood, Inflammation and Gun Shot Wounds," T. Bradford Publisher, Philadelphia, 1796.
2. Appley, M. H., and Trumbull, R.: On the Concept of Psychological Stress, in M. H. Appley and R. Trumbell (eds.), "Psychological Stress," Meredith Press, New York, 1967, p. 1.
3. Lazarus, R. S.: The Concepts of Stress and Disease, in L. Levi (ed.), "Society, Stress and Disease: The Psychosocial Environment and Psychosomatic Diseases," vol. 1, Oxford University Press, London, 1971, p. 53.
4. Mason, J. W.: A Review of Psychoendocrine Research on the Pituitary Adrenal Cortical System, *Psychosom. Med.*, 30:576, 1968.
5. Henry, J. P., and Ely, D. L.: Physiology of Emotional Stress: Specific Responses, *J. S.C. Med. Assoc.*, 75:501, 1979.
6. Von Holst, D.: Renal Failure as the Cause of Death in *Tupaia belangeri* (Tree Shrews) Exposed to Persistent Social Stress, *J. Comp. Physiol. Psychol.*, 78:236, 1972.
7. Lapin, B. A., and Cherkovich, G. M.: Environmental Changes Causing the Development of Neuroses and Corticovisceral Pathology in Monkeys, in L. Levi (ed.), "Society, Stress and Disease: The Psychosocial Environment and Psychosomatic Diseases," vol. 1, Oxford University Press, London, 1971, p. 266.
8. Ratcliffe, H. L., Luginbuhl, H., Schnarr, W. R., and Chacko, K.: Coronary Arteriosclerosis in Swine: Evidence of a Relation to Behavior, *J. Comp. Physiol. Psychol.*, 68:385, 1969.
9. Weber, H. W., and VanderWalt, J. J.: Cardiomyopathy in Crowded Rabbits: A Preliminary Report, *S. Afr. Med. J.*, 47:1591, 1973.
10. Miminoshvili, D. I., Magakian, G. O., and Kokaia, G. I.: Attempts to Obtain a Model of Hypertension and Coronary Insufficiency in Monkeys, in I. A. Utkin (ed.), "Theoretical and Practical Problems of Medicine and Biology in Experiments on Monkeys," Pergamon Press, New York, 1960, p. 103.
11. Ernst, F. A., Kordenat, R. K., and Snadman, C. A.: Learned Control of Coronary Blood Flow, *Psychosom. Med.*, 41:79, 1979.
12. Corley, K. C., Mauck, H. P., and Shiel, F. O. M.: Cardiac Responses Associated with "Yoked-Chair" Shock Avoidance in Squirrel Monkeys, *Psychophysiology*, 12:439, 1975.
13. Mason, J. W., Mather, J. T., Hartley, L. H., Mougey, E. H., Perlow, M. J., and Jones, L. G.: Selectivity of Corticosteroid and Catecholamine Responses to Various Natural Stimuli, in G. Serban (ed.), "Psychopathology of Human Adaptation," Plenum Publishing Corporation, New York, 1976, p. 147.
14. Russek, H. I.: Emotional Stress and Coronary Heart Disease in American Physicians, *Am. J. Med. Sci.*, 240:711, 1960.
15. Morris, J. N., Heady, J. A., and Barley, R. G.: Coronary Heart Disease in Medical Practitioners, *Br. Med. J.*, 1:503, 1952.
16. Lynch, J. J., Paskewitz, D. A., Gimbel, K. S., and Thomas, S. A.: Psychological Aspects of Cardiac Arrhythmia, *Am. Heart J.*, 93:645, 1977.
17. Jenkins, C. D.: Recent Evidence Supporting Psychologic and Social Risk Factors for Coronary Disease, *N. Engl. J. Med.*, 294:987, 1038, 1976.
18. Dimsdale, J. E.: Emotional Causes of Sudden Death, *Am. J. Psychiatry*, 134:1361, 1977.
19. Eliot, R. S.: "Stress and the Major Cardiovascular Disorders," Futura Publishing Company, Mt. Kisco, N.Y., 1979.
20. Celsus, A. C.: "DeMedicina," Liber III, 6, circa 30 A.D., quoted by C. F. T. East in "The Story of Heart Disease," William Dawson and Company, London, 1957.
21. Cannon, W. B.: Voodoo Death, *Psychosom. Med.*, 19:182, 1957.
22. Donlon, P. T., Meadow, A., and Amsterdam, E.: Emotional Stress as a Factor in Ventricular Arrhythmias, *Psychosomatics*, 20:233, 1979.
23. Buell, J. C., and Eliot, R. S.: The Clinical & Pathological Syndromes of Sudden Cardiac Death; An Overview, in F. Solomon, D. L. Perron, and P. B. Dews (eds.), "Biobehavioral Factors in Sudden Cardiac Death," National Academy Press, Washington, D.C., 1981, pp. 13–28.
24. Taggart, P., Gibbons, D., and Somerville, W.: Some Effects of Motor Car Driving on the Normal and Abnormal Heart, *Br. Med. J.*, 4:130, 1969.
25. Taggart, P., Carruthers, M., and Somerville, W.: EKG, Plasma Catecholamines and Lipids and Their Modification by Oxprenolol When Speaking before an Audience, *Lancet*, 2:341, 1973.
26. Engel, G. L.: Psychologic Stress, Vasodepressor (Vasovagal) Syncope and Sudden Death, *Ann. Intern. Med.*, 89:403, 1978.
27. Lown, B., DeSilva, R. A., and Lenson, R.: Roles of Psychologic Stress and Autonomic Nervous System Changes in Provocation of Ventricular Premature Complexes, *Am. J. Cardiol.*, 41:979, 1978.
28. Corbalan, R., Verrier, R., and Lown, B.: Psychological Stress and Arrhythmias during Myocardial Infarction in the Conscious Dog, *Am. J. Cardiol.*, 34:692, 1974.
29. Eliot, R. S., Clayton, F. C., Pieper, G. M., and Todd, G. L.: Influence of Environmental Stress on the Pathogenesis of Sudden Cardiac Death, *Fed. Proc.*, 36:1719, 1977.
30. Eliot, R. S., Todd, G. L., Clayton, F. C., and Pieper, G. M.: Experimental Catecholamine-Induced Acute Myocardial Necrosis, in V. Manninen and P. I. Halonen (eds.), "Advances in Cardiology," vol. 25, S. Karger, Basel, 1978, p. 107.
31. Raab, W.: Emotional and Sensory Stress Factors in Myocardial Pathology, *Am. Heart J.*, 72:538, 1966.
32. Myasnikov, A. L.: Influence of Some Factors on Development of Experimental Cholesterol Atherosclerosis, *Circulation*, 17:99, 1958.
33. Nerem, R.: "Social Environment as a Factor in Diet-Induced Aortic Atherosclerosis in Rabbits," Hugh Lofland Conference on Arterial Wall Metabolism, Boston, Mass., May, 1979.
34. Uhley, H. N., and Friedman, M.: Blood Lipids, Clotting and Coronary Artherosclerosis in Rats Exposed to a Particular Form of Stress, *Am. J. Physiol.*, 197:396, 1959.
35. Vlodaver, Z., Medalie, J., and Naufeld, H. N.: Coronary Arteries in Immature Monkeys, Preliminary Report of the Relationships to Activity and Diet, *J. Atheroscler. Res.*, 8:923, 1968.
36. Andrus, S. B., Portman, O. W., and Riopelle, A. J.: Comparative Studies of Spontaneous and Experimental Atherosclerosis in Primates: II. Lesions in Chimpanzees Including Myocardial Infarction and Cerebal Aneurysms, *Progr. Biochem. Pharmacol.*, 4:393, 1968.
37. Stout, L. C., and Bohorquez, F.: Significance of Intimal Arterial Changes in Nonhuman Vertebrates, in M. D. Altschule (ed.), "Symposium on Atherosclerosis," *Med. Clin. North Am.*, vol. 58, W. B. Saunders Company, Philadelphia, 1974, p. 245.
38. Steinberg, D., and Shafrir, E.: Cortisone Held "Vital" to Lipid Rise in Stress, *Med. News*, 6:1, 1960.
39. In Page, I. H.: Atherosclerosis: A Commentary, *Fed. Proc.*, 18(suppl. 3):47, 1959.
40. Raab, W., and Humphreys, R. J.: Drug Action upon Myocardial Epinephrine-Sympathin Concentration and Heart Rate: (Nitroglycerin, Papaverine, Priscol, Dibenamine Hydrochloride), *J. Pharmacol. Exp. Ther.*, 89:64, 1947.
41. Raab, W., Chaplin, J. P., and Bajusz, E.: Myocardial Necroses Produced in Domesticated Rats and in Wild Rats by Sensory and Emotional Stresses, *Proc. Soc. Exp. Biol. Med.*, 116:665, 1964.
42. Groover, M. R., Jr., Seljeskog, E. L., Haglin, J. J., and Hitchcock, C. R.: Myocardial Infarction in the Kenya Baboon without Demonstrable Atherosclerosis, *J. Angiol.*, 14:409, 1963.
43. Still, J. W., and Heiffer, M. H.: Blood Viscosity in Response to Various Stimuli, reported at Fed. Am. Soc. for Exp. Biol., April, 1958.
44. Haft, J. I.: Role of Blood Platelets in Coronary Artery Disease, *Am. J. Cardiol.*, 43:1197, 1979.
45. Rosenman, R. H., Brand, R. J., Jenkins, C. D., Friedman, M., Straus, R., and Wurm, M.: Coronary Heart Disease in the Western Collaborative Group Study: Final Follow-Up Experience of $8\frac{1}{2}$ Years, *JAMA*, 233:872, 1975.

46. Kopin, I. J., McCarty, R., and Yamaguchi, I.: Plasma Catecholamines in Human and Experimental Hypertension, *Clin. Exp. Hypertension,* 2(3–4);379, 1980.
47. Henry, J. P.: Coronary Heart Disease and the Arousal of the Adrenal Cortical Axis, in T. M. Dembroski, T. H. Schmidt, and G. Blümchen (eds.), "Biobehavioral Bases of Coronary Heart Disease," S. Karger, Basel, 1983, p. 365.
48. Goldie, R. G.: The Effects of Hydrocortisone on Response to an Extraneuronal Uptake of (−)-isoprenaline in Cat and Guinea-Pig Atria, *Clin. Exp. Pharmacol. Physiol.,* 3(3);225, 1976.
49. Davies, A. D., and Lefkowitz, R. J.: Corticosteroid-Induced Differential Regulation of Beta-Adrenergic Receptors in Circulating Human Polymorphonuclear Leukocytes and Mononuclear Leukocytes, *J. Clin. Endocrinol. Metab.* 51(3):599, 1980.
50. Kalbak, K.: Incidence of Arteriosclerosis in Patients with Rheumatoid Arthritis Receiving Long-Term Corticosteroid Therapy, *Ann. Rheum. Dis.,* 31(3):196, 1972.
51. Toxler, R. G., Sprague, E. A., Albanese, R. A., Fuchs, R., and Thompson, A. J.: The Association of Elevated Plasma Cortisol and Early Atherosclerosis as Demonstrated by Coronary Angiography, *Atherosclerosis,* 26(2);151, 1977.
52. Osler, W., and McCrae, T.: "Principles and Practice of Medicine," D. Appleton & Company, New York, 1920.
53. Friedman, M., and Rosenman, R. H.: Association of a Specific Overt Behavior Pattern with Increases in Blood Cholesterol, Blood Clotting Time, Incidence of Arcus Senilis and Clinical Coronary Artery Disease, *JAMA,* 169:1286, 1959.
54. Dembroski, T. M., MacDougall, J. M., and Shields, J. L.: Physiologic Reaction to Social Challenge in Persons Evidencing the Type A Coronary-Prone Behavior Pattern, *J. Hum. Stress,* 3:2, 1977.
55. Glass, D. C.: "Behavior Patterns, Stress and Coronary Disease," Lawrence Erlbaum Associates, Hillsdale, N.J., 1977.
56. Thomas, C. B., Ross, D. C., and Duszynski, K. R.: Youthful Hypercholesterolemia, Its Associated Characteristics and Role in Premature Myocardial Infarction, *Johns Hopkins Med. J.,* 136:193, 1975.
57. Bruhn, J. G., Paredes, A., Adsett, C. A., and Wolf, S.: Psychological Predictors of Sudden Death in Myocardial Infarction, *J. Psychosom. Res.,* 18:187, 1974.
58. Medalie, J. H., and Goldbourt, U.: Angina Pectoris among 10,000 Men: II. Psychosocial and Other Risk Factors as Evidenced by Multivariate Analysis of a Five-Year Incidence Study, *Am. J. Med.,* 60:910, 1976.
59. Cohen, J. B., Syme, S. L., Jenkins, C. D., Kagan, A.: The Cultural Context of Type A Behavior and the Risk of Coronary Heart Disease, *Am. J. Epidemiol.,* 102:434, 1975.
60. Vaillent, G. E.: Natural History of Male Psychologic Health: Effective Mental Health on Physical Health, *N. Engl. J. Med.,* 301:1249, 1979.
61. Henry, J. P., and Stevens, P. N.: "Health Stress and Social Environments," Springer-Verlag, New York, 1977.
62. Buell, J. C., and Sime, W. E.: Quantitation of Physiological Responses to Emotional Distress, *J. S.C. Med. Assoc.,* 75(11), 1979.
63. Rose, R. M., Jenkins, C. D., and Hurst, M. W.: "Air Traffic Controller Health Change Study," Report to the FAA, June, 1978.
64. Keys, A., Taylor, H., Blackburn, H., Brozek, J., Anderson, J., and Simonson, E.: Mortality and Coronary Heart Disease among Men Studied for 23 Years, *Arch. Intern. Med.,* 128:201, 1971.
65. Theorel, T., deFair, U., Schalling, D., Adamson, U., and Askevold, F.: Personality Traits and Psychophysiological Reaction to a Stressful Interview in Twins with Varying Degree of Coronary Heart Disease, *J. Psychosom. Res.,* 23:89, 1979.
66. Falkner, B., Kushner, H., Gaddo, O., and Angelikos, E. T.: Cardiovascular Characteristics in Adolescents Who Develop Essential Hypertension, *Hypertension,* 3:521, 1981.
67. Panin, L. Y., and Sokolov, V. P.: Psychophysiological and Biochemical Factors in the Development of Coronary Heart Disease and Arterial Hypertension in a Non-Resident Population of the Asiatic North, *J. Psychosom. Res.,* 24:39, 1980.
68. Sime, W. E., Buell, J. C., and Eliot, R. S.: Impact of Emotional Stress on Post MI Patients, *J. Hum. Stress,* 6(no. 3):39, 1980.
69. Eliot, R. S., and Buell, J. C.: The Role of the CNS in Cardiovascular Disorders, *Hosp. Practice,* 18(no. 5):189, 1983.
70. Eliot, R. S., Buell, J. C., and Dembroski, T. M.: Bio-Behavioural Perspectives on Coronary Heart Disease, Hypertension and Sudden Cardiac Death, *Acta Med. Scand.,* 660:203, 1982.
71. Harburg, E., Schull, W. J., Erfurt, J. C., and Schork, M.A.: A Family Set Method for Estimating Heredity and Stress: I. A Pilot Survey of Blood Pressure among Negroes in High and Low Stress Areas, Detroit, 1966–1967, *J. Chron. Dis.,* 23:69, 1970.
72. Gampel, B., Slome, C., Scotch, N., and Abramson, J. H.: Urbanization and Hypertension among Zulu Adults, *J. Chron. Dis.,* 15:67, 1962.
73. Ostfeld, A. M., Shekelle, R. B.: Psychological variables and blood pressure, in J. Stamler, R. Stamler, and T. N. Pullman (eds.), "Epidemiology of Hypertension," Grune & Stratton, N.Y., 1967, pp. 321–331.
74. Page, I. H.: Pathogenesis of Arterial Hypertension, *JAMA,* 140:451, 1949.
75. Alexander, F.: "Psychosomatic Medicine, Its Principles and Applications," W. W. Norton & Company, New York, 1950.
76. Esler, M., Julius, S., Zweifler, A., Randall, O., Harburg, E., Gardiner, H., and DeQuattro, V.: Mild High-Renin Essential Hypertension: Neurogenic Human Hypertension? *N. Engl. J. Med.,* 296:405, 1977.
77. deChamplain, J.: The Sympathetic System in Hypertension, in L. Landsberg (ed.), "Clinics in Endocrinology and Metabolism," vol. 6, "Catecholamines," W. B. Saunders Company, London, 1977, p. 633.
78. Light, K. C., Koepke, J. P., and Obriot, P. A.: Psychological Stress Induces Sodium and Fluid Retention in Men at High Risk for Hypertension, *Science,* 220:429, 1983.
79. Hartshorne, H.: On Heart Disease in the Army, *Am. J. Med. Sci.,* 48:89, 1864.
80. DaCosta, J. M.: On Irritable Heart: A Clinical Study of a Form of Functional Cardiac Disorder and Its Consequences, *Am. J. Med. Sci.,* 61:2, 1871.
81. Holmgren, A., Jonsson, B., Levander, L., Linderholm, H., Sjostrand, T., and Ström, G.: Low Physical Working Capacity in Suspected Heart Cases Due to Inadequate Adjustment of Peripheral Blood Flow (Vasoregulatory Asthenia), *Acta Med. Scand.,* 159:413, 1957.
82. Gorlin, R.: The Hyperkinetic Heart Syndrome, *JAMA,* 182:823, 1962.
83. Frohlich, E. D., Dustan, H. P., and Page, I. H.: Hyperdynamic Beta-Adrenergic Circulatory State, *Arch. Intern. Med.,* 117:614, 1966.
84. Cohen, M. E., Consolazio, F. C., and Johnson, R. E.: Blood Lactate Response during Moderate Exercise in Neurocirculatory Asthenia, Anxiety Neurosis or Effort Syndrome, *J. Clin. Invest.,* 26:339, 1947.
85. Wheeler, E. D., and Sheehan, D. V.: Emotional Stress: Cardiovascular Disease and Cardiovascular Symptoms, in J. W. Hurst, R. B. Logue, R. C. Schlant, and N. K. Wenger (eds.), "The Heart," 4th ed., McGraw-Hill Book Company, New York, 1978, p. 1802.
86. Christie, R. V.: Some Types of Respiration in the Neuroses, *Q. J. Med.,* 4:427, 1935.
87. Pitts, F. N., Jr., and McClure, J. N., Jr.: Lactate Metabolism in Anxiety Neurosis, *N. Engl. J. Med.,* 277:1329, 1967.
88. Kannel, W. B., Dawber, T. R., and Cohen, M. E.: The Electrocardiogram in Neurocirculatory Asthenia (Anxiety Neurosis or Neurasthenia): A Study of 203 Neurocirculatory Asthenia Patients and 757 Controls in the Framingham Study, *Ann. Intern. Med.,* 49:1351, 1958.
89. Levander-Lindgren, M.: Studies in Neurocirculatory Asthenia (DaCosta's Syndrome): 1. Variations with Regard to Symptoms and Some Pathophysiological Signs, *Acta Med. Scand.,* 172:665, 1962.
90. Moia, B.: Cardiac Neuroses: Recognition and Management,

in P. D. White (ed.), "International Cardiology," *Cardiovasc. Clin.* 2(3):221, 1971.
91. Friedman, M.: "Functional Cardiovascular Disease," The Williams & Wilkins Company, Baltimore, 1947.
92. Wooley, C. F.: Where Are the Diseases of Yesteryear? DaCosta's Syndrome, Soldier's Heart, the Effort Syndrome, Neurocirculatory Asthenia, and the Mitral Valve Prolapse Syndrome, *Circulation,* 53:749, 1976.
93. Boudoulas, H., Reynolds, J. C., Mazzaferri, E., and Wooley, C. F.: Metabolic Studies in Mitral Valve Prolapse Syndrome: A Neuroendocrine-Cardiovascular Process, *Circulation,* 61:1200, 1980.
94. Wolf, E., Braun, K., and Stern, S.: Effects of Beta-Receptor Blocking Agents Propranolol and Practolol on ST-T Changes in Neurocirculatory Asthenia, *Br. Heart J.,* 36:872, 1974.
95. Frohlich, E. D., Tarazi, R. D., and Dustan, H. P.: Hyperdynamic Beta-Adrenergic Circulatory State: Increased Beta-Receptor Responsiveness, *Arch. Intern. Med.,* 123:1, 1969.
96. Imhof, P., and Brunner, H.: The Treatment of Functional Heart Disorders with Beta-Adrenergic Blocking Agents, *Postgrad. Med. (Suppl.)* 46:96, 1970.
97. Vaisrub, S.: DaCosta Syndrome Revisited, *JAMA,* 232:164, 1975.
98. Wheeler, E. D., White, P. D., Reed, E. W., and Cohen, M. E.: Neurocirculatory Asthenia (Anxiety Neurosis, Effort Syndrome, Neurasthenia): A Twenty-Year Follow-Up Study of 173 Patients, *JAMA,* 142:878, 1950.
99. Wood, P.: "Diseases of the Heart and Circulation," 3d ed., J. B. Lippincott Company, Philadelphia, 1968, p. 1074.

82

Psychiatric Disorders in Cardiac Patients

Arthur M. Freeman III, M.D.
David G. Folks, M.D.

Impressive progress has been accomplished recently in the diagnosis and treatment of patients with coexisting psychiatric and cardiovascular disorders. Coronary artery disease, arrhythmia, mitral valve prolapse, end-stage cardiac disease, and hypertension are the major areas in which consultation psychiatrists have contributed to cardiology.[1] This chapter discusses each of these diagnostic entities as they are influenced by psychiatric disorders.

Myocardial Infarction and Angina

Various emotional characteristics of patients with angina and myocardial infarction (MI) have been noted by numerous observers.[2,3] Denial as a mechanism of psychological defense and mixed symptoms of anxiety and depression usually accompany the diagnosis of coronary artery disease, acute myocardial infarction, or recovery from an MI.

Instruments exist which are intended to measure psychological denial in patients with coronary disease. These scales utilize operational measures of reported fear and anxiety.[4] Denial, as we define it in cardiac patients, entails both suppression (conscious) and classical denial (unconscious). Investigators and clinicians, in attempting to examine the denial mechanism, run the risks of either eliciting more patient denial or disrupting the defense mechanism, thus distorting interpretation of the data. One way to view denial is as the inverse of overt anxiety.

The usefulness of the concept of denial becomes most apparent in the coronary care unit (CCU). Dimsdale et al.[4] and Gentry et al.[5] suggest that the ability to use denial in coping with an acute myocardial infarction is indispensable to the patient's initial prognosis and outcome. Those patients who are able to control their anxiety and remain hopeful have the best prognosis. The patient who uses positive denial is aware of the illness but minimizes the severity of the symptoms, remains hopeful about the outcome, and plans for the future. Physicians often encourage positive denial in the days immediately following an infarction and at other stressful times such as transfer from the coronary care unit or discharge from the hospital.

In contrast, negative or maladaptive denial is a defense mechanism which enables the patient to recognize that the illness exists but not to recognize its meaning or implications. This negative use of denial prevents the patient from seeking help, threatens the patient's survival in the coronary care unit, and interferes with cardiac rehabilitation. According to one study, as many as 20 percent of patients deny having had their first infarction.[6] Patients using negative denial were found to be less compliant, exhibiting early resumption of smoking, excessive eating, and premature return to work.

While we do not understand the mechanism of denial in precise terms, it is clearly of clinical significance. Further understanding of this mechanism may come from study of the personality types who deny or minimize their symptoms.

Although patients are likely to be impressed with medical technology in the coronary care unit, they are usually aware, at some level, of their precarious situation. Some degree of anxiety is useful or adaptive at all stages of an infarction by focusing a portion of patients' awareness on their illness and by alerting them to any potential complications.

Typically, the cardiac patient reacts to the experience of chest pain with major anxiety. If admitted to the hospital, the staff activity and monitoring equipment may even increase the symptoms of anxiety. Excessive anxiety may contribute to increased catecholamine secretion and potentially predispose the patient to the development of life-threatening arrhythmias. Anxiety almost always accompanies the patient's transfer from the unit to the general ward. Throughout this post-coronary care unit phase, anxiety persists in many patients, and, on discharge, persistent or excessive anxiety may disrupt adjustment to work and family life. The development of chronic anxiety is also commonly associated with a "homecoming depression."

For a variety of reasons, including the presence of denial, anxiety may be undertreated in patients who have experienced an MI. The conservative use of benzodiazepines with regularly scheduled office visits is often therapeutic, particularly for those patients in whom stress intensifies the symptoms. Anxiety may coexist with other emotional disorders such as phobias, panic attacks, depression, irritability, and passive-dependent behavior.

Anxiety and depression are usually found together. While anxiety occurs more during the acute course of the illness, depression has its onset typically in later stages. Denial may be more effective in reducing anxiety than preventing the onset of depression.[5] The "homecoming depression," occurring so frequently, resembles the grieving process. Depression causing dysfunction may occur in as many as 15 percent of MI patients.[7]

In some patients, the depressive symptoms occurring after an MI may have also preceded the event. Disruptions in marital, occupational, or social life are the cause of other depressive disorders. Some depressive states are "pseudodepressions" or states of weakness resulting from the patient's maintenance of the sick role. These more serious consequences of an infarction such as "pseudodepression" or "disability neurosis" can be just as threatening or destructive to rehabilitation as a "true" primary depression.[8]

A number of new treatment approaches exist for patients with postinfarction depression. Cardiac rehabilitation units may provide an environment in which formal and informal group therapy can flourish. Pharmacotherapy with psychotropic medications can improve the management of many patients who experience postinfarction depressions. Depression may be masked by anxiety, somatic complaints, personality traits, or the social status of some patients. In such patients, a significant postinfarction depression may go unrecognized and appropriate treatment not be instituted. Treatment of these more difficult cases usually requires careful diagnostic attention to all domains: biological, social, and psychological.

Coronary Bypass Surgery (see Chap. 45)

About 1 million coronary bypass operations have been performed. The operation relieves angina pectoris and prolongs the life of certain carefully selected patients with coronary disease.[9,10] The quality of life is improved in symptomatic patients who have the procedure compared to those treated medically.[11] Other considerations concerning the quality of life afforded by bypass surgery, as measured by overall psychosocial outcome and behavioral function, are also of major concern.[12] Psychiatric sequelae of coronary artery bypass surgery usually occur in three areas: affective, cognitive, and behavioral.

Coronary bypass patients may exhibit high levels of anxiety prior to surgery which can normally persist for 5 to 6 days postoperatively. In patients for whom symptoms of anxiety or depression existed prior to surgery, they usually will continue or, more commonly, exacerbate postoperatively. The long-term psychiatric symptoms, anxiety and depression, may be contrasted with the short-term cognitive symptoms which are more commonly observed in the immediate postoperative period.[13]

Symptoms of anxiety and depression tend to occur with increased frequency in patients exhibiting type A personality traits, in patients who experience forced retirement, and in patients with more severe coronary artery disease. An interesting study reported that a large percentage of bypass patients experience emotional impairment after surgery despite a good cardiac outcome.[14] Limited social life, lack of intimacy, unmet dependent strivings, and sexual dysfunction often coexist with symptoms of anxiety and depression.

Cognitive symptoms of confusion, disorientation, lability of affect, and hallucinations may occur transiently in bypass patients. Although numerous studies indicate a high incidence of such symptoms, improved surgical technique is probably responsible for a reduction in the incidence of cognitive impairment.[15] Postcardiotomy delirium is best understood according to a biopsychosocial model of illness. Some patients following surgery are confused and disoriented (biological). Others experience increased anxiety upon awakening in the coronary care unit which exacerbates the mild disorientation already present (psychological). Finally, some patients exhibit a clear interval for several days after surgery before developing a postoperative delirium (social, i.e., a reaction to the isolation of the hospital setting or intensive care unit environment). Other possible contributions to postoperative cognitive dysfunction include length of extracorporeal circulation, age, arterial pressure during surgery, postoperative cardiac output, type of heart disease, severity of preoperative illness, predisposing medications, and, perhaps the most important factor, the presence of emboli.

A study of the incidence of delirium in 100 inpatients who underwent coronary bypass surgery in the early 1970s revealed that disturbances of orientation, perception, and emotional responses were present in 28 percent with one-quarter of these patients developing a major episode of delirium.[16] The investigators found that the incidence of delirium was highly correlated with a previous history of infarction and the severity of the postoperative course in the recovery room.

Type A behavior continues to be a risk factor in the development of coronary artery disease; this behavioral pattern may also have implications for patients following coronary artery bypass surgery. Kahn et al.[17] reported that type A behavior ratings and a rise in intraoperative systolic and diastolic blood pressure from what was measured on admission were highly correlated. Medical complications (particularly arrhythmias), disabling anxiety, and significant depression have all been correlated with the presence of type A behavior in the coronary bypass patient. Hostility, assessed by a 50-item subscale of the Minnesota Multiphasic Personality Inventory, has also been shown to be associated with an increased risk of death, and preoperatively may contribute to the development of coronary atherosclerosis.[18–20]

Jenkins and colleagues, in studying behavioral changes and quality of life after bypass surgery, followed 318 patients for 6 months postoperatively at four university medical centers using 60 outcome measures.[21] In general, outcome was favorable at 6 months. Kornfeld and coworkers studied 100 patients up to 4½ years postoperatively and found that most of their patients had decreased angina and enhanced exercise capacity, resulting in increased general pleasure, as well as improvement in job and family roles. For as many as one-third of the patients, however, sexual adjustment was not improved.

Kornfeld and coworkers suggested that several areas of behavioral change occur in response to educational and group therapy programs. Smoking in their sample decreased from 39 percent preoperatively to 13 percent postoperatively.[16] A considerable number of patients increased their level of exercise. Other investigators have focused on ways to effect changes in type A behavior, especially in those patients exhibiting excessive levels of hostility or "pressured" personality patterns.[19]

Return to work has been extensively investigated in bypass patients. These studies have shown little agreement in terms of employment outcome.[22–25] In general, employment status prior to surgery, controlled for such factors as age, degree of angina, and educational level, still correlates best with postoperative return to work.[20–24,26–28] Absence of angina and dyspnea also correlate well with return to work.[12,24–30] Also, patients who see themselves as disabled preoperatively, or whose physicians support this belief, often will not attempt to return to work.[28]

Arrhythmias occur postoperatively in as many as 30 percent of coronary bypass patients.[31] Since intraoperative mortality and postoperative delirium are now seen less frequently, arrhythmias constitute the most significant immediate postoperative complication. The likelihood of arrhythmias occurring postoperatively may be increased by the presence of psychological distress. For example, Krantz et al.[32] and Zyzanski et al.[33] reported that type A behavior was associated with postoperative complications (mostly arrhythmias). Other studies have supported the hypothesis that psychological stress and arrhythmias are linked, perhaps by the mechanism of denial.[34] Lown[35] has demonstrated that psychologically induced stress can precipitate ventricular arrhythmias in predisposed patients.

Consistent with the findings relating type A behavior to perioperative arrhythmias, high ratings on factor H (hard-driving) of the Jenkins Activity Survey have been correlated with ventricular arrhythmias.[34] Of even greater importance is the possible relation of certain personality traits to all types of postoperative morbidity. The hostility scale and other previously mentioned behavioral findings support the opinion that therapeutic interventions in type A individuals with coronary artery disease should focus on the more destructive subcomponents of the personality behavior, such as hostility or the hard-driving component of the Jenkins Activity Survey.

Further Treatment Considerations

Treatment for patients recovering from myocardial infarction or cardiac surgery can be divided into psychosocial and psychopharmacological approaches. Cardiac rehabilitation programs emphasize exercise as the means to rehabilitation, but these centers also provide psychosocial support. Increased exercise tolerance leads to enhanced self-esteem, as does the companionship of others also participating in the rehabilitation. At times, more formal psychotherapy is indicated. If problems occur in the patient's marriage or family life, specific psychotherapies can address the patient's concerns. Individual psychotherapy may also be essential for some patients whose problems are more psychological.

Syndromes of combined anxiety and depression often respond to pharmacological treatment with anxiolytics or antidepressants. Benzodiazepines can be especially beneficial and are probably underutilized in this population. They are not cardiotoxic, and their only significant drug interaction is with other central nervous system depressants. Triazolobenzodiazepines, a new class of benzodiazepines, may also have specific antidepressant effects as well as anxiolytic effects.[36] Tricyclic antidepressants have been underused in cardiac patients because of physicians' fears about their potential toxicities. Much of the concern about these drugs is related to their effects following overdose rather than their effects in therapeutic concentrations. Instead of being arrhythmogenic, some of these compounds actually exert a quinidine-like effect on cardiac rhythm.[37] The tricyclic antidepressant drugs will only minimally depress the myocardium. Some delay of distal conduction occurs with these compounds. The only major clinical effect is orthostatic hypotension.[38] Side effects of the newer antidepressants, for example, exacerbation of preexisting ventricular arrhythmia by trazodone or precipitation of seizures by maprotiline, are rare; both of these drugs have added to our therapeutic potential. Nomifensine and bupropion are promising new antidepressants which may have even fewer cardiovascular side effects than currently available compounds.[39]

Cardiac Transplantation

Cardiac transplantation has been restored recently as a therapeutic option for some patients largely because of the use of cyclosporine A. Anxiety, depression, altered self-image, and organic mental symptoms have been reported in patients undergoing cardiac transplantation.[40,41] Potential compliance, substance abuse, family dysfunction, psychosis, and mental retardation are psychiatric issues which may influence the decision to transplant.[42,43] Some patients and their families may require psychotherapy.[44] Although steroid psychoses may become less frequent with the new immunosuppressive therapy, other psychiatric syndromes following cardiac transplantation will gain the attention of physicians.

Mitral Valve Prolapse

The development of the concept of mitral valve prolapse (MVP) syndrome from that of a neuropsychiatric disorder to that of an anatomic abnormality with pathophysiological findings spans the past decade.[45] Clinical knowledge of the mitral valve prolapse syndrome is still growing, and controlled studies have provided a better understanding of the cardiac symptoms and the importance of accompanying psychiatric symptoms.

DaCosta reported on "irritable heart" in his descriptions of cases of Civil War combatants who presented with symptoms of palpitations, chest pains, and syncope or near syncope precipitated by exertion. Levine, who participated in the British study of irritable heart or effort syndrome, suggested that this entity be termed *neurocirculatory asthenia.* Symptoms and their physiological correlates were later emphasized by a number of clinicians and the syndrome was renamed the *hyperdynamic beta-adrenergic circulatory state.* In 1963 Barlow et al.[46] related the auscultatory findings to the aneurysmal protrusion of the posterior leaflet of the mitral valve into the left atrium. This work resulted in numerous psychiatric and cardiologic studies of symptomatic mitral valve prolapse.

A high prevalence of mitral valve prolapse was initially reported as being found in patients with a variety of anxiety and sleep disorders.[47–49] There are several similarities between the epidemiology of MVP syndrome and that of anxiety neurosis. These include female predominance, an incidence of 5 to 10 percent, onset before age 35 in most cases, and evidence of a hereditary influence.[50,51] These similarities led to Wooley's[50] suggestion that many patients diagnosed with panic disorder are actually suffering from the MVP syndrome. Later studies demonstrated that the neuropsychiatric symptoms commonly attributed to MVP are as frequent among patients with MVP as without MVP.[52–57] Nonetheless, patients with primary MVP syndrome continue to be perceived by cardiologists as "anxious" or "depressed" more frequently than those patients with asymptomatic MVP or with cardiovascular disease without MVP. Thus, the multitude of reports demonstrating increased prevalence of panic disorder or anxiety neurosis in MVP patients may be due to selection bias to include highly symptomatic individuals.[54] Recent studies support the idea that two distinct syndromes exist, one a genuine cardiac disorder, the other an anxiety disorder.[52,58–60] Thus, searching for MVP syndrome in patients presenting with symptoms of anxiety is exceedingly important as it may help make a distinction between the psychological and physiological components of the presentation.[58,59]

Since recent psychobiological findings now point to a dual autonomic dysfunction in the MVP syndrome and support the hypothesis of an abnormality in adrenergic control mechanisms, optimal treatment may be tailored more specifically to the underlying disorder. The precise relation between the anatomic abnormality, autonomic adrenergic dysfunction, and psychiatric symptoms in these patients requires further clarification.

Education is probably the single most effective therapeutic maneuver for patients with the MVP syndrome. Rational explanation and reassurance may serve to allay disabling anxiety. Similarities in therapeutic approaches to MVP syndrome and panic disorder or anxiety neurosis include reassurance, support, and patient education. Treatment of MVP syndrome often includes pharmacological intervention aimed at modulation of abnormal sympathetic or parasympathetic activity.[60] An initial intervention of this type can then be followed by any additional psychiatric intervention required, including psychotherapy or pharmacotherapy with anxiolytics.

Hypertension

Compliance in patients treated with antihypertensive agents, psychological side effects of antihypertensive medications, and treatment of coexisting psychiatric illness in hypertensives are discussed in this section. Other behavioral aspects of hypertension, i.e., the psychological antecedents of the hypertensive state and the relationship between stress, personality type, and the development of hypertension are discussed in Chap. 49.

Compliance is defined as the extent to which an identified patient's behavior coincides with the prescriptions and proscriptions of a medical regimen.[61] *Noncompliance* is defined as any deviation from the medical regimen, including missing appointments, medication noncompliance, or failure to change harmful aspects of life-style. Fifty percent medication compliance may be the mean.[62–64] Two effective strategies which have been most helpful in increasing compliance are educational and behavioral.[61] Educational strategies are those that attempt to transmit information about the hypertensive illness and its treatment. Compliance often improves in response to health messages, written instructions, counseling by nurse specialists, or structured classes. Behavioral strategies are designed to increase compliance by an attempt to control the antecedents of compliance behavior or ultimately by rewarding and reinforcing compliance behavior. Feedback of serum drug levels, positive reinforcement of the taking of medications, and patient self-monitoring of medication-taking behavior or of symptom responsiveness have not been particularly effective practices for improving compliance.[65] Self-regulation with blood pressure checks and tailoring of drug regimens appear to be the more promising behavioral strategies for increasing compliance behavior.[61,63,65,66]

Psychiatric complications induced by antihypertensive medications are of great concern to clinicians treating hypertensive patients. Pseudodepression, which may be a serious side effect of some antihypertensive agents, is the psychological response to psychomotor retardation or sedation caused by an antihypertensive medication.[67] As many as three-fourths of the depressive episodes resulting from antihypertensive medications are likely to be pseudodepression.[68] True depressive syndromes have also been shown to occur about 5 months after the initiation of some antihypertensive agents, with reserpine being the most common offender. Other reports regarding psychological side effects or complications of antihypertensive agents have been reviewed and summarized by Paykel et al.[69] and Moss and Procci.[70] Unrecognized depression and sexual dysfunction resulting from antihypertensive agents are the most common psychiatric complications reviewed by these authors. Careful psychiatric history gathering before initiation of an antihypertensive agent can be preventative or predictive of psychiatric complications, as is determining any past history of depression or sexual dysfunction that might suggest a patient's vulnerability to complications with antihypertensive drug treatment. A family history of depression may also be a useful factor in identifying those patients at risk for developing an affective disorder. Other treatment for hypertension such as diet, salt restriction, exercise, or behavioral therapy may also be indicated for certain patients with coexisting hypertension and depression.

Physicians may expect that about 15 percent of patients who are psychiatrically disordered will also be hypertensive. Since drug treatment for hypertension has been shown to induce or exacerbate numerous psychiatric symptoms, consultations between treating physicians and psychiatrists should occur when assessing the relative benefits of antihypertensive and/or antidepressant treatment.[71] In a study of 452 psychiatric outpatients, major depression was three times as common among those with hypertension.[72] This difference was not accounted for by age, sex, chronic medical illness, or current antihypertensive medications. Thus, the higher rate of depression among hypertensive patients supports a clinically important relation between the two syndromes. In many studies the contrast between the 37 percent prevalence of depression in hypertensive patients and the 4 to 12 percent prevalence occurring in the general population has been presented.[72] In summary, four possible factors have been suggested by Huapaya and Ananth[67] to account for such a high prevalence of depression in hypertensive patients. These include (1) common etiology, (2) depression resulting from chronic illness, (3) depressive symptoms caused by antihypertensive medications, and (4) a chance association. The neurobiological linkage between antihypertensive medications and depressive illness, although partially understood, requires further elucidation.

Acknowledgments

We wish to express our appreciation to Lil Hicks and Vanna O'Neal for their help with manuscript preparation.

References

1. Freeman, A. M., and Folks, D. G.: Psychiatric Aspects of Cardiovascular Disease, in J. O. Cavenar and R. Michels (eds.), "Psychiatry," J. B. Lippincott, Philadelphia, in press.
2. Jenkins, C. D.: Recent Evidence Supporting Psychologic and Social Risk Factors for Coronary Disease (Second of Two Parts), *N. Engl. J. Med.*, 294:1033, 1976.
3. Stern, M. J., Pascale, L., and McLoone, J.: Psychosocial Adaptation following an Acute Myocardial Infarction, *J. Chron. Dis.*, 29:513, 1976.
4. Dimsdale, J. E., and Hackett, T. P.: Effect of Denial on Cardiac Health and Psychological Assessment, *Am. J. Psychiatry*, 139:11:1477, 1982.
5. Gentry, W. D., Foster, S., and Haney, T.: Denial as a Determinant of Anxiety and Perceived Health Status in the Coronary Care Unit, *Psychosom. Med.*, 34(1):39, 1972.
6. Croog, S. H., Shapiro, D. S., and Levine, S.: Denial among Male Heart Patients: An Empirical Study, *Psychosom. Med.*, 33:385, 1971.

7. Wishnie, H. A., Hackett, T. P., and Cassem, N. M.: Psychological Hazards of Convalescence following Myocardial Infarction, *JAMA,* 215:1292, 1971.
8. Ford, C. V.: Disability Syndromes, in "The Somatizing Disorders: Illness As A Way Of Life," Elsevier Biomedical, New York, 1984, p. 176.
9. Hall, R. J., Elayda, M. A., Gray, A., et al.: Coronary Artery Bypass: Long-Term Follow-Up of 22,284 Consecutive Patients, *Circulation,* 68(suppl. 2):20, 1983.
10. Schaff, H. V., Gersh, B. J., Pluth, J. R., et al.: Survival and Functional Status after Coronary Artery Bypass Grafting: Results 10 to 12 Years after Surgery in 500 Patients, *Circulation,* 68(suppl. 2):200, 1983.
11. CASS Principal Investigators and Their Associates: Coronary Artery Surgery Study (CASS): A Randomized Trial of Coronary Artery Bypass Surgery—Quality of Life in Patients Randomly Assigned to Treatment Groups, *Circulation,* 68:951, 1983.
12. LaMendola, W. F., and Pellegrini, R. V.: Quality of Life and Coronary Artery Bypass Surgery Patients, *Soc. Sci. Med.,* 13A:457, 1979.
13. Rabiner, C. J., and Willner, A. E.: Psychopathology Observed on Follow-Up after Coronary Bypass Surgery, *J. Nerv. Ment. Dis.,* 163:295, 1976.
14. Gundle, M. D., Reeves, B. R., Tate, S., Raft, D., and McLaurin, L. P.: Psychosocial Outcome after Coronary Artery Surgery, *Am. J. Psychiatry,* 137:1591, 1980.
15. Willner, A. E., and Rabiner, C. J.: Psychopathology and Cognitive Dysfunction Five Years after Open-Heart Surgery, *Compr. Psychiatry,* 20:409, 1979.
16. Kornfeld, D. S., Heller, S. S., Frank, K. A., Edie, R. N., and Corsa, J.: Psychological and Behavioral Responses after Coronary Artery Bypass Surgery, *Circulation,* 66(suppl. 3):24, 1982.
17. Kahn, J. P., Kornfeld, D. S., Frank, K. A., Heller, S. S., and Hoar, P. F.: Type A Behavior and Blood Pressure during Coronary Artery Bypass Surgery, *Psychosom. Med.,* 42:407, 1980.
18. Williams, R. B., Haney, T. L., Lee, K. L., Kong, Y. H., Blumenthal, J. A., and Whalen, R. E.: Type A Behavior, Hostility, and Coronary Atherosclerosis, *Psychosom. Med.,* 42:539, 1980.
19. Cottier, C., Adler, R., Vorkauf, H., Gerber, R., Hefer, T., and Hürney, C.: Pressured Pattern or Type A Behavior in Patients with Peripheral Arteriovascular Disease: Controlled Retrospective Exploratory Study, *Psychosom. Med.,* 45:187, 1983.
20. Shekelle, R. B., Gale, M., Ostfeld, A. M., and Oglesby, P.: Hostility, Risk of Coronary Heart Disease, and Mortality, *Psychosom. Med.,* 45:109, 1983.
21. Jenkins, C. D., Stanton, B., Savageau, J. A., and Harken, D. E.: Coronary Artery Bypass Surgery: Physical, Psychological, Social, and Economic Outcomes Six Months Later, *JAMA,* 250:782, 1983.
22. English, M. T., Logan, G. A., Eyer, K. M., Hammermeister, K. E., and Kennedy, J. W.: Employment following Coronary Artery Bypass Graft Surgery, *Circulation,* 51–52(suppl. 2):566, 1975.
23. Barnes, G. K., Ray, M. J., Oberman, A., and Kouchoukos, N. T.: Changes in Working Status of Patients following Coronary Bypass Surgery, *JAMA,* 238:1259, 1979.
24. Boulay, F. M., David, P. P., and Bourassa, M. G.: Strategies for Improving the Work Status of Patients after Coronary Artery Bypass Surgery, *Circulation,* 66(suppl. 3):43, 1982.
25. Zyzanski, S. J., Rouse, B. A., Stanton, B. A., and Jenkins, C. D.: Employment Changes among Patients following Coronary Bypass Surgery: Social, Medical, and Psychological Correlates, *Public Health Rep.,* 97:558, 1982.
26. Oberman, A., and Kouchoukos, N. T.: Working Status of Patients following Coronary Bypass Surgery, *Am. Heart,* 98:132, 1979.
27. Wayne, J. B., Oberman, A., Kouchoukos, N. T., Charles, E. D., Barnes, G. K., and Russell, R. O., Jr.: Occupation, Employment and Coronary Artery Disease, *Circulation,* 62(suppl. 3):353, 1980.
28. Almeida, D., Bradford, J. M., Wenger, N. K., King, S. B., and Hurst, J. W.: Return to Work after Coronary Bypass Surgery, *Circulation,* 68(suppl. 2):205, 1983.
29. Symmes, J. C., Lenkei, S. C., and Berman, N. D.: Influence of Aortocoronary Bypass Surgery on Employment, *Can. Med. J.,* 118:268, 1978.
30. Kimball, C.: A Predictive Study of Adjustment to Cardiac Surgery, *J. Thorac. Cardiovasc. Surg.,* 58:891, 1969.
31. Waldo, A. L., MacLean, W. A., Cooper, T. B., Kouchoukos, N. T., and Karp, R. B.: The Use of Temporarily Placed Epicardial Atrial Wire Electrodes for the Diagnosis and Treatment of Cardiac Arrhythmias following Open Heart Surgery, *J. Thorac. Cardiovasc. Surg.,* 76:500, 1978.
32. Krantz, D. S., Arabian, J. M., Davin, J. E., and Parker, J. S.: Type A Behavior and Coronary Bypass Surgery: Intraoperative Blood Pressure and Perioperative Complications, *Psychosom. Med.,* 44:273, 1982.
33. Zyzanski, S. J., Stanton, B. A., Jenkins, C. D., and Klein, M. D.: Medical and Psychosocial Outcomes in Survivors of Major Heart Surgery, *J. Psychosom. Res.,* 25:213, 1981.
34. Freeman, A. M., Fleece, L., Folks, D. G., Cohen-Cole, S. A., Waldo, A.: Psychiatric Symptoms, Type A Behavior and Arrhythmias following Coronary Artery Bypass Surgery, *Psychosomatics,* 25:586, 1984.
35. Lown, B., and DeSilva, R. A.: Role of Psychologic Stress and Autonomic Nervous System Changes in Provocation of Ventricular Premature Complexes, *Am. J. Cardiol.,* 41:979, 1978.
36. Feighner, J. P.: Open Label Study of Alprazolam in Severely Depressed Patients, *J. Clin. Psychiatry,* 44:332, 1983.
37. Bigger, J. T., Giardina, E. G., Perel, J., Kantor, S. J., and Glassman, A. H.: Cardiac Antiarrhythmic Effect of Imipramine Hydrochloride, *N. Engl. J. Med.,* 296:200, 1977.
38. Glassman, A. H., Johnson, L. L., Giardina, E. G. V., et al.: The Use of Imipramine in Depressed Patients with Congestive Heart Failure, *JAMA,* 250:1997, 1983.
39. Goldstein, B. J., Brauzer, B., Kentsmith, D., Rosenthal, S., and Charalampous, K. D.: Double-blind Placebo-Controlled Multicenter Evaluation of the Efficacy and Safety of Nomifensine in Depressed Outpatients, *J. Clin. Psychiatry,* 45:52, 1984.
40. Kraft, I.: Psychiatric Complications of Cardiac Transplantation, *Semin. Psychiatry,* 3:58, 1971.
41. Molish, B., Kraft, I., and Wiggins, P.: Psychodiagnostic Evaluation of the Heart Transplant Patient, *Semin. Psychiatry,* 3:46, 1971.
42. Freeman, A. M., Watts, D., and Karp, R.: Evaluation of Cardiac Transplant Candidates: Preliminary Observations, *Psychosomatics,* 25:197, 1984.
43. Watts, D., Freeman, A. M., McVay, R., Karp, R., Kirklin, J. K., and McGiffin, D. G.: Psychiatric Aspects of Cardiac Transplantation: Assessment and Management, *Heart Transplantation,* 3(3):243, 1984.
44. Christopherson, L.: Cardiac Transplantation Need for Patient Counseling, *Nurs. Mirror,* 143:34, 1976.
45. Wooley, C. F.: Where Are the Diseases of Yesteryear? DaCosta's Syndrome, Soldier's Heart, the Effort Syndrome, Neurocirculatory Asthenia and the Mitral Valve Prolapse Syndrome, *Circulation,* 53:749, 1976.
46. Barlow, J. B., Pocock, W. A., Marchand, P., and Denny, M.: The Significance of Late Systolic Murmurs, *Am. Heart J.,* 66:443, 1963.
47. Crowe, R. R., Pauls, D. L., Slymen, D. J., and Noyes, R.: A Family Study of Anxiety Neurosis: Morbidity Risk in Families of Patients with and without Mitral Valve Prolapse, *Arch. Gen. Psychiatry,* 37:77, 1980.
48. Pariser, S. F., Pinta, E. R., and Jones, B. A.: Mitral Valve Prolapse Syndrome and Anxiety Neurosis/Panic Disorder, *Am. J. Psychiatry,* 135:246, 1978.
49. Venkatesh, A., Pauls, D. L., Crowe, R., et al.: Mitral Valve Prolapse in Anxiety Neurosis (Panic Disorder), *Am. Heart J.,* 100:302, 1980.
50. Wooley, C. F.: The Mitral Valve Prolapse Syndrome, *Hosp. Practice,* 18(6):163, 1983.
51. Savage, D. D., Garrison, R. J., Devereux, R. B., et al.: Mitral

Valve Prolapse in the General Population. 1. Epidemiologic Features: The Framingham Study, *Am. Heart J.*, 106:571, 1983.
52. Uretski, B. F.: Does Mitral Valve Prolapse Cause Nonspecific Symptoms?, *Intl. J. Cardiology*, 1:435, 1982.
53. Szmuilowicz, J., and Flannery, J. G.: Mitral Valve Prolapse Syndrome and Psychological Disturbance, *Psychosomatics*, 21:419, 1980.
54. Hartman, W., Kramer, R., Brown, T., and Devereux, R. B.: Panic Disorder in Patients with Mitral Valve Prolapse, *Am. J. Psychiatry*, 139:669, 1982.
55. Mavissakalian, M., Salerni, R., Thompson, M. E., and Michelson, L.: Mitral Valve Prolapse and Agoraphobia, *Am. J. Psychiatry*, 140:1612, 1983.
56. Savage, D. D., Devereux, R. B., and Garrison, R. J.: Clinical Features: The Framingham Study, *Am. Heart J.*, 106:577, 1983.
57. Savage, D. D., Levy, D., and Garrison, R. J.: Dysrhythmias: The Framingham Study, *Am. Heart J.*, 106:582, 1983.
58. Weinstein, G., Allen, G., and Ford, C. V.: Anxiety and Mitral Valve Prolapse Syndrome, *J. Clin. Psychol.*, 43:33, 1982.
59. Folks, D. G.: Symptomatic Mitral Valve Prolapse and Diagnostic Considerations (letter), *South. Med. J.*, 77:479, 1984.
60. Coghlan, H. C., Phares, P., Cowley, M., et al.: Dysautonomia in Mitral Valve Prolapse, *Am. J. Med.*, 67:236, 1979.
61. Houpt, J. L., Orleans, C. S., George, L. K., and Brodie, H. K.: Lifestyle and Medical Illness: Noncompliance with Prescribed Medical Regimens, in "The Importance of Mental Health Services to General Health Care," Ballinger, Cambridge, 1979, p. 201.
62. Ksal, S. V.: Social-Psychological Characteristics Associated with Behaviors Which Reduce Cardiovascular Risk, in A. J. Enelow and J. B. Henderson (eds.), "Applying Behavioral Science to Cardiovascular Risk," American Hospital Association, Washington, 1975, p. 173.
63. Sackett, D. L., and Haynes, R. B. (eds.): "Compliance With Therapeutic Regimens," Johns Hopkins Press, Baltimore, 1976.
64. Sackett, D. L.: The Magnitude of Compliance, in A. C. Abbot et al. (ed.), "A Workshop/Symposium on Compliance," McMaster Medical Center, Hamilton, Ontario, 1977.
65. Epstein, L. H., and Cluss, P. A.: A Behavioral Perspective on Adherence to Long-Term Medical Regimens, *J. Consult. Clin. Psychol.*, 50:950, 1982.
66. Engel, B. T., Glasgow, M. S., and Gaarder, K. R.: Behavioral Treatment of High Blood Pressure: III. Follow-Up Results and Treatment Recommendations, *Psychosom. Med.*, 45:23, 1983.
67. Huapaya, L., and Ananth, J.: Depression Associated with Hypertension: A Review, *Psychiatr. J. Univ. Ottawa*, 5:58, 1980.
68. Goodwin, F. K., Ebert, M. H., and Bunney, W. E., Jr.: Mental Effects of Reserpine in Man, in R. I. Shader (ed.), "Psychiatric Complications of Medical Drugs," Raven Press, New York, 1972.
69. Paykel, E. S., Fleminger, R., and Watson, J. P.: Psychiatric Side Effects of Antihypertensive Drugs Other than Reserpine, *J. Clin. Psychopharm.*, 2:14, 1982.
70. Moss, H. B., and Procci, W. R.: Sexual Dysfunction Associated with Oral Antihypertensive Medication: A Critical Survey of the Literature, *Gen. Hosp. Psych.*, 4:121, 1982.
71. Goldberg, E. L., Comstock, G. W., and Graves, C. G.: Psychosocial Factors and Blood Pressure, *Psychol. Med.*, 10:243, 1980.
72. Rabkin, J. G., Charles, E., and Kass, F.: Hypertension and DSM-III Depression in Psychiatric Outpatients, *Am. J. Psychol.*, 140:1072, 1983.

83

Iatrogenic "Heart Disease"

Peter C. Gazes, M.D.   J. Willis Hurst, M.D.

In the last two decades there has been a tremendous growth of interest in electrocardiographic diagnosis and in the number and variety of electrocardiographs in use. In 1914, there was only one instrument of this kind in the State of Michigan, and this was not in operation; there were probably no more than a dozen electrocardiographs in the whole of the United States. Now there is one or more in almost every village of any size, and there are comparatively few people who are not in greater danger of having their peace and happiness destroyed by an erroneous diagnosis of cardiac abnormality based on a faulty interpretation of an electrocardiogram, than of being injured or killed by an atomic bomb.

Frank Wilson, 1951[1,*]

Iatrogenic "heart disease" implies that the patient has a condition that is physician-induced.[2–5] The word *iatro* is derived from the Greek word *iatros,* which means physician. The term *iatrogenic heart disease* is not a good one. It implicates the physician in an unfair way. Many patients who actually have no heart disease but assume they have heart disease after visiting a physician have emotional problems as the basis for their visit and their false assumptions. The same applies to many patients who, after visiting a physician, assume they are more disabled than they really are. The knowledge that emotionally disturbed patients are likely to misinterpret the words, actions, and demeanor of physicians and their personnel should, however, make physicians and the people who work with them sensitive to all that is done and said in the office and hospital. Iatrogenic heart disease that is the result of drugs or procedures is not necessarily the physician's fault. There is a definite complication rate related to the use of all drugs and procedures. Physicians try to keep these complications to a minimum, but the finest physi-

*Reproduced with permission from the publisher.

cians in the world will have a finite number of complications as a result of their treatment. The only way physicians can avoid the complications of modern medicine is to do nothing. This would, of course, prevent the physicians from bringing the benefits of modern medicine to their patients.

This discussion will deal with (1) iatrogenic heart disease resulting from statements or actions of physicians or their personnel; (2) iatrogenic heart disease related to the workup and treatment of patients; (3) patients with known heart disease who develop a cardiac phobia because of a physician, and (4) the prevention and treatment of iatrogenic heart disease.

Iatrogenic Heart Disease Resulting from the Statements or Actions of Physicians or Their Personnel

Whenever possible, patients should leave the physician's office or hospital feeling better about themselves than when they arrived. This goal is usually accomplished, but there are three reasons why it is not always accomplished. First of all, physicians may have to give bad news to patients and their families, and sometimes the ravages of disease continue on. Second, many patients are emotionally disturbed from the outset. This may be the real reason they seek medical advice. Some of these patients will misinterpret every word and action they hear and observe. They are likely to leave the office or hospital even more convinced that they have heart disease, or that their heart disease is worse than they thought it was, despite all the reassurance the physician gives. Third, the physician or the personnel may say or do something that would ordinarily cause no emotional reaction but does cause a reaction in an emotionally disturbed patient. Some examples of the responses these patients may have are given below.

An admitting clerk, trying to comfort a patient with small talk, once said, "Oh, I see you have heart disease. We will have you transported to the floor in a wheelchair." Hospital rules had demanded that the physician write down a "diagnosis" before admitting the patient. The physician had obtained a history from the patient on the telephone that suggested the presence of pulmonary edema and so admitted the patient to the hospital with a diagnosis of acute "heart failure." The patient, in reality, had hyperventilation. The emotionally disturbed patient remembered and doted on the admitting clerk's statement despite the physician's best efforts at reassurance.

The technician who records the ECG can make inappropriate remarks. One said, "You have funny looking T waves—do you feel all right?" The patient assumed she had serious heart disease. The patient chose to believe the technician rather than her physician because she thought her physician was trying to spare her the "bad news."

Some emotionally disturbed patients may be alarmed because the physician listens to their heart longer than usual, takes the blood pressure twice, takes the blood pressure in all four extremities, makes an ECG in the recumbent position and standing, repeats an x-ray of the chest, calls them on the telephone to see if they are feeling well, etc.

Some patients assume that they have serious heart disease because their physician looks over at an associate or house officer during the time he or she is examining the patient.

Patients are usually comforted by words such as *accurate, safe, gentle, definite,* and *protected.* They are disturbed by words and sentences such as, "We will have to *repeat the test,* the laboratory made another *error*"; "The monitor *won't work* and I am having a terrible time getting it repaired"; "It is a *rough procedure*"; "That's *not a safe test*"; "We *cannot be sure*"; "You have a *time bomb* in your chest"; *floppy valve; malignant hypertension; heart failure; physiological; organic;* and many others.

Patients with heart disease may assume they are more disabled than they are. This occurs because everyone is not aware of the emotional steps the patient goes through following a myocardial infarction or the discovery of a serious condition that requires an alteration of activity. Patients may exhibit the phase of denial, the phase of acceptance, the phase of anxiety and fear, the phase of dependence, the phase of depression, and the phase of realistic adaptation. The physician must recognize and assist the patient through all of these phases of recovery. Not to do so will allow the patients to assume that they are "sicker" than they are.

Many of the rules and regulations that are imposed by government agencies and private insurance companies compound the problem in that many patients will have a better financial "deal" when they accept medical disability and retirement than when they are permitted to work. When this occurs, it augments the patients' beliefs that they are more disabled than they are.

This short discussion is far from complete and includes only *examples* of the problems that can occur in sensitive patients as a result of the action, words, or demeanor of physicians and their personnel.

Iatrogenic Heart Disease Related to the Workup and Treatment of a Patient

The goal of all physicians is to work up and treat patients without causing harm. No physician is smart enough to be all-knowing and perfect. Therefore, despite the physician's best intentions and perfectly executed actions, there will be a few complications associated with the workup and treatment of patients. Here again, it is not always the physician's fault. The patient may discontinue the use of propranolol that is needed only to find the "rebound" effect on the heart is undesirable. A patient may postpone surgery that has been recommended until the risk of surgery is greater than it would have been earlier.

The Misinterpretations of Data

The misinterpretation of symptoms, signs, and laboratory data may create iatrogenic heart disease. (See Chaps. 7 to 13.)

Symptoms and Signs

It has been difficult for physicians to accept that their diagnosis of angina pectoris due to coronary atherosclerosis may be wrong when it is based solely on the analysis of the patient's symptoms. Ten to twenty percent of patients with angina pectoris produced by effort do not have atherosclerotic coronary heart disease. When the chest discomfort is not definitely related to effort, the diagnostic error rate is about 20 percent or more. The ability to diagnose angina pectoris due to atherosclerotic coronary heart disease in women is even poorer; error rates of 30 percent are common. The error is made when physicians assume that patients have atherosclerotic coronary heart disease when they do not have it. Accordingly, iatrogenic coronary heart disease has been very common in the past. However, iatrogenic coronary heart disease occurs less often now than formerly because coronary arteriography and other techniques have been developed and are commonly used to establish an accurate diagnosis.

Many patients with normal hearts complain of shortness of breath. Often their complaint is not dyspnea but inability to get enough air, described as a slow, deep, sighing respiration. Such dyspnea due to anxiety or dyspnea due to pulmonary disease may be incorrectly attributed to heart disease and treated with digitalis. Episodes of hyperventilation may be misdiagnosed as acute pulmonary edema.

Palpitation due to an occasional ectopic contraction may be disabling to a sensitive patient and thought to be ominous by the physician. Premature beats are very common, even in many persons without other evidence of heart disease. Benign arrhythmias, such as sinus arrhythmia, may be diagnosed as a serious abnormality of cardiac rhythm.

A diagnosis of essential hypertension may be made and the patient treated for it simply because the blood pressure is elevated on a single recording.

Kinking of the carotid artery may be misdiagnosed as an aneurysm of the artery.

Innocent murmurs are often attributed to heart disease. The midsystolic click and late systolic murmur of mitral valve prolapse may be considered to be an ominous condition, whereas it is usually benign.

Rales are not specific for heart failure and can be due to a variety of bronchorespiratory diseases. The wheezing of bronchitis may be misinterpreted as due to left-sided heart failure.

Hepatomegaly is not considered to be present unless the distance between the liver's flat, percussed upper border and its palpable lower edge is more than 11 cm. Right-sided heart failure is often misdiagnosed because the liver is palpable (due to a low diaphragm) and edema due to venous stasis is present. Peripheral edema is most unusual in heart failure unless cardiomegaly, hepatomegaly, and neck vein distension are present. Edema of the extremities secondary to obesity, hormonal administration, menopause, garters, or venous insufficiency may be wrongly attributed to congestive heart failure.

The Electrocardiogram

The normal range of the electrocardiogram is difficult to learn. A normal tracing does not exclude heart disease, and an abnormal tracing does not necessarily indicate heart disease. Many benign ST-T wave "abnormalities" at rest or with exercise are, unfortunately, attributed to heart disease. QRS conduction abnormalities, such as occur with the Wolff-Parkinson-White syndrome, may be misdiagnosed as myocardial infarction. Occasionally myocardial infarction may be correctly diagnosed by electrocardiography, but from a tracing that belongs to someone else. Reversal of the arm leads, if not recognized, can be misinterpreted as a disease state. Dr. Frank Wilson, one of the great contributors to electrocardiography, wrote the paragraph quoted at the beginning of this chapter in 1951, in order to emphasize his concern that erroneous and frightening diagnoses could result from the improper interpretation of the ECG. (See Chaps. 14 and 98.)

Chest X-Ray

Concentric hypertrophy may not be evident on chest x-ray. A normal transverse heart, especially in a poor inspiratory film, may be considered as being enlarged. In addition, the apparent enlargement may be due to a depressed sternum or an epicardial fat pad. The pulmonary artery may be normally prominent when the heart is vertically placed, and this may be misinterpreted as an abnormality. (See Chap. 15.)

The Echocardiogram and Doppler Echocardiography

There still remain patients in whom satisfactory echocardiograms cannot be obtained. The interpreter must have knowledge of the technique's limitations and capabilities, otherwise misinterpretations of tracings will occur. Physicians with inadequate training frequently overread tracings. In addition, the echocardiogram is now creating its own problems; for instance, a physician may overreact to the echocardiographic diagnosis of mitral valve prolapse, and this may lead to the disability of the patient.

Doppler echocardiography provides information concerning the direction and quality of blood flow at known sites within the heart and great vessels. As yet the significance of some flow disturbances in normal individuals has not been determined. The orifice of origin need not be anatomically abnormal, since abnormally high flow through a normal-sized orifice may cause a flow disturbance. Likewise the significance of mild regurgitant murmurs noted by Doppler in patients with no diagnostic physical findings needs further evaluation. Flow velocity profiles vary with the anatomic site as well as with severity of disease, and cross-sectional area measurement can be fraught with errors. These and other problems should be corrected with improvements in instrumentation. (See Chaps. 120 to 122.)

Radionuclide Studies
Radionuclide studies are now being performed in most hospitals. Unfortunately, inaccurate interpretation of such studies as a thallium stress test has led to the erroneous diagnosis of coronary disease. (See Chap. 109.)

Other Laboratory Studies
Elevation of the blood level of the "cardiac enzymes" by noncardiac conditions may be attributed to myocardial infarction.

The level of the serum cholesterol is often used in a frightening and unscientific manner.

Cardiac catheterization and Swan-Ganz catheterization data may be incorrect, and this can lead to misdiagnosis and incorrect treatment.

Complications Resulting from Medical Treatment

Digitalis
Digitalis may produce cardiac arrhythmias as well as anorexia, nausea, diarrhea, and yellow vision. Arrhythmias, especially atrial tachycardia with atrioventricular (AV) block and nonparoxysmal junctional tachycardia with AV dissociation, are common in patients who receive digitalis and who have a potassium deficit secondary to diuretic therapy. On the other hand, cardiac arrhythmias due to potassium intoxication may develop when potassium is given in moderate dosage, especially if a patient is also receiving a potassium-sparing diuretic. These arrhythmias may also occur if the potassium is continued after a diuretic is no longer effective or has been discontinued.

Several studies have indicated that it is not possible to determine the presence of digitalis toxicity on the basis of the serum level alone any more accurately than it can be determined on clinical grounds.[6] (See Chap 92.)

Antiarrhythmic Agents
Type I antiarrhythmic agents such as quinidine, procainamide, and disopyramide may prolong the QT interval and can precipitate torsades de pointes,[7] which is an unusual form of ventricular tachyarrhythmia. Quinidine sulfate may produce fever, diarrhea, and other side effects. Procainamide may produce a lupus erythematosus–like picture, including pericarditis. Disopyramide can precipitate urinary retention because of its anticholinergic effect. It also may aggravate or precipitate heart failure because of its negative inotropic effect. (See Chap. 89.)

Nitrates
Postural hypotension can occur with excessive use of nitroglycerin, especially in the elderly. Occasionally angina worsens with the use of nitroglycerin. When this occurs, the physician should look for severe aortic stenosis or idiopathic hypertrophic subaortic stenosis. (See Chap. 88.)

Beta Blockers
Beta-blocker drugs can aggravate or precipitate heart failure, asthma, and peripheral vascular insufficiency. Beta blockers may aggravate coronary spasm (which is frequently present in rest angina), for they allow unopposed coronary vasoconstrictor impulses to prevail. Hypoglycemia can be masked and prolonged in the diabetic. Sudden withdrawal of beta blockers can produce an exaggerated cardiac beta-adrenergic responsiveness which may precipitate more angina, cardiac arrhythmias, or acute myocardial infarction. (See Chap. 90.)

Calcium Channel Blockers
Such drugs can produce postural hypotension, headache, and peripheral edema. Verapamil (Calan, Isoptin) has a negative inotropic effect and can aggravate or precipitate heart failure in patients with left ventricular dysfunction. Nifedipine (Procardia), because of its potent peripheral vasodilator effect, can cause a reflex tachycardia, and this may precipitate more angina pectoris. Verapamil and possibly nifedipine may increase the serum digoxin level. (See Chap. 91.)

Diuretics
Vigorous diuresis may produce weakness, intravascular clotting, hypotension, and electrolyte imbalance. Diuretics can also produce skin rashes, hyperuricemia, hyperglycemia, blood dyscrasias, vasculitis, and lipid abnormalities. Acute hearing loss can occur with large doses of ethacrynic acid or furosemide, especially in patients with renal disease. In the presence of renal disease the potassium-sparing diuretics can produce hyperkalemia. Spironolactone, a corticosteroid, can produce gynecomastia. (See Chap 94.)

Thrombolytic Agents
Excessive hemorrhagic states (though infrequent) may occur with intravenous or intracoronary streptokinase. Arrhythmias can occur with myocardial reperfusion. As yet it has not been resolved whether patients may fare worse if the streptokinase intervention is unsuccessful in restoring coronary

flow when compared to no intervention at all. (See Chap. 117.)

Anticoagulants
Anticoagulants may cause hemopericardium and cardiac tamponade, hematuria, cerebrovascular hemorrhage, and many other types of hemorrhagic problems. (See Chap. 95.)

Antihypertensive Agents
Antihypertensive drugs, including thiazides, ganglionic blocking agents, and peripheral dilating agents, can produce postural hypotension and syncope. Beta blockers can produce a rise in triglycerides and a fall in high-density-lipoprotein cholesterol. However, these changes appear to be less with the more cardioselective beta-blocker agents.[8] (See Chap. 51.)

Platelet Inhibitors
Rarely, platelet inhibitors may precipitate hemopericardium in the presence of pericarditis. (See Chap. 95.)

Oral Contraceptives
Studies[9] suggest an increased risk of myocardial infarction, venous thromboembolic disease, and strokes in women age 35 years of age or older who are taking oral contraceptives. The effects on high-density lipoprotein (HDL) are related in part to the proportions of estrogen and progesterone. Estrogen raises HDL, and progesterone lowers it.[10]

Oral Antidiabetic Drugs
The University Group Diabetic Program (U.G.D.P.)[11] indicated that patients receiving tolbutamide and phenformin had an increased incidence of mortality from cardiovascular causes. This study has been criticized and the conclusions, until further investigation, must be regarded as questionable.

Toxic Agents
Psychotherapeutic agents and sedatives (e.g., phenothiazines and antidepressants), antineoplastic agents (e.g., adriamycin), antibiotics (e.g., penicillin and streptomycin), chemotherapeutic agents (e.g., antimalarials and emetine) and metallic compounds (e.g., arsenic, antimony, and cobalt) can produce myocardial changes and dysfunction. Endocardial fibrosis can result from the use of methysergide. (See Chap. 78.)

Complications of Procedures and Surgery

Cardiac Catheterization
Cardiac catheterization may precipitate cardiac arrhythmias. For example, all types of tachycardia may develop during the procedure, and complete heart block may develop in patients undergoing catheterization of the right side of the heart who initially have left bundle branch block and in patients undergoing catheterization of the left side of the heart who initially have right bundle branch block. The catheter may penetrate the right or left atrium and produce hemopericardium. On rare occasions an arteriovenous fistula may be produced by cardiac catheterization.[12] Endocarditis may occur on rare occasions as a result of cardiac catheterization. Aortography may cause arterial damage. Coronary arteriography may precipitate a cardiac arrhythmia, myocardial ischemia, and myocardial infarction. Local arterial complications such as occlusion, hematoma formation, false aneurysm, and infection can occur, namely, with the brachial approach. A venipuncture may lead to thrombophlebitis and may even introduce bacteria into the bloodstream. (See Chap. 108.)

Swan-Ganz Catheterization
Complications reported with the Swan-Ganz catheter include knotting of the catheter, ventricular arrhythmias and conduction blockage, pulmonary infarction, pulmonary artery rupture, balloon rupture, formation of thrombi on the balloon and catheter, and thrombophlebitis and infections at the cutdown site. (See Chap. 124.)

Percutaneous Transluminal Coronary Angioplasty
Complications due to percutaneous transluminal coronary angioplasty (PTCA) include death, myocardial infarction, coronary artery dissection, prolonged angina, arrhythmia, coronary spasm, hypotension, and ventricular fibrillation. Fortunately, death or serious complications are very rare. (See Chap. 117.)

Pacemakers
Physiological cardiac pacing is becoming popular and allows for improved cardiac hemodyamics. This need came about because of the "pacemaker syndrome,"[13] which is a collection of signs and symptoms related to the adverse hemodynamic and electrical consequences of normal ventricular demand pacing (VVI). Patients have such symptoms as weakness, dyspnea, palpitations, and syncope, and such signs as hypotension, cannon *a* waves, edema, rales, and arrhythmias. To overcome these syndromes several types of dual-chamber pacers have been developed. One such type, DDD pacing, has the ability to pace and sense in both the atrium and ventricle and has available multifunction programmability. However, these pacers do have limitations; they may induce a multiplicity of adverse and confusing pacemaker-mediated tachyarrhythmias. Physicians must be well versed in the new dual-chamber devices in order to interpret electrocardiographic-paced rhythms. (See Chaps. 28, 104, and 105.)

Cardioversion
Besides emboli and other major arrhythmias, further complications of dc shock are serum enzyme elevations and ECG changes. Rarely, acute pulmonary edema may occur after cardioversion of atrial fibrillation because the right atrium recovers prior

to the left atrium. The lung fields are flooded because the poorly functioning left atrium cannot receive the increased output from the right side. (See Chap. 103.)

Intraaortic Balloon Pump
The most common complication of balloon insertion is ischemia of the lower extremity due to thrombus formation distal to the insertion site. The second most common complication is groin wound infection. Dissection or perforation of aortic or iliac vessels can also occur. Thrombus formation on the balloon catheter with peripheral or visceral embolization has been reported. (See Chap. 129.)

Pericardiocentesis
Laceration of a coronary artery or right ventricle, perforation of the right atrium or ventricle, pneumothorax, arrhythmias, tamponade, hypotension, and ventricular fibrillation can occur with pericardiocentesis. (See Chap. 126.)

Cardiac Surgery
Peripheral emboli may occur during and after aortic and mitral valve surgical procedures. Iatrogenic coronary artery stenosis may occur following aortic valve replacement.[14] Bacterial endocarditis may develop after intracardiac surgical procedures. Complete heart block may result from surgical closure of an interventricular septal defect. Aortic regurgitation may develop as a complication of surgical treatment for aortic stenosis, and mitral regurgitation may result from the surgical treatment for mitral stenosis. The postoperative cardiotomy syndrome occurs in an unpredictable manner. Cardiac tamponade may develop in this setting. Cardiac arrhythmias may occur after thoracotomy and cardiac surgical procedures. Right vocal cord paralysis may occur following the use of an endotracheal tube during open heart operation. Arteritis may occur after correction of coarctation of the aorta. Surgical ligation of the inferior vena cava may lead to persistent edema and venous insufficiency. An arteriovenous fistula may be produced if the saphenous vein is accidentally attached to a coronary vein at the time of bypass surgery.[15] (See Chaps. 45 and 132.)

Cardiac Resuscitation
Cardiac resuscitation, utilizing external cardiac compression, may produce contusion of the heart and liver and fracture of the ribs. The use of a defibrillator may lead to cardiac arrhythmias and burns of the skin. (See Chap. 33.)

Patients with Known Cardiac Disease Who Develop a Cardiac Phobia Because of the Physician

Patients with organic heart disease may fear cardiac death and unnecessarily restrict their activities. Cardiac neurosis is more commonly seen in the patient with coronary disease, especially following an acute myocardial infarction. However, it can occur with any type of cardiac problem. The patient may restrict daily activities because of fear of death. Signs and symptoms of depression or anxiety may be subtle, and the physician should carefully interview both patient and family. Often these conditions are overlooked and may lead to a chronic hypochondriac behavior and eventually invalidism. The patient's reaction to the illness can often be altered by rehabilitation techniques.

The Prevention and Treatment of Iatrogenic Heart Disease

Physicians would like to prevent the creation of iatrogenic heart disease. They soon learn that they cannot always accomplish this goal. Their next hope is to successfully treat iatrogenic heart disease. Then they learn that they cannot always accomplish that goal. The difficulties encountered are largely those related to the emotional problems of some patients and the irreducible complication rates associated with modern medical and surgical treatment. Despite the difficulties encountered, physicians and all health workers must try to prevent and treat iatrogenic heart disease. Accordingly, an approach to the prevention and treatment of iatrogenic heart disease is discussed below.

The first step in the prevention and treatment of iatrogenic heart disease is to encourage physicians and the personnel who assist them to be exquisitely sensitive to the problem. Appropriate patient education will help prevent iatrogenic heart disease. The word *appropriate* is stressed here because poor patient education can be harmful. Anything that physicians and their personnel can do to decrease the anxiety of patients will help to decrease the incidence of iatrogenic heart disease. This includes proper instructions regarding procedures and therapy. Today a great deal of anxiety is provoked when patients are transported through the hospital to reach a strange place where strangers will perform a mysterious procedure. Patients usually arrive at their destination only to wait an unknown length of time. One could not design a more anxiety-provoking experience. This type of experience can only be stopped by teaching the hospital and office personnel how to relieve the anxiety of the patients.

Waiting rooms are often crowded with patients. This seems to occur sooner or later in every office and hospital. Patients talk to other patients while they are waiting to consult with the physician. Patients who wait become anxious, restless, and bored. The remedy for this, more waiting rooms, costs money. Most facilities need more private areas for patients and their families. In addition to this, every effort must be made to decrease the waiting periods.

Physicians must learn as much about disease processes as they possibly can. Physicians must learn the sensitivity, specificity, and predictive value of test results. This makes diagnostic work more reliable and decreases the amount of unnecessary testing, which in turn decreases the complication rate of procedures and the misinterpretation of data. The physician should use as few drugs as possible in order to decrease the cost of medical care and the number of drug reactions.

Physicians must always weigh the risks of what they do, with the associated complications, against the risk of what they do not do, with the associated discomfort and morbidity or mortality rates. Physicians must ask the following questions: Will the information gained from the diagnostic procedures be of sufficient value in the care of the patients to justify the risk involved? Will the potential benefit of drug therapy be worth the risk of drug complications in a certain clinical situation? Will the benefit of cardiac surgery with its risk be worthwhile for a patient?

Physicians must understand the stages of rehabilitation that patients may undergo after having a myocardial infarction or being told they have a serious cardiac disease that requires a modification of life-style. When physicians do not understand the stages of rehabilitation, patients may become more disabled than their heart disease warrants (see earlier discussion). Some modification of the workmen's compensation laws, disability insurance rules, and retirement rules are needed because many patients stop work for medical reasons when, in reality, there are other reasons. This leads them to believe that their heart disease is worse than it actually is.

When physicians recognize patients with iatrogenic heart disease, they must develop a carefully designed strategy of reassurance and rehabilitation. Physicians may believe that they have succeeded in accomplishing their goal only to find that their actions and instructions have also been misinterpreted by the patient. This may mark some of the patients as being emotionally ill. The proper management of such patients requires the use of psychological techniques, possibly for a long time. Emotionally stable patients, however, may accept the opinions of physicians who pronounce them well.

Many patients believe they are more disabled than they really are. Most patients in this category can be rehabilitated by their own physicians. Some patients in this group, however, may benefit from an organized and carefully supervised physical rehabilitation program.

Whenever physicians encounter patients who have had complications of a procedure, operation, or medication, they should explain to the patient that such complications may occur under the best of circumstances. No physician can condone poor work, but many complications are not the result of poor work. Whenever a complication is not the result of poor work, the physician must make this fact unmistakably clear to everyone concerned, since unscrupulous people may prey upon the fact that complications can occur in the setting of excellent work. Therefore, physicians must prepare patients for procedures, operations, and the use of drugs and be alert to the first sign of difficulty. Whenever a complication is discovered, the patient and family should be told and the condition should be managed promptly.

References

1. Wilson, F.: Foreword, in E. Lepeschkin (ed.), "Modern Electrocardiography," The Williams & Wilkins Company, Baltimore, 1951, vol. 1, p. v.
2. Aurbach, A., and Gliebe, P. A.: Iatrogenic Heart Disease: Common Cardiac Neurosis, *JAMA*, 129:338, 1945.
3. Weinberg, H. B.: Iatrogenic Heart Disease, *Ann. Intern. Med.*, 38:9, 1953.
4. Hart, A. D.: Iatrogenic Cardiac Neurosis: Critique, *JAMA*, 156:1133, 1954.
5. Wheeler, E. O., Williamson, C. R., and Cohen, M. E.: Heart Scare, Heart Surveys, and Iatrogenic Heart Disease: Emotional and Symptomatological Effects of Suggesting to 162 Adults That They Might Have Heart Disease, *JAMA*, 167:1096, 1958.
6. Ingelfinger, J. A., and Goldman, P.: The Serum Digitalis Concentration—Does It Diagnose Digitalis Toxicity?, *N. Engl. J. Med.*, 294:867, 1976.
7. Smith, W. M., and Gallagher, J. J.: "Les Torsades de Pointes": An Unusual Ventricular Arrhythmia, *Ann. Intern. Med.*, 93:578, 1980.
8. Day, J. L., Metcalfe, J., and Simpson, C. N.: Adrenergic Mechanisms in Control of Plasma Lipid Concentrations, *Br. Med. J.*, 284:1145, 1982.
9. Stadel, B. V.: Oral Contraceptives and Cardiovascular Disease, Parts 1 and 2, *N. Engl. J. Med.*, 305:612; 672, 1981.
10. Bradley, D. D., Wingerd, J., Petitti, D. B., et al.: Serum High Density Lipoprotein Cholesterol in Women Using Oral Contraceptives, Estrogen and Progestine, *N. Engl. J. Med.*, 299:17, 1978.
11. University Group Diabetes Program: A Study of the Effect of Hypoglycemic Agents on Vascular Complications in Patients with Adult Onset Diabetes: II. Mortality Results, *Diabetes (Suppl.)*, 19:789, 1970.
12. Lalljee, N.: Iatrogenic Arteriovenous Fistula: An Unusual Complication of Cardiac Catheterization, *J. Cardiovasc. Surg.*, 11(3):246, 1970.
13. Hass, J. K., and Strait, G. B.: Pacemaker-Induced Cardiovascular Failure: Hemodynamic and Angiographic Observations, *Am. J. Cardiol.*, 33:295, 1974.
14. Sethi, G. K., Scott, S. M., and Takaro, T.: Iatrogenic Coronary Artery Stenosis following Aortic Valve Replacement, *J. Thorac. Cardiovasc. Surg.*, 77(5):760, 1979.
15. Lawrie, G. M., Morris, G. C., Jr., and Winters, W. L.: Aortocoronary Saphenous Vein Autograft Accidentally Attached to a Coronary Vein: Follow-Up Angiography and Surgical Correction of the Resultant Arteriovenous Fistula, *Ann. Thorac. Surg.*, 22(1):87, 1976.

Section E

The Heart and Environmental Factors

84

The Influence of Environmental Factors on the Cardiovascular System

Robert F. Grover, M.D., Ph.D.
John T. Reeves, M.D.
Loring B. Rowell, Ph.D.
Claude A. Piantadosi, M.D.
Herbert A. Saltzman, M.D.

High Altitude

Each year millions of people visit the mountainous regions of the western United States for recreation. With modern transportation, rapid ascent to resort areas at an 8000- to 9500-ft altitude is a common occurrence. Major highways cross mountain passes above 11,000 ft, and during the summer season, a quarter of a million people drive to the summits of Pike's Peak and Mt. Evans, both exceeding 14,000 ft. Just how severe is the stress of such altitudes?

To begin with, ascent to high altitude means exposure to a decrease in total atmospheric pressure and a parallel decrease in the partial pressure of oxygen we breathe. At sea level, the inspired oxygen tension is 150 mmHg; it is 125 mmHg at 5000 ft, 100 mmHg at 10,000 ft, and about 80 mmHg at 14,000 ft. This is the atmospheric hypoxia to which people are exposed in the Rocky Mountains.

Circulatory Oxygen Transport

Arterial Oxygenation

Within the lung, the inspired oxygen tension is lowered by the presence of carbon dioxide. Furthermore, there is imperfect matching of blood flow to regional ventilation. Consequently, the arterial oxygen tension perfusing the body, which ranges from about 80 to 90 mmHg at sea level, is reduced to 45 to 50 mmHg at 14,000 ft.

Although the arterial oxygen tension on the summit of Pike's Peak is only half as great as at sea level, this does not mean that the quantity of oxygen in the blood has been reduced to one-half. That is because of the nonlinear oxygen-binding characteristics of hemoglobin. The relation between oxygen tension and oxygen saturation is defined by the hemoglobin-oxygen dissociation curve (Fig. 84-1).

FIGURE 84-1 As a consequence of the sigmoid shape of the hemoglobin-oxygen dissociation curve, the large decrease in arterial oxygen pressure (tension) on ascent from sea level to 14,000 ft (4300 m) altitude results in only a small decrease in hemoglobin saturation and blood oxygen content. (*From R. F. Grover, Man Living at High Altitudes, in J. D. Ives and R. G. Barry (eds.), "Arctic and Alpine Environments," Methuen & Co., London, 1974, p. 822. Reproduced with permission from the publisher and author.*)

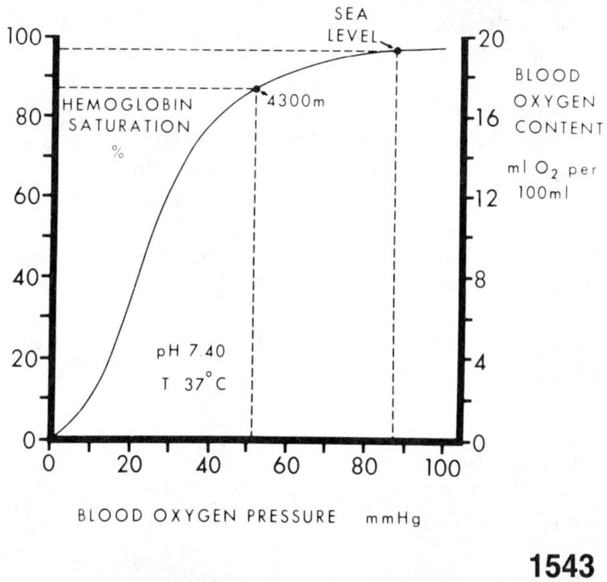

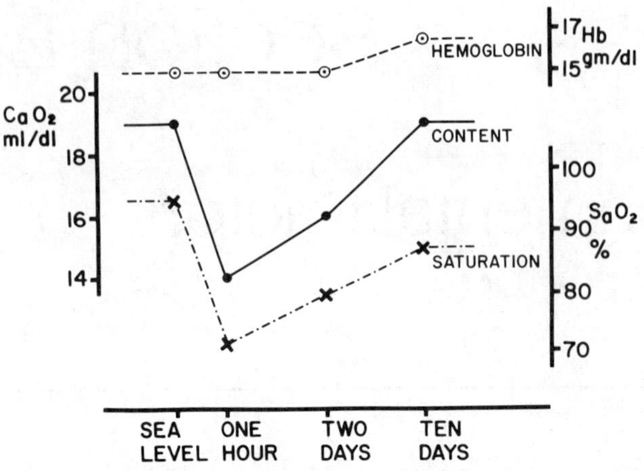

FIGURE 84-2 Arterial blood oxygenation during adaptation to high altitude. Following the initial fall, arterial saturation (SaO_2) improves with increasing ventilation. Concurrently, hemoconcentration increases the hemoglobin (Hb) concentration and hence the O_2-carrying capacity of the blood. The net result is restoration and arterial O_2 content (C_aO_2) to preascent values.

From this it can be seen that following adaptation to 14,000 ft, the arterial oxygen saturation is still 85 percent compared with 95 percent at sea level. Thus, a 50 percent decrease in arterial oxygen tension causes only a 10 percent reduction in saturation. At the more modest altitudes where the tourist and ski resorts are situated, the fall in saturation is even less. The moderate nature of this hypoxemia should be emphasized, since many of our concepts regarding high altitude are based upon much more severe hypoxic tests.

The effect of a decrease in saturation on the actual amount of oxygen in the blood (arterial O_2 content) depends upon the hemoglobin concentration. With a normal hemoglobin of 15 g/dl, when saturation falls to 85 percent, the arterial O_2 content is reduced from 19 to 17 ml/dl (Fig. 84-1). However, within the first few days at high altitude, plasma volume decreases while total red blood cell mass remains unchanged.[1] Consequently, hematocrit rises, and with it hemoglobin concentration, which increases the oxygen-carrying capacity of the blood. This offsets the fall in saturation and restores the arterial O_2 content to preascent values (Fig. 84-2). In other words, after a week at high altitude, even though the saturation is 85 percent, the quantity of oxygen in 100 ml of blood (ml O_2/dl) has been restored to normal. During heavy exercise, arterial oxygen content actually rises because there is further hemoconcentration which more than offsets any decrease in saturation.[2] True polycythemia, reflecting an increase in total red blood cell mass resulting from bone marrow stimulation, requires many weeks of residence at altitudes high enough to cause a sustained reduction in arterial saturation.

Cardiac Output

Since the transport of oxygen by the circulation depends not only on the quantity of oxygen in each

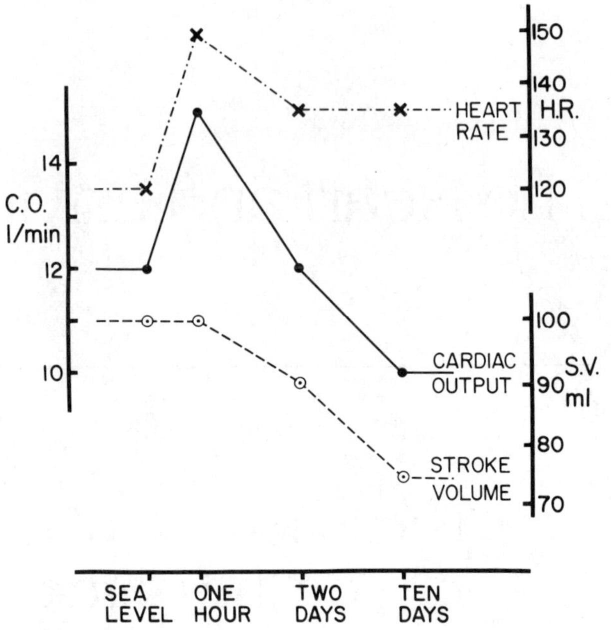

FIGURE 84-3 Time course of alterations in exercise heart rate (HR), stroke volume (SV), and cardiac output (CO) during adaptation to high altitude. After 10 days, CO is subnormal due to a significant decrease in SV.

unit of blood (arterial O_2 content) but also on the number of these units of blood pumped by the heart per minute, i.e., cardiac output, let us examine the latter, including its components, heart rate and stroke volume. With ascent to high altitude, heart rate

FIGURE 84-4 Oxygen transport (O_2T_r) by the systemic circulation during submaximal exercise. Upon ascent to high altitude, the fall in arterial blood O_2 content (C_aO_2) is offset by an increase in cardiac output (CO). Although C_aO_2 is restored within 10 days, the fall in CO to subnormal levels results in a net reduction in O_2T_r, which then requires greater O_2 extraction from the blood to preserve O_2 delivery.

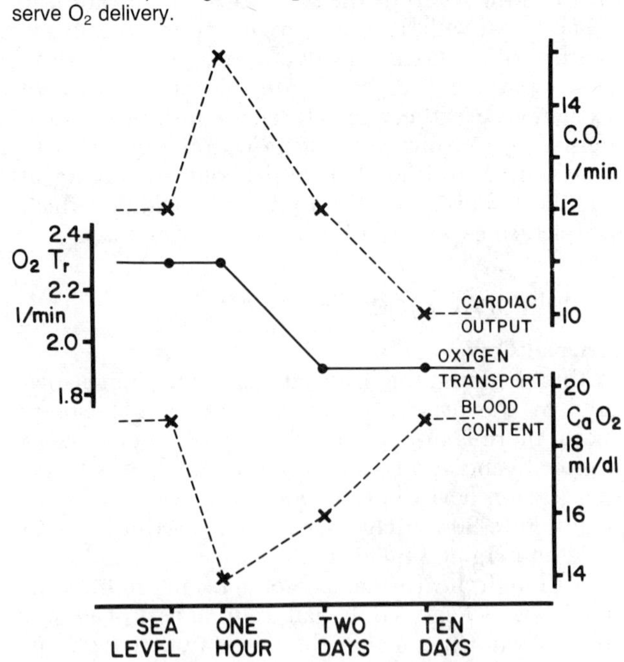

increases[3] due to hypoxic stimulation of the sympathetic nervous system combined with a decrease in parasympathetic activity.[4] This tachycardia increases cardiac output which offsets initial hypoxemia and preserves oxygen transport. However, this early tachycardia is not sustained. Within a day or two, resting heart rate returns to preascent values, and even the tachycardia of exercise diminishes[5] (Fig. 84-3). Surprisingly, cardiac stroke volume also decreases by as much as 25 percent during the first week at high altitude.[1] As a result of these circulatory adjustments, cardiac output, both at rest and during exercise, plateaus at levels about 20 percent below the corresponding values at sea level[1] (Fig. 84-3). Consequently, even though the quantity of oxygen in the arterial blood has been restored to normal by hemoconcentration, the amount of oxygen transported to the body is now reduced by the low cardiac output (Fig. 84-4). For the body to remain normally oxygenated, extraction of oxygen from arterial blood must be increased. Direct measurements in normal humans, both at rest and during exercise, confirm this increase in extraction (widening of the arteriovenous difference in blood O_2 content).[1]

Myocardial Function

By what mechanism does stroke volume decrease? Observations[6] made with M-mode echocardiography in normal individuals demonstrated a progressive decrease in both the end-diastolic and end-systolic diameters of the left ventricular chamber over the first week at high altitude. Volumes calculated from these diameters indicated a progressive decrease in stroke volume which was highly correlated with the decrease in end-diastolic volume while ejection fraction remained normal. Furthermore, the decline in diastolic volume paralleled the reduction in plasma volume from hemoconcentration. Thus, it appears that with a reduction in plasma volume, venous return and ventricular diastolic filling are reduced, and by the Frank-Starling mechanism, stroke volume is consequently decreased. All indices of contractility remained normal,[6] indicating that myocardial function is not compromised at high altitude, and the decrease in stroke volume reflects the operation of normal physiological mechanisms.

Coronary Circulation

In considering cardiovascular effects of high altitude, the stress on the coronary circulation is of prime importance. We are taught that hypoxia increases coronary blood flow. Evidence for this includes a study of 19 young men in whom breathing 10% oxygen nearly doubled coronary flow.[7] However, breathing 10% oxygen at sea level yields inspired oxygen tensions equivalent to sudden exposure to 18,000 ft, so such evidence does not apply directly to tourists ascending to 10,000 ft over several days. Here, again, the situation becomes clear when one thinks in terms of oxygen transport.

Oxygenation of the myocardium requires a balance between demand and supply. The primary determinants of demand are heart rate, systolic pressure (the so-called double product), and myocardial contractility. Ascent to high altitude increases myocardial oxygen demand, primarily through increased heart rate. Such increased demand must be met by an increase in oxygen supply. In general, this is accomplished by increasing coronary blood flow, since oxygen extraction from the coronary arterial blood (coronary arteriovenous difference) is always nearly maximal. If the altitude is sufficiently high to lower saturation and arterial oxygen content as well, less oxygen will be available for extraction, and compensation requires even greater flow. Hence, with initial ascent to high altitude, coronary blood flow will be increased in proportion to the increase in heart rate and the decrease in arterial saturation.

Increase in Oxygen Extraction

Within a few days at high altitude, heart rate will decrease and arterial oxygen content will be restored by hemoconcentration (Figs. 84-2 and 84-3). Both adjustments will tend to return coronary flow to preascent levels. In addition, a third important but subtle factor operates which permits coronary flow to decrease even further. This is a decrease in the affinity of hemoglobin for oxygen, which is another aspect of adaptation to high altitude. Within the red blood cell, the concentration of 2,3-diphosphoglycerate (2,3-DPG) increases, which produces a "right shift" in the hemoglobin dissociation curve,[8] lowering the saturation at any given tension. Because of the sigmoid shape of the dissociation curve, this right shift has little effect on arterial oxygen loading; however, it facilitates oxygen unloading from peripheral capillary blood.

Normal Decrease in Coronary Blood Flow

The coronary circulation is regulated to maintain the coronary sinus P_{O_2} constant at 18 mmHg. The corresponding saturation will be lowered from 34 percent at sea level to 22 percent at 10,200 ft as a consequence of the right shift in the dissociation curve.[9] Consequently, oxygen extraction from the coronary blood will increase significantly (wider coronary arteriovenous difference),[9] and less coronary blood flow will be needed to supply the myocardial oxygen requirements (Fig. 84-5). Literally, the right shift in the dissociation curve permits coronary flow to decrease. Direct measurements in normal humans studied first at sea level and again following adaptation to high altitude show a consistent decrease in coronary flow, both at rest and during exercise.[9] A decrease in coronary flow at high altitude is surprising but is entirely consistent with the operation of normal physiologic mechanisms designed to preserve the constancy of myocardial tissue P_{O_2} (coronary sinus blood P_{O_2}). The decrease in coronary flow is required to prevent a rise in coronary sinus P_{O_2}. There is no evidence of myocardial

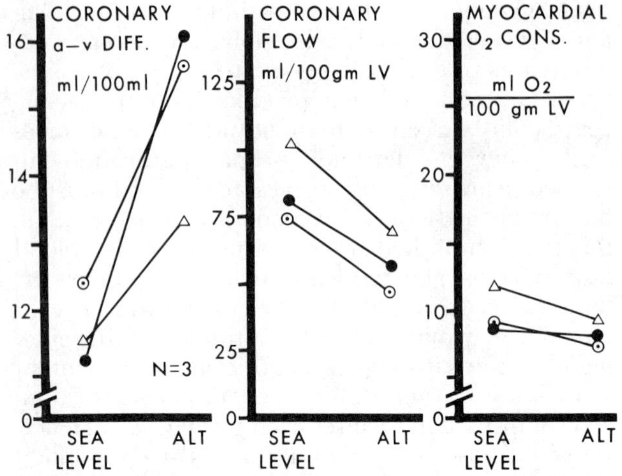

FIGURE 84-5 Alterations in the coronary circulation of the normal human heart following adaptation to 10,200-ft altitude. O_2 extraction from coronary blood increases, i.e., there is a significant widening of the coronary arteriovenous difference in O_2 content. This permits coronary flow (Q_{con}) to decrease while maintaining myocardial O_2 consumption unaltered. (*From R. F. Grover, Mechanisms of Augmenting Coronary Arterial Oxygen Extraction, in J. H. K. Vogel (ed.). "Myocardial Infarction: A New Look at an Old Subject," Advances in Cardiology, 9:97, S. Karger AG, Basel, 1973. Reproduced with permission from the publisher and author.*)

ischemia or hypoxia. Neither is there any impairment to increasing coronary flow when required to meet increased oxygen demands, as during exercise.

Coronary Artery Disease

Does visiting high altitudes pose a special risk for the patient with coronary artery disease? What do you advise the 50-year-old from Dallas who is contemplating a skiing vacation to Colorado? These are very practical questions, but well-controlled studies have not been conducted to provide definitive answers. However, clinical experience indicates no special risk from altitude, provided the patient continues to observe the same exercise limitations accepted at sea level. From discussions with physicians practicing in Aspen (7900 ft), Vail (8200 ft), and Breckenridge (9300 ft), the impression has been gained that occurrence of an acute myocardial infarction by a transient skier or summer tourist is an unusual event. This experience is in keeping with the known effects of altitude on the coronary circulation discussed above.

Okin[10] studied 11 men from Denver with documented coronary artery disease, 9 with previous myocardial infarction, and 4 with exertional angina. He subjected them to a standard exercise step test at 5300 ft, 8000 ft, and 10,400 ft, producing mean maximal heart rates of 119, 123, and 125 beats per minute, respectively. No patient developed symptoms or ECG signs of ischemia at the higher altitudes that had not been present at 5300 ft.

Using radiotelemetry, Grover and Tucker recorded ECGs from 149 men skiing at altitudes of 10,000 to 11,200 ft at Vail, Colorado. Of these, 92 were over 40, including 19 in their fifties and 5 in their sixties. While skiing, heart rates exceeded 150 beats per minute in over half the subjects, corresponding to over 80 percent of the age-adjusted predicted maximum rate. Despite tachycardia from strenuous exercise in the cold at high altitude, only one man developed ECG evidence of ischemia associated with angina; he had suffered a myocardial infarction 3 months earlier! Presumably such individuals are rare. We must conclude that among older men who engage in strenuous activities at high altitude, there is virtually no evidence to indicate an added risk beyond what one might expect at lower altitudes regarding the occurrence of a coronary event.

Not only does the limited available evidence indicate no increased risk of coronary insufficiency during a brief visit to high altitude, but also prolonged residence at high altitude may actually reduce mortality from coronary heart disease. Mortimer et al.[11] analyzed age-adjusted mortality rates for atherosclerotic heart disease in populations living at different altitudes in New Mexico. For males, although not for females, mortality rates declined progressively from low to high altitude; the rate above 6500 ft was only 72 percent of the rate below 3700 ft. This decline in rate was not explained by ethnic or socioeconomic factors and was concluded to be a true consequence of the higher altitude. The increased vascularity of the myocardium (and other tissues) in high-altitude residents may be a protective factor. In addition, left ventricular work may actually be less in high-altitude residents due to lower systemic arterial blood pressure[12] and lower heart rates.

Pulmonary Circulation

Pulmonary Hypertension

Airway hypoxia stimulates pulmonary vasoconstriction, but when hypoxia is induced acutely, alveolar oxygen tension must be reduced below 50 mmHg before a significant rise in pulmonary arterial pressure is seen.[13] This means that with ascent to high altitude, little or no pulmonary hypertension would be observed in the visitor to altitudes below 14,000 ft. However, when the airway hypoxia is sustained for months, as during residence at high altitude, impressive pulmonary hypertension does develop.[14] Among residents of Leadville, Colorado, living at 10,200 ft, pulmonary arterial pressures on the average are twice as high as at sea level. Mean pressures range from 11 to 45 mmHg at rest, and frequently exceed 60 mmHg during exercise.[15] This increased workload on the right ventricle is reflected in the ECG as a rightward shift in the mean QRS axis and right ventricular enlargement.[16] Although these findings differ from those usually encountered in normal sea level residents, the pulmonary hypertension of high altitude is generally benign, nonprogressive, and reversible with descent to lower altitude. Hence, it should not be considered cardiovascular disease, and the term *cor pulmonale* if used is misleading.

In special circumstances, the hypoxic pulmonary hypertension of high altitude may not be entirely benign. It may delay the usual postnatal resolution of the normally high pulmonary arterial pressure in the fetus,[17] and result in "persistent fetal circulation" of the newborn. Although high-altitude pulmonary hypertension appears well tolerated by the human right ventricle, it becomes so severe in cattle that heart failure develops, and the resulting edema produces what cattle raisers call *brisket disease*.[14] (See Chap. 52.)

High-Altitude Pulmonary Edema

Although the vast majority of people ascending to high altitude experience no pulmonary problems (apart from an awareness of the normal increase in ventilation), the occasional individual will develop acute high-altitude pulmonary edema (HAPE). The incidence is between 1 and 10 per 10,000 persons ascending rapidly to altitudes above 8000 ft.[18] Symptoms almost always appear during the first week at such altitudes. The patient has undue shortness of breath, cyanosis, tachycardia, moist rales, fatigue, and frequently a nonproductive cough. Untreated, HAPE tends to be progressive and fatal, whereas recovery is prompt upon descent to lower altitude. During the episode of HAPE, the heart is not enlarged and heart failure is absent. This is a form of noncardiac pulmonary edema which occurs in otherwise healthy and comparatively young individuals[18] with no underlying cardiovascular or pulmonary disease.[19] Despite intensive research, the pathogenesis of HAPE remains a mystery. The consensus is that HAPE is part of the spectrum of acute mountain sickness,[20] with relative hypoventilation and abnormal fluid retention as underlying factors.[21] Consequently, respiratory stimulation, as with acetazolamide, is both a rational and effective mode of prophylaxis for HAPE.

Although acute severe pulmonary hypertension is usually present during an episode of HAPE, the relation between these two conditions is not clear. Probably pulmonary hypertension per se does not precipitate the pulmonary edema. On the other hand, the increased pulmonary vascular reactivity in chronically hypoxic children living at high altitude may contribute to their predisposition to reentry HAPE.[22] (See Chap. 52.)

Heat Stress

Humans adjust to heat stress mainly by altering the vasomotor state of the skin to regulate heat exchange with the environment. Thermal balance is further modified by sweating or shivering. This section deals with adjustments of the systemic cutaneous and other regional circulations to regulate blood pressure and blood volume distribution along with body temperature. Reviews of this topic can be consulted for further details.[23,24]

Cutaneous Circulation

Reflex Control[25–27]

The skin receives only 5 to 10 percent of the cardiac output in normothermic individuals at rest but it can receive 50 to 70 percent during heat stress. Circulatory adjustments to thermal stress can be drastically modified by cutaneous sympathetic vasoconstrictor nerve fibers, which are the efferent arm of (1) thermoregulatory reflexes that originate principally in cutaneous thermoreceptors, (2) cardiopulmonary and arterial baroreflexes, and (3) reflex adjustments to upright posture and exercise. The body's efforts to maintain blood pressure and support metabolic demands of other organs competes with thermoregulatory needs for skin blood flow. The temperature we maintain in conditions other than supine rest is the result of these competing nervous influences on skin blood flow.

Human skin is unique in possessing an *active vasodilator* system, the dominant effector in human cardiovascular response to rising core temperature (not skin temperature), accounting for almost all the increase in skin blood flow. The mechanism of active cutaneous vasodilation is still unknown. It requires intact sympathetic innervation and is somehow functionally linked to sweat gland function inasmuch as patients with congenital absence of sweat glands (and intact sympathetic nerves) cannot vasodilate the skin or adequately regulate body temperature.[28] A rise in skin blood flow markedly increases the volume of blood within the compliant venous plexuses where it passes at reduced linear velocity just below the skin surface, increasing transcutaneous heat transfer. Cutaneous veins have a rich sympathetic nerve supply that reflexly controls the volume near the body surface in response to heat and cold. They are not responsive to baroreflexes, but they do constrict during exercise. As will be discussed, the shift in blood volume into cutaneous veins is the major regulatory problem in human cardiovascular adjustment to heat stress.

Circulatory Adjustments to Heat Stress

Supine Rest[23,24]

In normal resting individuals, heat stress can greatly increase cardiac output and total skin blood flow; however, responses vary widely because of differences in thermal conditions, duration of exposure, posture, internal temperature, and also methodology. During supine rest, the cardiovascular system's capacity to increase cardiac output and skin blood flow is great during direct, whole-body heating designed to generate a maximum response by raising body skin temperature, as shown in Fig. 84-6. Cardiac output increased by 6 to 7 liters/min, a rise of

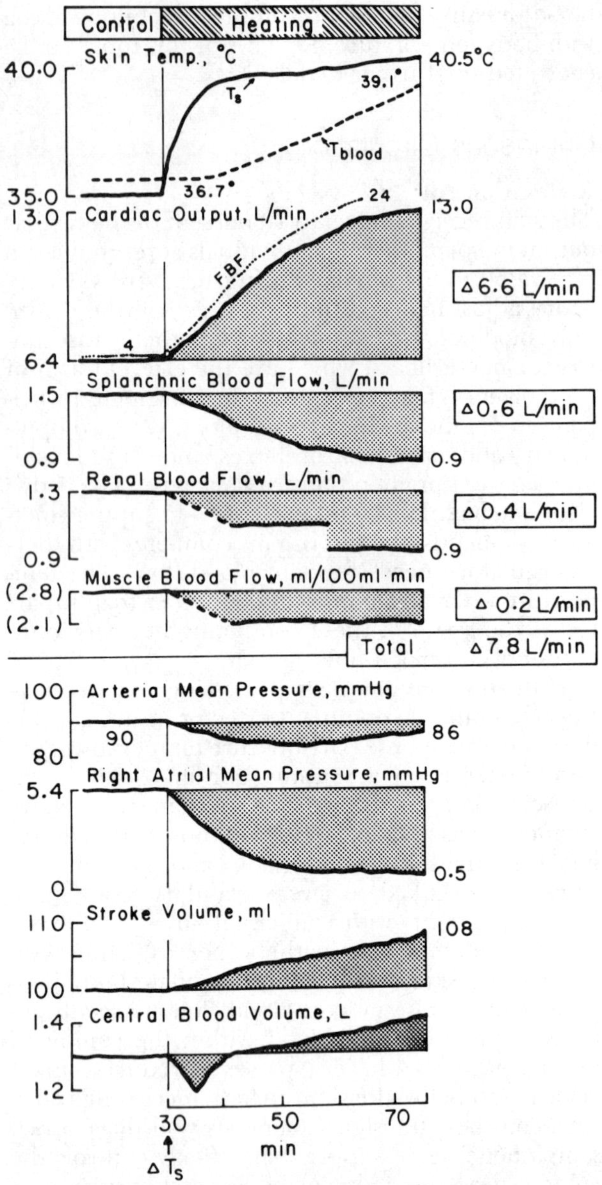

FIGURE 84-6 Average maximal circulatory responses to direct, whole-body heating. The initial and final values and time course are shown for skin temperature (T_s), rectal temperature (T_r), and T_{blood} (right atrium), and each cardiovascular variable. Contributions of increased cardiac output (in 12 men) and reduced regional blood flows to total skin blood flow (7.8 liters/min) are shown in boxes on the right. Note that arterial pressure is well maintained, but right atrial pressure fell markedly while stroke volume increased. (*From L. B. Rowell, Human Cardiovascular Adjustments to Exercise and Thermal Stress, Physiological Reviews, 54:75, 1974. Reproduced with permission from the publisher and author.*)

2.8 liters/min per °C increase in right atrial blood temperature. As blood flow to other major vascular beds decreases, the increase in cardiac output goes to skin as reflected by the increase in forearm skin blood flow in Fig. 84-6. Arterial blood pressure is well maintained. Similar changes in blood flow are seen in patients with erythroderma; their chronically high skin blood flow leads to high-output failure with edema, venous congestion, hepatomegaly, and cardiac enlargement along with renal and gastrointestinal abnormalities.[29] Paraplegic patients show blunted responses to increased core temperature.[30] The cause is unknown; loss of thermal sensors in the spinal cord may contribute.[24] The rise in skin blood flow is also subnormal in patients with diabetic neuropathy,[31] undoubtedly because of defective neural control of skin blood vessels.

Hyperthermia per se increases sympathetic nervous activity which causes regional vasoconstriction that, in turn, increases the fraction of cardiac output available for skin and alters the distribution of blood volume. Plasma norepinephrine concentration and plasma renin activity increase in proportion to core temperature; however, the renin-angiotensin system adds little to the neurogenic vasoconstriction elicited from thermoreceptors in the hypothalamus and spinal cord.[32]

Because high rates of skin blood flow increase the volume of blood in compliant cutaneous veins, translocation of blood volume from other regions is required to minimize the reduction in central blood volume (CBV) and cardiac filling pressure. The distribution of blood volume is altered most by splanchnic vasoconstriction which reduces the pressure within a capacious venous bed that contains approximately 20 percent of total blood volume. Since splanchnic veins are normally at their maximal compliance, large decrements in intravenous volume will accompany small pressure changes. Central mobilization of blood volume is enhanced by the fall in right atrial pressure (Fig. 84-6) caused by the large pressure gradient that develops between central and cutaneous veins at high rates of skin blood flow. We cannot say whether blood volume is actively expressed from visceral organs by venoconstriction, but the fall in right atrial pressure along with splanchnic vasoconstriction favors a *passive* mobilization. The increase in stroke volume under these conditions suggests an increase in myocardial contractile force. Since all the energy needed to force blood back to the heart is provided by the left ventricle (i.e., no muscle pump is active as in exercise), an increase in myocardial contractile force would be highly advantageous during heat stress. It follows that patients in mild congestive heart failure may develop acute left ventricular failure during heat stress.[33] Also, the reduction in filling pressure caused by cutaneous vasodilation creates severe problems for patients with stenotic valvular lesions and reduced ventricular compliance.

Standing at Rest[23,24]

When humans stand up, hydrostatic forces displace blood volume into dependent veins with approximately 600 ml moving into the legs.[34] In association with increases in skin blood flow and cutaneous venous compliance, blood volume in the legs increases an additional 200 ml.[34] This decreases further the return of blood to the heart and creates more severe orthostatic problems. CBV and filling pressure decrease as illustrated in Fig. 84-7. Right and left ventricular outputs can only be transiently maintained by depletion of preventricular sumps, i.e., thoracic and splanchnic veins and the pulmonary vasculature. Cardiac output falls as a result of the marked decrease in stroke volume. Without vasoconstriction in skin to supplement that occurring in other organs, syncope would occur rapidly. In short, we defend ourselves against heat syncope by cutaneous vasoconstriction, not venoconstriction; but vasoconstriction merely reduces the rate at which dependent cutaneous veins fill and thus delays rather than prevents syncope. In addition, vasoconstriction of the splanchnic region serves to minimize reduction in CBV (Fig. 84-7).

Exercise[23,24,35]

As during rest, cutaneous venous volume increases when heat stress and exercise are combined despite the pumping action of muscle contraction. In cool environments, the cutaneous veins of the legs refill so slowly after each compression by contracting muscle that their average pressure and volume remain low. In contrast, during heat stress these veins refill so rapidly after each contraction that average

FIGURE 84-7 Schematic illustration of effects of skin vasodilation (VD) upon preventricular volume sumps for right (RV) and left (LV) ventricles. As skin veins fill, venous return is transiently reduced so that preventricular sumps are depleted. CBV represents central or thoracic blood volume. Reduction in CBV is partially compensated by passive [caused by arteriolar vasoconstriction (VC)] expulsion of blood volume from splanchnic organs.

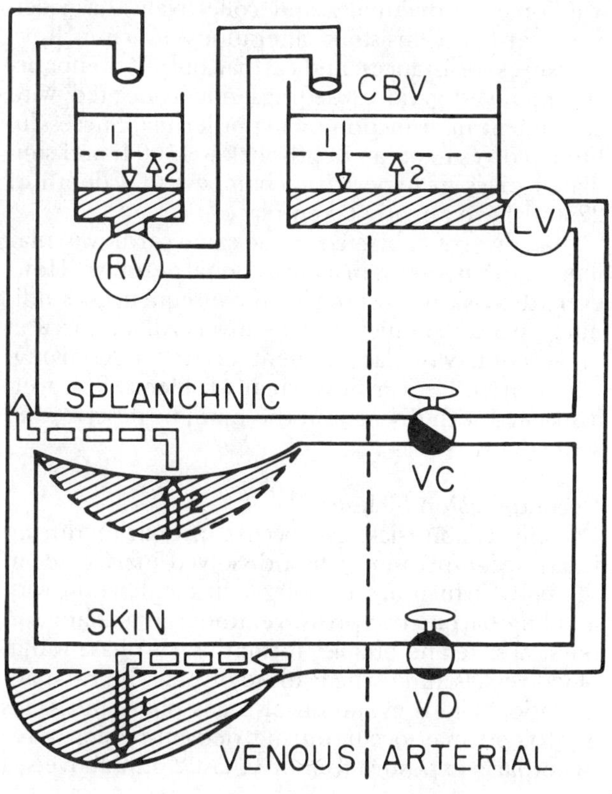

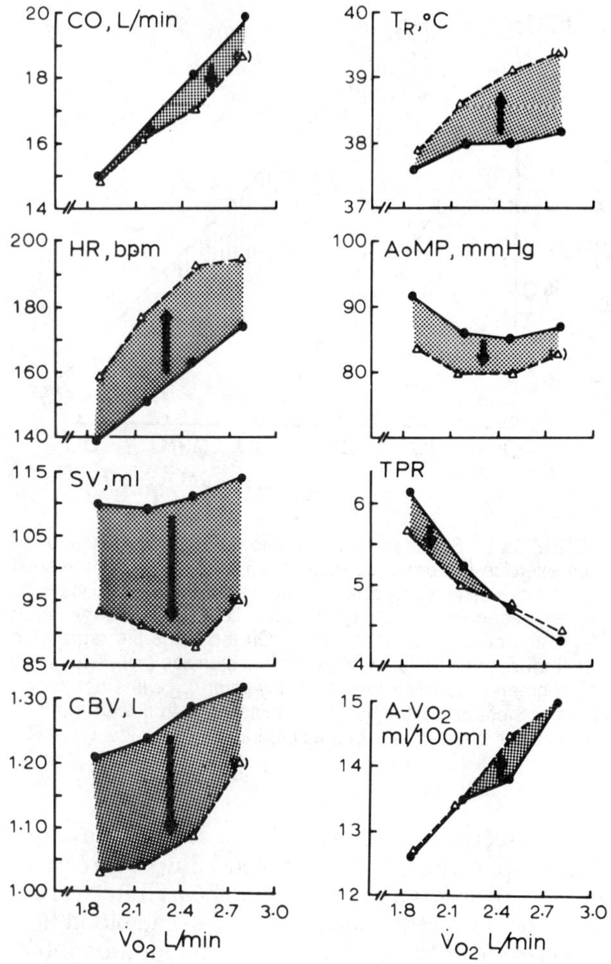

FIGURE 84-8 Summary of cardiovascular responses to graded exercise in hot (43.3°C, Δ----Δ) and neutral (25.6°C, ●—●) environments. Arrows show the direction of change in each variable with heating (variables coded as in Fig. 84-6). Average data from six men.

venous volume is increased markedly.[34] Venous volume is further increased by the loss of venoconstriction and the increase in compliance. Reductions in CBV, ventricular filling pressure, and stroke volume ensue, so that during moderate to heavy exercise, cardiac output is maintained by increased heart rate, but is *not* increased to meet the additional demands for skin blood flow (Fig. 84-8). Because of the decrease in stroke volume, heart rate approaches maximal values at submaximal levels of V_{O_2} so that eventually cardiac output is reduced below normal and demands for skin and muscle blood flow cannot be met. Even the most severe hyperthermia does not increase total skin blood flow to levels seen in supine individuals. Thus, cardiac output does not, as once thought, simply increase to raise skin blood flow until a maximal cardiac output is reached at submaximal levels of V_{O_2}. Again, this is prevented by the reduction in stroke volume.

The limited ability of the *normal* heart to meet the combined needs of skin and muscle is partly compensated for by redistribution of blood flow away

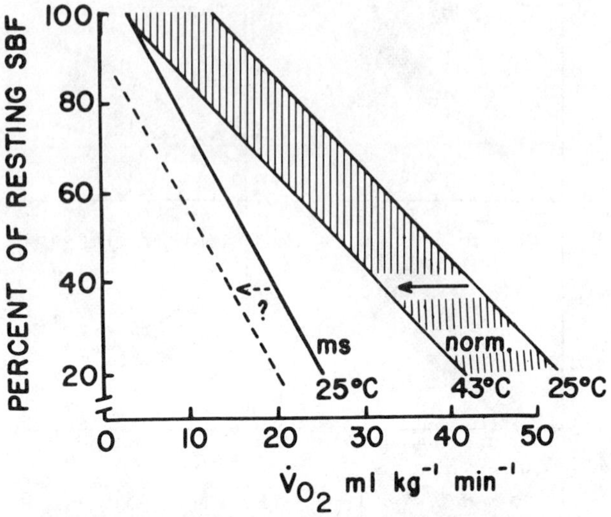

FIGURE 84-9 Summary of splanchnic vascular responses to upright exercise in normal subjects at 25 and 43°C environmental temperature. The shaded region marks the highly significant 20 percent reduction in splanchnic blood flow (SBF) at any given V_{O_2} in the heat in normal subjects. On the left is the regression line from seven patients with pure mitral stenosis (ms), who show much greater reduction in flow at any given V_{O_2}. It is not known whether these patients show further reduction in flow in the heat (dashed line shows result of predicted 20 percent reduction).[23,24]

from visceral organs (Fig. 84-9). In cool environments, splanchnic and renal blood flows decrease in inverse proportions to V_{O_2} and heart rate during exercise. This reduction in visceral organ blood flow is increased by heat stress so that an additional 600 to 800 ml of blood can be redistributed from these organs to skin each minute. During prolonged exercise in hot environments, splanchnic and renal blood flow decrease progressively so that function of these organs can be impaired. Reductions of 70 percent in splanchnic blood flow have been measured. The situation is analogous to that observed in cardiac patients who, being unable to raise their cardiac output adequately with exercise in cool environments, must rely instead on redistribution of cardiac output to perfuse working muscle.[36] Patients with pure mitral stenosis, for example, show marked reductions in splanchnic blood flow at low levels of work (Fig. 84-9).[37] If heat stress during exercise further reduces splanchnic blood flow in these patients (dashed line in Fig. 84-9), flow could reach critically low levels. The central lobular necrosis that can develop in such patients may result from frequent repetitions of visceral ischemia.

The cutaneous circulation does not escape the effects of increased sympathetic activity during exercise and heat stress. As core temperature rises above 38°C, the rate of rise of skin blood flow is reduced markedly and approaches an upper limit that is far below the values measured at the same core temperature in resting subjects. Skin blood flow, as measured in the initial stages of exercise, is reduced in patients with heart failure.[38] Cutaneous vasoconstriction can reduce or delay peripheral displacement of blood volume and help to maintain blood flow, but the price is augmented heat storage.

In the overall regulatory scheme, regulation of blood pressure during heat stress appears to have precedence unless core temperature rises beyond tolerable limits, at which point regulation fails. Such failure is most likely in patients with stenotic valvular lesions and reduced ventricular compliance because of the large reductions in cardiac filling pressure associated with heat stress. In addition, critical hepatic and renal functions are likely to be disrupted by increased diversion of their blood flow. This would be most likely in patients with low output whose perfusion of visceral organs is chronically reduced at rest.

Hyperbaric Pressure

Underwater Diving[39–45]

Underwater diving induces diverse but reasonably well defined changes in cardiovascular function. Under certain conditions catastrophes occur that are associated with profound alterations in cardiovascular function. We will describe the interacting physical factors leading to altered circulatory function and their pathological consequences.

Alterations in the physical environment by the diver breathing air include increases in barometric pressure, density of the breathing gas, the inspired P_{O_2}, the inspired pressure of nitrogen, and loss of body heat into the surrounding water. The most characteristic cardiovascular response to these physical forces, individually and collectively, has been bradycardia. Consistent alterations in circulatory pressures, resistances, and cardiac output do not occur in investigational settings not associated with equipment malfunction or hypothermia. Successful human dives to ocean depths below 1500 ft and simulated dives in hyperbaric chambers to a depth of 2250 ft have already taken place.[41]

The diver is subjected to the same cardiovascular illnesses that occur in conventional settings. However, the risk of ensuing fatal consequences is infinitely greater should an acute myocardial infarction or cerebral vascular accident occur while diving. There are other cardiovascular problems, however, associated with diving and these will be described in some detail.

Decompression Sickness[43]

Decompression sickness occurs primarily during rapid decompression when dissolved inert gases in the body, which are no longer in equilibrium with a falling barometric pressure, undergo a change in physical state and bubbles form; this gas phase within blood vessels and tissue leads to diverse clinical manifestations. This evolution of a gas phase in tissues and blood may occur during decompression after hyperbaric exposure to more than 2 atm above sea level or during a rapid simulated ascent from sea level (decompression to less than 0.5 atm above sea level). Explosive decompression is a familiar example of the latter circumstance. Factors more likely to be associated with decompression sickness include excessive body weight, prolonged exposure to a hyperbaric environment, and severe exercise, presumably because of an increased tissue uptake of inert gas. Other aggravating factors include increasing age, fatigue, and preexisting vascular disease, presumably because of associated relative impairment of gas transport from tissues to the external environment. Decompression sickness occurs less frequently with regular hyperbaric exposures.

Diverse secondary effects of gas phase formation complicate the pathophysiological evolution of decompression sickness. There is a loss of intravascular fluid volume, and platelet-red blood cell aggregation with release of active intermediate compounds such as serotonin and adenosine compounds. Clinical manifestations of decompression sickness reflect both sequestration of gas bubbles and secondary effects within vascular beds and extravascular spaces. Clinically evident symptoms and signs are likely to occur only when the bubbles lodge in regions wherein ischemia evolves with associated pain and/or perturbed function. For convenience, clinical manifestations are classified as being either minor (type 1) or severe (type 2). Recognition of diverse clinical patterns is important in formulating treatment programs appropriate to the severity in the individual patient. Both minor and severe manifestations of decompression sickness may be present in approximately one-third of these patients. Accordingly, a careful search for subtle type 2 manifestations is mandatory in every instance. Both the minor and severe manifestations of decompression sickness are listed in Table 84-1.

The most characteristic manifestation of mild decompression sickness is pain. Cutaneous or lymphatic involvement may occur as well. Pain is ordinarily localized within or near limb joints. After excursion dives in which compressed air is breathed, the pain is far more likely to occur in the upper rather than the lower limbs. After prolonged exposure to compressed air, as is the case for caisson workers, or after deep oxygen-helium saturation diving, pain typically occurs in the lower rather than the upper limbs. The initial symptom may be numbness. Characteristically, the discomfort becomes more severe in time and debilitating pain may evolve, requiring potent analgesic management. At times local edema may occur over the site of pain. Typically the pain subsides completely or lessens during prompt recompression and trial recompression may be employed diagnostically as well as therapeutically. Untreated limb pain will subside gradually, although complete disappearance of pain is likely to require several days. The cutaneous manifestations of mild decompression sickness include pruritus and patchy cutaneous vasodilatation, consistent with vascular stasis. Urticaria may occur as well. A relatively uncommon manifestation of mild decompression sickness is localized edema, perhaps related to lymphatic obstruction. Most patients also complain of malaise.

TABLE 84-1 Signs and Symptoms of Decompression Sickness

1. Type 1 (minor)
   a. Extremities
      (1) Pain (bends), paresthesia, numbness, edema
      (2) Skin (pruritus, mottling, rash, pallor, and urticaria)
2. Type 2 (severe)
   a. Central nervous system
      (1) Loss of consciousness, scintillating scotomas, Ménière's syndrome, vertigo, aphasia, staggering gait, spastic paralysis, sensory loss, bladder and bowel paralysis
   b. Cardiorespiratory
      (1) Substernal distress, paroxysmal coughing, tachypnea, asphyxia (chokes), shock, hemoconcentration, platelet-red blood cell aggregates
   c. Systemic
      (1) Extreme fatigue

Severe (type 2) decompression sickness is characterized by neural or cardiorespiratory involvement. Manifestations are diverse, multiple, and unpredictable. In the absence of recompression therapy, the natural history is variable. In fulminant cases, cardiorespiratory collapse and death may occur. Permanent serious neurological deficits including paraplegia may also occur. In other instances severe neurological deficits resolve gradually over intervals of weeks and months, despite the absence of appropriate treatment.

Severe decompression sickness involving the cardiorespiratory system is characterized by substernal discomfort, dyspnea, cough, tachypnea, and malaise. A sharp "catch" sensation during inhalation is characteristic. Divers refer to this symptom as the "chokes." Postural hypotension, oliguria, hemoconcentration, and hypovolemic shock may occur.

Neurological manifestations in severe decompression sickness generally involve the spinal cord, reflecting the consequences of the ischemic injury. The onset is often insidious with initial mild symptoms of limb paresthesia and weakness. Minutes or hours later paralysis is observed, commonly with severe impairment of bladder and bowel function. Girdle pains in the trunk are noteworthy early symptoms. Visual aberrations, headaches, abnormal behavior, and disturbed labyrinthine function with vertigo, nystagmus, nausea, and vomiting may develop as manifestations of upper central nervous system involvement. Migraine-like symptoms may occur, particularly in individuals with histories of true migraine headaches.

In a setting where decompression sickness is a serious diagnostic consideration, the most important alternative possibility is intraarterial air embolism.

The practical problem of management is simplified somewhat by the requirement for prompt recompression therapy in both instances. The generally distinctive manifestations of air embolism will be described later in this section.

Management of decompression sickness is straightforward and very successful. Prompt recompression in a hyperbaric chamber, alternately breathing air and 100% oxygen, leads to prompt relief of symptoms within a few minutes in most instances. With appropriate treatment the recovery rate approximates 95 percent. The rationale for treatment is based on the twin principles that (1) reexposure to hyperbaric pressures facilitates the return of free gas to the physically dissolved state, and (2) breathing pure oxygen lowers the concentrations of inert gas within blood, allowing more rapid removal from tissues. Clearly the best results with treatment are obtained with prompt intervention. In the more severe cases of decompression sickness other forms of ancillary therapy, including fluid repletion, colloid transfusions, and glucocorticoids, may be therapeutically beneficial. The details of treatment schedules are outlined fully in the U.S. Navy diving manual.[43] These tables represent standards employed throughout this country. Fortunately for the patient, even serious disability may respond to recompression therapy after a delay of some days. Furthermore, the prognosis for full recovery is good even when the initial response is incomplete. Complete recovery may require as long a period as 2 years in some cases.

Intraarterial Air Embolism[43–45]

In compressed air diving, arterial air (or gas) embolism may occur during ascent to the surface, particularly when the diver fails to exhale normally. Under these circumstances, as ambient pressure decreases during the ascent, gas within the lungs expands according to Boyle's law. Near the surface, small changes in depth result in large changes in gas volume. Failure to exhale may create a pressure gradient exceeding the distensibility of lung tissue. If the positive gradient of pressure between alveolar gas and the pulmonary interstitium leads to rupture of the tissue, free gas is likely to enter the bloodstream and travel through the left side of the heart into the arterial system. The amounts of disseminated gas may be very large. Air may distribute through the arterial circulation, including coronary and renal arteries; however, the most common clinical manifestations occur within the distribution of the carotid arterial system. The usual result is acute profound central nervous system dysfunction, characterized by loss of consciousness, seizures, and paralysis. This severe complication can readily occur after brief exposures or at very shallow depths, circumstances wherein decompression sickness is not a diagnostic consideration. A severe central nervous system deficit is more likely to be permanently disabling or lethal in the absence of adequate treatment than is decompression sickness.

TABLE 84-2 Hospital Procedures Sometimes Associated with Intraarterial Air Embolism

1. Deep venous catheter insertion and usage
2. Radiodiagnostic injections of contrast medium into the intraarterial system
3. Cardiovascular surgery
4. Diverse neural radiodiagnostic and surgical procedures, including myelography
5. Hemodialysis
6. Positive pressure ventilation
7. Transbronchial biopsy

Recompression therapy should commence within a very few minutes if an entirely satisfactory outcome is to be attained. The principles of treatment are similar to those elaborated for decompression sickness. The magnitude of hyperbaric exposure is likely to be greater, however, and adequate treatments may require several days of confinement within a pressure chamber. Some recent data[44] suggest that good results from treatment may be observed even after delays in excess of 24 h.

Serious intraarterial air embolism has also been reported as a consequence of explosive decompression of pressurized aircraft, after accidental trauma to the great vessels, and during blast injury of the thorax. The occurrence of intraarterial air embolism in the hospital setting is not infrequent but is often unrecognized as a complication of various diagnostic and therapeutic interventions (Table 84-2). Air may enter the arterial system directly, during cardiovascular surgery and arterial radiodiagnostic procedures, or after venous air embolism, when acute pulmonary hypertension permits air to cross a patent foramen ovale.

In the patient with serious underlying illness the presence of intraarterial air embolism imposes difficult therapeutic choices for the physician in many instances. Even when recompression therapy is practical, the prognosis is relatively guarded. The principles of treatment are the same as for the diver, however.

Hypoxic Injury

During underwater diving severe hypoxic injury may occur either from inhalation of water into the lungs (drowning) or from apnea, following depression of the central nervous system function. Air embolism or carbon dioxide retention are plausible etiologies for profound hypoventilation or apnea leading to hypoxia. The manifestations of hypoxia have been described elsewhere in this chapter. In a setting of underwater diving, the consequences of severe hypoxia are very likely to be lethal. Emphasis should be placed on prevention of circumstances in which hypoxia is likely to occur and on prompt treatment with oxygen of obtunded individuals seen immediately after a diving exposure.

Hyperbaric Oxygen Therapy

Hyperbaric oxygen therapy is defined as breathing 100% oxygen at greater than normal atmospheric pressures. This is achieved in special environmental chambers containing pressurized gas and at the same time providing adequate technological support for patient care. The importance of hyperbaric pressure is that it provides a means for overcoming a barrier to increased oxygen transport imposed by limited plasma solubility of oxygen. Whereas 100 ml of blood equilibrated at a normal P_{O_2} of 100 mmHg contains only 0.3 ml of physically dissolved oxygen, the latter amount can be increased to almost 6 ml at 3 atm above sea level by breathing 100% oxygen. In the latter circumstance the P_{O_2} in arterial blood will approach 2000 mmHg. The clinical rationale for employment of hyperbaric oxygen has been based on three concepts: (1) function of hypoxic vital organs can be maintained or restored even in the setting of reduced perfusion; (2) specific beneficial pharmacologic action of high oxygen pressures can be achieved; and (3) removal of bubbles within tissues can be expedited dramatically by the combined effect of increased hydrostatic pressure, reducing bubble size, and at the same time accelerating washout of dissolved inert gas by providing a much larger gradient for diffusive outward movement of inert gas molecules from the bubble. The latter principle is exploited fully in the treatment of decompression sickness and intraarterial air embolism, as outlined above. The second principle provides the rationale for use of hyperbaric oxygen in gas gangrene and other anerobic tissue infections. Application of the first principle, maintaining or restoring function of vital hypoxic tissues in a setting of reduced perfusion, is relevant in many cardiovascular diseases.

The potentially wide application of hyperbaric oxygen to the treatment of cardiovascular disease associated with ischemia has been greatly constrained by two major biological problems: (1) profound ischemia is likely to prevent delivery of oxygen to the hypoxic target, and (2) the toxic consequences of prolonged oxygen exposures rule out effective continuous application. As a practical matter, potential problems of neurological and pulmonary toxicity from oxygen are avoided by limiting exposures to generally less than 3 atm above sea level for intervals of time shorter than 90 to 120 min. In practice these intermittent, limited exposures are very well tolerated, and judgments of therapeutic efficacy are based on single or repetitive treatment profiles conforming to these criteria.

To a great extent observations concerning therapeutic application of hyperbaric oxygen to cardiovascular illnesses have been anecdotal. The applications listed in this section are currently not widely employed or accepted in clinical practice, except with carbon monoxide poisoning.

Cerebral Vascular Insufficiency[46–48]

The improvement of techniques for reestablishing arterial blood flow has led to renewed interest in surgical management of chronic cerebral arterial insufficiency. Surgeons have been reluctant to undertake risky interventions, however, in the absence of knowledge as to whether the neurological deficit could be reversed if arterial blood flow were restored. One approach to this difficult problem has been the diagnostic use of hyperbaric oxygen. Very limited observations to date suggest that reversal of neural impairment, associated with brief exposures to hyperbaric oxygen, identify a population of patients likely to respond well to cerebral vascular surgical intervention.

In a small fraction of patients suffering from acute cerebrovascular accidents, the neurological deficit has been reversed dramatically by exposure to hyperbaric oxygen. More often than not, however, the reversal has proved temporary; thereafter, in the absence of means for providing long-term benefit, widespread therapeutic employment has not seemed justifiable. It may be possible in the future, however, to employ prompt administration of hyperbaric oxygen with a therapy that will restore blood flow.

Peripheral Vascular Insufficiency

Medical management of atherosclerotic peripheral vascular insufficiency is associated with relatively limited benefit. Accordingly, there has been considerable interest in alternative therapy. The application of hyperbaric oxygen to this problem has yielded limited results, however, as might be expected when the fundamental problem of vascular insufficiency is not altered by the treatment modality. Therapeutic intervention with hyperbaric oxygen may be beneficial when superimposed acute problems occur such as infection or compromised skin grafts.

Vasculitis, involving the skin and extremities, is more reversible than atherosclerotic vascular insufficiency. Benefit from intermittent treatment with hyperbaric oxygen has been described for forms of vasculitis causing hypoxic injury, often with ulceration.

Ischemic Heart Disease[49]

The initial wave of enthusiasm for therapeutic hyperbaric oxygen generated hope for benefit in ischemic heart disease. One important early observation obtained largely from experimental animals was that hyperbaric oxygen exerted a predictable antiarrhythmic effect. Human observations have been sparse because alternative simple pharmacologic measures are generally successful and much easier to employ.

A concept of minimizing myocardial damage from myocardial infarction by the employment of therapeutic hyperbaric oxygen has been tested experimentally, with variable results. Aside from scattered anecdotal observations, only one controlled study has been performed in humans. In this series, overall mortality of patients treated with hyperbaric oxygen at 2 atm above sea level was lower than that of control patients. The diversity among the patients and comparable excellent results from other centers employing conventional management precluded definitive interpretation, however. At this time hyperbaric oxygen is viewed as being of unproved value in the treatment of ischemic heart disease. No benefit can be anticipated in the population having minimal myocardial injury, since these patients fare very well on conventional management. Significant benefits from hyperbaric oxygen also seem unlikely in that subpopulation suffering from severe cardiogenic shock, in view of the poor overall prognosis for this group. No adequate study has yet been performed in the group of greatest interest, i.e., patients with serious myocardial infarction, who have a substantial mortality when treated in a conventional manner.

Carbon Monoxide Poisoning[46,50]

Acute carbon monoxide (CO) poisoning impairs oxygen transport to tissue by two mechanisms. First, arterial oxygen content is reduced because hemoglobin binds CO with 200-fold greater affinity than oxygen. Second, carboxyhemoglobin shifts the oxyhemoglobin dissociation curve to the left, adversely affecting the release of O_2 from remaining oxyhemoglobin. The net result of high carboxyhemoglobin concentrations is tissue hypoxia with serious functional consequences in hypoxia-sensitive organs such as heart and brain. Clinical manifestations include headache, confusion, visual disturbances, unconsciousness, seizures, pulmonary edema, and, if untreated, death.

With mild forms of carbon monoxide intoxication, recovery is likely to occur with no specific treatment other than removal from the noxious gaseous environment. With more severe forms of intoxication, the outlook at the time of initial evaluation is uncertain. The severity of clinical illness may not correlate with absolute carboxyhemoglobin level. Patients with any form of central nervous system impairment or with carboxyhemoglobin levels above 25 percent merit vigorous therapeutic intervention. The rationale for treatment with high oxygen concentrations is based primarily on enhanced removal of carbon monoxide from blood and possible tissue sites. Because O_2 and CO compete for hemoglobin, hyperbaric oxygenation greatly accelerates CO elimination. Furthermore, O_2 dissolved in plasma under hyperbaric conditions effectively bypasses any impediment to oxygen transport caused by carboxyhemoglobin. Potentially lethal central nervous system injury may be averted as a consequence. Fifteen minutes of exposure to 2.5 atm above sea level of oxygen will effect a release of carbon monoxide from blood equivalent to that obtained after 5 h of breathing air. One hour of hyperbaric therapy is sufficient to reduce carboxyhemoglobin levels well below 10 percent. Prompt recovery is likely if treatment is initiated before irreversible brain damage has occurred.

Cyanide Poisoning[46]

Acute cyanide poisoning blocks mitochondrial electron transport at the terminal member of the respiratory chain, cytochrome A,A3. This rapid process is not competitive with oxygen. Consequently, reports of successful treatment of cyanide intoxication with hyperbaric oxygen are not explained by more rapid removal of cyanide from cytochrome A,A3. Nevertheless, oxygen may be a useful adjunct to the usual cyanide antidotes, sodium thiosulfate and sodium nitrite.

References

1. Alexander, J. K., Hartley, L. H., Modelski, M., and Grover, R. F.: Reduction of Stroke Volume During Exercise in Man following Ascent to 3100 m Altitude, *J. Appl. Physiol.*, 23:849, 1967.
2. Dempsey, J. A., Reddan, W. G., Birnbaum, M. L., Forster, H. V., Thoden, J. S., Grover, R. F., and Rankin, J.: Effects of Acute Through Life-Long Hypoxic Exposure on Exercise Pulmonary Gas Exchange, *Respir. Physiol.*, 13:62, 1971.
3. Vogel, J. A., and Harris, C. W.: Cardiopulmonary Responses of Resting Man during Early Exposure to High Altitude, *J. Appl. Physiol.*, 22:1124, 1967.
4. Hammill, S. C., Wagner, W. W., Jr., Latham, L. P., Frost, W. W., and Weil, J. V.: Autonomic Cardiovascular Control during Hypoxia in the Dog, *Circ. Res.*, 44:569, 1979.
5. Reeves, J. T., Grover, R. F., and Cohn, J. E.: Regulation of Ventilation during Exercise at 10,200 ft in Athletes Born at Low Altitude, *J. Appl. Physiol.*, 22:546, 1967.
6. Alexander, J. K., and Grover, R. F.: Mechanism of Reduced Stroke Volume at High Altitude, *Clin. Cardiol.*, 6:301, 1983.
7. Hellems, H. K., Ord, J. W., Talmers, F. N., and Christensen, R. C.: Effects of Hypoxia on Coronary Blood Flow and Myocardial Metabolism in Normal Human Subjects, *Circulation*, 16:893, 1957.
8. Eaton, J. W., Brewer, G. J., and Grover, R. F.: Role of Red Cell 2,3-Diphosphoglycerate in Adaptation of Man to Altitude, *J. Lab. Clin. Med.*, 73:603, 1969.
9. Grover, R. F., Lufschanowski, R., and Alexander, J. K.: Alterations in the Coronary Circulation of Man following Ascent to 3,100 m Altitude, *J. Appl. Physiol.*, 41:832, 1976.
10. Okin, J. T.: Response of Patients with Coronary Heart Disease to Exercise at Varying Altitude, in J. H. K. Vogel (ed.), "Hypoxia, High Altitude and the Heart, Advances in Cardiology," S. Karger A. G., Basel, Switzerland, vol. 5, 1970, p. 92.
11. Mortimer, E. A., Jr., Monson, R. R., and MacMahon, B.: Reduction in Mortality from Coronary Heart Disease in Men Residing at High Altitude, *N. Engl. J. Med.*, 296:581, 1977.
12. Maritocorena, E., Ruiz, L., Severino, J., Galvez, J., and Penaloza, D.: Systemic Blood Pressure in White Men Born at Sea Level: Changes after Long Residence at High Altitudes, *Am. J. Cardiol.*, 23:364, 1969.
13. Grover, R. F., Wagner, W. W., Jr., McMurtry, I. F., and Reeves, J. T.: Pulmonary Circulation, in J. T. Shepherd, F. M. Abboud, and S. R. Geiger (eds)., "Handbook of Physiology, Section 2: The Cardiovascular System," vol. 3, American Physiological Society, Bethesda, Maryland, 1983, p. 103.
14. Reeves, J. T., Wagner, W. W., Jr., McMurtry, I. F., and Grover,

R. F.: Physiological Effects of High Altitude on the Pulmonary Circulation, in D. Robertshaw (ed.), "Environmental Physiology: III. International Review of Physiology," vol. 20, University Park Press, Baltimore, 1979, p. 289.
15. Vogel, J. H. K., Weaver, W. F., Rose, R. L., Blount, S. G., Jr., and Grover, R. F.: Pulmonary Hypertension on Exertion in Normal Man Living at 10,150 Feet (Leadville, Colorado), in Robert F. Grover (ed.), "Normal and Abnormal Pulmonary Circulation," S. Karger, A. G., Basel, Switzerland, 1963, p. 269.
16. Pryor, R., Weaver, W. F., and Blount, S. G., Jr.: Electrocardiographic Observation of 493 Residents Living at High Altitude (10,150 feet), *Am. J. Cardiol.*, 16:494, 1965.
17. Reeves, J. T., and Grover, R. F.: High-Altitude Pulmonary Hypertension and Pulmonary Edema, in P. N. Yu and J. F. Goodwin (eds.), "Progress in Cardiology," vol. 4., Lea & Febiger, Philadelphia, 1975, p. 99.
18. Sophocles, A. M., Jr., and Bachman, J.: High-Altitude Pulmonary Edema among Visitors to Summit County, Colorado, *J. Family Practice*, 17:1015, 1983.
19. Grover, R. F., Hyers, T. M., McMurtry, I. F., and Reeves, J. T.: High-Altitude Pulmonary Edema, in A. P. Fishman and E. M. Renkin (eds.), "Pulmonary Edema," American Physiological Society, Bethesda, Maryland, 1979, p. 229.
20. Hultgren, H. N.: Medical Problems of High Altitude, *West. J. Med.*, 131:8, 1979.
21. Hackett, P. H., Rennie, D., Hofmeister, S. E., Grover, R. F., Grover, E. B., and Reeves, J. T.: Fluid Retention and Relative Hypoventilation in Acute Mountain Sickness, *Respiration*, 43:321, 1982.
22. Scoggin, C. H., Hyers, T. M., Reeves, J. T., and Grover, R. F.: High Altitude Pulmonary Edema in the Children and Young Adults of Leadville, Colorado, *N. Engl. J. Med.*, 297:1269, 1977.
23. Rowell, L. B.: Cardiovascular Aspects of Human Thermoregulation, *Circ. Res.*, 52:367, 1983.
24. Rowell, L. B.: Cardiovascular Adjustments to Thermal Stress, in J. T. Shepherd and F. M. Abboud (eds.), "Handbook of Physiology. Section 2: The Cardiovascular System. III: Peripheral Circulation and Oxygen Blood Flow," American Physiological Society, Bethesda, Maryland, 1983, p. 967.
25. Greenfield, A. D. M.: The Circulation through the Skin, in W. F. Hamilton and P. Dow (eds.), "Handbook of Physiology," vol. 2, American Physiological Society, Washington, D.C., 1963, p. 1325.
26. Shepherd, J. T.: "Physiology of the Circulation in Human Limbs in Health and Disease," W. B. Saunders Company, Philadelphia, 1963.
27. Rowell, L. B.: Reflex Control of the Cutaneous Vasculature, *J. Invest. Dermatol.*, 69:154, 1977.
28. Brengelmann, G. L., Freund, P. R., Rowell, L. B., Olerud, J. E., and Kraning, K. K.: Absence of Active Cutaneous Vasodilation Associated with Congenital Absence of Sweat Glands in Man, *Am. J. Physiol.*, 240:H571, 1981.
29. Shuster, S.: Systemic Effects of Skin Disease, *Lancet*, 2:907, 1967.
30. Freund, P. R., Brengelmann, G. L., Rowell, L. B., and Halar, E.: Attenuated Skin Blood Flow Response to Hyperthermia in Paraplegic Man, *J. Appl. Physiol.*, 56:1104, 1984.
31. Greeson, T. P., Freedman, R. I., Levan, N. E., and Wong, W. H.: Cutaneous Vascular Responses in Diabetics, *Microvas. Res.*, 10:8, 1975.
32. Escourrou, P., Freund, P. R., Rowell, L. B., and Johnson, D. G.: Spanchnic Vasoconstriction in Heat-Stressed Man—Role of the Renin-Angiotensin System, *J. Appl. Physiol.*, 52:1438, 1982.
33. Ansari, A., and Burch, G. E.: Influence of Hot Environment on the Cardiovascular System, *Arch. Intern. Med.*, 123:371, 1969.
34. Gauer, O. H., and Thron, H. I.: Postural Changes in the Circulation, in W. F. Hamilton and P. Dow (eds.), "Handbook of Physiology," vol. 3, American Physiological Society, Washington, D.C., 1965, p. 2409.
35. Rowell, L. B.: Competition between Skin and Muscle for Blood Flow during Exercise, in E. R. Nadel, "Problems with Temperature Regulation during Exercise," Academic Press, New York, 1977, p. 49.
36. Wade, O. L., and Bishop, J. M.: "Cardiac Output and Regional Blood Flow," Blackwell Scientific Publications, Oxford, 1962.
37. Blackmon, J. R., Rowell, L. B., Kennedy, J. W., Twiss, R. D., and Conn, R. D.: Physiological Significance of Maximal Oxygen Intake in Pure Mitral Stenosis, *Circulation*, 36:497, 1967.
38. Zelis, R., Mason, D. T., and Braunwald, E.: Partition of Blood Flow to the Cutaneous and Muscular Beds of the Forearm at Rest and during Leg Exercise in Normal Subjects and in Patients with Heart Failure, *Circ. Res.*, 24:799, 1969.
39. Bert, P.: "RLA Pression Barometrique," Masson, Paris, translated by M. A. Hitchcock, College Book Company, Columbus, 1943.
40. Bennett, P. B., and Elliott, D. H. (eds.): "The Physiology and Medicine of Diving and Compressed Air Work," 3d ed., Bailliere, Tyndall, London, Maxwell, New York, 1982.
41. Salzano, J. V., Stolp, B., Moon, R. E., and Camporesi, E. M.: Exercise at 47 and 66 Ata, in A. J. Bachrach and M. M. Matzen (eds.), "Underwater Physiology: VII. Proceedings of Seventh Symposium on Underwater Physiology," Undersea Med. Soc., Inc., Bethesda, Maryland, 1981, p. 181.
42. Boycott, A. E., Demant, G. C. C., and Haldane, J. S.: Prevention of Compressed Air Illness, *J. Hyg. (Camb.)*, 8:342, 1908.
43. U.S. Navy Diving Manual, NAV Ships, 0994–001–9010, Navy Department, Washington, 1973.
44. Miller, J. N., Fagraeus, L., Elliott, D. H., Shields, T. G., Grimstad, J., and Bennett, P. B.: Nitrogen-Oxygen Saturation Therapy in Serious Cases of Compressed Air Decompression Sickness, *Lancet*, 2:169, 1978.
45. Strauss, Richard H.: Diving Medicine, *Am. Rev. Respir. Dis.*, 119:001, 1979.
46. "Hyperbaric Oxygen Therapy," Undersea Med. Soc. Committee Report No. 30, CR (HBO), 1983.
47. Holbach, K. H., Wassman, H., and Banatelli, A. T.: A Method to Identify and Treat Reversible Alterations of Brain Tissue, in T. Schmiedek (ed.), "Microsurgery for Stroke," Springer-Verlag, New York, 1977.
48. Heyman, A., Saltzman, H. A., and Whalen, R. E.: The Use of Hyperbaric Oxygenation in the Treatment of Cerebral Ischemia and Infarction, *Circulation* 33(suppl. 2):20, 1966.
49. Thursda, J.: Myocardial Infarction, in J. C. Davis and T. K. Hunt (eds.), "Hyperbaric Oxygen Therapy," Undersea Med. Soc., Inc., Bethesda, Maryland, 1977, p. 315.
50. Kindwall, E. P.: Carbon Monoxide Poisoning Treated with Hyperbaric Oxygen, *Respir. Ther.*, 5:29, 1975.

Section F

Insurance, Legal, and Occupational Problems

85

Insurance Problems of Patients with Heart Disease

Joseph A. Wilber, M.D.

Insurance, n. An ingenious modern game of chance in which the player is permitted to enjoy the comfortable conviction that he is beating the man who keeps the table.

Ambrose Bierce, 1958[1]

Introduction

There are several aspects to the insurance problems of cardiac patients. All patients, including those with heart disease, usually have three kinds of insurance: life, health, and disability insurance (including social security). The amount and type of medical information needed for each type of insurance differ. To further complicate insurance problems, the physician may be called upon to submit medical evidence at two periods in time—when his or her patient is applying for insurance and/or at the time when claims are submitted to the insurance company for illness, disability, or death.

These different kinds of insurance and different purposes for requesting medical information lead to a great deal of misunderstanding. When the physician (or the physician's assistant) is filling out insurance forms he or she often is unaware of which kind of insurance the patient is applying for and is puzzled or even enraged when one patient with mitral valve prolapse (and a cardiac neurosis) is accepted for insurance without an extra premium for life insurance while another patient with the same diagnosis is charged an extra premium or "ridered" for health insurance and perhaps even declined for disability insurance.

Similarly, when claims are submitted for illness or disability, the physician is usually unaware of the terms of the insurance contract and thinks a diagnosis, e.g., angina pectoris, is sufficient information. Yet the claims specialist is working with specific rules and guidelines requiring detailed and objective evidence related to the diagnosis, e.g., frequency and type of chest pain, precipitating factors, response to therapy, and results of resting and stress ECGs, before the claim can be paid.

As a rule, the physician could save the patient time and trouble if he or she would consider the insurance company as a knowledgeable colleague who needs the same information that a consultant would need for diagnosis and treatment. In turn, insurance companies must make sure that their underwriters are very well trained and that their requests for information are clear, detailed, and reasonable, and include the type of insurance being applied for.

Mortality, Life Expectancy, Ratings, and Premiums

Most medical studies of prognoses are reported in terms of percentage dying or surviving over some time period of follow-up;[2] e.g., 15 percent mortality after myocardial infarction in the first year after discharge from the hospital. Usually we do not know the age distribution of the cohort of patients, the distribution of the severity of their disease, and, if there is no control group, we do not know what is the "normal" mortality for a group such as this. This makes comparison with other studies or treatments

TABLE 85-1 Relation of Mortality, Rating, Life Expectancy, and Premium in a 42-Year-Old Male Nonsmoker

			Representative Annual Premium per $100,000 Life Insurance	
Mortality Ratio, %	Table Rating	Life Expectancy in Years	Term Insurance, $	Ordinary Insurance, $
100	Standard	32	161	1,325
150	2	28	241	1,875
200	4	25	322	2,337
250	6	23	402	2,771
300	8	22	483	3,181
350	10	21	563	3,576
400	12	20	644	3,953

very difficult. In recent years, clinical researchers and epidemiologists are reporting more and more in actuarial or life insurance terms such as life table analyses and mortality ratios. Mortality ratios are very useful in describing risk. A mortality ratio may be defined as the number of *observed* deaths over the number of *expected* deaths for a cohort of a certain age and sex within a defined period of time. The *expected* deaths are the number of deaths occurring in a "healthy" population of the same sex and race or other characteristics who do not have the disease or impairment being studied. In life insurance studies, the *expected* death figures are based on 10-, 20-, or even 30-year follow-ups of large numbers of middle- and upper-class people who could afford a life insurance policy large enough to require a medical examination and who were found to be "healthy" or "standard" on that examination. Thus the life insurance population is quite different from the general population; it is better educated, has a higher income, and all those who have had known severe illness or who were found to be impaired have been excluded.

A mortality ratio of 100 percent is defined as the *standard;* 150 percent means 50 percent more deaths than expected, etc. Most companies will not insure anyone with an expected mortality ratio greater than 400 percent (Table 85-1), the reason being that the premium that must be charged for that high a risk becomes impractical.

While there is a direct relation, a 50 percent mortality does not mean a 50 percent decrease in life expectancy or a 50 percent higher price for the insurance. Table 85-1 illustrates the relation between mortality ratios, ratings, life expectancy, and annual premiums charged for a $100,000 term or ordinary life insurance policy by the average company for a 42-year-old male nonsmoker. These mortality ratios and life expectancy features are based on a 1965–1970 intercompany study. Life expectancy has improved 2 to 4 years since then for men and women.

Intercompany Variation

For many of the common chronic health problems of people who buy individual life insurance, such as overweight, elevated blood pressure, and diabetes mellitus, most life insurance companies base their underwriting on mortality studies of their own policyholders or on pooled data of several companies.[3–5] But for many other diseases and especially in order to keep up with newer diagnostic and treatment advances, the life insurance medical directors depend on current scientific medical literature[6] and consultation with authorities in the field.

If a case appears to involve extra risk, it usually is considered individually with consideration of family history, life-style, quality of medical care, and current research trends. In my opinion, many medical directors at this point in time think that an optimistic approach is warranted for some of the major killers, particularly cardiovascular disease.

Because of competition and company variation, it is always wise to get a second opinion if you are dissatisfied with the appraisal of risk for your patients or yourself—that is, if you are sure all the facts have been accurately presented to the life insurance medical director.

In the next sections of this chapter the *life* insurance aspects of the major cardiovascular disorders will be considered in detail. *Health* and *disability* insurance problems of patients with heart disease will be covered briefly toward the end of the chapter. It is my belief and hope that with better understanding and better communication between physician and insuror your patient's insurance needs can be fairly met.

Coronary Heart Disease

Coronary heart disease (CHD) is the leading cause of death in the insured population. The major advances in diagnosis and treatment of CHD in the past 20 years have stimulated a greater interest in prognosis and many clinical studies have reported on long-term survival after treatment, as well as better methods to differentiate the poor from the good risk patient.[7–11] Clinical researchers are interested in actuarial methods to evaluate these new therapies, not only in terms of improving care but also in terms of life expectancy and survival. The life insurance industry has benefited as well from this interest in prognosis and as a result can offer life insurance to most patients with known coronary heart disease at a reasonable though higher-than-average premium.

Survivor of Acute Myocardial Infarction

Approximately 50 to 60 percent of deaths from CHD are "sudden" and occur outside of hospitals or as DOAs in hospital emergency rooms.[12] Progress identifying those at risk of sudden death and preventing these deaths has as yet been limited. The majority of these prehospital deaths are mainly due to lethal ventricular arrhythmias, often without apparent precipitating cause.

Of those who reach the hospital alive, approximately 15 percent die during that admission. Of those discharged, another 15 percent die within 1 year—the majority in the first 6 months after discharge. Thereafter the mortality stabilizes at approximately 2 to 4 percent per year (almost four to eight times the mortality of a "healthy" population, depending on age). Because of these statistics most companies will not insure a myocardial infarction applicant until at least 3 and usually 6 months after the infarction, and if the applicant is under 65, most companies will not consider life insurance until the applicant returns to work or his or her usual occupation. The size of the increased premium will vary depending on factors that indicate low- or high-risk subgroups.

How do you identify the low- or high-risk myocardial infarction patient? The results of newer techniques in both invasive and noninvasive diagnosis testing are the key, if available, and are carefully evaluated by the medical underwriter. Hospital discharge summaries and physicians' records are sought to determine results of right and left heart catheterization, coronary angiograms, ambulatory and exercise electrocardiography, two-dimensional echocardiography, thallium scintigraphy, and nucleotide ventriculography. If done and made available, these test results enable the medical underwriter to accurately predict risk on an individual basis and offer the insurance applicant an equitable price for life insurance.

The major factors that the insurance underwriter considers are (1) the function of the ventricular muscle and (2) the extent and severity of the coronary artery obstructive disease. In general, the occurrence of congestive heart failure, marked cardiac enlargement, hypotension, an ejection fraction of less than 30 percent, large areas of ventricular wall dyskinesia or akinesia, or persistent ventricular ectopy indicate very high risk and most life insurance companies will decline the risk. A positive postinfarction exercise ECG (ST depression early or at Bruce stage 1 or 2), persistent resting tachycardia or ST depression, or inverted T waves are looked upon as indicators of poor risk. The presence of diabetes mellitus, hypertension, hyperlipidemia, or continued cigarette smoking also will result in a maximum high rating or decline. Postinfarction angina usually results in declination if it persists greater than 6 months.

Thus it is beneficial to the patient to have definitive diagnostic studies done prior to or shortly after discharge, not only for optimal treatment but also because the more data available the more accurate will be the risk assessment.

Bypass Surgery

Many of the major life insurance companies, by their underwriting policies and actions, indicate that they have decided to consider bypass surgery as a life-prolonging procedure.[13] While life insurance companies, like clinicians, prefer hard data from well-controlled clinical trials or long-term actuarial studies before attributing benefit to a new therapy, most medical directors tend to be prudently optimistic about the future of scientific progress.

Most companies, for example, will rate the patient who has had successful bypass surgery as a better risk than the unoperated patient with similar extent of disease and functions.

Angina Pectoris

It is usually much more difficult to evaluate and to accurately estimate prognosis in the insurance applicant with angina pectoris than in the applicant postinfarction. There usually is less diagnostic and prognostic information available and often the diagnosis is not documented by testing. The stable, controlled, and well-documented angina applicant, however, is usually considered a better risk than the postinfarction applicant and therefore is given a better (lower) extra premium rating. He or she is usually charged about half the extra premium of the postinfarction patient.

From reviewing many statements from attending physicians, it is apparent that angina pectoris is too often diagnosed without the classical pain and with little or no diagnostic testing. Inaccurate diagnosis may cause major employment and insurance problems for that unfortunate patient for many years. In my opinion, exercise electrocardiography at a minimum and other noninvasive studies are required to support the diagnosis and should be obtained whenever possible. In doubtful or difficult cases, cardiac catheterization and coronary angiography are justified, considering the implications of an exact diagnosis for treatment and prognosis.

Most insurance companies will insure the angina applicant 3 to 6 months after onset of angina pectoris if the disease appears to be stable in that pain is absent or very infrequent on medication, and the resting ECG is normal. The extra premium charged is usually about one-half or one-third less than the extra premium charged the postinfarction insured person. As in the infarction applicant, other risk factors such as cigarette smoking, hypertension, and overweight should be absent or controlled. Diabetes mellitus and angina are considered a very bad combination and usually result in a high rating or decline.

In both kinds of CHD, angina and myocardial infarction, the underwriter looks for the prescription of a good rehabilitation program including diet and exercise, and evidence from follow-up visits that the patient is trying to cooperate. Patients who get the best care usually benefit also from the lowest insurance premiums.

The decline in CHD mortality of approximately 25 percent since 1968[14] was not expected or predicted and has not been definitely attributed to any specific preventive or therapeutic advance but happily it seems to be real and continuing. This trend justifies an optimistic underwriting attitude and supports the prediction that the average American can expect a longer life expectancy.

Hypertension

The nature of the life insurance industry provides a unique opportunity for prospective studies on large numbers of individuals over long periods of time. Therefore it is not surprising that life insurance actuaries were the first to realize the value of the blood pressure measurement in evaluating risk. Physicians, aware of the liability of the casual blood pressure measurement, were initially quite skeptical of the life insurance data, but in the 1950s and 1960s, epidemiologic, prospective studies on general populations confirmed the insurance studies.

Since 1925, the life insurance industry has published five major comprehensive studies of mortality among insured lives according to variations in blood pressure. All of these show a direct, nearly linear relation between systolic and diastolic blood pressure and mortality. The higher the blood pressure, the greater the risk and the more premium that must be charged.

The latest study, the 1979 Blood Pressure Study,[15] dealt in the main with the mortality experience between 1954 and 1972 on about 4,350,000 policies issued to men and women aged 15 to 69. About 530,000 of the policies were issued to men and women with borderline and definite high blood pressure (up to 187 mmHg systolic, 112 mmHg diastolic). Mortality experience in this group was compared to the mortality experience of the remaining normotensive group. During the period of this study, the first effective treatment for high blood pressure was introduced in this country and thus the 1979 study, unlike the previous studies, was influenced by the increasing use of antihypertensive medication during this period. Comparing the 1979 (partially treated) to the 1959 (untreated) hypertensive group, it was seen that overall mortality in the recent study is definitely lower for any level of blood pressure but is especially lower for those with moderately high blood pressure.[15] "Mortality ratios" (previously defined as the *observed* mortality over the *expected* mortality) were approximately 20 percent lower for mild and moderate hypertensive individuals. In a subgroup of applicants taking antihypertensive medication at the time of entry and whose systolic and diastolic blood pressure on insurance examination appeared to be reduced to near normal; i.e., less than 145/less than 95 mmHg, mortality was nearly normal. It appeared that adequate treatment of high blood pressure in borderline and mild cases was most efficacious and reduced risk to that of individuals who did not have elevated blood pressure. For those with higher levels of blood pressure on treatment, mortality was still excessive though better than in 1959.

Untreated

With the great increase in screening and treatment for high blood pressure since 1972, undiagnosed elevated blood pressure discovered on application for life insurance is much less common and is not the problem it once was. If the usual three readings on examination average greater than about 160 mmHg systolic and/or 94 mmHg diastolic, most companies will request additional readings on one or more separate days. If these also are high, a rating (extra premium) is charged depending on age—higher at the younger ages. In general, the industry has become much more optimistic about elevated blood pressure because of the medical profession's greater ability in maintaining normal blood pressures and greater interest in treating even mild cases. If an untreated hypertensive is charged an extra premium initially, he or she can usually have this removed in 6 months to a year by presenting evidence (a physician's statement) that blood pressure has been brought under control and it is checked frequently. It should be rare today that a person continues to pay an extra premium for treated high blood pressure.

Treated

The applicant who admits treatment on examination and whose blood pressure is in the "normal" range (less than 140/90) will usually get standard insurance. Many companies routinely request an urinalysis and ECG in addition to a medical examination. They also write the attending physician to obtain representative readings and to assess adherence to the physician's recommendations. (The large national life insurance laboratories often screen urine specimens routinely for the presence of thiazide diuretics and/or beta-blocker type medications.)

Complicated

Any evidence of target organ damage (with the exception of slight cardiomegaly on x-ray) in an untreated or treated hypertensive applicant usually results in a high rating or a declination. The finding of proteinuria over 50 mg/dl, ST- and T-wave abnormalities on the ECG, or a blood creatinine greater than 1.5 mg/dl in combination with elevated blood pressure means a poor prognosis—often less than 10 years' life expectancy and usually the applicant is uninsurable.

Also, the presence or absence of other cardiovascular risk factors such as diabetes mellitus, hyperlipemia, cigarette smoking, obesity, and positive family history are noted in the assessment of risk in a hypertensive individual. If present, the risk and premium are exponentially increased.

Valvular Heart Disease

Ten years ago undiagnosed or poorly described heart murmurs found on insurance examinations or reported from attending physicians presented a common life insurance problem. These reports from examiners and private physicians often gave evidence that the physician was not well trained in cardiac function or physical examination. It was not too unusual to receive a report of a "functional" diastolic murmur or for a systolic murmur to be labeled "mitral stenosis." The most common problem was a report of a systolic murmur but no information about location, radiation, duration, or response to any maneuvers. As a result, particularly if there was a history of suspected rheumatic fever, systolic murmurs, many of them benign, were rated highly.

Today reports from pediatricians, family physicians, internists, and nearly all recently trained physicians doing life insurance examinations show a great improvement in the average physician's ability to examine the heart. This greater skill is shown by much more detailed descriptions of murmurs, as well as of heart sounds, gallops, clicks, and impulses. The family physician today is no longer satisfied to merely observe a murmur or "wait and see." Noninvasive and invasive diagnostic tests are ordered much earlier and more frequently. As a result, the asymptomatic child or adult with a heart murmur, with or without a history of rheumatic fever, has been or can usually be accurately classified and the risk appraised fairly.

Unfortunately, damage to the valves, whether congenital or from rheumatic fever or endocarditis, continues to impose a shortened life expectancy and therefore may lead to a high rating or declination for life insurance.

Mitral Valve Prolapse

Today this is the most common valve condition reported to insurance companies. Happily, most companies accept asymptomatic applicants at standard premium rates even though it is known that there is a slight increased risk of sudden death.[16] Cases of mitral valve prolapse with frequent chest pains and palpitations or with a holosystolic murmur and/or electrocardigraphic abnormalities may be rated moderately at one-and-one-half or two times average risk.

Congenital

Most companies postpone insuring an infant with known or suspected congenital heart disease until 1 or 2 years of age. Even then there must be a definitive proven diagnosis and surgically correctable lesions must have been repaired. In most cases of congenital heart disease, by age 16 most cases have been catheterized and surgery, if indicated, has usually been done. Cases still needing surgery are rarely seen by life insurance companies today. Many corrected defects, especially if the murmur is gone and heart size and ECG are normal or stable, can then be accepted at standard rates or with a relatively small extra rating that may be removed at a later date. These "best" cases include most atrial and ventricular septal defects, corrected pulmonic stenosis, patent ductus, and coarctation of the aorta. The latter is considered standard only if the arterial blood pressure returns to normal. Proven minor septal defects, unoperated (especially ventricular), are expected to close spontaneously and are also often accepted as standard risk.

In spite of tremendous advances in surgery for congenital and valvular heart disease, there still are some defects that even with correction leave the child or teenage individual with a life expectancy of only 20 to 30 years[17]—much too short to allow a reasonable insurance cost. These usually uninsurable cases include most cases of corrected tetralogy of Fallot, transposition of the great vessels, Ebstein's disease, anomalous venous return, and Eisenmenger's physiology or complex.

Congenital bicuspid aortic valve remains a difficult clinical and underwriting problem. The patient is usually a young or middle-aged adult with a murmur discovered years before, is asymptomatic, and the murmur is faint and may or may not radiate to the neck. Prognosis is extremely variable. Most companies will rate such a case as two to four times the average risk or will decline the risk, especially if the murmur is associated with any suspicion of left ventricular hypertrophy on physical examination, chest x-ray, or ECG.

Acquired

Acute rheumatic fever and rheumatic heart disease are becoming rare diseases in the United States. As a result, most insurance applicants with rheumatic heart disease today are middle-aged or are foreign-born applicants, particularly from Africa or Asia.

However, another form of acquired heart disease is seen with increasing frequency in the older applicant, that is, calcific aortic or mitral valve disease—the former sometimes superimposed on a congenitally abnormal valve.

Asymptomatic life insurance applicants with mitral or aortic valve disease are usually insurable with an extra premium in the absence of cardiac enlargement. In general, the older the applicant with significant heart murmurs, the lower the risk and the rating. For example, a 25-year-old applicant with the murmur of mitral regurgitation would be classified as four or six times the average risk, whereas a 60-year-old applicant with the same murmur might be taken at standard rates if the ECG and chest x-ray were normal. Many companies still decline the younger applicant with a history of rheumatic fever and typical murmurs of mitral stenosis, aortic stenosis, or regurgitation,[18] yet others may accept with a high rating. Most applicants with double murmurs are declined. A few companies are beginning to issue highly rated insurance 2 years after aortic or mitral valve replacement if there have been no complications.[19]

With any type of valvular heart disease, if there is more than mild cardiac enlargement, or if there is chronic atrial fibrillation or any history of past or present cardiac decompensation, the application is declined.

Other Heart Diseases

Space does not permit a detailed discussion of the insurability of all the various kinds of heart disease. Those that are usually diagnosed after serious symptoms appear; i.e., the congestive cardiomyopathies, scleroderma heart, and amyloidosis, are seldom seen by medical underwriters since these people are too sick to consider applying for life insurance.

With the advent of echocardiography and other noninvasive techniques, some diseases such as obstructive and nonobstructive cardiomyopathies are being diagnosed with increased frequency and in the early stages. Unfortunately, little is known as yet of the natural history of these cardiomyopathies, particularly the mild cases.[20,21] As a result most reports are of severe and fatal cases and most insurance companies decline to insure or rate highly anyone with echocardiographic or other evidence of ventricular obstruction or asymmetrical hypertrophy.

One or two episodes of paroxysmal atrial tachycardia or paroxysmal atrial fibrillation are usually accepted for insurance at standard rates if there is no other evidence of heart disease. Frequent and/or prolonged arrhythmias or chronic atrial fibrillation are usually declined.

Unexplained ECG abnormalities are a common problem and are often first discovered on an ECG obtained for life insurance purposes. In the absence of other evidence for heart disease, minor T-wave abnormalities are usually treated leniently. ST-segment abnormalities or frequent ventricular ectopic beats may cause the company to ask for an exercise or treadmill ECG. If there is no evidence of ischemic heart disease with exercise, most companies will issue standard insurance.

With all electrocardiographic abnormalities and particularly with bundle branch blocks, the medical underwriter attempts to obtain copies of or reports of any and all old ECGs. The longer the abnormality can be proven present and unchanged, the lower the rating. Right bundle branch block present several years in an applicant under 40 is usually considered a standard risk. Left bundle branch block is always rated, more so at the higher ages.

For large amounts of life insurance and with older applicants, ECGs and (less frequently) chest x-rays may be routinely requested in addition to an examination for underwriting purposes. About 2 percent of such chest x-rays show cardiomegaly of some degree.[22] This prompts a close scrutiny for any evidence of hypertension or other heart disease, yet only about 15 percent of these eventually are rated. If the cardiomegaly is less than 20 percent enlarged (Clark-Ungerleider tables) and there is no evidence of other disease, there is usually no rating.

Many companies have discontinued exercise ECGs as a routine requirement in applications for large amounts of insurance. A study by Ferrer[23] has shown that in the asymptomatic insurance population the treadmill test is no more sensitive than an adequately done Master's exercise ECG. Exercise ECGs are usually requested now because of a history of recent chest pains or because the resting ECG is abnormal. A negative treadmill ECG is helpful and reassuring. A positive treadmill ECG is usually rated even though it is realized that there is a relatively high incidence of false positives. I have seen on several occasions a positive treadmill ECG done for insurance purposes in an asymptomatic individual that resulted in coronary angiograms and subsequent bypass surgery. More often the angiograms are negative, the insurance is issued, and all parties are relieved.

Health and Disability Insurance

In general, the requirements for health and disability insurance are much more stringent than for life insurance. Common chronic disorders such as degenerative bone and joint disease, psychoneurosis, and chronic or frequently recurring genitourinary disorders, though seldom life-threatening, are usually ridered, rated, or declined because of the high risk of excess hospitalization and other medical costs.

For all practical purposes the patient with known heart disease of any kind is going to have difficulty obtaining standard *individual* health or disability insurance. His or her best opportunity is to obtain such insurance protection through employment or other groups. A major exception to the above is the well-controlled hypertensive person under regular medical supervision. He or she can frequently be accepted for health and disability insurance at standard rates.

Disability

The problem of deciding when a cardiac (or other) patient is disabled is a serious and complex problem. Patients are frightened and depressed after a heart attack or bypass surgery. Their family, friends, and even employers may urge them to retire prematurely and unnecessarily. The physician at this point plays a key role and has an obligation to make vigorous and repeated efforts to get that patient back to work for his or her own best interests. It is usually the family physician, who does not see as many cardiac patients as the specialist, who makes the error of encouraging the patient to retire. If there is a cardiac rehabilitation expert[24] or program nearby, all health insurors are willing and anxious to pay for rehabilitation.

The role of the attending physician is changing as disability determination becomes more scientific and specialized. Legal interpretations of disability based on medical tests and data are now common. Many insurors are no longer asking the physician his or her opinion on whether or not the patient is disabled and instead ask only for objective data and descriptions of illness. With the great advances in diagnosis and measurement of cardiac function, disability determination should become as accurate as estimating risk for death.

References

1. Bierce, A.: "The Devil's Dictionary," Dover Publications, New York, 1958.
2. Freis, J., and Ehrlich, G. (eds.): "Prognosis: Contemporary Outcomes of Disease," The Charles Press Publishers, Bowie, Maryland, 1981.
3. "Life Underwriting Manual," The North American Reassurance Company, 245 Park Avenue, New York, N.Y.
4. "Life Underwriting Manual," Connecticut General Life Insurance Company, Hartford, Conn.
5. "Life Underwriters Guide," American United Life, Indianapolis, Ind.
6. Singer, R., and Levinson, L. (eds.): "Medical Risks: Patterns of Mortality and Survival," Lexington Books, D. C. Heath and Company, Lexington, Mass., 1976.
7. Kannel, W. B., Sorlie, P., and McNamara, P. M.: Prognosis After Initial Myocardial Infarction. The Framingham Study, *Am. J. Cardiol.*, 44:53–59, 1979.
8. Multicenter Postinfarction Group: Risk Stratification and Survival After Myocardial Infarction, *N. Eng. J. Med.*, 309:331, 1983.
9. Schlant, R. C., Toman, S., Stamler, J., et al.: The Natural History of Coronary Heart Disease. Prognostic Factors after Recovery from Myocardial Infarction in 2,789 men. The 5 Year Findings of the Coronary Drug Project, *Circulation*, 66:401, 1982.

9a. CASS Principal Investigators and Associates: Coronary Artery Surgery Study (CASS): A Randomized Trial of Coronary Artery Bypass Surgery: Survival Data, *Circ.*, 68:939, 1983.

10. Weinblatt, E., Goldberg, J. D., Ruberman, W., Frank, C. W., Monk, M. A., and Chaudhory, B. S.: Mortality after First Myocardial Infarction. Search for a Secular Trend, *JAMA*, 247:1576, 1982.
11. Elveback, L. R., Connolly, D. C., and Kurland, L. J.: Coronary Heart Disease in Rochester, Minnesota, II. Mortality, Incidence and Survivorship, *Mayo Clinic Proc.*, 56:665, 1981.
12. Gettes, S.: "Candidates for Sudden Cardiac Death. Recognition and Prevention," Medical Section Proceedings, American Council of Life Insurance, 1982, p. 19.
13. Collins, J.: "Prognosis following Coronary Bypass Surgery," Transactions of The Association of Life Insurance Medical Directors of America, 65:72, 1982.
14. Havlik, R. J., and Feinleib, M.: "Proceeding of the Conference on The Decline in Coronary Heart Disease Mortality, Washington, D.C.," DHEW publ. no. NIH 79–1610, 1979.
15. Society of Actuaries and Association of Life Insurance Medical Directors of America: "Blood Pressure Study 1979," Recording and Statistical Corporation, 1980.
16. Khandheria, B., and Segal, B. L.: Sudden Death and Mitral Valve Prolapse, *Practical Cardiol.*, 10:160, 1984.
17. MacMahon, B., McKeown, T., and Record, R. G.: The Incidence and Life Expectation of Children with Congenital Heart Disease, *Br. Heart J.*, 15:121, 1953.
18. Spagnicolo, M., Kloth, H., Taranta, A., Doyle, E., and Pasternak, B.: Natural History of Rheumatic Aortic Regurgitation. Criteria Predictive of Death, Congestive Heart Failure and Angina in Young Patients, *Circulation*, 44:368, 1971.
19. Ellis, L. B., Singh, J. B., Morales, D. D., and Harken, D. E.: Fifteen to Twenty Year Study of One Thousand Patients undergoing Closed Mitral Valvuloplasty, *Circulation*, 48:357, 1973.
20. McKenna, W., Deanfield, J., Farugui, A., et al.: Prognosis in hypertrophic cardiomyopathy, *Circ. Res.*, 34(suppl.2):179, 1974.
21. Miller, D. H., and Borer, J. S.: The Cardiomyopathies, *Arch. Intern. Med.*, 143:2157, 1983.
22. Ferrer, M. I.: A Study of 6,000 Chest X-rays Obtained for Insurance Purposes, *J. Insurance Med.*, 14:12, 1983.
23. Ferrer, M. I.: Experience with 936 Exercise Electrocardiograms taken for Insurance Purposes, *J. Insurance Med.*, 14:10, 1983.
24. Wenger, N. K., et al.: Physician Practice in the Management of Patients with Uncomplicated Myocardial Infarction. Changes in the Past Decade, *Circulation*, 65:421, 1981.

86

Cardiac Examinations for Legal Purposes

Elliot L. Sagall, M.D.

Forensic medicine: *the specialty areas of medicine, medical science and technology concerned with investigation, preparation, and presentation of evidence and medical opinion in courts and other legal, correctional, and law-enforcement settings.*

William J. Curran, 1975[1]

In our modern society, heart disease and its ramifications constitute an ever-mounting legal as well as medical problem. Nationwide, claims instituted by heart patients and/or their beneficiaries alleging heart disorder, disability, and cardiac death as a workplace or accidental injury or as due to the negligent action of a health-care provider are burgeoning in number and scope. In many instances, the existence of a heart disorder is a key issue in the legal determinations of an individual's physical capacity to participate as a defendant or witness in a legal proceeding, to drive a motor vehicle, to pilot an airplane, to engage in gainful activity, to write a legally valid will or contract, or to enable an insurer to recover some of the moneys paid to a worker as compensation for a work-related injury.

The rapidly expanding interrelationships of heart disorders and the law necessarily will involve physicians who examine and treat cardiac patients more and more frequently in the legal processes concerned with resolution of disputed medical aspects of these claims in one or combinations of several roles. The physician may be a witness called upon to present factual observations personally made in history taking, in performing physical examinations and diagnostic studies, and in rendering treatment; the physician may be an "expert" medical witness called upon to present opinion testimony on the medical matters in issue; or he or she may be a defendant in a medical malpractice suit alleging professional negligence in the diagnostic and/or therapeutic management of a patient.

The question of a cardiac patient's eligibility for certain statutory or common law benefits is basically a legal rather than a medical problem, the ultimate determination of which is assigned to a court, jury, administrative agency, commissioner, referee or some other duly appointed person or persons referred to as a "fact finder." The legal resolution of disputed issues of a medical nature, however, almost invariably necessitates consideration of expert medical opinion by the legal fact finder. Crucial areas such as diagnosis, degree and duration of disability, "conscious" pain and suffering, reasonable costs of past and projected medical and surgical treatment, losses of bodily functions, reduction of life expectancy, prognosis, whether an "end-result" has been reached, and the many other factors that determine damages awarded to the victim of a cardiac injury or benefits available under covering workers' compensation or other legislative acts, and the relationship of each to the alleged injury, generally require that medical substantiation or refutation be presented for the fact finder's consideration in his or her resolution of controverted claims.

Legal Actions Requiring Cardiac Medical Evaluations

The spectrum of legal actions where medical questions relating to cardiology become key issues is vast and varied. Included are (1) claims brought under various state workers' compensation statutes and similar federal legislation (e.g., the Federal Longshoremen's and Harbor Workers' Compensation Act and the Federal Employees' Compensation Act) which allege cardiac disability, treatment, and death as a consequence of a work-related cardiac "injury"; (2) tort claims seeking damages for alleged cardiac injury due to negligence on the part of another person or persons, including suits for medical malpractice; (3) claims against insurers, including the Social Security Disability Insurance program, for pensions, covered medical expenses, losses of income, or accidental death benefits resulting from heart disease; (4) questions as to the fitness of a person with an alleged heart disorder to return to a specific job, to drive a motor vehicle, to operate machinery or other equipment, to pilot an airplane, to participate in a legal proceeding, to serve a prison sentence, or to prepare a will; and (5) claims instituted by insurers alleging preexistent heart disease as a basis for qualifying under "second injury funds" for reimbursement of workers' compensation benefits paid to an injured worker, the voiding of an insurance contract by reason of the applicant's fraudulent concealment of a preexisting heart disorder, or the nonpayment of special benefits provided in the insurance contract for death or injury due to an accident because of the contribution thereto by a preexistent cardiac disorder.

Although individual state and federal workers' compensation acts differ somewhat in requirements for eligibility and benefits provided to injured workers and their dependents with frequent legislative changes as well,[2] the fundamental social principle underlying all compensation statutes is the same, namely that the financial costs of work-related injuries should be assumed to a large extent by the employer as an expense of production and not by the injured worker, nor placed on the public dole. Without exception, all compensation acts embrace the basic concept that the right to compensation for work-incurred injury is afforded to the injured employee without regard to fault or demonstrable negligence of the employer. Legal defenses available under common law to employers to avoid or to mitigate liability such as "assumption of the risk" of the job by the employee's acceptance of the employment, or "contributory negligence" by the employee or fellow employees ("the fellow servant rule") are specifically excluded from workers' compensation. In turn, the benefits potentially accruing to an injured employee are generally limited to a portion of the lost wages plus allowances for dependents and reasonable and necessary medical expenses. Items such as pain and suffering, and loss of consortium, which may play a large role in the determination of an award to an injured person in actions for tort (negligence) under common law, are excluded.

In workers' compensation, legal liability attaches to the employer (or to his or her insurance carrier) for the consequences of an injury demonstrated to have occurred during "the course of" and to have arisen "out of" employment. Under some compensation statutes, this basic formula of compensable injury has been modified by specific legislative restrictive definitions that require that the alleged work injury be suffered "by accident," or be due to "unusual stress," or to "stress greater than normal nonwork stress." In many jurisdictions, an identified time and place of injury must be demonstrated for coverage to apply. And in one compensation act (Wyoming), a further restriction has been placed for acceptance of an alleged work-related cardiac injury by the requirement that no more than 4 h must have elapsed between the claimed time of injury and the first clinical manifestations of same.[3]

On the other hand, in many states the definitions of "personal injury" for purposes of compensation or for retirement under provisions of "accidental injury" have been modified for certain named occupational groups, particularly uniformed police and firefighters, by the legislative inclusion in the covering statutes of presumptions (theoretically rebuttable but practically most often not) to the effect that for these specifically named occupations disabling heart disease and/or hypertension are to be considered as job-related, presumably from the "stress" of these employments. In such instances, applicants for retirement under these statutes need only establish the existence of a disabling cardiac or hypertensive condition and not its causal relationship to work. Many of these statutes further define disability as an inability to perform "all" the duties and thereby further ease the probative requirements of the applicant. At the other end of the scale, one state (Nevada) has excluded in its compensation act recompense to a worker for injuries, disability or death due to coronary atherosclerosis, thereby eliminating by legislative action this category of heart disorder as an "occupational injury."[3]

Particularly important in adjudication of claims for cardiac injury, disability, or death under workers' compensation is the universal acceptance by compensation adjudicators of the common law precept that prior infirmity is no bar to benefits under the act even though the injured worker would not have suffered injury, as is the case in most cardiac claims, had he or she not been suffering from underlying heart disease, whether known or unknown. Legally, the injured worker is entitled to compensation benefits if it can be shown that the employment or some factor derived therefrom aggravated a preexisting condition to lead to injury, disability, or death sooner than otherwise would have been expected during the natural history of the underlying disorder.

Under actions in tort in common law, recovery of "damages" may be obtained when the plaintiff or those claiming through the plaintiff can show that the disorder and its consequences arose from or was aggravated by the negligent activity of another (commonly referred to as a "tortfeasor"). Unlike the doctrine of workers' compensation, liability in actions of tort is predicated on fault. To be awarded "damages," the injured party must show that (1) the defendant owed the plaintiff a duty, i.e., the duty to adhere to an accepted standard of medical or other care and the duty to refrain from negligence; (2) that the defendant's conduct breached that duty; (3) that the plaintiff suffered injuries or "harms"; (4) that the defendant's negligent conduct was the proximate cause of the damage (harms) allegedly suffered by the plaintiff and, generally, (5) that the victim's own negligence did not contribute to his or her harms ("the doctrine of contributory negligence").

Actions in tort alleging cardiac injury most commonly arise from motor vehicle accidents where it is claimed that a myocardial contusion, an acute coronary artery occlusion, or an acute cardiac ischemic episode in a person with known or previously unknown coronary atherosclerotic heart disease has resulted from mechanical or physical trauma or from the psychologic consequences of the accident. Most difficult in both medical and legal handling of such claims are those situations where it is alleged that a preexisting condition of angina pectoris has been aggravated, as evidenced by a change in the symptom complex manifested by an increase in the frequency and severity of attacks after an accident, or when new-onset angina allegedly occurs after an accident, but with no objective evidence to support the claimed symptomatology. Another commonly encountered vexing medicolegal problem in this area is whether a fatal cardiac episode was "the result of" or "the cause of" an accident—a determination also of import when insurance contracts provide double indemnity or other specified benefits for "accidental" death or injury.

Other frequently encountered actions in tort involving cardiac patients are those in which it is alleged that heart problems have stemmed from trauma or stress subsequent to negligent conduct, such as from falling objects, slipping and other accidentally induced falls, from exposure to food poisonings, from toxic fumes, from menacing animals, and from long-term psychologic "stress" claimed as a consequence of a chronic pain syndrome, or from an anxiety-producing situation of an injury such as the need for repeated hospitalizations, for surgery and/or from resulting financial hardships attributable to an original noncardiac injury.

Medical malpractice suits, often referred to as "professional negligence" to lessen the sting, fall within the province of actions in tort and are subject to the same legal considerations affecting all claims for "damages" due to "negligence." In malpractice cases, as with other actions in tort, the aggrieved patient or those acting through him or her has the burden of demonstrating by factual and opinion evidence (1) that the defendant doctor or other health-care provider named in the legal action breached a standard of care owed the plaintiff, and (2) that this breach did in fact cause the plaintiff "harms." In evidentiary proof, the plaintiff must define the standard of care alleged to have been breached by proferred expert medical opinion; the plaintiff must further establish the existence of alleged "harms" or "damage"; and also must then show, again by expert medical opinion, that the alleged deviation from the acceptable standard of care was the cause of the claimed "damages." Finally, in many jurisdictions the plaintiff must further demonstrate that his or her conduct did not negligently contribute to the claimed harms. Again, unless all these criteria are satisfied, the burden of proof legally assigned to the plaintiff will not be considered to have been met and a directed verdict for the defendant may be ordered by the judge, thereby effectively dismissing the plaintiff's legal action unless reversed by appeal to a higher court.

In some legal actions, existence of a prior cardiac disorder is of importance in assessment of financial awards. Under the so-called "Second Injury Funds" of the Federal Longshoremen's and Harbor Workers' Compensation Act and of many state workers' compensation acts, some financial relief is afforded the employer or insurer for disability payments to an injured worker if it can be demonstrated that the work incapacity following an accepted or assigned work injury was made substantially greater than would otherwise have been the case because of a preexistent medical condition, as for example, a prior myocardial infarction. In other instances, the demonstration of a heart disorder may be of key importance in a legal decision as to whether a worker can return to a prior job which an employer claims involves physical or psychologic stress potentially harmful to a person with known heart disease or where the operation of machinery by a person subject to sudden incapacity, as from an acute cardiac dysrhythmia, would endanger others; whether a person should be rejected from driving a motor vehicle, particularly one used in public transportation, or from piloting an airplane; whether a heart patient can participate in a court trial as a defendant or witness or serve a prison term, write a valid will, or be forced to pay alimony or other financial assessment; whether certain items claimed as income-tax-deductible medical expenses are medically justified as treatment; whether an insurance contract can be voided because of the applicant's fraudulent concealment of a known cardiac disorder in the original application for the policy; and in other situations where the question of preexistent heart disorder may be of importance for legal and insurance purposes.

A large area of litigation frequently involving heart disorder concerns the many applicants for disability benefits under the Social Security Disability Insurance Program, public welfare programs, the Veterans Administration service and nonservice-related pensions, and privately purchased disability, accident, and health insurance contracts. In most of these situations, the legal issue to be decided is the work capacity of the individual, based on a demonstrated medical condition, not the question of causation.

Miscellaneous legal actions that may require expert medical opinions on heart disorders and their consequences include determination of "conscious pain and suffering" as an element of tort "damages," losses of bodily functions under certain workers' compensation statutes, a reduction of life expectancy due to a cardiac disorder or worsening thereof, the projected reasonable medical expenses of future treatment in a cardiac patient, the relationship of a coronary artery bypass grafting to a compensable myocardial infarction, the prognosis, and other questions too numerous to list.

The Cardiologist in the Courtroom

It is in the role of an expert witness that physicians in cardiology most often find themselves involved with the legal profession. Any duly licensed physician, whether a general or family practitioner or a specialist, is considered legally qualified to present opinion testimony when the medical issues on the matter in hand are not patently discernible as a matter of common knowledge or are not within the recognized ken of a layperson, as in most cardiac cases. However, the appropriateness of a particular physician's competency to testify as an expert can be raised by either side to the dispute and put before the court or other legal body involved for its evaluation and acceptance or rejection. Once a physician has been accepted as an expert witness, his or her testimony can be received. The fact-finding body then determines the weight to be attached to the conclusions presented. As a practical matter, since the current state of scientific knowledge in cardiology does not enable, in many instances, clear-cut definitive answers to many of the courtroom medical questions raised in individual cases, there not infrequently is a difference between the conclusions reached by the expert witnesses called by the disputants in the litigation. In such instances, the legal fact finder can adopt as "factual" that opinion believed most likely to conform to the facts in the case and to reach a decision on that basis. In some jurisdictions, the fact finder may call upon an outside court-appointed physician or medical panel for an "impartial" opinion, but is not bound to accept the opinions so proferred.

The physician who testifies as an expert witness need not have personally examined the claimant, nor even have any personal knowledge of the claimant's medical condition prior to or following an alleged incident. The medical expert may reach conclusions solely from a review of the medical records of the claimant and other factual data that have been admitted into evidence. Alternatively, the expert may be presented with a hypothetical question that contains a set of facts to be assumed to be true and to be utilized as the factual basis for the conclusions reached and the opinions expressed. The law, however, does require that those facts put forth in the hypothetical question be supported by the evidence presented in the case. Thus, the fact finder cannot adopt the opinion expressed by an expert in answer to a hypothetical question unless the evidence on hand is sufficient to establish legally the truth of the underlying facts. When the factual evidence is conflicting, as is frequently the case, it is within the province of the fact finder to determine which evidence is to be believed and adopted as "factual." The hypothetical question posed to a medical expert in courtroom proceedings need not include all the evidence previously presented in the case. It may be limited to a partisan recital of that evidence most favorable to the proponent's side. However, the adversary party, in cross-examination of the expert, can propose a counter-hypothetical recital of alleged facts to provide facts omitted or now added to the original hypothetical question posed in direct examination. The medical expert can then be queried as to whether the newly assumed factual changes or additions alter or modify the opinions previously expressed. In this manner, both parties in the legal dispute have full opportunity to pose to medical experts respective versions of what they believe is factual. Again, however, the ultimate determination for legal purposes rests with the duly appointed fact finder.

Generally, it is not sufficient for an expert witness to present conclusions alone without supporting reasoning. The bases upon which he or she came to the opinion rendered also may be subject to attack in cross-examination so that they can be considered by the fact finder in reaching a decision as to which of conflicting medical opinions to adopt.

In formulating an opinion, the medical expert must appreciate the degree of certainty required in reaching medical conclusions when such opinions are to be expressed in the courtroom and not in a medical forum per se. The legal system recognizes the current inability of medical science to answer definitively and with absolute certainty many of the medical questions raised in individual cases. Yet, the legal body before which the claimant's case ultimately (often after long delay) has been placed for final legal resolution must answer as best it can all the issues raised at the time of trial. The law does not have the luxury of being able to defer resolution of controverted medical issues until medical science has advanced to the point of providing clear-cut answers to the questions on hand. Legal proof, therefore, cannot be equated with scientific proof. While pure science seeks absolute certainty or positive proof before reaching a determination, legal decisions necessarily are far less exacting in their demands for proof. In civil cases, decisions are based primarily upon such standards as "preponderance of the evidence," and "clear and convincing evidence," whereas in criminal matters, the requirements are more stringent, usually "beyond a reasonable doubt."

For answers to medical questions, the law generally requires that these be expressed in terms of "probability" rather than mere "possibility," which in essence means that the conclusions reached by an expert are, in his or her opinion, "more likely than not" true with a tilting of the balance scale to as little as 50.1 percent versus 49.9 percent sufficient to determine the courtroom outcome, although such a difference would not be acceptable to a body of scientists. In accord with legal philosophy, the medical expert is commonly asked to express his or her answers in terms of "reasonable medical certainty," when what is generally meant is in terms of "legal" certainty—a far less exacting criterion of proof than that required for rigid medical "scientific" certainty.

In cases involving cardiac claims, as in most civil cases, the burden of proof is placed upon the claimant who must show by a preponderance of supporting evidence, including expert opinion when necessary, that his or her contentions are true. For example, in a claim alleging a cardiac disorder and its consequences as a workplace injury, the claimant must provide the fact finder with sufficient supporting medical expert testimony attesting not only to the existence of a cardiac disorder but also its causal relationship to some element of the employment, otherwise the claim will fail. A claimant's burden of proof is not met when his or her medical expert merely acknowledges the "possibility" of the truth of the allegations rather than asserting their "probability"; nor is it sustained when the medical supportive conclusions are shown to be based upon speculation, surmise, or conjecture rather than on "reasonable medical certainty or probability"; nor when the medical expert admits that acceptance or denial of the allegations are equal possibilities which cannot be differentiated. In a few instances, as under the Federal Longshoremen's and Harbor Workers' Compensation Act, in some other compensation acts, and when the doctrine of *res ipsa loquitur* ("the thing speaks for itself") is applied legally in a medical malpractice case, the burden of proof in certain medical cause-and-effect determinations is shifted by a legal presumption establishing causation unless the contrary is established by the defendant.

When expert medical opinions presented by the respective litigants contradict or conflict, the fact finder may choose between them with his or her choice subject to reversal on appeal to a higher court only when blatantly against the weight of the evidence or resulting from an error in legal procedure, as with acceptance of evidence admissible under the law.

Commonly Requested Medicolegal Cardiac Evaluations

Medical examinations and evaluations performed specifically for legal and insurance reasons necessarily emphasize aspects of the medical situation not customarily addressed by physicians, since the primary purpose of such evaluations is the answering of legal questions and not the providing of medical care.

The scope of potential medicolegal questions in litigants whose heart disorder is germane to the litigation is too vast and varied for detailed discussion within the constraints of this chapter. Certain inquiries, however, are fundamental to most claims alleging cardiac injury, disorder, dysfunction, or death and warrant further consideration and elaboration. These are (1) the cardiac diagnosis that is to be accepted legally as established in a given claimant; (2) the time of onset of each specific cardiac lesion or dysfunction, particularly those with legal import; (3) the causal relationship, if any, between the factor or factors under legal examination and the cardiac disorder found or some aspect thereof; (4) the medical determination of the impairment to be assessed on the basis of the claimant's overall cardiovascular status and, more specifically, to each component of the cardiac condition that has legal significance in its derivation; and (5) the medical considerations in allegations of professional negligence in the physicians' and/or other health-care providers' handling of a cardiac patient as the basis of resulting harm.

Defining the Cardiac Diagnosis

From the medical viewpoint, the diagnosis (see Chap. 6) is the foundation upon which the treatment of the patient is constructed. From the legal viewpoint, the diagnosis is the foundation upon which many decisions and rulings are made concerning issues of causation, eligibility for disability and retirement pensions, awards for damages, and many other matters arising in the litigation on hand.

Although the diagnosis, in actuality, has to be made by a physician from medical data, legally the diagnosis is considered to be but one of the various factual determinations within the province of the fact-finding body assigned to adjudicate the case.

The diagnosis reached by a physician after the gathering, reviewing, and studying of the medical data is, in essence, merely an opinion based upon the individual examiner's specialized training, study, experience, and interpretation of the medical findings. As such, it is open to question both medically and legally as to reasonableness, accuracy, and completeness. Since the diagnostic conclusions in individual instances reached by a medical examiner may not be concurred in by other physicians evaluating the same data, opinions expressed in court concerning the diagnosis, as with all medical conclusions, are subject to interrogation by counsel during cross-examination.

The cardiac diagnosis[4] should be established in each instance as fully as possible in terms of (1) an *etiologic* diagnosis that describes the underlying disease processes basically responsible for the structural and functional disorders found in the patient/claimant, (2) an *anatomic* diagnosis that describes the specific structural abnormalities (lesions) found in the cardiovascular examination, (3) a *physiologic* diagnosis that describes the resulting physiologic disturbances of cardiovascular action, (4) cardiac status, and (5) prognosis. These should be delineated in generally accepted terminology, as recommended by the Criteria Committee of the New York Heart Association in the latest edition of that committee's publication, "Nomenclature and Criteria for Diagnosis of the Heart and Great Vessels."[4] (See Chap. 6.)

Because of varying connotations and implications, nonspecific terms, such as "heart attack," "coronary," "mild or massive heart attack," and "heart disease" without adequate qualification as to specific meaning should not be employed in the cardiac evaluator's written report or testimony. Similarly, umbrella terms, such as "unstable angina," "preinfarction angina," "acute coronary deficiency," and "acute coronary insufficiency," currently popular in medical jargon to designate certain symptom complexes encountered during the course of ischemic heart disease, should be avoided unless they are precisely defined.

The *etiologic diagnosis* should be reached after consideration of both the structural and functional disturbances found. If two or more etiologic bases for a person's heart disorder are present, each should be listed. Legally, the identification of the etiologic basis of a cardiac disorder or disorders becomes important in a causality assessment where an aggravation or worsening of a preexistent cardiac condition is claimed as a "personal injury" and must be differentiated from the expected natural progression of an underlying cardiac disorder and in legal actions where an estimation of life expectancy is of importance in determining awards for "damages" or in settlement proceedings.

The *anatomic diagnosis* comprises that component of the total cardiac diagnosis which describes the specific structural lesions of the heart and great vessels. A complete description of the anatomic alterations often constitutes an important aspect of the legal determinations of a cardiac "personal injury" and of disability. Thus, for example, there may be considerable difference in the benefits or awards available legally for the sustaining of an episode of prolonged ischemic cardiac pain when diagnosed as an intermediate coronary syndrome attack without new myocardial damage or when diagnosed as acute myocardial necrosis with resulting permanent new heart damage and a change in the preexistent condition.

Anatomic lesions of the heart and great vessels frequently can be delineated clinically on the basis of the history, the findings of physical examination, and the results of specialized cardiac diagnostic studies. Certain anatomic lesions, however, cannot be diagnosed with reasonable certainty by currently available cardiac studies. Thus, diagnoses of "coronary thrombosis" and "microscopic myocardial necrosis," terms not infrequently encountered in cardiac medicolegal reports and expert testimony, should be reserved for the pathologist after autopsy study. When more than one anatomic abnormality is found, each should be included in the final diagnosis.

The *physiologic diagnosis* specifies the alterations in cardiovascular dynamics that have resulted from the cardiac pathology. The physiologic diagnosis includes a description of the cardiac rhythm, and whether of normal or abnormal mechanism; disturbances in cardiac impulse conduction; disturbances in supravalvular, valvular, or subvalvular function; malfunctions of prostheses, homografts, and cardiac pacemakers; disturbances in myocardial pump functioning; disturbances in intravascular pressures; abnormal communications (shunts) in the heart or great vessels; and the anginal syndromes.

The *cardiac status* is determined by analyzing all the data collected on the patient. It is *not* determined by the patient's symptoms alone.[4]

The *prognosis* should be determined and graded according to the New York Heart Association.[4]

The physician performing a cardiac evaluation for legal purposes must determine if the patient-claimant had heart disease prior to the alleged potentially harmful exposure under legal consideration and, if so, whether there was a change in the preexistent cardiac status after the exposure. If a change is found, the physician must then define its nature, degree, and whether permanent or temporary.

Diagnoses presented to a legal forum must be established in terms of reasonable medical certainty which means in terms of "probability." "Possible," "potential," or "suspected" heart disorder has no place in the courtroom or in other legal determinations.

Timing the Onset of Cardiac Lesions and Dysfunctions

Determining the time of onset of a specific cardiac pathology or dysfunction is an essential part of most cardiac medicolegal evaluations, often the crux of an issue of causation or of eligibility for the benefits of an insurance contract. Because of the vagaries of clinical presentations, individual differences in response to and manifestations of illness, and the frequent initial "silent" development of many cardiac pathologies with no symptoms or abnormal signs evident until the process has progressed to an advanced state, the current state of the art frequently prevents medical science from timing the onset of cardiac pathologies and/or dysfunctions within the precise time framework sought by the law. Additionally, medical science may not be able even to delineate the sequence of development of the pathophysiologic processes underlying various pathologies such as an acute myocardial infarction. Yet, difficult though it may be in specific instances, the time of onset of cardiac lesions and dysfunctions must be defined by the cardiac examiner as best can be within frameworks of reasonable medical certainty and probability.

The time of occurrence of a single episode of angina pectoris is fairly easy to pinpoint since, in most cases, the symptoms of the attack are clear-cut and abrupt in onset, thereby enabling a reasonably accurate timing of the commencement of the individual attack. Similarly, the end of the attack is evidenced by the disappearance of symptoms, although some degree of subsiding myocardial ischemia may be present for a short time thereafter.

Delineating the time of onset of an episode of myocardial infarction is more difficult because of variable clinical presentations. The classic textbook presentation of sudden crushing anterior chest pain associated with profuse diaphoresis, dyspnea, weakness, and other cardinal symptomatology is a generally acceptable index of the occurrence at that time of discrete acute myocardial tissue necrosis, although the possibility of some degree of myocardial necrosis having occurred previously (silently or with atypical manifestations) cannot be excluded. In many patients, the process of acute myocardial infarction is an ongoing ischemic/necrotic process that may start minutes to hours to several days prior to the initial appearance of recognizable symptoms, signs, and laboratory or electrocardiographic abnormalities. In some patients, an acute myocardial infarction, although evident at a later date on an electrocardiogram or at postmortem examination, is clinically silent at the time of occurrence. In other patients, the clinical picture is one of waxing and waning ischemic symptoms or signs over the course of one or more days (a state often referred to as "unstable angina"), with or without culmination in a bout of classic, prolonged chest discomfort that heralds the infarction of a larger discrete mass of myocardium. In still other patients, the first anginal attack ("new onset angina") may actually represent an acute myocardial infarction. And in patients with previous angina pectoris, an acute myocardial infarction may be manifested by an anginal attack of greater severity and duration or with radiation and location different from that previously experienced.

It must further be appreciated that the time of occurrence of an acute myocardial infarction, if determinable, does not necessarily reflect the time of onset of underlying coronary atherosclerotic heart disease or the time of initiation of a thrombotic coronary artery occlusion or other pathophysiologic processes that result in infarction of the myocardium.

Clues to timing the onset of an acute myocardial infarction may be provided by the time of appearance of certain signs, laboratory findings, and the time sequence of development of electrocardiographic changes during the acute phases of the illness. Thus, a retrospective correlation of the time of the initial detection of abnormal cardiac enzyme and isoenzyme levels and the time of peak abnormal values with the clinical picture may enable a rough extrapolated determination of the time of occurrence of infarction of a significant degree to be so detected. Additional guides for such temporal extrapolations include the times of initial and peak leukocytosis, the development of postmyocardial infarction fever, the occurrence of a pericardial friction rub or of a rupture of infarcted myocardium, and of other potential concomitants of an acute myocardial infarction. From the viewpoint of the pathologist, the time of onset of a process of myocardial infarction can be roughly estimated by correlation of the gross and microscopic postmortem appearance of the involved tissue with those generally expected (on the basis of accumulated experience and knowledge) at different time periods after the beginning of the attack.

Unless otherwise determinable, the time of onset of a cardiac dysrhythmia generally is accepted as the time of occurrence of identifying symptoms such as palpitation or initial awareness of heartbeat irregularity, or of a sudden collapse as with a cardiac arrest due to ventricular tachycardia or fibrillation.

The time of onset of coronary atherosclerotic, valvular, hypertensive, and most other heart disorders generally cannot be determined medically with any greater accuracy than that the underlying etiologic condition must have been present for some time (usually only measurable in months or years) prior to the initial clinical manifestations or abnormality which led to its detection.

The occurrence of sudden collapse, acute pulmonary edema, cardiogenic shock, or severe pain provides an index of the time of rupture of an aortic aneurysm or of a cardiac valve, papillary muscle, chordae tendineae, or infarcted myocardium. However, the commencement of the pathophysiologic processes underlying such rupture most often cannot be pinpointed with accuracy because of subtle or silent initial clinical manifestations for a variable period of time preceding the end-stage catastrophic event.

Assessment of Causality

The determination of causation is vital to legal actions in which a heart disorder or its consequences is claimed as a compensable "work injury," as an injury due to someone's negligence, or as an "accident" under an insurance contract in which benefits are specifically provided for injury, disability, or death due to an "accident" rather than the result of "illness."

In such actions, claims of cardiac injury, dysfunction, disability, or death generally allege, as *a* or *the* cause, either (1) an isolated, specifically identified incident, event, accident, trauma, exposure, complication of medical or surgical treatment, or (as in a malpractice action) a negligent treatment or negligent failure to institute indicated treatment; or (2) a set of repetitive, cumulative factors which, although subliminal individually, have combined in additive effect to produce cardiovascular harm, such as a recent period of days, weeks, or months of mounting physical or psychologic stress as might be associated with unduly long work hours, an impending deadline or quota, trying business conditions, a forthcoming surgical procedure, or some other presumed stressful happenings; or (3) long-term "overall" job or situational physical or psychologic "stress"; or (4) a combination of one or more of the preceding.

In such actions, the claimant, in addition to establishing the existence of a cardiac disorder that can be accepted as an "injury" and the causal connection thereof to an item with attached liability, must also establish a causal connection between such "injury" and the alleged harmful consequences (disability, medical expenses, pain and suffering, death, and other items of "harm") for which benefits are claimed. The claimant usually has the further burden of disproving any contributions to his or her "harms" from intervening causes or from his or her own negligence should such allegation be raised by the defendant.

In disputed issues involving causality questions in medical disorders, the fact finder in reaching his or her legal decision must rely upon the evidence put forth by the respective litigants, particularly expert medical opinion testimony. Physicians presenting such testimony in cause-and-effect assessments must appreciate the different weights assigned by the legal profession to the various elements that comprise a legal causality determination from those assigned by the medical profession to a pure medical assessment of causality. Because of differences in training and orientation backgrounds, causation often means one thing to a physician and quite another to an attorney, judge, or administrative hearing official. It is not surprising, then, that on occasions medical opinion testimony based upon traditional medical concepts of causality differs dramatically from answers based primarily upon legal concepts utilized by a fact finder in reaching courtroom decisions.

The differences between the medical and legal approaches to solving causality problems are many.[5] The physician, for example, in viewing a patient's medical problems instinctively searches for the basic cause or causes underlying the overall disorder, whereas legal and judiciary professionals generally limit their concern to the one or more items under legal scrutiny as an "injury," independent of other causes. The physician generally defines "to cause" as the production of a new condition or a new pathology or dysfunction, whereas the law in its definition of "to cause" accepts the aggravation of an underlying disorder by the worsening, hastening, or acceleration of its progression to lead to impairment, bodily harm, or death sooner than otherwise would have occurred during the natural history of the preexisting condition without the claimed noxious exposure. The law thus includes in its framework of causation the "triggering" or "proximate-precipitation" of a new stage of pathology or of a new dysfunction in an underlying disorder.

Physicians are reluctant to assign causal responsibility when the degree of aggravation of a preexisting condition is small in overall relationship to the extent of the underlying abnormality or when the degree of hastening of an inevitable end result is minor in relation to the entire clinical condition. The law, on the other hand, emphasizes the fact of hastening or aggravation, not the quantitative aspects. The crux of legal causation thus is the occurrence of an aggravation of an underlying disorder, not the degree to which it was aggravated, or the hastening of an end result, not how much it was hastened.

Physicians in their assessments of causation are particularly impressed that the alleged injurious results, as is true in most cardiac cases, would not have occurred in the absence of a preexisting disorder which rendered the patient susceptible to harm from the alleged exposure. Legal fact finders, however, see it as immaterial that the event in question would not have caused injurious consequences had the victim been in good or average health. In all "personal injury" legal actions, the victim is "taken as he is found." Preexisting infirmity does not bar legal recovery, nor is it an acceptable excuse to relieve a defendant from legal responsibility nor mitigate the damages to be assessed. An illustration is the case of the proverbial "straw that broke the camel's back." To the physician, the proverb emphasizes the obvious predisposition to break down because of existing overload. The physician thus assigns the cause of the camel's collapse to the prior strain on his back, not to the added straw. The law, on the other hand, asserts that although loaded to the breaking point, the back had held up without breaking. Accordingly, the added straw must be viewed as the cause of the collapse and the person who placed the straw on that loaded back as legally responsible for the consequences. Most often, the assignment of legal liability in such situations is made without attempt to apportion a percentage harm between the triggering straw and the preload.

Unfortunately, the many current deficiencies in medical knowledge concerning the etiology and pathogenesis of most cardiac disorders and the limitations of presently available cardiac diagnostic testing procedures often prevent medical science from defining precisely the complete cardiac diagnosis, the nature and extent of the underlying pathology, the pathophysiologic mechanisms which have led to the end result, the sequence in which pathologic lesions have developed, the time of onset of certain lesions, and the answers to the many medical questions which may be of key importance in the legal matter on hand. The medical determination of causation is further made difficult because the very nature of most cardiac disorders categorized legally as "personal injuries" do not, in contrast to lesions such as burns or lacerations, present clinical or pathologic features pathognomonic of trauma or of an external cause. Thus, the question of whether some identified external element or stress played a contributory or precipitating role in their development or whether the disorder found stemmed from the natural, expected progression of an underlying cardiac disease unrelated to and unaffected by the item under legal scrutiny quite frequently is not amenable to clear-cut, noncontroversial answers nor to overall causality guidelines or criteria.

Similarly, differences in the provisions of the individual state and territorial workers' compensation acts under which most cardiac claims arise; differences in legal philosophy among the many persons assigned fact-finding roles in disputed litigation; the subtle differences in fact situations of claims which, at first glance, are seemingly identical; and the often diametrically opposed medical conclusions presented in a given case by equally competent medical experts, preclude the formulation of legal standards of causality that can uniformly be applied to cover all instances. Accordingly, each case must be decided, both medically and legally, on its own set of facts and medical testimony.

Certain precepts, however, should govern medical assessments of causality in cardiac claims. For an alleged causal connection to be accepted in a cardiac case as "probable" or with "reasonable medical certainty," the following criteria should be satisfied:

- The cardiac diagnosis should be delineated completely and established, as far as reasonably possible, by objective means, and those portions of the cardiac condition under consideration as potential "injuries" specified.

- The alleged causative element presented for legal consideration should be one that is currently recognized medically and scientifically as capable, under appropriate circumstances, of producing the heart disorder or injury found.
- Conversely, the cardiac condition or dysfunction diagnosed must be one generally recognized medically as a possible resultant of the alleged harmful exposure.
- The time interval elapsing between the alleged noxious exposure and the medically manifest evidence of heart damage or dysfunction must be consistent with currently accepted scientific concepts of pathogenesis.
- The proposed cause-and-effect relation, although not always fully explainable in terms of present-day scientific knowledge, must still be consistent with current scientific concepts.

As an aid to medical assessment of causality in coronary artery heart disease and its ischemic sequelae, the cardiac disorder by far the most frequent basis of heart claims, the reader is referred to the "Report of the American Heart Association's Committee on Stress, Strain, and Heart Disease." Although originally published in 1977,[6] the conclusions of this committee are currently valid without modification, have not been supplanted by any other formal set of medical causality guidelines, and are generally accepted by the medical profession. The conclusions pertinent to a medical assessment of causality in cardiac claims arising under workers' compensation are summarized below:

- Long-term repetitive physical effort, such as is inherent in many occupations, cannot currently be regarded medically as a causative element in the development of coronary atherosclerotic heart disease. Such activity, if playing any role in this disease process, is believed beneficial by preventing or slowing the rate of atherosclerotic progression.
- Long-term repeated physical effort of work and/or nonwork activities in persons with underlying heart disease theoretically may hasten the development of congestive heart failure by reason of the additional workload imposed upon an already weakened heart. However, it is not possible within the present state of medical knowledge to determine in any given heart patient when congestive heart failure would have occurred as the result of the expected natural progression of the underlying cardiac disorder in the absence of such exertional efforts, a causative role to such stress cannot be assigned with "reasonable medical certainty."
- Continued, protracted psychologic, emotional stress to which an individual may have been subjected over a long period of time has not been established scientifically as a causative or worsening agent in the genesis or acceleration of atherosclerotic disease, although the possibility of some contribution cannot be excluded in individual cases.
- A single, isolated, identified physical or emotional stress in individuals rendered susceptible to harm therefrom by reason of preexistent heart disease, whether or not previously known or symptomatic, if of sufficient intensity and duration, is capable of eliciting adverse cardiac responses which, in turn, can "trigger" or hasten certain cardiac lesions and dysfunctions such as an acute attack of angina pectoris or an acute myocardial infarction, a cardiac dysrhythmia (including sudden death therefrom), and a bout of acute congestive heart failure.
- The shorter the time interval between the exposure of an individual to a potentially noxious stimulus and the appearance of clinical or pathologic evidence of new heart disease or dysfunction, the more likely there is a causal relationship between the two. Conversely, the farther apart in time, the less likely is a cause-and-effect relation.
- The exposure of a person with underlying heart disease to a stimulus potentially capable of eliciting harmful cardiovascular responses does not mean that such will be elicited, even when such exposure would be advised against medically because of the possibility of ensuing harm.

The elements most often accepted by workers' compensation adjudicators in cardiac cases as work-related "competent-producing" causes of injury, disability, or death are physical work effort (usual, unusual, or of a degree greater than accustomed nonwork exertion, depending on the covering compensation act requirements); adverse work environments, e.g., excessive heat or cold, noxious fumes; an acute psychologic trauma such as a heated argument or a sudden fright; an accidental electric shock; a severe nonpenetrating blow or other mechanical injury to the chest cage; and adverse cardiac reactions to medical, surgical, corrective, and rehabilitative therapy of an industrial injury not originally involving the cardiovascular system. Allegations that overall job stress, tension, pressure, or overwork have hastened the progression of underlying coronary atherosclerotic heart disease, although accepted in isolated instances in some jurisdictions, have generally not been included in the category of "compensable injury."

So-called risk factors, such as cigarette smoking, elevated blood cholesterol, diabetes mellitus, hypertension, positive family history of coronary disease, and others are often referred to in causality assessments in coronary heart disease. In this regard, it should be recognized that risk factors are of importance primarily in epidemiologic studies applicable to groups, not to an individual. For any given person, the presence or absence of medical background risk factors does not necessarily indicate the premature development of this condition nor an escape therefrom. Thus, although statistically related to the presence of coronary heart disease, generally accepted risk factors for coronary atherosclerosis cannot be viewed medically as causative elements in the production of the disease. In any consideration of so-called personality types A and B as risk factors, it should further be recognized that, in addition to the practical impossibility of definitively separating human beings into type A or type B personalities, it must be kept in mind that the role of personality type, if any, in the pathogenesis of coronary atherosclerosis has not been scientifically established and, therefore, should not be presented to a court of law as within the realm of medical "probability" or "reasonable medical certainty."

Additionally, in medical causality assessments in coronary atherosclerotic heart disease, it must be appreciated that while physical stress may be definable quantitatively to some degree, emotional stress defies quantitative measurement. Nor can presumed long-term effects of an occupational endeavor or a presumed unpleasant life situation incident be separated from similar effects inherent in day-to-day life and interpersonal contacts. Finally, the effects of so-called psychologic stress are primarily, as with beauty, in the eyes of the beholder. A psychologic situation that may be harmful to one person may be but an exhilarating, stimulating challenge to another.

Not all cardiac claims require legal causality determinations. For example, in claims instituted under the Social Security Disability Insurance Program the primary issue is whether the applicant is unable to engage in substantial gainful employment as defined in the covering statute, not the medical or legal relationship of the disability to a particular causative element. Similarly, eligibility for benefits in most privately acquired insurance contracts is based upon the fact of disability, generally independent of cause unless the applicant must demonstrate that his or her disability stems from an "accident" rather than an illness, in which case the issue of causation has to be established.

For some applicants for disability benefits, legislative incorporation into a statute covering certain named categories of public employees of a presumption of causation to the job effectively relieves them of establishing job-causation of a disabling cardiac condition. Generally, these statutes, often referred to as "heart laws," have primarily been designed for members of police and fire departments, but in some states the legislative presumption of causation has been extended to prison guards, employees of registries of motor vehicles, liquor enforcement and control personnel, members of forestry and wildlife services, sewer department workers, and other categories of public employment. Although these statutes usually allow for a rebuttal of the causation presumption, the presumption, as a practical matter, can seldom be negated since the causes of most heart disorders are unknown and consequently a statutory requirement of offsetting "competent medical evidence to the contrary" for rebuttal cannot be satisifed.

Evaluation of Disability

Evaluation of disability for legal and insurance purposes is a complex process necessarily involving more than one professional discipline. At times the evaluation requires interrelating the fields of medicine, law, insurance, judiciary, vocational counseling, and rehabilitation. As a minimum, a cardiac disability evaluation is twofold: first, a medical assessment must be made of the extent of the patient-claimant's impairment in terms of what the patient can and cannot do and what the patient should not do by reason of the cardiac disorder and, second, there must be a legal translation of the medically determined impairments into the specific definition of disability incorporated in the applicable statute or insurance contract, the latter often involving questions of total vs. partial disability, permanent disability, etc.

As with most medicolegal evaluations, contested claims for disability benefits are decided by legal or administrative fact finders, with the physician's role limited to providing the fact finder with medical data and opinion testimony that can be utilized in reaching a conclusion.

As a minimum, the physician examining a patient-claimant for disability evaluation purposes should attempt to determine the following:

- The full cardiac diagnosis, including etiology when known, and all anatomic and functional derangements found, together with the supporting clinical evidence.
- The clinical manifestations of the disorder revealed by the medical examination, including all subjective complaints and, more important, all objective confirmatory findings of physical examination, x-ray, electrocardiogram, and laboratory and other studies which support the presence of a heart disease or disorder medically recognized as capable of producing the symptoms alleged as the basis for disability.
- The restrictions in the patient's physical activities and mental capacity that have resulted from the disorders found in terms of limitations of walking, stair climbing, standing, sitting, reaching, lifting, bending, pushing, pulling, gripping, running, work hours, work pace, ability to concentrate, and ability to work under conditions of tension, heat, cold, etc.
- Those restrictions of nonwork and work activities imposed to prevent an aggravation of the underlying heart disorder or to prevent further heart damage, such as advice to postmyocardial infarction patients not to subject themselves to sudden bursts of strenuous physical effort.

In those instances where the law requires that causation be apportioned between the parties (e.g., work-related vs. non-work-related disabilities), the physician may be asked to furnish an opinion as to the causation of each of the impairments found. For example, in claims based upon myocardial infarction, the physician may be asked what aspects of the impairments found are related to the underlying coronary atherosclerotic disease for which there may not be legal liability, and which are related to the myocardial infarction itself for which there may exist legal responsibility.

In those situations where a patient-claimant has impairments coexisting from cardiac as well as noncardiac disorders, the physician may be asked to separate the impairments due to each disorder, and, in assessing the overall combined impairments, whether noncardiac impairments, if present, magnify the impairment attributable to the heart disorder.

In reaching the conclusions expressed in the medical assessment of disability, the physician should utilize to the fullest extent all currently available objective means of diagnosis and measurement of cardiac function, within practical limits of risk to the patient, cost of the testing, and in terms of the information to be obtained relative to the assessment. Wherever feasible, medical evaluations of disability should be based upon objective findings to obviate depending only upon subjective complaints, which are often unreliable because they are self-serving.

Medical assessments of cardiac impairment are significantly hampered by (1) the necessary reliance in most cases upon subjective complaints; (2) the marked individual variations in symptoms, motivation, adjustment, and return-to-work desires among persons with similar cardiac abnormalities; (3) the paucity of currently available means for quantitative measurement of cardiac functional reserves; (4) the frequent discrepancy between objective findings and subjective complaints; (5) the practical difficulties in transferring the results of objective test measurements, such as those of exercise stress testing, under controlled environmental conditions, into the uncontrolled, variable environment of the workplace in which hostile environments, often immeasurable, may significantly affect the physiologic demands placed upon the heart; and (6) the fact that most cardiac impairments are rarely static and cannot be considered to have reached an end result, but are subject, because of the progressive nature of the underlying disorder and variations in therapeutic responses, to sudden change so that an impairment assessment or disability evaluation at a given date may be unpredictably rendered invalid for a later time.

As a guideline to the application of cardiac testing to disability determinations in patients with heart disease, the reader is referred to the cardiovascular system section in *A Handbook for Physicians*,[7] a booklet prepared and distributed by the Social Security Administration that presents the medical criteria used for evaluating disability under the Social Security Disability Insurance and the Supplemental Security Income programs.

As with causality assessments, medical and legal assessments of disability vary considerably in certain cases because of the difference in emphasis necessarily placed by each profession on individual aspects of the impairment in the disability rating process. While a physician might consider a patient not disabled and, therefore, employable, the fact finder may declare the same person disabled from work activity under the terms of the applicable law or insurance contract. In such instances, the physician must appreciate that in reaching the legal decision as to work capacity, the fact finder frequently has to include nonmedical elements such as age, sex, educational background, motivation, and prior work training and experience. Additionally, the fact finder's decision may be influenced by the availability of certain types of employment in the local or national labor market, the problems imposed by transportation to and from work sites, language or other communication problems, and other factors which, as a practical matter, so restrict a given person's opportunity for gainful employment as to make that individual actually disabled although medically cleared for work.

It is also important to recognize that because of differing statutory and contractual definitions, a person declared disabled and awarded benefits under one disability program may not be eligible for benefits under another program. Thus, an award for disability by one agency or insurer does not, by itself, bind another agency or insurer. Each insurance contract or other disability benefit program or statute must be considered individually and separately for each claim raised, although the claim in each instance is based upon the same medical disorders and impairments.

Determination of Malpractice[8]

The risk of a physician being sued for professional negligence should a patient suffer an untoward result during the course of diagnosis and treatment is an inescapable fact of today's professional life. Cardiology as a specialty increases this risk because of a variety of reasons, particularly because of: (1) the ever-present threat of sudden, unpredicted death due to the relentless progressive nature of most heart diseases independent of treatment or lack of treatment; (2) the adverse reactions often attributable to the narrow overlap between therapeutic and toxic ranges of commonly employed cardiac medications; (3) the inherent hazards and complications of exercise stress testing, invasive diagnostic procedures, and cardiac surgery; (4) the often-encountered lack of clear-cut diagnostic evidence in the early stages of an acute myocardial infarction, thereby leading to the "emergency room turn-away" of patients in the throes of an attack with later dire consequences; (5) the unavoidable mortality and morbidity associated with "last-ditch" heroic medical and surgical treatment of desperately ill patients in the end stages of heart disease; and (6) the many problems involved in obtaining "informed consent" for procedures beyond the understanding of most lay persons, particularly when frightened by the threats of a cardiac illness.

In medical malpractice cases, the aggrieved patient, or those acting through him or her, has the legal burden of demonstrating by factual and opinion evidence (1) that the defendant doctor or other health-care provider named in the suit owed a duty to the plaintiff as is legally and morally implied in the physician-patient relationship; (2) that the defendant violated that duty by breaching the standard of care owed; (3) that the patient suffered injury or harm; and (4) that the physician or other health-care provider's negligence was the proximate cause of that harm; and (5) in some jurisdictions, that the patient's conduct did not negligently contribute to the alleged harm (the doctrine of "contributory negligence"). Unless all these elements are established in the courtroom by the plaintiff, the legal action will fail.

The evidentiary proof required of the plaintiff in establishing the bases of his or her action generally necessitates that expert medical opinion be provided that (1) defines the standard of care due the plaintiff by the defendant(s), (2) establishes the breach or failure to conform to that standard of care, (3) defines the injuries or "harms" claimed, and (4) causally relates the harms found to the claimed negligent action or failure to act on the part of the defendant(s).

Should a patient suffer harm during the course of medical diagnosis and treatment, the physician and/or other health-care providers may be liable, separately or additionally, to two other legal actions besides that in tort. The first constitutes charges that the patient or those acting for him or her were not given sufficient information by the responsible professional persons to allow a legally valid "informed" consent to be made to a medically prescribed diagnostic test or treatment that resulted in injury, and that, therefore, performance of the procedure or treatment was legally an "assault," subject to evidentiary requirements less stringent than those required in actions in tort as well as protected by a differing statute of limitations. The second possible legal action is one based on alleged "breach of contract" should a particular result or cure allegedly promised and thereby "guaranteed" not be achieved. In both these actions supportive expert medical opinions may not be necessary to substantiate the claim since the legal issue in dispute often hinges on the factual determination of whether the defendant physician did or did not say what the patient alleges was actually said or not said in information imparted or in guarantee of results and not require a demonstration of professional negligence.

Medical evaluation of a malpractice claim requires a painstaking, thorough review of all the claimant's medical records with particular attention, first, to whether the defendant's professional actions were in accord with generally accepted and proper standards of professional conduct, and, secondly, determination of whether the alleged "harms" were causally related to the defendant's professional actions or failure to act.

In a medical evaluation of alleged professional negligence it is important to realize that the fact that a patient suffers injurious effects during or after a prescribed treatment or procedure does not by itself raise a legal presumption of negligence as a causative factor. A physician is not legally responsible for want of success in his or her professional endeavors unless it is proved that the want of success followed from want of professional care and diligence ordinarily possessed by others in the profession. The determination, however, must take due regard for the state of advancement of medical science at the time of the treatment or procedure performance. Nor is a physician legally responsible for errors in judgment in matters where reasonable doubt and uncertainty exist, if the physician has exercised his or her best judgment in the situation and has not performed any negligent act. As long as the professional judgment exercised does not represent a departure from the requirements of accepted medical practice or does not result in a failure to do something which accepted medical practice obligates or in doing something that accepted medical practice precludes, the physician is not guilty of malpractice.

The Medicolegal Cardiac Examination

The techniques employed in medicolegal cardiac examinations are essentially the same as in medical examinations performed for treatment purposes. Generally, the basic components of history taking, physical examination, a resting electrocardiogram, and chest roentgenogram, plus review and study of the available medical records suffice. In claims where the patient-claimant is not available for examination, the evaluation may have to be made entirely on the basis of medical records provided. Rarely do the legal questions require the employment of one or more of the specialized cardiac diagnostic techniques covered in Part VII of this book. In such cases, the recommending physician must keep in mind the principles which govern the use of the diagnostic testing selected, the information it can be expected to provide, the limitations of results, the pitfalls in interpretation, the availability and cost of the procedure, and the inherent risks and hazards to the patient. All must be weighed carefully against the legal need for the information to be obtained.

The basic tools of cardiac diagnosis are described in Part II of this book. However, because of the key role often played by the medical history in legal issues of liability and disability rating, and because the special components of such history taking are not generally appreciated or utilized by physicians primarily interested in treating the patient, specific discussion of history taking for medicolegal evaluations and its implications are warranted.

When cardiac disorders have legal consequences, the content of the medical history ultimately accepted by the legal arbiter of the claim frequently makes or breaks the action instituted by the plaintiff-claimant. For example, in many workers' compensation cases there often is no dispute legally concerning the presence of a disabling cardiac disorder for which benefits might be available under the law: rather, the key issue is medical, i.e., whether a work-connected factor played a role in precipitating, hastening, aggravating, or otherwise "causing" the disorder or disability for which benefits are claimed. The crucial element in such causality assessments frequently is the medical history that is to be accepted by the fact finder as depicting the sequence of events and circumstances surrounding the occurrence of cardiac symptoms and the findings claimed to represent an injury.

In those situations where it is alleged or where it can be anticipated that it will later be alleged that the patient's heart disorder arose in some part out of employment, thereby entitling the person to workers' compensation benefits for disability, loss of earning capacity, and medical expenses, the examining physician should inquire about and include in the written history the sequence of events preceding and leading to the onset of symptoms for which the patient sought medical attention. Inquiry should also be made as to the specific work activities engaged in before, during, and after an alleged cardiac incident; whether these were customary and usual for the employee or comprised unaccustomed, unusual activities; whether there were associated hostile environmental conditions that could have intensified the potential physiologic demands and thereby the cardiostressful attributes of the work effort, e.g., excessive heat or cold, humidity, dust or other respiratory irritants, or undue associated psychologic stress.

Similarly, in situations where mechanical trauma is alleged to be a cause of heart injury, as in tort cases involving motor vehicle accidents, inquiry should be directed to the exact type of mechanical forces involved, particularly the point or points of bodily contact; the effect on the patient's body such as jarring, whiplash, and dislodgment; the development and objective evidence of trauma such as cuts, lacerations, external bleeding, bruises, and ecchymoses; and the precise time and sequence of occurrence of symptoms and signs consistent with cardiac injury.

The list of potential questions that may be pertinent in the medicolegal history thus is virtually endless. In each case, therefore, the examiner's questioning must be tailored to provide the information needed to reach a reasonable medical conclusion for the facts on hand.

Hospital records generally contain more than one written history, depending upon the number of physicians involved in the care of the patient. Significant historical facts also sometimes appear in the progress notes, requests for consultations, consultants' reports, requisitions for diagnostic studies, and in the nurses' notes. Accordingly, the physician asked to make a medical evaluation for legal purposes should request from the referring party, when deemed appropriate, the complete hospital records rather than only the discharge summary, to have the benefits of all the histories contained therein.

Because the medical history is derived by a question-and-answer interview between a physician and a patient-claimant, simultaneously or later transposed into a written narrative record, it is subject to many limitations of content, distortion, and error which may affect its legal value. Many of these limitations stem from a failure of the interviewer to ask pertinent questions, a failure on the part of the interviewed patient to understand the questions asked or to respond appropriately, bias on the part of the interviewer, and self-serving motives of the interviewed patient. Typically, histories contained in hospital records are devoid of those items that later are of key importance in legal resolution of the claim. This is quite common in the history recorded at the time the patient is first seen with an actual or suspected acute myocardial infarction. In such situations, brevity in history taking is essential because of the urgent need to establish a diagnosis and institute lifesaving therapy rapidly. Characteristically, such histories make no mention of details relevant to causation that are crucial in later legal actions. In many instances, the attending physician, not aware of the potential legal actions that may stem from the patient's cardiac disorder, fails to record the detailed history necessary to resolve the legal aspects of the patient's illness, making it necessary that a detailed history be obtained at a later date at a time when the patient has become suspect as to reliability because of elements of financial or other gain associated with the institution of a claim for benefits.

The Medicolegal Report

The report prepared by the physician of the cardiac evaluation is an important document with far-reaching practical consequences. For the attorney or insurer to whom it is addressed, the report forms the basis for determining pretrial acceptance or denial of the claim, the consideration of settlement negotiations, the pretrial preparation, and the courtroom presentation of the medical aspects of the case. For the physician, the time put forth in compiling a comprehensive medical report of the examination findings, summary of medical records, and conclusions drawn therefrom will later provide a useful refresher for the marshalling of the pertinent medical findings and the bases for the conclusions reached should the matter come to trial at some later date when details of the original examination have been forgotten or have dimmed with the passage of time. Carelessly composed, poorly prepared, or obviously biased medical reports frequently prove damaging and embarrassing to the physician when called upon to testify at trial if they contain inaccuracies, inconsistencies, unwarranted medical conclusions, or if there are omissions.

The composition of a medical report for legal and insurance purposes differs from that of the usual medical report in that it often requires inclusion of information not directly related to the treatment of a patient but which is essential for answer to the various medical questions posed by the impending litigation. In most situations, the medicolegal report of a cardiac examination and findings is best presented in narrative form. As a minimum such a report should cover the following topics, preferably in the order listed:

- A recounting of the history personally related to the examining physician by the patient-claimant, or outlined in the medical records reviewed should the evaluation have to be made without opportunity to examine the claimant, with particular emphasis on the sequence of events leading to the seeking of medical attention. In a worker's compensation claim, adequate facts must be recorded in the medical history as to the overall job duties and requirements, including consideration of possible noxious occupational exposures and psychologic "stress," "pressures," and "tensions." There should also be detailed recounting of the work activity preceding, during, and after an alleged cardiac event. In an automobile accident or other situation where trauma is alleged as a cause of a cardiac "personal injury," there should be a description of the mechanical aspects of the contact or psychologic sequelae that are important in an evaluation of the competency of the alleged trauma or stress to precipitate cardiac lesions and/or dysfunctions. The significant past medical history should be detailed with particular reference to recognized background medical risk factors favoring premature development of coronary atherosclerotic heart disease and the existence of prior heart disorder or of other conditions that might affect the patient's susceptibility to cardiac injury and/or current medical status.
- A chronological listing, with summary of the contents deemed important, of the various hospital and medical reports and other data reviewed by the physician and utilized in the formulation of the opinions reached. And, if death has occurred, the pertinent findings of autopsy.
- A detailing of the physical examination findings with description of all the abnormalities detected as well as the important negatives.
- The results of the various diagnostic studies performed or utilized by the examining physician in reaching conclusions of the evaluation.
- A statement of the complete cardiac diagnosis with substantiating reasons if the diagnosis is questionable or not firmly established.
- The examiner's opinion concerning each of the various medicolegal questions posed in the individual case with substantiating reasons that support the conclusions expressed.

References

1. Curran, W. J.: Titles in the Medicolegal Field: A Proposal for Reform, *Am. J. Law Med.*, 1:1, 1975.
2. "Analysis of Workers' Compensation Laws," prepared and published annually by the Chamber of Commerce of the United States, 1615 H Street, N.W., Washington, D.C. 20062.
3. Sullivan, R. T.: Heart Injuries Under Workers' Compensation: Medical and Legal Considerations, *Suffolk University Law Review*, 14:1365, 1980.
4. The Criteria Committee of the New York Heart Association: "Nomenclature and Criteria for Diagnosis of Diseases of the Heart and Great Vessels," 8th ed., Little, Brown and Company, Boston, 1979.
5. Danner, D., and Sagall, E. L.: Medicolegal Causation: A Source of Professional Misunderstanding, *Am. J. Law Med.*, 3:303, 1977.
6. American Heart Association: Report of the Committee on Stress, Strain, and Heart Disease, *Circulation,* 55:825A, 1977.
7. "Disability Evaluation Under Social Security—A Handbook for Physicians," DHEW Publication 79-10089, U.S. Government Printing Office, Washington, D.C., 1979.
8. Sagall, E. L., and Lucas, I. (eds.): "Malpractice Hazards in Cardiology" (proceedings, symposium, Boston, May 12, 1971), Massachusetts Heart Association, Inc., Boston, 1973.

Suggested Reading

Committee on Rating of Mental and Physical Impairment, American Medical Association: "Guides to the Evaluation of Permanent Impairment," 2nd ed., American Medical Association, Chicago, 1984.

Holder, A. R.: "Medical Malpractice Law," 2d ed., John Wiley & Sons, New York, 1978.

"Proceedings of the Conference on Stress, Strain, Heart Disease and the Law," Boston, Jan 26–28, 1978, U.S. Government Printing Office, Washington, D.C., Publication 790-281-412/107, 1979.

Sagall, E. L., and Reed, B. C.: "The Heart and the Law—A Practical Guide to Medicolegal Cardiology," The Macmillan Company, New York, 1968.

Sagall, E. L., and Reed, B. C.: "The Law and Clinical Medicine," J. B. Lippincott Company, Philadelphia, 1970.

87

Occupation and Cardiovascular Disease

Nanette Kass Wenger, M.D.

It is extremely difficult to determine the real influence of employments upon health; for, on the one hand, employments closely resembling each other in character may be associated with very dissimilar habits of life; and, on the other, employments having nothing in common may be combined with some one bad habit which may be sufficiently powerful to render all of them unhealthy. Again, occupations, in themselves rather unhealthy than otherwise, may appear free from injurious results, in consequence of the temperate and regular habits of those who pursue them.

W. A. Guy, 1843[1]

Occupational Toxic Exposures and Cardiovascular Risk

General Considerations

Associations of occupations with cardiovascular diseases relate primarily to potential occupational toxic exposures.[2,3] Improved industrial hygiene and increased automation have decreased toxic occupational exposures; hazards result predominantly from leaks, blowouts, equipment breakdown, and the like. Occupational toxic exposures can be classified as physical, biological, and chemical. Physical exposures include extremes of oxygen pressure, barometric pressure, gravity, acceleration, noise, temperature, and humidity (see Chaps. 78 and 84). Biological agents are involved in laboratory-acquired infections or with work in an endemic area; allergy or hypersensitivity to medications or vaccines may be considered an iatrogenic toxic exposure (see Chaps. 57, 58, and 78). Many chemical agents enter the body by inhalation, skin absorption, or ingestion; these agents produce cardiovascular toxicity by a direct effect on the myocardium, by impairing the oxygen-carrying capacity of the blood, or (as with organic phosphorus insecticides) by cholinesterase inhibition, clinically evident as intense parasympathetic stimulation.[2]

Occupational toxic exposures may mimic cardiovascular disease.[4] Toxic gases or fumes can produce pulmonary edema with substernal pain or discomfort, mimicking myocardial infarction. Differentiation is important, as morphine is contraindicated because concomitant central nervous system toxicity and respiratory depression result from some chemical toxicities. Digitalis is generally ineffective and immediate therapy includes oxygen, bronchodilator and corticosteroid drugs, antibiotics for secondary infection, or tracheostomy if needed.[5]

South American miners working at high altitudes in the Andes who develop "high-altitude heart disease" (see Chap. 84) may be considered to have occupational heart disease.

Firefighters' chronic occupational exposure to carbon monoxide results in maximal allowable blood concentrations of carboxyhemoglobin, even in nonsmoking firefighters; serum enzyme level changes in one study suggested myocardial damage.[6] Carbon monoxide exposure with increased blood carboxyhemoglobin levels in steel and foundry workers has not been documented to accelerate atherogenesis; nevertheless, an increase in symptoms in patients known to have coronary disease has been clearly demonstrated with exposure to carbon monoxide.[7]

Exposure to halogenated hydrocarbons and fluorocarbons as solvents and propellants has been associated with cardiac arrhythmias[8] and sudden death.

Nitrate Exposure and Withdrawal

Employees with atherosclerotic coronary heart disease working in explosive factories using glyceric nitrol esters such as nitroglycol have an occupational hazard; nitroglycol is 180 times more volatile than nitroglycerin and is easily absorbed via the lungs and skin. Munitions workers developed angina during the weekend, that disappeared on returning to work; sudden death has occurred during the weekend, when there was deprivation of the nitroglycol vasodilation present during the workweek.[4]

Chest pain and even sudden death have occurred as "withdrawal symptoms" in persons without apparent coronary disease after prolonged nitroglycerin and other nitrate exposures; the time of increased risk is at 1 or 2 days after cessation of exposure, suggesting that rebound vasospasm may be etiologic. Exertional and emotional stimuli did not precipitate pain; coronary spasm, reversed by nitroglycerin, has been documented by angiography during nitrate withdrawal.[9] Another etiologic possibility is that chronic industrial vasodilator exposure provokes compensatory homeostatic vasoconstriction; its persistence during nitroglycerin withdrawal may result in a cardiac ischemic episode.

Carbon Disulfide

Epidemiologic studies have shown that workers involved in the manufacture of viscose rayon and of carbon tetrachloride, chronically exposed to carbon disulfide fumes, have an increased risk of coronary death.[7] The risk appears related to the sole effect of carbon disulfide exposure, although the risk is accentuated when concomitant hypertension and older age are present.[10] The mechanism of the toxic effect has not been elucidated.

Occupation and Vascular Hand Trauma

Repeated, prolonged occupational hand trauma, as encountered among machinists, welders, plumbers, iron and steel workers, and miners who use hand-held vibrating tools such as high-frequency pneumatic hammers and chain saws may result in severe ischemia of the digits (see Chap. 65). This traumatic vasospastic disease occurred almost predictably in 40 percent of lumberjacks after 3 to 5 years of occupational exposure.[11]

Cardiovascular changes similar to those encountered in endurance athletes have been described with vibration disease;[12] they include an increased left ventricular ejection fraction, mainly due to an increase in left ventricular end-diastolic dimension, and a decreased resting heart rate.

Atherosclerotic Coronary Heart Disease and Occupation

A number of studies relate the incidence and severity of clinical coronary disease to differences in occupational physical activity. The relation of emotional stress associated with occupational responsibilities to coronary atherosclerosis, as well as to hypertension, remains controversial (see Chaps. 42, 45, and 49).

Employment of the Cardiac Patient

General Considerations

Ramifications of employment or reemployment of cardiac patients relate to early rehabilitation; selective placement dependent on the type of heart disease and functional capacity; the effects of work and the work environment on the heart disease; patient, employer, labor union, and physician education; insurance, law, and workmen's compensation decisions; and industry's experience with cardiac patients as employees.[13]

The Council on Occupational Health of the American Medical Association has addressed the problem of employable patients with heart disease. The reader is referred to the article entitled "Employability of Workers Handicapped by Certain Diseases. A Guide for Employers and Physicians."[14] The following statement is reproduced with the permission of the publisher:

> Patients with cardiac disease can work. Most patients with cardiac disease should work, usually in gainful employment. Many patients with cardiac disease achieve satisfactory rehabilitation on their own. Many, however, achieve it only by painstaking attention to the varied factors of professionally guided rehabilitation. The extent of the pathologic symptoms and the apparent limitation of cardiac reserve are often not as important as the emotional factors and the resiliency with which the patient adjusts to his disease.
>
> The physician's alertness, ingenuity, flexibility, and maturity are needed to cope successfully with the variety of factors involved in any individual case. Many forms of assistance are available in the medical profession, in the industrial community, and among the social agencies. The great number of persons involved makes their successful rehabilitation important to industry, and community and to the nation.

Legislative Considerations (see also Chaps. 45, 85, and 86)

Social Security Disability

Policies and current regulations for the determination of cardiovascular disability under Titles II and XVI of the Social Security Act (P.L. 96–265, P.L. 96–473), published by the Social Security Administration[15,16] define severe impairment as resulting from one or more of three consequences of heart disease: congestive heart failure, ischemia of heart muscle, and conduction disturbances and/or arrhythmias resulting in cardiac syncope. Criteria are given for evaluating impairment and the documentation needed to support the evaluation is described.[16] Current legislation mandates review of all cases of nonpermanent disability at least every 3 years, and all other cases as deemed appropriate. Review determinations are based on contemporary definitions for disability for initial claims, rather than the policies at the time the disability benefits were awarded. Although the law does not mandate medical recovery for cessation of disability, some federal courts have required that medical improvement be shown before disability benefits are terminated.

Federal Motor Carrier Safety Regulations[17]

The Federal Highway Administration of the U.S. Department of Transportation requires a waiver to permit driving (Section 391.41) by individuals with a current clinical diagnosis of myocardial infarction, angina pectoris, coronary insufficiency, thrombosis, or cardiovascular disease known to be accompanied by or which is likely to cause syncope, dyspnea, collapse, or congestive cardiac failure. Suggestions for certification include a normal resting and stress electrocardiogram, no residual complications or physical limitations, and no use of medications likely to interfere with safe driving. Coronary bypass surgery and pacemaker implantation are considered remedial procedures and not cardiovascular conditions; thus they do not automatically disqualify drivers, but the final determination is based on the underlying cardiac condition. Specific blood pressure levels are defined which must be met for patients with hypertension to be eligible to drive; and antihypertensive medications must not be likely to interfere with alertness, judgment, coordination, and other prerequisites of driving.

Federal Aviation Administration

The flying status of pilots following successful coronary bypass surgery has generated considerable controversy and concern.[18] As of May 1982, no pilot with coronary artery disease significant enough to have required treatment is eligible for unrestricted medical certification by the National Transportation Safety Board (NTSB).

The NTSB, a nonmedical group, had previously ordered the Federal Aviation Administration (FAA) to medically certify pilots with surgically treated coronary disease, returning them to active private and commercial flight status without restriction.[19] These pilots were individuals with complete revascularization who had not had myocardial infarction and were asymptomatic after surgery; all their major risk factors had been reversed and their exercise electrocardiograms were normal. Under the new regulations, the FAA medical evaluation, as performed by the Federal Air Surgeon, may impose operational limitations on pilots after successful coronary bypass surgery and may specify requirements for subsequent medical evaluation. This latter approach is concordant with the recommendations of an American College of Cardiology Bethesda Conference on cardiovascular problems associated with aviation safety.[18]

The question of aircrew licensing after coronary bypass surgery will require serious review; Parker[19a] suggests a plan for follow-up evaluations. Conventional coronary risk factors appear to adversely affect the complication-free time after coronary bypass surgery.[19b]

Interim suggestions are also offered for licensing of persons for flying with congenital heart lesions that have a low risk of complications either before or after surgical correction.[19c]

Workmen's Compensation Considerations

Causal relation between occupation and heart disease from the viewpoint of workmen's compensation decisions and awards requires only that the employee be subjected to unusual or excessive physical or emotional strain in the course of work, prior to development of angina pectoris or an acute myocardial infarction. The administration of these "heart cases," however, differs widely among the states.[20] Compensation has also been awarded both on the basis of ordinary work activity as causally related to heart disease and on the basis that the cumulative physical and mental strain of a lifetime of work may culminate in an acute coronary episode.[21] Medical committees[13] properly emphasize that these attitudes often negate efforts to rehabilitate cardiac patients and hamper their employment or reemployment. (See also Chaps. 45, 85, and 86.)

References

1. Guy, W. A.: Contributions to a Knowledge of the Influence of Employments Upon Health, *J. R. Stat. Soc.*, 6:197, 1843.
2. Warshaw, L. J.: Cardiovascular Effects of Toxic Occupational Exposures, in L. J. Warshaw (ed.), "The Heart in Industry," Hoeber Medical Division, Harper & Row, Publishers, Inc., New York, 1960, p. 456.
3. Goldhaber, S. Z.: Cardiovascular Effects of Potential Occupational Hazards, *J. Am. Coll. Cardiol.*, 2:1210, 1983.
4. Weill, H.: Cardiorespiratory Effects of Inhalant Occupational Exposures, *Circulation*, 63:250A, 1981.
5. Kleinfeld, M.: Acute Pulmonary Edema of Chemical Origin, *Arch. Environ. Health*, 10:942, 1965.
6. Sammons, J. H., and Coleman, R. L.: Firefighters' Occupational Exposure to Carbon Monoxide, *J. Occup. Med.*, 16:543, 1974.
7. Rosenman, K. D.: Cardiovascular Disease and Environmental Exposure, *Br. J. Ind. Med.*, 36:85, 1979.
8. Speizer, F. E., Wegman, D. H., and Ramirez, A.: Palpitation Rates Associated with Fluorocarbon Exposure in a Hospital Setting, *N. Engl. J. Med.*, 292:624, 1975.
9. Klock, J. C.: Nonocclusive Coronary Disease after Chronic Exposure to Nitrates: Evidence for Physiologic Nitrate Dependence, *Am. Heart J.*, 89:510, 1975.
10. Nurminen, M., Mutanen, P., Tolonen, M., and Hernberg, S.: Quantitated Effects of Carbon Disulfide Exposure, Elevated Blood Pressure and Aging on Coronary Mortality, *Am. J. Epidemiol.*, 115:107, 1982.
11. Pyykko, I.: The Prevalence and Symptoms of Traumatic Vasospastic Disease among Lumberjacks in Finland. A Field Study, *Work Environ. Health*, 11:118, 1974.
12. Matoba, T., Itaya, M., Toyomasu, K., Tsuiki, T., Toshima, H., and Kuwahara, H.: Increased Left Ventricular Function as an Adaptive Response in Vibration Disease, *Am. J. Cardiol.*, 51:1223, 1983.
13. Report of the Committee on Stress, Strain, and Heart Disease, American Heart Association: *Circulation*, 55:825A, 1977.
14. Council Statement. Council on Occupational Health, American Medical Association: Employability of Workers Handicapped by Certain Diseases. A Guide for Employers and Physicians, *Arch. Environ. Health*, 17:389, 1968.
15. Department of Health and Human Services. Social Security Administration, 20 CFR Parts 404 and 416: Federal Old Age, Survivors, and Disability Insurance Benefits; Supplemental Security Income for the Aged, Blind, and Disabled, in *Federal Register*, vol. 45, no. 163, August 20, 1980, p. 55566.
16. Social Security Regulations: Rules for Determining Disability and Blindness, U. S. Department of Health and Human Services, Social Security Administration, SSA Pub. No. 64–014, June 1981, p. 34.
17. U. S. Department of Transportation, Federal Highway Administration: The Regulatory Criteria for Evaluation under Section 391.41 (b)(4), (b)(6), in *Federal Register*, November 23, 1977, revised October 1983 (nonsubstantive).
18. Cardiovascular Problems Associated with Aviation Safety. Eighth Bethesda Conference of the American College of Cardiology, April 25 and 26, 1975, Washington, D. C. Task Force III: Recommendations for Post-operative Patients with Ischemic Heart Disease, *Am. J. Cardiol.*, 36:610, 1975.
19. Sands, M. J., Jr.: Sounding Board. Aviator Medical Certification after Coronary-Artery Surgery, *N. Engl. J. Med.*, 307:52, 1982.
19a. Parker, D. J.: The Airline Pilot after Coronary Artery Bypass Grafting, *Eur. Heart J.*, 5(suppl. A):77, 1984.
19b. Hammond, I. W., Lee, E. T., Davis, A. W., and Booze, C. F., Jr.: Prognostic Factors Related to Survival and Complication-Free Times in Airmen Medically Certified after Coronary Surgery, *Aviat. Space Environ. Med.*, 55:321, 1984.
19c. Macartney, F. J.: Flying and Congenital Heart Disease, *Eur. Heart J.*, 5(suppl. A):147, 1984.
20. Barth, P. S., and Hunt, H. A. (eds.): "Workers' Compensation and Work-Related Illnesses and Diseases," The MIT Press, Cambridge, Mass, 1980, Chapter 4, p. 105.
21. Warshaw, L. J.: Heart Cases Under Workmen's Compensation Laws, *J. Occup. Med.*, 9:349, 1967.

PART VII

The Pharmacology of Cardiac Drugs and the Techniques of Special Procedures*

*See the introductions at the beginning of section A of Part VII and at the beginning of Sections B through H of Part VII.

Section A

The Pharmacology of Cardiac Drugs

The purpose of this section is to discuss the pharmacology of certain cardiac drugs. No attempt has been made to discuss every drug used in the treatment of cardiovascular disease, but the commonly used drugs are discussed in some detail. Discussing the details of drugs in this section makes it unnecessary to discuss such details in the individual chapters of the book. This arrangement prevents interruption of the thought process that could occur when a reader looks up a disorder or disease process and is mentally sidetracked by a lengthy discussion of pharmacology. Necessary information about specific drugs are, however, provided in chapters throughout the book. Should the reader wish to know more about a drug he or she can refer to a chapter in this section of the book where more details about a drug will be found.

88

Drugs Used to Control Vascular Resistance and Capacitance

Jay N. Cohn, M.D.

The traditional role in medicine for vasoactive drugs that alter vascular resistance and capacitance has been to influence arterial pressure. Thus, vasodilator drugs that reduce systemic vascular resistance have been used as a rational approach to the treatment of hypertension, and vasoconstrictor drugs that increase systemic vascular resistance have, at least in the past, been advocated for the treatment of hypotensive states. Although variable venous capacitance effects of these drugs have been known to result in differing acute hemodynamic responses, the importance of these capacitive effects in the use of these agents has not traditionally been emphasized.

The demand for more selectivity in the choice of drug therapy for specific vascular syndromes has led in recent years to more attention to the regional vascular effects of these drugs. In myocardial ischemic syndromes, it has become important to understand effects of drugs on the large coronary arteries, the coronary arterioles, and the collateral channels as well as on the systemic arteries and veins to gain insight into antianginal effectiveness. The specific action of drugs on the pulmonary circulation has taken on importance not only because of growing interest in the interactions between the right and left ventricles but also because of therapeutic attempts to use vasoactive drugs to counteract pulmonary hypertension. Effects of drugs on the renal, splanchnic, and skeletal muscle circulations have become important as we become more sophisticated in our approach to hypertension, shock, and heart failure.

A further development in recent years has been an emphasis on the role of peripheral vascular factors in influencing the performance of the heart and its metabolic requirements. This newly awakened recognition of the importance of the vascular component of the cardiovascular system has led to the need for studying the effects of vasoactive drugs on the arterial and venous beds and in carefully assessing the left ventricular response to these drugs.[1] Only through an understanding of the pharmacologic actions of these drugs is it possible to employ rational vasoactive therapy in managing hypertension, angina pectoris, and heart failure.

Hemodynamic Effects of Vasodilators

Role of Preload Changes in Cardiac Performance

The importance of preload (end-diastolic myocardial fiber length) in controlling stroke volume from the left ventricle has long been recognized from the classical Frank-Starling curves.[2] Several factors of particular importance when considering preload effects in the setting of heart disease must be considered:

- In the presence of myocardial disease the left ventricle may lose much of its sensitivity to preload, such that augmentation of preload may not result in much rise in stroke volume. A true descending limb of the Frank-Starling curve probably does not exist, however.[3]
- The dilated left ventricular chamber is not necessarily operating at a heightened preload, since much of the dilatation may reflect slippage of fibers rather than increased fiber length.[4]
- Changes in compliance of the ventricle may alter the relationship between diastolic pressure and volume and thus render change in filling pressure an unreliable guide to change in end-diastolic fiber length or preload.[5]
- Myocardial oxygen consumption is directly related to wall stress, which is a function of pressure and chamber diameter. Therefore, dilatation of the chamber should result in an increase in myocardial oxygen consumption. If the ventricle is operating on a flattened Starling curve, the increased oxygen consumption will not be accompanied by much increase in cardiac output (reduced external efficiency).[6]

Acute changes in ventricular preload may result from changes in vascular capacitance. Right ventricular preload is dependent on systemic venous capacitance as well as intravascular volume. Left ventricular preload is dependent on the capacitance of the pulmonary vascular bed as well as the output from the right ventricle. Interaction through the interventricular septum also may result in a direct effect on left ventricular compliance of changes in right ventricular filling.[7]

Role of Impedance Changes in Cardiac Performance

Although the normal left ventricle is able to maintain its performance in the face of a fairly wide range of outflow resistance (impedance), the damaged myocardium often loses this ability and ventricular performance becomes inversely related to impedance.[8] Thus, the impaired ventricle is characterized by reduced response to preload changes and heightened response to impedance changes.

In assessing the effects of drugs that alter impedance, consideration must be given to the following:

- Arteriolar resistance and arterial compliance are the major variables that influence impedance.[9] Afterload, or ventricular wall stress during ejection, is influenced by impedance, by the ventricular pressure generated by the force of ventricular contraction against a given impedance, by the end-diastolic chamber diameter, and by the shortening (stroke volume) during ejection. Vasoactive drugs may thus directly alter impedance but only secondarily influence afterload.
- Since increased impedance may decrease cardiac output in the presence of myocardial disease and at the same time result in increased pressure and volume and consequently increased myocardial oxygen consumption, the net effect of an increase in impedance is a decrease in cardiac efficiency.[10]
- Since vascular resistance and compliance are exquisitely sensitive to neurohumoral factors, changes induced by vasoactive drugs may be counteracted or magnified by reflex changes in activity of the sympathetic nervous system or the renin-angiotensin system.[11]
- Regional differences in effects of drugs on vascular tone influence peripheral distribution of blood flow. Cardiac output will respond to a change in total impedance, but the effects on flow to specific vascular beds relate to local vascular changes.[12]

Effects on Intravascular Volume

In addition to controlling resistance and capacitance, drugs that influence vascular tone influence the intravascular volume by altering capillary pressure, which determines the rate of capillary filtration. Since capillary pressure is influenced by the balance between precapillary arteriolar and postcapillary venular resistance, a drug that relaxes the venules would tend to lower capillary pressure, whereas one that lowered arteriolar resistance might increase it.[13] Changes in vascular volume become important, particularly when a therapeutic intervention is discontinued or during chronic administration of a drug. The concomitant use of diuretics with many of the vasoactive regimens will of course independently affect the intravascular volume.

Drugs That Directly Relax Vascular Smooth Muscle

A number of drugs that have been used to treat hypertension, angina pectoris, and congestive heart failure exert an effect on vascular smooth muscle that appears not to be dependent on receptor mechanisms. Some may depend for their effect on stimulation of cyclic guanosine monophosphate (GMP),[14] and with others the mode of action is not entirely clear.

Nitrates

Nitroglycerin and the various nitrates have been in use for the treatment of cardiac disease for more than 100 years. These agents have a profound venodilating effect which even in low doses results in an increase in vascular capacitance.[15] Although their effect on large-vessel compliance is more difficult to quantitate, considerable data indicate that even in relatively low doses these drugs increase the caliber and compliance of large conductance muscular arteries.[16] A reduction in arteriolar resistance appears to occur in some vascular beds but may be dependent on high doses of the drug and may be a relatively transient effect of the nitrates.[17] Evidence also exists that nitrates have a relaxing effect on collateral vascular channels, particular coronary collateral vessels, and this action may contribute to their beneficial effect in patients with angina pectoris.[18] The nitrates also appear to have a direct dilating effect on the pulmonary vasculature and therefore result in a lowering of pulmonary vascular resistance. The relative dilator effect of nitrates on various regional vascular beds is not entirely established, but it appears likely that the drugs have a prominent action on the cutaneous and skeletal muscle beds, with lesser effect on the visceral organs.[19]

Because of the diverse vascular actions of these agents they have found a place in the management of a variety of cardiovascular diseases. *Nitroglycerin* serves as the drug of choice to treat anginal attacks because of the rapid onset and magnitude of action after sublingual administration. The remarkable effectiveness of nitroglycerin in angina pectoris is dependent on several actions of the drug, including a relaxing effect on stenotic coronary arteries, a reduction of blood pressure, and an increase in vascular capacitance, with a consequent reduction of ventricular volume. An increase in collateral flow to ischemic myocardium also is likely.[20]

The major issues with the nitrates in recent years have been related to the relative efficacy and pharmacokinetics of various formulations, the efficacy of chronic administration, and the possibility of tolerance to the drug (Table 88-1). Sublingual administration of nitroglycerin is clearly effective, and it is now well established that oral administration of the nitrates, particularly *isosorbide dinitrate,* produces a predictable hemodynamic response.[21]

Considerable variability exists in the dosage requirement for a vascular action after oral administration; isosorbide dinitrate doses of 20, 40, or 60 mg orally given at 4 to 6 h may be necessary to produce a sustained hemodynamic effect. Newer formulations of the *5-mononitrate metabolite of isosorbide dinitrate* make available a longer-acting nitrate that appears to have similar circulatory effects.[22] Cutaneous administration of nitrates has long been utilized in ointment preparations that have been used for the treatment of angina.[23] More recently, formulations of nitroglycerin in matrix materials for skin absorption have become available.[24] Preliminary evidence suggests that absorption from these transdermal preparations is relatively modest and that large applications are necessary to produce hemodynamic effects comparable to what can be achieved with oral administration of nitrates.[25]

An unresolved issue is the appropriate dosing schedule for nitrate administration. Some investigators have suggested that fairly long drug-free intervals should be allowed each day for recovery of the vascular sensitivity to the nitrates.[26] Others have been less impressed with evidence of tolerance and continue to use the nitrates at frequent dosing intervals to maintain blood levels and circulatory effects. Carefully controlled studies to evaluate the relative merits of these two dosing regimens are necessary before a recommendation can firmly be made. Furthermore, there is reason to suspect that sensitivity and tolerance to the large arterial, arteriolar, and venous effects may not have the same time course. Therefore, appropriate dosing regimens for one clinical indication may not necessarily apply to other clinical indications.

TABLE 88-1 Effect of Commonly Used Nitrates

Drug	Route of Administration	Dosage	Onset of Effect	Duration of Effect	Reliability of Effect
Nitroglycerin (Nitrostate; Susadrin)	Sublingual	0.3–0.6 mg	30 s	15–30 min	High
Nitroglycerin (Nitrostat SR; Nitro-Bid)	Oral	2.5–19.5 mg	1 h	2–4 h	Low
Nitroglycerin (Nitro-Bid; Nitrodisc; Nitro-Dur; Nitrol ointment; Transderm)	Transdermal	1–2 in (ointment) 10–60 cm^2 (patches)	1 h	6–24 h	Medium
Nitroglycerin (Tridil)	Intravenous	10–200 μg/min	Immediate	—	High
Isosorbide dinitrate (Isordil; Sorbitrate; Dilatrate)	Sublingual	2.5–10 mg	5 min	1–2 h	High
Isosorbide dinitrate (Isordil; Sorbitrate; Dilatrate)	Oral	10–60 mg	30 min	4–6 h	High
Isosorbide 5-mononitrate (ISMO)	Oral	10–40 mg	30 min	8–21 h	High

Sodium Nitroprusside

Sodium nitroprusside is a potent smooth-muscle dilator that must be administered intravenously (see Table 88-2). It is likely that the cellular mechanism of action of nitroprusside is very similar to that of the nitrates and may be related to cyclic GMP stimulation.[27] Intravenous titration of nitroprusside can produce progressively increasing arteriolar dilation and therefore progressive reduction of systemic vascular resistance. This arteriolar dilation is accomplished in concert with considerable venodilation and an increase in vascular capacitance. The net result of infusion of sodium nitroprusside is a dose-dependent reduction of arterial pressure in patients with hypertension and a dose-dependent decrease of impedance in patients with congestive heart failure. The drug has been of particular value for acute short-term management of unstable patients in whom adjustment of pressure and/or cardiac output is essential to maintaining clinical integrity. It frequently is used to control arterial pressure in aortic dissection, hypertensive crisis, or in the postoperative cardiac patient, to produce hypotension during surgery, and to augment left ventricular performance in acute myocardial infarction or severe congestive heart failure.

The regional vascular effects of nitroprusside may be of importance in its use. Cerebral blood flow increases[28] and the drug has a pulmonary vasodilator effect,[29] but the systemic vasodilator effect does not favor the renal or splanchnic beds. Some experimental studies have suggested that myocardial ischemia may be aggravated by nitroprusside because of a coronary "steal" phenomenon,[30] but there is clinical evidence for efficacy of nitroprusside in myocardial ischemia.[31] In a carefully controlled multicenter study of acute myocardial infarction, early intervention with nitroprusside appeared to have a deleterious effect on mortality, whereas late intervention, when the goal was to improve persistently depressed cardiac function, had a beneficial effect.[32] Therefore, caution in administration of nitroprusside during the first 8 h after the onset of acute myocardial infarction is justified. Whether the same concern should apply to the use of nitroglycerin is not entirely clear.

During titration of nitroprusside infusion it is imperative that blood pressure be monitored closely and that infusion rate be carefully titrated. A wide variation in effective doses is noted, with some patients responding to doses as small as 20 to 40 μg/min, whereas others require as much as 600 to 800 μg/min. Toxicity of nitroprusside may be noted during prolonged administration of large doses of the drug, which may result in accumulation of thiocyanate that may lead to central toxicity.[33]

Hydralazine

Hydralazine exerts a dose-dependent arteriolar dilation that is effective in lowering systemic vascular resistance in patients with hypertension[34] and reducing impedance to left ventricular ejection in patients with heart failure[35] (see Table 88-3). Reflex cardiac stimulation with tachycardia is common in hypertensive patients but less often observed in patients with heart failure. Hydralazine exerts little if any effect on venous capacitance and therefore an increase in cardiac output is not counterbalanced by much decrease in ventricular filling.[35]

Dosage levels of oral hydralazine are restricted by side effects, which include nonspecific musculoskeletal symptoms and occasionally a full-blown syndrome of lupus erythematosus.[36] Toxicity from high-dose hydralazine is particularly prominent in individuals who are genetically slow acetylators and therefore tend to accumulate higher concentrations of the nonmetabolized drug in the blood. Angina may be precipitated by hydralazine, presumably in large part because of tachycardia, but also possibly related to coronary vascular effects precipitating maldistribution of flow in the myocardium or a direct effect to increase myocardial contractility.[37]

For treatment of hypertension the dose of hydralazine generally is kept below 300 mg daily to avoid side effects. It usually is preferable to admin-

TABLE 88-2 Effect of Direct-Acting Vasodilators

Drug	Route of Administration	Dosage	Onset of Effect	Duration of Effect	Large Arteries	Arterioles	Veins
Sodium nitroprusside (Nipride)	Intravenous	25–400 μg/min	Immediate	—	+	+++	+++
Nitroglycerin (Tridil)	Intravenous	10–200 μg/min	Immediate	—	++	+	+++
Isosorbide dinitrate (Isordil; Sorbitrate, Isobid; Isotrate; Sorate, Sorbide; Dilatrate)	Oral	20–60 mg	30 min	4–6 h	++	+	+++
Hydralazine (Apresoline)	Oral	50–100 mg	30 min	6–12 h	0	+++	±
Hydralazine (Apresoline)	IV or IM	5–40 mg	15 min	4–8 h	0	+++	±
Minoxidil (Loniten)	Oral	10–30 mg	30 min	8–12 h	0	+++	0
Diazoxide (Hyperstat)	Intravenous bolus	100–300 mg	Immediate	4–12 h	0	+++	±
Nifedipine (Procardia)	Oral	10–20 mg	20–30 min	2–4 h	++	+++	±
	Sublingual	10–20 mg	15 min	2–4 h	++	+++	±

TABLE 88-3 Effect of Drugs That Inhibit Neurohumoral Vasoconstriction

Drug	Route of Administration	Dosage	Onset of Effect	Duration of Effect	Myocardial Contractility	Plasma Norepinephrine	Plasma Renin Activity
Clonidine (Catapres)	Oral	0.1–0.3 mg	1 h	6–12 h	=	=	−
Guanabenz (Wytensin)	Oral	8–24 mg	1 h	6–12 h	=	=	−
Methyldopa (Aldomet)	Oral	250–1000 mg	2–4 h	6–12 h	−	−	±
Reserpine (Serpasil)	Oral	0.1–0.5 mg	2–4 h	12–24 h	−	0	0
Propranolol (Inderal)	Oral	20–80 mg	30 min	4–8 h	=	+	=
Guanethidine (Ismelin)	Oral	10–50 mg	1 h	24 h	−	+	±
Phentolamine (Regitine)	Intravenous	1–5 mg/min	Immediate	—	+	++	+
Prazosin (Minipress)	Oral	2–10 mg	30 min	4–8 h	0	±	+
Captopril (Capoten)	Oral	12.5–50 mg	30 min	4–8 h	0	−	++
Enalapril (MK421)	Oral	5–20 mg	1 h	12–24 h	0	−	++

ister hydralazine in conjunction with a diuretic and/or a beta-adrenoceptor blocker to minimize the reflex tachycardia and reflex increase in cardiac output. In patients with congestive heart failure similar doses of hydralazine may be employed although in some instances considerably higher doses may be necessary. Reflex tachycardia is attenuated in heart failure[38] and therefore it usually is not necessary to inhibit this response. For most clinical indications it is probably possible to administer hydralazine on a twice-daily schedule.

Minoxidil

Minoxidil is an arteriolar dilator similar to hydralazine but apparently more potent (see Table 88-2). The drug may be administered twice daily and in higher doses may produce a profound dilator effect that is effective in lowering blood pressures in severe hypertension resistant to other interventions.[39] Reflex cardiac stimulation and sodium retention, possibly because of the arteriolar dilating effect of the drug or possibly because of a direct antinatriuretic effect on the kidney, are the major complicating hemodynamic effects of minoxidil.[40] Stimulation of lanugal hair growth over the face, extremities, and trunk is a common side effect of minoxidil and makes the drug less well tolerated by female patients.

Diazoxide

Diazoxide is a nondiuretic thiazide derivative that exerts a potent arteriolar dilator effect when given intravenously (see Table 88-2). Its only place in cardiovascular therapy has been for acute management of hypertensive crisis, in which blood pressure lowering can be achieved quite rapidly and often can be maintained by continuous infusion or subsequent bolus injections. Sodium retention and hyperglycemia are common side effects of the drug and these complications limit its use. For acute management of severe hypertension, sodium nitroprusside is more reliable and more easily titrated with fewer side effects.

Calcium Antagonists

In recent years a number of vasodilator drugs have been identified that appear to have in common inhibition of transmembrane calcium transport across slow channels in both cardiac muscle and vascular smooth muscle (see Chap. 91). These drugs also appear to inhibit intracellular calcium release that in some vascular tissue plays an important role in increasing cytosol calcium concentration to stimulate muscle contraction.[41] Many of the drugs in this family of compounds are still undergoing investigation and are not yet available for general clinical use.

The first three agents to reach the marketplace in the United States are *verapamil, nifedipine,* and *diltiazem.* The vascular effect of all three of these agents is characterized by relaxation of vascular smooth muscle, particularly in the large conductance arteries and at the arteriolar level.[42] These drugs in general have less venous capacitance effect than the nitrates. Considerable individual differences exist in the responsiveness of various vascular beds to individual calcium antagonists. Some of these agents, such as nisoldipine and nifedipine (see Table 88-2), may produce considerable arteriolar dilatation in the coronary bed and cause an increase in coronary blood flow.[43,44] Others have a less profound arteriolar dilator effect. Some experimental agents appear to have selective actions favoring the renal bed and the cerebral bed, whereas others appear to have a more prominent effect on the skeletal muscle vascular bed.[45,46] The pulmonary vasculature appears to be particularly responsive to at least some of the calcium antagonists but less responsive to others.[47] The effects on the myocardium and the conducting system of the heart also are highly individual. Verapamil and diltiazem have a profound effect on the conducting system and are useful by the intravenous route for the management of supraventricular tachycardias. In contrast, nifedipine and the other dihydropyridines do not have an effect on the conducting system.

The negative inotropic effects of calcium antagonists also appear to vary considerably. Although all these agents may have a direct negative inotropic effect in isolated heart preparations, verapamil exerts a negative inotropic effect when administered systemically in humans, whereas diltiazem appears to have less of a negative inotropic effect, and drugs in the dihydropyridine group exhibit little if any negative inotropic activity. This freedom from negative inotropism could be related to differences in reflex sympathetic stimulation in response to these agents or could represent some change in baroreceptor function.[48]

Early clinical studies with calcium antagonists have been devoted primarily to their use in angina pectoris. In myocardial ischemia these drugs exert a number of actions that appear to have a favorable effect on myocardial perfusion: (1) they relax large conductance coronary artery caliber and therefore may reduce the severity of coronary stenoses; (2) they alter the resistance of coronary arterioles and coronary collateral channels and thus may augment myocardial perfusion in areas of ischemia; (3) they appear to inhibit reactive hyperemia in the coronary vascular bed and this inhibition of inappropriate vasodilation may have favorable effects on the intramyocardial distribution of blood flow; (4) they reduce systemic vascular resistance which may improve ventricular emptying, lower wall stress, and myocardial oxygen consumption; (5) they may produce a modest reduction of myocardial preload and thus further reduce myocardial oxygen consumption; and (6) they may reduce exercise-induced blood pressure and tachycardia, the major determinants of myocardial oxygen consumption.

In recent years these drugs have also been employed for the management of hypertension in both the systemic and pulmonary vascular beds.[49,50] The effectiveness of these drugs either with monotherapy or in combination with other agents to reduce vascular resistance has not yet been subjected to careful study. Nonetheless, these agents appear to be attractive because of the evidence for sustained effectiveness and the absence of severe side effects. Preliminary studies also have been carried out using these drugs in the management of subarachnoid hemorrhage, Raynaud's syndrome, migraine headache, etc.

Although interactions between calcium antagonists and other cardiovascular drugs have not been exhaustively studied, concern has been expressed for a possible additive negative inotropic effect of certain calcium antagonists and beta-adrenoceptor blockers. Caution thus must be exercised in the concomitant use of verapamil and beta blockers.[51] This caution does not appear to apply as strongly to the combined use of the other calcium antagonists with beta blockers. An interaction with digitalis also has been described with at least some of the calcium antagonists. It is therefore necessary to observe carefully for signs of digitalis toxicity when calcium antagonist therapy is initiated in the patient already receiving digitalis glycosides.

Sympathetic Vasoconstrictor Inhibitors

Maintenance of tone in vascular smooth muscle in arteries, arterioles, and veins is dependent at least in part on sympathetic vasoconstrictor activity mediated largely through alpha-adrenoceptor stimulation (see Table 88-3). Inhibition of this sympathetic vasoconstriction will result in a reduction in systemic vascular resistance, redistribution of peripheral blood flow, and an increase in venous capacitance. Sympathetic blockade also tends to produce orthostatic hypotension. Inhibition may be accomplished at numerous sites along the course of the sympathetic vasoconstrictor apparatus.

Central Inhibition

Stimulation of central $alpha_2$ receptors results in a decreased sympathetic outflow and reduced sympathetic vasoconstrictor activity. This mechanism appears to account for the antihypertensive activity of clonidine.[52] Another $alpha_2$ agonist, guanabenz, is also available for this purpose.[53] These agents have an effect on both arterial and venous responses and thus increase systemic capacitance as well as lowering vascular resistance. They also reduce sympathetic drive to the heart and therefore reduce heart rate and myocardial contractility. The negative inotropic effect of these drugs may limit their usefulness as vasodilator agents for the treatment of heart failure.[54]

Other antihypertensive drugs also may exert a central inhibiting effect on sympathetic discharge. The action of *methyldopa*[55] and *reserpine*[56] may at least in part be related to central inhibition, and a central action has even been implicated in the antihypertensive effect of beta-adrenoceptor blockers[57] (see Table 88-3).

Tolerance has not been a problem with these centrally acting agents, but side effects of drowsiness, lethargy, and orthostatic dizziness are frequent enough with some of the drugs to warrant a search for alternate agents in most patients with hypertension.

Ganglionic Blockade

Drugs that block sympathetic ganglia may be very effective in inhibiting sympathetic vasoconstriction, but the side effects of these drugs have practically eliminated them from clinical practice. Side effects of concomitant vagal blockade (constipation, urinary retention) and uncontrollable orthostatic hypotension are the most prominent complications of therapy.

Inhibition of Peripheral Norepinephrine Release

Guanethidine (see Table 88-3), *guanadrel*, *bethanidine*, and *bretylium* all inhibit postganglionic release of norepinephrine and thus reduce vascular tone and lower blood pressure. Since their action is accentuated when sympathetic tone is high, these agents all may produce orthostatic hypotension. Bethanidine and bretylium have an additional antiarrhythmic effect that has been useful in preventing and treating ventricular tachycardia/fibrillation.[58] Guanethidine is an attractive antihypertensive agent because of its potency and its once-a-day dosage. Guanadrel exerts similar effects but is shorter-acting. Tolerance does not develop to these agents and, when combined with a diuretic, they are capable of normalizing standing pressure in the most severe hypertensives. However, side effects of orthostatic hypotension and diarrhea often occur when attempts are made to increase the dose to normalize supine pressure; consequently these drugs are now reserved for unusual special circumstances when the better-tolerated agents prove ineffective.

Inhibition of Norepinephrine Synthesis

Tyrosine hydroxylase, the rate-limiting step in norepinephrine synthesis, may be inhibited by *metyrosine,* an orally effective drug that may reduce catecholamine biosynthesis by 35 to 80 percent.[59] Its use has been limited largely to patients with pheochromocytoma not amenable to immediate surgery.

Alpha-Adrenoceptor Blockers

Inhibition of sympathetic-mediated vasoconstriction by interference with the postganglionic alpha receptor has always appeared to be a rational approach to therapy of states in which the systemic vascular resistance is high. Early use of alpha-adrenoreceptor blockers was limited because the available agents, *phentolamine* (see Table 88-3) and *dibenzyline,* were poorly tolerated in clinical practice because of orthostatic hypotension and reflex tachycardia.[60] The introduction of *prazosin* (see Table 88-3) made it possible to utilize alpha-blocker therapy on a more chronic basis. The major difference between prazosin and the previously available alpha blockers appears to be related to the selectivity of effect on vascular alpha receptors. Whereas phentolamine and dibenzyline exert their action relatively nonselectively on both presynaptic and postsynaptic alpha receptors, prazosin's action is more highly localized to the postsynaptic alpha receptor.[61] This postsynaptic receptor, commonly referred to as the $alpha_1$ receptor, is the major mediator of sympathetic vasoconstriction of vascular smooth muscle. The presynaptic $alpha_2$ receptor appears to have a major effect on presynaptic release of norepinephrine.[62] Therefore $alpha_2$ stimulation tends to suppress norepinephrine release and $alpha_2$ blockade to enhance norepinephrine release. Therapeutic success with prazosin has therefore been attributed to the absence of inhibition of $alpha_2$ receptors and therefore the absence of enhanced norepinephrine release that might otherwise result in reflex tachycardia. Although prazosin may produce severe orthostatic hypotension after the first dose, this effect appears to wane with continued therapy.[63] The reason for tolerance to the orthostatic effects of prazosin has not been well explained, although it raises the possibility of some tolerance developing to the $alpha_1$-receptor blocking action of the drug. Several newer $alpha_1$-receptor blockers, including *indoramin* and *trimazosin,* also are undergoing clinical investigation.[64,65] These agents have been particularly advocated for use in hypertension and congestive heart failure.

Since sympathetic tone plays an important role not only on the arterial resistance vessels but also on the venous capacitance vessels it would be anticipated that alpha-adrenoceptor blockers would increase capacitance and reduce cardiac preload as well as reducing resistance. This appears to be the case with most of the alpha-adrenoceptor blockers that have been studied. The action of these alpha-adrenoceptor blockers on the renal vasculature and on renal tubular function is controversial. A sodium-retaining effect of alpha-adrenoceptor blockade perhaps related to reduction of perfusion pressure has been reported. On the other hand, data have been generated suggesting that $alpha_2$ receptors may have a direct effect on renal tubular sodium reabsorption and may therefore have an independent effect on renal sodium handling.[66] These effects should become clearer as additional studies are carried out with some of the newer alpha-adrenoreceptor blockers.

Converting Enzyme Inhibitors

Since angiotensin II is a potent constrictor of arteriolar resistance vessels the development of converting enzyme inhibitors provided an attractive means of inhibiting vasoconstriction by inhibiting the production of the vasoactive octapeptide angiotensin II from the decapeptide angiotensin I (see Table 88-3).[67] The action of *captopril* appears to be at least in large part related to its ability to inhibit production of angiotensin II; therefore, this drug has a vasodilator effect that lowers systemic vascular resistance and has in addition a natriuretic effect by inhibition of aldosterone secretion.[68] The effects of captopril (see Table 88-3) in lowering blood pressure in patients with essential hypertension, and particularly in patients with renovascular hypertension, and in lowering systemic vascular resistance and improving left ventricular performance in patients with congestive heart failure have now been well established.[69,70] Other actions of converting enzyme inhibitors also cannot be disregarded. Inhibition of degradation of bradykinin may lead to increased levels of circulating bradykinin that could also contribute to a vasodilator effect.[71] Since angiotensin II is an important stimulator of presynaptic norepinephrine release,[72] inhibition of production of angiotensin II also may reduce sympathetic vasomotor tone.[73] Central actions of angiotensin also may be important in influencing vascular resistance and salt and water balance; these actions may also be influenced by converting enzyme inhibition.[74,75]

Several new converting enzyme inhibitors are also undergoing clinical testing. *Enalapril* (see Table 88-3), an inhibitor of different structure and longer duration of action than captopril, appears to have a similar spectrum of activity in both hypertension and congestive heart failure. The absence of a sulfhydryl group on the enalapril molecule theoretically might reduce the incidence of captopril side effects, some of which have been attributed to the sulfhydryl structure. Studies to date have not convincingly demonstrated a significantly lower incidence of complications to enalapril than to captopril. Nonetheless, the longer duration of action of enalapril may provide some advantage for chronic therapy.

In general, the converting enzyme inhibitors appear to effectively block angiotensin-converting enzyme at relatively low doses. Higher doses of the drug therefore prolong the duration of inhibition rather than increase its peak effect. In early clinical testing, converting enzyme inhibition was utilized primarily for treatment of severe hypertension, particularly hypertension with high plasma renin activity, and for advanced stages of congestive heart failure. More recent data suggest that this approach to therapy might be useful also in milder forms of hypertension and milder states of congestive heart failure. Further experience is necessary before the ultimate place of this class of compounds in the management of these vascular disorders is established.

Vasoconstrictor Drugs

The use of vasoconstrictor agents for cardiovascular disorders has fallen into relative disrepute for several reasons. (1) Increases in vascular resistance may impair left ventricular output when the left ventricle is abnormal. Since an abnormality in left ventricular performance is common in shock and hypotensive states, administration of a vasoconstrictor drug may aggravate a flow deficiency in these syndromes even though it may at least temporarily support arterial pressure. (2) Vasoconstrictor drugs tend to redistribute peripheral blood flow away from vascular beds that are most sensitive to the vasoconstrictor effect of the administered agent. Since the renal bed may be particularly responsive to certain of these agents a reduction of renal blood flow, often an undesirable effect, may accompany the systemic administration of many of these agents. (3) Tolerance to the vasoconstrictor effect of drugs may develop within a short period of time and may make it particularly difficult to maintain the vascular tone desired.

Despite these theoretical disadvantages, however, there are certain clinical situations in which support of arterial pressure is so critically important that an agent that reliably raises blood pressure by increasing vascular tone may have a place in emergency therapy. The coronary vascular bed and cerebral vascular bed are particularly sensitive to perfusion pressure and the need for an adequate perfusion pressure is enhanced in the presence of stenotic lesions in the proximal coronary and cerebral vascular beds. Therefore, in circumstances when evidence of myocardial or cerebral ischemia accompanies syndromes in which arterial pressure is reduced, prompt restoration of blood pressure may be of great importance. Use of agents for this purpose is generally only temporary and can be replaced by more physiologic approaches to the circulatory disturbances as soon as the mechanism of the abnormality can be identified.

Sympathetic Agonists

Drugs which stimulate alpha adrenoceptors may produce both arterial and venous constriction and thus raise systemic vascular resistance and increase cardiac filling. Administration of these drugs generally also increases capillary pressure and results in intravascular depletion of plasma volume.[76] The major difference among these agents relates to their action on the heart. Drugs such as *norepinephrine* and *metaraminol* exert beta-agonistic as well as alpha-agonistic effects; the cardiac effect tends to support cardiac output in the face of peripheral vasoconstriction. In contrast, agents such as *phenylephrine* and *methoxamine* exert little direct positive inotropic effect, and therefore their actions are predominantly confined to peripheral constriction. These agents tend to raise blood pressure but at the expense of a reduction of cardiac output and considerable cardiac slowing. *Ephedrine* and the ephedrine-like analogs produce alpha constriction and beta cardiac stimulation but also produce beta vasodilatation in the skeletal muscle. Administration of ephedrine results in a variable effect on blood pressure, accompanied by considerable cardiac stimulation. Redistribution of blood flow away from vascular beds heavily endowed with alpha receptors, such as the renal bed, accompany the hemodynamic response to these agents.[77]

Angiotensin Analogs

Angiotensin is a potent vasoconstrictor which at one time was used clinically for support of blood pressure in hypotensive states.[78] The angiotensin amide previously marketed has been withdrawn from the market and is no longer available for clinical use. Angiotensin has a modest inotropic effect by virtue of augmented norepinephrine release but it also has a potent renal vasoconstrictor effect. There appears to be no clinical indication for specific administration of angiotensin in clinical conditions at the present time.

Vasopressin Analogs

Polypeptides of the *vasopressin* series are potent vasoconstrictor agents which exert an action on both the arterial and the venous bed. Some analogs have been developed that are essentially devoid of antidiuretic hormone properties and exert almost an exclusive action on the vasculature.[79] These agents are particularly effective on the coronary bed and have been used diagnostically to induce coronary spasm in susceptible individuals with atypical angina.[80] These agents also have a selective action on the mesenteric vascular bed and therefore have been used to control variceal bleeding by reduction of portal vein pressure.[81] Although the effectiveness of these agents in lowering portal pressure has been established, some question remains as to whether this vasoconstrictor effect persists during sustained administration and whether the portal pressure reduction can therefore be maintained. The action of these drugs on venous return and cardiac output appears to be somewhat species-dependent and the mechanism of the reduction of cardiac output is not entirely understood.

References

1. Cohn, J. N.: Vasodilator Symposium. Introduction: Marriage of the Heart and the Peripheral Circulation, *Prog. Cardiovasc. Dis.*, 24(3):189–190, 1981.
2. Sarnoff, S. J., and Berglund, E.: Ventricular Function. I. Starling's Law of the Heart Studied by Means of Simultaneous Right and Left Ventricular Function Curves in the Dog, *Circulation*, 9:706, 1954.
3. Katz, A. M.: The Descending Limb of the Starling Curve and the Failing Heart, *Circulation*, 32:871, 1965.
4. Linzbach, A. J.: Heart Failure from the Point of View of Quantitative Anatomy, *Am. J. Cardiol.*, 5:370, 1960.
5. Gaasch, W. H., Levine, H. F., Quinones, M. A., and Alexander, J. K.: Left Ventricular Compliance: Mechanisms and Clinical Implications, *Am. J. Cardiol.*, 38:645, 1976.
6. Sonnenblick, E. H., and Skelton, C. L.: Myocardial Energetics: Basic Principles and Clinical Implications, *N. Engl. J. Med.*, 285:668, 1971.
7. Ludbrook, P. A., Byrne, J. D., and McKnight, R. C.: Influence of Right Ventricular Hemodynamics in Left Ventricular Diastolic Pressure-Volume Relations in Man, *Circulation*, 59:21, 1979.
8. Cohn, J. N.: Vasodilator Therapy for Heart Failure: The Influence of Impedance on Left Ventricular Performance, *Circulation*, 48:5–8, 1973.
9. Milnor, W. R.: Arterial Impedance as Ventricular Afterload, *Circ. Res.*, 36:565, 1975.
10. Cohn, J. N., Mashiro, I., Levine, T. B., and Mehta, J.: Role of Vasoconstrictor Mechanisms in the Control of Left Ventricular Performance of the Normal and Damaged Heart, *Am. J. Cardiol.*, 44:1019–1022, 1979.
11. Moskowitz, R. M., and Cohn, J. N.: Hemodynamic Effects of Oxdralazine and Hydralazine in Hypertension, *Clin. Pharmacol. Ther.*, 27:773–778, 1980.
12. Cohn, J. N., Tristani, F. E., and Khatri, I. M.: Systemic Vasoconstrictor and Renal Vasodilator Effects of PLV-2 in Man, *Circulation*, 38:151–157, 1968.
13. Cohn, J. N.: Relationship of Plasma Volume Changes to Resistance and Capacitance Vessel Effects of Sympathomimetic Amines and Angiotensin in Man, *Clin. Sci.*, 30:267–278, 1966.
14. Schultz, G., Schultz, K. D., Bohme, E., and Kreye, V. A. W.: The Possible Role of Cyclic GMP in the Actions of Hormones and Drugs on Smooth Muscle Tone: Effects of Exogenous Cyclic GMP Derivatives, *Adv. Pharmacol. Ther.*, 3:113, 1978.
15. Wilkins, R. W., Haynes, F. W., and Weiss, S.: The Role of the Venous System in the Circulatory Collapse Induced by Sodium Nitrite, *J. Clin. Invest.*, 16:85, 1937.
16. Brown, B. G., Bolson, E., Peterson, R. B., Pierce, C. D., and Dodge, H. T.: The Mechanisms of Nitroglycerin Action: Stenosis Vasodilation as a Major Component of the Drug Response, *Circulation*, 64:1089, 1981.
17. Mason, D. J., and Braunwald, E. B.: The Effects of Nitroglycerin and Amyl Nitrite on Arteriolar and Venous Tone in the Human Forearm, *Circulation*, 32:755, 1965.
18. Fam, W. M., and McGregor, M.: Effect of Coronary Vasodilator Drugs on Retrograde Flow in Areas of Chronic Myocardial Ischemia, *Circ. Res.*, 15:355, 1964.
19. Vatner, S. F., Pagani, M., Rutherford, J. D., Millard, R. W., and Manders, W. T.: Effects of Nitroglycerin on Cardiac Function and Regional Blood Flow Distribution in Conscious Dogs, *Am. J. Physiol.*, 234:H–244, 1978.
20. McGregor, M.: The Nitrates and Myocardial Ischemia, *Circulation*, 66:689, 1982.
21. Franciosa, J. A., Mikulic, E., Cohn, J. N., and Fabie, A.: Hemodynamic Effects of Orally Administered Isosorbide Dinitrate in Patients with Congestive Heart Failure, *Circulation*, 50:1020–1024, 1974.
22. Chasseaud, L. F., Dawn, W. H., and Grundy, R. K.: Concentrations of the Vasodilator Isosorbide Dinitrate and its Metabolites in the Blood of Human Subjects, *Eur. J. Clin. Pharmacol.*, 8:157, 1975.
23. Davis, J. A., Wiesel, B. H., and Epstein, S. E.: The Treatment of Angina Pectoris with Nitroglycerin Ointment, *Am. J. Med. Sci.*, 230:259, 1955.
24. Olivari, M. T., and Cohn, J. N.: Cutaneous Administration of Nitroglycerin: A Review, *Pharmacotherapy*, 3:149–157, 1983.
25. Olivari, M. T., Carlyle, P. F., Levine, T. B., and Cohn, J. N.: Hemodynamic and Hormonal Response to Transdermal Nitroglycerin in Normal Subjects and in Patients with Congestive Heart Failure, *J. Am. Coll. Cardiol.*, 2:872–878, 1983.
26. Rudolph, W., Blasini, R., and Kraus, F.: Clinical Efficacy of Nitrates in the Treatment of Exertional Angina Pectoris, *Herz*, 7:286, 1982.
27. Cohn, J. N., and Burke, L. P.: Diagnosis and Treatment—Drugs Five Years Later: Nitroprusside, *Ann. Intern. Med.*, 91:752–757, 1979.
28. Ivankovich, A. D., Miletich, D. J., Albrecht, R. F., and Zaked, B.: Sodium Nitroprusside and Cerebral Blood Flow in the Anesthetized and Unanesthetized Goat, *Anesthesiology*, 44:21, 1976.
29. Pace, J. B.: Pulmonary Vascular Response to Sodium Nitroprusside in Anesthetized Dogs, *Anesth. Analg.*, 57:551, 1978.
30. Chiariello, M., Gold, H. K., Leinbach, R. C., Davis, M. A., and Maroko, P. R.: Comparison between the Effects of Nitroprusside and Nitroglycerin on Ischemic Injury during Acute Myocardial Infarction, *Circulation*, 54:766, 1976.
31. Awan, N. A., Miller, R. R., Vera, Z., DeMaria, A. N., Amsterdam, E. A., and Mason, D. T.: Reduction of ST Segment Elevation with Infusion of Nitroprusside in Patients with Acute Myocardial Infarction, *Am. J. Cardiol.*, 38:435, 1976.
32. Cohn, J. N., Franciosa, J. A., Francis, G. S., Archibald, D., Tristani, F., Fletcher, R., Montero, A., Cintron, G., Clarke, J., Hager, D., Saunders, R., Cobb, F., Smith, R., Loeb, H., and Settle, H.: Effect of Short-Term Infusion of Sodium Nitroprusside on Mortality Rate in Acute Myocardial Infarction Complicated by Left Ventricular Failure, *N. Engl. J. Med.*, 306:1129–1135, 1982.
33. McDowall, D. G., Keaney, N. P., Turner, J. M., Lane, J. R., and Okuder, Y.: The Toxicity of Sodium Nitroprusside, *Br. J. Anaesth.*, 46:327, 1974.
34. Freis, E. D., Rose, J. C., Higgins, T. F., et al.: The Hemodynamic Effects of Hypotensive Drugs in Man. IV. 1-Hydrazinopthalazine, *Circulation*, 8:199, 1953.

35. Franciosa, J. A., Pierpont, G., and Cohn, J. N.: Hemodynamic Improvement after Oral Hydralazine in Left Ventricular Failure: A Comparison with Nitroprusside Infusion in 16 Patients, *Ann. Intern. Med.*, 86:388–393, 1977.
36. Perry, H. M., Jr.,: Late Toxicity to Hydralazine Resembling Systemic Lupus Erythematosus or Rheumatoid Arthritis, *Am. J. Med.*, 54:58, 1973.
37. Khatri, I., Uemara, N., Notargiacomo, A., and Freis, E. D.: Direct and Reflex Cardiac Stimulating Effects of Hydralazine, *Am. J. Cardiol.*, 40:38, 1977.
38. Levine, T. B., Francis, G. S., Goldsmith, S. R., and Cohn, J. N.: The Neurohumoral and Hemodynamic Response to Orthostatic Tilt in Patients with Congestive Heart Failure, *Circulation*, 67:1070–1075, 1083.
39. DuCharme, D. W., Freyburger, W. A., Graham, B. E., and Carlson, R. G.: Pharmacologic Properties of Minoxidil: A New Hypotensive Agent, *J. Pharmacol. Exp. Ther.*, 184:662, 1973.
40. Koch-Weser, J.: Vasodilator Drugs in the Treatment of Hypertension, *Arch. Intern. Med.*, 133:1017, 1974.
41. Katz, A. M., Messineo, F. C., and Herbette, L.: Ion Channels in Membranes, *Circulation*, 65:1–2, 1982.
42. Fleckenstein, A.: Specific Pharmacology of Cardium in Myocardium, Cardiac Pacemakers and Vascular Smooth Muscle, *Annu. Rev. Pharmacol. Toxicol.*, 17:149, 1977.
43. Henry, P. D., Shuchleib, L. J., Borda, L. J., Roberts, R., Williamson, J. R., and Sobel, B. E.: Effects of Nifedipine on Myocardial Perfusion and Ischemic Injury in Dogs, *Circ. Res.*, 43:372, 1978.
44. Warltier, D. C., Meils, C. M., Gross, G. J., and Brooks, H. L.: Blood Flow in Normal and Ischemic Myocardium after Verapamil, Diltiazem, Nisuldipine—A New Dihydropyridine Calcium Antagonist, *J. Pharmacol. Exp. Ther.*, 218:296, 1981.
45. Shimizu, K., Ohta, T., and Toda, N.: Evidence for Greater Susceptibility of Isolated Dog Cerebral Arteries to Calcium Antagonists than Peripheral Arteries, *Stroke*, 11:261, 1980.
46. Kazda, S., Garthoff, B., and Knorr, A.: Nitrendipine and Other Calcium Entry Blockers (Calcium Antagonists) in Hypertension, *Fed. Proc.*, 42:196, 1983.
47. Young, T. E., Lundquist, L. J., Chesler, E., and Weir, E. K.: Comparative Effects of Nifedipine, Verapamil and Diltiazem as Pulmonary Hypertensives in the Anesthetized Dog, *Am. J. Cardiol.*, 49:942, 1982.
48. Millard, R. W., Lathrop, D. A., Grupp, G., Ashraf, M., Grupp, I. L., and Schwartz, A.: Differential Cardiovascular Effects of Calcium Channel Blocking Agents: Potential Mechanisms, *Am. J. Cardiol.*, 49:499, 1982.
49. Olivari, M. T., Bartorelli, C., Polese, A., Fiorentini, C., Moruzzi, P., and Guazzi, M. D.: Treatment of Hypertension with Nifedipine a Calcium Antagonist Drug, *Circulation*, 59:1056, 1979.
50. Olivari, M. T., Levine, T. B., Weir, E. K., and Cohn, J. N.: Hemodynamic Effects of Nifedipine at Rest and during Exercise in Primary Pulmonary Hypertension, *Chest*, 86:14–19, 1984.
51. Singh, B., Ellrodt, G., and Peter, C. T.: Verapamil: A Review of its Pharmacological Properties and Therapeutic Uses, *Drugs*, 15:169, 1978.
52. Raftos, J., Bauer, G. E., Lewis, R. G., et al.: Clonidine in the Treatment of Severe Hypertension, *Med. J. Aust.*, 1:786, 1973.
53. Baum, T., and Shropshire, A. T.: Studies on the Centrally Mediated Hypotensive Activity of Guanabenz, *Eur. J. Pharmacol.*, 37:31, 1976.
54. Giles, T. D., Iteld, B. J., Mautner, R. K., Rognoni, P. A., and Dillen Kaffer, R. L.: Short-term Effects of Intravenous Clonidine in Congestive Heart Failure, *Clin. Pharmacol. Ther.*, 30:724, 1981.
55. Henning, M.: Studies on the Mode of Action of α-Methyldopa, *Acta Physiol. Scand.*, 75(suppl. 322):1, 1969.
56. Shore, P. A.: Transport and Storage of Biogenic Amines, *Annu. Rev. Pharmacol.*, 12:209, 1972.
57. Tackett, R. L., Webb, J. G., and Privitera, P. J.: Cerebroventricular Propranolol Elevates Cardiospinal Fluid Norepinephrine and Lowers Arterial Pressure, *Science*, 213:911, 1981.
58. Bacaner, M. B., and Benditt, D. G.: Antiarrhythmic, Antifibrillatory, and Hemodynamic Actions of Bethanidine Sulfate: An Orally Effective Analog of Bretylium for Suppression of Ventricular Tachyarrhythmias, *Am. J. Cardiol.*, 50:728, 1982.
59. Engelman, K., Horwitz, D., Jequier, E., and Sjoerdsma, A.: Biochemical and Pharmacologic Effects of α-Methyltyrosine in Man, *J. Clin. Invest.*, 47:577, 1968.
60. Richards, D. A., Woodings, E. P., and Prichard, B. N. C.: Circulating and Alpha-Adrenoceptor Blocking Effects of Phentolamine, *Br. J. Clin. Pharmacol.*, 5:507, 1978.
61. Doxey, J. C., Smith, C. F. C., and Walker, J. M.: Selectivity of Blocking Agents for Pre- and Postsynaptic α-Adrenoceptors, *Br. J. Pharmacol.*, 62:91, 1977.
62. Constantine, J. E., Weeks, R. A., and McShane, W. K.: Prazosin and Presynaptic α-Receptors in the Cardioaccelerator Nerve of the Dog, *Eur. J. Pharmacol.*, 50:51, 1978.
63. Moulds, R. F. W., and Jauernig, R. A.: Mechanism of Prazosin Collapse, *Lancet*, 1:200, 1977.
64. Franciosa, J. A., and Cohn, J. N.: Hemodynamic Effects of Trimazosin in Patients with Left Ventricular Failure, *Clin. Pharmacol. Ther.*, 23:11–18, 1978.
65. Lewis, P. J., George, C. G., and Dollery, C. T.: Clinical Evaluation of Indoramin, a New Antihypertensive Agent, *Eur. J. Clin. Pharmacol.*, 6:211, 1973.
66. Bosanc, P., Dabb, J., Walker, B., Goldberg, M., and Agus, Z. S.: Renal Effects of Guanabenz: A New Antihypertensive, *J. Clin. Pharmacol.*, 16:631, 1976.
67. Cushman, D. E., Cheung, H. S., Sabo, E. F., and Ondetti, M. A.: Design of New Antihypertensive Drugs: Potent and Specific Inhibitors of Angiotensin-Converting Enzyme, *Prog. Cardiovasc. Dis.*, 21:176, 1978.
68. Bravo, E. L., and Tarazi, R. C.: Converting Enzyme Inhibition with an Orally Active Compound in Hypertensive Man, *Hypertension*, 1:39, 1979.
69. Brunner, H. P., Gavias, H., Wacker, B., et al.: Oral Angiotensin-Converting Enzyme Inhibitor in Long-Term Treatment of Hypertensive Patients, *Ann. Intern. Med.*, 90:19, 1979.
70. Captopril Multicenter Research Group: A Placebo-Controlled Trial of Captopril in Refractory Chronic Congestive Heart Failure, *J. Am. Coll. Cardiol.*, 2(4):755–763, 1983.
71. McCaa, R. E., Hall, J. E., and McCaa, C. S.: The Effects of Angiotensin I-Converting Enzyme Inhibitors on Arterial Blood Pressure and Urinary Sodium Excretion. Role of the Renal-Serum-Angiotensin and Kallikrein-Kinin Systems, *Circ. Res.*, 43:1–132, 1978.
72. Zimmerman, B. G., Gomer, S. K., and Lioa, J. C.: Action of Angiotensin on Vascular Adrenergic Nerve Endings: Facilitation of Norepinephrine Release, *Fed. Proc.*, 31:1344, 1972.
73. Antonaccio, M. J., and Kerwin, L.: Pre- and Postjunctional Inhibition of Vascular Sympathetic Function by Captopril in SHR. Implication of Vascular Angiotensin II in Hypertension and Antihypertensive Actions of Captopril, *Hypertension*, 3:1–54, 1981.
74. Share, L.: Interrelations between Vasopressin and Renin-Angiotensin System, *Fed. Proc.*, 38:2267, 1979.
75. Johnson, A. K., Mann, J. F. E., and Rosher, W.: Plasma Angiotensin II Concentrations and Experimentally Induced Thirst, *Am. J. Physiol.*, 240:R229, 1981.
76. Cohn, J. N.: Relationship of Plasma Volume Changes to Resistance and Capacitance Vessel Effects of Sympathomimetic Amines and Angiotensin in Man, *Clin. Sci.*, 30:267–278, 1966.
77. Goodyer, A. V. N., and Jaeger, C. A.: Renal Response to Non-shocking Hemorrhage: Role of the Autonomic Nervous System and of the Renal Circulation, *Am. J. Physiol.*, 180:69, 1955.
78. Cohn, J. N., and Luria, M. H.: Studies in Clinical Shock and Hypotension. II. Hemodynamic Effects of Norepinephrine and Angiotensin, *J. Clin. Invest.*, 44:1494–1504, 1965.
79. Cohn, J. N., Tristani, F. E., and Khatri, I. M.: Systemic Vasoconstrictor and Renal Vasodilator Effects of PLV-2 in Man, *Circulation*, 38:151–157, 1968.
80. Conti, C. R., Curry, R. C., Christie, L. G., and Pepine, C. J.: Clinical Use of Provocative Pharmacoangiography in Patients with Chest Pain, *Adv. Cardiol.*, 26:44, 1979.
81. Shaldon, S., Dolle, W., and Guevara, L.: Effect of Pitressin on the Splanchnic Circulation in Man, *Circulation*, 24:797, 1961.

89

Drugs Used to Treat Cardiac Arrhythmias

Warren M. Smith, M.B. Andrew G. Wallace, M.D.

"It's just a muscle," the Colonel said. "Only it is the main muscle. It works as perfectly as a Rolex Oyster Perpetual. The trouble is you cannot send it to the Rolex representative when it goes wrong. When it stops, you just do not know the time. You're dead."

Ernest Hemingway[1,*]

Many new antiarrhythmic drugs are becoming available for clinical investigation, reflecting the shortcomings of existing agents. This chapter will review the biochemistry, pharmacokinetics, pharmacology, and side effects of presently approved antiarrhythmic drugs and several promising investigational agents.

Classification of Antiarrhythmic Drugs

Although there is no universally accepted classification of antiarrhythmic drugs,[2] the format proposed by Vaughan Williams[3] and Brahma Singh[4] is perhaps the most widely used by clinicians (Table 89-1). Under this scheme, drugs with a class I action interfere directly with depolarization (subclassified according to their effect on action-potential duration—1A, prolongation; 1B, shortening; 1C, no effect). Class II drugs produce antisympathetic effects and class III drugs markedly prolong the duration of the action potential. A fourth class of action appears to relate to blockade of the slow inward depolarizing current. Some drugs possess more than one class of action.

An alternative classification has been proposed on the basis of the ionic currents associated with depolarization and repolarization. Drugs are classified according to their principal actions on the fast inward sodium current, the slow inward calcium current, and repolarization currents, and finally the relation between membrane currents and adrenergic receptor excitation and inhibition.[5] Quinidine, procainamide, lidocaine, mexiletine, and tocainide appear to reduce the fast inward current by reducing the number of sodium channels available. Diphenylhydantoin affects both fast and slow inward currents, while the latter is selectively blocked by verapamil. Both lidocaine and propranolol affect potassium repolarization currents. Thus, some correlation between the two classifications (Vaughan Williams[3] and ionic[5]) exists, although the ionic basis underlying the class II effect is not presently known.

*Ernest Hemingway, quoted from *Across the River and into the Trees.*

Class I Drugs

Quinidine

Quinidine is one of the alkaloids obtained by chemical extraction of cinchona bark and is the optical isomer of quinine. It was prepared and named by Pasteur in 1853 but was not introduced into western medicine until its antiarrhythmic effects were reported by Wenckebach (1914) and Frey (1918).

Pharmacokinetic Properties

Quinidine sulfate is rapidly and almost completely absorbed, with peak levels occurring about 1.5 h after ingestion (Table 89-2). About 80 percent (range 60 to 100 percent) of the dose is available to the systemic circulation, in contrast to the gluconate salt, which is more slowly absorbed, with peak levels at 4 h and 71 percent systemic availability (range 40 to 93 percent).[6] Eighty percent of the drug is bound to plasma albumin, and the half-life averages 5 to 7 h. Quinidine is partly excreted unchanged and partly metabolized by the liver, with the metabolites having little or no antiarrhythmic activity. Therapeutic levels range from 2.3 to 5 μg/ml.[7] Toxic effects are common with levels greater than 10 μg/ml.

Pharmacologic Properties

Electrophysiologic Effects Quinidine is principally concentrated in the cell membrane, where it decreases transmembrane permeability to sodium influx during phase 0 of the action potential. It depresses the maximum rate of depolarization (MRD) of the action potential and reduces the amplitude of the overshoot potential in all cardiac tissues.[8] These membrane effects are markedly lessened by hypokalemia and appear to be rate-related.[9] Quinidine also reduces phase IV depolarization and elevates the diastolic threshold of excitability. The effective refractory period (ERP) is markedly increased without a comparable increase in duration of the action potential. In awake dogs, serum concentrations of 5 to 10 mg/liter had little effect on atrioventricular (AV) node conduction but slowed conduction in

TABLE 89-1 Classification of Antiarrhythmic Drugs[3]

Class	IA	Quinidine, procainamide, disopyramide
	IB	Diphenylhydantoin, lidocaine, tocainide, mexiletine*
	IC	Encainide,* flecainide*
Class	II	Beta-adrenergic blocking drugs
Class	III	Bretylium
Class	IV	Verapamil, nifedipine, diltiazem*

*This drug has not been approved by the Food and Drug Administration of the United States at the time of publication.

TABLE 89-2 Pharmacokinetics of Antiarrhythmic Drugs

	Quinidine (Sulfate)	Procainamide	Disopyramide	Lidocaine	Diphenylhydantoin	Propranolol	Verapamil
Percent systemic availability	80	75–90	85	Low	95 (variable)	40 (variable)	10–22
Percent plasma protein bound	80	15	35–95*	60	70–95	90–96	90
Therapeutic range	2.3–5 μg/ml	4–10 μg/ml	2–5 μg/ml	1.5–5 μg/ml	10–20 μg/ml	40–100 ng/ml	?
Half-life, h	5–7	2.5–4.7	4.5 (IV)	1.2–2	6–32	4–6 (chronic dosage)	3–7
Route of excretion	Hepatic/renal	Hepatic/renal	Renal	Hepatic	Hepatic	Hepatic	Renal
Dosage:							
Oral	300–600 mg q 6 h	250–750 mg q 4 h	100–300 mg q 6 h		200–500 mg daily	10–100 mg q 6 h	30–180 mg q 6 h
IV	5–10 mg/kg†	10–15 mg/kg†		15–50 μg/kg/min infusion	10–15 mg/kg†	0.1 mg/kg†	0.145 mg/kg

*Concentration dependent. †Must be given very slowly. See text for discussion and references.

Purkinje tissue and prolonged ventricular activation.[10] Similar results have been reported in human beings, with decreased conduction and increased refractoriness of the atrium and His-Purkinje system[11] without significant effect on AV nodal conduction during sinus rhythm. However, shortening of the AH interval during atrial pacing was noted, together with shortening of the ERP of the AV node. These effects are consistent with an indirect (antivagal) action. The effects of quinidine on the ECG include prolongation of both the QRS complex and QT intervals.

Hemodynamic and Cardiovascular Effects Intravenous quinidine markedly depresses myocardial contractility and decreases systemic vascular resistance, primarily by alpha-adrenergic receptor blockade.[12] Although severe hypotension is a feature in reports from the older literature, more recent studies[13,14] with slow infusion rates have shown only minor falls in systolic blood pressure (5 to 15 mmHg).

Clinical Application and Toxicity

Quinidine may be used to suppress atrial and ventricular premature beats, which are often the initiating mechanism of paroxysmal tachycardia. It is also used to maintain sinus rhythm after successful reversion of atrial flutter and atrial fibrillation to sinus rhythm. Because quinidine is capable of slowing the rate of atrial flutter while enhancing conduction of the AV node, quinidine alone may result in atrial flutter with 1:1 AV conduction, thereby dangerously accelerating the ventricular rate. Most patients with atrial flutter/fibrillation should be given quinidine only after prior digitalization. The one exception to this rule is patients with the Wolff-Parkinson-White (WPW) syndrome, in whom quinidine prolongs refractoriness and slows conduction in the accessory pathways mediating the ventricular response to AF. The usual oral dosage is 300 to 600 mg every 6 h; intravenous administration is also possible, provided the infusion rate is slow.[13,14] Quinidine is contraindicated in the treatment of digitalis intoxication and relatively contraindicated in partial AV block because of the danger of asystole if progression to complete AV block occurs.

Unfortunately, side effects are frequent with quinidine, with gastrointestinal intolerance, particularly diarrhea, being the most common.[15] Large doses may cause cinchonism, a constellation of symptoms including tinnitus, blurred vision, and headache with gastrointestinal and cardiac toxicity in more advanced cases. Widening of the QRS complex is an indication of cardiac toxicity. Idiosyncratic reactions may result in thrombocytopenic purpura, and quinidine syncope,[16] commonly due to torsades dè pointes, appears to occur as a result of both individual susceptibility and excessive plasma concentration.[17] In the older literature fatalities from this complication were reported to occur in 2 to 4 percent of patients, although 0.5 percent has been cited in more recent reports.[15] Excessive prolongation of the QT interval may herald susceptibility to this complication. Because the normal range of QT prolongation with therapeutic quinidine levels has never been established, the actual values that constitute "excessive prolongation" are uncertain; we presently regard a QTc greater than 0.55 as undesirable and a value of 0.60 or more as an indication to discontinue therapy. The addition of quinidine may increase the plasma digoxin concentration by displacing digoxin from its tissue-binding sites.[18]

Procainamide (Pronestyl)

Procainamide was introduced in 1951 as a result of a systematic study of congeners of procaine.

Pharmacokinetic Properties

Absorption of procainamide is from 75 to 95 percent[19] in most subjects, with maximal plasma concentrations occurring about 60 min after ingestion (Table 89-2). Procainamide is extensively localized in body tissues, but its apparent volume of distribution varies among individual patients and is lower in patients with heart failure. At therapeutic concentrations, 15 percent of the drug is bound to plasma proteins. The biologic half-life is short, 3.5 h, with a range of 2.5 to 4.7 h. Procainamide is partly eliminated by the kidneys and partly acetylated by the liver to *N*-acetyl procainamide, which has antiarrhythmic actions in its own right and is almost entirely excreted by the kidneys. The half-life of this metabolite in patients with normal renal function is 6 to 8 h, and effective plasma levels range from 2 to 22 μg/ml.[20]

Pharmacologic Properties

Electrophysiologic Effects Procainamide has effects similar to quinidine, namely decreasing the amplitude of the MRD of phase 0 of the action potential. Unlike other class I drugs, these effects are independent of the external potassium concentration.[21] The ERP of Purkinje fibers is prolonged more than the duration of the action potential, diastolic threshold is increased, and phase IV depolarization is depressed. In Purkinje fibers with conduction disturbances due to enhanced phase IV depolarization, a biphasic effect of procainamide has been noted;[22] low procainamide concentrations (10 to 30 mg/liter) restored the diastolic membrane potential toward normal and improved conduction, whereas higher concentrations (60 to 120 mg/liter) usually further increased the conduction disturbance and actually enhanced automaticity. In studies on Purkinje fibers perfused with arterial blood from donor dogs in which therapeutic levels of procainamide had been attained, a rapid decrease in Purkinje fiber automaticity was seen, whereas slowing of conduction occurred later, simultaneously with changes in the duration of the QRS complex.[23] Membrane responsiveness was not significantly depressed until toxic plasma concentrations were reached.

Studies in humans have confirmed animal experiments, with minimal prolongation of AV nodal conduction, prolongation of His-Purkinje conduction and the relative refractory period of the His-Purkinje system, and increases in the atrial ERP being observed.[24] The ERP of the AV node was also noted to decrease, possibly through an anticholinergic effect of the drug. With therapeutic levels of procainamide, the QRS complex may be prolonged 5 to 10 percent, but usually remains within the normal range unless prior abnormality was present. The PR and QT intervals are also prolonged.

Hemodynamic and Cardiovascular Effects Procainamide decreases cardiac contractility and causes hypotension via peripheral vasodilation, probably mainly as a result of ganglionic blockade.[12] Cardiac toxicity is manifest by progressive QRS widening, ventricular arrhythmias, or electrical asystole and may be reversed by intravenous molar sodium lactate, while hypotension and impaired conduction may be improved by catecholamine infusion.[25]

Clinical Application and Toxicity

Procainamide is effective against a wide range of ventricular and supraventricular arrhythmias[26] but is probably best avoided in arrhythmias secondary to digitalis toxicity, where intensification of digitalis-related AV block may occur, together with enhancement of reentrant ventricular arrhythmias because of conduction delay. Procainamide may revert atrial fibrillation of recent onset to sinus rhythm, but acceleration of the ventricular response during atrial flutter, similar to quinidine, has been documented.[26]

Severe hypotension and fatalities have been recorded following intravenous procainamide.[27] The rate of intravenous administration should therefore be no greater than 50 mg/min;[19] in one study with administration of 100 mg every 5 min, hypotension and toxicity were not observed.[28] If an arrhythmia fails to revert after a total of 1 g intravenously, an alternative strategy, such as cardioversion, is preferable to the risk of inducing cardiovascular depression.

The short biologic half-life has required that procainamide be administered orally every 3 h if fluctuations greater than 50 percent in plasma concentration are to be avoided.[19] However, sustained-release preparations are now available that allow an 8-h dosage schedule. Oral dosages vary widely, largely because of variable absorption; plasma levels have a good relation to clinical effects. Initial therapy with 50 mg/kg divided into three hourly doses is a reasonable starting regimen, with recourse to estimation of the plasma levels if the desired therapeutic effect is not attained. Concentrations of 4 to 10 μg/ml are now accepted as therapeutic.[25,28] Toxic manifestations are common with levels greater than 12 μg/ml, and usual if levels exceed 16 μg/ml. Although procainamide prolongs the QT interval, in contrast to quinidine, torsade de pointes has only rarely been reported. Gastrointestinal intolerance is common. With prolonged therapy a syndrome resembling systemic lupus erythematosus (SLE) may develop in patients who are slow acetylators of the drug. Fifty to seventy percent of patients can be expected to develop positive antinuclear factor titers or the SLE cell phenomenon within weeks to months of therapy, although only one-third of these will develop a systemic lupus erythematosus-like syndrome. This acquired syndrome does not usually include renal and cerebral involvement, and there is no female predilection.

Disopyramide (Norpace)

The antiarrhythmic activity of disopyramide was described in 1962 by Mokler and Van Arman. The drug was first marketed in France in 1969, and was approved for use in the United States in 1977.

Pharmacokinetic Properties

Absorption is almost complete, with peak serum levels occurring 2 to 3 h after administration (Table 89-2). However, absorption may be lower in patients recovering from myocardial infarction. The major route of elimination is via urinary excretion, with 60 percent of the drug being recovered unchanged within 48 h. The protein binding of disopyramide is concentration-dependent in the therapeutic range, with the free fraction ranging from 0.05 to 0.65 at concentrations between 0.1 and 10 mg/ml.[29] The half-life is 4.5 h after intravenous disopyramide and 7 h after oral administration, with therapeutic plasma levels said to be from 2 to 5 μg/ml.[30]

Pharmacologic Properties

Electrophysiologic Effects Disopyramide's electrophysiologic properties resemble those of quinidine and procainamide so that the amplitude and MRD of phase 0 of the action potential are reduced, and there is a concentration-dependent decrease in the slope of phase IV depolarization.[31] Repolarization is altered so that action potentials with dissimilar durations recorded from the gate region and proximal and distal sites in the Purkinje fibers become equalized. In canine Purkinje fibers surviving experimental myocardial infarction, the duration of the action potential was augmented most in fibers with originally shorter action potentials, resulting in more homogeneous repolarization within the infarcted areas.[32] Studies in humans have shown no significant effect upon AV nodal or His-Purkinje conduction, although shortening of the ERP of the AV node has been noted, possibly as an indirect anticholinergic effect.[33]

Hemodynamic and Cardiovascular Effects In conscious dogs, intravenous disopyramide has been shown to decrease myocardial contractility.[34] In patients, intravenous infusion is generally well tolerated, provided left ventricular function is intact, but has caused profound hypotension in patients with left ventricular dysfunction.[35] With oral dosage the negative inotropic effects of 100 mg of disopyramide and 80 mg of propranolol have been shown to be comparable, although chronic disopyramide therapy (200 mg every 6 h for 1 week) had a greater negative inotropic effect than chronic propranolol therapy (80 mg every 8 h for 1 week).[36]

Clinical Application and Toxicity

Disopyramide appears effective against both ventricular and supraventricular arrhythmias and is useful in maintaining sinus rhythm after conversion from atrial fibrillation.[37] The usual oral dosage is 100 to 200 mg every 6 h. In patients with left ventricular dysfunction, the advisability of disopyramide therapy is a subject of controversy. Certainly, the drug appears contraindicated in patients with severe heart failure, as fatal electromechanical dissociation has resulted.[38] In patients with a past history of heart failure, Podrid and coworkers[39] found a very high recurrence rate following oral treatment and therefore consider the drug disproportionately depressant compared to current alternative agents. However, a recent multicenter study in patients with suspected acute myocardial infarction has failed to demonstrate a comparable effect.[40] Nonetheless, it seems prudent to monitor closely patients with cardiomegaly or a history of previous heart failure if disopyramide is preferred to alternative agents.

Side effects due to the drug's anticholinergic action are common and dose-dependent. Thus, dryness of the mouth, blurred vision, and urinary hesitancy are usually transient complications, although in patients at risk, glaucoma and acute urinary retention may be precipitated. Occasionally, severe hypoglycemia may occur and elderly patients or those with impaired hepatic or renal function may be more susceptible. Delayed repolarization arrhythmias (torsades de pointes) may occur with this drug, as with quinidine and procainamide, usually when marked QT prolongation has occurred.

Lidocaine (Lignocaine)

Lidocaine is a local anesthetic synthesized in 1946 and first used successfully as an antiarrhythmic drug in 1950.

Pharmacokinetic Properties

Lidocaine is 60 percent bound to plasma proteins and metabolized by the liver to monoethylglycine and xylidine, which necessitates parenteral administration (Table 89-2). Because the clearance of lidocaine approaches hepatic blood flow, drugs that reduce blood flow, such as propranolol and norepinephrine, will decrease lidocaine clearance and drugs that increase blood flow, such as isoproterenol, will increase lidocaine clearance.[41] Lidocaine clearance is also increased by phenobarbital, presumably by microsomal enzyme induction. Toxic accumulation of the drug may also occur in patients with severe liver disease. Plasma concentrations of lidocaine after bolus administration reflect a distribution phase and an elimination phase. Studies in monkeys have shown that within half a minute of bolus administration, 70 percent of the drug has left the blood and entered the lung, viscera, and muscle, while less than 1 percent has been metabolized.[42] Thereafter, as plasma levels fall, redistribution from tissues to plasma occurs, and elimination is determined by the hepatic clearance; the drug has a metabolic half-life of approximately 1.5 h (range 1.2 to 2.0 h). The duration of the antiarrhythmic effect following bolus injection approximates that of the distribution phase (10 to 20 min).

Pharmacologic Properties

Electrophysiologic Effects The effects of lidocaine on cardiac tissues vary according to the external potassium concentration. Initial studies performed using Tyrode's solution containing 2.7 to 3.0 meq of potassium per liter suggested that although lidocaine did reduce the MRD in canine Purkinje fibers, the required concentrations were so high as to be unlikely to contribute to the drug's antiarrhythmic action.[43] Subsequent experiments, however, showed that lidocaine at a concentration of 3 mg/liter produced a marked reduction in the MRD of atrial and ventricular potentials in 5.6 mmol KCl, whereas higher concentrations of lidocaine (5 mg/liter) had no effect in 3 mmol KCl.[44] Lidocaine also shortens the action-potential duration (APD) in ventricular muscle and Purkinje tissue, with the ratio of APD/ERP being less than unity. The magnitude of this effect varies with Purkinje fiber location within the specialized conduction system,[45] being greatest in those fibers with the longest action-potential durations situated in the "gate" region. Lidocaine depresses automaticity in Purkinje fibers by decreasing the slope of phase IV depolarization, an effect apparently due to an increase in membrane potassium conductance.[46]

In awake dogs, the administration of lidocaine produced no change in spontaneous heart rate or atrioventricular conduction time, although the conduction time in Purkinje tissue and the total ventricular activation time were slightly prolonged.[47] In dogs with heart block, a dose-dependent marked decrease in the ventricular escape rate was observed.

Therapeutic doses of lidocaine in patients with normal AV conduction produce minimal effects on heart rate and atrioventricular and intraventricular conduction,[48] with no consistent effect on the ERP of the atria or the AV node. However, significant shortening of the ERP of the AV node does occur in some individuals, and probably explains the acceleration of ventricular rate documented in some patients given lidocaine for atrial flutter.[49] Shortening of the ERP and relative refractory period of the His-Purkinje system has also been noted.[50] In contrast, in patients with impaired atrioventricular conduction, lidocaine has precipitated complete heart block[51] usually localized to the His-Purkinje system rather than the AV node. Similarly, in patients with sinus node dysfunction, sinus arrest has occurred following intravenous administration of the drug.[52] Lidocaine has no significant effect upon the QT interval.

Hemodynamic and Cardiovascular Effects Therapeutic doses of lidocaine cause little hemodynamic effect, although transient depression of myocardial function has been noted in patients with heart disease.[53] Animal studies suggest it is a mild cardiac depressant.

Clinical Application and Toxicity

The effectiveness of lidocaine, together with its rapid metabolism and limited toxicity, has resulted in its general use for the emergency treatment of ventricular arrhythmias complicating myocardial infarction and cardiac surgery. It also appears to be effective in controlling ventricular arrhythmias secondary to digitalis intoxication. It is less effective against atrial arrhythmias and should be avoided in atrial flutter, where enhancement of AV node conduction and slowing of the flutter rate may result in 1:1 AV conduction.

Therapeutic plasma levels are from 1.5 to 5 μg/ml. In patients with normal hepatic blood flow and function, plasma clearance is about 10 ml/kg/min.[20] As drug plasma concentration at a steady-state level equals the infusion rate divided by the plasma clearance, infusion rates of 15 to 50 μg/kg/min are appropriate. Toxic effects may occur if the infusion rate exceeds 50 μg/kg/min and blood levels exceed 5 μg/ml[54] although the levels associated with serious toxicity are usually around 9 to 10 μg/ml. In patients with heart failure, the volume of distribution is lower and hepatic clearance reduced, so that lower dosages should be used and serum levels carefully followed during maintenance infusion therapy. There also appears to be a progressive reduction in clearance with prolonged infusion, with the expected half-life of 100 min being prolonged up to 4 h in some patients receiving lidocaine after uncomplicated myocardial infarction.[55] The mechanism is unclear, but titration of the infusion rate to the antiarrhythmic effect rather than maintenance of constant rates seems prudent.

Although the common clinical practice is to administer a bolus injection of lidocaine, a single loading dose is unsatisfactory because the volume of distribution of lidocaine at equilibrium exceeds the initial volume of distribution by a factor of 3. This disadvantage may be avoided by giving either a series of smaller loading doses at approximately 8-min intervals (the half-life of the distribution phase) or a more rapid infusion (e.g., 120 μg/kg/min) for a short time preceding the standard maintenance infusion.[20] The maximum permissible loading dosage is not clearly established, although in one study up to 375 mg was given over an extended period of 30 min by intermittent bolus injection.[56] Certainly, the usual clinical dose is considerably less, of the order of 1 to 2 mg/kg. With overdosage, central nervous system symptoms occur, including drowsiness, disorientation, hearing loss, paresthesia, and convulsions.[25] Rarely, hypotension, sinus arrest, and death have been reported.

Diphenylhydantoin

Diphenylhydantoin was introduced as a treatment for convulsive disorders in 1938 and advocated for the treatment of acute ventricular arrhythmias in 1950.

Pharmacokinetic Properties

Absorption of diphenylhydantoin may be variable, but is usually almost complete (Table 89-2). It is 70 to 95 percent bound to plasma proteins, mainly albumin, and less than 5 percent is excreted unchanged in the urine. Most of the drug is parahydroxylated in the liver to an inactive metabolite and excreted as a glucuronic acid conjugate. The plasma half-life is approximately 24 h, but may vary enormously,[57] partly because the relationship of serum level to dose in any given patient is nonlinear. Effective plasma levels are between 10 and 20 μg/ml, with toxic effects usually seen at levels greater than 25 μg/ml. Toxic accumulation of the drug may occur in patients with severe hepatic disease. Drug interactions may occur with the warfarin anticoagulants and isonicotinic acid hydrazide when administered with para-aminosalicylic acid, both of which decrease diphenylhydantoin's metabolism, and with quinidine sulfate, whose half-life may be shortened by 50 percent.

Pharmacologic Properties

Electrophysiologic Effects The electrophysiologic effects of diphenylhydantoin depend upon the extracellular potassium concentration, the drug concentration, and state of the cardiac fiber being tested. Thus, experimentally, with low potassium (3.0 mg/liter) and drug (1 μg/ml) concentrations, no depressant effect upon ordinary atrial fibers has been noted,[58] whereas depression of membrane depolarization does occur with higher potassium and drug concentrations. In atrial fibers depressed by ouabain, enhancement of the rate of rise of phase 0 of the action potential is seen, and ouabain-induced sinoatrial block may be relieved.

In normal Purkinje fibers, diphenylhydantoin appears to have little or no effect upon the rate of the rise of the action potential or the size of the overshoot potential.[59] Repolarization in Purkinje fibers is accelerated. The slope of phase IV depolarization is moderately decreased but automaticity seldom abolished.

Studies in intact, awake dogs[60] have shown some shortening of the AV conduction time, although in cardiac denervated dogs, AV conduction time was prolonged by diphenylhydantoin, suggesting a direct depressant effect. Studies in humans have shown diphenylhydantoin to have no consistent effect on His-Purkinje or AV nodal conduction times.[61] Effects on the ECG include slight reduction of the PR interval and significant shortening of the QT interval.

Hemodynamic and Cardiovascular Effects Diphenylhydantoin appears well tolerated, although a slight fall in systolic blood pressure is usually seen with slow intravenous administration. With rapid administration cardiovascular collapse and death may occur.

Clinical Application and Toxicity

Diphenylhydantoin is a second-line drug rarely used alone. It is effective in controlling arrhythmias consequent to digoxin toxicity[62] and this is its main current use. It is reported to be variably effective against ventricular arrhythmias unrelated to digoxin toxicity.[63] Atrial arrhythmias respond rather poorly, and it is uniformly unsuccessful in reverting atrial flutter or fibrillation to sinus rhythm. Contraindications to its use include severe bradycardia and high-grade AV block.

The recommended intravenous dosage is 100 mg given every 5 min until the desired therapeutic effect occurs, or a total of 1000 mg has been given, or signs of toxicity (nystagmus) supervene.[64] If oral loading is desired, a reasonably rapid effect (24 h) may be achieved by administering 100 mg on day 1, 500 mg on days 2 and 3, and thereafter maintenance doses of 300 to 500 mg daily. Acute oral overdose produces central nervous system toxicity, predominantly referable to the cerebellum and vestibular system (nystagmus, ataxia, diplopia, and vertigo), although numerous other effects, including macrocytic anemia, systemic lupus erythematosus, and pseudolymphoma, are well documented with long-term therapy.

Class II Drugs: Beta-Adrenergic Receptor Antagonists

Propranolol

The synthesis in 1957 of dichloroisoproterenol, followed by pronethalol in 1962 and propranolol in 1964, drugs capable of blocking beta adrenoreceptors, finally vindicated Alquist's concept of two types of adrenergic receptors, alpha and beta.[65] Although many newer agents have been developed, including some with partial selectivity for cardiac beta receptors and/or partial agonist activity, propranolol, a nonselective beta blocker will be discussed as the index drug for the group. For more extensive discussion of beta-adrenergic receptor antagonists see Chap. 90.

Pharmacokinetic Properties

Propranolol (see Table 89-2) is well absorbed from the alimentary tract, but the systemic availability of an oral dose may be less than 30 percent because of high-affinity binding by the liver and subsequent metabolism before the drug enters the systemic circulation (first pass effect).[66] This results in a high degree of variability in plasma concentration of propranolol, so that a sevenfold range in plasma concentration has been documented in patients taking a single 80-mg dose.[67] Peak levels occur 1 to 2 h after oral administration, and the drug is 90 to 96 percent protein-bound. The half-life is 2 to 4 h, although with chronic oral administration this increases to 4 to 6 h because of some saturation of the excretion pathway. Therapeutic plasma levels range from 40 to 100 ng/ml.

Pharmacologic Properties

Electrophysiologic Effects The only electrophysiologic effect of propranolol in concentrations that inhibit cardiac beta adrenoreceptors is a reduction in the slope of the pacemaker potential of the sinus node, especially when this has been increased by catecholamines.[68] A second property of propranolol, completely unrelated to beta-adrenergic blockade, is a local anesthetic action, characterized by reduction in the MRD of the action potential and reduction in the overshoot potential. These changes are best explained by inhibition of the depolarizing inward sodium current, and considerable controversy has arisen over their relevance to the clinical antiarrhythmic effectiveness of propranolol and similar drugs. However, present evidence favors beta-adrenergic blockade as the mechanism of propranolol's antiarrhythmic actions when used in clinically realistic dosages. Arrhythmias have been shown to be suppressed by plasma propranolol concentrations one-fiftieth to one-hundredth of the level necessary to achieve membrane-depressant effects in isolated cardiac muscle while the dextro (+) isomer of propranolol, which has little beta-adrenergic blocking activity, is a weak antiarrhythmic drug even when patients receive five to ten times the effective dose of racemic (±) propranolol. In humans, intravenous propranolol given at a dosage of 0.1 mg/kg slowed the sinus rate, increased the AH interval, and prolonged both the functional and effective refractory periods of the AV node.[69] No significant effects were noted on conduction or refractoriness of the normal ventricular specialized conducting system. On the ECG the corrected QT interval is slightly shortened.

Hemodynamic and Cardiovascular Effects Propranolol decreases heart rate and stroke index in both normal subjects and patients with heart disease, some of whom have shown a significant rise in the left ventricular end-diastolic pressure[70] and indexes of myocardial contractility are also reduced. Blood flow to all tissues except the brain is reduced, and peripheral resistance is increased, probably as a reflex adjustment.

Clinical Application and Toxicity

Propranolol has proved more useful in treating supraventricular than ventricular arrhythmias. It slows the ventricular response in atrial fibrillation, particularly when combined with digoxin, and it often terminates acute reentrant supraventricular tachycardia when given intravenously. It may suppress ventricular premature beats and ventricular tachycardia and is particularly indicated for exercise-induced arrhythmias. Propranolol has been recommended for treating some digitalis intoxication arrhythmias, but diphenylhydantoin or lidocaine is preferable if partial AV block is present.

Propranolol may be given as an intravenous bolus at a dosage of 0.1 mg/kg with the injection rate not exceeding 1 mg/min. In patients with impaired left ventricular function, the drug should be given more slowly and atropine and isoproterenol should be available to treat AV block or excessive sinus bradycardia should they occur. The oral dosage of propranolol may range from 40 to 400 mg or more daily, in part due to the variable systemic availability. Side effects mainly relate to unwanted aspects of beta blockade. Heart failure may be precipitated but is reportedly uncommon.[71] Other side effects include excessive bradycardia, bronchoconstriction, hypoglycemia, and disturbed sleep. In patients with intermittent claudication or Raynaud's phenomenon, worsening of symptoms may occur, but sudden withdrawal in patients with ischemic heart disease has (rarely) led to increasing angina and acute myocardial infarction.

Class III Drugs

Bretylium

Bretylium, originally introduced as a hypotensive agent in 1959, was subsequently found to have antiarrhythmic properties.

Pharmacokinetic Properties

Oral absorption is unreliable, and the drug is usually given intramuscularly or intravenously. It is excreted without metabolic alteration, and the average half-life is 9.8 h (range 4 to 17 h). Therapeutic levels are stated to be 0.5 to 1 mg/liter.

Pharmacologic Properties

Electrophysiologic Effects Bretylium differs from most antiarrhythmic agents in that it fails to depress automaticity significantly. Although increased Purkinje fiber automaticity has been noted in normal dogs, this is most likely due to the release of catecholamines into the perfusing fluid from postganglionic sympathetic nerve endings, and is not seen in reserpine-pretreated animals. Bretylium does not appear to have class I effects. Further, the membrane response curve was not shifted in one group of experiments except at the highest concentration of bretylium studied (4.8×10^{-5} mol).[72] Bretylium does, however, exhibit a class III effect: it prolongs the action potential duration and ERP of canine Purkinje fibers in both normal and reserpine-pretreated dogs, which suggests that this is a direct effect. Bretylium also has marked antisympathetic actions, which include initial release of norepinephrine from adrenergic nerve endings with blockade of uptake of norepinephrine and epinephrine back into the nerve terminals and decreased release of norepinephrine by subsequent sympathetic nerve activity. Bretylium appears to have an important antifibrillatory action.[73] Dogs pretreated with bretylium are substantially protected against electrically induced ventricular fibrillation, and spontaneous defibrillation after drug administration has been observed.

Hemodynamic and Cardiovascular Effects Bretylium is said to increase contractility acutely and thus have a positive inotropic effect. However, this action is absent in animals treated with reserpine and can be abolished by beta-adrenergic receptor blockade with propranolol.[74] Given acutely in patients, bretylium may cause an initial rise in blood pressure accompanied by tachycardia, with later hypotension and bradycardia.[75]

Clinical Application and Toxicity

Preliminary reports of the use of bretylium in refractory ventricular tachycardia and ventricular fibrillation are encouraging.[75,76] There is some uncertainty as to the optimal dose and treatment intervals, although parenteral doses of 5 to 10 mg/kg given every 6 to 8 h have been most commonly used. Toxicity to date appears largely restricted to postural hypotension. Potentiation of concomitant catecholamine infusions can occur, and parotid pain has been reported in patients with chronic oral therapy.[75]

Class IV Drugs

Verapamil

Verapamil (see Chap. 91) is derived from papaverine and was first introduced as a smooth-muscle relaxant with peripheral and coronary vasodilator properties. Subsequently, it was found to also have antiarrhythmic effects.[77]

Pharmacokinetic Properties

Although gastrointestinal absorption is almost complete, systemic availability is low, being only 10 to 22 percent, suggesting substantial first pass metabolism in the liver (Table 89-2). Following both oral and intravenous administration, there is a biexponential decline in plasma levels with an initial rapid distribution phase lasting 18 to 35 min and a slower elimination phase lasting 3 to 7 h. The drug is 90 percent protein-bound, and up to 70 percent of an oral or intravenous dose is excreted via the kidneys.

Pharmacologic Properties

Electrophysiologic Effects Verapamil is thought to exert its antiarrhythmic effect by depressing the slow response.[78] It principally acts on the superficially located membrane storage sites for calcium and does not modify calcium uptake or binding or affect calcium-activated ATPase. Studies in humans show that verapamil exerts a selective effect upon conduction through the AV node, prolonging the AH interval, an effect only partly reversible with atropine.[79] In patients with paroxysmal supraventricular tachycardia, both intravenous and oral verapamil prolong the anterograde effective and functional refractory periods of the AV node.[80]

Hemodynamic and Cardiovascular Effects In patients with good left ventricular function, the negative inotropic action of intravenous verapamil is largely offset by the concomitant reduction of afterload via peripheral dilatation, so that the cardiac index remains unchanged. In patients with coronary artery disease or rheumatic valvular disease, a modest, transient fall in left ventricular *dP/dt* max was observed after intravenous injection.[81] Relatively few data are available for severely compromised patients. However, symptomatic deterioration following intravenous verapamil has been reported in three patients whose ventricular fractions were less than 0.35 and left ventricular end-diastolic pressures greater than 20 mmHg, suggesting the need for caution in such circumstances.[77] Verapamil is also a powerful coronary vasodilator.

Clinical Application and Toxicity

Verapamil appears to have a narrow antiarrhythmic spectrum. Given intravenously, it reliably terminates paroxysmal atrial tachycardia on the basis of reentry within the AV node or orthodromic reciprocating tachycardia (in which activation proceeds over the AV-node–His-bundle and returns via an accessory pathway). The ventricular response in atrial fibrillation and flutter is slowed.[82] In the WPW syndrome, verapamil has been reported to accelerate the ventricular response during atrial fibrillation in some patients.[83] Electrophysiologic testing prior to its use in such patients has therefore been recommended. Verapamil is usually ineffective against ventricular tachycardia. The usual intravenous dose is 10 mg (or 0.145 mg per kilogram of body weight) given over 15 to 60 s, which may be safely repeated after 30 min. Oral dosages are considerably higher because of the low systemic availability and range from 120 to 720 mg daily. When combined with beta-adrenergic antagonists, verapamil produces significant negative inotropic and chronotropic effects,[84] and such combination therapy is unwise in patients with impaired left ventricular function. Serious side effects are uncommon, but severe hypotension, bradycardia, and asystole have been reported following intravenous use, especially when the patient was receiving concurrent beta-adrenergic blocking drugs.[85] Calcium gluconate should always therefore be on hand when administering verapamil intravenously, as its prompt injection may ameliorate such severe reactions.

Newer Antiarrhythmic Drugs

Tocainide

Tocainide is a class I antiarrhythmic drug chemically similar to lidocaine but effective when given orally.[86]

Pharmacokinetic Properties

The drug is well absorbed and peak plasma levels are reached 30 min to 4 h after oral administration, with bioavailability approaching 100 percent. In contrast to lidocaine, 30 to 50 percent is excreted unchanged in the urine, with a further 25 percent excreted as a glucuronide conjugate. Plasma protein binding is similar to lidocaine (50 percent) and the elimination half-life is 12 to 15 h. Therapeutic levels range from 3.5 to 7.0 μg/ml with toxicity observed when levels are 10 to 15 μg/ml.

Pharmacologic Properties

Electrophysiologic Effects Intravenous tocainide has no important effects on atrioventricular or intraventricular conduction, with minor decreases occurring in the ERP of the atrium, AV node, and right ventricle.[87] The QTc is slightly decreased.

Hemodynamic and Cardiovascular Effects In humans tocainide appears to have little hemodynamic effect, with intravenous infusion of 7.5 to 11.3 mg/kg over 15 min causing transient slight increases in blood pressure and systemic vascular resistence.[88]

Clinical Application and Toxicity

Tocainide is effective for treating ventricular premature beats and ventricular tachycardia and may be particularly indicated when there has been demonstrated responsiveness to intravenous lidocaine or there is associated QT prolongation.[89] Oral dosage is 400 mg every 8 h, increasing to a maximum of 800 mg every 8 h. Side effects are common, comprising nausea and vomiting, and neurologic effects including tremor, light-headedness, paresthesia, and ataxia. Hepatitis and a lupus-like syndrome have been reported.

Mexiletine

Mexiletine is a class I antiarrhythmic agent structurally similar to lidocaine and tocainide.[90] It is a potent local anesthetic.

Pharmacokinetic Properties

Mexiletine is well absorbed with a systemic bioavailability of approximately 90 percent. Peak plasma concentrations occur within 2 to 4 h of ingestion, and the drug is approximately 70 percent plasma protein-bound. The metabolism of mexiletine is not fully understood, but appears principally hepatic, with only 10 percent of the drug being excreted unchanged in the urine. The plasma half-life after chronic oral administration is about 12 h but may be prolonged when hepatic blood flow is reduced (e.g., a half-life of 16 h in patients with acute myocardial infarction). Therapeutic levels are 0.75 to 2 μg/ml and side effects are likely when levels exceed 2 μg/ml.[90]

Pharmacologic Properties

Electrophysiologic Effects The overall effects are very similar to lidocaine, with reduction of the MRD of the action potential with little effect on resting membrane potential or sinus node automaticity, and a concentration-dependent reduction of action potential duration. In contrast to patients with normal sinus node function who show little change in resting heart rate or recovery times after overdrive pacing, patients with the sick sinus syndrome may develop severe bradycardia and abnormally prolonged recovery times.

Both increased and unchanged AV nodal and HV conduction times have been reported after drug administration and further studies are indicated to resolve these inconsistencies.

Hemodynamic and Cardiovascular Effects In patients with coronary artery disease 1.5 mg/kg of mexiletine intravenously caused a small increase in resting heart rate and left ventricular end-diastolic pressure without change in stroke volume.[90] Limited data suggest a dose-related depression of myocardial contractility in patients with preexisting ventricular impairment.

Clinical Application and Toxicity

Mexiletine appears to be effective in reducing ventricular premature beats after myocardial infarction, but variable success has been reported with ventricular tachycardia.[91,91a] Several cardiovascular drug interactions are described,[91b] including potentiation of antiarrhythmic efficacy with quinidine and beta-adrenergic blocking drugs. The usual oral dosage is 200 to 300 mg every 8 h.

Side effects occurred commonly in two long-term studies[91,92] and are principally neurologic and cardiovascular. The former include tremor, blurred vision, ataxia, drowsiness, and a toxic confusional state, and the latter hypotension, sinus bradycardia, widening of the QRS complex, and AV dissociation. Like tocainide, mexiletine is still undergoing evaluation, and its final role in the treatment of ventricular tachycardia is yet to be defined.

Amiodarone

Amiodarone is a benzofuran derivative developed in 1962 as an antianginal agent, but subsequently recognized to have important antiarrhythmic properties. Oral antiarrhythmic efficacy in humans was first reported in 1974.

Pharmacokinetic Properties

Knowledge of the pharmacokinetic actions of amiodarone is still incomplete despite its use for over a decade. In healthy volunteers oral absorption after a single dose is protracted up to 15 h (mean 6 h) with a low mean bioavailability of 35 percent. Amiodarone has an extended biphasic terminal elimination half-life which is much longer in patients on chronic therapy than after single-dose studies in volunteers (mean values of 53 and 25 days, respectively),[93] possibly due to time-dependent pharmacokinetics. Renal elimination is negligible and the principal metabolite is desethyl amiodarone, which, like amiodarone, may be assayed by high-pressure liquid chromatography. Drug concentrations of both compounds generally parallel dosage, but optimal plasma levels remain to be defined.

Pharmacologic Properties

Electrophysiologic Effects Amiodarone is not soluble in physiologic media, but intracellular recordings have been obtained in rabbits after long-term intraperitoneal administration of the drug.[94] These have shown no effect on the MRD, action potential amplitude, or resting membrane potential. A marked time-related increase in action potential duration occurred, however, such that the 90 percent repolarization time increased by 11 percent and 30 percent after 1 and 6 weeks' treatment, respectively. These repolarization effects were largely prevented by concomitant administraton of small doses of triiodothyronine (T_3). It seems possible, therefore, that the fundamental action of amiodarone is due to partially selective inhibition of the effects of T_3 on the myocardium,[94] a hypothesis that awaits testing.

Studies in humans are complicated by the fact that intravenous and oral amiodarone have disparate electrophysiologic effects.[95] After a single bolus injection only prolongation of the AH interval and the ERP of the AV node is observed with no significant prolongation of the QTc interval. In contrast, following sustained oral administration there is slowing of the heart rate, and prolongation of the HV interval, the ERP of atria, AV node and right ventricle, and the QTc interval. This latter effect is due to prolongation of the ventricular action potential duration. The cause of such disparity between acute and chronic effects is not yet explained, but is not due to differing myocardial drug concentrations.[94] Possibly, modification of the peripheral effects of T_3 is time-dependent and/or slowly formed active metabolites may be important. Furthermore, the basis of the acute effect on the AV node is unclear and possibly blockade of the slow channel is important.[94]

Hemodynamic and Cardiovascular Effects Amiodarone is a coronary and systemic vasodilator and appears to exhibit a moderate noncompetitive alpha and beta catecholamine receptor antagonism. In patients with normal ventricular function amiodarone appears well-tolerated. In patients with depressed left ventricular function, a transient mild negative inotropic effect was noted after intravenous administration,[96] although profound hypotension requiring inotropic support occurred in two patients with overt heart failure preinfusion. Data concerning the effects of chronic oral therapy are scanty, but it is alleged that aggravation of existing heart failure is uncommon.[96]

Clinical Application and Toxicity

Amiodarone is effective for both atrial and ventricular arrhythmias. Open trials have also shown it to be effective in patients resuscitated from sudden death or with otherwise refractory ventricular tachycardia.[97,98] Unfortunately, long-term use is associated with a very high incidence of side effects,[97,99] the most serious being pulmonary alveolitis, and proarrhythmic effects related to QT prolongation. So-called minor side effects, which may be disabling in individual patients, are at least partly dose-related and include photosensitivity, which may culminate in blue skin discoloration, nausea, hair loss, nightmares and insomnia, and corneal microdeposits. Asymptomatic transaminase elevation is common but clinical hepatitis rare, while similarly, clinically evident hyper- or hypothyroidism is uncommon despite frequently abnormal thyroid function tests. Neurologic side effects include tremor, paresthesia, and ataxia. The latter is occasionally disabling and requires cessation of treatment. Pulmonary toxicity has been observed in up to 7 percent of patients on long-term treatment,[99] and while usually responsive to drug withdrawal and corticosteroids if indicated, may be fatal.[100] Polymorphous ventricular tachycardia may occur[101] and isolated cases of sinus arrest have been reported.[102]

The relatively high incidence of pulmonary toxicity in the comparatively brief American experience compared with its virtual absence in the longer European exposure has prompted questions regarding the wisdom of high loading and maintenance doses of amiodarone.[103] While this problem cannot be said to be resolved, it would appear prudent to use moderate doses where clinical circumstances permit, of the suggested order of 800 to 1200 mg daily for 10 days, followed by 400 to 600 mg for 10 days, and subsequent reduction to 200 to 400 mg daily. Fully rational therapy awaits a more detailed understanding of the pharmacokinetics of amiodarone during the loading phase[104] and wider experience of the utility of serial estimations of plasma levels.

Two other aspects of amiodarone treatment deserve mention. The first concerns the frequency of drug interactions.[105] Amiodarone potentiates the anticoagulant effect of warfarin, which may occur after a few days or be delayed several weeks, and substantially elevates the serum digoxin level. Both mechanisms are unclear. Similarly, serum levels of quinidine and procainamide are enhanced: dosage reduction of all these drugs by one-third, or for digoxin by one-half, has therefore been recommended[105] when given concurrently with amiodarone.

The second aspect involves the latency in drug effectiveness: it is generally accepted that a variable period of 10 days to 3 weeks must elapse before a substantial drug effect is achieved. While the duration of this vulnerable period is partially dependent on the magnitude of the loading dose, there is an irreducible minimum of about 7 to 10 days, regardless of dosage protocol or rate of administration. Patients at risk of sudden death should therefore be monitored closely during this initial period, and a second antiarrhythmic drug such as procainamide may be temporarily added, recognizing that additive QT prolongation may enhance the risk of proarrhythmic effects.

In conclusion, amiodarone is undoubtedly a particularly valuable antiarrhythmic drug because of its broad spectrum, efficacy, and minimal negative inotropic effect. Indiscriminate usage, however, is inadvisable because of its toxicity during long-term administration. Continuing evaluation may permit the identification of patients at increased risk of serious toxic reactions. For the present, treatment is best restricted to patients with life-threatening arrhythmias or who prove refractory to conventional therapy.

References

1. Hemingway, E.: "Across the River and into the Trees," Penguin Books Ltd., England, 1966, p. 109.
2. Gettes, L. S.: On the Classification of Antiarrhythmic Drugs, *Mod. Concepts Cardiovasc. Dis.*, 48:13, 1979.
3. Vaughan Williams, E. M.: Classification of Antidysrhythmic Drugs, *Pharm. Ther.*, 1:115, 1975.
4. Singh, B. N., and Vaughan Williams, E. M.: A Fourth Class of Antiarrhythmic Action? Effect of Verapamil on Oubain Toxicity, on Atrial and Ventricular Intracellular Potentials and on Other Features of Cardiac Function, *Cardiovasc. Res.*, 6:109, 1972.
5. Hauswirth, O., and Singh, B. N.: Ionic Mechanisms in Heart Muscle in Relation to Genesis and the Pharmacological Control of Arrhythmias, *Pharmacol. Rev.*, 30:5, 1978.
6. Greenblatt, D. J., Pfeifer, H. J., Ochs, H. R., Franke, K., MacLaughlin, D. S., Smith, T. W., and Koch-Weser, J.: Pharmacokinetics of Quinidine after Intravenous, Intramuscular, and Oral Administration, *J. Pharmacol. Exp. Ther.*, 202:365, 1977.
7. Kessler, K.M., Lowenthal, D. T., Warner, H., Gibson, T., Briggs, W., and Reidenberg, M. M.: Quinidine Elimination in Patients with Congestive Heart Failure or Poor Renal Function, *N. Engl. J. Med.*, 290:706, 1974.
8. Prinzmetal, M., Ishikawa, K., Oishi, H., Ozkan, E., Wakayama, J., and Baines, J. M.: Effects of Quinidine on Electrical Behaviour in Cardiac Muscle, *J. Pharmacol. Exp. Ther.*, 157:659, 1967.
9. Johnson, E. A., and McKinnon, M. G.: Differential Effect of Quinidine and Pyrilamine on the Myocardial Action Potential at Various Rates of Stimulation, *J. Pharmacol. Exp. Ther.*, 120:460, 1957.
10. Wallace, A. G., Cline, R. E., Sealy, W. C., Young, W. G., and Troyer, W. G.: Electrophysiologic Effects of Quinidine. Studies Using Chronically Implanted Electrodes in Awake Dogs with and without Cardiac Denervation, *Circ. Res.*, 19:960, 1966.
11. Josephson, M. E., Seides, S. F., Batsford, W. P., Weisfogel, G. M., Akhtar, M., Caracta, A. R., Lau, S. H., and Damato, A. N.: The Electrophysiologic Effects of Intramuscular Quinidine on the Atrioventricular Conducting System in Man, *Am. Heart J.*, 87:55, 1974.
12. Hoffman, B. F., Rosen, M. R., and Wit, A. L.: Electrophysiology and Pharmacology of Cardiac Arrhythmias. VII. Cardiac Effects of Quinidine and Procainamide, B, *Am. Heart J.*, 90:117, 1975.
13. Conrad, K. A., Molk, B. L., and Chidsey, C. A.: Pharmacokinetic Studies of Quinidine in Patients with Arrhythmias, *Circulation*, 55:1, 1977.
14. Ueda, C. T., Hirschfield, D. S., Scheinmann, M. M., Rowland, M., Williamson, B. J., and Dzindzio, B. S.: Disposition Kinetics of Quinidine, *Clin. Pharmacol. Ther.*, 19:30, 1976.
15. Cohen, I. S., Hershel, J., and Cohen, S. I.: Adverse Reactions to Quinidine in Hospitalized Patients: Findings Based on Data from the Boston Collaborative Drug Surveillance Program, *Prog. Cardiovasc. Dis.*, 20:151, 1977.
16. Selzer, A., and Wray, H. W.: Quinidine Syncope, *Circulation*, 30:17, 1964.
17. Smith, W. M., and Gallagher, J. J.: Les Torsades de Pointes, *Ann. Intern. Med.*, 93:578, 1980.
18. Hager, W. D., Fenster, P., Mayersohn, M., Perrier, D., Graves, P., Marcus, F. I., and Goldman, S.: Digoxin-Quinidine Interaction Pharmacokinetic Evaluation, *N. Engl. J. Med.*, 300:1238, 1979.
19. Koch-Weser, J., and Klein, S. W.: Procainamide Dosage Schedules, Plasma Concentrations and Clinical Effects, *JAMA*, 215:1454, 1971.
20. Woosley, R. L., and Shand, D. G.: Pharmacokinetics of Antiarrhythmic Drugs, *Am. J. Cardiol.*, 41:986, 1978.
21. Rosen, M., Gelband, H., Merker, C., and Hoffman, B.: Effects of Procainamide on Electrophysiologic Properties of the Canine Ventricular Conducting System, *J. Pharmacol. Exp. Ther.*, 185:438, 1973.
22. Singer, D. H., Strauss, H. C., and Hoffman, B. F.: Biphasic Effects of Procainamide on Cardiac Conduction, *Bull. N.Y. Acad. Med.*, 43:1194, 1967.
23. Rosen, M. R., Gelband, H., and Hoffman, B. F.: Canine Electrocardiographic and Cardiac Electrophysiologic Changes Induced by Procainamide, *Circulation*, 46:528, 1972.
24. Josephson, M. E., Caracta, A. R., Ricauti, M. A., Lau, S. H., and Damato, A. N.: Electrophysiologic Properties of Procainamide in Man, *Am. J. Cardiol.*, 33:596, 1974.
25. Bigger, J. T., Jr., and Heissenbuttel, R. H.: The Use of Procainamide and Lidocaine in the Treatment of Cardiac Arrhythmias, *Prog. Cardiovasc. Dis.*, 11:515, 1969.
26. Kayden, H. J., Brodie, B. B., and Steele, J. M.: Procainamide—A Review, *Circulation*, 115:118, 1957.
27. Stearns, N. S., Callahan, E. J., and Ellis, L. B.: Value and Hazards of Intravenous Procainamide ("Pronestyl") Therapy, *JAMA*, 148:360, 1952.
28. Giardina, E. G. V., Heissenbuttel, R. H., and Bigger, J. T., Jr.: Intermittent Intravenous Procainamide to Treat Ventricular Arrhythmias, *Ann. Intern. Med.*, 78:183, 1973.
29. Harrison, D. C., Meffin, P. J., and Winkle, R. A.: Clinical Pharmacokinetics of Antiarrhythmic Drugs, *Prog. Cardiovasc. Dis.*, 20:217, 1977.
30. Koch-Weser, J.: Drug therapy. Disopyramide, *N. Engl. J. Med.*, 300:957, 1979.
31. Kus, T., and Sasyniuk, B. I.: Electrophysiological Actions of Disopyramide Phosphate on Canine Ventricular Muscle and Purkinje Fibers, *Circ. Res.*, 37:844, 1975.
32. Sasyniuk, B. I., and Kus, T.: Cellular Electrophysiologic Changes Induced by Disopyramide Phosphate in Normal and Infarcted Hearts, *J. Intern. Med. Res.*, 4(I):20, 1976.
33. Josephson, M. E., Caracta, A. R., Lau, S. H., Gallagher, J. J., and Damato, A. N.: Electrophysiological Evaluation of Disopyramide in Man, *Am. Heart J.*, 86:721, 1973.
34. Walsh, R. A., O'Rourke, R. A., Ludden, T., and Horwitz, L .D.: Adverse Hemodynamic Effects of Intravenous Disopyramide Compared to Quinidine in Conscious Dogs, *Am. J. Cardiol.*, 43:358, 1979 (Abstract).
35. Leach, A. J., Brown, J. E., and Armstrong, P. W.: Cardiac Depression by Intravenous Disopyramide in Patients with Left Ventricular Dysfunction, *Am. J. Med.*, 68:839, 1980.
36. Cathcart-Rake, W. F., Coker, J. E., Atkins, F. L., Huffman, D. H., Hassanein, K. M., Shen, D. D., and Azarnoff, D. L.: The Effect of Concurrent Oral Administration of Propranolol and Disopyramide on Cardiac Function in Healthy Man, *Circulation*, 61:938, 1980.
37. Morady, F., Scheinman, M. M., and Desai, J.: Diagnosis and Treatment. Drugs Five Years Later. Disopyramide, *Ann. Intern. Med.*, 96:337, 1982.
38. Desai, J., Hirschfeld, D., Peters, R., Scheinmann, M., and Gonzalez, R.: Electromechanical Dissociation Associated with

Disopyramide, *Circulation,* 58(suppl. II):II–178, 1978 (Abstract).
39. Podrid, P. J., Schoeneberger, A., and Lown, B.: Congestive Heart Failure Caused by Oral Disopyramide, *N. Engl. J. Med.,* 302:614, 1980.
40. U. K. Rhythmodan Multicentre Study Group. Oral Disopyramide after Admission to Hospital with Suspected Acute Myocardial Infarction, *Postgrad. Med. J.,* 60:98, 1984.
41. Branch, R. A., Shand, D. G., Wilkinson, G. R., and Nies, A. S.: The Reduction of Lidocaine Clearance by DL-Propranolol—An Example of a Hemodynamic Drug Interaction, *J. Pharmacol. Exp. Ther.,* 184:515, 1973.
42. Benowitz, N., Forsyth, R. P., Melmon, K. L., and Rowland, M.: Lidocaine Disposition Kinetics in Monkey and Man. I. Prediction by a Perfusion Model, *Clin. Pharmacol. Ther.,* 16:87, 1974.
43. Davis, L. D., and Temte, J. V.: Electrophysiological Actions of Lidocaine on Canine Ventricular Muscle and Purkinje Fibers, *Circ. Res.,* 24:639, 1969.
44. Singh, B. N., and Vaughan Williams, E. M.: Effect of Altering Potassium Concentration on the Action of Lidocaine and Diphenylhydantoin on Rabbit Atrial and Ventricular Muscle, *Circ. Res.,* 29:286, 1971.
45. Wittig, J., Harrison, L. A., and Wallace, A. G.: Electrophysiological Effects of Lidocaine on Distal Purkinje Fibers of the Canine Heart, *Am. Heart J.,* 86:69, 1973.
46. Weld, F. M., and Bigger, J. T., Jr.: The Effect of Lidocaine on Diastolic Transmembrane Currents Determining Pacemaker Depolarization in Cardiac Purkinje Fibers, *Circ. Res.,* 38:203, 1976.
47. Sugimoto, T., Schaal, S. F., Dunn, N. M., and Wallace, A. G.: Electrophysiologic Effects of Lidocaine in Awake Dogs, *J. Pharmacol. Exp. Ther.,* 166:146, 1969.
48. Rosen, K. M., Lau, S. H., Weiss, M. B., and Damato, A. N.: The Effect of Lidocaine on Atrioventricular and Intraventricular Conduction in Man, *Am. J. Cardiol.,* 25:1, 1970.
49. Marriott, H. J. L., and Bieza, C. F.: Alarming Ventricular Acceleration after Lidocaine Administration, *Chest,* 61:682, 1972.
50. Josephson, M. E., Caracta, A. R., Lau, S. H., Gallagher, J. J., and Damato, A. N.: Effects of Lidocaine on Refractory Periods in Man, *Am. Heart J.,* 84:778, 1972.
51. Roos, J. C., and Dunning, A. J.: Effects of Lidocaine on Impulse Formation and Conduction Defects in Man, *Am. Heart J.,* 89:686, 1975.
52. Cheng, T. O., and Wadhwa, K.: Sinus Standstill Following Intravenous Lidocaine Administration, *JAMA,* 223:790, 1973.
53. Schumaker, R. R., Lieberson, A. D., Childress, R. H., and Williams, J. F., Jr.: Hemodynamic Effects of Lidocaine in Patients with Heart Disease, *Circulation,* 37:965, 1968.
54. Gianelly, R., Van der Groeben, J. D., Spivack, A. P., and Harrison, D. C.: Effect of Lidocaine on Ventricular Arrhythmias in Patients with Coronary Heart Disease, *N. Engl. J. Med.,* 277:1215, 1967.
55. Le Lorier, J., Grenon, D., Caillé, Y., Dumont, G., Brosseau, A., and Sulignac, A.: Pharmacokinetics of Lidocaine after Prolonged Intravenous Infusions in Uncomplicated Myocardial Infarction, *Ann. Intern. Med.,* 87:700, 1977.
56. Wyman, M. G., Slaughter, R. L., Farolino, D. A., Gore, F., Cannom, D. S., Goldreyer, B. N., and Lalka, D.: Lignocaine: Therapeutic Use. Ventricular Arrhythmias, *J. Coll. Cardiol.,* 2:764, 1983.
57. Koch-Weser, J.: Pharmacokinetics of Antiarrhythmic Drugs, *Cardiol. Clin.,* 7:191, 1975.
58. Strauss, H. C., Bigger, J. T., Jr., Bassett, A. L., and Hoffman, B. F.: Actions of Diphenylhydantoin on the Electrical Properties of Isolated Rabbit and Canine Atria, *Circ. Res.,* 23:463, 1968.
59. Bigger, J. T., Jr., Bassett, A. L., and Hoffman, B. F.: Electrophysiological Effects of Diphenylhydantoin on Canine Purkinje Fibers, *Circ. Res.,* 22:221, 1968.
60. Rosati, R. A., Alexander, J. A., Schaal, S. F., and Wallace, A. G.: Influence of Diphenylhydantoin on Electrophysiological Properties of the Canine Heart, *Circ. Res.,* 21:757, 1967.
61. Caracta, A. R., Damato, A. N., Josephson, M. E., Ricciutti, M. A., Gallagher, J. J., and Lau, S. H.: Electrophysiologic Actions of Diphenylhydantoin, *Circulation,* 47:1234, 1973.
62. Hilmi, K. I., and Reagan, T. J.: Relative Effectiveness of Antiarrhythmic Drugs in Treatment of Digitalis-Induced Ventricular Tachycardia, *Am. Heart J.,* 76:365, 1968.
63. Mercer, E. N., and Osborne, J. A.: Current Status of Diphenylhydantoin in Heart Disease, *Ann. Intern. Med.,* 67:1084, 1967.
64. Bigger, J. T., Jr., Schmidt, D. H., and Kutt, H.: Relationship between the Plasma Level of Diphenylhydantoin Sodium and Its Cardiac Antiarrhythmic Effects, *Circulation,* 38:363, 1968.
65. Alquist, R. P.: A Study of the Adrenergic Receptors, *Am. J. Physiol.,* 153:586, 1948.
66. Conolly, M. E., Kesting, F., and Dollery, C. T.: The Clinical Pharmacology of Beta-Adrenoreceptor-Blocking Drugs, *Prog. Cardiovasc. Dis.,* 19:203, 1976.
67. Shand, D. G.: Individualization of Propranolol Therapy, *Med. Clin. North Am.,* 58:1063, 1974.
68. Singh, B. N., and Jewitt, D. E.: β-Adrenergic Receptor Blocking Drugs in Cardiac Arrhythmias, *Drugs,* 7:426, 1974.
69. Wit, A. L., Hoffman, B. F., and Rosen, M. R.: Electrophysiology and Pharmacology of Cardiac Arrhythmias. IX. Cardiac Electrophysiologic Effects of Beta Adrenergic Receptor Stimulation and Blockade. Part C, *Am. Heart J.,* 90:795, 1975.
70. Robin, E., Cowan, C., Puri, P., Ganguly, S., De-Boyne, E., Martinec, M., Stock, T., and Bing, R. J. A.: A Comparative Study of Nitroglycerine and Propranolol, *Circulation,* 36:175, 1967.
71. Goldstein, S.: Propranolol Therapy in Patients with Acute Myocardial Infarction: The Beta-Blocker Heart Attack Trial, *Circulation,* 67(suppl. I):I–53, 1983.
72. Wit, A. L., Steiner, C., and Damato, A. N.: Electrophysiological Effects of Bretylium Tosylate upon Single Fibers of the Canine Specialized Conducting System and Ventricle, *J. Pharmacol. Ther.,* 173:344, 1975.
73. Wenger, T. L., Lederman, S., Starmer, F., Brown, T., and Strauss, H. C.: A Method for Quantitating Antifibrillatory Effects of Drugs after Coronary Reperfusion in Dogs: Improved Outcome with Bretylium, *Circulation,* 69:142, 1984.
74. Markis, J. E., and Koch-Weser, J.: Characteristics and Mechanism of Inotropic and Chronotropic Actions of Bretylium Tosylate, *J. Pharmacol. Exp. Ther.,* 178:94, 1971.
75. Bernstein, J. G., and Koch-Weser, J.: Effectiveness of Bretylium Tosylate against Refractory Ventricular Arrhythmias, *Circulation,* 45:1024, 1972.
76. Holder, D. A., Sniderman, A. D., Fraser, G., and Fallen, E. L.: Experience with Bretylium Tosylate by a Hospital Cardiac Arrest Team, *Circulation,* 55:541, 1977.
77. Singh, B. N., Eilrodt, G., and Peter, C. T.: Verapamil: A Review of its Pharmacological Properties and Therapeutic Use, *Drugs,* 15:169, 1978.
78. Shigenobu, K., Scneider, J. A., and Sperelakis, N.: Verapamil Blockade of Slow Na^+ and Ca^{++} Responses in Myocardial Cells, *J. Pharmacol. Exp. Ther.,* 190:280, 1974.
79. Roy, P. R., Spurrell, R. A. J., and Sowton, G. E.: The Effect of Verapamil on the Conduction System in Man, *Postgrad. Med. J.,* 50:270, 1974.
80. Klein, G. J., Gulamhusein, S., Prystowsky, E. N., Carruthers, S. G., Donner, A. P., and Ko, P. T.: Comparison of the Electrophysiologic Effects of Intravenous and Oral Verapamil in Patients with Paroxysmal Supraventricular Tachycardia, *Am. J. Cardiol.,* 49:117, 1982.
81. Singh, B. N., and Roche, A. H. G.: Effects of Intravenous Verapamil on Hemodynamics in Patients with Heart Disease, *Am. Heart J.,* 94:593, 1977.
82. Heng, M. K., Singh, B. N., Roche, A. H. G., Norris, R. M., and Mercer, C. J.: Effects of Intravenous Verapamil on

Cardiac Arrhythmias and on the Electrocardiogram, *Am. Heart J.*, 90:487, 1975.
83. Gulamhusein, S., Ko, P., Carruthers, S. G., and Klein, G. J.: Acceleration of the Ventricular Response During Atrial Fibrillation in the Wolff-Parkinson-White Syndrome After Verapamil, *Circulation*, 65:348, 1982.
84. Packer, M., Meller, J., Medina, N., Yushak, M., Smith, H., Holt, J., Guerrero, J., Todd, G. D., McAllister, R. G., and Gorlin, R.: Hemodynamic Consequences of Combined Beta-Adrenergic and Slow Calcium Channel Blockade in Man, *Circulation*, 65:660, 1982.
85. Benaim, M. D.: Asystole after Verapamil, *Br. Med. J.*, 2:169, 1972.
86. Danilo, P.: Appraisal and Reappraisal of Cardiac Therapy. Tocainide, *Am. Heart J.*, 97:259, 1979.
87. Anderson, J. L., Mason, J. W., Winkle, R. A., Meffin, P. J., Fowles, R. E., Peters, F., and Harrison, D. C.: Clinical Electrophysiologic Effects of Tocainide, *Circulation*, 57:685, 1978.
88. Winkle, R. A., Anderson, J. L., Peters, F., Meffin, P. J., Fowles, R. E., and Harrison, D. C.: The Hemodynamic Effects of Intravenous Tocainide in Patients with Heart Disease, *Circulation*, 57:787, 1978.
89. Maloney, J. D., Nissen, G., and McColgan, B. S.: Open Clinical Studies at a Referral Center: Chronic Maintenance Tocainide Therapy in Patients with Recurrent Sustained Ventricular Tachycardia Refractory to Conventional Antiarrhythmic Agents, *Am. Heart J.*, 100:1023, 1980.
90. Chew, C. Y. C., Collett, J., and Singh, B. N.: Mexiletine: A Review of its Pharmacological Properties and Therapeutic Efficacy in Arrhythmias, *Drugs*, 17:161, 1979.
91. Heger, J. J., Nattel, S., Rinkenberger, R. L., and Zipes, D. P.: Mexiletine Therapy in 15 Patients with Drug Resistant Ventricular Tachycardia, *Am. J. Cardiol.*, 45:627, 1980.
91a. Stein, J., Podrid, P. J., Lampert, S., Hirsowitz, G., and Lown, B.: Long-Term Mexiletine for Ventricular Arrhythmia, *Am. Heart J.*, 107:1091, 1984.
91b. Bigger, J. T.: The Interaction of Mexiletine with Other Cardiovascular Drugs, *Am. Heart J.*, 107:1079, 1984.
92. Campbell, N. P. S., Pantridge, J. F., and Adgey, A. A. J.: Long-Term Oral Antiarrhythmic Therapy with Mexiletine, *Br. Heart J.*, 40:796, 1978.
93. Holt, D. W., Tucker, G. T., Jackson, P. R., and Storey, G. C. A.: Amiodarone Pharmacokinetics, *Am. Heart J.*, 106:840, 1983.
94. Singh, B. N.: Amiodarone: Historical Development and Pharmacologic Profile, *Am. Heart J.*, 106:788, 1983.
95. Wellens, H. J. J., Brugada, P., Abdollah, H., and Dassen, W. R.: A Comparison of the Electrophysiologic Effects of Intravenous and Oral Amiodarone in the Same Patient, *Circulation*, 69:120, 1984.
96. Schwartz, A., Shen, E., Morady, F., Gillespie, K., Scheinman, M., and Chatterjee, K.: Hemodynamic Effects of Intravenous Amiodarone in Patients with Depressed Left Ventricular Function and Recurrent Ventricular Tachycardia, *Am. Heart J.*, 106:848, 1983.
97. Morady, F., Sauve, M. J., Malone, P., Shen, E., Schwartz, A. B., Bhandari, A., Keung, E., Sung, R. J., and Scheinman, M. M.: Long-Term Efficacy and Toxicity of High-Dose Amiodarone Therapy for Ventricular Tachycardia or Ventricular Fibrillation, *Am. J. Cardiol.*, 52:975, 1983.
98. Nademanee, K., Singh, B. N., Cannom, D. S., Weiss, J., Feld, G., and Stevenson, W. G.: Control of Sudden Recurrent Arrhythmic Deaths: Role of Amiodarone, *Am. Heart J.*, 106:895, 1983.
99. Fogaros, R. N., Anderson, K. P., Winkle, R. A., Swerdlow, C. D., and Mason, J. W.: Amiodarone: Clinical Efficacy and Toxicity in 96 Patients with Recurrent, Drug-Refractory Arrhythmias, *Circulation*, 68:88, 1983.
100. Sobol, S. M., and Rakita, L.: Pneumonitis and Pulmonary Fibrosis Associated with Amiodarone Treatment: A Possible Complication of a New Antiarrhythmic Drug, *Circulation*, 65:819, 1982.
101. Sclarovsky, S., Lewin, R. S., Kracoff, O., Strasberg, B., Arditti, A., and Agmon, J.: Amiodarone Induced Polymorphous Ventricular Tachycardia, *Am. Heart J.*, 105:6, 1983.
102. McGovern, B., Garan, H., and Ruskin, J. N.: Sinus Arrest During Treatment with Amiodarone, *Br. Med. J.*, 284:160, 1982.
103. Rotmensch, H. H., Belhassen, B., and Ferguson, R. K.: Amiodarone—Benefits and Risks in Perspective, *Am. Heart J.*, 104:1117, 1982 (Editorial).
104. Siddoway, L. A., McAllister, C. B., Wilkinson, G. R., Roden, D. M., and Woosley, R. L.: Amiodarone Dosing: A Proposal Based on its Pharmacokinetics, *Am. Heart J.*, 106:951, 1983.
105. Marcus, F. I.: Drug Interactions with Amiodarone, *Am. Heart J.*, 106:924, 1983.

90

Beta-Adrenergic Blocking Drugs*

William H. Frishman, M.D. Edmund H. Sonnenblick, M.D.

Beta-adrenoceptor blocking drugs, which constitute a major pharmacotherapeutic advance, were initially conceived for the treatment of patients with angina pectoris and arrhythmias; however, they play a role in a diversity of clinical disorders including systemic hypertension, hypertrophic cardiomyopathy, mitral valve prolapse, migraine, glaucoma, and thyrotoxicosis.[1,2] Beta-blockers have been effective in treating unstable angina and in reducing the risk of cardiovascular mortality and perhaps reinfarction in patients who have survived an acute myocardial infarction.[3,4] Beta-blockers have also been suggested as a possible treatment modality for reducing the extent of myocardial injury and mortality during the hyperacute phase of myocardial infarction.[5,6]

In this chapter, the molecular and clinical pharmacology of beta-adrenergic blockers is reviewed. Also, the clinical actions of beta-adrenergic blockade are discussed.

The Beta-Adrenoceptor: Changing Concepts

Hormonal and Drug Receptors

The effects of an endogenous hormone or an exogenous drug depend ultimately on the physiochemical interactions with macromolecular structures of cells called receptors. Agonists interact with a receptor and elicit a response; antagonists interact with receptors and prevent the action of agonists.

In the case of catecholamine action, the circulating hormone or drug is the first "messenger," interacting with its specific receptor on the external surface of the target cells. The drug hormone–receptor complex activates the enzyme adenyl cyclase, on the internal surface of the plasma membrane of the target cell, which accelerates the intracellular formation of cyclic adenosine monophosphate (cyclic AMP)—the second "messenger" which then stimulates or inhibits various metabolic or physiologic processes.[7–9]

Until recently most research on receptor action bypassed the initial binding step and the intermediate steps and examined either the accumulation of cyclic AMP or the end step, the physiologic effect. Radioactive agonists or antagonists (*radioligands*) that attach to and label the receptors have been used to study binding and hormone action.[8,10]

The Beta-Adrenergic Receptor

The catecholamines norepinephrine and epinephrine are important regulators of many physiologic and metabolic effects. Norepinephrine acts primarily as a neurotransmitter released from sympathetic nerve terminals, and epinephrine functions as a circulating hormone released from the adrenal medulla.[8] Thirty-five years ago, Ahlquist characterized the receptors relative to the actions of epinephrine and norepinephrine, and defined two major types of receptors: alpha- and beta-adrenoceptors.[11] Adrenergic receptors have since been subclassified into discrete beta$_1$ and beta$_2$ as well as alpha$_1$ and alpha$_2$ subtypes. Others have emphasized the accompanying changes in the intracellular second "messengers." Radioligand-labeling techniques have greatly aided the investigation of adrenoreceptors.[8,10] and molecular pharmacologic techniques have identified the beta-adrenoceptor as a polypeptide with a molecular weight of 67,000.[12]

In contrast to the older classical concept of adrenoreceptors as static entities in cells which simply serve to initiate the chain of events, newer theories hold that the adrenoreceptors are subject to a wide variety of controlling influences which results in dynamic regulation of adrenoceptor sites and/or their sensitivity to catecholamines. Changes in tissue concentration of receptor sites are likely involved in mediating important fluctuations in tissue sensitivity to drug action.[10] These principles may have significant clinical and therapeutic implications. For example, an apparent increase in the number of beta-adrenoceptors, and thereby a supersensitivity to agonists, may be induced by chronic exposure to antagonists.[9,12] With prolonged adrenoceptor blocker therapy, receptor occupancy by catecholamines can be diminished and the number of available receptors increased.[13] When the beta-adrenoceptor blocker is suddenly withdrawn, an increased pool of sensitive receptors would be open to endogenous catecholamine stimulation. The resulting adrenergic stimulation could precipitate angina pectoris or a myocardial infarction.[14]

The concentration of beta-adrenoceptors in the membrane of mononuclear cells decreases significantly with age.[8] This could explain the progressive resistance to beta-adrenoceptor blocker therapy reported with increasing age of the hypertensive population. As shown in a recent study, a good response

*Dr. Frishman wrote the chapter "Beta-Adrenergic Blocking Agents," for *Clinical Essays on the Heart* in 1984. This updated version of the chapter is reproduced here for the convenience of the reader with the permission of McGraw-Hill Publishers and the author.

to beta-adrenoceptor blocker therapy occurred in 90 percent of hypertensive patients in their twenties, but the percentage of responders fell progressively with increasing age.[15]

Using radioligand techniques a decrease in beta-adrenoceptor sites in the myocardium has been demonstrated in patients with chronic congestive heart failure.[16,17] An apparent reduction in beta-adrenoceptors has also been associated with the development of refractoriness or desensitization to endogenous and exogenous catecholamines, a phenomenon caused by the prolonged exposure of these adrenoceptors to high levels of catecholamines.[16] This desensitization phenomenon is not caused by change in receptor formation or degradation, but rather by catecholamine-induced changes in the conformation of the receptor sites, thus rendering them ineffective.[10] These changes are reversible over a period of hours.[10] Beta-adrenoceptor blocking drugs do not induce desensitization or changes in the conformation of receptors, but do block the ability of catecholamines to desensitize receptors.[18]

Beta-Adrenoceptor Blocking Drugs: Basic Pharmacologic Differences

More than 15 beta-adrenoceptor blockers have been synthesized and over 15 are available worldwide.[19] Selectivity for two subgroups of the beta-adrenoceptor population has also been taken advantage of: $beta_1$ receptors in the heart and $beta_2$ receptors in the peripheral circulation and bronchi.[1,19] More controversial has been the introduction of beta-blocking drugs with alpha-adrenergic blocking actions, varying amounts of intrinsic sympathomimetic activity (partial agonist activity), and nonspecific membrane stabilizing effects.[2] There are also pharmacokinetic differences between beta-blocking drugs which may be of clinical importance.[1,19]

Eight beta-adrenoceptor blockers are now marketed in the United States: propranolol for angina pectoris, arrhythmias, systemic hypertension, migraine prophylaxis, hypertrophic cardiomyopathy, and for reducing the risk of cardiovascular mortality in survivors of an acute myocardial infarction; nadolol for hypertension and angina pectoris; timolol for hypertension and for reducing the risk of cardiovascular mortality and reinfarction in survivors of myocardial infarction, and in topical form for glaucoma; metoprolol for hypertension and for reducing the risk of cardiovascular mortality in survivors of myocardial infarction; atenolol and pindolol in hypertension; acebutolol for hypertension and ventricular arrhythmias; and labetalol for hypertension and in intravenous form for hypertensive emergencies.[1,2,20–23] Oxprenolol is approved for marketing in hypertension. Bevantolol, celiprolol, penbutolol, esmolol, and ACC-9089 are in the process of being approved for clinical use or in clinical trials.

Despite the extrinsic experience with beta blockers in clinical practice, there are no studies suggesting that one of these agents has major advantages or disadvantages in relation to another for treatment of cardiovascular diseases. When any available beta blocker is titrated properly, it can be effective in patients with arrhythmia, hypertension, or angina pectoris.[1,2,19–24] However, one agent may be more effective than others in reducing adverse reactions in some patients and clinical situations.

Potency

Beta-adrenoceptor blocking drugs are competitive inhibitors of catecholamine binding at beta-adrenoceptor sites. The dose-response curve of the agonist is shifted to the right; that is, a given tissue response requires a higher concentration of agonist in the presence of beta-blocking drugs.[1] $Beta_1$-blocking potency can be assessed by the inhibition of tachycardia produced by isoproterenol or exercise; potency varies from compound to compound (Table 90-1).[2] These differences in potency are of no therapeutic relevance; however, they do explain the different drug dosages needed to achieve effective beta-adrenergic blockade when initiating therapy in patients or when switching from one agent to another.[1,25]

Structure-Activity Relations

The chemical structures of most beta-adrenergic blockers have several features in common with the agonist isoproterenol (Fig. 90-1)—an aromatic ring with a substituted ethanolamine side chain linked to it by an $—OCH_2$ group.[1,2,26] The beta blocker timolol has a catecholamine-mimicking side chain but a more complex ring.

Most beta-blocking drugs exist as pairs of optical isomers and are marketed as racemic mixtures. Almost all the beta-blocking activity is found in the negative (−) levorotatory stereoisomer. The two stereoisomers of beta-adrenergic blockers are useful for differentiating between the pharmacologic effects of beta blockade and membrane-stabilizing activity (possessed by both optical forms). The positive (+) dextrorotatory stereoisomers of beta-blocking agents have no apparent clinical value.[1,25,26]

Membrane-Stabilizing Activity

In concentrations well above therapeutic levels, certain beta blockers have a quinidinelike or "local anesthetic" membrane-stabilizing effect on the cardiac action potential. This property is exhibited equally by the two stereoisomers of the drug and is unrelated to beta-adrenergic blockade and to any therapeutic antiarrhythmic effects. There is no evidence that membrane-stabilizing activity is responsible for any direct negative inotropic effects of beta-blocking drugs since drugs with and without this property equally depress left ventricular function.[1,27] Membrane-stabilizing activity can manifest itself clinically during massive beta-blocker intoxications.[2,28]

TABLE 90-1 Pharmacodynamic Properties of Beta-Adrenoceptor Blocking Drugs

Drug	β_1-Blockade Potency Ratio (Propranolol = 1.0)	Relative β_1 Selectivity	Intrinsic Sympathomimetic Activity	Membrane-Stabilizing Activity
Acebutolol	0.3	+	+	+
Atenolol	1.0	++	0	0
Esmolol (ASL-8052)	0.01	++	0	0
Labetalol*	0.3	0	+?	0
Metoprolol	1.0	++	0	0
Nadolol	1.0	0	0	0
Oxprenolol	0.5–1.0	0	+	+
Pindolol	6.0	0	++	+
Propranolol	1.0	0	0	++
Sotalol	0.3	0	0	0
Timolol	6.0	0	0	0
Isomer:				
D-Propranolol				++

*Labetalol has additional alpha-adrenergic blocking activity and direct vasodilatory actions. *Source:* Frishman, W. H.: "Clinical Pharmacology of the Beta-Adrenoceptor Blocking Drugs, 2d ed., Appleton-Century-Crofts, Inc., Norwalk, 1984, p. 15. Reproduced with permission from the publisher and author. Also, Frishman, W. H.: The Beta-Adrenergic Blocking Drugs, *Int. J. Cardiol.,* 2:166, 1982. Adapted and reproduced with permission from the publisher and author.

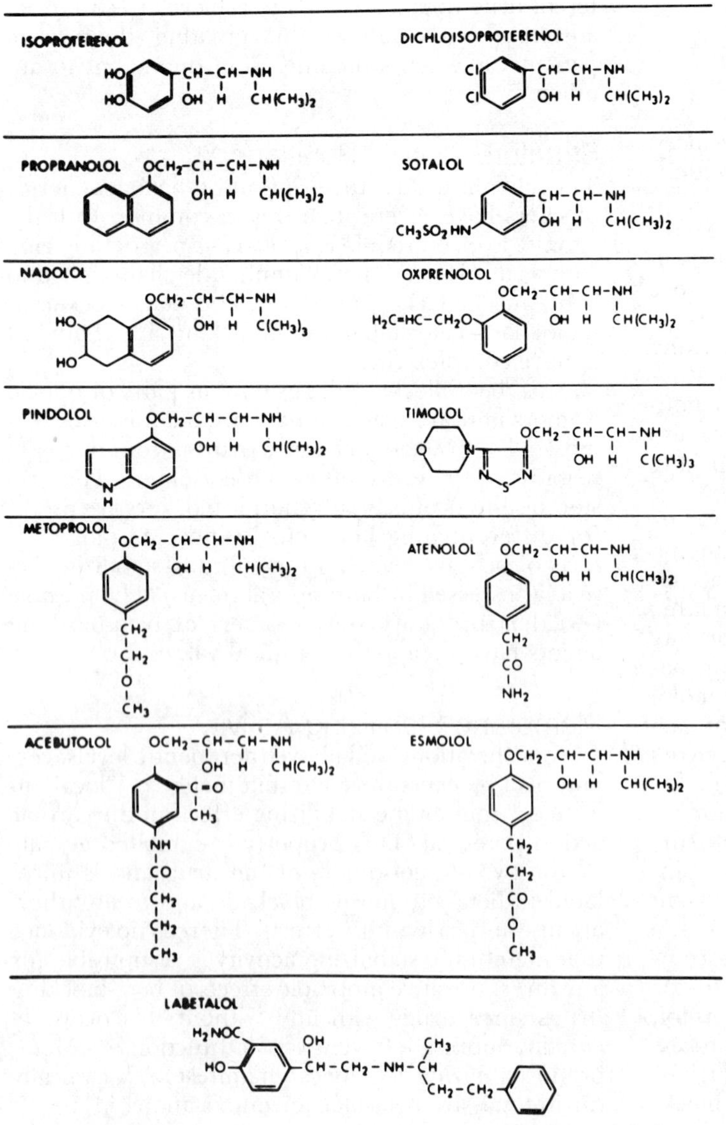

FIGURE 90-1 Molecular structure of the beta-adrenergic agonist isoproterenol and some beta-adrenergic blocking drugs. (*From W. H. Frishman: "Clinical Pharmacology of the β-Adrenoceptor Blocking Drugs," 2d ed., Appleton-Century-Crofts, Inc., 1984, p. 16. Reproduced with permission from the publisher and author.*)

Selectivity

Beta-adrenoceptor blockers may be classified as selective or nonselective according to their relative abilities to antagonize the actions of sympathomimetic amines in some tissues at lower doses than those required in other tissues.[1,20] When used in low doses, $beta_1$-selective blocking agents such as acebutolol, atenolol, and metoprolol inhibit cardiac $beta_1$ receptors but have less influence on bronchial and vascular beta-adrenoceptors ($beta_2$). In higher doses, however, $beta_1$-selective blocking agents will also block $beta_2$ receptors. Accordingly, $beta_1$-selective agents may be safer than nonselective ones in patients with obstructive pulmonary disease since $beta_2$ receptors remain available to mediate adrenergic bronchodilatation. However, even selective beta blockers may aggravate bronchospasm in certain patients, so that these drugs should generally not be used in patients with bronchospastic disease.

A second theoretical advantage is that unlike nonselective beta blockers, $beta_1$-selective blockers in low doses may not block the $beta_2$ receptors that mediate dilatation of arterioles. During infusion of epinephrine, nonselective beta blockers can cause a pressor response by blocking $beta_2$ receptor-mediated vasodilatation, since alpha-adrenergic vasoconstrictor receptors are still operative. Selective $beta_1$ antagonists may not induce this pressor effect in the presence of epinephrine and may lessen the impairment of peripheral blood flow. It is possible that leaving the $beta_2$ receptors unblocked and responsive to epinephrine may be functionally important in some patients with asthma, hypoglycemia, hypertension, or peripheral vascular disease treated with beta-adrenergic blocking drugs.[1,19,20]

Intrinsic Sympathomimetic Activity (Partial Agonist Activity)

Certain beta-adrenoceptor blocking drugs have intrinsic sympathomimetic activity (partial agonist activity). In a beta blocker, this property is identified as a slight cardiac stimulation which can be blocked by propranolol.[1,23,24] The beta-blocking drugs with this property slightly activate the beta receptor, in addition to preventing access of natural or synthetic catecholamines to the receptor (Fig. 90-2). Dichloroisoprenaline, the first beta-adrenoceptor blocking drug synthesized, exerted such marked partial agonist activity that it was unsuitable for clinical use.[24] However, compounds with less partial agonist activity are effective beta-blocking drugs. Partial agonist effects of beta-adrenoceptor blocking drugs such as pindolol, acebutolol, and oxprenolol differ from those of the agonist epinephrine or isoproterenol in that the maximum pharmacologic response that can be obtained is less, although the affinity for the receptor is high. In the treatment of patients with arrhythmia, angina pectoris of effort, or hypertension, drugs with mild to moderate partial agonist activity appear to be as efficacious as beta blockers

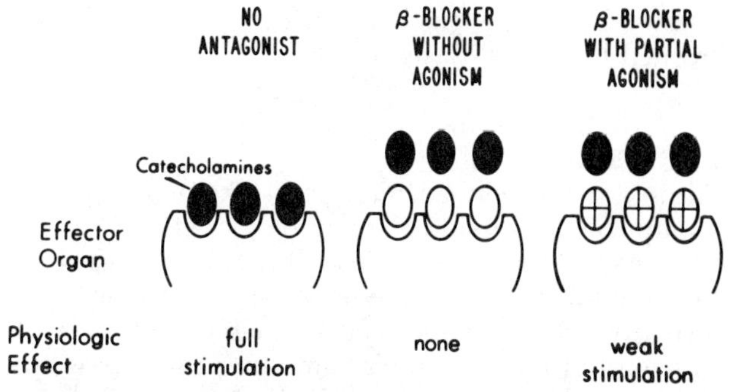

FIGURE 90-2 Physiologic effects of beta-adrenergic blocking drugs with and without partial agonist activity in the presence of circulating catecholamines. When circulating catecholamines (●) combine with beta-adrenergic receptors, they produce a full physiologic response. When these receptors are occupied by a beta blocker lacking partial agonist activity (o), no physiologic effects from catecholamine stimulation can occur. A beta-blocking drug with partial agonist activity (⊕) also blocks the binding of catecholamines to beta-adrenergic receptors, but in addition the drug also causes a relatively weak stimulation of the receptor. *(From W. H. Frishman: Pindolol: A New β-Adrenoceptor Antagonist with Partial Agonist Activity, N. Engl. J. Med., 308:941, 1983. Reproduced with permission from the publisher and author.)*

lacking this property. It is still debated whether the presence of partial agonist activity in a beta blocker constitutes an overall advantage or disadvantage in cardiac therapy.[23] Drugs with partial agonist activity cause less slowing of the heart rate at rest than propranolol or metoprolol, although the increments in heart rate with exercise are similarly blunted. They may reduce peripheral vascular resistance and may also depress atrioventricular conduction less than agents lacking this property.[23] Some investigators claim that partial agonist activity in a beta blocker protects against myocardial depression, bronchial asthma, and peripheral vascular complications.[23,29] The evidence supporting these claims is not definite and more definitive clinical trials will be necessary to resolve these questions.

Alpha-Adrenergic Blocking Activity

Labetalol is a beta blocker with antagonistic properties at both alpha- and beta-adrenoceptors, and has direct vasodilatory activity.[2,30] Labetalol has been shown to be six to ten times less potent than phentolamine at alpha-adrenoceptors, 1.5 to four times less potent than propranolol at beta-adrenoceptors, and is itself four to sixteen times less potent at alpha- then at beta-adrenoceptors.[2,30] Like other beta blockers, it is useful in the treatment of arrhythmias, hypertension, and angina pectoris.[2,31] However, unlike most beta-blocking drugs, the additional alpha-adrenergic blocking actions of labetalol lead to a reduction in peripheral vascular resistance which may maintain cardiac output.[2,30] Whether concomitant alpha-adrenergic blocking activity is actually advantageous in a beta-blocker remains to be determined.

An isomer of labetalol, dilevalol, a beta-blocking drug which has direct vasodilating activity and no alpha-adrenergic blocking effects, is now being studied in clinical trials.

Pharmacokinetics

Although the beta-adrenergic blocking drugs as a group have similar pharmacologic effects, their pharmacokinetics are markedly different (Tables 90-2, 90-3).[25,27,32,33] Their varied aromatic ring structures lead to differences in completeness of gastrointestinal absorption, amount of first pass hepatic metabolism, lipid solubility, protein binding, extent of distribution in the body, penetration into the brain, concentration in the heart, rate of hepatic biotransformation, pharmacologic activity of metabolites, and renal clearance of a drug and its metabolites which may influence the clinical usefulness of these drugs in some patients.[1,25,27] The desirable pharmacokinetic characteristics in this group of compounds are a lack of major individual differences in bioavailability and in metabolic clearance of the drug, and a rate of removal from the active tissue sites that is slow enough to allow longer dosing intervals.[1]

The beta-adrenergic blocking drugs can be divided by their pharmacokinetic properties into two broad categories: those eliminated by hepatic metabolism, which tend to have relatively short plasma half-lives; and those eliminated unchanged by the kidney, which tend to have longer half-lives.[1] Propranolol and metoprolol are both lipid-soluble, are almost completely absorbed from the small intestine, and are largely metabolized by the liver. They tend to have highly variable bioavailability and relatively short plasma half-lives.[1,20,25] A lack of correlation between the duration of clinical pharmacologic effect and plasma half-life may still allow these drugs to be administered once or twice daily.[1]

In contrast, agents such as atenolol and nadolol are more water-soluble, are incompletely absorbed through the gut, and are eliminated unchanged by the kidney.[21,22] They tend to have less variable bioavailability in patients with normal renal function, in addition to longer half-lives allowing one dose a day.[21,22] The longer half-lives may be useful in those patients who find compliance with beta-blocker therapy a problem.[21]

Recently, a long-acting, sustained-release preparation of propranolol was approved for marketing (Tables 90-2, 90-3).[34] The propranolol is part of a soluble matrix inside tiny spheroids made up of an insoluble membrane. Gastrointestinal fluid enters the spheroids and propranolol exits via a concentration gradient into the gut lumen and then the bloodstream.[34] Long-acting propranolol absorption is not dependent on gastric acidity or enzymatic action. Studies have shown that long-acting propranolol provides a much smoother curve of daily plasma levels than comparable divided doses of conventional propranolol.[35,36]

Ultra-short-acting beta blockers are now in the early stages of clinical testing and may be useful where a short duration of action is desired (e.g., in patients with questionable congestive heart failure). One of these compounds, esmolol (ASL-8052), a $beta_1$-selective drug (Tables 90-1–90-3), has been shown to be useful in treating supraventricular tachyarrhythmias. Another drug, ACC-9089, is now in clinical trials. The short half-life (approximately 15 min) relates to the rapid metabolism of the drug by blood tissue and hepatic esterases. Metabolism does not seem to be altered by disease states.[37–39]

TABLE 90-2 Pharmacokinetic Properties of Beta-Adrenoceptor Blocking Drugs

Drug	Extent of Absorption (% of dose)	Extent of Bioavailability (% of dose)	Dose-Dependent Bioavailability (Major First Pass Hepatic Metabolism)	Interpatient Variations in Plasma Levels	Beta-Blocking Plasma Concentrations	Protein Binding (%)	Lipid Solubility*
Acebutolol	≃70	≃50	No	7-fold	0.2–2.0 μg/ml	approx. 25	Moderate
Atenolol	≃50	≃40	No	4-fold	0.2–5.0 μg/ml	<5	Weak
Esmolol†	NA	NA	NA		0.3–1.0 μg/ml		
Labetalol	>90	≃33	Yes	10-fold	0.7–3.0 μg/ml	≃50	Weak
Metoprolol	>90	≃50	No	7-fold	50–100 ng/ml	12	Moderate
Nadolol	≃30	≃30	No	7-fold	50–100 ng/ml	≃30	Weak
Oxprenolol	≃90	≃40	No	5-fold	80–100 ng/ml	80	Moderate
Pindolol	>90	≃90	No	4-fold	5–15 ng/ml	57	Moderate
Propranolol	>90	≃30	Yes	20-fold	50–100 ng/ml	93	High
LA Propranolol (long-acting)	>90	≃20	Yes	10–20-fold	20–100 ng/ml	93	High
Sotalol	≃70	≃60	No	4-fold	0.5–4.0 μg/ml	0	Weak
Timolol	>90	≃75	No	7-fold	5–10 ng/ml	≃10	Weak

* = Determined by the distribution ratio between octanol and water.
† = Ultra-short-acting beta blocker only available in intravenous form.
NA = Not applicable. *Source:* Frishman, W. H.: "Clinical Pharmacology of the Beta-Adrenoceptor Blocking Drugs, 2d ed., Appleton-Century-Crofts, Inc., Norwalk, 1984, p. 21. Reproduced with permission from the publisher and author. Also, Frishman, W. H.: The Beta-Adrenergic Blocking Drugs, *Int. J. Cardiol.*, 2:171, 1982. Adapted and reproduced with permission from the publisher and author.

TABLE 90-3 Elimination Characteristics of Orally Active Beta-Adrenoceptor Blocking Drugs

Drug	Elimination Half-Life (n)	Total Body Clearance (ml/min)	Urinary Recovery of Unchanged Drug (% of Dose)	Total Urinary Recovery (% of Dose)	Predominant Route of Elimination*	Active Metabolites	Drug Accumulation in Renal Disease
Acebutolol	3–4	6–15	≈40	>90	RE	Yes	Yes
Atenolol	6–9	130	≈40	>95	RE	No	Yes
Esmolol†	≈10 min	285		>70	HM‡	No	No
Labetalol	3–4	2700	<1	>90	HN	No	No
Metoprolol	3–4	1100	≈3	>95	HM	No	No
Nadolol	14–24	200	70	70	RE	No	Yes
Oxprenolol	2–3	380	2–5	70–95	HM	No	No
Pindolol	3–4	400	≈40	>90	RE (≈40% unchanged and HM)	No	No
Propranolol	3–4	1000	<1	>90	HM	Yes	No
LA Propranolol (long-acting)	10	1000	<1	>90	HM	Yes	No
Sotalol	8–10	150	≈60	>90	RE	No	Yes
Timolol	4–5	660	≈20	65	RE (≈20% unchanged and HM)	No	No

* = RE denotes renal excretion and HM hepatic metabolism.
† = Ultra-short-acting beta blocker only available in intravenous form.
‡ = Metabolized by blood, tissue, and hepatic esterases. *Source:* Frishman, W. H.: "Clinical Pharmacology of the Beta-Adrenoceptor Blocking Drugs, 2d ed., Appleton-Century-Crofts, Inc., Norwalk, 1984, p. 22. Reproduced with permission from the publisher and author. Also, Frishman, W. H.: The Beta-Adrenergic Blocking Drugs, *Int. J. Cardiol.,* 2:172, 1982. Adapted and reproduced with permission from the publisher and author.

Specific pharmacokinetic properties of individual beta-adrenergic blockers (first pass metabolism, active metabolites, lipid solubility, and protein-binding) may be clinically important. When drugs with extensive first pass metabolism are taken by mouth, they undergo so much hepatic biotransformation that relatively little drug reaches the systemic circulation.[1,25,32] Depending on the extent of the first pass effect, an oral dose of beta blocker must be larger than an intravenous dose to produce the same clinical effects.[20,25,32] Some beta-adrenergic blockers are transformed into pharmacologically active compounds (acebutolol) rather than inactive metabolites. The total pharmacologic effect, therefore, depends on the amounts of both the drug administered and its active metabolites.[1,33] Characteristics of lipid solubility in a beta blocker have been associated with the ability of the drug to concentrate in the brain,[1] and many side effects of these drugs, which have not been clearly related to beta blockade, may result from their actions on the central nervous system (lethargy, mental depression, and hallucinations).[1,22] It is still not clear, however, whether drugs that are less lipid-soluble cause fewer of these adverse reactions.[21,22]

Relation between Dose, Plasma Level, and Efficacy

Attempts have been made to establish a relation between the oral dose, plasma level measured by gas chromatography, and pharmacologic effect of each beta-blocking drug. After administration of a certain oral dose, beta-blocking drugs that are largely metabolized in the liver show large interindividual variation in circulating plasma levels.[1] Many explanations have been proposed to explain wide individual differences in the relation between plasma concentrations of beta blockers and any associated therapeutic effect. First, patients may have different levels of "sympathetic tone" (circulating catecholamines and active beta-adrenoceptor binding sites), and may thus require different drug concentrations to achieve adequate beta blockade.[25] Second, many beta blockers have flat plasma drug level response curves.[33] Third, the active drug isomer and active metabolites are not specifically measured by many plasma assays. Fourth, the clinical effect of a drug may last longer than the period suggested by the drug's half-life in plasma,[25] since recycling of the beta blocker between receptor site and neuronal nerve endings may be occurring. Despite the lack of correlation between plasma levels and therapeutic effect, there is some evidence that a relationship does exist between the logarithm of the plasma level and the beta-blocking effect (blockade of exercise or isoproterenol-induced tachycardia).[20,25,33] Plasma levels have little to offer as therapeutic guides, except for ensuring compliance. Pharmacodynamic characteristics and clinical response should be used as guides in determining efficacy.

Clinical Effects and Therapeutic Applications

The therapeutic efficacy and safety of beta-adrenoceptor blocking drugs has been well established in patients with angina pectoris, cardiac arrhythmias, and hypertension, and for reducing the risk of mortality and possibly nonfatal reinfarction in survivors of acute myocardial infarction.[1,2,6] The drugs are also used for a multitude of other cardiac (Table 90-4)[2,40–52] and noncardiac (Table 90-5)[2,53–58] uses.

Cardiovascular Effects

Effects on Elevated Systemic Blood Pressure
Beta-adrenergic blockers are effective in reducing the blood pressure of many patients with systemic hypertension (Tables 90-6, 90-7). However, there is no consensus of opinion as to the mechanism(s) whereby these drugs lower blood pressure. It is probable that some, or all of the following proposed mechanisms play a part. Beta blockers appear to be more efficacious in white patients and younger patients than they are in the elderly and blacks.

Negative Chronotropic and Inotropic Effects Slowing of the heart rate and some decrease in myocardial contractility with beta blockers lead to a decrease in cardiac output, which in short and long term, may lead to a reduction in blood pressure.[1] It might be expected that these factors would be particularly important in treating hypertension related to high cardiac output,[59] and increased sympathetic tone.

Difference in Effects on Plasma Renin The relation between the hypotensive action of beta-blocking drugs and their ability to reduce to plasma renin activity remains controversial. Some beta-blocking drugs can antagonize sympathetically mediated renin release,[60] although adrenergic activity is not the only mechanism whereby renin release is mediated. Other major determinants are sodium balance, posture, and renal perfusion pressure.

The important question remains whether or not there is a clinical correlation between the beta-blocker effect on plasma renin activity and the lowering of blood pressure. Investigators[9] have found that "high-renin" patients respond well to propranolol; that "low-renin" patients do not respond or may even show a rise in blood pressure; and that "normal-renin" patients have less predictable responses. In the "high-renin" hypertensive patient, it has been suggested that renin may not be the only factor maintaining the high blood pressure state. At present, the exact role of renin reduction in blood pressure control is not well defined.

A Central Nervous System Effect There is now good clinical and experimental evidence to suggest that beta blockers cross the blood-brain barrier and enter the central nervous system.[61] Although there is little doubt that beta blockers with high lipophilicity (e.g.,

TABLE 90-4 Reported Cardiovascular Indications for Beta-Adrenoceptor Blocking Drugs

Hypertension*
Angina pectoris*
Supraventricular arrhythmias*
Ventricular arrhythmias*
Reducing the risk of mortality and reinfarction in survivors of acute myocardial infarction*
Hyperacute phase of myocardial infarction*
Dissection of the aorta
Hypertrophic cardiomyopathy*
Digitalis intoxication
Mitral valve prolapse
QT interval prolongation syndrome
Tetralogy of Fallot
Mitral stenosis
Congestive cardiomyopathy
Fetal tachycardia
Neurocirculatory asthenia

*Formally approved indications by FDA.

TABLE 90-5 Reported Noncardiovascular Indications for Beta-Adrenoceptor Blocking Drugs

Neuropsychiatric
Migraine prophylaxis*
Essential tremor
Anxiety
Alcohol withdrawal (delirium tremens)
Endocrine
Thyrotoxicosis*
Hyperparathyroidism
Other
Glaucoma*
Portal hypertension and gastrointestinal bleeding

*Formally approved indications by FDA.

TABLE 90-6 Proposed Mechanisms to Explain the Antihypertensive Actions of Beta Blockers

Reduction in cardiac output
Inhibition of renin
Central nervous system effects
Effects on prejunctional beta receptors—reductions in norepinephrine release
Reduction in peripheral vascular resistance
Reduction in venomotor tone
Reduction in plasma volume
Resetting of baroreceptor levels
Most important effects of beta blockers—prevents the pressor response to catecholamines with exercise and stress.

Source: Frishman, W. H.: "Clinical Pharmacology of the Beta-Adrenoceptor Blocking Drugs," 2d ed., Appleton-Century-Crofts, Inc., Norwalk, 1984, p. 28. Adapted and reproduced with permission from the publisher and author.

TABLE 90-7 Pharmacodynamic Properties and Cardiac Effects of Beta-Adrenoceptor Blockers

Drug	Relative β_1 Selectivity*	Partial Agonist Activity	Membrane-Stabilizing Activity	Resting Heart Rate	Exercise Heart Rate	Resting Myocardial Contractility	Resting Blood Pressure	Exercise Blood Pressure	Resting Atrioventricular Conduction	Anti-arrhythmic Effect
Acebutolol	+	+	+	↓	↓	↓	↓	↓	↓	+
Atenolol	+ +	0	0	↓	↓	↓	↓	↓	↓	+
Esmolol	+ +	0	0	↓	?	↓	↓	?	?	+
Labetalol‡	0	+ ?	0	↔	↓	↓ ↔	↓	↓ ↓	↓ ↔	+
Metoprolol	+ +	0	0	↓	↓	↓	↓	↓	↓	+
Nadolol	0	0	0	↓	↓	↓	↓	↓	↓	+
Oxprenolol	0	+	+	↓ ↔	↓	↓ ↔	↓	↓	↓ ↔	+
Pindolol	0	+ +	0	↓ ↔	↓	↓ ↔	↓	↓	↓ ↔	+
Propranolol	0	0	+ +	↓	↓	↓	↓	↓	↓	+
Sotalol	0	0	0	↓	↓	↓	↓	↓	↓	+
Timolol	0	0	0	↓	↓	↓	↓	↓	↓	+
Isomer										
D-Propranolol	0	0	+ +	↔	↔	↔ ↓ †	↔	↔	↔ ↓ †	+ +

*Beta$_1$-selectivity is only seen with low therapeutic drug concentrations. With higher concentrations, beta$_1$ selectivity is not seen.
†Effects of D-propranolol occur with doses in humans well above the therapeutic level. The isomer also lacks beta-blocking activity.
‡Labetalol has additional alpha-adrenergic blocking properties and direct vasodilatory activity.
+ + = Strong effect; + = modest effect; 0 = absent effect.
↑ = Elevation; ↓ = reduction; ↔ = no change.
Source: Frishman, W. H.: "Clinical Pharmacology of the Beta-Adrenoceptor Blocking Drugs," 2d ed., Appleton-Century Crofts, Inc., Norwalk, 1984, p. 32. Reproduced with permission from the publisher and author. Also, Frishman, W. H.: The Beta-Adrenergic Blocking Drugs, *Int. J. Cardiol.*, 2:167, 1982. Adapted and reproduced with permission from the publisher and author.

metoprolol, propranolol) enter the central nervous system in high concentrations, a direct antihypertensive effect mediated by their presence is not well defined. Also, those beta blockers which are less lipid-soluble, and less likely to concentrate in the brain, appear to be as effective in lowering blood pressure as propranolol.[21,22]

Peripheral Resistance Nonselective beta blockers have no primary action in lowering peripheral resistance and, indeed, may cause it to rise by leaving unopposed the alpha-stimulatory mechanisms.[62] The vasodilating effect of catecholamines on skeletal muscle blood vessels is beta$_2$-mediated, suggesting possible therapeutic advantages in using beta$_1$-selective blockers, agents with partial agonist activity, and drugs with alpha-blocking activity. Since beta$_1$-selectivity diminishes as the drug dosage is raised, and since hypertensive patients generally have to be given far larger doses than are required simply to block the beta$_1$-receptors alone, beta$_1$-selectivity[63] offers the clinician little if any real specific advantage in antihypertensive treatment.[20,63]

Effects on Prejunctional Beta Receptors Apart from their effects on postjunctional tissue beta receptors, it is believed that blockade of prejunctional beta receptors may be involved in the hemodynamic actions of beta-blocking drugs. Stimulation of prejunctional alpha$_2$ receptors leads to a reduction in the quantity of norepinephrine released by the postganglionic sympathetic fibers.[64,65] Conversely, stimulation of prejunctional beta receptors is followed by an increase in the quantity of norepinephrine released by postganglionic sympathetic fibers.[66–68] Blockade of the prejunctional beta receptors should, therefore, diminish the amount of norepinephrine released, leading to a weaker stimulation of postjunctional alpha receptors, an effect which would produce less vasoconstriction. Opinions differ, however, on the contributions of presynaptic beta blockade to both a reduction in the peripheral vascular resistance and the antihypertensive effects of beta-blocking drugs.

Other Proposed Mechanisms Less well documented effects of beta blockers that may possibly contribute to their antihypertensive actions are: favorable effects on venous tone and plasma volume,[2] membrane-stabilizing activity,[69,70] and resetting of baroreceptors.[71]

Effects in Angina Pectoris

Ahlquist[11] demonstrated that sympathetic innervation of the heart causes the release of norepinephrine-activating beta-adrenoreceptors in myocardial cells (Table 90-7). This adrenergic stimulation causes an increment in heart rate, isometric contractile force, and maximal velocity of muscle fiber shortening, all of which lead to an increase in cardiac work and myocardial oxygen consumption.[72] The decrease in intraventricular pressure and volume caused by the sympathetic mediated enhancement of cardiac contractility tends, on the other hand, to reduce myocardial oxygen consumption by reducing myocardial wall tension (law of LaPlace).[73] Although there is a net increase in myocardial oxygen demand, this is normally balanced by an increase in coronary blood flow. Angina pectoris is felt to occur when oxygen demand exceeds supply, i.e., when coronary blood flow is restricted by coronary atherosclerosis. Since the conditions which precipitate anginal attacks (exercise, emotional stress, food, etc.) cause an increase in cardiac sympathetic activity, it might be expected that blockade of cardiac beta adrenoreceptors would relieve the symptoms of the anginal syndrome. It is on this basis that the early clinical studies with beta-blocking drugs in angina were initiated.[74]

Three main factors—heart rate, ventricular systolic pressure, and the size of the left ventricle—contribute to the myocardial oxygen requirements of the left ventricle. Of these, heart rate and systolic pressure appear to be the most important (heart rate times systolic blood pressure product is a reliable index to predict the precipitation of angina in a given patient).[75,76]

The reduction in heart rate effected by beta blockade has two favorable consequences: (1) decrease in blood pressure, thereby reducing myocardial oxygen needs; and (2) a longer diastolic filling time associated with a slower heart rate, allowing for increased coronary perfusion. Beta blockade also reduces exercise-induced blood pressure increments, the velocity of cardiac contraction, and oxygen consumption at any patient workload.[75,76]

Studies in dogs have shown propranolol to cause a decrease in coronary blood flow.[77] However, subsequent experimental animal studies demonstrated beta-blocking-induced shunting to occur in the coronary circulation, maintaining blood flow to ischemic areas, especially in the subendocardial region.[78] In humans, concomitant with the decrease in myocardial oxygen consumption, beta blockers can cause a reduction in coronary blood flow and a rise in coronary vascular resistance.[79] However, on the basis of coronary autoregulation, the overall reduction in myocardial oxygen needs with beta blockers may be sufficient cause for this decrease in coronary blood flow.[75,76]

Virtually all beta blockers, whether or not they have partial agonist activity, alpha-blocking effects, membrane-stabilizing activity, general or selective beta-blocking properties, produce some degree of increased work capacity without pain in patients with angina pectoris. Therefore, it must be concluded that this results from their common property; blockade of cardiac beta receptors.[75] Both D- and L-propranolol have membrane-stabilizing activity, but only L-propranolol has significant beta-blocking activity. The racemic mixture (D- and L-propranolol) causes a decrease in both heart rate and force of contraction in dogs, while the D-isomer has hardly any effect.[80] In humans, D-propranolol, which has "membrane" activity but no beta-blocking properties, has been found to be ineffective in relieving angina pectoris, even with very high doses.[81]

Although exercise tolerance improves with beta blockade, the increments in heart rate and blood pressure with exercise are blunted, the rate-pressure product (systolic blood pressure times heart rate) achieved when pain occurs is less than that reached during a control run.[82] The depressed pressure-rate product at the onset of pain (about 20 percent reduction from control) is reported to occur with various beta-blocking drugs, probably related to decreased cardiac output. Thus, although there is increased exercise tolerance with beta blockade, patients exercise less than might be expected. This might also relate to the action of beta blockers to increase left ventricular size, causing increased left ventricular wall tension and an increase in oxygen consumption at a given blood pressure.[83]

Combined Use of Beta Blockers with Other Antianginal Therapies in Angina Pectoris

Nitrates Combined therapy with nitrates and beta blockers may be more efficacious for treating angina pectoris than either drug alone.[75,84] The primary effects of beta blockers are to reduce both resting heart rate and heart rate response to exercise. Since nitrates produce a reflex increase in heart rate owing to a reduction in arterial pressure, concomitant beta-blocker therapy will be extremely effective because it will block this reflex heart rate increment. Similarly, the preservation of diastolic coronary flow with a reduced heart rate will also be beneficial.[75] In patients with a propensity for myocardial failure who might have a slight increase in heart size with the beta blockers, the nitrates will counteract this tendency by reducing heart size due to its peripheral venodilatory effects. During the administration of nitrates, the reflex increase in contractility that is mediated through the sympathetic nervous system will be checked by the presence of beta blockers. Similarly, the increase in coronary resistance associated with beta-blocker administration can be ameliorated by the administration of nitrates.[75]

Calcium-Entry Blockers Calcium-entry blockers are a new group of antianginal drugs that block transmembrane calcium currents in vascular smooth muscle to cause arterial vasodilation (see Chapter 91). Some calcium-entry blockers (diltiazem, verapamil) will also slow the heart rate and reduce atrioventricular conduction. Combined therapy with beta-adrenergic and calcium-entry blockers can provide clinical benefits for patients with angina pectoris who remain symptomatic with either agent used alone.[75] Because adverse cardiovascular effects can occur, however, patients being considered for such treatment need to be carefully selected and observed.[75]

Angina at Rest and Vasospastic Angina

Clinical studies of beta-blocker therapy for angina at rest have been largely uncontrolled, with the rationale being that the pathogenesis of chest pain at rest is similar to that with exertion. However, angina pectoris can be caused by multiple mechanisms and coronary vasospasm appears responsible for ischemia in a significant proportion of patients with angina at rest.[75,85] Therefore, beta blockers that primarily reduce myocardial oxygen consumption, but fail to exert vasodilating effects on the coronary vasculature, may not be totally effective in patients in whom angina is caused or further increased by dynamic alterations in coronary luminal diameter.[75,86] Despite their theoretical dangers in rest and vasospastic angina, beta blockers have been successfully used alone and in combination with vasodilating agents in many patients.[75]

Antiarrhythmic Effects

Electrophysiologic Effects Beta-adrenoceptor blocking drugs have two main effects on the electrophysiologic properties of specialized cardiac tissue (Table 90-8).[2] The first results from specific blockade of adrenergic stimulation of cardiac pacemaker potentials. In concentrations causing significant inhibition of adrenergic receptors, the beta blockers produce little change in the transmembrane potentials of cardiac muscle. However, by competitively inhibiting adrenergic stimulation, beta blockers decrease the slope of phase 4 depolarization and the spontaneous firing rate of sinus or ectopic pacemakers, and thus decrease automaticity. Arrhythmias occurring in the setting of enhanced automaticity as seen in myocardial infarction, digitalis toxicity, hyperthyroidism, and pheochromocytoma, would therefore be expected to respond well to beta blockade.[2,87]

The second electrophysiologic effect of beta blockers is one of membrane-stabilizing action, also known as the "quinidine-like" or "local anesthetic" action, which is only observed at very high dose levels. This property is unrelated to inhibition of catecholamine action and is possessed equally by both the D- and L-isomers of the drugs (D-isomers have almost no beta-blocking activity).[87] Characteristic of this effect is a reduction in the rate of rise of the intracardial action potential without affecting the spike duration of the resting potential.[86] Associated features include an elevated electrical threshold of excitability, delay in conduction velocity, and a significant increase in the effective refractory period. This effect and its attendant changes have been explained by an inhibition of the depolarizing inward sodium current.[87]

TABLE 90-8 Antiarrhythmic Properties for Beta Blockers

Beta blockade
- Electrophysiology: depress excitability; depress conduction
- Prevention of ischemia: decrease automaticity; inhibit reentrant mechanisms

Membrane-stabilizing effects
- Local anesthetic, "quinidine-like" properties: depress excitability; prolong refractory period; delay conduction
- Clinically—probably not significant

Special pharmacologic properties (beta-cardioselectivity, intrinsic sympathomimetic activity) do not appear to contribute to antiarrhythmic effectiveness

Source: Frishman, W. H.: "Clinical Pharmacology of the Beta-Adrenoceptor Blocking Drugs," 2d ed., Appleton-Century-Crofts, Inc., Norwalk, 1984. p. 341. Reproduced with permission from the publisher and author.

Sotalol is unique among the beta blockers in that it alone possesses class III antiarrhythmic properties, causing prolongation of the action-potential period and thereby delaying repolarization.[2] Clinical studies have verified the efficacy of sotalol in control of arrhythmias,[88] but additional investigation will be required to determine whether its class III antiarrhythmic properties contribute significantly to its efficacy as an antiarrhythmic agent.

The most important mechanism underlying the antiarrhythmic effect of beta blockers (with the possible exclusion of sotalol) is felt to be beta blockade with resultant inhibition of pacemaker potentials. The contribution of membrane-stabilizing action does not appear to be clinically significant. In vitro experiments with human ventricular muscle have shown that the concentration of propranolol required for membrane stabilization is 50 to 100 times the concentration usually associated with inhibition of exercise-induced tachycardia and at which only beta-blocking effects occur.[87] Moreover, D-propranolol, which possesses membrane-stabilizing properties but no beta-blocking action, is a weak antiarrhythmic event in high doses, while beta blockers devoid of membrane-stabilizing action (atenolol, metoprolol, nadolol, pindolol, etc.) have been shown to be effective antiarrhythmic drugs.[2] *All* beta blockers are similarly effective at comparable levels of beta blockade. No superiority of one beta-blocking agent over another in the therapy of arrhythmias has been convincingly demonstrated.[2] Differences in overall clinical usefulness are related to their other associated pharmacologic properties.[2]

Therapeutic Uses in Cardiac Arrhythmias Beta-adrenergic blocking drugs have become an important treatment modality for various cardiac arrhythmias (Table 90-9).[2] While it has long been acknowledged that beta blockers are more effective in treating supraventricular arrhythmias than ventricular arrhythmias, it has only been recently appreciated that this may not be the case. These agents can be quite useful in the treatment of ventricular tachyarrhythmias in the setting of myocardial ischemia, mitral valve prolapse, and other cardiovascular conditions.[1,89–91]

Effects in Survivors of Acute Myocardial Infarction

Beta-adrenergic blockers have beneficial effects on many determinants of myocardial ischemia (Table 90-10).[2,76,92] The results of placebo-controlled long-term trials with some beta-adrenergic blocking drugs in survivors of acute myocardial infarction have demonstrated a favorable effect on total mortality, cardiovascular mortality, including sudden and

TABLE 90-9 Effects of Beta Blockers in Various Arrhythmias

Arrhythmia	Comment
Supraventricular	
Sinus tachycardia	Treat underlying disorder; excellent response to beta blocker, if need to control rate (e.g., ischemia).
Atrial fibrillation	Beta-blockers reduce rate, rarely restore sinus rhythm. May be useful in combination with digoxin.
Atrial flutter	Beta-blockers reduce rate, sometimes restore sinus rhythm.
Atrial tachycardia	Effective in slowing ventricular rate, may restore sinus rhythm. Useful in prophylaxis.
Ventricular	
PVCs	Good response to beta blockers (as effective as quinidine), especially digitalis-induced, exercise (ischemia)-induced, mitral valve prolapse, or hypertrophic cardiomyopathy.
Ventricular tachycardia	Effective as quinidine, most effective in digitalis toxicity or exercise (ischemia)-induced.
Ventricular fibrillation	Electrical defibrillation is treatment of choice. Beta blockers can be used to prevent recurrence in cases of excess digitalis or sympathomimetic amines. Appear to be effective in reducing the incidence of ventricular fibrillation and sudden death postmyocardial infarction.

Source: Frishman, W. H.: "Clinical Pharmacology of the Beta-Adrenoceptor Blocking Drugs," 2d ed., Appleton-Century-Crofts, Inc., 1984, p. 100. Reproduced with permission from the publisher and author.

TABLE 90-10 Possible Mechanisms by Which Beta Blockers Protect the Ischemic Myocardium

- Reduction in myocardial oxygen consumption
  - Reduction in heart rate, blood pressure, and myocardial contractility
- Augmentation of coronary blood flow
  - Increase in diastolic perfusion time by reducing heart rate
  - Augmentation of collateral blood flow
  - Redistribution of blood flow to ischemic areas
- Alterations in myocardial substrate utilization
- Decrease in microvascular damage
- Stabilization of cell and lysosomal membranes
- Shift of oxyhemoglobin dissociation curve to the right
- Inhibition of platelet aggregation

Source: Frishman, W. H.: "Clinical Pharmacology of the Beta-Adrenoceptor Blocking Drugs," 2d ed., Appleton-Century-Crofts, Inc., Norwalk, 1984, p. 306. Reproduced with permission from the publisher and author. Also, Braunwald, E., Muller, J. E., Kloner, R. A., and Maroko, P. R.: Role of Beta-Adrenergic Blockade in the Therapy of Patients with Myocardial Infarction, *Am. J. Med.*, 74:113, 1983. Reproduced with permission from the publisher and author.

nonsudden cardiac deaths, and on the incidence of nonfatal reinfarction. These beneficial results with beta-blocker therapy can be explained by both the antiarrhythmic (Table 90-9) and anti-ischemic effects of these drugs.[76,89,93] Two nonselective beta blockers, propranolol and timolol, and metoprolol, a beta$_1$-selective blocker, are approved by the Food and Drug Administration for this use when started 3 to 28 days postinfarction. Beta blockers have also been suggested as a treatment for reducing the extent of myocardial injury and mortality during the hyperacute phase of myocardial infarction,[40,94] but their role in this situation still remains unclear.[6,95]

Other Cardiovascular Applications

Although beta blockers have been studied extensively in patients with angina pectoris, arrhythmias, and hypertension, they have also been shown to be safe and effective for other cardiovascular conditions (Table 90-4). Some of these conditions are described below.

Hypertrophic Cardiomyopathy Beta-adrenoceptor blocking drugs have been proved to be efficacious in the therapy of patients with hypertrophic cardiomyopathy or idiopathic hypertrophic subaortic stenosis (IHSS).[43,96] These drugs are useful in controlling the symptoms: dyspnea, angina, and syncope.[2] Beta blockers have also been shown to lower the intraventricular pressure gradient, both at rest and with exercise.

The outflow pressure gradient is not the only abnormality in hypertrophic cardiomyopathy; more important is the loss of ventricular compliance which impedes normal left ventricular functioning. It has been shown by invasive and noninvasive methods that propranolol can improve left ventricular function in this condition.[97] The drug also produces favorable changes in ventricular compliance while it relieves patient symptoms. Propranolol is approved for this condition and may be combined with the calcium channel blocker verapamil in patients not responding to the beta blocker alone.

The salutary hemodynamic and symptomatic effects produced by propranolol derive from its inhibition of sympathetic stimulation to the heart.[98] However, there is no evidence that the drug alters the primary cardiomyopathic process; many patients remain in or return to their severely symptomatic state, and some die despite its administration.[43,96]

Mitral Valve Prolapse This auscultatory complex characterized by a nonejection systolic click, a late systolic murmur, or a midsystolic click followed by a late systolic murmur, has been studied extensively over the last 15 years.[99] Atypical chest pain, malignant arrhythmias, and nonspecific ST- and T-wave abnormalities have been observed with this condition. Beta-adrenergic blockers, by decreasing sympathetic tone, have been shown to be useful for relieving the chest pains and palpitations that many of these patients experience, and for reducing the incidence of life-threatening arrhythmias and other ECG abnormalities.[45]

Dissecting Aneurysms Beta-adrenergic blockade plays a major role in treating patients with acute aortic dissection. During the hyperacute phase, beta-blocking agents reduce the force and velocity of myocardial contraction (*dP/dt*) and hence, progression of the dissecting hematoma.[42] Moreover, such administration must be initiated simultaneously with the institution of other antihypertensive therapy that may cause reflex tachycardia and increases in cardiac output, factors which could aggravate the dissection process. Initially, propranolol is administered intravenously to reduce the heart rate below 60 beats per minute. Once a patient is stabilized and long-term medical management is contemplated, the patient should be maintained on oral beta-blocker therapy to prevent recurrence.[100]

Recently, it has been demonstrated that long-term beta-blocker therapy might also reduce the risk of dissection in patients prone to this complication (e.g., those with Marfan's syndrome). Systolic time intervals are used to assess the adequacy of beta blockade in children with Marfan's syndrome.

Tetralogy of Fallot By reducing the effects of increased adrenergic tone on the right ventricular infundibulum in tetralogy of Fallot, beta blockers have been shown to be useful for the treatment of severe hypoxic spells and hypercyanotic attacks.[47] With chronic use, the drugs have also been shown to prevent prolonged hypoxic spells.[47] These drugs should only be looked at as palliative, and definitive surgical repair of this condition is usually required.

QT Interval Prolongation Syndromes The syndrome of ECG QT interval prolongation is usually a congenital condition associated with deafness, syncope, and sudden death.[46] Abnormalities in sympathetic nervous system functioning in the heart have been proposed as explanations for the electrophysiologic aberrations seen in these patients.[46] Propranolol appears to be the most effective drug for treatment of this syndrome. It reduces the frequency of syncopal episodes in the majority of patients, and may prevent sudden death.[46] The drug will reduce the ECG QT interval.

Noncardiovascular Applications Beta-adrenergic receptors are ubiquitous in the human body, and their blockade affects a variety of organ and metabolic systems (Table 90-11).[2] Some noncardiovascular uses of beta blockers (glaucoma, migraine headache prophylaxis) are approved by the Food and Drug Administration.[1]

Adverse Effects of Beta Blockers

Evaluation of adverse effects is complex due to the use of different definitions of side effects, the kinds of patients studied, study design features, and different methods of ascertaining and reporting adverse side effects from study to study.[101] Overall, the types and frequencies of adverse effects attributed to various beta-blocker compounds appear similar.[102] The side effect profiles resemble those seen with concurrent placebo treatments, attesting to the remarkable safety margin of the beta blockers.[4,101]

Adverse effects fall in two categories: (1) those from known pharmacologic consequences of beta-

TABLE 90-11 Pharmacodynamic Properties and Noncardiac Effects of Beta-Adrenoceptor Blockers

Drug	Relative $Beta_1$ Selectivity*	Partial Agonist Activity	Membrane-Stabilizing Activity	Bronchial Tone	Platelet Aggregability	Plasma Renin Activity	Peripheral Vascular Resistance	RBF	GFR	HDL-CHOL	LDL-CHOL	VLDL-TRI
Acebutolol	+	+	+	↑↔↓		↓↔	↑↔	↓↔	↓↔	↔	↔	↔
Atenolol	+ +	0	0	↑↔↓		↓↔	↑↔	↓↔	↓↔	↔	↔	↔
Labetalol‡	0	+?	0	↑↔↓	↔	↓↔	↓	↔↑	↔	↔	↔	↔
Metoprolol	+ +	+ +	0	↑↔↓		↓↔	↑↔	↓↔	↓↔	↔↓	↔	↑↔
Nadolol	0	0	0	↔↓		↓↔	↑	↑	↑	?	?	?
Oxprenolol	0	+	+	↑↔↓	↓	↓↔	↑↔	↓↔	↓↔	?	?	?
Pindolol	0	+ +	0	↑↔↓	↓	↓↔↑	↔↓	↓↔	↓↔	↔	↔	↔
Propranolol	0	0	+ +	↔↓	↓	↓	↑	↓	↓	↓	↔	↑
Sotalol	0	0	0	↔↓		↓	↑	↓	↓	?	?	?
Timolol	0	0	0	↔↓	↓	↓	↑	↓	↓	?	?	?
Isomer												
D-Propranolol	0	0	+ +	↔	↓	↔	↔	↔	↔	?	?	?

*$Beta_1$ selectivity is only seen with low therapeutic drug concentrations. With higher concentrations, $Beta_1$ selectivity is not seen.
‡Labetalol has additional alpha-adrenergic blocking properties and direct vasodilatory activity.
+ + = Strong effect; + = modest effect; 0 = absent effect; ↑ = elevation; ↓ = reduction; ↔ = no change.
RBF = renal blood flow; GFR = glomerular filtration rate; HDL-CHOL = high-density lipoprotein cholesterol; LDL-CHOL = low-density lipoprotein cholesterol; VLDL-TRI = very low density lipoprotein triglycerides.
Source: Frishman, W. H.: "Clinical Pharmacology of the Beta-Adrenoceptor Blocking Drugs," 2d ed., Appleton-Century-Crofts, Inc., 1984, p. 36, 37. Reproduced with permission from the publisher and author.

adrenoceptor blockade; and (2) other reactions apart from beta-adrenoreceptor blockade.

The first type includes asthma, heart failure, hypoglycemia, bradycardia and heart block, intermittent claudication, and Raynaud's phenomenon. The incidence of these adverse effects varies with the beta blocker used.[2,101]

Side effects of the second category are rare. They include an unusual oculomucocutaneous reaction and the possibility of carcinogenesis.[2,101]

Adverse Cardiac Effects Related to Beta-Adrenoceptor Blockade

Congestive Heart Failure

Blockade of beta-receptors may cause congestive heart failure in an enlarged heart with impaired myocardial function where excessive sympathetic drive is essential to maintain the myocardium on a compensated Starling curve, and where left ventricular stroke volume is restricted and tachycardia is needed to maintain cardiac output.

Thus, any beta-blocking drug may be associated with the development of heart failure. Furthermore, heart failure may also be augmented by increases in peripheral vascular resistance produced by nonselective agents (e.g., propranolol, timolol, sotalol).[103] It has been claimed that beta blockers with intrinsic sympathomimetic activity are better in preserving left ventricular function and less likely to precipitate heart failure,[104] but there have been limited *in vivo* studies in humans to support this contention.[29]

In patients with impaired myocardial function who require beta-blocking agents, digitalis and diuretics can be used.

Sinus Node Dysfunction and Atrioventricular Conduction Delay

Slowing of the resting heart rate is a normal response to treatment with beta-blocking drugs with and without intrinsic sympathomimetic activity. Healthy individuals can sustain a heart rate of 40 to 50 without disability, unless there is clinical evidence of heart failure.[26] Drugs with intrinsic sympathomimetic activity do not lower the resting heart rate to the same degree as propranolol,[105] however, all beta-blocking drugs are contraindicated (unless an artificial pacemaker is present) in patients with the sick sinus syndrome.[86]

If there is a partial or complete atrioventricular conduction defect, use of a beta-blocking drug may lead to a serious bradyarrhythmia.[26] The risk of atrioventricular impairment may be less with beta blockers having intrinsic sympathomimetic activity.[106]

Overdosage

Suicide attempts and accidental overdosing with beta blockers are being described with increasing frequency. Since beta-adrenergic blockers are competitive pharmacologic antagonists, their life-threatening effects (bradycardia, myocardial and ventilatory failure) can be overcome with an immediate infusion of beta-agonist agents such as isoproterenol and dobutamine.[28] In situations where catecholamines are not effective, intravenous glucagon has been used.[28]

Close monitoring of cardiorespiratory function is necessary for at least 24 h after the patient responds to therapy. Patients who recover will usually have no long-term sequelae; however, they should be observed for the cardiac signs of sudden beta-blocker withdrawal.[28]

Beta-Adrenoceptor Blocker Withdrawal

Following abrupt cessation of chronic beta-blocker therapy, exacerbation of angina pectoris and, in some cases, acute myocardial infarction and death have been reported.[107–109]

Observations made in multiple double-blind randomized trials have confirmed the reality of a propranolol withdrawal reaction.[107–110] The exact mechanism for the propranolol withdrawal reaction is unclear. There is some evidence that the withdrawal phenomenon may be due to the generation of additional beta-adrenoceptors during the period of beta-adrenoceptor blockade. When the beta-adrenoceptor blocker is then withdrawn, the increased beta-receptor population readily results in excessive beta-receptor stimulation which will be clinically important when the delivery and use of oxygen is finely balanced, as occurs in ischemic heart disease. Other suggested mechanisms for the withdrawal reaction include heightened platelet aggregability,[109] an elevation in thyroid hormone activity,[111] and an increase in circulating catecholamines.[112]

Adverse Noncardiac Side Effects Related to Beta-Adrenoreceptor Blockade

Effect on Ventilatory Function

The bronchodilator effects of catecholamines on the bronchial $beta_2$-adrenoreceptors are inhibited by nonselective beta blockers (e.g., propranolol, nadolol).[113] Beta-blocking compounds with partial agonist activity,[23] $beta_1$ selectivity,[20,21] and alpha-adrenergic blocking actions[114] are less likely to increase airways resistance in asthmatics. $Beta_1$ selectivity, however, is not absolute, and may be lost with high therapeutic doses as shown with atenolol and metoprolol. It is possible in asthma to use a $beta_2$-selective agonist (such as albuterol) in certain patients with concomitant low-dose $beta_1$-selective blocker treatment.[115] In general, all beta blockers should be avoided in patients with bronchospastic disease.

Peripheral Vascular Effects (Raynaud's Phenomenon)

Cold extremities and absent pulses have been reported to occur more frequently in patients receiving beta blockers for hypertension, compared to treatment with methyldopa.[32] Among the beta blockers, the incidence was highest with propranolol and lower with drugs having $beta_1$ selectivity or intrinsic sympathomimetic activity. In some instances, vascular compromise has been severe enough to cause cyanosis and impending gangrene.[116] This is probaby due to the reduction in cardiac output and blockade of $beta_2$-adrenoceptor mediated skeletal muscle vasodilation, resulting in unopposed alpha-adrenoceptor vasoconstriction.[117] Beta-blocking drugs with $beta_1$ selectivity or partial agonist activity will not affect peripheral vessels to the same degree as propranolol.

Raynaud's phenomenon is one of the more common side effects of propranolol treatment.[118] It is more troublesome with propranolol than metoprolol, atenolol, or pindolol, probably due to the $beta_2$-blocking properties of propranolol.

Patients with peripheral vascular disease who suffer from intermittent claudication often report worsening of the claudication when treated with beta-blocking drugs.[119] Whether drugs with $beta_1$ selectivity or partial agonist activity can protect against this adverse reaction has yet to be determined.

TABLE 90-12 Drug Interactions That May Occur with Beta-Adrenoceptor Blocking Drugs

Drug	Possible Effects	Precautions
Aluminum hydroxide gel	Decreases beta-blocker absorption and therapeutic effect	Avoid beta blocker–aluminum hydroxide combination.
Aminophylline	Mutual inhibition	Observe patient's response.
Antidiabetic agents	Enhanced hypoglycemia: hypertension	Monitor for altered diabetic response.
Calcium channel inhibitors (e.g., verapamil, diltiazem)	Potentiation of bradycardia, myocardial depression, and hypotension	Avoid use, although few patients show ill effects.
Cimetidine	Prolongs half-life of propranolol	Combination should be used with caution.
Clonidine	Hypertension during clonidine withdrawal	Monitor for hypertensive response; withdraw beta blocker before withdrawing clonidine.
Digitalis glycosides	Potentiation of bradycardia	Observe patient's response; interactions may benefit angina patients with abnormal ventricular function.
Epinephrine	Hypertension; bradycardia	Administer epinephrine cautiously; cardioselective beta blocker may be safer.
Ergot alkaloids	Excessive vasoconstriction	Observe patient's response; few patients show ill effects.
Glucagon	Inhibition of hyperglycemic effect	Monitor for reduced response.
Halofenate	Reduced beta-blocking activity; production of propranolol withdrawal rebound syndrome	Observe for impaired response to beta blockade.
Indomethacin	Inhibition of antihypertensive response to beta blockade	Observe patient's response.
Isoproterenol	Mutual inhibition	Avoid concurrent use or choose cardiac selective beta blocker.
Levodopa	Antagonism of levodopa's hypotensive and positive inotropic effects	Monitor for altered response; interaction may have favorable results.
Lidocaine	Propranolol pretreatment increases lidocaine blood levels and potential toxicity	Combination should be used with caution; use lower doses of lidocaine.
Methyldopa	Hypertension during stress	Monitor for hypertensive episodes.
Monoamine oxidase inhibitors	Uncertain, theoretical	Manufacturer of propranolol considers concurrent use contraindicated.
Phenothiazines	Additive hypotensive effects	Monitor for altered response, especially with high doses of phenothiazine.
Phenylpropanolamine	Severe hypertensive reaction	Avoid use, especially in hypertension controlled by both methyldopa and beta blockers.
Phenytoin	Additive cardiac depressant effects	Administer IV phenytoin with great caution.
Quinidine	Additive cardiac depressant effects	Observe patient's response; few patients show ill effects.
Reserpine	Excessive sympathetic blockade	Observe patient's response.
Tricyclic antidepressants	Inhibits negative inotropic and chronotropic effects of beta blockers	Observe patient's response.
Tubocurarine	Enhanced neuromuscular blockade	Observe response in surgical patients, especially after high doses of propranolol.

Source: Frishman, W. H.: "Clinical Pharmacology of the Beta-Adrenoceptor Blocking Drugs," 2d ed., Appleton-Century-Crofts, Inc., Norwalk, 1984, p. 160, 161. Reproduced with permission from the publisher and author. Also, Missri, J. C.: How Do Beta-Blockers Interact with Other Commonly Used Drugs? *Cardiovasc. Med.,* 8:668, 1983. Adapted and reproduced with permission from the publisher and author.

Hypoglycemia and Hyperglycemia

Several clinicians have described severe hypoglycemic reactions during therapy with beta-adrenergic blocking drugs.[120] Some of the patients affected were insulin-dependent diabetics, while others were nondiabetic. Studies of resting normal volunteers have demonstrated that propranolol produces no alteration in blood glucose values,[121] although the hyperglycemic response to exercise is blunted.

The enhancement of insulin-induced hypoglycemia and its hemodynamic consequences may be less with $beta_1$ selective agents (where there is no blocking effect on $beta_2$ receptors) and agents with intrinsic sympathomimetic activity (which may stimulate $beta_2$ receptors).[122]

There is also a marked diminution in the clinical manifestations of sympathetic discharge associated with hypoglycemia (tachycardia).[123] These findings suggest that beta blockers interfere with compensatory responses to hypoglycemia and can mask certain "warning signs" of this condition. Other hypoglycemic reactions, such as diaphoresis, are not affected by beta-adrenergic blockade.

Central Nervous System Effects

Dreams, hallucinations, insomnia, and depression can occur during therapy with beta blockers.[118,124] These symptoms are evidence of drug entry into the central nervous system (CNS) and are especially common with the highly lipid-soluble beta blockers (propranolol, metoprolol) which presumably penetrate the CNS better. It has been claimed that beta blockers with less lipid solubility (atenolol, nadolol) will cause fewer CNS side effects.[21,22] This claim is intriguing, but its validity must be corroborated with more extensive clinical experiences.

Miscellaneous Side Effects

Diarrhea, nausea, gastric pain, constipation, and flatulence have been seen occasionally with all beta blockers (2 to 11 percent of patients).[125]

Hematologic reactions are rare: rare cases of purpura[126] and agranulocytosis[127] have been described with propranolol.

A devastating blood pressure rebound effect has been described in patients who discontinued clonidine while being treated with nonselective beta-

TABLE 90-13 Clinical Situations That Would Influence the Choice of a Beta-Blocking Drug

Condition	Choice of Beta Blocker
Asthma, chronic bronchitis with bronchospasm	Avoid all beta blockers if possible; however, small doses of $beta_1$-selective blockers (e.g., acebutolol, atenolol, metoprolol) can be used. $Beta_1$ selectivity is lost with higher doses. Drugs with partial agonist activity (e.g., pindolol, oxprenolol) and labetalol with alpha-adrenergic blocking properties can also be used.
Congestive heart failure	Drugs with partial agonist activity and labetalol might have an advantage, although beta blockers are usually contraindicated.
Angina	In patients with angina at low heart rates, drugs with partial agonist activity probably contraindicated. Patients with angina at high heart rates but who have resting bradycardia might benefit from a drug with partial agonist activity. In vasospastic angina, labetalol may be useful; other beta blockers should be used with caution.
Atrioventricular conduction defects	Beta blockers generally contraindicated but drugs with partial agonist activity and labetalol can be tried with caution.
Bradycardia	Beta blockers with partial agonist activity and labetalol have less pulse-slowing effect and are preferable.
Raynaud's phenomenon, intermittent claudication, cold extremities	$Beta_1$-selective blocking agents, labetalol, and those with partial agonist activity might have an advantage.
Depression	Avoid propranolol. Substitute a beta blocker with partial agonist activity.
Diabetes mellitus	$Beta_1$-selective agents and partial agonist drugs are preferable.
Thyrotoxicosis	All agents will control symptoms but agents without partial agonist activity are preferred.
Pheochromocytoma	Avoid all beta blockers unless an alpha blocker is given. Labetalol may be used as a treatment of choice.
Renal failure	Use reduced doses of compounds largely eliminated by renal mechanisms (nadolol, sotalol, atenolol) and of those drugs whose bioavailability is increased in uremia (propranolol, alprenolol). Also consider possible accumulation of active metabolites (alprenolol, propranolol).
Insulin and sulphonylurea use	Danger of hypoglycemia. Possibly less using drugs with $beta_1$ selectivity.
Clonidine	Avoid sotalol (other nonselective beta blockers). Severe rebound effect with clonidine withdrawal.
Oculomucocutaneous syndrome	Stop drug. Substitute any other beta blocker.
Hyperlipidemia	Avoid nonselective beta blockers; use agents with partial agonism, $beta_1$ selectivity, or labetalol.

Source: Frishman, W. H.: "Clinical Pharmacology of the Beta-Adrenoceptor Blocking Drugs," 2d ed., Appleton-Century-Crofts, Inc., Norwalk, 1984, p. 162. Reproduced with permission from the publisher and author. Also, Frishman, W. H.: The Beta-Adrenoceptor Blocking Drugs, *Int. J. Cardiol.*, 2:173, 1982. Reproduced with permission from the publisher and author.

blocking agents. The mechanism for this may be related to an increase in circulating catecholamines and an increase in peripheral vascular resistance.[128] Whether $beta_1$-selective or partial agonist beta blockers have similar effects following clonidine withdrawal, remains to be determined. It has not been a problem with labetalol.[129]

Adverse Effects Unrelated to Beta-Adrenoceptor Blockade

Oculomucocutaneous Syndrome A characteristic immune reaction, the oculomucocutaneous syndrome, affecting singly or in combination eyes, mucous and serous membranes, and the skin, often in association with a positive antinuclear factor, has been reported in patients treated with practolol and has led to curtailment of its clinical use.[130] Close attention has been focused on this syndrome because of fears that other beta-adrenoreceptor blocking drugs may be associated with this syndrome. In 19 patients with such a reaction with practolol, the lesions healed after switching to atenolol treatment.[21]

Drug Interactions

Beta blockers are commonly employed and the list of commonly used drugs with which they interact is extensive (Table 90-12).[2,131,132] The majority of reported interactions have been associated with propranolol, the best studied of the beta blockers, and may not necessarily apply to other drugs in this class.

How to Choose a Beta Blocker

The various beta-blocking compounds given in adequate dosage appear to have comparable, antihypertensive, antiarrhythmic, and antianginal effects. Therefore, the beta-blocking drug of choice in an individual patient is determined by the pharmacodynamic and pharmacokinetic differences between the drugs, in conjunction with the patient's other medical conditions (Table 90-13).[2,19]

References

1. Frishman, W. H.: Beta-Adrenoceptor Antagonists: New Drugs and New Indications, *N. Engl. J. Med.*, 305:500, 1981.
2. Frishman, W. H.: "Clinical Pharmacology of the Beta-Adrenoceptor Blocking Drugs" (2d ed), Appleton-Century-Crofts Inc., Norwalk, 1984.
3. The Norwegian Multicenter Study Group: Timolol Induced Reduction in Mortality and Reinfarction in Patients Surviving Acute Myocardial Infarction, *N. Engl. J. Med.*, 304:801, 1981.
4. Beta-Blocker Heart Attack Trial Research Group: A Randomized Trial of Propranolol in Patients with Acute Myocardial Infarction. I. Mortality Results, *JAMA*, 247:1707, 1982.
5. Braunwald, E.: Treatment of the Patient after Myocardial Infarction, *N. Engl. J. Med.*, 302:290, 1980.
6. Frishman, W. H., Furberg, C. D., and Friedewald, W. T.: Beta-Adrenergic Blockade for Survivors of Acute Myocardial Infarction, *N. Engl. J. Med.*, 310:830, 1984.
7. Sutherland, E. W., Robinson, G. A., and Butcher, R. W.: Some Aspects of the Biological Role of Adenosine 3′5′-Monophosphate (Cyclic AMP), *Circulation*, 37:279, 1968.
8. Motulsky, H. J., and Insel, P. A.: Adrenergic Receptors in Man: Direct Identification, Physiologic Regulation, and Clinical Alterations, *N. Engl. J. Med.*, 307:18, 1982.
9. Lefkowitz, R. J., and Michel, T.: Plasma Membrane Receptors, *J. Clin. Invest.* 72(4):1185–1189, 1983.
10. Lefkowitz, R.: Direct Binding Studies of Adrenergic Receptors: Biochemical, Physiologic and Clinical Implications, *Ann. Intern. Med.*, 91:450, 1979.
11. Ahlquist, R. P.: A Study of Adenotropic Receptors, *Am. J. Physiol.*, 53:586, 1948.
12. Cerione, R. A., Strulovici, B., Benovic, J. L., Lefkowitz, R. J., and Caron, M. G.: Pure Beta-Adrenergic Receptor: The Single Polypepticle Confirms Catecholamine Responsiveness to Adenyl Cyclase, *Nature*, 306:562, 1983.
13. Glaubiger, G., and Lefkowitz, R. J.: Elevated Beta-Receptor Number after Chronic Propranolol Treatment, *Biochem. Biophys. Res. Commun.*, 78:720, 1977.
14. Shand, D. G., and Wood, A. J. J.: Propranolol Withdrawal Syndrome—Why? *Circulation*, 58:202, 1978.
15. Buhler, F. R., Bukart, F., Benno, L. E., King, M., Marbet, G., and Pfisterer, M.: Antihypertensive Beta-blocking Action as Related to Renin and Age. A Pharmacological Tool to Identify Pathogenic Mechanisms in Essential Hypertension, *Am. J. Cardiol.*, 36:653, 1975.
16. Bristow, M. R., Ginsberg, R., Minobe, W., et al.: Decreased Catecholamine Sensitivity and Beta-Adrenergic Receptor Density in Failing Human Hearts, *N. Engl. J. Med.*, 307:205, 1982.
17. Colucci, W. S., Alexander, R. W., Williams, G. H., et al.: Decreased Lymphocyte Beta-Adrenergic Receptor Density in Patients with Heart Failure and Tolerance to the Beta-Adrenergic Agonist Parbuterol, *N. Engl. J. Med.*, 305:185, 1981.
18. Frishman, W. H.: Clinical Pharmacology of the New Beta-Adrenergic Blocking Drugs. Part 13. The Beta-Adrenergic Blocking Drugs: A Perspective, *Am. Heart J.*, 99:665, 1980.
19. Frishman, W. H.: The Beta-Adrenoceptor Blocking Drugs. *Int. J. Cardiol.*, 2:165, 1982.
20. Koch-Weser, J.: Metoprolol, *N. Engl. J. Med.*, 301:698, 1979.
21. Frishman, W. H.: Atenolol and Timolol, Two New Systemic Beta-Adrenoceptor Antagonists, *N. Engl. J. Med.*, 306:1456, 1982.
22. Frishman, W. H.: Nadolol: A New Beta-Adrenoceptor Antagonist, *N. Engl. J. Med.*, 305:678, 1981.
23. Frishman, W. H.: Pindolol: A New Beta-Adrenoceptor Antagonist with Partial Agonist Activity, *N. Engl. J. Med.*, 308:940, 1983.
24. Frishman, W., and Silverman, R.: Clinical Pharmacology of the New Beta-Adrenergic Blocking Drugs. Part 3. Comparative Clinical Experience and New Therapeutic Applications, *Am. Heart J.*, 98:119, 1979.
25. Frishman, W.: Clinical Pharmacology of the New Beta-Adrenergic Blocking Drugs. Part 1. Pharmacokinetic and Pharmacodynamic Properties, *Am. Heart J.*, 98:663, 1979.
26. Conolly, M. E., Kersting, F., and Dollery, C. T.: The Clinical Pharmacology of Beta-Adrenoceptor Blocking Drugs. *Prog. Cardiovasc. Dis.*, 19:203, 1976.
27. Opie, L. H.: Drugs and the Heart. 1. Beta-Blocking Agents, *Lancet*, 1:693, 1980.
28. Frishman, W., Jacob, H., Eisenberg, E., and Ribner, H.: Clinical Pharmacology of the New Beta-Adrenergic Blocking Drugs. Part 8. Self-Poisoning with Beta-Adrenoceptor Blocking Drugs: Recognition and Management, *Am. Heart J.*, 98:798, 1979.
29. Taylor, S. H., Silke, B., and Lee, P. S.: Intravenous Beta-Blockade in Coronary Heart Disease: Is Cardioselectivity or Intrinsic Sympathomimetic Activity Hemodynamically Useful? *N. Engl. J. Med.*, 306:631, 1982.

30. Frishman, W., and Halprin, S.: Clinical Pharmacology of the New Beta-Adrenergic Blocking Drugs. Part 7. New Horizons in Beta-Adrenoceptor Blocking Therapy: Labetalol, *Am. Heart J.*, 98:660, 1979.
31. Frishman, W. H., Strom, J., Kirschner, M., et al.: Labetalol Therapy in Patients with Systemic Hypertension and Angina Pectoris: Effects of Combined Alpha- and Beta-Adrenergic Blockade, *Am. J. Cardiol.*, 48:917, 1981.
32. Waal-Manning, H. J.: Hypertension: Which Beta-Blocker? *Drugs*, 12:412, 1976.
33. Johnsson, G., and Regardh, C. G.: Clinical Pharmacokinetics of Beta-Adrenoceptor Blocking Drugs, *Clin. Pharmacokinet.*, 1:233, 1976.
34. Frishman, W. H., Teicher, M.: Long-acting Propranolol, *Cardiovasc. Rev. Rep.*, 4:1100, 1983.
35. Halkin, H., Vered, I., Saginer, A., and Rabinowitz, B.: Once-daily Administration of Sustained Release Propranolol Capsules in the Treatment of Angina Pectoris, *Eur. J. Clin. Pharmacol.*, 16:387, 1979.
36. Parker, J. O., Porter, A., and Parker, J. D.: Propranolol in Angina Pectoris: Comparison of Long-acting and Standard Formulation Propranolol, *Circulation*, 65:1351, 1982.
37. Zaroslinski, J., Borgman, R. J., O'Donnel, J. P., et al.: Ultra-short Acting Beta-Blockers: A Proposal for the Treatment of the Critically Ill Patient, *Life Sci.*, 31:899, 1982.
38. Gorczyski, R. J., Shaffer, J. E., Lee, R. J., and Vuong, A.: Pharmacology of ASL-8052, A Novel Beta-Adrenergic Receptor Antagonist with an Ultra-short Duration of Action, *J. Cardiovasc. Pharmacol.*, 5:668, 1983.
39. Murthy, V. S., Hwang, T. F., Zagar, M. E., et al.: Cardiovascular Pharmacology of ASL-8052. An Ultra-short-acting Beta-Blocker. *Eur. J. Pharmacol.*, 94:43, 1983.
40. Hjalmarson, Å., Ehnfeldt, D., Herlitz, J., et al.: Effect of Mortality of Metoprolol in Acute Myocardial Infarction, *Lancet*, 2:823, 1981.
41. Cohn, J. N.: Nitroprusside and Dissecting Aneurysms of Aorta, *N. Engl. J. Med.*, 295:567, 1976.
42. Wheat, M. W., Jr.: Treatment of Dissecting Aneurysms of the Aorta: Current Status, *Prog. Cardiovasc. Dis.*, 16:87, 1973.
43. Cohen, L. S., and Braunwald, E.: Amelioration of Angina Pectoris in Idiopathic Hypertrophic Subaortic Stenosis with Beta-Adrenergic Blockade, *Circulation*, 35:847, 1967.
44. Turner, J. R. B.: Propranolol in the Treatment of Digitalis-Induced and Digitalis-Resistant Tachycardia, *Am. J. Cardiol.*, 18:450, 1966.
45. Winkle, R. A., Lopes, M. G., Goodman, D. S., et al.: Propranolol for Patients with Mitral Valve Prolapse, *Am. Heart J.*, 93:422, 1970.
46. Vincent, G. M., Abildskov, J. A., and Burgess, M. J.: Q-T Interval Syndromes, *Prog. Cardiovasc. Dis.*, 16:523, 1974.
47. Shah, P. M., and Kidd, L.: Circulatory Effects of Propranolol in Children with Fallot's Tetralogy. Observations with Isoproterenol Infusion, Exercise and Crying, *Am. J. Cardiol.*, 19:653, 1967.
48. Meister, S. G., Engel, T. R., Feitosa, G. S., et al.: Propranolol in Mitral Stenosis During Sinus Rhythm, *Am. Heart J.*, 94:685, 1977.
49. Bhatia, M. L., Shrivastava, S., and Roy, S. G.: Immediate Haemodynamic Effects of a Beta-Adrenergic Blocking Agent—Propranolol—in Mitral Stenosis at Fixed Heart Rates, *Br. Heart J.*, 34:638, 1972.
50. Svedberg, K., Hjalmarson, A., and Waagstein, F.: Beneficial Effects of Long-Term Beta-Blockade in Congestive Cardiomyopathy, *Br. Heart J.*, 44:117, 1980.
51. Teuscher, A., Bossi, E., Imhof, P., et al.: Effect of Propranolol on Fetal Tachycardia in Diabetic Pregnancy, *Am. J. Cardiol.*, 42:304, 1978.
52. Furberg, C., and Morsing, C.: Adrenergic Beta-Receptor Blockade in Neurocirculatory Asthenia, *Pharmacologia Clinica*, 1:168, 1969.
53. Weber, R. B., and Reinmuth, O. M.: The Treatment of Migraine with Propranolol, *Neurology*, 22:366, 1972.
54. Young, R. R., Growdon, J. H., and Shahani, B. T.: Beta-Adrenergic Mechanisms in Action Tremor, *N. Engl. J. Med.*, 293:950, 1975.
55. Granville-Grossman, K. L., and Turner, P.: The Effect of Propranolol on Anxiety, *Lancet*, 1:788, 1966.
56. Sellers, E. M., Degani, N. C., Silm, D. H., and MacLeod, S. M.: Propranolol Decreased Noradrenaline Secretion and Alcohol Withdrawal, *Lancet*, 1:94, 1976.
57. Ingbar, S. H.: The Role of Antiadrenergic Agents in the Management of Thyrotoxicosis, *Cardiovasc. Rev. Rep.*, 2:683, 1981.
58. Caro, J. F., Castro, J. H., Glennon, J. A.: Effect of Long-term Propranolol Administration on Parathyroid Hormone and Calcium Concentration in Primary Hyperparathyroidism, *Ann. Intern. Med.*, 91:740, 1979.
59. Frohlich, E. D.: Hyperdynamic Circulation and Hypertension, *Postgrad. Med. J.*, 5:64, 1972.
60. Laragh, J. H.: Vasoconstriction-Volume Analysis for Understanding and Treating Hypertension: The Use of Renin and Aldosterone Profiles, *Am. J. Med.*, 55:261, 1973.
61. Myers, M. G., Lewis, P. J., Reid, J. L., and Dollery, C. T.: Brain Concentration of Propranolol in Relation to Hypotension Effects in the Rabbit with Observations on Brain Propranolol Levels in Man, *J. Pharmacol. Exp. Ther.*, 192:327, 1975.
62. Prichard, B. N. C.: Propranolol as an Antihypertensive Agent, *Am. Heart J.*, 79:128, 1970.
63. Imhof, P. R.: Characterization of Beta-Blockers as Antihypertensive Agents in the Light of Human Pharmacology Studies, in Schweizer, W. (ed.), "Beta-Blockers—Present Status and Future Prospects," Huber, Bern, 1974, pp. 40–50.
64. Langer, S. Z.: Presynaptic Receptors and their Role in the Regulation of Transmitter Release, *Br. J. Pharmacol.*, 60:481, 1977.
65. Berthelsen, S., and Pettinger, W. A.: A Functional Basis for Classification of Alpha-Adrenergic Receptors, *Life Sci.*, 21:77, 1977.
66. Yamaguchi, N., de Champlain, J., and Nadeau, R. L.: Regulation of Norepinephrine Release from Cardiac Sympathetic Fibers in the Dog by Presynaptic Alpha- and Beta-Receptors, *Circ. Res.*, 41:108, 1977.
67. Stjarne, L., and Brundin, J.: Beta-Adrenoceptors Facilitate Noradrenaline Secretion from Human Vasoconstrictor Nerves, *Acta. Physiol. Scand.*, 97:88, 1976.
68. Majewski, H. J., McCulloch, M. W., Rand, M. J., and Story, D. F.: Adrenaline Activation of Pre-junctional Beta-Adrenoceptors in Guinea Pig Atria, *Br. J. Pharmacol.*, 71:435, 1980.
69. Waal, H. J.: Hypotensive Action of Propranolol, *Clin. Pharmacol. Ther.*, 7:558, 1966.
70. Rahn, K. H., Hawlina, A., Kersting, F., and Planz, G.: Studies on the Antihypertensive Action of the Optical Isomers of Propranolol in Man, *Naunyn Schmiedebergs Arch. Pharmacol.*, 286:319, 1974.
71. Pickering, T. G., Gribbin, B., Peterson, E. S., et al.: Effects of Autonomic Blockade on the Baroreflex in Man at Rest and During Exercise, *Circ. Res.*, 30:177, 1972.
72. Sonnenblick, E. H., Ross, J., Jr., and Braunwald, E.: Oxygen Consumption of the Heart. Newer Concepts of its Multifactorial Determination, *Am. J. Cardiol.*, 22:328, 1968.
73. Sonnenblick, E. H., and Skelton, C. L.: Myocardial Energetics: Basic Principles and Clinical Implications, *N. Engl. J. Med.*, 285:668, 1971.
74. Black, J. W., and Stephenson, J. S.: Pharmacology of a New Adrenergic Beta-Receptor Blocking Compound (Nethalide), *Lancet*, 2:311, 1962.
75. Frishman, W. H.: Beta-Adrenergic Blockade in the Treatment of Coronary Artery Disease, in "Clinical Essays on the Heart" vol. 2, Hurst, J. W. (ed.), McGraw-Hill Book Co., Inc., New York, 1983, p. 25.
76. Frishman, W. H.: Multifactorial Actions of Beta-Adrenergic Blocking Drugs in Ischemic Heart Disease: Current Concepts, *Circulation*, 67(suppl. 1):11, 1983.
77. Parratt, J. R., and Grayson, J.: Myocardial Vascular Reactivity after Beta-Adrenergic Blockade, *Lancet*, 1:388, 1966.
78. Becker, L. C., Fortuin, N. J., and Pitt, B.: Effects of Ischemia and Antianginal Drugs on the Distribution of

Radioactive Microspheres in the Canine Left Ventricle, *Circ. Res.*, 28:263, 1971.
79. Wolfson, S., and Gorlin, R.: Cardiovascular Pharmacology of Propranolol in Man, *Circulation*, 40:501, 1969.
80. Barrett, A. M.: A Comparison of the Effect of (±) Propranolol and (+) Propranolol in Anesthetized Dogs: Beta-Receptor Blocking and Hemodynamic Action, *J. Pharm. Pharmacol.*, 21:241, 1969.
81. Bjorntorp, P.: Treatment of Angina Pectoris with Beta-Adrenergic Blockade, Mode of Action, *Acta Med. Scand.*, 184:259, 1968.
82. Gianelly, R. S., Goldman, R. H., Triester, B., and Harrison, D. C.: Propranolol in Patients with Angina Pectoris, *Ann. Intern. Med.*, 57:1216, 1967.
83. Robinson, B. F.: The Mode of Action of Beta-Antagonists in Angina Pectoris, *Postgrad. Med. J.*, 47(suppl. 2):451, 1971.
84. Parmley, W. W.: The Combination of Beta-Adrenergic Blocking Agents and Nitrates in the Treatment of Stable Angina Pectoris, *Cardiol. Rev. Rep.*, 3:1425, 1982.
85. Maseri, A., L'Abbate, A., Ballestra, A. M., et al.: Coronary Vasospasm in Angina Pectoris, *Lancet*, 1:713, 1977.
86. Parodi, O., Simonetti, I., L'Abbate, A., and Maseri, A.: Verapamil Versus Propranolol for Angina at Rest, *Am. J. Cardiol.*, 50:923, 1982.
87. Singh, B. N., and Jewitt, D. E.: β-Adrenoceptor Blocking Drugs in Cardiac Arrhythmias, in Avery, G. (ed.): "Cardiovascular Drugs," vol. 2, University Park Press, Baltimore, 1977 pp. 141–142.
88. Latour, Y., Dumont, G., Brousseau, A., and LeLorie, J.: Effects of Sotalol in Twenty Patients with Cardiac Arrhythmias, *Int. J. Clin. Pharmacol.*, 15:275, 1977.
89. Pratt, C., and Lichstein, E.: Ventricular Anti-arrhythmic Effects of Beta-Adrenergic Blocking Drugs: A Review of Mechanism and Clinical Studies, *J. Clin. Pharmacol.*, 22:335, 1982.
90. Rydén, L., Ariniego, R., Arnman, K., et al.: A Double-Blind Trial of Metoprolol in Acute Myocardial Infarction: Effects on Ventricular Tachyarrhythmias, *N. Engl. J. Med.*, 308:614, 1983.
91. Lichstein, E., Morganroth, J., Harrist, R., and Hubble, E.: Effect of Propranolol on Ventricular Arrhythmias—The Beta-Blockers: Preliminary Data from the Heart Attack Trial Experience, *Circulation*, 67(suppl. 1):I–32, 1983.
92. Braunwald, E., Muller, J. E., Kloner, R. A., and Maroko, P. R.: Role of Beta-Adrenergic Blockade in the Therapy of Patients with Myocardial Infarction, *Am. J. Med.*, 74:113, 1983.
93. Furberg, C. D., Hawkins, C. M., and Lichstein, E.: Effect of Propranolol in Post-Infarction Patients with Mechanical or Electrical Complications, *Circulation*, 69:761, 1984.
94. International Collaborative Study Group. Reduction of Infarct Size with the Early Use of Timolol in Acute Myocardial Infarction, *N. Engl. J. Med.*, 310:9, 1984.
95. Muller, J., Roberts, R., Stone, P., et al.: Failure of Propranolol Administration to Limit Infarct Size in Patients with Acute Myocardial Infarction, *Circulation*, 68(suppl. III):294, 1983, (Abstract.)
96. Swan, D. A., Bell, B., Oakley, C. M., and Goodwin, J.: Analysis of Symptomatic Course and Prognosis and Treatment of Hypertrophic Obstructive Cardiomyopathy, *Br. Heart J.*, 33:671, 1971.
97. Hubner, P. J. B, Ziady, G. M., Lane, G. K., et al.: Double-Blind Trial of Propranolol and Practolol in Hypertrophic Cardiomyopathy, *Br. Heart J.*, 35:1116, 1973.
98. Epstein, S. E., Henry, W. L., Clark, C. E., et al.: Asymmetric Septal Hypertrophy, *Ann. Intern. Med.*, 81:650, 1974.
99. Jeresaty, R. M.: Mitral Valve Prolapse Syndrome, *Prog. Cardiovasc. Dis.*, 15:623, 1973.
100. Slater, E. E., and DeSanctis, R.: Dissection of the Aorta, *Med. Clin. North Am.*, 63:141, 1979.
101. Friedman, L. M.: How do the Various Beta-Blockers Compare in Type, Frequency, and Severity of their Adverse Effects? *Circulation*, 67(suppl. I):89, 1983.
102. Frishman, W., Silverman, R., Strom, J., et al.: Clinical Pharmacology of the New β-Adrenoceptor Blocking Drugs. Part 4. Adverse Effects. Choosing a β-Adrenoceptor Blocker, *Am. Heart J.*, 98:256, 1979.
103. Vaughan Williams, E. M., Baywell, E. E., and Singh, B. N.: Cardiospecificity of Beta-Receptor Blockade. A Comparison of the Relative Potencies on Cardiac and Peripheral Vascular Beta-Adrenoceptors of Propranolol, of Practolol and its Ortho-Substituted Isomer and of Oxprenolol and its Para-Substituted Isomer, *Cardiovasc. Res.*, 7:226, 1973.
104. Frishman, W. H., and Kostis, J.: The Significance of Intrinsic Sympathomimetic Activity in β-Adrenoceptor Blocking Drugs, *Cardiovasc. Rev. Rep.*, 4:503, 1982.
105. Frishman, W., Kostis, J., Strom, J., et al.: Clinical Pharmacology of the New Beta-Adrenergic Blocking Drugs. Part 6. A Comparison of Pindolol and Propranolol in Treatment of Patients with Angina Pectoris. The Role of Intrinsic Sympathomimetic Activity, *Am. Heart J.*, 98:526, 1979.
106. Giudicelli, J. F., and Lhoste, F.: β-Adrenoceptor Blockade and Atrioventricular Conduction in Dogs. Role of Intrinsic Sympathomimetic Activity, *Br. J. Clin. Pharmacol.*, 13(suppl. 2):167, 1982.
107. Alderman, E. L., Coltart, D. J., Wettach, G. E., and Harrison, D. C.: Coronary Artery Syndromes after Sudden Propranolol Withdrawal, *Ann. Intern. Med.*, 81:925, 1974.
108. Miller, R. R., Olson, H. G., Amsterdam, E. A., and Mason, D. T.: Propranolol Withdrawal Rebound Phenomenon: Exacerbation of Coronary Events after Abrupt Cessation of Anti-anginal Therapy, *N. Engl. J. Med.*, 293:416, 1975.
109. Frishman, W. H., Christodoulou, J., and Weksler, B., et al.: Abrupt Propranolol Withdrawal in Angina Pectoris: Effects on Platelet Aggregation and Exercise Tolerance, *Am. Heart J.*, 95:169, 1978.
110. Frishman, W. H., Klein, N., Strom, J., et al.: Comparative Effects of Abrupt Propranolol and Verapamil Withdrawal in Angina Pectoris, *Am. J. Cardiol.*, 50:1191, 1982.
111. Kristensen, B. O., Steiness, E., and Weeke, J.: Propranolol Withdrawal and Thyroid Hormones in Patients with Essential Hypertension, *Clin. Pharmacol. Ther.*, 23:624, 1978.
112. Rangno, R., and Nattel, S.: Prevention of Propranolol Withdrawal Phenomena by Gradual Dose Reduction, *Clin. Res.*, 28:214A, 1980.
113. Dunlop, D., and Shanks, R. G.: Selective Blockade of Adrenoceptive Antagonist with Partial Agonist Activity, *N. Engl. J. Med.*, 308:940, 1983.
114. George, R. B., Manocha, K., Burford, J., et al.: Effects of Labetalol in Hypertensive Patients with Chronic Obstructive Pulmonary Disease, *Chest*, 83:457, 1983.
115. Benson, M. K., Berrill, W. T., Cruickshank, J. M., and Sterling, G. S.: A Comparison of Four Adrenoceptor Antagonists in Patients with Asthma, *Br. J. Clin. Pharmacol.*, 5:415, 1978.
116. Frohlich, E. D., Tarazi, R. C., and Dustan, H. P.: Peripheral Arterial Insufficiency: A Complication of Beta-Adrenergic Blocking Therapy, *JAMA*, 208:2471, 1969.
117. Lundvall, J., and Jarhult, J.: Beta-Adrenergic Dilator Component of the Sympathetic Vascular Response in Skeletal Muscle, *Acta Physiol. Scand.*, 96:180, 1976.
118. Simpson, F. O.: β-Adrenergic Receptor Blocking Drugs in Hypertension, *Drugs*, 7:85, 1974.
119. Rodger, J., Sheldon, C. D., Lerski, R. A., and Livingston, W. R.: Intermittent Claudication Complicating Beta-Blockade, *Br. Med. J.*, 1:1125, 1976.
120. Reveno, W. S., and Rosenbaum, H.: Propranolol Hypoglycemia, *Lancet*, 1:920, 1968.
121. Allison, S. P., Chamberlain, M. I., and Miller, J. E.: Effects of Propranolol on Blood Sugar, Insulin, and Free Fatty Acids, *Diabetologia*, 5:339, 1969.
122. Deacon, S. P., and Barnett, D.: Comparison of Atenolol and Propranolol during Insulin-Induced Hypoglycaemia, *Br. Med. J.*, 2:7, 1976.
123. Lloyd-Mostyn, R. H., and Oram, S.: Modification by Propranolol of Cardiovascular Effects of Induced Hypoglycaemia, *Lancet*, 2:1213, 1975.
124. Frishman, W. H., Razin, A., Swencionis, C., and Sonnenblick, E. H.: Beta-Adrenoceptor Blockade in Anxiety States:

A New Approach to Therapy? *Cardiovasc. Rev. Rep.*, 2:447, 1981.
125. Jacob, H., Brandt, L. J., Farkas, P., and Frishman, W.: Beta-Adrenergic Blockade and the Gastrointestinal System, *Am. J. Med.*, 74:1042, 1983.
126. Stephen, S. A.: Unwanted Effects of Propranolol. *Am. J. Cardiol.*, 18:463, 1966.
127. Nawabi, I. U., and Ritz, N. D.: Agranulocytosis Due to Propranolol, *JAMA*, 223:1376, 1973.
128. Bailey, R., and Neale, T. J.: Rapid Clonidine Withdrawal with Blood Pressure Overshoot Exaggerated by Beta-Blockade, *Br. Med. J.*, 1:942, 1976.
129. Agabiti-Rosei, E., Brown, J. J., Lever, A. F., et al.: Treatment of Phaeochromocytoma and Clonidine Withdrawal Hypertension with Labetalol, *Br. J. Clin. Pharmacol.*, 3(suppl.3):809, 1976.
130. Wright, P.: Untoward Effect Associated with Practolol Administration. Oculomucocutaneous Syndrome, *Br. Med. J.*, 1:595, 1975.
131. Missri, J. C.: How Do Beta-Blockers Interact with Other Commonly Used Drugs? *Cardiovasc. Med.*, 8:668, 1983.
132. Hansten, P.: "Drug Interactions," 4th ed., Lea & Febiger, Philadelphia, 1979, pp. 13–24.

91

Calcium Channel Blockers

William H. Frishman, M.D.

Edmund H. Sonnenblick, M.D.

The new group of compounds classified as calcium channel antagonists are a heterogeneous group of drugs with widely variable effects on heart muscle, sinus node function, atrioventricular (AV) conduction, peripheral blood vessels, and coronary circulation.[1,2] Three of these drugs, nifedipine, verapamil, and diltiazem, which have recently been approved in the United States, will be discussed here. Other drugs in this class, which include bepridil, gallopamil, lidoflazine, nicardipine, niludipine, nimodipine, nisoldipine, and nitrendipine, are now being evaluated.

Physiologic Background

The Calcium Channel Blockers: Basic Principles

Calcium ions play a fundamental role in the activation of cells. An influx of calcium ions into the cell through specific ion channels is required for myocardial contraction, for determining peripheral vascular resistance through calcium dependent-regulated tone of vascular smooth muscle, and for helping to initiate the pacemaker tissues of the heart, which are activated largely by the slow calcium current.[2]

The concept of calcium channel inhibition began in 1960 when it was noted that prenylamine, a newly developed coronary vasodilator, depressed cardiac performance in canine heart-lung preparations.[3] Initial studies with verapamil showed that it exerted a negative inotropic effect on the isolated myocardium in addition to its vasodilator properties.[4] These potent negative inotropic effects seemed to distinguish these drugs from the classical coronary vasodilators, such as nitroglycerin and papaverine, which are potent vasodilators, but have little if any myocardial depressant effect. Unlike beta-adrenergic antagonists, this new group of compounds depressed cardiac contractility without altering the height or contour of the monophasic action potential, and thus acted as uncouplers of excitation-contraction coupling.[5] Reversible closing of specific calcium ion channels in the membrane of the mammalian myocardial cell was suggested to explain the observed effects.[6]

Subsequently, the effects of verapamil on atrial and ventricular intracellular potentials were studied.[7] A classification of antiarrhythmic compounds was arrived at, of local anesthetics which decreased the maximum rate of depolarization, beta blockers, and a third class which prolonged the duration of the cardiac action potential.[8] However, none of these effects explained the antiarrhythmic effect of verapamil.[8] Thus, a fourth class of antiarrhythmic drug was proposed, typified by verapamil, with effects separate from those of sodium channel inhibitors and beta blockers.[7] The antiarrhythmic actions and negative inotropic effects of verapamil were suggested to act through interference with calcium conductance.[7]

Chemical Structure and Pharmacodynamics

Structure of the Calcium Channel Blockers

The structures of the three slow-channel blockers approved by the Food and Drug Administration are shown in Fig. 91-1. Diltiazem is a benzothiazepine derivative that is structurally unrelated to other vasodilators.[1] Nifedipine is a dihydropyridine deriv-

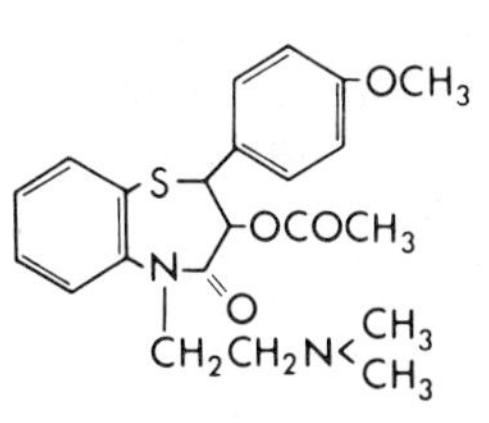

DILTIAZEM

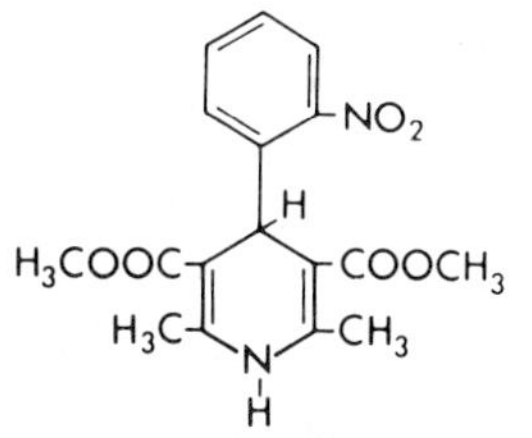

NIFEDIPINE

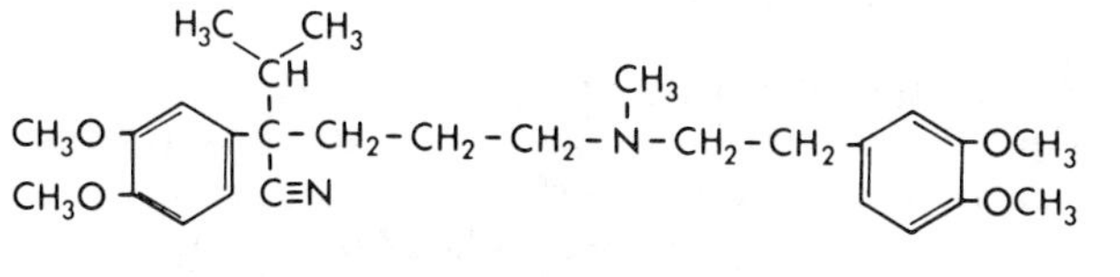

VERAPAMIL

FIGURE 91-1 Chemical structures of diltiazem (a benzothiazepine derivative), nifedipine (a dihydropyridine derivative), and verapamil (structurally similar to papaverine).

ative unrelated to the nitrates, and is lipophilic and inactivated by light.[1,9] Several other dihydropyridine derivatives (niludopine, nimodipine, nisoldipine, nitrendipine, and nicardipine) are now under investigation. Verapamil ({±} verapamil) has some structural similarity to papaverine.[1]

Differential Effects on Slow Channels

The predominant effect of calcium antagonist drugs is on the slow channels of the cell membrane. These calcium channels permit entry of some sodium in addition to calcium, and are activated much slower than the fast channels through which sodium predominantly enters to cause the initial rapid rise in the action potential.

Nifedipine has been shown to depress the slow inward calcium ion current in a dose-dependent manner in isolated cat papillary muscles under voltage clamp conditions. At concentrations of 10^{-7} to 10^{-5} *M*, there was no effect on the fast inward Na^+ current or on the rate of activation, inactivation, or recovery of the slow currents.[2,10–12] This action of nifedipine is similar to that of tetrodotoxin on the sodium channels and thus nifedipine is thought to "plug" the Ca^{2+} ion channels, leaving their control mechanisms unaffected, thus explaining its dose-dependent effect. However, further research is required to define the specific site of action of nifedipine.

Verapamil is a racemic mixture of the (R) (+)-enantiomer and the (S) (−)-enantiomer, each having different electrophysiologic effects.[1] The (+)-isomer depresses the maximal rate of rise of the action potential and has additional effects on the plateau phase and overall shape of the action potential. The (−)-isomer depresses the plateau phase of the action potential. Both of these effects are frequency-dependent, being much more pronounced at a stimulus rate of 90 per minute than at 15 per minute.[13] These effects are markedly enhanced by increasing the length of exposure to the drug.[14] In contrast to nifedipine, verapamil alters the kinetics of the slow channels, slowing both activation and, more markedly, recovery from inactivation.[15] The effects of verapamil are thus quite complex since it is a mixture of (+)- and (−)-enantiomers, each with different actions. The drug cannot be thought of as only a selective blocker of the slow inward current.[16]

Diltiazem lowers the plateau and shortens the duration of the action potential.[17] High concentrations also reduce the maximal rate of rise of the action potential, suggesting that diltiazem is primarily an inhibitor of the slow channel at low concentrations (2.2×10^{-6} *M*), but exerts fast (sodium) channel inhibitory effects at higher concentrations (2.2×10^{-5} *M*). It has been proposed that there are two sets of calcium channels: potential-operated channels and receptor-operated channels.[18] These two sets of channels are believed to exist because of their selective sensitivities to D-600 (a verapamil analog) and because they are additive. There is also felt to be a passive influx of calcium into smooth muscle (most noticeable in sodium-free media), which is insensitive to D-600. Diltiazem does not seem to inhibit calcium extrusion from the cell, but does inhibit calcium entry through both types of calcium channels.[19]

In conclusion, each of the calcium channel blockers differs in apparent mode of action, time course of action, concentration-effect relation, and pharmacologic action in different tissues.[1]

Intracellular Effects

In addition to their effects on the slow channels, calcium channel antagonists can inhibit the availability of calcium ions for excitation coupling at intracellular sites. Such an interaction may take place at the inner surface of the sarcolemma, sarcoplasmic reticulum, mitochondria, or at any site where calcium may be made available as an excitation-response messenger.[2,20]

Cardiovascular Effects

Effects on Muscular Contraction

Calcium is the primary ionic link between neurological excitation and mechanical contraction of cardiac, smooth, and skeletal muscle.[2] Actin and myosin are the protein filaments which slide past one another in the adenosine triphosphate (ATP)-dependent contractile process of all muscle cells. In myocardial cells, the regulatory proteins tropomyosin and troponin inhibit this process. When the myocardial cell membrane repolarizes, calcium enters the cell and triggers the release of additional calcium from internal stores within the sarcoplasmic reticulum. Calcium released from this large intracellular reservoir then initiates contraction by combining with the inhibitors troponin and tropomyosin. Previously hidden active sites on actin molecules are then available for binding by myosin.[2]

Effects on Coronary and Peripheral Arterial Blood Vessels (Table 91-1)

The contraction of vascular smooth muscle such as that found in the coronary arteries is slightly different from cardiac and skeletal muscles. Myosin must be phosphorylated, and calmodulin is the regulatory protein to which calcium binds.[2] In addition, vascular smooth muscle cells have significantly less intracellular calcium stores than do the myocardial cells and so rely more heavily on the influx of extracellular calcium.[2]

The observation that calcium channel blockers are significantly more effective in inhibiting contraction in coronary and peripheral arterial smooth muscle than in cardiac and skeletal muscle is of great clinical importance. This differential effect is explained by the observation that arterial smooth muscle is more dependent on external calcium entry for contraction, whereas cardiac and skeletal muscle rely on a recirculating internal pool of calcium.[2] Because calcium-entry blockers are membrane-active drugs, they reduce the entry of calcium into cells, and therefore exert a much larger effect on vascular wall contraction.[2,21] This preferential effect allows calcium-entry blockers to dilate coronary arteries in doses that do not severely affect myocardial contractility and that have little, if any, effect on skeletal muscle.

TABLE 91-1 Cardiovascular Effects of Calcium-Entry Blockers

Effect	Verapamil	Nifedipine	Diltiazem
Decreased Ca ion influx into cells	+	+	+
Effect on fast channels	+	0	+
Local anesthetic effect	+	0	+
Slowing of AV conduction	+	0	+
Prolongation of refractory period in AV node	+	0	+
Reduction myocardial O_2 consumption	+	+	+
Negative inotropic effect	+	+ (0)*	+
Negative chronotropic effect	+	+ (0)*	+
Peripheral vasodilator effect	+	++	+
Coronary vasodilator effect	+	+	+
Pulmonary artery vasodilator effect	+	+	+
Activation of baroreceptor reflexes	+	++	+

Note: + = Effect present with drug; ++ = Strong effect with drug; 0 = No effect with drug; * = In vivo.

Source of data: D. Keefe and W. H. Frishman: Clinical Pharmacology of the Calcium-Channel Blocking Drugs, in M. Packer, W. H. Frishman (eds.), "Calcium Channel Antagonists in Cardiovascular Disease," Appleton-Century-Crofts, Norwalk, 1984, p. 13. Reproduced with permission from the publisher, editor, and author. T. T. Zsoter and J. G. Church: Calcium Antagonists—Pharmacodynamic Effects and Mechanism of Action, *Drugs*, 25:104, 105, 1983. Reproduced with permission from the publisher and author. W. H. Frishman and T. LeJemtel: Electropharmacology of Calcium Channel Antagonists in Cardiac Arrhythmias, *Pace*, 5:402, 1982. Reproduced with permission from the publisher and author.

Effects on Veins

The calcium channel blockers seem to be less active in veins than in arteries, and are ineffective at therapeutic doses (in contrast to nitrates) for decreasing venous capacitance.[20]

Effects on Myocardial Contractility (Table 91-1)

Force generation during cardiac muscle contraction depends in part on calcium influx during membrane depolarization.[22] In isolated myocardial preparations, all calcium channel antagonists have been demonstrated to exert potent negative inotropic effects.[23] In guinea pig atria exposed to drug concentrations of 10^{-6} *M*, the order of potency for depressing the maximal rate of force development during constant pacing was nifedipine > verapamil > diltiazem.[24] In dog papillary muscle, developed tension was also decreased most markedly by nifedipine, the relative potencies (on a weight basis) of verapamil and diltiazem being 1/15 and 1/40, respectively.[25]

The negative inotropic effects of the calcium channel antagonists are dose-dependent.[26] The excitation-contraction coupling of vascular smooth muscle is three to ten times more sensitive to the action of calcium channel antagonists than that of myocardial fibers.[23,26] Hence, the relatively low doses of these drugs used in vivo to produce vasodilation or beneficial antiarrhythmic effects may not produce significant negative inotropic effects.[26,27] Furthermore, in intact animals and humans, the intrinsic negative inotropic properties of these compounds are greatly modified by a baroreceptor-mediated reflex augmentation of beta-adrenergic tone, consequent to vasodilation and a decrease in blood pressure.[28,29] Nifedipine, which exerts the greatest vasodilator effect of these agents, accordingly produces the strongest reflex beta-adrenergic response and one most likely to offset the drugs' negative inotropic activity, and to lead to enhancement of ventricular performance.[30] While this mechanism plays an important role in patients with normal or near-normal left ventricular function, it is unlikely to play a similar role in patients with severe congestive heart failure in whom the baroreceptor sensitivity is markedly attenuated.[27,31]

Electrophysiologic Effects

While verapamil, nifedipine, and diltiazem all depress cardiac contractility with only quantitative differences, their effects (see Tables 91-1 to 91-3) on the electrophysiology of the heart are different quantitatively.[20,32] Local anesthetic actions of diltiazem and particularly of verapamil may account for some of these differences.[34] Nifedipine has a more

TABLE 91-2 Effects of Verapamil on Cardiac Electrophysiology

Tissue	Effect of Verapamil
SA node	
Spontaneous rate	↓
Corrected node recovery time	↑
Atrium	
Conduction	↔
Effective refractory period	↔
AV node	
Conduction	↓
Effective refractory period	↑
His-Purkinje system	
Conduction	↔
Effective refractory period	↔
Ventricle	
Conduction	↔
Effective refractory period	↔
Anomalous pathway (WPW)	
Conduction	↔
Effective refractory period	↔

Note: ↓ = Decrease; ↔ = No apparent effect; ↑ = Increase.
Source: W. H. Frishman and T. LeJemtel: Electropharmacology of Calcium Channel Antagonists in Cardiac Arrhythmias, *Pace,* 5:404, 1982. Reproduced with permission from the publisher and author.

selective action at the slow channels, while verapamil and diltiazem, at least at higher doses, also inhibit currents in the fast channels like the local anesthetics.[35]

Verapamil and diltiazem prolong the conduction and refractoriness in the AV node; the AH interval is lengthened more than the HV interval.[36] In therapeutic concentrations, there are no demonstrable actions on the rate of depolarization or on the repolarization phases of the action potentials in atrial, ventricular, or Purkinje fibers.[33] The rate of discharge of the sinus node, which depends on the calcium ion current, is depressed by all calcium channel blockers. In vivo, this effect can be compensated or overcompensated for by activation of baroreceptor reflexes which increase sympathetic nervous activity.[33]

TABLE 91-3 Effects of Verapamil on the Surface and His Bundle Electrocardiographic Intervals

Interval	Effect of Verapamil
R-R	↔ ↓
P-R	↑
QRS	↔
Q-Tc	↔
A-H	↑
H-V	↔

Note: ↓ = Decrease; ↔ = No apparent effect; ↑ = Increase.
Source: W. H. Frishman and T. LeJemtel: Electropharmacology of Calcium Channel Antagonists in Cardiac Arrhythmias, *Pace,* 5:404, 1982. Reproduced with permission from the publisher and author.

The antiarrhythmic actions of verapamil relate to its effects on nodal cardiac tissues.[33] In sinoatrial (SA) and AV nodal cells, the drug modifies slow-channel electropotentials in three ways: First, there is a decrease in the rate of rise and slope of diastolic slow depolarization and an increase in the membrane threshold potential, which reduces the rate of firing in the cell;[37] second, the action-potential upstroke is decreased in amplitude, which slows conduction;[38] third, the action-potential duration is increased.[37] These electrophysiologic effects are dose-related, and above the clinical range, electrical standstill may occur in SA and AV nodal cells.[36] These observations and others support the concept that slow-channel activity is important in the generation of pacemaker potential in the SA node. Verapamil also exerts a depressant effect on the AV node, and in low concentrations prolongs the effective refractory period.[38,39] Unlike beta-adrenergic blocking drugs and vagomimetic interventions, which depress AV node transmission by altering autonomic impulse traffic, verapamil prolongs AV nodal refractoriness directly.[39] However, verapamil may have some additional vagomimetic effects.[33]

Effects on Nonvascular Tissues

Calcium ions are required for contraction in all smooth muscles and these drugs can inhibit contractions in the gastrointestinal tract.[40] Calcium is also important in excitation-secretion coupling. However, there is no evidence that these drugs have any significant effects on the endocrine glands in clinical doses.[41,42] Although antiadrenergic effects of some calcium-entry blockers have been suggested, further studies are needed.[20,43,44]

Some calcium-entry blockers may partially inhibit adenosine diphosphate (ADP) and epinephrine-induced platelet aggregation and thromboxane release from platelets.[45–50]

Pharmacokinetics

Although classified together, calcium-entry blockers have differences in their pharmacokinetic properties (see Tables 91-4 and 91-5).[1,51,52] Differences in completeness of gastrointestinal absorption, amount of first pass hepatic metabolism, protein-binding, extent of distribution in the body, and the pharmacologic actions of different metabolites may influence the clinical usefulness of these drugs in different patients.[1,51]

Dosage and Therapeutic Levels

After administration of a certain oral dose, the calcium-entry blocking drugs, which are largely metabolized in the liver, show large interindividual variation in circulating plasma levels.[51–53] In angina pectoris, wide individual differences also exist in the relation between plasma concentrations of calcium-

TABLE 91-4 Pharmacokinetics of the Calcium Channel Blockers

Agent	Synonyms	Absorption, %	Bioavailability, %	Protein-Binding, %	Volume of Distribution, 1/kg	t, (β) h	Clearance, ml/min/kg
Diltiazem	Cardizem	> 90	24–43	78	7.6	4.1–5.6	46
Nifedipine	Procardia (Adalat)	> 90	65	90		≈5	
Verapamil	Calan Isoptin	> 90	10–20	90	4.3	6 ± 4 IV 8 ± 6 PO	13 ± 7

$t_{J}(\beta)$ = Elimination of half-life of oral preparations

Source: D. Keefe and W. H. Frishman: Clinical Pharmacology of the Calcium-Channel Blocking Drugs, in M. Packer, and W. H. Frishman (eds.), "Calcium Channel Antagonists in Cardiovascular Disease," Appleton-Century-Crofts, Norwalk, 1984, p. 7. Reproduced with permission from the publisher, editor, and author.

TABLE 91-5 Clinical Use of Calcium Channel Blockers

	Dosage		Onset of Action		Therapeutic Plasma		Excretion,
	Oral	IV	Oral	IV	Concentration	Metabolism	%
Diltiazem	30–90 mg q 6–8 h	75–150 μg/kg (10–20 mg)	< 30 min	< 10 min	50–200 ng/ml	Deacetylation *N*-demethylation *O*-demethylation	60 fecal
Nifedipine	10–40 mg q 6–8 h	5–15 μ/kg	< 20 min	— (3 min sublingual)	25–100 ng/ml	A hydroxycarboxylic acid and a lactone with no known activity	20–40 fecal 50–80 renal
Verapamil	80–120 mg q 6–12 h	150 μg/kg (10–20 mg)	< 30 min	< 5 min	> 100 ng/ml	*N*-dealkylation *N*-demethylation Major hepatic first-pass effect	15 fecal 70 renal

Source: D. Keefe and W. H. Frishman: Clinical Pharmacology of the Calcium-Channel Blocking Drugs, in M. Packer and W. H. Frishman (eds.), "Calcium Channel Antagonists in Cardiovascular Disease," Appleton-Century-Crofts, Norwalk, 1984, p. 8. Reproduced with permission from the publisher, editor, and author.

entry blockers and the associated therapeutic effect.[53]

Usual doses of diltiazem are 30 to 90 mg every 6 to 8 h orally, although higher doses may be required. Intravenous dosage is 75 to 150 μg/kg or 10 to 20 mg over several minutes. Therapeutic plasma concentrations are estimated to be 50 to 200 ng/ml. Nifedipine is usually administered in doses of 10 to 40 mg every 6 to 8 h. Intravenous doses are about one-tenth the oral doses or 10 to 30 μg/kg. Therapeutic plasma concentrations are estimated to be 25 to 150 ng/ml. Usual doses of verapamil are 80 to 160 mg orally every 6 to 8 h, which may be lengthened to every 8 to 12 h during chronic therapy; and 5 to 20 mg slowly administered intravenously in divided doses. Therapeutic plasma concentrations range from 15 to 100 ng/ml at trough levels, although higher (100 to 400 ng/ml) peak or mean levels may correlate with successful therapy of supraventricular arrhythmias and angina pectoris.[1]

Clinical Applications

The calcium channel blockers are now available in the United States for the treatment of angina pectoris (diltiazem, nifedipine, and verapamil) and for supraventricular arrhythmias (verapamil). The drugs are now under consideration for approval in hypertension and arrhythmia prophylaxis and are also being evaluated for a multitude of other cardiovascular (Table 91-6) and noncardiovascular conditions.

Angina Pectoris

The antianginal mechanisms of calcium-entry blockers are complex (Table 91-7).[1,2,54–57] The drugs exert vasodilator effects on the coronary and peripheral vessels as well as depressant effects on cardiac contractility and conduction, all actions which may be important in mediating the drugs' antianginal effects.[2,54–57] The drugs are only mild dilators of epicardial vessels not in spasm, but they markedly attenuate sympathetically-mediated and ergonovine-induced coronary vasoconstriction; these actions provide a rational basis for the drugs' effectiveness in vasospastic ischemic syndromes.[2,56] In patients with exertional angina pectoris, the peripheral vasodilator actions of diltiazem and verapamil and the inhibitory effects on the sinus node, serve to attenuate the increases in double product that normally accompany, and serve to limit, exercise.[55]

TABLE 91-6 Cardiovascular Uses of Calcium Channel Blockers

Angina pectoris*
- Effort angina
- "Rest" angina
- Prinzmetal's variant

Arrhythmias (acute* and chronic†)—verapamil
Systemic hypertension†
Hypertensive emergencies†
Hypertrophic cardiomyopathy—verapamil
Congestive heart failure—nifedipine
Myocardial infarction (containing size of infarct)
Myocardial preservation during open-heart surgery
Primary pulmonary hypertension
Peripheral vascular disease
- Raynaud's phenomenon
- Intermittent claudication
- Cerebral arterial spasm (subarachnoid hemorrhage)—nimodipine
- Mesenteric insufficiency
- Migraine headache prophylaxis

Deacceleration of atherosclerosis
Prevention of cardiomyopathy

*Approved use by the Food and Drug Administration.
†Use under consideration for approval by the Food and Drug Administration.

Stable Angina Pectoris

Multiple double-blind, placebo-controlled studies have clearly confirmed the efficacy of diltiazem,[58–60] nifedipine,[61,62] and verapamil[63–68] in stable angina, reducing attacks of pain and nitroglycerin consumption while improving exercise tolerance. Calcium-entry blockers appear to be as safe and effective as beta blockers and nitrates when used as monotherapies in patients.[69–76]

In attempting to choose between a calcium channel antagonist and a beta-adrenergic blocking drug in the management of patients with effort-related symptoms, it is apparent that some patients do better with one drug than with the other. Unfortunately, we know little about how to predict with confidence the superior agent in a specific patient short of a therapeutic trial. However, verapamil and diltiazem can be used as an effective alternative in patients who remain symptomatic despite therapy with propranolol, and as a first-time antianginal drug in patients with contraindications to beta blockade; the use of nifedipine as a first-line drug is likely limited by the reflex tachycardia that may accompany its use.[75]

The comparative effects of abrupt withdrawal of verapamil and propranolol in patients with angina pectoris have been compared.[44] Ten percent of patients with stable effort-related symptoms experienced a severe clinical exacerbation of their anginal syndrome upon withdrawal of propranolol; no patient experienced rebound symptoms when verapamil was abruptly discontinued.[44]

TABLE 91-7 Hemodynamic Effects of the Calcium-Entry Blockers on Myocardial O_2 Supply and Demand

Verapamil	Nifedipine	Diltiazem	
			DEMAND
↑ ↔	↔ (reflex)	↔	Wall tension
↓	↓	↓	Systolic blood pressure
↑	↔	↔	Ventricular volume
↓*	↑ (reflex)	↓ ↔	Heart rate
↓ ↓	↓	↓	Contractility
			SUPPLY
↑	↑ ↑	↑	Coronary blood flow
↓	↓ ↓	↓	Coronary vascular resistance
↓	↓	↓	Spasm
↑	↓	↑ ↔	Diastolic perfusion time
↔	↑	↑	Collateral blood flow

Note: ↑ = Increase; ↓ = Decrease; ↔ = No apparent effect; * = Heart rate may increase acutely but decreases with chronic use.

Angina at Rest

Patients with angina at rest comprise a wide spectrum of disorders, ranging from those with variant angina (ST elevation) associated with angiographically normal coronary arteries, to those with unstable angina with ST depression or elevation associated with multivessel coronary artery disease.[55,57,77] The studies of Maseri et al. suggest that the coronary vasospasm plays a major role in the pathogenesis of ischemia in most patients with angina at rest, regardless of the coronary anatomy.[78] In clinical trials, calcium channel antagonists were effective in this syndrome because of their ability to block spontaneous and drug-induced spasm.[79–85]

The comparative efficacy of verapamil and propranolol was assessed in a randomized blinded crossover trial in rest angina. Only verapamil reduced symptomatic and asymptomatic episodes of ischemia. These findings are consistent with the concept that coronary vasospasm plays a crucial role in patients with angina at rest; in contrast, rather than provide any benefit, propranolol may exacerbate vasospastic phenomena.[86]

Another study assessed the comparative efficacy of verapamil and nifedipine. Both verapamil and nifedipine proved equally effective, and neither drug depressed ventricular function, either at rest or during exercise.[87] Accordingly, in managing patients with variant angina, the choice of a calcium antagonist is likely to be determined not so much by which drug is more effective, but by which agent is better tolerated by an individual patient.

The usefulness of calcium channel antagonists in the long-term management of unstable angina has recently been demonstrated in a double-blind, randomized clinical trial, showing that the addition of nifedipine to patients receiving nitrates and propranolol reduced the number of patients with unstable anginal syndromes requiring surgery for relief of pain; the incidence of sudden death and myocardial infarction was similar in the two groups.[88]

TABLE 91-8 Hemodynamic Effects of Calcium-Entry Blockers, Beta Blockers, and Combination Treatment

	Ca^{2+} Blockers	Beta Blockers	Combination
Heart rate	↓ ↔ ↑ (reflex)	↓	↓ ↔
Contractility	↓ ↔ (reflex)	↓	↓ ↔
Wall tension	↓	↔	↓
Systolic blood pressure	↓	↓	↓
Left ventricular volume	↓ ↔	↑	↑ ↔
Coronary resistance	↓	↑ ↔	↓ ↔

Note: ↓ = Decrease; ↔ = No change; ↑ = Increase.
Source: W. H. Frishman: Beta-adrenergic Blockade in the Treatment of Coronary Artery Disease, in J. W. Hurst (ed.), "Clinical Essays on The Heart," vol. 2, McGraw-Hill Book Co., New York, 1984, p. 48. Reproduced with permission from the publisher and author.

Of interest, however, is the fact that clinical benefits were largely confined to patients whose pain was accompanied by ST segment elevation.

Unlike the established cardioprotective effects of the beta-blocking drugs,[89] there is no evidence available to show that long-term therapy with any of the calcium channel antagonists prevents recurrent myocardial infarction or reduces the incidence of cardiac-related deaths in patients who have recently experienced an acute myocardial infarction. A long-term study with diltiazem in myocardial infarction survivors is now in progress to address this issue.

Combination Therapy

Combination therapy with nitrates and/or beta blockers may be more efficacious for treatment of angina pectoris than one drug used alone.[53,55,57,71,90,91] The hemodynamic effects of a calcium-blocker beta-blocker combination are shown in Table 91-8.[71] Because adverse effects can occur from this combination (heart block, severe bradycardia, congestive heart failure), patients need careful selection and observation.[92,93] The hemodynamic effects of combined nitrate/calcium channel blocker therapy are shown in Table 91-9. Hypotension should be avoided. Different calcium blockers may also be combined (nifedipine with verapamil or diltiazem) with added benefit and side effects seen when compared to monotherapy.

Arrhythmias (Table 91-10)

Atrial Fibrillation

Except in rare situations, verapamil is ineffective in converting acute and chronic atrial fibrillation to normal sinus rhythm. However, verapamil is an effective agent for decreasing and controlling ventricular rate during atrial fibrillation, by prolonging AV nodal conduction and refractoriness and thereby increasing AV block. Clinical trials which have evaluated slow-channel blockade during atrial fibrillation have shown that verapamil's ability to decrease ventricular rate appears to be unrelated to chronicity, etiology, or patient's age.[94–97] However, verapamil appears more effective than digoxin in slowing down the rapid ventricular rate in response to physical activity.[98] The drug can be used orally in combination with digoxin when treating acute and chronic atrial fibrillation and flutter.[33]

TABLE 91-9 Hemodynamic Rationale for Combining Nitrates and Calcium-Entry Blockers in Angina Pectoris

	Nitrates	Calcium Blockers	Combination
Heart rate	↑ (reflex)	±	↑ (reflex)
Blood pressure	↓	↓	↓ ↓
Heart size	↓ /0	±/↑	0
Contractility	↑ (reflex)	↓	0
Venomotor tone	↓	0	↓
Peripheral resistance	↓	↓	↓ ↓ ?
Coronary resistance	↓	↓	↓ ↓ ?
Coronary blood flow	↑	↑	↑ ↑ ?
Collateral blood flow	↑	↑	↑ ↑ ?

Note: ↓ ↓ = Questionable additive effects; ↓ = Decrease; ↔ = No change; ↑ = Increase.
Source: W. H. Frishman: Beta-adrenergic Blockade in the Treatment of Coronary Artery Disease, in J. W. Hurst (ed.), "Clinical Essays on The Heart," vol. 2, McGraw-Hill Book Co., New York, 1984, p. 48. Reproduced with permission from the publisher and author.

Paroxysmal Supraventricular Tachycardia

Virtually all cases of supraventricular tachycardia due to intranodal reentry or those related to circus movement type of tachycardia in preexcitation respond promptly and predictably to intravenous verapamil, whereas only about two-thirds of ectopic

TABLE 91-10 Effects of Verapamil in Treatment of Common Arrhythmias

Effective	Ineffective
Supraventricular tachycardia	Sinus tachycardia
AV nodal reentrant PSVT	Nonparoxysmal automatic atrial tachycardia
Accessory pathway reentrant PSVT	Atrial fibrillation and flutter in WPW syndrome (Ventricular rate may not decrease.)
SA nodal reentrant PSVT	Ventricular tachyarrhythmias*
Atrial reentrant PSVT	
Atrial flutter (Ventricular rate decreases but arrhythmia will only occasionally convert.)	
Atrial fibrillation (Ventricular rate decreases but arrhythmia will only occasionally convert.)	

* = Only limited experience in this area.
PSVT = Paroxysmal supraventricular tachycardia.
Source: W. H. Frishman and T. LeJemtel: Electropharmacology of Calcium Channel Antagonists in Cardiac Arrhythmias, *Pace*, 5:407, 1982. Reproduced with permission from the publisher and author.

atrial tachycardia convert to sinus rhythm after adequate doses of the drug.[33,99,100] Intravenous verapamil is highly efficacious in reentry paroxysmal supraventricular tachycardia, regardless of etiology or age.[33,100]

The recommended dosage range of verapamil for terminating paroxysmal supraventricular tachycardia in adults is 0.075 to 0.15 mg/kg infused over 1 to 3 min, with a maintenance infusion of 0.005 mg/kg/min or 5 to 10 mg over 1 to 3 min, repeated at 30 min.[33] In patients with myocardial dysfunction, the dose should be reduced. Children have safely been treated with the 0.075-to-0.15-mg/kg regimen.[33]

There have been few clinical studies comparing intravenous verapamil with other standard regimens in the treatment of paroxysmal supraventricular tachycardia.[101] However, there are a number of clinical situations where verapamil might offer an advantage over either digitalis or beta-adrenergic blockers. For instance, verapamil would be preferable in cases where there is an urgent need to terminate paroxysmal supraventricular tachycardia, since it can produce therapeutic responses within 3 min of infusion, whereas digoxin's effects are not evident for approximately 30 min.[33] Also, should drug therapy fail to achieve normal sinus rhythm, verapamil's short duration of action permits earlier cardioversion without some of the dangers that accompany electric cardioversion during digoxin therapy. Verapamil also offers distinct advantages over beta-adrenergic blocking drugs in patients whose arrhythmias are associated with chronic obstructive lung disease and/or peripheral vascular disease.[33]

There is a growing clinical experience with oral verapamil for prophylaxis against paroxysmal supraventricular tachycardia in doses of 160 to 480 mg/day, and the results of these trials have yielded, for the most part, favorable results.[102,103]

Atrial Flutter

The immediate effects of intravenous verapamil in atrial flutter in most patients is an increase in AV block that slows the ventricular response, rarely followed by a return to sinus rhythm.[33,97] In some, the response is via development of atrial fibrillation with a controlled ventricular response.[33] A single intravenous dose of verapamil has been found to be of diagnostic value in differentiating rapid atrial flutter from paroxysmal supraventricular tachycardia when these two arrhythmias are indistinguishable on the electrocardiogram. If the rhythm is atrial flutter, the AV block increases immediately, revealing the true nature of the arrhythmia.[95] Oral verapamil has also been used to convert paroxysmal atrial flutter or to reduce rapid ventricular rates associated with this arrhythmia.[104]

Preexcitation

Verapamil has been found to induce reversion of most cases of accessory pathway supraventricular tachycardia.[99] Using intracardiac recordings of electrical activity during programmed electrical stimulation of the heart, data have become available regarding the actions of verapamil on the electrophysiologic properties of the accessory pathway in overt cases of the Wolff-Parkinson-White (WPW) syndrome.[104,105] The drug has minimal effect on the antegrade and retrograde conduction times and on the refractory period.[33,37,106] Verapamil, therefore, terminates accessory pathway paroxysmal supraventricular tachycardia in the same manner as it does AV nodal reentrant paroxysmal supraventricular tachycardia, by slowing AV nodal conduction and increasing refractoriness. The minimal effects of verapamil on the electrophysiologic properties of the bypass tract is consistent with the observation that the drug is ineffective in atrial fibrillation, complicating WPW syndrome in which fibrillatory impulses, as with digoxin, conduct predominantly through the anomalous pathway.[95]

Ventricular Arrhythmias

Intravenous verapamil has no apparent benefit in ventricular arrhythmias except in acute myocardial infarction.[37,107]. Presently, oral verapamil has no demonstrated role in the management of ventricular tachyarrhythmias.

Precautions in Treating Arrhythmias

A diseased SA node is much more sensitive to slow-channel blockers and may be depressed to the point of atrial standstill.[108] Sinus arrest can also occur without overt evidence of sick sinus syndrome.[33] Second, calcium channel blockade may suppress potential AV nodal escape rhythms that need to arise should atrial standstill occur.[33] In patients with the brady–tachy form of sick sinus syndrome, either digoxin or beta-adrenoceptor blocking drugs should probably not be combined with verapamil in the prophylaxis of tachyarrhythmias unless a demand ventricular pacemaker is first inserted.[33]

Systemic Hypertension

Calcium channel blockers have recently been used to treat systemic hypertension and some appear to be effective.[109] The possible mechanisms of action are shown in Table 91-11. There are many ongoing trials in the United States evaluating the efficacy and safety of diltiazem,[110] nifedipine, verapamil,[111] and other calcium channel blockers[112] in patients with hypertension. Conventional verapamil tablets appear to be useful in twice-daily dosing,[111] and sus-

TABLE 91-11 Antihypertensive Effects of Calcium-Entry Blockers

1. Peripheral vasodilator
2. Antiadrenergic effects (possible)
3. Natriuretic effects (possible)
4. Direct negative inotropic effects (possible)

tained-release preparations of diltiazem, nifedipine, and verapamil for once-daily use are now being investigated in clinical trials.[113] The drugs reduce both systolic and diastolic pressures with a minimal amount of side effects, including orthostasis.[104] Some drugs in this class may also have additional antiadrenergic and natriuretic activity.[109] They can be used in combination with other antihypertensive drugs, if necessary.[109] The drugs do not lower the pressure of normotensive patients.

The drugs may be shown to be most useful in elderly patients, and in patients with low-renin, salt-dependent hypertension.[114,115]

Hypertensive Emergencies
Calcium channel blockers have also been shown to be beneficial and safe in patients with severe hypertension and hypertensive crisis.[109,116,117] Single oral, sublingual, and intravenous doses of these drugs have rapidly and smoothly reduced blood pressure in adults and children without significant untoward effects.[116,117] The absolute reduction in blood pressure with treatment appears to be inversely correlated with the height of the pretreatment blood pressure level, and few episodes of hypotension have been reported.[116] Continuous hemodynamic monitoring of patients does not seem necessary in most patients.[116] The place of calcium-entry blockers in the treatment of hypertensive emergencies still needs to be established in relation to other available approved drug regimens for this condition.

Hypertrophic Cardiomyopathy

For many years, propranolol has been the therapeutic agent for symptomatic patients with hypertrophic cardiomyopathy. The beneficial effects produced by propranolol derive from its inhibition of sympathetic stimulation to the heart.[118]

Clinical studies have shown that the administration of verapamil improves exercise capacity and symptoms in many patients with hypertrophic cardiomyopathy.[119–122] The exact mechanism by which verapamil produces its beneficial effects is not known. Acute and chronic verapamil administration reduces left ventricular outflow obstruction, but examination of indices of left ventricular systolic function during chronic therapy shows that this effect does not result from a reduction in left ventricular hypercontractility.[119] Since patients with hypertrophic cardiomyopathy also exhibit abnormal diastolic function, it is likely that improvement in diastolic filling may be responsible in part for verapamil's benefit.[119] Enhanced early diastolic filling and an improvement in the diastolic pressure-volume relation might be expected to result in an increase in left ventricular end-diastolic volume which would decrease the Venturi forces which act to move the anterior mitral valve leaflet across the outflow tract toward the septum.[119] The decrease would cause a diminution of obstruction, reducing left ventricular pressure and myocardial wall stress, thereby raising the threshold at which symptoms occur.[119]

In a large study[119] of patients with hypertrophic cardiomyopathy refractory to beta blockers, verapamil proved to be effective on a long-term basis, with almost 50 percent showing either a significant improvement in exercise tolerance or an improvement in symptoms. Approximately 50 percent of patients considered candidates for surgery because of moderately severe symptoms unresponsive to propranolol showed significant improvement on verapamil and surgery was no longer considered necessary.[119] With long-term therapy, there was no clear changes in left ventricular wall thickness during echocardiographic studies.[119]

There may be serious and fatal complications of verapamil treatment in patients with hypertrophic cardiomyopathy.[119] These result from either accentuated hemodynamic or electrophysiologic effects of the drug. It is not clear whether the fatal complications occur as a result of verapamil-induced reduction in blood pressure with a resultant increase in left ventricular obstruction, or the negative inotropic effects of the drug.[119] The drug should probably not be used in patients with clinical congestive heart failure. The loss of sequential atrial ventricular depolarization due to the drug's electrophysiologic effects could also compromise cardiac function. The adverse electrophysiologic effects are often transient; however, they could prevent the use of larger drug doses which might provide more optimal relief.[119]

If verapamil's calcium-entry blocking effects are responsible for its therapeutic actions in hypertrophic cardiomyopathy, then other drugs in this class may be useful. However, the preliminary results of a double-blind trial comparing verapamil to nifedipine indicate that verapamil was more effective than nifedipine in improving exercise tolerance and clinical symptoms.[123]

Congestive Heart Failure

The potent systemic vasodilator action of nifedipine makes it potentially attractive for use as an afterload-reducing agent in patients with left ventricular failure.[24,124,125] Unlike other vasodilator drugs, however, nifedipine also exerts a direct negative inotropic effect on the myocardium consistent with its ability to block transmembrane calcium transport in cardiac muscle cells.[24,55] The successful use of nifedipine as a vasodilator in patients with left ventricular failure is dependent on its effects of reducing afterload exceeding its direct negative inotropic actions and leading to an improvement in hemodynamics and forward flow.[55]

Studies evaluating the hemodynamics effect of nifedipine in patients with heart failure uniformly demonstrate significant reductions in systemic vascular resistance, usually associated with increases in cardiac output.[126] Our group[127] and others[128] have found resting ejection fractions also to rise with nifedipine therapy. Reflex increases in heart rate have been reported,[127] but most investigators have found heart rate to remain the same[128,129] and in isolated cases, to fall.[130] Left ventricular filling pressures usually decrease[128,129] or do not change significantly,[126,130] but there are instances where pulmonary capillary wedge pressures rise with use of nifedipine in heart failure.[131,132] Patients with left ventricular afterload, i.e., disproportionately low wall stress and those with intrinsic fixed mechanical interference to forward flow, e.g., aortic stenosis, appear most likely to have unfavorable hemodynamic responses to nifedipine therapy.[124,125] Most of the published data report only on the acute hemodynamic effects of the agent after single sublingual dosing, with little work done on the use of the agent as chronic oral therapy for left ventricular failure.

The total clinical experience with use of nifedipine and other calcium blockers in heart failure is limited.[124,125] Therefore, the evidence at present would not support use of the drug as a ventricular unloading agent of first choice because there are other vasodilators available which do not have negative inotropic activity.[125] Use of nifedipine as acute vasodilator therapy in patients with left ventricular failure should be considered only if additional clinical reasons for its administration exist, i.e., angina pectoris and systemic hypertension, and particularly if these conditions play important contributory roles in the development or exacerbation of left ventricular dysfunction. The drug should be administered only after careful assessment of the clinical situation and preferably with invasive monitoring of pulmonary artery or pulmonary capillary wedge pressure.[124,125] Further clinical experience, including controlled clinical trials, will ultimately help define the precise role of nifedipine, as well as other calcium channel antagonists, in the acute and chronic treatment of heart failure.

Myocardial Preservation in Surgery and during Infarction

Several experimental studies have indicated that nifedipine and diltiazem can reduce the size of myocardial necrosis induced in experimental ischemia.[133–136] Ischemia can lead to diminished ATP production. This depression in ATP synthesis can eventually affect the sodium and calcium ion pumps with the ultimate consequence of calcium ion accumulation in the cytoplasm and calcium overload in mitochondria. Calcium channel blockers can diminish myocardial oxygen consumption and inhibit the influx of calcium ions to the myofibrils and thus favorably influence the outcome of experimental coronary occlusion.[20,134] These experimental observations have suggested the use of calcium channel blockers for reducing or containing the extent of myocardial infarction during acute coronary artery occlusions in humans, and as an adjunct to cardioplegia during open-heart surgery. However, there are no adequate studies in human beings to support these approaches.

Primary Pulmonary Hypertension

Primary pulmonary hypertension is an entity characterized by excessive pulmonary vasoconstriction and increased pulmonary vascular resistance induced by unknown stimuli.[137] Typically, the affected patient is a young to middle-aged woman presenting with fatigue, dyspnea, chest discomfort, or syncope. Despite many attempts to develop effective therapy, the results of drug treatment have been generally unsatisfactory, and the syndrome continues to bear a poor prognosis.[137]

Based on the presently available data, it may be concluded that some calcium channel antagonists provide beneficial responses in selected patients with pulmonary hypertension.[138–141] In general, patients with less severe pulmonary hypertension appear to respond better than those with more advanced disease.[142] Furthermore, early treatment may serve to attenuate progression of the disease.

Cerebral Arterial Spasm

A major complication of subarachnoid hemorrhage is cerebral arterial spasm which may occur several days after the initial event.[143] Such spasm may be a focal or diffuse narrowing of one or more of the large cerebral vessels, which may cause additional ischemic neurologic deficits. Though the exact etiology of this spasm is unknown, a combination of various blood constituents and neurotransmitters has been postulated to produce a milieu that enhances the reactivity of the cerebral vasculature.[143] The final pathway for the vasoconstriction, however, involves an increase in the free intracellular calcium concentration.[144] Accordingly, it is reasonable to postulate that the calcium channel antagonists might have a beneficial effect in reducing cerebral spasm.[145]

Although verapamil and nifedipine have been shown to prevent cerebral arterial spasm in experimental animals,[146,147] nimodipine, a nifedipine analogue, has demonstrated a preferential cerebrovascular action in this disorder.[148] Nimodipine's lipid solubility enables it to cross the blood-brain barrier; this may account for its more potent cerebrovascular effects. In a recent multicenter, placebo-controlled study involving 125 patients,[143] it was demonstrated that nimodipine significantly reduced the occurrence of severe neurologic deficits following angiographically demonstrated cerebral arterial spasm. All patients had a documented subarachnoid hemorrhage and a normal neurological status within 96 h of entry into the study. While 8 of 60 placebo-treated patients developed a severe neurologic deficit, only 1 of 55 nimodipine-treated patients suffered such an outcome. These results are encouraging and suggest that nimodipine could be considered a standard therapy for patients who are neurologically stable

TABLE 91-12 Noncardiovascular Uses* of Calcium Channel Blockers

Bronchial asthma
Esophageal spasm
Dysmenorrhea
Premature labor

*Indications not yet approved by the Food and Drug Administration.

after a subarachnoid hemorrhage in order to prevent subsequent cerebral arterial spasm.

Other Cardiovascular Uses

Calcium channel blockers have been shown to be effective in some patients with Raynaud's phenomenon, migraine headache, mesenteric insufficiency, and intermittent claudication (Table 91-9).[145,149] They have also been shown in experimental studies to be effective in arresting the atherosclerotic process.[150]

Recently, it has been shown that coronary artery vasospasm may be an important pathophysiologic mechanism in cardiomyopathy.[151] Verapamil treatment has been shown experimentally to reduce vasospasm in response to myocarditis and by this mechanism to prevent the development of cardiomyopathy heart failure.[152]

Noncardiovascular Applications

Calcium-entry blockers are now undergoing clinical trials in the treatment of bronchial asthma, esophageal spasm, dysmenorrhea, and premature labor (Table 91-12).[145,149] The pathophysiology of these conditions may be influenced in part by abnormalities in calcium ion transport across cell membranes, thereby explaining the potential application of calcium channel blockers.

Adverse Effects

In addition to their widely varying effects on cardiovascular function, these three agents also have differing spectra of adverse effects (Table 91-13).[1,55,153] Nifedipine has a very high incidence of minor adverse effects (approximately 40 percent) but serious adverse effects are uncommon.[154] The most frequent adverse effects reported with nifedipine use are headache, pedal edema, flushing, paresthesias, and dizziness. The most serious adverse effects of this drug are exacerbation of angina, which may occur in up to 10 percent of patients, and occasional hypotension.[75] Both diltiazem and verapamil can exacerbate sinus node dysfunction and impair AV nodal conduction, particularly in the patient with underlying conduction system disease.[1,55,153] The most frequent adverse effect of verapamil is constipation.[1,55,153] The drug may also worsen congestive heart failure, particularly when used in combination with beta blockers or disopyramide.[1,55,153] Most of the adverse effects noted with diltiazem have been cardiovascular, with occasional headache and gastrointestinal complaints.[1,55,153]

TABLE 91-14 Cardiovascular Toxicity of Verapamil and Recommendations for Treatment

Effect*	Suggested Treatment
Profound hypotension	1. 10% calcium gluconate or calcium chloride 2. Norepinephrine or dopamine
Severe left ventricular dysfunction	1. 10% calcium gluconate or calcium chloride 2. Isoproterenol or dobutamine 3. Glucagon 4. Norepinephrine or dopamine
Profound bradycardia Sinus bradycardia SA node and AV node block Asystole	1. Atropine sulfate (not always effective) 2. 10% calcium gluconate or calcium chloride 3. Isoproterenol or dobutamine 4. External cardiac massage and cardiac pacing (if above measures fail)

* = These effects are seen more frequently in patients who have underlying myocardial dysfunction and/or cardiac conduction abnormalities, and who are receiving concomitant beta-adrenergic blocker treatment.

Source: W. H. Frishman, N. A. Klein, S. Charlap, P. Klein, M. N. Cohen, and H. H. Rotmensch: Recognition and Management of Verapamil Poisoning, in M. Packer and W. H. Frishman (eds.), "Calcium Channel Antagonists in Cardiovascular Disease," Appleton-Century-Crofts, Norwalk, 1984, p. 368. Reproduced with permission from the publisher, editor, and author.

TABLE 91-13 Adverse Effects of the Calcium Channel Blockers

	Overall	Headache	Dizziness	GI	Flushing	Paresthesia	Decreased AV Conduction	Congestive Heart Failure	Hypotension	Pedal Edema	Worsening of Angina
Diltiazem	≈5%	+	+	+	+	0	3+	+	+	+	0
Nifedipine	40%	3+	3+	+	3+	3+	0	1+	2+	2+	+
Verapamil	8%	+	+	3+	0	0	3+	2+	+	+	0

Note: 0 = No report; + = Rare; 2+ = Occasional; 3+ = Frequent.

Source: D. Keefe and W. H. Frishman: Clinical Pharmacology of the Calcium-Channel Blocking Drugs, in M. Packer and W. H. Frishman (eds.), "Calcium Channel Antagonists in Cardiovascular Disease," Appleton-Century-Crofts, Norwalk, 1984, p. 14. Reproduced with permission from the publisher, editor, and author.

Drug Withdrawal

There have been serious problems reported with abrupt withdrawal of long-term beta-blocker therapy in patients with angina, which appear related to heightened adrenergic activity.[44] Preliminary clinical experiences with calcium-entry blocker withdrawal would suggest that although patients with angina get worse after calcium-entry blocker treatment is stopped abruptly, there is no evidence of an "overshoot" in anginal symptoms.[44]

Drug Overdose

Calcium-entry blocker overdosage has been described with increasing frequency. The cardiovascular problems associated with this condition are hypotension, left ventricular conduction, bradycardia, nodal blocks, and asystole. Treatment approaches are described in Table 91-14.[155]

Drug Interactions

There is as yet little data on the interactions of diltiazem with other drugs.[1] Both nifedipine and verapamil increase serum digoxin levels. Verapamil has been reported to increase serum digoxin levels by approximately 70 percent,[156,157] apparently by decreasing renal clearance,[156] the nonrenal clearance, and the volume of distribution.[157,158] Studies of the time course of this effect show that it begins with the first dose, and reaches steady state within 1 to 4 weeks. Nifedipine also has been reported to increase serum digoxin concentrations in patients, but to a lesser extent (about 45 percent).[159] The mechanism for this effect is unclear. Nifedipine has been reported to have no significant effect on digoxin levels in normal volunteers.[160] Verapamil[157] and diltiazem[161] have additive effects on AV conduction in combination with digitalis. They can be used to cause further decreases in heart rate compared to digitalis alone when patients are in atrial fibrillation.

Combinations of propranolol with nifedipine or verapamil have been extensively studied for the therapy of angina pectoris.[55,71] Several studies have shown improved efficacy for the combinations as compared to any of the drugs alone.[90,91] Hemodynamic studies have shown mild negative inotropic effects of verapamil in patients on a beta blocker.[92] There are also slight decreases in heart rate, cardiac output, and left ventricular ejection fraction.[92] Both combinations of nifedipine and propranolol or metoprolol, and of verapamil and propranolol are well tolerated by patients with normal left ventricular function, but there may be a greater potential for hemodynamic compromise in patients with impaired left ventricular function with combined verapamil-propranolol treatment.[92] Combinations of diltiazem, nifedipine, or verapamil with nitrates are well tolerated and clinically useful.[55]

Conclusion

Each of the new calcium antagonists—diltiazem, nifedipine, and verapamil—exert their effects through inhibition of slow channel-mediated calcium transport. However, each of the drugs appears to accomplish this by different mechanisms, and each has differing effects on target organs. These differences allow the clinician to select the particular drug most suitable for the specific needs of his or her patient. In addition, the side effect profiles of each of these drugs (with little overlap between them) assure that most patients will tolerate at least one of these agents.

References

1. Keefe, D., and Frishman, W. H.: Clinical Pharmacology of the Calcium-Channel Blocking Drugs, in M. Packer, and W. H. Frishman, (eds.), "Calcium Channel Antagonists in Cardiovascular Disease," Appleton-Century-Crofts, Norwalk, 1984, p. 3.
2. Braunwald, E.: Mechanism of Action of Calcium-Channel Blocking Agents, *N. Engl. J. Med.*, 307:1618, 1983.
3. Lindner, E.: Phenyl-Propyl-Diphenyl-Propyl-Amin, a New Substance with a Dilating Action in the Coronary Vessels, *Arzneim. Forsch.*, 10:569, 1960.
4. Haas, H., and Hartfelder, G.: α-Isopropyl-α(N-methylhomoveratryl)-8-Aminopropyl)-3,4-Dimethoxy-Phenylacetonitrol, a Substance with Vasodilating Properties, *Arzneim. Forsch.*, 12:549, 1962.
5. Fleckenstein, A., Kammermeier, H., Doring, H., and Freund, H. J.: On the Action Mechanism of New Coronary Dilators with Oxygen Sparing Myocardial Effects—Prenylamin and Iproveratril, *Z. Kreislaufforsch.*, 56:716, 1967.
6. Fleckenstein, A.: Control of Myocardial Metabolism by Verapamil: Sites of Action and Therapeutic Effects, *Arzneim. Forsch.*, 20:1317, 1970.
7. Singh, B. N., and Vaughan Williams, E. M.: A Fourth Class of Antidysrhythmic Action? Effect of Verapamil on Ouabain Toxicity, on Atrial and Ventricular Intracellular Potentials, and on Other Features of Cardiac Function, *Cardiovasc. Res.*, 6:109, 1972.
8. Vaughan Williams, E. M.: Classification of Antiarrhythmic Drugs, in E. Sande, E. Flensted-Jensen, and K. H. Olsen (eds.), "Symposium on Cardiac Arrhythmias," A. B. Astra, Elsinore, Denmark, Sodertalje, Sweden, 1970, pp. 449–501.
9. Ebel, V. S., Schutz, H., and Hornitschek, A.: Studies on the Analysis of Nifedipine Considering in Particular Transformation Products Formed by Light Exposure. *Arzneim. Forsch.*, 28:2188, 1978.
10. Bayer, R., Rodenkirchen, R., Kaufman, R., Lee, J. H., and Hennekes, R.: The Effects of Nifedipine on Contraction and Monophasic Action Potential of Isolated Cat Myocardium, *Naunyn Schmiedebergs Arch. Pharmacol.*, 301:29, 1977.
11. Bayer, R., and Ehara, T.: Comparative Studies on Calcium Antagonists, *Prog. Pharmacol.*, 2:31, 1978.
12. Kolhardt, M., and Fleckenstein, A.: Inhibition of the Slow Inward Current by Nifedipine in Mammalian Ventricular Myocardium, *Naunyn Schmiedebergs Arch. Pharmacol.*, 298:267, 1977.
13. Bayer, R., Kalusche, D., Kaufmann, R., and Mannhold, R.: Inotropic and Electrophysiological Actions of Verapamil and D600 in Mammalian Myocardium: III. Effects of the Optical Isomers on Transmembrane Action Potentials, *Naunyn Schmiedebergs Arch. Pharmacol.*, 290:81, 1975.
14. Ehara, T., and Kaufmann, R.: The Voltage and Time-Dependent Effects of (−) Verapamil on the Slow Inward Current in Isolated Cat Ventricular Myocardium, *J. Pharmacol. Exp. Ther.*, 207:49, 1978.

15. Kohlhardt, M., Krause, H., Kübler, M., and Herdey, A.: Kinetics of Inactivation and Recovery of the Slow Inward Current in the Mammalian Ventricular Myocardium, *Pfluegers Arch.*, 355:1, 1975.
16. Henry, P. D.: Comparative Pharmacology of Calcium Antagonists: Nifedipine, Verapamil and Diltiazem, *Am. J. Cardiol.*, 46:1047, 1980.
17. Saikawa, T., Nagamoto, Y., and Arita, M.: Electrophysiologic Effects of Diltiazem, a New Slow Channel Inhibitor, on Canine Cardiac Fibers, *Jpn. Heart J.*, 18:235, 1977.
18. Meisheri, K. D., Hwang, O., and van Breeman, C.: Evidence of Two Separate Ca^{2+} Pathways in Smooth Muscle Plasmalemma, *J. Membr. Biol.*, 59:19, 1981.
19. van Breeman, C., Mangel, A., Fahim, M., and Meisheri, K.: Selectivity of Calcium Antagonistic Action in Vascular Smooth Muscle, *Am. J. Cardiol.*, 49:507, 1982.
20. Zsotér, T. T., and Church, J. G.: Calcium Antagonists—Pharmacodynamic Effects and Mechanism of Action, *Drugs* 25:93, 1983.
21. Braunwald, E.: Calcium-Channel Blockers: Pharmacologic Considerations, *Am. Heart J.*, 104:665, 1982.
22. Millard, R. W., Lathrop, D. A., Grupp, G., Ashraf, M., Grupp, J. L., and Schwartz, A.: Differential Cardiovascular Effects of Calcium Channel Blocking Agents: Potential Mechanisms, *Am. J. Cardiol.*, 49:499, 1982.
23. Fleckenstein, A.: Specific Pharmacology of Calcium in Myocardium, Cardiac Pacemakers, and Vascular Smooth Muscle, *Annu. Rev. Pharmacol. Toxicol.*, 17:149, 1977.
24. Henry, P. D., Borda, L., and Schuchleib, R.: Chronotropic and Inotropic Effects of Vasodilators, in P. R. Lichtlen, E. Kmura, and N. Taira (eds.), "International Adalat Panel Discussion: New Experimental and Clinical Results," Excerpta Medica, Amsterdam, 1979, pp. 14–21.
25. Cohn, J. N., and Franciosa, J. A.: Vasodilator Therapy of Cardiac Failure, *N. Engl. J. Med.*, 297:27, 1977.
26. Henry, P. D.: Comparative Pharmacology of Calcium Antagonists: Nifedipine, Verapamil and Diltiazem, *Am. J. Cardiol.*, 46:1047, 1980.
27. Himori, N., Ono, H., and Taira, N.: Simultaneous Assessment of Effects of Coronary Vasodilators on the Coronary Blood Flow and the Myocardial Contractility by Using the Blood Perfused Canine Papillary Muscle, *Jpn. J. Pharmacol.*, 26:427, 1976.
28. Singh, B. N., Hecht, H. S., Nademanee, K., and Chew, C. Y. C.: Electrophysiologic and Hemodynamic Effects of Slow Channel Blocking Drugs, *Prog. Cardiovasc. Dis.*, 25:103, 1982.
29. Braunwald, E.: Calcium Channel Blocking Agents in the Treatment of Cardiovascular Disorders: Part II: Hemodynamic Effects and Clinical Applications, *Ann. Intern. Med.*, 93:886, 1980.
30. Ellrodt, G., Chew, C. Y. C., and Singh, B. N.: Therapeutic Implications of Slow-Channel Blockade in Cardiocirculatory Disorders, *Circulation*, 62:669, 1980.
31. Beiser, G. D., Epstein, S. E., Stampfer, M., and Goldstein, R. E.: Impaired Heart Response to Sympathetic Nerve Stimulation in Patients with Cardiac Decompensation, *Circulation*, 37–38(suppl. VI):40, 1984. (Abstr.)
32. Mitchell, L. B., Schroeder, J. S., and Mason, J. W.: Comparative Clinical Electrophysiologic Effect of Diltiazem, Verapamil and Nifedipine—a Review. *Am. J. Cardiol.*, 49:629, 1982.
33. Frishman, W. H., and LeJemtel, T.: Electropharmacology of Calcium Channel Antagonists in Cardiac Arrhythmias, *Pace*, 5:402, 1982.
34. Singh, B. N., Chew, C. Y. C., Hecht, H., Collett, J., and Ormiston, J.: Effects of Intravenously Administered Verapamil on Hemodynamic Variables and Ventricular Function in Acute Myocardial Infarction, *Clin. Invest. Med.*, 3:73, 1980.
35. Nayler, W. G., and Poole-Wilson, P. H.: Calcium Antagonists: Definition and Mode of Action, *Basic Res. Cardiol.*, 76:1, 1981.
36. Yamaguchi, I., Obayashi, K., and Mandel, W. J.: Electrophysiological Effects of Verapamil, *Cardiovasc. Res.*, 12:597, 1978.
37. Singh, B. N., Collet, J., and Chew, C. Y. C.: New Perspectives in the Pharmacologic Therapy of Cardiac Arrhythmias, *Prog. Cardiovasc. Dis.*, 22:243, 1980.
38. Wit, A., and Cranefield, P.: The Effects of Verapamil on the Sinoatrial and Atrioventricular Nodes of the Rabbit and the Mechanisms by Which It Arrests Reentrant AV Nodal Tachycardia, *Circ. Res.*, 35:413, 1974.
39. Zipes, D. P., and Fischer, J. C.: Effects of Agents Which Inhibit the Slow Channel on Sinus Node Automaticity and Atrioventricular Conduction in the Dog, *Circ. Res.*, 34:184, 1974.
40. Triggle, C. R., Swamy, V. C., and Triggle, D. J.: Calcium Antagonists and Contractile Responses in Rat Vas Deferens and Guinea Pig Ileal Smooth Muscle, *Can. J. Physiol., Pharmacol.*, 57:804, 1979.
41. Frishman, W. H., Klein, N. A., Charlap, S., et al.: Comparative Effects of Verapamil and Propranolol on Parathyroid Hormone and Serum Calcium Concentration, in M. Packer and W. H. Frishman (eds.), "Calcium Channel Antagonists in Cardiovascular Disease," Appleton-Century-Crofts, Norwalk, 1984, p. 343.
42. Shamoon, H., Baylor, P., Kambosos, D., Charlap, S., and Frishman, W.: Effects of Oral Verapamil Therapy on Glucose-Induced Changes in Insulin and Counter-Regulatory Hormone Secretion, *Diabetes*, 33(suppl. 1):340A, 1984. (Abstr.)
43. Zelis, R., Wichmann, T., and Starke, K.: Inhibition of Vascular Noradrenaline Release by Diltiazem, *Circulation*, 66:II–139, 1982.
44. Frishman, W. H., Klein, N., Strom, J., et al.: Comparative Effects of Abrupt Withdrawal of Propranolol and Verapamil in Angina Pectoris, *Am. J. Cardiol.*, 50:1191, 1982.
45. Chierchia, S., Crea, F., Bernini, W., et al.: Antiplatelet Effects of Verapamil in Man, *Am. J. Cardiol.*, 47:399, 1981.
46. Pumphrey, C. W., Fuster, V., Dewanjee, M. K., Chesebro, J. H., Vlietstra, R. E., and Kaye, M. P.: Comparison of the Antithrombotic Action of Calcium Antagonist Drugs with Dipyridamole in Dogs, *Am. J. Cardiol.*, 51:591, 1983.
47. Tai, E., Berezow, J., Weksler, B., Klein, N., LeJemtel, T., and Frishman, W. H.: Comparative Effects of Oral Verapamil and Propranolol on Platelet Activation in Angina Pectoris: A Placebo-Controlled Double Blind Crossover Study, *Circulation*, 66(II):323, 1982. (Abstr.)
48. Burns, F. R., and Frishman, W. H.: The Anti-Platelet Effects of Calcium Channel Blockers Add to Their Antianginal Properties, *Int. J. Cardiol.*, 4:372, 1983.
49. Burns, E. R., Frishman, W. H., Klein, N. A., Tai, E., and Weksler, B.: Calcium Channel Blocking Drugs as Platelet Antagonists in Ischemic Heart Disease, in M. Packer, and W. H. Frishman (eds.), "Calcium Channel Antagonists in Cardiovascular Disease," Appleton-Century-Crofts, Norwalk, 1984, p. 351.
50. Barnathan, E. S., Addonizio, V. P., and Shattil, S. J.: Interaction of Verapamil with Human Platelet α-Adrenergic Receptors, *Am. J. Physiol.*, 242:H19, 1982.
51. McAllister, R. G.: Clinical Pharmacology of Slow Channel Blocking Agents, *Prog. Cardiovasc. Dis.*, 25:83, 1982.
52. Kates, R.: Calcium Antagonists—Pharmacokinetic Properties, *Drugs*, 25:113, 1983.
53. Frishman, W. H., Kirsten, E., Klein, M. et al.: Clinical Relevance of Verapamil Plasma Levels in Stable Angina Pectoris, *Am. J. Cardiol.*, 50:1180, 1982.
54. Singh, B. N., Chew, C. Y. C., Josephson, M. A., and Packer, M.: Hemodynamic Mechanisms Underlying the Antianginal Actions of Verapamil, *Am. J. Cardiol.*, 50:886, 1982.
55. Singh, B. N., Ellrodt, G., and Nademanee, K.: Calcium Antagonists: Cardiocirculatory Effects and Therapeutic Actions, in J. W. Hurst (ed.), "Clinical Essays on the Heart," McGraw-Hill Book Co., New York, 1984, p. 65.
56. Stone, P. H., Antman, E. M., Muller, J. E., and Braunwald, E.: Calcium Channel Blocking Agents in the Treatment of Cardiovascular Disorders: Part II. Hemodynamic Effects and Clinical Applications, *Ann. Intern. Med.*, 93:886, 1980.
57. Theroux, P., Taeymans, Y., and Waters, D.: Calcium Antagonists: Clinical Use in the Treatment of Angina, *Drugs*, 25:179, 1983.

58. Hossack, K. F., Pool, P. E., and Steele, P.: Efficacy of Diltiazem in Angina of Effort—a Multicenter Trial, *Am. J. Cardiol.,* 49:567, 1982.
59. Strauss, W. E., McIntyre, K. M., Parisi, A. R., and Shapiro, W.: Safety and Efficacy of Diltiazem Hydrochloride for the Treatment of Stable Angina Pectoris—Report of a Cooperative Trial, *Am. J. Cardiol.,* 49:560, 1982.
60. Ono, K.: Clinical Effect of Herbesser on Ischemic Heart Disease—Double-Blind Studies with Inactive Placebo in Par, *Jpn. J. Clin. Exp. Med.,* 49:2304, 1972.
61. Moskowitz, R. M., Piccini, P. A., Nacarelli, G. V., and Zelis, R.: Nifedipine Therapy for Stable Angina Pectoris: Preliminary Results of Effects on Angina Frequency and Treadmill Exercise Response, *Am. J. Cardiol.,* 44:811, 1979.
62. Mueller, H. S., and Chahine, R. A.: Interim Report of Multicenter Double-Blind Placebo-Controlled Studies of Nifedipine in Chronic Stable Angina, *Am. J. Med.,* 71:645, 1981.
63. Bala Subramanian, V., Parmasivan, R., Lahiri, A., and Raftery, E. B.: Verapamil in Chronic Stable Angina—A Controlled Study with Computerized Multistage Treadmill Exercise, *Lancet,* 1:841, 1980.
64. Pine, M. B., Citron, P. D., Bailly, D. J., et al.: Verapamil Versus Placebo in Relieving Stable Angina Pectoris. *Circulation,* 65(suppl. I):17, 1982.
65. Weiner, D. A., and Klein, M. D.: Verapamil Therapy for Stable Exertional Angina, *Am. J. Cardiol.,* 50:1153, 1982.
66. Frishman, W. H., and Charlap, S.: Verapamil in the Treatment of Chronic Stable Angina, *Arch. Intern. Med.,* 143:1407, 1983.
67. Frishman, W. H., and Charlap, S.: Calcium Channel Blockade in Cardiovascular Therapy: Effects of Verapamil on Myocardial Ischemia and Other Disorders, *Cardiovasc. Med.,* 7:773, 1982.
68. Scheidt, S., Frishman, W. H., Packer, M., Mehta, J., Parodi, O., and Bala Subramanian, V.: Long-term Effectiveness of Verapamil in Stable and Unstable Angina Pectoris. One Year Follow-up of Patients Treated in Placebo-Controlled Double-Blind Randomized Clinical Trials, *Am. J. Cardiol.,* 50:1185, 1982.
69. Livesley, B., Catley, P. F., Campbell, R. C., and Oram, S.: Double-Blind Evaluation of Verapamil, Propranolol and Isosorbide Dinitrate Against Placebo in the Treatment of Angina Pectoris, *Br. Med. J.,* 1:375, 1973.
70. Frishman, W. H., Klein, N. A., Strom, J. A., et al.: Superiority of Verapamil to Propranolol in Stable Angina Pectoris—A Double-Blind Randomized Crossover Trial, *Circulation,* 65(suppl. I):51, 1982.
71. Frishman, W. H.: Beta-Adrenergic Blockade in the Treatment of Coronary Artery Disease, in J. W. Hurst (ed.), "Clinical Essays on the Heart," vol. 2, McGraw-Hill Book Co., New York, 1984, p. 25.
72. Lynch, P., Dargie, H., Krikler, S., and Krikler, D.: Objective Assessment of Antianginal Treatment: A Double-Blind Comparison of Propranolol, Nifedipine, and Their Combination, *Br. Med. J.,* 48:131, 1981.
73. Kenmure, A. C. F., and Scruton, J. H.: A Double-Blind Controlled Trial of the Anti-Anginal Efficacy of Nifedipine Compared with Propranolol, *Br. J. Clin. Pract.,* 8:49, 1980.
74. Bala Subramanian, V., Bowles, M. J., Davies, A. B., and Raftery, E. B.: Comparative Effectiveness of Verapamil and Propranolol in Angina of Effort, *Am. J. Cardiol.,* 50:1158, 1982.
75. Bala Subramanian, V., Bowles, M. J., Khupml, N. S., Davies, A. B., and Raftery, E. B.: Comparative Effectiveness of Verapamil and Nifedipine in Stable Angina Pectoris, *Am. J. Cardiol.,* 50:1173, 1982.
76. Frishman, W. H., Klein, N., Klein, P., et al.: Comparison of Oral Propranolol and Verapamil for Combined Systemic Hypertension and Angina Pectoris. A Placebo-Controlled Double-Blind Randomized Crossover Trial, *Am. J. Cardiol.,* 50:1164, 1982.
77. Silverman, K., and Grossman, W.: Angina Pectoris: Natural History and Strategies for Evaluation and Management, *N. Engl. J. Med.,* 310:1712, 1984.
78. Maseri, A., L'Abbate, A., Chierchia, S., et al.: Significance of Spasm in the Pathogenesis of Ischemic Heart Disease, *Am. J. Cardiol.,* 44:788, 1979.
79. Johnson, S. M., Mauitson, D. R., Willerson, J. T., and Hillis, L. D.: A Controlled Trial of Verapamil for Prinzmetal's Variant Angina, *N. Engl. J. Med.,* 304(15):862, 1981.
80. Mehta, J., and Conti, C. R.: Calcium Channel Antagonists in the Treatment of Unstable Angina, *Am. J. Cardiol.,* 50:919, 1982.
81. Theroux, P., Waters, D. D., Affaki, G. S., Critten, J., Bonan, R., and Mizgala, H. F.: Provocative Testing with Ergonovine to Evaluate the Efficacy of Treatment with Calcium Antagonists in Variant Angina, *Circulation,* 60:504, 1979.
82. Antman, E., Muller, J. E., and Goldberg, S.: Nifedipine Therapy for Coronary Artery Spasm Experience in 127 Patients, *N. Engl. J. Med.,* 302:1269, 1980.
83. Schroeder, J. S., Feldman, R. L., Griles, T. D., et al.: Multiclinic Controlled Trial Diltiazem for Prinzmetal's Angina, *Am. J. Med.,* 72:227, 1982.
84. Feldman, R. L., Pepine, C. J., Whittle, J., and Conti, C. R.: Short- and Long-Term Responses to Diltiazem in Patients with Variant Angina, *Am. J. Cardiol.,* 49:554, 1982.
85. Goldberg, S., Reichek, N., Wilson, J., Hirshfeld, Jr., J. W., Muller, J., and Kastor, J. A.: Nifedipine in the Treatment of Prinzmetal's (Variant) Angina, *Am. J. Cardiol.,* 44:804, 1979.
86. Parodí, O., Simonetti, I., L'Abbate, A., and Maseri, A.: Comparative Effectiveness of Verapamil and Propranolol in Angina at Rest, *Am. J. Cardiol.,* 50:923, 1982.
87. Johnson, S. M., Mauritson, D. R., Willerson, J. T., and Hillis, D. L.: Comparison of Verapamil and Nifedipine in the Treatment of Variant Angina Pectoris—Preliminary Observations in 10 Patients, *Am. J. Cardiol.,* 47:1295, 1981.
88. Gerstenblith, G., Ougang, P., Achuff, S., et al.: Nifedipine in Unstable Angina. A Double-Blind Randomized Trial, *N. Engl. J. Med.,* 306:885, 1982.
89. Frishman, W. H., Furberg, C. D., and Friedewald, W. T.: β-Adrenergic Blockade in Survivors of Acute Myocardial Infarction, *N. Engl. J. Med.,* 310:830, 1984.
90. Subramanian, B., Bowles, M. K., Davies, A. B., and Raftery, E. B.: Combined Therapy with Verapamil and Propranolol in Chronic Stable Angina, *Am. J. Cardiol.,* 49:125, 1982.
91. Dargie, H. J., Lynch, P. G., Krikler, D. M., Harris, L., and Krikler, S.: Nifedipine and Propranolol: A Beneficial Drug Interaction, *Am. J. Med.,* 71:676, 1981.
92. Packer, M., Leon, M. B., Bonow, R. O., Kieval, J., Rosing, D. R., and Bala Subramanian, V.: Hemodynamic and Clinical Effects of Combined Therapy with Verapamil and Propranolol in Ischemic Heart Disease, *Am. J. Cardiol.,* 50:903, 1982.
93. Packer, M., and Frishman, W. H.: Calcium Channel Antagonists in Perspective, in M. Packer, and W. H. Frishman (eds.), "Calcium Channel Antagonists in Perspective," Appleton-Century-Crofts, Norwalk, 1984, XVII.
94. Schamroth, L., Krikler, D. M., and Garrett, C.: Immediate Effects of Intravenous Verapamil in Cardiac Arrhythmias, *Br. Med. J.,* 1:660, 1972.
95. Heng, M. K., Singh, B. N., Roche, A. H. G., and Norris, R. M.: Effects of Intravenous Verapamil on Cardiac Arrhythmias and on the Electrocardiogram. *Am. Heart J.,* 90:487, 1975.
96. Klein, H. O., Pauzner, H., DiSegni, E., David, D., and Kaplinsky, E.: The Beneficial Effects of Verapamil in Chronic Atrial Fibrillation, *Arch. Intern. Med.,* 139:747, 1979.
97. Weiner, I.: Verapamil Therapy for Atrial Flutter and Fibrillation, in M. Packer, and W. H. Frishman (eds.), "Calcium Channel Antagonists in Cardiovascular Disease," Appleton-Century-Crofts, Norwalk, 1984, p. 257.
98. Klein, H. O., and Kaplinsky, E.: Comparative Effectiveness of Verapamil and Digoxin in Atrial Fibrillation, *Am. J. Cardiol.,* 50:894, 1982.
99. Krikler, D. M., and Spurrel, R. A. J.: Verapamil in the Treatment of Paroxysmal Supraventricular Tachycardia, *Postgrad. Med. J.,* 50:447, 1974.
100. Singh, B. N., Nademanee, D., and Baky, S.: Calcium Antagonists: Uses in the Treatment of Cardiac Arrhythmias, *Drugs,* 25:125, 1983.

101. Hartel, G., and Hartikainen, M.: Comparison of Verapamil and Practolol in Paroxysmal Supraventricular Tachycardia, *Eur. J. Cardiol.*, 4:87, 1976.
102. Tonkin, A. M., Aylward, P. E., Joel, S. E., and Heddle, W. F.: Verapamil in Prophylaxis of Paroxysmal Atrioventricular Nodal Reentrant Tachycardia, *J. Cardiovasc. Pharmacol.*, 2:473, 1980.
103. Mauritson, D. R., Winniford, M. D., Walker, W. S., Rude, R. E., Cary, J. R., and Hillis, L. D.: Oral Verapamil for Paroxysmal Supraventricular Tachycardia: A Long-Term, Double-Blind, Randomized Trial, *Ann. Intern. Med.*, 96:409, 1982.
104. Spurrell, R. A. J., Krikler, D. M., and Sowton, G. E.: The Effect of Verapamil on the Electrophysiological Properties of the Anomalous Atrioventricular Connections in Wolff-Parkinson-White Syndrome, *Br. Heart J.*, 36:256, 1974.
105. Matsuyama, E., Konishi, T., Okazaki, H., Matsuda, H., and Kawai, C.: Effects of Verapamil on Accessory Pathway Properties and Induction of Circus Movement Tachycardia in Patients with the Wolff-Parkinson-White Syndrome, *J. Cardiovasc. Pharmacol.*, 3:11, 1981.
106. Shigenobu, K., Schneider, J. A., and Sperelakis, N.: Verapamil Blockade of Slow Na^{+} and Ca^{++} Responses in Myocardial Cells, *J. Pharmacol. Exp. Ther.*, 190:280, 1974.
107. Gotsman, M., Lewis, B., Bakst, A., and Mitha, S.: Verapamil in Life-threatening Tachyarrhythmias, *South. Afr. Med. J.*, 46:2017, 1972.
108. Carrasco, H. A., Fuenmayor, A., Barboza, J., and Gonzalez, G.: Effect of Verapamil on Normal Sino-Atrial Node Dysfunction and on Sick Sinus Syndrome, *Am. Heart J.*, 96:760, 1978.
109. Spivack, C., Ocken, S., and Frishman, W. H.: Calcium Antagonists: Clinical Use in Treatment of Systemic Hypertension, *Drugs,* 25:154, 1983.
110. Inouye, I. K., Massie, B. M., Benowitz, N., Simpson, P., and Loge, D.: Antihypertensive Effect of Diltiazem and Comparison with Hydrochlorthiazide, *Am. J. Cardiol.*, 53:1588, 1984.
111. Charlap, S., Kimmel, B., Monuszko, E., et al.: Efficacy and Safety of Twice-Daily Oral Verapamil in Systemic Hypertension, *Clin. Res.*, 32:329A, 1984. (Abstr.)
112. Charlap, S., Kimmel, B., Lazar, E., et al.: Twice Daily Nicardipine in the Treatment of Essential Hypertension, *J. Clin. Hypertension,* 1985 (Dec.).
113. Schutz, E., Ha, H. R., Buhler, F. R., and Follath, F.: Serum Concentration and Antihypertensive Effect of Slow Release Verapamil, *J. Cardiovasc. Pharmacol.*, 4:S346, 1982.
114. Buhler, F. R., Hulthen, U. L., Kiowski, W., and Bolli, P.: Greater Antihypertensive Efficacy of the Calcium Channel Inhibitor Verapamil in Older and Low Renin Patients, *Clin. Sci.*, 63:439S, 1982.
115. Erne, P., Bolli, P., Bertel, O., et al.: Antihypertensive Monotherapy with Calcium Antagonists Relates to Older Age, Liver Pretreatment Renin and Higher Blood Pressure: Comparison of Nifedipine and Verapamil, *Hypertension,* 5(suppl. II):97, 1983.
116. Frishman, W. H., Weinberg, P., Peled, H., Kimmel, B., Charlap, S., and Beer, N.: Calcium-Entry Blockers for the Treatment of Severe Hypertension and Hypertensive Emergencies, *Am. J. Med.*, 77(2B):35, 1984.
117. Beer, N., Gallegos, I., Cohen, A., Klein, N., Sonnenblick, E. H., and Frishman, W. H.: Efficacy of Sublingual Nifedipine in the Acute Treatment of Systemic Hypertension, *Chest,* 79:571, 1981.
118. Cohen, L. S., and Braunwald, E.: Amelioration of Angina Pectoris in Idiopathic Hypertrophic Subaortic Stenosis with Beta-Adrenergic Blockade, *Circulation,* 35:847, 1967.
119. Rosing, D. R., Bonow, R. O., Packer, M., and Epstein, S. E.: Verapamil Therapy for the Management of Hypertrophic Cardiomyopathy, in M. Packer, and W. H. Frishman (eds.), "Calcium Channel Antagonists in Cardiovascular Disease," Appleton-Century-Crofts, Norwalk, 1984, p. 313.
120. Kaltenbach, M., Hopf, R., Kober, G., Bussman, W. D., Keller, M., and Petersen, Y.: Treatment of Hypertrophic Obstructive Cardiomyopathy with Verapamil, *Br. Heart J.*, 42:35, 1979.
121. Rosing, D. R., Kent, K. M., Maron, B. J., Epstein, S. E.: Verapamil Therapy—A New Approach to the Pharmacologic Treatment of Hypertrophic Cardiomyopathy: II. Effects on Exercise Capacity and Symptomatic Status, *Circulation,* 60:1209, 1979.
122. Rosing, D. R., Kent, K. M., Borer, J. S., Seides, S. F., Maron, B. J., and Epstein, S. E.: Verapamil Therapy—A New Approach to the Pharmacologic Treatment of Hypertrophic Cardiomyopathy: I. Hemodynamic Effects, *Circulation,* 60:1201, 1979.
123. Rosing, D. R., Cannon, R. O., Watson, R. M., Kent, K. M., Lakatos, E., and Epstein, S. E.: Comparison of Verapamil and Nifedipine Effects on Symptoms and Exercise Capacity in Patients with Hypertrophic Cardiomyopathy, *Circulation,* 66(suppl. II):II–24, 1982. (Abstr.)
124. Charlap, S., Kimmel, B., and Frishman, W. H.: Calcium-Channel Blockers in Heart Failure, in N. K. Wenger (ed.), "Cardiology, vol. IV, Heart Failure," Butterworths, Ltd., London, 1985 (in press).
125. Charlap, S., and Frishman, W. H.: Nifedipine in Heart Failure, *Int. J. Cardiol.*, 6:665, 1984.
126. Elkayam, U., Weber, L., Torkan, B., McKay, C. R., and Rahimtoola, S. H.: Comparison of Hemodynamic Responses to Nifedipine and Nitroprusside in Severe Chronic Congestive Heart Failure, *Am. J. Cardiol.*, 53:1321, 1984.
127. Losardo, A. A., Klein, N. A., Beer, N., Strom, J. A., Wexler, J. P., Sonnenblick, E. H., and Frishman, W. H.: Beneficial Effects of Sublingual Nifedipine in Patients with Ischemic Heart Disease and Depressed Left Ventricular Function, *Angiology,* 33:811, 1982.
128. Klugmann, S., Salvi, A., and Camerini, F.: Haemodynamic Effects of Nifedipine in Heart Failure, *Br. Heart J.*, 43:440, 1980.
129. Polese, A., Fiorentini, C., Olivari, M. T., and Guazzi, M. D.: Clinical Use of a Calcium Antagonistic Agent (Nifedipine) in Acute Pulmonary Edema, *Am. J. Med.*, 66:825, 1979.
130. Fifer, M. A., Colucci, W. S., Barry, W. H., Wynne, J., and Lorelli, B. H.: Comparative Hemodynamic and Neuroendocrine Effects of Nitroprusside and Nifedipine in Heart Failure, *Circulation,* 68(suppl. III):8, 1983. (Abstr.)
131. Brooks, N., Cattell, M., Pidgeon, J., and Balcon, R.: Unpredictable Response to Nifedipine in Severe Heart Failure. *Br. Med. J.*, 281:1324, 1980.
132. Elkayam, U., Weber, L., McKay, C., and Rahimtoola, S.: Variable, Unpredictable, and Deleterious Hemodynamic Response to Oral Nifedipine in Severe Chronic Heart Failure: An Experience in 32 Patients, *J. Am. Coll. Cardiol.*, 3:478, 1984. (Abstr.)
133. Millard, R. W., Lathrop, D. A., Grupp, G., Ashraf, M., Grupp, I. L., and Schwartz, A.: Differential Cardiovascular Effects of Calcium Channel Blocking Agents: Potential Mechanisms, *Am. J. Cardiol.*, 49:499, 1982.
134. Nayler, W. G.: Cardioprotective Effects of Calcium Ion Antagonists in Myocardial Ischemia, *Clin. Invest. Med.*, 3:91, 1980.
135. Selwyn, A. P., Welman, E., Fox, K., Horlock, P., Pratt, T., and Klein, M.: The Effects of Nifedipine on Acute Experimental Myocardial Ischemia and Infarction in Dogs, *Circ. Res.*, 44:16, 1979.
136. Maroko, P. R.: Experimental Infarction Studies, *Clin. Invest. Med.*, 3:139, 1980.
137. Fein, S., and Frishman, W. H.: Primary Pulmonary Hypertension: Modern Approaches to an Old Problem, *Lung,* 158:113, 1980.
138. Olivari, M. T., Cohn, J. N., Carlyle, P., and Levine, B.: Beneficial Hemodynamic and Exercise Response to Nifedipine in Primary Pulmonary Hypertension, *J. Am. Coll. Cardiol.*, 1:735, 1983. (Abstr.)
139. Rubin, L. J., Nicod, P., Hillis, D., and Firth, B. G.: Hemodynamic Effects of Nifedipine in Primary Pulmonary Hy-

pertension, *J. Am. Coll. Cardiol.*, 1:735, 1983. (Abstr.)
140. Kambara, H., Fujimoto, K., Wakabayashi, A., and Kawai, C.: Primary Pulmonary Hypertension: Beneficial Therapy with Diltiazem, *Am. Heart J.*, 101:230, 1981.
141. DeFeyter, P. J., Kerkkamp, H. J. J., and deJong, J. P.: Sustained Beneficial Effect of Nifedipine in Primary Pulmonary Hypertension, *Am. Heart J.*, 105:333, 1983.
142. Packer, M., Medina, N., and Yushak, M.: Adverse Hemodynamic and Clinical Effects of Nifedipine in Patients with Primary Pulmonary Hypertension, *J. Am. Coll. Cardiol.*, 1:736, 1983. (Abstr.)
143. Allen, G. S., Ahn, H. S., Preziosi, T. J., et al.: Cerebral Arterial Spasm—a Controlled Trial of Nimodipine in Patients with Subarachnoid Hemorrhage, *N. Engl. J. Med.*, 308:619, 1983.
144. Towart, R.: The Pathophysiology of Cerebral Vasospasm and Pharmacological Approaches to its Management, *Acta Neurochir.*, 62:253, 1982.
145. Bussey, H. I., and Talbert, R. L.: Promising Uses of Calcium-Channel Blocking Agents, *Pharmacotherapy*, 4:137, 1984.
146. Allen, G. S., and Bahr, A. L.: Cerebral Arterial Spasm. Part 10: Reversal of Acute and Chronic Spasm in Dogs with Orally Administered Nifedipine, *Neurosurgery*, 4:43, 1979.
147. Allen, G. S., and Banghart, S. B.: Cerebral Arterial Spasm: Part 9: In Vitro Effects of Nifedipine on Serotonin, Phenylephrine and Potassium-Induced Contractions of Canine Basilar and Femoral Artery, *Neurosurgery* 4:37, 1979.
148. Kazda, S., and Towart, R.: Nimodipine: A New Calcium Antagonistic Drug with a Preferential Cerebrovascular Action, *Acta Neurochir.*, 63:259, 1982.
149. Schwartz, M. L., Rotmensch, H. H., Frishman, W. H., and Vlasses, P. H.: Potential Applications of Calcium-Channel Antagonists in the Management of Noncardiac Disorders, in M. Packer, and W. H. Frishman (eds.), "Calcium Channel Antagonists in Cardiovascular Disease," Appleton-Century-Crofts, Norwalk, 1984, p. 371.
150. Fleckenstein, A., and Fleckenstein-Grun, G.: Protection by Calcium Antagonists against Experimental Arterial Calcinosis, in K. Pyorala, E. Rapaport, K. Konig, G. Schletter, C. Diehm (eds.), "Secondary Prevention of Coronary Heart Disease," Thieme-Stratton, New York, 1983.
151. Factor, S. M., Minase, T., Cho, S., et al.: Microvascular Spasm in the Cardiomyopathic Syrian Hamster. A Preventable Cause of Focal Myocardial Necrosis, *Circulation*, 66:342, 1982.
152. Factor, S. M., and Sonnenblick, E. H.: Microvascular Spasm as a Cause of Cardiomyopathies, *Cardiovasc. Rev. Rep.*, 9:1177, 1983.
153. Lewis, J. G.: Adverse Reactions to Calcium Antagonists, *Drugs*, 25:196, 1983.
154. Terry, R. W.: Nifedipine Therapy in Angina Pectoris: Evaluation of Safety and Side Effects, *Am. Heart J.*, 104:681, 1982.
155. Frishman, W. H., Klein, N. A., Charlap, S., Klein, P., Cohen, M. N., and Rotmensch, H. H.: Recognition and Management of Verapamil Poisoning, in M. Packer, and W. H. Frishman (eds.), "Calcium Channel Antagonists in Cardiovascular Disease," Appleton-Century-Crofts, Norwalk, 1984, p. 365.
156. Klein, H. O., Lang, R., Weiss, E., et al.: The Influence of Verapamil on Serum Digoxin Concentrations, *Circulation*, 65:998, 1982.
157. Schwartz, J. B., Keefe, D., Kates, R. E., Kirsten, E., and Harrison, D. C.: Acute and Chronic Pharmacodynamic Interaction of Verapamil and Digoxin in Atrial Fibrillation, *Circulation*, 65:1163, 1982.
158. Pedersen, K. E., Dorph-Pedersen, A., Hvidt, S., Klitgaard, N. A., and Nielsen-Kudsk, F.: Digoxin-Verapamil Interaction, *Clin. Pharmacol. Ther.*, 30:311, 1981.
159. Belz, G. G., Aust, P. E., and Munkes, R.: Digoxin Plasma Concentrations and Nifedipine, *Lancet*, 1:844, 1981.
160. Pedersen, K. E., Dorph-Pedersen, A., Hvidt, S., Klitgaard, N. A., Kjaer, K., and Nielsen-Kudsk, F.: Effect of Nifedipine on Digoxin Kinetics in Healthy Subjects, *Clin. Pharmacol. Ther.*, 32:562, 1982.
161. Mitchell, L. B., Jutzy, K. R., Lewis, S. J., Schroeder, J. S., and Mason, J. W.: Intracardiac Electrophysiologic Study of Intravenous Diltiazem and Combined Diltiazem-Digoxin in Patients, *Am. Heart J.*, 103:57, 1982.

92

Digitalis

Frank I. Marcus, M.D.

Shoei K. Huang, M.D.

Digitalis is a term used to designate the entire class of cardiac glycosides, one of the most important and widely used groups of drugs in clinical medicine. Cardiac glycosides of medicinal importance are obtained from the plants, *Digitalis purpurea* (digitoxin, gitalin) and *Digitalis lanata* [digoxin, lanatoside-C (Cedilanid), deslanoside (Cedilanid-D), acetyldigitoxin (Acylanid), digitoxin].

Chemistry

Cardiac glycosides have a characteristic ring structure known as an aglycone or genin coupled with one to four sugar molecules (Fig. 92-1). The aglycone portion of the glycoside consists of a steroid nucleus and a five- or six-membered α,β unsaturated lactone ring at the C_{17} position of the steroid nucleus. A beta-oriented hydroxyl substitution is usually present at the C_3 and C_{14} position. The sugar portion of the glycoside is attached to the steroid nucleus, usually through a hydroxyl group at the C_3 position. The most commonly used cardiac glycoside, digoxin, differs from digitoxin only by the presence of a C_{12} hydroxyl group.

Structure Activity Relations

Molecular requirements for potent cardiac effects include the unsaturated lactone ring, the C_{14} hy-

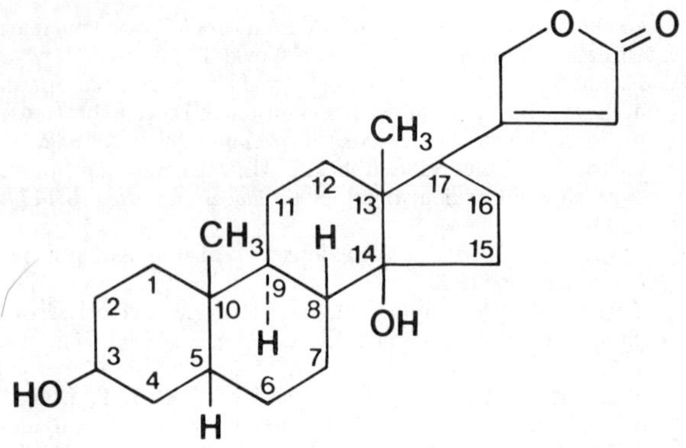

	12 position	Sugar(s) at 3 position
Acetyldigitoxin	—	**acetyltridigitoxose**
Deslanoside	OH	**tridigitoxose - glucose**
Digitoxin	—	**tridigitoxose**
Digoxin	OH	**tridigitoxose**

FIGURE 92-1 Comparative structures of cardiac glycosides. The aglycone is pictured. Digitoxose sugar has the molecular structure $C_6H_{10}O_3$. (This diagram was constructed after studying several sources.)

droxyl group, and the spatial (*cis*) configuration of the C-D ring structures containing carbons 8 through 17 (Fig. 92-1).[1] This particular *cis* configuration differentiates this steroid ring structure from those of endogenous steroids from mammalian species. Saturation of the lactone ring yields the dihydro derivative, a much less potent compound. Increasing the number of hydroxyl groups on the aglycone increases polarity and decreases lipid solubility which, in turn, is associated with decreased absorption. The number of sugars influences the pharmacokinetics more than they alter the potency. As the number of sugars attached to the genin of digitoxin (and presumably digoxin) diminishes, the greater is the metabolism to water-soluble metabolites and shorter the half-life.[2–4] In general, the more lipid-soluble cardiac glycosides, such as digitoxin, are metabolized before excretion while the more polar cardiac glycosides, such as digoxin, deslanoside, and lantoside-C are excreted primarily by the renal route, mostly in unchanged form.

Pharmacokinetics

The pharmacokinetics of the two most widely used cardiac glycosides, digitoxin and digoxin, are summarized in Table 92-1.[5–15] In comparison with digitoxin, digoxin is much less bound to plasma proteins, has a nearly tenfold larger volume of distribution and has a half-life four times as rapid as digitoxin.

Cardiac glycosides are widely distributed in body tissues. The highest concentrations are found in the kidney, followed by cardiac muscle.[16] The concentration of digoxin in skeletal muscle is less than in cardiac muscle, but since skeletal muscle represents approximately 40 percent of the total body weight, digoxin is distributed principally to this tissue. About 60 percent of digoxin is excreted in the urine.[17] Until recently it was thought that digoxin was excreted primarily in unchanged form, but a variety of metabolites have now been identified, particularly the dihydro derivative of digoxin.[18,19] Only about 15 percent of digitoxin is excreted unchanged in the urine, although an equal amount is excreted in unchanged form in the feces.

Special Considerations of Digoxin Pharmacokinetics

An understanding of the alterations that occur with digoxin pharmacokinetics is important because alterations in digoxin kinetics mandate a change in digoxin dosage.

Digoxin Bioavailability

Digoxin is unstable in acidic solutions. Significant hydrolysis of digoxin occurs if the intragastric pH is below 2, particularly if there is delayed gastric

TABLE 92-1 Pharmacokinetics of Digoxin and Digitoxin in Humans with Normal Renal Function*

Glycoside	Absolute Bioavailability, %	Plasma Protein-Binding, %	Volume of Distribution, 1/kg	Biological Half-Life, Days
Digoxin		25 (20–30)†	5 (4–8)	1.7 (1.1–1.9)
Tablet	60 (50–80)			
Elixir	70 (60–80)			
Capsules††	85 (80–100)			
Digitoxin	90 (80–100)	93 (80–97)	0.46 (0.4–0.65)	7.0 (5–10)

*Data from normal subjects and patients.
†( ) range.
††Lanoxicaps.

emptying time.[20] In addition, digoxin may be extensively metabolized in the gut to dihydro derivatives, and this has been found in approximately one of every ten subjects studied.[21] In some patients, extensive biotransformation of digoxin to dihydro metabolites in the intestines may account for resistance to therapy and unusually high digoxin requirements.[19] The use of a highly bioavailable preparation such as an encapsulated liquid concentrate of digoxin minimizes metabolic inactivation in those subjects with extensive intraintestinal metabolism of digoxin to dihydro derivatives.[22]

Infants and Children

Infants have been found to absorb digoxin in solution at the same rate and to the same extent as adults.[23] However, binding of digoxin to several tissues appears to be more extensive in infants than in adults, as exemplified by a larger volume of distribution. This may account for the clinical observation that larger doses, calculated on the basis of body weight or surface area, need to be administered to infants and children than to adults to achieve similar serum concentrations of digoxin. In infants (except neonates) the elimination half-life of digoxin is shorter than in adults. Infants and children appear to tolerate higher serum concentrations of digoxin without manifestations of toxicity.

Elderly Patients

The pharmacokinetic alterations of digoxin in the elderly are in a direction opposite to that of the infant.[24–26] This is a decrease in the apparent volume of distribution, principally due to a decrease in skeletal mass. There is also a decrease in the renal clearance of digoxin due to aging. This accounts for the well-known observation that the loading dose and maintenance dose of digoxin needs to be decreased in the elderly.

Obesity

The kinetics of digoxin are little altered in the obese individual since the concentration of digoxin in fatty tissue is quite low.[27,28] Thus, the dosage of digoxin should be calculated on the basis of lean body mass rather than on total body weight.

Renal Failure

Impaired kidney function is the most important condition that influences digoxin pharmacokinetics. Digoxin is excreted primarily by the kidneys.[29] It would seem reasonable to assume that patients with renal failure would have a decrease in digoxin clearance, with a consequent increase in half-life, and thus require a smaller dose. Indeed, this has been borne out in numerous studies.[30–32] Although the fecal excretion of digoxin is increased in patients with renal failure as well as in anephric patients, this does not compensate for the diminished renal excretion of digoxin.[31] There is no change in the pattern of digoxin metabolites, including the amount of dihydrodigoxin excreted in patients with renal failure as compared with subjects with normal renal function.[33] Although there is no marked change in the biotransformation of digoxin, a 35-to-50 percent decrease in the apparent volume distribution of digoxin subjects with severe renal insufficiency has been documented.[7,34] The mechanism of this decrease in the apparent volume of distribution is not clear. A recent study indicates that binding of digoxin to skeletal muscle is not decreased, since the ratio of skeletal muscle to serum digoxin concentration in patients with renal failure is not significantly different from this ratio in subjects with normal renal function.[35] Possible explanations for the decreased volume of distribution are either reduction of tissue mass or reduced digoxin binding to organs other than skeletal muscle.[36] Whatever the explanation, this decrease in volume of distribution indicates that a smaller-than-usual loading dose should be given to patients with severe renal insufficiency.[34,37]

Hepatic Failure

The pharmacokinetics of digoxin are not significantly altered in patients with acute hepatitis[38] or in patients with chronic liver disease due to alcoholic cirrhosis.[39]

Pregnancy

It is not clear whether serum levels of digoxin are altered during pregnancy. Rogers et al.[40] found that the serum digoxin levels in five pregnant patients were lower at delivery than 1 month later. On the other hand, Luxford and Kellaway[41] observed a significantly higher digoxin level in the third trimester compared to the postpartum period in 16 women who were maintained on the same dose of digoxin during this interval. The latter observation of a higher digoxin concentration during pregnancy is puzzling since Luxford and Kellaway found that there was an increase in creatinine clearance, in digoxin renal clearance and in the 24-hour excretion of digoxin during pregnancy than postpartum. They postulated that an increased absorption of digoxin during pregnancy may account for their findings.

Paired cord and maternal blood samples obtained at parturition showed lower digoxin levels in cord blood than in maternal blood.[42] This is of interest because occasionally one may need to treat supraventricular tachycardia in the fetus with digoxin and this suggests that higher concentrations of digoxin should be given to the mother to obtain a therapeutic effect in the fetus. However, daily maintenance doses of digoxin, 0.125 to 0.5 mg given to the mother, have successfully treated fetal supraventricular tachycardia.[43] Although the concentration of digoxin in breast milk is approximately equal to the unbound plasma digoxin concentration, the quantity of digoxin ingested daily by infants is estimated to be between $\frac{1}{100}$ to $\frac{1}{20}$ of the recommended maintenance dose.[44] Therefore, breastfeeding may safely be permitted in lactating mothers receiving digoxin therapy.

Hypothyroidism and Hyperthyroidism

In 1966, Doherty and Perkins[45] studied digoxin metabolism in hypothyroidism and hyperthyroidism. They found that serum digoxin levels were lower after an intravenous dose of digoxin in hyperthyroid patients and higher in hypothyroid patients as compared to euthyroid patients. They could not explain these changes. There was no statistical difference in the excretion of a single dose of tritiated digoxin among hypothyroid or euthyroid patients. In studies in dogs with altered thyroid function there was no difference in the tissue concentration when the serum levels showed their greatest differences. In addition, they found they could not document a difference in absorption or excretion after oral administration. Despite extensive studies by several other investigators of the pharmacokinetics of digoxin in altered states of thyroid function,[46–48] we are now no closer to an explanation for the effects observed by Doherty nearly 20 years ago. Since it is not clear whether end-organ susceptibility to alterations in thyroid function are present, it would seem reasonable to maintain serum digoxin concentration within the therapeutic range.

Pharmacological Actions

William Withering[49] emphasized the diuretic action of digitalis, since this was an effect that was desirable and readily measurable. Only relatively recently was it established that the primary action by which digitalis improves the circulation in patients with heart failure is its inotropic effect.[50] Over the past 40 years, there have been literally hundreds of investigations attempting to clarify the actions of digitalis, including its action at the subcellular level,[51–53] and these have resulted in tremendous advances in our understanding of the effects of digitalis in humans. The action of digitalis is complex and involves several mechanisms, including an inotropic effect that can be demonstrated in both the normal and abnormal myocardium, an enhancement of the vagal and diminution of the sympathetic effect on the heart, and finally, direct arterial vasoconstriction.

Inotropic Effect

Digitalis enhances contractility by increasing the amount of calcium available during excitation-contraction coupling. The precise mechanism by which this occurs has not been clearly defined. Cardiac glycosides bind to Na^+, K^+, activated membrane adenosine triphosphatase (ATPase) of various tissues, including the heart. There are two hypotheses to account for the increase in calcium induced by Na^+, K^+-ATPase binding. The first is that digitalis binding to the sodium pump directly results in enhanced calcium influx. Another hypothesis is that the glycoside acts by causing a decrease in sodium pump activity. Intracellular sodium concentration increases, and this favors the influx of calcium. The net result is that digitalis causes an increase of intracellular calcium that results in enhanced myocardial contractility.

Enhancement of Parasympathetic Activity

Digitalis increases the sensitivity of the arterial baroreceptor reflex so that afferent signals are augmented, resulting in increase of vagal and a decrease in sympathetic efferent activity.[54] Digitalis also acts in the central vagal nuclei and nodose ganglia to enhance efferent signals.[55] Digitalis alters the electrical excitability of efferent vagal fibers and impulse transmission in autonomic ganglia.[56] Finally, there is evidence that digitalis may increase the sensitivity of cardiac fibers to the actions of acetylcholine.[57] These parasympathomimetic effects are primarily responsible for the therapeutic efficacy of digitalis in the treatment of supraventricular arrhythmias.

Diminution of Sympathetic Activity

Digitalis, through sensitization of the baroreceptor reflexes, causes some decrease in efferent sympathetic activity, and this decrease contributes to the decrease in sinus rate and prolongation of the atrioventricular (AV) nodal refractory period.[58]

Direct Vasoconstrictor Effect of Digitalis

Digoxin induces contraction in isolated human arteries and veins which are not diminished by α-adrenoceptor blockade, but are abolished by a calcium antagonist.[59] A neurogenic vasoconstrictor effect of digitalis on coronary vascular resistance has also been reported.[60] The vasoconstrictor effect of digitalis can result in an increase in systemic resistance as well as pulmonary resistance[61] which can worsen failure, particularly when given as a bolus.[62,63] The increase in the vasoconstrictor effect, which is rapid in onset, may precede the inotropic effect on the heart.

Electrophysiologic Effects of Digitalis

The influences of digitalis on the electrophysiologic properties of the heart are quite complex. These effects vary with dose, type of cardiac tissue involved, and autonomic activity. It has direct effects on the transmembrane action potentials by inhibition of $Na^+ = K^+ =$ ATPase (sodium pump).[64] Its most important properties in the treatment of superventricular arrhythmias are indirect and dependent upon vagal and antiadrenergic neural mechanisms. The electrophysiologic effects of digi-

TABLE 92-2 Electrophysiologic Effect of Digitalis on Cardiac Tissue

	Automaticity	Excitability	Conduction Velocity	Effective Refractory Period	(Delayed After-depolarization)
SA node					
Therapeutic	↔ (or ↓)	-	↓*	-	-
Toxic	↔ or ↑ (↑)	-	↓↓*	-	-
Atrial muscle					
Therapeutic	↔	↔	↔ (↑)	↔ (↓**)	-
Toxic	↑	↓	↔ or ↓ (↓)	↑	+
AV node					
Therapeutic	↔	-	↓	↑	-
Toxic	↑	-	↓↓	↑↑	-
Purkinje fibers					
Therapeutic	↔	↑	↔ or ↓	↔ or ↑ (↑)	-
Toxic	↑	↓	↓	↓	+
Ventricular muscle					
Therapeutic	↔	Variable	↔ or ↓	↓	-
Toxic	↑	↓	↓	↓	+
Accessory pathway					
Therapeutic	-	-	↑	↔ or ↓	-
Toxic	-	-	↑	↓	-

Note: Phrase or symbol inside parentheses indicates observations made only in animal studies.
* = Sinoatrial conduction: ** = Increase after atropine; + = present; - = absent or not applicable; ↑ = increase; ↓ = decrease; ↔ = no effect; ↑↑ = markedly increased; ↓↓ = markedly decreased.

talis vary according to the animal species studied. These effects are summarized in Table 92-2.

Sinoatrial Node

In mammalian species, administration of therapeutic doses of digitalis causes little chronotropic effect on the sinoatrial (SA) node.[55,65–68] Administration of digitalis to patients with ventricular failure often results in slowing of the sinus rate. This is largely explained by the fact that digitalis improves ventricular performance with a decrease in sympathetic tone. If digitalis is given to subjects without heart failure, the sinus rate remains unchanged. Digitalis can be administered to most patients with sinus bradycardia or asymptomatic sinus pauses without further decreasing sinus rate or accentuating the post-tachycardia pauses.[69–71] However, the patient with sick sinus syndrome may have accentuation of symptoms due to secondary pauses after digitalis administration. If digitalis therapy is indicated for heart failure in patients with sick sinus syndrome, an electrophysiologic study is indicated. The findings of a corrected sinus node recovery time of over 1000 ms has been found to be predictive of further lengthening of pauses in some, but not all patients.[72] Twenty-four hours ambulatory ECG recordings also should be done before and after digitalis administration in patients with sick sinus syndrome.

Atrium

The electrophysiologic effects of digitalis on atrial tissue are highly variable and are influenced by an interplay between drug concentration and the level of autonomic tone. In most intact animal studies, therapeutic concentrations of digitalis appear to have a predominant vagal action that results in shortening of atrial effective refractory period and acceleration of conduction.[64,73,74] After denervation or atropine, digitalis increases atrial effective refractory period and slows conduction.[73,74] Therapeutic doses of cardiac glycosides cause either no change[75,76] or an increase in atrial refractory periods in humans.[67,77] Atrial conduction velocity, as measured by the PA interval, has been found to be increased[67] or show no change[69] following digitalis administration. These conflicting findings have been partially clarified by Hayward et al.[78] who showed that the observed changes are time-dependent. They observed a biphasic electrophysiologic response to methyldigoxin in the human right atrium. There was initial prolongation of the action potential, which was maximal at 20 min after infusion and was associated with an increase in atrial effective refractoriness and vulnerability to atrial tachyarrhythmia induction. During the later phase (30 to 40 min) of infusion, atrial action potential shortened with a decrease in effective refractoriness and vulnerability to tachyarrhythmias. Atropine reduced the magnitude of both early and late components of the biphasic action-potential response to digitalis. These observations of a time-dependent effect on atrial tachycardia induction are important when electrophysiologic testing is performed for the evaluation of digitalis effect on the supraventricular tachyarrhythmias.

Atrioventricular Node

Digitalis causes a prolongation of conduction and refractory periods of the AV node.[79] These effects are predominantly due to the vagal and antiadrenergic influence of digitalis.[56,66] Wu et al.[75] have shown that ouabain increases the effective refractory periods of both the fast and slow AV nodal pathways in the anterograde direction. The effect of digitalis on retrograde conduction and the retrograde refractory period in the AV node is variable.[68]

Purkinje Fibers and Ventricular Muscle

There are little neural (indirect) effects of digitalis in therapeutic concentrations on Purkinje fibers and ventricular muscle.[80,81] Digitalis shortens the effective refractory period in the ventricle.[76]

Accessory Pathway

In human studies, there is a variable effect of digitalis on the anterograde effective refractory period of the accessory pathway in Wolff-Parkinson-White (WPW) syndrome.[82–84] Jedeikin found that digitalis shortened this interval by more than 40 ms in nearly 40 percent of children.[85] The retrograde effective refractory period of the accessory pathway is generally not affected by digitalis.[83,84]

Use of Digitalis

Digitalis has two major uses: (1) treatment of congestive heart failure, and (2) treatment as well as the prevention of supraventricular arrhythmias. At present, the trend is to not completely rely on digitalis for treatment of acute congestive heart failure since there are more potent inotropic drugs available for parenteral use. For treatment of acute or chronic heart failure, diuretics may be administered intravenously or orally and can effectively relieve symptoms and signs of heart failure. Moreover, vasodilating drugs such as captopril, hydralazine, and prazosin are effective in relieving symptoms of congestive heart failure, as well as increasing exercise tolerance. However, digitalis has many advantages as a drug for the treatment of chronic congestive heart failure. It is an inotropic drug that can be given orally once a day, has excellent short- and long-term tolerance, does not exhibit tachyphylaxis, and is inexpensive. It remains to be determined whether treatment for chronic congestive heart failure should be initiated with digitalis, diuretics, or vasodilators alone or in combination. In the United States the most common practice is to start therapy for congestive heart failure with digitalis in combination with diuretics. Vasodilators are considered a second line of therapy.

To a large extent, digitalis has been replaced by the calcium channel blocking drugs, verapamil and diltiazem, for treatment of paroxysmal supraventricular tachycardia. Digitalis is still the drug choice for treatment of this condition in the patient who is also receiving beta-blocking drugs or who has known sick sinus syndrome, since the calcium channel blocking drugs may result in marked asystole after conversion. In addition, certain calcium channel blocking drugs such as verapamil decrease cardiac contractility, thereby giving digitalis an advantage in treating paroxysmal supraventricular tachycardia in the presence of congestive heart failure. Finally, digitalis is effective in preventing atrial fibrillation, whereas the calcium channel blocking drugs are not.

Heart Failure

Left Ventricular Failure in Patients with Acute Myocardial Infarction

Digitalis has minimal and unpredictable effects in patients with heart failure due to acute myocardial infarction,[86] and other drugs are preferable. When ouabain was compared with furosemide in patients with myocardial infarction who had an increase in pulmonary arterial pressure, furosemide caused a greater decrease in pulmonary arterial diastolic pressures than did ouabain. Cardiac output was not markedly decreased with furosemide.[87] A comparison of dobutamine and digoxin in patients with acute myocardial infarction and cardiac failure showed that dobutamine markedly increased cardiac output, decreased filling pressure, and relieved pulmonary congestion, whereas digoxin did not affect either preload or afterload.[88] Thus, an inotropic drug alone and/or with a diuretic is the preferred treatment for patients with acute myocardial infarction who have congestive heart failure. However, an alternate mode of therapy would be to combine digoxin and an afterload-reducing agent such as nitroprusside. When nitroprosside was used alone in patients with congestive heart failure complicating acute myocardial infarction, there was a decrease in the wedge pressure as well as an increase in cardiac output. The addition of digoxin further increased cardiac output and decreased systemic vascular resistance.[89]

Right Heart Failure Due to Cor Pulmonale

Digitalis has not been shown to be beneficial in these patients,[90] but one should not overlook the possibility that patients who have cor pulmonale may also have left heart failure which may benefit from digitalis. Determination or radionuclide left and right ventricular ejection fraction may be helpful in clarifying the presence or absence of left heart failure. Not only is digitalis not beneficial in patients with right heart failure due to cor pulmonale, but it may be especially hazardous since such patients are sensitive to digitalis intoxication even in the absence of hypokalemia.[91]

Heart Failure Due to Left-to-Right Shunt in Infants and Children

There is serious question as to whether the majority of infants and children with left-to-right shunt due to a ventricular septal defect or patent ductus arteriosus are benefited by digitalis.[92–94] There are no controlled trials which document the efficacy of digitalis for infants with left-to-right shunts who may have normal left ventricular contractility and whose symptoms of heart failure may be due to circulatory overload.[95]

Maintenance Digitalis and Chronic Heart Failure
Despite 200 years of digitalis use, its proper therapeutic role in congestive heart failure with sinus rhythm is not known. It is firmly established that digoxin has a long-term inotropic effect in patients with normal sinus rhythm.[96] There are few rigorously designed studies that have utilized a placebo-controlled, double-crossover design to determine the value of digitalis in chronic heart failure.[96–98] Dobbs et al. found that 16 of 46 (35 percent) of clinically stable patients deteriorated when a placebo was substituted for digoxin. Lee et al. treated outpatients with clinical and radiographic evidence of heart failure with digoxin. Fourteen of twenty-five patients who completed the protocol improved clinically with digoxin. It appeared that the patients who improved had more severe heart failure, particularly an S_3 gallop. However, this should not imply that patients who do not have an S_3 gallop can be safely withdrawn from this drug. In the study by Lee, most patients with appreciable heart failure treated with digoxin deteriorated clinically when digoxin was discontinued. On the other hand, half of the patients with little evidence of heart failure while taking digoxin deteriorated clinically. Therefore it appears that we cannot now identify which patients may be safely withdrawn from digoxin on the basis of clinical information.

Somewhat at odds with this study is that report by Fleg[97] which concluded that chronic digoxin therapy was of no clinical benefit in patients with stable congestive heart failure because none of the 30 patients completing the protocol deteriorated clinically during 3 months of placebo administration. Of particular note are the results of the study by Arnold et al.[99] who found that digitalis withdrawal was accompanied by deterioration of left ventricular function in all nine patients who were in chronic heart failure. After digitalization was reinstated, the effectiveness of digitalis was again demonstrated hemodynamically by invasive methods. It can be concluded that some patients with chronic left heart failure may deteriorate clinically and hemodynamically after digitalis withdrawal despite continuation of diuretic therapy.

As yet it is unclear how to accurately identify patients in whom digitalis can be safely withdrawn. If the reason for initial digitalization was acute heart failure associated with myocardial infarction, pneumonia, or heart failure associated with surgery, and signs of congestive heart failure have not recurred, it would seem reasonable to stop digitalis. One must be alert to the fact that an appreciable number of patients who have signs and symptoms of heart failure may have circulatory failure because of diastolic dysfunction and digitalis is not likely to benefit these patients. These individuals may be identified by having a normal left ventricular ejection fraction in the presence of congestive heart failure.

Possible Enhanced Mortality in Patients on Chronic Digitalis Therapy after Myocardial Infarction
Until recently it has been assumed that the benefits of digitalis in chronic congestive heart failure outweigh its possible harmful effects. However, the controversy of the harmful effects of digitalis has been heightened by several reports which indicate that there may be an increase in mortality associated with digitalis treatment in the early months following an acute myocardial infarction.[100–102] The reported increase in mortality associated with digoxin therapy was present even after adjustment for major cardiac covariates such as left ventricular ejection fraction and ventricular ectopic beat frequency.[102] Other investigators have not been able to document an increase in mortality associated with digitalis, either after an infarction or in patients with chronic coronary artery disease.[103,104] Nevertheless, the possible increased mortality associated with digitalis after infarction should cause the physician to carefully evaluate the need for digitalis therapy, particularly within the first year after myocardial infarction.

Treatment of Arrhythmias

Paroxysmal Supraventricular Tachycardia
Most paroxysmal supraventricular tachycardias (PSVT) are due to reentry involving the AV node. By its modification of the critical relation between conduction time and refractory period of the slow and fast pathways in the AV node, digitalis can terminate paroxysmal AV nodal reentrant tachycardias.[75,105] Digitalis alone or in combination with other beta blockers or calcium channel blocking agents is also useful in preventing paroxysmal supraventricular tachycardias. Prior to therapy with digitalis for PSVT, digitalis intoxication should be excluded as a cause of the arrhythmia.

Atrial Fibrillation or Flutter
Digitalis is commonly used to treat atrial fibrillation or flutter with a rapid ventricular rate. Digitalis can decrease ventricular rate, both at rest and during moderate exercise, by increased concealed conduction into the AV node, decreased conduction velocity, and prolonged refractoriness of the AV node.[106–108] Conversion to normal sinus rhythm may occur in the course of digitalization. Addition of calcium channel or beta-blocking agents may be useful when the ventricular rate is difficult to control by digitalis alone.

Multifocal Atrial Tachycardia
Digitalis is generally not effective in either abolishing this rhythm or slowing the ventricular response. In addition, since this arrhythmia is usually associated with severe obstructive pulmonary disease, a condition in which there is increased sensitivity to digitalis toxicity, the use of digitalis should be avoided in the treatment of multifocal atrial tachycardia unless there is concomitant congestive heart failure.[109]

Ventricular Ectopy
The use of digitalis in treating ventricular arrhythmias is not impressive.[110] However, Lown et al.[111] reported that the frequency and grade of ventricular premature beats were reduced in 46 percent of patients receiving acetylstrophanthidin, unchanged in 26 percent, and increased in 28 percent. They concluded that the antiarrhythmic action of acetylstrophanthidin did not appear to be related to its positive inotropic action. Other observers[112,113] have found that digoxin was ineffective in suppressing complex ventricular ectopy and the reduction in frequency of ectopy was found primarily in patients with normal ejection fraction. There is general agreement that digitalis should not be withheld in patients with congestive heart failure and ventricular ectopy not due to digitalis intoxication.

Wolff-Parkinson-White Syndrome
The beneficial electrophysiologic effects seen in AV nodal reentrant paroxysmal supraventricular tachycardia may also apply to patients with WPW syndrome who have narrow QRS paroxysmal circus movement tachycardia. In this type of tachycardia the anterograde conduction occurs by the AV node and the impulse returns to the atrium by way of the accessory pathway. However, Dhingra et al.[83] found that sustained tachycardia was still inducible in 89 percent of the 19 patients after administration of intravenous ouabain. This suggests that digitalis alone may be of benefit only in a minority of patients who have this type of tachycardia. Combination therapy with type I drugs, such as procainamide or quinidine, or propranolol, may be more effective in preventing recurrent tachycardia.[114] Digitalis is hazardous in the WPW syndrome since it can increase the ventricular response via the accessory pathway and may result in ventricular fibrillation and sudden death.[115] Sellers et al.[84] found that treatment with digitalis was temporally related to the onset of ventricular fibrillation resulting from atrial fibrillation in nine of 21 patients. Each of these patients had short RR intervals (220 ms or less) during atrial fibrillation in the control state. For this reason, it is suggested that digitalis not be used in patients with WPW syndrome. If it must be used, an electrophysiologic study should be performed before institution of long-term therapy.

Choice of a Digitalis Preparation and Dosing

There are only two cardiac glycosides in common use in the United States at this time, digoxin and digitoxin. Ouabain is no longer available commercially. A loading dose of digoxin is usually not necessary unless there is urgency in achieving digitalis effect. In the absence of a loading dose, steady-state serum and tissue concentrations are achieved in 5 to 7 days. The usual oral maintenance dose is 0.25 mg. Generally, it is half that amount in the elderly or in patients with severe renal insufficiency. In some patients, particularly those who have a large, lean body mass, the dose may be 0.5 mg. The average oral loading dose of digoxin ranges from 1.25 to 1.5 mg given in divided doses over a 24-h period. The oral loading dose for Lanoxicaps, a formulation of digoxin in an encapsulated gel form, is 0.8 to 1.2 mg, while the usual daily maintenance dose with this preparation if 0.1 to 0.4 mg. Intravenous doses are approximately 70 percent of the oral dose recommended for the tablet.

Digitalization with digitoxin is usually started with a loading dose since it would require approximately a month to achieve a steady state. The loading dose ranges from 0.8 to 1.2 mg in 24 h, given in divided doses. The maintenance dose is usually 0.1 to 0.15 mg of digitoxin daily. The dose for the intravenous drug is the same as that for oral administration.

Drug Interactions with Digitalis

Of great importance is the recognition that the serum levels of digoxin or digitoxin can be altered by coadministration of other medicines. Drug interactions with digoxin are listed in Table 92-3. Although drug interactions which alter the serum levels of digoxin are well recognized, and the pharmacokinetic mechanisms of the interactions have been defined, it is not clear whether or to what extent the effectiveness of digoxin changes when the serum levels are altered. Quantitation of the concentration of cardiac glycosides in the heart would not resolve the question because most of the cardiac glycoside in heart muscle is nonspecifically bound to membrane lipids and other sites where it does not exert a pharmacological effect. It is extremely difficult to relate serum concentration of cardiac glycoside and effective occupancy of specific receptors in heart muscle. Until further investigations clarify the clinical significance of serum levels as altered by concomitantly administered drugs, we must assume that digoxin serum concentration reflects the intensity of the action of digoxin and strive to keep the serum levels within the accepted therapeutic range.

TABLE 92-3 Clinically Significant Pharmacokinetic Interactions with Digoxin

Interfering Drugs	Change in Steady State Serum Digoxin Levels, %	Mechanism of Interaction	Comments	Ref.
Cholestyramine (Questran)	− 30	Physical binding to resin	Avoid by dosing cholestyramine bid, 8 h from digoxin administration	116,117
Metoclopramide (Reglan)	− 36	↓ Bioavailability by ↑ intestinal motility	(?) Administer digoxin as elixir or as Lanoxicaps	118
Propantheline (Pro-Banthine)	+ 27	↑ Bioavailability by ↓ intestinal motility	(?) Administer digoxin as elixir or as Lanoxicaps	
Sulfasalazine (Azulfidine)	− 20	↓ Bioavailability		117
Erythromycin or Tetracycline*	+ 72	↑ Bioavailability due to inactivation of gut flora	Measure serum digoxin with coadministration of these antibiotics with digoxin	119
Neomycin	− 28	↓ Bioavailability	Measure serum digoxin levels	119
Chemotherapy	− 50	↓ Bioavailability (?) due to damage to intestinal mucosa	Measure serum digoxin levels	120
Amiodarone (Cordarone)	+100	↓ In renal and total body clearance of digoxin	↓ Digoxin dose by one-half	121,122,123
Quinidine	+100	(?) ↑ Absorption ↓ vol. of distribution ↓ renal and total body clearance of digoxin	↓ Digoxin dose by one-half	124,125,126,127
Quinine	+ 75	↓ Renal clearance of digoxin	↓ Digoxin dose by one-half	128
Verapamil	+ 75	↓ Renal and total body clearance of digoxin	↓ Digoxin dose by one-half	129,130

*Expected to occur in 10 percent of patients; those who have substantial conversion in gut of digoxin to dihydro derivatives.

Digitalis Toxicity

Intoxication with digitalis continues to be a frequent complication of therapy because of the narrow toxic therapeutic ratio. The signs and symptoms of digitalis toxicity are well known. Among the most common manifestations are anorexia, fatigue, visual disturbances, and, in the elderly, confusion. Although these symptoms are not specific, their onset or exacerbation should raise the suspicion of digitalis toxicity. The physician should reevaluate whether the dose prescribed is appropriate and should carefully review whether or not the patient is actually taking the prescribed amount. Patients can readily become confused when they are taking multiple drugs for treatment of congestive heart failure. Inadvertently they may take several times the daily dose of digitalis that has been prescribed. Other frequent causes of toxicity are drugs concomitantly prescribed that raise serum digoxin levels (Table 92-3),[116–130] as well as diuretic-induced hypokalemia. Worsening heart failure may result in a decrease in renal function with consequent decrease in renal and extrarenal excretion of digoxin with resultant digoxin accumulation. Under these circumstances the half-life of digoxin can approach that of digitoxin.

The therapeutic serum concentration of digoxin in adults is 1.0 to 2.0 ng/ml. Digoxin serum levels are frequently helpful in confirming the clinical suspicion of digitalis toxicity, especially if the serum digoxin level is greater than 3.0 ng/ml. A review of 19 reports showed that, in intoxicated patients, the mean serum digoxin concentration was 3.6 ng/mg in the absence of hypokalemia.[131] If a serum digoxin level is less than 1.5 ng/ml in a patient who does not have hypokalemia and who is suspected of digoxin toxicity, the clinician must search for another explanation for the patient's symptoms since digitalis intoxication is unlikely. If the serum digoxin level is less than 1.0 in a normokalemic patient, digitalis toxicity is sufficiently rare so as to exclude this diagnosis.

Electrocardiographic manifestations of digitalis toxicity are protean, are not diagnostic of this condition, and depend in part upon the state of the myocardium. For example, accentuation of the vagal effects of digitalis are more commonly seen in healthy individuals with suicidal digitalis overdose. In contrast, digitalis-intoxicated patients with advanced cardiac disease often develop ventricular ectopy at doses and blood levels below those required to produce AV conduction disturbances in patients without intrinsic cardiac disease.[132] The arrhythmogenic effects of digitalis are complex, and their etiology has not been fully elucidated in humans. Possible mechanisms include delayed afterpotentials, enhanced diastolic depolarization, and reentry. These mechanisms have recently been reviewed in detail by Smith and coworkers.[133]

Digitalis-induced arrhythmias may be best understood by considering those manifestations which are due predominantly to excessive parasympathomimetic effects and those which are related to enhanced ectopy. Manifestations of enhanced vagal effect (or diminished sympathetic effect) include sinus bradycardia or SA exit block and AV nodal block usually of the Wenckebach type. Examples of digitalis-induced ectopy include atrial premature beats, junctional tachycardia, and ventricular ectopic activity. Death may be due to digitalis-induced ventricular tachycardia and/or ventricular fibrillation. Ectopy may be combined with signs of excessive vagal effects to produce the ECG patterns of atrial tachycardia with AV block or junctional tachycardia with AV block.

Therapy of digitalis toxicity will depend upon numerous factors, including the time of the last dose ingested which may allow determination of peak effect, the total amount of digitalis taken, the state of health of the patient, and the nature of the electrocardiographic manifestations of toxicity. For example, temporary discontinuation of digoxin is sufficient if the last dose of digoxin was taken longer than 6 h before examination, the dose was not massive, and the ECG manifestations are primarily vagal with an adequate ventricular response to maintain circulation. A temporary pacemaker must be inserted if there is inadequate circulation due to severe bradycardia or complete heart block. Correction of hypokalemia in addition to stopping the drug may be all that is needed to control digitalis-induced tachyarrhythmia. Digitalis-induced atrial, junctional, or ventricular tachycardia should be treated by antiarrhythmic drugs. Diphenylhydantoin may be given intravenously in 100-mg doses every 5 min until the arrhythmia is abolished, until 1000 mg is administered, or until drowsiness, nystagmus, vertigo, or nausea occur.[134] Diphenylhydantoin has been used successfully to suppress not only atrial and ventricular ectopy induced by digitalis but also may restore AV conduction. Lidocaine is effective, particularly in diminishing the severity and frequency of digitalis-induced ventricular ectopy. Quinidine should be avoided since it may displace digoxin from its binding sites to raise serum digoxin levels and will decrease both the renal and nonrenal excretion of digoxin. Procainamide may be used. Beta-adrenergic blocking drugs should generally be avoided in treating digitalis toxicity in a patient with a history of heart failure.

The fact that only vagal manifestations of toxicity are present in a patient who has ingested a massive amount of digitalis does not permit complacency and preparations must be made to immediately rid the body of nonabsorbed digoxin, as well as to administer digoxin antibodies to reverse anticipated lethal toxicity.

Therapy of massive overdose with digitalis has been revolutionized by the extraordinary success obtained with the administration of digoxin-specific sheep Fab fragments.[135] This clinical study grew out of a substantial body of experimental evidence accumulated over the past decade showing that digitalis-specific antibodies are effective in reversing toxic effects of cardiac glycosides.[136] These highly specific antibodies are made in response to injection of a digoxin protein conjugate to rabbits or sheep. The affinity of these antibodies is up to 50 times higher than that for digitoxin. The digoxin-specific antibodies bind and neutralize not only digoxin but also the major cardioactive metabolites of digoxin. The digoxin antibody globulin can be split into two Fab fragments and one Fc fragment by enzymatic digestion with papaine. The haptene-binding capacity of the Fab fragments is fully preserved and the smaller molecular size of the Fab fragments may enable more rapid diffusion to cellular digoxin-binding sites than complete antibody molecules. The intravenous administration of specific Fab fragments binds to digoxin and rapidly accelerates the removal of digoxin from cellular membranes. This causes a marked increase in serum digoxin concentration; however, the digoxin is bound and therefore is pharmacologically inactive. Due to the smaller molecular weight, Fab fragments pass glomerular membranes, resulting in rapid renal excretion and a biological half-life of less than 5 h. Thus the Fab fragments are capable of rapidly reversing digoxin-induced toxicity and the glycoside is promptly eliminated by the renal route, much of it in the protein-bound form.[137] Administration of digoxin-specific Fab fragments are effective in the treatment of toxicity due to digitoxin, even though the affinity of the antibody is much less for digitoxin than for digoxin.

The safety and efficacy of the digoxin-specific Fab antibody fragments was demonstrated in 26 cases reported by Smith and colleagues. All patients had an initial favorable response to the administration of the Fab fragments, and there were no adverse reactions to treatment. Twenty-one of the twenty-six patients with advanced life-threatening digoxin or digitoxin toxicity survived to make a full recovery. On the basis of this favorable experience it would appear reasonable to extend this treatment to patients who have digitalis toxicity but who do not have life-threatening arrhythmias. The major concern in using the Fab fragments for these less severely intoxicated patients is that immunogenicity is a potential problem, particularly if the patient requires a second administration of the antibody fragments.

Ancillary treatment for both digoxin and digitoxin toxicity includes the administration of activated charcoal with an initial dose of 50 to 100 g, repeated at a dose of 20 g every 6 h. Activated charcoal enhances the rate of drug diffusion from the body into the gastrointestinal tract by efficiently absorbing the drug from gastrointestinal fluids. This maximizes the concentration gradient and permits the further diffusion of drug into the lumen.[138] Charcoal may decrease the absorption of digoxin, even when given 1 to 4 h after the glycoside.[139,140]

Activated charcoal has been shown to decrease the half-life of digitoxin in several patients who have taken an overdose of this medication.[141] It is yet to be determined if activated charcoal will decrease the half-life of digoxin under these circumstances. Cholestyramine has been advocated for the treatment of both digoxin and digitoxin toxicity since it binds these glycosides and prevents reabsorption. Although cholestyramine has been reported to decrease the half-life of both digoxin and digitoxin after an overdose with these drugs, the decrease in half-life is variable. Cholestyramine should be used as an adjunct, particularly for non-life-threatening overdose with the cardiac glycosides.[142,143]

The removal of digoxin or digitoxin by hemoperfusion is controversial. Theoretically, this procedure should be more effective for removing an overdose of digitoxin since the plasma concentrations of digitoxin are tenfold higher compared with digoxin, indicating a smaller volume of distribution and a smaller tissue-bound fraction of the body load. Indeed, it has been used to successfully treat a patient with massive digitoxin overdose.[144] However, it should be minimally effective, if at all, for digoxin.[145] Uniform success has not been the experience of using hemoperfusion to treat digoxin poisoning.[146] If this method is used at all, hemoperfusion with XAD-4 resin appears more efficient than with charcoal hemoperfusion.[147]

References

1. American Hospital Formulary Service: Current Drug Therapy: Cardiac Glycosides, *Am. J. Hosp. Pharm.,* 35:1495, 1978.
2. Gierke, K. D., Graves, P. E., Perrier, D., Marcus, F. I., Mayersohn, M., and Goldman, S.: Metabolism and Rate of Elimination of Digoxigenin Bisdigitoxoside in Dogs before and during Chronic Azotemia. *J. Pharmacol. Exp. Ther.,* 212:448, 1981.
3. Graves, P. E., Fenster, P. E., MacFarland, R. T., Marcus, F. I., and Perrier, D.: Pharmacokinetics of Digitoxin and the Bis and Monodigitoxosides of Digitoxigenin in Normal Subjects, *Clin. Pharmacol. Exp. Ther.,* 36:601, 1984.
4. Graves, P. E., Fenster, P. E., MacFarland, R. T., Marcus, F. I., and Perrier, D.: Pharmacokinetics of Digitoxin and the Bis and Monodigitoxosides of Digitoxigenin in Renal Insufficiency, *Clin. Pharmacol. Exp. Ther.,* 36:607, 1984.
5. Lukas, D. S., and DeMartino, A. G.: Binding of Digitoxin and Some Related Cardenolides to Human Plasma Protein, *J. Clin. Invest.,* 48:1141, 1969.
6. Lukas, D. S.: Some Aspects of Distribution and Disposition of Digitoxin in Man, *Ann. N.Y. Acad. Sci.,* 179:338, 1971.
7. Reuning, R. H., Sams, R. A., and Notari, R. E.: Role of Pharmacokinetics in Drug Dosage Adjustment. I. Pharmacological Effect, Kinetics and Apparent Volume of Distribution of Digoxin, *J. Clin. Pharmacol.,* 13:127, 1973.
8. Huffman, D. H., Manion, C. V., and Azarnoff, D. L.: Inter-Subject Variation in Absorption of Digoxin in Normal Volunteers, *J. Pharm. Sci.,* 64:433, 1975.
9. Rabkin, S. W., and Grupp, G.: A Two-Compartment Open Model for Digoxin Pharmacokinetics in Patients Receiving a Wide Range of Digoxin Doses, *Acta Cardiol. (Brux.),* 30:343, 1975.
10. Marcus, F. I., Dickerson, J., Pippins, S., Stafford, M., and Bressler, R.: Digoxin Bioavailability: Formulations and Rates of Infusion, *Clin. Pharmacol. Ther.,* 20:253, 1976.
11. Ilsalo, E.: Clinical Pharmacokinetics of Digoxin, *Clin. Pharmacokinetics,* 2:1, 1977.
12. Perrier, D., Mayersohn, M., and Marcus, F. I.: Clinical Pharmacokinetics of Digitoxin, *Clin. Pharmacokinetics,* 2:292, 1977.
13. Storstein, L.: Protein Binding of Cardiac Glycosides in Disease States, *Clin. Pharmacokinetics,* 2:220, 1977.
14. Ochs, R., Greenblatt, D. J., Bodem, G., and Harmatz, J. F.: Dose-Independent Pharmacokinetics of Digoxin in Humans, *Am. Heart J.,* 96:507, 1978.
15. Doherty, J. E., Marcus, F. I., and Binnion, P. F.: A Multicenter Evaluation of Absolute Bioavailability of Digoxin Dosage Forms, *Curr. Ther. Res.,* 35(2):301, 1984.
16. Doherty, J. E., Perkins, W. H., and Flanigan, W. J.: The Distribution and Concentration of Tritiated Digoxin in Human Tissues. *Ann. Intern. Med.,* 66:116, 1967.
17. Marcus, F. I., Burkhalter, L., Cuccia, C., Pavlovich, J., and Kapadia, G. G.: Administration of Tritiated Digoxin with and without a Loading Dose. A Metabolic Study, *Circulation,* 34:865, 1966.
18. Gault, M. H., Longerich, L. L., Loo, J. C. K., Ko, P. T. H., Fine, A., Vasdev, F. C., and Dawe, M. A.: Digoxin Biotransformation. *Clin. Pharmacol. Ther.,* 35:74, 1984.
19. Peters, U., Falk, L., and Kalman, S. M.: Digoxin Metabolism in Patients, *Arch. Intern. Med.* 138:1074, 1978.
20. Gault, H., Kalra, J., Ahmed, M., Kepkay, D., Longerich, L., and Barrowman, J.: Influence of Gastric pH on Digoxin Biotransformation: II. Extractable Urinary Metabolites, *Clin. Pharmacol. Ther.,* 29:181, 1981.
21. Lindenbaum, J., Rund, D. G., Butler, V. P., Jr., Tse-Eng, D., and Ranjan Saha, J.: Inactivation of Digoxin by the Gut Flora: Reversal by Antiobiotic Therapy, *N. Engl. J. Med.,* 305:789, 1981.
22. Rund, D. G., Lindenbaum, J., Dobkin, J. F., Butler, V. P., Jr., and Saha, J. R.: Decreased Digoxin Cardioinactive-Reduced Metabolites after Administration as an Encapsulated Liquid Concentrate, *Clin. Pharmacol. Ther.,* 34:738, 1983.
23. Wettrell, G., and Anderson, K. E.: Clinical Pharmacokinetics of Digoxin in Infants, *Clin. Pharmacokinetics,* 2:17, 1977.
24. Ewy, G. A., Kapadia, G. G., Yao, L., Lullin, M., and Marcus, F. I.: Digoxin Metabolism in the Elderly, *Circulation,* 39:449, 1969.
25. Cusack, B., Kelly, J., O'Malley, K., Noel, J., Lavan, J., and Horgan, J.: Digoxin in the Elderly: Pharmacokinetic Consequence of Old Age: *Clin. Pharmacol. Ther.,* 25:772, 1979.
26. Reid, J., Kennedy, R. D., and Caird, F. I.: Digoxin Kinetics in the Elderly, *Age Aging,* 12:29, 1983.
27. Ewy, G. A., Groves, B. M., Ball, M. S., Nimmo, L., Jackson, B., and Marcus, F. I.: Digoxin Metabolism in Obesity, *Circulation,* 44:810, 1971.
28. Abernethy, D. R., Greenblatt, D. J., and Smith, T. W.: Digoxin Disposition in Obesity: Clinical Pharmacokinetic Investigation, *Am. Heart J.,* 740, 1981.
29. Bloom, P. M., and Nelp, W. B.: Relationship of the Excretion of Tritiated Digoxin to Renal Function. *Am. J. Med. Sci.,* 251:133, 1966.
30. Doherty, J. E., Perkins, W. H., and Wilson, M. C.: Studies with Tritiated Digoxin in Renal Failure, *Am. J. Med.,* 37:536, 1964.
31. Marcus, F. I., Peterson, A., Salel, A., Scully, J., and Kapadia, D. G.: The Metabolism of Tritiated Digoxin in Renal Insufficiency in Dogs and Man, *J. Pharmacol. Exp. Ther.,* 152:372, 1966.
32. Doherty, J. E., Flanigan, W. J., Perkins, W. H., and Ackerman, G. L.: Studies with Tritiated Digoxin in Anephric Human Subjects, *Circulation,* 35:298, 1967.
33. Gault, M. H., Sugden, D., Maloney, C., Ahmed, M., and Tweeddale, M.: Biotransformation and Elimination of Digoxin with Normal and Minimal Renal Function, *Clin. Pharmacol. Ther.,* 25:499, 1979.
34. Aronson, J. K., and Grahame-Smith, E. G.: Altered Distribution of Digoxin in Renal Failure—A Cause of Digoxin Toxicity? *Br. J. Clin. Pharmacol.,* 3:1045, 1976.
35. Jogestrand, T., and Ericsson, F.: Skeletal Muscle Digoxin

Binding in Patients with Renal Failure, *Brit. J. Clin, Pharmacol.*, 16:109, 1983.
36. Jusko, W. J., and Weintraub, M.: Myocardial Distribution of Digoxin and Renal Function, *Clin. Pharmacol. Ther.*, 16:449, 1974.
37. Gault, M. H., Churchill, D. N., and Kalra, J.: Loading Dose of Digoxin in Renal Failure, *Br. J. Clin. Pharmacol.*, 9:593, 1980.
38. Zilly, W., Richter, E., and Rietbrock, N.: Pharmacokinetics and Metabolism of Digoxin- and β-Methyl-Digoxin-12α-^{3}H in Patients with Acute Hepatitis, *Clin. Pharmacol. Ther.*, 17:303, 1975.
39. Marcus, F. I., and Kapadia, G. G.: The Metabolism of Tritiated Digoxin in Cirrhotic Patients, *Gastroenterology*, 47:517, 1964.
40. Rogers, M. C., Willerson, J. T., Goldblatt, A., and Smith, J. W.: Serum Digoxin Concentration in the Human Fetus, Neonate and Infant, *N. Engl. J. Med.*, 287:1010, 1972.
41. Luxford, A. M. E., and Kellaway, G. S. M.: Pharmacokinetics of Digoxin in Pregnancy, *Eur. J. Clin. Pharmacol.*, 25:117, 1983.
42. Chan, V., Jse, T. F., and Wong, V.: Transfer of Digoxin across the Placenta and into Breast Milk, *Br. J. Obstet. Gynecol.*, 85:605, 1978.
43. King, C. R., Mattioli, L., Goertz, K. K., and Snodgrass, W.: Successful Treatment of Fetal Supraventricular Tachycardia with Maternal Digoxin Therapy, *Chest*, 85:573, 1984.
44. Loughlan, P. M.: Digoxin Excretion in Breast Milk, *J. Pediatr.*, 92:1019, 1978.
45. Doherty, J. E., and Perkins, W. H.: Digoxin Metabolism in Hypo- and Hyperthyroidism, *Ann. Intern. Med.*, 64:489, 1966.
46. Shenfield, G. M., Thompson, J., and Horn, D. B.: Plasma and Urinary Digoxin in Thyroid Dysfunction, *Eur. J. Clin. Pharmacol.*, 12:437, 1977.
47. Lawrence, J. R., Sumner, D. J., Kalk, W. J., Ratcliffe, A., Whiting, B., Gray, K., and Lindsay, M.: Digoxin Kinetics in Patients with Thyroid Dysfunction, *Clin. Pharmacol. Ther.*, 22:7, 1977.
48. Eichelbaum, M.: Drug Metabolism in Thyroid Disease, *Clin. Pharmacokinetics*, 1:339, 1976.
49. Withering, W.: "An Account of the Foxglove," C. G. J. and J. Robinson, Paternoster-Row, London, 1785.
50. Gold, H., and Cattell, M.: Mechanism of Digitalis Action in Abolishing Heart Failure, *Arch. Intern. Med.*, 65:263, 1940.
51. Repke, K., and Portius, H. J.: Uber die identitat der Ionenpumpen-ATPase in der bel Zellmembran des Herzmuskels mit einem Digitalis-Rezeptorenzym, *Experientia*, 19:452, 1963.
52. Akera, T., and Brody, T. M.: The Role of Na^+, K^+-ATPase in the Inotropic Action of Digitalis, *Pharmacol. Rev.*, 29:187, 1978.
53. Matsui, H., and Schwartz, A.: Mechanism of Cardiac Glycoside Inhibition of the (Na+-K+)-Dependent ATPase From Cardiac Tissue, *Biochim. Biophys. Acta*, 151, 655, 1968.
54. Pace, D. G., and Gillis, R. A.: Neuroexcitatory Effects of Digoxin in the Cat, *J. Pharmacol. Exp. Ther.*, 199:583, 1976.
55. Chai, C. Y., Wang, H. H., Hoffman, B. F., and Wang, S. C.: Mechanisms of Bradycardia Induced by Digitalis Substances, *Am. J. Physiol.*, 212:26, 1967.
56. Ten Eick, R. E., and Hoffman, B. F.: The Effect of Digitalis on the Excitability of Autonomic Nerves, *J. Pharmacol. Exp. Ther.*, 169:95, 1969.
57. Toda, M., and West, T. C.: The Action of Ouabain on the Function of the Atrioventricular Node in Rabbits, *J. Pharmacol. Exp. Ther.*, 169:287, 1969.
58. Ten Eick, R. E., and Hoffman, B. F.: Chronotropic Effect of Cardiac Glycosides in Cats, Dogs and Rabbits, *Circ. Res.*, 25:365, 1969.
59. Mikkelsen, E., Andersson, K. E., and Lederballe Pedersen, O.: Effects of Digoxin on Isolated Human Peripheral Arteries and Veins, *Acta Pharmacol. Toxicol.*, 45:249, 1979.
60. Hamlin, N. P., Willerson, J. T., Garan, H., and Powell, W. J., Jr.: The Neurogenic Vasoconstrictor Effect of Digitalis on Coronary Vascular Resistance, *J. Clin. Invest.*, 53:288, 1974.
61. Mikkelsen, E.: Effects of Digoxin on Isolated Human Pulmonary Vessels, *Acta Pharmacol. Toxicol.*, 45:139, 1979.
62. Haustein, K. E., Assmann, I., and Fiehring, H.: Problems of Rapid Digitalization in Severe Congestive Heart Failure, *Eur. J. Cardiol.*, 11:135, 1980.
63. DeMots, H., Rahimtoola, S. H., McAnulty, J. H., and Porter, G. A.: Effects of Ouabain on Coronary and Systemic Vascular Resistance and Myocardial Oxygen Consumption in Patients without Heart Failure, *Am. J. Cardiol.*, 41:88, 1978.
64. Rosen, M. R., Wit, A. L., and Hoffman, B. F.: Electrophysiology and Pharmacology of Cardiac Arrhythmias: IV. Cardiac Antiarrhythmic and Toxic Effects of Digitalis, *Am. Heart J.*, 89:391, 1975.
65. Toda, N., and West, T. C.: Influence of Ouabain on Cholinergic Responses in the Sinoatrial Node, *J. Pharmacol. Exp. Ther.*, 153:104, 1966.
66. Mendez, C., Aceves, J., and Mendez, R.: Inhibition of Adrenergic Cardiac Acceleration by Cardiac Glycosides, *J. Pharmacol. Exp. Ther.*, 131:191, 1961.
67. Dhingra, R. C., Amet-Y-Leon, F., Wyndham, C., Wu, D., Denes, P., and Rosen, K. M.: The Electrophysiological Effects of Ouabain on Sinus Node and Atrium in Man, *J. Clin. Invest.*, 56:555, 1975.
68. Kugler, J. D., Garson, A., Jr., and Gillette, P. G.: Electrophysiologic Effect of Digitalis on Sinoatrial Nodal Function in Children, *Am. J. Cardiol.*, 44:1344, 1979.
69. Engel, T. R., and Schaal, S. F.: Digitalis in the Sick Sinus Syndrome, *Circulation*, 48:1201, 1973.
70. Vera, Z., Miller, R. R., McMillin, D., and Mason, D. T.: Effects of Digitalis on Sinus Nodal Function in Patients with Sick Sinus Syndrome, *Am. J. Cardiol.*, 41:318, 1978.
71. Reiffel, J. A., Bigger, J. T., and Cramer, M.: Effects of Digoxin on Sinus Nodal Function before and after Vagal Blockade in Patients with Sinus Nodal Dysfunction, *Am. J. Cardiol.*, 43:983, 1979.
72. Perrot, G., Houppe, J. P., Ethevenot, G., Cherrier, F., and Faivre, G.: Actions des Digitaliques sur le Noeud Sinusal Pathologique, *Arch. Mal. Loeur.*, 6:259, 1983.
73. Mendez, C., and Mendez, R.: The Action of Cardiac Glycosides on the Refractory Period of Heart Tissues, *J. Pharmacol. Exp. Ther.*, 107:24, 1953.
74. Mendez, C., and Mendez, R.: The Action of Cardiac Glycosides on the Excitability and Conduction Velocity of the Mammalian Atrium, *J. Pharmacol. Exp. Ther.*, 121:402, 1957.
75. Wu, D., Wyndham, C., Amat-Y-Leon, F., Denes, P., Dhingra, R. C., and Rosen, K. M.: The Effects of Ouabain on Induction of Atrioventricular Nodal Re-entrant Paroxysmal Supraventricular Tachycardia, *Circulation*, 52:201, 1975.
76. Gomes, J. A. D., Dhatt, M. S., Akhtar, M., Carambas, C. R., Rubenson, D. S., and Damato, A. N.: Effects of Digitalis on Ventricular Myocardial and His-Purkinje Refractoriness and Re-Rentry in Man, *Am. J. Cardiol.*, 42:931, 1978.
77. Engel, T. R., and Gonzales, A. D. C.: Effects of Digitalis on Atrial Vulnerability, *Am. J. Cardiol.*, 42:570, 1978.
78. Hayward, R. P., Hamer, J., Taggart, P., and Emanuel, R.: Observations on the Biphasic Nature of Digitalis Electrophysiological Actions in the Human Right Atrium, *Cardiovasc. Res.*, 17:533, 1983.
79. Schaal, S. F., Sugimoto, T., Wallace, A. G., and Sealy, W. C.: Effects of Digitalis on the Functional Refractory Period of the AV Node: Studies in Awake Dogs with and without Cardiac Denervation, *Cardiovasc. Res.*, 4:356, 1968.
80. Hoffman, B. F., and Singer, D. H.: Effects of Digitalis on Electrical Activity of Cardiac Fibers, *Prog. Cardiovasc. Dis.*. 7:226, 1964.
81. Rosen, M. R., Gelband, H., and Hoffman, B. F.: Correlation between effects of Ouabain in the Canine Electrocardiogram and Transmembrane Potentials of Isolated Purkinje Fibers, *Circulation*, 47:65, 1973.
82. Wellens, H. J. J., and Durrer, D.: Effect of Digitalis on Atrioventricular Conduction and Circus-Movement Tachycardias in Patients with Wolff-Parkinson-White Syndrome, *Circulation*, 47:1229, 1973.

83. Dhingra, R. C., Palileo, E. V., Strasberg, B., Swiryn, S., Bauernfeind, R., Wyndham, C., and Rosen, K. M.: Electrophysiologic Effects of Ouabain in Patients with Preexcitation and Circus Movement Tachycardia, *Am. J. Cardiol.*, 47:139, 1981.
84. Sellers, T. D., Jr., Bashore, T. M., and Gallagher, J. J.: Digitalis in the Pre-Excitation Syndrome. Analysis during Atrial Fibrillation, *Circulation*, 56:260, 1977.
85. Jedeikin, R., Gillette, P., and Zinner, A.: Effect of Ouabain on the Antegrade Effective Refractory Period of Accessory Atrioventricular Connections in Children, *Circulation*, 66:II, 171, 1982. (Abstract.)
86. Hodges, M., Friesinger, G. C., Riggins, R. C. K., and Dagenais, G. R.: Effects of Intravenously Administered Digoxin on Mild Left Ventricular Failure in Acute Myocardial Infarction in Man, *Am. J. Cardiol.*, 29:749, 1972.
87. Sjogren, A.: Left Heart Failure in Acute Myocardial Infarction, *Acta Med. Scand.* 510 (suppl.):1, 1970.
88. Goldstein, R. A., Passamani, E. R., and Roberts, R.: A Comparison of Digoxin and Dobutamine in Patients with Acute Infarction and Cardiac Failure, *N. Engl. J. Med.*, 303:846, 1980.
89. Raabe, D. S.: Combined Therapy with Digoxin and Nitroprusside in Heart Failure Complicating Acute Myocardial Infarction, *Am. J. Cardiol.*, 43:990, 1979.
90. Mathur, P. N., Powles, P., Pugsley, S. O., McEwan, M. P., and Campbell, E. J. M.: Effect of Digoxin on Right Ventricular Function in Severe Chronic Airflow Obstruction, *Ann. Intern. Med.*, 95:283, 1981.
91. Baum, G. L., Dick, M. M., Shotz, S., and Gumpel, R. C.: Digitalis Toxicity in Chronic Cor Pulmonale, *South. Med. J.*, 49:1037, 1956.
92. Berman, W., Jr., Dubynsky, O., Whitman, V., Friedman, Z., and Maisels, N. J.: Digoxin Therapy in Low-Birth-Weight Infants with Patent Ductus Arteriosus, *J. Pediatr.*, 93:652, 1978.
93. Berman, W., Jr., Yabek, S. M., Dillon, T., Niland, C., Corlew, S., and Christensen, D.: Effects of Digoxin in Infants with a Congested Circulatory State due to a Ventricular Septal Defect, *N. Engl. J. Med.*, 308:363, 1983.
94. Lundell, B. P. W., and Boreus, L. O.: Digoxin Therapy in Left Ventricular Performance in Premature Infants with Patent Ductus Arteriosus, *Acta Paediatr. Scand.*, 72:339, 1983.
95. White, R. D., and Lietman, P. S.: Commentary: A Reappraisal of Digitalis for Infants with Left-to-Right Shunts and "Heart Failure," *J. Pediatr.*, 92:867, 1978.
96. Dobbs, S. M., Kenyon, W. I., and Dobbs, R. J.: Maintenance Digoxin after an Episode of Heart Failure: Placebo-Controlled Trial in Outpatients, *Br. Med. J.*, 1:749, 1977.
97. Fleg, J. L., Gottlieb, S. H., and Lakatta, E. G.: Is Digoxin Really Important in Treatment of Compensated Heart Failure? *Am. J. Med.*, 73:244, 1982.
98. Lee, D. C., Johnson, R. A., Bingham, J. B., Leahy, M., Dinsmore, R. E., Goroll, A. H., Newell, J. B., Strauss, H. W., and Haber, E.: Heart Failure in Outpatients: A Randomized Trial of Digoxin vs. Placebo, *N. Engl. J. Med.*, 306:699, 1982.
99. Arnold, S. B., Byrd, R. C., Meister, W., Melmon, K., Cheitlin, M. D., Bristow, J. D., Parmley, W. W., and Chatterjee, K.: Long-Term Digitalis Therapy Improved Left Ventricular Function in Heart Failure, *N. Engl. J. Med.*, 303:1443, 1981.
100. Moss, A. J., Davis, H. T., Conard, D. L., DeCamilla, J. J., and Odoroff, C. L.: Digitalis-Associated Cardiac Mortality after Myocardial Infarction, *Circulation*, 64:1150, 1981.
101. Bigger, J. T., Jr., Weld, F. M., Rolnitzky, L. M., and Ferrick, K. G.: Is Digitalis Treatment Harmful in the Year after Acute Myocardial Infarction? *Circulation*, 64(suppl. 4):83, 1981. (Abstract.)
102. Moss, A. J., Davis, H. T., Odoroff, C. L., Bigger, J. T., and the Multicenter Postinfarction Research Group: Digitalis-Associated Mortality in Postinfarction Patients, *Circulation*, 68(suppl. 3):368, 1983. (Abstract.)
103. Madsen, E. B., Gilpin, E., Henning, H., Ahnve, S., LeWinter, M., Mazur, J., Shabetai, R., Collins, D., and Ross, J., Jr.: Prognostic Importance of Digitalis after Acute Myocardial Infarction, *J. Am. Coll. Cardiol.*, 3:681, 1984.
104. Ryan, T. J., Bailey, K. R., McCabe, C. H., Luk, S., Fisher, L. D., Mock, M. B., and Killip, T.: The Effects of Digitalis on Survival in High-Risk Patients with Coronary Artery Disease: The Coronary Artery Surgery Study (CASS), *Circulation*, 67:735, 1983.
105. Wellens, H. J. J., Durrer, D. R., Liem, K. L., and Lie, K. I.: Effect of Digitalis in Patients with Paroxysmal Atrioventricular Nodal Tachycardia, *Circulation*, 52:779, 1975.
106. Redfors, A.: Digoxin Dosage and Ventricular Rate at Rest and Exercise in Patients with Atrial Fibrillation, *Acta Med. Scand.*, 190:321, 1971.
107. Aberg, H., Strom, G., and Werner, I.: The Effect of Digitalis on the Heart Rate during Exercise in Patients with Atrial Fibrillation, *Acta Med. Scand.*, 191:441, 1972.
108. Meijler, F. L., Kroneman, J., Van Der Tweel, I., Herbschleb, J. N., Heethaar, R. M., and Borst, C.: Nonrandom Ventricular Rhythm in Horses with Atrial Fibrillation and Its Significance for Patients, *J. Am. Coll. Cardiol.*, 4:316, 1984.
109. Wang, K., Goldfarb, B. L., Gobel, F. L., and Richman, H. G.: Multifocal Atrial Tachycardia, *Arch. Intern. Med.*, 137:161, 1977.
110. DeMey, C., and Snoeck, J.: Review of the Use of Digitalis Glycosides in Ventricular Dysrhythmias, *Acta Cardiol.*, 35:153, 1980.
111. Lown, B., Grayboys, T. B., Podrid, P. J., Cohen, B. H., Stockman, M. B., and Ganghan, C. E.: Effect of Digitalis Drug on Ventricular Premature Beats, *N. Engl. J. Med.*, 296:301, 1977.
112. Blumberg, J., Hayes, J. G., Stevens, M., Sullivan, G., and Killip, T.: Digitalis in Treatment of Ventricular Extrasystoles in the Otherwise Normal Heart, *Circulation*, 48(suppl. 4):18, 1973. (Abstract.)
113. Gradman, A. H., Bergen, H., Cunningham, M., Harbison, M., Zaret, B.: Effects of Oral Digoxin on Ventricular Ectopy and its Relation to Left Ventricular Function, *Am. J. Cardiol.*, 51:765, 1983.
114. Wu, D., Amat-Y-Leon, F., Simpson, R. J., Latif, P., Wyndham, C. R. C., Denes, P., and Rosen, K. M.: Electrophysiological Studies with Multiple Drugs in Patients with Atrioventricular Re-entrant Tachycardia Utilizing an Extranodal Pathway, *Circulation*, 56:727, 1977.
115. Dreifus, L. S., Hait, R., Watanabe, Y., Arriaga, J., and Reitman, N.: Ventricular Fibrillation: A Possible Mechanism of Sudden Death in Patients with Wolff-Parkinson-White Syndrome, *Circulation*, 43:520, 1971.
116. Brown, D. D., Juhl, R. P., and Warner, S. L.: Decreased Bioavailability of Digoxin due to Hypocholesterolemic Interventions, *Circulation*, 58:164, 1978.
117. Juhl, R. P., Summers, R. W., Guillory, J. K., Blaug, S. M., Cheng, F. H., and Brown, D. D.: Effect of Sulfasalazine on Digoxin Bioavailability, *Clin. Pharm. Ther.*, 20:387, 1976.
118. Manninen, V., Melin, J., Apajalahti, A., and Karesoja, M.: Altered Absorption of Digoxin in Patients Given Propantheline and Metoclopramide, *Lancet*, 1:398, 1973.
119. Lindenbaum, J., Maulitz, R. M., and Butler, V. P., Jr.: Inhibition of Digoxin Absorption by Neomycin, *Gastroenterology*, 71:399, 1976.
120. Kuhlmann, J., Zilly, W., and Wilke, J.: Effects of Cytostatic Drugs on Plasma Level and Renal Excretion of β-acetyldigoxin, *Clin. Pharm. Ther.*, 30:518, 1981.
121. Moysey, J. O., Jaggarao, N. S. V., Grundy, E. N., and Chamberlain, D. A.: Amiodarone Increases Plasma Digoxin Concentrations, *Br. Med. J.*, 282:272, 1981.
122. Nager, G., and Nager, F.: Interaktion Zwischen Amiodaron und Digoxin, *Schweiz. Med. Wschr.*, 113:1727, 1983.
123. Fenster, P. E., and White, N. W., Jr.: Pharmacokinetic Evaluation of the Digoxin-Amiodarone Interaction, *J. Am. Coll. Cardiol.*, 5:108, 1985.
124. Ejvinsson, G.: Effect of Quinidine on Plasma Concentrations of Digoxin, *Br. Med. J.*, 1:279, 1978.
125. Hager, W. D., Fenster, P. E., Mayersohn, M., Perrier, D., Graves, P., Marcus, F. I., and Goldman, S.: Digoxin-Quinidine Interaction, *N. Engl. J. Med.*, 300:1238, 1979.

126. Hager, W. D., Mayersohn, M., and Graves, P. E.: Digoxin Bioavailability During Quinidine Administration, *Clin. Pharm. Ther.*, 30:594, 1981.
127. Pedersen, K. E., Christiansen, B. D., Klitgaard, N. A., and Nielsen-Kudsk, F.: Effect of Quinidine on Digoxin Bioavailability, *Eur. J. Clin. Pharmacol.*, 24:41, 1983.
128. Aronson, J. K., and Carver, J. G.: Interaction of Digoxin with Quinine, *Lancet*, 1:1418, 1981.
129. Klein, H. O., Lang, R., DiSegni, E., and Kaplinsky, E.: Verapamil-Digoxin Interaction, *N. Engl. J. Med.*, 303:160, 1980.
130. Pedersen, K. E., Dorph-Pedersen, A., Hvidt, S., Anders Klitgaard, N., and Nielsen-Kudsk, F.: Digoxin-Verapamil Interaction, *Clin. Pharmacol. Ther.*, 30:311, 1981.
131. Lee, T. H., and Smith, T. W.: Serum Digoxin Concentration and Diagnosis of Digitalis Toxicity: Current Concepts, *Clin. Pharmacokinetics*, 8:279, 1983.
132. Smith, T. W., and Willerson, J. T.: Suicidal and Accidental Digoxin Ingestion: Report of 5 Cases with Serum Digoxin Level Correlations, *Circulation*, 44:29, 1971.
133. Smith, T. W., Antman, E. M., Friedman, P. L., Blatt, C. M., and Marsh, J. D.: Digitalis Glycosides: Mechanisms and Manifestations of Toxicity, *Prog. Cardiovasc. Dise.*, 26:413, 495, 1984.
134. Bigger, T. J., Schmidt, D. H., and Kutt, H.: Relationship between the Plasma Level of Diphenylhydantoin Sodium and its Cardiac Antiarrhythmic Effects, *Circulation*, 38:363, 1968.
135. Smith, T. W., Butler, V. P., Jr., Haber, E., Fozzard, H., Marcus, F. I., Bremner, W. F., Schulman, I. C., and Phillips, A.: Treatment of Life-Threatening Digitalis Intoxication with Digoxin-Specific Fab Antibody Fragments, *N. Engl. J. Med.*, 307:1357, 1982.
136. Butler, V. P., Jr., Watson, J. F., Schmidt, D. H., Gardner, J. D., Mandel, W. J., and Skelton, C. L.: Reversal of the Pharmacological and Toxic Effect of Cardiac Glycosides by Specific Antibodies, *Pharmacol. Rev.*, 25:239, 1973.
137. Butler, V. P., Jr., Schmidt, D. H., Smith, T. W., Haber, E., Raynor, B. D., and Demartini, P.: Effects of Sheep Digoxin-Specific Antibodies and their Fab Fragments on Digoxin Pharmacokinetics in Dogs, *J. Clin. Invest.*, 59:345, 1977.
138. Levy, G.: Gastrointestinal Clearance of Drugs with Activated Charcoal, *N. Engl. J. Med.*, 307:676, 1982.
139. Neuvonen, P. J., Elfving, S. M., and Elonen, E.: Reduction of Absorption of Digoxin, Phenytoin and Aspirin by Activated Charcoal in Man, *Eur. J. Clin. Pharmacol.*, 13:213, 1978.
140. Reissell, P., and Manninen, V.: Effect of Administration of Activated Charcoal and Fibre on Absorption, Excretion and Steady State Blood Levels of Digoxin and Digitoxin. Evidence for Intestinal Secretion of the Glycosides, *Acta Med. Scand.*, 668 (suppl.):88, 1982.
141. Pond, S., Jacobs, M., Marks, J., Garner, J., Goldschlager, N., and Hansen, D.: Treatment of Digitoxin Overdose with Oral Activated Charcoal, *Lancet*, 2:1177, 1981.
142. Baciewitz, A. M., Isaacson, M. L., and Lipscomb, G. L.: Cholestyramine Resin in the Treatment of Digitoxin Toxicity, *Drug Intelligence and Clinical Pharmacy*, 17:57, 1983.
143. Fresard, F., Balant, L., Noble, J., Garcia, B., and Muller, A. F.: Cholestyramine et Intoxication a la Digoxine: Efficacite Therapeutique? *Schweiz. Med. Wschr.*, 109:431, 1979.
144. Gilfrich, H. J., Kasper, W., Meinertz, T., Okonek, S., and Bork, R.: Treatment of Massive Digitoxin Overdose by Charcoal Haemoperfusion and Cholestyramine, *Lancet*, 1:505, 1978.
145. Gilfrich, H. J., Okonek, S., Manns, M., and Schuster, C. J.: Digoxin and Digitoxin Elimination in Man by Charcoal Hemoperfusion, *Klin. Wochenschr.*, 56:1179, 1978.
146. Bismuth, C., Wattel, F., Gosselin, B., Lambert, H., Genestal, M., and Galliot, M.: L'Hemoperfusion sur scharbon Active Enrobe. Experience des Centres Anti-poisons Francais: 60 Intoxications, *Nouv. Presse. Med.*, 8:1235, 1979.
147. Hoy, W. E., Gibson, T. P., Rivero, A. J., Jain, V. K., Talley, T. T., Bayer, R. M., Montondo, D. F., and Freeman, R. B.: XAD-4 Resin Hemoperfusion for Digitoxic Patients with Renal Failure, *Kidney Int.*, 23:79, 1983.

93

Nondigitalis Cardiac Inotropic Agents

Thierry H. LeJemtel, M.D.

Edmund H. Sonnenblick, M.D.

As the limited therapeutic benefits of digitalis have been increasingly recognized in the treatment of severe congestive heart failure, the search for more potent cardiotonic agents has intensified and also focused on the rationale and safety of such pharmacologic intervention.[1] The use of inotropic agents for the treatment of heart failure is predicated on the existence of a residual myocardial function in the depressed ventricle and the supposition that this residual myocardial function can be mobilized in a sustained manner without producing further myocardial damage. The therapeutic aims of positive inotropic therapy also vary according to the clinical setting. In acute left ventricular failure, which may occur in an evolving myocardial infarction, therapy is aimed at improving left ventricular performance as manifested by increased cardiac output accompanied by decreased ventricular filling pressures without worsening myocardial ischemia or enhancing ventricular irritability. In chronic longstanding congestive heart failure, positive inotropic stimulation is aimed not only at improving left ventricular performance but also at enhancing blood flow to essential organs, i.e., kidneys, brain, and skeletal muscle during exercise. When long-term therapy is sought, is is also particularly relevant to determine whether positive inotropic stimulation can be sustained without attenuation of hemodynamic effects, whether the central benefits are translated into improvement of peripheral organ function, and whether the natural history of underlying cardiac disease is altered.

Regulation of the Contractile Process and Possible Sites of Action of Positive Inotropic Agents

The rapidity of action of inotropic agents makes it unlikely that their effects could be mediated through structural changes in the contractile process or alteration of myosin ATPase activity.[2] Increased delivery of activating Ca^{2+} to the contractile apparatus and/or increased affinity of the contractile apparatus for Ca^{2+} are therefore likely to mediate their positive inotropic actions. While most of the Ca^{2+}, which enters the cell during the plateau phase of the action potential, is stored in the subsarcolemmal cisternae of the sarcoplasmic reticulum, a small portion triggers the release of Ca^{2+} from the intracellular stores into the cytosol to activate the contractile apparatus.[3] Once the level of Ca^{2+} into the cytosol falls below the resting level following reuptake and storage of Ca^{2+} by sarcoplasmic reticulum and activation of the Na^+-Ca^{2+} exchange system, relaxation occurs. Control of the cytoplasmic Ca^{2+}, which plays a major role in the regulation of the contractile process, can be influenced through several mechanisms by the different nondigitalis cardiotonic agents presently available. The precise events leading to the increase in cytoplasmic Ca^{2+} which represents the final common pathway of action of all cardiotonic agents will be reviewed separately with each class of these agents. The extent to which they may also modify the affinity of the contractility apparatus for Ca^{2+} will also be discussed.

Classification of Nondigitalis Cardiotonic Agents

Nondigitalis cardiotonic agents can be classified in two major groups. The first one includes the catecholamines, i.e., norepinephrine, dopamine, and their derivatives, such as dobutamine and isoproterenol (Fig. 93-1). At the present time they are the only nondigitalis inotropic agents approved by the Food and Drug Administration, and are only available for parenteral use, which considerably limits their usefulness. Other artificially synthesized catecholamines (e.g., aramine), act to some extent by releasing catecholamines from endogenous stores.[4] The new oral catecholamine derivatives which are presently available for clinical investigation (i.e., pirbuterol, prenalterol), do not appear to be of great therapeutic interest for the treatment of chronic congestive heart failure, due to excess $beta_2$-receptor stimulation (see below), tachycardia, tachyphylaxis, arrhythmias, and adverse peripheral circulatory responses.[5,6]

The second group of nondigitalis cardiotonic agents is characterized by inhibition of myocardial cellular phosphodiesterase. However, their positive inotropic action may not entirely be due to phosphodiesterase inhibition. These newer inotropic agents which are orally active, also produce direct peripheral arterial vasodilation, which in certain instances may be the predominant factor in improving cardiac performance. The prototype of these newer inotropic agents is amrinone (Fig. 93-2) and the list keeps increasing to include milrinone (WIN 47203), sulmazole (ARL 115BS), posicor (RO 13-6438), fenoximone (MDL 17043), and piroximone (MDL 19025).[7–12]

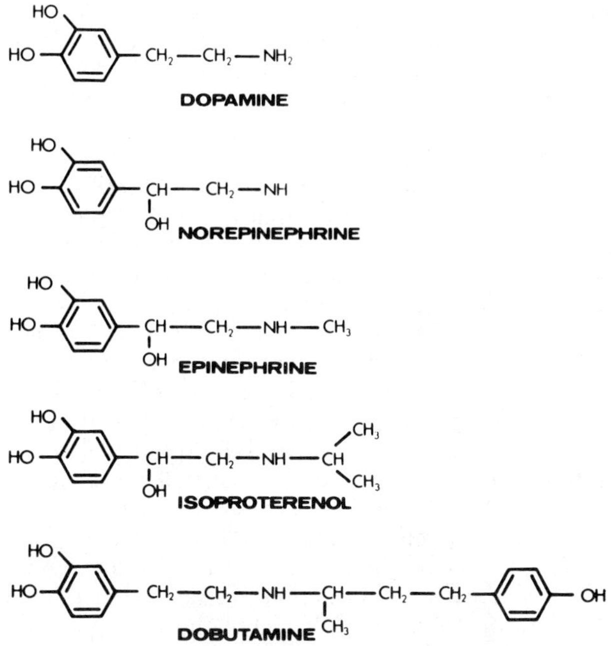

FIGURE 93-1 Chemical structure of dopamine, norepinephrine, epinephrine, isoproterenol, and dobutamine.

Catecholamines and Their Derivatives

Dopamine, a naturally occurring precursor of norepinephrine, and norepinephrine itself, may be used to increase myocardial contractility. However, both dopamine in high doses and norepinephrine constrict the peripheral arterioles, which limit their use.

FIGURE 93-2 Chemical structure of amrinone 5-amino[3,4′-bipyridine]-6(1H)-one and milrinone 1,6-dihydro-2-methyl-6-oxo-[3,4′-bipyridine]-5-carbonitrate.

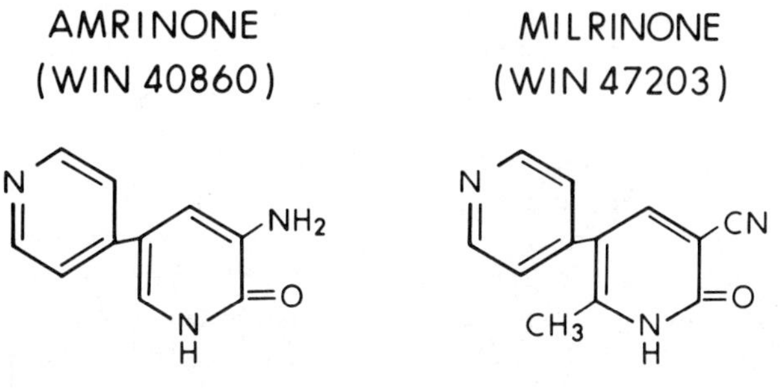

Dobutamine, which is a synthesized catecholamine derivative without vasoconstrictive activity, has become the most widely used as a positive inotropic agent for intravenous use.

Biochemistry, Regulation of Intracellular Calcium, and Pharmacokinetics

The endogenous catecholamines include dopamine, norepinephrine, epinephrine, and their derivatives. Norepinephrine is synthesized and stored in granules in sympathetic nerve endings and released with nerve stimulation, diffusing then to receptors located on the cell surface. Activation of the inotropic receptor results, in turn, in activation of adenyl cyclase which then catalyzes the conversion of ATP to 3′5′ cyclic AMP. Thereafter, phosphorylation of multiple membrane systems occurs, leading to an increasing number of Ca^{2+} channels so that the Ca^{2+} influx into the cell is increased. Phosphorylation also favors the accumulation of the Ca^{2+} by the sarcoplasmic reticulum which enhances relaxation.[13] The half-life of endogenous catecholamines in the human plasma is brief, on the order of minutes.

Most inactivation of norepinephrine takes place normally from reuptake into the sympathetic nerve endings. Norepinephrine is also inactivated by two enzymes, catechol O-methyltransferase (COMT) and monoamine oxidase (MAO), and the products are mostly excreted in the urine. The former mechanism in the heart is severely compromised in congestive failure,[14] although the adrenergic receptors on the cardiac cells remain active (see below). Dobutamine has a half-life of 2 min and is metabolized in inactive glucuronide conjugates and 3-O methyldobutamine in the liver. These metabolites are mostly excreted in the urine.

Pharmacologic Actions

Endogenous catecholamines and dobutamine have different physiologic actions which result from their relative specificity for the various adrenoceptors. These receptors are classified as alpha and beta receptors.[15] Alpha receptors include alpha$_1$ receptors which are postsynaptic and are located either in the vascular smooth muscle or the myocardium. The smooth muscle alpha$_1$ receptors are responsible for vasoconstriction, while the myocardial alpha$_1$ receptors mediate relatively weak positive inotropic and negative chronotropic responses. The alpha$_2$ adrenoreceptors are mostly presynaptic and responsible for decreasing norepinephrine release in the peripheral nerve terminals and decreasing the sympathetic outflow in the central nervous system.[16] In addition, alpha$_2$-adrenergic receptors may be located in the smooth muscle and may be responsible for vasoconstriction in some vascular beds.[17]

Beta-adrenergic receptors are, in turn, classified in beta$_1$ receptors which are located in the myocardium and are responsible for positive inotropic, chronotropic, and dromotropic responses. They respond preferentially to neuronally released norepinephrine. Beta$_2$ adrenoreceptors are located in the smooth muscle and mediate vasodilatation. Beta$_2$ receptors may, however, also be located in the sinoatrial node and also be responsible for positive chronotropy.[18] Beta$_2$ receptors respond preferentially to circulating norepinephrine released from the adrenal medulla and to exogenous catecholamines. In addition, there are specific dopaminergic receptors in the mesenteric and renal vascular bed which are responsible for arterial vasodilatation.[19] The physiologic actions of the endogenous catecholamines and their derivatives are thus determined by their specificity for the alpha$_1$, beta$_1$, and beta$_2$-adrenergic receptors (Table 93-1).

TABLE 93-1 Receptor Activity of Sympathomimetic Amines

	α_1	β_1	β_2	Dopaminergic
Norepinephrine	++++	++++	0	0
Epinephrine	++++	++++	++	0
Dopamine	++++	++	+	++++
Isoproterenol	0	++++	++++	0
Dobutamine	+++	++++	++	0

Dobutamine

The synthesis of dobutamine resulted from systematic modification to the chemical structure of isoproterenol. Tuttle and Mills demonstrated on the intact dog that dobutamine produces a potent positive inotropic action with little change on heart rate or vascular resistance.[20] It is generally accepted that the positive inotropic action of dobutamine is mediated through direct stimulation of beta$_1$-adrenergic receptors in the myocardium which, in turn, increases cyclic AMP.[21] In addition, unlike dopamine, it does not stimulate the heart indirectly by releasing norepinephrine from the nerve endings. The relative lack of positive chronotropic effect of dobutamine is, however, not well understood. Either the chronotropic response to catecholamine may be mediated not by beta$_1$ but by beta$_2$ adrenoreceptors, which are only partially activated by dobutamine, or some of the positive inotropic action of dobutamine could result from stimulation of alpha$_1$-myocardial receptor.[22] The latter possibility would account for the predominant inotropic action of dobutamine, since alpha$_1$ receptors also mediate a negative chronotropic response by decreasing the upstroke of phase IV of the action potential.

Independent of its exact mechanism of action, dobutamine is presently the cardiotonic agent which exerts the most potent inotropic action without producing unwanted effects of heart rate or blood pressure. In the setting of acute myocardial infarction, complicated by symptomatic left ventricular dysfunction, dobutamine is the cardiotonic agent of choice unless severe hypotension is present.[21] If systemic arterial pressure is substantially reduced, stimulation of beta$_2$ adrenoreceptors may be detrimental, and administration of dopamine at high doses or norepinephrine may be required to maintain adequate blood pressure through $alpha_1$ vasoconstriction. Since dobutamine, while improving cardiac output, reduces left ventricular filling pressure, it tends to decrease heart size. This effect more than offsets the effect of augmented myocardial contractility to increase myocardial oxygen requirements. In addition, dobutamine improved coronary perfusion by increasing diastolic perfusion time, due to a reduction in heart rate mediated by withdrawal of sympathetic tone. Dobutamine also increases the pressure gradient which drives blood flow into the ischemic tissue by reducing left ventricular diastolic pressure without affecting aortic diastolic pressure.

Administration of dobutamine to patients with acute myocardial infarction and left ventricular dysfunction is safe and most often improves cardiac performance without overtly worsening myocardial ischemia.[23] The *rate of infusion* should start at 3 μg/kg/min and be titrated up to obtain an optimal cardiac output, if this measurement is available. If not available, heart rate and blood pressure should be closely monitored to avoid tachycardia or major changes in blood pressure. The most serious side effect of dobutamine is the precipitation of ventricular arrhythmias which may require drug dose reduction or even discontinuation.

In chronic congestive heart failure, administration of dobutamine is useful either during acute decompensation precipitated by a concomitant illness or for intermittent inotropic support which may require short-term hospitalization or be carried out on an outpatient basis with a small portable infusion pump.[24] Although patients with severe congestive heart failure have a decreased density and affinity for catecholamines of myocardial beta-adrenergic receptors,[25] they do experience a hemodynamic and clinical improvement following administration of dobutamine. Moreover, this improvement is sustained during long-term therapy despite some initial attenuation of the peak hemodynamic effects. Indeed, while a decrease in the number of active beta receptors (i.e., down regulation) does not seem to occur with the use of a specific agonist, it might complicate therapy with nonselective beta agonists and may explain the lack of sustained benefit.[26] Concomitant *infusion* of dopamine at doses of 3 μg/kg/min or less may be useful to obtain dopaminergic renal arterial vasodilatation, to increase renal blood flow and thus promote sodium excretion.

Nondigitalis, Noncatecholamine Cardiac Inotropic Agents

Amrinone (Inocor) is the prototype of a new class of cardiotonic agents which do not act through the cellular mechanisms attributed to digitalis or catecholamines, but do inhibit phosphodiesterase activity, resulting in increasing levels of cyclic AMP in cardiac tissue. These new cardiotonic agents include milrinone (Milnicor), fenoximone (MDL 17043), piroximone (MDL 19025), posicor (RO 13-6438), and sulmazole (ARL 175BS).[8–12] At the present time only the parenteral form of amrinone has been approved by the Food and Drug Administration for use in congestive heart failure. The phosphodiesterase activity appears more selective within the cardiac cell than that produced by papaverine or theophylline. Such selectivity may contribute to the relatively greater inotropic action of amrinone when compared to the conventional phosphodiesterase inhibitors. The positive inotropic action of these new cardiotonic agents may also result from increased sensitivity of contractile proteins for Ca^{2+} phenomena documented by Fabiato with theophylline.[27] Of therapeutic interest, the positive inotropic action of these new agents may vary with the level of cyclic AMP present in the cardiac cell and may be, therefore, more apparent after $beta_1$-adrenergic stimulation, such as during physical exercise or administration of exogenous catecholamines.

Independent of their positive inotropic actions, all the new cardiotonic agents exert direct arteriolar vasodilating properties which are demonstrated experimentally in the hind limb preparation. However, the dose response of the positive inotropic and vasodilating actions is probably different for each of these cardiotonic agents. For some, the direct vasodilating properties are present even at low doses, while for others, the dilating properties are only observed at high doses.

Pharmacologic Actions

In vitro preparations of amrinone cause a dose-dependent increase in papillary muscle developed tension.[28] In anesthetized and unanesthetized dogs, amrinone increases cardiac contractile force and the rate of left ventricular pressure rise while it produces only small changes in heart rate or blood pressure.[28] Amrinone does not alter the action potential of driven or spontaneously beating canine Purkinje fibers. However, amrinone shortens the functional refractory period and the conduction time of the canine atrioventricular (AV) node.[29] In experimental models of heart failure, amrinone increases cardiac output and reduces left ventricular filling pressures with minimal changes in heart rate or blood pressure. These hemodynamic improvements are accompanied by a decrease in myocardial oxygen consumption.[30] In healthy dogs, amrinone enhances regional blood flow to the kidneys, spleen, and liver.

Pharmacokinetics

In patients with congestive heart failure, the half-life of amrinone usually ranges from 5 to 8 h with a considerable patient variation from 3 to 13 h. Amrinone is metabolized via conjugative pathways. However, in humans, up to 40 percent of amrinone is excreted unchanged in the urine. Preliminary information indicates that the half-life of milrinone is shorter than amrinone, on the order of 2 h.

Therapy with amrinone should be initiated with an intravenous bolus at a dose ranging from 0.75 to 3 mg/kg and followed by a continuous infusion at a rate ranging from 5 to 10 μg/kg/min. In patients with severe renal insufficiency, this rate of infusion should be subsequently decreased to avoid toxic plasma levels of amrinone, and adverse potential reactions such as ventricular arrhythmias and hypotension.

Use in Congestive Heart Failure

Amrinone, like all the new nondigitalis, noncatechol cardiotonic agents, consistently increases cardiac output, which reduces left ventricular filling pressure in patients with severe chronic congestive heart failure without associated tachycardia or change in arterial pressure. The changes in myocardial contractility, as evidenced by the rate of left ventricular pressure rise, are quite variable from patient to patient. Consequently, in patients experiencing minimal changes in myocardial contractility, arteriolar vasodilatation induced by amrinone contributed substantially to improve left ventricular performance. These hemodynamic benefits are accompanied by a decrease in myocardial oxygen requirements.[31]

These beneficial effects may be summated with those of vasodilators. Moreover, peripheral vasodilatation may occur in different beds. For example, angiotensin-converting enzyme inhibitors dilate the renal arterial bed but not skeletal muscle beds, while milrinone does the converse.[32] While these agents are orally active, side effects of amrinone have limited its use in this fashion. The other agents in this group of drugs are currently being studied in clinical trials and if side effects do not limit their use, they should be important therapeutic agents in the balanced treatment of heart failure.

Whether survival will be altered is unknown and may well reflect spontaneous advancement of underlying pathology, concomitant life-threatening arrhythmias, and the effects of the agents to improve contractility, while perhaps placing as yet undefined loads on an already compromised myocardium. Further work is needed to resolve these questions.

References

1. Sonnenblick, E. H., and LeJemtel, T. H.: Newer Inotropic Agents, in E. Braunwald, M. B. Mock, and J. Watson (eds.): "Congestive Heart Failure: Current Research and Clinical Applications," Grune & Stratton, New York, 1982, p. 291.
2. Scheuer, J., and Bhan, A. K.: Cardiac Contractile Proteins, Adenosine Triphosphatase Activity and Physiological Function, *Circ. Res.*, 45:1, 1979.
3. Fabiato, A., and Fabiato, F.: Calcium and Cardiac Excitation-Contraction Coupling, *Am. Rev. Physiol.*, 41:473, 1979.
4. Harrison, D. C., Chidsey, C. A., and Braunwald, E.: Studies on the Mechanism of Action of Metaraminol (Aramine), *Ann. Intern. Med.*, 59:297, 1963.
5. Weber, K. T., Andrews, V., Janicki, J. S., Likoff, M., and Reichek, N.: Pirbuterol, an Oral Beta-Adrenergic Receptor Agonist in the Treatment of Chronic Cardiac Failure, *Circulation*, 66:1262, 1982.
6. Lambertz, H., Meyer, J., and Erbel, R.: Long-Term Hemodynamic Effects of Prenalteral in Patients with Severe Congestive Heart Failure, *Circulation*, 69:298, 1984.
7. Benotti, J. R., Grossman, W., Braunwald, E., Davolos, D. D., and Alousi, A. A.: Hemodynamic Assessment of Amrinone: A New Inotropic Agent, *N. Engl. J. Med.*, 299:1373, 1978.
8. Maskin, C. S., Sinoway, L., Chadwick, B., Sonnenblick, E. H., and LeJemtel, T. H.: Sustained Hemodynamic and Clinical Effects of a New Cardiotonic Agent WIN 47203 in Patients with Severe Congestive Heart Failure, *Circulation*, 67:1065, 1983.
9. Diedien, W., and Weisenberg, H.: Studies on the Mechanism of Positive Inotropic Action of ARL-115BS, a New Cardiotonic Drug, *Arzn. Forschung. Drug*, 3:129, 1981.
10. Daly, P., Viquerat, C., Curran, D., Dobras, F., and Parmley, W.: Improved Left Ventricular Function without Increased Metabolic Cost with RO 13-6438 a Non-Glycoside, Non-Catecholamine Inotrope Vasodilator, *Clin. Res.*, 32:158A, 1984.
11. Uretsky, B. F., Generalovich, T., Reddy, P. S., Spangenberg, R. B., and Follansbee, W. P.: The Acute Hemodynamic Effects of a New Agent MDL 17043 in the Treatment of Congestive Heart Failure, *Circulation*, 67:823, 1983.
12. Petein, M., Levine, B. T., and Cohn, J. N,: Hemodynamic Effects of a New Inotropic Agent, Piroximone (MDL 19025) in Patients with Chronic Heart Failure, *J. Am. Coll. Cardiol.*, 4:364, 1984.
13. Katz, A. M.: Excitation-Contraction Coupling, in A. M. Katz, "*Physiology of the Heart*," Raven Press, New York, 1977, p. 137.
14. Chidsey, C. A., Braunwald, E., and Morrow, A. G.: Catecholamine Excretion and Cardiac Stores of Norepinephrine in Congestive Heart Failure, *Am. J. Med.*, 39:442, 1965.
15. Ahlquist, R. P.: A Study of the Adrenotropic Receptors, *Am. J. Physiol.*, 135:586, 1948.
16. Langer, S. Z.: Presynaptic Receptors and Their Role in the Regulation of Transmitter Release. Sixth Gaddum Memorial Lecture, *Br. J. Pharmacol.*, 60:481, 1977.
17. Hoffman, B. B., and Lefkowitz, R. J.: Alpha-Adrenergic Receptor Subtypes, *N. Engl. J. Med.*, 302:1390, 1981.
18. Carlsson, E. C., Dahlof, A., Hedberg, H., Persson, H., and Tangstrand, B.: Differentiation of Cardiac Chronotropic and Inotropic Effects of Beta-Adrenergic Agonists, *Naunyn Schmiedebergs Arch. Pharmacol.*, 300:101, 1977.
19. Goldberg, L. I.: Cardiovascular and Renal Actions of Dopamine: Potential Clinical Applications, *Pharmacol. Rev.*, 24:1, 1972.
20. Tuttle, R. R., and Mills, J.: Dobutamine: Development of a New Catecholamine to Selectively Increase Cardiac Contractility, *Circ. Res.*, 36:185, 1975.
21. Sonnenblick, E. H., Frishman, W. H., and LeJemtel, T. H.: Dobutamine: A New Synthetic Cardioactive Sympathetic Amine, *N. Engl. J. Med.*, 300:17, 1979.
22. Williams, R. S., and Bishop, T.: Selectivity of Dobutamine for Adrenergic Receptor Subtypes. In Vitro Analysis by Radioligand Binding, *J. Clin. Invest.*, 67:1703, 1981.
23. Keung, E., Siskind, S. J., Sonnenblick, E. H., Ribner, H. S., Schwartz, W. J., and LeJemtel, T. H.: Dobutamine, a Substitute for Dopamine-Nitroprusside Therapy in Patients with Severe Left Ventricular Dysfunction and Hypotension Complicating Acute Myocardial Infarction. *JAMA*, 245:144, 1981.
24. Applefeld, M. M., Newman, K. A., Grove, W. R., Sutton, F. J., Roffman, D. S., Pharm, D., Reed, W. P., and Linberg, S. E.: Intermittent, Continuous Outpatient Dobutamine Infusion in the Management of Congestive Heart Failure, *Am. J. Cardiol.*, 51:455, 1983.
25. Bristow, M. R., Ginsburg, R., Minobe, W., Cubiciotti, R. S., Sageman, W. S., Lurie, K., Billingham, M. E., Harrison, D. C., and Stinson, E. B.: Decreased Catecholamine Sensitivity and Beta-Adrenergic Receptor Density in Failing Human Hearts, *N. Engl. J. Med.*, 307:205, 1982.
26. Colucci, W. S., Alexander, W. R., Williams, G. H., Rude, R. E., Holman, B. L., Konstman, M. A., Wynne, J., Mudge, G. H., and Braunwald, E.: Decreased Lymphocyte Beta-Ad-

renergic Receptor Density in Patients with Heart Failure and Tolerance to the Beta-Adrenergic Agonist Pirbuterol, *N. Engl. J. Med.*, 305:185, 1981.
27. Fabiato, A.: Effects of Cyclic AMP and Phosphodiesterase Inhibitors on the Contractile Activation and the Ca^{2+} Transient Detected with Aequorin in Skinned Cardiac Cells from Rat and Rabbit Ventricles, *J. Gen. Physiol*, 78:15A, 1981.
28. Alousi, A. A., Farah, A. E., Lesher, G. Y., and Opalka, C. J.: Cardiotonic Activity of Amrinone-WIN 40680 [5-Amino-3,4'-Bipyridin-6(1H)-One], *Circ. Res.*, 45:666, 1979.
29. Nusrat, A., Tepper, D., Hertzberg, J., Sonnenblick, E. H., and Aronson, R. S.: Effects of Amrinone on Atrioventricular Conduction in the Intact Canine Heart, *J. Clin. Pharmacol*, 23:257, 1983.
30. Jentzer, J. H., LeJemtel, T. H., Sonnenblick, E. H., and Kirk, E. S.: Beneficial Effect of Amrinone on Myocardial Oxygen Consumption during Acute Left Ventricular Failure in Dogs. *Am. J. Cardiol.*, 48:75, 1981.
31. Benotti, J. R., Grossman, W., Braunwald, E., and Carabello, B. A.: Effects of Amrinone on Myocardial Energy Metabolism and Hemodynamics in Patients with Severe Congestive Heart Failure due to Coronary Artery Disease, *Circulation*, 62:28, 1980.
32. LeJemtel, T. H., Maskin, C. S., Mancini, D., Sinoway, L., Feld, H., and Chadwick, B.: Comparative Systemic and Regional Hemodynamic and Metabolic Effects of Angiotensin Inhibition with Captopril and Inotropic Therapy with Milrinone in Heart Failure, *Clin. Res.* 32:542A, 1984.

94

Diuretics

Vera Delaney, M.D.   Edmund Bourke, M.D.

In 1919 a diligent nurse recorded an increase in urine output following administration of a mercury-containing antisyphilitic agent. She reported to the prescribing medical student who passed the information on to the skeptical attending physician. This observation was followed by the birth of the mercurial diuretics[1] and a new chapter in the management of edema.

Diuretics have become one of our most powerful pharmacological tools. Their development was paralleled by and interdependent on other major advances in our understanding of the renal regulation of salt and water. About 1.5 kg of salt, some fivefold of the total body content, leaves the circulation daily through the glomeruli into the proximal tubules. It is a paradox of evolutionary physiology that most of the oxygen consumed by the kidneys is expended in retrieving over 99 percent back into the circulation through the peritubular capillaries.[2] The sodium finally excreted is fine-tuned to the amount ingested, and external balance is achieved. A further very small increase in the fractional tubular reabsorption of sodium tips the scales of this delicate balance and is the ultimate cause of all forms of generalized edema. Clinical states of excess total body sodium—whether cardiac, hepatic or preeclamptic, endocrine, iatrogenic, or idiopathic—are all ultimately of renal origin. With the exception of end-stage renal disease, where the cause is the negligible quantities filtered, all other situations are due to excessive or inappropriate tubular sodium reabsorption. Diuretics block the reabsorption of some of the filtered sodium, causing an increase in urinary excretion. They act at the level of the renal tubular cell.

By blocking the transport of salt at the renal tubular cell, diuretics act at sites removed from the pathogenic stimulus to excess tubular reabsorption. The renal tubular cells possess little intrinsic capacity to adapt salt reabsorption to the body's needs.[3] Rather, the factors that determine the amount of salt reabsorbed and, by extension, the development of edema, are to be found in the peritubular environment. The hydrostatic pressure in the peritubular capillaries can play a crucial role in certain clinical circumstances. For example, impairment of cardiac function may lead to an alteration in renal blood flow distribution, resulting in decreased peritubular hydrostatic pressure and enhanced sodium reabsorption.[4] Second, the oncotic pressure of the peritubular plasma proteins which can be altered by changes in the filtration fraction may also play a role in the enhanced salt reabsorption of cardiac edema.[5] Third, hormones play an important role in the physiology of renal salt and water regulation, although their importance in the pathogenesis of edema requires elucidation.

"Secondary aldosteronism" is important to electrolyte balance and to diuretic efficacy (see below) but does not cause edema.[6] On the other hand, the evidence for the existence of a "natriuretic hormone" is compelling,[7] and it is likely that diminished activity of this hormone plays a role in the pathogenesis of some edematous states. The more general statement can be reiterated that the pathogenesis of the excessive salt reabsorption, the ultimate cause of edema, is to be found in the altered nature of the peritubular environment. By contrast, the diuretics which we use to treat edema act at a step distinct from this pathogenic defect, namely at the level of the renal tubular cell. Diuretics then counter-regulate rather than correct the altered physiology.

The Biochemical Structure and Structural Activity Relations of Diuretics

Inhibitors of Carbonic Anhydrase

When sulfonamide was being used as an antimicrobial, side effects included inhibition of carbonic anhydrase and the development of metabolic acidosis. Subsequent studies established the role of carbonic anhydrase in renal tubular transport and explained the interrelationship between these two side effects. Inhibition of carbonic anhydrase in the proximal tubule decreases bicarbonate reabsorption. The resultant bicarbonaturia causes acidosis. Since some sodium reabsorption accompanies bicarbonate, increased sodium excretion is the practical consequence.[8] Acetazolamide is the prototype of this class of diuretics. It inhibits carbonic anhydrase via adenyl cyclase stimulation.[9]

The Benzothiadiazines (Thiazides) and Related Diuretics

These are also sulfonamide derivatives. They were synthesized as an outgrowth of studies on inhibitors of carbonic anhydrase. Modifying the structure was found to change radically the characteristics of the diuresis. The natriuresis of the thiazides is accompanied by a predominant chloriuresis rather than bicarbonaturia.[10] The diuresis induced by the thiazides and related sulfonamide diuretics, chlorthalidone and metolazone, is largely independent of this carbonic anhydrase-inhibiting effect. The precise cellular mechanism of action is unclear. Inhibition of Na-K-ATPase does not seem to be a factor. The renal extraction of fatty acid, a potential metabolic fuel, is inhibited by chlorothiazide in the dog,[11] but the relevance of this to its natriuretic action has not been established. Numerous thiazide diuretics are commercially available (Table 94-1). They all have the same mechanism of action and differ only in dosage and duration of action.

The High-Ceiling "Loop" Diuretics

These drugs are grouped together by virtue of their distinctive pattern of action. Two of them, furosemide and bumetanide, are sulfonamide derivatives; ethacrynic acid is chemically distinct. The in vitro carbonic anhydrase inhibitory effect of furosemide is less than the thiazides, negligible with bumetanide,[12] and nonexistent with ethacrynic acid.[13] Although a transient bicarbonaturia is observed at the peak of diuresis with the former two, all these agents produce a predominant chloriuresis. Many studies have suggested possible molecular mechanisms of action, but their significance requires further study. Inhibition of Na-K-ATPase has been demonstrated but not consistently correlated with diuretic action.[14] Interpretation is further complicated by our current understanding that this enzyme relates to cation transport whereas the high-ceiling diuretics act primarily on chloride cotransport (see below). The demonstration that ethacrynic acid inhibits renal prostaglandin dehydrogenase,[15] an enzyme which metabolizes prostaglandins, is of interest since prostaglandin E_2 inhibits chloride reabsorption in the medullary segment of the thick ascending limb of the loop of Henle.[16] It is of further interest in view of the blunted response to high-ceiling diuretics induced by the prostaglandin synthetase-inhibiting, nonsteroidal anti-inflammatory drugs.[17]

The Potassium-Sparing Diuretics

These agents do not represent a family, either chemically or in terms of mechanism of action, but have a similar final effect on urinary electrolytes, with the production of a mild natriuresis and a decrease in urinary potassium and hydrogen excretion.[18] They are spironolactone, triamterene, and amiloride.

Spironolactone is the diuretic whose precise mechanism of action we are closest to understanding. It was developed as an outgrowth of the observation that progesterone was natriuretic provided aldosterone was present.[18] Spironolactone, a homologue of the mineralocorticoid aldosterone, is a specific competitive inhibitor of the initial binding step of aldosterone to its receptor protein in the renal tubular cell cytoplasm. Normally, aldosterone which is bound in this way is carried to the nucleus where it causes the transcription of messenger RNA which in turn codes for the production of proteins involved in the transport of Na and K. Although spironolactone promptly blocks the initial binding step, events already set in action beyond this blockade will continue. This explains, in part, the delayed onset of action of up to 60 h frequently seen with this drug.

Triamterene, a pteridine derivative, has a structure resembling folic acid. Its action, presumed to be directly on the tubular cell, does not require aldosterone.[18] Amiloride is an organic base which specifically decreases sodium permeability at the level of the tubular luminal cell membrane.[19]

The Site of Action of Diuretics in the Renal Tubule

The noninvasive renal clearance techniques by which we localize diuretic action in humans have been validated by studies in isolated perfused nephron segments (Fig. 94-1).[19] Thus, since the bulk of bicarbonate and phosphate are reabsorbed in the proximal tubule, an increased excretion of these anions following administration of a diuretic favors a proximal tubular site of action. The thick ascending limb

TABLE 94-1 Doses and Duration of Action of the Commonly Used Diuretics

Type of Agent	Generic Name	Trade Name	Market Preparation (Tablets, mg)	Average Daily Effective Dose (mg)	Duration of Action (h)
Carbonic anhydrase inhibitor	Acetazolamide	Diamox	125, 250	250–500	8–12
Loop diuretics*	Ethacrynic acid	Edecrin	25, 50	25–150	4–6
	Furosemide	Lasix	20, 40, 80	20–160	4–6
	Bumetanide	Bumex	0.5, 1	0.5–3	4–6
Thiazides and related drugs†	Chlorothiazide	Diuril	250, 500	500–1500	6–12
	Benzthiazide	Exna	50	50–200	6–12
	Hydroflumethiazide	Diucradin Saluron	25, 50	25–50	6–12
	Bendroflumethiazide	Naturetin	2.5, 5.0	2.5–15	18–24
	Hydrochlorothiazide	Esidrix Oretic Hydrodiuril	25, 50, 100	50–150	12–24
	Trichlormethiazide	Metahydrin, Naqua	2, 4	2–4	18–24
	Methyclothiazide	Enduron	2.5, 5.0	5.0–10.0	18–24
	Polythiazide	Renese	1, 2, 4	2–8	18–24
	Cyclothiazide	Anhydron	2	2–6	18–24
	Chlorthalidone	Hygroton	25, 50, 100	50–100	24–48
	Quinethazone	Hydromox	50	50–150	24–48
	Metolazone	Diulo Zaroxolyn	2.5, 5.0, 10.0	2.5–20	24–48
Potassium-sparing diuretics	Spironolactone	Aldactone	25, 100	50–200	48–72
	Triamterene	Dyrenium	50, 100	100–200	6–8
	Amiloride	Midamor	5	5–20	12–24

*The high doses of loop diuretics are required mainly in patients with renal insufficiency.
†In hypertension management the low doses of thiazides are generally effective with fewer side effects.

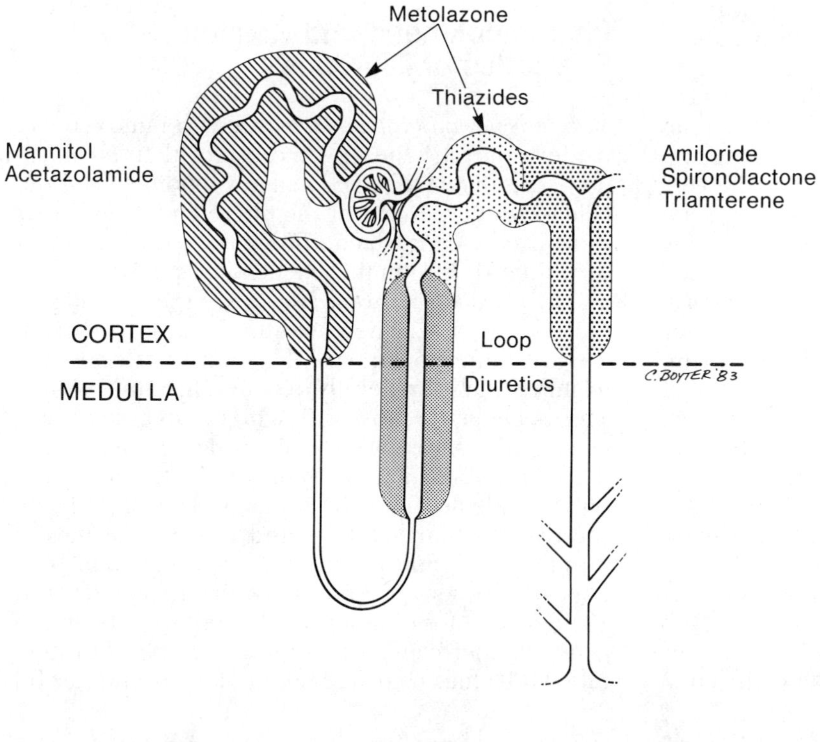

FIGURE 94-1 Approximate sites of action of diuretics within the nephron.

of the loop of Henle is located partly in the renal medulla and partly in the renal cortex. The medullary segment is the site of production of a hyperosmotic medullary interstitial space, an essential prerequisite for the formation of a concentrated urine. The cortical segment of the ascending limb and early part of the adjoining distal convoluted tubule represent the major diluting segments of the nephron. Diuretic-induced impairment of urinary concentrating and/or diluting capacity localizes its site of action to these segments. Since the late distal tubule and cortical collecting duct are the sites of potassium and hydrogen ion secretion, diuretics which reduce kaliuresis and acid excretion act at these tubular sites.

The *carbonic anhydrase inhibitors,* such as acetazolamide, decrease bicarbonate and sodium reabsorption in the proximal tubules. Increased delivery of poorly reabsorbed anion (HCO_3^-) to more distal sites is the major explanation for (1) their diuretic properties, since there is an accompanying obligatory natriuresis; and (2) the observed kaliuresis, since the increased HCO_3^- in the distal nephron promotes increased K^+ secretion down the steeper electrochemical gradient.[19]

The *thiazides and related diuretics* chlorthalidone and metolazone decrease the capacity to generate free water (C_{H_2O}) or, in other words, to form a maximally dilute urine, indicating that their major site of action is in the cortical segment of the ascending limb of the loop of Henle and the adjoining early distal convoluted tubule.[19] They also have a small proximal tubular effect as evidenced by phosphaturia and bicarbonaturia, attributable to carbonic anhydrase-inhibiting activity. The kaliuresis seen with these diuretics is a consequence of increased electronegativity due in turn to enhanced sodium reabsorption in the late distal convoluted tubule and cortical collecting duct. The fact that chloride, the predominant urinary anion in thiazide diuresis, is more permeable than bicarbonate at these distal sites explains why potassium loss is less with thiazides than with acetazolamide.

The *high-ceiling diuretics* act throughout the cortical and medullary segment of the ascending limb of the loop of Henle, hence their alternate name, "loop diuretics." This conclusion in humans is based on the demonstration that they decrease the capacity to form solute free water (C_{H_2O}) during water diuresis and negative free water ($T^c_{H_2O}$), i.e., a concentrated urine, during hydropenia.[20,21] This site of action has been confirmed for the "loop" diuretics ethacrynic acid, furosemide, and bumetanide by in vitro microperfusion of thick ascending limbs.[22] The transepithelial potential difference across the thick ascending limb is lumen-positive. This landmark observation[23,24] led to the conclusion that active transport of chloride occurs in this nephron segment with sodium following passively. An extension of this conclusion is that diuretics which act on part (e.g., thiazides) or all (e.g., the high-ceiling diuretics) of this segment do so by inhibition of chloride transport. The fact that these agents inhibit chloride transport in this segment in vitro in the absence of sodium (e.g., choline chloride) supports this contention. A provocative analysis of the experimental data suggest, however, that such a passive role for sodium transport in this nephron segment, which has the highest concentration of Na-K-ATPase, may represent an oversimplification.[25] Chloride and sodium and potassium cotransport is currently viewed as the most likely mechanism.

Furosemide and bumetanide, but not ethacrynic acid, cause bicarbonaturia and phosphaturia at the peak of diuresis, indicating an additional minor action at the level of the proximal tubule.[20,21] The same passive forces account for the kaliuresis seen with the loop diuretics as obtained in the case of the thiazides.

The site of action of the *potassium-sparing diuretics* has been clarified. It was formerly believed that aldosterone and its antagonist, spironolactone, acted on the distal convoluted tubule, but recent studies have shown that the negative potential difference in this part of the nephron is independent of mineralocorticoids. In vitro microperfusion studies have now localized the site of action of aldosterone and spironolactone to the cortical collecting duct.[19] Triamterene also acts at this site, whereas amiloride acts on both the late distal convoluted tubule and the cortical collecting duct. By reducing reabsorption of sodium, luminal electronegativity is decreased, and the passive secretion of potassium and hydrogen is reduced. Hence, mild natriuresis, increase in urine pH, and decreased kaliuresis follow administration of these drugs.

Pharmacokinetic and Related Properties of Diuretics

The *carbonic anhydrase inhibitors* have a minor role in modern diuretic therapy because of their weak action, the maximal fractional excretion of sodium being about 3 percent of the filtered load, and their short-lived effect, which in turn is a consequence of the induced self-limiting metabolic acidosis.

The *thiazides and related drugs* are the mainstay of diuretic therapy. They are rapidly absorbed from the gastrointestinal tract with a diuretic effect within 90 min, which is generally over by 6 h. Some of these agents, generally those with a higher degree of protein-binding and slower excretion rate, have a longer duration of action.[18] Bendroflumethiazide and polythiazide act for approximately 18 and 24 h, respectively. Chlorthalidone and metolazone have a duration of action up to 48 h. The maximal fractional excretion of sodium with these agents is 10 percent of the amount of filtered.[13] They are generally ineffective when the glomerular filtration rate (GFR) falls below 20 ml/min and are not useful diuretics in patients with renal failure. An exception to this is metolazone, where high doses may induce a diuresis in advanced renal insufficiency.[26] Metolazone has a wider dose response curve than other agents in this group, a property that enables it to play a role in refractory edema (see below).

The *high-ceiling diuretics* are readily absorbed from the gastrointestinal tract and show considerable protein-binding but are nonetheless rapidly excreted in the urine, predominantly by secretion through the probenecid-sensitive organic acid secretory path in the proximal tubule.[18] They are thus carried in the lumen of the nephron to their site of action in the loop of Henle. A diuretic effect is apparent within an hour of oral and 5 min of intravenous administration. Bumetanide, the most recently introduced of these agents, is effective in a dose of about 2 percent that of furosemide or ethacrynic acid,[27] but the maximum effect of these agents is similar. The maximal fractional sodium excretion with all high-ceiling diuretics is about 20 percent of the amount filtered.[12,13] All three agents are effective when GFR is low. The diuretic effect of this group of drugs may be additive to that of other less potent agents, including the thiazides,[28] but they are not additive to each other. Metabolic alkalosis may result from the use of high-ceiling diuretics. Initially this is attributable to a contraction of plasma volume, so-called contraction alkalosis. With prolonged use, the increased chloriuresis relative to natriuresis and the increased excretion of potassium and hydrogen maintain the alkalosis. Metabolic alkalosis does not impair diuretic responsiveness.[20,29]

The *potassium-sparing diuretic,* triamterene, is rapidly absorbed and rapidly excreted. The duration of action is about 6 h.[30] Most of the drug in the urine is in the form of metabolites. After oral administration the absorption of amiloride is about 20 percent, but nearly all of this is excreted unchanged in the urine. The diuretic action is more prolonged than triamterene, up to about 24 h. The overall magnitude of the diuresis is also slightly greater,[31] but this difference is not clinically important. Although spironolactone is adequately absorbed by the oral route and rapidly reaches its renal site of action, the onset of the peak diuretic effects may not become apparent for 2 to 3 days.[13] This is partly due to the fact that the changes in cellular function set in motion by aldosterone prior to its blockade take time to run their course (see above). The potassium-sparing diuretics are weak diuretic agents, the maximal fractional sodium excretion being about 2 percent of the amount filtered.[13] The effects of spironolactone with either triamterene or amiloride are additive, indicating their distinctive mechanisms of action. The combination is generally contraindicated clinically due to the potential hazard of dangerous hyperkalemia. These drugs are more effective in combination with diuretics which increase sodium delivery to the site of action of potassium-sparing diuretics. The corollary of this is seen in some states of secondary aldosteronism where more potent diuretics fail to result in a diuresis until spironolactone is added. Most commonly the potassium-sparing diuretics are used as adjuncts to other diuretics with emphasis placed on their potassium-sparing properties as implied by their group name.

The Clinical Uses of Diuretics

The Management of Edema

Cardiac Failure

The primary therapeutic emphasis in congestive failure is on improving myocardial performance with digitalis or other cardiotropic drugs. Diuretics are nonetheless indicated sooner or later to mobilize edema fluid and to relieve symptoms of dyspnea.

Extreme dietary sodium restriction is usually not indicated since compliance is not readily achieved. On the other hand an unrestricted sodium intake is self-defeating if diuretics are necessary. Added salt should be omitted from meal trays with overall intake approximating a 4½ g salt (2 g sodium) diet.

Body weight is the best way to confirm that an appropriate diuretic response is taking place. Daily weight changes of more than 0.25 kg can be assumed to result from changes in total body water and can be used to determine the type, dose, and interval of administration of the diuretic. Monitoring of clinical symptoms, signs, and exercise tolerance is important during diuretic therapy in the cardiac patient.

A thiazide is the recommended initial drug of choice, but low-dose loop diuretics may also be employed. Secondary hyperaldosteronism does not usually play an important role in mild to moderate congestive failure, and spironolactone is not necessary. A combination of a thiazide with amiloride or triamterene helps prevent diuretic-induced hypokalemia in predisposed patients. Hypokalemia is most likely to occur during phases of rapid mobilization of edema fluid. It should be prevented or promptly treated in patients on digitalis since it increases the sensitivity of the myocardium to glycoside-induced toxicity. Overly vigorous diuresis in cardiac failure decreases plasma volume and, as a consequence, cardiac output and tissue perfusion. This is most readily recognized by a rise in blood urea nitrogen (BUN), indicating reduced renal blood flow. Diuretics are generally unnecessary when ankle edema is minimal and pulmonary congestion is absent. In advanced congestive failure secondary aldosteronism may play a significant role, and addition of spironolactone may be of benefit. In very advanced cases, with refractory cardiac edema, the superimposition of diuretics on low-dose dopamine[32] may induce a favorable response.

In *acute pulmonary edema* the high-ceiling diuretic, furosemide, has therapeutic effects other than those resulting from decreased tubular sodium reabsorption. Furosemide increases venous capacitance, decreases cardiac preload, and, in consequence, decreases left ventricular end-diastolic pressure and pulmonary congestion in acute pulmonary edema. This effect occurs prior to the onset of diuresis. It has been proposed that furosemide induces the release of a vasodilator such as prostaglandin to mediate this effect.[33]

Cirrhosis with Ascites

In this situation[34] secondary aldosteronism is frequent and spironolactone is the initial drug of choice to induce natriuresis while minimizing hypokalemia. Hypokalemia is undesirable since it stimulates renal ammonia production[35] in excess of the diseased liver's capacity to convert it to urea, often precipitating hepatic encephalopathy. The role of diuretics in cirrhotic ascites is to provide comfort from increased intraabdominal tension and elevated diaphragms rather than elimination of ascites. It is important to stop short of this and to avoid rapid diuresis lest volume contraction precipitate acute renal insufficiency. Such a hepatorenal syndrome is readily provoked since the renal vasculature is in a state of heightened responsiveness to vasoconstrictor stimuli. Weight loss of 2 to 3 kg a week represents adequate diuresis. If spironolactone is inadequate, metolazone is a suitable alternative or additive. In refractory cases intravenous albumin infusion may be necessary to initiate diuresis.

The Nephrotic Syndrome

Specific management of the nephrotic syndrome requires knowledge of the cause and of the associated structural lesions.[36] With regard to the edema per se, similar principles to those used in cirrhosis generally apply when the nephrotic syndrome is accompanied by normal renal function. When the glomerular filtration rate is substantially reduced, a loop diuretic is usually required as the primary diuretic agent, using spironolactone and/or metolazone as important adjuncts.

Idiopathic Edema of Females

The precise etiopathogenesis of this syndrome[37] remains an enigma. Factors such as carbohydrate binges, alcohol abuse, excess salt ingestion, psychoneurotic disorders, and, occasionally, oral contraceptives, may play an etiologic or aggravating role. Many patients use diuretics excessively. Exaggerated antinatriuresis on diuretic withdrawal may aggravate the syndrome. More importantly, diuresis and remission may follow a period of several days off diuretics, implicating them in its pathogenesis. Diuretics should, if possible, be avoided in this condition and the patient reassured as to its benign nature.

Preeclamptic Edema

The current majority view in obstetrical practice is that diuretics should be avoided where possible in pregnancy.

Chronic Renal Failure with Edema

The high-ceiling diuretics are the mainstay of therapy and furosemide is the most widely used.[38] Metolazone in more limited clinical experience has produced impressive results.[26] Conventional doses of these drugs may not be adequate. The renal tubular secretory pathway for organic acids is saturated in chronic renal failure due to the accumulation of other organic acids in the plasma. Doses four or more times those normally employed may be required to promote diuresis. The potassium-sparing diuretics are generally contraindicated in chronic renal failure because of the danger of hyperkalemia and their relative ineffectiveness as diuretics.

Refractory Edema

Refractory edema may be cardiac, renal, or hepatic. It is present if a patient is not progressively losing weight on twice the conventional doses of high-ceiling diuretics yet (1) is not taking added salt at meals or other sources of unsuspected salt intake, (2) is not on sodium-retaining drugs, and (3) is not hypokalemic.

Time is well spent rechecking for surreptitious or iatrogenic excess salt intake. If the urinary sodium in an edematous patient exceeds 100 meq per day without weight loss, sodium intake is too high. High-dose sodium penicillin or carbenicillin may cause edema in predisposed patients.

Drugs which may promote sodium retention include steroids; estrogen preparations in some patients; calcium channel blockers; antihypertensives, particularly vasodilators; anticonvulsants; and nonsteroidal anti-inflammatory drugs. The latter by virtue of their prostaglandin synthetase-inhibitory effect reduce renal production of the natriuretic prostaglandin E_2 and are thus antinatriuretic.[17] They also blunt the action of high-ceiling diuretics on the loop of Henle.[17] Furthermore, aspirin inhibits spironolactone-induced natriuresis.[39]

Hypokalemia in refractory edema implies that the diuretic was effective in blocking sodium reabsorption, with subsequent increased sodium delivery to the late distal tubule and cortical collecting duct, promoting excessive potassium secretion. A kaliuresis thus replaces the intended natriuresis. The addition of a potassium-sparing diuretic to a high-ceiling diuretic may overcome refractoriness in this instance.

It is a common observation that patients, hospitalized because of failure to control edema, are discharged 1 week later, edema-free, despite little change in the diuretic regimen. Better compliance contributes, but of equal importance is the assumption of the recumbent position with increased renal blood flow and GFR and decreased plasma renin and aldosterone secretion. This improves diuretic responsiveness in a number of cases of refractory edema. In this regard, some patients with edema respond better to administration of diuretics at bedtime.

The persistence of diuretic unresponsiveness despite these measures is an indication for hospitalization. Impaired absorption from an edematous intestine is a possibility indicating a trial by the intravenous route. Intravenous albumin infusion in selected cases of the nephrotic syndrome or cirrhosis may initiate a diuresis. It may also restore diuretic responsiveness even though correction of hypoalbuminemia is short-lived. In cirrhosis with ascites the volume-expanding effect appears to be the critical factor and 5 percent albumin is ideal.[34] In the nephrotic syndrome, on the other hand, it is the plasma albumin concentration achieved, not the quantity infused, that determines responsiveness. In the latter situation the infusion must be of sufficient quantity and rate to significantly elevate the plasma albumin concentration, and 25 percent albumin solutions are preferable.

Based on knowledge of the mechanisms of renal tubular sodium reabsorption and the sites of diuretic action within the tubule the approach to management of refractory edema is facilitated by sequential measurements of 24-h urinary Na^+ and K^+ excretions. Data on patients hospitalized with the two major patterns of refractory edema are summarized in Fig. 94-2. The patient in the upper half had low basal electrolyte excretions which were essentially unaltered following the combination of a thiazide and the more distally acting amiloride. The response to oral furosemide, 80 mg once daily, was clinically inadequate to mobilize edema. A threefold increase in the oral dose achieved a satisfactory diuresis. This response was much greater than when the same quantity of drug was given in divided doses.

These findings permit the following interpretation: Failure of diuretic blockade in the ascending limb, the distal tubule, and the collecting duct with furosemide, thiazide, and amiloride suggest a prox-

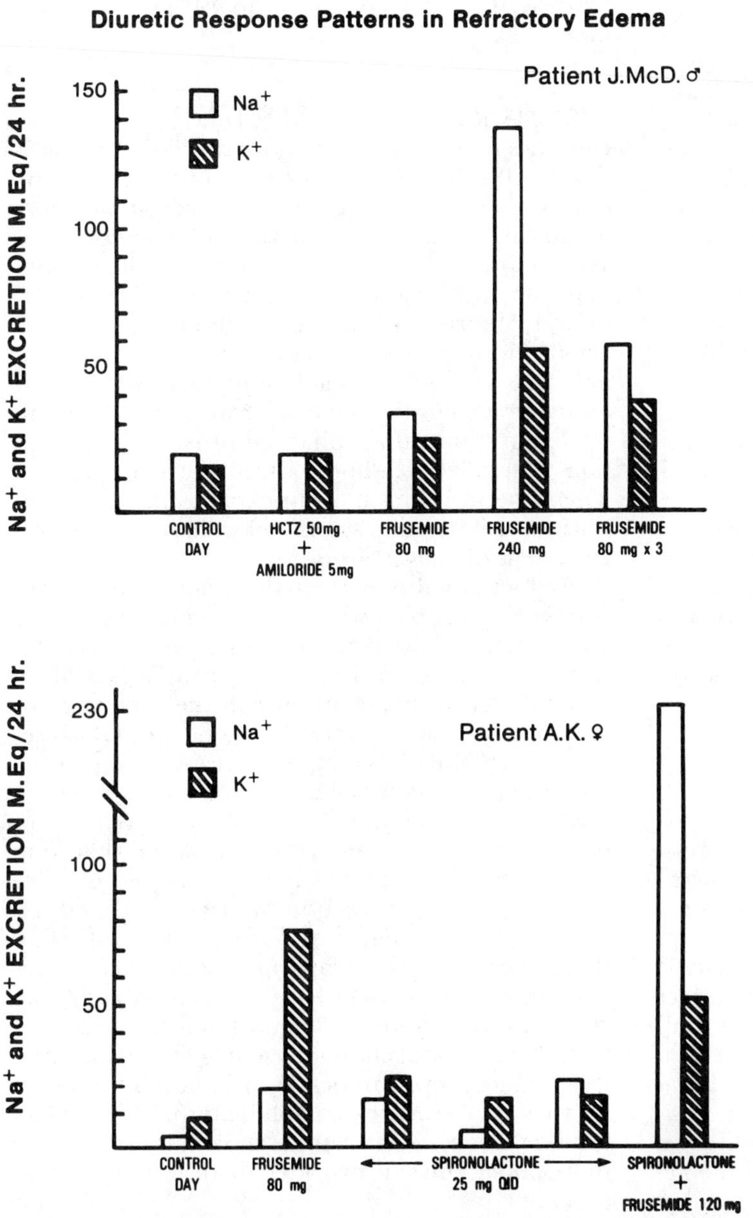

FIGURE 94-2 Natriuretic and kaliuretic response pattern in two patients hospitalized with refractory edema (see text for interpretation); HCTZ = hydrochlorothiazide. (*From E. Bourke, The Rational Approach to the Management of Edema, Ir. J. Med. Sci., 144:86, 1975. Reproduced and modified with permission from the publisher and author.*)

imal tubular site of enhanced sodium reabsorption. The response to the more "pharmacological" dose of furosemide is attributable to a significant proximal effect of the drug at such doses. This additional proximal effect was not achieved when divided doses were used.

A different pattern of refractory edema is summarized in the lower half of Fig. 94-2. Avid basal sodium retention was present with reversal of the normal urinary Na:K ratio. Furosemide (80 mg PO daily) was more kaliuretic than natriuretic. Such a response would ultimately induce hypokalemia but, unless sodium intake were markedly restricted, would not mobilize edema. Conventional doses of spironolactone were weakly natriuretic, but when combined with furosemide at a dose that was only 50 percent higher than originally employed, a substantial natriuresis ensued, and potassium excretion was less than that observed with furosemide alone. The data are explicable on the basis of secondary aldosteronism with most of the increased distal sodium delivery induced by furosemide being subsequently reabsorbed in the collecting duct under the influence of aldosterone. Spironolactone alone was not effective because insufficient sodium reached the collecting duct in the absence of furosemide. The combination of both diuretics would predictably result in resolution of edema. These examples illustrate the value of 24-h urine collections in the management of refractory edema.

Metolazone is particularly useful when excessive proximal reabsorption appears to be a major cause of refractoriness.[41] When proximal reabsorption is avid but increased delivery of filtrate from this site is reabsorbed back at the more distal sites, the diuretic triad of metolazone, furosemide, and spironolactone in combination may result in prompt diuresis and resolution of edema.

Finally, and for poorly understood reasons, removal of edema fluid by dialysis may restore responsiveness to conventional therapy. Peritoneal dialysis in refractory edema is clearly not the first step but nor should it be seen as a final step. It may be a helpful interim maneuver to restore diuretic responsiveness.

Diuretics in the Management of Hypertension

The thiazides or related sulfonamide diuretics represent the greatest single contribution to the management of hypertension and remain the cornerstone of modern antihypertensive therapy (see Chap. 50). The average decrease in blood pressure caused by these agents is 21/10 mmHg.[42] The initial effect is attributable to the natriuresis and consequent fall in plasma volume. Over succeeding weeks plasma volume is reconstituted yet diminished peripheral vascular resistance persists. Although the mechanism whereby this effect is produced remains to be established, a diminished sodium content of the arterial wall has been proposed.[43,44] Thiazides alone provide adequate control for many cases of mild hypertension.

Another important role of thiazides in hypertension management is prevention of secondary salt retention and possible pseudotolerance produced by many antihypertensive agents, particularly the vasodilators. Furosemide is less effective in the treatment of mild hypertension, the decrease in blood pressure being about half that obtained with thiazides.[42] It does have a role, however, (1) as an adjunct in the parenteral therapy of hypertensive crises because of its rapidity of action, (2) in moderate to severe renal failure where thiazides are relatively ineffective natriuretic agents, and (3) as an adjunct in the treatment of resistant hypertension. The potassium-sparing diuretics have a secondary role in the management of hypertension, namely prevention or correction of hypokalemia. The exception is primary aldosteronism where spironolactone may assume the major role in nonsurgical management.

Miscellaneous Uses of Diuretics

Diuretics have found several useful clinical applications[45] whose detailed discussion is outside the scope of this text. Thiazides (but not spironolactone) ameliorate the clinical manifestations of *nephrogenic diabetes insipidus.* They do so by inducing mild sodium depletion with consequent enhanced proximal sodium reabsorption. This results in decreased delivery of filtrate to the collecting duct and decreased polyuria. Thiazides ameliorate *proximal (type 2) renal tubular acidosis* by the same mechanism, mild sodium depletion stimulating enhanced proximal reabsorption generally including bicarbonate reabsorption. The same mechanism again explains the increased calcium reabsorption associated with thiazides in the treatment of *idiopathic hypercalciuria.*

High-ceiling diuretics, on the other hand, are calciuretic and coupled with volume replacement have an important role in the management of *acute hypercalcemia.* They also have a contributory role in helping control hyponatremia in the syndrome of inappropriate antidiuretic hormone (ADH) secretion *(SIADH).* By blocking NaCl reabsorption in the ascending limb, they reduce the hypertonicity of the medullary interstitium. The capacity of ADH to induce excess water reabsorption from the collecting duct is thereby impaired and the degree of dilutional hyponatremia seen in SIADH is reduced.

The hyperuricemia and uricosuria following therapy of myelo- or lymphoproliferative disorders may result in *intratubular urate crystallization* and acute renal failure. Although allopurinol is the predominant therapeutic agent in this setting, increased urine flow induced by diuretics is an important adjunct. In view of the increased solubility of uric acid in alkaline urine, acetazolamide in conjunction with a more potent diuretic provides an ideal combination.

Diuretics have a contributory role to play in the management of a variety of *intoxications.* Bromide, fluoride, and iodide are particular examples. Furosemide cannot distinguish these halides from chloride and markedly enhances their excretion. The excretion of many toxins is accelerated nonspecifically by increased urine flow rate, reducing the time for reabsorption. The loop diuretics by virtue of their greater potency are the most useful in this situation. Acetazolamide accelerates the rate of elimination of weak lipid-soluble organic acids, such as salicylates and phenobarbital, by promoting an alkaline urine. In patients with *acute oliguria* where volume replacement is deemed adequate and yet such indices as urine osmolality, fractional urinary sodium excretion, and urine:plasma creatinine ratios suggest a "prerenal" cause, high-dose intravenous furosemide may reestablish a diuresis and thereby simplify management. Finally, carbonic anhydrase inhibitors have an established role in the long-term treatment of *glaucoma.*

Complications of Diuretic Therapy

These can be classified into three groups:

1. Allergic reactions ranging from skin rashes to blood dyscrasias. These may be seen with any drug and are not discussed further except to point out that the majority of diuretics are related to the original sulfonamide molecule and cross-reactions may be seen.
2. Metabolic complications and those due to fluid-electrolyte, acid-base disorders.
3. Miscellaneous complications.

Fluid-Electrolyte, Acid-Base, and Metabolic Complications[45,46]

Volume Depletion

Chronic volume depletion of significant degree does not occur in most patients even with prolonged usage since counterregulatory mechanisms abolish the continuation of diuresis when edema is resolved and mild salt depletion ensues. It can occur, however, when impaired renal function does not permit these protective mechanisms to come into play or when extrarenal fluid loss occurs in parallel. Prerenal uremia is the consequence, diuretic withdrawal and fluid replacement the treatment. Decreased effective circulatory volume may complicate unduly rapid diuresis even in the presence of marked edema. This in turn results in a decrease in cardiac output and renal perfusion with the same consequence, prerenal uremia.

Hypokalemia

This complication occurs in some patients on diuretics and may result in significant complications, particularly when cardiac glycosides are also used, or hepatocellular insufficiency is present. On the other hand, the degree of potassium depletion and the incidence of hypokalemia in patients receiving diuretics is small. It is more likely during mobilization of edema than during its subsequent control. Except in certain subsets of patients it usually does not become significant during treatment of hypertension unless unduly high doses are used. The hazards of the injudicious use of potassium supplements have been emphasized.[47] If diuretics are used in nonedematous states, potassium supplements or potassium-sparing diuretics are unnecessary unless severe hypokalemia is demonstrated (less than 3 meq/liter) or the patient is prone to digitalis intoxication or hepatic encephalopathy.

Metabolic Alkalosis

This is more likely to be seen with the high-ceiling diuretics than with thiazides due to volume contraction acutely and to multifactorial reasons, outlined above, with chronic use.

Metabolic Acidosis

This is classically seen with acetazolamide and may also occur with spironolactone, triamterene, and amiloride.

Hyponatremia

This can occur with the loop diuretics or thiazides since they impair urinary diluting ability. It may be aggravated by diuretic-induced volume contraction, which increases ADH release. Furthermore, significant potassium depletion causes sodium shifts into cells with hyponatremia. It is particularly likely when water intake is excessive since the excretion of a water load is impaired by these drugs. Hyponatremia is not clinically significant in most patients on diuretics. In an occasional patient profound hyponatremia occurs. A particularly severe defect in water excretion appears to be the explanation. It may recur on rechallenge, so careful vigilance is necessary if diuretic therapy is resumed.

Hypercalcemia

Mild elevations within the normal range are not infrequent with thiazides due to their hypocalciuric effect. Occasionally, substantial hypercalcemia is seen, particularly if hyperparathyroidism or vitamin D supplementation are also present.

Hypomagnesemia

This is not infrequently attributable to chronic diuretic therapy. Increased urinary losses of zinc may occur, but the significance of this is not established.

Hyperglycemia

Carbohydrate intolerance, especially in patients with latent or previously mild diabetes, has been most frequently reported with thiazides and occasionally with furosemide. The mechanisms involved are multifactorial and complex. The incidence is not clear.

There is some risk of decreasing diabetic control in noninsulin and insulin-dependent diabetics. Precipitation of nonketotic hyperosmolar coma has also been reported.

Hyperuricemia
This is common with most diuretics. Two mechanisms are responsible for it: competition for the common organic acid secretory path in the proximal tubule, decreasing secretion; and the enhanced proximal reabsorption of filtrate, which generally follows mild volume depletion. It is usually asymptomatic, but clinical gout is occasionally seen.

Hyperlipidemia
Reports indicate that the disturbances in lipid metabolism seen after the institution of diuretic therapy are short-lived[48] and thus of no clinical consequence.

Miscellaneous Complications[18,45,46]
Triamterene stones and megaloblastosis have been reported with triamterene. Calcium phosphate stones and acceleration of anticonvulsant-induced osteomalacia have been reported with acetazolamide. Gynecomastia, diminished libido, and irregular menses may complicate spironolactone therapy. Cholecystitis, pancreatitis, interstitial nephritis, impotence, and thrombocytopenia have been reported with the thiazides. Pancreatitis and interstitial nephritis have also occurred with furosemide. The loop diuretics are potentially ototoxic. Although generally reversible, permanent deafness has been reported with ethacrynic acid and furosemide. Bumetanide is the least ototoxic.[49] Finally, in patients receiving lithium therapy, diuretics may increase plasma concentration[50] and result in toxicity. When both agents are indicated, serum lithium levels should be monitored.

References

1. Vogel, A.: The Discovery of the Organic Mercurial Diuretics, *Am. Heart J.*, 39:881, 1950.
2. Cohen, J. J., and Barac-Nieto, M.: Renal Metabolism of Substrates in Relation to Renal Function, in R. W. Berliner and J. Orloff (eds.), "Handbook of Physiology," American Physiological Society, Washington, D.C. 1973, Section 8, p. 909.
3. Morgan, T., and Berliner, R. W.: In Vitro Perfusion of Proximal Tubules of the Rat: Glomerulotubular Balance, *Am. J. Physiol.*, 217:992, 1971.
4. Barger, A. C., and Herd, J. A.: Renal Vascular Anatomy and Distribution of Blood Flow, in R. W. Berliner and J. Orloff (eds.), "Handbook of Physiology," American Physiological Society, Washington, D.C., 1973, Section 8, p. 249.
5. Falchuk, K. H., Brenner, B. M., Tadokaro, M., and Berliner, R. W.: Osmotic and Hydrostatic Pressures in Peritubular Capillaries and Fluid Reabsorption by the Proximal Tubule, *Am. J. Physiol.*, 220:1427, 1971.
6. Seldin, D. W., Eknoyan, G., Suki, W. N., and Rector, F. C., Jr.: Localization of Diuretic Action from the Pattern of Water and Electrolyte Excretion, *Ann. N.Y. Acad. Sci.*, 139:328, 1966.
7. de Wardener, H. E.: The Natriuretic Hormone (Proceedings 8th Int. Cong. Nephrol.), S. Karger, Basel, 1981, p. 47.
8. Kunan, R. T., Jr.: The Influence of Carbonic Anhydrase Inhibitor on the Reabsorption of Chloride, Sodium and Bicarbonate in the Proximal Tubule of the Rat, *J. Clin. Invest.*, 51:294, 1972.
9. Rodriguez, H. J., Walls, J., Yates, J., and Klahr, S.: Effects of Acetazolamide on the Urinary Excretion of Cyclic AMP, *J. Clin. Invest.*, 50:617, 1974.
10. Beyer, K. H., and Baer, J. E.: Physiological Basis for the Action of Newer Diuretic Agents, *Pharmacol. Rev.*, 13:517, 1961.
11. Barac-Nieto, M., and Cohen, J. J.: Nonesterified Fatty Acid Uptake by Dog Kidney: Effects of Probenecid and Chlorothiazide, *Am. J. Physiol.*, 215:98, 1968.
12. Bourke, E.: Some Aspects of the Renal Action and Clinical Pharmacology of Oral Bumetanide in Man, *Postgrad. Med.*, 51:23, 1975.
13. Anderton, J. L., and Kincaid-Smith, P.: Diuretics 1: Physiological and Pharmacological Consideration, *Drugs*, 1,54, 1971.
14. Nechay, B. R.: Biochemical Basis of Diuretic Action, *J. Clin. Pharmacol.*, 17:626, 1977.
15. Wright, J. T., Jr., Corder, C. N., and Taylor, R.: Studies on Rat Kidney 15-Hydroxy-Prostaglandin Dehydrogenase, *Biochem. Pharmacol.*, 25:1669, 1976.
16. Stokes, J. B.: Effect of Prostaglandin E_2 on Chloride Transport across the Rabbit Thick Ascending Limb of Henle. Selective Inhibition of the Medullary Portion, *J. Clin. Invest.*, 64:495, 1979.
17. Brater, D. C.: Resistance to Diuretics: Emphasis on a Pharmacological Perspective, *Drugs* 22:477, 1981.
18. Mudge, G. H.: Diuretics and Other Agents Employed in the Mobilization of Edema Fluid, in L. S. Goodman and A. G. Gilman (eds.), "The Pharmacological Basis of Therapeutics," 6th ed., Macmillan, Inc., New York, 1980, p. 892.
19. Jacobson, H. R., and Kokko, J. P.: Diuretics: Sites and Mechanisms of Action, *Ann. Rev. Pharmacol.*, 16:201, 1976.
20. Goldberg, M.: The Renal Physiology of Diuretics, in R. W. Berliner and J. Orloff (eds.), "Handbook of Physiology," American Physiological Society, Washington, 1973, Section 8, p. 1003.
21. Bourke, E., Asbury, M. J. A., O'Sullivan, S., and Gatenby, P. B. B.: The Sites of Action of Bumetanide in Man, *Eur. J. Pharmacol.*, 23:283, 1973.
22. Imai, M.: Effect of Bumetanide and Furosemide on the Thick Ascending Limbs of Henle's Loop of Rabbits and Rats Perfused In Vitro, *Eur. J. Pharmacol.*, 41:409, 1977.
23. Rocca, A. S., and Kokko, J. P.: Sodium Chloride and Water Transport in the Medullary Thick Ascending Limb of Henle, *J. Clin. Invest.*, 52:612, 1973.
24. Burg, M. B., and Green, N.: Function of the Thick Ascending Limb of Henle's Loop, *Am. J. Physiol.*, 224:659, 1973.
25. Westenfelder, C., and Kurtzman, N. A.: Bartter's Syndrome: A Disorder of Active Sodium and/or Passive Chloride Transport in the Thick Ascending Limb of Henle's Loop, *Mineral and Elect. Metab.*, 5:135, 1981.
26. Dargie, H. J., Allison, M. E. M., Kennedy, A. C., and Gray, M. J. B.: High Dose Metolazone in Chronic Renal Failure, *Br. Med. J.*, 4:196, 1972.
27. Asbury, M. J. A., Gatenby, P. B. B., O'Sullivan, S., and Bourke, E.: Bumetanide: Potent New Loop Diuretic, *Br. Med. J.*, 1:211, 1972.
28. Wollam, G. L., Tarazl, R. C., Bravo, E. L., and Dustan, H. P.: Diuretic Potency of Combined Hydrochlorothiazide and Furosemide Therapy in Patients with Azotemia, *Am. J. Med.*, 72:929, 1982.
29. Bourke, E., Counihan, T. B., Keelan, P., and Ryan, M.: Clinical Trial of a New Diuretic, Ethacrynic Acid, *J. Ir. Med. Assoc.*, 56:1, 1965.
30. Bourke, E., Counihan, T. B., Farrell, I., and Keelan, P.: Clinical Trial of the Diuretic Triamterene, *Ir. J. Med. Sci.*, 6:57, 1965.
31. Lant, A. F., Smith, A. J., and Wilson, G. M.: Clinical Evaluation of Amiloride, a Potassium Sparing Diuretic, *Clin. Pharmacol. Ther.*, 10:50, 1969.
32. Mason, D. T., Miller, R. R., Williams, D. O., De Maria,

A. N., Segal, L. D., and Amsterdam, E. A.: Management of Chronic Refractory Congestive Heart Failure, in D. T. Mason (ed.), "Congestive Heart Failure," Yorke Medical Books, New York, 1976, p. 293.
33. Bourland, W. A., Day, D. K., and Williamson, H. E.: The Role of the Kidney in the Early Nondiuretic Action of Furosemide to Reduce Elevated Left Atrial Pressure in the Hypervolemic Dog, *J. Pharm. Exp. Ther.*, 282:221, 1977.
34. Galambos, J. T.: "Cirrhosis," W. B. Saunders, Philadelphia, 1979, p. 323.
35. Tannen, R. L.: Relationship of Renal Ammonia Production and Potassium Homeostasis, *Kidney Int.*, 11:453, 1977.
36. Hutt, M. P., and Glassock, R. J.: Proteinuria and the Nephrotic Syndrome, in R. W. Schrier (ed.), "Renal and Electrolyte Disorders," 2d ed., Little, Brown and Co., Boston, 1980, p. 501.
37. Feely, J.: The Many Faces of Idiopathic Edema of Women, *Postgrad. Med. J.*, 58:229, 1982.
38. Allison, M. E., and Kennedy, A. C.: Diuretics in Chronic Renal Failure: A Study of High-dose Furosemide, *Clin. Sci.*, 41:171, 1971.
39. Tweeddale, M. G., and Ogilvie, R. L.: Antagonism of Spironolactone Induced Natriuresis by Aspirin in Man, *N. Engl. J. Med.*, 289:198, 1973.
40. Bourke, E.: The Rational Approach to the Management of Edema, *Ir. J. Med. Sci.*, 144:86, 1975.
41. Epstein, M., Lepp, B. A., Hoffman, D. S., and Levinson, R.: Potentiation of Furosemide by Metolazone in Refractory Edema, *Curr. Ther. Res.*, 21:656, 1977.
42. McMahon, F. G.: "Management of Essential Hypertension," Futura Publishing Company, New York, 1978, p. 21.
43. Tobian, L.: Why do Thiazides Lower Blood Pressure in Essential Hypertension? *Ann. Rev. Pharmacol.*, 7:399, 1967.
44. Shah, S., Khatri, S., and Fries, F. P.: Mechanism of Antihypertensive Effect of Thiazide Diuretics, *Am. Heart J.*, 95:611, 1978.
45. Reineck, H. J., and Stein, J. H.: Mechanisms of Action and Clinical Uses of Diuretics, in B. M. Brenner and F. C. Rector, Jr. (eds.), "The Kidney," 2d ed., W. B. Saunders, Philadelphia, 1981, p. 1097.
46. Francisco, L. L., and Ferris, T. F.: The Use and Abuse of Diuretics, *Arch. Intern. Med.*, 142:28, 1982.
47. Harrington, J. T., Isner, J. M., and Kassirer, J. P.: Our National Obsession with Potassium, *Am. J. Med.*, 73:155, 1982.
48. Williams, W. R., Borhani, N. O., Schnafer, H. W., Schneider, K. A., and Slotkoff, L.: The Relationship between Diuretics and Serum Cholesterol in HDFP Participants, *J. Am. Coll. Cardiol.*, 1:623, 1983.
49. Bourke, E.: Furosemide, Bumetanide and Ototoxicity, *Lancet*, 1:917, 1976.
50. Kerry, R. J., Ludlow, J. M., and Owen, G.: Diuretics Are Dangerous with Lithium, *Br. Med. J.*, 2:371, 1980.

95

Anticoagulants, Platelet-Controlling Drugs, and Thrombolytic Agents

Sol Sherry, M.D. Arthur Belber, M.D.

I am beginning to believe that nothing can ever be proved. These are reasonable hypotheses which take the facts into account: but I am too well aware that they come from me, that they are simply a way of unifying my own knowledge.
Jean-Paul Sartre, La Nauseé, 1938[1]

Anticoagulants

Heparin

Heparin, a naturally occurring polysaccharide, is obtained most commonly from preparations of beef lung and pork mucosa; it is available in both the sodium and calcium salts.

Mechanism of Action

Heparin exerts its action by binding to the epsilon aminolysyl moieties on antithrombin III, a protease inhibitor found in normal plasma. The heparin–antithrombin III complex is much more active and immediately neutralizes the serine proteases formed during blood coagulation, i.e., thrombin (IIa), as well as factors XIIa, XIa, IXa, and Xa, the activated forms of their respective proenzymes. Since thrombin is inactivated, the formation of fibrin from fibronogen is inhibited; and the inactivation of the earlier-acting clotting enzymes markedly slows the coagulation cascade. Heparin thus prevents the initiation as well as propagation of thrombi formed by blood coagulation.

Since the action of heparin is more readily demonstrable by its effects on the intrinsic coagulation pathway, adequacy of therapy is usually measured with the activated partial thromboplastin time. An activated partial thromboplastin time (PTT) between $1\frac{1}{2}$ to $2\frac{1}{2}$ times the control value indicates that therapeutic anticoagulation has been achieved.[2]

Therapeutic Regimens

Two commonly used types of heparin dosing are "full-dose" intravenous and "minidose" subcutaneous heparin. Full-dose intravenous heparin is used when evidence exists for thrombus formation. The purpose of full-dose heparin is to prevent the propagation of an established thrombus; here, higher concentrations are necessary to inactivate the causative thrombin. Clinically, full-dose heparinization is accomplished via a continuous infusion or with intermittent bolus injections.

When a continuous infusion is employed, the patient is given a bolus of heparin of 5,000 to 10,000 units (the USP unit is used in the United States; it is approximately 15 percent more active than the IU used abroad) intravenously and a heparin drip (1000 units per hour) is then started via a constant infusion pump. Activated PTTs are drawn frequently, with adjustments of the infusion rate, until the steady state occurs, usually 6 to 8 h. When therapeutic levels are achieved, a PTT determination is made on a daily basis and dosage adjusted accordingly. When the intermittent bolus technique is used, 5,000 to 10,000 units of heparin are given intravenously every 4 h. Adequacy of anticoagulation is determined from blood drawn for a PTT 5 min before the next bolus. The bolus dose is adjusted to achieve a PTT $1\frac{1}{2}$ to $2\frac{1}{2}$ times normal before the next dose is given.

Because of its ability to induce an immediate state of anticoagulation, heparin is the agent of choice for initiating therapy when an immediate antithrombotic effect is desired. Also, many investigators believe that when used in appropriate dosages so as to prolong and maintain the PTT to $1\frac{1}{2}$ to $2\frac{1}{2}$ times normal, heparin induces a more powerful anticoagulant state than that achieved with effective Warfarin (Coumadin) therapy; therefore, they employ the former until the thrombus is well anchored to the vessel wall so as to prevent embolization, i.e., for periods of up to 7 to 10 days, and to delay the initiation of Warfarin therapy for several days. Evidence for this superiority is lacking. Accordingly, many physicians are starting Warfarin therapy with the onset of heparin therapy, or shortly thereafter, as was done years ago, and discontinuing heparin therapy as soon as the prothrombin time is adequately prolonged by the oral therapy.

Low-dose subcutaneous heparin administration has a totally different rationale. Since small amounts of the early activated coagulation enzymes, i.e., factors IXa, Xa, and XIa, eventually lead to large amounts of thrombin, low doses of heparin activate sufficient amounts of antithrombin III to effectively prevent initiation of clotting. Patients who are at risk for developing venous thrombosis, but in whom thrombosis is not clinically detectable, are given subcutaneous heparin in doses of 5000 units every 8 to 12 h; these doses are generally too low to prolong the PTT or to produce clinical bleeding. While this form of low-dose therapy has proven effective in the primary prevention of venous thrombosis and pulmonary embolism in patients undergoing thoracoabdominal surgery, postmyocardial infarction, etc., it has not been proven to be a satisfactory preventive when there is a strong thrombogenic stimulus, as in patients subjected to extensive bone surgery (hip arthroplasty, etc.), abdominal prostatectomy, or in the secondary prevention of recurrent venous thrombosis, unless adjustments are made in the dosage of heparin to prolong the PTT to $1\frac{1}{2}$ times normal. Also, evidence has not been provided that, following a large transmural infarct, low-dose heparin as commonly practiced will prevent an endocardial mural thrombus or its subsequent embolization.

Adverse Reactions

The most common adverse effect of heparin is bleeding. Three of the four prospective randomized trials[3–5] that studied intermittent versus continuous heparin administration concluded that the intermittent administration of heparin was associated with an increased incidence of major bleeding. In the dissenting study,[6] more heparin was given by the continuous infusion than by intermittent administration.

Bleeding from heparin may be spontaneous, or secondary to some predisposing factor. Perhaps the most important of the latter is a preexisting hemostatic defect. Patients with a history of aspirin use, or those who consume alcoholic beverages also may be at increased risk of bleeding while receiving heparin.[7] A predisposition to bleeding is frequently cited in elderly females; data from prospective randomized trials do not confirm this observation. Whether heparin-induced thrombocytopenia leads to an increased bleeding risk remains to be clarified. Ecchymoses, gastrointestinal bleeding, hematuria, and retroperitoneal bleeding are the most common types of hemorrhage, and a high clinical index of suspicion of a bleeding complication is necessary when managing patients receiving heparin therapy.

Heparin-associated thrombocytopenia has been recognized with increasing frequency and has varied between 2 to 30 percent in various studies. Most commonly, platelet counts fall within the first 10 days of heparin administration, with 90 percent of the affected patients having platelet counts below 50,000. Steroid therapy does not appear to alter the course of thrombocytopenia, but discontinuation of heparin reverses the process. The pathogenic mechanism(s) for heparin-associated thrombocytopenia are not known with certainty. When the effects on platelets are very severe, the heparin-induced thrombocytopenia may be accompanied by intense platelet aggregation with the formation of white thrombi sufficient to cause vascular occlusions or to trigger a disseminated intravascular clotting syndrome.[8]

The plasma levels of antithrombin III, the major natural inhibitor of the active coagulation enzymes, become progressively reduced during heparin therapy.[9] Whether this effect increases the risk of a thrombotic event when heparin is discontinued remains to be evaluated.

Rarely, heparin-induced osteoporosis has been reported. This serious problem may be due to enhanced collagenase activity and appears to occur primarily in patients who are treated with heparin for a prolonged time. If a patient is to be treated with full-dose heparin for a protracted period (more than 4 months in reported cases), the complaint of back pain should alert physicians to evaluate the possibility of heparin-induced osteoporosis.

Indications
Heparin is the agent of choice for initiating an antithrombotic state in all patients in whom a diagnosis is made of an acute thromboembolic event, unless there is an indication for instituting therapy with a thrombolytic agent (see "Thrombolytic Agent" below). Thus, the indications for its use include all forms of deep vein thrombosis, pulmonary embolism, arterial thrombosis, and systemic embolism. Contraindications to heparin therapy include the presence of an active bleeding lesion, the presence of known hemostatic defects (either congenital or acquired), disease states which will predispose to bleeding (advanced renal or hepatic failure, accelerated hypertension, etc.), and known allergy to heparin.

New Developments
Separation of heparin according to the molecular size of its mucopolysaccharide components has yielded two active heparin fractions (low- and high-molecular-weight fractions) with differing effects on platelets and, when complexed with antithrombi III, on thrombin inactivation, suppression of Xa activity, and possibly bleeding and thrombotic complications.[10] Currently, clinical studies evaluating the low-molecular-weight fraction are being carried out.

Coumarins
Long-term oral anticoagulation therapy is accomplished by drugs of the coumarin and indanedione classes. Dicoumarol, the first of these compounds, was identified as the hemorrhagic agent present in spoiled sweet clover and subsequently synthesized. Currently, warfarin is the most widely used oral anticoagulant.

Mechanism of Action
Warfarin and related compounds act by interfering with the metabolism of vitamin K. Vitamin K is reduced in the liver to its hydroxyquinone form in a reaction requiring NADH or NADPH. It is then oxidized to the epoxide form in a coupled reaction which carboxylates the glutamic acid residues on the vitamin K-dependent coagulation proteins II, VII, IX, and X (all precursor proteases of the coagulation cascade except for VII). The major action of warfarin as an anticoagulant is to interfere with the carboxylation reaction by inhibiting the reduction of vitamin K epoxide. The lack of carboxyl groups on factors II, VII, IX, and X prevents them from binding calcium; this results in a retardation of thrombin formation in both the intrinsic and extrinsic pathways.

In recent years, other actions of warfarin have been identified; these include (1) incomplete synthesis of protein C, and (2) increased levels of antithrombin III. Protein C is a plasma proteolytic proenzyme which is activated by thrombin; once activated, it rapidly degrades factors V and VIII, thus turning off the coagulation cascade. Conceptually, the activation of protein C can be viewed as a check to excessive coagulation and a way of limiting fibrin formation to a localized area. The synthesis of protein C by the liver is dependent on vitamin K and, in the presence of warfarin, inadequate carboxylation of its glutamic residues occurs; this impairs calcium binding and its enzymatic activity. While the warfarin-induced action on protein C would appear to temper the state of anticoagulation, its importance during therapy remains to be evaluated.

Antithrombin III levels are increased during warfarin therapy but the mechanism by which this occurs is still unclear. While some investigators believe this contributes significantly to the antithrombotic effect produced by warfarin, this aspect remains to be elucidated.

The rapidity with which warfarin acts depends not only on the extent of inhibition of the hepatic synthesis of the vitamin K-dependent clotting factors but on the half-lives of these coagulation factors. Factor VII has the shortest half-life, approximately 5 h; prothrombin (factor II) has the longest half-life (100 h); and the half-lives of factors IX and X are intermediate. For this reason, loading doses of warfarin, which were formerly popular, are no longer recommended. They prolong the prothrombin time very quickly due to a rapid fall in factor VII but, while this may enhance the risk of a bleeding complication, it does not slow the rate of formation of thrombin, the primary objective of anticoagulation. The latter occurs when the levels of vitamin K-dependent factors in the coagulation cascade, which have a longer half-life (II, IX, X), are reduced significantly.

Therapeutic Regimens
Oral anticoagulation usually is initiated in the following way. Warfarin, 10 to 15 mg orally, is given on the first day and daily prothrombin times are obtained. Most patients will require 2 to 3 days of the 10-mg dosage before the prothrombin time usually starts to prolong. When the prothrombin time is in the range of 14 to 16 s, a smaller dose of warfarin is given; the warfarin dosage is then titrated to maintain a prothrombin time $1\frac{1}{2}$ to $2\frac{1}{2}$ times the normal control time. Most patients require 5 to $7\frac{1}{2}$ mg of warfarin daily for control. When a steady state of anticoagulation is reached, prothrombin times are taken every 1 to 2 weeks and adjustments in the warfarin dosage are made as necessary.

Indications

Cardiomyopathy Cardiomyopathy is defined as primary disease of the heart muscle arising from diverse etiologies;[11] it may be further subdivided into dilated cardiomyopathy and hypertrophic cardiomyopathy. In patients with dilated cardiomyopathy, there is an appreciable incidence of mural thrombosis and systemic and pulmonary embolism.

Fuster et al.[12] studied the natural history of 104 patients with idiopathic dilated cardiomyopathy. Eighteen percent of patients had systemic emboli during the period of follow-up, or an incidence of 4 percent per year among such patients. In contrast, no systemic emboli were reported in 32 patients while they were taking oral anticoagulants. Patients who had atrial fibrillation tended to have more embolic episodes than those in sinus rhythm, but this difference was not statistically significant. Demakis and colleagues[13] followed 57 patients with dilated cardiomyopathy presumably due to alcoholism. During clinical follow-up, the subgroup of 15 patients who showed clinical improvement had no episodes of systemic or pulmonary emboli. Two of 12 patients with stable disease and 10 of 30 patients with clinical deterioration experienced pulmonary emboli. Interestingly, no systemic emboli were reported. Seven patients were autopsied—all seven had mural thrombosis present in the left ventricle. This group also reported evidence of systemic or pulmonary thromboembolism in nine of 27 patients with peripartum myopathy.[14]

Recommendation: In patients with moderate or severe symptomatic dilated cardiomyopathy, oral anticoagulation is a reasonable therapeutic intervention.

Mitral Valvular Heart Disease Arterial thromboembolism is a major cause of morbidity and mortality in patients with valvular heart disease, especially among those with rheumatic heart disease.

Daley and colleagues[15] reviewed their experience with systemic emboli in 194 patients with rheumatic heart disease from 1923 to 1950. Of these, 26 percent had isolated mitral stenosis, 32 percent had combined mitral stenosis and mitral regurgitation, 10 percent had pure mitral regurgitation, and 3 percent had other than mitral involvements; the rest had mitral valvular disease associated with other lesions. These data suggest that in patients with rheumatic heart disease, mitral valvular involvement with some element of stenosis is seen in most patients who have thromboembolism. However, the exact incidence of systemic emboli in patients with rheumatic heart disease is difficult to determine, for it depends on the method of investigation, as well as the follow-up interval and cardiac rhythym. When all the available evidence is examined, it appears that approximately 20 percent of patients with rheumatic valvular disease will experience a thromboembolic episode at some time. Several factors have been determined to influence the individual's risk of thromboembolism; these include the presence of atrial thrombus, cardiac rhythm, age, platelet survival, and, possibly, the severity of valvular disease.

An atrial thrombus has been identified three times more frequently in patients with systemic emboli as compared to patients without systemic emboli. The pathogenesis of atrial thrombi appear to be intimately related to atrial fibrillation; atrial fibrillation was noted to occur in 87 percent of patients with an atrial thrombus.[16] Atrial fibrillation, whether paroxysmal or chronic, was associated with an increased number of embolic events. Of 1075 patients, 7 percent with normal sinus rhythm experienced systemic emboli, while 30 percent of 1127 patients with atrial fibrillation had an embolus.[16] When patients had emboli, the rhythm was atrial fibrillation 82 percent of the time.

Patients over the age of 40 have a higher propensity for an atrial thrombus and also have a higher risk for embolization. This increased risk with age appears to be independent of the presence or absence of atrial fibrillation.

The severity of valvular disease has been thought to influence the risk of systemic embolization. Most studies on this aspect have involved patients with mitral stenosis. While it appears that a positive correlation exists for the severity of mitral stenosis and the presence of an atrial thrombus, no correlation has been established between the severity of mitral stenosis and clinical embolization. This has important clinical implications, for the patient with mildly symptomatic mitral stenosis with atrial fibrillation is still at substantial risk for a disabling systemic embolus.

In contrast to the usually accepted associations noted above, Greenwood et al. in their study[17] found no predictive value of age, severity of disease, or atrial fibrillation in determining which patients would have an embolic episode during a prospective 5-year follow-up.

Clinically significant systemic emboli most frequently affect the cerebral, peripheral, and renal circulations. Selzer and Cohn, in their review of the natural history of mitral stenosis,[18] noted that up to three-quarters of all clinical embolic episodes may involve the cerebral circulation.

Kellogg et al.[19] determined the number of clinical embolic episodes in each of 42 patients with systemic emboli. The majority of their patients had one embolus, but one-quarter had multiple embolic episodes. A necropsy study by Daley[15] revealed one embolus in half of their patients and multiple emboli in the rest.

Systemic embolization carries with it a definite risk of mortality, let alone morbidity. Rowe et al.[20] reported on the causes of death in 110 patients with mitral stenosis; arterial embolization accounted for 19 percent of the fatalities. Coulshed et al.[21] analyzed systemic emboli in 839 patients with mitral valve disease. During the follow-up period, 65 patients died, 10 as a direct consequence of their embolus.

While anticoagulant use in valvular heart disease has never been tested in a randomized prospective clinical trial, several studies among patients who had suffered a previous embolic episode were undertaken between 1950 and 1965. Despite their shortcomings (controls not carefully matched, nonrandomized patient selection, patients serving as their own controls), they all showed fewer thromboembolic events while on anticoagulants.

Recommendation: Unless a specific contraindication exists, anticoagulant therapy can be recommended for several groups with valvular heart disease. These include patients with a history of mitral valvular disease and prior embolic episode, and patients with mitral valvular disease (particularly mitral stenosis) who have atrial fibrillation, congestive heart failure, or echocardiographic evidence of left atrial thrombus.

Aortic Valvular Heart Disease In the absence of endocarditis, thromboembolism from the aortic valve is a relatively uncommon event. Only five patients in Daley's series of 194 patients with systemic emboli had isolated aortic valve disease,[15] and the most common etiologies of isolated aortic valvular disease are nonrheumatic. Holley et al.[22] reviewed the necropsy material from 165 patients with calcific aortic stenosis of diverse causes. They found pathologic evidence of calcific emboli in 18 percent of the patients, and the most common sites for embolization were the coronary, renal, and cerebral arteries. Their pathologic descriptions suggested that all the emboli were calcific in nature. While no studies have been performed to study the effects of anticoagulation on aortic valve embolization, the calcific nature of the emboli suggest that anticoagulant therapy may not be protective.

Prosthetic Valves Thromboembolism arising from prosthetic heart valves can cause significant morbity and mortality, and is a particularly important consideration for those patients whose hemodynamic derangements have been improved by valve replacement. Anticoagulant therapy adds its own risk of bleeding and must be included in any discussion of prosthetic valves. The valves with the most complete clinical follow-up include the Starr-Edwards ball valve, the Bjork-Shiley tilting disk valve, and the bioprostheses.

Starr-Edwards Valves. Fuster and associates[23] followed 302 patients with several models of Starr-Edwards valves in the mitral and aortic position for 10 to 19 years. Thromboembolism continued to be a problem both early and during late follow-up. After 15 years, only 59 percent of the aortic valve group and 56 percent of the mitral valve group remained free of systemic embolism. In their study, cerebral emboli accounted for 80 percent of all emboli; half of these emboli led to a permanent neurologic deficit, and 10 percent of these patients died as a result of the embolism. This study evaluated the adequacy of anticoagulation, and found a higher and statistically significant difference in the incidence of embolic episides in mitral valve recipients who were not undergoing anticoagulation (14.2 events per 100 patient years) compared with those who were undergoing anticoagulation (6.4 events per 100 patient years). Adequacy of anticoagulation was less important in patients with aortic valve replacement. Fewer thromboembolic complications appeared to occur with the newer Starr-Edwards valve models, probably because the cloth interface was extended to the edge of the inlet surface.

Bjork-Shiley Valves. Cheung et al.[24] followed patients with Bjork-Shiley valves in the aortic position for a total of 1925 patient years. They noted a total of 1.8 thromboembolic events per 100 patient years. A potentially lethal complication noted with Bjork-Shiley valves has been thrombosis of the valve itself.[25] In the mitral position, Lepley et al.[26] found an incidence for four thromboembolic events per 100 patient years. This is similar to and slightly lower than anticoagulated Starr-Edwards valves in the mitral position.

Biologic Valves. Various biologic valves have been used as valve replacements because of favorable hemodynamic features and a low thromboembolic rate. In the aortic position, the biologic valves appear to be less thrombogenic than their mechanical counterparts,[27] and patients are usually treated with anticoagulants for 6 to 12 weeks until endothelialization of the valve occurs.

In the mitral position, the bulk of evidence suggests that atrial fibrillation and a dilated left atrium continue to pose a risk of thromboembolism, regardless of valve type. For bioprostheses, the thromboembolism risk has been approximated at two to six embolic events per 100 patient years.

Summary. In summary, the indications for anticoagulation are as follows: (1) Give anticoagulants to all patients with mechanical prostheses; (2) give anticoagulants to patients with biologic valves in the mitral position with a history of atrial fibrillation, dilated left atrium, or previous thromboembolic episode; (3) give anticoagulants for 6 to 12 weeks to patients with biologic valves in the aortic position (anticoagulants can be stopped then if the patient is in normal sinus rhythm); and (4) when anticoagulation fails to prevent a thromboembolic episode, supplement anticoagulation with an antiplatelet agent (see below).

Atrial Fibrillation In patients with atrial fibrillation who have concomitant mitral valvular disease, especially rheumatic mitral stenosis, the available evidence favors the use of prophylactic anticoagulants. Hinton et al.[28] evaluated the influence of the etiology of atrial fibrillation on the incidence of systemic embolization. They found a 41 percent prevalence of emboli in patients with atrial fibrillation and mitral valvular disease, but also noted that 35 percent of 171 patients with atrial fibrillation and ischemic heart disease had embolic episodes. A group of control patients with ischemic heart disease and normal sinus rhythm had a 7 percent incidence of emboli. Hurst et al.[29] found systemic emboli in similar percentages of patients with mitral valvular disease and in coronary artery disease. This was confirmed by

Aberg[30] in a study of 642 cases with atrial fibrillation. These studies suggest that the incidence of systemic embolism in nonvalvular heart disease with atrial fibrillation is higher than expected; these patients should also be considered for prophylactic anticoagulant therapy.

Cardioversion There is a small but definite risk of thromboembolic complications during cardioversion. Bjerkelund and Örning[31] studied the influence of anticoagulant therapy in 572 attempted cardioversions. Overall, 3 percent of the patients had embolic episodes, 0.8 percent in the anticoagulated group and 5.3 percent in the nonanticoagulated group ($p < 0.02$). This difference appeared to occur irrespective of the presence of mitral valvular disease. Lown[32] described the course of 456 episodes of atrial fibrillation treated by dc cardioversion and found embolic episodes in 1.2 percent but no episodes occurred in the 100 patients who received anticoagulants. Mancini and Goldberger[33] have reviewed these and several other studies and have found an overall incidence of systemic emboli after cardioversion approaching 2 percent.

Recommendation: Although controlled prospective studies have not yet been performed, our recommendations concur with those of Mancini; anticoagulation for 2 to 3 weeks prior to attempted cardioversion and for 2 weeks post cardioversion is indicated.

Congestive Heart Failure Regardless of cause, patients who are immobilized because of protracted severe congestive heart failure are at risk of developing venous thromboembolism, probably related to stasis of blood in the deep veins of their lower extremities. Most of the data on incidence were obtained before the advent of more potent and aggressive therapy for circulatory congestion when the clinical diagnosis of pulmonary embolism in patients hospitalized with severe heart failure varied from 6 percent to 16 percent, and as high as 35 percent to 66 percent in autopsied patients dying from heart failure. While the magnitude of the venous thromboembolic problem today is considerably less, patients with severe biventricular failure, prolonged bed rest, history of previous phlebitis, or low cardiac output syndromes are still at considerable risk.

A large number of older studies found a significant reduction in the incidence of venous thromboembolism in patients treated prophylactically with anticoagulation; accordingly, the following recommendations can be made: For those hospitalized with a severe bout of congestive failure, institute low-dose heparin prophylaxis (5000 units subcutaneously two to three times daily). Patients who remain incapacitated as a result of chronic failure should, while at home, and in the absence of contraindications, be maintained on warfarin therapy adjusted to maintain a prothrombin time of only $1\frac{1}{2}$ times normal so as to reduce the number of bleeding complications.

Acute Transmural Myocardial Infarction Warfarin has been used in patients at high risk of having a myocardial infarction. This includes patients with chronic coronary disease, previous myocardial infarction, and unstable angina. Prospective studies on the use of anticoagulation in preventing myocardial infarction have been inconclusive[34] and led to an abandonment of its use as a preventive measure. Despite this, several retrospective studies deserve comment. Tonascia, Gordis, and Schmerler[35] examined information on all patients in the state of Maryland with myocardial infarction for a 1-year period. In-hospital mortality was $2\frac{1}{2}$ times higher in patients who did not receive anticoagulants than in those who did ($p < 0.0001$). This difference remained in both university and community hospital subgroups, regardless of CCU care, and was also independent of prevalence of arrhythmias, heart failure, or shock. A similar study evaluated 2330 patients hospitalized in Israel for the first definite myocardial infarction during 1966.[36] They found a 21-day mortality rate of 8.3 percent in those receiving anticoagulant versus 27.3 percent in those not receiving anticoagulant therapy.

Horwitz and Feinstein[37] approached the question in a different way. They used patients hospitalized at Yale-New Haven Hospital from 1974 until 1978. Although the study was retrospective, the anticoagulated group was defined using the principles of a randomized controlled trial. They also used case control sampling from a cohort population. Using this methodology, there were 151 fatalities, 151 survivors of similar age, sex, and race. Anticoagulants were used in 28 percent of fatalities and 50 percent of the survivors, for a protective odds ratio of 2.5 to 1 ($p < 0.001$).

Although the studies above suffer the limitations of retrospective uncontrolled trials, the results are provoking, especially since recent observations (1) reestablish the importance of acute coronary thrombosis in the pathogenesis of acute transmural infarction;[38,39] (2) provide data from the pooled results of randomized trials which claim that long-term anticoagulation of myocardial infarction survivors resulted in a reduction in mortality of 16 percent and (3) interpret data from the pooled results of randomized trials involving the use of platelet-controlling drugs as also showing a 16 percent reduction in mortality.[41]* These observations will reopen the question of anticoagulant use, either alone or in combination with a platelet-controlling drug.

Treatment. Following an acute transmural myocardial infarction a substantial number of patients

*Studies involving pooled data are based on the premise that current trial sizes are inadequate to establish statistically significant differences, and only by pooling data can a signficant effect be demonstrated. While a 16 percent reduction is not a major effect, the numbers of infarcts per year are so large that even a modest reduction in mortality represents a large number of lives.

will have a left ventricular mural thrombus, particularly those with large infarcts and significant akinesis or dyskinesis of part of the ventricle. Ansinger et al.[42] performed echocardiograms in 70 consecutive patients with myocardial infarction—35 with inferior wall myocardial infarction, and 35 with anterior myocardial infarction. None of the patients with inferior wall motion abnormalities developed a left ventricular thrombus, but 12 out of 35 patients (34 percent) with an anterior myocardial infarction had thrombus visualized. All the patients with left ventricular thrombus had akinesis of the apex in addition to the anterior wall. The seeming importance of akinesis or dyskinesis of the apex in the pathogenesis of a left ventricular thrombus is poorly understood, but it probably is related to circulatory stasis as well as endocardial injury.

Clinical methods of detecting left ventricular thrombi have been evaluated only recently. At the Mayo Clinic, Reeder and associates[43] reviewed the ventriculographic accuracy of the presence of thrombus in 100 consecutive patients with left ventricular aneurysmectomy. For the detection of left ventricular thrombi, they found ventriculograms to be 31 percent sensitive, 75 percent specific, with a predictive accuracy of only 54 percent. In an echocardiographic study, Stratton et al.[44] found a sensitivity of 95 percent, specificity of 86 percent, and a predictive value of 72 percent for the detection of left ventricular thrombi. The predictive value of a negative study was 89 percent. At the present time, echocardiography appears to be the single best diagnostic test for detecting a left ventricular thrombus. Two other methods, namely scanning for thrombus with ^{111}I-labeled autologous platelets[45] and computed tomography (CT) scanning with electrocardiogram (ECG) gaiting[46] await widespread clinical evaluation.

The most important complication of a ventricular thrombus, systemic embolization, usually takes place in the second to third weeks. The reported incidence has varied considerably. In a large Veterans Administration study,[47] which tested the efficacy of anticoagulants in preventing embolization, the incidence of definite systemic embolism during the first 30 days among the 499 control patients was 4.8 percent; these 24 episodes included 16 strokes, 2 renal and 6 peripheral emboli (this rate for systemic embolism may be higher than commonly encountered).

Patients with an acute transmural infarction are also at high risk of developing deep-vein thrombosis and its complication, pulmonary embolism. Deep vein thrombosis can be demonstrated in approximately 22 percent of patients after myocardial infarction when the sensitive ^{125}I-fibrinogen scanning test is used,[48] and this incidence is greater in the presence of shock or heart failure. The majority of the thrombi occur in the calf veins and are probably of little significance unless they extend to involve one or more deep veins (approximately one in five instances); this latter group is at significant risk of pulmonary embolism. Unfortunately, the clinical diagnosis of pulmonary embolism in the setting of myocardial infarction is quite difficult because it can be confused with recurrent infarction, angina pectoris, pneumonia, and heart failure; however, its clinical incidence is estimated at approximately 5 percent[49] and may be an important contributing cause of death (30 percent of patients dying after myocardial infarction who did not receive anticoagulant therapy have pulmonary emboli at autopsy,[50]) and approximately one in 20 hospital deaths following an infarct can be ascribed to a pulmonary embolus.

Despite the controversy over the value of anticoagulants in reducing mortality after an acute myocardial infarction, all trials have shown a reduction in thromboembolic complications both clinically and at autopsy. In the Veterans Administration study,[47] the incidence of certain systemic embolism was reduced from 4.8 percent (control) to 0.8 percent (treated) and the incidence of proven pulmonary emboli from 2.6 percent (control) to 0.2 percent (treated).

Recommendation: Following an acute transmural infarction and in the absence of contraindications, oral anticoagulation can be recommended for: (1) patients with apical akinesis or dyskinesis demonstrated by two-dimensional echocardiography or more advanced techniques, and associated with a recent anterior myocardial infarction; (2) patients known to be at increased risk because of advanced age, recurrent infarction, or evidence of extensive infarction (shock, congestive heart failure, very high enzyme levels); and (3) patients with persistent congestive heart failure.

Treatment with warfarin in conventional doses should be carried out for a minimum of 30 days unless a definite ventricular aneurysm follows. Initiation of anticoagulation with heparin does not appear necessary. Low-dose heparin may be useful in preventing deep-vein thrombosis and pulmonary embolism but its value in preventing mural thrombosis and systemic embolism has never been documented.

Ventricular Aneurysm The ventricular aneurysms which follow a transmural infarct are frequently complicated by local thrombus formation and an increased risk for systemic embolization. At autopsy, emboli have been found in 4 to 52 percent of patients, and the clinical incidence in various series has varied from 0 to 36 percent.

The value of anticoagulation for ventricular aneurysms has been somewhat controversial. Cabin and Roberts[51] found a low frequency of thromboembolic events among patients with well-defined ventricular aneurysms. They make the point, however, that their definition of left ventricular aneurysm requires ventriculography, and that "the difficulty in diagnosing aneurysm in the absence of angiography leads us to suggest their (anticoagulant) use in most patients with severe, chronic congestive heart failure after healing of acute myocardial infarction." Similarly, Simpson et al.[52] found a low incidence of systemic embolization in 58 patients with thrombi and left ventricular aneurysms and no difference in embolization rates despite anticoagulation. Reeder et al.[43] found that anticoagulation for at least 1 month did not seem to affect the incidence of thrombus found at surgery (50 percent versus 47 percent not on anticoagulants) but that a longer length of anticoagulation was associated with a lower incidence. In his series of 100 patients, five had an embolic episode and four of these has received no anticoagulant. Also, as is well known, recurrent embolization in a patient known to have had a previous myocardial infarction should lead one to suspect the presence of a ventricular aneurysm with a superimposed thrombus.

When considering the benefit of anticoagulation in this situation, one must also consider the risk of bleeding while on anticoagulant therapy. Edmunds[27] found between 0 and 1.1 fatal complications per 100 patient years, with a weighted mean of 0.17 fatal complications per 100 patient years. Nonfatal serious bleeding complications occurred at a rate of 0.5 to 6.3 per 100 patient years with a weighted mean of 2.2 occurrences.

Recommendation: Our recommendation is for long-term warfarin anticoagulation in (1) patients with a "functional" aneurysm (protrusion during ventricular systole)[51] and the presence of left ventricular thrombus; and (2) patients with a known aneurysm and a documented episode of systemic embolism.

Coronary Artery Bypass Surgery Graft occlusion after coronary artery bypass surgery has been a persistent problem. Anticoagulant therapy after bypass has been evaluated in two prospective randomized trials.[53,54] Both studies evaluated warfarin versus control and either aspirin or aspirin and dipyramidole starting on the third or fourth postoperative day. Both studies failed to demonstrate statistically significant differences in graft patency with anticoagulation therapy.

A variety of mechanisms may limit the effectiveness of anticoagulant therapy in preventing coronary artery graft occlusion. Endothelial damage begins when the vein graft is harvested and may be aggravated by surgical techniques, time delays before implantation, as well as its insertion into the arterial system;[55] early formation of platelet aggregates has been demonstrated on the vein endothelial surface. For these reasons, therapy directed at decreasing bypass-graft occlusion needs to be started prior to operation. In this regard, the two-step technique of warfarin therapy recently developed by Francis et al.[120] could have application for this purpose.

Adverse Reactions

The most common adverse effect of oral anticoagulant therapy is bleeding. Various studies indicate that bleeding is related both to the intensity of anticoagulation (excessive prolongation of prothrombin time) and to the presence of underlying lesions. Major bleeding episodes are reported to occur in approximately 5 percent of patients taking oral anticoagulants, and increases significantly as prothrombin time increases. Coon and Willis[56] noted that two-thirds of the bleeding episodes occurred when the prothrombin time was greater than $2\frac{1}{2}$ times control, underscoring the need for careful monitoring of anticoagulated patients.

Several factors appear to influence the activity of oral anticoagulants. Absorption from the gastrointestinal tract may be impeded by binding resins, such as cholestyramine (cholestyramine also binds vitamin K, but its affinity for warfarin is stronger). The net effect of concomitant cholestyramine and warfarin administration is to return the prothrombin time toward normal. Once oral anticoagulants are absorbed, they are transported in the blood bound to albumin. If a patient is given another drug with a higher affinity for albumin, e.g., oral hypoglycemic agents, and sulfinpyrazone, warfarin is displaced and transported as the free drug. This results in a higher prothrombin time since it is the free drug which affects the hepatic synthesis of the vitamin K-dependent factors. Many drugs interfere with the metabolism of oral anticoagulants. Barbiturates, for example, induce enzymes in the rough endoplasmic reticulum which increase the rate of warfarin degradation. Diphenylhydantoin and chlorpropamide, on the other hand, are degraded by the same enzyme system and increase the half-life of warfarin.

Consequently, physicians and patients should be aware that a great many drugs affect the action of warfarin; patients should be advised not to take other or new drugs without informing the physician responsible for the warfarin therapy, and the physician should have ready access to information on all known drug interactions. Patient compliance, a good laboratory, and physician monitoring are essential components for effective and safe oral anticoagulation.

Therapeutic approaches to the patient with clinical bleeding while on oral anticoagulant therapy depend on the prothrombin time, severity of bleeding, and underlying diseases. If the prothrombin time is markedly prolonged, the administration of fresh frozen plasma will replenish normal factors for use in the coagulation cascade. Vitamin K administration has a much slower onset of action and may make the patient refractory to re-anticoagulation. If a patient has significant bleeding from the gastrointestinal or genitourinary tracts while on anticoagulants, a search for underlying lesions should be undertaken once the patient is stabilized clinically.

New Developments

The observation that low-dose heparin therapy can prevent thrombus formation by interfering with the earlier steps of the coagulation cascade has raised questions about the possible effectiveness of lower-intensity warfarin therapy. It appears that this may be so but for a different reason. The recommendation that prothrombin time be prolonged to twice normal (about 20 percent of normal prothrombin) during oral anticoagulant therapy was based on observations made using a highly sensitive human brain thromboplastin in the prothrombin time assay. Rabbit brain thromboplastin, in use in almost all clinical laboratories today, is much less sensitive to the effect induced by Coumadin; thus it appears that a prolongation of the prothrombin time to 1.4 times normal, when a rabbit brain thromboplastin is used, may be as effective an anticoagulant state as the 2.0 times normal level originally recommended with human brain thromboplastin. Support for the use of lower-intensity warfarin therapy has now been obtained in experimental and clinical studies;[57] in the clinical study, low-intensity warfarin therapy proved to be as effective as the more conventional therapy in preventing recurrent venous thrombosis, but with a much lower incidence of bleeding complications.

Platelet-Controlling Drugs

In high-pressure, rapid-flow systems, as is present in the arterial circulation, thrombosis is initiated by an interaction between the vessel wall and circulating blood platelets. Under normal circumstances the vessel wall protects itself from initiation of the thrombotic process by producing prostacyclin (PGI_2),[58] a prostaglandin which inhibits platelet aggregation (also a powerful vasodilator). However, when denudation of the endothelium takes place, platelets adhere to exposed collagen fibers and basement membrane through the formation of a complex between collagen-bound von Willebrand factor and a glycoprotein (glycoprotein I) on the platelet surface.

When the injury to the vessel wall is more extensive or other stimuli are also present (thrombin, ADP, platelet-activating factor, epinephrine, etc.), platelets are activated to undergo aggregation through complex processes which mediate their linking to each other through an interaction between platelet surface glycoproteins II and III and fibrinogen. Activation of the platelet is associated with formation of the prostaglandin, thromboxane A_2 (derived from arachidonic acid released from surface phospholipids during the activation process). Thromboxane A_2, besides being a potent vasoconstrictor, serves to simulate the various processes leading to platelet aggregation; these include the breakdown of cyclic adenosine monophosphate (AMP), initiation of the platelet contractile mechanism and the release of platelet adenosine diphosphate (ADP). The latter greatly accelerates the rate and extent of platelet aggregation (secondary wave of aggregation). Many drugs inhibit platelet aggregation by interfering with one or more of the mechanisms leading to this process.

Types of Drugs

Inhibitors of Thromboxane Production
Aspirin and many other nonsteroidal anti-inflammatory compounds (naproxyn, ibuprofen, fenoprofen, indomethacin) inhibit platelet aggregation by competitively inhibiting or inactivating the cyclooxygenase which converts arachidonic acid to the precursor endoperoxides which lead ultimately to the formation of the biologically active regulatory prostaglandins. The same is true for sulfinpyrazone, an analogue of butazolidin but without the latter's anti-inflammatory property. Certain imidazole compounds are more selective; they inhibit thromboxane synthetase, the enzyme responsible for the synthesis of thromboxane A_2, but not of the other active prostaglandins (prostacyclin, etc.).

Inhibitors of Cyclic AMP Metabolism
Dipyridamole is an inhibitor of platelet phosphodiesterase, an enzyme responsible for the conversion of adenosine triphosphate (ATP) to ADP; consequently, when this enzyme is inhibited, ATP and cyclic AMP levels are kept high. Since the breakdown of cyclic AMP is necessary for the platelet contractile mechanism and the release reaction to be operative, sustained high levels of cyclic AMP in the platelet membrane impair the ability of platelets to aggregate. While dipyridamole by itself does not appear to be a potent inhibitor of platelet aggregation, it significantly augments the action of prostacyclin, the prostaglandin produced by endothelial cells which inhibits platelet aggregation by maintaining high levels of cyclic AMP in platelets.

Currently the most widely used and evaluated platelet-controlling drugs have been aspirin (best dosage unknown, currently recommended dose 0.3 g daily), sulfinpyrazone (current recommended dose 0.8 g daily), and dipyridamole (current recommended dose 0.1 to 0.4 g daily along with aspirin), and these substances, referred to as the first-generation platelet antiaggregants, form the basis of the clinical discussion which follows; the details of their pharmacology and pharmacokinetics have been reviewed recently.[59] Thromboxane synthetase inhibitors are still in the early stages of clinical investigation,[60] while prostacyclin, because of its short half-life and the need to give it intravenously, has had a limited application for the prevention of platelet-initiated cardiovascular disorders.[61] However, there is interest in the development of prostacyclin analogues which might circumvent these difficulties.

Possible Clinical Cardiac Uses for Platelet-Controlling Drugs

Platelet aggregation and platelet-derived vasoactive substances have been implicated in a wide variety of important clinical events. Included in this category are (1) changes in arterial blood flow due to vasospasm or transient mechanical obstruction by platelet masses[62,63] (these processes may be implicated in unstable angina); (2) release of small fibrin platelet emboli, as are responsible for episodes of transient ischemic attacks, and have been implicated as an initiating event in sudden cardiac death;[64,65] (3) acute arterial thrombotic occlusion, probably the most common pathogenetic mechanism in acute transmural myocardial infarction, strokes, early occlusion of bypass grafts and synthetic shunts; and (4) emboli from diseased native or prosthetic valves. In addition to these events, platelets adhering to an injured vessel wall probably contribute to the initiation or pathogenesis of atherosclerosis by releasing platelet-derived growth factor; this protein(s) has been shown to be responsible for smooth-muscle cell proliferation.[66]

The clinical evaluation of platelet-controlling drugs has been complicated by a lack of certainty of the most effective dose; by differences in response by sex and trial design; and by their effect during different time frames in the natural history of the illness.[67] Also, in several situations, studies evaluating the usefulness of these agents have not provided any results as yet; these include the primary prevention of cardiovascular disease (two studies with aspirin, one by English and one by American physicians are underway), and a secondary prevention study by the Mayo Clinic of aspirin in patients with stable angina. The cardiac problems, where the preventive potential of antiplatelet agents has been studied, follow (reference 67 is a recent, more extensive, and detailed review of this subject).

Prosthetic Valve and Rheumatic Heart Disease Thromboembolism

Patients with prosthetic valves in either the mitral or aortic position experience thromboembolic events, and although anticoagulant therapy is beneficial, thromboembolism has remained an important clinical problem. Evidence for enhanced platelet activity in patients with prosthetic valves was noted by Weily and Genton.[68] They evaluated platelet survival time and platelet adhesiveness and aggregation in patients with prosthetic mitral valves, and found platelet survival time diminished in 15 of 16 patients. Patients with prosthetic valve replacements and shortened platelet survival times were found to have a higher frequency of thromboembolic events, and only patients with shortened platelet survival time preoperatively had postoperative thromboembolism.[69] Sulfinpyrazone in doses of 800 mg/day corrected the platelet survival time to normal. Similarly, Harker and Slichter[70] found decreased platelet survival time in patients with prosthetic valves, and also found that prosthetic mitral recipients had shorter platelet survival times than those with aortic prostheses. In a small number of patients, they noted normalization of platelet survival time with dipyridamole, 400 mg/day, or dipyridamole, 100 mg/day with aspirin, 0.6 g/day. Sullivan, Harken, and Gorlin[71] gave dipyridamole 400 mg/day or placebo to 163 anticoagulated patients with prosthetic valves. After 1 year of therapy, a significant difference favoring dipyridamole therapy was noted.

Steele and colleagues[72] prospectively studied a group of patients with prosthetic valve replacement and shortened platelet survival time. These patients were then treated with warfarin and sulfinpyrazone, and compared to patients who had normal platelet survival times and did not receive sulfinpyrazone. When platelet survival remained shortened despite sulfinpyrazone therapy, thromboembolic events occured subsequently. However, in patients whose platelet survival was normalized by sulfinpyrazone, no thromboembolic events were observed.

More recently, Chesebro et al.[73] performed a prospective randomized trial of warfarin and aspirin or dipyridamole in patients with prosthetic heart valves. They found an unacceptably high incidence of gastrointestinal bleeding with the warfarin-aspirin combination, but the group taking warfarin and dipyridamole showed a trend toward lower thromboembolic rates with no increase in gastrointestinal bleeding.

The available information on the subject of thromboembolism from prosthetic valves indicates that oral anticoagulation significantly reduces the incidence of embolic complications, that platelet-controlling drugs alone have little effect, and that the addition of an antiplatelet agent to patients on warfarin, while posing hazards, further reduces the incidence of embolic events. At present, the patient who benefits mostly from combined therapy would appear to be those with a significantly shortened platelet survival time. Since platelet survival times are not readily adapted to clinical practice, further clinical studies are necessary to define those patients who would benefit from combined therapy.

Recommendation: Our recommendation is for the addition of a platelet-controlling drug to chronic warfarin anticoagulation for patients with prosthetic valves who have an embolus while receiving oral anticoagulants, or in those who have valve models with a history of frequent thromboembolism. When aspirin is combined with anticoagulants, a dose of 0.3 g is recommended; careful monitoring of the prothrombin time is necessary when either aspirin or sulfinpyrazone is used.

In the absence of a prosthesis, patients with rheumatic valvular disease and embolic episodes also have been shown to have shortened platelet survival times.[69] When anticoagulants fail to prevent further embolic events, the addition of a platelet-controlling drug deserves consideration.

Coronary Artery Bypass Graft Occlusion

With the increased use of coronary bypass surgery, occlusion of bypass grafts has become a significant problem. Early postoperative occlusions appear to be thrombotic in nature, and interventions with antiplatelet agents have been under investigation.

Most studies show little or no benefit.[53,54,74,75] Importantly, in these studies antiplatelet agents were not started preoperatively or very early in the postoperative period. In contrast, a recent Mayo Clinic study[76] in which dipyridamole (400 mg/day) was begun 2 days preoperatively and aspirin (975 mg/day) started 7 h after surgery, reported improved graft patency. This prospective double-blind study randomized 507 patients; 268 received aspirin and dipyridamole, while 239 patients received a placebo. Angiography was repeated at a median of 1 year postoperatively. The treatment group had 50 percent fewer graft occlusions than the placebo group, and the frequency of graft occlusions in the treated group was one-third that of the control group.

Since thrombosis is the major cause of early occlusions, pretreatment with platelet-controlling agents may be of critical importance in lowering the rate of graft occlusions. In this regard, a Mayo Clinic study involving the preoperative use of aspirin is in progress.

Unstable Angina Pectoris

Folts and associates[62,63] have provided evidence that in canine circumflex coronary arteries made stenotic, cyclical reduction in coronary blood flow occurs. This was shown to be due to formation of platelet masses in the stenosed lumen, which then broke loose to be carried downstream. This cyclical flow reduction was prevented by treatment with aspirin, dipyridamole, and sulfinpyrazone.

In addition, patients with unstable angina have been shown to have increased levels of beta thromboglobulin and platelet factor 4[77] and increased levels of coronary sinus thromboxane B_2[78] (the breakdown products of thromboxane A_2).

A recently completed multicenter study by the United States Veterans Administration[78a] evaluated the effect of 324 mg of buffered aspirin versus placebo in 1266 men with unstable angina pectoris over a 12-week period. They found a 51 percent decrease in death or acute myocardial infarction, 55 percent decrease in fatal or nonfatal acute myocardial infarction, and a 51 percent reduction in nonfatal acute myocardial infarction: These values were all statistically significant. As for death alone, there was a 51 percent reduction during this study (3.3 percent in the placebo group versus 1.6 percent in the treated group), but in terms of numbers this did not reach statistical significance ($p = 0.054$). The use of a buffered aspirin preparation in this study did not cause gastrointestinal bleeding or upper gastric discomfort more than the placebo. The results of this study suggest that aspirin therapy has a beneficial effect in the treatment of unstable angina.

Myocardial Infarction

The effects of antiplatelet agents on post-myocardial infarction mortality and reinfarction have been evaluated in nine recent clinical trials[79–87] (Table 95-1). The results of one (PARIS II) are not yet available. These trials are all multicenter, random-

TABLE 95-1 Use of Platelet-Inhibiting Drugs after Myocardial Infarction: Prospective, Randomized, Double-Blind Trials with Placebo Control

Trial	Total Number of Patients	Average Follow-up (Months)	Treatment Drug (mg/day)	End Points	Results of Therapy
Elwood et al.[79]	1239	12	Aspirin (300)	Total mortality	Favorable trend
Coronary Drug Project[80]	1529	22	Aspirin (972)	Total and CAD mortality, MI and other cardiovascular events	Favorable trend
German-Austrian Study[81]	946	24	Aspirin (1500) Phenprocoumon	Total and CAD mortality, sudden death and nonfatal MI	Favorable trend
Elwood and Sweetnam[82]	1682	12	Aspirin (900)	Total mortality	Favorable trend
Aspirin-Myocardial Infarction Study (AMIS)[83]	4524	38	Aspirin (1000)	Total and CAD mortality, MI and other cardiovascular events	No benefit
Persantine-Aspirin Reinfarction Study (PARIS I)[84]	2026	44	Aspirin (972)	Total and CAD mortality, coronary incidence	Favorable trend
			Aspirin (972) plus Dipyridamole (225)		Favorable trend
Anturane Reinfarction Trial (ART)[85]	1558	16	Sulfinpyrazone (800)	CAD mortality	Favorable trend
Anturane Italian Reinfarction Study (ARIS)[86]	727	19	Sulfinpyrazone (800)	Fatal and nonfatal CAD events, other thromboembolic events	Positive effect
Persantine-Aspirin Reinfarction Study (PARIS II)[87]			Aspirin (972) plus dipyridamole (225)	Total and CAD mortality, coronary incidence	In progress

Note: CAD = coronary artery disease; MI = myocardial infarction.

ized, double-blind, and placebo-controlled, but differ in respect to drug tested, drug dosage, end points evaluated, number of patients enrolled, and time from index myocardial infarction to randomization. These differences may have important implications for trial outcome. For example, it is known that mortality post-myocardial infarction is highest in the immediate post-myocardial infarction period, then progressively decreases over the next 7 months when it reaches a constant rate for the next 5 years or more.[67] Most deaths in the immediate post-myocardial infarction period appear to be related to pump failure. During the period from hospital discharge to 7 months post-myocardial infarction, electrical instability with sudden death is the major problem. After 7 months, mortality approximates only 3 percent per year, and the causes of mortality are similar to those of chronic ischemic heart disease. If the time from the index myocardial infarction to trial randomization is greater than 7 months, the period of maximal benefit for mortality reduction has been exceeded.

As shown in Table 95-1, all completed studies except the National Institute of Health sponsored AMIS trial show a trend toward decreased mortality or coronary incidence with antiplatelet agents. When these trials are examined with respect to early versus late effects, the major effect of antiplatelet agents appears to occur within 6 months of hospital discharge (Table 95-2). Indeed, the PARIS II trial, currently in progress, is evaluating only patients with a recent myocardial infarction.[87] Evaluation of the pooled results from these trials indicates that platelet-controlling drugs reduce mortality by 16 percent but this is not enough to reach statistical significance in individual studies with trial sizes as currently employed;[41] a similar conclusion had been reached previously for anticoagulant therapy.[40] Perhaps trials employing a combination of a platelet-controlling drug and an anticoagulant should now receive serious consideration.

Recommendation: At the present time, the use of platelet-controlling drugs early after myocardial infarction, e.g., following discharge from the hospital, and for a period of at least 6 to 7 months, appears reasonable. The PARIS II study should provide further information about the combined use of dipyridamole and aspirin soon after myocardial infarction.

Adverse Reactions to Platelet-Controlling Drugs

Aspirin

Other than the usual concerns and contraindications associated with aspirin use, the interaction of aspirin with oral anticoagulants so as to increase the latter's effects should be borne in mind. Also, patients on chronic aspirin administration may develop hyperuricemia and/or an elevated blood urea nitrogen.[73]

Sulfinpyrazone

This drug also interacts with warfarin, displacing the latter from its binding sites on albumin; the higher free levels of warfarin result in a more profound effect on the vitamin K-dependent blood clotting factors. Similarly, sulfinpyrazone may produce a more striking hypoglycemic effect when oral hypoglycemic agents are used. Since the drug is a potent uricosuric agent, it is important at the beginning of its use to maintain a high urine output so as to avoid the possibility of a uric acid nephropathy. Hypersensitivity reactions, including a transient interstitial nephritis, have been described.

Dipyridamole

Except for headaches, its use has been generally free of toxicity or drug interactions.

Thrombolytic Agents

Two thrombolytic agents, streptokinase and urokinase, whose techniques of administration are described in Chap. 118, are currently available for use in the dissolution of thrombi and emboli. Approved indications for the use of streptokinase include deep-vein thrombosis, pulmonary embolism, arterial thrombosis and embolism, coronary thrombosis (by intracoronary perfusion), and for the lysis of clotted arteriovenous cannulae (dialysis shunts, etc.). The approved indications for urokinase are pulmonary

TABLE 95-2 Observed Effect in Various Trials of Risk by Period following an Acute Myocardial Infarction

Study	Drug	Early Postrecovery Period	Late Postrecovery Period
Elwood (1974)[79]	Aspirin	+	−
Elwood (1979)[82]	Aspirin	+	−
German-Austrian trial[81]	Aspirin	+	−
AMIS[83]	Aspirin	−	−
PARIS I[84]	Persantine-aspirin	+	−
	Aspirin	+	−
ART[85]	Sulfinpyrazone	+	−
ARIS[86]	Sulfinpyrazone	+	+

embolism, coronary thrombosis (by intracoronary thrombolysis), and for intravenous catheter clearance (central lines, Hickman catheters, etc.). Two new agents, tissue plasminogen activator and acylated streptokinase-plasminogen activator complex, are under active development and clinical investigation.

Available Drugs

Streptokinase

Streptokinase (SK) is produced from cultures of Lancefield Group C beta-hemolytic streptococci and has a molecular weight of 47,000 daltons. SK does not directly cleave plasminogen but activates plasminogen indirectly via the formation of an intermediate. The intermediate, a stoichiometric 1:1 complex of human plasminogen or plasmin and SK, then converts plasminogen into active plasmin.

In the utilization of streptokinase for therapeutic purposes, variable amounts of circulating antistreptokinase antibody, consequent to previous streptococcal infections, must be overcome. The cumbersome dose titrations employed in the past to determine the amount of streptokinase to neutralize such antibodies are no longer performed. Clinical experience with large numbers of patients has shown that a loading dose of 250,000 units given intravenously is sufficient to overcome the antibody level in 95 percent of patients. The exceptions are those patients who have been treated recently with streptokinase or have had a hemolytic streptococcal infection within the previous 6 months or have maintained a high antibody level.

The antigenic response to SK has been well studied. Antibody titers may rise even during the first day and peak in very high titers from day 7 to 10. High titers persist for 3 months and then slowly decline. By 7 months after a course of therapy, an initial loading dose of 250,000 units is generally sufficient for initiating another course of therapy. In vivo, there are two half-lives for SK, a rapid one of 16 min which represents antibody complexing and its removal, and a slower one of about 83 min, representing the biologic half-life of this protein, its complex with plasminogen or plasmin and their degradation products. However, the half-life of the active moieties (free streptokinase and the activator complex) is shorter than the latter though its duration has not been clearly defined as yet.

The administration of streptokinase results in the activation of both plasma plasminogen and thrombus plasminogen; the latter action is primarily responsible for the thrombolytic activity[88] while the former, which also occurs rapidly and extensively, results in a transient state of hyperplasminemia.[89] The level of this hyperplasminemia and its duration depend upon the rate of plasminogen activation, the concentration of α_2 antiplasmin (normally there is sufficient α_2 antiplasmin to inactivate about half of all the plasmin which can be formed from plasma plasminogen), the rate of inactivation of plasmin by the slower nonstoichiometric and progressive but reversible inhibitor complex formed with α_2 macroglobulin, and the rate of clearance of plasmin by the reticuloendothelial system. Thus, the state of hyperplasminemia and its effects varies considerably among patients and is primarily observed during the period when plasminogen is being rapidly activated (first few hours). Subsequently, when plasma plasminogen has been reduced to very low levels, plasmin activity progressively declines to near-zero levels despite the continuation of the streptokinase infusion.

During the period of brisk hyperplasminemia, which is usually well tolerated by the patient, most of the fibrinogen is partially degraded; fragment X (a poorly clottable fibrinogen derivative with strong antithrombin activity) appears early but later there is the progressive appearance of such incoagulable fragments as Y, D, and E which have the ability to slow the formation of fibrin polymers.[90] In addition to the effects of the fibrinogen breakdown products on the coagulation mechanism, the degradation of fibrinogen also interferes with the ability of platelets to aggregate normally. These changes plus the associated hypofibrinogemia and the partial degradation of factors V and VIII induce a hemostatic defect which resolves slowly as the therapy is continued. This aberration and the dissolution of fibrin previously laid down at sites of invasive procedures place the patient at increased risk of a bleeding event (the major adverse reaction encountered during therapy).

In vitro, the rate of clot lysis has been shown to be a direct function of the concentrations of both the plasminogen activator concentration in the immediate proximity of the thrombus and of clot plasminogen.[88] However, there is evidence that other mechanisms such as the action of circulating plasmin and the activation of plasma plasminogen perfusing a clot may also contribute as well. Thus, the total effect during streptokinase therapy is a combination of both internal and external lysis of the thrombus.

Urokinase

Urokinase (UK), presently synthesized from human fetal kidney cell cultures or isolated from urine, exists in two forms with molecular weights of 54,000 and 31,600 daltons; the former is believed to be the native form, the latter an active fragment. UK, an active protease, directly cleaves plasminogen to plasmin. Of the two forms of plasminogen, activation of lys-plasminogen proceeds more rapidly than with glu-plasminogen. Of interest is that UK, while a native human plasminogen activator, is different from the activator(s) appearing in plasma following stimulation of the intrinsic or extrinsic mechanisms of fibrinolysis. This suggests that the urinary source of urokinase is from local production in the kidney rather than by excretion from plasma. The in vivo half-life of UK is approximately 16 min. The most frequently used loading dosage to initiate a thrombolytic state is 2000 units per lb of body weight. Since the methods for standardizing urokinase and streptokinase are different, their units are not the same; in practice, the in vivo activity of 3 units of UK is comparable to 1 of SK.

UK has several theoretical advantages as a thrombolytic agent in clinical practice: (1) it is nonantigenic, and true allergy is not seen; (2) for the same reason, there are no anti-UK antibodies present to interfere with drug action, though variability in the rates of inactivation and clearance of UK occurs; and (3) UK, as compared to SK, has a greater affinity for fibrin-bound plasminogen than it has for plasma plasminogen. Theoretically, this increased propensity for fibrin-bound plasminogen should result in more clot lysis at lower levels of hyperplasminemia. Nevertheless, in studies comparing UK with SK, the following observations have been made with currently recommended dosage schedules: no significant difference in clinical efficacy between UK and SK exists, nor are there significant differences in the incidence of hemorrhagic complications[91] (bleeding complications are most frequently due to the lysis of hemostatic plugs at the sites of recent invasive procedures and not to the hematologic changes). Also, while SK, a streptococcal protein, elicits antibodies and may cause pyrogenic and allergic reactions, these are managed easily in practice and cause little significant morbidity. These facts, coupled with far lower cost, have resulted in SK being the more commonly used thrombolytic agent in clinical medicine today.

Once a thrombolytic state is established with either of these agents, there is little correlation with the level of circulating plasma activity and the rate or extent of thrombolysis. The latter are dependent on local factors in and around the thrombus; these include the accessibility of the activator to the thrombus, the surface area of the clot exposed to the plasminogen activator, the concentration of fibrin-bound plasminogen within the clot as well as the activator concentration surrounding the thrombus, and the age of the clot (fresh clots dissolve more readily than older ones).

Rationale and Indications

Deep-Vein Thrombosis

While anticoagulation is the mainstay of therapy for deep-vein thrombosis, it serves only as a secondary preventive measure, i.e., it slows or stops the underlying thrombotic process and, in so doing, inhibits extension of the venous thrombus and decreases the likelihood of pulmonary embolism or its recurrence. However, anticoagulation has no acute demonstrable effect on the original thrombus, i.e., it does not alter the acute hemodynamic disturbance, nor does it prevent the late or chronic abnormalities which may result from the original thrombus or embolus.

Serial venographic studies carried out during the first week in patients treated with heparin following an attack of thrombophlebitis involving the popliteal and/or more proximal vessels (femoral, ileofemoral, etc.), have shown that complete resolution of the thrombosis occurs during this time frame in 10 percent or less of patients, some resolutions may be evident in approximately another 15 percent, while the remainder (75 percent) show either no resolution or some progression of the underlying process.[92,93] Pathological and radiological studies have shown that large venous thrombi which do not undergo rapid resolution within the first week to 10 days undergo organization and subsequent recanalization but the new channel contains no valves or, where valves remain, they are functionally inadequate due to cicatricial changes and anatomical disfiguration; thus the vast majority of patients are left with persistent venous hypertension in the affected extremity. While the appearance of an overt and disabling postphlebitic insufficiency syndrome may be relatively uncommon, most of these patients will remain symptomatic (bouts of pain, swelling, etc.) and be at permanent high risk of recurrent thrombophlebitis once anticoagulation is stopped. In a study by Elliott and his associates,[94] it was observed that of 25 cases treated with adequate anticoagulation alone for proximal thrombophlebitis, two died of pulmonary embolism and two others subsequently died of malignant disease. Of the remaining 21 who were available for 2-year follow-up studies, 19 were still symptomatic, with four having gone on to develop venous claudication and one suffered from venous ulcers. In Arnesen's study,[95] where patients were followed for an average of 6.5 years, similar results were obtained.

These consequences can be avoided if therapy is aimed at removing the offending thrombus first, so as to restore the circulation and anatomy to normal, and then preventing recurrence. The latter cannot be accomplished in the vast majority of cases by anticoagulation alone but requires the removal of the thrombus either by a surgical procedure or enzymatic lysis. Unfortunately, the usefulness of surgical thrombectomy has been very limited because recurrence of thrombosis usually follows. On the other hand, a successful enzymatic thrombectomy can be accomplished in a majority of the cases,[96] particularly when the lesion is less than 72 h old; this has resulted in a more rapid and satisfactory clinical improvement over that observed with heparin for proximal deep-vein thrombosis.[97] More importantly, when successful enzymatic lysis is followed by anticoagulation to prevent recurrence, many of the late consequences described above for the more conventional therapy of thrombophlebitis are avoided.[94,95]

Recommendation: At present, thrombolytic therapy can be recommended for all cases of adequately documented (usually by venography) proximal deep-vein thrombosis of the lower and upper extremities, provided that the benefit/risk ratio in each individual case favors its use.

Pulmonary Embolism
The natural history of pulmonary embolism in anticoagulated patients is not as innocuous as formerly believed. Despite the view that the ultimate disappearance of the perfusion defect on lung scanning in approximately 80 percent of patients suggests that the pulmonary vascular bed usually returns to normal, both anatomically and physiologically, this interpretation is probably misleading; the course of pulmonary emboli, particularly when large or extensive, is not very dissimilar from that of venous thrombi from which they arise.

There is evidence that when pulmonary hypertension is associated with an embolic episode, it is not acutely affected by heparin therapy.[98] Equally important is the observation that the acute pulmonary hypertension, though moderating with time, is still present when patients are restudied 3 to 5 years later[99] and that patients with persistent pulmonary hypertension, secondary to a pulmonary embolism, have a poor long-term prognosis.[100] Furthermore, autopsy studies frequently have demonstrated the presence of recurrent pulmonary emboli in different stages of organization and recanalization, and, in patients dying of other causes, fibrous webs and bands in the pulmonary arteries resulting from previous embolic episodes are often evident.[101] Even in cases where the perfusion defect has ultimately resolved, permanent hemodynamic disturbances due to an increased pulmonary vascular resistance is evident on examination.[99] Finally, the observation of Sharma et al.[102] on a permanent defect in pulmonary capillary blood volume which follows an acute embolic episode in patients treated with anticoagulation alone provides additional evidence that anticoagulation by itself is a limited form of therapy and leaves a modest but permanent handicap.

Ideal therapy requires removal of the embolus, restoration of the circulation to normal, and then prevention of recurrence with anticoagulation. The former may be achieved either by a surgical or enzymatic embolectomy. Surgical embolectomy, because of its high morbidity and mortality, has very restricted indications and presents logistical problems. Successful enzymatic lysis can be achieved in the majority of cases safely; the acute clinical effects are considerably better than that observed with anticoagulation alone,[103,104] as are the late consequences.[92]

Recommendation: Recommended indications for thrombolytic therapy, barring significant contraindications, include any one of the following circumstances: (1) pulmonary embolism with evidence of acute pulmonary hypertension, (2) pulmonary embolism associated with protracted shock, and (3) pulmonary embolism with a perfusion defect (single or multiple) equivalent to one lobe or more.[105]

Arterial Thrombosis and Embolism
When feasible, rapid removal of an acute thrombotic or embolic arterial obstruction has always been considered a therapeutic objective so as to avoid tissue necrosis or permanent impairment of the circulation. Thrombolytic therapy provides an alternative to surgery. Nevertheless, because many successful surgical techniques are immediately available for managing acute arterial thromboembolic problems in the extremities, *systemic* thrombolytic therapy, as commonly practiced, is usually restricted to those situations where an operative procedure is refused or not likely to be tolerated, or when the lesion is not accessible, e.g., in the more distal vessels. Therapeutic radiologists and vascular surgeons[106,107] have extended the indications and usefulness of thrombolytic therapy by placing catheters in the immediate proximity of an acute thrombus or embolus and locally perfusing the vessel with clot-dissolving agents. The advantages of local perfusion appear to be (1) delivery of the agent to the intended site is assured; (2) higher local concentration of the plasminogen activators are achieved with lower dosage schedules, thus maximizing rates of clot lysis while minimizing systemic effects; and (3) the duration of therapy can be shortened and effectively tailored to the desired therapeutic objective. The application of this approach has extended the indications for this therapy to all lesions accessible to local perfusion, and has allowed vascular surgeons to use both surgery and lytic therapy to best advantage in the total management of more complex problems.

Coronary Thrombosis (by Intracoronary Perfusion)
While a number of cardiac situations, e.g., clotted prosthetic valves and bypass grafts, have been successfully lysed by streptokinase and urokinase, the major cardiac use of thrombolytic therapy lies in its potential for reducing infarct size in patients during the early stages of an evolving transmural infarction. The rationale for its use for this purpose is based on (1) unequivocal evidence that an acute coronary thrombosis is present and pathogenetic in most cases of acute transmural myocardial infarction;[38,39] (2) clotted coronary arteries usually can be recanalized in approximately 75 to 80 percent of cases within 20 to 30 min by the local perfusion of streptokinase or urokinase;[108,109] and (3) evidence that early restoration of the obstructed coronary artery within the first few hours following the onset of chest pain by coronary thrombolysis has resulted in reduction of infarct size by thallium scanning[110]

and improved function of areas of the myocardium which otherwise would have been expected to proceed to a permanent loss of contractility.[111,112] While the value of this therapy remains to be established, the current state of information has been reviewed recently, including studies to determine whether similar results can be accomplished with high-dose, brief-duration, intravenously administered infusions of streptokinase.[108] The latter is now being extensively investigated.

Clotted Dialysis Shunts and Catheters
Thrombolytic agents have been shown to be useful in the recanalization of clotted arteriovenous cannulae[113] and in the clearing of clotted catheters.[114]

Types of Regimens for Thrombolytic Therapy and Specifics of Administration

This subject is discussed in detail in Chapter 118.

New Developments

The activation of plasma plasminogen when streptokinase or urokinase is present in the circulating blood usually leads to a significant hemostatic defect (fibrinogen reduced, fibrinogen breakdown products increased, impaired platelet function, etc.). In contrast, the activator made by endothelial cells, fibroblasts, tumor cells, etc., requires fibrin as a cofactor for the activation of plasminogen. Thus, when this type of human activator, referred to as tissue-type plasminogen activator (TPA), is introduced into the bloodstream, no hemostatic abnormalities ensue; its activity is restricted to activation of the fibrin-bound plasminogen, the most sensitive mechanism for thrombolysis. Currently, an extensive investigation is under way to evaluate TPA. Originally the material was obtained in tissue culture from a human melanoma cell line; preliminary studies on the lysis of venous and coronary thrombi with this preparation have been encouraging.[115–117] Currently, the material is being made in tissue culture by recombinant DNA technique (rTPA) utilizing a mammalian cell line.

Another development involves the acylation of the streptokinase-plasminogen activator complex; this inactivates the SK activator so that upon its introduction into the bloodstream no hemostatic abnormalities are produced. However, after the acylated compound binds to fibrin, deacylation takes place, releasing the original activator complex so as to activate the plasminogen bound to fibrin. Though animal studies with such preparations have been very encouraging,[118] more recent observations in humans indicate that the presently used substances are deacylating in the general circulation and inducing a hemostatic defect.[119]

References

1. Sartre, J. P.: "Nausea" (translated by Lloyd Alexander), New Directions, New York, 1959.
2. Basu, D., Gallus, A., and Hirsch, J., et al.: A Prospective Study of the Value of Monitoring Heparin Treatment with the Activated Partial Thromboplastin Time, *N. Engl. J. Med.*, 287:324, 1972.
3. Salzman, E. W., Deykin, D., Shapiro, R. M., and Rosenberg, R. D.: Management of Heparin Therapy. Controlled Prospective Trial, *N. Engl. J. Med.*, 292:1046, 1975.
4. Glazier, R. L., and Crowell, E. B.: Randomized Prospective Trial of Continuous versus Intermittent Heparin Therapy, *JAMA*, 236:1365, 1976.
5. Wilson, J. R., and Lampman, J.: Heparin Therapy: A Randomized Prospective Study, *Am. Heart J.*, 97:155, 1979.
6. Mant, M. J., Thong, K. L., Birtwhistle, R. D., O'Brien, B. D., Hammond, G. W., and Grace, M. G.: Hemorrhagic Complications of Heparin Therapy, *Lancet*, 1:1133, 1977.
7. Walker, A. M., and Gick, H.: Predictors of Bleeding during Heparin Therapy, *JAMA*, 244:1209, 1980.
8. Klein, H. G., and Bell, W. R.: Disseminated Intravascular Coagulation during Heparin Therapy, *Ann. Intern. Med.*, 80:477, 1974.
9. Rao, A. K., Niewiarwoski, S., Guzzo, J., and Day, H. J.: Antithrombin-III Levels during Heparin Therapy, *Thromb. Res.*, 24:181, 1981.
10. Rosenberg, R. D.: Heparin-Antithrombin System, in R. W. Colman, J. Hirsh, V. J. Marder, and E. W. Salzman (eds.), "Hemostasis and Thrombosis," J. P. Lippincott, Philadelphia, Toronto, 1982, p. 962.
11. Johnson, R. A., and Palacios, N. I.: Dilated Cardiomyopathies of the Adults, *N. Engl. J. Med.*, 307:1051, 1982.
12. Fuster, V., Gersh, B. J., Giuliani, E. R., Tajik, A. J., Brandenberg, R. O., and Frye, R. L.: The Natural History of Idiopathic Dilated Cardiomyopathy, *Am. J. Cardiol.*, 47:525, 1981.
13. Demakis, J. G., Proskey, A., Rahimtoola, S. H., et al.: The Natural Course of Alcoholic Cardiomyopathy, *Am. Intern. Med.*, 80:283, 1974.
14. Demakis, J. G., Rahimtoola, S. H., Sutton, G. C., et al.: Natural Course of Peripartum Cardiomyopathy, 44:1053, 1971.
15. Daley, R., Mattingly, T. W., Holt, C. L., Bland, E. F., and White, P. D.: Systemic Arterial Embolism in Rheumatic Heart Disease, *Am. Heart J.*, 42:566, 1951.
16. Abernathy, W. S., and Willis, P. W., III: Thromboembolic Complications of Rheumatic Heart Disease, *Cardiovasc. Clin.*, 5:131, 1973.
17. Greenwood, W. F., Aldridge, H. E., and McKelvey, A. D.: Effective Mitral Commissurotomy on Duration of Life, Functional Capacity, Hemoptysis, and Systemic Embolism, *Am. J. Cardiol.*, 11:348, 1963.
18. Selzer, A., and Cohn, K. E.: Natural History of Mitral Stenosis: A Review, *Circulation*, 45:878, 1972.
19. Kellogg, F., Liu, C. K., Fishman, W., and Larson, R.: Systemic and Pulmonary Emboli before and after Mitral Commissurotomy, *Circulation*, 24:263, 1961.
20. Rowe, J. C., Bland, E. F., Sprague, H. B., and White, P. D.: The Course of Mitral Stenosis without Surgery: Ten and Twenty Year Perspectives, *Ann. Intern. Med.*, 52:741, 1960.
21. Coulshed, N., Epstein, E. J., McKendrick, C. S., Galloway, R. W., and Walker, E.: Systemic Embolism in Mitral Valve Disease, *Br. Heart J.*, 32:26, 1970.
22. Holley, K. E., Bahn, R. C., McGoon, D. C., and Mankin, H. T.: Spontaneous Calcific Embolization Associated with Calcific Aortic Stenosis. *Circulation*, 27:197, 1963.
23. Fuster, V., Pumphrey, C. W., McGoon, M. D., Chesebro, J. H., Pluth, J. R., and McGoon, D. C.: Systemic Thromboembolism in Mitral and Aortic Starr-Edwards Prostheses: A 10–19 Year Follow-up, *Circulation*, 66(suppl. I):I-157, 1982.
24. Cheung, D., Flemma, R. J., Mullen, D. C., Lepley, D., Jr., Anderson, A. J., and Weirauch, E.: Ten Year Follow-up in

Aortic Valve Replacement Using the Bjork-Shiley Prosthesis, *Ann. Thorac. Surg.*, 32:138, 1981.

25. Copans, H., Lakier, J. B., Kinsley, R. H., Coisen, T. R., and Barlowe, B. J.: Thrombosed Bjork-Shiley Mitral Prostheses, *Circulation,* 61:169, 1980.
26. Lepley, Jr., D., Flemma, R. J., Mullen, D. C., et al.: Long-term Follow-up of the Bjork-Shiley Prosthetic Valve Used in the Mitral Position, *Ann. Thorac. Surg.*, 30:164, 1980.
27. Edmunds, Jr., L. H.: Thromboembolic Complications of Current Cardiac Valvular Prostheses, *Ann. Thorac. Surg.*, 34:96, 1981.
28. Hinton, R. C., Kistler, J. P., Fallon, J. T., Friedlich, A. L., and Fisher, C. M.: Influence of Etiology of Atrial Fibrillation on Incidence of Systemic Embolism, *Am. J. Card.*, 40:509, 1977.
29. Hurst, J. W., Paulk, E. A., Protor, H. D., et al.: Management of Patients with Atrial Fibrillation, *Am. J. Med.*, 37:728, 1964.
30. Aberg, H.: Atrial Fibrillation: I. A Study of Atrial Thrombosis and Systemic Embolism in Necropsy Material, *Acta Med. Scand.*, 185:373, 1969.
31. Bjerkelund, C. J., and Orning, O. M.: The Efficacy of Anticoagulant Therapy in Preventing Embolism Related to D.C. Electrical Conversion of Atrial Fibrillation, *Am. J. Cardiol.*, 23:208, 1969.
32. Lown, B.: Electrical Reversion of Cardiac Arrhythmias, *Br. Heart J.*, 29:469, 1967.
33. Mancini, G. B. J., and Goldberger, A. L.: Cardioversion of Atrial Fibrillation: Consideration of Embolization, Anticoagulation, Prophylactic Pacemaker, and Longterm Success. *Am. Heart J.*, 104:617, 1982.
34. Rogers, P. H., and Sherry, S.: Current Status of Antithrombotic Therapy in Cardiovascular Disease, *Prog. Cardiovasc. Dis.* 19:235, 1976.
35. Tonascia, J., Gordis, L., Schmerler, H.: Retrospective Evidence Favoring Use of Anticoagulant for Myocardial Infarction, *N. Engl. J. Med.*, 292:1362, 1975.
36. Modan, B., Shani, M., Schor, S., et al.: Reduction of Hospital Mortality from Acute Myocardial Infarction by Anticoagulant Therapy, *N. Engl. J. Med.*, 292:1359, 1975.
37. Horwitz, R. I., and Feinstein, A. R.: The Application of Therapeutic-Trial Principles to Improve the Design of Epidemiologic Research: A Case-Control Study Suggesting that Anticoagulants Reduce Mortality in Patients with Myocardial Infarction, *J. Chronic Dis.* 34:575, 1981.
38. Phillips, S. J., Kongtahworn, C., Zeff, R., et al.: Emergency Coronary Artery Revascularization: A Possible Therapy for Acute Myocardial Infarction, *Circulation,* 60:241, 1979.
39. DeWood, M. A., Spores, J., Notske, R., et al.: Prevalence of Total Coronary Occlusion During the Early Hours of Transmural Myocardial Infarction, *N. Engl. J. Med.*, 303:897, 1980.
40. Chalmers, T. C., Matta, R. J., Smith, H., et al.: Evidence Favoring the Use of Anticoagulants in the Hospital Phase of Acute Myocardial Infarction, *N. Engl. J. Med.*, 297:1091, 1977.
41. Unsigned Editorial: Aspirin after Myocardial Infarction, *Lancet,* 1:1172, 1980.
42. Ansinger, R. W., Mikell, F. L., Elsberger, J., and Hodges, M.: Incidence of Left Ventricular Thrombosis after Acute Transmural Myocardial Infarction, *N. Engl. J. Med.*, 305:297, 1981.
43. Reeder, G. S., Lengyel, M., Tajik, A. J., Seward, J. B., Smith, H. C., and Danielson, G. K.: Mural Thrombus in Left Ventricular Aneurysm. *Mayo Clin. Proc.*, 56:77, 1981.
44. Stratton, J. R., Lighty, G. W., Jr., Pearlman, A. S., and Ritchie, J. L.: Detection of Left Ventricular Thrombus by Two Dimensional Echocardiography: Sensitivity, Specificity, and Causes of Uncertainty, *Circulation,* 66:156, 1982.
45. Ezekowitz, M. D., Wilson, D. A., Smith, E. O., et al.: Comparison of Indium 111 Platelet Scintigraphy and Two Dimensional Echocardiography In the Diagnosis of Left Ventricular Thrombi, *N. Engl. J. Med.*, 306:1509, 1982.
46. Tomada, H., Hoshiae, M., Furuya, H., et al.: Evaluation of Left Ventricular Thrombus with Computed Tomography, *Am. J. Cardiol.*, 48:573, 1981.
47. Ebert, R. V.: Anticoagulants in Acute Myocardial Infarction; Results of a Cooperative Clinical Trial, *JAMA,* 225:724, 1973.
48. Wray, R., Maurer, B., and Shillingford, J.: Prophylactic Anticoagulant Therapy in the Prevention of Calf-Vein Thrombosis after Myocardial Infarction, *N. Engl. J. Med.*, 288:815, 1973.
49. Report of the Working Party on Anticoagulant Therapy in Coronary Thrombosis to the Medical Research Council, *Br. Med. J.*, 1:335, 1969.
50. Hilden, T., Iverson, K., Raaschon, F., et al.: Anticoagulation in Acute Myocardial Infarction, *Lancet,* 2:327, 1961.
51. Cabin, H., S., and Roberts, W. C.: Left Ventricular Aneurysm: Intraaneurysmal Thrombus and Systemic Embolus in Coronary Heart Disease, *Chest,* 77:586, 1980.
52. Simpson, M. T., Oberman, A., Kouchoukos, N. T., and Rogers, W. J.: Prevalence of Mural Thrombi and Systemic Embolization with Left Ventricular Aneurysm, *Chest,* 77:463, 1980.
53. Pantely, G. A., Goodnight, S. H., Jr., Rahimtoola, S. H., et al.: Failure of Antiplatelet and Anticoagulant Therapy to Improve Patency of Graft after Coronary Artery Bypass, *N. Engl. J. Med.*, 301:962, 1979.
54. McEnany, M. T., Salzman, E. W., Mundth, E. D., et al.: The Effect of Antithrombotic Therapy on Patency Rates of Saphenous Vein Coronary Artery Bypass Grafts, *J. Thorac. Cardiovasc. Surg.*, 83:81, 1982.
55. Chesebro, J. H., and Fuster, V.: Drug Trials in Prevention of Occlusion of Aorta-Coronary Artery Vein Grafts, *J. Thorac. Cardiovasc. Surg.*, 83:90, 1982.
56. Coon, W. W., and Willis, P. W., III: Hemorrhagic Complications of Anticoagulant Therapy, *Arch. Intern. Med.*, 133:386, 1974.
57. Hull, R., Hirsch, J., Jay, R., et al.: Different Intensities of Oral Anticoagulant Therapy in the Treatment of Proximal-Vein Thrombosis, *N. Engl, J. Med.*, 307:1676, 1982.
58. Moncada, S., and Vane, J. R.: Arachidonic Acid Metabolites and the Interaction between Platelet and Blood Vessel Walls, *N. Engl. J. Med.*, 300:1142, 1979.
59. FitzGerald, G. A., and Sherry, S.: Pharmacology and Pharmacokinetics of Platelet Active Drugs under Current Clinical Investigation, in J. Oates (ed.), "Prostaglandins and the Cardiovascular System (vol. 10, Advances in Prostaglandin, Thromboxane and Leukotriene Research)", Raven Press, New York, 1982, p. 107.
60. Gresele, P., Arnout, J., Janssens, W., et al.: BM 13.177, a Selective Blocker of Platelet and Vessel Wall Thromboxane Receptors, is Active in Man, *Lancet,* 1:991, 1984.
61. Higgs, E. A., Moncado, S., and Vane, J. R.: The Biological Importance and Therapeutic Potential of Prostacyclin, in H. L. Conn, E. De Felice, and P. T. Kuo (eds.), "Prostaglandins, Platelets, Lipids: New Developments in Atherosclerosis," Elsevier/North Holland, 1981, p. 1.
62. Folts, J. D., Crowell, E. B., and Rowe, G. G.: Platelet Aggregation in Partially Obstructed Vessels and its Elimination with Aspirin, *Circulation,* 54:365, 1976.
63. Folts, J. D., and Beck, R. A.: Inhibition of Platelet Plugging in Stenosed Dog Coronary Arteries with Sulfinpyrazone, in M. McGregor, J. F. Mustard, M. F. Oliver, and S. Sherry (eds.), "Cardiovascular Actions of Sulfinpyrazone: Basic and Clinical Research," Symposia Specialists, Miami, Florida, 1980, p. 211.
64. Jorgensen, L., Rowsell, H. C., Hovig, T., Glynn, M. F., and Mustard, J. F.: Adenosine Diphosphate-Induced Platelet Aggregation and Myocardial Infarction in Swine, *Lab. Invest.*, 17:617, 1967.
65. Haerem, J. W.: Platelet Aggregates in Intramyocardial Vessels of Patients Dying Suddenly and Unexpectedly of Coronary Artery Disease, *Atherosclerosis,* 19:529, 1974.
66. Ross, R. J., and Glomset, A.: The Pathogenesis of Atherosclerosis, *N. Engl. J. Med.*, 295:369, 420, 1976.
67. Sherry, S.: Effects of Prostaglandin Mediated Platelet Sup-

pressant Drugs on Acute Cardiovascular Catastrophies, in J. A. Oates, (ed.), "Prostaglandins and the Cardiovascular System (vol. 10, Advances in Prostaglandin, Thromboxane and Leucotriene Research)," Raven Press, New York, 1982, p. 173.
68. Weily, H. S., and Genton, E.: Altered Platelet Function in Patients with Prosthetic Mitral Valves, *Circulation*, 42:967, 1970.
69. Weily, H. S., Steele, P. P., Davies, H., Pappas, G., and Genton, E.: Platelet Survival in Patients with Substitute Heart Valves, *N. Engl. J. Med.*, 290:534, 1974.
70. Harker, L. A., and Slichter, S. J.: Studies of Platelet and Fibrinogen Kinetics in Patients with Prosthetic Heart Valves, *N. Engl. J. Med.*, 283:1302, 1970.
71. Sullivan, J. M., Harken, D. E., and Gorlin, R.: Pharmacologic Control of Thromboembolic Complications of Cardiac Valve Replacement, *N. Engl. J. Med.*, 284:1391, 1971.
72. Steele, P., Rainwater, J., and Vogel, R.: Platelet Suppressant Therapy in Patients with Prosthetic Cardiac Valves, *Circulation*, 60:910, 1979.
73. Chesebro, J. H., Fuster, V., Elveback, L. R., et al.: Trial of Combined Warfarin Plus Dipyridamole or Aspirin Therapy in Prosthetic Heart Valve Replacement: Danger of Aspirin Compared with Dipyridamole, *Am. J. Cardiol.*, 51:1537, 1983.
74. Baur, H. R., Van Tassel, R. A., Pierach, C. A., and Gobel, F. L.: Effects of Sulfinpyrazone on Early Graft Closure after Myocardial Revascularization, *Am. J. Cardiol.*, 49:420, 1982.
75. Sharma, G. V. R. K., Khuri, S. F., Josa, M., Folland, E. D., and Parisi, A. F.: The Effect of Antiplatelet Therapy on Saphenous Vein Coronary Artery Bypass Patency, *Circulation*, (part II)68:II–218, 1983.
76. Chesebro, J. H., Fuster, V., Elveback, L. R., Clements, I. P., et al.: Effect of Dipyramidole and Aspirin in Late Vein Graft Patency after Coronary Bypass Operations, *N. Engl. J. Med.*, 310:209, 1984.
77. Smitherman, T. C., Milam, M., Wod, J., Willerson, J. T., and Frenkel, E. P.: Elevated Beta Thromboglobulin in Peripheral Venous Blood of Patients with Acute Myocardial Ischemia: Direct Evidence for Enhanced Platelet Reactivity in Vivo, *Am. J. Cardiol.*, 48:395, 1981.
78. Hirsch, P. D., Hillis, L. D., Campbell, W. B., Firth, B. G., and Willerson, J. T.: Release of Prostaglandins and Thromboxane into the Circulations in Patients with Ischemic Heart Disease, *N. Engl. J. Med.*, 304:685, 1981.
78a. Lewis, H. D., Jr., Davis, J. W., Archibald, D. G., et al.: Protective Effects of Aspirin Against Acute Myocardial Infarction and Death in Men with Unstable Angina, *N. Engl. J. Med.*, 309:396, 1983.
79. Elwood, P. C., Cochrane, A. L., Burr, M. L., et al.: A Randomized Controlled Trial of Acetylsalicylic Acid in the Secondary Prevention of Mortality from Myocardial Infarction, *Br. Med. J.*, 1:436, 1974.
80. The Coronary Drug Project Research Group: Aspirin in Coronary Heart Disease, *J. Chronic Dis.*, 29:625, 1976.
81. Breddin, K., Loew, D., Lechner, K., Uberla, K., and Walter, E.: Secondary Prevention of Myocardial Infarction: Comparison of Acetylsalicylic Acid, Phenprocoumon and Placebo, *Thromb. Haemost.*, 40:225, 1979.
82. Elwood, P. C., and Sweetnam, P. M.: Aspirin and Secondary Mortality After Myocardial Infarction, *Lancet*, 2:1313, 1979.
83. Aspirin Myocardial Infarction Study Research Group: A Randomized Controlled Trial of Aspirin in Persons Recovered from Myocardial Infarction, *JAMA*, 243:661, 1980.
84. The Persantine-Aspirin Reinfarction Study Research Group: Persantine and Aspirin in Coronary Heart Disease, *Circulation*, 62:449, 1980.
85. The Anturane Reinfarction Trial Research Group: Sulfinpyrazone in the Prevention of Sudden Death after Myocardial Infarction, *N. Engl. J. Med.*, 302:250, 1980.
86. Anturane Reinfarction Italian Study Group: Sulfinpyrazone in Post-myocardial Infarction, *Lancet*, 1:237, 1982.
87. The Persantine-Aspirin Reinfarction Study II: (personal communication).
88. Alkjaersig, N., Fletcher, A. P., and Sherry, S.: The Mechanism of Clot Dissolution by Plasmin, *J. Clin. Invest.*, 38:1086, 1958.
89. Fletcher, A. P., Alkjaersig, N., and Sherry, S.: The Maintenance of a Sustained Thrombolytic State in Man: I. Induction and Effects, *J. Clin. Invest.*, 38:1096, 1959.
90. Marder, V. J., and Budzynski, Z. A.: Fibrinogen and its Derivatives. Hereditary and Acquired Abnormalities, *Schweiz. Med. Wochenschr.*, 104:1338, 1974.
91. Urokinase-Streptokinase Pulmonary Embolism Trial Study Group: Urokinase-Streptokinase Pulmonary Embolism Trial. Phase II Results. A National Cooperative Study, *JAMA*, 229:1606, 1974.
92. Arnesen, H., Heilo, A., Jakobsen, E., et al.: A Prospective Study of Streptokinase and Heparin in the Treatment of Venous Thrombosis, *Acta Med. Scand.*, 203:457, 1978.
93. Marder, V. J., Soulen, R. L., and Atichartakarn, V.: Quantitative Venographic Assessment of Deep Vein Thrombosis in the Evaluation of Streptokinase and Heparin Therapy, *J. Lab. Clin. Med.*, 89:1018, 1977.
94. Elliot, M. S., Immelman, E. J., Jeffery, P., et al.: A Comparative Randomized Trial of Heparin Versus Streptokinase in the Treatment of Acute Proximal Venous Thrombosis: An Interim Report of a Prospective Trial, *Br. J. Surg.*, 66:838, 1979.
95. Arnesen, H., and Hoiseth, A.: Streptokinase or Heparin in the Treatment of Deep Vein Thrombosis. Follow-up Results of a Prospective Study, in G. Trubestein, and F. Etzel (eds.), "Fibrinolytic Therapy," F. K. Schattauer Verlag, Stuttgart-New York, 1983, p. 283.
96. Sherry, S.: Why Thrombolytic Therapy, *Western J. Med.*, 134:149, 1981.
97. Robertson, B. R.: On Thrombosis, Thrombolysis and Fibrinolysis, *Acta Chir. Scand.* [*Suppl.*], 421:5, 1971.
98. Urokinase Pulmonary Embolism Trial Study Group: The Urokinase Pulmonary Embolism Trial. A National Cooperative Study. *Circulation*, 47(suppl. II):II–1, 1973.
99. de Soyza, N. D. B., and Murphy, M. L.: Persistent Post Embolic Pulmonary Hypertension, *Chest*, 62:665, 1972.
100. Riedel, M., Stanek, V., Widimsky, J., and Prervosky, I.: Longterm Follow-up of Patients with Pulmonary Thromboembolism, *Chest*, 81:151, 1982.
101. Frieman, D. G.: Venous Thromboembolic Disease in Medical and Malignant States, in S. Sherry, K. M. Brinkhous, E. Genton, and J. M. Stengle (eds.), "Thrombosis," National Academy of Sciences, Washington, D. C., 1969, p. 5.
102. Sharma, G. V. R. K., Burleson, V. A., and Sasahara, A. A.: Effect of Thrombolytic Therapy on Pulmonary Capillary Blood Volume in Patients with Pulmonary Embolism, *N. Engl. J. Med.*, 303:842, 1980.
103. Miller, G. A. H., Hall, R. C. J., and Paneth, M.: Pulmonary Embolectomy, Heparin and Streptokinase; Their Place in the Treatment of Acute Massive Pulmonary Embolism, *Am. Heart J.*, 93:568, 1977.
104. Ly, B., Arnesen, H., Eie, H., et al.: A Controlled Trial of Streptokinase and Heparin in the Treatment of Major Pulmonary Embolism, *Acta Med. Scand.*, 203:405, 1978.
105. Sherry, S., Bell, W. R., Duckert, F. H., et al.: Thrombolytic Therapy in Thrombosis: A National Institutes of Health Consensus Development Conference, *Ann. Intern. Med.*, 93:141, 1980; also *Br. Med. J.*, 1:1585, 1980.
106. Katzen, B. T., and Van Breda, A.: Low Dose Streptokinase in the Treatment of Arterial Occlusions, *AJR* 136:1171, 1981.
107. Chaise, L., Comerota, A., Soulen, R. K., and Rubin, R. N.: Selective Intraarterial Streptokinase Therapy in the Immediate Postoperative Period, *JAMA*, 247:2397, 1982.
108. Spann, J. F., and Sherry, S.: Coronary Thrombolysis for Evolving Myocardial Infarction, *Drugs* 28:465, 1984.
109. Tennant, S. N., Dixon, J., Venable, T. C., et al.: Intracoronary Thrombolysis in Patients with Acute Myocardial Infarction: Comparison of the Efficacy of Urokinase with Streptokinase, *Circulation*, 69:756, 1984.
110. Markis, J. E., Malagold, M., Parker, A., et al.: Myocardial Salvage after Intracoronary Thrombolysis with Streptoki-

nase in Acute Myocardial Infarction, *N. Engl. J. Med.*, 305:777, 1982.

111. DeFeyter, P. J., van Eenign, M. J., van der Wall, E. E., et al.: Effects of Spontaneous and Streptokinase-induced Recanalization on Left Ventricular Function after Myocardial Infarction, *Circulation,* 67:1039, 1983.
112. Ong, L., Reiser, P., Coromilas, J., Scherr, L., and Morrison, J.: Left Ventricular Function and Rapid Release of Creatine Kinase MB in Acute Myocardial Infarction. Evidence for Spontaneous Reperfusion, *N. Engl. J. Med.*, 309:1, 1983.
113. Lawson, J., Bottino, J. C., Hurtubsie, M. R., and McCredie, K. B.: The Use of Urokinase to Restore the Patency of Occluded Central Venous Catheters, *Am. J. IV Ther. Clin. Nutr.*, 9:29, 1982.
114. Data on file. Hoechst-Roussel Pharmaceuticals, Somerville, N.J., 08876.
115. Weimer, W., Stibbe, J., Van Seyen, A. J., et al.: Specific Lysis of an Iliofemoral Thrombus by Administration of Extrinsic (Tissue Type) Plasminogen Activator, *Lancet,* 2:1018, 1980.
116. Sobel, B. E., Geltman, E. M., Tiefenbrunn, A. J., et al.: Improvement of Regional Myocardial Metabolism after Coronary Thrombolysis Induced with Tissue-type Plasminogen Activator of Streptokinase, *Circulation,* 69:983, 1984.
117. Van de Werf, F., Ludbrook, P. A., Bergmann, S. R., et al.: Coronary Thrombolysis with Tissue-Type Plasminogen Activator in Patients with Evolving Myocardial Infarction, *N. Engl. J. Med.,* 310:609, 1984.
118. Dupe, R. J., English, P. D., Smith, R. A. G., and Green, J.: Acyl-Enzymes as Thrombolytic Agents in Dog Models of Venous Thrombosis and Pulmonary Embolism. *Thromb. Haemost.*, 51:248, 1984.
119. Walker, I. D., Davidson, J. F., Rae, A. P., Hutton, I., and Laurie, T. D. V.: Acylated Streptokinase-Plasminogen Complex in Patients with Acute Myocardial Infarction, *Thromb. Haemost.*, 51:204, 1984.
120. Francis, C. W., Marder, V. J., Evarts, C. M., and Yaukoolbodi, S.: Two Step Warfarin Therapy. Prevention of Post-Operative Venous Thrombosis without Excessive Bleeding, *JAMA,* 249:374, 1983.

Sections B through H

Techniques of Special Procedures

The introduction to Part II emphasizes that the cardiovascular problems of most patients can be diagnosed by obtaining the history, performing the physical examination, and studying the chest roentgenogram and electrocardiogram. When these methods of examination do not permit the physician to diagnose the patient's problem, the physician should pause and ask whether or not the problem should be further clarified. If the answer is yes, the physician must state his or her questions clearly. Not to do so prohibits the proper selection of the best procedure which must be chosen from an array of diagnostic techniques. The questions themselves will usually fall into one or more of the following categories.

- Is there an abnormality of cardiovascular structure and blood flow?
- Is there an abnormality of cardiac function and myocardial contractility?
- Is there an abnormality of cardiac rhythm or cardiac conduction (electrical abnormality)?
- Is there a metabolic abnormality such as myocardial ischemia?

The strategy of work up (including the use of various diagnostic procedures), which permits the physician to answer the questions, is discussed in Part III.

In Sections B through H of Part VII, these specialized diagnostic techniques are described in terms of the principles that govern their use, the measurements obtained, and the equipment utilized. The results of the tests serve as illustrations for disease states and disorders which are discussed in Parts IV, V, and VI. We deferred discussion of the details of the techniques of specialized diagnostic tests until Section B or Part VII in an effort to emphasize our contention that a perceptive physician should have the questions in mind that he or she hopes to answer before obtaining laboratory tests which may be expensive, painful, or give misleading results. When the questions are clearly in mind, it is wise to select the diagnostic test that will yield a result with an acceptable predictive value.

The therapeutic management of a patient may require the use of a technique that has been mastered by only a few physicians. This is not the place to describe the details of the performance of the procedures. Accordingly, we highlight the techniques in Part VII (Sections B through H) in such a way that the principles of the procedure can be easily understood. For example, all physicians should know the type of information cardiac catheterization can yield, and medical cardiologists should know what the cardiac surgeon does when he or she operates on the heart.

Section B

Techniques of Vectorcardiography, Specialized Electrocardiography, Electrophysiology, and Electrical Treatment of Arrhythmias

96

Technique of Vectorcardiography

A. Calhoun Witham, M.D.

Be Not the First by Whom the New are Tried Nor yet the Last to Lay the Old Aside.

Alexander Pope[1]

Vector analysis of cardiac electrical forces was first employed by Einthoven.[2] Later, Mann and others manually constructed single planar images, or "monocardiograms," from the QRS complex of simultaneously recorded limb leads. The first vectorcardiograms (VCG), which performed this task electronically, followed the invention of the cathode ray oscilloscope, and were published in 1931.[3]

What Is the Vectorcardiogram?

The VCG loop is a derivative of two simultaneously recorded scalar ECGs. It is formed by a beam of electrons focused on an oscilloscope and deflected simultaneously along two perpendicular axes by two pairs of charged plates set at 90° to each other. The plates are charged by the rise and fall of voltage during one cardiac cycle, sensed by two scalar ECGs, whose lead axes are designed also to be at right angles to each other across the thorax. Thus, the two lead axes are rectilinear coordinates defining a plane and the QRS loop represents a continuous XY analogue plot of voltages projecting on that plane during one cycle. The mean direction of depolarization fronts at each instant is also obvious in the loop display. The VCG is ordinarily recorded successively in three planes of the body using combinations of three scalar leads (Fig. 96-1). The orientations of these lead axes approximate those of the familiar ECG leads I (horizontal or X), aV_F (vertical or Y), and V_2 (sagittal or Z). The frontal plane requires the XY combination, the horizontal or transverse plane utilizes X and Z, and the sagittal is formed by Z and Y (Fig. 96-1). Timing is achieved by modulating the intensity of the beam with a sawtooth wave form oscillating at a fixed frequency so that the loop is interrupted at known intervals (usually 2.5 or 4 ms).

The most popular of the many complex electrical networks designed to produce X, Y, and Z leads is that offered by Frank.[4] It consists of a belt, carrying five strategically placed electrodes, which are wrapped around the chest. Their outputs, individually weighted, are averaged to produce X and Z leads. Y is determined principally by a bipolar system of electrodes on the neck and leg. Their output also influences X and Z slightly.

Although the dipole theory upon which vectorcardiography is based is an oversimplification, it is doubtful that the diagnostic content of the 12-lead ECG exceeds that of X, Y, and Z leads. It is ironic, therefore, that interest in VCG has waned, for reasons noted below, while newer technology would

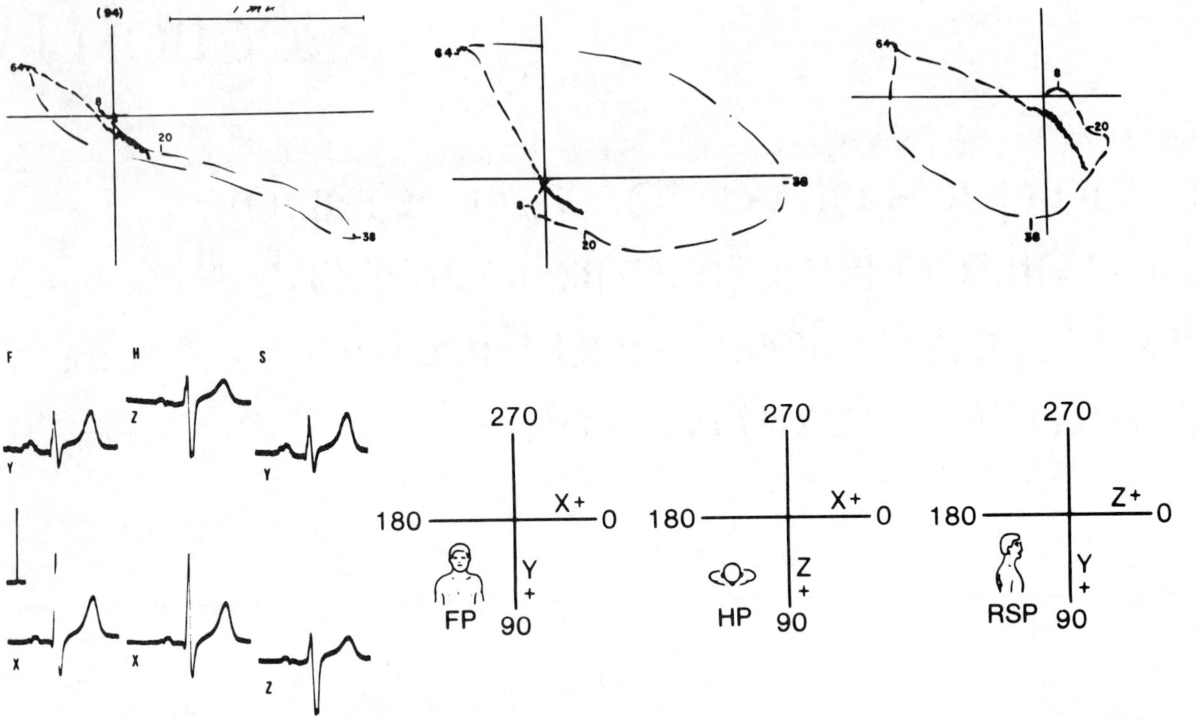

FIGURE 96-1 Scalar tracings of X, Y, and Z leads, as well as loops, obtained from a normal young male subject are displayed in the appropriate pairs for frontal, horizontal, and right sagittal projections. The ECG exhibited the S_1, S_2, S_3 variant. The diagram at lower right shows the arbitrarily designated polarities and the lead axes in each plane. Only the positive poles are marked.

The loops are interrupted every 4 ms and the sharp ends of the dashes indicate direction of transcription. The numbers refer, in milliseconds, to total QRS duration (94) and the timing of the major turning points, labeled Q (8), R (38), and S (64) vectors.

The normal features of timing, direction, and sequence of transcription, or "rotation," seen in these loops are described in the text. Their anatomic origins are also discussed. (*From A. C. Witham, "A System of Vectorcardiographic Interpretation," Year Book Medical Publishers, Inc., Chicago, copyright © 1975. Modified and reproduced with permission from the publisher and author.*)

permit combining the virtues of scalar and vector electrocardiography in one record—a strip of directly recorded X, Y, and Z leads for intervals and arrhythmias followed by loop displays for detailed QRS analysis.

Current Position of Vectorcardiography

The enthusiasm for VCG has declined because newer modalities have eroded its value. Enlargement of the cardiac chambers can be demonstrated directly by anatomical images created by echocardiography, radionuclear scintigraphy, and other techniques. Healed myocardial infarction can be confirmed by perfusion defects and wall motion abnormalities exposed by these methods, and the "gold standard," coronary arteriography, is used more freely. The VCG's contributions were always limited; for example, it rarely embellished the diagnosis of ordinary intraventricular conduction defects or acute myocardial infarction. Its relative demise has been hastened further because VCG recorders are no longer so easily obtained. They are expensive "orphan" devices and currently available only on special order or assembled locally. The electrocardiogram, of course, also suffers by comparison with imaging but its convenience, cheapness, and familiarity have kept it competitive.

Although the role of the VCG has diminished, it is not yet extinguished. Most who teach electrocardiography still believe "the vector approach" and loop displays are important to learning their subject as is attested by their continued inclusion in in-depth treatments of the ECG. The high price of angiography and cardiac imaging, several hundred dollars more than that of the VCG, must also be considered. The VCG can be a cost-effective alternative, an extender of the ECG interpretation, in certain circumstances. These include nondiagnostic hints of prior myocardial infarction, nonstereotyped intraventricular blocks, left anterior fascicular block which may mimic or mask myocardial infarction, and slurred initial QRS complexes which raise the suspicion of preexcitation.

Description of the Normal Adult QRS Loop

The *spatial* QRS loop normally exhibits three major turning points, labeled Q, R, and S vectors, in order of appearance. Their average characteristics follow and can be appreciated in the three planar displays in Fig. 96-1, but most easily in the horizontal projection. Q appears at about 10 ms, averages 0.1 mV, and aims anteriorly and to the right. R, the most leftward point, is in midloop at approximately

40 ms, averages 1.6 mV, and is slightly anterior or posterior. The terminal vector S appears at 60 ms, averages 0.4 mV, and is posterior, slightly to right or left. The sequence of transcription is consistently counterclockwise in the horizontal plane, clockwise in the right sagittal plane, but variable in the frontal plane. Q reflects left-to-right septal depolarization but is modified by two opposing forces; depolarization of the septum from right to left and of the endocardial shell of the left ventricle. R is principally left ventricular in origin but is foreshortened and its position altered by oppositely directed right ventricular forces and continued migration of the septal wave front posterobasally. The late vector, S, arises in this area of the septum but is also affected by small, variable contributions from paraseptal myocardium of the two ventricles.

Every abnormal QRS pattern, ECG or VCG, is a consequence of changes in timing, voltage, or direction of these three vectors or by rearrangement of their relationship to each other. If the triple anatomical origin of each are considered, a sound explanation of the abnormal pattern is usually possible. For example, left ventricular hypertrophy causes vector R to increase in size, and point more toward this chamber (posteriorly). The stronger contributions of the left ventricle to Q and S move these vectors to the left also. In contrast, increased right ventricular mass pulls S to the right and anterior, where this chamber lies, while canceling some of the voltage of R. The rationality of this type of explanation explains its appeal to teachers. Many expert electrocardiographers analyze difficult tracings by dissecting out the initial, mid-, and terminal vectors from the ECG and, in effect, constructing a crude VCG.

Quantitative, detailed criteria for VCG diagnosis as well as the uses of P and T loops are described in the fifth edition of this book and in the general references cited.[5,6]

Healed Myocardial Infarction

Since the commonest use of the VCG now is in resolving the question of prior myocardial infarction, this will be covered briefly for the two most common areas.

The general principle is that a localized mass of electrically inert tissue causes a shift of vectors away from this area, as the electrical field becomes dominated by normal muscle on the opposite side of the heart. With inferior and anterior infarction that involves the initial forces (Q vector) or those immediately following Q because the septal or paraseptal myocardium is almost always involved. With inferior infarction, two distinctive patterns, whose specificity exceeds 90 percent in the absence of ventricular hypertrophy, are possible.[7] In the first, Q is directed superiorly and the superior forces sweep clockwise above the X-axis (frontal plane) for at least 26 ms. The VCG is more sensitive than the ECG in this pattern because it offers more precise timing and direction of the initial and early forces recorded as Q waves in the inferior ECG leads, and adds the characteristic clockwise transcription of this segment. The second pattern exhibits a downward initial force, which, however, shifts abruptly above the X-axis in about 10 ms, and thereafter duplicates the first pattern. This is particularly interesting as no Q waves are possible in the inferior ECG leads because the initial forces are normal—presumably the septum is spared—and it is only the post-Q forces which confirm the pathology (Fig. 96-2). In either type, the diagnosis is not confounded by the presence of left anterior fascicular block as is often true with the ECG.

FIGURE 96-2 The ECG, obtained from a male with stable angina pectoris, exhibits an apparently uncomplicated pattern of left anterior fascicular block. There are normal R waves in the inferior and precordial leads.

The loops are interrupted every 4 ms, and the sharp end of the dash indicates direction of transcription. The numbers indicate, in milliseconds, QRS duration (92) and timing of Q (8), R (40), and S (56–58) vectors. In the frontal plane (*left*), there is a normally directed initial vector (8), aimed inferiorly and to the right, which is consonant with the R waves in II, III, and aV_F. The post-Q forces, however, turn sharply upward and sweep clockwise above the X-axis. This feature is compatible with inferior myocardial infarction but is not apparent in the ECG, presumably because the inferior septum is not involved. The loop in the horizontal plane is normal except for the first 20 ms. Q (8) is abnormally rightward but anterior forces do not develop until 20 ms. This configuration is known as "destruction of the normal Q loop." For comparison, note the normal Q loop in Fig. 96-1. The expected pathology is scarring in the anterior paraseptal area of the left ventricle. The abnormality is not reflected in the ECG. If V_2 and V_3 complexes are derived from this loop, assuming the electrodes are just to the left of the Z-axis, initial negativity instead of positivity would have been expected. The discrepancy is probably explained by the downward direction of the initial forces, as seen in the frontal plane, which are directed toward electrodes below the dipole, as discussed in the text. *(From A. C. Witham, "A System of Vectorcardiographic Intepretation," Year Book Medical Publishers, Inc., Chicago, copyright © 1975. Modified and reproduced with permission from the publisher and author.)*

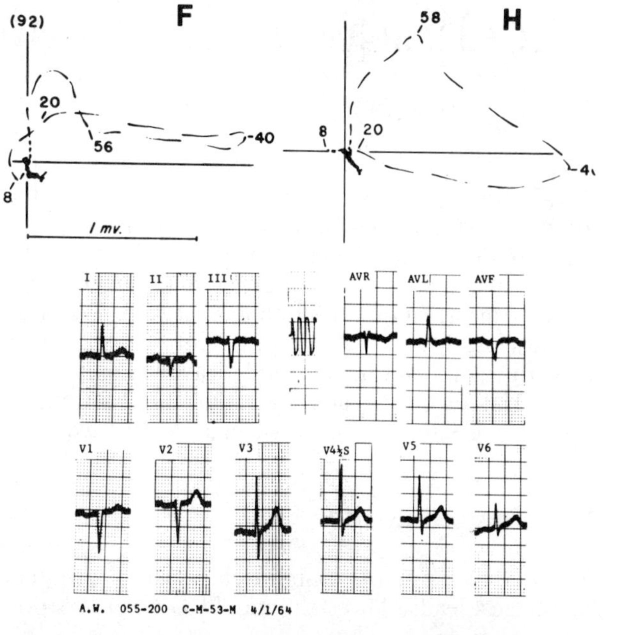

With anterior infarction a variety of patterns can be present but the common denominator is abnormality of Q or post-Q forces.[8] Thus, in the horizontal plane all anterior forces may be absent. The deficit, however, may be confined to disappearance of the normally right-anterior Q vector. Finally a normal Q may be followed by a failure of the expected subsequent anterior evolution but only for 10 to 20 ms. Any of these morphologies may be accompanied by an ECG showing diagnostic precordial Q waves, only the nonspecific "poor R wave progression," or normal R waves. Why do not the scalar precordial leads consistently reflect the loop abnormalities? The fault is in the assumption that the chest leads are always directly in front of the cardiac dipole, i.e., at the same vertical level as this hypothetical origin of the QRS complex. This is not always true. Therefore, the influence of any significant superior or inferior tilt of these vectors on the precordial complex is ignored. This geometric imperfection may cause Q waves when anterior forces are present or R waves when there are none. For example, anterior but sharply superior initial vectors might appear as negative initial deflections if electrode V_2 is well below the dipole, and suggest infarction where none exists (false positive). On the other hand, if the electrode is low, and initial vectors are posterior but sharply downward, this movement will be transcribed as initial positivity (R waves) and infarction will not be suspected (false negative). Other misinformation is possible with "high" electrodes. The precordial artifacts of left anterior fascicular block (Q or R′ in V_{1-2}, loss of normal Q and persistent S in $V_{5,6}$) are of this nature because of shift in position of the dipole and are frequently misinterpreted, but have no counterpart in the VCG.[6,9]

This short resume only scratches the surface of the subject of misleading ECGs in patients thought to have had myocardial infarction, which may be clarified by VCG. It has been extensively reviewed.[9]

References

1. Pope, A.: Quoted from Bartlett, J.: "Familiar Quotations," 12th ed., C. Morley and D. Everett (eds.), Little, Brown and Co., Boston, 1948, p. 211.
2. Einthoven, W.: The Different Forms of the Human ECG and Their Significance, *Lancet*, 1:853, 1912.
3. Mann, H.: Interpretation of Bundle Branch Block by Means of the Monocardiogram, *Am. Heart J.*, 6:447, 1931.
4. Frank, E.: An Accurate, Clinically Practical System for Spatial Vectorcardiography, *Circulation*, 13:737, 1956.
5. Chou, T. D., Helm, R. A., and Kaplan, S.: "Clinical Vectorcardiography," 2d ed., Grune & Stratton, Inc., New York, 1974.
6. Witham, A. C.: "A System of Vectorcardiographic Interpretation," Year Book Medical Publishers, Inc., Chicago, 1975.
7. Starr, J. W., Wagner, G. S., Behar, V. S., Walston, A., and Greenfield, J. C.: Vectorcardiographic Criteria for the Diagnosis of Inferior Myocardial Infarction, *Circulation*, 49:829, 1974.
8. Starr, J. W., Wagner, G. S., Draffin, R. M., Reed, J. B., Walston, A., and Behar, V. S.: Vectorcardiographic Criteria for the Diagnosis of Anterior Myocardial Infarction, *Circulation*, 53:229, 1976.
9. Witham, A. C.: VCG Patterns of Myocardial Scarring in the Absence of Diagnostic Q Waves, in R. C. Schlant, and J. W. Hurst (eds.), "Advances in Electrocardiography," Grune & Stratton, New York, 1976, p. 245-262.

97

Technique of Esophageal Electrocardiography

Ross D. Fletcher, M.D.   Robert C. Saunders, M.D.

P-wave timing and occasionally vector are needed to analyze disturbances of cardiac rhythm. Accordingly, many approaches have been developed to detect atrial activity (Table 97-1).[1–20] Standard electrocardiogram (ECG) and bipolar chest leads often do not disclose P waves and invasive intracardiac atrial recording may not be practical or available. Recording atrial electrical activity from the esophagus, however, is simple, noninvasive, and effective.

Esophageal Leads

Recent developments facilitate clinical application of esophageal leads. Three-channel ECG recorders now in general use permit simultaneous surface and esophageal recording. Filtered preamplifiers and bipolar recording eliminate baseline drift. Recording electrodes are small, easily positioned, and tolerated by the patient.

While other systems are useful, the esophageal pill electrode developed by Arzbaecher is also easily swallowed and well tolerated.[21] This insulated lead system consists of long, filamentous wires connected to a cylinder 3 mm in diameter and 1.9 cm long with a 6-mm electrode on each end (Fig. 97-1, lower panel). A gelatin capsule encloses the electrode and dissolves in the stomach. The pill may be swallowed with liquid or embedded in ice cream, although many patients swallow it without capsule or liquid. The

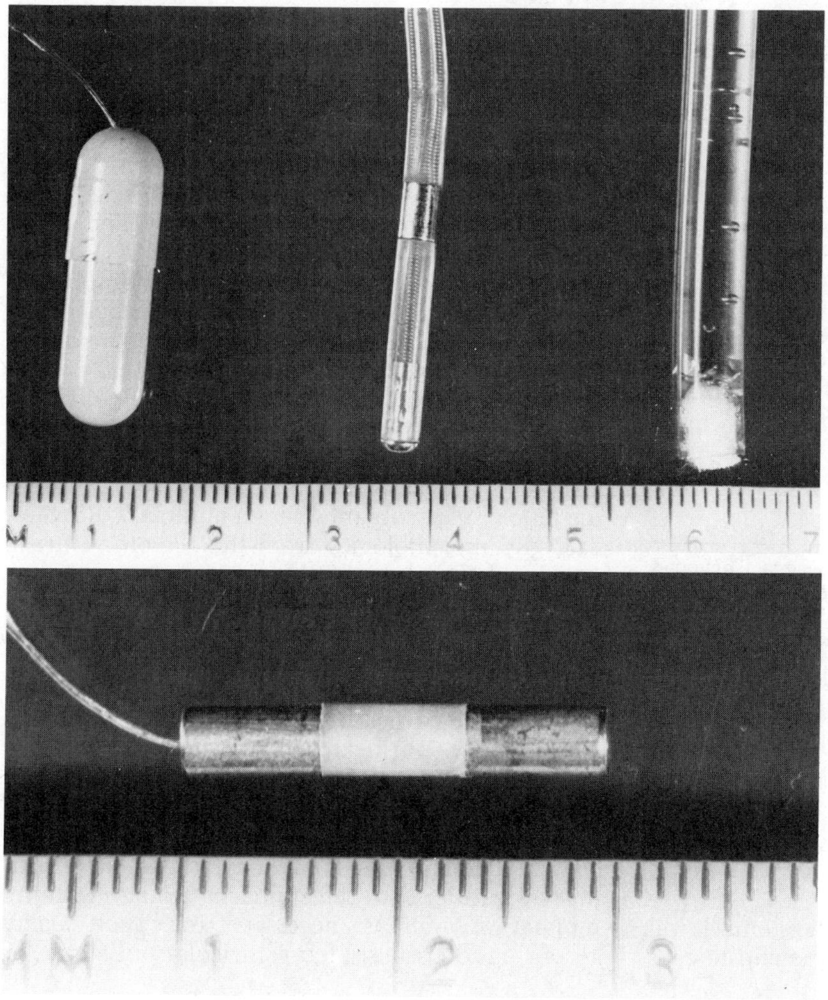

FIGURE 97-1 Upper panel compares the encapsulated pill electrode, an implantable pacemaker lead, and a conductive-gel-filled nasogastric tube with cotton plug. The pill is swallowed. The others are inserted by the nasal route. Lower panel enlarges the pill electrode without its gelatin capsule. (*From R. Fletcher and R. Saunders, Esophageal Electrocardiography—1981, in J. W. Hurst (ed.), "Update V—The Heart," McGraw-Hill, New York, 1981. Reproduced with permission from the publisher and author.*)

TABLE 97-1 Methods for Detecting Atrial Activity

1 Jugular venous pulse tracings
2 Standard electrocardiographic leads (II, V_1, aV_R)
3 Bipolar chest leads
  a Lewis lead
  b Right parasternal bipolar leads
4 Intracavitary atrial electrocardiogram
  a Pacing electrode catheter
  b Saline-filled polyethylene tubing
  c Temporary atrial pacing electrode
  d Quadripolar catheter for pacing and recording
  e Zucker catheter with lumen
  f Balloon-tipped, flow-directed catheter with electrodes 25–30 cm from the catheter tip
5 Esophageal electrode
  a Solid nasogastric tube with multiple electrodes: Nyboer tube
  b Standard nasogastric tube with conductive paste and cotton wick
  c Silastic bipolar pacemaker lead
  d Esophageal "pill" electrode
6 Echocardiography: detection and timing of right and left AV valve with dual echocardiogram

Source: R. Fletcher and R. Saunders, Esophageal Electrocardiography—1981, in J. W. Hurst (ed.), "Update V—The Heart," McGraw-Hill, New York, 1981. Reproduced with permission from the publisher and author.

wires are usually comfortable, but may produce a scratchy sensation relieved with anesthetic gargle. The pill is swallowed to 45 cm, noted by a marker on the wire. The leads are connected to a single or three-channel ECG recorder. Permanent pacemaker leads are also effective and not subject to lead fracture. Simultaneous unipolar and bipolar esophageal recording is achieved with an implantable lead designed for bipolar pacing and endocardial shock.

Recording Systems

While all recording systems described in Table 97-2 are effective, a three-channel recorder in the lead I-II-III position with the Arzco preamplifier consistently provides a useful record. The preamplifier sends a moderately filtered bipolar esophageal signal to channel I, a normal lead II to channel II, and a compound signal (bipolar and esophageal) to channel III (Fig. 97-2). The distal and proximal esophageal leads may be attached directly to the right and left arm leads of an ECG patient cable, producing a bipolar esophageal trace in channel I (no low-frequency filtering) and a compound left leg-

TABLE 97-2 Esophageal Recording Systems

1 Single-channel recorder
  a Unipolar: attach to V lead
  b Bipolar: attach distal to left arm and proximal to right arm: record lead I
2 Standard three-channel ECG recorder
  a Unipolar
    (1) V_2: normal position
    (2) V_2: distal esophageal electrode
    (3) V_3: proximal esophageal electrode
  b Bipolar
    (1) Lead I: bipolar esophageal (attach as single-channel bipolar)
    (2) Lead II: compound leg and proximal electrode
    (3) Lead III: compound leg and distal electrode
3 Standard three-channel ECG recorder with preamplifier
  a Lead I: bipolar esophageal
  b Lead II: standard lead II
  c Lead III: compound esophageal and lead II

Source: R. Fletcher and R. Saunders, Esophageal Electrocardiography—1981, in J. W. Hurst (ed.), "Update V—The Heart," McGraw-Hill, New York, 1981. Reproduced with permission from the publisher and author.

esophageal trace on channels II and III. Proximal and distal unipolar tracings are obtained simultaneously with V leads using a three-channel recorder (Fig. 97-3).

Lead Positions

Careful withdrawal of the pill from the stomach will yield deflections from the left ventricle and low interatrial septum. As the electrode is positioned 35 to 42 cm from incisor teeth, maximal atrial deflection with minimal ventricular contamination is seen on the bipolar trace. In this position, remote ventricular activity is recorded on both unipolar leads. During bipolar recording the similar ventricular deflections cancel when proximal and distal electrodes are assigned positive and negative polarity and added algebraically by the differential ECG amplifier.[17,22,23] Figure 97-4 presents a bipolar esophageal trace with lead II, recorded as the pill was placed at different distances from the incisors. Low in the esophagus the ventricular deflection is larger than the atrial deflection. As the pill passes the atrioventricular (AV) groove to the atrium (37 cm), the atrial deflection is enlarged. The best position for bipolar atrial monitoring in this patient is at 36 cm, where the bipolar electrogram writes a minimal QRS. Similar QRS morphologies from the remote ventricle are canceled and the local atrial deflection is accentuated. While atrial activity recorded from the lowest possible lead position may be the goal in some studies, usually the largest atrial deflection is desired. In one report, the most distal lead position recorded the earliest retrograde atrial electrogram (46 ± 6 cm), but the largest P waves were recorded between 37 ± 6 cm and 41 ± 4 cm from the incisors.[20]

Tracing artifacts can be minimized in several ways.[24] The baseline is often erratic when recordings are made from the stomach. Contact with the esophageal wall is necessary for good-quality recordings. Peristalsis, left ventricular pulsations, or

FIGURE 97-2 Bipolar lead. A standard bedside, three-channel ECG recorder, patient cable harness attached to a preamplifier and esophageal lead. In lead selection position I-II-III, this system inscribes a 5-Hz filtered, double-standard amplified bipolar esophageal electrogram on channel I, a surface lead II on channel II, and a compound lead (distal esophageal electrode to lead II) on channel III.

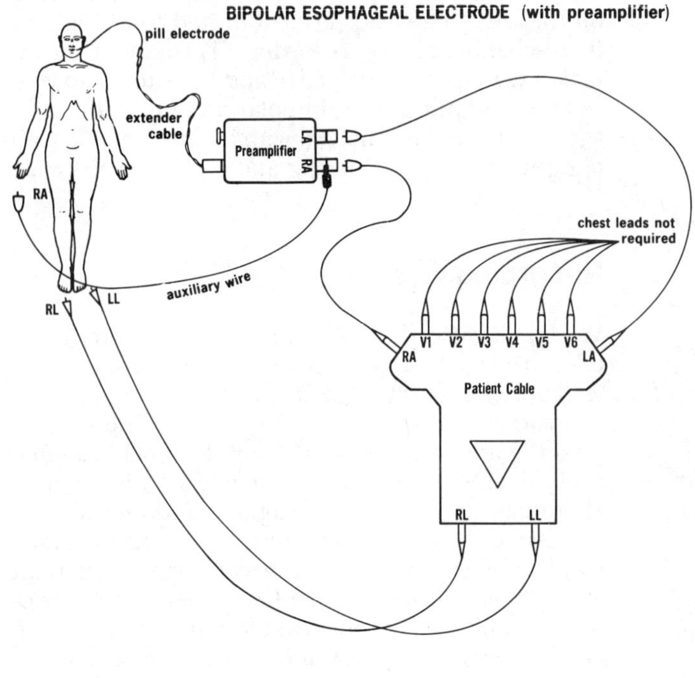

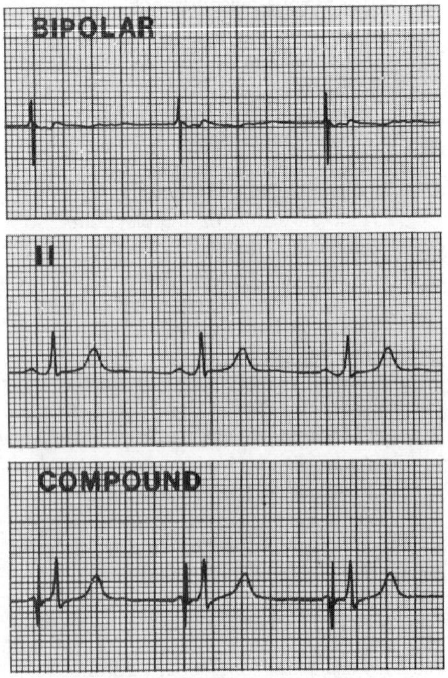

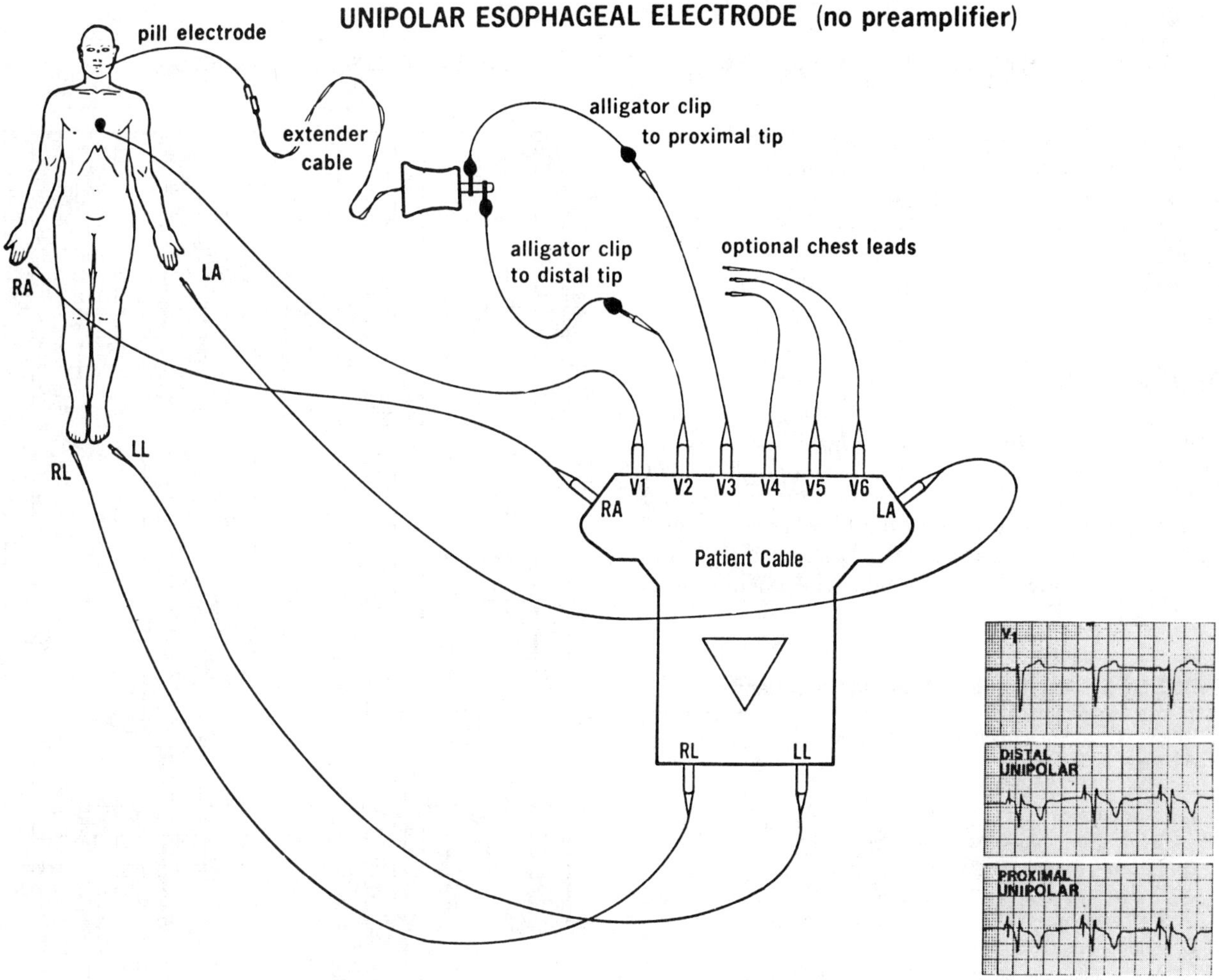

FIGURE 97-3 Unipolar leads. Using the recorder and lead harness shown in Fig. 97-2, the diagram shows necessary attachments to inscribe simultaneous distal and proximal unipolar esophageal leads and lead V_1. Record in lead selection position V_1-V_2-V_3.

FIGURE 97-4 Recording at intervals of 39 to 33 cm from the teeth during withdrawal of the bipolar esophageal electrode (BEE) shows pure left atrial activity (with smallest QRS) to occur at 36 cm in this patient. (*From R. Fletcher and R. Saunders, Esophageal Electrocardiography—1981, in J. W. Hurst (ed.), "Update V—The Heart," McGraw-Hill, New York, 1981. Reproduced with permission from the publisher and author.*)

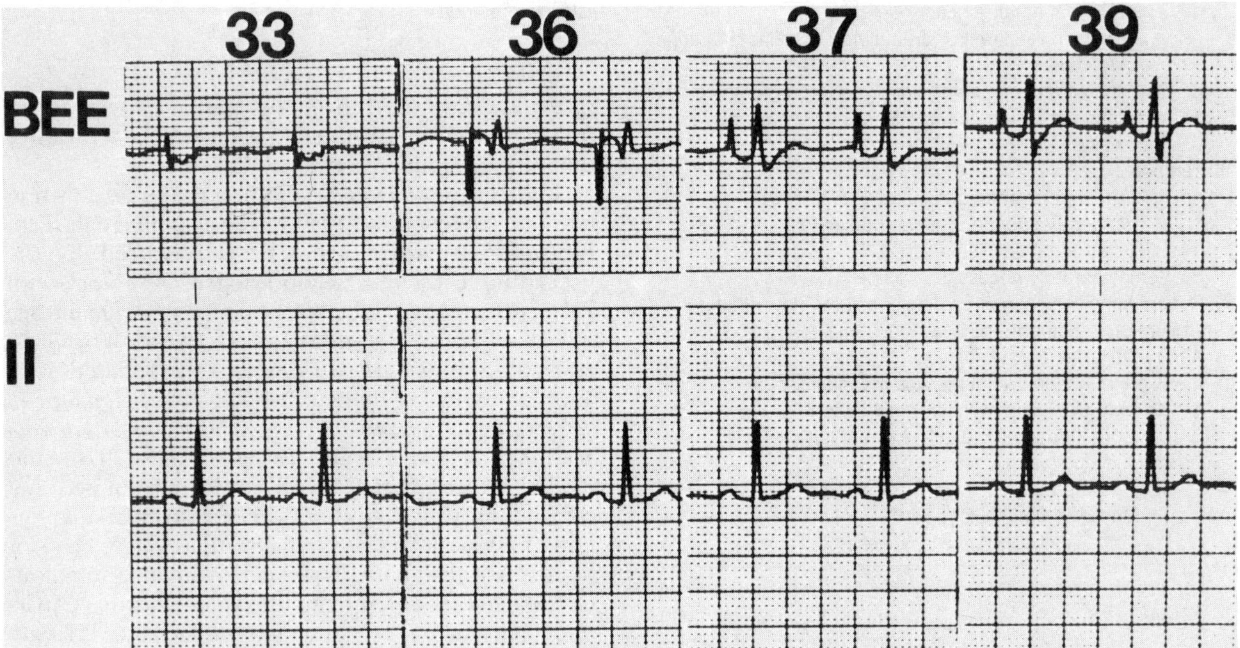

aortic pulsations may cause artifacts which are minimized with mild filtering. Low-frequency filters, commonplace with intracavitary recording,[25,26] were adapted for esophageal recording by Barold[18] and later by Arzbaecher, who incorporated mild (5-Hz) low-frequency filters into a preamplifier.

Applications

Esophageal recordings have many applications (Table 97-3), particularly when P-wave activity cannot be delineated on an external tracing. The presence of *atrial tachycardia* is revealed on a bipolar esophageal electrogram while external lead II showed no rapid atrial activity (Fig. 97-5). Rapid atrial pacing easily restored sinus rhythm in this patient, favoring intraatrial circus movement like atrial flutter rather than an automatic focus.

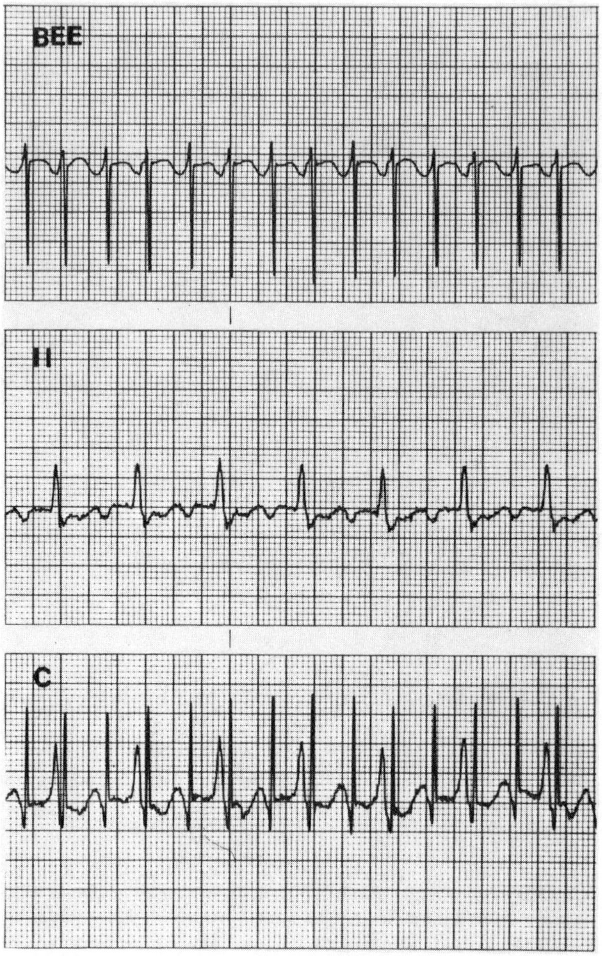

FIGURE 97-5 Simultaneous bipolar esophageal electrogram (BEE), standard lead II, and compound lead. Atrial tachycardia of 200 beats per minute is clearly seen on the bipolar esophageal trace. (*From R. Fletcher and R. Saunders, Esophageal Electrocardiography—1981, in J. W. Hurst (ed.), "Update V—The Heart," McGraw-Hill, New York, 1981. Reproduced with permission from the publisher and author.*)

TABLE 97-3 Application of Esophageal Leads

- I Detect or confirm inapparent atrial activity
  - A Atrial tachycardias
    - 1 Flutter
    - 2 Fibrillation
    - 3 Reentrant atrial AV nodal tachycardia
  - B Pauses: Detect P wave in the pause
    - 1 Blocked premature atrial beat
    - 2 Inapparent AV block with 2:1 conduction
  - C Anomalous QRS beats
    - 1 Atrial activity controlling aberrant ventricular depolarization
    - 2 Ventricular depolarization dissociated from atrial activity
    - 3 Ventricular tachycardia with 1:1 retrograde conduction to atrium: dissociated or blocked with carotid sinus pressure or propranolol
  - D Pauses during atrial pacing
    - 1 Confirms atrial capture but with AV block
    - 2 Confirms lack of atrial capture by pacemaker
      - *a* Normal atrial refractory period
      - *b* Hidden reentrant or premature P making the atrium refractory
  - E Detect atrial activity during noninvasive programmed stimulation of atrium or ventricle using permanent pacemakers
- II Temporary pacing
  - A Atrium: 70 percent successful at 20–30 mA
    - 1 Temporary support of atrial bradycardias
    - 2 Revert atrial tachycardias
  - B Ventricle: rarely necessary: 50 mA
- III Record specific posterior cardiac structures (low atrial septum on left atrium)
  - A Dissimilar atrial rhythms
    - 1 Right and left atrial tachycardia mimicking atrial flutter
    - 2 Right sick sinus with left atrial flutter
  - B Measure intraatrial and left atrium to left ventricle conduction times
  - C Timing of retrograde P wave obscured by QRS
    - 1 Junctional ventricular beats
    - 2 Wolff-Parkinson-White syndrome

Source: R. Fletcher and R. Saunders, Esophageal Electrocardiography—1981, in J. W. Hurst (ed.), "Update V—The Heart," McGraw-Hill, New York, 1981. Reproduced with permission from the publisher and author.

The nature of *pauses* seen on a surface recording may be determined using the esophageal lead. Blocked premature atrial beats obscured by the preceding T wave or second degree AV block with 2:1 conduction may be seen on an esophageal trace but missed with a standard surface lead. The presence or absence of atrial activity associated with anomalous QRSs helps *differentiate beats initiated in the ventricles from beats of supraventricular origin with aberrant conduction to the ventricles* (Figs. 97-6 and 97-7).[27] Antecedent P waves, with prolonged AV conduction times, confirm the supraventricular origin of anomalous QRSs occurring as single beats or bursts. Atrial activity dissociated from an anomalous QRS tachycardia confirms the diagnosis of ventricular tachycardia. Atrial activity associated 1:1 with sustained anomalous QRS tachyarrhythmia is seen

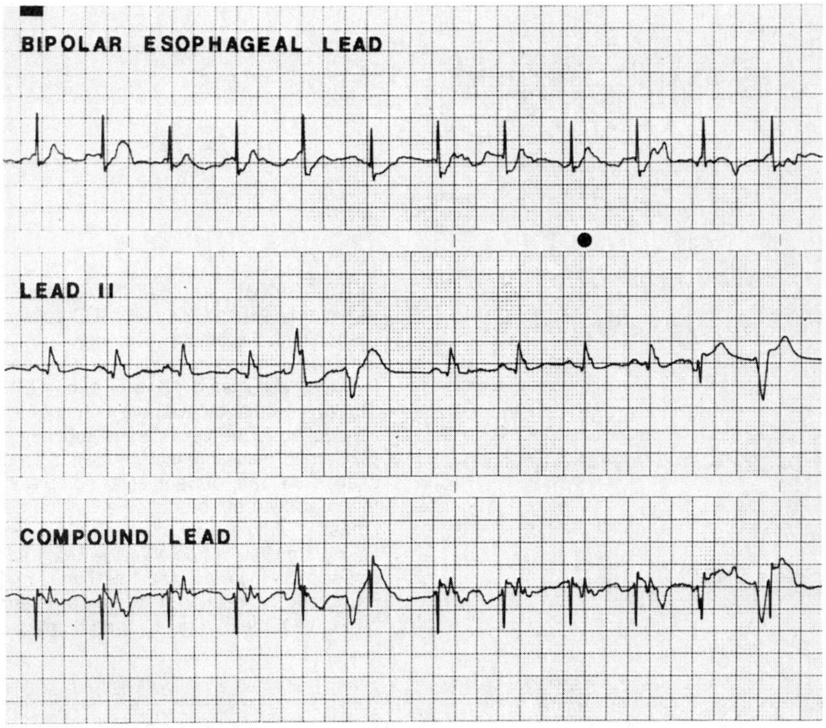

FIGURE 97-6 A multiform, anomalous QRS couplet is seen on lead II. Ventricular origin of these beats is confirmed on the bipolar esophageal trace by the presence of regular, dissociated atrial activity marching through the couplet. (*From R. Fletcher and R. Saunders, Esophageal Electrocardiography—1981, in J. W. Hurst (ed.), "Update V—The Heart," McGraw-Hill, New York, 1981. Reproduced with permission from the publisher and author.*)

with supraventricular rhythms but can also be present during ventricular tachycardia with 1:1 retrograde conduction to the atrium. Vagal maneuvers, IV propranolol, or IV verapamil may increase retrograde block or dissociate the atrium from the ventricle, making more firm the diagnosis of ventricular tachycardia.

Difficulty discerning these rhythms is illustrated by a patient we studied. A tentative diagnosis of supraventricular tachycardia was established because a triphasic rsR′ was seen on lead MCL_1 and the esophageal lead showed P waves associated with every QRS (Fig. 97-8*A*). Carotid sinus pressure, however, eliminated all atrial activity for a short period after which P waves reappeared with 3:1 retrograde conduction and finally 1:1 with the QRS (Fig. 97-8*B*). Atrial activity was altered without any change in the anomalous QRS tachyarrhythmia, confirming a ventricular rhythm independent of the atrium. The 1:1 relation of P wave to QRS was due to retrograde conduction. Although uncommon, this rhythm could be junctional with aberrant conduction. In this patient, ventricular tachycardia was confirmed by intracavitary recording in which no antecedent His bundle deflection was seen before the anomalous QRS (Fig. 97-8*C*, upper panel). Note the change in

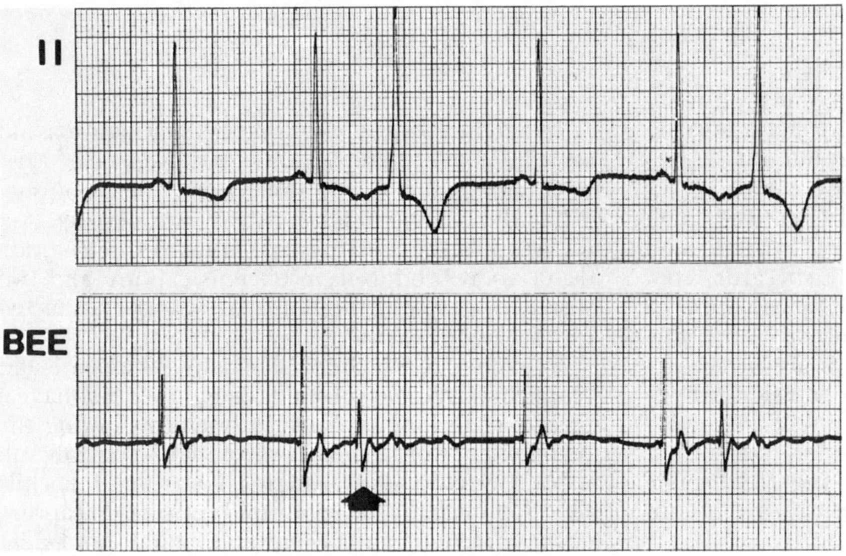

FIGURE 97-7 Suspected from lead II but seen clearly on the bipolar esophageal electrogram (BEE), an antecedent P wave (arrow) identifies the anomalous QRS as aberrant conduction.

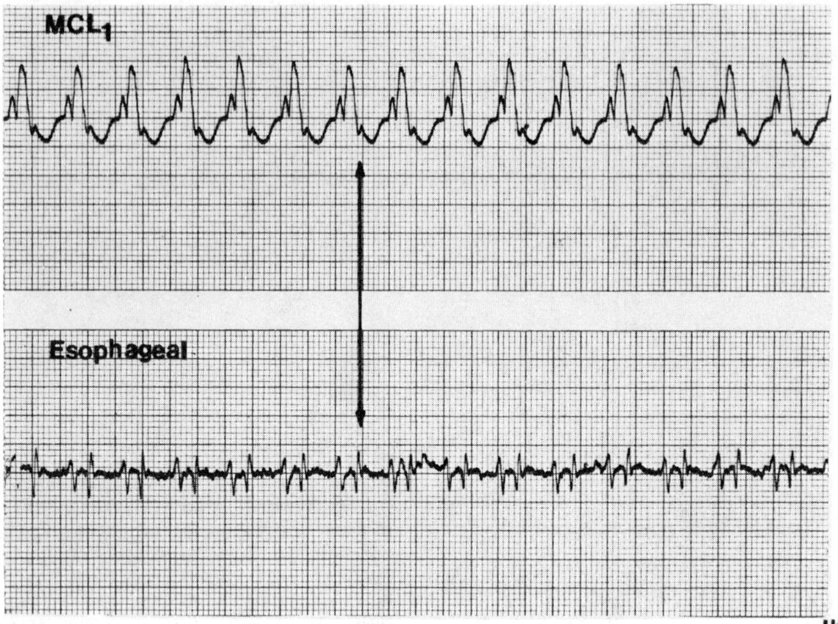

A

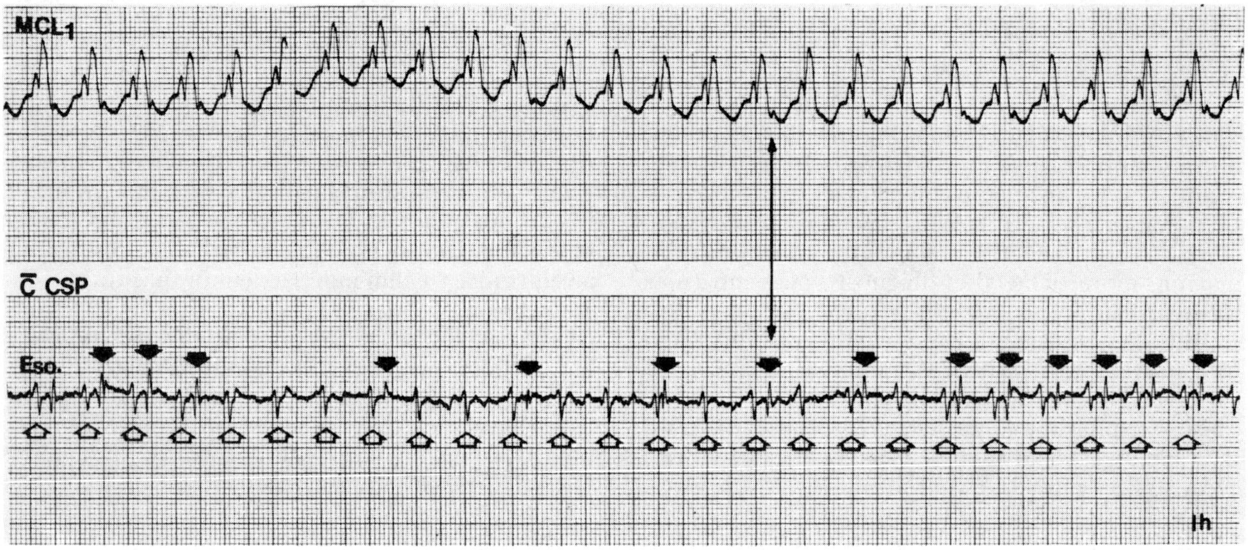

B

FIGURE 97-8 *A*. Lead MCL_1 shows tachycardia with a wide rsR′ QRS pattern. A simultaneous bipolar esophageal trace recorded from the transitional zone shows P waves associated 1:1 with each QRS. Supraventricular tachycardia with aberrant conduction to the ventricles is suggested. *B*. Carotid sinus pressure (CSP) did not change the rate of ventricular complexes (open arrows) but produced a striking decrease in atrial activity (black arrows), confirming complete retrograde (VA) block and dissociation followed by 2:1 and finally 1:1 retrograde conduction. P waves are seen on the MCL_1 lead (double-ended arrow).

sequence of atrial activation from normal antegrade conduction (high right atrium, His bundle electrogram, esophageal lead) to retrograde conduction (His bundle electrogram, bipolar esophageal lead, high right atrium). A simultaneous record of MCL_1 and a true V_1 lead during ventricular tachycardia contrasts the deceptive rsR′ seen on MCL_1 with the QRS in V_1, the latter being more suggestive of the true rhythm (Fig. 97-8*C*, lower panel). It also shows abrupt loss of retrograde capture. The rsR′ and 1:1 P-QRS relation led this patient's physicians to exhaust the armamentarium employed to treat supraventricular tachycardia before 100 mg of lidocaine IV promptly reverted ventricular tachycardia to sinus rhythm.

In another patient with wide QRS tachycardia and association between atrium and ventricle (Fig. 97-9*A*), carotid pressure slowed only the atrial rate. While the change in atrial activity was best seen on the esophageal electrogram, transient retrograde dissociation produced an obvious capture and two fusion beats pathognomonic of ventricular tachycardia (Fig. 97-9*B*).

Situations in which atrial activity disappears and reappears can be clarified using the esophageal recording technique. Surface tracings showing the reappearance of normal P waves may be equally valuable. Certainty of a changing P-wave vector while the rhythm changed from rapid retrograde capture of the atrium to sinus rhythm, although not essen-

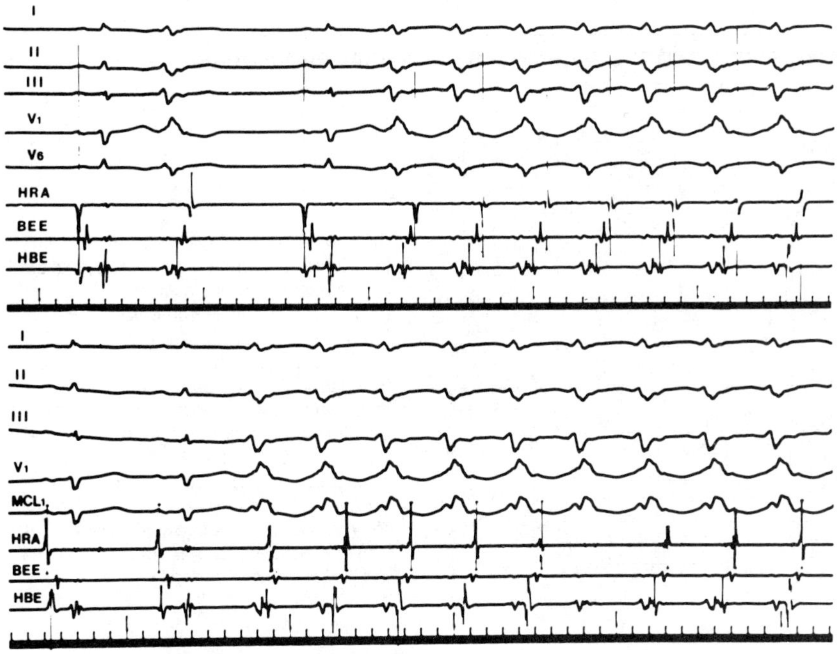

C

FIGURE 97-8 (*Continued*) *C. Upper panel:* Onset of the anomalous QRS tachycardia without antecedent P wave or His bundle deflection identifies ventricular tachycardia. Recorded sequence of depolarization with antegrade conduction is high right atrium (HRA), His bundle electrogram (HBE), and bipolar esophageal electrogram (BEE). The order changes during retrograde conduction to the atrium: HBE, BEE, and then HRA. *Lower panel:* Anomalous QRS patterns recorded simultaneously in V_1 and MCL_1 are contrasted. In MCL_1, the triphasic rsR′ suggests right bundle branch block. In the true V_1, QRS morphology is suggestive of ventricular tachycardia. The sixth QRS in the run displays retrograde block induced by CSP. (*From R. Fletcher and R. Saunders, Esophageal Electrocardiography—1981, in J. W. Hurst (ed.), "Update V—The Heart," McGraw-Hill, New York, 1981. Reproduced with permission from the publisher and author.*)

FIGURE 97-9 *A.* The esophageal lead reveals one P wave for each QRS representing 1:1 antegrade conduction with first degree block or 1:1 retrograde conduction in a patient with ventricular or junctional tachycardia. *B.* Carotid sinus pressure (CSP) produced ventriculoatrial dissociation which allowed one pure capture (C) and two fusion beats (F) to reveal the diagnosis of ventricular tachycardia.

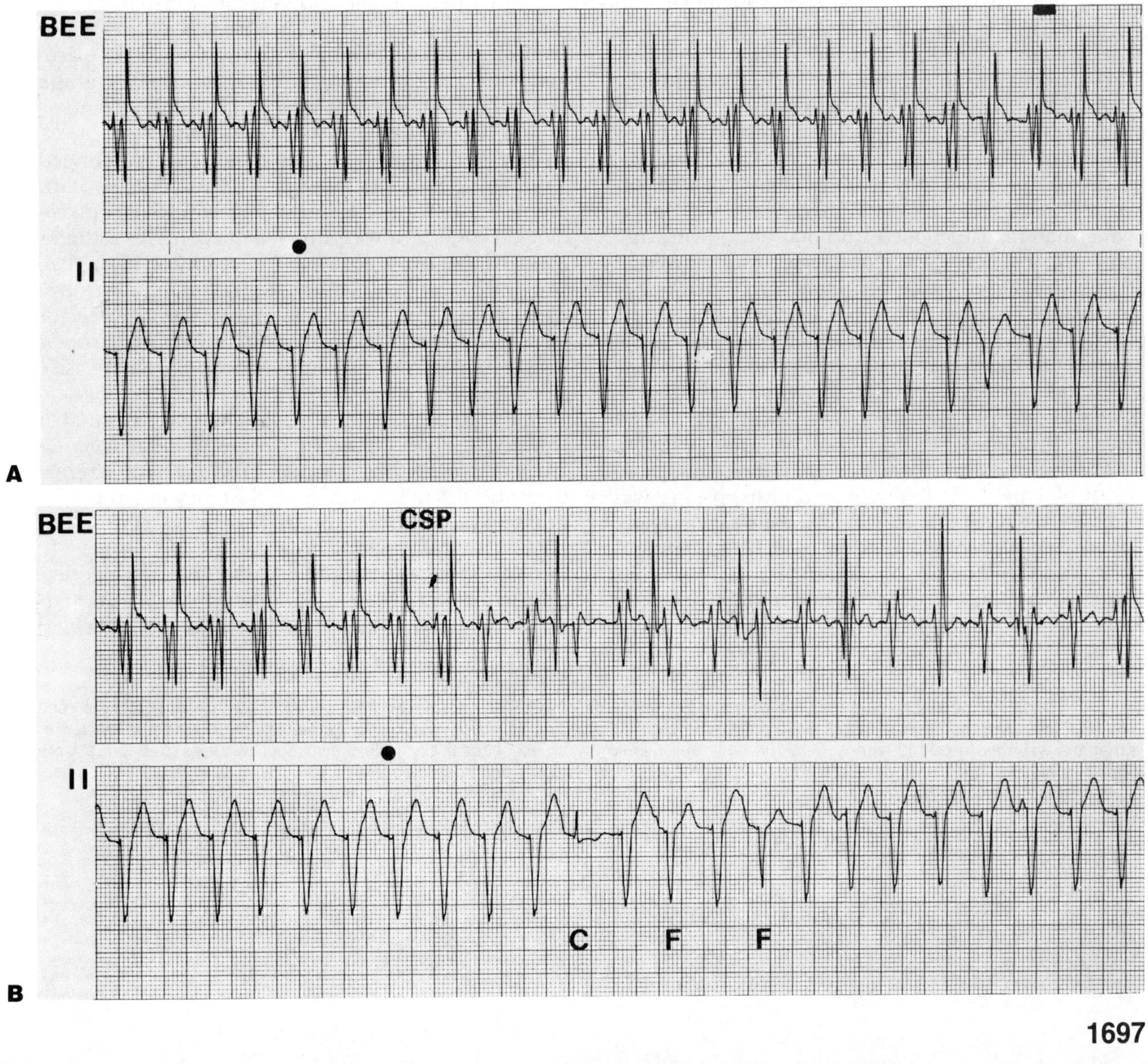

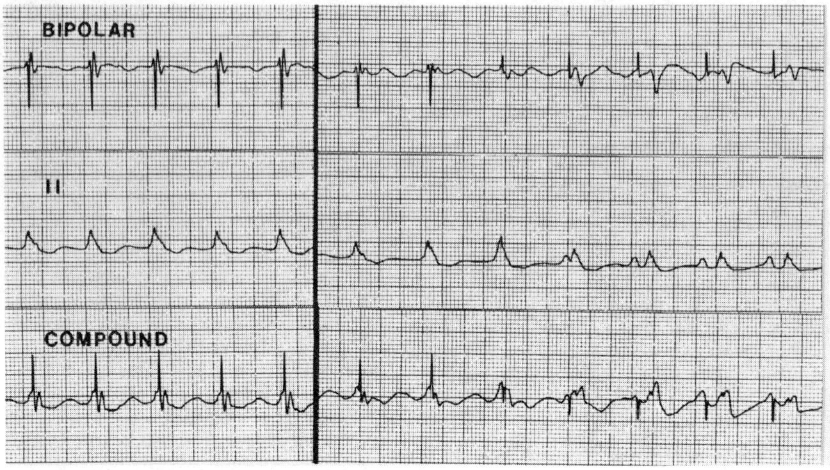

FIGURE 97-10 P waves not apparent in lead II are recorded by the esophageal lead 0.07 s after onset of the wide QRS. Change in P vector when RR interval slows confirms first retrograde then sinus origin of the P waves. When atrium eventually controls ventricles, the same anomalous QRS is inscribed, confirming that initial beats were accelerated junctional rhythm with bundle branch block. (*From R. Fletcher and R. Saunders, Esophageal Electrocardiography—1981, in J. W. Hurst (ed.), "Update V—The Heart," McGraw-Hill, New York, 1981. Reproduced with permission from the publisher and author.*)

tial, strongly confirmed in one patient the diagnosis of accelerated junctional rhythm with bundle branch block (Fig. 97-10).

Sustained atrial pacing should be accomplished by the intracardiac route, but the esophageal lead may provide *temporary atrial pacing or pace out of atrial tachycardias.*[28–33] A patient with bradycardia-tachycardia syndrome illustrates this and other applications of the esophageal lead. The patient had reentrant supraventricular tachycardia using a concealed Kent bundle defined by previous electrophysiologic study. A permanent coronary sinus pacemaker treated occasional sinus bradycardia. The pacemaker had malfunctioned with marked slowing and failure to capture. An esophageal lead permitted temporary, noninvasive, demand atrial pacing at 25 mA, and avoided potential displacement of the permanent intracavitary lead by a temporary pacing wire and morbidity from an invasive procedure while the patient awaited generator change (Fig. 97-11). Using a 2-cm spaced bipolar electrode, the lowest pacing threshold (12 mA) was achieved using a 7-ms stimulus, while 19 mA are required for a pulse width of 1 ms.[34] At lower pulse widths, pacing was only 70 percent reliable.[35,36] The esophageal route for *ventricular pacing* has been used by Lubell and by Burack and Furman at even higher current levels (50 mA).[37,38] This is accomplished in lower lead positions where, using the bipolar configuration, large ventricular deflections are recorded. Pacing from the esophagus is not yet proved innocuous and should be limited to short-term supportive pacing for bradycardias and conversion of atrial arrhythmia.

In this patient, the esophageal electrogram also reveals the reason for an absent QRS during acceleration of a programmable permanent atrial pacemaker at rates of more than 110 beats per minute (Fig. 97-12). The esophageal lead showed no atrial activity after the pacing spike, rather than AV block. Failure to capture was caused not by a prolonged atrial refractory period, but a premature, perhaps reentrant P wave. In usual invasive electrophysiology laboratory procedures, a quadripolar catheter records the presence of atrial capture from two proximal electrodes after bipolar pacing from two distal electrodes. In this patient, esophageal leads were equivalent to the proximal atrial electrodes, thus providing information similar to an invasive study.

Another patient, with a dual-chamber pacemaker inserted for sick sinus syndrome, experienced recurrent pacemaker-mediated tachycardia. Premature atrial activity occurring just beyond the programmed postventricular atrial refractory period (PVARP) was presumed to initiate this arrhythmia. In fact, PMT was established because failure to capture the atrium, seen clearly on the esophageal lead, permitted an atrial escape beat to occur at the critical

FIGURE 97-11 Permanent coronary sinus pacemaker placed for bradycardia-tachycardia syndrome. First three pacing outputs recorded on lead II indicate generator failure (28 beats per minute). The third pacing deflection fails to capture the atrium. In the same sequence, the atrium was then paced (20-mA output; 104 beats per minute) by an esophageal electrode previously positioned to record a large bipolar atrial deflection (A). (*From R. Fletcher and R. Saunders, Esophageal Electrocardiography—1981, in J. W. Hurst (ed.), "Update V—The Heart," McGraw-Hill, New York, 1981. Reproduced with permission from the publisher and author.*)

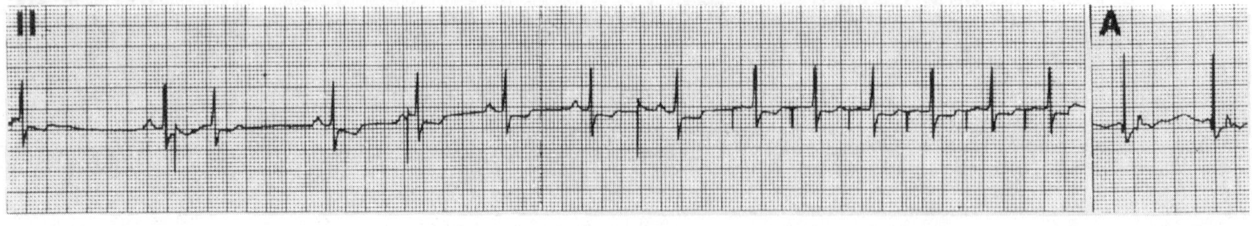

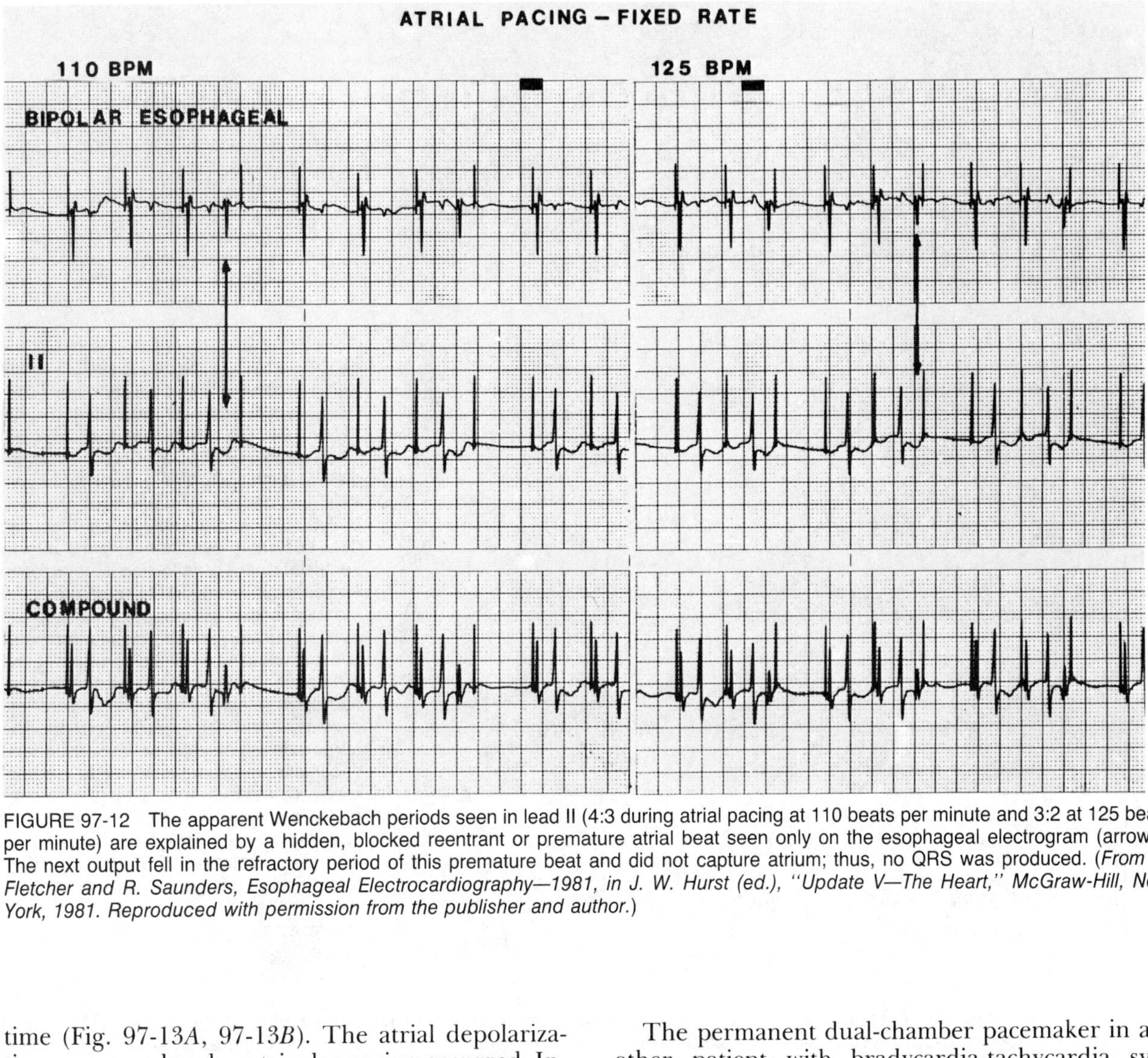

FIGURE 97-12 The apparent Wenckebach periods seen in lead II (4:3 during atrial pacing at 110 beats per minute and 3:2 at 125 beats per minute) are explained by a hidden, blocked reentrant or premature atrial beat seen only on the esophageal electrogram (arrows). The next output fell in the refractory period of this premature beat and did not capture atrium; thus, no QRS was produced. (*From R. Fletcher and R. Saunders, Esophageal Electrocardiography—1981, in J. W. Hurst (ed.), "Update V—The Heart," McGraw-Hill, New York, 1981. Reproduced with permission from the publisher and author.*)

time (Fig. 97-13*A*, 97-13*B*). The atrial depolarization was sensed and ventricular pacing occurred. Intact ventriculoatrial conduction with VA conduction time exceeding the PV-ARP allowed perpetuation of the tachycardia. Atrial capture was ensured and recurrence prevented by reprogramming atrial output from 0.4 ms/4 mA to 1.0 ms/10 mA (Fig. 97-13*C*).

Commercially available, programmable, permanent atrial and AV synchronous pacemakers allow complete *testing for inducible tachycardia and for pace out* with test made pacing rates above 300 beats per minute. This testing requires simultaneous recording of atrial activity for evidence of retrograde conduction, dissociation, atrial tachycardia, and atrial capture during rapid atrial stimulation. A patient had sick sinus syndrome with recurrent atrial tachycardia and episodes of profound bradycardia treated with a permanent atrial pacemaker. The tachycardia responded to overdrive pacing when capture was clearly demonstrated by esophageal recording (Fig. 97-14, lower). Lack of capture was evident during the unsuccessful attempt to pace out this tachycardia (Fig. 97-14, upper).

The permanent dual-chamber pacemaker in another patient with bradycardia-tachycardia syndrome was temporarily programmed for noninvasive electrophysiologic testing to evaluate recurrent pacemaker-mediated tachycardia. Bipolar and unipolar esophageal electrograms (BEE and UEE) recorded left atrial activity. Since dual AV drive is more likely to reveal retrograde conduction,[39] an eight-beat atrial and ventricular pacing drive (S_1S_1) was followed with a single ventricular extrastimulus with S_1S_2 of 380 ms (Fig. 97-15). Pacemaker-mediated tachycardia ensued. Atrial deflection polarity changed on UEE with the first P wave recorded after S_2 and remained changed during the tachycardia. The unipolar esophageal electrogram confirmed that a reentrant P wave initiated this tachycardia and enabled precise VA conduction time measurement. Postventricular atrial refractory period reprogrammed to exceed the measured VA time prevented the tachycardia. The simultaneous bipolar and unipolar esophageal recording technique, suggested by Andrew Cohen[40] was achieved with an intracardiac defibrillation catheter passed into the patient's esophagus.

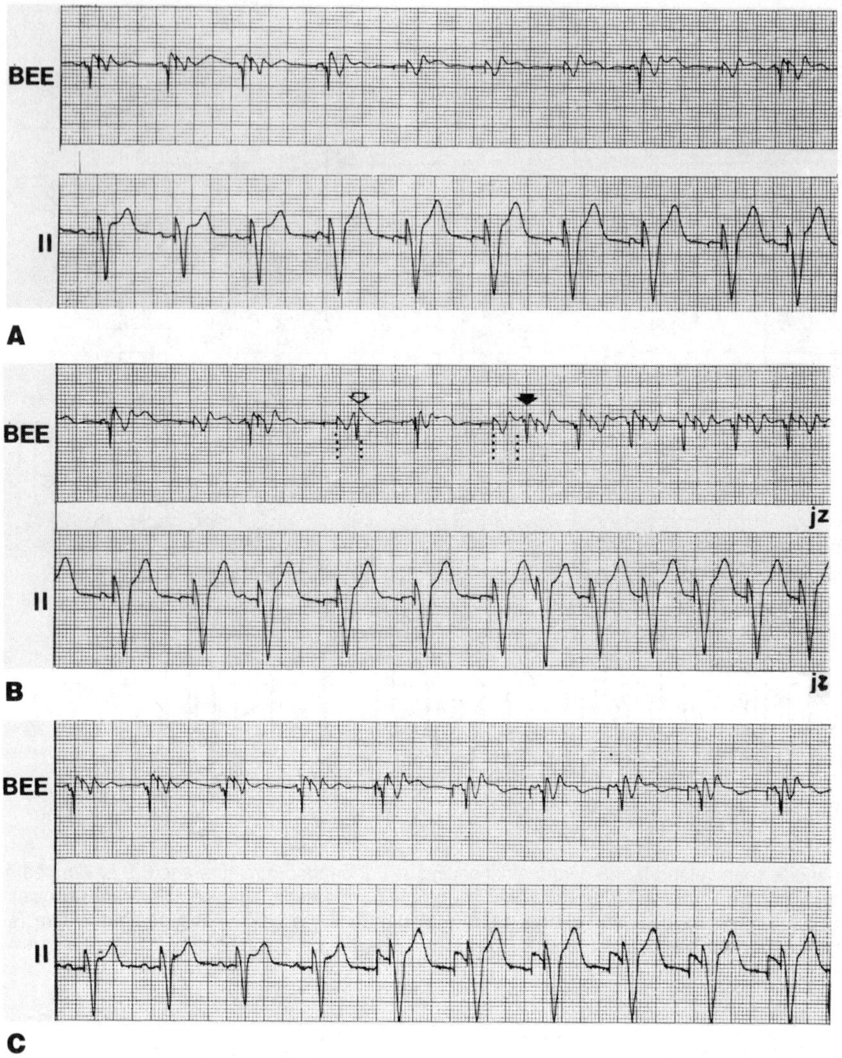

FIGURE 97-13 *A.* Failure to capture atrium with a programmable dual-chamber pacemaker is followed by a slow atrial escape rhythm seen on the bipolar esophageal electrogram (BEE). *B.* Pacemaker-mediated tachycardia (PMT) is initiated by an atrial escape beat. Atrial refractory period is 250 ms in this patient. An atrial escape beat occurring less than 250 ms after a ventricular pacing deflection is not sensed and does not initiate PMT (open arrow). An atrial deflection occurring just outside the atrial refractory period (closed arrow) is sensed, causing ventricular pace at the programmed AV interval. Retrograde conduction is intact and VA conduction time exceeds the atrial refractory period. The retrograde atrial capture is sensed and pacemaker-mediated tachycardia is established. *C.* Atrial capture is assured and recurrence prevented by reprogramming atrial output to 1.0 ms/10 mA. Note the time from left atrial depolarization (P wave on BEE) to ventricular pacing output is 130 ms when ventricle tracks native P waves, but is shortened to nearly 0 ms when atrium is paced.

FIGURE 97-14 *Upper:* Unsuccessful pace out of atrial tachycardia using a programmable permanent atrial pacemaker. The bipolar esophageal electrogram (BEE) reveals failure to capture. *Lower:* The 1:1 capture of atrium recorded on the esophageal lead predicts successful pace out of the atrial tachycardia. (*From R. Fletcher and R. Saunders, Esophageal Electrocardiography—1981, in J. W. Hurst (ed.), "Update V—The Heart," McGraw-Hill, New York, 1981. Reproduced with permission from the publisher and author.*)

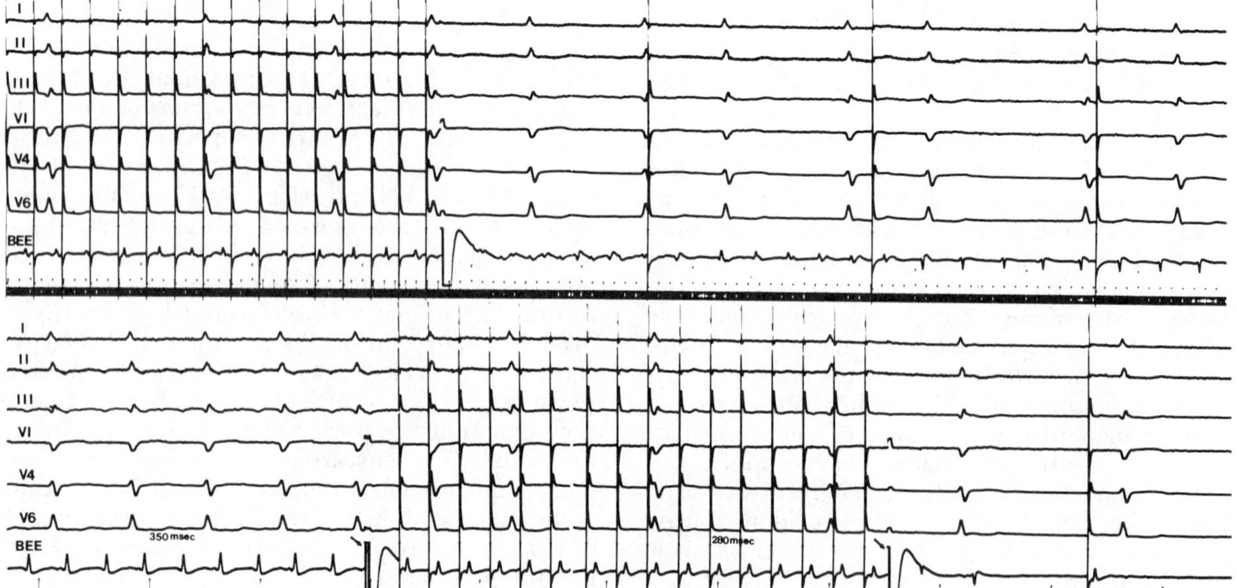

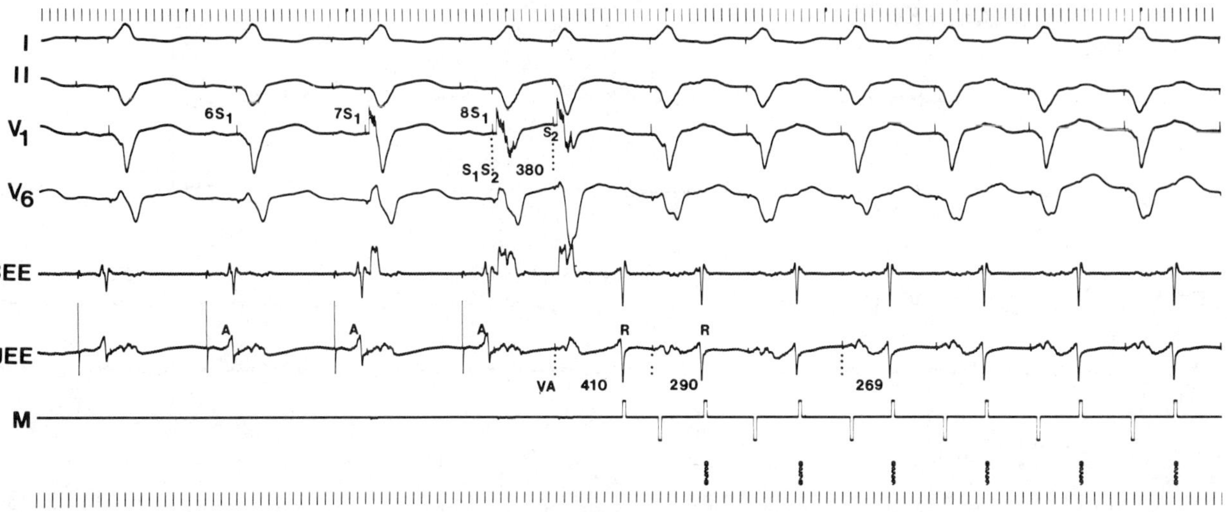

FIGURE 97-15 Bipolar and unipolar esophageal electrograms (BEE and UEE) are recorded simultaneously during a noninvasive test for pacemaker-mediated tachycardia. A permanent DDD pacemaker is driven with synchronized programming to produce eight AV sequential S_1's followed by an S_2 in the ventricle. Vector of the atrial depolarization following S_2, seen on the bipolar lead at 410 ms, is changed to retrograde, a change apparent only on the unipolar lead. Antegrade P waves (A) shift to retrograde (R). The sensed retrograde P, with initial VA conduction of 410 ms, triggers ventricular pacing and produces sustained pacemaker-mediated tachycardia. Reprogramming the post-V atrial refractory period to exceed the stabilized VA conduction time of 269 ms eliminates retrograde P sensing and prevents this pacemaker tachycardia.

The hemodynamic effect of dual-chamber pacing is influenced by the programmed AV delay but may be enhanced by controlling the relation of left atrial to left ventricular events,[41] a relation not always predictable from knowledge of the right atrium to left ventricular time (i.e., AV delay). *Intraatrial and left atrium to left ventricle timing* may be determined by using the BEE to record left atrial events.[42] Right atrial timing is marked by the beginning of programmed AV delay, seen in the DVI mode as an atrial pacing output or, in the VDD mode, as a sensed local right atrial depolarization which may be revealed by a telemetered right atrial electrogram (A-EGM) available from some permanent single- or dual-chamber pacemakers. Simultaneous recording of left atrial activity from the esophagus and a right atrial appendage electrogram (A-EGM) telemetered from a temporarily nonsensing dual-chamber pacemaker inserted for complete heart block reveals a 70-ms delay from the sensed right atrial event to left atrial depolarization (Fig. 97-16). This right atrial-left atrial delay is not apparent on surface lead V_1. At a constant AV delay, simultaneous recording of right and left atrial events revealed shortening of the left atrium

FIGURE 97-16 Right atrial to left atrial delay of 70 ms (arrow) is recorded in a patient with a nonsensing programmable pacemaker inserted for complete heart block. The right atrial electrogram (A-EGM) is telemetered from the pacemaker and left atrial events are seen on the bipolar esophageal electrogram (BEE).

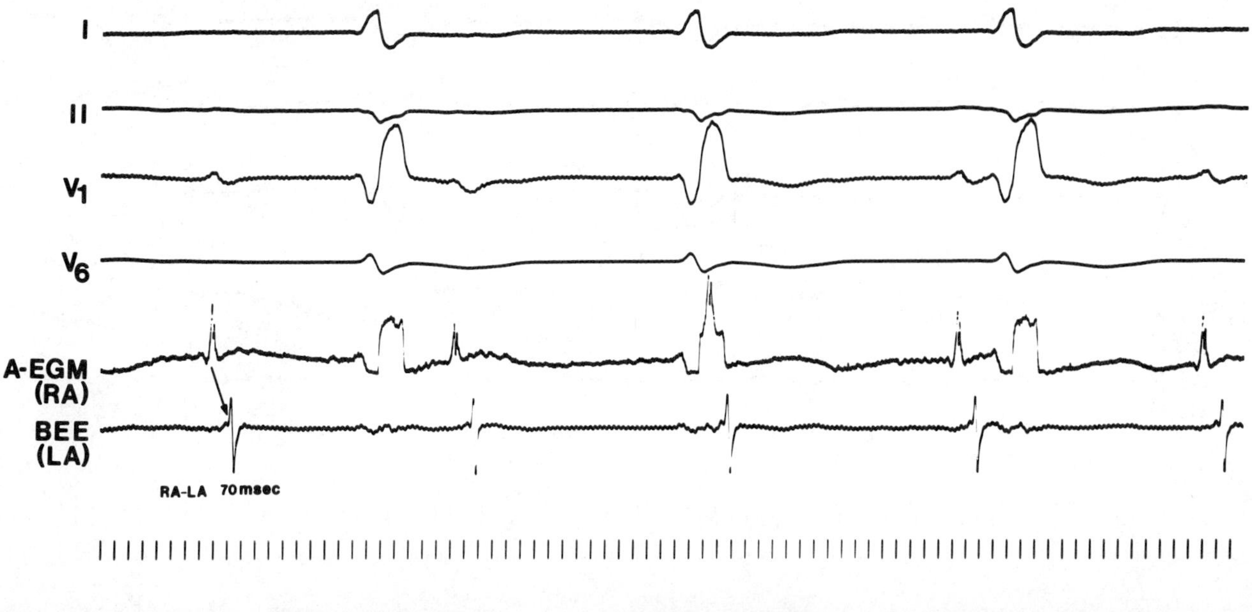

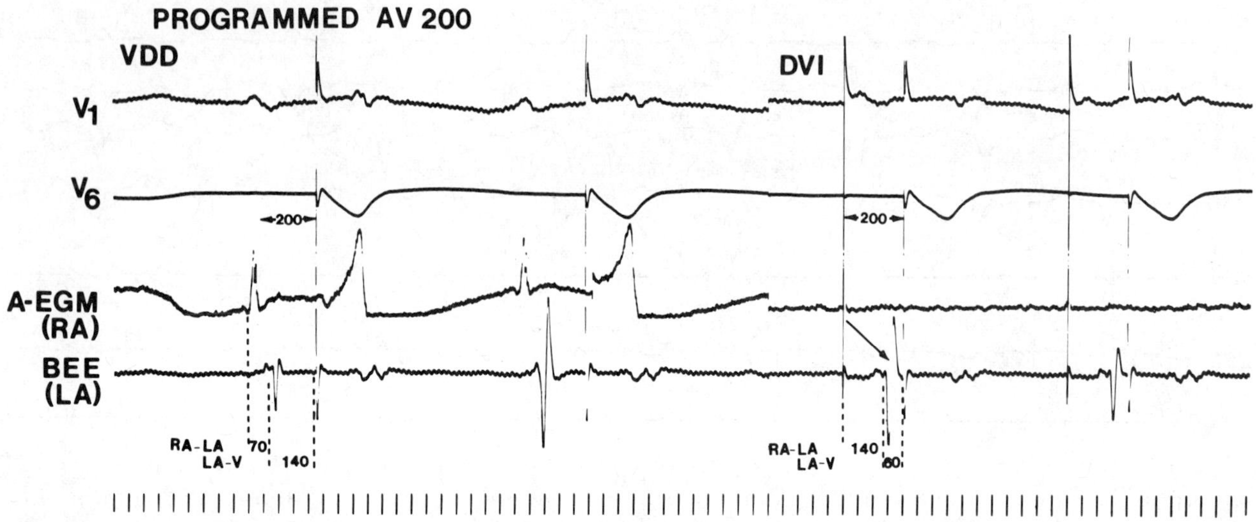

FIGURE 97-17 In a patient paced for complete heart block, variations in intraatrial (RA-LA) and left atrium to ventricular pacing spike (LA-V) conduction times were visualized noninvasively by simultaneous recording of the telemetered right atrial electrogram (A-EGM) from a DDD pacemaker and left atrial activity from a bipolar esophageal electrogram (BEE). Atrial tracking in the VDD mode produced LA-V of 140 ms. With DVI pacing, LA-V is foreshortened to 60 ms. While programmed AV delay remains 200 ms whether in the VDD or DVI mode, the relation of left atrial to left ventricular events varies.

to left ventricle delay of 80 ms when the mode changed from atrial tracking (VDD) to atrial pacing (DVI) (Fig. 97-17). In addition, an ectopic atrial beat prolonged the left atrium to left ventricle delay 55 ms with no change in right atrium-right ventricle delay (Fig. 97-18).

Variations in RA-LA and LA-LV timing, which may be seen by esophageal recording, will have increased clinical importance as dual-chamber pacing becomes widely employed.

Summary

The inexpensive and noninvasive esophageal recording technique will have wide application in clin-

FIGURE 97-18 LA-V is increased from 100 ms to 155 ms in association with a foreshortened RA-LA time. This occurs because atrial depolarization spreading from an ectopic focus arrives at the right atrial appendage and left atrium at nearly the same time, but it takes 55 ms longer to traverse from the ectopic focus to LA (155 ms) than from right atrial appendage to LA (100 ms). In each case, AV delay is 150 ms. An apparent disparity between RA-V (RA-LA plus LV-V) and the AV delay is seen because in the VDD mode, AV delay begins with right atrial sensing (*downslope* of right atrial P wave), but RA is marked at the *beginning* of the right atrial P wave.

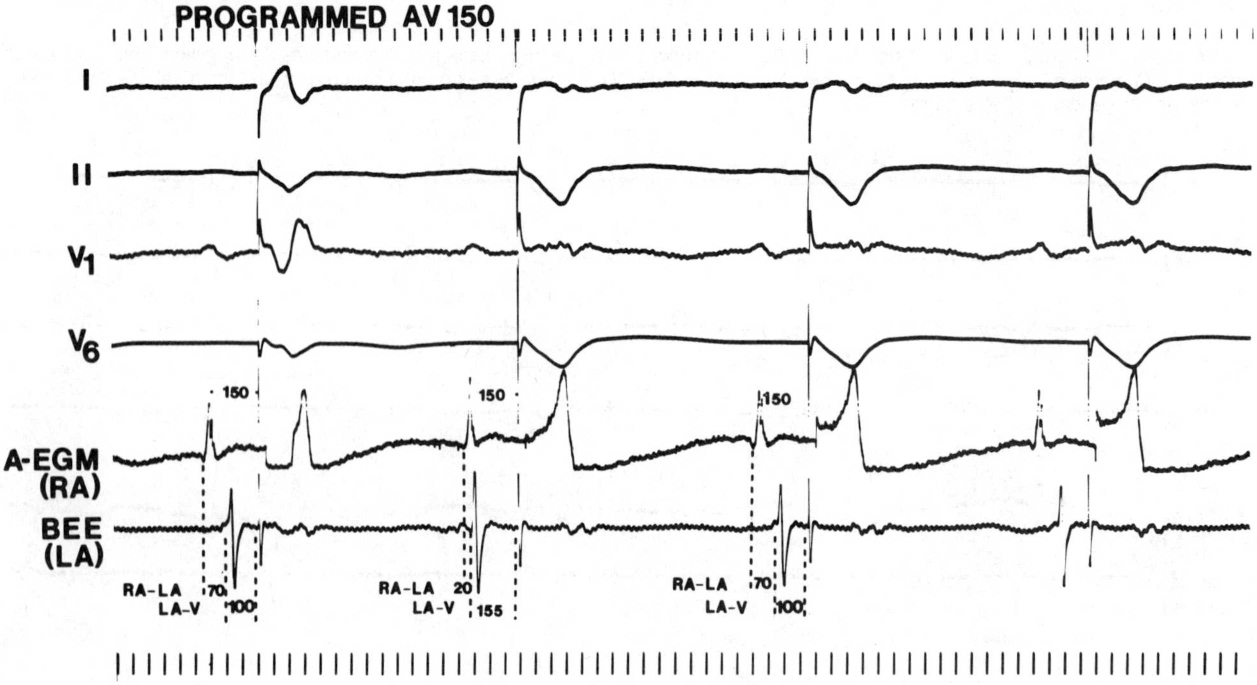

ical cardiology. Bipolar recording, signal filtering, and general use of three-channel recorders, plus small, well-tolerated recording electrodes make it a practical tool. Noninvasive detection of left atrial activity with the esophageal electrogram is an appealing, effective aid to manage native and pacemaker-related arrhythmia.

References

1. Cremer, M.: Ueber die direkte Ableitung der Akionsstrome des menslichen Herzens vom Oesophagus und uber das Elektrokardiogramm des Fotus, *Munch. Wochenschr.*, 53:811, 1906.
2. Brown, W. H.: A Study of the Esophageal Lead in Clinical Electrocardiography: Parts 1 and 11, *Am. Heart J.*, 12:1, 307, 1936.
3. Smith, C.: An Endo-oesophageal Stethoscope, *Anesthesiology*, 15:566, 1954.
4. Matsumoto, M., Oka, Y., Lin, Y. T., Strom, J., Sonnenblick, E. H., and Frater, R. W. M.: Transesophageal Echocardiography for Assessing Ventricular Performance, *N.Y. State J. Med.*, 79:19, 1979.
5. Wenckebach, E. F.: Ueber Verkehrsstorungen in Herzen, *Wien. Med. Wochenschr.*, 77:1307, 1927.
6. Lewis, T., Meakings, J., and White, P. D.: The Excitatory Process in the Dog's Heart. Part 1: The Auricle, *Philos. Trans. R. Soc. Lond.* [Biol.], 205:375, 1914.
7. Wilson, F. N., McLeod, A. G., and Baker, P. S.: The Order of Ventricular Excitation in Human Bundle Branch Block, *Am. Heart J.*, 7:305, 1931.
8. Vogel, J. H. K., Tabari, K., Averile, K. H., and Blount, S. G.: A Simple Technique for Identifying P Waves in Complex Arrhythmias, *Am. Heart J.*, 67:158, 1964.
9. Dreifus, L. S., Najmi, M., Domerantz, D., and Novack, P.: The Right Atrial Electrogram: A Bedside Procedure for the Diagnosis of Cardiac Arrhythmias, *Dis. Chest*, 48:617, 1965.
10. Berens, S. C., Kolin, A., MacAlpin, R. N., and Lenz, M. W.: New Stable Temporary Atrial Pacing Loop, *Am. J. Cardiol.*, 34:325, 1974.
11. Zucker, R., Rothfeld, E., and Bernstein, A.: A New Multipurpose Cardiac Catheter, *Am. J. Cardiol.*, 15:45, 1965.
12. Chatterjee, K., Swan, H. J. C., Ganz, W., Gray, R., and Albus, J.: Multipurpose Flotation Electrode Catheter—A New Catheter for Arrhythmia and Intracardiac Pressure Monitoring, *Am. J. Cardiol.*, 33:130, 1974.
13. Wilson, F. N.: The Distribution of the Potential Differences Produced by the Heart Beat within the Body and at Its Surface, *Am. Heart J.*, 5:599, 1930.
14. Goldberger, E.: A Simple, Indifferent Electrocardiographic Electrode of Zero Potential and a Technique of Obtaining Augmented, Unipolar Extremity Leads, *Am. Heart J.*, 23:483, 1942.
15. Hamilton, J. G. M., and Nyboer, J.: The Ventricular Deflections in Myocardial Infarction. An Electrocardiographic Study Using Esophageal and Precardial Leads, *Am. Heart J.*, 15:414, 1938.
16. Brody, D. A., Harris, T. R., and Romans, W. E.: A Simple Method for Obtaining Esophageal Electrocardiograms of Good Diagnostic Quality, *Am. Heart J.*, 50:923, 1955.
17. Copeland, G. D., Tullis, E. F., and Brody, D. A.: Clinical Evaluation of a New Esophageal Electrode, with Particular Reference to the Bipolar Esophageal Electrocardiogram, *Am. Heart J.*, 57:862, 1959.
18. Barold, S. S.: Filtered Bipolar Esophageal Electrocardiography, *Am. Heart J.*, 57:862, 1972.
19. Zipes, D. P., and DeJoseph, R. L.: Dissimilar Atrial Rhythms in Man and Dog, *Am. J. Cardiol.*, 32:618, 1973.
20. Prystowsky, E. N., Pritchett, E. L. C., and Gallager, J. J.: Origin of the Atrial Electrogram Recorded from the Esophagus, *Circulation*, 61:1017, 1980.
21. Arzbaecher, R.: A Pill-Electrode for the Study of Cardiac Arrhythmia, *Med. Instrum.*, 12:277, 1978.
22. Luisada, A.: Derivazioni elettive per le correnti di origine atriale, *Cuore Circ.*, 19:77, 1935.
23. Kistin, A. D., and Bruce, J. C.: Simultaneous Esophageal and Standard Electrocardiographic Leads for the Study of Cardiac Arrhythmias, *Am. Heart J.*, 53:65, 1957.
24. Oblath, R., and Karpman, H.: The Normal Esophageal Lead Electrogram, *Am. Heart J.*, 41:369, 1951.
25. Lister, J. W., Delman, A. J., Stein, E., Greenwald, R. P., and Robinson, G.: Dominant Pacemaker of the Human Heart: Antegrade and Retrograde Activation of the Heart, *Circulation*, 35:22, 1967.
26. Lister, J. W., Cohen, I. S., Bernstein, W. H., and Samet, P.: Treatment of Supraventricular Tachycardia by Rapid Atrial Stimulation, *Circulation*, 38:1044, 1968.
27. Rubin, L., Jagendorf, B., and Goldberg, A. L.: The Esophageal Lead in the Diagnosis of Tachycardias with Aberrant Ventricular Conduction, *Am. Heart J.*, 57:19, 1959.
28. Montoyo, J. V., Angel, J., Valle, V., and Gausi, C.: Cardioversion of Tachycardias by Transesophageal Atrial Pacing, *Am. J. Cardiol.*, 32:85, 1973.
29. Hartzler, G. O., and Maloney, J. D.: Transesophageal Atrial Pacing in the Wolff-Parkinson-White Syndrome, *Mayo Clin. Proc.*, 52:576, 1977.
30. Gallagher, J. J., Smith, W., Kerr, C., Kassel, J., Cook, L., Reiter, M., Sterba, R., and Harte, M.: Esophageal Pacing: A Diagnostic and Therapeutic Tool, *Circulation*, 65:336, 1982.
31. Critelli, G., Grassi, G., Perticone, F., Coltorti, F., Monda, V., and Condorelli, M.: Transesophageal Pacing for Prognostic Evaluation of Preexcitation Syndrome and Assessment of Protective Therapy, *Am. J. Cardiol.*, 51:513, 1983.
32. Benson, D. W., Dunnigan, A., Sterba, R., Benditt, D. G.: Atrial Pacing from the Esophagus in the Diagnosis and Management of Tachycardia and Palpitations, *J. Pediatr.*, 102(1):40, 1983.
33. Kerr, C. R., Gallagher, J. J., Smith, W. M., Sterba, R., German, L. D., Cook, L., and Kasell, J. H.: The Induction of Atrial Flutter and Fibrillation and the Termination of Atrial Flutter by Esophageal Pacing, *Pace*, 6(1 Pt. 1):60, 1983.
34. Gallagher, J. J., Kasell, J., Reiter, M., Smith, W. M., Benson, D. W., Cook, L., and Kopp, D.: Esophageal Pacing: A Diagnostic and Therapeutic Tool, *Circulation*, 62:111, 1980.
35. Shafiroff, B. G. P., and Linder, J.: Effects of External Electrical Pacemaker Stimuli on the Human Heart, *J. Thorac. Surg.*, 33:544, 1957.
36. Arzbaecher, R., Collins, S., and Brown, D.: Transesophageal Recording and Pacing with a New Pill Electrode, *Circulation*, 58:ii, 1978. (Abstract.)
37. Lubell, D. L.: Cardiac Pacing from the Esophagus, *Am. J. Cardiol.*, 27:641, 1971.
38. Burack, B., and Furman, S.: Transesophageal Cardiac Pacing, *Am. J. Cardiol.*, 23:469, 1969.
39. Mahmud, R., Lehmann, M., Denker, R., Gilbert, C., Akhtar, M.: Atrioventricular Sequential Pacing: Differential Effect on Retrograde Conduction Related to Level of Impulse Collision, *Circulation*, 68:(1)23, 1983.
40. Cohen, A. I.: Personal communication.
41. Wish, M., Gottdiener, J., Cutler, D. J., Cohen, A., Gay, J., Chauvin, L., and Fletcher, R.: Optimal Hemodynamic Programming of Dual Chamber Pacemakers Using 2D-Doppler Echocardiography, *J. Am. Coll. Cardiol.*, 3:507, 1984. (Abstract.)
42. Brinkley, P. F., Bush, C. A., Kolibash, A. J., Magorien, R. D., Hamlin, R. L., and Leier, C. V.: The Anatomic Relationship of the Esophageal Lead to the Left Atrium, *Pace*, 5(6):853, 1982.

98

Techniques of Exercise Testing

Robert F. DeBusk, M.D.

New things are made familiar, and familiar things are made new.

Samuel Johnson, 1779[1]

Major changes have occurred in the utilization of exercise testing during the past decade. These include:

1. Increasing emphasis on *prognostic stratification* of patients with established ischemic heart disease, especially soon after acute events such as myocardial infarction and coronary artery bypass graft (CABG) surgery.
2. Increasing utilization for evaluating *functional capacity,* including the effects of therapeutic interventions such as antianginal and antiarrhythmic medication and CABG surgery. This includes the *provision of guidelines for physical activity,* including prescription of exercise conditioning regimens and clearance for resumption of customary activities, including return to work.
3. Increasing use of exercise testing along with imaging techniques to charactrize the *pathophysiologic mechanisms* underlying ischemic heart disease, i.e., myocardial ischemia and left ventricular dysfunction. Thallium myocardial perfusion scintigraphy has been used to localize and quantitate myocardial ischemia; radionuclide ventriculography has been used to detect regional wall motion abnormalities and to quantitate left ventricular ejection fraction (LVEF) at rest and during exercise.

These newer indications have considerably expanded the role of exercise testing in the clinical management of patients. They supplement rather than supplant the more traditional *diagnostic* role of exercise testing in the evaluation of chest pain.

The term *coronary artery disease* as used here refers to angiographically demonstrated coronary lesions, i.e., an *anatomic* abnormality. In contrast, the term *ischemic heart disease* refers to the *functional consequences* of this anatomic abnormality (Fig. 98-1). These functional consequences, mediated by myocardial ischemia, i.e., a disparity between myocardial oxygen supply and demand, include clinical syndromes of angina pectoris, myocardial infarction, and sudden cardiac death.

Studies of cardiac function during exercise have documented a good prognosis in patients whose mechanical response to exercise (i.e., peak treadmill workload, heart rate, and cardiac output) is well preserved despite moderate to severe anatomic coronary disease.[2–5] Indeed, in patients with chronic ischemic heart disease, peak left ventricular ejection fraction during exercise correlates better with prognosis than does the extent of angiographic coronary lesions. An exercise-induced increase in LVEF is a clinically important mechanical expression of myocardial ischemia. Such a response correlates well with parameters of myocardial ischemia such as exercise-induced angina pectoris and reversible myocardial perfusion defects.[7,8]

FIGURE 98-1 Relation between coronary artery disease and ischemic heart disease. Tl = thallium; LVEF = left ventricular ejection fraction.

CORONARY ARTERY DISEASE (FUNCTIONAL ABNORMALITY)

ISCHEMIC HEART DISEASE (PHYSIOLOGIC ABNORMALITY)

MYOCARDIAL ISCHEMIA
- EXERCISE-INDUCED
  - ST DEPRESSION
  - ANGINA PECTORIS
  - REVERSIBLE TL DEFECTS

ISCHEMIC LEFT VENTRICULAR DYSFUNCTION
- EXERCISE-INDUCED
  - WALL MOTION ABNORMALITIES
  - UNCHANGED OR DECREASED LVEF
  - LOW PEAK HEART RATE, PRESSURE, WORKLOAD

Modes of Exercise Testing

Dynamic Lower Extremity Testing (Treadmill, Cycle Ergometer)

Treadmill testing is the most widely used method for exercise testing in the United States. Technical refinements such as quieter treadmills, low-impedance electrocardiogram (ECG) electrodes, and signal averaging of the QRS complex have minimized the former disadvantages of treadmill testing compared to cycle ergometry, namely ECG motion artifact, difficulty in recording blood pressure by sphygmomanometer, etc. Americans are less familiar with cycling than with walking and climbing—their peak cycle exercise workload is often limited by fatigue of the quadriceps and/or knee problems. However, cycle ergometry is often favored for obese or poorly coordinated patients who cannot perform even low-intensity treadmill exercise. Cycle ergometry is the only method of exercise used with radionuclide ventriculography and is the only practicable method for carrying out dynamic exercise during cardiac catheterization.

Diagnostic sensitivity is comparable for treadmill exercise and cycle ergometry, although peak heart rate is higher and peak systolic and diastolic pressure are lower with the former.[9]

Dynamic Upper Extremity Testing

Arm ergometry, which elicits a peak workload which is only 60 to 80 percent that of leg ergometry, is less sensitive than leg ergometry for eliciting exercise-induced ischemic and arrhythmic abnormalities.[10] However, this technique may be useful in patients with peripheral vascular disease, orthopedic abnormalities, and other limitations to lower extremity effort.[11]

Static Effort

Static effort, e.g., handgrip or forearm lifting, is much less effective than dynamic effort in eliciting ischemic and arrhythmic abnormalities.[12,13]

Exercise Test Protocols

The overall objective of exercise testing is to disclose diagnostically and prognostically important abnormalities. *Mechanical* abnormalities include a low peak heart rate, blood pressure, and workload; *ischemic* abnormalities include angina pectoris and ischemic ST-segment depression, and *electrical* abnormalities include ventricular ectopic activity.

Symptom-limited testing is generally preferred to heart rate-limited or "submaximal" testing. The greater heart rate, blood pressure, and workload elicited by symptom-limited testing is more likely than submaximal testing to disclose diagnostically and prognostically important abnormalities. Symptom-limited testing is carried to the point of *limiting symptoms* of angina pectoris, generalized fatigue, dyspnea, and local muscular fatigue, or until the appearance of other abnormalities which may compromise the safety of continued exercise. The latter include marked ischemic ST-segment depression of 0.3 mV or more; exercise-induced hypotension, i.e., 10 mm Hg or more fall in systolic pressure compared to blood pressure measured during a previous stage of exercise; and complex ventricular ectopic activity, i.e., three or more consecutive PVCs. Whether test safety is enhanced by terminating exercise at the onset of lesser ischemic or arrhythmic abnormalities is unknown.

Treadmill Protocols

Since all protocols elicit a similar *peak oxygen consumption,* the choice of protocol is guided primarily by the expected effort tolerance of the patient. A protocol with a low initial workload and small work increments such as the Naughton test (Fig. 98-2*A*) is optimal for testing patients soon after myocardial infarction or CABG surgery, debilitated patients, and those who are moderately limited by angina pectoris or other symptoms. A protocol with a relatively higher initial workload and greater work increments, e.g., the Bruce test (Fig. 98-2), is preferred for evaluating patients with little or no symptomatic limitation. The objective of all protocols is to elicit a symptom-limited response within 6 to 15 minutes of effort. A briefer test may fail to demonstrate ischemic responses;[14] a longer one may be limited primarily by muscular fatigue rather than by myocardial ischemia.

FIGURE 98-2 Treadmill exercise test protocols. METs = metabolic equivalents, i.e., multiples of resting oxygen consumption in ml/kg/min. Functional class = New York Heart Association functional classification. (*From S. M. Fox III, J. Naughton, and W. L. Haskell, Physical Activity and the Prevention of Coronary Heart Disease, Ann. Clin. Res., 3:404–432, 1971. Adapted and reproduced with permission from the publisher and author.*)

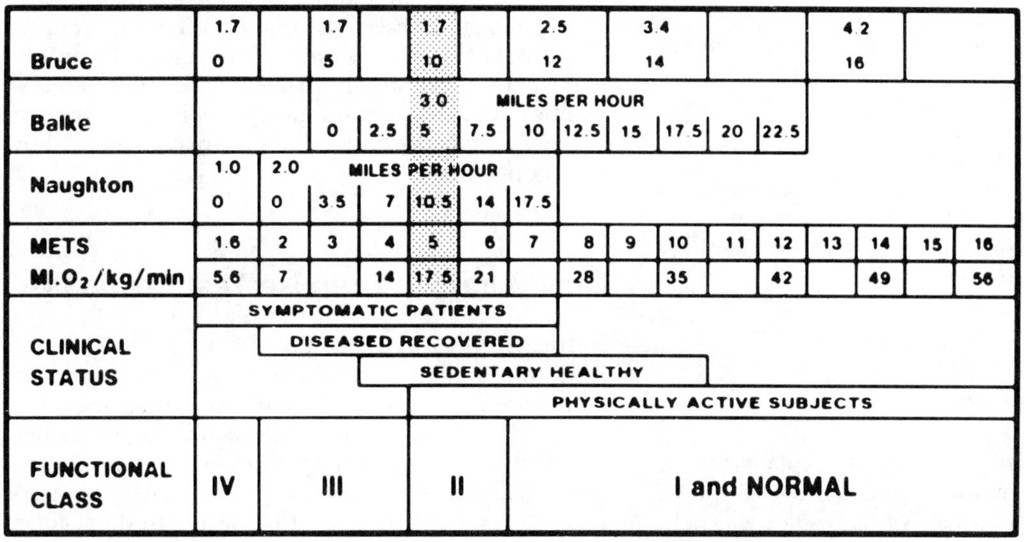
Bruce
1.7 0
1.7 5
1.7 10
2.5 12
3.4 14
4.2 16
Balke
3.0 MILES PER HOUR
0 2.5 5 7.5 10 12.5 15 17.5 20 22.5
Naughton
1.0 0
2.0 0
MILES PER HOUR
3.5 7 10.5 14 17.5
METS
1.6 2 3 4 5 6 7 8 9 10 11 12 13 14 15 16
Ml.O₂/kg/min
5.6 7 14 17.5 21 28 35 42 49 56
CLINICAL STATUS
SYMPTOMATIC PATIENTS
DISEASED RECOVERED
SEDENTARY HEALTHY
PHYSICALLY ACTIVE SUBJECTS
FUNCTIONAL CLASS
IV
III
II
I and NORMAL

WORKLOAD Kg. Meters/Min.	150	300	450	600	750	900	1050	1200	1500	1800
WATTS (approx.)	25	50	75	100	125	150	175	200	250	300
OXYGEN USED INCLUDING BASAL Ml./Min. (approx.)	600	900	1200	1500	1800	2100	2400	2700	3300	3900
KILOCALORIES/Min (approx.)	3	4-1/2	6	7-1/2	9	10-1/2	12	14	17	20
OXYGEN USED Ml./Min. per Kg. OF BODY WEIGHT										
FOR: Lbs. 88 Kg. 40	15	22-1/2	30	37-1/2	45	52-1/2	60	67-1/2	82-1/2	97-1/2
110 50	12	18	24	30	36	42	48	54	66	78
132 60	10	15	20	25	30	35	40	45	55	65
154 70	8-1/2	13	17	21-1/2	25-1/2	30	34-1/2	38-1/2	47	55-1/2
176 80	7-1/2	11	15	19	22-1/2	26	30	34	41	49
198 90	6-2/3	10	13-1/3	16-2/3	20	23-1/3	26-2/3	30	36-2/3	43-1/3
220 100	6	9	12	15	18	21	24	27	33	39
242 110	5-1/2	8	11	13-1/2	16-1/2	19	22	24-1/2	30	35-1/2
264 120	5	7-1/2	10	12-1/2	15	17-1/2	20	22-1/2	27-1/2	32-1/2

FIGURE 98-3 Oxygen requirements of bicycle ergometric workloads. (*From S. M. Fox III, J. Naughton, and W. L. Haskell, Physical Activity and the Prevention of Coronary Heart Disease, Ann. Clin. Res. 3:404–432, 1971. Adapted and reproduced with permission from the publisher and author.*)

A convention which facilitates comparison of treadmill protocols is referred to as the *MET*. This term, derived from the work *metabolic,* is used to describe the energy cost of physical activity. One MET, the energy cost of sitting quietly at rest, is approximately equal to an oxygen consumption of 3.5 ml/kg/min. The first stage of the standard Bruce protocol, the third stage of the Balke protocol, and the fifth stage of the Naughton protocol all elicit a metabolic response of five METs, or five times the resting energy cost (17.5 ml/kg/min) as shown in the shaded column of Fig. 98-2*A*. This workload also marks the boundary between New York Heart Association class II and III. The peak workload in METs is the highest treadmill speed and grade which the patient can tolerate for at least 2 min. Values of peak oxygen consumption estimated from treadmill workload, i.e., speed and grade, correlate well with measured values as long as patients do not grasp the handrail.

Whereas the metabolic response to treadmill exercise is relatively independent of body mass, the metabolic requirements of ergometric workloads are inversely related to body mass. For example, a 600-kg/min (100-watt) cycle workload represents 21.5-ml/kg/min oxygen uptake for a 70-kg man, approximating six METs, whereas this same cycle workload approximates only 5 METs (16.7 ml/kg/min) for a 90-kg man (Fig. 98-3).

Preparation of the Patient for Exercise Testing

Informed consent and a thorough explanation of the test indications, methods, and interpretation of the test results are essential. A brief *history* will help to exclude patients at unusually high risk, i.e., those with heart failure, unstable angina pectoris, and recent syncope. Similarly, a brief *physical examination* will help to establish the presence of these conditions and/or other limitations to physical effort, such as pulmonary disease and obstructive vascular disease, which may significantly influence interpretation of the test results. A *standard 12-lead ECG* using limb and chest electrodes is important in evaluating previous myocardial infarction. Adequate skin preparation is important to assure optimal recording of the ECG. Low-impedance, disposable ECG electrodes are commercially available. The preferred ECG lead configuration depends on the purpose of the test. Twelve-lead ECGs are preferred for evaluating patients with known ischemic heart disease in which myocardial ischemia may be present in certain leads but not others (Fig. 98-4). On the other hand, a single MCL-5 bipolar lead appears adequate for evaluating exercise-induced myocardial ischemia in patients with atypical chest pain.[15]

Patients should not eat or smoke for at least 2 h before the test. They should wear comfortable clothing, including rubber-soled shoes for good traction. Whether medication should be discontinued before testing depends on the purpose of the test. If the test is performed primarily to evaluate *functional consequences* of ischemic heart disease, including response to medications, these should be continued. If the purpose of the test is *diagnostic,* e.g., to evaluate the cause of obscure chest pain, cardiac medications should be withdrawn before testing in order not to influence the ST-segment response to exercise.

Before testing, patients should be told to expect breathlessness and fatigue, especially at higher levels of effort. Reassurance and encouragement of patients during the test help assure a truly symptom-limited exercise test performance.

Patients should be reexamined immediately after testing, with cardiac auscultation performed in the left lateral decubitus position to detect exercise-induced, i.e., ischemic abnormalities such as new S_3 or S_4 gallops, mitral regurgitation murmurs reflecting papillary muscle dysfunction, and left ventricular aneurysmal bulging. Detection of these abnormalities helps to corroborate the ischemic nature of ST-segment depression which is unaccompanied by angina pectoris.

Monitoring the Exercise Test Response

Symptomatic Endpoints

Symptom-limited exercise testing is preferred to "submaximal" testing in almost all circumstances except very soon (i.e., 10 to 14 days) after acute cardiac events such as myocardial infarction and CABG surgery. Symptom-limited testing has been safely performed as soon as 72 h after the last episode of chest

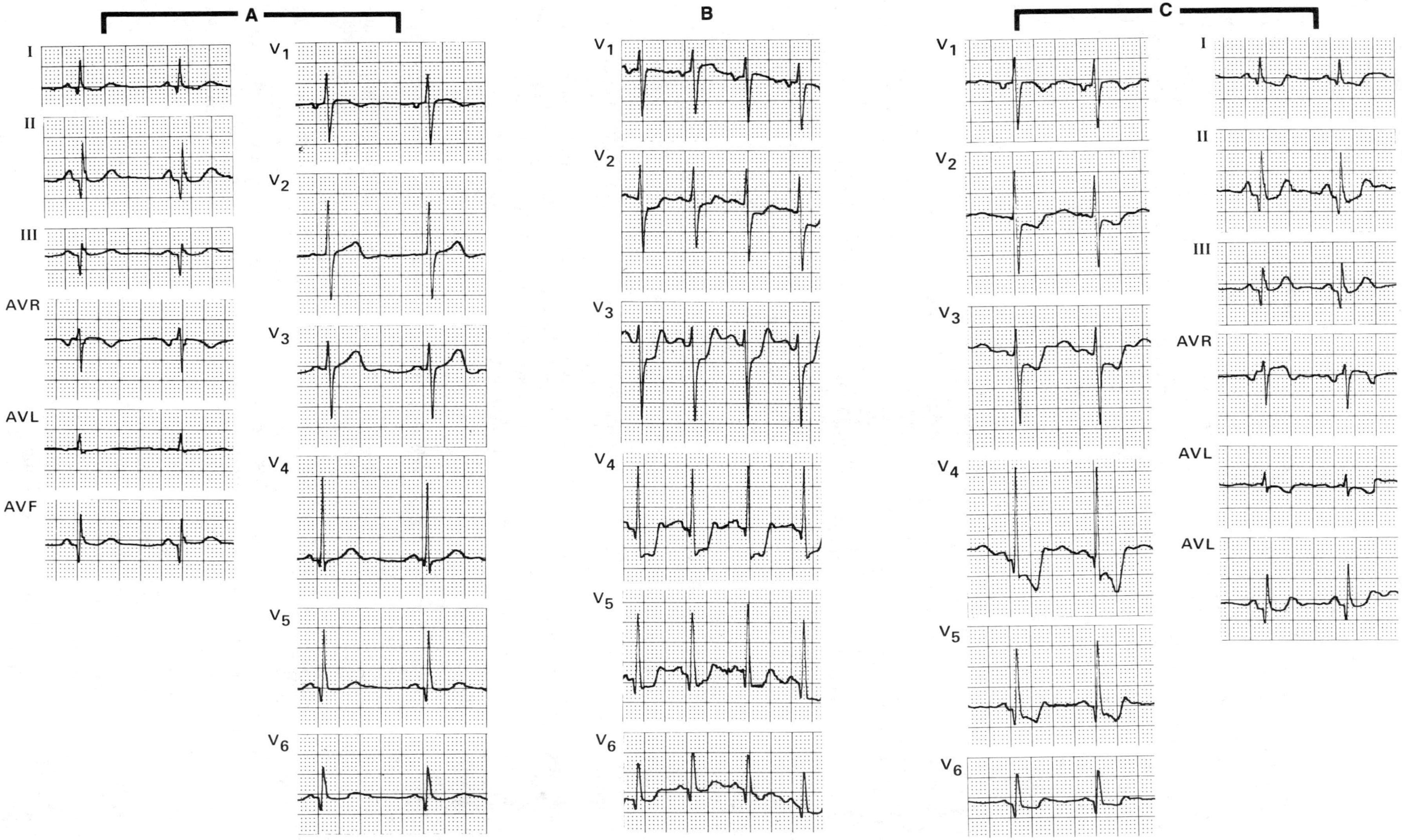

FIGURE 98-4 (A) Rest, (B) exercise, and (C) recovery ECGs in a 59-year-old man who underwent treadmill testing to evaluate increasingly severe angina pectoris in the 6 months preceding testing. Inferior myocardial infarction had occurred 6 years previously. The resting ECG demonstrates old inferolateral infarction and left atrial abnormality. Exercise was terminated by exertional angina pectoris at a peak heart rate of 110 beats per minute and peak workload of 6 METs. Ischemic ST-segment depression is noted during exercise in leads V_2–V_5, maximally (0.5 mV) in lead V_4. Postexertional T-wave inversion is noted in V_2–V_5 accompanied by ischemic ST-depression maximally 0.4 mV in lead V_4. Major lesions in the three major coronary arteries were surgically bypassed. The patient had been largely asymptomatic and without recurrent infarction during the 6 years following initial infarction; an exercise test performed 6 months previously demonstrated similar ST-segment abnormalities at a peak heart rate of 145 and peak workload of 9 METs. Beta blockers were withdrawn 72 h prior to testing.

pain in patients admitted to hospital for unstable angina pectoris (myocardial infarction ruled out).

The use of "submaximal" exercise testing which is discontinued upon attainment of an arbitrary heart rate or workload is often predicated on the mistaken assumption that such testing is safer than symptom-limited testing. On the contrary, patients with the most serious underlying cardiac disease are those most likely to experience marked exercise-induced myocardial ischemia and complex ventricular ectopic activity at a relatively low heart rate, e.g., below 75 to 85 percent of age-predicted maximum. *There is no arbitrary submaximal heart rate below which serious ischemic, mechanical, and electrical abnormalities are absent.*

Angina Pectoris

The distinction between angina pectoris and other kinds of chest pain is often clarified by close questioning of patients during exercise testing. Patients should be encouraged to continue exercise to the point where angina increases to moderate severity, i.e., 3 on a scale of 4.

Dyspnea and Fatigue

Although limiting dyspnea and fatigue are seemingly subjective, the peak heart rate and workload associated with these limiting symptoms are highly reproducible.[16,17] Close observation and encouragement of patients are necessary to assure that dyspnea and fatigue are truly limiting.

Leg Fatigue, Claudication, Joint Pain

Limitation of effort due to peripheral vascular disease or orthopedic abnormalities precludes measurement of the peak cardiac response to exercise. The pretest history will usually disclose these abnormalities. It is often clinically important to determine whether patients' limitations are primarily cardiac or noncardiac in origin.

Blood Pressure

Blood pressure should be measured at the end of each 3-min stage of exercise and at 1-m intervals when the blood pressure fails to increase by 10 mmHg compared to an earlier stage of exercise. A fall of 10 mmHg in systolic pressure compared to an earlier stage of exercise or rest is an indication to terminate the test. A falling pressure during exercise may indicate severe ischemic left ventricular dysfunction, especially if it is accompanied by angina pectoris or occurs at a low workload.[18] In contrast, an exercise-induced fall in pressure in a patient receiving a beta blocker or one which occurs only at a high workload and heart rate, especially in the absence of angina pectoris, may have little functional or prognostic significance.

For practical purposes, an "excessive" blood pressure, i.e., greater than 280 mmHg, is rarely the sole indication to cease exercise and has not been associated with cardiac complications of exercise testing.

ECG Abnormalities

ST-Segment Depression

Flat or downsloping exercise-induced ST-segment depression of 0.1 mV or more compared to rest, especially if accompanied by angina, is considered diagnostic of myocardial ischemia. If the test is being performed to evaluate prognosis or functional capacity, i.e., to quantitate myocardial ischemia, it is important to continue effort until the onset of limiting symptoms, a fall in systolic pressure, or the onset of potentially serious ventricular arrhythmia. It is prudent to terminate exercise upon the appearance of marked ischemic ST-segment depression of 0.3 mV or more.

Ventricular Ectopic Activity

The appearance of three or more consecutive PVCs, i.e., ventricular tachycardia, is a well-accepted although infrequent cause of exercise test termination. Premature termination of exercise because of putatively "malignant" arrhythmias such as bigeminy or couplets may not contribute to test safety, especially since most episodes of ventricular tachycardia occur after, not during, exercise.

Cardiac Signs

The flushed skin and warm perspiration observed during middle stages of exercise are succeeded at near-maximal effort by a gray coloration and a cold, clammy touch. These findings indicate a symptom-limited or even "supramaximal" performance. A *staggering gait, mental confusion, or glazed facies* reflect critical cerebrovascular insufficiency. These signs rarely occur if the patient is closely observed and the blood pressure properly monitored.

Anticipated Results of Exercise Testing

Exercise testing discloses three major kinds of abnormalities: (1) myocardial ischemia, (2) left ventricular dysfunction, and (3) ventricular ectopic activity. Important relationships exist between these: exercise-induced myocardial ischemia manifested by ST-segment displacement and/or angina pectoris is often accompanied by a poor exercise tolerance which reflects exercise-induced left ventricular dysfunction.[6,7] Exercise-induced ventricular ectopic activity is more frequent and complex in patients with significant resting and/or exercise-induced left ventricular wall motion abnormalities than in those without such abnormalities.[19,20]

The clinician must realize that there is no such thing as a "positive" or "negative" test—all three primary test abnormalities lie on a continuum of functional severity. This is true even for apparent dichotomies such as the presence or absence of exercise-induced angina pectoris or ischemic ST-segment depression. The clinical significance of these abnormalities is significantly modified by the heart rate, blood pressure, and workload at which they occur and at which the test is terminated. In general, prognosis is better in patients whose ischemic ST-segment depression and/or angina pectoris occur at a relatively high heart rate and workload.[2–5]

Myocardial Ischemia

Exercise-Induced "Ischemic" ST-Segment Depression

The most widely used ECG criterion for exercise-induced myocardial ischemia is 0.1 mV or more of flat or downsloping ST-segment depression at 0.08 s after the J point. This criterion represents an optimal trade-off between diagnostic sensitivity and specificity.[21] The configuration and extent of ischemic ST-segment depression have diagnostic and prognostic significance: ST-segment depression which is marked, i.e., 0.2 mV or more flat or downsloping, appearing in many leads and accompanied by T-wave inversion, is more serious than an upsloping ST-segment configuration appearing in a single lead and unaccompanied by T-wave inversion.[22,23]

The clinical significance of ischemic ST-segment abnormalities is also modified by the *functional* accompaniments (heart rate[24] and workload[25]) at which they appear, whether they are accompanied by exercise-induced angina[26] or hypotension,[27] the peak heart rate and workload which is achieved,[28] and their persistence during recovery.[29] For example, only ST-segment depression of 0.2 mV or occurring at a heart rate of less than 135 was found to be prognostically significant in postinfarction patients undergoing symptom-limited exercise testing 3 weeks after infarction. ST-segment depression of 0.2 mV or more occurring at a heart rate of 135 or over was not prognostically significant.[30] Similarly, exercise-induced angina pectoris had no independent prognostic significance apart from its association with exercise-induced ST-segment depression.

Most research on exercise testing has addressed the question of whether the exercise test predicts the presence or absence of disease as assessed by coronary arteriography. Most such studies have been cross-sectional in nature, i.e., the relation between the exercise test and the coronary arteriogram is established at one point in time. While cross-sectional studies have helped elucidate the relation between anatomic disease and exercise test results, they have largely failed to document the outcome of patients with narrowings in two or more coronary arteries: such a finding is simply assumed to be "significant." However, the extent of coronary artery lesions bears only a rough relation to symptomatic limitation or prognosis, i.e., the risk of myocardial infarction or death. This relation is too imprecise to be of much value in the management of the individual patient unless exercise-induced angina pectoris is so severe as to constitute an adequate basis for performing CABG surgery or coronary angioplasty. In this instance, the coronary angiogram is used to localize the lesions for the surgeon or coronary angioplasty operator, rather than as a test to determine whether these procedures are indicated. In other words, exercise testing is more useful for identifying functionally and prognostically important myocardial ischemia, irrespective of the number of affected coronary arteries, than for predicting the number of vessels which are affected.[2–4]

Hence, the appropriate clinical question is not whether the exercise test predicts the anatomy, but whether the anatomy predicts the outcome. Prognosis is the true "gold standard." In the few reports in which longitudinal follow-up has been performed in patients who have undergone coronary arteriography and exercise testing, the exercise test results have correlated well with prognosis. Indeed, prognosis is more closely related to clinical and exercise test characteristics than to the number of diseased coronary arteries.[4]

Reliance upon an *anatomic* rather than a *physiologic* standard of performance has tended to disparage the clinical value of exercise testing. In the anatomic context, an exercise test is "falsely negative" if ischemic ST-segment depression and other abnormalities are absent in patients with one or more coronary artery lesions. Similarly, patients with exercise test abnormalities in the absence of coronary artery lesions are said to have "falsely positive" tests. However, the clinical significance of falsely negative and falsely positive responses to exercise depends on the extent of *functional impairment* which accompanies these responses. For example, if peak treadmill heart rate and workload are high, patients with falsely negative tests have a good prognosis despite coronary lesions. Conversely, patients with falsely positive ST-segment responses to exercise may experience congestive heart failure, angina pectoris, or cardiac death even in the absence of coronary artery lesions: Falsely positive exercise tests are often an early marker of progressive myocardial disease.[31]

Falsely negative tests, i.e., absence of "ischemic" ST-segment depression despite "significant" coronary lesions, reflect both anatomic and functional conditions. Anatomic explanations include disease in single vessels,[32] especially in vessels such as the left circumflex which supply electrically silent areas of myocardium, and vessels supplying infarcted myocardial segments which are incapable of generating "ischemic" ST-segment abnormalities.[33] Functional reasons include a level of stress inadequate to elicit myocardial ischemia. This may reflect left ventricular dysfunction, poor motivation, and termination of a test short of limiting cardiac symptoms, or be due to noncardiac limitations to exercise, e.g., orthopedic or pulmonary disease or the effect of drugs such as beta blockers, calcium antagonists, and nitrates, which ameliorate myocardial ischemia.

Reasons for falsely positive tests, i.e., "ischemic" ST-segment depression occurring in the absence of "significant" coronary lesions, include a variety of conditions resulting in *myocardial fibrosis* (myocarditis, left ventricular hypertrophy); abnormal myocardial metabolism; the effects of *drugs*, especially digitalis; and *electrolyte abnormalities*, especially hypokalemia; and *intraventricular conduction abnormalities* such as the Wolff-Parkinson-White syndrome and left bundle branch block. Most of these conditions produce resting ST-segment abnormalities, but falsely positive ischemic ST-segment abnormalities may appear only during or after exercise.

Utilized for the purpose of functional and prognostic assessment, exercise testing is an extremely valuable guide to the management of patients with ischemic heart disease. Except in patients with unstable angina pectoris or heart failure, exercise testing should be routinely performed before coronary arteriography. In patients who achieve a heart rate of 160 or more or enter the fourth stage of the Bruce test (equivalent to 13 METs), the annual mortality is less than 1 percent, irrespective of the extent of ST-segment depression or the number of coronary arteries which are found to be narrowed at arteriography.[2] Attainment of the third stage of the Bruce test with less than 0.1 mV ischemic ST-segment depression is similarly associated with an annual mortality of less than 1 percent.[4] It is in these very low risk patients that it is most difficult to demonstrate the beneficial effects of medical or surgical therapy on prognosis. Hence, coronary arteriography can generally be avoided in patients whose exercise test performance indicates a very good prognosis.

Exercise testing is often helpful in indicating the need for coronary artery surgery or angioplasty in patients who have undergone coronary arteriography. Among patients with three-vessel disease and well-preserved left ventricular function, those with a high treadmill capacity have a nearly normal prognosis while those with a low capacity have a poorer prognosis (Fig. 98-5). Similarly, the prognosis of ischemic ST-segment depression depends on the extent of mechanical impairment, i.e., limitation of treadmill capacity, which accompanies it (Fig. 98-6).

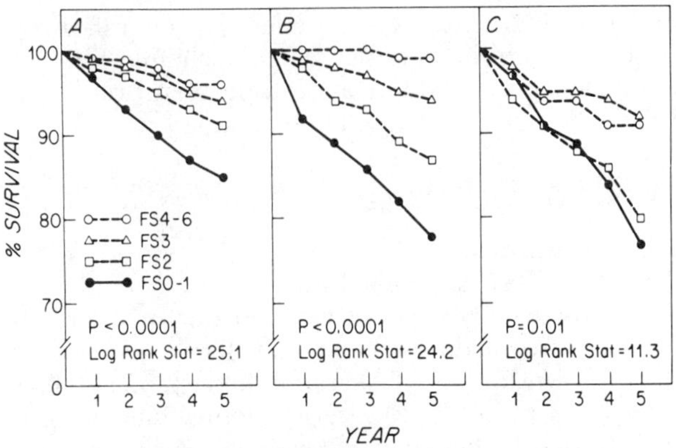

FIGURE 98-6 Final exercise stage (FS) and prognosis according to extent of ischemic ST-segment depression. For any extent of ischemic ST-segment depression survival is directly related to the final stage of treadmill exercise (Bruce protocol). (*From D. A. Weiner, T. J. Ryan, C. H. McCabe, B. R. Chaitman, L. T. Sheffield, J. C. Ferguson, L. D. Fisher, and F. Tristani, Prognostic Importance of a Clinical Profile and Exercise Test in Medically Treated Patients with Coronary Artery Disease, J. Am. Coll. Cardiol., 3:772–779, 1984. Reprinted with permission from the American College of Cardiology and the author.*)

FIGURE 98-5 Final exercise stage (FS) and prognosis. Survival at 4 years is directly related to the final stage of treadmill exercise (Bruce protocol) attained by patients undergoing exercise testing and coronary arteriography in the CASS study. (*From D. A. Weiner, T. J. Ryan, C. H. McCabe, B. R. Chaitman, L. T. Sheffield, J. C. Ferguson, L. D. Fisher, and F. Tristani, Prognostic Importance of a Clinical Profile and Exercise Test in Medically Treated Patients with Coronary Artery Disease, J. Am. Coll. Cardiol., 3:772–779, 1984. Reprinted with permission from the American College of Cardiology and the author.*)

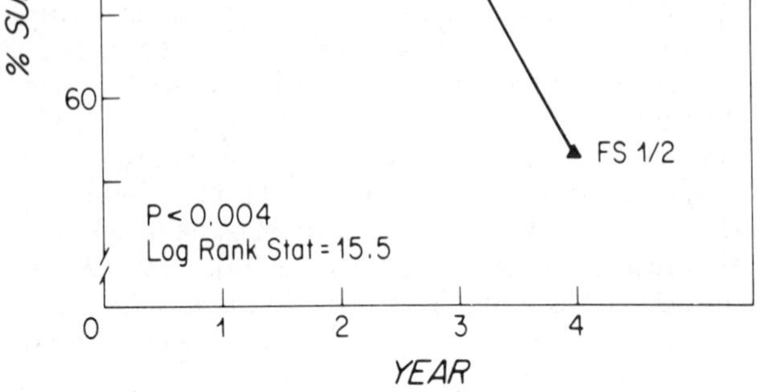

Exercise-Induced ST-Segment Elevation

This usually occurs in one of two settings: (1) in ECG leads demonstrating Q waves at rest, reflecting wall motion abnormalities and/or periinfarctional ischemia;[34,35] and (2) in ECG leads reflecting very severe, i.e., transmural exercise-induced myocardial ischemia associated with critically severe, fixed coronary stenoses[36] or coronary artery spasm. These responses are ordinarily observed in leads V_1 and aV_L.[36] Exercise-induced ST-segment elevation occurs in 10 to 20 percent of patients with Prinzmetal's angina. It is observed in the same leads which demonstrate ST-segment elevation during spontaneous attacks of angina pectoris.

Left Ventricular Dysfunction

The peak exercise workload attained during symptom-limited exercise testing is a clinically important measure of functional limitation due to cardiac or noncardiac conditions such as obesity, orthopedic or pulmonary vascular disease, general debility, or deconditioning. In the absence of these noncardiac conditions, a low peak exercise workload during symptom-limited testing usually represents one or more of the following: (1) "fixed" left ventricular dysfunction resulting from infarction or other myocardial disease, (2) exercise-induced myocardial ischemia, and (3) the functional consequences of valvular or pericardial disease. The functional capacity

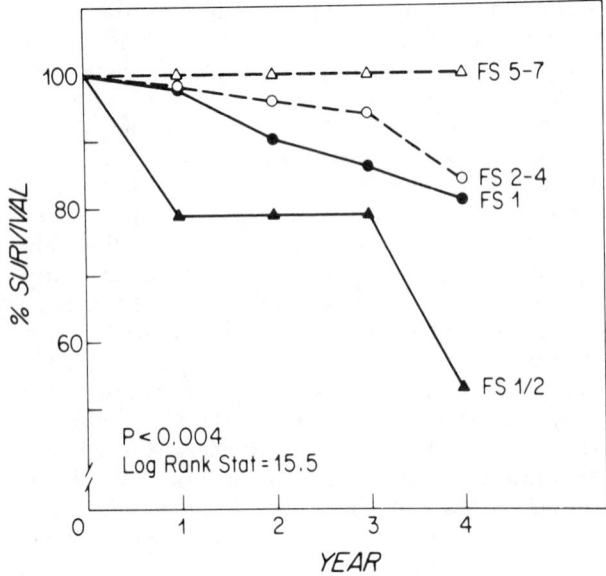

therefore provides an integrated measure of exercise impairment which is useful in evaluating the need for and the response to medical and surgical therapy.

Exercise-induced hypotension, which usually reflects severe ischemic left ventricular dysfunction in patients with chronic ischemic heart disease, has a different mechanism and a different prognostic implication in the postinfarction patient. Depression of peak exercise heart rate during the first 7 weeks after myocardial infarction (MI) contributes to exercise-induced hypotension and to the diminished peak workload observed during this interval.[17] A decreasing frequency of exercise hypotension and an increase in functional capacity—both of which occur spontaneously in the first 7 weeks after infarction—reflect an increase in the peak exercise heart rate.[17] It is important, therefore, not to equate exercise-induced hypotension during the early post-MI testing with severe ischemia, for it is largely a nonspecific response of little independent prognostic importance.

An abnormally low peak exercise heart rate, i.e., less than 95th percentile for age, is known as *chronotropic incompetence.*[37] Many patients with this abnormality have occult left ventricular dysfunction manifested by a diminished peak workload. Prognosis is relatively poor, especially in the absence of ischemic abnormalities such as ST-segment depression or angina pectoris.[38]

Exercise testing is helpful in assessing the symptomatic response to CABG surgery, coronary angioplasty, antianginal medical therapy, and exercise training. Such testing is primarily useful for assessing the functional consequences of such therapy rather than for its prognostic implication. It is not surprising that exercise testing following CABG surgery and coronary angioplasty has relatively little prognostic value, for most of the prognostic information is already established on the basis of the coronary angiogram and left ventriculogram, the number of vessels treated, and the presence or absence of myocardial infarction in the perioperative procedure period.[39,40]

Ventricular Ectopic Activity

The frequency, complexity, and clinical significance of exercise-induced ventricular arrhythmia reflect the clinical severity of underlying heart disease, especially the extent of regional wall motion abnormalities and global left ventricular dysfunction.[19,20] In individuals with known or suspected heart disease, the prevalence of PVCs at rest, during, and following exercise is as high as 40, 60, and 80 percent, respectively.[41] Couplets and ventricular tachycardia and other "complex" forms of PVCs are preferentially enhanced by exercise compared to unifocal or "simple" PVCs.[42] The prevalence and reproducibility of PVCs increase when exercise is carried to a symptom-limited maximum as opposed to a "submaximal" heart rate.[43]

Treadmill testing is less sensitive than ambulatory electrocardiography for the diagnosis of PVCs but complex arrhythmias noted on exercise tests are usually present on ambulatory electrocardiograms.[42] The absence of treadmill-induced PVCs is no guarantee of the absence of PVCs on ambulatory electrocardiography, however.[42]

Exercise-induced ventricular arrhythmia is not predictive of cardiac events, especially in asymptomatic individuals.[44] In patients with manifest ischemic heart disease, exercise-induced PVCs have demonstrated independent prognostic significance in some studies[45] but not in others.[46] Even "complex" PVCs recorded on exercise ECGs may have little independent prognostic significance in post-myocardial-infarction patients who are free of clinically significant left ventricular dysfunction.[47]

Complications of Exercise Testing

Serious complications of exercise testing are relatively infrequent: death rates range from 1/10,000 to 1/50,000 tests.[48] Nonfatal myocardial infarction is a much less frequent complication of exercise testing, approximately 1/100,000 tests.[49]

The most important single contributor to test safety is *patient selection,* i.e., the clinical severity of underlying heart disease. In general, patients with clinically manifest left ventricular dysfunction, clinically severe angina pectoris, and a history of cardiac syncope are at substantially higher risk for complications of exercise testing than patients without these abnormalities. The clinician's primary obligation is to assure that the diagnostic and prognostic information to be obtained from exercise testing outweighs the potential risks, especially in clinically high-risk patient subsets.

After patient selection, the safety of exercise testing is most dependent upon the early detection of incipient left ventricular failure. As noted above, exercise-induced pump failure is reflected in a falling systolic pressure and/or cerebrovascular insufficiency manifested by a staggering gait or mental confusion.

The third line of defense in assuring the safety of exercise testing is adequate provision for prompt cardiac resuscitation in the event of exercise-induced cardiac arrest. Testing of patients who are perceived to be at high risk, e.g., 10 to 14 or less days after acute myocardial infarction, requires the presence of a physician. Specially trained nurses or physicians' assistants have increasingly taken on the role of exercise test supervision in lower risk patients. Experienced nonphysician personnel perform effectively in all aspects of exercise testing, including immediate and appropriate responses to potentially serious cardiac abnormalities arising in the course of exercise testing. Policies which reserve exercise testing to physicians usually have a historical rather than a medical basis. It is axiomatic that defibrillators must be kept in working order and that crash carts must be fully stocked with appropriate medications. As with other aspects of exercise test laboratory supervision, these functions are best carried out by specially trained nurses or physicians' assistants.

Evaluation of Patients with Clinically Manifest Ischemic Heart Disease

General Considerations

The principal syndromes of ischemic heart disease include: chronic stable angina pectoris, unstable angina pectoris (myocardial infarction ruled out), documented myocardial infarction, status postcoronary angioplasty, and status post-CABG surgery. Management of these diverse clinical syndromes fundamentally involves evaluation of prognosis, assessment of functional capacity, and reassurance of patients regarding their ability to resume their customary physical activity such as occupational work. Although these aspects of management are often treated as separate issues, in reality all reflect the clinician's ability to assess the extent of myocardial ischemia and left ventricular dysfunction and to provide a treatment program which minimizes the impact of these on prognosis and functional capacity.

Exercise testing has important diagnostic, prognostic, and therapeutic applications to these management issues. For example, much of the disability resulting from acute myocardial infarction reflects patients' uncertainty about prognosis and the safe limits for physical activity.[50,51] Even those with an excellent prognosis, no cardiac symptoms, and a well-preserved functional capacity may needlessly restrict their physical activities. Exercise testing, performed within 3 weeks of the acute clinical event, provides explicit reassurance to patients about their capacity to resume their customary activities with safety.[52] This reassurance results from successful completion of the exercise test and from the physician's explanation of the implications of the test results for subsequent management, including the need for further diagnostic evaluation and treatment and for resumption of customary activity such as return to work.

Evaluation of Prognosis

This is the cornerstone of management in ischemic heart disease. Prognosis reflects the extent of myocardial ischemia and left ventricular dysfunction resulting from myocardial infarction and/or myocardial ischemia. Clinical heart failure and medically unresponsive angina pectoris portend a poor prognosis in patients with ischemic heart disease. Exercise testing is not required to establish this fact and the risk of such testing may outweigh the benefits.

In patients without clinically evident congestive heart failure or myocardial ischemia, exercise testing may disclose prognostically important *latent* left ventricular dysfunction and/or myocardial ischemia. Exercise testing performed alone or in conjunction with radionuclide imaging techniques has proven more sensitive than coronary arteriography for the prediction of subsequent cardiac events in patients with chronic stable angina pectoris[4] and in those recovering from myocardial infarction.[53,54]

The clinical characteristics of the population to which the test is applied are a crucial consideration in the use of any specialized test, including the exercise test.[55,56] What is most important to the clinician is the *predictive value* of a "positive" or "negative" test, i.e., the possibility that a patient with an abnormal test will develop a subsequent cardiac event such as infarction or death which might be prevented by timely therapy. It is also important to quantitate the risk of subsequent cardiac events in patients with normal tests, for the risk of subsequent cardiac events in such patients may be so low that there is little realistic possibility for improvement with medical or surgical therapy. For example, in post-myocardial-infarction patients the risk of subsequent cardiac events within the first year (death, reinfarction, CABG surgery) almost never exceeds 50 percent, even in those classified as "high risk" based upon markedly abnormal exercise electrocardiograms,[57] radionuclide ventriculograms,[58] thallium perfusion scintigrams,[53] and coronary arteriograms.[59] In patients with "low-risk" test responses, the risk is as low as 5 to 10 percent.

Functional Evaluation

Assessment of Functional Severity of Heart Disease

Quantitation of the extent of functional impairment by means of symptom-limited exercise testing often obviates unnecessary cardiac catheterization and/or coronary angiography. This is especially true in patients with chronic valvular disease such as mitral stenosis and insufficiency and aortic regurgitation. The exercise test performance is often found to be markedly diminished in patients with few symptoms, reflecting a progressive voluntary limitation of physical activity in these patients. Conversely, the exercist test performance is often found to be well preserved in patients who report severe symptoms.[60] When disparities exist between symptoms and exercise test performance, the latter usually correlates better than the former with abnormalities at cardiac catheterization.[61] Similarly, exercise testing is often required to determine the functional severity of angiographically demonstrated coronary artery disease, especially when the anatomic disease is unexpectedly mild. There are few circumstances in which exercise testing should not precede coronary angiography in patients with stable chronic ischemic heart disease.

A wide variety of conditions diminish the effort tolerance of patients with ischemic heart disease, including exposure to cold[62] and cigarette smoke,[63] ingestion of food,[64] and the performance of static (isometric) effort.[65] Exposure to psychological stress and sexual activity may also precipitate angina pectoris in susceptible individuals.[66,67] It is impractical to simulate these conditions in the exercise laboratory. A practical alternative for assessing the capacity of patients to tolerate these conditions is to elicit a peak cardiovascular response (heart rate, double product, workload) by means of symptom-limited exercise testing. Symptom-limited treadmill or cycle exercise reveals an incidence of ischemic and arrhythmic abnormalities which is similar to that observed when such testing is combined with these environmental and psychological stressors.[62,68]

In practical terms, myocardial ischemia is more likely to occur during a symptom-limited test than during most customary activities. Patients who are free of prognostically or functionally significant abnormalities during symptom-limited exercise testing do not require restriction of their physical activity. In patients who *do* manifest significant ischemic abnormalities, the first priority of management is provision of therapy which may improve functional status and/or prognosis. Although restriction of physical activity may decrease symptoms in such patients, it provides no guarantee against subsequent cardiac events.

Exercise Prescription

The role of exercise training for improving prognosis in patients with ischemic heart disease has waned with the advent of potent medical and surgical therapy. However, exercise training is effective in increasing functional capacity and in diminishing cardiac symptoms, even in relatively high-risk coronary patients.[69–71] The exercise training intensity is usually based upon a training heart rate which approaches 70 to 85 percent of the peak heart rate achieved with symptom-limited exercise testing.[72] An even lower intensity of exercise training is effective in augmenting functional capacity within the first 3 months after clinically uncomplicated myocardial infarction.[73,74] Exercise training may safely commence as soon as 3 weeks after infarction in clinically low-risk patients and under certain circumstances may be carried out at home.[74] Since most episodes of training-induced cardiac arrest occur at heart rates exceeding the prescribed range,[75] portable heart rate monitors are helpful in regulating the intensity of exercise training within the prescribed range.[74]

Evaluation of Individuals with Suspected Ischemic Heart Disease—Asymptomatic Individuals

The primary goal of exercise testing of asymptomatic persons is to institute prophylactic therapy in those who are identified as having a high risk for future cardiac events. However, this goal is unfulfilled on every count, since (1) exercise testing is insensitive for the detection of "significant" coronary artery lesions in these individuals;[76,77] (2) even in asymptomatic individuals with such lesions the rate of cardiac events is low;[78,79] and (3) neither medical nor surgical therapy is of proven benefit in improving the prognosis of persons with asymptomatic coronary artery disease. For example, in asymptomatic individuals with abnormal exercise test responses and one or more "significant" coronary lesions by arteriography, only one-quarter manifested overt signs of ischemic heart disease during the next 5 years.[79] The remaining 75 percent would be considered "falsely positive" responders if the coronary angiogram were considered as a "test result" and the development of ischemic heart disease were considered as an "event." Moreover, in most of these individuals the presenting manifestation of ischemic heart disease was angina pectoris rather than myocardial infarction or death.[79]

Although exercise testing has proved useful in identifying asymptomatic individuals with an increased risk of subsequent cardiac events, the proportion of these individuals is quite small. Even in the 1 percent of 2365 clinically healthy men who were identified as "high risk" on the basis of conventional risk factors and exercise test abnormalities, only 33 percent experienced angina pectoris, myocardial infarction, or cardiac death during the next 5 years.[80]

Only among individuals with one or more conventional risk factors was the risk of cardiac events increased by the presence of two or more exertional risk factors, including ischemic ST-segment depression of more than 0.1 mV, heart rate impairment of 10 percent or more, peak exercise duration less than 6 min (7 METs), and chest discomfort on maximal exertion.[80] Although the rate of cardiac events was higher in patients with two or more exertional risk factors than in those with fewer exertional risk factors (52 percent versus 39 percent), the proportion of patients with *either* response was less than 2 percent. Thus, specialized testing, including exercise testing, radionuclide imaging techniques, and coronary arteriography plays a small role in identifying asymptomatic individuals with an increased risk of cardiac events.

Exercise testing to provide "clearance" for sedentary middle-aged persons to undertake exercise training is a related issue. Exercise testing is ineffective for this purpose, because of the very low rate of exercise-induced deaths: 1 in 396,000 hours of jogging in one study.[81] Although this rate is seven times the estimated death rate from ischemic heart disease during more sedentary activities, it is still too low to justify a policy of routine exercise testing before exercise training in asymptomatic individuals—identifying one potential victim of an exercise-related death would require between 2,000 and 13,000 screening exercise tests. Moreover, even among patients dying suddenly during exercise, as many as one-third manifested prior evidence of ischemic heart disease, e.g., angina or myocardial infarction on a resting electrocardiogram. This would have obviated the need for exercise testing to make the diagnosis of ischemic heart disease. Finally, the relative risk of jogging-induced death *decreases* as age increases, reflecting an increase in the number of deaths occurring during activities less vigorous than jogging.[81]

Evaluation of Chest Discomfort of Possible Ischemic Origin

Clinical characteristics of chest pain are good predictors of the extent of coronary artery disease. In patients with pain characterized as "nonischemic," "probable angina," and "definite angina," the prevalence of anatomic disease is 10 percent, 50 percent, and 90 percent, respectively.[82] If the primary objective of exercise testing is to establish the presence rather than the functional severity of disease, it is in patients with atypical chest pain that exercise testing is of greatest value.

References

1. Johnson, S.: "Lives of the Poets," 1779, cited in "Bartlett's Familiar Quotations," 14th ed., Little, Brown and Company, Boston, 1968, p. 428.
2. McNeer, J., Margolis, J. R., Lee, K. L., et al.: The Role of the Exercise Test in the Evaluation of Patients for Ischemic Heart Disease, *Circulation*, 57:64, 1978.
3. Podrid, P., Graboys, T. B., and Lown, B. L.: Prognosis of Medically Treated Patients with Coronary Artery Disease with Profound ST-segment Depression during Exercise Testing, *N. Engl. J. Med.*, 305:1111, 1981.
4. Weiner, D., Ryan, T. J., McCabe, C. H., et al.: Prognostic Importance of a Clinical Profile and Exercise Test in Medically Treated Patients with Coronary Artery Disease, *J. Am. Coll. Cardiol.*, 3:772, 1984.
5. Gohlke, H., Samek, L., Betz, P., and Roskamm, H.: Exercise Testing Provides Additional Prognostic Information in Angiographically Defined Subgroups of Patients with Coronary Artery Disease, *Circulation*, 68:979, 1983.
6. Pryor, D., Harrell, F. E., Jr., Lee, K. L., et al.: Prognostic Indicators from Radionuclide Angiography in Medically Treated Patients with Coronary Artery Disease, *Am. J. Cardiol.*, 53:18, 1984.
7. Higginbotham, M., Coleman, R. E., Jones, R. H., and Cobb, F. R.: Mechanism and Significance of a Decrease in Ejection Fraction during Exercise in Patients with Coronary Artery Disease and Left Ventricular Dysfunction at Rest, *J. Am. Coll. Cardiol.*, 3:88, 1984.
8. Upton, M., Rerych, S. K., Newman, G. E., Port, S., Cobb, F. R., and Jones, R. H.: Detecting Abnormalities in Left Ventricular Function during Exercise before Angina and ST-segment Depression, *Circulation*, 62:341, 1980.
9. Wicks, J., Sutton, J. R., Oldridge, N. B., and Jones, N. L.: Comparison of the Electrocardiographic Changes Induced by Maximum Exercise Testing with Treadmill and Cycle Ergometer, *Circulation*, 57:1066, 1978.
10. DeBusk, R., Valdez, R., Houston, N., and Haskell, W. L.: Cardiovascular Responses to Dynamic and Static Effort Soon after Myocardial Infarction. Application to Occupational Work Assessment, *Circulation*, 58:368, 1978.
11. Shaw, D., Crawford, M. H., Karliner, J. S., et al.: Armcrank Ergometry: A New Method for the Evaluation of Coronary Artery Disease, *Am. J. Cardiol.*, 33:801, 1974.
12. Hung, J., McKillop, J., Savin, W., et al.: Comparison of Cardiovascular Response to Combined Static-dynamic Effort, to Postprandial Dynamic Effort and to Dynamic Effort Alone in Patients with Chronic Ischemic Heart Disease, *Circulation*, 65:1043, 1982.
13. Ferguson, R., Cote, P., Bourassa, M. G., and Corbara, F.: Coronary Sinus Blood Flow during Isometric and Dynamic Exercise in Angina Pectoric Patients, *J. Cardiac. Rehab.*, 1:21, 1981.
14. Redwood, D., Rosing, D. R., Goldstein, R. E., Beiser, G. D., and Epstein, S. E.: Importance of the Design of an Exercise Protocol in the Evaluation of Patients with Angina Pectoris, *Circulation*, 43:618, 1971.
15. Chaitman, B., and Hanson, J.: Comparative Sensitivity and Specificity of Exercise Electrocardiographic Lead Systems, *Am. J. Cardiol.*, 47:1335, 1981.
16. Smokler, P., MacAlpin, R. N., Alvara, A., and Kattus, A. A.: Reproducibility of a Multistage Near Maximal Treadmill Test for Exercise Tolerance in Angina Pectoris, *Circulation*, 48:346, 1973.
17. Haskell, W., and DeBusk, R.: Cardiovascular Responses to Repeated Treadmill Exercise Testing Soon after Myocardial Infarction, *Circulation*, 60:1247, 1979.
18. Thomson, P., and Kelemen, M. H.: Hypotension Accompanying the Onset of Exertional Angina, *Circulation*, 52:28, 1975.
19. Crawford, M., O'Rourke, R. A., Ramakrishna, N., Henning, H., and Ross, J.: Comparative Effectiveness of Exercise Testing and Continuous Monitoring for Detecting Arrhythmias in Patients with Previous Myocardial Infarction, *Circulation*. 50:301, 1974.
20. Califf, R., McKinnis, R. A., McNeer, J. F., et al.: Prognostic Value of Ventricular Arrhythmias Associated with Treadmill Exercise Testing in Patients Studied with Cardiac Catheterization for Suspected Ischemic Heart Disease, *J. Am. Coll. Cardiol.*, 2:1060, 1983.
21. Martin, C., and McConahay, D. R.: Maximal Treadmill Exercise Electrocardiography. Correlations with Coronary Arteriography and Cardiac Hemodynamics, *Circulation*, 46:956, 1972.
22. Goldschlager, N., Selzer, A., and Cohn, K.: Treadmill Stress Tests as Indicators of Presence and Severity of Coronary Artery Disease, *Ann. Intern. Med.*, 85:277, 1976.
23. Ellestad, M., and Wan, M. K. C.: Predictive Implications of Stress Testing. Follow-up of 2700 Subjects after Maximum Stress Testing, *Circulation*, 51:363, 1975.
24. Bartel, A., Behar, V. S., Peter, R. H., Orgain, E. S., and Kong, Y.: Graded Exercise Stress Tests in Angiographically Documented Coronary Artery Disease, *Circulation*, 49:349, 1974.
25. Schneider, R., Seaworth, J. F., and Dohrmann, M. L.: Anatomic and Prognostic Implications of an Early Positive Treadmill Exercise Test, *Am. J. Cardiol.*, 50:682, 1982.
26. Cole, J., and Ellestad, M. H.: Significance of Chest Pain during Treadmill Exercise: Correlation with Coronary Events, *Am. J. Cardiol.*, 41:227, 1978.
27. Hamby, R., Davison, E. T., Hilsenrath, J., et al.: Functional and Anatomic Correlates of Markedly Abnormal Stress Tests, *J. Am. Coll. Cardiol.*, 3:1375, 1984.
28. Chaitman, R., Bourassa, M. G., Wagniart, P., Corbara, F., and Ferguson, R. S.: Improved Efficiency of Treadmill Exercise Testing Using a Multiple Lead ECG System and Basic Hemodynamic Exercise Response, *Circulation*, 57:71, 1978.
29. Weiner, D., McCabe, C. H., and Ryan, T. J.: Identification of Patients with Left Main and Three Vessel Coronary Disease with Clinical and Exercise Test Variables, *Am. J. Cardiol.*, 46:21, 1980.
30. DeBusk, R., Kraemer, H. C., and Nash, E.: Stepwise Risk Stratification Soon after Acute Myocardial Infarction, *Am. J. Cardiol.*, 52:1161, 1983.
31. Erikssen, J., Dale, J., Rootwelt, K., and Myhre, E.: False Suspicion of Coronary Heart Disease: A 7 Year Follow-up Study

of 36 Apparently Healthy Middle-aged Men, *Circulation,* 68:490, 1983.
32. Bartel, A., Behar, V. S., Peter, R. H., Orgain, E. S., and Kong, Y.: Graded Exercise Stress Tests in Angiographically Documented Coronary Artery Disease, *Circulation,* 49:348, 1974.
33. Kramer, N., Susmano, A., and Shekelle, R. B.: The "False Negative" Treadmill Exercise Test and Left Ventricular Function, *Circulation,* 57:763, 1978.
34. Chahine, R., Raizner, A. E., and Ishimoni, T.: The Clinical Significance of Exercise-Induced ST-Segment Elevation, *Circulation,* 54:209, 1976.
35. Dunn, R., Baily, I. K., Uren, R., and Kelly, D. T.: Exercise-Induced ST-segment Elevation. Correlation of Thallium-201 Myocardial Perfusion Scanning and Coronary Arteriography, *Circulation,* 61:989, 1980.
36. Dunn, R., Freedman, B., Kelly, D. T., Bailey, I. K., and McLaughlin, A.: A Predictor of Anterior Myocardial Ischemia and Left Anterior Descending Coronary Artery Disease, *Circulation,* 63:1357, 1981.
37. Ellestad, M.: "Stress Testing" (appendix), 2d ed., F. A. Davis, Philadelphia, 1980, p. 403.
38. Hammond, H., Kelly, T. L., and Froelicher, V.: Radionuclide Imaging Correlatives of Heart Rate Impairment during Maximal Exercise Testing, *J. Am. Coll. Cardiol.,* 2:826, 1983.
39. Lawrie, G., and Morris, G. C., Jr.: Factors Influencing Late Survival after Coronary Bypass Surgery, *Ann. Surg.,* 187:665, 1978.
40. Lawrie, G., Morris, G. C., Jr., Calhoon, J. H., et al.: Results of Coronary Bypass in 500 Patients at Least Ten Years after Operation, *Circulation,* 64(suppl. IV):IV–91, 1981.
41. Jelinek, M., and Lown, B.: Exercise Stress Testing for Exposure of Cardiac Arrhythmias, *Prog. Cardiovasc. Dis.,* 16:497, 1974.
42. Ryan, M., Lown, B., and Horn, H.: Comparison of Ventricular Ectopic Activity during 24-Hour Monitoring and Exercise Testing in Patients with Coronary Heart Disease, *N. Engl. J. Med.,* 292:224, 1975.
43. Sami, M., Kraemer, H., and DeBusk, R.: The Reproducibility of Exercise-induced Ventricular Arrhythmias following Myocardial Infarction, *Am. J. Cardiol.,* 43:724, 1979.
44. Froelicher, V., Jr., Thomas, M. M., Pillow, C., et al.: Epidemiologic Study of Asymptomatic Men Screened by Maximal Treadmill Testing for Latent Coronary Artery Disease, *Am. J. Cardiol.,* 34:770, 1974.
45. Udall, J., and Ellestad, M. H.: Predictive Implications of Ventricular Premature Contractions Associated with Treadmill Stress Testing, *Circulation,* 56:985, 1977.
46. Nair, C., Aronow, W. S., Sketch, M. H., et al.: Diagnostic and Prognostic Significance of Exercise-induced Premature Ventricular Complexes in Men and Women: A Four Year Follow-up, *J. Am. Coll. Cardiol.,* 1:1201, 1983.
47. DeBusk, R., Davidson, D., Houston, N., and Fitzgerald, J.: Serial Ambulatory Electrocardiography and Treadmill Exercise Testing following Uncomplicated Myocardial Infarction, *Am. J. Cardiol.,* 45:547, 1980.
48. Rochmis, P., and Blackburn, H.: A Survey of Procedures, Safety and Litigation Experience in Approximately 170,000 Tests, *JAMA,* 217:1061, 1971.
49. Stuart, R., and Ellestad, M. H.: National Survey of Exercise Stress Testing Facilities, *Chest,* 77:94, 1980.
50. Wishnie, H., Hackett, T. P., and Cassem, N. H.: Psychological Hazards of Convalescence following Myocardial Infarction, *JAMA,* 215:1292, 1971.
51. Klein, R., Dean, A., Willson, M., and Bogdonoff, M. D.: The Physician and Postmyocardial Infarction Invalidism, *JAMA,* 194:123, 1965.
52. Ewart, C., Taylor, C. B., Reese, L. B., and DeBusk, R. F.: The Effects of Early Post Infarction Exercise Testing on Self Perception and Subsequent Physical Activity, *Am. J. Cardiol.,* 51:1076, 1983.
53. Gibson, R., Watson, D. D., Craddock, G. B., et al.: Prediction of Cardiac Events after Uncomplicated Myocardial Infarction: A Prospective Study Comparing Predischarge Exercise Thallium-201 Scintigraphy and Coronary Angiography, *Circulation,* 68:321, 1983.
54. DeFeyter, P., van Eenige, M. J., Dighton, D. H., Visser, F. C., de Jong, J., and Roos, J. P.: Prognostic Value of Exercise Testing, Coronary Angiography and Left Ventriculography 6–8 Weeks after Myocardial Infarction, *Circulation,* 66:527, 1982.
55. Rifkin, R., and Hood, W. B.: Bayesian Analysis of Electrocardiographic Exercise Stress Testing, *N. Engl. J. Med.,* 297:681, 1977.
56. Diamond, G., and Forrester, J. S.: Analysis of Probability as an Aid to the Clinical Diagnosis of Coronary Artery Disease, *N. Engl. J. Med.,* 300:1350, 1979.
57. Theroux, P., Waters, D. D., Halphen, C., Debaisieux, J-C., and Mizgala, H. F.: Prognostic Value of Exercise Testing Soon after Myocardial Infarction, *N. Engl. J. Med.,* 301:341, 1979.
58. Corbett, J., Dehmer, G. J., Lewis, S. E., et al.: The Prognostic Value of Submaximal Exercise Testing with Radionuclide Ventriculography before Hospital Discharge in Patients with Recent Myocardial Infarction, *Circulation,* 64:535, 1981.
59. Taylor, G., Humphries, J. O., Mellits, E. D., et al.: Predictors of Clinical Course, Coronary Anatomy and Left Ventricular Function after Recovery from Acute Myocardial Infarction, *Circulation,* 62:960, 1980.
60. Parran, T., Hellerstein, H., Cohen, D., and Goldston, E.: Results of Studies at the Work Classification Clinic of the Cleveland Area Heart Society, in F. F. Rosenbaum and E. L. Belnap (eds.), "Work and the Heart," Paul B. Hoeber, Inc., New York, 1959, p. 330.
61. Patterson, J., Naughton, J., Pietras, R. J., and Gunnar, R. M.: Treadmill Exercise in Assessment of the Functional Capacity of Cardiac Patients with Cardiac Disease, *Am. J. Cardiol.,* 30:757, 1972.
62. Lassvik, C., and Areskog, N. H.: Angina Pectoris during Inhalation of Cold Air. Reactions to Exercise, *Br. Heart J.,* 43:661, 1980.
63. Aronow, W., and Cassidy, J.: Effect of Carbon Monoxide in Maximal Treadmill Exercise, *Ann Intern. Med.,* 83:469, 1975.
64. Goldstein, R., Redwood, D. R., Rosing, D. R., Beiser, G. D., and Epstein, S. E.: Alterations in the Circulatory Response to Exercise following a Meal and Their Relationship to Postprandial Angina Pectoris, *Circulation,* 44:90, 1971.
65. DeBusk, R., Pitts, W., Haskell, W. L., and Houston, N.: A Comparison of Cardiovascular Responses to Combined Static-dynamic and Dynamic Effort Alone in Patients with Chronic Ischemic Heart Disease, *Circulation,* 59:977, 1979.
66. Littler, W., Honour, A. J., Sleight, P., and Stott, F. D.: Direct Arterial Pressure to the Onset of Pain in Angina Pectoris, *Circulation,* 48:125, 1973.
67. Hellerstein, H., and Friedman, E. H.: Sexual Activity and the Postcoronary Patient, *Arch. Intern. Med.,* 125:987, 1970.
68. Taylor, C., Davidson, D. D., Houston, N., Agras, W. S., and DeBusk, R. F.: The Effect of a Standardized Psychological Stressor on the Cardiovascular Response to Physical Effort Soon after Uncomplicated Myocardial Infarction, *J. Psychosom. Res.,* 26:263, 1982.
69. Ferguson, R., Petitclerc, R., Choquette, G., et al.: Effect of Physical Training on Treadmill Exercise Capacity, Collateral Circulation and Progression of Coronary Disease, *Am. J. Cardiol.,* 34:764, 1974.
70. Paterson, D., Shepard, R. K., and Cunningham, D.: Effects of Physical Training on Cardiovascular Function following Myocardial Infarction, *J. Appl. Physiol.,* 47:482, 1979.
71. Lee, A., Ice, R., Blessey, R., et al.: Long-term Effects of Physical Training on Coronary Patients with Impaired Ventricular Function, *Circulation,* 60:1519, 1979.
72. Hellerstein, H., and Franklin, B. A.: Exercise Testing and Prescription, in H. K. Hellerstein and N. K. Wenger (eds.), "Rehabilitation of the Coronary Patient," John Wiley & Sons, New York, 1978, p. 149.
73. DeBusk, R., Houston, H., Haskell, W., Parker, M., and Fry,

G.: Exercise Training Soon after Myocardial Infarction, *Am. J. Cardiol.*, 44:1223, 1979.
74. Miller, N., Haskell, W. L., Berra, K., and DeBusk, R. F.: Home Versus Group Exercise Training for Increasing Functional Capacity after Myocardial Infarction, *Circulation*, 70:645, 1984.
75. Hossack, K., and Hartwig, R.: Cardiac Arrest Associated with Supervised Cardiac Rehabilitation, *J. Card. Rehab.*, 2:402, 1982.
76. Froelicher, V., Thompson, A. J., Wolthuis, R., et al.: Angiographic Findings in Asymptomatic Aircrewmen with Electrocardiographic Abnormalities, *Am. J. Cardiol.*, 39:32, 1977.
77. Borer, J., Brensike, J. F., Redwood, D. R., et al.: Limitations of the Electrocardiographic Response to Exercise in Predicting Coronary Artery Disease, *N. Engl. J. Med.*, 293:367, 1975.
78. Langou, R., Huang, E. K., Kelley, M. J., and Cohen, L. S.: Predictive Accuracy of Coronary Artery Calcification and Abnormal Exercise Test for Coronary Artery Disease in Asymptomatic Men, *Circulation*, 62:1196, 1980.
79. Hickman, J., Jr., Uhl, G. S., Cook, R. L., Engel, P. J., and Hopkirk, A.: A Natural History Study of Asymptomatic Coronary Disease, *Am. J. Cardiol.*, 45:422, 1980. (Abstract.)
80. Bruce, R., DeRouen, T. A., and Hossack, K. F.: Value of Maximal Exercise Tests in Risk Assessment of Primary Coronary Heart Disease in Healthy Men. Five Years' Experience of the Seattle Heart Watch Study. *Am. J. Cardiol.*, 46:371, 1980.
81. Thompson, P., Stern, M. P., Williams, P., Duncan, K., Haskell, W. L., and Wood, P. D.: Death during Jogging or Running. A Study of 18 Cases, *JAMA*, 242:1265, 1979.
82. Weiner, D., Ryan, T. J., McCabe, C. H., et al.: Correlations among History of Angina, ST-segment Response and Prevalence of Coronary Artery Disease in the Coronary Artery Surgery Study (CASS). *N. Engl. J. Med.*, 301:230, 1979.

99

Technique of QRS Signal Averaging

Paul F. Walter, M.D.
Scott J. Pollak, M.D.

We have seen that a family of powerful new techniques, both biomathematical and electronic are now available to extract the essential temporal pattern out of a variety of ordinarily variable noisy measures of physiologically important function.
Otto H. Schmitt, 1964[1,*]

A major problem in recording small, bioelectric cardiac signals is interference from extraneous noise. The purpose of signal averaging is to improve the signal-to-noise ratio of highly amplified bioelectric events. This technique allows detection of signals that are otherwise masked by random noise. Ventricular late potentials, His bundle activation, and sinus node potentials have been recorded from the body surface.[2–4] In recent years, ventricular late potentials have received major attention, and they will serve as the focus of the remaining discussion.

Principles of Signal Averaging

Noise that conceals the small electrical events of the heart has three principal sources: (1) physiologic noise from skeletal muscles; (2) electronic noise from electrodes and amplifiers; and (3) 60-Hz noise with higher frequency harmonics.[5] The problem of noise contamination is partially solved when signal averaging techniques are used.[1,6] This technique averages together multiple samples of a repeating waveform and randomly occurring noise is diminished. Several requirements must be met before signal averaging can reduce noise: (1) The signal of interest and the noise must be independent in time; (2) characteristics of both noise and signal must remain independent throughout the signal processing; (3) the noise should be random with a Gaussian distribution; and (4) a suitable reference time must be found so that the computer can average together multiple points of a repeating waveform.[6,7]

Intercostal muscle noise is easily averaged to zero, since respiration is not synchronous with the cardiac cycle. Isolation amplifiers and proper grounding reduce 60-Hz interference from power lines. Ectopic ventricular beats produce artifact and must be rejected by the computer before averaging. The reduction of noise is primarily dependent upon the number of cycles to be summed. The signal-to-noise ratio improves in proportion to the square root of the number of averaged cycles.[5] Following signal averaging, the electrocardiogram is high-pass filtered to reduce low-frequency signals contained in the QRS complex and ST segment.

Recording Technique and Signal Processing

Signal averaging can be performed at the patient's bedside. From the patient's perspective, the recording process is similar to that of a scalar electrocar-

*Reproduced with the permission from the publisher and author.

diogram (ECG), and recording time is less than 12 min. The signal processing, hardware, and methods used at our institution are identical to those described by Simson.[2] Bipolar X, Y, and Z leads are recorded. The bipolar lead signals are amplified, prefiltered, and digitally sampled into a microcomputer. Each bipolar lead is subsequently signal averaged after passing through a template recognition program to reject ectopic or excessively noisy beats. Approximately 200 beats are averaged. A reference time for the averaging process is derived from a bipolar lead at a point where the QRS complex slope is rapid. Each averaged lead is then high-pass filtered with a 25-Hz bidirectional filter. The filtered signals for the three leads are combined into a vector magnitude, $\sqrt{x^2 + y^2 + z^2}$.

Conventional high-pass filters may ring or create an artifact after a large-amplitude signal. Impulse ringing impairs the detection of low-amplitude potentials after the QRS complex. Simson eliminated this problem by developing a bidirectional digital filter.[2] This filter processes the signal forward in time until the middle of the QRS complex, and then processes backward in time until the same midpoint of the QRS complex is reached.

Value of QRS Signal Averaging

Ventricular Late Potentials

The initial clinical application of signal averaging was recording the His-Purkinje ECG.[8] Emphasis changed in 1978 when Berbari et al. recorded low-level potentials during the ST segment of a surface averaged lead in a canine myocardial infarction model.[9] These late potentials were thought to originate from areas of delayed ventricular activation. At this point, interest in recording late potentials in patients with ventricular tachycardia began to increase.

Delayed ventricular activation has been recorded directly from infarcted and ischemic myocardium in animals and humans.[10–13] In patients with recurrent ventricular tachycardia, fragmented ventricular activation may extend beyond the T wave and herald the onset of ventricular tachycardia.[14] Most patients with a ventricular aneurysm demonstrate delayed depolarization in the subendocardial margin of the aneurysm, and the extent and severity of signal fragmentation is greatest in those with recurrent ventricular tachycardia.[15] The most plausible source of late potentials recorded from the body surface is delayed, fragmented electrocardiographic activity (Fig. 99-1).[16] Late potentials correlate temporally with delayed endocardial electrograms, and may disappear after subendocardial resection for control of ventricular tachycardia.[7] Endocardial tissue removed at surgery shows muscle bundles consisting of normal and abnormal cells that are widely separated by dense connective tissue.[17] Low-amplitude, fragmented extracellular electrograms may result from the weak interconnection of muscle bundles, and the abnormal membrane properties of many of the surviving cells.

Using the technique developed by Simson, nearly all normal volunteers can be identified properly by using a combination of (1) filtered QRS duration less than 110 ms; and (2) voltages greater than 25 microvolts (μV) in the last 40 ms of the QRS (Fig. 99-2).[18] Serial recordings in normal subjects and patients with recurrent ventricular tachycardia show reproducible results.[19] Approximately 80 percent of patients with recurrent ventricular tachycardia after myocardial infarction have less than 25 μV of high-frequency voltage in the last 40 ms of the QRS (Fig. 99-3).[2,18] This low-level signal, a late potential, has

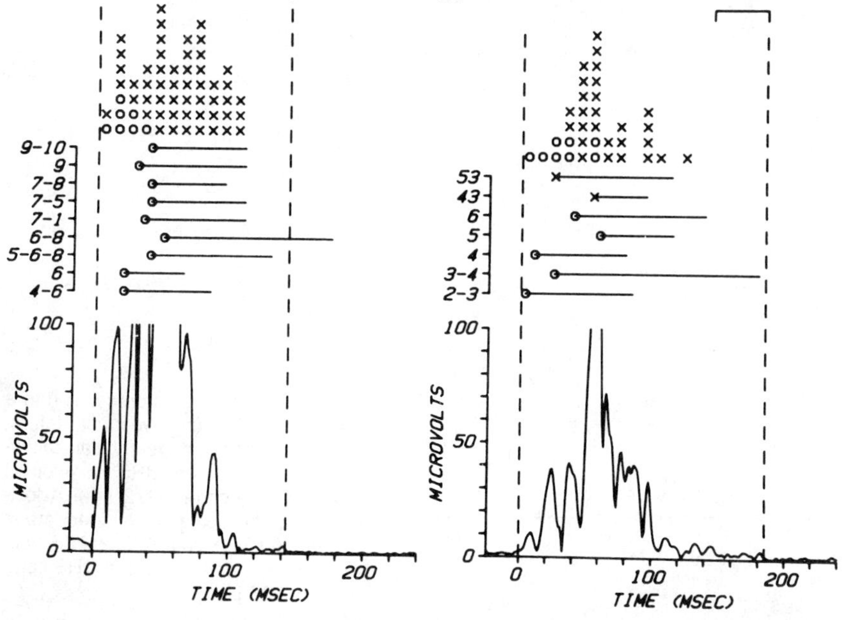

FIGURE 99-1 (*A* and *B*) Temporal relation between epicardial and endocardial electrograms and the filtered QRS complex in two patients with ventricular tachycardia. The brackets indicate the last 40 ms of the filtered QRS complex. The symbols on top show the timing of the electrograms. An X represents an epicardial electrogram and a circle represents an endocardial electrogram. Fragmented electrograms are depicted with a line which indicates the onset and duration of the electrograms. During the last 40 ms of the QRS complex, the low-amplitude body surface signal corresponds to fragmented electrograms. Normal electrograms are seen at an earlier time in the QRS complex. (*From M. B. Simson, W. J. Untereker, S. R. Spielman, et al., Relation between Late Potentials on the Body Surface and Directly Recorded Fragmented Electrograms in Patients with Ventricular Tachycardia, Am. J. Cardiol., 51:105, 1983. Reproduced with permission from the publisher and author.*)

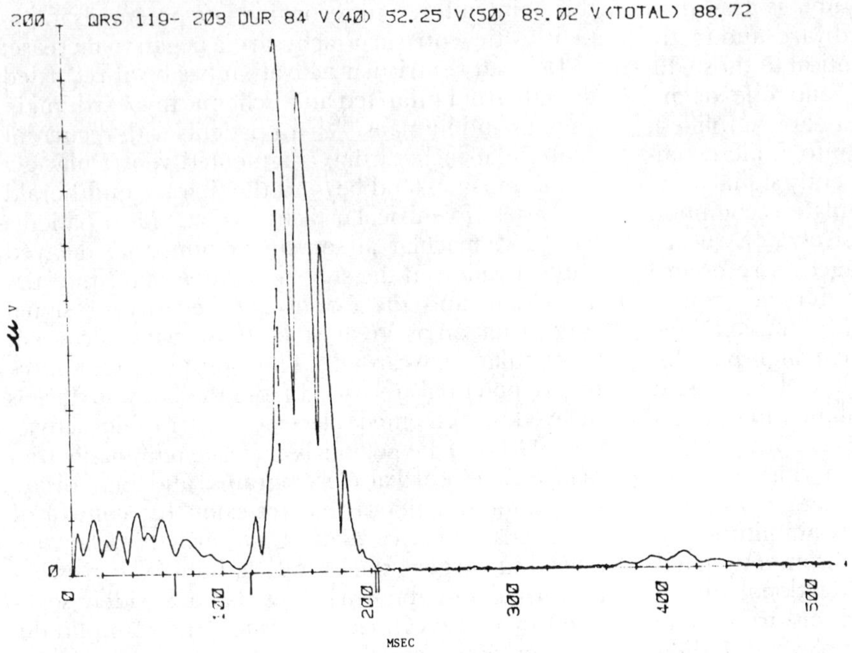

FIGURE 99-2 Signal processing in a normal volunteer. The filtered QRS duration is 84 ms, and the voltage in the last 40 ms of the filtered QRS complex is 52.25 μV.

an amplitude that varies from 1 to 20 μV. Ventricular late potentials lengthen the filtered QRS duration, and over 70 percent of patients with ventricular tachycardia have a QRS duration exceeding 110 ms. Several investigators, using a variety of signal averaging techniques, have recorded late potentials in patients with ventricular tachycardia.[4,20,21] Marcus et al. identified delayed ventricular potentials during normal sinus rhythm or atrial pacing in one-third of patients with arrhythmogenic right ventricular dysplasia.[22]

Late potentials are not found in all patients with recurrent ventricular tachycardia. In some instances, the fragmented activity may be too brief or the late potential may be masked by bundle branch block. Delayed, diastolic electrical activity is probably related to reentrant ventricular arrhythmias, but other potential mechanisms of ventricular tachycardia, increased automaticity and triggered activity, may not be associated with late potentials. Patients with ventricular tachycardia in the absence of demonstrable structural heart disease rarely have late potentials.[23]

Class I antiarrhythmic drugs and amiodarone increase the duration of the filtered QRS complex, but do not abolish late potentials.[7] Late potentials dis-

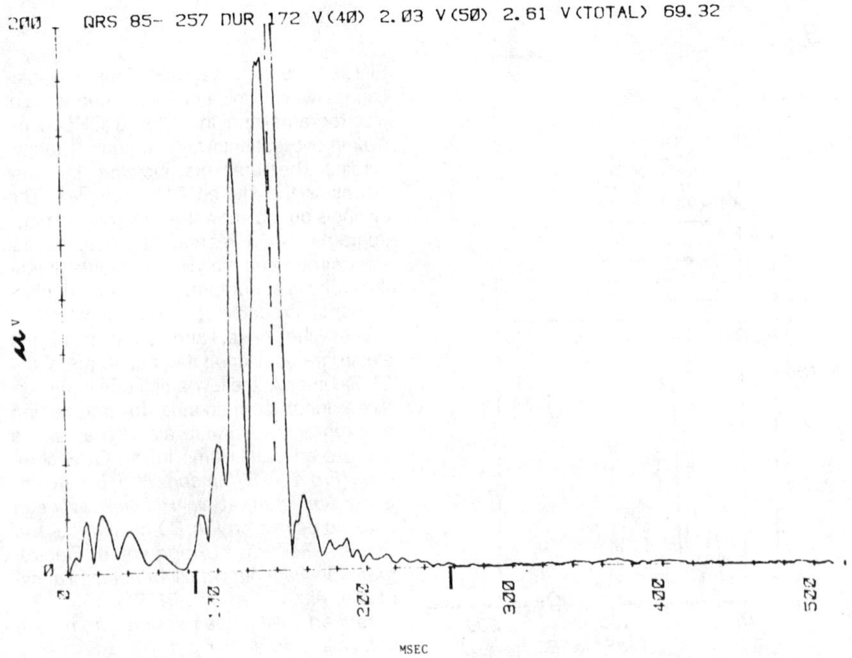

FIGURE 99-3 Signal processing in a patient with inferior myocardial infarction and recurrent ventricular tachycardia. The filtered QRS duration is markedly prolonged (172 ms). A low-amplitude late potential is seen late in the filtered QRS complex, and the voltage in the last 40 ms of the QRS complex is 2.03 μV.

appear in approximately 50 percent of patients after subendocardial resection. Ventricular tachycardia may be controlled despite the persistence of late potentials, suggesting that a successful operation need not abolish all slow-conducting tissue. Breithardt et al. found late potentials in some patients with left ventricular dysfunction but without a history of ventricular tachycardia.[21] However, late potentials occurred with a higher prevalence and had a longer duration in patients with ventricular tachycardia.

Limitation of the Technique

Much remains to be learned about the uses and limitations of signal averaging. A potentially fruitful application is the use of signal averaging as a screening procedure for vulnerability to ventricular tachycardia. It is known that some postmyocardial infarction patients without a history of ventricular tachycardia have late potentials. Whether these patients are prone to ventricular tachycardia requires further study. The technique is new. Therein lies its limitation. It does show promise and it is for this reason included in this edition of *The Heart*.

References

1. Schmitt, O. H.: Averaging Techniques Employing Several Physiologic Variables, *Ann. N.Y. Acad. Sci.*, 115:952, 1964.
2. Simson, M. B.: Use of Signals in the Terminal QRS Complex to Identify Patients with Ventricular Tachycardia after Myocardial Infarction, *Circulation*, 64:235, 1981.
3. Flowers, N. C., Hand, R. C., Orander, P. C., Miller, C. B., Walden, M. O., and Horan, L. G.: Surface Recording of Electrical Activity from the Region of the Bundle of His, *Am. J. Cardiol.*, 33:284, 1974.
4. Hombach, V., Braun, V., Hopp, H. W., et al.: The Applicability of the Signal Averaging Technique in Clinical Cardiology, *Clin. Cardiol.*, 5:107, 1982.
5. Berbari, E. J., Lazzara, R., Samet, P., and Scherlag, B. J.: Noninvasive Technique for Detection of Electrical Activity during the P-R Segment, *Circulation*, 48:1005, 1973.
6. Evanich, M. J., Newberry, A. O., and Partridge, L. D.: Some Limitations on the Removal of Periodic Noise by Averaging, *J. Appl. Physiol.*, 33:536, 1972.
7. Simson, M. B.: Clinical Application of Signal Averaging, *Cardiology Clinics*, 1:109, 1983.
8. Berbari, E. J., Lazzara, R., El-Sherif, N., and Scherlag, B. J.: Extracardiac Recording of His Purkinje Activity during Conduction Disorders and Junctional Rhythms, *Circulation*, 51:802, 1975.
9. Berbari, E. J., Scherlag, B. J., Hope, R. R., and Lazzara, R.: Recording from the Body Surface of Arrhythmogenic Ventricular Activity during the S-T Segment, *Am. J. Cardiol.*, 41:697, 1978.
10. Boineau, J. P., and Cox, J. L.: Slow Ventricular Activation in Acute Myocardial Infarction: A Source of Reentrant Premature Ventricular Contraction, *Circulation*, 48:702, 1973.
11. Scherlag, B. J., El-Sherif, N., Hope, R., and Lazzara, R.: Characterization and Localization of Ventricular Arhythmias Resulting from Myocardial Ischemia and Infarction, *Circ. Res.*, 35:372, 1974.
12. Waldo, A. L., and Kaiser, G. A.: A Study of Ventricular Arrhythmias Associated with Acute Myocardial Infarction in the Canine Heart, *Circulation*, 47:1222, 1973.
13. Josephson, M. E., Horowitz, L. N., Farshidi, A., Spielman, S. R., Michelson, E. L., and Greenspan, A. M.: Sustained Ventricular Tachycardia: Evidence for Protected Localized Reentry, *Am. J. Cardiol.*, 42:416, 1978.
14. Josephson, M.E., Horowitz, L. N., and Farshidi, A.: Continuous Local Electrical Activity: A Mechanism of Recurrent Ventricular Tachycardia, *Circulation*, 57:659, 1978.
15. Weiner, I., Mindich, B., and Pitchon, R.: Determinants of Ventricular Tachycardia in Patients with Ventricular Aneurysms: Results of Intraoperative Epicardial and Endocardial Mapping, *Circulation*, 65:856, 1982.
16. Simson, M. B., Untereker, W. J., Spielman, S. R., et al.: Relation between Late Potentials on the Body Surface and Directly Recorded Fragmented Electrograms in Patients with Ventricular Tachycardia, *Am. J. Cardiol.*, 51:105, 1983.
17. Fenoglio, J. J., Pham, T. D., Harken, A. H., Horowitz, L. N., Josephson, M. E., and Wit, A. L.: Recurrent Sustained Ventricular Tachycardia: Structure and Ultrastructure of Subendocardial Regions in Which Tachycardia Originates, *Circulation*, 68:518, 1983.
18. Simson, M. B., Falcone, R. A., Dresden, C. A., and Josephson, M. E.: Identification of Patients with Ventricular Tachycardia after Myocardial Infarction from the Signal Averaged Electrocardiogram, *J. Am. Coll. Cardiol.*, 3:622, 1984. (Abstract.)
19. Denes, P., Santarelli, P., Hauser, R. G., and Uretz, E. F.: Quantitative Analysis of the High-Frequency Components of the Terminal Portion of the Body Surface QRS in Normal Subjects and in Patients with Ventricular Tachycardia, *Circulation*, 67:1129, 1983.
20. Rozanski, J. J., Mortara, D., Myerburg, R. J., and Castellanos, A.: Body Surface Detection of Delayed Depolarizations in Patients with Recurrent Ventricular Tachycardia and Left Ventricular Aneurysm, *Circulation*, 63:1172, 1981.
21. Breithardt, G., Borggrefe, M., Karbenn, U., Abendroth, R. R., Yeh, H. L., and Seipel, L.: Prevalence of Late Potentials in Patients with and without Ventricular Tachycardia: Correlation with Angiographic Findings, *Am. J. Cardiol.*, 49:1932, 1982.
22. Marcus, F. I., Fontaine, G. H., Guiraudon, G., et al.: Right Ventricular Dysplasia: A Report of 24 Adult Cases, *Circulation*, 65:384, 1982.
23. Simson, M. B., Dresden, C., Falcone, R., Buxton, A., Josephson, M.: Signal Averaged ECG in Patients with Ventricular Tachycardia, Normal Coronary Arteries, and Normal Ventriculograms, *Circulation*, 68 (suppl. III): 428, 1983. (Abstract.)

100

Techniques of Long-Term Continuous Electrocardiographic Recording

R. Joe Noble, M.D. Douglas P. Zipes, M.D.

Long-term electrocardiographic recording (Holter monitoring) is a method of recording the electrocardiogram (ECG) for extended periods of time; the tape is subsequently analyzed for rhythm and ST-T alterations.[1–3] Technological advances in the past few years have provided a diversity of recording and analysis systems.

The indications for long-term ECG recording are discussed in Chaps. 27 and 45, as well as the information provided by extended ECG recording, and the sensitivity and specificity of the technique. This chapter will be concerned with the technical aspects of long-term ECG recording: the recording systems, analyzer systems, comparison of different techniques, optimal duration of recording, and artifacts and errors in long-term ECG recording and analysis.

Recording Techniques

Three methods of recording are currently available: continuous recorders, event markers, and microcomputers (or combinations of these techniques).

Continuous Recorders

The ECG may be recorded continuously on tape, either reel-to-reel or cassette. The tape recorder is a battery-powered miniaturized device with very slow tape speed and is small enough to be suspended by a strap over the shoulder or around the waist. Most current systems provide channels sufficient to record at least two ECG leads, which are essential in differentiating between ventricular ectopy and supraventricular ectopy with aberrancy, and also to assess ST-T segments. The frequency response of older models was limited in the lower ranges, so that accurate ST-T configuration could not be recorded;[4,5] current model systems should conform to accepted ECG standards.[6] Most current recorders are equipped with a digital clock, synchronized to the recorder; the patient illuminates the digital clock and also marks one of the channels for easy recognition during playback. The patient carries a diary in which are entered any symptoms experienced during the recording period, the patient's activities, and the time at which the symptoms occurred.

The lead systems on recorders vary from one manufacturer to another. As mentioned, at least two leads should be simultaneously recorded, either V_1 and V_5, or a bipolar limb and unipolar chest lead. Meticulous attention must be paid to placing the electrodes on the patient's chest, since poor electrode contact will produce technically inadequate recordings (Fig. 100-1).

Event Recorders

An alternative method records only *abnormalities* in rhythm or conduction; or records when the patient senses symptoms. There are two types of event recorders. In the first, the rhythm is monitored continuously. Operators select those parameters they wish the recorder to recognize as abnormal, and hence print out, such as a maximum or minimum rate, a premature complex, or a pause exceeding the predetermined limit. Most instruments incorporate a "memory" in that a delay loop records information several seconds before and after the recognized event. Patients may also activate the unit when they experience symptoms.

In the second variety, the rhythm is not monitored continuously. Instead, the patient has a miniature, solid-state recorder (sufficiently small to fit into his or her pocket or purse) with which the rhythm can be recorded, whenever symptomatic, by the patient simply placing the unit on the precordium. The recorded data are stored in memory until the patient transmits the information either directly or transtelephonically to an ECG receiver where it is recorded. The information on the patient's tape is then erased, and subsequent data recorded and transmitted, to facilitate the recording of the rhythm and pattern during several symptomatic episodes.

Microcomputers

When incorporated into an ambulatory recording system, sophisticated microcomputers and microelectronic circuits sample the cardiac rhythm at real time when it is being recorded, convert the analog signal into a digital signal, and analyze the data in terms of maximal or minimal rates, RR intervals, and changes in RR intervals. Selected, brief segments of the patient's ECG, e.g., 6- to 10-s intervals, can also be stored. Within minutes of disconnection from the patient, the information can be retrieved in the form of a histogram covering the entire recording period and a write-out in real time of selected segments. Thus, this instrument records the analysis of the entire recording period, which in this sense is similar to continuous tape recording. It is

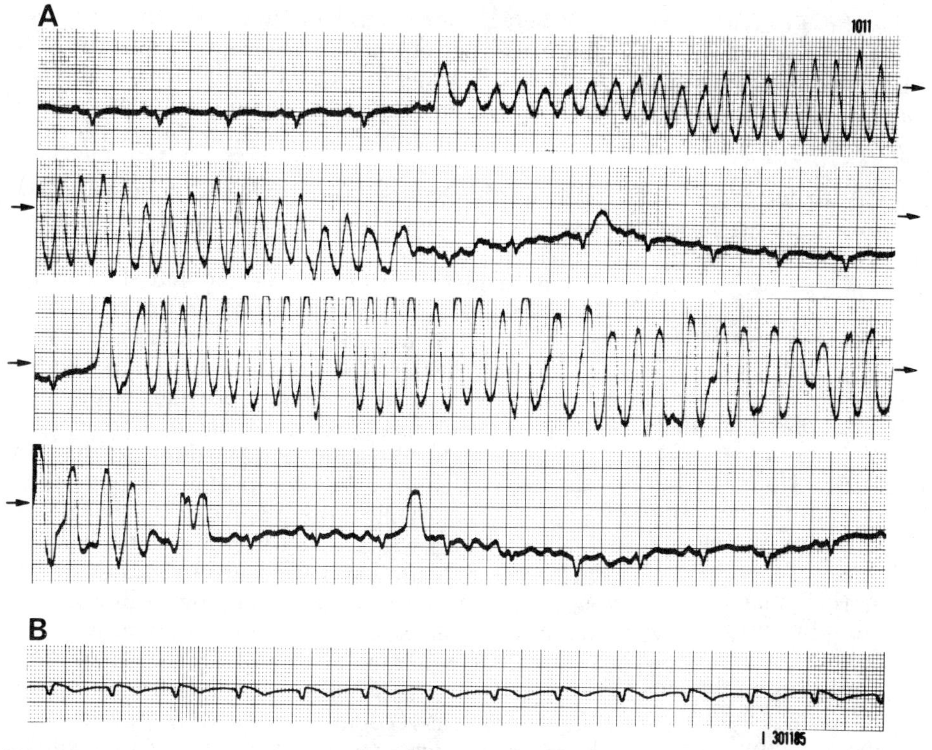

FIGURE 100-1 Artifact recorded on Holter monitor. A loose electrode was responsible for the artifactual tracing mimicking ventricular flutter-fibrillation recorded by the monitor in *A*. A simultaneous ECG (*B*) confirmed continuous sinus rhythm, and the patient remained asymptomatic.

dissimilar in that the actual ECG has not been recorded on tape. Microcomputers have been developed which can analyze electronic data over prolonged periods—even several days.

Scanning and Analysis Techniques

The recording may be analyzed by scanning the tape at high speed, by writing it out directly, or as in the case of microcomputers, by processing during the recording and writing out the analysis at the termination of the sampling.

Scanning techniques include technician-dependent analysis, in which a technician interprets the cardiac rhythm as it is played back at high speed on an oscilloscope at 30 to 120 times real time. One commonly used method of scanning superimposes each QRS complex on the immediately preceding complex, so that identical QRS contours present as a stationary image. Variations in QRS contour then become readily apparent. Simultaneously displayed on the oscilloscope for each cardiac cycle is a vertical bar graph, the height of which is directly proportional to each RR interval and QRS morphology. Thus, the occurrence of a premature ventricular extrasystole would alter the stationary image by producing a variation in the QRS contour, would alter the pitch and sound of the audio signal, and would shorten the vertical bar reflecting cycle lengths. When such an abnormal event is noted, the tape can be played in real time for analysis on a standard ECG.

To minimize the human factor and provide accurate quantitative data, the tape may be analyzed by a semiautomated electronic analyzer, which quantitates the number of abnormalities it recognizes. The accuracy of the system depends upon the system's ability to distinguish abnormal from normal.

A computer may be interfaced with the scanner to quantitate the data even more accurately. The playback analysis may be as rapid as 240 times real time. Electronic analyzers and computers, as well as the scanner, can be "taught" to recognize the patient's own QRS complex and then to recognize any deviation from the normal. The computer program can provide summaries of heart rates, frequency of premature atrial or ventricular extrasystoles, coupling intervals, runs of tachycardia or other arrhythmias, and variations in QRS, ST, or T patterns during any time period; hard copies can be written out for verification. When arrhythmias or pattern changes are detected, automatic ECG write-out can be triggererd by the event marker or by the computer.

Scanning services are available, which can generally provide reasonably accurate analysis at less cost than can small institutions or offices with smaller volumes of long-term ECG recordings. Recorders may be purchased, leased, or rented.

An alternative method to scanning is the *direct*

write-out of the entire record. The ECG is compressed so as to reduce the amount of paper which the physician must examine. By directly writing out the entire ECG, the need for a trained technician and scanners may be obviated.

Since *microcomputers* assess the ECG in real time, as it is recorded, there is no need for a scanner or expert technician when the results are written out. The physician evaluates the trend chart or any recorded rhythm strip.

Comparison of Techniques for Prolonged ECG Recording

Operator-dependent, high-speed audiovisual analysis of the tape, without direct write-out or electronic analysis, probably recognizes serious rhythm disturbances. However, the operator may miss as many as one-third to two-thirds of ventricular and supraventricular arrhythmias.[7] Operator-dependent systems are affected by the capabilities of this person. If quantitation is unimportant, this system of analysis is quite adequate.

Electronic analysis systems improve upon the sensitivity and specificity of interpretation of long-term ECG recordings. Computer analysis systems are said to be 90 to 95 percent accurate in quantitating ectopic complexes;[7–9] both electronic and computer analysis systems increase cost.

Both because of the cost and the problems inherent in semiautomated and computer systems of analysis, the current trend is toward "full disclosure"—i.e., hard-copy write-out of the entire record. A visual analysis of the record immediately identifies complex disturbances, such as ventricular tachycardia or prolonged asystolic intervals. In addition, it is often useful to have hard-copy data available (as opposed to analyzed data) with which to compare subsequent records. The direct write-out does not quantitate the actual number of events. Assuming care in interpretation, the direct write-out may be more sensitive than high-speed, operator-dependent, and semiautomated systems, and probably more accurate than computer-based systems in identifying pairs or triplets of consecutive ectopic complexes.[7]

An event recorder does not require a scanner or an experienced technician. However, the continuous-event recorder itself is more expensive than a continuous tape recorder. The recorder, which the patient applies only when symptomatic, without continuous tape recording capability, is less expensive. Both types of event recorders provide an ECG record more quickly than a system which requires scanning,[10] but neither records a long-term record of the ECG during asymptomatic intervals. The automatic event recorder is limited by the accuracy and sensitivity of the algorithm used to detect abnormalities. Either event recorder clearly allows correlation between the patient's symptoms and the rhythm.

When a more rapid identification of a rhythm abnormality is essential, such as in the patient with a potentially dangerous rhythm disturbance, a new development permits frequent and automatic transtelephonic transmission of the ambulatory record to a hospital telemetry receiver. The monitor technician can then quickly identify a serious rhythm abnormality, and arrange for the patient's proper management.

Those microcomputers which analyze the rhythm in real time, simultaneous with the recording, should theoretically prove more accurate than other high-speed, playback analysis systems. More importantly, longer periods can be monitored than is practical for other systems. The cost of the analysis is independent of the duration of recording, so that patient cost should be less for prolonged periods of monitoring. Finally, the analysis of the entire recording and the actual write-out of the specific ECG segment are available within minutes of the recording. On the other hand, only limited segments of actual ECG records are generally available, and the accuracy of abnormal rhythm or pattern recognition remains dependent upon the computer algorithm; this recognition is far from perfect, since many problems of computer analysis of complex rhythm disturbances remain unsolved.

The ultimate selection of a long-term ECG recording system depends upon individual patient needs. If a precise count of ectopy is required, then a continuous recorder with computer-based analysis is essential. On the other hand, if the purpose of the recording is to detect ventricular tachycardia or asystole, then an event recorder, a microcomputer, or direct write-out of the entire record would be excellent choices. A microcomputer provides an opportunity to monitor over prolonged periods of time, and it is beneficial to the patient whose rhythm disturbance occurs infrequently. When the goal is to correlate the patient's rhythm or ECG pattern with symptoms that are very infrequent (at weekly intervals or less) then the patient-applied and activated recorder is the optimal choice. This and the direct write-out are less expensive for an individual physician or small clinic's use.

Except with large scanning services, it is impractical for an individual physician to have available all the monitoring techniques for each individual patient's needs. Hence, the physician's selection of a system is based upon his or her own patient population, the frequency of using this test, the availability of dependable scanning services, and his or her own cost analysis. The physician would do well to realize that any or all of the above systems are available alone or in combination. The more detailed and precisely quantitated the final report, generally the more expensive the equipment and personnel required. All systems recognize ventricular tachycardia or marked bradycardia, and qualitatively, at least, detect ectopy. For clinical purposes, this amount of information is usually sufficient.

The practicing physician does not really require precise quantitation since the therapeutic and prognostic significance of such quantitation is not yet known. In short, technology exceeds clinical assimilation of the results at the present time.

Duration of Recording

A standard resting ECG, which records less than 1 min of cardiac rhythm, detects ventricular premature systoles in about 8 percent of patients with known coronary artery disease; this frequency doubles if the recording period is extended to 12 h.[11] A 24-h ECG recording period detects additional and more complex ventricular arrhythmias and supraventricular tachyarrhythmias and also displays the character and frequency of rhythm disturbances during sleep as well as during awake periods.

Arrhythmias may be evanescent, occurring only rarely. In such patients, 24-h ECG recordings are unlikely to detect the abnormal rhythm. Even when arrhythmias are frequent, marked variation in the frequency and complexity of the rhythm disturbance is expected, with variations occurring during and between days. Spontaneous reduction in the frequency of ventricular ectopy of 50 to 90 percent is common.[12,13] For screening purposes, 24-h ECG tape recording seems an optimal compromise between the practical limits of recording and the point of diminishing return.[11,14,15]

If a reduction in total number of premature ventricular complexes (PVCs) is the goal of antiarrhythmic therapy, then more than one control 24-h ECG recording and several recordings on therapy are required to prove efficacy. The total number of PVCs must be reduced by about 80 percent.[12,13,16] However, since it has not yet been demonstrated that reducing the total number of PVCs necessarily implies an elimination of more dire ventricular rhythm disturbances or sudden death, this is often not the goal of the physician. Instead, simply preventing sustained, symptomatic ventricular tachycardia may be the therapeutic goal,[17] in which case multiple 24-h recordings are less essential.

The ideal duration of recording varies from patient to patient, depending upon the physician's goals. If the objective is to correlate the cardiac rhythm or pattern with a symptom such as syncope, palpitations, or chest pain, then the recording period must be extended sufficiently to incorporate a symptomatic period, whether these intervals occur with a frequency of hours or days.

ST-T Recordings

For several reasons, both technical and physiological, long-term ECG recording devices do not provide the same degree of reliability in the interpretation of the pattern of the ST segment and T wave as in the detection of rhythm disturbances. Technical limitations have included unsatisfactory low-frequency responses, which have precluded accurate display of the very low frequency ST segment and T waves.[4,5] Another limitation has been the use of a one-lead system. Just as a single lead on a standard ECG might not record "ischemic" ST and T changes with myocardial ischemia, so a single lead is inadequate for this purpose with prolonged recording. Technical improvements in more recently developed models, including the expansion of the lower-limit frequency response and the use of two leads, have enhanced the reliability of QRS-T pattern interpretation with long-term recording.

Even more important than these technical considerations, however, are certain physiological limitations. For instance, standing, hyperventilation, eating, anxiety, drugs, or change in heart rate are all daily events which may result in depression of the ST segment or inversion of the T wave to simulate ischemic changes. Striking ST-segment elevation has been recorded during prolonged recording in patients without organic heart disease.[18]

Despite these limitations, preliminary evaluations of the technique of prolonged ECG recording to detect ischemic heart disease have indicated in some instances (1) that patients who display ischemic ST-T changes are more likely to develop overt manifestations of ischemic heart disease subsequently than those who do not display such alterations, and (2) that a similar ECG pattern during recording correlates with angiographic evidence of coronary artery disease.[19–21] However, the sensitivity and specificity of the technique remains to be determined.

Long-term ECG recording proves superior to exercise testing in detecting angina at rest accompanied by ST-segment elevation, which cannot be reproduced with exercise (Prinzmetal's variant angina). Another potential use of prolonged ECG recording is to correlate symptoms which occur during normal daily activity with ECG evidence of ischemia. In this setting, the demonstration of significant ST-T wave alterations which cannot be reproduced by hyperventilation or change in position, particularly when reinforced by documentation in the patient's diary of simultaneous symptoms of angina, prove highly suggestive of ischemic heart disease. In still other patients, in whom exercise testing is precluded by physical disability, ambulatory recording could be helpful; or, in patients in whom exercise testing produces negative results and yet symptoms highly suggestive of myocardial ischemia continue with other specific activities, prolonged ECG recording provides useful information.

Artifacts and Errors

Virtually every variety of supraventricular and ventricular bradycardia and tachycardia have been

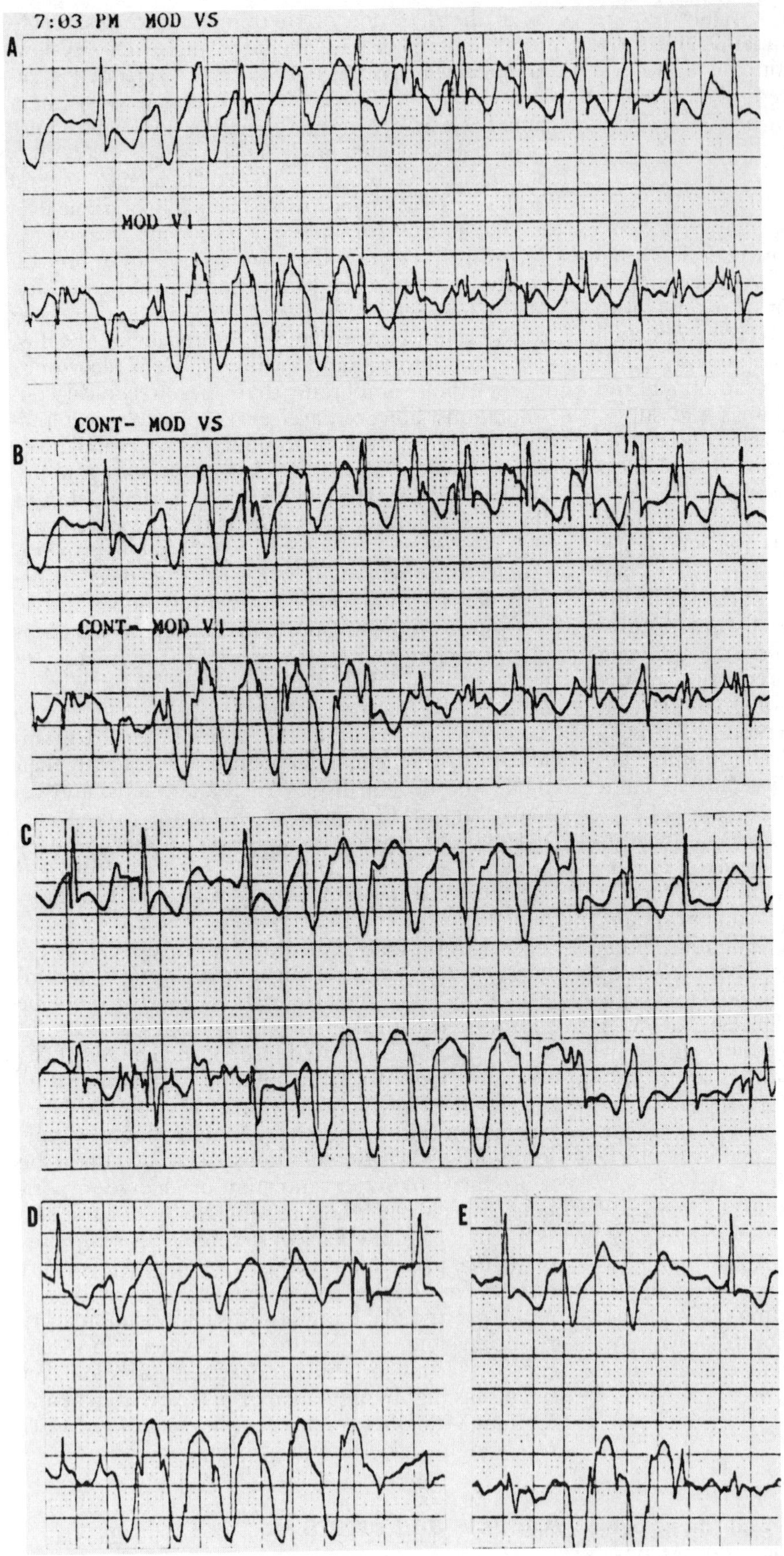

FIGURE 100-2 Mechanical stimulation of electrodes mimicking ventricular tachycardia. Regular, rapid (160 per minute) broad QRS complexes were repeatedly recorded in both leads V_1 and V_5 and interpreted as ventricular tachycardia (*A* through *D*) or pairs of PVCs (*E*); antiarrhythmic therapy was administered. However, the clue to the artifactual recording is the normal QRS "marching through" the "ventricular tachycardia"; and the fact that the coupling interval between the last normal complex preceding the "tachycardia" and the first complex following it are often so short as to be unphysiological. Intense pruritus from the electrodes elicited scratching, which explained the artifacts.

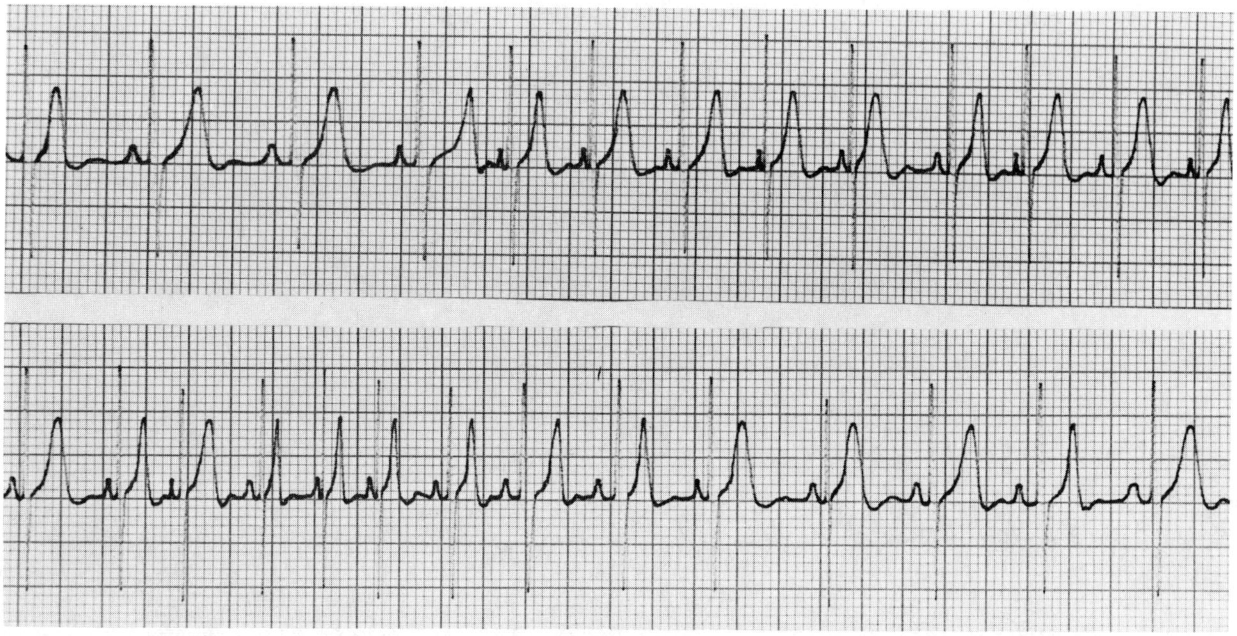

FIGURE 100-3 Deceleration of tape during recording. Supraventricular tachycardia is simulated toward the end of the top and beginning of the second trace, as the tape, which transiently slowed due to battery failure during recording, was played back on recording paper at proper speed. Note the foreshortening of the duration of the P wave, PR interval, QRS complex, and QT interval.

mimicked and consequently misdiagnosed as a result of artifacts registered during prolonged ECG recording.[22,23] Most of these artifacts are identical to those plaguing standard 12-lead electrocardiography but are simply detected more frequently due to the length of the recording; however, many are unique to extended recording by virtue of the magnetic tape recorder.

Probably the most common artifact is that resulting from a loose electrode (Fig. 100-1) or mechanical "stimulation" of the electrode. In Fig. 100-2, ventricular tachycardia is simulated by the patient "scratching" the electrodes. Failure of either the battery or the motor of the recorder generally results in a slowing of the tape speed as the ECG is recorded. When played back, the heart rate will appear elevated, i.e., it will mimic a tachycardia (Fig. 100-3). However, the concomitant reduction in all ECG intervals (PR, QRS, QT, and RR) and decrease in QRS voltage serve to alert the interpreter to the artifact. Conversely, transient slowing or sticking of the tape during playback will suggest bradycardia or atrioventricular (AV) or intraventricular conduction disturbances (Fig. 100-4). Recording an ECG on a previously used tape which is incompletely erased results in the simultaneous registration of two ECGs and perhaps the misinterpretation of a "parasystolic" ectopic rhythm (Fig. 100-5).

The technician and/or physician who interprets prolonged ECG recordings must have a working knowledge of these and other potential artifacts in order to interpret the records properly.

FIGURE 100-4 Deceleration of tape during playback. Slowing or sticking of the tape during playback spreads out the P wave, PR interval, and QRS complex to resemble sinus deceleration, or transient atrioventricular or intraventricular conduction delay. (Fifth complex in top trace; sixth complex in bottom trace.)

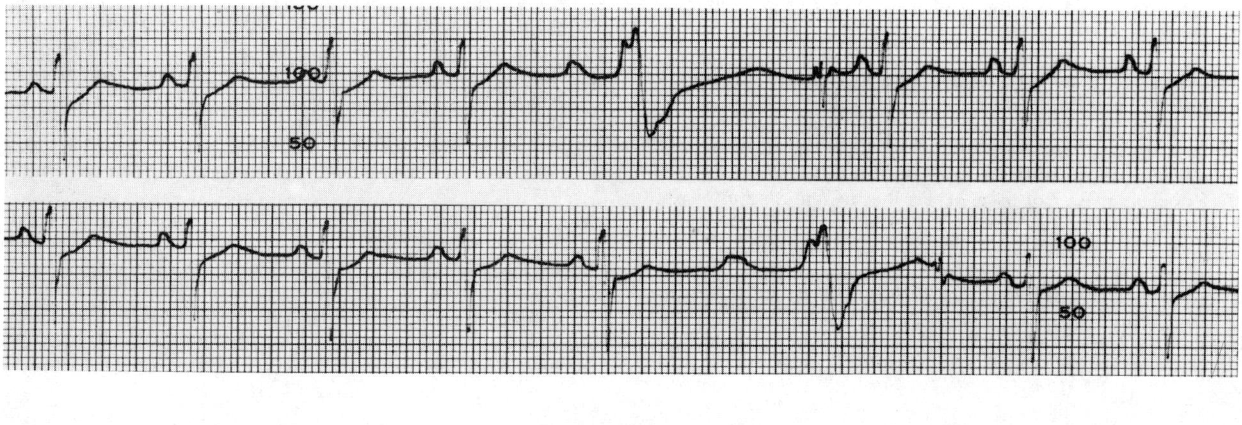

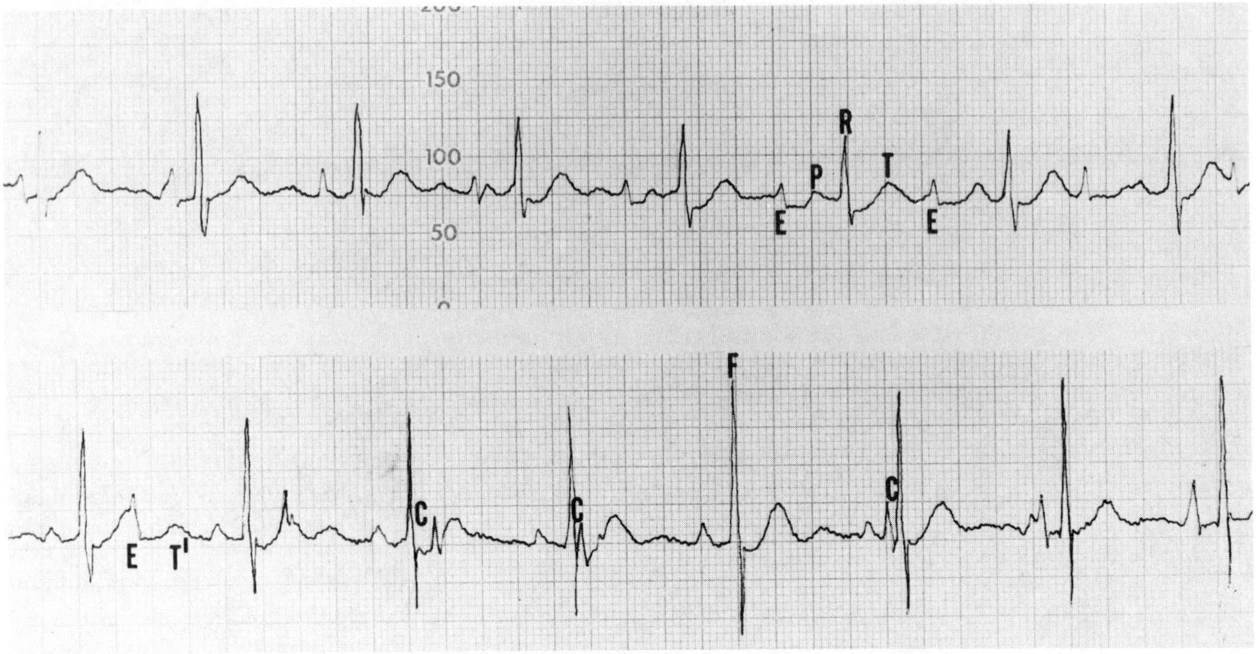

FIGURE 100-5 Incomplete erasure of tape. Two independent ventricular rhythms are identified: a larger QRS, labeled R, whose P wave and T wave are also labeled, and a smaller QRS, considered "ectopic," and labeled E; its T wave is labeld T′. The sequence could be recorded with a piggyback heart transplant, or in Siamese twins. Alternately, ectopic complex E might be misinterpreted to represent a parasystolic rhythm even fusing with complex R at F. The very short coupling intervals (C) preclude this possibility and indicate that the ECG record of one patient is superimposed on that of another.

References

1. Holter, N. J.: New Method for Heart Studies: Continuous Electrocardiography of Active Subjects over Long Periods Is Now Practical, *Science,* 134:1214, 1961.
2. Gilson, J. S., Holter, N. J., and Glassock, W. R.: Clinical Observations Using This Electrocardiocorder—AVSEP Continuous Electrocardiographic System, *Am. J. Cardiol.,* 14:204, 1964.
3. Winkle, R. A.: Curriculum In Cardiology, Current Status of Ambulatory Electrocardiography, *Am. Heart J.,* 102:757, 1981.
4. Hinkle, L. E., Jr., Meyer, J., Stevens, M., and Carver, S. T.: Recordings of the ECG of Active Men, *Circulation,* 36:752, 1967.
5. Crawford, M. H., Mendoza, C. A., O'Rourke, R. A., White, D. H., Boucher, C. A., and Gorwit, J.: Limitations of Continuous Ambulatory Electrocardiogram Monitoring for Detecting Coronary Artery Disease, *Ann. Intern. Med.,* 89:1, 1978.
6. Report of Committee on Electrocardiography, American Heart Association: Recommendations for Standardization of Leads and of Specifications for Instruments in Electrocardiography and Vectorcardiography, *Circulation,* 35:583, 1967.
7. Stein, I. M., Plunkett, J., and Troy, M.: Comparison of Techniques for Examining Long-Term ECG Recordings, *Med. Instr.,* 14:69, 1980.
8. Fitzgerald, J. W., Spitz, A. L., Winkle, R. A., and Harrison, D.C.: Quantitation of Ambulatory Electrocardiograms, *Circulation,* 56(suppl. 3):178, 1977. (Abstract.)
9. Knoebel, S. B., Lovelace, D. E., Rasmussen, S., and Wash, S. E.: Computer Detection of Premature Ventricular Complexes: A Modified Approach, *Am. J. Cardiol.,* 38:440, 1976.
10. Dreifus, L. S., and Pennock, R.: Newer Techniques in Cardiac Monitoring, *Heart Lung,* 4:568, 1975.
11. Lown, B., and Wolf, M.: Approaches to Sudden Death from Coronary Heart Disease, *Circulation,* 14:130, 1971.
12. Winkle, R. A.: Antiarrhythmic Drug Effect Mimicked by Spontaneous Variability of Ventricular Ectopy, *Circulation,* 57:1116, 1978.
13. Morganroth, J., Michelson, E. L., Horowitz, L. N., Josephson, M. E., Pearlman, A. S., and Dunkman, W. B.: Limitations of Routine Long-Term Ambulatory Electrocardiographic Monitoring to Assess Ventricular Ectopic Frequency, *Circulation,* 58:408, 1978.
14. Lopes, M. G., Runge, P., Harrison, D. C., and Schroeder, J. S.: Comparison of 24 versus 12 Hours of Ambulatory ECG Monitoring, *Chest,* 67:269, 1975.
15. Kennedy, H. L., Chandra, V., Sayther, K. L., and Caralis, D. G.: Effectiveness of Increasing Hours of Continuous Ambulatory Electrocardiography in Detecting Maximal Ventricular Ectopy, *Am. J. Cardiol.,* 42:925, 1978.
16. Sami, M., Kraemer, H., Harrison, D. C., Houston, N., Shimasaki, C., and DeBusk, R. F.: A New Method for Evaluating Antiarrhythmic Drug Efficacy, *Circulation,* 62:1172, 1980.
17. Winkle, R. A., Alderman, E. L., Fitzgerald, J. W., and Harrison, D.C.: Treatment of Recurrent Symptomatic Ventricular Tachycardia, *Ann. Intern. Med.,* 85:1, 1976.
18. Golding, B., Wolf, E., Tzivoni, D., and Stern, S.: Transient S-T Elevation Detected by 24-Hour ECG Monitoring during Normal Daily Activity, *Am. Heart J.,* 86:501, 1973.
19. Stern, S., and Tzivoni, D.: Early Detection of Silent Ischaemic Heart Disease by 24-Hour Electrocardiographic Monitoring of Active Subjects, *Br. Heart J.,* 36:481, 1974.
20. Wolf, E., Tzivoni, D., and Stern, S.: Comparison of Exercise Tests and 24-Hour Ambulatory Electrocardiographic Monitoring in Detection of ST-T Changes, *Br. Heart J.,* 36:90, 1974.
21. Stern, S., and Tzivoni, D.: Dynamic Changes in the ST-T Segment during Sleep in Ischemic Heart Disease, *Am. J. Cardiol.,* 32:17, 1973.
22. Krasnow, A. Z., and Bloomfield, D. K.: Artifacts in Portable Electrocardiographic Monitoring, *Am. Heart J.,* 91:349, 1976.
23. Malek, J., and Glushien, A.: To The Editor: Artifacts in Portable ECG Monitoring, *Ann. Intern. Med.,* 77:1004, 1972.

101

Techniques of His Bundle Recordings: Clinical Value and Indications

Douglas L. Packer, M.D.
John J. Gallagher, M.D.
Andrew G. Wallace, M.D.

The ability to obtain intracavitary recordings from specialized cardiac conduction tissue has greatly advanced the understanding of the human atrioventricular (AV) conduction system. Since the first clinical applications of the His bundle catheter technique to record electrical activity from tissue previously inaccessible to routine electrocardiographic leads,[1-3] not only have prior noninvasive observations been confirmed, but further understanding of conduction disturbances has been facilitated as well. The recording of the His bundle deflection that divides the PR interval into segments that reflect impulse propagation through the AV node and conduction via the His-Purkinje system has also given access to both diagnostic and prognostic information useful in managing patients with conduction defects. Additional refinements of this technique have also elucidated the mechanisms of cardiac arrhythmias.

Techniques of His Bundle Recording

Recording the His bundle electrogram requires not only the technical skill to position the electrode catheter safely but also the laboratory equipment for monitoring during catheter manipulation and for permanently recording the electrograms. This equipment should include an electrocardiographic preamplifier with variable gain and filter settings to permit amplification of the His bundle electrogram within the desired frequencies. In addition, the system should include an oscillographic display with sweep speeds of up to 100 to 200 mm/s. For permanent recording, electrograms are either written out on a recording device at similar speeds or stored on magnetic tape. These recording speeds, which are four to eight times faster than the standard 25-to-50-mm/s speed of the surface electrocardiogram (ECG), allow enhanced signal separation. The entire system, including x-ray and pacing equipment, should be grounded to guard against the hazards of current leakage.

Introduction of the electrode catheter into the right side of the heart for recording the His bundle electrogram is typically performed through the right femoral vein. After the right inguinal region is shaved, prepped, and draped in a sterile fashion, an area 1.5 to 2 cm below the inguinal ligament and medial to the femoral artery is anesthetized. A tripolar electrode catheter with a preformed curve is introduced into the right femoral vein and advanced under fluoroscopic control via the inferior vena cava across the tricuspid valve into the right ventricle. The appropriate bipolar electrodes are then connected to the ac input of the electrocardiographic preamplifier and recordings are filtered at 40 to 50 Hz to 500 to 1000 Hz. This permits electrocardiographic, as well as fluoroscopic, control as the catheter is further positioned.

The anatomy of the AV conduction system must be appreciated to understand further catheter positioning. The compact portion of the AV node lies just below the endocardial surface of the inferomedial portion of the right atrium, anterior to the coronary sinus orifice near the membranous septum and the septal attachment of the tricuspid valve. The penetrating portion of the AV bundle (or bundle of His) exits from the distal portion of the compact AV node and pierces the central fibrous body (which unites the mitral, tricuspid, and aortic valve annuli) to enter the lower confines of the membranous septum and course along the summit of the muscular interventricular septum. Here it gives off a sheet of fibers which travels down the left side of the septum to form the left bundle branch. The remaining distinct cord continues as the right bundle branch and runs superficially down the right side of the septum to the moderator band and on to the Purkinje-ventricular ramifications. As the catheter crosses the tricuspid valve annulus, it comes into close proximity with the penetrating portion of the His bundle and right bundle branch, thus allowing recording of electrical activity.

With the catheter positioned well into the right ventricle, a large ventricular deflection with no accompanying atrial activity will be observed (Fig. 101-1, panel 1). Gentle clockwise torque will then bring the catheter tip into close proximity with the interventricular septum. As it is carefully withdrawn, with continuing torque, the catheter approaches the right bundle branch where its potential may be recorded (Fig. 101-1, panel 2). This is a small, sharp biphasic or triphasic deflection, typically 10 to 12 ms in duration, that precedes the onset of ventricular activity by 10 to 25 ms. At this point, typically no atrial deflection is evident. Upon further withdrawal of the catheter, the size of the atrial de-

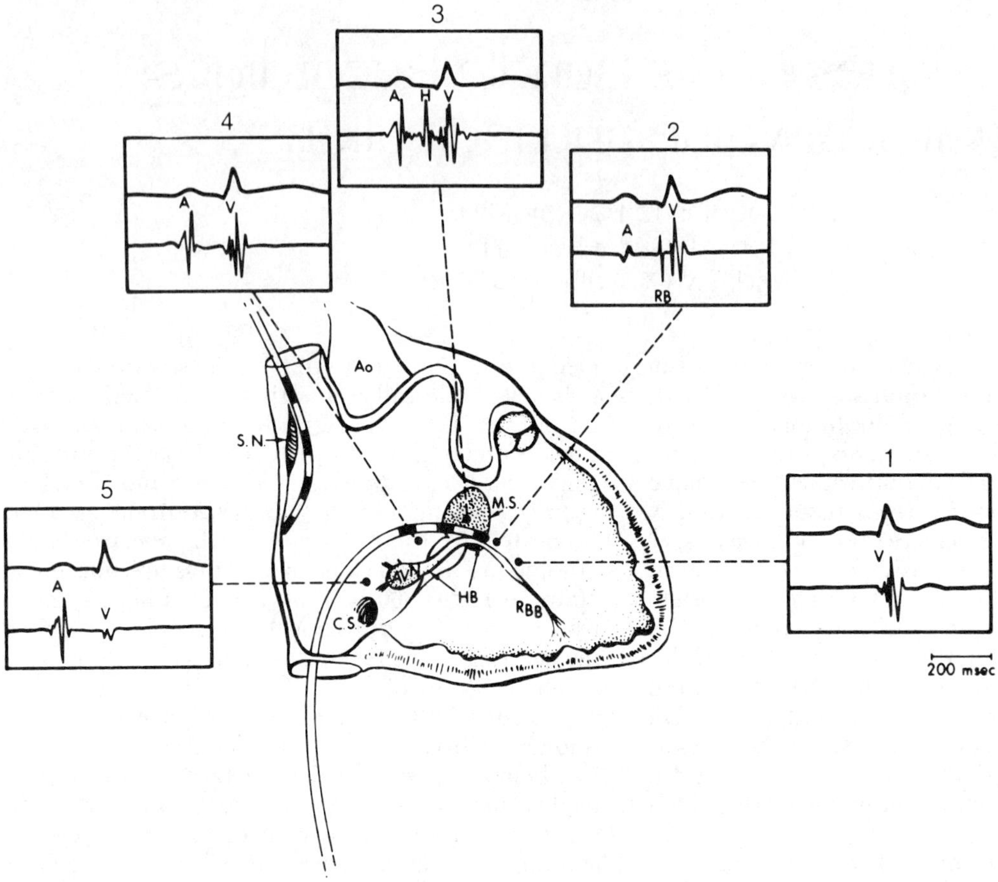

FIGURE 101-1 Pullback of the electrode catheter from the right ventricular cavity. A cutaway view of the heart demonstrating the electrode catheter lying across the tricuspid valve. The intracavitary electrograms obtained during progressive withdrawal of the catheter are shown in inserts 1 to 5. SN = sinus node; CS = orifice of the coronary sinus; AVN = atrioventricular node; HB = His bundle; MS = membranous septum; RBB = right bundle branch; A = atrial electrogram; H = His bundle electrogram; V = ventricular electrogram. (*From J. J. Gallagher and A. N. Damato, Technique of Recording His Bundle Activity in Man, in W. Grossman (ed.), "Cardiac Catheterization and Angiography," 2d ed., Lea & Febiger, Philadelphia, 1980, p. 285.*)

flection increases as the ventricular deflection decreases. In addition, a larger sharp biphasic or triphasic His deflection of 15-to-20-ms duration appears between the atrial and ventricular deflections, preceding the ventricular deflection by 30 to 55 ms (Fig. 101-1, panel 3). Additional withdrawal results in a further increase in the atrial and decrease in the ventricular deflections as well as the loss of the His bundle potential (Fig. 101-1, panel 4). The catheter tip, if withdrawn too far, will slip back into the atrium, recording only atrial electrical activity (Fig. 101-1, panel 5). Fine-tuning can be accomplished by carefully advancing or withdrawing the catheter while maintaining the clockwise torque. If the His and atrial deflections are decreasing in size, minimal catheter withdrawal should reestablish an optimal His deflection. In contrast, an increasing atrial deflection with a diminishing His deflection indicates that the catheter is positioned too proximally. This in turn may be corrected by careful catheter advancement.

Several other problems may be encountered during catheter placement and His bundle electrogram recordings. On occasion, large atrial and ventricular deflections may appear without any intervening His activity. This may indicate that the coronary sinus has been inadvertently entered, although this is less likely to occur with the femoral vein approach. In addition, inasmuch as the right bundle branch is superficially located on the right side of the interventricular septum, catheter manipulation in this area may traumatize either the His bundle or the right bundle branch.[4] Although this is usually transient, complete AV block may occur, particularly in patients with preexistent left bundle branch block. Any catheter manipulation, especially in patients with preexisting left bundle branch block, must be carefully performed and equipment for ventricular pacing must be readily available should this complication occur.

In some instances it may not be possible to use the right femoral vein approach; for example, in patients with (1) significant vascular disease of the lower extremities, including thrombophlebitis; (2) infection at the catheter site; (3) marked edema or obesity, making femoral catheterization technically difficult; and (4) iliac or inferior vena caval disease, thrombosis, or obstruction. In these cases an antecubital vein approach can be used to obtain His bundle electrograms safely and consistently.[5] It is also possible to obtain His bundle electrograms from the arterial side, by passing a catheter via a femoral artery through the aorta into the noncoronary cusp of the aortic valve to the left of the interventricular septum.[6] By further advancing the catheter 1 to 2 cm below the aortic valve, the left bundle potential may also be recorded. There is some additional risk with this approach.

As with any invasive vascular procedure, His bundle catheterization may be complicated by local or systemic infection or vascular damage, including hematoma formation, thrombophlebitis, or possible arteriovenous fistula formation. In addition, catheter manipulation may result in transient ventricular ectopy although this is rarely a significant problem. Nevertheless, the laboratory in which this procedure is performed should be equipped with standard resuscitation equipment including a dc cardioversion unit.

Validation of His Bundle Recordings

In order to ensure against interpretation errors from improper catheter position, it is important to verify that the activity being recorded is actually from the His bundle and not the right bundle branch. Proper catheter position can be confirmed in several ways. (1) The HV interval obtained with the catheter in the appropriate proximal His position is typically more than 35 ms, whereas the right bundle branch V interval is usually less than 30 ms. (2) A prominent atrial deflection should be present with the catheter properly positioned, whereas a smaller (or absent) atrial electrogram is consistent with a more distal right bundle branch position. (3) His bundle pacing with the catheter in the proper position should yield an HV interval of more than 30 ms with a QRS morphology similar to that present during sinus rhythm. In contrast, pacing the right bundle branch region is more likely to yield a wide QRS complex. (4) If necessary, a His bundle recording may be obtained simultaneously from the arterial side with a catheter positioned in the noncoronary cusp of the aortic valve near the central fibrous body. Simultaneous right- and left-sided deflections suggest that the proximal His bundle position is being recorded from the venous catheter site.

Nomenclature and Normal Values

The His bundle electrogram recorded from the region of the tricuspid annulus is composed of three separate bipolar deflections. These include an atrial deflection or electrogram (A) reflecting atrial activity originating in the region of the low interatrial septum, the His bundle deflection (H), and finally, the ventricular deflection (V) from the high inter-

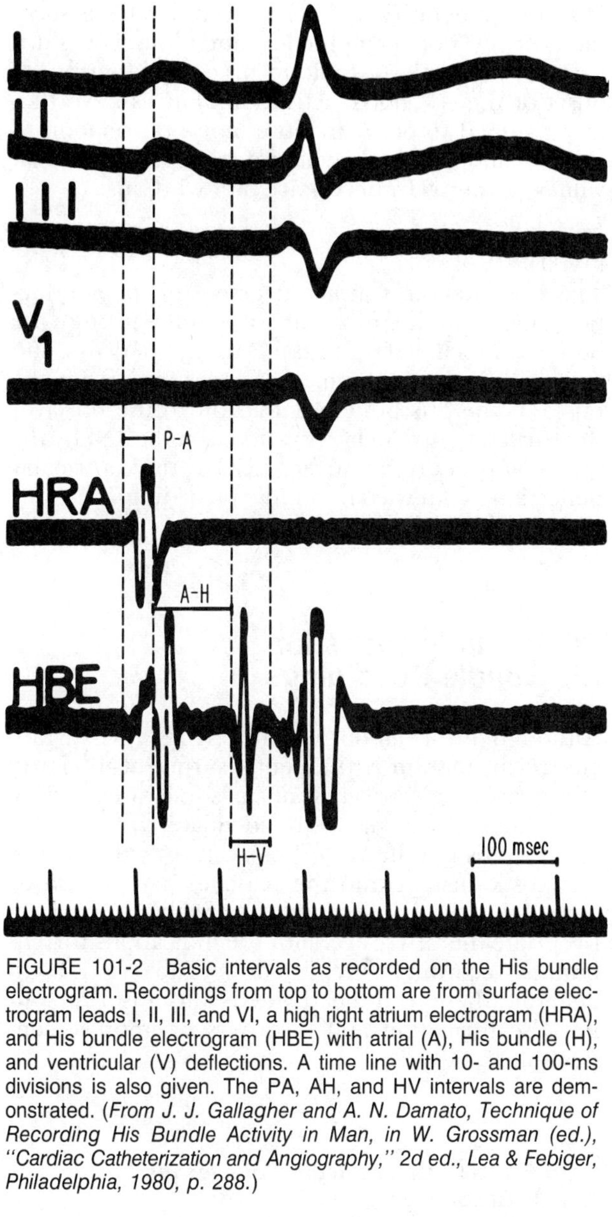

FIGURE 101-2 Basic intervals as recorded on the His bundle electrogram. Recordings from top to bottom are from surface electrogram leads I, II, III, and VI, a high right atrium electrogram (HRA), and His bundle electrogram (HBE) with atrial (A), His bundle (H), and ventricular (V) deflections. A time line with 10- and 100-ms divisions is also given. The PA, AH, and HV intervals are demonstrated. (*From J. J. Gallagher and A. N. Damato, Technique of Recording His Bundle Activity in Man, in W. Grossman (ed.), "Cardiac Catheterization and Angiography," 2d ed., Lea & Febiger, Philadelphia, 1980, p. 288.*)

ventricular septal region (Fig. 101-2). These distinct deflections along with the surface P waves simultaneously recorded from three or four surface electrocardiographic leads (such as I, II, III, and V_1) allow the division of the PR segment into three smaller intervals.

PA Interval

This interval begins with the onset of the P wave recorded on the surface electrocardiogram and extends to the first rapid deflection of the atrial electrogram. This interval reflects intraatrial conduction time and has normal values of 24 to 45 ms.

AH Interval

The AH interval is taken from the first rapid deflection of the atrial electrogram to the onset of the

His bundle deflection. This is an indirect measurement of AV nodal conduction time, however, since it is not presently possible to precisely identify the onset of the AV nodal activation. This is nevertheless assumed to occur in close temporal relation to the activation of the low interatrial septum. Normal values of the AH interval are 60 to 140 ms.

HV Interval

The HV interval is a measurement of the conduction time from the proximal His bundle through the bundle branch system to the Purkinje network and ventricular myocardium. It is measured from the onset of the His bundle deflection to the onset of the earliest ventricular activation as indicated by the QRS complex on the surface ECG or the ventricular deflection (V) of the His bundle recording. The normal range of values is 35 to 55 ms.

Clinical Indications for His Bundle Recordings

Although information available from the surface electrocardiogram is frequently sufficient to clarify many cardiac electrical events, in some cases surface recordings alone may be inadequate. In these instances, His bundle recordings can provide further diagnostic insight into the patient's arrhythmia or conduction disturbance and thus facilitate more appropriate therapy. Several of the indications for His bundle recordings are listed in Table 101-1. In general, these can be divided into disorders of impulse formation and disorders of impulse conduction.

TABLE 101-1 Clinical Indications for His Bundle Recordings

1. Disorders of impulse formation
   a. Differentiation of ventricular from supraventricular rhythms with aberrancy
2. Disorders of impulse conduction
   a. AV block
      (1) Type I second degree AV block, persistent 2:1 AV block, and complete AV block associated with bundle branch block or intraventricular conduction delay
      (2) Apparent type II second degree AV block with other surface ECG evidence suggestive of concealed junctional premature beats
      (3) Apparent type II second degree AV block associated with a normal QRS complex
   b. Chronic bifascicular block in symptomatic patients
   c. (?) New bundle branch block following an acute anteroseptal myocardial infarction
   d. Syncope of undetermined etiology
3. Other
   a. Evaluation of patients with the preexcitation syndromes
   b. Classification of repetitive ventricular responses

Disorders of Impulse Formation

A common clinical problem is determining the origin of wide complex arrhythmias. Observations based on QRS morphology, width, and axis on the surface ECG may assist in differentiating supraventricular tachycardia with aberrancy from ventricular tachycardia.[7] The additional presence of AV dissociation and fusion or capture beats allows a more certain diagnosis of ventricular tachycardia. Frequently, the surface ECG alone is inadequate to make this critically important determination with certainty and a His bundle electrogram is required. A His potential preceding the ventricular deflection with a normal or greater than normal HV interval indicates a supraventricular origin, while no preceding His deflection or an HV interval less than normal is consistent with a ventricular site of origin.[8] Overdrive atrial pacing to produce fusion or capture beats with normalization of the HV interval may also indicate a ventricular origin of tachycardia. Analysis of the HV interval is similarly useful in determining the origin of sporadic wide complex beats as may be observed during atrial fibrillation. Since these determinations in each case are dependent on the HV relation, proper positioning of the recording catheter and validation of the His deflection during some normally conducted beats are mandatory.

His bundle recordings are also a critical part of a multiple catheter electrophysiology study used to more completely define the mechanism of both supraventricular and ventricular arrhythmias. In patients with a preexcitation syndrome, His bundle recordings not only assist in determining the presence and the location of an accessory AV pathway but also facilitate demonstrating its participation in an observed reentrant rhythm.[9] A His bundle recording is also required in the interpretation of repetitive ventricular responses following premature ventricular extrastimuli that are introduced during programmed stimulation in patients with ventricular arrhythmias. The recordings may help differentiate His bundle reentry or reentry in the bundle branch system from that occurring within the ventricles. Recordings made from the His catheter also allow characterization of automaticity, conduction, and refractoriness of the AV conduction system in response to various antiarrhythmic medications used in drug studies.

Disorders of Conduction

The disturbances of impulse propagation in the AV conduction system have traditionally been classified as first, second, or third degree AV block based on the presence of, respectively, prolongation of conduction without actual interruption, intermittent failure to conduct, or persistent conduction failure of a temporary or a permanent variety. Each of these may occur at any level of the AV conduction system. Second degree AV block has been further subdivided into Möbitz type I and II based on the behavior of the PR interval before and after the dropped beat.

The further division of conduction disturbances into those occurring in the AV node and those occurring within or below the His-Purkinje system has the added advantage of providing prognostic information which can be used as a guide to therapy. Conduction disturbances occurring within the AV node, although infrequently progressing to complete heart block, are usually associated with a stable escape rhythm originating in the His-Purkinje system if block does occur. As a result the overall outcome of block at this level is good. In contrast, those patients with a conduction disturbance in or below the His bundle are at higher risk for abruptly developing complete heart block with an inadequate lower-level escape rhythm. Syncope or sudden death may occur.

Usually the site of the conduction disturbance can be deduced from the surface ECG and the clinical setting in which the disturbance occurs. In the case of first degree AV block with a narrow QRS complex, the site of delay is usually the AV node, although on rare occasions the conduction delay may occur in the His bundle. Analysis of the PR interval does not allow discrimination between those two sites. Furthermore, conduction delay within the bundle branch system, which typically results in a wide complex QRS morphology, could be indistinguishable from first degree AV block occurring in the AV node in the setting of preexistent disease in lower levels of the conduction system. A His bundle recording may be necessary to make the distinction.

The approach to patients with second degree AV block is dictated by the patient's symptoms and the level of block within the conduction system. Those patients with prominent symptoms from bradycardia due to higher-grade block should undergo pacemaker implantation regardless of the location of the conduction abnormality. In contrast, the treatment of asymptomatic patients or those with symptoms not clearly related to AV block depends more on the level of the conduction disturbance. This can usually be satisfactorily predicted from the surface ECG and analysis of the QRS morphology, behavior of the PR interval, and rate of the escape rhythm if present. Patients with typical Wenckebach periodicity and a narrow QRS morphology are most likely to have a type I conduction defect confined to the AV node.[10] A conduction disturbance at this level is further indicated by an increase in block with carotid sinus massage or by total resolution of block with atropine.[11] Since type I block in the AV node generally does not progress to more advanced AV block,[12] pacemaker therapy in these patients is unlikely to be of benefit.

In contrast, patients with both a Mobitz type II pattern of block on a surface ECG and typical wide complex QRS morphology are much more likely to have block below the AV node in the His-Purkinje system.[10,13] Block at this level is not likely to be diminished with atropine nor increased with carotid sinus massage.[11] In fact, carotid sinus massage may decrease and atropine may increase the degree of block. In view of the increased risk of complete heart block and Stokes-Adams attacks,[14] patients with conduction defects in the His-Purkinje system can appropriately be considered pacemaker candidates.[15]

In other patients with second degree AV block the level of block cannot be determined from the ECG alone. Patients with episodic second degree AV block in the setting of chronic underlying bundle branch block,[15,16] those with ECG evidence of concealed junctional premature beats[17] mimicking Mobitz type II block, and those with apparent Mobitz type II block and normal QRS morphology may require His bundle recordings to differentiate relatively benign block within the node from block below the node where pacemaker implantation is appropriate. This differentiation may be further facilitated by the use of atropine[11] and atrial pacing during His bundle recordings to further "stress" the AV conduction system. The final group likely to benefit from such a study are patients with fixed 2:1 AV block. Patients in this subgroup who have normal QRS morphology are likely to have block within the node, while those who have wide QRS complexes may have block either within or below the AV node. This differentiation can only be made by His bundle recordings.

Patients with chronic bifascicular block as a group are also at risk for the development of complete heart block.[19–21] Although it would be of theoretical importance to identify individual patients at particular risk for developing higher-grade AV block, the incidence of such progression is low enough[18,19] that invasive His bundle studies for this purpose cannot be recommended in asymptomatic patients. His bundle recordings may nevertheless be of potential benefit in the evaluation of the subgroup of patients with transient neurological symptoms such as syncope or presyncope occurring in the absence of noninvasive documentation of higher-grade block. The development of infranodal block demonstrated on the His bundle electrogram during the added stress of atrial pacing has been shown to be associated with a higher risk of progression to complete heart block.[18] As a result, these patients may be considered for pacemaker therapy.

The usefulness of the HV interval in predicting subsequent progression to complete heart block has been more controversial, however. While several initial studies have shown no correlation between a prolonged HV interval and either sudden death or progression to complete heart block,[18,22,23] others have demonstrated a higher risk for such progression.[20,21] This is especially true in patients with HV intervals of more than 100 ms, in whom a 24 percent rate of progression to high-grade block over a 22-month follow-up period has been observed.[20] The difference between these reports is likely related to the difference in the prevalence of trifascicular conduction system disease in the populations being studied as suggested by differences in age, underlying cardiac disease, and the presence or absence of neurological symptoms.

That a prolonged HV interval is predictive of subsequent complete heart block is further supported by a more recent clinical investigation.[19] In a study of more patients with longer follow-up, an increase in spontaneous progression to trifascicular block (defined as second or third degree AV block distal to this His bundle recording rate) in patients with chronic bifascicular block and a prolonged HV interval was demonstrated. This is particularly important since earlier reports from this group failed to show any such correlation.[18,23] Thus, in those patients with chronic bifascicular block and recurrent syncope, a prolonged HV interval may indicate intermittent trifascicular block as the cause of symptoms, and pacemaker therapy may therefore be appropriate. It should be stressed, however, that although such treatment may be successful in alleviating transient neurological symptoms,[20] it has not been shown to decrease the incidence of sudden death, nor increase longevity in this patient population.[20] Sudden death and overall mortality, in turn, appear to be more closely related to the severity of the underlying disease and an increased prevalence of malignant ventricular arrhythmias in this patient population.[24]

Finally, although decisions regarding pacing in patients with new Mobitz type II or bifascicular block during the periinfarct period are usually made on a clinical basis alone, a prolonged HV interval in the setting of a new bundle branch block following an acute anteroseptal myocardial infarction may be helpful in identifying those patients who are at an increased risk of developing third degree AV block.[25] It is unclear whether this determination provides independent prognostic information, however.

Therapeutic Utility of the His Bundle Catheter

Since the first His bundle potentials were successfully recorded, the His bundle catheter has been used exclusively as a diagnostic tool. More recently the catheter has been used in animals[26,27] and humans[28,29] to deliver a direct current shock to the His bundle to create AV block without demonstrable damage to the intraatrial or ventricular septum or tricuspid valve apparatus. Closed-chest catheter ablation of the AV conduction system is now the procedure of choice for the creation of AV block in patients with medically refractory supraventricular arrhythmias and has obviated the need and risk of an open surgical procedure for this purpose in most patients. Although stable escape rhythms may be present following His ablation, those patients in whom complete AV block is induced are assumed to be pacemaker-dependent.

In performing a catheter His ablation, the standard tripolar catheter used for His bundle recordings is positioned across the tricuspid valve in the region of the His bundle and unipolar His electrograms are filtered at 0.5 to 1000 Hz.[28] The catheter is then further positioned to record the largest amplitude His deflection. After appropriate switching from recording to current delivery modes, a direct current shock of 200 to 400 J is delivered from a conventional cardioversion unit via the distal catheter unipole to a back paddle positioned adjacent to the left scapula.[29] The catheter position is obviously critical as a malpositioned catheter may result in inappropriate delivery of energy to the myocardium or bundle branch system. To date, catheter His ablation has been carried out without evidence of untoward structural damage or increased ventricular ectopy from the ablation site. Nevertheless, the risks are of sufficient concern that this procedure should be performed only by those with appropriate experience with this technique.

Recently, laser energy directed by a standard His bundle catheter has been successfully applied to interrupt the AV conduction system in animals.[30,31] This suggests that a pervenous laser catheter system may also be useful in the future treatment of supraventricular arrhythmias.

Noninvasive His Bundle Recordings

Much effort has been directed toward developing a reliable noninvasive means of recording electrical activity from the specialized AV conduction system at the body surface. By using multiple leads, esophageal electrodes, or signal averaging, several groups have successfully recorded what appears to be the His bundle deflection in the PR interval.[32-34] Thus far, however, the usefulness of these techniques is limited by the continued difficulty in isolating the small-amplitude His bundle potential from noise originating in skeletal muscle activity, as well as amplifier and electrode sources. It has also been difficult to clearly separate His bundle from terminal atrial activity. Nevertheless, with additional technological advances, a satisfactory system for this purpose will likely be developed.

References

1. Scherlag, B. J., Lau, S. H., Helfant, R. H., Berkowitz, W. D., Stein, E., and Damato, A. N.: Catheter Technique for Recording His Bundle Activity in Man, *Circulation*, 39:13, 1969.
2. Damato, A. N., Lau, S. H., Berkowitz, W. D., Rosen, K. M., and Lisi, K. R.: Recording of Specialized Conducting Fibers (A-V Nodal, His Bundle, and Right Bundle Branch) in Man Using an Electrode Catheter Technique, *Circulation*, 39:435, 1969.
3. Gallagher, J. J., and Damato, A. N.: Technique of Recording His Bundle Activity in Man, in W. Grossman (ed.), "Cardiac

Catheterization and Angiography," Lea & Febiger, Philadelphia, 1980, p. 283.
4. Jacobson, L. B., and Scheinman, M.: Catheter Induced Intra-Hisian and Intrafascicular Block During Recording of His Bundle Electrogram: A Report of Two Cases, *Circulation*, 49:579, 1974.
5. Gallagher, J. J., Damato, A. N., Lau, S. H., Towar, A. J., Caracta, A. R., Varghese, P. J., and Josephson, M. E.: Antecubital Vein Approach for Recording His Bundle Activity in Man, *Am. Heart J.*, 85:199, 1973.
6. Narula, O. S., Javier, R. P., Samet, P., and Maramba, L. C.: Significance of His and Left Bundle Recordings from the Left Heart in Man, *Circulation*, 42:385, 1970.
7. Wellens, H. J. J., Bar, F. W., and Lie, K. I.: The Value of the Electrocardiogram in the Differential Diagnosis of a Tachycardia with a Wide QRS Complex, *Am. J. Med.*, 64:27, 1978.
8. Castor, J. A., Horowitz, L. N., Harkins, A. H., and Josephson, M. E.: Clinical Electrophysiology of Ventricular Tachycardia, *N. Engl. J. Med.*, 304:1004, 1981.
9. Gallagher, J. J., Pritchett, E. L. C., Sealy, W. C., Kasell, J., and Wallace, A. G.: The Preexcitation Syndrome, *Prog. Cardiovasc. Dis.*, 20:285, 1978.
10. Damato, A. N., Lau, S. H., Helfant, R., Stein, E., Patton, R. D., Scherlag, B. J., and Berkowitz, W. D.: A Study of Heart Block in Man Using His Bundle Recordings, *Circulation*, 39:297, 1969.
11. Mangiardi, L. M., Bonamini, R., Conte, M., Gaita, F., Orzan, F., Presbitero, P., and Brusca, A.: Bedside Evaluation of Atrioventricular Block with Narrow QRS Complexes: Usefulness of Carotid Sinus Massage and Atropine Administration, *Am. J. Cardiol.*, 49:1136, 1982.
12. Strasberg, B., Amat-y-Leon, F., Dhingra, R. D., Palileo, E., Swiryn, S., Bauernfeind, R., Wyndham, C., and Rosen, K. M.: Natural History of Chronic Second-Degree Atrioventricular Nodal Block, *Circulation*, 63:1043, 1981.
13. Narula, O. S., and Samet, P.: Wenckebach and Mobitz Type II A-V Block Due to Block Within the His Bundle and Bundle Branches, *Circulation*, 41:947, 1970.
14. Langendorf, R., and Pick, A.: Atrioventricular Block, Type II (Mobitz): Its Nature and Clinical Significance, *Circulation*, 38:819, 1968.
15. Dhingra, R. C., Denes, P., Wu, D., Chuquimia, R., and Rosen, K. M.: The Significance of Second Degree Atrioventricular Block and Bundle Branch Block. Observations regarding Site and Type of Block, *Circulation*, 49:638, 1974.
16. Zipes, D. P.: Second-Degree Atrioventricular Block, *Circulation*, 60:465, 1979.
17. Rosen, K. M., Rahimtoola, S. H., and Gunnar, R. M.: Pseudo A-V Block Secondary to Premature Non-Propagated His Bundle Depolarizations: Documentation by His Bundle Electrocardiography, *Circulation*, 42:367, 1970.
18. Dhingra, R. C., Wyndham, C., Bauernfeind, R., Swiryn, S., Deedwania, P. C., Smith, T., Denes, P., and Rosen, K. M.: Significance of Block Distal to the His Bundle Induced by Atrial Pacing in Patients with Chronic Bifascicular Block, *Circulation*, 60:1455, 1979.
19. Dhingra, R. C., Palileo, E., Strasberg, B., Swiryn, S., Bauernfeind, R., Wyndham, C. R. C., and Rosen, K. M.: Significance of the HV Interval in 517 Patients with Chronic Bifascicular Block, *Circulation*, 64:1265, 1981.
20. Scheinman, M. M., Peters, R. W., Sauve, M. J., Desai, J., Abbott, J. A., Cogan, J., Wohl, B., and Williams, K.: Value of the H-Q Interval in Patients with Bundle Branch Block and the Role of Prophylactic Permanent Pacing, *Am. J. Cardiol.*, 50:1316, 1982.
21. Altschuler, H., Fisher, J. O., and Furman, S.: Significance of Isolated H-V Interval Prolongation in Symptomatic Patients Without Documented Heart Block, *Am. Heart J.*, 97:19, 1979.
22. McAnulty, J. H., Rahimtoola, S. H., Murphy, E., DeMots, H., Ritzman, L., Kanarek, P. E., and Kauffman, S.: Natural History of "High Risk" Bundle-Branch Block: Final Report of a Prospective Study, *N. Engl. J. Med.*, 307:137, 1982.
23. Denes, P., Dhingra, R. C., Wu, D., Chuquimia, R., Amat-y-Leon, F., Wyndham, C., and Rosen, K. M.: H-V Interval in Patients with Bifascicular Block (Right Bundle Branch Block and Left Anterior Hemiblock): Clinical Electrocardiographic and Electrophysiologic Correlations, *Am. J. Cardiol.*, 35:23, 1975.
24. Denes, P., Dhingra, R. C., Wu, D., Wyndham, C. R., Amat-y-Leon, F., and Rosen, K. M.: Sudden Death in Patients with Chronic Bifascicular Block, *Arch. Intern. Med.*, 137:1005, 1979.
25. Lie, K. I., Wellens, H. J., Schuilenburg, R. M., Becker, A. E., and Durher, D.: Factors Influencing Prognosis of Bundle Branch Block Complicating Acute Antero-Septal Infarction: The Value of His Bundle Recordings, *Circulation*, 50:935, 1974.
26. Bardy, G. J., Ideker, R. E., Kasell, J., Worley, S. J., Smith, W. M., German, L. D., and Gallagher, J. J.: Transvenous Ablation of the Atrioventricular Conduction System in Dogs: Electrophysiologic and Histologic Observations, *Am. J. Cardiol.*, 51:1775, 1983.
27. Gonzalez, R., Scheinman, M., Margaretten, W., and Rubinstein, M.: Closed Chest Electro-Catheter Technique for His Bundle Ablation in Dogs, *Am. J. Physiol.*, 241:H283, 1981.
28. Gallagher, J. J., Svenson, R. H., Kasell, J. H., German, L. D., Bardy, G. H., Broughton, A., and Critelli, G.: Catheter Technique for Closed Chest Ablation of the Atrioventricular Conduction System, *N. Engl. J. Med.*, 306:194, 1982.
29. Scheinman, M. M., Morady, F., Hess, D. F., and Gonzalez, R.: Catheter-Induced Ablation of the Atrioventricular Junction to Control Refractory Supraventricular Arrhythmias, *JAMA*, 248:851, 1982.
30. Abela, G. S., Griffin, J. C., Hill, J. A., Normann, S., and Conti, C. R.: Transvascular Argon Laser-Induced Atrioventricular Conduction Ablation in Dogs, *Circulation*, 68(suppl.III):145, 1983.
31. Narula, O. S., Bharati, S., Chan, M. C., Embi, A. A., and Lev, M.: Micro-Transection of the His Bundle with Laser Radiation through a Pervenous Catheter: Correlation of Histologic and Electrophysiologic Data, *Am. J. Cardiol.*, 54:186, 1984.
32. Flowers, N. C., Hand, R. C., Orander, P. C., Miller, C. B., Walden, M. O., and Horan, L. G.: Surface Recording of Electrical Activity from the Region of the Bundle of His, *Am. J. Cardiol.*, 33:384, 1974.
33. Mehra, R., Kelen, G. J., Zeiler, R., Zephiran, D., Fried, P., Gomez, J. A., and El-Sherif, N.: Non-Invasive His Bundle Electrogram: Value of Three Vector Lead Recordings, *Am. J. Cardiol.*, 49:344, 1982.
34. Hombach, V., Behrenbeck, D. W., and Hilger, H. H.: Esophagal sternal and Esophagal Apical Leads for Registration of Surface His-Bundle Potentials, *Z. Kardiol.*, 66:565, 1977.

102

Techniques of Programmed Stimulation, Atrial Pacing, and Electrical Assessment of Drug Therapy

Harold C. Strauss, M.D.
Lawrence D. German, M.D.
Andrew G. Wallace, M.D.

Background

The development of clinical electrophysiologic techniques has led to a more rational approach to the diagnosis and management of patients with brady- and tachyarrhythmias (Table 102-1). These techniques have been used to: (1) characterize the electrophysiologic properties of different tissues in the heart; (2) establish the mechanisms, site, and severity of a bradycardia; (3) establish the mechanisms and site of origin of a tachycardia; (4) uncover latent arrhythmias whose intermittent manifestations result in diagnostic problems; and (5) evaluate the beneficial and potentially harmful effects of different therapeutic programs.

Three general categories of electrophysiologic testing can be distinguished. The first consists of programmed stimulation techniques used to evaluate the function of the sinoatrial (SA) node and atrioventricular (AV) conduction system (AV node, His-Purkinje system, accessory pathway). The second consists of programmed stimulation techniques used to induce and terminate supraventricular and ventricular arrhythmias. The third consists of mapping techniques used to determine the tachycardia pathways.

Technical Methods

The number of catheter electrodes, their position inside the heart, and the type of programmed pulse sequence will vary depending upon the purpose of the study.[1,2] Nonetheless, all features have certain common elements. Like most invasive procedures, electrophysiologic studies should be performed in the fasting state. Concurrent medications should be in a steady state, and unless antiarrhythmic therapy is being evaluated, drugs with antiarrhythmic properties should be discontinued for at least three half-lives before the procedure. These procedures are generally performed under local anesthesia (lidocaine or procaine). Overuse of these agents can result in therapeutic blood levels. If needed, sedation with diazepam, lorazepam, and meperidine can be used. The technique of catheter placement and the recording apparatus are described in Chap. 101.

TABLE 102-1 Indications for Electrophysiologic Studies

Diagnosis	
	Syncope, presyncope
	Complex arrhythmias
Preoperative assessment	
	Preexcitation syndromes
	Ventricular tachycardia
Guiding therapy	
	Assessment of antiarrhythmic drug therapy
	Evaluation for antitachycardia pacemakers

The number of electrocardiogram (ECG) and electrogram recordings needed will depend on the type of study being performed. Sinus node function is evaluated with multiple surface ECG leads and electrogram recordings from the high right atrium and the His bundle. Complex mapping studies may require four or more catheters to be in place at one time. When mapping ventricular tachycardia, we routinely use catheters in the coronary sinus, right atrium, His bundle region, and right ventricle in addition to a left ventricular catheter. In contrast, simple induction studies may be performed with only one or two catheters.

The complexity of the stimulator unit will vary depending upon the type of electrophysiologic study planned. Atrial pacing for determination of sinus node recovery times requires only a temporary pacemaker unit. Introduction of premature beats at preselected times in the cardiac cycle for determination of refractoriness requires a programmable stimulator. Regardless of the type of stimulator used, it is mandatory to have the output isolated from ground to minimize current leakage from the stimulator to the patient.

The range of normal values for many of the electrophysiologic variables is provided in Table 102-2.

Sinus Node

Although noninvasive evaluation (ambulatory ECG monitoring) of sinus node function has proved to be invaluable in establishing diagnosis and guiding therapy, the results obtained using this approach may be inconclusive.[3–5] Further, it may be preferable to evaluate the potential adverse drug effects in a control setting so that if needed, cardiac pacing can be promptly instituted.[3–5] In either instance, provocative invasive investigation may prove helpful.

Three stimulation techniques have been designed to assess the two pathophysiologic mechanisms underlying sinus node dysfunction.[3,4] Rapid atrial pacing is used to evaluate disturbances of automaticity, while premature atrial stimulation and constant atrial pacing are used to evaluate disturbances of SA conduction.[6,7] While it is desirable to distinguish disturbances of automaticity from disturbances of conduction, this may not always be possible since disturbances of conduction may preclude accurate evaluation of sinus node automaticity.

Rapid Atrial Pacing Technique

In principle, this technique measures the degree of suppression of sinus node automaticity following a period of imposed atrial overdrive (Fig. 102-1).[3,4] Following cessation of pacing, the interval between the last paced atrial electrogram and the first spontaneous atrial electrogram is measured and is termed the sinus node recovery time (SNRT). A period of overdrive pacing of 1 min is used with multiple pacing rates being evaluated starting at a rate slightly faster than the spontaneous sinus rate and increasing in 20 beats per minute increments up to 150 or 170 beats per minute. In general, the degree of suppression depends on the inherent automaticity of the sinus node, the number of paced impulses reaching the node, and the autonomic tone at the time of study. Normally, SNRT increases as the pacing rate increases, reaching a maximum value ($SNRT_{max}$) between 118 and 130 beats per minute. At faster pacing rates, a decrease in SNRT may be seen due to the development of sinus node entrance block.[6] In patients with sick sinus syndrome, the pacing rate at which $SNRT_{max}$ occurs may fall outside the range seen in normal patients, emphasizing the need for repeated determinations of SNRT at different pacing rates.

FIGURE 102-1 Effects of rapid atrial pacing on spontaneous sinus cycle length are shown for a patient with sinus node dysfunction. ECG leads I and V_1 are shown during the period (heart rate: *A*, 90 beats per minute and *B*, 130 beats per minute) and the postpacing cycles following termination of pacing (indicated by dashed line between the panels). In panel *A* the first postpacing atrial cycle length is 1.3 s. In panel *B*, at the more rapid pacing rate 2:1 AV block occurred. The first postpacing atrial cycle is prolonged at 2.2 s (note the intervening junctional escape beat). Note also prolongation of the subsequent postpacing atrial cycles (secondary pauses).

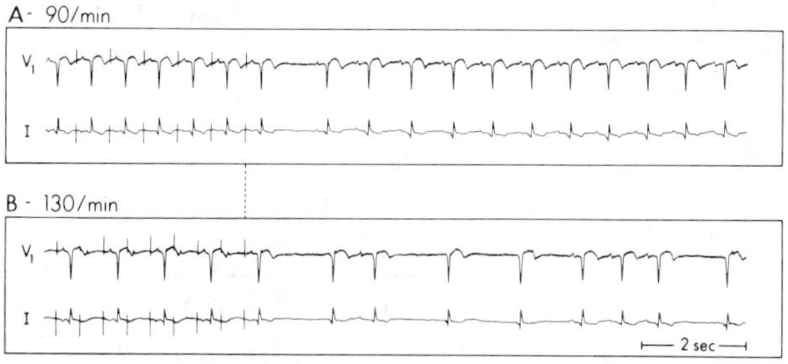

In normal subjects, $SNRT_{max}$ is dependent on prepacing cycle length and is therefore usually corrected for heart rate by subtracting the spontaneous cycle length from the sinus node recovery time, yielding the corrected sinus node recovery time (CSNRT). Normal values for CSNRT range between 375 to 533 ms, being 525 ms in our institution. The sinus node recovery time may also be expressed as a ratio of the spontaneous cycle length. The normal ratio is up to 1.61 for spontaneous atrial cycle lengths ranging between 600 and 800 ms, and up to 1.83 for spontaneous cycle lengths greater than 800 ms.

Abnormal responses to rapid atrial pacing may be detected in cycles subsequent to the first and criteria for their detection have been established. Analysis of the first 10 postpacing cycles rather than analysis of only the first postpacing cycle improves the sensitivity of the rapid atrial pacing technique for the detection of sinus node dysfunction.

Premature Atrial Stimulation and Constant Atrial Pacing Techniques

Estimation of the SA conduction time (SACT) may be performed using either the premature atrial stimulation or constant atrial pacing techniques.[3,4] Both methods make the same assumption regarding sinus node activity. During deployment of the premature atrial stimulation technique, a premature stimulus is introduced following every eighth spontaneous sinus cycle. The coupling interval between the last spontaneous atrial electrogram and the premature stimulus is varied in 5-to-10-ms steps so that the excitable portion of diastole is scanned. Late premature beats are followed by compensatory return cycles, presumably due to collision between the paced beat and the emerging sinus node impulse. Earlier premature beats are followed by less-than-compensatory return cycles, presumably because they penetrate and reset the sinus node. The duration of the less-than-compensatory atrial return cycle is determined by the retrograde conduction time of the premature beat into the node, the sinus node return cycle, and the antegrade conduction time back to the atrium. If the sinus node return cycle is not altered by the premature beat and remains equal to the basic sinus node cycle, then the difference between the atrial return cycle and the spontaneous sinus cycle should equal the sum of the retrograde and antegrade SA conduction times ($SACT_{A+R}$). This approximation of the true SA conduction time is expressed as the sum of the antegrade and retrograde conduction times since they may not be equal. The mean value of $SACT_{A+R}$ is derived from the analysis of many such pulse sequences and in our laboratory is considered to be prolonged if it exceeds 206 ms.

The constant atrial pacing technique employs a brief period of atrial pacing (8 beats) at a rate less than 10 beats per minute faster than the spontaneous rate. The SACT is calculated by subtracting the spontaneous cycle length prior to pacing from the atrial return cycle following pacing. A consistent correlation between the premature atrial stimulation and constant atrial pacing techniques has not been confirmed experimentally, and indirect estimates of SACT are usually obtained with the premature atrial stimulation technique. Direct measurements of SA conduction time using sinus node electrogram recording may prove to be an important addition to the assessment of SA conduction.

In our hands, both of these methods for estimating SACT have proven to be less sensitive than the rapid atrial pacing technique in establishing the diagnosis of sinus node dysfunction, and in unmasking latent disturbances of sinus node function, in guiding therapy and in predicting adverse drug responses.[3]

These techniques are particularly useful in patients with sick sinus syndrome in whom syncope or presyncope is suspected to be due to intermittent sinus node dysfunction, or to test for possible adverse effects of drugs used to treat other rhythm disturbances.

Evaluation of AV Node Function

The anatomy of the AV node allows one to record electrical activity directly from tissue that is proximal (low right atrium) and distal (His bundle) to the AV node. Measurements of AV nodal conduction time (AH interval) and His-Purkinje conduction time (HV interval) during spontaneous sinus rhythm have enabled electrophysiologists to confirm diagnoses made indirectly from ECG analysis and to examine the prognostic and therapeutic significance of their findings.[1,2,7–9] In some patients, however, further information bearing on the AV conduction system is desirable and can be obtained by incremental atrial pacing and programmed atrial stimulation.

Incremental Atrial Pacing Technique

In principle, this technique stresses the AV conduction system to unmask latent disturbances of conduction.[1] Pacing is performed from the high right atrium. Pacing is started at a cycle length that is just below the spontaneous cycle length and is decreased every 60 s in 50-to-100-ms steps until a minimum value of 300 ms is attained. In normal patients, as the pacing cycle length decreases, the AH interval increases, until second degree AV block with Wenckebach periodicity appears. The pacing cycle length at which second degree AV nodal block appears usually ranges between 500 and 350 ms. Differences in autonomic tone may cause block to appear outside this range of values. Block occurring in the AV node generally does not require intervention. During incremental atrial pacing the HV interval is usually unchanged. In a symptomatic individual, the development of HV interval prolongation or block within the His-Purkinje system at any pacing cycle length is usually an abnormal finding.[1,2,7–9]

Programmed Atrial Stimulation Technique

This technique is used to measure the refractoriness of the AV conduction system, principally of the AV node, but also of the His-Purkinje system if the refractoriness of the AV node is short enough.[1,2] The high right atrium is paced at a constant cycle length and a premature stimulus is introduced following every eighth driven cycle. The coupling interval of the premature stimulus is decreased to 10-to-20-ms steps until the excitable portion of atrial diastole is scanned. Measurement of the intervals in the electrogram recordings obtained from sites proximal and distal to the tissue under study permits the determination of the effective, relative, and functional refractory periods of that tissue (Fig. 102-2). For example, in the AV node, the effective refractory period is the longest atrial premature interval in which the atrial premature beat fails to propagate to the His bundle. The relative refractory period is the atrial

FIGURE 102-2 Atrial and AV refractory period determination. The filled squares represent a plot of the atrial response A_1–A_2 (*y* axis) versus the premature stimulus coupling interval S_1–S_2 (*x* axis). The point at which latency develops results in a departure from the line of identity which determines the relative refractory period (RRP) of the atrium. The point at which failure to capture occurs is the effective refractory period (ERP) of the atrium. The open circles represent a plot of the His bundle response H_1–H_2 (*y* axis) versus A_1–A_2 (*x* axis). The longer refractory period of the AV node than in the atrium results in deviation from the line of identity at a longer premature beat coupling interval. The functional refractory period (FRP) of the AV node is the shortest H_1–H_2 interval obtained. The ERP of the AV node is the point at which A_2 fails to propagate to the ventricle. The scale on both axes is in milliseconds.

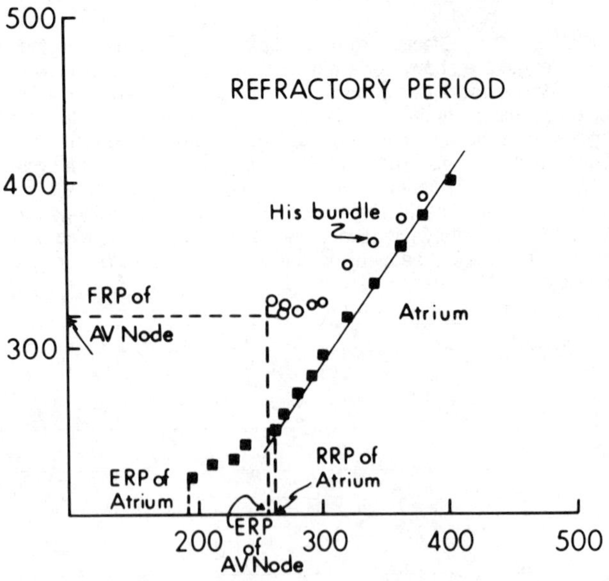

TABLE 102-2 Range of Normal Values

Interval	Value, ms
PA	20–50
AH	50–130
HV	30–50
His duration	10–25
CSNRT	< 525
SACT	< 206
ERP	
RA	170–300
AVN	230–425
His-Purkinje	330–450
Ventricle	170–290

premature interval associated with the first detectable increase in the AH interval of the premature response compared to the regular driven response. The functional refractory period is the shortest interval between His bundle responses resulting from premature atrial stimulation. The range of normal values reported for the refractory periods of the AV node and His-Purkinje system is wide (Table 102-2). While determination of refractoriness is currently of research interest in the evaluation of patients with disturbances in the AV conduction system, its role in the routine evaluation of patients has not been demonstrated.

Arrhythmia Induction and Termination

Two pacing techniques are used routinely for the induction and termination of supraventricular and ventricular arrhythmias; premature stimulation and rapid pacing of the atria or the ventricles[1,2,10–16] (Figs. 102-3 and 102-4). During premature stimulation one to four premature stimuli are introduced during diastole either following a drive-train of paced beats or following a predetermined number of sinus beats. Premature stimuli are initially delivered late in diastole and then the coupling interval is progressively decreased until refractoriness is reached and/or an arrhythmia results. If single premature stimuli fail to elicit the arrhythmia, additional multiple premature stimuli are used. As refractoriness decreases after a premature stimulus, subsequent premature beats can be elicited at shorter coupling intervals than that following the first extrastimulus. Rapid pacing may take the form of a continuous period of pacing at rates faster than the spontaneous sinus rate followed by abrupt cessation of pacing, or may involve burst pacing using short periods of pacing at rapid cycle lengths (generally from 360 to 240 ms) or until one-to-one capture of the chamber being paced cannot be maintained. Burst pacing can be synchronous, that is, beginning at a set interval during diastole, or asynchronous, beginning randomly in diastole.

Rapid pacing and burst pacing are especially effective for inducing atrial flutter or fibrillation. In addition, arrhythmias that depend on the development of conduction delay in the AV nodes such as reciprocating tachycardia due to AV nodal reentry and the various preexcitation syndromes are often induced by burst pacing of the atria or ventricles. Ventricular tachycardia may be induced by burst pacing in some patients, although in our experience, premature stimulation using multiple premature stimuli is a more effective and controlled method. Rapid repetitive stimulation has been used to terminate atrial flutter, supraventricular tachycardia, and ventricular tachycardia. For the latter arrhythmia, it is used less often because of the risk of inducing ventricular fibrillation or accelerating ventricular tachycardia.

The initiation of the tachycardia is evaluated to establish the relation of the P wave to the QRS complex and to determine whether its onset is related to delay in AV nodal conduction times (AV nodal tachycardia). The tachycardia itself is evaluated to determine the relation of the P wave to the QRS complex, the pattern of retrograde atrial activation, and the effects of premature atrial and ventricular beats on the cycle length of tachycardia. The demonstration that the ventricle forms an integral part of the reentry circuit indicates that an accessory pathway must be part of the circuit. This is determined by the demonstration of (1) an increase in cycle length of the tachycardia following development of ipsilateral bundle branch block (spontaneous or induced), and (2) the preexcitation of the atrium and advancement of the tachycardia by a ventricular premature beat when the His bundle is refractory. The functional characteristics of the AV

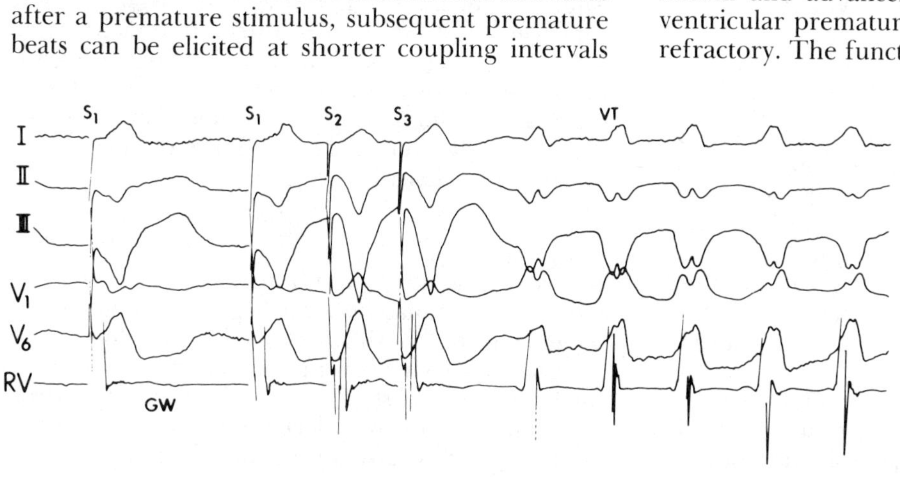

FIGURE 102-3 Initiation of ventricular tachycardia by programmed stimulation. Right ventricular (RV) pacing (S_1) at a cycle length of 600 ms is followed by two premature stimuli (S_2, S_3) resulting in the induction of ventricular tachycardia (VT).

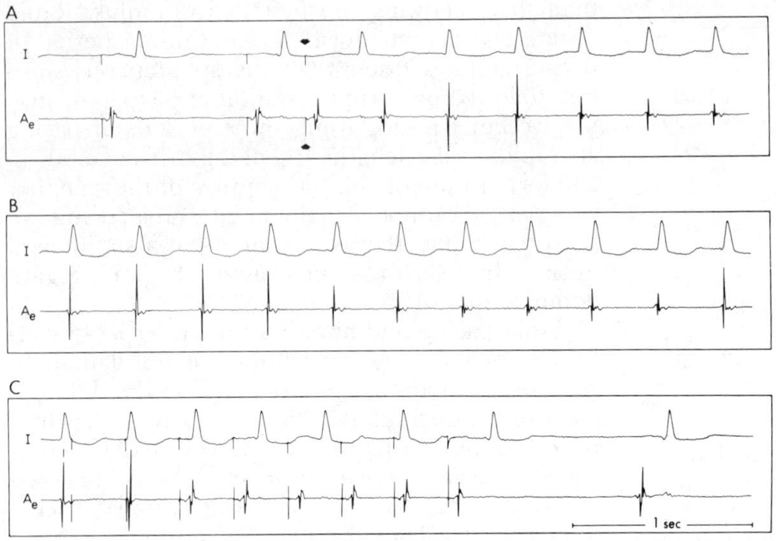

FIGURE 102-4 Initiation and termination of a paroxysmal supraventricular tachycardia in a patient with recurrent palpitations. ECG lead I and high right atrial electrogram (A_e) are shown in the top and bottom traces of each panel. In panel *A* with the pacing catheter in the coronary sinus an atrial premature depolarization (indicated by the arrow) initiates the tachycardia. In panel *B* the tachycardia is shown just prior to the onset of overdrive pacing. Overdrive pacing (*C*) is initiated and following atrial capture the tachycardia is terminated. Sinus rhythm resumes following termination of pacing.

node and accessory pathway should be evaluated during programmed atrial and ventricular stimulation to determine the echo zone and the refractoriness of the accessory pathway. If refractoriness is extremely short in the accessory pathway, then the development of atrial fibrillation could result in frequent impulse transmission through this pathway to the ventricles, possibly leading to ventricular fibrillation.

Programmed stimulation of the ventricle using multiple premature stimuli at various drive cycle lengths is most often used in the study of patients with ventricular tachycardia (Fig. 102-3). Although criteria were developed to identify those instances where reentry was the underlying mechanism, recent information suggests this goal may not be attainable.[17] At this time, the primary purpose of the stimulation protocols is in the ability to repetitively induce ventricular arrhythmias so that, if need be, they can be mapped and the effects of drugs on induction and termination can be assessed. Careful correlation of arrhythmia morphology with documented spontaneously occurring arrhythmia is mandatory.

Mapping

One of the more useful applications of electrophysiologic testing has been in the localization of the pathway of the arrhythmia.[11,17] The techniques described above may be used to repeatedly induce tachycardia and, when coupled to the systematic mapping of the activation sequence of the cardiac chambers using electrode catheters, has enabled us to precisely localize the accessory AV pathways, and the origins of ventricular tachycardia, as well as the sites of the automatic tachycardia to direct surgical intervention.

The mapping of atrial arrhythmias is accomplished by using a multipolar electrode catheter introduced from the left subclavian vein into the coronary sinus to record electrical activity from the left atrium around the mitral annulus and special mapping catheters introduced from the femoral vein to record electrical activity from predetermined sites in the right atrium.

The mapping of patients with AV reentrant tachycardias is performed by paying particular attention to the presence or absence of retrograde ventriculoatrial conduction, the route of retrograde conduction (via the His bundle and AV node or accessory pathways as indicated by an eccentric activation sequence), the presence of preexcitation during antegrade pacing or sinus rhythm, or the effect of premature stimuli during the tachycardia. In addition, the effects of functional bundle branch block during reciprocating tachycardia may give important evidence for the localization of accessory pathways, since a lengthening of VA intervals with ipsilateral bundle branch block indicates an accessory pathway on that side. Differentiation of reciprocating tachycardia due to accessory pathways from that due to reentry in the AV node is also possible and has important therapeutic implications.

Localization of the site of ventricular tachycardia is more difficult. Multiple sites in the right and left ventricles must be sampled during the tachycardia and approximate localization is possible using biplane fluoroscopy. Pacing from suspected sites of tachycardia initiation may also allow comparison of the paced QRS morphology with the ECG recorded during the tachycardia.

Drug Testing

In addition to studying the mechanism of localization of arrhythmias, both the beneficial and arrhythmogenic effects of drugs on the arrhythmia can be studied with induction and termination techniques used in the control study.[1,2,12] Acute intravenous drug administration during electrophysiologic study can be performed to assess potentially effective antiarrhythmic agents. Serial testing on oral regimens is facilitated by leaving an indwelling catheter for repeat stimulation studies. Repeat stimulation should be performed with knowledge of drug levels and with plasma drug concentrations at steady state.

Anticipated Results

In patients with sinus node disease, electrophysiologic testing is often unrewarding. Tests of sinus node function (especially SNRT) are highly specific when clearly abnormal but not highly sensitive. The decision to implant a pacemaker for symptoms of syncope or presyncope due to sinus node disease is often more readily made on the basis of ambulatory recordings than invasive stimulation testing.

Syncope may be the result of sinus node dysfunction or atrial arrhythmias in addition to transient ventricular arrhythmias or conduction abnormalities. When noninvasive tests fail to disclose an etiology for syncope, electrophysiologic testing may be expected to produce a diagnosis in approximately half of patients with organic heart disease, and fewer patients with no heart disease. Syncope will frequently be found to be the result of ventricular tachycardia. Vasodepressor reactions producing syncope are also frequently found in patients with sinus node dysfunction and other arrhythmias. Symptoms may be exacerbated by inappropriate antiarrhythmic therapy, and may not be helped by pacemaker implantation. Therefore, careful exclusion of hypotensive episodes due to abnormal vagal tone is necessary as part of the electrophysiologic evaluation in patients with syncope.

Mapping studies for supraventricular arrhythmias including ectopic tachycardias, Wolff-Parkinson-White (WPW) syndrome, and rare variants of the preexcitation syndromes, as well as ventricular tachycardia, are highly useful in experienced hands. These studies are mandatory before considering surgical treatment of these arrhythmias.

The use of electrophysiologic testing to induce arrhythmias and to test antiarrhythmic medications is one of the most widespread applications at this time. Numerous reports have attested to the superiority of antiarrhythmic regimens chosen on the basis of serial drug testing over empiric therapy in treating ventricular tachycardia. The best results can be expected in patients with ischemic heart disease and documented sustained ventricular tachycardia. If it can be shown that the clinically documented arrhythmia is suppressed by one or more antiarrhythmic regimens, a high degree of success can be expected.

Arrhythmia induction studies are critical in evaluating antitachycardia pacemakers. These devices may be extremely effective in controlling the recurring episodes of supraventricular tachycardia and to a lesser extent than the treatment of ventricular tachycardia. The mechanism of the arrhythmia must be known and the safety and efficacy of the proposed pacing modality tested before the permanent device can be implanted. In particular, one needs to ensure that the stable ventricular tachycardia is not converted to a hemodynamically unstable form of ventricular tachycardia or to ventricular fibrillation during pacing.

Complications

Complications of electrophysiologic testing can be divided into three major categories: those related to arrhythmias, those related to catheterization, and those related to the administration of drugs. Generally, the purpose of the electrophysiologic study is to elicit arrhythmias and as such cannot be regarded as a complication. There is, however, always the potential to precipitate an unwanted or unexpected arrhythmia. Bradyarrhythmias are rarely produced during catheter studies. However, an occasional patient with sinus node dysfunction may develop prolonged pauses in rhythm on termination of rapid atrial pacing which may require resumption of pacing. In addition, development of catheter-induced right bundle branch block in a patient with preexisting left bundle branch block may produce complete heart block. Adverse reactions to pain or apprehension may also develop during the invasive studies. This may be associated with hypotension and nausea as well as bradycardia. Ventricular fibrillation or unstable ventricular tachycardia may develop from catheter manipulation in the ventricle or during programmed stimulation. Rarely, rapid, sustained ventricular arrhythmias are induced during simple refractory period determinations in apparently normal patients. In patients with WPW syndrome, the induction of atrial fibrillation or flutter may be associated with a rapid ventricular rate leading to hypotension and possibly ventricular fibrillation. Patients with hypertrophic cardiomyopathy or aortic stenosis often tolerate rapid arrhythmias poorly.

Mechanical complications are the most serious potential of catheter electrophysiologic studies. Perforation of the right ventricle, the right atrium, and the coronary sinus may produce cardiac tamponade. Trauma to vessels during catheter introduction may involve the subclavian and femoral veins, and the subclavian and femoral arteries. In addition, the risk of pneumothorax is present with subclavian puncture. Infection and thrombosis are possible with puncture sites, especially in the femoral vein. Heparin is usually administered during longer studies to minimize this complication.

When antiarrhythmic drugs are administered during electrophysiologic studies, the potential for drug reactions is always present. A careful drug history before the procedure helps minimize these complications.

Therapeutic Applications of Atrial Pacing

Bradyarrhythmias

Symptomatic bradyarrhythmias occurring in patients with SA or AV node dysfunction are treated with permanent pacemaker implantation.[2] In general, the majority of these patients will do well with a ventricular pacemaker. However, in those patients with SA node dysfunction in whom atrial pacing may be indicated, AV conduction should be assessed to determine whether or not this pacing site may be used. In a small group of patients, AV sequential pacing may be indicated. Patients with the bradycardia-tachycardia syndrome may require pacemaker implantation so that drugs can be used to control the tachyarrhythmias. A ventricular pacemaker would not be expected to reduce the frequency of attacks of supraventricular arrhythmias, but would prevent the bradyarrhythmic effects of antiarrhythmic drugs. Atrial pacing has been shown to reduce the frequency of supraventricular arrhythmias in some of these patients. Permanent atrial pacing may be accomplished through the use of a specially designed pervenous catheter electrode placed in the coronary sinus or the right atrial appendage, or through an atrial epicardial electrode implanted at thoracotomy.

Tachyarrhythmias

Patients with recurrent episodes of supraventricular tachycardia who are unresponsive to vigorous pharmacologic therapy may be treated by a variety of antitachycardia pacing techniques.[16,18] Devices are available which perform patient-activated burst pacing for the termination of paroxysmal supraventricular tachycardia, as well as more sophisticated devices that automatically sense tachycardias and respond with bursts or critically timed extrastimuli. Many of these devices also have incorporated backup pacing capability if termination of tachycardia is followed by a period of bradycardia. Since atrial pacing may convert the tachycardia to atrial fibrillation, these patients should undergo prior electrophysiologic study to exclude the presence of an accessory AV pathway with a short refractory period.

Patients with recurrent ventricular tachycardia or fibrillation may be refractory to pharmacologic therapy alone. In a small number of patients it has been recognized that overdrive pacing at relatively rapid rates may be a useful adjunct to the management of this group of patients with intractable or recurrent life-threatening arrhythmias. Recent studies have advocated the use of pervenous coronary sinus atrial pacemakers in this group of patients to keep the cardiac output at as high a level as possible because of the rapid rates generally employed, and to minimize the likelihood of mechanical and electrical stimuli from a ventricular pacemaker contributing to a ventricular irritability.[14]

In general, most of the complications associated with atrial pacing are similar to the complications associated with ventricular pacing. The complications or problems are related to the insertion of the pacemaking system, the type of electrode and pacemaker generator selected, pacing site selected, and precipitation of other arrhythmias.

Potential problems with atrial pacing include dislodgment, perforation, development of high pacing threshold, unreliable atrial sensing, and induction of atrial arrhythmias. Particular problems associated with atrial pacing from the coronary sinus include ventricular pacing if too high a current is used, and sensing of ventricular depolarization. Although thrombosis of the coronary vein has not been reported with the use of this pacing site, the number of patients in which long-term coronary sinus pacing has been performed are so few that the risk of occurrence of this complication is remote.

References

1. Josephson, M. E., and Seides, S. F.: "Clinical Cardiac Electrophysiology: Techniques and Interpretations," Lea & Febiger, Philadelphia, 1979.
2. Scheinman, M. M., and Morady, F.: Invasive Cardiac Electrophysiologic Testing: The Current State of the Art, *Circulation,* 67:1169, 1983.
3. Kerr, C. R., Grant, A. O., Wenger, T. L., and Strauss, H. C.: Sinus Node Dysfunction, in D. P. Zipes (ed.), "Arrhythmias II. Cardiology Clinics," W. B. Saunders Co., Philadelphia, 1983, p. 187.
4. Bonke, F. I. M. (ed.): "The Sinus Node: Structure, Function and Clinical Relevance," Martinus Nijhoff, The Hague, 1978.
5. LaBarre, A., Strauss, H. C., Scheinman, M. M., Evans, G. T., Bashore, T., Tiedeman, J. S., and Wallace, A. G.: Electrophysiologic Effects of Disopyramide Phosphate on Sinus Node Function in Patients with Sinus Node Dysfunction, *Circulation,* 59:226, 1979.
6. Kerr, C. R., and Strauss, H. C.: The Nature of Atriosinus Conduction during Rapid Atrial Pacing in the Rabbit Heart, *Circulation,* 63:1149, 1981.
7. Denes, P., Wu, D., Dhingra, R., Pietras, R., and Rosen, K. M.: The Effects of Cycle Length on Cardiac Refractory Periods in Man, *Circulation,* 49:32, 1974.
8. Dhingra, R. C., Palileo, E., Strasberg, B., Swiryn, S., Bauernfeind, R. A., Wyndham, C. R. E., and Rosen, K. M.: Significance of HV Interval in 517 Patients with Chronic Bifascicular Block, *Circulation,* 64:1265, 1981.
9. Scheinman, M. M., Peters, R. W., Sauve, M. J., Desai, J., Abbott, J. A., Cogan, J., Wohl, B., and Williams, K.: Value of the HQ Interval in Patients with Bundle Branch Block and the Role of Prophylactic Permanent Pacing, *Am. J. Cardiol.,* 50:1316, 1982.
10. Wellens, H. J. J.: Value and Limitations of Programmed Electrical Stimulation of the Heart in the Study and Treatment of Tachycardia, *Circulation,* 57:845, 1978.
11. Gallagher, J. J., Pritchett, E. L. C., Sealy, W. C., Kasell, J., and Wallace, A. G.: The Preexcitation Syndromes, *Prog. Cardiovas. Dis.,* 20:285, 1978.
12. Mason, J. D., and Winkle, R. A.: Electrode-Catheter Arrhythmia Induction in the Selection and Assessment of Antiarrhythmic Drug Therapy for Recurrent Ventricular Tachycardia, *Circulation,* 58:971, 1978.

13. Waldo, A. L., and MacLean, W. A. H.: "Diagnosis and Treatment of Cardiac Arrhythmias Following Open Heart Surgery. Emphasis on the Use of Atrial and Ventricular Epicardial Wire Electrodes," Futura Publishing Co., Mt. Kisco, N.Y., 1980.
14. Camm, A. J., and Ward, D. E.: "Pacing for Tachycardia Control," Butler and Tanner, Ltd., Rome and London, 1983.
15. Fisher, J. D., Kim, S. A., Furman, S., and Matos, J. A.: Role of Implantable Pacemakers in Control of Recurrent Ventricular Tachycardia, *Am. J. Cardiol.*, 49:194, 1982.
16. German, L. D., and Strauss, H. C.: Electrical Termination of Tachyarrhythmias by Discrete Pulses, *PACE*, 7(part II):54–521, 1984.
17. Josephson, M. E., Horowitz, L. N., Waxman, H. L., Spielman, S. R., Untereker, W. J., and Marchlinski, F. E.: Role of Catheter Mapping in Evaluation of Ventricular Tachycardia, in M. E. Josephson (ed.), "Ventricular Tachycardia: Mechanisms and Management," Futura Publishing Co., Mt. Kisco, N.Y., 1982, pp. 309.
18. Spurrell, R. A. J., Nathan, A. W., Bexton, R. S., Hellestrand, K. J., Nappholz, T., and Camm. A. J.: Implantable Automatic Scanning Pacemaker for Termination of Supraventricular Tachycardia, *Am. J. Cardiol.*, 49:753, 1982.

103

Cardioversion and Defibrillation

Bernard Lown, M.D.
Regis A. de Silva, M.D.

Cardioversion and *defibrillation* refer to the use of synchronized and unsynchronized direct current (dc) electrical discharge respectively to terminate cardiac arrhythmias.[1,2] The essential electrical circuitry consists of a resistance, an inductance, and a capacitor (R-L-C circuit) in series. The capacitor stores a charge and closing the switch results in the discharge of a single pulse. The majority of units utilize a half-sinusoidal waveform; some units use a trapezoidal waveform, as do implantable defibrillators. Energy is measured in watt-seconds (W·s) or joules (J); 1 W·s equals 1 J. The majority of devices store 300 to 400 J but the delivered energy may be 80 percent or less than the stored amount. There is no evidence that devices which store more than 400 J are clinically necessary, and indeed use of such a device may result in arrhythmias and cardiac damage.[3,4] Cardioversion is accomplished through electrode paddles measuring 8 to 10 cm in diameter, one of which is the anode and the other the cathode. The objective is to deliver an electrical discharge transthoracically so as to envelop a significant portion of the heart during passage of the current through the chest. Electrode position is thus an important determinant of the amount of energy used and the success or failure of the procedure.

The physiological basis for cardioversion derives from several principles: (1) First, the provocation of tachyarrhythmias, be they atrial, junctional, or ventricular, is related to the operation of a multiplicity of interacting factors, some of which are transient. Once initiated, however, the abnormal mechanism can be self-sustaining. (2) When such a disorder is momentarily terminated, the sinus node, possessing the highest level of automaticity in the heart, resumes function as the dominant pacemaker. (3) The majority of tachyarrhythmias in humans are due either to macroreentry or microreentry; the electrical discharge depolarizes the so-called excitable gap separating the "head" of the recirculating wave front of excitation from its "tail."[2] (4) The heart can be depolarized across the intact chest by an adequate electrical discharge. In the case of ventricular fibrillation, it was originally assumed by Wiggers[5] that complete depolarization of the heart is essential for abolishing the arrhythmia. However, evidence indicates that partial depolarization of the heart by low levels of energy may suffice to terminate ventricular fibrillation.[4] None of these considerations sheds light on why arrhythmias such as atrial flutter and ventricular tachycardia require lower energy levels for reversion than atrial fibrillation and ventricular fibrillation, or why the same arrhythmias may require differing levels of energy for reversion at different times.

Method of Cardioversion

Cardioversion should be performed following an overnight fast or, in more urgent cases, after withholding the previous meal. Careful explanation to the patient of the simplicity and safety of the procedure will avoid anxiety and thereby facilitate reversion. Serum levels for digoxin and electrolytes should be obtained on the day preceding cardioversion. Digitalis need not be withheld unless overdosage is suspected. Anticoagulation is unnecessary except with atrial fibrillation which has persisted for longer than a few days, in which case warfarin (Coumadin) should be administered for a period of at least 3 weeks. Cardioversion should be carried out, preferably early in the day, in a room equipped for cardiopulmonary resuscitation. An intravenous infusion is started for drug administration. Blood pressure and the electrocardiogram (ECG) are monitored during and for at least 1 h following the procedure. Sedation is provided by administering 100 mg of phenobarbital intramuscularly or orally an hour before cardioversion. At the time of cardioversion, diazepam is administered intravenously in a dose of 5 mg followed by 2.5 mg every 2 min with monitoring of blood pressure and respiratory rate. The objective is to achieve sedation and amnesia. Generally, 10 to 30 mg of diazepam suffice for this purpose.

Monitoring of the ECG with the tallest R-wave configuration is necessary to avoid accidental triggering of ventricular fibrillation. Improper synchronization may result when there are artifactual spikes, in the presence of very prominent T waves, or bundle branch block with the R′ wave taller than the R wave. Although the likelihood of a synchronized shock provoking ventricular fibrillation is less than 5 percent, this risk may be enhanced in the presence of hypokalemia, digitalis or quinidine intoxication, or acute myocardial ischemia. The electrodes must be completely covered with conductive gel or paste, particularly around the edges, to prevent skin burns.

Both anteroposterior and anterolateral electrode positions may be employed for cardioversion. The anterior electrode is held firmly to the right of the sternum at the level of the second and third intercostal spaces, and the posterior electrode is placed at the angle of the left scapula. With devices equipped with anterior and anterolateral electrode paddles, the second paddle is placed at the level of the cardiac apex at the midaxillary line. The path of current flow is thus along the long axis of the heart, encompassing the greater part of the cardiac mass. Lown et al. and others have suggested that the anterior-posterior electrode configuration reduces energy requirements for cardioversion of atrial arrhythmias as compared to anterior-lateral placement.[6,31] Other investigators have not found such a difference.[32,33] Kerber and colleagues demonstrated that the two electrode positions provide equivalent success rates and that energy levels required were not significantly altered for reversion of atrial fibrillation and flutter.[33] Electrodes should not be placed over the sternum, vertebral column, or scapula because bony tissue has high impedance and will lower effectiveness of the shock. Placement of electrodes side by side should be avoided because the shock will not be transthoracic and such positioning may short-circuit the discharge due to bridging between the electrodes by the conductive paste, rendering the shock ineffective. Proper technique provides a greater assurance of success and reduces cardiac damage and other complications.[6]

Energy titration is employed during elective cardioversion to utilize the minimum required for restoring sinus rhythm. The initial setting should be 10 J, and if reversion fails, the procedure is continued using stepwise increases of 25, 50, 100, 200, 300, and 400 J until reversion occurs. After each discharge, electrocardiographic monitoring of lead II and especially lead V_1 is necessary to define resumption of sinus rhythm. The latter lead is important because immediately following reversion, P waves may be diminutive in the limb leads, and if the rhythm is irregular, the mistaken interpretation is that atrial fibrillation is still ongoing. This leads to unnecessary and repeated shocks while the patient is already in sinus rhythm. If ventricular arrhythmias emerge after electrical discharge, without restoration of a normal rhythm, a 50 to 100-mg bolus of lidocaine is administered and energy titration is cautiously continued.

Treatment of Specific Arrhythmias

The energy requirements for treatment of arrhythmias depend on the specific arrhythmia. A knowledge of the mean energy level required for each arrhythmia is helpful in selecting an initial dose if energy titration is not used. Table 103-1 summarizes approximate mean energy levels and ranges for reversion of various arrhythmias.

Atrial Fibrillation

Pretreatment with quinidine sulfate, 1.2 g daily in four divided doses, is begun 24 to 48 h before cardioversion for atrial fibrillation. Our experience indicates that such pretreatment improves the patient's chances of remaining in normal sinus rhythm immediately after reversion, reduces the number of shocks necessary, decreases the energy level required to restore sinus rhythm, and diminishes the incidence of postreversion arrhythmias. Furthermore, one obtains a small dividend of drug-induced reversions to sinus rhythm in 10 to 15 percent of patients having sustained atrial fibrillation. If the patient is intolerant of quinidine, disopyramide may be substituted. Anticoagulation should be started 3 weeks before cardioversion and is continued for at least 4 weeks thereafter to prevent embolism.

We have achieved a success rate of 94 percent in

TABLE 103-1 Approximate Mean Energy Doses and Ranges for Reversion of Specific Arrhythmias

Arrhythmia	Range
Atrial flutter	5–50 (mean 25 J)
Ventricular tachycardia	5–100 J
Atrial fibrillation	10–400 (mean 100 J)
Supraventricular tachycardia	100–400 (mean 200 J)
Ventricular fibrillation	50–400 J

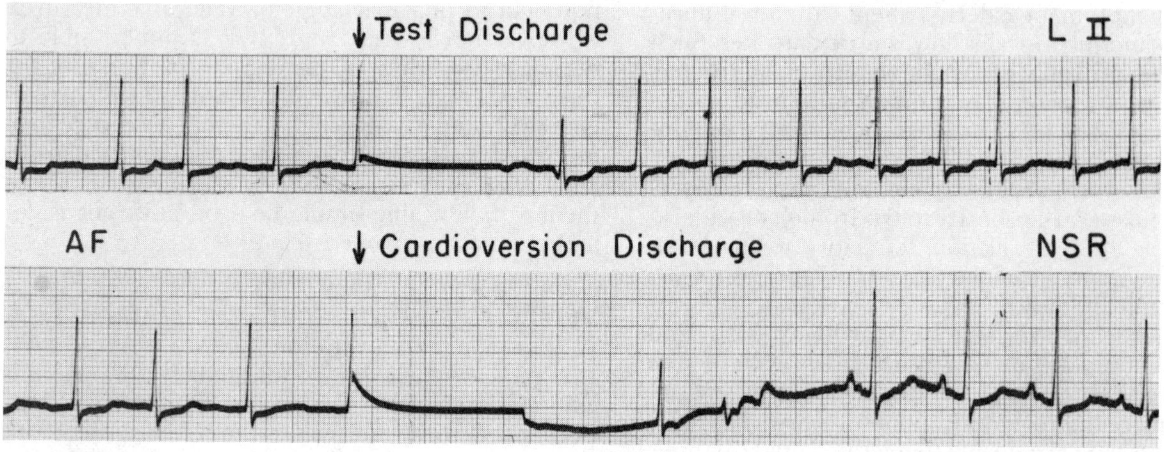

FIGURE 103-1 Patient with atrial fibrillation of 1-year duration. An initial test discharge with 25 W-s is without effect. A repeat shock of 50 W-s results in normal sinus rhythm after 3.8 s. A ventricular escape beat precedes the onset of the sinus mechanism.

456 episodes of atrial fibrillation in 350 patients.[2] When anterior-posterior electrode placement is used, the mean energy level for terminating atrial fibrillation is 100 J, and 40 percent of patients are reverted to sinus rhythm with 50 J or less, while success in 95 percent of patients may be achieved with 200 J or less (Fig. 103-1). The duration of the rhythm disorder is a major determinant of both the success of the procedure and the energy level at which reversion occurs. When atrial fibrillation has been present for 3 months or less, the success rate is 98 percent and the mean energy level required 87 J. When atrial fibrillation has been present for over a year, not only is there an increase in energy requirement for reversion, but early relapse is also frequent.[2] However, such patients deserve at least one cardioversion attempt since sinus rhythm persists in an occasional patient.

The energy requirement and success of cardioversion appear to be related to the size of the fibrillation (f) wave in lead V_1. Higher energy levels are also required for atrial fibrillation of long duration, for "lone" atrial fibrillation, for patients with preexcitation syndrome, and for those with cardiomyopathy, congestive heart failure, and myocardial infarction. In the presence of cardiac decompensation, the electrical energy requirement may be high, success is not ensured, and recurrence of atrial fibrillation may ensue within minutes. In such cases, pretreatment with a rapidly acting glycoside such as ouabain intravenously will serve to reduce pulmonary congestion and permit prompt cardioversion. In patients with acute myocardial infarction, treatment of pump failure with digitalis is often successful in abolishing the rhythm disorder, thereby obviating the need for cardioversion. However, if rapid atrial fibrillation occurs in the absence of heart failure or is the result of atrial infarction, prompt reversion and antiarrhythmic drug treatment are desirable to present further compromise of jeopardized myocardium. It must be emphasized that these patients are difficult to maintain in sinus rhythm. The best compromise may be to achieve a slow ventricular rate with drug therapy in atrial fibrillation.

Following reversion of atrial fibrillation, the sinus rate is slow and first degree atrioventricular (AV) block is frequently present. Atrial ectopic activity is common and resumption of sinus rhythm may be delayed. In some patients the sinus node requires a warm-up period during which junctional rhythm prevails and a sinus mechanism emerges slowly to become dominant only after one or more minutes. This phenomenon has been designated the "somnolent sinus syndrome."[2] Other patients, generally those with long duration of atrial fibrillation following cardioversion, exhibit bradycardia chaotically alternating with multiform atrial tachycardia, miniparoxysms of fibrillation, and junctional rhythm while the P waves demonstrate variable morphology. This abnormal state has been designated the "sick sinus syndrome" and usually augurs recurrence of atrial fibrillation.[2]

Before cardioversion is undertaken, one needs to assess whether the procedure will be successful and whether maintenance of sinus rhythm is likely. Cardioversion is unlikely to succeed or is relatively contraindicated in the following groups of patients:

- Patients who have had atrial fibrillation of over a year's duration. Although one attempt at cardioversion is worthwhile, sustained sinus rhythm is unlikely.
- Patients who have mitral valve disease, especially mitral regurgitation, with a giant left atrium. The presence of extensive atrial fibrosis precludes sustaining sinus rhythm. If valve replacement has been performed, the chances of success are remote.
- Patients who have lone atrial fibrillation, which occurs in the presence of a structurally normal heart and in the absence of thyrotoxicosis. Such patients generally have a normal-sized heart, small f waves in lead V_1, and relatively slow ventricular rates. Energy requirements for reversion are high and sinus rhythm is frequently not sustained.

- The symptomatic elderly patient with atrial fibrillation and intrinsically slow ventricular rates. Such patients probably have conduction system disease, and cardioversion may result in sinus bradycardia with episodes of sinus arrest which may require implantation of a cardiac pacemaker.
- Patients with chaotic, recurrent atrial tachyarrhythmias (Parkinson-Papp syndrome), or with recurrent atrial fibrillation refractory to drugs. in such patients, sustained atrial fibrillation is the arrhythmia of choice.[7]
- Patients who have congestive cardiomyopathy and left ventricular failure. In such cases, even the use of large energy levels for cardioversion may result in only temporary resumption of sinus rhythm.
- Patients who are unable to tolerate antiarrhythmic medications. In this group of patients, atrial fibrillation may be accepted as the preferred rhythm, and suitable rate control is achieved with the use of digitalis glycoside, beta-adrenergic blocking agents, or verapamil.[7]

Atrial Flutter

This arrhythmia is one of the most difficult to treat pharmacologically. Atrial flutter may have serious and life-threatening consequences if the ventricular rate is rapid and the patient has significant myocardial impairment. Administration of antiarrhythmic drugs often merely shows the flutter rate. Digitalis treatment promotes the emergence of atrial fibrillation, which then may lead to resumption of sinus rhythm. The advent of cardioversion has greatly facilitated reversion of atrial flutter, for which it is the treatment of choice. Atrial flutter is one of the easiest arrhythmias to terminate electrically as it requires low-energy shocks and success rates range up to 100 percent.[2,4,8] In a large series, the mean energy level required was 25 J and usually only one shock sufficed.[2] With shocks of 50 J or less, 95 percent of cases can be reverted to sinus rhythm. When energy levels of 10 J or less are administered, instead of achieving sinus rhythm, atrial fibrillation may be precipitated in as many as 67 percent of patients.[8] The finding is of some importance in patients who have recurrent atrial flutter and whose ventricular rate is refractory to slowing. Atrial fibrillation is then the preferred rhythm since it almost invariably permits proper regulation of the ventricular response with one or more drugs.

Supraventricular Tachycardia

The majority of patients with supraventricular tachycardia does not require cardioversion since this rhythm is often reverted pharmacologically or by vagal maneuvers.[9] In those cases where digitalis intoxication is the cause for the abnormal mechanism, cardioversion is contraindicated. When supraventricular tachycardia occurs in patients with severe myocardial impairment, the rapid rate further compromises cardiac function. When the arrhythmia does not yield to pharmacologic or vagotonic measures, cardioversion is employed. If it is not possible to determine whether excess digitalis is the cause for the arrhythmia, cardioversion is utilized with careful energy titration. If low-energy discharges expose high grades of atrioventricular block and ventricular arrhythmias, digitalis intoxication is suggested. Treatment with lidocaine should be prompt if ventricular arrhythmia is provoked.

Ventricular Tachycardia

If lidocaine administration fails to restore sinus rhythm, cardioversion is indicated. If the patient is clinically stable, elective cardioversion should be performed with energy titration. Energy levels as low as 1 J can terminate ventricular tachycardia, and over 90 percent of cases can be reverted with 10 J or less.[10] Only rarely is more than 100 J necessary. When ventricular tachycardia is rapid and the QRS complex is wide and indistinguishable from the T wave, synchronization has an equal chance of occurring on either of these. In such a circumstance, the instrument should be switched to the defibrillator mode and an unsynchronized shock of 100 J delivered, thereby reducing or avoiding entirely the danger of ventricular fibrillation.

Ventricular Fibrillation

The use of the cardioverter in the unsynchronized mode is referred to as *defibrillation*. The setting is used only for ventricular fibrillation or, at times, for emergency treatment of ventricular tachycardia. Although the ideal electrode positions for defibrillation in humans have not been established, the same electrode configurations are employed as for cardioversions of atrial arrhythmias. The initial energy setting should be between 300 to 400 J, which is the maximum output for most devices. The use of single or rapid sequential shocks with energy levels lower than 300 J is successful in over 95 percent of cases.[11,12] However, an approach utilizing sequential low-energy shocks is recommended only if the resuscitation team is highly experienced in this method of defibrillation.

The mean energy doses required for human defibrillation is still undefined since energy titration cannot be performed as readily as in cardioversion. Studies in animals and one retrospective clinical study indicate that the energy dose for defibrillation is a function of body weight.[13,14] As a result of these data, it was suggested that conventional defibrillators storing 300 to 400 J were inadequate to defibrillate heavy adults. Prospective studies since have shown that clinical defibrillation can be achieved with energy levels of less than 400 J and that even lower energy levels are successful in over 95 percent of cases.[3,11,12,15–18] Thus, the use of energy levels in excess of 400 J is unwarranted. The use of low-energy levels of the order of 10 to 100 J is recommended for pediatric defibrillation. The success of defibrillation is related less to the particular energy level of discharge than to other factors such as the presence of myocardial damage, duration of fibrillation, severity of acid-base imbalance, the existence of hypotensive shock prior to onset of ventricular fibrillation, and the technique employed. When maximum available energy settings are utilized, improper electrode placement is a common cause of failure to defibrillate on the first attempt.

Cardioversion during Digitalis Therapy

Digitalization of the heart lowers the threshold for the emergence of ventricular tachycardia and fibrillation.[19,20] In the presence of digitalis toxicity ventricular fibrillation and death may occur as an early or late complication.[21–23] There is, however, no evidence that in the absence of digitalis toxicity that cardioversion, properly performed, poses such a hazard. In animal studies, a 2000-fold increase in sensitivity to electric shock is seen after induction of ouabain toxicity, as judged by the emergence of repetitive ventricular activity.[19] In humans, Kleiger and Lown[20] found that when the precardioversion ECG had ventricular premature beats, atrial tachycardia with block, junctional rhythm with or without AV dissociation, or first degree heart block, significant postcardioversion ventricular arrhythmia occurred. The severity of the complicating arrhythmia was a function of the discharge energy level. In a study of 21 patients, 17 of whom were receiving quinidine, propranolol, or lidocaine, it was found that none developed ventricular tachycardia after cardioversion.[24] None of the patients were considered to be digitalis-toxic. There was no consistent difference in the frequency of ventricular premature beats before and after cardioversion despite a wide range of serum digoxin levels.

In the absence of clinical evidence for digitalis toxicity, digoxin need be held only on the day of cardioversion. If clinical evidence for digitalis toxicity, suspected digitalis toxicity, or quinidine-digoxin interaction is present, it is safest to withhold digoxin for several days before cardioversion is attempted. However, if cardioversion cannot be deferred, it is safest to pretreat the patient with a lidocaine bolus of 50 to 100 mg immediately before the shock. Energy titration should be employed to detect the early emergence of ventricular arrhythmia. If life-threatening arrhythmias are not suppressed by lidocaine, attempts at cardioversion should be discontinued and pharmacologic treatment attempted.

Complications

Repeated use of high-energy shocks may produce both morphological and functional cardiac damage. It is thus advisable to limit the discharge to the lowest energy level essential for restoring a sinus mechanism. Following electric shock, creatinine phosphokinase (CK), or other enzymes, acetylcholine, and catecholamines are released.[4] The level of CK elevation following cardioversion does not usually obscure the diagnosis of myocardial infarction, for only with repeated shocks of high energy is there a rise in this enzyme; even then the elevation is transient.[25,26] While total CK and lactic dehydrogenase increases may follow cardioversion, myocardial fractions of both enzymes are only rarely observed. Electric shock also releases cardiac potassium, and this release is accentuated in digitalized subjects.[27] Electrocardiographic changes of hyperkalemia are at times detected after repeated high-energy shocks, and in these instances, the potassium derives from traumatized skeletal muscles subjacent to the electrode paddles.

Diverse cardiac arrhythmias may result from cardioversion. By and large, these are transient and innocuous. Most frequent are ventricular, junctional, or atrial ectopic beats. Occurrences of serious arrhythmias are related to the following factors: the level of discharge, the presence of overdigitalization, the severity of the heart disease, and existence of electrolyte derangements. We have never encountered life-threatening rhythm disorders with discharges of 100 J or less, except in patients who were unsuspectingly overdigitalized.

When ventricular fibrillation is a complication of cardioversion, it is most often the result of improper synchronization, with the discharge being delivered during the vulnerable period. The arrhythmia begins instantly after the shock. When onset of ventricular fibrillation is delayed for minutes or even hours after cardioversion, it is the consequence of digitalis, quinidine, or both, in toxic or near-toxic doses.[21–23] Experimental evidence suggests that these arrhythmias may be secondary to potassium efflux occurring as a result of the effects of electric shock upon excessively digitalized myocardium.[27] Prolonged periods of asystole occur after cardioversion if high-energy levels are used. In the ischemic or infarcted heart, this may lead to the emergence of ventricular arrhythmias, including ventricular tachycardia and fibrillation.

Pulmonary edema as a consequence of cardioversion has been noted immediately following cardioversion or several hours thereafter.[28] The cause of this complication is unknown. It has most often been noted in the presence of mitral and aortic valvular disease or left ventricular dysfunction. It is likely that acute alterations or disparities in atrial or ventricular mechanical function consequent to electrical discharge may precipitate pulmonary congestion. Delayed return of left atrial function and pulmonary embolism have been suspected as other possible mechanisms for pulmonary edema.

Systemic embolism is one of the major complications of cardioversion in patients with atrial fibrillation. Pharmacologic or electrical reversion of this arrhythmia both result in an approximately 1.2-

to-1.5-percent incidence of embolism.[2,29] Resumption of left or right atrial function may be delayed for days or even weeks after cardioversion, which accounts for late embolic complications. This complication is reduced or avoided by anticoagulation as discussed above. Some miscellaneous complications are observed rarely. Unexplained hypotension may occur and last for hours after cardioversion. Usually no treatment is necessary because the condition resolves spontaneously. Generally, electric shock does not damage implanted pacemakers. Cardioversion during pregnancy has been safely performed, and fetal death as a direct consequence of cardioversion has not been reported.[30] Nonetheless, in the interest of safety, monitoring of fetal heart rate and rhythm should be performed whenever possible.

Despite these reported complications, when properly utilized, the use of electrical energy for reversion of diverse cardiac arrhythmias is safely accomplished with an extremely low incidence of serious adverse reactions.

References

1. Lown, B., Amarasingham, R., and Neuman, J.: New Method for Terminating Cardiac Arrhythmias. Use of Synchronized Capacitor Discharge, *JAMA*, 182:548, 1962.
2. Lown, B.: Electrical Reversion of Cardiac Arrhythmias, *Br. Heart J.*, 29:469, 1967.
3. Lown, B., Crampton, R. S., DeSilva, R. A., and Gascho, J. A.: The Energy for Ventricular Defibrillation—Too Little or Too Much? *N. Engl. J. Med.*, 298:1252, 1978.
4. DeSilva, R. A., Graboys, T. B., Podrid, P. J., and Lown, B.: Cardioversion and Defibrillation, *Am. Heart J.*, 100:881, 1980.
5. Wiggers, C. J.: The Physiologic Basis for Cardiac Resuscitation from Ventricular Fibrillation—Method of Serial Defibrillation, *Am. Heart J.*, 20:418, 1940.
6. Lown, B., Kleiger, R., and Wolff, G.: Technique of Cardioversion, *Am. Heart J.*, 67:282, 1964.
7. Kowey, P., DeSilva, R. A., and Lown, B.: Sustained Atrial Fibrillation as a Rhythm of Choice, *Circulation*, 59,60(suppl. 2):253, 1979.
8. Guiney, T. E., and Lown, B.: Electrical Conversion of Atrial Flutter to Atrial Fibrillation. Flutter Mechanism in Man, *Br. Heart J.*, 34:1215, 1972.
9. Margolis, B., DeSilva, R. A., and Lown, B.: Episodic Drug Treatment in the Management of Paroxysmal Arrhythmias, *Am. J. Cardiol.*, 45:621, 1980.
10. Lown, B., Temte, J. V., and Arter, W. J.: Ventricular Tachyarrhythmias. Clinical Aspects, *Circulation*, 47:1364, 1973.
11. Gascho, J. A., Crampton, R. S., Cherwek, M. L., et al.: Determinants of Ventricular Defibrillation in Adults, *Circulation*, 60:231, 1979.
12. Campbell, N. P. S., Webb, S. W., Adgey, A. A. J., and Pantridge, J. F.: Transthoracic Ventricular Defibrillation in Adults, *Br. Med. J.*, 2:1379, 1977.
13. Geddes, L. A., Tacker, W. A., Rosborough, J. P., Moore, A. G., and Cabler, A. S.: Electrical Dose for Ventricular Defibrillation of Large and Small Animals Using Precordial Electrodes, *J. Clin. Invest.*, 53:310, 1974.
14. Tacker, W. A., Galioto, F., Guiliani, E., Geddes, L. A., and McNamara, D. G.: Energy Dosage for Human Transchest Defibrillation, *N. Engl. J. Med.*, 290:214, 1974.
15. DeSilva, R. A., and Lown, B.: Energy Requirement for Defibrillation of a Markedly Overweight Subject, *Circulation*, 57:827, 1978.
16. Adgey, A. A. J.: Electrical Energy Requirements for Ventricular Defibrillation, *Br. Heart J.*, 40:1971, 1978.
17. Pantridge, J. F., Adgey, A. A. J., Webb, S. W., and Anderson, J.: Electrical Requirements for Ventricular Defibrillation, *Br. Med. J.*, 2:313, 1975.
18. Gascho, J. A., Crampton, R. S., Sipes, J. N., Cherwek, M. L., Hunter, F. P., and O'Brien, W. M.: Energy Level and Patient Weight in Ventricular Defibrillation, *JAMA*, 242:1380, 1979.
19. Lown, B., Cannon, R. L., III, and Rossi, M. A.: Electrical Stimulation and Digitalis Drugs: Repetitive Response in Diastole, *Proc. Soc. Exp. Biol. Med.*, 126:698, 1967.
20. Kleiger, R., and Lown, B.: Cardioversion and Digitalis. II. Clinical Studies, *Circulation*, 33:878, 1966.
21. Rabbino, M. D., Likoff, W., and Dreifus, L. S.: Complications and Limitations of Direct Current Countershock, *JAMA*, 190:147, 1964.
22. Ross, E. M. Cardioversion Causing Ventricular Fibrillation, *Arch. Intern. Med.*, 114:811, 1964.
23. Castellanos, A., Lamberg, L., Gilmore, H., and Johnson, D.: Countershock Exposed Quinidine Syncope, *Am. J. Med. Sci.*, 260:254, 1965.
24. Ditchey, R. V., and Karliner, J. S.: Safety of Electrical Cardioversion in Patients without Digitalis Toxicity, *Ann. Intern Med.*, 95:676, 1981.
25. Ehsani, A., Ewy, G. A., and Sobel, B. E.: Effects of Electrical Countershock on Serum Creatinine Phosphokinase (CPK) Isoenzyme Activity, *Am. J. Cardiol*, 37:12, 1976.
26. Reiffel, J. A., McCarthy, D. M., and Leakey, E. B.: Does DC Cardioversion Affect Isoenzyme Recognition of Myocardial Infarction? *Am. Heart J.*, 97:810, 1974.
27. Regan, T. J., Markov, A., Oldewurtel, H. A., and Harman, H. A.: Myocardial K^+ Loss after Countershock and the Relation to Ventricular Arrhythmias after Nontoxic Doses of Acetyl Strophanthidin, *Am. Heart J.*, 77:367, 1969.
28. Resnekov, L., and McDonald, L.: Complications in 220 Patients with Cardiac Dysrhythmias Treated by Phased Direct Current Shock and Indications for Electroversion, *Br. Heart J.*, 29:926, 1967.
29. Goldman, M. J.: The Management of Chronic Atrial Fibrillation: Indications for and Method of Conversion to Sinus Rhythm, *Prog. Cardiovasc. Dis.*, 2:465, 1960.
30. Schroeder, J. S., and Harrison, D. C.: Repeated Cardioversion during Pregnancy, *Am. J. Cardiol.*, 27:445, 1971.
31. Morris, J. J., Jr., Kong, Y., North, W. C., and McIntosh, H. D.: Experience with "Cardioversion" of Atrial Fibrillation, *Am. J. Cardiol.*, 14:94, 1964.
32. Resnekov, L., and McDonald, L.: Appraisal of Electroconversion in Treatment of Cardiac Dysrhythmias, *Br. Heart J.*, 30:786, 1968.
33. Kerber, R. E., Jensen, S. R., Grayzel, J., Kennedy, J., and Hoyt, R.: Elective Cardioversion: Influence of Paddle-Electrode Location and Dose on Success Rates and Energy Requirements, *N. Engl. J. Med.*, 305:658, 1981.

104

Artificial Cardiac Pacemakers: Transvenous Implantation Techniques

Harry G. Mond, M.D.

We started with the experiments on total implant of pacemakers in 1956 on dogs, and we made our first implantation in man in October, 1958. The first patient was a 40 year old electronic engineer. . . . He told, when he looked at the electronic circuit of a pacemaker that we "have no idea about electronics."

From Ake Senning, M.D., the implanter of the first pacemaker in man, writing to David Schechter, M.D.[1]

The evolution of a permanent pacemaker implantation protocol from the highly complicated, time-consuming procedure practiced by Senning and his contemporaries to the highly technical, rapid, and relatively uncomplicated transvenous routine practiced today has been very dramatic. Major reasons for this improvement include local anesthesia, small pulse generators, and sophisticated transvenous lead systems with a stiffening and directing stylet. The implantation of an epimyocardial lead, however, still necessitates surgical exposure of the epicardial surface of the heart. Consequently, pacemaker lead implantation by the transvenous route has become the practiced routine in most pacemaker centers. In this chapter a standard method of permanent implantation using transvenous atrial and ventricular leads will be presented.

Transvenous Ventricular Lead Implantation

Transvenous pacemaker implantation surgery is simple and the complications are inversely proportional to the experience, skill, and interest of the operator. Irrespective of whether a cardiologist or surgeon performs the implant, such surgery should only be performed by skilled and specifically trained personnel in specialized centers able to perform at least 30 implants a year.

Preoperative Assessment and Preparation

Prior to pacemaker implantation, the patient should meet with a member of the operating team who should carefully explain the procedure and reassure the patient. A check should be made of the patient's medications, and, in particular, anticoagulant drugs should be stopped or reversed. The patient must fast for at least 4 h before the procedure and the bladder must be emptied. The surgical site is shaved and prepared with povidone iodine or any other suitable antiseptic. The surgical area should be covered with a clean or sterile towel and the patient dressed in an operating gown. An appropriate premedication is given, although atropine should not be added to the premedication as dryness in the mouth may irritate the patient, and if atrioventricular conduction is intact sinus tachycardia may make lead threshold measurements difficult.

Preoperative prophylactic antibiotics are not universally recommended although they are used by most surgeons who implant prosthetic devices. In a prospective trial, prophylactic antibiotics reduced the incidence of pacemaker wound infections.[2] It is preferable to use a single dose or a very short, intensive, broad-spectrum course; the regimen depends on the expected sensitivity patterns relevant to that institution or geographic location. A recommended antibiotic regimen includes parenteral gentamycin and an antistaphyloccocal penicillinase-stable penicillin derivative such as flucloxacillin.

Rapid venous access via an intravenous infusion or simple intravenous line is essential during the operation. Although an intravenous infusion may prevent dehydration, it may also cause fluid overload in the patient, leading to pulmonary edema, troublesome venous bleeding, and a distended bladder during surgery. A temporary transvenous pacing lead is not essential as a routine preoperative procedure. A temporary pacing lead, if inserted, should be well away from the routine permanent implant site.

Operating Room Personnel and Equipment

All operating room staff should be trained in general operating room procedures, sterility techniques, and emergency resuscitation as well as those pacemaker procedures pertaining to their employment. The operator, whether a cardiologist or surgeon, must have training in general surgical skills and a working understanding in lead manipulation, fluoroscopic techniques, and operative lead and pulse generator measurements. An experienced operating room or cardiac catheterization nurse or technician may perform lead and pulse generator testing. Biomedical engineers and anesthesiologists are not required to attend routine initial pacemaker implants performed under local anesthesia unless they are trained to perform lead and pulse generator testing. The practice of inviting the local pacemaker manufacturer representative to attend each implant to "aid" the implanter and to test the lead and pulse generator should be discouraged.

The operating room should have a controlled atmosphere with air conditioning and a filtered exhaust. Fluoroscopy, ECG monitoring, and good surgical lighting are essential. The room should have a unipotential ground and be regularly inspected for electrical hazards. A pacing system analyzer and resuscitative equipment, including a defibrillator, oxygen, and suction should be available. In an adjoining room there should be updated records of all patients as well as comprehensive pacemaker stock, including a range of lead types, pulse generators, and accessory items. A member of the pacemaker team should be responsible for rotating such stock and reordering.

Vein Isolation

On arrival in the operating room, the patient is placed on the fluoroscopy operating table and monitoring leads attached. A 5-to-6-cm incision line is marked on the chest wall. The line is 1 cm below and parallel to the clavicle. For isolation of the cephalic vein, the junction of the lateral third and middle third of this line should lie over the deltopectoral groove. For the routine subclavian puncture technique, the incision should be more medial. The position of the subclavian vein where it crosses the inferior border of the clavicle at the junction of its medial and middle thirds should be marked in all cases, even when the cephalic vein is to be used. An incision for cephalic vein isolation has been described which is parallel to the deltopectoral groove.[3] Such an incision would be unsuitable if subclavian puncture is required.

Before surgery, the dressings covering a temporary lead, if present, are removed and the lead exposed at its insertion site. It is then covered with a sterile dressing. This is to allow easy removal of the temporary lead later in the procedure. The operation area is prepared with povidone iodine or another suitable antiseptic solution and the drapes applied. Plastic sheeting over the operation site is useful but should not be applied until the local anesthetic has been injected. A local anesthetic agent such as lidocaine 1% is injected along the line of the incision deep to the deltopectoral groove and over the area of the pulse generator pocket. The pacing system analyzer cables are prepared for lead and pulse generator testing and the analyzer turned on in the event that emergency pacing is required.

The Cephalic Vein

The cephalic vein lies with the acromioclavicular artery in the infraclavicular triangle or fossa between the deltoid muscle lateral, the clavicular head of the pectoralis major muscle medial, and the inferior border of the clavicle superior. The vein is usually of sufficient size to accept one or more standard pacing leads. Occasionally, the cephalic vein is very small, thrombosed, composed of a plexus of small vessels, or appears to bifurcate one or more times while lying in the infraclavicular fossa. Careful dissection down to the pectoralis minor muscle and deep to the most lateral fibers of the clavicular head of the pectoralis major muscle usually reveals an acromial or pectoralis minor branch which joins the small cephalic vein to produce a vein which is acceptable for cannulation and lead implantation. Occasionally, the vein may not be large enough to accept a pacing lead except where it enters the subclavian vein. Although this area can be adequately exposed, it is potentially hazardous and thus dissection and lead introduction requires considerable skill and experience. Many operators at this point proceed directly to subclavian puncture.

Once isolated and cleaned, the distal end of the cephalic vein is ligated and the proximal end secured. A small transverse incision is made with fine scissors and the intima observed or free bleeding seen. Using a catheter introducer (Becton-Dickinson, New Jersey), the pacing lead with stylet fully inserted is placed within the vein. For tined or flange tip leads, gentle rotation assists venous entry. The lead is passed to the subclavian vein. If difficulty is experienced in entering this vein, the stylet is withdrawn 1 or 2 cm and the lead advanced again with rotation. If obstruction is still encountered, gentle traction on the distal ligature will straighten the cephalic vein and this may facilitate subclavian entry. Continuing obstruction necessitates careful dissection along the cephalic vein to ensure that the lead is not lodged in a tributary. Finally, the shoulder can be moved to alter the angle of attachment of the cephalic vein to the subclavian vein.

The Subclavian Vein

Percutaneous subclavian vein puncture is an excellent and popular method of transvenous pacemaker lead insertion. The method was originally applied in cases of failed cephalic vein insertion, but now many operators use this method of entry as their first choice. Because the technique is potentially more dangerous than cephalic vein insertion, experience and understanding of the local anatomy are key factors in success.[4,5] The subclavian vein, which is 1 to 2 cm in diameter, arches over the first rib deep to the medial third of the clavicle. To distend the subclavian vein the patient should be in the Trendelenberg position. A pillow or rolled towel should be placed under the patient's thoracic vertebrae to force the shoulders back, thus elevating the subclavian vein from the apex of the lung. The incision for pacemaker insertion using the subclavian puncture technique is the same length as that used for cephalic vein isolation but lies more medial. Some operators prefer to make a very small skin incision and extend this after the vein has been punctured.

The puncture set and pacemaker lead are prepared. A commonly used system is the peel-away introducer set sold by most pacemaker manufacturers. The dilator sheaths are available in a number of sizes and the appropriate catalog from the manufacturers lists the kit size for most pacing leads. Prior to insertion, the pacemaker lead should be passed through the sheath to confirm that its passage will be smooth and unimpeded. For tined leads, the electrode and tines should not be passed through the distal end of the sheath as retracting it may damage the tines.

To puncture the subclavian vein, the needle and syringe are placed immediately below the inferior border of the clavicle at the junction of the medial and middle thirds. With the patient performing a Valsalva maneuver, the needle is advanced under the clavicle with the tip aimed at the sternal notch, keeping the syringe parallel at all times to the anterior chest wall. The operator should gently aspirate the syringe until venous blood is freely obtained. Firmly securing the needle, the syringe is removed and the J wire passed into the vein, again with the patient performing a Valsalva maneuver. Before the needle is removed, fluoroscopy should confirm that the guide wire has passed into the superior vena cava. Over the guide wire, the vein dilator and sheath are passed to the subclavian vein, using moderate pressure and a twisting motion. Using finger pressure to control bleeding, the guide wire and dilator are removed and the pacemaker lead introduced into the superior vena cava.

Using fluoroscopic control the sheath can be peeled away and removed when the electrode has reached the right atrium or after positioning in the right ventricle. The guide wire may be left within the sheath during lead insertion in order to pass a second dilator and sheath for two-lead, dual-chamber pacing.[6] To prevent guide wire embolization, the exteriorized end of the guide wire should be clamped with a pair of forceps. Once the sheath has been removed from the vein the Trendelenberg position can be corrected and the rolled towel between the scapulae removed.

Reported and potential complications of subclavian puncture include pneumothorax,[5] wound hematoma,[7] subclavian arterial puncture,[5,7] hemopneumomediastinum, air embolism, arteriovenous fistula, thoracic duct injury, subcutaneous emphysema, infection, and nerve injury. Most of these complications are preventable. Difficulties may occur in patients with a previous fractured clavicle or with chronic obstructive airway disease.

Other Veins

Other venous entry sites have very little place in transvenous lead insertion. The external jugular vein was a common site for transvenous lead insertion, but the technique has many disadvantages, including difficult venous cannulation and lead manipulation. Two incisions are required for pacemaker implantation and the formation of a loop of the lead in the neck may lead to conductor fracture or lead erosion and is both uncomfortable and unsightly if the lead is superficial. The internal jugular vein, anterior pectoral veins, and femoral vein have all been used for transvenous lead insertion, particularly when cephalic vein isolation proved unsuccessful. With the success of the subclavian route, these venous entry sites are very rarely used today.

Lead Positioning

Once in the subclavian vein, the lead with stylet slightly withdrawn is passed, usually without difficulty, to the right atrium. Occasionally the lead fails to negotiate the subclavian–innominate venous junction but rather passes superior into the internal jugular vein. By partially withdrawing the stylet, a loop of lead can be produced which is guided into the innominate vein. If difficulty persists, the stylet shape can be altered or the shoulder or neck moved to alter the angle of the subclavian innominate venous junction. Similar principles apply if the lead, after venous insertion, inadvertently passes distal from the subclavian vein to the axillary vein. At other times, with insertion from the right side, the lead passes from the right to the left innominate vein at their junction with the superior vena cava. Again, by partially withdrawing the stylet, a loop can be formed which is then directed into the superior vena cava. By gently reinserting the stylet the electrode falls toward the right atrium. On rare occasions, congenital anomalies of the superior vena cava are encountered and these present particular problems to the unsuspecting implanter.[8] Other venous abnormalities occasionally encountered include major venous thrombosis[9] and stenosis.[10] They usually follow previous lead implantation on the ipsilateral side, and occasionally the new lead can be passed to the right atrium via large collaterals or through the stenosis. A thrombosis may be "silent" although evidence of superficial venous engorgement can usually be found.[9]

Once in the right atrium, the proximal portion of lead must be directed across the tricuspid valve into the right ventricle and positioned at the apex of the right ventricle. To prevent perforation of the right ventricle, the stylet tip should remain at a position just beyond the tricuspid valve as the lead is advanced. Leads without an anchoring or fixation device can usually be passed without difficulty. Using the direct approach, the coronary sinus will be entered in a significant proportion of cases and the electrode then lies within a cardiac vein. To prevent this the lead with curved stylet fully inserted is pushed against the lateral atrial wall, producing a loop directed toward the tricuspid valve. By partially withdrawing the stylet, rotating the lead and withdrawing and advancing the lead, the electrode can be directed across the tricuspid valve and positioned in the right ventricular outflow tract or pulmonary artery. Using a straight stylet inserted just beyond the tricuspid valve, the lead is gradually retracted until the electrode is directed toward the right ventricular apex. The lead with stylet retracted 2 or 3 cm is advanced and the electrode positioned at the apex.

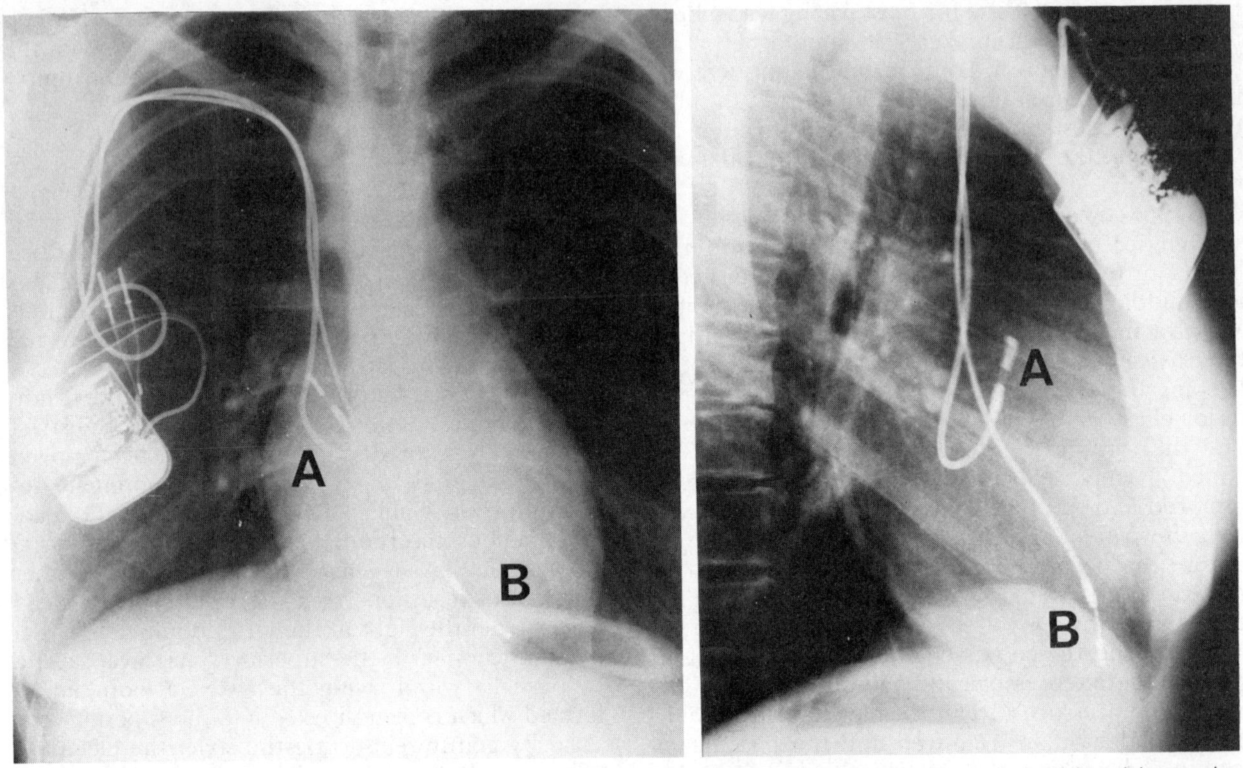

FIGURE 104-1 Posteroanterior (*left*) and lateral (*right*) chest radiographs illustrating two bipolar leads, one in the right atrial appendage (A) and the other at the apex of the right ventricle (B). In the lateral view both leads pass anterior. Only one lead is attached to the pulse generator and the remaining lead has its terminal pins insulated with Silastic caps.

During the lead manipulation from right atrium to right ventricle, atrial and ventricular arrhythmias are common. Atrial arrhythmias may be troublesome with the sick sinus syndrome but are of no consequence with complete heart block. In most cases, they are short-lived but occasionally overdrive pacing or rarely electrical reversion may become necessary. Ventricular arrhythmias are common during lead manipulation although ventricular fibrillation is rare. Once positioned at the right ventricular apex, the electrode should be stable throughout the cardiac cycle. If a tined lead is used, it should be gently retracted to demonstrate lead entrapment beneath or between right ventricular trabeculae. Other endocardial lead fixation devices should now be activated.

To exclude inadvertent coronary venous pacing the lateral fluoroscopic view should be used. In the posteroanterior view, a lead in the coronary sinus is directed superiorly toward the left shoulder and is different to the position of the lead at the right ventricular apex.[11] Electrodes in the middle or posterior cardiac veins, however, are directed inferior and mimic the right ventricular apical position in the posteroanterior view.[11] In the lateral view, right ventricular leads are directed anterior (Fig. 104-1), whereas those in the coronary venous system lie posterior.[11] A lead positioned in the coronary sinus will usually give atrial pacing depending on the position of the electrode in the sinus, whereas an electrode in a cardiac vein will pace the ventricle. Other distinguishing features of cardiac vein or coronary sinus pacing include an elevated pacing threshold[12] and a characteristic endocardial electrogram.[8]

Lead Testing

Lead electrical studies at the time of pacemaker implantation allow for selection of the optimal electrode stimulation and sensing site. Using pacing system analyzers, such testing has become simple and routine. The threshold voltage and current, R-wave sensitivity, system impedance, and integrity of the pulse generator can all be determined. Following electrode placement, the lead should be temporarily fixed to the vein or surrounding tissues to prevent inadvertent dislodgment. With unipolar systems the lead pin is attached to the negative or cathode terminal of the pacing system analyzer cable. The positive or anode terminal is attached to exposed subcutaneous tissue or skeletal muscle. With bipolar systems, the distal or tip electrode is the cathode and the proximal ring the anode.

The most likely parameter to be inadequate, thus requiring lead repositioning, is R-wave size and this should be measured first. The R wave should also be measured prior to pacing as, on occasion, pacemaker dependence occurs immediately, making it very difficult to reestablish a satisfactory spontaneous rhythm after measuring pacing thresholds. A value greater than 4 mV is required for adequate pulse generator sensing. A level less than 4 mV requires repositioning. On occasion, despite repeated lead repositioning, levels of 3 to 4 mV are persistently measured. If the lead is bipolar, conversion to a unipolar system should be considered if the R-wave size is improved. In general, levels of 3 to 4 mV will be adequately sensed by conventional pulse generators but if such levels are finally accepted, a programmable pulse generator with a range of high sensitivity values is advisable. Another method of determining R-wave size is to directly measure the recorded potential from an intracardiac electrogram using the implanted lead. Standard electrophysiological measuring equipment of high impedance, high paper speed, and suitable frequency response should be used.

Another measurement obtained from the sensed R wave is the slew rate. This is the maximum rate of voltage change (*dv/dt*) in the ventricular electrogram and represents the steepness of the slope over a 2-mV voltage excursion. The slew rate can often be measured by the pacing system analyzer or directly from the intracardiac electrogram. Adequate R-wave slew rates are of the order of 1 to 4 V/s and the minimum usually required to inhibit a pulse generator is 0.5 V/s. An intracardiac electrogram showing current of injury pattern should also be recorded.

To measure lead threshold, the pacing system analyzer is set at 5 V and the pacing rate increased until steady, regular pacing is achieved. A pulse duration is chosen. The voltage output is slowly reduced until loss of capture occurs (consistent pacing not present). This is referred to as the "stimulation threshold."[13] The voltage and resultant current are noted. The voltage output is then increased until consistent pacing is reestablished. This is referred to as the "pacing threshold."[13] There is often a difference in the two threshold levels, the pacing threshold being higher by about 0.1 to 0.3 V. There is no convention on which value to record. When measuring the voltage and current threshold it is essential to choose a pulse duration similar to that of the proposed pulse generator. For multiprogrammable pulse generators, however, a range of pulse duration recordings are required. As a routine, voltage and current thresholds for 0.2-, 0.5-, 1.0-, and 2.0-ms pulse durations are advisable. The higher the pulse duration the lower the threshold voltage and current. The usual acceptable range for acute threshold recordings is from 0.3 to 1.0 V with a current of 0.3 to 2.0 mA. If the pacing system analyzer records a variable and erratic current threshold, then the electrode position may be unstable and mobile or because of myocardial perforation lies on the epicardial surface. Repositioning should be considered.

To measure the impedance (resistance) of the implanted system, the heart is paced at 5 V. If a direct measurement is not available on the pacing system analyzer, the current is recorded and the impedance calculated using the formula,

$$\text{Impedance (ohm)} = \frac{\text{voltage (V)}}{\text{current (A)}}$$

For example, a recorded current of 10 mA (0.01 A) will give an impedance of 500 ohm. It is important to use a voltage level of about 5 V. If a voltage near threshold is chosen, the results may be inaccurate due to the relative effects of polarization potentials at the electrode myocardial interface.[14] The usual range for impedance is from 250 to 1000 ohm. Low impedance levels are found with older style leads, having large electrodes with a surface area of 25 to 100 m^2. High impedance levels of up to 1000 ohm occur with electrode surface areas as low as 6 mm^2.

During pacing system analysis it is desirable to determine a diaphragmatic pacing threshold. The ventricle is paced at 10 V and diaphragmatic contractions observed by fluoroscopy. If such stimulations occur, the pacing voltage should be reduced and the diaphragmatic pacing threshold determined. A low threshold of 4 to 5 V usually necessitates repositioning of the lead. In all cases where diaphragmatic contractions occur, irrespective of the acutal threshold level, output programmable pulse generators must be used.

While the testing data are being collected, the patient may become pacemaker-dependent. This is of no consequence if a temporary pacemaker lead is present, but when termination of pacing causes a Stokes-Adams attack, the pacing system analyzer should be used to pace the patient at a very slow rate, such as 40 beats per minute, until a spontaneous rhythm reemerges.

Once satisfactory lead testing data have been obtained, the lead is examined by fluoroscopy to determine if sufficient loop or slack is left in the atrium and across the tricuspid valve. The lead is then secured to the vein or surrounding tissues using two to three nonabsorbable ligatures. Lead manufacturers recommend using the anchoring sleeve supplied with the lead to prevent the suture material damaging the lead insulator. Once secured, the lead should be brought to the pulse generator implantation site. For cephalic vein or subclavian techniques, the pulse generator is implanted in a subclavicular pocket immediately inferior and deep to the incision and only one incision is required. For jugular or femoral approaches, the lead is transferred to the pulse generator site by subcutaneous tunneling.

Transvenous Atrial Lead Implantation

Atrial J Lead

The majority of atrial J leads used today are thin and have polyurethane insulation and two to four small tines. Prior to venous insertion, the terminal part of the J should be straightened with a stylet.

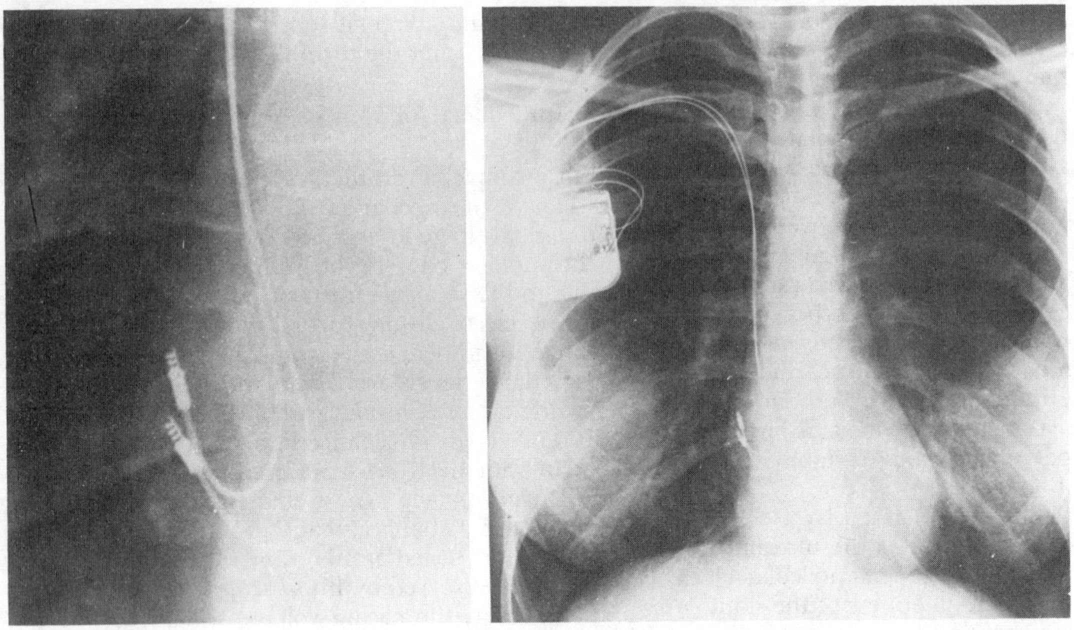

FIGURE 104-2 Posteroanterior chest radiograph illustrating two atrial active fixation screw-in leads (Medtronic Bisping) attached to the anterolateral wall of the right atrium. The left illustration is a magnified view of the point of attachment of the two electrodes to the atrial wall.

With the lead in the right atrium, the stylet should be withdrawn sufficiently to partially reform the J. The electrode is then positioned adjacent to the tricuspid valve and should lie anterior and to the left. The lead is gradually retracted so that the electrode moves superior into the right atrial appendage. Radiographic appearances in the posteroanterior and lateral positions of a right atrial J lead are shown in Fig. 104-1.

Once in the right atrial appendage, retracting the lead straightens the J, confirming correct positioning. The J also demonstrates a characteristic rocking or swaying lateral to medial motion with each atrial and ventricular contraction. Further confirmation of right atrial appendage positioning can be seen by twisting the lead gently clockwise and anticlockwise for about 180° in either direction. With the electrode in the right atrial appendage any rotating movement is impeded. Finally, the lead should be jerked upward to anchor the tines well into the appendage. The patient should then be asked to perform a deep inspiration and by fluoroscopy the J should straighten slightly but should not take on an L configuration. Lead stability can be assessed by vigorous coughing. A number of other active and passive fixation leads can be placed in the right atrial appendage, and in particular a standard tined ventricular lead positioned using a J-shaped stylet.

The lead is tested for adequate atrial sensing and pacing. Unlike ventricular potentials, atrial signals are small but fortunately most multiprogrammable pulse generators now cater to the specific sensing needs of the atrium. Atrial signals are usually biphasic and the pacing system analyzer should record values of 2 to 3 mV. On the electrogram, however, peak-to-peak amplitudes are usually up to 3.5 mV.[15] The slew rates of the atrial electrogram are also lower than those recorded for the ventricle. The atrial threshold for pacing should, where possible, be measured. Unless a well-recognized P wave or a QRS (intact conduction) follows the atrial stimulus artifact, accurate determination of threshold is difficult. Threshold voltage at 0.5-ms pulse duration ranges from about 0.6 to 2.0 V and the resultant current, 1.0 to 3.0 mA.[15] The remainder of the atrial implant procedure is identical to ventricular lead implantation.

Atrial Screw-In Lead

Atrial active fixation screw-in leads have been discussed in Chap. 28. The major advantage of the screw-in lead is that virtually any position in the atrium can be chosen. The interatrial septum is preferred because of the fear of perforation on the free walls. Using the stylet appropriately curved, the distal tip of the lead is positioned on the atrial wall at the selected site. According to the design of the lead, the proximal connector pin or even the whole lead has to be rotated during screwing. Once performed, the lead is gently retracted to confirm attachment. Full pacing system analysis measurements are made. Because of endomyocardial trauma, the initial levels may be unsuitable and it may be necessary to wait a few minutes and repeat the testing. If results remain unsuitable then the lead is unscrewed and another position sought. The atrial screw-in lead may also be positioned in the atrial appendage using the J-shaped stylet. Irrespective of the electrode position in the atrium, it is important to leave a generous loop of lead in the atrium to compensate for atrial position changes when standing or during deep inspiration (Fig. 104-2).

Coronary Sinus Lead

Coronary sinus pacing is only rarely performed today. Specialized coronary sinus leads should be passed via a left-sided venous entry site. After the lead is passed to the right atrium, the tip is moved against the interatrial septum and then usually without difficulty into the coronary sinus. The tip is seen to pass up toward the left shoulder. Confirmation of coronary sinus positioning is made by fluoroscopic observation in the lateral position. Threshold testing shows values higher than in the right atrium and atrial signals can only be accurately assessed by an electrogram because of the proximity of the ventricle.

Dual-Chamber Pacing

Because of the success of atrial endocardial leads, thin polyurethane insulation, miniature electronic circuits, long-life lithium power sources and programmability, dual-chamber systems will play a major role in future pacing. A dual-chamber pacing system can be created by inserting two leads, one in the atrium and the other in the ventricle. To date, a simple and successful single-pass lead for both atrial and ventricular pacing and sensing has not been achieved. When two thin polyurethane leads are implanted in the same procedure, it is usually possible to insert both leads through the same cephalic vein. Once the thick distal end of the atrial lead has been passed into the vein, the remainder of the body of the lead is much thinner and small tined ventricular leads can often be passed into the same venous incision with surprising ease. If this is unsuccessful, subclavian puncture is necessary, unless another vein can be found within the same incision. Lead insertion using the external jugular vein is not recommended. Some operators use a single subclavian puncture and two introducer sheaths for both lead insertions.[6] The order in which dual-chamber leads should be inserted and positioned depends on the preferences of the operator. However, while manipulating one lead, the other should have a stylet partially inserted and secured at the venous entry site by the assistant so as to prevent dislodgment. A frequent problem during manipulation is entanglement of an atrial J lead with the ventricular lead dislodging it. This is less likely to occur with atrial screw-in leads. Only when both leads are positioned are lead measurements taken.

Pulse Generator Implantation

With the introduction of new, small lithium pulse generators, the subclavicular area has become an ideal pulse generator implantation site. Positioned medially, the pulse generator rarely erodes. It is comfortable even for patients with little subcutaneous fat and is accessible to the physician and technician for magnet testing and reprogramming. When preparing the pulse generator pocket, it is important to find a plane deep to adipose tissue and superficial to the pectoralis major fascia. Although the plane can initially be defined with forceps and scissors, it is best to actually prepare the pocket using blunt dissection with fingers. The pocket size should be larger than the pulse generator, so that when the pulse generator is inserted, the superior border should lie inferior to the incision line. While waiting for hemostasis the pulse generator can be tested using the pacing system analyzer. The data obtained are compared with the manufacturer's prior to packaging and shipment. With modern pacing system analyzers, the pulse repetition rate, voltage output, current output, pulse duration, sensitivity level, and refractory period can all be documented.

When attaching the pulse generator to the lead, the terminal pin is impelled into the receiving port of the pulse generator; if difficulty is experienced because of friction, a lubricant is used. Using the appropriate Allen key screwdriver the lead pin is secured to the pulse generator by a small set screw. If necessary, the set screw is insulated with a small plastic cap. For bipolar systems, the procedure is repeated for the second connector and pacing will start if the patient's intrinsic rate is slower than the repetition rate of the pulse generator. For unipolar systems, pacing will start only if the indifferent plate is placed against subcutaneous tissues. If a temporary pacemaker is in situ, temporary pacing should be continued until the permanent system is functional. Many manufacturers use a soft silicone rubber entry hole for the pulse generator terminal. Nonabsorbable suture material can be used around this entry hole to prevent fluid migration into the connector.

The pulse generator is buried in the prepared pocket and the redundant lead placed deep so as not to be inadvertently cut during reoperation. For unipolar systems, the indifferent plate should lie against the subcutaneous tissue to prevent muscle stimulation. Some pulse generators are not coated with silicone rubber and thus the whole of the metal container acts as the indifferent plate. If this causes muscle stimulation, then a silicone rubber boot can be used to insulate the muscle side. Pacing should be confirmed and the lead position checked by fluoroscopy. The temporary lead can now be removed. The wound is closed in layers, cleaned, and covered.

Pulse Generator Replacement

The general surgical principles, patient preparation, and operation room procedures are similar to

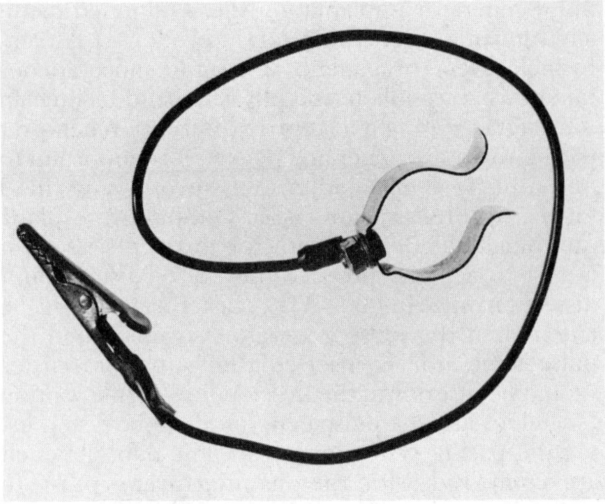

FIGURE 104-3 Indifferent clamp used to maintain pacing with a unipolar pulse generator removed from its implantation pocket.

that described for the initial implantation. The wound is opened along the line of the original incision and, if necessary, the scar excised. The deeper tissues are opened using blunt dissection or fine scissors. A major concern is damage to the insulation and even conductor of the lead. The pulse generator is delivered and with unipolar pacing, the ECG observed for spontaneous rhythm. An indifferent clamp which connects the indifferent plate of the pulse generator to the pulse generator pocket may be used if necessary (Fig. 104-3). Using an appropriate Allen key, the screw or screws holding the pulse generator to the lead pin are loosened and the lead withdrawn from the pulse generator terminal. The pulse generator and lead are tested by the pacing system analyzer. The pacing threshold will have risen from the time of implant, but levels of 3.5 V and 6 mA are acceptable. If high normal or unacceptable levels are found, it is advisable to use a multiprogrammable pulse generator with a high voltage output capability. The lead should be carefully checked for damage to the insulation. Occasionally it is advisable to replace the lead connector. The old connector is cut with wire cutters and a new one applied as directed by the manufacturers.

If the patient is pacemaker-dependent, the replacement of the connector on a unipolar lead can be hazardous. To overcome the problem of asystole and Stokes-Adams attacks, a 25-gauge needle can be inserted through the insulator at some point from the connector and contact made with the conductor. The temporary pulse generator cables are attached to the metal part of the needle and pacing maintained through this until the connector is replaced.[16] The hole in the insulator must be repaired with a small amount of silicone adhesive. Once the lead connector is regarded as satisfactory, the new pulse generator is chosen, tested, and implanted.

Postoperative Care

Following return to the ward, the patient is observed at half-hourly intervals for 4 h and then at 2- or 4-h intervals for up to 24 h. In patients who have had an initial pacemaker implant, a low blood pressure and poor output state may indicate cardiac tamponade and hemopericardium. The wound should be observed for bleeding or tense hematoma. ECG monitoring is advisable for 24 h. The patient can be mobilized as soon as the effects of the premedication have worn off. Prior to discharge, the pacemaker system should be tested, a full 12-lead ECG taken and posteroanterior and lateral overpenetrated radiographic views of the chest performed. For subclavian puncture patients a pneumothorax should be excluded postoperatively. For programmable pulse generators, the desired parameters should be programmed.

In general, patients who have had endocardial leads inserted under local anesthesia are ready for hospital discharge on the second postoperative day. At the time of discharge the patient should be given information regarding the identification of the pacing system, the results of the initial testing, and, if programmable, the parameters chosen.

References

1. Schechter, D. C.: Background of Clinical Cardiac Electrostimulation: VII. Modern Era of Artificial Cardiac Pacemakers, *N.Y. State J. Med.*, 72:1175, 1972.
2. Muers, M. F., Arnold, A. G., and Sleight, P.: Prophylactic Antibiotics for Cardiac Pacemaker Implantation, *Br. Heart J.*, 46:539, 1981.
3. Feldman, S., Yahini, J. H., and Neufeld, N. H.: An Improved Method for Implantation of Permanent Endocardial Electrode through the Cephalic Vein, *PACE*, 3:370. 1980. (Abstract.)
4. Linos, D. A., Mucha, P., and VanHeerdon, J. A.: Subclavian Vein. A Golden Route, *Mayo Clin. Proc.*, 55:315, 1980.
5. Miller, F. A., Holmes, D. R., Gersh, B. J., and Maloney, J. D.: Permanent Transvenous Pacemaker Implantation via the Subclavian Vein, *Mayo Clin. Proc.*, 55:309, 1980.
6. Bellot, P. H.: A Variation on the Introducer Technique for Unlimited Access to the Subclavian Vein, *PACE*, 4:43, 1981.
7. Janchuck, S. J., Gill, B. S., and Petty, A. H.: Permanent Cardiac Pacing through the Subclavian Vein, *Br. J. Surg.*, 61:373, 1974.
8. Mond, H. G.: "The Cardiac Pacemaker: Function and Malfunction," Grune & Stratton, New York, 1983.
9. Gillmer, D. J., Vythilingum, S., and Mitha, A. S.: Problems Encountered during Insertion of Permanent Endocardial Pacing Electrodes, *PACE*, 4:212, 1981.
10. Mathews, D. M., and Fosfar, J. C.: Superior Vena Caval Stenosis: A Complication of Transvenous Endocardial Pacing, *Thorax*, 34:412, 1979.
11. Kaul, T. K., and Bain, W. H.: Radiographic Appearances of Implanted Transvenous Endocardial Pacing Electrodes, *Chest*, 72:323, 1977.
12. Gulotta, S. J.: Transvenous Cardiac Pacing. Techniques for Optimal Electrode Positioning and Prevention of Coronary Sinus Placement, *Circulation*, 42:701, 1970.

13. Smyth, N. P. D.: Techniques of Implantation: Atrial and Ventricular Thoracotomy and Transvenous, *Prog. Cardiovasc. Dis.*, 23:435, 1981.
14. Byrd, C.: Permanent Pacemaker Implantation Techniques, in P. Samet and El-Sherif (eds.), "Cardiac Pacing," 2d ed., Grune & Stratton, New York, 1980, p. 229.
15. Sutton, R., and Elsberry, D.: Stimulation Threshold Waveform Analysis of Atrial Endocardial Leads in Atrial Pacemaker Design, in C. Meere (ed.) (proceedings of the VIth World Symposium on Cardiac Pacing), Montreal, Chapter 34.12, 1979.
16. Bahadir, I., Koopot, R., and Diethrich, E. B.: Technique for Continuous Electrical Pacing during Pulse Generator Replacement, *Am. J. Cardiol.*, 42:1061, 1978. (Letter.)

105

Artificial Cardiac Pacemakers: Testing Methods

Harry G. Mond, M.D.

Exhaustion of the battery supply is signaled by a slow rise in the pulse rate taking place over a period of weeks so that ample warning is given.

Greatbatch and Chardack referring to implantable pulse generators.

David Schechter, M.D., 1972[1]

Until the early 1970s, the safety of a pacemaker implant was dependent on the rapid detection and correction of malfunctions as they arose. The electrocardiogram (ECG) helped confirm an intact pacing system and the oscilloscope was used to visualize the stimulus artifact and help establish end of life characteristics.[2] In practice, these testing methods were often unpredictable and many pacing centers explanted pulse generators on an elective basis, rather than waiting until end of life characteristics emerged.

Modern routine pacemaker testing is remarkably simple, quick, and highly accurate. Some older testing methods such as vector analysis have been abandoned, whereas other tests such as fluoroscopy, oscilloscopic examination, and chest wall stimulation, although not routine, nevertheless remain valuable investigative tools for suspected malfunction. In this chapter, testing methods have been divided into two sections: the routine postoperative follow-up procedures, and the investigative procedures for suspected pacemaker malfunction.

Routine Follow-Up Procedures

Prior to discharge from hospital, a 12-lead ECG in pacing rhythm and a chest radiograph should be performed. These are baseline procedures and need not be repeated unless there is suspected pacemaker malfunction. Baseline electronic pulse generator testing is essential. This includes the pulse repetition rate and pulse duration. In some clinics the oscilloscopic analysis of the stimulus artifact wave form is also performed.

The Pacemaker Follow-Up Clinic

For successful long-term management of pacemaker patients, a well-organized follow-up clinic is essential. A number of different clinic structures have been described. The most important common feature is a central reviewing clinic. This is conducted by a physician and nursing staff experienced in pacemaker work and most patients will be tested by this central clinic. Although the major function of the clinic is a mechanical one with pacemaker testing, nevertheless, the physician must be able to cope with other medical problems. Following discharge from hospital, the pacemaker patient should be reviewed within 2 weeks of implantation. The operation site is inspected, sutures removed when necessary, and the system checked. It is probably safe to review the patient again in 2 to 3 months and then every 6 months. Toward the end of the power source life, more frequent review becomes necessary. This was a difficult and unpredictable period for the pacemaker-dependent patient with a zinc-mercury-powered pulse generator. An elective replacement was often preferred. For patients with a lithium-powered pulse generator, the remaining power reserve even at the predicted end of life allows these latter visits to be every 2 or 3 months.

For patients who live far from a pacemaker clinic, a number of other systems have been devised. The most common of these is the transtelephone pacemaker clinic.[2] By the use of the telephone, confirmation of pacing by ECG and the status of the power source can be determined without the patient leaving home. This convenient system allows more frequent evaluation than the standard clinic follow-up and, in an emergency, review can be performed any time. There is, however, a limitation on the amount of information than can be transmitted. It is possible to transmit the ECG, peripheral pulse wave form, and to measure the asynchronous pulse repetition rate and pulse duration. For a transtelephone pace-

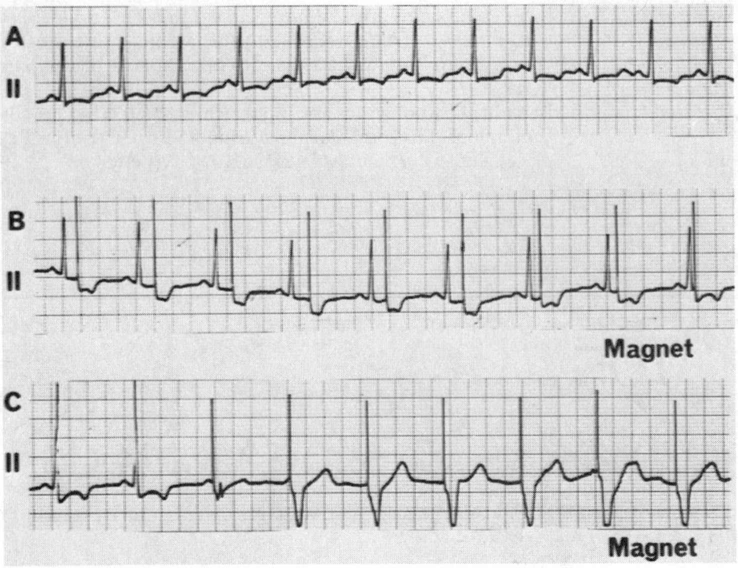

FIGURE 105-1 ECG lead II demonstrating the use of a magnet to confirm cardiac pacing. *A.* Synchronous mode. Sinus rhythm with no evidence of cardiac pacing. *B.* On application of magnet, the asynchronous discharge of the pulse generator is shown but cardiac pacing is not demonstrated as each stimulus artifact falls in the refractory period of the sinus beats. *C.* On reapplying the magnet the stimulus artifacts are now earlier and the first four beats are fusion beats. Regular cardiac pacing then occurs.

maker monitoring system to be successful, the patient equipment must be simple and inexpensive. The patient or a responsible relative must be instructed in placing the magnet over the pulse generator and correctly applying the transmitter module. Although apparently simple to the manufacturers and physicians, such equipment may be very difficult for the elderly to operate.

On occasion, the transtelephone transmitting equipment may be at a regional pacemaker clinic such as the office of a local primary physician or small hospital. A group of local residents having pacemakers can attend at regular intervals and the information sent to the central clinic. The cost of a transtelephone monitoring service run by a hospital with only a small pacemaker clinic can be exorbitant. Large, central, commercial telephone monitoring services have been established, particularly in the United States, and have been successful in detecting impending power source depletion and other pacemaker malfunctions.[3] A disadvantage of the transtelephone pacemaker clinic is the lack of direct communication between patient and physician, especially if a commercial company is involved.

The traveling pacemaker clinic is another means of monitoring patients who live long distances from the central clinic.[4] In this system pacemaker personnel from the central clinic travel to a regional clinic where patients attend two or more times a year. Patient self-testing is a controversial issue. With the zinc-mercury power source, patients were instructed in taking their pulse and notifying the clinic of any change. Frequently, however, this led to problems such as confusion between sensed and paced beats, causing significant fear, apprehension, and panic. Because of the reliability of modern pacing systems, patients are now frequently advised not to regularly take their peripheral pulse rate. However, the patient and relatives should be taught to do so if the patient suspects pacemaker malfunction. Because pulse repetition rate counters are now inexpensive and freely available, this will in the future become a means of home self-testing.

Routine Pacemaker Electrocardiography

Confirmation of pacing using the ECG is an essential function of the pacemaker clinic. This must be performed in the synchronous (demand or base) mode as well as the asynchronous (fixed rate or magnet) mode. The ECG lead II is the best lead to confirm pacing. In cases where pacing is not clear or pacemaker malfunction is suspected, long strips of as many ECG leads as necessary should be taken. With magnet testing, the specific magnet supplied by the company should be used. It is gently positioned over the implanted pulse generator and orientated according to the manufacturer's recommendations. Bar, crescent, or horseshoe magnets must be aligned correctly so as to trigger the reed switch. In obese patients, or in patients where the pulse generator lies deep or is relatively inaccessible, the magnet may not trigger the reed switch. In these cases, two or more similar magnets should be used. The ECG in Fig. 105-1 demonstrates the correct use of a magnet to confirm cardiac pacing. Because of competitive rhythms when using a magnet, most manufacturers now use a magnet rate faster than the base rate to override spontaneous rhythms. In these cases, pulse repetition rates of 90 to 100 beats per minute are usually used.

Pacemaker Electronic Testing

Measurement of the interval between stimulus artifacts, both in the synchronous and asynchronous modes, can be rapidly determined using a variety of relatively inexpensive and highly accurate rate counters. The interval in milliseconds is automatically converted to beats per minute. The equipment need only be placed on the chest and a reading is immediately given provided the four electrodes on the undersurface make contact with skin and the patient is pacing. As well as the pacing rate, the equipment can also measure the pulse duration (atrium and ventricle) and the atrioventricular delay with dual-chamber systems. As with ECG recordings, pacemaker clinic personnel must have a comprehensive knowledge of the changes that occur with the pulse repetition rate and pulse duration, both in the synchronous and asynchronous modes.

Testing parameter changes that are incorporated into the pulse generator as the power source depletes vary from manufacturer to manufacturer and may even be different between models from the same manufacturer. Most companies, particularly with rate programmable pacemakers, use the magnet mode to demonstrate the pulse repetition rate changes. These changes, especially with the lithium-iodine power source, may be gradual throughout life or may occur abruptly toward the end of life. In general, the pulse duration increases as the voltage output falls. This is used to maintain a steady pulse generator energy output. Once the testing data have been recorded there should be an immediate comparison with previous recordings. In some clinics, this information is computerized and a printout obtained comparing all previous tests.

Other Procedures Used in Routine Pacemaker Follow-Up

Oscilloscopic Analysis of the Stimulus Artifact Waveform

Described in the early 1960s, this was the first method used to evaluate battery status.[5] Using a standard high-speed storage oscilloscope and ECG limb leads, the calibrated stimulus artifact from leads I, II, and III is displayed on the screen and a permanent record made.[6] A fall in height of the stimulus artifact (voltage) from previous recordings may indicate impending power source depletion. Unfortunately, this is unreliable and routine oscilloscopic analysis of the stimulus artifact waveform never found widespread usage. Some clinics, however, perform baseline oscilloscopic measurements for comparison with recordings taken at a later date in evaluating patients with suspected malfunction.

Stimulus Artifact Frontal Plane Vector Analysis

First described in 1968,[7] the analysis never found widespread usage. The technique involved calculating the frontal plane vector of the oscilloscopic stimulus artifact waveform. Vector analysis was found to be valuable in detecting a break in the conductor or insulator. In this situation gross changes in the vector occurred.

Computer Assessment

With the increasing use of computers in medicine, it is not surprising that pacemaker clinics have used this facility to document patient records and to assist in follow-up. Advantages include rapid retrieval of information, reliability, efficiency of large clinics, automatic pacemaker physician reports, and alerting the clinic physician to test abnormalities.

Threshold Measurements

As a means of assessing pacemaker lead function, threshold measurements are valuable. Either the voltage or pulse duration threshold can be measured using special features of multiprogrammable pulse generators. Threshold levels are useful when using low-energy outputs on multiprogrammable pulse generators or in patients who have high thresholds for pacing. The various systems available have been reviewed by the author.[6]

Reprogramming

Routine pulse generator reprogramming can be performed to assess lead pacing threshold, to evaluate underlying rhythms, or to test the programming functions of the pulse generator. This will be further discussed in the investigative procedures for suspected pacemaker malfunction.

Investigative Procedures for Suspected Pacemaker Malfunction

In assessing a patient with suspected pacemaker malfunction, every attempt must be made to diagnose and even correct the malfunction without the need for surgical intervention. In many cases, the diagnosis can be made by routine testing and simple investigations. When confronted with a patient with suspected pacemaker malfunction, the physician should follow a set investigative protocol. All abnormal data must be repeated or confirmed by another method. Not infrequently, abnormal data represent a pseudomalfunction where the abnormality results from faulty testing equipment or incorrect recording of data. The remainder of this chapter briefly outlines an investigative troubleshooting protocol for pacemaker malfunction.

Clinical Findings

The symptomatic pacemaker patient must be seen by a physician and the clinical findings carefully evaluated. In many cases, the symptoms are not related to the pacemaker system. A number of symptoms mimic those seen in patients before pacemaker insertion. In particular, dizziness may reflect vertebrobasilar insufficiency or postural hypotension. However, should the history indicate the recurrence of symptoms experienced before the pacemaker implantation, then the possibility of pacemaker malfunction, even intermittent, should be entertained.

Routine Testing Methods

The most important tests to establish pacemaker malfunction are those used for routine testing. These include electronic testing and the ECG rhythm strip, both in the synchronous and asynchronous modes. These tests establish the presence or absence of normal pacing at the time of testing. Electronic testing confirms the delivery of a normal stimulus artifact at the correct pulse repetition rate to the myocardium, but does not confirm a myocardial response. Marked changes in the asynchronous pulse repetition rate or pulse duration may signify impending power source depletion. The pacemaker rhythm strip confirms pacing or a myocardial response at the time the ECG is taken. The finding of normal test data by routine methods does not exclude intermittent pacemaker malfunction. If the symptoms suggest an intermittent pacemaker problem, it may be appropriate to repeat the ECG during monitoring or provocative movements.

Noninvasive Investigations

Chest Radiography and Fluoroscopy

This is an important investigation for suspected or confirmed pacemaker malfunction. Visualization of the pacing system by radiographic means will help confirm a lead fracture. Electrode position is assessed using the posteroanterior and lateral views. Fluoroscopy also allows provocative movements to be performed while observing the lead and pulse generator.

Oscilloscopic Examination

With modern pacemaker testing, the main value of the oscilloscopic examination is to assess the abnormal stimulus artifact. An abnormal stimulus artifact may be due to an electronic malfunction or a break in the pacemaker-patient electrical circuit and in particular a fracture in the lead system with contact between the fractured ends. As with other investigative tools, provocative movements may be useful during oscilloscopic examination.

Reprogramming and Telemetry

Most of the programmable functions of multiprogrammable pulse generators have become useful in both investigation and treatment of patients with suspected pacemaker malfunction. The pulse repetition rate can be increased to confirm pacing in situations when the spontaneous rhythm inhibits the pulse generator and the ECG in the magnet or asynchronous mode is confusing because of the competitive rhythm and fusion beats. The pulse repetition rate can be reduced to allow a spontaneous rhythm to emerge to confirm sensing. Output mode reprogramming assists in evaluating lead threshold, whereas the sensitivity and refractory period programs are used in the investigation of suspected sensing problems. Reprogramming is essential in assessing dual-chamber systems.

It is expected that the recent introduction of telemetry will aid considerably in the evaluation of suspected malfunction. Battery and lead status can now be obtained. Threshold values can be rapidly measured and electrograms recorded noninvasively. Marker channels can be telemetered simultaneously with endocardial electrograms onto multichannel ECG machines (Fig. 105-2). These marker channels confirm sensing and pacing and can be used for suspected pacemaker malfunction.

Chest Wall Stimulation

The use of external pulsed electrical stimulations to the chest wall has been a valuable tool both in the assessment of the sensing function of implanted pulse generators and for inspecting underlying spontaneous rhythms.[8] The technique involves the application to the chest wall of two electrodes which are attached to a standard external pulse generator set at about 70 beats per minute and the voltage from 1 to 5 V or current 2 to 10 mA. With an ECG recording being observed, the external pulse generator is turned on. Small stimulus artifacts will be seen on

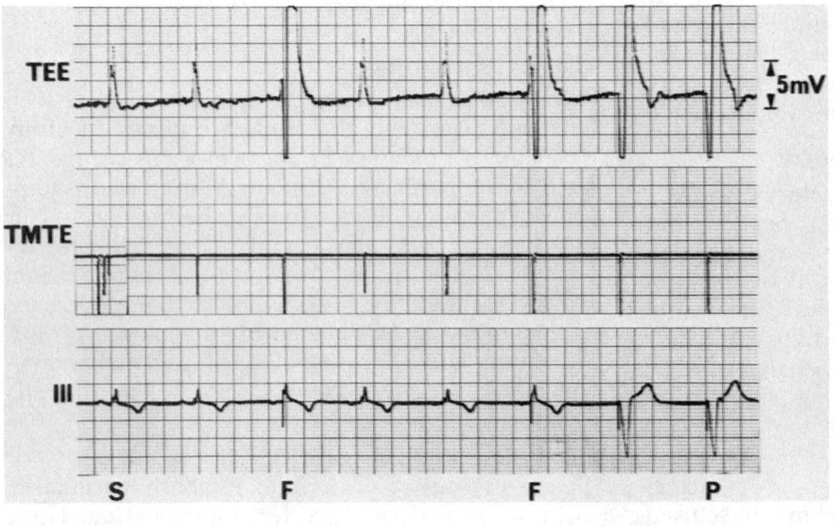

FIGURE 105-2 Simultaneous recording. TEE = telemetered endocardial electrogram (calibrated); TMTE = telemetered main timing events. Lead III of the surface ECG (Telectronics, Optima MPT). The ECG shows QRS complexes of sinus origin (S), paced beats (P), and fusion beats (F). The simultaneous electrogram shows a 6-to-8-mV QRS of sinus origin and paced beats which are markedly deformed by the stimulus artifact. There are three main timing events with the calibrations at the left edge. The largest deflection is due to paced beats, the middle size to sensed beats, and the smallest to sensed events within the refractory period of the pulse generator. Such telemetered information is very valuable in evaluating pacing rhythms and in the investigation of suspected pacemaker malfunction.

the ECG which represent the external energy being delivered to the chest wall and heart. The stimulus artifacts are too weak to affect the heart but are large enough to be sensed by the implanted pacemaker system. Failure to inhibit an implanted atrial inhibited (AAI) or ventricular inhibited (VVI) pulse generator by chest wall stimulation will occur with a malfunctioning sensing circuit and will help differentiate problems such as undersensing caused by a small P or R wave.

Electrocardiographic Monitoring
Prolonged ECG monitoring of pacemaker patients is a very valuable investigation for cases of suspected intermittent pacemaker malfunction. Systems include continuous 24-h or even longer ambulatory monitoring (Holter), event recorders, ECG telemetry, direct bedside monitoring, and telephone transmission of the ECG. A major disadvantage of all these systems is the inability to identify and adequately record the stimulus artifact, but this is expected to improve in future designs of this equipment.

Provocative Movements
In patients with a suspected or documented inoperative pacemaker system, fluoroscopy may fail to demonstrate a break in the pacemaker electrical circuit. In these cases, provocative movements may separate the broken ends, thus confirming the diagnosis and pinpointing the site of lead fracture. Provocative movements are performed during a testing procedure and both ECG documentation and resuscitation facilities must be available. Provocative movements may also demonstrate skeletal muscle inhibition and failure of the pulse generator set screw to make firm contact with the lead pin. Examples of provocative movements include abruptly pushing on the implanted pulse generator, forced inspiration, shoulder movements, and unusual postures. To document skeletal myopotential inhibition, rapid arm movements and isometric exercises are necessary.

Noninvasive Threshold Measurements
The value of noninvasive threshold measurements has already been discussed. This technique can be used to diagnose a high threshold of pacing and for follow-up assessment of such patients.

Echocardiography
Echocardiography has been used in the diagnosis of pacing lead complications and in particular lead displacement and perforation of the right ventricle.[9]

Environmental Testing
In the highly technological and industrialized world there are only a few hazards which consistently interfere with pacemaker function and once recognized, the patient should be appropriately warned. However, on occasion significant symptomatic pulse generator inhibition may occur in the working or home environment. These can usually be diagnosed with ambulatory monitoring but environmental testing at the location of the symptoms may become necessary.

Carotid Sinus Pressure
Carotid sinus pressure can be used to slow a sinus rhythm which prevents analysis of pacing rhythm. The procedure must be performed gently, never on both sides simultaneously, and resuscitation equipment should be available as severe bradycardia may occur in the event of pacemaker malfunction.

Invasive Investigations

Surgical Exploration
The requirements of the operating room and the reoperation surgical principles have been discussed in Chap. 104. Pacemaker records and previous operation notes are essential. At operation, the pulse generator and lead system are mobilized and inspected; both are tested using the pacing system analyzer and an intracardiac electrogram is performed when indicated. The lead system is carefully observed under fluoroscopy and where necessary traction is applied to demonstrate fractured ends. Any site where nonabsorbable suture material is tied around the lead should be very carefully inspected. Any area where there is an acute angle bend, such as in the neck with an external jugular venous entry approach, is a likely site of lead fracture. Blood inside the lead insulation suggests an insulation break and a possible site for current leakage.

Pacing System Analysis
Table 105-1 summarizes the pacing system analysis of a number of more common pacemaker malfunctions. Such malfunctions are related to the pulse generator, the lead, the myocardium, or a combination of these. The inoperative pacemaker can be easily differentiated into a lead or pulse generator fault. The finding of a high-voltage threshold, low current, and very high impedance suggests a lead fracture with current conduction due to contact of the fractured ends or a fluid bridge. A high-voltage threshold also occurs with lead displacement or exit block and in both of these situations the impedance remains normal. Lead displacement and exit block can be differentiated with fluoroscopy. A lead insulation break results in a low impedance due to current leak and thus high current requirements. A thorough review of these complications of pacing is available.[6]

Intracardiac Electrography
The intracardiac electrogram is an endocardial ECG recording taken at the time of pacemaker implantation or at reoperation and is particularly valuable in troubleshooting. A complete review of the technical aspects and normal appearances is available.[6]

TABLE 105-1 Pacing System Analysis of Common Pacemaker Malfunctions

	Variable Voltage—0.5-ms Pulse Duration				
	Voltage Threshold	**Resultant Current**	**Impedance**	**Recorded P or R Wave Value**	**Pulse Generator Testing**
Normal range (chronic lead)	Less than 3.5 V	Less than 6 mA	250–1000 ohm	Greater than 4 mV (ventricle) and 2 mV (atrium)	5 V-output 2-mV sensing
Lead fracture (no conduction)	Pacing not possible	Pacing not possible	Infinity	0	Normal
Lead fracture (intermittent conduction)	High	Low	Very high	Normal (if retained)	Normal
Lead displacement	Very high (if pacing possible)	Very high (if pacing possible)	Normal	Variable	Normal
Exit block	High	High	Normal	Variable	Output may be low
Lead insulation break	Normal or low	High	Low	Usually low	Output may be low (high current drain)
Undersensing (synchronous)	Normal	Normal	Normal	Low (myocardial cause)	Sensing fault (pulse generator cause)
Oversensing (synchronous)	Normal	Normal	Normal	Normal (may sense large P or T waves)	Normal (unless programmed very sensitive)
Pulse generator inoperative	Normal	Normal	Normal	Normal	No output
Reduced pulse repetition rate (asynchronous)	Normal	Normal	Normal	Normal	Low output (power source depletion)

The most common appearance of the ventricular electrogram is a biphasic wave with the S wave usually dominant (Fig. 105-3).

Once contact is made with the endocardium, ST elevation and T-wave inversion occurs. In comparison, the epicardial ventricular pattern (coronary sinus tributary or lead perforation of the right ventricle) almost always has a dominant R wave without the ST elevation and T-wave inversion. The calibrated electrogram can also be used to measure the QRS or P-wave size and slew rate for problems with undersensing.

Testing the Explanted Pulse Generator

In conjunction with a biomedical engineering department all explanted pulse generators should be tested to document the pulse generator malfunction under investigation. Similarly, pulse generators removed for other reasons such as patient death should also undergo thorough testing. If a fault is found, the pulse generator should be returned to the manufacturers.

References

1. Schechter, D.C.: Background of Clinical Cardiac Electrostimulation. VII. Modern Era of Artificial Cardiac Pacemakers, *N.Y. State J. Med.*, 72:1166, 1972.
2. Furman, S.: Cardiac Pacing and Pacemakers VIII. The Pacemaker Follow-up Clinic, *Am. Heart J.* 94:795, 1977.
3. Hurzeler, P., Morse, D., Leach, C., Sands, M. J., Pennock, R., and Zinberg, A.: Longevity Comparison among Lithium An-

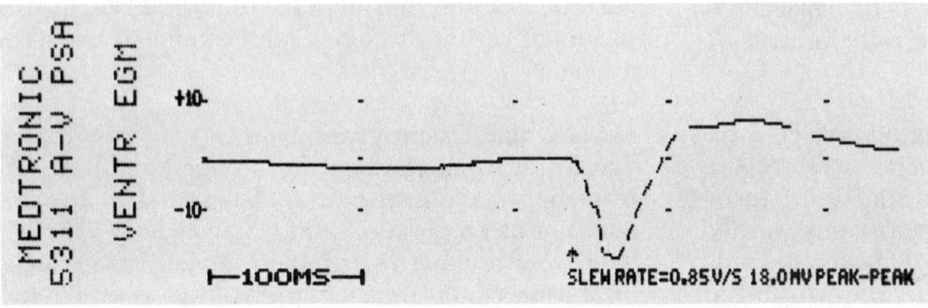

FIGURE 105-3 Normal endocardial ventricular electrogram taken at the time of lead insertion (Medtronic 5311 pacing system analyzer). The QRS is purely an S wave, has a slew rate of 0.85 V per second, a peak-to-peak size of 18 mV, and is followed by ST elevation.

ode Power Cells for Cardiac Pacemakers, *PACE,* 3:555, 1980.
4. Mond, H., Gerloff, D., Flower, D., Kertes, P., and Hunt, D.: The Travelling Pacemaker Clinic—A Ten Year Appraisal, *PACE,* 6:A–30, 1983. (Abstract.)
5. Knuckey, L., McDonald, R., and Sloman, G.: A Method of Testing Implanted Cardiac Pacemakers, *Br. Heart J.* 27:483, 1965.
6. Mond, Harry G.: "The Cardiac Pacemaker; Function and Malfunction," Grune & Stratton, New York, 1983.
7. Green, G. D., Forbes, W., Bain, W. H., and Shaw, G. B.: Detecting Break in Insulation in Negative Pacemaker Lead, *Br. Med. J.* 4:645, 1968. (Letter to editor.)
8. Barold, S. S., Pupillo, G. A., Gaidula, J. J., and Linhart, J. W.: Chest Wall Stimulation in Evaluation of Patients with Implanted Ventricular-inhibited Demand Pacemakers, *Br. Heart J.,* 32:783, 1981.
9. Nanda, N. C., and Barold, S. S.: Usefulness of Echocardiography in Cardiac Pacing, *PACE,* 5:222, 1982.

106

The Implantable Cardioverter-Defibrillator

M. Mirowski, M.D.

The advantages and disadvantages of the (automatic implantable defibrillator) approach . . . to the prevention of sudden coronary death merit careful study. One would hope that the time necessary for establishing its feasibility and practicality will be brief, as we have very little else to offer today to patients with high-risk of dying suddenly. . . .

M. Mirowski et al., 1970[1,*]

Termination of ventricular fibrillation and of most hemodynamically unstable ventricular tachycardias requires application of a sufficiently strong electrical countershock to the heart. The effectiveness of this maneuver, however, depends upon the immediate availability of specialized personnel and equipment. Because such preconditions are rarely satisfied outside the hospital, sudden cardiac death continues to exact a heavy toll of lives.

The difficulties in managing malignant ventricular arrhythmias in the community prompted the development of the automatic implantable cardioverter-defibrillator (AICD).[1–7] A self-contained diagnostic-therapeutic system, the AICD continuously monitors the heart, identifies ventricular fibrillation or tachycardia, and then delivers corrective discharges to restore normal rhythm. Since the device performs its functions promptly and automatically, the constraints of time and the need for trained personnel—the two stumbling blocks in conventional out-of-hospital resuscitation—are eliminated.

Description of the Device

The AICD weighs 298 g and occupies a volume of 162 cm^3 (Fig. 106-1). A pair of transcardiac electrodes serves for both defibrillation and sensing. One electrode is located on a catheter placed in the superior vena cava and the other is a flexible patch covering the apex of the heart. An additional bipolar right-ventricular electrode catheter or two epicardial screw-in electrodes provide rate determination and R-wave synchronization signals. The device has an estimated 2- to 3-year monitoring life or the capability of delivering about 100 discharges.

The AICD diagnoses the arrhythmia by morphological and heart rate criteria. When ventricular fibrillation occurs, a 25-J pulse is delivered within 15 to 20 s; when ventricular tachycardia faster than a preset heart rate is diagnosed, the pulse is R-wave synchronized. If a discharge is ineffective, the device can recycle as many as three times, with the strength of each additional pulse increased to 30 J. Noninvasive communication with the implanted device is made possible through magnetically triggered, coded audio signals and an external analyzer.

Patient Population and Surgical Technique

In the group of some 300 patients who underwent implantation of the device as of April 1984, left ventricular dysfunction was common (mean ejection fraction of less than 40 percent). Coronary artery disease was the most frequent underlying disorder with various types of cardiomyopathies present in about one-fourth of the patients. The initial implantees were required to have survived at least two arrhythmic cardiac arrests not associated with acute myocardial infarction; one of these episodes must have occurred despite presumably effective drug therapy, and one must have been electrocardiographically documented. As the clinical experience grew, these criteria were somewhat relaxed; the latest

*Reproduced with permission from the publisher.

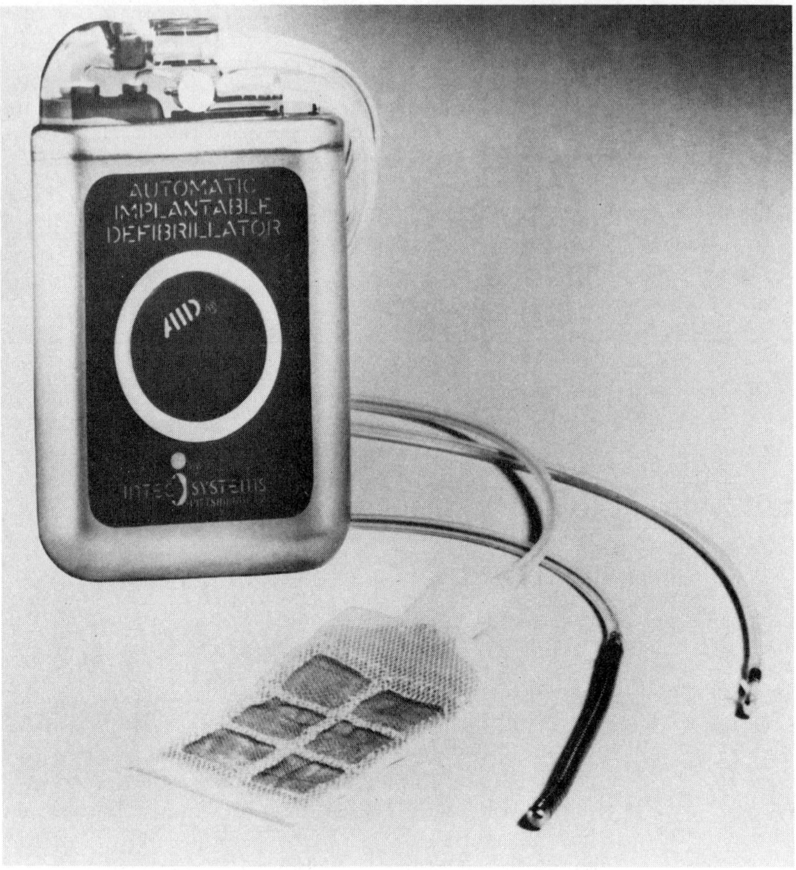

FIGURE 106-1 The automatic implantable cardioverter-defibrillator with, *right* to *left*, bipolar right ventricular, superior vena cava, and apical patch electrodes. For more details see text.

protocol requires only a history of a single ventricular fibrillation or hypotensive ventricular tachycardia without acute myocardial infarction, and evidence of incomplete protection despite antiarrhythmic therapy.

At first, placement of the apical electrode was always made through a thoracotomy with the remaining electrodes being inserted transvenously. More recently, a subxiphoidal approach obviating a thoracotomy has been developed and has become the preferred approach.[8] The pulse generator is usually implanted subcutaneously in a left paraumbilical pocket. Thoracotomy is always performed if the patient has had previous cardiovascular surgery or when AICD implantation is associated with endocardial resection or coronary bypass grafting.

Results and Complications

The clinical experience indicates that the AICD can monitor cardiac rhythm for extended periods of time and reliably detect ventricular fibrillation and tachycardias; the diagnostic accuracy is 99 percent for the former and 98 percent for the latter. The conversion effectiveness is also excellent and one 25-J discharge is generally sufficient to restore normal rhythm (Fig. 106-2). Rarely, ventricular tachycardia will accelerate to a faster rhythm or to ventricular fibrillation; if this occurs, the device recognizes the new arrhythmia and corrects it with a subsequent discharge. Potential risks also include surgical complications, infection, thromboembolism, lead dislodgment or fracture, premature battery depletion,

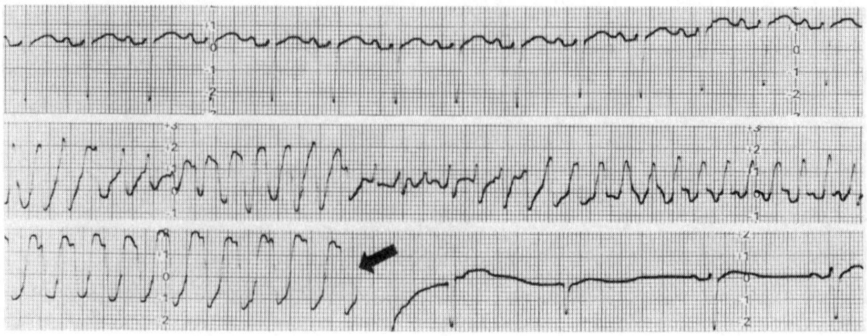

FIGURE 106-2 Automatic conversion of ventricular flutter-fibrillation to sinus rhythm. *Upper strip*: baseline rhythm recorded prior to cardiac arrest. *Middle strip*: ventricular flutter-fibrillation. *Lower strip*: 25-J internal discharge restores normal rhythm (arrow) some 20 s after onset of the arrhythmia. The strips are not continuous.

and random component failure; the frequency and severity of these complications is similar to those observed with electronic pacemakers. The internal discharges are generally well tolerated; false-positive shocks, sometimes triggered by supraventricular tachyarrhythmias, may represent a problem, but they are clinically benign and have never induced serious arrhythmias.

Impact on Mortality

The total 1-year mortality in the initial 52 implantees was decreased by 52 percent, and the sudden death mortality was only 8.5 percent.[9] In 70 patients who received a more recent model of the device, the 1-year sudden death mortality was reduced to 1.8 percent.[10] Since patients with malignant ventricular arrhythmias refractory to therapy usually have an incidence of sudden death in excess of 30 percent per year, the observed improvement in survival is substantial indeed.

Conclusion

The clinical use of the AICD has resulted in a marked decrease in the mortality rate of the implantees. Further broadening of the indication to include other subgroups of high-risk patients appears to be warranted.

References

1. Mirowski, M., Mower, M. M., Staewen, W. S., Tabatznik, B., and Mendeloff, A. I.: Standby Automatic Defibrillator: An Approach to Prevention of Sudden Coronary Death, *Arch. Intern. Med.,* 126:158, 1970.
2. Mirowski, M., Mower, M. M., Staewen, W. S., Denniston, R. H., and Mendeloff, A. I.: The Development of the Transvenous Automatic Defibrillator, *Arch. Intern. Med.,* 129:773, 1972.
3. Mirowski, M., Mower, M. M., Langer, A., Heilman, M. S., and Schreibman, J.: A Chronically Implanted System for Automatic Defibrillation in Active Conscious Dogs: Experimental Model for Treatment of Sudden Death from Ventricular Fibrillation, *Circulation,* 58:90, 1978.
4. Mirowski, M., Mower, M. M., Bhagavan, B. S., et al.: Chronic Animal and Bench Testing of the Implantable Automatic Defibrillator (proceedings, VIth world symposium on cardiac pacing, Montreal, Oct., 1979), *Pacesymp,* Canada, 1979.
5. Mirowski, M., Reid, P. R., Mower, M. M., et al.: Termination of Malignant Ventricular Arrhythmias with an Implanted Automatic Defibrillator in Human Beings, *N. Engl. J. Med.,* 303:322, 1980.
6. Reid, P. R., Mirowski, M., Mower, M. M., et al.: Clinical Evaluation of the Internal Automatic Cardioverter-Defibrillator in Survivors of Sudden Cardiac Death, *Am. J. Cardiol.,* 51:1608, 1983.
7. Winkle, R. A., Bach, S. M., Echt, D. S., et al.: The Automatic Implantable Defibrillator: Local Ventricular Bipolar Sensing to Detect Ventricular Tachycardia and Fibrillation, *Am. J. Cardiol.,* 52:265, 1983.
8. Watkins, L., Mirowski, M., Mower, M. M., et al.: Implantation of the Automatic Defibrillator: The Sub-Xiphoid Approach, *Ann. Thorac. Surg.,* 34:515, 1982.
9. Mirowski, M., Reid, P. R., Winkle, R. A., et al.: Mortality in Patients with Implanted Automatic Defibrillators, *Ann. Intern. Med.,* 98:585, 1983.
10. Echt, D. S., Armstrong, K., Schmidt, P., Oyer, P. E., Stinson, E. B., and Winkle, R. A.: Clinical Experience, Complications, and Survival in 70 Patients with the Automatic Implantable Cardioverter-Defibrillator, *Circulation,* 71(2):289, 1985.

Section C

Techniques of Diagnostic Radiography, Nuclear Cardiology, Radiographic Guided Intervention, and Nuclear Magnetic Resonance

107

Technique of Cardiac Fluoroscopy

James T. T. Chen, M.D.

Cardiac roentgenography deals primarily with anatomic details by filming at short exposure times that stop the motion. Cardiac fluoroscopy, on the other hand, explores the dynamic features of the organ that are discernible only in motion.[1] The two techniques are mutually complementary.

Technical Methods[2]

A good-quality image intensifier is a prerequisite for the proper performance of cardiac fluoroscopy. The modern intensifier with the use of cesium iodide phosphors has increased the brightness of the fluoroscopic image by at least 10,000 times. Television viewing permits cone vision under dim light with bettter perception of detail. The attached videotape or videodisk recorder provides a means for instant playback as well as future analysis of the fluoroscopic observation.

The milliamperage and the kilovoltage of the fluoroscope should be adjusted according to the patient's size in different projections. The milliamperage ranges from 1.5 to 3.5 and the kilovoltage varies between 90 and 120. Too high a kilovoltage tends to reduce the contrast, and excessive milliamperage will blur off the margin of the image. The shortest fluoroscopic time and the smallest shutter opening are to be employed in order to reduce the dose of radiation to the minimal. The average examining time for this author is 3.5 min.

The patient is routinely examined in the erect position with four views. The patient should be asked to stop breathing during the brief moment of fluoroscopy. A barium meal is given only after a thorough search for cardiac calcifications is completed. Occasionally a recumbent position is used for better visualization of small calcifications, as well as for a critical evaluation of cardiac asynergy. The cardiac output increases and the heart rate decreases upon assuming recumbency, thereby giving a truer and more representative picture of the left ventricular contractility. In obese patients, the thick layer of soft tissues over the thorax will be compressed and pushed aside, thereby improving the fluoroscopic image significantly.

Anticipated Results

When properly performed, cardiac fluoroscopy is quite useful in the following areas of investigation: (1) assessment of cardiovascular dynamics, (2) detection of small cardiovascular calcifications, (3) visualization of important anatomic landmarks, e.g., subepicardial fat stripes, (4) differentiation of cardiac from noncardiac diseases, (5) evaluation of cardiac valve prostheses, pacemakers, and radiopaque foreign bodies.

Complications

Both the patient and the examiner should be protected from excessive radiation. Even with an image intensifier a routine cardiac fluoroscopy still involves more radiation than does two-view chest roentgenography. Therefore, the fluoroscopist should be well prepared to accomplish the task within the shortest possible period of time. Although all aspects of the heart are briefly surveyed, one should emphasize special areas of interest for each patient as suggested by the baseline radiographs. If coarctation of the aorta is suspected in a patient older than 40 years, particular attention should be paid to finding calcium in the aortic valve.

General Application

Assessment of Cardiovascular Dynamics[3-6]

The chest roentgenogram which is taken at random largely records the diastolic image of the heart. Fluoroscopy, on the other hand, provides a continuous vision of the pulsating organ throughout the entire cardiac cycle. Upon becoming familiar with the normal cardiovascular movements, any deviation from the norm will become obvious to the fluoroscopist.

The telltale x-ray signs of many cardiac lesions manifest themselves only in ventricular systole. Therefore, what may be missed on the film is often readily seen and diagnosed under the fluoroscope. For instance, left ventricular enlargement may be the only radiographic abnormality of severe aortic insufficiency in children or young adults. On fluoroscopy, however, the aorta is vigorously expanding in systole and rapidly collapsing in diastole. This dynamic alteration is characteristic of aortic insufficiency (Fig. 107-1). Other examples in the same vein include mild mitral insufficiency, mitral valve prolapse, left ventricular dyskinesia, or broad-based left ventricular aneurysm.

In valvular pulmonary stenosis, vigorous pulsation of the pulmonary trunk in its left branch is in bold contrast to the diminished pulsation of the right pulmonary artery.[5] Increased pulsation of diffusely enlarged pulmonary arteries is characteristic of left-to-right shunts. When marked discrepancy in size and pulsation is noted between the central and peripheral vessels, Eisenmenger's syndrome should be considered. Exaggerated left atrial expansion in ventricular systole is a reliable sign of mitral insufficiency.[6]

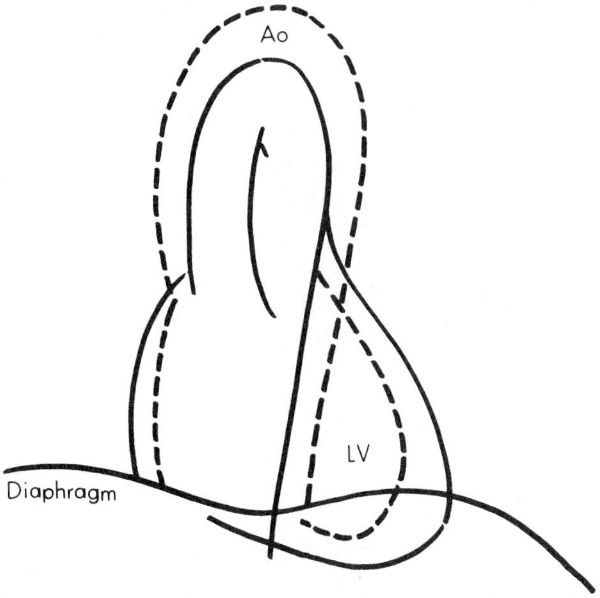

FIGURE 107-1 Schematic representation of dynamic changes of aortic insufficiency. Interrupted lines represent images in systole; solid lines, those in diastole.

Detection of Cardiovascular Calcifications[7]

Heavy calcifications of the heart and vessels are easily detected by chest roentgenography, particularly in the lateral and oblique views (Fig. 107-2). Small calcifications, on the other hand, can be registered only by fluoroscopy by virtue of their rhythmic movements from the pulsating heart. Detection of even tiny coronary artery calcifications is of vital

FIGURE 107-2 Lateral view shows heavy railroad-track-like calcification of all three major coronary arteries: r = right coronary artery; a = anterior descending coronary artery; c = circumflex coronary artery. Note the ringlike densities representing vessels viewed on end.

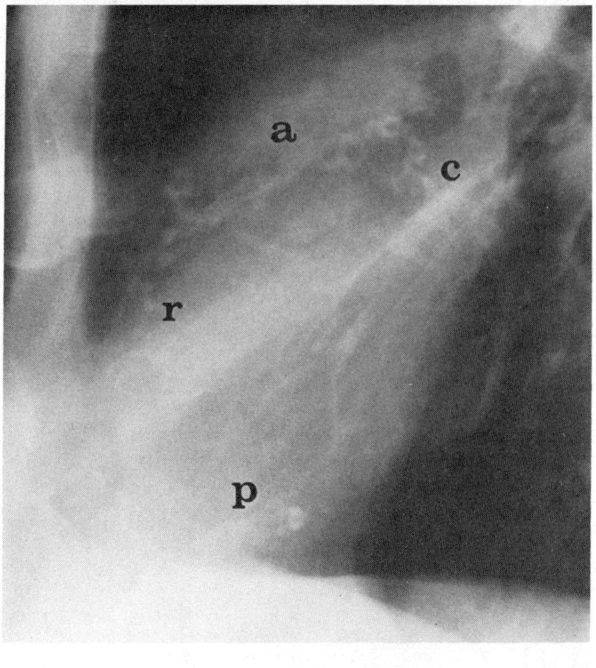

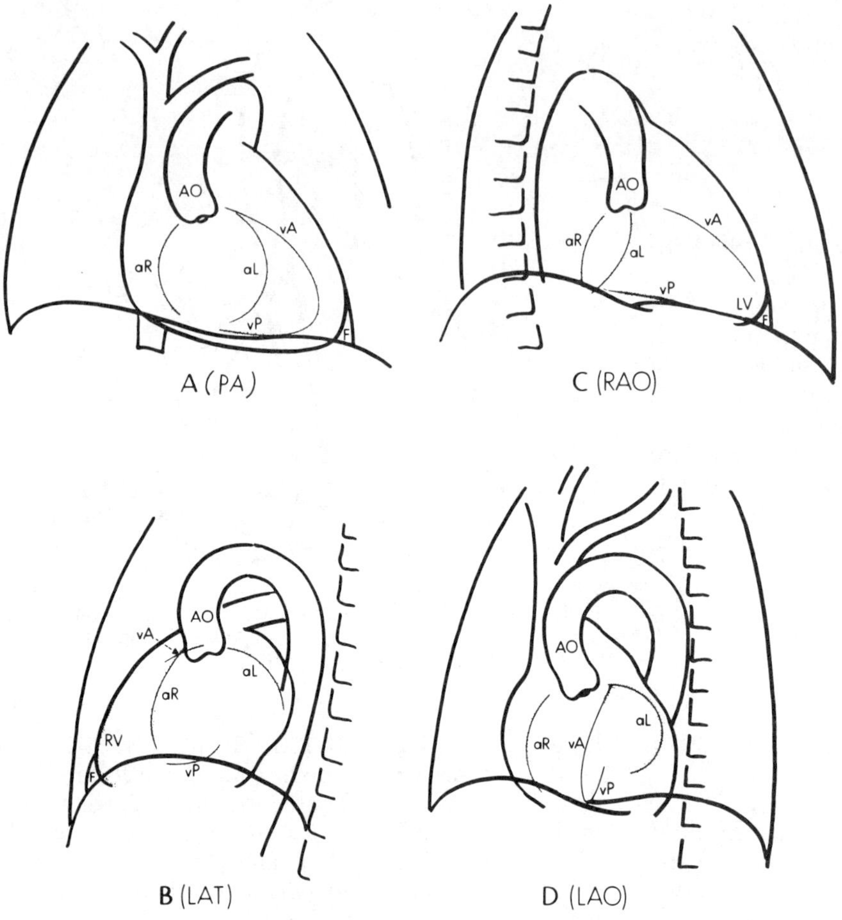

FIGURE 107-3 Schematic representation of the subepicardial fat stripes in relation to major coronary arteries. *A.* Posteroanterior (PA) view. *B.* Lateral (LAT) view. *C.* Right anterior oblique (RAO) view. *D.* Left anterior oblique (LAO) view. Abbreviations: aL = left atrioventricular groove (circumflex); aR = right atrioventricular groove (right); vA = anterior interventricular groove (anterior descending); vP = posterior interventricular groove (posterior descending).

FIGURE 107-4 Subepicardial fat stripe in the diagnosis of pericardial effusion. *A.* Lateral view in a patient 3 weeks after coronary bypass procedure showing a normal pericardium as a hairline density (arrow) sandwiched between the subepicardial fat stripe interiorly and the mediastinal fat exteriorly. Also note the metallic sutures in the sternum and a surgical clip marking the origin of a venous graft in the ascending aorta. *B.* Lateral view of the same patient who developed postpericardiotomy syndrome 5 weeks after operation. Note the subepicardial fat stripe (arrow) to be displaced interiorly by the widened pericardium. The fat stripe became more distinct in the presence of pericardial effusion.

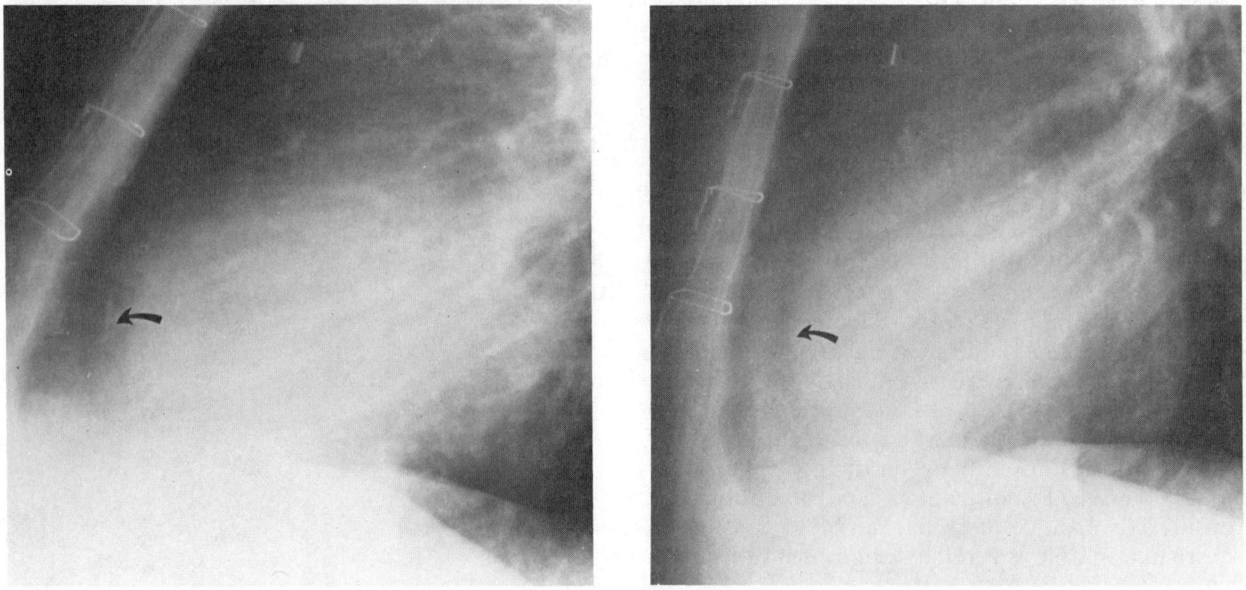

A **B**

practical importance. The combination of chest pain and coronary calcification results from major vascular obstruction 94 percent of the time.[7] Since the major coronary arteries are embedded in the subepicardial fat stripes in the grooves between cardiac chambers (Fig. 107-3), such fat stripes can be used effectively to locate the calcified arteries. Under the fluoroscope the fat stripes present as pulsating radiolucent (bright) lines in contrast to the accompanying pulsating radiopaque (dark) lines of calcified coronary arteries. If the artery coincides with the fat line within the left atrioventricular groove (aL), it portrays the circumflex coronary artery. The right coronary artery is moving synchronously and within the right atrioventricular groove (aR). The anterior descending artery coincides with the anterior interventricular groove (Va), as does the posterior descending artery with the posterior interventricular groove (Vp).

The lateral view is the best or the only view for the detection of a calcified right coronary artery. The left anterior oblique view at 20 to 30 degrees is the most suitable for localizing the bifurcation of the left coronary artery. In this view, the left coronary artery is brought into relief between the hilar shadow anteriorly and the spinal column posteriorly. A ringlike density is frequently seen in this view, representing the end-on image of the calcified anterior descending artery. The right anterior oblique angle is used to view the calcified left main coronary artery. If both the anterior descending and the circumflex branches are also calcified, a Y-shaped density may be seen. The calcified cardiac valves, the myocardium, and the pericardium are easily confirmed by fluoroscopy.[3]

Visualization of Subepicardial Fat Stripes

The subepicardial fat lines are an important landmark in the diagnosis of heart disease. The fat stripe is a cushionlike structure separating the myocardium from the pericardium. Normally it is difficult to see the fat line because of the adjacent similar radiolucency of the air-filled lung. The in-between hairline density of the normal pericardium is delicate and also difficult to see except in the left lateral view (Fig. 107-4*A*). In the presence of pericardial effusion or thickening, the subepicardial fat line is displaced interiorly and becomes more visible because of the added background of water density (Fig. 107-4*B*). The subepicardial fat pulsates with the contracting myocardium within the immobile band of pericardial fluid. This is diagnostic of pericardial effusion.[8] In contrast, when pericardial thickening alone is present, the exterior border of the heart will pulsate with the fat line. This in turn suggests the diagnosis of pericardial constriction.

Differentiation of Cardiac from Noncardiac Disease

When respiration is suspended, any structures that are moving are likely to be cardiovascular in nature. Conversely, noncardiac structures are immobile. This is exemplified by one bullet in the heart versus another in the chest wall. A pulmonary varix or an azygos vein will collapse on Valsalva maneuver, with exaggerated pulsation following release of the breath. Enlarged nodes in these areas, on the other hand, will not change with such a maneuver.

Evaluation of Valve Prostheses and Pacemakers

The normal movements of cardiac valve prostheses are parallel between the two phases of cardiac cycle. If a significant angle of tilt (more than 12) is formed between the two phases, instability of the valve with associated insufficiency is nearly almost always present[4,9] (Fig. 107-5).

FIGURE 107-5 Intercalative roentgenograms showing a normal and abnormal movement of the prosthetic valves. *A.* Intercalative roentgenogram showing a normally functioning mitral valve prosthesis. Note that the base of the valve in systole (white arrows) is parallel to that in diastole (black arrows). *B.* Intercalative roentgenogram showing a leaking aortic valve prosthesis. Note that the base of the valve in systole (white ring) is obviously unparallel to that in diastole (black ring). LA = left atrium; LV = left ventricle; DAO = descending aorta; D = diaphragm; SP = spine; LHB = left heart border. *(From J. T. T. Chen, H. D. McIntosh, M. P. Capp, et al., Intercalative Angiocardiography: A Method for Recording Cardiovascular Dynamics on a Single Film, Radiology, 93:499, 1969. Reproduced with permission from publisher and author.)*

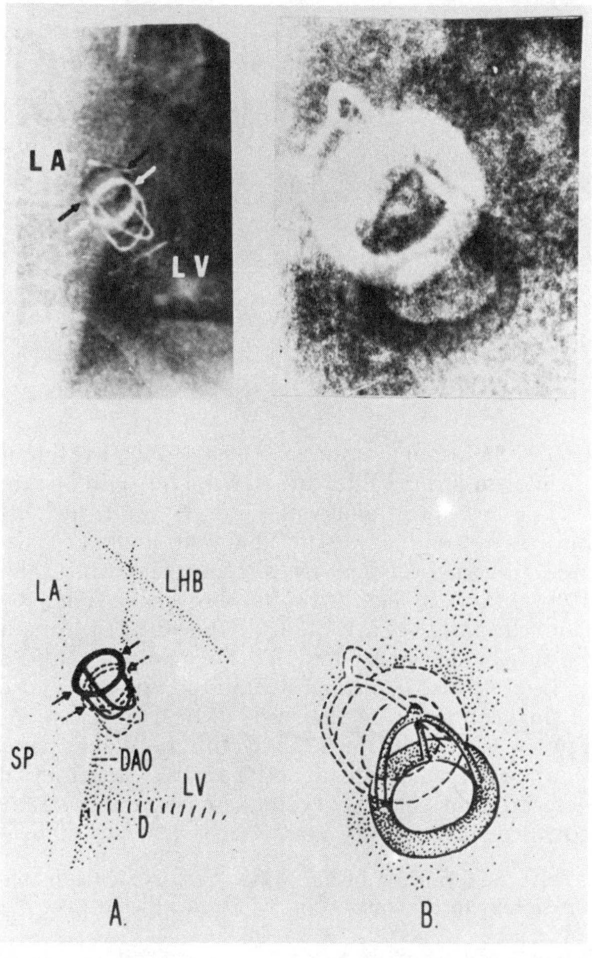

The position of the pacemaker can be promptly determined under the fluoroscope and recorded on the film.[10] The subepicardial fat line overlies the myocardium and underlies the pericardium. If the pacing catheter is found within the fat stripe it may have passed through the coronary sinus and entered one of the major cardiac veins. If the tip of the catheter is seen outside the fat stripe it may have perforated the myocardium and thus lies in the pericardium.[10] While the wires and electrodes of a transmediastinal pacemaker may look normal on the films, minor breakage can only be appreciated in ventricular systole by aid of fluoroscopy.[10]

References

1. Jefferson, K., and Rees, S. (eds.), "Clinical Cardiac Radiology," 2d ed., Butterworths, London, 1980.
2. Cooley, R. N.: "Radiology of the Heart and Great Vessels," 3d ed., Williams & Wilkins Company, Baltimore, 1978.
3. Chen, J. T. T.: Cardiac Fluoroscopy, in M. J. Kelley (ed.), "Symposium on Chest Radiography for the Cardiologist," *Cardiol. Clin. North Am.,* 1:565, 1983.
4. Chen, J. T. T., McIntosh, H. D., Capp, M. P., Morris, J. J., Canent, R. V., and Lester, R. G.: Intercalative Angiocardiography: A Method for Recording Cardiovascular Dynamics on a Single Film, *Radiology,* 83:499, 1969.
5. Chen, J. T. T., Robinson, A. E., Goodrich, J. K., and Lester, R. G.: Uneven Distribution of Pulmonary Blood Flow between Left and Right Lungs in Isolated Valvular Pulmonary Stenosis, *Am. J. Roentgenol.,* 107:343, 1969.
6. Chen, J. T. T., Lester, R. G., and Peter, R. H.: Posterior Wedging Sign of Mitral Insufficiency, *Radiology,* 113:451, 1974.
7. Bartel, A. G., Chen, J. T. T., Peter, R. H., Behar, V., Kong, Y., and Lester, R. G.: The Significance of Coronary Calcification Detected by Fluoroscopy. A Report of 360 Patients, *Circulation,* 49:1247, 1947.
8. Jorgens, J., Kundel, R., and Lieber, A.: The Cinefluorographic Approach to the Diagnosis of Pericardial Effusion, *Am. J. Roentgenol. Ther. Nucl. Med.,* 87:911, 1962.
9. Gimenez, J. L., Soulen, R. L., and Davila, J. C.: Prosthetic Valve Detachments; Its Roentgenographic Recognition. Report of Cases, *Am. J. Roentgenol.,* 103:595, July 1968.
10. Sorkin, R. P., Schuurmann, B. J., and Simon, A. B.: Radiographic Aspects of Permanent Cardiac Pacemakers, *Radiology,* 119:281, 1976.

108

Techniques of Cardiac Catheterization Including Coronary Arteriography

Robert H. Franch, M.D.
Spencer B. King III, M.D.
John S. Douglas, Jr., M.D.

A valuable suggestion may remain unexploited on the grounds of a preconceived opinion.

G. Liljestrand, 1956[1,*]

In 1929 Werner Forssman (1904–1979), a resident surgeon at Eberswalde, catheterized his right atrium from a left antecubital vein cutdown, utilizing self-fluoroscopy with a mirror. The position of the catheter tip was verified by a roentgenogram (Fig. 108–1).[2,3] The extensive use of the catheter by Cournand in the early 1940s in the study of human cardiovascular physiology led his group and those of Dexter, McMichael, and Bing to explore the use of this technique for the study of heart disease.[4] At Emory University in 1945 Brannon, Weens, and Warren described the hemodynamics of atrial septal defect in four patients.[5] From these beginnings steady advances in methods have occurred.[6–13] Catheterization has spread from the laboratory to the bedside, where it yields physiological data that guide treatment, and its use in balloon valvuloplasty or dilating arteries or, in other instances, closing them seems a promising therapeutic intervention.[14,15]

*At the awarding of the Nobel Prize in Medicine and Physiology to Forssman, Cournand, and Richards.

Preparations for Cardiac Catheterization

The patient should be in the hospital the afternoon prior to study. A relaxed meeting with the patient and the patient's family serves to lessen long-standing apprehension, to correct any misunderstanding, and to establish rapport. Since catheterization is frequently the first major step on the road to cardiac surgery, a tolerable experience now fosters an optimistic attitude in the patient and his or her family toward future events. The physician who is to do the catheterization should obtain the history, examine the patient, and review the current chest x-ray, electrocardiogram, echocardiogram, and past catheterization and surgical records and angiocardiograms. A clinical diagnosis is made and a catheterization protocol is designed to answer pertinent specific questions. The catheterization protocol may then be intelligently modified as various data become available during the procedure.

A patient's education booklet, *Your Cardiac Catheterization* (Fig. 108–2), has usually been read by the patient prior to securing informed consent. Anticoagulants are stopped and the prothrombin time is brought to less than 20 s before a percutaneous arterial catheterization. Breakfast is withheld for a morning procedure; for an afternoon procedure coffee or juice is permitted and lunch is withheld. In our experience prophylactic antibiotics are not necessary. General anesthesia is not used in our laboratory. A combination of 6.25 mg of promethaxine (Phenergan), 6.25 mg of chlorpromazine (Thorazine), and 25 mg of meperidine hydrochloride (Demerol) per milliliter of mixture provides excellent sedation.[16] The intramuscular dose for a child is 0.5 to 2.0 ml, depending on the age and weight, and is given 1 h before the procedure. The mixture is not given intravenously, nor is it given again after the initial loading dose. If additional sedation is required, small doses of intravenous Demerol or diazepam may be used. In the neonate, or in the very sick infant, no premedication is used. In the adult, diazepam (Valium) 2.5 to 10 mg is given intravenously. Subcutaneous 0.5 to 2 percent lidocaine (Xylocaine) is given, depending on the age of the patient. Occasionally, particularly in the adult, vagal slowing of the pulse, nausea, and perspiration are noted. Intravenous atropine is antidotal.

FIGURE 108-1 Forssman catheterized his own right atrium in 1929. This was the first documented catheterization of the right side of the heart: "Der Katheter reicht von der linken Vena cephalica herabkommend bis in die rechte Vorkammer." (*From W. Forssman: Die Sondierung des rechten Herzens, Berl. Klin. Wochenschr., 8:2085, 1929. Reproduced with permission from the publisher.*)

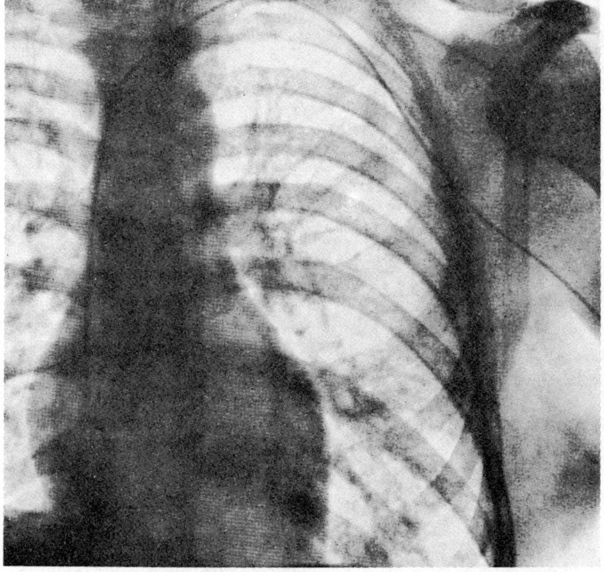

Patient Education Booklet (Contents)	Page
Definition and purpose	6–7
Admission to the hospital	8–9
Preparation for catherization	10
Cardiac catheterization lab	11–12
Catheter insertion	13
Injection of dye	14–15
After catheterization	16–19
Leg artery	16–17
Arm artery	18
General precautions and information	19
Getting out of bed	20
Results of catheterization	21
Going home	22
Recommendations for treatment	22
Medications	23
Activities	24–25
Surgery	26
Angioplasty	27–28
Appendix (other diagnostic tests)	
EKG (electrocardiogram)	30
Treadmill or stress test	31–32
Echo (echocardiogram)	33
Nuclear scanning	34–35

FIGURE 108-2 Table of contents of the patient's education booklet used at Emory University Hospital prior to cardiac catheterization. [*From Cardiac Catheterization (and other Cardiac Diagnostic Tests and Radiological Procedures), Pritchett & Hull Associates, Inc., Atlanta, Georgia, 1982. A booklet for patient education. Reproduced with permission from the publisher and authors.*]

It is desirable that the laboratory be involved daily in diagnostic work. General efficiency is increased, costly equipment and space are utilized, and, most important, all personnel become confident and knowledgeable with experience. Certainly the most important ingredient in the laboratory is the thoroughly experienced technical-professional team. The procedure must move briskly. No data should be obtained until pulse, respiration, and blood pressure are completely stable. The primary objective is to make an accurate diagnosis at one sitting, with the least possible risk and discomfort to the patient.

Outpatient left heart and coronary artery studies require careful selection of patients and an experienced support team.[17]

Techniques

Catheterization of the Right Side of the Heart

Percutaneous Venous

Percutaneous femoral or median cubital vein catheterization usually permits reuse of the vein.[18] To extend the range of the percutaneous technique, a thin tubular polyester sheath is advanced over a short introducer catheter into the lumen of the vein (Fig. 108–3). This temporary conduit may then be used

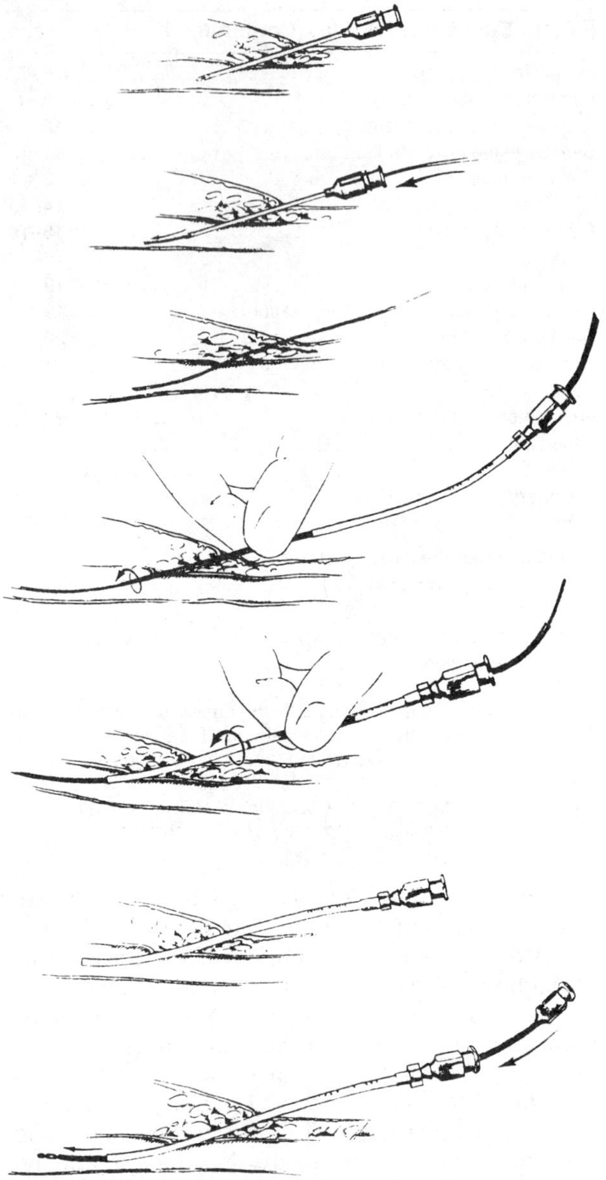

FIGURE 108-3 Percutaneous sheath catheterization of the femoral vein is illustrated. Following venous puncture, a spring guide wire is introduced into the vein. The needle is withdrawn, leaving the guide in the vein. A Teflon dilator–venous sheath assembly is advanced in a rotary motion over the guide into the vein. The Teflon dilator and the guide wire are removed, leaving the flexible sheath in the vein. Various types of catheters, including closed-tip side-hole catheters, can now be inserted using the sheath as a conduit. (*Courtesy of Drs. W. H. Neches and C. E. Mullins.*)

to introduce a variety of closed-tip catheters.[19] Two catheters can be inserted through a single femoral vein puncture site by initially placing two guide wires through the femoral vein sheath; the maneuver is repeated to insert an additional catheter.[20] If the hepatic portion of the inferior vena cava is absent, the azygos vein channels the catheter tip into the right superior vena cava and thence into the right atrium (Fig. 108–4). In order to cross the tricuspid valve, bending or looping the catheter tip against the right atrial wall may be required. If atrial ectopy occurs, the catheter tip can be looped in a hepatic vein and then advanced into the right atrium. A balloon-tipped catheter produces little ectopy since the advancing force is distributed over the surface of the balloon. The internal jugular vein or the subclavian vein may also be used to insert a balloon catheter percutaneously.

Venous Cutdown

If, in the older child or adult, the cutdown approach is necessary, the right basilic or median cubital vein is preferred. In the infant, the saphenous vein or the superficial femoral vein distal to its junction with a deep femoral vein is used. If a common femoral vein cutdown is used, temporary coldness, blueness, and edema of the leg may follow complete interruption of this vein. Superficial radial, ulnar, or accessory brachial arteries may be initially mistaken for veins. If the superficial veins are small, the venae comitantes of the brachial artery may be used. From the left arm, the catheter tip may enter a persistent left superior vena cava, exiting via the coronary sinus into the right atrium in an awkward position for entering the right ventricle. A deep inspiration will often enable the catheter tip to pass the subclavian vein–brachiocephalic vein junction. The seating of a conventional catheter tip in the pulmonary artery wedge position may be difficult if severe pulmonary artery hypertension or if extreme enlargement of the right side of the heart is present. A flow-directed balloon catheter may then be used. Clues to inadvertent coronary sinus catheterizations are (1) the acute angle that the catheter shaft makes as it enters the coronary sinus, especially in the right anterior oblique position; (2) the marked desaturation of

FIGURE 108-4 Selective opacification of the azygos vein. If the hepatic portion of the inferior vena cava is absent, the catheter tip enters the right atrium superiorly via the azygos vein.

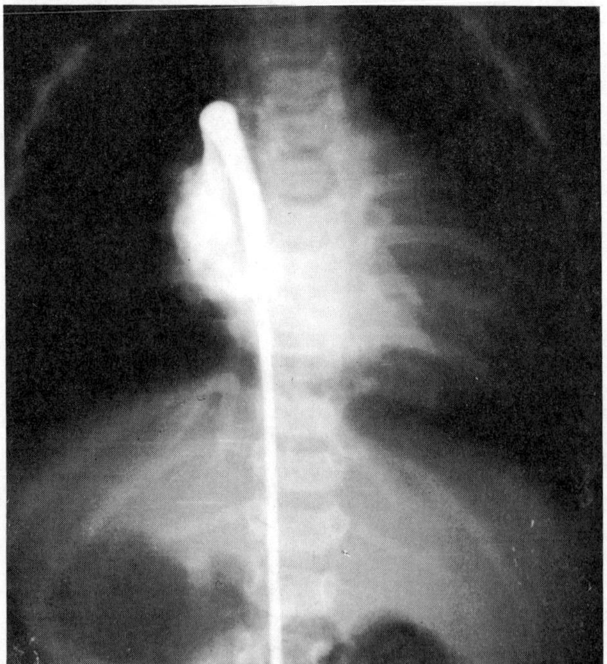

coronary sinus blood; and (3) the posterior position of the catheter.

In order to enter the pulmonary artery in patients with transposition of the great arteries and intact ventricular septum, a balloon catheter is passed across the inevitably present interatrial communication to the left atrium and then superiorly looped in the left ventricular outflow tract from which it enters the pulmonary artery readily. In the postsurgical patient with pulmonary valve atresia the pulmonary artery may also be entered via a subclavian (Blalock) or aorticopulmonary (Waterston) or Potts' shunt.

Catheterization of the Left Side of the Heart

Percutaneous Technique

In 1953, Sven Ivar Seldinger of the Department of Radiology of the Karolinska Sjurhuset described the use of a flexible metal leader to introduce a polyethylene tube into the artery. The Seldinger technique is commonly used in the femoral and less often in the axillary or brachial arteries in carrying out catheterization of the left side of the heart. The puncture site for the femoral artery is 3 cm below the midinguinal point, where the femoral artery is compressible against the head of the femur. In the obese patient the groin crease may be below the inguinal ligament; too high a puncture is more likely to occur in the thin patient. External rotation of the leg and slight adduction helps fixate the artery. The artery is punctured at a 45° angle transfixing the anterior and posterior wall. The guide wire is inserted only when the needle spurt is maximal. Resistance to insertion usually means an intramural or extravascular position of the needle or entry into a side branch artery by the guide. The catheter is inserted into the artery over the guide wire, or a sheath assembly may be used, facilitating catheter introduction in the very obese patient or if scar tissue is superficial to the artery (Fig. 108–5). The catheter sheath reduces bleeding during manipulation and reduces discomfort during catheter changes.[20,21] An arterial pressure may be monitored through a side port in the sheath. The guide tip is kept at the level of the diaphragm, and the catheter is advanced to this level. The catheter is aspirated and then flushed with heparinized saline solution. Occasionally, small particles of plaque material may be found in the aspirate. On catheter pullout, aspirate vigorously and permit a single spurt. The femoral and foot pulses are palpated prior to withdrawal. The artery is compressed manually for 10 to 15 min, maintaining normal ankle pulses. The brachial artery is punctured with an 18-gauge needle and a no. 7 French 80-cm multipurpose catheter is advanced to the ascending aorta over an 0.032-in J-guide. Five thousand units of heparin is then given. A sheath is not routinely used nor is protamine given. An arm board is applied for 6 h. One significant complication occurred in 70 procedures: A woman required thrombectomy after inadvertent catheterization of an aberrant ulnar artery. Simultaneous puncture of the brachial vein overlying the artery may result in an arteriovenous fistula.

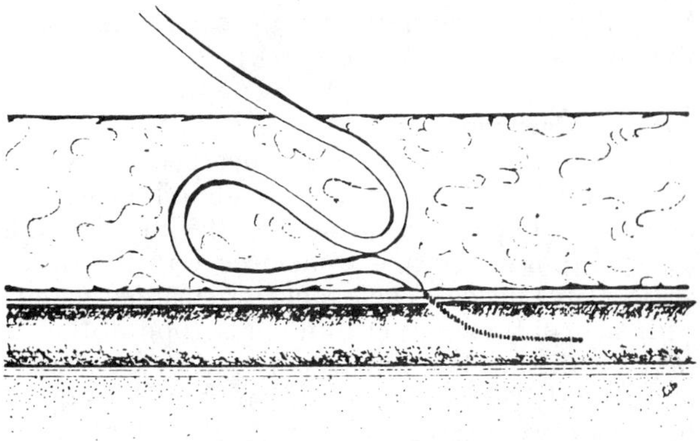

CATHETER CURLS IN THE SOFT TISSUE

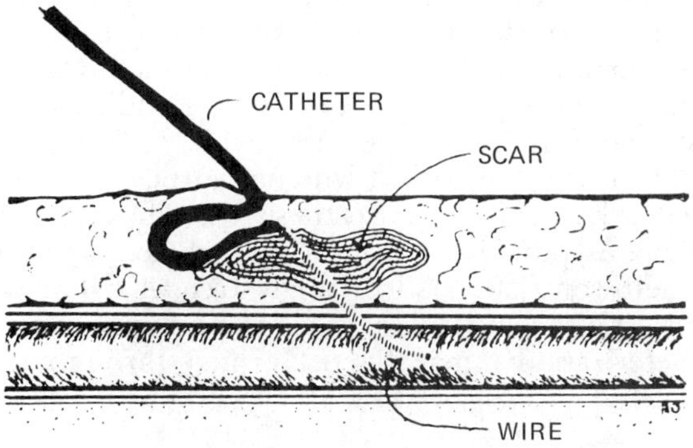

CATHETER TIP CURLS SUPERFICIAL TO THE SCAR

FIGURE 108-5 Occasionally the catheter tip will not follow the guide wire into the femoral artery in the obese patient or in the case of an overlying scar. A larger-caliber guide wire or a sheath dilation assembly should be used. *(From S. Swamy, L. I. Segal, and S. Mouli, "Percutaneous Angiography," Charles C Thomas, Publisher, Springfield, Illinois, 1977. Reproduced with permission from Charles C Thomas, Springfield, Illinois, editor, and author.)*

Percutaneous left heart catheterization via an aortofemoral synthetic bypass graft has been surprisingly free of complications. Potential hazards include disruption of the pseudointima with subsequent thrombosis, infection, or separation of the catheter on withdrawal if a thin-walled no. 5 French catheter unsupported by a guide wire is used. The normal aortic valve is easily crossed retrogradely with the catheter tip. Even in aortic valve stenosis the left ventricle is entered in nearly all cases. By slowly withdrawing the catheter tip from its looped position in the left aortic sinus, wall-to-wall exploration of the severely stenotic valve is possible. A straight guide wire may enhance this maneuver.

Left and right Judkins, left Amplatz, and pigtail catheters with a 145° bend 7 cm from the tip have all been used to center the guide wire in the aortic root for more effective probing of the stenotic orifice.[22]

In cases with both femoral and axillary artery disease, selective coronary arteriography has been performed via a translumbar approach utilizing a sheath.[23]

Arterial Cutdown
The cutdown technique for left heart study usually utilizes the brachial artery. After administering 100 units/kg of heparin intravenously, the anterior wall of the exposed artery is punctured with the tip of an 18-gauge needle. The opening is enlarged slightly with a small forceps, permitting insertion of the tapered catheter. The arteriotomy is closed by either a previously placed, very small purse string loop or by one or two interrupted sutures. If brisk bleeding does not occur from both proximal and distal artery segments, thrombectomy is performed with a balloon catheter. Rarely, the right subclavian artery will rise aberrantly as the last root vessel of a left aortic arch, precluding easy access to the ascending aorta from the right brachial artery.

In the selected patient who has aortic and mitral valve disk or ball-valve prosthesis, a brief direct percutaneous puncture through the palpable apex of the left ventricle is surprisingly free of complications. Left ventricular angiography and aortic catheterization[24] may be performed through the cannula.

Transseptal Approach Transseptal catheterization may be used to enter the left atrium. From the right femoral vein, percutaneously, a long needle with a curved tip is advanced through a thin-walled catheter in a posteromedial direction so as to puncture the lower third of the atrial septum or preferably higher, beneath the ledge of the limbus fossae ovalis. Biplane fluoroscopy, a catheter in the aortic root, and knowledge of the size and position of the left atrium following pulmonary artery angiography may be helpful in positioning the transseptal needle. The left atrial pressure is checked, and a blood sample is obtained. The catheter tip is advanced with the needle until it is free in the left atrium. The needle is withdrawn, and the footward-curved catheter tip may be advanced across the mitral valve into the left ventricle. The left atrium is difficult to enter if there is deformity of the thoracic or lumbar spine or if there is a very large right atrium. Other relative contraindications to transseptal catheterization included marked dilatation of the aortic root, myxoma of the left atrium, and a history of recent systemic artery embolization. A long Teflon sheath may be placed in the left atrium over a dilator catheter.[25] This permits various closed-tipped catheters to be passed into the left ventricle or a carbon-dioxide-filled balloon catheter to be passed from the left atrium to the left ventricle to the ascending aorta.[26,27] Occasionally the portion of the right atrial septum lying within the fossa ovalis can be punctured by the needle-stiffened catheter alone. Retrograde catheterization of the left atrium from the left ventricle was reported to be successful in 84 percent of cases with dominant mitral stenosis, and in 97 percent of cases of mitral regurgitation.[28] The tapered flexible catheter forms a clockwise loop in the left ventricle as it passes to the left atrium. The patient is in a 25° right anterior oblique position. A no. 8 French pigtail catheter has been similarly used.[29]

Equipment

Catheters
Disposable, single-use catheters in a wide range of sizes, shapes, and lengths with end and/or side holes are available for diagnostic use. The ideal nonpreformed catheter is soft enough to permit bending as required, has memory to hold its shape, and has enough strength or body to permit the curve of the tip to be advanced intact. Torque control is improved by incorporating a thin wire braid in the walls. Torque is damped by a tortuous artery, so that the response of the tip may even be reversed. Preformed catheters are made to serve a specific function with a minimum of manipulation. Catheters should have smooth, regular surfaces to reduce thrombogenicity. Atrial septostomy with a fluid-filled balloon catheter or with a controlled folding surgical blade at the catheter tip[30] improves shunting and increases systemic arterial saturation in patients with transposition of the great arteries. A precompressed ivalon plug inserted by catheter has been used to close the patent ductus arteriosus. Loop-snare catheters are used for nonthoracotomy retrieval of intraluminal cardiovascular foreign bodies.[31] A catheter-tip electromagnetic probe is used to measure blood flow velocity.[32] Stroke volume is derived utilizing the diameter of the aorta, angiographically determined.

A 1.8-mm-diameter intravascular fiberoptic scope inserted either directly in the operating room or via a no. 10 French guiding catheter is under trial as a tool for visualizing the coronary arteries and heart valves.[33] Small no. 5 French preformed "shepherd's crook" coronary artery ostial seeking catheters have been designed for pediatric use.[34] A silica fiber in the lumen of a cardiac catheter may become clinically useful in transmitting laser energy to reduce the size of an arterial plaque or to decrease valvular stenosis.[35]

Used in treating valvular pulmonic stenosis[36,37] and coarctation of the aorta,[38] pulmonary valvuloplasty and aortic angioplasty balloons up to 4 cm long with inflation diameter up to 20 mm are made of high tensile strength polyethylene. Inflation to 3 to 4 atm with a 20-ml plastic syringe is usual. The lumen between the no. 8 or 9 French catheter and the balloon is large, permitting deflation in less than 7 s, decreating the occlusion time.[39]

Endomyocardial bioptome catheters acquire a 1-to-3-mm specimen of ventricular muscle for light and electron microscopy, biochemical and immunofluorescent studies, and for viral culture.[40] These studies are clinically useful in detecting cardiac allograft rejection and antineoplastic drug cardiotoxicity and in assessing the presence, activity, and occasionally the etiology of myocardial diseases.[41]

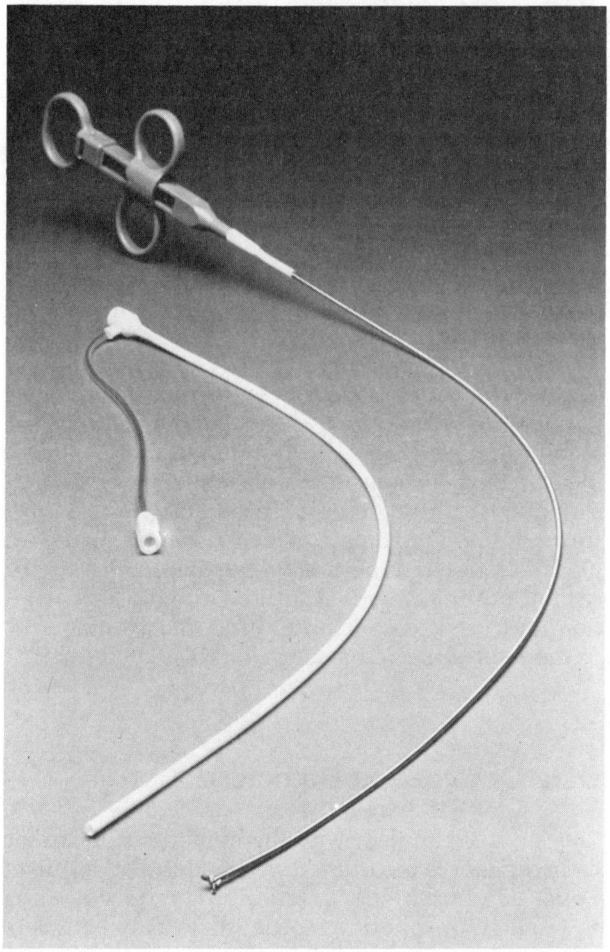

A

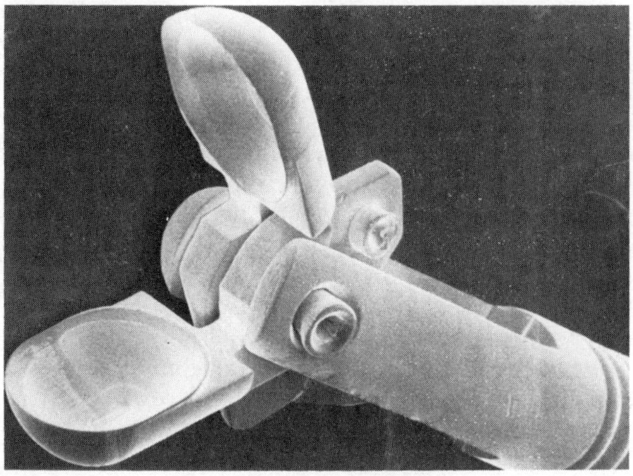

B

FIGURE 108-6 *A.* Photograph of the 98-cm long, radiopaque polyethylene guiding sheath and the 104-cm long, no. 6 French bioptome instrument used for endomyocardial ventricular biopsy via the femoral approach. *B.* Scanning electron microscopic photograph of the stainless steel cutting jaws at the tip of the disposable endomycardial bioptome shown in *A.* (*Reproduced with permission from the Cordis Corporation.*)

Contraindications to the procedure include bleeding disorders, mural thrombus, and anticoagulant therapy. Biopsy specimens should be properly received and processed; skilled microscopic interpretation is mandatory. The right ventricle is more commonly biopsied. The Stanford technique uses a short no. 9 French introducer sheath placed in the right internal jugular vein through which a 50-cm, no. 9 French bioptome with one fixed and one movable jaw is directed across the tricuspid valve in order to obtain three to five samples from the apical portion of the interventricular septum of the right ventricle.[42] No deaths have occurred in over 5000 biopsies; the morbidity is less than 1 percent. Six cases of hemopericardium were treated by pericardiocentesis and/or surgery. In a Mayo study of 114 right ventricular biopsies, three cases of ventricular tachycardia occurred, one of whom required cardioversion.[43] Right ventricular biopsy has been performed in infants 3 to 20 months of age.[44]

At Emory University Hospital left ventricular biopsy is performed via the femoral artery using a long sheath introduced into the left ventricle over a pigtail catheter.[45] A disposable no. 6 French bioptome catheter with two movable jaws at the tip is used (Figs. 108–6*A* and *B*). The final advance beyond the sheath to the septal wall of the apical portion of the left ventricle is made with the jaws open to lessen the chance of ventricular perforation. Fluoroscopy in two planes is used; the posterobasal left ventricle is avoided as a biopsy site. No embolism, arrhythmia, or perforation have been noted in 20 cases.

Radiation Exposure

A qualified radiologic physicist should check the catheterization facilities, and secondary or scattered radiation should be minimized. Radiation intensity varies inversely as the distance, i.e., if the distance to the source is doubled the amount of radiation will only be one-quarter as much. One should select the smallest possible collimation and keep the image intensifier as close to the patient as possible. The U-arm position that places the x-ray tube to the examiner's side of the table causes the greatest exposure as a result of scattered radiation from the patient. Two film badges should be worn, one at the belt beneath the 0.5-mm equivalent lead apron and the other at the collar level outside the apron. The eyes, gonads, and red bone marrow have a whole-body limit of 5 rem (roentgen equivalent man) per year; any specific organ, such as the thyroid or skin, has a yearly limit of 15 rem. Lead glass spectacles, a thyroid collar, and a floating or preferably a floor-length screen provide adequate shielding to the operator.[46] If possible, women of childbearing age should have studies done within 10 days after the onset of menstruation.

Pressure-Recording System

If the heart rate is 60 beats per minute, the frequency of the basic wave is 1 per second. The first 10 harmonic components of the pressure wave occur up to a rate of 10 Hz and are important to detect

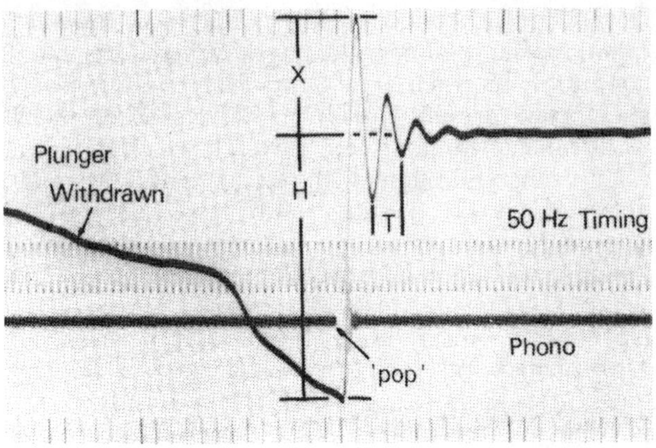

FIGURE 108-7 In order to measure the frequency response of a catheter transducer system, an abrupt transient input pressure is applied to the catheter tip (a plunger is pulled free of an air-filled syringe); the pressure oscillations are recorded at a fast paper speed and measured. X = height of the initial overshoot; H = end height of the recorded deflection; T = period of free oscillation, 0.08 s. The natural frequency is 13 Hz; the useful range, 4 Hz. If this underdamped system is optimally damped by the addition of a narrow-bore tube between catheter and transducer, X/H is reduced to 0.06 and the useful frequency range is increased to 12.5 Hz. (*Reproduced with permission of Irex Corporation.*)

without phase lag or amplitude distortion since they contribute to the steeply rising or falling parts of the pressure curve. A properly responding pressure-recording system should have a high natural frequency and optimal damping. A high natural frequency is obtained by using a bubble-free, saline solution–filled system of minimum length, whose catheter and connector tubings have stiff walls and wide bores. This system requires that a damping needle or tube be placed between the catheter and the transducer so that a uniform frequency response (i.e., input = output ± 5 percent) is extended as close to the natural frequency as possible. The frequency response of the system is tested in vitro by a square wave pressure input to the catheter tip created by a plunger pulled from a syringe (Fig. 108-7) or a flame-popped balloon or from a sine wave pressure generator. A 5 to 7 percent overshoot in the square waveform is optimal. This means that frequencies below the natural or resonant frequency will be properly recorded. For clinical cardiac catheterization a manometer system with a uniform dynamic response up to 6 to 10 Hz is adequate.

An additional limiting factor in pressure recording is the superimposition of artifacts on the pressure pulse by the accelerating and decelerating movements imparted to the fluid-filled cardiac catheter by the beating heart. Distortion of the catheter-obtained phasic pressure waveform by motion artifact is avoided by the use of a catheter-tip, side-mounted, ultraminiature, semiconductor gauge.

Oxygen Analysis

The total oxygen content of the blood may be determined by the classical Van Slyke manometric technique, or, more rapidly, by gas chromatography, mass spectrometry, or by a detection cell that generates an electric current proportional to the oxygen absorbed. Direct oximetry of unhemolyzed, undiluted blood by flow through cuvettes connected directly to the catheter avoids blood loss. Small samples of blood from a syringe may also be analyzed in these cuvettes, or by a membrane electrode, or after hemolysis, by a precision spectrophotometer. A fiberoptic reflection oximeter catheter permits intracardiac oxygen saturation measurements without withdrawal of blood.[47]

Analysis of expired air for oxygen and carbon dioxide may be made by extraction techniques, paramagnetic analyzers, closed-circuit methods, or membrane electrodes.[48] In infants and children, ideally, oxygen consumption should be measured continuously throughout the procedure using a flow-through hood technique. The atrioventricular (AV) O_2 difference and thermal or dye dilution values for cardiac output can be substituted into the Fick equation and used to check the direct measurement of oxygen consumption against the calculated one.

Data Obtained at Catheterization

One must be familiar with the limitations of cardiac catheterization in order to avoid mistakes in diagnosis. There may be technical errors in obtaining the data, or properly recorded data may be misinterpreted or may not be specific.

Pressure Measurements

High-fidelity phasic pressure curves are usually not obtained from the ventricles or great arteries by conventional recording systems. The underdamped curve gives falsely high systolic and falsely low diastolic readings, and the overdamped curve has a smooth shape with disappearance of the incisura. The shape of the ventricular or great artery pressure trace is occasionally of diagnostic aid. An abrupt fall in pressure in early diastole (early diastolic dip) followed by a sudden rise to a high end-diastolic pressure plateau occurs in abnormal compliance states such as constrictive pericarditis and restrictive cardiomyopathy. In isolated pulmonic stenosis the configuration of the right ventricular pressure curve is frequently peaked or triangular, but it is trapezoidal if a large ventricular septal defect is associated with the pulmonic stenosis.

In valvular pulmonic stenosis, the pulse pressure is frequently greater in the left pulmonary artery than in the right pulmonary artery because flow is preferentially directed into the left pulmonary artery and kinetic energy is translated into lateral pressure. In bilateral branch pulmonary artery stenosis, the proximal main pulmonary artery shows a wide pulse pressure with a low dicrotic notch (Fig.

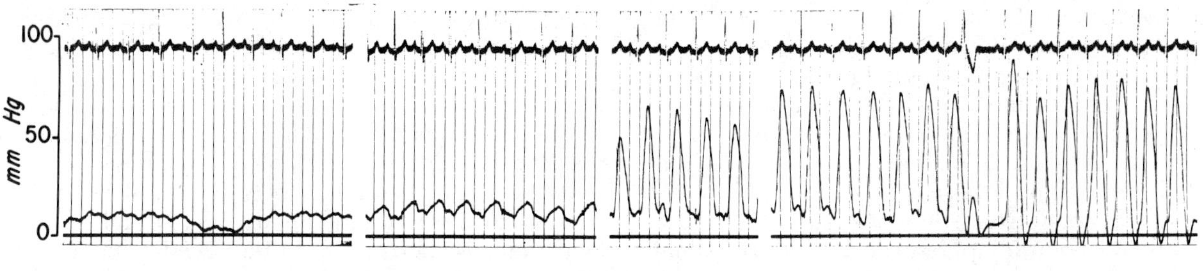

FIGURE 108-8 Pressure record in multiple congenital stenosis of the right and left pulmonary artery branches, illustrating a systolic pressure differential between the distal, proximal, and main pulmonary artery. There are systolic hypertension and a wide pulse pressure in the proximal right and main pulmonary arteries, related to a reduction in the capacity of the pulmonary artery compression chamber.

108–8). In supravalvular aortic stenosis, the coanda effect makes the right brachial and right carotid artery peak pressures greater than those on the left. A giant A wave in the right atrium is characteristic of valvular pulmonic stenosis but not of tetralogy of Fallot. A large atrial V wave, when present, is indicative of significant mitral or tricuspid regurgitation.

Left ventricular end-diastolic pressure (LVEDP) is recorded on a high-sensitivity scale, and is measured where the downslope of the A wave in the left ventricle coincides with the initial upstroke of the left ventricular pressure. LVEDP may be measured at the peak of the R wave of the ECG. An elevated LVEDP reflects an alteration in the ventricular pressure-volume relation or a decrease in diastolic compliance of the ventricle. An increased LVEDP occurs commonly with a dilated failing left ventricle, but may also be noted in the small ventricular cavity with thick walls or in the normal-size left ventricular cavity during an acute ischemic attack.

In order to measure the maximal rate of rise of left ventricular pressure, or peak *dP/dt*, a high-fidelity pressure record is needed, obtained ideally via a catheter-tip transducer (Fig. 108–9).[49] This value is influenced by preload and muscle hypertrophy in addition to the contractile state. Another preejection period index, V_{ce}, is the instantaneous velocity of shortening of contractile elements in muscle lengths per second.

$$V_{ce} = \frac{(dP/dt)}{KP}$$

V_{ce} may be plotted with the aid of a computer as a function of P, the developed left ventricular pressure at various points during isovolumic systole. This relation is relatively insensitive to changes in preload or afterload. Deviations from the control state during inotropic interventions may be monitored and changes in the left ventricular contractility before and after aortic valve surgery documented.[50] In daily practice, however, ejection phase indexes derived from the conventional left ventricular angiogram are used to assess left ventricular function.[51] The ejection fraction is commonly employed as an index of ventricular contractility but is sensitive to changes in preload and afterload as well.

A satisfactory pulmonary artery wedge pressure provides a good estimate of left atrial mean pressure. Some change in waveform and phase shift (0.06-s time delay) occurs in the transmitted signal when compared with the direct left atrial pressure record. Pulmonary artery diastolic pressure measured from a properly recorded curve provides an indirect estimate of mean left atrial pressure if the pulmonary vascular resistance is normal. Pulmonary vein wedge pressure does not give an accurate estimate of the pulmonary artery pressure in the presence of pulmonary artery hypertension.

Pressure recording permits measurement of either the peak or the mean pressure differential across a stenotic semilunar or AV valve or a segmentally narrowed blood vessel. If possible, simultaneous pressure recordings across a valve should be obtained, especially if there is atrial fibrillation. If the pulmonary artery wedge is used as an estimate of left atrial mean pressure, the waveform and amplitude should be confirmed at a second site. The error in assessing the mitral valve area in mitral stenosis may be large when the measured pressure differential is

FIGURE 108-9 Left ventricular high-fidelity pressure tracing and corresponding rate of force development (*dP/dt*) and velocity of shortening of the contractile elements (V_{ce}) in a patient with normal left ventricular function. AoP = aortic pressure; LVP = left ventricular pressure; *dP/dt* = first derivative of LVP; ECG = electrocardiogram; ML = muscle lengths; V_{CE} = instantaneous velocity of shortening of contractile elements in muscle lengths per second. *(From H. A. Krayenbuehl, O. M. Hess, and J. Turina, Assessment of Left Ventricular Function, J. Cardiovasc. Med., 3:883, 1978. Reproduced with permission from the publisher and author.)*

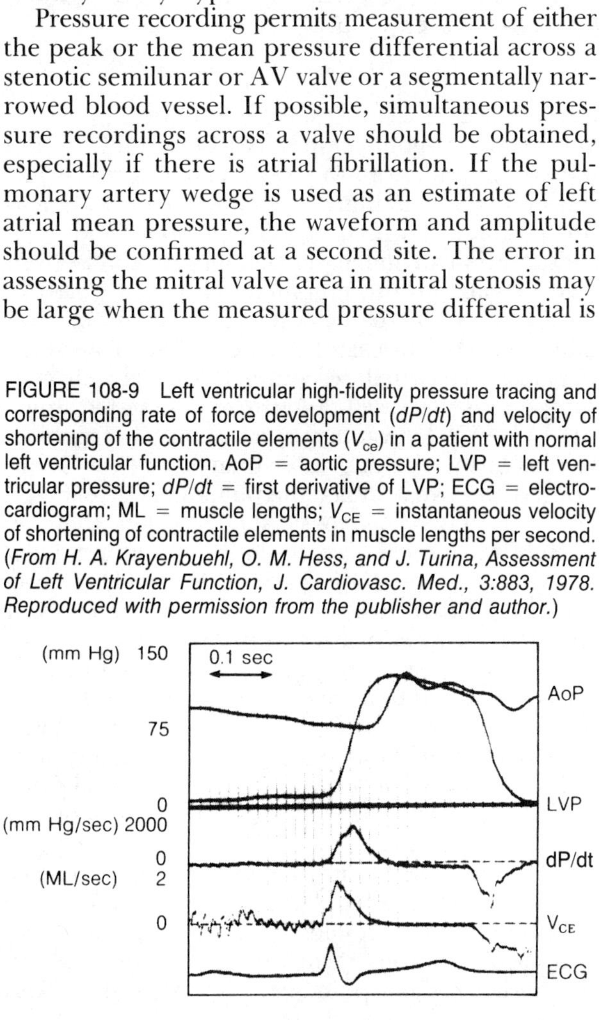

small. Because of the slow fall of the y descent in the wedge position, the mitral valve gradient may be overestimated by 3 to 4 mmHg when compared to the gradient obtained with a direct left atrial pressure.[52] A pullback record across a semilunar valve performed with a catheter having multiple paired side holes may show a false zone of composite ventricular and great artery pulses resulting from the simultaneous recorded pressures through proximal and distal side holes. Occasionally a gradient may be overlooked if the catheter tip cannot be advanced well into the ventricle so that it washes into the aorta in systole and falls into the left ventricle diastole. In a case of proximal infundibular pulmonic stenosis, if the pullback is at the cranial aspect of the tricuspid valve, the catheter may fall back into the right atrium from the right ventricular outflow tract quickly, missing the gradient.

Left ventricular cavity obliteration with catheter entrapment may result in spurious pressure gradient. To detect an intraventricular gradient the left ventricular pressure should be checked in the inflow and outflow, i.e., submitral and subaortic, positions simultaneously and in the apical versus the inflow or outflow positions simultaneously. These recordings enable one to detect the delay in fall of left ventricular systolic pressure that may occur when the catheter is entrapped.[53]

Interventions during Catheterization

Our bicycle ergometer handles loads of 0 to 450 watts (W) in steps of 5 W; the level of effort remains constant by maintaining a monitor pointer at a neutral position. The regression equation for oxygen consumption in milliliters per minute for a given load in watts on this ergometer is: $V_{O_2} = 13.16$ W + 254 ml. An increase in cardiac output of 0.6 liter/min or greater for each 100 ml of oxygen consumed presumes a normal response. If the oxygen consumption is increased 200 to 250 ml/min by supine use of a bicycle ergometer, an increase of arteriovenous difference of greater than 30 ml/liter is considered abnormal. When the pulmonary artery oxygen saturation falls to substantially less than 30 percent during exercise, the upper limit of circulatory stress is being approached. Normally, during exercise LVEDP falls and stroke work increases; if left ventricular performance is impaired, LVEDP rises and stroke work rises; and in severe dysfunction, stroke work fails to increase as an increase in LVEDP occurs. Isometric handgrip exercise increased heart rate, systemic mean pressure, and cardiac output. A fall in left ventricular stroke work and a sharp rise in LVEDP during the grip test indicate poor left ventricular reserve.

All patients with mitral stenosis who have normal or mildly increased pulmonary artery and wedge pressures at rest should have the mitral gradient and cardiac output rechecked during exercise. In the normal patient pulmonary artery pressure with exercise rises minimally, usually no higher than 25 mmHg mean. In a patient with a repaired ventricular septal defect and residual pulmonary vascular disease, the pulmonary artery pressure may be at the upper limits of normal or slightly increased at rest but may double with low-level exercise.

Rapid atrial pacing may be used as a stress intervention. In normal individuals, LVEDP falls as the heart rate is increased. If the paced patient with coronary artery disease is unable to meet the increased myocardial oxygen demands, the LVEDP rises in the early postpacing period and excess lactate is noted in coronary sinus blood. In patients with tetralogy of Fallot atrial pacing produces a drop in arterial oxygen saturation and an increase in right-to-left shunting by increasing dynamic right ventricular outflow tract obstruction.

In hypertrophic subaortic stenosis, isoproterenol, amyl nitrite, exercise, tilting, and the Valsalva maneuver intensify or provoke a systolic pressure differential; a purely vasopressor amine, angiotensin, ameliorates it and may reduce associated mitral regurgitation.

Blood Oxygen Measurements

An oxygen content step-up in the chambers of the right side of the heart in excess of the normal variation in oxygen content on serial sampling is used as evidence of a left-to-right shunt (Fig. 108–10). Thus an oxygen step-up from superior vena cava (SVC) to right atrium in excess of 1.9 volume per-

FIGURE 108-10 Sites of blood sampling during catheterization of the right side of the heart. Catheter introduced from the left basilic vein into the right pulmonary artery. INN. V = innominate vein (brachiocephalic vein); SVC = superior venae cavae; HRA, MRA, LRA = high, mid-, and low right atria; RVI, RVO = right ventricular inflow and outflow tracts; TV, PV = tricuspid and pulmonary valves; MPA, RPA = main and right pulmonary arteries; PAWP = pulmonary artery wedge position.

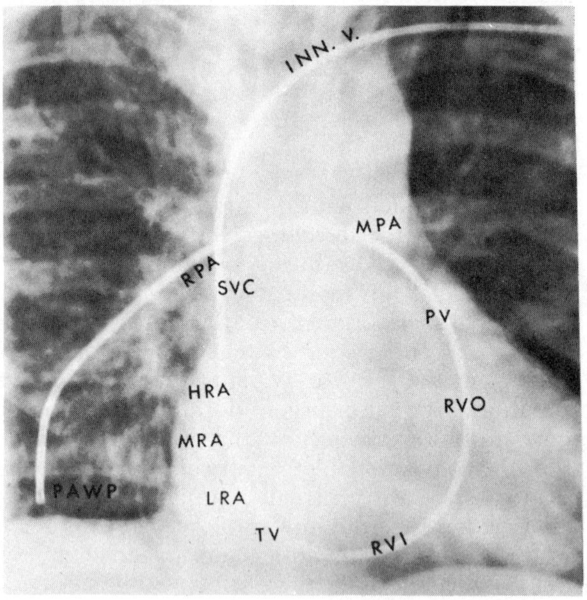

cent indicates shunting into the right atrium; a step-up from right atrium to right ventricle of 0.9 volume percent or greater and a step-up from the right ventricle to the pulmonary artery of 0.5 volume percent or greater indicates a left-to-right shunt at the right ventricular and pulmonary artery level, respectively. By these criteria, false-positive results are rare, but false-negative results occur in patients with small shunts. In the anemic or polycythemic patient, the detection of shunting is best reflected by the step-up in percent oxygen saturation rather than the step-up in volume percent, since the latter is dependent on the hemoglobin concentration.[54,55]

Studies show that sensitivity in detecting left-to-right shunts is improved if numerous serial blood samples are withdrawn in rapid succession for oximetry. If two sets of interrupted samples are taken from the superior vena cava, right atrium, right ventricle, and pulmonary artery, then a 9 percent saturation increase indicates an atrial shunt; 5 percent saturation increase, a ventricular shunt; and 3 percent saturation increase, a pulmonary artery shunt. Sensitivity can be improved if blood samples are obtained in multiple pairs in a rapid serial sweep without flushing with saline solution between samples. The rise in oxygen saturation step-up for a given left-to-right shunt is related to the saturation of mixed venous blood (MVB). For example, if the MVB is 84 percent, a 5 percent step-up represents a 2:1 shunt; if MVB is 75 percent, a 10 percent step-up is needed; if the MVB is 65 percent, a 15 percent step-up indicates a 2:1 shunt. The results of the blood oxygen analysis should be reviewed before the catheterization is completed. Left-to-right shunts less than 20 percent of pulmonary flow are not detectable by oximetry. Since no oximetric criteria exist for exclusion of a shunt, selective angiography and/or the use of hydrogen electrode provide maximal sensitivity and reliability in excluding small shunts. The presence of an increased oxygen step-up in the right side of the heart should be closely correlated with angiographic findings.

Catheter Position

The catheter position may be useful in identifying the anatomic location of an intracardiac defect (Fig. 108–11). In crossing a membranous ventricular septal defect in the anteroposterior view the catheter passes from the arm into the ascending aorta from the right ventricle in a hairpin loop and enters the pulmonary artery from the right ventricle in a wider U loop (Fig. 108–12). A patent ductus arteriosus is frequently entered as the tip of the catheter points to the "roof" of the junction of the main and left pulmonary arteries. Failing direct catheter passage, a flexible-spring guide wire, introduced while the venous catheter tip rests in the main pulmonary artery, readily passes through the ductus into the descending aorta; in aorticopulmonary septal defect

FIGURE 108-11 *A.* The catheter tip passes from the right superior vena cava to the right atrium, thence to the coronary sinus, thence to the left superior vena cava. *B.* The catheter tip passes from the left superior vena cava to an anomalous left upper lobe pulmonary vein.

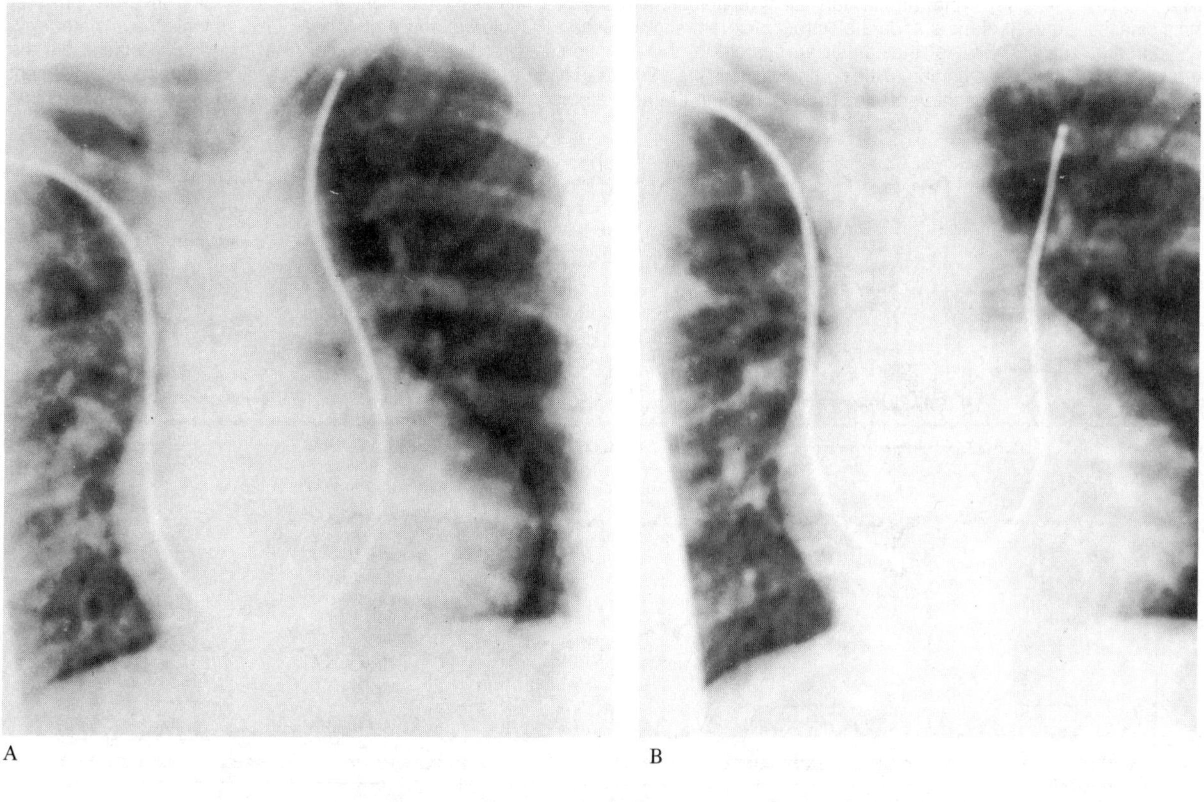

A B

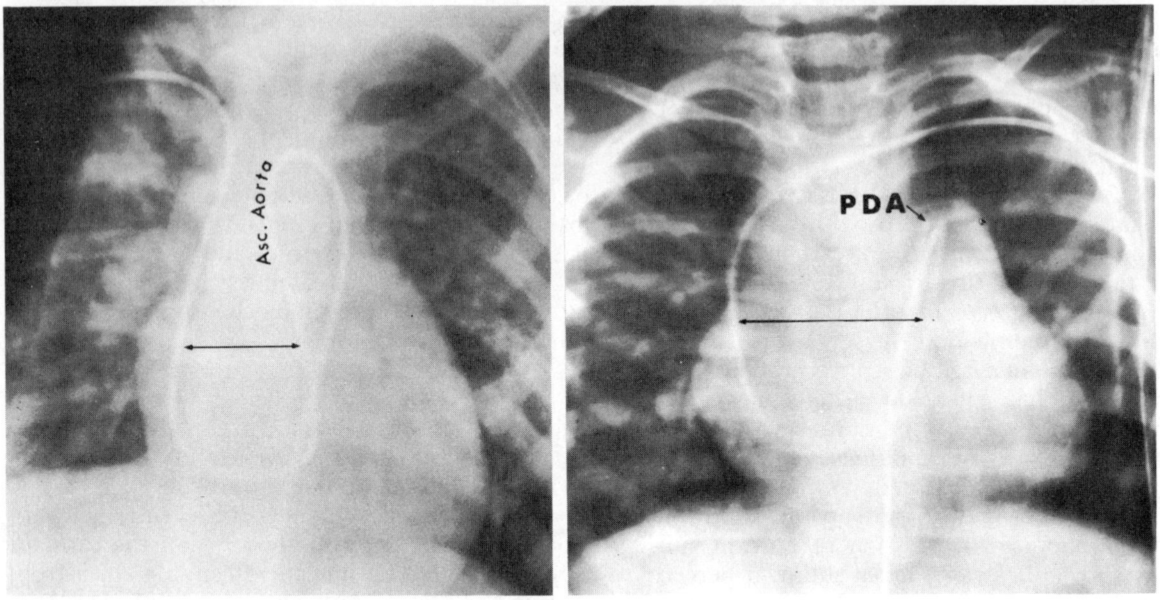

A B

FIGURE 108-12 Anteroposterior roentgenograms to demonstrate the difference in width of the catheter loop when (*A*) the catheter tip passes in a hairpin loop (arrow) from the right ventricle to the ascending aorta via a ventricular septal defect; (*B*) the catheter tip passes in a wide U loop (arrow) from the right ventricle to the pulmonary artery, thence to the descending thoracic aorta via a patent ductus arteriosus (PDA).

the tip passes directly up the ascending aorta from the main pulmonary artery. When the catheter tip enters a pulmonary vein within the heart shadow, angiography or a dye curve is necessary to ascertain whether the pulmonary vein drains into the left or the right atrium. A secundum atrial septal defect is more easily crossed from the leg approach, a sinus venosus defect from an arm approach, and an ostium primum defect is easily crossed from either approach. If the tricuspid valve is congenitally displaced into the right ventricle, the pressure transition from right ventricle to right atrium may occur

FIGURE 108-13 The use of the intracavitary electrocardiogram (I.C. EKG) and simultaneous pressure recording in a diagnosis of Ebstein's disease. Lead III of the standard electrocardiogram shows a short PQ interval and a prolonged QRS complex associated with WPW syndrome. The I.C. EKG of the "atrialized portion" of the right ventricle resembles the I.C. EKG of the right ventricle, but the pressure pulse of the atrialized portion of the right ventricle is the same as that of the right atrium proper. This finding suggests displacement of the tricuspid valve into the right ventricle. The I.C. EKG in the right atrium proper shows characteristic peaked biphasic P waves and reduction in voltage of the QRS.

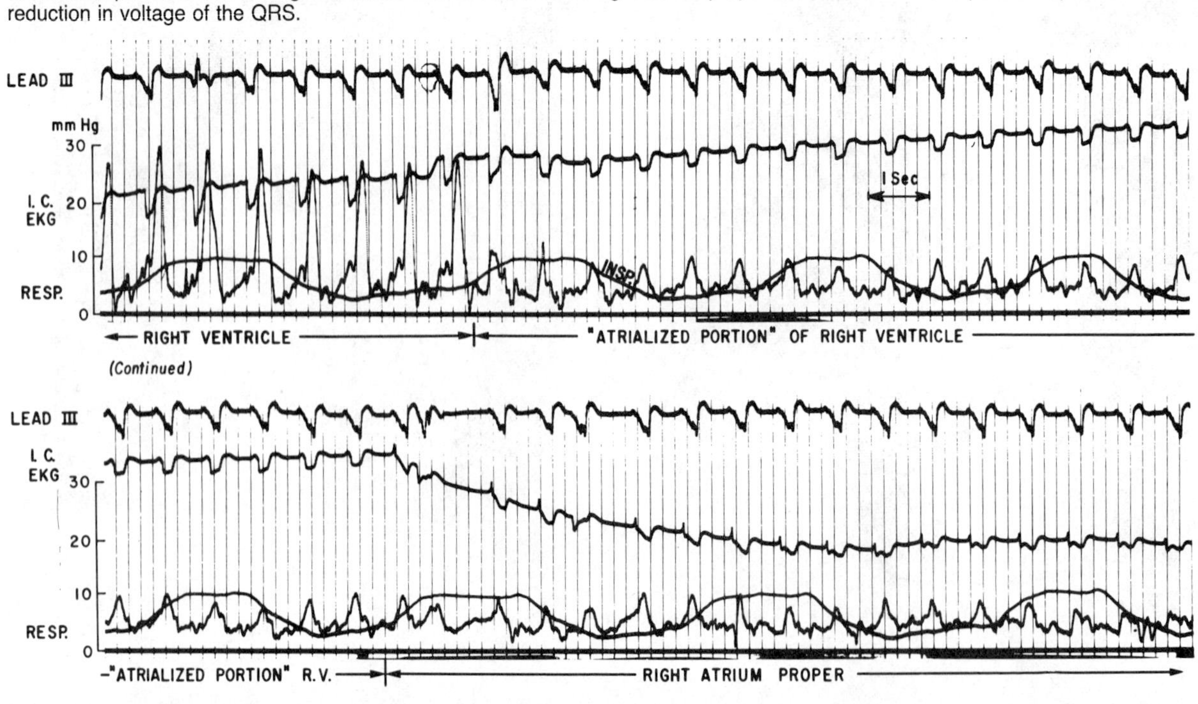

while the catheter tip is far to the left of the spine. Simultaneous intracardiac electrocardiography is confirmatory (Fig. 108–13).

Flow and Shunt Calculations

Fick Method

Cardiac Output In 1870 Adolph Fick expounded a theory for the measurement of blood flow that he never used in the laboratory: "The total uptake or release of a substance by an organ is the product of the blood flow to the organ and of the arteriovenous concentration of the substance." The cardiac output may be calculated given the following three values: total oxygen consumption is 300 ml/min; arterial blood oxygen content is 19 ml per deciliter of blood; and mixed venous blood oxygen content is 14 ml per deciliter of blood. The cardiac output, in liters per minute, is equal to the oxygen consumption divided by the arteriovenous oxygen difference multiplied by 10 (to convert the latter to liters). In this case the cardiac output equals 6.0 liters/min. Cardiac output may be related to the body surface area (BSA) as the cardiac index. Assuming a BSA of 2.0 m^2, the cardiac index would be $\frac{6}{2}$ or 3 liters/min/m^2. The normal range is from 2.6 to 4.2 liters/min/m^2. Because of laminar flow from the coronary sinus and the cavae, mixed venous blood is best obtained from the pulmonary artery. Under conditions of exercise a minimum of 3 min is usually required to obtain a steady state preliminary to expired air and blood collection. In a given person, repeated measurements of the cardiac output at rest by the Fick technique may vary to a maximum of ± 17 percent, presuming a continued steady state.

Shunt Calculations Shunt calculations utilizing the Fick principle tend to be approximations since complete mixing of venous and shunted blood may not occur. Too, as the arteriovenous oxygen narrows, small errors in the analysis or in the collection of blood samples make large variations in the calculated pulmonary blood flow possible. The calculation of shunt flow, however, is useful; it provides a quantitative index that is combined with clinical findings to determine whether surgery is advisable.

Numerous formulas have been developed, but those listed below are most often used. The oxygen capacity is the maximal amount of oxygen that will combine with hemoglobin at a high P_{O_2}. One gram of hemoglobin fully loaded combines with 1.34 ml of oxygen. Oxygen content is related to both the hemoglobin concentration and the oxygen saturation. The oxygen content = 1.34 × Hb (g%) × O_2 sat (%)/100.

1. Calculation of left-to-right shunt:

Total oxygen consumption (V_{O_2})	240 ml/min
Pulmonary artery blood oxygen content (PA_{O_2})	17 ml/dl blood
Mixed venous blood oxygen content (MV_{O_2})	15 ml/dl blood
Arterial blood oxygen content (Sa_{O_2}) (assumed to equal pulmonary venous oxygen content)	19 ml/dl blood

$$\text{Pulmonary flow } (Q_p) = \frac{V_{O_2}}{Sa_{O_2} - PA_{O_2}} = \frac{240}{19 - 17(10)} = 12 \text{ liters/min}$$

$$\text{Systemic flow } (Q_s) = \frac{V_{O_2}}{Sa_{O_2} - MV_{O_2}} = \frac{240}{19 - 15(10)} = 6 \text{ liters/min}$$

a. Pulmonary flow/systemic flow ratio = Q_p/Q_s = $\frac{12}{6}$ = 2.

b. If one substitutes for Q_s and Q_p in the above formula, and reduces to a common denominator, the pulmonary flow/systemic flow ratio is obtained from a formula requiring only the oxygen saturation. Assuming an oxygen capacity of 20 volumes percent, the following blood oxygen saturations for the above samples are Sa = 95%, PA = 85%, and MV = 75%.

$$Q_p/Q_s = \frac{Sa_{O_2}\% - MV_{O_2}\%}{Sa_{O_2}\% - PA_{O_2}\%} = \frac{95 - 75}{95 - 85} = 2$$

c. Left-to-right shunt may also be expressed as the percentage of total pulmonary flow that originates from the left heart. The 2:1 Q_p/Q_s ratio above then represents a 50 percent left-to-right shunt.

2. Calculation of right-to-left shunt:

$$V_{O_2} = 240 \text{ ml/min}$$
$$MV_{O_2} = 13 \text{ ml/dl blood}$$
$$Sa_{O_2} = 17 \text{ ml/dl blood}$$

Pulmonary vein blood oxygen content is as follows:

$$PV_{O_2} = 19 \text{ ml/dl blood}$$

(Assumed to be 98% of oxygen capacity + 0.3 ml of dissolved oxygen)

$$Q_p = \frac{V_{O_2}}{PV_{O_2} - MV_{O_2}} = \frac{240}{19 - 13(10)} = 4 \text{ liters/min}$$

$$Q_s = \frac{V_{O_2}}{Sa_{O_2} - MV_{O_2}} = \frac{240}{17 - 13(10)} = 6 \text{ liters/min}$$

Pulmonary/systemic flow ratio = Q_p/Q_s = 0.7

3. Calculation of bidirectional shunt:

$$V_{O_2} = 240 \text{ ml/min}$$
$$PA_{O_2} = 15 \text{ ml/dl blood}$$
$$MV_{O_2} = 13 \text{ ml/dl blood}$$
$$Sa_{O_2} = 18 \text{ ml/dl blood}$$
$$PV_{O_2} = 19 \text{ ml/dl blood}$$

$$Q_p = \frac{V_{O_2}}{PV_{O_2} - PA_{O_2}} = \frac{240}{19 - 15(10)} = 6 \text{ liters/min}$$

$$Q_s = \frac{V_{O_2}}{Sa_{O_2} - MV_{O_2}} = \frac{240}{18 - 13(10)} = 4.8 \text{ liters/min}$$

$$Q_{ep}{}^* = \frac{V_{O_2}}{PV_{O_2} - MV_{O_2}} = \frac{240}{19 - 13(10)} = 4.0 \text{ liters/min}$$

$$\text{Left-to-right shunt} = Q_p - Q_{ep} = 6 - 4 = 2 \text{ liters/min}$$

$$\text{Right-to-left shunt} = Q_s - Q_{ep} = 4.8 - 4.0 = 0.8 \text{ liters/min}$$

Indicator-Dilution Technique

Cardiac Output: Dye Method The cardiac output, or the mean volume rate of flow, may be determined by using a modification of the standard concentration equation used for the determination of a static fluid volume such as the blood volume:

*Effective pulmonary flow, Q_{ep}, is that volume of mixed venous blood which, after returning to the right atrium, finally reaches the pulmonary capillaries.

$$V = \frac{I}{C}$$

where V = fluid volume, ml
I = indicator added to fluid, mg
C = concentration of indicator in each milliliter of fluid, mg/ml

For determination of a moving fluid volume,

$$\text{Cardiac output} = \frac{I}{Ct}$$

where t = the time required for all indicator-fluid mixture to pass the sampling site once

If the indicator particles are injected into the circulation as a bolus and measured in the initial passage at a downstream site, they distribute themselves in a time-concentration plot of grossly predictable form called an *indicator-dilution curve* (Fig. 108–14). The descending limb of the indicator-dilution curve is distorted by indicator-blood mixture that has begun a second circulation. To exclude recirculating indicator, the concentration is plotted logarithmically against time. The early portion of the disappearance slope is linearly extrapolated on semilogarithmic paper to obtain a primary curve, on the premise that if indicator-blood mixing is complete, the washout of indicator is an exponential function of time. A cuvette densitometer is used to obtain a continuous arterial time-concentration curve. Thus:

$$\text{Cardiac output (in liters/min)} = \frac{I \times 60 \text{ s}}{Ct}$$

where C = mean concentration of indicator in one circulator passage, mg/liter
t = time, s

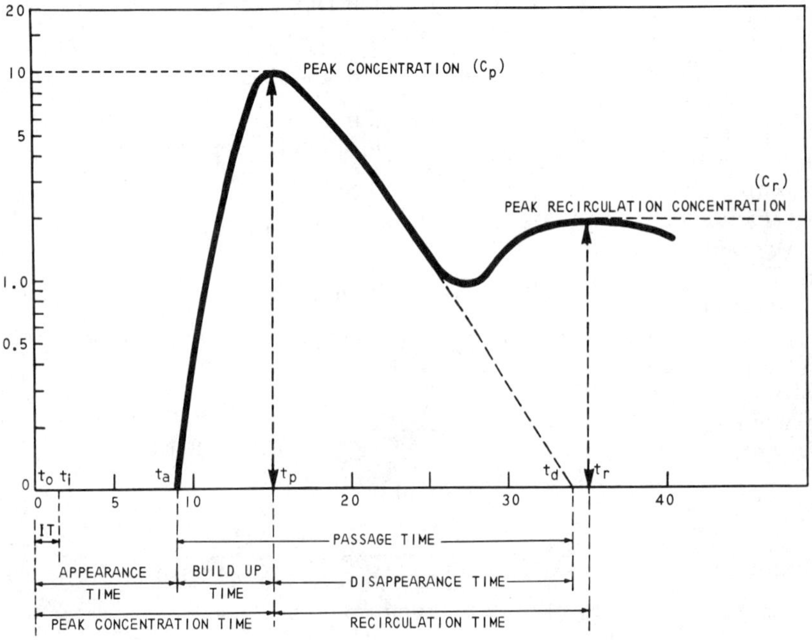

FIGURE 108-14 Time and concentration components of a normal indicator-dilution curve that has been replotted semilogarithmically, with extrapolation of the declining slope of concentration to eliminate the effect of recirculated indicator. The logarithm of the concentration on the ordinate is plotted against time on the abscissa. t_o = time of onset of injection of the indicator slug; t_i = time from t_o to the end of injection; t_a = time from t to the first detectable appearance of indicator at the sampling site; t_p = time from t_o to the peak (maximal) concentration of the indicator; t_d = time when the declining concentration of indicator reaches a minimally detectable value; t_r = time from t_o to the time of the secondary concentration peak due to systemic recirculation of indicator. IT = the injection time. (*From E. H. Wood and H. J. C. Swan, Definition of Terms and Symbols for Description of Circulatory Dilution Curves, J. Appl. Physiol. 6:797, 1954. Modified and reproduced with permission from the publisher and author.*)

The cardiac output is falsely high if some indicator is lost. If some indicator is counted twice, i.e., if undetected recirculation occurs, the cardiac output is falsely low. A small analog computer provides rapid calculation of cardiac output from dye-dilution curves and detects whether logarithmic decay of indicator concentration has occurred. The Stewart-Hamilton formula assumes constant heart rate and stroke volume and a linear runoff in the pulmonary artery. Values for cardiac output obtained with the indicator-dilution technique compare closely with those obtained by the Fick method.[56]

In the absence of shunt, the indicator-dilution curve shows an uninterrupted buildup slope, a sharp concentration peak, a steep disappearance slope, and a prominent recirculation peak. Two major types of distortion are produced by central shunting. In a left-to-right shunt, there is decreased peak concentration of dye, a gentle disappearance slope (prolonged disappearance time), and absence of the recirculation peak. These alterations are produced by the recirculation of indicator particles through the lungs, resulting in a slow release of indicator to the peripheral circulation. The typical curve produced by a venoarterial, or right-to-left, shunt shows deformity of the buildup slope by an abnormal or early-appearing hump, or reflection, representing indicator that has been shunted from right to left. The distortion in contour of the indicator-dilution curve in valvular regurgitation is similar to that occurring with left-to-right shunts. Efforts have been made to predict all or part of the curve from certain other curve components. The cardiac output obtained by the forward-triangle method compares favorably with the classical Hamilton method. In this technique, the initial portion of the indicator-dilution curve is considered to be a triangle. The area of this triangle multiplied by a constant gives the area of the primary dilution curve.

Cardiac Output: Thermodilution Technique The thermodilution technique was introduced by Fegler in 1953 in order to measure volume flow rate.[57] A precalibrated bead thermistor-tipped catheter or a multiple-lumen, flow-directed thermistor catheter is placed in the pulmonary artery. A slug of ice-cold dextrose solution is injected via a second catheter or a second lumen into the right atrium. As the cold dextrose-blood mixture is initially ejected from the right ventricle, the pulmonary artery temperature drops maximally and then progressively rises in a beat-to-beat disappearance slope as the cold dextrose-blood mixture is washed out of the ventricle. A derived factor is used to correct for negative heat loss between the injection site and the right atrial delivery site. At room temperature, 25°C, injectate temperature will rise $\frac{1}{3}$°C in 15 s if there is a delay in injecting. The recirculation phase is negligible. The area under the resulting temperature-time curve is obtained, and cardiac output is calculated by the Stewart-Hamilton method. Since there is no gold standard for cardiac output, the results are compared with the dye-dilution and Fick techniques and are noted to correlate well.[58] Electronic integration and computation by means of a battery-powered unit provides an instant display of the cardiac output.

Quantification of Shunts by Indicators The forward-triangle method of indicator-dilution curve analysis may be used to quantitate *left-to-right* shunts. The percent left-to-right shunt may be obtained by simultaneously recording a peripheral and a central dilution curve. Following the injection of indicator into the distal pulmonary artery, simultaneous dilution curves are obtained by withdrawing blood from the proximal pulmonary artery and from a systemic artery. The total pulmonary blood flow and the fraction of pulmonary blood due to shunted blood may then be calculated from the respective curves. In another method, Carter has estimated the percentage of left-to-right shunt from a peripheral arterial or earpiece densitometer dilution curve following an indicator injection into the right side of the heart. The amplitude of the curve at peak concentration of indicator is related to the amplitude at a point on the curve taken at either once or twice the buildup time beyond the peak concentration. The deflections are measured directly from the recorded dilution curve without conversion to absolute units of concentration. Similar determinations of shunt ratio have been made from thermodilution curves.[59] In infants, erroneously large left-to-right shunts are obtained by the usual indicator-dilution calculation. A formula developed by Krovetz shows improved correlation with oximetric results.[60]

The estimation of a *right-to-left* shunt by indicator-dilution techniques is based on the supposition that the area under the early-appearing hump of the dilution curve is proportional to the volume of shunt flow. The ratio of shunt area to total area gives the percentage of right-to-left shunt, and sampling is by cuvette from a peripheral artery or by earpiece densitometer (Fig. 108–15).

Detection of Shunts by Indicators A peripheral *dye-dilution curve* recorded following a central injection is highly successful in detecting a small right-to-left shunt (less than 5 percent of the systemic flow). A right-to-left shunt at the atrial level is best detected by injecting the inferior vena cava in order to take advantage of preferential streaming toward the atrial septal opening.

The configuration of the peripheral dye-dilution curve is not usually altered by a left-to-right shunt of less than 20 percent of pulmonary flow. Following an injection into a distal lobar pulmonary artery catheter, a left-to-right shunt as small as 5 percent of pulmonary flow may be detected by a second proximal catheter, sampling from the main pulmonary artery. For localization of the level of left-to-right shunting, the sampling site is moved retrogradely from the pulmonary artery until early dye

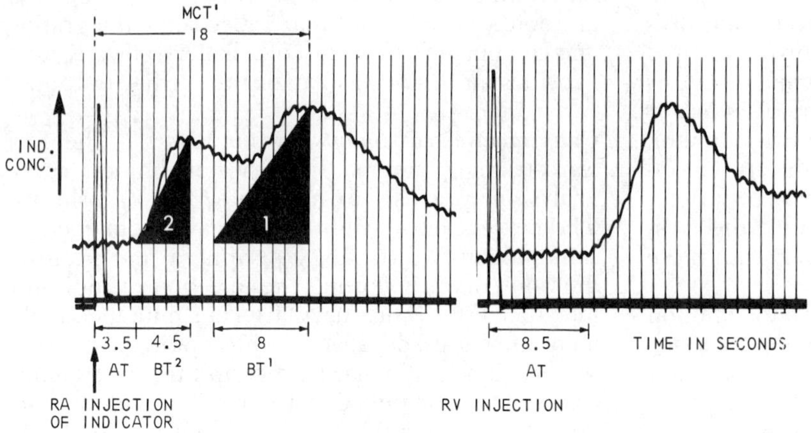

FIGURE 108-15 The use of buildup triangles for the calculation of right-to-left shunt in a patient with reversal of flow through an atrial septal defect. There is early appearance of indicator following right atrial injection. Note the normal appearance time following right ventricular injection of indicator. Triangles 1 and 2 represent the areas of the buildup triangles of the primary and secondary curves, respectively. BT^1 is theoretically derived (BT^1 = 0.44 MCT^1). AT = appearance time; BT^1 and BT^2 = buildup times of primary and secondary curves; MCT^1 = maximal concentration time. The peak concentration of the primary and secondary curves is measured directly from the record. The quotient (area of triangle 2 divided by the area of triangles 1 plus 2) times 100 equals the right-to-left shunt in percentage of systemic flow. In this example, 30 percent of the systemic flow was shunted from the venous side.

is no longer detected. The detection and quantitation of left-to-right cardiac shunts with radionuclide angiography is obtained by a gamma scintillation camera connected to a digital computer.[61]

The *hydrogen electrode* utilizes the principle of potentiometry in measuring the direct voltage between a silver and a platinum electrode. Hydrogen gas (dissolved in blood) yields, reversibly, two hydrogen ions plus two electrons on contact with a platinum surface. The potential developed (300 to 400 mV) is easily recorded. The hydrogen electrode is sensitive to other redox substances, such as ascorbic acid. The adult inhales hydrogen gas from a conductive bag; the infant inhales the gas via nasal prongs connected to a small stiff balloon (Fig. 108–16). Inhaled gas is dissolved in the alveolar capillary blood and enters the left side of the heart. If a left-to-right shunt is present, the hydrogen gas will be detected within 4 s of the time of inhalation at the site of shunt or downstream from it (Fig. 108–17). The site of shunt can be detected by varying the position of the platinum electrode–tipped catheter. Rapid circulation as a cause of early-appearing hydrogen can be excluded by a simultaneous recording from a peripheral artery electrode. An intravenous injection of hydrogen dissolved in saline solution or blood is completely cleared in one passage through the lung. Hydrogen or ascorbic acid detected early in the aorta or its branches is due to right-to-left shunt. The hydrogen-electrode system is extremely sensitive and is easy to use. Inhalations may be repeated numerous times.

Ventricular Volume Measurements

Left ventricular volume is estimated by selective injection of contrast medium into the left ventricle or into the left atrium. The image of the opacified left ventricular cavity is obtained either by a large film changer or by cineangiography. Biplane views used include frontal and lateral, or right and left anterior oblique, or half-axial left anterior oblique and conventional right anterior oblique.[62–64] A single-plane mode using the frontal or the right anterior oblique projection is adequate.[65,66] In the classic biplane technique each shadow of the left ventricular cavity is treated as an ellipse. The long axis of the ventricle (L_m) and the two mutually perpendicular short axes

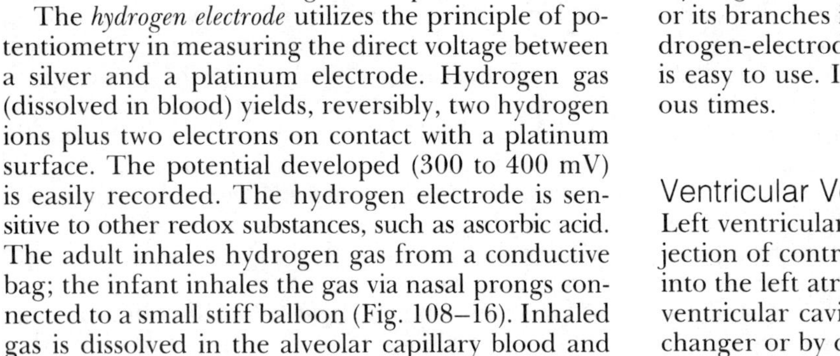

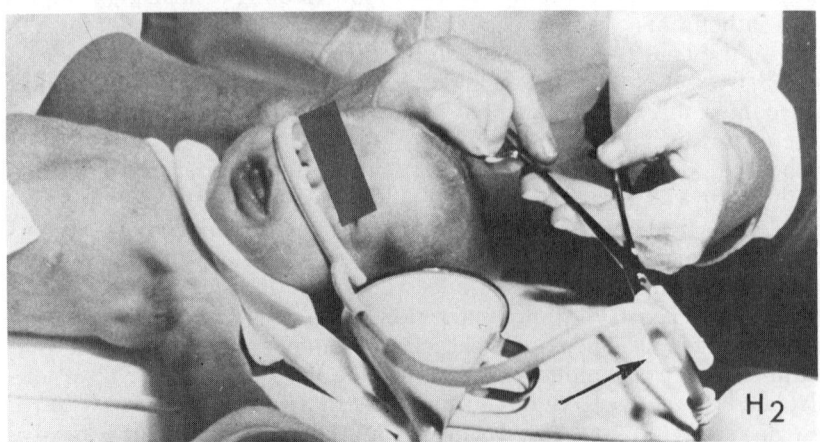

FIGURE 108-16 The method shown is used in our laboratory to deliver a bolus of hydrogen gas (H_2) to the infant in order to detect a left-to-right shunt by a catheter electrode. A latex Penrose drain connected to nasal prongs by rubber tubing is ballooned with H_2 while the tubing is clamped. The clamp is released (arrow) to deliver the gas in early inspiration. If the respiratory rate is extremely rapid, random release is effective in most cases.

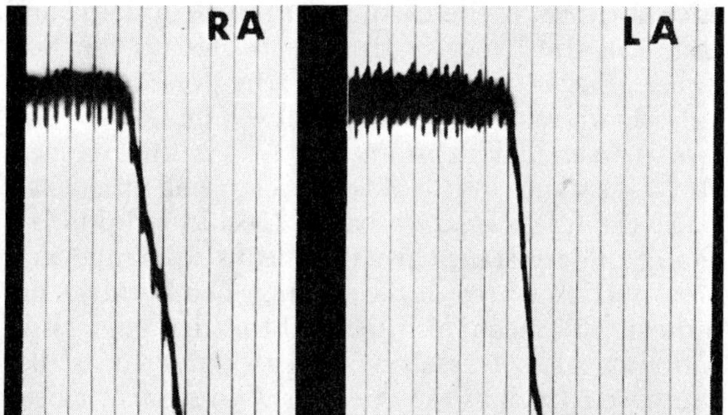

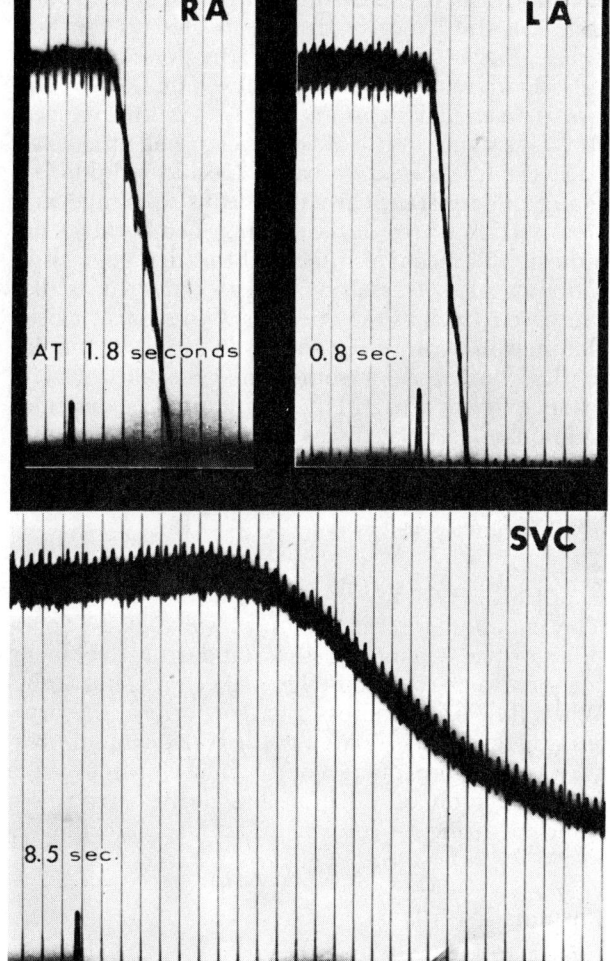

FIGURE 108-17 Use of the platinum electrode catheter in the detection and localization of left-to-right shunts. Note the abnormal early appearance of inhaled hydrogen gas at the right atrial level in a patient with atrial septal defect. A normal venous circulation curve is noted in the superior vena cava.

at its midpoint (D_a and D_1) are measured, and the volume (V) is calculated from the formula for volume of an ellipsoid:

$$V = \frac{4}{3}\pi \times \frac{D_a}{2} \times \frac{D_1}{2} \times \frac{L_m}{2}$$

or

$$V = \frac{\pi}{6} \times D_a \times D_1 \times L_m$$

In the single-plane method, the long axis and one short axis are measured; the second nonvisible short axis is assumed to equal the first; thus

$$V = \frac{\pi}{6} \times L_m \times D_1^2$$

More often, in either the biplane or single-plane method, the short-axis dimension is derived from the measured long axis and the area (A) of the left ventricular shadow, treated as an ellipse (area-length method of Dodge) (Fig. 108–18):

$$A = \pi L_m \frac{D}{4}$$

Corrections are made for magnification due to the divergence of the x-ray beam and, in the cine technique, for the possibility of more magnification at the periphery than in the center of the field (pincushion effect). A calibrated grid is filmed at the estimated level of the left ventricle. Geometric and nongeometric, count-based radionuclide techniques for calculation of ventricular volumes are well validated.[67]

If the left ventricle of a postmortem heart specimen is filled with contrast material and filmed, the calculated estimate of the volume of the left ventricle is higher than the known volume of the left ventricle. An appropriate regression equation for both single-plane[65,66] and biplane[62,64] techniques has been derived to adjust for this initial overestimate. The left ventricular end-diastolic volume is normally 70 ± 20 ml/m^2, and the end-systolic volume is 24 ± 10 ml/m^2. The forward stroke volume obtained by left ventriculography agrees well with indicator dilution and Fick determinations. The ejection fraction of the left ventricle is 0.67 ± 0.08; values below 0.5 are usually considered abnormal. Diastolic left ventricular wall thickness by angiography is 9 mm for women and 12 mm for men, and left ventricular wall mass is 76 g/m^2 for women and 99 g/m^2 for men.[68]

The total stroke volume obtained by left ventriculography is used to assess the severity of mitral and aortic valve regurgitation. Total stroke volume minus forward stroke volume equals regurgitant stroke volume. The regurgitant fraction equals regurgitant stroke volume divided by total stroke volume. Se-

FIGURE 108-18 Dimensions of the left ventricular (LV) cavity in end diastole used for the calculation of the ventricular volume by the area-length method, biplane technique. A-P = anteroposterior plane; A_a, A_1 = area, A-P and area lateral plane (planimetry); L_a, L_1 = length or long axis of the left ventricle, A-P and lateral plane (measured); D_a, D_1 = diameter of short axis, A-P and lateral plane (derived); L_m = maximum length or long axis whether from the A-P or lateral plane; h = wall thickness, LV. See text for formulas. (*Left and middle portion of figure from H. Sandler and H. T. Dodge, The Use of Single Plane Angiocardiograms for the Calculation of Left Ventricular Volume, Am. Heart J., 75:325, 1968. Right portion of figure from H. T. Dodge, Hemodynamic Aspects of Cardiac Failure, Hosp. Prac., January 1971, p. 91. Illustration by B. Tagawa and A. Miller. Reproduced with permission from the publishers and authors.*)

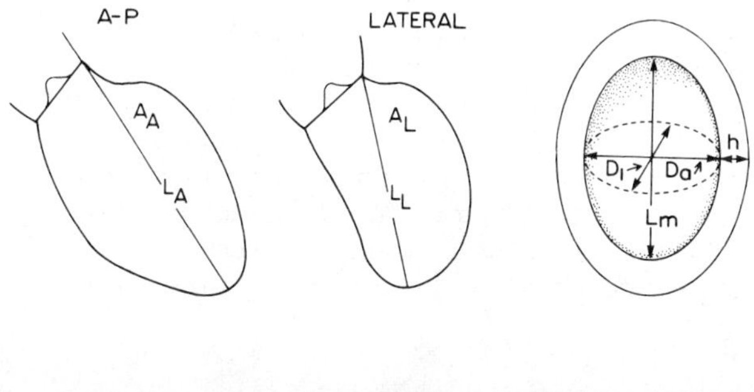

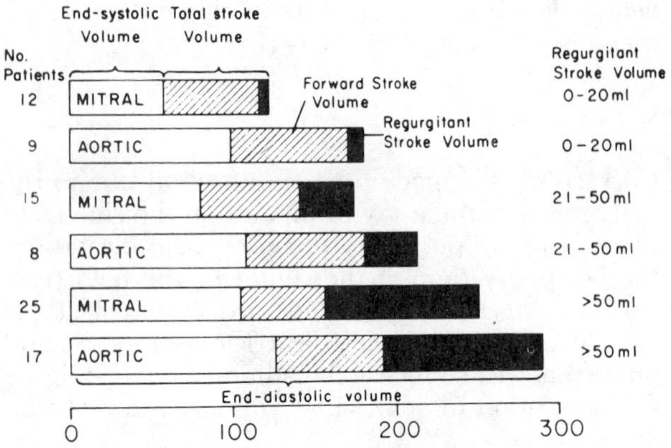

FIGURE 108-19 The mean values for left ventricular volumes obtained by ventriculography in patients with minimal, moderate, and marked aortic and mitral valve regurgitation. The entire bar represents the end-diastolic volume in milliliters. The total stroke volume equals the forward plus the regurgitant stroke volume. (*From J. W. Jones, C. E. Rackley, R. A. Bruce, H. T. Dodge, L. A. Cobb, and H. Sandler, Left Ventricular Volumes in Valvular Heart Disease, Circulation, 29:887, 1964. Reproduced with permission from the American Heart Association, Inc. and the author.*)

vere valvular regurgitation has a regurgitant fraction of 0.50 or greater (Fig. 108–19).

Right ventricular volume is estimated by applying Simpson's rule or the area-length method to the cavity silhouettes following biplane angiography.[69] The end-diastolic volume of the right ventricle in normal persons is 81 ± 12 ml/m^2.[70] The opacified left atrial shadow is represented as an ellipsoid so that left atrial volume can also be calculated in the biplane mode; the normal left atrial maximal volume is 63 ml ± 16 ml with mean volume of 35 + 8.7 ml.[71]

Resistance

By Poiseuille's law the flow varies directly with the fourth power of the radius of a tube; resistance varies inversely with the fourth power of the radius. Vascular resistance to blood flow in systemic, pulmonary, or regional vascular beds is estimated by analogy to Ohm's law:

$$\text{Resistance} = \frac{\text{pressure (in volts)}}{\text{flow (in amperes)}}$$

or

$$\text{Resistance} = \frac{\text{mean pressure differential across the vascular bed}}{\text{blood flow}}$$

To obtain the pressure difference across the pulmonary bed subtract the pulmonary artery wedge pressure from the pulmonary artery mean pressure; for the systemic pressure difference subtract the central venous pressure from the mean aortic pressure. Conversion into centimeter-gram-second (cgs) units (dyn·s/cm^5) does not add to the intrinsic significance of the measurements. Resistance may be expressed simply as R in units = pressure difference divided by the cardiac output. In infants and children, the pressure drop is related to the flow index, thus: R in units × m^2 = the pressure difference divided by the cardiac index. The normal pulmonary vascular resistance = 1 to 2 units. Generally, 1 resistance unit = 80 dyn·s/cm^5. In a physiologic sense the term *resistance* avoids specific definition. A change in resistance usually means a change in a cross-sectional area of the vascular bed but does not indicate the mechanism behind the change. Passive widening of the vessels by increases in intravascular pressure as well as the opening of previously closed channels may produce changes in resistance similar to those of active vasomotion. Clinically, the resistance figure is useful in quantitating the extent of pulmonary vascular disease; thus a patient with pulmonary vascular resistance values of 10 units × m^2 would not likely benefit from closure of a septal defect.

Calculation of Valve Areas

The equation for calculation of valve area (Torricelli's orifice equation) uses a standard hydrokinetic formula for a rounded-edge orifice or a short tube. When flow occurs across a narrow orifice, the pressure differential is related to the conversion of pressure energy into kinetic energy. The Gorlin formula for calculation of valve area is derived from two standard orifice formulas, describing flow and velocity.[72]

Formula I

$$F = AVC_c$$

where F = volume rate of flow during the time the valvular orifice is open, ml/s of diastole or systole
A = area of fixed orifice, cm^2
V = velocity flow, cm/s
C_c = coefficient of orifice contraction compensating for the physical phenomenon of reduction of the orifice stream to an area less than the area of the actual orifice

Formula II

$$V^2 = C_v^2\, 2gh \quad \text{or} \quad V = C_v\sqrt{2gh}$$

where V = as above
C_v = coefficient of velocity (allowing for some loss in conversion of pressure energy to velocity)
g = gravity acceleration (980 cm/s/s)
h = pressure head or differential across the orifice, cmH$_2$O

Combining I and II

$$A = \frac{F}{C_c \times C_v\sqrt{2gh}} \qquad A = \frac{F}{C \times 44.3\sqrt{P_1 - P_2}}$$

where C = discharge coefficient (an orifice constant obtained by comparing calculated with measured valve areas at postmortem, which combined C_c, C_v, conversion factor, mmHg to cmH_2O, other unknown factors)

$44.3 = \sqrt{2g} = \sqrt{1960}$

$h = P_1 - P_2$

= pressure differential across the orifice, mmHg

The duration of ventricular filling or emptying is measured in seconds from pullback or simultaneous pressure records obtained immediately upstream and downstream to the valve. The systolic or diastolic time per beat multiplied by the heart rate gives the number of seconds in each minute during which either filling or emptying occurs across the valve. Thus the volume rate of flow in milliliters per second of systole or diastole is the mean volume rate of flow (cardiac output, in milliliters per minute) divided by the filling or emptying time in seconds per minute.

A sample calculation of mitral valve area is as follows:

Cardiac output (CO) = 5000 ml/min
Diastolic filling period (DFP) beat = 0.38 s/beat
Pulse rate = 90 beats/min
DFP/min = 34 s/min
Left atrial mean diastolic pressure (LAP) = 30 mmHg
Left ventricular mean diastolic pressure (LVDP) = 5 mmHg
C = 0.85 (orifice constant for the mitral valve)[73]

$$\text{Mitral valve flow (MVF)} = \frac{\text{CO}}{\text{DFP/min}} = \frac{5000 \text{ ml/min}}{34 \text{ s/min}}$$

147 ml/s of diastole

Mitral valve orifice area (MVA)

$$= \frac{\text{MVF}}{0.85 \times 44.5\sqrt{\text{LAP} - \text{LVDP}}} = \frac{147}{38\sqrt{25}} = 0.8 \text{ cm}^2$$

The calculation for the aortic valve area is as follows:

$$\text{AVA (in cm}^2) = \frac{F}{C \times 44.5\sqrt{P_1 - P_2}} = \frac{\text{aortic valve flow (ml/systolic sound)}}{1 \times 44.5\sqrt{\text{LVS} - \text{ASP}}}$$

where LVS = left ventricular systolic mean pressure, mmHg

ASP = aortic systolic mean pressure, mmHg

C = orifice constant coefficient (value of 1 for the aortic valve)

Similarly, orifice areas may be calculated for the tricuspid and pulmonary valves, using an orifice constant of 1.0. The approximations and systematic errors in the formula do not detract from their usefulness in providing objectivity in the classification of patients with valvular disease. If flow is normal, reducing the orifice diameter to less than half or the cross-sectional area to one-fourth is required to offer significant obstruction. A critically reduced mitral valve area is 1 cm^2; aortic valve area, 0.7 cm^2.

Calculation of the orifice area of a stenotic valve in the presence of associated valvular regurgitation must take into consideration the added regurgitant flow, or the severity of the stenosis will be overestimated. In order to obtain an estimate of mitral or aortic regurgitant volume, the forward stroke volume (Fick) should be subtracted from total angiographic left ventricular stroke volume.

Selective Angiography

Since 1947, when contrast medium was first injected through a rubber catheter placed in the right ventricle,[74] the technique of selective angiography has been continually refined to the point that it now assumes the principal role in the diagnostic laboratory. A catheter with a large lumen facilitates rapid low-pressure delivery of a single bolus of the contrast agent. A closed-end catheter with laterally directed openings reduced recoil. A balloon-tipped angiographic catheter with proximal side holes is easy to manipulate and induces less ectopy than conventional catheters (Fig. 108–20). A power injector delivers the desired volume of contrast media at a preselected maximal flow rate; the time to reach peak flow is adjusted to reduce recoil.

Contrast Media

All contrast media contain three iodine molecules attached to a fully substituted benzene ring. The fourth position, in the standard ionic agent, is taken up by sodium or methylglucamine as cation; the remaining two positions of the benzene ring have side chains of diatrizoate or metatrizoate or iothalamate. All media are excreted predominantly by glomerular filtration. Normal half-time of excretion is 20 min; biliary excretion is 1 percent. A dose of 1 ml/kg of medium may be scaled up or down in relation to total body weight, size of the heart chambers, systemic blood flow, degree of left-to-right shunting, severity of pulmonary vascular disease, and the clinical status of the patient. Since significant hemodynamic changes may rapidly follow the administra-

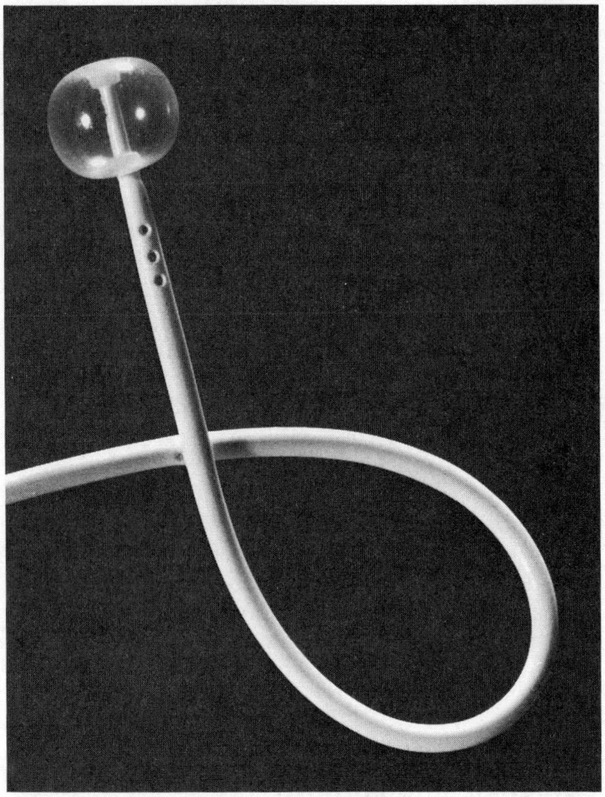

FIGURE 108-20 A Berman balloon angiographic catheter permits easy access to the right ventricle, pulmonary artery, and, if an atrial septal defect is crossed, to the left ventricle and even to the aorta. Maximum flow rates of contrast media are 5, 14, and 20 ml/s for nos. 5, 6, and 7 French catheters respectively; myocardial staining and ventricular ectopy are reduced by this method. *(Courtesy of Critikon, A Johnson & Johnson Company.)*

tion of contrast media, serial injections should ideally be spaced in time as the clinical status of the patient dictates. Marked peripheral vasodilatation occurs within 30 s, accompanied by transient hypotension and tachycardia returning to control or slightly higher levels within 1 or 2 min.[75] An early increase in cardiac output of 50 percent may occur, and an increase in left ventricular ejection time index (LVETI) is noted within 1 min, reflecting the transient increase in stroke volume modified by the negative inotropic effect of the contrast medium. In 1 to 2 min the plasma volume increases 2 to 14 percent, and the plasma osmolality 3 to 9 percent. Transient hypervolemia causes increased ventricular preload and is in part responsible for the elevation of the left atrial and left ventricular end-diastolic pressure and for the rise in pressure differential across the stenotic valve.

To reduce the osmotic effects of contrast medium, the number of dissolved particles must be decreased.[76] Nonionic contrast agents have the same viscosity and iodine content, but are not charged and have only one third to one half the osmolality of the ionic agents, e.g., metrizamide and iopamidol, 580 and 796 mosmol/kg H_2O, respectively, versus 1689 mosmol for Renografin-76.[77] Advantages of the nonionic agents include less renal toxicity, less hemodynamic loading,[78–80] less binding of ionic calcium,[81] and less depression of cardiac contractility; a disadvantage is the high cost. The principal use of nonionic agents may be in the very ill patient, especially the infant in heart failure[82] and in adults with severe cardiorenal disease. The current role of these new agents is being assessed in light of the known adverse effects of the ionic agents.

Filming Methods

A single or biplane roll or cut-film changer provides films at a programmed rate of up to 12 per second. These studies have the advantage of excellent detail; disadvantages are the high film costs and, in practice, the inability to monitor the injection.

A second technique, cineangiography, uses intensification and amplification fluoroscopy and provides for inexpensive, trouble-free filming by a 35-mm movie camera as well as television monitoring and tape recording.[83] Though the detail of the individual cine frame lacks the total resolution of the conventional roentgenogram, the motion itself increases visual perception by noise averaging and use of the integrating (5 frames per second) or persistence ability of the eye (0.2 s). The circular image of the phosphor is usually overframed on relatively slow 35-mm film with an 18- × -24-mm useful film area. Finally, meticulous attention to film processing is essential to obtaining a quality image. A spot-film fluorographic camera using roll film is employed as an adjunct to cineangiography. The frame rates are 1 to 12 per second; the 105-mm films permit direct viewing. Biplane cineangiography with biplane video recording is highly desirable in the study of complex congenital heart defects, especially in infancy. The total amount of contrast medium is significantly reduced, and chamber and great-vessel relations are better defined.

To perform computer-enhanced digital radiography the catheterization laboratory image intensifier and video camera are linked to an analog-to-digital converter, a computer system, and digital storage device (Fig. 108–21). The analog video signal is digitized into a series of separate numeric values that represent continuous voltage fluctuation storable on disks. The computer controls the rate at which images are obtained and the x-rays pulsed. The operator, via a console, interacts with the computer to enhance spatial and contrast resolutions of the angiographic image. Interfering background details can be electronically subtracted. The image is transferred to a video screen and can be recorded on x-ray film. Selective high-quality aortic or left ventricular angiograms can be obtained with 7 ml of contrast media rather than 40 ml, permitting the use of small catheters and repeat studies during pacing, exercise, or drug interventions. Coronary ar-

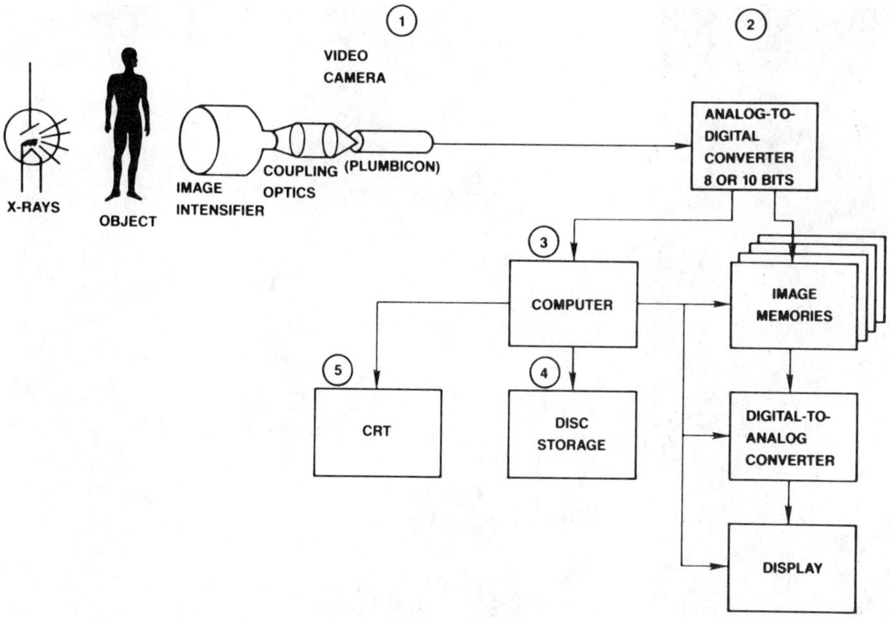

FIGURE 108-21 Diagram of the components of a digital radiography system. CRT = communication terminal. (*Reproduced with permission from ADAC Laboratories.*)

teriography and pediatric angiography[84] may also be performed with smaller doses of contrast media and decreased radiation dosage.

Second-generation digital radiographic left heart imaging with true digital storage, performed via venous or selective right heart angiography, demands the same rate of delivery and a total volume of contrast agent less than used in standard angiographic procedures.[85,86] Since motion of the subject produces artifact in image reproduction, a cooperative patient is desirable. A poor image may result from slowed levophase delivery of contrast media due to low cardiac output.

Cardiovascular computed x-ray transmission tomography (CT) with intravenous contrast media enhancement is useful in the diagnosis of dissecting aneurysm and is capable of identifying patent coronary artery grafts.

Positioning

Universal positioning capability of the x-ray and intensifier tubes by using stands of L-, U-, or C-arm configuration permit angled views of the supine patient. Thus a 45° left anterior oblique (LAO) view with 40° cranial angulation sees the four heart chambers without superimposition, and the atrial and posterior interventricular septa lie in the same plane. This very important view localizes septal and AV canal defects. An elongated right anterior oblique (RAO) view, useful for seeing the right ventricular infundibulum and supracristal ventricular septal defect is obtained by moderate right anterior oblique and 40° caudal angulation. The main pulmonary artery and its bifurcation are seen in the frontal position with 30° of cranial angulation. Patient positioning for angulated views using a fixed horizontal tube and vertical biplane tubes has been elegantly outlined.[87]

A successful procedure results when a rapid injection of the proper volume of contrast medium is made through an adequate-sized catheter, properly positioned, with detailed attention to radiologic technique and position of the patient in regard to the information needed.

Uses of Angiography

Right atrial angiography is useful in defining (1) the tricuspid valve in Ebstein's anomaly and tricuspid atresia or stenosis, (2) myxoma or thrombus, (3) juxtaposition of right atrial appendage in cyanotic congenital heart disease, (4) the right atrial border in effusion or tumor, and (5) atrial septal defect with right-to-left shunting or occasionally an anomalous pulmonary vein by reflux. In the lateral position a right ventricular injection is used in order to study the caliber and the level of obstruction to right ventricular outflow and the relation of the great vessels to the right ventricle (Figs. 108–22 and 108–23). A pulmonary artery injection may be used to fill the left side of the heart in order to detect a left-to-right shunt and to detect the site of partial (Fig. 108–24) or total anomalous venous drainage of the pulmonary veins and to visualize the pulmonary artery and its branches. An atrial septal defect is best defined by selectively injecting the right upper-lobe pulmonary vein rather than the left atrium itself. To identify the pulmonary arteries in cases of pulmonary atresia with ventricular septal defect (VSD) or to identify one pulmonary artery in cases where a shunt procedure has inadvertently produced discontinuity between right and left branches, a selective pulmonary vein wedge contrast-medium hand injection will frequently retrogradely opacify the pulmonary ar-

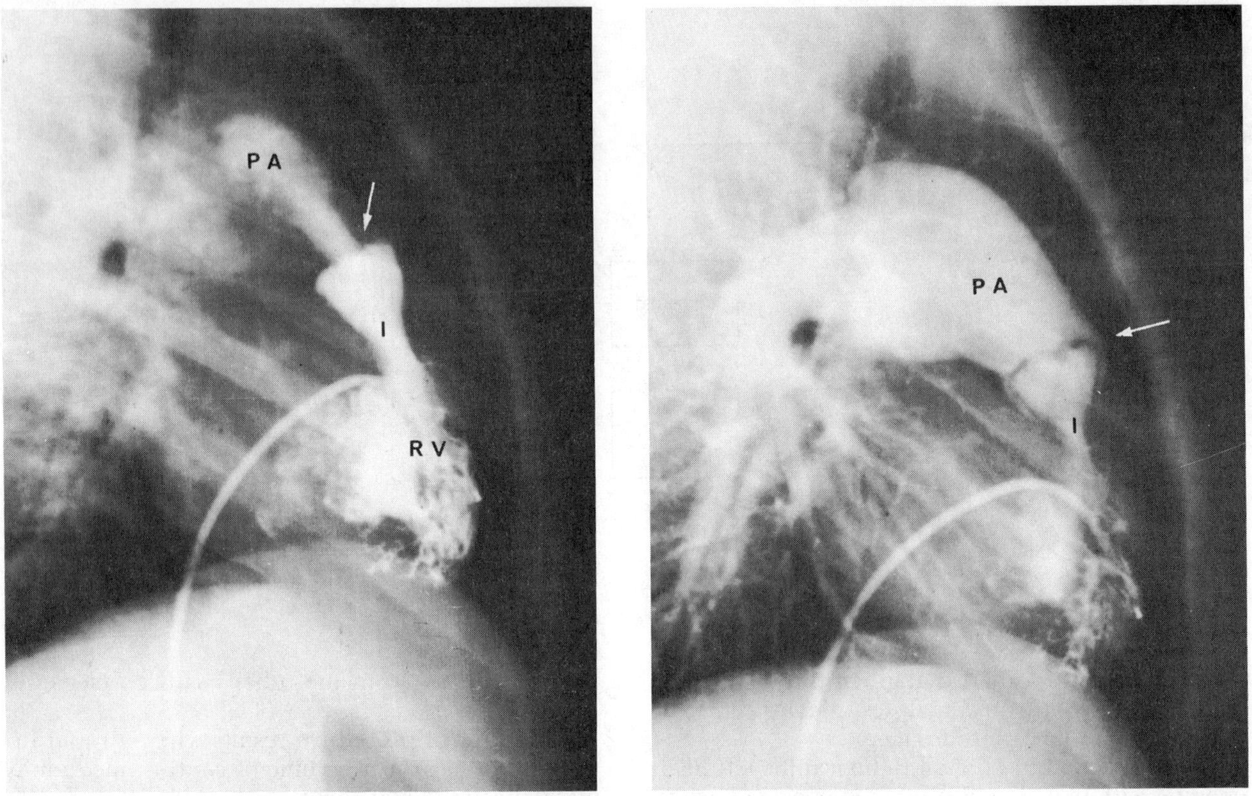

A B

FIGURE 108-22 *A.* Valvular pulmonary stenosis (lateral view). Right ventricular injection of opaque medium. Contrast material exits through central orifice of pulmonary valve in form of a jet (arrow). RV = right ventricle; I = infundibulum of right ventricle; PA = pulmonary artery. *B.* Valvular pulmonary stenosis (lateral view). Right ventricular injection of opaque medium reveals bulging of fused cusps (arrow) into dilated pulmonary artery and narrowing of infundibulum of right ventricle.

terial tree (Fig. 108–25).[88] A left brachial artery countercurrent injection in infants demonstrates an aorticopulmonary window, aortic valve atresia, patent ductus arteriosus, and coarctation of the aorta (Fig. 108–26).

Valve Regurgitation

Injections made above the aortic valve serve to detect aortic regurgitation. In milder degrees of aortic regurgitation, a regurgitant jet is noted; opacification is limited to the left ventricular outflow tract, clearing with each systole (grade 1), or faint, persistent, incomplete opacification of the left ventricular cavity (grade 2) occurs. In grades 3 and 4, no distinct jet is seen, and dense complete opacification of the left ventricle occurs, either progressively or in one or two diastolic cycles; and so left ventricular

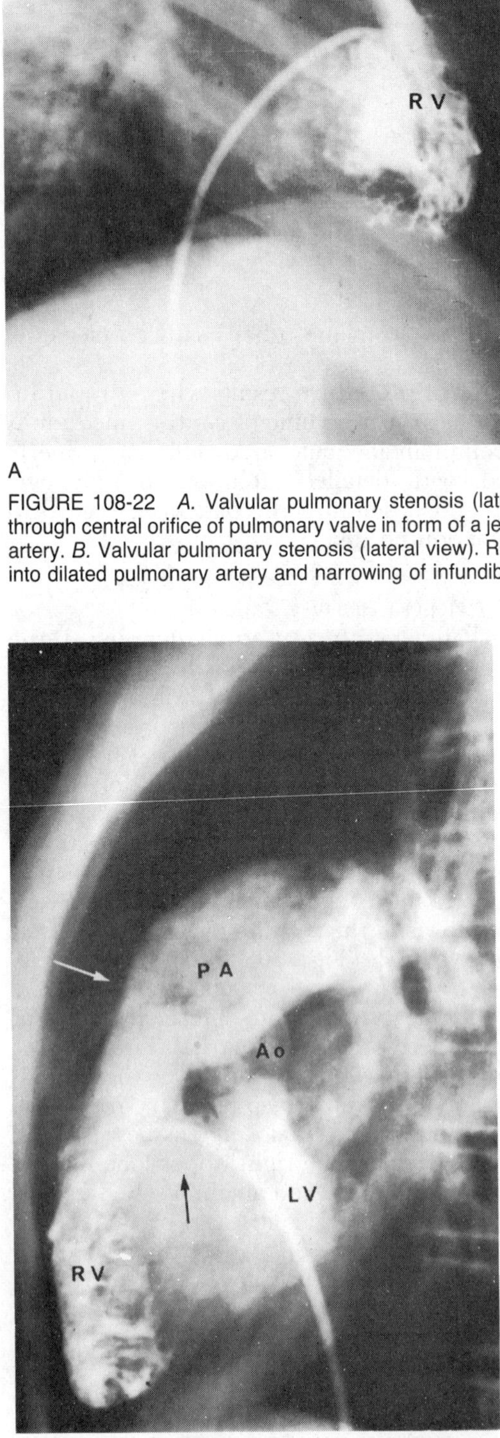

FIGURE 108-23 Ventricular septal defect and pulmonary hypertension (lateral view). Right ventricular injection reveals normal outflow and moderate-sized ventricular septal defect (bottom arrow) in membranous portion of ventricular septum. Contrast material passes into the aorta. Observe large size of main pulmonary artery and normal pulmonary valve (top arrow). PA = pulmonary artery; Ao = aorta; RV = right ventricle; LV = left ventricle.

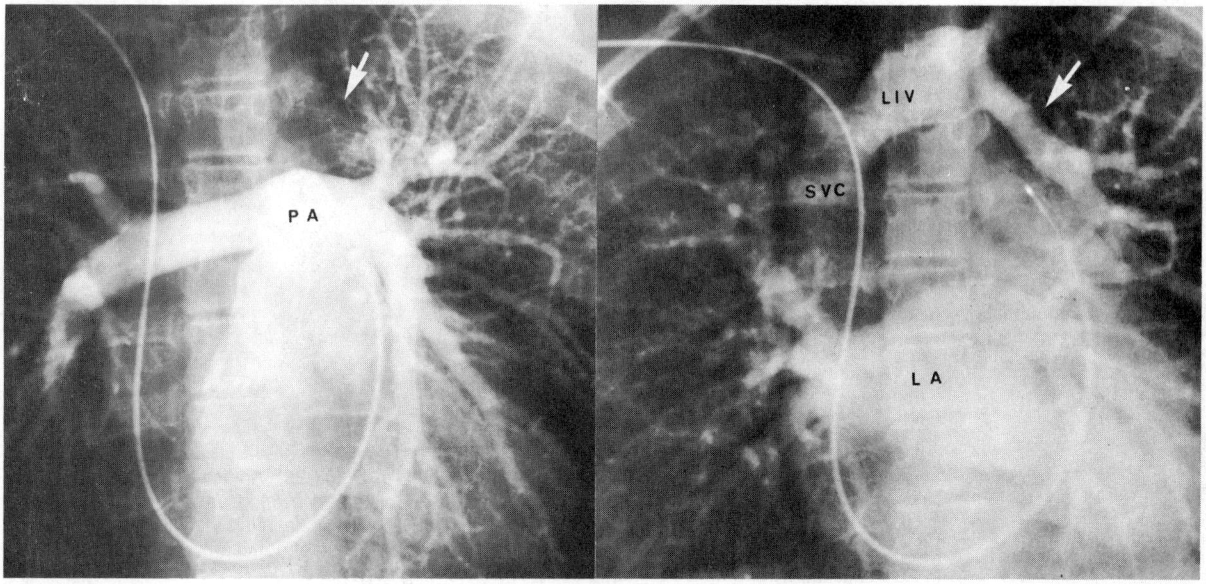

A B

FIGURE 108-24 Partial anomalous drainage of pulmonary veins (frontal view). *A.* The catheter has been introduced into the right atrium and ventricle and positioned in the main pulmonary artery (PA), where selective injection is performed. *B.* Pulmonary venous phase. A large pulmonary vein (arrow) drains the upper lobe of the left lung, with anomalous venous return to the left brachiocephalic vein. SVC = superior vena cava; LA = left atrium.

density exceeds aortic density in the severe case. Following an aortic injection, the size and mobility of a stenotic aortic valve may be visualized by negative-contrast washout of the opacified aorta with non-opaque ventricular blood. In the LAO view the mouthlike opening of a bicuspid aortic valve is seen. A left ventricular injection may display the level of obstruction to left ventricular outflow. And in the patient with endocardial cushion defect, the frontal view may show a radiolucent notch in the anterior mitral valve leaflet; the left ventricular outflow tract has an elongated or gooseneck appearance in early diastole.

Left ventricular injection in the RAO view is used to detect and to grossly quantitate mitral regurgitation. The angiographic criteria for grading mitral

FIGURE 108-25 Selective angiograms of a 5-year-old girl with pulmonary valve atresia, single ventricle, and levo transposition of the aorta. A side-to-side ascending aorta-to-right pulmonary artery (RPA) shunt was done at 1 week of age. *A.* The selective ascending aortogram shows no filling of the left pulmonary artery (LPA). A segmental area of narrowing in the proximal RPA occurs at the site of the Waterston shunt. *B.* A no. 6 French end-hold catheter passes across the foramen ovale to the left atrium (LA), thence into a left upper-lobe pulmonary vein wedge (PVW) position. A hand injection of 4 ml of contrast medium fills the LPA by retrograde flow through the pulmonary vascular bed.

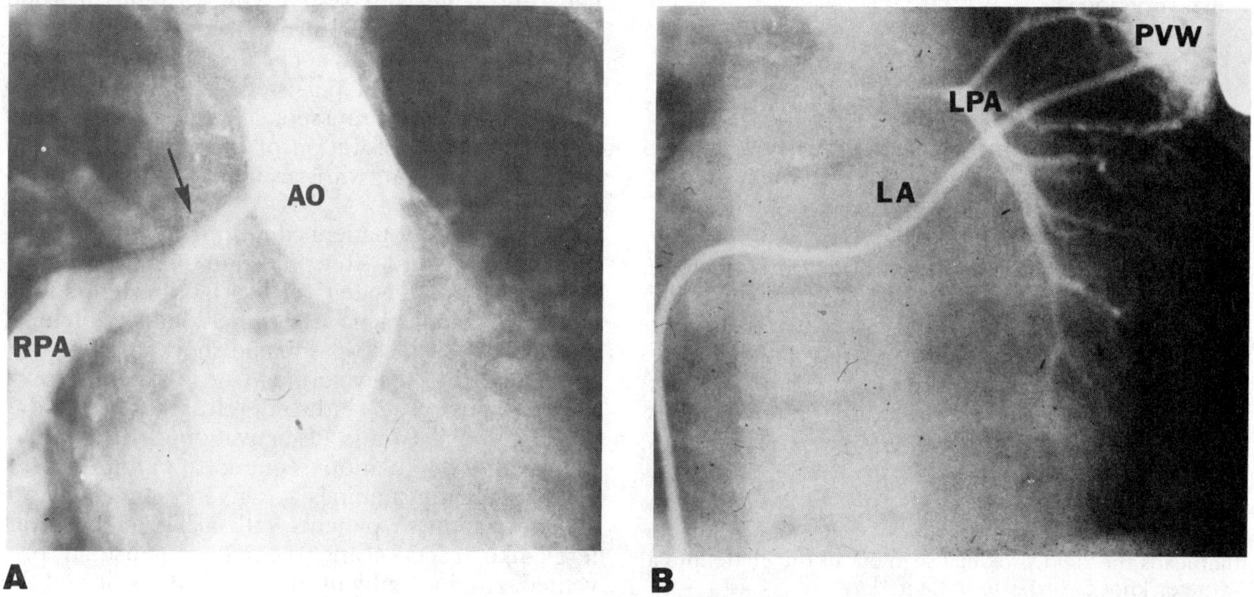

A **B**

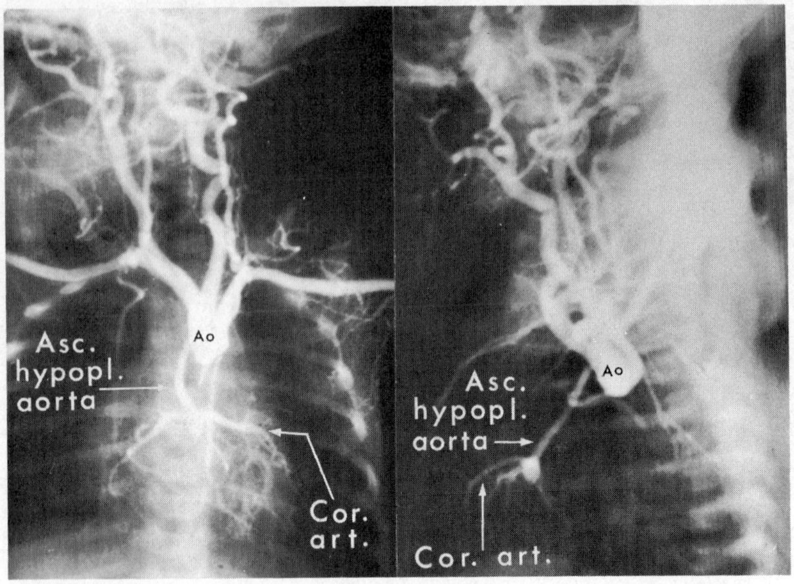

FIGURE 108-26 Aortic valvular atresia (frontal and lateral views). Contrast medium injected through cannula in left brachial artery. Excellent opacification of aortic arch, hypoplastic ascending aorta, and coronary arteries.

regurgitation are somewhat subjective, and so disagreement may arise between observers in assessing the degree of reflux. In grades 1 and 2 mitral regurgitation, a narrow-to moderate-width regurgitant jet of slight to moderate density is noted; minimum to moderate opacification of the left atrium clears quickly. In grades 3 and 4, a well-defined jet is absent, and left atrial opacification is intense, immediate, and lingering; and so the left atrium appears denser than the left ventricle or aorta in grade 4 mitral regurgitation. In mitral valve prolapse, shown best in a lateral projection with slight cranial angulation, all or a portion of one or both leaflets balloon above the mitral annulus in systole with or without associated mitral valve regurgitation. A normal mitral valve may leak if ectopic beating occurs. Unlike valves with poppets, prosthetic tissue valves can be crossed with the catheter tip without interfering with valve function.

Complications of Cardiac Catheterization and Angiography

The experienced operator can carry out catheterization of the right side of the heart without difficulty in practically all cases. Complications may include knotting of the catheter;[89]* breakage of the guide wire; excessive blood loss in infants; perforation of the atrium, ventricle, or coronary vein; and pulmonary infarction or hemorrhage.[91] Complete heart block may be induced if left bundle branch block is already present, or if prolonged catheter manipulation is required in the cyanotic infant. Prolonged ventricular or atrial arrhythmia may occur.

In the catheterization of the left side of the heart thrombosis or bleeding may occur at the percutaneous puncture site or into the mediastinum or retroperitoneum if perforation occurs at a tortuous subclavian or pelvic arterial site. Of 23,000 patients (72 percent males) at Emory University Hospital who had coronary artery angiography via the percutaneous femoral approach using a no. 8 French multipurpose catheter, 14 patients (12 female and 2 male) required femoral artery thrombectomy. The smaller femoral artery of the female is more prone to thrombotic occlusion than that of the male. Arteriovenous fistula and false aneurysm occur uncommonly. Cerebral embolism may result from plaque dislodgment or fibrin clot. In 30,000 coronary artery and left ventricular catheterizations, 35 patients had central nervous system complications (carotid distribution in 15, vertebrobasilar in 20, two cases, diffuse encephalopathy). The deficit resolved in one half of all cases and persisted in one half. There were two deaths. Transseptal puncture may result in inadvertent perforation of the aorta or the free wall of the atrium, with resultant cardiac tamponade.

Ten percent of patients develop nausea and vomiting immediately after injection of contrast medium, probably related to direct brainstem stimulation. Adverse reactions also include hives, itching, angioedema, bronchospasm, and shock.[93] These may be related to (1) development of a true allergy or hypersensitivity, (2) induced release of histamine, (3) chemotoxicity, and (4) activation of the complements and coagulation sequences. Parenteral steroids and antihistamines are given $\frac{1}{2}$ to 1 h before catheterization to patients with a history of an allergic-like reaction, and recurrence is usually prevented. Angiography in the elderly diabetic and the

*The Lunderquist exchange guide wire (0.038 in in diameter, 120 cm long) has an 8-cm flexible spring tip that leads the rigid proximal segment of the guide into a catheter knot in order to untie it.[90]

juvenile-onset diabetic both with nephropathy (creatinine 5 mg/dl or greater) is usually followed by the onset of acute renal failure that is probably due to acute tubular cell injury, increased urate and oxalate excretion, and an antidiuretic hormone (ADH)-like response.[94,95] Pulmonary edema following angiography may be caused by sodium and volume overload, negative inotropic effect, classical anaphylaxis, or rarely by a nonimmunologic direct effect on the pulmonary capillary endothelium.[96] In desperately ill, cyanotic infants or in those with marked ventricular dysfunction or severe valvular obstruction the desire for films that display the cardiac anatomy spectacularly should be tempered by the potential consequences of large doses of contrast medium in this setting.

Coronary Arteriography and Left Ventriculography

Coronary arteriography remains the standard by which all methods of diagnosing coronary artery disease are measured. It is the sole method of defining coronary anatomy in the living patient. To accomplish this in a safe, reliable, and reproducible manner, adherence to certain principles of performance and interpretation is required. This chapter will address itself to the techniques of coronary arteriography, the information gained from these techniques, and the limitations and risk of coronary arteriography.

Information To Be Gained

Coronary arteriography provides not only an anatomic map of the coronary arteries, including the site and severity of stenotic lesions, but also the characteristics of distal vessels in terms of size, presence of atherosclerotic disease, mass of myocardium served, a rough index of differential coronary flow, identification of collateral vessels, and an estimate of their functional importance.[97–107] In addition, the presence of coronary spasm can be ascertained by provocative maneuvers.[108–113] Left ventricular catheterization makes possible measurements of the left ventricular pressure at rest, with exercise, or after pharmacologic agents. Left ventriculography enables one to make a visual analysis of wall motion. Ventricular systolic and diastolic volume and ejection fraction can be calculated. Careful correlation of the coronary arteriogram and left ventriculogram permits identification of those stenotic and potentially bypassable arteries serving viable myocardium. Left ventricular wall motion can be further evaluated by the addition of stress such as atrial pacing or exercise. Augmenting left ventricular contraction by the use of nitrates, catecholamines, or postextrasystolic beats may permit the identification of left ventricular wall segments which have a potential for improved function following revascularization surgery.[114–116] The presence of associated valvular heart disease may be determined. In patients who have undergone surgery previously, patency of grafts and status of the native coronary arteries can be ascertained. In certain children with congenital heart disease, the location of the coronary arteries can be determined as an aid to planning surgical correction.[117,118]

Techniques of Coronary Arteriography

Mason Sones ushered in the modern era of coronary arteriography in 1958 when he developed a safe and reliable method of selective coronary arteriography.[97] The Sones technique utilizes an antecubital incision over the brachial artery. The artery is exposed and a woven Dacron catheter (Sones USCI) is passed into the brachial artery and maneuvered through the axillary and subclavian arteries into the ascending aorta. Manipulation techniques depend on deflecting the soft, tapered catheter tip off the aortic valve cusps up to the coronary orifices. The Sones technique has stood the test of time. Advantages are that it requires only one catheter, aortoiliac disease is avoided, and the operator is close to the aortic root and therefore gets the best feel of the catheter tip. Disadvantages are that an antecubital dissection, arteriotomy, and arterial closure are needed. Manipulation skills and precise knowledge of the aortic root anatomy are required. A detailed description of the Sones technique has been recently published.[119]

Percutaneous arterial catheterization described in 1953 by Seldinger[120] (Fig. 108–3) was first used to study the coronary arteries as reported by Rickets and Abrams in 1962.[121] Modification of catheters was made by Amplatz[122] and by Judkins[123] in 1967. The Judkins technique requires three preformed catheters: one for each coronary artery and a pigtail catheter for the left ventricular injection. The Judkins technique is much easier to learn, and, paradoxically, this may be its major drawback. The femoral artery is punctured below the inguinal ligament, and a left coronary artery catheter is passed over the guide wire into the aorta. After the catheter is flushed and good pressure tracings are obtained from the tip, the catheter is advanced until it engages the left coronary orifice. The preformed shape of the catheter holds it against the inside of the aortic curve, enabling the tip to spring into the left coronary orifice. The tip is made in four lengths, for use with different-sized aortic roots. After the left catheter is removed, the appropriate-sized right coronary catheter is inserted over a guide wire and positioned above the right coronary orifice, where it is rotated clockwise. The tip will descend and will be held against the outside curve of the aorta, causing it to spring into the right coronary orifice. Left ventricular studies are performed by replacing the coronary catheters with the pigtail catheter. A detailed description of the Judkins technique has been recently published.[124]

This technique has the advantages of a percutaneous approach; the disadvantages are the requirement for multiple catheter exchanges and a potential increased risk of emboli to the coronary or cerebral circulation. Complications may arise from the ease of entry of the catheter tip into the coronary arteries. Some poorly trained angiographers have applied this technique without proper appreciation for the devastating consequences of catheter obstruction of the left main coronary artery. Methods of avoiding serious complications of catheter emboli, including systemic heparinization and catheter debriding techniques, have reduced complications in active centers.

In an attempt to combine the advantages of the Sones and Judkins techniques, the single-catheter percutaneous femoral approach was first applied by Schoonmaker in 1968, and the use of this technique was reported by Schoonmaker and King.[125] Since 1972, this technique has been the principal one employed and taught to cardiology fellows at Emory University Hospital, and since then over 25,000 studies have been performed.

Performance of Coronary Arteriography

The description of our technique of coronary arteriography is brief. A more detailed description has been recently published.[126] It is the authors' belief that one cannot become expert in performing any coronary arteriography method simply by reading. Only through training in an active laboratory performing hundreds of coronary arteriograms under close supervision can the physician gain a proper appreciation for the potential hazards of coronary arteriography so that they can be avoided.

A close physician-patient relationship is essential to reduce fear of the examination. The patient is seen the day before the procedure, and a thorough history, physical examination, and description of the procedure are completed. Propranolol and nitrates are usually continued up to and through the procedure. An intravenous line is routinely started for administration of 0.6 mg of atropine and 5 to 10 mg of diazepam when sedation is needed. The intravenous line is also essential as a port for administration of additional drugs during the procedure as needed if pain or hypotension occur or if congestive failure is aggravated. Electrocardiographic monitoring is performed throughout the procedure. Atropine, lidocaine, propranolol, furosemide, corticosteroids, an antihistamine, nitroglycerin, epinephrine and other vasopressors, and narcotics should be readily available for intravenous administration. Heparin and antibiotics are not routinely administered in our laboratory. Patients with a history of anaphylactoid reactions to contrast media are pretreated with antihistamines and corticosteroids.

A three-way stopcock manifold is connected to lines for pressure monitoring, contrast medium, and heparinized saline solution. A clear catheter is maintained by intermittent flushing with saline solution and contrast medium. The femoral artery is catheterized by the Seldinger technique, and a multipurpose polyurethane (Cordis) or woven Dacron (USCI) catheter is inserted into the descending aorta, where it is flushed before being advanced around the aortic arch without a guide wire. The catheter is advanced to the left ventricle, where, following pressure measurements and test injections to exclude catheter-tip entrapment, left ventricular injection with 32 to 40 ml of contrast medium is made over 4 s. This slow injection allows adequate visualization without recoil of the end-hole and side-hole catheter. Filming is routinely done in the right anterior oblique view or in a biplane mode using right anterior and left anterior oblique views.

Essential to any coronary arteriographic technique is a thorough knowledge of aortic root anatomy (Fig. 108–27). Usually the left coronary orifice arises from the left sinus of Valsalva, which is posterior and to the left. The right coronary artery usually arises from the right sinus of Valsalva, which is anterior. Because of extensive variation in the position, size, and number of orifices, considerable experience is required to avoid failure to identify and study one of the arteries. Left coronary cannulation is performed in the following manner: The tip of the catheter is placed in the noncoronary cusp which lies posterior and to the left (toward the spine in the right anterior oblique view). As the catheter is advanced with a slight clockwise rotation, the tip flips up into the left coronary ostium or into the left cusp. From the left coronary cusp, the catheter tip can be rotated posteriorly and advanced superiorly into the left coronary ostium (Fig. 108–27). An alternative method is to advance the catheter tip in the right cusps. It curls into the right orifice. Right coronary artery catheterization is done by positioning the tip of the catheter above the left coronary cusp and rotating clockwise so that the tip sweeps along the

FIGURE 108-27 *Left.* A 30° right anterior oblique view of the aortic root demonstrating the left coronary orifice. *Right.* A 60° left anterior oblique view of the aortic root demonstrating location of the right coronary orifice. (*From F. W. Schoonmaker and S. B. King, Coronary Arteriography by the Single Catheter Percutaneous Femoral Technique, Circulation, 50:737, 1974. Reproduced with permission from the American Heart Association, Inc., and the author.*)

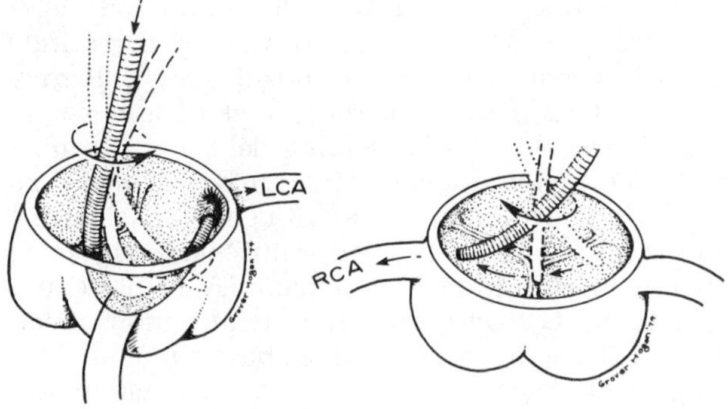

anterior aortic root until it reaches the right coronary ostium (Fig. 108–27). When the operator is unsuccessful in reaching one or the other coronary orifice, the catheter is removed and replaced by an appropriate Judkins or other preformed catheter.

All injections into the coronary arteries are preceded by aspiration of a small amount of contrast medium into the hand-held syringe (to exclude the possibility of air embolism) and are monitored visually until the contrast medium clears. Pressure monitoring is done following these injections. Hypotension following coronary injection usually clears spontaneously or with coughing, which transiently increases aortic pressure and enhances clearing of contrast medium. If hypotension lasting more than a few seconds occurs, especially in a patient with severe proximal coronary artery disease, a pressor agent in an adequate dose to obtain a quick response is started promptly. Adequate coronary perfusion pressure is essential in these patients. If congestive heart failure is aggravated by the effect of contrast medium, the first drug used is sublingual nitroglycerin; furosemide may be needed, however. When chest pain occurs, nitrates are given sublingually or intravenously and the catheter is repositioned in the left ventricle to monitor left ventricular end-diastolic pressure. If pain continues or ST-segment elevation occurs, coronary injection may reveal coronary spasm. Intracoronary nitroglycerin or sublingual nifedipine usually provides prompt relief. If severe end-diastolic pressure elevation occurs, the patient may be propped up and given additional nitrates and oxygen. When tachycardia accompanied by adequate or elevated blood pressure develops during angina, 1-mg increments of propranolol may be given intravenously, producing dramatic relief. Hypertension is treated with nifedipine, 5 to 10 mg sublingual. Narcotics are used for pain which is not promptly relieved by nitroglycerin, nifedipine, and propranolol. Ventricular fibrillation, a rare occurrence, is promptly corrected with the defibrillator. All laboratory personnel must be thoroughly trained in cardiopulmonary resuscitation, as unstable patients may develop life-threatening arrhythmias before, during, and after angiography. Minor anaphylactoid reactions are treated with antihistamines; more serious reactions are treated with the addition of epinephrine and corticosteroids.[127] Maximal safety of the procedure is obtained when an expert angiographer performs a brief but complete study, obtaining all clinically pertinent information with a minimal number of injections. Because of the osmotic diuresis induced by the contrast media, intravenous and oral fluid supplements are required post catheterization and postural hypotension must be checked for when the patient is allowed up.

Interpretation of the Coronary Arteriogram

Once of interest to angiographers and surgeons only, the viewing and interpretation of coronary angiograms should now be of vital interest to cardiologists if they are to make informed decisions about their patients.

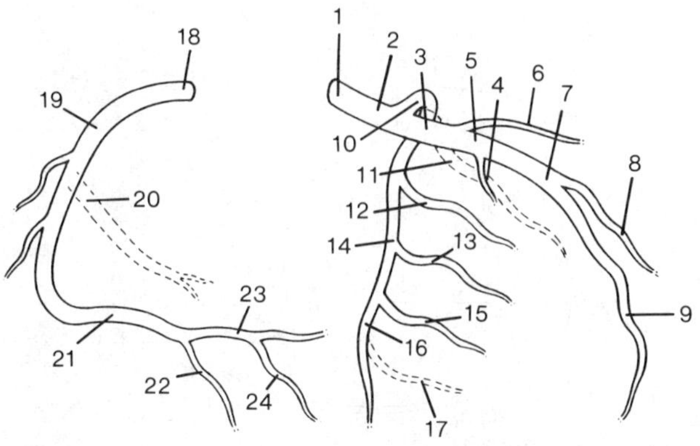

FIGURE 108-28 Diagram of the coronary circulation. Each arterial segment is evaluated carefully in all views and the degree of stenosis is determined. Left main coronary artery 1, 2; left anterior descending coronary artery 3, 5, 7, 9; diagonal branches 6, 8; major septal perforating branch 4; circumflex coronary artery in the atrioventricular groove 10, 14, 16; ramus intermedius 11; obtuse marginal branches 12, 13, 15; posterior descending branch of the circumflex coronary artery if present 17; right coronary artery in the atrioventricular groove 18, 19, 21, 23; large right ventricular branch of the right coronary artery 20; posterior descending branch of the right coronary artery 22; left ventricular branch of the right coronary artery 24. *(From S. B. King III and J. S. Douglas, Jr., "Coronary Arteriography and Angioplasty," McGraw-Hill Book Company, New York, 1985, p. 363. Reproduced with permission from the publisher and authors.)*

The coronary arteriogram should be viewed in a systematic fashion. Because coronary anatomy can be quite variable, one needs to view the films with an eye toward making sure the entire left ventricular epicardial surface and septum are adequately supplied and that no gaps exist. If significant gaps are found, then an occluded or anomalous artery is likely. The coronary arteries should be viewed one at a time, and some division of arterial segments such as suggested by the American Heart Association[128] should be made (Fig. 108–28). Areas of foreshortening and overlap should be examined in other views to convince the observer that there is not a hidden lesion. It is helpful for several observers to study the arteriogram. As each segment is viewed, a systematic scoring and recording system is mandatory if consistency is to be maintained and no segments are to be overlooked.

Angiographic Views

Filming is done in a number of projections such that all coronary arteries can be visualized throughout their lengths and significant disease can be detected and quantified. Multiple views in the transverse plane (Figs. 108–29 to 108–31) were utilized until 1973 when Bunnell reported the advantages of obtaining views incorporating sagittal angulation of the x-ray

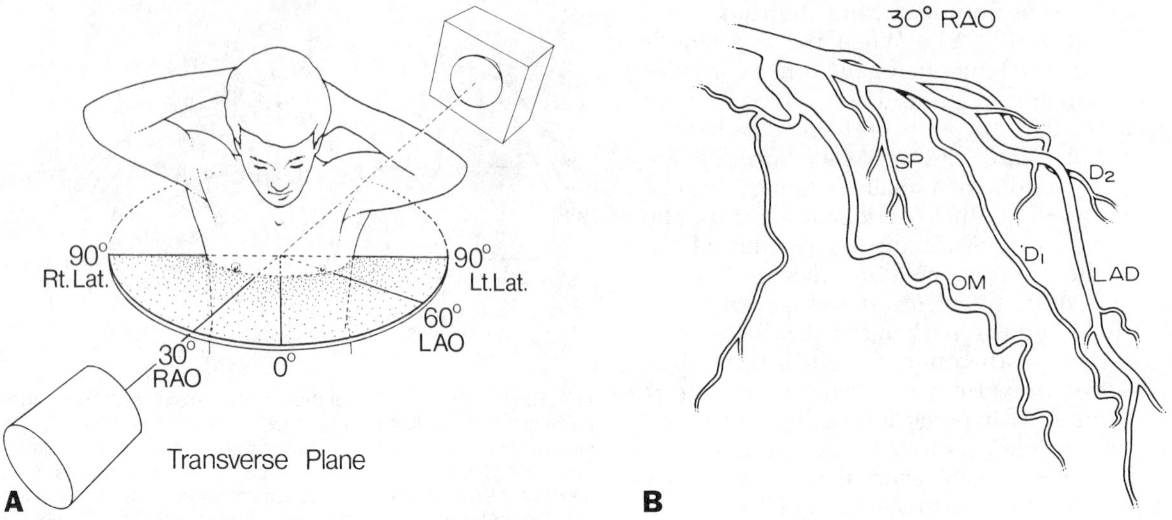

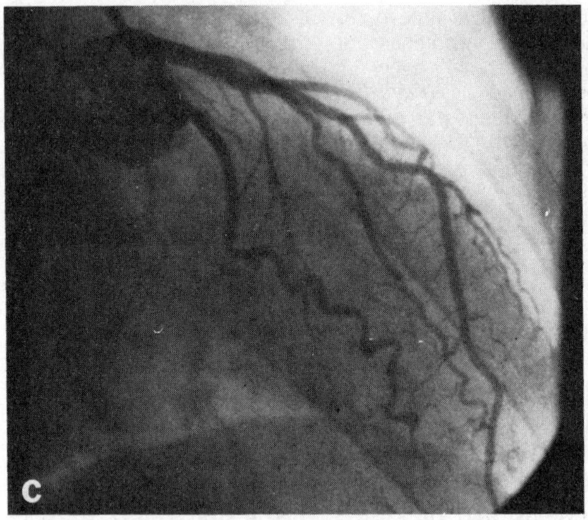

FIGURE 108-29 Diagrammatic representation of the standard right anterior oblique (RAO) view of the left coronary angiogram, the direction of the x-ray beam, and the position of the overhead image intensifier. Most of the left coronary artery is well visualized in this projection, although there is considerable overlap of the mid left anterior descending artery and the diagonal branches. When the left main, circumflex, and diagonal branches have a leftward initial course, the long axis of these arterial segments is projected away from the image intensifier, preventing optimal visualization from the RAO view. The image intensifier is placed anteriorly in an RAO position relative to the patient. *(From S. B. King III, J. S. Douglas, Jr., and D. C. Morris, New Angiographic Views for Coronary Arteriography, in J. W. Hurst (ed.), Update IV: The Heart, McGraw-Hill Book Company, New York, 1981, p. 203. Reproduced with permission from the publisher, editor, and author.)*

beam along the long axis of the body (Fig. 108–32). The use of these views (Figs. 108–33 and 108–34) greatly enhances the ability to visualize the proximal left coronary artery, unmasking lesions that would otherwise be missed in up to 20 percent of patients and significantly improving diagnosis in an additional 30 to 40 percent.[129–131] The evolution of a new generation of x-ray equipment to obtain these views has revolutionized coronary arteriography.[132] In most laboratories, standard views of the left coronary artery are the frontal view, 30° RAO, 45° LAO, 45° LAO with 30° cranial angulation, 30° RAO with 30° cranial, and 30° RAO with 15° caudal angulation. Other views may be needed to separate overlapping vessels or to focus in on a particular problem area. The right coronary artery is usually visualized in the right and left oblique projections, and sagittally angulated views are frequently helpful in evaluating the proximal posterior descending artery (Figs. 108–35 and 108–36). The use of sagittally angulated views, extensively reviewed recently,[132] also provides for improved visualization of left ventricular wall motion and mitral valve motion and for evaluation of the left ventricular outflow tract.

The Left Coronary Artery

The ostium of the left coronary artery originates from the left sinus of Valsalva near the sinotubular ridge. The main left coronary usually courses to the left and slightly anterior. After a quite variable length, it gives rise at near right angles to the circumflex artery and continues in a straight line as the anterior descending artery (Figs. 108–37 and 108–38). The left orifice and the left main coronary artery are best seen in a direct frontal view or in a shallow LAO or RAO projection or shallow LAO with 30° cranial angulation. The diagonal artery may arise between the circumflex and anterior descending arteries as a trifurcation of the left main coronary artery, or the diagonal branch may originate from the anterior descending artery and course over the anterolateral free wall of the left ventricle. The diagonal branches are seen on side in the RAO view; however the origin is obscured by overlap with the anterior descending artery (Figs. 108–29, 108–37, and 108–38). The LAO view separates the anterior descending artery and diagonals somewhat; however, because of the frequent horizontal orientation of these arteries, there may be considerable foreshortening.

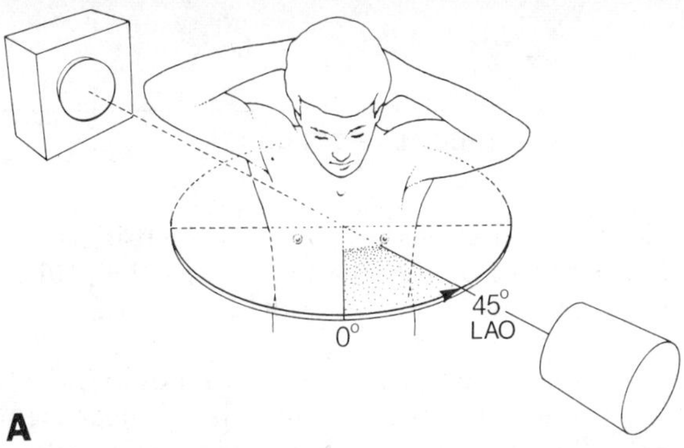

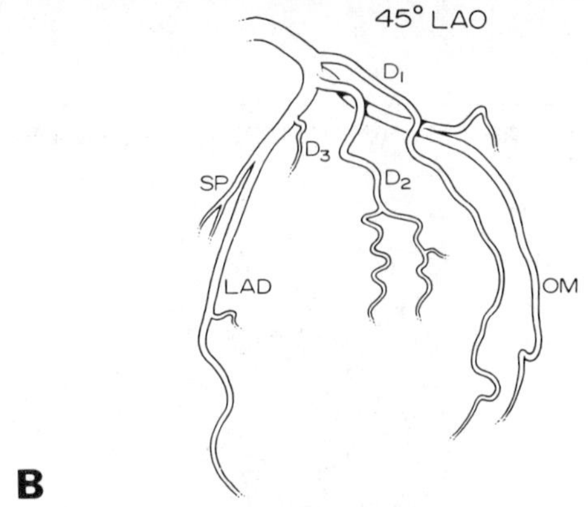

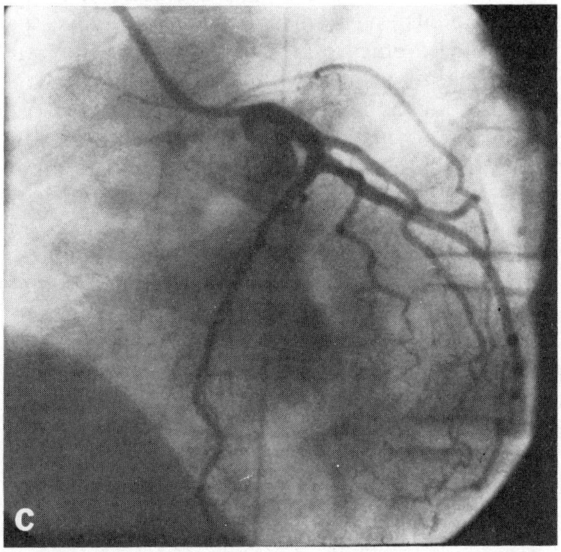

FIGURE 108-30 Diagrammatic representation of the left anterior oblique (LAO) left coronary angiogram and the direction of the x-ray beam in this view. The value of this view depends in large part on the orientation of the long axis of the heart. When the heart is relatively horizontal, the left anterior descending (LAD) coronary artery and diagonal branches are seen end-on throughout much of the course. In this illustration, the longitudinal axis is an intermediate position, and there is moderate foreshortening of the anterior descending and diagonal branches in their proximal portions (compare with Fig. 108-33). The LAO projection is frequently inadequate to visualize the proximal LAD and its branches; the left main segment, which is directed toward the image tube and therefore foreshortened; and the proximal circumflex coronary artery, which may be obscured by overlapping vessels, as in this illustration. The LAO projection is frequently used to visualize the distal LAD and its branches, the mid-circumflex coronary artery in the atrioventricular (AV) groove, and the distal right coronary artery that is filling via collaterals from the left coronary artery. The image intensifier is above the patient in an LAO position. *(From S. B. King III, J. S. Douglas, Jr., and D. C. Morris, New Angiographic Views for Coronary Arteriography, in J. W. Hurst (ed.), Update IV: The Heart, McGraw-Hill Book Company, New York, 1981, p. 204. Reproduced with permission from the publisher, editor, and author.)*

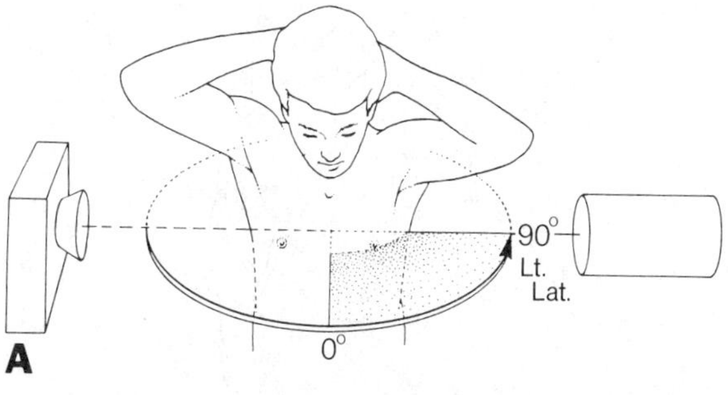

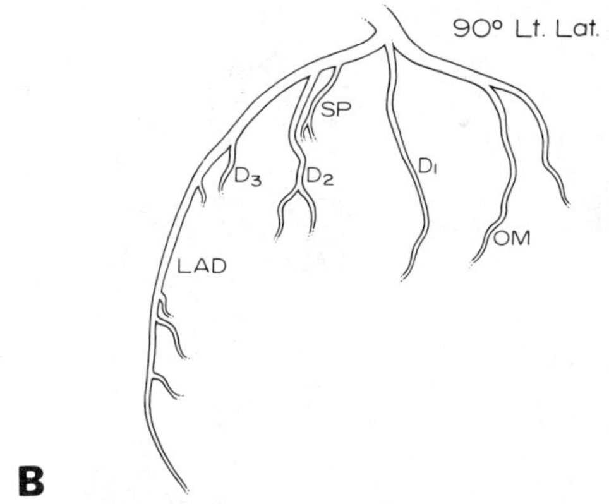

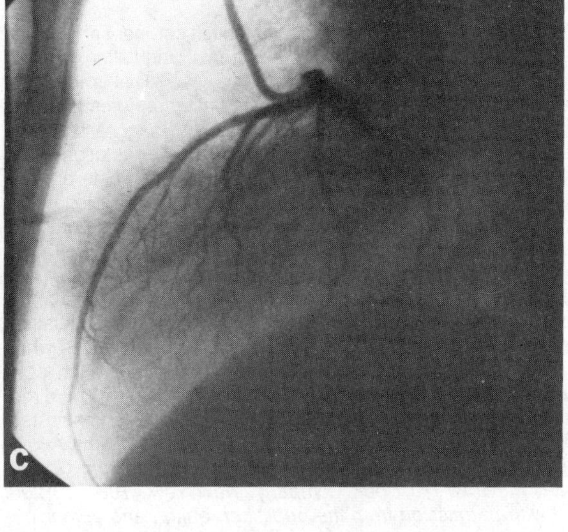

FIGURE 108-31 Diagrammatic illustrations of the left lateral or 90° LAO view of the left coronary arteriogram and direction of the x-ray beam. The left lateral view of the left coronary artery is most useful for analyzing the proximal and mid-LAD by avoiding overlap with the diagonal branches, which commonly take an inferior course from the LAD in this projection. The most proximal portion of the diagonal branches may not be well visualized since the long axis of these segments may be in the direction of the x-ray beam. The leftward-directed left main segment is foreshortened in this view (compare with Fig. 108-30). In this view, the image intensifier is placed on the patient's left, and the x-ray beam has a right-to-left direction in the horizontal plane. (*From S. B. King III, J. S. Douglas, Jr., and D. C. Morris, New Angiographic Views for Coronary Arteriography, in J. W. Hurst (ed.), Update IV: The Heart, McGraw-Hill Book Company, New York, 1981, p. 205. Reproduced with permission from the publisher, editor, and author.*)

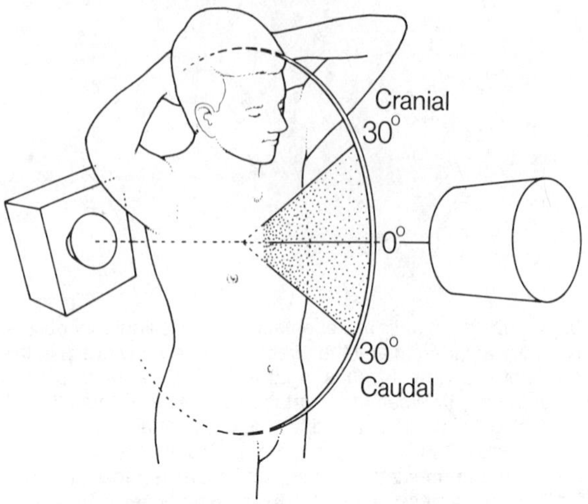

FIGURE 108-32 Illustration of sagittal angulation of x-ray beam in coronary arteriography. (*From S. B. King III, J. S. Douglas, Jr., and D. C. Morris, New Angiographic Views for Coronary Arteriography, in J. W. Hurst, (ed.), Update IV: The Heart, McGraw-Hill Book Company, New York, 1981, p. 205. Reproduced with permission from the publisher, editor, and author.*)

Cranial angulation of the overhead intensifier with shallow LAO or RAO rotation is most helpful in separating the proximal anterior descending artery and its diagonal branches (Figs. 108–33 and 108–35). The anterior descending artery continues in the AV groove toward the apex, giving rise at near-right angles to the septal perforating arteries that go deep into the muscular septum. The first septal perforator may arise before or after the first diagonal, and is usually the largest septal artery. The septal vessels differ from the epicardial arteries in that they are straighter and move little with cardiac action, in contrast to the buckling of epicardial arteries that frequently occurs with systole. The left anterior descending artery usually continues around the apex but may end short of the apex in association with an unusually long posterior descending artery. The anterior descending artery is usually best visualized in the RAO view and in a cranially angulated shallow oblique view unless the orientation of the anterior descending artery is unusually superior, in which case a caudally angulated LAO view or a straight lateral view may be helpful.

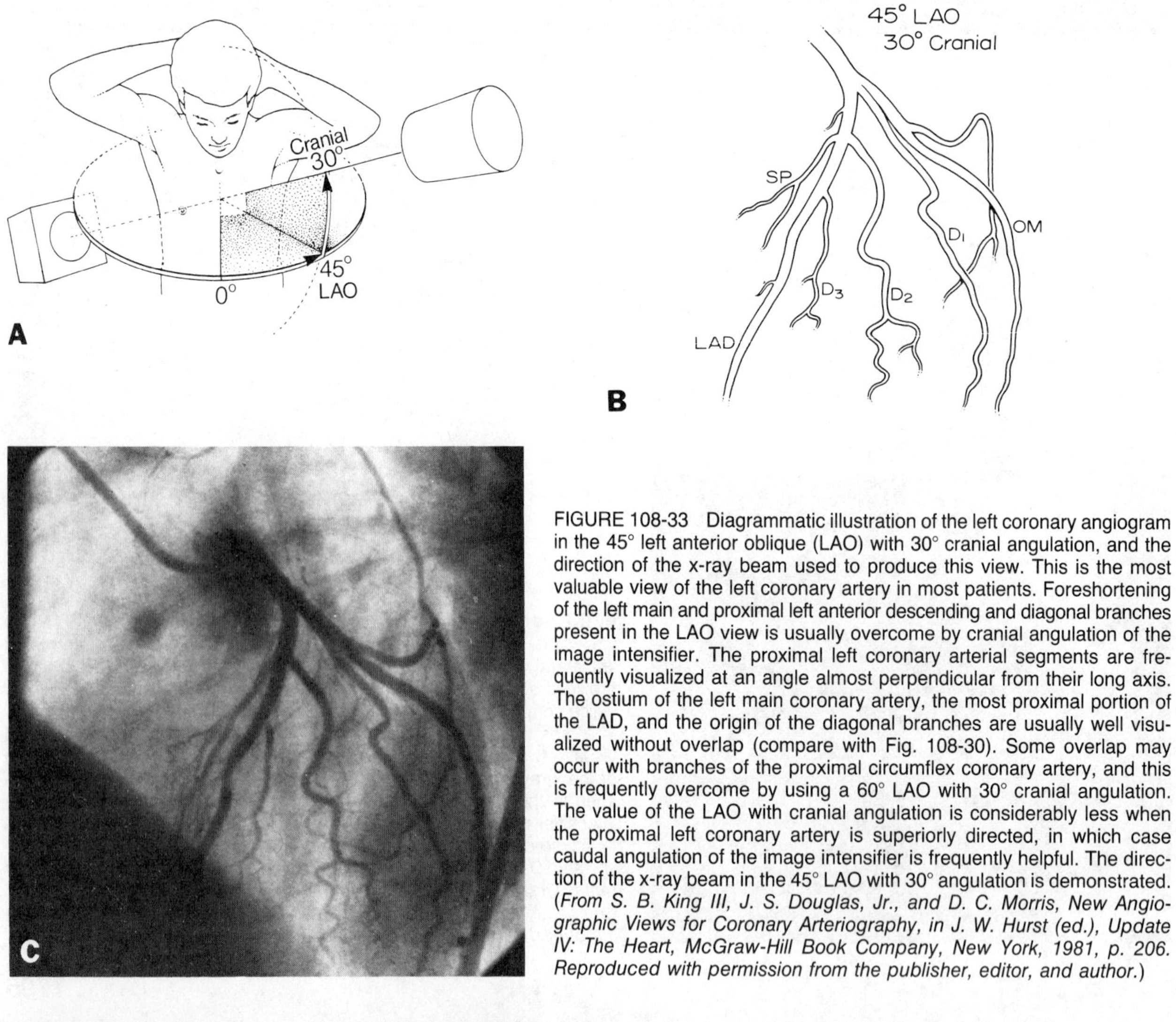

FIGURE 108-33 Diagrammatic illustration of the left coronary angiogram in the 45° left anterior oblique (LAO) with 30° cranial angulation, and the direction of the x-ray beam used to produce this view. This is the most valuable view of the left coronary artery in most patients. Foreshortening of the left main and proximal left anterior descending and diagonal branches present in the LAO view is usually overcome by cranial angulation of the image intensifier. The proximal left coronary arterial segments are frequently visualized at an angle almost perpendicular from their long axis. The ostium of the left main coronary artery, the most proximal portion of the LAD, and the origin of the diagonal branches are usually well visualized without overlap (compare with Fig. 108-30). Some overlap may occur with branches of the proximal circumflex coronary artery, and this is frequently overcome by using a 60° LAO with 30° cranial angulation. The value of the LAO with cranial angulation is considerably less when the proximal left coronary artery is superiorly directed, in which case caudal angulation of the image intensifier is frequently helpful. The direction of the x-ray beam in the 45° LAO with 30° angulation is demonstrated. (*From S. B. King III, J. S. Douglas, Jr., and D. C. Morris, New Angiographic Views for Coronary Arteriography, in J. W. Hurst (ed.), Update IV: The Heart, McGraw-Hill Book Company, New York, 1981, p. 206. Reproduced with permission from the publisher, editor, and author.*)

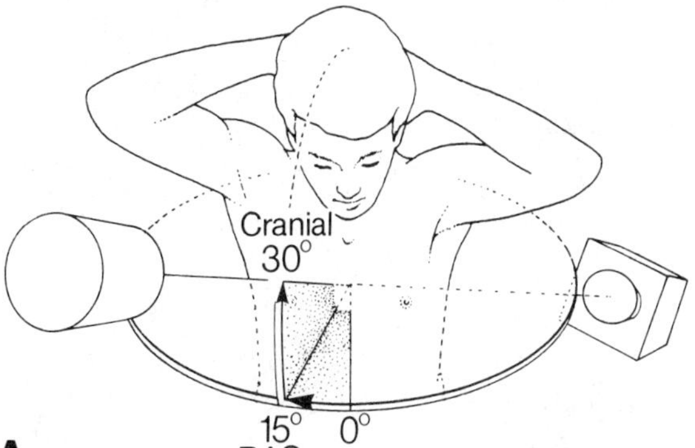

A

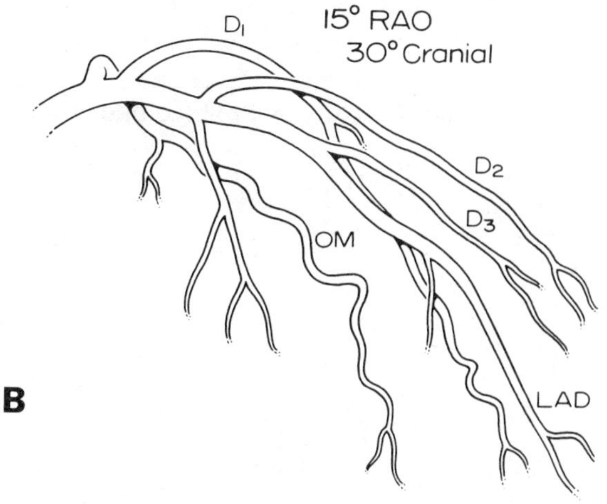

B

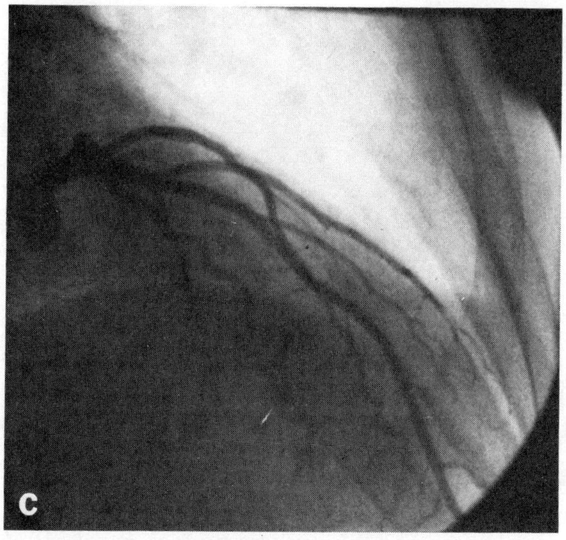

C

FIGURE 108-34 Diagrammatic illustration of the left coronary angiogram in the 15° RAO with 30° cranial angulation, and the direction of the x-ray beam. This view is particularly helpful in analyzing the mid-left anterior descending artery and the diagonal branch points. Overlap with diagonal branches is usually avoided. The origin of the circumflex artery may be well seen, as in this illustration. *(From S. B. King III, J. S. Douglas, Jr., and D. C. Morris, New Angiographic Views for Coronary Arteriography, in J. W. Hurst (ed.) Update IV: The Heart, McGraw-Hill Book Company, New York, 1981, p. 208. Reproduced with permission from the publisher, editor, and author.)*

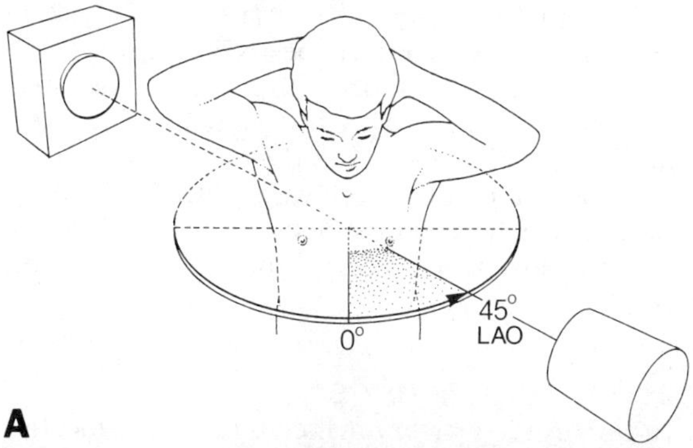

A

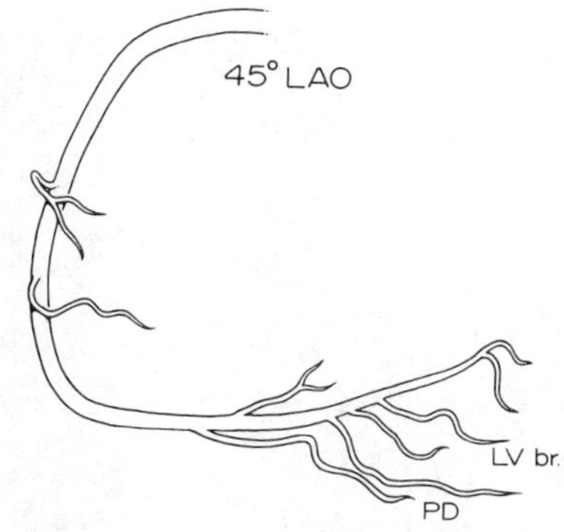

B

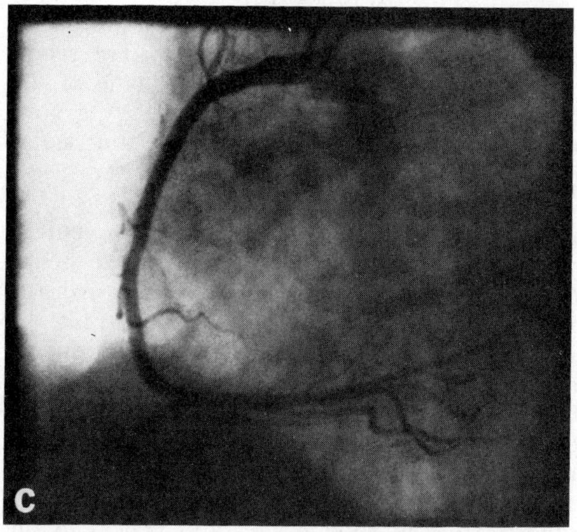

C

FIGURE 108-35 Diagrammatic illustration of the right coronary artery in the 45° LAO projection and direction of the x-ray beam. This view is excellent for visualizing the proximal mid and distal right coronary artery in the AV groove since the direction of the x-ray beam is perpendicular to these arterial segments. Ostial lesions of the right coronary artery are not well visualized if the proximal right coronary artery takes an anterior direction from the aorta and therefore originates in a direction parallel to the x-ray beam. This can usually be overcome by turning to a more severe left oblique projection. The posterior descending and left ventricular branches of the right coronary artery, which pass down the posterior aspect of the heart toward the apex, are severely foreshortened since the long axis of these vessels is in the same direction as the x-ray beam. The proximal posterior descending branches can be visualized by cranial angulation of the overhead intensifier (see Fig. 108-36) or from a right oblique view. The image intensifier is in the standard LAO position. *(From S. B. King III, J. S. Douglas, Jr., and D. C. Morris, New Angiographic Views for Coronary Arteriography, in J. W. Hurst (ed.), Update IV: The Heart, McGraw-Hill Book Company, New York, 1981, p. 208. Reproduced with permission from the publisher, editor, and author.)*

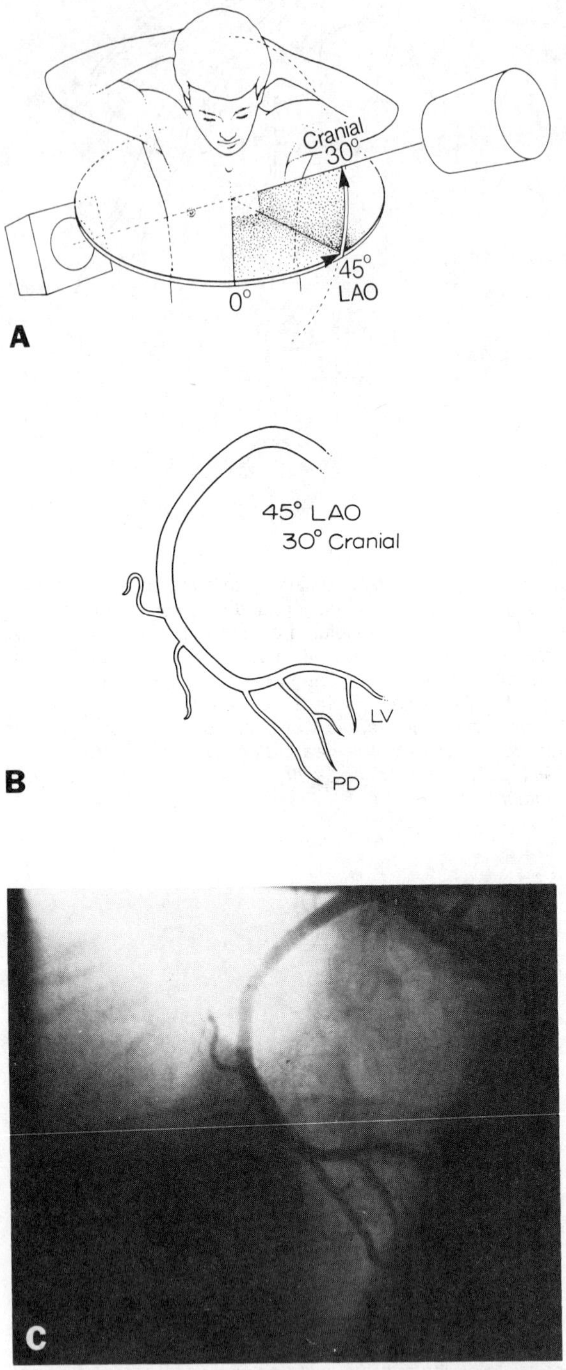

FIGURE 108-36 Diagrammatic illustration of the right coronary artery in 30° LAO with 30° cranial angulation and direction of the x-ray beam. Cranial angulation of the image intensifier overcomes the problem of foreshortening of the posterior descending and left ventricular branches observed in Fig. 108-35. Lesions in the posterior descending or left ventricular branches can be well visualized. When the right coronary artery originates anteriorly from the aorta, the proximal portion of the vessel is frequently well seen in this projection. With anomalous origin of the left anterior descending artery from the right coronary artery, this view is helpful since the standard LAO view produces considerable foreshortening of the anomalous artery. The direction of the x-ray beam is the same as in Fig. 108-33. *(From S. B. King III, J. S. Douglas, Jr., and D. C. Morris, New Angiographic Views for Coronary Arteriography, in J. W. Hurst (ed.), Update IV: The Heart, McGraw-Hill Book Company, New York, 1981, p. 210. Reproduced with permission from the publisher, editor, and author.)*

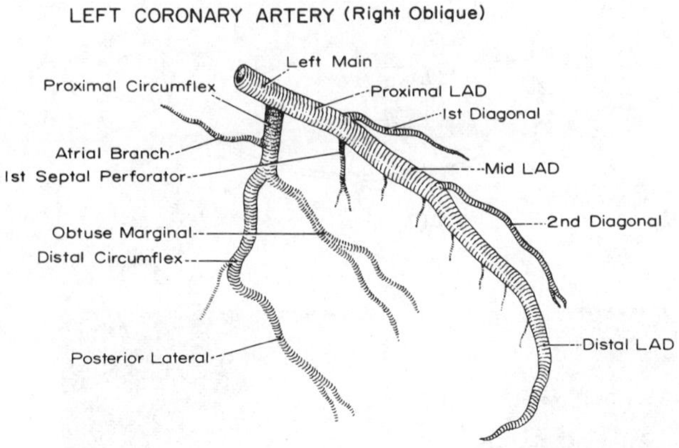

FIGURE 108-37 Anatomy of the left coronary tree in the right oblique view.

The circumflex coronary artery, after its right-angle origin from the left anterior descending (LAD) artery, travels in the AV groove. Its course is quite variable. The artery may terminate in one or more large, obtuse marginal branches which course over the lateral to posterolateral left ventricular free wall, or it may continue as a large artery in the AV groove and in 10 to 15 percent of cases give rise to a posterior descending artery as more commonly occurs from the right coronary artery (Fig. 108–39). When the circumflex artery supplies the major posterior descending artery, it is commonly referred to as a *dominant circumflex artery*. The circumflex artery in the atrioventricular groove is best seen in the LAO view, but surgically more important marginal branches are visualized best in the RAO view. Occasionally proximal stenoses in the circumflex artery are best viewed in an RAO view with 15° caudal angulation, which produces a view as though looking from the superior aspect of the liver toward the left shoulder.

The Right Coronary Artery

The right coronary artery orifice is normally located in the right sinus of Valsalva. It may be high near the sinotubular ridge or above it, or in the mid sinus, or occasionally low near the aortic valve. The artery commonly courses upward from the plane of the aortic valve and then travels in the right AV groove as a conduit to reach the posterior left ventricular wall (Figs. 108–40 and 108–41). Along the way, several vessels arise. The conus branch and sinus node branches arise first, followed by small right ventricular branches. At the acute margin of the heart, there is usually a large branch that courses over the right ventricle. In some cases this may supply the apical portion of the interventricular septum and therefore be of greater importance. The posterior descending artery usually arises before the right coronary artery reaches the crux of the heart (junction of the interventricular and interatrial septa). The posterior descending artery arises from the right coronary artery at right angles and travels in the

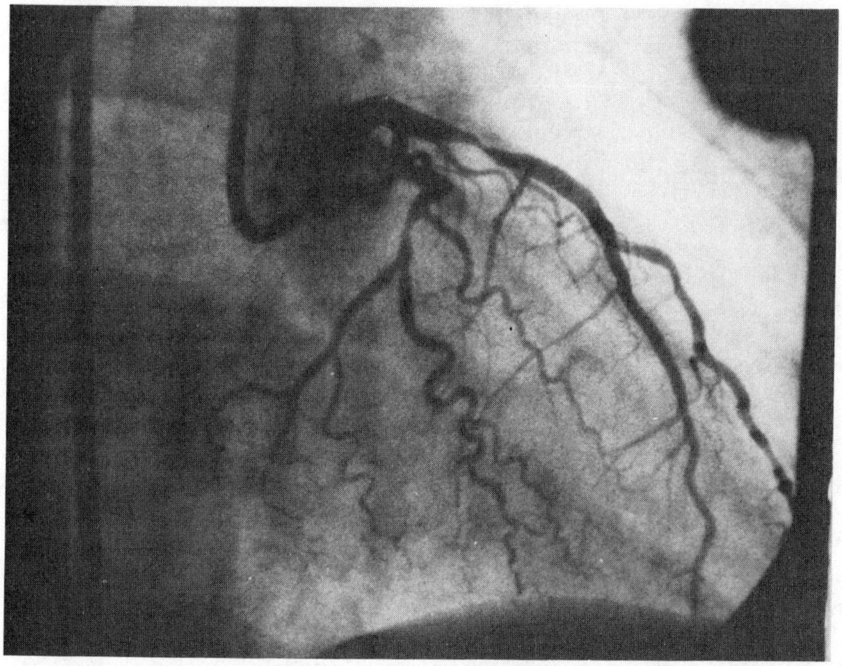

FIGURE 108-38 Right anterior oblique view of the left coronary artery showing high-grade stenosis of the left anterior descending proximal to the first septal perforating branch.

posterior interventricular groove, supplying the perforating branches to the basal and posterior one-third of the septum. A right coronary artery that supplies the major posterior descending branch has been referred to as a *dominant right coronary artery.*

FIGURE 108-39 LAO view of left coronary artery demonstrating dominant circumflex coronary artery giving rise to the posterior descending artery.

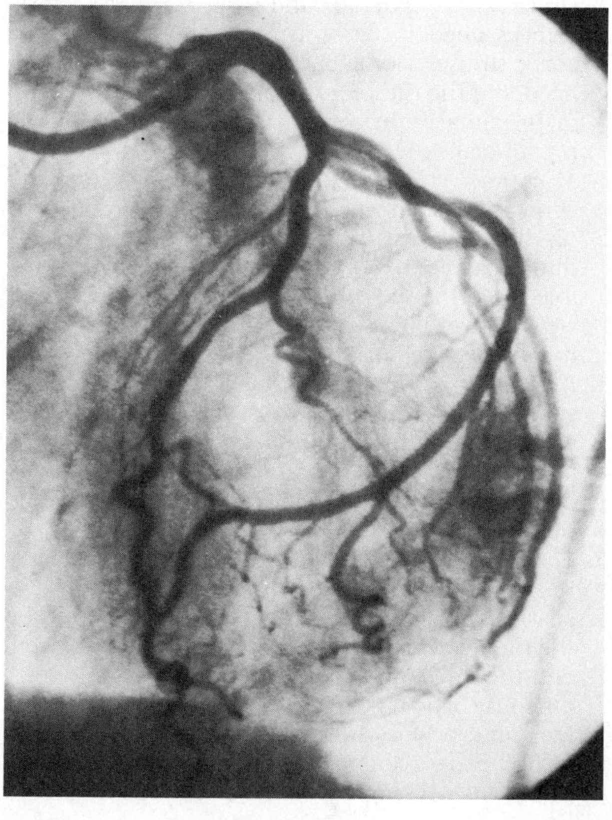

The posterior descending artery usually stops before reaching the apex, but it may curl around the apex in association with a short anterior descending artery to form the loop previously described. After giving rise to the posterior descending artery, the right coronary artery becomes intramyocardial at the crux, gives rise to the atrioventricular node artery, and subsequently returns to the surface, making an inverted U curve (Fig. 108–41). The left ventricular branches of the right coronary artery are variable and cover the same area as the posterolateral branches of a large circumflex system. The proximal conduit portion of the right coronary artery is well seen in standard RAO and LAO views. However, because of its horizontal orientation, the origin of the posterior descending artery is well seen in the RAO

FIGURE 108-40 Anatomy of the right coronary tree.

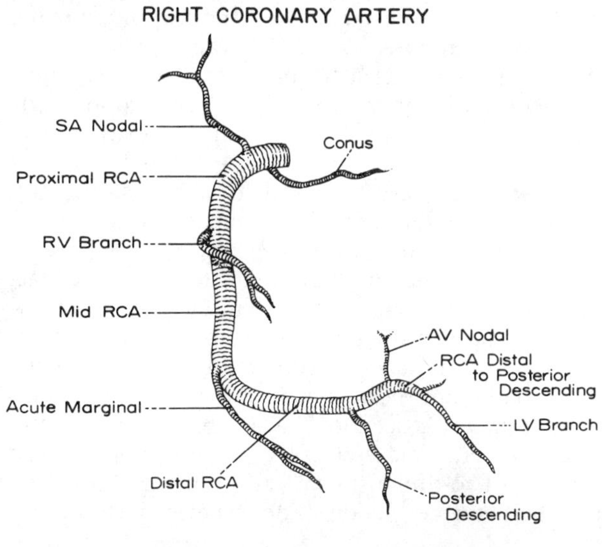

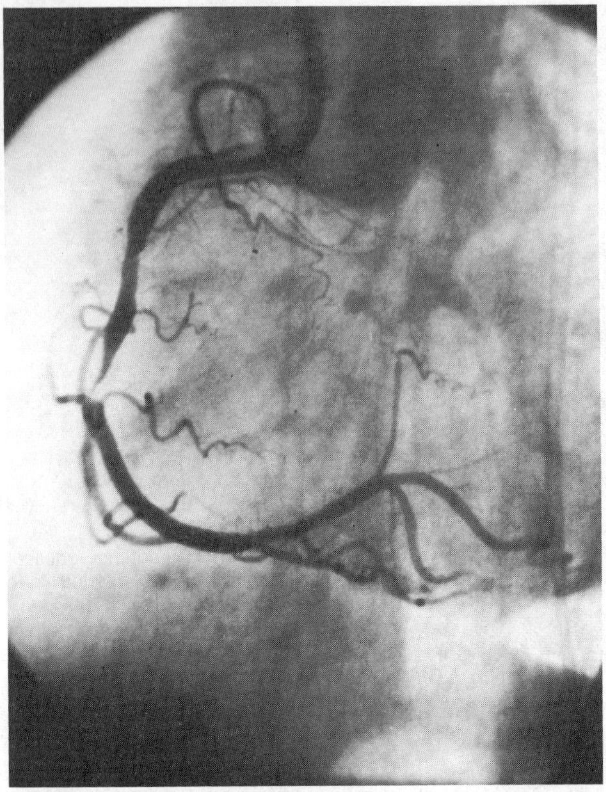

FIGURE 108-41 LAO view of the right coronary artery (RCA) with high-grade lesion in its midportion.

view but foreshortened in the LAO view; to overcome this, cranial angulation of the intensifier is necessary. Pathologic studies indicate that lesions at the takeoff of the posterior descending artery are frequently overlooked if standard oblique views in the transverse plane are used.

Grading Stenoses

Visual inspection of the coronary arteriogram has traditionally been used to assess the severity of coronary artery stenosis. In our laboratory, a system of analyzing each arterial segment has been used and the degree of stenosis recorded as reduction in lumen diameter or cross-sectional area expressed as a percent, with total occlusion being 100 percent. Diseased segments are observed in all views, and the greatest diameter reduction is measured and compared with normal-appearing adjacent segments. Arterial segments are classified into one of six categories: (1) normal, (2) less than 50 percent cross-sectional area reduction, (3) 50 to 74 percent reduction, (4) 75 to 90 percent reduction, (5) greater than 90 percent reduction, and (6) total obstruction. Although cross-sectional area reduction is the measurement that is obviously important, it is true that in a two-dimensional figure, one can see only the diameter reduction. The American Heart Association has recommended that the diameter method be adopted for grading coronary artery stenosis.[128] A 50 percent diameter reduction is equivalent to a 75 percent cross-sectional area reduction and a 75 percent diameter reduction is equal to a 90 percent cross-sectional area reduction. It is readily apparent that it is of great importance to identify which method of expressing stenosis is used. From the standpoint of surgically significant lesions, it has been our practice to consider lesions with greater than 50 percent diameter reduction or 75 percent cross-sectional area reduction as lesions that may produce myocardial ischemia. Lesions in series or long stenoses are of added importance. Quantitative computerized methods of calculating coronary artery stenoses have been devised but have not been applied widely for routine clinical coronary arteriography.[133]

Pitfalls in Coronary Arteriography

There are a number of pitfalls in coronary arteriography that should be looked for and avoided.

1. *Short left main or double left coronary orifices.* When the left main orifice is very short or absent, selective injection of the anterior descending or circumflex arteries may be made (Fig. 108–42). If on viewing an arteriogram, no circumflex or anterior descending artery is seen either filling primarily or through collaterals from the right coronary artery, then the possibility that the artery was missed by subselective injection must be suspected.
2. *Orifice lesions.* The left and right coronary artery orifices need to be seen on a tangent with the aortic sinuses. Some backflow from the orifices is needed if the catheter is lying within the left main or proximal right coronary artery to avoid missing an orifice lesion.
3. *Myocardial bridges.* The anterior descending, diagonal, and marginal branches not uncommonly dip intramyocardially, and the overlying myocardium may act to compress the artery during systole (Fig. 108–43). If the coronary artery is not viewed carefully in diastole, this bridging may give the appearance of an area of stenosis.[134–137]
4. *Foreshortening.* When possible, avoid reading lesions in segments that are seen only coming toward or away from the image intensifier. Dense opacification of segments seen end on may produce the appearance of a lesion in an intervening segment.
5. *Coronary spasm.* Catheter-induced spasm may give the appearance of a lesion (Fig. 108–44). When spasm is suspected (usually at the catheter tip in the right coronary artery), nitrates should be given and the injection repeated in 5 to 10 min. Spontaneous coronary artery spasm is a separate problem, and when this is suspected, nitrates and atropine are avoided since the atropine may play a role in blocking coronary artery spasm. Prov-

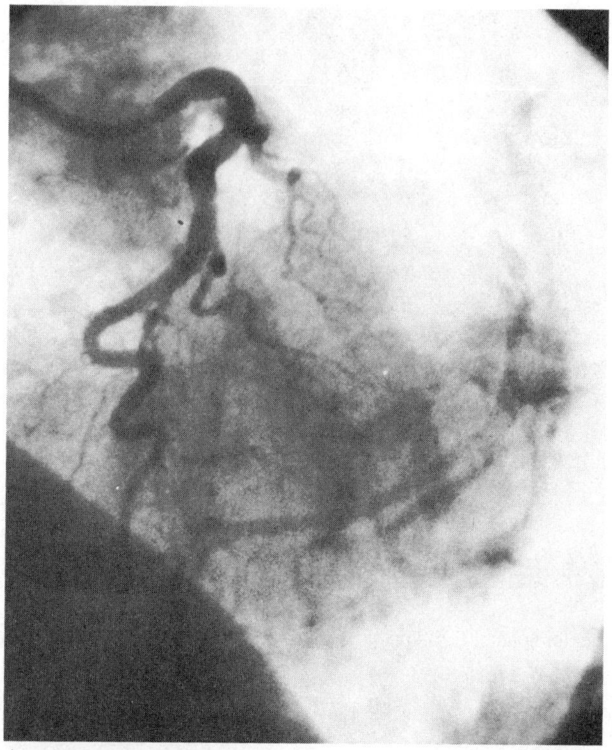

A

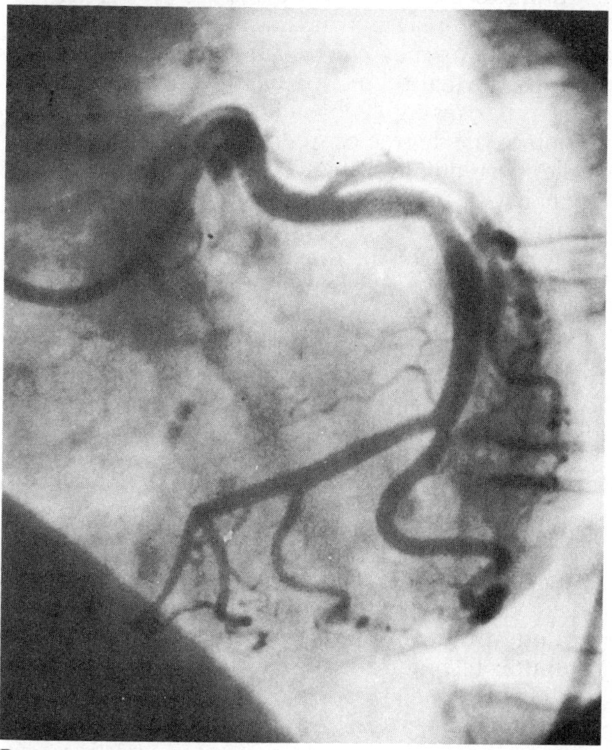

B

FIGURE 108-42 *A.* LAO view of selective injection into left anterior descending (LAD) artery. *B* LAO view of selective injection into circumflex artery.

ocation with ergot derivatives will identify most patients with spontaneous coronary artery spasm.[108–112]

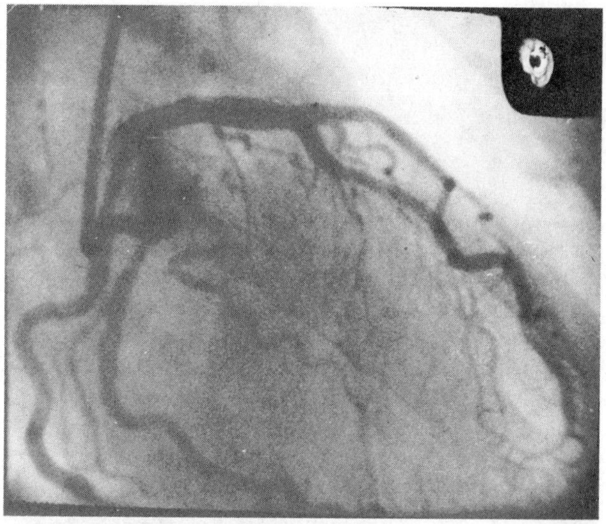

A

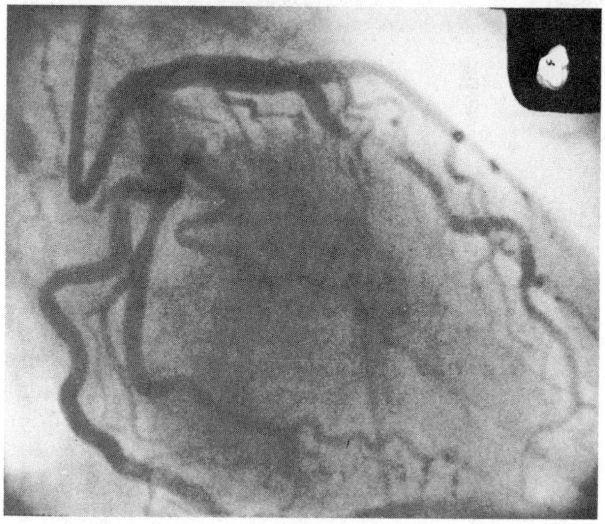

B

FIGURE 108-43 RAO view of left coronary artery system. *A.* Diastolic appearance of anterior descending artery showing smooth lumen. *B.* Systolic appearance showing obliteration of the lumen by an overriding muscular bridge.

6. *Anomalous coronary arteries.* Coronary arteries may arise from ectopic locations, or a single coronary artery may be present.[138–157] Only by ensuring that the entire epicardial surface has an adequate arterial supply can one be confident that all branches have been visualized.
7. *Totally occluded arteries or vein grafts.* Absence of vascularity in a portion of the heart may indicate total occlusion of its arterial supply. Usually, however, collateral channels permit visualization of the distal occluded artery unless it is an acute occlusion.[158–162] Vessels filled solely by collaterals have very little pressure supporting their walls and may appear smaller than their actual lumen size, giving a false sense of pessimism about the possibilities for surgical anastomosis.

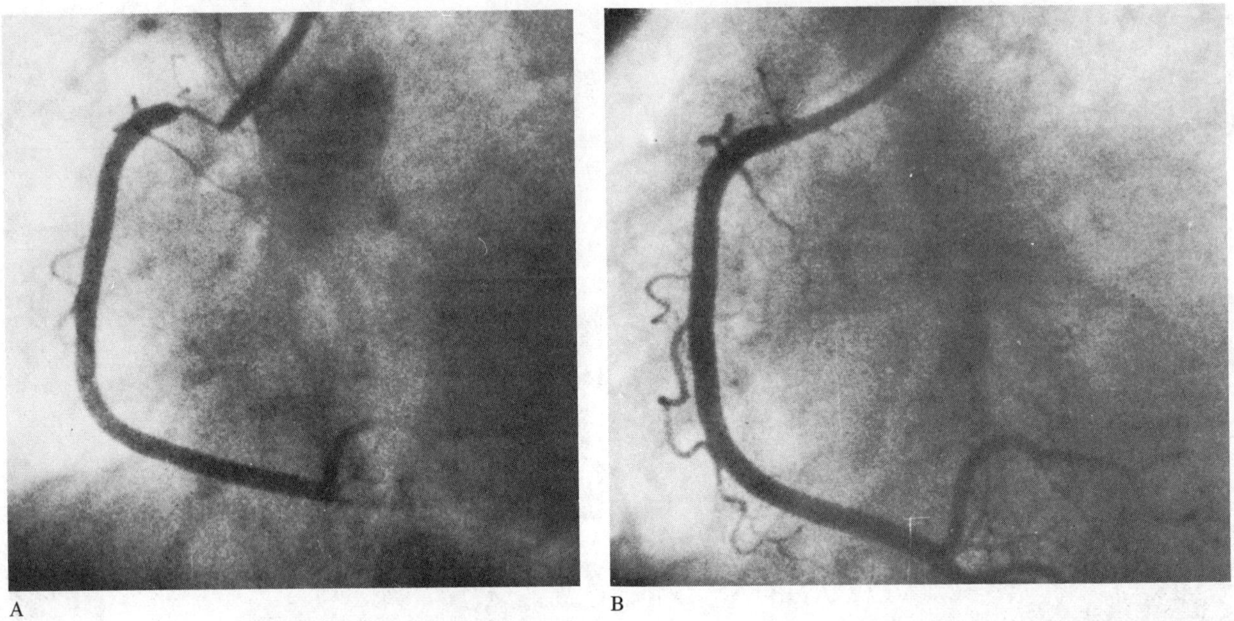

FIGURE 108-44 *A.* LAO view of right coronary injection showing pericatheter spasm. *B.* Same view following nitroglycerin showing relief of spasm.

Limitations of Coronary Arteriography

In spite of significant improvements in the quality of coronary arteriographic studies as a result of more sophisticated x-ray imaging systems, there remain a number of limitations of the method that one must not lose sight of. Film interpretation is subjective. Different angiographers may interpret the same film differently, and the same angiographer may render a different interpretation at a time remote from the first reading.[163,164] It has been reported that the average standard deviation of estimation of any segmental stenosis by experienced angiographers may be as high as 20 percent and that disagreement about the number of major vessels with 70 percent stenosis may occur 30 percent of the time.[164] These reported studies, however, utilized only views in the transverse plane, imposing greater interpretive burdens than are encountered when sagittally angulated views are obtained. Further studies using sagittally angulated views would be expected to show less variability in interpreting coronary arteriograms. The interobserver and intraobserver variability in interpreting coronary arteriograms is not unlike the interpretive differences in chest x-rays or other diagnostic studies involving human error and judgment. Routine use of several readers has been shown to reduce interpretive error.[164] Although correlation of angiography with postmortem findings has been acceptable in most studies,[165–176] certain coronary pathologic-anatomic factors may favor angiographic underestimation of the degree of stenosis present in any arterial segment. In large part, this is due to the tendency for diffuse atheromatous narrowing of the coronary arteries to occur. In attempting to grade stenosis of an obviously narrow segment, one may not have a normal segment for comparison or may choose for comparison an apparently normal segment which in fact has diffuse tabular narrowing.[168–170] This leads to underestimation of the degree of stenosis present. Pathologic studies currently available probably overestimate the frequency of this problem since the pathologic material available for study represents the severest end of the spectrum of the disease. Eccentric atherosclerotic plaques also may be underestimated unless the minor axis of the stenotic lumen is visualized. Sagittally angulated views are particularly valuable in this regard. Very discrete membrane-like lesions, fortunately rare, may be missed unless they are visualized directly in the plane of the lesion. Recent preliminary pathologic studies show poor correlation between left main coronary stenosis at autopsy and that at angiography, especially in the presence of a short left main coronary artery, and point up the importance of sufficient angiographic views and excellent interpretive skills in evaluating this critical portion of the coronary circulation.[171] Quantitative computer techniques have shown excellent correlation between the cross-sectional luminal area of stenotic lesions at arteriography and direct planimetered measurements of distended postmortem specimens.[172] Dynamic phenomena, not active at the time of the study, may be important. "Hit and run" events such as coronary embolization or thrombosis with subsequent resolution, coronary artery spasm, and even primary coronary artery dissection may leave left ventricular scars but not result in coronary angiographic findings.

Risk of Coronary Arteriography

As with any invasive procedure, there is a finite risk to the patient undergoing coronary arteriography. The magnitude of the risk is influenced by certain factors definable prior to the procedure (skill of the angiographer and instability of clinical symptoms) but primarily by the extent of the disease found at coronary arteriography and left ventriculography.[99,125,173,174] Physicians referring patients for coronary arteriograms must be aware of the complication rate in a given laboratory and, when practical, should achieve stability of clinical symptoms prior to study. That is not to say that unstable patients should not be studied, but the physician must balance the risk of the procedure and potential benefit against the risk of not doing the procedure (see Chap. 45). The frequency of major complications has decreased in active centers (Table 108–1).

Major complications are of two types. *Local arterial complications* consist of arterial occlusion or stenosis, hematoma formation, false aneurysm, and infection. These occur more frequently with the brachial approach. The other and more lethal group of complications relates to *thromboembolic events* or depression of myocardial function due to infarction or acute ischemia. Thromboemboli are more commonly due to multiple catheter and guide wire exchanges during which thrombus material is stripped from the catheter surface at the puncture site only to be deposited on a subsequent catheter, as suggested by Takaro and associates.[180] The addition of systemic heparinization was felt to have reduced thromboembolic complications in some laboratories. However the early CASS report[174] and that by Abrams and Adams[173] found that the use of heparin did not influence complication rates. Of equal or more importance may be the routine use of catheter debriding techniques with vigorous aspiration and flushing of the catheter in the abdominal aorta to dislodge any retained thrombus material. Minor allergic reactions to contrast media in the form of urticaria occur commonly, but anaphylactic and pyrogenic reactions are exceedingly rare.[177–179] Radiation exposure to the patient, estimated as 20 to 45 R, has little risk unless multiple restudies are needed.

Reported mortality rates related to coronary arteriography range from 0.05 to 4 percent, and virtually all deaths occur in patients with severe, multivessel coronary disease or left main coronary artery stenosis.[125,173,174] A widely quoted acceptable mortality rate for coronary arteriography is 0.1 percent. Case selection, however, may play an important role in determining mortality. Studies in predominantly stable patients will result in a very low mortality rate. On the other hand, if a broad spectrum of patients is studied—including those with preinfarction angina, acute myocardial infarction, and complications of myocardial infarction such as heart failure, cardiogenic shock, ruptured interventricular septum, and ruptured papillary muscle—complication rates will be higher, depending on the frequency with which sicker patients are studied. The overall mortality rate in the CASS reports was 0.07 to 0.2 percent; however it was 0.8 percent in patients with left main coronary artery stenosis.[174,175] The point to be made is that laboratory and surgical teams must be prepared to act in the best interest of severely ill patients and not be overly concerned with an arbitrary mortality figure.

Left Ventriculography

Left ventriculography is the standard method for evaluating left ventricular performance in the coronary angiography laboratory. The normal pattern of left ventricular contraction is a uniform and almost concentric inward movement of all points along the endocardial surface during systole. Harrison[181] introduced the term *asynergy,* which has been used to indicate a disturbance of the normal contraction pattern. The Ad Hoc Committee for Grading of Coronary Artery Disease of the American Heart Association[128] has recommended that five RAO segments and two LAO left ventricular segments be defined and characterized as to wall motion (Figs. 108–45 and 108–46). Herman and coworkers[182]

TABLE 108–1 Complications of Coronary Arteriography

	CASS*		SOC CARD Angiography†[176]	Abrams and Adams[173]			
				Femoral		Brachial	
	1979[174]	1983[175]		H	NH	H	NH
Death	0.0020	0.0007	0.0014	0.0016	0.0015	0.0010	0.0030
Myocardial infarction	0.0025	0.0027	0.0007	0.0018	0.0023	0.0014	0.0023
Cerebral emboli	0.0003	0.0007	0.0007	0.0008	0.0010	0.0008	0.0009
Arterial complications	0.0080	0.0082	0.0057				
Ventricular fibrillation	0.0063	0.0038	0.0056				

*CASS = Coronary Artery Surgery Study.
†Society for Cardiac Angiography (includes noncoronary procedures).
Note: H = systemic heparin; NH = no systemic heparin.

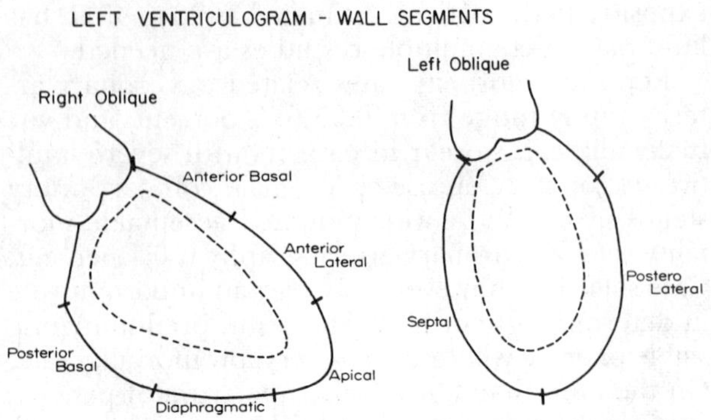

FIGURE 108-45 Left ventricular wall silhouette in RAO and LAO views.

classified left ventricular asynergy according to the severity of the contractile abnormality, and a similar classification of a left ventricular wall motion was recommended by the Ad Hoc Committee; normal (normal wall motion of the indicated ventricular segment), reduced (reduced velocity and/or amplitude of indicated wall segment), none (absence of appropriate wall motion of indicated ventricular segment), dyskinetic (paradoxical wall motion of the indicated segment), aneurysmal (bulging during systole and diastole with sharply defined margins of indicated ventricular segment), and/or undefined wall motion. Many angiographers use the term *akinesis* when no wall motion is present and the term *hypokinesis* when the wall motion is reduced.

FIGURE 108-46 Left ventriculography performed with biplane technique. *A.* RAO of left ventricle (LV) at end diastole. *B.* RAO of left ventricle at end systole. (Notice contraction abnormality of anterior wall.) *C.* LAO at end diastole. *D.* LAO at end systole.

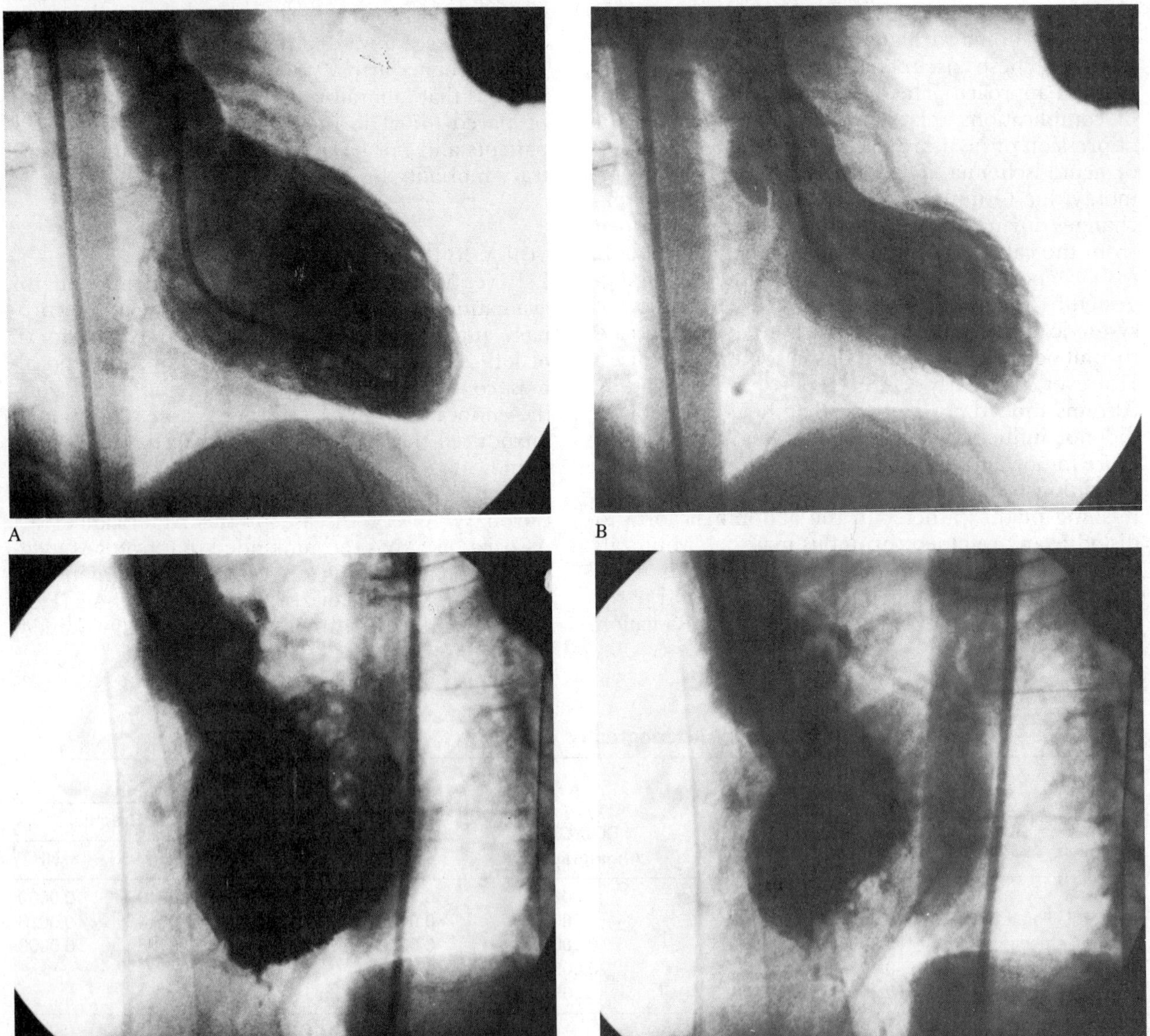

The ability of the left ventricle to function as a pump is best analyzed by left ventricular volume determinations. If it is assumed that the left ventricular chamber is ellipsoid and if the area-length method of Dodge and his associates is employed,[183] left ventricular volumes may be calculated and regression equations utilized to correct the consistent overestimation that occurs. Single-plane and biplane volume determinations may differ significantly in patients with coronary artery disease and nonhomogeneous contraction patterns. In particular, the single-plane right anterior oblique or lateral left ventriculogram frequently underestimates overall left ventricular contraction because it selectively visualizes the anterior and inferior free walls of the left ventricle, which are most commonly involved in myocardial infarction. Vogel et al.[184] found that the single-plane RAO left ventriculogram underestimated ejection fraction in 70 percent of patients with coronary artery disease. For this reason, biplane left ventriculography is frequently desirable in evaluating patients with coronary artery disease.

References

1. Liljestrand, G.: In "Le Prix Nobel en 1956," Nobel Foundation, Stockholm, 1957.
2. Steckelberg, J. M., Ulietstra, R. E., Ludwig, J., and Mann, R. J.: Werner Forssman (1904–1979) and His Unusual Success Story, *Mayo Clin. Proc.*, 54:746, 1979.
3. Forssman, W.: Die Sondierung des rechten Herzens, *Berl. Klin. Wochenschr.*, 8:2085, 1929.
4. Cournand, A.: Cardiac Catheterization: Development of the Technique, Its Contribution to Experimental Medicine and Its Initial Application to Man, *Acta Med. Scand. Suppl.*, 579:7, 1975.
5. Brannon, E. S., Weens, H. S., and Warren, J. V.: Atrial Septal Defect: Study of Hemodynamics by the Technique of Right Heart Catheterization, *Am. J. Med. Sci.*, 210:480, 1945.
6. Grossman, W. (ed.): "Cardiac Catheterization and Angiography," 2d ed., Lea & Febiger, Philadelphia, 1980.
7. Johnsrude, I. S., and Jackson, D. C.: "A Practical Approach to Angiography," 1st ed., Little, Brown and Company, Boston, 1979.
8. Friesinger, G. C., Adams, D. F., Bourassa, M. G., et al.: Optimal Resources for Examination of the Heart and Lungs: Cardiac Catheterization and Radiographic Facilities, *Circulation*, 68: 893A, 1983.
9. Rowe, R. D.: "Cardiac Catheterization in Heart Disease in Infancy and Childhood," 3d ed., The Macmillan Company, New York, 1978, chap. 6, p. 81.
10. Shabetai, R., and Adolph, R. J.: Principles of Cardiac Catheterization, in N. O. Fowler (ed.), "Cardiac Diagnosis and Treatment," 3d ed., Harper & Row, Hagerstown, Md., 1980.
11. Swamy, S., Segal, L. I., and Mouli, S.: "Percutaneous Angiography," Charles C. Thomas, Publisher, Springfield, Ill., 1977.
12. Yang, S. S., Bentivoglio, L. G., Maranhao, V., and Goldberg, H.: "From Cardiac Catheterization Data to Hemodynamic Parameters," F. A. Davis Company, Philadelphia, 1980.
13. Levin, D. C., and Dunham, L.: New Equipment Considerations for Angiographic Laboratories, *Am. J. Roentgenol.*, 139:775, 1982.
14. Athanasoulis, C. A.: Therapeutic Application of Angiography, *N. Engl. J. Med.*, 302:1117, 1174, 1980.
15. Swan, H. J. C., and Ganz, W.: Hemodynamic Measurements in Clinical Practice: A Decade in Review, *J. Am. Coll. Cardiol.*, 1:303, 1983.
16. Ruckman, R. N.: Sedation for Cardiac Catheterization: A Controlled Study, *Pediatr. Cardiol.*, 1:263, 1980.
17. Fierens, E.: Outpatient Coronary Arteriography, *Catheter. Cardiovasc. Diagn.*, 10:27, 1984.
18. Mathews, R. A., Park, S. C., Neches, W. H., Fricher, F. J., Lenox, C. C., and Zuberbuhler, J. R.: Iliac Venous Thrombosis in Infants and Children after Cardiac Catheterization, *Catheter. Cardiovasc. Diagn.*, 5:67, 1979.
19. Hillis, L. D.: Percutaneous Left Heart Catheterization and Coronary Arteriography Using a Femoral Artery Sheath, *Catheter. Cardiovasc. Diagn.*, 5:393, 1979.
20. Cooper, M. W.: A Simple Method for Insertion of Multiple Catheters through a Single Venipuncture Site, *Catheter. Cardiovasc. Diagn.*, 8:305, 1982.
21. Endrys, J.: Percutaneous Catheterization in New Infants and Older Children, *Pediatr. Cardiol.*, 1:269, 1980.
22. Baur, H. R., Mruz, G. L., Erickson, D. L., and Van Tassel, R. L.: New Technique for Retrograde Left Heart Catheterization in Aortic Stenosis, *Catheter. Cardiovasc. Diagn.*, 8:299, 1982.
23. Nath, P. H., Soto, B., Holt, J. H., and Salter, L. F.: Selective Coronary Angiography by Translumbar Aortic Puncture, *Am. J. Cardiol.*, 52:425, 1983.
24. Wong, P. H. C., Choco, J. S. F., Chen, W. W. C., and Miller, G. A. H.: Aortic Catheterization via Percutaneous Left Ventricular Puncture, *Catheter. Cardiovasc. Diagn.*, 9:421, 1983.
25. Duff, D. F., and Mullins, C. E.: Transseptal Left Heart Catheterization in Infants and Children, *Catheter. Cardiovasc. Diagn.*, 4:213, 1978.
26. Lam, W., Juska, J., and Pietras, R.: Transseptal Balloon Catheterization of the Left Ventricle in Adult Valvular Heart Disease, *Am. Heart J.*, 107:147, 1984.
27. Kotoda, K., Hosegawa, T., Mizumo, A., and Saigusa, M.: Transseptal Left Heart Catheterization with Swan-Ganz Flow Directed Catheter, *Am. Heart J.*, 105:436, 1983.
28. Shirey, E. K., and Sones, M. F.: Retrograde Transaortic and Mitral Valve Catheterization, *Am. J. Cardiol.*, 18:745, 1966.
29. Iskandrian, A. S., Bemis, C. E., Kimbiris, D., and Owens, J.: Retrograde Catheterization of Left Atrium, *Br. Heart J.*, 42:715, 1979.
30. Park, S. C., Neches, W. H., Zuberbuhler, J. R., et al.: Clinical Use of Blade Atrial Septostomy, *Circulation*, 58:600, 1978.
31. Fisher, R. G., and Ferreyro, R.: Evaluation of Current Techniques for Nonsurgical Removal of Intravascular Iatrogenic Foreign Bodies, *Am. J. Radiol.*, 130:541, 1978.
32. Nichols, W. W., Pepine, C. J., Conti, C. R., Christie, L. G., and Feldman, R. L.: Evaluation of a New Catheter Mounted Electromagnetic Velocity Sensor during Cardiac Catheterization, *Catheter. Cardiovasc. Diagn.*, 6:97, 1980.
33. Spears, J. R., Marais, H. J., Serier, J., et al.: In Vivo Coronary Angioscopy, *J. Am. Coll. Cardiol.*, 1:1311, 1983.
34. Takahashi, M., Schieber, R. A., Wishner, S. H., et al.: Selective Coronary Arteriography in Infants and Children, *Circulation*, 68:1021, 1983.
35. Abela, G. S., Normann, S., Cohen, D., Feldman, R. L., Geiser, E. A., and Conti, C. R.: Effects of Carbon Dioxide, Nd-Yag, and Argon Laser Radiation on Coronary Atheromatous Plaques, *Am. J. Cardiol.*, 50:1199, 1982.
36. Rocchini, A. P., Kveselis, D. A., Crowley, D., MacDonald, D., and Rosenthal, A.: Percutaneous Balloon Valvuloplasty for Treatment of Congenital Pulmonary Valvar Stenosis in Children, *J. Am. Coll. Cardiol.*, 3:1005, 1984.
37. Kan, J. S., White, R. I., Jr., Mitchell, S. E., Anderson, J. H., and Gardner, J. J.: Percutaneous Transluminal Balloon Valvuloplasty for Pulmonary Valve Stenosis, *Circulation*, 69:554, 1984.
38. Lock, J. E., Bass, J. L., Amplatz, K., Fuhrman, B. P., and Castaneda-Zunigo, A.: Balloon Dilatation Angioplasty of

Aortic Coarction in Infants and Children, *Circulation*, 68:109, 1983.
39. Mitchell, S. E., White, R. I., Jr., Kan, J., and Tolkoff, J.: Improved Balloon Catheters for Large Vessel and Valvular Angioplasty, *Am. J. Roentgenol.*, 142:571, 1984.
40. Richardson, D. J.: Kings Endomyocardial Bioptome, *Lancet*, 1:660, 1974.
41. Fenoglio, J. J., Jr., Ursell, P. C., Kellogg, C. F., Drusen, R. E., and Weiss, M. B.: Diagnosis and Classification of Myocarditis by Endomyocardial Biopsy, *N. Engl. J. Med.*, 308:12, 1983.
42. Mason, J. W.: Techniques for Right and Left Ventricular Endomyocardial Biopsy, *Am. J. Cardiol.*, 41:887, 1978.
43. Nippoldt, T. B., Edwards, W. D., Holmes, D. R., Reeder, G. S., Hartzler, G. O., and Smith, H. C.: Right Ventricular Endomyocardial Biopsy: Clinico-Pathologic Correlates in 100 Consecutive Patients, *Mayo Clin. Proc.*, 57:407, 1982.
44. Richardson, P. J.: Endocardial Biopsy: Technique and Evaluation of the New Long Sheath and Disposable Cardiac Biopsy Forceps, International Workshop on Viral Heart Disease, Munich, 1983. (Abstract.)
45. Brooksby, I. A. B., Swanton, R. H., Jenkins, B. S., and Webb-Peploe, M. M.: Long Sheath Technique for Introduction of Catheter Tip Manometer or Endomyocardial Bioptome into Left or Right Heart, *Br. Heart J.*, 36:908, 1974.
46. Gertz, E. W., Wisneski, J. A., Gould, R. G., and Akin, J. R.: Improved Radiation Protection for Physicians Performing Cardiac Catheterization, *Am. J. Cardiol.*, 50:1283, 1982.
47. Krovetz, L. J., Brenner, J. I., and Polanyi, M.: Application of an Improved Intracardiac Fiber Optic System, *Br. Heart J.*, 40:1010, 1978.
48. Dehmer, G. J., Firth, B. G., and Hillis, L. D.: Oxygen Consumption in Adult Patients during Cardiac Catheterization, *Clin. Cardiol.*, 5:436, 1982.
49. Nichols, W. W., Pepine, C. J., and Millar, H. D.: Percutaneous Left Ventricular Catheterization with an Ultra-miniature Catheter Tip-Pressure Transducer, *Cardiovasc. Res.*, 12:566, 1978.
50. Krayenbuehl, H. P., Turina, M., Hess, O. M., Rothlin, M., and Senning, A.: Pre and Postoperative Left Ventricular Contractile Function in Patients with Aortic Valve Disease, *Br. Heart J.*, 41:204, 1979.
51. Dodge, H. T., and Sheehan, F. H.: Quantitative Contrast Angiography for Assessment of Ventricular Performance in Heart Disease, *J. Am. Coll. Cardiol.*, 1:73, 1983.
52. Hosenpud, J. D., McAnulty, J. H., and Morton, M. J.: Overestimation of Mitral Valve Gradients Obtained by Phasic Pulmonary Artery Wedge Pressure, *Catheter. Cardiovasc. Diagn.*, 9:283, 1983.
53. Falicov, R. E., and Resnekov, L.: Mid Ventricular Obstruction in Hypertrophic Cardiomyopathy, *Br. Heart J.*, 39:701, 1977.
54. Freed, M. D., Miettinen, O. S., and Nadas, A. S.: Oximetric Detection of Intracardiac Left-to-Right Shunts, *Br. Heart J.*, 42:690, 1979.
55. Antiman, E. M., Marsh, J. D., Green, L. H., and Grossman, W.: Blood Oxygen Measurements in the Assessment of Intracardial Left to Right Shunts: A Critical Appraisal of Methodology, *Am. J. Med.*, 46:265, 1980.
56. Bloomfield, D. A.: "Dye Curves: The Theory and Practice of Indicator Dilution," University Park Press, Baltimore, 1974.
57. Levett, J. M., and Replogle, R. L.: Thermodilution Cardiac Output: A Critical Analysis and Review of the Literature, *J. Surg. Res.*, 27:392, 1979.
58. Fischer, A. P., Benis, A. M., Jurado, R. A., Seely, E., Teirstein, P., and Litwak, R. S.: Analysis of Errors in Measurement of Cardiac Output by Simultaneous Dye and Thermal Dilution in Cardiothoracic Surgical Patients, *Cardiovasc. Res.*, 12:190, 1978.
59. Morady, F., Brundage, B. H., and Gelberg, H. J.: Rapid Method for Determination of Shunt Ratio using a Thermodilution Technique, *Am. Heart J.*, 106:369, 1983.
60. Krovetz, L. J., and Gessner, I. H.: A New Method Utilizing Indicator Dilution Technics for Examination of Left to Right Shunts in Infants, *Circulation*, 32:772, 1965.
61. Treves, S.: Detection and Quantitation of Cardiovascular Shunts with Commonly Available Radionuclides, *Semin. Nucl. Med.*, 10:16, 1980.
62. Dodge, H. T., Sandler, H., Ballew, D. W., and Lord, J. D., Jr.: The Use of Biplane Angiocardiography for the Measurement of Left Ventricular Volume in Man, *Am. Heart J.*, 60:762, 1960.
63. Als, A. V., Paulin, S., and Aroesty, J. M.: Biplane Angiographic Volumetry Using the Right Anterior Oblique and Half-Axial Left Anterior Oblique Technique, *Radiology*, 126:511, 1978.
64. Wynne, J., Green, L. H., Mann, T., Levin, D., and Grossman, W.: Estimation of Left Ventricular Volumes in Man from Biplane Cineangiograms Filmed in Oblique Projections, *Am. J. Cardiol.*, 41:726, 1978.
65. Sandler, H., and Dodge, H. T.: The Use of Single Plane Angiocardiograms for the Calculation of Left Ventricular Volume in Man, *Am. Heart J.*, 75:325, 1968.
66. Kennedy, J. W., Trenholme, S. E., and Kasser, I. S.: Left Ventricular Volume and Mass from Single Plane Cineangiocardiograms, *Am. Heart J.*, 80:343, 1970.
67. Siegel, J. A., Maurer, A. H., Wie, R. K., et al.: Absolute Left Ventricular Volume by an Iterative Build Up Factor Analysis of Gated Radionuclide Images, *Radiology*, 151:477, 1984.
68. Kennedy, J. W., Baxley, W. A., Figley, M. M., Dodge, H. T., and Blackmon, J. R.: Quantitative Angiocardiography. I. The Normal Left Ventricle in Man, *Circulation*, 34:272, 1966.
69. Shimazaki, Y., Kawashima, Y., Mori, T., and Beppie, S.: Angiographic Volume Estimation of Right Ventricle, *Chest*, 77:390, 1980.
70. Gentzler, R. O., II, Briselli, M. F., and Gault, J. H.: Angiographic Estimation of Right Ventricular Volume in Man, *Circulation*, 50:324, 1974.
71. Murray, J. A., Kennedy, J. W., and Figley, M. M.: Quantitative Angiocardiography. II. The Normal Left Atrial Volume in Man, *Circulation*, 37:800, 1968.
72. Gorlin, R., and Gorlin, G.: Hydraulic Formula for Calculation of Area of Stenotic Mitral Valve, Other Cardiac Valves and Central Circulatory Shunts, *Am. Heart J.*, 41:1, 1951.
73. Cohen, M. V., and Gorlin, R.: Modified Orifice Equation for the Calculation of Mitral Valve Area, *Am. Heart J.*, 84:839, 1972.
74. Chavez, I., Dorbecker, N., and Celis, A.: Direct Intracardiac Angiocardiography: Its Diagnostic Value, *Am. Heart J.*, 33:560, 1947.
75. Brown, R., Rahimtoola, S. H., David, G. D., and Swan, H. J. C.: The Effects of Angiocardiographic Contrast Medium on Circulatory Dynamics in Man: Cardiac Output during Angiocardiography, *Circulation*, 31:234, 1965.
76. Almen, T.: Experience from 10 Years of Development of Water Soluble Nonionic Contrast Media, *Invest. Radiol.*, 15:S283, 1980.
77. Bettmann, M. A.: Angiographic Contrast Agents: Conventional and New Media Compared, *Am. J. Roentgenol.*, 139:787, 1982.
78. Peck, W. W., Slutsky, R. A., Hackney, D. B., et al.: Effects of Contrast Media on Pulmonary Hemodynamics: Comparison of Ionic and Non-ionic Agents, *Radiology*, 149:371, 1983.
79. Gwilt, D. J., and Nagle, R. E.: Contrast Media for Left Ventricular Angiography: A Comparison between Cardio-conray and Iopomidol, *Br. Heart J.*, 51:427, 1984.
80. Mancini, G. B. J., Ostrander, D. R., Slutsky, R. A., et al.: Intravenous Versus Left Ventricular Injection of Ionic Contrast Material: Hemodynamic Implications for Digital Subtraction Angiography, *Am. J. Roentgenol.*, 140:425, 1983.
81. Morris, T. W., Sahler, L. G., Violante, M., et al.: Reduction of Calcium Activity by Radiopaque Contrast Media, *Radiology*, 148:55, 1983.
82. Dissessa, T. G., Zednikova, M., Hiraishi, S., et al.: The Car-

diovascular Effects of Metrizamide in Infants, *Radiology,* 148:687, 1983.
83. Levin, D. C., Dunham, L. R., and Stueve, R.: Causes of Cine Image Quality Deterioration in Cardiac Catheterization Laboratories, *Am. J. Cardiol.,* 52:881, 1983.
84. Levin, A. R., Goldberg, H. L., Borer, J. S., et al: Digital Angiography in the Pediatric Patient with Congenital Heart Disease: Comparison with Standard Methods, *Circulation,* 68:374, 1983.
85. Buonocore, E., Pavaliceh, W., Modec, M. T., et al.: Anatomic and Functional Imaging of Congenital Heart Disease with Digital Subtraction Angiography, *Radiology,* 147, 1983.
86. Saddekni, S., Sos, T. A., Sniderman, K. W., et al.: Optimal Injection Technique for Intravenous Digital Subtraction Angiography, *Radiology,* 150:655, 1984.
87. Bargeron, L. M., Jr., Elliott, L. P., Soto, B., Bream, P. R., and Curry, G. C.: Axial Cineangiography in Congenital Heart Disease. I. Concept, Technical and Anatomic Considerations, *Circulation,* 56:1081, 1977.
88. Nihill, M. R., Mullins, C. E., and McNamara, D. G.: Visualization of the Pulmonary Arteries in Pseudotruncus by Pulmonary Vein Wedge Angiography, *Circulation,* 58:140, 1978.
89. Thomas, H. A., and Stevers, R. E.: Nonsurgical Reduction of Arterial Catheter Knots, *Am. J. Roentgenol.,* 132:1018, 1979.
90. Lo, W. W. M.: Use of Lunderquist Exchange Guide Wire for Nonsurgical Elimination of Angiographic Catheter Knots, *Radiology,* 145:835, 1982.
91. Pope, L. A., Hoffajee, C. I., and Alpert, J. S.: Fatal Pulmonary Hemorrhage after Use of the Flow-Directed Balloon-Tipped Catheter, *Ann. Intern. Med.,* 90:344, 1979.
92. Furlan, A. J., and Brever, A. C.: Central Nervous System Complications of Open Heart Surgery, *Curr. Conc. Cerebrovasc. Dis.,* 19:7, 1984.
93. Lalle, A. F.: Contrast Media Reactions: Data Analysis and Hypothesis, *Radiology,* 134:1, 1980.
94. Weinrauch, L. A., Healy, R. W., Leland, O. S., and D'elia, J. A.: Coronary Angiography and Acute Renal Failure in Diabetic Nephropathy, *Ann. Intern. Med.,* 86:56, 1977.
95. Katzberg, R. W., Morris, T. W., and Schulman, G.: Reactions to Intravenous Contrast Media, *Radiology,* 147:327, 1983.
96. Greganti, M. A., and Flowers, W., Jr.: Acute Pulmonary Edema after the Intravenous Administration of Contrast Media, *Radiology,* 132:583, 1979.
97. Sones, F. M., Jr., and Shirey, E. K.: Cine Coronary Arteriography, *Mod. Concepts Cardiovasc. Dis.,* 31:735, 1962.
98. Abrams, H. L., and Adams, D. F.: The Coronary Arteriogram. I and II. Structural and Functional Aspects, *N. Engl. J. Med.,* 281:1276, 1336, 1969.
99. Conti, E. R.: Coronary Arteriography, *Circulation,* 55:227, 1977.
100. Gorlin, R.: Coronary Collaterals. *Major Probl. Intern. Med.,* 11:59, 1976.
101. Verani, M. S.: The Functional Significance of Coronary Collateral Vessels: Anecdote Confronts Science, *Catheter. Cardiovasc. Diagn.,* 9:333, 1983.
102. Schwarz, F., Schuler, G., Hoffmann, M., and Kubler, W.: Recruitment of Collaterals following Acute Coronary Occlusion Reduces Infarct Size in Man, *J. Am. Coll. Cardiol.,* 1:591, 1983.
103. Hamby, R. I., Aintablian, A., and Schwartz, A.: Reappraisal of the Functional Significance of the Coronary Collateral Circulation, *Am. J. Cardiol.,* 38:305, 1976.
104. Nohara, R., Kambara, H., Murakami, T., et al.: Collateral Function in Early Acute Myocardial Infarction, *Am. J. Cardiol.,* 52:955, 1983.
105. Mehmel, H. C., Schwarz, F., Schuler, G., Maurer, W., Tillmanns, H., Senges, J., and Kubler, W.: The Functional Result of Intracoronary Streptokinase Therapy after Myocardial Infarction may be Determined by Collaterals, *Circulation,* 64(suppl. IV):IV–194, 1981.
106. Rentrop, P., Merx, W., Mathey, D., Blanke, H., Rutsch, W., and Karsch, K. R.: Functional Results of Streptokinase-Reperfusion in Relation to Collaterals and Duration of Symptoms, *Circulation,* 64(suppl. IV):IV–194, 1981.
107. Helfant, R. H., Vokonas, P. S., and Gorlin, R.: Functional Importance of the Human Coronary Collateral Circulation, *N. Engl. J. Med.,* 284:1277, 1971.
108. Heupler, F. A., Jr.: Syndrome of Symptomatic Coronary Arterial Spasm with Nearly Normal Coronary Arteriograms, *Am. J. Cardiol.,* 45:873, 1980.
109. Curry, R. C., Pepine, C. J., Sabom, M. C., et al.: Effects of Ergonovine in Patients with and without Coronary Artery Disease, *Circulation,* 56:803, 1977.
110. Conti, C. R., Curry, R. C., Christie, L. G., et al.: Clinical Use of Provocative Pharmacoangiography in Patients with Chest Pain, *Adv. Cardiol.,* 26:44, 1979.
111. Oliva, P., Potts, D., and Pluss, R.: Coronary Arterial Spasm in Prinzmetal Angina: Documentation by Coronary Arteriography. *N. Engl. J. Med.,* 288:746, 1973.
112. Waters, D. D., Szlachcic, J., and Bonan, R.: Comparative Sensitivity of Exercise, Coldpressor and Ergonovine Testing in Provoking Attacks of Variant Angina in Patients with Active Disease, *Circulation,* 67:310, 1983.
113. Maseri, A., Severi, S., DeNes, M., et al.: "Variant" Angina: One Aspect of a Continuous Spectrum of Vasospastic Myocardial Ischemia. Pathogenic Mechanisms, Estimated Incidence and Clinical and Arteriographic Findings in 138 Patients, *Am. J. Cardiol.,* 42:1019, 1978.
114. Helfant, R. H., Pine, R., Meister, S. G., Feldman, M. S., Trout, R. G., and Banka, V. S.: Nitroglycerin to Unmask Reversible Asynergy: Correlation with Post Coronary Bypass Ventriculography, *Circulation,* 50:108, 1974.
115. Horn, H. R., Teicholz, L. E., Cohn, P. F., Herman, M. V., and Gorlin, R.: Augmentation of Left Ventricular Contraction Pattern in Coronary Artery Disease by Inotropic Catecholamine: The Epinephrine Ventriculogram, *Circulation,* 49:1063, 1974.
116. Dyke, S. H., Cohn, P. F., Gorlin, R., and Sonnenblick, E. H.: Detection of Residual Myocardial Function in Coronary Artery Disease Using Post Extrasystolic Potentiation, *Circulation,* 50:694, 1974.
117. Formanek, A., Nath, P. H., Zollikofer, C., and Moller, J. H.: Selective Coronary Arteriography in Children, *Circulation,* 61:84, 1980.
118. Dabizzi, R. P., Caprioli, G., Aiazzi, L., Castelli, C., Baldrighi, G., Parenzan, L., and Baldrighi, V.: Distribution and Anomalies of Coronary Arteries in Tetralogy of Fallot, *Circulation,* 61:95, 1980.
119. Heupler, F. A., Jr.: Coronary Arteriography and Left Ventriculography: Sones Technique, in S. B. King, III, and J. S. Douglas, Jr. (eds.), "Coronary Arteriography," McGraw-Hill Book Company, New York, 1984.
120. Seldinger, S. I.: Catheter Replacement of the Needle in Percutaneous Arteriography: A New Technique, *Acta. Radiol.,* 39:368, 1953.
121. Ricketts, H. J., and Abrams, H. L.: Percutaneous Selective Coronary Cine Arteriography, *JAMA,* 181:620, 1962.
122. Amplatz, K., Formanck, G., Stranger, P., and Wilson, W.: Mechanics of Selective Coronary Artery Catheterization via Femoral Approach. *Radiology,* 89:1040, 1967.
123. Judkins, M. P.: Selective Coronary Arteriography. I. A. Percutaneous Transfemoral Technique, *Radiology,* 89:815, 1967.
124. Judkins, M. P., and Judkins, E. J.: The Judkins Technique, in S. B. King, III, and J. S. Douglas, Jr. (eds.), "Coronary Arteriography," McGraw-Hill Book Company, New York, 1984.
125. Schoonmaker, F. W., and King, S. B., III: Coronary Arteriography by the Single Catheter Percutaneous Femoral Technique: Experience with 6,800 Cases, *Circulation,* 50:735, 1974.
126. King, S. B., III, and Douglas, J. S., Jr.: Catheterization Techniques in Coronary Arteriography and Left Ventriculography: Multipurpose Techniques, in S. B. King, III, and J. S. Douglas, Jr. (eds.), "Coronary Arteriography," McGraw-Hill Book Company, New York, 1984.

127. Douglas, J. S., Jr., and King, S. B., III: Complications of Coronary Arteriography: Management During and Following the Procedure, in S. B. King, III, and J. S. Douglas, Jr. (eds.), "Coronary Arteriography," McGraw-Hill Book Company, New York, 1984.
128. Austin, W. G., Edwards, J. E., Frye, R. L., Gensini, G. G., Gott, V. L., Griffith, L. S. C., McGoon, D. C., Murphy, M. L., and Rose, B. B.: A Reporting System on Patients Evaluated for Coronary Artery Disease: Report of the Ad Hoc Committee for Grading Coronary Artery Disease, Council on Cardiovascular Surgery, American Heart Association, *Circulation,* 51(suppl. 4):30, 1975.
129. Bunnell, L. I., Greene, D. G., Tandon, R. N., and Arani, D. T.: The Halfaxial Projection: A New Look at the Proximal Left Coronary Artery, *Circulation,* 48:1151, 1973.
130. Aldridge, H. E., McLoughlin, M. J., and Taylor, K. W.: Improved Diagnosis in Coronary Cine Arteriography with Routine Use of 110 Oblique Views and Cranial and Caudal Angulations, *Am. J. Cardiol.,* 36:468, 1975.
131. Frederick, P. R., Fry, W. H., Russell, J. G., and Marshall, H. W.: Longitudinal Angulation in Coronary Arteriography: Apparatus and Evaluation, *Catheter. Cardiovasc. Diagn.,* 3:305, 1977.
132. King, S. B., III, Douglas, J. S., Jr., and Morris, D. C.: New Angiographic Views for Coronary Arteriography, in J. W. Hurst (ed.), "Update IV: The Heart," McGraw-Hill Book Company, New York, 1980.
133. McMahon, M. M., Brown, B. G., Cukingnan, R., Rolett, E. L., Bolson, E., Frimer, M., and Dodge, H. T.: Quantitative Coronary Angiography: Measurement of the "Critical" Stenosis in Patients with Unstable Angina and Single Vessel Disease without Collaterals, *Circulation,* 60:106, 1979.
134. Kramer, J. R., Kitazume, H., Proudfitt, W. L., and Sones, F. M., Jr.: Clinical Significance of Isolated Coronary Bridges: Benign and Frequent Condition Involving the Left Anterior Descending Artery, *Am. Heart J.,* 103:283, 1982.
135. Ishimori, T., Raizner, A. E., Chahine, R. A., et al.: Myocardial Bridges in Man: Clinical Correlations and Angiographic Accentuations with Nitroglycerin, *Catheter. Cardiovasc. Diagn.,* 3:59, 1977.
136. Kitazume, H., Kramer, J. R., and Krauthamer, D.: Myocardial Bridges in Obstructive Hypertrophic Cardiomyopathy, *Am. Heart J.,* 106:131, 1983.
137. Brugada, P., Bar, F. W. H. M., DeZwaan, C., et al.: "Saw-Fish" Systolic Narrowing of the Left Anterior Descending Coronary Artery: An Angiographic Sign of Hypertrophic Cardiomyopathy, *Circulation,* 66:80, 1982.
138. Engel, H. J., Torres, C., and Page, H. L.: Major Variations in Anatomical Origin of the Coronary Arteries, *Catheter. Cardiovasc. Diagn.,* 1:157, 1975.
139. Chaitman, B. R., Lesperance, J., Saltiel, J., and Bourassa, M. G.: Clinical, Angiographic, and Hemodynamic Findings in Patients with Anomalous Origin of the Coronary Arteries, *Circulation,* 53:122, 1976.
140. Donaldson, R. M., Raphael, M., Radley-Smith, R., Yacoub, M. H., and Ross, D. N.: Angiographic Identification of Primary Coronary Anomalies Causing Impaired Myocardial Perfusion, *Catheter. Cardiovasc. Diagn.,* 9:237, 1983.
141. Ogden, J. A.: Congenital Anomalies of the Coronary Arteries, *Am. Cardiol.,* 25, 474, 1970.
142. Benge, W., Martins, J. B., and Funk, D. C.: Morbidity Associated with Anomalous Origin of the Right Coronary Artery from the Left Sinus of Valsalva, *Am. Heart J.,* 99:96, 1980.
143. Antopol, W., and Kugel, M. A.: Anomalous Origin of the Left Circumflex Coronary Artery, *Am. Heart J.,* 8:802, 1933.
144. Donaldson, R. M., and Raphael, M. J.: Missing Coronary Artery. Review of Technical Problems in Coronary Arteriography Resulting from Anatomical Variants, *Br. Heart J.,* 47:62, 1982.
145. Kimbiris, D., Iskandrian, A. S., Segal, B. L., and Bemis, C. E.: Anomalous Aortic Origin of the Coronary Arteries, *Circulation,* 58:606, 1978.
146. Page, H. L., Jr., Engel, H. J., Campbell, W. B., and Thomas, C. S., Jr.: Anomalous Origin of the Left Circumflex Coronary Artery. Recognition, Angiographic Demonstration, and Clinical Significance, *Circulation,* 50:768, 1974.
147. Levin, D. C., Fellows, K. E., and Abrams, H. L.: Hemodynamically Significant Primary Anomalies of the Coronary Arteries, Angiographic Aspects, *Circulation,* 58:25, 1978.
148. Moodie, D. S., Gill, C., Loop, F. D., and Sheldon, W. C.: Anomalous Left Main Coronary Artery Originating from the Right Sinus of Valsalva. Pathophysiology, Angiographic Definition, and Surgical Approaches, *J. Thorac. Cardiovasc. Surg.,* 80:198, 1980.
149. Mustafa, I., Gula, G., Radley-Smith, R., Durrer, S., and Yacoub, M.: Anomalous Origin of the Left Coronary Artery from the Anterior Aortic Sinus: A Potential Cause of Sudden Death. Anatomic Characterization and Surgical Treatment, *J. Thorac. Cardiovasc. Surg.,* 82:297, 1981.
150. Chaitman, B. R., Lesperance, J., Saltiel, J., and Bourassa, M. G.: Clinical, Angiographic and Hemodynamic Findings in Patients with Anomalous Origin of the Coronary Arteries, *Circulation,* 53:122, 1976.
151. Liberthson, R. R., Dinsmore, R. E., and Fallon, J. T.: Aberrant Coronary Artery Origin from the Aorta. Report of 18 Patients. Review of Literature and Delineation of Natural History and Management, *Circulation,* 59:748, 1979.
152. Thompson, S. I., Vieweg, W. V., Alport, J. S., and Hagan, A. D.: Anomalous Origin of the Right Coronary Artery from the Left Sinus of Valsalva with Associated Chest Pain. Report of Two Cases, *Catheter. Cardiovasc. Diagn.,* 2:397, 1976.
153. Roberts, W. C., Siegel, R. J., and Zipes, D. P.: Origin of the Right Coronary Artery from the Left Sinus of Valsalva and its Functional Consequences: Analysis of 10 Necropsy Patients, *Am. J. Cardiol.,* 49:863, 1982.
154. Brandt, B., III, Martins, J. B., and Marcus, M. L.: Anomalous Origin of the Right Coronary Artery from the Left Sinus of Valsalva, *N. Engl. J. Med.,* 309:596, 1983.
155. Ogden, J. A., and Goodyer, A. V. N.: Patterns of Distribution of the Single Coronary Artery, *Yale J. Biol. Med.,* 43:11, 1970.
156. Sharbaugh, A. H., and White, R. S.: Single Coronary Artery. Analysis of the Anatomic Variation, Clinical Importance, and Report of Five Cases, *JAMA,* 230:243, 1974.
157. Lipton, M. J., Barry, W. H., Obrez, I., Silverman, J. F., and Wexler, L.: Isolated Single Coronary Artery: Diagnosis, Angiographic Classification, and Clinical Significance, *Radiology,* 130:39, 1979.
158. Gorlin, R.: Coronary Collaterals. *Major Probl. Intern. Med.,* 11:59, 1976.
159. Verani, M. S.: The Functional Significance of Coronary Collateral Vessels: Anecdote Confronts Science. *Catheter. Cardiovasc. Diagn.,* 9:333, 1983.
160. Hamby, R. I., Aintablian, A., and Schwartz, A.: Reappraisal of the Functional Significance of the Coronary Collateral Circulation, *Am. J. Cardiol.,* 38:305, 1976.
161. Morales, A. R., Romanelli, R., and Boucek, R. J.: The Mural Left Anterior Descending Coronary Artery, Strenuous Exercise and Sudden Death, *Circulation,* 62:230, 1980.
162. Levin, D. C.: Pathways and Functional Significance of the Coronary Collateral Circulation, *Circulation,* 50:831, 1974.
163. Zir, L. M., Miller, J. W., Dinsmore, R. E., Gilbert, J. P., and Harthorne, J. W.: Interobserver Variability in Coronary Arteriography, *Circulation,* 53:627, 1976.
164. DeRouen, T. A., Murray, J. A., and Owen, W.: Variability in the Analysis of Coronary Arteriograms, *Circulation,* 55:324, 1977.
165. Schwartz, J. N., King, Y., Hackel, D. B., and Bartel, A. G.: Comparison of Angiographic and Postmortem Findings in Patients with Coronary Artery Disease, *Am. J. Cardiol.,* 36:174, 1975.
166. Kemp, H. G., Evans, H., Elliott, W. C., and Gorlin, R.: Diagnostic Accuracy of Selective Coronary Cinearteriography, *Circulation,* 36:526, 1967.
167. Grandin, C. M., Dyrda, I., Pastemac, A., Campeau, L., Dourossa, M. G., and Lesperance, J.: Discrepancies between

Cineangiographic and Postmortem Findings in Patients with Coronary Artery Disease and Recent Myocardial Revascularization, *Circulation,* 49:703, 1974.
168. Roberts, W. C.: The Coronary Arteries and Left Ventricle in Clinically Isolated Angina Pectoris. A Necropsy Analysis, *Circulation,* 54:388, 1976.
169. Arnett, E. N., Isner, J. M., Redwood, D. R., Kent, K. M., Baker, W. P., Ackerstein, H., and Roberts, W. C.: Coronary Artery Narrowing in Coronary Heart Disease: Comparison of Cine Angiographic and Necropsy Findings, *Ann. Intern. Med.,* 91:350, 1979.
170. Roberts, C. S., and Roberts, W. C.: Cross-Sectional Area of the Proximal Portions of the Three Major Epicardial Coronary Arteries in 98 Patients with Different Coronary Events. Relationship to Heart, Weight, Age, and Sex, *Circulation,* 62:953, 1980.
171. Isner, J. M., Kishel, J., Kent, K. M., Ronan, J. A., Ross, A. M., and Roberts, W. C.: Inaccuracy of Angiographic Determination of Left Main Coronary Arterial Narrowing: Angiographic-Histologic Correlative Analysis of 29 Patients, *Circulation,* 59, 60(suppl. 2):II–161, 1979.
172. Brown, B. G., Bolson, E., Frimer, M., and Dodge, H. T.: Quantitative Coronary Arteriography. Estimation of Dimensions, Hemodynamic Resistance, and Atheroma Mass of Coronary Artery Lesions Using the Arteriogram and Digital Computation, *Circulation,* 55:329, 1977.
173. Abrams, H. L., and Adams, D. F.: The Complications of Coronary Arteriography, *Circulation,* 52(suppl. 2):27, 1975.
174. Davis, K., Kennedy, J. W., Kemp, H. G., Jr., Judkins, M. P., Gosselin, A. J., and Killip, T.: Complications of Coronary Arteriography from the Collaborative Study of Coronary Artery Surgery (CASS), *Circulation,* 59:1105, 1979.
175. Gersh, B. J., Kronmal, R. A., Frye, R. L., et al.: Coronary Arteriography and Coronary Bypass Surgery: Morbidity and Mortality in Patients Ages 65 Years or Older. A Report from the Coronary Artery Surgery Study, *Circulation,* 67:483, 1983.
176. Kennedy, J. W.: Symposium on Catheterization. Complications Associated with Cardiac Catheterization and Angiography, *Catheter. Cardiovasc. Diagn.,* 8:5, 1982.
177. Patterson, R., and Anderson, J.: Allergic Reactions to Drugs and Biologic Agents, *JAMA,* 248:2637, 1982.
178. Lieberman, P., Siegle, R. L., and Taylor, W. W.: Anaphylactoid Reactions to Iodinated Contrast Material, *J. Allergy Clin. Immunol.,* 62:174, 1978.
179. Madowitz, J. S., and Schweiger, M. J.: Severe Anaphylactoid Reaction to Radiographic Contrast Media, *JAMA,* 241:2813, 1979.
180. Takaro, T., Hultgren, H. N., Littman, D., and Wright, E. C.: An Analysis of Deaths Occurring in Association with Coronary Arteriography, *Am. Heart J.,* 86:587, 1973.
181. Harrison, T. R.: Some Unanswered Questions Concerning Enlargement and Failure of the Heart, *Am. Heart J.,* 69:100, 1965.
182. Herman, M. V., Henile, R. A., Klein, M. D., and Gorlin, R.: Localized Disorders in Myocardial Contraction, *N. Engl. J. Med.,* 227:222, 1967.
183. Dodge, H. T., Sandler, H., Ballew, D. W., and Lord, J. D.: The Use of Biplane Angiocardiography for the Measurement of Left Ventricular Volume in Man, *Am. Heart J.,* 60:762, 1960.
184. Vogel, J. H. K., Cornish, D., and McFadden, R. B.: Underestimations of Ejection Fraction with Single Plane Angiography in Coronary Artery Disease. Role of Biplane Angiography, *Chest,* 64:217, 1973.

109*

Techniques of Nuclear Cardiology

Barry L. Zaret, M.D.   Harvey J. Berger, M.D.

Previous studies have shown that the arm to arm circulation time can be measured in man by injecting the active deposit of radium into the antecubital vein of one arm and subsequently, by means of a suitable detecting device, noting its time of arrival in the arteries about the elbow of the other arm. It seemed that if the procedure for measuring the arm to arm circulation time could be adapted to the measurement of the pulmonary circulation time in man, the information obtained would be valuable for the following reasons. 1. Information would be secured about a fundamental aspect of the pulmonary circulation hitherto unstudied in man. 2. The pulmonary circulation could be studied under both normal and pathological conditions without in any way interfering with the phenomena under observation. 3. The method could be quantitative, objective, and require no cooperation from the patient. 4. The effect of the variability of the peripheral capillary circulation would be obviated.

H. L. Blumgart and S. Weiss, 1927[1,†]

Nuclear cardiology techniques are based upon the ability to detect, define, and quantify radiation emanating from cardiac structures with externally placed radiation detection instrumentation. When

**Note:* This chapter, "Techniques of Nuclear Cardiology," by Drs. Zaret and Berger, initially appeared in the fifth edition of *The Heart* (1982). A much shorter version on the same subject by Dr. Zaret appeared in the 16th edition of *Cecil's Textbook of Medicine* edited by Wyngaarden and Smith and published by Saunders in 1982. This current chapter has been extensively updated. It is published here with the permission of the publishers of the two books, McGraw-Hill and Saunders, and the authors.

†Reproduced from the *Journal of Clinical Investigation,* 1927, 4, 399, with permission from The American Society for Clinical Investigation.

applied to the study of cardiac disease, these techniques have two general advantages. First, they are relatively noninvasive and generally require only the intravenous injection of relatively short-lived radionuclides. Thus, studies can be repeated on several occasions without undue concern about radiation safety. Second, studies often provide relevant physiologic data concerning myocardial perfusion, viability, and metabolism which cannot be examined by other techniques, whether they are invasive or noninvasive.

At the onset, one may ask whether these techniques, in the appropriate clinical setting, are clinically efficacious and whether they have a meaningful effect on patient diagnosis and therapy. Goldman et al.[2] analyzed the first 171 consecutive nuclear cardiology studies performed at Yale–New Haven Hospital from August to November 1977. The physicians ordering the tests felt that 72 percent of studies were useful and 28 percent contributed directly to changes in patient management. In addition, 15 of 171 studies altered decisions concerning performance of cardiac catheterization, and 3 studies influenced decisions concerning patient suitability for cardiac surgery. Thus, even at this relatively early stage in the clinical application of these techniques, nuclear cardiology was shown to provide relevant information. Since that time numerous clinical studies and reports in the literature have established the clinical utility of nuclear cardiology examinations. It is within the context of current and potential clinical relevance that the field of nuclear cardiology will be reviewed.

Nuclear cardiology techniques generally can be divided into two generic categories. The first involves the assessment of cardiac performance. For these studies radioactive tracers which remain within the intravascular space during the period of study are employed. The second category involves the study of myocardial perfusion, viability, and metabolism. In this instance, radioactive tracers are employed that pass through the myocardial capillary network and are accumulated intracellularly. These individual tracers are distributed within the myocardium in response to a variety of stimuli, ranging from regional myocardial blood flow to the degree of myocardial necrosis. In addition, new techniques involving biologically active substances, such as radiolabeled blood cells (platelets and leukocytes), antibodies, and metabolites, have been developed. The use of specific positron-labeled substances has provided a means of studying regional myocardial metabolism in a noninvasive fashion. This chapter will concentrate on noninvasive techniques and will not deal with specific invasive approaches involving cardiac catheterization, such as myocardial blood flow measurements following the intracoronary injection of radioactive xenon[3] or static imaging following the direct intracoronary injection of radiolabeled particles.[4]

Historical Background

The use of radioactive tracers to study cardiovascular dynamics was reported initially by Blumgart and Weiss in 1927.[1] These workers used radon gas injected intravenously and employed a modified cloud chamber to measure circulation time in humans. It was not until 20 years later that Prinzmetal et al. described the gross characteristics of the first pass radiocardiogram using ^{22}Na and a Geiger-Müller counter positioned over the precordium.[5] In the 1960s, instrumentation advances occurred that led to an improved ability to assess cardiac performance. Donato et al. analyzed the quantitative aspects of the radiocardiogram using a newly developed shielded and collimated scintillation probe.[6] This allowed definition of both cardiac dynamics and myocardial blood flow. During that decade, prototype scintillation cameras were developed. Initial studies using a multicrystal scintillation camera (autofluoroscope) were performed by Bender and Blau in 1963.[7] In 1965, Anger and colleagues demonstrated the ability to define cardiac transit with analogue images obtained from the prototype single-crystal scintillation camera.[8] In the early 1970s, the concept of electrocardiographic gating of the equilibrium cardiac blood pool was proposed as a means of evaluating both regional wall motion and global left ventricular performance as measured by ejection fraction.[9,10] At roughly the same time, Van Dyke et al. described the first transit technique using the scintillation camera for measuring left ventricular function.[11] In the late 1970s, additional advances involved the application of computer techniques to the equilibrium cardiac blood pool and first-transmit studies and the addition of exercise stress to the assessment of ventricular performance.[12,13]

The assessment of myocardial perfusion and viability has followed a parallel developmental course. Carr et al. were the first to demonstrate that potassium analogues would be suitable for imaging myocardial perfusion.[14] Initial studies were performed with radioactive cesium. Following this demonstration, radioactive potassium and rubidium were employed.[15–17] In 1973, exercise myocardial perfusion imaging using ^{43}K for assessing transient ischemia was introduced.[18] In 1973, ^{201}Tl was introduced as a potassium analogue with physical characteristics more suitable for conventional scintillation camera imaging.[19] In 1978 an initial tomographic approach to ^{201}Tl imaging employing a seven-pinhole collimator system was developed.[20] This approach has since been superseded by tomographic studies involving rotating scintillation camera detectors and sophisticated computer systems. These are currently undergoing intense evaluation.

The concept of imaging myocardial infarction as a zone of increased radioactivity was first reported in 1962 by Carr et al. using radiolabeled chlormerodrin.[21] It was not, however, until 1973 that Holman et al. reported on the efficacy of ^{99m}Tc-labeled tetracycline imaging as a means of demonstrating acute myocardial infarction in humans.[22] Shortly thereafter, Bonte et al. and Parkey et al. demonstrated the applicability of pyrophosphate imaging for defining acute myocardial infarction in animals and humans.[23,24]

Instrumentation

Virtually all nuclear cardiology imaging studies performed today involve a scintillation camera and computer system. There are variations of these components which will determine the type and quality of studies performed. The basic characteristics of these instruments will be reviewed briefly. For a more detailed discussion, the reader is referred to several recent reviews dealing with instrumentation and nuclear medicine physics.[25–27]

Anger Scintillation Camera

The Anger scintillation camera provides an image of the overall distribution of radioactivity within the body. This instrument is composed of a single large, flat sodium iodide ($\frac{1}{4}$-to-$\frac{1}{2}$-in-thick) crystal that is optically coupled to a series of photomultiplier tubes, generally arranged in a hexagonal array. The exact number of photomultiplier tubes depends in part on the size of the field of view. With a standard field of view camera (250 to 300 mm in diameter) a minimum of 37 photomultiplier tubes is required. With the large field of view cameras (400 to 500 mm in diameter) there often are 61 or 75 tubes to provide better spatial resolution. Because of the size of the heart, detectors less than 300 mm in diameter frequently are used for cardiac studies. Gamma rays from the patient interact with the sodium iodide crystal and are converted to light. Subsequently, the scintillations are translated by the photomultiplier tubes into voltage pulses, which are used to calculate the position of the interaction, as well as the spectrum of the gamma emission. The intensity of the energy signal is amplified substantially, such that the output pulse from the photomultiplier tube is proportional to the total energy absorbed within the field of view of the tube.

Electronic circuits compute the precise X and Y coordinates of the interaction, defining the location of the initial photon interaction with the crystal in a two-dimensional array. The photons emanating from the patient subsequently are displayed on a matrix oriented anatomically consistent with their occurrence within the patient. In addition to these X and Y pulses, the Z pulse is defined, which determines the energy of the event. A multichannel analyzer assesses whether the energy signal is a primary event or a low-energy scatter event. For example, ^{99m}Tc has a primary photopeak of 140 keV with a spectrum window of ± 20 percent. Scattered events have energies below the lower limit cutoff (i.e., 126 keV in this example) and are not accepted.

The collimator is a critical component of the camera system and functions similarly to a camera lens. It usually is made of lead which absorbs gamma rays. The only way a gamma ray can reach the crystal is by passing through the holes within the collimator. For radionuclides generally used in nuclear cardiology (i.e., ^{99m}Tc and ^{201}Tl) low-energy collimators are used. For radionuclides such as ^{195m}Au or ^{111}In, which also have been employed in nuclear cardiology, medium-energy collimators are required. The major difference between these two classes of collimators is the amount of lead in the collimator and the thickness of the septa separating the holes (higher energy tracers require thicker collimators and crystals).

In general, for both low and medium energies, parallel hole collimators are utilized. Most collimators are designed with a trade-off between spatial resolution (resolving capacity) and detector sensitivity (counting capacity). High-resolution parallel hole collimators have the highest resolution but the lowest sensitivity. The major use of high-sensitivity collimators is for first pass dynamic studies, in which the number of photons emitted is severely limited, and the primary determinant of the quality of this study is the maximal count rate achieved, rather than intrinsic resolution.

In addition to sensitivity and spatial resolution, other important characteristics which determine performance of the Anger scintillation camera include field uniformity, energy resolution, and count rate linearity. Using National Electrical Manufacturers Association (NEMA) standards, most state-of-the-art scintillation cameras have a spatial resolution of approximately 4 mm and a count rate linearity up to approximately 75,000 counts per second. Field flood uniformity should be approximately ± 5 percent.

Multicrystal Scintillation Camera

The multicrystal camera consists of 294 individual sodium iodide crystals arranged in a rectangular array of 14 × 21 crystals. There are 35 photomultiplier tubes optically coupled to the crystals by means of a complex light pipe system. A photon interaction is located within the field of view by the crystal in which it is detected. The overall design allows the system to operate at high counting rates with a linear response. This means that as the amount of radioactivity seen by the detector increases, there is a comparable relative increase in detected counts. This system has been designed to process scintillation events extremely rapidly, providing a maximal count rate of approximately 400,000 counts per second, which is approximately five times faster than most standard Anger cameras. Thus, this system is optimally designed for dynamic flow studies, such as first pass radionuclide angiocardiography.

A disadvantage of this detector design is the relatively poor intrinsic spatial resolution. There also is much poorer energy resolution with this system than with the conventional Anger camera. However, for first pass cardiac studies the system has been found to provide a reliable analysis of cardiac function.

Recently, a new mobile version of the multicrystal camera has been developed. This system has a single sodium iodide detector, but one that has been optically divided into 400 components, which are coupled to 115 photomultiplier tubes. Integrated hybrid circuits on each photomultiplier tube transform the signal to a digital pulse which is the input into a digital positioning logic and a dual window pulse height analyzer. With this new design, maximal count rates are enhanced even further, providing linearity up to approximately 800,000 counts per second. Energy resolution and edge resolution also have been improved substantially.

Nonimaging Single Probe Detector

The scintillation probe is a microprocessor-controlled single detector system which is well suited to analyze left ventricular function at the bedside. This instrument is portable, very small, and lightweight. It provides determination of left ventricular ejection fraction, as well as other indices of global systolic and diastolic left ventricular function. The detector is composed of a single sodium iodide crystal 3 in in diameter and 1 in thick. Because of this design, the detector is extremely sensitive to emitted photons, allowing accumulation of extremely high count rates. Because there are no images to guide the operator in determining the region of interest to be sampled by the probe, operator routines and microprocessor algorithms have been designed to help in determining the correct left ventricular background positions. Appropriate training and experience are required in order to obtain accurate and reliable results. Data can be displayed in a beat-to-beat fashion on a strip chart recorder or on a computer console.

Recently, smaller probe systems have been developed using cadmium telluride and mercuric iodide semiconductor detectors, rather than sodium iodide.[28–30] Based upon preliminary work, it may be possible to monitor ventricular performance sequentially over many hours after affixing the probe to the patient's chest.

Single Photon Tomographic Imaging Systems

A major limitation of routine planar imaging is the overlap of different regions within an organ, as well as the overlap of the structure with background. There are two general techniques for performing single photon emission computed tomography: limited angle and transaxial. The limited angle technique is a form of collimator-based tomography, in which either the seven-pinhole or rotating slant hole collimator provides different views of an organ in the longitudinal plane parallel to the long axis of the body. This approach involves utilization of a special collimator attached to a routine Anger camera. However, depth resolution is extremely poor, and this technique is not used widely at this time. On the other hand, transaxial tomography provides far better depth resolution and appears to allow quantification of the distribution of radioactivity within an organ. This approach utilizes a gamma scintillation camera which rotates on a gantry and acquires planar images (32 to 64) at frequent intervals around the circumference of the patient over a 180° to 360° arc. It is important to point out that a minimum of 180° of data are required in order to use back projection reconstruction methods. Transaxial tomograms are obtained in the same orientation as x-ray computed tomography.

Most of the clinical studies performed to date with tomographic studies have utilized a single detector rotating around the patient. However, new camera designs including dual- or triple-headed systems may increase the sensitivity and accuracy of the method. With presently available cameras, the detector rotates in a circular orientation around the patient. A recent development is body contour rotation around the organ of interest. For example, when imaging the heart, these new systems will allow elliptical rotation around the chest. This would decrease the distance between the heart and the collimator, which should improve the resolution and sensitivity of the technique substantially.

Computer Systems

Scintillation data derived from the imaging devices must be organized and analyzed in a quantitative manner. To achieve this goal, a variety of data processing systems have been developed and interfaced to scintillation cameras. At this time the computer component of nuclear imaging system is the most important factor in determining the system's capabilities. Briefly, the nuclear medicine computer contains a central processing unit, image memory, interactive terminals, and high-speed, high-capacity mass storage, such as floppy or hard disks and magnetic tape. In addition, many of the newer systems include array processors for faster image manipulation. These computers generally are fully programmable, allowing definition of specific algorithms for quantitative analysis. The computer should be adequate for all types of nuclear cardiology studies, including first pass equilibrium radionuclide angiocardiography. In general, a matrix size of at least 256 × 256 picture elements (pixels) is required. The capabilities for high temporal resolution (50 frames per second) also are important. In order to perform single photon emission computed tomography, the systems must have software for tomographic reconstruction (filtered back projection), image filtering, and allow for rotation of the gamma camera. This requires a dedicated interface with necessary support software. In order to perform and review tomographic studies well, specific software for quality control and image display are necessary.

A recent development in camera-computer design involves full computer control of the gamma camera. This minimizes the necessity for duplicate analog and digital electronics and provides for better automated camera quality control. Another advantage of the digital camera design is the capability for higher count rates, comparable to that achieved with the multicrystal camera.

Cardiac Performance

Assessment of cardiac performance with radionuclides is currently the most widely employed study in nuclear cardiology. This assessment can be performed in one of two ways: (1) by analysis of the first transit through the central circulation (first pass technique), or (2) by analysis of the entire blood pool after intravascular labeling (equilibrium gated technique).

First Pass Radionuclide Angiocardiography

The general technique of first pass radionuclide angiocardiography has been applied to the assessment of global and regional function of right and left ventricles.[31] The technique involves the rapid intravenous injection of an intact bolus of radioactivity. The high-frequency characteristics of the passage of the radioactivity through the individual cardiac chambers are recorded. Quantitative analysis of the data is based upon application of conventional indicator-dilution principles. It is assumed that there is homogeneous mixing of the radioactive indicator with blood, such that changes in radioactive count rates are proportional reflections of corresponding changes in chamber volumes. Since there is temporal and anatomic separation of the radioactivity within each cardiac chamber, quantitative evaluation of both right and left ventricular function can be made from a single study. Direct assessment can be made of transit times, ventricular ejection fractions, and ejection and relaxation rates. From traced outlines of ventricular silhouettes, measurement of ventricular volume can be made. Regional wall motion can be assessed in both qualitative and quantitative fashions.

Technical Considerations

The choice of scintillation camera for these studies is an important aspect. A major factor limiting studies on conventional single-crystal Anger cameras is the relatively low count rates achieved. Above approximately 75,000 counts per second, current systems generally are no longer linear in terms of their response. Because of lack of linearity and dead-time losses, there is distortion of data accumulation. In order to overcome this inherent limitation, substantial statistical manipulation and processing of the data are necessary. An alternative approach for obtaining first pass data involves the use of a computerized multicrystal scintillation camera which can accumulate high count rates up to 450,000 counts per second without major dead-time losses. Using appropriate collimation, a 25-mCi dose of ^{99m}Tc can result in over 400,000 counts per second during the first transit, with count densities of approximately 500 counts per square centimeter in the region of the left ventricle.

A major aspect of the adequate performance of these studies involves the appropriateness of the injection technique. A compact radionuclide bolus is essential. Slow streaming of the incoming radioactivity will result in artifacts and invalidation of study results. Injections are usually made into an antecubital vein or external jugular vein and need not be made centrally. The medial basilic system is the preferred site of injection when the upper extremity is used since this will provide the most direct route to the superior vena cava. In general, an indwelling polyethylene catheter is inserted in the vein prior to injection. An intravenous infusion is established and continued prior to injection to ensure patency. To facilitate optimal bolus injection, the polyethylene catheter is attached to an extension tube of small volume into which the actual radionuclide bolus is loaded. When the study is performed, the bolus is flushed in rapidly with 20 ml of either saline solution or dextrose in water contained in a separate syringe that is attached to the distal end of the extension tubing. This general design ensures the introduction of a compact radionuclide bolus into the central circulation.

Radiopharmaceuticals labeled with ^{99m}Tc are presently used for first pass studies. The radiopharmaceuticals remain primarily within the intravascular space long enough for the less than 30 s required for completion of the first pass study. Each first pass study requires a separate radionuclide injection. When multiple studies are to be performed on the same day, a number of different individual technetium compounds can be employed in addition to free ^{99m}Tc, such that each will be cleared rapidly from the blood pool by a different mechanism. This allows for repeated study without excessive residual background radioactivity and without excessive radiation burden to any one organ. For example, ^{99m}Tc can be complexed with sulfur colloid, which will be cleared rapidly by the reticuloendothelial system, or with diethylenetriaminepentaacetic acid (DTPA), which will be cleared by the kidneys. In addition, if a pyrophosphate infarct image is to be done also, the ^{99m}Tc stannous pyrophosphate can be injected as a bolus, allowing for initial measurement of ventricular function and subsequent assessment of infarct size and site. Generally, 8 to 20 mCi are used for each injection, with a total dose on any one day usually not exceeding 35 mCi for an adult. The radiopharmaceutical preparations might be of high specific activity; that is, the radioactivity must be contained in a relatively small volume (generally less than 1 ml). This will ensure an adequate injection bolus.

Although ^{99m}Tc radiopharmaceuticals are currently used for first pass studies, they are not ideal because they have a physical half-life of 6 h and the number of repeated studies obtainable in one day is limited. Short-lived generator-produced radionuclides would add significantly to performance of multiple first pass studies. One such generator system, involving ^{195m}Hg–^{195m}Au has undergone recent testing.[32,33] The short-lived radionuclide ^{195m}Au with a physical half-life of 30.5 s is utilized for repeat high-activity, high count rate, first pass studies. The tracer is produced from its mercury parent in a small tabletop generator. Multiple serial studies have been obtained in patients and experimental animals. The higher energy of ^{195m}Au (262 keV) mandates additional instrumentation requirements in comparison with lower energy ^{99m}Tc (140 keV). The rapid decay of short-lived tracer allows its use in combination with ^{201}Tl perfusion imaging during a single exercise study.

Computer processing of data is a necessary part of the first pass study. Data generally are acquired in frame mode and are stored on high-speed magnetic disks at framing rates sufficient to produce data at 10- to 50-ms intervals. At slower heart rates, framing can be at 50-ms intervals. At the more rapid heart rates encountered during exercise, framing intervals should be shorter (10 to 30 ms). Using any one of a variety of computer light pen systems, regions of interest are selected over either right or left ventricle. A fixed region of interest corresponding to the end-diastolic image is employed. Methods for standardizing selection of the region of interest have been reported and involve both isocount contours and color coding.[31] Errors introduced in the selection of the region of interest can influence results substantially. Activity is analyzed during the time when the bolus is only in the cardiac chamber of interest (Fig. 109-1). This temporal separation of radioactivity, first in the right side of the heart and then in the left side of the heart, allows utilization of imaging positions such as the anterior or right anterior oblique positions, which under other circumstances would result in overlapping activity from the two ventricles.

Background corrections are employed for both right and left ventricular measurements. Background results from scattered and overlying radioactivity from adjacent structures. The methods of background correction have varied in individual laboratories. For the left ventricle, background corrections employed include utilization of the time-activity curve to provide a fixed background, or selection of a visually determined background region around the left ventricle. Utilization of an appropriate background correction is critical. Over- or

FIGURE 109-1 Sequential 1-s images obtained during first pass of the radionuclide bolus through the central circulation. The normal temporal and anatomic separation of radioactivity within the cardiac chambers and great vessels is present. The right ventricle and pulmonary artery are best identified in frame 3; the left ventricle and ascending aorta are seen well in frames 7 and 8. (*From H. J. Berger, R. A. Matthay, L. M. Pytlik, A. Gottschalk, and B. L. Zaret, First-Pass Radionuclide Assessment of Right and Left Ventricular Performance in Patients with Cardiac and Pulmonary Disease, Semin. Nucl. Med., 9:275, 1979. Reproduced with permission from the publisher and author.*)

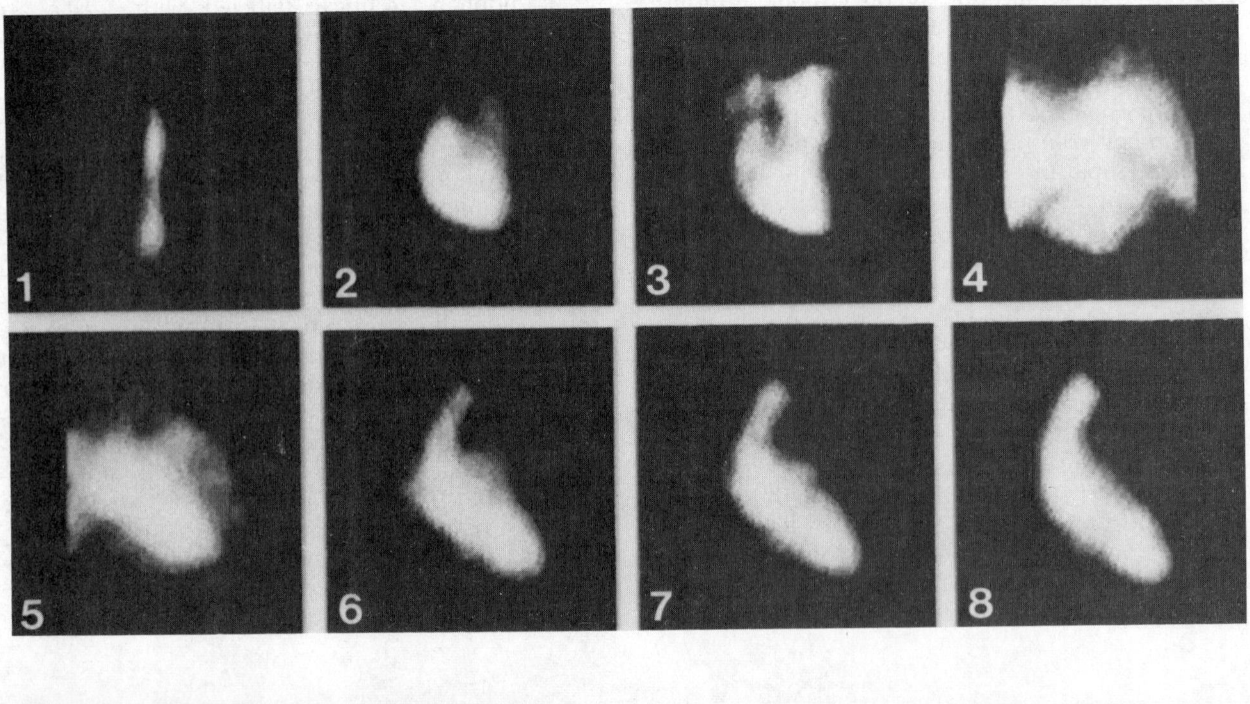

undercorrection for background will introduce major errors in the measurement of ventricular ejection fraction.

The background-corrected time-activity curve from the ventricular region of interest is used for assessment of ventricular function (Fig. 109-2). Since the radioactivity is in equilibrium with blood, peak activity is equivalent to peak (end-diastolic) volume, and valley activity is equivalent to minimal (end-systolic) volume. For the left ventricle, 3 to 6 beats at the peak of the time-activity curve generally are available for analysis. Left ventricular ejection fraction is determined from data from these individual beats. The data are summed to form a single representative cardiac cycle which is analogous to a relative ventricular volume curve. Left ventricular ejection fraction is calculated as the difference between background-corrected end-diastolic and end-systolic counts divided by end-diastolic counts. This is the same formula employed routinely in contrast angiographic assessment of ventricular volumes. Since only a few beats are available for analysis, it can be appreciated that substantial arrhythmias or premature beats can limit the accuracy of a single study.

In addition to ejection fraction, global measures of performance, such as ejection rate, velocity of circumferential fiber shortening, and assessment of the first third of ejection can be made from these studies. Ejection fraction measured by the first pass technique, using either single-crystal or multicrystal scintillation camera, correlates well with that measured by contrast left ventricular angiography.[34–37] In addition, first pass ejection fraction data correlate closely with ejection fraction obtained by multigated equilibrium cardiac blood pool imaging (Fig. 109-3).[38,39] The technique has a relatively low intrinsic variability. In a group of 20 stable volunteers studied on three separate days, the mean variability of ejection fraction measurements was ±4.6 percent.[40] Inter- and intraobserver reproducibility in the measurement of ejection fraction with this technique is excellent.[37]

FIGURE 109-2 Right ventricular (RV) and left ventricular (LV) time-activity curves obtained in 20 frames per second with the computerized multicrystal scintillation camera. Note the extremely high count rates achieved. Ejection fraction and other indexes of global ventricular performance are calculated from these time-activity curves. (*From H. J. Berger, R. A. Matthay, L. M. Pytlik, A. Gottschalk, and B. L. Zaret, First-Pass Radionuclide Assessment of Right and Left Ventricular Performance in Patients with Cardiac and Pulmonary Disease, Semin. Nucl. Med., 9:275, 1979. Reproduced with permission from the publisher and author.*)

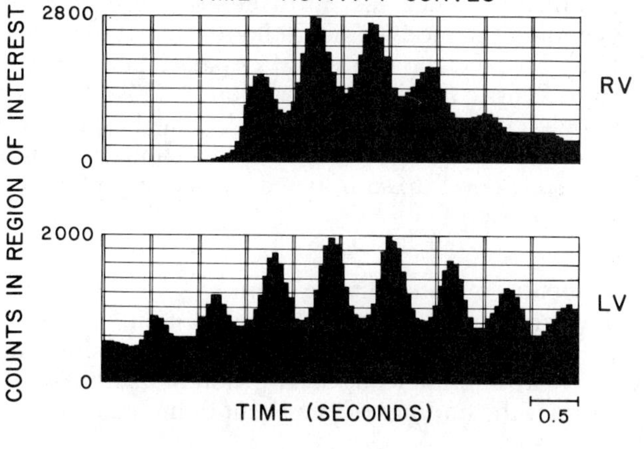

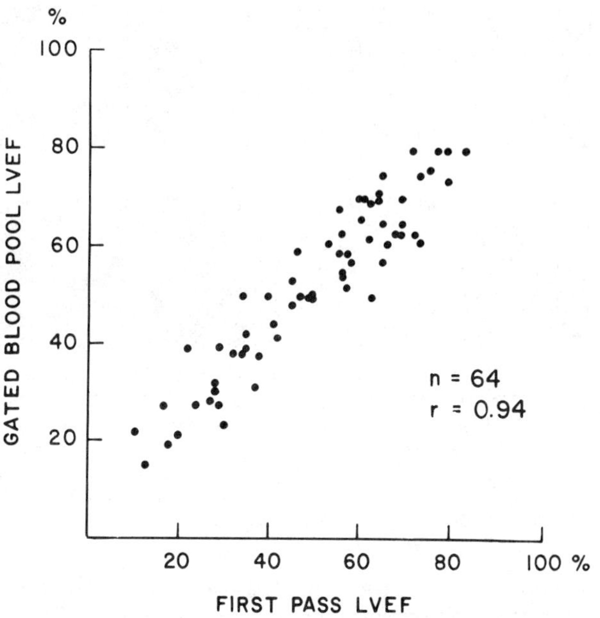

FIGURE 109-3 Left ventricular ejection fraction (LVEF) obtained in 64 patients initially by the first pass technique and then by multiple gated cardiac blood pool imaging. Note the excellent correlation between the two methods over a wide range of ejection fractions. (*From F. J. Wackers, H. J. Berger, D. E. Johnstone, et al., Multiple Gated Cardiac Blood Pool Imaging for Left Ventricular Ejection Fraction: Validation of the Technique and Assessment of Variability, Am. J. Cardiol., 43:1159, 1979. Reproduced with permission from the publisher and author.*)

Measurement of ventricular volumes can be obtained with this technique using principles employed in conventional contrast left ventricular angiography. It is difficult to measure volumes on a count-based method with the first pass technique. From an outline of the end-diastolic silhouette, left ventricular volumes can be determined by conventional area-length analysis. Volumes measured in this manner on the multicrystal camera correlate well with those obtained by contrast angiography.[41]

Assessment of Regional Left Ventricular Performance

Regional left ventricular performance also can be assessed from the first pass study. The summed representative cardiac cycle provides quantitative data analogous to a relative volume curve. Assessment of the visual data in this temporal series of images, each formed from a 10- to 50-ms portion of the cardiac cycle, provides a qualitative assessment of regional contraction patterns.[35–37] This entire cycle can be viewed in a continuous endless-loop cine display (Fig. 109-4). The data can be quantified using a hemiaxial approach comparable to that employed in conventional contrast angiography.[36] The end-diastolic pe-

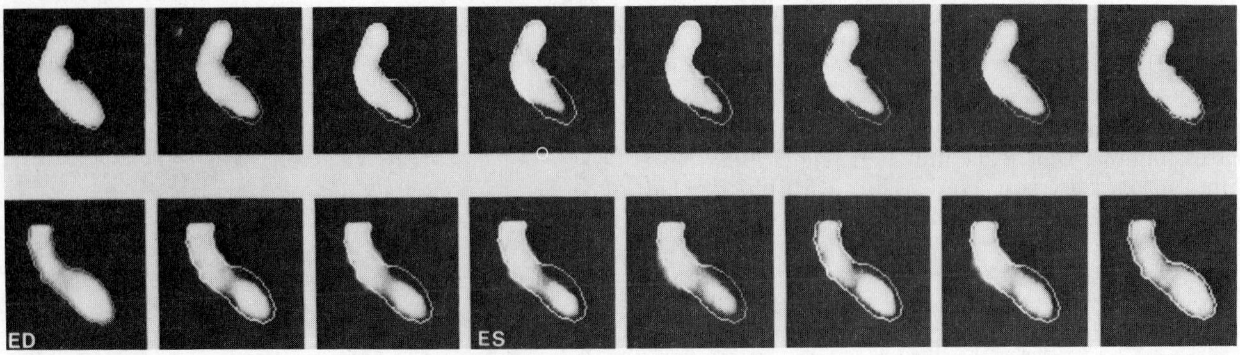

FIGURE 109-4 Selected serial 50-ms left ventricular images through the cardiac cycle shown superimposed over the end-diastolic perimeters generated by computer technique. The first frame in each series represents end-diastole (ED) and the fourth frame end-systole (ES). The upper row of images was obtained at rest, the lower row during maximal bicycle exercise, in a patient with coronary artery disease. The two series are displayed at the same heart rate. Regional wall motion is normal at rest. With exercise, inferoapical hypokinesis develops. (*From H. J. Berger, R. A. Matthay, L. M. Pytlik, A. Gottschalk, and B. L. Zaret, First-Pass Radionuclide Assessment of Right and Left Ventricular Performance in Patients with Cardiac and Pulmonary Disease, Semin. Nucl. Med., 9:275, 1979. Reproduced with permission from the publisher and author.*)

rimeter can be superimposed upon either the end-systolic image or perimeter, thereby providing a static assessment of wall motion. In addition, digital images can provide a functional display, known as the ejection fraction image.[42–44] This image provides an isofunctional map of the relative contributions of different regions to the total ejection fraction. With this technique, quantitative data concerning regional contraction patterns can be obtained in a nontangential manner. This approach has several potential advantages, particularly in asymmetric ventricles and in ventricles in which there is an extensive degree of intrinsic rotation associated with cardiac contraction patterns.

Assessment of wall motion can only be made in one position for each radionuclide injection. It is clear that in the instance of coronary artery disease it may be necessary to obtain an assessment of wall motion in more than one position. This requires the utilization of several radionuclide injections or the application of dual-angle bilateral collimators, which may allow simultaneous acquisition of data in two positions.

Right Ventricular Performance

With the use of techniques comparable to those employed for the assessment of left ventricular function, right ventricular global performance can also be measured. A high-frequency time-activity curve is generated from the right ventricular region of interest, either in the anterior or right anterior oblique position. With the multicrystal scintillation camera, studies obtained in the anterior position have employed a background correction obtained at the region of the tricuspid valve plane. This background accounts for the degree of right atrial–right ventricular overlap encountered in this anatomic position. Subtraction of the background time-activity curve from that obtained in the ventricular region of interest results in a high-count-rate, background-corrected right ventricular time-activity curve from which right ventricular ejection fraction can be measured directly (Fig. 109-2).[45]

Right ventricular studies have also been performed with conventional Anger scintillation cameras. In one approach, a routine time-activity curve is obtained, which then is analyzed following background correction.[46] This approach is limited because of the lack of statistical reliability of this low-count-rate data. More recently, a gated first pass technique has been introduced.[47] With this technique, first pass data are acquired in synchrony with the patient's electrocardiogram and stored temporally. Several beats are summed during the right ventricular phase, forming a representative cardiac cycle. This provides relatively reliable higher-count-rate data.

Normal values of right ventricular ejection fraction have been established (Fig. 109-5).[45] Unlike the case of the left ventricle, an adequate contrast angiographic standard against which radionuclide data can be compared for the right ventricle does not currently exist. The technique has been standardized based upon (1) establishment of a normal range using a large number of normal subjects, (2) demonstrably lower inter- and intraobserver variation in measurements, (3) reproducibility on repeated study, and (4) appropriate response to inotropic stimulation, such as intravenous isoproterenol. Combined hemodynamic-radionuclide studies have demonstrated the marked afterload dependence of right ventricular ejection fraction.[48] This afterload dependence can be utilized such that the presence of an abnormal right ventricular ejection fraction is relatively good presumptive evidence of pulmonary hypertension.[49]

Detection of Intracardiac Shunts

The first pass study can be used to define intracardiac shunts.[50] Visual inspection of the radionuclide angiocardiogram leads to suspicion of a left-to-right shunt if the findings of persistent pulmonary activity

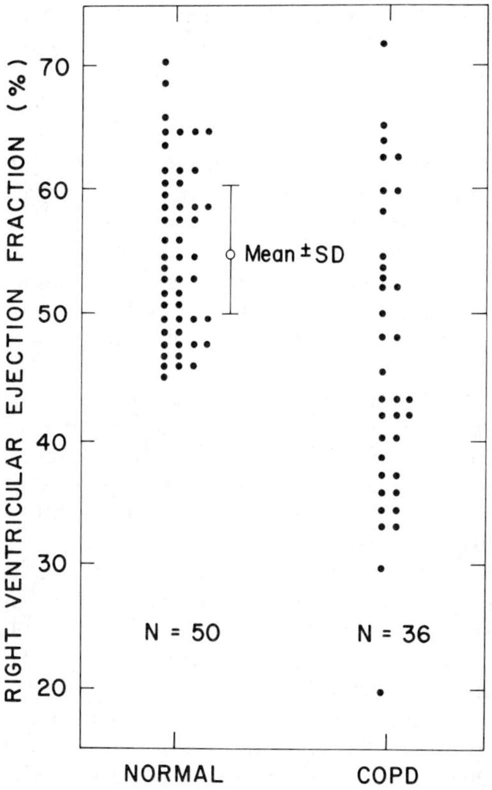

FIGURE 109-5 Resting right ventricular ejection fraction in 50 normal control subjects without cardiopulmonary disease (*left*) and in 36 patients with chronic obstructive pulmonary disease (COPD) (*right*). The mean ± 1 standard deviation is shown. The lower limit of normal is 45 percent. Note the broad range of right ventricular ejection fractions obtained in patients with COPD. (*From H. J. Berger, R. A. Matthay, J. Loke, R. C. Marshall, A. Gottschalk, and B. L. Zaret, Assessment of Cardiac Performance with Quantitative Radionuclide Angiography: Right Ventricular Ejection Fraction with Reference to Findings in Chronic Obstructive Pulmonary Disease, Am. J. Cardiol., 41:897, 1978. Reproduced with permission from the publisher and author.*)

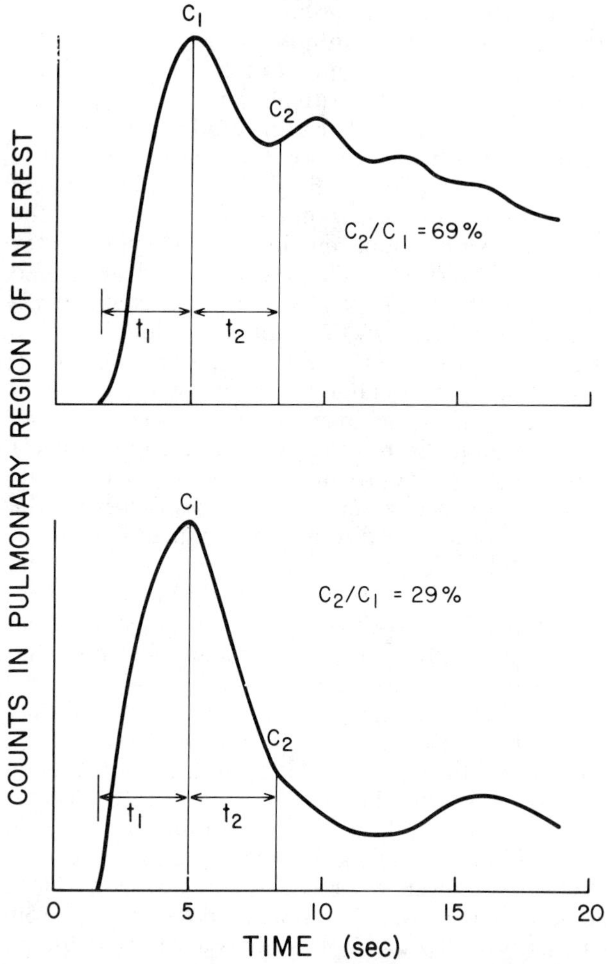

FIGURE 109-6 Pulmonary time-activity curves obtained in a normal subject (*lower panel*) and in a patient with a left-to-right shunt (*upper panel*). Note the delayed washout of pulmonary activity and the abnormally elevated C_2/C_1 ratio in the presence of a left-to-right shunt.

and poor visualization of the left side of the heart are observed. This is generally of value in shunts in which the pulmonary/systemic flow ratios exceed 1.6. The quantitative approach to shunt detection is far more meaningful and accurate. With this technique, a region of interest is selected over the lung fields. The pulmonary time-activity curve from this region is analyzed. Under normal circumstances, there is an initial sharp rise in radioactivity as the bolus reaches the pulmonary capillary bed, followed by a sharp decline as the bolus leaves. There is a second lower-amplitude peak occurring later. This is due to normal recirculation. In the presence of left-to-right shunting, persistent high activity remains in the lungs. There is early reappearance of radioactivity and interruption of the usual exponential decrease in activity that follows the initial peak. The ratio between peak activity (C_1) and activity (C_2) at a point after peak activity equal in time to the period between initial appearance and peak activity (C_2/C_1 ratio) provides a reliable qualitative statement concerning the presence or absence of a left-to-right shunt (Fig. 109-6). It is not sufficient for quantitative determination of the degree of shunting. By deconvolution of the pulmonary time-activity curve using a gamma-variate model, the magnitude of shunting can be quantified. Excellent correlations have been obtained between the pulmonary/systemic flow ratio measured by the radionuclide technique and that measured by oximetry at the time of cardiac catheterization. It should be noted that accurate assessment of left-to-right shunting with this technique can be made only in the presence of relatively normal ventricular function. In the presence of abnormal left ventricular function, pulmonary transit may be delayed substantially, thereby presenting a false appearance of a shunt in the pulmonary time-activity curve.

For right-to-left shunting, insights can be obtained from a qualitative assessment of the first transit revealing early appearance of activity in the aorta. Quantitative analysis of the time-activity curves generated from the left ventricle can aid in the detection of significant right-to-left shunts.

Advantages and Limitations of the First Pass Technique

The first pass technique can be performed extremely rapidly. The patient can pass through the laboratory for a simple resting study in a matter of minutes. The actual period of data acquisition is less than 30 s. This allows definition of rapidly changing physiologic states and is optimal for the study of the acutely ill who cannot remain in a stable position for long periods of time. The technique is ideally suited for use with *upright* exercise and in specific patients unable to exercise in the supine position. This is a significant advantage. Assessment of individual cardiac chambers is obtained without potential contamination from activity in adjacent ventricles. The first pass technique is the most appropriate approach for assessing right ventricular function and currently provides the best noninvasive means of assessing the presence of intracardiac shunts and quantifying their magnitude.

The technique is limited in that regional wall motion can only be assessed in one view per study. Multiple measurements cannot be made following a single radionuclide injection (as can be made with the equilibrium multigated technique). This difficulty could be overcome with the use of short half-life tracers such as ^{195m}Au. Since analysis is based on only a small sampling of cardiac cycles, the occurrence of ectopic beats or arrhythmias during data acquisition can make data analysis impossible. The data are of lower count density when compared with data obtained with the multigated technique. From a technical standpoint, it is necessary to have an impeccable injection technique. On occasion, the absence of appropriate venous injection sites can limit the ability to perform this first pass study.

First pass techniques are best obtained on a multicrystal scintillation camera. In the past this instrument was not portable. This objection will be overcome, at least in part, with the advent and availability of newly designed instruments. In addition, newly developed high-count-rate cameras which are portable currently are available. Therefore, this technology now can be brought to the bedside in an intensive care unit environment.

Equilibrium Radionuclide Angiocardiography

In the equilibrium gated blood pool technique, electrocardiographic events are used to establish meaningful temporal relations between the times of data acquisition and the mechanical activity of the heart.[51] Repetitive sampling from physiologically selected phases of the cardiac cycle is obtained over multiple heartbeats until data are acquired at sufficient count density to allow analysis. When the technique was first introduced in 1971, left ventricular outlines were drawn manually and the silhouettes were analyzed quantitatively to assess left ventricular ejection fraction and wall motion in a manner comparable to that employed in contrast left ventricular angiograms.[9,10] Major advances in computer technology recently have been applied to this method.[27,52]

Technique

As opposed to the first pass study, the gated equilibrium study samples and sums several hundred cardiac cycles. In order to obtain meaningful data, cardiac performance must be relatively stable during this relatively long period of data accumulation. The patient must remain relatively still beneath the detector so that motion artifacts are minimized. The radionuclide must remain in a stable manner within the intravascular space during the period of study. Framing intervals must be short enough to provide adequate temporal resolution of the data at varying heart rates, while the duration of the study must be sufficiently long to provide appropriate counting statistics to assure adequate spatial resolution.

The radiopharmaceuticals used for blood pool labeling in equilibrium studies all involve ^{99m}Tc. The entire intravascular space must be labeled in a stable manner. Studies were performed initially with ^{99m}Tc-labeled human serum albumin. However, at the present time, examinations are performed almost exclusively with ^{99m}Tc labeling of the patient's own red blood cells. This has provided a relatively stable blood pool label with a biologic half-life of approximately 4 h. Blood pool labeling is accomplished by either in vitro or in vivo techniques. When the in vitro technique is employed, the patient is injected with 1 to 3 mg of unlabeled stannous pyrophosphate 15 min prior to administration of ^{99m}Tc pertechnetate. Labeling occurs directly within the intravascular space. The in vitro approach involves labeling a small volume of blood in a sterile vial, in a manner similar to other kits. Recently, a modified in vivo technique has been proposed. With this approach the tin is injected intravenously as in the in vivo method. However, the labeling is then performed in a sterile closed system of syringe and extension tubing directly connected to the patient.[53] This later method appears to provide the best labeling and is the preferred approach in our laboratory. This radiopharmaceutical labeling provides a higher target-to-background ratio than obtained previously with labeled albumin. This allows the acquisition of higher-resolution images over a shorter period of time. Serial imaging following a single injection can be obtained for periods ranging from 6 to 12 h.

Equilibrium studies are performed currently with Anger scintillation cameras. These instruments are now available as portable equipment and consequently can be brought to the bedside of the acutely ill patient. Studies are performed with parallel-hole collimators. Studies obtained in the resting state should use a high-resolution or all-purpose collimator. A slant-hole collimator has also been developed.[54] This collimator provides additional caudal angulation, allowing greater separation of left ventricle from left atrium. For exercise or rapid-inter-

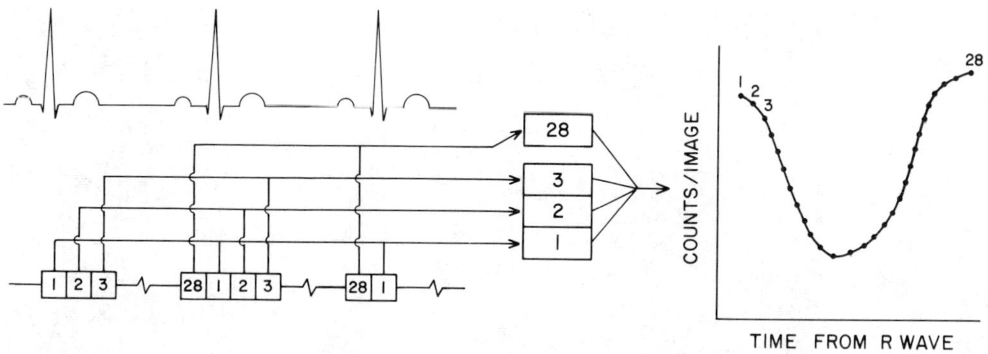

FIGURE 109-7 Schematic representation of the data processing involved in generation of a summed left ventricular time-activity curve with the multigated equilibrium technique. In this example, the cardiac cycle has been divided into 28 segments. Data occurring during the specific time intervals shown below are stored in computer memory for several hundred individual cardiac cycles. Following background subtraction, these individual data points are displayed as a relative volume curve as indicated on the right.

vention imaging, an all-purpose collimator with a greater sensitivity should be employed.

To perform the routine study the R wave of the electrocardiogram is employed as the triggering signal for the computer system.[12,55] This signal is most desirable since generally it is easy to obtain from the routine electrocardiogram, it bears a general relation to the contractile events of the left ventricle, and generally occurs in appropriate size and shape once per cardiac cycle. Specific artifacts can be introduced into the gating portion of the study in patients with relatively small R waves or high spiked T waves (as might be encountered in hyperkalemia). Further sources of gating artifacts involve pacemaker spikes which may or may not result in effective mechanical activity, movement artifacts, and artifacts relating to the occurrence of spontaneous transient arrhythmias during the period of data acquisition.

Data analysis is performed by computer and frequently requires significant operator interaction. All radionuclide data are collected and segregated temporally, based upon synchrony with the electrocardiographic trigger (Fig. 109-7). The RR interval is divided into 16 to 28 equal subdivisions, depending upon the heart rate. Generally, a framing interval of 40 to 50 ms is used at rest and 20 to 30 ms during exercise or with heart rates that are more rapid than usual. Short framing intervals are required for the high temporal resolution studies necessary for resolution of diastolic events. Data occurring during consecutive time intervals are sorted into the computer bin whose location in the temporal sequence is determined by the time elapsed from the onset of the R wave. When the next R wave is reached, the sorting process is reset and begun again. Studies require from 2 to 10 min for completion. The end result is a single sequence spanning the cardiac cycle which is the sum of data from several hundred individual heartbeats. Studies may be acquired to a present left ventricular count density or to a given level of total counts in the entire image.

A left ventricular time-activity curve, analogous to a relative ventricular volume curve and suitable for assessment of ejection fraction and rates of filling and relaxation, is based upon analysis of only the left anterior oblique position study. This is the only position in which there is adequate separation of the two ventricles. A count-based approach then can be employed to measure ejection fraction directly from the volume curve according to standard formulas. Ejection fraction measured in this manner correlates well with measurements made at the time of contrast left ventricular angiography.[12,38,52] In instrumented animals, radionuclide measurements correlate well with independent hemodynamic assessment.[56] It is mandatory to correct for background contributions to the left ventricular radioactivity. This contribution comes from overlying and adjacent structures, most notably lungs, left atrium, and chest wall. Although there is substantial overlap between the left atrium and left ventricle, the atrium contributes relatively little to left ventricular activity because of its distance from the detector (Fig. 109-8). Semiautomated methods have been developed for determination of the left ventricular region of interest. The techniques of edge detection generally are of two types: (1) threshold and (2) second derivative or maximal gradient. Neither will work perfectly well for all patients. Advances in edge detection techniques are necessary. One promising new approach involves application of the principles of artificial intelligence to computerized recognition of left ventricular margins, particularly when there is chamber overlap.[57] Operator quality control and interaction when appropriate is mandatory. For optimal performance of gated studies, a variable region of interest should be employed, rather than a fixed region of interest such as is utilized in the first pass technique.[58]

Regional wall motion cannot be analyzed adequately from the left anterior oblique image alone. To obtain an adequate assessment of wall motion, at least three views and preferably four views should be obtained. These generally are the anterior, 45° left anterior oblique, and left lateral and left posterior oblique images. Choice of the degree of left anterior obliquity to employ in each study must be

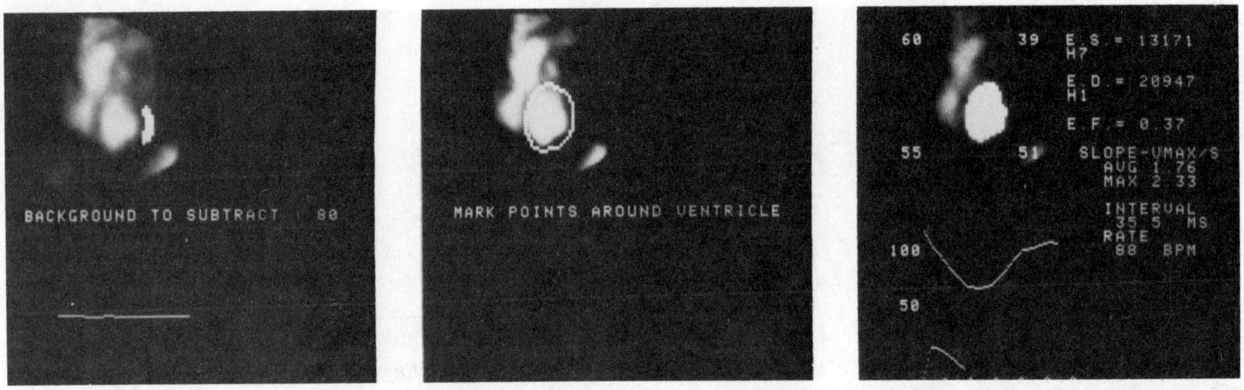

FIGURE 109-8 A series of images illustrating some of the technical aspects involved in multigated equilibrium blood pool studies. All images represent the cardiac blood pool in the left anterior oblique position. The image on the left shows the background region selected and the corresponding flat time-activity curve. The image in the middle panel shows the left ventricular region of interest. The image on the right demonstrates the actual display of the data on the oscilloscope screen, indicating the ejection fraction (EF) and displaying the relative volume curve from which the ejection fraction is demonstrated. (*From H. J. Berger, A. Gottschalk, and B. L. Zaret, Radionuclide Assessment of Left and Right Ventricular Performance, Radiol. Clin. North Am., 18:441, 1980. Reproduced with permission from the publisher and author.*)

individualized, based upon visual assessment of the adequacy of separation of both ventricles. Analysis of regional wall motion abnormalities can be made from comparison of static images at end-diastole and end-systole, but is more effective from visualization of an endless-loop radionuclide cineangiogram (Fig. 109-9). The anterior and apical walls can be evaluated well in the anterior images. The inferior wall

FIGURE 109-9 Serial images obtained from a multigated equilibrium blood pool study using 16 frames in a single cardiac cycle. All images are displayed in the left anterior oblique position. End-diastole (ED) is shown in the upper left-hand corner. The temporal sequence is read from left to right. The seventh image is end-systole (ES). In this study, normal uniform ventricular contraction can be appreciated throughout the cardiac cycle. (*From H. J. Berger, A. Gottschalk, and B. L. Zaret, Radionuclide Assessment of Left and Right Ventricular Performance, Radiol. Clin. North Am., 18:441, 1980. Reproduced with permission from the publisher and author.*)

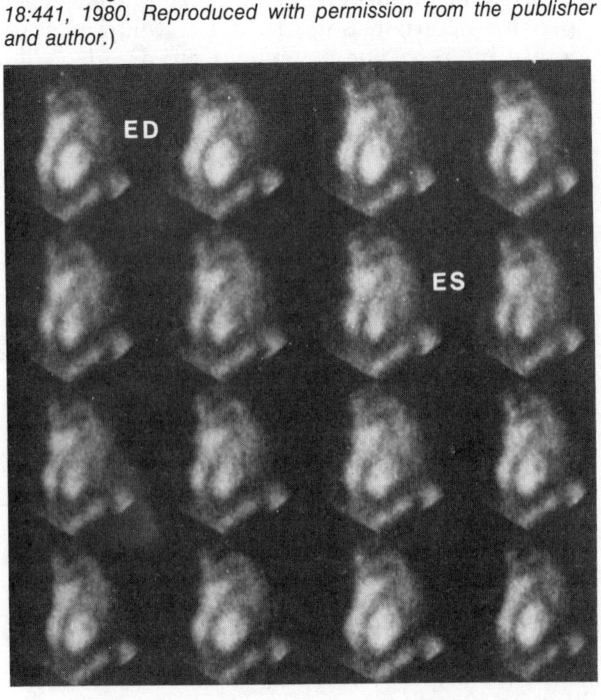

is best evaluated in the left lateral image or a very steep left anterior oblique image.[59,60] The posterolateral and septal walls are best assessed in the left anterior oblique image. Assessment of large anterior wall aneurysms requires multiple views, since in the left anterior oblique view the false impression of diffuse hypokinesis will be obtained frequently (Figs. 109-10 and 109-11). Analysis of regional function need not be only qualitative. Simple semiquantitative analysis can be employed using a reproducible 5-point scoring system for each segment, grading from dyskinesis, through akinesis, hypokinesis, and normal. Computer programs have been and are being developed currently for assessing regional contraction patterns based on measurement of hemiaxes, radials, or regional ejection fractions[61] (Fig. 109-12). In addition, techniques developed for contrast left ventriculography such as the "center-line method" may be adopted to nuclear data.[62] Other techniques involve the ejection fraction functional imaging approach similar to that discussed above in the section dealing with first pass radionuclide angiocardiography and Fourier phase imaging.[63]

Recently, the equilibrium technique has been applied to measurement of left ventricular volumes. Left ventricular volumes may be measured in two ways. First, the conventional contrast angiographic area-length methods may be used. With this method good correlations with measurement made at the time of contrast left ventricular angiography have been noted.[51] However, this approach has significant limitations. The second approach is based upon quantification of radioactivity emanating from the left ventricle. Since radioactivity is proportional to volume (at equilibrium), it should be possible to establish a meaningful relation between ventricular volume and counts in the ventricular region of interest once a blood sample is obtained as a counting standard. Initial studies using this method did not deal with the quantitative problems of radiation at-

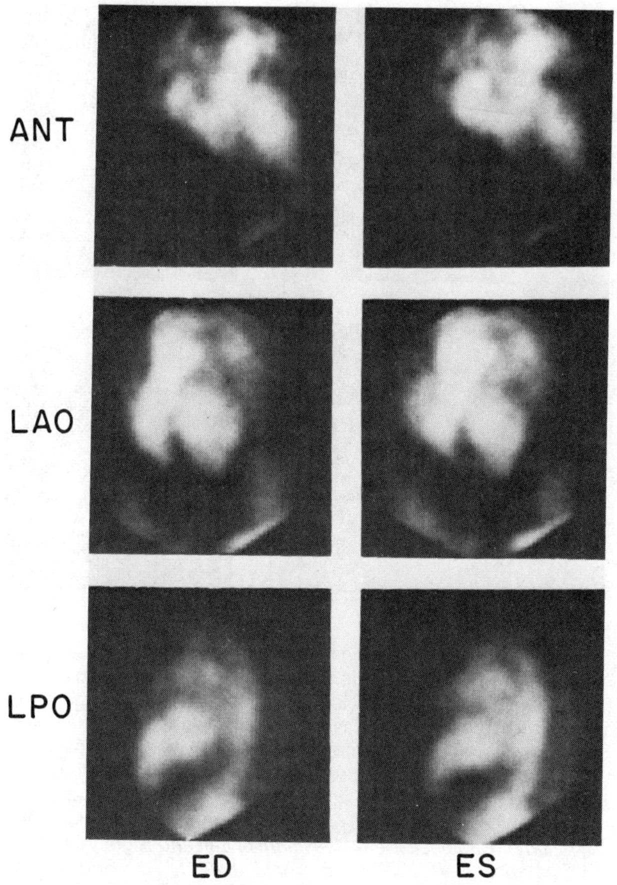

FIGURE 109-10 Multigated equilibrium blood pool images in the anterior (ANT), left anterior oblique (LAO), and left posterior oblique (LPO) positions at end-diastole (ED) and end-systole (ES) in a patient with an anteroapical aneurysm. The aneurysm can be appreciated in the anterior position but is not seen well in the left anterior oblique position. It is best seen in the LPO position. (*From H. J. Berger, A. Gottschalk, and B. L. Zaret, Radionuclide Assessment of Left and Right Ventricular Performance, Radiol. Clin. North Am., 18:441, 1980. Reproduced with permission from the publisher and author.*)

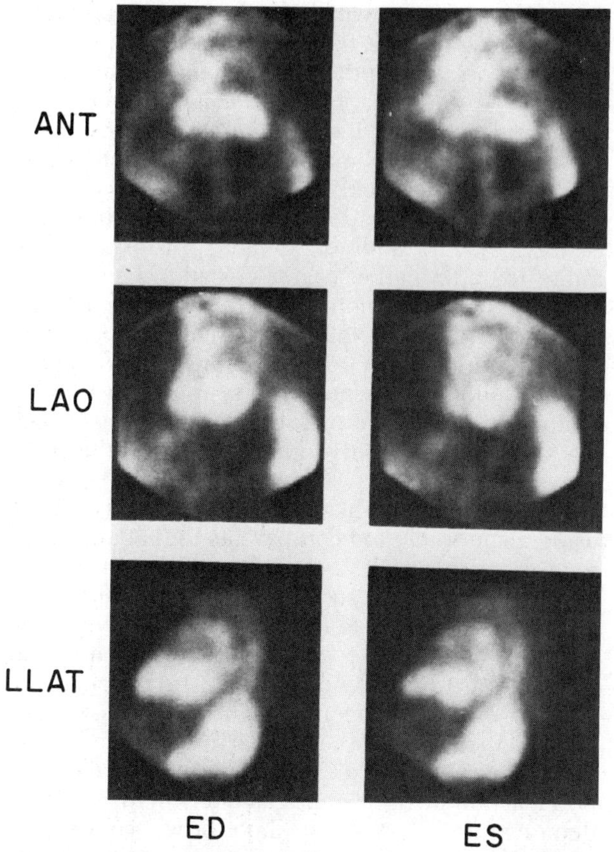

FIGURE 109-11 Multigated equilibrium cardiac blood pool images in a patient with a posterobasal aneurysm. Images are shown in the anterior (ANT), left anterior oblique (LAO), and left lateral (LLAT) positions at end-diastole (ED) and end-systole (ES). The aneurysm is best appreciated in the LLAT position. This study clearly indicates the need to obtain multigated studies in multiple positions in order to define aneurysms or significant regional wall motion abnormalities. (*From H. J. Berger, A. Gottschalk, and B. L. Zaret, Radionuclide Assessment of Left and Right Ventricular Performance, Radiol. Clin. North Am., 18:441, 1980. Reproduced with permission from the publisher and author.*)

FIGURE 109-12 Ventricular volume curve (*left*) and regional ejection fraction (*right*) in a patient with an anteroseptal infarction. Data were obtained in the left anterior oblique position. The image on the left shows the ventricular volume curve and regions of interest for the left ventricle; the ejection fraction of 39 percent. On the right, the left anterior oblique left ventricular region of interest is divided into five distinct sectors. The upper sector, representing the valve plane area, is not included. As can be seen, the septal and apical segments have depressed ejection fractions of 30, 34, and 34 percent, respectively. In contrast, the inferolateral and posterolateral segments have ejection fractions of 51 and 49 percent. This approach provides a nongeometric means of evaluating regional ventricular function.

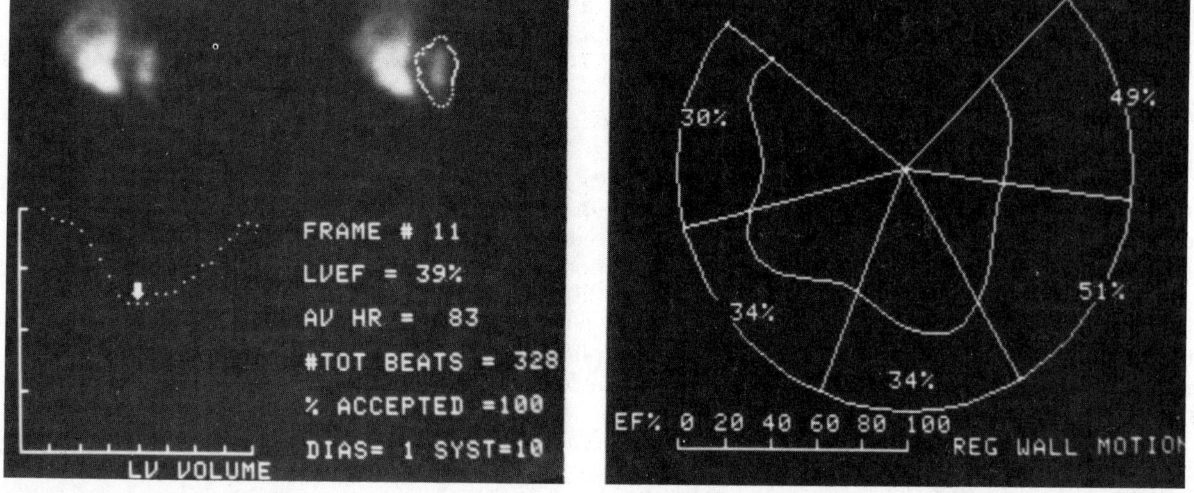

tenuation. Left ventricular counts (or volume, if counts are converted to volume based upon activity measured in the standard blood sample) calculated from regression equations have correlated well with measured angiographic volumes.[64] This approach has the advantage of making a measurement somewhat independent of ventricular geometry. More recently, the problem of attenuation also has been addressed. The addition of an appropriate technique for attenuation correction adds significantly to the value of this nongeometric volume measurement.[65] In general, volumetric analysis appears to be quite important. Measurement of end-systolic volume allows assessment of systolic function by evaluation of systolic pressure-volume data, which may be a more sensitive index of contractile function.[66]

Calculation of right ventricular ejection fraction using a count method comparable to that employed for the left ventricle is somewhat more difficult. A problem resides in underlying right atrial activity and its contribution to the apparent right ventricular time-activity curve, making the right ventricular ejection fraction erroneously low. In patients with small or minimally enlarged right ventricles, the relative contribution of the right atrium is greatest. Although an ability to measure right ventricular ejection fraction with the multigated technique has been demonstrated,[67] in all likelihood it will continue to be simpler and more accurate to measure right ventricular function with the first pass technique (either gated first pass or routine first pass methods).

Concomitant assessment of relative stroke volume counts of both the right and left ventricle at equilibrium allows an assessment of the presence and extent of valvular regurgitation. If regions of interest corresponding to each ventricle are defined accurately, then the stroke volume counts of each chamber should be equal. In the presence of valvular regurgitation involving the aortic or mitral valve, this will not be the case, and left ventricular stroke volume counts will exceed significantly that generated from the right ventricle. Relations have been established for the application of this technique for both detection of regurgitation and measurement of the degree of aortic or mitral regurgitation.[68] Data have been correlated with regurgitant fraction measured at cardiac catheterization. In addition, studies in animals have demonstrated the accuracy of this approach under the experimental conditions of acute aortic regurgitation.[69] However, significant error can be introduced into this measurement, particularly in the presence of ventricular enlargement and dysfunction and cardiac arrhythmia.[70] In addition there often are problems in distinguishing mild degrees of regurgitation from the normal heart.

Since at equilibrium the entire intravascular blood pool is radioactively labeled, a wide range of additional useful information can be obtained. The relative size of each cardiac chamber can be assessed.

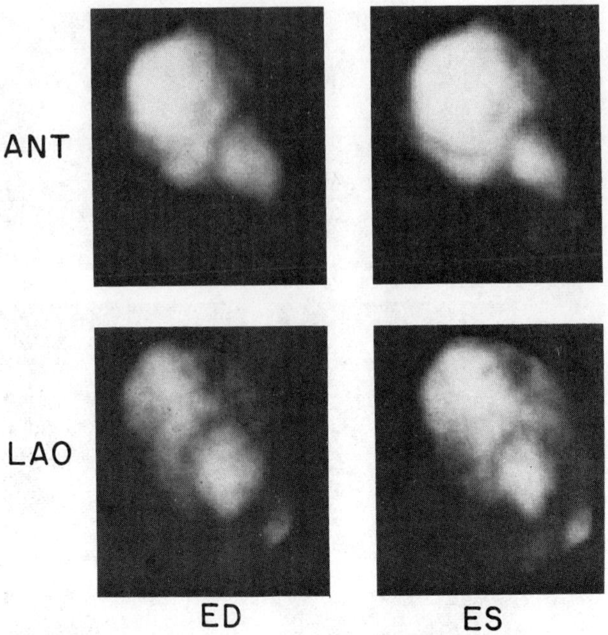

FIGURE 109-13 Multigated equilibrium blood pool images in the anterior (ANT) and left anterior oblique (LAO) positions at end-diastole (ED) and end-systole (ES) in a patient with a large aneurysm of the proximal aorta. Note the relatively normal left ventricular and right ventricular size and the massive aneurysm above the aortic valve. This study demonstrates the additional information available in an equilibrium study concerning anatomic features of the cardiovascular system. (*From H. J. Berger, A. Gottschalk, and B. L. Zaret, Radionuclide Assessment of Left and Right Ventricular Performance, Radiol. Clin. North Am., 18:441, 1980. Reproduced with permission from the publisher and author.*)

The relative adequacy of contraction patterns of right and left ventricle can be assessed directly in a qualitative sense. The size and relative orientation of the great vessels can be appreciated. Dilatation of the pulmonary artery or aorta, aortic aneurysms, and extracardiac vascular structures and anomalies can be appreciated (Fig. 109-13). The presence of intracardiac masses can be detected.[71] Insights into specific pathologic entities can be obtained by assessing the relative sizes of the individual cardiac chambers. Relative thickness of the interventricular septum can be appreciated, and the diagnosis of hypertrophic cardiomyopathy can be inferred.[72]

Quantitative data also can be obtained from a number of regional circulations. This approach has been employed in the study of relative changes in pulmonary blood volume. Using the equilibrium technique, Okada et al. noted changes in blood volume in patients exercising to levels of myocardial ischemia.[73] Increased pulmonary blood volume was noted in 90 percent of patients with coronary artery disease studied during supine exercise, while these changes were not seen in normal persons. This implies an element of reversible pulmonary congestion associated with exercise in coronary disease.

In a similar fashion, the capacity of the peripheral circulation also has been assessed. This technique may be of particular importance in view of the current emphasis upon utilization of pharmacologic agents that alter left ventricular preload by affecting the capacitance circulation in humans. Since at equilibrium counts are proportional to volume, relative changes in counts in the extremity will reflect relative changes in the blood volume of this extremity. Rutlen et al. demonstrated this relation in both the upper and lower extremities of humans and correlated radioactivity changes with concomitant changes in volume as measured by plethysmographic techniques.[74] Increases in extremity blood volume were appropriately evident in response to physical and pharmacologic (nitroglycerin) maneuvers, and decreases in capacity were demonstrated following elevation of the extremity. The same principles have been applied to the study of the splanchnic capacitance circulation in both animals and humans.[75,76]

Advantages and Limitations of the Equilibrium Gated Technique and Comparison with First Pass Approach

The equilibrium study has several distinct advantages. Multiple studies can be performed over several hours following a single radionuclide injection. Therefore, regional wall motion can be assessed in as many views as is necessary for adequate evaluation. In addition, data during a variety of physiologic or pharmacologic interventions can be obtained sequentially over sustained time periods. This serial assessment may provide meaningful information that would be lost if observations were made only at the beginning (or control) and at a solitary endpoint. The ability to obtain multiple studies is thus a significant advantage over the first-pass technique, where each study requires an individual radionuclide injection. Again, this problem of the first-pass technique may be obviated with the availability of generator-produced short-lived tracers.

The high count density of the equilibrium study also presents an advantage in terms of the statistical reliability of assessing regional wall motion, particularly when dealing with more subtle abnormalities. The ability to view the entire cardiovascular blood pool has both advantages and disadvantages. In a positive sense, direct comparisons are available immediately concerning qualitative aspects of right and left ventricular size and function, atrial size, and position of the great vessels. In a negative sense, this additional activity may detract from direct assessment of the left ventricle, which generally is the main purpose for performance of the study. In comparison, the first pass study allows direct assessment of each ventricle without distracting superimposed activity from the other. The equilibrium study is less prone to invalidation because of transient arrhythmias than is the first pass technique, where analysis is limited to only a few cardiac cycles. However, if ectopic beats occur more than 20 percent of the time, the equilibrium study may be of no value unless computational ability exists to screen out data from irregularly occurring cardiac cycles.

A disadvantage of the equilibrium study, in relation to first pass studies, is the duration of the examination. Equilibrium gated studies require 2 to 10 min of patient time beneath the scintillation camera, whereas first pass studies are completed in 15 to 30 s. This seems particularly relevant when dealing with acutely ill patients and rapidly changing physiologic states. Exercise ventricular performance can be assessed with either technique. However, with the first pass approach, upright exercise is more readily and reproducibly obtained, while equilibrium studies are performed predominantly in the supine position. The position in which exercise is performed may influence results because of differing preload and afterload effects in the upright and supine positions and the patient's inability to exercise adequately in the supine position. Right ventricular performance has been evaluated with equilibrium technique. However it is likely that a more discriminating, reproducible, and technically satisfactory study can be obtained with the first pass technique.

In summary, it can be appreciated that each approach to assessment of cardiac performance has specific virtues and limitations. Any one laboratory should perform that type of study with which it is most familiar, which makes optimal use of available equipment, and which is most suitable to the patient population available for study.

Clinical Applications of Ventricular Performance Assessment

Both first pass and equilibrium techniques have been employed in a variety of clinical conditions both at rest and during exercise stress.

Resting Ventricular Performance

Measurement of right and left ventricular performance in patients with suspected or documented heart failure is of value in distinguishing a cardiac from a pulmonary etiology for dyspnea, in defining ventricular dysfunction that may be amenable to surgical therapy (such as left ventricular aneurysm or pseudoaneurysm), and in designing and following appropriate pharmacologic therapy, such as positive inotropic or afterload-reducing agents. In this latter clinical instance, assessment of ventricular volumes is of major importance.[77] In terms of etiology of heart failure, radionuclide studies provide distinct patterns in primary congestive cardiomyopathy (biventricular enlargement with diffuse dysfunction), hypertrophic cardiomyopathy, and ischemic cardiomyopathy.[78] The presence of an enlarged left ventricle with normal or near-normal ejection fraction suggests volume overload, as can be seen, for example, in aortic or mitral insufficiency or renal failure.

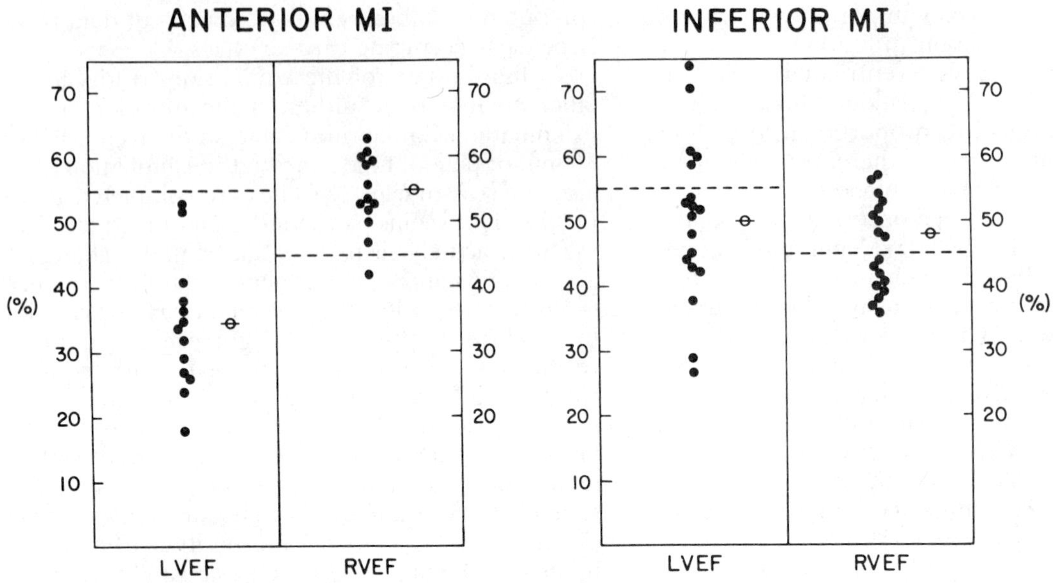

FIGURE 109-14 Left ventricular ejection fraction (LVEF) and right ventricular ejection fraction (RVEF) in 31 patients with acute transmural myocardial infarction (MI). Note that right ventricular ejection fraction was abnormal in 9 of 18 patients with inferior infarction but was normal in 12 of 13 patients with anterior infarction. The lower limits of normal are shown by the dashed horizontal lines. (*From L. A. Reduto, H. J. Berger, L. S. Cohen, A. Gottschalk, and B. L. Zaret, Sequential Radionuclide Assessment of Left and Right Ventricular Performance After Acute Myocardial Infarction, Ann. Intern. Med., 89:441, 1978. Reproduced with permission from the publisher and author.*)

Several studies of ventricular performance in the resting state have dealt with the patient following myocardial infarction. Using radionuclide techniques, Dymond et al. and Rigo et al. were able to differentiate between postinfarction left ventricular aneurysm and diffuse hypokinesis.[79,80] Reduto et al. evaluated the interrelationship between right and left ventricular function over the course of hospitalization for acute myocardial infarction.[81] In this study, 31 hemodynamically stable patients with a first transmural myocardial infarct without additional cardiac disease or antecedent angina pectoris were studied sequentially. The first measurements were obtained an average of 16 h following the onset of chest pain (Fig. 109-14). Anterior wall myocardial infarction resulted in greater depression in left ventricular ejection fraction than did inferior wall myocardial infarction. When right ventricular ejection fraction was analyzed, an opposite result was observed: inferior wall myocardial infarction resulted in greater reduction of right ventricular ejection fraction than did anterior wall infarcts. In fact, in anterior wall infarcts, right ventricular dysfunction was extremely unusual. Thus, based upon radionuclide studies, it is evident that the site of infarction impacts significantly upon the type and degree of ventricular dysfunction observed. These same observations continued throughout the course of hospitalization. Furthermore, there was no tendency for the group as a whole toward improvement or deterioration of ventricular performance during the period of evaluation.

These studies were confirmed by Tobinick et al., who also noted the relatively frequent occurrence of right ventricular dysfunction in patients with inferior wall myocardial infarction.[46] These clinicians also related abnormal right ventricular function to abnormal pyrophosphate myocardial accumulation. Observations of marked right ventricular dysfunction in the course of inferior infarction have also been made by Rigo et al.[82] and Sharpe et al.[83] using the equilibrium gated technique. Several studies since have evaluated both global and regional ventricular function following infarction.[84–89] In addition, several recent reports have emphasized the prognostic impact of abnormal ejection fraction following infarction. This parameter appears to be the single best index of survival following infarction.[90–92] Finally, the prognostic impact of postinfarction functional aneurysm formation recently has also been reported.[93] This assessment can be made readily from the multiview equilibrium study.

Exercise Stress

Assessment of exercise ventricular performance can be obtained with either first pass or equilibrium techniques. As noted above, with the equilibrium technique, exercise generally is performed in the supine position, while first pass studies are performed in either upright or supine positions. Appropriate ergometer bicycles are available for exercise in either position. In addition, a variety of exercise tables have been developed commercially with appropriate stabilized construction such that patients can be studied during supine exercise with a minimum of excess upper-torso motion (which would introduce significant artifact). The widest application of exercise function studies has been in coronary artery disease.

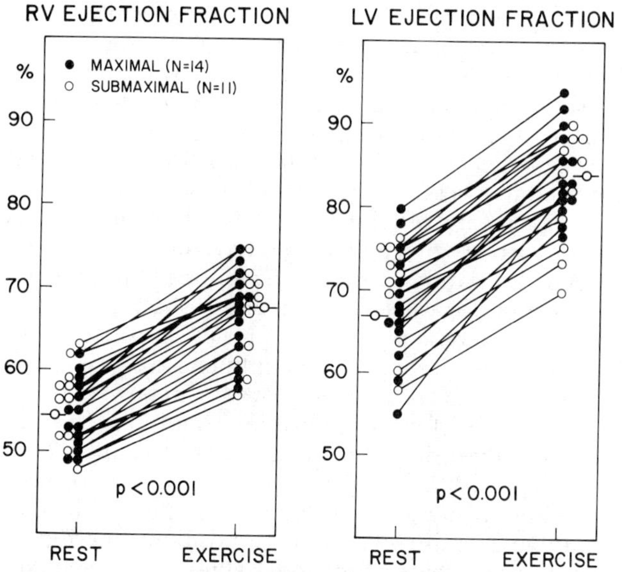

FIGURE 109-15 Right ventricular (RV) and left ventricular (LV) ejection fraction obtained during exercise in 25 normal control subjects. Individual subjects who exercised maximally are indicated by the closed circles, while those who exercised submaximally using a single-stage protocol are indicated by the open circles. Means for each group are shown at the sides of each panel. Ejection fraction increased by at least 5 percent in all subjects, irrespective of the exercise protocol. (*From R. A. Matthay, H. J. Berger, R. A. Davies, et al., Radionuclide Assessment of Right and Left Ventricular Exercise Performance in Chronic Obstructive Pulmonary Disease, Ann. Intern. Med., 93:234, 1980. Reproduced with permission from the publisher and author.*)

The normal response to bicycle exercise involves an absolute increase of at least 5 percent in the ejection fraction of both right and left ventricles (Fig. 109-15). This is associated with normal regional wall motion and little if any increase in ventricular volume. In patients with coronary disease, left ventricular ejection fraction generally falls or remains unchanged (within ± 5 percent of the resting value) with exercise. Abnormal global responses are frequently associated with the development of abnormal segmental wall motion contraction patterns and substantial ventricular dilatation.[13,41,94–96] These responses have been noted in approximately 85 to 90 percent of patients with coronary artery disease and appear to be related to the extent of the underlying pathologic process. In a series of 60 patients with documented coronary disease, Berger et al. noted an abnormal left ventricular response to exercise in all 30 patients with electrocardiographic evidence of myocardial ischemia, and in only 18 out of 30 patients without electrocardiographic evidence of ischemia in whom exercise was limited by fatigue (Fig. 109-16).[94] Regional wall motion abnormalities appear to occur less frequently than an abnormal ejection fraction response; however, their occurrence is more specific for coronary artery disease.[85,97]

Recently, Rozanski et al. reported a decrease in specificity of exercise radionuclide studies when a recent series from the same laboratory was compared to the initial group of normal subjects evaluated in that laboratory when the technique was first implemented.[98] The difference was attributed to differences in the selection of the normal populations during the two periods of evaluation. The first group of normal subjects was derived from those with an extremely low likelihood of disease who were frequently volunteers, laboratory personnel, etc. The second group of normal subjects was derived from patients studied in the cardiac catheterization laboratory and determined to have no major coronary anatomic lesions. This latter group had a much higher pretest probability of coronary disease. The posttest referral bias contributed as well to the decline in specificity since all patients with a positive exercise response were referred for subsequent evaluation at cardiac catheterization. It should be noted that identification of patients with abnormal exercise responses and otherwise normal coronary arteries may not be a limitation or artifact of the test. Rather, this may be the uncovering of a heretofore-unrecognized cardiac condition involving supply-demand imbalances that require new definition and classification.

FIGURE 109-16 Exercise left ventricular (LV) function in 60 patients with documented coronary artery disease. Individual patients are shown by closed circles; means are shown by open circles at the sides of each panel. Patients are divided based upon their exercise endpoints: electrocardiographic evidence of myocardial ischemia (*left*) and symptom-limiting fatigue (*right*). All 30 patients with ischemia had normal left ventricular function at rest and demonstrated abnormal exercise reserve. Of 30 patients who exercised to fatigue, 22 demonstrated either abnormal exercise reserve or abnormal ejection fraction at rest. (*From H. J. Berger, L. A. Reduto, D. E. Johnstone, et al., Global and Regional Left Ventricular Response to Bicycle Exercise in Coronary Artery Disease: Assessment by Quantitative Radionuclide Angiocardiography, Am. J. Med., 66:13, 1979. Reproduced with permission from the publisher and author.*)

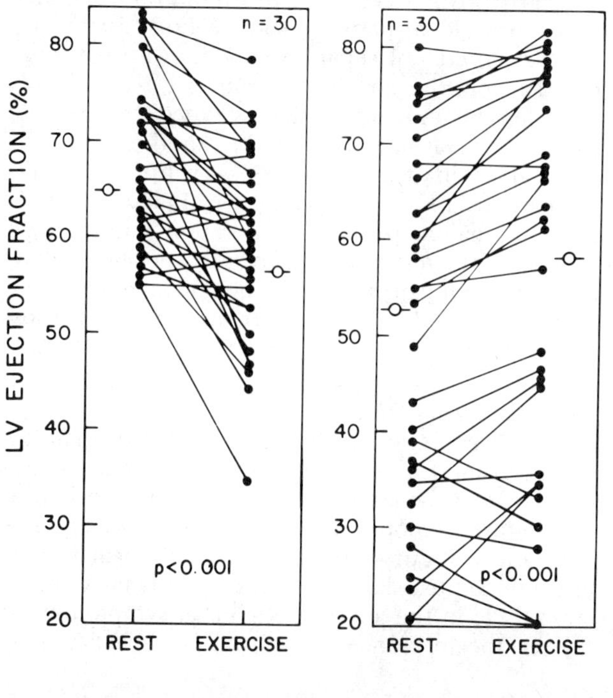

There are other patient subsets in whom the usual criteria for normal exercise increment of at least 5 percent may not be suitable. These include patients with elevated resting left ventricular ejection fractions of more than 70 to 75 percent. In addition, female patients do not appear to augment ejection fraction to the same degree as do males.[99] The elderly population has been noted to have an abnormal exercise response frequently even in the absence of coronary artery disease.[100] Finally, in order to maximize the specificity of an exercise radionuclide study it is important to exclude patients who may have ventricular dysfunction for reasons other than coronary disease. In contrast, in our experience, hypertension alone is not associated with an abnormal left ventricular exercise response.[101]

It is clear that the level of exercise stress is of major importance in inducing left ventricular dysfunction. Studies at subcritical myocardial oxygen requirements, whether related to therapy (i.e., propranolol) or inability to exercise, may demonstrate normal performance. Exercise techniques have also been used to assess the effects of a variety of potential therapies for coronary disease, including bypass surgery, drugs such as nitroglycerin or propranolol, and physical conditioning.[102–105] Abnormalities in exercise right ventricular performance are also noted in coronary artery disease. In this instance, abnormal reserve seems to be more dependent upon concomitant left ventricular function than intrinsic coronary anatomy.[106]

Although bicycle exercise has been the most common form of stress employed, other potent physiologic means of stressing the ventricle are available. Bodenheimer et al. employed isometric handgrip and noted that 90 percent of patients with coronary disease manifested abnormal regional left ventricular performance during stress.[43] The responses to handgrip stress were more profound on a regional than on a global basis. Global ejection fraction responses could not separate patients with coronary disease from those without coronary disease. Reflex hypertension and tachycardia associated with the cold pressor test has been proposed as another stress circumstance in which to assess ventricular performance.[107] This test has the advantage of not requiring major patient cooperation and effort. However, the test is not sufficiently specific to allow separation of coronary patients from normal patients and should not be used clinically for diagnostic purposes.[108]

Valvular Heart Disease

Rest and exercise ventricular performance studies are relevant for defining functional status in patients with valvular heart disease.[109] Most work in this area has centered about the study of patients with aortic regurgitation in whom abnormal exercise left ventricular responses have been demonstrated (1) in the absence of clinical symptoms and (2) in the presence of normal ventricular performance at rest.[110,111] Borer et al. noted abnormal performance in 9 of 22 asymptomatic patients studied at exercise;[110] 21 of these 22 patients had normal resting function. Abnormal exercise responses have often reverted to normal following aortic valve replacement.[112] Further follow-up studies are required to assess the utility of exercise function studies as a means of establishing operability in patients with aortic regurgitation who have not as yet developed the symptom state conventionally used as an indication for valve replacement. It should be noted that the exercise performance results in patients with aortic regurgitation may be influenced significantly by the type of exercise employed: supine versus upright. The difference in loading conditions encountered in these two exercise conditions will affect both the degree of valvular regurgitation and ventricular dilatation. In a group of patients studied with comparable exercise levels in both positions, there generally was greater functional abnormality with supine as opposed to upright exercise.[113]

The assessment of ventricular performance at rest may also be of value in defining operability in patients with mitral regurgitation. Specifically, the finding of relatively intact left ventricular function suggests a primary valvular problem, suitable for surgical therapy, while severe left ventricular dysfunction suggests that the mitral regurgitation may be secondary to primary myocardial disease or that the lesion has progressed beyond the point where valve replacement would be of value.

Monitoring of Drug-Induced Cardiotoxicity

An additional potential application of radionuclide function techniques involves the assessment of doxorubicin cardiotoxicity. Doxorubicin is a commonly employed antineoplastic drug. Unfortunately, therapy may be associated with development of a cardiomyopathy that may be irreversible and often fatal. A group of 55 patients in whom serial first pass studies were obtained over a 1½-year period was studied by Alexander et al.[113a] Concomitant systolic time interval measurements were obtained. Cardiotoxicity was determined from clinical findings and from analysis of the radionuclide left ventricular function data. Severe cardiotoxicity was defined by the clinical presence of heart failure and an ejection fraction of less than 30 percent. Moderate cardiotoxicity occurred in the absence of symptoms and was associated with an absolute decrease in ejection fraction of at least 15 percent to a level less than 45 percent. This finding was predictive of subsequent congestive heart failure if doxorubicin was continued. Mild cardiotoxicity was defined by the absence of symptoms or signs and a fall in ejection fraction of 10 percent or more without fulfilling criteria for moderate toxicity. No patient developed heart failure after demonstrating only mild toxicity. In the course of the study, five patients developed heart failure; all demonstrated moderate toxicity (Fig. 109-17). Subsequently, six additional

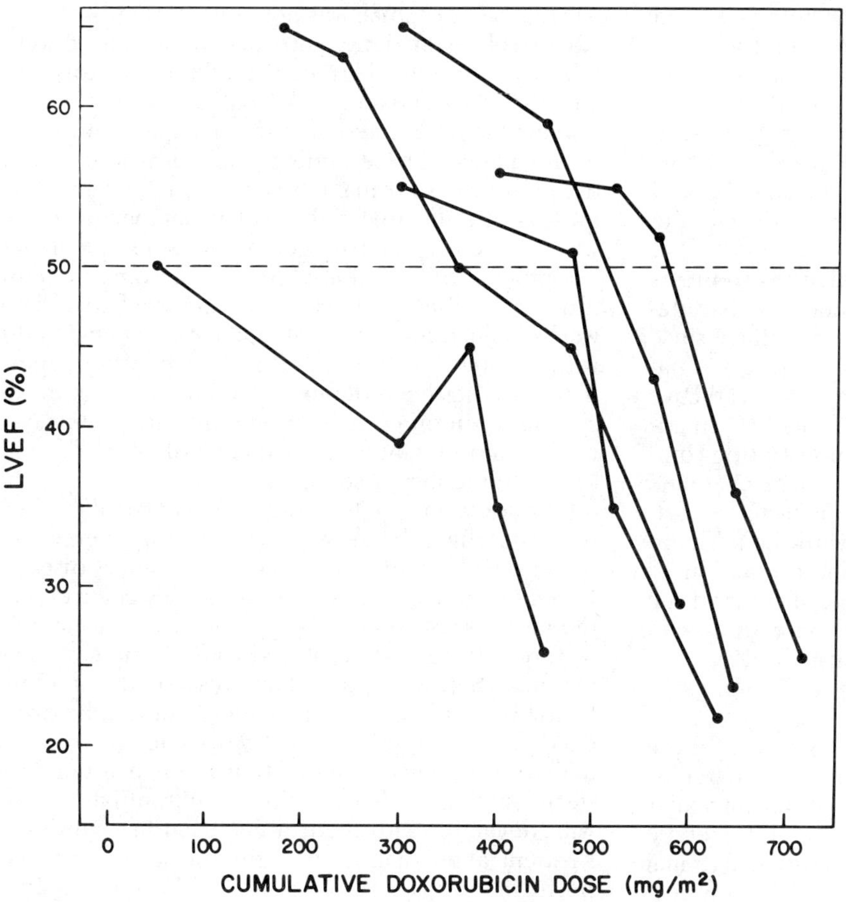

FIGURE 109-17 Sequential measurement of left ventricular ejection fraction (LVEF) in five patients who developed severe cardiotoxicity with congestive heart failure during doxorubicin therapy. Note how each of these patients initially passed through a phase of moderate cardiotoxicity which was detected with serial ejection fraction measurements. (*From J. Alexander, N. Dainiak, H. J. Berger, et al., Serial Assessment of Doxorubicin Cardiotoxicity with Quantitative Radionuclide Angiocardiography, N. Engl. J. Med., 300:278, 1979. Reproduced with permission from The New England Journal of Medicine and author.*)

FIGURE 109-18 Sequential measurement of left ventricular ejection fraction (LVEF) in six patients in whom doxorubicin was discontinued after demonstration of moderate cardiotoxicity. Follow-up measurements in each patient are shown in *B*. Note that LVEF increased modestly in all patients after discontinuation of doxorubicin. These data stand in direct contrast to those in Fig. 97-17, where further falls in ejection fraction were noted as doxorubicin was continued. (*From J. Alexander, N. Dainiak, H. J. Berger, et al., Serial Assessment of Doxorubicin Cardiotoxicity with Quantitative Radionuclide Angiocardiography, N. Engl. J. Med., 300:278, 1979. Reproduced with permission from The New England Journal of Medicine and author.*)

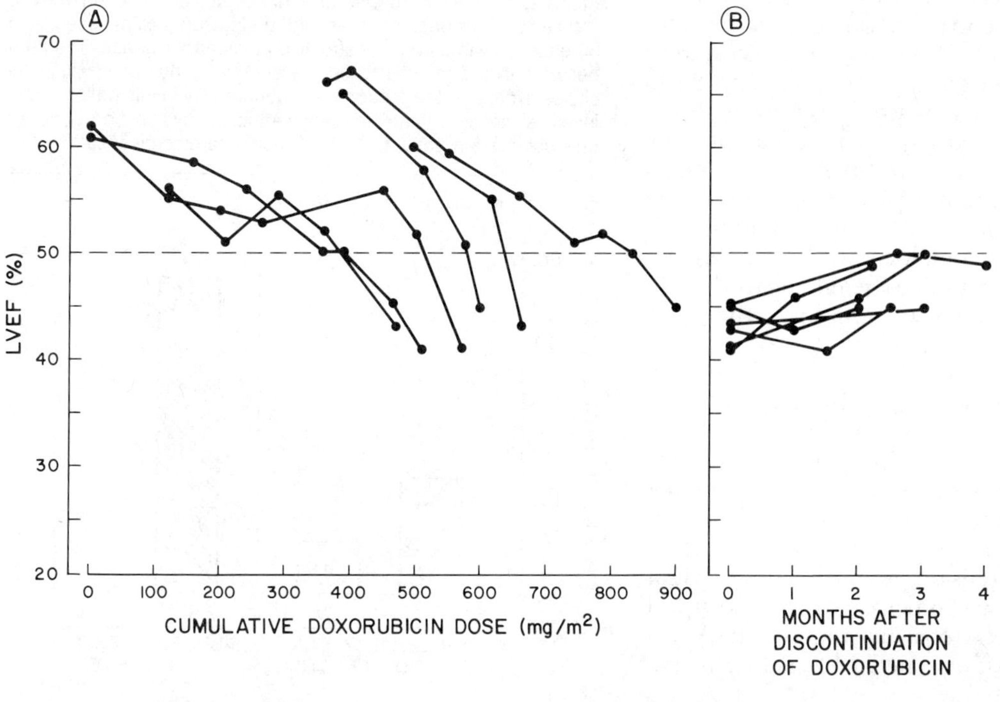

patients demonstrated moderate cardiotoxicity and had doxorubicin discontinued. None of these patients developed heart failure over a sustained follow-up period (Fig. 109-18). This study demonstrates the potential utility of standardized radionuclide techniques for defining cardiac abnormalities prior to major clinical manifestations and indicates how they may be employed in developing appropriate therapeutic guidelines. It is of note that in this series, systolic time interval measurements were poorly predictive of subsequent cardiac decompensation or its absence. These data have since been amplified in a substantially larger group of patients studied in the same laboratory. The predictive ability of the resting study was confirmed.[114] In addition, data have been obtained demonstrating comparable reliability in patients with abnormal baseline function who are receiving doxorubicin.[115] Improved sensitivity has been noted with the addition of exercise stress to the radionuclide evaluation.[116] However, the issue of decreased specificity and the suitability of performing serial exercise studies in this patient population must be considered.

Congenital Heart Disease

Studies in congenital heart disease primarily have involved shunt detection employing the first pass technique. However, assessment of biventricular performance under conditions of rest and exercise may be of value in assessing patients with congenital heart disease preoperatively as well as following corrective cardiac surgery. A prototype study of this type has been performed in asymptomatic patients following surgical repair of tetralogy of Fallot.[117] In a group of 16 postoperative patients studied an average of 10 years following total correction, 13 manifested abnormal right ventricular performance in association with exercise stress, whereas 15 of the 16 had normal right ventricular function in the resting state. Left ventricular function was intact under conditions of rest and exercise in each patient. Such postoperative studies, demonstrating abnormal performance in the absence of symptoms, may play an increasing role in the future in the long-term management of patients with complex congenital anomalies who undergo corrective surgery early in life. Studies have since been obtained evaluating ventricular function in a variety of congenital heart disease patient groups, including transposition of the great vessels, atrial septal defects, etc.[117–119]

Chronic Obstructive Pulmonary Disease

The major hemodynamic burden in chronic obstructive pulmonary disease falls upon the right ventricle. This chamber is quite dependent upon the afterload state imposed by the pulmonary vasculature. In the presence of pulmonary vasoconstriction or pulmonary hypertension, abnormalities in right ventricular function are anticipated. In a group of 36 patients with chronic obstructive pulmonary disease studied in the resting state, abnormal right ventricular performance was noted in 19 (Fig. 109-5).[45] Abnormalities in right ventricular performance were related to both the degree of ventilatory impairment and arterial hypoxemia. All patients with cor pulmonale demonstrated abnormal right ventricular performance. These findings generally occurred in the presence of normal left ventricular function. The finding of abnormal right ventricular performance was frequently a harbinger of the subsequent development of cardiopulmonary decompensation during a follow-up period. Similar predictive data were obtained in a group of ambulatory young adults with cystic fibrosis.[120] Right ventricular performance has been demonstrated to augment in response to therapeutic intervention, such as intravenous aminophylline, oral theophylline,[121,122] and other pulmonary vasodilators.[123]

In addition, right and left ventricular performance have been measured during exercise in patients with chronic obstructive pulmonary disease. Exercise in patients with chronic obstructive pulmonary disease should be performed in a manner different from that employed routinely in coronary patients. Since in pulmonary disease the limiting factor is ventilatory status, patients should be exercised only to a submaximal workload in order to maintain an aerobic state. If patients are not in a steady-state aerobic condition, a substantial acidosis will develop, with concomitant additional independent abnormalities in right and left ventricular performance as a result of the acidosis alone. In a group of 30 patients with chronic obstructive pulmonary disease assessed during exercise, abnormal right ventricular function was noted in 80 percent (Fig. 109-19).[124] Abnormal right ventricular func-

FIGURE 109-19 Incidence of right ventricular (RV) and left ventricular (LV) dysfunction at rest and during submaximal exercise in 30 patients with chronic obstructive pulmonary disease. The number of patients in each group is shown by numbers within the circles. Note that the predominant abnormality in this patient group involves the right ventricle. Left ventricular dysfunction generally only occurred in patients with additional cardiac disease.

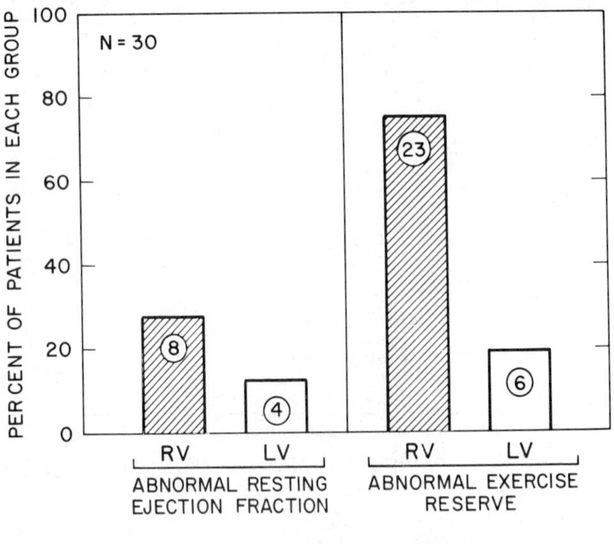

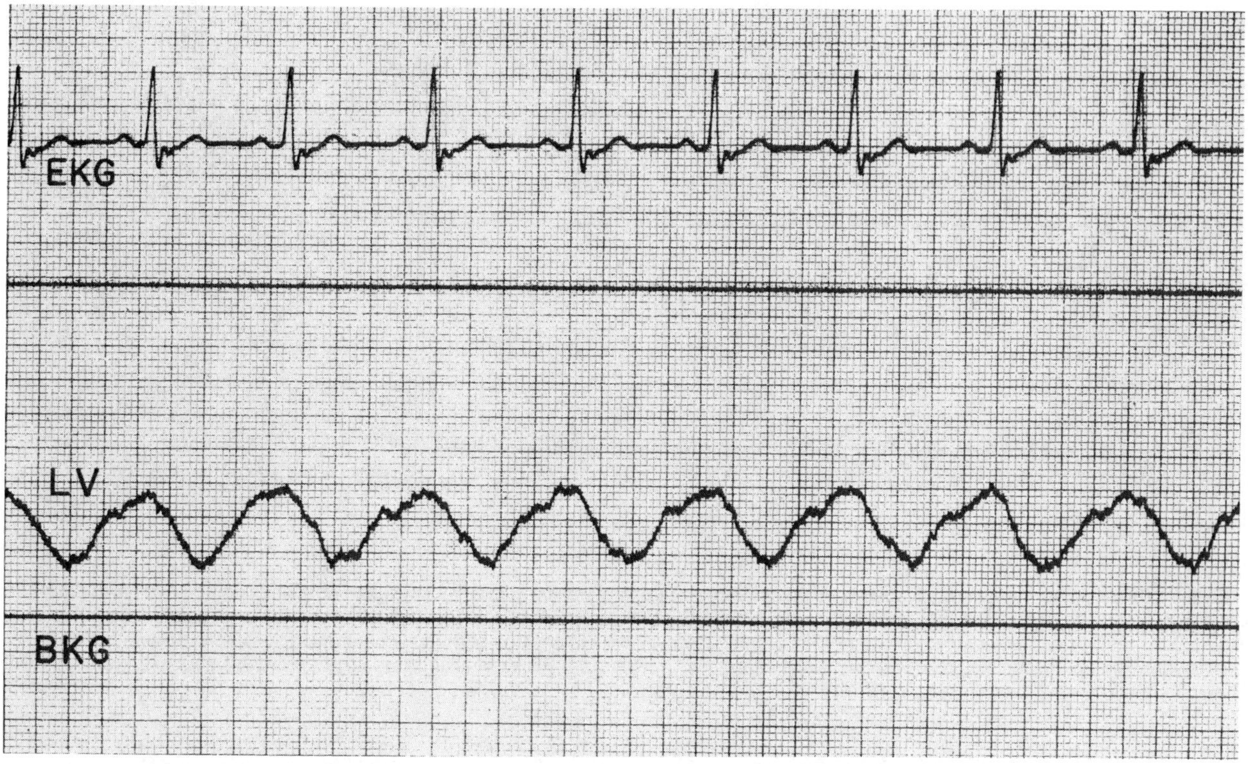

FIGURE 109-20 Representative strip-chart recording of the beat-to-beat display of the background (BKG) activity level and the left ventricular (LV) volume curve generated by the computerized nuclear probe, and the electrocardiogram (EKG) in a patient with normal sinus rhythm and normal LV function. Note the constancy and uniform periodicity of the curve. (*From H. J. Berger, R. A. Davies, W. P. Batsford, et al., Beat to Beat Left Ventricular Performance Assessed from the Equilibrium Cardiac Blood Pool Using a Computerized Nuclear Probe, Circulation, 63:133, 1981. Reproduced with permission from the American Heart Association, Inc., and the author.*)

tion was evident during exercise even in patients with mild disease. This abnormal right ventricular exercise response may not be an indicator of intrinsic right ventricular dysfunction, but rather may be a normal response to abnormal afterload changes induced either by pulmonary vasoconstriction or changes in intrathoracic pressure. In contrast, the left ventricular exercise response generally was normal in these patients. Because of the afterload dependence of the right ventricle, abnormal right ventricular ejection fraction may be used as an indirect index of pulmonary hypertension in pulmonary patients.[49]

Nonimaging Nuclear Probe

Nonimaging nuclear probes were first employed using first pass techniques.[6] Recent modification of the probe technique so that it can be employed in equilibrium studies has produced a major advance.[125] By the use of special collimation and a dedicated microprocessor, equilibrium data can be obtained concerning global left ventricular function, namely ejection fraction, ejection rate, relative cardiac output, and volumes. These data are generated in the conventional gated mode. In comparison to the scintillation camera, this instrument has the advantages of decreased cost, portability, and increased sensitivity. Because of the increased sensitivity, gated summed data over short time periods, such as 15 to 60 s, can be obtained.

Perhaps as important, data can be obtained and analyzed on a beat-to-beat basis without gating. Data concerning the continuous beat-to-beat relative ventricular volume curve can be displayed simultaneously with the electrocardiogram (Fig. 109-20).[126,127] Analysis of the data allows the addressing of specific issues that cannot be dealt with using conventional scintillation camera instrumentation. For example, the immediate physiologic consequences of cardiac arrhythmias, cardiac reflexes, and acute pharmacologic interventions can be studied (Fig. 109-21).[128–130] In addition, the high temporal resolution and high sensitivity of the probe allows rapid, direct assessment of diastolic filling. The probe concept presents an attractive means of monitoring ventricular performance during unstable clinical periods in an attempt to optimize hemodynamic status. A definite role for such monitoring is envisioned in the intensive care unit environment.

Data concerning left ventricular ejection fraction on a beat-to-beat basis correlate well with those measured by conventional first pass techniques (Fig. 109-22).[127] Furthermore, the inter- and intraobserver variation and intrinsic variability of sequential measurements are sufficiently low to allow meaningful criteria and investigational application.[127]

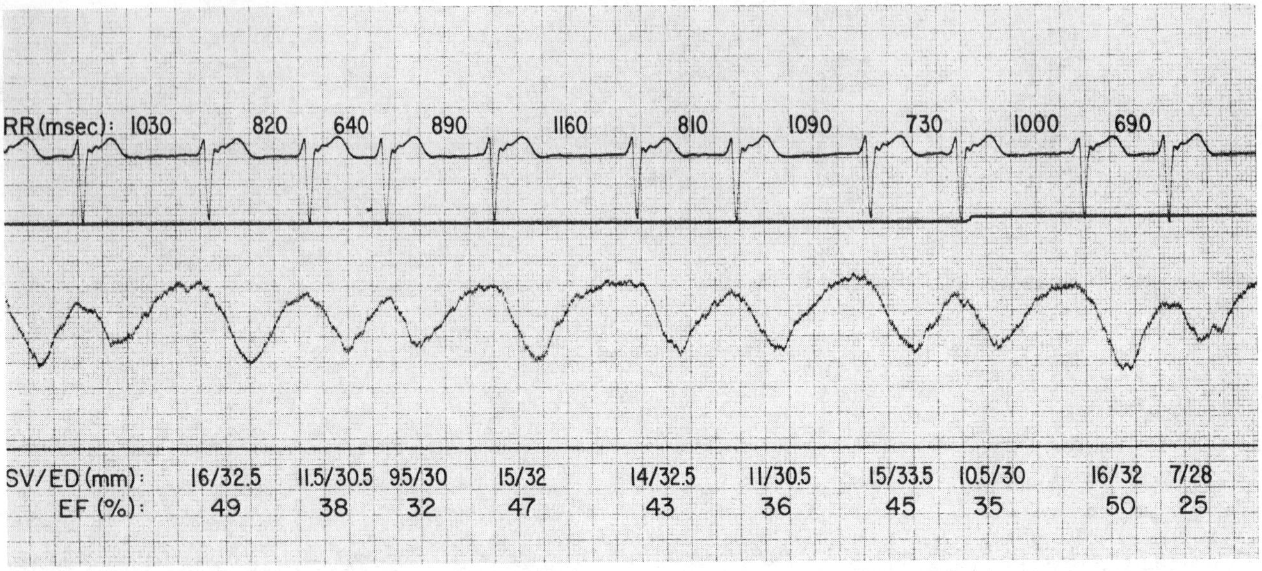

FIGURE 109-21 Beat-to-beat relative left ventricular volume curve in a patient with atrial fibrillation obtained with the nuclear probe. The display format is the same as in Fig. 109-20. The individual RR intervals in milliseconds (msec) are shown for each cardiac cycle. Relative stroke volume (SV) and end-diastolic volume (ED) as measured by the dimensions of the volume curve are given in millimeters (mm) for each beat. Ejection fraction (EF) also is shown. Note the relation between the RR interval and cardiac performance, suggesting a significant Starling effect.

FIGURE 109-22 Comparison of left ventricular ejection fraction measured by first pass radionuclide angiocardiography and the beat-to-beat nuclear probe technique. The probe ejection fraction is the average of 10 individual beats calculated from the strip-chart recording. Note the excellent correlation over a wide range of ejection fraction values. (*From H. J. Berger, R. A. Davies, W. P. Batsford, et al., Beat to Beat Left Ventricular Performance Assessed from the Equilibrium Cardiac Blood Pool Using a Computerized Nuclear Probe, Circulation, 63:133, 1981. Reproduced with permission from the American Heart Association, Inc., and the author.*)

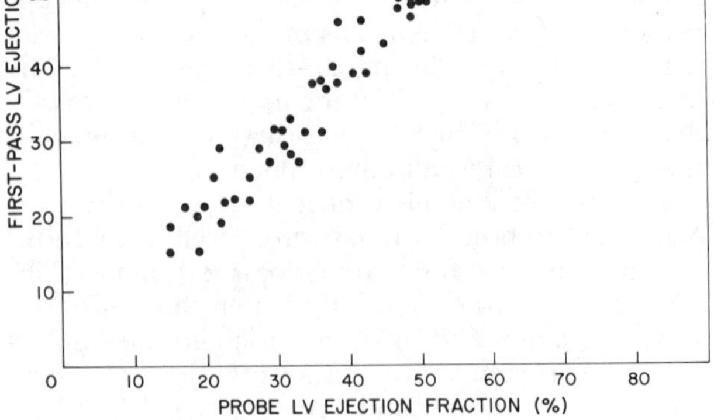

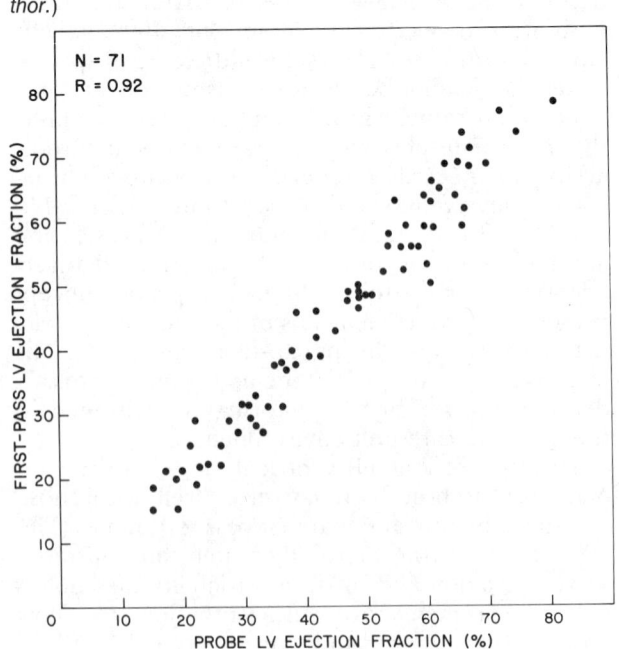

However, the technique has limitations. Only global left ventricular function is measured. No insights are obtained into left ventricular regional wall motion or right ventricular function. Since there are no images to guide the operator, appropriate algorithms and operator routines have been developed for probe positioning with respect to the ventricular region of interest and background. This makes the technique somewhat more difficult to carry out than the routine gated scintillation camera equilibrium study. However, with appropriate training and experience, reliable, precise, and reproducible data can be obtained.

Diastolic Function

Evaluation of diastolic function also may be obtained from the equilibrium radionuclide ventricular volume curve. Evaluation of the diastolic portion of the volume curve is more difficult than systole since there is greater variability with respect to changes in cycle length noted in diastole. For this reason it is necessary to employ specific computer approaches to the processing of the diastolic portion of the curve. These problems can, in part, be obviated with the use of the high-sensitivity, high-temporal resolution, nonimaging nuclear probe. Using radionuclide techniques, peak filling rate and time to peak filling rate can be measured accurately. Peak filling rate is the maximal rate of change in counts occurring within early to middiastole. The measurement is normalized to end-diastolic volume. Time to peak filling rate is the time from end-systole (minimum number of counts) to peak filling rate. The actual relation of these volumetric indices of diastolic function to the more complex pressure-volume assessment of diastole remain to be defined.

Abnormal diastolic function has been noted in this manner in a substantial number of patients with coronary artery disease studied at rest, even in the absence of systolic dysfunction. In one study, abnormal peak filling rates were noted in 85 percent of such coronary patients.[131] These findings occurred in the absence of myocardial infarction and clinically evident myocardial ischemia. These parameters are capable of dynamic change. Improvement in filling parameters has been noted following successful coronary angioplasty or institution of antianginal therapy with verapamil.[132,133] Abnormal diastolic function also has been noted in patients with clinical congestive heart failure but normal systolic function.[134] Measurement of diastolic function appears to offer a substantial new dimension to radionuclide ventricular functional assessment.

Thallium-201 Myocardial Perfusion Studies at Rest and during Exercise

Myocardial imaging with ionic tracers provides information concerning relative regional myocardial perfusion, regional viability, and qualitative anatomic data concerning relative left ventricular cavity size and wall thickness.[135] Currently, ionic ^{201}Tl is employed as the radionuclide tracer. The rationale for using thallium is based upon its ability to substitute biologically for ionic potassium, thereby accumulating rapidly within viable myocardial cells. Thallium-201 was introduced in 1975 as a potassium analogue with physical properties more suitable for imaging with conventional scintillation cameras.[19] Thallium-201 is a cyclotron-produced radionuclide with a physical half-life of 73 h. It has a relatively low energy spectrum, and imaging is usually carried out using a window centered around the 80 keV mercury x-ray photopeak. Additional gamma-ray photopeaks occur at 135 keV and 167 keV, but these are substantially less abundant and are not employed in clinical imaging.

Physiology of Thallium Uptake

Thallium distribution within the myocardium is dependent upon several factors, the most important of which are regional myocardial perfusion and cellular viability. The amount of ^{201}Tl present in a myocardial region at any time represents the net result of several kinetic factors that determine the influx and efflux characteristics of the radionuclide. Thallium is extracted rapidly and effectively by myocardium. The first pass extraction efficiency is 88 percent.[136] The initial thallium distribution within the myocardium generally is proportional to regional myocardial blood flow as measured by the radioactive microsphere technique. This correlation has been observed in both acute canine coronary occlusion preparations and 24-h-old infarct preparation.[137,138] However, the relation between thallium myocardial deposition and regional blood flow is not linear over the entire flow range encountered in experimental and clinical situations. In reactive hyperemia, regional thallium deposition will underestimate substantially the degree of flow augmentation.[137] This underestimation of flow is less than noted previously in a similar model with potassium-43.[139] Nevertheless, it is clear that ^{201}Tl is an imperfect flow marker in the high-flow range. In extremely low flow situations, ^{201}Tl activity tends to overestimate perfusion. This phenomenon is due to presumed augmented extraction efficiency resulting from prolonged regional residence time. However, within the wide range of coronary blood flows between the two extremes, ^{201}Tl distributions correlate well with regional blood flow.

Since ^{201}Tl is moving rapidly from extracellular to intracellular space, it is not surprising that its distribution is also affected by metabolic events that impact upon intracellular ion flux. Factors such as intracellular pH and intact Na-K-ATPase systems affect ^{201}Tl accumulation.[140] Pharmacologic agents which alter metabolic function, such as propranolol and digitalis, may also affect ^{201}Tl distribution.[141]

Three to four percent of the injected dose of ^{201}Tl is accumulated initially in the myocardium.[137] Approximately 8 to 10 percent of the injected intravenous dose is deposited in the lungs. This proportion can be augmented significantly in the presence of prolonged pulmonary transit time, as is seen in congestive heart failure.[142]

Important concepts concerning ^{201}Tl imaging have been advanced based upon understanding of ^{201}Tl kinetics. Pohost et al. have described thallium kinetics on a cellular level in the form of a three-compartment model: vascular, interstitial, and cellular.[140] This model has been applied to ^{201}Tl kinetics in both the intact animal and the fetal mouse heart in organ culture. At any one time, ^{201}Tl myocardial uptake represents the net result of both continuous extraction and release of ^{201}Tl by myocytes. Initially, normal myocardial cells accumulate ^{201}Tl to an extent that far exceeds efflux of the ion. Some time thereafter the cellular release of the ion will be greater than its accumulation, with the result of myocardial-tracer washout. When viewed in serial images, these physiologic findings will be translated into an initial myocardial accumulation and subsequent efflux of ^{201}Tl from nonischemic zones associated with thallium accumulation in previously ischemic zones that initially accumulated relatively less tracer. In clinical imaging, this is termed the *redistribution* phenomenon.[143]

Imaging Technique

Thallium images must be obtained with current state-of-the-art scintillation cameras possessing optimal imaging characteristics. Imaging generally is performed using a high-resolution collimator. The injected dose is approximately 1.5 mCi. Images should be obtained with high count densities (200,000–400,000 counts per image) in at least three positions. These three positions should include anterior, 45° left anterior oblique, and either steep left anterior oblique or left lateral images. If left lateral images are to be performed, it is essential that they be obtained with the patient lying on the right side. Lateral images obtained with the patient supine frequently result in artifacts simulating inferior wall perfusion defects.[144]

When imaging is performed in association with exercise stress, it is critical that the exercise laboratory be sufficiently close to the nuclear laboratory such that imaging can begin approximately 10 min after injection of the intravenous tracer. If longer time periods are allowed to elapse, it is possible that thallium redistribution will begin prior to or during imaging. This can result in an apparent false-negative imaging study. The most commonly employed stress has been treadmill or bicycle exercise.[145–148] For exercise studies, an intravenous infusion is begun prior to exercise. Patients then exercise to the point of rate-limiting symptoms. Prior to conclusion of exercise, the thallium is injected rapidly into the infusion line, and exercise is then continued for an additional 45 to 60 s. This continuation of exercise allows the major portion of the injected dose to be distributed during the appropriate physiologic state.

The left anterior oblique position image generally is obtained first, since this view provides the maximum separation of individual myocardial segments, and coronary vascular beds without overlap. If redistribution studies are to be performed, they are obtained 3 to 4 h following injection.

Data can be interpreted directly from analog images or following processing with a variety of computer techniques. These computer techniques involve background correction, contrast enhancement of the image data, and quantification of regional radioactivity.

Normal Thallium Image

In normal subjects, the ^{201}Tl perfusion image demonstrates a homogeneous distribution of radioactivity within the left ventricular myocardium.[149] Generally, thallium uptake in the right ventricular myocardium is not appreciated on resting studies, except when right ventricular hypertrophy, acute increases in right ventricular afterload, or tachycardia are present. This is in contrast to findings in exercise studies, where right ventricular thallium accumulation is seen routinely, presumably as a result of augmented right ventricular blood flow associated with exercise. Thallium images demonstrate a central zone of relatively decreased tracer accumulation which corresponds to the region of the left ventricular cavity. This central zone is increased in the presence of ventricular dilatation and decreased in patients with compensated hypertrophic states. In approximately 20 percent of normal persons, there is a small apical defect due to the anatomic variant of relative thinning of left ventricular myocardium at the apex. In cases of ventricular dilatation, the apical defect can be quite pronounced.[150] This finding is not necessarily an indication of a perfusion abnormality, and must be recognized as such.

Images must be obtained in multiple views in order to define perfusion defects appropriately (Fig. 109-23). In the anterior position, the anterolateral, apical, and inferior walls can be identified and defined. In the left anterior oblique position, septal, inferoapical, and posterolateral walls are defined. In the left lateral position, the anterior wall, the apex, and the entire extent of the inferior wall, including the posterobasal segment, are defined. Confidence in the identification of a perfusion deficit is enhanced if the abnormality is seen in more than one position. It should be emphasized that because of thallium's relatively low energy spectrum, myocardial radioactivity will be attenuated easily. This is especially evident in patients with thick chests, large breasts, or inappropriately placed electrocardiographic electrodes. Unrecognized attenuation of thallium activity is a frequent cause of either technically poor images or images containing substantial

FIGURE 109-23 Normal ^{201}Tl images obtained in the anterior (ANT), left anterior oblique (LAO), and left lateral (LL) positions. Relation to left ventricular anatomy is shown to the left of each image. Note the homogeneous distribution in the left ventricular wall and a central area corresponding to the left ventricular cavity. (*From F. Wackers, E. Busemann, S. Sokole, S. Samson, and J. B. Van der Schoot, Atlas of ^{201}Tl Myocardial Scintigraphy, Clin. Nucl. Med., 2:64, 1977. Reproduced with permission from the publisher and author.*)

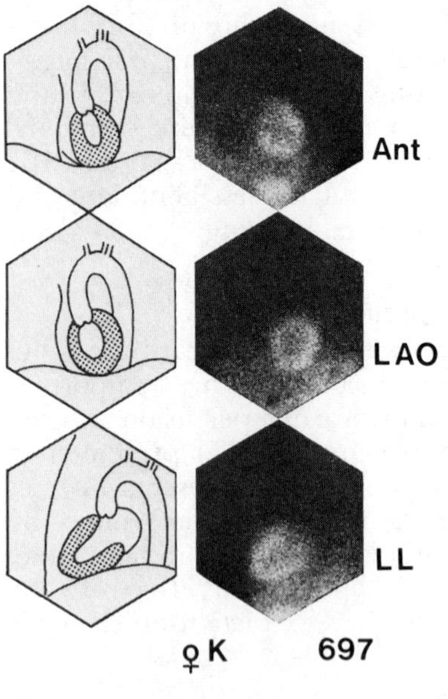

artifacts. The finding of apparent perfusion defects that do not correspond anatomically to the distributions of coronary vascular beds should immediately raise the possibility of the presence of attenuation artifacts.[151]

Thallium Imaging at Rest

Thallium-201 images at rest have been performed in patients with acute myocardial infarction (Figs. 109-24 and 109-25). Initial studies in this setting were obtained by Wackers et al. who evaluated 200 consecutive patients with acute myocardial infarction.[152] In this series, 165 of 200 patients (82 percent) demonstrated abnormal images defined by myocardial regions with a relative decrease in radionuclide uptake. This study also established a definite relation between the frequency of positive imaging results following infarction and the time interval between the onset of symptoms and imaging. All 44 patients studied within 6 h of the onset of chest pain had positive images. Eighty-eight percent of 52 patients studied between 6 and 24 h after the onset of chest pain demonstrated perfusion defects. Of the 104 patients imaged later than 24 h after the onset of symptoms, only 72 percent demonstrated perfusion defects. For the entire series, 88 percent of the patients with acute transmural infarction had positive images, while 63 percent of those with nontransmural infarction had positive images. The influence of the temporal imaging sequence upon imaging results appeared most pronounced in those patients with relatively small infarcts. All patients studied within 6 h of the onset of nontransmural infarcts or enzymatically small infarcts had abnormal images. Between 6 and 24 h after infarction, the incidence of positive images decreased to 57 percent in patients with enzymatically small infarcts and 70 percent in those with nontransmural infarcts. Twenty-four hours after infarction and later, the incidence of positive results in this group decreased further. In contrast, in patients with transmural infarction, all studies were positive within 6 h and 97 percent were positive between 6 and 24 h. After 24 h, 78 percent still remained positive. These initial observations have been confirmed by other investigators in various studies, including one large multicenter study.[148] Animal studies also have supported these observations. Umbach et al. studied serial thallium images in dogs subjected to an acute anterior wall myocardial infarction who underwent quantitative imaging following individual thallium injections 4 h and again 24 h after the onset of infarction.[153] A decrease in size of the imaged thallium defect was noted in 10 of 13 animals. The imaged infarct zone averaged 34 percent of the left ventricular thallium distribution at 4 h, and 22 percent at 24 h ($p < 0.001$).

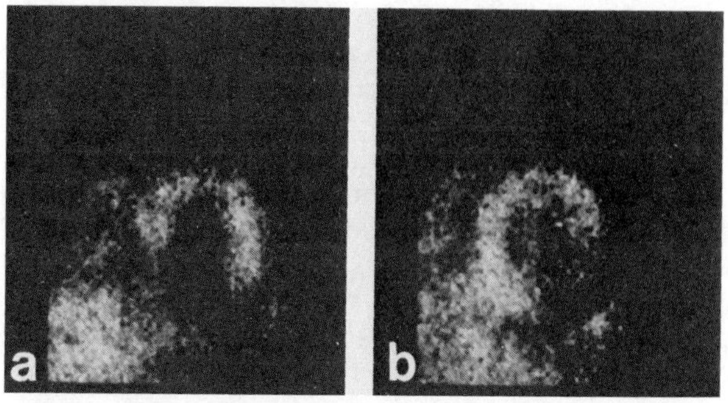

FIGURE 109-24 Thallium-201 images obtained in the anterior (*a*) and left anterior oblique (*b*) positions in a patient with a large inferoapical myocardial infarction. Note the large perfusion defect in both positions.

In addition to providing potential relevant diagnostic data, ^{201}Tl defects in the acute phase of myocardial infarction also may have prognostic significance. Observations by Silverman et al. in a series of 42 patients with acute myocardial infarction studied within 15 h of the onset of symptoms indicate that the presence and size of the thallium perfusion defect can be related meaningfully to ultimate patient survival. A quantitative score based on the thallium image was more predictive than conventional variables either alone or in combination.[154] These data were confirmed subsequently by a follow-up study from the same laboratory by Becker et al.[155]

FIGURE 109-25 Thallium-201 images at rest in the anterior (ANT), left anterior oblique (LAO), and left lateral (LLAT) positions in a patient with an anteroseptal infarct. Note the large perfusion defect in all three positions.

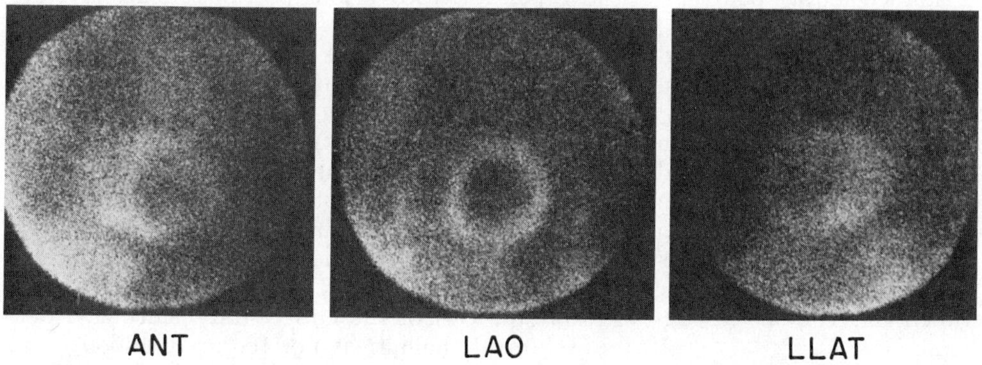

Thallium imaging, following both intracoronary and intravenous administration, has been proposed for assessment of the efficacy of reperfusion following thrombolytic therapy as a means of salvaging ischemic but viable myocardium. Using dual injection techniques, significant improvement in perfusion patterns have been noted following successful thrombolysis.[156] However, the kinetics of thallium accumulation in recently reperfused myocardium, particularly when administered intracoronary, is a complex, as yet not completely understood phenomenon.[157]

Because of the high sensitivity of thallium imaging in the early hours of myocardial infarction, the radionuclide technique has been proposed as a potential means of screening patients for admission to the coronary care unit.[158] A pilot study assessing the efficacy of this approach was carried out in 203 patients in whom the diagnosis of infarction was unclear at the time of admission. Of these patients, 17 percent (34 patients) subsequently manifested evidence of acute infarction. Thallium images were positive in 30 of these 34 patients (88 percent). Abnormal images also were obtained in 10 of 47 patients with unstable angina without infarction, and in 9 of 24 patients with a previous infarct but no new acute infarct. Thus, early thallium imaging in patients with atypical complaints or equivocal clinical findings may be of value. This finding will require further confirmation prior to consideration of early thallium imaging for broad clinical application.

Thallium-201 imaging in the acute stage of infarction appears to be sensitive; however, the study lacks specificity. Differentiation between old and acute myocardial infarction cannot be made unless prior images are available for comparison.[159] In addition, conditions resulting in transient myocardial ischemia may also produce abnormal thallium-uptake patterns at rest. Perhaps the most dramatic demonstration of this occurs in patients with coronary spasm studied either following a spontaneous clinical event or following coronary spasm induced by intravenous ergonovine maleate.[160] In these instances, dramatic perfusion defects are detected which correspond to the region of myocardium supplied by the spastic coronary artery. Abnormalities also have been noted at rest in patients with unstable angina pectoris. Patients studied *during* pain episodes usually will have abnormal images. However, 98 patients with unstable angina were evaluated during a pain-free period within 18 h of the last anginal attack; 40 percent had abnormal images.[161] The incidence of abnormal images was higher in those studied within 6 h of the chest pain as opposed to those studied at longer intervals thereafter. In patients with unstable angina, demonstrable resting perfusion abnormalities may result from either severe reduction of coronary flow at rest or possible regional metabolic dysfunction secondary to repeated and ongoing ischemia.

Recent quantitative data indicate that resting ^{201}Tl perfusion defects can be defined in a quantitative sense in patients with severe coronary stenosis and stable as well as unstable angina.[162] In a series of 29 patients, 26 manifested perfusion abnormalities at rest, while only 14 had electrocardiographic evidence of infarction. Furthermore, when these patients were studied sequentially, perfusion abnormalities tended to normalize on delayed redistribution images. Roughly two-thirds of 91 segments with diminished initial thallium uptake demonstrated redistribution. The data could also be expressed quantitatively, allowing definition of regional thallium kinetics. This analysis was concordant with visual assessment of the serial images. Furthermore, the perfusion abnormalities were frequently reversed following effective coronary bypass surgery. These observations are consistent with other data reported by Gewirtz et al.[163]

Exercise Imaging

It has long been apparent that evaluating the patient at rest generally is not sufficient for assessment of coronary reserve in the setting of transient ischemia or suspected angina pectoris. The majority of patients with arteriosclerotic heart disease and no myocardial infarction will not have perfusion abnormalities demonstrable in the resting state. There are physiologic reasons for this observation. At rest, regional coronary blood flow tends to remain intact, even in the presence of significant coronary stenosis, until the degree of obstruction is almost total. The major pathophysiologic abnormality involves diminished coronary vascular reserve and a limited ability to augment blood flow appropriately in response to increased oxygen demands. Thallium-201 is extracted rapidly from blood. Therefore, it can be injected intravenously during a period of exercise stress when there is maximal heterogeneity of regional myocardial blood flow in patients with significant coronary artery disease. Blood flow, and hence initial ^{201}Tl deposition, will be maximal in myocardium supplied by normal coronary arteries, whereas there will be substantially less radionuclide deposition in zones supplied by stenotic coronary vessels. The relative ^{201}Tl myocardial distribution will indicate relative perfusion in various portions of the myocardium.

Comparison of images obtained immediately after exercise with those obtained either at a serial redistribution study 2 to 4 h later or a totally separate study at rest allows assessment of the reversible relative hypoperfusion that characterizes transient ischemia. The findings of Pohost et al. concerning redistribution studies generally have allowed an effective substitution of the redistribution study for a separate rest study.[143] This has decreased considerably the cost of the entire study, since a second injection of thallium is not required. Blood et al.

compared redistribution images at 4 h with separate rest images.[164] They found comparable data in 80 percent of patients studied. In patients without prior infarction in whom adequate redistribution does not occur by 4 h, a second rest study should be performed.

The following scheme should be used when qualitatively comparing exercise images with either redistribution or separate rest images. Perfusion abnormalities present on the exercise study but not at redistribution or rest are indicative of transient myocardial ischemia. For clinical purposes, when evaluating images qualitatively in a purely visual manner, if the initial exercise study is normal, there is no need to obtain further follow-up images. Perfusion defects present at exercise that are unchanged at rest or redistribution are most consistent with previous infarction and scar without ischemia. Finally, exercise perfusion abnormalities that are substantially larger than defects present at redistribution or rest are consistent with ischemia superimposed upon previous infarction and scar (Figs. 109-26, 109-27, and 109-28).

Exercise perfusion imaging has been evaluated in many laboratories since its introduction in 1973. Initially, ^{43}K was the radionuclide employed.[18] From 1976 to 1979, a total of 1077 patients in whom ^{201}Tl exercise imaging was performed were reported in the literature. The cumulative data comparing the results of exercise imaging with coronary arteriographic findings and exercise electrocardiography indicate that perfusion imaging has a sensitivity of 82 percent and a specificity of 90 percent for the detection of angiographically documented significant coronary artery stenosis.[140] In comparison, exercise electrocardiograms obtained during the radionuclide studies demonstrated a diagnostic sensitivity of only 61 percent and a specificity of 82 percent. Both differences between exercise imaging and electrocardiography are statistically significant.[140]

Perfusion defects can be correlated anatomically with the geographic location of specific vascular beds. Ideally, a perfusion defects should be detected in the same myocardial segment in more than one view. Defects seen in the septum on the left anterior oblique images are attributable to left anterior descending stenosis arising proximal to the first septal perforator. Other left anterior descending lesions may appear as defects in the anterior wall or apex in multiple views. Stenosis of the right coronary artery appears as an inferior wall defect seen on the anterior and left lateral views. Circumflex lesions generally are manifest as perfusion defects in the posterolateral region seen in the left anterior oblique view. There may be substantial variation in each of

FIGURE 109-26 Thallium-201 images obtained immediately following exercise (*upper row*) and at redistribution (*lower row*) in the anterior (ANT), left anterior oblique (LAO), and left lateral (LLAT) positions. Note the large perfusion defect involving the apex and anteroseptal walls present during exercise, with substantial normalization (filling in) on the 4-h redistribution studies. This is consistent with exercise-induced transient myocardial ischemia.

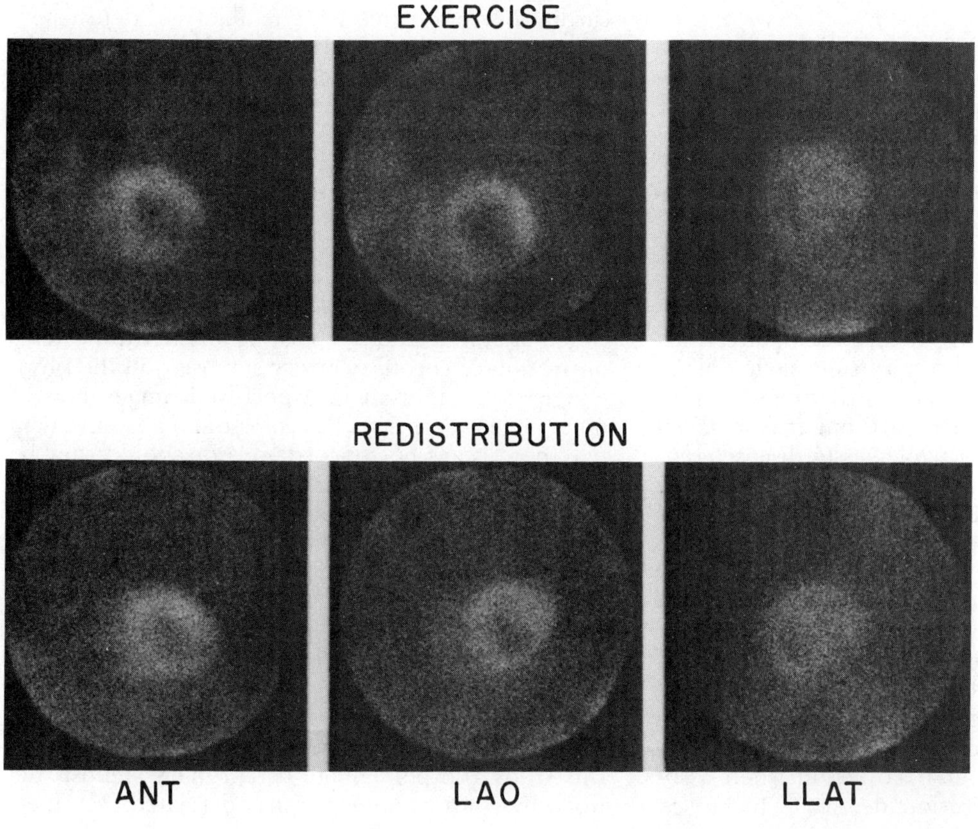

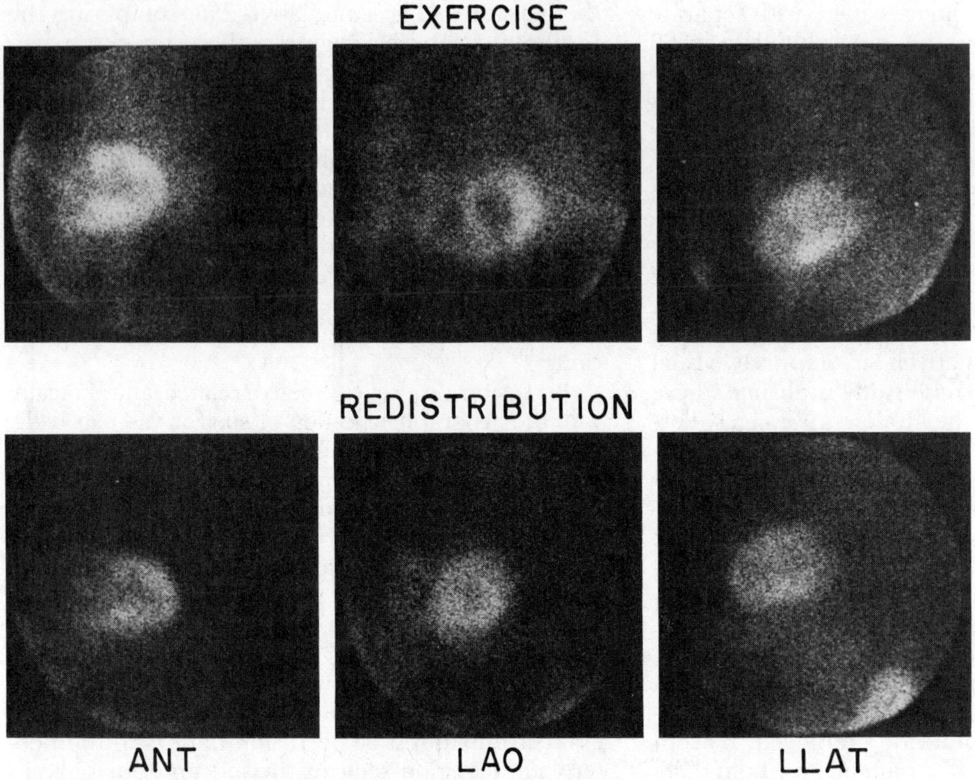

FIGURE 109-27 Exercise and redistribution ^{201}Tl images in a patient with transient myocardial ischemia. The formal is the same as in Fig. 109-26. Note the prominent anteroseptal perfusion defect best seen in the left anterior oblique (LAO) position immediately following exercise, with complete normalization (filling in) on the 4-h redistribution study.

these patterns based upon the expected variation in coronary anatomy.

In a qualitative sense left anterior descending stenosis can be predicted with a sensitivity of approximately 75 percent and specificity of 90 percent. Right coronary stenosis can be detected with a sensitivity of approximately 70 percent and specificity of 85 percent. Circumflex stenosis is associated with poor sensitivity (38 percent) and a specificity of 91 percent. Because of the high specificity noted in the analysis of individual vascular beds, defects in multiple vascular beds strongly suggest multivessel disease.[165,166] Rigo et al. have described a pattern associated with left main coronary stenosis involving perfusion defects in multiple distributions.[167] This pattern is sensitive (92 percent), but may be seen frequently in double- or triple-vessel disease, rendering it relatively nonspecific. However, the absence of this pattern speaks against the presence of left main coronary artery disease.

Markedly increased ^{201}Tl pulmonary uptake may be encountered in exercise images (Fig. 109-29).[142] This is a clue to significant underlying disease producing transient heart failure during exercise. Left ventricular failure at the time of exercise is suggested by a lung-to-myocardium ratio of greater than 0.5. Increased pulmonary uptake is indicative of ischemic-related ventricular dysfunction when associated with a focal perfusion defect.[168] Increased pulmonary uptake may at times also obscure a myocardial perfusion defect. The ability to detect perfusion abnormalities is also dependent upon the exercise endpoint achieved. Patients exercising to modest workloads with limited increase in heart rate and double product tend to have a higher incidence of false-negative images.[169] In addition, propranolol therapy may be associated with a significant incidence of false-negative images. This may occur independently of the propranolol effect on heart rate.

It should be emphasized that comparisons between anatomic data such as the angiographic demonstration of coronary artery stenosis and the physiologic data inherent in a perfusion image may at times be inappropriate. Physiologic and anatomic data may not always be concordant, nor should they be expected to be. Furthermore, there are potential interpretive difficulties inherent in coronary angiography. Interobserver variation in evaluating coronary angiography is notoriously high. What may appear to be a so-called subcritical lesion on coronary arteriography may in fact be responsible for a major physiologic perfusion deficit, and a high-grade angiographic lesion may have limited physiologic consequences as a result of collaterals, etc. This was emphasized in the recent study of White et al.[170] In this study the percentage of coronary stenosis defined by contrast angiography correlated extremely

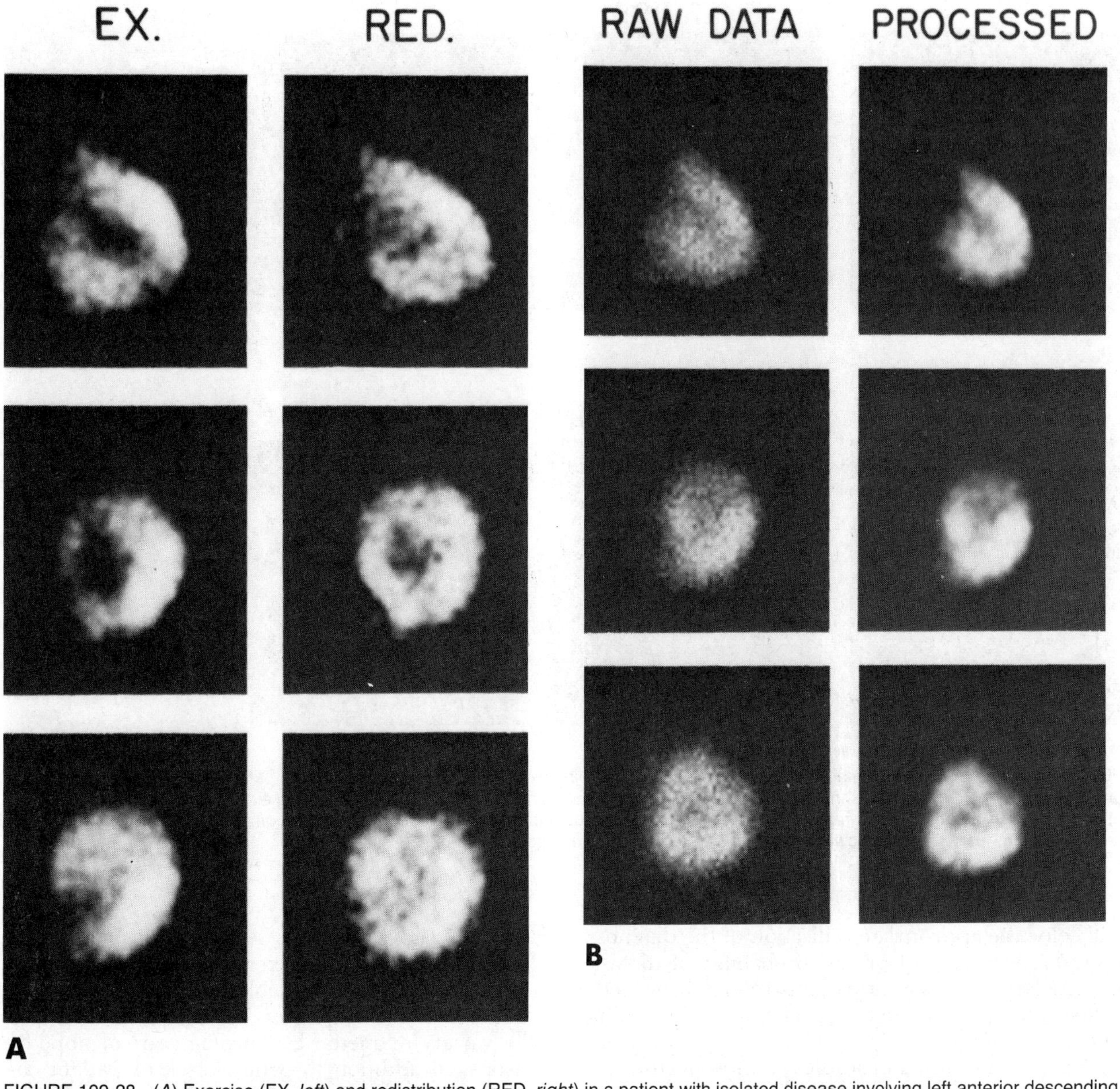

FIGURE 109-28 (*A*) Exercise (EX, *left*) and redistribution (RED, *right*) in a patient with isolated disease involving left anterior descending coronary artery. The upper images are obtained in the anterior position, the middle images in left anterior oblique position, and the lower images in the left lateral position. A prominent septal defect is seen in the left anterior oblique position and an apical defect in the anterior and lateral positions. The redistribution images show normalization of the exercise abnormalities. (*B*) Exercise images obtained in the same patient following successful coronary angioplasty. Images on the left are the raw data while those on the right are processed images. Anterior images are on the upper panel, left anterior oblique images in the middle panel, and left lateral images in the lower panel. Note that this exercise study following successful coronary angioplasty is associated with total reversal of the previous abnormality.

poorly with a physiologic index in the same vessel, namely the reactive hyperemic response measured intraoperatively with a Doppler flow technique.

There are a number of clinical indications for the use of exercise perfusion imaging. These include situations where exercise electrocardiography is difficult to interpret, as may occur with digitalis therapy, or with an abnormal baseline electrocardiogram, and in the asymptomatic patient with a positive exercise electrocardiogram; the symptomatic patient with an equivocal exercise test; the patient being assessed for postoperative coronary bypass graft patency; the patient evaluated following transluminal coronary angioplasty; or the patient evaluated as part of a routine preoperative assessment.

From a diagnostic standpoint, the population in whom ^{201}Tl exercise studies is most valuable is one with a pretest probability of disease in the range of 30 to 70 percent.[171] In such a population, a positive test increases the post-test probability to approximately 90 percent and a negative test decreases the probability to 10 percent. In any patient, based upon probability analysis, the pretest likelihood of coronary disease may range from 1 percent (35-year-old asymptomatic female) to 94 percent (65-year-old male with typical angina). These pretest probabilities clearly

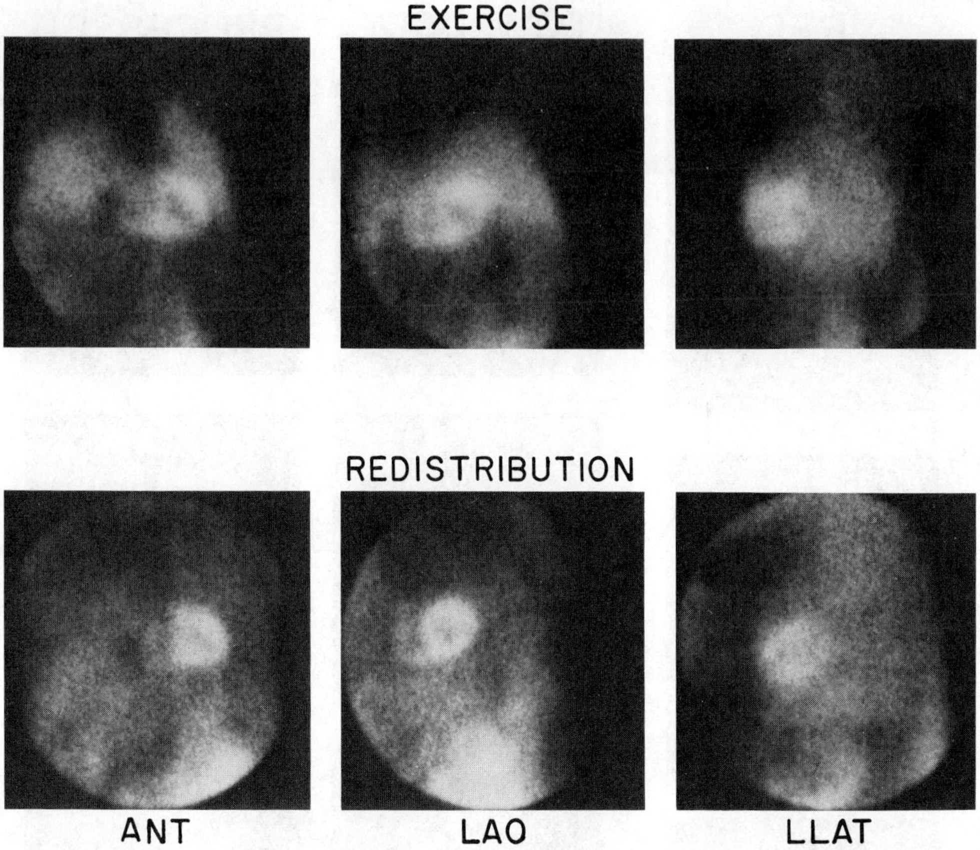

FIGURE 109-29 Thallium-201 images obtained immediately following exercise and at redistribution in a patient with multivessel coronary artery disease. The format is the same as in Fig. 109-26. Note the substantial pulmonary uptake following exercise. This uptake decreases at redistribution, at which time greater ^{201}Tl activity is seen in subdiaphragmatic structures. In addition, there is a suggestion of an anteroseptal perfusion defect following exercise. The redistribution images are normal.

will color the appropriate utilization of the diagnostic test. Awareness of pretest probability of disease is necessary for triage of patients referred for laboratory and appropriate interpretation of the results obtained.

A growing number of studies are now performed to help evaluate the results of angiographic studies. In this instance, the exercise perfusion images are employed after the invasive study, to provide additional physiologic insights into what may be a somewhat unclear anatomic situation. It should be apparent that there are many instances where exercise electrocardiography by itself may provide the appropriate information. Except in a setting in which the exercise electrocardiogram frequently is nondiagnostic (for example, in patients receiving digitalis or patients with abnormal baseline electrocardiograms), it is recommended that a conventional exercise test be performed initially. If this does not provide the appropriate information, then an exercise radionuclide study should be considered. A setting in which exercise imaging should be helpful is that of left bundle branch block. However, this condition appears to be associated with apparent "false-positive" perfusion abnormalities in the absence of coronary disease.[172]

Pharmacologic Stress Imaging

Certain patients cannot exercise to a workload sufficient to provoke detectable heterogeneity of regional blood flow responses. This may occur because of a variety of medical, neurologic, or orthopedic reasons, in addition to general lack of patient cooperation. Under these circumstances, it would be of value to have a nonexercise form of physiologic stress. This can be performed with atrial pacing, a known stress that increases myocardial oxygen demand. However, this is an invasive procedure which substantially limits its routine use. Another approach that has been reasonably attractive involves the use of a pharmacologic stress capable of increasing myocardial blood flow. The agent employed for pharmacologic stress imaging is dipyridamole.[173] This drug, when either infused intravenously or given orally, produces maximal coronary vasodilatation. Albro et al. have employed ^{201}Tl imaging following dipyridamole administration in 62 patients undergoing coronary arteriography and compared results with exercise imaging.[174] The sensitivity of ^{201}Tl imaging for detecting significant coronary artery disease was equal in both instances: after dipyridamole administration and after exercise stress. Defects were detected in 67 percent of patients with significant coronary stenosis by each of the techniques. Infusion of dipyridamole resulted in a modest increase in heart rate and decrease in blood pressure. Of note, angina and electrocardiographic evidence of myocardial ischemia occurred far more frequently with exercise than with dipyridamole. Significant ST-segment depression was noted in only 3 percent of patients following dipyridamole administration, suggesting that images diagnostic of heterogeneity of myocardial perfusion were obtained without the induction of significant myocardial ischemia. Thus, pharmacologic coronary vasodilatation appears to be an effective means of assessing myocardial perfusion abnormalities with ^{201}Tl imaging. This approach appears to be as effective as maximal exercise. Use of dipyridamole ^{201}Tl scintigraphy also has been employed following acute myocardial infarction. In a recent study by Leppo et al. this evaluation was shown to have significant prognostic impact.[175] Fifty-one patients recovering from acute myocardial infarction were studied. Twelve died or experienced reinfarction during a follow-up period that averaged 19 months. Eleven of these twelve patients had manifested abnormal redistribution dipyridamole ^{201}Tl images prior to hospital discharge. In addition, 24 of 51 patients required readmission for management of angina pectoris. Twenty-two of these twenty-four patients also showed redistribution on the dipyridamole study. In this study, dipyridamole–^{201}Tl imaging proved to be a more sensitive indicator of subsequent cardiac events than submaximal electrocardiographic stress testing.

Thallium-201 Quantification

One of the major drawbacks of ^{201}Tl image interpretation is its subjectivity. There is a great need for standardization of image interpretation and quantification of results. Quantitative ^{201}Tl imaging involves assessment of ^{201}Tl uptake, both spatially and temporally.[176] As described earlier, high spatial resolution images should be obtained immediately following exercise and 2 to 4 h later. The precise time of delayed imaging should be recorded, as this is needed to calculate normalized regional washout. Careful attention must be paid to precise replication of the imaging positions and obliquities, so that the initial and delayed images can be compared directly after apical realignment. Background subtraction usually involving a bilinear interpolation is performed to correct for activity from adjacent and superimposed structures (lung and liver). Thereafter, a profile of myocardial activity is obtained. This profile may be circumferential or linear, and it may involve mean or maximal activity at each point. Today, most programs involve circumferential analysis. A curve representing myocardial activity at each location in the myocardial profile is obtained for exercise and delayed imaging. The washout then is calculated as exercise activity minus redistribution activity divided by exercise activity and is expressed as a percent. This also may be displayed for each location along the profile. Comparison of each of these three curves with a normal range allows definition of areas of normal myocardial perfusion (Fig. 109-30).

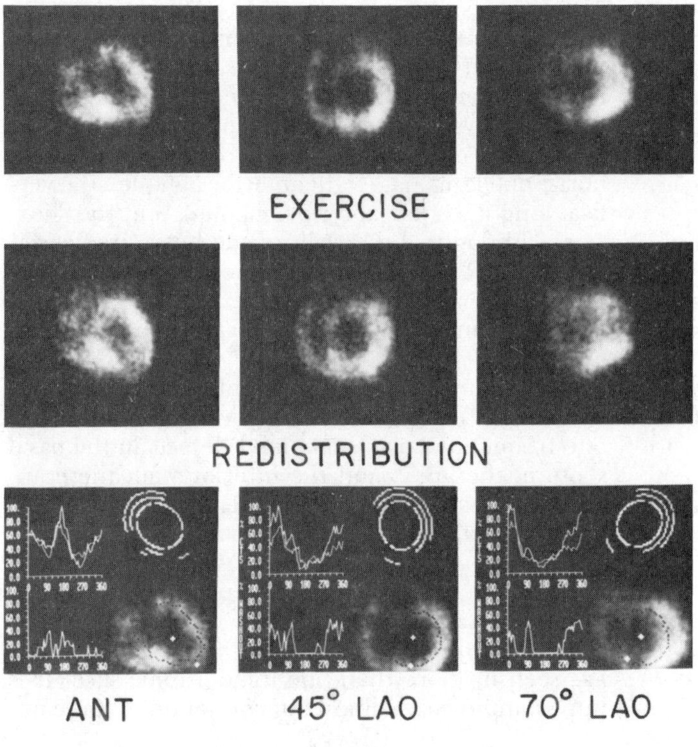

FIGURE 109-30 Visual images obtained at exercise and redistribution (*upper panels*) and quantitative washout data (*lower panel*) in a patient with multivessel disease. Visual interpretation of the images shows a significant reversible anteroseptal defect. The quantitative washout data demonstrate diffuse slow washout consistent with the anatomic finding of significant triple-vessel disease.

These quantitative methods depend heavily on precise correction for background. Since the bilinear interpolative background correction method does not solve all the problems associated with background correction from two-dimensional imaging, this represents an area of ongoing research. In addition, excessive contrast enhancement and smoothing may result in a decrease in specificity. Thallium-201 washout also may be affected by the degree of exercise and problems with ^{201}Tl injection. For example, the quantitative standards for washout kinetics are based upon reaching at least 85 percent of the predicted maximal heart rate. At lower levels of exercise, different normal standards need to be developed since the same quantitative analysis of washout cannot be used. Furthermore, markedly delayed washout will be seen in patients in whom the dose has infiltrated even partially. Thus, it is helpful to obtain an image over the injection site to determine whether or not there is substantial residual activity. Both this information, as well as the heart rate achieved, need to be taken into account when analyzing quantitative washout data.

Reversible perfusion defects will be seen as abnormalities in the exercise and washout curves, but with normal delayed profiles. Persistent defects are associated with abnormalities in the stress and delayed curves, but have normal washout. Furthermore, the presence of washout in the absence of visually apparent perfusion defects represents an important finding which is consistent with ischemia. Abnormal ^{201}Tl washout is defined either as washout below the lower limit of normal, or nonhomogeneous washout within the absolute normal range. Importantly, diffuse myocardial ischemia often may not be apparent from visual interpretation of images, because no region is actually normal. In this instance, diffuse slow washout may occur and may be apparent only through quantitative analysis of ^{201}Tl images. Such patients with multivessel disease may have falsely normal qualitative images, but definitely abnormal quantitative studies.

Quantitative ^{201}Tl imaging has become routine in many laboratories. The smoothed background corrected images have a far better contrast than routine planar images. For visual analysis, this also may be beneficial. Although the overall sensitivity and specificity of quantitative and qualitative ^{201}Tl imaging for *detection* of disease are relatively comparable, the quantitative technique appears superior in determining the extent and location of disease. In several studies, this approach has added to the ability of ^{201}Tl imaging to define multivessel disease, as well as high-risk patients following myocardial infarction.[176–178]

Tomographic Thallium Imaging

Planar ^{201}Tl imaging results in substantial superimposition of myocardial regions. Small defects and/or multiple defects may be obscured because of overlap with normal myocardium. The obvious advantage offered by thallium tomography would be avoidance of such areas of regional overlap and potential definition of abnormalities limited to the subendocardium, a portion of myocardium highly susceptible to regional ischemia. For rotational tomography, a gamma scintillation camera rotates on a specially designed gantry around the patient and acquires images at frequent intervals around the circumference of the thorax.[179–183] Generally, 32 to 64 images are obtained over 180° arc from the right anterior oblique to the left posterior oblique positions. Because of the dependence of tomography on the count rates achieved, it is recommended to utilize 3.0 to 3.5 mCi of ^{201}Tl for these studies. The overall acquisition time is approximately 20 to 25 min. There are two modes of data acquisition, specifically, step-and-shoot and continuous. With the step-and-shoot approach, there is a short interval between acquisition of each individual planar image. Using 32 images, each is acquired for 40 s. Thus, the total time of acquisition is the same as for three routine high-resolution planar images. Although the potential problem of rapid redistribution is often mentioned, this does not appear to be a real limitation. Data acquisition over 360° is not used because this includes substantial data from the posterior portion of the heart, which is severely attenuated. Better-quality images are obtained using 180° acquisition. Initially, transaxial tomograms are obtained. However, because the long axis of the heart is not parallel to the long axis of the body and is oriented upward to the left, it is preferable to reorient the transaxial images relative to the heart's true axis.

Using new computer techniques, oblique angle reconstruction is performed as a subsequent step in data analysis. Appropriate quality control measures should be undertaken to minimize problems associated with (1) uniformity errors, (2) incorrect center of rotation, (3) incorrect planar view data (sinogram displays), and (4) the detector not being parallel to the axis of rotation. Image review involves the horizontal long axis (right anterior oblique), the vertical long axis (left anterior oblique), and the short axis. Although all the walls of the heart are viewed theoretically from the multiple short-axis tomograms, in many cases particular regions are better viewed or imaged using the displays in other orientations.

The normal tomographic thallium image is homogeneous throughout the myocardium. However, one frequently encounters mild defects in the basal septum, the apex, and the inferior wall; these appear to be normal variants. When comparing stress and redistribution images, their appearance generally is comparable. Focally increased activity often is noted in the posterolateral wall, probably due to the posterolateral papillary muscle. Abnormal regions are defined as areas of decreased ^{201}Tl uptake, which are seen in more than one tomographic slice. It is important to base clinical interpretation of these im-

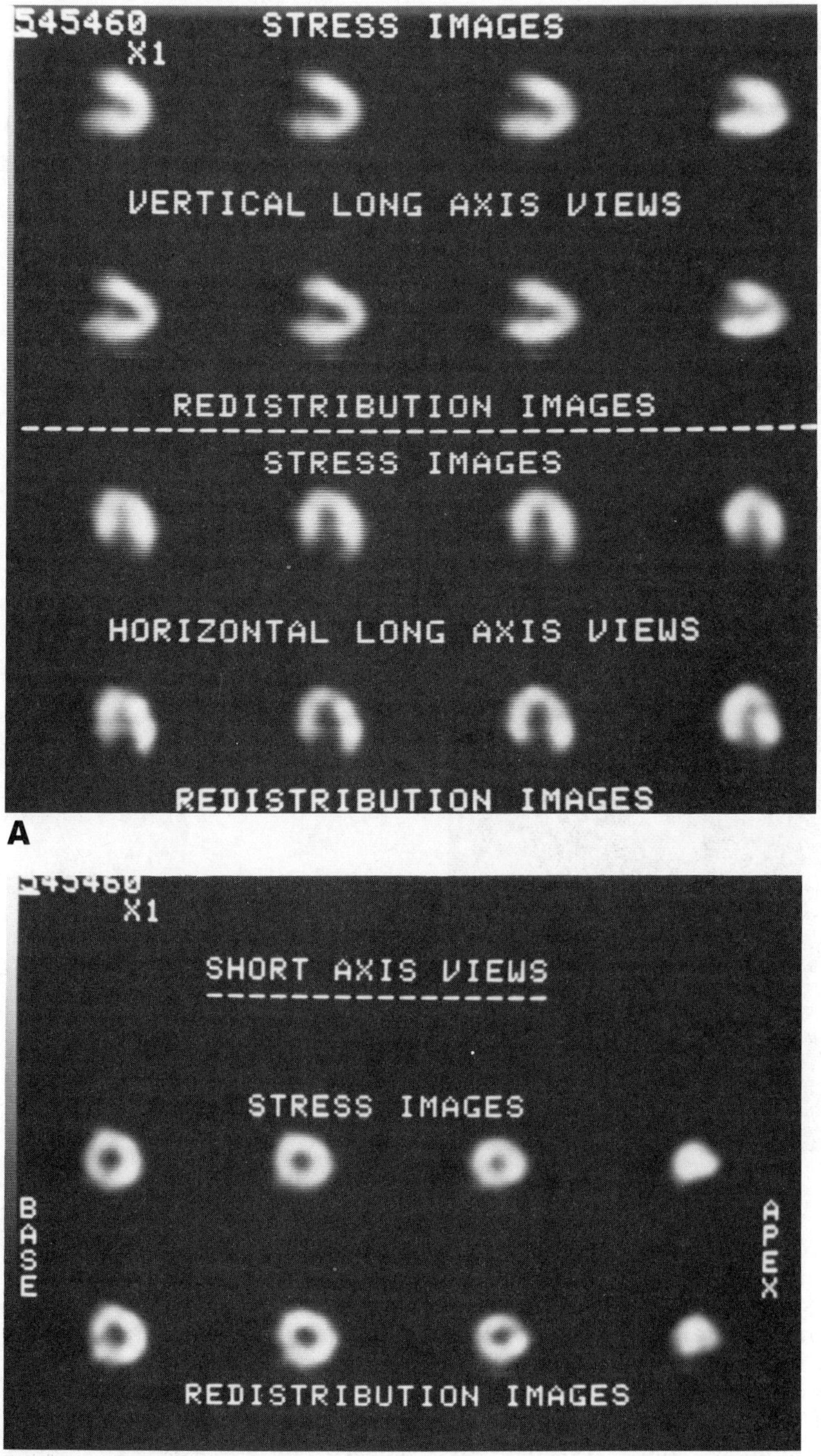

FIGURE 109-31 Thallium-201 tomographic studies obtained in a normal individual. Long-axis exercise and redistribution tomographic slices are shown in *A* and short-axis views are shown in *B*. Note the homogeneous distribution of thallium within the myocardium in all slices.

ages upon multiple orientations and multiple slices (Figs. 109-31 and 109-32; also see front and back endpapers).

New quantitative methods involving circumferential profile algorithms similar to those used for planar imaging now have been developed for quantitative assessment of tomographic thallium distribution and washout. Using the short-axis data, each of the tomograms is subjected to a circumferential analysis in which the maximal counts per pixel in each of approximately 40 to 60 sectors are plotted against angular position. Thereafter, using new dis-

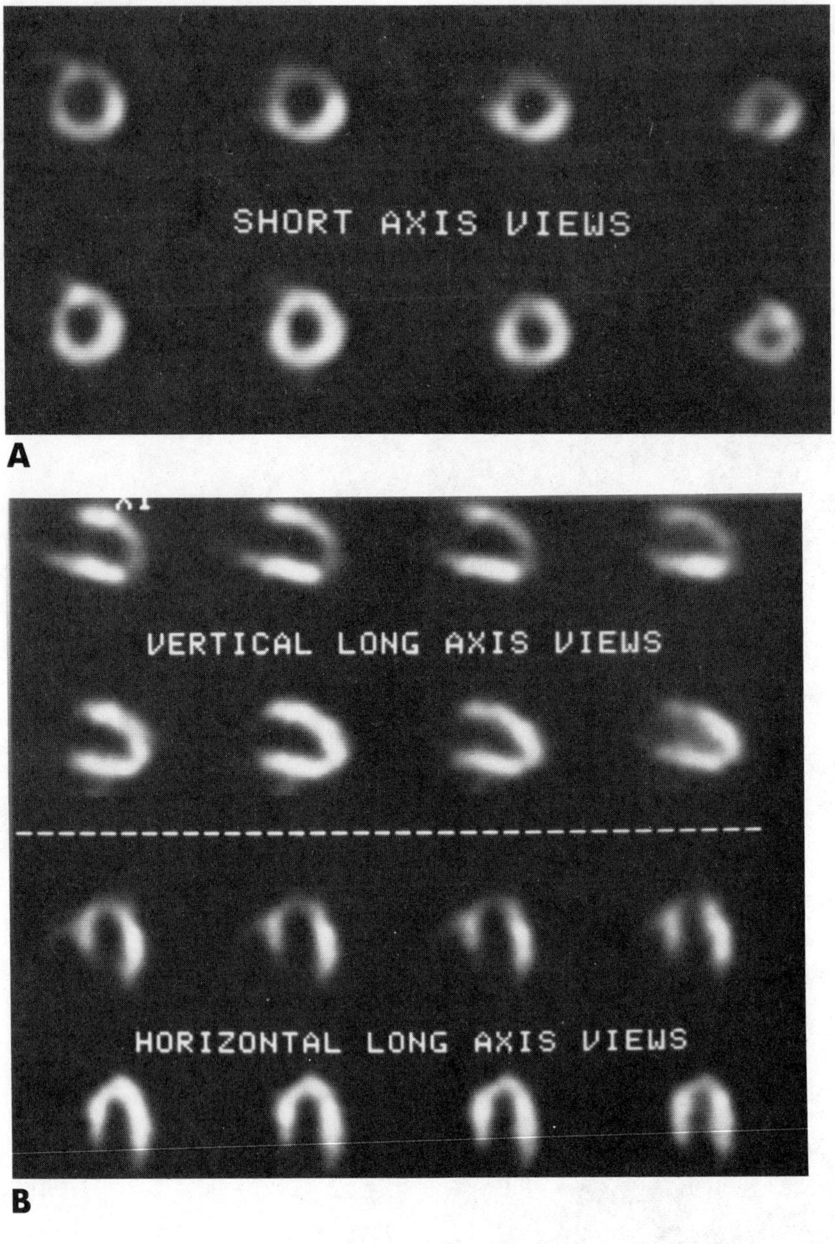

FIGURE 109-32 Thallium-201 tomographic slices obtained during exercise in a patient with ischemic heart disease. The short-axis views are shown in *A* and long-axis views in *B*. Exercise images are above and redistribution images below. Note the significant perfusion defect with reversal at the redistribution studies.

play techniques, a series of tomographic data at rest and/or at exercise can be displayed in a single functional image.

It is likely that quantitative tomographic ^{201}Tl imaging will undergo further development and validation. Several recent clinical studies have suggested that tomographic thallium imaging has a greater sensitivity for detecting myocardial infarction and ischemia than conventional planar imaging.[179–181] Thallium tomography appears to improve topographic localization of perfusion abnormalities. However, detailed comparisons between state-of-the-art quantitative planar imaging and tomographic imaging have not yet been performed.

Comparison of Exercise Thallium-201 and Exercise Left Ventricular Function Studies

It is not totally clear presently which exercise approach should be used in the initial assessment of patients with known or suspected coronary artery disease. Only a few studies have performed concomitant evaluation of both techniques in the same patients. Johnstone et al. studied 48 patients with exercise first pass left ventricular function and exercise ^{201}Tl studies;[184] 39 had angiographically documented coronary artery disease and 9 had normal coronary arteries. The 9 normal persons had both normal exercise ^{201}Tl images and normal exercise functional responses. Electrocardiographic evidence of myocardial ischemia was demonstrated in 17 of 39 patients with coronary disease (44 percent). New or augmented perfusion defects were detected in 62 percent of patients with coronary disease, compared with abnormal left ventricular exercise reserve in 85 percent ($p < 0.05$) (Fig. 109-33). There was close concordance between exercise-induced perfusion defects and induced regional wall motion abnormalities. The magnitude of change in ejection frac-

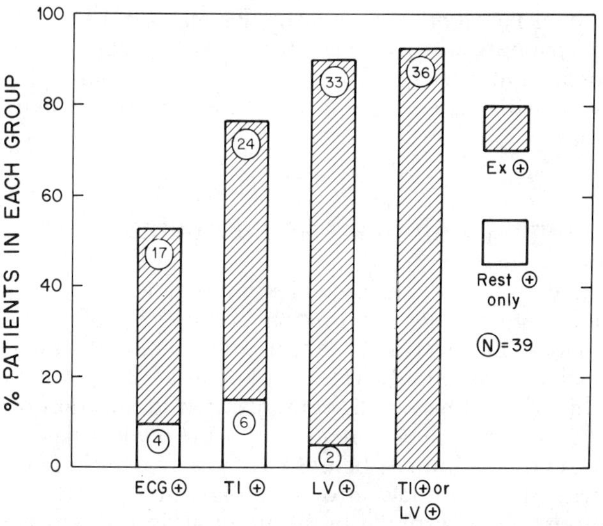

FIGURE 109-33 Comparison of concomitant evaluation of the electrocardiogram (ECG), ^{201}Tl imaging, and left ventricular function studies (LV) in 39 patients with angiographically confirmed coronary artery disease. Abnormalities present at exercise are indicated by the cross-hatched portions of the columns, while abnormalities present only at rest are indicated by the open portions of the columns. Numbers within the circles refer to the number of patients. Note that abnormal exercise LV reserve occurred significantly more frequently than exercise-induced perfusion defects. *(From D. E. Johnstone, M. J. Sands, H. J. Berger, et al., Comparison of Exercise Radionuclide Angiocardiography and Thallium-201 Myocardial Perfusion Imaging in Coronary Artery Disease, Am. J. Cardiol., 45:1113, 1980. Reproduced with permission from the publisher and author.)*

tion from rest to exercise was significantly greater in patients with abnormal ^{201}Tl imaging results as compared to those with normal perfusion patterns. Both radionuclide studies were abnormal in 54 percent of patients with coronary disease, while both were normal in only three patients, all of whom had single-vessel disease. Abnormalities at rest or exercise were present on ^{201}Tl imaging in 77 percent and left ventricular function studies in 90 percent of these patients.

Similar observations were reported by Caldwell et al., who evaluated 52 patients undergoing coronary angiography.[97] Of the 52 patients, 41 had significant coronary artery disease. Within this group, the exercise ejection fraction measurement was more sensitive than that of the thallium technique (93 percent versus 71 percent). When the two techniques were combined, coronary artery disease was detected appropriately in all patients. However, the specificity of the exercise left ventricular function studies was substantially lower than that of the thallium examination. Comparable data have also been reported by Jengo et al.[185]

Thus, it appears that exercise left ventricular function studies presently are a more sensitive means of detecting angiographically documented coronary artery disease than are exercise ^{201}Tl studies. However, they are also somewhat less specific. These comparisons must, however, be reevaluated with new state-of-the-art quantitative ^{201}Tl imaging techniques. Abnormal exercise left ventricular function studies occur in a variety of conditions, such as valvular disease, administration of cardiotoxic agents, and healed myocarditis, which may lead to a false impression of underlying coronary artery disease. The decision as to which type of study to employ should be based on the available equipment and the experience of the laboratory, as well as the clinical subset into which a given patient falls. There generally will be a trade-off between greater sensitivity (function studies) and greater specificity (^{201}Tl studies). Exercise left ventricular function studies often require a greater degree of instrumentation than do exercise ^{201}Tl studies. A computer is mandatory for the performance of exercise function studies, while this currently is not absolutely necessary for the performance of exercise thallium images.

There are definite clinical situations where exercise function studies should *not* be the first approach. One such situation involves patients with known baseline arrhythmias or exercise-induced arrhythmias in whom it may not be possible to get an adequate functional assessment because of artifacts introduced by the arrhythmia during the period of data sampling. Another involves the extremely anxious patient who enters the laboratory with augmented performance at rest as a result of high sympathetic tone. An abnormally high ejection fraction at baseline will make it potentially difficult to interpret exercise ejection fraction responses. In patients with associated valvular disease, it would be difficult to determine if an abnormal ventricular performance response was due to coronary or valvular disease. In patients such as the postoperative bypass patient, or postangioplasty patient where assessment of a specific vascular bed is at issue, exercise thallium imaging would appear the better study. If a major clinical suspicion concerning the presence of coronary disease persists after the performance of an initial study, it is worthwhile performing a second study using the alternative exercise technique. Several series have now demonstrated that negative results by both exercise techniques speak strongly against the presence of major multivessel coronary artery disease.[97,184]

Resting Thallium-201 Imaging as a Means of Defining Anatomic Structure

Thallium-201 imaging can provide substantial insight into cardiac anatomy. Left ventricular dilatation can be appreciated. Left ventricular hypertrophy can be assessed qualitatively by perception of a thickened myocardial wall and decreased cavity size. Asymmetric septal hypertrophy also can be identified from the resting thallium image.[186] While echocardiography clearly remains the optimal modality for diagnosing this disease entity, imaging data also may be helpful and should be recognized if obtained during the course of routine evaluation.

As stated above, ^{201}Tl uptake generally is not appreciated in right ventricular myocardium at rest in

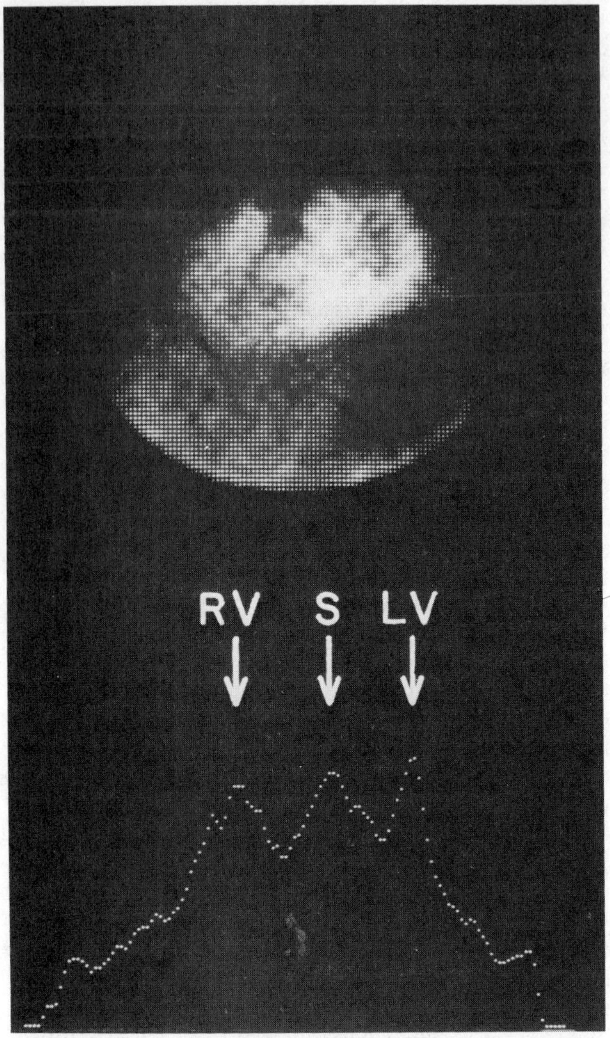

FIGURE 109-34 Thallium-201 image obtained in the left anterior oblique position in a patient with marked right ventricular hypertrophy. Note the marked uptake of ^{201}Tl in the right ventricle at rest. Below the image, a profile through the mid portion of the heart is shown, indicating the left ventricular (LV) free wall, interventricular septum (S), and right ventricular (RV) free wall. (*From L. A. Reduto, H. J. Berger, D. E. Johnstone, et al., Radionuclide Assessment of Right and Left Ventricular Exercise Reserve after Total Correction of Tetralogy of Fallot, Am. J. Cardiol., 45:1013, 1980. Reproduced with permission from the publisher and author.*)

the absence of either right ventricular hypertrophy or right ventricular volume overload (Fig. 109-34). In the latter case, abnormal uptake is related to an increase in right ventricular blood flow associated with loading conditions. In a group of 53 patients Khaja et al. related right ventricular visualization to right ventricular systolic pressure at the time of cardiac catheterization.[187] Right ventricular systolic pressure was significantly higher in patients with right ventricular visualization (57.4 mmHg) than in those with nonvisualization (21.2 mmHg). Right ventricular visualization occurred frequently in the absence of right ventricular enlargement or electrocardiographic evidence of right ventricular hypertrophy. Similar observations have been made by others.[188] Abnormal right ventricular uptake may also be noted in patients with marked postinfarction congestive heart failure where there is both abnormal right ventricular pressure and decreased left ventricular mass.

Imaging with Infarct-Avid Agents

Imaging acute myocardial infarction with infarct-avid agents allows definition of the zone of acute myocardial necrosis as an area of increased radioactivity, commonly referred to as a *hot spot.* Although Holman et al. demonstrated localization of ^{99m}Tc tetracycline in regions of acute myocardial infarction in human beings,[22] it was not until 1975 with the introduction of imaging with ^{99m}Tc stannous pyrophosphate by Bonte et al. in the experimental animal[23] and its subsequent assessment in humans by Parkey et al.[24] that infarct-avid imaging was performed to any great extent. Thereafter, there was a brief period of wide utilization of this technique. More recently, it has become clear that there are only certain specific instances where the pyrophosphate infarct-imaging approach has substantial clinical value. For this reason, in most laboratories infarct-avid imaging is the least frequently employed of the currently available clinical nuclear cardiology techniques. However, with the current interest in thrombolytic therapy, the need to assess zones of myocardial necrosis and to estimate infarct size may lead to renewed intense interest in infarct-avid imaging.

Mechanisms of Pyrophosphate Uptake

Technetium-99m stannous pyrophosphate accumulation in zones of acute myocardial necrosis is the result of a complex series of pathophysiologic events. This radiopharmaceutical is used routinely for bone imaging. It was noted initially that pyrophosphate accumulation was linked closely to calcium deposition.[189] Histochemically, calcium accumulation within the peripheral zones of myocardial infarction can be demonstrated readily, with maximal accumulation at 48 to 72 h after the event. Electron microscopic studies demonstrate calcium deposition within mitochondria as well as within the cytoplasm of necrotic cells.[190] The temporal sequence of calcium accumulation within infarcted myocardium parallels closely that seen with pyrophosphate, and there is also a topographic relation between areas where calcium accumulates maximally, namely the periphery of the infarct, and the site of maximal pyrophosphate deposition. However, detailed experiments have failed to show a quantitative relation between the magnitude of calcium deposition in a given area of ischemic necrosis and the magnitude of pyrophosphate deposition.[190]

An additional operative mechanism involves pyrophosphate binding to denatured proteins or other macromolecules which become uniquely accessible to radionuclides during the course of the necrotic process. Dewanjee et al. demonstrated with in vitro experiments that there is substantial pyrophosphate binding to macromolecules.[191] Riba et al. noted in a rabbit endocarditis model that there was major pyrophosphate binding to the endocarditis lesion, which consisted primarily of denatured protein and bacteria.[192] The major cellular site of pyrophosphate accumulation appears to be not in the mitochondrial fraction, as was initially postulated based upon the calcium hypothesis, but rather in the cytoplasm.[190] Uptake of pyrophosphate is not related to leukocyte infiltration since abnormal images are noted in animals in whom leukopenia is induced pharmacologically.[193]

Regional accumulation of pyrophosphate also is dependent upon regional myocardial blood flow. Maximal accumulation of pyrophosphate within an infarct zone occurs in regions where flow is approximately 30 to 40 percent of normal.[194] In regions with flow below this level, pyrophosphate uptake actually falls, even though the degree of myocardial necrosis is more intense. In regions with flow greater than 30 to 40 percent of normal, pyrophosphate accumulation does follow an inverse linear relation to blood flow. Pyrophosphate myocardial deposition thus requires appropriate delivery of the radionuclide to zones of necrosis. In extremely low flow zones delivery is limited, thereby leading to decreased myocardial radionuclide accumulation even though these are the regions of maximal necrosis. It is clear from these observations that assessment of the actual intensity of pyrophosphate accumulation in a myocardial region will not provide direct quantitative data concerning the degree of necrosis in the region.

Imaging Technique and Interpretation

Imaging presently is performed almost exclusively with ^{99m}Tc stannous pyrophosphate. Care must be taken to ensure an appropriate radiopharmaceutical preparation. Poor labeling of the phosphate compounds with ^{99m}Tc or rapid breakdown of the label in the vial or syringe will result in poor clearance of the radionuclide and subsequent labeling of the blood pool, resulting in images which might be interpreted incorrectly. Radiopharmaceuticals must be tested routinely for labeling efficiency. The routine radionuclide dose is 15 mCi of ^{99m}Tc tagged to 5 mg of stannous pyrophosphate. Studies generally should be performed 60 to 90 min after injection. Pyrophosphate compounds are cleared from the blood by a renal mechanism, directly related to glomerular filtration rate.[195] In the presence of decreased renal function, as might be seen in congestive heart failure or in intrinsic renal disease, the time for imaging should be delayed to 3 to 4 h following injection.

Imaging should be performed in at least three positions: anterior, left anterior oblique, and left lateral. Images generally are obtained for 400,000 counts. Interpretation involves a grading scheme based upon both the site of abnormal myocardial accumulation and its intensity. The site is generally described as being either focal (localized to one myocardial region) or diffuse (poorly localized to any one region of the left or right ventricle). Intensity is generally graded by relating activity in the myocardium to that in the sternum according to a system proposed by Parkey et al.[24] In this system, zero represents no uptake and 4 + most intense uptake. A 1 + represents minimal activity, and 2 + represents definite myocardial activity less than that of the sternum; 3 + activity is visually equal in intensity to that seen in the sternum, while 4 + activity is greater in intensity than that seen in the sternum. The 2 + pattern of uptake is generally considered equivocal and nonspecific; 3 + and 4 + activity are considered diagnostic and specific for myocardial necrosis. Attempts should always be made to distinguish myocardial uptake from that due to residual blood pool activity. This generally is not a problem when dealing with the focal uptake patterns, but difficulties may be encountered with diffuse uptake patterns. A reasonable aid in distinguishing residual blood pool activity from true diffuse myocardial uptake involves additional imaging of other vascular structures. If activity is seen in the region of the great vessels or at the bifurcation of the aorta, then residual blood pool activity is still present and imaging should be repeated in 2 h.

Pyrophosphate imaging should be performed roughly 48 to 72 h after the onset of infarction. This is the time of the greatest likelihood of achieving a positive result. Infarct images generally become negative approximately 7 to 10 days after the infarct. However, it has been noted that in many patients a good deal of time is necessary for the image to return totally to normal, and positive patterns persist. The persistently positive patterns are generally less intense than those noted during the acute infarct period and often may be diffuse. Olson et al. noted a return to normal in only 43 percent of a group of patients with infarction evaluated 6 to 37 weeks after the acute event.[196] Persistently positive images have been associated with the distinct pathologic finding of myocytolysis.[197]

In order to make a diagnosis of myocardial infarction and relate it to a specific left ventricular wall, relation between the myocardial accumulation and bony uptake must be made (Fig. 109-35).[198] These relations to extracardiac structures are critical since, unlike thallium images, there is no uptake in normal myocardium to serve as a system of anatomic reference (Figs. 109-36 and 109-37). In large anterior wall myocardial infarctions, abnormal uptake patterns with a central infarct zone of relatively decreased pyrophosphate accumulation are often noted. This phenomenon has been termed the *doughnut sign.* It is associated with large infarcts and appears to be associated with a poor prognosis.[199]

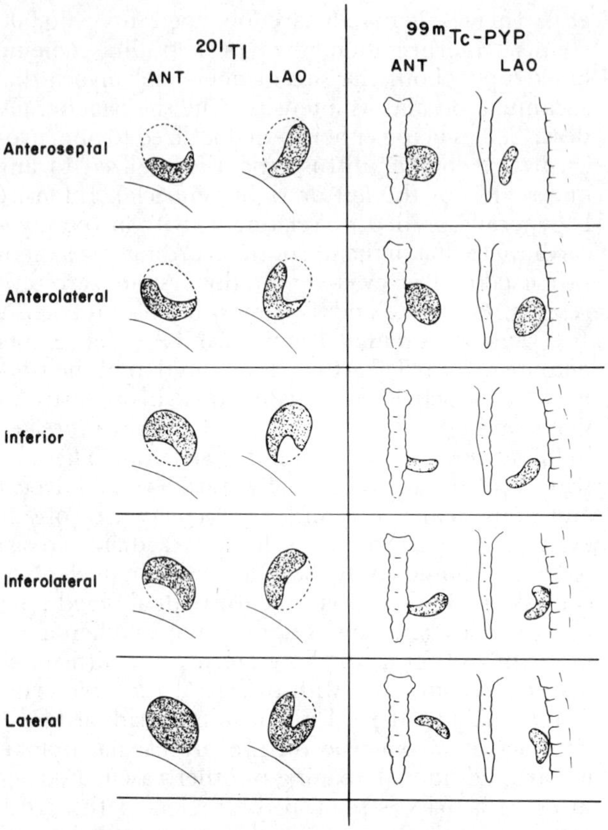

FIGURE 109-35 Schematic representation of various abnormal image patterns encountered with ^{201}Tl and ^{99m}Tc pyrophosphate (^{99m}Tc-PYP) imaging in the anterior (ANT) and left anterior oblique (LAO) positions in a different types of myocardial infarction. Note that for the pyrophosphate images, comparison must be made to activity in skeletal structures. With ^{201}Tl images, anatomic localization is achieved by comparison with uptake in normal myocardium. (*From H. J. Berger, A. Gottschalk, and B. L. Zaret, Dual Radionuclide Study of Myocardial Infarction: Comparison of Thallium-201 and Technetium-99m Stannous Pyrophosphate Imaging in Man, Ann. Intern. Med., 88:145, 1978. Reproduced with permission from the publisher and author.*)

The mechanism of its occurrence probably relates to a large central infarct area with extremely low residual myocardial blood flow.

Clinical Imaging Results

A large number of published series have appeared defining the potential utility of pyrophosphate imaging. In initial reports describing the technique it appeared to be both highly sensitive and specific.[200–202] In a compilation of 22 different series involving approximately 935 patients with acute infarction, infarct imaging was positive in 93 percent of the cases.[203] In an additional group of 1334 patients in whom infarction was not present, the pyrophosphate images were negative in approximately 83 percent. Within this compilation, patients with unstable angina had a relatively high incidence of positive results (78 percent) in the absence of infarction. These patients generally manifested a diffuse pattern. Thus, pyrophosphate imaging is a relatively sensitive but somewhat less specific technique. It should be noted that sensitivity appears to be substantially lower in patients with relatively small and nontransmural infarcts.[204] In canine preparations the lower limit of infarct detection is approximately 3 g of infarcted tissue.[205] It is not clear that such sensitive definition can be obtained in humans. Sensitivity and specificity determinations are also dependent upon criteria employed for grading of positive images.[206] A 2 + diffuse pattern is commonly seen in patients with unstable angina. If this is considered an equivocal result, then sensitivity will be lower and specificity higher. Likewise, if these images all are considered positive, then sensitivity will be much higher and specificity much lower. However, in the correlative pathologic study of Poliner et al. there was excellent correlation between pathologic evidence of myocardial necrosis and associated abnormal pyrophosphate uptake in 52 patients coming to necropsy evaluation.[207] This relation was noted in patients with both acute myocardial infarction and unstable angina pectoris.

A number of clinical conditions other than acute myocardial infarction may be associated with abnormal pyrophosphate accumulation. These conditions include: skeletal abnormalities of any type (such as fractures), calcified costal cartilage, left ventricular aneurysms, intracardiac calcifications, skeletal muscle damage, postcardioversion changes in both skel-

FIGURE 109-36 Technetium-99m pyrophosphate images obtained in a normal (N) patient without myocardial infarction (*left*), in a patient with a large anterior (A) myocardial infarction (*middle*), and in a patient with an inferior (I) myocardial infarction (*right*). Images were obtained in the anterior (ANT), left anterior oblique (LAO), and left lateral (LL) positions. Note the expected skeletal uptake in the patient without infarction and the areas of substantial myocardial accumulation of the radionuclide in the patients with the two types of infarction.

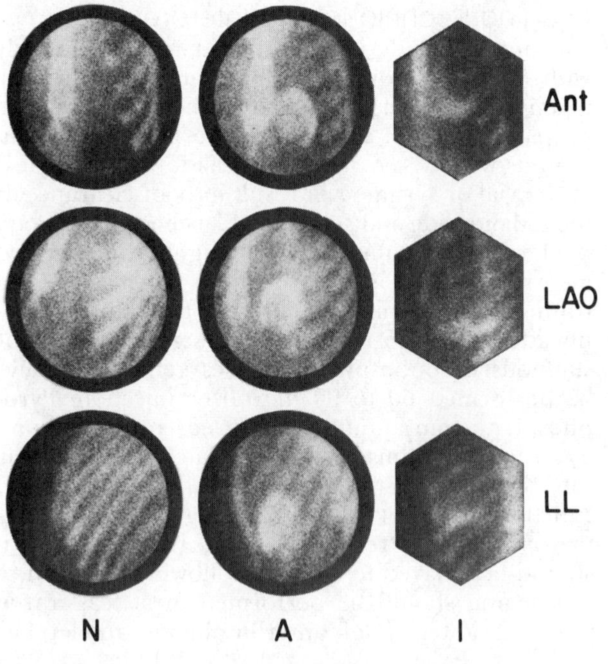

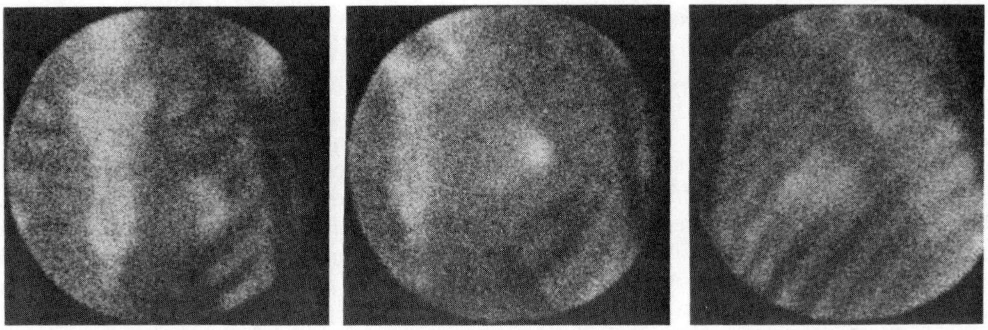

FIGURE 109-37 Technetium-99m pyrophosphate images in a patient with a lateral wall myocardial infarction obtained in the anterior (*left panel*), left anterior oblique (*middle panel*), and left lateral (*right panel*) positions. Note the abnormal area of uptake superimposed on skeletal structures.

etal or cardiac muscle, contusion of the myocardium, breast tumors, tumors metastatic to the myocardium, cardiomyopathy, and overlying skin lesions.[203] Abnormal uptake has also been reported with high frequency in unstable angina pectoris.[208]

Indications for Pyrophosphate Imaging

Pyrophosphate imaging as a means of detecting acute infarction has potential clinical uses. It would appear to be most valuable in defining acute myocardial infarction in patients who present several days after the acute event at a time when conventional indexes of myocardial necrosis, such as the electrocardiogram and enzyme analysis, will either be negative or nonspecific. In addition, pyrophosphate imaging might be of help in patients in whom the initial appropriately timed clinical evaluation produces equivocal results. In patients with major conduction system abnormalities in whom conventional electrocardiographic manifestation of infarction is difficult, imaging may be of benefit occasionally. Pyrophosphate imaging also allows definition of right ventricular myocardial necrosis by demonstrating abnormal accumulation anterior to the interventricular septum (Fig. 109-38).[209] Pyrophosphate studies in the perioperative period following coronary artery surgery allow definition of acute necrosis while conventional assessment with electrocardiogram and enzyme studies generally is nonspecifically abnormal.[210,211] In other than a diagnostic sense, pyrophosphate imaging may provide insight into overall infarct size, and this may have prognostic implications.[212,213] The demonstration of a persistently positive infarct pattern following infarction may also have prognostic significance.[197]

Place of Pyrophosphate Imaging in the Coronary Care Unit

It is clear that the majority of patients presenting to the coronary care unit with acute myocardial infarction do not require pyrophosphate imaging for

FIGURE 109-38 Comparative ^{201}Tl and ^{99m}Tc pyrophosphate (^{99m}Tc-PYP) images obtained in a patient with a small inferior wall myocardial infarction and a large right ventricular infarct. Note that in the ^{201}Tl images, a perfusion defect is apparent primarily in the left lateral (LL) image. On the left anterior oblique (LAO) pyrophosphate image, there is a large area of abnormal right ventricular accumulation extending anteriorly adjacent to the sternum. This is diagnostic of major right ventricular infarction (*From F. J. Wackers, K. I. Lie, E. Busemann-Sokole, J. Res., J. B. Van der Schoot, and D. Durrer, Prevalence of Right Ventricular Involvement in Inferior Wall Infarction Assessed with Myocardial Imaging with Thallium-201 and Technetium-99m Pyrophosphate, Am. J. Cardiol., 42:358, 1978. Reproduced with permission from the publisher and author.*)

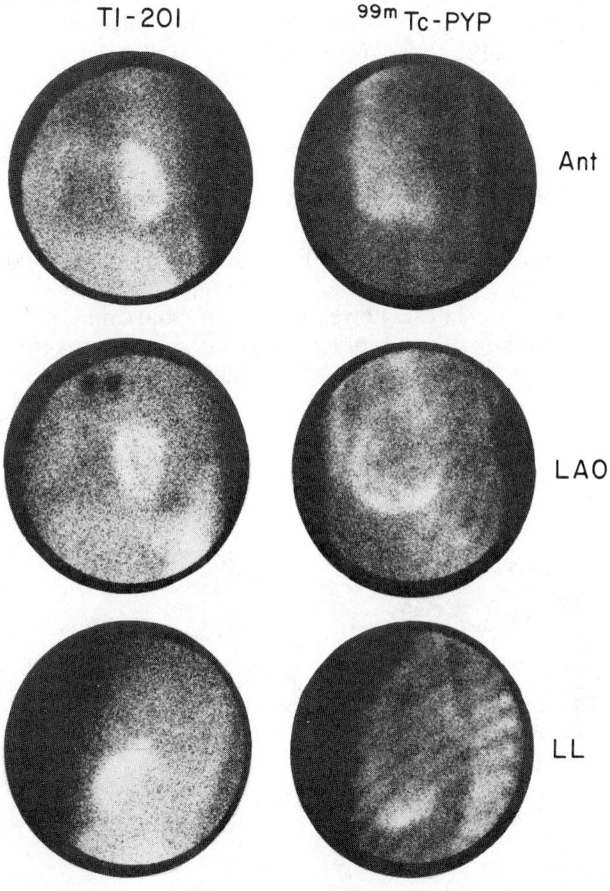

diagnostic purposes. Selected clinical situations as defined above do occur where this imaging approach may have diagnostic value. Imaging data obtained with this approach may have prognostic implications. However, the prognostic value of pyrophosphate imaging must be compared directly with that of thallium imaging and left ventricular function assessment, both of which have also been shown to provide prognostic data. When used in the coronary care unit, the appropriate temporal sequence of imaging must be appreciated. In the initial hours of infarction, pyrophosphate imaging clearly would not be the proper approach, while thallium imaging would be. When used prudently, dual imaging with thallium and pyrophosphate may provide meaningful complementary data in individual patients.

Infarct Sizing

Several investigators have shown that an estimate of infarct size correlating well with histopathologic assessment can be obtained with pyrophosphate imaging.[205,212,214–217] These estimates have been derived from conventional planar imaging as well as tomographic and three-dimensional reconstruction techniques. However, this experimental measurement can only be obtained with reliability in a temporal sequence allowing best definition at approximately 48 h after infarction. Therefore, these measurements can be made only after the maximal amount of myocardial necrosis has already occurred, and they are not suitable for serial study assessing interventions.

New Techniques

A number of new techniques have been proposed recently for studying specific pathophysiologic processes. These newer techniques have been developed on a firm biologic basis and involve imaging with radiolabeled blood cells, antibodies, and metabolites.

Indium-111–Labeled Platelet Imaging

Since platelet aggregation serves as an initiating focus for thrombosis in regions of high blood flow and stress, it has been proposed that labeled platelets may serve as an appropriate means of imaging cardiac thrombosis. Platelets have been labeled with ^{111}In in a manner that makes them suitable for use as imaging agents.[218] Indium-111 is a radionuclide with high-energy gamma emissions with energies of 173 and 247 keV, which are well suited for detection with conventional scintillation cameras. It has a physical half-life of 2.8 days, permitting imaging over several days after a single injection. Indium-111 complexed with 8-hydroxyquinoline (oxine) forms a lipid-soluble compound which labels platelets by passive diffusion without altering their functional characteristics. Labeled platelets have a life span of approximately 8 days.

Riba et al. have studied ^{111}In platelet imaging in several animal models. Indium-111 platelets were shown to be an extremely effective imaging agent for detecting the lesion of experimental aortic valve endocarditis in rabbits.[219] In its acute phase this lesion is composed primarily of platelets. From 48 to 72 h after the platelet administration, in vivo imaging demonstrated abnormal uptake in the region of the aortic valve in a distinct anatomic pattern. Images of the excised heart demonstrated abnormal discrete cardiac uptake conforming to the in vivo images. Radionuclide accumulation in the aortic valve vegetation was 240 times that in normal myocardium and 99 times greater than that present in blood.

Platelet imaging also was demonstrated to be a feasible means of detecting experimental coronary artery thrombosis in the dog.[220] Uptake was routinely defined in animals imaged 2 h after the induction of thrombosis. Serial imaging of acutely formed thrombi over 22 h after the administration of labeled platelets showed no significant change in the scintigraphic appearance (Fig. 109-39). However, 24-h-old coronary artery thrombosis failed to reveal enhanced activity within the region of the thrombus-containing coronary artery. Others have demonstrated the efficacy of ^{111}In-labeled platelets for imaging experimental acute pulmonary

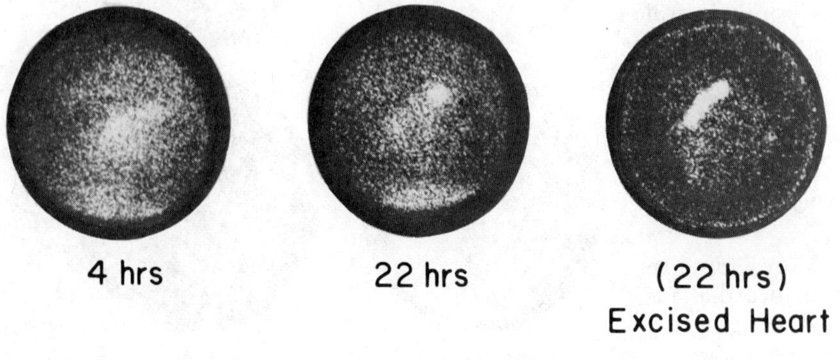

FIGURE 109-39 Indium-111 labeled platelet images obtained in a dog 4 and 22 h after thrombus induction. The images on the left and in the middle were obtained in situ, while the image on the right was obtained after the heart was excised. Note the regions of increased platelet uptake corresponding to the coronary thrombosis. All images were obtained with a pinhole collimator. *(From A. L. Biba, M. L. Thakur, A. Gottschalk, and B. L. Zaret, Imaging Experimental Coronary Artery Thrombosis with Indium-111 Platelets, Circulation, 60:767, 1979. Reproduced with permission from the American Heart Association, Inc., and the author.)*

embolism[221] and acute platelet deposition at the site of saphenous vein coronary bypass anastomosis in the dog.[222]

Studies now have been obtained in humans as well. Recent observations indicate that ^{111}In-labeled platelets are suitable for detecting intracardiac thrombosis in regions of left ventricular aneurysms.[223,224] Davis et al. used the labeled-platelet imaging technique for detecting platelet deposition in regions of carotid artery atherosclerosis.[225] Platelet deposition was noted in 61 percent of sites of angiographically demonstrable atherosclerotic lesions. The frequency of positive scintigraphic results was slightly higher in patients not treated with antithrombotic agents than in those on such drugs (70 percent versus 57 percent). Platelet deposition has been imaged at sites of significant peripheral vascular disease as well as at vascular prostheses.[226] The effects of antiplatelet drugs have been evaluated.[227] More recently, platelet deposition has been imaged early after transluminal balloon angioplasty in peripheral vessels.[228] The relation of this finding to subsequent restenosis is an area of considerable interest. Ezekowitz et al. have also demonstrated the efficacy of platelet imaging as a means of defining zones of acute deep-vein thrombosis.[229] In this context, as opposed to arterial thrombosis, heparin will significantly inhibit imaged platelet deposition. This technique can potentially provide highly relevant data, particularly in understanding the role of platelets in vascular stenosis and occlusion and the impact of various therapeutic strategies.

Indium-111 Polymorphonuclear Leukocyte Imaging

Indium-111 oxine can also be used to label polymorphonuclear leukocytes. Cells labeled in this manner retain biologic activity and may be used to study cardiac inflammatory responses, particularly following acute myocardial infarction. Thakur et al. have evaluated this in dogs subjected to anterior wall myocardial infarction.[230] Abnormal radiolabeled leukocyte accumulation was noted in discrete anatomic areas in all animals studied within 24 to 96 h after infarction. All images obtained 120 h after infarction were negative. Polymorphonuclear leukocyte infiltration was maximal in areas of lowest flow. Maximal epicardial infiltration occurred within the first 24 h after infarction, while maximum endocardial infiltration occurred at 72 h after infarction. Davies et al. have extended these observations to leukocyte imaging in human beings.[231] Positive leukocyte images were present in 58 percent of patients evaluated. The incidence of positive images was greatest in the first 48 h after infarction.

Indium-111–labeled leukocytes as a means of studying cardiac inflammation requires further evaluation. It clearly is not meant to be a replacement of other infarct-avid imaging techniques. In selected instances, this imaging study may provide additional relevant pathophysiologic data concerning the inflammatory response and may serve as a means of monitoring this response during therapy. Also, this may provide a means of assessing additional inflammatory reactions such as pericarditis or myocarditis.

Radiolabeled Myosin-Specific Antibody

Purified radiolabeled antibody against cardiac myosin has been proposed as an additional means of detecting regions of acute myocardial necrosis following myocardial infarction.[232] Initial studies were done with intact antibodies. More recently imaging has been obtained with antibody fragments (Fab). Inverse relationships have been noted between regional myocardial blood flow and uptake of the antibody.[233] Maximal activity has been noted in the lowest flow zones. Imaging of radiolabeled antibody distributions within regions of myocardial infarction recently has been accomplished. Patients have now been studied with this imaging technique. Initial results are encouraging.[234]

Positron and Metabolic Imaging

Positron-emission computed tomography is a new technique with potential for assessment of myocardial blood flow and myocardial metabolism.[235–237] This particular approach involves specific unique capabilities. These capabilities include (1) an imaged distribution of radionuclides displayed in a three-dimensional fashion, (2) spatial resolution which is independent of depth, and (3) independence from attentuation effects. Positron annihilation is associated with the generation of two 511-keV photons leaving a site of interaction in opposite directions. Simultaneous emission of these photons is detected by pairs of opposing scintillation detectors. Only interactions occurring within the range of the pair of detectors are recorded. This feature forms the basis for relative independence from depth.

Radionuclides specific for a variety of metabolic pathways can be synthesized with positron-emitting radiolabels. The radionuclides most frequently employed are ^{15}O, ^{11}C, and ^{13}N. These substances can be incorporated into compounds without altering their biologic activity. Fluorine-18 has also been used to label chemical analogues with altered biologic properties, such that the synthesized compounds will be trapped after entering the cell.[238]

Nitrogen-13 ammonia and rubidium-82 have been used as markers of regional myocardial blood flow in a manner comparable to ^{201}Tl. Within the range of physiologically encountered blood flows, tissue accumulation of these radionuclides is related linearly to myocardial blood flow. Assessment of myocardial perfusion using ^{13}N and positron tomography has been evaluated both in animals and in human beings.[239,240] Studies are now under way evaluating generation-produced ^{82}Rb as a means of directly measuring regional blood flow and perfusion.[241]

Myocardial metabolic studies have involved primarily two radiolabeled metabolites to date. Carbon-11 palmitate has been described as a myocardial imaging agent suitable for assessing fatty acid metabolism and sizing myocardial infarction both in animals and in humans.[242–244] Total uptake and turnover rates in the myocardium provide a measure of the rate of fatty acid metabolism. In addition to assessing metabolism directly in ischemic and infarcted states, ^{11}C fatty acid imaging and kinetics has been shown to be of value in defining myocardial viability of salvage following thrombolysis.[245] Recent studies involving carbohydrate metabolism have employed 2-fluoro-2-deoxyglucose. When administered intravenously, this substance behaves initially in a manner similar to glucose. Within the myocardial cell, it is phosphorylated by hexokinase to fluorodeoxyglucose-6-phosphate. It then becomes trapped metabolically without further metabolism. Metabolically unbound fluorodeoxyglucose clears from the myocardium, and images obtained at equilibrium reflect regional utilization rates of exogenous glucose. Studies demonstrating increased accumulation of radiolabeled glucose, consistent with inefficient substrate utilization secondary to ischemia, have been noted in experimental models as well as in humans with unstable angina.[246] Abnormal patterns of glucose utilization and/or fatty acid metabolism also have been reported in primary cardiomyopathies.[247,248]

Finally, ^{11}C carbon monoxide may be used to label the blood pool following binding to hemoglobin after inhalation of small amounts of the radioactive gas. This then allows positron tomographic assessment of regional and global left ventricular function.

The ultimate clinical application of positron tomography studies in humans remains to be defined. The investigational potential of the techniques is enormous. Clearly, the cost of these studies is great. Instrumentation is expensive, and because of the short-lived nature of the radionuclide employed, onsite cyclotrons or accelerators are a necessity. In the future, compact, less-expensive cyclotrons, such as are being prepared for ^{82}Rb, may be available for medical use. Generator systems may become available as well, thereby obviating the need for an onsite cyclotron. It is clear the physiologic data available through use of this technique are unique.

A major future area for nuclear cardiology involves metabolic imaging. The information that can be obtained in this manner is unique and potentially of major clinical importance. Definition of myocardial viability in acute ischemic syndromes, definition of altered myocardial metabolism in cardiomyopathy, and definition of the metabolic consequences of functional derangements are all of extreme importance. Interdigitation of metabolic data with the classical structure-function relations represents the next stratum of nuclear cardiologic investigations.

Although the major thrust of metabolic imaging has involved positron techniques, a number of recent studies also have emphasized the possibility of single photon studies of fatty acid metabolism. It is of interest that one of the first reports of cardiac imaging involved the attempt by Evans et al. to employ iodinated oleic acid to image myocardial infarction.[249] For the most part, single photon radioiodinated free fatty acid studies have involved the use of ^{123}I as the radioactive label with a number of varying length fatty acids employed as the radioactive metabolic substrate. Abnormalities have been detected in myocardial infarction, ischemia, and cardiomyopathy.[250–254] In addition to looking at direct images, investigators have attempted to define regional washout curve characteristics as a representation of regional myocardial utilization of the radioactive metabolite. However, problems have arisen in the interpretation of the data in these washout curves because of the associated release of iodine from the fatty acid, leading to a high level of nonmetabolic background radioactivity which can complicate any attempt at regional kinetic analysis.[255] Currently, attempts are under way to derive new fatty acid radioactive tracers which will not be subject to the same difficulties of the previously labeled radioiodinated tracers. Principles of metabolic trapping comparable to that employed with fluorodeoxyglucose are currently being tested.

References

1. Blumgart, H. L., and Weiss, S.: Studies on the Velocity of Blood Flow. VII. The Pulmonary Circulation Time in Normal Resting Individuals, *J. Clin. Invest.*, 4:399, 1927.
2. Goldman, L., Feinstein, A. R., Batsford, W. P., Cohen, L. S., Gottschalk, A., and Zaret, B. L.: Ordering Patterns and Clinical Impact of Cardiovascular Nuclear Medicine Procedures, *Circulation*, 62:680, 1980.
3. L'Abbatte, A., and Maseri, A.: Xenon Studies of Myocardial Blood Flow: Theoretical, Technical and Practical Aspects, *Semin. Nucl. Med.*, 10:2, 1980.
4. Hamilton, G. W.: Myocardial Imaging with Radioactive Particles, in H. W. Strauss and B. Pitt (eds.), "Cardiovascular Nuclear Medicine," The C. V. Mosby Company, St. Louis, 1979, p. 214.
5. Prinzmetal, M., Corday, E., and Sprizler, R. J.: Radiocardiography and Its Clinical Applications, *JAMA*, 139:617, 1949.
6. Donato, L.: Basic Concepts of Radiocardiography, *Semin. Nucl. Med.*, 3:111, 1973.
7. Bender, M. A., and Blau, M.: The Evaluation of Renal and Cardiac Dynamics with the Autofluoroscope, *J. Nucl. Med.*, 4:186, 1963.
8. Anger, H. O., Van Dyke, D. C., Gottschalk, A., Yano, Y., and Schaer, L. R.: The Scintillation Camera in Diagnosis and Research, *Nucleonics*, 23:51, 1965.
9. Zaret, B. L., Strauss, H. W., Hurley, P. J., Natarajan, T. K., and Pitt, B.: A Noninvasive Scintiphotographic Method for Detecting Regional Ventricular Dysfunction in Man, *N. Engl. J. Med.*, 284:1165, 1971.
10. Strauss, H. W., Zaret, B. L., Hurley, P. J., Natarajan, T. K., and Pitt, B.: A Scintiphotographic Method for Measuring Left Ventricular Ejection Fraction in Man without Cardiac Catheterization, *Am. J. Cardiol.*, 28:575, 1971.

11. Van Dyke, D. C., Anger, H. O., Sullivan, R. W., Vetter, W. R., Yano, Y., and Parker, H. G.: Cardiac Evaluation from Radioisotope Dynamics, *J. Nucl. Med.,* 13:585, 1972.
12. Burow, R. D., Strauss, H. W., Singleton, R., Pond, M., Rehn, T., Bailey, I. K., Griffith, L. S. C., Nickoloff, E., and Pitt, B.: Analysis of Left Ventricular Function from Multiple Gated Acquisition Cardiac Blood Pool Imaging, *Circulation,* 56:1024, 1977.
13. Borer, J. S., Bacharach, S. L., Green, M. V., Kent, K. M., Epstein, S. E., and Johnston, G. S.: Real-Time Radionuclide Cineangiography in the Noninvasive Evaluation of Global and Regional Left Ventricular Function at Rest and during Exercise in Patients with Coronary Artery Disease, *N. Engl. J. Med.,* 296:839, 1977.
14. Carr, E. A., Walker, B. J., and Bartlett, J.: The Diagnosis of Myocardial Infarcts by Photoscanning after Administration of Cesium-131, *J. Clin. Invest.,* 42:922, 1963.
15. Romhilt, D. W., Adolph, R. J., Sodd, V. C., Levenson, N. I., August, L. S., Mishiyana, H., and Berke, R. A.: Cesium-129 Myocardial Scintigraphy to Detect Myocardial Infarction, *Circulation,* 48:1242, 1973.
16. Hurley, P. J., Cooper, M., Reba, R. C., Poggenburg, K. J., and Wagner, H. N.: ^{43}KC1: A New Radiopharmaceutical for Imaging the Heart, *J. Nucl. Med.,* 12:516, 1971.
17. Martin, N. D., Zaret, B. L., McGowan, R. L., Wells, H. P., and Flamm, M. D.: Rubidium-81: A New Myocardial Scanning Agent, *Radiology,* 111:651, 1974.
18. Zaret, B. L., Strauss, H. W., Martin, N. D., Wells, H. P., and Flamm, M. D.: Noninvasive Regional Myocardial Perfusion with Radioactive Potassium: Study of Patients at Rest, with Exercise and during Angina Pectoris, *N. Engl. J. Med.,* 288:809, 1973.
19. Lebowitz, E., Greene, M. W., Bradley-Moore, P., Atkins, H., Ansari, A., Richards, P., and Belgrave, E.: ^{201}Tl for Medical Use, *J. Nucl. Med.,* 14:421, 1973.
20. Vogel, R. A., Kirch, D., LeFree, M., and Steele, P.: A New Method of Multiplanar Emission Tomography Using a Seven Pinhole Collimator and an Anger Scintillation Camera, *J. Nucl. Med.,* 19:648, 1978.
21. Carr, E. A., Carfuny, E. J., and Bartlett, J. D.: Evaluation of ^{203}Hg-Chlormerodrin in the Demonstration of Human Myocardial Infarcts by Scanning, *Univ. Mich. Med. Bull.,* 29:27, 1963.
22. Holman, B. L., Lesch, M., Zweiman, F. G., Temte, J., Lown, B., and Gorlin, R.: Detection and Sizing of Acute Myocardial Infarcts with ^{99m}Tc (Sn) Tetracycline, *N. Engl. J. Med.,* 291:159, 1974.
23. Bonte, F. J., Parkey, R. W., Graham, K. D., Moore J., and Stokely, E. M.: A New Method for Radionuclide Imaging of Myocardial Infarcts, *Radiology,* 110:473, 1974.
24. Parkey, R. W., Bonte, F. J., Meyer, S. L., Atkins, J. M., Curry, G. L., Stokely, E. M., and Willerson, J. T.: A New Method for Radionuclide Imaging of Acute Myocardial Infarction in Humans, *Circulation,* 50:540, 1974.
25. Budinger, T. F.: Physics and Physiology of Nuclear Cardiology, in J. T. Willerson (ed.), "Nuclear Cardiology," F. A. Davis Company, Philadelphia, 1979, p. 9.
26. Buddemeyer, E. V., Bacharach, S. L., and Mitchell, T. G.: Instrumentation in Nuclear Cardiology, in H. W. Strauss and B. Pitt (eds.), "Cardiovascular Nuclear Medicine," The C. V. Mosby Company, St. Louis, 1979, p. 3.
27. Bacharach, S. L., Green, M. V., and Borer, J. S.: Instrumentation and Data Processing in Cardiovascular Nuclear Medicine: Evaluation of Ventricular Function, *Semin. Nucl. Med.,* 9:257, 1980.
28. Hoffer, P., Berger, H., Steidley, J., Brendel, A., Gottschalk, A., and Zaret, B. L.: Miniaturized Cadmium Telluride Detector Module for Continuous Monitoring of Left Ventricular Performance, *Radiology,* 138:477, 1981.
29. Lahiri, A., Crawley, J., Jones, R. I., Bowles, M. J., and Raftery, E. B.: A Noninvasive Technique for Continuous Monitoring of Left Ventricular Function Using a New Solid State Mercuric Iodide Radiation Detector, *Clin. Sci.,* 66:551, 1984.
30. Wilson, R. A., Sullivan, P. J., Moore, R. H., Zielonka, J. F., Alpert, N. M., Boucher, C. A., McKusick, K. A., and Strauss, H. W.: An Ambulatory Ventricular Function Monitor: Validation and Preliminary Clinical Results, *Am. J. Cardiol.,* 52:601, 1983.
31. Berger, H. J., Matthay, R. A., Pytlik, L. M., Gottschalk, A., and Zaret, B. L.: First-Pass Radionuclide Assessment of Right and Left Ventricular Performance in Patients with Cardiac and Pulmonary Disease, *Semin. Nucl. Med.,* 9:275, 1979.
32. Wackers, F. J., Giles, R. W., Hoffer, P. B., Lange, R. C., Berger, H. J., and Zaret, B. L.: Gold 195-m: A New Generator Produced Short-Lived Radionuclide for Sequential Assessment of Ventricular Performance by First-Pass Radionuclide Angiocardiography, *Am. J. Cardiol.,* 50:89, 1982.
33. Wackers, F. J., Stein, R., Pytlik, L., Plankey, M. W., Lange R., Hoffer, P., Sands, M. J., Zaret, B. L., and Berger, H. J.: Gold-195m for Serial First-Pass Radionuclide Angiocardiography During Upright Exercise in Patients with Coronary Artery Disease, *J. Am. Coll. Cardiol.,* 2:497, 1983.
34. Slutsky, R., Gordon, D., Karliner, J., Battler, A., Walaski, S., Verba, J., Pfisterer, M., Peterson, K., and Ashburn, W.: Assessment of Early Ventricular Systole by First Pass Radionuclide Angiography, *Am. J. Cardiol.,* 44:459, 1979.
35. Hecht, H. S., Mirell, S. G., Rolett, E. L., and Blahd, W. H.: Left Ventricular Ejection Fraction and Segmental Wall Motion by Peripheral First-Pass Radionuclide Angiography, *J. Nucl. Med.,* 19:17, 1978.
36. Bodenheimer, M. M., Banka, V. S., Fooshee, C. M., Hermann, G. A., and Helfant, R. H.: Quantitative Radionuclide Angiography in the Right Anterior Oblique View: Comparison with Contrast Ventriculography, *Am. J. Cardiol.,* 41:718, 1978.
37. Marshall, R. C., Berger, H. J., Costin, J. C., Freedman, G. S., Wolberg, J., Cohen, L. S., Gottschalk, A., and Zaret, B. L.: Assessment of Cardiac Performance with Quantitative Radionuclide Angiocardiography: Sequential Left Ventricular Ejection Fraction, Normalized Left Ventricular Ejection Rate, and Regional Wall Motion, *Circulation,* 56:820, 1977.
38. Wackers, F. J., Berger, H. J., Johnstone, D. E., Goldman, L., Reduto, L. A., Langou, R. A., Gottschalk, A., and Zaret, B. L.: Multiple Gated Cardiac Blood Pool Imaging for Left Ventricular Ejection Fraction: Validation of the Technique and Assessment of Variability, *Am. J. Cardiol.,* 43:1159, 1979.
39. Folland, E. D., Hamilton, G. W., Larson, S. M., Kennedy, J. W., Williams, D. L., and Ritchie, J. L.: The Radionuclide Ejection Fraction: A Comparison of Three Radionuclide Techniques with Contrast Angiography, *J. Nucl. Med.,* 18:1159, 1977.
40. Marshall, R. C., Berger, H. J., Reduto, L. A., Gottschalk, A., and Zaret, B. L.: Variability in Sequential Measures of Left Ventricular Performance Assessed with Radionuclide Angiocardiography, *Am. J. Cardiol.,* 41:531, 1978.
41. Rerych, S. K., Scholz, P. M., Newman, G. E., Sabiston, D. C., and Jones, R. H.: Cardiac Function at Rest and Exercise in Normals and Patients with Coronary Disease: Evaluation by Radionuclide Angiocardiography, *Ann. Surg.,* 187:449, 1978.
42. Shad, N.: Nontraumatic Assessment of Left Ventricular Wall Motion and Regional Stroke Volume after Myocardial Infarction, *J. Nucl. Med.,* 18:333, 1977.
43. Bodenheimer, M. M., Banka, V. S., Fooshee, C. M., Gillespie, J. A., and Helfant, R. H.: Detection of Coronary Heart Disease Using Radionuclide Determined Regional Ejection Fraction at Rest and during Handgrip Exercise: Correlation with Coronary Arteriography, *Circulation,* 58:640, 1978.
44. Williams, B., Berger, H., Wackers, F., Brendel, A., Lewis, S., Gottschalk, A., and Zaret, B.: Left Ventricular Ejection Fraction Functional Images at Rest and Bicycle Exercise: Definition of Normal and Abnormal Regional Responses in Coronary Artery Disease. *J. Nucl. Med.,* 21:P65, 1980. (Abstract.)

45. Berger, H. J., Matthay, R. A., Loke, J., Marshall, R. C., Gottschalk, A., and Zaret, B. L.: Assessment of Cardiac Performance with Quantitative Radionuclide Angiocardiography: Right Ventricular Ejection Fraction with Reference to Findings in Chronic Obstructive Pulmonary Disease, *Am. J. Cardiol.*, 41:897, 1978.
46. Tobinick, E., Schelbert, H. R., Henning, H., LeWinter, M., Taylor, A., Ashburn, W. L., and Karliner, J. S.: Right Ventricular Ejection Fraction in Patients with Acute Anterior and Inferior Myocardial Infarction Assessed by Radionuclide Angiography, *Circulation*, 57:1078, 1978.
47. McKusick, K. A., Bingham, J. B., and Strauss, H. W.: The Gated First Pass Radionuclide Angiogram, *Circulation*, 58:II-6, 1978. (Abstract.)
48. Brent, B. N., Berger, H. J., Matthay, R. A., Mahler, D., Pytlik, L., and Zaret, B. L.: Physiologic Correlates of Right Ventricular Ejection Fraction in Chronic Obstructive Pulmonary Disease: A Combined Radionuclide and Hemodynamic Study, *Am. J. Cardiol.*, 50:255, 1982.
49. Brent, B. N., Mahler, D., Matthay, R. A., Berger, H. J., and Zaret, B. L.: Noninvasive Diagnosis of Pulmonary Hypertension in Chronic Obstructive Pulmonary Disease; Utility of Resting Right Ventricular Ejection Fraction, *Am. J. Cardiol.*, 53:1349, 1984.
50. Treves, S.: Detection and Quantitation of Cardiovascular Shunts with Commonly Available Radionuclides, *Semin. Nucl. Med.*, 10:16, 1980.
51. Strauss, H. W., McKusick, K. A., Boucher, C. A., Bingham, J. B., and Pohost, G. M.: Of Linens and Laces: The Eighth Anniversary of the Gated Blood Pool Scan, *Semin. Nucl. Med.*, 9:296, 1979.
52. Zaret, B. L., and Berger, H. J.: Radionuclide Studies of Ventricular Performance in Coronary Artery Disease in P. N. Yu and J. F. Goodwin (eds.), "Progress in Cardiology," Lea & Febiger, Philadelphia, 1983, pp. 33–66.
53. Callahan, R. J., Froelich, J. W., McKusick, K. A., Leppo, J., and Strauss, H. W.: A Modified Method for the In Vivo Labeling of Red Blood Cells with Tc-99m: Concise Communication, *J. Nucl. Med.*, 23:315, 1982.
54. Parker, J. A., Uren, R. F., Jones, A. G., Maddox, D. E., Zimmerman, R. E., Neill, J. M., and Holman, B. L.: Radionuclide Left Ventriculography with the Slant Hole Collimator, *J. Nucl. Med.*, 18:848, 1977.
55. Bacharach, S. L., Green, M. V., Borer, J. S., Douglas, M. A., Ostrow, H. G., and Johnston, G. S.: A Real-Time System for Multi-image Gated Cardiac Studies, *J. Nucl. Med.*, 18:79, 1977.
56. Green, M. V., Ostrow, H. G., Scott, R. N., Douglas, M. A., Bailey, J. J., and Johnston, G. S.: A Comparison of Simultaneous Measurements of Systolic Function in the Baboon by Electromagnetic Flowmeter and High Frame Rate ECG-Gated Blood Pool Scintigraphy, *Circulation*, 60:312, 1979.
57. Duncan, J. S.: "Intelligent Detection of Left Ventricular Boundaries in Gated Nuclear Medicine Image Sequences," IEEE Seventh International Conference on Pattern Recognition Proceedings, 1984, p. 875.
58. Williams, D. L., and Hamilton, G. W.: The Effect of Errors in Determining Left Ventricular Ejection Fraction from Radionuclide Counting Data, in S. L. Bacharach, N. M. Alpert, and D. M. Shames (eds.), "Nuclear Cardiology: Selected Computer Aspects," Society of Nuclear Medicine, New York, 1978, p. 107.
59. Freeman, M. R., Berman, D. S., Staniloff, H. M., et al.: Improved Assessment of Inferior Segmental Wall Motion by the Addition of a 70 Degree Left Anterior Oblique View in Multiple Gated Equilibrium Scintigraphy, *Am. Heart J.*, 101:169, 1981.
60. Kelly, M. J., Giles, R. W., Simon, T. S., Berger, H. J., Zaret, B. L., and Wackers, F. J.: Multigated Equilibrium Radionuclide Angiocardiography: Improved Detection of Left Ventricular Wall Motion Abnormalities and Aneurysms with the Addition of the Left Lateral View, *Radiology*, 139:167, 1981.
61. Maddox, D. E., Wynne, J., Uren, R., Parker, J. A., Idoine, J., Siegel, L. C., Neill, J. M., Cohn, P. F., and Holman, B. L.: Regional Ejection Fraction: A Quantitative Index of Left Ventricular Performance, *Circulation*, 59:984, 1979.
62. Sheehan, F. H., Matthey, D. G., Schofer, J., Kreber, H. J., and Dodge, H. T.: Effect of Interventions in Salvaging Left Ventricular Function in Acute Myocardial Infarction: A Study of Intracoronary Streptokinase, *Am. J. Cardiol.*, 52:431, 1983.
63. Botvinick, E., Dunn, R., Freis, N., O'Connell, W. M., Shosa, D., Herkens, R., and Scheinman, M.: The Phase Image: Its Relationship to Patterns of Contraction and Conduction, *Circulation*, 65:551, 1982.
64. Dehmer, G. J., Lewis, S. E., Hillis, L. D., Twieg, D., Falkoff, M., Parkey, R. W., and Willerson, J. T.: Nongeometric Determination of Left Ventricular Volumes from Equilibrium Blood Pool Scans, *Am. J. Cardiol.*, 45:293, 1980.
65. Links, J. M., Becker, L. C., Shindledecker, J. G., et al.: Measurement of Absolute Left Ventricular Volume From Gated Blood Pool Studies, *Circulation*, 65:82, 1982.
66. Carabello, B. A., and Spann, J. F.: The Uses and Limitations of End-systolic Indexes of Left Ventricular Function, *Circulation*, 69:1058, 1984.
67. Maddahi, J., Berman, D. S., Matsuoka, D. T., Waxman, A. D., Stankus, K. E., Forrester, J. S., and Swan, H. J. C.: A New Technique for Assessing Right Ventricular Ejection Fraction Using Multiple-Gated Equilibrium Cardiac Blood Pool Scintigraphy: Description, Validation and Findings in Chronic Coronary Artery Disease, *Circulation*, 60:581, 1979.
68. Rigo, P., Alderson, P. O., Robertson, R. M., Becker, L. C., Wagner, H. N.: Measurement of Aortic and Mitral Regurgitation by Gated Cardiac Blood Pool Scans, *Circulation*, 60:306, 1979.
69. Baxter, R. H., Becker, L. C., Alderson, P. O., Rigo, P., Wagner, H. N., and Weisfeldt, M. L.: Quantification of Aortic Valvular Regurgitation in Dogs by Nuclear Imaging, *Circulation*, 61:404, 1980.
70. Lam, W., Pavel, D., Byrom, E., Sheikh, A., Best, D., and Rosen, K.: Radionuclide Regurgitant Index: Value and Limitations, *Am. J. Cardiol.*, 47:292, 1981.
71. Pohost, G. M., Pastore, J. O., McKusick, K. A., Chiotellis, P. N., Kapellakis, G. Z., Myers, G. S., Dinsmore, R. E., and Block, P. C.: Detection of Left Atrial Myxoma by Gated Radionuclide Cardiac Imaging, *Circulation*, 55:88, 1977.
72. Pohost, P. C., Vignola, P. A., McKusick, K. A., Block, P. C., Myers, G. S., Walker, H. J., Copen, D. L., and Dinsmore, R. E.: Hypertrophic Cardiomyopathy: Evaluation by Gated Cardiac Blood Pool Scanning, *Circulation*, 55:92, 1977.
73. Okada, R. D., Pohost, G. M., Kirshenbaum, H. D., Kushner, F. G., Boucher, C. A., Block, P. C., and Strauss, H. W.: Radionuclide-Determined Change in Pulmonary Blood Volume with Exercise: Improved Sensitivity of Multigated Blood-Pool Scanning in Detecting Coronary Artery Disease, *N. Engl. J. Med.*, 301:569, 1979.
74. Rutlen, D. L., Wackers, F. J., and Zaret, B. L.: Radionuclide Assessment of Peripheral Intravascular Capacity: A New Technique to Measure Intravascular Volume Changes in the Capicitance Circulation in Man, *Circulation*, 64:146, 1981.
75. Bell, L., Zaret, B. L., and Rutlen, D. L.: Influence of Alpha Adrenergic Receptor Stimulation on Splanchnic Intravascular Volume and Cardiac Output in the Intact Dog, *Clin. Res.* 32:150A, 1984.
76. Bell, L., Zaret, B. L., and Rutlen, D. L.: Influence of Alpha Adrenergic Receptor Stimulation on Splanchnic Intravascular Volume as Determined by Quantitative Radionuclide Imaging in Conscious Humans, *Clin. Res.*, 32:150A, 1984.
77. Fritch, B. G., Dehmer, G. J., Markham, R. V., Willerson, J. T., and Hillis, L. D.: Assessment of Vasodilator Therapy in Patients with Severe Congestive Heart Failure: Limitations of Measurements of Left Ventricular Ejection Fraction and Volume, *Am. J. Cardiol.*, 50:954, 1982.
78. Nichols, A. B., McKusick, K. A., Strauss, H. W., Dinsmore,

R. E., Block, P. G., and Pohost, G. M.: Clinical Utility of Gated Cardiac Blood Pool Imaging in Congestive Heart Failure, *Am. J. Med.*, 65:785, 1978.
79. Dymond, D. S., Jarritt, P. H., Britton, K. E., and Spurrell, R. A. J.: Detection of Postinfarction Left Ventricular Aneurysms by First-Pass Radionuclide Ventriculography Using a Multicrystal Gamma Camera, *Br. Heart J.*, 41:68, 1979.
80. Rigo, P., Murray, M., Strauss, H. W., and Pitt, B.: Scintiphotographic Evaluation of Patients with Suspected Left Ventricular Aneurysm, *Circulation,* 50:985, 1974.
81. Reduto, L. A., Berger, H. J., Cohen, L. S., Gottschalk, A., and Zaret, B. L.: Sequential Radionuclide Assessment of Left and Right Ventricular Performance after Acute Myocardial Infarction, *Ann. Intern. Med.*, 89:441, 1978.
82. Rigo, P., Murray, M., Taylor, D. R., Weisfeldt, M., Kelly, D. T., Strauss, H. W., and Pitt, B.: Right Ventricular Dysfunction Detected by Gated Scintigraphy in Patients with Acute Inferior Infarction, *Circulation,* 52:268, 1975.
83. Sharpe, D. N., Botvinick, E. H., Shames, D., Schiller, N. B., Massie, B. M., Chatterjee, K., and Parmley, W. W.: The Noninvasive Diagnosis of Right Ventricular Infarction, *Circulation,* 57:483, 1978.
84. Schelbert, H. R., Henning, H., Ashburn, W. L., Verba, J. W., Karliner, J. S., and O'Rourke, R. A.: Serial Measurements of Left Ventricular Ejection Fraction by Radionuclide Angiography Early and Late after Myocardial Infarction, *Am. J. Cardiol.*, 38:407, 1976.
85. Rigo, P., Strauss, H. W., Taylor, D., Kelly, D., Weisfeldt, M., and Pitt, B.: Left Ventricular Function in Acute Myocardial Infarction Evaluated by Gated Scintigraphy, *Circulation,* 50:678, 1974.
86. Battler, A., Slutsky, R., Karliner, J., Froelicher, V., Ashburn, W., and Ross, J.: Left Ventricular Ejection Fraction and First Third Ejection Fraction Early after Acute Myocardial Infarction: Value for Predicting Mortality and Morbidity, *Am. J. Cardiol.*, 45:197, 1980.
87. Shah, P. K., Pichler, M., Berman, D. S., Singh, B. N., and Swan, H. J. C.: Left Ventricular Ejection Fraction Determined by Radionuclide Ventriculography in Early Stages of First Transmural Myocardial Infarction: Relation to Short Term Prognosis, *Am. J. Cardiol.*, 45:542, 1980.
88. Nicod, P., Corbett, J. R., Sanford, C. F., Mukharji, J., Dehmer, J. G., Croft, C. H., Rude, R. E., Lewis, S., and Willerson, J. T.: Comparison of the Influence of Acute Transmural and Nontransmural Myocardial Infarction on Ventricular Function, *Am. Heart J.*, 107:28, 1984.
89. Ohsuzu, F., Boucher, C. A., Newell, J. B., Yasuda, T., Gold, H. K., Leinbach, R. C., McKusik, K. A., Okada, R. D., Rosenthal, S., Pohost, G. M., and Strauss, H. W.: Relation of Segmental Wall Motion to Global Left Ventricular Function and Acute Myocardial Infarction, *Am. J. Cardiol.*, 51:1275, 1983.
90. The Multicenter Postinfarction Research Group. Risk Stratification and Survival After Myocardial Infarction, *N. Engl. J. Med.*, 309:331, 1983.
91. Norris, R. M., Barnaby, P. F., Brandt, P. W. T., Grayson, G. G., Whitlock, R. M. L., Wild, C. J., and Barratt-Boyes, B. G.: Prognosis After Recovery From First Acute Myocardial Infarction: Determinants of Reinfarction and Sudden Death, *Am. J. Cardiol.*, 53:408, 1984.
92. Sanz, G., Kastener, A., Betriu, A., Magrina, J., Rois, E., Coll, S., Pare, J. C., and Navarro-Lopez, F.: Determinants of Prognosis in Survivors of Myocardial Infarction: A Prospective Clinical Angiographic Study, *N. Engl. J. Med.*, 306:1065, 1982.
93. Meizlish, J., Berger, H. J., Plankey, R. T., Errico, D., Levy, W., and Zaret, B. L.: Functional Left Ventricular Aneurysm Formation Following Acute Anterior Transmural Myocardial Infarction: Incidence, Natural History and Prognostic Implications, *N. Engl. J. Med.*, 311:101, 1984.
94. Berger, H. J., Reduto, L. A., Johnstone, D. E., Borkowski, H., Sands, J. M., Cohen, L. S., Langou, R. A., Gottschalk, A., and Zaret, B. L.: Global and Regional Left Ventricular Response to Bicycle Exercise in Coronary Artery Disease: Assessment by Quantitative Radionuclide Angiocardiography, *Am. J. Med.*, 66:13, 1979.
95. Jengo, J. A., Oren, V., Conant, R., Brizendine, M., Nelson, T., Uszler, J. M., and Mena, I.: Effects of Maximal Exercise Stress on Left Ventricular Function in Patients with Coronary Artery Disease Using First-Pass Radionuclide Angiocardiography, *Circulation,* 59:60, 1979.
96. Slutsky, R., Karliner, J., Ricci, D., Schuler, G., Pfisterer, M., Peterson, K., and Ashburn, W.: Response of Left Ventricular Volume to Exercise in Man Assessed by Radionuclide Equilibrium Angiography, *Circulation,* 60:565, 1979.
97. Caldwell, J. H., Hamilton, G. W., Sorensen, S. G., Ritchie, J. L., Williams, D. L., and Kennedy, J. W.: The Detection of Coronary Artery Disease with Radionuclide Techniques: A Comparison of Rest-Exercise Thallium Imaging and Ejection Fraction Response, *Circulation,* 61:610, 1980.
98. Rozanski, A., Diamond, G. A., Berman, D., Forrester, J. S., Morris, D., and Swan, H. J. C.: The Declining Specificity of Exercise Radionuclide Ventriculography, *N. Engl. J. Med.*, 309:518, 1983.
99. Gibbons, R. H., Lee, J. L., Cobb, F. R., and Jones, R. H.: Ejection Fraction Response to Exercise in Patients with Chest Pain and Normal Coronary Arteriograms, *Circulation,* 64:952, 1981.
100. Port, S., Cobb, R. R., Coleman, R. E., and Jones, R. H.: Effect of Age on the Response of the Left Ventricular Ejection Fraction to Exercise, *N. Engl. J. Med.*, 303:1133, 1980.
101. Francis, C. K., Cleman, M., Berger, H. J., Davies, R. A., Giles, R. W., Black, H. R., Zito, R. A., and Zaret, B. L.: Left Ventricular Systolic Performance During Upright Bicycle Exercise in Patients with Essential Hypertension, *Am J. Med.*, 75:40, 1983.
102. Kent, K. M., Borer, J. S., Green, M. V., Bacharach, S. L., McIntosh, C. L., Conkle, D. M., and Epstein, S. E.: Effects of Coronary-Artery Bypass on Global and Regional Left Ventricular Function during Exercise, *N. Engl. J. Med.*, 298:1434, 1978.
103. Borer, J. S., Bacharach, S. L., Green, M. V., Kent, K. M., Johnston, G. S., and Epstein, S. E.: Effect of Nitroglycerin on Exercise-Induced Abnormalities of Left Ventricular Regional Function and Ejection Fraction in Coronary Artery Disease, *Circulation,* 57:314, 1978.
104. Port, S., Cobb, F. R., and Jones, R. H.: Effects of Propranolol on Left Ventricular Function in Normal Men, *Circulation,* 61:358, 1980.
105. Rerych, S. K., Scholz, P. M., Sabiston, D. C., and Jones, R. H.: Effects of Exercise Training on Left Ventricular Function in Normal Subjects: A Longitudinal Study by Radionuclide Angiography, *Am. J. Cardiol.*, 45:244, 1980.
106. Berger, H. J., Johnstone, D. E., Sands, J. M., Gottschalk, A., and Zaret, B. L.: Response of Right Ventricular Ejection Fraction to Upright Bicycle Exercise in Coronary Artery Disease, *Circulation,* 60:1292, 1979.
107. Kurz, R. G., Brady, T. J., Besozzi, M. D., Thrall, J. H., and Pitt, B.: Cold Pressor Radionuclide Ventriculography, *Clin. Res.*, 28:189A, 1980. (Abstract.)
108. Jordan, L. J., Borer, J. S., Zullo, M., Hayes, D., Kubo, S., Moses, J. W., and Carter, J.: Exercise Versus Cold Temperature Stimulation During Radionuclide Cineangiography: Diagnostic Accuracy in Coronary Artery Disease, *Am J. Cardiol.*, 51:1091, 1983.
109. Boucher, C. A., and O'Kada, R. D.: Radionuclide Angiography in Valvular Heart Disease, in P. N. Yu and J. F. Goodwin (eds.), "Progress in Cardiology," Lea & Febiger, Philadelphia, 1983, pp. 5–32.
110. Borer, J. S., Bacharach, S. L., Green, M. V., Kent, K. M., Henry, W. L., Rosing, D. R., Seides, S. F., Johnston, G. S., and Epstein, S. E.: Exercise-Induced Left Ventricular Dysfunction in Symptomatic and Asymptomatic Patients with Aortic Regurgitation: Assessment by Radionuclide Cineangiography, *Am. J. Cardiol.*, 42:351, 1978.
111. Lewis, S. M., Riba, A. L., Berger, H. J., Davies, R. A., Wackers, F. J., Alexander, J., Cohen, L. S., and Zaret, B. L.: Radionuclide Angiographic Exercise Left Ventric-

ular Performance in Chronic Aortic Regurgitation: Relationship to Resting Echocardiographic Dimensions and Systolic Wall Stress Index, *Am. Heart J.*, 103:498, 1982.
112. Borer, J. S., Rosing, D. R., Kent, K. M., Bacharach, S. L., Green, M. V., McIntosh, C. J., Morrow, A. G., Epstein, S. E.: Left Ventricular Function at Rest and during Exercise after Aortic Replacement in Patients with Aortic Regurgitation, *Am J. Cardiol.*, 44:1297, 1979.
113. Marx, P., Borkowksi, H., Sands, M. J., Wolfson, S., Berger, H. J., and Zaret, B. L.: Exercise Left Ventricular Performance in Aortic Regurgitation: Dissimilar Responses in Supine and Upright Positions, *Circulation*, 66:II–354, 1982.
113a. Alexander, J., Dainiak, N., Berger, H. J., Goldman, L., Johnstone, D., Reduto, L., Duffy, T., Schwartz, P., Gottschalk, A., and Zaret, B. L.: Serial Assessment of Doxorubicin Cardiotoxicity with Quantitative Radionuclide Angiocardiography, *N. Engl. J. Med.*, 300:278, 1979.
114. Schwartz, R. G., McKenzie, W. B., D'Souza, A. W., Sager, P. T., Alexander, J., Surkin, L. A., Schwartz, P., Wackers, F. J., Berger, H. J., and Zaret, B. L.: Utility of Monitoring Doxorubicin Cardiotoxicity with Resting First Pass Radionuclide Angiocardiography for Prevention of Irreversible Congestive Heart Failure: A Seven Year Experience in 1115 Patients, *J. Am. Coll. Cardiol.*, 5:452, 1985.
115. Choi, B. W., Berger, H. J., Schwartz, P. E., Alexander, J., Wackers, F. J., Gottschalk, A., and Zaret, B. L.: Serial Radionuclide Assessment of Doxorubicin Cardiotoxicity in Cancer Patient with Abnormal Baseline Resting Left Ventricular Performance, *Am. Heart J.*, 106:638, 1983.
116. Gottdeiner, J. S., Mathisen, D. J., Borer, J. S., et al.: Doxorubicin Toxicity: Assessment of Late Left Ventricular Dysfunction by Radionuclide Cineangiography, *Ann. Intern. Med.*, 94:430, 1981.
117. Reduto, L. A., Berger, H. J., Johnstone, D. E., Hellenbrand, W., Wackers, F. J., Whittemore, R., Cohen, L. S., Gottschalk, A., and Zaret, B. L.: Radionuclide Assessment of Right and Left Ventricular Exercise Reserve after Total Correction of Tetralogy of Fallot, *Am J. Cardiol.*, 45:1013, 1980.
118. Parrish, M. D., Graham, T. V., Bender, H. W., Jones, J. P., Patton, J., and Partain, C. L.: Radionuclide Angiographic Evaluation of Right and Left Ventricular Function during Exercise after Repair of Transposition of the Great Arteries: Comparison with Normal Subjects and Patients with Congenitally Corrected Transposition, *Circulation*, 67:178, 1983.
119. Liberthson, R. R., Boucher, C. A., Strauss, H. W., Dinsmore, R. E., McKusick, K. A., and Pohost, G. M.: Right Ventricular Function in Adult Atrial Septal Defect: Preoperative and Postoperative Assessment and Clinical Implications, *Am. J. Cardiol.*, 47:56, 1981.
120. Matthay, R. A., Berger, H. J., Loke, J., Dolan, T. F., Fagenholz, S. A., Gottschalk, A., and Zaret, B. L.: Right and Left Ventricular Performance in Ambulatory Young Adults with Cystic Fibrosis, *Br. Heart J.*, 43:474, 1980.
121. Matthay, R. A., Berger, H. J., Loke, J., Gottschalk, A., and Zaret, B. L.: Effects of Aminophylline on Right and Left Ventricular Performance in Chronic Obstructive Pulmonary Disease: Noninvasive Assessment by Radionuclide Angiocardiography, *Am J. Med.*, 65:903, 1978.
122. Matthay, R. A., Berger, H. J., Davies, R., Loke, J., and Zaret, B. L.: Improvement in Cardiac Performance by Oral Long-Acting Theophylline in Chronic Obstructive Pulmonary Disease, *Am. Heart J.*, 104:1022, 1982.
123. Brent, B. N., Berger, H. J., Matthay, R. A., Mahler, D., Pytlik, L., and Zaret, B. L.: Contrasting Acute Effects of Vasodilators Upon Right Ventricular Performance in Patients with Chronic Obstructive Pulmonary Disease and Pulmonary Hypertension, *Am J. Cardiol.*, 51:1682, 1983.
124. Matthay, R. A., Berger, H. J., Davies, R. A., Loke, J., Mahler, D. A., Gottschalk, A., and Zaret, B. L.: Radionuclide Assessment of Right and Left Ventricular Exercise Performance in Chronic Obstructive Pulmonary Disease, *Ann. Int. Med.*, 93:234, 1980.
125. Wagner, H. N., Wake, R., Nickoloff, E., and Natarajan, T. K.: The Nuclear Stethoscope: A Simple Device for Generation of Left Ventricular Volume Curves, *Am J. Cardiol.*, 38:747, 1976.
126. Camargo, E. E., Harrison, K. S., Wagner, H. N., Bourguignon, M. H., Reid, P. R., Alderson, P. O., and Baxter, R. H.: Noninvasive Beat to Beat Monitoring of Left Ventricular Function by a Nonimaging Nuclear Detector during Premature Ventricular Contractions, *Am J. Cardiol.*, 45:1219, 1980.
127. Berger, H. J., Davies, R. A., Batsford, W. P., Hoffer, P. B., Gottschalk, A., and Zaret, B. L.: Beat to Beat Left Ventricular Performance Assessed from the Equilibrium Cardiac Blood Pool Using a Computerized Nuclear Probe, *Circulation*, 63:133, 1981.
128. Schneider, J., Berger, H. J., Sands, M., Lachman, A., and Zaret, B. L.: Beat to Beat Left Ventricular Performance in Atrial Fibrillation: Radionuclide Assessment with the Computerized Nuclear Probe, *Am. J. Cardiol.*, 51:1189, 1983.
129. Giles, R. W., Berger, H. J., Barash, P. G., et al.: Continuous Monitoring of Left Ventricular Performance with the Computerized Nuclear Probe during Laryngoscopy and Intubation Prior to Coronary Artery Bypass Surgery, *Am J. Cardiol.*, 50:735, 1982.
130. Giles, R. W., Marx, P., Berger, H. J., and Zaret, B. L.: Importance of Rapid Sequential Sampling of Left Ventricular Function during the Cold Pressor Test by Beat-to-Beat Assessment with the Computerized Nuclear Probe, *J. Nucl. Med.*, 22:P47, 1981.
131. Bonow, R. O., Bacharach, S. L., Green, M. V., et al.: Impaired Left Ventricular Diastolic Filling in Patients with Coronary Artery Disease: Assessment with Radionuclide Angiography, *Circulation*, 64:315, 1981.
132. Bonow, R. O., Kent, K. M., Rosing, D. R., Lipson, L. C., Bacharach, S. L., Green, M. V., and Epstein, S. E.: Improved Left Ventricular Diastolic Filling in Patients with Coronary Artery Disease After Percutaneous Transluminal Coronary Angioplasty, *Circulation*, 66:1159, 1982.
133. Bonow, R. O., Leon, M. B., Rosing, D. R., et al.: Effects of Verapamil and Propranolol on Left Ventricular Systolic Function and Diastolic Filling in Patients with Coronary Artery Disease: Radionuclide Angiographic Studies at Rest and during Exercise, *Circulation*, 65:1337, 1981.
134. Soufer, R., Wohlgelernter, D., Vita, N. A., Amuchestegui, M., Sostman, D. H., Berger, H. J., and Zaret, B. L.: Intact Systolic Left Ventricular Function in Clinical Congestive Heart Failure, *Am. J. Cardiol.*, 55, 1985.
135. Zaret, B. L.: Myocardial Imaging with Radioactive Potassium and Its Analogs, *Prog. Cardiovasc. Dis.*, 20:81, 1977.
136. Welch, H. F., Strauss, H. W., and Pitt, B.: Myocardial Extraction Fraction of Thallium-201, *Circulation*, 56:188, 1977.
137. Strauss, H. W., Harrison, K., Langan, J. K., Lebowitz, E., and Pitt, B.: Thallium-201 for Myocardial Imaging: Relation of Thallium-201 to Regional Myocardial Perfusion, *Circulation*, 51:641, 1975.
138. DiCola, V. C., Downing, S. E., Donabedian, R. K., and Zaret, B. L.: Pathophysiologic Correlates of Thallium-201 Myocardial Uptake in Experimental Infarction, *Cardiovasc. Res.*, 11:141, 1977.
139. Prokop, E. K., Strauss, H. W., Shaw, J., Pitt, B., and Wagner, H. N.: Comparison of Regional Myocardial Perfusion Determined by Ionic Potassium-43 to That Determined by Microspheres, *Circulation*, 50:978, 1974.
140. Pohost, G. M., Alpert, N. A., Ingwall, J. S., and Strauss, H. W.: Thallium Redistribution: Mechanisms and Clinical Utility, *Semin. Nucl. Med.*, 10:70, 1980.
141. Costin, J. C., and Zaret, B. L.: Effect of Propranolol and Digitalis upon Radioactive Thallium and Potassium Uptake in Myocardial and Skeletal Muscle, *J. Nucl. Med.*, 17:535, 1976. (Abstract.)
142. Kushner, F. G., Okada, R. D., Kirshenbaum, H. D., Boucher, C. A., Strauss, H. W., and Pohost, G. M.: Lung Thallium-201 Uptake after Stress Testing in Patients with Coronary Artery Disease, *Circulation*, 63:341, 1981.
143. Pohost, G. M., Zir, L. M., Moore, R. H., McKusick, K. A., Guiney, T. E., and Beller, G. A.: Differentiation of Tran-

siently Ischemic from Infarcted Myocardium by Serial Imaging after a Single Dose of Thallium-201, *Circulation,* 55:294, 1977.
144. Johnstone, D. E., Wackers, F. J., Berger, H. J., Kelley, M. J., Gottschalk, A., and Zaret, B. L.: Effect of Patient Positioning on Left Lateral Thallium-201 Myocardial Images, *J. Nucl. Med.,* 20:183, 1979.
145. Bailey, I. K., Griffith, L. S. C., Rouleau, J., Strauss, H. W., and Pitt, B.: Thallium-201 Myocardial Perfusion Imaging at Rest and during Exercise: Comparative Sensitivity to Electrocardiography in Coronary Artery Disease, *Circulation,* 55:79, 1977.
146. Botvinick, E. H., Taradash, M. R., Shames, D. M., and Parmley, W. W.: Thallium-201 Myocardial Perfusion Scintigraphy for the Clinical Clarification of Normal, Abnormal and Equivocal Electrocardiographic Stress Tests, *Am. J. Cardiol.,* 41:43, 1978.
147. Ritchie, J. L., Trobaugh, G. B., Hamilton, G. W., Gould, K. L., Narahara, K. A., Murray, J. A., and Williams, D. L.: Myocardial Imaging with Thallium-201 at Rest and during Exercise: Comparison with Coronary Arteriography and Resting and Stress Electrocardiography, *Circulation,* 56:66, 1977.
148. Ritchie, J. L., Zaret, B. L., Strauss, H. W., Pitt, B., Berman, D. S., Schelbert, H. R., Ashburn, W. L., Berger, H. J., and Hamilton, G. W.: Myocardial Imaging with Thallium-201: A Multicenter Study in Patients with Angina Pectoris or Acute Myocardial Infarction, *Am. J. Cardiol.,* 42:345, 1978.
149. Cook, D. J., Bailey, I., Strauss, H. W., Rouleau, J., Wagner, H. N., and Pitt, B.: Thallium-201 Myocardial Imaging: Appearance of the Normal Heart, *J. Nucl Med.,* 17:583, 1976.
150. Gewirtz, H., Grotte, G. J., Strauss, H. W., O'Keefe, D. D., Atkins, C. W., Daggett, W. M., and Pohost, G. M.: The Influence of Left Ventricular Volume and Wall Motion on Myocardial Images, *Circulation,* 59:1172, 1979.
151. Dunn, R. F., Wolff, L., Wagner, S., and Botvinick, E. H.: The Inconsistent Pattern of Thallium Defects: A Clue to the False Positive Perfusion Scintigram, *Am. J. Cardiol.,* 48:224, 1981.
152. Wackers, F. J., Busemann-Sokole, E., Samson, G., van der Schoot, J. B., Lie, K. I., Liem, K. L., and Wellens, H. J. J.: Value and Limitations of Thallium-201 Scintigraphy in the Acute Phase of Myocardial Infarction, *N. Engl. J. Med.,* 295:1, 1976.
153. Umbach, R. E., Lange, R. C., Lee, J. C., and Zaret, B. L.: Temporal Change in Sequential Thallium-201 Imaging Following Myocardial Infarction in Dogs: Comparison of Four and Twenty-Four Hour Infarct Images, *Yale J. Biol. Med.,* 51:597, 1978.
154. Silverman, K. J., Becker, L. C., Bulkley, B. H., Burow, R. D., Mellits, E. D., Kallman, C. H., and Weisfeldt, M. L.: Value of Early Thallium-201 Scintigraphy for Predicting Mortality in Patients with Acute Myocardial Infarction, *Circulation,* 61:996, 1980.
155. Becker, L. D., Silverman, K. J., Bulkley, B. H., Kallman, S., Mellits, E., and Weisfeldt, M.: Comparison of Early Thallium-201 Scintigraphy and Gated Blood Pool Imaging for Predicting Mortality in Patients with Acute Myocardial Infarction, *Circulation,* 67:1272, 1983.
156. Markis, J. E., Malagold, M., Parker, J. A., Silverman, K. J., Barry, W. H., Als, A. V., Pauline S., Grossman, W., and Braunwald, D. E.: Myocardial Salvage After Intracoronary Thrombolysis with Streptokinase in Acute Myocardial Infarction: Assessment by Intracoronary Thallium-201, *N. Engl. J. Med.,* 305:777, 1981.
157. Melin, J. A., Becker, L. C., and Bulkley, B. H.: Differences in Thallium-201 Uptake in Reperfused and Nonreperfused Myocardial Infarction, *Circ. Res.,* 53:414, 1983.
158. Wackers, F. J., Lie, K. I., Liem, K. L., Busemann-Sokole, E., Samson, G., van der Schoot, J., and Durrer, D.: Potential Value of Thallium-201 Scintigraphy as a Means of Selecting Patients for the Coronary Care Unit, *Br. Heart J.,* 41:111, 1979.
159. Wackers, F. J.: Thallium-201 Myocardial Scintigraphy in Acute Myocardial Infarction and Ischemia, *Semin. Nucl. Med.,* 10:127, 1980.
160. Maseri, A., Parodi, O., Severi, S., and Pesola, A.: Transient Transmural Reduction of Myocardial Blood Flow, Demonstrated by Thallium-201 Scintigraphy as a Cause of Variant Angina, *Circulation,* 54:280:1976.
161. Wackers, F. J., Lie, K. K., Liem, K. L., Busemann-Sokole, E., Samson, G., van der Schoot, J. B., and Durrer, D.: Thallium-201 Scintigraphy in Unstable Angina Pectoris, *Circulation,* 57:738, 1978.
162. Berger, B. C., Watson, D. D., Burwell, L. R., Crosby, I. K., Wellons, H. A., Teates, C. D., and Beller, G. A.: Redistribution of Thallium at Rest in Patients with Stable and Unstable Angina and the Effect of Coronary Artery Bypass Surgery, *Circulation,* 60:1114, 1979.
163. Gewirtz, H., Beller, G. A., Strauss, H. W., Dinsmore, R. E., Zir, L. M., McKusick, K. A., and Pohost, G. M.: Transient Defects of Resting Thallium Scans in Patients with Coronary Artery Disease, *Circulation,* 59:707, 1979.
164. Blood, D. K., McCarthy, D. M., Sciacca, R. R., and Cannon, P. J.: Comparison of Single-Dose and Double-Dose Thallium-201 Myocardial Perfusion Scintigraphy for the Detection of Coronary Artery Disease and Prior Myocardial Infarction, *Circulation,* 58:777, 1978.
165. Berman, D. S., Garcia, E. V., and Maddahi, J.: Thallium-201 Myocardial Scintigraphy in the Detection and Evaluation of Coronary Artery Disease, in D. S. Berman, and D. T. Mason, (eds.), "Clinical Nuclear Cardiology," Grune & Stratton, 1981, pp. 86–93.
166. Dunn, R., Freedman, B., Bailey, I. K., et al.: Non-invasive Prediction of Multivessel Disease after Myocardial Infarction, *Circulation,* 62:726, 1980.
167. Rigo, P., Bailey, I. K., Griffith, L. S. C., et al.: Value and Limitations of Segmental Analysis of Stress Thallium Myocardial Imaging for Localization of Coronary Artery Disease, *Circulation,* 61:973, 1980.
168. Gibson, R. S., Watson, D. O., Carabello, B. A., et al.: Clinical Implication of Increased Lung Uptake of Thallium-201 during Exercise Scintigraphy 2 Weeks after Myocardial Infarction, *Am. J. Cardiol.,* 49:1586, 1982.
169. McLaughlin, P. R., Martin, R. P., Doherty, P., Daspit, S., Goris, M., Haskell, W., Lewis, S., Kriss, J. P., and Harrison, D. C.: Reproducibility of Thallium-201 Myocardial Imaging, *Circulation,* 55:497, 1977.
170. White, C. W., Wright, C. B., Doty, D. B., Hiratza, L. F., Eastham, C. L., Harrison, D. G., and Marcus M. L.: Does Visual Interpretation of the Coronary Arteriogram Predict the Physiologic Importance of a Coronary Stenosis? *N. Engl. J. Med.,* 310:819, 1984.
171. Hamilton, G. W., Trobaugh, G. B., Ritchie, J. L., Gould, R. L., DeRowen, T. A., and Williams, D. L.: Myocardial Imaging with ^{201}Thallium: An Analysis of Clinical Usefulness Based on Bayes' Theorem, *Semin. Nucl. Med.,* 8:358, 1978.
172. Hirzel, H. O., Senn, M., Nuesch, K., Buettner, C., Pfeiffer, A., Hess, O. M., and Krayenbuehl, H. P.: Thallium-201 Scintigraphy in Complete Left Bundle Branch Block, *Am. J. Cardiol.,* 53:764, 1984.
173. Gould, K. L.: Noninvasive Assessment of Coronary Stenosis by Myocardial Perfusion Imaging during Pharmacologic Vasodilatation. I. Physiologic Basis and Experimental Validation, *Am. J. Cardiol.,* 41:267, 1978.
174. Albro, P. C., Gould, K. L., Westcott, R. J., Hamilton, G. W., Ritchie, J. L., and Williams, D. L.: Noninvasive Assessment of Coronary Stenoses by Myocardial Imaging during Pharmacologic Coronary Vasodilatation III. Clinical Trial, *Am. J. Cardiol.,* 42:751, 1978.
175. Leppo, J. A., O'Brian, J., Rothendler, J. A., Getchell, J. D., and Lee, V. W.: Dipyridamole-Thallium-201 Scintigraphy in the Prediction of Future Cardiac Events after acute Myocardial Infarction, *N. Engl. J. Med.,* 310:1014, 1984.
176. Maddahi, J., Garcia, E. V., Berman, D. S., et al.: Improved Noninvasive Assessment of Coronary Artery Disease by Quantitative Analysis of Regional Stress Myocardial Dis-

tribution and Washout of Thallium-201, *Circulation*, 64:924, 1981.
177. Gibson, R. S., Watson, D. D., Taylor, G. J., et al.: Prospective Assessment of Regional Myocardial Perfusion before and after Coronary Revascularization Surgery by Quantitative Thallium-201 Scintigraphy, *J. Am. Coll. Cardiol.*, 1:804, 1983.
178. Gibson, R. S., Taylor, G. J., Watson, D. D., et al.: Predicting the Extent and Location of Coronary Artery Disease during the Early Post-infarction by Quantitative Thallium-201 Scintigraphy, *Am. J. Cardiol.*, 47:1010, 1981.
179. Tamaki, N., Mukai, T., Ishii, Y., et al.: Clinical Evaluation of Thallium-201 Emission Myocardial Tomography Using a Rotating Gamma Camera: Comparison with 7 Pinhole Tomography, *J. Nucl. Med.*, 22:849, 1981.
180. Tamaki, S., Nakajima, H., Murakami, T., Yui, Y., Kambara, H., Kadota, K., Yoshida, A., Kawai, C., Tamaki, N., Mukai, T., Ishii, Y., and Torizuka, K.: Estimation of Infarct Size by Myocardial Emission Computed Tomography with Thallium-201 and Its Relation to Creatine Kinase-MB Release after Myocardial Infarction in Man, *Circulation*, 66:994, 1982.
181. Ritchie, J. L., Williams, D. L., Harp, G., Stratton, J. L., and Caldwell, J. H.: Transaxial Tomography with Thallium-201 for Detecting Remote Myocardial Infarction: Comparison with Planar Imaging, *Am. J. Cardiol.*, 50:1236, 1982.
182. Coleman, R. E., Jaszczak, R. J., and Cobb, F. R.: Comparison of 180-Degree and 360-Degree Data Collection in Thallium-201 Imaging Using Single Photon Emission Computerized Tomography (SPECT), *J. Nucl. Med.*, 23:655, 1982.
183. Budinger, T. F.: Physical Attributes of Single-Photon Tomography, *J. Nucl. Med.*, 21:579, 1980.
184. Johnstone, D. E., Sands, M. J., Berger, H. J., Reduto, L. A., Lachman, A. B., Wackers, F. J., Cohen, L. S., Gottschalk, A., and Zaret, B. L.: Comparison of Exercise Radionuclide Angiocardiography and Thallium-201 Myocardial Perfusion Imaging in Coronary Artery Disease, *Am. J. Cardiol.*, 45:1113, 1980.
185. Jengo, J. A., Greeman, R., Brizendine, M., and Mena, I.: Detection of Coronary Artery Disease: Comparison of Exercise Stress Radionuclide Angiocardiography and Thallium Stress Perfusion Scanning, *Am. J. Cardiol.*, 45:535, 1980.
186. Bulkley, B. H., Rouleau, J., Strauss, H. W., Pitt, B.: Idiopathic Hypertrophic Subaortic Stenosis: Detection by Thallium-201 Myocardial Perfusion Imaging, *N. Engl. J. Med.*, 293:1113, 1975.
187. Khaja, F., Alam, M., Goldstein, S., Anbe, D. T., and Marks, D. S.: Diagnostic Value of Visualization of the Right Ventricle Using Thallium-201 Myocardial Imaging, *Circulation*, 59:182, 1979.
188. Ohsuzu, F., Handa, S., Kondo, M., Yamazaki, H., Tsugu, T., Kubo, A., Takagi, Y., and Nakamura, Y.: Thallium-201 Myocardial Imaging to Evaluate Right Ventricular Overloading, *Circulation*, 61:620, 1980.
189. Buja, L. M., Parkey, R. W., Dees, J. H., Stokely, E. M., Harris, R. A., Bonte, F. J., and Willerson, J. T.: Morphologic Correlates of Technetium-99m Stannous Pyrophosphate Imaging of Acute Myocardial Infarcts in Dogs, *Circulation*, 52:596, 1975.
190. Buja, L. M., Tofe, A. J., Kulkarni, P. V., Mukherjee, A., Parkey, R. W., Francis, M. D., Bonte, F. J., and Willerson, J. T.: Sites and Mechanisms of Localization of Technetium-99m Phosphorus Radiopharmaceuticals in Acute Myocardial Infarcts and Other Tissues, *J. Clin. Invest.*, 60:724, 1977.
191. Dewanjee, M. K., and Kahn, P. C.: Mechanism of Localization of ^{99m}Tc-Labeled Pyrophosphate and Tetracycline in Infarcted Myocardium, *J. Nucl. Med.*, 17:639, 1976.
192. Riba, A. L., Downs, J., Thakur, M. L., Gottschalk, A., Andriole, V. T., and Zaret, B. L.: Technetium-99m Stannous Pyrophosphate Imaging of Infective Endocarditis, *Circulation*, 58:111, 1978.
193. Coleman, R. E., Klein, M. S., Ahmed, S. A., Weiss, E. S., Buchholz, W. M., and Sobel, B. E.: Mechanisms Contributing to Myocardial Accumulation of Technetium-99m Stannous Pyrophosphate after Coronary Artery Occlusion, *Am. J. Cardiol*, 39:55, 1977.
194. Zaret, B. L., DiCola, V. C., Donabedian, R. K., Puri, S., Wolfson, S., Freedman, G. S., and Cohen, L. S.: Dual Radionuclide Study of Myocardial Infarction: Relationships between Myocardial Uptake of Potassium-43, Technetium-99m Stannous Pyrophosphate, Regional Myocardial Blood Flow and Creatine Phosphokinase Depletion, *Circulation*, 53:422, 1976.
195. Schneider, R. M., Hayslett, J. P., Downing, S. E., Berger, H. J., Donabedian, R. K., and Zaret, B. L.: Effect of Methylprednisolone upon Technetium-99m Pyrophosphate Assessment of Myocardial Necrosis in the Canine Countershock Model, *Circulation*, 56:1029, 1977.
196. Olson, H. G., Lyons, K. P., Aranow, W. S., Brown, W. T., and Greenfield, R. S.: Follow-Up Technetium-99m Stannous Pyrophosphate Myocardial Scintigrams after Acute Myocardial Infarction, *Circulation*, 56:181, 1977.
197. Buja, L. M., Poliner, L., Parkey, R. W., Pulido, J., Hutcheson, D., Platt, M. R., Mills, L., Bonte, F. J., and Willerson, J. T.: Clinicopathologic Study of Persistently Positive Technetium-99m Stannous Pyrophosphate Myocardial Scintigrams and Myocytolytic Degeneration after Acute Myocardial Infarction, *Circulation*, 56:1016, 1977.
198. Berger, H. J., Gottschalk, A., and Zaret, B. L.: Dual Radionuclide Study of Myocardial Infarction: Comparison of Thallium-201 and Technetium-99m Stannous Pyrophosphate Imaging in Man, *Ann. Intern. Med.*, 88:145, 1978.
199. Rude, R., Parkey, R. W., Bonte, F. J., Twieg, D., Lewis, S., Pulido, J., Buja, L. M., and Willerson, J. T.: Clinical Implications of the "Doughnut" Pattern of Uptake in Technetium-99m Stannous Pyrophosphate Myocardial Scintigrams in Patients with Acute Myocardial Infarction, *Circulation*, 59:721, 1979.
200. Willerson, J. T., Parkey, R. W., Bonte, F. J., Meyer, S. L., Atkins, J. M., and Stokely, E. M.: Technetium-99m Stannous Pyrophosphate Myocardial Scintigrams in Patients with Chest Pain of Varying Etiology, *Circulation*, 51:1046, 1975.
201. Willerson, J. T., Parkey, R. W., Bonte, F. J., Meyer, L. S., and Stokely, E. M.: Acute Subendocardial Myocardial Infarction in Patients; Its Detection by Technetium-99m Stannous Pyrophosphate Myocardial Scintigrams, *Circulation*, 51:436, 1975.
202. Parkey, R. W., Bonte, F. J., Buja, L. M., Stokely, E. M., and Willerson, J. T.: Myocardial Infarct Imaging with Technetium-99m Phosphates, *Semin. Nucl. Med.*, 7:15, 1977.
203. Wynne, J., and Holman, B. L.: Acute Myocardial Infarct Scintigraphy with Infarct-Avid Radiotracers, *Med. Clin. North Am.*, 64:119, 1980.
204. Massie, B. M., Botvinick, E. H., Werner, J. A., Shames, D., Chatterjee, K., and Parmley, W. W.: Myocardial Infarction Scintigraphy with Technetium-99m Stannous Pyrophosphate: An Insensitive Test for Nontransmural Myocardial Infarction, *Am. J. Cardiol.*, 43:186, 1979.
205. Stokely, E. M., Buja, L. M., Lewis, S. E., Parkey, R. W., Bonte, F. J., Harris, R. A., and Willerson, J. T.: Measurement of Acute Myocardial Infarcts in Dogs with Technetium-99m Stannous Pyrophosphate Scintigrams, *J. Nucl. Med.*, 17:1, 1976.
206. Prasquier, R., Taradash, M. R., Botvinick, E. H., Shames, D. M., and Parmley, W. W.: The Specificity of the Diffuse Pattern of Cardiac Uptake in Myocardial Infarction Imaging with Technetium-99m Stannous Pyrophosphate, *Circulation*, 55:61, 1977.
207. Poliner, L. R., Buja, L. M., Parkey, R. W., Bonte, F. J., and Willerson, J. T.: Clinico-Pathologic Findings in 52 Patients Studied by Technetium-99m Stannous Pyrophosphate Myocardial Scintigrams, *Circulation*, 59:257, 1979.
208. Donsky, M. S., Curry, G. C., Parkey, R. W., Meyer, S. L., Bonte, F. J., Platt, M. R., and Willerson, J. T.: Unstable

Angina Pectoris: Clinical, Angiographic and Myocardial Scintigraphic Observations, *Br. Heart J.*, 38:257, 1976.
209. Wackers, F. J., Lie, K. I., Busemann-Sokole, E., Res, J., van der Schoot, J. B., and Durrer, D.: Prevalence of Right Ventricular Involvement in Inferior Wall Infarction Assessed with Myocardial Imaging with Thallium-201 and Technetium-99m Pyrophosphate, *Am. J. Cardiol.*, 42:358, 1978.
210. Righetti, A., O'Rourke, R. A., Schelbert, H., Henning, H., Hardarson, T., Daily, P. O., Ashburn, W., and Ross, J.: Usefulness of Preoperative and Postoperative Tc-99m (Sn)-Pyrophosphate Scans in Patients with Ischemic and Valvular Heart Disease, *Am. J. Cardiol.*, 39:43, 1977.
211. Platt, M. R., Parkey, R. W., Willerson, J. T., Bonte, F. J., Shapier, W., and Sugg, W. L.: Technetium Stannous Pyrophosphate Myocardial Scintigrams in the Recognition of Myocardial Infarction in Patients Undergoing Coronary Artery Revascularization, *Ann. Thorac. Surg.*, 21:311, 1976.
212. Willerson, J. T., Parkey, R. W., Stokely, E. M., Bonte, F. J., Lewis, S. F., Harris, R. A., Blomquist, C. G., Poliner, L., and Buja, L. M.: Infarct Sizing with Technetium-99m Stannous Pyrophosphate Scintigraphy in Dogs and Man: The Relationship between Scintigraphic and Precordial Mapping Estimates in Infarct Size in Patients, *Cardiovasc. Res.*, 11:291, 1977.
213. Holman, B. L., Chisholm, R. J., and Braunwald, E.: The Prognostic Implication of Acute Myocardial Infarct Scintigraphy with ^{99m}Tc-Pyrophosphate, *Circulation*, 57:320, 1978.
214. Botvinick, E. H., Shames, D., Lappin, H., Tyberg, J. V., Townsend, R., and Parmley, W. W.: Noninvasive Quantitation of Myocardial Infarction with Technetium-99m Pyrophosphate, *Circulation*, 52:909, 1975.
215. Keyes, J. W., Leonard, P. F., Brody, L. S., Svetkoff, D. J., Rogers, W. L., and Lucchesi, B. R.: Myocardial Infarct Quantification in the Dog by Single Photon Emission Computerized Tomography, *Circulation*, 58:227, 1978.
216. Kronenberg, M. W., Ettinger, V. R., Wilson, G. A., Schenk, E. A., Cohn, J.: A Comparison of Radiotracer and Biochemical Methods for the Quantitation of Experimental Myocardial Infarct Weight: In Vitro Relationships, *J. Nucl. Med.*, 20:224, 1979.
217. Lewis, M., Buja, L. M., Saffer, S., Michelvich, D., Stokely, E., Lewis, S., Parkey, R., Bonte, F., and Willerson, J. T.: Experimental Infarct Sizing Utilizing Computer Processing and a Three-Dimensional Model, *Science*, 197:167, 1977.
218. Thakur, M. L., Welch, M. J., Joist, J. H., and Coleman, R. E.: Indium-111 Labeled Platelets: Studies on Preparation and Evaluation of In Vitro and In Vivo Functions, *Thromb. Res.*, 9:345, 1976.
219. Riba, A. L., Thakur, M. L., Gottschalk, A., Andriole, V. T., and Zaret, B. L.: Imaging Experimental Infective Endocarditis with Indium-111 Labeled Blood Cellular Components, *Circulation*, 59:336, 1979.
220. Riba, A. L., Thakur, M. L., Gottschalk, A., and Zaret, B. L.: Imaging Experimental Coronary Artery Thrombosis with Indium-111 Platelets, *Circulation*, 60:767, 1979.
221. McIlmoyle, G., Davis, H. H., Welch, M. J., Primeau, J. L., Sherman, L. A., and Siegel, B. A.: Scintigraphic Diagnosis of Experimental Pulmonary Embolism with In-111 Labeled Platelets, *J. Nucl. Med.*, 18:910, 1977.
222. Dewanjee, M. K., Fuster, V., Kaye, M. P., and Josa, M.: Imaging Platelet Deposition with ^{111}In-Labeled Platelet in Coronary Artery Bypass Grafts in Dogs, *Mayo Clin. Proc.*, 53:327, 1978.
223. Ezekowitz, M. D., Leonard, J., Smith, E. O., Allen, E. W., and Taylor, F. B.: Identification of Left Ventricular Thrombi in Man Using Indium-111 Labeled Autologous Platelets, A Preliminary Report, *Circulation*, 63:803, 1981.
224. Ezekowitz, M. D., Wilson, D. A., Smith, E. O., Burow, R. D., Harrison, L. H., Parker, D. E., Elkins, R. C., Peyton, M., and Taylor, F. B.: Comparison of Indium-111 Platelet Scintigraphy and Two-Dimensional Echocardiography in Diagnosis of Left Ventricular Thrombi, *N. Engl. J. Med.*, 306:1509, 1982.
225. Davis, H. H., Siegel, B. A., Sherman, L. A., Heaton, W. A., Naidich, T. P., Joist, J. H., and Welch, M. J.: Scintigraphic Detection of Carotid Atherosclerosis with Indium-111 Labeled Autologous Platelets, *Circulation*, 61:982, 1980.
226. Stratton, J. R., Thiele, B. L., and Ritchie, J. L.: Platelet Deposition on Dacron Aortic Bifurcation Grafts in Man: Quantitation with Indium-111 Platelet Imaging, *Circulation*, 66:1287, 1982.
227. Pumphrey, C. W., Chesebro, J. H., Dwanjee, M. K., Wahner, H. W., Hollier, L. H., Pairolero, P. C., and Fuster, V.: In Vivo Quantitation of Platelet Deposition on Human Peripheral Arterial Bypass Grafts Using Indium-111 Platelets: Effect of Dipyridamole and Aspirin, *Am. J. Cardiol.*, 51:796, 1983.
228. Pope, C. F., Ezekowitz, M. D., Smith, E. O., et al.: Detection of Platelet Deposition at the Site of Peripheral Balloon Angioplasty Using Indium-111 Platelet Scintigraphy, *Am. J. Cardiol.*, 55:495, 1985.
229. Ezekowitz, M. D., Pope, C. F., Sortman, D., et al.: Indium-111 Platelet Scintigraphy for the Diagnosis of Deep Vein Thrombosis. Correlation with Venography, *Clin. Res.*, 32:307A, 1984.
230. Thakur, M. L., Gottschalk, A., and Zaret, B. L.: Imaging Experimental Myocardial Infarction with Indium-111 Labeled Autologous Leukocytes: Effects of Infarct Age and Residual Myocardial Blood Flow, *Circulation*, 60:297, 1979.
231. Davies, R. A., Thakur, M. L., Berger, H. J., Wackers, J. T., Gottschalk, A., and Zaret, B. L.: Imaging the Inflammatory Response to Acute Myocardial Infarction in Man Using Indium-111 Labeled Autologous Leukocytes, *Circulation*, 63:826, 1981.
232. Khaw, B. A., Beller, G. A., Haber, E., and Smith, T. W.: Localization of Cardiac Myosin-Specific Antibody in Myocardial Infarction, *J. Clin. Invest.*, 58:439, 1976.
233. Khaw, B. A., Beller, G. A., and Haber, E.: Experimental Myocardial Infarct Imaging Following Intravenous Administration of Iodine-131 Labeled Antibody $(Fab')_2$ Fragment Specific for Cardiac Myosin, *Circulation*, 57:743, 1978.
234. Khaw, B. A., Gould, H. K., Yasuda, T., Leinbach, R. C., Strauss, H. W., Fallon, J. T., Kahill, S. L., and Hayberg, E.: Acute Myocardial Infarct Imaging with Technetium-99m DTPA-Antimyosin Fab, *Circulation*, 66, II–272, 1982.
235. Schelbert, H. R., Phelps, M. E., Hoffman, E., Huang, S., Kuhl, D. E.: Regional Myocardial Blood Flow, Metabolism and Function Assessed Noninvasively by Positron Emission Tomography, *Am. J. Cardiol.*, 46:1269, 1980.
236. Phelps, M. E.: Emission Computed Tomography, *Semin. Nucl. Med.*, 7:337, 1977.
237. Goldstein, R. A., Mullani, N. A., and Gould, K. L.: Quantitative Myocardial Imaging with Positron Emitters, in P. N. Yu and J. F. Goodwin (eds.), "Progress in Cardiology," Lea & Febiger, Philadelphia, 1983, pp. 147–192.
238. Phelps, M. E. Hoffman, E. J., Selin, C., Huang, S. C., Robinson, G., MacDonald, N., Schelbert, H. R., and Kuhl, D. E.: Investigation of ^{18}F-2-Fluoro-2-Deoxyglucose for the Measure of Myocardial Glucose Metabolism, *J. Nucl. Med.*, 19:1311, 1978.
239. Gould, K. L., Schelbert, H. R., Phelps, M. E., and Hoffman, E. J.: Noninvasive Assessment of Coronary Stenosis by Myocardial Perfusion Imaging during Pharmacologic Coronary Vasodilatation. V. Detection of 47% Diameter Coronary Stenosis with Intravenous N-13 Ammonia and Emission Computed Tomography in Intact Dogs, *Am. J. Cardiol.*, 43:200, 1979.
240. Schelbert, H. R., Phelps, M. E., Huang, S. C., MacDonald, N. S., Hansen, H., Selin, N. C., and Kuhl, D. E.: N-13-Ammonia as an Indicator of Myocardial Blood Flow, *Circulation*, 63:1259, 1981.
241. Goldstein, R. A., Mullani, M. A., Marani, S. K., Fischer, D. J., Gould, K. L., and O'Brien, H. A.: Myocardial Perfusion with Rubidium-82: Effects of Metabolic and Pharmacologic Interventions, *J. Nucl. Med.*, 24:907, 1983.

242. Weiss, E. W., Hoffman, E. J., Phelps, M. E., Welch, M. J., Henry, P. D., Ter-Pogossian, M. M., and Sobel, B. E.: External Detection and Visualization of Myocardial Ischemia with ^{11}C-Palmitic Acid, *Circ. Res.*, 39:24, 1976.
243. Weiss, E. S., Ahmed, S. A., Welch, M. J., Williamson, J. R., Ter-Pogossian, M. M., and Sobel, B. E.: Quantification of Infarction in Cross Sections of Canine Myocardium in Vivo with Positron Emission Transaxial Tomography and ^{11}C-Palmitate, *Circulation*, 55:66, 1977.
244. Ter-Pogossian, M. M., Klein, M. S., Markham, J., Roberts, R., and Sobel, B. E.: Regional Assessment of Myocardial Metabolic Integrity in Vivo by Positron-Emission Tomography with ^{11}C-Labeled Palmitate, *Circulation*, 61:242, 1980.
245. Bergman, S. R., Lerch, R. A., Fox, K. A., Ludbrook, P. A., Welch, M. J., Ter-Pogossian, M. M., and Sobel, B. E.: Temporal Dependence of Beneficial Effects of Coronary Thrombolysis Characterized by Positron Tomography, *Am. J. Med.*, 73:573, 1982.
246. Marshall, R. C., Tillisch, J. H., Phelps, M. E., Huang, S. C., Carson, R., Henze, E., and Schelbert, H. R.: Identification of and Differentiation of Resting Myocardial Ischemia and Infarction in Man with Positron Computed Tomography, ^{18}F-labeled Fluorodeoxyglucose and N-13 Ammonia, *Circulation*, 67:766, 1983.
247. Perloff, J. K., Henze, E., and Schelbert, H. R.: Alterations in Regional Myocardial Metabolism, Perfusion and Wall Motion in Duchenne Muscular Dystrophy Studied by Radionuclide Imaging, *Circulation*, 69:33, 1984.
248. Lerch, R. A., Bergmann, S. R., Ambas, H. D., Welch, M. J., Ter-Pogossian, M. M., and Sobel, B. E.: Effective Flow-Independent Reduction of Metabolism on Regional Myocardial Clearance of ^{11}C-Palmitate, *Circulation*, 65:731, 1982.
249. Evans, J. R., Phil, D., Gunton, R. W., Baker, R. G., Beanlands, D. S., and Spears, J. C.: Use of Radioiodinated Fatty Acid for Photoscans of the Heart, *Circ. Res.*, 16:1, 1965.
250. van der Wall, E. E., Hollander, W. den, Westera, G., Majid, P. A., and Roos, J. P.: Dynamic Myocardial Scintigraphy with I-123 Labeled Free Fatty Acids in Patients with Myocardial Infarction, *Eur. J. Nucl. Med.*, 6:383, 1981.
251. van der Wall, E. E., Heidendal, G. A. K., Hollander, W. den, Westera, G., and Roos, J. P.: Metabolic Myocardial Imaging with I-123 Labeled Heptadecanoic Acid in Patients with Angina Pectoris, *Eur. J. Nucl. Med.*, 6:391, 1981.
252. Hoeck, A., Freundlieb, C., Vyska, K., Loesse, B., Erbel, R., and Feinendegen, L. E.: Myocardial Imaging and Metabolic Studies with [17-I-123] Iodoheptadecanoic Acid in Patients with Idiopathic Congestive Cardiomyopathy, *J. Nucl. Med.*, 24:22, 1983.
253. van der Wall, E. E., Westera, G., Hollander, W. den, Visser, F. C., Roos, J. P., and Heidendal, G. A. K.: The Effect of Pindolol on Myocardial Uptake of Free Fatty Acids in the Dog, *Curr. Ther. Res.*, 33:591, 1983.
254. Rella, J. S., Corbett, J. R., Kuokarni, P., Morgan, C., Devous, M. D., Buja, L. M., Busch, L., Parkey, R. W., Willerson, J. T., and Lewis, S. E.: Iodine-123 Phenylpentadecanoic Acid: Detection of Acute Myocardial Infarction and Injury in Dogs Using an Iodinated Fatty Acid and Single-Photon Emission Tomography, *Am. J. Cardiol.*, 52:1326, 1983.
255. Visser, F. C., van Eenige, M. J., van der Wall, E. E., and Roos, J. P.: The Mechanism of the Elimination of Rate of 123I-Heptadecanoic Acid from the Myocardium, *J. Am. Coll. Cardiol.*, 3:476, 1984.

110

The Use of Digital Subtraction Imaging in Cardiac Disease

William J. Casarella, M.D.

Digital subtraction angiography is a relatively new technique which has proven itself useful in the evaluation of the carotid and renal arteries following an intravenous injection of contrast material.[1–4] Clinical applications of the method to the heart and great vessels have been somewhat limited in comparison to its wide use in the evaluation of the peripheral circulations. The intent of this chapter is to review the current status of digital vascular imaging in the heart and great vessels.

Physical Basis for Digital Subtraction Angiography

The primary radiographic information is recorded on an image intensifier which can vary in diameter from 6 to 14 in. Optimally, the image intensifier must be of high quality with an intrinsic resolution of 3 to 4 line pairs per millimeter. The image intensifier is then linked to a television camera, usually of the Plumbicon type, with at least a 200:1 signal-to-noise ratio. The signal output of the Plumbicon tube is then logarithmically processed and digitized with an 8- or 10-bit analog to digital convertor using a 512 × 512 pixel matrix. The data are then stored in a digital memory. The first preinjection digitized fluoroscopic image is stored to be used as a subtraction mask. Later, real-time data are stored in a second memory to form a series of static images from which the mask containing only background information can be subtracted. With most systems dynamic studies at 60 frames per second may be enhanced and later converted to analog form. Instead of utilizing vast amounts of digital data storage, some systems use an analog storage method although pure digital storage is becoming the most popular medium as the cost of digital memory devices continues to fall.

The images stored in the digital memory represent a map of iodine distribution isolated by time subtraction. The vascular image is then multiplied digitally by a factor of 8 to 16 in order to enhance the iodine contrast. The multiplication occurs before the data are then reconverted to an analog form for viewing and final storage prior to visualization or further manipulation. The stored analog data may be redigitized for further processing or remasking if there is a necessity for postprocessing or further quantification and manipulation of the data. During the final step errors in registration of the first mask with the later vascular images may be corrected by shifting pixels in order to re-register the mask on the new image. It is also possible to subtract one image from another during the course of the angiogram in order to obtain quantitative data relative to change in shape of the blood vessel or ventricle, and to obtain semiquantitative measures of blood flow.

The main advantage of digital manipulation of the vascular images lies in increasing the visibility of the vascular structures and the contrast resolution of what are intrinsically poor images with insufficient amount of iodine in order to obtain diagnostic studies. The end result is a marked increase in the signal-to-background ratio by a factor of approximately 200.

Since the main thrust of digital subtraction is to convert an intrinsically poor image to a good one, the system allows arteriograms of diagnostic quality to be obtained following the intravenous injection of large boluses of contrast material or the intraarterial injection of very small quantities of iodinated contrast.

Use of the intravenous route for arterial opacification avoids the hazards of arterial catheterization and allows more patients to be evaluated without having to admit them to the hospital. Digital subtraction angiography performed from the arterial side allows for a marked decrease in the dose of contrast material, and produces images of generally higher quality than the intravenous approach.

Diseases of the Aorta

Since the aorta is a rather large structure that can be visualized at a relatively low intrinsic resolution, it would be expected that it would become an ideal subject for digital subtraction angiography. In his review of 315 cases, Boxt[5] found the technique to be adequate for aneurysms, dissections, coarctations, atherosclerosis, and postoperative assessment of the thoracic and abdominal aorta. Several limitations were identified which included motion artifacts, overlap of vessels, lack of contrast in patients with poor cardiac output, and a degraded image secondary to excessive variation in contrast density in the chest. Most of these limitations can be partially overcome by excellent technique and filtering of the image. However, excessive patient motion and poor cardiac output are severe limitations. Nonetheless, it appeared evident that a simple peripheral intravenous injection followed by digital subtraction angiography was an acceptable method of evaluating the thoracic and abdominal aorta in patients with major lesions of that structure.

Guthaner and Miller[6] specifically studied aortic dissection in six patients and claimed excellent results with good visualization of both the true and false channels using the technique. They felt that digital subtraction angiography (DSA) was a complementary study to computerized tomography in that it provided a more conventional angiographic image to complement the cross-sectional format obtained during computerized tomography. Sahn et al.[7] used DSA in evaluating anomalies of the aortic arch and reported their results in two cases.

It is evident from the reported series that intravenous DSA for evaluation of the aorta appears to have clinical utility, and in most cases will produce a diagnostic study. In our experience, we have found that arterial DSA of the thoracic aorta has been a better choice than the use of routine intravenous studies since the quality of the images is superior and an excellent study may be obtained with 10 to 15 ml of contrast material instead of the 40 to 45 ml necessary for the intravenous approach. Since it is possible to use 15 ml of contrast material diluted to 45 ml with normal saline, it is very easy to inject the dilute material of low viscosity through no. 4 French or no. 5 French catheters and obtain an excellent study. Advantages of this approach lie in the marked reduction of contrast load to the kidneys and decrease in pain and patient motion secondary to the contrast material itself. Because most examinations of the aorta require at least two views to rule out significant pathology, the intraarterial route is preferred since virtually all digital subtraction angiography systems are single-plane, and multiple peripheral injections would be necessary to completely evaluate the aorta in several views.

Quantitative Digital Subtraction Angiography in the Assessment of the Left Ventricle

Since it provides an adequate, already digitized image of the left ventricle from a peripheral injection of contrast material, DSA has been extensively studied as a means to evaluate left ventricular function.[8–12] The investigators of DSA in left ventricular function have taken two different approaches. One has utilized the peripheral injection of contrast material either in the antecubital fossa or the vena cava with visualization of the left ventricle on the levophase of the injection. Other clinicians[10,11] have attempted to determine how small an injection of contrast material is needed to produce diagnostically accurate ventriculograms following selective catheterization of the left ventricle. The studies utilizing primarily the intravenous route[8,9,12] demonstrated that intravenous DSA was equal to conventional left ventriculography in the measurement of ejection fraction, cardiac output, and stroke volume. Correlation with regional wall motion abnormalities was not quite as high as with the other measurements. This result, however, may be due to a higher standard error of the measurements rather than any intrinsic difference between the two imaging modalities.

Other studies showed basically the same results following the selective injection of either 7 ml[10] or 10 ml[11] of contrast material directly into the left ventricle. The study by Nichols et al.[10] demonstrated that 7 ml of contrast material diluted to a volume of 45 ml by the addition of dextrose and saline produced ventriculograms of equal quality to those performed by conventional means following the injection of 45 ml of undiluted contrast material (Figs. 110-1 to 110-4). Additional benefits of the low-dose digital left ventriculogram are the significant reduction in the hemodynamic effects that result from the injection of conventional doses of contrast. It can be argued that the quantitative aspects of left ventriculography are more accurately assessed without the negative inotropic effects of large doses of contrast material. Furthermore, the selective injection of contrast material into the left ventricle allows for the assessment of mitral regurgitation, a lesion which could not be identified on the intravenous studies.

The quality of digital left ventriculograms permits also the identification of left ventricular aneurysms,[13] and adequately studies the aortic valve.

Coronary Artery Disease

Clearly, the main goal of DSA is the noninvasive depiction of coronary artery anatomy. So far this ambition has not been fully realized. The intravenous approach to coronary artery visualization has failed largely because of intrinsic difficulties with resolving vessels of the size of coronary arteries and because of the inherent problems of superimposition of the coronary arteries on the contrast-filled left ventricle.

Moderate success has been obtained in the nonselective injection of the aortic root with digital subtraction recording of the resultant coronary im-

FIGURE 110-1 A comparison of digital left ventriculogram (*top*) with 7 ml of contrast and conventional ventriculograms (*bottom*) with 45 ml of contrast material. (*From D. J. Sahn, L. M. Valdes-Cruz, T. W. Ovitt, et al., Two Dimensional Echocardiography and Intravenous Digital Video Subtraction Angiography for Diagnosis and Evaluation of Double Aortic Arch, Am. J. Cardiol., 50:342, 1982. Reproduced with permission from the publisher and author.*)

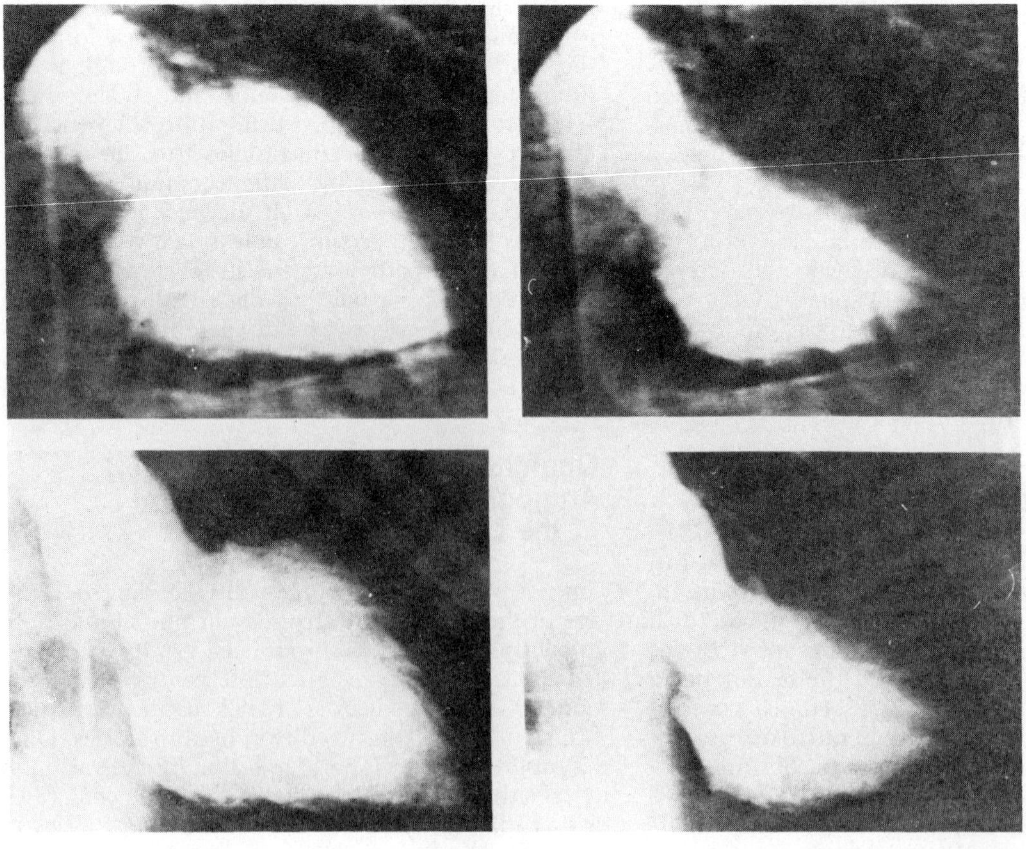

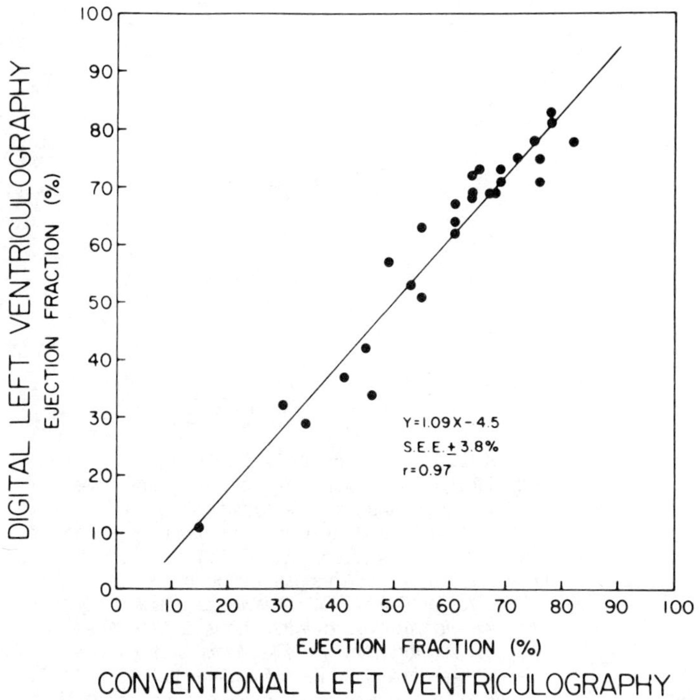

FIGURE 110-2 Data demonstrating the very high correlation between ejection fractions measured from digital and conventional left ventriculograms. (*From D. J. Sahn, L. M. Valdes-Cruz, T. W. Ovitt, et al., Two Dimensional Echocardiography and Intravenous Digital Video Subtraction Angiography for Diagnosis and Evaluation of Double Aortic Arch, Am. J. Cardiol., 50:342, 1982. Reproduced with permission from the publisher and author.*)

ages.[14] Although this method seems to work very well in experimental animals, it has not been particularly useful in clinical trials. There clearly is very little advantage to recording coronary angiography on digital subtraction devices if selective catheterization and injection of contrast material directly into the coronary arteries is required for adequate studies. This important area of clinical endeavor is still awaiting further advances and subsequent clinical trials.

Pediatric Angiocardiography

DSA is theoretically an excellent method for imaging cardiac lesions in infants and children. It offers the potential for a relatively less invasive study than selective cardiac catheterization and has the potential advantage of markedly reducing the contrast load. Furthermore, a significant reduction in radiation dose should be possible. In their study of 42 patients, Levin et al.[15] showed that diagnostic information on

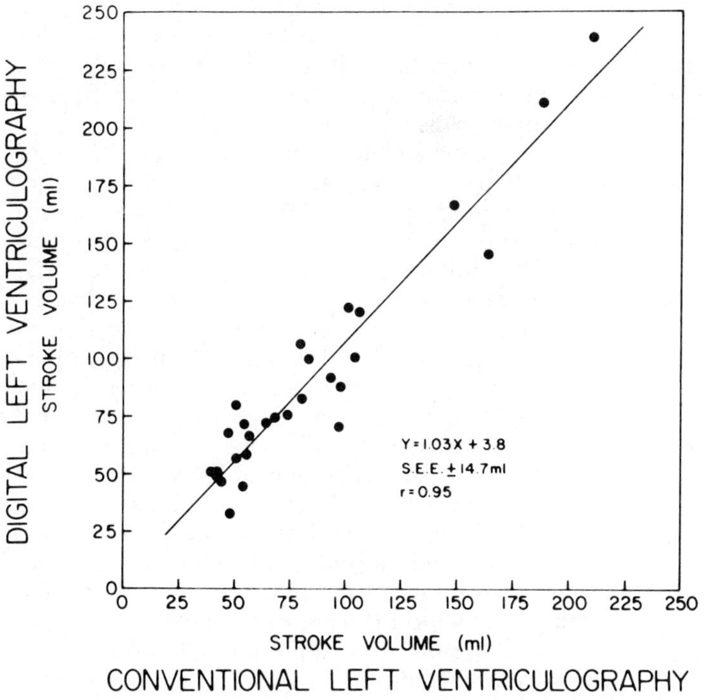

FIGURE 110-3 Stroke volume data reveals nearly identical results from digital and conventional left ventriculogram. (*From D. J. Sahn, L. M. Valdes-Cruz, T. W. Ovitt, et al., Two Dimensional Echocardiography and Intravenous Digital Video Subtraction Angiography for Diagnosis and Evaluation of Double Aortic Arch, Am. J. Cardiol., 50:342, 1982. Reproduced with permission from the publisher and author.*)

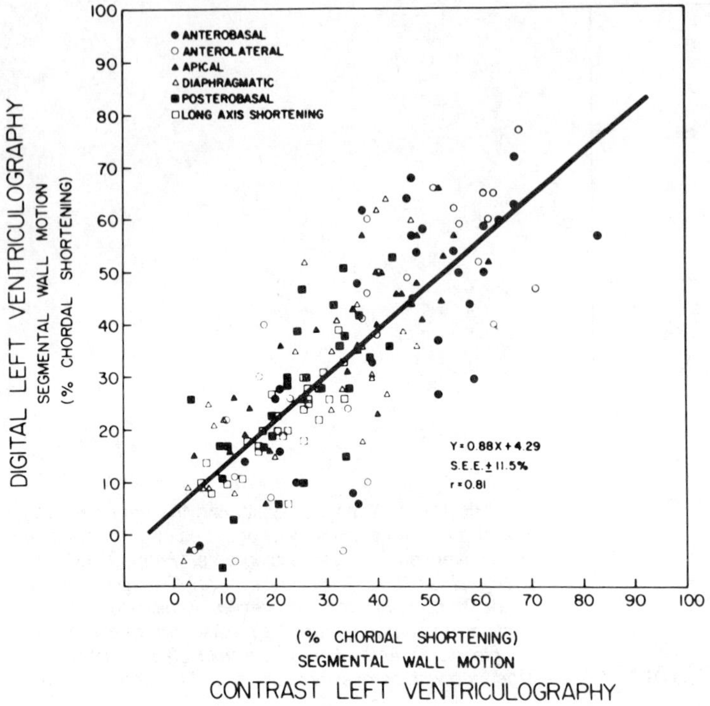

FIGURE 110-4 Segmental wall motion studies comparing digital left ventriculography and contrast left ventriculography. Note that there is considerable scatter of data points. Higher standard error of the measurement and different inotropic effects of high and low doses of contrast material may explain the difference. (*From D. J. Sahn, L. M. Valdes-Cruz, T. W. Ovitt, et al., Two Dimensional Echocardiography and Intravenous Digital Video Subtraction Angiography for Diagnosis and Evaluation of Double Aortic Arch, Am. J. Cardiol., 50:342, 1982. Reproduced with permission from the publisher and author.*)

DSA was equal to that obtained on selective angiocardiography in 81 of 87 studies. Five other studies were technically suboptimal, indicating that in 81 of 92 total digital angiocardiograms, information obtained was equal to that using conventional means.

One significant disadvantage of DSA in the pediatric population is its limitation to single-plane filming instead of the conventional biplane approach. There was no saving in contrast material when the injections were made from a peripheral location. However, a 58 to 73 percent reduction in injected contrast material was possible when selective injections were made. The radiation dose was markedly reduced over conventional cine runs resulting in a tenfold reduction using DSA. This factor may be especially important in children since Martin et al.[16] have shown that conventional doses employed during cardiac catheterization cause a 20-fold increase in risk for the development of subsequent thyroid carcinoma in infants and children.

It seems evident, therefore, that digital subtraction techniques could be used to supplement conventional filming in pediatric cardiology where single-plane filming would be considered adequate, and when diagnostic information might be limited to specific questions of anatomy. Reduction in contrast dose and in radiation are the major advantages of this technique in the pediatric population.

Pulmonary Angiography

Following the experimental studies of Chiles et al.[17] and Witte et al.[18] which demonstrated that pulmonary emboli as small as 2 mm in size could be visualized by DSA, several clinical trials using the method in detection of pulmonary emboli have appeared. Kollath and Riemann[19] studied 220 patients and claimed a diagnostic study in 98 percent. However, there were no controls using radionuclide scanning or conventional pulmonary angiographic techniques. Their technique was an exceedingly simple one utilizing a total of 25 ml of contrast material injected at 10 ml into the antecubital vein. The lack of adequate controls makes this study somewhat questionable. In addition, the clinicians only concern themselves with the diagnosis of pulmonary emboli that were visible in first- and second-order pulmonary branches. Their technique, however, was so relatively simple and noninvasive that further evaluation seems indicated.

In a somewhat later study, Ferris et al.[20] evaluated 40 patients by means of conventional pulmonary angiography and DSA. Of 26 patients with positive pulmonary angiograms, 20 were identified using DSA following injections of contrast material into the vena cava. Serious questions could be raised regarding the wisdom of accepting a reduction in diagnostic accuracy for the slight advantage in performing an injection in the vena cava rather than in the pulmonary artery and employing conventional filming. Goldhaber et al.[21] have pointed out this shortcoming of the technique, and also emphasized that digital pulmonary angiograms require at least 15 s of strict breath holding on the patient's part and should be done only with a 14-in-large field image intensifier in order to capture the entire pulmonary circulation during each injection. It seems evident, therefore, that although digital subtraction angiography following nonselective injection of contrast material may be adequate for detecting large pulmonary emboli, the decrease in diagnostic accuracy obtained may be too high a price to pay for the small savings in invasiveness and contrast material gained from utilizing the digital approach.

Summary

Currently, digital subtraction angiography provides a useful adjunct to conventional filming in the performance of left ventriculography and aortography. It clearly is an excellent way to perform quantitative left ventriculography using either very low doses of contrast material, or peripheral injections of conventional amounts of contrast material. Evaluation of the aortic arch and its major branches is also well accomplished by means of digital subtraction angiography. The pulmonary circulation is not as accurately assessed using current digital methods in comparison to cut film angiography. The true promise of digital subtraction angiography lies in the future assessment of the coronary circulation with anatomic precision that rivals conventional cine angiography. Presently, DSA represents a useful albeit costly supplement to the standard filming capabilities of the regular catheterization laboratory.

References

1. Myerowitz, P. D.: Digital Subtraction Angiography: Present and Future Uses in Cardiovascular Diagnosis, *Clin. Cardiol.*, 5:623, 1982.
2. Chilcote, W. A., Modic, M. T., Pavlicek, W. A., Little, J. R., Furlow, A. J., and Duchesseau, P. M.: Digital Subtraction Angiography of the Carotid Arteries: Comparative Study in 100 Patients, *Radiology*, 139:287, 1981.
3. Meaney, T. F., Weinstein, M. A., and Buonocore, E., et al.: Digital Subtraction Angiography of the Human Cardiovascular System, *AJR* 135:1153, 1980.
4. Mistretta, C. A., and Crummy, A. B.: Diagnosis of Cardiovascular Disease by Digital Subtraction Angiography, *Science*, 214:761, 1981.
5. Boxt, L. M.: Intravenous Digital Subtraction Angiography of the Thoracic and Abdominal Aorta, *Cardiovasc. Intervent. Radiol.*, 6:205, 1983.
6. Guthaner, D. F., and Miller, D. C.: Digital Subtraction Angiography of Aortic Dissection, *AJR* 141:157, 1983.
7. Sahn, D. J., Valdes-Cruz, L. M., Ovitt, T. W., et al.: Two Dimensional Echocardiography and Intravenous Digital Video Subtraction Angiography for Diagnosis and Evaluation of Double Aortic Arch, *Am. J. Cardiol.*, 50:342, 1982.
8. Mancini, G. B. J., Higgins, C. B., Norris, S. L., and Slutsky, R. A.: Cardiac Imaging with Digital Subtraction Angiography, *Cardiovasc. Intervent. Radiol.*, 6:252, 1983.
9. Tobis, J., Nalcioglu, O., Johnston, W. D., et al.: Left Ventricular Imaging with Digital Subtraction Angiography Using Intravenous Contrast Injections and Fluoroscopic Exposure Controls, *Am. Heart J.*, 104:20, 1982.
10. Nichols, A. B., Martin, E. C., Fles, T. P., et al.: Validation of the Angiographic Accuracy of Digital Left Ventriculography, *Am. J. Cardiol.*, 51:224, 1983.
11. Tobis, J. M., Nalcioglu, O., Johnston, W. D., et al.: Correlation of 10-Milliliter Digital Subtraction Ventriculograms Compared with Standard Cineangiograms, *Am. Heart J.*, 105:946, 1983.
12. Goldberg, H. L., Borer, J. S., Moses, J. W., Fisher, J., Cohen, B., and Skelly, N. T.: Digital Substraction Intravenous Left Ventricular Angiography: Comparison with Conventional Intraventricular Angiography, *J. Am. Coll. Cardiol.*, 1:858, 1983.
13. Yiannikas, J., Moddie, D. S., Sterba, R., and Gill, C. C.: Intravenous Digital Subtraction Angiography to Assess Aneurysms of the Ventricular and Atrial Septum Pre- and Postoperatively, *Am. J. Cardiol.*, 53:383, 1984.
14. Myerowitz, P. D., Turnipseed, W. D., Swanson, D. K., et al.: Digital Subtraction Angiography as a Method of Screening for Coronary Artery Disease during Peripheral Vascular Angiography, *Surgery*, 92:1042, 1982.
15. Levin, A. R., Goldberg, H. L., Borer, J. S., et al.: Digital Angiography in the Pediatric Patient with Congenital Heart Disease: Comparison with Standard Methods, *Circulation*, 68:374, 1983.
16. Martin, E. C., Olson, A. P., Steeg, C. N., and Casarella, W. J.: Radiation Exposure to the Pediatric Patient during Cardiac Catheterization and Angiocardiography. Emphasis on the Thyroid Gland, *Circulation*, 64:153, 1981.
17. Chiles, C., Guthaner, D. F., and Djang, W. T.: Detection of Pulmonary Emboli in Dogs Using Digital Subtraction Angiography, *Invest. Radiol.*, 18:507, 1983.
18. Witte, G., Maas, R., Grabbe, R. E., Obermöller, U., Höhne, K. H., and Hageman, J.: Digital Venous Subtraction Angiography of Pulmonary Embolism in Dogs, *Acta Radiol. (Diagn.)*, 24:101, 1983.
19. Kollath, J., and Riemann, H.: Pulmonary Digital Subtraction Angiography, *Cardiovasc. Intervent. Radiol.*, 6:233, 1983.
20. Ferris, E. J., Holder, J. C., Lim, W. N., et al.: Angiography of Pulmonary Emboli: Digital Studies and Balloon-Occlusion Cineangiography, *AJR* 142:369, 1984.
21. Goldhaber, S. Z., and Markisz, J.: Digital Subtraction Pulmonary Angiography—an Internist's and Radiologist's View, *Cardiovasc. Intervent. Radiol.*, 6:239, 1983.

111

Computed Tomography of the Heart

Murray G. Baron, M.D.

Introduction

Since 1972, when the first clinical computed tomography (CT) unit was put into use, CT has become an integral part of imaging of almost every part of the body, except for the heart. Its usefulness in cardiac diagnosis has been limited because the required exposure times, even though reduced in newer models to 2 to 4 s, is still too long to produce stop-motion images of the beating heart. This problem has been largely overcome by electrocardiogram (ECG) gating and, more recently, by advances in scanner design, so that the true potential of cardiac CT is first being realized.

CT images, similar to standard x-ray images, are a graphic representation of the intensity of an x-ray beam after it has been attenuated by passing through the body. The various tissues and organs cast shadows of different densities because they differ in their capacity to absorb x-rays from the incident beam. CT measures the intensity of the transmitted x-ray beam directly, with a bank of radiation detectors, rather than an intensifying screen-film combination as in standard radiography. The incident x-ray beam of the CT scanner is collimated to a fine slit and rotates around the patient during the exposure, thus irradiating only a thin "slice," usually about 1 cm in thickness. The intensity measurements of the exiting x-ray beam from the many angular views are fed into a computer which calculates the attenuation values for as many as a quarter of a million points within the cross-sectional area. These attenuation values are assigned shades of gray, along a scale where bone is white and air is black, and the final image is generated on the screen of a cathode ray tube.

CT has two main advantages over other imaging methods for the study of heart disease. First, it provides very sharp, cross-sectional images with a spatial and density resolution far greater than that of ultrasound or nuclear imaging. Furthermore, these images can be reconstructed by the computer from the primary data so that the heart can be viewed in the coronal, sagittal, or oblique planes. Second, the CT scanner can measure extremely small increments of radiation. It is 6 to 10 times more sensitive to differences in the x-ray density of structures than other radiographic techniques. Excellent differentiation between blood and myocardium is possible with relatively small intravenous infusions of contrast material. In addition to the anatomic information provided by the CT scan, because the data are stored in digital form, they are readily manipulated to provide real-time measurements of physiological events (Fig. 111-1).

With scan times of 2 to 4 s, data are collected over two or more cardiac cycles. The final picture, therefore, represents a summation of multiple views of the beating heart during different phases of the cardiac cycle. The computed image is that of the heart at end-diastole,[1] because this is the longest part of the cardiac cycle and, therefore, the period during which most of the data were collected. The images of the heart during systole cannot be specifically identified and are represented only by some blurring of the margins of the moving cardiac structures.

Cardiac motion can be stopped, for practical purposes, if the length of exposure does not exceed one-tenth of a cardiac cycle.[2] However, with almost every scanner, the data collected during such a short period are insufficient for construction of an adequate image. One solution is to gate the CT scanner from the ECG, allowing repeated, short exposures to be made at the same time in multiple cardiac cycles, while the heart is in the same position. The data are then combined to produce a stop-motion image of the heart at a chosen point in its cycle of contraction and relaxation.

Unfortunately, gating is not a simple matter. CT images are generated from numerous measurements that are accumulated as the x-ray source rotates around the body. In essence, the data are collected from multiple angular views of the heart. If the input from some of these views is missing, the image is degraded and is distorted by streak artifacts. Gated x-ray exposures, although synchronized with the heart, are related purely by chance to the position of the x-ray tube in its orbit around the patient. In order to compensate for this random data acquisition, many cardiac cycles must be scanned in order to include the required angular views. The time required to accomplish this would entail an unacceptable radiation exposure for the patient and could not be completed while the patient held his or her breath. For this reason, retrospective gating, with selection of appropriate images from previously recorded data, has not proven feasible.[3]

Newer techniques utilize prospective gating. The scanner is still linked to, and triggered by, the ECG, but the motion of the x-ray tube is controlled by a computer. This monitors the angular views that have been obtained and determines when to launch the x-ray tube for the next exposure,[4,5] thus minimizing the amount of data missing from the completed scan.

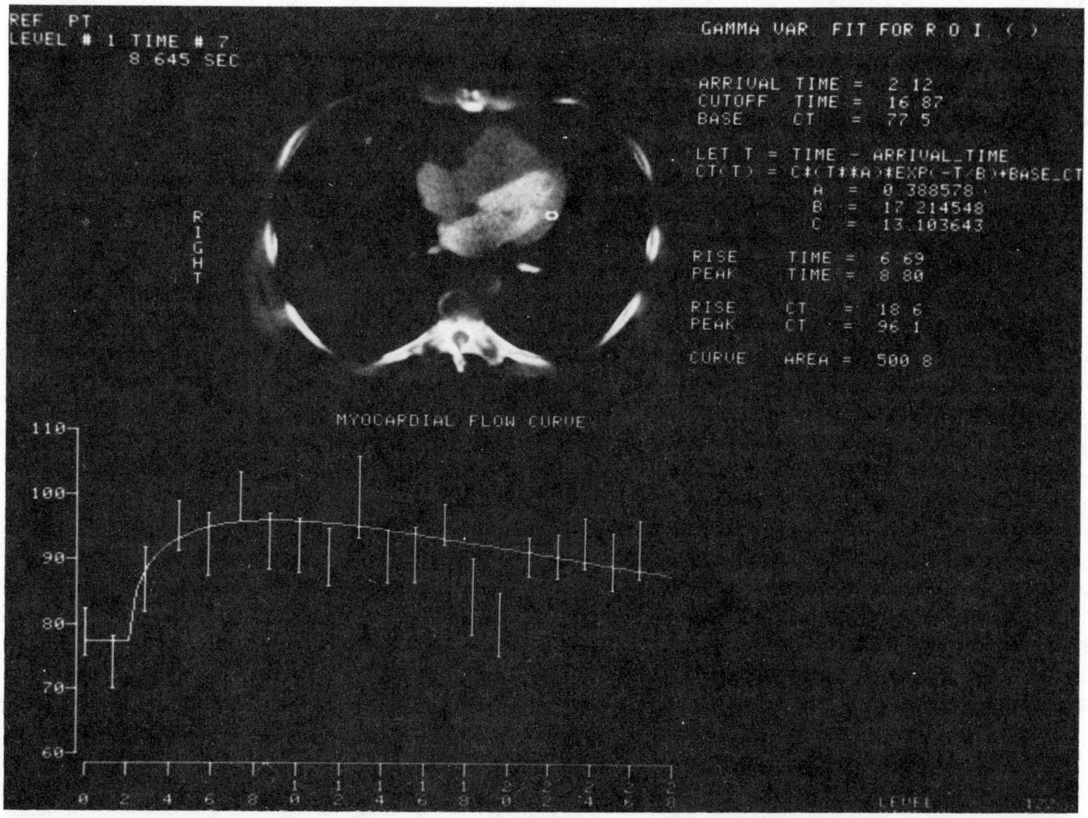

A

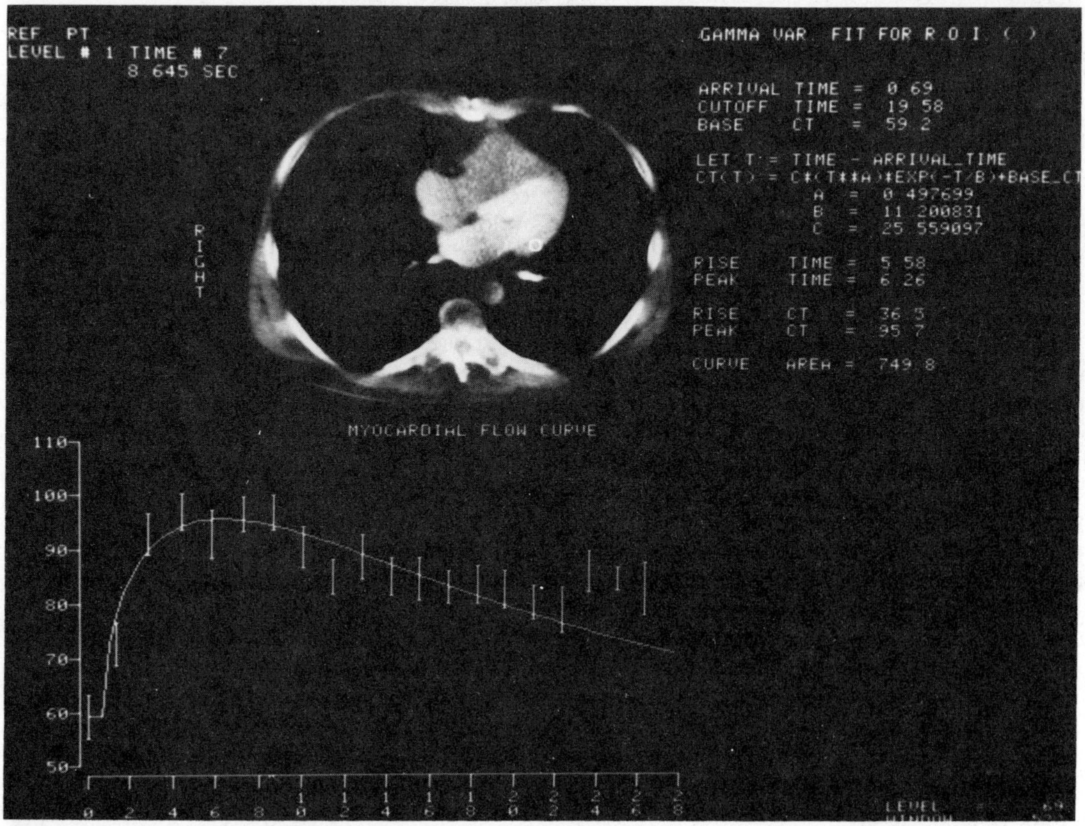

B

FIGURE 111-1 Myocardial blood flow. Patient with previous anterolateral infarction (arrow). Following an intravenous bolus of 25 ml of contrast material, the density changes at specific areas in the myocardium are measured at the identical point in 20 cardiac cycles. The time-density curve is then corrected for recirculation by a gamma-variate curve fit. *A.* The cursor is positioned at the edge of the infarct. The rise in CT number of only 18.6 indicates diminished blood flow through this region. *B.* Sampling the myocardium further removed from the infarct shows a considerably greater flow with an increase in CT number of 36.5. The cardiac output can be calculated from a similar density curve in the left ventricle or ascending aorta. (*Courtesy D. Boyd, Imatron Corporation.*)

In this manner, successfully gated scans have been obtained within a period of 12 s.[6] Although some of the required angular views are missing, they are evenly distributed and can be compensated for by averaging data from adjacent views.[4]

More recently, a cardiac CT scanner with exposure times in the millisecond range has become available. Instead of driving the x-ray tube around the gantry, rotation of the x-ray source is achieved electronically. Two contiguous 8-mm-thick slices, 8 mm apart, can be obtained from one 50-msec exposure.[7] The interscan time is extremely short, and rigid, repetitive scans can be obtained. The potential of this equipment for collecting both anatomic and physiological cardiac data seems great (Fig. 111-1).

Technique

In order to accentuate the distinction between the blood in the heart and the cardiac wall, cardiac scans are usually performed in conjunction with an intravenous injection of angiographic contrast media. The amount and concentration of the contrast utilized, and the rate of injection, are determined by the purpose for the scan, as well as the age, size, and condition of the patient.

There are basically two protocols for scanning the heart. When anatomic information is the primary goal, scans are made at successive levels so that the entire heart and the proximal portions of the great vessels are included. An infusion of 150 to 300 ml of 30 percent contrast material, for adults, dripped in over 7 to 10 min, provides satisfactory opacification of the entire blood pool.

More rapid, dynamic scanning is utilized for rapidly moving structures or when the needed information is dependent on blood flow (Fig. 111-2). A single scan level is chosen and, following the bolus intravenous injection of 76 percent contrast material, or its equivalent, multiple scans are obtained at a rate of 10 to 20 per minute. A sufficiently rapid injection of contrast material can usually be accomplished manually, through an 18-gauge needle.

The risks of CT scanning of the heart are essentially those associated with the intravascular injection of iodinated contrast material. The radiation dosage with current equipment is well within acceptable limits, about 1 rad being delivered to the thin cross-section of the thorax imaged for each "slice." The radiation exposure to the gonads and other sensitive organs is low because of the extreme collimation of the x-ray beam.

Quantitation

The methodology for determining cardiac chamber volumes from multiple CT sections through the heart has been shown to be valid and accurate.[8] End-diastolic volumes can be adequately calculated from ungated, contrast-enhanced scans, but gating is required in order to obtain end-systolic measurements.[9]

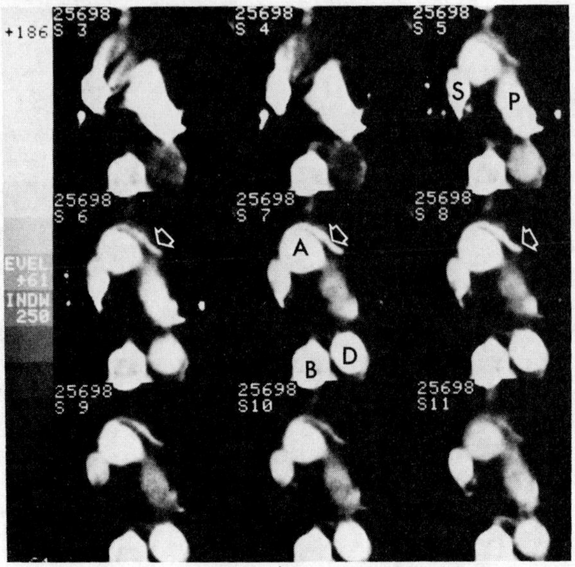

FIGURE 111-2 Coronary bypass graft, dynamic scan at level of the aortic root. Following a rapid intravenous injection of 25 ml of contrast material, the bypass graft (open arrow) is visualized arising from the anterior surface of the aorta (A) and running transversely in the plane of the section. S = superior vena cava, P = pulmonary artery, B = vertical body, D = descending aorta. *(From M. J. Lipton and C. B. Higgins, Evaluation of Ischemic Heart Disease by Computerized Transmission Tomography, Radiol. Clin. North Am., 18:557, 1980. Reproduced with permission from the publisher and author.)*

Ejection fraction, stroke output, and other volume-dependent parameters can then be easily calculated.

The sharp delineation of the myocardium between the opacified blood within the heart and the radiolucent air in the lungs, and fat around the heart, allow an accurate measurement of ventricular muscle mass to be made from the CT scan.[10] On gated scans, regional thickening of the myocardium can be measured throughout the cardiac cycle[9,11] and plotted, providing a graphic means for evaluating segmental ventricular function. CT measurements have been used to demonstrate the limitation of myocardial contractility in ischemic heart disease in animals, and its relation to the degree of coronary narrowing.[12] Global or eccentric thickening associated with ventricular hypertrophy or a cardiomyopathy has also been well documented.[13]

Blood flow can be estimated from the serial images of a dynamic CT scan, much in the same way as with other indicator dilution techniques. The density of an area within the cross-sectional image of a vessel or cardiac chamber is measured on each of the series of sequential scans. A time-density curve can be developed from these data to provide an indication of the rate of appearance of an intravenous bolus of contrast material and the rate of clearing (Fig. 111-1). Such measurements made over the root of the aorta have been used to evaluate cardiac output.[14] Because of the newness of this technique it has, as yet, not been adequately validated in a clinical setting.

The lungs are routinely visualized on the same sections as the heart. By simple computer manipulation, an accurate measurement of lung density can be obtained from the cardiac scans.[15,16] A significant portion of the radiodensity of the lung is due to its water content. The density increases in proportion to the increase in intrapulmonary fluid. The CT scan, therefore, can be used as an indicator of congestive heart failure. The density of the lung correlates well with plain film findings, increasing as the pulmonary changes progress from minimal venous hypertension to frank alveolar edema.[17] However, after the chest has returned to normal in treated patients, there still may be CT evidence of increased lung water. CT is considerably more sensitive to the presence and degree of congestive failure than plain radiographs of the chest and also, it appears, to measurements of peripheral venous pressure and circulation time.[17]

Congenital Heart Disease

Other than rare, specific instances usually related to anomalies of the great vessels, CT scanning has not proven to be of practical value for the diagnosis of congenital heart disease. This is particularly true with infants and young children in whom, because of the small size of the heart and the rapid pulse rate, it is almost impossible to get sufficiently thin sections with adequate detail for diagnostic purposes. Large ventricular septal defects have been demonstrated in older children and adults by reformatting the image in an oblique plane, perpendicular to the ventricular septum. However, these examples are anecdotal and the needed clinical information must still be obtained by cardiac catheterization and angiography.

Coronary Artery Disease

Calcification of the Coronary Arteries

Because of its greater contrast resolution, CT is more sensitive for the detection of intimal calcific plaques than other radiographic techniques. Calcific plaques can be seen with scan times extending over more than one cardiac cycle, because they usually occur within the proximal portions of the coronary arteries at the base of the heart—an area that undergoes limited motion during the cardiac cycle. There are no adequate data regarding the sensitivity of CT for detection of coronary calcification as compared to that of carefully performed cardiac fluoroscopy. However, the radiation dosage to the patient will almost always be less with CT, and the success of the examination is not as dependent on the individual expertise and patience of the examining physician as is fluoroscopy. Cardiac CT, for the detection of coronary calcification, should be considered in younger patients with atypical chest pain, in whom the possibility of coronary artery disease is not sufficiently strong to warrant catheterization.

Myocardial Infarction

It is possible to detect and to quantify areas of myocardial ischemia on cross-sectional CT images. Edema of the myocardium is one of the first changes following coronary artery occlusion. Because the x-ray attenuation of the waterlogged tissue is significantly less than normal, the ischemic area can be demonstrated on unenhanced CT scans as a zone of increased radiolucency in the heart wall. This has been demonstrated in dogs within 2 h of occlusion of a coronary artery.[18] At first, the interface between the ischemic and normal myocardium is indistinct, but it becomes considerably sharper over the next 48 h.[19]

Infarcts as small as 1 cm in diameter have been demonstrated in dogs, and subendocardial infarcts distinguished from transmural ones.[20] If the infarct size is calculated from the zone of radiolucency, it will be underestimated by about 25 percent.

Visualization of an infarct is considerably improved by performing the scan with contrast enhancement. If radiopaque material is injected as a compact bolus and the heart scanned within 60 to 90 s, the contrast material acts as a perfusion marker. The normal myocardium shows an increase in density as it is perfused by the contrast-laden blood, while the infarct appears as a relatively radiolucent area.[21] The findings are comparable to those obtained with ^{201}Tl myocardial imaging. Both methods will routinely underestimate infarct size.[22]

About 2 to 3 min after the bolus injection, the infarct itself begins to enhance and becomes more radiopaque than the surrounding normal myocardium. This effect seems to reach a peak at 10 to 15 min.[11,23] The enhancement effect is not seen in infarcts younger than 2 h and seems to be due to a loss of integrity of the myocardial cell membrane, so that the iodinated contrast agent can enter the damaged cell.[24,25] The distribution of contrast material in the myocardium and infarct is similar to that using ^{99m}Tc pyrophosphate.[26]

Persistent contrast enhancement of the infarct has been demonstrated in lesions at least 30 days old. Thus, it is a sign of myocardial damage but not an indicator of the acuteness of the lesion. If the zone of enhancement is considered a part of the infarct, estimation of infarct size and volume is very accurate[23,27] and more reliable than estimations using scintigraphic techniques.[22] In dogs with a patchy or subendocardial infarct, a zone of enhancement often cannot be defined. However, in these cases, the infarcts usually become apparent as perfusion defects during the first pass of a bolus of contrast material.[23]

Gated scans that provide end-systolic and end-diastolic images can be used to evaluate myocardial function.[9,12,28] In dogs, as the coronary flow falls below 33 percent of normal, a decrease in systolic wall thickening can be demonstrated in the ischemic area as well as a compensatory thickening of the normal myocardium. The changes are progressive as coronary flow is further limited. With severe, acute ischemia, thinning of the involved ventricular wall in systole, as well as diastole, occurs.

Almost all the above work has been done with laboratory animals, although limited experience with patients is confirmatory.[4] There are several practical drawbacks to the use of CT for the study of patients with acute myocardial infarction. The patient must be transported from the intensive care unit, and it is necessary for him or her to be able to lie relatively flat and still for at least a half-hour. Furthermore, the patient must be able to tolerate the infusion of a sizable volume of iodinated contrast material. Experimental data, however, suggest that the CT examination may provide important information regarding the viability of the damaged myocardium. When studied with contrast-enhanced scans, animals with irreversible myocardial changes all showed persistent zones of contrast enhancement in the periphery of the ischemic area, while those with myocardial injury due to more transient ischemia did not.[29]

Ventricular Aneurysm

The advantages of CT for the study of ventricular aneurysms as compared to echocardiography or radionuclide studies lie in its considerably greater spatial resolution and the ability to reformat the cross-sectional images along other body planes. In this manner, the relation of the aneurysm to the normal ventricular wall can be completely mapped out. An infusion of contrast material is needed to delineate the wall of the aneurysm and to evaluate the surrounding myocardium. This will also serve to highlight the presence of thrombi within the aneurysm.

Coronary Artery Bypass

Although portions of the coronary arteries can be seen on contrast-enhanced scans, especially when they course in the plane of the section, CT, for the most part, is of no value for detection of lesions of the native coronary circulation. However, it is of considerable use for evaluation of the patency of coronary bypass grafts. The grafts can be routinely visualized on scans, because they are not tortuous and course vertically so that they are viewed in cross-section. The grafts are usually of greater caliber than the coronary arteries and can be imaged near the root of the aorta, where blurring due to cardiac motion is minimal.

The preferred level for scanning is in the region of the aortic root, above the level of the native coronary arteries. The coronary arteries are excluded to prevent mistaking one for a graft. Determination of the scan level is greatly simplified if ostial markers were affixed at the time of surgery. Adequate studies can be obtained with routine scanning protocols, but dynamic scanning is preferred (Fig. 111-2). Although only the proximal portion of the graft is visualized, a valid estimation of patency can be made because, despite the level at which a graft is occluded, there almost always is retrograde thrombosis back to its aortic origin. The bypass graft usually cannot be identified without the injection of contrast material. If the graft is patent, its density will increase and become maximum at, or close to, the time of peak of opacification of the ascending aorta. Absence of opacification is presumptive evidence of graft closure. Both false-positive and false-negative results have been reported.[30] In general, a diagnosis of graft patency seems to be more reliable than one of graft occlusion.

The accuracy rate of CT in evaluating graft patency in recently reported series varies between 79 percent and 97 percent of grafts studied, using angiography as the standard. However, since many patients have multiple grafts, the percentage of patients who are completely and correctly evaluated is significantly smaller. CT is most accurate in evaluating grafts to the left anterior descending coronary artery[31] and least accurate with circumflex coronary grafts, particularly when they are routed behind the aorta.[30]

CT evaluation of internal mammary artery bypasses is not as satisfactory as the evaluation of vein grafts.[32] The artery is smaller than a vein graft and is often partially obscured by the radiopaque surgical clips used to occlude its intercostal branches.

There are several drawbacks to the use of CT for the evaluation of graft patency. Although complete obstruction of the main graft can be recognized in the majority of cases, the distal portion of the graft is not visualized. Thus, one limb of a Y-graft or one segment of a jump-graft may be occluded without any abnormality being noted on the CT scan. Furthermore, because the scan does not show the entire length of the graft, significant stenosis can be present and go completely undetected.[31] Serial densitometric measurements on a dynamic scanner have been used to predict blood flow within the graft, but this technique is still under study.[32]

Despite the success rate of CT in assessing the patency of coronary grafts, its associated error rate and the limited information regarding flow within the graft and local stenoses make it an inappropriate technique for the study of symptomatic patients. The role of CT, at present, appears to be primarily that of a noninvasive screening method for evaluating patency of grafts in asymptomatic patients.[33,34]

Intracardiac Masses

Tumors

Echocardiography is considered to be the diagnostic procedure of choice for evaluation of cardiac tumors. It is of most value with pedunculated lesions such as atrial myxomas which exhibit considerable motion during the cardiac cycle. The accuracy of echocardiography decreases when dealing with malignant tumors that infiltrate the myocardium and do not produce a sizable intraluminal component. These lesions can be reliably demonstrated by cardiac CT. In addition, CT will show the extent of the tumor and its distribution[35,36] and may provide an indication as to the tissue type.

Thrombi

CT has proven to be considerably more sensitive in the detection of intracardiac thrombi than two-dimensional echocardiography.[37,38] Contrast-enhanced scans are required for a satisfactory study, the thrombi appearing as lucent filling defects within the opacified chamber. Although clots that present as intraluminal masses are equally detected by CT and ultrasound, CT is also able to reliably identify mural thrombi which conform to the curve of the cardiac wall. The same is true of thrombi in the left atrial appendage, an area very difficult to evaluate by echocardiography.

Pericardium

The normal pericardium appears on a CT scan as a curvilinear structure, about 2 mm in thickness, best seen anteriorly, in front of the right ventricle. Its soft tissue density is visible between the more radiolucent mediastinal fat outside the pericardium and the epicardial fat between the visceral pericardium and the myocardium. The thickness of the pericardial stripe thus represents the combined shadows of the visceral layer of pericardium, the parietal pericardium, and the fluid present in the pericardial sac (Fig. 111-3). The normal pericardium can be identified on about 95 percent of scans.[33,40] It is least likely to be visualized in children or in adults with sparse mediastinal fat.

Pericardial Effusion

Although echocardiography remains the prime diagnostic method for the detection of pericardial fluid, CT should be considered, at the least, a valuable adjunct. The sensitivity of CT in detection of pericardial effusion is comparable to that of echocardiography.[41] Experimentally, as little as 50 ml of fluid in the pericardial sac can be reliably demonstrated.[42] With the patient supine, small amounts of pericardial fluid tend to localize behind the left ventricle. As the volume of fluid increases, it extends laterally and anteriorly, eventually enveloping the heart. Fluid in the anterior portion of the pericardial space is seen as a thickened pericardial stripe between the mediastinal and epicardial fat layers. Measurement of the radiodensity of the fluid can provide an indication of its nature. Blood and exudates have a high attenuation coefficient and have densities approaching that of soft tissue, while transudates and chyle are considerably less radiodense.[43]

False-positive results from echocardiography can occur when soft tissue is interposed between the epicardial surface of the heart and the adjacent lung. Erroneous echocardiographic diagnoses of pericardial effusion have been reported from metastatic disease involving the pericardium, and pleural effusions and hernias, among others.[41,44] All these conditions will be correctly identified on a CT scan. The scan is also of use as a guide for pericardiocentesis, especially in the postoperative patient where the fluid is frequently loculated due to adhesions (Fig. 111-4).[45]

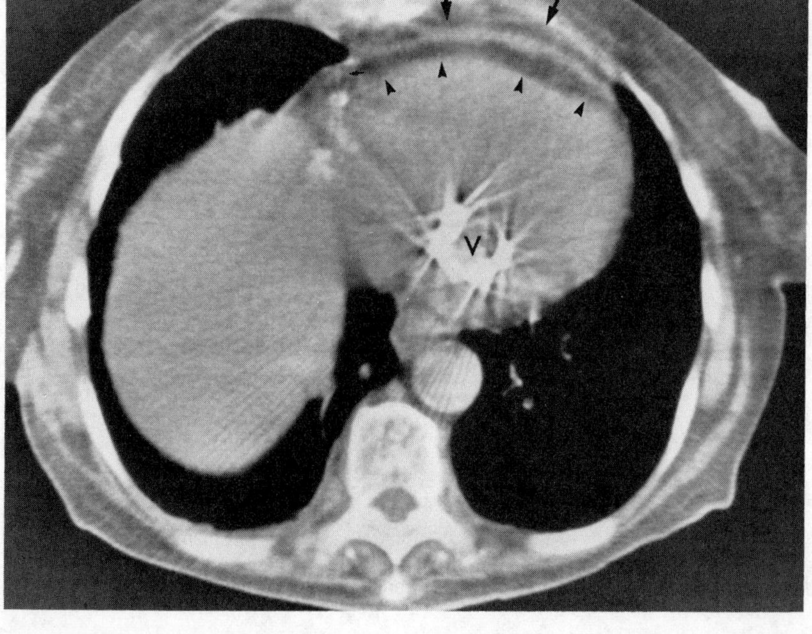

FIGURE 111-3 Pericardial thickening. Seventy-seven-year-old female, post-mitral valve replacement. A scan at the level of the mitral heterograft (V) shows thickening of the anterior pericardium between the more lucent epicardial fat (arrowheads) and retrosternal fat (arrows).

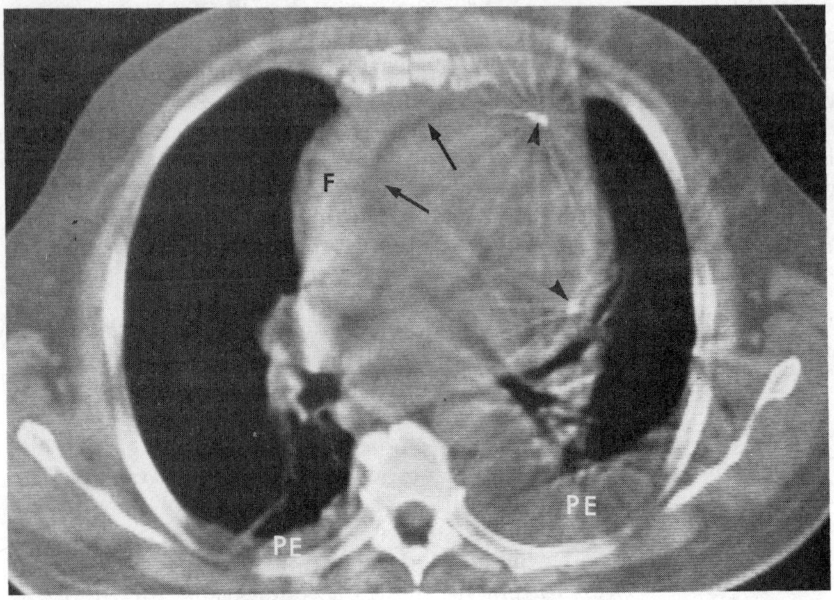

FIGURE 111-4 Loculated pericardial effusion. Fifty-three-year-old male examined because of suspected mediastinitis, 2 weeks following coronary bypass surgery. There is a loculated collection of fluid in the right side of the pericardial space (F), outlined by the air-containing lung laterally and the epicardial fat (arrows) medially. Bilateral pleural effusions are also present (PE). The two densities (arrowheads) with streak artifacts are surgical clips.

Constrictive Pericarditis

The normal pericardium becomes somewhat thicker near its caudal insertion and may measure between 3 to 4 mm in this area.[46] Short segments of local thickening are encountered normally, but diffuse thickening of the pericardium greater than 4 mm is definitely abnormal (Fig. 111-5). Although such thickening is most often the result of inflammatory disease, it can also be caused by Hodgkin's disease, metastatic involvement of the pericardium, or radiation reaction.[39] In some instances, it is difficult to distinguish between a thickened pericardium and a small collection of pericardial fluid on the CT scan.

Differentiation between constrictive pericarditis and a restrictive cardiomyopathy is often not possible on clinical grounds. Although echocardiographic findings have been described for each condition, there is considerable overlap, and they cannot be considered specific for either disease.[47] Even cardiac catheterization may not be able to conclusively demonstrate whether the impaired diastolic filling of the ventricles is due to encasement by a thickened pericardium or to the limited distensibility of a diseased myocardium. The key diagnostic determinant between the two conditions is the presence or absence of thickening of the pericardium. CT scans in constrictive pericarditis demonstrate significant and, usually, diffuse pericardial thickening, while the pericardium tends to be normal in cases of cardiomyopathy.[40,46,47]

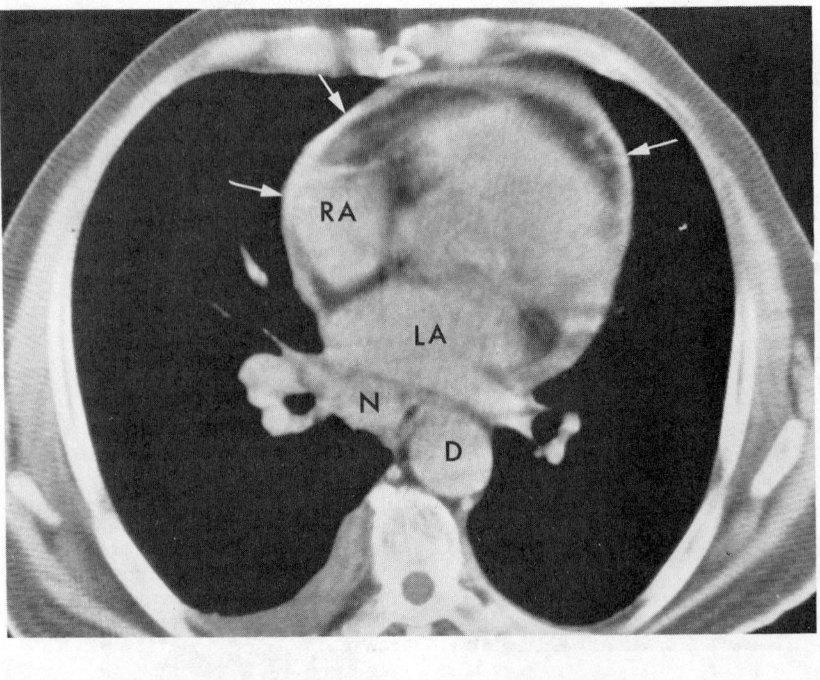

FIGURE 111-5 Chronic pericarditis. Fifty-five-year-old patient with bronchogenic carcinoma. A section at the level of the left atrium (LA) shows the pericardium as a thickened rind (arrows) surrounding the heart. At surgery, the pericardium was markedly thickened due to chronic inflammatory disease. A small effusion was also present. There was no evidence of neoplasm involving the pericardium. LV = left pulmonary vein, RA = right atrium, D = descending aorta, N = enlarged subcarinal nodes.

The converse, however, is not true. It is not possible to predict from the CT appearance of a thickened pericardium whether or not the hemodynamic manifestations of constrictive pericarditis are present. Not uncommonly, patients with fairly marked thickening of the pericardium are completely asymptomatic relative to the heart.

In constrictive pericarditis, the inferior vena cava is often considerably dilated. Normally, the cava, near its entance into the right atrium, is the same size as, or only slightly larger than, the descending aorta at that level. Cavae as large as three times the diameter of the aorta have been reported in cases of constrictive pericarditis.[40] A similar finding can be seen with pericardial effusion if the fluid is sufficient to produce cardiac tamponade. Distension of the superior vena cava is much less noticeable.

Congenital Lesions

Unless a pericardial cyst is positioned so that it is accessible to examination by ultrasound, it is rarely possible to establish a secure diagnosis preoperatively except by CT scanning. This is particularly true with a mass in the cardiophrenic angle. These may represent a pericardial cyst, collections of mediastinal fat, or an enlarged lymph node involved with malignant lymphoma or metastatic disease. They can be distinguished by their CT densities.[48]

The pericardial cyst appears as a circumscribed mass abutting on the cardiac silhouette and filled with a fluid that has a radiodensity similar to that of water. A lipoma or collection of mediastinal fat will be more radiolucent than water, while an enlarged node is considerably denser.

Several cases of partial absence of the pericardium that have been examined by CT have been reported.[46,49] The findings, however, were appreciated only in retrospect, and it is not certain whether they are valid or reliable.

Great Vessels

Dissecting Aneurysm

Until recently, selective aortography was the only reliable technique for establishing, or excluding, the diagnosis of dissecting aneurysm. This can now be accomplished, in most cases, with equal accuracy by contrast-enhanced CT scans.[50,51] Although the correct diagnosis can often be made from serial scans through the thorax during the infusion of contrast material, multiple rapid sections at a fixed level, such as the mid-ascending aorta, following a bolus injection of contrast media, are preferable.[52]

The CT criteria for the diagnosis of dissecting aneurysm are essentially the same as those used with aortography.[53] Demonstration of two opacified channels within the aorta separated by a radiolucent line of dissected intima is pathognomonic (Fig. 111-6). Actually, visualization of the intimal flap, even though opacification of a second channel is uncertain, has the same significance. The dissected intima would not be seen as a lucent line unless there was opacified blood in both channels.[54] If there is no demonstrable flow in the false channel, the distinction between a fusiform aneurysm with lamellar thrombus and a dissecting hematoma may be difficult, unless calcific plaques are present to indicate the position of the aortic intima.[55] The cross-sectional view of the aorta, however, is helpful, as a lamellar thrombus usually tends to follow the curve of the aortic wall, while a dissected hematoma is more likely to bulge inward and deform the contrast-filled lumen. Inward displacement of intimal calcification, indicating an abnormally thickened aortic wall, is a

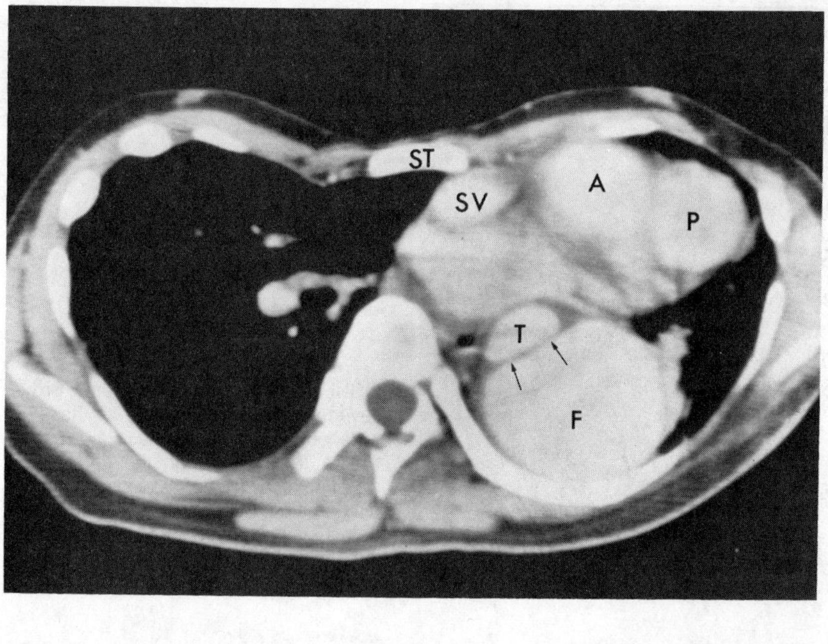

FIGURE 111-6 Type III dissecting aneurysm, contrast-enhanced scan. Nineteen-year-old male with Marfan's syndrome. A section through the aortic root. The descending aorta is markedly dilated and is divided into two channels, separated by a strip of soft tissue (arrows) representing the dissected intima. The false channel (F) lies posteriorly and to the left and compresses the true lumen (T). The ascending aorta (A) is not involved. The heart is displaced because of the severe pectus deformity. SV = superior vena cava, P = pulmonary trunk, ST = sternum.

valid sign of dissection. However, this sign cannot be applied with equal certainty to all parts of the aorta. Because of partial volume averaging, a calcific plaque which is actually located at a slightly different level may be projected on sections through the aortic arch[52] and mimic inward displacement of the intima. The sign is reliable, however, when seen in the ascending or descending aorta, where the vessel is viewed in cross-section.

The major advantage of CT over aortography is that it is a noninvasive procedure. In addition, its greater sensitivity to density differences allows the detection of small amounts of opacified blood in the false channel, thus indicating flow when none can be detected on the aortogram. However, the aortogram does provide more data. The extent of the dissection and its extension into major arterial branches are easily evaluated, the relation of the arteries to the true and false channels can be determined, the intimal tears can often be located, and the presence and severity of aortic valvular regurgitation documented. Furthermore, in patients with severe aortic insufficiency or those who are in shock, the forward flow of blood into the aorta may be quite slow, so that opacification from an intravenous bolus is less than optimal.

Because of these considerations, aortography is still considered the diagnostic method of choice for the acutely ill patient for whom surgery is considered, or the patient in shock. In other patients, CT will provide an equivalent diagnostic yield. Because it is noninvasive, CT is the ideal method for serially following patients after surgical or medical treatment.[56]

Anomalies

Although anomalies of the aortic arch and great arteries can be demonstrated on CT scans,[57] simpler and less costly methods, such as a chest film with barium in the esophagus, are adequate for most purposes. The main exception is in the diagnosis of a double aortic arch. The two levels of the arch tend to lie in a cross-sectional plane and can be well delineated as they encircle the trachea and esophagus (Fig. 111-7).[57,58] It is important, however, to be familiar with the appearance of arch anomalies on the CT scan, as they are often unsuspected in patients being studied because of a widened mediastinum.[59]

Azygos continuation of the inferior vena cava most often occurs as an isolated anomaly, although it may be part of the spectrum of abnormalities associated with polysplenia. The azygos vein is considerably dilated and often is mistaken for a mass in the right tracheobronchial angle on a frontal chest film. The correct diagnosis is obvious on a CT scan, even without the use of contrast material. A large azygos vein can be identified just in front of the spine to the right of the aorta at the level of the diaphragm or slightly higher. Just above the carina, the vein is seen to arch forward to enter the superior vena cava.[60] Cuts through the upper abdomen, above the level of the renal vein, will show an absence of the inferior vena cava.

References

1. Ringertz, H. G., Skioldebrand, C. G., Refsum, H., Tyberg, J. V., Napel, S. A., and Lipton, M. J.: A Comparison between the Information in Gated and Nongated Cardiac CT Images, *J. Comput. Assist. Tomogr.*, 6:933, 1982.
2. Moore, S. C., Judy, P. F., Garnic, J. D., Kambic, G. X., Bonk, F., Cochran, G., Margosian, P., McCroskey, W., and Foote, F.: Prospectively Gated Cardiac Computed Tomography, *Med. Phys.*, 10:945, 1983..
3. Berninger, W. H., Redington, R. W., Doherty, P., Lipton, M. J., and Carlsson, E.: Gated Cardiac Scanning: Canine Studies, *J. Comput. Assist. Tomogr.*, 5:155, 1979.
4. Oyama, Y., Uji, T., Hirayama, T., Inada, Y., Ishikawa, T., and Fujii, M.: Gated Cardiac Imaging Using a Continuously

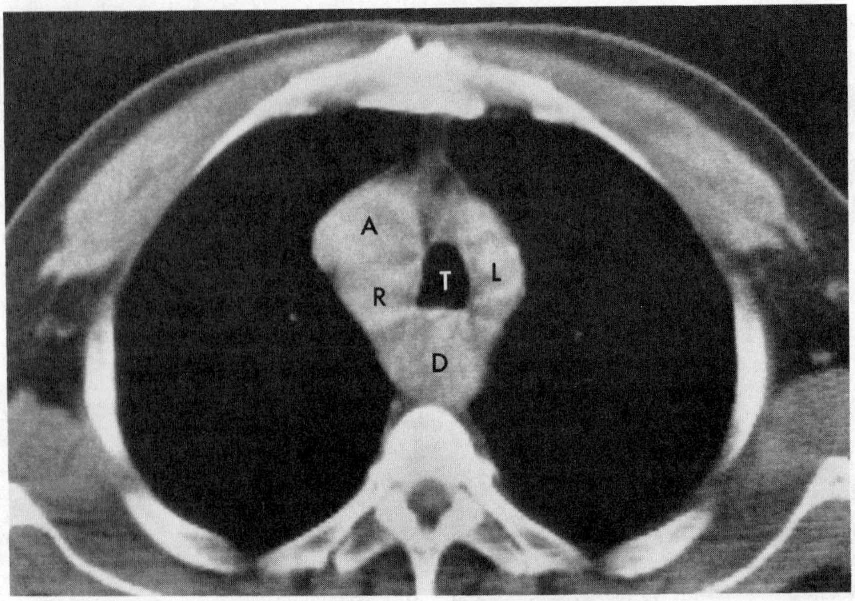

FIGURE 111-7 Double aortic arch. Sixty-seven-year-old male found to have a widened mediastinum on a routine chest film. A section through the upper mediastinum shows a normal-sized right arch (R) and a smaller left arch (L). Both arise from the ascending aorta (A) and encircle the trachea (T) to join the descending aorta (D).

Rotating CT Scanner: Clinical Evaluation of 91 Patients, *AJR,* 141:865, 1984.

5. Garnic, J. D., Moore, S. C., Judy, P. F., Harrington, D. P., Lois, J., and Levin, D. C.: Prospectively Gated Cardiac CT. Preliminary Results in Normal and Postinfarction Animal Models, *Invest. Radiol.,* 18:419, 1983.
6. Cipriano, P., Nassi, M., and Brody, W. R.: Clinically Applicable Gated Cardiac Computed Tomography, *AJR,* 140:604, 1983.
7. Boyd, D. P., Gould, R. G., Quinn, J. R., Sparks, R., Stanley, J. H., and Herrmannsfeldt, W. B.: A Proposed Dynamic Cardiac 3-D Densitometer for Easy Detection and Evaluation of Heart Disease, *I.E.E. Trans. Nucl. Sci.,* 26:2724, 1979.
8. Lipton, M. J., Hayashi, T. T., Boyd, D. P., and Carlsson, E.: Measurement of Left Ventricular Cast Volume by Computed Tomography, *Radiology,* 129: 419, 1978.
9. Mattrey, R. F., Slutsky, R. A., Long, S. A., and Higgins, C. B.: In Vivo Assessment of Left Ventricular Wall and Chamber Dynamics during Transient Myocardial Ischemia Using Prospectively ECG-gated Computerized Transmission Tomography, *Circulation,* 67:1245, 1983.
10. Skioldebrand, C. G., Lipton, M. J., Mavroudis, C., and Hayashi, T. T.: Determination of Left Ventricular Mass by Computed Tomography, *Am. J. Cardiol.,* 49:63, 1982.
11. Skioldebrand, C. G., Ovenfors, C.-O., Mavroudis, C., and Lipton, M. J.: Assessment of Ventricular Wall Thickness in Vivo by Computed Transmission Tomography, *Circulation,* 61:960, 1980.
12. Mattrey, R. F., and Higgins, C. B.: Detection of Regional Myocardial Dysfunction during Ischemia with Computerized Tomography. Documentation and Physiologic Basis, *Invest. Radiol.,* 17:329, 1982.
13. Lackner, K., Hahn, N., Reske, S. N., Eichelkraut, W., and Thurn, P.: Der Experimentelle Myokardinfarkt im Computertomogramm, *RoFo,* 137:152, 1982.
14. Herfkens, R. J., Axel, L., Lipton, M. J., Napel, S., Berninger, W., and Redington, R.: Measurement of Cardiac Output by Computed Transmission Tomography, *Invest. Radiol.,* 17:550, 1982.
15. Wegener, O. H., Koeppe, P., and Oeser, H.: Measurement of Lung Density by Computed Tomography, *J. Comput. Assist. Tomogr.,* 2:263, 1978.
16. Rosenblum, L. J., Mauceri, R. A., Wellenstein, D. E., Thomas, F. D., Bassano, D. A., Raasch, B. N., Chamberlain, C. C., and Heitzman, E. R.: Density Patterns in the Normal Lung as Determined by Computed Tomography, *Radiology,* 137:409, 1980.
17. Morooka, N., Watanake, S., Masuda, Y., and Inagaki, Y.: Estimation of Pulmonary Water Distribution and Pulmonary Congestion by Computed Tomography, *Jpn. Heart J.,* 23:697, 1982.
18. Jennings, R. B., Sommers, H. M., Kaltenbach, J. P., and West, J. J.: Electrolyte Alterations in Acute Myocardial Ischemic Injury, *Circ. Res.,* 14:260, 1964.
19. Higgins, C.B., Siemers, P. T., Schmidt, W., and Newell, J. D.: Evaluation of Myocardial Ischemic Damage at Various Ages by Computerized Transmission Tomography. Time-Dependent Effects of Contrast Material, *Circulation,* 60:284, 1979.
20. Lipton, M. J., and Higgins, C.B.: Evaluation of Ischemic Heart Disease by Computerized Transmission Tomography, *Radiol. Clin. North Am.,* 18:557, 1980.
21. Doherty, P. W., Skioldebrand, C. G., Redington, R. W., Berninger, W. H., and Lipton, M. J.: Measurement of Regional Changes in Myocardial Perfusion using Dynamic Computed Tomography and Contrast Medium, *Acta Radiol. Diagn.,* 24:297, 1983.
22. Gerber, K. H., and Higgins, C. B.: Quantitation of Size of Myocardial Infarctions by Computerized Transmission Tomography. Comparison with Hot-spot and Cold-spot Radionuclide Scans, *Invest. Radiol.,* 18:238, 1983.
23. Doherty, P. W., Lipton, M. J., Berninger, W. H., Skoldebrand, C. G., Carlsson, E., and Redington, R. W.: Detection and Quantitation of Myocardial Infarction in Vivo Using Transmission Computed Tomography, *Circulation,* 63:597, 1981.
24. Abraham, J. L., Higgins, C. B., and Newell, J. D.: Uptake of Iodinated Contrast Material in Ischemic Mycoardium as an Indicator of Loss of Cellular Membrane Integrity, *Am. J. Pathol.,* 101:319, 1980.
25. Newell, J. D., Higgins, C. B., and Abraham, J. L.: Uptake of Iodinated Contrast Material by the Ischemically Damaged Myocardial Cell, *Invest. Radiol.,* 17:61, 1982.
26. Higgins, C. B., Hagen, P., Newell, J. D., Schmidt, W., and Haigler, F.: Contrast Enhancement of Myocardial Infarction: Dependence on Necrosis and Residual Blood Flow and the Relationship to Distribution of Scintigraphic Imaging Agents, *Circulation,* 65:739, 1982.
27. Slutsky, R. A., Mattrey, R. F., Long, S. A., and Higgins, C. B.: In Vivo Estimation of Myocardial Infarct Size and Left Ventricular Function by Prospectively Gated Computerized Transmission Tomography, *Circulation,* 67:759, 1983.
28. Lackner, K., and Thurn, P.: Computed Tomography of the Heart: ECG-gated and Continuous Scans, *Radiology,* 140:413, 1981.
29. Newell, J. D., Mayr, W., Gerber, K. H., and Higgins, C. B.: Computerized Tomographic (CT) Appearance of the Myocardium after Reversible and Irreversible Ischemic Injury, *Invest. Radiol.,* 17:544, 1982.
30. Godwin, J. D., Califf, R. M., Korobkin, M., Moore, A. V., Breiman, R. S., and Kong, Y.: Clinical Value of Coronary Bypass Graft Evaluation with CT, *AJR,* 140:649, 1983.
31. Daniel, W. G., Dohring, W., Stender, H.-S., and Lichtlen, P. R.: Value and Limitations of Computed Tomography in Assessing Aortocoronary Bypass Graft Patency, *Circulation,* 67:983, 1983.
32. Brundage, B. H., Lipton, M. J.: What is the Role of CT Scanning of the Heart? Controversies in Coronary Artery Disease, *Cardiovasc. Clin.,* 13:91, 1983.
33. Ullyot, D. J., Turley, K., McKay, C. R., Brundage, B. H., Lipton, M. J., and Ebert, P. A.: Assessment of Saphenous Vein Graft Patency by Contrast-Enhanced Computed Tomography, *J. Thorac. Cardiovasc. Surg.,* 83:512, 1982.
34. Albrechtsson, V., Stahl, E., and Tylen, V.: Evaluation of Coronary Artery Bypass Graft Patency with Computed Tomography, *J. Comput. Assist. Tomogr.,* 5:822, 1981.
35. Niehues, B., Heuser, L., Jansen, W., and Hilger, H. H.: Noninvasive Detection of Intracardiac Tumors by Ultrasound and Computed Tomography, *Cardiovasc. Intervent. Radiol.,* 6:30, 1983.
36. Godwin, J. D., Axel, L., Adams, J. R., Schiller, N. B., Simpson, Jr., P. C., and Gertz, E. W.: Computed Tomography: A New Method for Diagnosing Tumor of the Heart, *Circulation,* 63:448, 1981.
37. Nair, C. K., Sketch, M. H., Mahoney, P. D., Lynch, J. D., Mooss, A. N., and Kenney, N. P.: Detection of Left Ventricular Thrombi by Computerized Tomography. A Preliminary Report, *Br. Heart J.,* 45:535, 1981.
38. Tomoda, H., Hoshai, M., Furuya, H., Kuribayashi, S., Ootaki, M., Matsuyama, S., Koide, H., Kawada, S., and Shotsu, A.: Evaluation of Intracardiac Thrombus with Computed Tomography, *Am. J. Cardiol.,* 51:843, 1983.
39. Silverman, P. M., Harell, G. S., Korobkin, M.: Computed Tomography of the Abnormal Pericardium, *AJR,* 140:1125, 1983.
40. Doppman, J. L., Rienmuller, R., Lissner, J., Cyran, J., Bolte, H.-D., Strauer, B. E., and Hellwig, H.: Computed Tomography in Constrictive Pericardial Disease, *J. Comput. Assist. Tomogr.,* 5:1, 1981.
41. Isner, J. M., Carter, B. L., Bankoff, M. S., Konstam, M. A., and Salem, D. N.: Computed Tomography in the Diagnosis of Pericardial Disease, *Ann. Intern. Med.,* 97:473, 1982.
42. Wong, B. Y. S., Lee, K. R., and MacArthur, R. I.: Diagnosis of Pericardial Effusion by Computed Tomography, *Chest,* 81:177, 1982.
43. Tomoda, H., Hoshai, M., Furuya, H., Oeda, Y., Matsumoto, S., Tanabe, T., Tamachi, H., Sasamoto, H., Koide, S., Kuribayashi, S., and Matsuyama, S.: Evaluation of Pericardial

Effusion with Computed Tomography, *Am. Heart J.*, 99:701, 1980.
44. Come, P. C., Riley, M. F., and Fortuin, N. J.: Echocardiographic Mimicry of Periocardial Effusion, *Am. J. Cardiol.*, 47:365, 1981.
45. Higgins, C. B., Mattrey, R. F., and Shea, P.: CT Localization and Aspiration of Postoperative Pericardial Fluid Collection, *J. Comput. Assist. Tomogr.*, 7:734, 1984.
46. Moncada, R., Baker, M., Salinas, M., Demos, T. C., Churchill, R., Love, L., Reynes, S. C., Hale, D., Cardoso, M., Pifarre, R., and Gunnar, R. M.: Diagnostic Role of Computed Tomography in Pericardial Disease: Congenital Defects, Thickening, Neoplasms and Effusions, *Am. Heart J.*, 103:203, 1982.
47. Isner, J. M., Carter, B. L., Bankoff, M. S., Pastore, J. O., Ramaswamy, K., McAdam, K. P. W. J., and Salem, D. N.: Differentiation of Constrictive Pericarditis from Restrictive Cardiomyopathy by Computed Tomographic Imaging, *Am. Heart J.*, 105:1019, 1983.
48. Modic, M. T., and Janicki, P. C.: Computed Tomography of Mass Lesions of the Right Cardiophrenic Angle, *J. Comput. Assist. Tomogr.*, 4:521, 1980.
49. Baim, R. S., MacDonald, I. L., Wise, D. J., and Lenkei, S. C.: Computed Tomography of Absent Left Pericardium, *Radiology,* 135:127, 1980.
50. Thorsen, M. K., San Dretto, M. A., Lawson, T. L., Foley, W. D., Smith, D. F., and Berland, L. L.: Dissecting Aortic Aneurysms: Accuracy of Computed Tomographic Diagnosis, *Radiology,* 148:773, 1983.
51. Parienty, R. A., Couffinhal, J.-C., Wellers, M., Farge, C., and Pradel, J.: Computed Tomography Versus Aortography in Diagnosis of Aortic Dissection, *Cardiovasc. Intervent. Radiol.*, 5:285, 1982.
52. Godwin, J. D., Breiman, R. S., and Speckman, J. M.: Problems and Pitfalls in the Evaluation of Thoracic Aortic Dissection by Computed Tomography, *J. Comput. Assist. Tomogr.*, 6:750, 1982.
53. Heiberge, E., Wolverson, M., Sundaram, M., Connors, J., and Susman, N.: CT Findings in Thoracic Aortic Dissection, *AJR*, 136:13, 1981.
54. Baron, M. G.: Use of the Contrast Interface in Angiocardiography, *Circulation,* 43:311, 1971.
55. Godwin, J. D., and Korobkin, M.: Acute Disease of the Aorta. Diagnosis by Computed Tomography and Ultrasonography, *Radiol. Clin. North Am.*, 21:551, 1983.
56. Guthaner, D. F., Brody, W. R., and Miller, D. C.: Intravenous Aortography after Aortic Dissection Repair, *AJR*, 137:1019, 1981.
57. Webb, W. R., Gamsu, G., Speckman, J. M., Kaiser, J. A., Federle, M. P., and Lipton, M. J.: CT Demonstration of Mediastinal Aortic Arch Anomalies, *J. Comput. Assist. Tomogr.*, 6:445, 1982.
58. McLoughlin, M. J., Weisbrod, G., Wise, D. J., and Yeung, H. P. H.: Computed Tomography in Congenital Anomalies of the Aortic Arch and Great Vessels, *Radiology,* 138:399, 1981.
59. Baron, R. L., Levitt, R. G., Sagel, S. S., and Stanley, R. J.: Computed Tomography in the Evaluation of Mediastinal Widening, *Radiology,* 138:107, 1981.
60. Breckenridge, J. W., and Kinlaw, W. B.: Azygous Continuation of Inferior Vena Cava: CT Appearance, *J. Comput. Assist. Tomogr.*, 4:392, 1980.

112

Studies of the Carotid Artery and Its Branches

Ira F. Braun, M.D.
J. Timothy Fulenwider, M.D.
Robert B. Smith III, M.D.

A new ultrasonic technique for arterial visualization has been developed. . . . The method has some advantages over x-ray angiography in that it is completely free of risk and discomfort, is cheaper, and provides views that are unobtainable by any other means.

Mozersky, Hokanson, Baker, Sumner, and Strandness, 1971[1]

Brief Background

A variety of diagnostic tests are presently offered for the investigation of the patient with suspected cerebrovascular insufficiency, and innovations in both angiography and noninvasive vascular laboratory studies are being introduced with ever-increasing rapidity. While angiography remains the "gold standard," it is not infallible in carotid imaging. Indeed, some of the newer noninvasive examinations have allowed the question to be asked: "Is routine angiography necessary prior to carotid endarterectomy?"[2] Certainly, the responsible clinician should be well informed concerning the various diagnostic modalities available before ordering any of these expensive and, in some cases, risk-laden manipulations.

Technical Methods

Cerebral Angiography

In the patient with cerebrovascular disease, cerebral angiography is performed primarily to obtain anatomic information with regard to the morphology of the lesion, its surgical accessibility, and the presence or absence of collateral circulation.[3] Proper preoperative evaluation of patients should not be limited to a single carotid artery or to the extracranial circulation alone; a complete examination is desirable in most circumstances. In addition to visualization of the effects of atherosclerotic disease, angiography can also diagnose less common causes of arterial stenosis and occlusion such as fibromuscular dysplasia and spontaneous carotid dissection—rare but important causes of cerebral ischemia.[4–7] Opacification of the carotid arterial tree, whether by means of conventional angiography, intravenous digital subtraction angiography (IVDSA) or intraarterial digital subtraction angiography (IADSA), is the only means by which all the above can be accomplished.

Stenotic lesions secondary to atherosclerosis usually occur at vessel origins and bifurcations, the most common extracranial sites being internal and external carotid origins and the vertebral origin. Common intracranial sites include the carotid siphon, the basilar artery, and the proximal portion of the middle cerebral artery. In instances of flow-limiting carotid stenoses or occlusions, the phenomenon of collateralization can be seen angiographically. Occlusion of the common carotid usually recruits collaterals from the thyrocervical trunk and muscular branches of the vertebral artery anastomosing with external carotid branches. In instances of vertebral artery occlusion, the flow reverses in these tributaries. A commonly seen collateral pathway in internal carotid occlusion is supply to the ophthalmic artery from the distal internal maxillary artery, a branch of the external carotid system. The circle of Willis also provides important collateral pathways in these cases.

Visualization of the intracranial circulation is an essential part of a complete cerebrovascular examination and can influence decisions regarding therapy. A siphon stenosis, for example, may be of higher grade than the proximal lesion at the bifurcation (tandem lesions), in which case operation upon the extracranial carotid will fail to increase total cerebral blood flow. In addition to demonstration of intracranial stenoses and collaterals, Berry aneurysms or other vascular lesions may be visualized, the presence of which may alter the surgical approach; these lesions are themselves the source of distal emboli in some patients.[8]

Conventional angiography (Fig. 112-1) is usually performed via percutaneous puncture of the femoral artery followed by selective catheterization. The retrograde brachial and axillary routes and direct carotid puncture provide alternate methods in patients with occluded iliofemoral vessels. Digital subtraction angiography is a relatively new imaging technique which uses the fluoroscopic x-ray tube and intensifier rather than the film-screen combination. The image is read by a television camera, amplified, digitized, and stored into computer memory. Individual images containing contrast may then be electronically subtracted from others without contrast, instantaneously allowing visualization of vascular structures with exclusion of background bone and soft tissue. Intravascular contrast levels of as little as 2 percent may be detected, whereas conventional angiography requires up to 50 to 60 percent concentrations.[9] Intraarterial digital subtraction angiography (Fig. 112-2) has allowed a substantial reduction in the time involved per examination, the duration of which correlates directly with angiographic morbidity.[10] The superior contrast resolution of digital subtraction angiography over conventional angiography allows one to decrease the rate, volume, and concentration of contrast material. In addition to lessened renal toxicity, reduced cerebral toxicity is also likely in patients with an altered blood-brain barrier. Moreover, there is considerable saving in film costs: approximately $10 per examination using digital subtraction angiography, compared to $175 for conventional angiography. The diagnostic accuracy of intraarterial digital subtraction angiography compares quite favorably with conventional angiography. In a large study of 247 vessels, intraarterial digital subtraction angiography was felt to approach the quality of conventional angiography for

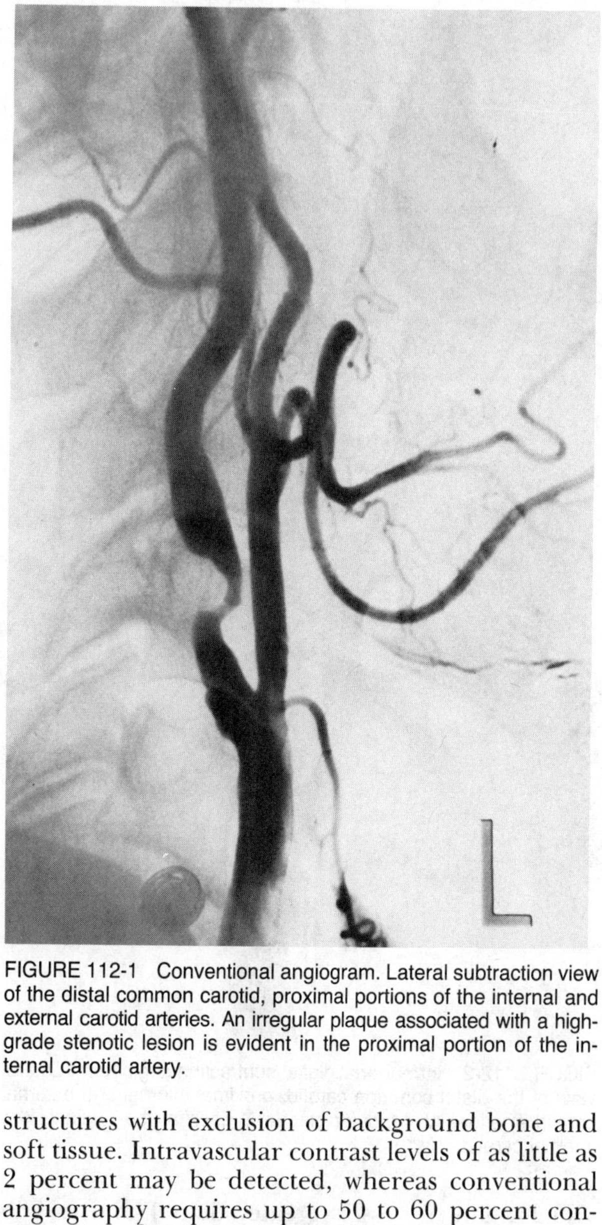

FIGURE 112-1 Conventional angiogram. Lateral subtraction view of the distal common carotid, proximal portions of the internal and external carotid arteries. An irregular plaque associated with a high-grade stenotic lesion is evident in the proximal portion of the internal carotid artery.

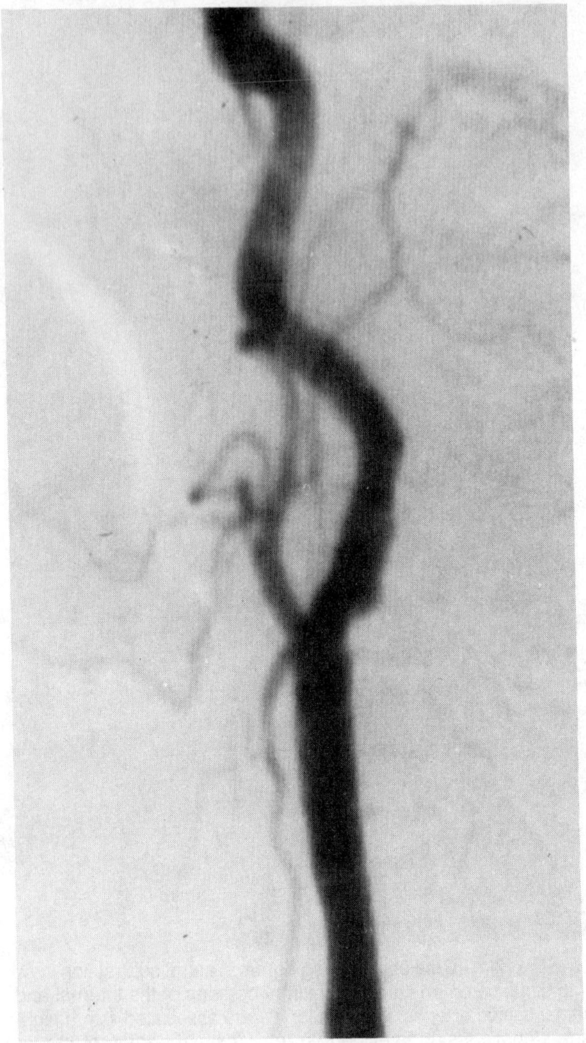

FIGURE 112-2 Intraarterial digital subtraction angiogram. Lateral view of the distal common carotid, proximal internal and external carotid arteries. An irregular plaque is seen at the origin of the internal carotid artery.

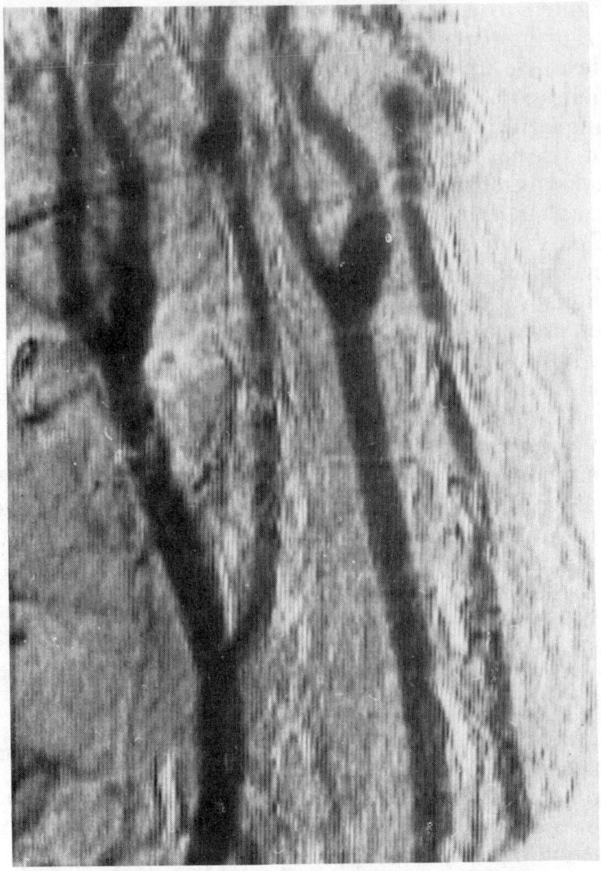

FIGURE 112-3 Intravenous digital subtraction angiogram. Oblique view of the cervical cephalic vessels. Note that all the arterial branches are visualized and imaged simultaneously with the intravenous technique. No definite abnormalities are demonstrated.

visualization of vessels greater than 1 mm in 236 instances.[11]

Intravenous digital subtraction angiography, on the other hand, has a limited role in the evaluation of patients with suspected cerebrovascular disease. This method involves the high-pressure bolus injection of a larger amount of contrast material into a central vein followed by fluoroscopic exposures. Inherent in the technique is simultaneous opacification of the carotid and vertebral systems, making vessel superimposition unavoidable (Fig. 112-3).[12] A reflex urge to swallow after injection of the bolus of contrast produces laryngeal motion and results in severe degradation of the image in many patients. This motion artifact usually obscures the carotid bifurcation and results in poor imaging of small irregularities. Clarity may also be degraded in patients with low cardiac output in whom slow circulation time causes progressive dilution of the contrast bolus. For these reasons, much of the initial enthusiasm for intravenous digital subtraction angiography as a screening method has abated.

Computed Tomography of the Head

The most important role of computed tomography (CT) in evaluating the patient with acute brain disease is to detect intracranial hemorrhage. This is easily accomplished in most patients and permits appropriate therapeutic measures to be deployed rapidly. The CT scan can often differentiate between bland and hemorrhagic cerebral infarct and may allow determination of the age of the infarct: acute, subacute, or chronic; an important consideration since both angiography and surgery may carry greater risk in the acute and subacute stages (Fig. 112-4).[13]

Although the exact role of the CT scan in the workup of cerebrovascular insufficiency is presently unsettled, the authors feel that most patients presenting with a neurologic deficit should have a CT scan performed prior to more invasive procedures, such as angiography. Patients with transient ischemic attacks (TIAs) may also benefit from a CT scan to exclude other, less common, causes for transient ischemic attacks such as tumor, large aneurysms, or arteriovenous malformation.

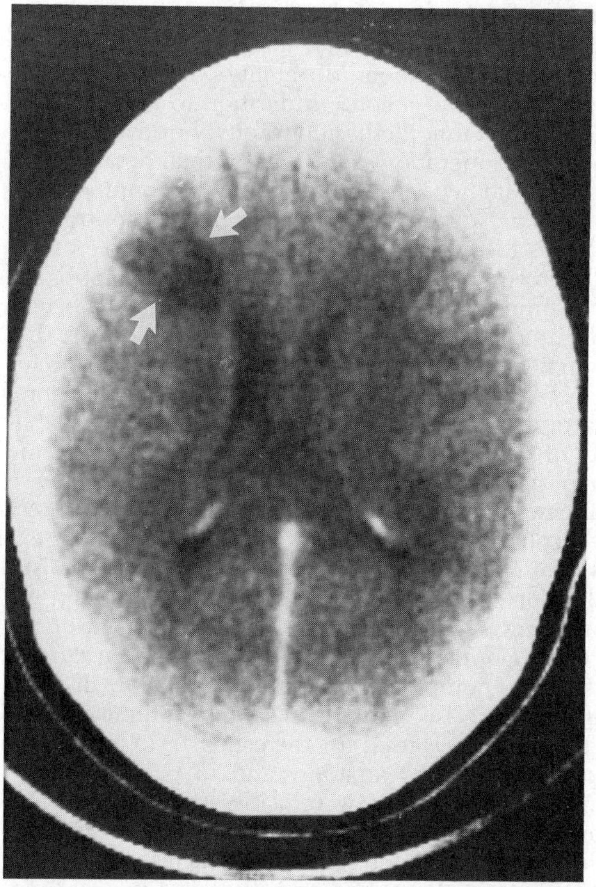

FIGURE 112-4 Noncontrast axial CT scan demonstrating a cortically oriented, wedge-shaped lucency situated in the right frontal lobe (arrows).

Noninvasive Vascular Laboratory Tests

Noninvasive vascular laboratory (NIVL) tests are designed primarily to detect flow-reducing stenoses (50 percent diameter reduction or 75 percent reduction of lumen area) by either indirect or direct modalities. Indirect noninvasive vascular laboratory tests rely on changes in the ophthalmic and supraorbital arterial pressures and flow directions. Theoretically, pressure-reducing stenoses of the carotid system should reduce the ophthalmic systolic pressure (OSP); however, any hemodynamically significant stenosis occurring between the aortic valve and the ophthalmic artery may also reduce the ophthalmic systolic pressure. In addition to the deficiency of anatomic specificity, the indirect noninvasive vascular laboratory tests may be normal even with severe carotid stenosis or occlusion since multiple craniocerebral collaterals may fully compensate for an obstructing carotid lesion. Direct noninvasive vascular laboratory tests interrogate the extracranial carotid bifurcation transcutaneously, usually employing ultrasonography for imaging with or without analysis of complex audiofrequency Doppler signals. While the indirect tests provide assessment of collateral carotid circulation, direct tests focus on the extracranial carotid artery and are insensitive in detecting intracranial flow-reducing lesions and assessing collateral circulation. Nonetheless, the direct tests are more sensitive to noncritical stenoses which are not flow-limiting. Neither direct nor indirect noninvasive vascular laboratory tests enjoy 100 percent accuracy in assessment of carotid stenoses, and neither reliably discriminate between the atherosclerotic, fibromuscular dysplastic or aneurysmal dissection etiologies responsible for carotid arterial flow reduction. Whether combinations of tests yield additive sensitivity while maintaining cost-effectiveness remains controversial. As Laing has stated, the increasing numbers of diagnostic procedures have created situations in which marginal benefits accrue from massive additional expenditures.[14]

Appropriate choices of noninvasive vascular laboratory cerebrovascular diagnostic tests are dependent upon knowledge of the diagnostic accuracy of each test (sensitivity, specificity) and the inherent limitations of the test chosen. Sensitivity refers to the probability that the test will be positive when the disease is present (true positive); specificity is the probability that the test will be negative when the disease is absent (true negative). In a population with a low prevalence of carotid disease, a screening test with high specificity is desirable to avoid unnecessary arteriography; however, when the prevalence of carotid occlusion is high, a screening test with high sensitivity should be chosen to avoid missing significant disease. A combination of tests dependent upon different principles is theoretically appealing; however, criteria of positivity for the "test battery" when individual tests disagree may enhance sensitivity at the expense of specificity; whereas criteria of "test battery" positivity which depend upon each test's being positive may enhance specificity at the expense of sensitivity. Obviously, the physician's choice depends upon the need to minimize false-negative results as opposed to false-positive results in a given clinical situation.

From the list of clinically employed noninvasive vascular laboratory tests, those found most useful include oculopneumoplethysmography (OPG) and B-mode ultrasound carotid arteriography with real-time frequency analysis of Doppler signals (duplex scan). The past decade has seen gradual replacement of older noninvasive vascular laboratory cerebrovascular tests such as thermography, ophthalmodynamometry, carotid compression tomography, forehead skin blood pressure determination, and carotid phonoangiography. More recently, the value of the periorbital directional Doppler examination has also been questioned because of limited sensitivity.[15,16]

Oculopneumoplethysmography, introduced by William Gee in 1973, records ophthalmic artery systolic pressure and compares the ophthalmic artery systolic pressure with the higher brachial systolic pressure (BSP)[17,18] Following topical anesthesia of the conjunctivae, plastic suction cups are applied to both lateral sclerae (Fig. 112-5). Negative ocular pres-

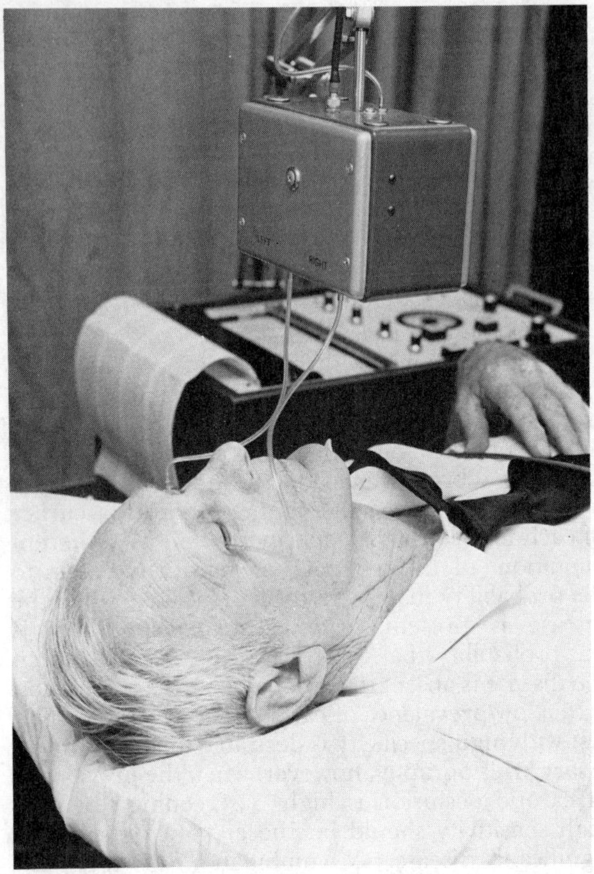

FIGURE 112-5 OPG in progress with suction cups in place on the anesthetized sclerae bilaterally. (*Reproduced with permission from the subject.*)

sures of 300 to 500 mmHg are applied simultaneously over 3 to 5 s and then slowly reduced to ambient pressure. Intraocular pressures rise in linear fashion as increasing suction distorts the globes. When intraocular pressure exceeds ophthalmic artery systolic pressure, retinal arterial flow ceases, resulting in transient visual loss. As the applied suction decreases, retinal arterial flow resumes at ophthalmic systolic pressure, which is recorded as the first of serially increasing systolic deflections on the plethysmographic strip chart recorder. The ophthalmic systolic pressure for each eye is estimated from standard graphic correlates of applied suction and compared with a reference line of hemodynamic significance determined by Gee. In general, positive criteria for oculopneumoplethysmography are the the following: (1) ophthalmic systolic pressure $\geqslant 5$ mmHg less than the contralateral ophthalmic systolic pressure, (2) ophthalmic systolic pressure/brachial systolic pressure < 0.66 when ophthalmic systolic pressures differ by 1 to 4 mmHg, (3) ophthalmic systolic pressure/brachial systolic pressure < 0.60 when both ophthalmic systolic pressures are equal. With carotid stenoses of more than 60 percent (diameter reduction), the accuracy of the oculopneumoplethysmography is excellent (sensitivity 70 to 95 percent, specificity 96 to 100 percent).[15] Major advantages of oculopneumoplethysmography include its safety, reproducibility, technical simplicity, low cost, and equipment durability. Systemic anticoagulation is not a contraindication to performance of oculopneumoplethysmography; however, lack of patient cooperation, glaucoma, retinal detachment, intraocular lens implantation, active conjunctivitis, or ocular surgery within 6 months are contraindications to this test. Complications seen in less than 2 percent of cases include transient chemosis or subconjunctival hemorrhage. Unfortunately, oculopneumoplethysmography cannot discriminate between high-grade carotid stenoses and total occlusions—essential points for the surgeon contemplating carotid revascularization. Additionally, the reliability of oculopneumoplethysmography with extreme hypertension and severe bilateral carotid occlusive disease has been questioned.

Probably the most versatile direct test of the extracranial carotid artery is the *duplex scanner*. Visualization of the common carotid artery and its branches is performed using B-mode ultrasound. Pulsed Doppler ultrasonography and spectral analysis is also employed for detection of flow disturbances in precise, midstream sample volumes. A single scan head is used for the echoarteriogram, both to survey carotid anatomy and to produce information regarding flow velocities (Fig. 112-6). The pulsed Doppler component allows interrogation of flow in the center stream from which the spectrum of velocities is analyzed and displayed in real time. Determinations of the peak systolic frequency, spectral broadening, and spectral "window" have proven useful in the detection of minor carotid stenoses and in categorizing obstructing lesions into grades of severity. Hemodynamically insignificant stenoses pro-

FIGURE 112-6 B-mode ultrasound imaging of the carotid bifurcation by means of a duplex scanner. (*Reproduced with permission from the subjects.*)

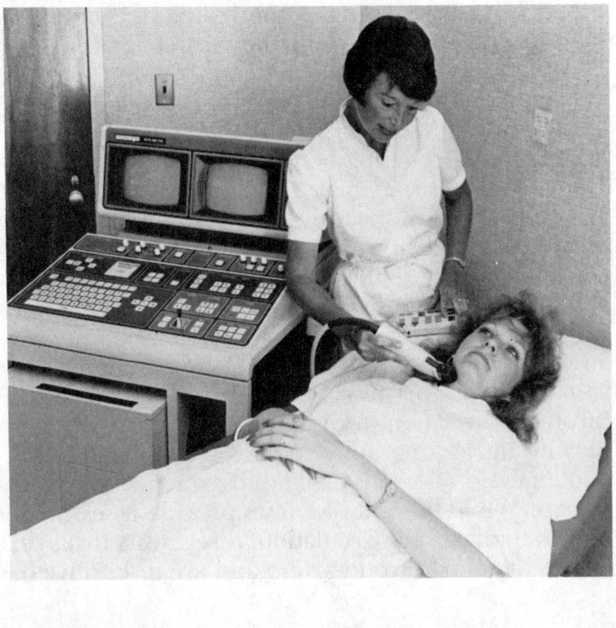

duce widening of the spectrum, especially in the deceleration phase of systole, while the peak frequency remains unchanged. Significant stenoses (greater than 50 percent diameter reduction) produce additional spectral broadening with obliteration of the spectral window, and progressive increases in peak systolic frequency. Duplex scanning can also reliably separate high-grade carotid stenosis from total occlusion.[19] Conditions that limit usefulness of the duplex technique include vessel tortuosity and extensive collateralization, both of which impair precise vessel insonation, and extensive calcification, which reflects much of the ultrasound energy. Additional disadvantages include the substantial cost of the study and the extreme dependency upon the technologist's skill for accurate test performance. Since the examination may prove lengthy, it is difficult to apply to large patient populations as a screening method.

Complications

For practical purposes the complications of noninvasive studies are of little consequence and can be disregarded. The complications of angiography relate to the technical performance of the procedure as well as to allergic reactions to the contrast agent. One of the highest angiographic complication rates in neuroradiology occurs in patients with cerebral occlusive disease (1.2 to 1.9 percent) in comparison with lower rates among patients undergoing cerebral angiography for suspected tumor, seizure, or headache (0.35 percent).[20] Patients with recent strokes or frequent transient ischemia attacks have a relatively higher incidence of serious neurologic complications during and following angiography.[21] Morbidity is known to increase directly with the duration of the study, strongly suggesting that intraarterial digital subtraction angiography, which allows for a more rapid examination, should be the procedure of choice.

Although intravenous digital subtraction angiography is generally regarded as a benign and minimally invasive procedure, a complete study requires four to six times the contrast load compared to intraarterial digital subtraction angiography, placing the patient at greater risk of renal toxicity. In addition, the central venous catheter used for injection can perforate the superior vena cava, allowing contrast to be injected into the mediastinum. Minor untoward effects such as nausea and vomiting frequently follow the intravenous administration of contrast material. Major reactions, however, are much less common. These complaints are quite rare following intraarterial injection of contrast. It is felt that this difference relates to the release of a histamine-like substance by the lung in the first pass of the relatively undiluted venous contrast as it proceeds through the pulmonary circulation.

All contrast media used for angiography contain iodine and are both hyperbaric and hypertonic. Preexisting damage to the blood-brain barrier, such as exists in cerebral infarction, may permit intravascular contrast material to escape and allow neurons to be bathed by the neurotoxic agent. Angiography and contrast-enhanced CT, therefore, should not ordinarily be performed acutely following a cerebrovascular accident.

Applications

In the selection of carotid diagnostic studies a number of factors come into consideration: clinical relevance of the examination, sensitivity and specificity of the test, patient comfort and safety, cost effectiveness, and whether or not the examination can be done on an outpatient basis. Too often, unnecessary tests are performed because of improper sequencing or the erroneous notion that all tests available in the noninvasive vascular laboratory should be run as a "carotid battery." Cost-effectiveness demands that the most direct and highest-yield study be selected when operation is contemplated. In the setting of hemispheric neurologic symptoms, noninvasive tests to ascertain hemodynamic significance are largely superfluous since the majority of complaints are thought to relate to embolization from ulcerated plaques, not to obstructed blood flow. Accordingly, if the patient has transient ischemic attacks or amaurosis fugax, the definitive first examination should be complete cerebral angiography, preferably intraarterial digital subtraction angiography. One may justifiably question the role of noninvasive vascular laboratory testing in this setting, as none currently in use reliably detects the minimally stenotic, ulcerative atheroma which could be the source for cerebral embolism. If, on the other hand, the patient has experienced a recent cerebrovascular accident with good recovery and is considered a candidate for carotid endarterectomy, it would be appropriate to obtain a CT scan first, and then proceed with cerebral angiography nearer the time of the contemplated operative procedure. Noninvasive tests, specifically oculopneumoplethysmography and duplex scanning, are used in these situations adjunctively to assess collateralization and to establish a preoperative baseline in order to compare results of postoperative examinations.

Contrariwise, in the patient with an asymptomatic carotid bruit or the individual with nonhemispheric neurologic symptoms, noninvasive vascular laboratory studies should be done first for screening to establish the hemodynamic significance of extracranial carotid lesions. Angiography in this setting is ordered only if the lesion is found to be flow-limiting, and if the patient would be willing to permit endarterectomy should a threatening stenosis be found. Unfortunately, bruits are not always dependable markers for carotid stenosis and may be absent in the more severe degrees of obstruction.

Selected noninvasive vascular laboratory tests are quite useful in the postoperative follow-up of patients after carotid endarterectomy or in the periodic evaluation of asymptomatic "second side" lesions discovered at the time of initial angiographic workup. With the general availability of oculopneumoplethysmography and duplex scanning, the older periorbital Doppler examination and carotid phonoangiography have become studies of historic interest only in many centers.

References

1. Mozersky, D. J., Hokanson, D. E., Baker, D. W., Sumner, D. S., and Strandness, D. E. J.: Ultrasonic Arteriography, *Arch. Surg.*, 103:663, 1971.
2. Ricotta, J. J., Holen, M. D., Schenk, E., et al.: Is Routine Angiography Necessary Prior to Carotid Endarterectomy? *J. Vasc. Surg.*, 1:96 1984.
3. Kilgore, B. B., and Fields, W. S.: Arterial Occlusive Disease in Adults, in R. H. Newton and D. G. Potts (eds.), "Radiology of the Skull and Brain—Angiography," vol. 2, book 4, C. V. Mosby Co., St. Louis, 1974, p. 2314.
4. Strole, W. E., Jr., Clark, W. H., Jr., and Isselbacher, K. J.: Progressive Arterial Occlusive Disease: A Frequently Fatal Cutaneosystemic Disorder, *N. Engl. J. Med.*, 276:195, 1967.
5. Grollman, J. H., Jr., and Hannah, V. S.: The Roentgen Diagnosis of Takayasu's Arteritis, *Radiology*, 83:387, 1964.
6. Taveras, J. M.: Multiple Progressive Intracranial Arterial Occlusions: A Syndrome of Children and Young Adults, *AJR*, 106:235, 1969.
7. Ehrenfeld, W. K., Stoney, R. J., and Wylie, E. J.: Fibromuscular Hyperplasia of the Internal Carotid Artery, *Arch. Surg.*, 95:284, 1967.
8. Cohen, M. M., Hemalatha, C. P., D'Addario, R. T., and Goldman, H. W.: Embolization from a Fusiform Middle Cerebral Artery Aneurysm, *Stroke*, 2:158, 1980.
9. Kelly, W., Brant-Zawadski, M., and Pitts, L. H.: Arterial Injection-digital Subtraction Angiography, *Journal of Neurosurgery*, 58:851, 1983.
10. Mani, R. L., and Eisenberg, R. L.: Complications of Catheter Cerebral Angiography: Analysis of 5,000 Procedures: III. Assessment of Arteries Injected, Contrast Medium Used, Duration of Procedure, and Age of Patient, *AJR*, 131:871, 1978.
11. Davis, P. C., and Hoffman, J. C., Jr.: Work in Progress. Intraarterial Digital Subtraction Angiography: Evaluation of 150 patients, *Radiology*, 148:9, 1983.
12. Turski, P. A., Zwiebel, W. J., Strother, C. M., Crummy, A. B., Celesia, G., and Sackett, J. R.: Limitations of IVDSA, *AJNR*, 4:271, 1983.
13. Graber, J. N., Vollman, R. W., Johnson, W. C., et al.: Stroke After Carotid Endarterectomy: Risk as Predicted by Preoperative Computerized Tomography, *Am. J. Surg.*, 147:492, 1984.
14. Laing, W.: Cost Effectiveness, *J. Med. Eng. Technol.*, 3:113, 1979.
15. Kempczinski, R. F., and Yao, J. S. T.: "Practical Noninvasive Vascular Diagnosis," Year Book Medical Publishers, Inc., Chicago, pp. 164 and 374.
16. Lye, C. R., Sumner, D. S., Strandness, D. E.: The Accuracy of the Supraorbital Doppler Examination in the Diagnosis of Hemodynamically Significant Carotid Occlusive Disease, *Surgery*, 79:42, 1976.
17. McDonald, K. M., Gee, W., Kaupp, H. A., and Bast, R. G.: Screening for Significant Carotid Stenosis by Ocular Pneumoplethysmography, *Am. J. Surg.*, 137:244, 1979.
18. Bernstein, E. F., (ed.): "Noninvasive Diagnostic Techniques in Vascular Diseases," 2d ed., C. V. Mosby Co., St. Louis, 1982, pp. 57–76; 220–230.
19. Blackshear, W. M., Phillips, D. J., Thiele, B. L., and Bast, R. G.: Detection of Carotid Occlusive Disease by Ultrasonic Imaging and Pulsed Doppler Spectrum Analysis, *Surgery*, 86:698, 1979.
20. Mani, R. L., and Eisenberg, R. L.: Complications of Catheter Cerebral Angiography: Analysis of 5,000 Procedures: II. Relation of Complication Rates to Clinical and Arteriographic Diagnoses, *AJR*, 131:867, 1978.
21. Earnest, F., Forbes, G., Sandok, B. A., and Bast, R. G.: Complications of Cerebral Angiography: Prospective Assessment of Risk, *AJNR*, 4:1191, 1983.

113

Radionuclide Lung Imaging and Pulmonary Angiography

Peter J. Sones, M.D. William A. Fajman, M.D.

Radionuclide Lung Imaging

The diagnosis of pulmonary embolism is difficult, and its diagnosis based on clinical information alone is fraught with error. Blood gases may be helpful, but they are in no way specific.[1] Given this diagnostic problem, objective evidence of pulmonary embolism becomes more important prior to embarking on therapy with anticoagulants or vena caval filter.

Indications

The clinical use of radionuclide lung imaging is almost exclusively devoted to the evaluation of patients with suspected PE. The modern radionuclide lung study consists of two parts, ventilation and perfusion. The perfusion portion of the study by itself is highly sensitive but nonspecific. A positive perfusion study may result from a variety of lesions such as tumors, vasculitis, bullous lesions, pneumonias, physiological shunting away from areas of poor ventilation, or any other factor which causes changes in the perfusion pattern.[2] The ventilation study adds specificity to the examination.

Technique

Perfusion imaging is performed using ^{99m}Tc labeled macroaggregates of albumin or albumin microspheres, particulates which have a size of 10 to 40 μm and temporarily occlude approximately $\frac{1}{1000}$ of the arteriolar-capillary units in the lung. Once the material is injected into the patient, images are obtained in at least six views.

The technique for performing *ventilation studies* is dependent upon the availability of a variety of isotopes. The most commonly used agent is the radioactive gas xenon, ^{133}Xe. Typically, this agent is used to perform a ventilation study prior to the perfusion study because the energy of the emissions from this isotope are lower than those of the ^{99m}Tc used for perfusion images. This avoids the problem of scattered radiation interfering with the ventilation imaging. The imaging sequence usually includes an image of a "single breath," one of an equilibrium phase, and one each minute during the washout phase for an average of 6 min. The obvious disadvantage of this radioisotope is the fact that ventilation is performed before perfusion. In the majority of instances, the ability to correlate the ventilatory status of an area of abnormal perfusion is paramount in interpretation. It would thus be much more effective to perform ventilation after the perfusion scan. Other isotopes which surmount this problem are available to a limited extent. ^{127}Xe has a high-energy emission and can be used to perform directed postperfusion images, but is not readily available. ^{81m}Kr, another gas which may be used postperfusion, has a very short half-life (13 s) and must be supplied daily; it is, therefore, too costly for most centers. Apparatus has become commercially available which allows deposition of aerosolized particles of ^{99m}Tc DTPA deep in the lung. The prolonged retention time of the aerosol allows multiview assessment of pulmonary ventilation.

Complications

Perfusion lung imaging is an extremely safe procedure. There is the potential for allergic reaction to the injected protein, and a rare death has been reported in association with severe pulmonary hypertension. We have performed several thousand studies at our center and have not observed any untoward effects from the procedure.

Interpretation

Adequate interpretation of the ventilation-perfusion study requires correlation with a good quality chest roentgenogram, which must be obtained almost simultaneously with the radionuclide study. Because several entities may cause abnormalities in lung perfusion, attempts have been made to develop criteria by which lung images can be categorized relative to the probability of PE as the cause of a particular ventilation-perfusion pattern.

Although minor differences exist in diagnostic criteria, it is generally accepted that a negative perfusion study excludes the diagnosis of pulmonary embolism. This may, in fact, be the most useful pattern, since it obviates further testing of the diagnosis of embolic disease. Low probability is typically assigned to studies in which there is a clear perfusion abnormality with abnormal ventilation (a ventilation-perfusion match) or a single subsegmental defect with normal ventilation.[2–4] Depending upon the observer, high probability may be assigned to even one area involving 75 percent of an anatomic segment with normal ventilation (a ventilation-perfusion mismatch).

The remaining ventilation-perfusion patterns are categorized as of moderate probability or indeterminate. This group includes patients who have greater than 50 percent of the lung involved by severe obstructive lung disease[5] or who have infiltrates corresponding to the perfusion abnormality. This latter group can be divided into further categories, however. An infiltrate with a corresponding perfusion defect which is much larger than the area of infiltrate is a pattern of high probability. Conversely, a perfusion defect which is smaller than the area of infiltrate shows low probability of pulmonary embolism. Densities on the roentgenogram with equivalent perfusion defects have an approximately 25 percent chance of being secondary to PE.[6] The presence of diffuse disease such as pulmonary edema or interstitial fibrosis should not result in the a priori assumption of an indeterminate radionuclide study, since in almost three-fourths of these patients, the study may be normal or near normal and thus exclude the diagnosis of pulmonary embolism.[7]

Clinical Use of Radionuclide Lung Imaging

The radionuclide lung study should be used as an aid in clinical decision making. A low or high probability study in the appropriate circumstance may be sufficient to allow institution of appropriate therapy. The clinician, however, should not defer further study, regardless of the lung scan interpretation, if the overall clinical circumstance is discordant.

Follow-up radionuclide studies may also be helpful. The majority of abnormalities due to pulmonary embolism will show some change in the perfusion pattern within 1 to 2 weeks, although failure to change does not exclude the diagnosis.[8] The radionuclide lung study also serves as a guide to suspicious areas if pulmonary angiography is required.

Pulmonary Angiography

Pulmonary angiography has been and continues to be recognized as the "gold standard" for the diagnosis of pulmonary embolism. There is widespread agreement that most experts would treat patients with a positive pulmonary angiogram and would not treat patients with a negative pulmonary angiogram.[1] In a study utilizing data from a national cooperative study, Bell and Simon[9] found consistent interobserver agreement on the angiographic diagnosis and estimation of severity of pulmonary embolism.

Indications

A normal pulmonary perfusion scan, for all practical purposes, excludes pulmonary embolism. The primary indication for pulmonary angiography is a patient with a high clinical suspicion of embolus and a ventilation-perfusion radionuclide scan showing either low or moderate probability. While those patients with a high probability radionuclide scan might reasonably be treated with anticoagulants, any clinical contraindication to anticoagulants, such as coagulopathy, and gastrointestinal bleeding, might require that pulmonary angiography be performed for a definitive diagnosis. In all patients in whom a caval filter is considered, a definitive angiographic diagnosis is required.

Findings on conventional radiographs of the chest may include wedge-shaped peripheral pulmonary infiltrates, pleural thickening and/or effusion, areas of oligemia, and/or enlargement of the proximal pulmonary arteries as a result of acute pulmonary hyptertension. Unfortunately, the chest x-ray is frequently normal in patients with pulmonary embolism. The described positive findings would, of course, heighten one's suspicion of pulmonary embolism. The overall accuracy of the chest film in detecting pulmonary embolism is 40 percent.[10] Pneumonia, which might easily be confused with pulmonary embolism, can be distinguished from infarction due to pulmonary embolism by angiographic demonstration of the embolus.[11]

Findings on the radionuclide scan can be extremely helpful. Specifically, those areas of defect on the perfusion scan must be carefully scrutinized angiographically. Special views or techniques may be utilized to facilitate optimal visualization of the arteries supplying any area in question on the nuclide scan.

Technique

The femoral vein, at the groin, is the site usually preferred by patients and is, in our opinion, the easiest and safest route of access to the venous system for pulmonary angiography. Right heart and main pulmonary artery pressures are essential to evaluate the extent of pulmonary disease and evaluate the safety of injection of contrast medium into the pulmonary artery.

Various clinicians have suggested that the main pulmonary artery not be injected if the mean pressure exceeds 50 mmHg. Usually, even with elevated pulmonary artery pressure, a limited modified study can be obtained. The critical factor is that only a small quantity of contrast medium be used, preferably selectively in a pulmonary artery branch supplying an area of deficit indicated on the perfusion lung scan.

The main right pulmonary artery and its proximal branches are best visualized in the straight anterior-posterior projection. The left main pulmonary artery and its proximal branches are best visualized in the right posterior oblique projection. Two different views of each lung are essential to exclude a pulmonary embolus. Superimposition of vessels may otherwise obscure emboli. If routine views of the lung demonstrate no emboli, selective injection into pulmonary artery branches supplying any area of defect on the radionuclide perfusion scan are indicated. Magnification filming of such a sub-

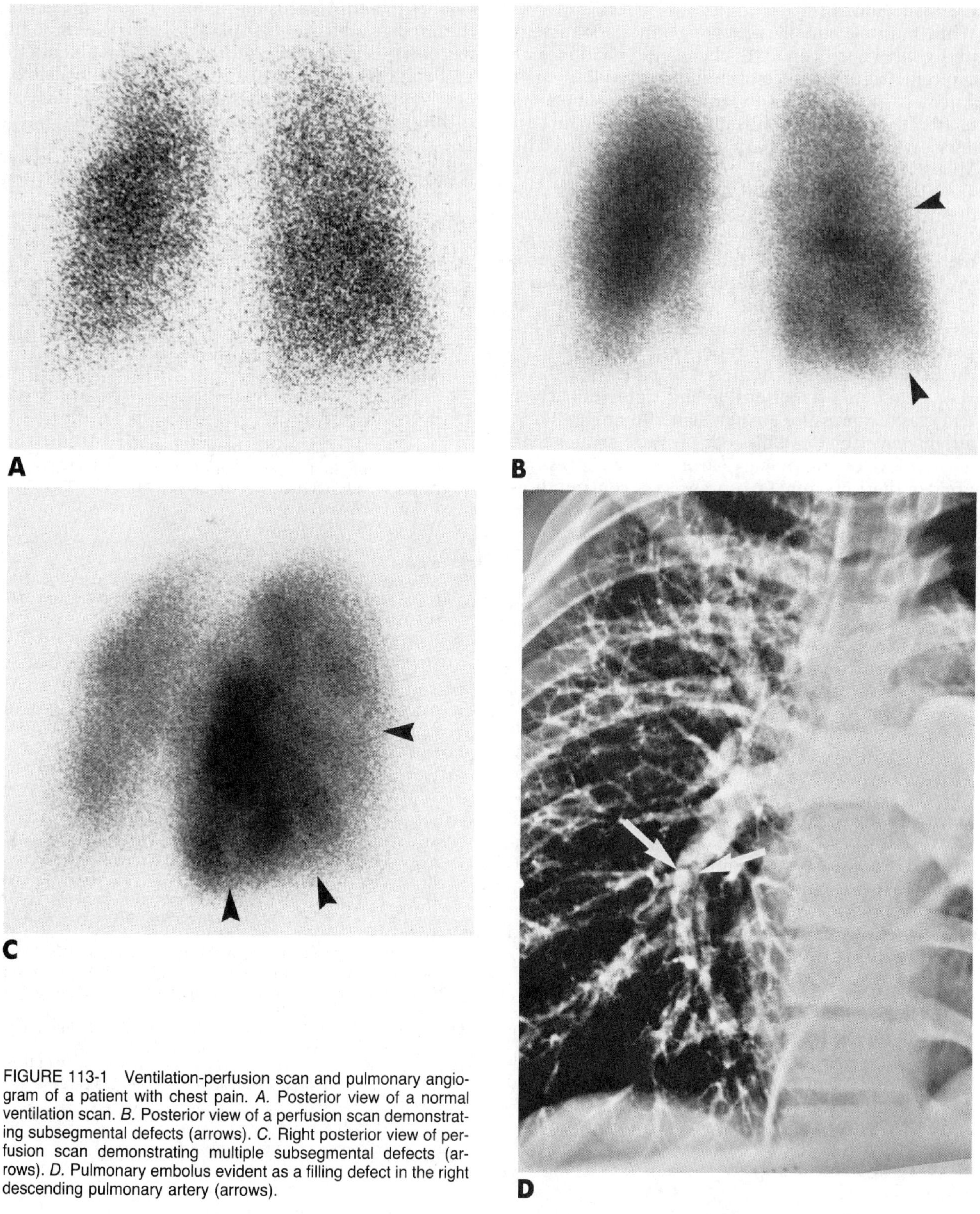

FIGURE 113-1 Ventilation-perfusion scan and pulmonary angiogram of a patient with chest pain. *A.* Posterior view of a normal ventilation scan. *B.* Posterior view of a perfusion scan demonstrating subsegmental defects (arrows). *C.* Right posterior view of perfusion scan demonstrating multiple subsegmental defects (arrows). *D.* Pulmonary embolus evident as a filling defect in the right descending pulmonary artery (arrows).

selective injection will further facilitate the identification of emboli. In some patients with multiple small recurrent emboli resulting in pulmonary hypertension, the emboli may be too small to be visualized angiographically.[9]

Digital subtraction angiography (DSA) has been suggested as an alternative to conventional radiographic filming of pulmonary angiography.[12] In patients who are able to cooperate by remaining motionless and holding their breath throughout the filming sequence, this technique may indeed demonstrate large pulmonary embolism involving the main pulmonary artery through third-order branches. In our opinion, conventional filming should be available without moving the patient if DSA is to be employed, and should be used if DSA is normal.

Complications

While multiple complications of pulmonary angiography have been reported, the overall incidence of clinically significant complications was less than 1 percent in a national cooperative study.[9] The mortality rate in this series was less than 0.5 percent. In a series of 1350 pulmonary angiograms reported by Mills et al.,[13] the overall morbidity was 3 percent and the death rate was 0.2 percent. Contrast medium reactions occur with the same low rate of incidence as in peripheral venous injections of contrast media. Cardiac arrhythmias represent a potential problem, and the angiographer should be prepared to treat arrhythmias which develop. The greatest risk factor is clearly significant pulmonary artery hypertension. In the series reported by Mills et al.,[13] the only three deaths occurred in patients with severe pulmonary hypertension and right ventricular end diastolic pressure greater than 20 mmHg. Thus, a right ventricular end diastolic pressure greater than 20 mmHg or pulmonary artery mean pressure greater than 50 mmHg represents a contraindication to injection of the pulmonary artery.

Interpretation

Decreased perfusion of a portion of the lung manifested by delayed arterial filling, areas of oligemia or avascularity, "pruning" of the distal arteries, or delayed venous filling all indicate decreased perfusion and are indirect signs suggesting the possibility of pulmonary embolism. One cannot make a definitive diagnosis, however, unless the embolus as such is demonstrated angiographically.[14,15] Emboli manifest themselves as a filling defect within a pulmonary artery or by abrupt cutoff of a pulmonary artery with angiographic evidence of the trailing edge of the embolus (Fig. 113-1). Adhering to these criteria, one will rarely encounter a false-positive pulmonary angiogram for pulmonary embolism. The described indirect signs of pulmonary embolism can be further evaluated with subselective injection and magnification of the areas in question.

Clinical Use of Pulmonary Angiography

Surgical intervention to remove pulmonary emboli is occasionally undertaken in cases of massive pulmonary embolism. This procedure is accompanied by high morbidity and mortality in this group of very ill patients. Infusion of fibrinolytic agents via the angiographic catheter placed within the embolus has been successful in a few cases. Adequate data to evaluate this procedure are not presently available. One may attempt to aspirate embolic material through an especially shaped catheter.[15]

References

1. Robin, E. D.: Overdiagnosis and Overtreatment of Pulmonary Embolism: The Emperor May Have No Clothes, *Ann. Intern. Med.*, 87:775, 1977.
2. Neuman, R. D., Sostman, H. D., and Gottschalk, A.: Current Status of Ventilation-Perfusion Imaging, *Semin. Nucl. Med.*, 10:198, 1980.
3. McNeill, B. J.: Ventilation-Perfusion Studies and the Diagnosis of Pulmonary Embolism: Concise Communication, *J. Nucl. Med.*, 21:319, 1980.
4. Biello, D. R., Mattar, A. G., McKnight, R. C., and Siegel, B. A.: Ventilation-Perfusion Studies in Suspected Pulmonary Embolism, *A.J.R.*, 133:1033, 1979.
5. Alderson, P. O., Biello, D. R., Sachariah, K. G., and Siegel, B. A.: Scintigraphic Detection of Pulmonary Embolism in Patients with Obstructive Pulmonary Disease, *Radiology*, 138:661, 1981.
6. Biello, D. R., Mattar, A. G., Osei-Wusu, A., Alderson, P. O., McNeill, B. J., and Siegel, B. A.: Interpretation of Indeterminate Lung Scintigrams, *Radiology*, 133:189, 1979.
7. Newman, G. E., Sullivan, D. C., Gottschalk, A., and Putnam, C. E.: Scintigraphic Perfusion Patterns in Patients with Diffuse Lung Disease, *Radiology*, 143:227, 1982.
8. Alderson, P. O., Dzebolo, N. N., Biello, D. R., Seldin, D. W., Martin, E. C., and Siegel, B. A.: Serial Lung Scintigraphy: Utility in Diagnosis of Pulmonary Embolism, *Radiology*, 149:797, 1983.
9. Bell, W. R., and Simon, T. L.: A Comparative Analysis of Pulmonary Perfusion Scans with Pulmonary Angiograms, *Am. Heart J.*, 92:700, 1976.
10. Greenspan, R. H., Ravin, C. E., Polansky, S. M., and McLoud, T. C.: Accuracy of the Chest Radiograph in Diagnosis of Pulmonary Embolism, *Invest. Radiol.*, 17:539, 1982.
11. Bookstein, J. J., Alazraki, N. P., and Jassy, L. N.: Subselective Magnification Angiography of Experimental Pneumonia, *Cardiovasc. Intervent. Radiol.* 6:41, 1983.
12. Reilley, R. F., Smith, C. W., Price, R. R., Patton, J. A., and Diggs, J.: Digital Subtraction Angiography: Limitations for the Detection of Pulmonary Embolism, *Radiology*, 149:379, 1983.
13. Mills, S. R., Jackson, D. C., Older, R. A., Heaston, D. K., and Moore, A. V.: The Incidence, Etiologies and Avoidance of Complications of Pulmonary Angiography in a Large Series, *Radiology*, 136:295, 1980.
14. Sagel, S. E., and Greenspan, R. H.: Nonuniform Pulmonary Arterial Perfusion, *Radiology*, 99:541, 1970.
15. Viamonte, M., Jr., Koolpe, H., Janowitz, W., and Hildner, F.: Pulmonary Thromboembolism—Update. *JAMA*, 243:2229, 1980.

114

Phlebography

Renate L. Soulen, M.D.

Things are seldom what they seem, skim milk masquerades as cream.

W. S. Gilbert, 1878[1]

Indications

Radiographic visualization of the venous system is useful as a road map for venous sampling; for delineation of tumors or vascular malformations; for assessment of trauma, venous insufficiency, and the suitability of veins for bypass grafting or shunts; and above all for the diagnosis of venous thrombosis. This chapter will consider only the latter.

Deep vein thrombosis remains a common cause of serious morbidity and mortality yet eludes reliable diagnosis on the bases of history and physical examination alone.[2] While radionuclide and noninvasive techniques have contributed greatly to the diagnosis, phlebography remains the "gold standard" and, when properly performed, has an accuracy approaching 100 percent.[3,4]

Technique

Upper Extremity and Mediastinal Phlebography

Contrast medium, 30 ml of a 60 percent aqueous solution, is injected relatively slowly (e.g., 5 ml/s) through a needle in the dorsum of the hand or, when the problem is clearly intrathoracic, in the basilic or brachial vein while serial films of the extremity and chest are obtained with the patient supine. At the completion of injection, while filming the axilla and chest, the arm is elevated to an angle of 90°, thereby creating a good bolus and promoting emptying of the arm. If the mediastinum is of interest, both upper extremities are injected simultaneously and both are elevated in order to avoid spurious filling defects from unopacified blood. We prefer hand injection so that the injection site is kept in view and injection can be stopped immediately should extravasation be seen. An adequate study can be obtained even when the medium is hand-injected through a 23-gauge needle. A leaded shield and distance permitted by extra connecting tubing protect the operator. The veins are further cleared of contrast medium by infusion of saline solution or 5 percent glucose in water through the same needle while the films are processed.

Lower Extremity Phlebography

Though unanimity is lacking as to the optimal method, variations of the technique of Rabinov and Paulin[5] are the most widely accepted. The key features of their technique are that the patient is semierect, the leg of interest is non-weight-bearing, and the injection of contrast medium is made with no tourniquet on. This requires a tilt table as well as hand grips and axillary support for patients unable to bear weight on the contralateral leg. Contrast medium is injected into as distal and medial a vein as possible. Retrograde insertion of the needle facilitates filling of the foot veins and thereby the deep calf veins into which they drain. We inject 100 ml by hand, taking a lateral film of the foot and ankle after 25 ml, anteroposterior, lateral, and internal oblique views of the calf and knee after 75 ml, anteroposterior and lateral views of the thigh after completion of injection, and an anteroposterior film of the abdomen and pelvis immediately following elevation of the leg and calf massage during infusion of saline solution or 5 percent glucose in water. The table is then immediately lowered to the horizontal, and infusion of the flush solution is continued while the films are processed. Operator protection is as previously described. Excellent opacification of the entire deep venous system is obtained without fluoroscopy (Fig. 114-1). In the presence of many superficial varicosities, stereoscopic views of the calf may be helpful, or an ankle tourniquet may be used to reduce opacification of the superficial veins. Retrograde injection into a superficial vein of the lower leg, with a tourniquet just below the knee, may provide an alternative to venous cutdown in patients with no available foot veins. We give 30 to 50 mg lidocaine through the same venipuncture site immediately before the contrast medium in order to reduce discomfort and protect the venous endothelium.[6]

The Rabinov-Paulin technique avoids artifacts due to layering of the contrast medium and to extrinsic compression of intrinsically normal veins by tourniquet or muscle contraction. Consequently, failure to opacify a major deep vein can confidently be attributed to obstruction *providing* the feeding foot veins have been adequately filled. The foot film serves three important purposes: (1) it permits determination of this filling, (2) it documents presence or absence of injection site extravasation, and (3) it demonstrates disease if present. Deep vein thrombosis limited to pedal veins has been reported in 10 percent of patients whose phlebograms include

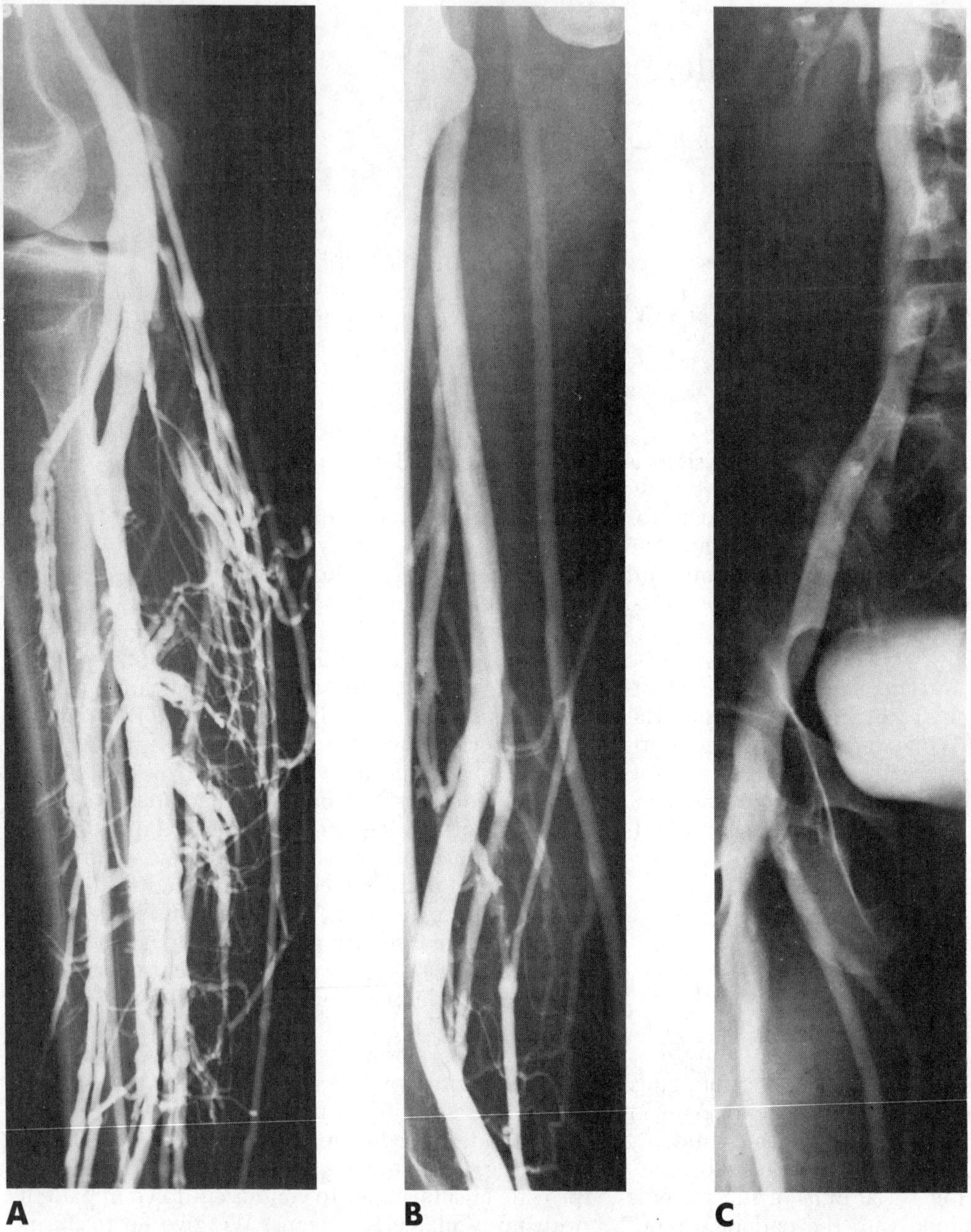

FIGURE 114-1 Normal phlebogram. Note excellent opacification of the entire deep venous system. *A.* Lateral film of the lower leg. *B.* The thigh. *C.* Abdomen and pelvis. Film of the foot and additional views of the calf and thigh, included in all examinations, are not shown.

the foot and has been associated with pulmonary embolism.[7]

Though a large calf hematoma or other mass could lead to extrinsic obstruction, in the great majority of patients failure to opacify a deep vein, in whole or in part, equates with thrombotic occlusion of indeterminate age. Presence of collaterals lends further support to this diagnosis. Demonstration of a broad intraluminal filling defect, characteristically with a tapered antegrade tail, permits diagnosis of acute deep vein thrombosis. Destruction of valves and irregular filling defects reflect the postphlebitic state and deep vein incompetence.

Complications

In a large prospective study, adverse reactions to contrast media occurred in 2.7 percent of patients undergoing phlebography and ranged from nausea to cardiovascular collapse. Less than 33 percent of these required therapy; less than 2 percent required hospitalization; 0.017 percent was fatal.[8] Though patients with a positive allergy history have twice the incidence of untoward reactions of those without, these reactions are unpredictable and may occur on first exposure to contrast medium or following prior uneventful exposure.

The hyperosmolality of all intravascular agents currently approved by the FDA produces an increase in plasma volume, endothelial injury, and variable degrees of discomfort during injection. The large volume of contrast medium needed for lower limb phlebography thus can cause pulmonary edema in patients in borderline or frank cardiac failure. If phlebography is deemed urgent in such a high-risk patient, pretreatment with intravenous furosemide (Lasix) is recommended. The endothelial injury leads to a mural inflammatory response which in turn promotes thrombosis. The variation in the reported incidence of postphlebography thrombosis from negligible to 48 percent[9,10] is the result of widely disparate phlebographic techniques and criteria for the postphlebographic diagnosis. There is general agreement, however, that (1) damage is lessened by keeping endothelial exposure time minimal, (2) a newly positive fibrinogen uptake test post phlebography reflects mural inflammation, not necessarily with clot, (3) there is poor correlation between the postphlebography syndrome of pain and swelling and evidence of deep vein thrombosis on objective reexamination, and (4) there is need for contrast medium with more physiological osmolality. The incidence of postphlebography syndrome and of newly positive fibrinogen uptake test, and the magnitude of discomfort during injection, have all been reduced by dilution of standard contrast agents[11] and, most dramatically, by new nonionic agents not yet approved in the United States.[9] The osmolality of these new agents approaches that of blood; FDA approval appears imminent. Heparin has been advocated as a preventive measure[12] but has not proved protective in our hands.[13] Transient renal failure induced by contrast medium may follow phlebography in patients with preexisting impaired renal function. Good hydration minimizes this risk.

Extravasation of contrast medium at the puncture site causes a chemical cellulitis which may progress to ulceration, necrosis, and, very rarely, to gangrene requiring amputation. The likelihood of necrosis is greater in the presence of arterial or venous insufficiency and if the extravasation provokes regional vascular spasm. The importance of constant puncture site monitoring cannot be overemphasized. Immediate cessation of injection, elevation, and warm soaks will minimize injury.

Relation to Other Tests

Doppler ultrasound, impedance plesythmography, and phleborheography share the advantages of bedside capability and no risk and the disadvantages of being nonspecific and dependent upon alterations in flow for diagnosis. Consequently the false-negative rate for clots limited to the lower leg is high, extrinsic disease cannot be distinguished from intrinsic venous disease, and nonthrombotic diseases which alter venous flow, such as severe arterial insufficiency or heart failure, may render studies uninterpretable. The fibrinogen uptake test is also a bedside exam with virtually no risk and has high sensitivity for clots forming below the knee. However, reliable interpretation requires at least a 24-h delay from the time of radionuclide injection, clot outside a vein cannot be distinguished from clot inside a vein (limiting its use in the high-risk orthopedic surgery group), and edema, cellulitis, and arthritis also produce high counts. In comparison, phlebography is not a bedside exam and carries small though potentially serious risks; it is, however, the only technique which is specific, highly accurate, and provides an immediate definitive answer. Therefore in the setting of possible deep vein thrombosis, phlebography is recommended whenever the clinical picture and noninvasive results are discordant, routinely 5 to 7 days following hip surgery or knee replacement, and for differentiation of intrinsic from extrinsic compromise of axillary, subclavian, and mediastinal veins.

References

1. Gilbert, W. S.: "H.M.S. Pinafore," Act I, 1878.
2. Kakkar, V. V.: Deep Vein Thrombosis: Detection and Prevention, *Circulation*, 51:8, 1975.
3. Hull, R., Hirsh, J., Sackett, D. L., et al.: Clinical Validity of a Negative Venogram in Patients with Clinically Suspected Venous Thrombosis, *Circulation*, 64:622, 1981.
4. Lea Thomas, M.: Thromboembolism, in "Phlebography of the Lower Limb," Churchill Livingstone, London, 1982, p. 85.
5. Rabinov, K., and Paulin, S.: Roentgen Diagnosis of Venous Thrombosis in the Leg, *Arch. Surg.*, 104:134, 1972.
6. Ritchie, W. G. M., Lynch, P. R., and Stewart, G. J.: The Effect of Contrast Media on Normal and Inflammed Canine Veins, *Invest. Radiol.*, 9:444, 1974.
7. Lea Thomas, M., and O'Dwyer, J. A.: A Phlebographic Study of the Incidence and Significance of Venous Thrombosis in the Foot, *AJR*, 130:751, 1978.
8. Shehadi, W. H., and Toniolo, G.: Adverse Reactions to Contrast Media, *Radiology*, 137:299, 1980.
9. Albrechtsson, U., and Olsson, C. G.: Thrombosis after Phlebography: A Comparison of Two Contrast Media, *Cardiovasc. Radiol.*, 2:9, 1979.
10. Lea Thomas, M.: Complications, in "Phlebography of the Lower Limb," Churchill Livingstone, London, 1982, p. 54.
11. Bettman, M. A., Salzman, E. W., Rosenthal, D., et al.: Reduction of Venous Thrombosis Complicating Phlebography, *AJR*, 134:1169, 1980.
12. Laerum, F. and Holm, H. A.: Postphlebographic Thrombosis, *Radiology*, 140:651, 1981.
13. Ritchie, W. G. M., Soulen, R. L., and Rogers, P. W.: Effect of Phlebography on the ^{125}I Uptake Test, *AJR*, 133:855, 1979.

115

Magnetic Resonance Imaging of the Heart and Great Vessels

William J. Casarella, M.D. Harvey J. Berger, M.D.

During the past 20 years, new imaging techniques have revolutionized the practice of cardiology. Angiography, ultrasound, and radionuclide imaging have all become indispensable tools in cardiovascular diagnosis. Magnetic resonance imaging (MRI), formerly called nuclear magnetic resonance imaging (NMR), is a new, high-technology modality that has great promise of being more precise and less invasive than the other three. A typical clinical system is shown in Fig. 115-1. A major advantage of this technique is the lack of any ionizing radiation associated with the procedure. The purpose of this chapter is to outline the current status of MRI in the cardiovascular system.

Basic Physical Considerations in Cardiovascular MRI

Certain atomic nuclei with an odd number of protons or neutrons have an asymmetric distribution of charge and are said to have magnetic moment. When placed in a magnetic field, some of the nuclei tend to align themselves in the direction of the field.

Radio frequency signals of a specific energy and frequency imposed on a given field can induce the nuclei to align themselves against the field. As the excited nuclei in the magnetic field return to their resting state, they emit specific radio frequency signals. The location of the signals from the relaxing nuclei is determined by the presence of a second, low-strength gradient field along the longitudinal axis of the static major field. This gradient field causes changes in the resonant frequencies emitted by the relaxing nuclei along the gradient field. Localization of MRI signals thus is achieved by tuning-in a frequency corresponding to a given cross section. Utilizing these basic principles and reconstruction algorithms developed for x-ray computed tomography (CT), Lauterbur[1] achieved the first two-dimensional images based on MRI signals.

Because hydrogen (^{1}H) is the most prevalent odd-numbered nucleus in the body, it is best suited for MRI. However, the physiological and biochemical significance of the much less abundant nuclei (^{31}P, ^{23}Na, ^{15}O, ^{13}C, etc.) have stimulated investigators to contemplate further development of MRI and spectroscopy incorporating these nuclei as well as the ubiquitous hydrogen nucleus.[2–8] For assessment of myocardial metabolism, utilization of exogenous ^{13}C-labeled substrates as tracers appears promising.[5] At least for the foreseeable future, it is likely that high-resolution imaging will be performed using only proton techniques. It may be possible to obtain regional spectroscopy using surface coil methods but relying on proton images for spatial localization of these spectra.

The intensity of the proton MRI signal that is manipulated by the computer to reconstruct an image is based primarily on the concentration of protons, their relaxation rates (T_1 and T_2), and flow. The two relaxation times refer to the interval required for the nuclei to return to their initial aligned position in the longitudinal plane (T_1) and to lose net transverse energy (T_2). The times T_1 and T_2 are also called spin-lattice and spin-spin relaxation times, respectively. The final magnetic resonance image is derived using one of a series of different pulse sequences, each producing variable degrees of contrast because of emphasis on different factors. For example, spin-echo imaging weights an image with T_2, while saturation recovery emphasizes T_1 and proton density.[9,10] It is likely that the relaxation times as depicted on MRI will provide important insights into the characteristics of tissues themselves (i.e., myocardium or pericardial fluid). This may allow identification of patients with cardiomyopathies as well as differentiation among types of myopathic processes.

In performing MRI spectroscopy, the same nuclei in a given sample relax at slightly different speeds, depending on their molecular position and environment. The familiar multiple peaks of a myocardial ^{31}P spectrum result from such variations, allowing quantification of inorganic phosphate, phosphocreatine, and ATP. Spectroscopy has many potential applications to clinical medicine. Using topical magnetic resonance surface coil techniques, the abnormal phosphate metabolism associated with exercise in McArdle's syndrome has been demonstrated.[11] Stringent homogeneity of very high magnetic field strengths (probably greater than 1.5 to 2.0 T) is required for in vivo spectroscopy. Such requirements have not yet been met for routine clinical use in cardiac diagnosis.

Other variables are important in the analysis and reconstruction of magnetic resonance images of the heart and great vessels. Cardiac and respiratory motion markedly degrade the image, since data acquisition times are in the range of minutes rather than

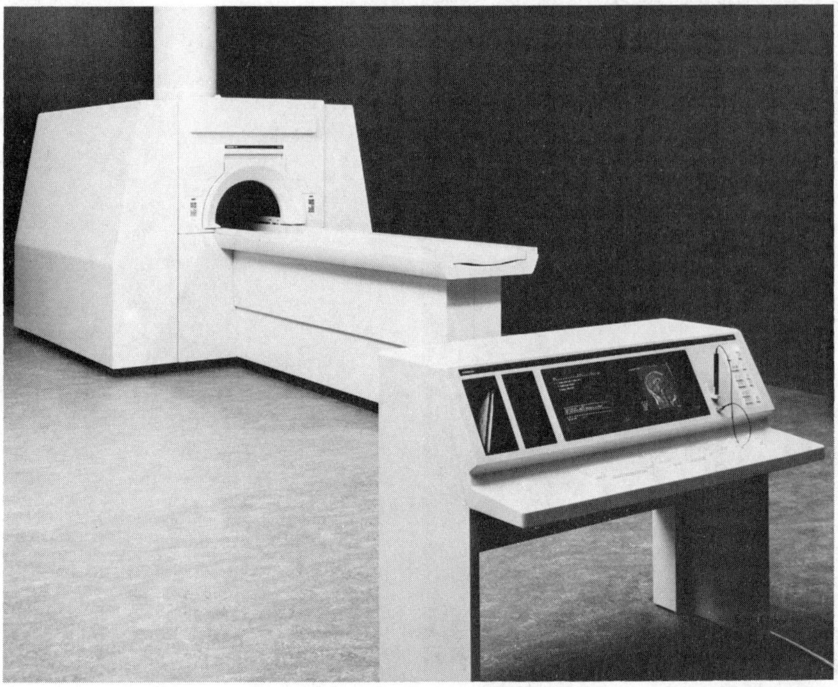

FIGURE 115-1 A typical clinical MRI system. The superconductive large field magnet and patient table are evident. The operator's console is essentially a specialized computer terminal almost identical to the now familiar CT console. The large cylinder on the top of the magnet covering is the conduit for liquid helium and nitrogen needed to cool the magnet. (*Courtesy of Philips Medical Systems, Inc., Shelton, Conn.*)

milliseconds. The simplest solution is use of a finger-pulse plethysmograph to trigger the radio frequency pulse.[12] This technique is relatively imprecise, and a superior method is to trigger the signal off the electrocardiographic R wave, which has been telemetrically transmitted outside of the magnetic field.[12,13] Various radio frequency pulse sequences may also be used to synchronize imaging events to the cardiac cycle.[14] Ungated imaging is possible, but there tends to be very poor contrast between the myocardium and blood. Using a superconductive magnet system, multiplanar gated MRI of the heart requires approximately 6 to 8 min, with the exact time depending upon the heart rate and resolution desired. The limitations of temporal resolution may be overcome by the echo-planar technique being developed by Mansfield and colleagues. The entire tomographic image can be obtained in less than 100 ms without gating. Although the resolution of these images is less than optimal at this time, this innovative technique may lead to cine-MRI of the heart in the future.[15]

Because cohorts of energized nuclei in flowing blood are swept out of the sensitive field before they can contribute to the generation of the magnetic resonance image, blood vessels usually appear black (no signal) on magnetic resonance images.[9,16] Thus, naturally occurring, moving materials provide an intrinsic contrast material for the heart and blood vessels.

The strength of the magnetic field plays a major role in the type and quality of the MRI signals produced.[10,17] In general, the higher-strength magnets are much more costly, both in initial purchase and in maintenance. Magnets greater than 0.35 tesla in strength are usually of the superconductive type that require cooling with expensive liquid helium and nitrogen. Site preparation is more difficult with high-strength magnets. Greater shielding is required for environmental safety, and heavy, nonferrous structural support of the magnet is necessary. Improved signal-to-noise ratio and short data acquisition times are the major advantages of the high field strength magnets. Useful biological information from nuclei other than hydrogen will almost certainly require the use of magnetic fields greater than 1.5 tesla. Other, less expensive types of magnets with lower field strengths are available; these include resistive and permanent magnet systems. In both instances, field strengths are limited to less than 0.35 tesla, compared with 1.5 to 2.0 tesla for the superconductive magnet systems. Most cardiac studies to date have been obtained with superconductive magnet systems.

In addition to magnetic shielding to keep electromagnetic forces confined to the imaging laboratory, radio frequency shielding must be provided to keep ambient radio signals out. The MRI site must also be configured to prevent the unsuspecting person with an implanted cardiac pacemaker from being adversely affected. Loose metal objects must be excluded by means of remote metal detectors and controlled access to the MRI scanner in order to prevent accidents caused by flying metal objects attracted to the magnet with great force. To preserve the exquisite homogeneity of the magnetic field, it also must be isolated from moving, large metal objects such as elevators and moving vehicles. Therefore, site selection and preparation are critical and almost certainly very costly.

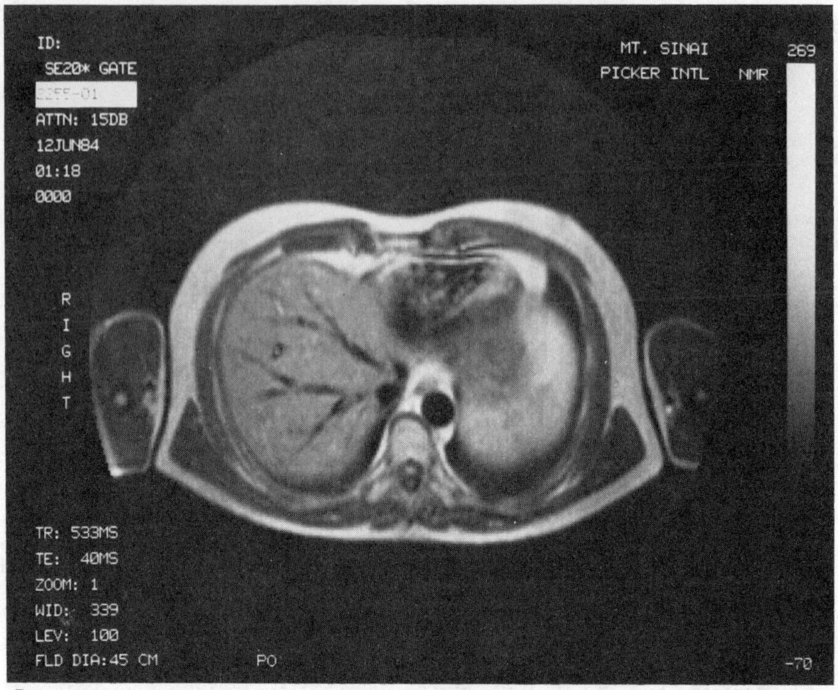

A

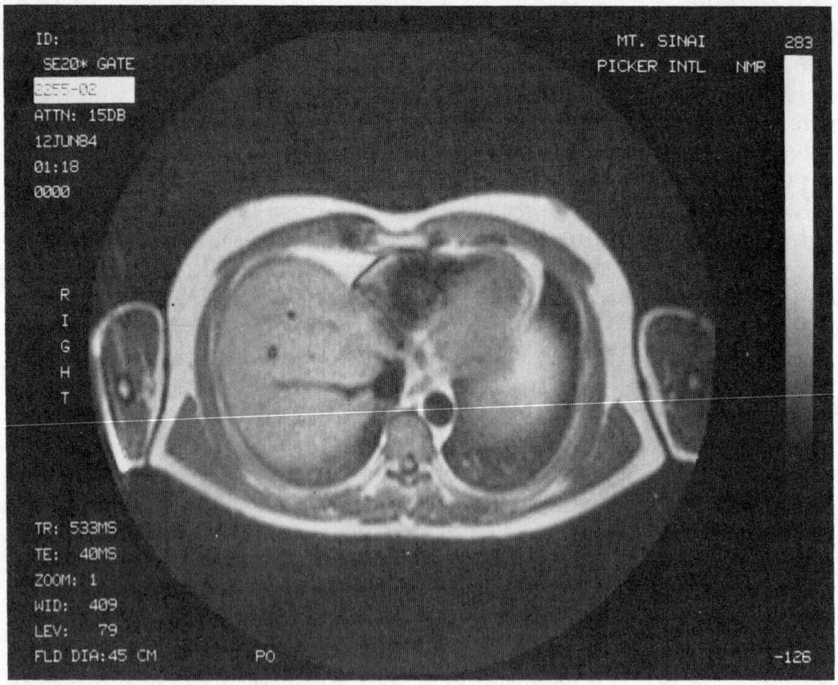

B

Clinical Experience

Acquired Lesions of the Heart and Aorta

Magnetic resonance images generally are displayed in the transaxial plane similar to x-ray CT, but they also can be reoriented to the sagittal and coronal planes (Figs. 115-2 and 115-3). Natural contrast between flowing blood and the myocardium or vessel wall is one of the great advantages of MRI over x-ray CT and permits the clear demonstration of lesions of the left ventricle and aorta. The epicardium and endocaridum are well visualized, with high contrast compared to the cavity. Intrinsic resolution is adequate to identify moderator bands, papillary muscles, valve leaflets, and proximal coronary arteries. Dissecting aneurysms,[18] atherosclerotic aneurysms and plaques,[19] and ventricular aneurysms[20] have all been imaged by high-resolution multiplanar

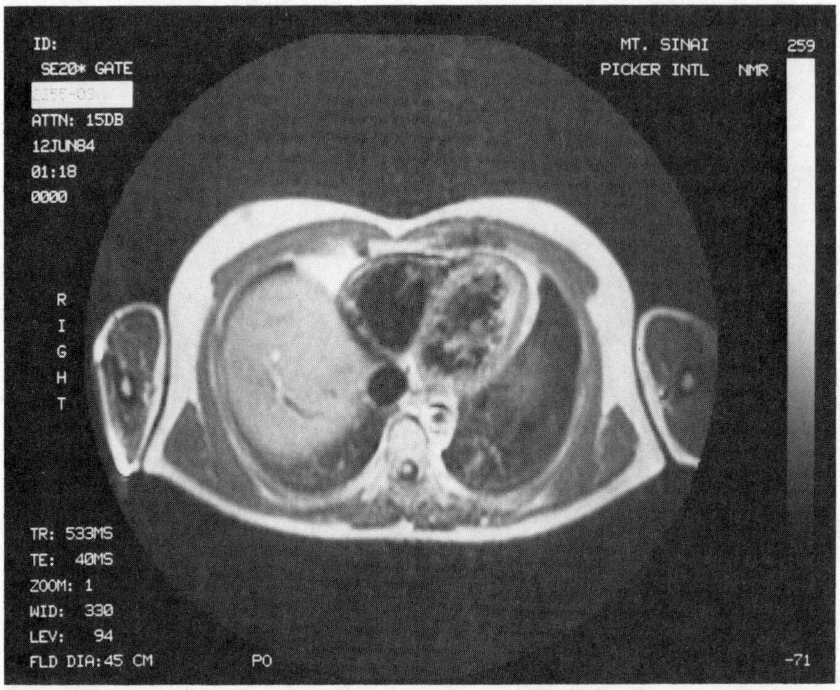

C

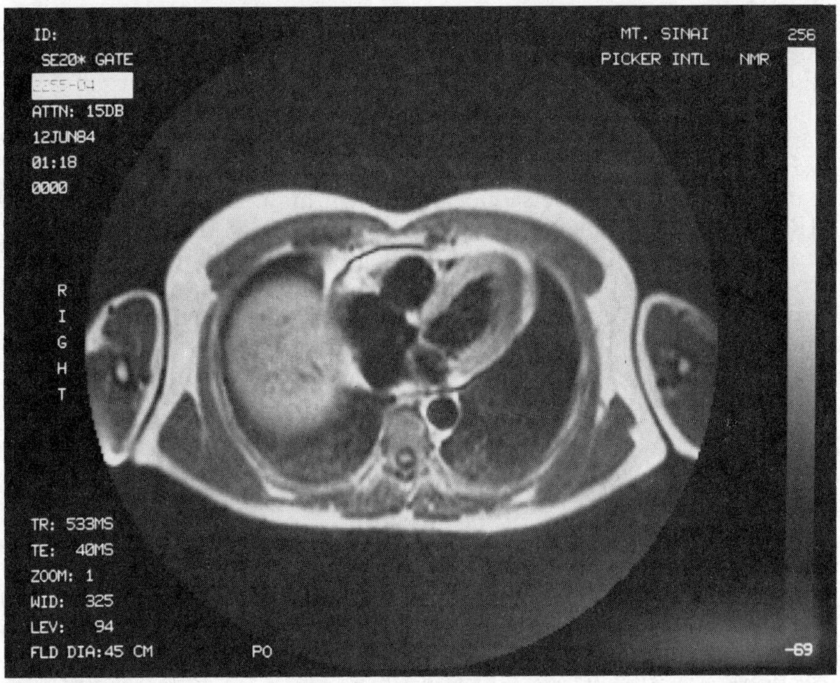

D

FIGURE 115-2 Four MRI images in a normal volunteer. Total time for imaging and reconstruction for the four images was 7 min. *A.* Transverse MRI section through the base of the heart in middiastole. This is a gated image using spin-echo multislice technique. *B.* The same individual imaged in early diastole. *C.* At end diastole, note the enhanced signal in the descending aorta, as well as the pulmonary vasculature. *D.* In late systole, the left ventricular myocardium, moderator band in the right ventricle, and atrioventricular valves are well seen. Note the absence of signal from the descending aorta. (*Courtesy of Dr. Roderic Pettigrew, Picker International, and Dr. Stephen Wiener, Mt. Sinai Hospital, Cleveland, Ohio.*)

MRI. Examples of arteriovenous malformations, mural thrombi in the aorta and left ventricle, and the location and patency of coronary artery bypass grafts are all detectable by MRI and have been illustrated in the pioneering work of Higgins and his colleagues.[18–22]

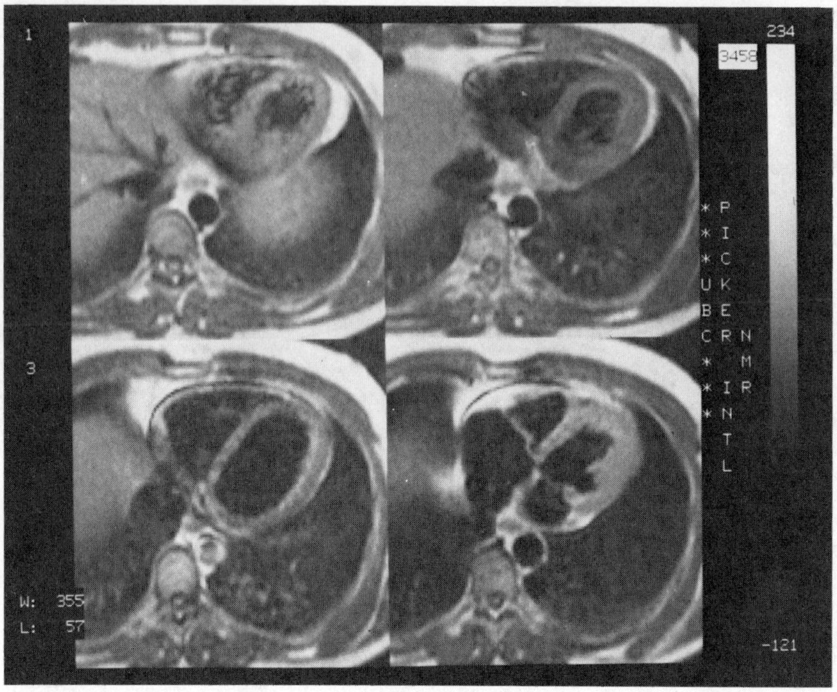

FIGURE 115-3 Four cross-sectional images in a normal volunteer again demonstrate cardiac anatomy of all four chambers, the atrioventricular valves, pericardium, and variation of blood flow in the descending aorta. *(Courtesy of Dr. Roderick Pettigrew, Picker International, Cleveland, Ohio, and Dr. David Li, University of British Columbia, Vancouver, B.C., Canada.)*

It has been possible to define lesions of the pericardium with great accuracy[23] and to identify lesions of the thorax and mediastinum.[24] Multislice[25,26] high-resolution images and elegant three-dimensional reconstruction techniques[27] have been applied to the quantitative assessment of ventricular size and function, as well as to the demonstration of congenital lesions. Although it is unlikely that MRI will be the most cost-effective means of evaluating left ventricular performance, it may be possible to obtain these data routinely as part of any cardiac magnetic resonance study taking advantage of new image-processing algorithms and gated acquisition.

Demonstration of Abnormal Flow Patterns

Several abnormalities of blood flow have been recognized by MRI. Using variations of spin-echo MRI techniques, Herfkens et al. demonstrated intense echoes from an occluded vascular graft.[21] They contrasted the abnormal graft with the absence of signal from a comparable vessel with free flow. Variations in flow velocity are also important in detecting the true and false channels of aortic dissections. Areas of atherosclerosis in vessels may be visualized because their lipid content is different from that of adjacent endothelium and flowing blood.[9]

The possibility of quantifying blood flow has been explored by several investigators. Following Singer's early work,[28] Kaufman et al.[9] have shown that laminar flow with a velocity of 10 to 15 cm/s produces no detectable MRI signal in the region of the vessel. However, when a second cross-sectional image is obtained distal to the first section, paradoxical enhancement of the MRI signal may occur in the region of the flowing blood. Most likely, this phenomenon occurs because new blood-borne nuclei arrive in the image region and become fully magnetized and thereby are out of phase with the stationary nuclei that are already undergoing depolarization and relaxation. It is, therefore, difficult to quantitate blood flow solely on the basis of MRI signal intensity. Gore[29] suggested that changes in pulse sequencing which highlight flow, rather than proton density, may make flow imaging more feasible. In addition, other radio frequency and gradient field pulse-sequencing patterns have been suggested by Kaufman.[9] Most likely, turbulent flow, as well as absent or decreased flow, will be detectable by MRI. True clinical quantification of blood flow seems to be possible but has yet to be achieved.

Congenital Cardiac Disease

A spectrum of congenital cardiac anomalies involving the heart and great vessels has been studied thus far. In a series of 19 patients with congenital cardiac disease, Fletcher et al.[12] obtained diagnostic information in 17 and demonstrated that MRI information was superior to that obtained with x-ray CT. They were less convinced of its superiority to two-dimensional, echocardiography. Detailed comparison studies of MRI, angiocardiography, and echocardiography in pediatric cardiac lesions has yet to be done. However, the imaging techniques currently available and the capability for three-dimensional reconstruction[27] will almost certainly be successfully utilized in the diagnosis of congenital cardiac lesions.

Myocardial Ischemia

In vitro studies have demonstrated varying relaxation times between normal and necrotic myocardium.[30] These studies have subsequently been confirmed in vivo.[31] Values of T_2 derived using spin-echo imaging clearly discriminated between normal and infarcted zones. Areas of myocardial necrosis were identified by increased MRI signal due to augmentation in T_2 and proton density (both related to increased water content). Using gated, multislice spin-echo techniques, Higgins et al.[32] studied 10 patients with proven myocardial infarction and compared them with 8 normal controls. They were able to demonstrate the endocardial surface, as well as the epicardium and pericardial fat and lung. Cross sections of the coronary arteries also were obtained. The magnetic resonance images correlated well with left ventriculograms and two-dimensional echocardiograms. Three left ventricular aneurysms and two mural thrombi also were identified. Thinning of the myocardium or global hypokinesis was shown in 9 of the 10 patients with myocardial infarction. A positive image with increased T_2 in the infarct similar to that obtained in the animal studies already described was not obtained in the patients. Although this study represents the most extensive clinical experience with myocardial infarction yet reported, many questions remain unanswered. Whether or not MRI can differentiate viable myocardium, reversible ischemia and completed infarction is still unclear. Furthermore, the clinical applicability of MRI for visualizing the coronary arteries remains to be elucidated. At this time, only the proximal coronaries have been clearly delineated.[18,25]

The role of surface coils and in vivo regional ^{31}P spectroscopy to detect early changes in the myocardium, such as shifts in intracellular pH or high-energy phosphate metabolism, is still unknown.[2,3,6,7,33] Of interest, one preliminary report has described increased sodium accumulation during prolonged coronary artery occlusion in cats using ^{23}Na imaging in a high-field prototype system.[34] These early studies, as well as others, should provide the basis for the application of NMR techniques to the study of myocardial metabolism in vivo.

Pericardial Disease

Diseases of the pericardium are well studied by MRI.[18,22,23] Chronic thickening of the pericardium in constrictive pericarditis is detectable, as is the high signal intensity produced by active inflammatory lesions. Markedly increased signals from inflammatory pericardial effusions suggest that MRI may be able to judge the activity of pericarditis and other inflammatory diseases, as well as merely detect their presence. Pericardial cysts and tumors also have been detected in isolated instances.

Paramagnetic Contrast Agents

Although MRI has intrinsic high tissue contrast based on the properties already discussed, considerable work has been done to artificially enhance the contrast level by extrinsic means. MRI contrast agents function indirectly by altering the magnetic properties of nuclei. Paramagnetic agents enhance relaxation times (T_1 and T_2) and thus change image contrast. The physicochemical basis of this phenomenon lies in the unpaired electrons in paramagnetic species. In most molecules, electrons are distributed in pairs which have opposite spins that effectively cancel each other and result in a diamagnetic species. When electrons in a given orbit are unpaired, a net electron spin results which generates a local magnetic field that can shorten T_1 and T_2 of neighboring protons. Since the paramagnetic effect of unpaired electrons is almost 700 times that of the magnetic moment of a proton, considerable influence on relaxation times can be achieved by close contact between the water molecules and the paramagnetic contrast agents.[35,36]

Most paramagnetic species are heavy metal ions with incompletely filled electron orbitals which can bind directly to water molecules (Table 115-1). Other paramagnetic species include nitroxide stable free radicals and molecular oxygen, with its two unpaired electrons.

Paramagnetic contrast agents may provide a means of performing myocardial perfusion imaging using MRI techniques (Table 115-1). Manganese appears to be ideally suited, because it is distributed according to regional myocardial blood flow (similar to ^{210}Tl.[37] Early in vivo imaging studies demonstrated enhancement of the MRI signal from normal myocardium and thus better delineation of the margins of healed infarcts.[38]

The delayed clearance of metallic ions from the body and their potential toxicity may exclude them from routine clinical use. Paramagnetic chelates such as manganese, chromium, or gadolinium ethylenediaminetetracetic acid (EDTA) or diethylenetriaminepentaacetic acid (DTPA) probably have the most potential for human use. Gadolinium DTPA has been most extensively studied.[39–41] It appears to be well tolerated in animal studies and is strongly paramagnetic due to the seven unpaired electrons in gadolinium. It is readily excreted by the kidneys, with a

TABLE 115-1 Paramagnetic Species

Metallic ions
Titanium (T_1^{3+})
Iron (Fe^{3+})
Vanadium (V^{4+})
Cobalt (Co^{3+})
Chromium (Cr^{3+})
Nickel (Ni^{3+})
Manganese (Mn^{2+})
Copper (Co^{2+})
Gadolinium (Gd^{3+})
Praseodynium (Pr^{3+})
Nitroxide stable free radicals
Pyrrolidine and piperidine derivatives
Molecular oxygen (O_2)

20-min half-life in the body. Furthermore, it is very hydrophilic, and therefore allows for close attachment between the proton-rich water molecules, and is stable in vivo. Marked MRI enhancement of brain tissue and renal parenchyma, as well as myocardium, have been achieved in experimental animals and patients.

One of the most innovative uses of paramagnetic agents has been the attempt to direct them to specific tissues with monoclonal antibodies. Preliminary work by Brady et al. utilizing monoclonal antibodies to myosin loaded with manganese indicates the potential for this approach in the detection of myocardial infarction.[42] This work is the outgrowth of studies which have been proceeding for several years in which a radioactively labeled antimyosin antibody has been used to image acute myocardial infarcts. Clinical trials of these paramagnetic agents have not yet been reported.

Inhalation of molecular oxygen has theoretical use in enhancing magnetic resonance images, especially in the cardiovascular system. Differentiation of oxygenated arterial blood from deoxygenated venous blood is enhanced, and T_1 values of blood and myocardium are altered by this attractive, simple method. More work in this area will be forthcoming. Nitroxide stable free radicals of the pyrrolidine and piperidine groups are also promising.[43] Two excellent reviews of the current status of contrast agents in MRI are available.[35,36]

Possible Hazards in MRI

Possible harmful effects of MRI could result from the high static magnetic field, the radio frequency field, or the rapidly switching magnetic gradient fields. There have been no clearly documented adverse biological effects from these variables, either in experimental systems or in MRI workers.

Major areas of concern lie in the interaction of extrinsic factors with the MRI system itself. Magnetic foreign bodies such as pacemakers,[44] surgical clips, and metallic implants[45] are affected by the energy levels used in MRI. Pacemakers appear to function erratically in the presence of an MRI system. Heat may be generated in metallic prostheses, and aneurysm clips may be loosened or dislodged in high magnetic fields.[35] Development of nonferrometallic pacemakers, surgical clips, and prostheses is possible and will probably occur as the modality's efficacy becomes more proven. Potential hazards and safe levels of magnetic and radio frequency energy levels have been well summarized by Budinger.[46]

Summary

Cardiovascular MRI is still in its infancy. The technique is very costly and complex, but it has potential to be of great significance in the diagnosis of cardiac and vascular disease. During the past 2 years, multislice imaging techniques have been developed, and positive early clinical experience has been recorded. Attempts at measuring blood flow alterations have been made. New contrast agents have been studied in vivo. Advancements in hardware and software design are being produced in numerous laboratories around the world. The proliferation of MRI facilities in more medical centers will serve to advance the field of cardiovascular MRI and to define its future role relative to other noninvasive imaging techniques.

However, major emphasis thus far has been placed on the utility of MRI in morphological assessment of the heart and vessels. In the future, it is likely that the emphasis will shift to evaluation of myocardial metabolism by analysis of endogenous substrates and metabolic tracers.

References

1. Lauterbur, P. C.: Image Formation by Induced Local Interactions: Examples Employing NMR, *Nature,* 242:190, 1973.
2. Haselgrove, J. C., Subramanian, V. H., Leigh, J. S., Gyulai, L., and Chance, B.: In Vivo One-Dimensional Imaging of Phosphorus Metabolites by Phosphorus-31 Nuclear Magnetic Resonance, *Science,* 220:1170, 1983.
3. Nunnally, R. L., and Bottomley, P. A.: 31P NMR Studies of Myocardial Ischemia and Its Response to Drug Therapies, *J. Comput. Assist. Tomogr.,* 5:296, 1981.
4. Burt, C. T., and Koutcher, J. A.: Multinuclear NMR Studies of Naturally Occurring Nuclei, *J. Nucl. Med.,* 25:237, 1984.
5. Alger, J. R., Sillerud, L. O., Behar, K. L., Gillies, R. J., and Shulman, R. G.: In Vivo Carbon-13 Nuclear Magnetic Resonance Studies of Mammals, *Science,* 214:660, 1981.
6. Fossel, E. T., Morgan, H. E., and Ingwall, J. S.: Measurement of Changes in High-Energy Phosphates in the Cardiac Cycle Using Gated P-31 NMR, *Proc. Natl. Acad. Sci.,* 77:3654, 1980.
7. Nunnally, R. L., and Bottomley, P. A.: Assessment of Pharmacological Treatment of Myocardial Infarction by Phosphorus-31 NMR with Surface Coils, *Science,* 211:177, 1981.
8. DeLayre, J. L., Ingwall, J. S., Malloy, C., and Fossel, E. T.: Gated Sodium-23 Nuclear Magnetic Resonance Images of an Isolated Perfused Working Rat Heart, *Science,* 212:935, 1981.
9. Kaufman, L., Crooks, L., Sheldon, P., Hricak, H., Herfkens, R., and Banks, W.: The Potential Impact of Nuclear Magnetic Resonance Imaging on Cardiovascular Diagnosis, *Circulation,* 67:251, 1983.
10. Harms, S. E., Morgan, T. J., Yamanashi, W. S., Harle, T. S., and Dodd, G. D.: Principles of Nuclear Magnetic Resonance Imaging, *RadioGraphics,* 4:26, 1984.
11. Ross, B. D., Radda, G. K., Gadian, D. G., Rocker, G., Esiri, M., and Falconer-Smith, J.: Examination of a Case of Suspected McArdle's Syndrome by P-31 NMR, *N. Engl. J. Med.,* 304:1338, 1981.
12. Fletcher, B. D., Jacobstein, M. D., Nelson, A. D., Riemenschneider, T. A., and Alfidi, R. J.: Gated Magnetic Resonance Imaging of Congenital Cardiac Malformations, *Radiology,* 150:137, 1984.
13. Lanzer, P., Botvinick, E. H., Schiller, N. B., et al.: Cardiac Imaging Using Gated Magnetic Resonance, *Radiology,* 150:121, 1984.
14. van Dijk, P.: Direct Cardiac NMR Imaging of Heart Wall and Blood Flow Velocity, *J. Comput. Assist. Tomogr.,* 8:429, 1984.

15. Orlidge, R. J., Mansfield, P., Doyle, M., and Coupland, R. E.: "Real-time" Movie Images by NMR, in R. L. Witcofski, N. Karstaedt, and C. L. Partain (eds.), "Proceedings of the International Symposium in NMR Imaging," (Bowman Gray School of Medicine, Winston-Salem, North Carolina, 1982, p. 89.) *Br. J. Radiol.*, 55:729, 1982.
16. Ratner, A. V., Okada, R. D., and Brady, T. J.: Nuclear Magnetic Resonance Imaging of the Heart, *Semin. Nucl. Med.*, 13:339, 1983.
17. Doutcher, J. A., Burt, C. T., Lauffer, R. B., and Brady, T. J.: Contrast Agents and Spectroscopic Probes in NMR, *J. Nucl. Med.*, 25:506, 1984.
18. Higgins, C. B., Lanzer, P., Stark, D., et al.: Nuclear Magnetic Resonance Imaging of Atherosclerosis, *RadioGraphics*, 4:137, 1984.
19. Higgins, C. B., Herfkens, R., Hricak, H., et al.: Nuclear Magnetic Resonance Imaging in Atherosclerosis, *RadioGraphics*, 4:137, 1984.
20. Herfkens, R. J., Higgins, C. B., Hricak, H., et al.: Nuclear Magnetic Resonance Imaging of the Cardiovascular System: Normal and Pathologic Findings, *Radiology*, 147:749, 1983.
21. Herfkens, R. J., Higgins, C. B., Hricak, H., et al.: Nuclear Magnetic Resonance Imaging in Atherosclerotic Disease, *Radiology*, 148:161, 1983.
22. Higgins, C. B., Hricak, H., Gamsu, G., et al.: Clinical Nuclear Magnetic Resonance Imaging of the Body, *Semin. Nucl. Med.*, 13:347, 1983.
23. Stark, D. D., Higgins, C. B., Lanzer, P., et al.: Magnetic Resonance Imaging of the Pericardium: Normal and Pathologic Findings, *Radiology*, 150:469, 1984.
24. Brasch, R. C., Gooding, C. A., Lallemand, D. P., and Wesbey, G. E.: Magnetic Resonance Imaging of the Thorax in Childhood, *Radiology*, 150:463, 1984.
25. Higgins, C. B., Stark, D., McNamara, M., Lanzer, P., Crooks, L. E., and Kaufman, L.: Multiplane Magnetic Resonance Imaging of the Heart and Major Vessels: Studies in Normal Volunteers, *Am. J. Radiol.*, 142:661, 1984.
26. Crooks, L. E., Hoenninger, J., Arakawa, M., et al.: High-Resolution Magnetic Resonance Imaging, *Radiology*, 150:163, 1984.
27. Herman, G. T., Udupa, J. K., Kramer, D. M., Lauterbur, P., Rudin, A. M., and Schneider, J. S.: Three-Dimensional Display of Nuclear Magnetic Resonance Images, *Optical Eng.*, 21:923, 1982.
28. Singer, J. R.: Blood Flow Measurements in NMR, in L. Kaufman, L. E. Crooks, and A. R. Margulis (eds.), "NMR Imaging in Medicine," Igaku-shoin, New York, 1981, Chap. 8.
29. Gore, J. C.: The Meaning and Significance of Relaxation in NMR Imaging, in R. L. Witcofski, N. Karstaedt, and C. L. Partain (eds.), "Proceedings of the International Symposium in NMR Imaging," Bowman Gray School of Medicine, Winston-Salem, North Carolina, 1981, p. 15.
30. Williams, E. S., Kaplan, J. L., Thatcher, F., Zimmerman, G., and Krobel, S. B.: Prolongation of Proton Spin—Lattice Relaxation Times in Regionally Ischemic Tissue from Dog Hearts, *J. Nucl. Med.*, 21:449, 1980.
31. Higgins, C. B., Herfkens, R., Lipton, M. J., et al.: Nuclear Magnetic Resonance Imaging of Acute Myocardial Infarction in Dogs: Alterations in Magnetic Relaxation Times, *Am. J. Cardiol.*, 52:184, 1983.
32. Higgins, C. B., Lanzer, P., Stark, D., et al.: Imaging by Nuclear Magnetic Resonance in Patients with Chronic Ischemic Heart Disease, *Circulation*, 69:523, 1984.
33. Ruigrok, T. J. C., van Echteld, C. J. A., de Kruijff, B., Borst, C., and Meijler, F. L.: Protective Effect of Nifedipine in Myocardial Ischemia Assessed by Phosphorus Nuclear Magnetic Resonance, *J. Am. Coll. Cardiol.*, 1:666, 1983.
34. Cannon, P. J., Maudsley, A., Hilal, S. K., Simon, H. E., and Cassedy, F.: NMR Imaging of Na-23 in Myocardium following Coronary Artery Occlusion, *Circulation*, 68(suppl. 3): III–177, 1983. (Abstract.)
35. Runge, V. M., Clanton, J. A., Lukehart, C. M., Partain, C. L., and James, E. A.: Paramagnetic Agents for Contrast-Enhanced NMR Imaging: A Review, *Am. J. Radiol.*, 141:1209, 1983.
36. Wolf, G. L., and Baum, S.: Nuclear Magnetic Resonance Contrast Agents for Proton Imaging, *RadioGraphics*, 4:66, 1984.
37. Chauncey, D. M., Jr., Schelbert, H. R., Halpern, S. E., Delans, F., McKegney, M. L., Ashburn, W. L., and Hagan, P. L.: Tissue Distribution on Studies with Radioactive Manganese: A Potential Agent for Myocardial Imaging, *J. Nucl. Med.*, 18:933, 1977.
38. Brady, T. J., Goldman, M. R., Pykett, I. L., et al.: Proton Nuclear Magnetic Resonance Imaging of Regionally Ischemic Canine Hearts: Effect of Paramagnetic Proton Signal Enhancement, *Radiology*, 144:343, 1982.
39. Brady, T. J., Rosen, B. R., Gold, H. K., et al.: Selective Decrease in T_1 Relaxation Time of Infarcted Myocardium with the Use of a Manganese Labeled Monoclonal Antibody, Antimyosin ["Proceedings, Society of Magnetic Resonance in Medicine," Second Annual Meeting, San Francisco, 1983, p. 10. (Abstract).] *Magn. Res. M.*, 1(2):286, 1984.
40. Brasch, R. C.: Work in Progress: Methods of Contrast Enhancement for NMR Imaging and Potential Applications, *Radiology*, 147:781, 1983.
41. Brasch, R. C., Weinmann, H. J., and Wesbey, G. E.: Contrast-Enhanced NMR Imaging: Animal Studies Using Gandolinium-DTPA Complex, *Am. J. Radiol.*, 142:625, 1984.
42. Brady, T. J., Rosen, B. R., Gold, H. K., et al.: Selective Decrease in T_1 Relaxation Time of Infarcted Myocardium with the Use of a Manganese Labeled Monoclonal Antibody, Antimyosin, Proceedings, Society of Magnetic Resonance in Medicine, Second Annual Meeting, San Francisco, 1983, p. 10. (Abstract.)
43. Brasch, R. C., London, D. A., Wesbey, G. E., et al.: Work in Progress: Nuclear Magnetic Resonance Study of a Paramagnetic Nitroxide Contrast Agent for Enhancement of Renal Structures in Experimental Animals, *Radiology*, 147:773, 1983.
44. Paclicek, W., Geisinger, M., Castle, L., et al.: The Effects of Nuclear Magnetic Resonance on Patients with Cardiac Pacemakers, *Radiology*, 147:149, 1983.
45. New, P., Rosen, B. R., Brady, T. J., et al.: Potential Hazards and Artifacts of Ferromagnetic and Nonferromagnetic Surgical and Dental Materials and Devices in Nuclear Magnetic Resonance Imaging, *Radiology*, 147:139, 1983.
46. Budinger, T. F.: Nuclear Magnetic Resonance (NMR) *in vivo* Studies: Known Thresholds for Health Effects, *J. Comput, Assist. Tomogr.*, 5:800, 1981.

116

Radiologically Guided Intervention in the Heart and Great Vessels

William J. Casarella, M.D.

Percutaneous interventional techniques developed in the past 7 years for increasing blood flow to the heart and other organs have been extremely successful. Going in the reverse direction, methods of selective embolization therapy have been applied to the management of hemorrhage, tumor ablation, trauma, and other instances where a regional decrease in blood flow is essential. This chapter will describe the current status of angioplasty and embolization techniques in the management of various cardiovascular problems.

Selective Embolization in the Pulmonary Circulation

Usually, instances of acute hemoptysis result from chronic pulmonary disease with bleeding from hypertrophied bronchial vessels. Occasionally, this clinical problem may result from lesions of the pulmonary arteries themselves. Surgery is extremely difficult in critically ill patients with massive hemoptysis from the pulmonary artery. Reports[1,2] describe the use of coils and Gelfoam in the management of a hemorrhaging Rasmussen aneurysm of the pulmonary artery and of a large mycotic pulmonary aneurysm occluded with a detachable balloon. Szarnicki et al.[3] had also described the technique of selective embolization of systemic pulmonary artery collaterals using guidewire coils in a group of patients following corrective surgery for pulmonary atresia. Other reports describe the use of detachable silicone balloons in the closure of unneeded Blalock-Taussig shunts in patients who have undergone total repair of tetralogy of Fallot but no longer need the subclavian artery to pulmonary artery anastomosis, which was left intact at the time of total corrective surgery.[4,5] In similar cases, wire coils have also been used, with comparable results.

The availability of large stainless steel coils and detachable balloons which can be inserted through small catheters to occlude relatively large vessels have made possible occlusion of relatively large vessels, which communicate between the right and left sides of the circulation, without the danger of inadvertent passage of the embolization material into the systemic circulation. Some of the most difficult lesions to treat in the pulmonary circulation are arteriovenous malformations which typically have large fistulous connections between the pulmonary arteries and veins. Taylor et al.[6] reported the first successful closure of a single pulmonary arteriovenous malformation using stainless steel coils. A year later the technique was extended to the successful closure of multiple diffuse bilateral pulmonary arteriovenous malformations using multiple coils.[7] Although this technique was successful in a few case reports, the lack of precise control in placement of the coils and the fear of systemic embolization stimulated the development of detachable balloons for solution of this difficult clinical problem.

White et al. developed an elegant technique for the precise placement of variously sized detachable silicone balloons using coaxial selective catheterization.[8] It allows for the precise placement of the balloons and the verification of their position prior to detachment from the balloon catheter. Development of the detachable balloons led to the classic article by Terry et al.[9] which described the balloon embolization of multiple pulmonary arteriovenous malformations in a 55-year-old male with hereditary hemorrhagic telangiectasia. In this particular case, nine balloons were properly positioned in the region of the arteriovenous fistulas. Following the procedure the patient's oxygen saturation increased from 73 to 90 percent, and his clinical picture markedly improved. Other case reports have appeared[10–12] describing good results using balloon occlusion of pulmonary arteriovenous malformations.

The group at Johns Hopkins followed up their initial success with a series of five patients who had a total of 16 pulmonary arteriovenous malformations, all of which were treated with balloon occlusion.[13] Four of those five patients did extremely well. One patient could not be successfully embolized because of the presence of a fistula too large to be closed with the available balloons. There were two pulmonary infarctions in this series. Of the 15 arteriovenous malformations that were obliterated, 14 were shown to be still occluded on follow-up studies 6 months to 2 years after the original procedure. In a later report,[14] the same group described 10 patients where 58 of 71 visible arteriovenous malformations were embolized with detachable balloons. In this group, 9 of 10 patients showed significant functional improvement with increase in arterial oxygen saturation from an average of 43 mmHg to 64 mmHg, and an increase in oxygen saturation from 79 to 92 percent. One other group briefly described the use of detachable deBrun latex balloons in the management of multiple pulmonary arteriovenous malformations.[15] Since approximately 60 percent of patients with this lesion have bilateral disease with multiple fistulas and subsequent oxygen desaturation, corrective surgery may be very difficult or even impossible without resection of considerable pulmonary parenchyma. The ingenious technique of embolization of pulmonary arteriovenous malformations with detachable balloons has allowed for the successful percutaneous management of what previously had been a debilitating disease with a very poor surgical prognosis.

Complications reported in this application of selective embolization have been extremely low and are considerably lower than the complications of paradoxical systemic emboli, hemorrhage, and infection that can result from the untreated form of the disease.

Applications of Percutaneous Angioplasty Techniques in the Heart and Great Vessels

Ever since the reports of the successful management of peripheral vascular and coronary artery disease by means of balloon angioplasty, investigators have been eager to attempt the technique in coarctation of the aorta. Lock and his colleagues[16] developed an animal model in newborn lambs based on wedge resections and partial ligation of the descending aorta. Of 13 animals that subsequently underwent percutaneous transluminal angioplasty of the artificially induced coarctation, 12 did well with permanent dilatation of the stricture and eventually healing of damaged intima. One animal suffered a ruptured aorta during overdilatation with a large balloon catheter. Success in this particular animal model presaged subsequent clinical experience in the management of postoperative coarctations, and did not predict the mixed results in the management of primary coarctation in infants.

In Singer's report of a dilatation of a restenosis following repair of a coarctation in a newborn, successful relief of the aortic pressure gradient was achieved using a no. 5 French, 5-mm Gruentzig balloon catheter.[17] However, a long-term follow-up was lacking in this particular case.

In two cases reported by Sperling et al.[18] the procedure was totally ineffective in a 3-week-old infant and was successful in an 11-month-old child with a primary coarctation. Lababidi[19] reported the successful dilatation of a severe *coarctation* in a 5-week-old infant using a no. 5 French catheter with a 5-mm balloon. Follow-up at 1 month demonstrated a normal infant with no evidence of a hemodynamically significant coarctation. In this particular case, the balloon was inflated four times for at least 10-s intervals. This suggests that a temporary relief may be obtained which could allow an infant with coarctation to grow sufficiently in size so that a definitive repair could be undertaken with greater safety.

Conversely, Finley and his group reported more disappointing results in four infants, in three of whom the angioplasty was attempted as the first method of correcting a severe coarctation.[20] In all three infants, the coarctation recurred after 7 days. One patient died of a ruptured aorta during the procedure.

The most optimistic report has been made by Kan et al.[21] in their series of seven patients with restenosis of the aorta following primary surgical repair for coarctation. These seven patients ranged in age from 10 months to 17 years. The average pressure gradient across the restenosis was 58 mmHg in the preangioplasty patient and 13 mmHg following balloon dilatation. Follow-up period has lasted from 1 to 14 months with continued patency of the repair. One patient in this group died 6 h following the angioplasty. At autopsy there was no damage to the aorta, and signs of intimal proliferation with dilatation and small intimal tears were evident.

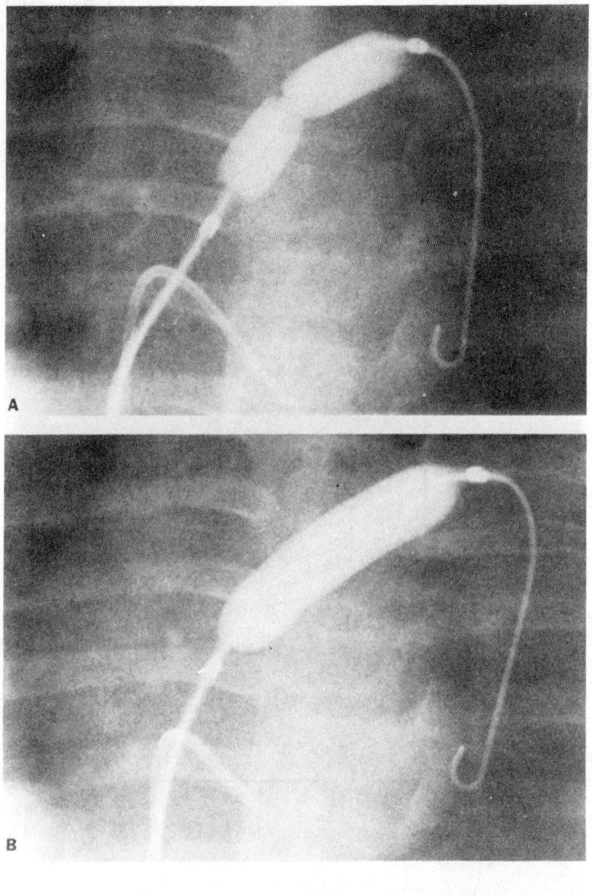

FIGURE 116-1 *A.* Balloon angioplasty in pulmonary valvular stenosis. A large-lumen 15-mm balloon catheter was passed across the stenotic pulmonary valve and inflated to 6 atm of pressure. *B.* The valvular impression on the balloon is eliminated indicating disruption of the valve leaflets and relief of the transvalvular pressure gradient. (*From J. S. Kan, R. I. White, Jr., S. E. Mitchell, J. H. Anderson and T. J. Gardner: Percutaneous Transluminal Balloon Valvuloplasty for Pulmonary Valve Stenosis, Circulation, 69:556, 1984. Reproduced with permission from the American Heart Association, Inc., and the author.*)

The results of Kan's group were substantiated by Lock et al.[22] in their series of eight infants who underwent angioplasty of coarctations of the aorta. In three of the patients, percutaneous transluminal angioplasty (PTA) was attempted as the primary method of repair. All three of these patients subsequently failed and required surgery. However, the five patients that had angioplasty for restenosis following surgery did well, with an average increase in aortic lumen diameter from 4.7 to 7.7 mm. A single case report of balloon angioplasty in an adult with coarctation of the aorta[23] indicates that there might be a place for this technique in the older age group. Preliminary results in children indicate excellent success in the management of postoperative restenosis of coarctations and very limited success in the use of angioplasty for the primary management of coarctation of the aorta.

One of the lesions that has attracted considerable attention as possibly being amenable to percutaneous balloon dilatation is *pulmonary valvular stenosis* (Fig. 116-1). The development of a new series of catheters by White and his colleagues[24] has stimulated work in this field. They have designed catheters with large balloons measuring 18 to 20 mm in diameter with a large second lumen for the balloon that allows for rapid inflation and deflation. Using this type of large balloon and standard techniques of cardiac catheterization and balloon angioplasty, a series of single case reports have appeared describing the successful dilatation of pulmonary valvular stenosis in three patients.[25–27] A particularly well-documented case was reported by Pepine et al.[28] using a catheter with a 20-mm balloon in a 59-year-old female. In this particular patient, a 140-mmHg gradient across the pulmonary valve was reduced to a 38-mmHg gradient. The clinicians postulated that right-to-left shunting via a catheter-patent foramen ovale might be helpful in decompressing the right side of the heart during total occlusion of the pulmonary artery with the balloon inflated. In all of these individual cases, the catheter was inflated for about 5 to 10 s.

The best documented series of cases has been reported by Kan and White.[29] Twenty patients were reported with follow-up catheterization available in eleven. The average systolic gradient across the pulmonary valve was decreased from 68 to 23 mmHg. Patients ranged in age from 8 months to 56 years. There were no complications in this entire group. Eighteen patients had successful valvuloplasties (Fig. 116-2). There were two failures, one due to hypoplasia of the right ventricular outflow tract and the other to severely deformed dysplastic valve leaflets. All of these patients were discharged within 2 days of the procedure, and so far, 90 percent have had a successful outcome for periods of up to 2 years.

A more difficult problem for both the interventional cardiologist and the surgeon has been that of *peripheral pulmonary stenosis.* An animal model developed by Lock and his colleagues[30] was used for an experimental study of peripheral pulmonary angioplasty. Although the stenosis was artificially induced by surgery, significant increase in diameter of the pulmonary artery was achieved in nine lambs that underwent surgical stricture of the pulmonary ar-

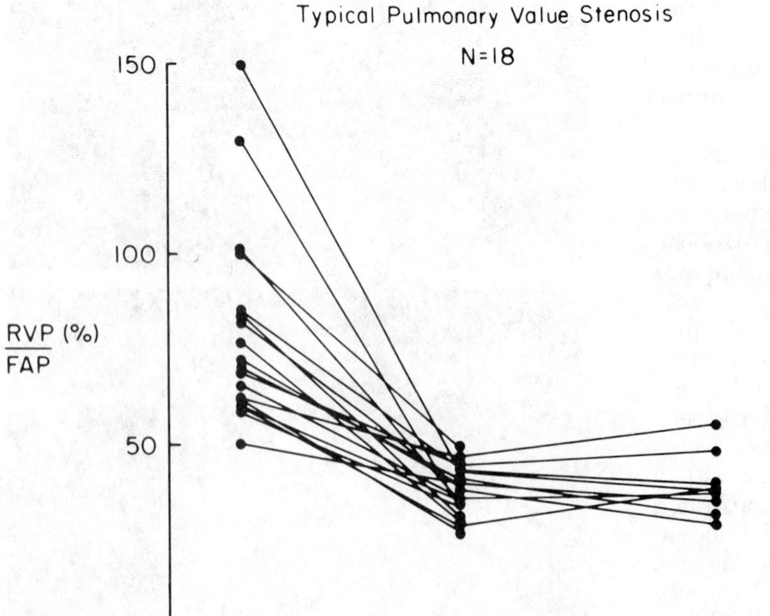

FIGURE 116-2 The results in 18 patients who underwent balloon angioplasty of the pulmonary valve. Intermediate follow-up data reveals persistence of the repair. (*From J. S. Kan, R. I. White, Jr., S. E. Mitchell, J. H. Anderson and T. J. Gardner: Percutaneous Transluminal Balloon Valvuloplasty for Pulmonary Valve Stenosis, Circulation, 69:557, 1984. Reproduced with permission from the American Heart Association, Inc., and the author.*)

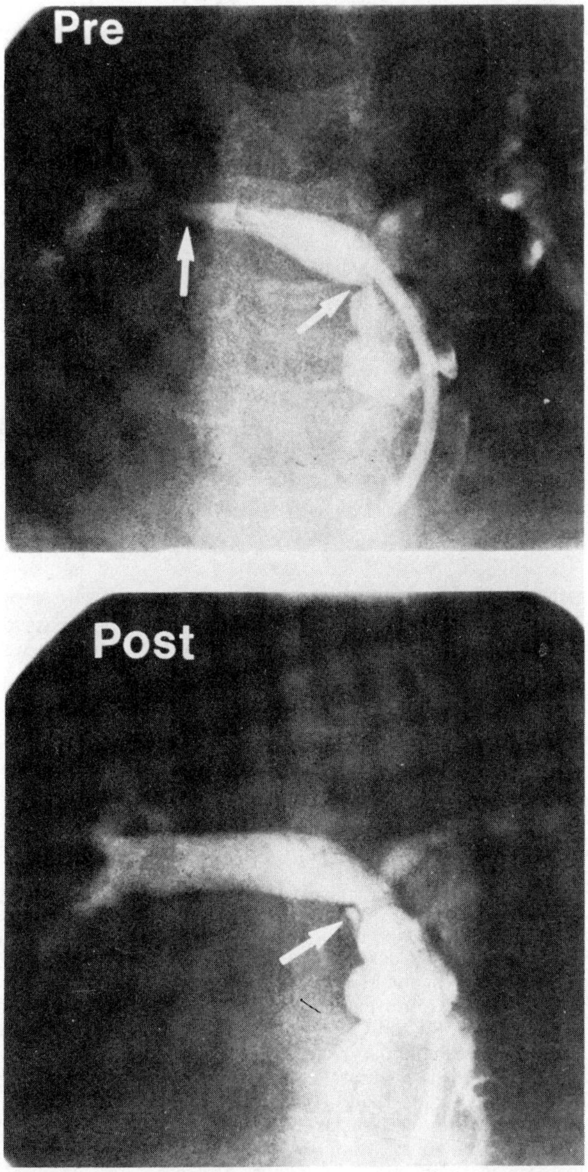

FIGURE 116-3 A child with inoperable peripheral pulmonary stenosis is successfully managed with balloon angioplasty. An intimal tear is present at the bifurcation of the main pulmonary artery, and the right pulmonary artery is now widely patent proximal to its division into lobar branches. (*From J. E. Lock, W. R. Castaneda-Zuniga, B. P. Fuhrman, and J. L. Bass: Balloon Dilation Angioplasty of Hypoplastic and Stenotic Pulmonary Arteries, Circulation, 67:965, 1983. Reproduced with permission from the American Heart Association, Inc., and the author.*)

tery and subsequent angioplasty. This moderately encouraging experimental result led to a clinical trial in seven patients with peripheral pulmonary stenosis, all of whom either were deemed to be inoperable or had had previous surgery[31] (Fig. 116-3). Two of the seven resulted in technical failures. However, five of the seven showed considerable improvement, with average gradient fall from 61 to 22 mmHg following angioplasty. There were no reported complications in this group, although the clinicians felt that overdilatation of the vessels was necessary in order to produce a good dilatation and lasting result. I have used the technique with success in two patients with postoperative pulmonary artery stricture (Fig. 116-4).

It is apparent from preliminary studies that pulmonary valvular stenosis may be well managed by angioplasty techniques. Peripheral pulmonary vascular lesions are more difficult to dilate and may not do quite as well as valvular lesions. However, the surgical results are also very disappointing, so further clinical trials are probably indicated.

Conclusions

Selective percutaneous interventional techniques have been ingeniously applied to the solution of different clinical problems in the cardiovascular system. Selective embolization with detachable balloons has become the treatment of choice in the management of multiple pulmonary arteriovenous malformations. Pulmonary valvular stenosis and restenosis of coarctations of the aorta following surgery are very well managed with percutaneous transluminal angioplasty techniques. The efficacy of similar techniques in critical aortic stenosis, primary coarctation of the aorta, and peripheral pulmonary stenosis requires further evaluation.

FIGURE 116-4 *A.* An oblique projection of a right ventricular angiocardiogram revealing stenosis at the anastomotic site of the distal (right) end of a pulmonary Dacron arteriograft. A similar lesion was present on the left. The ring of the Hancock valve is noted.

A

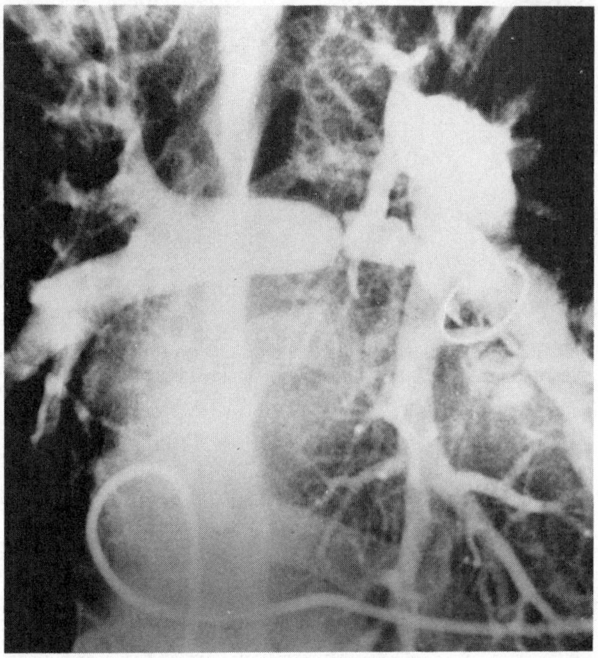

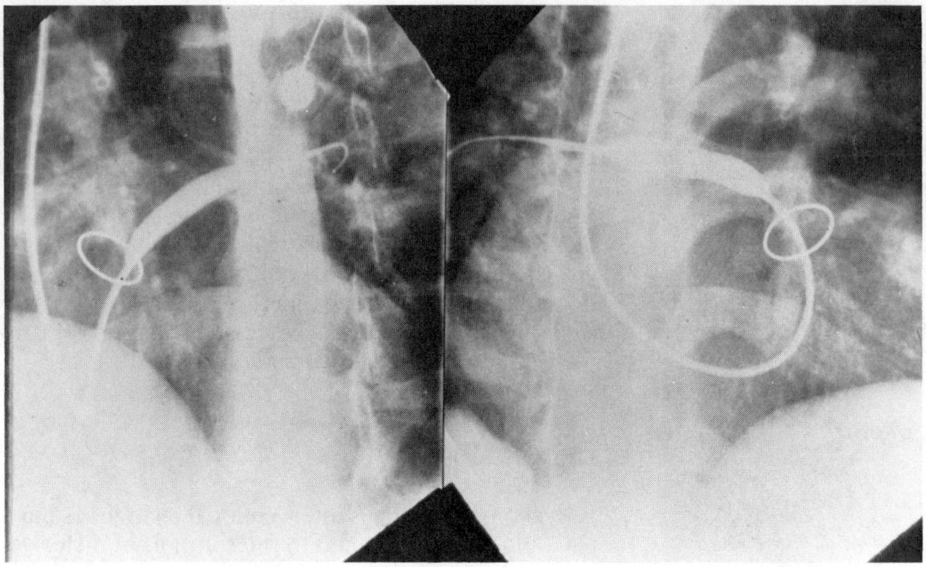

B

FIGURE 116-4 (*continued*) *B.* Dilatation of the stenosis of the Dacron pulmonary graft. Ten-millimeter balloon catheters were passed across both lesions and inflated to 8 atm of pressure. Left film displays the dilated balloon in the left pulmonary artery. Right film displays the dilated balloon in the right pulmonary artery.

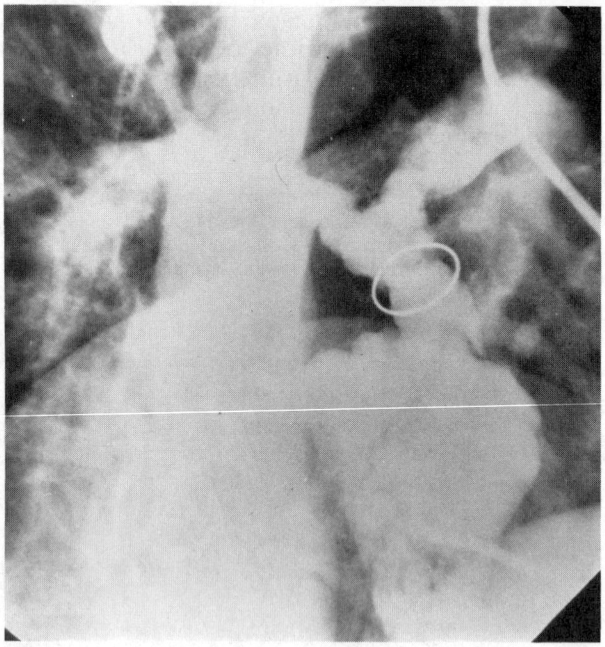

C

FIGURE 116-4 (*continued*) *C.* The 80-mm pressure gradient was eliminated and an 8-mm lumen was achieved by dilatation.

References

1. Remy, J., Smith, M., Lemaitre, L., Marache, P., and Fournier, E.: Treatment of Massive Hemoptysis by Occlusion of a Rasmussen Aneurysm, *AJR,* 135:605, 1980.
2. Renie, W. A., Rodeheffer, R. J., Mitchell, S., Balke, W. C., and White, R. I., Jr.: Balloon Embolization of a Mycotic Pulmonary Artery Aneurysm, *Am. Rev. Respir. Dis.,* 126:1107, 1982.
3. Szarnicki, R., Krebber, H. J., and Wack, J.: Wire Coil Embolization of Systemic-Pulmonary Artery Collaterals following Surgical Correction of Pulmonary Atresia, *J. Thorac. Cardiovasc. Surg.,* 8:124, 1981.
4. Reidy, J. F., Baker, E., and Tynan, M.: Transcatheter Occlusion of a Blalock-Taussig Shunt with a Detachable Balloon in a Child, *Br. Heart J.,* 50:101, 1983.
5. Florentine, M., Wolfe, R. R., and White, R. I., Jr.: Balloon Embolization to Occlude a Blalock-Taussig Shunt, *J. Am. Coll. Cardiol.,* 3:200, 1984.
6. Taylor, B. G., Cockerill, E. M., Manfredi, F., and Klatte, E. C.: Therapeutic Embolization of the Pulmonary Artery in Pulmonary Arteriovenous Fistula, *Am. J. Med.,* 64:360, 1978.
7. Hatfield, D. R., and Fried, A. M.: Therapeutic Embolization of Diffuse Pulmonary Arteriovenous Malformations, *AJR,* 137:861, 1981.
8. White, R. I., Jr., Kaufman, S. L., Barth, K. H., DeCaprio, V., and Strandbert, J. D.: Embolotherapy with Detachable Silicone Balloons: Technique and Clinical Results, *Radiology,* 131:619, 1979.
9. Terry, P. B., Barth, K. H., Kaufman, S. L., and White, R. I., Jr.: Balloon Embolization for Treatment of Pulmonary Arteriovenous Fistulas, *N. Engl. J. Med.,* 302:1189, 1980.
10. Jonsson, K., Hellekant, C., Olsson, O., and Holen, O.: Percutaneous Transcatheter Occlusion of Pulmonary Arteriovenous Malformation, *Ann. Radiol.,* 23:335, 1980.
11. Castaneda-Zuniga, W., Epstein, M., Zollikofer, F., et al.: Embolization of Multiple Pulmonary Artery Fistulas, *Radiology,* 134:309, 1980.
12. Rankin, R. N., McKenzie, F. N., and Ahmad, D.: Embolization of Arteriovenous Fistulas and Aneurysms with Detachable Balloons, *Can. J. Surg.,* 26:317, 1983.
13. Barth, K. H., White, R. I., Jr., Kaufman, S. L., Terry, P. B., and Roland, J. M.: Embolotherapy of Pulmonary Arteriovenous Malformations with Detachable Balloons, *Radiology,* 142:599, 1982.
14. Terry, P. B., White, R. I., Jr., Barth, K. H., Kaufman, S. L., and Mitchell, S. E.: Pulmonary Arteriovenous Malformations. Physiologic Observations and Results of Therapeutic Balloon Embolization, *N. Engl. J. Med.,* 308:1197, 1983.
15. Rankin, R. N.: Multiple Pulmonary Arteriovenous Fistulas, *J. Thorac. Cardiovasc. Surg.,* 84:933, 1982. (Letter.)
16. Lock, J. E., Niemi, T., Burke, B. A., Einzig, S., and Castaneda-Zuniga, W. R.: Transcutaneous Angioplasty of Experimental Aortic Coarctation, *Circulation,* 66:1280, 1982.
17. Singer, M. I., Rowen, M., and Dorsey, T. J.: Transluminal

Aortic Balloon Angioplasty for Coarctation of the Aorta in the Newborn, *Am. Heart. J.*, 103:131, 1982.
18. Sperling, D. R., Dorsey, T. J., Rowen, M., and Gazzaniga, A. B.: Percutaneous Transluminal Angioplasty of Congenital Coarctation of the Aorta, *Am. J. Cardiol.*, 51:562, 1983.
19. Lababidi, Z.: Neonatal Transluminal Balloon Coarctation Angioplasty, *Am. Heart. J.*, 106:752, 1983.
20. Finley, J. P., Beaulieu, R. G., Nanton, M. A., and Roy, D. L.: Balloon Catheter Dilatation of Coarctation of the Aorta in Young Infants, *Br. Heart J.*, 50:411, 1983.
21. Kan, J. S., White, R. I., Jr., Mitchell, S. E., Farmlett, E. J., Donahoo, J. S., and Gardner, T. J.: Treatment of Restenosis of Coarctation by Percutaneous Transluminal Angioplasty, *Circulation,* 68:1087, 1983.
22. Lock, J. E., Bass, J. L., Amplatz, K., Fuhrman, B. P., and Castaneda-Zuniga, W.: Balloon Dilatation Angioplasty of Aortic Coarctation in Infants and Children, *Circulation,* 68:109, 1983.
23. Lababidi, Z., Madigan, N., Wu, J. R., and Murphy, T. J.: Balloon Coarctation Angioplasty in an Adult, *Am. J. Cardiol.*, 53:350, 1984.
24. Mitchell, S. E., White, R. I., Jr., Kan, J., and Tolkoff, J.: Improved Balloon Catheters for Large-Vessel and Valvular Angioplasty, *AJR,* 142:571, 1984.
25. De Vega, N. G., Ferreiros Mur, J. M., and Guti'errez de Loma, J.: Transpulmonary Valvulotomy Using Balloon Catheter (Preliminary Report). A New Technic for the Treatment of Severe Pulmonary Stenosis in Infants, *Rev. Esp. Cardiol.*, 35:175, 1982.
26. Fontes, V. F., Sousa, J. E., Pimentel Filho, W. A., Buchler, J. R., da Silva, M. V., and Bembom, M. C.: Pulmonary Balloon Valvuloplasty. Report of a Case, *Arq. Bras. Cardiol.*, 41:49, 1983.
27. Lababidi, Z., and Wu, J. R.: Percutaneous Balloon Pulmonary Valvuloplasty, *Am. J. Cardiol.*, 52:560, 1983.
28. Pepine, C. J., Gessner, I. H., and Feldman, R. L.: Percutaneous Balloon Valvuloplasty for Pulmonic Valve Stenosis in the Adult, *Am. J. Cardiol.*, 50:1442, 1982.
29. Kan, J. S., White, R. I., Jr., Mitchell, S. E., Anderson, J. H., and Gardner, T. J.: Percutaneous Transluminal Balloon Valvuloplasty for Pulmonary Valve Stenosis, *Circulation,* 69:554, 1984.
30. Lock, J. E., Niemi, T., Einzig, S., Amplatz, K., Burke, B., and Bass, J. L.: Transvenous Angioplasty of Experimental Branch Pulmonary Artery Stenosis in Newborn Lambs, *Circulation,* 64:886, 1981.
31. Lock, J. E., Castaneda-Zuniga, W. R., Fuhrman, B. P., and Bass, J. L.: Balloon Dilatation Angioplasty of Hypoplastic and Stenotic Pulmonary Arteries, *Circulation,* 67:962, 1983.

117

Technique of Percutaneous Transluminal Angioplasty of the Coronary, Renal, Mesenteric, and Peripheral Arteries

David Petrie Hall, M.D.   Andreas R. Gruentzig, M.D.

While invasive angiography began with Forssmann's experimentation in 1929[1,2] it was not until Dotter and Judkin's intervention in peripheral vascular disease in 1964[3] that efforts were focused on therapy. These clinicians described an original technique whereby stepwise passage of a coaxial double catheter resulted in luminal enlargement.[3] Despite skepticism of the medical community concerning their techniques, some early success along with contributions by the German radiologists Porstmann[4] and Zeitler[5] enabled the method to survive. In 1974, continued problems with initial trauma prompted a major advance with the incorporation of a distensible tip.[6] Further modification and miniaturization of the system by Gruentzig in 1976 led to experimental use in the coronary circulation[7] and, subsequently, the first clinical application in September 1977.[8] Rapid technical evolution has resulted in improved success and a broadened application of the technique in both atherosclerotic and nonatherosclerotic disease.[9,10,11] Today, percutaneous angioplasty is utilized in a myriad of vascular beds and is considered the method of choice in some patients with obstructive disease and a therapeutic alternative to surgery in others.

The rationale behind the technique is simply that of improving reduced blood flow by increasing the luminal diameter of the diseased segment.[8] This goal is achieved through application of a lateral force against the vessel wall by means of a distensible (balloon) tip. The "controlled injury" that results yields a gamut of histological changes that in atherosclerotic disease may include compression or redistribution of the plaque as well as mural stretching and disruption.[12–17] Consequent to the localized trauma, phagocytosis, retraction, and incorporation lead to the removal of the exposed debris that had been previously walled off by the fibrous cap.[14,15,18,19] Early fears concerning prohibitive embolization of plaque constituents were resolved with intraoperative studies using millipore filters.[20] In conjunction with plaque mobilization, endothelialization occurs and a wider channel often results.[14,15,18,19,21] The healing of the dilated segment has been demonstrated in hemodynamic, angiographic, and histological follow-up studies.[19,21]

Documentation of the effects of successful dilatation has been established far beyond mere anatomic improvement or symptom relief. Preliminary work in peripheral disease first demonstrated the rise in distal pressure consequent to translesional gradient reduction.[3] Later, successful dilatation of obstructed renal vessels was shown to reverse the pathophysiologic state associated with renovascular hypertension.[22] The greatest investigative effort has focused on coronary dilatation and its role in reducing or eliminating the manifestations of myocardial ischemia.

Beginning on a cellular level, reduction or reversal of the pathophysiological state has been confirmed by measurements of oxygen consumption and lactate extraction.[23–25] Proceeding to clinical trials, investigation has been extremely thorough, particularly concerning the effects of percutaneous transluminal coronary angioplasty (PTCA) on exercise-induced systolic dysfunction. Confirmation of improved ventricular performance and increased work capacity has been repeatedly demonstrated by myocardial scintigraphy,[26,27] as well as by serial exercise testing.[28–30] Even diastolic function has been studied, revealing improved filling at rest after successful dilatation.[31] In research utilizing more direct measurements of coronary flow such as ^{201}Tl imaging,[32,33] thermodilution,[34] and computer-derived techniques,[35] improvement or normalization of perfusion has also been shown. Finally, in examining the clinical expression of this reclaimed functional capacity, benefits are readily apparent as evidenced by both employment and recreation patterns after successful dilatation.[36]

Coronary Angioplasty

Patient Selection

Discussion of candidacy for coronary angioplasty should at first emphasize the important role team experience should play in governing case selection. Despite its obvious similarities to diagnostic angiography, PTCA demands additional skills and judgment in manipulation of the guidewire and catheters.[37] As with coronary angiography, the acquisition of these skills requires time and training. A seasoned surgical team is of primary importance and must be immediately available.[37] Even in experienced hands, urgent bypass grafting is occasionally necessary, and an efficient, coordinated effort is important in protecting jeopardized myocardium.

While the candidacy spectrum has evolved over the past several years, some criteria remain unchanged. Foremost among these is the absolute requirement of surgical eligibility.[8] This characterization is based on clinical status, ventricular function, vascular anatomy, and willingness to undergo the procedure.

Clinical Considerations

Eligibility for coronary angioplasty on a clinical basis involves several considerations. The first of these is symptomology; the ideal candidate has well-defined, limiting ischemic symptoms despite good medical therapy. Therapeutic results are better defined in patients with discrete symptoms. Second, the length of symptoms deserves review, because long-standing angina is often associated with harder stenoses,[38,39] though segregation on this basis is certainly not absolute. The age of the patient should also be considered. While advanced age does not preclude dilatation if clinically warranted,[40,41] it should be recognized that, should bypass surgery prove necessary, it is associated with a somewhat higher morbidity in this group.[42]

Single Vessel Disease

Isolated discrete single-vessel disease remains the classic angiographic indication for PTCA[43] (Fig. 117-1). Within this subgroup, however, there are several important anatomic considerations. The first of these concerns the demonstration of critical fixed disease. While the procedure is technically feasible in patients with spasm as the primary disease component, symptoms on this basis frequently persist postdilatation and are often accompanied by restenosis.[44]

FIGURE 117-1 Left coronary artery in a 61-year-old man with unstable angina. *A.* The RAO projection shows a severe concentric stenosis of the proximal left anterior descending coronary artery. *B.* Guidewire in distal artery and inflated balloon positioned across the stenosis. *C.* Immediate postangioplasty angiogram after successful dilatation.

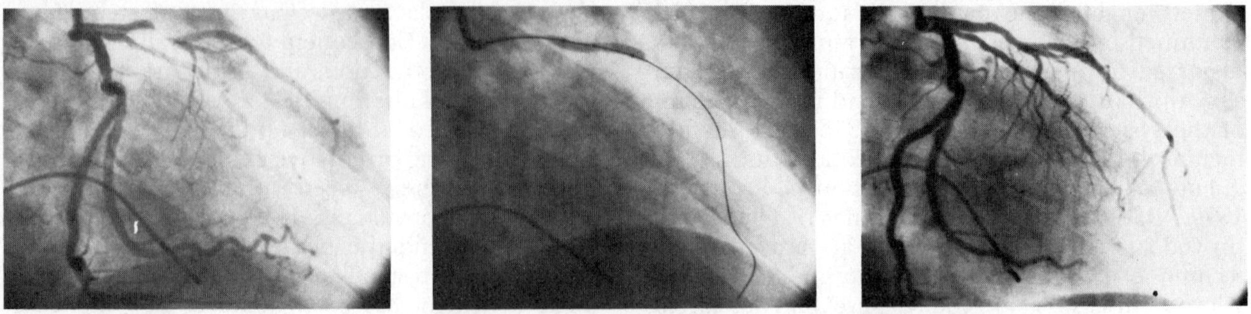

A B C

The second important morphological attribute is that of location. Though PTCA was previously confined to proximal disease, the advent of the steerable system made most lesions in the proximal two-thirds of the coronary circulation accessible for dilatation. Despite their location, ostial lesions represent one exception to this rule, as they are typically resistant to dilatation and are associated with a high recurrence rate.[45] Additionally, stenoses of the left mainstem are unacceptable for dilatation, unless a distal bed is grafted because of the life-threatening hazard of dissection.[43]

Geometry and complexity of the stenosis also have an impact on the selection process. Angioplasty should not be performed in mild disease (< 60 percent diameter stenosis) because of the uncertain natural history of these lesions coupled with the risk of acceleration of the disease process.[46] Extremely tight stenoses, on the other hand, are associated with an increased risk of dissection,[47] particularly if long (> 10 mm) and/or eccentric.[48] Evidence of vascular calcification in the stenotic area suggests a stenosis more resistant to dilatation and more likely to evidence significant intimal disruption, but it does not preclude the procedure. The ideal lesion demonstrates a smooth-walled hourglass configuration, while angiographic evidence of preexisting intimal disruption or thrombus formation is undesirable.[49]

Post Coronary Artery Bypass Grafting

Despite the efficacy of coronary bypass grafting, disease progression leads to recurrent or worsening symptoms in 5 to 10 percent of postoperative patients annually,[50–52] resulting in reoperation in up to 10 percent of individuals followed long-term.[53–55] In selected patients, PTCA represents an alternative to an often technically difficult second bypass procedure.[56–60] Following guidelines previously described, several sites have proven favorable for dilatation. These include (1) vessels not previously bypassed, (2) vessels jeopardized by graft closure, (3) lesions distal to implanted grafts, (4) lesions proximal to patent grafts but compromising flow to other branches, and (5) distal anastomoses (vein to coronary artery junction).[56,57] Proximal anastomoses (saphenous vein to aorta junction) represent less favorable sites for dilatation due to technical difficulties with guiding catheter support and higher recurrence rates.[56,57] The latter problem also accompanies dilatation of graft body stenoses (saphenous vein independent of anastomoses), where early studies have demonstrated good preliminary success but intermediate-term recurrence rates of approximately 50 percent.[56,57]

Double-Vessel Disease

The growth of experience and technology has led to the inclusion of a subset of individuals with double-vessel disease as candidates for PTCA. Selection from this group requires a particularly cautious approach, excluding individuals with high-risk lesions at either site. Timing of the procedures is of primary importance, with the lesion whose location and severity is most ominous dilated first. Any uncertainty as to the outcome of the first procedure should result in postponement of the second. This approach can reduce the hazard of simultaneously jeopardizing two vascular beds.[45]

Occluded Vessels

Experience in recanalizing occluded vessels has grown rapidly, with success rates reported to range between 53 and 76 percent in selected cases.[61–63] As in other candidacy groups, the target vessel should subtend viable myocardium responsible for persistent symptoms. An additional clinical consideration is the length of time since occlusion, as long-standing occlusions (> 6 months) are associated with significantly lower success rates. Important angiographic parameters include mandatory visualization of the distal vessel to define the length of the occluded segment and, ideally, the presence of a "funnel-shaped" entrance port to channel the guidewire along the original lumen.[45] Extremely long occlusions (> 15 mm) are unacceptable for dilatation owing to the risks of dissection or distal embolization. Recurrence rates in this subgroup appear to exceed those seen after dilatation of stenotic disease,[63] but series are small and further definition is needed.

Post Streptokinase Therapy

Thrombolytic therapy frequently yields individuals in need of urgent definitive revascularization. While several groups have reported success in combining PTCA with thrombolysis acutely,[64–67] experience has been limited. Obvious benefits to be derived from prompt dilatation include improved reperfusion of the ischemic myocardium by reduction of the residual stenosis and a diminished risk of reocclusion.[65] On the basis of current data, however, the present recommendation is to postpone routine dilatation for approximately 3 days after thrombolytic therapy, while acknowledging the fact that reocclusion may occasionally prompt earlier action.

Nonatherosclerotic Disease

Percutaneous dilatation of the coronary arteries is not limited only to those afflicted with atherosclerotic disease. Angioplasty has been successfully performed on a repeated basis in many vascular beds for segmental disease secondary to a variety of causes including fibromuscular dysplasia and arteritis.[11,68] With the presently available technology, PTCA should be considered as a therapeutic option in any individual with focal obstructive coronary disease regardless of cause.

Technology and Technique

Radionuclide Equipment

Angioplasty often demands significantly greater angiographic information than the capability afforded by many laboratories. The basic requirements are high resolution in delineating the diseased segment and in monitoring catheter manipulation, and rapid visualization of the coronary circulation from several different projections. The following are radiologic capabilities considered optimal for the performance of coronary angioplasty: (1) an x-ray tube–image intensifier configuration capable of multiangular projections, including cranial and caudal angulation, which is easily positioned and preferably biplanar, (2) a high-resolution image intensifier and monitor chain providing definition of steerable, 0.012-in diameter guidewire (> 1000 lines of resolution), (3) multimode image intensification including 4- to 5-in, 6- to 7-in, and 8- to 9-in (10- to 13-cm, 15- to 18-cm, and 20- to 23-cm) field sizes, and (4) high-resolution freeze-frame video capacity through a recorder or disk so that at least two guide projections can be displayed constantly for comparison with real-time images (four monitors are necessary).[43]

Catheter System

Since the technology was first introduced in 1977,[8] the catheter system utilized in coronary angioplasty has become increasingly sophisticated. The goals of this evolution have been to maximize the safety and applicability of the procedure by improved hemodynamic monitoring and by the development of more responsive catheters. The basic components include (1) the guiding catheter with an outer diameter of no. 8 or 9 French and (2) the dilatation catheter with an outer diameter of no. 4 French (Fig. 117-2).

The larger guiding catheter is a bonded composite of three layers—the outer layer of polyurethane for memory, the middle layer of fine wire mesh for torque control, and the inner surface of Teflon utilized for its coefficient of friction.[69] With relatively stiff shafts, these catheters have been designed to provide the longitudinal support necessary to maintain tip stability in the coronary ostium. These preformed guiding catheters are available in a variety of shapes with nontapered tips (to permit unimpeded dilatation catheter passage) and lengths of 100 or 80 cm for the femoral or brachial approach. Present selection includes (1) modified Judkins left and right forms with in- or out-of-plane configurations, (2) Amplatz curves for the femoral approach, (3) a multipurpose curve form, and (4) a flexible tip brachial catheter.[69,70] Vented right coronary forms are also available for use in the event that the guiding catheter wedges. All catheters are used in conjunction with Y connectors to enable both pressure measurement and contrast medium injection.

Dilatation catheters of the latest generation are 135 cm long with two lumina. The central lumen is used for pressure measurement, supraselective contrast medium injection, and to accommodate the guidewire; the second, eccentric lumen is used for balloon inflation and deflation.[69] Located at the distal tip of the catheter, the balloon is composed of either polyvinylchloride or polyethylene and is designed to tolerate up to 5 atm of inflation pressure. Most balloons are 20–25 mm in length, while inflated diameters range from 2 to 4.2 mm. Outer diameters are somewhat dependent on inflation pressure, as a great variety of pressure-diameter relations have been demonstrated.[71]

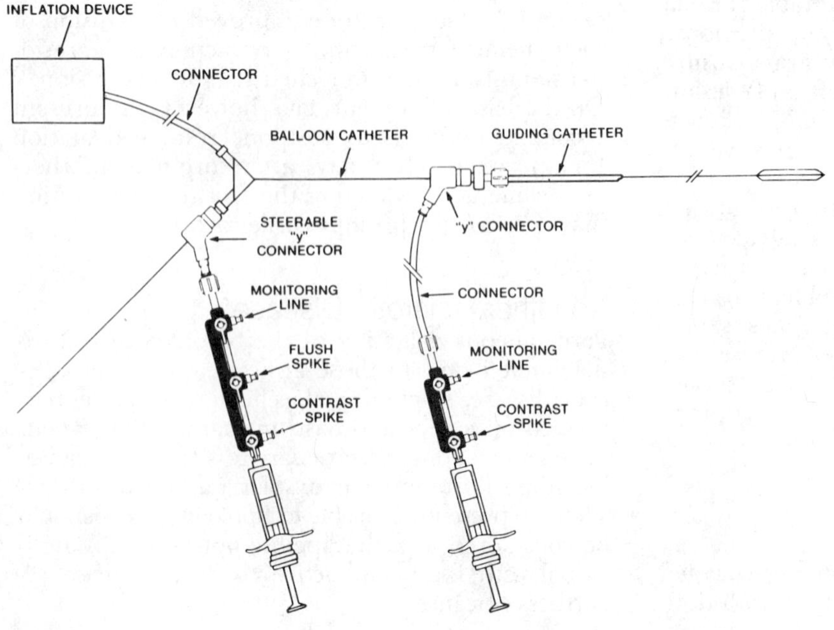

FIGURE 117-2 Catheter assembly—guidewire, balloon catheter, and guiding catheter with associated connections necessary for the steerable dilatation catheter system.

Continued efforts to minimize intimal trauma during balloon placement have led to the recent development of softer, more flexible catheter tips with longer, more gradual balloon tapers. Also recently available are tandem configurations with a small 2.0-mm distal balloon and a 3.0-mm proximal balloon. All dilatation catheters are connected proximally to specially designed Y connectors to accommodate the central guidewire and to permit pressure measurement and contrast medium injection.

Steerable guidewires are 175 cm in length, range in size from 0.012 to 0.016 in in diameter, and are available with either straight or J-tip (30° curve) configurations. These characteristics are desirable: distal flexibility to minimize intimal trauma, tip formability to allow necessary preshaping, and torque control. Also available are 300-cm wires for use in the event of the need for catheter exchange.

Procedure (Femoral Approach)

Preparations begin with the acquisition of informed consent, with careful explanation of the nature of the procedure and the risks, including the possibility of abrupt surgical intervention. In addition to the history, physical, and routine admission laboratory work, the patient is typed and screened for 4 units of whole blood and 2 units of packed cells. Baseline parameters of cardiac status are obtained in the form of an admission cardiac x-ray and ECG, a blood sample for creatine kinase (CK) level, and an exercise test of antianginal medications (clinical status permitting). Testing is often done in conjunction with nuclear imaging, particularly in patients with double-vessel disease. Five grains of acetylsalicyclic acid are administered the evening prior to dilatation.

The procedure is carried out with the patient in the fasting state after surgical backup has been made available for the day. Upon arrival of the patient at the laboratory, ECG monitoring is begun and a good-caliber intravenous line is secured. After the patient is sedated with intravenous diazepam, local anesthesia is achieved with 2 percent lidocaine. The femoral vein is cannulated and a no. 5 French pacing catheter advanced to the right ventricular apex, both as a precaution in the event of bradyarrhythmias and to serve as a spatial marker between times of contrast medium injection. Once capture has been assured, arterial puncture is performed and appropriate femoral insertion is made on the basis of aortic and coronary ostial anatomy and anticipated backup needs (no. 7 French provides more longitudinal support). If an acceptable preformed guiding catheter cannot be found, reshaping of the catheter can be accomplished by using the 0.063-in (1.6-mm) guidewire to overbend the catheter tip, briefly passing it under a heating gun, then promptly immersing it in saline solution for quick cooling. Subsequently, the guiding catheter is advanced retrograde into the ascending aorta over a 0.063-in (1.6-mm) guidewire, the catheter is aspirated, and baseline aortic pressure recorded. At this point several medications are administered to prevent thrombosis (10,000 units of heparin given intravenously) and to counteract spasm (sublingual nitroglycerin and nifedipine).

Angiograms of the stenotic vessel are obtained to define several important considerations of coronary anatomy. These include (1) adequate seating of the guide catheter in the coronary ostium to ensure stability but avoid wedging and its hemodynamic consequences, (2) clear demonstration of lesion geometry including length and possible eccentricity, (3) definition of the arterial path to the lesion to define proximal disease and display the origins of alternative channels, (4) visualization of any uninvolved side branches in the region of the stenosis (and so temporarily occluded by the balloon) or branches compromised by and arising from the stenotic segment, and (5) visualization of the distal vessel and its ramifications.[43]

Commonly utilized projections for left anterior descending (LAD) artery lesions are an left anterior oblique (LAO) cranial view to demonstrate vessel take-off and provide diagonal separation, a right anterior oblique (RAO) projection for septal perforator separation, and the lateral projection to complement definition of the stenosis. Extremely proximal LAD lesions occasionally require an extremely steep, shallow LAO projection. RAO and LAO projections are most commonly used for the right coronary artery while RAO caudal and LAO cranial projections usually provide the best definition of circumflex disease. Projections should be well centered, as it is often necessary to visualize both the vessel ostium and its distal extent simultaneously during the procedure. The angulation and skew of each projection are recorded so that the identical projection may be subsequently repeated should it prove necessary to temporarily reposition the image intensifiers during the case. The initial angiograms are reviewed and guiding frames are chosen for reference during the case.

Balloon selection is based on several considerations. The most important of these include the caliber of the vessel adjacent to the stenotic segment and the severity of the stenosis. The inflated diameter of the balloon should approximate vessel diameter; if the vessel size falls between presently available catheters, slight undersizing is desirable. Selection is also affected by the degree of stenosis, as extremely tight lesions are often difficult to cross with the standard dilatation catheter. In these instances, the newer "low-profile" catheters are advantageous because of their more gradually tapered deflated profile. Rarely it is necessary to use a markedly undersized tapered balloon to initially cross and dilate and then, using a 300-cm (117-in) wire, to exchange to a larger catheter. In addition to severe stenoses, there are several other clinical and angiographic clues that passage might require a low-profile configuration. These include (1) a long history of angina, (2) poor guiding catheter seating, (3) presence of calcium in the stenosis, (4) tortuous proximal vessel or stenotic segment, (5) distal lesions, and (6) long stenoses (> 10 mm).

Dilatation catheter preparation is begun by flushing the central lumen with heparinized saline and then evacuating the balloon by applying suction for approximately 1 min using a mixture of contrast medium and heparinized saline solution. In an attempt to balance maximum visualization with acceptable viscosity (which determines deflation time), various mixtures are used. In the standard balloons, 50:20 concentrations (contrast medium: saline solution) are used while 50:50 blends are utilized in larger (4.2-mm) and low-profile balloons because of unacceptable deflation times with the standard concentration. After evacuation, a trial inflation is observed to insure competency, and the balloon is connected to the inflation device. A repeat inflation to 5 atm is performed followed by an assessment of deflation time (prompt deflation mandatory). The dilatation catheter is then passed through the "nonsteerable" Y connector, and the central wire is inserted prior to loading into the guiding catheter.

Disconnecting the three-port manifold from the guider, the dilatation catheter is slowly advanced in the larger catheter while a check is continually made for a blood return so as to avoid air trapping. With the guiding catheter outside the coronary orifice, the nonsteerable Y connector is then connected to the guiding catheter and the balloon advanced to its distal tip under fluoroscopic guidance. Both catheters are then flushed and baseline pressures obtained to ensure that there is no significant intrinsic gradient.

The coronary ostium is again engaged, and the balloon is advanced within the guiding catheter with the steerable wire extending about 8 to 10 cm beyond the distal end of the dilatation catheter. Using repeated contrast medium injections through the guiding catheter as well as the "frozen" guiding frames, the 0.016-in (0.4-mm) wire is advanced slowly into the coronary ostium. If difficulties are encountered in entering the desired vessel, three tacks are possible. These include (1) careful rotation of the guiding catheter to better direct its orifice toward the desired vessel (e.g., counterclockwise rotation for most LADs), (2) withdrawing the dilatation catheter and exaggerating the J-tip curve in its original plane, and (3) changing to a different guiding catheter that demonstrates better subselective orientation.

Once the appropriate channel has been entered, 200 μg of nitroglycerin is given in the coronary artery to minimize spasm associated with intimal trauma. Wire tip freedom should be continuously demonstrated during passage so as to exclude the possibility of intimal violation. When approaching the lesion, special care should be taken to hug the appropriate wall if eccentricity has been demonstrated. The guidewire should never be advanced if resistance is felt or appreciated on fluoroscopy by alteration of the J tip. After the stenosis is crossed, the wire should be advanced well distally in the primary artery to aid somewhat in anchoring of the system when the balloon is passed and to afford a margin of safety in the event of intimal disruption and need for recrossing the stenosis with the balloon. The dilatation catheter is then advanced while the guidewire is simultaneously withdrawn. Often the patient evidences signs and symptoms of ischemia as the lesion is approached, which dictates efficient movement.[43]

Only when the correct balloon position is assured should inflation be performed; if indecision exists, the catheter should be withdrawn until its hemodynamic consequences are no longer in evidence. Ideally, the balloon should symmetrically bridge the stenosis to reduce the likelihood of the dilatation catheter slipping at the time of inflation. Once positioned, the guiding catheter should be slightly withdrawn from the coronary orifice to maximize flow. With the balloon in place, the initial gradient is quickly recorded and inflation begun. For future reference, it is important to note the adequacy of collateral flow evidenced by the distal occlusion pressure and the sensitivity of the monitored electrocardiographic leads for signs of ischemia.

Care is taken to note the deformity imposed by the lesion on the balloon to further confirm the correct positioning. Inflation pressure is increased in stepwise fashion until altered balloon deformity indicates a response. Duration of the first inflation is usually 15 to 30 s, determined in part by the patient's symptoms or other evidence of myocardial ischemia. After complete deflation of the balloon has been assured, the residual gradient is determined and small quick distal injections are made to assure good distal flow. Subsequent inflations are usually to pressure levels at or slightly above that at which the first response was noted. Inflations are repeated at appropriate intervals (to allow interim recovery) until further reductions in the gradient are not apparent or until the value falls below approximately 16 mmHg[72] (Fig. 117-3).

When it appears that adequate dilatation has been accomplished, the wire is advanced simultaneously with dilatation catheter withdrawal so that the wire remains distal to the stenosis and the balloon is positioned proximal to the site of the original stenosis. Under no circumstances should the lesion be recrossed with the guidewire, as the risk of dissecting the freshly dilated area is prohibitively high. Injections are performed through both the guiding and balloon catheters to define the status of the dilated vessel segment in several projections. With favorable results, the balloon catheter is removed after a short period of observation, and an angiogram is repeated utilizing the original projections. If, however, there appears to be a significant residual obstruction, the lesion is recrossed by advancing the balloon over the steerable wire and additional inflations are per-

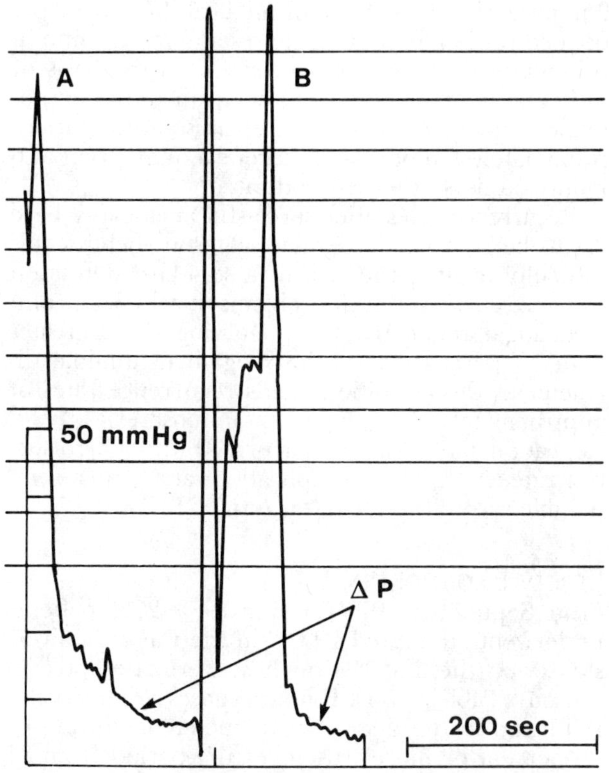

FIGURE 117-3 Pressure gradient recordings before, during, and after balloon inflation. *A.* Pressure representing first inflation, after which an initial gradient of 85 mmHg fell to 6 mmHg. *B.* A second balloon inflation reduced the gradient to its final reading of 4 mmHg.

formed. Upon completion of the procedure, the inner cannulas are inserted into the femoral sheaths and carefully secured, and the patient is transported to the nursing unit.[43]

Postangioplasty Care

Routine postangioplasty care is designed to monitor the patient closely for signs or symptoms of myocardial ischemia. On return from the laboratory, the patient is placed on telemetry, a 12-lead ECG is obtained, and blood is drawn for CK levels. If the angiographic result was a well-defined success and the patient received the routine 10,000 units of heparin, the femoral sheaths are pulled approximately 2 h after the procedure. If, however, there is angiographic evidence of significant intimal disruption, anticoagulation in the form of a continuous heparin drip is maintained until the following morning. Telemetry is continued for 18 h and serial ECGs and CK values are obtained. Routine medications for the immediate post-PTCA period include 325 mg of acetylsalicylic acid daily, sublingual and transdermal nitrates, and a calcium antagonist. The patient is allowed to ambulate at will the morning following the procedure, and repeat exercise testing is performed on the second day postangioplasty.

Before discharge, all factors defining the results of intervention are reviewed. These include (1) pre- and postangioplasty exercise tests, (2) stenosis measurement pre- and postprocedure, (3) initial and final gradients, (4) serial ECGs, and (5) serial CK values. The patient is counseled at the time of discharge on the advisability of cessation of tobacco abuse and the need to maintain a high activity level. Routine discharge medication consists of nifedipine, 40 mg/day in divided dosage, and aspirin, 325 mg/day.[43]

Complications

Since its introduction in 1976 as an investigative procedure, coronary angioplasty has undergone many refinements with a resultant fall in procedural morbidity and mortality. These changes are due in part to technical advances but perhaps more importantly have resulted from the growth of collective and individual experience.[73] While coronary dilatation can be performed with a low complication rate, the procedure has both inherent and associated risks.[73] Recognition of these potential problems is the first step toward improved safety of the procedure.

The most frequent major complication of PTCA is acute embarrassment of coronary flow. Reported in approximately 5 percent of patients,[74] this problem may be manifest as prolonged angina or coronary occlusion leading to infarction. The most common basis for this difficulty is coronary artery dissection as a result of guidewire trauma or balloon inflation. While present technology does not permit elimination of this hazard or even recognition of all high-risk individuals, several unfavorable morphologic attributes have been identified. These angiographic characteristics include (1) high-grade obstruction (> 90 percent),[47] (2) lesion eccentricity,[48] (3) excessive lesion length (> 15 mm), (4) a tortuous or bifurcating diseased segment,[74] and (5) a "complicated" angiographic morphology. Combinations of these factors further increase the risk of dissection.

Mechanisms other than dissection of the stenotic segment may also result in myocardial ischemia. Coronary spasm has been reported in approximately 4 percent of patients either as an isolated problem or in combination with other complications.[73] Additional serious but less common bases for diminished flow include coronary embolization (plaque or air) and intimal trauma caused by the guiding catheter. Side branch occlusion can occasionally cause ischemia, though the risk of such event is small (14 percent) even when the branch is involved in the disease process.[75] Ischemia arising in the first few hours after the effects of heparin have waned is often due to thrombosis, though spasm may play a role.

Appropriate management of the patient with abrupt reduction in coronary flow requires a careful but rapid assessment. With the goal of myocardial preservation, initial therapy should begin with oxygen administration,[76] repeat dosing with sublingual nifedipine, and, if needed, additional heparin. If the patient has already returned to the nursing unit he or she should be taken immediately to the catheterization laboratory, sheaths should be exchanged, and a repeat angiogram obtained. In the event of coronary obstruction, therapy should continue with intracoronary nitroglycerin (200 μg). If no response is achieved, the diseased segment should be recrossed and repeat angioplasty attempted.[77] Persistent inadequacy of perfusion associated with symptoms or other evidence of ischemia should dictate prompt surgical revascularization in appropriate cases.

In the interim prior to surgery additional therapy may be warranted. Continuous infusion of intravenous nitroglycerin should be used empirically[78] if the hemodynamic status permits. Intravenous propranolol may also be valuable in reducing myocardial oxygen demand.[79,80] If cardiac output is embarrassed, intraaortic balloon pumping should be initiated utilizing existing arterial access.[81]

Other potential complications of percutaneous coronary angioplasty include (1) ventricular fibrillation (incidence 1 percent)[74] most commonly encountered in right coronary artery dilatation; (2) vascular complications including hematoma formation, retroperitoneal blood loss, and development of a pseudoaneurysm; (3) central nervous system events; and (4) allergic reactions. The nature of the procedure accounts for increased risk of the first two problems listed, while with proper precautions the latter two events should not exceed the low occurrence rate seen with diagnostic procedures.

Mortality associated with dilatation in single-vessel disease has been approximately 1 percent.[73] This figure largely reflects operator experience, being significantly lower in large individual series. Other factors of primary importance in reducing the risk of death include prudent case selection and facilities and staff available for expedient surgical revascularization.[82]

Recurrent Stenosis after Successful Dilatation

While the majority of individuals continue to demonstrate sustained angiographic and clinical improvement after successful dilatation, a certain number of cases will evidence recurrent stenosis.[74,83–87] Recurrences may be partial or complete, or may even surpass the degree of initial stenosis.[46] The basis for recurrent disease is unknown but in part is probably due to fibrocellular proliferation that exceeds other late pathologic mechanisms of angioplasty. At present no definite angiographic, hemodynamic, or clinical predictors of recurrent disease have been established. Importantly, restenosis usually manifests itself as recurrent angina,[74] most often appearing between 2 and 4 months (peak 3 months) after the procedure and only rarely after 9 months.[74,83–87] Because of medical therapy or patient education, infarction represents an uncommon presentation of recurrent disease. On the basis of the data above, routine follow-up in the asymptomatic patient should include exercise testing at approximately 3 months and a repeat angiogram at 6 months unless otherwise indicated.

Recurrence rates after successful angioplasty have yet to be completely defined. Reasons behind this difficulty include the lack of a standard definition of recurrence as well as problems in achieving complete angiographic follow-up. Utilizing loss of greater than 50 percent of the initial gain in luminal diameter as the definition yields recurrence rates of approximately 25 to 35 percent in most series.[74,83,87] Repeat dilatation can be performed with a high success rate,[74,83,84] a low complication rate[84] and a comparable secondary recurrence rate.[84]

Emory Experience

From September 1977 through 1983, 2785 patients underwent attempted PTCA in the Emory University series (the first 194 of these were attempted in Zurich) (Table 117-1). Primary success (defined as a reduction in the degree of diameter narrowing by 20 percent or more) rose over the period from 81 to 91 percent. Concomitant with this improvement in initial success, the frequency of all major complications fell. Emergency coronary bypass grafting, which was necessary in 6.7 percent of the Zurich patients, dropped to 1.9 percent in 1983. Q-wave infarction, which was evidenced in 2.6 percent of the original group, also fell to 1.9 percent in 1983. There has been a total of three deaths in the series.[88]

Angioplasty in Peripheral Vascular Disease

Since its introduction in 1964,[3] Dotter's innovative approach to peripheral vascular disease has undergone numerous refinements. Early problems led to the development first of the "caged" balloon catheter by Porstmann in 1973[4] and later of a rigid balloon by Gruentzig and Hopff in 1974.[89] Favorable experience with this latest catheter in peripheral

TABLE 117-1 Results of PTCA in the Emory University Hospital Series

	Zurich	1980–81	1982	1983	Total
Patients	194	518	813	1260	2785
Lesions	194	540	896	1424	3054
PS (lesion), %	81.0	82.0	91.0	91.0	89.0
EM CABG, %	6.7	5.6	3.2	1.9	3.2
MI—Q wave, %	2.6	3.6	1.7	1.9	2.2
Death, %	0	0	1	2	3

Notes: PS = primary success; EM CABG = emergency bypass surgery; MI = myocardial infarction.

vessels led to widespread use, first in Europe and later in the United States. Today percutaneous transluminal angioplasty (PTA) represents an effective means of restoring regional blood flow in a variety of peripheral beds.

Case Selection

Patients considered for PTA must undergo the same preliminary testing that precedes vascular surgical procedures. This begins with a careful history to define the degree of ischemia and is followed by a comprehensive physical examination. Particular emphasis should be placed on defining possible coexistent coronary and cerebral disease as they represent important sources of morbidity and mortality in this group.[90] Noninvasive testing should include recording of appropriate peripheral pulses along with segmental Doppler pressures at rest and, if necessary, after exercise or reactive hyperemia. Invasive testing should include arteriography with biplane filming if possible and intraarterial pressure measurement.[91]

Angiographic criteria for peripheral dilatation in some ways parallel those utilized in the coronary angioplasty. Short discrete lesions (< 5 cm) associated with limited distal vessel involvement and good runoff are favorable characteristics.[74,91–94] Total occlusions selected for dilatation should also be short, as those longer than 10 cm are associated with poor success at the outset and subsequent high recurrence rates.[94,95] Total obstructions in the iliac vessels represent a relative contraindication to the procedure because of the uncertainty of the course of the common and external iliac arteries.[91] In general, iliac dilatation yields better long-term patency rates than angioplasty in the femoral popliteal arteries.[92,94–97] The exception to this rule is disease occurring in the iliacs near the aortic bifurcation.[74]

Technology and Technique

The balloon catheter utilized in peripheral disease is a double-lumen, single-end-hole no. 7 to 8 French catheter. Composed of polyvinylchloride, it is smoothly tapered from tip to hub to minimize thrombogenicity. The distal balloon segment is filled via a second lumen or longitudinal groove cut along the outer surface of the inner catheter. A variety of balloon lengths (2 to 10 cm) and expanded diameters (4 to 10 mm) are available.[95]

A number of Teflon-coated guidewires are manufactured for use with these double-lumen catheters. Configurations include straight-tip, movable-core, and fixed J types. Wire sizes vary from 0.032 to 0.038 in.

After informed consent has been obtained, the patient is brought to the radiology laboratory. Arterial puncture technique is determined by the site of the dilatation. Bilateral femoral artery puncture (retrograde contralateral and antegrade ipsilateral) is usually performed in iliac disease. The following discussion, however, relates to the ipsilateral common femoral approach, which is the most common approach utilized in superficial femoral dilatation.[91]

With a no. 7 or 8 French Teflon catheter with a single end hole, dilute contrast material is injected under fluoroscopy so that the rough limits of obstruction can be marked. Angiography is then performed (10 to 20 ml undiluted contrast medium) to demonstrate the limits of the diseased segment, assess collaterals, and define the status of the distal vasculature. The guidewire is then manipulated through the stenosis using a Y connector and repeated dye injections. After luminal patency is assured with dilute contrast medium injection, the Teflon catheter is passed over the wire in preparation for the dilatation catheter. Following passage, heparin (5000 units) and a vasodilator [e.g., tolazoline (Priscoline), 25 mg, or adenosine triphosphate, 25 mg] are injected through the catheter into the distal vessels.[95,97,98]

While the wire is carefully maintained distal to the occlusion, the Teflon catheter is then exchanged for the dilatation catheter. This process should begin with careful balloon evacuation and folding around the inner catheter (to avoid enlargement of the puncture hole). Care should be taken to keep the guidewire stationary during catheter positioning. Bridging first the distal aspect of the obstruction, the balloon is expanded with 3.5 to 5.0 atm of pressure to its maximum diameter. Inflation is usually maintained for 30 to 60 s. After evacuation of the balloon it is withdrawn to the adjacent proximal portion of the diseased segment and the process repeated. When the entire segment has been dilatated, the wire is removed and a repeat angiogram is obtained. Evaluation should include not only the site of the original stenosis but also distal vasculature to exclude the possibility of embolization. Any significant residual stenosis is redilatated.[95,97,98]

Distal pressure can be monitored during the procedure to aid in defining the effects of intervention. When satisfactory hemodynamic results have been obtained, the procedure should be terminated (Fig. 117-4). Continued dilatation for "vascular cosmetics" may result in distal embolization.[95]

Management after the procedure is designed to carefully monitor distal perfusion. This begins with documentation of distal pressure immediately postdilatation and serial measurements thereafter. Adjunctive medical therapy consists of warfarin (Coumadin) and sulfinpyrazone (Anturane), 200 mg, four times daily (the latter begun 4 days prior to the procedure). Long-term anticoagulation of this type has been shown to reduce the reocclusion rate by one-half in several follow-up studies.[99,100] We are using 315 mg aspirin daily only. Finally, modification of risk factors is emphasized, particularly the cessation of tobacco abuse. Patients are usually discharged from the hospital on the next day postprocedure though, in selected individuals, angioplasty of lower extremity arteries can be done on an ambulatory basis.[101]

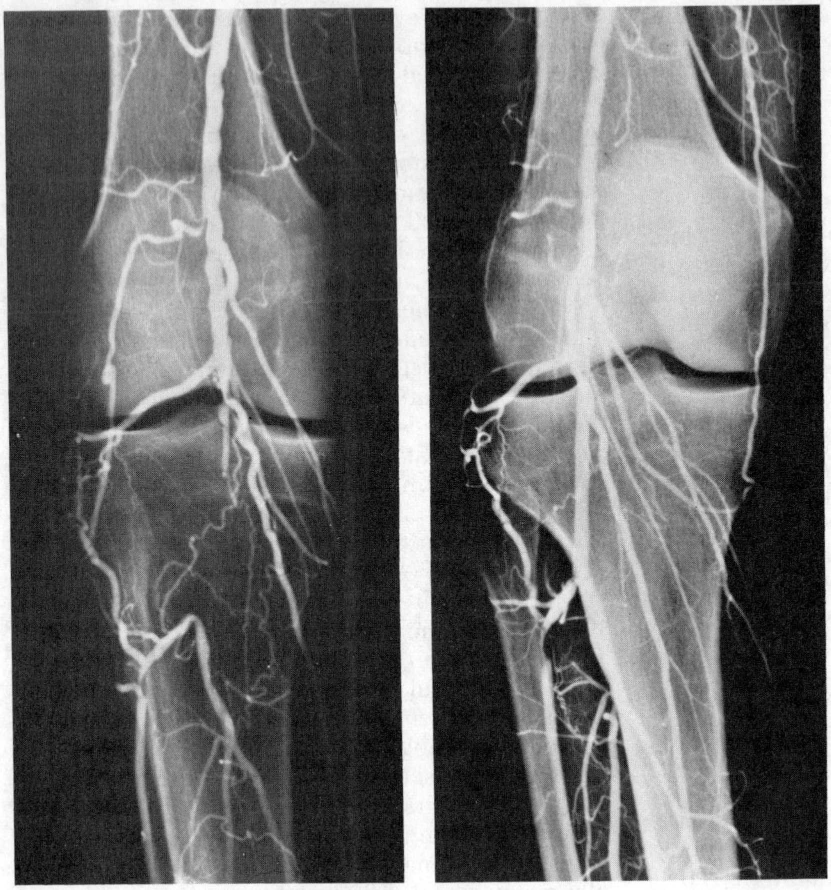

A B

FIGURE 117-4 Popliteal artery occlusion in a 56-year-old male. *A*. Before recanalization with a 4-mm angioplasty balloon (balloon length 10 cm). *B*. After recanalization.

Complications

The morbidity of percutaneous transluminal angioplasty for obstructive disease of the iliac, femoral, and popliteal arteries is less than that of surgical treatment.[74,98] Most series reveal complication rates of approximately 10 percent, consisting primarily of groin hematomas.[74,92] Angiographically evident distal embolization occurs in approximately 5 percent of patients and usually carries no clinical significance.[74,102] Vessel rupture at the time of balloon inflation is also a rare complication. Approximately 5 percent of patients experience one of the following problems: intimal flap with obstruction, thrombosis, arterial spasm, arteriovenous fistula or false aneurysm formation, arterial perforation, hematoma and hemorrhage at the puncture site, or reaction to contrast material.[74] One hazard conspicuously absent from this method of revascularization is that of damage to sympathetic nerve fibers subserving genital function.[103]

Surgical intervention is required in some form in approximately 3 percent of patients. Extensive disease and acute illness appear to be associated with a higher risk of complications. There is a small mortality rate (approximately 0.5 percent) related directly to or associated with the procedure.[74,104]

Results

Clinical and angiographic success rates for percutaneous dilatation of the iliac arteries range from 80 to 90 percent at 1 year and 70 to 85 percent in 2 to 3 years after the procedure.[74,98,103,105] Rates for dilatation of the femoral and popliteal arteries are 70 to 80 percent and 60 to 75 percent respectively.[74,98,103,105] These rates approximate those for saphenous vein graft surgery and aortoiliac endarterectomy.[74]

Renal Angioplasty

Of the estimated 23 million people in the United States with established hypertension,[106] approximately 4 percent, or 1 million persons, are believed to have potentially correctable renovascular disease as a basis.[107] Though the benefits of surgical correction over medical therapy have been demonstrated in this group, morbidity and mortality of this intervention have been high (5.8 to 9 percent in reported series).[108] In 1978, Gruentzig and associates reported a successful renal angioplasty using their newly miniaturized coaxial catheter system.[22] Subsequently, renal angioplasty has been shown to be an effective long-term therapy for a subset of patients with hypertension secondary to renal artery stenosis.[74,108]

Patient Selection

In general, candidacy for renal angioplasty is based on the same considerations as those defining surgical eligibility. Diagnostic criteria include (1) pharmacologically resistant hypertension due to an accessible, angiographically documented renal artery stenosis, (2) a functioning ipsilateral kidney, (3) an ipsilateral to contralateral renal vein renin ratio greater than 1.5, and (4) eligibility for surgical therapy or dialysis in the event of complications.[10,74] These guidelines may be amended in the occasional patient who is unable to tolerate medical therapy or demonstrates deteriorating renal function.

Etiology and location of the lesion are important factors in determining eligibility for dilatation. Obstructive disease can be divided into atherosclerotic and nonatherosclerotic types, including fibromuscular dysplasia and postsurgical (e.g., posttransplant) disease. Candidacy appears improved in patients in these latter groups relative to those afflicted with atherosclerosis.[74,108,109] As is the case in other vascular beds, discrete focal disease responds most favorably to dilatation. The continued exception to this rule is ostial lesions which respond poorly and demonstrate high recurrence rates.[109]

Technology and Technique

Balloon catheters for percutaneous renal artery dilatation may be either coaxial catheters or single catheters with double lumen. Selection is usually made on the basis of accessibility and vessel size. Large coaxial catheters are often used when a branch stenosis requires treatment, but in the majority of cases disease of the main trunk deserves use of a double-lumen catheter. Commonly utilized balloons range from 4 to 6 mm.[110,111]

Three different percutaneous angiographic techniques are available for renal artery dilatation. These include use of (1) the guided coaxial catheter system (femoral approach), (2) the femoral balloon catheter system inserted through the axillary approach, and (3) the femoral balloon catheter system utilizing the femoral approach.[111] Whereas the guided coaxial system is similar to the coronary technique and need not be repeated, the latter technique will be described in this section.

The common femoral artery is punctured and a no. 6 French cobra catheter is introduced by the Seldinger technique. After heparin administration, the orifice of the renal artery is selected and an initial angiogram is obtained to define the stenosis. Under fluoroscopic control, a 0.89-mm Teflon-coated movable-core J guidewire is passed across the stenosis and into the distal vessel. The catheter is then advanced across the lesion and the guidewire is withdrawn. At this point, a small amount of dilute contrast material is injected to confirm the position of the catheter and to demonstrate the intraluminal position of the catheter. The guide wire is reinserted, and the appropriate dilatation catheter is introduced (without a femoral sheath) and positioned under fluoroscopic guidance. Serial inflations are performed for periods of 30 to 60 s monitored, as in all procedures, by the balloon configuration and periodic test injections. At the completion of the procedure, complete deflation of the balloon should be assured by the application of negative pressure prior to removal[109,111] (Fig. 117-5).

Blood pressure is monitored closely for the first 24 h following the procedure because of the risk of

FIGURE 117-5 Percutaneous angioplasty of the right renal artery in a 14-year-old male. *A*. Arteriogram before dilatation. *B*. Arteriogram after dilatation.

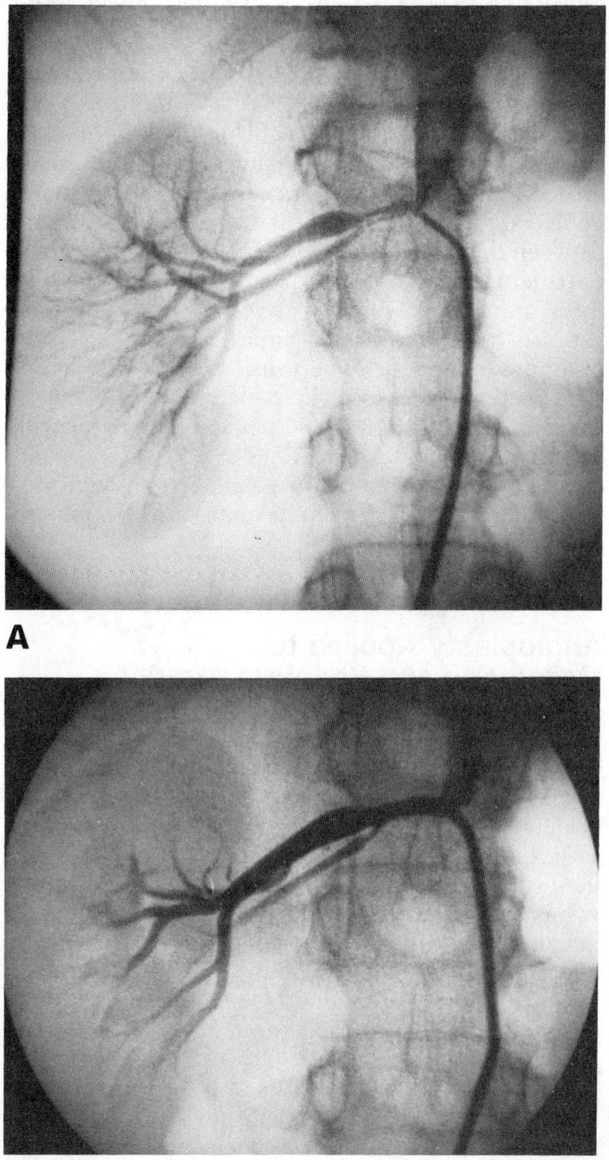

A

B

profound hypotension that may develop after a good result.[74,109,111] Additional monitoring of renal function may consist of serial blood urea nitrogen and creatinine determinations as well as repeat isotope perfusion studies. While some investigators recommend low-dose heparin for 1 to 3 days post dilatation, benefits of this therapy have not been proved. Patients can generally be discharged from the hospital within 3 to 5 days. All patients should receive acetylsalicylic acid for 6 months following dilatation unless contraindicated.

Complications

Complications after attempted renal artery dilatation are similar in nature and frequency to those described for peripheral angioplasty. Emergency surgical intervention is necessary in approximately 1 percent of patients.[74] Specific hazards include subsegmental infarction and deterioration of renal function. Reactions to contrast material are seen more often in patients with impaired renal function.[74]

Results

The efficacy of renal artery dilatation is difficult to assess because of varied selection criteria and an assortment of reporting methods in the available series. Pooled data reveal technical success rates ranging between 83 and 100 percent,[108,110,111] being highest in patients with fibromuscular disease and lowest in those individuals with extensive or ostial atherosclerotic disease.[74] Short-term clinical success (remission or improvement of hypertension at 1 year) is approximately 75 percent in patients with fibromuscular disease[112] and 50 to 60 percent in patients with atherosclerotic involvement.[74,108,109] Recurrent stenoses are low (3-year follow-up) in fibromuscular disease but exceed 50 percent in some series of patients with atherosclerosis.[74]

Angioplasty Applied to Mesenteric and Vertebral Arteries

As a result of its success in peripheral and coronary disease, percutaneous angioplasty has been applied in an increasing number of vascular beds. In 1980, Gruentzig and associates[113] first reported successful dilatation of a superior mesenteric artery in a patient with abdominal angina. Subsequently, other investigators have published reports of similar success in patients with this affliction.[114] Both double-lumen and coaxial catheter techniques have been utilized in obstructions at this site. No significant complications have been reported though total experience has been limited.

While carotid dilatation has not been attempted in atherosclerotic disease owing to fear of cerebral embolization, experience has been gained in the vertebral system.[115] Results with the double-lumen catheter in these vessels have been encouraging, though the number of procedures has been small. Most disease approached has been confined to the origin of the vertebral vessels where angiographically the lesions appear small and nonulcerated.[115] Pending further investigation, angioplasty appears to be a viable therapeutic alternative in selected patients from this group.

Summary

Rapid and broad technical advances have been achieved since therapeutic catheter technology was introduced 20 years ago. Most importantly, however, experience gained with balloon angioplasty has resulted in improved success and a dramatic fall in procedural morbidity and mortality. While we await the discovery of effective preventive therapy in atherosclerosis, this approach to vascular disease offers effective palliation at a reduced cost in terms of physical and emotional suffering as well as hospital expense and loss of income.[116]

References

1. Hurst, J. W.: History of Cardiac Catheterization, in S. B. King and J. S. Douglas (eds.), "Coronary Arteriography and Angioplasty, McGraw-Hill Book Company, New York, 1985, p. 1.
2. Forssman, W.: Die Sondierung des Rechten Herzens, *Klin. Wachenschr.*, 8:2085, 1929.
3. Dotter, C. T., and Judkins, M. P.: Transluminal Treatment of Arteriosclerotic Obstruction: Description of a New Technique and a Preliminary Report of its Application, *Circulation*, 30:654, 1964.
4. Porstmann, W.: Ein Neuer Korsett-Ballonkatheter zur Transluminalen Rekanalisation nach Dotter unter Besonderer Beruchsichtigung von Obliterationen an den Beckerarterien, *Radiol. Diagn. (Berl.)*, 14:239, 1973.
5. Zeitler, E., Schniodtke, J., and Schoop, W.: Die Perkutane Behandlung von Arteriellen Durchblutungsstorungen der Extremitaten mit Katheter, *Vasa*, 2:401, 1973.
6. Gruentzig, A. R.: Die Perkutane Rekanalization Chronisher Arterieller Verschlusse (Dotter-Prinzip) mit Einem Doppelluminger Dilatations-Katheter, *ROFO*, 124:80, 1976.
7. Gruentzig, A. R., Turina, M. I., and Schneider, J. A.: Experimental Percutaneous Dilatation of Coronary Artery Stenosis, *Circulation*, 54(*suppl. 2*):81, 1976. (Abstract 0319.)
8. Gruentzig, A., Senning, A., and Siegenthaler, W.: Nonoperative Dilatation of Coronary Artery Stenosis: Percutaneous Transluminal Coronary Angioplasty (PTCA), *New Eng. J. Med.*, 301:61, 1979.
9. Saddekni, S., Sniderman, K. W., and Hilton, S.: Percutaneous Transluminal Angioplasty of Nonatherosclerotic Lesions. *Am. J. Roentgenol.*, 135:975, 1980.
10. Novelline, R. A.: Percutaneous Transluminal Angioplasty: Newer Applications, *Am. J. Roentgenol.*, 135:983, 1980.
11. Martin, E. C., Diamond, N. G., and Casarella, W. J.: Percutaneous Transluminal Angioplasty in Non-atherosclerotic Disease, *Diagn. Radiol.* 135:27, 1980.
12. Lee, G., Ikeda, R. M., Joye, J. A., Bogren, H. G., DeMaria, A. N., and Mason, D. T.: Evaluation of Transluminal Angioplasty of Chronic Coronary Artery Stenosis. Value and Limitations Assessed in Fresh Human Cadaver Hearts, *Circulation*, 61:77, 1980.

13. Block, P. C., Fallon, J. T., and Elmer, D.: Experimental Angioplasty: Lessons from the Laboratory, *AJR,* 135:907, 1980.
14. Casteneda-Zuniga, W. R., Formanek, A., Tadavarthy, M., Vlodavar, Z., Edwards, J. E., Zollikofer, C., Amplatz, K.: The Mechanism of Balloon Angioplasty, *Radiology,* 135:565, 1980.
15. Block, P. C., Baughman, K. L., Pasternak, R. C., and Fallon, J. T.: Transluminal Coronary Angioplasty: Correlation of Morphologic and Angiographic Findings in an Experimental Model, *Circulation,* 61:778, 1980.
16. Baughman, K. L., Pasternak, R. C., Fallon, J. T., and Block, P. C.: Transluminal Coronary Angioplasty of Postmortem Human Hearts, *Am. J. Cardiol.,* 48:1044, 1981.
17. Block, P. C., Myler, R. K., Sretzer, S., and Fallon, J. T.: Morphology after Transluminal Angioplasty in Human Beings, *N. Eng. J. Med.,* 305:382, 1981.
18. Leu, H. J., and Gruentzig, A.: Histopathologic Aspects of Transluminal Recanalization, in E. Zeitler, A. Gruentzig, and W. Schoop (eds.), "Percutaneous Vascular Recanalization," Springer, Heidelberg, 1978, p. 39.
19. Rapaport, E.: Percutaneous Transluminal Coronary Angioplasty. *Circulation,* 60:969, 1979. (Editorial.)
20. Gruentzig, A. R., Myler, R. K., Hanna, E. H., and Turina, M. I.: Coronary Transluminal Angioplasty, *Circulation,* 55(suppl. 3):84, 1977. (Abstract.)
21. Gruentzig, A. R.: "Die Perkutane Transluminale Rekanalisation Chronischer Arterienverschlusse mit einem Neuen Dilatationstechnik," G. Witzstrock, Baden-Baden, 1977.
22. Gruentzig, A., Kuhlmann, U., Vetter, W., Luetolf, U., Meier, B., and Siegenthaler, W.: Treatment of Renovascular Hypertension with Percutaneous Transluminal Dilatation of a Renal Artery Stenosis, *Lancet,* II:801, 1978.
23. Williams, D. O., Riley, R. S., Singh, A. K., Most, A. S.: Restoration of Normal Coronary Hemodynamic and Myocardial Metabolism after Percutaneous Transluminal Coronary Angioplasty, *Circulation,* 62:653, 1980.
24. Rothman, M., Baim, D., Simpson, J., Harrison, D.: Improved Hemodynamic and Metabolic Indices after Percutaneous Transluminal Coronary Angioplasty (PTCA), *Circulation,* 64(suppl 4):253, 1981. (Abstract.)
25. Williams, D. O., Riley, R. S., Singh, A. K., and Most, A. S.: Coronary Circulatory Dynamics before and after Successful Coronary Angioplasty, *J. Am. Coll. Cardiol.,* 1:1268, 1983.
26. Kent, K. M., Bentivoglio, L. G., Block, P. C., Cowley, M. J., Dorros, C., Gosselin, A. J., Gruentzig, A. R., Myler, R. K., Simpson, J., Stertzer, S. H., Mullin, S. M., and Mock, M. B.: Percutaneous Transluminal Coronary Angioplasty: Report from the Registry of the National Heart, Lung and Blood Institute, *Am. J. Cardiol.,* 49:2011, 1982.
27. Sigwart, U., Grbic, M., Essinger, A., Bischof-Delaloye, A., Sadeghi, H., and Rivier, J. L.: Improvement of Left Ventricular Function after Percutaneous Transluminal Coronary Angioplasty, *Am. J. Cardiol.,* 49:651, 1982.
28. Meier, B., Gruentzig, A., Siegenthaler, W. E., and Schlumpf, M.: Long-Term Exercise Performance after Percutaneous Transluminal Coronary Angioplasty and Coronary Artery Bypass Grafting, *Circulation,* 68:796, 1983.
29. Kaltenback, M., Kober, G., Satter, P., Gruentzig, A. R., Myler, R., and Stertzer, S.: Koronare Eingefaberkrankung. *Verh. Stdch. Ges Herz Kreislauttorsch.,* 46:130, 1980.
30. "Proceeding of the Workshop on Percutaneous Transluminal Coronary Angioplasty, June 15–16, 1979." U.S. Department of Health, Education and Welfare, Public Health Service, National Institutes of Health, NIH Publ. No. 80:2030, 1980.
31. Bonow, R. O., Kent, K. M., Rosing, D. R., Lipson, L. C., Bacharach, S. L., Green, M. V., and Epstein, S. E.: Improved Left Ventricular Diastolic Filling in Patients with Coronary Artery Disease after Percutaneous Transluminal Coronary Angioplasty, *Circulation,* 66:1159, 1982.
32. Hirzel, H., Neusch, K., Gruentzig, A., and Luetolf, U.: Short- and Long-Term Changes in Myocardial Perfusion after Percutaneous Transluminal Coronary Angioplasty Assessed by Thallium-201 Exercise Scintigraphy, *Circulation,* 63:1001, 1981.
33. Scholl, J. M., Chaitman, B. R., David, P. R., Dupras, G., Brevers, G., Val, P. G., Crepeau, J., Lesperance, J., and Bourassa, M. G.: Exercise Electrocardiography and Myocardial Scintigraphy in the Serial Evaluation of the Results of Percutaneous Transluminal Coronary Angioplasty, *Circulation,* 66:380, 1982.
34. Williams, D.O., and Korr, K. S.: Beneficial Effect of Percutaneous Transluminal Coronary Angioplasty on Coronary Circulatory Dynamics, *Circulation,* 64(suppl.4):254, 1981. (Abstract.)
35. Aueron, F., and Gruentzig, A.: Effects of Successful Percutaneous Transluminal Coronary Angioplasty (PTCA) on Acute Chronic Coronary Flow Reserve, *Circulation,* (suppl. 2)68:III–31, 1983. (Abstract.)
36. Holmes, D. R., Vlietstra, R. E., Mock, M. B., Smith, H. C., Dorros, G., Cowley, M. J., Kent, K. M., Hammes, L. N., Janke, L., Elveback, L. R., and Vetrovec, G. W.: Employment and Recreation Patterns in Patients Treated by Percutaneous Transluminal Coronary Angioplasty: A Multicenter Study, *Am. J. Cardiol.,* 52:710, 1983.
37. Williams, D. O., Gruntzig, A., Kent, K. M., Myler, R. K., Stertzer, S. H., Bentivoglio, L., Bourassa, M., Block, P., Cowley, M., Detre, K., Dorros, G., Gosselin, A., Simpson, J., Passamani, E., and Mullin, S.: Guidelines for the Performance of Percutaneous Transluminal Coronary Angioplasty, *Circulation,* 66:693, 1982.
38. Gruentzig, A., and Meier, B.: Percutaneous Transluminal Coronary Angioplasty. The First Five Years and the Future, *Int. J. Cardiol.* 2:319, 1983.
39. Hamby, R. I., and Katz, S.: Percutaneous Transluminal Coronary Angioplasty: Its Potential Impact on Surgery for Coronary Artery Disease, *Am. J. Cardiol.,* 45:1161, 1980.
40. McCallister, B. D., Hartzler, G. O., Rutherford, B. D., and McConahay, D. R.: Palliative Percutaneous Transluminal Coronary Angioplasty for Unstable Angina in Patients Over 70 Years of Age, *Circulation,* (suppl. 4):255, 1981. (Abstract.)
41. Hall, D. P., and Morris, D. C.: Coronary Disease in the Elderly, in J. W. Hurst (ed.), "Clinical Essays on The Heart," McGraw-Hill Book Company, New York, 1984, vol. 3, p. 3.
42. Knapp, W. S.: Efficacy of Coronary Artery Bypass Grafting in Elderly Patients with Coronary Artery Disease, *Am. J. Cardiol.,* 47:923, 1981.
43. Hall, D. P., and Gruentzig, A.: Percutaneous Transluminal Coronary Angioplasty—Current Procedure and Future Direction, *AJR,* 142(1):13, Jan. 1984.
44. David, P., Waters, D., Scholl, J., Crepeau, J., Szlachcic, J., Lesperance, J., Hudon, G., and Bourassa, M. G.: Percutaneous Transluminal Coronary Angioplasty in Patients with Variant Angina, *Circulation,* 66:695, 1982.
45. Hall, D. P., and Gruentzig, A. R.: Selection of Patients for Percutaneous Transluminal Coronary Angioplasty, *Practical Cardiol.,* 1984.
46. Ischinger, T., Gruentzig, A., Hollman, J., King, S., Douglas, J., Meier, B., Bradford, J., and Tankersley, R.: Should Coronary Arteries with Less than 60% Diameter Stenosis be Treated by Angioplasty? *Circulation,* 68:148, 1983.
47. Kent, K. M., Bentivoglio, L. G., Block, P. C., Cowley, M. J., Dorros, G., Gosselin, A. J., Gruentzig, A. R., Myler, R. K., Simpson, J., Stertzer, S. H., Mullin, S. M., and Mock, M. B.: Percutaneous Transluminal Coronary Angioplasty: Report from the Registry of the National Heart, Lung and Blood Institute, *Am. J. Cardiol.,* 49:2011, 1982.
48. Meier, B., Gruentzig, A., Hollman, J., Ischinger, T., and Bradford, J. M.: Does Length or Eccentricity of Coronary Stenoses Influence the Outcome of Transluminal Dilatation? *Circulation,* 67:497, 1983.
49. Levin, D. C., Fallon, J. T.: Significance of the Angiographic Morphology of Localized Coronary Stenosis Histopathologic Correlations, *Circulation,* 66:316, 1982.
50. Campeau, L., Lesperance, J., Hermann, J., Corbara, F., Grondin, C. M., and Bourassa, M. G.: Loss of Improvement

of Angina between 1 & 7 Years after Aortocoronary Bypass Surgery. Correlations with Changes in Vein Grafts and in Coronary Arteries, *Circulation* 60(suppl. 1):1, 1979.
51. Seides, S. F., Borer, J. S., Kent, K. M., Rosing, D. R., McIntosh, C. L., and Epstein, S. E.: Long-Term Anatomic Fate of Coronary Bypass Grafts and Functional Status of Patients Five Years after Operation, *N. Engl. J. Med.*, 298:1213, 1978.
52. Guthaner, D. F., Robert, E. W., Alderman, E. L., and Wesler, L.: Long-Term Serial Angiographic Studies after Coronary Bypass Surgery, *Circulation,* 60:250, 1979.
53. Lawrie, G. M., Morris, G. C., Jr., Calhoun, J. H., et al.: Clinical Results of Coronary Bypass in 500 Patients at Least 10 Years after Operation, *Circulation,* 66(suppl. 1):1, 1982.
54. Loop, F. D., Sheldon, W. C., Lytle, B. W., Cosgrove, D. M. III, and Proudfit, W. L.: The Efficacy of Coronary Artery Surgery, *Am. Heart J.*, 101:86, 1981.
55. Schaff, H. V., Gersh, B. J., and Pluth, J. R.: Survival and Functional Results after Coronary Artery Bypass Grafting; Results 10-12 Years Post-operatively in 500 Patients, *Circulation,* 66(suppl.2):246, 1982. (Abstract.)
56. Douglas, J., Gruentzig, A., King, S. B., III, Hollman, J., Ischinger, T., Meier, B., Craver, J. M., Jones, E. L., Waller, J. L., Bone, D. K., and Guyton, R.: Percutaneous Transluminal Coronary Angioplasty in Patients with Prior Coronary Bypass Surgery, *J. Am. Coll. Cardiol.*, 2:745, 1983.
57. Hall, D. P., Corzo, O., Douglas, J. S., and Gruentzig, A. R.: Percutaneous Transluminal Coronary Angioplasty in Patients with Prior Coronary Bypass Surgery, *Internat. J. Cardiol.*, 6:645, 1984.
58. Alpert, J. R., Ring, E. J., Berkowitz, H. D., Freiman, D. B., Oleaga, J. A., Gordon, R., and Roberts, B.: Treatment of Vein Graft Stenosis by Balloon Catheter Dilatation. *JAMA* 242:2769, 1979.
59. Ford, W. B., Wholey, M. H., Zikria, E. A., Miller, W. H., Samadani, S. R., Koimattur, A. G., and Sullivan, M. E.: Percutaneous Transluminal Angioplasty in the Management of Occlusive Disease Involving the Coronary Arteries and Saphenous Vein Bypass Grafts. *J. Thorac. Cardiovasc. Surg.*, 79:1, 1980.
60. Jones, E. L., Craver, J. M., Gruentzig, A. R., King, S. B., III, Douglas, J. S., Bone, D. K., Guyton, R. G., and Hatcher, C. R., Jr.: Percutaneous Transluminal Coronary Angioplasty: Role of the Surgeon, *Ann. Thorac. Surg.*, 34:493, 1982.
61. Dervan, J. P., Baim, D. S., Cherniles, J., and Grossman, W.: Transluminal Angioplasty of Occluded Coronary Arteries: Use of a Movable Guide Wire System, *Circulation,* 68:776, 1983.
62. Libow, M., Hall, D. P., and Gruentzig, A. R.: Coronary Angioplasty (PTCA) in Patients with Chronic Total Occlusion, in press. (Abstract.)
63. Aueron, F., and Gruentzig, A.: Outcome of Patients Waiting to Undergo Percutaneous Transluminal Coronary Angioplasty (PTCA), *Circulation,* 68:(suppl. 3):96, 1983. (Abstract.)
64. Meyer, J., Merx, W., Dorr, R., Lambertz, H., Bethge, C., and Effert, S.: Successful Treatment of Acute Myocardial Infarction Shock by Combined Percutaneous Transluminal Coronary Recanalization (PTCR) and Percutaneous Transluminal Coronary Angioplasty (PTCA), *Am. Heart J.*, 103:132, 1982.
65. Meyer, J., Merx, W., Schmitz, H. J., Erbel, R., Kiesslich, T., Dorr, R., Lambertz, H., Bethge, C., Krebs, W., Bardos, P., Minale, C., Messmer, J., and Effert, S.: Percutaneous Transluminal Coronary Angioplasty Immediately after Intracoronary Streptolysis of Transmural Myocardial Infarction, *Circulation,* 66:905, 1982.
66. Goldberg, S., Urban, P. L., Greenspon, A., Lebenthal, M., Walinsky, P., Maroko, M. B., Harbord, T., and Calcagno, J.: Combination Therapy for Evolving Myocardial Infarction: Intracoronary Thrombolysis & Percutaneous Transluminal Angioplasty, *Am. J. Med.*, 72:994, 1982.
67. Serruys, P. W., Wijns, W., Van Den Brand, M., Ribeiro, V., Fioretti, P., Simoons, M. L., Kooijman, C. J., Reiber, J. H., and Hugenholtz, P. H.: Is Transluminal Coronary Angioplasty Mandatory after Successful Thrombolysis? *Br. Heart J.*, 50:257, 1983.
68. Fallon, J. T.: Pathology of Arterial Lesions Amenable to Percutaneous Transluminal Angioplasty, *AJR*, 135:913, 1980.
69. Myler, R. K., Gruentzig, A. R., and Stertzer, S. H.: Coronary Angioplasty, in E. Rappaport (ed.), "Text Cardiology Update: Review for Physicians," Elsevier Publishing Co., New York, 1983, p. 1.
70. Dorros, G., Stertzer, S. H., Bruno, M. S., Kaltenbach, M., Myler, R. K., and Spring, D. A.: The Brachial Artery Method to Transluminal Coronary Angioplasty, *Cathet. Cardiovasc. Diagn.*, 8:233, 1982.
71. Thornton, M. A., Gruentzig, A. R., Brown, J. E., Arnold, T. C., and Hesser, F.: Characteristics of Coronary Balloon Dilatation Catheters, *Circulation,* 68(suppl. 3):347, 1983. (Abstract.)
72. Aueron, F., and Gruentzig, A.: Effects of Successful Percutaneous Transluminal Coronary Angioplasty (PTCA) on Acute and Chronic Coronary Flow Reserve, *Circulation,* 68(suppl. 3):30, 1983. (Abstract.)
73. Dorros, G., Cowley, M., Simpson, J., Bentivoglio, L., Block, P., Bourassa, M., Detre, K., Gosselin, A., Gruentzig, A., Kelsey, S. F., Kent, K. M., Mock, M. B., Mullin, S., Myler, R., Passamani, E., Stertzer, S., Williams, D. O.: Percutaneous Transluminal Coronary Angioplasty: Report of Complications from the National Heart, Lung, and Blood Institute PTCA Registry, *Circulation,* 67:723, 1983.
74. Health and Public Policy Committee, American College of Physicians: Percutaneous Transluminal Angioplasty, *Ann. Intern. Med.*, 99:864, 1983.
75. Meier, B., Gruentzig, A., King, S. B., Douglas, J. S., Hollman, J., Ischinger, T., Auron, F., and Galan, K.: Risk of Side Branch Occlusion During Coronary Angioplasty, *Am. J. Cardiol.*, 53:10, 1984.
76. Maroko, P. R., Radvany, P., Braumwald, E., and Hale, S. L.: Reduction of Infarct Size by Oxygen Inhalation following Acute Coronary Occlusion, *Circulation,* 52:360, 1975.
77. Hollman, J., Gruentzig, A. R., Douglas, J. S., King, S. B., Ischinger, T., and Meier, B.: Acute Occlusion after Percutaneous Transluminal Coronary Angioplasty—A New Approach, *Circulation,* 68:725, 1983.
78. Bussman, W., Passek, D., Seidel, W., and Kaltenbach, M.: Reduction of CK and CK-MB Indexes of Infarct Size by Intravenous Nitroglycerin, *Circulation,* 63:615, 1981.
79. Gold, H. K., Leinbach, R. C., Maroko, P. R.: Propranolol-Induced Reduction of Signs of Ischemic Injury During Acute Myocardial Infarction, *Am. J. Cardiol.*, 38:689, 1976.
80. Peter, T., Norris, R. M., Clarke, E. D., Heng, M. K. J., Singh, B. N., Williams, B., Howell, D. R., and Ambler, P. K.: Reduction of Enzyme Levels by Propranolol after Acute Myocrdial Infarction, *Circulation,* 57:1091, 1978.
81. Alcan, K. E., Stertzer, S. H., Wallsh, E., De Pasquale, N., and Bruno, M. S.: The Role of Intraaortic Balloon Counterpulsation in Patients Undergoing Percutaneous Transluminal Coronary Angioplasty, *Am. Heart J.*, 105:517, 1983.
82. Jones, E. L., Douglas, J. S., Gruentzig, A. R., Craver, J. M., King, S. B., Guyton, R. G., and Hatcher, C. R.: Percutaneous Saphenous Vein Angioplasty to Avoid Reoperative Bypass Surgery, *Ann. Thorac. Surg.*, 36:389, 1983.
83. Scholl, J. M., David, P. R., Chaitman, J., Lesperance, J., Crepeau, I., Dyrda, M. G., and Bourassa, M. G.: Recurrence of Stenosis following Percutaneous Transluminal Coronary Angioplasty, *Circulation,* 64(suppl.4):193, 1981. (Abstract.)
84. Gruentzig, A. R., Knudston, M., and Schlumpf, M.: Repeated Coronary Angioplasty (PTCA) after Recurrence of Stenosis, *Circulation,* 64(suppl. 4):108, 1981.
85. Mabin, T. A., Holmes, D. R., Smith, H. C., Reeder, G. S., Bresnahan, J. F., Bove, A. A., Hammes, L., Orszulak, T. A.: Long-Term Follow-Up after Percutaneous Transluminal Coronary Angioplasty (PTCA), *Circulation,* 68(suppl. 3):97, 1983. (Abstract.)
86. Renkin, J., David, P. R., Dangoisse, V., Lesperance, J., and

Bourassa, M. G.: Coronary Angiographic Results 6 and 18 Months after Successful Percutaneous Transluminal Angioplasty in 53 Consecutive Patients, *Circulation*, 68(suppl. 3):314, 1983.

87. Levine, S., Ewels, C. J., Rosing, D. R., Kent, K. M.: Restenosis (R) Following Transluminal Coronary Angioplasty (TCA), *Circulation*, 68(suppl 3):96, 198.
88. Emory University Cardiac Data Bank, Atlanta, Ga.
89. Gruentzig, A. R., and Hopff, H.: Perkutane Rekanalisation Chronischer Arterieller Verschlusse mit einem Neuen Dilatationskatheter. Modification der Dotter-Technik, *Dtsch. Med. Wochenschr*, 99:2502, 1974.
90. Gordon, G., and Kannel, W. B.: Predisposition to Atherosclerosis in the Head, Heart and Legs. The Framingham Study, *JAMA* 221:661, 1972.
91. Sos, T. A., and Sniderman, K. W.: Percutaneous Transluminal Angioplasty, *Semin. Roengenol.*, 16:26, 1981.
92. Motarjeme, A., Keifer, J. W., and Zuska, A. J.: Percutaneous Transluminal Angioplasty and Case Selection, *Diagn. Radiol.*, 135:574, 1980.
93. Martin, E. C., Frankuchen, E. I., Karlson, K. B., Dolgin, C., Collins, R. H., Voorhees, A. B., and Casarella, W. J.: Angioplasty for Femoral Artery Occlusion: Comparison with Surgery, *AJR*, 137:915, 1981.
94. Zeitler, E., Richter, E. I., Roth, F. J., Schoop, W.: Results of Percutaneous Transluminal Angioplasty, *Radiology*, 146:57, 1983.
95. Gruentzig, A. R., and Kumpe, D. A.: Technique of Percutaneous Transluminal Angioplasty with the Gruentzig Balloon Catheter, *AJR*, 132:547, 1979.
96. Zeitler E: Die Perkutane Rekanalisation Arterieller Obliterationen mit Katheter nach Dotter (Dotter-Technik), *Dtsch. Med. Wochenschr.*, 97:1392, 1972.
97. Katzen, B. T., and Chang, J.: Percutaneous Transluminal Angioplasty with the Gruentzig Balloon Catheter, *Radiology*, 130:623, 1979.
98. Katzen, B. T., Chang, J., and Knox, W. G.: Percutaneous Transluminal Angioplasty with the Gruentzig Balloon Catheter. A Review of 70 Cases, *Arch. Surg.*, 114:1389, 1979.
99. Zeitler, E.: Drug Treatment before and after Percutaneous Transluminal Recanalization, in E. Zeitler, A. R. Gruentzig, and W. Schoop, (eds.), "Percutaneous Vascular Recanalization," Berlin, Springer-Verlag, 1978, p. 73.
100. Schmidtke, I., Zeitler, E., Schoop, W.: Late Results of Percutaneous Catheter Treatment (Dottler's Technique) in Occlusion of the Femoropopliteal Arteries, Stage II, in E. Zeitler, A. R. Gruentzig, and W. Schoop, (eds.), "Percutaneous Vascular Recanalization," Berlin, Springer-Verlag, 1978, p. 99.
101. Manashil, G. B., Thunstrom, B. S., Thorpe, C. D., Lipson, S. R.: Outpatient Transluminal Angioplasty, *Radiology*, 147:7, 1983.
102. Gruentzig, A. R.: Percutaneous Balloon Catheter Angioplasty. Presented at the Annual Meeting of the Society of Cardiovascular Radiology, New Orleans, 1978.
103. Andel, G. J.: Transluminal Iliac Angioplasty Long-Term Results, *Radiology*, 135:607, 1980.
104. Glover, J. L., Benedick, P. J., Dilley, R. S.: Efficacy of Balloon Catheter Dilatation for Lower Extremity Atherosclerosis, *Surgery*, 91:560, 1982.
105. Dotter, C. T.: Transluminal Angioplasty: A Long View, *Radiology*, 135:561, 1980.
106. Stokes, J. B., Payne, G. H., Cooper, T.: Hypertension Control: The Challenge of Patient Education, *N. Eng. J. Med.*, 289:1369, 1973.
107. Hunt, J. C., and Strong, C. G.: Renovascular Hypertension Mechanisms: Natural History and Treatment, *Am. J. Cardiol.* 32:562, 1973.
108. Kuhlmann, U., Vetter, W., Furrer, J., Luetolf, U., Siegenthaler, W. and Gruentzig, A.: Renovascular Hypertension: Treatment by Percutaneous Transluminal Dilatation. *Ann. Intern. Med.* 92:1, 1980.
109. Sos, T. A., Saddekni, S., Sniderman, K. W., Weiner, M., Beinart, C., Pickering, T. G., Cade, D. B., Vaughan, D., and Laragh, J. H.: Renal Artery Angioplasty: Techniques and Early Results. *Urol. Radiol.* 3:223, 1982.
110. Casarella, W. J.: Percutaneous Transluminal Angioplasty of the Renal and Iliac Arteries, in J. J. Bergon and H. S. Yao (eds.), "Surgery of the Aorta and Its Body Branches," Grune & Strattan, New York, 1979.
111. Tegtmeyer, C. J., Dyer, R., Teates, C. D., Ayers, C. R., Carey, R. M., Wellons, H. A., and Stanton, L. W.: Percutaneous Transluminal Dilatation of the Renal Arteries, *Radiology*, 135:589, 1980.
112. Schwarten, D. E.: Transluminal Angioplasty of Renal Artery Stenoses: 70 Experiences, *AJR*, 135:969, 1980.
113. Furrer, J., Gruentzig, A., Kugelmeier, J., Goebel, N.: Treatment of Abdominal Angina with Percutaneous Dilatation of an Arteria Mesenterica Superior Stenosis, *Cardiovasc. Intervent. Radiol.*, 3:43, 1980.
114. Golden, D. A., Ring, E. J., McLean, G. K., and Freiman, D. B.: Percutaneous Transluminal Angioplasty in the Treatment of Abdominal Angina, *AJR*, 139:247, 1982.
115. Motarjeme, A., Keifer, J. W., Zuska, A. J.: Percutaneous Transluminal Angioplasty of the Vertebral Arteries, *Radiology*, 139:715, 1981.
116. Jang, G. C., Block, P. C., Cowley, M. J., Gruentzig, A. R., Dorros, G., Holmes, D. R., Kent, K. M., Leatherman, L. L., Myler, R. K., Stertzer, S. H., Sjolander, M., Willis, H., Vetrovech, E. W., and Williams, D. O.: Comparative Cost Analysis of Coronary Angioplasty and Coronary Bypass Surgery: Results from a National Cooperative Study, *Circulation* 66(suppl. 2):124, 1982.

118

Techniques of Achieving Pulmonary, Peripheral, and Coronary Thrombolysis

James F. Spann, Jr., M.D.
Sol Sherry, M.D.
Ronald N. Rubin, M.D.

Indications for the use of thrombolytic therapy in deep vein thrombosis, pulmonary embolism, peripheral arterial disease, and acute myocardial infarction have been discussed in detail in Chaps. 45, 54, 65, 68, and 95, as have the pathophysiology and diagnosis of these conditions. The following is a technical discussion of current methods of safely and effectively delivering thrombolytic agents to patients with these diagnoses and indications.

General Considerations

With either systemic or local streptokinase (Streptase or Kabikinase) infusions, patient selection, patient care, and technique of therapy are important to lessen the incidence of both minor and major hemorrhage. Undue patient manipulation and invasive procedures should be avoided. Fibrin at sites of recent hemostatic plugs, such as those formed at venipuncture and arterial puncture sites and cutdowns, can be expected to dissolve, and normal hemostasis will not take place during therapy. Accordingly, invasive procedures are to be avoided as far as possible. Bed rest is suggested to avoid accidental trauma to patients, and diagnostic procedures should be avoided if possible. No intramuscular injections should be given, and other antithrombotic agents, such as aspirin and heparin, should not be administered during lytic therapy. However, some investigators are administering heparin during and immediately after lytic therapy, particularly when intravascular catheters are being used, rather than waiting to initiate anticoagulant therapy.

Lytic agents are most effective in fresh clots, so in general only patients with clots of less than 7 to 10 days duration should be offered therapy. With older clots there is less efficacy, yet the patient is exposed to the side effects of bleeding. In acute myocardial infarction there is even less time, since the "window" of time for myocardial salvage seems no greater than 6 h after onset of pain. In general, whenever thrombolysis is indicated, the sooner therapy can be initiated, the better chance for clot lysis.

High titer streptokinase antibody will neutralize streptokinase and render it ineffective. Patients with a high titer of streptokinase antibody will not respond to therapy; they account for about 5 percent of cases. Predictors of high streptokinase antibody levels are recent streptococcal infection and prior streptokinase therapy within 6 months. In these instances, urokinase (Abbokinase) is the drug of choice.

Patients likely to bleed should not receive streptokinase. The various contraindications are discussed below.

Specifics of Administration

Systemic Intravenous Infusions for Pulmonary Embolism or Proximal Deep Vein Thrombosis

The following steps should be followed in administering a lytic agent by systemic intravenous infusion:

- Administer streptokinase or urokinase via an infusion pump to ensure accurate, timed dosages.
- Minimize allergic and pyrogenic reactions by premedicating patients with hydrocortisone, 100 mg intravenously, if streptokinase is the drug used. This can be repeated every 8 h if needed (it is usually not necessary during the period of streptokinase administration).
- Obtain baseline coagulation tests. The best tests for following the condition of a patient on thrombolytic agents are the fibrinogen level and thrombin time. The activated partial thromboplastin time (APTT) is a less sensitive measure. Some investigators use the fibrinogen assay but also obtain an APTT for later changeover to heparin.
- Give a "loading" dose of 250,000 international units of streptokinase by infusion over 30 min. This dose neutralizes low-titer streptokinase antibodies arising from previous streptococcal infections and initiates an active clot-dissolving state. Such loading doses are effective in establishing systemic clot lysis in 95 percent of patients. For urokinase, the loading dose is 2000 units/lb given intravenously over 30 min. (Units of urokinase and streptokinase are standardized by different methods and are not comparable.)
- Begin a maintenance infusion of streptokinase, 100,000 international units/h, and continue it for the duration of treatment. For urokinase, the maintenance infusion is 2000 units/lb/h.

- Continue treatment for pulmonary embolism for 24 h. For proximal deep vein thrombosis, continue treatment for 24 to 72 h, depending upon the restoration of blood flow as judged by noninvasive techniques such as impedance phlethysmography, Doppler ultrasound, and phleborrhaphy. Serial venograms are not recommended because of the increased risk of rethrombosis.

Monitoring of Therapy

During the second through fourth hour of treatment, the fibrinogen assay or measurement of thrombin time is repeated. The fibrinogen level should be significantly lowered or the thrombin time prolonged. With streptokinase, the fibrinogen will be lowered to half or less; the thrombin time will be twice the baseline or greater. Milder changes are observed with urokinase. Such values confirm the presence of a systemic thrombolytic state, and the infusion is then continued for the duration of the treatment. However, since the thrombolytic agent achieves clot lysis primarily by activating fibrin-bound plasminogen, the tests do not measure events in the thrombus and are of limited usefulness in judging the effectiveness of clot lysis. If a thrombolytic state has not been induced although the patient is receiving the proper dosage and the infusion apparatus is working correctly, the physician should consider aborting the infusion and switching to heparin or another thrombolytic agent.

Following completion of the infusion, the coagulation tests are repeated. At this time, the fibrinogen level or thrombin time has usually improved toward normal, as compared with the test done during therapy. Heparin therapy to prevent rethrombosis should be instituted when the APTT is within the therapeutic range ($1\frac{1}{2}$ to $2\frac{1}{2}$ times baseline). A sustaining infusion of heparin, without a loading dose, is started and maintained according to conventional methods. If the APTT is more than $2\frac{1}{2}$ times baseline, there should be a wait of 2 to 3 h, after which the APTT should be repeated. Once APTT is in the therapeutic range, heparin therapy should be started, as previously described. If the APTT is less than $1\frac{1}{2}$ times baseline, a small loading dose of heparin is employed at the start of the sustaining infusion. The heparin protocol may vary in myocardial infarction patients, as will be discussed later.

Efficacy, defined as significant (greater than 80 percent) venographic improvement, is in the 50 to 70 percent range for deep venous thrombosis.[1,2] Serious bleeding incidence has been in the 4 to 9 percent range.[3] Pulmonary embolism patients treated with lytic agents almost uniformly manifest prompt clinical improvement and physiological improvement, as determined by serial angiography and pulmonary pressures.[4] Long-term morbidity seems improved, as compared with that of heparin-treated patients,[5] but further documentation is required.

Local Infusions for Thrombosis of Peripheral Arteries

The above comments regarding using infusion pumps, pretreating with steroids if streptokinase is used, and obtaining baseline coagulation tests also apply to local infusions. Streptokinase has been the lytic agent used most frequently for local infusion of peripheral arteries.

The catheter is placed as for routine angiography. After the angiogram documents the presence of a thrombus, the catheter tip is positioned at the proximal border of the thrombus in preparation for local perfusion of lytic agent.

For peripheral vascular diseases many dose forms have been used, ranging from 5000 to 50,000 international units of streptokinase per hour. Rubin et al. have found that after 6 to 12 h almost all doses initiate a systemic fibrinolytic state,[6] but more rapid rates of lysis may be expected with the higher doses. Once started, the infusion should be continued for 4 to 6 h. Efficacy should be checked by repeat arterial injections of contrast agent. Doppler pressure-wave monitoring is also performed hourly.

Optimal results occur when the infusion catheter is in place at the proximal edge of the clot. As time progresses and clot lysis occurs, the catheter should be repositioned distally to the new edge of the clot.

When clot lysis is occurring, therapy should continue until Doppler pressure and arteriograms stabilize. Therapy is then stopped.

If no effect is seen after 4 to 6 h although techniques are proper (i.e., catheter in appropriate position and pump functioning well), the infusion should be aborted.

After an appropriate delay, as described above, fibrinogen and APTT are measured. The catheter is removed if fibrinogen is greater than 100 mg/dl. If persistent hypofibrinogenemia results, cryoprecipitate is administered to elevate levels of fibrinogen and clotting factors and to lessen chances for puncture-site hematoma. Systemic anticoagulation with heparin is then instituted as described above.

Efficacy ranges from 60 to 90 percent. Bleeding incidence ranges from 5 to 15 percent.[7–9]

Intracoronary Infusion for Acute Myocardial Infarction

The intracoronary catheter is placed in the femoral artery via a catheter sheath. Occlusion of the infarct artery is then determined by angiography. Although the incidence of coronary artery spasm is 5 percent or less, intracoronary or intravenous nitroglycerin is given to exclude spasm. Streptokinase or urokinase is infused through the coronary catheter. Subselective infusion is rarely done. Streptokinase is given at a rate of 2000 to 4000 international units/min. Urokinase is given at a rate of 6000 units/min. At least 1 h of total infusion is generally given, and in some studies intracoronary infusion has been continued for an additional 30 min. to 1 h following clot lysis. Clot lysis generally occurs within the first 30 min of infusion. Periodic injection of the infarct artery with contract dye is used to determine reperfusion. Patients with reperfusion are generally maintained on a systemic infusion of heparin, 800 to 1200 units/h, for 2 to 7 days. The catheter sheath is generally left in place for 24 h to aid hemostasis at the puncture site.

Reperfusion occurs in an average of 75 percent of treated patients, varying from 60 to 90 percent.[10–12] Reocclusion occurs with an average frequency of 17 percent. Significant bleeding has occurred in an average of 4.8 percent of patients.[10] Most of this bleeding occurs at the site of catheter placement.

When appropriate regional techniques for evaluation of the jeopardized myocardium before and after reperfusion were utilized, significant salvage of myocardium was indicated by recovery of contractile function in patients who were reperfused during the first 6 h of myocardial infarction.[13,14] Myocardial labeling with ^{201}Tl is dependent on intact coronary flow and uptake of isotope by functional cells. Improved regional perfusion and ^{201}Tl uptake have been observed following successful reperfusion.[15,16]

The time from onset of severe ischemia to achievement of reperfusion determines extent of myocardial salvage in experimental animals; 6 h is thought to be the maximum duration of severe ischemia which is consistent with myocardial salvage.[17] Myocardial salvage is better when reperfusion occurs. However, some believe later reperfusion is also beneficial.[18]

The Western Washington Randomized Trial reported by Kennedy et al. studied the effect of thrombolysis on mortality.[19] In this study, 134 patients were randomly assigned to a group receiving intracoronary streptokinase therapy, and 116 patients were randomly assigned to a placebo group. Each patient had left ventricular angiography and coronary arteriography performed before streptokinase infusion. Of the 116 control patients, 13 died within the first 30 days (11.2 percent), while 5 of the 134 streptokinase-treated patients died (3.7 percent, $p < 0.02$). The 6-month mortality rate in the control group was 14.7 percent (17 of 116); it was 3.7 percent (5 of 134) in the streptokinase-treated group ($p = 0.0025$).

Urokinase in doses of 6000 units/min by intracoronary infusion has been reported to have an effectiveness similar to that of streptokinase in achieving coronary thrombolysis.[20]

Systemic Intravenous Infusion for Acute Myocardial Infarction

Although intracoronary thrombolysis is an exciting new therapy, a number of major difficulties limit its widespread application. The intracoronary procedure requires rapid access to specially trained personnel and complex, expensive equipment. Making the procedure available to large numbers of patients would necessitate the establishment of high-cost facilities in many locations.

High-dose brief-duration intravenous streptokinase, given within the first few hours of symptoms of myocardial infarction, is simple to administer and may prove to be as effective as local intracoronary perfusion. Early administration may increase incidence of successful recanalization. Brief administration of a high dose ensures high concentrations of streptokinase in the coronary circulation and avoids a protracted period of circulating hyperplasminemia. The risk of bleeding may therefore be reduced.

An infusion pump is used, and hydrocortisone is given as described above. Streptokinase is administered through a peripheral vein in doses which have varied from 750,000 international units given in 20 min to 1,500,000 international units given in 60 min. One recent study gave 500,000 international units as a bolus, followed by 200,000 international units/h for 4 h.[21] While it is not clear which dose is correct, it appears that a dose larger than 500,000 international units should be administered during a 1-h infusion; we continue to utilize 1,500,000 international units in a 1-h infusion.

In the absence of coronary arteriography before and after streptokinase administration, it is difficult to determine with certainty whether reperfusion has occurred. Since many patients who achieve reperfusion should have coronary angiography to determine if bypass surgery or percutaneous transluminal coronary angioplasty is needed, it is important to determine which patient has achieved reperfusion. Findings suggestive of reperfusion are sudden pain relief, ventricular reperfusion arrhythmias, and rapid return of the ST-segment elevation toward the baseline. When these events occur within the first 2 h after intravenous infusion of streptokinase, and if the muscle brain-creatine kinase (MB-CK) value peaks within the first 13 h, one should consider the possibility that the patient has had early reperfusion. A sudden, early rise in hourly CK levels has been used by some to indicate reperfusion.[22]

Early reports suggested that high-dose brief-duration administration of streptokinase could lyse intracoronary clot in acute myocardial infarction in 46 to 60 percent of patients.[23–25] Coronary angiography has been performed on 155 patients before and after high-dose brief-duration intravenous streptokinase.[23,24,26–28] Of the 155 patients 79 patients (51 percent) achieved coronary reperfusion within 1 h of initiation of the infusion, and the percentage of patients achieving reperfusion was quite consistent (52, 60, 49, 46, and 44 percent). A recent report has shown a higher rate of reperfusion (81 percent) and documented this result by early angiography.[21] Another report which lacked early angiographic proof believed that 96 percent of patients had reperfusion.[22]

In the first five studies, in which 237 patients were treated with systemic intravenous infusion for acute myocardial infarction, serious bleeding occurred in 2 patients (0.8 percent).[10]

Three studies of high-dose brief-duration intravenous streptokinase given early reported data on ventricular function before and after streptokinase administration.[23,24,26] Early and sustained reperfusion was associated with significant improvement of ventricular function in each study, but randomized trials are needed.

A major unanswered question is whether early high-dose brief-duration intravenous streptokinase decreases the acute and long-term mortality in acute myocardial infarction. As yet, no randomized and controlled trial has been reported, although a major randomized and controlled trial testing the efficacy of early high-dose brief-duration intravenous streptokinase in reducing mortality of acute myocardial infarction is currently underway in a multicenter study involving 21 German and Swiss hospitals.

Systemic intravenous use of urokinase in acute myocardial infarction has not yet been reported.

Stabilization following Either Intracoronary or Intravenous Coronary Thrombolysis

The incidence of reocclusion at the second angiogram, 2 to 4 weeks after reperfusion by intracoronary streptokinase, varied from 9 to 29 percent in four studies of 82 patients, and the average incidence of reocclusion was 17 percent. The incidence of reocclusion at angiography 2 to 4 weeks after reperfusion by intravenous streptokinase varied from 5 to 26 percent in four studies of 159 patients and averaged 18 percent.[10] Many such patients sustained reinfarction or extension of the original infarction.

In all patients with early coronary reperfusion, a sustained intravenous infusion of heparin (800 to 1200 units/h) should begin when the APTT is 50 s or less. Following recatheterization or after 7 to 14 days, all patients judged to have persistent coronary reperfusion should be maintained on oral warfarin sodium (Coumadin). The specifics for optimal antithrombotic prevention of rethrombosis (by anticoagulants, platelet-controlling drugs, etc.) remain unclear. In one study, 5000 to 10,000 units of heparin was administered before the streptokinase and a sustaining heparin infusion was started immediately after the streptokinase infusion, regardless of APTT level.[22] The potential for substantially increased bleeding with such vigorous use of heparin appears real since serious bleeding occurred in 12.3 percent of these patients.[22]

A two-step therapy, aimed first at immediate salvage of myocardium by thrombolysis and second at improving coronary artery anatomy to stabilize the situation and preserve the salvaged myocardium, may be necessary in many patients. Three studies have now reported early percutaneous transluminal angioplasty, and three have reported early coronary bypass surgery following either intracoronary or intravenous thrombolysis.[26,29–33] How to judge which patient should have a second and stabilizing intervention following myocardial salvage is currently unknown and requires additional research.

Adverse Reactions and Their Management

Adverse Reactions

Allergic reactions occur because streptokinase is a foreign, bacteria-derived protein. Streptokinase antibody titers clearly occur after treatment with streptokinase and are significant by day 7. They persist for 3 to 6 months, then decline. Such antibodies may interfere with efficacy and may cause allergic side effects if streptokinase is given again. True allergic side effects occur in 1 to 2 percent of cases; they include angioneurotic edema, hypotension, and bronchospasm. Milder "allergic" phenomena including rash, urticaria, and flushing are more common, occurring in up to 5 to 10 percent of patients. These milder reactions can be almost completely abolished by premedication of patients with 100 mg hydrocortisone; this can be repeated at 6 to 12 h intervals. Most investigators continue streptokinase therapy despite the presence or persistence of minor reactions. In the unusual instance of an anaphalactoid type of allergic reaction, therapy should be stopped. Allergy to urokinase, a human-derived protein, is extremely unusual.

On occasion, patients with preexisting high titers of streptokinase antibody are encountered. These neutralizing antibodies come about by recent streptococcal infections or recent streptokinase exposure. In such patients, ordinary doses of streptokinase are unable to overcome the antibody effects and therapy is ineffective. Such patients are a small minority, perhaps 5 percent of patients being considered for streptokinase. These are the patients who do not manifest a systemic lytic state and who should be treated with urokinase instead.

Fever occurs in streptokinase-treated patients; incidence rates as high as 30 percent have been reported. Again, pretreatment with steroid can effectively reduce this incidence to less than 5 percent. With urokinase, fevers may also occur in 1 to 2 percent of patients, although the mechanism is obscure.

Bleeding is the major and most serious complication associated with lytic therapy. Incidence is variable and is contingent upon the investigator's definition of "bleeding." Some have defined bleeding as all bleeding episodes, including minor cutdown or venipuncture oozing, others have considered only transfusion-dependent episodes, and still others only life-threatening episodes. Attention to proper technique and patient selection are also critical variables which determine incidence of bleeding.

In thrombolytic treatment of pulmonary embolism, deep venous thrombosis and peripheral arterial occlusion, major bleeding (defined as intracranial, retroperitoneal, or gastrointestinal bleeding) occurs in 2 percent of patients. Less major bleeding (defined as a puncture site hematoma which requires transfusion, hematuria, or a spreading ecchymosis which requires transfusion) occurred in 9 percent of patients. These figures compare with an approximately 5 percent incidence of hemorrhage when full-dose heparin is given to similar patients.[34]

Most bleeding episodes are minor. Nuisance bleeding, such as venipuncture oozing, is to be expected because hemostatic plugs are lysed during therapy. Such bleeding is easily managed by pressure and local care. Therapy should not be stopped for this type of minor bleeding. Minor bleeding, and often major bleeding, is directly related to the number and types of invasive procedures undertaken before and during therapy as well as technique and attention to detail.

Bleeding requiring either transfusion or surgical repair of the site of arterial puncture occurred in 31 of 640 patients (4.8 percent) in nine studies of intracoronary streptokinase therapy.[10] No patient died from bleeding or had major intracranial hemorrhage.

Bleeding requiring transfusion occurred in 2 of 237 patients (0.8 percent) in the first five studies of systemic intravenous streptokinase for myocardial infarction.[10]

The best approach to the hemorrhage problem associated with thrombolytic therapy is to prevent its occurrence. This is best achieved by proper patient selection and the avoidance of unnecessary invasive procedures or other traumatic testing before or during therapy.

Proper patient selection includes a properly established diagnosis. Only patients likely to benefit (proper indication, recent thrombosis) should be treated. Careful consideration of contraindications is vital. Absolute contraindications include actively bleeding lesions and intracranial disorders with potential for hemorrhage, such as recent stroke, intracranial tumor, or uncontrolled severe hypertension. Relative contraindications include major surgery less than 10 days previously, postpartum state, recent cardiopulmonary resuscitation, recent biopsy or needle puncture of poorly compressible areas, and concomitant hypocoagulable states. Some studies of systemic intravenous thrombolytic therapy for acute myocardial infarction have excluded patients greater than 70 years of age.

Attention to technique and detail is very important. Patients will bleed from invasive procedures. Thus, as far as possible, arterial and deep venous puncture, biopsies, and cutdowns are to be avoided.

Distal extremities should be used when either venous or arterial access is necessary since they provide easily compressible sites. Bed rest should be strictly enforced to avoid trauma.

Since systemic hyperplasminemia and bleeding complications have been observed with both systemic and local routes of administration and in all of the above indications for thrombolytic therapy, these precautions and principles for decreasing the incidence of bleeding apply to all uses of thrombolytic therapy.

Management of Adverse Reactions

Management of allergic reactions to streptokinase depends upon their severity. Mild-to-moderate rash, itching, and urticaria can be effectively managed with antihistamines and/or steroids. Streptokinase therapy should be continued. More severe anaphylactoid reactions require vigorous and immediate therapy with steroids and possibly epinephrine, and the immediate cessation of streptokinase infusion.

Pyrexia is variously managed. Some physicians prophylactically administer nonaspirin antipyretics or a combination of nonaspirin antipyretics and steroids. Others treat any fevers which occur with nonaspirin antipyretics.

Bleeding is managed variously depending on degree and nature. The common nuisance oozing is easily managed by local pressure and streptokinase therapy should be continued.

Transfusion-dependent bleeding or bleeding into inaccessible sites (gastrointestinal, central nervous system, and retroperitoneal bleeding) requires immediate cessation of streptokinase infusion. Within a few hours very little streptokinase remains in the circulation. However, since it takes several additional hours for the body to remove the breakdown products of fibrinogen and fibrin and to synthesize new coagulation factors depleted by the therapy, the return of hemostatic function is delayed. If a more rapid return of hemostatic function is desirable, this can be obtained by administering fresh frozen plasma and cryoprecipitate. These are both excellent sources of fibrinogen and factors V and VIII. In catastrophic situations such as central nervous system hemorrhage, the effects of the thrombolytic agents can be immediately stopped by use of fibrinolytic inhibitors. The most common is aminocaproic acid (Amicar). Because of the low incidence of such hemorrhage, there is limited experience with such drastic measures. However, anecdotal reports indicate that the use of such measures can restore hemostatic function to bleeding patients within 2 h.

Lidocaine (Xylocaine), by bolus and/or infusion at 2 mg/min, is generally initiated prior to streptokinase use in acute myocardial infarction and continued as an infusion following streptokinase infusion. While many patients have a transient period of ventricular irritability at the time of coronary recanalization, ventricular arrhythmias have not usually proved to be a serious problem and have not limited the therapy.

New Drugs

Tissue-Type Plasminogen Activators

Infusion of a tissue-type plasminogen activator, similar to native endothelial cell activator, does not result in systemic hyperplasminemia and its attendant hemostatic and coagulation dysfunction. Theoretically it would initiate fibrinolysis only on the surface of a thrombus.[35] Once the infused tissue-type plasminogen activator is bound to an existing thrombus and no longer circulating, a new thrombus could form to prevent bleeding at new sites of trauma. This might result in a more specific lysis of the clot with less risk of bleeding complications. Preliminary reports on the use of this material in patients with acute myocardial infarction and deep venous thrombosis have been encouraging.[36,37] It is now being made by recombinant DNA technique in mammalian cells, and trials with this material have now been initiated.

References

1. Marder, V. J., Soulen, R. L., and Atichartakarn, V., et al.: Quantitative Venographic Assessment of Deep Vein Thrombosis in the Evaluation of Streptokinase and Heparin Therapy, *J. Lab. Clin. Med.*, 89:1018, 1977.
2. Eliot, M. S., Immelman, E. J., and Jeffery, P., et al.: A Comparative Randomized Study of Heparin versus Streptokinase in the Treatment of Acute Proximal Venous Thrombosis: An Interim Report of a Prospective Trial, *Br. J. Surg.*, 66:838, 1979.
3. Marder, V. J., and Bell, W. R.: Fibrinolytic Therapy, in R. Coleman, J. Hirsh, V. J. Marder, and E. Salsman (eds.), "Hemostasis and Thrombosis," Lippincott, Philadelphia, 1982, p. 1000.
4. A National Cooperative Study: Urokinase-Streptokinase Pulmonary Embolism Trial: Phase 2 Results: A Cooperative Study, *JAMA*, 229:1606, 1974.
5. Sharma, G. V., Burleson, V. A., and Sasahara, A. A.: Effect of Thrombolytic Therapy on Pulmonary-Capillary Blood Volume in Patients with Pulmonary Embolism, *New Engl. J. Med.*, 303:842, 1980.
6. Rubin, R., Comerota, A., and Soulen, R.: Systemic Coagulation Effects Associated with Intraarterial Infusions of Low Doses of Streptokinase for Peripheral Arterial Occlusions, *Vasc. Diagn. Ther.*, in press.
7. Hess, H., Ingrisch, H., Mietaschk, A., and Rath, H.: Local Low Dose Thrombolytic Therapy of Peripheral Arterial Occlusions, *New Engl. J. Med.*, 307:1627, 1982.
8. Rubin, R. N., Comerota, A., Soulen, R., Tyson, R., Budzynski, A., and Sherry, S.: Intra Arterial Thrombolytic Therapy for Peripheral Artery Disease, *Blood*, 60:221(a), 1982.
9. Marbet, G. A., Eichlisberger, F., Duckert, F., et al.: Side Effects of Thrombolytic Treatment with Porcine Plasma and Low Dose Streptokinase, *Thromb. Haemost.*, 48:196, 1982.
10. Spann, J. F., and Sherry, S.: Coronary Thrombolysis for Evolving Myocardial Infarction, *Drugs*, 28:465, 1984.
11. Rentrop, P., Blanke, H., Karsch, K. R., Kaiser, H., Kostering, H., and Leitz, K.: Selective Intracoronary Thrombolysis in Acute Myocardial Infarction and Unstable Angina Pectoris, *Circulation*, 63:307, 1981.
12. Ganz, W., Buchbinder, N., Marcus, H., et al.: Intercoronary Thrombolysis in Evolving Myocardial Infarction, *Am. Heart J.*, 101:4, 1981.
13. Anderson, J. L., Marshall, H. W., Bray, B. E., et al.: A Randomized Trial of Intracoronary Streptokinase in the Treatment of Acute Myocardial Infarction, *New Engl. J. Med.*, 308:1312, 1983.
14. Stack, R. S., Phillips, H. R., Grierson, D. S., et al.: Functional Improvement of Jeopardized Myocardium following Intracoronary Streptokinase Infusion in Acute Myocardial Infarction, *J. Clin. Invest.*, 72:84, 1983.
15. Markis, J. E., Malagold, M., Parker, A., et al.: Myocardial Salvage after Intracoronary Thrombolysis with Streptokinase in Acute Myocardial Infarction, *New Engl. J. Med.*, 305:777, 1981.
16. Simoons, M. L., Wijns, W., Balakumaran, K., et al.: The Effect of Intracoronary Thrombolysis with Streptokinase on Myocardial Thallium Distribution and Left Ventricular Function Assessed by Blood-Pool Scintigraphy, *Eur. Heart J.*, 3:433, 1982.
17. Rude, R. E., Muller, J. E., and Braunwald, E.: Efforts to Limit the Size of Myocardial Infarcts, *Ann. Int. Med.*, 95:736, 1981.
18. Smalling, R. W., Fuentes, F., Matthews, M. W., et al.: Sustained Improvement in Left Ventricular Function and Mortality by Intracoronary Streptokinase Administration during Evolving Myocardial Infarction, *Circulation*, 63:131, 1983.
19. Kennedy, J. W., Ritchie, J. L., Davis, K. B., and Fritz, J. K.: Western Washington Randomized Trial of Intracoronary Streptokinase in Acute Myocardial Infarction, *New Engl. J. Med.*, 309:1477, 1983.
20. Tennant, S. N., Dixon, J., Venable, T. C., et al.: Intracoronary Thrombolysis in Patients with Acute Myocardial Infarction: Comparison of the Efficacy of Urokinase with Streptokinase, *Circulation*, 69:756, 1984.
21. Taylor, G. J., Mikell, F. L., Moses, H. W., et al.: Intravenous vs. Intracoronary Streptokinase Therapy for Acute Myocardial Infarction: Advantages of Intravenous Streptokinase in Community Hospitals, *Am. J. Cardiol.*, 54(3):256, 1984.
22. Ganz, W., Geft, I., Shah, P. K., et al.: Intravenous Streptokinase in Evolving Acute Myocardial Infarction, *Am. J. Cardiol.*, 53:1209, 1984.
23. Neuhaus, K. L., Tebbe, U., Sauer, G., Kreuzer, H., and Kostering, H.: High Dose Intravenous Streptokinase in Acute Myocardial Infarction, *Clin. Cardiol.*, 6:426, 1983.
24. Schroder, R., Biamino, G., Enz-Rudiger, L., et al.: Intravenous Short-Term Infusion of Streptokinase in Acute Myocardial Infarction, *Circulation*, 63:536, 1983.
25. Spann, J. F., Sherry, S., Carabello, B. A., et al.: High-Dose, Brief Intravenous Streptokinase Early in Acute Myocardial Infarction, *Am. Heart J.*, 104:939, 1982.
26. Spann, J. F., Sherry, S., Carabello, B. A., et al.: Coronary Thrombolysis by Intravenous Streptokinase in Acute Myocardial Infarction: Acute and Follow-Up Studies, *Am. J. Cardiol.*, 53:655, 1984.
27. Rogers, W. J., Mantle, J. A., Hood, W. P., et al.: Prospective Randomized Trial of Intravenous and Intracoronary Streptokinase in Acute Myocardial Infarction, *Circulation*, 68:1051, 1983.
28. Schwarz, F., Hoffman, M., Schuler, G., and Kubler, W.: Combined Intravenous and Intracoronary versus Intracoronary Streptokinase in Acute Myocardial Infarction, *J. Am. Coll. Cardiol.*, 1:615, 1983. (Abstract.)
29. Goldberg, S., Urban, P. L., Greenspon, A., Lebenthal, M., Walinsky, P., and Maroko, P.: Combination Therapy for Evolving Myocardial Infarction: Intracoronary Thrombolysis and Percutaneous Transluminal Angioplasty, *Am. J. Med.*, 72:994, 1982.
30. Mathey, D. G., Rodewald, G., Rentrop, P., et al.: Intracoronary Streptokinase Thrombolytic Recanalization and Subsequent Surgical Bypass of Remaining Atherosclerotic Stenosis in Acute Myocardial Infarction: Complementary Combined Approach Effecting Reduced Infarct Size, Preventing Reinfarction and Improving Left Ventricular Function, *Am. Heart J.*, 102:1194, 1981.
31. Messmer, B. J., Merx, W., Meyer, J., Bardos, P., Minale, C., and Effert, S.: New Developments in Medical-Surgical Treatment of Acute Myocardial Infarction, *Ann. Thorac. Surg.*, 35:70, 1983.

32. Meyer, J., Merx, W., Schmitz, H., et al.: Percutaneous Transluminal Coronary Angioplasty Immediately after Intracoronary Streptolysis of Transmural Myocardial Infarction, *Circulation,* 66:905, 1982.
33. Serruys, P. W., Wigns, W., and van den Brand, M.: Is Transluminal Coronary Angioplasty Mandatory after Successful Thrombolysis? Quantitative Coronary Angiographic Study, *Br. Heart J.,* 50:257, 1983.
34. Rubin, R. N.: Update on Heparin Therapy, *Philadelphia Med.,* 80:294, 1984.
35. Collen, D., and Verstraete, M.: Systemic Thrombolytic Therapy of Acute Myocardial Infarction, *Circulation,* 68:462, 1983.
36. Van de Werf, F., Ludbrook, P. A., Bergmann, S. R., et al.: Coronary Thrombolysis with Tissue-Type Plasminogen Activator in Patients with Evolving Myocardial Infarction, *New Engl. J. Med.,* 310:609, 1984.
37. Weimer, W., Stibbe, J., Van Seyen, A. J., et al.: Specific Lysis of an Iliofemoral Thrombus by Administration of Extrinsic (Tissue Type) Plasminogen Activator, *Lancet,* 2:1018, 1980.

119

The Use of the Laser in the Treatment of Coronary Artery Obstruction

George S. Abela, M.D. C. Richard Conti, M.D.

The acronym *laser* stands for *l*ight *a*mplification by *s*timulated *e*mission of *r*adiation. The principle of laser theory was described by Albert Einstein in 1917.[1] In 1958, Townes and Schawlow further expanded the laser theory which eventually led to the construction of the first laser system in 1960.[2]

The laser is an amplified monochromatic and coherent light that has several properties that allow its use in biology and medicine. These properties include the ability to photocoagulate tissue, to be selectively absorbed, to be precisely directed, and to be transmitted through an optical fiber. All of these qualities suggest that the laser, when used appropriately, will be a suitable instrument to recanalize obstructed blood vessels or widen channels through partially obstructive lesions within the vascular system. The parameters can be varied by changing the medium through which lasing is performed (e.g., blood versus saline solution), the optical fiber through which it is delivered, the pulse duration and power, or the radiation wavelength that is utilized.[3]

Three types of lasers are being used for medical purposes at this time, the argon laser, the carbon dioxide (CO_2) laser, and the neodymium-yttrium-aluminum garnet (Nd:YAG) laser. The argon laser emits light at wave lengths of 488 and 514.5 nm. This radiation is poorly absorbed by water but well absorbed by hemoglobin and retinal pigments. Thus this laser is suitable for the treatment of neovascularization and for repairing retinal tears. In contrast, the radiation emitted by the CO_2 laser, at a wavelength of 10,600 nm, is well absorbed by the water in the plasma and in red blood cells. This feature makes it a less-efficient energy source for ablating tissues through a water or blood medium because the laser energy is absorbed by the fluid. The Nd:YAG laser's wavelength is intermediate between those of the argon and CO_2 lasers—this laser emits radiation at 1064 nm. This wavelength is partially absorbed by water in plasma and in red blood cells but remains an effective means of ablating tissues through a saline or blood medium. Because of their absorption characteristics, the argon and Nd:YAG lasers have become more commonly used than CO_2 lasers for intravascular application.

Experimental Studies

Several investigators have reported attempts to recanalize atherosclerotic blood vessels in human cadavers and experimental animal models.[3–6] Most of these investigations revealed that all three lasers, i.e., CO_2, Nd:YAG, and argon were suitable for use in recanalizing occluded blood vessels.

Investigations indicate that the degree of vaporization of the atherosclerotic plaque depends on the total energy delivered and the duration of exposure.[3,7] Histological and gross examination show that laser radiation ablates the atherosclerotic plaque, resulting in a smooth-walled channel which is free of debris and surrounded by zones of thermal and possible acoustic injury (Fig. 119-1).

Studies using laser radiation to recanalize vascular obstructions in live animal models (New Zealand White rabbits fed a high-cholesterol diet) have shown that both the Nd:YAG and the argon lasers were effective in reducing vascular stenoses. In these experiments, the laser radiation was delivered at various intensities and durations to the site of the ob-

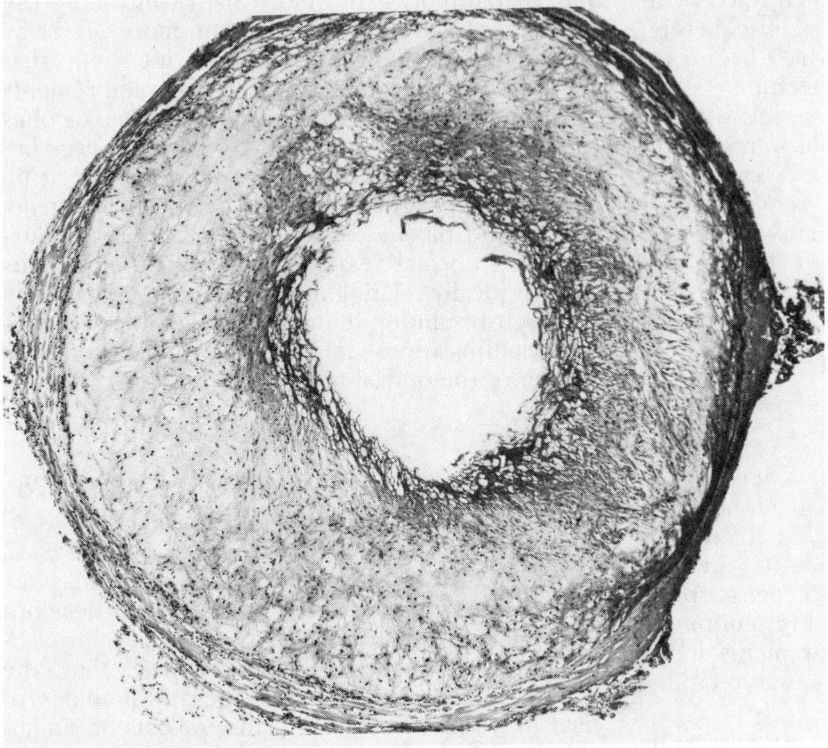

FIGURE 119-1 Histological section from an atherosclerotic occlusion of a rabbit femoral artery recanalized by an argon laser at a total of 30 J (3 W × 10 s). Prior to lasing, the vessel was totally occluded by intimal proliferation. The laser vaporized the central portion of the plaque creating a new lumen. A thin zone of charring is seen at several sites at the lumen edge. The surrounding tissue is disrupted and vacuolized which probably represents a zone of acoustic shock.

struction until the vascular stenoses were reduced. On occasion, high-energy lasing increased the risk of perforating the vessel wall. There was a significant overlap between laser energy required for recanalization and that which caused perforation. In these experiments emboli in distal vessels were not noted by angiographic study.[8] One must conclude from experiments such as these that the precise power and duration of laser exposure necessary for recanalization needs better definition.

Additional experiments, using human atherosclerotic coronary arteries transplanted to the femoral artery of the dog, revealed that the argon laser could recanalize the totally occluded vascular lumen without evidence of distal embolization. Figure 119-2 illustrates one such experiment. However, in all of these experiments, perforation of the vessel wall remained the major acute complication. Perforation occurs because of misdirection of the optical fiber, with penetration of the blood vessel by the fiber, or because of excessive laser energy.[9]

Because of the possibility of laser exposure of the normal portion of blood vessels, immediate and long-term effects of laser radiation on normal vascular tissues were examined.[10] Lased vascular sites in the dog femoral or carotid arteries were biopsied at 2, 4, 7, 14, and 30 days, and specimens were examined by both light, scanning, and transmission electron microscopy. Results indicated that the artery heals almost completely within 1 month. The initial laser

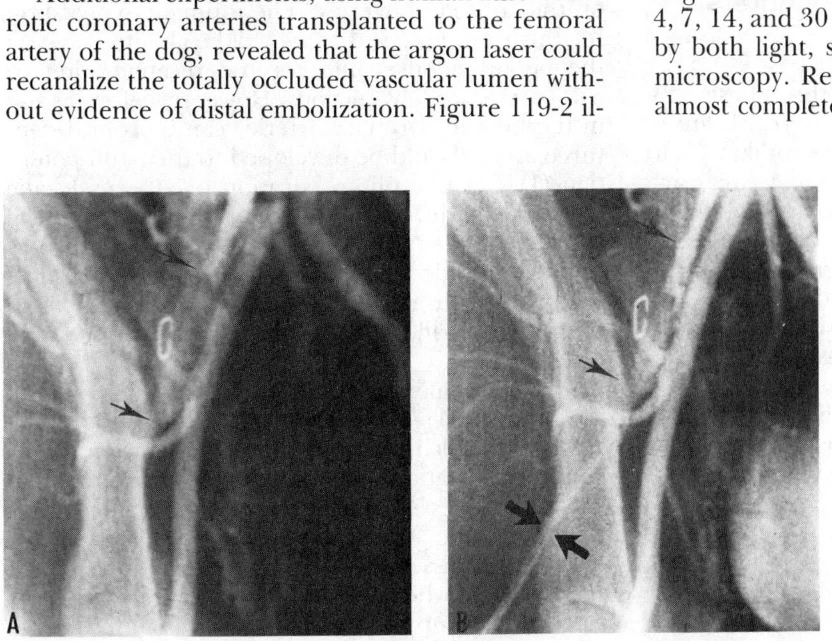

FIGURE 119-2 Pre- and post-lasing femoral angiograms of a dog with a human coronary artery xenograft (small arrows). *A.* A vessel which is completely obstructed, prior to lasing. The occluded vessel segment (to right of marker clip) stains with contrast material. *B.* Post-lasing angiogram. After 15 bursts of laser radiation (total energy of 135 J), the occluded segment is opacified and the distal artery fills with contrast medium (large arrows). (*From G. S. Abela, C. R. Conti, S. Normann, R. L. Feldman, and C. J. Pepine, A New Model for Investigation of Transluminal Recanalization: Human Atherosclerotic Coronary Artery Xenografts, Am. J. Cardiol., 54:200–205, 1984. Reproduced with permission from the publisher and authors.*)

impact site forms a crater which is then filled by a coagulum of blood elements. This is subsequently covered by a surface endothelium which begins to appear 10 to 14 days after lasing. The same experiment was performed on the blood vessels of atherosclerotic monkeys, and similar results were found. In addition there was no evidence of acceleration of the atherosclerotic process when vessels were examined 2 months after lasing.[11] Gerrity et al. reported similar data using an atherosclerotic pig model.[7]

Observations in Patients with Vascular Obstruction

Ginsberg et al. reported "salvage of an ischemic limb by laser angioplasty."[12] The patient had a totally occluded superficial femoral artery and 95 percent stenosis of the deep femoral artery. Following percutaneous lasing, using 2 W of delivered energy from an argon laser source, the patient had resolution of symptoms and Doppler flow measurements indicated that posterior tibial blood flow was reestablished.

Geschwind et al. reported on three patients with obstructed femoral or popliteal arteries that were recanalized using an Nd:YAG laser coupled to optical fibers.[13] The optical fiber was inserted into an inflated balloon catheter, and the fiber tip was placed 3 mm beyond the catheter tip against the atherosclerotic plaque. One femoral artery was enlarged from 1 to 4 mm and two occluded arteries were recanalized. These investigators report that the only side effect was a burning sensation in the limb during laser emission.

Potential Hazards and Complications, and Measures to Limit Them

Three potential problems exist: (1) thrombosis, (2) embolization, and (3) perforation of the vessel. From the animal experiences cited, it seems unlikely that thrombosis will be a problem.[14] Healing occurs normally and there is reendothelialization of the blood vessel wall. Distal embolization with serious consequences is not likely to occur. In contrast, perforation still remains a problem that needs to be solved, especially if the technique is to be used in the coronary circulation by the percutaneous approach. In the peripheral circulation, perforation of an artery, although serious, would not be as life-threatening as perforation of a coronary artery. In the latter instance, pericardial tamponade may result, with catastrophic consequences.

In order to minimize the problem of perforation, efforts must be directed (1) to developing new ways to control position of the optical fiber within the blood vessel, (2) to defining the energy ranges required to vaporize plaques, (3) to controlling the direction of the emitted laser beam more precisely, and (4) to developing a photosensitizing agents that localize in plaque and decrease energy requirements for plaque ablation.[15] These agents can then be photochemically activated by low-level laser energy because they selectively absorb the laser energy at the emitted wavelength. The result is a selective destruction of the plaque without an effect on the surrounding normal vessel wall. Other developments not specifically relating to the laser, e.g., angioscopy and high-resolution fluoroscopy, may diminish vascular complications simply by allowing better positioning of the optical fibers.

Potential Applications in Man: What We Can Expect in the Next Five Years

Although the use of laser radiation to recanalize occluded vessels is still in the early stages of development, its use in human beings is rapidly approaching. It seems reasonable to expect that the development of this potential therapy should proceed in a fashion similar to that of balloon angioplasty, that is, by a careful stepwise approach in which investigators study its effect and gather experience by using it in the peripheral circulation under direct vision in the operating room. One such clinical trial has begun. When more information is obtained, reported, and confirmed, percutaneous techniques may be more widely applied in the peripheral circulation. This type of approach will allow the investigators to develop new technology as well as to understand potential hazards of the technique, and they will gain confidence with the approach. Once this level of competence is achieved, similar investigations should be carried out in the operating room on the coronary arteries. The ultimate expectation for this technique is that we will be able to use it by the percutaneous route for the recanalization of coronary artery obstructions. However, before its use in the human coronary arteries can be considered, three areas should be developed to their full potential: (1) selective photoactivation of atherosclerotic plaques, (2) development of more suitable optical fibers, (with regard to flexibility and beam dispersion), and (3) development of a device that will allow the operator to direct the tip of the optical fiber as precisely as balloon angioplasty catheters are now directed.

Laser recanalization has the following potential advantages: (1) it can be used in totally occluded vessels; (2) calcification of the plaque does not prevent recanalization; (3) results will be immediate; (4) small distal vessels can be approached; and (5) the atherosclerotic plaque is ablated rather than disrupted and dissected.

However, when the use of the laser reaches its full potential application in man, it is unlikely that it will replace balloon angioplasty or coronary bypass surgery. It will instead be used as adjunctive therapy with both of these well-established procedures.

References

1. Einstein, A.: Zur Quantentheorie der Strahlung, *Phy. S.Z.*, 18:121, 1917.
2. Goldman, L.: "Biomedical Aspects of the Laser," Springer-Verlag, New York, 1967, p. 1.
3. Abela, G. S., Normann, S., Cohen, D., Feldman, R. L., Geiser, E. A., and Conti, C. R.: Effects of Carbon Dioxide, Nd-YAG and Argon Laser Radiation on Coronary Athermatous Plaques, *Am. J. Cardiol.*, 50:1199, 1982.
4. Lee, G., Ikeda, R. M., Herman, I., Dwyer, R. M., Bass, M., Hussein, H., Hussein, H., Kozina, J., and Mason, D. T.: The Qualitative Effects of Laser Irradiation on Human Arteriosclerotic Disease, *Am. Heart J.*, 105:885, 1983.
5. Eldar, M., Battler, A., Neufeld, H.N., Gaton, E., Arieli, R., Akelrod, S., Levite, A., and Katzin, A.: Transluminal Carbon Dioxide–Laser Catheter Angioplasty for Dissolution of Atherosclerotic Plaques, *J. Am. Coll. Cardiol.*, 3:135, 1984.
6. Choy, D. S. J., Stertzer, S., Rotterdam, H., and Burns, M. S.: Laser Coronary Angioplasty. Experience with Nine Cadaver Hearts, *Am. J. Cardiol., 50:1206, 1982.*
7. Gerrity, R. G., Loop, F. D., Golding, L. A. R., Ehrhart, L. A., Argenyi, Z. B.: Arterial Response to Laser Operation for Removal of Atherosclerotic Plaques, *J. Thorac. Cardiovasc. Surg.*, 85:409, 1983.
8. Abela, G. S., Cohen, D., Feldman, R. L., Geiser, E. A., Normann, S., and Conti, C. R.: Use of Laser Radiation to Recanalize Stenosed Arteries in a Live Animal Model, *Circulation,* 66(suppl. 2):366, 1982. (Abstract.)
9. Abela, G. S., Conti, C. R., Normann, S., Feldman, R. L., and Pepine, C. J.: A New Model for Investigation of Transluminal Recanalization: Human Atherosclerotic Coronary Artery Xenografts, *Am. J. Cardiol.*, 54:200–205, 1984.
10. Abela, G. S., Staples, E. D., Conti, C. R., Pepine, C. J., Faro, R. S., Knauf, D. G., Alexander, J. A., Hay, D. A., and Roberts, A. J.: Immediate and Long-Term Effects of Laser Radiation on the Arterial Wall: Light and Electron Microscopic Observation, *Surg. Forum,* 34:454, 1983.
11. Abela, G. S., Franzini, D., Crea, F., Pepine, C. J., and Conti, C. R.: No Evidence for Accelerated Atherosclerosis following Laser Radiation, *Circulation,* 70(suppl. 2):323, 1984.
12. Ginsburg, R., Kirr, D.-S., Guthaner, P., Toth, J., and Mitchell, R. S.: Salvage of an Ischemic Limb by Laser Angioplasty: Description of a New Technique, *Clin. Cardiol.*, 7:54, 1984.
13. Geschwind, H., Bonssignac, G., Teisseire, B., Vieilledent, C., Gaston, A., Becquenin, J. P., and Mayiolini, P.: Percutaneous Transluminal Laser Angioplasty in Man, *Lancet,* 1:844, 1984. (Letter.)
14. Abela, G. S., Normann, S., Hay, D. A., Feldman, R. L., Faro, R. A., Pepine, C. J., and Conti, C. R.: Immediate and Long Term Effects of Laser Radiation on the Arterial Wall: Light and EM Observation, *J. Am. Coll. Cardiol.* 1(2): 691, 1983. (Abstract.)
15. Spears, R. J., Serur, J., Shropshire, D., and Paulin, S.: Fluorescence of Experimental Atheromatous Plaques with Hematoporphyrin Derivative, *J. Clin. Invest.*, 71:395, 1983.

Section D

Echocardiography and Doppler Techniques

120

Echocardiography

Joel M. Felner, M.D.

One of the most important noninvasive techniques for cardiovascular diagnosis that provides reliable information together with patient safety is ultrasound. Ultrasound is defined as sound above the upper threshold of human hearing (20,000 Hz). Ultrasonics, the technology of high-frequency sound waves, deals with the transmission of these high-frequency pressure waves through a medium. The high-frequency vibrations are created by striking an appropriate piezoelectric crystal with alternating electric current. A short burst or pulse of high-frequency, low-intensity sound is then emitted and directed through the human body to detect boundaries between structures of different acoustic impedance. This technique is termed *pulsed-reflected ultrasound.*

Ultrasound in the millions of cycles per second range (MHz) has become well established as a medical diagnostic tool primarily because of its harmless nonionizing radiation and its ability to detect the position of both stationary and moving structures within the body. Ultrasound can not only determine the depth and position of echoes (reflected sonic waves) returned from the body but also can accurately record the motion of structures over a period of time. Since the movement patterns of the various cardiac components are related to function and have been found to change in pattern consistent with specific diseases, the heart is ideally suited for ultrasonic examination. The transmission of pulsed-reflected ultrasound through the heart, with detection of the returning echoes detailing the position and movement of the cardiac acoustic interfaces, is termed *cardiac ultrasound* or *echocardiography.*

Cardiac ultrasound presently consists of three interrelated modalities: M-mode echocardiography, two-dimensional echocardiography, and Doppler echocardiography. M-mode echocardiography (where M stands for motion), the original ultrasonic technique developed for cardiac examination, uses a narrow ultrasound beam to depict a one-dimensional slice of the target structure. Two-dimensional echocardiography is a system for recording a spatially correct image of the heart. Two-dimensional units scan the heart in an arclike motion, resulting in cross-sectional (tomographic) slices (planes) of cardiac structures. Doppler ultrasound tracks the velocity of blood flow through the heart and great vessels. It will be discussed in Chapter 121.

The advantages of echocardiography over other noninvasive diagnostic tests are as follows:

1. It is painless and can be employed in any setting without patient preparation, discomfort, or inconvenience.
2. It is extremely safe, even in children and pregnant women, and does not have cumulative effects.
3. The equipment is mobile and, therefore, can be operated at the patient's bedside or in the office.
4. It takes only 15 to 30 min to perform a complete examination.
5. It is a valuable screening device for early diagnosis.
6. It is useful for following serial changes over an extended period of time.

Information gleaned from this study can be used to pinpoint certain specific abnormalities and malfunctions and to furnish direction for diagnostic studies and treatment.

Historical Perspectives

Echo sounding, a technique used by certain birds and animals for distance perception, was first applied by human beings in the 1920s for depth recordings in oceanograpic studies and submarine detection. The principles of diagnostic ultrasound have their roots in navy sonar, which uses sound impulses to detect objects and measure distance in water. The use of high-frequency ultrasonic waves as a diagnostic tool in medicine is a relatively recent development. In 1950, Keidel was one of the first investigators to use ultrasound to examine the heart.[1] It was not until the mid-1950s, however, that Edler and Hertz pioneered the use of pulsed ultrasonic techniques in the description of certain aspects of cardiac anatomy.[2,3] Echocardiography was popularized in the United States by Holmes in 1957.[4] Initially, this technique was used for the assessment of mitral stenosis,[5,6] but more widespread interest followed its application in the diagnosis of pericardial effusion and the assessment of cardiac chamber size.[7,8]

A major development in the field of cardiac ultrasound was the introduction of two-dimensional echocardiography. The investigators most active in this area were Ebina et al.,[9] who developed ultrasound cardiotomography in the mid-1960s, and Bom, who developed the multielement cardiac scanner.[10] This technique took a static image of cardiac anatomy and provided recognizable images of cardiac structure in real time.

The next significant milestone in the evolution of cardiac ultrasound was the addition of the pulsed Doppler device, initially investigated by Baker.[11] This technique, which has emerged in the 1980s, "adds sound to the echocardiographic picture." The latest step in the evolutionary spectrum of echocardiography appears to be "digital" ultrasound, which enhances the ultrasound images for such applications as quantitative analysis and tissue characterization.[12,13]

Basic Principles of Ultrasound

The ability to perform and interpret echocardiograms and to appreciate fully the capabilities, advantages, and limitations of this technique depends upon an understanding of the basic principles of ultrasound.[14–16] M-mode and two-dimensional echocardiography are both based on the same fundamental ultrasonic principles. The basic circuitry of the pulsed-reflected ultrasound system causes the transducer, which contains one or more crystals with piezoelectric properties, to function as both a transmitter and a receiver of ultrasound. After the transducer is applied to the patient's skin over the area to be studied, a timer in the transmitter regulates the duration and frequency of the ultrasonic impulse. During the transmitting cycle the electronic circuit provides a very short burst or pulse (500 to 1500 pulses per second) of alternating current, causing the piezoelectric crystal to vibrate at a very high frequency. During the much longer receiving cycle, the same piezoelectric crystal detects the ultrasound vibrations and transforms them back into an electric signal that can be amplified and appropriately displayed and recorded. Any boundary or interface between materials having different acoustic impedances, or acoustic mismatch, will produce a sound reflection, or echo, back to the crystal. The difference between the M-mode and two-dimensional techniques is that the M-mode ultrasonic beam is aimed in one direction and therefore depicts only a single dimension of the target structure in an image that does not resemble cardiac structures, whereas the two-dimensional beam sweeps in an arc to yield a panoramic view of the heart that results in cross-sectional images that are anatomically recognizable.

Clinical echocardiography requires ultrahigh-frequency sound (2 to 5 MHz) so that it can be transmitted as a narrow beam and directed along a rather well-defined path through the soft tissues of the body. As the sound strikes a cardiac structure, a portion is reflected back to the receiver. Since the speed of sound in the body is known (approximately 1540 m/s), the time it takes for sound to travel to a cardiac structure and return to the receiver allows determination of the structure's distance from the transmitter.

The amount of ultrasound energy passing through the tissue is minimal, since the transducer acts as a transmitter less than 1 percent of the time and as a receiver more than 99 percent of the time. Tissue damage could be produced by very long exposure to high-energy ultrasound, because ultrasound excites molecules to move back and forth and to generate heat. Woodward et al. have shown, however, that there is a wide margin of safety, despite much greater than normal exposure to sound vibrations, that is not likely to be reached in a routine clinical ultrasound study.[17] No adverse effect of clinical echocardiography has been reported to date.

When an ultrasound pulse of sufficient energy travels through a medium and meets an acoustic interface, an echo of the sound wave may be produced. Sound waves lose energy or become attenuated when they pass through any medium. The strength of the echo returning to the transducer from the boundary, therefore, depends on several factors:

1. The degree of acoustic mismatch between the two media. Since echoes are generated only at interfaces of tissues with different acoustic impedances, no echoes are produced while the beam traverses a homogenous medium.
2. The absorption of the transmitted ultrasonic waves as they meet the interface.
3. The character of the interface (i.e., rough, smooth, calcified).

4. The resolution, penetration, and frequency of the ultrasound. *Resolution* is the ability to differentiate and recognize structures that are close to each other.[18] With the sound frequencies used clinically, two structures that are 1 to 2 mm apart within the heart can be differentiated. If two structures are not separated by at least this distance, they will appear as one on the oscilloscope face. *Penetration* is the ability to transmit sufficient ultrasonic energy into the chest to provide a satisfactory image. Both resolution and penetration are affected by the frequency of sound transmitted by the transducer. High-frequency sound (greater than 3.5 MHz) gives an excellent image at the expense of penetration, whereas low-frequency sound (1 to 3.5 MHz) penetrates better but has poorer resolving power. Therefore, for each patient examined the transducer chosen must balance the importance of resolution with the need for penetration.

The processed data from within the body can be displayed in three modes, A, B, and M, in order to present the clinical information in the most meaningful way. In A (amplitude) mode echoes are displayed as vertical spikes along the abscissa or horizontal axis. The distance between spikes (echoes) represents time required for echo return. The amplitude (height) of the spike there corresponds to the relative intensity (strength) of the echo; its position along the horizontal axis indicates the depth of the structure. The A mode was the earliest presentation used in ultrasonic diagnosis and is currently used in echoencephalography and ophthalmology. It is not, by itself, suitable for use in echocardiography because it does not show motion, but it provides sufficient information so that most M-mode designated systems provide the option of an A-mode display. In the past, A mode was preferred by many operators, at least during the exploratory phase of the procedure. In the B (brightness) mode the horizontal baseline remains unchanged, but the echoes are now displayed as dots rather than spikes. The more intense the echo, the greater the brightness of the dot.

M (motion) mode or TM (time-motion) mode is achieved by sweeping a B-mode display across the oscilloscope at a uniform speed. In this presentation the depth of an echo is shown along the vertical axis and the time is represented along the horizontal axis. The intensity of an echo is still proportional to its brightness, but the dots now appear as undulating lines. In effect, an M-mode recording is a continuous graph of the depth of the structures with respect to time. It provides an ideal means of following motion of cardiac structures.[19,20]

Ultrasonic Instrumentation

The basic ultrasonic equipment in current use is an echocardiograph which consists of an oscilloscope, a transducer, and a photographic or video recorder. In a pulsed-echo system the echocardiograph transducer usually emits bursts of ultrasound energy for 1 μs; the echocardiograph transmits, receives, and electronically processes the data. These data, along with other physiologic parameters such as the electrocardiogram and respiratory cycle, are displayed on an oscilloscope monitor and fed into a physiologic recorder.

M-mode echocardiographic instruments use a transducer containing one crystal that emits a single beam of sound. This produces a very narrow "ice-pick" image of cardiac structures, but the spatial resolution (1 to 2 mm along the axis of the sound beam) is the highest of any widely available, noninvasive cardiac diagnostic technique. Since this high-resolution image is obtained over a very short interval (it repeats its transmit-receive cycle about 1000 times per second), there is also a very high degree of temporal resolution. Therefore, if one is imaging a moving structure, its motion will be small compared to the interval of sampling by the M-mode ultrasound beam, and an accurate high-resolution representation of motion can be obtained (these motions include valve opening, closing, fluttering, and subtle wall motion abnormalities). Despite this high degree of axial and temporal resolution, there is no simultaneous field of view lateral to the transducer beam. This shortcoming prompted the development of two-dimensional echocardiography.

Two-dimensional instruments use a transducer containing one or more crystals that are mechanically rotated or electronically fired sequentially. This creates a fan-shaped, 60 to 90° image of the heart. Transmitting and receiving discrete beams through a 60 to 90° sector take substantially longer than pulsing a single M-mode beam (120 versus 1 individual beams are needed for an image). Therefore, building up a tomographic plane for two-dimensional images takes time and results in a limited frame rate—about 30 to 60 times per second rather than 1000 per second, as with M mode. These frame rates are fast enough to be integrated by the eye into a real-time presentation, but there is a substantial decrease in resolution. In addition, if the structure to be imaged is more than 16 cm from the transducer, the frame rate is reduced even further and resolution decreases even more.

M-Mode Echocardiographic Equipment

Most modern ultrasound systems integrate M-mode and two-dimensional imaging in a convenient, easy-to-use, mobile unit. These units can display the two-dimensional image alone or simultaneously with an M-mode image, since one or two cursors are usually available to select from the two-dimensional sector the acoustic scan line(s) to be displayed in M-mode. The availability of complementary and simultaneous M-mode displays, from known locations and orientations, has increased the sophistication and meaning of real-time M-mode studies by providing them with more accurate spatial orientation. A full range of adult, pediatric, and neonatal cardiac applications can be satisfied with most systems. There are, however, many solely designated M-mode machines still in use today.

The Transducer

The selection of the appropriate transducer for either an M-mode or a two-dimensional examination is of vital importance to the performance of a satisfactory echocardiogram. One of the most widely used transducers for adult M-mode echocardiography utilizes a piezoelectric crystal with a diameter of 13 mm, emits a sound signal with a frequency of 2.25 MHz, and focuses the ultrasonic beam at a depth of 4 to 8 cm. This transducer is designed for maximum penetration. It is useful for scanning deep-seated (far-field) structures and examining patients of above-average body size. It permits an examination of 20 cm of tissue depth with a resolution of about 1 mm. In emphysematous patients or obese adults the desired effects of greater resolution must be compromised to achieve the necessary penetration. In such instances a transducer with a lower-frequency response (e.g., 1.6 MHz), larger crystal diameter (e.g., 19 mm), and greater focal length may be required.

The 3.5-MHz transducer, similar in design to the 2.25-MHz transducer, is especially useful for scanning patients of normal body size, since it offers an excellent combination of penetration and resolution. In young children and infants a smaller transducer is usually preferable, however, because penetration is much less important than resolution, since the heart is close to the transducer. The common transducers used in pediatric echocardiography have either a 3.5- or 5-MHz frequency, a 10-mm diameter, and short or medium focal length. For neonates and premature infants, a 5-MHz 7-mm-diameter nonfocused transducer is especially useful when maximum resolution is desired.[21] The optimal choice of transducer for any sonographic study is, therefore, a balance between tissue penetration and resolution.

Special-purpose transducers are used occasionally. A hammer-shaped M-mode transducer has been designed to facilitate echocardiographic examination from the suprasternal notch.[22] The special M-mode pericardiocentesis transducer, which has a central hole, allows the examiner to follow the needle as it enters the pericardial space.[23]

Recording Methods

In clinical medicine it is imperative to provide a hard-copy record of the procedure for both future study and the patient's record. There are essentially two ways of recording M-mode echocardiograms, by oscilloscope cameras and by physiologic recorders. In the early days of echocardiography, the M-mode image was recorded directly from the cathode ray tube with a suitable Polaroid camera. The major disadvantage of this record was that it was limited to a few cardiac cycles; it has since been replaced by the strip-chart recorder. This is a graphic recording instrument that provides paper copies of continuous strips of M-mode data collected during real-time scanning. This recording method makes it possible for records that represent hundreds of cardiac cycles to be produced, thus enhancing the probability of recording the often fleeting echoes produced during the procedure.

A prerequisite of the recorder is the capability for variable paper speeds. Strip-chart recorder speeds of 25 to 50 mm/s are usually adequate for most of the echocardiographic examination. Faster paper speeds (75 or 100 mm/s) are necessary when time intervals are being measured, as for example, the preejection and ejection periods on the aortic valve echocardiogram. Abnormal septal wall motion is also better demonstrated at fast paper speeds, since they permit easy correlation of septal wall motion with that of the left ventricular posterior wall. Slower paper speeds (10 mm/s) are used to record "condensed" apex-to-base sweeps that afford a way of relating various cardiac structures to each other. The presence of *gray scale,* standard on most oscilloscopes and strip-chart recorders, is essential for obtaining the highest possible resolution of the echocardiographic tracing. This device makes possible detailed resolution of close or juxtaposed tissues because the center of the signal is more intense than the edges. Without the various shades of gray the entire signal would be of equal intensity; if the edges touched, the two echoes would bleed into each other and appear as one.[24] A multichannel recorder that provides simultaneous recording of the electrocardiogram, the phonocardiogram, external pulse tracings, and the respiratory cycle along with the echocardiogram is also available and may provide additional diagnostic information.

Echocardiographic Controls

The controls on most machines, whether they are designed solely for M mode or for combined two-dimensional mode and M mode, can be grouped as follows: those affecting image size and position, and those affecting image quality and intensity.[16,19,20] The *depth control,* in centimeters, governs the maximum range of the ultrasonic field and hence the depth to which the beam travels as well as the size of the image of the cardiac structures. The *position control* enables the operator to vary the position of the image on the oscilloscope, thus providing an area for recording other physiologic parameters.

The majority of echocardiographic controls affect the image quality and intensity. Since ultrasound decreases in intensity as it travels through the body, echoes returning from the far field are weaker than those returning from the near field. If this normal attenuation were not corrected for before the image was displayed, the deeper structures would always appear less intense than the near-field structures even though the structures might be equivalent in size, mass, and reflectivity. To overcome this limitation all echocardiographs have a circuit for suppressing near-field echoes and enhancing far-field echoes; it is referred to as *time gain compensation* (TGC). These controls (a series of levers or knobs) refine the image observed on the display screen by increasing or decreasing amplification of selected portions of the image. They must be adjusted for each patient and are frequently altered during the study.

An echocardiograph also has *power controls* (i.e., controls called the transmit, sensitivity, gain, reject, and damping controls) that uniformly decrease or amplify the intensity of the echoes as they are received. Increasing one of the power controls increases the amplitude of the ultrasonic waves transmitted into the tissue and results in a general brightening of the displayed image, enabling weaker reflective structures to come into view on the display. If the gain is too high, the brightness of the brightest structures may increase so much that weaker structures are difficult to distinguish. Approximately 30 different shades of gray can be obtained from the large variety of returning sound intensities, but overuse of the power controls can eliminate some of the subtle texture differences useful in diagnosis.

Two-Dimensional Echocardiographic Equipment

The systems that have been developed to generate two-dimensional echocardiograms can be divided into static and real-time categories. The static machines, used mainly in the 1970s, were called "B-scanning machines."[25] They employed an ultrasonic transducer articulated to a fixed arm that limited its motion to one plane. This equipment has not gained wide popularity because it is technically difficult and time-consuming to use, but it is very similar to current methods used to image abdominal structures.

Real-time systems currently available include the multiple-crystal scanner, designed by Bom;[10] the single-crystal mechanical scanner, designed by Griffith;[26] and the phased-array electronically steered scanner, adapted for cardiac imaging by von Ramm and Thurstone.[27,28] The basic requirement of these systems is that distance information (x axis) as well as height information (y axis) in the plane of the image can be displayed for echo targets semiquantitatively at image rates rapid enough to simulate real-time motion.

Two-Dimensional Scanners

Mechanical scanners may contain either a single crystal or a series of rotating crystals. The single-crystal mechanical scanners are similar to the M-mode units. The principal difference is that in two-dimensional systems the transducer is not moved solely by hand, it is mounted on a head containing a motor and a drive assembly that mechanically oscillates the crystal(s). The crystal used is of about the same diameter as those used in conventional M-mode transducers, but the housing is larger and may vibrate. The mechanical scanners usually operate at a pulse repetition frequency of about 4000 per second, so that each frame contains about 133 lines when a frame rate of 30 per second is used. The quality of the individual frames, because of the high line density, is considerably better than that obtained with the multielement system. The remainder of the ultrasonic system is identical to that used in M-mode echocardiography with the addition of a videotape recorder. These units are mobile and can be used for bedside examinations.

Electronic scanners contain multiple crystals and may be linear- or phased-array systems. The fixed-beam linear-array system developed by Bom uses a large transducer, usually 6 to 8 cm in length, that consists of 20 small ultrasonic elements.[10] The elements are fired rapidly and sequentially, and the end result is a virtually simultaneous firing of the individual elements. This forms a well-columned ultrasonic beam that is electronically swept along the length of the array and goes through the sequence rapidly (up to 60 times per second). The transducer is designed to image objects that lie just beneath each element. A linear scan of the heart produces a large rectangular image, so structures lying near the chest wall are displayed more completely than is possible with other scanners. Although it has not gained widespread acceptance, it is particularly advantageous in congenital heart disease, since right-side heart structures are well seen.[29] These units are small and allow portability to the bedside.

The *phased-array scanner* is the most advanced device for obtaining two-dimensional images of the heart.[27,28] This electronic device provides an image similar to that obtained with mechanical scanners, but it differs in the manner in which beam scanning is accomplished. The fan-shaped beam is electronically swept through the body tissue between 17 and 64 times per second. The applicator is small (2.5 mm in diameter), but the crystal is composed of 32 to 64 individual elements arranged linearly. A motor housing is not required, and there is no vibration. Free mobility and angulation of the transducer are possible. The scanning angle is adjustable and may be extended up to 90° for wide-angle viewing of a large portion of the heart. Frame rates up to 30 per second are utilized, and images are recorded on videotape.

In operation, the phased-array transducer is held stationary while the individual elements are excited sequentially, with a small delay interposed in the activation of individual crystals. This system is considerably more complex than mechanical sector scanners and therefore requires a computer or microprocessor for control of the individual elements. The phased-array principle can also be used to focus the beam, and accomplishes it better than focusing done with acoustic lenses. The result is a marked improvement in the width of the beam, and therefore of lateral resolution throughout the area of interest. In addition, the phased-array machines are the only instruments that can derive high-quality M-mode information from any angle on the sector scanner simultaneously with the real-time image. Phased-array systems are expensive, however, and some are rather large; some of them may not be transportable to the bedside, although the newest ones are mobile.

Digital Scan Converter

The addition of a digital scan converter to currently available ultrasound systems has resulted in major advances in image processing, display, and storage.[30] This device changes the ultrasound signal from analog to digital format. Digital data are then placed in the memory of a microprocessor, frame by frame, and can be read out in a real-time television format through a video recorder. In the absence of a digital scan converter some image degradation may occur when the unprocessed ultrasound data is fed through the television camera for the video image.

In addition to producing better image quality, the digital scan converter can manipulate measurements, store large amounts of data, and freeze the ultrasound image. The two-dimensional images, therefore, can be viewed as they are continuously updated on the screen in real time, can be frozen and recorded on videotape, or can be obtained as copies of individual freeze-frames of real-time or videotaped images produced with a strip-chart recorder or Polaroid camera. The scan converter also allows a variety of pre- and postprocessing curves to be selected for additional image refining (e.g., curves for enhancing boundaries, for optimizing gray-scale presentation, and for studying tissue texture). *Postprocessing* can be applied to the real-time image or can be applied to the frozen images after digital storage, thus providing additional flexibility in adjusting image characteristics. Postprocessing can also affect videotaped material. Despite the advantages of the digital format over the standard analog format, recording of ultrasound signals on videotape may result in degradation of image quality with either technique. In some videotape systems only half of the scan lines displayed in real time are exhibited during stop-frame imaging.

Other Features

Other features of the echocardiograph are an *alphanumeric keyboard, electronic calipers* (e.g., light pen or joystick), and an *electrocardiographic trigger,* which permits images to be frozen in preselected portions of the cardiac cycle (e.g., end systole and end diastole). These features provide considerable flexibility in documentation (e.g., recording patient identification, date, time, and tape number), making measurements on the frozen images (e.g., measuring the mitral valve orifice or determination of left ventricular volumes), and automatically displaying the calculated results.

Techniques for Performing the Examination

The acquisition of comprehensive and technically adequate echocardiographic studies requires a thorough knowledge of cardiac anatomy, physiology, and spatial orientation, since echocardiography requires immediate on-line interpretative evaluation. Unless the type and significance of abnormal structures, motion, and function are recognized, adequate views and complete anatomy will not be recorded and the study may not be adequate for diagnostic purposes. For these reasons, and so that the study can be directed along clinically relevant lines, certain information about the patient is necessary prior to the beginning of the examination. This includes height and weight (to determine body surface area), age, and cardiac findings. A complete echocardiographic examination, however, should be performed on all patients studied regardless of the clinical suspicions.

Both M-mode and two-dimensional echocardiographic examinations are performed with the patient in the supine position. This position serves to standardize the values for cardiac dimensions and also enables cardiac relations to be interpreted more consistently. Varying the position of the patient, however, may enhance the recording of the echoes from certain portions of the chest and should be a routine part of each study. Another position that is commonly employed is to have the patient lie in left lateral decubitus with the trunk raised about 30 to 45°. This enables the interventricular septum, and consequently the left ventricle, to be more accurately recorded, but it may distort right ventricular dimensions; interpretations may be erroneous if this is not appreciated. Therefore, we routinely examine the patient first in the supine position and then in the left lateral position. Pediatric patients frequently require sedation. For children aged 3 to 7 years, oral chloral hydrate in a dose of 50 to 100 mg/kg should be given about 30 min before the study;[31] intramuscular phenobarbital, however, yields the best results in uncooperative patients. For infants we offer a sugar nipple or sugar water.[21]

The application of an electrocardiographic lead (usually II or III) is critical, not only for timing purposes and analyzing the echocardiogram but also because certain arrhythmias or conduction defects may cause motion abnormalities that may be confused with other cardiac abnormalities if the electrocardiogram is unknown.

We perform the echocardiographic examination from the patient's left side so that the transducer is at the long axis of the heart. When the patient is in a steep left lateral position, which is preferable for apical imaging, reaching across from the right side of the bed is much more difficult than working from the left, and if the patient is quite large or obese it is harder to palpate and impossible to visualize the apex impulse. The direction from which the patient is approached, however, really does not matter as long as the examination is consistently performed and the scanning posture permits freedom of transducer movement, adequate room for reaching the controls, and an unimpeded view of the video screen.

The examination involves both hands. Usually the transducer is held in the left hand while the right hand is used to manipulate the controls of the echocardiograph and recorder. Alternatively, the left hand may be used as a stabilizing hand, with the forearm and hand resting on the patient, while the right hand is used to angulate and rotate the transducer as well as to operate the controls of the machine. Maintaining the transducer in a stable precordial position without excessive pressure or loss of image is critical; therefore, many echocardiographers rest the heel of the hand and some of the fingers on the patient's chest wall, whereas others prefer an arm rest to prevent the arm from becoming fatigued. A foot switch that manipulates the freeze-frame, strip-chart, and videotape controls is also extremely useful during two-dimensional scanning.

There must be airless contact between the transducer and the skin. Since the ultrasound beam is scattered in air, a liquid coupling medium (glycol-based or water-based) must be generously applied either over the area of the skin to be scanned or directly to the transducer head. Insufficient coupling medium can result in poor images. It is preferable to have the patient on a firm foam mattress approximately 8 in thick with a semicircular hole cut out on the left side. The patient is then positioned so that the cardiac apex is directly over this cutout, which facilitates apical imaging.

The examination is begun by placing the transducer on the skin overlying the precordium and moving it about in order to locate the best acoustic window. Since body size, structures, and organ positions vary considerably, the acoustic windows will be slightly different for each patient, making an initial search necessary. The best acoustic windows have little, if any, lung tissue or bony structures interposed between the skin and the heart, since both the air-tissue and the calcium-tissue interfaces almost totally reflect ultrasound, preventing it from reaching the deeper structures. This problem is not present in infants, since the ribs and sternum are cartilaginous. Once the desired image has been obtained, hold the transducer firmly over the area, being careful not to let the transducer slip.

M-mode echocardiography has gained wide popularity as an excellent noninvasive technique, but since it is one-dimensional it provides only an ice-pick view of the heart. Two-dimensional echocardiography overcomes many of the limitations of M mode by providing a spatial orientation of the cardiac structures. Since these two imaging modalities are combined in the modern ultrasound system, the quality of the M-mode recording is significantly improved by employing simultaneous two-dimensional imaging to identify the precise location and direction of the M-mode cursor. This flexibility can provide more information about cardiac structures and function than either system could alone. Therefore, the M-mode and two-dimensional studies should be performed simultaneously or in sequence as part of the same echocardiographic examination, and measurements and interpretative information from both recordings should be incorporated into a single report. Nevertheless, since there are many designated M-mode machines in use today, the M-mode and two-dimensional examinations will be discussed separately.

The M-Mode Examination

There are several positions on the chest wall for transducer placement when an M-mode echocardiogram is being performed. The most useful diagnostic imaging information, however, is usually recorded from the parasternal location. The standard echo windows are between the second and fifth intercostal spaces, within 3 cm of the left sternal border. A high transducer placement (second left intercostal space) is occasionally used in obese or postoperative patients, whereas a low transducer placement (fifth left intercostal space) is used for thin individuals with vertical hearts. Additional ultrasound windows for the M-mode examination include (1) the apical location to study motion of prosthetic heart valves and the inferior left ventricular wall in patients with ischemic heart disease; (2) the subxyphoid approach for patients with chronic lung disease or barrel chests;[32,33] (3) the suprasternal notch to examine the aorta, right pulmonary artery, and cephalocaudal diameter of the left atrium and to evaluate patients with aortic ball-valve prostheses or congenital heart disease;[19,21] and (4) just to the right of the sternum for patients with dextrocardia or for evaluation of the right atrium or interatrial septum.

After establishing the best acoustic window and patient position, survey the heart to establish the depth of the most posterior cardiac structure. Although the left ventricle usually occupies the posterior position, a pericardial effusion or a dilated left atrium, in patients with mitral disease, may be located even more posteriorly. The bottom part of the screen and recorder should be occupied by lung tissue or reserved for a left pleural effusion. On occasion the depth of the image field will have to be markedly compressed for examination of a very large patient.

The principal use of M-mode echocardiography is to direct the ultrasound beam toward a specific structure or group of structures and to record a so-called ice-pick view of the motion pattern exhibited by that structure. Even today M mode is still the major method of making echocardiographic diagnoses in patients with valvular heart disease. It became apparent, however, that not only the motion pattern of isolated structures and areas but also the interrelation of these structures and areas are important. This led to the development of the *M-mode scan.*[20,34] A scan refers to rotating or angling the ultrasonic beam while the strip chart is constantly recording. The ultrasonic beam is usually moved in a sector format, meaning that the point of the transducer remains stationary while only the angle changes. A slow apex-to-base or base-to-apex scan, referred to as a condensed M-mode scan, is obtained using a very slow paper speed (10 cm/s) for recording.[34] Prior to two-dimensional echocardiography, M-mode scans constituted an essential part of the echocardiographic examination. They afforded a way of relating various cardiac structures to each other and provided an excellent overall picture of left ventricular geometry, especially if scans were obtained from several different transducer locations. The clinical application of the M-mode scan, especially the condensed scan, was greatest in patients with ischemic heart disease or pericardial effusion. Today, much of the information that once was gleaned from the M mode is better obtained from two-dimensional studies.

The Normal M-Mode Echocardiogram

The M-mode echocardiogram should usually be performed in conjunction with the two-dimensional study. The following discussion, however, will be focused solely on the M-mode examination, assuming that in many circumstances it is the only method available. Figure 120-1 is a schematic diagram of a cross section of the heart, showing how the ultrasonic beam can be swept in an arc between the cardiac apex and the base of the heart for structure identification. With the transducer at the third left intercostal space and angled toward the left hip, the ultrasonic beam traverses first the skin-transducer interface and then the chest wall, anterior right ventricular free wall, right ventricular cavity, interventricular septum, left ventricle, and posterior left ventricular wall. As the transducer tilts progressively cephalad, the posterior papillary muscles are imaged, then the mitral valve leaflets are traversed, and finally the aorta, aortic valve, and left atrial cavity are seen. In order to image the tricuspid and pulmonic valves, the ultrasound beam must angle between the right hip and left shoulder.

Figure 120-2 is a diagrammatic presentation of the M-mode scan as the transducer is swept from the cardiac apex toward the base of the heart. The letters correspond to the direction of the transducer in Fig. 120-1. These two illustrations demonstrate the relations of the heart valves and cardiac chambers to each other. For example, the left ventricle is about 2 to $2\frac{1}{2}$ times as large as the right ventricle, the aorta and left atrium are roughly equal in size, the septum is in continuity with the anterior aortic wall, and the anterior mitral leaflet is in continuity with the posterior aortic wall.

Begin the M-mode examination with a search for the mitral valve by placing the transducer 1 to 2 cm to the left of the sternal border in the third or fourth intercostal space and pointing it almost directly pos-

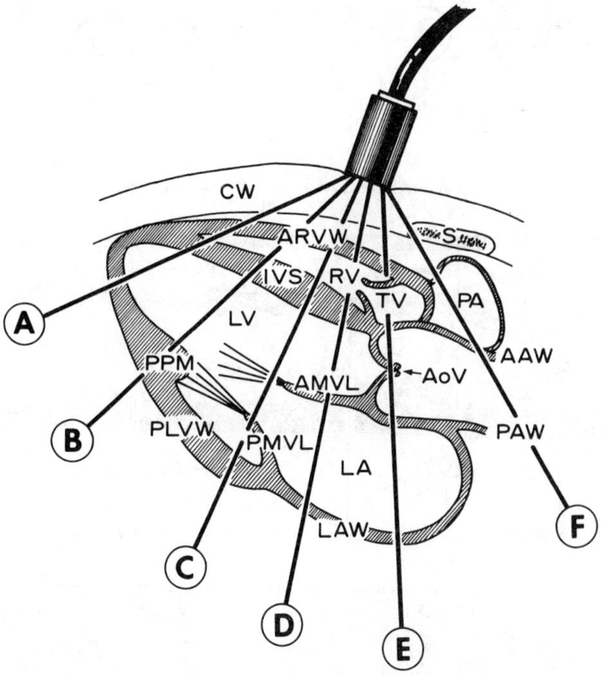

FIGURE 120-1 A cross section of the heart. Lines A through F show how the ultrasonic beam is swept in an arc between the apex and the base of the heart. With the transducer at A, the ultrasonic beam traverses the skin-transducer interface, chest wall (CW), anterior right ventricular wall (ARVW), right ventricle (RV), intraventricular septum (IVS), left ventricle (LV) at the apex, and posterior left ventricular wall (PLVW). As the transducer is tilted progressively cephalad, the following structures are imaged: at B, the left ventricle at the posterior papillary muscle (PPM); at C, anterior (AMVL) and posterior (PMVL) mitral valve leaflets; at D, anterior mitral leaflet at the junction of posterior left ventricular wall and left atrial wall (LAW): at E, tricuspid valve (TV), anterior (AAW) and posterior (PAW) aortic walls, aortic valve (AoV), and left atrium (LA); at F, pulmonary artery (PA). *(From J. M. Felner and R. C. Schlant, "Echocardiography: A Teaching Atlas," Grune & Stratton, Inc., New York, 1976. Reproduced with permission from the publisher and author.)*

terior (perpendicular to the chest wall). The anterior leaflet of the mitral valve will be quite distinctive and easily recognizable, even by the beginner, and provides a useful landmark in most patients (Fig. 120-3). To understand the echocardiographic pattern produced by the anterior mitral leaflet, keep in mind that all motion is indicated relative to a fixed point on the anterior chest wall. The point of maximum excursion of the anterior leaflet is designated E, and the nadir of the initial diastolic closing valve is designated F. The middiastolic closing motion, referred to as the EF slope, represents the velocity of blood moving from the left atrium into the left ventricle. It is reduced by conditions producing mitral valve obstruction (e.g., mitral stenosis or left atrial myxoma) or elevated left ventricular end-diastolic pressure (e.g., hypertrophic cardiomyopathy or aortic stenosis). With atrial systole, blood is propelled through the mitral orifice and the leaflets reopen. The peak of this reopening is designated A; with atrial relaxation, the valve begins to close again. Complete closure, point C, occurs following the on-

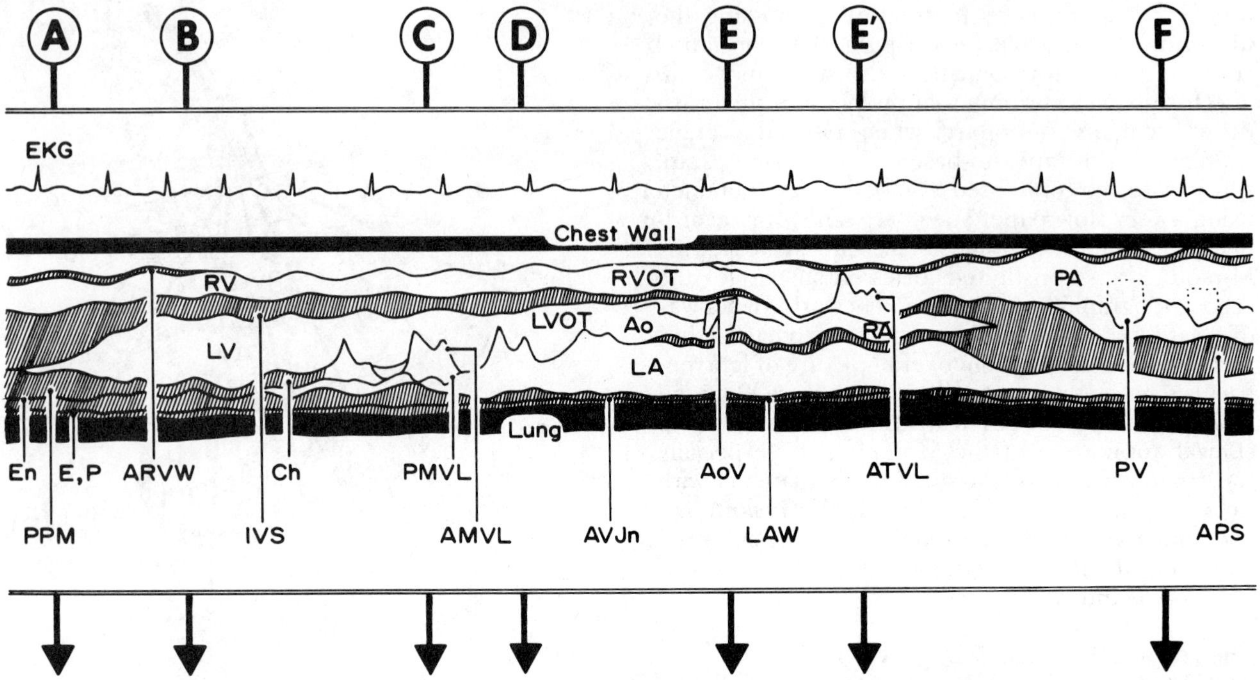

FIGURE 120-2 Representation of an M-mode echocardiographic recording as the ultrasonic beam is swept in an arc from the apex to the base of the heart. The arrows labeled A through F correspond approximately to the transducer positions in Fig. 120-1. An electrocardiogram is shown for timing. The ultrasound beam traverses the following structures: at A, the homogeneous, stationary echo of the chest wall (CW), anterior right ventricular wall (ARVW), right ventricle (RV), muscular portion of the interventricular septum (IVS), left ventricle (LV) at the level of the posterior papillary muscle (PPM), free left ventricular wall myocardium, consisting of endocardium (En) and epicardial (E) and pericardial (P) interface and lung; at B, left ventricle at the level of the chordae tendineae (Ch); at C, the right and left ventricles at the level of the anterior (AMVL) and posterior (PMVL) mitral valve leaflets; at D, the left ventricular outflow tract (LVOT) anterior to the mitral valve; at E, the right ventricular outflow tract (RVOT), ascending aorta (Ao), aortic valve (AoV), left atrium (LA), and left atrial wall (LAW); at E, the right ventricle, anterior tricuspid valve leaflet (ATVL), right atrium (RA), and left atrium; at F, the pulmonary artery (PA), pulmonic valve (PV), atriopulmonic sulcus (APS), and left atrium. (*From J. M. Felner and R. C. Schlant, "Echocardiography: A Teaching Atlas," Grune & Stratton, Inc., New York, 1976. Reproduced with permission from the publisher and author.*)

set of ventricular systole. The anterior mitral leaflet in diastole resembles the letter *M*, while the mirror-image posterior leaflet resembles the letter *W*. Once the mitral valve has been imaged, it serves as the focal point for locating the other valves and chambers.

The base-to-apex or apex-to-base scan should be obtained following identification of the mitral valve (Fig. 120-3). To record echoes from the base of the heart, rotate the transducer medially and superiorly away from the mitral valve (toward the right shoulder) until the anterior leaflet of the mitral valve smooths out in appearance and becomes the posterior wall of the aorta (anatomic posterior continu-

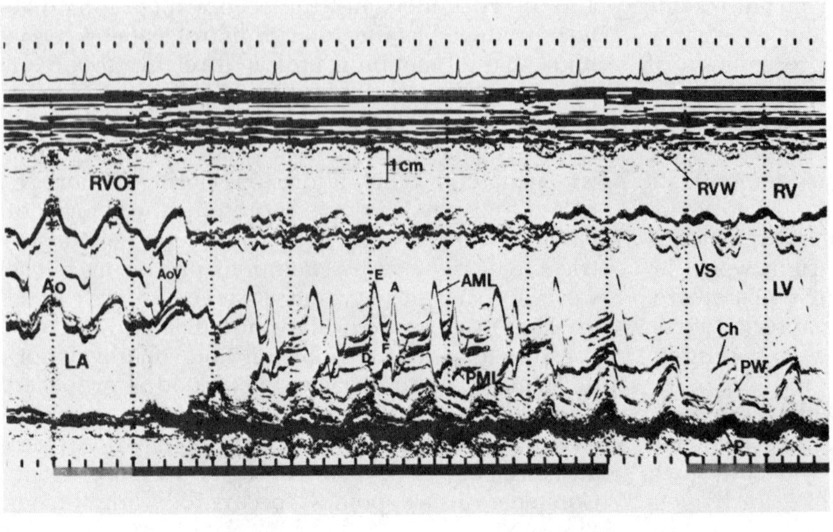

FIGURE 120-3 A normal M-mode echocardiographic base-to-apex scan. The leaflets of the boxlike aortic valve (AoV) open widely in systole, whereas in diastole they coapt and are midway between the anterior and posterior aortic walls. The aorta (Ao) and left atrium (LA) are equal in size. There is normal anterior continuity between the anterior aortic wall and the interventricular septum (VS), and normal posterior continuity between the posterior aortic wall and the anterior mitral leaflet (AML). The mitral valve has a characteristic M-shaped anterior leaflet and W-shaped posterior leaflet (PML). Onset of mitral valve opening is designated by the letter D, full opening of the anterior leaflet by E, middiastolic closure by F, atrial systole by A, and valve closure by C. RVW = right ventricular wall; RVOT = right ventricular outflow tract; Ch = chordae tendineae; LV = left ventricle.

ity); simultaneously the interventricular septum becomes the anterior wall of the aorta (anatomic anterior continuity). The two aortic walls will move parallel to each other (anteriorly in systole and posteriorly in diastole) and have a characteristic echo appearance. The leaflets of the aortic valve form a boxlike structure within the walls of the aorta (Fig. 120-3). The anterior (right coronary) and posterior (noncoronary) cusps can consistently be recorded, but the middle (left coronary) cusp, which is parallel to the ultrasound beam, is only occasionally seen. Posterior to the aorta is the left atrium. The left atrial posterior wall usually does not move at this level because it is attached to the mediastinum. To image the left ventricle at the level of the papillary muscles and/or the chordae tendineae, gradually rotate the transducer, with minimal shifting, inferiorly from the mitral valve position toward the left hip. Turning the patient into the left lateral position facilitates this maneuver because the heart is dropped laterally from underneath the sternum, posteriorly displacing the septum and making cardiac structures more accessible. The left ventricular cavity is bordered by the interventricular septum anteriorly and the left ventricular free wall posteriorly. Both of these walls move, toward each other during systole and away from each other during diastole. A portion of the right ventricular cavity lies between the nonmoving chest wall and the septum; frequently the right ventricular free wall can be seen just beneath the chest wall echo.

At the mitral valve level tilt the transducer medially (toward the right hip "underneath" the sternum) to locate the anterior leaflet of the tricuspid valve or laterally and superiorly (toward the suprasternal notch) to image the pulmonary artery and the pulmonic valve. Because of the oblique angle of the beam only the posterior (left) pulmonic cusp is recorded. In infants and young children, because of the small heart and the cartilaginous sternum, the transducer may be placed directly over the valve in question in order to obtain an optimal image.

M-Mode Echocardiographic Measurements

The American Society of Echocardiography (ASE) has attempted to standardize the common M-mode measurements and has recommended that they be made by use of the *leading edge* method.[35] That is, measurements from one structure to another should be made from the leading edge of the last echo produced by the anterior structure to the leading edge of the first echo produced by the posterior structure. It is also recommended that all measurements be obtained by averaging five cardiac cycles recorded at end expiration, since inspiration causes an increase in right ventricular and a decrease in left ventricular volume. The attempt to determine left ventricular dimensions from M-mode echocardiograms using the criteria advocated by the American Society of Echocardiography has met with a diversity of opinion. There are data supporting their results from one group,[36] whereas another group believes that the recommendations are not clearly superior to other currently available techniques.[37]

The timing and locations of the various M-mode measurements, suggested by the American Society of Echocardiography and supported by us, are shown in Fig. 120-4. Measurements should be made as follows:

1. The aortic root, the distance between the anterior edges of the two aortic walls, at end diastole.
2. The left atrium, the distance between the anterior portion of the posterior aortic wall and the anterior surface of the posterior left atrial wall, at end systole.
3. The left ventricle, the distance between the left side of the interventricular septum and the posterior left ventricular endocardium at the level of the chordae tendineae, except infants and young children, where it is best determined at the level of the mitral valve. Transducer position should be standard (i.e., perpendicular to the chest wall with very slight angulation),[38] since an abnormally low transducer placement may spuriously decrease left ventricular internal dimensions by producing a falsely thick septum. End diastole is defined as the onset of the QRS, and end systole is determined by the most posterior position of the septum. When septal motion is abnormal, the most anterior position of the posterior wall identifies end systole. Percent fractional shortening

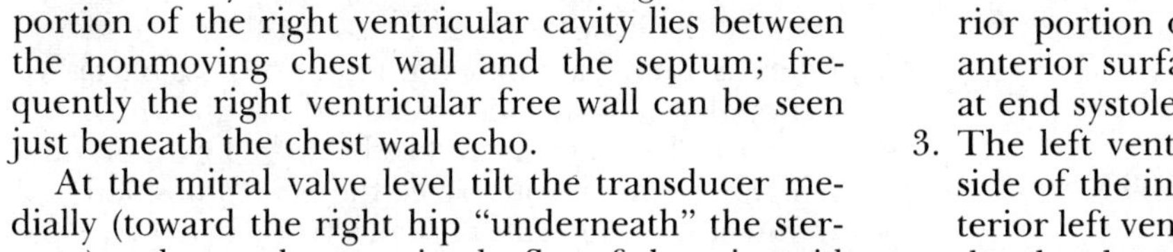

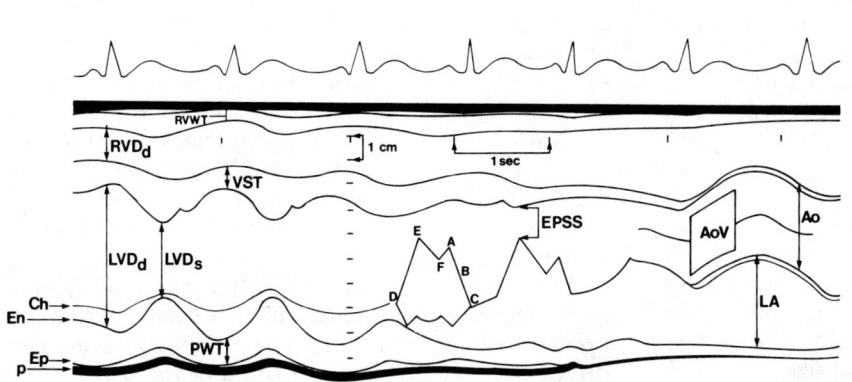

FIGURE 120-4 Schematic M-mode echocardiographic apex-to-base scan illustrating the location for determining intracardiac measurements. The anterior mitral leaflet is labeled A through F. See text for details. The mitral valve E point–ventricular septal separation (EPSS) is shown. RVWT = right ventricular wall thickness; RVD_d = right ventricular dimension, end diastole; LVD_d = left ventricular dimension, end diastole; LVD_s = left ventricular dimension, end systole; Ch = chordae tendineae; En = endocardium; Ep = epicardium; P = pericardium; VST = ventricular septal thickness; PWT = posterior wall thickness; AoV = aortic valve; Ao = aorta; LA = left atrium.

TABLE 120-1 Normal Values

	Mean ± Standard Deviation	Range	Mean ± Standard Deviation	Range
No. of patients	25		50	
Age, years	10 ± 3	4–18	24 ± 6	18–47
BSA, M^2	1.33 ± 0.38	0.72–2.04	1.81 ± .34	1.10–2.53
LVIDd, mm	44 ± 6	32–50	50 ± 3	42–60
LVIDs, mm	28 ± 7	20–34	33 ± 2	22–43
Δ D or FSLV	34 ± 4	25–42	33 ± 3	28–37
V_{cf}, circ/s	1.09 ± 0.12	0.82–1.30	1.26 ± 0.3	0.95–1.60
Max_s PMV, mm/s	42 ± 10	32–55	60 ± 13	40–78
Max_d PMV, mm/s	137 ± 30	91–204	160 ± 48	110–280
IVS thickness, mm	8 ± 2	5–10	9 ± 1	7–12
IVS excursion, mm	7 ± 1	5–9	5 ± 1	3–6
PW_d thickness, mm	7 ± 2	4–9	9 ± 1	7–12
PW_s thickness, mm	12 ± 3	8–17	16 ± 2	13–20
Δ thickening PW	0.70 ± 0.25	0.41–0.95	0.50 ± 0.19	0.32–0.69
PW excursion	9 ± 2	7–14	11 ± 2	9–17
RVD_d supine, mm			15 ± 6	7–22
RVD_d left lateral, mm			20 ± 8	10–37
$Aorta_d$, mm	23 ± 4	15–27	28 ± 5	26–36
LAD_s, mm	25 ± 5	20–31	27 ± 6	12–35

Source: J.M. Felner, and R.C. Schlant. "Echocardiography: A Teaching Atlas," Grune and Stratton, New York, 1976. Reproduced with permission from the publisher and author.

(percent delta D) of the left ventricle is determined as follows:

$$\frac{\text{End-diastolic dimension} - \text{End-systolic dimension}}{\text{End-diastolic dimension}} \times 100$$

4. The right ventricle, the distance between the anterior right ventricular free wall and the right side of the septum, at end diastole. The right ventricular dimension is subject to significant error because only a small portion of it is actually visualized and because the dimension varies depending upon patient position and beam orientation.[19,20]
5. Septal wall thickness, the distance between the anterior right septal echo and the anterior left septal echo, at end diastole.
6. Posterior wall thickness, the distance between the anterior endocardial echo and the anterior surface of the epicardial echo, at end diastole.
7. The right ventricular free wall thickness, the distance between the anterior epicardial and anterior endocardial surfaces, at end diastole.
8. E point septal separation (EPSS), the distance between the E point of the anterior mitral leaflet and the left margin of the ventricular septum should not exceed 7 mm.[39,40]

Normal values for these M-mode echocardiographic measurements are shown in Table 120-1. These values, however, change during aging.[41,42] For example, increasing age correlates with increased aortic root diameter, left ventricular wall thickness, and left atrial size.

The Two-Dimensional Examination

There is almost a limitless number of possible cross-sectional (tomographic) planes through which the heart can be viewed or sliced.[24,43,44] This potential is highly advantageous, since the heart's position and architecture vary substantially from patient to patient. The American Society of Echocardiography has attempted to standardize the two-dimensional examination by recommending a nomenclature for the various cardiac sections based on the position of the transducer (i.e., parasternal, apical, subcostal, and suprasternal positions) and the plane of cardiac anatomy being imaged (i.e., long-axis, short-axis, and four-chamber planes).[45]

The long-axis plane is the tomographic section that transects the heart parallel to the long (major) axis of the left ventricle (Fig. 120-5). The short-axis plane is obtained by rotating the sector 90° and transecting the heart perpendicular to the plane of the long axis (Fig. 120-6). The four-chamber plane transects the heart approximately parallel to the dorsal and ventral surfaces of the body (Fig. 120-7). Each of these orthogonal planes, however, is actually a series or family of planes that can be generated by moving the transducer from side to side, from top to bottom, or clockwise to counterclockwise. For example, the long axis describes a family of planes parallel to the long axis of the heart and within 45° of the plane perpendicular to the dorsal and ventral surfaces of the body.

The American Society of Echocardiography also recommends that an index mark be placed on every two-dimensional transducer in order to indicate the direction in which the ultrasound beam is being an-

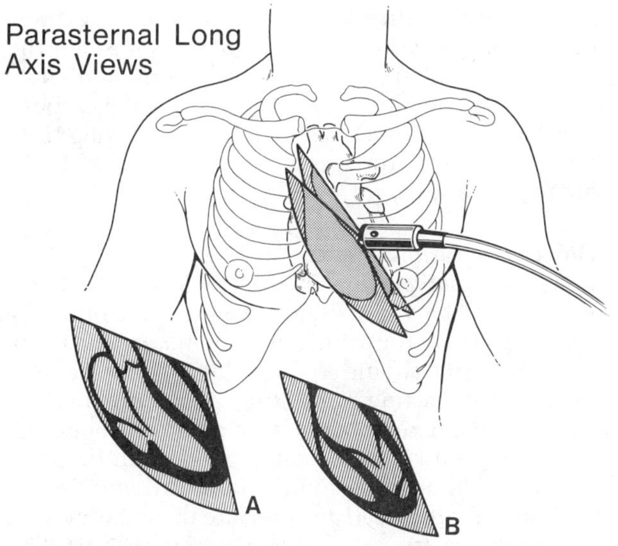

FIGURE 120-5 Anatomic reference drawing showing the position and inclination of the parasternal long-axis examining planes obtained with the transducer in the third intercostal space and the index mark (black dot) cephalad. *A.* Oriented with the sector beam between the right shoulder and left hip to show predominately structures of the left side of the heart. *B.* Oriented with the sector beam tilted medially and slightly inferiorly toward the right hip to show predominately structures of the right side of the heart. In real-time imaging, these two long-axis views are inverted and displayed as though the observer were viewing them from the patient's left side. (*The cardiac ultrasound examination—some commonly recorded views. Slightly modified and reproduced with permission from Hewlett-Packard.*)

FIGURE 120-6 Anatomic reference drawing showing the position and inclination of some of the many parasternal short-axis examining planes obtained with the transducer in the third intercostal space and the index mark (black dot) to the patient's left. The short-axis planes shown are obtained by gradually tilting the transducer from base to apex. *A.* Aortic valve level. *B.* Mitral valve level. *C.* Papillary muscle level. *D.* Cardiac apex. In real-time imaging the apex image (*D*) is inverted. (*The cardiac ultrasound examination—some commonly recorded views. Slightly modified and reproduced with permission from Hewlett-Packard.*)

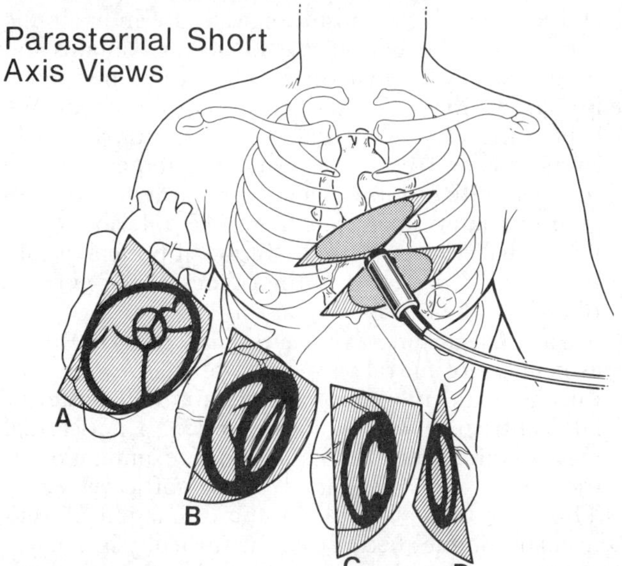

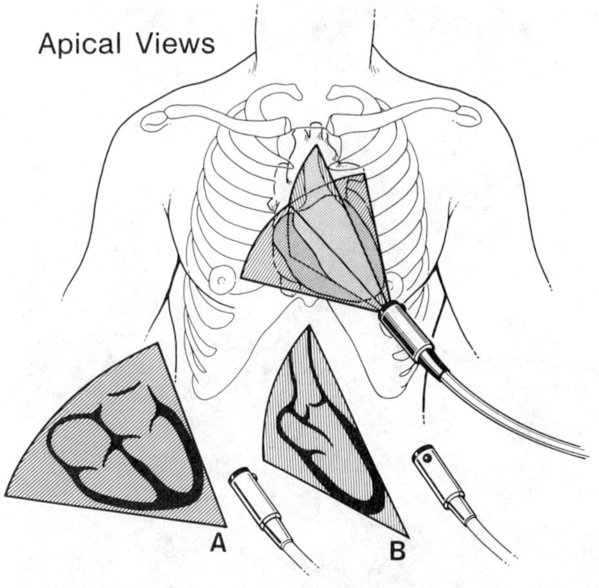

FIGURE 120-7 Anatomic reference drawing showing the position and inclination of two of the family of apical examining planes. *A.* Four-chamber view obtained with the index mark to the patient's left. *B.* Long-axis view obtained with the index mark cephalad. In real-time imaging the apical views are inverted and displayed as though the observer were looking down the heart. (*The cardiac ultrasound examination—some commonly recorded views. Slightly modified and reproduced with permission from Hewlett-Packard.*)

gled (Fig. 120-5, 120-6, and 120-7).[45] Its main purpose, however, is to identify the portion of the image plane that will appear on the right side of the display as the viewer faces the video screen. For example, if the index mark is pointing cephalad toward the right shoulder, in the direction of the aorta in a parasternal long-axis view, the aorta would appear on the right side of the video display. In addition, when the images are viewed on the screen, the signals returning from the structures located near the surface of the transducer should appear at the top of the screen in the narrowest part of the sector, while the structures located farthest from the transducer should appear at the bottom on the screen in the widest part of the sector wedge. If the equipment is provided with an image inversion switch, the operator can reverse the image; the structures near the surface (close to the transducer) will then appear at the bottom of the image and the more distant structures will appear at the top of the display, without producing a change in the left-right orientation of the image. For best orientation, the transducer index mark should always be pointed either in the direction of the patient's head or to the patient's left side.

There are several techniques used in two-dimensional echocardiography that are not used in M-mode echocardiography. *Sliding* moves the transducer over the precordium, passing the sector into various positions within the heart. This maneuver is most helpful for evaluation of the size and shape of the heart and for preliminary estimation of the general direc-

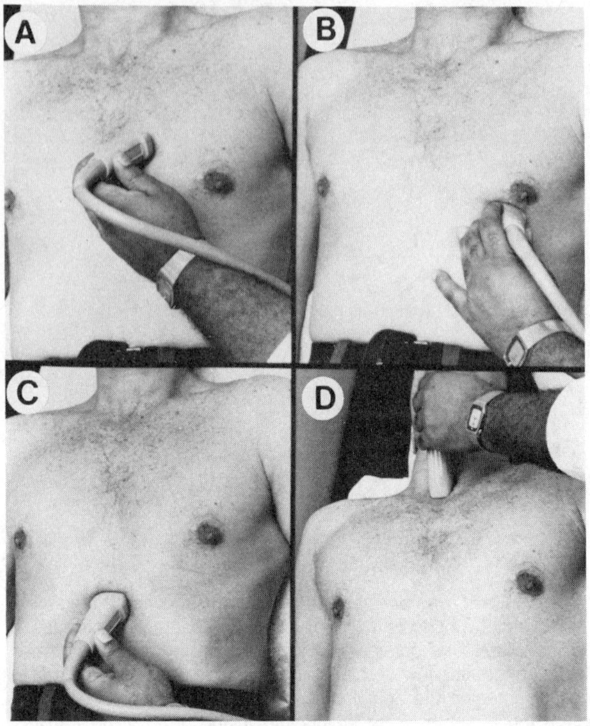

FIGURE 120-8 Commonly used transducer positions for the two-dimensional examination. *A.* Parasternal position at the third or fourth left intercostal space. *B.* Apical position directly over the palpable apex impulse. *C.* Subcostal position facilitated by flexing the patient's knees. *D.* Suprasternal notch position facilitated by placing a pillow behind the patient's neck and shoulders.

tion of specific planes within the heart. *Angulation* extends the view of the heart obtained by a particular sector and involves scanning the fan-shaped examination plane along its arc or width, thereby sequentially increasing the longitudinal extent of the area under study. *Tilting* displaces the sector in a direction perpendicular to its width and is useful for changing the plane of study and for development of three-dimensional spatial orientation of structures in a particular scanning plane. *Pivoting* is a rotational motion that changes the direction of the axis of the sector scan in relation to intracardiac structures. It is accomplished by rotating the transducer on its longitudinal axis while retaining a known target in the sector.

The two-dimensional examination begins with the patient usually positioned in the supine or left lateral position and the transducer (2.5, 3.5, or 5.0 MHz) placed at an acoustic window identical to that used for the M-mode examination. This examination, however, is usually performed using all four of the basic transducer positions: parasternal, apical, subcostal and suprasternal (Fig. 120-8).[43] Recordability of parasternal views is highly influenced by body build and age. In normal children and young adults cardiac echoes are usually obtained from the second to fifth left intercostal spaces, but in elderly patients and in those with some degree of pulmonary emphysema the echocardiographic window shrinks in size so that only the lower intercostal spaces are usable. From this position the sector image of the heart along its long and short axes can be obtained. Additional transducer positions have also proved useful, including imaging from the right side of the sternum and in the mid and low precordium.

The Tomographic Views

The *parasternal long-axis view* of the left ventricle extends from the right shoulder to the left hip. The index mark on the transducer points cephalad toward the right shoulder (Fig. 120-5). This plane is an excellent starting point, since it is comparable to the long-axis scan obtained from an M-mode examination and resembles an angiogram in the right anterior oblique projection. Therefore, most echocardiographers already appreciate the anatomy and motion of structures in this plane (Fig. 120-9). This two-dimensional image allows examination of the size and shape of the left ventricle, right ventricular outflow tract, left atrium, and aortic root, as well as examination of the motion of the mitral and aortic valves (Fig. 120-10). The point of the fan-shaped sector is occupied by the transducer artifact and the chest wall. In the middle of the sector almost the entire length of the left ventricle can be examined, although the cardiac apex is usually not seen in this view. The septum appears to become gradually thinner from the inferior (muscular) portion to the more superior (membranous) portion, where it is in anatomic continuity with the anterior wall of the aorta. Anterior to the aortic root and beneath the chest wall echo is the right ventricular outflow tract. The posterior wall of the aorta is in anatomic continuity with the large anterior mitral leaflet; the smaller posterior leaflet originates at the atrioventricular groove. Only the anterior (right coronary) and the posterior (noncoronary) cusps of the aortic valve are seen during systole. During diastole the cusps of the aortic valve coapt as a single line. The left atrium and left ventricular posterior walls are in anatomic continuity. The bottom of the sector contains the posterior cardiac structures. The descending aorta is a large, circular, echo-free structure immediately behind the left atrium. The coronary sinus is a small, circular, echo-free structure medial and anterior to the descending aorta, which is recorded in the region of the atrioventricular groove anterior to the pericardial echo. A pleural effusion, if present, would be recorded posterior to the echoes of the pericardium and the descending aorta.

Parasternal long-axis views have been useful in assessment of mitral valve apparatus, assessment of thickness and motion of the septum and posterior left ventricular wall, identification of a pericardial effusion and other fluid collections, examination of the aorta, and assessment of the aortic valve.[24,46] This view is not useful for the estimation of ventricular volumes because of the difficulty in recording the true cardiac apex. In order to record the

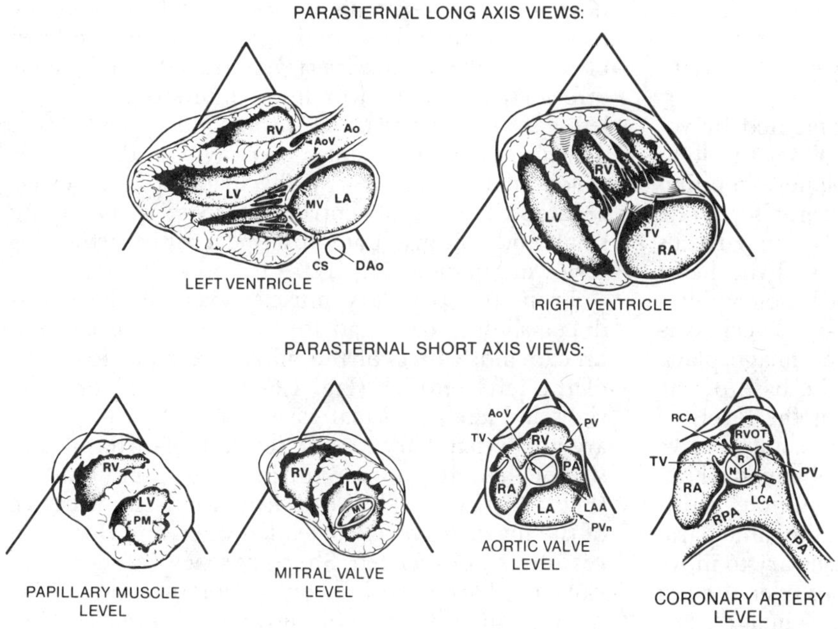

FIGURE 120-9 Anatomic drawings of the parasternal imaging planes oriented as they would be seen on the video screen. The two long-axis views illustrate the plane of the left ventricle (LV) and surrounding structures and the plane of the right ventricular inflow tract. The four short-axis views illustrate the left ventricle at the papillary muscle (PM) and mitral valve (MV) levels and the levels of the great vessels and coronary arteries. RV = right ventricle; AoV = aortic valve; Ao = aorta; LA = left atrium; CS = coronary sinus; DAo = descending aorta; TV = tricuspid valve; RA = right atrium; PV = pulmonic valve; PA = pulmonary artery; LAA = left atrial appendage; PVn = pulmonary vein; RCA = right coronary artery; LCA = left coronary artery; R = right coronary cusp; L = left coronary cusp; N = noncoronary cusp; RVOT = right ventricular outflow tract; RPA = right pulmonary artery; LPA = left pulmonary artery. [*From D. J. Sahn and F. Anderson, "Two-Dimensional Anatomy of the Heart. An Atlas for Echocardiographers," copyright © 1982 John Wiley & Son, New York. (Except figures in right upper and right lower portion of the illustration.) Adapted and reproduced with permission from John Wiley & Sons, Inc., and the author.*]

apex in the parasternal long-axis view the transducer must be moved to a lower interspace. Frequently a pseudo apex is recorded when the ultrasound beam transects the medial wall of the left ventricle, producing a foreshortened image.

From the parasternal long-axis view of the left ventricle the transducer can be angled medially to image the long axis of the right ventricle and right atrium (Fig. 120-5). In this *right ventricular inflow tract view* the main orientation is through the right ventricle, tricuspid valve, and right atrium. The aorta has disappeared, and only a small portion of the left

FIGURE 120-10 Two-dimensional parasternal long-axis views from a normal subject. *A*. Long-axis plane of the ventricle (LV) in diastole. The aorta (Ao) and left atrium (LA) are to the right of the sector image, and the apex of the left ventricle to the left of the sector image. The outflow tract portion of the right ventricle (RV) appears anteriorly, at the top or narrowest part of the fan-shaped image, while the posterior walls of the left ventricle and left atrium appear near the bottom or widest portion of the image. The coronary sinus (CS) and descending aorta (DAo) are the most posterior structures. *B*. Enlargement of view *A* in systole excludes the most posterior structures and shows that the leaflets of the aortic valve (AoV) open to the periphery, while the leaflets of the mitral valve (MV) are closed. The left ventricle is two to three times the size of the right ventricle. *C*. Right ventricular inflow tract view shows the right atrium (RA), right ventricle, tricuspid valve (TV), and a small portion of the left ventricle.

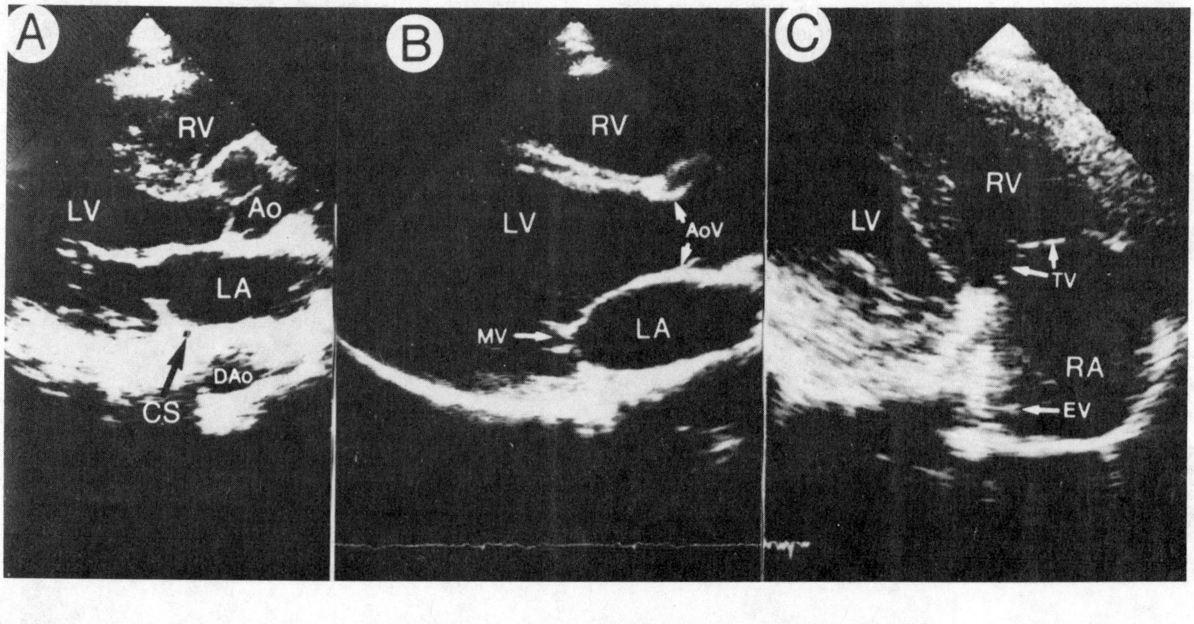

ventricle and a portion of the membranous septum are visualized (Fig. 120-9). The inflow portion of the right ventricle is bordered by the septum and anterior right ventricular wall. This view is useful for evaluating the tricuspid valve and for detecting right atrial masses.[24]

The *parasternal short-axis view* is obtained by rotating the transducer 90° clockwise from the long axis of the heart, parallel to the plane extending from the left shoulder toward the right hip. The index mark on the transducer points to the patient's left side (Fig. 120-6). Short-axis views of the heart are unique to two-dimensional echocardiography—they are impossible to obtain with M-mode echocardiography or angiography. When the image plane is swept from the cardiac apex to the base of the heart, a series of short-axis planes at the levels of the true cardiac apex, papillary muscles, mitral valve orifice, and great arteries can be obtained (Figs. 120-6 and 120-9). Although these multiple short-axis views can often be recorded from the same parasternal interspace, it is frequently necessary to move the transducer into different locations over the left precordium to obtain all the short-axis images. For example, a more cephalad location (second interspace) may be advantageous in visualizing the great arteries, whereas a more caudad location (fourth or fifth interspace) is used to visualize the cardiac apex.[24,43,46]

Begin the short-axis examination with the transducer in the third interspace pointing directly posteriorly and locate the left ventricle and the papillary muscles as they project into the ventricular cavity (Fig. 120-11). The left ventricle will appear circular if the tomographic plane is truly perpendicular to the major axis of the heart. The posteromedial papillary muscle is located at 7–8 o'clock, while the anterolateral papillary muscle is located at 3–4 o'clock. Pathological conditions of the papillary muscles, including hypertrophy, calcification, and rupture, can now be visualized; this is not possible with other techniques, including angiography. From the level of the papillary muscles, if the transducer is tilted inferiorly or moved to a lower interspace, the true left ventricular apex will be imaged in short axis. The size of the left ventricular cavity at this level is much smaller, and the trabeculations more exaggerated. The right ventricular cavity is now quite small and will gradually disappear with further inferior angulation (Fig. 120-11).

From the papillary muscle level tilt the transducer slightly cephalad to image the chordae tendineae and leaflets of the mitral valve in the center of the left ventricle (Fig. 120-11). At this level the right and left ventricular cavities are larger than they are at the papillary muscle level. The difference in size of the left ventricle during systole and diastole (Fig. 120-12), as well as the "fish mouth" appearance of the mitral valve as the leaflets open and close, can readily be appreciated. Short-axis views at the mitral valve level are useful for evaluation of regional wall motion, quantification of mitral orifice area, and observing various causes of mitral regurgitation. Portions of the right ventricle, tricuspid valve apparatus, ventricular septum, and left ventricular outflow tract are visualized anteriorly and to the left of the mitral valve. From this position, angling the transducer toward the right ventricle will more optimally record tricuspid valve motion.

As the transducer is tilted superiorly from the mitral valve area, the left ventricular outflow tract and then the great arteries at the base of the heart are sectioned transversely. The circular aorta containing the aortic valve is seen in the middle of the image (Figs. 120-6, 120-9, and 120-11). In diastole, the three aortic cusps usually form a Y configura-

FIGURE 120-11 Two-dimensional parasternal short-axis views from a normal subject. *A.* The level of the cardiac apex shows a small, thick-walled left ventricle (LV) and only a very small portion of the right ventricle (RV). *B.* Left ventricle at the level of the papillary muscles (P). The right ventricle is larger and the left ventricular cavity is uniformly round and larger than at the apical level. *C.* Left ventricle, at the level of the partially opened mitral valve (MV), is larger than at the papillary muscle level. *D.* Diastolic frame at the base of the heart shows the closed aortic valve, with the right (RC), left (LC), and noncoronary (NC) cusps resembling the letter Y. The tricuspid (TV) and pulmonic (PV) valves are identified. *E.* Systolic frame at the same level as *D* shows the open aortic valve. IAS = interatrial septum; LA = left atrium; RA = right atrium; LAA = left atrial appendage; PVn = pulmonary vein.

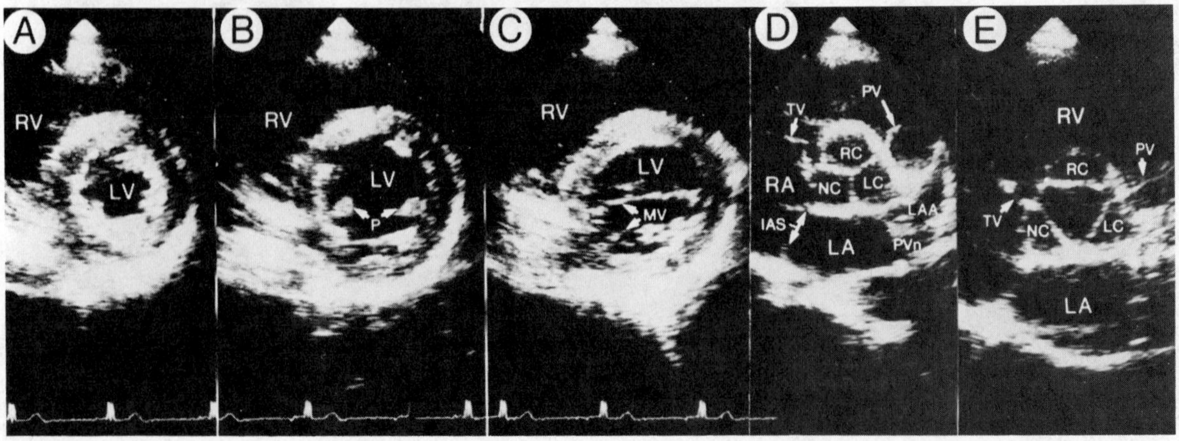

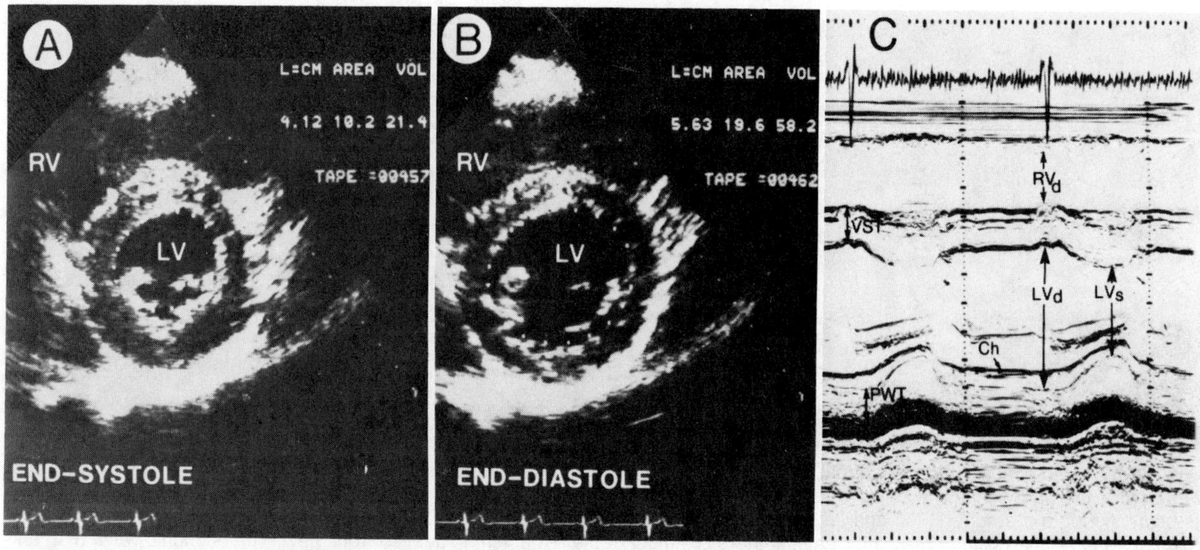

FIGURE 120-12 *A.* Two-dimensional parasternal short-axis view at end systole. *B.* Two-dimensional parasternal short-axis view at end-diastole. *C.* A simultaneously obtained M-mode view of the left ventricle (LV) at the level of the chordae tendineae (Ch). The two-dimensional echograms demonstrate the method of calculating left ventricular volumes with a modern ultrasound system. The left ventricular endocardium is outlined (circular dots) permitting the on-line computer to calculate volume (VOL) shown at the upper right portion of the sector images. The ejection fraction is calculated to be 63 percent. RV = right ventricle, RV_d = right ventricle, end diastole; LV_d = left ventricle, end diastole; LV_s = left ventricle, end systole; VST = ventricular septal thickness; PWT = posterior wall thickness.

tion. Occasionally, the posterior junction, between the left and noncoronary cusps, is difficult to image because it is parallel to the plane of sound. When this occurs, only two of the three diastolic lines may be seen simultaneously, resulting in a V rather than a Y pattern. The anterior (right coronary) cusp is seen between the tricuspid and pulmonic valves. The left coronary cusp lies between the pulmonic valve and the left atrium; the posterior (noncoronary) cusp lies between the left atrium and the tricuspid valve opposite the interatrial septum. The right ventricle appears sausage-shaped in this view as it courses anteriorly around the aorta to reach the pulmonary artery. The pulmonic valve, at 2 o'clock on the aortic circle, separates the right ventricular outflow tract from the main pulmonary artery. The left atrial appendage, occasionally seen in this view, may be mistaken for a portion of the main pulmonary artery when the transducer beam is oriented so that a pulmonary vein is seen entering the left atrium. With slight medial angulation the septal and anterior tricuspid valve leaflets, at 10 o'clock on the aortic circle, form the transition between the right ventricle and the right atrium.

From the parasternal short-axis view at the base, tilting the transducer laterally toward the left shoulder identifies the pulmonary artery branches and a portion of the left main coronary artery, which originates at 4 o'clock on the aortic circle, just inferior to the pulmonic valve (Fig. 120-9). This tomographic plane affords an excellent view of the right ventricular outflow tract, pulmonic valve, main pulmonary artery, and bifurcation of right and left pulmonary arteries (Fig. 120-13). Most of the left atrium is detected from this view. A portion of the tricuspid valve and right atrium are seen.

These two imaging planes at the base of the heart are best for evaluating the aortic valve, aortic root, and left atrium and are the primary views for assessing the relative positions of the great vessels. In addition, the tricuspid and pulmonic valves can be analyzed and the diameter of the pulmonary artery and its branches can be determined. The origin of the coronary arteries can also be visualized.

The *apical views* are a family of planes obtained with the transducer positioned at the cardiac apex. The *apical four-chamber* view is the classic and most important of these.[24,46] To optimally obtain this view, turn the patient to a steeper left lateral position, place the transducer directly over the palpable apex impulse and direct the beam toward the base of the heart (Fig. 120-7). The plane of the beam will be perpendicular to the septum while passing through the plane of the atrioventricular valves. The index mark is to the patient's left, so that the left ventricle is to the right and the right ventricle is to the left on the video screen.

The apical four-chamber view displays all four cardiac chambers, permits evaluation of the ventricular and atrial septa, and images the septal (medial) and anterior (lateral) leaflets of the tricuspid valve and the anterior (medial) and posterior (lateral) leaflets of the mitral valve (Figs. 120-14 and 120-15). A useful anatomic landmark is the central fibrous body (called the crux of the heart) where the interatrial and interventricular septa and atrioventricular valves meet. It appears as a high-intensity echo in the middle to posterior portion of the sector. Although side-by-side dimensions of the ventricles are obtainable, the left ventricle usually occupies more of the apical image than does the right ventricle, and the true right ventricular apex may not be imaged. The left

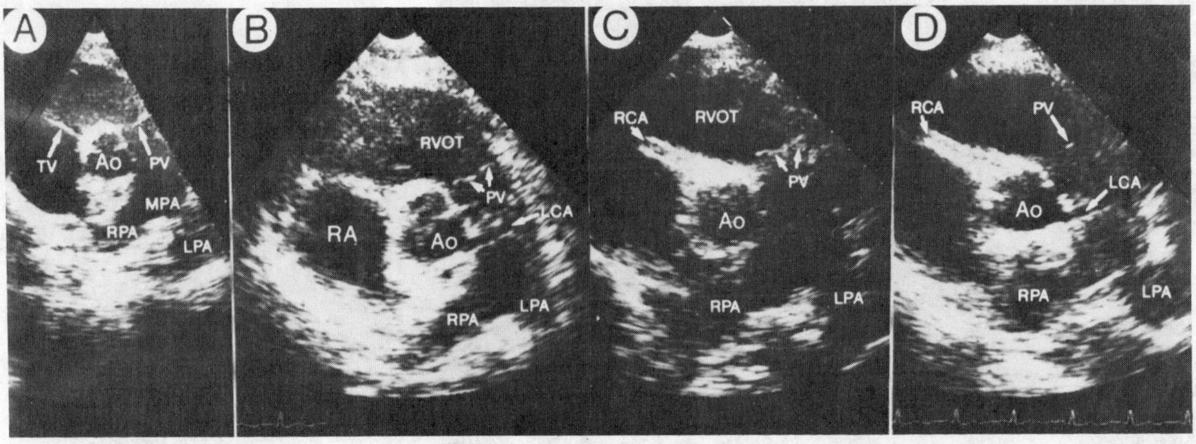

FIGURE 120-13 Two-dimensional parasternal short-axis views at the base of the heart with significant leftward angulation of the sector beam to identify the right ventricular outflow tract, main pulmonary artery, and coronary arteries. *A.* The main pulmonary artery (MPA) and its bifurcation into the right (RPA) and left (LPA) pulmonary arteries are seen. The sector beam is angled through the ascending aorta (Ao) superior to the plane of the aortic leaflets, therefore most of the left atrium is deleted from view. The pulmonic valve (PV) and portions of the tricuspid valve (TV) and right atrium (RA) are present. *B.* Enlargement of view *A*, with slight inferior angulation of the ultrasound beam, allows imaging at the proximal portion of the left coronary artery (LCA). This view provides an excellent opportunity to obtain a high-quality M-mode recording of two of the cusps of the pulmonic valve. *C.* Slight superior angulation of the transducer from position shown in *A* images the proximal portion of the right coronary artery (RCA). *D.* The right (RCA) and left (LCA) coronary arteries can occasionally be imaged simultaneously when the transducer is directed toward the bifurcation of the right and left pulmonary arteries.

ventricular free wall is the lateral wall and the right ventricular free wall is the anterior wall. The ventricles can be differentiated by the following: (1) the endocardial outline of the left ventricle is finer than that of the right ventricle; (2) the right ventricle has coarser trabeculations and has the moderator band near its apex; and (3) the septal tricuspid leaflet is anchored in a slightly more inferior (apical) position with reference to the anterior mitral leaflet. Occasionally a portion of the aorta is seen at the junction formed by the interventricular septum, interatrial septum, anterior mitral leaflet, and septal tricuspid leaflet. This is then referred to as the *apical five-chamber view* (Fig. 120-15).

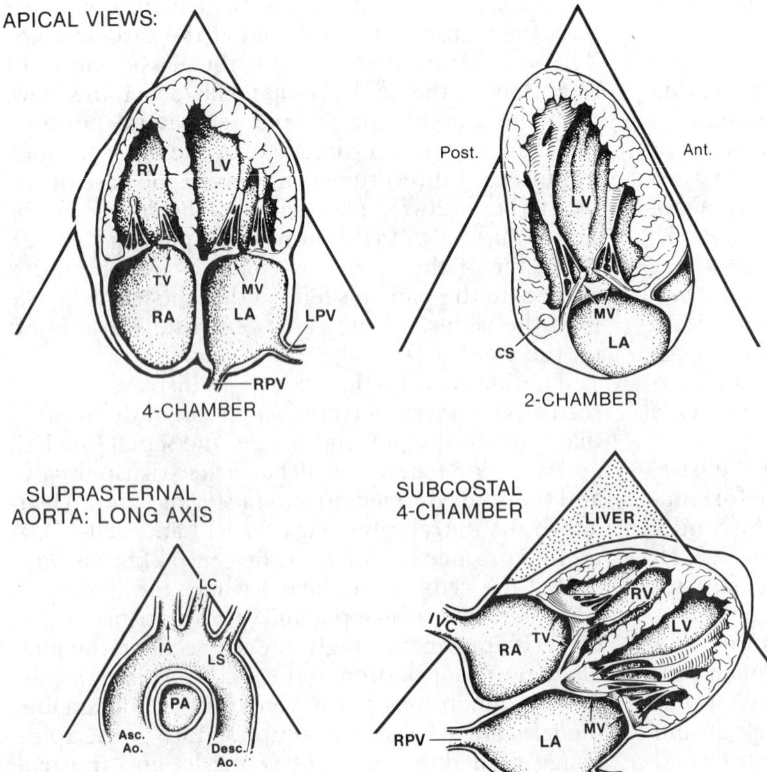

FIGURE 120-14 Anatomic drawings of some of the commonly obtained apical, suprasternal, and subcostal imaging planes oriented as they would be seen on the videoscreen. RV = right ventricle; LV = left ventricle; MV = mitral valve; RA = right atrium; LA = left atrium; LPV = left pulmonary vein; RPV = right pulmonary vein; Post. = posterior; Ant. = anterior; CS = coronary sinus; Asc Ao = ascending aorta; Desc. Ao = descending aorta; PA = pulmonary artery; IA = brachiocephalic (innominate) artery; LC = left carotid artery; LS = left subclavian artery; IVC = inferior vena cava. *(From D. J. Sahn and F. Anderson, "Two-Dimensional Anatomy of the Heart. An Atlas for Echocardiographers," copyright © 1982. John Wiley & Son, New York. Adapted and reproduced with permission from John Wiley & Sons, Inc., and author.)*

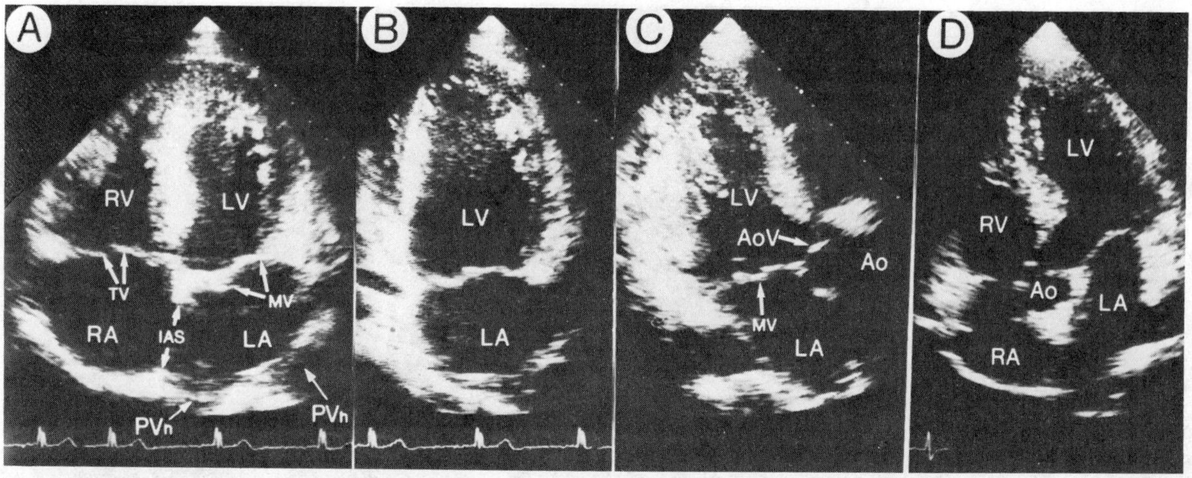

FIGURE 120-15 The family of two-dimensional apical views from a normal subject. *A*. Systolic frame of the four-chamber view shows the relations of the cardiac chambers, atrioventricular valves, and the interatrial and interventricular septa to each other. Note that the insertion of the tricuspid valve (TV) is inferior (more apical) to that of the mitral valve (MV) and that the common problem of partial drop-out of the midportion of the interatrial septum (IAS) is apparent. The entry of the pulmonary veins (PVn) into the left atrium (LA) is clearly seen. *B*. Systolic frame of the two-chamber view shows the left ventricle and left atrium with the closed mitral valve. *C*. Systolic frame of the long-axis view shows the aortic valve (AoV) and the proximal portion of the ascending aorta (Ao). The anterolateral and posteromedial walls of the left ventricle (LV) and the left atrium are also seen. The posteromedial papillary muscle, arising near the apex, may be seen in this view. *D*. Five-chamber view includes a portion of the aorta (Ao) seen at the junction formed by the cardiac septa and atrioventricular valves, as well as the right (RA) and left atria and right (RV) and left ventricles.

For total assessment of ventricular function and anatomy in patients with coronary artery disease the four-chamber view is essential.[24,25,47] It is the view best suited for examination of the left ventricular apex, where aneurysms and thrombi are usually located. This view is also useful for identifying the entry of the right and left inferior pulmonary veins into the left atrium and for showing the distribution of pericardial fluid. It is the best view for confirming the diagnosis of mitral valve prolapse. In patients with congenital heart disease this is also one of the most helpful views, since defects in the atrial and ventricular septa may be seen directly and the relation of the cardiac chambers to each other determined. The midportion of the interatrial septum is frequently not imaged, however, because: (1) the region of the fossa ovalis is thin; (2) the sound beam is perpendicular to this portion of the septum; and (3) the distance from the transducer to this structure is great.[46]

When the transducer is rotated 90° counterclockwise from the apical four-chamber plane the *apical long-axis view* is obtained. The plane of the beam is parallel to the ventricular septum and left ventricle, and therefore, the left atrium, left ventricular outflow tract, aortic valve, and proximal portion of the ascending aorta are imaged (Figs. 120-7 and 120-15). This view approximates the left ventricular silhouette seen on the right anterior oblique ventriculogram. In addition, it is quite similar to the image of the left ventricle in the parasternal long-axis view and may be an adequate substitute if a parasternal long-axis view is unobtainable. This view is particularly useful for examination of the left ventricle in patients with ischemic heart disease, since the cardiac apex as well as the septum and lateral walls are well seen.

If the transducer is rotated counterclockwise just 45° from the apical four-chamber image the *apical two-chamber view* is obtained. The ultrasound beam is nearly parallel to the septum in this plane, but the view does not include the aorta or right ventricle and is considered to be a variant of the apical long-axis view (Figs. 120-14 and 120-15). Since this plane passes through the anterior and posterior left ventricular walls it, too, is extremely useful for the evaluation of segmental wall motion abnormalities in patients with ischemic heart disease.[24,43,46]

The *subcostal or subxyphoid approach* allows imaging of the heart, great vessels, and several infradiaphragmatic structures (Fig. 120-14). This approach is best accomplished with the patient supine (head not elevated) with knees flexed so the abdominal muscles are relaxed. The transducer is placed in the upper epigastrium, pressed firmly back, and directed toward the patient's head with a little posterior and leftward tilt. By rotating the transducer inferiorly and rightward along the horizontal plane it is possible to visualize the inferior vena cava–right atrial junction and the drainage of the hepatic veins into the inferior vena cava (Fig. 120-16). The most suitable patient is thin, with a scaphoid abdomen and lax abdominal wall. This location provides a higher diagnostic yield in patients with chronic pulmonary disease because hyperinflation of the lungs and a low diaphragm usually preclude examination of the precordial and apical windows. Pulmonary emphysema may actually facilitate subcostal echocardiography by lowering the diaphragm, thereby bringing the heart closer to the transducer.

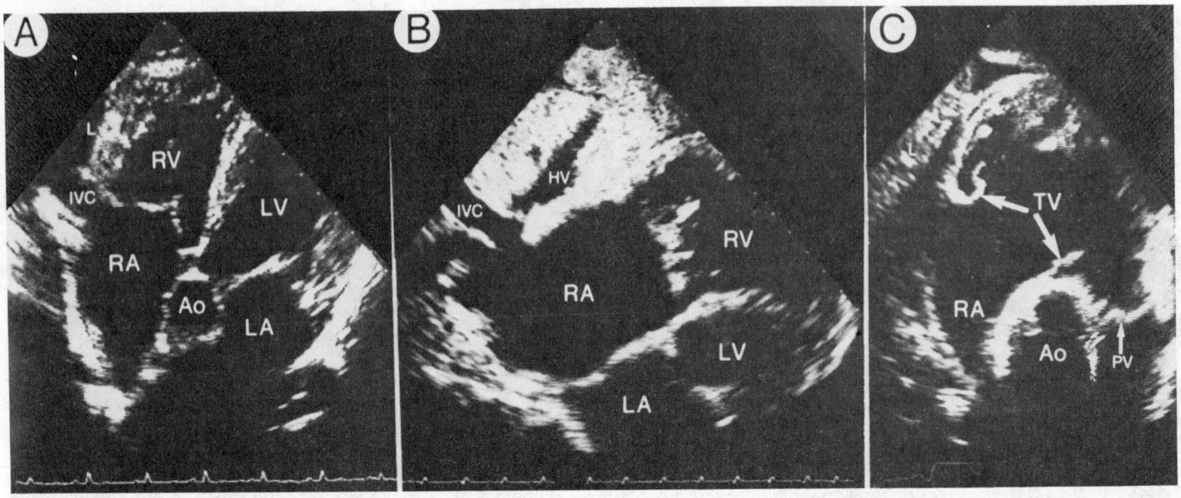

FIGURE 120-16 Two-dimensional subcostal views from a patient with chronic obstructive lung disease. The liver (L) is seen anteriorly in each frame. *A.* Five-chamber view, directed to include a portion of the inferior vena cava (IVC) at its junction with the right atrium (RA), shows the aorta (Ao) between the cardiac septa and atrioventricular valves in addition to the right and left (LA) atria and right (RV) and left (LV) ventricles. The cardiac apex is not seen in this view. *B.* Enlargement of the four-chamber view to best show the junction of the inferior vena cava (IVC) and the right atrium. The hepatic vein (HV) empties into the inferior vena cava. Complete imaging of the interatrial septum is appreciated in this view. *C.* Diastolic frame of the short-axis right ventricular outflow tract plane. The aorta (Ao) occupies the central portion of the image. Two of the open leaflets of the tricuspid valve (TV) and the closed pulmonic valve (PV) are identified. The pulmonic valve and pulmonary artery, often in the far field in this plane, may not be imaged as well as in the parasternal short-axis plane, but the subvalvular portion of the right ventricular outflow tract is more easily appreciated.

The subcostal approach allows images to be recorded from both short-axis and four-chamber planes (Fig. 120-16). A series of short-axis views can be recorded by sweeping the ultrasound beam from base to apex in a manner similar to obtaining images from the parasternal transducer location. With the transducer pointed cranially and the index mark toward the patient's head, the *right ventricular outflow tract plane*, the most useful of the short-axis planes, is obtained. The sound beam passes across the aorta, which appears as a circle or semicircle near the bottom of the image. The right ventricular outflow tract wraps around the aorta, and frequently all three tricuspid leaflets are seen as well as two of the pulmonic leaflets. The left ventricle can be seen in short axis if the transducer is rotated toward the patient's left shoulder with the index mark to the patient's left. The left ventricle appears circular as it did in the parasternal short-axis image, but the papillary muscles are now at 8 and 11 o'clock and the right ventricle is to its right or anteriorly.

If the transducer is rotated 90° clockwise from the right ventricular outflow tract short-axis plane, with the ultrasound beam imaging between the patient's shoulders, a *subcostal four-chamber view*, similar to the apical four-chamber view, is obtained. The cardiac apex is to the right side of the video screen, although the true apex is usually not imaged. Since the interatrial septum is now perpendicular to the ultrasound beam, the most complete visualization of the interatrial septum and right atrium is possible. The right and left superior pulmonary veins can be seen as they enter the left atrium; more of the left atrium is visualized in the subcostal four-chamber view than in the apical four-chamber view. The hepatic structures are usually interposed between the transducer and the right ventricular free wall anteriorly. With slight anterior angulation the aorta and left ventricular outflow tract are seen in a *subcostal five-chamber view*.

The subcostal view is most useful for evaluating the right ventricular free wall and the inferior vena cava and for the diagnosis of tricuspid regurgitation and atrial and ventricular septal defects. Positioning the right ventricular wall perpendicular to the M-mode cursor in the four-chamber view makes possible accurate recordings of right ventricular wall thickness. Since the ultrasonic beam is now perpendicular to the atrial septum, the entire length of the septum can be scanned for the presence and location of atrial septal defects.[48,49] It is also important to record the inferior vena cava in both four-chamber and short-axis views in order to assess its diameter and observe respiratory effects.[43,46] A special utility of this examining plane occurs in patients with a left pleural effusion, which complicates the ultrasonic diagnosis when the heart is viewed from the standard precordial positions.

The *suprasternal notch approach* visualizes mediastinal structures posterior to the sternum, including the ascending aorta, aortic arch, origin of the brachiocephalic vessels, and descending thoracic aorta (Fig. 120-14). Tomographic imaging from this transducer position, however, is more difficult than it is from any of the other locations. Therefore, make the patient as comfortable as possible by placing a pillow underneath the shoulders and upper back. This will extend the neck and facilitate manipula-

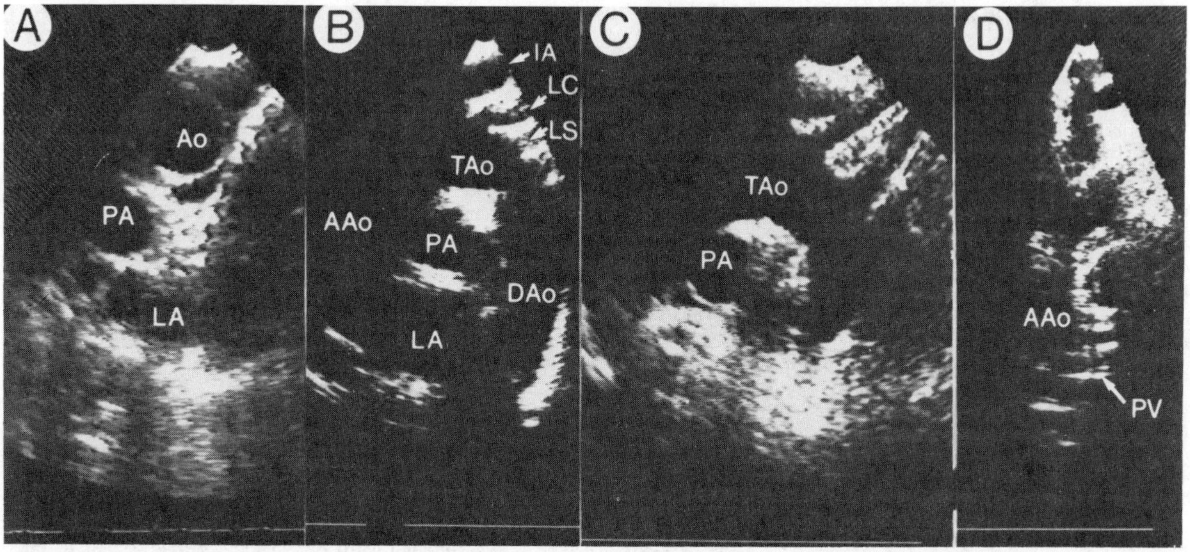

FIGURE 120-17 Two-dimensional suprasternal views of the great vessels from a normal subject. *A*. Short-axis plane shows the circular appearance of the transverse aorta (Ao). A portion of the long axis of the pulmonary artery (PA) is imaged beneath the aorta with the left atrium (LA) posterior to the pulmonary artery. In this view, with more medial angulation, the left and right brachiocephalic (innominate) veins may be seen entering the superior vena cava. *B*. Long-axis plane shows the ascending (AAo), transverse (TAo), and descending (DAo) aorta and the pulmonary artery, which appears to be circular because it is now seen in short-axis view. Arch vessels emerging from the transverse aorta are identified as the brachiocephalic (innominate) (IA), left common carotid (LC), and left subclavian (LS) arteries. *C*. Enlargement of view *B* to more clearly show the transverse aorta and arch vessels. *D*. Right supraclavicular transducer position enables one to rotate the imaging plane more anteriorly in order to image more of the ascending aorta and show its relation with the pulmonary artery and pulmonic valve (PV).

tion of the transducer, which should be pressed firmly back in the groove just above the manubrium-sternum and clavicles (Fig. 120-8).

The *suprasternal long-axis view* images the ascending aorta, the transverse aorta with the origins of the major arterial branches (brachiocephalic innominate, left carotid, and left subclavian) and the descending aorta (Fig. 120-17). Proper transducer orientation with the index mark cephalad places the descending aorta on the right of the video screen. Posterior to the aortic arch, the right pulmonary artery is seen as a circle in short axis. The mainstem bronchus, being air-filled, is a densely reflective structure between the aorta and the pulmonary artery. The left atrium is recorded posterior to the pulmonary artery. When the transducer is rotated 90° from this plane, the ascending aorta is seen in this *suprasternal short-axis view* as a circular, pulsating structure anteriorly, while the right pulmonary artery is imaged inferiorly in its long axis (Fig. 120-17). The superior vena cava–right atrial junction may be seen with slight anterior angulation. The right supraclavicular approach is an alternative plane that provides a view much like the suprasternal one (Fig. 120-17). It is used mainly for visualizing the motion of prosthetic aortic valves, particularly the Starr-Edwards ball valve, which is not well imaged from the precordium.

Echocardiographic examination from the suprasternal notch facilitates detection of aortic root abnormalities (e.g., saccular aneurysm, dissecting aneurysm, and coarctation), whereas elevation of the pulmonary artery and its branches may detect a patent ductus arteriosus.[31,43,46,50]

Two-Dimensional Echocardiographic Measurements

Two-dimensional echocardiographic measurements should be made using the leading-edge method.[51,52] Preliminary data suggest that values for diastolic and systolic left ventricular diameters, systolic left atrial diameters, fractional shortening of the left ventricle, and left ventricular posterior and septal wall thicknesses are similar to those obtained with M-mode echocardiography.[43,51,53] The accepted echocardiographic views and locations for common two-dimensional measurements are shown in Fig. 120-18. Normal two-dimensional measurements for various intracardiac chambers and great vessels have been determined by several clinicians; a compilation of their findings is shown in Table 120-2.

The dimensions of the left ventricle and the thicknesses of both the interventricular septum and posterior wall are made at the level of the chordae tendineae in either the parasternal long-axis or short-axis views. The papillary muscles should not be included in assessment of wall thickness. Although M-mode echocardiography appears to be very sensitive for detection of true anatomic hypertrophy,[54,55] two-dimensional echocardiography is superior for quantitative assessment of left ventricular mass.[56] The shape and dimension of the left atrium varies in each tomographic view. The inferior-superior dimension is slightly greater than the anterior-poste-

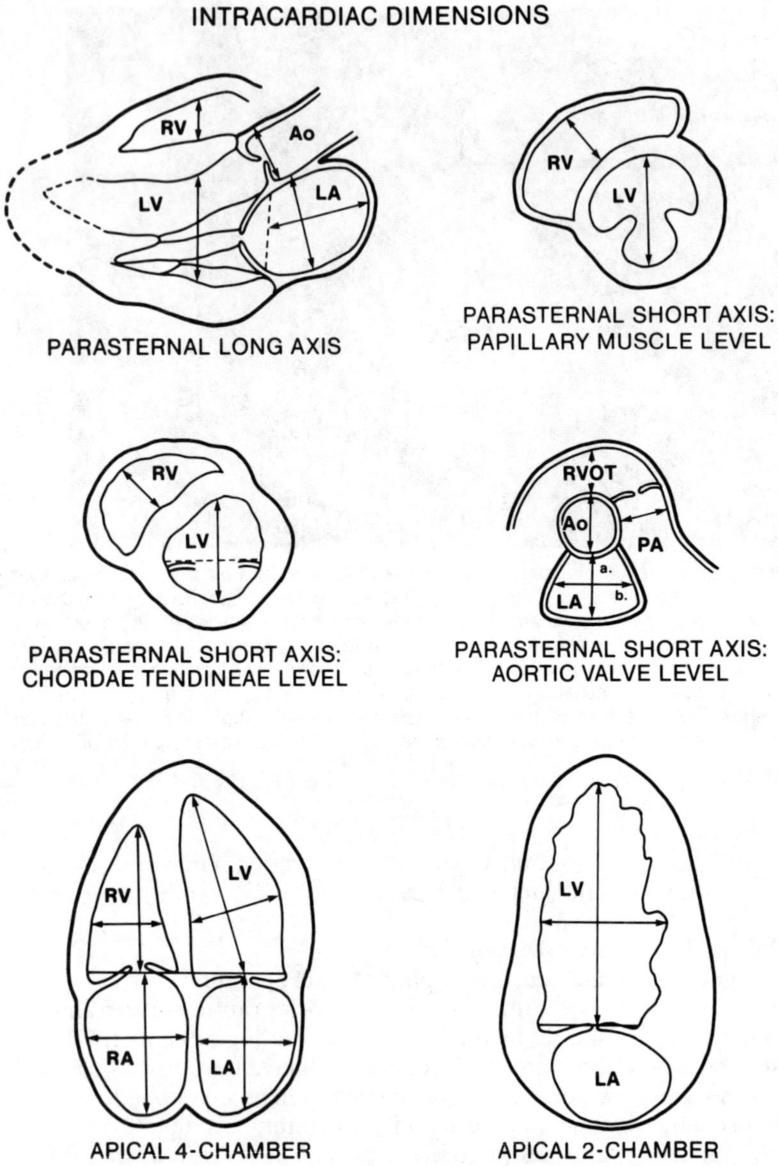

FIGURE 120-18 Some of the two-dimensional echocardiographic planes and locations for determining intracardiac dimensions. The left atrium (LA) is measured in both the anteroposterior (a) and inferolateral (b) dimensions, perpendicular to each other, from the parasternal long-axis, short-axis and apical four-chamber views (as illustrated in the parasternal short-axis view). The right atrium (RA) is measured in the apical four-chamber view and also in the parasternal long-axis right ventricular inflow tract view which is not shown. The major axis of each ventricle is measured in the four-chamber view from the atrioventricular plane to the apical endocardium. The left ventricular major axis is also measured in the two-chamber view. The minor axis of each ventricle is taken perpendicular to its major axis. This measurement may be taken at two-thirds of the length of the major axis (from the apical endocardium), as shown in the four-chamber view, or at the midpoint of the major axis, as shown in the two-chamber view. RV = right ventricle; LV = left ventricle; RVOT = right ventricular outflow tract; Ao = aorta; PA = pulmonary artery. (*From A. E. Weyman, "Cross-Sectional Echocardiography," Lea & Febiger, Philadelphia, 1982, and I. Schnittger, E. P. Gordon, P. J. Fitzgerald, and R. L. Popp, Standardized Intracardiac Measurements of Two-Dimensional Echocardiography, J. Am. Coll. Cardiol., 2:934, 1983. Drawn after studying multiple sources.*)

rior dimension in both the apical four-chamber and apical long-axis views.[43] The right ventricular and right atrial chambers are best evaluated from the apical four-chamber view.[57] The thickness of the right ventricular wall, however, is best determined from the subcostal four-chamber view by directing the M-mode cursor perpendicular to the right ventricular free wall.[58]

M-mode echocardiography has been useful for determining left ventricular volumes in patients with nonsegmental disease and has been easily quantitated, since it involves only making measurements on a strip-chart recording.[59–66] It is limited, however, since it is not spatially correct and has not been reliable in the presence of asynergy.[67,68] In addition, several assumptions must apply when M-mode dimensions are used to calculate left ventricular volumes: (1) the left ventricle approximates a prolate ellipse; (2) the major (long) axis of the left ventricle is twice the length of the minor (short) axis; and (3) the left ventricular wall motion sampled by the ultrasound beam is representative of the entire left ventricular chamber.[19] Although quantitative two-dimensional echocardiography is still in its infancy, its reliability has been documented for both segmental and nonsegmental diseases. It thus appears superior to M mode for quantitative estimation of left ventricular volumes, because it directly measures all three hemiaxes, by imaging from apical as well as parasternal windows.[69–75]

Left ventricular volumes and left atrial volumes have been determined by two-dimensional echocardiography in a normal adult population and validated by angiography, radionuclide studies, and pathological measurements.[76–80] There are several ways of calculating left ventricular volumes, including the biplane area–length method, the single-plane ellipse method, and the modified Simpson's

TABLE 120-2 Cardiac Dimensions by Two-Dimensional Echocardiography

Cardiac Feature	Range	Mean	Index, cm/m^2
Apical Four-Chamber View			
LV_d major	6.9–10.3 cm	8.6 cm	4.1–5.7
LV_d minor	3.3–6.1 cm	4.7 cm	2.2–3.1
LV_s minor	1.9–3.7 cm	2.8 cm	1.3–2.0
LV_d area	21.2–40.2 cm^2	31.2 cm^2	
LV_s area	8.0–21.1 cm^2	14.2 cm^2	
RV major	6.5–9.5 cm	8.0 cm	3.8–5.3
RV minor	2.2–4.4 cm	3.3–3.5 cm	1.0–2.8
RV_d area	12.0–22.2 cm^2	18.6–2.1 cm^2	
RV_s area	5.4–14.6 cm^2	9.9 cm^2	
LA major	4.1–6.1 cm	5.1 cm	2.3–3.5
LA minor	2.8–4.3	3.5 cm	1.6–2.4
LA area	10.2–17.8	14.7 cm^2	
RA major (inf-sup)	3.5–5.5 cm	4.3–4.5 cm	2.0–3.1
RA minor	2.5–4.9	3.7 cm	1.7–2.5
RA area	11.3–16.7 cm^2	13.8–14 cm^2	
Apical Two-Chamber View			
LV_d major	6.8–9.4 cm^2	8.0 cm^2	
LV_d minor	3.8–5.7 cm^2	4.6 cm^2	
LV_d area	19.4–48.0 cm^2	35.6 cm^2	
LV_s	8.9–27.0	14.3 cm^2	
Parasternal Long-Axis View			
LV_d	3.5–6.0 cm	4.8 cm	2.3–3.1
LV_s	2.1–4.0 cm	3.1 cm	1.4–2.1
RV	1.9–3.8 cm	2.8 cm	1.2–2.0
LA (A-P)	2.7–4.5 cm	3.6 cm	1.6–2.4
LA (S-I)	3.1–5.5 cm	4.4 cm	
LA area	9.0–19.3 cm^2	13.8 cm^2	
Ao	2.2–3.6 cm	2.9 cm	1.4–2.0
Parasternal Short-Axis View			
Ao	2.3–3.7	3.0–2.3 cm	1.6–2.4
RVOT	1.9–2.2 cm	2.7 cm	
PA	1.5–2.5 cm	1.9–2.2 cm	
LA	2.6–4.5 cm	3.6 cm	1.6–2.4
LA area	7.2–13.0 cm^2	10.8 cm^2	
LV_d (PM level)	3.5–5.8 cm	4.7 cm	2.2–3.1
LV_s (PM level)	2.2–4.0 cm	3.1 cm	1.4–2.2
LV_d area (PM level)	16.0–31.2 cm^2	22.2 cm^2	
LV_s area (PM level)	5.2–13.4 cm^2	8.5 cm^2	
LV_d (Ch. level)	3.5–6.2	4.8 cm	2.3–3.2
LV_s (Ch. level)	2.3–4.0 cm	3.2 cm	1.5–2.2
LV_d area (Ch. level)	16.4–32.3 cm^2	22.5 cm^2	
LV_s area (Ch. level)	6.1–16.8	10.7 cm^2	
Subcostal View			
IVC diameter	—	1.8 cm	

Source: The values shown in this table represent a compilation of data from three sources:

I. Schnittinger, E. P. Gordon, P. J. Fitzgerald, and R. L. Popp: Standardized Intracardiac Measurements of Two-Dimensional Echocardiography, *J. Am. Coll. Cardiol.*, 5:934, 1983.

M. Triulzi and A. Weyman: Normal Cross-Sectional Measurements in Adults, in A. Weyman (ed.), "Echocardiography," Lea & Febiger, Philadelphia, 1982, p. 497.

A. D. Hagan, T. G. DiSessa, C. M. Bloor, and H. B. Calleja: "Two-Dimensional Echocardiography. Clinical-Pathological Correlations in Adult and Congenital Heart Disease," Little, Brown and Company, Boston, 1983, p. 553.

rule.[43,53,74] The modified Simpson's rule, originally developed for biplane angiography, appears to be a very reliable method, since it makes no assumptions about the geometry of the ventricles and is relatively unaffected by segmental wall motion abnormalities.[43,53,74] This method divides the left ventricle into slices of known thickness and the volume of the left ventricle is then equal to the sum of the volumes of this series of slices. There are several two-dimensional adaptations of Simpson's rule requiring different tomographic sections including: (1) apical four-chamber view and parasternal short-axis views at mitral and papillary muscle levels,[79] (2) apical four- and two-chamber views,[80] and (3) apical two-chamber view and parasternal short-axis view at the papillary muscle level.[74] The single apical plane analysis of Silverman et al. is especially useful when technical difficulties prevent adequate orthogonal long-axis views required by the Simpson's rule algorithm.[78] Although there seems to be a consistent underestimation of left ventricular volumes using two-dimensional echocardiography as compared with volumes determined by angiography, these measurements have proved reliable when tested by interobserver and intraobserver methods.[74] Ejection fraction, however, correlates well with cineangiographic data, since two-dimensional echocardiography underestimates end-diastolic volume and end-systolic volume equally.[81,82]

The determination of right ventricular volume is more difficult than that of left ventricular volume.[83–85] While the left ventricle resembles a prolate ellipse (a convenient volumetric model), the right ventricle has a complex shape, defying geometric description. The problem is compounded by irregular trabeculations, a separate infundibulum, and variations in shape with physiologic conditions (e.g., respiration).

Additional Echocardiographic Techniques

Echophonocardiography

Echophonocardiography is the simultaneous recording of echocardiograms, usually M-mode data, and heart sounds on multichannel recorders.[86] Together with pulse tracings, the combination of echocardiography and phonocardiography increases the information available above that from both tests performed separately. Precise timing of heart sounds and movements of cardiac structures with those heart sounds is possible through this combined technique. Research into the origin and significance of heart sounds and murmurs has been greatly advanced with this procedure.[87] Clinically, it has greatly improved the noninvasive evaluation of prosthetic heart valves[88] and has proved useful in identifying the site of origin of systolic honks and murmurs.[89]

Systolic time intervals (STIs) can be derived from the M-mode echocardiogram.[19,90] Left-side STIs can be determined from either the aortic valve echocardiogram or a combination of the electrocardiogram, phonocardiogram, and carotid pulse tracing. We presently use a combination of echocardiography and phonocardiography to substantiate our results. Commonly determined intervals include the left ventricular ejection time and the preejection period. Because of the ability of STIs to detect early changes in left ventricular dysfunction, the ease with which they are obtained, and their reproducibility, STIs are ideally suited for serially following patients, especially those receiving such cardiotoxic chemotherapy as doxorubicin hydrochloride (Adriamycin).[91] Right-side STIs can be derived only by imaging the pulmonic valve.[92] They are used to assess and follow pulmonary artery pressure and pulmonary vascular resistance.[93,94]

Contrast Echocardiography

Contrast echocardiography has played an important role in the development of cardiac ultrasound. Initially, it was used to validate various structures by M-mode echocardiography.[95–97] More recently, contrast methods have been used with two-dimensional echocardiography to delineate structures not readily seen by M-mode examination (e.g., the superior and inferior venae cavae,[98] descending aorta, and coronary arteries[99]) as well as to evaluate intracardiac shunts,[100] regurgitant lesions,[101,102] and complex congenital heart problems.[103–105]

The contrast substance that has been used clinically consists of the microbubbles that occur with the injection of fluid into the intravascular system.[19,20] Almost any liquid contains expended microbubbles and will produce a contrast effect when injected. The addition of small amounts of gas to the liquid prior to injection will provide a maximal contrast effect. The contrast agents used most frequently are normal saline solution and indocyanine green dye. The latter substance has a very low surface tension, so that small bubbles stay suspended longer. Virtually any peripheral venous injection, even the handling of closed intravenous lines, will produce some echocardiographic contrast effect.[106] As the time from injection increases and the gases are gradually absorbed into the blood, the contrast effect diminishes. It further dwindles as the gas is absorbed during passage through the pulmonary and systemic capillary system, which act as filters. The diameter of pulmonary capillary bed is so small that contrast microbubbles capable of traversing this bed will dissolve owing to surface tension effects.[107] Therefore, contrast substance is not seen in the left side of the heart of normal subjects following the intravenous injections of fluids.

The actual performance of contrast echocardiography in the clinical setting is quite simple, and it can be employed either at the patient's bedside or in the echocardiographic laboratory. We use a three-way stopcock attached to a scalp-vein intravenous line with two 10-ml syringes, each filled with 6 to 8 ml of saline solution, attached to the open ports of the stopcock. The saline solution becomes cloudy in appearance when vigorously injected back and forth between the two syringes, indicating that the amount of suspended air to be delivered is adequate. Then 6 ml of fluid from one syringe is injected rapidly and with extreme force into the vein. This procedure consistently produces an optimal contrast effect but obviously requires two individuals—one to perform the echocardiogram and the second to inject the bolus of fluid.

After the injection of saline solution and visualization of a satisfactory contrast effect, another contrast effect can often be obtained by raising the patient's arm over his or her head and then massaging the inner aspect of the upper arm toward the central circulation. This second contrast bolus, almost equal in intensity to the first, presumably is due to the release of residual contrast substance within the peripheral venous circulation. Echocardiographic contrast studies are best recorded during held respiration, although basic flow changes during respiration sometimes yield interesting physiologic information. The Valsalva maneuver should be performed in patients suspected of having a small atrial septal defect or patent foramen ovale, since a momentary right-to-left shunt may be produced during the release phase.[107]

The widest use of contrast echocardiography is in the evaluation of blood flow patterns, specifically the demonstration of intracardiac shunting and valvular regurgitation. Once injected, echocardiographic contrast microbubbles flow with the blood and surface in markers that are easily imaged. Since these microbubbles do not pass through the lungs, the appearance of contrast echoes in a chamber of the left side of the heart following a peripheral venous injection confirms the presence of an abnormal right-to-left shunt. Two-dimensional echocardiography, however, must be used for accurate identification of the defect, because the precise site of a shunt cannot be visualized on the M-mode echocardiogram. The optimal imaging planes include the apical or subcostal four-chamber views, because either enables one to image the atria, ventricles, and interatrial and interventricular septa simultaneously. This has permitted the detection of even small numbers of microbubbles crossing a right-to-left shunt (Fig. 120-19).[108]

Most clinicians have found that contrast echocardiography is extremely sensitive and specific for evaluating patients with right-to-left shunts, since the diagnosis is confirmed if only a few microbubbles of the millions injected cross the defect.[100,109] Contrast echocardiography appears to be more sensitive than oximetry and at least as sensitive as dye dilution techniques in the detection of right-to-left shunts as small as 3 percent at the atrial, ventricular, or aortic levels. It is thus often sufficiently sensitive to disclose small right-to-left shunts in patients with a patent foramen ovale or surgically repaired atrial septal defects when other techniques show no such abnormalities.[108] When a large right-to-left shunt is suspected it is best to limit the number of injections of contrast substance given. While undue effects of contrast substance administration are very rare, there are a few reported instances of central nervous system symptoms that have occurred in the setting of a large right-to-left shunt. In all cases, signs and symptoms were reversible.[110]

In addition to disclosing right-to-left shunts, contrast echocardiography can be extremely useful in demonstrating predominately left-to-right shunts using peripheral venous injections. It has been found that the majority of patients with predominately left-to-right shunts through an atrial septal defect also have small, transient right-to-left shunts. These transient right-to-left shunts can often be evoked by having the patient perform the Valsalva and/or Müller maneuvers, which alter intrathoracic and cardiac pressures sufficiently to cause some blood, and therefore contrast substance, to cross an atrial septal defect in a right-to-left direction.[107] In addition, a number of reports have demonstrated a *negative contrast effect* that is seen exclusively in patients with left-to-right shunts.[111] For example, if a left-to-right shunt exists at the atrial level, nonopacified blood from the left atrium will wash contrast microbubbles away from the interatrial area, yielding a contrast-free area or negative contrast effect.

Contrast echocardiography has proved to be of diagnostic value in the recognition of valvular regurgitation. From a noninvasive standpoint, the tricuspid valve is the only structure that can be conveniently assessed by this technique. When the inferior vena cava is imaged from the subcostal view in patients with a significant degree of tricuspid regurgitation, contrast substance may be observed to reflux into this vessel from the right atrium during

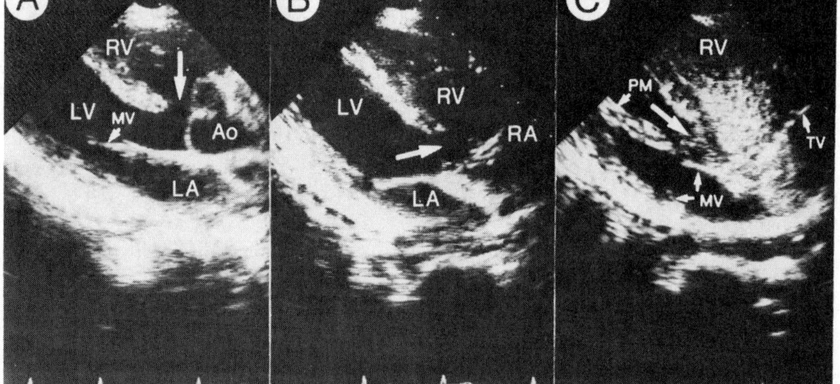

FIGURE 120-19 Two-dimensional echocardiogram from a patient with tetralogy of Fallot. *A*. Parasternal long-axis view demonstrates the aorta (Ao) overriding a large ventricular septal defect (arrow). *B*. Precordial four-chamber view shows the large ventricular septal defect (arrow). *C*. Same as view *B*, obtained during injection of aerated saline into an arm vein. Microbubbles, acting as contrast substance, virtually occlude the right atrium and right ventricle (RV), cross the ventricular septal defect (arrow), and enter the left ventricle (LV). MV = mitral valve; RA = right atrium; LA = left atrium; TV = tricuspid valve; PM = papillary muscle.

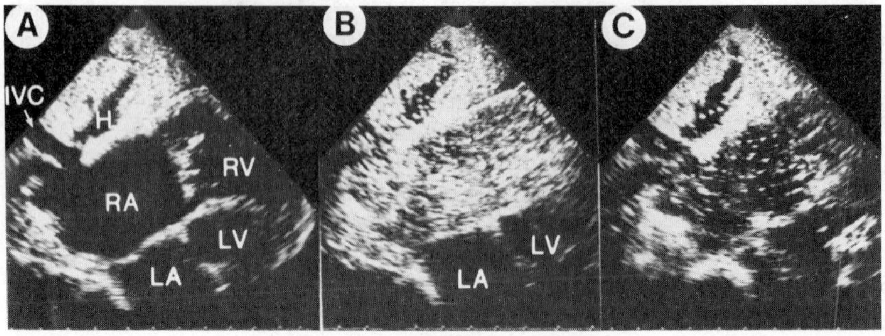

FIGURE 120-20 Two-dimensional subcostal four-chamber views, angled to show the junction between the inferior vena cava (IVC) and the right atrium (RA), the hepatic vein (H), and the right ventricle (RV), from a patient with severe tricuspid regurgitation. *A*. Prior to a peripheral intravenous injection of aerated saline solution. *B*. During the injection, microbubbles, acting as contrast substance, virtually occlude the inferior vena cava, hepatic vein, right atrium, and right ventricle. *C*. More than 30 s after the injection, microbubbles are still present in the hepatic vein, inferior vena cava, and right atrium. LA = left atrium; LV = left ventricle.

systole following installation of the injectate into a peripheral vein.[112] The persistent reflux of large amounts of contrast substance into the inferior vena cava represents an accurate indication of tricuspid regurgitation, especially if the bubbles are seen to pass into the hepatic vein (Fig. 120-20).[101,102] This is an excellent technique for diagnosis of tricuspid regurgitation, despite the fact that transient, minor reflux of a few microbubbles into the inferior vena cava during atrial contraction may be observed in normal subjects. Analysis of the moment of appearance of the contrast substance bolus in the inferior vena cava, after an upper-extremity vein injection, also aids in the diagnosis or exclusion of tricuspid regurgitation. If contrast microbubbles appear in the inferior vena cava in synchrony with the V wave of the atrial pressure curve, the diagnosis of tricuspid regurgitation can be made with a great degree of accuracy. Two-dimensional echocardiography has been used in this instance but may lead to a false-positive diagnosis because the timing of the appearance of contrast substance is less accurate than it is with M-mode recordings. Analysis of contrast echocardiograms should, therefore, include timing of appearance, pattern of opacification, duration of opacification (clearance time), intensity of contrast, and negative contrast effects.[113]

New developments in contrast echocardiography include (1) quantitation of the contrast effect with specifically designed contrast agents whose gas content and size are controlled;[114] (2) specialized microbubbles capable of transit through the pulmonary vascular bed and thereby capable of opacification of the left side of the heart;[115] and (3) direct intracoronary injection of renograffin, peroxide, and saline solution to delineate the coronary perfusion territory of individual coronary arteries. These injections result in formation of microbubbles and marked increase in myocardial brightness by echocardiography, which may determine the area at risk in coronary-prone patients.[116–118]

Exercise Echocardiography

Supine (bicycle) or upright (treadmill) exercise has been used in conjunction with echocardiography during or immediately after the stress. The application of ultrasound to the study of exercise left ventricular dynamics was begun in the early 1970s.[119,120] Crawford et al. reported a 50 percent success rate in obtaining adequate M-mode tracings during supine and upright bicycle exercise in a group of normal subjects.[121] In 1979 Wann et al. demonstrated the feasibility of using two-dimensional echocardiography during exercise to detect myocardial ischemia.[122] In the 1980s exercise two-dimensional echocardiography is beginning to assume a clinical role in the evaluation and management of patients with ischemic disease, since it can (1) analyze both ventricles,[123] (2) accurately detect regional wall motion abnormalities, (3) determine the extent of regional myocardial thickening, and (4) measure global ejection fraction.

The success in obtaining images of diagnostic quality with exercise two-dimensional echocardiography ranges between 71 and 100 percent, but has depended on the modality of exercise, the position of the patient, and the cardiac window utilized. Since ischemic regional wall motion abnormalities persist for several minutes following cessation of treadmill exercise, and since the left ventricle is adequately visualized in the first 30 to 60 s after exercise, echocardiography immediately after exercise gives excellent images because it avoids the technical problems of chest wall motion and hyperventilation.[122–126] If multiple left ventricular views are obtained in the first 5 min after exercise, success ranges from 85 to 100 percent. The apical window, with use of the four-chamber and two-chamber views, appears to be the best transducer position,[123,126] although the subcostal four-chamber view may also be useful.[127] The sensitivity of exercise echocardiography varies between 66 and 93 percent, but is influenced by the prevalence of multivessel coronary artery disease. Its specificity varies between 69 and 100 percent.[122–126]

Comparison of exercise two-dimensional echocardiography with either stress-electrocardiography or radionuclide techniques is quite favorable to the echocardiographic technique. Sensitivity of exercise two-dimensional echocardiography is actually higher than that of radionuclide techniques if right ventricular wall motion abnormalities are included.[123] The specificities of the two techniques are virtually identical.[125] Two-dimensional echocardiography may, in fact, be more accurate in measuring ejection fraction than is radionuclide angiography, since the nuclear technique requires 2 to 3 min of average cardiac cycles for computing the ejection fraction, whereas two-dimensional echocardiography examines individual cardiac cycles.[127] Two-dimensional echocardiography has other practical advantages over nuclide angiography, including the following: (1) Analysis of beat-to-beat images of many cardiac cycles from multiple views gives inherently better resolution; (2) some areas of the heart are examined better with echocardiography than with radionuclide angiography; (3) there is a cost saving because two-dimensional echocardiography is less expensive than nuclear studies; (4) with echocardiography there is no need for intravenous injections or radiation hazard; and (5) two-dimensional echocardiography can be easily added to routine treadmill testing. The major limitation of two-dimensional echocardiography is the need for extensive observer interaction for reproducibility of measurements and observations. Computer-assisted methods for image enhancement and endocardial border recognition, however, may overcome this limitation and provide more objective quantitation of global and regional myocardial performance.[128]

Pharmacologic and Physiologic Interventions

Pharmacologic and physiologic interventions can influence left ventricular performance and valve motion while a patient is being monitored echocardiographically. The most clinically useful pharmacologic agent is amyl nitrite, since it can provoke systolic anterior motion of the mitral valve in patients with hypertrophic cardiomyopathy and systolic posterior motion of the mitral valve in patients with mitral valve prolapse.[129,130]

The Valsalva maneuver (forced expiration) and the Müller maneuver (forced inspiration) may be used during the echocardiographic examination to "bring out" diagnostic abnormalities in patients with hypertrophic cardiomyopathy or congestive heart failure and may demonstrate the patency of the foramen ovale or detect a small atrial septal defect.[131] Echocardiograms performed while the patient is standing or squatting may also be useful, but are technically difficult.

Invasive Echocardiography

Although echocardiography is primarily a noninvasive technique, it has been used in a variety of invasive procedures including: (1) contrast echocardiography requiring an intravenous injection, (2) intracardiac echocardiography, (3) transesophageal echocardiography, and (4) intraoperative echocardiography, performed directly on the surface of the heart.

Intracardiac Echocardiography

Contrast echocardiography has been used in the catheterization laboratory by injecting saline solution or indocyanine green through an intracardiac catheter with simultaneous echocardiography. Its major advantage is to obviate the need for cineangiography in young, critically ill patients, in pregnant women, in individuals allergic to iodine dye, and in patients not permitted a high osmotic load (e.g., uremic patients). Contrast echocardiography has also been used as a supplement to angiographic studies, especially in the neonate, since it helps provide a better control of the number and site of angiographic injections. When contrast medium is delivered to the left or right atrium through surgically placed pressure-monitor catheters, contrast echocardiographic studies in the postoperative period have proved useful in testing the effectiveness of surgical repair of anatomic and functional defects.[97] In many instances contrast echocardiography can be superior to standard angiography.[132] Intracardiac echocardiography has also been used to obtain histologic information in studies in which a very high frequency transducer is placed at the tip of an intracardiac catheter and the catheter is positioned against a myocardial wall.[133]

Transesophageal Echocardiography

Transesophageal echocardiography (TEE) has been used by several investigators, initially with M mode and more recently with two-dimensional scanning.[134–137] This approach has the advantage of providing an unobstructed view of the heart because there is no interference by chest wall structures. Ultrasonic single or multielement transducers can easily be placed on the tip of esophageal catheters or incorporated into the tip of a commercially available gastroscope. The small, flexible tube and transducer are easily swallowed, and although the transducer is moved rapidly there is no loss of esophageal wall contact. A barium x-ray examination of the esophagus must be performed prior to the ultrasound examination in order to exclude a diverticulum. The patient should fast for 8 h and should receive 0.5 mg atropine 1 h prior to the examination in order to avoid bradycardia or hypersalivation. The transesophageal study is done while the patient is in a supine position. The positional controls of the gastroscope allow the transducer to show multiple and reproducible views of the heart. No complications have been reported in over 150 patients studied by Hanrath et al.[136a]

There are unique applications of transesophageal echocardiography that cannot be satisfactorily achieved from the precordial positions, including (1) ability to image technically difficult patients, (2) detailed assessment of mediastinal and retrocardiac anatomy (e.g., thoracic aorta), (3) assessment of left ventricular performance during dynamic upright exercise, (4) continuous intraoperative monitoring of the left ventricle, and (5) postoperative observation of the heart. Measurements of left ventricular

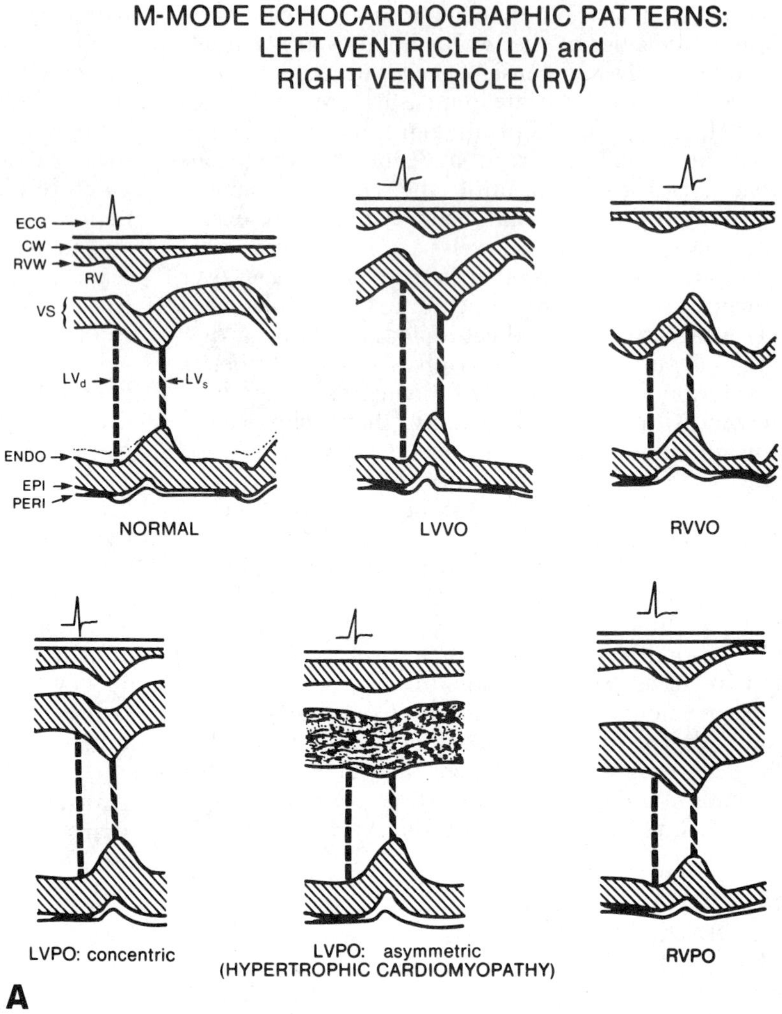

dimensions with the transesophageal technique correlate excellently with those using the transthoracic method.[136] Transesophageal echocardiography has been used to determine cardiac anatomy and function before, during, and after induction of anesthesia in high-risk patients, during operative procedures on patients with cardiac problems, and in the intensive care unit.[137] Unlike conventional transthoracic echocardiography this system can record cardiac images continuously from base to apex as the transducer is being withdrawn or advanced in the esophagus.

Intraoperative Echocardiography

Echocardiography has been used for scanning open-chested patients before and after surgical correction.[138–141] Intraoperative scanning through the right atrioventricular junction or through the right atrium provides a unique view of the right ventricular inflow tract and tricuspid valve morphology. It has been helpful in diagnosing unsuspected tricuspid stenosis in patients with rheumatic heart disease and assessing the effects of tricuspid angioplasty in patients with tricuspid regurgitation.[140] In patients with hypertrophic cardiomyopathy, the technique has defined the tunnel of muscle resected during myotomy and myectomy and defined the absence of residual systolic anterior motion in conjunction with hemodynamic measurements.[141] Some investigators have used intraoperative echocardiography to evaluate the mitral valve after mitral commissurotomy.[139] Excellent images of the coronary arteries have also been obtained with this technique. Cardiac surgeons have used a very high frequency ultrasonic probe, held directly on the surface of the heart, for exploring abnormalities within the coronary arteries prior to the insertion of bypass grafts.[140,141] The excellent resolution and the display of the image of vessel size appears to exceed the detail provided by current coronary angiographic techniques and bears a close relationship to the pathological anatomy. This technique may be invaluable in the decision of whether or not to bypass individual coronary arteries and may be useful in evaluating the graft-vessel anastomosis.

Clinical Application of Echocardiography

Echocardiography is an integral part of the cardiovascular data base of many patients. In order to ac-

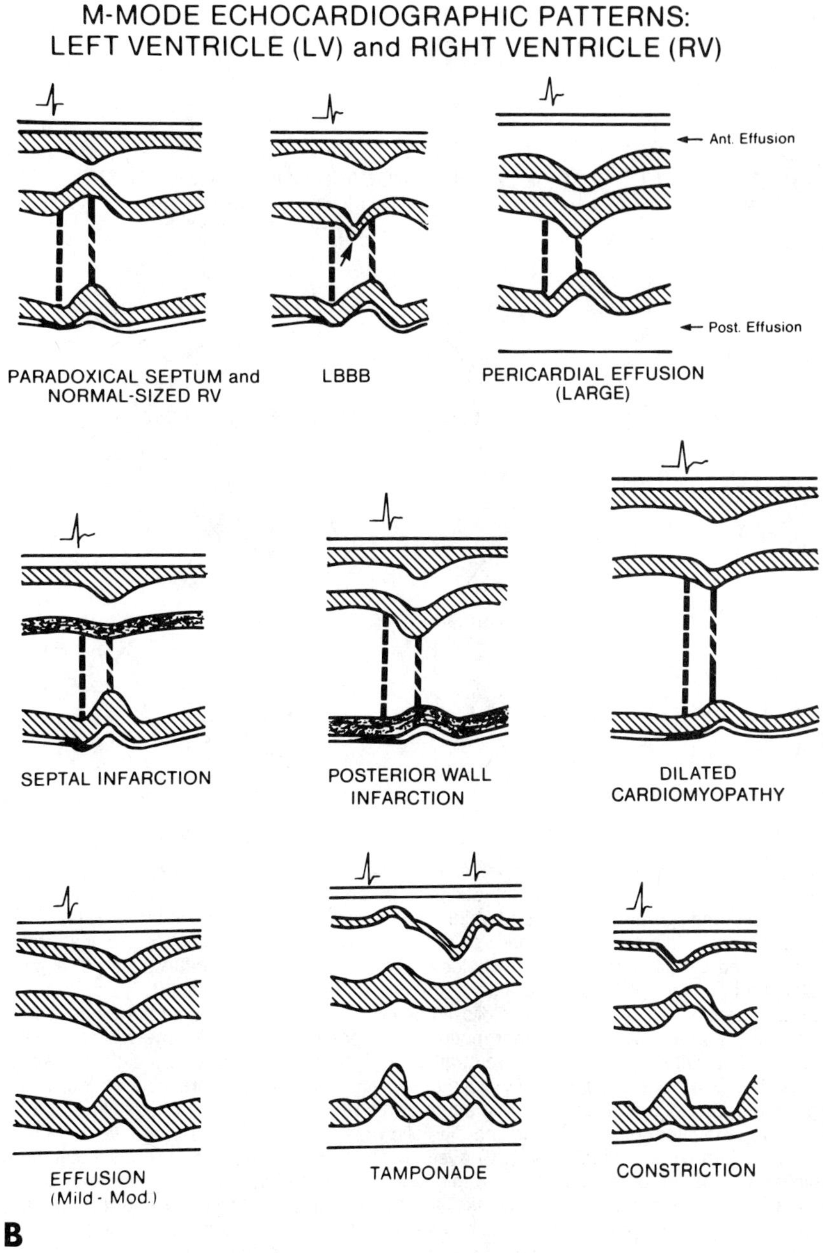

FIGURE 120-21 *A.* (*facing page*) Schematic M-mode echocardiographic patterns of the left and right ventricles. The left ventricular dimensions at end diastole (LV_d) and end systole (LV_s) are identified by the broken vertical lines. A left ventricular volume overload (LVVO) lesion (e.g., aortic regurgitation and mitral regurgitation) is characterized by a dilated left ventricle and hyperdynamic ventricular septal (VS) and posterior wall motion. A right ventricular volume overload (RVVO) lesion (e.g., atrial septal defect and tricuspid regurgitation) is characterized by a dilated right ventricle (RV) and paradoxical septal motion. A left ventricular pressure overload (LVPO) lesion may have concentric hypertrophy (e.g., aortic stenosis and systemic arterial hypertension) or asymmetric septal hypertrophy (e.g., hypertrophic cardiomyopathy). Right ventricular hypertrophy is usually present in both groups. A right ventricular pressure overload (RVPO) lesion (e.g., valvular pulmonic stenosis and tetralogy of Fallot) is characterized by right ventricular hypertrophy and asymmetric septal hypertrophy. CW = chest wall; RVW = right ventricular wall; Endo = endocardium; Epi = epicardium; Peri = pericardium. *B.* Paradoxical septal motion with a normal-sized right ventricle (RV) may be seen in patients with myocardial ischemia or infarction of the interventricular septum and patients after open heart surgery. Left bundle branch block (LBBB) is characterized by early posterior septal motion (arrow) followed by paradoxical septal motion. Pericardial effusions are classified as large if there is significant anterior and posterior fluid, moderate (mod) if there is significant posterior and small anterior fluid, and small (mild) if only posterior fluid is present. Myocardial infarction may demonstrate hypokinesis or akinesis of the septum or posterior wall with absence of systolic thickening. Congestive (dilated) cardiomyopathy is characterized by a dilated left ventricle with hypokinetic septal and posterior wall motion. Cardiac tamponade is characterized by anterior and posterior pericardial fluid with respiratory variation in chamber size and wall motion. Pericardial constriction is characterized by paradoxical septal motion and parallel movement of the epicardium and pericardium.

curately describe its many uses and indications a thorough analysis of each application as to sensitivity, specificity, reproducibility, and quantitation would be necessary. Although this is not the purpose of this chapter, some insight into these variables will be enumerated.

During the last several years the relative roles of two-dimensional and M-mode echocardiography has shifted, and the two-dimensional technique, which previously was only a small component of the echocardiographic examination, has now become the primary imaging modality. Two-dimensional echocardiography appears to be faster and easier to use than M-mode echocardiography and is superior for most clinical applications. Since it provides a more comprehensive cardiac image and accurate spatial relationships of the cardiac structures, it is especially valuable in patients with segmental disease. M-mode recordings, however, yield a more convenient and accessible permanent record, give better detail and analysis of complex valve and wall motion patterns, and are more suitable for measuring cardiac chamber dimensions, wall thicknesses, and the slopes and amplitudes of the valve leaflets and myocardial walls. M-mode echocardiography also facilitates analysis of time relations with other simultaneously recorded physiologic variables (e.g., electrocardiograms, heart sounds, and pulse tracings). Since an understanding of the M-mode image is still essential for echocardiographic interpretation, a series of representative diagrams is shown in Figs. 120-21, 120-22, and 120-23. In a modern, well-equipped diagnostic labo-

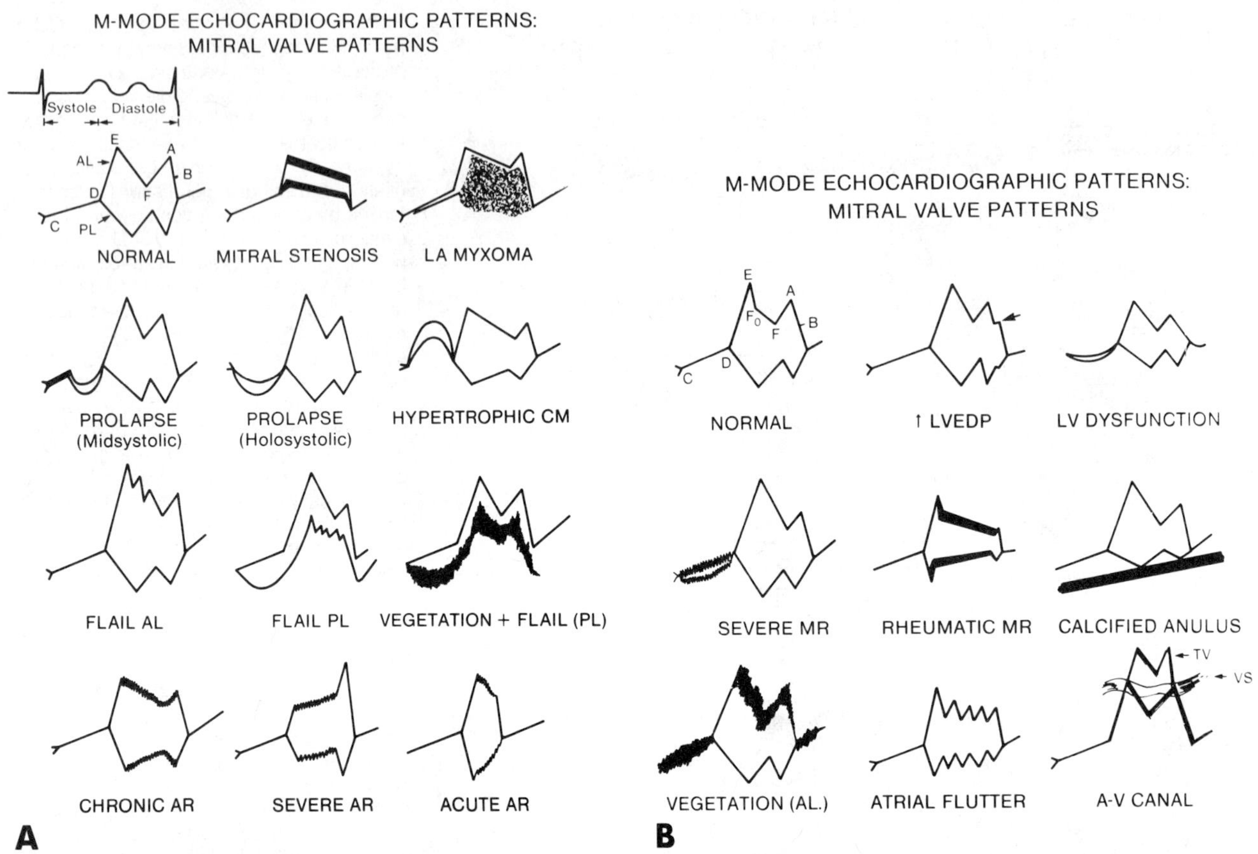

FIGURE 120-22 *A*. Schematic M-mode echocardiographic patterns of the mitral valve. The anterior leaflet is designated by letters A to F (see Fig. 120-4). Mitral stenosis is characterized by thickened (calcified or fibrotic) leaflets with reduced diastolic (EF) slope, diminished excursion of the anterior leaflet, and paradoxical motion of the posterior leaflet. Left atrial (LA) myxoma is characterized by a tumor mass that occludes the mitral valve orifice. The clear space in early diastole corresponds to the time required for the tumor to prolapse from left atrium to left ventricle. Mitral prolapse is characterized by either midsystolic or holosystolic posterior bowing of the posterior and/or anterior leaflets. Hypertrophic cardiomyopathy (CM) is characterized by systolic anterior motion and reduced diastolic (EF) slope of the anterior mitral leaflet. A flail anterior leaflet (AL) is characterized by coarse diastolic fluttering on the anterior leaflet, whereas a flail posterior leaflet (PL) is characterized by holosystolic prolapse and diastolic anterior motion of the posterior leaflet. A vegetation on a flail posterior leaflet may mimic mitral valve prolapse or a left atrial myxoma. Aortic regurgitation (AR) is characterized by high-frequency diastolic fluttering of the mitral leaflets. Severe aortic regurgitation may significantly elevate left ventricular diastolic pressure so that initial opening of the valve is absent or reduced, or the valve may close prematurely as in acute aortic regurgitation. *B*. The diastolic slope of the normal mitral valve may be designated EF or EF_0. Elevated left ventricular end-diastolic pressure (LVEDP) is characterized by a shoulder on the closing slope referred to as a B notch (arrow). Left ventricular (LV) dysfunction is characterized by a double-diamond configuration of the mitral valve in diastole and slight hammocking of the leaflets in systole. Mitral regurgitation (MR), if severe, may show systolic fluttering of the mitral valve. If regurgitation is due to rheumatic heart disease, the leaflets may be thickened and the anterior leaflet may have a "ski-slope" appearance. A dense band of calcium is posterior to the valve in patients with a calcified mitral anulus. Vegetations on the anterior leaflet (AL) appears as hazy, dense echoes in systole and diastole. So-called flutter waves may be seen on the valve in patients with atrial flutter. The anterior mitral leaflet appears to "move through" the ventricular septum (VS) and merge with the tricuspid valve (TV) in patients with partial (ostium primum atrial septal defect) or complete atrioventricular (AV) canal.

ratory a comprehensive echocardiographic study should utilize both M-mode and two-dimensional recordings to provide information about cardiac anatomy and physiology for optimal patient care.[142–145]

Specific Cardiac Lesions

The echocardiographic examination is extremely useful in the differential diagnosis of a variety of cardiac signs, symptoms, and laboratory abnormalities including chest pain, certain heart murmurs, and the enlarged cardiac silhouette on chest x-ray. In patients with an enlarged cardiac silhouette on chest x-ray, echocardiography can separate those with pericardial effusion from those with true cardiomegaly, accurately identify the specific cardiac chamber enlarged, and distinguish cavitary dilatation from myocardial hypertrophy.

The diagnosis of *pericardial effusion* was one of the first medical uses for echocardiography,[7] and this technique is now considered the method of choice in patients with a suspected pericardial effusion.[146,147] M-mode echocardiography is superior in qualitative diagnosis (e.g., small effusions, constrictive hemodynamics, and pericardial thickening), whereas two-dimensional echocardiography is superior for assessing the amount, distribution, and loc-

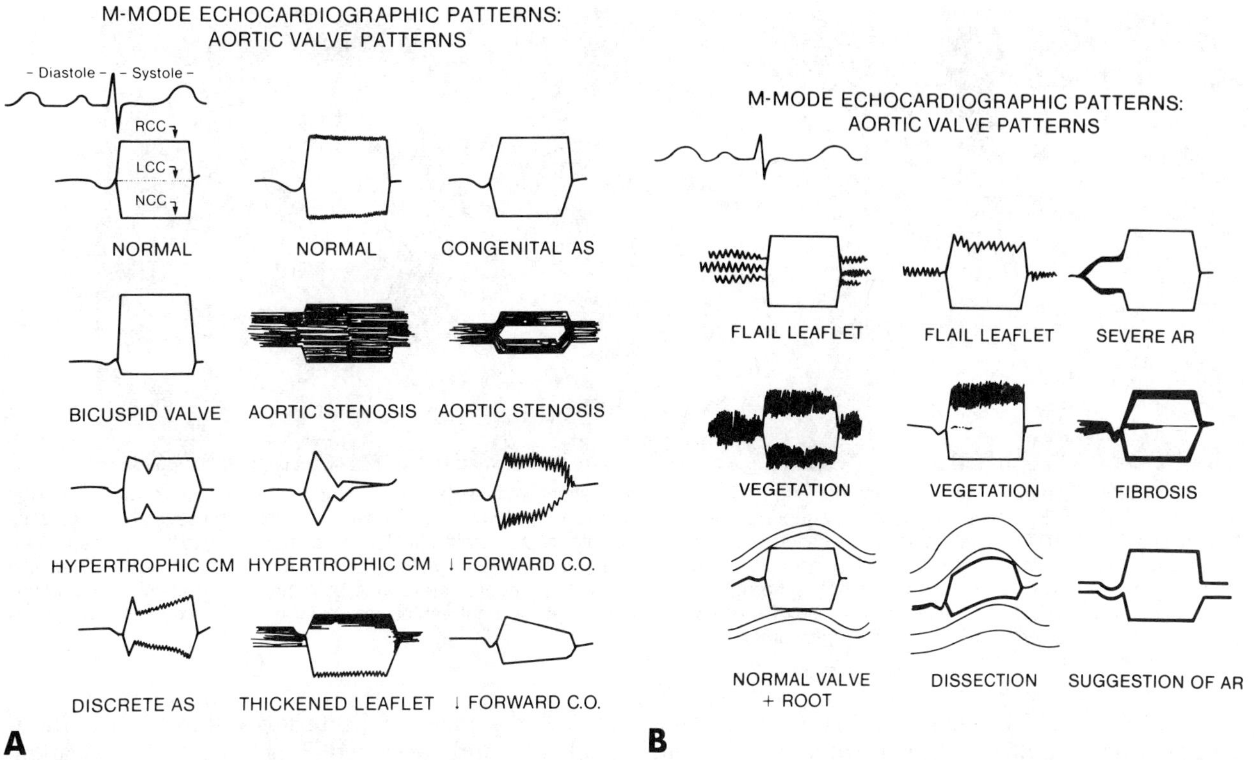

FIGURE 120-23 *A.* Schematic M-mode echocardiographic patterns of the aortic valve. The anterior or right coronary (RCC) and posterior or noncoronary (NCC) cusps are usually seen, but the middle or left coronary (LCC) cusp is parallel to the beam of sound and is not usually seen. The normal valve may occasionally exhibit high-frequency systolic vibrations. The valve may appear normal in patients with congenital aortic stenosis (AS), because the actual valve opening is out of the plane of the ultrasonic beam. A bicuspid aortic valve has eccentric diastolic closure. Calcific aortic stenosis, characterized by dense echoes (calcification) in systole and diastole and a reduced or absent valve orifice, must be differentiated from the thickened (fibrotic) leaflets of aortic valve sclerosis. Hypertrophic cardiomyopathy (CM) with obstruction has partial (notch) or complete midsystolic aortic valve closure, whereas discrete (membranous) subaortic stenosis has partial (notch) early systolic closure. Reduced forward cardiac output (CO), as seen with mitral regurgitation or left ventricular dysfunction, may show high-frequency systolic fluttering and gradual systolic closure. *B.* A flail aortic leaflet is characterized by coarse fluttering in systole and/or diastole. Premature opening of the aortic valve is evidence of elevated left ventricular diastolic pressure and is seen in severe aortic regurgitation (AR). Vegetations appear as dense, shaggy echoes on the leaflet(s) in systole and/or diastole. Separation of the leaflets in diastole of more than 3 mm is suggestive, but not diagnostic, of aortic regurgitation. The normal aorta is characterized by two parallel lines, each 1 to 3 mm thick, that move anteriorly in systole and posteriorly in diastole. The aortic leaflets normally open to the periphery of the aortic walls. Dissection of the aorta is characterized by a dilated aortic root (more than 42 mm), widened anterior or posterior (more than 9 mm) aortic walls, and thin aortic leaflets that open to the periphery of the inner lumen.

ulation of pericardial fluid and is particularly useful in avoiding diagnostic pitfalls.[146–150] In addition, two-dimensional echocardiography can detect fibrous strands, fibrin clots, and tumor implants on the pericardium or in the fluid.[151] Furthermore, two-dimensional echocardiography now appears to provide reliable criteria for the diagnosis of *cardiac tamponade.*[152–154] Although this is still primarily a clinical and hemodynamic bedside diagnosis, the collapse of the right ventricular and/or right atrial walls during diastolic filling (a time when the right ventricle should be increasing in volume and dimensions) has been commonly seen on two-dimensional examination in patients with tamponade (Fig. 120-24). Wall motion reverts to normal after pericardiocentesis in these patients. Although right ventricular diastolic collapse appears to be a relatively reliable sign of impending tamponade, there are factors that affect its sensitivity and specificity. Therefore, diastolic right ventricular collapse should best be considered only as a marker of the equalization of the right ventricular diastolic and pericardial pressures. Its absence should not exclude tamponade, but in the setting of an otherwise normal right ventricle this absence makes the diagnosis of tamponade very unlikely.

Echocardiography also appears to be useful in minimizing the hazards of pericardiocentesis.[155,155a] The pericardiocentesis needle can be identified in the scanning plane, and the position of the needle tip can be confirmed by contrast echocardiography (Fig. 120-24). The position of the needle or catheter should be monitored continuously during the procedure and it should be repositioned if necessary. Percutaneous pericardial biopsy, under two-dimensional echocardiographic guidance, has been recently introduced without complications reported to date.[156]

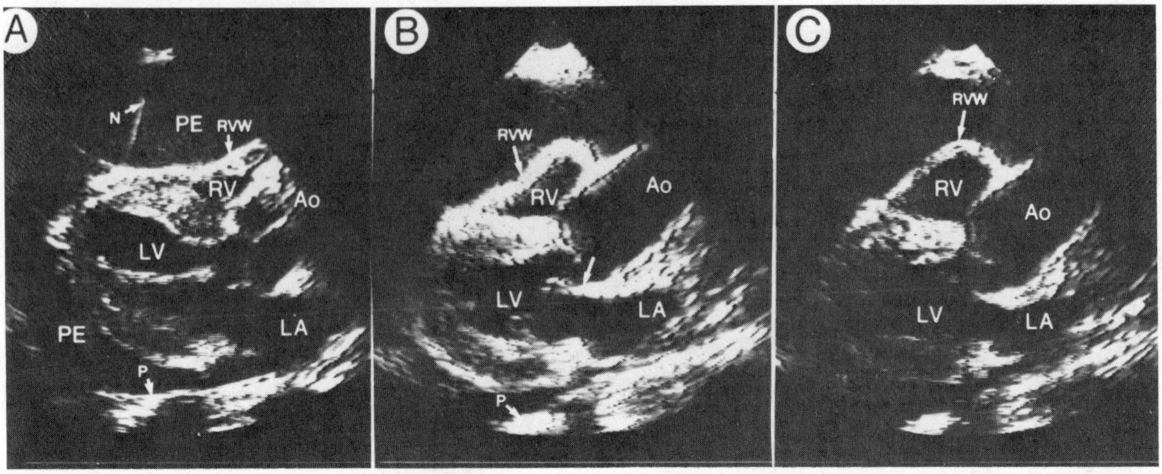

FIGURE 120-24 Two-dimensional parasternal long-axis views from a patient with cardiac tamponade. *A*. Diastolic frame shows a large pericardial effusion (PE) that almost completely surrounds the heart up to the atrioventricular groove posteriorly and severely compresses the right ventricle (RV). The pericardiocentesis needle (N) is seen in the anterior pericardial effusion in close proximity to the right ventricular wall (RVW). Left ventricular hypertrophy is present. *B*. Middiastolic frame shows the mitral valve (arrow) partially closed. The right ventricular cavity is slightly increased in size, but the right ventricular wall still indents the cavity. Left and right ventricular hypertrophy are evident. *C*. Systolic frame obtained after removal of 850 ml shows that the right ventricular cavity has fully expanded. LV = left ventricle; Ao = aorta; LA = left atrium; P = pericardium.

Echocardiography provides precise information about cardiac chamber enlargement and the extent of functional impairment. Determination of ventricular cavity dimensions, wall thickness, and systolic and diastolic function allows classification of the cardiomyopathies into three types: dilated, hypertrophic, and restrictive types. *Idiopathic congestive (dilated) cardiomyopathy* consists of dilatation of all four cardiac chambers, usually in a predictable, symmetrical pattern (Figs. 120-21*B* and 120-25).[157] Left ventricular function is diminished, as evidenced by reduced septal and posterior wall motion, reduced delta D, and increased E point–septal separation. The cardiac valves are usually normal, but the excursion of the mitral and aortic valves is frequently diminished.

Echocardiography is extremely sensitive and undoubtedly the best method of diagnosing *hypertrophic cardiomyopathy*.[158,159,159a] Severe left ventricular hypertrophy may have a recognizable cause, such as aortic stenosis or systemic hypertension, or it may be seen in the familial disorder known as

FIGURE 120-25 Two-dimensional echocardiogram from a patient with a congestive cardiomyopathy. *A*. Parasternal long-axis view shows a markedly dilated left ventricle (LV) and moderately dilated left atrium (LA) and right ventricle (RV). Although there appears to be a rounded apex, this is a foreshortened view and the true cardiac apex is not seen. In this end-systolic frame, the closed mitral valve (MV) is more than 30 mm from the septum, consistent with a markedly reduced ejection fraction. *B*. Parasternal short-axis view at end systole (identified by the electrocardiographic trigger at the bottom of the frame), shows that the septum and posterior wall appear thin in comparison with the dilated left ventricle. *C*. Apical four-chamber view shows that both ventricles cannot be imaged simultaneously because the left ventricle is very large. There appears to be slight compression of the right ventricle by the left ventricle. Interatrial septal drop-out, common in this view, is apparent between the dilated atria. *D*. M-mode echocardiogram obtained from the parasternal short-axis view with the cursor across the left ventricle at the level of the chordae tendineae. The left ventricle measures 88 mm at end diastole, the walls are thin and markedly hypokinetic, and the delta D is 9 percent. Ao = aorta; RA = right atrium.

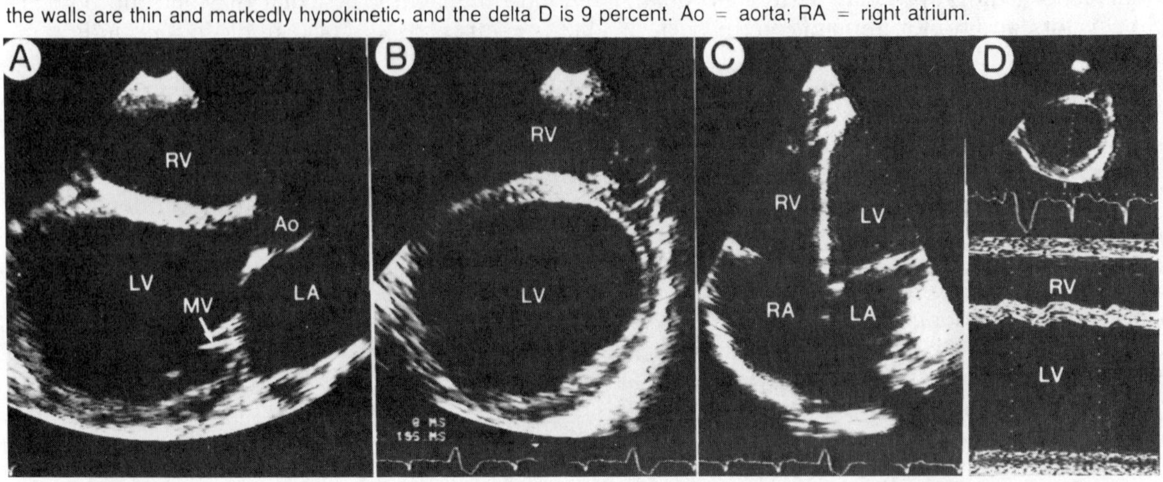

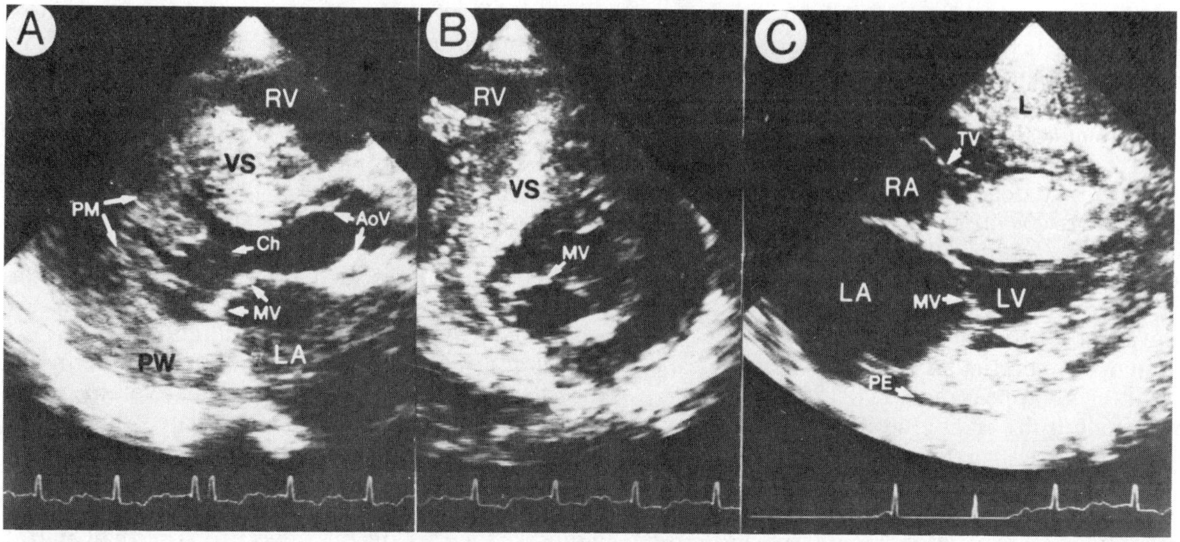

FIGURE 120-26 Two-dimensional echocardiogram from a patient with hypertrophic cardiomyopathy. *A*. Parasternal long-axis view in systole demonstrates asymmetric septal hypertrophy. The thickness of the ventricular septum wall (VS) is 31 mm and that of the posterior wall (PW) is 20 mm. Characteristic brightening of the septal echoes is evident. The papillary muscles (PM) and chordae tendineae (Ch) are also hypertrophied. The left ventricular outflow tract, between the mitral valve (MV) and septum, is narrowed and the left atrium (LA) is dilated. In diastole, not shown, the free edge of the anterior mitral leaflet and chordal structures were in apposition to the septum. *B*. Parasternal short-axis view at the level of the mitral valve shows that the septal hypertrophy involves both the anterior and posterior portions of the interventricular septum. *C*. Subcostal four-chamber view in systole shows the disproportionate septal hypertrophy best, because the septum is perpendicular to the ultrasound beam. Note the right ventricular hypertrophy (arrow), slitlike right ventricular cavity, and dilated left atrium. A small pericardial effusion (PE) is evident. AoV = aortic valve; RV = right ventricle; RA = right atrium; TV = tricuspid valve; L = liver.

idiopathic hypertrophic subaortic stenosis (IHSS). The pathognomonic finding in IHSS is asymmetric septal hypertrophy (ASH) in which the ratio of the septal to posterior wall thickness is greater than 1.3:1.0 (Figs. 120-21*A* and 120-26). Symmetric hypertrophy, however, can be seen in a small percentage of patients. Systolic anterior motion of the mitral valve is also characteristically seen in these patients (Fig. 120-22*B*). The left ventricular cavity is usually decreased in size, while the left atrium is

FIGURE 120-27 Two-dimensional echocardiogram from a patient with confirmed amyloid heart disease. *A*. Parasternal long-axis view in diastole shows right ventricular hypertrophy, concentric left ventricular hypertrophy, and bright reflectors of the interventricular septum (VS), characteristic of amyloid involvement of the myocardium. The left ventricular (LV) cavity is normal in size, but the left atrium is dilated. The mitral valve (MV) appears thickened. *B*. Short-axis view at the level of the hypertrophied papillary muscles (P) also shows right ventricular hypertrophy, concentric left ventricular hypertrophy, and a general increase in refractile pattern. *C*. Apical four-chamber view again shows the general increase in the refractile pattern of the septum and the hypertrophied papillary muscle (P) and chordae tendineae. The fact that the interatrial septum does not have significant dropout suggests that it, too, is hypertrophied. RV = right ventricle; CS = coronary sinus; PW = posterior wall; AoV = aortic valve; Ao = aorta; RA = right atrium.

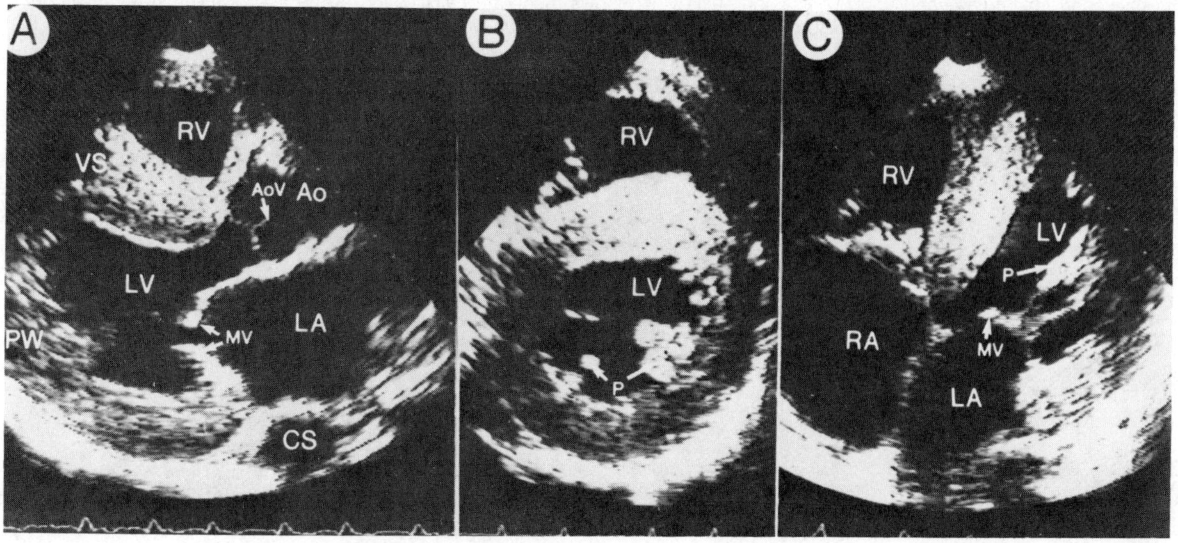

dilated. The most reliable sign of left ventricular outflow tract obstruction is midsystolic partial (notch) or complete closure of the aortic valve (Fig. 120-23*A*).

Restrictive (infiltrative) cardiomyopathies have a multiplicity of causes and only amyloidosis can be diagnosed with any degree of certainty. In general, there is concentric ventricular hypertrophy, normal or decreased left ventricular cavity size, and decreased left ventricular function both in systole and diastole. In the case of cardiac amyloidosis the valves and interatrial septum are thickened, and the hypertrophied left ventricular walls may have an abnormal glittering appearance (Fig. 120-27).[160]

Echocardiography is unique in its ability to examine cardiac valve structure and motion and therefore is of great value for determining both the causes and severity of valvular heart disease. Criteria for valve stenosis and regurgitation and specific indications for surgical intervention are emerging based on two-dimensional echocardiographic findings. Direct detection and quantitation of stenotic cardiac valves are virtually limited to the echocardiographic approach. In *mitral stenosis* leaflet motion is restricted, the orifice is reduced, and calcification is usually present (Figs. 120-22*A* and *B* and 120-28). Echocardiography is the most sensitive and most specific noninvasive method for diagnosing mitral stenosis.[19,20,161] Published data have documented the usefulness of two-dimensional measurement of mitral valve area in patients with rheumatic mitral stenosis (Fig. 120-28).[162,163] Planimetry of the mitral valve orifice is accomplished by use of the parasternal short-axis view. Care must be taken to assess the mitral valve at the level of its leaflet tips; therefore, recordings must be obtained that slowly scan the body of the mitral valve apically toward the chordae tendineae. After the proper level is located, the image is slowly played until it demonstrates the largest mitral valve orifice size seen in early diastole. This area is then planimetered using computer-assisted area assessment. Echocardiography is also useful for confirming mitral stenosis in the presence of associated abnormalities such as left or right ventricular dysfunction, aortic or tricuspid valve disease, and pulmonary hypertension (Fig. 120-29).

Mitral regurgitation is frequently suggested by indirect signs including a left ventricular volume overload pattern characterized by a dilated, hypercontractile left ventricle and an increased ejection fraction or delta D and systolic expansion of an enlarged left atrium (Fig. 120-21*A*).[164] However, the etiologic diagnoses, such as mitral valve prolapse, flail mitral leaflet, and calcified mitral anulus, are best determined by analysis of the motion and configuration of the mitral valve itself.[165]

Mitral valve prolapse can be considered the boon or bane of echocardiography (Fig. 120-22*A*). A very large number of patients are referred "to rule out" this condition, and substantial overdiagnosis seems to have become the rule. To provide better diagnostic definition of mitral valve prolapse, examine not only valve motion but also valve morphology.[166,166a,167,167a,167b] Two-dimensional echocardiograms in patients with auscultatory and phonocardiographic evidence of mitral valve prolapse reveal a wide spectrum of valve types. Some valves are voluminous, thick, and redundant and prolapse re-

FIGURE 120-28 Two-dimensional echocardiogram from a patient with moderate mitral stenosis. *A*. Parasternal long-axis view in diastole demonstrates doming (arrow) of the anterior leaflet, commonly seen in rheumatic mitral stenosis in the absence of marked valvular calcification. The leaflet tips are only moderately calcified, and the left atrium (LA) is moderately dilated. The extent of leaflet tip separation of the mitral valve (MV) is beneficial for identifying the true orifice in the parasternal short-axis plane and is also helpful as a rough guide to judge whether the parasternal short-axis image is precisely through the leaflet tips. *B*. Parasternal short-axis view through the tips of the mitral leaflets demonstrates the technique for determining mitral valve area. Planimetry of the valve area (dotted line) is performed at the onset of diastole when the orifice appears the largest; the valve orifice measures 1.2 cm.² *C*. Parasternal short-axis view in systole shows the thickened leaflet tips coapted. *D*. Apical long-axis view shows moderate calcification at the tips of the mitral leaflets, less significant disease at the base of the valve, and bowing of the anterior leaflet due to predominant involvement at the free edge of the valve. Marked left atrial enlargement is apparent. LV = left ventricle; RV = right ventricle; Ao = aorta; AoV = aortic valve.

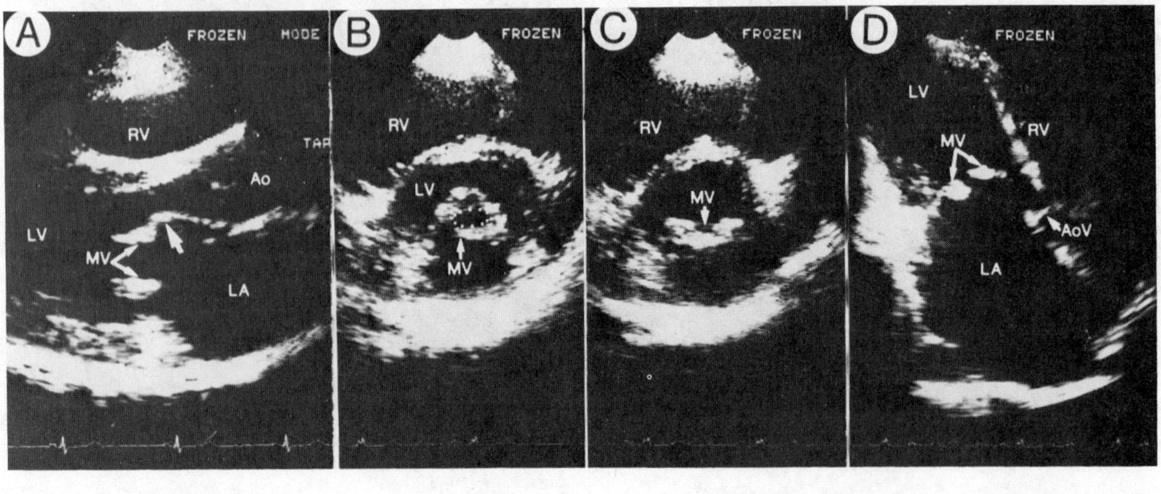

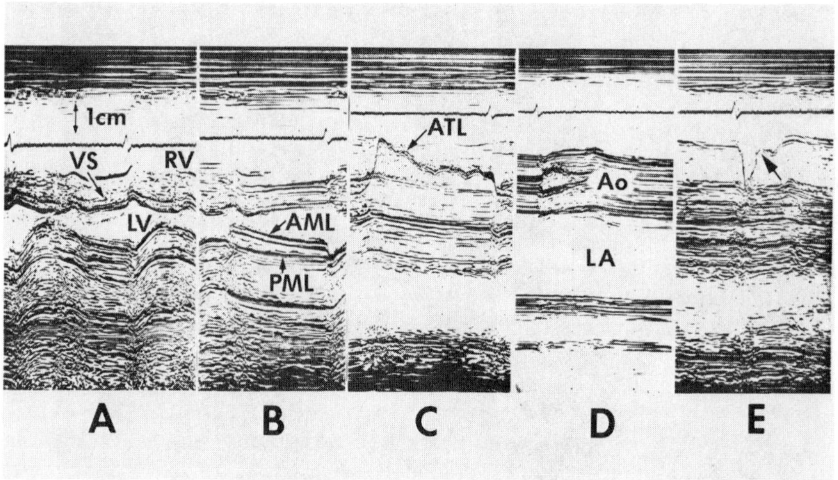

FIGURE 120-29 M-mode echocardiogram from a patient with moderately severe mitral stenosis. *A*. At the level of the papillary muscles the left ventricle (LV) is reduced in size and the right ventricle (RV) is dilated. Ventricular septal (VS) motion is reduced. *B*. Moderately thickened mitral valve with reduced diastolic (EF) slope of the anterior leaflet (AML) and paradoxical motion of posterior leaflet (PML). *C*. Anterior tricuspid leaflet (ATL) shows evidence of atrial fibrillation with a long diastole, but is otherwise normal. *D*. Aorta (Ao) is normal in size, but the aortic valve is thickened with reduced excursion suggestive of aortic stenosis. The left atrium (LA) is dilated. *E*. The pulmonic valve shows evidence of pulmonary hypertension with a flat diastolic slope and midsystolic closure (arrow).

gardless of the view (Fig. 120-30), whereas others are small, thin, and normal in appearance and prolapse in mid or late systole only in one view. It appears that diagnostic criteria using motion and morphology can separate patients with and without prolapse with a high degree of sensitivity and specificity. Mitral valve prolapse is occasionally associated with tricuspid valve prolapse and/or aortic valve prolapse.[168,168a] In patients with a *flail mitral leaflet* the tips of the valve, which remain within the ventricle in prolapse, are displaced into the left atrium during systole.[169,170]

The sensitivity and specificity of ultrasound for identifying cardiac calcification are excellent. The echocardiographic pattern of *mitral annular calcification* is virtually diagnostic.[171] Echocardiography is more sensitive than chest roentgenography or fluoroscopy for detecting mitral annular calcification.

Aortic regurgitation produces high-frequency diastolic fluttering of the mitral leaflets and occasionally of the interventricular septum, best seen on M-mode examination. The left ventricle is dilated with the characteristic volume overload pattern.[171a] M-mode echocardiography can frequently separate acute from chronic aortic regurgitation, since the former may show premature closure of the mitral valve, a sign of hemodynamically severe disease (Fig. 120-22*A*).[172] In the patient who has an apical diastolic rumbling murmur, echocardiography can determine the cause from among mitral stenosis, aortic regurgitation (Austin Flint murmur), left atrial myxoma, and mitral regurgitation.[19]

The aortic valve in patients with *valvular aortic stenosis* may show thickening, calcification, and reduced mobility of the leaflets (Figs. 120-23*A* and 120-31). Aortic stenosis is usually associated with concentric left ventricular hypertrophy and a dilated aortic root. Although two-dimensional echocardiography is not quite as accurate in quantitating aortic valve area as it is with mitral valve area, its ability to distinguish mild from severe aortic stenosis is often adequate for clinical purposes.[173,174] Problems in diagnosis occur in elderly patients, especially those with hypertension, who may show aortic leaflet thickening (fibrosis, sclerosis, or annular calcification).

A *bicuspid aortic valve* is best diagnosed by two-dimensional visualization of the aortic valve, since this technique offers the advantage of being able to determine leaflet morphology as well as cusp num-

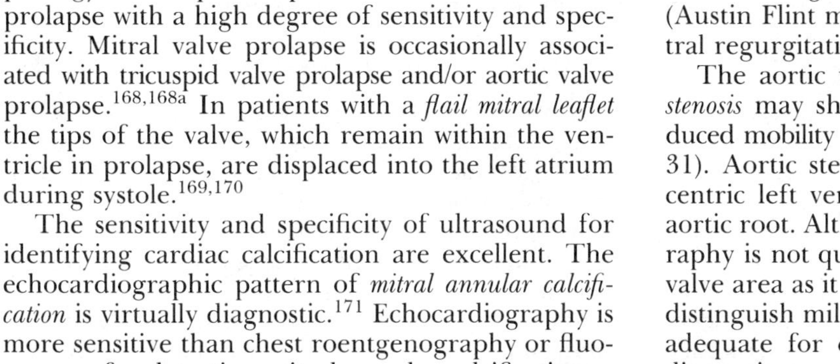

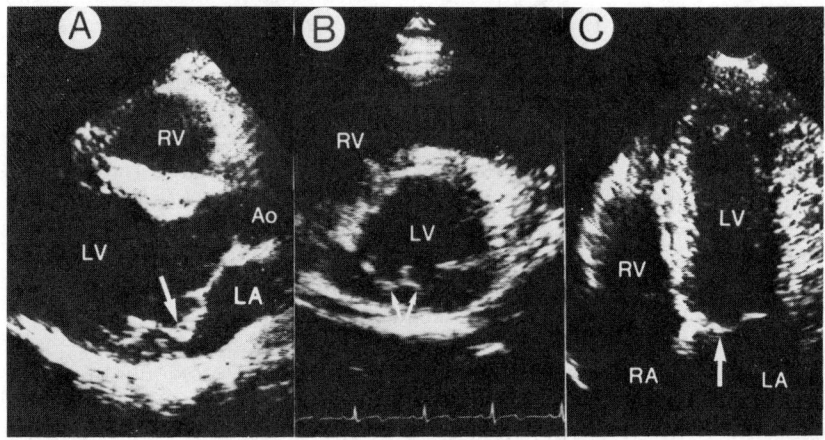

FIGURE 120-30 Two-dimensional echocardiogram from a patient with severe mitral valve prolapse. *A*. Parasternal long-axis view in systole shows the anterior and posterior leaflets arching posteriorly (arrow), above the level of the atrioventricular groove and behind the normal coaptation point into the left atrium. *B*. Parasternal short-axis view, at the level of the mitral valve and left ventricular outflow tract in systole, shows the anterior leaflet buckling posteriorly (arrows). *C*. The apical four-chamber view in systole shows the classic image of a prolapsing anterior mitral leaflet (arrow). RV = right ventricle; LV = left ventricle; Ao = aorta; RA = right atrium.

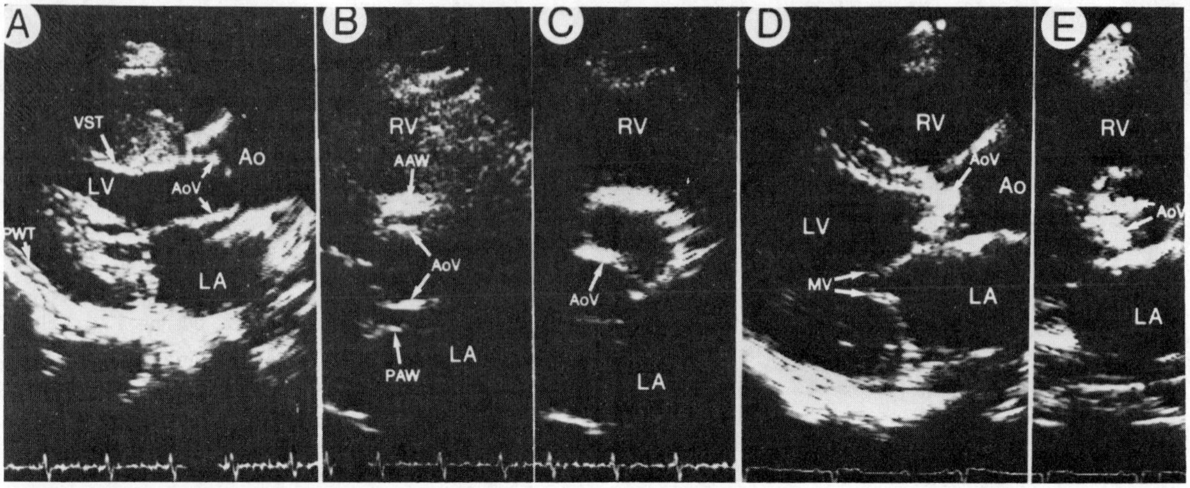

FIGURE 120-31 Two-dimensional echocardiograms from two patients with severe aortic stenosis, one with a bicuspid valve (*A,B,C*) and the other with a calcified trileaflet valve (*D,E*). *A*. Parasternal long-axis view shows systolic doming of anterior and posterior cusps of the aortic valve (AoV). During diastole, not shown, the aortic cusps prolapsed (bulged inferiorly) into the left ventricular outflow tract. Left ventricular hypertrophy is present, and the left atrium (LA) is dilated. *B*. Parasternal short-axis view, at the level of the aortic valve in systole, shows only two aortic cusps that are parallel to the anterior (AAW) and posterior (PAW) aortic walls. *C*. Same as view *B*, in diastole, shows that the closure of the aortic valve is represented by an abnormal, dominant, single echo, which appears S-shaped. *D*. Parasternal long-axis view in systole shows a dense mass of calcium totally obscuring the leaflets and orifice of the aortic valve (AoV). *E*. Parasternal short-axis view, at the level of the aorta in systole, shows a heavily calcified trileaflet aortic valve with markedly reduced opening. VST = ventricular septal thickness; PWT = posterior wall thickness; Ao = aorta; RV = right ventricle.

ber (Fig. 120-31).[175] The sensitivity (78 percent) and specificity (96 percent) of the two-dimensional diagnosis of a bicuspid valve has been determined.[176] Analysis of the aortic valve can also establish the diagnosis of a flail aortic leaflet[177] and aortic valve prolapse.[178] Two-dimensional echocardiography can visualize the entire thoracic aorta[179] and therefore is extremely valuable in diagnosing abnormalities of the aorta (e.g., dissecting aneurysm,[180,181] saccular aneurysm,[182,183] and coarctation[184]).

Currently, echocardiography is the only technique available that can visualize a vegetation, except for cardiac surgery. *Infective vegetations* have been described on all four of the cardiac valves.[185–188] They appear as bright, mobile, echo-dense structures attached to the valve leaflets. They are usually 2 to 40 mm in size and often move in a direction and speed different from that of the leaflet itself (Figs. 120-22*A* and 120-23*B*). The presence of a vegetation allows confirmation of the diagnosis and provides localization of involvement. There is substantial controversy, however, as to its meaning when detected by echocardiography.[15,187] For instance, the mere presence of a vegetation is not, by itself, an indication for surgery; nor is its size. The absence of a vegetation on echocardiography does not rule out endocarditis, since normal studies may be obtained with M mode in more than half of the patients with clinically diagnosed infective endocarditis. Two-dimensional echocardiography, however, is much more sensitive, imaging vegetations in 70 to 85 percent of cases.[189] Two-dimensional echocardiography can not only estimate vegetation size, shape, and mobility but also can detect some of the complications of endocarditis, such as leaflet destruction and valve ring abscess.[190] If significant leaflet involvement is found, serial studies should be performed, since echocardiography is useful in assessing the extent of damage and the hemodynamic consequences. Serial echocardiograms, however, are not generally useful in assessing antibacterial therapy, since vegetations may persist for months to years after initial infection and bacteriologic cure.[19] A predischarge echocardiogram should be obtained to provide a baseline study, especially in drug-abuse patients, since recurrences are likely.

Two-dimensional echocardiography has become the technique of choice for identifying *intracardiac masses,* since this method allows display of intracardiac structures in a spatial manner and visualizes areas of the heart that are not accessible by other noninvasive techniques (e.g., right atrium and left atrial appendage). Cardiac tumors, including atrial myxomas (Fig. 120-22*A*), sarcomas, and metastases as well as thromboembolic material have been identified in each of the cardiac chambers.[191–199]

Echocardiography has been useful in patients with suspected *ischemic heart disease* for the evaluation of chest pain, determination of left ventricular performance, and diagnosis of acute myocardial infarction and its complications.[200–203a] The two-dimensional mode has become the principal echocardiographic technique in these patients,[204–209] but M-mode echocardiography is a useful adjunct because it can accurately record wall motion. M-mode echocardiography, however, cannot quantitate the amount of abnormally moving myocardium and cannot image all of the areas of the left ventricle

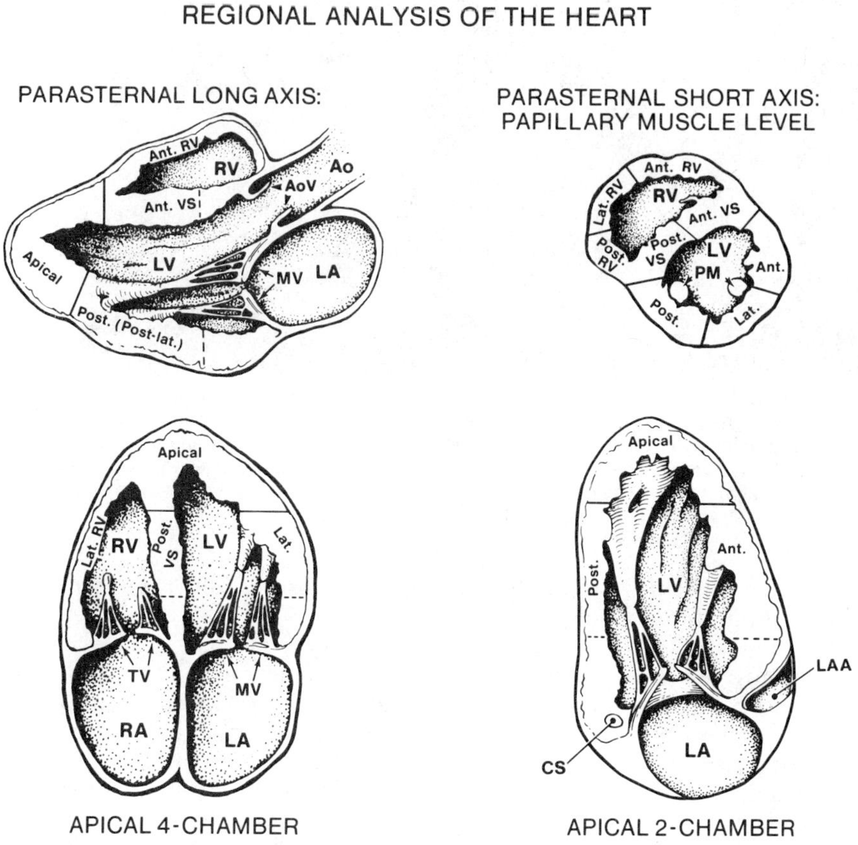

FIGURE 120-32 Some of the two-dimensional echocardiograms used to identify the regional anatomy of the ventricles and the method of subdividing the myocardial walls into three regions of equal length. Each level extends approximately one-third of the distance from base to apex. The parasternal long-axis view shows the approximate location of the cardiac apex, since it is usually not seen in this plane. The apical, mid, and basal portions of the anterior septum (Ant. VS) and the posterior (Post.) walls are illustrated. The posterolateral (Post-Lat) wall may be obtained with slight change in transducer orientation. The right ventricular free wall is the anterior wall (Ant. RV). The parasternal short-axis view of the left ventricle, at the level of the papillary muscle, is shown as an example of the short-axis views (i.e., apex and mitral valve levels) that should also be evaluated. The left ventricular (LV) wall is divided into five segments, the septum into anterior and posterior segments, and the right ventricular wall into anterior, lateral, and posterior segments. The apical four-chamber view identifies the apical, mid, and basal portions of the posterior septum (Post. VS) and the left ventricular lateral (Lat) wall. The right ventricular free wall is the lateral wall (Lat. RV). The apical two-chamber view identifies the apical, mid, and basal portions of the anterior (Ant.) and posterior (Post.) walls of the left ventricle. (Posterior is synonymous with inferior). *(From D. J. Sahn and F. Anderson, "Two-Dimensional Anatomy of the Heart. An Atlas for Echocardiographers," copyright © 1982 John Wiley & Son, New York. Adapted and reproduced with permission from John Wiley & Sons, Inc., and the author.)*

(e.g., the apex and lateral wall). If images of suitable quality are obtained, it is possible with two-dimensional echocardiography to analyze ventricular wall motion on a regional basis and to apply quantitative descriptions to each segment of the myocardium.[202,205] A variety of methods have been used to divide the left and right ventricles anatomically.[46–49,56] One method of *regional analysis* and nomenclature that may be of considerable help in the evaluation of patients with suspected coronary artery disease is shown in Fig. 120-32. In patients with suspected ischemic heart disease all segments of the left ventricle must be evaluated systematically and related one to another in order to build a true three-dimensional image.

Echocardiographic abnormalities occurring in patients with ischemic heart disease include changes in structure, such as thinning of the myocardial walls, and changes in wall motion (i.e., hypokinetic, akinetic, and dyskinetic changes). Visual assessment of the absence of myocardial wall thickening or actual thinning of the wall are specific, but not sensitive, signs of the presence of myocardial infarction.[210–213] They are, however, more specific than are wall motion abnormalities, and they are especially useful when conduction abnormalities such as left bundle branch block are associated with the infarction. The simplest method of assessing wall motion is to note the differences between normal and abnormal adjacent segments.[214] Extensive regional wall motion abnormalities on two-dimensional echocardiography in patients with myocardial ischemia have predictive value and are useful in identifying high-risk patients.[208] Because of differences in views, however, it is often difficult to make size comparisons between two-dimensional and angiographic assessments of wall motion abnormalities. Wall motion studies are extremely useful in excluding transmural myocardial infarction, since virtually all areas of transmural infarction will show akinesis or dyskinesis. Not all wall motion abnormalities are associated with demonstrable pathology, however, and subendocardial infarction may exist with an apparently normal echocardiogram.

Echocardiography also has prognostic value in patients with myocardial infarction, because it shows the relation and the extent of echocardiographic asynergy and the outcome of the infarction.[208] The

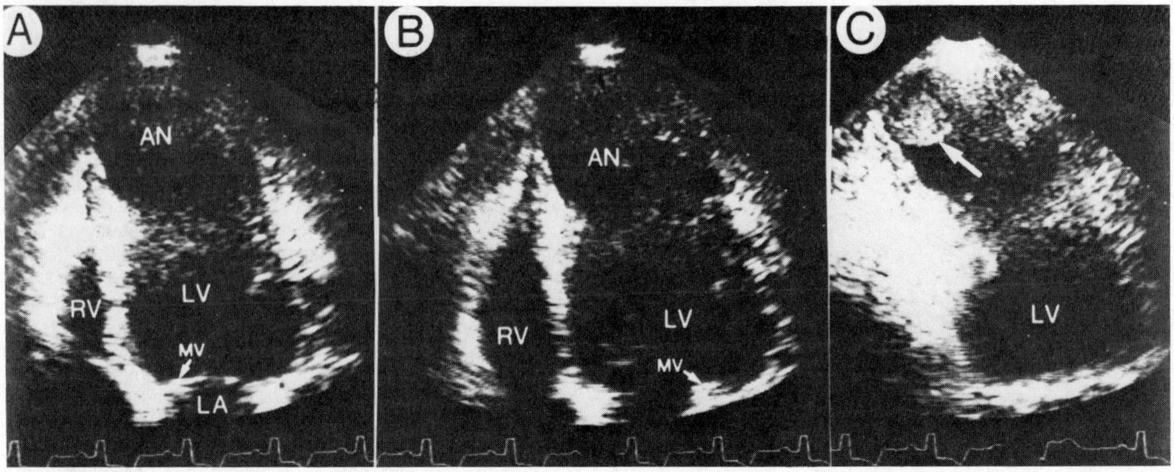

FIGURE 120-33 Two-dimensional echocardiogram from a patient with a recent anterior myocardial infarction. *A*. Systolic frame of the apical four-chamber view. *B*. Diastolic frame of the same view. Both show a large apical aneurysm (AN). The left ventricle (LV) is moderately dilated at its base, but there is extensive thinning of the apical wall. The aneurysm has a wide neck and fundus. *C*. Apical two-chamber view shows a round mass (arrow) partially filling the aneurysm as it extends from the surface of the akinetic wall, indicative of a mural thrombus. RV = right ventricle; LA = left atrium; MV = mitral valve.

extent of ischemic damage,[215] the presence of right ventricular infarction,[216] and certain complications such as left ventricular dysfunction,[217] aneurysm,[218] pseudoaneurysm,[219] and left ventricular thrombi,[220] as well as ventricular septal defect [221] and papillary muscle rupture,[222] can be accurately diagnosed by two-dimensional echocardiography. *Left ventricular aneurysms* are thin-walled dyskinetic segments readily detected by two-dimensional echocardiography. They are typically located at the apex and show systolic expansion while the rest of the functioning myocardium contracts inwardly (Fig. 120-33). *Left ventricular thrombi* are frequently seen in patients with acute anterior myocardial infarction, particularly within a left ventricular aneurysm.[223] They are found usually at the left ventricular apex but are always in an area of decreased wall motion (Fig. 120-33). Appropriate use of the gain controls, together with multiple tomographic views, is very important if false-positive and false-negative results are to be avoided. Two-dimensional echocardiography has been reported to be the best method for detection of left ventricular thrombi associated with myocardial infarction, but age or activity cannot be determined.[196,223,224]

Two-dimensional echocardiography is also capable of directly visualizing the proximal portions of the coronary arteries.[224a] Both the right and left coronary arteries have been identified but are difficult to image, since they are constantly moving in and out of the plane of examination (Fig. 120-13). Left main coronary artery disease has been detected in some patients by two-dimensional echocardiography, but the sensitivity and specificity of the technique for this purpose has not been established.[225] In addition, patients with coronary artery disease may have high-intensity echoes, originating from the proximal portion of the left main coronary artery, that may be difficult to distinguish from surrounding structures.

The ability to image the cardiac structural relations and the lack of reliance on ionizing radiation have made echocardiography extremely useful in evaluating patients with congenital heart disease.[21,31,53,225a,225b] Valvular heart disease (e.g., bicuspid aortic valve and pulmonic stenosis) can be diagnosed, great vessel abnormalities (e.g., coarctation of the aorta) can be identified, and atrial and ventricular septal defects can be visualized directly and by contrast echocardiography.[226,227] Cyanotic heart lesions also readily lend themselves to echocardiographic recognition.[19–21,31,46,54] Even complex congenital heart lesions have been detailed noninvasively using deductive two-dimensional echocardiography and accurate identification of the great arteries, atrioventricular and semilunar valves, interatrial and interventricular septa, and orientation of the ventricles.[228,228a]

Ventricular Function

The assessment of cardiac performance, especially global and regional function of the left ventricle, is one of the most valuable clinical applications of echocardiography. Cardiac chamber size can be accurately measured by both M-mode and two-dimensional echocardiography. Left ventricular internal dimensions at end systole and end diastole provide a reliable index of left ventricular chamber size, are subject to the least interobserver variability, and are the most reproducible (Figs. 120-12 and 120-21*A*).[229–231] Virtually all indexes of left ventricular pump performance have been derived from measurements of volume and pressure. The indexes derived from volume measurements, however, have proved to be of greatest clinical value.[229] Left ventricular volumes can be calculated by M mode but are not valid in asynergic ventricles.[67,230–232] Two-dimensional echocardiography offers considerable advantage over M mode for quantitating volumes because a variety of tomographic slices of the left ventricle can be analyzed. The correlations between volumes determined by angiography and by two-dimensional echocardiography in patients with and without asynergy have been excellent (r = 0.8 to 0.9).[69–77]

Dynamic measurements of left ventricular function include (1) percent fractional shortening, (2) mean circumferential fiber shortening, (3) ejection fraction, (4) mitral E point–interventricular septal separation, (5) percent systolic wall thickening, and (6) wall motion analysis (i.e., hypokinesis, akinesis, dyskinesis). *Percent fractional shortening* of the left ventricle (percent delta D) is a valuable index of the overall left ventricular contractile state. This simple dimensional change, however, is valid only if regional contraction abnormalities are minimal or absent. Determination of mean circumferential fiber shortening (V_{CF}), calculated in the same manner as percent delta D except that ejection time is taken into consideration, is also a useful index of left ventricular performance but does not offer any practical advantages over percent delta D in characterizing left ventricular function. The *mitral E point–septal separation* (EPSS) has proved to be a sensitive and specific indicator of global left ventricular performance (Fig. 120-4).[39,40] EPSS is independent of left ventricular size and is not influenced by regional wall motion abnormalities. *Ejection fraction* is the most useful single index of left ventricular function because it correlates best with the patient's clinical outcome.[81,82] M-mode ejection fraction, however, offers no advantage over the simpler percent delta D expression of contractility and may give spurious information in patients with segmental wall abnormalities. The ejection fraction derived from two-dimensional echocardiographic volumes, however, has been shown to have a more consistent relation to angiographic ejection fraction whether or not asynergy is present.

Two-dimensional echocardiography appears to be the ideal modality for analyzing left ventricular motion, since virtually all segments of the myocardium are accessible with the variety of tomographic planes available. Several specific views, however, apply particularly to wall motion analysis because they reproducibly outline left ventricular anatomy. These are the parasternal long-axis view, the parasternal short-axis view at both the mitral and papillary muscle levels, and the apical four-chamber and two-chamber views (Fig. 120-32). Analysis of regional endocardial wall motion (i.e., hypokinesis, akinesis, and dyskinesis), as well as regional wall thickening, is necessary for discriminating between normal and ischemic or infarcted zones of myocardium. M-mode echocardiography is considerably restricted in analyzing regional left ventricular function, since it images only in the septal-posterolateral plane, and is unreliable in the presence of asynergy. Nevertheless, because of its high resolution (1 to 2 mm), regional wall motion analysis, including amplitude and rate of motion from end diastole to peak systole and measurements of thickening of both the left side of the septum and the posterior wall are even better than those obtained by radionuclide angiography.

The evaluation of right-sided cardiac chambers and function has not been reliable using M-mode echocardiography but has been greatly enhanced by two-dimensional echocardiography.[43,53,83–85] The right-sided structures are well seen in the parasternal long-axis right ventricular inflow tract view, since the anteroposterior dimension of the right ventricle and most of the right atrium are well visualized. Parasternal short-axis views of the left ventricle at the level of the chordae tendineae and parasternal short-axis views of the aortic root provide additional views of the right ventricle. The apical four-chamber view, however, appears to be the single most important view for evaluating the size and function of the right ventricle and the right atrium. Subcostal imaging of the inferior vena cava also provides useful information about the functional status of the right ventricle and right atrium.

Cardiac performance can also be evaluated indirectly by analyzing the motion of the heart valves with M-mode echocardiography. Mitral valve analysis can relate hemodynamic information as follows: (1) reduction in the diastolic (EF) slope suggests a reduced rate of left ventricular filling (Fig. 120-22*B*);[19,20] (2) premature closure suggests elevated left ventricular diastolic pressure, especially in patients with acute aortic regurgitation (Fig. 120-22*A*);[172] (3) increased EPSS inversely correlates with ejection fraction; (4) reduced E point amplitude or delayed valve opening with an accentuated A wave suggests elevated left ventricular early diastolic pressure, especially in patients with severe chronic aortic regurgitation (Fig. 120-22*A*);[19,20] and (5) a prominent shoulder (B notch) on the closing (AC) slope or a PR minus AC interval of less than 0.06 s suggests elevated left ventricular end-diastolic pressure (Fig. 120-22*B*).[20] The rate of left atrial emptying (or left ventricular filling) is reflected by the slope of the posterior aortic root in early diastole. It is another useful indirect measurement of left ventricular function. A flat posterior aortic wall in early diastole suggests reduced left ventricular filling.[233]

The area of opening of the aortic valve and the pattern of leaflet motion provide qualitative information about left ventricular stroke volume.[19,20] Among structurally normal aortic valves, cusp separation is a function of initial forward left ventricular stroke volume, whereas the distance between cusps throughout systole and the time the cusps remain separated are affected by aortic flow volume, velocity, and heart rate. In low-output states or with significant mitral regurgitation, the aortic leaflets tend to open abruptly but close gradually throughout sys-

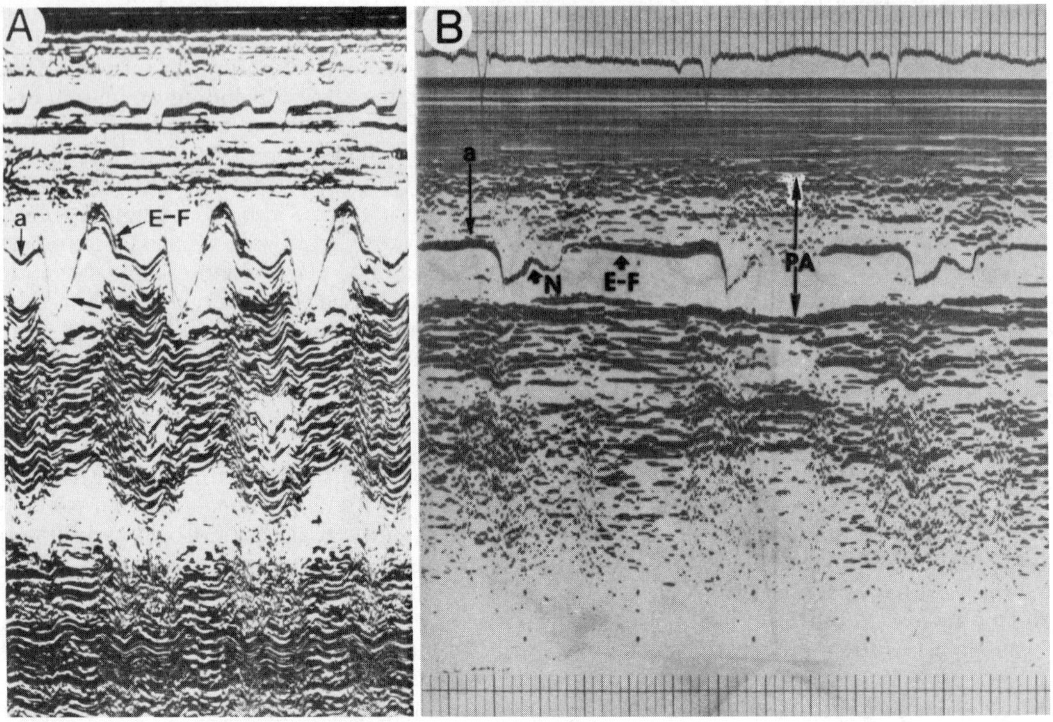

FIGURE 120-34 M-mode echocardiograms of the pulmonic valve from two patients. *A*. The normal posterior leaflet shows an *a* dip (arrow a) of 5 mm, a diastolic (EF) slope of 30 mm/s, and abrupt systolic opening and closing. *B*. The posterior leaflet from a patient with pulmonary hypertension shows an absent *a* dip (arrow a), flat EF slope, and notch (N) due to partial midsystolic closure. PA = pulmonary artery. (*A from J. M. Felner and R. C. Schlant, "Echocardiography: A Teaching Atlas," Grune & Stratton, Inc., New York, 1976, p. 34. Reproduced with permission from the publisher and author.*)

tole (early partial aortic valve closure) and, therefore, have a systolic pattern that more closely resembles a bullet than the usual parallelogram (Fig. 120-23*A*).[19] Premature opening of the aortic valve suggests markedly elevated left ventricular diastolic pressure, especially in patients with very severe aortic regurgitation (Fig. 120-23*B*).[234] Very early systolic partial closure (notch) is evidence of outflow tract obstruction in patients with discrete membranous subvalvular aortic stenosis, whereas early to midsystolic partial (notch) or complete closure is evidence of obstruction in patients with hypertrophic cardiomyopathy (Fig. 120-23*A*).[19,20]

Analysis of pulmonic valve motion may reveal the hemodynamic status of the right heart. Pulmonary arterial hypertension is suggested by a combination of reduced or absent *a* dip, midsystolic notch, flat EF slope and/or abnormal right-sided systolic time intervals (Fig. 120-34).[19,20] An abnormally large *a* dip suggests valvular pulmonic stenosis, whereas coarse systolic fluttering suggests infundibular pulmonic stenosis. However, a normal *a* dip may be seen in patients with pulmonary hypertension complicated by right heart failure, whereas an absent *a* dip may be seen in patients with valvular pulmonic stenosis and a fibrotic pulmonic valve. Tricuspid valve motion is also influenced by the functional status of the structures of the right side of the heart. For example, a prominent B notch on the tricuspid closing slope is evidence of elevated right ventricular end-diastolic pressure.[19,20]

Limitations of Echocardiography

As with all diagnostic procedures, echocardiography has its problems as well as its advantages.[235–239] The interpretation of echocardiograms is extremely difficult, and many technical as well as clinical factors may lead to erroneous or inaccurate diagnoses. The most important limitation of echocardiography is the inability to obtain a complete diagnostic examination in all patients referred for study; the delineation of all the important cardiac structures is achieved only 80 to 90 percent of the time.[19,20,53] Since ultrasound travels poorly, if at all, through bone, lung, and thick chest walls, ultrasonic examination of the heart may be very difficult or even impossible in certain patient groups, including: (1) elderly subjects, especially those with skeletal abnormalities such as pectus excavatum, (2) patients with severe pulmonary disease, especially those with emphysema, since the lung can be an insurmountable barrier to the cardiac examination because the air it contains is a very potent attenuator of ultrasonic energy, and (3) extremely obese patients, because the thick chest wall may attenuate the ultrasonic energy to the point where the return is indistinguishable from the background artifact.

The most notable limitation of *M-mode echocardiography* is its confining, ice-pick view of the heart.[20] Since the M-mode view lacks lateral projection, the spatial orientation of intracardiac structures cannot be readily appreciated. While it is possible to obtain useful information concerning intracardiac spatial relationships with an M-mode scan, it cannot be assumed that these time-motion recordings represent a true picture of the spatial relations between the targets. The resulting images are distorted by both the time that it takes to perform the sweep and the constantly changing transducer-to-target distance. The inability to image some of the cardiac structures (e.g., the cardiac apex, right atrium, and inferior and lateral left ventricular walls) is another limitation of M mode.

A major limitation of *two-dimensional echocardiography* is the anatomic analysis. Classic tomographic slices of the heart have been made mostly in planes that parallel or cross the major axes of the trunk, not in those that consistently relate one intracardiac structure to another.[43,46] In addition, a variety of planes are needed to describe the anatomy, since small changes in the scanning planes are made during the examination. Furthermore, near structures that occupy the narrow portion of the fan-shaped image are stretched to accommodate the rectangular format of strip-chart recorders.

Misinterpretation of an ultrasound study is commonly due to technical limitations. There is a real danger of mistaking artifacts or extraneous echoes, which result from the aberrent or unexplained behavior of reflected ultrasound, for evidence of cardiac pathology.[238] It is possible for ultrasound to be reflected twice from a cardiac structure and appear on the echocardiographic tracing as an abnormal echo. These reverberatory or "phantom echoes" are the most common artifacts. They result from multiple reflections of acoustic energy and affect both the M-mode display and the two-dimensional images.[235] Careful measurement shows that these artifacts give the false impression of a second interface virtually twice as far from the transducer as the true echo (first interface), and their amplitude will be twice as large.[18,238,239] These reechoes may also occur between structures within the heart, resulting in an apparent deepening of the position of the structure and inversion of the phase of its motion pattern. Reverberations also occur within a fibrotic or calcified valve. This might partially explain the multilayered appearance of the mitral valve in patients with mitral stenosis and invalidates the thickness measurements. Another example of reverberations are the lung echoes that often obscure the entire image during inspiration. These shallow echoes are simply multiple reflections between the transducer and the lung or between the chest wall and the lung. Reverberations may also be recorded from intracardiac catheters, pacing wires, or prosthetic valves.[235,239] Ultrasound reflected from the plastic casing of the scan head of two-dimensional transducers tends to appear within the left ventricular image near its apex, thus mimicking a mural thrombus.

Artifactual echoes may also be produced by incorrect use of the echocardiographic controls.[238] Inappropriately high gain settings cause targets to "bloom" (i.e., appear larger and more distorted than their actual size and shape). This may result in valve orifices appearing reduced on two-dimensional echocardiographic studies when they are compared with the other targets. Other problems resulting from excessive gain include (1) false-negative diagnoses because of obliteration of the echo-free space, as might be seen in the presence of a pericardial effusion; (2) reduction in left ventricular cavity size by lengthening the trailing edge of the left-sided septal echo.[14,16] Since an interface is best displayed by the leading edge of its echo and not by its trailing edge, the use of high-gain settings to visualize the septum will lengthen the trailing edge of the left-sided septal echo; (3) cloudlike noise in cardiac cavities, which may be misread as intracardiac thrombi. Artifacts can also be produced by inappropriate use of the near-gain compensation control and time-gain compensation (TGC) control. The most common error introduced by incorrect use of these echocardiographic controls is the elimination of a portion of the echoes from the right side of the interventricular septum or even from the entire septum itself. This kind of artifact can be avoided by a judicious use of the TGC control, even if this results in unwanted echoes in the right ventricle.[236,237]

All transducers have beam patterns that contain "side lobe" artifacts. These weaker beams of ultrasound energy are adjacent to the main beam and are generated from the edges of the individual transducer elements. They appear as an arclike, hazily bordered, lateral extension of a prominent echo-producing structure.[238,239] Characteristically, side lobe artifacts produce extended echoes from strong reflecting surfaces such as pericardium, calcified valves, or prostheses and are depicted throughout the full sector image. Although these phantom echoes are generally weaker in intensity than those reflected from the main beam, they may occasionally be confused with true anatomic structure. Side lobe artifacts can usually be diminished or eliminated by decreasing the gain settings or increasing the reject level of the ultrasound instruments.

One of the most serious limitations of the echocardiographic systems in current use is the width of the ultrasound beam, which determines lateral resolution.[20,42,43,238,239] Ultrasound energy cannot be accurately focused over the entire depth range of the beam but spreads over a finite angle. This causes some echoes to appear as if they are from structures in the central beam, whereas, in fact, they are echoes from structures off the main or display axis. These nonstructural spurious echoes are displayed at a site where there is no directly corresponding anatomic structure and may result in misinterpretation of clinical tracings. An echo from a target on the edge of the ultrasound beam may be displayed as if it were in the middle and will, therefore, not represent the true location of the target. The intensity of echoes from reflecting structures may vary widely, since they depend on several physical factors such as distance traveled, acoustic impedance, and angle of incidence of the sound beam. Thus, only structures that are relatively perpendicular to the ultrasonic beam will be accurately recorded, and target "dropout" results when the transducer-to-target relation is not maintained. Target dropout is quite common in two-dimensional echocardiography, because the multiple ultrasonic beams that are directed from the transducer are reflected from irregular cardiac targets, only some of which may be perpendicular to the interrogating beam.[46,238] Dropouts of the interventricular septum may falsely suggest the existence of an interventricular septal defect, whereas endocardial dropouts hamper the correct identification of the true ventricular wall contour in stop-frame images.

Two-dimensional images are displayed on a cathode ray tube during the examination and recorded on videotape, using a standard television camera or a digital scan converter, for a permanent record and subsequent analysis. This process may deteriorate image quality. In most systems only half of the scan lines, and thus only one-half of the information available during real-time study, is available for all off-line analyses. In addition, there is loss of information when the video format is displayed in stop-action. Furthermore, videotape remains a difficult, expensive, and cumbersome medium for data storage and retrieval. The television format itself can produce ghosts (persistent artifacts of structures that had appeared on the screen a moment before and had not quite faded away when the next image arrived).[43,238]

Electrical interference elsewhere in the building can also produce artifacts that appear as irregular, fine, linear markings on the tracing, with abrupt onset and cessation.[16,43,238] They should not be mistaken for the microbubbles produced by saline solution injections in contrast echocardiography or for swirling intracavitary blood in patients with low-cardiac-output syndromes.

Pitfalls may also be related to improper examination technique. Most of these limitations are related to M-mode echocardiography, since transducer position on the chest wall influences motion patterns on M-mode echocardiograms.[38] When the transducer is at a higher than standard interspace, the anterior aortic wall is closer to the transducer than the septum is, and a false pattern of aortic-septal discontinuity may be recorded. A high transducer position can also give a pattern suggestive of mitral valve prolapse in normal subjects because the mitral leaflets move away from the transducer during systole when the base of the left ventricle moves toward the apex.

For most cardiac diseases clinical information is highly valuable for making intelligent echocardiographic conclusions. Professional interpretation of the echocardiogram should not be separated from the individual conducting the study, and interpretation should be based only on what can be definitely identified. Making judgments from incomplete echoes or in the absence of electrocardiographic reference should be avoided.[236–238] As an example, paradoxical septal motion is not a specific abnormality and is seen in many conditions, such as right ventricular volume overload lesions and myocardial infarction and after open heart surgery or in the presence of left bundle branch block as shown by electrocardiogram. Changing sensitivity and specificity of various echocardiographic criteria must also be known. For instance, asymmetric septal hypertrophy, once believed specific for hypertrophic cardiomyopathy, now is known to occur in newborns and in patients with systemic hypertension, aortic stenosis, pulmonary hypertension, and a variety of congenital heart diseases.

Future of Echocardiography

Several developments that are presently under investigation offer an exciting future for echocardiography. These include computerizing ("digitizing") the ultrasonic image, ultrasound tissue characterization, and three-dimensional echocardiography. Most of the newer ultrasound equipment presently displays the echocardiographic images in a digital rather than analog format.[240,241] *Digital image processing* improves the image and allows for manipulation and evaluation of echoes by computer. Its main clinical uses include (1) ability to obtain quantitative information, (2) structure enhancement and identification that make regional wall motion abnormalities more apparent,[242] (3) three-dimensional reconstructing, and (4) detailed acoustic analysis of tissue.

Ultrasound tissue characterization is the study of using ultrasound to gain information about tissues beyond simply locating the positions of major cardiac structures and studying their motion patterns.[243] Clinical areas in which echocardiography has recognized alterations in cardiac tissue include the detection of fibrosis and calcification and the identification of myocardial scar.[244] Scarred areas of the myocardium, for example, are more echo-intense and thinner than normal muscle. An alteration in the myocardial echoes has also been noted in patients with hypertrophic cardiomyopathy and amyloid heart disease.[245] Thus far, most of the observations using echocardiography for the analysis of tissue type have been qualitative in nature. Conversion of the gray-scale image to color, which enhances the differences in the returning echoes and permits better identification of tissue types, has been performed, is commercially available, and may provide the impetus for further advancement in this area.[246] The increasing use of computer analysis of echocardiographic data should help develop a quantative method for identifying subtle changes in acoustic properties, whether they be in color or various shades of gray.

Reconstructed three-dimensional echocardiography may provide an enhanced appreciation for spatially oriented data. Several techniques are available for assessing the position and angle of the ultrasonic transducer, which is all that is necessary for the reconstruction of multiple two-dimensional images into a three-dimensional display.[247,248] Irrespective of how a three-dimensional echocardiogram is obtained, it theoretically should provide a more accurate spatial image of the heart and thus provide more accurate quantitative and qualitative information.

References

1. Keidel, W. D.: Uber eine Methode zur Registriering der Volumanderungen des Herzens am Menschen: 2. *Z. Kreisl-Forsch*, 39:257, 1950.
2. Edler, I., and Hertz, C. H.: The Use of Ultrasonic Reflectoscope for the Continuous Recording of Movement of Heart Walls, *Kungl Fysiogr Sallski Fund Forhandl*, 24:5, 1954.
3. Edler, I.: Diagnostic Use of Ultrasound in Heart Disease, *Acta. Med. Scand.*, 308:32, 1955.
4. Holmes, J. H., Howry, D. H., Posakony, G. J., et al.: Ultrasonic Visualization of Soft Tissue Structures in Human Body, *Trans. Am. Clin. Climatol. Assoc.* 66:208, 1955.
5. Edler, I., and Gustafson, A.: Ultrasound Cardiogram in Mitral Stenosis, *Acta. Med. Scand.* 159:85, 1957.
6. Joyner, C. R., Reid, J. M., and Bond, J. P.: Reflected Ultrasound in the Assessment of Mitral Valve Disease, *Circulation*, 27:503, 1963.
7. Feigenbaum, H., Waldhausen, J. A., and Hyde, P. P.: Ultrasound Diagnosis of Pericardial Effusion, *JAMA*, 191:107, 1965.
8. Joyner, C. R., Jr., and Reid, J. M.: Application of Ultrasound in Cardiology and Cardiovascular Physiology, *Progr. Cardiovasc. Dis.*, 5:482, 1963.
9. Ebina, T., Oka, S., Tanaka, M., Kosaka, S., et al.: The Ultrasonotomography of the Heart and Great Vessels in Living Human Subjects by Means of Ultrasonic Reflection Technique, *Jpn. Heart J.* 8:331, 1967.
10. Bom N., Lancee, C. T., Jr., Van Zwieten, G., Kloster, F. E., and Roelandt, J.: Multiscan Echocardiography: I. Technical Description, *Circulation*, 48:1066, 1973.
11. Baker, D. W.: Pulsed Ultrasonic Doppler Blood-Flow Sensing, *IEEE Trans. Sonics Ultrasonics*, 1970, vol. SU-17, no. 3.
12. Skorton, D. J., McNary, C. A., Child, J. S., et al.: Real-Time Computerization of Two-Dimensional Echocardiography, *Am. Heart J.*, 101:783, 1981.
13. Garcia, E., Gueret, P., Bennet, M., et al.: Digital Image Processing of Two-Dimensional Echocardiograms: Identification of the Endocardium, *Am. J. Cardiol.*, 48:479, 1981.
14. Wells, P. N. T.: "Physical Principles of Ultrasonic Diagnosis," Academic Press, London, 1969.
15. Kremkau, F. W.: Physical Principles of Ultrasound, *Semin. Roentgenol.* 10:259, 1975.
16. Hillard, W.: Basic Physics of Ultrasound, in J. Schapira, Y. Charuzi, R. M. Davidson (eds.), "Two-Dimensional Echocardiography," The Williams & Wilkins Company, Baltimore, 1982, p. 319.
17. Woodward, B., Pond, J. B., and Warwick, R.: How Safe is Diagnostic Sonar? *Br. J. Radiol.*, 43:719, 1970.
18. Roelandt, J., van Dorp, W. C., Bom, N., Laird, J. D., and Hugenholta, P. G.: Resolution Problems in Echocardiography: A Source of Interpretation Error, *Am. J. Cardiol.*, 37:256, 1976.
19. Felner, J. M., and Schlant, R. C.: "Echocardiography: A Teaching Atlas," Grune and Stratton, Inc., New York, 1976.
20. Feigenbaum, H.: "Echocardiography," 2d ed., Lea & Febiger, Philadelphia, 1976.
21. Meyer, R. A.: "Pediatric Echocardiography," Lea & Febiger, Philadelphia, 1977.
22. Goldberg, B. B.: Suprasternal Ultrasonography, *JAMA*, 215:245, 1971.
23. Goldberg, B. B., and Pollack, H. M.: Ultrasonically Studied Pericardiocentesis, *Am. J. Cardiol.*, 31:490, 1973.
24. Weyman, A. E.: "Cross-Sectional Echocardiography," Lea & Febiger, Philadelphia, 1982.
25. King, D. L.: Cardiac Ultrasonography: A Stop-Action Technique for Imaging Intracardiac Anatomy, *Radiology*, 103:387, 1972.
26. Griffith, J. M., and Henry, W. L.: A Sector Scanner for Real Time Two-Dimensional Echocardiography, *Circulation*, 49:1147, 1974.
27. von Ramm, O. T., and Thurstone, R. L.: Cardiac Imaging Using a Phased Array Ultrasonic System: I. System Design, *Circulation*, 53:258, 1976.
28. Thurstone, F. L., and von Ramm, O. T.: Electronic Beam Steering for Ultrasonic Imaging, in M. de Vlieger, D. N. White, and V. R. McCready (eds.), "Ultrasound in Medicine," American Elsevier Publishing Company, Inc., New York, 1974, p. 304.
29. Nishimura, K., Hibi, N., Fukui, T., et al.: Real-Time Observation of Cardiac Movement and Structures in Congenital and Acquired Heart Disease Employing High-Speed Ultrasonocardiotomography, *Am. Heart J.*, 92:340, 1976.
30. Henry, W. L.: Evaluation of Left Ventricular Function Using Two-Dimensional Echocardiography, *Am. J. Cardiol.*, 49:319, 1982.
31. Silverman, N. H., and Snider, A. R.: "Two-Dimensional Echocardiography in Congenital Heart Disease," Appleton-Century-Crofts, Inc., Norwalk, 1982.
32. Chang, S., and Feigenbaum, H.: Subxyphoid Echocardiography, *J. Clin. Ultrasound*, 1:14, 1973.
33. Starling, M. R., Crawford, M. H., O'Rourke, R. A., Groves, B. M., and Amon, K. W.: Accuracy of Subxiphoid Echocardiography for Assessing Left Ventricular Size and Performance, *Circulation*, 61:367, 1980.
34. Chang, S., Feigenbaum, H., and Dillon, J. C.: Condensed M-Mode Echocardiographic Scan of the Symmetrical Left Ventricle, *Chest*, 68:93, 1975.
35. Sahn, D., DeMaria, A., Kisslo, J., and Weyman, A.: Recommendations Regarding Quantitation in M-Mode Echocardiography: Results of a Survey of Echocardiographic Measurements, *Circulation*, 58:1072, 1978.
36. Friedman, M., Roeske, W. R., Sahn, D. J., Larson, D., and Goldberg, S. J., Accuracy of M-Mode Echocardiographic Measurements of the Left Ventricle, *Am. J. Cardiol.*, 49:716, 1982.
37. Crawford, M. H., Grant, D., O'Rourke, R. A., Starling, M. R., and Groves, B. M.: Accuracy and Reproducibility of New M-Mode Echocardiographic Recommendations for Measuring Left Ventricular Dimensions, *Circulation*, 61:137, 1980.
38. Popp, R., Filly, K., Brown, O. R., and Harrison, D. C.: Effect of Transducer Placement on Echocardiographic Measurement of Left Ventricular Dimension, *Am. J. Cardiol.*, 35:537, 1975.
39. Massie, B. M., Schiller, N. B., Ratshin, R. A., and Parmley, W. W.: Mitral-Septal Separation: New Echocardiographic Index of Left Ventricular Function, *Am. J. Cardiol.*, 39:1008, 1977.
40. Child, J. S., Krivokapich, J., and Perloff, J. K.: Effect of Left Ventricular Size on Mitral E Point to Ventricular Septal Separation in Assessment of Cardiac Performance, *Am. Heart J.*, 101:797, 1981.
41. Gardin, J. M., Henry, W. L., Savage, D. D., Ware, J. H., Burn, C., and Borer, J. S., Echocardiographic Measurements in Normal Subjects: Evaluation of an Adult Population without Clinically Apparent Heart Disease, *J. Clin. Ultrasound*, 7:439, 1979.
42. Henry, W. L., Gardin, J. M., and Ware, J. H.: Echocardiographic Measurements in Normal Subjects from Infancy to Old Age, *Circulation*, 62:1054, 1980.
43. Tajik, A. J., Seward, J. B., Hagler, D. J., Mair, D. D., and Lie, J. T.: Two-Dimensional Real-Time Ultrasonic Imaging of the Heart and Great Vessels. Technique Image Orientation, Structure, Identification, and Validation, *Mayo. Clin. Proc.*, 53:271, 1978.

44. DeMaria, A. N., Bommer, W., Joye, J. A., and Mason, D. T.: Cross-Sectional Echocardiography: Physical Principles, Anatomic Planes, Limitations and Pitfalls, *Am. J. Cardiol.*, 46:1097, 1980.
45. Henry, W. L., DeMaria, A., Gramiak, R., et al.: Report of the American Society of Echocardiography Committee on Nomenclature and Standards in Two-Dimensional Echocardiography, *Circulation*, 62:212, 1980.
46. Sahn, D. J., and Anderson, F.: "Two-Dimensional Anatomy of the Heart. An Atlas for Echocardiographers," John Wiley and Son, New York, 1982.
47. Edwards, W. D., Tajik, A. J., and Seward J. B.: Standardized Nomenclature and Anatomic Basis for Regional Tomographic Analysis of the Heart, *Mayo. Clin. Proc.*, 56:479, 1981.
48. Bierman, F. Z., and Williams, R. G.: Subxiphoid Two-Dimensional Imaging of the Interatrial Septum in Infants with Congenital Heart Disease, *Circulation*, 60:80, 1979.
49. Shub, C., Dimopoulos, I. N., Seward, J. B., Callahan, J. A., et al.: Sensitivity of Two-Dimensional Echocardiography in the Direct Visualization of Atrial Septal Defect Utilizing the Subcostal Approach: Experience With 154 Patients, *J. Am. Coll. Cardiol.*, 2:127, 1983.
50. Snider, R. A., and Silverman, N. H.: Suprasternal Notch Echocardiography: A Two-Dimensional Technique for Evaluating Congenital Heart Disease, *Circulation*, 63:165, 1981.
51. Schnittger, I., Gordon, E. P., Fitzgerald, P. J., and Popp, R. L.: Standardized Intracardiac Measurements of Two-Dimensional Echocardiography, *J. Am. Coll. Cardiol.*, 2:934, 1983.
52. Wyatt, H. L., Haendchen, R. V., Meerbaum, S., and Corday, E., Assessment of Quantitative Methods for Two-Dimensional Echocardiography, *Am. J. Cardiol.*, 52:396, 1983.
53. Hagan, A. D., DiSessa, T. G., Bloor, C. M., and Calleja, H. B.: "Two-Dimensional Echocardiography. Clinical-Pathological Correlations in Adult and Congenital Heart Disease," Little, Brown and Company, Boston, 1983.
54. Reicheck, N., and Devereaux, R. B., Left Ventricular Hypertrophy: Relationship of Anatomic, Electrocardiographic, and Echocardiographic Findings, *Circulation*, 63:1391, 1981.
55. Woythaler, J. N., Singer, S. L., Kwan, O., Meltzer, R. S., Reubner, B., Bommer, W., and DeMaria, A.: Accuracy of Echocardiography versus Electrocardiography in Detecting Left Ventricular Hypertrophy: Comparison with Postmortem Mass Measurements, *J. Am. Coll. Cardiol.*, 2:305, 1983.
56. Reicheck, N., Helak, J., Plappert, T., St. John-Sutton, M., and Weber, K. T.: Anatomic Validation of Left Ventricular Mass Estimates from Clinical Two-Dimensional Echocardiography. Initial Results, *Circulation*, 67:348, 1983.
57. Bommer, W., Weinert, L., Neumann, A., Mason, D. T., and DeMaria, A.: Determination of Right Atrial and Right Ventricular Size by Two-Dimensional Echocardiography, *Circulation*, 60:91, 1979.
58. Prakish, R.: Echocardiographic Diagnosis of Right Ventricular Hypertrophy: Correlation with ECG and Necropsy Findings in 248 Patients, *Cathet. Cardiovasc. Diagn.*, 7:179, 1981.
59. Feigenbaum, H.: Echocardiographic Examination of the Left Ventricle, *Circulation*, 51:1, 1975.
60. Feigenbaum, H., Popp, R. L., Wolfe, S. B., Troy, B. L., Pombo, J. F., Haine, C. L., and Dodge, H. T.: Ultrasound Measurements of the Left Ventricle: A Correlative Study with Angiography, *Arch. Intern. Med.*, 129:461, 1972.
61. Belenkie, I., Nutter, D. O., Clark, D. W., McGraw, D. B., and Raizner, A. E.: Assessment of Left Ventricular Dimensions and Functions by Echocardiography, *Am. J. Cardiol.*, 31:755, 1973.
62. Bennett, D. H., and Evans, D. W.: Correlation of Left Ventricular Mass Determined by Echocardiography with Vectorcardiographic and Electrocardiographic Voltage Measurements, *Br. Heart J.*, 36:981, 1974.
63. Fortuin, N. J., Hood, W. P., Jr., and Craige, E.: Evaluation of Left Ventricular Function by Echocardiography, *Circulation*, 46:26, 1972.
64. Gibson, D. G.: Estimation of Left Ventricular Size by Echocardiography, *Br. Heart J.*, 35:128, 1972.
65. Ludbrook, P., Karliner, J. S., Peterson, K., Leopold, G., and O'Rourke, R. A.: Comparison of Ultrasound and Cineangiographic Measurements of Left Ventricular Performance in Patients with and without Wall Motion Abnormalities, *Br. Heart J.*, 35:1026, 1973.
66. Murray, J. A., Johnston, W., and Reed, J.: Echocardiographic Determination of Left Ventricular Dimension, Volumes and Performance, *Am. J. Cardiol.*, 30:252, 1972.
67. Teichholz, L. E., Kruelen, T. H., Herman, M. V., and Gorlin, R.: Problems in Echocardiographic Volume Determinations: Echo-Angiographic Correlation, *Circulation*, 46:1175, 1972.
68. Abdulla, A. M., Frank, M. J., Canedo, M. L., and Stefadouros, J. A.: Limitations of Echocardiography in the Assessment of Left Ventricular Size and Function in Aortic Regurgitation, *Circulation*, 61:148, 1980.
69. Starling, M. R., Crawford, M. H., Sorensen, S. G., Levi, B., Richards, K. L., and O'Rourke, R. A.: Comparative Accuracy of Apical Biplane Cross-Sectional Echocardiography and Gated Equilibrium Radionuclide Angiography for Estimating Left Ventricular Size and Performance, *Circulation*, 63:1075, 1981.
70. Bommer, W., Chun, T., Kwan, O. L., Newmann, A., Mason, D. T., and DeMaria, A. N.: Biplane Apex Echocardiography versus Biplane Cineangiography in the Assessment of Left Ventricular Volume and Function: Validation by Direct Methods, *Am. J. Cardiol.*, 45:471, 1980.
71. Erbel, R., Schweizer, P., Meyer, J., Grenner, H., Krebs, W., and Effert, S.: Left Ventricular Volume and Ejection Fraction Determination by Cross-Sectional Echocardiography in Patients with Coronary Artery Disease: A Prospective Study, *Clin. Cardiol.*, 3:377, 1980.
72. Tortoledo, F. A., Quinones, M. A., Fernandez, G. C., Waggoner, A. D., and Winters, W. L.: Quantification of Left Ventricular Volumes by Two-Dimensional Echocardiography: A Simplified and Accurate Approach, *Circulation*, 67:579, 1983.
73. Gordon, E. P., Schnittger, I., Fitzgerald, P. J., Williams, P., and Popp, R. L.: Reproducibility of Left Ventricular Volumes by Two-Dimensional Echocardiography, *J. Am. Coll. Cardiol.*, 2:506, 1983.
74. Wahr, D. W., Wang, Y. S., and Schiller, N. B.: Left Ventricular Volumes Determined by Two-Dimensional Echocardiography in a Normal Adult Population, *J. Am. Coll. Cardiol.*, 1:863, 1983.
75. Parisi, A. F., Moynihan, P. F., Folland, E. D., and Feldman, C. L.: Quantitative Detection of Regional Left Ventricular Contraction Abnormalities by Two-Dimensional Echocardiography: II. Accuracy in Coronary Artery Disease, *Circulation*, 63:761, 1981.
76. Schiller, N. B., Acquatella, H., Ports, T. E., et al.: Left Ventricular Volume from Paired Biplane Two-Dimensional Echocardiography, *Circulation*, 60:547, 1979.
77. Helak, J., and Reichek, N.: Quantitation of Human Left Ventricular Mass and Volume by Two-Dimensional Echocardiography: In Vitro Anatomic Validation, *Circulation*, 63:1398, 1981.
78. Gutman, J., Wang, Y. S., Wahr, D., and Schiller, N. B.: Normal Left Atrial Function Determined by Two-Dimensional Echocardiography, *Am. J. Cardiol.*, 51:336, 1983.
79. Folland, E. D., Parisi, A. F., Moynihan, P. F., Jones, D. R., Feldman, C. L., and Tow, D. E.: Assessment of Left Ventricular Ejection Fraction and Volumes by Real-Time, Two-Dimensional Echocardiography and Radionuclide Techniques, *Circulation*, 60:760, 1979.
80. Silverman, M. H., and Schiller, N. B.: Apex Echocardiography, *Circulation*, 57:503, 1978.
81. Baran, A. O., Rogal, G. J., and Nanda, N. C.: Ejection Fraction Determination without Planimetry by Two-Di-

mensional Echocardiography: A New Method, *J. Am. Coll. Cardiol.,* 1:1471, 1983.
82. Quinones, M. A., Waggoner, A. D., Reduto, L. A., et al.: A New Simplified and Accurate Method for Determining Ejection Fraction with Two-Dimensional Echocardiography, *Circulation,* 64:744, 1981.
83. Levine, R. A., Gibson, T. C., Aretz, T., Gillam, L. D., et al: Echocardiographic Measurement of Right Ventricular Volume, *Circulation,* 69:497, 1984.
84. Watanabe, T., Katsume, H., Matsukubo, H., Furukawa, K., and Ijichi, H.: Estimation of Right Ventricular Volume With Two-Dimensional Echocardiography, *Am. J. Cardiol.,* 49:1946, 1982.
85. Starling, M. R., Crawford, M. H., Sorensen, S. G., and O'Rourke, R. A.: A New Two-Dimensional Echocardiographic Technique for Evaluating Right Ventricular Size and Performance in Patients with Obstructive Lung Disease, *Circulation,* 66:612, 1982.
86. Mills, P., and Craige, E.: Echophonocardiography, *Prog. Cardiovasc. Dis.,* 20:337, 1978.
87. Burggraf, G. W.: The First Heart Sound in Left Bundle Block: An Echocardiographic Study, *Circulation,* 63:429, 1981.
88. Felner, J. M., and Miller, D. D.: Echocardiographic Characteristics of Normally and Abnormally Functioning Mechanical Prosthetic Heart Valves, *Echo: Rev. Cardiovasc. Ultrasound,* 1:300, 1984.
89. Felner, J. M., Harwood, S., Mond, H., Plauth, W., Brinsfield, D., and Schlant, R. C.: Systolic "Honks" in Young Children, *Am. J. Cardiol.,* 40:206, 1977.
90. Stefadouros, M. A., and Witham, A. C.: Systolic Time Intervals by Echocardiography, *Circulation,* 51:115, 1975.
91. Ewy, G. A., Jones, S. E., and Friedman, M. J.: Echocardiographic Detection of Adriamycin Heart Disease, *Proc. Am. Soc. Clin. Oncol.,* 16:228, 1975.
92. Hirschfeld, S., Meyer, R. A., Schwartz, D. C., Korfhagen, J., and Kaplan, S.: Measurement of Right and Left Ventricular Systolic Time Intervals by Echocardiography, *Circulation,* 51:304, 1975.
93. Silverman, N. H., Snider, A. R., and Rudolph, A. M.: Evaluation of Pulmonary Hypertension by M-Mode Echocardiography in Children with Ventricular Septal Defect, *Circulation,* 61:1125, 1980.
94. Riggs, T., Hirschfeld, S., Borkat, G., Knoke, J., and Liebman, J.: Assessment of the Pulmonary Vascular Bed by Echocardiographic Right Ventricular Systolic Time Intervals, *Circulation,* 57:939, 1978.
95. Gramiak, R., Shah, P. M., and Kramer, D. H.: Ultrasound Cardiography: Contrast Studies in Anatomy and Function, *Radiology,* 92:939, 1976.
96. Seward, J. B., Tajik, A. J., Spangler, J. G., and Ritter, D. G.: Echocardiographic Studies. Initial Experience, *Mayo Clin. Proc.,* 50:163, 1975.
97. Tajik, A. J., and Seward, J. B.: Contrast Echocardiography, in M. N. Kotler and B. L. Segal (eds.), "Clinical Echocardiography," and A. N. Brest (ed.), "Cardiovascular Clinics," F. A. Davis Company, Philadelphia, 1978, p. 317.
98. Wise, N. K., Myers, S., Fraker, T. D., Stewart, J. A., and Kisslo, J. A.: Contrast M-Mode Ultrasonography of the Inferior Vena Cava, *Circulation,* 63:1100, 1981.
99. Weyman, A., Feigenbaum, H., Dillon, J., Johnston, K., and Eggleton, R. C.: Noninvasive Visualization of the Left Main Coronary Artery by Cross-Sectional Echocardiography, *Circulation,* 54:169, 1976.
100. Valdes-Cruz, L. M., and Sahn, D. J.: Ultrasonic Contrast Studies for the Detection of Cardiac Shunts, *J. Am. Coll. Cardiol.,* 3:978, 1984.
101. DePace, N. L., Ross, J., Iskandrian, A. S., Nestico, P. F., et al.: Tricuspid Regurgitation: Noninvasive Techniques for Determining Causes and Severity, *J. Am. Coll. Cardiol.,* 3:1540, 1984.
102. Meltzer, R. S., Hoogenhuyze, D. V., Serruys, P., Haalebos, M. M. P., Hugenholtz, P. G., and Roelandt, J.: Diagnosis of Tricuspid Regurgitation by Contrast Echocardiography, *Circulation,* 63:1093, 1981.
103. Seward, J. B., Tajik, A. J., and Hagler, D. J.: Peripheral Venous Contrast Echocardiography, *Am. J. Cardiol.,* 39:202, 1977.
104. Truman, A. T., Syamasundar, Rao P., and Kulangara, R. J.: Use of Contrast Echocardiography in Diagnosis of Anomalous Connection of Right Superior Vena Cava to Left Atrium, *Br. Heart J.,* 4:718, 1980.
105. Silverman, N. H., Snider, A. R., Colo J., et al.: Superior Vena Caval Obstruction after Mustard's Operation: Detection by Two-Dimensional Echocardiography, *Circulation,* 64:392, 1981.
106. Meltzer, R., Tickner, E. G., Sahines, T. P., et al.: The Source of Ultrasonic Contrast Effects, *JCU,* 8:121, 1980.
107. DeMaria, A. N., Bommer, W., Takeda, P., Mason, D. T., Kwan, O. L., and Rasor, J.: Value and Limitations of Contrast Echocardiography in Cardiac Diagnosis, in N. O. Fowler (ed.), "Noninvasive Diagnostic Methods in Cardiology," F. A. Davis Company, Philadelphia, 1983, p. 167.
108. Valdes-Cruz, L. M., Pieroni, D. R., Roland, J. M. A., et al.: Recognition of Residual Postoperative Shunts by Contrast Echocardiographic Techniques, *Circulation,* 55:148, 1977.
109. Pieroni, D. R., Varghese, P. J., Freedom, R. M., et al.: The Sensitivity of Contrast Echocardiography in Detecting Intracardiac Shunts, *Cathet. Cardiovasc. Diagn.,* 5:19, 1979.
110. Bommer, W. J., Shah, P. N., Allen, H., Meltzer, R., and Kisslo, J.: The Safety of Contrast Echocardiography: Report of the Committee on Contrast Echocardiography in the American Society of Echocardiography, *J. Am. Coll. Cardiol.,* 3:6, 1984.
111. Weyman, A. E., Wann, L. S., Caldwell, R. L., Hurwitz, R. A., Dillon, J. C., and Feigenbaum, H.: Negative Contrast Echocardiography: A New Method for Detecting Left-to-Right Shunts, *Circulation,* 59:498, 1979.
112. Lieppe, W., Behar, V. S., Scallion, R., et al.: Detection of Tricuspid Regurgitation with Two-Dimensional Echocardiograhy and Peripheral Vein Injections, *Circulation,* 57:128, 1978.
113. Meltzer, R. S., Vered, Z. V. I., Roelandt, J. O. S., and Neufeld, H. N.: Systematic Analysis of Contrast Echocardiograms, *Am. J. Cardiol.,* 52:375, 1983.
114. Smith, M. D., Kwan, O. L., Reiser, H. J., and DeMaria, A. N.: Superior Intensity and Reproducibility of SHU-454, a New Right Heart Contrast Agent, *J. Am. Coll. Cardiol.,* 3:992, 1984.
115. Ten Cate, F. J., Feinstein, S., Zwehl, W., Meerbaum, S., Fishbein, M., Shah, P. M., and Corday, E.: Two-Dimensional Contrast Echocardiography: II. Transpulmonary Studies, *J. Am. Coll. Cardiol.,* 3:21, 1984.
116. Maurer, G., Ong, K., Haendchen, R., Torres, M., Tei, C., Woods, F., et al.: Myocardial Contrast Two-Dimensional Echocardiography: Comparison of Contrast Disappearance Rates in Normal and Underperfused Myocardium, *Circulation,* 69(2):418, 1984.
117. Armstrong, W. F., Mueller, T. M., Kinney, E. L., Tickner, E. G., Dillon, J. C., and Feigenbaum, H.: Assessment of Myocardial Perfusion Abnormalities with Contrast Enhanced Two-Dimensional Echocardiography, *Circulation,* 66:166, 1982.
118. Sakamaki, T., Tei, C., Meerbaum, S., Shimoura, K., et al.: Verification of Myocardial Contrast Two-Dimensional Echocardiographic Assessment of Perfusion Defects in Ischemic Myocardium, *J. Am. Coll. Cardiol.,* 3:34, 1984.
119. Kraunz, R. F., and Kennedy, J. W.: Ultrasonic Determinaton of Left Ventricular Wall Motion in Normal Man: Studies at Rest and after Exercise, *Am. Heart J.,* 79:36, 1970.
120. Smithen, C. S., Wharton, C. F. P., and Wowton, E.: Independent Effects of Heart Rate and Exercise on Left Ventricular Wall Movement Measured by Reflected Ultrasound, *Am. J. Cardiol.,* 30:43, 1972.

121. Crawford, M. H., White, S. H., and Amon, W. K.: Echocardiographic Evaluation of Left Ventricular Size and Performance during Handgrip and Supine and Upright Bicycle Exercise, *Circulation,* 59:1188, 1979.
122. Wann, L. S., Faris, J. V., Childress, R. H., Dillon, J. C., Weyman, A. E., and Feigenbaum, H.: Exercise Cross-Sectional Echocardiography in Ischemic Heart Disease, *Circulation,* 60:1300, 1979.
123. Maurer, G., and Nanda, N. C.: Two-Dimensional Echocardiographic Evaluation of Exercise-Induced Left and Right Ventricular Asynergy: Correlation with Thallium Scanning, *Am. J. Cardiol.,* 48:720, 1981.
124. Morganroth, J., Chen, C. C., David, D., et al.: Exercise Cross-Sectional Echocardiographic Diagnosis of Coronary Artery Disease, *Am. J. Cardiol.,* 47:20, 1981.
125. Visser, C. A., van der Wieken, R. L., Kan, G., et al.: Comparison of Two-Dimensional Echocardiography with Radionuclide Angiography during Dynamic Exercise for the Detection of Coronary Artery Disease, *Am. Heart J.,* 106:528, 1983.
126. Limacher, M. C., Quinones, M. A., Lawrence, P. R., et al.: Detection of Coronary Artery Disease with Exercise Two-Dimensional Echocardiography. Description of a Clinically Applicable Method and Comparison with Radionuclide Ventriculography, *Circulation,* 67:1211, 1983.
127. Crawford, M. H., Petru, M. A., Amon, K. W., Vance, W. S., et al.: Comparative Value of Two-Dimensional Echocardiography and Radionuclide Angiography for Quantitating Changes in Left Ventricular Performance during Exercise Limited by Angina Pectoris, *Am. J. Cardiol.,* 53:42, 1984.
128. Quinones, M. A.: Exercise Two-Dimensional Echocardiography, *Echo: Rev. Cardiovasc. Ultrasound,* 1:151, 1984.
129. Burggraf, G. W., and Parker, J. D.: Left Ventricular Volume Changes after Amyl Nitrite and Nitroglycerin in Man as Measured by Ultrasound, *Circulation,* 49:136, 1974.
130. Winkle, R. A., Goodman, D. J., and Popp, R. L.: Simultaneous Echocardiographic-Phonocardiographic Recordings at Rest and during Amyl Nitrite Administration in Patients with Mitral Valve Prolapse, *Circulation,* 51:522, 1975.
131. Parisi, A. F., Harrington, J. J., Askenazi, J., Pratt, R. C., and McIntyre, K. M.: Echocardiographic Evaluaton of the Valsalva Maneuver in Healthy Subjects and Patients with and without Heart Failure, *Circulation,* 54:921, 1976.
132. Waldman, J. D., Rummerfield, P. S., Gilpin, E. A., et al.: Radiation Exposure to the Child during Cardiac Catheterization, *Circulation,* 64:158, 1981.
133. Glassman, E., and Kronzon, I.: Transvenous Intracardiac Echocardiography, *Am. J. Cardiol.,* 47:1255, 1981.
134. Frazin, L., Talano, J. V., Stephanides, L., Loeb, H. S., Kopel, L., and Gunnar, R. M.: Esophageal Echocardiography, *Circulation,* 54:102, 1976.
135. Matsumoto, M., Oka, Y., Strom, J., Frishman, W., Kadish, A., Becker, R. M., Frater, R. W. M., and Sonnenblick, E. H.: Application of Transesophageal Echocardiography to Continuous Intraoperative Monitoring of Left Ventricular Performance, *Am. J. Cardiol.,* 46:95, 1980.
136. Schulter, M., Hinrichs, A., Wolfgang, T., Kremer, P., et al.: Transesophageal Two-Dimensional Echocardiography: Comparison of Ultrasonic and Anatomic Sections, *Am. J. Cardiol.,* 53:1173, 1984.
136a. Hanrath, P., Schluter, M., Langenstein, B. A., Polster, J.: Transesophageal Horizontal and Sagittal Imaging of the Heart with a Phased Array System. Initial Clinical Results, in P. Hanrath, W. Bleifeld, and J. Souquet (eds.), "Cardiovascular Diagnosis by Ultrasound. Transesophageal, Computerized, Contrast, Doppler Echocardiography," Martinus Nijhoff Publ., The Hague, 1982, p. 188.
137. Schiller, N. B.: Evaluation of Cardiac Function during Surgery by Transesophageal Two-Dimensional Echocardiography, in P. Hanrath, W. Bleifeld, and J. Souquet (eds.), "Cardiovascular Diagnosis by Ultrasound. Transesophageal, Computerized, Contrast, Doppler Echocardiography," Martin Nijhoff Publ., The Hague, 1982, p. 289.
138. Duff, H. J., Buda, A. J., Kramer, R., Strauss, H. D., David, T. E., and Berman, N. D.: Detection of Entrapped Intracardiac Air with Intraoperative Echocardiography, *Am. J. Cardiol.,* 46:255, 1980.
139. Spotnitz, H. M.: Two-Dimensional Ultrasound and Cardiac Operations, *J. Thorac. Cardiovasc. Surg.,* 83:43, 1982.
140. Sahn, D. J., Copeland, J. G., Temkin, L. P., Wirt, D. P., Mammana, R., and Gleen, W.: Anatomic-Ultrasound Correlations for Intraoperative Open Chest Imaging of Coronary Artery Atherosclerotic Lesions in Human Beings, *J. Am. Coll. Cardiol.,* 3:1169, 1984.
141. Sahn, D. J., Barratt-Boyes, B., Graham, K., et al.: Ultrasonic Imaging of the Coronary Arteries in Open Chest Humans: Evaluation of Coronary Atherosclerotic Lesions during Heart Surgery, *Circulation,* 66:1034, 1982.
142. Popp, R. L., Rubenson, D. S., Tucker, C. R., and French, J. W.: Echocardiography: M-Mode and Two-Dimensional Methods, *Ann. Intern. Med.,* 93:844, 1980.
143. Kotler, M. N., Mintz, G. S., Segal, B. L., and Parry, W. R.: Clinical Uses of Two-Dimensional Echocardiography, *Am. J. Cardiol.,* 45:1061, 1980.
144. Markiewicz, W., Peled, B., Hammerman, H., Grief, Z. V. I., Hir, J., and Riss, E.: Contribution of M-Mode Echocardiography in Cardiac Diagnosis, *Am. J. Med.,* 65:803, 1978.
145. Bansal, R. C., Tajik, A. J., Seward, J. B., and Offord, K. P.: Feasibility of Detailed Two-Dimensional Echocardiographic Examination in Adults: Prospective Study of 200 Patients, *Mayo Clin. Proc.,* 55:291, 1980.
146. Horowitz, M. S., Schultz, C. S., Stinson, E. B., Harrison, D. C., and Popp, R. L.: Sensitivity and Specificity of Echocardiographic Diagnosis of Pericardial Effusion, *Circulation,* 50:239, 1974.
147. Martin, R. P., Rakowski, H., French, J., et al.: Localization of Pericardial Effusion with Wide Angle Phased-Array Echocardiography, *Am. J. Cardiol.,* 42:904, 1978.
148. Martin, R. P., Bowden, R., and Filly, K.: Intrapericardial Abnormalities in Patients with Pericardial Effusion: Findings by Two-Dimensional Echocardiography, *Circulation,* 61:568, 1980.
149. Schnittger, I., Bosden, R. E., Abrams, J., et al.: Echocardiography: Pericardial Thickening and Constrictive Pericarditis, *Am. J. Cardiol.,* 42:388, 1978.
150. Tei, C., Child, J. S., Tanaka, H., et al.: Atrial Systolic Notch on the Interventricular Septal Echogram: An Echocardiographic Sign of Constrictive Pericarditis, *J. Am. Coll. Cardiol.,* 1:907, 1982.
151. Chandraratna, P. A. N., and Aronow, W. S.: Detection of Pericardial Metastases by Cross-Sectional Echocardiography, *Circulation,* 63:197, 1981.
152. Singh, S., Wann, S., Schuchard, H., Kopfenstein, S., Leimbruger, P. P., Keelan, M. H., Jr., and Brooks, H. L.: Right Ventricular and Right Atrial Collapse in Patients with Cardiac Tamponade—A Combined Echocardiographic and Hemodynamic Study. *Circulation,* 70:966–971, 1984.
153. Armstrong, W. F., Schilt, B. F., Helper, D. J., Dillon, J. C., and Feigenbaum, H.: Diastolic Collapse of the Right Ventricle with Cardiac Tamponade: An Echocardiographic Study, *Circulation,* 65:1491, 1982.
154. Gilliam, L. D., Guyer, D., King, M. E., et al.: Hydrodynamic Compression of the Right Atrial Free Wall, a New Highly-Sensitive Echocardiographic Sign of Cardiac Tamponade, *Am. J. Cardiol.,* 49:1010, 1982.
155. Chandraratna, P. A. N., First, J., Langevin, E., et al.: Clinical Usefulness of Echocardiographic Contrast Studies during Pericardiocentesis, *Ann. Intern. Med.,* 87:199, 1977.
155a. Callahan, J. A., Seward, J. B., Nishimura, R. A., et al: Two-Dimensional Echocardiographically Guided Pericardiocentesis: Experience in 117 Consecutive Patients. *Am. J. Cardiol.,* 55:476–479, 1985.
156. Cikes, I.: New Echocardiographic Possibilities in the Etiological Diagnosis and Therapy of Pericardial Diseases, in P. Hanrath, W. Bleifeld, and J. Souquet, (eds.), "Cardiovascular Diagnosis by Ultrasound. Transesophageal, Computerized, Contrast, Doppler Echocardiography," Martinus Nijhoff Publ., The Hague, 1982, p. 188.

157. Corya, B. C., Feigenbaum, H., Rasmussen, S., and Black, M. J.: Echocardiographic Features of Congestive Cardiomyopathy Compared with Normal Subjects and Patients with Coronary Artery Disease, *Circulation,* 49:1153, 1974.
158. Henry, W. L., Clark, C. E., and Epstein, S. E.: Asymmetric Septal Hypertrophy (ASH): Echocardiographic Identification of the Pathognomonic Anatomic Abnormality of IHSS, *Circulation,* 47:225, 1973.
159. Martin, R. P., Rakowski, H., French, J., and Popp, R. L.: Idiopathic Hypertrophic Subaortic Stenosis Viewed by Wide-Angle, Phased-Array Echocardiography, *Circulation,* 59:206, 1979.
159a. Topol, E. J., Traill, T. A., and Fortuin, N. J.: Hypertensive Hypertrophic Cardiomyopathy of the Elderly. *N. Engl. J. Med.,* 312:277–283, 1985.
160. Siqueira-Filho, A. G., Cunha, C. L. P., Tajik, A. J., Seward, J. B., Schattenbert, T. T., and Giuliani, E. R.: M-Mode and Two-Dimensional Echocardiographic Features in Cardiac Amyloidosis, *Circulation,* 63:188, 263, 1973.
161. Glover, M. U., Warren, S. E., Vieweg, W. V. R., Hagen, A. D., and Ceretto, W. J.: M-Mode and Two-Dimensional Echocardiographic Correlation with Findings at Catheterization and Surgery in Patients with Mitral Stenosis, *Am. Heart J.,* 105:98, 1983.
162. Wann, L. S., Weyman, A. E., Feigenbaum, H., Dillon, J. C., Johnston, K. W., and Eggleton, R. C.: Determination of Mitral Valve Area by Cross-Sectional Echocardiography, *Ann. Intern. Med.,* 88:337, 1978.
163. Martin, R. P., Rakowski, H., Kleiman, J. H., Beaver, W., London, E., and Popp, R. L.: Reliability and Reproducibility of Two-Dimensional Echocardiographic Measurement of Stenotic Mitral Valve Orifice Area, *Am. J. Cardiol.,* 43:560, 1979.
164. Felner, J. M., and Williams, B. R.: Noninvasive Evaluation of Left Ventricular Overload and Cardiac Function, *Prac. Cardiol.,* 5:158, 1979.
165. Mintz, G. S., Kotler, M. N., Segal, B. L., and Parry, W. R.: Two-Dimensional Echocardiographic Evaluation of Patients with Mitral Insufficiency, *Am. J. Cardiol.,* 44:670, 1979.
166. Shah, P. M.: Update of Mitral Valve Prolapse Syndrome: When is Echo Prolapse a Pathological Prolapse, *Echo: Rev. Cardiovasc. Ultrasound,* 1:87, 1984.
166a. Alpert, M. A., Carney, R. J., Flaker, G. C., Sanfellipo, J. F., Webel, R. R., and Kelly, D. L.: Sensitivity and Specificity of Two-Dimensional Echocardiographic Signs of Mitral Valve Prolapse. *Am. J. Cardiol.,* 54:792–796, 1984.
167. Levine, R. A., and Weyman, A. E.: Mitral Valve Prolapse: A Disease in Search Of, or Created By, Its Definition, *Echo: Rev. Cardiovasc. Ultrasound,* 1:3, 1984.
167a. Chandraratna, P. A. N., Nimalasuriya, A., Kawanishi, D., Dunchan, P., Rosin, B., and Rahimtoola, S. H.: Identification of the Increased Frequency of Cardiovascular Abnormalities Associated with Mitral Valve Prolapse by Two-Dimensional Echocardiography. *Am. J. Cardiol.,* 54:1283–1285, 1984.
167b. Abbasi, A. S., DeCristofaro, D., Anabtawi, J., and Irwin, L.: Mitral Valve Prolapse: Comparative Value of M-Mode, Two-Dimensional and Doppler Echocardiography. *J. Am. Coll. Cardiol.,* 2:1219–1223, 1983.
168. Morganroth, J., Jones, R. H., Chen, C. C., and Naito, M.: Two-Dimensional Echocardiography in Mitral, Aortic and Tricuspid Valve Prolapse, *Am. J. Cardiol.,* 46:1164, 1980.
168a. Stewart, W. J., King, M. E., Gillam, L. G., Guyer, D. E., and Weyman, A. E.: Prevalence of Aortic Valve Prolapse with Bicuspid Aortic Valve and Its Relation to Aortic Regurgitation: A Cross-Sectional Echocardiographic Study. *Am. J. Cardiol.,* 54:1277–1282, 1984.
169. Mintz, G. S., Kotler, M. M., Parry, W. R., and Segal, B. L.: Statistical Comparison of M-Mode and Two-Dimensional Echocardiographic Diagnosis of Flail Mitral Leaflets, *Am. J. Cardiol.,* 45:253, 1980.
170. Child, J. S., Skorton, D. J., Taylor, R. D., et al.: M-Mode and Cross-Sectional Echocardiographic Features of Flail Posterior Mitral Leaflets, *Am. J. Cardiol.,* 44:1383, 1979.
171. D'Cruz, I., Panetta, F., Cohen, H., and Glick, G.: Submitral Calcification or Sclerosis in Elderly Patients; M-Mode and Two-Dimensional Echocardiography in "Mitral Anulus Calcification," *Am. J. Cardiol.,* 44:31, 1979.
171a. Vandenbossche, J.-L., Kramer, B. L., Massie, B. M., Morris, D. L., and Karliner, J. S.: Two-Dimensional Echocardiographic Evaluation of the Size, Function, and Shape of the Left Ventricle in Chronic Aortic Regurgitation: Comparison with Radionuclide Angiography. *J. Am. Coll. Cardiol.,* 4:1195–1206, 1984.
172. Botvinick, E. H., Schiller, N. B., Wickramasekaran, R., Klausner, S. C., and Gertz, E.: Echocardiographic Demonstration of Early Mitral Valve Closure in Severe Aortic Insufficiency. Its Clinical Application, *Circulation,* 51:836, 1975.
173. DeMaria, A. N., Bommer, W., Joye, J., Lee, G., Bouteller, J., and Mason, D. T.: Value and Limitations of Cross-Sectional Echocardiography of the Aortic Valve in the Diagnosis and Quantification of Valvular Aortic Stenosis, *Circulation,* 62:304, 1980.
174. Godley, R. W., Green, D., Dillon, J. C., Rogers, E. W., Feigenbaum, H., and Weyman, A. E.: Reliability of Two-Dimensional Echocardiography in Assessing the Severity of Valvular Aortic Stenosis, *Chest,* 79:657, 1981.
175. Fowles, R. E., Martin, R. P., Abrams, J. M., Schapira, J. N., French, J. W., and Popp, R. L.: Two-Dimensional Echocardiographic Features of Bicuspid Aortic Valve, *Chest,* 75:4, 1979.
176. Brandenburg, R. O., Tajik, A. J., Edwards, W. D., Reeder, G. S., Shub, C., and Seward, J. B.: Accuracy of Two-Dimensional Echocardiographic Diagnosis of Congenitally Bicuspid Aortic Valve: Echocardiographic-Anatomic Correlation in 115 Patients, *Am. J. Cardiol.,* 5:1469, 1983.
177. Krivokapich, J., Child, J. S., and Skorton, D. J.: Flail Aortic Valve Leaflets: M-Mode and Two-Dimensional Echocardiography, *Am. Heart J.,* 99:425, 1980.
178. Mardelli, T. J., Morganroth, J., Naito, M., and Chen, C. C.: Cross-Sectional Echocardiograph Detection of Aortic Valve Prolapse, *Am. Heart J.,* 101:295, 1980.
179. Seward, J. B., and Tajik, A. J.: Noninvasive Visualization of the Entire Thoracic Aorta: A New Application of Wide-Angle Two-Dimensional Sector Echocardiography, *Am. J. Cardiol.,* 43:387, 1979.
180. Okumachi, F., Yoshikawa, J., Kato, H., Yanagihara, K., Takagi, Y., Yoshida, K., and Asaka, T.: Usefulness and Limitations of Two-Dimensional Echocardiography in the Diagnosis of Acute Dissecting Aneurysm of the Aorta, *J. Cardiogr.,* 11:1169, 1981.
181. Victor, M. E., Mintz, G. S., Kotler, M. N., Wilson, A. R., and Segal, B. L.: Two-Dimensional Echocardiographic Diagnosis of Aortic Dissection, *Am. J. Cardiol.,* 48:1155, 1981.
182. Iliceto, S., Antonelli, G., Biasco, G., and Rizzon, P.: Two-Dimensional Echocardiographic Evaluation of Aneurysms of the Descending Thoracic Aorta, *Circulation,* 66:1045, 1982.
183. DeMaria, A., Bommer, W., Neumann, A., Weinert, L., Borgen, H., and Mason, D. T.: Identification of Aneurysms of the Ascending Aorta by Cross-Sectional Echocardiography, *Circulation,* 59:755, 1979.
184. Weyman, A. E., Caldwell, R. L., Hurwitz, R. A., Girod, D. A., Dillon, J. C., Feigenbaum, H., and Green, D.: Cross-Sectional Echocardiographic Detection of Aortic Obstruction: 2. Coarctation of the Aorta, *Circulation,* 57:498, 1978.
185. Pratt, C., Whitcomb, C., and Newmann, A.: Relationship of Vegetations on Echocardiograms to the Clinical Course in Systemic Emboli and Bacterial Vegetations (? Endocarditis), *Am. J. Cardiol.,* 61:374, 1980.
186. Stewart, J. A., Silimperi, D., Harris, P., Wise, N. K., Fraker, T. D., Jr., and Kisslo, J. A.: Echocardiographic Documentation of Vegetative Lesions in Infective Endocarditis: Clinical Implications, *Circulation,* 61:374, 1980.
187. Melvin, E. T., Berger, M., Lutzker, L. G., Goldberg, E., and Mildvan, D.: Noninvasive Methods for Detection of Valve Vegetations in Infective Endocarditis, *Am. J. Cardiol.,* 47:271, 1981.

188. Berger, M., Delfin, L. A., Jelvehm, M., and Goldberg, E.: Two-Dimensional Echocardiography Findings in Right-Sided Infective Endocarditis, *Circulation,* 61:855, 1980.
189. Mintz, G. S., Kotler, M. N., Segal, B. L., and Parry, W. R.: Comparison of Two-Dimensional and M-Mode Echocardiography in the Evaluation of Patients with Infective Endocarditis, *Am. J. Cardiol.,* 43:738, 1979.
190. Scanlan, J. G., Seward, J. B., and Tajik, A. J.: Valve Ring Abscess in Infective Endocarditis: Visualization with Wide Angle Two-Dimensional Echocardiography, *Am. J. Cardiol.,* 49:1794, 1982.
191. Ports, T. A., Cogan, J., Schiller, N. B., and Rapaport, E.: Echocardiography of Left Ventricular Masses, *Circulation,* 58:528, 1978.
192. DePace, N. L., Soulen, R. L., Kotler, M. N., and Mintz, G. S.: Two-Dimensional Echocardiographic Detection of Intraatrial Masses, *Am. J. Cardiol.,* 48:954, 1981.
193. DeMaria, A. N., Vismara, L. A., Miller, R. R., Neuman, A., and Mason, D. T.: Unusual Echocardiographic Manifestations of Right and Left Heart Myxomas, *Am. J. Med.,* 59:713, 1975.
194. Ports, T. A., Schiller, N. B., and Strunk, B. L.: Echocardiography of Right Ventricular Tumors, *Circulation,* 56:439, 1977.
195. Felner, J. M., and Knopf, W.: Intracardiac and Extracardiac Masses Diagnosed by Two-Dimensional Echocardiography, *Echo: Rev. Cardiovasc. Ultrasound,* 2:3, 1985.
196. Stratton, J. R., Lighty, G. W., Jr., Pearlman, A. S., and Ritchie, J. L.: Detection of Left Ventricular Thrombus by Two-Dimensional Echocardiography: Sensitivity, Specificity, and Causes of Uncertainty, *Circulation,* 66:156, 1982.
197. Felner, J. M., Churchwell, A., and Murphy, D.: Right Atrial Thromboemboli: Clinical, Echocardiographic and Pathophysiologic Manifestations, *J. Am. Coll. Cardiol.,* 4:1041, 1984.
198. Schweizer, P., Bardos, F., Erbel, R., et al.: Detection of Left Atrial Thrombi by Echocardiography, *Br. Heart J.,* 45:148, 1981.
199. Herzog, C. A., Bass, D., Kane, M., and Asinger, R.: Two-Dimensional Echocardiographic Imaging of Left Atrial Appendage Thrombi, *J. Am. Coll. Cardiol.,* 3:1340, 1984.
200. Kerber, R. E., and Abboud, F. M.: Echocardiographic Detection of Regional Myocardial Infarction, *Circulation,* 47:997, 1973.
201. Kisslo, J. A., Robertson, D., Gilbert, B. W., von Ramm, O. T., and Behar, V. S.: A Comparison of Real-time, Two-Dimensional Echocardiography and Cineangiography in Detecting Left Ventricular Asynergy, *Circulation,* 55:936, 1976.
202. Morganroth, J., Chen, C. C., David, D. D., Naito, M., and Mardelli, T. J.: Echocardiographic Detection of Coronary Artery Disease: Detection of Effects of Ischemia on Regional Myocardial Wall Motion and Visualization of Left Main Coronary Artery Disease, *Am. J. Cardiol.,* 46:1178, 1980.
203. Parisi, A. F., Moynihan, P. F., Folland, E. D., Strauss, W. E., Sharama, G. V. R. K., and Sasahara, A. A.: Echocardiography in Acute and Remote Myocardial Infarction, *Am. J. Cardiol.,* 46:1205, 1980.
203a. Nishimura, R. A., Tajik, A. J., Shub, C., Miller, F. A., Jr., Ilstrup, D. M., and Harrison, D. C.: Role of Two-Dimensional Echocardiography in the Prediction of In-Hospital Complications after Acute Myocardial Infarction. *J. Am. Coll. Cardiol.,* 4:1080–1087, 1984.
204. Parisi, A. F., Moynihan, P. F., Folland, E. D., and Feldman, C. L.: Quantitative Detection of Regional Left Ventricular Contraction Abnormalities by Two-Dimensional Echocardiography: II, Accuracy in Coronary Artery Disease, *Circulation,* 63:761, 1981.
205. Gibson, R. S., Bishop, H. L., Stamm, R. B., Crampton, R. S., Beller, G. A., and Martin, R. P.: Value of Early Two-Dimensional Echocardiography in Patients with Acute Myocardial Infarction, *Am. J. Cardiol.,* 49:1110, 1982.
206. Heger, J. J., Weyman, A. E., Wann, L. S., Dillon, J. C., and Feigenbaum, H.: Cross-Sectional Echocardiography in Acute Myocardial Infarction: Detection and Localization of Regional Left Ventricular Asynergy, *Circulation,* 60:531, 1979.
207. Horowitz, R. S., Morganroth, J., Parrotto, C., Chen, C. C., Soffer, J., and Pauletto, F. J.: Immediate Diagnosis of Acute Myocardial Infarction by Two-Dimensional Echocardiography, *Circulation,* 65:323, 1982.
208. Nishmura, R. A., Reeder, G. S., Miller, J. A., Ilstrup, D. M., Shub, C., et al.: Prognostic Value of Predischarge Two-Dimensional Echocardiogram after Acute Myocardial Infarction, *Am. J. Cardiol.,* 53:429, 1984.
209. Henschke, C. I., Risser, T. A., Sandor, T., Hanlon, W. B., Neumann, A., and Wynne, J.: Quantitative Computer-Assisted Analysis of Left Ventricular Wall Thickening and Motion by Two-Dimensional Echocardiography in Acute Myocardial Infarction, *Am. J. Cardiol.,* 52:960, 1983.
210. Likoff, M., Reichek, N., St. John-Sutton, M., Macovick, J., and Harken, A.: Epicardial Mapping of Segmental Myocardial Function: An Echocardiographic Method Applicable in Man, *Circulation,* 66:1050, 1982.
211. Kerber, R. E., and Marcus, M. L.: Evaluation of Regional Myocardial Function in Ischemic Heart Disease by Echocardiography, *Prog. Cardiovasc. Dis.,* 20:41, 1978.
212. Pandian, N., and Kerber, B.: Two-Dimensional Echocardiography in Experimental Coronary Stenosis: I. Sensitivity and Specificity in Detecting Transient Myocardial Dyskinesis: Comparison with Somomicrometers, *Circulation,* 66:597, 1982.
213. Nieminen, M., Parisi, A., O'Boyle, J. E., Folland, E. D., Khuri, S., and Kloner, R. A.: Serial Evaluation of Myocardial Thickening and Thinning in Acute Experimental Infarction: Identification and Quantification Using Two-Dimensional Echocardiography, *Circulation,* 66:174, 1982.
214. Nixon, J. V., Brown, C. N., and Smitherman, T. C.: Identification of Transient and Persistent Segmental Wall Motion Abnormalities in Patients with Unstable Angina by Two-Dimensional Echocardiography, *Circulation,* 65:1497, 1982.
215. Heger, J. J., Weyman, A. E., Rogers, E. W., Dillon, J. C., and Feigenbaum, H.: Cross-Sectional Echocardiographic Analysis of the Extent of Left Ventricular Asynergy in Acute Myocardial Infarction, *Circulation,* 66:1113, 1980.
216. D'Arcy, B. J., Gondi, B., Nanda, N. C., Gatewood, R. P., and Biddle, T.: Real-Time Two-Dimensional Echocardiography in Right Ventricular Infarction, *Am. J. Cardiol.,* 45:436, 1980.
217. Pandian, N., Koyanagi, S., Skorton, D., Collins, S., Marcus, M., and Kerber, R.: Serial Quantification of Myocardial Dyskinesis in Acute Myocardial Infarction by Two-Dimensional Echocardiography, *J. Am. Coll. Cardiol.,* 1:619, 1983.
218. Visser, C. A., Kan, G., David, G. K., Lie, K. I., and Durrer, D.: Echocardiographic-Cineangiographic Correlation in Detecting Left Ventricular Aneurysm: A Prospective Study of 422 Patients, *Am. J. Cardiol.,* 50:337, 1982.
219. Catherwood, E., Mintz, G. S., Kotler, M. N., Parry, W. R., and Segal, B. L.: Two-Dimensional Echocardiographic Recognition of Left Ventricular Pseudoaneurysm, *Circulation,* 62:294, 1980.
220. Asinger, R. W., Mikell, F. L., Sharma, B., and Hodges, M.: Observations on Detecting Left Ventricular Thrombus with Two-Dimensional Echocardiography: Emphasis on Avoidance of False Positive Diagnosis, *Am. J. Cardiol.,* 47:145, 1981.
221. Farcot, J. C., Boisante, L., Rigaud, M., Bardet, J., and Bourdarias, J. P.: Two-Dimensional Echocardiographic Visualization of Ventricular Septal Rupture after Acute Myocardial Infarction, *Am. J. Cardiol.,* 45:370, 1980.
222. Erbel, R., Schweizer, P., Bardos, P., and Meyer, J.: Two-Dimensional Echocardiographic Diagnosis of Papillary Muscle Rupture, *Chest,* 79:595, 1981.
223. Reeder, G. S., Lengyel, M., Tajik, A. J., Seward, J. B., Smith, H. C., and Danielson, G. K.: Mural Thrombus in Left Ventricular Aneurysm. Incidence, Role of Angiog-

raphy, and Relation between Anticoagulation and Embolization. *Mayo Clin. Proc.*, 56:77, 1981.
224. Weinreich, D. J., Burke, J. F., and Pauletto, F. J.: Left Ventricular Mural Thrombi Complicating Acute Myocardial Infarction. Long Term Follow-up with Serial Echocardiography, *Ann. Intern. Med.*, 100:789, 1984.
224a. Meyer, R. A.: Echocardiography in Assessing Cardiac Anatomy: Summary and Discussion. *J. Am. Coll. Cardiol.*, 5:44S–47S, 1985.
225. Rink, L. D., Feigenbaum, H., Godley, R. W., Weyman, A. E., Dillon, J. C., Phillips, J. F., and Marshall, J. E.: Echocardiographic Detection of Left Main Coronary Artery Obstruction, *Circulation*, 65:719, 1982.
225a. Gutgesell, H. P.: Echocardiographic Assessment of Cardiac Function in Infants and Children. *J. Am. Coll. Cardiol.*, 5:95S–103S, 1985.
225b. Bierman, F. Z.: Two-Dimensional Echocardiography in the Older Child. *J. Am. Coll. Cardiol.*, 5:37S–43S, 1985.
226. Capelli, H., Andrade, J. L., and Somerville, J.: Classification of the Site of Ventricular Septal Defect by Two-Dimensional Echocardiography, *Am. J. Cardiol.*, 51:1474, 1983.
227. Felner, J. M.: Echocardiography: Acyanotic Congenital Heart Lesions, in M. N. Kotler and B. L. Segal (eds.), "Clinical Echocardiography," and A. N. Brest (ed.), "Cardiovascular Clinics," F. A. Davis Company, Philadelphia, 1978, p. 251.
228. Solinger, R., Elbl, F., and Minhas, K.: Deductive Echocardiographic Analysis in Infants with Congenital Heart Disease, *Circulation*, 50:1072, 1974.
228a. Williams, R. G.: Echocardiography in the Neonate and Young Infant. *J. Am. Coll. Cardiol.*, 5:30S–36S, 1985.
229. Kreulen, T. M., Bove, A. A., McDonough, M. T., et al.: The Evaluation of Left Ventricular Function in Man. A Comparison of Methods, *Circulation*, 51:677, 1975.
230. Popp, R. L., Alderman, E. I., Brown, O. R., and Harrison, D. C.: Sources of Error in Calculation of Left Ventricular Volumes by Echocardiography, *Am. J. Cardiol.*, 31:152, 1973.
231. Felner, J. M., Blumenstein, B. A., Schlant, R. C., et al.: Sources of Variability in Echocardiographic Measurements, *Am. J. Cardiol.*, 45:995, 1980.
232. Felner, J. M.: The Value and Limitations of Echocardiography, in J. W. Hurst (ed.), "Update I: The Heart," McGraw-Hill Book Company, New York, 1979, p. 47.
233. Dreslinski, G. R., Frohlich, E. D., Dunn, F. G., Messerli, F. H., Suarez, D. H., and Reisin, E.: Echocardiographic Diastolic Ventricular Abnormality in Hypertensive Heart Disease: Atrial Emptying Index, *Am. J. Cardiol.*, 47:1087, 1981.
234. Pietro, D. A., Parisi, A. F., Harrington, J. J., and Askenazi, J.: Premature Opening of the Aortic Valve: An Index of Highly Advanced Aortic Regurgitation, *JCU*, 6:179, 1978.
235. Kotler, M. N., Segal, B. L., Mintz, G. S., and Parry, W. R.: Pitfalls and Limitations of M-Mode Echocardiography, *Am. Heart J.*, 94:227, 1977.
236. Felner, J. M.: Common Errors Made in Echocardiography, *Med. Times*, 107:93, 1979.
237. O'Rourke, R. A., and Crawford, M. H.: How to Avoid Errors in Use of Echocardiography, *Cardiovasc. Med.*, 4:1079, 1979.
238. Roelandt, J., and Lubse, J.: Limitations and Pitfalls of M-Mode and Two-Dimensional Echocardiography, in J. Roelandt (ed.), "The Practice of M-Mode and Two-Dimensional Echocardiography," Martinus Nijhoff Publ., The Hague, 1983, p. 53.
239. Latson, L. A., Cheathan, J. P., and Gutgesell, H. P.: Resolution and Accuracy in Two-Dimensional Echocardiography, *Am. J. Cardiol.*, 48:106, 1981.
240. Buda, A. J., Delp, E. J., Meyer, C. R., Jenkins, J. M., Smith, D. N., Bookstein, F. L., and Pitt, B.: Automatic Computer Processing of Digital Two-Dimensional Echocardiograms, *Am. J. Cardiol.*, 52:384, 1983.
241. Garcia, E., Gueret, P., Bennett, M., et al.: Real Time Computerization of Two-Dimensional Echocardiography, *Am. Heart J.*, 101:783, 1981.
242. Collins, S. M., Skorton, D. J., Geiser, E. A., Nichols, J. A., Conetta, D. A., Pandian, N. G., and Kerber, R. E.: Computer-Assisted Edge Detection in Two-Dimensional Echocardiography: Comparison with Anatomic Data, *Am. J. Cardiol.*, 53:1380, 1984.
243. Skorton, D. J., Collins, S. M., Nichols, J., et al.: Quantitative Texture Analysis in Two-Dimensional Echocardiography: Application to the Diagnosis of Experimental Myocardial Contusion, *Circulation*, 68:217, 1983.
244. Cohen, R. D., Mottley, J. G., Miller, J. G., et al.: Detection of Ischemic Myocardium in Vivo through the Chest Wall by Quantitative Ultrasonic Tissue Characterization, *Am. J. Cardiol.*, 50:838, 1982.
245. Fraker, T. D., Jr., Nelson, A. D., Arthur, J. A., and Wilkerson, R. D.: Altered Acoustic Reflectance on Two-Dimensional Echocardiography as an Early Predictor of Myocardial Infarct Size, *Am. J. Cardiol.*, 53:1699, 1984.
246. Bhandair, A. K., and Nanda, N. C.: Myocardial Texture Characterization by Two-Dimensional Echocardiography, *Am. J. Cardiol.*, 51:817, 1983.
247. Matsumoto, M., Inoue, M., Tamura, S., et al.: Three-Dimensional Echocardiography for Spatial Visualization and Volume Calculations of Cardiac Structures, *JCU*, 9:156, 1981.
248. Geiser, E. A., Ariet, M., Conetta, D. A., et al.: Dynamic Three-Dimensional Reconstruction of the Human Left Ventricle in Vivo: Technique and Initial Observation in Patients, *Am. Heart J.*, 103:1056, 1982.

121

Doppler Methods for Analysis of Arterial and Venous Disorders

D. E. Strandness, Jr., M.D.

The introduction of ultrasonic methods in clinical medicine has permitted the characterization of both normal flow states and the abnormal flow states associated with a variety of cardiovascular diseases.[1] The most useful method of evaluating arterial and venous disorders has been with Doppler ultrasound, which can be used to evaluate those vessels outside the confines of the thorax.[2,3] The use of this method has been possible because of the ease of access of ultrasound to large- and medium-sized vessels and to the small arteries of the digits as well.

Since the initial human studies in the 1960s, considerable improvements have been made in the Doppler systems themselves. There is also greater understanding of the pathophysiology of the effects of disease on the pressure-flow changes that occur on both the arterial and the venous sides of the circulation.

Instrumentation

The types of devices available and currently in use vary from simple pocket-sized units to complex systems that combine B-mode with pulsed Doppler systems; these are currently in the forefront of the entire field. Furthermore, it is clear that progress in the analysis of the velocity data will become extremely important in the detection of the early lesions of atherosclerosis and in the study of their progression over time.[4]

Continuous Wave System

For clinical purposes, sound waves transmitted in a continuous mode have found the widest application.[5] The transmitted frequency used depends upon the intended applications. For evaluation of the peripheral vascular system, frequencies in the range of 5 to 10 MHz are most suitable. These frequencies are satisfactory both in terms of achieving the necessary depth of penetration and of obtaining Doppler frequency shifts that are satisfactory for auditory interpretation and analog recording. Every moving item in the path of the sound beam produces a frequency shift, and it is necessary to filter the lower frequencies (those below 200 Hz) that occur with vessel wall motion. It is also essential that the physician or technologist using the system be familiar with the anatomy of the vascular segments being evaluated.

Shortly after implementation of this method for clinical studies, it became apparent that there are directional changes in flow on both the arterial and venous sides of the circulation that are of importance. Thus, the current systems have the dual capability of detecting changes in flow velocity and of defining the time-varying directional changes which are so critical in distinguishing normal from abnormal patterns of flow.[6]

Pulsed Doppler System

Because of the need in some areas of the circulation to selectively examine the flow patterns from single vessels, pulsed systems have been developed[7] (Fig. 121-1). Bursts of ultrasound are sent out, and it is possible, by time gating, to sample flow at any point within the vessel in the path of the sound beam. The instrumentation for such a system is complex, but it is very useful in evaluating such areas as the carotid bifurcation.

Combined B-Mode and Pulsed Doppler System

The B-mode systems can visualize specific arterial segments, defining the anatomy and identifying the lesions which develop secondary to atherosclerosis. By combining the B-mode and Doppler methods, it is now possible both to visualize in real time the vessels being examined and to selectively assess the flow patterns from any particular region of interest.[4] As will be discussed, this approach is currently used for the detection of extracranial atherosclerosis.

Arterial System

Normal Physiology, Peripheral Arteries

Arterial pressure measurements show a slight decrease in the mean pressure but an amplification of the systolic pressure in going from the level of the central aorta to the pedal arteries. Thus, the systolic pressure recorded at the ankle is normally greater than that recorded from the arm. This ankle-arm index is therefore normally 1.0 or greater.[8]

The velocity patterns show three basic directional changes with each pulse cycle: (1) forward flow during systole, (2) transient flow reversal in early diastole, and (3) a small, forward flow component in middiastole to late diastole.[9] This pattern is nor-

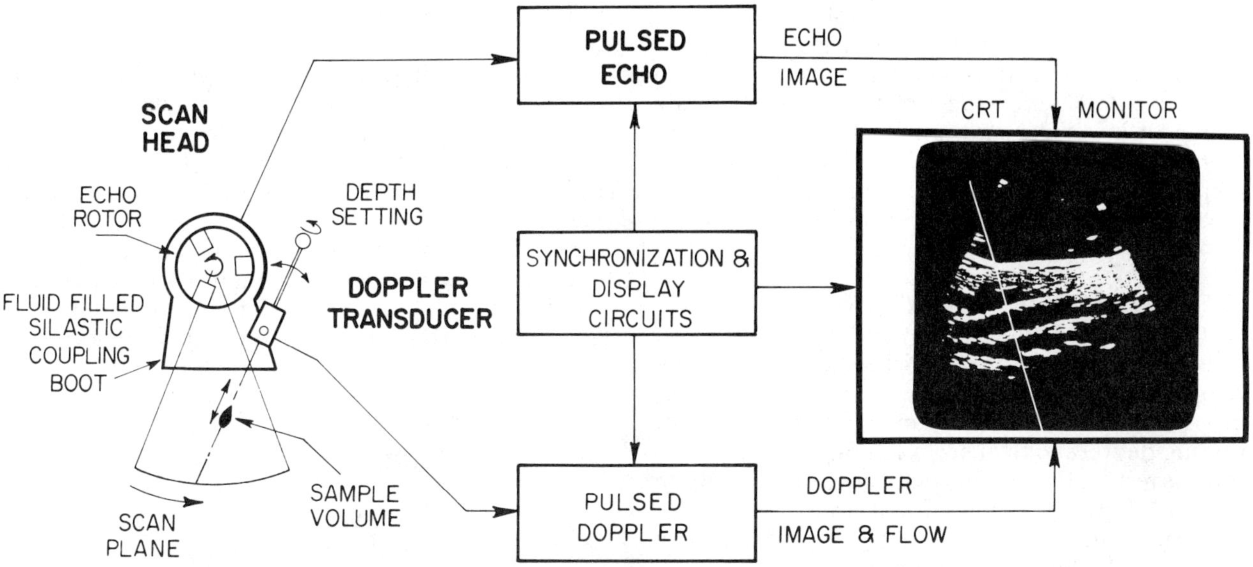

FIGURE 121-1 Block diagram of the ultrasonic duplex scanner system. The echoes from the tissue in the scan plane are shown in real time on the television monitor. The path of the Doppler beam is displayed as a white line and can be varied by moving the transducer. The position at which the velocity is being detected (termed the *sample volume*) can also be varied.

mally found from the level of the common femoral artery down to and including the pedal arteries.

Following exercise, the systolic pressure at the ankle normally either will show no change or will increase in the poststress period.[10] At very high workloads (near maximum) there may be a transient fall in systolic pressure at the ankle, but there is a rapid return to normal after cessation of walking (within 1 to 2 min).

Effects of Arterial Narrowing and Occlusion, Peripheral Arteries

With the development of atherosclerosis, there is progressive narrowing and eventual occlusion of the arteries, which force the blood through high-resistance collateral channels. This results in a fall in the pulse and the mean blood pressure distal to the occlusion.[8] Under these circumstances, the continuous wave Doppler systems can be used to indirectly measure the systolic pressure from the pedal arteries both at rest and following exercise.

Flow through the high-resistance collaterals results in loss of pressure energy, with a fall in the ankle-arm index. The magnitude of the decrease is a reflection of the extent of the disease. Values between 0.5 and 1.0 are seen with occlusion of a single segment; values below 0.5 are observed with multilevel disease.[8] After treadmill exercise, the ankle pressure falls and requires an abnormally long recovery time; this is a reflection of the degree of ischemia and the extent of the functional disability.[10]

The velocity patterns distal to sites of disease are also altered, with a loss of the reverse flow component, a reduction in peak velocity, and a monophasic signal which is above zero flow levels.[11] The standard sites from which these recordings are made include the common femoral, superficial femoral, popliteal, and pedal arteries (see Chap. 65). The Doppler frequency shift is most commonly processed using a zero-crossing detector and a direct current recorder. While there are inherent problems with this type of signal processing, it is inexpensive and does work well for a qualitative inspection of the time-varying characteristics of arterial flow.[12]

It is now possible, using the duplex scanner shown in Fig. 121-1, to examine the arterial system from the level of the aorta to below the knee. An area of occlusion can be detected by the presence of a plaque in the artery and lack of flow in the region. Stenoses can be recognized by the increase in flow velocity through the narrowed segment. The velocity patterns are best displayed by a fast Fourier transform spectrum analyzer which permits an analysis of peak velocity and an analysis of the degree to which the spectrum is broadened because of turbulence. This method assists in the selection of patients for transluminal angioplasty and direct arterial surgery. The same technique is useful for long-term follow-up studies.

Normal Physiology, Extracranial Arterial System

Flow in the extracranial arteries has characteristics which are entirely different from those observed in the peripheral arteries. The common carotid artery supplies blood to the external carotid artery; this is a relatively high-resistance circuit as compared with the internal carotid artery, which is in a low-resistance bed. Thus, flow to the brain is quasi-steady and is normally above zero. On the other hand, the flow pattern in the external carotid artery often goes to or approaches zero in late systole and diastole. It has been noted, using pulsed Doppler studies, that flow through the normal carotid bulb is complex, with the development of boundary-layer separation in the posterolateral aspect of the sinus. This is a region of low shear and is the site where the atheromatous plaque first develops. These flow phenomena can now be examined noninvasively to study the effects of early disease on velocity patterns.[13]

Effects of Arterial Narrowing and Occlusion, Extracranial Arteries

The most common site at which atherosclerosis develops is at the carotid bifurcation. This leads to progressive changes that range from stenosis of varying degrees to total occlusion of the internal carotid artery. The velocity patterns in the common carotid artery will retain their quasi-steady flow until the stenosis in the internal carotid approaches total occlusion. Under these circumstances, flow in the common carotid artery will commonly go to zero or may even reverse in early diastole.

The flow velocity through the stenosis will increase by an amount related to the degree of narrowing. The backscattered frequency from the area of stenosis will show a greater Doppler shift, because of the greater flow velocity. The amount of shift also depends on the transmitted frequency and the cosine of the angle of incidence of the sound beam. A further observation is that as flow becomes disturbed or turbulent because of changes in lumen diameter, the usual narrow band of frequencies normally associated with systole will become widened, producing spectral broadening. Knowledge of these relations and of the operating characteristics of the Doppler system used permits estimates of the degree of stenosis to be made with an acceptable degree of accuracy.

Considerable experience with the application of duplex scanning to the carotid arteries is now available. When used to study the carotid bifurcation, the test will give a sensitivity of 98 percent and a specificity of 84 percent. Stenoses can be easily detected and distinguished from total occlusion—a fact of considerable clinical importance.

The technique can be used in the following applications: (1) screening of asymptomatic patients with cervical bruits, (2) evaluation of the carotid bifurcation in patients undergoing major arterial procedures and aortocoronary bypass grafting, (3) assessment of patients with symptoms suggestive of transient cerebral ischemia, and (4) long-term follow-up.

Since progression of atherosclerosis results in further narrowing of the carotid artery, it can be monitored by changes in the velocity patterns across the area of involvement. It has been noted that the degree of stenosis may predict the clinical outcome. For example, stenoses of greater than 80 percent in terms of diameter reduction are frequently associated with the development of transient ischemic attacks, stroke, and total occlusion of the internal carotid artery.

In addition, it is possible to monitor the outcome after carotid endarterectomy. In approximately 19 percent of patients, a high-grade restenosis may develop secondary to myointimal hyperplasia. These lesions are smooth, in contrast to the atherosclerotic plaque, and do not appear to be associated with the development of transient ischemic attacks in most circumstances. Duplex scanning has been useful for monitoring these changes, in order to relate the degree of progression of disease to the clinical outcome.

Venous System

Normal Physiology

Under resting conditions, venous return is largely determined by the intrathoracic and intraabdominal pressure changes that accompany respiration.[3] Normally, flow in the major leg veins decreases or goes to zero with inspiration, because the intraabdominal pressure exceeds venous pressures. With expiration, venous pressures exceed intraabdominal pressures and flow increases. In the presence of competent valves, coughing, deep breathing, or a Valsalva maneuver does not result in flow reversal in the major veins of the limbs.

Effects of Venous Occlusion and Valvular Incompetence

Acute venous thrombosis, which is a common inhospital problem, alters the flow pattern in a predictable manner. Since the obstructed segment offers added resistance, flow is diverted via collateral channels in proportion to the extent of the resistance change, depending also on the location of the occlusion. The presence of venous obstruction and its effect on the physiology of flow can be evaluated with a 5-MHz continuous wave Doppler system.

It is critically important that the flow characteristics of the same veins be compared and that these include the external iliac, common femoral, superficial femoral, popliteal, and posterior tibial veins. With complete occlusion no flow will be detected from the involved vein. Distal to sites of acute occlusion, venous flow loses its phasic quality and becomes continuous. This technique can be successfully used if the examiner understands the normal venous anatomy and its relation to the adjacent arteries.[3]

When the valves are destroyed and rendered incompetent secondary to venous thrombosis, there is reversal of flow with cough, Valsalva maneuver, or limb compression proximal to the site of the damaged valve or valves. In establishing the site and extent of involvement, it is important not only to assess the deep veins in the usual location, but to assess the superficial veins as well. In practice, the greater and lesser saphenous veins are examined as well as the perforating veins, which empty into the posterior arch vein in the lower one-third of the leg.

Since venous thrombosis results in hypertension below sites of occlusion, it is possible to test the impairment in emptying that occurs. This can be done using either an impedance or a strain gauge plethysmograph. When a thigh cuff is inflated to 50 mmHg, venous congestion occurs. With sudden deflation of the cuff, the rate of venous emptying from the calf can be calculated and plotted against venous capacitance. The value obtained can be compared to a discriminant line which is predictive of the physiologic derangement that is diagnostic of acute venous thrombosis.[14] This method is very accurate for detection of thrombi that develop proximal to the level of the popliteal vein.

The accuracy of Doppler ultrasound and plethysmography for the detection of major venous thrombosis is in the range of 90 percent. With involvement of the tibial veins, the sensitivity of the plethysmographic methods alone is below 50 percent; however, sensitivity is higher (approximately 80 percent) with the Doppler method.[15]

It is clear that the noninvasive tests can be used to screen patients suspected of having acute venous thrombosis. In fact, it is now acceptable to treat patients on the basis of a positive test and to withhold anticoagulants when the results are unequivocally negative. This represents a major advance in this field.

References

1. Satomura, S.: Study of Flow Patterns in Peripheral Arteries by Ultrasonics, *J. Acoust. Soc. Jpn.,* 15:151, 1959.
2. Strandness, D. E., Jr., McCutcheon, E. P., and Rushmer, R. F.: Application of Transcutaneous Doppler Flowmeter in Evaluation of Occlusive Arterial Disease, *Surg. Gynecol. Obstet.,* 22:1039, 1966.
3. Strandness, D. E., Jr., and Sumner, D. S.: Ultrasonic Velocity Detector in Diagnosis of Thrombophlebitis, *Arch. Surg.,* 104:180, 1972.
4. Longlois, Y. E., Roederer, G. O., Chan, A., Phillips, D. J., Beach, K. W., Martin, D. C., and Strandness, D. E., Jr.: Evaluating Carotid Artery Disease: The Concordance between Pulsed Doppler/Spectrum Analysis and Angiography, *Ultrasound Med. Biol.,* 9:51, 1983.
5. Strandness, D. E., Jr., Schultz, R. D., Sumner, D. S., and Rushmer, R. F.: Ultrasonic Flow Detection: A Useful Technic in the Evaluation of Peripheral Vascular Disease, *Am. J. Surg.,* 113:311, 1967.
6. Jager, K. A., Longlois, Y. E., Roederer, G. O., and Strandness, D. E., Jr.: Noninvasive Assessment of Lower Extremity Ischemia, in J. J. Bergan, and J. S. T. Yao (eds.), "Evaluation and Treatment of Upper and Lower Extremity Circulatory Disorders," Grune & Stratton, Inc., Orlando, 1984, p. 97.
7. Phillips, D. J., Powers, J. E., Eyer, M. K., Blackshear, W. M., Bodily, K. C., and Strandness, D. E., Jr.: Detection of Peripheral Vascular Disease Using the Duplex Scanner III, *Ultrasound Med. Biol.,* 6:205, 1980.
8. Carter, S. A.: Role of Pressure Measurements in Vascular Disease, in E. F. Bernstein (ed.), "Noninvasive Diagnostic Techniques in Vascular Disease," The C.V. Mosby Co., St. Louis, 1978, p. 261.
9. Strandness, D. E., Jr., and Sumner, D. S.: "Ultrasonic Techniques in Angiology," Hans Huber Publishing Company, Bern, 1975, p. 13.
10. Strandness, D. E., Jr.: Exercise Testing in the Evaluation of Patients Undergoing Direct Arterial Surgery, *J. Cardiovasc. Surg.,* 11:192, 1970.
11. Knox, R. A., and Strandness, D. E., Jr.: Ultrasound Techniques for Evaluation of Lower Extremity Arterial Occlusion. *Semin. Ultrasound* 2:265, 1981.
12. Johnston, K. W., Maruzzo, B. C., and Cobbold, R. S. C.: Errors and Artifacts of Doppler Flowmeters and Their Solution, *Arch. Surg.,* 112:1335, 1977.
13. Phillips, D. J., Greene, F. M., Jr., Langlois, Y. E., Roederer, G. O., and Strandness, D. E., Jr.: Flow Velocity Patterns in the Carotid Bifurcations of Young, Presumed Normal Subjects. *Ultrasound Med. Biol.,* 9:39, 1983.
14. Wheeler, H. B.: A Modern Approach to Diagnosing Deep Venous Thrombosis, *J. Cariovasc. Med.,* 5:217, 1980.
15. Barnes, R. W.: Doppler Ultrasonic Diagnosis of Venous Disease, in E. F. Bernstein (ed.), "Noninvasive Diagnostic Techniques in Vascular Disease," The C.V. Mosby Company, St. Louis, 1978, p. 344.

122

The Use of Doppler in the Evaluation of Cardiac Disorders and Function

Alan S. Pearlman, M.D.

He who trusts the statements of text-books will not think that the recognition of a given valvular defect is difficult; for so many and such definite signs are given and the recognition of these signs is so simple that even one who is but little skilled can scarcely miss the correct diagnosis. Such is the opinion of the young physician; but he who has grown old at the bedside and who has learned what the autopsy table teaches thinks otherwise. He knows how deceptive is the interpretation of these phenomena which are by no means so easily recognized.

—Theodor von Jurgensen, 1908[1]

In spite of their important clinical uses, M-mode and two-dimensional echocardiography are limited by their inability to "image" blood within the cardiac chambers; these techniques provide only indirect clues about hemodynamic disorders. In contrast, Doppler echocardiography allows direct evaluation of intracardiac blood flow. Blood flow analysis (Doppler) and structural imaging (echocardiography) are complementary, and noninvasive laboratories are finding it increasingly sensible to use Doppler, two-dimensional, and M-mode echocardiography in an integrated fashion.

Technique

This chapter is oriented primarily toward reviewing the clinical applications of Doppler echocardiography, but a brief review of Doppler principles and instrumentation appears warranted. More complete discussions of this topic are found elsewhere.[2,3] Doppler echocardiography evaluates blood flow by virtue of ultrasound scattered by red blood cells, much as light is scattered by fog droplets. When ultrasound encounters red blood cells, some of the ultrasound energy is scattered back toward the transducer. If the blood cells are moving, the frequency of this backscattered sound will be altered in comparison with the ultrasound frequency originally emitted by the transducer. The change in frequency between the emitted and the return ultrasound signals is known as the *Doppler shift*, and its magnitude is determined by both the direction and the velocity of blood flow.

This relation is expressed mathematically by the Doppler equation

$$V = \frac{c(f_r - f_t)}{2f_t\,(\cos\theta)}$$

where V = blood flow velocity
c = speed of sound in soft tissue (approximately 1540 m/s)
f_r = frequency of return signal
f_t = frequency of transmitted signal
θ = intercept angle between direction of blood flow and ultrasound beam

The quantity $(f_r - f_t)$ is the Doppler shift, or Δf. Note that f_t is a constant frequency determined by the ultrasonoscope, while c is essentially uniform in soft tissue. When these constant terms are combined in a constant k, the Doppler equation can be transposed to give

$$\Delta f = kV\cos\theta$$

Angle θ must therefore be determined in order to calculate blood flow velocity from the measured Doppler shift. Many devices integrate Doppler with two-dimensional echocardiography, but tomographic views demonstrate cardiac structures in only two dimensions, and actual blood flow cannot be imaged. Thus, angle θ cannot be measured in three-dimensional space. The cosine function is a maximum (1.0) when θ = 0°; as θ increases from 0°, its cosine decreases. Therefore, most investigators try to align the Doppler beam with the presumed direction of flow and then adjust angulation so as to record the maximum Doppler shifts. When no higher shifts can be detected despite diligent searching from multiple orientations, a near-zero intercept angle presumably has been achieved.

Doppler shifts are recorded from groups of red blood cells moving through the ultrasound beam. Normally, red blood cells move essentially in the same direction and with the same velocity as their neighbors. The Doppler shifts recorded from these organized groups of red blood cells are relatively uniform at each instant, although Doppler shifts do increase and decrease as blood flow accelerates and decelerates during the cardiac cycle. In a number of abnormal situations, however, blood flow becomes *disturbed;* red blood cells move in differing directions and with different velocities than those of their neighbors. These differing directions and velocities generate a broad variety of simultaneous Doppler shifts at any instant in the cardiac cycle. Blood flow velocity cannot be calculated accurately from the Doppler shifts in a flow disturbance.

Two different sampling modes have been developed, pulsed and continuous wave Doppler. Pulsed

Doppler uses a single piezoelectric element alternately as transmitter and receiver. A brief burst of ultrasound is emitted by the transducer, which then functions in receive mode until signals from the depth of interest have returned to the receiver. The cycle then repeats. The sampling rate is inversely related to the transit time from the transducer to the depth of interest and back. The return signal is analyzed for Doppler shifts only during a brief time period, the onset of which can be adjusted in relation to the time at which the burst was emitted. Accordingly, Doppler shifts in frequency can be determined at specific points along the ultrasound beam. The region of Doppler sampling is known as the *sample volume;* its position is indicated along a cursor line superimposed on a two-dimensional image of the heart (Fig. 122-1). The strength of pulsed Doppler lies in its ability to record flow at specific regions within the heart. However, its relatively slow sampling rate limits pulsed Doppler for quantitating high flow velocities.

In continuous wave Doppler, two piezoelectric elements are used; one as transmitter and the other as receiver. Ultrasound energy is transmitted continuously, and backscattered signals are also sampled continuously. Since the timing relation between transmitted and received ultrasound cannot be defined, continuous Doppler has no range resolution; that is, one cannot determine from which point along the ultrasound beam the recorded return signals originated. On the other hand, its very high sampling rates make continuous wave Doppler an ideal technique for recording high flow velocities.

Doppler shift frequencies can be played through loudspeakers. An appreciation of the pitch, timing, and quality of the signals helps in both performing the measurement and interpreting the Doppler findings. More precise timing and quantitation of Doppler frequencies and, hence, of flow velocities can be obtained from a graphic output. The Doppler findings are displayed by plotting flow velocity (or occasionally, Doppler frequency shift) as a function of time (Fig. 122-1). Flow toward the transducer is plotted above the baseline, while flow away from the transducer is plotted below the baseline. The strength of the Doppler signal is depicted in gray scale.

A Doppler examination is best performed in conjunction with two-dimensional echocardiography, which provides an anatomic orientation. Proper transducer positioning will depend upon the information sought. To measure flow velocity, one needs to use examining windows that align the ultrasound beam with the direction of blood flow. To detect regions of flow disturbance, which are characterized by multiple directions of the red blood cells, a variety of examining windows can be used.

Clinical Applications

Measurement of Ventricular Performance

Doppler velocity measures can be used to assess ventricular performance. For example, ventricular stroke volume and cardiac output can be calculated.[4] In theory, this approach is straightforward; one can determine the volume of flow per beat (i.e., the stroke volume) if one knows the cross-sectional area of flow and the distance per beat traveled by an average red blood cell (Fig. 122-2). For example, left ventricular stroke volume is ejected into the ascending aorta, which is relatively circular in cross section. Accordingly, during systole, a cylindrically shaped volume of blood is ejected into the aorta. The volume of this cylinder can be calculated from its cross-sectional area and its length. The cross-sectional area of the aorta is calculated from aortic diameter, assuming the vessel to be circular. The length of aorta filled during systole is measured as the product of the average velocity of flow over systole, in centimeters per second, and the duration of systole, in seconds. This product, expressed in centimeters, is easily measured by integrating the area under the aortic systolic flow velocity curve (Fig. 122-1).

The aortic systolic velocity curve can be recorded from the apical or suprasternal windows, by orient-

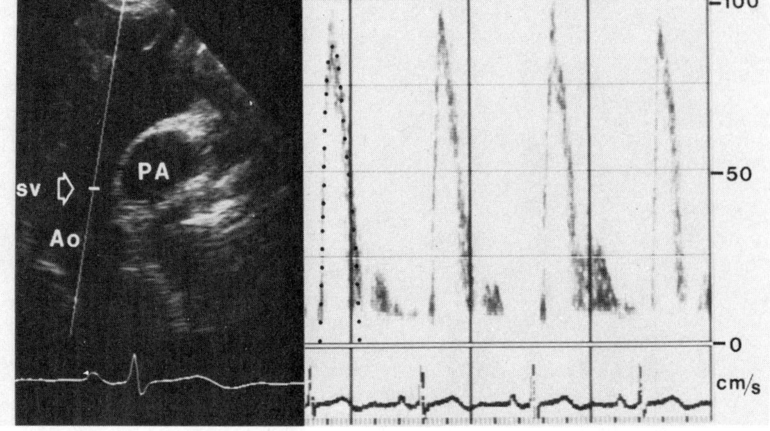

FIGURE 122-1 Aortic flow, suprasternal notch approach. *Left.* The Doppler beam (cursor line) is directed down the ascending aorta (Ao); the sample volume (SV) is indicated by the open arrow. PA = pulmonary artery. *Right.* The Doppler velocity waveform demonstrates laminar flow toward the transducer (upright waveform). The area under the curve (dotted line) is the flow velocity integral. See text for discussion.

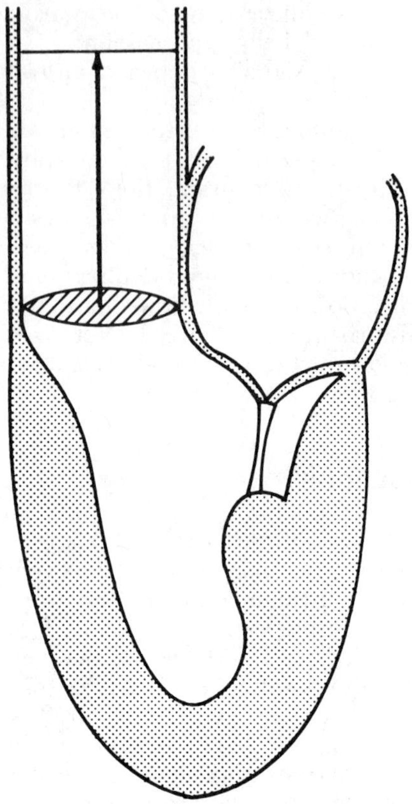

FIGURE 122-2 Determination of aortic stroke volume. The volume of blood ejected into the aorta is the product of the aortic cross-sectional area (cross-hatched circle) and the length traveled during systole by an average red blood cell (arrow).

ing the ultrasound beam parallel to the aortic centerline; aortic diameter can be measured from the two-dimensional echocardiographic images or by conventional M mode technique. However, this approach makes a number of assumptions.[5] It assumes that flow follows the walls of the aorta, and that flow velocities are relatively uniform across the aorta. It also assumes that the aorta is circular in cross section, that its true diameter can be measured, and that aortic expansion and recoil during systole are negligible. These are reasonable approximations, but none is strictly true.

Other intracardiac locations can also be used for echocardiographic and Doppler determination of stroke volume.[6–9] Pulmonary artery flow and diameter can be recorded from the high parasternal position (Fig. 122-3). Accurate measurement of pulmonary artery diameter is not always easy, however. Volume flow can also be measured in the mitral orifice, using an apical approach to record the flow velocity waveform (Fig. 122-4). The orifice area can be determined by recording the maximum mitral valve opening in early diastole at the mitral leaflet tips, using a short-axis image. Since the mitral leaflet separation varies as a function of time during diastole, a correction factor relating the mean to the maximum diastolic separation is determined from the mitral M-mode tracing.[6] This correction factor is then used to compute the average mitral opening during diastole. Alternatively, one can assume that the average mitral orifice area is approximated by the cross-sectional area of the mitral annulus.[7] Annular diameter can be measured from apical four-chamber (Fig. 122-4), apical long-axis, or parasternal long-axis views, and the cross-sectional area can be computed by assuming that the orifice is circular. For tricuspid valve flow, the flow velocity waveform is recorded using the apical four-chamber, parasternal short-axis, or right ventricular inflow views. Annular diameter is used to determine the cross-sectional flow area.

Doppler measures of volume flow in the aorta, pulmonary artery, mitral orifice, and tricuspid orifice have been compared with independent cardiac output or stroke volume determinations by Fick, thermodilution, or roller pump techniques in both experimental and clinical studies.[4,6–12] As performed by experienced investigators, Doppler measures have shown good correspondence with reference standard determinations. Preliminary reports have suggested that volume flow measures also can be made from flow velocity curves and diameters recorded high in the right and left ventricular

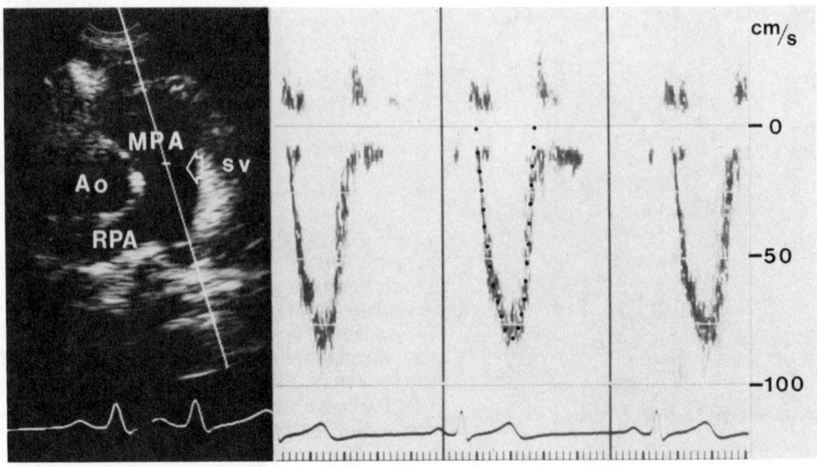

FIGURE 122-3 Pulmonary flow, high left parasternal approach. *Left.* The Doppler beam (cursor line) is directed along the main pulmonary artery (MPA); the sample volume (SV) is indicated by the open arrow. Ao = ascending aorta; RPA = right pulmonary artery. *Right.* Laminar flow away from the transducer (inverted waveform) is evident. The flow velocity integral is denoted by the dotted line.

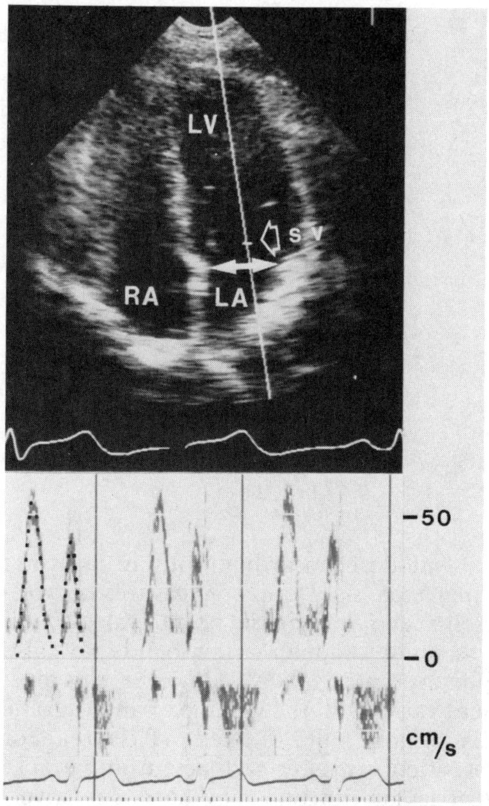

FIGURE 122-4 Mitral flow, apical approach. *Above.* The Doppler sample volume (SV, open arrow) is positioned just proximal to the mitral annular plane (double-headed arrow). LA = left atrium; RA = right atrium. *Below.* The flow velocity waveform (dotted line) shows early and late peaks, separated by a period of diastasis. The negative deflections in systole represent left ventricular (LV) outflow.

outflow tracts.[7,9] In normal individuals, stroke volume determinations from different measuring sites should be equivalent. In patients with intracardiac shunts or valvular regurgitation, the differences between volume flows measured at different sites permit calculation of the pulmonary/systemic flow ratio or the regurgitant fraction. These applications are discussed below.

The velocity and time course of ventricular ejection also provide valuable insight about global ventricular systolic function. Exercise-induced increases in left ventricular ejection dynamics are accompanied by increases in the peak velocity of ejection and increased rates of acceleration of flow into the aorta; in contrast, the failing ventricle ejects blood at a lower peak velocity and with a slower acceleration than normal.[13] Changes in Doppler measures of peak velocity and acceleration have been used successfully to follow the effects of vasodilator therapy in patients with heart failure.[14]

This approach to quantitating global ventricular performance is particularly attractive. First, the aortic velocity curve is fairly easy to record, using either the suprasternal or apical approaches. Second, alterations in the velocity and acceleration of ventricular ejection are indicators of *global* systolic ventricular performance and are independent of abnormalities of *regional* function. Accurate quantitation of left ventricular systolic performance by M-mode and even two-dimensional echocardiography is rendered difficult, if not impossible, by the geometric distortion of a large apical aneurysm, for example. In contrast, reductions in peak ejection velocity and acceleration will remain accurate indicators of the degree of global left ventricular impairment. Third, the pulmonary artery flow velocity waveform provides unique information about global right ventricular systolic performance. Ejection velocity and acceleration are reduced with right ventricular impairment, while acceleration is increased and the time to peak velocity is shortened with pulmonary hypertension.[15] These Doppler approaches have particular promise for analyzing the global systolic performance of the right ventricle, which heretofore has been difficult because of the complexities of right ventricular geometry.

Assessment of Valvular Function

Echocardiographic techniques have been of enormous use in demonstrating the presence and anatomy of valvular lesions, but they have significant limitations in evaluating the stenotic aortic valve and demonstrate only indirect evidence for valvular regurgitation. In contrast, Doppler echocardiography allows direct evaluation of the hemodynamic alterations that accompany valvular heart disease. Thus, in the assessment of valvular function, echocardiographic images and Doppler flow records are often complementary.

Valvular Stenosis

Flow through a stenotic valve has characteristic fluid-dynamic alterations.[16] Proximal to the valve, blood flow is laminar; adjacent red cells move in similar directions and with similar velocities. Within the stenotic orifice, the velocity of blood flow increases in order to maintain volume flow. In this high-velocity jet, blood flow remains laminar. Beyond the stenotic orifice, vortices of flow move in radial directions away from the centerline of the net-flow vector. The flow velocities also decrease as one moves away from the jet. Farther downstream, flow direction and velocities return to normal. Both the high-velocity jet and the region of postjet flow disturbance are useful indicators of valvular stenosis.

The velocity of flow through a stenotic valve varies with the severity of stenosis. The Bernoulli equation relates the drop in pressure across a stenosis to several fluid dynamics terms. If the stenosis is discrete, the major determinant of the pressure drop (ΔP) is the peak flow velocity (V_{max}) within the jet. Hatle and her colleagues[17] have shown that the Bernoulli equation can be simplified to $\Delta P = 4(V_{max})^2$. Hence, the pressure difference across a discrete stenosis can be determined by measuring the peak flow velocity in the stenotic orifice, squaring it, and mul-

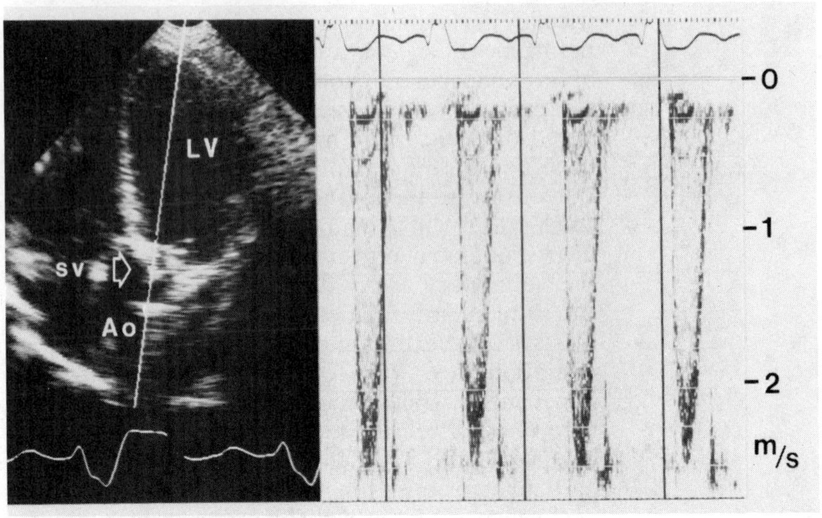

FIGURE 122-5 Mild aortic stenosis, apical approach. *Left.* The pulsed Doppler sample volume (SV, open arrow) is positioned in the high-velocity jet. Ao = aorta; LV = left ventricle. *Right.* When the sampling rate is doubled, a peak velocity of approximately 2.6 m/s is recorded, predicting a peak instantaneous gradient of 27 mmHg.

tiplying by the constant 4. Since the velocity measurement is instantaneous, the corresponding pressure drop would represent an instantaneous pressure difference, rather than the peak-to-peak pressure gradient that is generally measured at catheterization.

In patients with aortic stenosis, several investigators have used the equation $\Delta P = 4(V_{max})^2$ to calculate instantaneous peak pressure gradients that correspond well with peak-to-peak[18,19] or peak instantaneous[20] gradients measured at catheterization (Figs. 122-5 and 122-6). The mean gradient can also be determined from instantaneous gradient measurements over the course of systole. Most workers have employed continuous wave Doppler, although some have used modified pulsed Doppler techniques.[21] These observations are particularly exciting because of the limitations of two-dimensional and M-mode echocardiography in assessing aortic valvular stenosis. Doppler measures of pressure gradients across stenotic mitral valves, pulmonic valves, and pulmonary artery bands have also proved to be accurate.[17,19,22–24] However, the pressure gradient varies with the volume of anterograde flow across a stenotic valve of fixed orifice area. For example, a patient with low cardiac output because of poor ventricular function may have a relatively low pressure gradient as measured both by Doppler and invasive hemodynamic measures, despite severe aortic stenosis. Thus, a pressure gradient is not invariably an accurate indicator of the degree of stenosis.

Some investigators have used Doppler measures of pressure gradient and volume flow to develop a modification of the Gorlin equation, in order to compute the area of the orifice of the stenotic valve.

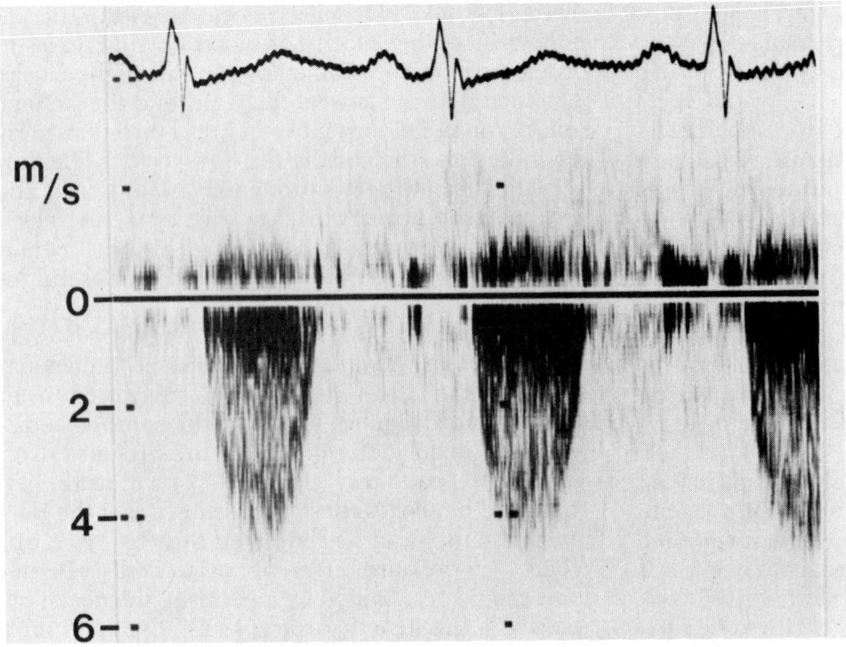

FIGURE 122-6 Severe aortic stenosis, apical approach. The waveform, recorded using a nonimaging continuous wave Doppler device, shows flow away from the transducer with a peak velocity of approximately 4.6 m/s, predicting a peak pressure gradient of 86 mmHg.

Volume flow cannot be measured accurately beyond the stenotic valve because of the multiple flow directions and velocities in the postjet flow disturbance. Accordingly, forward flow measured in the pulmonary artery has been coupled with the estimated mean aortic pressure gradient to calculate the aortic valve orifice area.[25] Conversely, pulmonary gradients and aortic flows have been used to compute orifice areas for stenotic pulmonary valves. Unfortunately, this approach is limited when significant regurgitation is combined with stenosis, since forward flow across another valve would not be equal to that across the stenotic valve.

In mitral stenosis, a particularly attractive approach using Doppler methods to measure the valve orifice area is the *pressure half-time* measurement.[26] The rate at which the left atrial–left ventricular pressure gradient falls during diastole is determined by the rate of left atrial emptying, which decreases as the mitral orifice area decreases. The time required for the peak early diastolic pressure difference to fall to one-half of its initial value, known as the pressure half-time, is thus inversely related to the stenotic mitral valve area. Empirical studies have demonstrated that the pressure half-time is approximately 220 ms when the mitral orifice area is 1.0 cm^2. Thus, the mitral valve area can be derived by dividing the measured pressure half-time, in milliseconds, into 220 ms/cm^2 (Fig. 122-7). The pressure half-time accurately predicts the mitral orifice area in patients with mitral stenosis,[19,26] regardless of transmitral volume flow.

A final Doppler approach to the severity of valvular stenosis is the quantitative analysis of turbulence parameters. Using pulsed Doppler, several investigators have found that by measuring the area filled by the disturbed flow signals in patients with aortic or mitral stenosis, mild, moderate, and severe degrees of obstruction can be separated.[27]

Regurgitant Lesions

Doppler techniques can be used to detect and estimate the severity of regurgitant valvular lesions. In valvular regurgitation a high-pressure area communicates with a low-pressure chamber through a relatively small orifice in the incompetent valve. Accordingly, there is usually a high-velocity laminar jet of flow in the regurgitant orifice itself and a flow disturbance in the chamber receiving the regurgitant flow. The corresponding Doppler findings are (1) retrograde flow across the regurgitant valve, generally of increased velocity and (2) spectral broadening in the chamber proximal to the regurgitant valve (Figs. 122-8 and 122-9).

Studies using both continuous wave and pulsed techniques have demonstrated that the presence or absence of these Doppler findings accurately indicates the presence or absence of valvular regurgitation, with angiography used as a reference standard.[28] Moreover, Doppler findings are still accurate indicators of the presence or absence of valvular incompetence even when a second valve is diseased. For example, Doppler can be used to identify coexisting aortic insufficiency in a patient with rheumatic mitral stenosis,[29] with an accuracy exceeding that of clinical auscultation. Obviously, this can be especially helpful in patients with complicated multivalvular disease.

Doppler findings sometimes suggest valvular incompetence when clinical evidence of regurgitation is absent or, at most, unimpressive. When there is a discrepancy between Doppler and clinical auscultation as regards suspected valvular incompetence, angiographic results generally support the Doppler findings.[30] For example, of 72 patients with aortic incompetence shown by aortic root angiography, we found that nearly 25 percent did not have diagnostic auscultatory findings; in contrast, Doppler findings correctly predicted the presence of aortic incompetence in 97 percent of proven cases. Doppler findings were also highly specific, being normal in 95 percent of 22 patients without aortic incompetence. We have had similar experience with mitral and tricuspid incompetence. Accordingly, we find Doppler echocardiography extremely helpful in screening for valvular regurgitation. The Doppler findings may help in planning a catheterization procedure by alerting the physician to an otherwise "silent" lesion.

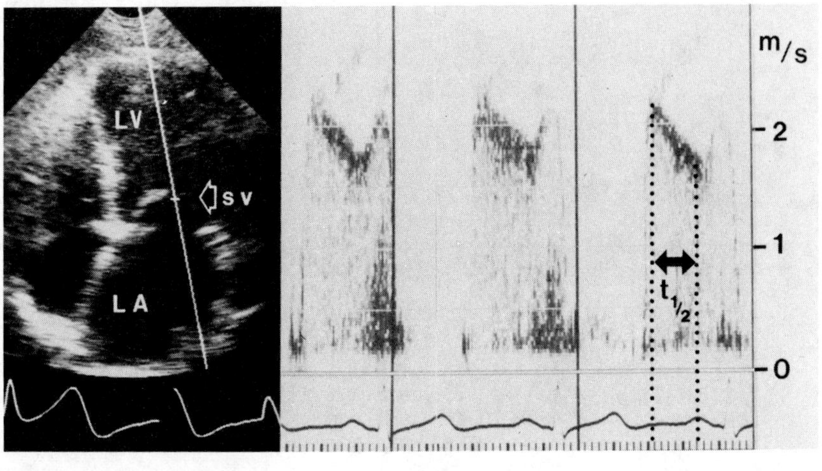

FIGURE 122-7 Mitral stenosis, apical approach. *Left.* The Doppler sample volume (SV, open arrow) is positioned in the stenotic mitral valve orifice. LA = left atrium; LV = left ventricle. *Right.* The flow velocity curve shows an increased peak of approximately 2.2 m/s, predicting a peak early diastolic gradient of 19 mmHg. The pressure half-time ($t_{1/2}$, double-headed arrow) is 260 ms, predicting a mitral valve area of 220/260 = 0.8 cm^2. See text for discussion.

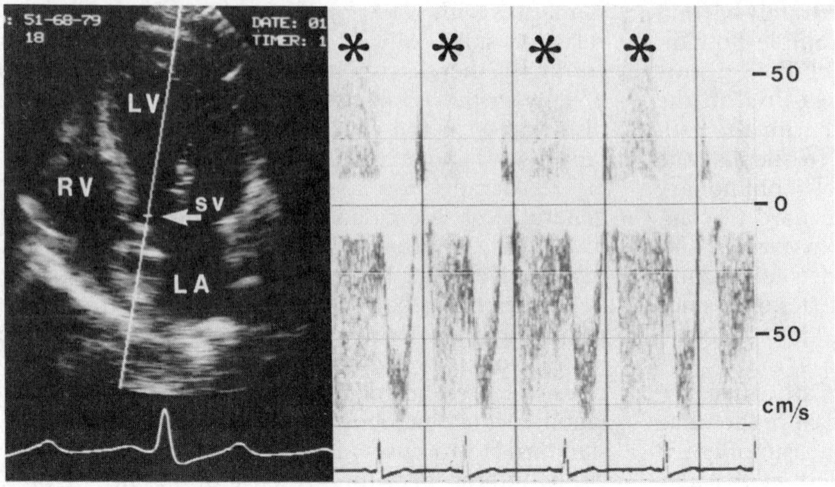

FIGURE 122-8 Aortic regurgitation, apical approach. *Left.* The sample volume (SV, arrow) is positioned just proximal to the plane of the closed aortic leaflets, high in the left ventricular (LV) outflow tract. LA = left atrium; RV = right ventricle. *Right.* The flow waveform shows laminar systolic outflow; diastolic spectral broadening (asterisks) indicates the flow disturbance of aortic regurgitation.

Doppler echocardiography appears particularly useful if one plans to send a patient for valve-replacement surgery without catheterization, on the basis of clinical and noninvasive evaluation.

Several methods can be used to estimate the degree of valvular regurgitation. One such method, known as *flow mapping,* requires pulsed Doppler.[3] By successively placing the Doppler sample volume in different regions of the appropriate chamber, this technique defines the spatial distribution of the regurgitant flow disturbance as an indicator of severity. As illustrated in Fig. 122-10, the flow disturbance is localized to an area near the plane of the regurgitant valve in mild insufficiency, is distributed widely throughout the chamber in severe insufficiency, and is intermediate in degree in moderate insufficiency. In general, the semiquantitative results of Doppler flow mapping have showed concurrence with selective cineangiographic findings in distinguishing among mild, moderate, and severe degrees of regurgitation.[3]

A narrow jet and a broad front of regurgitation can both travel the same distance from the valve, although the regurgitant volume flow is smaller in the former than the latter case. Thus, the distance from the valve plane over which the regurgitant flow disturbance can be mapped is an oversimplified expression of the spatial distribution of valvular regurgitation. The regurgitant flow fills a three-dimensional volume within the receiving chamber, but only two of these dimensions can be defined in a single two-dimensional echocardiographic plane. For this reason, we try to map regurgitation in at least two approximately orthogonal planes.[31] For example, in mitral regurgitation, mapping in both apical four-chamber and long-axis planes allows assessment of the lateral-medial and anteroposterior extent of the flow disturbance. Owing to the multiple directions of red blood cells in the regurgitant vortices, flow disturbances can be recorded from the precordial echocardiographic windows as well as from the apex. This allows placement of the Doppler sample volume closer to the transducer, hence limiting the attenuation of ultrasound strength with increasing depth. We find the parasternal long- and short-axis views are helpful for detecting and mapping regurgitant flow.

Regurgitant flow can also be quantitated by measuring volume flow at multiple sites within the heart and great vessels. When a valve is regurgitant,

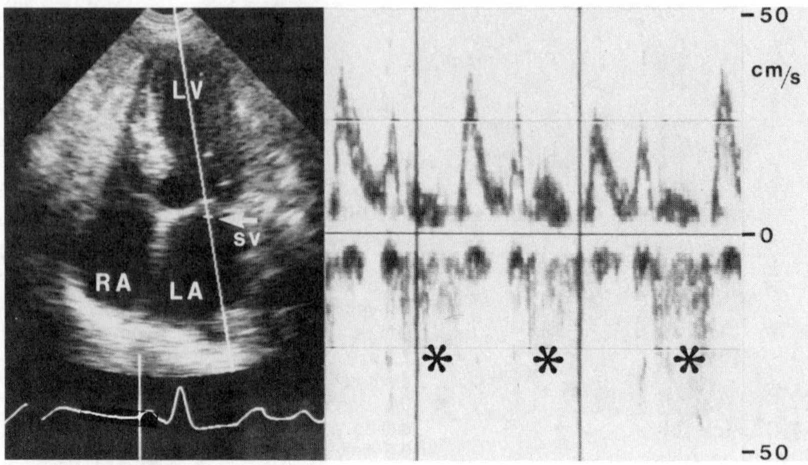

FIGURE 122-9 Mitral regurgitation, apical approach. *Left.* The sample volume (SV, arrow) is positioned just to the left atrial (LA) side of the closed mitral leaflets in systole. LV = left ventricle; RA = right atrium. *Right.* The flow waveform shows laminar diastolic emptying of the left atrium; a systolic flow disturbance (asterisks) is diagnostic of mitral regurgitation.

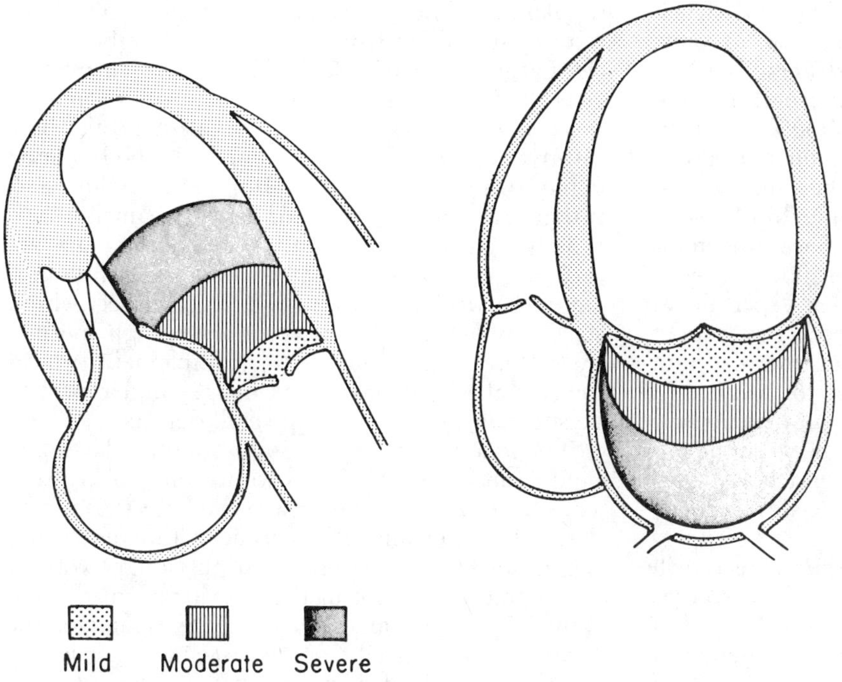

FIGURE 122-10 Flow mapping of regurgitant valves, apical approach. *Left.* Aortic regurgitation. *Right.* Mitral regurgitation. The spatial distribution of regurgitant flow increases as the severity of regurgitation increases. See text for discussion.

anterograde flow across that valve will exceed net forward flow (measured elsewhere) by an amount equal to the regurgitant flow. For example, in aortic regurgitation, the difference between the systolic aortic and pulmonary artery stroke volumes would represent the regurgitant stroke volume, while the ratio of regurgitant to total (aortic) stroke volume would represent the regurgitant fraction. Preliminary studies have demonstrated the feasibility of this approach.[7,32] The volume of regurgitant flow across other valves can be measured in a similar manner, if (1) *anterograde* flow across the incompetent valve is relatively laminar, (2) normal forward flow can be measured at another site, and (3) the cross-sectional flow area can be measured accurately. This latter requirement is often the hardest to meet.

A final approach entails estimating both forward and retrograde flow. In aortic insufficiency, the suprasternal notch approach can be used to record flow in the proximal descending thoracic aorta. The volume of flow recorded during systole (the systolic flow velocity integral multiplied by the cross-sectional area of the aorta) reflects forward flow through this area, while the volume of retrograde flow (the diastolic flow velocity integral multiplied by the cross-sectional area of the aorta) reflects regurgitant volume flow. Since the cross-sectional area of the aorta is approximately the same during systole and diastole, the ratio of reverse (diastolic) to forward (systolic) flow velocity integrals provides a Doppler index that corresponds well to angiographic regurgitant fraction.[33] Similarly, flow velocity waveforms from the middle hepatic vein (recorded from the subcostal window) allow estimation of the relative volume of anterograde flow (away from the transducer during diastole) and regurgitant flow (toward the transducer during systole). These data provide a useful index of tricuspid regurgitation.[34]

Regurgitant volumes are particularly sensitive to ventricular preload and afterload. Thus, comparisons of Doppler techniques with other methods for quantitating regurgitation are difficult to interpret when measures have not been simultaneous and loading conditions have not been defined. Notwithstanding these difficulties in validating their accuracy, Doppler techniques have allowed us to segregate patients with mild, moderate, and severe degrees of regurgitation, and this information has helped us manage individual patients.

Prosthetic Valve Dysfunction

Using Doppler to detect and define the severity of prosthetic valve dysfunction is particularly attractive, in part because of the limitations of other noninvasive techniques. The fluid-dynamic alterations of prosthetic valve stenosis and regurgitation are similar to those of native valves. Accordingly, prosthetic valve stenosis is manifested as anterograde flow of increased velocity, and the peak flow velocity does reflect the instantaneous pressure drop across the prosthesis.[35] Prosthetic valve regurgitation is accompanied by retrograde flow across the prosthesis and by a flow disturbance in the chamber receiving the regurgitant flow.[36] Detection of these abnormalities by continuous and pulsed wave Doppler has been reported in patients with malfunctioning prostheses.

Unfortunately, investigation of valvular prostheses using any ultrasound technique is difficult because of their design and construction. Mechanical valves have echogenic plastic and metal parts that attenuate substantially the strength of ultrasound passing through them. Bioprostheses, while less of a problem, do contain echogenic sewing rings and struts. Moreover, the many prosthesis types and designs each have their own functional and hemodynamic characteristics. The velocity of anterograde flow through a specific prosthetic valve should vary with the valve's size and position of implantation and with volume flow across it. In light of these influences, adequate "ranges of normal" Doppler findings in patients with prosthetic valves have not yet been established. Finally, the direction of flow through prosthetic valves can be quite complex, especially in valves with noncentral orifices or eccentric poppet opening.[37] In diseased bioprostheses, the direction of blood flow may also be difficult to predict. In these instances, accurate measurement of true flow velocity may be technically difficult, because the angle between the ultrasound beam and blood flow must be known in order to calculate flow velocity from the measured Doppler shifts.

Some prosthetic valves normally regurgitate a small volume of blood, especially mechanical prostheses whose poppets do not close as briskly as the leaflets of a normal valve. The amount of this normal back flow varies with loading conditions and heart rate.[38] We do not have sufficient experience yet to distinguish "normal" from subtle cases of "pathological" regurgitation in patients with valvular prostheses.

To summarize, Doppler techniques for measuring the velocity of forward flow and detecting the presence of regurgitant flow provide useful diagnostic information in many patients with suspected prosthetic stenosis or regurgitation. This information clearly supplements and complements other noninvasive tests, but additional work is needed before Doppler findings can confidently separate subtle cases of abnormality from the range of normal in patients with valvular prostheses.[39]

Assessment of Shunt Lesions

In general, intracardiac shunt lesions are detected by demonstrating flow through the abnormal communication, the direction of which is (by definition) abnormal, and the velocity of which is usually increased. The severity of shunting is determined from volume flows measured at different locations within the heart and great vessels.

Ventricular Septal Defect

Ventricular septal defect can be detected by demonstrating systolic flow through the ventricular septum, using either pulsed or continuous Doppler techniques. Since flow in ventricular septal defect is generally from left to right, the precordial echocardiographic windows are particularly useful for demonstrating shunt flow toward the transducer. Many locations of the defect are possible, however, and in some individuals subcostal views are also helpful. Even ventricular septal defects too small to be imaged can be detected by their accompanying flow disturbances. In general, flow through small ventricular septal defects is high in velocity, since there is a pressure drop from the left to the right ventricle. Large ventricular septal defects, which may be associated with equalization of pressure, do not always cause increased flow velocities. A postjet flow disturbance within the right ventricular body can be demonstrated using pulsed Doppler; this flow disturbance frequently extends downstream into the right ventricular outflow tract and pulmonary artery. In comparison with angiographic findings, Doppler can detect ventricular septal defect with a sensitivity of 95 to 100 percent and a high specificity.[40] Doppler findings clearly complement two-dimensional echocardiographic images, and appear to be superior in patients with small defects.

The amount of flow through a ventricular septal defect cannot be measured within the defect itself, since the cross-sectional area of the defect cannot be determined reliably. Flow distal to the ventricular septal defect is nonlaminar, so pulmonary volume flow is measured not in the pulmonary artery but rather in the mitral valve orifice. Systemic volume flow can be measured from the ascending aortic flow velocity curve and aortic diameter. The ratio between pulmonary (mitral) and systemic (aortic) flow volumes has correlated well to catheterization measures of the Q_P/Q_S ratio in both experimental and clinical studies.[8,10,12] These results support the role of Doppler in estimating the degree of shunting through a ventricular septal defect.

Atrial Septal Defect

Atrial septal defect is usually best detected from subcostal windows, which align the ultrasound beam with the direction of shunting. Flow from the left atrium into the right atrium (toward the transducer) can often be detected both in late systole and diastole; with pulsed techniques, this flow appears to have some disturbed characteristics. Greatly increased velocities are generally not present, owing to the small pressure drop between the two atrial chambers. The majority of atrial septal defects are relatively large and can be imaged directly by two-dimensional echocardiography, but the atrial septum does "drop out" normally in certain views, so that Doppler findings provide a helpful adjunct in assessing the presence of an atrial septal defect. Venous inflow into the right atrium from the superior vena cava can frequently be recorded high along the interatrial septum, and care should be taken not to mistake this normal phenomenon for an interatrial shunt. When there is a question about the Doppler findings, a contrast two-dimensional echocardiographic study may help resolve the issue.

The magnitude of the shunt can be quantitated by measuring pulmonary volume flow in the pulmonary artery and systemic volume flow in the aorta. The ratio between these two measures corresponds well to the Q_P/Q_S ratio as determined at catheterization in both experimental models and patients.[11,12] It appears that Doppler can distinguish shunts requiring closure from those sufficiently small that operation can be avoided.

Patent Ductus Arteriosus

Persistent patency of the ductus arteriosus, although infrequent in adults, is a common problem in the newborn nursery. One of the most common cardiac causes for neonatal respiratory distress is left-to-right shunting through a ductus arteriosus, and the medical or surgical management of this lesion requires its accurate diagnosis. Unfortunately, many cases are not accompanied by diagnostic clinical findings.

Left-to-right flow through a patent ductus arteriosus is detected reliably by examining flow in the pulmonary artery,[41] usually from a high parasternal approach. In normal individuals, systolic flow from the right ventricle into the pulmonary artery is directed away from the transducer. During diastole, no appreciable back flow toward the transducer is recorded. In the patient with a patent ductus arteriosus, retrograde flow from the aorta into the pulmonary artery is recorded reliably.[41] Moreover, patients without pulmonary hypertension have persistent ductal flow through diastole, while those with significant pulmonary hypertension have abbreviated ductal flow that does not persist through diastole.

In patent ductus arteriosus, flow in the pulmonary artery is disturbed, therefore volume flow cannot be measured in this region. Moreover, volume flow in the ascending aorta represents both forward and shunt flow. Accordingly, to quantitate the Q_P/Q_S ratio, systemic flow is measured from the flow velocity integral and diameter of the right ventricular outflow tract (which is relatively cylindrical). Pulmonary flow can be measured in either the mitral orifice or the ascending aorta, since the total volume of shunt flow passes through these regions. Several investigators have reported good correlation between estimates of pulmonary/systemic flow ratios made by Doppler and made by catheterization in both experimental aorta-pulmonary connections and children with patent ductus arteriosus.[9,12]

Limitations of Doppler Echocardiography

Doppler echocardiography is subject to a number of technical limitations. Doppler makes use of low-amplitude signals, since the amount of ultrasonic energy backscattered from red cells is substantially smaller than that reflected from large myocardial-to-blood interfaces. Distinction of Doppler signals from background noise is sometimes difficult, particularly in patients with so-called poor ultrasound penetration, or when flow is examined at a great distance from the transducer (where depth-related attenuation becomes a factor). Second, the frequency shifts measured by Doppler do not always correspond directly to blood flow velocities. The ultrasound beam must be oriented parallel to the direction of blood flow in three-dimensional space, and since blood flow cannot actually be imaged, this sometimes requires a time-consuming trial-and-error approach. Third, Doppler shifts recorded from a single sample volume provide a spatially limited view of flow in a given cardiac chamber or vessel. Doppler mapping must be used to assess flow in three dimensions. This is tedious, and furthermore, it is of limited use when flow volume varies from beat to beat (as during an arrhythmia). Finally, Doppler is a technically demanding technique that requires the examiner to have a good ear for the Doppler frequencies, a knowledge of hemodynamics, and a great deal of patience.

General Recommendations

Since Doppler provides direct information about intracardiac hemodynamics while two-dimensional and M-mode echocardiography provide structural information, these techniques supplement each other and provide intrinsic checks. For example, Doppler can be used to determine if apparent echo drop-out in the ventricular or atrial septum actually represents a septal defect, while the echocardiographic images help determine how to aim the Doppler beam and where to place the sample volume. Similarly, direct measurement of the mitral orifice area by two-dimensional echocardiography can be checked against pressure half-time results determined by Doppler. Hence, Doppler echocardiography should be used in conjunction with two-dimensional and M-mode echocardiography, as part of the comprehensive ultrasonic evaluation of the patient with known or suspected heart disease. In our laboratory, we use Doppler routinely, making those flow measures that appear important in the context of the clinical presentation and other examination findings. We begin by familiarizing ourselves with the structural abnormalities, and then we use imaging and Doppler in an interactive manner. At the present time, we believe that Doppler echocardiography is clinically useful in (1) detecting and estimating the severity of valvular stenoses or discrete narrowings in cardiac chambers and great vessels (i.e., hypertrophic cardiomyopathy, pulmonary artery bands); (2) demonstrating valvular insufficiency and estimating its severity; and (3) establishing the presence and determining the significance of an intracardiac shunt. We feel that the use of Doppler for measuring absolute volume flow is promising but believe that technical problems, especially in accurate measurement of the cross-sectional area through which flow occurs, still require additional work. We do think it reasonable to use the Doppler flow velocity integral to follow changes in volume flow in individual patients, especially in the appropriate clinical context. Finally, we consider the technically demanding nature of Doppler echocardiography to require continued comparison of Doppler results with those of other diagnostic modalities, as an intrinsic check.

Additional applications for Doppler echocardiography are on the horizon. Doppler velocity measures in regurgitant tricuspid jets have allowed accurate prediction of the right ventricular–right atrial pressure gradient and thence of peak systolic right ventricular (and pulmonary arterial) pressure. Aortic regurgitant velocities, while more difficult to record, have allowed prediction of left ventricular end-diastolic pressure. Doppler measures of left ventricular inflow velocities have promise for defining global left ventricular diastolic properties. Finally, the recently introduced technique of *color flow imaging,* using multigate pulsed Doppler and phased-array beam steering, appears particularly interesting. This technique provides tomographic color images of Doppler shifts superimposed upon two-dimensional echocardiographic views of cardiac structure.[42] Regurgitant jets can be imaged directly, and impressive visualization of shunt flow through the ventricular septum (either left-to-right or right-to-left) has been demonstrated. However, the sensitivity of this technique to various lesions and its ability to quantitate blood flow velocities (given the inherent limitations in pulsed Doppler sampling rates) have yet to be defined. Ultimately, however, this technique may allow evaluation of blood flow in a three-dimensional fashion.

References

1. Von Jurgensen, T.: Valvular Disease, in G. Dock (ed.), "Diseases of the Heart," W. B. Saunders Company, Philadelphia, 1908, p. 328.
2. Hatle, L., and Angelsen, B.: "Doppler Ultrasound in Cardiology: Physical Principles and Clinical Applications," 2nd ed., Lea & Febiger, Philadelphia, 1985.
3. Pearlman, A. S., Scoblionko, D. P., and Saal, A. K.: Assessment of Valvular Heart Disease by Doppler Echocardiography, *Clin. Cardiol,* 6:573, 1983.
4. Huntsman, L. L., Stewart, D. K., Barnes, S. R., Franklin, S. B., Colocousis, J. S., and Hessel, E. A.: Non-invasive Doppler Determination of Cardiac Output in Man–Clinical Validation, *Circulation,* 67:593, 1983.
5. Pearlman, A. S.: Evaluation of Ventricular Function Using Doppler Echocardiography, *Am. J. Cardiol.,* 49:1324, 1982.
6. Fisher, D. C., Sahn, D. J., Friedman, M. J., et al.: The Mitral Valve Orifice Method for Non-invasive Two-Dimensional Echo Doppler Determinations of Cardiac Output, *Circulation,* 67:872, 1983.
7. Lewis, J. F., Kuo, L. C., Nelson, J. G., Limacher, M. C., and Quinones, M. A.: Pulsed Doppler Echocardiographic Determination of Stroke Volume and Cardiac Output: Clinical Validation of Two New Methods Using the Apical Window, *Circulation,* 70:425, 1984.
8. Sanders, S. P., Yeager, S., and Williams, R. G.: Measurement of Systemic and Pulmonary Blood Flow and Q_P/Q_S Ratio Using Doppler and Two-Dimensional Echocardiography, *Am. J. Cardiol.,* 51:952, 1983.
9. Meijboom, E. J., Valdes-Cruz, L. M. Horowitz, S., et al.: A Two-Dimensional Doppler Echocardiographic Method for Calculation of Pulmonary and Systemic Flow in a Canine Model with a Variable-Sized Left-to-Right Extracardiac Shunt, *Circulation,* 68:437, 1983.
10. Valdes-Cruz, L. M., Horowitz, S., Mesel, E., et al.: A Pulsed Doppler Echocardiographic Method for Calculation of Pulmonary and Systemic Flow: Accuracy in a Canine Model with Ventricular Septal Defect, *Circulation,* 68:597, 1983.
11. Valdes-Cruz, L. M., Horowitz, S., Mesel, E., Sahn, D. J., Fisher, D. C., and Larson, D.: A Pulsed Doppler Echocardiographic Method for Calculating Pulmonary and Systemic Blood Flow in Atrial Level Shunts: Validation Studies in Animals and in Initial Human Experience, *Circulation,* 69:80, 1984.
12. Barron, J. V., Sahn, D. J., Valdes-Cruz, L. M., et al.: Clinical Utility of Two-Dimensional Doppler Echocardiographic Techniques for Estimating Pulmonary to Systemic Blood Flow Ratios in Children with Left to Right Shunting Atrial Septal Defect, Ventricular Septal Defect or Patent Ductus Arteriosus, *J. Am. Coll. Cardiol.,* 3:169, 1984.
13. Gardin, J. M., Iseri, L. T., Elkayam, U., et al.: Evaluation of Dilated Cardiomyopathy by Pulsed Doppler Echocardiography, *Am. Heart J.,* 106:1057, 1983.
14. Elkayam, U., Gardin, J. M., Berkley, R., Hughes, C. A., and Henry, W. L.: The Use of Doppler Flow Velocity Measurement to Assess the Hemodynamic Response to Vasodilators in Patients with Heart Failure, *Circulation,* 67:377, 1983.
15. Kitabatake, A., Inoue, M., Asao, M., et al.: Non-invasive Evaluation of Pulmonary Hypertension by a Pulsed Doppler Technique, *Circulation* 68:302, 1983.
16. Kececioglu-Draelos, Z., Goldberg, S. J., Areias, J., and Sahn, D. J.: Verification and Clinical Demonstration of the Echo Doppler Series Effect and Vortex Shed Distance, *Circulation,* 63: 1422, 1981.
17. Hatle, L., Tromsdal, A., and Angelsen, B.: Non-invasive Assessment of Pressure Drop in Mitral Stenosis by Doppler Ultrasound, *Br. Heart J.,* 40:131, 1978.
18. Hatle, L., Angelsen, B. A., and Tromsdal, A.: Non-invasive Assessment of Aortic Stenosis by Doppler Ultrasound, *Br. Heart J.,* 43:284, 1980.
19. Stamm, R. B., and Martin, R. P.: Quantification of Pressure Gradients across Stenotic Valves by Doppler Ultrasound, *J. Am. Coll. Cardiol.,* 2:707, 1983.
20. Berger, M., Berdoff, R. L., Gallerstein, P. E., and Goldberg, E.: Evaluation of Aortic Stenosis by Continuous Wave Doppler Ultrasound, *J. Am. Coll. Cardiol.,* 3:150, 1984.
21. Stevenson, J. G., and Kawabori, I.: Non-invasive Determination of Pressure Gradients in Children: Two Methods Employing Pulsed Doppler Echocardiography, *J. Am. Coll. Cardiol.,* 3:179, 1984.
22. Holen, J., and Simonsen, S.: Determination of Pressure Gradient in Mitral Stenosis with Doppler Echocardiography, *Br. Heart J.,* 41:529, 1979.
23. Lima, C. O., Sahn, D. J., Valdes-Cruz, L. M., et al.: Non-invasive Prediction of Transvalvular Pressure Gradient in Patients with Pulmonary Stenosis by Quantitative Two-Dimensional Echocardiographic Doppler Studies, *Circulation,* 67:866, 1983.
24. Valdes-Cruz, L. M., Horowitz, S., Sahn, D. J., Larson, D., Lima, C. O., and Mesel, E.: Validation of a Doppler Echocardiographic Method for Calculating Severity of Discrete Stenotic Obstructions in a Canine Preparation with a Pulmonary Arterial Band, *Circulation,* 69:1177, 1984.
25. Kosturakis, D., Allen, H. D., Goldberg, S. J., Sahn, D. J., and Valdes-Cruz, L. M.: Non-invasive Quantification of Stenotic Semilunar Valve Areas by Doppler Echocardiography, *J. Am. Coll. Cardiol.,* 3:1256, 1984.
26. Hatle, L., Angelsen B., and Tromsdal, A.: Non-invasive Assessment of Atrioventricular Pressure Half-Time by Doppler Ultrasound, *Circulation,* 60:1096, 1979.
27. Richards, K. L., Cannon, S. R., Crawford, M. H., and Sorensen, S. G.: Noninvasive Diagnosis of Aortic and Mitral Valve Disease with Pulsed-Doppler Spectral Analysis, *Am. J. Cardiol.,* 51:1122, 1983.
28. Pearlman, A. S., and Lighty, G. W., Jr.: Clinical Applications of Two-Dimensional/Doppler Echocardiography, *Cardiovasc. Clin.,* 13:201, 1983.
29. Saal, A. K., Gross, B. W., Franklin, D. W., and Pearlman,

A. S.: Non-invasive Detection of Aortic Insufficiency in Patients with Mitral Stenosis by Pulsed Doppler Echocardiography, *J. Am. Coll. Cardiol.*, 5:176, 1985.
30. Esper, R. J.: Detection of Mild Aortic Regurgitation by Range-Gated Pulsed Doppler Echocardiography, *Am J. Cardiol.*, 50:1037, 1982.
31. Bas, S., Manin, J. P., Veyrat, C., Abitbol, G., and Kalmanson, D.: Pulsed Doppler Calculation of a Three-Dimensional Index of Severity of Mitral Regurgitation with Pathophysiological Implications, in C. T. Lancee (ed.), "Ultrasonoor Bulletin, Fifth Symposium on Echocardiology," Bohn, Scheltema and Holkema, Utrecht/Antwerpen, 1983, p. 101. (Abstract.)
32. Stewart, W. J., Palacios, I., Jiang, L., Dinsmore, R. E., and Weyman, A. E.: Doppler Measurement of Regurgitant Fraction in Patients with Mitral Regurgitation: A New Quantitative Technique, *Circulation*, 68(suppl. 3):III-111, 1983. (Abstract.)
33. Boughner, D. R.: Assessment of Aortic Insufficiency by Transcutaneous Doppler Ultrasound, *Circulation*, 52:874, 1975.
34. Diebold, B., Touati, R., and Blanchard, D.: Quantitative Assessment of Tricuspid Regurgitation Using Pulsed Doppler Echocardiography, *Br. Heart J.*, 50:443, 1983.
35. Holen, J., Simonsen, S., and Froysaker, T.: An Ultrasound Doppler Technique for the Non-invasive Determination of the Pressure Gradient in the Bjork-Shiley Mitral Valve, *Circulation*, 59:436, 1979.
36. Caputo, G. R., Pearlman, A. S., Namay, D., and Dooley, T. K.: Detection of Prosthetic Valve Incompetence Using Pulsed Doppler Echocardiography, *Circulation*, 52(suppl. 3): III-252, 1980. (Abstract.)
37. Bruss, K.-H., Reul, H., VanGilse, J., and Knott, E.: Pressure Drop and Velocity Fields at Four Mechanical Prostheses: Bjork-Shiley Standard, Bjork-Shiley Concave-Convex, Hall-Kaster and St. Jude Medical, *Life Support Systems*, 1:3, 1983.
38. Dellsperger, K. C., Wieting, D. W., Baehr, D. A., Bard, R. J., Brugger, J.-P., and Harrison, E. C.: Regurgitation of Prosthetic Heart Valves: Dependence on Heart Rate and Cardiac Output, *Am. J. Cardiol.*, 51:321, 1983.
39. Pearlman, A. S.: Doppler Echocardiography: A Promising Method for Investigating Prosthetic Valve Dysfunction, *Echocardiography*, 1:257, 1984.
40. Stevenson, J. G., Kawabori, I., Dooley, T., and Guntheroth, W. G.: Diagnosis of Ventricular Septal Defect by Pulsed Doppler Echocardiography, *Circulation*, 58:322, 1978.
41. Stevenson, J. G., Kawabori, I., and Guntheroth, W. G.: Pulsed Doppler Echocardiographic Diagnosis of Patent Ductus Arteriosus: Sensitivity, Specificity, Limitations, and Technical Features, *Cathet. Cardiovasc. Diagn.* 6:255, 1980.
42. Miyatake, K., Okamoto, M., Kinoshita, N., et al.: Clinical Applications of a New Type of Real-Time Two-Dimensional Doppler Flow Imaging System, *Am. J. Cardiol.*, 54:857, 1984.

Section E

Phonocardiography and Pulse Wave Tracing

123

Technique of Phonocardiography and Pulse Wave Tracings

Ernest Craige, M.D.

Thus we may conclude that the human hearing mechanism alters or distorts logarithmically, with respect to frequency, the relative intensities of the components of the sounds that are transmitted to the tympanum of the ear by the stethoscope.

Maurice B. Rappaport and
Howard B. Sprague, 1942[1,*]

The term *phonocardiography* as used in this chapter encompasses not merely the recording of heart sounds and murmurs but also the recording of combinations of acoustic phenomena and pulsatile tracings of carotid, apex, and jugular venous origin. These graphic methods provide a permanent visual confirmation of the physical signs that may have been perceived by bedside techniques of inspection, palpation, and auscultation. Despite their apparent advantages, these graphic methods have suffered a decline in popularity along with the unfortunate but widespread tendency to pass over time-honored methods of personal observation in favor of using elaborate technological devices for cardiac diagnosis. Thus, one currently finds that phonocardiography is routinely practiced only in those relatively few institutions where there has been a traditional emphasis on the physical examination. This trend represents a failure to appreciate the enhanced utility of phonocardiography resulting from two recent developments: (1) investigations which have provided an improved understanding of the physiological basis of heart sounds, murmurs, and pulse tracings,[2–7] and (2) improvements in instrumentation which permit the simultaneous registration on high-speed, sensitized paper of the M-mode echocardiogram *with* phonocardiograms, pulse tracings, and the ECG. The information thus obtained has multiplied the diagnostic utility of noninvasive methods in cardiology.[7,8]

In the author's opinion, the practice of requesting a phonocardiogram in isolation is, indeed, obsolete. Our preference is to make an initial bedside assessment utilizing traditional methods of history, physical examination, electrocardiogram (ECG), and chest x-ray and then, if indicated, plan a noninvasive assessment. Depending on the preliminary differential diagnosis, this would require an appropriate combination of echo- and phonocardiograms with apex, carotid, or jugular venous pulse tracings, systolic time intervals, etc., designed to resolve certain clearly defined questions. Thus, for example, in a suspected case of mitral valve prolapse, the auscultatory phenomena would be displayed along with an echocardiogram of the mitral valve. The observation of click and murmur on the phonocardiogram occurring simultaneously with the apparent collapse of the valve leaflet on the echocardiogram would add significantly to the credibility of either of these findings alone in a diagnostic situation notorious for problems in interpretation of borderline and false-positive manifestations.

*Reproduced with permission from the publisher.

Facilities and Equipment

Recording Environment

One reason for disappointment with phonocardiography is the presence of background noises which appear as artifacts on the finished tracing. A completely soundproof room is not necessary, however. An adequately conditioned room can easily be obtained by the judicious use of absorbent tiles on walls, ceiling, and door; drapes over windows; and a rug on the floor.

A comfortable bed equipped with a device for elevating the head is necessary. Wedge-shaped pillows, readily available through radiological supply sources, provide a convenient method of supporting the patient in a laterally tilted position when indicated.

A rack on the wall near the head of the bed can be used to hold the transducers for sound and pulse recording. This simple bit of carpentry keeps the delicate instruments safe and readily available and helps to avoid a disagreeable tangle of wires.

Lighting should be controlled by a rheostat so that subdued light can be maintained during periods when the oscilloscope is monitored.

Instrumentation

Recorder

The recorder is the most important piece of equipment in the phonocardiographic laboratory. The choice of a recorder depends on several factors: (1) the graphic phenomena that one hopes to record, (2) price, (3) portability, (4) dependability, and (5) availability of service. Usually a five- or six-channel instrument is required in order to record combinations of, for example, an ECG, phonocardiograms from two locations on the chest, a pulse tracing, and an M-mode echocardiogram. There are a variety of methods for registering the graphic information. A photographic method provides the most brilliant contrast of black and white images, suitable for teaching demonstrations and publications. It requires, however, a dark room and an automatic processor, and the paper is very expensive. The instantly developed paper is cheaper and requires less personnel time. However, the product inevitably lacks contrast and yields dull reproductions. Both of the above methods are suitable for combinations of echocardiograms, phonocardiograms, and pulse tracings, but there is a vast range of quality in the phonocardiograms obtained from commercially available recorders that are well known for their echocardiographic capability. If one wishes to restrict the recordings to phonocardiograms and pulse tracings with an ECG, a jet ink writer is quite satisfactory. Such an instrument with multiple paper speeds including 100 mm/s is ideal for measurement of systolic time intervals (ECG with carotid pulse tracing and phonocardiogram), and the cost of the paper is relatively low. The principal drawback of the jet ink writer is that it cannot be used for echocardiography.

One should avoid recorders that consist essentially of a direct-writing ECG modified to produce a rudimentary pulse and sound tracing for calculation of systolic time intervals. The poor quality of recorded vibrations and the slow paper speed of such instruments preclude their use for any type of serious work. For appreciation of the details of a phonocardiogram, such as the separation of A_2 to P_2 or A_2 to opening snap, or for measurement of systolic time intervals, a paper speed of 100 mm/s is most satisfactory. The recorder, however, should have the capability of recording at slower speeds such as 25 and 50 mm/s.

Microphones and Amplifiers

Two types of microphones are generally available for recording heart sounds—the *contact* and the *air-coupled* types. The contact microphone consists of a small circular plate which receives vibrations from the chest wall and transmits them to a sensing device—a crystal or moving coil. The microphone itself is held firmly attached to the chest wall by a rubber strap. When room noise is a problem, the contact microphone may be advantageous. The air-coupled microphone, which we prefer, is attached to the chest by a rubber strap or with suction provided by a rubber bulb.* An airtight seal is necessary. The air-coupled microphone is activated by vibrations which emanate from the chest wall and subject the enclosed volume of air to pressure changes which, in turn, deflect a thin diaphragm attached to a crystal sensing element.

The minute electric impulses from the microphone are amplified and filtered for display on an oscilloscope and for permanent recording. A variety of methods of filtration are used, but in general they serve to modify the raw vibrations such that the final product will more nearly approximate the spectrum appreciated by the human ear. This is accomplished by selectively diminishing the lower frequencies, whose greater strength would otherwise result in the domination of the tracing.

Pulse Transducers

The piezoelectric crystal type of pulse transducer is the one most commonly used for registration of carotid, apex, and venous pulse tracings. Formerly there was a problem with many of the commercially available pulse transducers of this type in that they suffered from too short a time constant. This resulted in a systematic distortion of the recorded tracing such that a sustained plateau in an apex cardiogram, for instance, might appear as an inverted V and a shallow trough might become a deep crevasse. Tem-

*Leatham microphone, Irex Corp., Ramsey, New Jersey.

poral landmarks were likewise distorted.[9,10] Because of this problem, some laboratories turned to strain gauge transducers with a time constant of infinity. This recourse is not necessary any longer since a number of quite satisfactory transducers are available. The most common design includes a funnel for application to the pulsatile area under study, with air transmission to the sensitive crystal provided via a short rubber tube, preferably of rather stiff consistency to avoid damping. Air leaks must be scrupulously avoided.

Respiration

It is frequently desirable to record a respiratory tracing in conjunction with the phonocardiogram. One commonly used probe is the nasal thermistor, which is inserted into the nostril and held in place by adhesive tape. The difference in temperature between inhaled and exhaled air is sensed by this device, amplified, and displayed in conjunction with acoustic and pulsatile events.

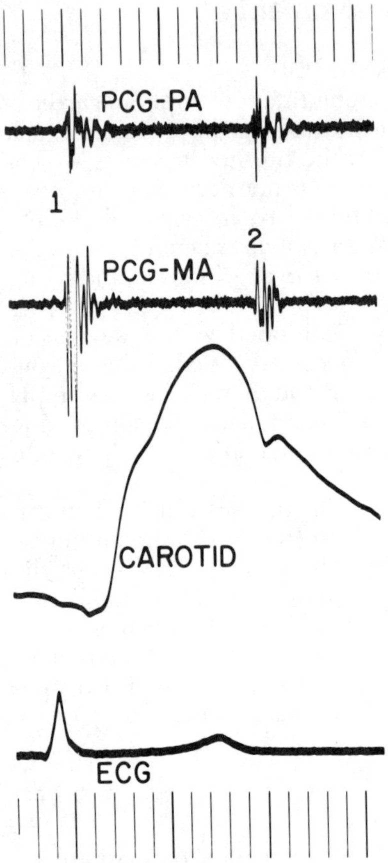

FIGURE 123-1 Normal carotid tracing. There is a swift upstroke and a well-formed incisura immediately following S_2 of the phonocardiogram. PCG-PA and PCG-MA = phonocardiograms in the pulmonary and mitral areas, respectively.

Recording Technique

It should be explained to paitents that their heart sounds will be recorded for diagnostic purposes and that the procedure will be painless and harmless. The patient should disrobe from the waist up and be asked to lie comfortably on the bed with the head elevated as required for comfort.

Preliminary Examination

Before transducers are applied to the chest wall, it is recommended that a brief physical examination of the cardiovascular system be performed so that the optimal combinations of sites of the chest wall for microphones and pulse transducers can be selected. Decisions must be made regarding the position of the patient—supine or left lateral decubitus—as well as appropriate combinations of phonocardiograms, pulse tracings, and, we would recommend, echocardiograms. Examples of recommended combinations of acoustic, pulsatile, and ultrasonic phenomena for particular suspected diagnoses are listed at the end of this chapter. If, in taking a phonocardiogram, one merely places the microphones in standard positions on the chest wall without any particular objective or protocol in mind, the results will be disappointing and frequently quite misleading.

Application of Electrodes and Microphones for Phonocardiogram

ECG electrodes are attached to the extremities with good contact required, as in routine electrocardiography, to avoid artifacts. The quality of the ECG should be monitored on the oscilloscope. For phonocardiography, the microphone or (preferably) two microphones are placed on the chest wall in the location(s) determined by preliminary auscultation[11] (Fig. 123-1). The advantage afforded by recording two phonocardiograms simultaneously is that it is easy to demonstrate that certain sounds in one area are identical with or distinct from others. For instance, a tracing from the second left intercostal space will show details of the second heart sound (A_2,P_2), while a simultaneous tracing from lower on the precordium might demonstrate another sound, slightly later—an opening snap or third sound. It may be necessary to shave small areas to eliminate acoustic artifacts caused by hairs. The presence of hair has the additional disadvantage of disrupting the seal necessary for the air-coupled microphone. A thin layer of petroleum jelly facilitates the maintenance of the airtight seal.

Operators should take advantage of the stethophone that is provided with most recorders so that they can monitor the signal by listening as well as by watching the oscilloscope. This precaution helps to eliminate artifacts that might be produced by the percussive impact of a hyperdynamic cardiac impulse on the sensitive microphone, or noises from hairs or crossed wires—artifacts that can occur rhythmically with the heartbeat, thus simulating heart sounds, clicks, rubs, etc. Auscultation easily verifies the quality of such extraneous noises as artifactual, although their source may not be apparent in the finished recording. Listening through the stethophone at the same time that one monitors the vibrations on the oscilloscope also provides an opportunity to adjust the filters on the recorder for optimal appreciation of acoustic phenomena.

Carotid Pulse

To record the carotid pulse, have the patient lie with head elevated and neck slightly hyperextended. This can be accomplished by placing a pillow underneath the shoulders so that the head falls backward to some extent. This position, with the neck convex anteriorly, places the carotid pulse in prominent profile, where it is usually visible and easily palpable. The area of most accessible and obvious pulsation is located by palpation. Then the funnel of the transducer is firmly placed over the pulse, achieving a tight air seal between the rim of the funnel and the skin. That the pulse is of adequate quality for permanent registration can be determined from inspection of the oscilloscope. The features one should look for are a swift upstroke, a well-marked incisura, and a gradual decline during diastole (Fig. 123-1). Obviously, these manifestations may be altered by aortic valve disease. If large presystolic waves are seen, the tracing may be suffering from contamination by the venous pulse. Elevating the patient's head to a greater degree may be useful in eliminating this problem. If the carotid pulse tracing is to be used in the calculation of systolic time intervals, a paper speed of 100 mm/s is optimal to minimize errors in measurement.[12]

Jugular Venous Pulse

During the brief physical examination that precedes the recording of the phonocardiogram and pulse tracings, the jugular venous pulse should have been identified in the manner described in Chap. 9. This may require changing the degree of elevation of the head of the bed so that the pulsating column of blood in the internal jugular vein may be optimally visible. Many experienced clinicians despair of interpreting the morphological details of the rapid, kaleidoscopic, pulsatile phenomena at the base of the neck that constitute the venous pulse. However, the practice of confirming one's clinical impression with graphic records will result in greater confidence and will enhance the diagnostic yield of physical examination.

Graphic methods for recording the jugular venous pulse have generally been of two types—the sensing of *volume* changes in the internal jugular system and the sensing of *pressure* changes. In order to appreciate volume changes one would need a completely weightless transducer, such as an electronic beam, which would detect movements of the profile of the vein with the cardiac cycle without distorting the pulsation by its own contact. Although such devices are available, the transducer-recorder method, more generally employed in the United States, reflects pressure changes. These mimic closely the pressure pulse in the right atrium. The same transducer can be used as for the carotid pulse and the apexcardiogram. The funnel leading to a piezoelectric crystal through a short stiff rubber tube is applied to the fossa above the clavicle between the two heads of the sternocleidomastoid muscle. The patient should be comfortable and relaxed, with the head in a position that will avoid torsion or pressure on the area under observation. Even though the venous pulse may not be visible in this supraclavicular location, the funnel may be in close contact with the jugular bulb. One has to monitor the oscilloscope closely since interfering anterial pulsations are easily picked up in this location; they can be recognized by their systolic upstroke and dicrotic notch. It is often rewarding to press the funnel of the transducer downward and in a medial direction in order to exclude arterial pulsations and to obtain an uncontaminated signal of venous origin. A satisfactory waveform can be appreciated by the presence of diastolic peaks—the *a* and *v* waves and the descent waves *x* and *y*. Even though these pulsations can only be interpreted qualitatively, in their morphology they simulate the analogous curves from the right atrium[13] (Fig. 123-2).

Apexcardiogram

The apexcardiogram is a graphic tracing which represents precordial movements resulting from the

FIGURE 123-2 Jugular venous pulse (JVP) tracing from a normal subject. The phonocardiograms illustrate a trivial systolic murmur. The principal waves of the JVP are identified (see text).

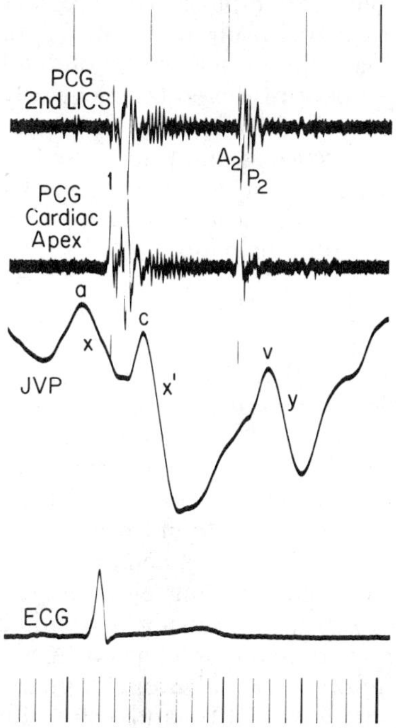

heartbeat. The technique dates from the 1860s when Marey produced quite satisfactory tracings using a capsule transducer, which is the precursor of the tambour still widely used in Europe and the United States.[14] The technique and apparatus for apexcardiography can also be used for the registration of other precordial pulsatile activity such as thrusts at the left sternal edge, reflecting right ventricular hypertrophy, or ectopic pulsations over the midprecordium, resulting from aneurysms or bulges of the anterior surface of the left ventricle. Although a number of methods are available for recording pulsatile movements of the precordium,[15] (kinetocardiography, impulse cardiography,[16] etc.), we will confine our description to the technique of apexcardiography.[17] Each of these methods has contributed to our understanding of precordial pulsations. However, there has been a confusing multiplicity of published records from different laboratories, using various types of apparatus and methodology, which may have contributed to a lessening of interest in recordings of precordial movement. Apexcardiography is a technique by which one senses the excursion of the movable diaphragm of the transducer (or the skin acting as a diaphragm) relative to the rim of the sensing head, with the patient lying on his or her left side. The technique of kinetocardiography[15] utilizes a transducer attached to a fixed point in space. Thus, it records the "absolute" movement of the chest wall from various points on the thorax, with the patient lying supine.

It should be realized that none of these methods reflect exactly the events that are palpated at the bedside. Unfortunately, the mechanoreceptors in the human fingertips are relatively insensitive to the small, low-frequency movements which make up the cardiac impulse.[18] In normal subjects one perceives by palpation only the outward impulse which occurs during the brief period of isovolumic contraction. Diastolic events such as filling in early diastole and with atrial systole are not appreciated unless greatly exaggerated, as in disease.[16] Therefore, the apexcardiogram should be recorded and interpreted in its own right as a portion of a noninvasive assessment rather than as an attempt to reproduce precisely what one perceives by palpation.

Physiological Correlations of the Apexcardiogram

One of the principal uses of the apexcardiogram is as a temporal marker for intracardiac events. Its upstroke begins at almost precisely the same instant as the analogous event in the left ventricular pressure pulse.[19] Its initial peak (point E) occurs approximately at the onset of ejection of blood from the left ventricle (Fig. 123-3). A gradual decline in the apex tracing during systole occurs during ejection, followed by an almost vertical fall during isovolumic relaxation. A nadir (zero point) is reached at approximately the time of mitral valve opening, followed by a rapid-filling wave (RFW) and a slow-filling wave (SFW). The A wave (A) resulting from the additional ventricular filling provided by atrial systole is of small dimensions in normal subjects.

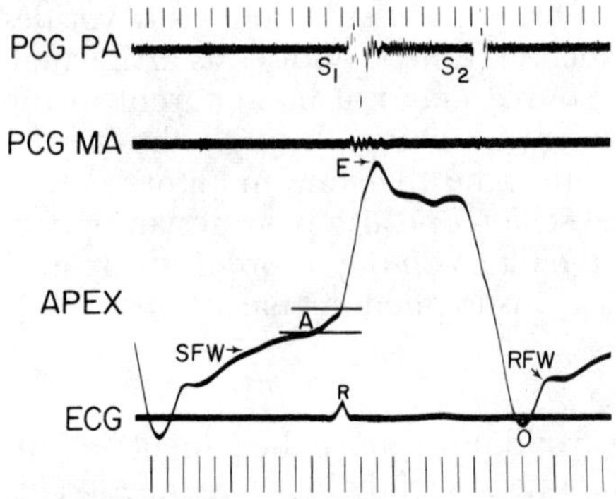

FIGURE 123-3 Normal apexcardiogram. A brisk outward movement occurs immediately after the R wave, during the isovolumic portion of systole. It culminates in the E point at approximately the time of onset of ejection. There is an inward movement manifested by a decline of the curve during systole with a more rapid fall beginning just before the second heart sound (S_2). A nadir (0) is reached at approximately the time of opening of the mitral valve. This is followed by a rapid-filling wave (RFW) and a slow-filling wave (SFW). The A wave (A) is small in comparison with the total amplitude of the apexcardiogram. (*From E. Parker, E. Craige, and W. P. Hood, Jr., The Austin Flint Murmur and the A Wave of the Apex Cardiogram in Aortic Regurgitation, Circulation, 43:349, 1971. Reproduced with permission from the American Heart Association, Inc., and authors.*)

The utility of the apexcardiogram lies in two main areas: (1) identification of heart sounds and other events of the cardiac cycle and (2) derivation of physiological information from patterns of systolic movement.

Identification of Heart Sounds In view of the close temporal relationship between certain landmarks on the apex tracing and intracardiac events, the external record can be very useful in identification of questionable heart sounds. The A wave of the apex tracing, for instance, is the palpable counterpart of the atrial or fourth heart sound (refer to Fig. 123-4). These two phenomena, the fourth heart sound and the A wave of the apexcardiogram, are of similar origin and are dependent on low-frequency vibrations resulting from distension of the ventricle following atrial systole. Therefore, it is often helpful to have an apexcardiogram to sort out a complex of sounds in close proximity to the expected time of the first heart sound.

The identity in timing of the systolic upstroke of the apexcardiogram and the left ventricular pressure curve makes it possible to dissect the preejection period (PEP) into its two major subdivisions—the electromechanical interval and the isovolumic contraction time.

In early diastole, the nadir or zero point occurs roughly at the time of mitral valve opening, so it may be used to distinguish an opening snap from a broadly split second heart sound or a prominent third heart sound. A combined echophonocardiogram, however, provides a more precise correlation

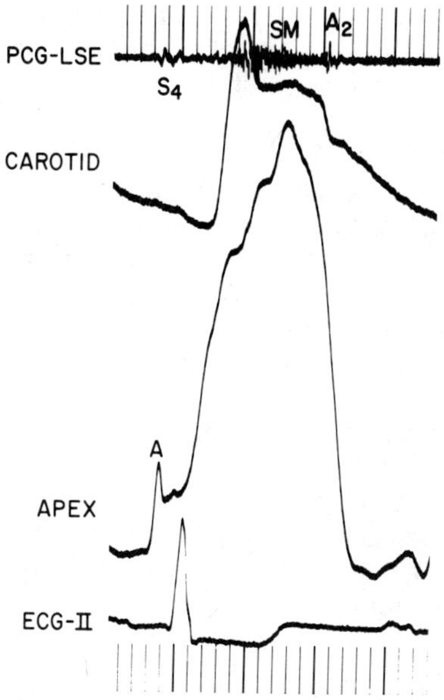

FIGURE 123-4 Apexcardiogram in hypertrophic cardiomyopathy. This shows a sustained type of systolic wave corresponding with the heaving apical impulse. Often in this condition the apexcardiogram has two distinct peaks. The A wave is exaggerated in height and sharp in configuration. It corresponds in time with the S_4. The carotid tracing shows a swift upstroke and a second prolonged hump. There is a midsystolic murmur (SM). LSE = left sternal edge. (*From E. Craige, The Value of Apex Cardiography in Cardiac Diagnosis, in N. O. Fowler, "Diagnostic Methods in Cardiology," F. A. Davis Company, Philadelphia, 1975. Reproduced with permission from the publisher and author.*)

between the halting of the mitral valve in its opening movement and its auscultatory manifestation, the opening snap.

The third heart sound occurs precisely at the peak of the rapid-filling wave of the apexcardiogram. Thus, the apex tracing can be very useful in the identification of extra sounds in early diastole.

Physiological Information There are three basic types of systolic curves registered in the apexcardiogram: (1) normal, (2) hyperdynamic, and (3) sustained. The *normal* tracing has been briefly described above. *Hyperdynamic* curves differ from normal curves in amplitude but not in basic morphology. A much larger systolic rise provides a graphic counterpart of the exaggerated apical impulse, which has long been known to be characteristic of conditions in which there is a large stroke volume, as occurs in mitral regurgitation.[20] Unfortunately, quantitation of the height of the apexcardiogram is technically quite difficult. Therefore, an estimation of amplitude remains rather crude. However, a frequent accompaniment of the hyperdynamic systolic movement is an increased rapid-filling wave in early diastole peaking at the time of a third heart sound. A *sustained* type of apex impulse is a graphic representation of a systolic "heave" or "thrust" (Fig. 123-4). It displays an augmented height, but a more important feature is its plateau (horizontal) or rising shape during systole. This type of movement is found in aortic stenosis, systemic hypertension, or any condition characterized by hypertrophy of the left ventricle. In hypertrophic cardiomyopathy, a variant of this pattern is seen, with a brisk initial upstroke followed by a larger sustained second hump during the remainder of systole.

As noted above, there are a number of situations where the apexcardiogram, in conjunction with other noninvasive techniques, can be of help in cardiac diagnosis. Continuing investigations in several centers give promise of establishing with greater precision the physiological correlates which would further enhance the apexcardiogram's utility.[21–23] The limitations of apexcardiography include difficulty in quantitation, lack of specificity of most of the patterns that are obtained, and problems of reproducibility owing to differences in technological devices among laboratories as well as to unavoidable variations in the application of transducers to the chest wall even by the same individual.

Technique of Apexcardiography

The same piezoelectric transducer that is used for recording pulsations of the carotid artery and jugular vein can be used for apexcardiography. The importance of an adequate time constant for the transducer-recording system has been previously mentioned.

The patient should be examined before any transducers are applied so that the point of maximal impulse can be determined. This can be marked on the chest wall for ready reference. Usually a maximal excursion of the apex impulse can be obtained with the patient in the left lateral decubitus. This position can be comfortably maintained with the support of a wedge-shaped radiological pillow under the back. The sensing head of the transducer is held firmly by hand or with an elastic strap over the point of maximum impulse. The exact site can usually be located with some practice, and satisfactory records can be obtained in about four out of five individuals referred for noninvasive assessment. If the transducer is held over a position away from the center of the maximal thrust, an inverted or distorted type of movement may be recorded, which will be misleading. Enlarged or hypertrophied hearts make contact with the chest wall over a larger area than do normal hearts and are thus easier to record. Difficulty is encountered with obese or emphysematous patients. Pulsations in other localities over the chest wall may be recorded in similar manner. This would apply to ectopic movements due to ventricular or aortic aneurysms, right ventricular hypertrophy, dilated pulmonary artery, or even twitches of intercostal muscles due to pacemaker stimuli.[17,24] The position of the patient can be altered to bring out the phenomenon under observation to best advantage. Occasionally in older individuals with chronic lung disease, the area just beneath the xiphoid may be the only site of palpable (and recordable) movement.

Examples of Combinations of Noninvasive Parameters Where Certain Common Clinical Situations Are Suspected

Aortic Stenosis

Physical examination may have revealed a midsystolic murmur consistent with aortic stenosis. An appropriate combination of noninvasive observations might include the following:

1. A phonocardiogram may demonstrate the murmur, an ejection sound, possible reversal of A_2 and P_2, or atrial sound in presystole.
2. A recording of the carotid pulse will show the rate of rise of the pulse wave and, in combination with ECG and phonocardiogram, the systolic time intervals.
3. The apexcardiogram may be used to check for an exaggerated A wave and a sustained type of movement in systole.
4. If, as recommended above, an echocardiogram is performed in conjunction with the above observations, there may be evidence of eccentricity or calcification of the aortic valve. The thickness of the walls of the left ventricle may supply information of value in assessing severity of outflow obstruction, particularly in children.
5. The jugular venous pulse may disclose an exaggerated *a* wave, reflecting the effects of septal hypertrophy on the filling characteristics of the right ventricle.

Aortic Regurgitation

Phonocardiographic microphones recording simultaneously at the left sternal edge and the cardiac apex may confirm the presence of a decrescendo diastolic blowing murmur and an Austin Flint murmur. The presence or absence of a first heart sound may be of importance in assessing the severity of acute regurgitation (see Chap. 37).

A carotid pulse tracing may display an exaggerated amplitude, bisferiens shape in systole, and absence of a dicrotic notch.

An apexcardiogram can demonstrate the hyperdynamic apical impulse and exaggerated rapid-filling wave.

An accompanying echocardiogram will be invaluable in providing information regarding chamber size and vibrations of the anterior leaflet of the mitral valve and, in the syndrome of acute aortic regurgitation, evidence of premature closure of the mitral valve or possibly of vegetations or flail-like disruption of the aortic valve itself.

Mitral Stenosis

The phonocardiogram with the microphone at the cardiac apex and the patient in the left lateral decubitus may confirm the diastolic murmur as well as a loud S_1 and opening snap of the mitral valve. A phonocardiogram at the upper left sternal edge may show an increased intensity of P_2 or an ejection sound of pulmonary valve origin, suggesting the presence of pulmonary hypertension. The jugular venous pulse may show an exaggerated *a* wave if the patient is in sinus rhythm, which is consistent with the effects of right ventricular hypertrophy. In advanced cases a 1/C wave may indicate the presence of tricuspid regurgitation.

The apexcardiogram will show a diminished rapid-filling wave because of the obstruction at the mitral valve. Precordial movement at the left sternal edge may consist of a thrust of right ventricular hypertrophy.

The above phonocardiographic findings in conjunction with a characteristic echocardiographic picture should provide a very informative noninvasive assessment of mitral stenosis.

Mitral Regurgitation

Phonocardiograms at the cardiac apex will confirm the presence of the systolic murmur and give some details regarding its timing—whether it is pansystolic or confined to early or late systole (Fig. 123-5). A third sound and middiastolic rumbling murmur may be recorded in more severe cases. The carotid pulse, in conjunction with the ECG and phonocardiogram, can be used to measure systolic time intervals. The apexcardiogram will demonstrate a hyperdynamic excursion in systole and heightened rapid-filling wave. An accompanying echocardiogram will provide information regarding chamber size and possibly the type of mitral valve disorder, whether rheumatic, prolapsed, or flail (Fig. 123-5).

Other Conditions

Similar protocols can be constructed which may provide the maximum yield in suspected cases of cardiomyopathy (either of the dilated or hypertrophic variety), constrictive pericarditis, myxoma, etc. In every case an individualized approach will be most productive. One should realize that the routine type of examination that might be appropriate for recording an ECG or chest roentgenogram is fruitless in the noninvasive cardiac laboratory. Whether technician, physician, or a combined team, the operator or operators must have some idea of the questions being asked so that a well-thought-out protocol involving type and location of transducers, position of patient, use of filters, paper speed, etc., can be constructed in accordance with the problem as perceived from a preliminary survey. In response to information flowing from the recording devices, the procedure may have to be modified in midstream. This requires experience and imagination as well as a thorough grounding in cardiac anatomy and physiology and the modifications that may occur from disease states, surgery, and pharmacologic agents. The results, however, can be very gratifying in terms of diagnostic yield. The absence of trauma

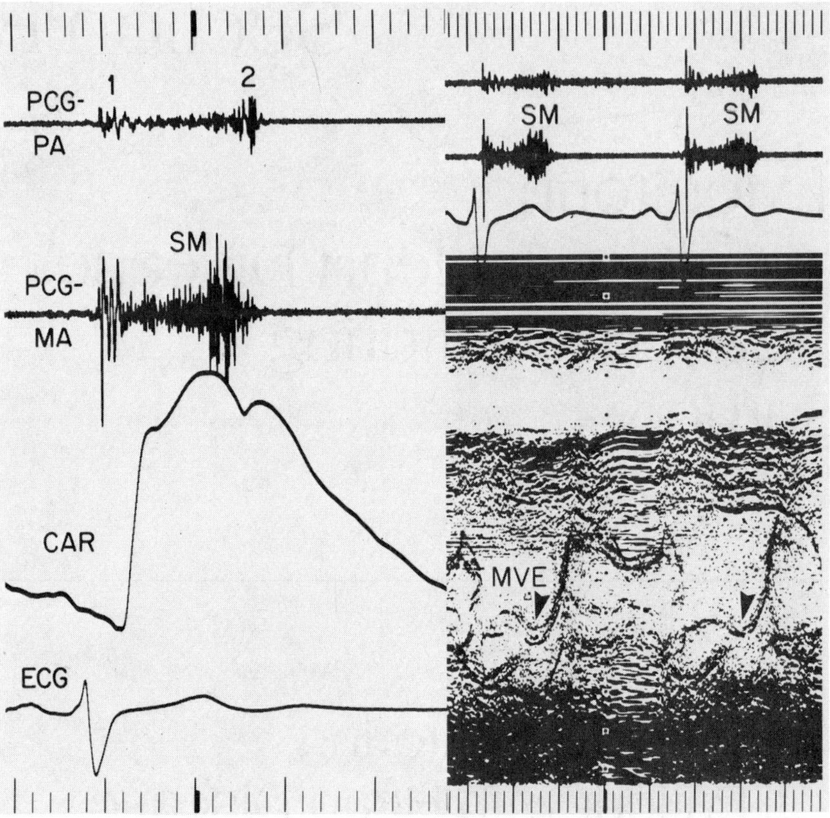

FIGURE 123-5 Severe mitral regurgitation due to ruptured chordae tendinae. *Left.* Phonocardiogram shows a crescendo pansystolic murmur maximal at the mitral area. *Right.* The combined echophonocardiogram (at 50 mm/s paper speed) shows that the late systolic accentuation of the murmur corresponds with the obvious prolapse of the mitral valve (arrow).

and the relatively low cost of the procedure, as well as the ability to repeat the observations ad libitum, all contribute to the advantages of a modern noninvasive cardiac diagnostic assessment.

References

1. Rappaport, M. B., and Sprague, H. B.: The Graphic Registration of the Normal Heart Sounds, *Am. Heart J.*, 23:591, 1942.
2. Craige, E.: Echocardiography in Studies of the Genesis of Heart Sounds and Murmurs, in P. N. Yu and J. F. Goodwin (eds.), "Progress in Cardiology," Lea & Febiger, Philadelphia, 1975.
3. Waider, W., and Craige, E.: First Heart Sound and Ejection Sounds, *Am. J. Cardiol.*, 35:346, 1975.
4. Mills, P. G., Brodie, B., McLaurin, L., Schall, S., and Craige, E.: Echocardiographic and Hemodynamic Relationships of Ejection Sounds, *Circulation*, 56:430, 1977.
5. Ozawa, Y., Smith, D., and Craige, E.: Origin of the Third Heart Sound: I. Studies in Dogs, *Circulation*, 67:393, 1983.
6. Ozawa, Y., Smith, D., and Craige, E.: Origin of the Third Heart Sound: II. Studies in Human Subjects, *Circulation*, 67:399, 1983.
7. Craige, E.: Phonocardiography and Pulse Tracings, *Int. J. Cardiol.*, 4:1, 1983.
8. Mills, P., and Craige, E.: Echophonocardiography, *Prog. Cardiovasc. Dis.*, 20:337, 1978.
9. Mashimo, K., Tanabe, Y., Kinoshita, S., Sakamoto, S., and Tsaushima, N.: An Instrumental Aspect of Apex Cardiography: Decay Characteristic of Transducers and Its Clinical Implication, *Jpn. Heart J.*, 7:536, 1966.
10. Kesteloot, H., Willems, J., and Van Vollenhoven, E.: On the Physical Principles and Methodology of Mechanocardiography, *Acta Cardiol. Brux.*, 24:147, 1969.
11. Leatham, A.: "Auscultation of the Heart and Phonocardiography," Churchill Livingstone, 1975.
12. Lewis, R. P., Rittgers, S. E., Forester, W. F., and Boudoulas, H.: A Critical Review of the Systolic Time Intervals, *Circulation*, 56:146, 1977.
13. Constant, J.: The X Prime Descent in Jugular Contour Nomenclature and Recognition, *Am. Heart J.*, 88:372, 1974.
14. Marey, E. J.: Études physiologiques sur les caractères du battement de coeur et les conditions qui le modifrent, *J. d'Anatomie et de Physiologie*, 2:276, 416, 1865.
15. Eddlemen, E. E.: Ultra Low Frequency Precordial Movements—Kinetocardiograms, *Am. J. Cardiol.*, 4:649, 1959.
16. Mounsey, J. P. D.: Inspection and Palpation of the Cardiac Impulse, *Prog. Cardiovasc. Dis.*, 10:187, 1967.
17. Craige, E.: Apex Cardiogram, in A. M. Weissler (ed.), "Noninvasive Cardiology," Grune & Stratton, Inc., New York, 1974.
18. Smith, D., and Craige, E.: Enhancement of Tactile Perception as Employed in Palpation, *Circulation*, 62:1114, 1980.
19. Willems, J. L., DeGeest, H., and Kesteloot, H.: On the Value of Apex Cardiography for Timing Intracardiac Events, *Am. J. Cardiol.*, 28:59, 1971.
20. Sutton, G. C., Prewitt, T. A., and Craige, E.: Relationship between Quantitated Precordial Movement and Left Ventricular Function, *Circulation*, 41:179, 1970.
21. Denef, B., DeGeest, H., and Kesteloot, H.: The Clinical Value of the Calibrated Apical A Wave and Its Relationship to the Fourth Heart Sound, *Circulation*, 60:1412, 1979.
22. Upton, M. T., and Gibson, D. G.: The Study of Left Ventricular Function from Digitized Echocardiograms, *Prog. Cardiovasc. Dis.*, 20:359, 1978.
23. Manolas, J., Krayenbuehl, H. P., and Rutishauser, W.: Use of Apexcardiography to Evaluate Left Ventricular Diastolic Compliance in Human Beings, *Am. J. Cardiol.*, 43:939, 1979.
24. Kesteloot, H., and Willems, J.: Relationship between the Right Apexcardiogram and the Right Ventricular Dynamics, *Acta Cardiol. Brux.*, 22:64, 1967.

Section F

Techniques of Monitoring Seriously Ill Patients with Heart Disease and Computer-Based Monitoring after Cardiac Surgery

124

Techniques of Monitoring the Seriously Ill Patient with Heart Disease (Including Use of Swan-Ganz Catheter)

H. J. C. Swan, M.D., Ph.D.

Whatever is true . . . think about such things . . . put it into practice.

Phillippians 4:8, 9[1]

Wisdom is supreme; therefore, get wisdom. Though it cost you all you have, get understanding.

Proverbs 4:7[1]

In the critically ill patient, changes in the cardiovascular system and in its control mechanisms are so sudden, and their consequences may be so grave, that direct measurements of the principal determinants and consequences of cardiac performance are frequently necessary for optimal care. Such variables include the heart rate and rhythm and the systemic arterial blood pressure. In addition, the importance of ventricular input pressure (preload), outflow resistance (afterload), and quantitative blood flow to the body (cardiac output) are now recognized as critical. The level of these values and the direction of their changes are not readily identifiable from clinical examination alone. These data, defined almost a century ago, were initially measured in humans by diagnostic cardiac catheterization, the significance of which was identified by the award of the 1956 Nobel prize for Physiology and Medicine to Cournand, Richards, and Forssman.

Balloon-flotation catheters[2,3] were developed to allow application of diagnostic catheterization to those clinical settings in which such data is vitally needed. These include the anesthesia suite,[4] operating room, and recovery area; medical, respiratory, and cardiac intensive care units; shock, burn, and trauma management facilities; and the cardiac catheterization laboratory.[5]

Modification of catheter specifications ensures that the technique can be applied in the absence of facilities for fluoroscopic guidance and with a minimum of significant complications. Further, collection of those data elements which are *critical* to the understanding of the underlying disease was a prime objective in the developmental phase. In addition, the qualities of simplicity, practicality, and ready applicability in the appropriate clinical environment are considered paramount.

Effective and safe hemodynamic monitoring is best achieved if all aspects of technique employed in a given institution are as uniform and consistent as is practical. Variation between units or physicians is to be deplored. This uniformity extends to equipment, data display and recording, and procedures. A wide range of catheter sizes are available from several manufacturers for a variety of monitoring (and pacing) purposes. A manual of procedures and practices for *all* personnel should be maintained and should be consistent among the differing disciplines within a given institution.

Systemic Arterial Pressure

The measurement of systemic arterial blood pressure is a mainstay of decision making in the treatment of critically ill cardiac and noncardiac patients. The measurement, by traditional indirect methods or by direct recordings of intraarterial pressure, provides numerical values describing the phasic and mean levels of pressure in the systemic arterial bed. It is a function not only of cardiac output but also of the resistance or impedance offered by the small arterial vessels to the outflow of blood from the central arterial tree. In critically ill patients, large swings in vasomotor tone occur, with constriction of systemic arterials; this degree of constriction may differ between body organs. While mean arterial pressure falls progressively from the aortic root to the peripheral arteries, phasic peak systolic pressure normally increases while diastolic pressure falls in comparison with that of the central aorta. This increase is not just a function of the vessel in which the arterial pressure is measured. Also, the magnitude of systolic amplification is enhanced when regional vasodilatation is present and is reduced or even seriously damped when vasoconstriction occurs in patients with profound shock. The phasic recording of direct arterial blood pressure may be extremely important for effective synchronization of diastolic augmentation of intraaortic pressure using devices such as the intraaortic balloon.

Complications

Complications of intraarterial cannulation include vasospasm, local hematoma, pseudoaneurysm, and infection. Severe arterial trauma in smaller vessels, such as the radial artery, may result from intraarterial catheterization, but gangrene or loss of a limb secondary to arterial puncture is rare. Major complications in a trauma unit may be 27 percent[6] and are less frequent when the femoral side is used.

Catheterization of the Right Side of the Heart

Conventional, semistiff, woven catheters should not be used. Flexible flow-guided devices minimize endocardial trauma and potentially life-threatening arrhythmias.

Insertion Technique

Percutaneous insertion at the site of a large central venous channel is recommended. The selection of the exact site will depend upon prior skills and assessment of need. Probably the most uniformly desirable location is the right internal jugular vein, since potential application includes patients undergoing intrathoracic surgery. The right or left subclavian vein is also suitable. The femoral vein, right or left, is less desirable, although it is appropriate for patients undergoing short-term diagnostic catheterization procedures. The exact point of venous insertion should be accurately predetermined by a probing no. 22 needle, followed by strict adherence to one of the established techniques using the guidewire-sheath insertion procedure. Supervised performance is required before an individual undertakes these techniques alone, since complications may be serious and are, in general, associated with inexperience. Direct antecubital fossa venostomy—widely practiced by cardiologists—immobilizes the arm and is associated with a higher frequency of catheter displacement and migration.

The catheter is advanced to the region of the right atrium, where its position may be recognized by intravascular pressure fluctuations concordant with the respiratory cycle. The catheter is then advanced 3 to 5 cm, depending upon body build (1 to 2 cm if inserted from the femoral vein), and the guidance balloon is inflated to the volume recommended. The catheter is then slowly but consistently advanced and, because a catheter of appropriate flex is used, the balloon is deflected medially through the tricuspid valve to the mid or outflow portion of the right ventricle. The propulsive effects of right ventricular contraction will then drive the balloon catheter into the pulmonary artery, its progress continuing until it impacts in a vessel slightly smaller than the diameter of the distended balloon. A permanent record of intravascular pressures and cardiac rhythms during the advancement is recommended. Records of at least one complete respiratory cycle should be obtained in the right atrium and in the pulmonary capillary wedge position. The balloon is then deflated, and a final recording of pulmonary artery pressure through one to two respiratory cycles is obtained.

The catheter should not be advanced too rapidly during insertion or, in particular, as the balloon enters the pulmonary artery, since redundant loops may form in the right atrium or right ventricle. If care is taken on balloon deflation, the catheter tip will then locate in the right or left main branch of the pulmonary artery or in the main pulmonary artery itself. If the pressure trace on inspiration suggests right ventricularization, the balloon should be reinflated slowly and allowed to advance with insertion of 1 to 2 cm of additional catheter shaft. The catheter should be placed, with the balloon deflated, in a central pulmonary artery and not in a distal branch. When recordings of wedge pressure are to be obtained, inflation of the balloon is intended to *float* the catheter out to a distal vessel and *not* to occlude acutely the pulmonary artery from a fixed tip location. Care in ensuring an optimal position of the catheter in the pulmonary artery is the most important single factor in minimizing complications.

The catheter shaft should then be anchored securely at the site of its skin insertion, with due attention to appropriate sterile techniques. Under no circumstance should advancement of a catheter be anticipated once the sterile component of the procedure is completed. Several packaging devices are now available which allow the insertion of flotation catheters in a nonsurgical environment with a minimum likelihood of infection.

Data Collection

Great Vessel and Intracardiac Pressures

Pressures measured by flotation catheters must be referenced to an appropriate zero point. This is usually the level of the tricuspid valve orifice, the point of lowest potential energy in the circulation. With careful establishment and maintenance of the zero reference point and appropriate calibrations, pressure may be measured with an accuracy of ±2 mmHg under clinical circumstances. Appropriate corrections for the influences of respiration, particularly under conditions of positive pressure ventilation, are essential. The influence of intrathoracic pressures should be minimized at the time of pressure recording. Dynamic response characteristics and inertial artifacts are similar to those associated with conventional (stiff) fluid-filled catheters. A frequency response, flat to 8 or 10 Hz with a rapid attenuation of greater frequencies, provides an optimal record of right-sided heart pressures.

Cardiac Output

Thermodilution is the most frequently used technique for the measurement of cardiac output in human beings because of simplicity of application and inherent precision. The fluid injected into the right atrium is harmless. Detection of the change in temperature is accomplished by a thermistor located 4 cm from the catheter tip. No blood is withdrawn from the body, as it is for the determination of concentration of indicator dyes. The procedure may be carried out at the bedside by a single individual, and the relevant data may be displayed immediately. The thermodilution technique satisfies the assumptions underlying Fick's principle, provided that the cold indicator passes through two valves and one contracting chamber to attain uniformity of mixing. A minimal amount of negative heat transfer to the walls of the cardiac chambers during initial passage of the bolus of cold fluid is promptly returned to the flowing bloodstream and recognized by the detecting thermistor. Loss of "indicator" (cold) to the injection catheter system is compensated for in most computational devices. These devices allow for uniformity in the recognition and calculation of the transient changes in blood temperature at the detecting site.

Precision, i.e., the variability between repeated measurements of the same value, determines the significance of observed differences in cardiac output. Precision in such determinations is dependent upon exact attention to the performance of the thermodilution technique. In a series of triplicate determinations obtained from patients in a steady state, the sum of methodologic and biologic variance was 3.9 percent[7] (the lowest attained by any technique commonly used for the measurement of cardiac output in human beings). A review of 22 comparisons of estimation of cardiac output by thermodilution and by a variety of other methods showed a correlation exceeding 0.90 in 17 separate studies, and exceeding 0.95 in 11 of them.[8] Thus, changes from a previous value of ±10 percent are directionally significant. Nevertheless, if conditions violate steady state assumptions and if details of the procedure are not followed precisely, methodologic variations may be expected so that changes of 15 percent above or below an initial value may not truly establish validity even of the direction of the change.

The physiologic significance of derived variables is presented in Table 124-1.

Indications for Balloon Flotation Catheterization[9]

Application of this technique is indicated in any situation in which the therapeutic decision making will be substantively improved by the availability of critical hemodynamic data. This implies an ability to carefully apply the technique with a minimum of complications and an ability to identify and assess the relevant data in the light of the underlying pathophysiology. In addition, most importantly, a clear therapeutic plan based upon the derived data must be a possibility. In those institutions, situations,

TABLE 124-1 Physiologic Significance of Catheterization Data

Measured or Derived Variables	Physiologic Interpretation
Cardiac output	Total body perfusion; oxygen delivery
Systemic vascular resistance	Geometry of systemic arterioles
Systemic artery pressure	Perfusion head; afterload left ventricle
Pulmonary capillary wedge pressure	Preload left ventricle; hydrostatic gradient pulmonary capillary–interstitial space
Pulmonary vascular resistance	Geometry of pulmonary arterioles
Pulmonary artery pressure	Afterload right ventricle
Right atrial pressure	Preload right ventricle; venous pressure-volume relations

and medical conditions in which clear programs of potentially beneficial interventions are absent or impossible, hemodynamic monitoring is absolutely contraindicated.

In the management of the high-risk surgical patient, flotation catheters are used throughout anesthesia and during the early phases of recovery. The patients include those in whom the surgical procedure contemplated carries a higher risk than usual and those who, because of intrinsic cardiac disease, are faced with a higher than average hazard. Examples of these situations include resection of aortic aneurysm, active angina pectoris in patients with prior myocardial infarction, and prostatic resection in elderly patients, who may experience relatively large fluid shifts. The objective of monitoring is to minimize cardiovascular stress during induction and maintenance of anesthesia and during the critical phases of the surgical procedure and thus to reduce mortality and, more importantly, postoperative morbidity.

In medical, cardiac, and respiratory intensive care units, hemodynamic monitoring is currently confined to the critically ill and potentially moribund patients. Application of hemodynamic data to appropriate decision making is discussed in other chapters of this text. Nevertheless, the potential of hemodynamic monitoring for identifying favorable therapeutic options should not be ignored. Hemodynamic monitoring is not generally recommended for all patients with acute myocardial infarction[10] but is utilized for decision making relative to the appropriate treatment of, for example, established and severe heart failure. In the future, a more aggressive approach in the early phases of a potentially large infarct is likely to be justified, since it is evident that the true magnitude of circulatory deficit is not apparent in the initial hours on clinical grounds alone. Such a patient may be a candidate for early myocardial revascularization, intraaortic balloon counterpulsation, or dissolution of intracoronary thrombi, with restoration of a sufficient blood flow. In such circumstances more intense early monitoring may be indicated.

The general diagnostic categories in which hemodynamic monitoring may be used with benefit are listed in Table 124-2.[11]

TABLE 124-2 Indications for Hemodynamic Monitoring

In the Surgical Setting
Cardiac surgery
Valve replacement (multiple, elderly)
Severe associated pulmonary disease (mitral stenosis)
Coronary artery bypass grafting
Resection of ventricular aneurysm
Preoperative congestive heart failure
Vascular procedures
Dissecting aneurysm
Resection of thoracic aneurysm
Prostatic resection
Extensive intraabdominal resection (tumor)
Prolonged orthopedic procedures (elderly)
Severe burns
Multiple injuries
In the Medical Setting
Acute cardiac conditions
Acute myocardial infarction—complicated
Right ventricular infarction
Perforated ventricular septum, mitral regurgitation
Postinfarction angina
Acute bacterial endocarditis
Acute cardiac tamponade
Chronic cardiac insufficiency
Congestive cardiomyopathy
End-stage cardiac failure (therapy)
Constrictive pericarditis, tamponade
Acute respiratory disorders
Acute pulmonary edema (nonmyocardial infarction)
Pulmonary embolus
Cor pulmonale with pneumonia
Fat embolism (trauma)
Ventilator management
Miscellaneous indications
Severe noncardiac hypotension
Extensive multisystem infections
Dialysis
Overdose of drugs
Intraaortic balloon support
Acute vasodilator therapy
Research
Development of physiologic subsets
Therapeutic responses

Source: H. J. C. Swan and W. Ganz, Measurement of Right Atrial and Pulmonary Arterial Pressures and Cardiac Output: Clinical Application of Hemodynamic Monitoring, in G. H. Stollerman et al. (eds.), "Advances in Internal Medicine," vol. 27, Year Book Medical Publishers, Chicago, 1982, p. 27. Copyright © 1982 by Year Book Medical Publishers, Inc., Chicago. Reproduced with permission from the publisher, editor, and authors.

Complications of Balloon Flotation Catheterization

Complications Associated with Insertion

Complications associated with insertion of the catheter include vascular damage, venous or arterial hematoma, localized infection, and thrombosis. Inexperience in vascular puncture procedures and poor attention to sterile techniques favor such complications. Difficulty may be encountered in patients with diseases of the cervical spine or with a tortuous carotid arterial system. Pneumothorax is a particular complication, occurring in 1 to 4 percent of patients when the subclavian vein is to be catheterized. The frequency of this complication is inversely related to the experience of the operator.

Complications Associated with Advancement

Complications associated with advancement of the catheter include atrial (rare) and ventricular (uncommon) ectopy. The inflated balloon serves to minimize the forces which may initiate arrhythmias by stimulation of the subendocardial myocardium. Careful, continuous advancement of the catheter ensures that the locus of the ectopic impulses is rapidly changed and a sustained ectopy is not generated. Nevertheless, reports of ventricular tachycardia (usually brief and self-limited) and of at least four episodes of fatal ventricular fibrillation have been published. Dysrhythmias other than ventricular premature beats are rare. Complete heart block has been reported in association with left bundle branch block. Care should be used in patients known to have disease of the conduction system. Pulmonary infarction is probably a frequent complication of balloon flotation catheterization. It is usually associated with prolonged wedging of a catheter and possibly of an infusion of a hyperosmotic solution into a pulmonary segment. The great majority of these occurrences are not productive of symptoms.

Complications Associated with Maintenance

Significant pulmonary vascular damage is uncommon, and pulmonary artery rupture is rare. Nevertheless, this most serious complication appears to be specific to the technique, since the majority of cases were fatal because of intractable pulmonary hemorrhage.[12] Erosion of a pulmonary artery branch may be caused by continuous impaction and leverage of the tip of the catheter. Inappropriate inflation of the balloon carried at the catheter tip when it lies in a vessel of 3-mm diameter or less causes the forces within the balloon to be borne by the thin walls of the small pulmonary arteries, and physical rupture is possible. These complications appear to be more common in elderly patients and in those with evidence of pulmonary hypertension. Experimentally, it is difficult to rupture a pulmonary artery in animal models or small human pulmonary vessels at autopsy.

Other late complications include thrombosis around the shaft of the catheter, particularly in patients in whom a thrombotic tendency exists. Ventricular ectopy due to migration of the catheter tip into the outflow tract of the right ventricle may occur. Failure of catheter performance because of luminal occlusion or fractured leads may also occur. Prolonged maintenance of intravascular catheters appears to favor the development of bacteremia and endocarditis. This is particularly true in patients in whom ventilators are utilized as part of the therapy.

Nevertheless, since the number of insertions of balloon catheters for monitoring exceeds several million, the incidence of complications appears to remain small. Recognition of the possibility of complications and attention to specific details, as well as restriction of the application of these techniques to a limited number of trained, skillful, and well-informed professional and paraprofessional personnel, will do much to maximize the effective application of the balloon flotation catheter system and proper safety of hemodynamic monitoring.

Several prospective studies of the nature and incidence of the complications of hemodynamic monitoring are now available. Minor complications such as nonsustained arrhythmias and infections appear common (15 to 40 percent). Major complications—pneumothorax, arrhythmias, septicemia, and pulmonary complications—occur in 3 to 4.4 percent of critically ill patients.[13,14] It has been concluded that the risk/benefit ratio is small.

Summary and General Comments

A major application of hemodynamic monitoring is during elective surgery in higher risk patients. In a nonconcurrent, nonrandomized comparison, Rao et al.[15] studied the incidence of perioperative myocardial reinfarction in patients undergoing cardiac surgery for noncardiac causes. The reinfarction rate was 7.7 percent in nonmonitored patients and 1.9 percent in monitored patients. The risk was highest (as was the benefit) in patients operated on within 6 months of the first infarction, those who experienced angina pectoris, and those with congestive heart failure. Rao et al. suggested that preoperative optimization of the patient's status, aggressive invasive monitoring, and prompt treatment of hemodynamic alterations utilizing vasodilators and beta blockade extensively were of benefit; however, the structure of the study does not allow an absolute statement.

It has been suggested that not all patients undergoing cardiac bypass surgery require hemodynamic monitoring. Those with a preoperative ejection fraction greater than 0.50 without angiographically demonstrable dyssynergy preoperatively could possibly be managed by measurement of central venous pressure alone.[16] These conclusions have been debated in that, in many coronary patients with good preoperative left ventricular function, relatively severe abnormalities in pulmonary capillary wedge pressure, cardiac index, and systemic vascular resistance occurred during anesthesia and were missed in 65 percent of instances by experienced cardiac anesthesiologists "blinded" to the actual data.[17]

A number of reports have documented the frequency with which a diagnosis has been changed and a therapeutic plan altered by reason of availability of the hemodynamic data. Again, these reports are observational only and suffer from absence of a randomization protocol and frequently of a concurrent control group. Nevertheless, such comparisons indicate the inadequacy of clinical evaluation for both magnitude of hemodynamic derangement and optimal therapeutic intervention. In a group of critically ill patients without acute myocardial infarction, pulmonary capillary wedge pressure was predicted correctly only 42 percent of the time and cardiac index only 44 percent of the time within three rather broad categories (low, normal, and high).[18] Serious misinterpretation occurred in more than 40 percent of instances, and the physicians would have been more correct to assume gross abnormalities in all cases than to attempt any evaluation on a clinical basis alone. The ejection fraction in patients with acute myocardial infarction is poorly related to the initial clinical classification when the evaluation has been made within 12 h.[19] Late evaluation (after the time of potential intervention) is substantively more accurate. In surgical patients, similar diagnostic errors occurred with 20 percent of patients requiring blood volume support prior to the induction of anesthesia. Thirty-eight percent of patients exhibited important changes before the initiation of cardiopulmonary bypass.[20] In a general medical intensive care unit, 60 percent of physicians made at least one major therapeutic change, 32 percent made two or more, and 13 percent made three or more alterations in therapy based on catheterization data on the right side of the heart. Early congestive heart failure proved to be the most difficult diagnosis to predict.

References

1. Holy Bible, New International Version, Zoundervan Publishing House, Grand Rapids, 1978.
2. Swan, H. J. C., Ganz, W., Forrester, J., Marcus, H., Diamond, G., and Chonette, D.: Catheterization of the Heart in Man with the Use of Flow-Directed Balloon-Tipped Catheters, *N. Engl. J. Med.*, 283:447, 1970.
3. Chatterjee, K., Swan, H. J. C., Ganz, W., Gray, R., Loebel, H., Forrester, J., and Chonette, D.: Use of Balloon-Tipped Flotation Electrode Catheter for Cardiac Monitoring, *Am. J. Cardiol.*, 36:56, 1975.
4. Pace, N. L.: A Critique of Flow-Directed Pulmonary Artery Catheterization, *Anesthesiology,* 47:455, 1977.
5. Steele, P., and Davies, H.: The Swan-Ganz Catheter in the Cardiac Laboratory, *Br. Heart J.*, 35:647, 1973.
6. Soderstram, C. A., Wasserman, D. H., and Cowley, R. A.: Arterial Monitoring Catheters. A Prospective Study of Use and Complications, *Crit. Care Med.*, 9:203, 1981. (Abstract.)
7. Forrester, J. S., Ganz, W., Diamond, G., McHugh, T., Chonette, D., and Swan, H. J. C.: Thermodilution Cardiac Output Determination with a Single Flow-Directed Catheter, *Am. Heart J.*, 83:306, 1972.
8. Riedenger, M. D., and Shellock, F.: Technical Aspects of the Thermodilution Method for Measuring Cardiac Output, *Heart Lung,* 13:215, 1984.
9. Swan, H. J. C.: The Role of Hemodynamic Monitoring in the Management of the Critically Ill, *Crit. Care Med.*, 3:38, 1975.
10. Shaver, J. A.: Hemodynamic Monitoring in the Critically Ill Patient, *N Engl. J. Med.*, 308:277, 1983.
11. Swan, H. J. C., and Ganz, W.: Measurement of Right Arterial and Pulmonary Arterial Pressure and Cardiac Output: Clinical Application of Hemodynamic Monitoring, *Adv. Intern. Med.*, 27:453, 1982.
12. Pape, L. A., Haffajee, C. I., Markis, J. E., Ockene, I. S., Paraskos, J. A., Dalen, J. E., and Alpert, J. S.: Fatal Pulmonary Hemorrhage after Use of the Flow-Directed Balloon-Tipped Catheter, *Ann. Intern Med.*, 90:344, 1979.
13. Shakford, S. R.: Complications of the Flow-Directed Pulmonary Artery Catheter: A Prospective Analysis in 219 Patients, *Crit. Care Med.*, 9:315, 1981.
14. Boyd, K. D., Thomas, S. J., Gold, J., and Boyd, A. D.: A Prospective Study of Complications of Pulmonary Artery Catheterization in 500 Consecutive Patients, *Chest,* 84:245, 1983.
15. Rao, T. L. K., Jacobs, K. H., and El-Eter, A. A.: Reinfarction following Anesthesia in Patients with Myocardial Infarction, *Anesthesiology,* 59:499, 1983.
16. Mangano, D. T.: Monitoring Pulmonary Arterial Pressure in Coronary Artery Disease, *Anesthesiology,* 53:364, 1980.
17. Waller, J. L., Johnson, S. P., and Kaplin, J. A.: Usefulness of Pulmonary Artery Catheters during Aortic Coronary Bypass Surgery, *Anesth. Analg.*, 61:221, 1982.
18. Connors, A. F., McCaffree, D. R., and Gray, B. A.: Evaluation of Right Heart Catheterization in the Critically Ill Patient without Acute Myocardial Infarction, *N. Engl. J. Med.*, 308:263, 1983.
19. Shah, P. K., Pichler, M., Berman, D., Maddahi, J., Waxman A., Singh, B. N., and Swan, H. J. C.: Left Ventricular Ejection Fraction Determined by Radionuclide Ventriculography in Early Stages of First Transmural Myocardial Infarction and Its Relationship to Short-Term Morbidity and Mortality, *Am. J. Cardiol.*, 45:542, 1980.
20. Davies, M. D., Cronin, K. D., and Domaingue, C. M.: Pulmonary Artery Catheterization in Assessment of Risks and Benefits in 220 Surgical Patients, *Anesth. Intensive Care,* 10:9, 1982.

125

Techniques of Computer-Based Monitoring after Cardiac Surgery

Louis C. Sheppard, Ph.D.

Concepts

Monitoring

Monitoring of critically ill patients with the aid of computers has been explored intensively for nearly two decades.[1–4] However, clinical usefulness has been elusive in some instances. Hence, we must question whether the objectives have been realistic and clinical requirements adequately defined. In the larger view, which includes all the components of patient care, monitoring is only one of several areas wherein computers may be useful. Other aspects of patient care which warrant consideration include the frequent acquisition of clinical measurements, the detection and reporting of clinically significant events, data storage and retrieval, medical record preparation, and structured analysis of the clinical data according to rules and logic, the latter allowing more accurate assessment of the status of the patient as well as clinical decision making. Additionally, since 1967 we have utilized computer control of blood infusion to maintain left atrial pressure automatically,[5] and since 1974 the computer has been used in the closed-loop control of hypotensive agents to lower and regulate the mean arterial pressure of hypertensive patients in the early hours following cardiac surgical procedures.[6]

Structured Care

The style of care delivery in the particular critical care unit is a crucial issue. Highly structured care procedures are amenable to automation, but unstructured, ill-defined, and especially impromptu care practices are not. Computer-based systems are more likely to be successfully applied in units wherein the care procedures are well defined and highly organized because the nurses and physicians are better able to adapt to the relatively rigid and repetitive processes imposed by the system. In a less organized unit the personnel may be unwilling to accept the system which imposes discipline and the requirement to follow operating procedures explicitly.

Systematic Decision Making

Following a major cardiac surgical procedure, the patient may be considered as a complex system composed of a number of separate but interrelated subsystems. The care of such a patient can be accomplished effectively utilizing a "system analysis" approach.

With this approach, as proposed by Kirklin,[7] each organ subsystem is analyzed separately by assessing all available information relative to the present performance of the system, the adequacy of this performance relative to the requirements of the patient as an integrated system, and the used and unused reserves of the subsystem. Analysis of the cardiovascular subsystem performance and therapeutic decision making can be organized so that rules and logic can be applied to objective data, preferably numerical data.[7]

Technology in Critical Care

Systems and devices which allow observation, measurement, evaluation, treatment, and life support are needed to provide the nurses and physicians with the proper tools with which to track and alter the clinical course of the patient. Techniques and instrumentation for acquiring the essential measurements must function well when subjected to the stress of clinical use. The measurement and decision-making procedures can be incorporated within a system which employs biomedical electronics and computer technology. Closing the loop to directly involve the system in control of interventions to regulate physiological variables is feasible in certain instances.

Computer-Based Systems

Monitoring of Arrhythmias

Common to nearly all monitoring systems are the display and processing of the electrocardiogram, particularly in the operating room, the recovery room, the cardiothoracic or general surgical intensive care unit, and in coronary care and shock trauma units. Since this readily available bioelectric signal can be acquired with electrodes placed noninvasively, many attempts to perfect systems for computerized monitoring of arrhythmias have been made.[8] Recent advances in commercially available systems have resulted in improvements in the ability to distinguish between patterns which should be detected and events which should be ignored.

Respiratory Measurements

Another class of variables which can be monitored noninvasively is respiratory measurements; these are particularly useful for adjusting respirators and detecting leaks, incorrect settings, and malfunctions. Additionally the measurements may be useful in evaluating the clinical status of the patient and in clinical decision making.[9] Automation of the measurement of these variables may require the use of costly transducers and devices to ensure signal fidelity and measurement reliability. Hence the clinical application of computer-based systems has been on a somewhat smaller scale in respiratory intensive care than in cardiovascular intensive care.

Cardiovascular Measurements

Apart from monitoring the electrocardiogram, cardiovascular measurement techniques are mainly applied to patients in whom invasive methods must be employed in order to obtain reliable measurements. The present state of technology seems to limit the application of these systems to critically ill patients in whom the added risk of invasive maneuvers is justified because accurate and reliable data are required for the correct diagnosis of complex problems and for the selection of proper treatment modalities.

System Design

Requirements Analysis

Computer systems development has often suffered from inadequate requirements analysis. Design and implementation have generally begun before the designers and users reached a sufficient understanding of needs and functional requirements. *Requirements definition* states why a system is needed, what functions the system must accomplish, and how the system is to be constructed.

To benefit clinical users, the system must perform useful functions that are otherwise time-consuming or difficult to accomplish; it must be flexible, must be easy to learn and use, and must protect the data. Inspection and evaluation of existing prototypes are useful in the requirements analysis phase because they provide concrete, working examples, from which potential users can discern how others use computer systems, what functions can be performed, and how computer technology might be applied to their problems.

Equipment and Programming

Computer-based systems are usually composed of the biomedical monitoring equipment, the computer hardware, and the computer programs that operate the system. The computer programs can be divided into two categories: (1) programming systems for operating the computer's input/output devices and for compiling the programs and (2) applications programs that tailor the computer to the particular monitoring duties and data manipulation desired.

Staffing and Procedures

Consistent and reproducible application of present knowledge to the care of acutely ill patients requires a highly organized, multidisciplinary staff of competent, well-trained personnel and explicit procedures for the implementation of this knowledge to achieve effective operation of the intensive care unit.

Strong professional leadership by someone who commands the respect and allegiance of nursing staff and physicians in the unit is imperative. The intent of this person must be that the system will be utilized effectively and the staff will be held accountable for maintaining the operational integrity of the system (i.e., electrode contact with skin, catheter patency, signal fidelity, etc.). To this end, there should be adequate support staff to facilitate interconnection of the system to patients, to maintain bioelectronic devices, and to provide programming support. Additionally, well-organized procedures are required for the proper application of the electrodes and sensors and for routine maintenance to ensure measurement accuracy and signal fidelity.

Objectives

The aim should be to completely integrate the computer-based functions and all other care-related tasks into a cohesive clinical system. This should include routine use of data and records produced by the system in actual patient management. By this means the clinical personnel will rely on the computer-based system to play a unique role in the care processes; it will not be a redundant or superfluous adjunct to care. The intent should be to avoid duplication of computer-based functions with continuing dependence on parallel manual procedures.

Measurements

The care of patients following open intracardiac operations employing extracorporeal circulatory support requires periodic measurement of certain variables to assess the status of the patients during the early postoperative period. For example, in the Cardiac Surgical Intensive Care Unit (CICU) at the University Hospital, University of Alabama at Birmingham (UAB), monitoring of the electrocardiogram (ECG), radial artery pressure (ART), right atrial pressure (RAP), left atrial pressure (LAP) and, intermittently, cardiac index (CI) provides the basis for clinical assessment of cardiovascular system performance. In our experience, measurement of CI by green dye dilution or by thermodilution combined with ART and mean LAP measurements allows a more accurate assessment of cardiac function and the response to therapeutic interventions than does measurement of ART and central venous pressure without CI. Additionally, measurement of chest tube drainage, urine output, rectal temperature, arterial blood gases, and respiratory variables enables the clinical staff to detect potential problems. Intravascular and intracardiac pressure measurements are most useful in optimizing the care of critically ill patients, particularly in those with diminished cardiac performance.[10]

Clinical Functions Afforded by the System

At 2-min intervals the automated measurements are acquired and displayed at the bedside. Measurements for two patients in adjacent beds are combined in a single frame and displayed on each of the video monitors positioned between each pair of beds. These measurement variables are transferred from computer memory to the disk storage unit at 5-min intervals. Manually entered data and data derived therefrom, such as the blood gas measurements and base excess, as well as computer-aided measurements, such as cardiac output, are logged to the disk.

Tabular listings of the clinical data are printed as each full page of measurements accumulates. Once each day these records are verified, signed, and inserted in the patient's charts. Since most patients are transferred from the CICU to a semiprivate room on the day following operation, less than 24 h of data storage is required for the majority of patients.

Previous and current values of the automated measurements are retrieved and displayed at the bedside in tabular form on demand. Excessive rate of blood loss for 1 h, 2 h, and 3 h in succession, and cumulative loss at 4 h and 5 h (also 6 h for infants) constitute the basis for recommending reoperation. If any value exceeds the appropriate limit, the recommendation CONSIDER REOPERATION is displayed.

The manual administration of pharmacologic agents requires the computation of dosages according to a specified protocol for each drug. These protocols have been implemented on the computer system to aid the nurses and the physicians in the error-free determination of the correct concentration (in 5% dextrose in water) and infusion rate (ml/h) for a specified dose (μg/kg/min) of a particular drug [sodium nitroprusside, trimethaphan camsylate, isoproterenol, dopamine, dobutamine, norepinephrine, epinephrine, or lidocaine (Xylocaine)].

Computer Control of Interventions

Well-established physiological principles were applied in the development of the procedure for automatic blood infusion.[2] The infusion is controlled by the computer system based on end-expiratory mean LAP, which is related to stroke volume (SV) and, hence, cardiac output. An LAP limit is specified by the physician to represent that level which is associated with the optimal SV. If after infusion of a volume of blood (250 to 1000 ml of blood per square meter of body surface area), the LAP fails to increase above the limit, the total volume of blood to be infused is limited to a multiple (typically 2, 2.5, or 3) of the cumulative blood loss measurement to prevent overinfusion.

The blood pressure of hypertensive patients is controlled automatically with a computer-programmed proportional-integral-derivative (PID) regulator, which is augmented by a decision table to limit the incremental increase of the rate of infusion of peripheral vasodilating agents and to bias the controller in favor of decreasing the rate of infusion.[6] For sodium nitroprusside, the MAP measurement is fed back at 1-min intervals and the computer-controlled infusion pump* is adjusted to maintain the MAP near the desired level by increasing, holding constant, or decreasing the rate of infusion by an incremental amount specified by the deviation of the MAP from the target and the rate of change of the MAP.

Trends

Manufacturers of monitoring systems are exploiting recent advances in microcircuit technology by adopting designs that use microprocessors, programmable read-only memory chips and random-access memories in the bedside monitors and central stations. Infusion device companies have opted to employ this technology as well. Hence, more and more the intelligence heretofore residing in the mainframe minicomputer is being distributed among the bedside monitors and devices.

Data communications issues are arising with increasing frequency. Most, if not all, of the critical care monitoring systems are designed around some type of communications structure that may be viewed as a kind of local area network (LAN). Unfortunately each company has its own proprietary LAN specifications and protocols; communication among vendors is virtually nil. However, interconnecting critical care systems with other systems (clinical laboratory, pharmacy, catheterization laboratory) and the hospital mainframe computer to achieve true integration promises to become reality.

Increasing computing power poised at the bedside affords an enormous opportunity to explore the usefulness of artificial intelligence. The subset called "expert systems" may be applicable to assessment of patient status and decision making with respect to treatment.

*IMED, San Diego, Calif.

Further Reading

In an excellent paper on computer monitoring, Glaeser and Thomas[11] give a broad but in-depth review, including definitions, systems, techniques, and concepts. A more recent review article focuses mainly on cardiac surgical intensive care.[12] Both articles address the evaluation of impact on care, clinical benefits, and economics. Katona[13] reviews computer control of therapeutic interventions.

References

1. Weil, M. H., Shubin, H., and Rand, W.: Experience with a Digital Computer for Study and Improved Management of the Critically Ill, *JAMA,* 198:1011, 1966.
2. Sheppard, L. C., Kouchoukos, N. T., Kurtts, M. A., et al.: Automated Treatment of Critically Ill Patients Following Operation, *Ann. Surg.,* 168:596, 1968.
3. Osborn, J. J., Beaumont, J. O., Raison, J. C., et al.: Computation for Quantitative On-Line Measurements in an Intensive Care Ward, *Comput. Biomed. Res.,* 3:207, 1969.
4. Robicsek, F., Masters, T. N., Reichertz, R. L., et al.: Three Year's Experience with Computer-Based Intensive Care of Patients Following Open Heart and Major Vascular Surgery, *Surgery,* 81:12, 1977.
5. Sheppard, L. C., and Kirklin, J. W.: Cardiac Surgical Intensive Care Computer System, *Fed. Proc.,* 33:2326, 1974.
6. Sheppard, L. C., Kouchoukos, N. T., Shotts, J. F., et al.: "Regulation of Mean Arterial Pressure by Computer Control of Vasoactive Agents in Postoperative Patients," Computers in Cardiology, IEEE-75CH1018-1C, Rotterdam, The Netherlands, October 2–4, 1975, p. 91.
7. Kirklin, J. W.: "Systems Analysis in Surgical Patients with Particular Attention to the Cardiac and Pulmonary Systems," 15th Macewen Memorial Lecture, University of Glasgow, 1970.
8. Cox, J. R., Nolle, F. M., Fozzard, H. A., et al.: Aztec, a Preprocessing Program for Real-Time ECG Rhythm Analysis, *IEEE Trans. Biomed. Eng.,* 15:128, 1968.
9. Osborn, J. J.: "The Evolution of Monitoring into Quantitative Measurement on the Intensive Care Unit," Second Henry Ford International Symposium on Cardiac Surgery, Sec. IV, Chapter 23, p. 148.
10. Kouchoukos, N. T., and Karp, R. B.: Management of the Postoperative Cardiovascular Surgical Patient, *Am. Heart J.,* 92:513, 1976.
11. Glaeser, D. H., and Thomas, L. J.: Computer Monitoring in Patient Care, *Annu. Rev. Biophys. Bioeng.* 1:449, 1975.
12. Sheppard, L. C.: The Computer in the Care of Critically Ill Patients, *Proc. IEEE.,* 67:1300, 1979.
13. Katona, P. G.: Automated Control of Physiological Variables and Clinical Therapy, *CRC Crit. Rev. Biomed. Eng.,* 8:281, 1982.

Section G

Cardiovascular Surgical Techniques

126

Surgical Management of Pericardial Disease*

Joseph I. Miller, Jr., M.D.

Life is short; The art is long; The occasion instant; The experiment perilous; The decision difficult.

Hippocrates[1]

Operative Treatment of the Pericardium

There are generally three operative procedures performed on the pericardium: (1) pericardiocentesis, (2) pericardiotomy for biopsy, exploration, and drainage, and (3) pericardiectomy.

Pericardiocentesis

Pericardiocentesis is generally done for four reasons: (1) to attempt to establish a diagnosis of pericardial disease by diagnostic studies of pericardial fluid,[2] (2) to relieve acute cardiac tamponade, (3) to study physiologic elevation of venous pressure,[2] and (4) to aid anesthetic management of the perioperative decompensated patient requiring pericardiectomy. The first two are by far the most common.

Pericardiocentesis ideally should be carried out in the cardiac catheterization laboratory, with equipment capable of cardiac monitoring. When carried out at the bedside, it should be done with electrocardiographic monitoring by experienced personnel. The individual performing the procedure should have knowledge of the surgical anatomy of the heart and pericardium, the technique, and its complications.

The two anatomic surgical approaches for pericardiocentesis are the subxiphoid approach and the parasternal approach. The subxiphoid is the approach of choice and also the safest (Fig. 126-1). The patient is given adequate sedation, and generally atropine (0.5 mg to 1 mg) is given intravenously to prevent vasovagal reactions. If time permits, the patient should fast for 3 to 4 h prior to the procedure in case emergency surgery is necessitated.

The subxiphoid approach (Fig. 126-1) is as follows: The patient is placed in a semi-Fowler's position at an angle of 45 degrees. A point 2 cm inferior to the tip of the xiphoid and just to the left of the midline is anesthetized with a local anesthetic solution. A small gauge needle, such as a no. 21 spinal needle, at least 6 in long and filled with anesthetic solution is introduced under electrocardiographic monitoring and is slowly advanced toward the left shoulder. The needle will be felt to meet some resistance as it passes through the diaphragm and as it passes into the pericardium—a sensation of "popping through" will often be felt. If the needle touches the right ventricular epicardium, the V lead connected to the epicardium will show ST-segment elevation;[3] rarely the right atrium will be contacted, and PR-segment elevation is recorded. The operator may feel a scratch sensation as the needle touches the epicardium. The distance from the skin to the heart is 6 to 8 cm in an adult, and 5 cm or less in a child.[4] Initially, only 3 to 5 ml of fluid should be removed; if it is grossly bloody, it should be tested to see if it clots. If the aspirated blood clots, the right ventricle has been entered and the fluid is not from the pericardial aspiration. If the pericardial space is easily localized, a large no. 16 lumbar puncture needle

Note: The discussion of this subject by Dr. Joseph I. Miller and Dr. Charles R. Hatcher, Jr., first appeared in J. W. Hurst (ed.), *Update III: The Heart*, McGraw-Hill Book Company, New York, 1980, p. 147. The material was brought up to date by the authors in the previous edition of *The Heart*. It is again made current in this edition. The text, tables, and figures that are identical to the previous publications have been reproduced with the permission of the publisher, editor, and authors.

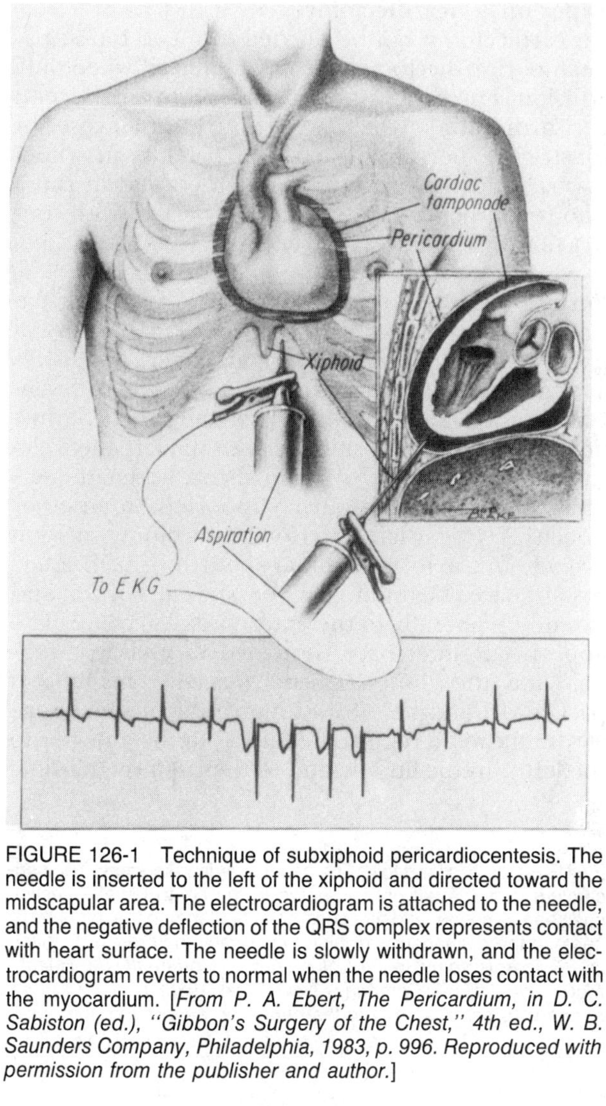

FIGURE 126-1 Technique of subxiphoid pericardiocentesis. The needle is inserted to the left of the xiphoid and directed toward the midscapular area. The electrocardiogram is attached to the needle, and the negative deflection of the QRS complex represents contact with heart surface. The needle is slowly withdrawn, and the electrocardiogram reverts to normal when the needle loses contact with the myocardium. [*From P. A. Ebert, The Pericardium, in D. C. Sabiston (ed.), "Gibbon's Surgery of the Chest," 4th ed., W. B. Saunders Company, Philadelphia, 1983, p. 996. Reproduced with permission from the publisher and author.*]

is introduced along the same pathway. Aspiration is done and the fluid is sent for appropriate studies. All possible fluid should be removed.

If the fluid is removed for diagnosis, it may be helpful to inject air into the pericardium at the completion of the procedure. Follow-up x-rays will then indicate the thickness of the pericardium, the presence of myocardial masses, the size of the heart, and the amount of residual fluid present.[2]

At the completion of the procedure, it may be helpful to leave a plastic Intracath in the pericardial space to allow further drainage and to prevent the recurrence of tamponade. Intrapericardial steroids can be introduced if the diagnosis and underlying condition should so indicate.

The complications that may occur with pericardiocentesis are laceration of a coronary artery or right ventricle, perforation of the right atrium or ventricle, perforation of stomach or colon, pneumothorax, arrhythmias, tamponade, hypotension, and ventricular fibrillation.

Pericardiotomy

In certain clinical situations, pericardiotomy is a simple but effective procedure for pericardial biopsy and for exploration and drainage of the pericardium. When pericardiocentesis is not feasible, or when a diagnosis is still in doubt, direct open biopsy of the pericardium for tissue and fluid removal is a safe, reliable method for establishing a diagnosis. It has been utilized most often in cases of recurrent effusion in which previous studies of fluid have not revealed a diagnosis and examination of tissue is needed.

The two approaches most commonly used are the subxiphoid approach and the left parasternal approach in the left fourth and fifth intercostal space. The approach of choice is subxiphoid, unless one needs to perform a large pericardial window into the left chest for drainage, or unless constrictive pericarditis is suspected. In the latter two instances, incision at the left fourth or fifth intercostal space is preferred.

Technique of Subxiphoid Pericardiotomy

General anesthesia is preferred, but the procedure may be carried out under local anesthesia with adequate sedation if the clinical situation so dictates. A small, 6- to 8-cm incision is made in the midline beginning at the top of the xiphoid process and extended inferiorly about 3 cm below the tip of the xiphoid. The linea alba is divided in the midline, and the cleavage plane between the posterior wall of the sternum and the anterior pericardium is developed by blunt finger dissection. The correct plane is identified by the smooth, silky plane of the fascia on the posterior aspect of the sternum. The xiphoid process is then resected in toto with the electric Bovie. With blunt dissection, the fat lying anterior to the peritoneum and the diaphragm is swept away with a sponge stick, and the lower anterior pericardium and diaphragm are identified. With downward traction, with two Kocher clamps utilized on the diaphragm, the pericardium easily comes into view. It is incised with a no. 15 knife blade. A 4- to 6-cm^2 area of pericardium can be removed for tissue examination. Appropriate catheters may be inserted for pericardial drainage and brought out through separate stab wounds. The incision is closed in layers.

Pericardiectomy

The surgical indications for pericardiectomy are as listed in Table 126-1. Pericardiectomy may consist of two types: (1) parietal pericardiectomy, which is the procedure done in most cases involving recurrent pericardial effusion, and (2) visceral pericardiectomy, which is required along with parietal pericardiectomy in cases of constrictive pericarditis.

Four operative incisions provide access to the pericardium for pericardiectomy; each has its advantages and disadvantages. The approaches are as

TABLE 126-1 Surgical Indications for Pericardiectomy

I. Congenital problems
  A. Congenital anomalies and defects
  B. Cysts and diverticula
II. Acute and chronic pericarditis
  A. Predominant effusion with and without tamponade
    1. Idiopathic recurrent
    2. Uremic
    3. Infectious
      a. Pyogenic (purulent)
      b. Tuberculous
      c. Viral
    4. Neoplastic
    5. Associated with systemic disease (connective tissue disease)
    6. Traumatic
    7. Radiation-caused
  B. Predominant constriction with and without effusion
    1. Idiopathic (nonspecific)
    2. Infectious
    3. Following cardiac surgery

Source: J. I. Miller, Jr., Pericardiectomy, in J. W. Hurst (ed.), "Update III: The Heart," McGraw-Hill Book Company, New York, 1980, p. 153. Reproduced with permission from the publisher, editor, and author.

follows: (1) subxiphoid, (2) bilateral anterior thoracotomy, (3) left anterior thoracotomy, and (4) median sternotomy.

The subxiphoid approach is generally indicated for diagnostic purposes, in life-threatening situations, or in the extremely debilitated patient. Its advantages are that it is quick and easy to perform and is associated with a low morbidity rate. Potential disadvantages include problems with subsequent recurrent effusions and the possibility of future constriction. It is contraindicated in patients with constrictive pericarditis.

Bilateral anterior thoracotomy is the least utilized of the four approaches because of its higher associated morbidity. Its main advantage is that it provides the greatest exposure of the pericardium. It is generally indicated when a patient has had a previous operative procedure on the pericardium and repeat median sternotomy is not feasible.

A left anterior thoracotomy is the most common approach used in our institution for pericardiectomy, excluding those cases of constrictive pericarditis. It has the advantages of being quick to perform, providing good exposure, having minimal morbidity, and allowing removal of approximately 60 to 75 percent of the parietal pericardium. It is the approach of choice, except in constrictive pericarditis.

Median sternotomy is the fourth approach to the pericardium and is the approach of choice in constrictive pericarditis. When constriction is present, open heart pump standby is always available, but is seldom needed.

Types of Pericardiectomy

Pericardiectomy can be divided into two types: parietal pericardiectomy, which is required when only effusion is present without constriction; and visceral pericardiectomy, which is necessary "in all cases of constrictive pericarditis both in patients in whom visceral and parietal layers are fused and in those who retain pericardial effusion associated with constriction by the visceral layer only."[2]

Parietal Pericardiectomy The heart following parietal pericardiectomy is shown in Fig. 126-2. All patients are monitored by radial artery pressures and measurement of cardiac hemodynamics by Swan-Ganz catheters. After appropriate anesthetic induction, the patient is positioned with the left chest elevated to 30 degrees by rolled sheets under the left flank and with the left arm supported on an ether screen. A 10-cm left anterior thoracotomy incision is made in the inframammary fourth or fifth intercostal space, beginning at the sternal border and extending laterally to the anterior axillary line. The appropriate interspace is opened with electric cautery and the chest retractor placed. The lung is packed off and held by a lung retractor. The pericardium can be removed easily from the anterior to the left phrenic bundle and to the right mediastinal

FIGURE 126-2 Heart following parietal pericardiectomy. The pericardium from the left phrenic nerve to the right pleural reflection has been removed, and all pericardium posterior to the left phrenic nerve to the pulmonary vasculature is removed. [*From J. I. Miller, Jr., Pericardiectomy, in J. W. Hurst (ed.), "Update III: The Heart," McGraw-Hill Book Company, New York, 1980, p. 151. Reproduced with permission from the publisher, editor, and author.*]

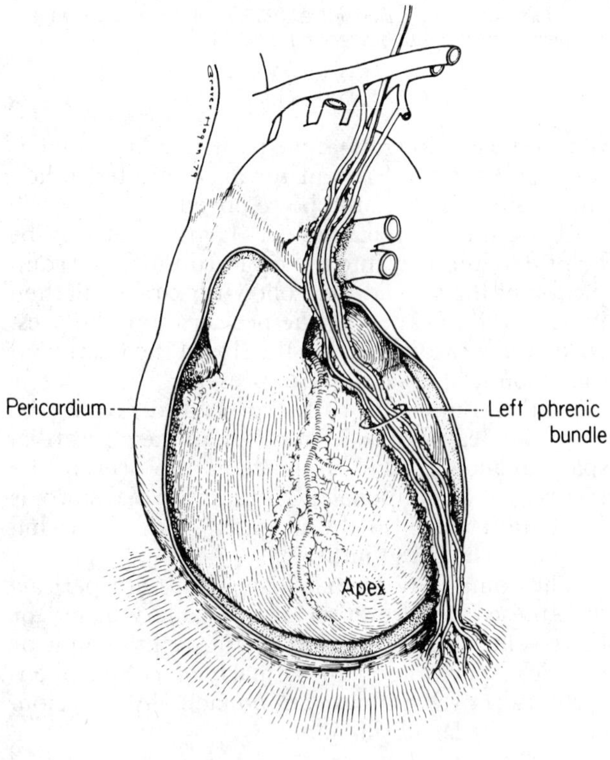

pleural reflection; with further retraction, it can be removed all the way to the right phrenic bundle. The pericardium posterior to the left phrenic bundle is then removed to the level of the pulmonary vasculature. A 1-in bridge of tissue containing the phrenic nerve, artery, and vein is preserved. All pericardium is removed with the coagulation mode of the electric cautery; this provides good hemostasis and minimal postoperative bleeding. Care must be taken to preserve the phrenic nerve as it leaves the pericardium and branches out into the diaphragm.

With this technique, 50 to 75 percent of the parietal pericardium can be removed. Two suction catheters are left in the chest, and the incision is closed in layers.

Visceral Pericardiectomy "Visceral pericardiectomy is necessary in all cases of constrictive pericarditis."[2] Because of the high risk of myocardial tear and excessive blood loss, the procedure is always performed with cardiopulmonary bypass on standby. Our preference is to perform the procedure without the utilization of cardiopulmonary bypass, if possible, but when circumstances necessitate bypass, it should be immediately available, set up, and ready to go. This is in contrast to the feelings of other groups who prefer to do the entire procedure routinely on cardiopulmonary bypass.[5]

After appropriate monitoring lines have been inserted and the patient anesthetized, a standard median sternotomy incision is made (Fig. 126-3). This is the incision we prefer for constrictive pericarditis. It allows for good control of bleeding should the myocardium or cardiac chamber be inadvertently entered and allows quick access to cardiopulmonary bypass should this be needed.

The initial point of exposure is around the apex of the left ventricle.[6] There is generally an area of pericardium around the apex of the heart which is not too adherent or calcified and which will allow one to establish exposure in this area. Two traction sutures of no. 2-0 silk are then taken 1 cm apart over the anterior wall of the left ventricular pericardium. An incision is then made with a no. 15 knife blade through the thickened pericardium down to the myocardium, where the muscle fibers can be recognized. A plane can generally be developed between the epicardium and the pericardium. By use of a combination of traction on the flaps of pericardium and retraction on the heart, combined with sharp and blunt dissection, the constrictive pericardium can be removed. It is extremely important that the pericardium overlying the left ventricle be removed before the right ventricle is freed; otherwise, the increased flow of blood transferred to the constrictive left ventricle will result in significant pulmonary edema and profound congestive heart failure. Areas of calcification embedded in the myocardium and not easily removed should be left alone, so long as there is no sizeable area of involvement

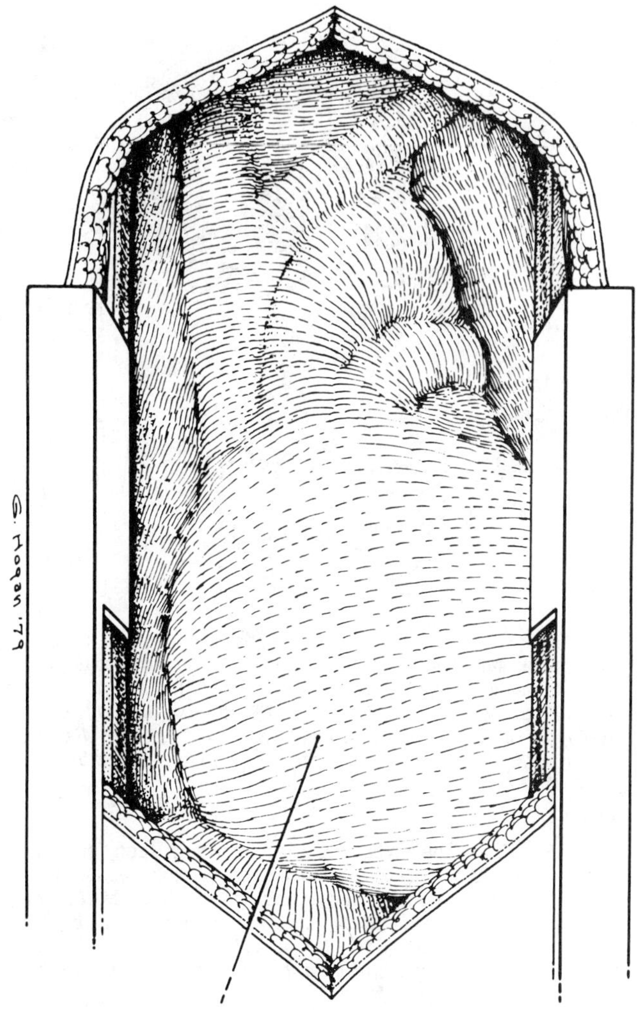

FIGURE 126-3 Heart encased in constrictive pericardium as viewed through median sternotomy approach. [*From J. I. Miller, Jr., Pericardiectomy, in J. W. Hurst (ed.), "Update III: The Heart," McGraw-Hill Book Company, New York, 1980, p. 151. Reproduced with permission from the publisher, editor, and author.*]

over either ventricle. The pericardium is removed over both left and right ventricles to the phrenic bundle (Fig. 126-4). If dissection permits, a phrenic bridge of tissue containing artery, nerve, and vein is left and the pericardium removed to the pulmonary hilus. No attempt is made to remove the pericardium from the atrioventricular groove or left atrium. The pericardium is removed from the pulmonary outflow tract, but removal is not carried out onto the pulmonary artery. The diaphragmatic pericardium is removed and the right ventricle decorticated. If the right ventricle is entered, it is repaired with Teflon felt–pledget sutures. The right atrioventricular groove is not decorticated. If the superior vena cava and inferior vena cava are involved, they are decorticated. If there is no involvement of the venae cavae, they are left alone. If significant ascites is present, decortication of the inferior vena cava at its entrance into the right atrium will

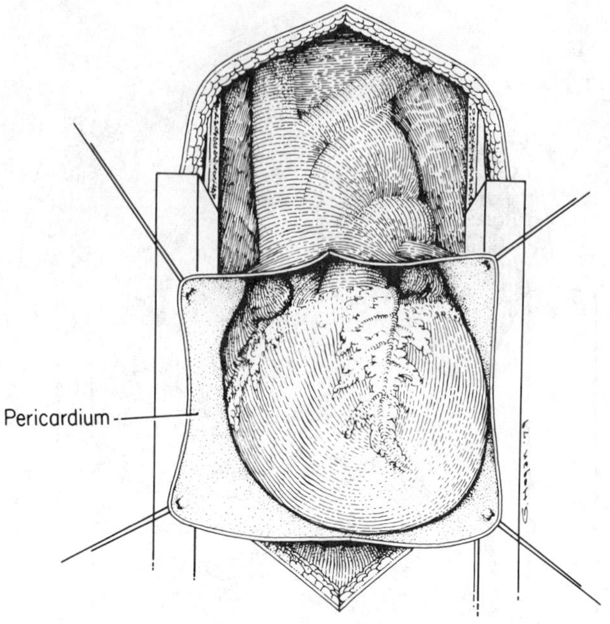

FIGURE 126-4 The left and right ventricles have been freed of the constricting pericardium, and removal of the pericardium laterally to each phrenic bundle is accomplished. [*From J. I. Miller, Jr., Pericardiectomy, in J. W. Hurst (ed.), "Update III: The Heart," McGraw-Hill Book Company, New York, 1980, p. 152. Reproduced with permission from the publisher, editor, and author.*]

FIGURE 126-5 The myocardium is completely freed following visceral pericardiectomy. All constricting pericardium has been removed anteriorly, inferiorly, and around the great vessels. [*From J. I. Miller, Jr., Pericardiectomy, in J. W. Hurst (ed.), "Update III: The Heart," McGraw-Hill Book Company, New York, 1980, p. 152. Reproduced with permission from the publisher, editor, and author.*].

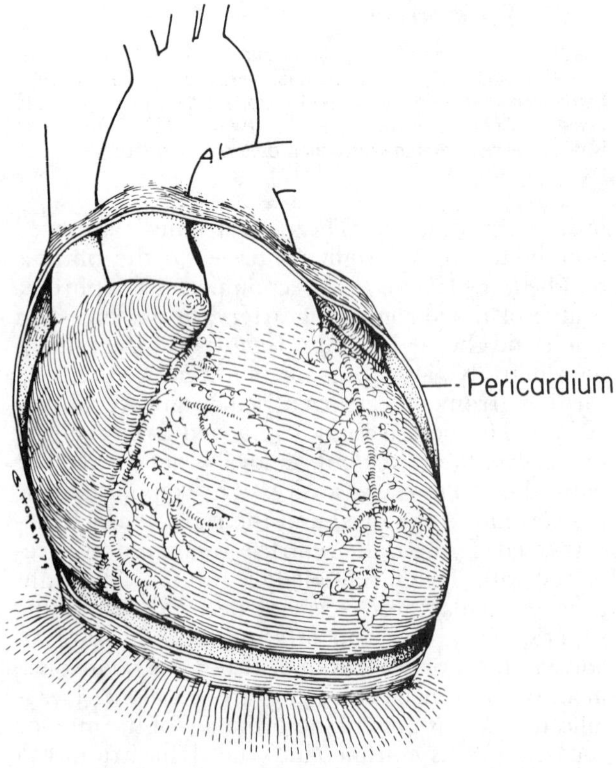

generally be necessary. One must be extremely careful with areas of calcification in the right atrium; these are best left alone unless a significant area is involved. The dissection is not carried past the right phrenic bundle since this is not generally necessary. It is extremely important that no constricting epicardium be left behind (Fig. 126-5). At the completion of the procedure, good muscular contractions from both ventricles should be evident.[4] If any significant constricting pericardium is left, the result may be inadequate and recurrence may result. Adequate hemostasis is achieved and drainage tubes inserted and connected to Pleurovac suction.

Postoperative Complications

The most common postoperative complications of pericardiectomy are congestive heart failure, which occurs in 30 to 35 percent of patients undergoing pericardiectomy for constrictive pericarditis; arrhythmias, in 15 to 20 percent; infection, in 1 to 3 percent; significant bleeding, in less than 1 percent, and the postpericardiotomy syndrome.

Emory University Experience with Pericardiectomy

Table 126-2 reflects the author's experience with pericardiectomy at Emory University Affiliated Hospitals during the 10-year period from 1974 to 1984. Part of this experience has been previously reported.[7] The majority of procedures were performed for recurrent effusions with tamponade due to a number of causes. The most common indication during this period has been neoplastic pericardial disease. In this group, the most common primary tumor was of the breast, followed by lymphoma and tumor of the lung. We prefer a left thoractomy for malignant effusions due to breast tumor and lymphoma, as the expected outcome is quite good. However, when the malignant effusion is due to a lung tumor, we prefer a subxiphoid approach, as the prognosis is limited. Uremic pericarditis contin-

TABLE 126–2 Indications for Pericardiectomy, 1974 to 1984

Cause	Constrictive	Effusive	Number
Neoplastic	0	32	32
Uremic	0	25	25
Idiopathic	6	21	27
Tuberculous	3	8	11
Infectious	1	6	7
Radiation-caused	2	4	6
Rheumatoid	3	0	3
Following open heart surgery	27*	0	27
Traumatic	0	1	1
Drug-induced	0	1	1
Totals	42	98	140

*Includes cases of three Emory surgeons.

ues to be the second most common indication for pericardiectomy in our center.

Constrictive pericarditis accounts for approximately 25 percent of patients undergoing pericardiectomy. The most common cause of constrictive pericarditis in our center is prior open heart surgery.

In this series of patients, there were 10 hospital deaths, for an overall hospital mortality of 7.1 percent.

From a technical standpoint, we believe that all cases of predominant effusive pericarditis should be approached through a left anterior thoracotomy; all cases of constrictive pericarditis, through a median sternotomy with cardiopulmonary bypass standby (although it will be required only rarely). The subxiphoid approach is reserved for those patients too ill for the above, or in whom only a piece of pericardium is needed for biopsy and simple drainage.[7]

References

1. Hippocrates: Aphorisms, in F. Adams (trans.), "The Genuine Works," The Williams & Wilkins Company, Baltimore, sec. I, no. 1, 1939.
2. Hancock, E. W.: Management of Pericardial Disease, *Mod. Concepts Cartiovasc. Dis.*, 47:1, 1979.
3. Bishop, L. H., Jr., Estes, E. H., Jr., and McIntosh, H. D.: Electrocardiograms as a Safeguard in Pericardiocentesis, *JAMA*, 162:264, 1956.
4. Baue, A. E., and Blakemore, W. S.: The Pericardium, *Ann. Thorac. Surg.*, 143:81, 1972.
5. Copeland, J. G., Stinson, E. B., Griepp, R. B., and Shumway, N. E.: Surgical Treatment of Chronic Constrictive Pericarditis Using Cardiopulmonary Bypass. *J. Thorac. Cardiovasc. Surg.*, 69:236, 1975.
6. Miller, J. I.: Pericardiectomy, in J. W. Hurst (ed.), "Update III: The Heart," McGraw-Hill Book Company, New York, 1980, p. 147.
7. Miller, J. I., Mansour, K. A., and Hatcher, C. R., Jr.: Pericardiectomy: Current Indications, Concepts, and Results in a University Center, *Ann. Thorac. Surg.*, 34:40, 1982.

127

Treatment of Tachycardia by Cardiac Surgery

Edward L. C. Pritchett, M.D.   Andrew G. Wallace, M.D.

Treatment of tachycardia by cardiac surgery was a relatively late frontier in the operative treatment of heart disease. Indirect procedures for the treatment of tachycardia have included sympathectomy, implantation of pacemakers, and coronary artery bypass surgery. Direct procedures for controlling tachycardia (such as division of congenital conduction abnormalities, removal of diseased myocardium, and division of specific conduction tissue) required development of techniques for preoperative and intraoperative demonstration of the electrophysiologic abnormalities causing the arrhythmia. Rational application of these operations demands rigorous preoperative study using intracardiac recordings and programmed stimulation (Chaps. 101 and 102). In almost all cases, intraoperative electrophysiologic study is required also.

Technique of Intraoperative Electrophysiologic Study

Intraoperative electrophysiologic study is used to define precisely the location for operative intervention. The study uses programmed stimulation and recordings of electrograms from the epicardium, endocardium, or myocardium. Reference electrograms for timing are recorded from plaque electrodes sutured to the atrium and the ventricle. A probe with bipolar electrodes is used to explore endocardial and epicardial sites. Surface electrocardiograms (ECGs), electrograms from the reference electrodes, and electrograms from the probe are recorded and displayed as analog data. Systematic exploration of the epicardium and endocardium with the probe is used to generate maps that display the sequence of electrical activation. Epicardial mapping of ventricular activation has been used extensively in the intraoperative study of patients with the Wolff-Parkinson-White (WPW) syndrome (Fig. 127-1).[1] Atrial activation during ventricular pacing and during reentrant arrhythmias also is studied by epicardial mapping in patients with this syndrome. In contrast to epicardial mapping, endocardial mapping is more commonly used in patients with ventricular tachycardia due to ventricular aneurysms. It also is used to locate the His bundle so that it can be protected during operative interruption of accessory pathways located in the right atrioventricular (AV) groove.

Electrophysiologic study using the methods described above is limited to the study of electrical events recorded on the cardiac surfaces and to the study of stable cardiac rhythms. Special recording tools

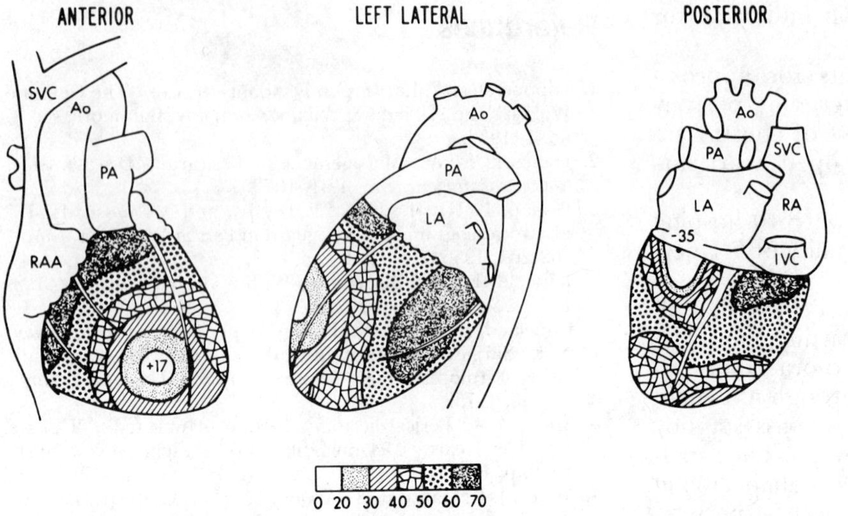

FIGURE 127-1 Epicardial map of ventricular activation during sinus rhythm in a patient with the Wolff-Parkinson-White (WPW) syndrome. Numbers indicated by shading are the time intervals after the onset of the QRS complex. The earliest epicardial activation was recorded at the base of the left ventricle 35 ms before the onset of the QRS complex. Epicardial activation initiated by the normal conduction system began on the surface of the right ventricle 17 ms after the onset of the QRS complex.

such as needles with multiple recording electrodes (plunge electrodes) and cloth mesh with multiple surface electrodes have been developed for the study of intramyocardial activation and unstable arrhythmias.[2]

Technique of Operative Treatment of Tachycardia

There are case reports of treatment of focal atrial tachycardia by excision of the focus, of ventricular tachycardia by cryoablation of the focus, of tachycardia due to reentry in the AV node by partial incision of the AV node, and numerous other tachycardias by a variety of creative operations. There are relatively few operations that have been tested in a series of consecutive patients and published with operative results and long-term follow-up. These latter operations are emphasized in this section. All these procedures should be reserved for severely symptomatic patients whose arrhythmia has not been controlled by rigorous medical management.

Division of Accessory Conduction Pathways

Operative division of accessory pathways in patients with the WPW syndrome is the best operative procedure for the treatment of tachycardia.[3] A successful operation restores the ECG to normal and prevents AV reentrant tachycardia. In patients with atrial fibrillation, it prevents rapid AV conduction over the accessory pathway.

The location of the incision to divide an accessory pathway is determined by the intraoperative electrophysiologic study. In the conventional operation, cardiopulmonary bypass is required. If the accessory pathway is located in the right AV groove, then a high right atriotomy is made to expose the endocardium near the annulus of the tricuspid valve. The annulus is identified by inspection and palpation. The accessory pathway is divided by incising the endocardium 2 mm above the annulus in the location defined by the intraoperative electrophysiologic study. The fat in the AV groove is dissected from the top of the ventricle and the outer surface of the atrium.[4] Since accessory pathways may course through the fat, it is essential that this entire area be meticulously cleaned with a nerve hook.

Access to the endocardium at the left annulus is gained by opening the interatrial groove with the same incision used to replace the mitral valve. Dividing an accessory pathway in the posterior septum is more difficult because of the large amount of fat in this space.

An alternative to the conventional operation combines sharp dissection and cryosurgery from the epicardial side. This new procedure, which appears promising, avoids cardiopulmonary bypass and reduces perioperative morbidity. With either procedure, the success rate for dividing accessory pathways should be approximately 95 percent with a mortality rate less than 1 percent. Since most patients are young and free of other cardiac disease, the operation restores patients to a full lifetime of productivity.

Operative Treatment of Ventricular Tachycardia

Operative treatment of ventricular tachycardia is an important option for many patients with this disabling arrhythmia. The highest success rate is now achieved in patients with coronary artery disease and left ventricular aneurysms.[5] In this procedure an incision in the aneurysm is used to enter the ventricle and expose the endocardium. The endocardium is then mapped during tachycardia to locate diseased areas. The diseased endocardium is resected and a conventional aneurysmectomy is done. If indicated, coronary artery bypass surgery may be done at the same time.

The vast majority of patients having this procedure remain free from their arrhythmia, do not require antiarrhythmic drug therapy, and survive for many years. Late deaths have not been due to arrhythmias. Autopsies performed after late deaths have found new endothelium covering the site denuded at surgery.

Arrhythmogenic right ventricular dysplasia also appears amenable to operative treatment. In this rare, congenital syndrome the right ventricle is thin and contains multiple sacculations resembling many small aneurysms. The coronary arteries and left ventricle are commonly normal. Operative procedures have included simple ventriculotomy, cryoablation of abnormal myocardium, and total exclusion of the right ventricle. Any of these procedures may be effective antiarrhythmic therapy in specific cases.[6]

Division of the AV Node and His Bundle

Division of the AV node and His bundle is used to prevent a rapid ventricular rate during atrial arrhythmias or to interrupt the reentry circuit in patients with AV reentrant tachycardia.[7,8] In patients with the latter tachycardia, it is a far less desirable alternative than cutting the accessory pathway. A successful operation results in complete heart block. The average rate of the escape rhythm following this procedure is 48 beats per minute, and the QRS morphology recorded during the escape rhythm is normal. A permanent ventricular pacemaker is always implanted at the time of this palliative surgery. The need for this procedure has been reduced by the introduction of catheter ablation techniques.[9]

References

1. Gallagher, J. J., Kasell, J., Sealy, W. C., Pritchett, E. L. C., and Wallace, A. G.: Epicardial Mapping in the Wolff-Parkinson-White Syndrome, *Circulation,* 57:854, 1978.
2. Ideker, R. E., Smith, W. M., Wallace, A. G., Kasell, J., Harrison, L. A., Klein, G. J., Kinicki, R. E., and Gallagher, J. J.: A Computerized Method for the Rapid Display of Ventricular Activation during Intra-Operative Study of Arrhythmias, *Circulation,* 59:449, 1979.
3. Sealy, W. C., Gallagher J. J., and Pritchett, E. L. C.: The Surgical Anatomy of Kent Bundles Based on Electrophysiological Mapping and Surgical Exploration, *J. Thorac. Cardiovasc. Surg.,* 76:804, 1978.
4. Sealy, W. C., Gallagher, J. J., and Wallace, A. G.: The Surgical Treatment of Wolff-Parkinson-White Syndrome: Evaluation of Improved Methods for Identification and Interruption of the Kent Bundle, *Ann. Thorac. Surg.,* 22:443, 1976.
5. Horowitz, L. N., Harken, A. H., Kastor, J. A., and Josephson, M. E.: Ventricular Resection Guided by Epicardial and Endocardial Mapping for Treatment of Recurrent Ventricular Tachycardia, *N. Engl. J. Med.,* 302:589, 1980.
6. Fontaine, G., Guiraudon, G., Frank, R., Vedel, J., Grosgogeat, Y., Cabrol, C., and Facquet, J.: Stimulation Studies and Epicardial Mapping in Ventricular Tachycardia: Study of Mechanism and Selection for Surgery, in H. E. Kulbertus (ed.), "Reentrant Arrhythmias," MTP Press, Lancaster, England, 1977, p. 334.
7. Sealy, W. C., Hackel, D. B., and Seaber, A. V.: A Study of Methods for Surgical Interruption of the His Bundle, *J. Thorac. Cardiovasc. Surg.,* 73:424, 1977.
8. Klein, G. J., Sealy, W. C., Pritchett, E. L. C., Harrison, L., Hackel, D. B., Davis, D., Kasell, J., Wallace, A. G., and Gallagher, J. J.: Cryosurgical Ablation of the Atrioventricular Node-His Bundle: Long-Term Follow-Up and Properties of the Junctional Pacemaker, *Circulation,* 61:8, 1980.
9. Gallagher, J. J., Svenson, R. H., Kasell, J., German, L. D., Bardy, G. H., and Broughton, A.: Catheter Technique for Closed Chest Ablation of the Atrioventricular Conduction System in Man: A Therapeutic Alternative for the Treatment of Refractory Supraventricular Tachycardia, *N. Engl. J. Med.,* 306:194, 1982.

128

Techniques for Insertion of Epicardial Pacemakers

Kamal A. Mansour, M.D.

The endocardial (or pervenous) pacemaker implantation has evolved as the primary approach for cardiac pacing owing to improvement of the endocardial electrode tip, which has lowered the incidence rate of electrode displacement. However, there remains an important place for epicardial pacemaker implantation in certain situations. Epicardial pacing is the primary approach for implantation in the newborn and during open heart surgery. It should also be employed whenever endocardial pacing fails, in patients with endocarditis of the tricuspid valve, and in patients with right ventricular apical electrical silence. Anatomic anomalies of the right atrium and right ventricle may dictate epicardial implantation—these include right atrial enlargement; too small, too large, or anteriorly displaced right ventricle; persistent left superior vena cava; and septal defects.

Epicardial Pacemaker Implantation

A temporary endocardial electrode may be used preoperatively to maintain pacing during the procedure.[1] General anesthesia is usually administered.

For atrial epicardial implantation a sutured or short, sutureless screw-in electrode (model 6917A)* may be used on the atrial appendage. For ventricular epicardial implantation the sutureless screw-in electrode (model 6917)* (Fig. 128-1) is most commonly used. Recently a new "stab-in" (fish-hook) electrode (Model 4951)* has been developed for atrial and ventricular epicardial implantation (Fig. 128-2). The electrode head is about 60 percent smaller than the standard epicardial screw-in ventricular leads and is affixed to the lateral atrial wall or ventricle by a simple stab-in procedure. Suture holes are also provided if additional fixation is desired.

Standard Approach

There are several techniques for epicardial pacemaker implantation (Fig. 128-3). The standard approach is a left anterior or anterolateral thoractomy incision (Fig. 128-4). The patient is placed in the supine position with the left side of the chest slightly elevated; the pleural space is usually entered through the fifth or sixth interspace; the pericardium is opened parallel and anterior to the phrenic bundle. One (unipolar) or two (bipolar) electrodes should be inserted; the electrodes should be at least 2 cm apart in bipolar implantation. The electrodes are inserted into a relatively avascular area of the left ventricular myocardium near the apex. Stimulation and sensitivity thresholds are then measured using a pacing system analyzer. After satisfactory measurements are obtained, the pericardium is loosely sutured over the electrodes. Care is taken to keep the phrenic nerve out of the immediate vicinity of the electrode to avoid diaphragmatic stimulation. The electrode leads are usually tunneled subcutaneously or subcostally. The pulse generator is then attached and placed in a subcutaneous pocket or in a pocket beneath the external oblique aponeurosis muscle in the left lower quadrant of the abdomen. It may also be placed subcutaneously in the pectoral area.

In order to avoid entrance into the pleural cavity, several more limited surgical approaches have been advocated:

- An upper abdominal–lower-sternum-splitting incision[2]
- An upper abdominal retrosternal approach[3]
- A subcostal transdiaphragmatic incision[4]
- Dissection of the fifth and sixth costal cartilages under local anesthesia[5]

With the introduction of the sutureless screw-in electrode, the midline subxiphoid approach[6,7,8] and the left subcostal approach[9,10] have become most popular.

FIGURE 128-1 Sutureless (screw-in) electrode tip.

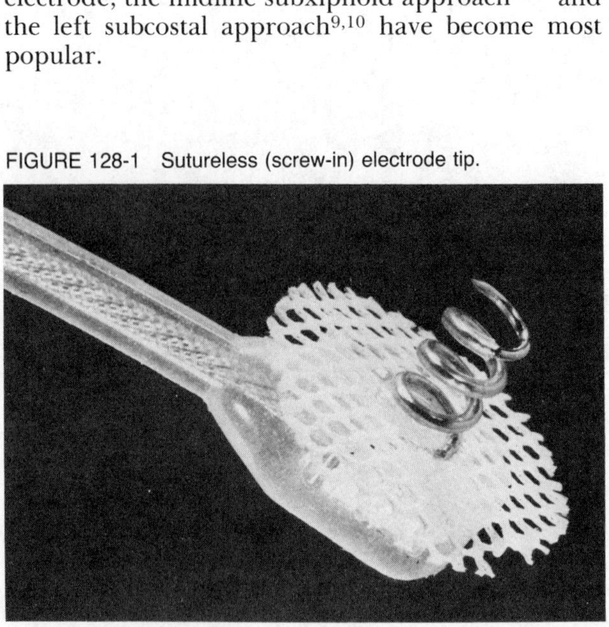

*Manufactured by Medtronic, Inc., Minneapolis, Minn.

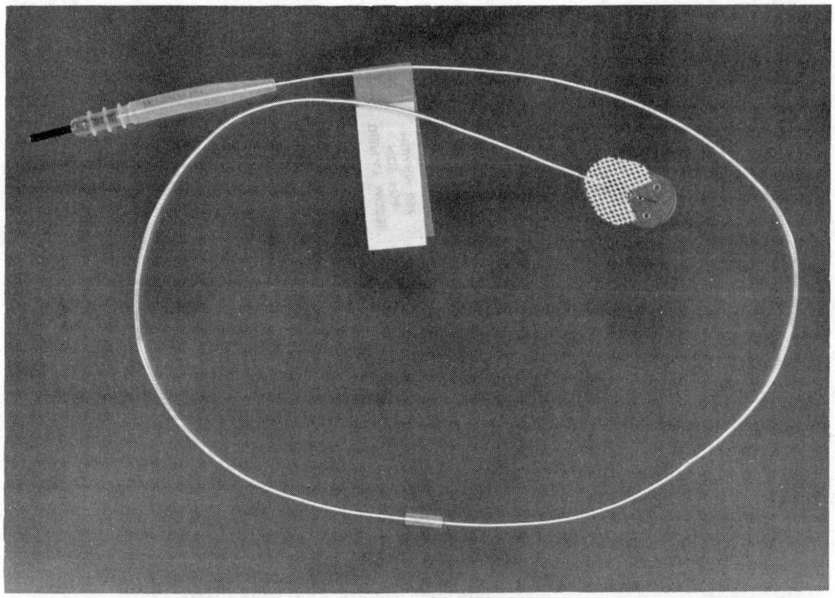

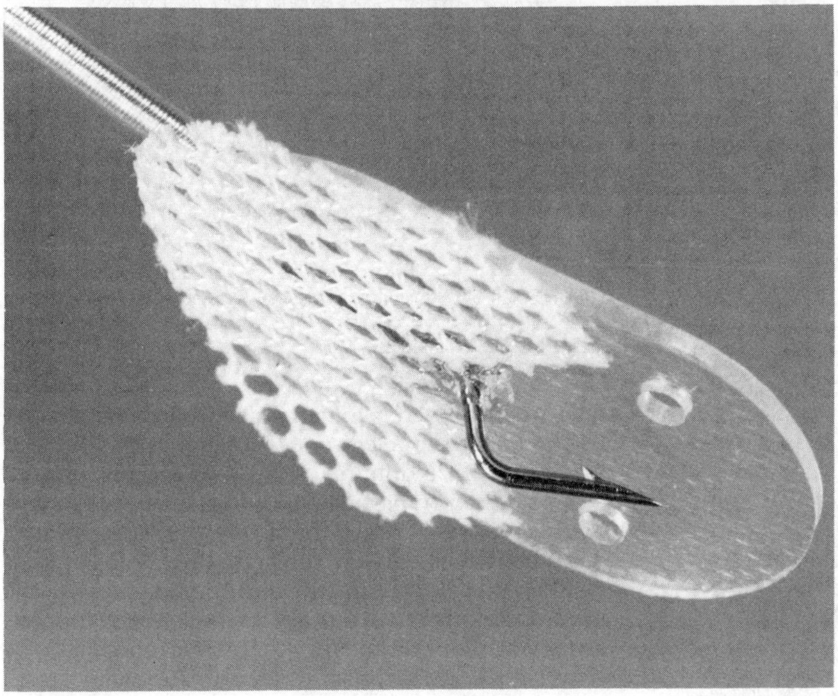

FIGURE 128-2 Stab-in (fish-hook) electrode.

Subxiphoid Approach

The subxiphoid approach (Fig. 128-5) has simplified the epicardial implantation by reducing the operative time and avoiding violation of the pleural space. A midline incision is made over the xiphoid process, extending about 1 in above and 2 in below, and is carried down through the skin and subcutaneous tissues in the linea alba. The xiphoid process is grasped with a Kocher clamp, and the attachments of the abdominal muscles and the sternal portion of the diaphragm are divided. After the sternum is retracted forward and the diaphragm downward, the pericardium is easily identified. By blunt dissection, the prepericardial fat and both pleural reflections are dissected away from the pericardium. The pericardium is then incised inferiorly along its attachment to the diaphragm. The diaphragmatic surface of the right and left ventricles is readily exposed through this approach. A healthy-looking area of myocardium, free of scarring and coronary vessels, is chosen for electrode insertion. While the diaphragmatic surface of the heart is being stabilized, two screw-in (sutureless) electrodes are usually inserted—one 4 mm long for the right ventricle and one 6 mm long for the left ventricle. After satisfactory insertion, pacing and sensitivity thresh-

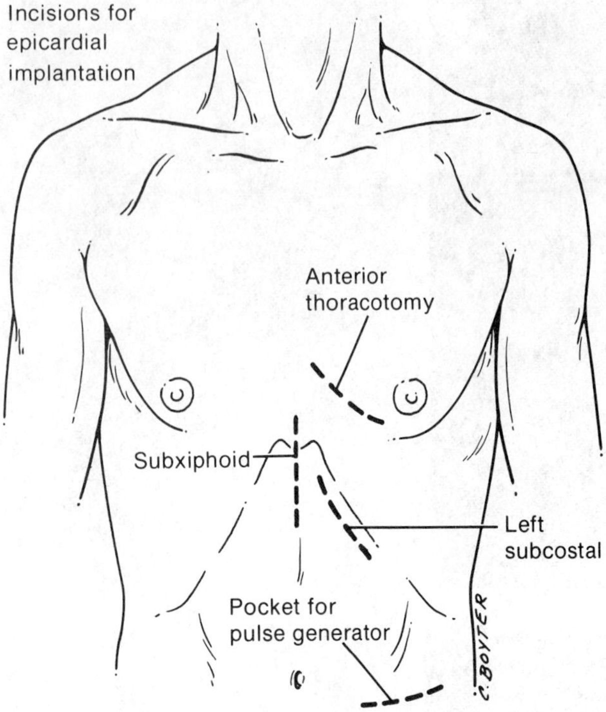

FIGURE 128-3 Incisions for epicardial pacemaker implantation.

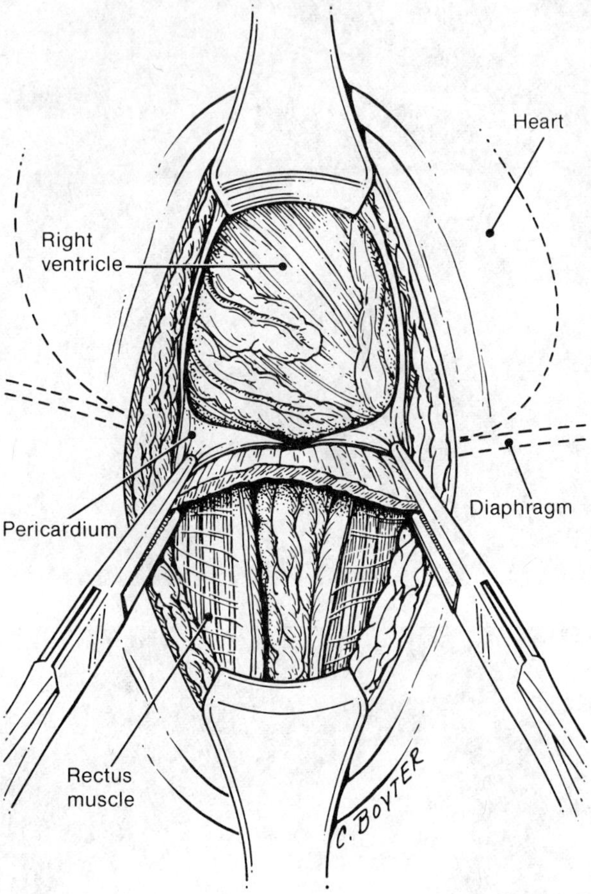

FIGURE 128-5 Subxiphoid approach for epicardial pacing.

FIGURE 128-4 Anterior thoracotomy approach for epicardial pacing.

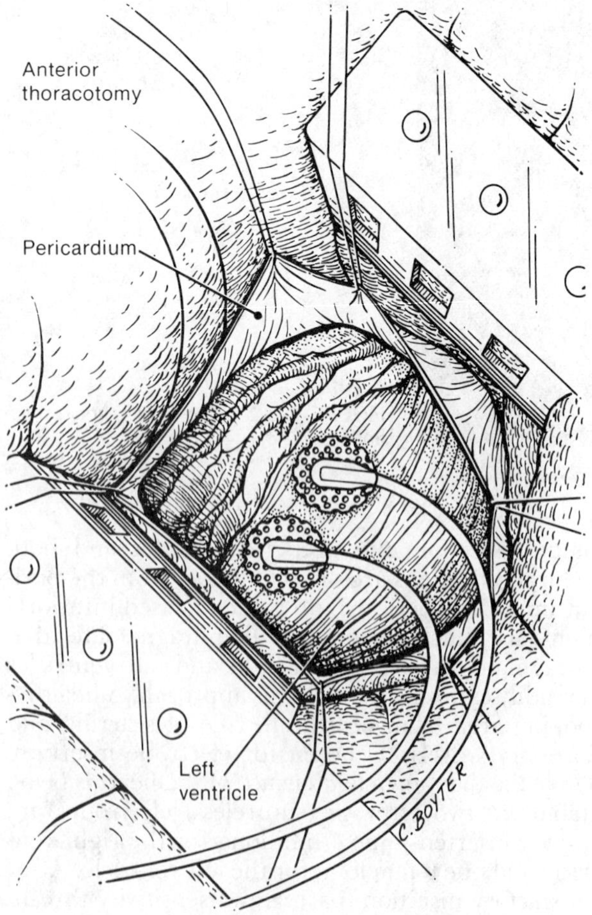

olds are measured using an appropriate system analyzer. Following electrode insertion, attention is turned to the abdominal portion of the procedure. A 2- to 3-inch transverse incision is made to the left of the umbilicus and lateral to the rectus sheath. The incision is carried through the subcutaneous tissues, and the external oblique aponeurosis muscle is incised along the length of the incision. A pocket is then developed beneath the external oblique muscle for housing the pulse generator. A small incision is made in the anterior rectus sheath, and a specially prepared probe is passed from the abdominal incision and guided with the other hand into the midline incision. With use of the probe, the lead with the lower threshold is connected to the pulse generator of a unipolar system or to the cathodal end of a bipolar system. The electrode leads should be arranged in a strain-relieving loop to prevent traction at the point of attachment of the electrode to the epicardium. Sharp bends and kinks must be avoided. No sutures should be placed around the lead wires. The excess length of the lead is carefully wrapped around the pulse generator before the pulse generator is inserted in the pocket. The pocket is usually closed without drainage and prophylactic antibiotic therapy is given.

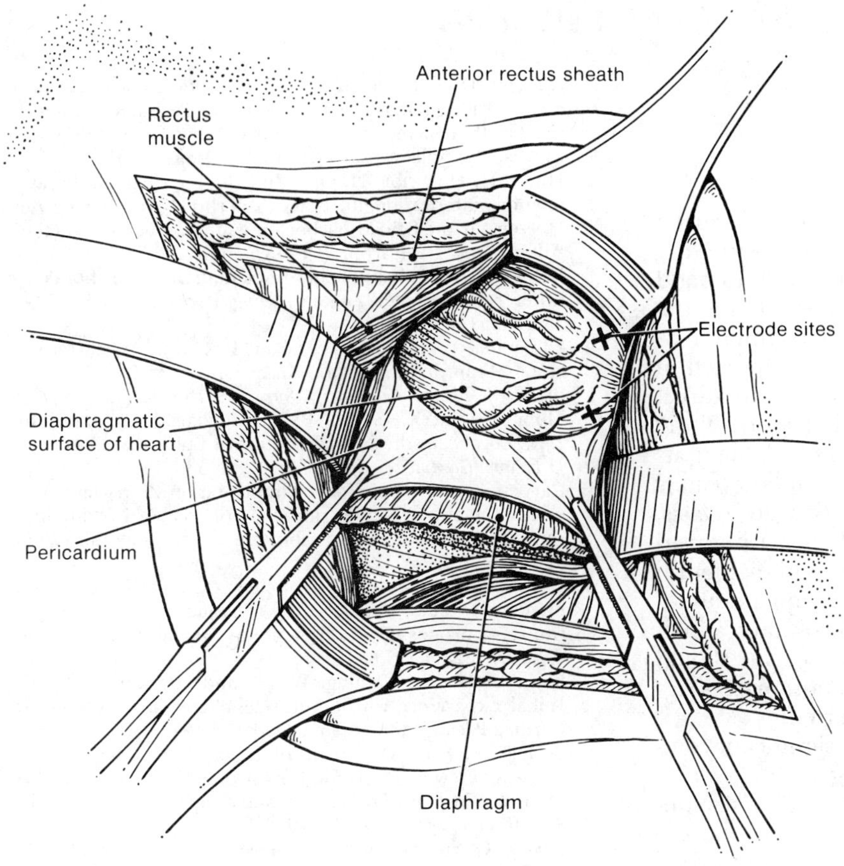

FIGURE 128-6 Left subcostal approach for epicardial pacing.

Left Subcostal Approach

The procedure can be performed by a left subcostal approach (Fig. 128-6) under local anesthesia in the poor-risk patient; however, general anesthesia is customary.

A 3- to 4-inch incision begins below the costal margin and is extended obliquely to the proximal midline. It is carried down through the skin and subcutaneous tissues and through the anterior sheath of the rectus abdominis muscle. The borders of the anterior sheath are retracted, exposing the underlying rectus muscle, which is then separated away from the posterior rectus sheath and incised along the length of the incision. Care is taken not to open the posterior rectus sheath, which during closure provides an additional supportive element to the wound.

Using blunt dissection, the surgeon separates the intact posterior sheath and diaphragm away from the inferior border of the wound. The xiphoid process is identified. The wound is then retracted, allowing identification of the pericardium within the space of Larrey. The anterior and inferior borders of the pericardium are isolated and the pericardium is opened to expose the ventricles and provide a suitable site for implantation of the screw-in electrodes into either ventricle. Unipolar or bipolar leads can be used. The leads are tested and secured to the pulse generator, which is placed in a pocket fashioned in conjunction with the single incision.

Dual-Chamber Pacing

A P-wave synchronous (VAT) pacemaker or an atrial synchronous–ventricular inhibited (VDD) pacemaker requires an additional electrode to sense the atrial potential. The atrioventricular sequential (DVI) pacemaker and the fully automatic (DDD) pacemaker have the capability of stimulating both chambers and of sensing either the ventricle or both chambers. The most commonly practiced epicardial approach for installation of the dual-chamber system is a left anterolateral thoracotomy through the fifth interspace. The lung is retracted posteriorly, the pericardium is incised anteriorly and parallel to the phrenic bundle. The left atrial appendage is exposed and an atrial electrode is inserted. Good experience has been reported with the atrial stab-in electrode.[11] A screw-in sutureless electrode is inserted in the apex of the left ventricle. After stimulation and sensitivity thresholds are checked, the two electrode leads are tunneled beneath the costal margin, brought into the abdominal incision, and connected to the pulse generator in the same manner used for ventricular epicardial implantation.

The stab-in electrode can be used for both atrial

and ventricular implantations through a subxiphoid approach.[12]

Complications of Epicardial Implantation

Complications of epicardial implantations have been those inherent in the thoracotomy itself and the opening of the pericardium.[13] Risk will depend therefore upon the condition of the patient, the technique of the surgeon, and the technique of anesthesia. Lead dislodgment has been reported in few patients. Wires do break secondary to direct trauma to the wire or to repeated flexion of the electrode close to the pulse generator or near its insertion at the heart if sufficient redundant lead is not left in these spaces. Postoperative atelectasis, pneumonitis, and pleural effusion do occur but usually resolve without untoward effect. Either pleural space may be inadvertently entered and pneumothorax may develop with lateral subcostal or subxiphoid approaches. A postoperative chest x-ray should make the diagnosis and, if the pneumothorax is significant, a chest tube should be inserted.

Pericarditis proves to be the most significant complication. It occurs with varying degrees of severity and usually necessitates mild analgesics for its control. In about 5 percent of cases pericarditis may be severe and may require indomethacin or steroids.[14]

Ventricular lacerations can occur, usually owing to roughness at the time of electrode implantation or implantation of the electrode in a friable area of the myocardium. Bleeding can be severe enough to require suturing for its control. Pericardial tamponade, though rare, may occur and may require reoperation for its relief.

Diaphragmatic stimulation can also occur owing to the proximity of the implanted electrodes to the phrenic nerve. This can be corrected by switching the electrodes, by crushing the nerve, by transposition of the nerve,[15] by reducing the stimulus amplitude if this is feasible, or by interposing a sheet of nonconductive material such as Teflon felt between the electrode tip and the phrenic bundle.

References

1. Abelson, D. S., Samet, P., Rand, G., and Moraca, J.: Endocardial Pacemaking and Insertion of a Permanent Internal Cardiac Pacemaker; A Dual Approach in a Case of Repeated Cardiac Asystole, *N. Engl. J. Med.*, 625:692, 1961.
2. Hirsh, H. H., Scior, H., and Zipf, K. E.: Uber die Pericardiotomia inferior longitudinalis (Sauerbruch) als Zugang zum Herzen fur die Schrittmacher implantation beim Morgagni-Adams-Stokes Syndrom, *Beitr. Klin. Chir.*, 208:446, 1964.
3. Behrends, W.: Schrittmacher implantation: Transthorakaler order retrosternaler Zugang? *Langenbecks Arch. Klin. Chir.*, 313:632, 1965.
4. Parsonnet, V., Gilbert, L., Zucker, I. R., and Assefi, I.: Subcostal Transdiaphragmatic Insertion of a Cardiac Pacemaker, *J. Thorac. Cardiovasc. Surg.*, 49:739, 1965.
5. Mobin-Uddin, K., Smith, P. E., Lombardo, C., and Jude, J. R.: Local Anesthesia for Insertion of Epicardial Electrodes, *J. Thorac. Cardiovasc. Surg.*, 55:112, 1968.
6. Carpentier, A.: Technique d'implantation de pacematers a electrodes epicardiaques par une voie d'abord abdominale sous-xiphoidienne extraperiotneale et extrapleurale, *Presse Med.*, 76:75, 1968.
7. Castellani, L., Barsotti, J., Fauchier, J., and Greco, J.: Implantation d'un stimulateur cardiaque par voie epigastrique—a propos de 72 observations. *Ann. Chir. Thorac. Cardiovasc.* 10:299, 1971.
8. Mansour, K. A., Fleming, W. H., and Hatcher, C. R., Jr.: Initial Experience with a Sutureless Screw-in Electrode for Cardiac Pacing, *Ann. Thorac. Surg.*, 16:127, 1973.
9. O'Neill, T. J. E.: Discussion of Initial Experience with Sutureless Screw-in Electrode for Cardiac Pacing by Kamal A. Mansour, William H. Fleming and Charles R. Hatcher, Jr., *Ann. Thorac. Surg.*, 16:127, 1973.
10. Lawrie, G. M., Morris, G. C., Howell, J. F., and DeBakey, M. E.: Left Subcostal Insertion of the Sutureless Myocardial Electrode, *Ann. Thorac. Surg.*, 21:350, 1976.
11. Bognolo, D., Stokes, K., Wiebisch, W., Vijaganagar, R., Eckstein, P., and Cromartie, S.: Experimental and Clinical Study of a New Permanent Myocardial Atrial Sutureless Pacing Lead, *PACE*, 4:A-35, 1981.
12. Ott, D. A., Gillette, P. C., and Cooley, D. A.: Atrial Pacing via the Subxyphoid Approach, *Texas Heart Institute Journal*, 9(2):149, 1982.
13. Mansour, K. A., Dorney, E. R., Tyras, D. H., and Hatcher, C. R., Jr.: Cardiac Pacemakers: Comparing Epicardial and Pervenous Pacing, *Geriatrics*, 28:151, 1973.
14. Mansour, K. A., Miller, J. I., Symbas, P. N., and Hatcher, C. R., Jr.: Further Evaluation of the Sutureless, Screw-in Electrode for Cardiac Pacing, *J. Thorac. Cardiovasc. Surg.*, 77:858, 1979.
15. Sprinkle, J. D., Takaro, T., and Scott, S. M.: Phrenic Nerve Stimulation as a Complication of the Implantable Cardiac Pacemaker, *Circulation*, 28:114, 1963.

129

Techniques of Using the Intraaortic Balloon Pump

Joseph M. Craver, M.D. Charles R. Hatcher, Jr., M.D.

The intraaortic balloon pump (IABP) is the most widely used form of mechanical circulatory assist. A nonocclusive balloon catheter device positioned in the descending thoracic aorta causes diastolic pressure augmentation by balloon inflation in diastole and afterload reduction by deflation during ventricular systole. This system for counterpulsation was first described by Mouloupoulos et al. in 1962.[1]

Since balloon counterpulsation permits the elevation of diastolic aortic pressure and augmentation of coronary blood flow while reducing the load against which the systolic heart must pump, it has been employed in the following circumstances:

1. It has been used in cardiogenic shock to try to maintain viable perfusion pressure in the patient whose heart is highly damaged, but in whom recovery is still possible.
2. It has been used as an adjunct to the therapy of the intermediate syndromes in which the balance between ischemia and infarction has not been established in the presence of impending myocardial infarction. In such a circumstance, where vasodilators and perhaps beta blockers have already been utilized, counterpulsation has been of added use in further reducing oxygen needs of the heart while augmenting coronary perfusion. Indeed, in some institutions this is a therapy of choice in order to stabilize the patient prior to further therapy.
3. It has been used in the postoperative period to aid ventricular performance so that the patient can be weaned from bypass. As improvements in bypass technique have occurred and less cardiac damage has ensued following the use of hypothermia and cardiac arrest, the need for this type of support in the postoperative period has been reduced.
4. It has been used effectively in supporting patients prior to emergency coronary bypass surgery when percutaneous coronary angioplasty fails and is complicated by refractory myocardial ischemia.[2]

Balloon Counterpulsation

Balloon counterpulsation offers both diastolic and systolic advantages. By inflating during diastole, the balloon displaces a volume of blood equal to its own volume, thereby raising aortic diastolic pressure and augmenting coronary perfusion, which occurs primarily during diastole. In systole, balloon deflation is made to occur just prior to the next aortic valve opening and abruptly reduces aortic pressure, thereby allowing the left ventricle to eject against a greatly reduced arterial impedance. This may lead to decreased systolic and diastolic ventricular volumes. Myocardial pressure work, and therefore myocardial oxygen consumption, is reduced.[3,4] If ventricular function is complicated by mitral regurgitation or by ventricular septal defects (e.g., after acute myocardial infarction), the reduced ventricular volumes and pressure improve hemodynamic function by reducing the regurgitant flow or left-to-right shunt, respectively.[5–7]

The Intraaortic Balloon

Significant advances have been made in the design and manufacture of the intraaortic balloon and catheter. First, an additional lumen has been incorporated into the catheter, through which can be passed a flexible guidewire over which balloon catheter insertion can be directed. This second lumen is also available to monitor central aortic pressure after insertion is completed and the wire removed. Second, reduction in the diameter of the catheter despite incorporation of the second lumen has enabled a balloon 40 cm^3 in volume to be wrapped around the central catheter and yet maintain an overall unit diameter that can be inserted through a no. 11.5 French sheath.

There are three IABP systems available at the present time: Datascope System 83, Kontron Model-10, and S.M.E.C. model 1300 M. Each company manufactures a variety of balloon catheters for percutaneous or surgical insertion. The Datascope and Kontron balloons can be used with either the Datascope or Kontron pump consoles, while the S.M.E.C. balloons can be used with all consoles. Balloons manufactured for percutaneous insertion incorporate a single-chambered 40-cm^3 displacement balloon mounted on a double-lumen catheter. Although manufactured for percutaneous insertion, this is the most widely utilized balloon regardless of the technique of insertion. The Datascope model, Percor DL, has the advantage of being mounted on a 10.5 French catheter, which is smaller than the other percutaneous models. S.M.E.C. percutaneous balloons range from 30 cm^3 to 50 cm^3, but these are available only on single-lumen catheters which range from 11.5 to 12.5 French.

Balloons available for surgical insertion vary widely among the manufacturers. Datascope offers balloons for surgical insertion in a range of sizes with volume displacement from 10 to 40 cm^3, with custom-made sizes available on request. Datascope surgical balloons come in single- or dual-chamber models. The dual-chamber "unidirectional" balloon has a short distal chamber which inflates first and occludes the aorta; then a proximal longer chamber inflates. This two-step inflation is thought to cause most of the augmented flow to travel proximally toward the coronary and cerebral vessels. Kontron surgical insertion balloons are available in volume displacements of 20, 30, and 40 cm^3, with catheters sized down to 9.5 French. All have three chambers. With the Kontron trisegmented balloon, inflation begins in the middle segment, followed by inflation of both end segments. Thus, this balloon exerts its influence in both directions equally. S.M.E.C. balloons for surgical insertion range from 6 to 60 cm^3 in volume displacement. All are single-chamber and mounted on single-lumen catheters. Datascope and S.M.E.C. balloons are manufactured from polyurethane, while the Kontron balloon material is Cardiothane-51. All have low-thrombogenic surface properties and excellent durability. All systems now inflate the balloons with helium.

Balloon Insertion

Insertion of the IABP balloon catheter is accomplished by one of three routes: (1) retrograde insertion through a sheath placed in the femoral artery by the Seldinger technique,[3,8,9] (2) insertion via a side arm graft sewn to the femoral artery, or (3) insertion through a graft attached to the ascending aorta.

Retrograde insertion of the IABP balloon catheter through a sheath in the femoral artery is the most commonly used method at this time and is applicable and practical under local anesthesia in virtually any location in which electrocardiogram (ECG) and arterial monitoring are possible. Once the ECG and arterial monitoring devices are functioning, the patient's groins are bilaterally prepared and draped. The common femoral artery having the strongest palpable pulse is selected. The technique is applied by percutaneously cannulating the femoral artery, with a flexible guidewire then passed through the cannula well up into the lower abdominal aorta. The arterial puncture is enlarged by passing progressively larger arterial dilators over the wire until a no. 14 French sheath can be introduced into the artery. The length of the balloon catheter to be inserted is measured by placing the balloon tip at the angle of Louis and marking with a ligature the location on the catheter at which it would exit the femoral artery. The single-chambered balloon is tightly and smoothly wrapped around the catheter, inserted through the sheath, and passed over the guidewire into the thoracic aorta. The balloon must be inserted without untwisting the wrap if it is to pass through the small sheath. Once it is in the thoracic aorta, the balloon is carefully unwrapped prior to connection of the catheter to the pump console; counterpulsation can now begin. Once the system is in place the balloon catheter must be securely fastened to the leg by separate heavy suture. Correct position is checked by portable chest x-ray or fluoroscopy, and any adjustment is made.

Modification of this technique for balloon insertion has been helpful when the patient is still on cardiopulmonary bypass, when femoral pulses are absent, or when percutaneous femoral cannulation is felt to be hazardous. In these situations surgically exposing the common femoral artery enables the operator to cannulate that artery under direction vision. Direct visualization during cannulation may avoid tangential arterial laceration, subintimal insertion, or excessive hematoma formation which may lead to unsuccessful arterial cannulation.[10]

Prior to the development and refinement of a balloon catheter which could be inserted by the Seldinger technique, extensive experience was attained in inserting the balloon via a side arm graft sewn to the femoral artery. This technique is still employed in many centers and can be applied also under local anesthesia wherever ECG and arterial monitoring are possible. After both groins are prepared and draped, a 5-cm segment of common femoral artery just above the origin of the deep femoral artery is exposed and isolated between cotton vascular tapes, which are later used as tourniquets. Formerly the largest possible size of balloon (20, 30, or 40 cm^3) was selected, based on the size of the femoral artery. Now the 40 cm^3 balloon used in the percutaneous technique is often selected for all vessels, since its total catheter diameter is smaller than that of even the former 20-cm^3 surgical balloon catheter. Development is continuing into even smaller balloon catheters for use in extremely small femoral vessels. The balloon catheter is then passed through a 10-cm length of 10-mm woven Dacron graft, which will later be sewn to the femoral artery. The balloon length to be inserted is measured as above. The patient is heparinized 3 min before the artery is opened. The femoral artery is occluded using both vascular tourniquets and then is opened for 1 cm. A flexible guidewire is inserted proximally into the aorta, and then the deflated, wrapped balloon catheter is inserted over the guidewire into the aorta until the length marked with the ligature is reached. The proximal vascular tourniquet is again tightened, the balloon is unwrapped, and counterpulsation can begin. The Dacron graft is sutured to the femoral arteriotomy. Heavy silk ligatures are tied around the graft and catheter to prevent bleeding. The tourniquets are then released and blood flow restored to the leg. The balloon catheter is separately secured to the leg with heavy suture. The wound is then checked for hemostasis, irrigated, and closed in layers over the graft and insertion site. Balloon position is checked as noted above.

The employment of a flexible wire passed into the aorta, over which the double-lumen balloon catheter can be passed during insertion, has been a major improvement in the ease, safety, and success of balloon insertion. With young patients in whom femoral blood flow is excellent, employment of the guidewire may not be necessary. However, with the elderly population and in all patients with aortoiliac obstructive disease utilization of the guidewire can reduce problems associated with balloon passage that may be related not only to obstructive atheroma in these vessels but also to the extreme tortuosity that can be present even when flow is not impaired.

Should obstruction be encountered in the aorto-iliac vessels which prevents passage either of the guidewire or of the balloon catheter over the guide-wire with reasonable pressure, the opposite femoral artery should be tried. If balloon passage meets obstruction in this second site as well, the femoral route is abandoned. Forcing the balloon past a vascular obstruction greatly increases the risk of major vascular complications and embolization.

The majority of intraoperative balloon insertions are performed during or after an open heart surgical procedure.[11,12] General anesthesia makes it easier to expose higher segments of the iliac artery system should obstructive atheroma be encountered in the femoral area. Also, having the heart and great vessels exposed for the cardiac surgical procedure provides an opportunity to attach the graft to the ascending aorta for anterograde balloon insertion should retrograde passage prove impossible.[13]

Timing of Intraaortic Balloon Pump

Proper timing is essential if counterpulsation is to provide effective ventricular assist. The initial timing of IABP is done with the balloon at half volume and in the 1:2 mode. This enables one to see an unaugmented beat compared with a balloon-augmented beat. Ideally, the balloon should inflate immediately after aortic valve closure. If one is recording a central aortic pressure, this can be established accurately. If, however, a radial artery pressure trace is utilized, there will be a 50-ms delay in the waveform propagation. Therefore, balloon inflation is set to occur just before the dicrotic notch on the radial arterial pressure curve. As the proper timing interval for inflation is reached, one will see the obliteration of the dicrotic notch and a maximal height of the diastolic augmented peak (Fig. 129-1).

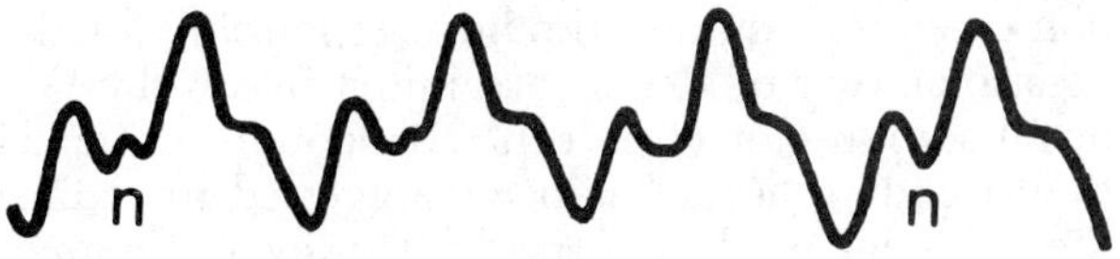

FIGURE 129-1 Timing of balloon inflation is adjusted to obliterate the dicrotic notch (n) on radial artery pressure curve.

Adjustment of the deflation timing is equally important, in order to provide the maximum length of diastolic augmented interval and the greatest reduction in arterial impedance. Again, use of the 1:2 mode will allow one to look at normal and augmented diastolic curves. By moving the deflation point closer to the ensuing systole, one seeks to achieve a waveform in which the end-diastolic dip is 10 to 15 mm below the level of the unaugmented diastolic level. Also one should see a maximal reduction in the height of the systolic peak which follows the augmented diastolic interval, when it is compared with the peak following an unaugmented beat (Fig. 129-2).

Complications of Intraaortic Balloon Pump

Complications occur in approximately 5 to 35 percent of balloon insertions.[12,14–20] Ischemia of the extremity distal to the femoral insertion site is the most common complication of IABP and may be more frequent when the percutaneous insertion technique is employed.[20] Early removal of the catheter with thrombectomy is effective in most cases. Cross-over grafts from the opposite femoral artery to a site distal to balloon insertion have been used as an alternative to removing the balloon when assist is still required.[19] Progressive ischemia requiring amputation of toes, the foot, or the lower leg has occurred in 1 to 2 percent of cases.[12,14–19]

Wound infection of the groin insertion site is the second most common complication, occurring in 3 to 4 percent of patients. These infections usually present themselves several days after the balloon has been removed and heal with topical care and systemic antibiotics. Deep infection requiring removal of the graft remnant is less frequent.[15–18]

Dissection or perforation of aortic, iliac, renal, or mesenteric vessels has been observed in 2 to 4 percent of patients and is usually suspected to stem from "difficult" balloon insertions.[12,18,20] Localized dissec-

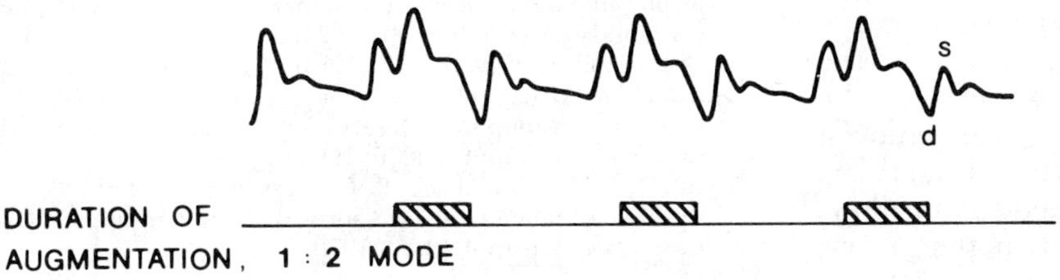

FIGURE 129-2 Timing of balloon deflation is adjusted to provide an end-augmentation diastolic dip (d) of 10 to 15 mmHg and to maximize reduction of ensuing ventricular systole (s).

tion or emboli are also thought responsible for the occasional case of spinal cord injury or small bowel or renal infarction (1 percent). Balloon insertion via the ascending aorta has been suggested to reduce the problem of dissection.[13,15] However, cannulation of visceral arteries with bowel infarction has been reported with this route.[21]

Thrombus formation on the balloon catheter with peripheral or visceral embolization has been reported.[7] Minidose heparin or infusion of low-molecular-weight dextran can prevent this but may cause bleeding complications.

Inability to pass the balloon catheter has been an important limitation of this technique in the past. Data regarding the frequency of this limitation are generally not available.[17] Utilization of the flexible guidewire to negotiate tortuous iliac vessels and obstructive atheromatous plaques in the femoral techniques and the use of the ascending aorta as a site for insertion may reduce the incidence of nonpassage.

Weaning from the Intraaortic Balloon Pump

IABP is continued in the 1:1 mode with the balloon at full volume until the patient's ventricular function appears satisfactorily restored and the need for the inotropic infusions has decreased. Weaning from IABP can then be accomplished over 6 to 12 h by systematic stepwise reductions of the assist mode from 1:1 to 1:2 and eventually to 1:8.[21] At each step, cardiac function must be carefully assessed and time allowed to elapse (4 to 6 h per step) so that an accurate hemodynamic response is observed before further reduction in IABP assist is made. Measurements of cardiac index, arterial gas tensions, urine output, and pulmonary capillary wedge pressure along with careful clinical assessment of the patient's well-being serve as guides for further weaning or reinstitution of IABP assist. When hemodynamic independence of IABP assist is established, with the patient on 1:8 for 4 to 6 h, the balloon may be removed.

Balloon Removal

The procedure for balloon removal can be performed under local anesthesia in the intensive care unit. Removal of balloons inserted surgically is accomplished by reexposing the femoral insertion site. If the balloon was inserted through a sheath the deflated balloon is withdrawn to the level of the sheath, then the sheath and balloon are removed simultaneously, while the femoral artery distal to the insertion site is temporarily occluded. This allows any thrombus that may be present in the artery, around the catheter or sheath or on the balloon itself, to exit via the insertion arteriotomy rather than to embolize distally in the artery. A careful prophylactic proximal and distal catheter embolectomy reduces retention of clot in the artery. Repair of the site can usually be performed with a few simple vascular sutures, rarely a vein patch repair may be needed if the vein is severely atherosclerotic. If a side arm graft was employed the removal procedure is the same, with the graft usually being cut off near the insertion site and oversewn. Removal of the graft and primary arterial repair or vein patch repair of the anastomotic site can be done but usually is unnecessary.

Percutaneously inserted balloons are removed by similar techniques, simply by withdrawing the deflated balloon catheter to the level of the sheath and then removing both together while applying firm pressure to the femoral area just distal to the insertion site. Firm pressure just distal to the percutaneous insertion site is felt to reduce distal embolization of any clot or debris that may accompany balloon removal. Any such material will egress from the artery with the balloon catheter. After the balloon is removed, firm pressure over the femoral insertion site for 30 min to 1 h is essential, as is a normal coagulation profile, to avoid major groin hematoma. It may be that routine surgical removal and prophylactic proximal and distal catheter embolectomy may prove to be advisable on removal of percutaneously inserted balloons as well.[22]

When the balloon is inserted via an ascending aortic graft, usually the graft has been tunneled substernally into the epigastric subcutaneous tissue, allowing balloon removal by a similar procedure under local anesthesia. The end of the graft is then oversewn, buried in the wound, and allowed to clot. If the balloon cannot be removed or if a short graft has been used, reopening of the sternotomy will be necessary.

References

1. Mouloupoulos, S. D., Topaz, S., and Kolff, W. J.: Diastolic Balloon Pumping (with Carbon Dioxide) in the Aorta: Mechanical Assistance to the Failing Circulation, *Am. Heart J.*, 63:669, 1962.
2. Murphy, D. A., Craver, J. M., Jones, E. L., et al.: Surgical Management of Acute Myocardial Ischemia following Percutaneous Transluminal Coronary Angioplasty: Role of the Intraaortic Balloon Pump, *J. Thorac. Cardiovasc. Surgery*, 87(3):332, 1984.
3. Weber, K. T., and Janicki, J. S.: Intra-aortic Balloon Counterpulsation: A Review of Physiologic Principles, Clinical Results, and Device Safety, *Ann. Thorac. Surg.*, 17:602, 1974.
4. Braunwald, E., Covell, J. W., Maroko, P. R., and Ross, J., Jr.: Effects of Drugs and of Counterpulsation on Myocardial Oxygen Consumption: Observation on the Ischemic Heart, *Circulation*, 40(suppl. 4):220, 1969.
5. Buckley, M. J., Leinbach, R. C., Kastor, J. A., et al.: Hemodynamic Evaluation of Intra-aortic Balloon Pumping in Man, *Circulation*, 41(suppl. 2):30, 1970.

6. Phillips, P. A., and Bregman, D.: Intra-operative Application of Intra-aortic Balloon Counterpulsation Determined by Clinical Monitoring of the Endocardial Viability Ratio, *Ann. Thorac. Surg.*, 23:45, 1977.
7. Dunkman, W. B., Leinbach, R. C., Buckley, M. J., et al.: Clinical and Hemodynamic Results of Intraaortic Balloon Pumping and Surgery for Cardiogenic Shock, *Circulation*, 46:465, 1972.
8. Seldinger, S. I.: Catheter Replacement of the Needle in Percutaneous Arteriography: A New Technique, *Acta Radiol. (Stockh.)*, 39:368, 1953.
9. Bregman, D., and Casarella, W. J.: Percutaneous Intra-aortic Balloon Pumping: Initial Clinical Experience, *Ann. Thorac. Surg.*, 29(2):153, 1980.
10. Shahian, D. M., Neptune, W. B., and Ellis, F.H.: Intraaortic Balloon Pump Morbidity: A Comparative Analysis of Risk Factors between Percutaneous and Surgical Techniques, *Ann. Thorac. Surg.*, 36(6):644, 1983.
11. Buckley, M. J., Craver, J. M., Gold, H. K., et al.: Intra-aortic Balloon Pump Assist for Cardiogenic Shock after Cardiopulmonary Bypass, *Circulation*, 46/47(suppl. 3):90, 1973.
12. Craver, J. M., Kaplan, J. A., Jones, E. L., Kopchak, J., and Hatcher, C. R.: What Role Should the Intraaortic Balloon Pump Have in Cardiac Surgery? *Surgery*, 189(6):769, 1979.
13. Gueldner, G. L., and Lawrence, G. H.: Intra-aortic Balloon Assist through Cannulation of the Ascending Aorta, *Ann. Thorac. Surg.*, 19:88, 1975.
14. Bechman, C. B., Geha, A. S., Hammond, G.L., et al.: Results and Complications of Intra-aortic Balloon Counterpulsation, *Ann. Thorac. Surg.*, 24(6):550, 1977.
15. Macoviak, J., Stephenson, L. W., Edmunds, L. H., Jr., Harken, A., and MacVaugh, H., III: The Intraaortic Balloon Pump: An Analysis of Five Years' Experience, *Ann. Thorac. Surg.*, 29(5):451, 1980.
16. Balooki, H.: "Clinical Application of the Intra-aortic Balloon Pump," Futura Publishing Company, Inc., Mount Kisco, N.Y., 1977.
17. Lefemine, A. A., Kosowsky, B., Madoff, I., et al.: Results and Complications of Intra-aortic Balloon Pumping in Surgical and Medical Patients, *Am. J. Cardiol.*, 40:416, 1977.
18. McEnany, M. T., Kay, H. R., Buckley, M. J., et al.: Clinical Experience with Intra-aortic Balloon Pump Support in 728 Patients, *Circulation*, 58(suppl. 1):124, 1978.
19. Alpert, J., Parsonnet, V., Goldenkranz, R. J., et al.: Limb Ischemia during Intra-aortic Balloon Pumping: Indications for Femorofemoral Cross-Over Graft, *J. Thorac. Cardiovasc. Surg.*, 79:729, 1980.
20. Biddle, T. L., Stewart, S., and Stuart, I. D.: Dissection of Aorta Complicating in Intra-aortic Balloon Counterpulsation, *Am. Heart J.*, 92:781, 1976.
21. Kaplan, J. A., and Craver, J. M.: Assisted Circulation, in J. A. Kaplan (ed.), "Cardiac Anesthesia," Grune & Stratton, Inc., New York, 1979.
22. Goldberg, M. J., Kantrowitz, A., et al.: Intra-aortic Balloon Pump Insertion: A Randomized Study Comparing Percutaneous and Surgical Techniques, *J. Am. Coll. Cardiol.*, 3(2):505, 1984.

130

Techniques of Cardiopulmonary Bypass

Robert A. Guyton, M.D.
Willis H. Williams, M.D.
Charles R. Hatcher, Jr., M.D.

. . . delivery of the correct amount of appropriately oxygenated blood to the tissues of the whole body without attendant or ensuing adverse physiologic effects.

P. M. Galleti and
G. A. Brecher, 1962[1,*]

The Development of Cardiopulmonary Bypass

Early Landmarks

As early as 1812, LeGallois first suggested that infusion of blood into organs could maintain viability.[2] In the 1850s Brown-Séquard demonstrated that black blood could be turned red by whipping and that severed animal parts could be reactivated by blood perfusion. A bubble oxygenator was constructed by von Schroder in 1882. A film oxygenator was devised by von Frey and Gruber in 1884. In 1890, Jacoby constructed an organ perfusion device.[1,3]

In the first two decades of the 1900s two major advances facilitated the development of cardiopulmonary bypass. In 1900, Landsteiner proposed the ABO blood group system, and, in 1916 to 1918, McLean, Howell, and Hope used heparin for anticoagulation. In 1934, DeBakey developed the roller pump which is still the most commonly used pump today.[1,3]

Cardiopulmonary Bypass

The critical animal experiment was conducted in 1937. Gibbon was motivated by the catastrophic sequelae of pulmonary embolism and struggled to develop a system for removal of this fatal plug. In 1937, he successfully bypassed the hearts of dogs during pulmonary occlusion. His device was a ro-

*Reproduced with permission from the publisher and author.

tating vertical-cylinder oxygenator with multiple pulsatile pumps, valves, and pressure controls.[4] Cardiopulmonary bypass in humans seemed just around the corner, but years were to pass.

The world was immersed in World War II and cardiopulmonary bypass was of lesser importance. But even during the war in Holland, Kolff built his artificial kidney and observed that oxygenation could occur across membranes. After the war, the struggle continued with the first attempts at cardiopulmonary bypass in human beings. But it was not Gibbon or the pioneers at the University of Minnesota who first succeeded. This was a worldwide effort. The first successful application of cardiopulmonary bypass in a human being occurred in Torino, Italy, with bypass of the right heart for removal of a mediastinal tumor by Dogliotti.[5]

American efforts followed quickly. In the same year (1951) Dennis, at the University of Minnesota, attempted total cardiopulmonary bypass in a 6-year-old girl for closure of an intracardiac abnormality. He used a rotating-screen oxygenator in an attempt to close an endocardial cushion defect. Unfortunately, the surgeons were frustrated by complex anatomy, and the allowable time for bypass was only 40 min. The patient did not survive.[6]

Finally, in 1953, an intracardiac defect was successfully repaired by Gibbon, some 16 years after his first reported cardiopulmonary bypass in animals.[7] But the flush of success was all too brief and failures followed for Gibbon. An army of others came forward to carry on. In 1956, Kirklin reported the successful use of Gibbon's apparatus in a series of 40 patients from the Mayo Clinic. Within only a few years, the technique spread around the country. New clinical oxygenators appeared. In 1955, De Wall's helical bubble oxygenator kept Minnesota at the forefront of development. Clowes and Kolff developed membrane oxygenators for clinical use. The disk oxygenator of Kay and Cross was widely used because it allowed oxygenation of up to 4 liters of venous blood per minute. Not far behind was the disposable plastic bag oxygenator, the forerunner of today's disposable equipment.[1,3]

Goals of Cardiopulmonary Bypass

Galletti and Brecher wrote a classic text on cardiopulmonary bypass in 1962 and stated that the ideal goal of bypass was "delivery of the correct amount of appropriately oxygenated blood to the tissues of the whole body without attendant or ensuing adverse physiologic effects."[1] But try as we may, we cannot escape the fact that cardiopulmonary bypass is a major derangement of physiology. We cannot eliminate the derangement, rather we must try to eliminate the adverse sequelae. Virtually every aspect of cardiopulmonary bypass is a threat to homeostasis.

The Mechanics of Cardiopulmonary Bypass

Anticoagulation

Anticoagulation with heparin has been the standard technique since the beginning of cardiopulmonary bypass efforts. After heparin is administered, the activated clotting time is used to verify anticoagulation. Antithrombin III deficiency may make anticoagulation difficult, particularly after prolonged preoperative heparin infusion. A patient with antithrombin III deficiency may require the infusion of massive doses of heparin.

Reversal of heparinization is accomplished by protamine. Protamine must be infused slowly to avoid hemodynamic deterioration, which can be disastrous in marginal patients. Protamine can also cause an anaphylactic reaction, with marked histamine release and capillary leakage.[8]

The Blood Pump

A roller pump, which delivers a calibrated volume of blood regardless of afterload pressure, is used at most institutions. The occlusion of the pump is adjusted to allow a very slight backward leak to minimize hemolysis. Centrifugal pumps cause less trauma to blood elements, but pump output is dependent upon afterload.

Cannulation Technique

Arterial return to the body is accomplished through the ascending aorta, by placement of a purse string suture in the aorta and insertion of the cannula through a central stab wound. Care must be taken to avoid atherosclerotic areas in the aorta, and the systemic blood pressure is usually lowered at the time of cannulation and decannulation to decrease the possibility of aortic dissection. An effort is made to avoid clamps on the ascending aorta whenever possible. When aortic cannulation is impossible because of operative considerations, groin cannulation is accomplished via the common femoral artery, and the artery is repaired at the end of the procedure.

The venous drainage is also usually accomplished centrally. Peripheral venous drainage of the inferior vena cava via a cannula placed in the common femoral vein is associated with an increased incidence of deep venous thrombosis postoperatively. Double venous cannulation via the atrium allows more complete isolation of the heart and is more effective in maintaining cardiac hypothermia, but placement of a single venous cannula is adequate for most cardiac procedures, including most coronary bypass operations.

Oxygenators

There are three basic types of oxygenators. The film oxygenator exposes the blood to air while the blood is allowed to flow over a surface. The bubble oxygenator bubbles an oxygen and carbon dioxide mixture through the blood. Both bubble and film oxygenators necessarily have a blood-air interface, which damages blood elements and requires a defoaming chamber. The membrane oxygenator avoids this problem by separating blood from air by a membrane porous to oxygen and carbon dioxide. The membrane oxygenator causes less damage to blood elements, but it requires a large surface area and is more expensive than bubble oxygenators.[1,3]

Heat Exchange

Systemic cooling and warming is accomplished by a heat exchanger, which may be a separate unit within the extracorporeal circuit or may be built into the oxygenator. The water temperature is maintained within 10°C of blood temperature to avoid hemolysis and the formation of gas bubbles because of solubility changes.

Perfusion Technique

Hemodilution

The extracorporeal circuit is ordinarily primed with a physiologic crystalloid solution with or without an oncotically active component. The hematocrit usually decreases to approximately 18 to 20 as the patient is placed on cardiopulmonary bypass. This decrease in hematocrit ordinarily causes no impairment of systemic oxygen delivery, but it can cause regional myocardial ischemia in the presence of coronary pathology.[9] Hemodilution allows the performance of open heart surgery with minimal blood usage. At the end of the procedure, the blood from the extracorporeal circuit is returned to the patient either directly or after hemoconcentration.

Hypothermia

The systemic temperature is usually decreased during cardiopulmonary bypass to facilitate myocardial protection and allow safe conduct of the operation. Decreasing the systemic temperatures allows a lower perfusion rate because the metabolic rate is decreased. If the temperature is reduced below 20°C, total circulatory arrest may be accomplished. In infants, we have used a body temperature of 18°C with a total circulatory arrest interval of 1 h safely for large numbers of operations. In adults, for unusual operations such as reconstruction of the aortic arch, total circulatory arrest may be used at temperatures as low as 12°C.

There are potential hazards with hypothermia, because the oxygen affinity of hemoglobin increases with hypothermia and the ability of local tissues to autoregulate their own blood supply is eliminated. This may cause regional ischemia despite the reduction in metabolic rate, particularly if hypothermia is combined with hypotension.[8,9]

Flow Rate and Arterial Pressure

In general, flow rate is adjusted to maintain a cardiac index of 2.4 liters/min/m^2. Adequate renal perfusion is usually confirmed by a urine output greater than 0.5 ml/kg/h. Adequate systemic perfusion may be verified by measurement of the oxygen saturation of the venous drainage from the body. If oxygen saturation is greater than 60 to 65 percent, average systemic tissue perfusion is adequate. A fall in mixed venous oxygen saturation with an adequate cardiopulmonary bypass flow rate usually is related to increased systemic oxygen consumption because of a light anesthesia or inadequate muscle paralysis. Metabolic acidosis is, of course, another indicator that perfusion of some part of the body is inadequate.

Arterial pressure is important in the presence of cerebrovascular disease. In this circumstance, we make an attempt to maintain mean systemic arterial pressure above 9.3 kPa (70 torr) using alpha agonists (phenylephrine, methoxamine, and norepinephrine) as necessary. Continuous monitoring of the electroencephalogram is possible in unusually precarious situations.

As the systemic temperature is decreased, flow rate can be safely reduced to one-half or even one-quarter of normal flow. It must be noted, however, that the use of alpha agonists to artificially elevate blood pressure is not necessarily a benign maneuver. In dogs with a collateralized region of myocardium, the use of an alpha agonist to elevate blood pressure can be associated with subendocardial ischemia.[9]

Myocardial Protection during Ischemic Arrest

Basic Concepts of Myocardial Protection

The surgeon seeks a quiet, bloodless field to facilitate the performance of the operation. Cessation of myocardial contraction can be accomplished by metabolic poisoning, profound cooling, or simple ischemic arrest. The most widely used method of myocardial protection today is a combination of hypothermia and metabolic poisoning. Using these techniques, metabolic requirements are greatly reduced as the heart is isolated from its blood supply. Upon reperfusion, the heart's recovery is determined by attention to the details of myocardial protection. Myocardial protection involves not only infusion of a cardioplegic agent but also hemodynamic and pharmacologic preparation, profound hypothermia, and manipulation of the reperfusate.[9]

Preparation of the Heart for Ischemic Arrest

Cardiopulmonary bypass represents a major derangement of homeostasis. Cardiopulmonary bypass causes hypotension, hemodilution, and hypothermia. In addition, ventricular fibrillation or ventricular distension may increase myocardial ischemia. The surgeon should attempt to maintain perfusion pressure at 10.0 to 10.6 kPa (75 to 80 torr) as the heart is being cooled and to prevent ventricular distension. This becomes critically important in patients with aortic regurgitation. If the heart should fibrillate and distend, the aortic cross-clamp must be placed immediately, and the aortic root must be opened for infusion of a cardioplegic agent into the coronary ostia.

The heart may be pharmacologically prepared for arrest by decreasing the metabolic rate of the myocardium. Propranolol has been proved to be effective in this role, and pretreatment with propranolol leads to improved functional and metabolic recovery after arrest. Calcium channel blockers have also been shown to be effective in improving myocardial tolerance to ischemic arrest when used either alone or as adjuncts to cold cardioplegic arrest.[9]

Hypothermia

Myocardial hypothermia reduces oxygen consumption in the beating heart, in the fibrillating heart, and in the chemically arrested heart. A reduction in the temperature of the myocardium reduces the damage caused by ischemic arrest in all experimental models. The most effective way to cool the heart is by infusion of cold solutions into the coronary ostia, but the surgeon must keep in mind that this is often a heterogeneous infusion because of coronary pathology. A variation of myocardial temperatures of 10°C is not uncommon after perfusion hypothermia and, indeed, in regions distal to a critical stenosis, myocardial temperature may fall only minimally. Attempts to overcome this problem include infusion of cardioplegic solutions at pressures up to 20.0 kPA (150 torr) and at temperatures as low as 2°C. After each distal anastomosis is performed, additional cardioplegic solution may be infused into the vein graft. Vein grafts are first constructed to regions of myocardium supplied by the most critically stenosed arteries. Systemic hypothermia prior to perfusion hypothermia allows the heart to cool uniformly and affords additional protection. Local hypothermia produced by flooding the pericardium with cold lactated Ringer's solution also improves the homogeneity of cooling and prevents rewarming of the myocardium during the ischemic arrest interval.[9]

Cardioplegia

Cardioplegic solutions are metabolic poisons. They prevent the contraction of the myocyte and thereby reduce oxygen consumption. It is important that this poison be reversible. Chemical asystole can be achieved by a number of different methods. The most popular method is hyperkalemia, achieved by infusing a solution with a potassium concentration of approximately 25 meq/liter. In general, a balanced electrolyte solution or a blood-based solution is optimal because it causes less derangement of homeostasis. Intracellular solutions have been utilized, but hearts infused with intracellular solutions are much more susceptible to variations in volume of cardioplegic agent infused. There is general agreement that ischemic arrest is better tolerated if the acid milieu, which is the consequence of anaerobic metabolism, can be prevented or at least delayed by an alkaline solution. The osmotic pressure of the cardioplegic solution should be slightly hyperosmolar. Hypoosmolar solutions may increase cell swelling; hyperosmolar solutions may cause cellular dehydration. The optimal oncotic pressure of cardioplegic solutions is a subject of debate. Some studies have shown increased cellular water with crystalloid solutions. In our own laboratory, however, we have found that if the myocyte recovers, autoregulation of cellular water is quickly restored. Obviously, if there is myocardial damage, increased myocardial water content is to be expected.[9]

Oxygen Delivery

Oxygen can be delivered to the myocardium by both blood and crystalloid solutions. An oxygenated, cold crystalloid solution delivers approximately 3 to 4 ml oxygen per 100 ml solution to the myocardium. Blood solutions deliver approximately the same quantity of oxygen to the myocardium, primarily because the affinity of hemoglobin for oxygen is greatly increased at the cold temperatures used for myocardial protection. A potential advantage of blood cardioplegia, however, is a better buffering system than that available in most crystalloid solutions. In our own clinical practice, we have found the oxygenated crystalloid system to be simple, inexpensive, and very effective.[9,10]

Reperfusion

The circumstances of reperfusion can increase or decrease myocardial injury after cardioplegic or ischemic arrest. The coronary vasculature is abnormal, with absent autoregulation and some local myocardial swelling. The optimum perfusion pressure appears to be approximately 10.6 kPa (80 torr). A slightly elevated oncotic pressure (particularly if achieved by addition of mannitol) is beneficial. The calcium concentration of the reperfusate should not be elevated because myocardial contracture can be increased by temporarily increasing calcium availability. There is general agreement that the reperfusate should be alkaline, or at least not acidic, and that myocardial recovery is improved if the heart is rested for 15 to 30 min after the ischemic arrest interval. Several experimental studies have also shown that chemical asystole during reperfusion may be beneficial and that substrate enhancement to restore high-energy phosphate levels may be useful during this interval. In our clinical practice, we maintain reperfusion pressure at approximately 10.6 kPa (80 torr), use an alkaline reperfusate, and infuse mannitol into the heart-lung circuit prior to reperfusion. The heart is rested for 20 to 30 min before an attempt is made to force it to work.[9]

Complications of Cannulation for Cardiopulmonary Bypass

Arterial cannulation is a major threat to the patient during cardiopulmonary bypass. Because atherosclerotic disease may be present both in the ascending aorta and in the common femoral artery, dissection from either cannulation site is possible. Dissection of the ascending aorta, if recognized early, may be treated by local repair without replacement of the entire ascending aorta. Dissection of the ascending aorta usually originates from the site of aortic cannulation, from clamps placed on the ascending aorta, or from proximal coronary vein graft anastomoses. Dissection can be recognized by discoloration of the ascending aorta and bleeding from multiple suture sites in the area of discoloration. A sudden elevation in the pressure in the arterial perfusion line indicates extensive dissection. If dissection can be recognized while it is still a local event, it can be repaired by deep sutures beneath a partial occlusion clamp. Such treatment leads to improved operative survival, as compared to the more extensive procedure of replacing the ascending aorta.[11]

Systemic embolization from cannulation of the ascending aorta is particularly devastating if cerebral damage occurs. The aorta is carefully palpated prior to choice of a cannulation site and the placement of clamps on the ascending aorta is avoided when possible. If the ascending aorta is calcified, arterial perfusion may be carried out from the groin. Bypass of coronary arteries may be accomplished by attaching proximal anastomoses to the brachiocephalic vessels or by utilizing internal mammary artery grafts.[8]

Future Considerations

Great advances have been made in techniques of cardiopulmonary bypass over the last three decades. Systems have been standardized which allow excellent recovery for the vast majority of patients. In the unusual patient with unusual pathology, or in whom abnormal responses to cardiopulmonary bypass occur, problems still exist. Technology for monitoring, for detection, and for treatment of these unusual situations are possible, but expensive. Our expanding technology has become a monumental structure. But as we face the era of cost effectiveness in medicine, our goal must be not only to make our techniques fail-safe but also to simplify them and seek economy of effort and of material.

References

1. Galleti, P. M., and Brecher, G. A.: "Heart-Lung Bypass, Principles and Techniques of Extracorporeal Circulation," Grune & Stratton, Inc., New York, 1962.
2. LeGallois, J. J. C.: "Experience sur le Principe de la Vie," D'Hautel, Paris, 1812.
3. Nose, Y.: "Manual on Artificial Organs, The Oxygenator," the C. V. Mosby Company, St. Louis, 1973, vol 2.
4. Gibbon, J. H., Jr.: Artificial Maintenance of Circulation during Experimental Occlusion of Pulmonary Artery, *Arch. Surg.*, 34:1105, 1937.
5. Dogliotti, A. M.: Clinical Use of the Artificial Circulation with a Note on Intra-arterial Transfusion, *Bull. Johns Hopkins Hosp.* 90:131, 1952.
6. Dennis, C., Spreng, D. S., Jr., Nelson, G. E., et al.: Development of a Pump-Oxygenator to Replace the Heart and Lungs: An Apparatus Applicable to Human Patients and Application to One Case, *Ann. Surg.*, 134:709, 1951.
7. Gibbon, J. H., Jr.: Application of a Mechanical Heart and Lung Apparatus to Cardiac Surgery, *Minn. Med.* 37:171, 1954.
8. Utley, J. R.: "Pathophysiology and Techniques of Cardiopulmonary Bypass," The Williams & Wilkins Company, Baltimore, 1982, vol. 1.
9. Guyton, R. A.: Method and Magic in Myocardial Preservation, in J. W. Hurst, (ed.), "Clinical Essays of the Heart," McGraw-Hill Book Company, New York, 1983, vol. 1, p. 183.
10. Guyton, R. A., Dorsey, L. M. A., Craver, J. M., Bone, D. K., Jones, E. L., Murphy, D. A., and Hatcher, C. R., Jr.: Improved Myocardial Recovery after Cardioplegic Arrest with an Oxygenated Crystalloid Solution, *J. Thorac. Cardiovasc. Surg.*, June 1985.
11. Murphy, D. A., Craver, J. M., Jones, E. L., Bone, D. K., Guyton, R. A., and Hatcher, C. R., Jr.: Recognition and Management of Ascending Aortic Dissection Complicating Cardiac and Surgical Operations, *J. Thorac. Cardiovasc. Surg.*, 85:247, 1984.

131

Techniques of Valvular Surgery

Robert A. Guyton, M.D. Charles R. Hatcher, Jr., M.D.

Historical Perspective

The forbidden territory inside the heart was first explored in 1923 with a bold attempt at mitral valvotomy by Cutler and Levine.[1] After an initial success, failure followed and the field of endeavor remained quiescent until after World War II. Harken and Bailey in the late 1940s proved digital mitral commissurotomy to be safe and effective.[2,3] The development of the Tubbs dilator in the 1950s led to a more reliable technique of closed mitral commissurotomy.[4]

Replacement of valves with prostheses awaited the development of cardiopulmonary bypass in the mid-1950s. As early as 1953, however, Hufnagel and Harvey placed a ball valve in the descending aorta, which allowed some improvement in patients with aortic regurgitation.[5] Open debridement of the aortic valve and partial replacement of leaflets were performed in the late 1950s. Prosthetic replacement of the aortic valve was accomplished by Harken in 1960 and in 1961 by Lillihei and by Muller.[6–8] The mitral valve was first replaced with the ball valve of Starr and Edwards in 1961. Prosthetic replacement of the tricuspid valve was accomplished in 1963 by Starr and colleagues.[9]

The Aortic Valve

Preoperative Evaluation

As the surgeon approaches the patient with aortic valve disease, careful review of preoperative data allows him or her to be technically and emotionally prepared for the task at hand. In the examination of the patient, one must pay particular attention to peripheral and cerebral vascular disease, examining the femoral vessels for potential cardiopulmonary bypass access or intraaortic balloon pump insertion and examining the carotid vessels for cerebrovascular disease, the signs and symptoms of which may be masked by aortic valve disease. Examination of the chest x-ray allows one to assess cardiac chamber enlargement and enlargement of the ascending aorta. A cineangiogram reveals further information about the size of the ascending aorta and possible calcification. One can also determine proximity of the ascending aorta to the posterior table of the sternum and possible fixation of the aorta to the sternum, a deadly trap when the sternum is cut. Coronary angiography (performed in our institution in women over the age of 50, in men over the age of 40, and in all patients with angina) discloses possible concomitant coronary disease. Even in the absence of coronary disease, it is important for the surgeon to be aware of the coronary anatomy for the purposes of cardioplegic protection. The length of the left main coronary artery should be known to avoid selective infusion of cardioplegic solution either into the left anterior descending or the circumflex artery. The distribution of the right coronary artery should be known to determine the need for separate infusion of cardioplegic solution into the right coronary ostium. A complete catheterization of the right side of the heart should be performed to evaluate the possibility of pulmonary vascular disease and right ventricular dysfunction. In some instances, retrograde catheter passage across the aortic valve is impossible. In this instance, it is prudent to assess the mitral valve echocardiographically to prevent the appearance of silent mitral stenosis as an intraoperative surprise. The mitral valve can, of course, be evaluated by transseptal catheterization, but this is not usually necessary.

If there is a clinical suspicion of subaortic stenosis, the subaortic region should be examined both angiographically and echocardiographically prior to operative intervention. Echocardiography can also be useful in determining the size of the ascending aorta when the need for root replacement is considered.

The Operative Technique

A standard median sternotomy allows superior exposure of the ascending aorta and aortic valve. Enlargement of the ascending aorta secondary to intrinsic disease of the aorta, aortic stenosis, or aortic regurgitation often places the ascending aorta very close to the posterior table of the sternum and, indeed, erosion of the posterior table can occur. When preoperative evaluation has suggested such an occurrence, the sternum is carefully sawed with an oscillating saw after the femoral artery is exposed for possible groin cannulation. After the pericardium has been opened, the aorta is carefully examined and palpated. The enlarged aorta is often thin in the area midway between the aortic valve and the brachiocephalic artery. The aorta is usually thicker and of normal diameter near the brachiocephalic artery. Cannulation is therefore best accomplished just proximal to the brachiocephalic artery or just to the leftward side of the artery in an area in which the aorta is felt to be of good quality. Venous cannulation is usually accomplished via the right atrium, using an inferior vena caval and a superior vena caval cannula. Some surgeons prefer a single venous cannula with an atrial and an inferior vena caval opening, but we prefer double cannulation, which would allow isolation of the heart if a more extensive procedure should become necessary.

As the patient is placed on cardiopulmonary bypass, a purse string suture is placed in the right superior pulmonary vein for placement of a ventricular vent. Systemic cooling is accomplished. Intravenous propranolol is administered, both as an adjunct to myocardial protection and to prevent ventricular fibrillation as the patient is cooled. In patients with aortic regurgitation, it is particularly important that the heart remain beating during cooling because the aorta must usually be clamped to prevent sudden ventricular distension when the heart fibrillates. The heart is much better protected if it has been cooled to 25 or 23° C prior to aortic cross-clamping, particularly since, with aortic regurgitation, it is usually several minutes after the clamp is placed before protective solutions can be infused down each coronary artery and cold cardioplegic arrest can be accomplished. While the patient is cooled, dissection of the aortic root may be accomplished, but it is important not to manipulate the ventricle and thereby trigger ventricular fibrillation. The left ventricular vent is not introduced until the left atrial pressure begins to rise, since air can be introduced into the heart by attempted placement of the vent when atrial pressure is low. The vent is not directed into the left ventricle until fibrillation has occurred. If aortic regurgitation is minimal, systemic cooling can continue after ventricular fibrillation has occurred, but if the heart cannot be decompressed because of aortic regurgitation, the aortic clamp must be placed at once.

Myocardial protection is accomplished by systemic cooling, local irrigation with cold solution, and intracoronary infusion of cold cardioplegic solutions. If aortic regurgitation is minimal, cardioplegic solution can be infused into the aortic root after placement of the aortic clamp. Because the left ventricle is vented, care must be taken to avoid air being sucked into the ascending aorta below the cross clamp prior to infusion of cardioplegic solution. This is usually achieved by temporarily turning the vent off as the ascending aorta is filled with cardioplegic solution. If a patient has moderate or severe aortic regurgitation, the ascending aorta is opened and a soft, sponge-tipped Silastic catheter is inserted into each coronary orifice for infusion of cardioplegic solution. The volume of infusion is based upon the surgeon's knowledge of the coronary anatomy in each particular patient; into each coronary artery a volume proportional to the amount of muscle supplied by that vessel is infused. Ordinarily, we infuse approximately 700 ml into the left main coronary artery and 300 to 400 ml into the right coronary artery. The pericardium is continuously irrigated with 2°C lactated Ringer's solution during the cross-clamping interval.

An oblique aortotomy, beginning about 2 cm cephalad to the commissure between the right and left coronary cusps and spiraling down into the sinus of the noncoronary cusp, is standard. Excision of the valve is extremely important. The most convenient location to begin the excision is at the commissure between the right and noncoronary cusps. If this region is heavily calcified, however, a different beginning site should be chosen lest the surgeon cut too deeply and find the bundle of His in the top of the septum. Calcification in the right coronary cusp can usually be peeled away from the annulus, with scissor tips used to elevate the calcium as the valve is excised. This is similarly true for the leftward half of the left coronary cusp. The calcium in the noncoronary cusp and the rightward half of the left coronary cusp is often continuous with calcium in the anterior leaflet of the mitral valve, and it may be necessary to cut across calcified deposits in this region. Care must be taken to carefully debride loose calcium deposits to prevent subsequent systemic emboli. At this stage in the procedure, the ventricle and the annulus are rinsed clean with cold lactated Ringer's solution, with the left coronary ostium protected from debris with a sucker tip or a cardioplegia infusion cannula.

Sutures are next placed around the aortic annulus. Sutures may be placed in a simple, horizontal mattress fashion or a figure-of-eight fashion and then passed through the valve. The use of horizontal mattress sutures reinforced with Teflon pledgets (placed on the ventricular side of the annulus) has virtually eliminated perivalvar leaks in our institution. Particular care is taken to avoid placing sutures into muscle underneath the right coronary cusp, as complete heart block may result with a deep suture in this location. If, as the valve is excised, a transmural tear occurs through the wall of the aorta or through the annulus, this tear may be repaired with the sutures used to replace the valve. After the valve is lowered and tied in place, both coronary ostia are again inspected or infused with cardioplegic solution to be certain that they are free of obstruction. The aortic root is irrigated with saline solution while the ventricular cavity is aspirated with the ventricular vent. If a significant perivalvar leak is present, the saline solution is quickly sucked into the ventricle.

The aortotomy may be closed with either a two-layer or a single-layer closure with a running monofilament suture. Occasionally, the suture line must be reinforced with a strip of Teflon felt along either side. Ventricular venting is stopped, and the ascending aorta is allowed to fill with blood as the suture line is completed. A vent hole for air evacuation is placed in the most superior aspect of the aorta. Unfortunately, the most superior aspect of the aorta is usually the thinnest part of the aorta. The cross clamp is removed. Air is evacuated by rolling the patient from side to side while the ventricle is ejecting and the heart is vigorously massaged. The large vent hole in the ascending aorta may be left open until the patient is off cardiopulmonary bypass, but if the aorta is unusually thin, it may be prudent to repair the vent hole while the patient is still on cardiopulmonary bypass and the pressure of the ascending aorta may be decreased while sutures are tied.

After the patient has been weaned from cardiopulmonary bypass, the patient often requires an elevated end-diastolic pressure because of the thick, noncompliant left ventricle. Ventricular function is usually excellent. Transient supraventricular arrhythmias are common in the early postoperative period. All patients are treated with digoxin for this reason.

Operative Management of the Small Aortic Annulus

Preoperative evaluation should alert the surgeon that the aortic annulus may be too small for placement of an adequate prosthesis. In an average man, a no. 23 bioprosthesis or a no. 21 tilting disk prosthesis is the smallest prosthesis which can be inserted without a significant postoperative gradient. The problem of a small aortic annulus is even more common in children, as one wishes to place the largest possible prosthesis to allow for growth. There are three major techniques for insertion of a prosthesis larger than the annulus of the original valve. First, one may simply tilt the prosthetic valve so that one can place a larger prosthesis in the root without enlargement of the annulus. Usually, the valve is sewn to the original annulus beneath the left and right coronary ostia, and it is placed several millimeters above the annulus in the noncoronary cusp.[10,11] The second technique involves extension of the aortotomy down to or into the annulus in the region of the noncoronary cusp and enlargement of the aorta with a patch of pericardium or cloth. This incision can be extended down into the anterior leaflet of the mitral valve if the annulus is unusually small. The valve is then sewn to the annulus underneath the right and left coronary ostia and to the aorta and the new patch above the noncoronary cusp. This technique allows placement of a valve two to three sizes larger than that originally measured.[12,13] Finally, in a few situations, it is necessary to perform an extensive operation to enlarge a small aortic annulus. The Konno or Rastan operation involves incision of the aorta between the left and right coronary ostia, cutting into the ventricular septum and into the right ventricle. The newly created ventricular septal defect is repaired with a cloth patch, and the annulus can be enlarged by three to four valve sizes as the left coronary ostium is moved away from the right coronary ostium. This technique requires a vertical aortic incision and therefore should be planned prior to aortotomy.[14,15] Most techniques of aortic annular enlargement require a more lengthy period of cardiac arrest than does simple aortic valve replacement. This does not usually present a problem when pathological conditions of the coronary arteries are not present. When pathological conditions are present, however, cardioplegic myocardial protection is difficult and a compromise must often be reached between placement of a large prosthesis and the need for a relatively short cardioplegic arrest interval.

The Mitral Valve

Mitral Commissurotomy

Closed mitral commissurotomy was the first effective intervention in valvular heart disease. With the refinement of cardiopulmonary bypass and myocardial protection techniques, closed mitral commissurotomy is now an unusual operation in the United States. In other countries, however, it remains a lifesaving operation for large numbers of carefully selected patients. The ideal patient for closed mitral commissurotomy is a young woman with no calcium in a stenotic mitral valve with no preoperative mitral regurgitation. Closed mitral commissurotomy is usually performed through the left chest; the surgeon places a finger in the left atrium through a purse string suture and a dilator through the apex of the ventricle. The dilator is guided with the finger into the center of the valve and expanded, enlarging the orifice to a predetermined size.

Open mitral valvuloplasty allows more precise reconstruction of the mitral valve than does the closed technique. With the use of cardiopulmonary bypass and cardioplegic myocardial protection, the mitral valve is exposed and the commissures examined and carefully incised. Fused chordae, as well as papillary muscles, can be split. Results of open mitral valvuloplasty for mitral stenosis have been excellent. Open mitral valvuloplasty is the procedure of choice for any patient in whom the valve is not heavily calcified and in whom subvalvar chordal infusion is not extensive.

The treatment of mitral regurgitation by open valvuloplasty has become increasingly successful as techniques have been refined. Notable advances have been made by Kay and Carpentier. Chordae may be shortened, flail segments of the posterior leaflet may be excluded, and the mitral annulus may be shortened by use of a Carpentier ring or a DeVega type of purse string suture around the mitral annulus. Reattachment of an entire ruptured papillary muscle is, in general, not successful, especially in the acute situation.[16–18]

Mitral Valve Replacement

Replacement of the mitral valve is best performed through a median sternotomy, although replacement can be accomplished through the right chest or left chest in unusual circumstances. Dissection of the superior vena cava up to the level of the azygos vein and dissection of the inferior vena cava toward the hepatic veins allow greater mobility of the right side of the heart and facilitate exposure of the left atrium.[19] Dual atrial cannulation is necessary for isolation of the heart and to allow retraction of the right side of the heart without compromising venous return. Cardiopulmonary bypass is utilized to cool the patient systemically to approximately 25°C. The aorta is cross-clamped, and cardioplegic solution is infused to protect the myocardium and to facilitate exposure of the valve. If an atrial thrombus is present, it is carefully dissected away from the atrium; a plane of dissection is established just beneath the endocardium in order to leave as smooth a surface as possible in the atrium. The valve is pulled upward into the wound and is excised, leaving a 3-mm rim of valve tissue attached to the annulus. Heavy calcification is often encountered in the commissures. This calcification is usually removable. The chordae are excised through the tips of the papillary muscles, but deep excision of the papillary muscles is avoided as is extensive excision of the chordae of the posterior leaflet which lend some support to the ventricular free wall. Sutures are placed around the annulus, usually reinforced with Teflon felt pledgets placed on either the atrial or ventricular side of the annulus. The sutures are passed through the sewing ring of the valve and the valve is lowered in place and tied. There are several potential dangers in valve excision and suture placement. If one numbers the mitral annulus like the face of a clock, as the surgeon sees it, with 12 o'clock being directly toward the sternum, then a deep suture in the region between 12 o'clock and 3 o'clock could damage the bundle of His and cause complete heart block. Deep excision or suturing along the posterior leaflet from 4 o'clock to 8 o'clock could lead to dissection of the atrioventricular (AV) groove with lethal hemorrhage. An especially deep suture in the region from 5 o'clock to 8 o'clock could penetrate or encircle the circumflex coronary artery, which is only a few millimeters away in the AV groove. A deep suture between 9 o'clock and 12 o'clock could tear the noncoronary cusp of the aortic valve and cause postoperative aortic regurgitation.[20–22]

After the valve is tied into position, the aortic cross clamp is removed while air is vented from the ascending aorta. The right coronary artery is occluded with the surgeon's finger as the cross clamp is removed to prevent air embolism into the right coronary artery. The mitral valve is kept incompetent. In the case of a porcine valve a large chest tube or vent is placed across the valve into the ventricle, and in the case of a mechanical valve a small Foley catheter prevents seating of the disk or ball. The left atriotomy is then closed as the heart begins to recover. Air is carefully evacuated from the left atrium and left ventricle as the vent or Foley catheter is removed and the ventricle begins to eject. The patient is rewarmed and weaned from cardiopulmonary bypass.

Postoperative Care

In patients with pulmonary hypertension consequent to mitral valve disease, special difficulties may arise in the postoperative period. Pulmonary end-diastolic pressure may not accurately reflect left atrial pressure; use of a left atrial catheter is often advisable in these situations. Right ventricular dysfunction can be a major problem, especially if air has been introduced into the right coronary artery during infusion of cardioplegic solution or as the aortic cross clamp was removed. Pulmonary vasodilation is often necessary using either nitroglycerin or sodium nitroprusside. Some patients have an increase in pulmonary vascular resistance as they are subsequently weaned from mechanical ventilation, and long-term use of vasodilators (such as nitroglycerin paste or long-acting nitrates) is helpful.

The Tricuspid Valve

Organic versus Functional Disease

The most common cause of tricuspid regurgitation is dilatation of the tricuspid annulus secondary to pulmonary hypertension and right ventricular dysfunction in the presence of disease of the left-sided valves. This "functional" tricuspid regurgitation is exacerbated by loss of the atrial contribution to the cardiac work cycle. Rheumatic disease of the tricuspid valve is very rare in the absence of disease of the mitral valve, and usually some element of tricuspid stenosis exists in addition to tricuspid regurgitation. Endocarditis of the tricuspid valve is becoming an increasing problem as intravenous drug abuse becomes more prevalent.

Tricuspid Repair

Repair of valve dysfunction on the left side of the heart often leads to a marked improvement in functional tricuspid regurgitation. If a patient has chronic symptoms of tricuspid regurgitation (ascites, hepatomegaly, chronic edema), however, then repair or replacement of the tricuspid valve is usually beneficial. Tricuspid regurgitation can be assessed digitally at the time of operation by insertion of a finger into the right atrium as the patient is being prepared for cardiopulmonary bypass. The surgeon should be aware at this time of the patient's fluid status and pulmonary artery pressure. If the patient is excessively dry with low pulmonary pressures, then the amount of tricuspid regurgitation palpated at the beginning of the operation may underestimate the problem.

The tricuspid valve is exposed via a right atriotomy. The functionally regurgitant tricuspid valve looks quite normal with thin, delicate leaflets. The septal leaflet ordinarily has not been elongated and the annulus is stretched only along the anterior and posterior leaflets. Both the DeVega annuloplasty and the Carpentier prosthesis are designed to shorten this portion of the annulus.[23,24] The DeVega annuloplasty is performed by insertion of a continuous monofilament suture from the cephalad end of the septum, in-and-out through the tissue of the anterior and posterior portions of the annulus, to the caudal end of the septum. A no. 33 or no. 31 valve sizer is then inserted into the annulus and the suture is tied snugly to shorten the annulus. Palpation of the valve after the operation allows an evaluation of the success of the procedure, again with the patient's fluid status and pulmonary artery pressure taken into account. If the patient derives sustained relief from repair of valve dysfunction on the left side of the heart, then further problems with the tricuspid valve are unusual.

Tricuspid Replacement

The need for tricuspid valve replacement is unusual but certainly can occur in the case of bacterial endocarditis, organic tricuspid regurgitation, or severe functional tricuspid regurgitation. Mechanical prostheses have not functioned well in this position and the porcine or pericardial bioprosthesis is used. The valve is sutured to the septal leaflet of the tricuspid valve, with care being taken not to place sutures into the myocardium of the ventricular septum because of proximity of AV conduction tissue. Attempts to insert a large mitral prosthesis and a large tricuspid prosthesis can also compress the AV conduction system between the valves and cause complete heart block.

Results of Valve Surgery

Aortic Valve Replacement

Replacement of the aortic valve as an isolated procedure currently has approximately a 2 to 5 percent operative mortality and a 80 to 85 percent 5-year survival.[25–27] Major determinants of the results of aortic valve replacement include the age of the patient, the presence of coexisting coronary artery disease, and the functional state of the left ventricle. Deterioration of left ventricular function is manifested by a decrease in ejection fraction and left ventricular enlargement. Minimal deterioration of ventricular function may be reversed after valve replacement for either aortic stenosis or aortic regurgitation, but more severe deterioration of left ventricular function is not reversible and compromises long-term survival.

Mitral Valve Replacement

Operative survival for isolated mitral valve replacement ranges between 3 and 10 percent and 5-year survival is about 70 to 85 percent.[26–28] Once again, the major determinants of operative survival are the age of the patient, coexistence of coronary disease, and the status of ventricular function. In addition, the presence or absence of pulmonary hypertension importantly influences operative survival, long-term survival, and relief of symptoms postoperatively.

Multiple Valve Replacement[29]

Combined replacement of the aortic and mitral valves has an operative mortality only slightly higher than replacement of the mitral valve alone, ranging from 5 to 15 percent. Five-year survival, however, is considerably reduced, at approximately 50 to 60 percent. Concomitant disease of the tricuspid valve or stenoses of the coronary arteries further increase operative mortality.

Choice of the Prosthetic Valve

Each type of prosthetic valve has deficiencies and advantages. The individual patient must be carefully assessed and the prosthetic valve chosen for that individual. The porcine or pericardial bioprosthesis has a low thromboembolism rate in both the aortic and mitral position (about 1 per 100 patient-years) but the long-term durability of the valve remains a question; one should plan for valve survival averaging about 7 years in young adults (less than 35 years old) and 10 years in older patients, although some reports are more encouraging. In children, deterioration of the porcine valve appears to be even further accelerated. Anticoagulation is not necessary in patients in normal sinus rhythm.[27,30–32]

The Bjork-Shiley tilting disk prosthesis has excellent long-term durability but has a higher rate of thromboembolism (about 5 per 100 patient-years) and a significant rate of thrombosis in the mitral position. In the aortic position, the thrombosis and thromboembolism rate is acceptable (about 1 per 100 patient-years) with proper anticoagulation.[27,31,33]

The Starr-Edwards ball valve prosthesis offers excellent long-term durability and a moderately low rate of valve thrombosis or thromboembolism (aortic, 4 or 5 per 100 patient-years; mitral, 1 to 8 per 100 patient-years). But in the mitral position, it requires a large ventricle, and in the aortic position, a significant transvalvar gradient can exist compared with the Bjork-Shiley valve or bioprostheses of similar size.[27,31]

New tilting disk prostheses such as the St. Jude valve or Hall Medtronic valve offer possibilities for superior hemodynamic performance combined with a low incidence of thromboembolism and thrombosis. Long-term evaluation will be necessary to properly determine the role of these prostheses.[27,31,34,35]

In the final analysis, the choice of the valve prosthesis should be a joint decision of the patient, the surgeon, and the patient's permanent physician. Difficulty with anticoagulation is a strong argument against a mechanical prosthesis. Patients under the age of 35, in general, should receive a mechanical prosthesis because of rapid deterioration of bioprostheses. But there are occasional young women who are so anxious to bear children that a bioprosthesis is appropriate, with recognition that the valve will need to be replaced within 10 years. When considering placement of a bioprosthesis in a young person, one must evaluate the risk of reoperation. The risk is generally low when the operation is carried out under elective circumstances, but becomes as high as 50 percent when the reoperation is an emergency.[36,37] Porcine valves deteriorate slowly, and if the patient and the patient's permanent physician are cautious, reoperation can usually be carried out in an elective situation. Mechanical valve dysfunction is more frequently catastrophic and emergency valve reoperation is necessary.

Summary

An understanding of the technical aspects of valve surgery is important for the cardiologist in helping the surgeon achieve a preoperative knowledge of all important pathological conditions. Operative techniques will vary from surgeon to surgeon as each surgeon seeks those methods best suited to his own strengths and weaknesses. The timing of operative intervention in valve disease will always be a topic of debate—superior operative results are obtainable with early intervention, but the valve prostheses themselves carry significant yearly morbidity and mortality. As valve prostheses are improved and reoperative mortality is diminished, earlier intervention in the course of cardiac valve disease becomes increasingly appropriate.

References

1. Cutler, E. C., and Levine, S. A.: Cardiotomy and Valvulotomy for Mitral Stenosis, *Boston Med. Surg. J.*, 188:1023, 1923.
2. Harken, D. E., Ellis, L. B., Ware, P. F., and Norman, L. R.: The Surgical Treatment of Mitral Stenosis, *N. Engl. J. Med.*, 239:801, 1948.
3. Bailey, C. P.: The Surgical Treatment of Mitral Stenosis (Mitral Commissurotomy), *Dis. Chest,* 15:377, 1949.
4. Logan, A., and Turner, R.: Surgical Treatment of Mitral Stenosis with Particular Reference to the Transventricular Approach with a Mechanical Dilator, *Lancet,* 2:874, 1959.
5. Hufnagel, C. A., and Harvey, W. P.: The Surgical Correction of Aortic Regurgitation: Preliminary Report, *Bull. Georgetown U. Med. Ctr.*, 6:60, 1953.
6. Harken, D. E., Sorof, H. S., Taylor, W. J., Lefemine, A. A., Gupta, S. K., and Lunzer, S.: Partial and Complete Prostheses in Aortic Insufficiency, *J. Thorac. Cardiovasc. Surg.*, 40:744, 1960.
7. Lillihei, C. W., Barnard, C. N., Long, D. M.: Aortic Valve Reconstruction and Replacement by Total Valve Prosthesis, in K. A. Merendino (ed.), "Prosthetic Heart Valves for Cardiac Surgery," Charles C Thomas, Springfield, Ill., 1961, p. 527.
8. Muller, W. H., Jr., Littlefield, J. B., and Dammann, J. F.: Subcoronary Prosthetic Replacement of the Aortic Valve, in K. A. Merendino (ed.), "Prosthetic Heart Valves for Cardiac Surgery," Charles C Thomas, Springfield, Ill., 1961, p. 493.
9. Starr, A., McCord, G. W., and Wood, J.: Surgery for Multiple Valve Disease, *Ann. Surg.*, 160:596, 1964.
10. David, T. E., and Uden, D. E.: Aortic Valve Replacement in Adult Patients with Small Aortic Annuli, *Ann. Thorac. Surg.*, 36:577, 1983.
11. Olin, C. L., Bomfim, V., Halvazulis, V., Holmgren, A. G., and Lamke, B. J.: Optimal Insertion Technique for the Bjork-Shiley Valve in the Narrow Aortic Ostium, *Ann. Thorac. Surg.*, 36:567, 1983.
12. Manoguian, S., and Seybold-Epting, W.: Patch Enlargement of the Aortic Valve Ring by Extending the Aortic Incision into the Anterior Mitral Leaflet: New Operative Technique, *J. Thorac. Cardiovasc. Surg.*, 78:402, 1979.
13. Piehler, J. M., Orszulak, T. A., Schaff, H. V., and Shub, C.: Enlargement of the Aortic Root or Annulus with Autogenous Pericardial Patch during Aortic Valve Replacement: Long-Term Follow-up, *J. Thorac. Cardiovasc. Surg.*, 86:350, 1983.
14. Rastan, H., and Koncz, J.: Aortoventriculoplasty: A New Technique for the Treatment of Left Ventricular Outflow Tract Obstruction, *J. Thorac. Cardiovasc. Surg.*, 71:920, 1976.
15. Misbach, G. A., Turley, K., Ullyot, D. J., and Ebert, P. A.: Left Ventricular Outflow Enlargement by the Konno Procedure, *J. Thorac. Cardiovasc. Surg.*, 84:696, 1982.
16. Laschinger, J. C., Cunningham, J. N., Jr., Baumann, F. G., Isom, O. W., Catinella, F. P., Mendelsohn, A., Adams, P. X., and Spencer, F. C.: Early Open Radical Commissurotomy: Surgical Treatment of Choice for Mitral Stenosis, *Ann. Thorac. Surg.*, 34:287, 1982.
17. Bonchek, L. I.: Current Status of Mitral Commissurotomy: Indications, Techniques and Results, *Am. J. Cardiol.*, 52:411, 1983.
18. Carpentier, A.: Cardiac Valve Surgery—the "French Correction," *J. Thorac. Cardiovasc. Surg.*, 86:323, 1983.
19. Pifarre, R., Balderman, S., Sullivan, H. J., Montoya, A., and Bakhos, M.: Technique to Facilitate Mitral Valve Exposure, *Ann. Thorac. Surg.*, 33:92, 1982.
20. Cobbs, B. W., Hatcher, C. R., Jr., Craver, J. M., Jones, E. L., and Sewell, C. W.: Transverse Midventricular Disruption after Mitral Valve Replacement, *Am. Heart J.*, 99:33, 1980.
21. Gosalbez, F., de Linera, F. A., Cofiño, J. L., Naya, J. L., Rodriguez, J., and Ortuña, A.: Isolated Mitral Valve Replacement and Ventricular Rupture: Presentation of 6 Patients, *Ann. Thorac. Surg.*, 31:105, 1981.
22. Virmani, R., Chun, P. K. C., Parker, J., and McAllister, H. A.: Suture Obliteration of the Circumflex Coronary Artery in Three Patients Undergoing Mitral Valve Operation, *J. Thorac. Cardiovasc. Surg.*, 84:774, 1982.
23. Burr, L. H., Krayenbuhl, C., and Sutton, M.: The Mitral Plication Suture: A New Technique of Mitral Valve Repair, *J. Thorac. Cardiovasc. Surg.*, 73:589, 1977.
24. Carpentier, A., Deloche, A., and Hanania, G.: Surgical Management of Acquired Tricuspid Valve Disease, *J. Thorac. Cardiovasc. Surg.*, 67:53, 1974.
25. Crosby, I. K., and Muller, W. H., Jr.: Acquired Disease of the Aortic Valve, in D. C. Sabiston, Jr., and F. C. Spencer (eds.) "Gibbon's Surgery of the Chest" 4th ed., W. B. Saunders Company, Philadelphia, 1983, p. 1280.
26. Craver, J. M., Jones, E. L., McKeown, P., Bone, D. K., Hatcher, C. R., Jr., and Kandrach, M.: Porcine Cardiac Xenograft Valves: Analysis of Survival, Valve Failure, and Explantation, *Ann. Thorac. Surg.*, 34:16, 1982.
27. Bonchek, L. I.: Current Status of Cardiac Valve Replacement: Selection of a Prosthesis and Indications for Operation, *Am. Heart J.*, 101:96, 1981.
28. Spencer, F. C.: Acquired Disease of the Mitral Valve, in D. C. Sabiston, Jr., and F. C. Spencer (eds.) "Gibbon's Surgery of the Chest" 4th ed., W. B. Saunders Company, Philadelphia, 1983, p. 1225.
29. West, P. N., Ferguson, T. B., and Clark, R. E.: Multiple Valve Replacement: Changing Status, *Ann. Thorac. Surg.*, 26:32, 1978.

30. Dunn, J. M.: Porcine Valve Durability in Children, *Ann. Thorac. Surg.*, 32:357, 1981.
31. Edmunds, L. H., Jr.: Thromboembolic Complications of Current Cardiac Valvular Prostheses, *Ann. Thorac. Surg.* 34:96, 1982.
32. Angell, W. W., Angell, J. D. and Kosek, J. C.: Twelve-Year Experience with Glutaraldehyde-Preserved Porcine Xenografts, *J. Thorac. Cardiovasc. Surg.* 83:493, 1982.
33. Murphy, D. A., Levine, F. H., Buckley, M. J. Swinski, L., Daggett, W. M., Atkins, C. W., and Austen, W. G.: Mechanical Valves: A Comparative Analysis of the Starr-Edwards and Bjork-Shiley Prostheses, *J. Thorac. Cardiovasc. Surg.* 86:746, 1983.
34. Cohn, L. H.: The Long-Term Results of Aortic Valve Replacement, *Chest*, 85:387, 1984.
35. Nitter-Hauge, S., Semb, B., Abdelnoor, M., and Hall, K. V.: A 5 Year Experience with the Medtronic-Hall Disc Valve Prosthesis, *Circulation*, 68(suppl. 2) 169, 1983.
36. Huseby, D. G., Pluth, J. R., Piehler, J. M., Schaff, H. V., Orszulak, T. A., Puga, F. J., and Danielson, G. K.: Reoperation on Prosthetic Heart Valves: An Analysis of Risk Factors in 552 Patients, *J. Thorac. Cardiovasc. Surg.*, 86:543, 1983.
37. Wideman, F. E., Blackstone, E. H., Kirklin, J. W., Karp, R. B., Kouchoukos, N. T., and Pacifico, A. D.: Hospital Mortality of Re-replacement of the Aortic Valve: Incremental Risk Factors, *J. Thorac. Cardiovasc. Surg.*, 82:692, 1981.

132

Techniques for the Surgical Treatment of Atherosclerotic Coronary Artery Disease and Its Complications

Ellis L. Jones, M.D.   Charles R. Hatcher, Jr., M.D.

The purpose of this chapter, which has been written for physicians who are not cardiac surgeons, is to define the technical factors important in the performance of coronary bypass surgery and to discuss the surgical treatment of ventricular rupture, septal rupture, papillary muscle rupture, and ventricular aneurysm.

Performance of Coronary Bypass Surgery

Techniques of Cardiopulmonary Bypass

So that the surgeon may operate on a quiet heart, the pumping function of the ventricles is assumed by an external mechanical pump. Hypothermia is utilized to arrest the heart in diastole and reduce myocardial oxygen needs and thus avoid ischemic damage. Venous flow is returned to the pump with separate caval cannulas to avoid premature warming of the right side of the ventricular septum, which occurs with a single atrial cannula. Reduced cardiac temperatures can be more adequately maintained with cannulas placed in the superior and inferior venae cavae, thereby improving the efficacy of the hypothermic technique. Systemic cooling to a nasopharyngeal temperature of 28°C is accomplished in order to reduce myocardial oxygen requirements. As the beating heart cools, stroke volume initially increases but then rapidly decreases, so that left ventricular distension and elevation of pulmonary artery pressure may occur in some patients. To avoid ventricular distension, the left ventricle may be vented through the right superior pulmonary vein. A significant disadvantage of left ventricular venting is the introduction of air into the cardiac chambers. In spite of every effort to remove air bubbles at the conclusion of the operation, instances of neurologic injury continue to occur. Accordingly, there has been a trend away from the venting technique in recent years. Alternatively, pulmonary artery pressure can be monitored carefully, and if there is no concomitant aortic regurgitation, venting may not be necessary.

Choice of Graft for Coronary Bypass Operation

Autogenous veins and arteries have been used to connect the aorta with distal portions of narrowed or occluded coronary arteries.[1] The reversed saphenous vein graft from the calf has been the choice for most vascular arterial conduits in recent years (Fig. 132-1). This vein, taken from ankle to knee, is usually superior to a vein in the thigh because of its closer approximation in size to that of the coronary arteries. Where there has been prior stripping and ligation, the lesser saphenous vein has usually been found intact and offers a satisfactory alternative. If the lesser saphenous system is inadequate or nonexistent, the cephalic vein from the arm may be used.

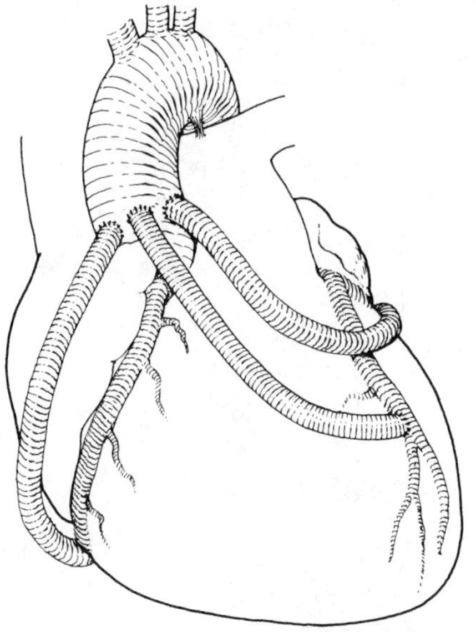

FIGURE 132-1 Reversed autogenous saphenous vein aortocoronary bypass grafts to left anterior descending, marginal circumflex, and right coronary arteries.

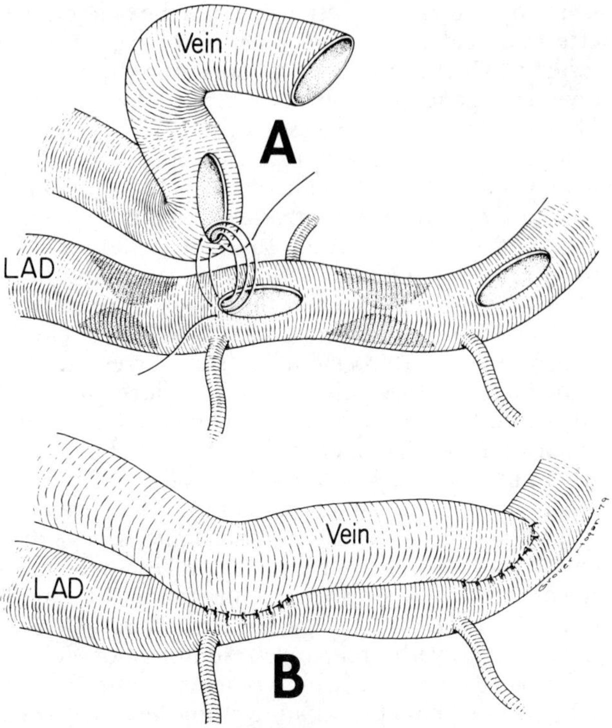

FIGURE 132-2 Sequential grafting for multiple lesions of the anterior descending coronary artery. (*From E. L. Jones, Coronary Artery Bypass Grafting: Simplification and Refinement of Surgical Technique, Ann. Thorac. Surg., 30:84, 1980. Reproduced with permission from the publisher and author.*)

Extremes in diameter of the veins used for bypass grafting can present some problems. Varicose segments are excluded whenever possible. Diameters of at least 2.0 mm are necessary to ensure adequate flow through the bypass graft.

Sequential grafting is often performed for multiple lesions of a single artery and diagonal branches of the anterior descending coronary artery (Fig. 132-2). Rarely are there more than two distal anastomoses for any single vein segment. The possibility of proximal graft failure and kinking or angulating of the graft on its way to the aorta generally limits multiple anastomoses using a single vein segment.

The internal mammary artery offers an excellent alternative to the saphenous vein as an arterial conduit, particularly for grafting to the left anterior descending coronary artery. The internal mammary artery provides an artery-to-artery graft which results in excellent long-term patency rates which have approximated 95 percent after many years.[1,2] Disadvantages and limitations in the use of the internal mammary graft are that it must have adequate size and flow, and it requires a finite period of time for the retrosternal dissection in its preparation. The latter may limit the use of the internal mammary artery in patients with unstable angina pectoris where operating time is a critical factor. In addition, the mammary artery is frequently very small in female patients.

In recent years, an autogenous radial artery has been used as a free graft between the aorta and coronary artery. Poor results have been universally experienced, however, primarily because of proximal stenosis and high early occlusion rates, so that the technique has been largely abandoned.[3]

In the preparation of the venous segment to be employed, autologous heparinized blood or buffered electrolyte solution (Normosol) is injected into the vein at moderate pressure while the venous branches are ligated. It is important to minimize the trauma of distension during the injection and removal of the venous segment from the leg to reduce the incidence of late stenosis of the grafts.

Technique of Myocardial Preservation

Once coronary flow has been interrupted by cross-clamping the aorta, a hyperosmolar potassium solution* at 4°C is injected into the ascending aorta to arrest the heart. Asanguineous cardioplegia has been preferred because of its greater simplicity and because it affords the ability to operate at lower myocardial temperatures without increased viscosity and provides a coronary vascular bed free of formed elements. Myocardial temperature is usually lowered to between 15 and 20°C, where metabolic activity is usually reduced well below half that at normothermia. In addition to the protection afforded by reduced myocardial temperature, electromechanical dissociation induced by the high potassium content may aid in the preservation of myocardial glycogen and high-energy phosphate stores. The al-

*Contents of the solution (concentrations in milliequivalents per liter): K = 28, HCO_3 = 9.3, Na = 95.7; dextrose (50%) = 3.2 ml, mannitol (15%) = 200 ml with H_2O to 1000 ml; pH = 8.1, osmolality = 415 mosmol at room temperature.

kaline nature of the solution combats the deleterious effect of acid metabolites on intracellular enzyme systems, whereas the hyperosmolality reduces both myocardial and endothelial cellular edema induced by the anoxic arrest.[4–7] Cessation of all electrical activity is usually observed after injection of approximately 200 to 300 ml. An additional 150 to 200 ml of solution reduces the myocardial temperature to approximately 15 to 16°C. Injection of larger volumes or use of solutions with higher concentrations of potassium frequently produces troublesome bradyarrhythmias, consisting of bundle branch block, atrioventricular dissociation, or sinus arrest, in the immediate postoperative period. Failure or difficulty with the cardioplegic technique is usually seen when there is incompetency of the aortic valve or where there is marked left ventricular hypertrophy secondary to long-standing hypertension, hypertrophic subaortic stenosis, or concomitant valve disease. Excessive noncoronary collateral flow may produce difficulties during the operation by rapid clearing of the cardioplegic solution from the coronary arteries with premature resumption of electrical activity or by obscuring vision as a result of the large flow of blood emanating from the open coronary arteries.

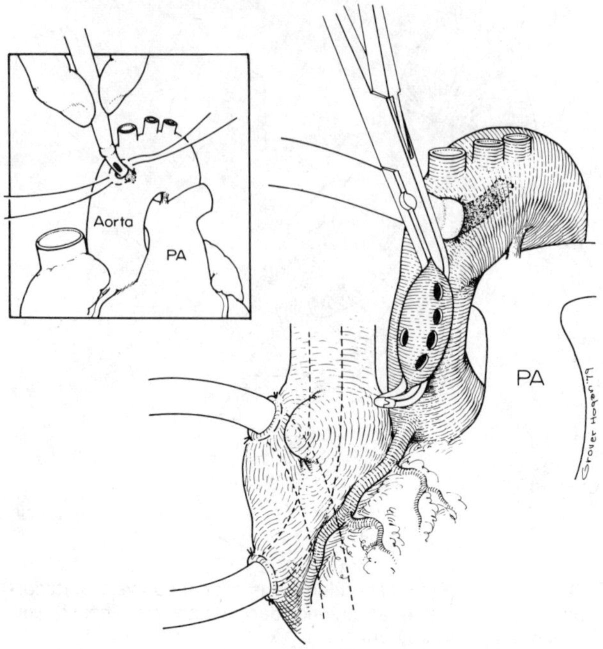

FIGURE 132-3 Construction of multiple graft sites along ascending aorta. (*From E. L. Jones, Coronary Artery Bypass Grafting: Simplification and Refinement of Surgical Technique, Ann. Thorac. Surg., 30:84, 1980. Reproduced with permission from the publisher and author.*)

Technique of Dissection and Anastomosis

The epicardium is dissected from the coronary artery only in the area to be used for anastomosis. The surrounding epicardial attachments are left intact to prevent angulation and distortion at the area of the anastomosis. Intramyocardial coronary arteries may be difficult to locate at times but often can be identified along the obtuse margin of the heart as a thin, pale pink line just visible beneath the epicardial surface. Intramyocardial left anterior descending arteries may be more difficult to find and usually lie beneath a visible epicardial groove running cephalad from the apex or may be found by tracing the diagonal branch of the left anterior descending artery (LAD) proximally. Intramyocardial arteries lack the usual thickness of vessel wall and may be delicate and fragile when the anastomosis is performed. However, intramyocardial arteries are usually free of atheromatous disease.

Currently the choice of a coronary anastomotic site has moved to a more distal location since the most extensive obstruction occurs proximally. As optical magnification and surgical techniques have improved, access to smaller, more disease-free peripheral arteries has become easier. Patency rates have been very acceptable in arteries 1.25 mm or greater in diameter. At Emory University Hospital endarterectomy has been largely abandoned as an effective treatment for obstructive coronary disease.

Conclusion of Operation

Once all distal anastomoses have been completed, rewarming is begun, coronary perfusion is reestablished by removing the aortic clamp, and the heart is electrically defibrillated if spontaneous conversion has not occurred. The proximal ends of the graft are sutured to the aorta using a single application of a large side-biting clamp. As many as six separate grafts may be constructed to the side of the aorta without difficulty (Fig. 132-3). One of the most important aspects of the operation is accurate adjustment of the length of the graft so that there is a symmetrical, graceful curve of the bypass vein. Proper adjustment of the graft length is best performed by transiently retarding the venous line to the oxygenator, thereby distending the pulmonary artery. Air is evacuated from the aorta and vein grafts, and the patient is removed from cardiopulmonary bypass.

Relation of Arteriogram to Gross Findings at Operation

Arteries less than 1 mm in diameter by arteriographic measurements are usually not satisfactory for bypass grafting. Akinesis determined by ventriculographic analysis is not necessarily a contraindication for bypass grafting provided that the distal vessels are suitable in size and quality and ischemic but viable myocardium is present in the region. However, when akinesis of a ventricular segment is present, there is usually a concomitant reduction in the size, quality, and distribution of the arteries supplying this region. Preservation of the artery to a segment of myocardium is usually indicative of the existence of viable, but poorly functioning, muscle.

Proximally occluded vessels are usually found adequate for bypass grafting if the area which they supply has normal or near-normal angiographic wall motion. This is true even when the totally occluded vessel cannot be adequately visualized at the time of catheterization. However, when the artery can be well visualized and is shown to be very small, irregular, and diffusely diseased, this has usually been the finding at the time of operation. Arteries which are difficult to revascularize are the circumflex artery in the atrioventricular groove, which frequently lies under the great cardiac vein and is inaccessible, and large septal perforators, which frequently have a long area of obstructive disease at their takeoff from the anterior descending coronary artery. Vigorous exploration to locate septal perforating branches may often lead to extensive bleeding and sometimes entry into the right ventricular cavity. In addition, the origins of the septal perforators are proximal and thus in the area of greatest disease. Another area which may be somewhat difficult to expose is the distal right coronary artery well below the takeoff of the posterior descending branch. This area is frequently buried deep within the fat and becomes intramyocardial toward the crux of the heart.

The decision to revascularize areas demonstrated to be angiographically akinetic may be difficult, but certain guidelines have been helpful. Preservation of adequate size and quality of the artery supplying the akinetic segment usually means that significant distal regional vascular bed and its associated dependent muscle mass remain viable and worthy of bypass grafting. Postoperative angiography in several patients has shown patent grafts into the posterior descending branch of the right coronary artery supplying a large distribution of blood to the posterior one-third of the ventricular septum while the base and inferior segments of the heart remain noncontractile. In patients with totally obstructed anterior descending arteries distal to the first septal perforator, the anterior wall may be noncontractile, while the septum and cardiac base are seen to move satisfactorily. A graft of the proximal LAD may be beneficial in this situation.

Some patients have a profound depression of left ventricular function as determined by the ejection fraction but have little difficulty in the postoperative period after coronary bypass grafting. Such patients may obtain striking relief of angina and heart failure symptoms. Arteriography in such patients usually demonstrates total proximal obstruction of one or more major coronary arteries, with satisfactory distal vessels filling late through collaterals. The ejection fraction represents left ventricular function at only one point in time, and to exclude patients with low calculated values and adequate distal vessels is unjustified. Conversely, if segmental muscle mass has been replaced with scar tissue, and little or no viable muscle remains, the size of the artery supplying this area usually diminishes proportionately.

Complications of the Coronary Bypass Operation

Postoperative complications of this operation are similar to those seen in any patients undergoing cardiac surgery with cardiopulmonary bypass. Such problems consist of aortic dissection, cerebral embolus or ischemia, anastomotic bleeding, perioperative infarction, deep mediastinal infection, and requirements for inotropic drugs in order to discontinue cardiopulmonary bypass.

Aortic dissection continues to account for significant mortality in performance of the coronary bypass operation. Patients at increased risk are the elderly, those with a long history of hypertension, and patients with occult medial cystic necrosis or severe atherosclerotic involvement of the ascending aorta. Treatment is difficult, and the problem is most effectively handled by prophylactic maneuvers to avoid this lethal complication. Preventive maneuvers consist of reducing central aortic pressure each time a clamp is applied or removed from the aorta, minimizing the frequency with which clamps are placed on the ascending aorta, meticulous incorporation of all layers of the aorta into the proximal graft suture line, and pharmacologic prevention of wide swings in systemic blood pressure once the operation has been completed.

Central nervous system damage such as strokes or transient postoperative neurologic sequelae have occurred in less than 1 percent of patients at our institution. This may be due to air or particulate embolization from the aorta to the cerebral circulation. Air may be introduced into the systemic circulation at the time of left ventricular venting or by dislodgment of air which is trapped beneath the edge of the side-biting aortic clamp once resumption of cardiac activity has occurred. Because of the trend away from cardiac venting during the bypass operation, the incidence of this phenomenon appears to have been reduced. Air is usually vented from the aorta through a small hole, with the patient in the head-down position. Embolization of particulate matter usually occurs from left ventricular mural thrombus or calcific debris dislodged at the time the proximal aortic clamp is released. Platelet-fibrin deposition on the aortic suture line may also be a cause of early or late embolization. However, the occurrence of this latter phenomena is sufficiently infrequent that routine anticoagulation is unjustified. Neurologic deficits secondary to air embolism are usually transient and resolve completely at a variable rate during the postoperative period. Embolization of particulate matter, on the other hand, is usually more devastating, and resolution, if it occurs, requires a more prolonged period of time.

Anastomotic bleeding is usually seen when grafts have been placed to arteries of marginal quality and the vessel wall is friable and thin, particularly where a posterior atherosclerotic plaque terminates anteriorly and laterally. Repairing sutures are frequently necessary, often resulting in compromise of the vessel lumen. For this reason, the ultimate decision of whether to graft questionable coronary arteries must be reserved until the moment of surgery.

The frequency of perioperative myocardial infarction is not statistically related to extent of vessel disease, abnormality of left ventricular function, or inability to achieve complete revascularization.[8] We have rarely seen perioperative new Q-wave formation in the distribution of an artery which was not bypassed. The reason for this finding is unknown but may be related to a reperfusion injury. Since routine employment of better myocardial preservation techniques by most cardiac surgical centers, the incidence of perioperative infarction has diminished significantly.

The prevention of deep mediastinal wound infections requires constant attention to antiseptic detail. Introduction of organisms through intravenous or intraarterial monitoring lines or at the time of operation must be meticulously avoided. Streptococcus and staphylococcus are the most frequently offending organisms. Gram-negative infections are more prevalent in patients with chronic obstructive pulmonary disease.

The need for inotropic drugs to permit discontinuation of cardiopulmonary bypass has progressively decreased over the years as techniques of myocardial preservation have improved and technical proficiency has increased. If left ventricular function is abnormal, the need for inotropic drugs is significantly increased.

We use the principles enumerated in this text to manage patients having the coronary bypass operation, and our present operative mortality in the last 3479 consecutive patients has been 0.8 percent. Precise definition and understanding of factors important in the technical performance of this procedure have made it one of the safest major operations in recent surgical history.

Mechanical Defects Complicating Acute Myocardial Infarction

Mechanical defects occurring as a result of myocardial infarction are usually catastrophic and result in high mortality. Patients in cardiogenic shock following myocardial infarction should be carefully assessed for the presence of such mechanical defects, which include (1) rupture of the ventricular free wall, (2) rupture of the ventricular septum, and (3) rupture of papillary muscle.

Acute Rupture of the Ventricular Free Wall

Rupture of the ventricular free wall is described in more detail in Chap. 45. Cardiac rupture accounts for 10 to 15 percent of deaths from infarction.[9] Of ventricular ruptures, 84 percent occur in the first week, and 33 percent within the first 24 h of infarction.[10]

Ventricular rupture is usually abrupt and is difficult to distinguish from postinfarction cardiogenic shock without rupture. The anterior left ventricular wall is three times more likely to be involved than is the inferior wall. Sudden death is usual but there may be tamponade of an irregular rupture by hematoma, adhesions, or false aneurysm formation, which may allow stabilization of hemodynamic status for a period of time.[11]

Surgical Treatment

When rupture is suspected, prompt pericardiocentesis should be performed to establish the diagnosis and improve hemodynamic status. Continuous drainage through a soft catheter with side holes may allow time for transport of the patient to the operating room. Once the diagnosis is confirmed, the patient should be placed on cardiopulmonary bypass and the defect repaired. If cardiopulmonary bypass is used, infarctectomy and closure of viable ventricular wall is performed. Late deaths have resulted from cardiogenic shock, recurrent rupture, or myocardial infarction.

Rupture of the Ventricular Septum

Chapter 45 describes rupture of the ventricular septum. Septal rupture occurs in approximately 1 percent of patients who die as a result of myocardial infarction. The majority of these ruptures occur within the first week, and 20 to 30 percent develop as early as the first 24 h after the onset of initial symptoms of infarction. Of patients with septal rupture, 50 percent die within the first week, and 85 percent die by the end of the second week following rupture. Because of the inordinately high mortality with medical management, surgical repair should be considered in most patients.

The blood supply to the septum arises from branches of the left anterior descending coronary artery, the posterior descending branch of the right coronary artery, or the circumflex artery when it is dominant. Approximately 60 percent of septal ruptures occur with infarction of the anterior wall and 40 percent with infarction of the posterior or inferior wall.[12]

When septal rupture is recognized, administration of digitalis and intravenous administration of sodium nitroprusside may improve pump function by decreasing afterload, ventricular filling, and regurgitant flow. If hypotension is present, an inotropic drug is also utilized. If there is not prompt hemodynamic stabilization, which is usually the case, an intraaortic balloon assist device should be inserted prior to cardiac catheterization and eventual surgery. The benefit of intraaortic balloon pumping is twofold: (1) reduction in afterload with a decrease in left-to-right shunting, and (2) diastolic augmentation with an increase in coronary blood flow resulting in improvement in the oxygen supply/demand ratio. This aggressive approach often results in temporary stabilization of these extremely ill patients, but, in general, the benefits achieved are disappointingly brief. Therefore, early diagnostic evaluation and rapid surgical intervention should usually be planned. Only about 15 percent of patients can be controlled by conventional medical measures for the period of 3 to 6 weeks, after which surgery can be performed at a greatly reduced risk.

Surgical Treatment
Surgical repair of postinfarction ventricular septal defect was first reported by Cooley in 1957.[13] The approach used at that time was to approach the defect through a right ventriculotomy, much as a congenital defect would be corrected today. Since then, extensive modifications in surgical technique have occurred and at present the site of ventriculotomy is through the area of infarction.[14] This allows optimal exposure of the defect while minimizing damage to functional myocardium.

Operative mortality is directly related to the interval between infarction and surgical repair. If repair is performed 3 weeks or more after infarction, operative mortality is approximately 20 percent; if surgery is performed prior to this time, mortality approaches 50 percent.[15]

The technique of closure of these defects has resulted in several ingenious procedures. The procedure utilized is determined by the location of the defect. Most defects are anteroapical, and closure utilizes a technique of buttressing the defect with viable muscle from the adjacent anterior left ventricular wall. Small chronic defects located high in the ventricular septum and the larger defects are closed with a Dacron patch.[16]

The less common high posterior septal or inferior defect is approached through the inferior portion of the heart, usually in the distribution of the posterior descending branch of the right coronary artery. The incision is made in the area of maximal infarction, which is usually on the right ventricular side of the septum. A well-proven principle of repair of these defects is synthetic patch closure without tension.[17]

Papillary Muscle Rupture
Mitral regurgitation following myocardial infarction reflects loss of structural and functional integrity of the papillary muscle apparatus and is said to occur with an autopsy incidence of approximately 1 percent. The anterolateral papillary muscle receives its blood supply from the obtuse marginal branch of the circumflex artery, while the posteromedial papillary muscle is dependent on the right coronary artery. Injury to the posteromedial papillary muscle is significantly more frequent than injury to the anterolateral papillary muscle. Interference with this blood supply may result in frank infarction and rupture or gradual replacement with fibrosis, both of which will impair function of the mitral apparatus. Principles of management include all measures to improve left ventricular function and decrease regurgitant flow. The spectrum of therapeutic intervention may include administration of digitalis, diuretics, and sodium nitroprusside; infusion of inotropic agents; and intraaortic balloon assistance.

Surgical Treatment
At best, the surgical treatment of these patients is difficult and carries with it a mortality of between 10 and 25 percent, depending on the extent of impairment of left ventricular function. Surgical exposure of the mitral valve is often difficult because of the small left atrium uniformly noted in patients with acute mitral regurgitation. The goal of surgical intervention is to provide the patient with a competent, nonstenotic mitral valve, and this can be reliably accomplished with prosthetic valve replacement. Annuloplastic techniques are usually not applicable in these emergency situations.[18,19]

Left Ventricular Aneurysm (see Chap. 45)

Indications for Surgery
Primary indications for surgical treatment of left ventricular aneurysm consist of left ventricular failure, angina pectoris, thromboembolism, and tachyarrhythmias. In recent years the primary indication for resection of left ventricular aneurysm has been angina pectoris associated with prior myocardial infarction and multivessel coronary artery disease. Persistent severe left ventricular failure, as a result of multiple infarctions or a single massive infarction, is less of an indication today.

Endocardial thrombosis frequently accompanies transmural myocardial infarction, and mural thrombus is usually identified at the time of aneurysm resection. One potential complication of left ventricular aneurysm is thromboembolism. However, the occurrence of this complication has probably been overstated in the past and rarely is an indication by itself for aneurysm resection.

Surgical Treatment
Once cardiopulmonary bypass is instituted the heart is decompressed and cooled. The heart is allowed to cool until it fibrillates. Resection of the aneurysm may then be performed without cross-clamping the aorta and prolonging ventricular ischemic time. At very cold temperatures (25°C) left ventricular fibrillation is probably not injurious to the myocardium. A left ventricular vent is inserted across the right superior pulmonary vein into the left ventricle to minimize distension. In addition, this allows precise delineation of the aneurysmal sac and adjacent viable myocardium. Care should be taken not to embolize thrombus from the left ventricular endocardium by excessive manipulation of the heart prior to fibrillation. A linear incision is made in the collapsed aneurysm and all thrombus removed. The left ventricular endocardium is wiped clean of re-

sidual thrombus and the left ventricular cavity irrigated copiously with iced saline solution. The aneurysm is closed with multiple layers of running zero and 3-0 monofilament suture, reinforced with strips of Teflon felt. Once the aneurysm is closed, coronary bypass can then be performed in routine fashion.[20]

Technical complications of closure primarily involve tearing of the myocardium at the base of the suture line. For this reason an adequate margin of fibrous left ventricular aneurysm, which retains sutures well, should be left. The extent of placement of the initial sutures is determined by vital structures such as epicardial circumflex arteries, as well as the muscular components of the mitral valve apparatus.

Aneurysm resection performed with modern techniques can be done with mortalities well below 5 percent at the present time. The risk of operation is determined by the quality of residual left ventricular myocardial function.[21]

References

1. Loop, F. D., Irarrazaval, M. J., Bredee, J. J., Siegel, W., Taylor, P. C., and Sheldon, W. C.: Internal Mammary Artery Graft for Ischemic Heart Disease, Effect of Revascularization on Clinical Status and Survival, *Am. J. Cardiol.*, 39:516, 1977.
2. Kay, E. B., Naraghipour, H., Beg, R. A., DeManey, M., Tambe, A., and Zimmerman, H. A.: Internal Mammary Artery Bypass Graft. Long-Term Patency Rate and Follow-up, *Ann. Thorac. Surg.*, 18:269, 1974.
3. Carpentier, A., Guermonprez, J. L., Deloche, A., Frechette, C., and DuBost, C.: The Aorta-to-Coronary Radial Artery Bypass Graft, *Ann. Thorac. Surg.*, 16:111, 1973.
4. Leaf, A.: Cell Swelling, *Circulation*, 48:455, 1973. (Editorial.)
5. Willerson, J. T., Powell, W. J., Guiney, T., Stark, J. J., Sander, C. A., and Leaf, A.: Improvement in Myocardial Function and Coronary Blood Flow in Ischemic Myocardium after Mannitol, *J. Clin. Invest.*, 51:2989, 1972.
6. Leaf, A.: On the Mechanism of Fluid Exchange of Tissues in Vitro, *Biochem. J.*, 62:241, 1956.
7. Jones, E. L., Tyras, D. H., King, S. B., Logue, R. B., and Hatcher, C. R.: Myocardial Revascularization Combined with Intracoronary Infusion of Hyperosmolar Solution in the Early Management of Post Infarction Ventricular Septal Defect. Report of a Case, *Circulation*, 52:170, 1975.
8. Jones, E. L., Craver, J. M., King, S. B., Douglas, J. S., Bradford, J. M., Brown, C. M., Bone D. K., and Hatcher, C. R.: Clinical, Anatomic and Functional Descriptors Influencing Morbidity, Survival and Adequacy of Revascularization following Coronary Bypass, *Ann. Surg.*, 192(3):390, 1980.
9. Bates, R. J., Bentler, S., Resnekov, L., and Anagnostopoulos, C. E.: Cardiac Rupture—Challenge in Diagnosis and Management, *Am. J. Cardiol.*, 40:429, 1977.
10. Rasmussen, S., Leth, A., Kjoller, E., Pèdersen, A.: Cardiac Rupture in Acute Myocardial Infarction. A Review of Seventy-Two Consecutive Cases, *Acta Med. Scand.* 205:11, 1979.
11. VanTassel, R. A., and Edwoods, J. E.: Rupture of the Heart Complicating Myocardial Infarction, *Chest*, 61:104, 1972.
12. Swithinback, J. M.: Perforation of the Intraventricular Septum in Myocardial Infarction, *Br. Heart J.*, 21:562, 1959.
13. Cooley, D. A., Belmonte, B. A., Zeis, L. B., Schnur, S.: Surgical Repair of Ruptured Inter-ventricular Septum following Acute Myocardial Infarction, *Surgery*, 41:930, 1957.
14. Kitamura, S., Mendez, A., and Kay, J. H.: Ventricular Septal Defect following Myocardial Infarction: Experience with Surgical Repair through a Left Ventriculotomy and Review of the Literature, *J. Thorac. Cardiovasc. Surg.*, 61:186, 1971.
15. Daggett, W. M., Guyton, R. A., Mundth, E. D., et al.: Surgery for Post-myocardial Infarct Ventricular Septal Defect, *Ann. Surg.*, 186:260, 1977.
16. Daggett, W. M., and Buckley, M. J.: The Surgical Treatment of Post Infarction Ventricular Septal Defect. Indications, Techniques and Results, in J. Moran and L. L. Michaelis (eds.), "Surgery for the Complications of Myocardial Infarction," Grune & Stratton, Inc., New York, 1980, p. 211.
17. Daggett, W. M.: Surgical Technique for Early Repair of Posterior Ventricular Septal Rupture, *J. Thorac. Cardiovasc. Surg.*, 84:306, 1982.
18. Austen, W. G., Sokol, D. M., DeSanctis, R. W., and Sanders, C. A.: Surgical Treatment of Papillary Muscle Rupture Complicating Myocardial Infarction, *N. Engl. J. Med.*, 278:1137, 1968.
19. Gerbode, F. L., Hetzer, R., and Krebber, H. J.: Surgical Management of Papillary Muscle Rupture, *World J. of Surg.*, 2:791, 1978.
20. Harken, A. H.: Left Ventricular Aneurysm, in D. C. Sabiston, Jr., and F. C. Spencer (eds.), "Gibbons Surgery of The Chest," W. B. Saunders Company, 1983, vol. 2, p. 1480.
21. Jones, E. L., Craver, J. W., Hurst, J. W., et al.: Influence of Left Ventricular Aneurysm on Survival following the Coronary Bypass Operation, *Ann. Surg.*, 193:733, 1981.

133

Techniques of Surgical Treatment of Diseases of the Aorta

Panagiotis N. Symbas, M.D.

Charles R. Hatcher, Jr., M.D.

During the last three decades the development of reliable and safe methods of cardiopulmonary bypass and aortography, along with improved construction of prosthetic grafts and the accumulation of knowledge of the hemodynamic and pathological changes associated with various aortic lesions and their management, have resulted in radical improvement of surgical treatment of aortic diseases. The common aortic lesions which are amenable to surgical treatment are aneurysms of the aorta, dissection of the aorta, blunt and penetrating injuries of the aorta, coarctation of the aorta, and double aortic arch.

Aneurysms of the Aorta

Aneurysms of the aorta may involve the sinuses of Valsalva (with or without involvement of the ascending aorta), the ascending aorta, the aortic arch, and the descending aorta. The surgical treatment of the aortic aneurysm is dependent upon the site and the patient's general condition.

When the risk of resection of the aneurysm is great, either because of coexisting medical diseases or because of age, then wrapping of the aneurysm could provide satisfactory protection from future rupture of the aneurysm.[1,2] A woven or knitted Dacron graft is incised along its axis, and two or more of these grafts are sutured together to increase the diameter of the graft to a size greater than the diameter of the aneurysm. After satisfactory exposure and dissection of the aneurysm from the surrounding structures, the graft is wrapped around the aorta, including the aneurysm and a small segment of the proximal and distal aorta. The graft is then snugly sutured to enclose the aneurysm without causing compression.

Sinus of Valsalva Aneurysms

The surgical treatment of sinus of Valsalva aneurysms is accomplished under total cardiopulmonary bypass, moderate hypothermia to 25°C, and myocardial protection from ischemia with intermittent intracoronary injection of cold (4 to 6°C) cardioplegic solution.

When there is a sinus of Valsalva fistula without an aneurysm, the ascending aorta is cross-clamped, just proximal to the brachiocephalic artery, after total cardiopulmonary bypass has been instituted and the left ventricle vented. Cardioplegic solution is injected into the coronary ostia, and the fistula is sutured, preferably at both ends, through an aortotomy and cardiotomy.

When an aneurysm of the sinuses of Valsalva is present, the cardioplegic solution is injected and the aneurysm is incised along its axis. If aortic regurgitation is present, the valve is replaced and the continuity of the aorta is then restored with the interposition of the appropriate-sized, tubular, woven microporous Dacron graft. Depending upon the pathological-anatomic changes of the aortic root, the proximal aortic anastomosis is constructed in one of two ways:

1. If the aneurysm is relatively small, and the segment of the sinus of Valsalva between the coronary ostia and the aortic valve annulus is neither greatly dilated nor thin-walled, the anastomosis is performed just above the aortic annulus adjacent to the coronary ostia.
2. When this is not the case, and aortic regurgitation is present (Fig. 133-1), the aortic valve substitute is first sutured to the aortic graft (Fig. 133-2*A*), and then the aortic graft with the valve is sutured to the aortic valve annulus (Fig. 133-2*B*).

The continuity of the coronary arteries is then established, either by suturing the coronary ostia to the aortic graft (Fig. 133-2*C*) or by the interposition of a saphenous vein graft between the aortic graft and the coronary arteries, with subsequent suturing of the coronary ostia. The distal end of the aortic graft is then sewn to the distal aorta, the air in the left side of the heart and the ascending aorta is appropriately expelled from the systemic circulation, and cardiopulmonary bypass is terminated.[3]

Aneurysms of the Ascending Aorta[4]

Resection of an ascending aortic aneurysm is performed through a median sternotomy under cardiopulmonary bypass (Fig. 133-3), with moderate systemic hypothermia to 25°C. The myocardium is protected with intermittent intracoronary injection of cold (4 to 6°C) cardioplegic solution.

A circumferential segment of the aorta, just proximal to the brachiocephalic artery, is dissected for cross-clamping, with special care being taken to avoid injury of the main or right pulmonary artery. The aorta is cross-clamped at this level, and the left ventricle is decompressed by a left ventricular catheter,

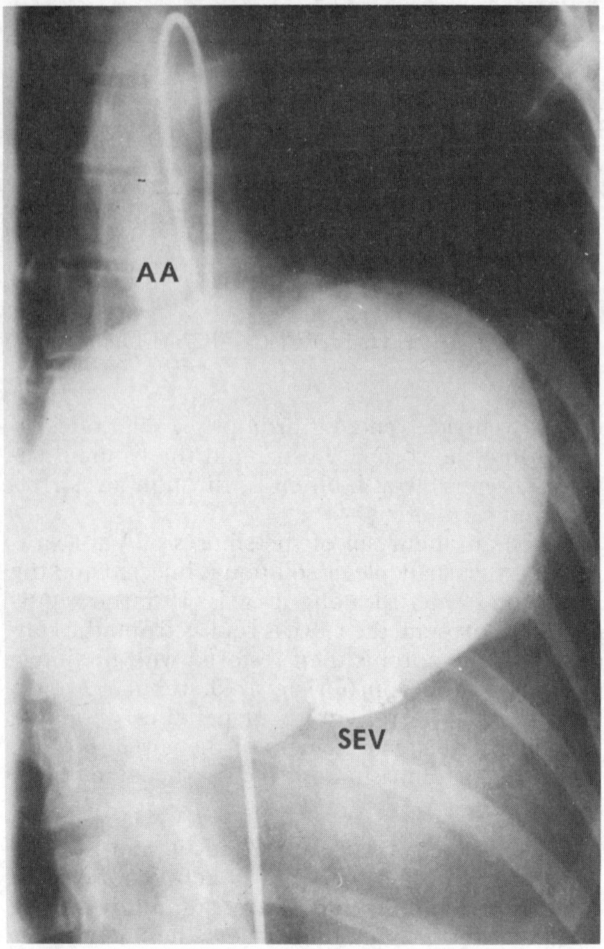

FIGURE 133-1 Aortogram showing giant sinus of Valsalva aneurysms. SEV = Starr-Edwards aortic valve inserted; AA = ascending aorta, replaced a few years earlier. (*From P. N. Symbas, A. E. Raizner, D. H. Tyras, et al., Aneurysms of All Sinuses of Valsalva in Patients with Marfan's Syndrome: An Unusual Late Complication following Replacement of Aortic Valve and Ascending Aorta for Aortic Regurgitation and Fusiform Aneurysm of Ascending Aorta, Ann. Surg., 174:902, 1971. Reproduced with permission from the publisher and authors.)*

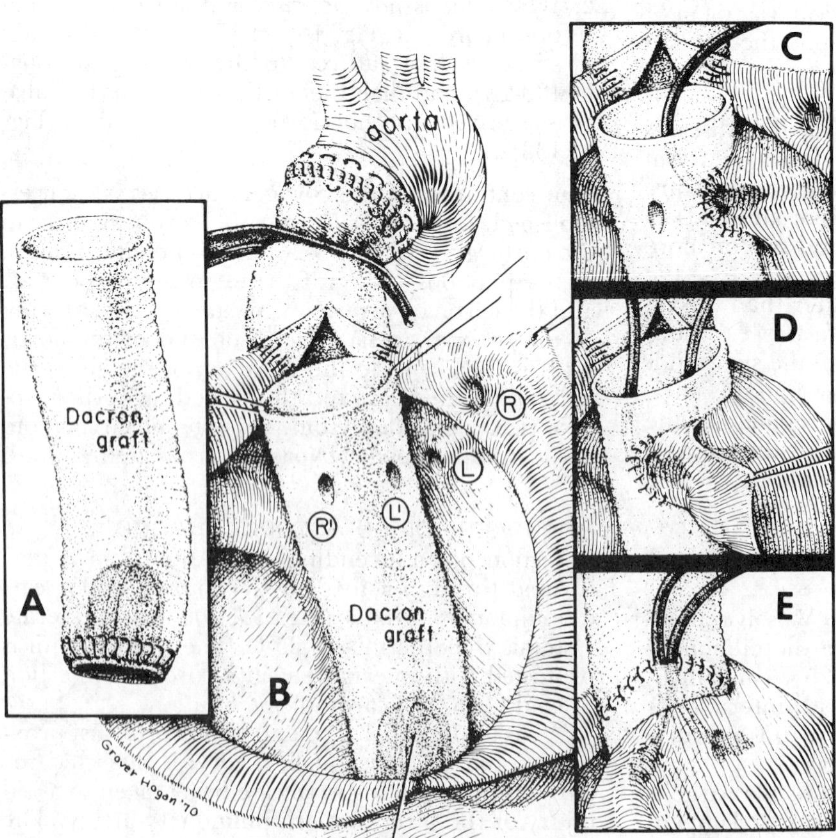

FIGURE 133-2 Repair of sinus of Valsalva aneurysms. R = right coronary artery; L = left coronary artery; R′ = opening for right coronary artery; L′ = opening for left coronary artery. (*From P. N. Symbas, A. E. Raizner, D. H. Tyras, et al., Aneurysms of All Sinuses of Valsalva in Patients with Marfan's Syndrome: An Unusual Late Complication following Replacement of Aortic Valve and Ascending Aorta for Aortic Regurgitation and Fusiform Aneurysm of Ascending Aorta, Ann. Surg., 174:902, 1971. Reproduced with permission from the publisher and authors.)*

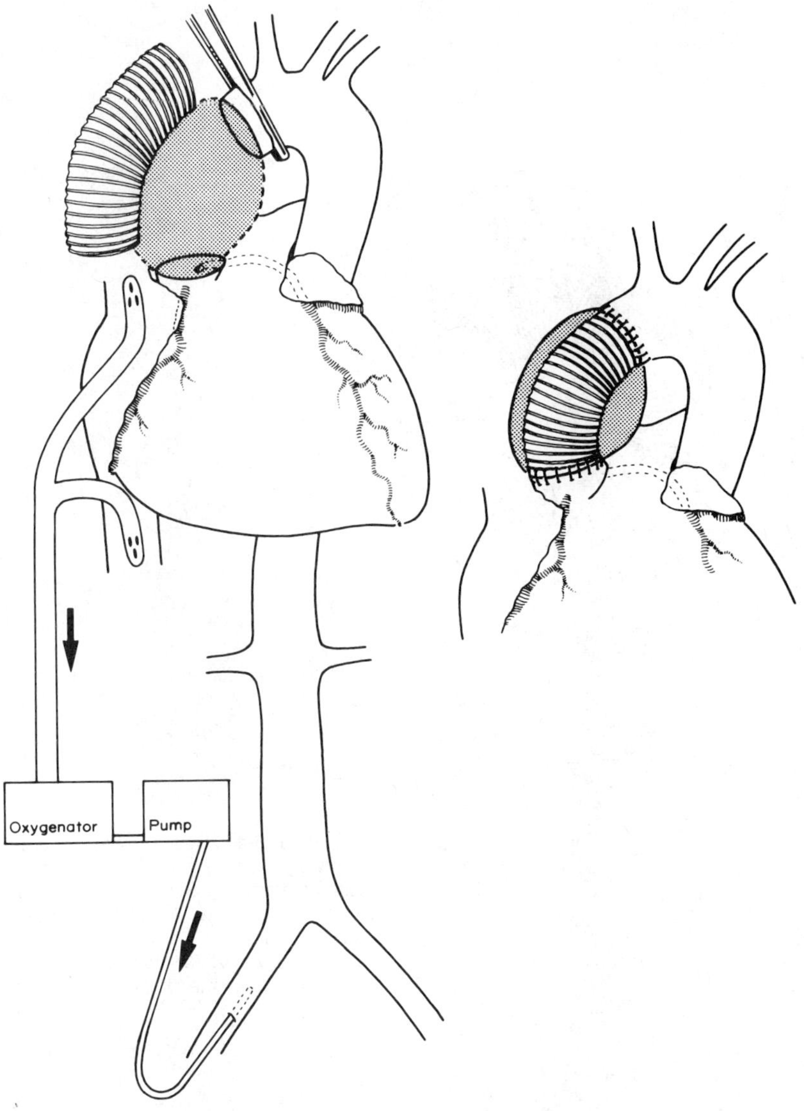

FIGURE 133-3 Repair of ascending aortic aneurysm. [*From P. N. Symbas, Treatment of Thoracic Surgical Aortic Diseases, in J. Lindsay, Jr., and J. W. Hurst (eds.), "The Aorta," Grune & Stratton, Inc., New York, 1979. Reproduced with permission from the publisher and author.*]

inserted through the right superior pulmonary vein. The aneurysm is opened anteriorly and longitudinally, and the aorta is transected proximal to the brachiocephalic artery.[5,6] The wall of the aneurysm is left in situ, to prevent injury of the pulmonary artery and/or the superior vena cava, to which the aneurysm is frequently densely adherent. The aortic valve, if insufficient, is replaced. A microporous woven Dacron tubular graft, tailored to match the aorta, is sutured just above the coronary ostia and to the distal transected aorta (Fig. 133-3). The air is appropriately evacuated from the ascending aorta, the aortic clamp is removed, and cardiopulmonary bypass is discontinued after rewarming is accomplished.

Aortic Arch Aneurysms

The resection of an arch aneurysm is a complex operative procedure, requiring perfusion of the carotid arteries and many anastomotic suture lines, some of which are quite difficult to approach through one thoracotomy incision.[7–9] The patient is prepared, with the left thorax elevated to about 30°, and draped to the level of the anterior margin of the left latissimus dorsi. The operative procedure is accomplished through a median sternotomy incision, and, with the patient so positioned, an additional left anterolateral incision can be made through the third or fourth intercostal space if the performance of the distal anastomosis is unsatisfactory through the median sternotomy incision. The arch aneurysms are treated either by resection or by bypass and exclusion. The resection of these aneurysms, like those of the ascending aorta, is performed under total cardiopulmonary bypass and moderate hypothermia (20 to 25°C). In the past, in this group of patients, in addition to the conventional cannulation for total cardiopulmonary bypass, the brachiocephalic and left common carotid arteries were separately cannulated and perfused, to protect the brain from ischemic injury during their cross-clamping (Fig. 133-4). The carotid blood flow

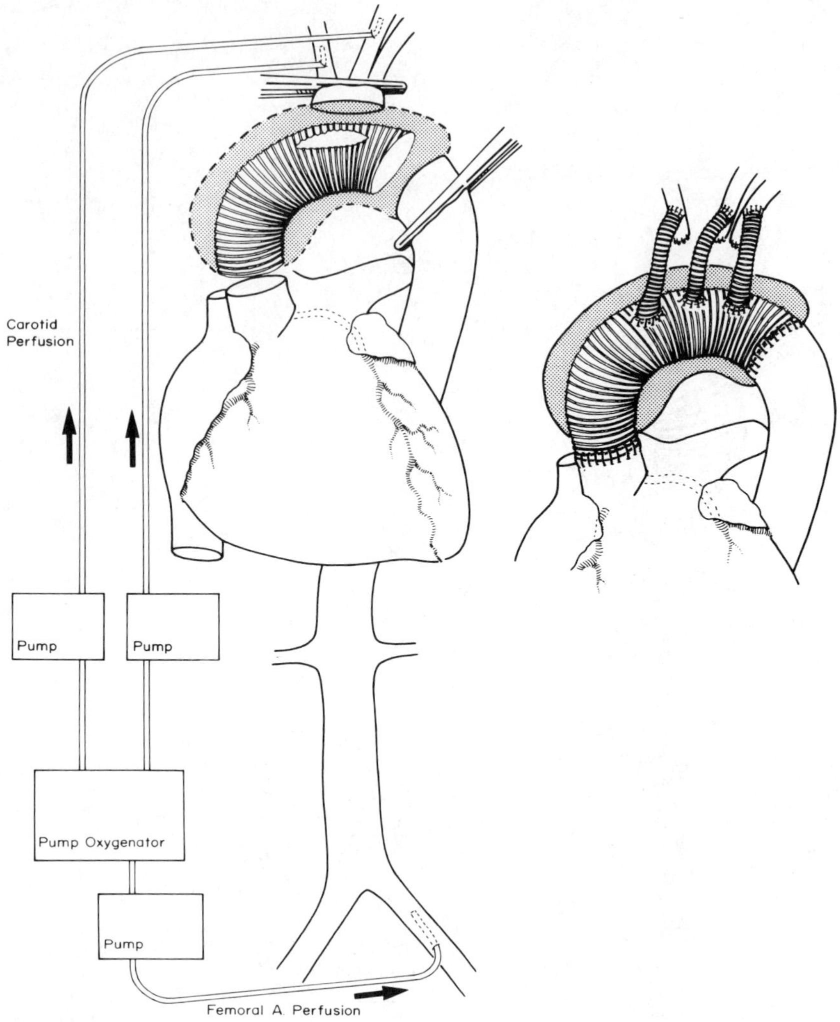

FIGURE 133-4 Repair of aortic arch aneurysm. [*From P. N. Symbas, Treatment of Thoracic Surgical Aortic Diseases, in J. Lindsay, Jr., and J. W. Hurst (eds.), "The Aorta," Grune & Stratton, Inc., New York, 1979. Reproduced with permission from the publisher and author.*]

was maintained at a rate of 250 to 300 ml/min for each carotid artery. Currently, however, the operative procedure is usually done under deeper hypothermia (18°C) and without perfusion of the carotid arteries.[10–12] Myocardial protection from ischemic injury is provided by intermittent intracoronary injection of cold cardioplegic solution and by local hypothermia. The descending aorta, just distal to the left subclavian artery, and the brachiocephalic vessel are dissected, circled with tape, and cross-clamped. The aneurysm is incised along its long axis, and if it does not extend into the origin of the brachiocephalic vessels, a large cuff of aortic wall is excised, including the origin of these three arch vessels (Fig. 133-4). The aorta is transected just distal to the origin of the left subclavian artery and proximally as far as the aneurysm extends into the ascending aorta. The continuity of the aorta is restored with an appropriate-sized microporous, tubular woven Dacron graft, and the aortic cuff, with the origin of the brachiocephalic vessels, is anastomosed to the newly created aortic arch (Fig. 133-4). If the aneurysm extends into the origin of the brachiocephalic vessels, then the brachiocephalic and left common carotid arteries are ligated at their origin and a woven Dacron graft is interposed between them and the newly created aortic arch (Fig. 133-4). The clamp placed on the descending aorta is first removed, and the air trapped in the arch and carotid vessels is appropriately evacuated. The clamps on the carotid arteries are then removed, rewarming is accomplished, and cardiopulmonary bypass is terminated.

The exclusion and bypass of the arch aneurysm is approached in the same manner, but no cardiopulmonary bypass is required. An appropriate-sized preclotted woven Dacron graft is anastomosed end to side to the ascending and descending aorta, and then appropriate-sized grafts are similarly anastomosed end to side to the arch graft and end to side to the brachiocepahlic and carotid arteries. The air is evacuated from the newly created arch and brachiocephalic vessels, and blood flow through the graft is begun. The aorta is then transected and sutured proximally and distally to the aneurysms. Similarly, the brachiocephalic vessels are transected and sutured just cephalad to their origin from the arch.

Aneurysms of Descending Aorta

Although the indications and surgical approach to descending thoracic aneurysms is well established[6,13] whether the repair of the lesion should be performed under some form of bypass is somewhat controversial. Some investigators feel that some form of bypass is essential and should be provided for perfusion of the abdominal viscera and spinal cord during the resection of the descending aortic aneurysm, particularly if the time required for aortic cross-clamping will exceed 30 min.[9,14,15] Others contend that the results of the resection of these aneurysms without any form of bypass to provide perfusion to the visceral organs are better than when some form of bypass is utilized.[16]

In order to facilitate the exposure and resection of descending thoracic aneurysms and prevent injury to the lung from excessive traction, a Garlens or Shaw's orotracheal tube is utilized so that during the resection of the aneurysm, the ventilation is carried out only through the right lung, while the left lung is completely collapsed.

The descending thoracic aneurysm is approached through a posterolateral thoracotomy incision through the bed of the fifth rib. The aorta proximal and distal to the aneurysm is dissected and encircled with tape, and femoral vein-to-femoral artery partial cardiopulmonary bypass, or bypass through an external temporary shunt (Fig. 133-5), is then instituted. After the aneurysm is isolated between the clamps, its anterior wall is incised longitudinally, the orifices of the intercostal arteries present in the aneurysm are sutured and ligated, and the continuity of the aorta is restored with the interposition of the appropriate size of woven, microporous tubular Dacron graft. After aortic continuity has been reestablished, the distal aortic clamp is removed. The air is aspirated from the graft, the proximal aortic clamp is removed, and the bypass is terminated.

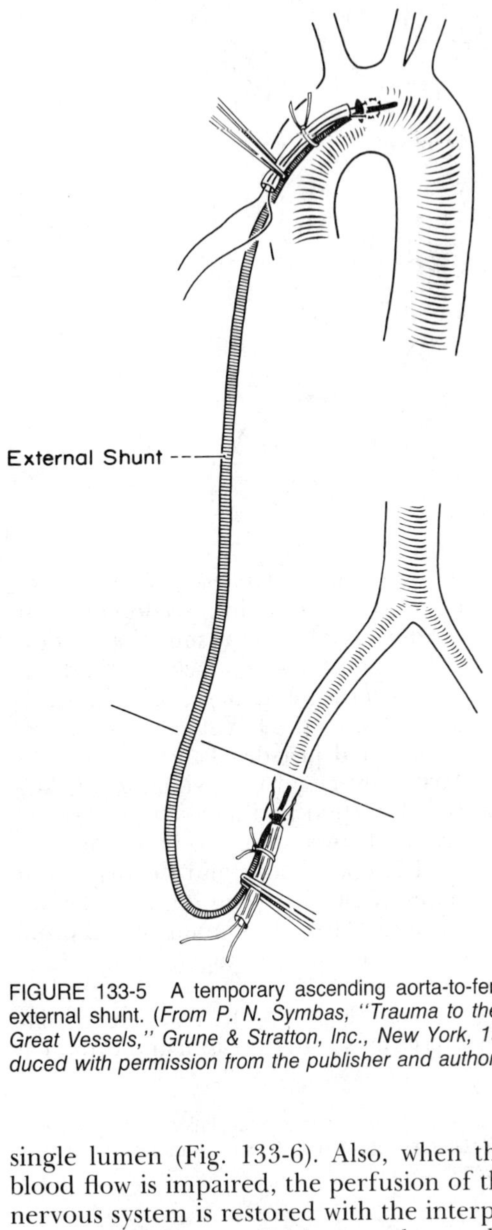

FIGURE 133-5 A temporary ascending aorta-to-femoral artery external shunt. *(From P. N. Symbas, "Trauma to the Heart and Great Vessels," Grune & Stratton, Inc., New York, 1978. Reproduced with permission from the publisher and author.)*

Dissecting Aneurysms

The method of surgical treatment of these aneurysms depends on the site and extent of the dissection.[17–19] The surgical procedure for the repair of the type II dissecting aneurysm is similar to that employed for the resection of other types of ascending aortic aneurysms. The surgical procedure for type I dissecting aneurysms without aortic regurgitation is similar to the procedure used for the repair of ascending aortic aneurysms without aortic valve incompetence, with the exceptions described below. When the distal false lumen extends beyond the point of transection of the ascending aorta, it is first obliterated by suturing together, with or without enforcement by Teflon felt strips, the edges of the inner and outer walls, and then a microporous, tubular woven Dacron graft is anastomosed to the single lumen (Fig. 133-6). Also, when the carotid blood flow is impaired, the perfusion of the central nervous system is restored with the interposition of a woven tubular graft between the newly created ascending aorta and the involved carotid artery. Although the aortic regurgitation associated with other ascending aortic aneurysms is managed with aortic valve replacement, aortic valve incompetence with dissection can be repaired in many patients; in others the valve is replaced. The repair of the valve is accomplished by reattaching the valve commissures with pledgeted sutures with or without interposition of a Teflon felt patch between the two aortic walls and in the false lumen (Fig. 133-7). The edges of the inner and outer walls with the interposed patch are sutured together, and then microporous, tubular woven Dacron graft is anastomosed to the proximal and distal single lumina of the aorta.

The surgical procedure for the repair of the type III dissecting aneurysm, for the most part, is similar to the surgical procedure utilized for the resection of other types of descending thoracic aneurysms.

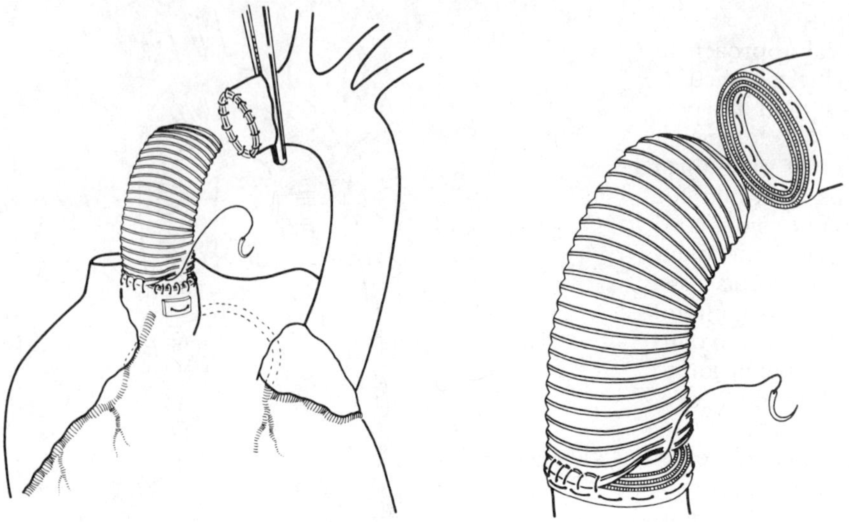

FIGURE 133-6 Repair of type I dissecting aneurysm. [*From P. N. Symbas, Treatment of Thoracic Surgical Aortic Diseases, in J. Lindsay, Jr., and J. W. Hurst (eds.), "The Aorta," Grune & Stratton, Inc., New York, 1979. Reproduced with permission from the publisher and author.*]

After the appropriate dissection and cannulation for perfusion are accomplished, as in resection of other types of descending aortic aneurysms, the aorta is cross-clamped between the left subclavian and left common carotid arteries. The descending aorta is then cross-clamped, as is the left subclavian artery. The aorta is transected just distal to the origin of the left subclavian artery, just proximal to the site of origin at the dissection and 5 to 10 cm distally. The aortic segment between the two points of transection is incised longitudinally, and the orifices of intercostal arteries originating from this segment are sutured and ligated. The false lumen of the distal aorta is obliterated by suturing together the edges of the inner and outer walls with or without the use of Teflon felt strips (Fig. 133-8). A woven tubular graft is then anastomosed to the distal and proximal single lumen (Fig. 133-8). Although usually all of the descending as well as the abdominal aorta is involved in the dissecting process, it is advisable to resect only a small proximal descending aortic segment to prevent the sacrifice of many intercostal arteries and to avoid paraplegia from spinal cord ischemia. Unusual forms of dissection, e.g., intimo-intimal intussusception and type III dissection with both forward and backward dissection, are handled appropriately.[18]

Aortic Trauma

Penetrating aortic injuries manifesting by massive and/or sustained blood loss are managed by exploratory thoracotomy and repair of the wound after

FIGURE 133-7 Correction of aortic regurgitation from dissecting aneurysm. [*From P. N. Symbas, Treatment of Thoracic Surgical Aortic Diseases, in J. Lindsay, Jr., and J. W. Hurst (eds.), "The Aorta," Grune & Stratton, Inc., New York, 1979. Reproduced with permission from the publisher and author.*]

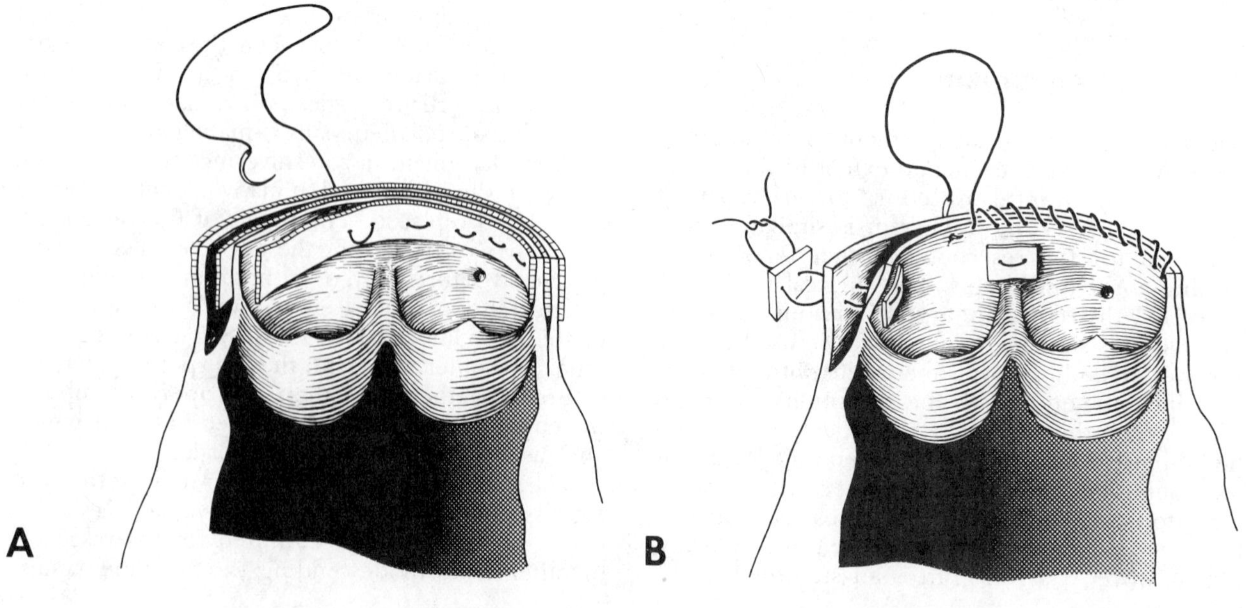

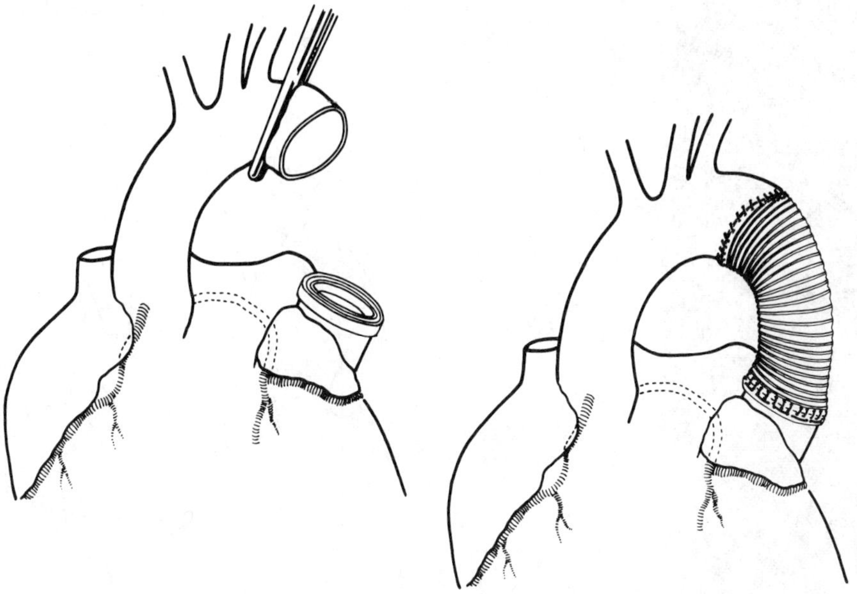

FIGURE 133-8 Repair of type III dissecting aneurysm. [*From P. N. Symbas, Treatment of Thoracic Surgical Aortic Diseases, in J. Lindsay, Jr., and J. W. Hurst (eds.), "The Aorta," Grune & Stratton, Inc., New York, 1979. Reproduced with permission from the publisher and author.*]

tangential occlusion or after cross-clamping of the aorta. The type of thoracotomy and mode of management of penetrating aortic injuries manifesting with mediastinal hematoma, aortocardiac fistula, or fistula from aorta-to-venous channels are selected after aortographic demonstration of the site and type of injury.[20,21]

Injuries of the ascending aorta or aortic arch are best approached through a midsternotomy incision, whereas wounds of the descending aorta are repaired through a posterolateral thoracotomy at the fifth intercostal space. Repair of the aortic wounds can be performed after tangential clamping of the aorta, when feasible, or after cross-clamping. When cross-clamping of the aorta proximal to the left common carotid artery is required for the repair of an aortic wound or for an aortocardiac or an aortopulmonary fistula, this is done under total cardiopulmonary bypass, moderate hypothermia to 25°C, and protection of the myocardium from ischemic injury by intermittent intracoronary injection of cold cardioplegic solution.

Similarly, when cross-clamping of the descending aorta is required for longer than 20 to 30 min, a temporary external shunt is utilized to protect the spinal cord from ischemic injury.[15,22,23]

Rupture of the Aorta

Rupture of the aorta just distal to the left subclavian artery from blunt trauma is usually amenable to surgical treatment. This type of injury is exposed through a posterolateral left thoracotomy, and the repair is preferably done under some form of bypass, femoral vein–to–femoral artery bypass or temporary external shunt from the ascending aorta to the femoral artery, in order to protect the spinal cord from ischemic injury. The temporary external shunt should be exclusively utilized in patients with rupture of the aorta when systemic heparinization is contraindicated, particularly in patients with coexisting central nervous system injury.[20,24] The repair may be done without any form of bypass if the aortic cross-clamping period is less than 20 to 30 min.

After the aortic injury is exposed and bypass commenced, the left subclavian artery and the aorta just proximal to the left subclavian artery and distal to the injury are dissected, encircled with tape, and cross-clamped. The mediastinal hematoma is opened and evacuated, the site of aortic rupture is identified, and the rupture is repaired either with end-to-end anastomosis or, as is usual, with the interposition of microporous woven Dacron graft.[20,24]

Coarctation of the Aorta[2]

The operative procedure for repair of coarctation of the aorta is dependent upon the patient's age and the type of coarctation. The ideal age for surgical repair of the postductal type of coarctation is just as soon as the aorta has reached or is approaching its full growth. However, this lesion is usually repaired either during the neonatal period, in infants presenting with congestive heart failure, or between the ages of 6 and 12 years.[25–27]

The operation is accomplished through a left posterolateral thoracotomy incision at the fourth intercostal space. In adults, subperiosteal resection of the fifth rib and thoracotomy through its bed is a preferable approach. The parietal pleura is incised longitudinally over the descending aorta, distal aortic arch, and left subclavian artery, and the pleura is reflected medially. The left subclavian artery, the aortic arch between the common carotid artery, and the descending aorta distal to the coarctation are

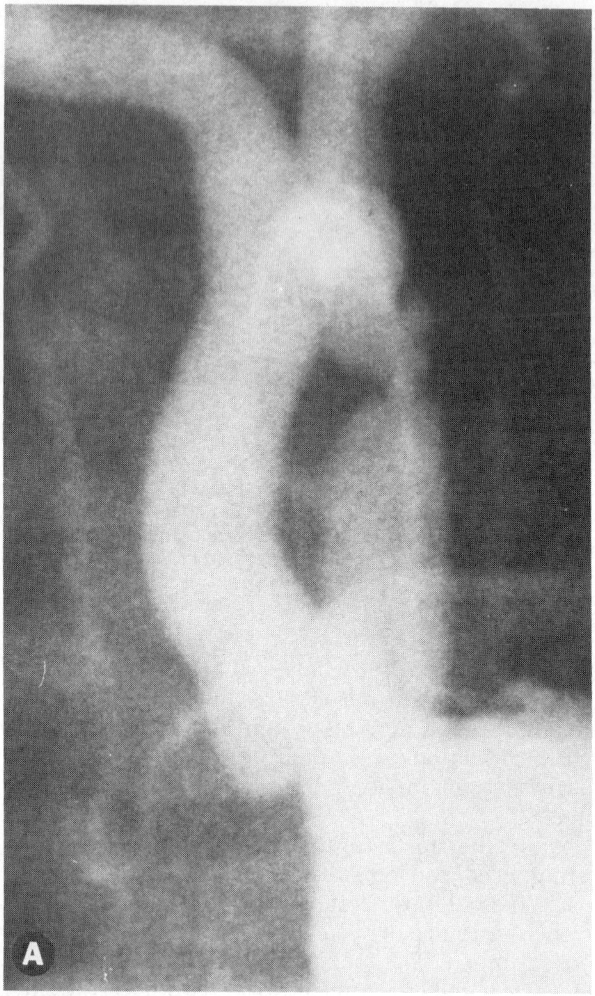

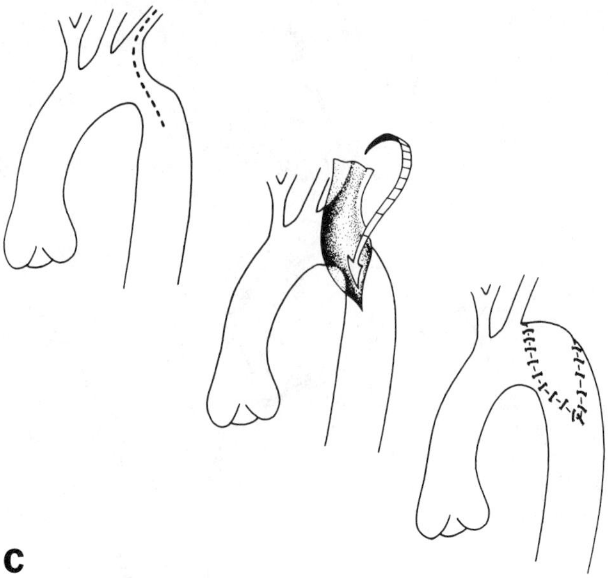

C

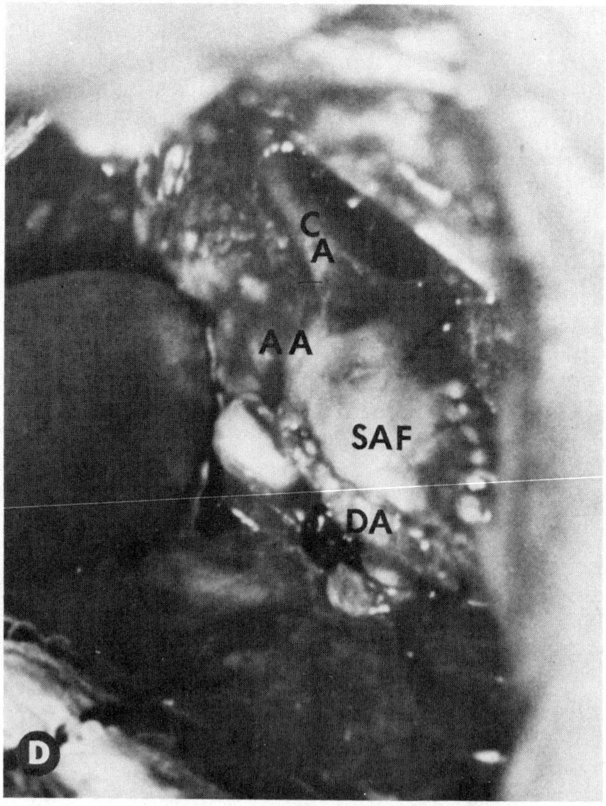

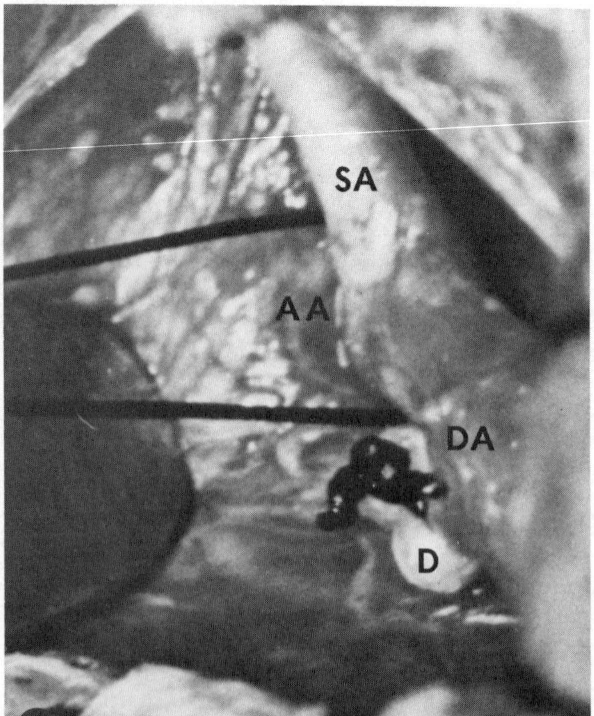

FIGURE 133-9 *A.* Aortogram showing postductal coarctation of the aorta. *B.* Photograph of coarctation of same child. *C.* Diagram depicting the repair of coarctation with the use of proximal left subclavian artery as a flap. *D.* Photograph after the repair. AA = aortic arch; SA = subclavian artery; DA = descending aorta; D = ligated and divided ductus; C_A = left common carotid artery; SAF = subclavian artery flap. [*From P. N. Symbas, Treatment of Thoracic Surgical Aortic Diseases, in J. Lindsay, Jr., and J. W. Hurst (eds.), "The Aorta," Grune & Stratton, Inc., New York, 1979. Reproduced with permission from the publisher and author.*]

encircled with umbilical tape (Figs. 133-9*A* and 133-9*B*), and the coarcted aortic segment and ligamentum arteriosus are dissected. In patients in whom the repair of the coarctation is being performed for the first time, the patent ductus arteriosus or the ligamentum arteriosis is ligated and divided. If needed, one intercostal artery pair, adjacent to the coarctation, is then ligated and divided by gently lifting the aorta by the umbilical tapes. These intercostal arteries are frequently aneurysmally dilatated and very friable and, as a result, can be quite easily injured. After the aorta is sufficiently mobilized, it is cross-clamped proximal and distal to the coarctation. The entire coarcted segment is then removed and the aortic continuity restored with end-to-end anastomosis or with the interposition of a woven Dacron tubular graft, if the two ends cannot be brought together without tension.

In children, there is experimental evidence that continuous suture may prevent growth of the aorta at the site of the anastomosis.[28,29] Accordingly, its anterior part may be sutured with interrupted horizontal mattress sutures, using either nonabsorbable synthetic suture or (preferably) absorbable suture. Another method for repair of the coarctation is to use the proximal segment of the left subclavian artery as a flap to enlarge the coarcted segment of the aorta (Fig. 133-9*C* and *D*). At the completion of the repair, the distal clamp is removed first, the air from the aorta is evacuated, and then the proximal aortic clamp is slowly released while volume expanders are administered.

When resection of the aorta is too hazardous, such as in the presence of persistent coarctation after previous resection, bypass of the stenosed area is the procedure of choice. The aorta proximal and distal to the coarctation is clamped tangentially without altering its blood flow, a lineal incision is made in the excluded aortic segment, and a suitable graft is sutured end to side. Also, in selected cases, instead of excision of the coarcted segment, the stenosed area is incised longitudinally and the aortic lumen is enlarged by suturing a prosthetic patch graft of appropriate size.

Double Aortic Arch

Surgical correction of this anomaly is best accomplished through a left posterolateral incision at the fourth intercostal space. In type I double aortic arch, the smaller of the two patent arches is divided. The division of the arch is always performed distal to the origin of the left common carotid artery so that this vessel is left to receive blood from the ascending aorta, rather than from the descending aorta where the orifice at the point of junction of the arch to the descending aorta might be small. In type II double aortic arch, the atretic segment is divided and the diverticulum of the aorta obliterated. Should the proximal segment of the left aortic arch still appear to be compressing the trachea, it is lifted from the trachea and is sutured through its adventitia to the posterior aspect of the sternum. Because of the possibility of tracheal collapse with the loss of external tissue support, the dissection around the trachea should be minimal, leaving all the supportive tissue.[30,31]

References

1. Robicsek, F., Daugherty, H. K., Mullen, D. C., et al: Is There a Place for Wall Reinforcement in Modern Aortic Surgery? *Arch. Surg.*, 105:824, 1972.
2. Robicsek, F., Perkins, R. S., and Mullen, D. C., et al.: Fusiform Aneurysm of the Entire Aortic Arch, *J. Thorac. Cardiovasc. Surg.*, 63:756, 1972.
3. Symbas, P. N., Raizner, A. E., Tyras, D. H., et al.: Aneurysms of All Sinuses of Valsalva in Patient with Marfan's Syndrome: An Unusual Late Complication following Replacement of Aortic Valve and Ascending Aorta for Aortic Regurgitation and Fusiform Aneurysm of Ascending Aorta, *Ann. Surg.*, 174:902, 1971.
4. Krause, A. H., Ferguson, T. B., and Weldon, C. S.: Thoracic Aneurysmectomy Utilizing the TDMAC-Heparin Shunt, *Ann. Thorac. Surg.*, 14:123, 1972.
5. Bahnson, H. T., and Spencer, F. C.: Excision of Aneurysm of the Ascending Aorta with Prosthetic Replacement during Cardiopulmonary Bypass, *Ann. Surg.*, 151:879, 1960.
6. DeBakey, M. E., Cooley, D. A., and Creech, O., Jr.: Aneurysms of the Aorta Treated by Resection: Analysis of Three Hundred Thirteen Cases, *JAMA*, 163:1439, 1957.
7. DeBakey, M. E., Diethrich, E. B., Noon, G. P., et al.: Surgical Management of Aortic Arch Aneurysms, *Circulation*, 38(suppl. 6):64, 1968.
8. Muller, W. H., Warren, W. D., and Blanton, F. S., Jr.: A Method for Resection of Aortic Arch Aneurysm, *Ann. Surg.*, 151:225, 1960.
9. Stranahan, A., Alley, R. D., Sewell, W. H., et al.: Aortic Arch Resection and Grafting for Aneurysm Employing an External Shunt, *J. Thorac. Surg.*, 29:54, 1955.
10. Griepp, R. B., Stinson, E. D., Hollingsworth, J. F., et al.: Prosthetic Replacement of the Aortic Arch, *J. Thorac. Cardiovasc. Surg.*, 70:1051, 1975.
11. Cooley, D. A., Ott, D. A., Frazier, O. H., et al.: Surgical Treatment of Aneurysms of Transverse Aortic Arch: Experience with 25 Patients Using Hypothermic Techniques, *Ann. Thorac. Surg.*, 32:260, 1981.
12. Lindsay, J. J., Cooley, D. A., Reul, G. J., et al.: Resection of Aortic Arch Aneurysms: A Comparison of Hypothermic Techniques in 60 Patients, *Ann. Thorac. Surg.*, 36:19, 1983.
13. DeBakey, M. E., and Cooley, D. A.: Successful Resection of Aneurysm of Thoracic Aorta and Replacement by Graft, *JAMA*, 152:673, 1953.
14. Kahn, D. R., Vathayanon, S., and Sloan, H.: Resection of Descending Thoracic Aneurysms without Left Heart Bypass, *Arch. Surg.*, 97:336, 1968.
15. Symbas, P. N., Pfaender, L. M., Drucker, M. H., et al.: Effects of Cross-Clamping of the Descending Aorta, *J. Thorac. Cardiovasc. Surg.*, 85:300, 1983.
16. Crawford, E. S., Synder, D. M., Cho, G. C., and Roehm, J. O. F., Jr.: Progress in Treatment of Thoracoabdominal and Abdominal Aortic Aneurysms Involving Celiac, Superior Mesenteric and Renal Arteries, *Ann. Surg.*, 188:404, 1978.
17. DeBakey, M. E., Henly, W. S., Cooley, D. A., et al.: Surgical Management of Dissecting Aneurysm of the Aorta, *J. Thorac. Cardiovasc. Surg.*, 49:130, 1965.
18. Symbas, P. N., Kelly, T. F., and Vlasis, S. E.: Intimointimal Intussusception and Other Unusual Manifestations of Aortic Dissection. *J. Thorac. Cardiovasc. Surg.*, 79:926, 1980.
19. Wheat, M. W., Jr., Harris, P. D., Malm, J. R., et al.: Acute

Dissecting Aneurysms of the Aorta: Treatment and Results in 64 Patients, *J. Thorac. Cardiovasc. Surg.*, 58:344, 1969.
20. Symbas, P. N.: "Trauma to the Heart and Great Vessels," Grune & Stratton, Inc., New York, 1979.
21. Symbas, P. N., Kourias, E., Tyras, D. H., et al.: Penetrating Wounds of the Great Vessels, *Ann. Surg.*, 179:757, 1974.
22. Eisemann, B., and Summer, W. B.: Factors Affecting Spinal Cord Ischemia during Aortic Occlusion, *Surgery*, 38:1063, 1955.
23. Gerbode, F., Braimbridge, M., Osborn, J. J., et al.: Traumatic Thoracic Aneurysms: Treatment by Resection and Grafting with the Use of an Extracorporeal Bypass, *Surgery*, 42:975, 1957.
24. Symbas, P. N., Tyras, D. H., Ware, R. E., et al.: Traumatic Rupture of the Aorta, *Ann. Surg.*, 178:6, 1973.
25. Crawford, C., and Nylin, G.: Congenital Coarctation of the Aorta and Its Surgical Treatment, *J. Thorac. Surg.*, 14:347, 1945.
26. Glass, I. H., Mustard, W. T., and Keith, J. D.: Coarctation of the Aorta in Infants. A Review of Twelve Years' Experience, *Pediatrics*, 26:109, 1960.
27. Olsson, P., Oderlung, S., Dubiel, W. T., et al.: Patch Grafts or Tubular Grafts in the Repair of Coarctation of the Aorta. A Follow-up Study, *Scand. J. Thorac. Cardiovasc. Surg.*, 10:139, 1976.
28. Hurwitt, E. S., and Rosenblatt, M. A.: Observations on the Growth of Aortic Anastomoses in Puppies, *Arch. Surg.*, 70:491, 1955.
29. Johnson, J., Kirby, C. K., Allam, M. W., and Hagan, W.: The Growth of Vascular Anastomoses with Continuous and Interrupted Anterior Silk Suture, *Surgery*, 29:721, 1951.
30. Mustard, W. T.: Vascular Rings Compressing the Esophagus and the Trachea, in C. D. Benson, W. T. Mustard, and M. M. Ravitch (eds.), "Pediatric Surgery," Year Book Medical Publishers, Chicago, 1962, vol. 1, p. 427.
31. Symbas, P. N., Shuford, W. H., Edwards, F. K., et al.: Vascular Ring, *J. Thorac. Cardiovasc. Surg.*, 61:149, 1971.

134

Technique of Carotid Artery Surgery

Robert B. Smith III, M.D.

When such attacks [hemiplegia and blindness] are associated with internal carotid obstruction it is possible that they may be abolished by removing the obstruction to the internal carotid artery.

H. H. G. Eastcott,
G. W. Pickering,
and C. G. Rob, 1954[1,*]

Atheromatous plaque in the carotid bifurcation is the most frequent cause of cerebral ischemia. The majority of transient cerebral ischemic attacks (TIAs) and fixed neurologic deficits are thought to result from embolization of material from ulcerated plaques, but reduced regional blood flow related to a severely stenotic or totally occluded internal carotid artery also accounts for some ischemic deficits (Fig. 134-1). Over the past 30 years, carotid endarterectomy has become a widely accepted, generally effective, and relatively safe operation for direct intervention in the stroke-prone patient. It is now one of the most frequently performed surgical procedures within the scope of general vascular surgery.

Technical Methods

In preparation of the patient for carotid endarterectomy, vigorous neck scrubs are not performed prior to operation lest mechanical dislodgment of embolic material result in a neurologic deficit. Male patients are told to shave as usual on the morning of operation; women require no special skin preparation. Prophylactic antistaphylococcal antibiotic coverage is administered intravenously in the operating room prior to commencement of the procedure. Most carotid operations are performed with the patient under general endotracheal anesthesia, but some surgeons prefer local or cervical block anesthesia.[2] Since the carotid artery is an accessible structure in the neck and very little relaxation is needed, a cooperative patient, especially one with a thin neck, can be done under local anesthesia with considerable ease. Both surgeon and anesthesiologist, however, may proceed in a more relaxed environment with better control of the patient when general anesthesia is given. If unexpected technical difficulties occur, such as presence of a plaque which extends unusually high into the internal carotid with necessity to enlarge the incision, having the patient asleep greatly facilitates the extra maneuvers.

After the chosen method of anesthesia has been induced, the patient is positioned supine with the neck slightly extended and the head rotated comfortably to the opposite side. An iodoform skin treatment is performed over the proposed field and appropriate surgical drapes applied. The surgeon then makes one of two standard incisions—either a vertical incision parallel to the anterior border of the sternocleidomastoid muscle or an obliquely

*Reproduced with permission from the publisher.

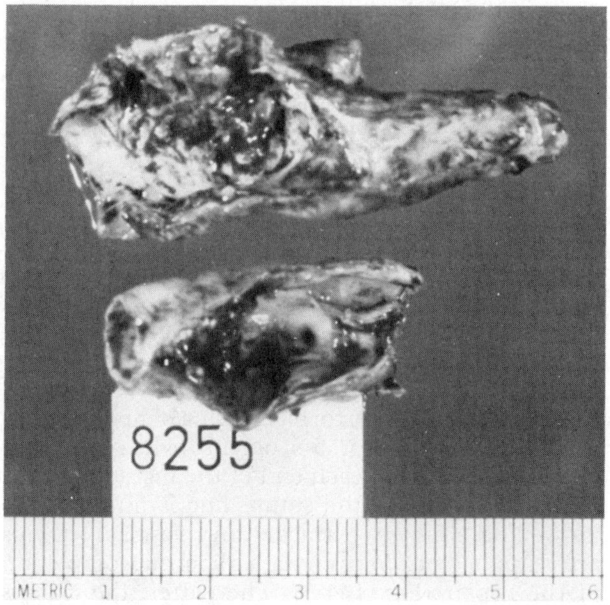

FIGURE 134-1 Ulcerated atheromatous carotid plaque removed from a patient with TIAs.

transverse one corresponding to the skin lines of the neck. The former incision has the advantage of better exposure and is especially useful if a long plaque must be removed from the common carotid artery as well as from the bifurcation. The oblique incision is now preferred by many experienced surgeons, however, because of its superior cosmetic appearance postoperatively. The skin incision is deepened through the subcutaneous adipose tissue and the platysma muscle, while hemostasis is preserved by electrocoagulation of small bleeders. One or more branches of the external jugular vein may be encountered and should be divided and ligated. Care must be exercised to preserve the greater auricular nerve at the posterocephalad end of the incision in order to avoid postoperative numbness of the ear lobe. If the incision is properly placed, there should be little risk of direct injury to the mandibular branch of the facial nerve, but trauma from a self-retaining retractor is a potential threat to that structure. Dissection is carried around the anterior border of the sternocleidomastoid muscle, which is then retracted laterally to expose the carotid sheath. At this time the internal jugular vein is easily visible through the thin fascial envelope. The sheath is entered sharply along the medial border of the vein, dissecting with care in case the vagus nerve should happen to be located anterior to its usual course. As the dissection proceeds cephalad, it is necessary to divide and to ligate the facial vein, which is a useful landmark because it generally crosses in the immediate vicinity of the carotid bifurcation. Once the artery has been identified gentle, meticulous technique is used to expose the common carotid artery and its external and internal carotid branches. It is said that when properly done "the patient is dissected away from the carotid," rather than the reverse. Rough handling of the vessel or careless sponging in the field must be avoided because of the possibility of causing an intraoperative embolic complication.

As vascular tapes are being passed around the internal and external carotid branches near the bifurcation, the carotid sinus may be stimulated. If bradycardia and hypotension result and are not immediately responsive to intravenous atropine, the carotid sinus should be infiltrated with a few drops of plain lidocaine. Systemic heparinization is then effected by the administration of 100 units of heparin per kilogram body weight. Vascular clamps are applied to the three major arterial trunks and a vertical arteriotomy is made in the common carotid artery below the bifurcation (Fig. 134-2). With fine scissors, the arterial incision is carried cephalad into the first portion of the internal carotid artery to a point just beyond the upper end of the visible plaque. If an indwelling plastic shunt is to be used during the endarterectomy, it is inserted at this time, first into the internal carotid artery and then, after air has been flushed out by retrograde blood flow, into the common carotid vessel (Fig. 134-3). The operative field is thus kept dry while blood flows through the shunt, which is secured in place by tourniquet-like fasteners on encircling tapes.

The endarterectomy plane is usually developed

FIGURE 134-2 Location of the arteriotomy incision in the carotid bifurcation.

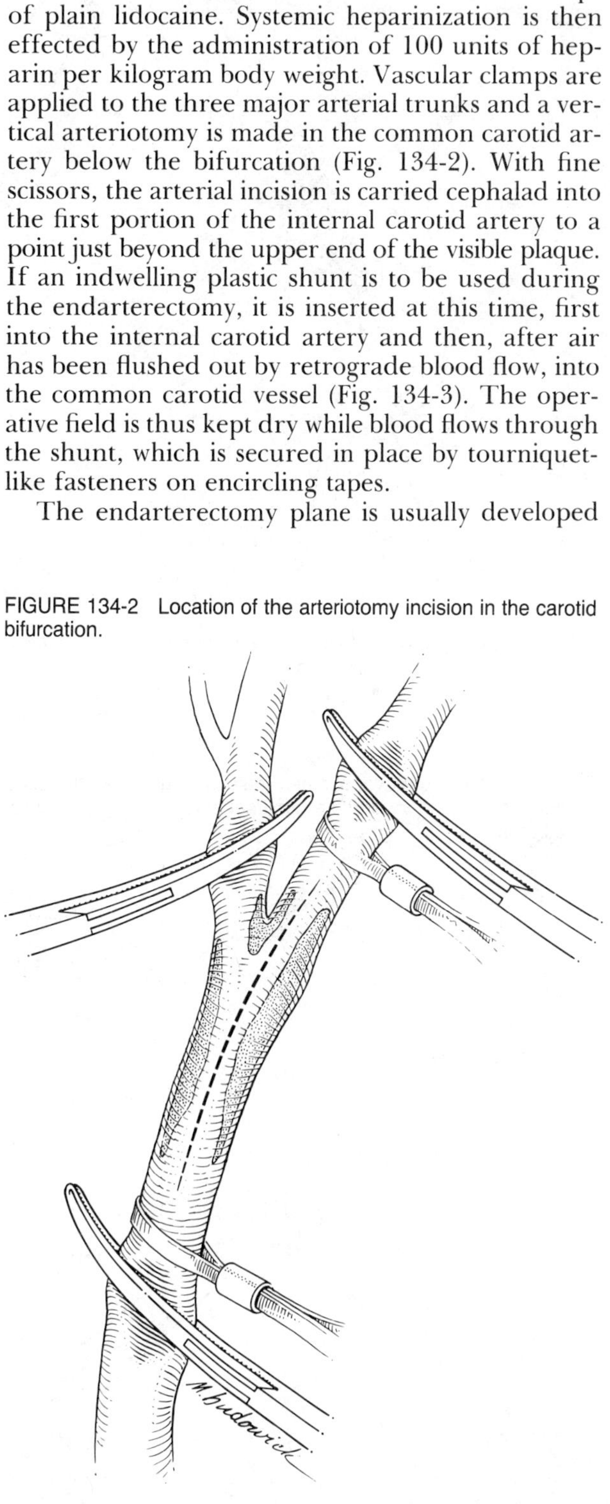

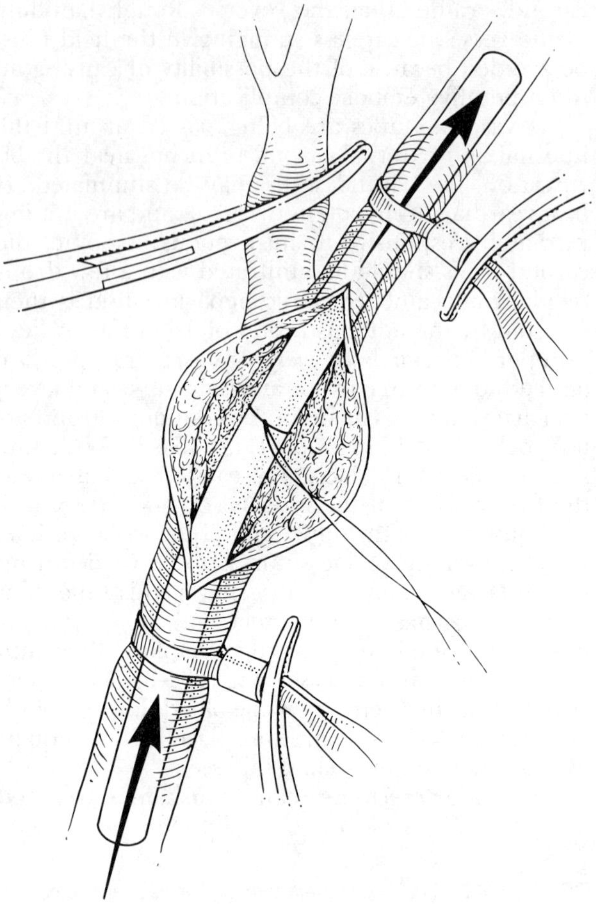

FIGURE 134-3 Indwelling shunt in place to preserve internal carotid flow during the endarterectomy.

FIGURE 134-4 Removal of atheromatous plaque from the distal common carotid artery and the proximal external and internal carotid branches.

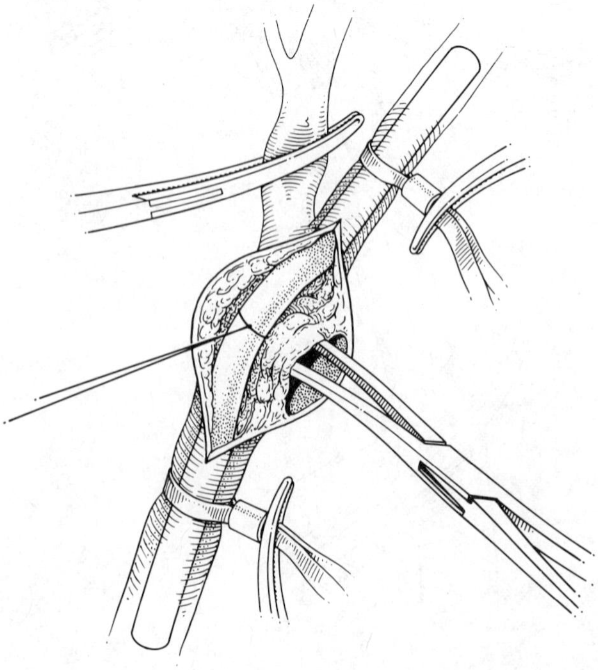

easily in the media, which allows removal of the atheromatous material from the common carotid artery first, the external vessel next, and the internal last (Fig. 134-4). In most cases the plaque feathers to a smooth edge as it releases from the cephalad end, leaving adherent intima as an endpoint in the internal carotid artery. Rarely, circumferential tacking sutures may be necessary to secure an unusually thick or loosened intimal flap. Thereafter, attention is returned to the endarterectomy field, which is thoroughly inspected for fragments of loosened media that might embolize if allowed to remain. The use of operating telescopes to magnify the field greatly assists in this aspect of the procedure. Closure of the arteriotomy is performed with a simple, continuous suture of 5-0 or 6-0 polypropylene, the surgeon suturing from each end of the incision toward the middle. Before the suture line is finished, the indwelling shunt is extracted and vascular clamps are reapplied just long enough to permit completion of the repair (Fig. 134-5). Thereafter, the clamps are removed in sequence, with flow restored to the internal carotid last as protection against any debris or air bubbles that might remain in the vessel. The majority of surgeons proceed at this stage with preparations to close the wound; some delay closure to perform complete angiography or intraoperative ultrasound imaging of the vessel to assure that no technical deficiencies exist. Reapproximation of the incision is done in two layers—the platysma is sutured with interrupted absorbable sutures, and the skin with a continuous monofilament plastic. The wound can be drained by means of a closed suction drain for 24 h according to the surgeon's preference; ordinarily, heparin is not reversed by use of protamine in these operations.

Generally, carotid endarterectomy patients are observed in an intensive care setting for 24 h. In both the recovery room and the intensive care unit, careful attention must be given to fluctuations in blood pressure. Appropriate pharmacologic therapy is begun promptly if any trend is observed toward significant hypotension or hypertension, since either can be associated with an increased incidence of postoperative neurologic deficit. A dilute phenylephrine (Neo-Synephrine) drip should correct hypotension if the blood volume is normal; either a nitroglycerine or nitroprusside drip may be used for treatment of elevated pressure levels. Most patients require little in the way of postoperative analgesia and are able to be out of bed and to return to a regular diet the morning after operation. The majority are discharged from the hospital on the fourth day; usually sutures are removed on the day of release from the hospital. Both aspirin and dipyridamole are prescribed for their antiplatelet effect during the first several weeks following operation.

Among practitioners of carotid endarterectomy the one technical feature that produces the most controversy is whether or not to insert an indwelling shunt intraoperatively. Some surgeons use a shunt on every operation, some on selected patients only;

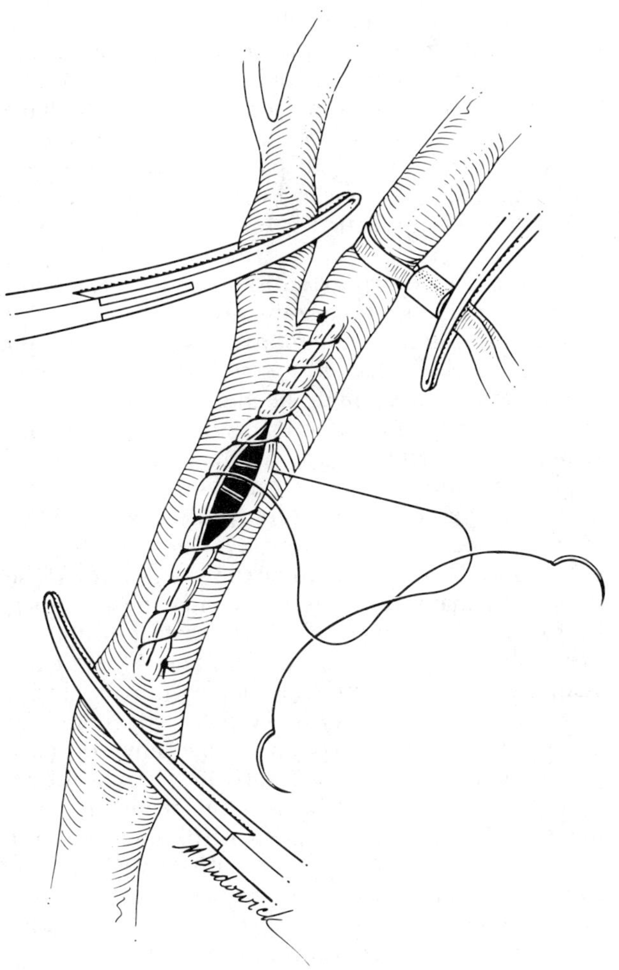

FIGURE 134-5 Completion of the arteriotomy closure after removal of the internal shunt.

a minority never use a shunt but depend entirely on collateral circulation via the circle of Willis. Proponents of the shunt feel that it can be placed with little risk and that it essentially eliminates concern about hemispheric undercirculation during the period of clamping. Opponents of shunting cite the risk of embolization or of intimal injury associated with insertion of the device and also the suboptimal visualization of the endarterectomy field with the plastic tube in place. Those who shunt selectively base the decision upon (1) the patient's response to a trial period of clamping under local anesthesia, (2) actual measurement of back pressure in the internal carotid artery, or (3) changes in intraoperative electroencephalography following carotid clamping.[3–5] It is generally felt that as many as 80 percent of patients can be operated on safely without the use of a shunt; the remaining 20 percent constitute the potentially threatened group. Among surgeons who are not inclined to shunt routinely, it is acknowledged that a shunt should be used in patients with total occlusion of the opposite internal carotid artery and those with a history of previous cerebrovascular accident.

Anticipated Results

Carotid endarterectomy in properly selected candidates provides successful prophylaxis against cerebrovascular accidents. Once the endarterectomy has been performed and the plaque responsible for hemispheric symptoms has been removed, the risk of subsequent stroke in that distribution is greatly reduced. In the patients with TIAs related to a large ulcerative lesion, the risk of stroke falls from approximately 6 percent per year to 1 percent per year following a successful operation.[6] Fields et al. described a randomized series in which operated patients sustained an overall stroke rate of 4 percent compared with 12.4 percent among control patients during the same interval.[7] Other clinicians have reported similar experiences following treatment for transient ischemic attacks, but opinions differ widely and recommendations are far from uniform concerning asymptomatic lesions and those associated with more severe or unstable neurologic states.

Extended follow-up of operated patients has shown a recurrent stenosis rate in the range of 10 percent at the operative site over a period of years.[8] A few patients have an accelerated build-up of myointimal hyperplasia in the operated segment and develop recurrent symptoms leading to early reoperation.[9] The most frequent cause of late death among carotid patients is myocardial infarction; late stroke is a less common source of mortality. Inherent in these long-term results is the clear need for close follow-up of carotid endarterectomy patients in the effort to detect and to treat appropriately their carotid disease and their associated cardiovascular complications.

Complications

Early postoperative morbidity related to carotid endarterectomy can be divided between central nervous system complications and all other problems. The incidence of perioperative stroke is quite low in the hands of experienced surgeons, but even the most senior operator has an occasional unexpected neurologic complication.[10] Fortunately, the majority are focal and transient; they are due presumably to microscopic embolization occurring during the operative procedure or immediately thereafter. All that is necessary in these situations is supportive treatment, since the majority of small deficits clear completely within a few days. Approximately 1 percent of patients, however, have evidence of a more severe hemispheric deficit upon recovering from anesthesia or as a new event developing hours or days following the procedure. Those that occur immediately postoperatively can often be attributed to thrombosis of the arteriotomy site, perhaps due to technical deficiency in the closure or to an unrecognized intimal flap. Such patients can be helped by immediate return to the operating room for reexploration of the arteriotomy.[11]

If the vessel is occluded it should be reopened and a thrombectomy accomplished, probably with the addition of a vein patch angioplasty. If, on the other hand, the artery is pulsating normally throughout its course, an operative angiogram should be performed to search for a correctable defect. When the arteriogram demonstrates an intracerebral embolus, but the arteriotomy site itself is clean, no further surgery is indicated; supportive care is the course to follow in such patients. Hemispheric neurologic deficits occurring later in the hospital stay are more ominous in nature and usually less responsive to reoperation. If the patient is stable, however, a repeat angiogram should be done promptly in the radiology department in order to exclude an actively progressing lesion such as a vessel partially occluded by intraluminal thrombus.

Local complications related to the cervical wound are variable in frequency and severity. Postoperative cervical hematomas are rather common but are generally of little consequence and rarely require surgical evacuation. Wound infections are extremely unusual. Cranial nerve injuries due to transection of such major nerves as the vagus or hypoglossal nerves are rare complications among virgin endarterectomy procedures; they occur with significant frequency among carotid reoperations or in patients with previous scarring of the region.[12] Lesser neural injuries such as those produced by retractor trauma are much more common, if sought, but usually the effects are reversible within a few days. Death in the hospital following endarterectomy is most often attributable to myocardial infarction or to complications of a perioperative stroke. A mortality rate of 1 percent is acceptable, as is a serious neurologic morbidity rate of 1 percent. Even these low rates must be scrutinized carefully, however, in centers where carotid endarterectomy is undertaken in asymptomatic patients. In order to justify preventive surgery of this type, the team must be satisfied that the procedure in their hands carries an extremely low risk of undesirable consequences.

General Applications

Atheromatous plaque disease localized to the carotid bifurcation falls into three distinct clinical categories: (1) asymptomatic stenosis or ulceration; (2) hemispheric or monocular TIAs or fixed neurologic deficits; and (3) nonhemispheric ischemic symptoms. There is general agreement that the subgroup which has the clearest indication for surgical intervention includes patients with hemispheric TIAs or amaurosis fugax, before a permanent neurologic or visual deficit occurs. A second cohort that clearly stands to gain from the procedure includes patients who have had a recent cerebrovascular accident traceable to a carotid source, but who have made a good recovery and would benefit from protection against a recurrent event in the same distribution. Judgment is required in this latter category, however, to restrict the operation to patients with a reasonable life expectancy and a neurologic status worth the risk of operation to preserve. Patients who have had acute strokes are not considered suitable candidates for operation, but patients with "crescendo TIAs" and selected ones with "stroke-in-evolution" are felt to be appropriate for operation by some surgical groups.[13]

Even more controversial is surgery on asymptomatic individuals who are discovered to have large carotid ulcerations or hemodynamically significant stenoses (greater than 50 percent diameter reduction). Such patients might be identified by the presence of an asymptomatic bruit, by positive noninvasive carotid tests, or as an incidental finding on an angiogram done for an associated lesion. If prophylactic endarterectomy is offered to the patient in this circumstance, the referring physician and the surgeon must be confident that the operation can be done with maximum safety and that the patient is fit for the procedure.[14,15] Otherwise it would be preferable simply to observe the patient for the development of TIAs, mindful that an individual with a carotid atheroma very likely also has generalized atherosclerotic manifestations, especially coronary artery disease.[16] The combination of significant carotid and coronary occlusions not infrequently raises the question of proper sequencing of operations for both conditions. The experience of Craver et al. has confirmed that the two procedures may be done jointly under the same anesthesia, if necessary, with no significant change in overall morbidity.[17]

A final category of patients that might be considered for carotid surgery includes individuals with nonhemispheric or global symptoms, such as dizziness, lightheadedness, near syncope, or progressive mental deterioration. In general, this group responds less dramatically to operation, but with careful workup the occasional suitable candidate can be identified with gratifying surgical results.[18]

References

1. Eastcott, H. H. G., Pickering, G. W., and Rob, C. G.: Reconstruction of Internal Carotid Artery in a Patient with Intermittent Attacks of Hemiplegia, *Lancet,* 2:994, 1954.
2. Peitzman, A. B., Webster, M. W., Loubeau, J. M., et al.: Carotid Endarterectomy under Regional (Conductive) Anesthesia, *Ann. Surg.,* 196:59, 1982.
3. Moore, W. S., Yee, J. M., and Hall, A. D.: Collateral Cerebral Blood Pressure: An Index of Tolerance to Temporary Carotid Occlusion, *Arch. Surg.,* 106:520, 1973.
4. Kwaan, J. H. M., Peterson, G. J., and Connolly, J. E.: Stump Pressure; An Unreliable Guide for Shunting during Carotid Endarterectomy, *Arch. Surg.,* 115:1083, 1980.
5. Sundt, T. M., Jr., Sharbrough, F. W., Piepgras, D. G., et al.: Correlation of Cerebral Blood Flow and Electroencephalographic Changes during Carotid Endarterectomy, *Mayo Clin. Proc.,* 56:533, 1981.
6. Moore, W. S.: Surgical Significance and Management of the Ulcerated Carotid Plaque, in J. J. Bergan and J. S. T. Yao

(eds.), "Cerebrovascular Insufficiency," Grune & Stratton, New York, 1983, p. 199.
7. Fields, W. S., Maslenikov, V., Meyer, J. S., et al.: Joint Study of Extracranial Arterial Occlusion, *JAMA*, 211:1993, 1970.
8. DeWeese, J. A.: Long-Term Results of Surgery for Carotid Artery Stenosis, in J. J. Bergan and J. S. T. Yao (eds.), "Cerebrovascular Insufficiency," Grune & Stratton, New York, 1983, p. 507.
9. Stoney, R. J., and String, S. T.: Recurrent Carotid Stenosis, *Surgery*, 80:705, 1976.
10. Thompson, J. E.: Complications of Carotid Endarterectomy and Their Prevention, *World J. Surg.*, 3:155, 1979.
11. Perdue, G. D.: Management of Postendarterectomy Neurologic Deficits, *Arch. Surg.*, 117:1079, 1982.
12. Hertzer, N. R., Feldman, B. J., Beven, E. G., et al.: A Prospective Study of the Incidence of Injury to the Cranial Nerves during Carotid Endarterectomy, *Surg. Gynecol. Obstet.*, 151:781, 1980.
13. Goldstone, J., and Moore, W. S.: A New Look at Emergency Carotid Artery Operations for the Treatment of Cerebrovascular Insufficiency, *Stroke*, 9:599, 1978.
14. Busuttil, R. W., Baker, J. D., Davidson, R. K., et al.: Carotid Artery Stenosis—Hemodynamic Significance and Clinical Course, *JAMA*, 245:1438, 1981.
15. Riles, T. S., Imparato, A. M., Mintzer, R., et al.: Comparison of Results of Bilateral and Unilateral Carotid Endarterectomy Five Years after Surgery, *Surgery*, 91:258, 1982.
16. Heyman, A., Wilkinson, W. E., Heyden, S., et al.: Risk of Stroke in Asymptomatic Persons with Cervical Arterial Bruits; A Population Study in Evans County, Georgia, *N. Engl. J. Med.*, 302:838, 1980.
17. Craver, J. M., Murphy, D. A., Jones, E. L., et al.: Concomitant Carotid and Coronary Artery Reconstruction, *Ann. Surg.*, 195:712, 1982.
18. Haynes, C. D., Gideon, D. A., King, G. D., et al.: The Improvement of Cognition and Personality after Carotid Endarterectomy, *Surgery*, 80:699, 1976.

135

Technique of Surgical Treatment of Peripheral Vascular Disease

Robert B. Smith III, M.D.

It was conceived that if arterial defects were bridged by prostheses constructed of fine mesh cloth, leakage of blood through the walls of the prosthesis would be terminated by the formation of fibrin plugs and would thus allow the cloth tubes to conduct arterial flow.

A. B. Voorhees, Jr.,
A. Jaretzki III,
and A. H. Blakemore, 1952[1,*]

Both the aortoiliac and femoropopliteal arterial systems are especially liable to gradual development of intraluminal atherosclerosis producing segmental partial or complete obstruction. Chronic arterial ischemia of the lower extremities is the result (see Chap. 65). This condition is responsible for a major portion of patients described as having "peripheral vascular disease." Generally, collateral anastomoses in the trunk and limbs provide alternate pathways for blood flow and preserve viability of distal parts as the main vessels become progressively occluded. Eventually, however, atheromatous plaques may produce multiple levels of obstruction or cause interruption of collateral pathways, resulting in limb-threatening ischemia. Although atherosclerosis accounts for the vast majority of patients with symptomatic, chronic arterial insufficiency of the lower extremities, other disorders occasionally come into consideration—congenital anomalies, trauma, embolic occlusion, fibromuscular dysplasia, thromboangiitis obliterans, and a variety of vasculitides.

Typically the patient with arterial insufficiency of the lower limb experiences intermittent claudication as the first symptom, but sedentary persons may have no awareness of occlusive complaints despite total absence of pulses in one or both limbs. Progression of the disorder is slow, but inevitable, over a period of years. Patients may later develop signs and symptoms of more severe arterial insufficiency, such as rest pain or tissue loss. Male patients sometimes experience vasculogenic impotence as a result of aortic or iliac artery occlusion. In the large group of older persons with atherosclerotic peripheral vascular disease there is a high incidence of associated diabetes, atherosclerotic heart disease, and cerebrovascular insufficiency. It is vitally important, therefore, to evaluate each patient's general medical status carefully in order to assess comorbidity and to determine the risk of operation versus other methods of therapy. An alternative form of treatment that is being used with increasing frequency, percutaneous transluminal balloon angioplasty, is especially useful in some patients with localized stenotic lesions of the terminal aorta or iliac arteries.[2]

Once surgical treatment has been chosen, appro-

*Reproduced with permission from the publisher and author.

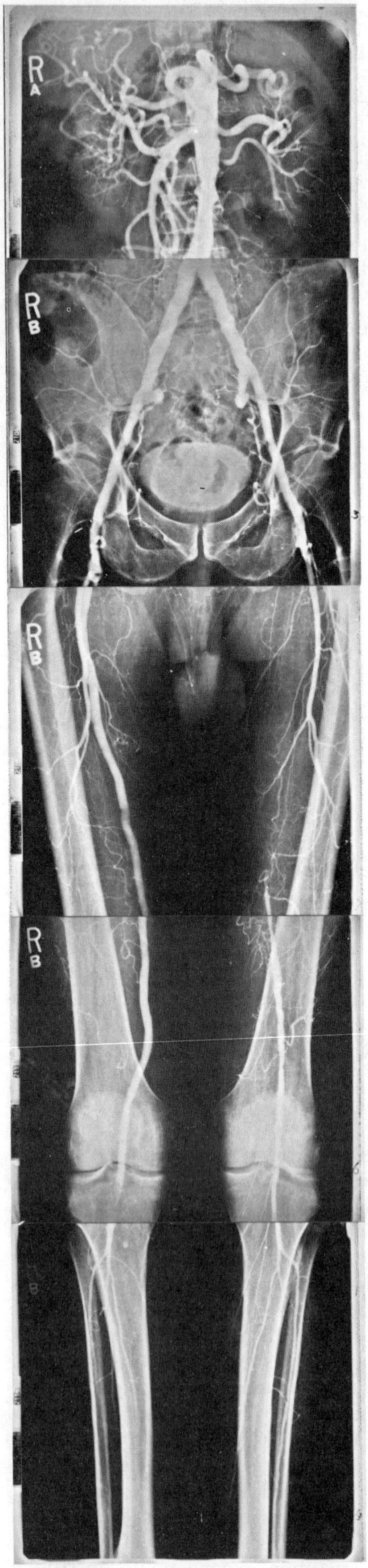

priate preoperative evaluation includes complete angiography of the abdominal aorta with visualization of arterial runoff to the level of the foot (Fig. 135-1). Oblique views of the pelvis and groin may be helpful to evaluate fully the external iliac and deep femoral arteries. In addition to the anatomic assessment by means of angiography, the patient should also undergo physiologic studies in the noninvasive vascular laboratory preoperatively; Doppler segmental pressures, ankle/brachial index, and pulse volume recordings should be obtained in both legs to confirm the suspected arterial insufficiency and to serve as a baseline for postoperative follow-up.[3] If there is a discrepancy between the patient's symptoms and the noninvasive studies at rest, a treadmill exercise test may help discriminate. It should demonstrate a postexercise drop in ankle/brachial index if significant arterial occlusion exists.

Technical Methods

Aortoiliac Endarterectomy

This procedure, first proposed by dos Santos in 1946, is appropriate for selected patients with very localized segmental stenosis or occlusion of the infrarenal abdominal aorta or proximal iliac arteries.[4,5] The vessels are exposed via a standard laparotomy incision and transperitoneal approach. In addition to the aorta itself and the iliac branches, it is necessary to control the respective lumbar arteries and the inferior mesenteric artery in order to minimize back-bleeding at the time of arteriotomy. After the patient has been systemically heparinized the vessels are clamped and the segment to be disobliterated is opened. A localized endarterectomy is then performed with the thin adventitial layer left to constitute the arterial wall (Fig. 135-2). Care must be taken to assure adherence of the distal intima in order to avoid postoperative thrombosis caused by subintimal dissection; intimal tacking sutures or a prosthetic patch angioplasty are acceptable methods to preserve patency of the runoff. The arteriotomy is closed with continuous polypropylene suture, and blood flow is restored to the lower limbs. The operation is then completed by reapproximation of the posterior peritoneum over the aorta and closure of the abdominal wall. The chief advantage of aortoiliac endarterectomy is avoidance of a large Dacron graft with its possible late complications of infection or false aneurysm; disadvantages of this technique relate to the greater extent of periaortic dissection necessary and the longer duration of operation as compared to bypass.

FIGURE 135-1 Aortogram demonstrating generalized atherosclerotic plaque disease with total occlusion of the left superficial femoral artery.

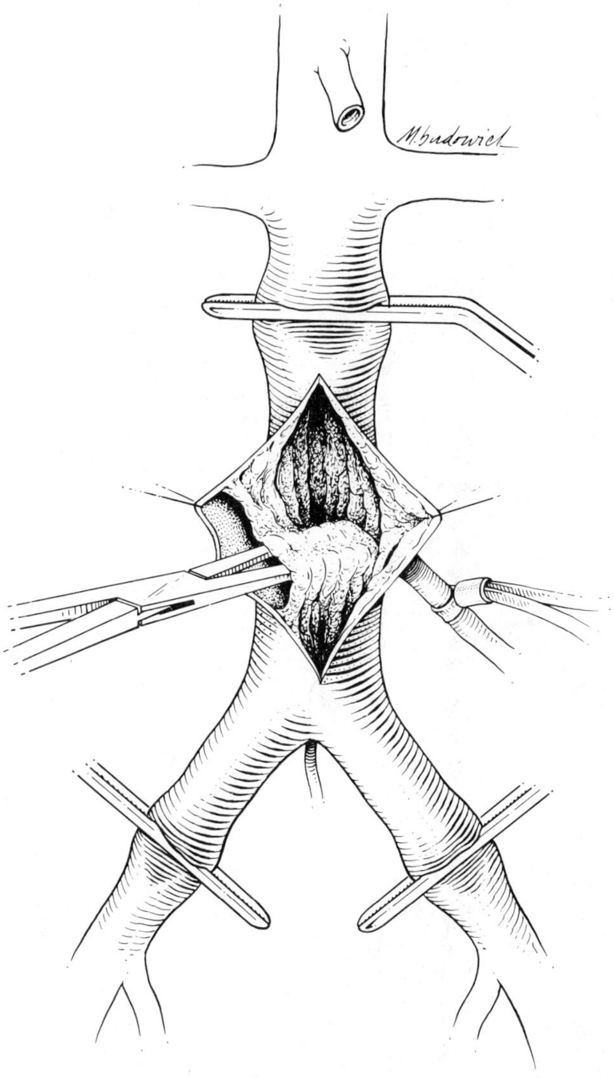

FIGURE 135-2 Aortoiliac endarterectomy may be performed for localized stenosis or occlusion of the aorta or common iliac branches.

Aortofemoral Bypass

This operative technique is selected by the majority of vascular surgeons to revascularize the patient with aortoiliac occlusive disease. Approach to the abdominal aorta is usually made via a long midline incision; the common femoral arteries are also exposed by means of a vertical incision in each groin. Dissection of the aorta is kept at a minimum to reduce unnecessary blood loss and to avoid injury to sympathetic nerves which contribute to sexual function in the male patient. A short segment of infrarenal aorta is mobilized to permit an end-to-end proximal anastomosis with the Dacron bifurcation graft (Fig. 135-3). The diseased aortic segment is not removed but is simply oversewn and bypassed by the iliac limbs of the graft, which are passed via retroperitoneal tunnels into the groin incision on each side. An end-to-side anastomosis is then made between the limbs of the graft and the common femoral arteries bilaterally. Blood flow is restored to the lower extremities slowly in order to minimize declamping hypotension. Before the abdominal incision is closed it is advisable to interpose parietal peritoneum or a flap of omentum between the Dacron graft and the duodenum in order to protect against subsequent graft-intestine erosion. Modifications of the standard aortofemoral bypass procedure are often necessary, including one or more of the following: concomitant patch profundaplasty to enhance runoff from the graft, reimplantation of the inferior mesenteric artery to preserve colonic blood flow, and simultaneous revascularization of the renal or superior mesenteric artery branches.[6,7] The chief advantage of the aortobifemoral bypass is its relative simplicity

FIGURE 135-3 Aortobifemoral bypass procedure, with a Dacron bifurcation graft inserted end to end to the infrarenal aorta and end to side to the common femoral arteries.

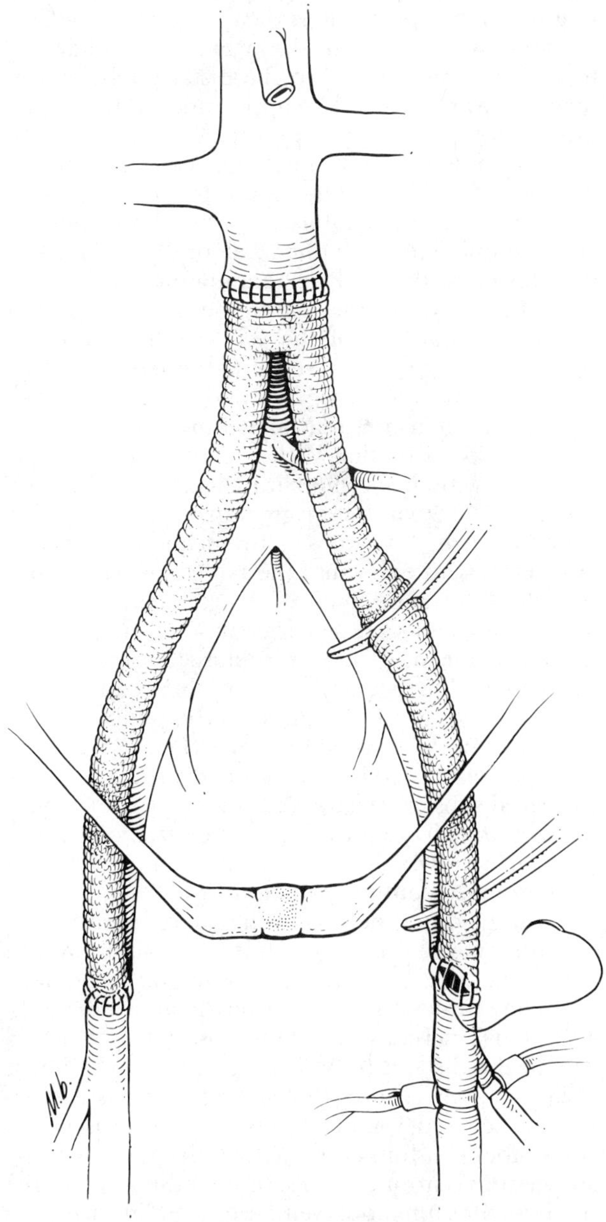

with lessened dissection, shortened operating time, and reduced blood loss. Delayed graft-related problems, especially perigraft infections and anastomotic false aneurysms, are the main disadvantages of this technique, but the incidence of these complications is acceptably low in good hands.

Femoropopliteal Bypass

For occlusive disease distal to the inguinal ligament, revascularization by means of a bypass graft is the preferred surgical approach and autogenous saphenous vein is the conduit of choice.[8] If the subject's own saphenous vein is not suitable or when it is necessary to minimize the operating time because of the patient's general condition, alternative graft materials, such as human umbilical vein, polytetrafluoroethylene (PTFE), or knitted Dacron, may be used. After the conduit has been selected the next important decision to be made is the location of the distal anastomosis, whether to the proximal popliteal artery above the knee or to the distal popliteal segment below the knee. The appearance of the angiogram and the surgeon's personal preference both influence this choice. If autogenous saphenous vein is to be used, a vertical incision is made in the groin over the common femoral artery and the saphenous vein identified at the saphenofemoral junction. It is then dissected distally by extending the skin incision along the course of the vein in the medial aspect of the thigh. Branches of the vein are ligated and a sufficient length of the vessel harvested. After the vein is removed it is irrigated and gently distended with cold, heparinized lactated Ringer's solution to detect leaks. Attention is then returned to the arterial dissection for mobilization of the common femoral artery via the original groin incision. The popliteal artery is exposed by means of a medial approach, with entry into the popliteal space above or below the knee joint. The proximal and distal arterial segments chosen for anastomosis are connected by means of a deep subfascial tunnel. Once the patient has been systemically heparinized, the reversed vein graft is sutured to the popliteal arteriotomy in an end-to-side manner (Fig. 135-4). The graft is then passed into the groin via the previously prepared subsartorial tunnel and the proximal anastomosis done in identical end-to-side fashion. At this point it is advisable to perform an intraoperative angiogram to confirm patency of the system and to rule out technical defects in the anastomosis.

Under certain conditions it is necessary to extend the level of the distal anastomosis to one of the tibial branches rather than to the popliteal artery itself. Additional incisions may be necessary to permit access to the distal aspect of the peroneal or anterior tibial arteries. Autogenous graft reconstruction should be used for tibial bypass, if at all possible, since other conduits carry high failure rates over the succeeding year or two. A recent modification in the method of saphenous vein use, the "in-situ technique," has permitted more successful performance of distal tibial bypasses.[9] In this operation the saphenous vein is allowed to remain in its bed but the valves are incised, thus allowing blood to flow in a direction that permits anastomosis of the larger, proximal end of the vein to the femoral artery and the smaller, distal end to one of the tibial branches.

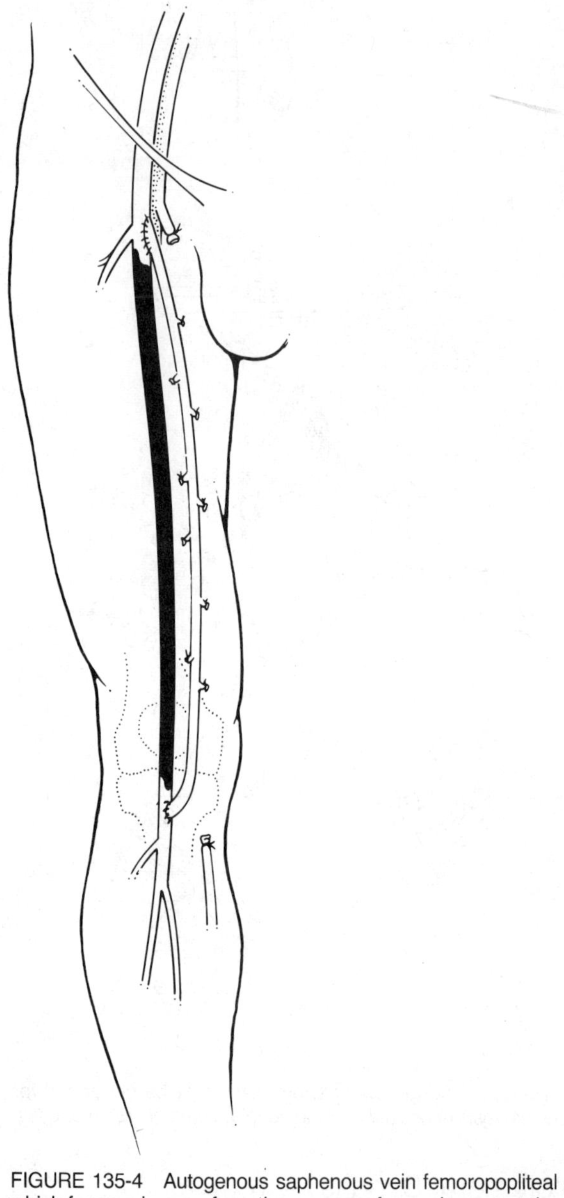

FIGURE 135-4 Autogenous saphenous vein femoropopliteal graft, which forms a bypass from the common femoral artery at the groin to the popliteal artery below the knee.

Postoperatively, the patient is encouraged to begin early ambulation but is cautioned to avoid extremes of knee joint flexion. Frequent elevation of the limb minimizes postoperative lymphedema. If a material other than autogenous saphenous vein has been used for the bypass, aspirin and dipyridamole are prescribed postoperatively for their antiplatelet effect. Regardless of the type of operation performed, the patient is urged to give up tobacco, to follow a low-animal-fat diet, and to maintain optimal control of blood pressure. The vascular surgeon is obligated to follow all such patients periodically on a permanent basis.

Extraanatomic Bypass

In the subgroup of patients with severe ischemia of the leg who are not candidates for direct aortoiliac reconstruction because of extreme comorbidity, an extraanatomic bypass should be considered.[10] These techniques include axillofemoral, axillobifemoral, and femorofemoral bypasses. All three are relatively low-stress procedures in which prosthetic grafts are passed through subcutaneous tunnels to conduct blood from a superficial donor artery to the recipient vessel. Some reduction in long-term patency is traded for a distinctly improved risk at the time of the operative procedure.

Lumbar Sympathectomy

Lumbar sympathectomy is capable of increasing blood flow through a vascular graft to the leg. For that reason it may be performed as an adjunct to bypass in selected patients with severely impaired runoff or those with ischemic lesions of the skin.[11] Sympathetic ganglionectomy may also be offered in the rare patient with advanced occlusive disease in whom definitive revascularization is not possible, but skin blood flow is one of the main concerns. This operation, however, has no place as the primary method of treatment for intermittent claudication, since sympathectomy does not increase muscle blood flow.[12]

Anticipated Results

Aortofemoral revascularization by means of endarterectomy or Dacron bypass results in an excellent long-term patency, exceeding 90 percent over 5 years. Patency rates for reconstructions distal to the inguinal ligament are significantly lessened because of the reduced vessel diameter and the more severely impaired runoff. Bypasses from the groin to the above-the-knee popliteal segment, either of autogenous vein or of one of the substitutes, produce a 5-year patency in the range of 60 to 70 percent. More distal bypasses result in progressively reduced success as the smaller tibial vessels are used; a 2-year patency of 30 to 40 percent is commonly quoted for femorotibial bypasses. Operative mortality for aortic procedures and femoropopliteal reconstructions should not exceed 2 to 3 percent; for distal tibial bypasses, 5 to 6 percent. Perhaps of more significance in terms of patient selection is the fact that these elderly persons with atherosclerotic disease have a diminished life expectancy when compared with age-matched peers from the population at large. Overall, more than one-half of patients followed with severe peripheral occlusive disease are dead within 10 years.[13]

Complications

Revascularization by means of endarterectomy or bypass graft may fail early as a result of arterial thrombosis due to technical difficulties, hypercoagulability, or poor choice of operation related to impaired inflow or outflow. Late graft thrombosis is usually attributable to progression of the atheromatous disease with reduced volume of blood flow. In either the early or late variety of graft occlusion, patency generally can be restored and maintained by prompt intervention. More serious graft-related complications include retroperitoneal perigraft sepsis, aortoenteric erosions, and false aneurysms of the host-graft suture lines.[14,15] When these problems are promptly and correctly diagnosed, they can be treated effectively; otherwise, life and limb may be in severe jeopardy. Less severe complications that occur with greater frequency include lower extremity lymphedema in patients who undergo femoral dissections and almost a 50 percent incidence of disturbance in sexual function among male patients who undergo extensive periaortic dissection.[16]

The majority of cases of morbidity among vascular surgical procedures, both in the hospital and remote from the time of operation, is caused by atherosclerotic heart disease. The responsible surgeon is well advised, therefore, in a patient with severe or unstable coronary artery disease to refer the individual for consideration of myocardial revascularization prior to any contemplated peripheral reconstruction. Since the vascular surgical procedures of greater magnitude carry the risk of serious complications related to blood loss, especially in a setting of preexisting heart disease, it is particularly important to maintain normovolemia intraoperatively and to protect against extreme fluctuations in blood pressure and afterload. Postoperative renal insufficiency, formerly a serious threat in major aortic procedures, has been largely eliminated by maintenance of the hydration of the patient and avoidance of prolonged hypotension.

General Application

Since arterial surgery for peripheral atherosclerotic occlusive disease is palliative in nature, the patient must be carefully selected and the operation individually tailored. Results of the revascularization effort must be superior to the natural history of the disorder over a period of years, and there should be an acceptable risk/benefit ratio in terms of operative morbidity. The principal indication for lower extremity revascularization is limb salvage, although rapidly progressive or disabling claudication may be an acceptable indication in selected patients. In the case of threatened limb loss, retention of a functional, comfortable limb for 1 year or longer is considered successful palliation. Prophylaxis against subsequent amputation, however, is not a legitimate excuse for bypass in the claudicant, as experience has shown that fewer than 10 percent of such patients, untreated, progress to amputation over a period of years.[17] Extended femorotibial bypass and complex operations for multilevel obstructions are not justified for claudication alone, for the reason that long-term patency following these procedures does not support interventions of this magnitude.

In patients who have tandem levels of occlusion of arterial supply to the leg it is important to repair the proximal obstruction first. When there is uncertainty as to the relative contribution of aortoiliac versus femoropopliteal occlusions, the impact of each can be ascertained by noninvasive tests, by transarterial pressure determinations, or by the use of papaverine vasodilation to simulate exercise effect.[18]

References

1. Voorhees, A. B., Jr., Jaretzki, A., III, and Blakemore, A. H.: The Use of Tubes Constructed from Vinyon "N" Cloth in Bridging Arterial Defects; A Preliminary Report, *Ann. Surg.*, 135:332, 1952.
2. Lu, C. T., Zarins, C. K., Yang, C. F., et al.: Percutaneous Transluminal Angioplasty for Limb Salvage, *Radiology*, 142:337, 1982.
3. Kempczinski, R. F., and Yao, J. S. T. (eds.): "Practical Noninvasive Vascular Diagnosis," Yearbook Medical Publishers, Inc., Chicago, 1982.
4. dos Santos, J. C.: Sur la Desobstruction des thromboses arterielles anciennes, *Mem. Acad. Chir.*, 73:409, 1947.
5. Wylie, E. J.: Thromboendarterectomy for Arteriosclerotic Thrombosis of Major Arteries, *Surgery*, 32:275, 1952.
6. Leeds, F. H., and Gilfillan, R. S.: Importance of Profunda Femoris in the Revascularization of the Ischemic Limb, *Arch. Surg.*, 82:25, 1931.
7. Brewster, D. C., Buth, J., Darling, R. C., et al.: Combined Aortic and Renal Artery Reconstruction, *Am. J. Surg.*, 131:457, 1976.
8. Dale, W. A., DeWeese, J. A., and Scott, W. J. M.: Autogenous Venous Shunt Grafts, *Surgery*, 46:145, 1959.
9. Leather, R. P., Shah, D. M., Buchbinder, D., et al.: Further Experience with the Saphenous Vein Used in Situ for Arterial Bypass, *Am. J. Surg.*, 142:506, 1981.
10. Mannick, J. A., Williams, L. E., and Nabseth, D. C.: The Late Results of Axillofemoral Grafts, *Surgery*, 68:1038, 1970.
11. de Takats, G.: Place of Sympathectomy in the Treatment of Occlusive Arterial Disease, *Arch. Surg.*, 77:655, 1958.
12. Rutherford, R. B., and Valenta, J.: Extremity Blood Flow and Distribution: The Effects of Arterial Occlusion, Sympathectomy and Exercise, *Surgery*, 69:332, 1971.
13. DeWeese, J. A., and Rob, C. G.: Autogenous Venous Grafts Ten Years Later, *Surgery*, 82:775, 1977.
14. Goldstone, J., and Moore, W. S.: Infection in Vascular Prostheses: Clinical Manifestations and Surgical Management, *Am. J. Surg.*, 128:225, 1974.
15. Szilagyi, D. E., Smith, R. F., Elliott, J. P., et al.: Anastomotic Aneurysms after Vascular Reconstruction: Problems of Incidence, Etiology, and Treatment, *Surgery*, 78:800, 1975.
16. May, A. G., DeWeese, J. A., and Rob, C. G.: Changes in Sexual Function following Operation on the Abdominal Aorta, *Surgery*, 65:41, 1969.
17. Boyd, A. M.: The Natural Course of Arteriosclerosis of the Lower Extremities, *Proc. R. Soc. Med.*, 55:591, 1963.
18. Hutchison, K. J., Thiele, B. L., Bodily, K. C., et al.: Evaluation of the Accuracy of Pulsed Doppler Femoral Artery Waveform Patterns in Predicting Hemodynamically Significant Disease in the Aortoiliac Segment, in D. E. M. Taylor and A. L. Stevens (eds.), "Blood Flow: Theory and Practice," Academic Press, New York, 1983.

136

Technique of Cardiac Transplantation

John C. Baldwin, M.D.
Edward B. Stinson, M.D.
Philip E. Oyer, M.D., Ph.D.
Stuart W. Jamieson, M.D.
Norman E. Shumway, M.D., Ph.D.

The concept of cardiac transplantation, with its potential appeal for the treatment of patients with end-stage heart failure, has existed for many years. However, its realization as a surgical technique depended on the achievement of several milestones. These included the development of proper surgical technique, the advent of safe cardiopulmonary bypass, the understanding of myocardial preservation, and the acquisition of means for diagnosing and treating rejection.

The first reported cardiac transplant operation was carried out in 1905 by Alexis Carrel, who described vascular surgical technique and performed a canine heterotopic cardiac transplant.[1] Technical refinements were contributed by Mann in the 1930s.[2] In the 1950s, using dogs, Demikhov performed a series of important experiments in which the second heart was placed within the thorax and the recipient heart was excluded from the circulation, so that the total circulation of the dog was assumed by the transplanted heart.[3]

The development of safe cardiopulmonary bypass in the early 1950s made orthotopic transplantation feasible, and in 1960, Lower and Shumway reported the first successful series of canine orthotopic cardiac transplants.[4] Principal elements of their technique included the excision and implantation of the donor heart at the midatrial level and the preservation of graft function using topical hypothermia with saline solution at 4°C.

The problems of diagnosis and treatment of rejection were addressed during this period of laboratory investigation. Immunosuppressive techniques which had been used in renal transplantation were successfully applied in the animal model.[5] Prompt diagnosis of rejection of an orthotopic cardiac transplant is of obvious importance to host survival, and the loss of electrocardiographic voltage, as well as the occurrence of supraventricular and ventricular arrhythmias, was found to be an effective noninvasive means of diagnosing rejection.[6]

The first orthotopic cardiac transplant in a human was carried out in 1964, when Hardy transplanted a chimpanzee heart into a 68-year-old man.[7] Barnard performed the first orthotopic homotransplant in late 1967,[8] and the long laboratory experience of Shumway and his colleagues at Stanford was implemented in a clinical program beginning in January of 1968.

Early widespread enthusiasm for the operation led to the performance of more than 100 cardiac transplants in 1968, but dismal clinical results soon dampened the interest. The clinical program at Stanford continued with parallel supportive efforts in the laboratory, and as of early 1985, more than 350 cardiac transplant operations had been performed at Stanford. The clinical cardiopulmonary transplantation program began in 1981, and 24 such operations have been performed at Stanford as of this writing.

Technique

Several criteria have been established for selection of recipients for cardiac transplantation. Patients should be less than 60 years old and have end-stage heart failure. Life expectancy should be measured in weeks or months, and there should be agreement that all other medical and surgical modalities have been exhausted. There should be no irreversible disease of other organ systems; prerenal azotemia and passive hepatic congestion are frequently seen and generally fall into the category of reversible disease. There should be no active infection. Recent pulmonary infarction is a contraindication, because of the risk involved in anticoagulation for cardiopulmonary bypass and the possibility of infection. Insulin-requiring diabetes mellitus is a contraindication, because of the expected exacerbation with steroid therapy. Pulmonary vascular resistance greater than 8 Wood units precludes heart transplantation because of the inability of the donor right ventricle to sustain function in this setting. The vast majority of patients fulfilling these criteria will fall into the two major categories of end-stage coronary artery disease and cardiomyopathy.

Brain-dead organ donors should be less than 35 years old and have no prior history of cardiac disease. There should be no severe chest trauma likely to have resulted in significant cardiac contusion. Prolonged cardiopulmonary resuscitation rules out the possibility of organ donation. There should be no evidence of infection in the donor.

Proper donor management includes attentive and aggressive intensive care management, with particular emphasis on adequate volume replacement, treatment of diabetes insipidus with intramuscular vasopressin, and weaning of the donor from inotropic support. Inability to wean the donor from pressor support usually signifies unsuitability of the donor heart for transplantation.

The recipient is treated preoperatively with a single dose of cyclosporine orally (18 mg/kg). No other preoperative immunosuppression is given.

The technique used in excision of the donor heart is of critical importance to the success of the operation. A standard median sternotomy incision is performed, and the great vessels are fully dissected. The venae cavae are encircled. Heparin (30,000 units) is administered via the superior vena cava, and a 14-gauge catheter is attached to a bubble-free solution of crystalloid potassium cardioplegia. The superior vena cava is ligated, and the inferior vena cava is clamped. The heart is allowed to beat for three or four cycles to empty, and the aorta is clamped, with immediate commencement of instillation of cardioplegic solution. The inferior vena cava and right superior pulmonary vein are quickly incised to exclude any possibility of distension. Distension constitutes one of the major potentially injurious occurrences for the donor heart. Topical hypothermia with saline solution at 4°C is applied during instillation of crystalloid cardioplegia solution. The heart is then excised, beginning with division of the cavae, followed by division of the aorta at the level of the brachiocephalic artery, the pulmonary veins directly on the pericardium, and the pulmonary artery at its bifurcation.

Since the advent in 1977 of techniques for distant procurement of donor hearts, more than 125 transplants have been carried out at our institution with grafts removed at other hospitals.[9] Simple topical hypothermia with saline solution at 4°C is used for transport; it is our practice to limit donor ischemic periods to less than 4 h.

The original orthotopic technique described by Lower and Shumway has remained largely unmodified and is shown in Fig. 136-1. Standard median sternotomy is employed, and, after heparinization, cannulation of the ascending aorta is carried out in standard fashion. The venae cavae are individually cannulated using a somewhat lateral approach on the right atrium to provide for an adequate right atrial cuff. Snares are placed around the

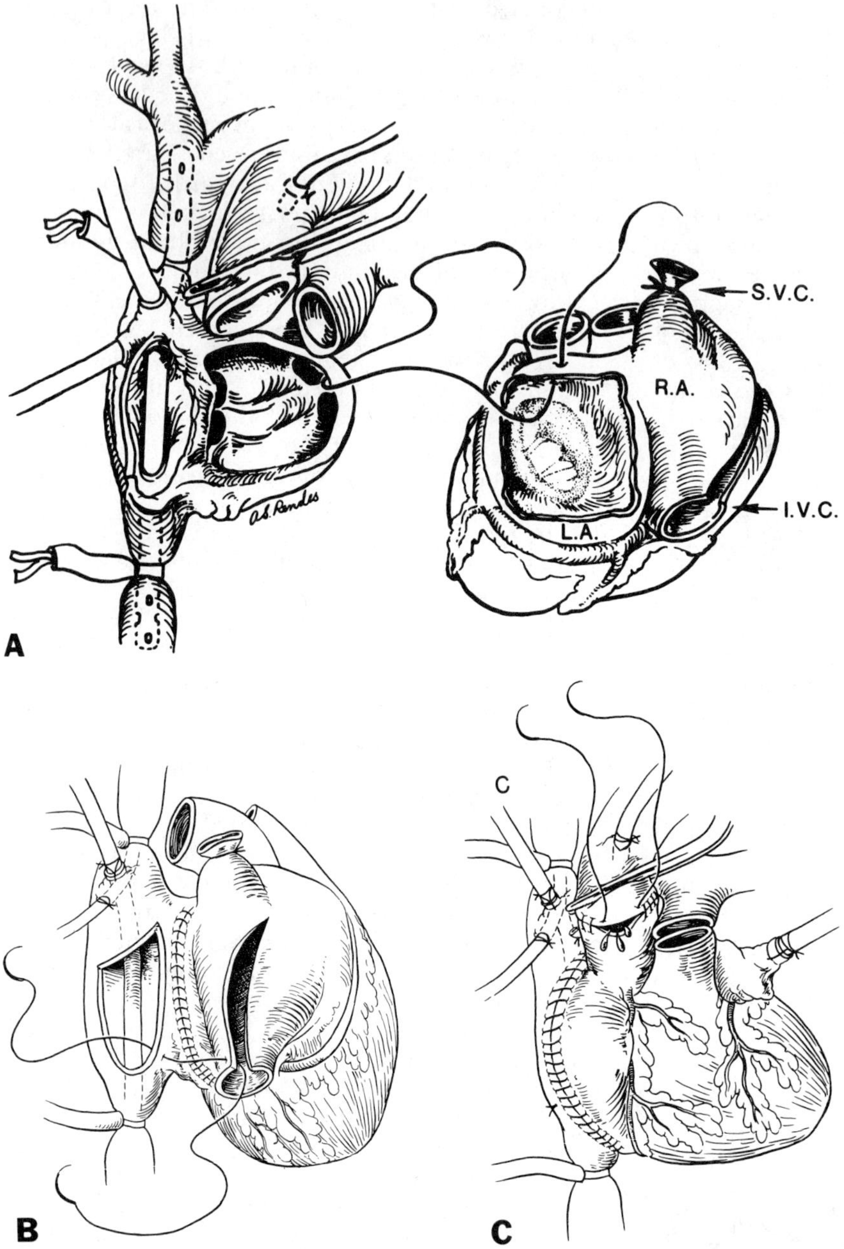

FIGURE 136-1 *A.* The left atrial anastomosis is commenced at the recipient left superior pulmonary vein and the donor left atrial appendage. *B.* The left atrial anastomosis is completed, and the right atrial anastomosis is begun. Note that the incision in the donor right atrium begins through the inferior vena cava and then curves anteromedially, to avoid injury to the SA node. *C.* The atrial anastomoses are complete, and the aortic anastomosis is near completion. The pulmonary arterial anastomosis is carried out last, after removal of the aortic clamp.

venae cavae. The donor heart is prepared by interconnecting the pulmonary veins to form a continuous left atrial circumference and trimming the pulmonary artery and aorta appropriately for the recipient vessels. Cardiopulmonary bypass is instituted, and systemic cooling to 28°C is begun. Caval snares are tightened, and the aortic cross clamp is applied. The right atrium is incised—inferiorly, along the atrioventricular groove to enter the left atrium via the septum, and superiorly, posterior to the right atrial appendage. The aorta and pulmonary artery are divided at the immediate supravalvular level, and the excision of the heart is completed with excision of the left atrium just posterior to the left atrial appendage.

The left atrial anastomosis is commenced at the recipient left superior pulmonary vein and the donor left atrial appendage and completed with a running polypropylene anastomosis. Continuous topical cold saline solution at 4°C is instituted, and a second bubble-free infusion of cold saline solution is commenced into the left atrial appendage to enhance endomyocardial cooling and, more important, to aid in exclusion of air from the graft. The right atrial anastomosis is commenced in the area of the midatrial septum and is carried out with continuous polypropylene suture. The aortic anastomosis is done next, using an end-to-end technique with continuous polypropylene suture. At the commencement of the aortic anastomosis, systemic warming is begun. At the conclusion of the aortic anastomosis, the aortic cross clamp is removed with careful attention to the evacuation of air from the graft (Fig. 136-1*C*).

The pulmonary arterial anastomosis is carried out with the aortic clamp off, using an end-to-end anastomosis with continuous polypropylene suture. The heart is gradually resuscitated, and the patient is weaned from cardiopulmonary bypass.

Clinical experience indicates that donor hearts function best when chronotropic and inotropic support with low-dose isoproterenol is continued for 3 to 5 days postoperatively. Extubation should be accomplished as early as possible, usually on the first postoperative day. Early removal of drains and catheters and early mobilization of the patient are desirable.

Current immunosuppression involves only the use of steroids and cyclosporine. Methylprednisolone, 500 mg, is administered intravenously shortly after discontinuation of cardiopulmonary bypass, and three additional doses of methylprednisolone, 125 mg intravenously, are given at 8-h intervals. Oral prednisone is then begun at 1 mg/kg/day, given in two divided doses. Weaning from steroids is begun immediately, with a schedule gradually tapering to approximately 0.7 kg/mg/day at 1 week and 0.5 mg/kg/day at 2 weeks post transplantation. Patients are generally discharged on a regimen of approximately 0.2 mg/kg/day at 3 to 6 weeks post transplantation.

Cyclosporine is given orally or via nasogastric tube on the first postoperative day at a dose of 16 to 18 mg/kg/day in two divided doses. Dosage should be reduced in the face of impaired renal and/or hepatic function. Cyclosporine levels are monitored biweekly and should be maintained in a range of 200 to 250 ng/ml.

Antithymocyte globulin is not given routinely; its use is restricted in our program to patients with evidence of severe acute rejection or rejection which is resistant to standard steroid therapy.

In patients treated with cyclosporine, previously used clinical criteria for rejection, such as the presence of overt congestive heart failure, gallops, and loss of electrocardiogram (ECG) voltage, may be absent. This is possibly related to the frequent absence of interstitial myocardial edema as a histological finding in cyclosporine-treated patients with rejection. Therefore, the right ventricular endomyocardial biopsy has taken on singular importance in the management of these patients. This technique has been well described,[10] and the apparatus used for percutaneous biopsy under local anesthesia is indicated in Fig. 136-2. Biopsy is carried out 1 week postoperatively and at weekly intervals during the initial hospitalization, so long as rejection does not intervene.

When rejection with evidence of myocyte necrosis occurs, treatment initially consists of methylprednisolone, 1 g intravenously per day for 3 days, and cessation of the weaning from oral prednisone. Rebiopsy is carried out 4 days after treatment. If resolution of histological rejection has occurred, the program of weaning from oral prednisone and weekly biopsy is resumed. If persistent rejection is found, the 3-day treatment with intravenous methylprednisolone is repeated. Cyclosporine dosage is not altered in the face of rejection but rather is adjusted strictly according to serum levels and renal and hepatic function, as indicated previously.

Patients are discharged 3 to 6 weeks postoperatively on cyclosporine and low-dose prednisone, and outpatient follow-up and biopsies are individualized according to individual circumstances.

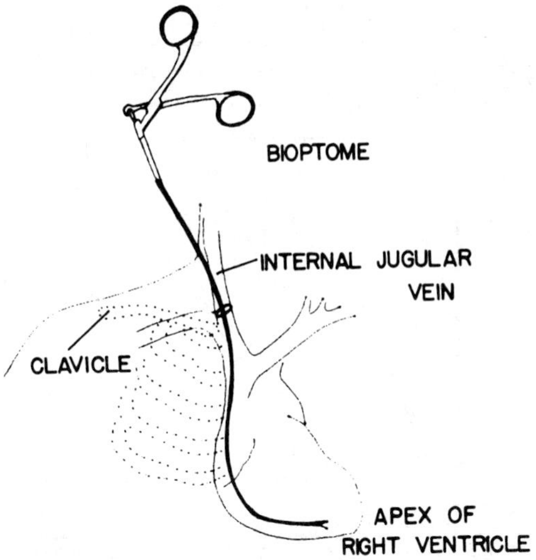

FIGURE 136-2 The bioptome is inserted by a percutaneous Seldinger technique via the right internal jugular vein, advanced under fluoroscopy, and apposed against the interventricular septum for biopsy.

Results

As of this writing, more than 350 heart transplant operations have been carried out at this institution. As indicated in Fig. 136-3, there has been progressive and substantial improvement in survival during the development of this program. Figure 136-4 indicates survival curves for several groups of patients in the cardiac transplant program. The curve in solid squares indicates survival among patients for whom no donor is found. The curve in solid circles describes survival among the first patients receiving transplants in this program. The curve in open circles shows survival associated with the introduction of antithymocyte globulin therapy. The curve in open squares reflects survival since the insitution of cyclosporine immunosuppression therapy in December 1980.

One-year survival has now reached 88 percent. It is of particular importance to note that, in this group of young patients with disease principally limited to cardiac failure and directly associated pathophysiology, full rehabilitation is achieved in more than 80 percent of one-year survivors.

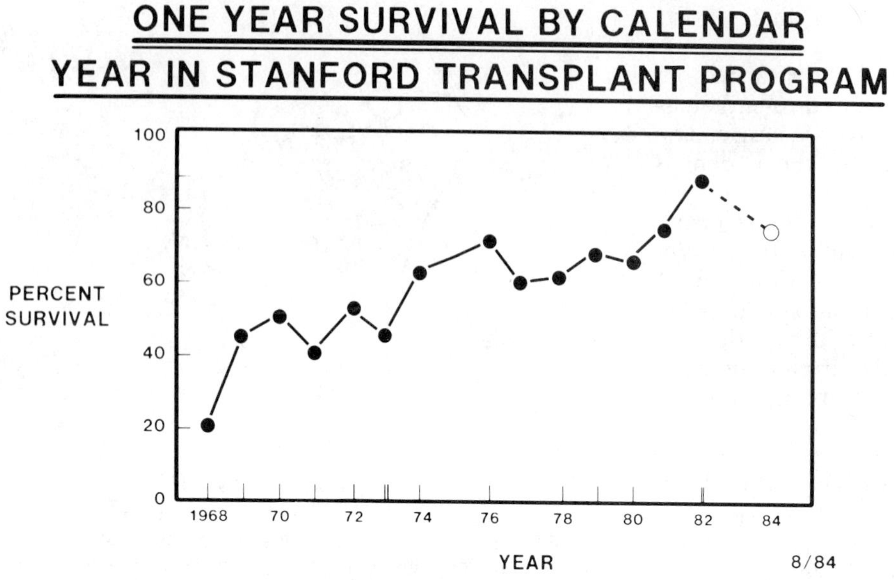

FIGURE 136-3 Percentage of patients surviving cardiac transplantation each year at Stanford. Total operated on is more than 325.

Complications

The primary causes of death in 170 patients who died after cardiac transplantation are indicated in Fig. 136-5. Infection and rejection remain the principal complications in these patients. Rejection is of particular importance in morbidity and mortality during the early period after transplantation. Approximately one-half of the patients will have had an episode of rejection by 1 month postoperatively, and 80 percent of patients will have had rejection by 3 months postoperatively. The methods used for treatment of rejection are described above. In cases of acute severe rejection which is refractory to standard modes of therapy, including cyclosporine, high-dose steroids, and antithymocyte globulin, retransplantation may be necessary. At our institution, five patients with acute rejection have been treated with retransplantation. Three of these patients have survived more than 3 months.

Infection remains the major cause of death in this group, particularly after the immediate postoperative period. The recent experience with infectious episodes, outlined in Fig. 136-6, continues to show a broad range of infections, with pulmonary infections being the most common. As noted in Fig. 136-7, bacterial infections are most commonly seen, but viral, fungal, protozoan, and nocardial infections all occur in this population. The incidence of infection since the institution of cyclosporine immunosuppression has not diminished in a statistically significant fashion, but it is the clinical impression that patients treated with cyclosporine immunosuppression are more responsive to treatment for infectious episodes when they do occur.

Graft atherosclerosis remains a major problem occurring after cardiac transplantation. The bases for this occurrence are not well understood, but two factors which have been correlated with graft atherosclerosis are the age of the heart donor and

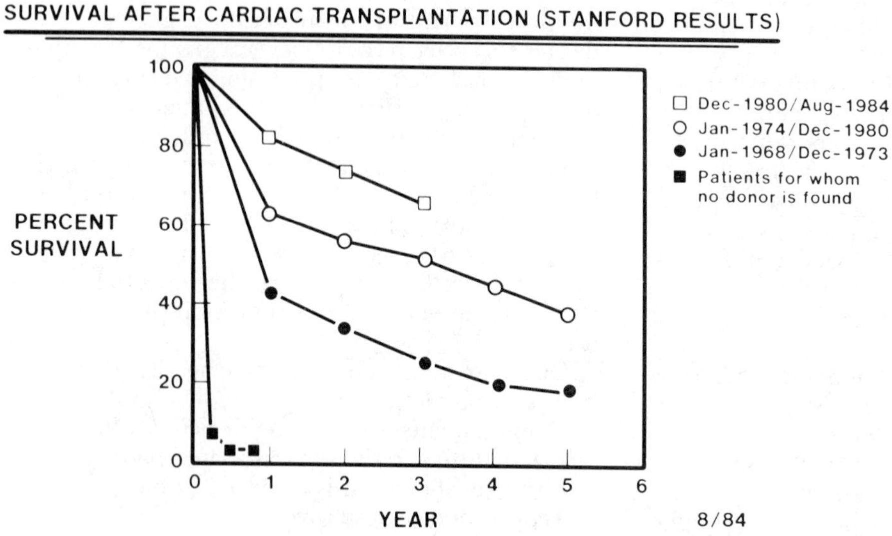

FIGURE 136-4 Survival curves for three groups of patients who have received cardiac transplants, grouped according to time frame in which the procedure was performed.

(n = 307 PATIENTS)	
INFECTION	93
REJECTION	30
CORONARY ARTERIOSCLEROSIS	18
MALIGNANCY	12
PULMONARY HYPERTENSION	7
SUDDEN DEATH	6
STROKE	3
PULMONARY EMBOLUS	2
CEREBRAL EDEMA	1
MYOPATHY	1
SUICIDE	1
ACUTE GRAFT FAILURE	2
HEPATIC FAILURE	1
TOTAL	177

8/84

FIGURE 136-5 Cause of death after cardiac transplantation.

the compatibility of the donor and recipient at the HLA-A2 antigen. It is postulated that an immunologically mediated endothelial injury may result in platelet adherence and formation of atherosclerotic lesions in the the allograft. Dietary lipid restriction and use of antiplatelet agents are of unproven benefit. It is of considerable interest that the incidence of graft atherosclerosis appears to be similar in patients with cardiomyopathy and in those with coronary artery disease as the presenting illness at the time of initial transplantation. The atherosclerotic vessel disease which occurs in these patients is particularly aggressive and prone to be diffuse, involving small vessels. These factors make consideration of coronary artery bypass grafting impractical in this population, and when follow-up catheterization reveals severe atherosclerotic lesions, retransplantation should be contemplated. Fifteen retransplantations have been carried out in our program for graft atherosclerosis.

Heart and Lung Transplantation

The history of clinical efforts in pulmonary and cardiopulmonary/transplantation has frequently included disappointing results.[11,12] Long-standing interest has existed in the area of cardiopulmonary transplantation, and the operation was successfully carried out in laboratory animals in our institution in the late 1950s and early 1960s.[13] Prolonged survival was principally limited by respiratory failure and the interrelated problems of surgical interruption of the lymphatics, pulmonary edema, and rejection. Steady improvement in surgical and immunosuppressive techniques for cardiopulmonary transplantation, good results in nonhuman primates, and clinical success with cyclosporine in heart transplantation prompted the initiation of a clinical cardiopulmonary transplantation program at our hospital.[14,15]

FIGURE 136-6 Sites of infection among cardiac transplant recipients.

December 15, 1980 - March 31,1984	
Pulmonary	50
Septicemia	20
Urinary Tract	20
Mediastinum	8
Retinitis	2
Empyema	1
C.N.S.	1

December 15, 1980 - March 31, 1984	
BACTERIAL	89
VIRAL	63
FUNGAL	17
PROTOZOAN	3
NOCARDIA	3

FIGURE 136-7 Organisms causing infections among cardiac transplant recipients.

The diseases associated with end-stage pulmonary vascular pathological changes are notoriously difficult to treat medically. This spectrum of diseases is broad, and many conditions associated with such pathological changes are not clinically apparent until the pathophysiology is irreversible. Therapy has therefore been devoted in large part to palliation. Two major examples are primary pulmonary hypertension, which is a progressive and fatal illness, and Eisenmenger's syndrome, which cannot be treated by cardiac transplantation alone because of the inability of the donor right ventricle to function with elevated pulmonary vascular resistance. Cardiopulmonary transplantation may represent the best available therapy for these and other conditions associated with end-stage pulmonary vascular disease. The technique for this operation has been described previously; important features of the surgery relate to the safe removal of the recipient cardiopulmonary axis, with preservation of the vagi, the phrenic nerves, and the recurrent laryngeal nerve.[16,17] Meticulous hemostasis, particularly with respect to the bronchial circulation, is of paramount importance, because of the propensity of these vessels to bleed and because of their inaccessibility after implantation of the graft. Topical hypothermia, potassium crystalloid cardioplegic solution, and pulmonary artery perfusion with modified Collins solution are used in preservation of the graft. Implantation of the graft involves a continuous polypropylene tracheal anastomosis, and anastomoses of the same type for the right atrium and aorta.

The immunosuppressive techniques used at our institution are similar to those used for cardiac transplantation, although steroid therapy is avoided during the first 2 weeks postoperatively.

As of this writing, 24 combined heart and lung transplant operations in 23 patients have been performed in our institution, and 14 patients are surviving at intervals of 8 months to 48 months. Early deaths have been related to hemorrhage, renal and hepatic failure, and sepsis. Only one late death has occurred, and this was due to graft atherosclerosis.

Cardiac catheterization carried out 12 months postoperatively has shown normal intracardiac pressures, normal cardiac indices, and normal pulmonary vascular physiology. Initial spirometry and blood gas measurements have been normal, although late follow-up data suggest that some patients may develop both obstructive and restrictive disease in the transplanted lungs.

Summary

Cardiac and cardiopulmonary transplantation have been developed in conjunction with the advances in vascular and cardiothoracic surgery in this century. Because of problems of rejection and its associated complications, the cardiac and cardiopulmonary transplant effort has drawn upon the developments which have occurred in cardiology, immunology, and treatment of infectious disease.

Cardiac transplantation has emerged as a standard mode of clinical therapy, with broad applicability and excellent outlook for survival and rehabilitation. Cardiopulmonary transplantation remains an investigational technique as of this writing. The breadth of its potential application remains to be defined. Improved management of postoperative cardiopulmonary transplant patients will require better understanding of the process of pulmonary rejection and the complex interrelation of pulmonary edema, denervation, and surgical interruption of lymphatic drainage. Furthermore, the long-term pathophysiological sequelae of cardiopulmonary transplantation, particularly in terms of pulmonary function, remain unknown.

Like cardiac transplantation, this modality depends entirely upon the availability of suitable organ donors. Increased public awareness of this need and improved ability of physicians to identify and to manage potential organ donors will facilitate broader clinical application.

References

1. Carrel, A., and Guthrie, C. C.: The Transplantation of Veins and Organs, *Am. J. Med.,* 11:1101, 1905.
2. Mann, F. C., Priestley, J. T., Markowitz, J., and Yaker, W. M.: Transplantation of the Intact Mammalian Heart, *Arch. Surg.,* 26:219, 1933.
3. Demikhov, V. P.: "Experimental Transplantation of Vital Organs," Basil Haigh (trans.), Consultants' Bureau, New York, 1962, p. 126.
4. Lower, R. N., and Shumway, N. E.: Studies on the Orthotopic Homotransplantation of the Canine Heart, *Surg. Forum,* 11:18, 1960.
5. Reemtsma, K., Williamson, W. E., Jr., Iglesias, F., Pena, E., Sayegh, S. F., and Creech, O., Jr.: Studies in Homologous Canine Heart Transplantation: Prolongation of Survival with a Folic Acid Antagonist, *Surgery,* 52:127, 1962.
6. Lower, R. R., Dong, E., Jr., and Glazener, F. S.: Electrocardiograms of Dogs with Heart Homografts, *Circulation,* 33:455, 1966.
7. Hardy, J. D., Chavez, C. M., Karnes, F. D., et al.: Heart Transplantation in Man, *JAMA,* 188:1132, 1964.
8. Barnard, C. N.: The Operation, *S. African Med. J.,* 41:1271, 1967.
9. Watson, D. C., Dong., E., Jr., and Shumway, N. E.: Distant Heart Procurement for Transplantation, *Surgery,* 86:56, 1979.
10. Caves, P. K., Stinson, E. B., Billingham, M., and Shumway, N. E.: Percutaneous Transvenous Endomyocardial Biopsy in Human Heart Recipients, *Ann. Thorac. Surg.,* 16:325, 1973.
11. Wildevuur, R. C. H., and Benfield, J. R.: A Review of 23 Human Lung Transplantations by Twenty Surgeons, *Ann. Thorac. Surg.,* 9:515, 1970.
12. Cooley, D. A., Bloodwell, R. D., Hallman, G. L., et al.: Organ Transplantation for Advanced Cardiopulmonary Disease, *Ann. Thorac. Surg.,* 8:30, 1969.
13. Lower, R. R., Stofer, R. C., Hurley, E. J., et al.: Complete Homograft Replacement of the Heart and Both Lungs, *Surgery,* 50:842, 1961.
14. Reitz, B. A., Burton, N. A., Jamieson, S. W., Bieber, C. P., Pennock, J. L., Stinson, E. B., and Shumway, N. E.: Heart and Lung Transplantation: Autotransplantation and Allotransplantation in Primates with Extended Survival, *J. Thorac. Cardiovasc. Surg.,* 80:360, 1980.
15. Jamieson, S. W., Burton, N. A., Oyer, R. E., et al.: Cardiac Allograft Survival in Primates Treated with Cyclosporin A., *Lancet,* 1:545, 1979.
16. Baldwin, J. C., Jamieson, S. W., Stinson, E. B., Oyer, P. E., and Shumway, N. E.: Cardiopulmonary Transplantation: *Cardiovasc. Rev. Results,* 5(2):148, 1984.
17. Jamieson, S. W., Baldwin, J. C., Reitz, B. A., et al.: Combined Heart and Lung Transplantation, *Lancet,* 1:1130, 1983.

137

Technique of Using the Mechanical Heart

William C. DeVries, M.D.

History of Development of the Total Artificial Heart

On December 1, 1982, in Salt Lake City, Utah, an artificial heart was placed in the chest of a 61-year-old man suffering from end-stage cardiomyopathy (Fig. 137-1). This patient lived 112 days before expiring of complications of antibiotic therapy.[1–4] This represented one additional step in a long history of assisted circulation, which began with experimental prototypes as suggested by Lindberg,[5] Dale and Shuster,[6] and DeBakey.[7] Akutsu and Kolff[8] placed a pneumatically driven artificial heart made of polyvinyl chloride in dogs' chests as early as 1957. One animal survived 90 min. Over 400 sheep and calves at the University of Utah School of Medicine have had artificial hearts implanted within the last 15 years. Several have survived for periods longer than 9 months with no evidence of infection or significant degradation of blood products.[9,10] In vitro testing of the device has shown only moderate degeneration in mock circulations driven continuously for up to 4 years.[5]

A temporary pneumatic artificial heart was implanted by Cooley, in 1969, in a 47-year-old man who could not be weaned from cardiopulmonary bypass after resection of a large ventricular aneurysm. The patient lived 64 h with the artificial heart and died of overwhelming pneumonia shortly after a heart transplant.[11] Dr. Cooley implanted another model of a pneumatic artificial heart into a young Dutch patient who had sustained a cardiac arrest in the surgical intensive care unit after three-vessel coronary artery bypass grafting in July 1981. This patient survived 72 h before a heart transplant could be performed. The patient expired several days thereafter.[12] These two experiments demonstrated the feasibility of the pneumatic heart as an interim life-sustaining device for the patient awaiting cardiac transplant.

Within the past 20 years, more than 200 million dollars in federal funds have been expended in the United States in research leading to the development of a clinically available artificial heart.

Technical Methods

The current model of the Utah Artificial Heart (Jarvik 7) has been developed over a 20-year period and has involved input from over 250 investigators. The device consists of separate right and left ventricles composed of rigid polyurethane cases with flexible polyurethane pumping diaphragms and four size-29 Medtronic Hall valves with pyrolytic carbon disks (two inflow and two outflow) (Fig. 137-2). It displaces 680 cm^3 of chest volume. A maximum stroke volume of approximately 100 ml may be developed from each side; this varies with inflow pressures and thereby responds in a Frank-Starling manner. The device is inherently sensitive to preload and afterload. Inflow pressures of 5 to 7 mmHg will generate a cardiac output of 4 to 5 liters/min while inflow pressures of 10 to 15 mmHg will automatically result in cardiac outputs of 12 to 13 liters/min without a change of heart rate[5,12] The pump is connected to an external drive system by two $\frac{3}{8}$-in tubes 2.46 m in length. The heart is designed with anatomic transitions to the intact right and left atrium and great vessels via Dacron grafts. Specially designed skin buttons allow tissue ingrowth at the junction of the skin sites and the drive lines. These buttons have been shown to be successful in the prevention of infection of the prosthesis in many animals.[13]

The driving system delivers compressed air or nitrogen from standard hospital outlets or auxillary air tanks. Electric output and air pressures are backed up by alternate sources that compensate immediately in the event of power or air pressure failure. The heart rate may be pulsed from 0 to 299 beats per minute. The left and right ventricular pressures and rates may be varied independently. The air pressure from the driving system can be increased or decreased and subsequently causes the ventricular blood pressure to vary directly with this change. The present drive system weighs 113 kg (250 lb) and is approximately the size and mobility of an intraaortic balloon pump (Fig. 137-3). By utilizing a pneumotachograph on the exhausts of the drive system, instantaneous stroke volumes (and subsequently cardiac outputs) may be determined (Figs. 137-4 and 137-5). This method is unique and was recently developed by the University of Utah Institute for Biomedical Research for use in the Utah artificial heart drive system. A portable drive system will be used for the next patient on a temporary basis. This drive system weighs approximately 5.4 kg (12 lb) and has a rechargeable battery life of up to 4 h (Fig. 137-6).

Surgical Implantation

The patient is anesthetized, the chest is opened through a standard median sternotomy, and the patient is placed on cardiopulmonary bypass. The pa-

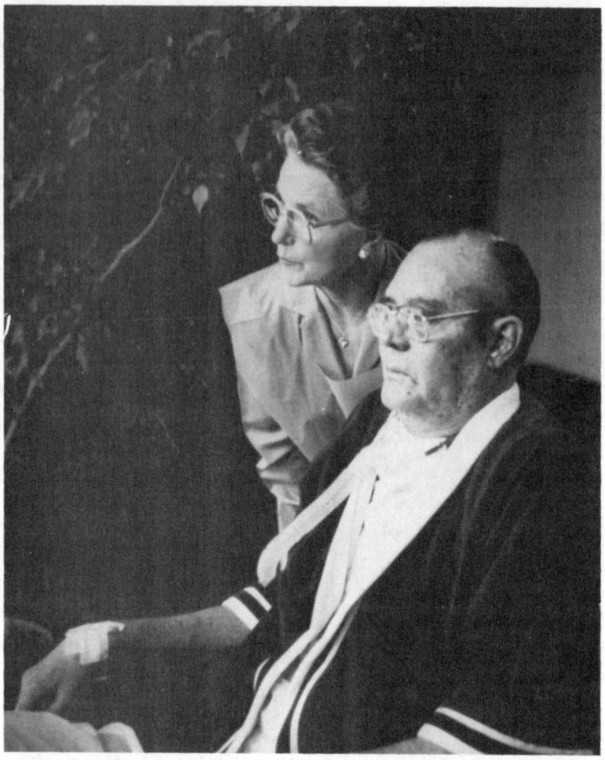

FIGURE 137-1 Dr. Barney B. Clark, with Mrs. Clark, in postoperative period. (*Reproduced with permission of Mrs. Barney B. Clark.*)

tient's diseased right and left ventricles are removed by separating these chambers from the atrium at the atrioventricular (AV) groove. The pulmonary artery and the aorta are each divided above the valves and the four Dacron cuffs of the artificial prosthesis are sewn into position with prolene sutures (Fig. 137-2). The two drive lines are brought through separate stab wounds in the left periumbilical area. The patient is weaned from bypass, and the chest is closed.

Expected Results

The preoperative and postoperative chest x-rays are shown in Figs. 137-7 and 137-8. The patient with the total artificial heart demonstrates remarkably "natural" hemodynamics (Fig. 137-9). The prosthesis is sensitive to preload and afterload, which results in various stroke volumes depending upon the volume in the natural atrium. In the case of the first patient at Utah, cardiac outputs were adjusted to 6.5 liters/min with a cardiac index of 3.2 liters/min/m^2. The heart rate was 95 beats per minute; systemic blood pressure was 124/60 mmHg, with a left atrial mean pressure of 12 mmHg, a pulmonary artery pressure of 36/20 mmHg, and a right atrial pressure of 12 mmHg. A postoperative ejection fraction of 77 percent was reported by radionuclide angiocardiogram, as opposed to a preoperative value of 8 percent. During the second month of life with the artificial heart, it became increasingly difficult to vary the cardiac output and arterial pressures by manipulating the drive system. In the early postoperative days, small intravascular infusions of fluid (300 ml) would result in 1- to 2-liter/min changes in cardiac output or corresponding increases in the systemic arterial pressures. During the second month, changes of up to 2 liters in intravascular volume

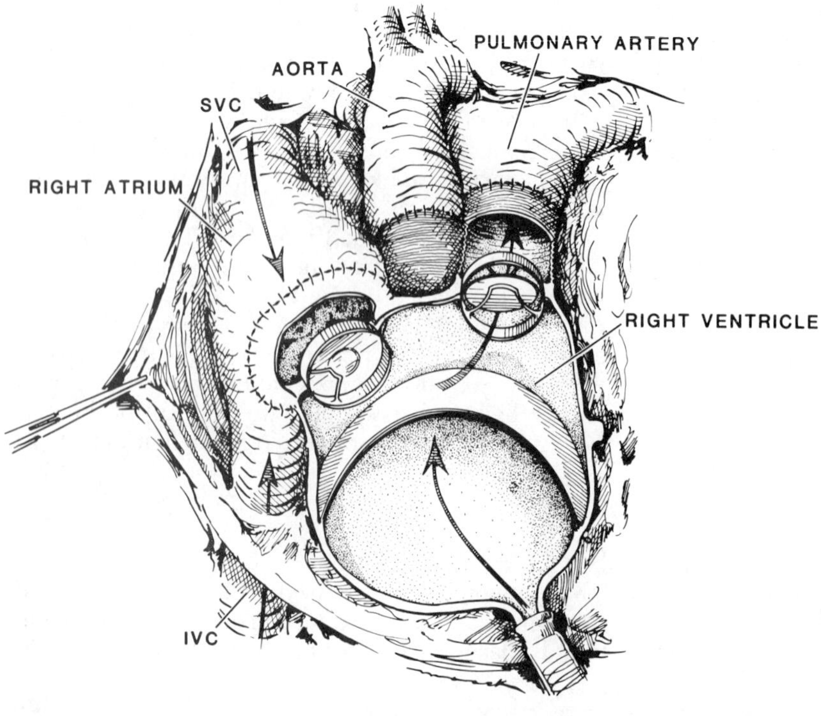

FIGURE 137-2 Cut-away drawing of the implanted right ventricle.

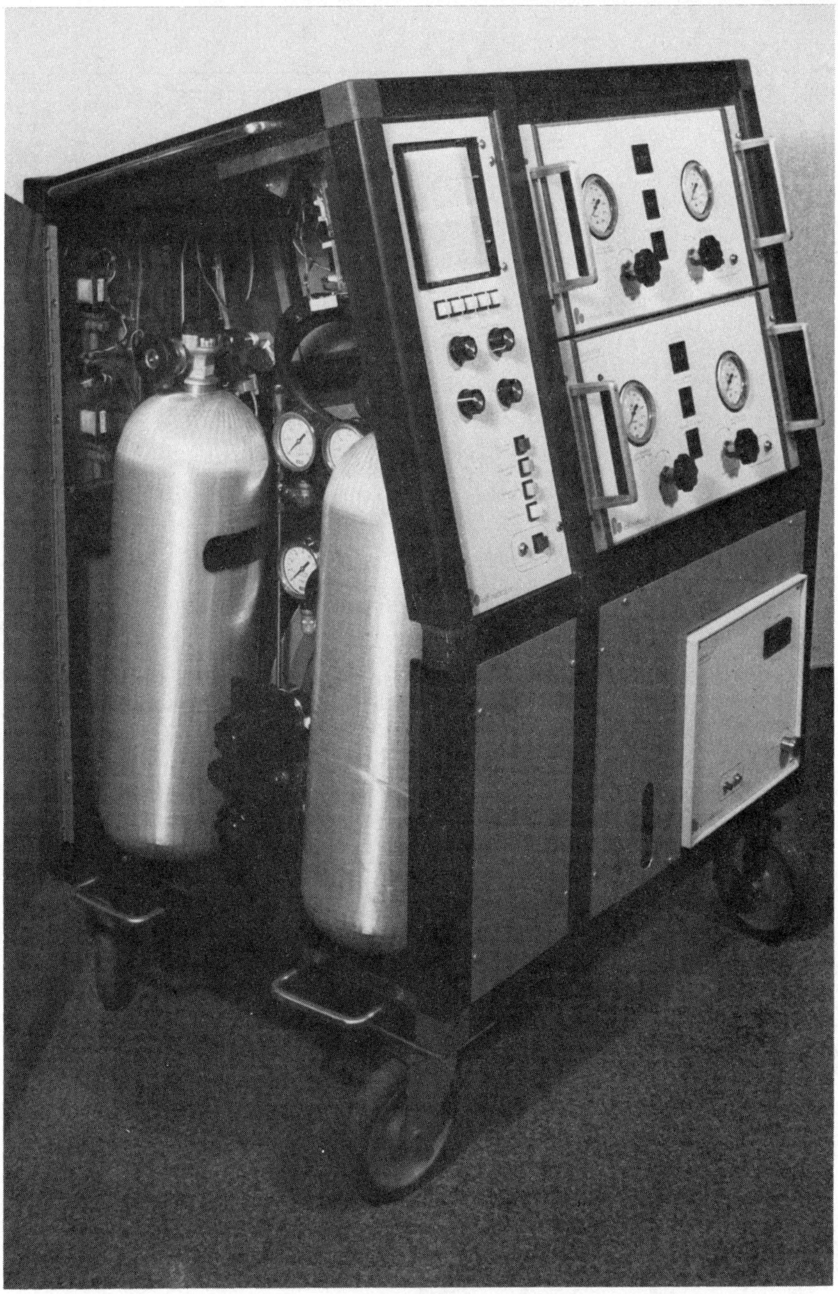

FIGURE 137-3 Utah external drive system.

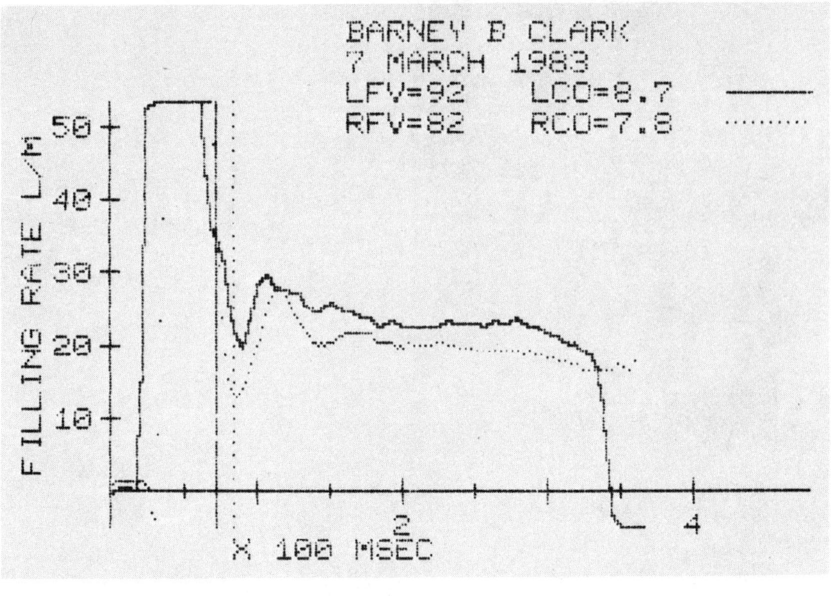

FIGURE 137-4 Recording of simultaneous stroke volumes of left and right ventricles as determined by measurement of exhausted gas. (*This record, showing Barney B. Clark's name, is reproduced with the permission of Mrs. Barney B. Clark.*)

1	95	L	85	8.1	R	72	6.8	84 %
2	95	L	87	8.3	R	69	6.6	79 %
3	95	L	77	7.3	R	63	6	81 %
4	95	L	92	8.7	R	86	8.2	93 %
5	95	L	60	5.7	R	47	4.5	78 %
6	95	L	27	2.6	R	47	4.5	174%
7	95	L	86	8.2	R	66	6.3	76 %
8	95	L	13	1.2	R	32	3	246%
9	95	L	94	8.9	R	76	7.2	80 %
10	95	L	86	8.2	R	66	6.3	76 %
AVERG		L	70	6.7	R	62	5.9	88 %

FIGURE 137-5 Continuous record of stroke volumes and cardiac output as the patient stands erect. First column represents stroke count; second column, heart rate; third column, ventricle side; fourth column, stroke volume (ml); fifth column, cardiac output (liters/min); sixth column, ventricle side; seventh column, stroke volume (ml); eighth column, cardiac output (liters/min); ninth column, percentage of left to right side outputs.

would not change the cardiac output or blood pressure. The peripheral vascular circulation became exceedingly reactive with recovery. Small elevations in blood pressure would result in vascular dilatation and homeostatic return to premanipulation levels. This phenomenon had not been noticed before in animals. These observations were not confirmed with physiological measurements of peripheral and systemic vascular resistances because of our reluctance to reinstrument the patient at this time. Such invasive studies seemed unwarranted in view of our overall objective of survival and desire to establish an adequate quality of life for this, the first patient in our series of artificial heart implantations.

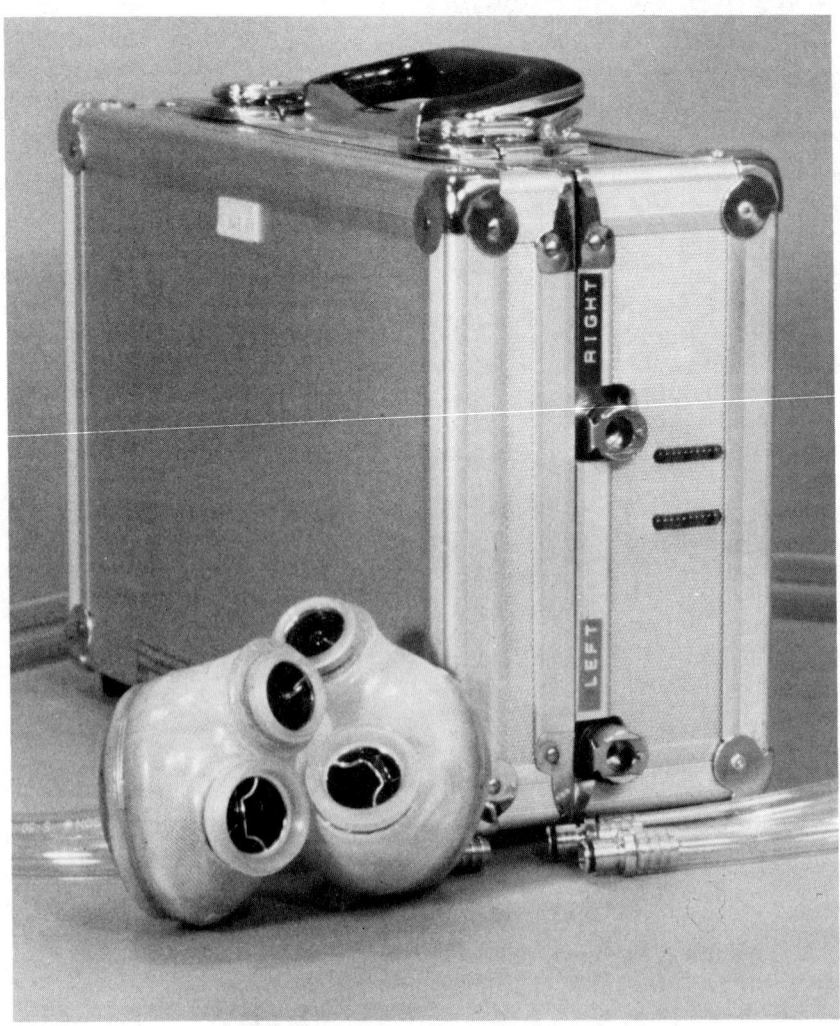

FIGURE 137-6 Heimes portable drive system.

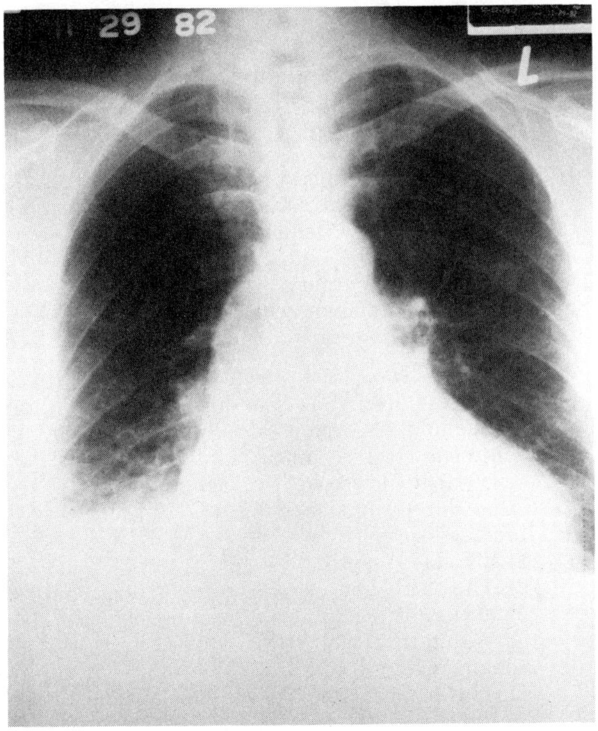

FIGURE 137-7 Preoperative chest x-ray.

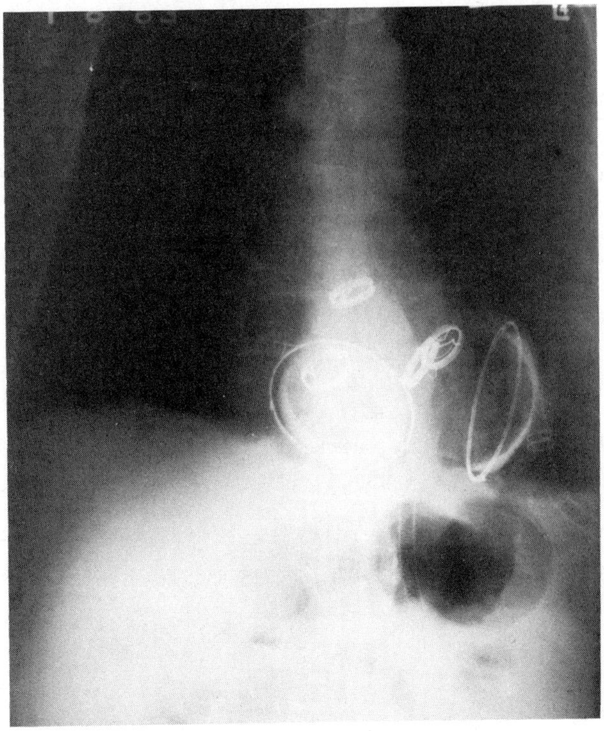

FIGURE 137-8 Postoperative chest x-ray.

A very useful therapy in patient care is the ability to vary the output of the right side of the heart independent of that of the left. Pulmonary edema may be avoided by simply turning down cardiac output of the right side and increasing cardiac output of the left.

Hematologically, platelet counts are initially suppressed by the cardiopulmonary bypass, but usually by day 20 counts have returned to normal (Fig. 137-10). Levels of lactic acid dehydrogenase (LDH) are initially elevated because of the cardiopulmonary bypass but stabilize at 300 to 400 units for most of the postoperative course. The plasma hemoglobin levels rapidly return to normal. Daily hematocrits vary but usually remain at 30 to 34 percent without transfusion. The level of hemolysis caused by the device appears to be well tolerated by the reticuloendothelial system (Fig. 137-11). Patients with artificial hearts may expect a low level of well-compensated disseminated intravascular coagulation.

The patient will surely undergo significant changes in lifestyle. He or she will be taken from a stage IV cardiac patient to stage II with the device. The patient must, however, be content with a life tethered to a machine, with all the mechanical and psychological restrictions involved.

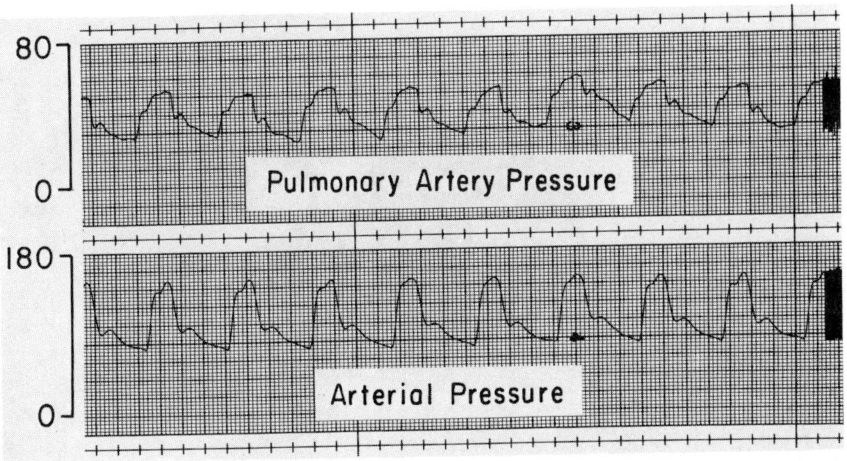

FIGURE 137-9 Postoperative aortic and pulmonary arterial pressure waveforms.

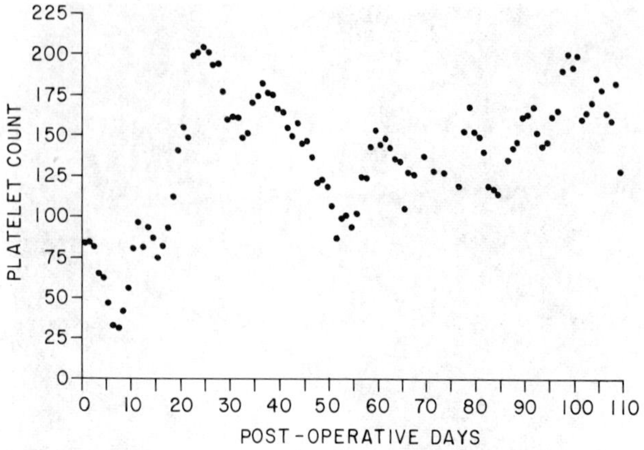

FIGURE 137-10 Daily platelet counts during hospital course.

FIGURE 137-11 Daily hematocrit, LDH, and plasma hemoglobin values.

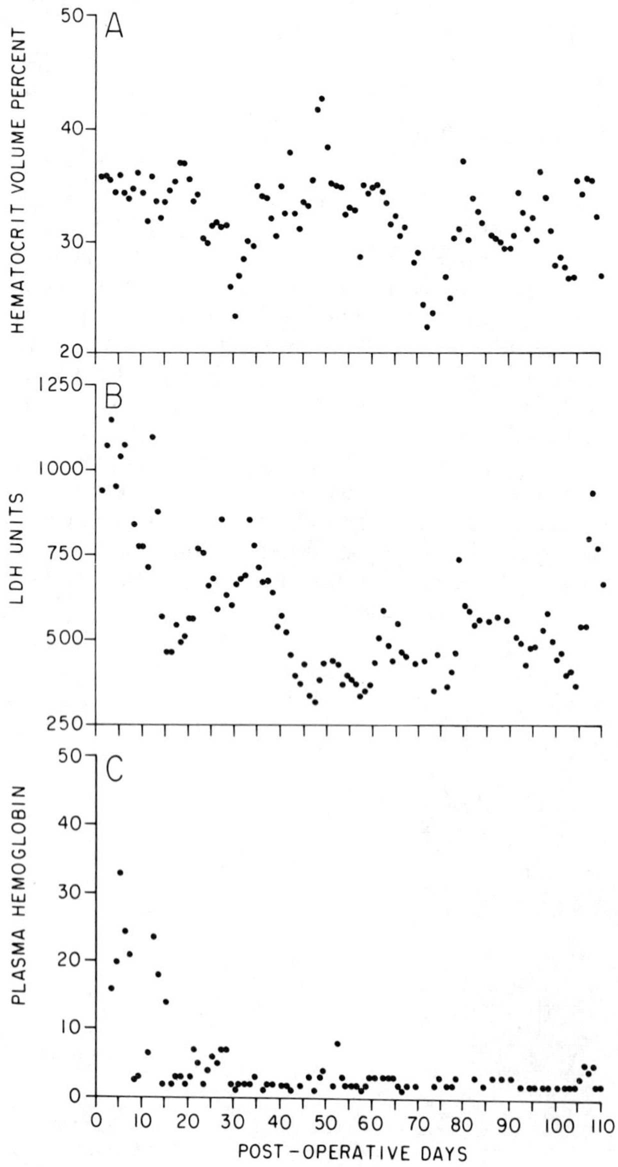

Complications

A review of the possible complications may be obtained by referring to the following paragraphs of the patient consent form.

> I have also been informed of the substantial risks involved in cardiovascular surgery and the administration of general anesthesia, and understand that there are additional risks beyond those normally associated with cardiovascular surgery, as a result of a Total Artificial Heart implantation, which may result in serious bodily impairment, or death. These risks include:

(a) Emboli or blood clots which may lead to stroke, kidney loss, liver, bowel or lung dysfunction, or damage to other organs or body functions.
(b) Malfunction or mechanical failure of the Total Artificial Heart device or breakage of the Total Artificial Heart valves. [See Fig. 137-12.]
(c) Infection of:
  (1) My blood (sepsis)
  (2) The drive lines to the Total Artificial Heart device, or
  (3) Within the Total Artificial Heart itself
(d) Hemorrhage resulting from:
  (1) The action of the Total Artificial Heart upon the vessels
  (2) Surgery to expose the natural heart
  (3) Deficiencies in the blood clotting mechanisms secondary to the Total Artificial Heart
  (4) Anticoagulation medication
(e) Damage to:
  (1) The red blood cells (that carry oxygen and carbon dioxide)
  (2) The platelets (that cause blood to clot)
  (3) White blood cells (that act as scavengers against foreign substances and provide for immunization) which might cause a change in my blood immune system or anemia
(f) Pneumothorax (air in the chest cavity from my lungs or as a result of leakage from the Total Artificial Heart itself). This may result in breathing difficulties requiring a separate tube(s) to be placed in my chest or an operation to treat the defect.
(g) Seizures or convulsions due to emboli, metabolic

FIGURE 137-12 Broken Bjork-Shiley valve strut with embolus of valve disk.

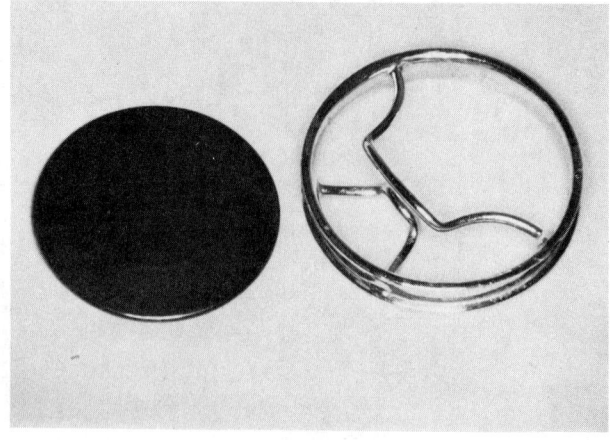

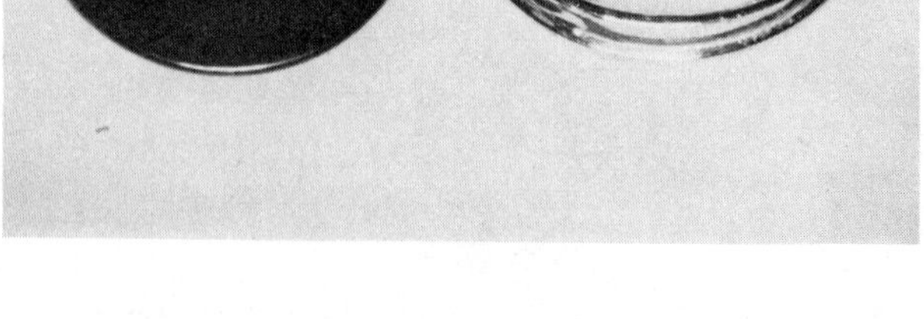

imbalance or blood flow imbalances from the Total Artificial Heart placed in my chest.

(h) Renal failure or inability of my kidneys to excrete metabolic waste products or fluids.

(i) Pulmonary insufficiency causing shortness of breath or necessitating prolonged respirator support.

Because this is a highly experimental procedure other unforseeable risks may arise, and the above listed potential problems should be considered only as illustrative, and not all inclusive.

I further recognize that this procedure is *experimental*. Similar Total Artificial Heart devices have been implanted in two patients in other institutions as temporary emergency, life-prolonging procedures until heart transplants could be obtained. The devices used in these patients were not the model of the Total Artificial Heart which will be used in my case. With these two patients the artificial heart was removed and a heart transplant performed, and both of these patients died within one week from complications.

On December 1, 1982, a 61 year old dentist, Dr. Barney Clark, had his failing natural heart removed and a Total Artificial Heart implanted. His Total Artificial Heart was similar to the one that I will have implanted in me, except that the heart valves are a different type. Dr. Clark lived for 112 days in the University Hospital until his death which resulted from infection. During his life with the Total Artificial Heart, Dr. Clark experienced kidney and lung problems, a pneumothorax (air in the lung cavity), valve breakage, seizures, bleeding complications and depression. He remained hospitalized during the entire 112 day period. The medical team at the University of Utah have thoroughly discussed Dr. Clark's case with me and have answered all of my questions concerning the case to my satisfaction.

General Applications

A review of the significant advances within the last 5 years of experimentation with the total artificial heart in animals is impressive. Animals with total artificial hearts implanted appeared to be normal in all aspects (except for their tethers). Development in mechanical drive systems has shown significant trends in reduction of size, portability, noise reduction, and durability. Animal experimental yield appeared at a plateau at the University of Utah Medical Center. Human experimentation was the next natural step in the development of the clinically usable artificial heart.

Approval was obtained for the use of the total artificial heart in a clinical series of seven patients from the University of Utah Institutional Review Board and the Federal Drug Administration after approximately $2\frac{1}{2}$ years of negotiation and clinical protocol changes. Two main groups of candidates have been identified. The first group is represented by a high-risk patient failing to be weaned from cardiopulmonary bypass after cardiac surgery. After a specific resuscitation protocol has been met in a patient who had previously signed the consent form for the artificial heart, the natural heart would be removed and the total artificial heart would be implanted. Under this protocol, four patients have been taken to surgery, but none of the four required total artificial heart implantation. The second group is represented by the patient with end-stage chronic congestive failure. This general group requires a patient to be in a class IV progressive chronic congestive heart failure with a ventricular ejection fraction under 18 percent and percutaneous myocardial biopsy showing no active disease, thereby dismissing the possibility of recoverable failure. There must be no significant surgically correctable lesions present. There must be no other significant medical illness present. The patient must be at least 18 years of age. Additionally the candidate must demonstrate a stable home situation with a reliable spouse, sibling, or other person to help with care (Fig. 137-1). The patient must demonstrate a good history of medical compliance and be able to deal with illnesses with sound psychological mechanisms. The Federal Drug Administration had further stipulated that the patient must not be a candidate for a heart transplant. Each candidate must be approved by an evaluation committee consisting of the author, two clinical cardiologists, a social worker, a psychiatrist, and a nurse, along with a monitor from the Institutional Review Board. Of fundamental importance is that the patient must have the ability and the opportunity for accurate informed consent. The informed consent form is signed by the patient and re-signed after a 24-h waiting period, reconfirming the intent to participate in the experiment.

The Utah patient further demonstrates several important aspects of the selection process for clinical artificial heart experimentation. Because of his age (61 years) and pulmonary hypertension, he was *not* a candidate for a heart or heart-lung transplantation as determined by any transplantation center protocol available to us. There was no competing device (such as a left ventricular assist device) or medical therapy available to this patient. The patient had had an extensive and well-documented medical workup, which included the use of experimental inotropic drugs and endomyocardial biopsy studies. No question could be raised as to whether further medical therapy should be used effectively. Finally, the patient was immediately preterminal, as manifested by the frequency and nature of his arrhythmias. No consultants available could question the possibility of this patient's being minutes to hours from death.

It must be also emphasized that this initial experience has been classified as "human experimentation" (not "innovative therapy") in all documentation and considerations for the patient. The endpoints of this experiment have been clearly demonstrated: The artificial heart can feasibly be implanted in a patient for at least 112 days without significant localized infection and consumption of blood products; the patient can expect a reasonable quality of life (as clearly stated by this patient himself) with the implanted device (as compared to the preoperative quality); many new complex interrelations between the heart and circulatory system have been demonstrated; and new impetus has been developed for making the prosthetic system more acceptable for clinical uses. The importance of this clinical model in the determination of the sites of action of many cardiovascular drugs is obvious.

There are many extremely important aspects requiring exploration for future cases. Questions raised in socioeconomic, ethical, medical, surgical, biochemical, engineering, and administrative fields require meticulous consideration. On a snowy night on the first of December, 1982, one brave man and his family began to open these doors. This chapter is dedicated respectfully to his memory.

Acknowledgment

The editor-in-chief wishes to express his appreciation to Mrs. Clark for permitting us to reproduce the text, tables, and figures that relate to Dr. Barney B. Clark's illness. Dr. Clark and his wife have attained a place in medical history and we are grateful to them.

At the time of this writing four additional artificial hearts have been implanted. Three have been implanted in Louisville, Kentucky, and one in Stockholm, Sweden.

References

1. DeVries, W. C., Anderson, J. L., Joyce, I. D., et al.: Clinical Use of the Total Artificial Heart, *N. Engl. J. Med.*, 310:273, 1984.
2. Joyce, L. D., DeVries, W. C., Hastings, W. L., et al.: Response of the Human Body to the First Permanent Implant of the Jarvik-7 Total Artificial Heart, *Trans. Am. Soc. Artif. Intern. Organs,* 29:81, 1983.
3. DeVries, W. C., and Joyce, L. D.: The Artificial Heart, *Clin. Symp.*, 35:4, 1983.
4. Anderson, F. L., DeVries, W. C., Anderson, J. L., et al.: Evaluation of Total Artificial Heart Performance in Man, *Am. J. Card.*, in press.
5. Jarvik, R. K.: The Total Artificial Heart, *Sci. Am.,* 224(1):66, 1981.
6. Dale, H. H., and Schuster, E. A.: A Double Perfusion Pump, *J. Physiol.,* 64:356, 1928.
7. DeBakey, M. E.: A Simple Continuous Flow Blood Transfusion Instrument, *New Orleans Med. Surg. J.,* 87:386, 1934.
8. Akutsu, T., and Kolff, W. J.: Permanent Substitutes for Valves and Hearts, *Trans. Am. Soc. Artif. Intern. Organs,* 4:230, 1958.
9. Hastings, W. L., Aaron, J. L., Deneris, J., et al. A Retrospective Study of Eight Calves Surviving Five Months on the Pneumatic Total Artificial Heart, *Trans. Am. Soc. Artif. Intern. Organs,* 27:71, 1981.
10. Olsen, D. B., Nielsen, M., Lunn, J., et al. Total Artificial Heart Performance in the Calf. *Am. J. Cardiol.,* 37:160, 1976.
11. Cooley, D. A., Liota, D., and Hallman, G. L.: Orthotopic Cardiac Prosthesis for Two-Staged Cardiac Replacement, *Am. J. Cardiol.,* 24:730, 1969.
12. Cooley, D. A., Akutsu, T., Norman, J. C., et al.: Total Artificial Heart in Two-Staged Cardiac Transplantation, *Cardiovasc. Dis., Bull. Texas Heart Inst.,* 8(3):305, 1981.
13. DeVries, W. C.: The Total Artificial Heart, in D. C. Sabiston (ed.), "Gibbon's Surgery of the Chest," 4th ed., W. B. Saunders Company, Philadelphia, 1983, p. 1629.

Section H

Opening the Heart at Necropsy

138

Examining the Heart at Necropsy

William C. Roberts, M.D.

Numerous publications have appeared describing methods of examining the heart at necropsy.[1–32] Despite the many methods described, most hearts, irrespective of the disease present, appear to be opened the same way. This approach consists of opening each of the four cardiac chambers according to the flow of blood. An incision generally is made from the orifice of the superior vena cava to that of the inferior vena cava or vice versa. Either the lateral or posterior wall of right atrium is incised. The incision is extended through the tricuspid valve ring and into the right ventricle to its apex. The incision is then extended up the anterior wall of the right ventricle and out into the pulmonary trunk. The left atrium is opened, usually by an incision extending from a right to a left pulmonary vein or vice versa. The left atrium, mitral valve, and left ventricle are opened by an incision either in the lateral or posterior wall down to the apex of the left ventricle. The incision then turns toward the base of the heart anteriorly and out the left ventricular outflow tract through the aortic valve and into the ascending aorta.

Although the technique described above is the one most commonly employed by pathologists in the United States, it actually provides poor demonstration of most gross structural alterations. This approach converts all four cardiac chambers and valves from three-dimensional to two-dimensional structures, and the "space" of the chambers is completely lost. Thereafter, determining chamber or valvular orifice sizes is fraught with error. This technique may be analogous to studying an automobile tire by cutting it transversely at one site and spreading out the two cut ends until the tire is converted from a circle to a straight line—it no longer looks like a tire.

The technique described above was advocated in the latter part of the nineteenth century because the "water test" previously used was considered unreliable and the measurement of valvular anuli was considered an objective means of determining whether or not a valve orifice was stenotic, incompetent, or normal.[4] Previously, the performance of the water test at necropsy had made mandatory the retaining of the valves intact. (Competency of a valve had been determined by injecting water into either great artery or ventricle and thereafter observing the upstream chamber—atrium or ventricle—to determine whether water regurgitated.) Only recently has it become evident that the measurement of valve anuli is, with the exception of valves of patients with mitral valve prolapse,[33] a waste of time. Another problem with the technique of opening described above is that the heart is opened when it is fresh. Opening the heart when it is fresh may provide some quick answers, but the three-dimensional relations are gone forever.

Certain principles regarding the study of the heart at necropsy have proved useful to me, and they are described in the remainder of this chapter.

First Principle

Do not, except under rare circumstances, open the heart when it is fresh. After excising the heart at necropsy, fix it in formalin or in another firming and preserving solution for at least 24 h before opening. To preserve its shape, place small crumbled-up bits of paper (such as paper towels) *loosely* in the atria and in the great arteries, but not in the ventricles. Do not "stuff" the chambers, for that distorts or enlarges their size. The sizes of the ventricles at necropsy correspond to their sizes during ventricular systole during life. Thus, to retain that systolic size, it is important *not* to fill either of these chambers with any material at necropsy.

The fixing of the specimen before opening it is the key to preserving the three-dimensional configuration of the heart. However, convincing prosectors of the usefulness of fixing the heart before opening it is difficult. Most prosectors take for granted that the brain should be fixed before it is opened, and the same is true for the heart. The neuropathologists have done a better job than cardiovascular pathologists have in convincing prosectors of the value of fixation before incision.

Second Principle

X-ray the heart after fixation if cardiac disease is thought to be present. Of course, postmortem clot and the crumbled bits of paper should be removed from the intact specimen before radiographs are taken. An industrial type of film is ideal because its contrast is far better than that of the film used for live patients. Radiographs of the cardiac specimen are useful to determine the presence of and the extent of calcific deposits and to visualize the relative sizes of the cardiac chambers in proportion to the thicknesses of the cardiac walls including the septa.

Third Principle

The method used to open the heart is determined by the type of cardiac disease that is present or suspected. The method most commonly used to open the heart in a patient with coronary heart disease is usually not ideal for the study of the heart of a patient with valvular or congenital heart disease. The methods used to study the various types of cardiac diseases are described below.

Coronary Heart Disease

The chief purposes of the cardiac examination in coronary heart disease are to determine the type of, and extent of, coronary arterial disease and to determine the presence of, and extent of, foci of myocardial fibrosis, necrosis, or both. The epicardial or extramural coronary arteries may be studied best by excising the main trunks, including the coronary ostia, from the surface of the heart. The adipose tissue is then excised from the surfaces of these arteries, which are then x-rayed again. The arteries are then fixed in formalin for at least another 24 h, and if calcific deposits are present they are decalcified (the formic acid–sodium citrate method is preferred). At this point the arteries are sectioned at 5-m intervals at right angles to their longitudinal axes and examined for degrees of luminal narrowing and for the presence of absence of intraluminal thrombus and/or plaque hemorrhage and/or dissection. Ideally, of course, each 5-mm segment is processed in alcohol and xylene and embedded in paraffin, and a histological section is prepared. The amount of narrowing of the luminal cross-sectional area is classified into five categories: 0 to 25 percent; 26 to 50 percent, 51 to 75 percent, 76 to 95 percent, and 96 to 100 percent.

In patients with conduits between the aorta and one or more coronary arteries, the aorta containing the graft anastomosis is excised; this allows retention of the grafts with the native coronary arteries, which are excised from the specimen. Measuring the total length of each of the bypass conduits is useful. Also, it is useful to measure the total lengths (from the aortic ostia) of the native coronary arteries. The length of the left anterior descending coronary artery plus the left main coronary artery may be 12 cm and the graft anastomosis may be 7 cm downstream from the aortic ostium of the native coronary artery. The degree of luminal narrowing of the native coronary artery at, and distal to, the graft-coronary anastomosis is determined. The grafts are sectioned in the same manner as the native coronary arteries.

After excision of the epicardial coronary arteries (and grafts), the ventricles are cut in "breadloaf" fashion. The cuts are made parallel to the posterior atrioventricular (AV) sulcus beginning at the apex at intervals of about 1 cm in width, and ending about 2 cm caudal to the AV sulcus. The location of foci of fibrosis or necrosis are identified.

Valvular Heart Disease without a Substitute Valve

The chief purposes of the cardiac examination in this condition are to determine the type of and the severity of the valvular disease, the effect of the valvular disease on the rest of the heart, and the presence or absence of associated cardiac disease. The best way to determine the type of valve lesion at necropsy is to study the valve when it is intact. The size of the valve orifice cannot be determined accurately after the valve has been opened. The valves are studied from both their inflow and outflow aspects. Photographing a semilunar valve from the ventricular aspect rarely produces a good picture. The semilunar valves are best studied by excising the pulmonary trunk and aorta just above, or at the level of, the cephalad extension of the valve commissures. The tricuspid and mitral valvular inflow surfaces can be studied by opening the atria laterally—the right one by an incision extending from the orifice of the superior vena cava to a level just above the tricuspid valve annulus at its lateral wall. (Never make an incision from the orifice of the superior to that of the inferior vena cava because the orifice of the latter provides a good landmark for orientation purposes.) The left atrium can be opened initially by an incision extending from one of the right to one of the left pulmonary veins, and then by an extension of this incision down the left lateral wall of the left atrium to just above the annulus of the mitral valve. An alternative method of studying the inflow portions of the AV valves is to excise the atrial free walls and atrial septum. The AV valves can be studied from below either by breadloafing the cardiac ventricles or by opening the ventricles along their lateral and anterior walls without extending either incision into either cardiac valve.

After the valves are studied intact, the heart can be opened in longitudinal or coronal fashion, or incisions can be made along the lateral and anterior walls of the ventricles. The longitudinal incision is usually made to correspond to the long-axis view utilized in echocardiography. The incision is actually an anterior-posterior one, and it is made by an incision extending through the right and left aortic valve cusps and left atrial walls and caudally between the two left ventricular papillary muscles just lateral to the cardiac apex. The key in studying hearts with valvular disease, to reemphasize, is first to study and photograph the intact valve and not to incise the valve until its intact structure has been carefully documented.

Valvular Heart Disease with a Substitute Cardiac Valve

Many patients with severe valvular heart disease have had one or more cardiac valves replaced with prosthetic (or bioprosthetic) valves, most of which have rigid or semirigid types of supporting frames.[31] A major purpose of the necropsy in a patient with a prosthetic cardiac valve is to evaluate the prosthesis and its relation to surrounding structures. Is there enough room in the ventricle or ascending aorta to freely accommodate the prosthesis? Is movement of the occluder inhibited by its contact with adjacent structures? Is thrombus present? Is the sewing ring intact, or are one or more peribasilar leaks present? Does a structure interfere with poppet movement or closure? Is there evidence of degeneration or wear of the prosthesis?

To answer these and other questions the prosthesis must be studied by examining it in relation to its surrounding structures. In the case of a prosthesis in either the mitral or tricuspid valve position, it is best to breadloaf the ventricles by incisions parallel to the posterior AV sulcus. These cuts allow these prostheses to be studied in relation to their surrounding intact structures. In the case of a prosthesis in the aortic valve position, it is best to excise the aorta just above the prosthesis so that the size of the prosthesis can be compared to the size of the aorta into which it was inserted. Examination of the inflow surfaces of the prostheses also is important. The atrial aspects of a prosthesis in the mitral or tricuspid valve position can be examined by incising or excising the atria as described previously; the ventricular aspect of an aortic prosthesis can be examined also by opening the ventricles by almost any method described previously.

Congenital Malformations of the Heart or Great Vessels

Examination of the heart with either coronary or valvular heart disease is more standardized than is the examination of the congenitally malformed heart. The relative sizes of the chambers and the origin and courses of the coronary arteries should be studied first simply by examining the epicardial surface of the heart. The method of examining the interior of the malformed heart is highly dependent on the anomaly suspected. Congenital heart disease in essence consists of "holes" in septa, anomalous communications between vessels or between vessels and cardiac chambers, obstructions at or near valves, or combinations of holes, abnormal communications, and obstructions. No single method of examination can be used to study such anomalies. The same principles discussed under valvular heart disease are applicable to obstructive lesions that are congenital in origin. Anomalous communications between vessels or between vessels and chambers are best demonstrated and illustrated before the interior of the heart is exposed. Longitudinal incisions can be used to demonstrate the relations between defects in the atrial or ventricular septa and adjacent structures. Histological sections usually are not beneficial when studying congenitally malformed hearts. Histological study in these patients should be directed toward the examination of the lungs. It is beneficial to keep the lungs attached to the heart, at least initially.

Myocardial Heart Disease (Not Resulting from Coronary Arterial Disease) and Systemic Hypertension

Some of the best demonstrations of specimens with the dilated or hypertrophic forms of cardiomyopathy and with systemic hypertension have come from longitudinal incisions of the heart. One corresponds to the echocardiographic long-axis view and the second to the echocardiographic four-chamber view. The major disadvantage of the latter method is that the incision at necropsy for this demonstration is posterior to the aortic valve, and therefore neither semilunar valve is retained with the anatomically appropriate one-half of the specimen. These incisions demonstrate the relations between the thicknesses of the ventricular septum and the right and left ventricular free walls and also the comparative relations between the amount of ventricular myocardium and the sizes of the ventricular chambers (also atrial chambers). Sectioning the ventricles transversely, i.e., parallel to the posterior AV sulcus, also is useful in demonstrating these chamber size–wall thickness relations.

Pericardial and Pulmonary Heart Diseases

A good method for demonstrating and photographing these conditions is by fixing the heart and lungs en bloc and thereafter incising both together either longitudinally (coronally) or transversely.

Summary

Three principles should be kept in mind when the heart is examined at necropsy.

- *Principle 1* is to fix the heart in formalin or in some other preserving and firming medium before opening it. Fixation of the specimen before incision allows retention of the three-dimensional configuration of the heart and permits more meaningful comparisons between chamber sizes, wall thicknesses, valve orifices, etc.
- *Principle 2* is to x-ray the fixed heart specimen before opening it. Radiographs reduce the three-dimensional intact heart to a two-dimensional structure and provide additional means of visualizing chamber sizes and wall thicknesses.
- *Principle 3* is that the method chosen to open the heart is determined by the type of cardiac disease that is present or suspected. There is no single way to open the heart, and, in general, hearts with different diseases require different methods of opening.

Opening hearts according to the flow of blood, a common practice, is usually the least desirable method of incising hearts.

References

1. Delafield, F., and Prudden, T. M.: "A Handbook of Pathological Anatomy and Histology," William Wood & Company, New York, 1885.
2. Virchow, R.: "Post-mortem Examination with Especial Reference to Medico-legal Practice," 4th German ed., T. P. Smith (trans.), P. Blakiston Son & Company, Philadelphia, 1885.
3. Hektoen, L.: "The Technique of Post-mortem Examination," The W. S. Keener Company, Chicago, 1894.
4. Mallory, F. B., and Wright, J. H.: "Pathological Technique: A Practical Histology and Bacteriology, Including Directions for the Performance of Autopsies and for Clinical Diagnosis by Laboratory Methods,' W. B. Saunders Company, Philadelphia, 1897.
5. Box, C. R.: "Post-mortem Manual. A Handbook of Morbid Anatomy and Post-mortem Technique," J. & A. Churchill, Ltd., London, 1910.
6. Oppenheimer, B. S.: A Routine Method of Opening the Heart with Conservation of the Bundle of His and the Sino-auricular Node, *JAMA*, 59:937, 1912.
7. Gross, L., Antopol, W., and Sacks, B.: A Standardized Procedure Suggested for Microscopic Studies on the Heart: With Observations on Rheumatic Hearts, *Arch. Pathol.*, 10:840, 1930.
8. Gross, L., and Leslie, E.: Paraffin Infiltration of Hearts: A Permanent Method for Preservation, *Am. Heart J.*, 6:665, 1931.
9. Saphir, O.: "Autopsy Diagnosis and Technique," Raul B. Hoeber, Inc., New York, 1937.
10. Kramer, F. M.: Dry Preservation of Museum Specimens: A Review, with Introduction of Simplified Technique, *J. Technol. Methods*, 18:42, 1938.
11. Schlesinger, M. J.: An Injection plus Dissection Study of Coronary Artery Occlusions and Anastomoses, *Am. Heart J.*, 15:528, 1938.
12. Rodriguez, F. L., and Reiner, L.: A New Method of Dissection of the Heart, *Arch. Pathol.*, 63:160, 1957.
13. Saphir, O.: Gross Examination of the Heart: Injection of Coronary Arteries; Weight and Measurements of Heart, in S. E. Gould (ed.), "Pathology of the Heart," 2d ed., Charles C Thomas, Publisher, Springfield, Ill., 1960, p. 1043.
14. U.S. Department of Defense, Army Department: "Autopsy Manual," U.S. Government Printing Office, Washington, 1960.
15. Lev, M., Rowlatt, U. F., and Rimondi, H. J. A.: Pathologic Methods for Study for Congenitally Malformed Heart. Methods for Electrocardiographic and Physiologic Correlation, *Arch. Pathol.*, 72:493, 1961.
16. Glagov, S., Eckner, F. A. O., and Lev, M.: Controlled Pressure Fixation Apparatus for Hearts, *Arch. Pathol.*, 76:640, 1963.
17. Chapman, C. B.: On the Study of the Heart. A Comment on Autopsy Techniques, *Arch. Intern. Med.*, 113:318, 1964.
18. Lumb, G., and Hardy, L. B.: Technique for Dissection and Perfusion of Heart, *Arch. Pathol.*, 77:233, 1964.
19. Robbins, S. L., and Fish, S. J.: A New Angiographic Technique Providing a Simultaneous Permanent Cast of the Coronary Arterial Lumen, *Am. J. Clin. Pathol.*, 42:309, 1966.
20. Layman, T. E., and Edwards, J. E.: A Method for Dissection of the Heart and Major Pulmonary Vessels, *Arch. Pathol.*, 82:314, 1966.
21. Roberts, W. C., and Morrow, A. G.: Cardiac Valves and the Surgical Pathologist, *Arch. Pathol.*, 82:309, 1966.
22. Brody, G., Belding, A., Belding, M., and Feldman, S.: The Identification and Delineation of Myocardial Infarcts, *Arch. Pathol.*, 84:312, 1967.
23. Roberts, W. C., and Morrow, A. G.: Anatomic Studies of Hearts Containing Caged-Ball Prosthetic Valves, *Johns Hopkins Med. J.*, 121:271, 1967.
24. Reiner, L.: Gross Examination of the Heart, in S. E. Gould (ed.), "Pathology of the Heart and Blood Vessels," 3d ed., Charles C Thomas, Publisher, Springfield, Ill, 1968, p. 1111.
25. McVie, J. G.: Postmortem Detection of Inapparent Myocardial Infarction, *J. Clin. Pathol.*, 23:203, 1970.
26. Roberts, W. C.: Examining the Precordium and the Heart, *Chest*, 57:567, 1970.
27. Suberman, C. O., Suberman, R. I., Dalldorf, F. G., and Orlando, F. G.: Radiographic Visualization of Coronary Arteries in Postmortem Hearts: A Simple Technique, *Am. J. Clin. Pathol.*, 53:254, 1970.
28. Lie, J. T., Holley, K. E., Kampa, W. R., and Titus, J. L.: New Histochemical Method for Morphologic Diagnosis of Early Stages of Myocardial Ischemia, *Mayo Clin. Proc.*, 46:319, 1971.
29. Lie, J. T., and Ludwig, J.: Heart and Vascular System, in J. Ludwig (ed.), "Current Methods of Autopsy Practice," 2d ed., W. B. Saunders Company, 1979, pp. 21–50.
30. Lichtig, C., Glagov, S., Feldman, S., and Wissler, R. W.: Myocardial Ischemia and Coronary Artery Atherosclerosis: A Comprehensive Approach to Post-mortem Studies, *Med. Clin. North Am.*, 57:79, 1973.
31. Roberts, W. C.: Choosing a Substitute Cardiac Valve: Type, Size, Surgeon, *Am. J. Cardiol.*, 38:633, 1976.
32. Waller, B. F., Morrow, A. G., Maron, B. J., Del Negro, A. A., Kent, K. M., McGrath, F. J., Wallace, R. B., McIntosh, C. L., and Roberts, W. C.: Etiology of Clinically Isolated, Severe, Chronic, Pure Mitral Regurgitation: Analysis of 97 Patients Over 30 Years of Age Having Mitral Valve Replacement, *Am. Heart J.*, 104:276, 1982.
33. Bulkley, B. H., and Roberts, W. C.: Dilatation of the Mitral Anulus. A Rare Cause of Mitral Regurgitation, *Am. J. Med.*, 59:457, 1975.

EPILOGUE

The Future of Cardiology

J. Willis Hurst, M.D.

The future will be here when we are not.

J. Willis Hurst, 1985

The prologue and the epilogue act as bookends for this edition of *The Heart.* The prologue, "The Growth of Knowledge," written by Dr. Howard Burchell, illuminates the path that has led us to where we are today. The book itself shows the present. The epilogue, "The Future of Cardiology," is designed to shine a light into the future so that we can find the path we should follow in the decades ahead.

The who, where, what, when, and how of *past* events are difficult to ascertain with accuracy. The *present,* a complex of actions on many fronts, is not easy to encompass. The *future,* where all that we can imagine may happen, is difficult to predict. Accordingly, I will only consider three broad areas of development and change that I believe will take place in the years ahead.

The Growth of Technology

High technology will invade medicine as it has all other areas of our lives. There is no way to stop it. The forces that create high technology are bigger than the forces that wish to stop it. I, for one, would not wish to stop it, for it will bring many useful procedures to our profession and will benefit our patients. For example, who would deny the value of cardiac catheterization now? Yet, in the beginning, the technique was considered to be dangerous and the concept was thought to be foolish.

The high technology of the future will come in larger and larger waves and we cannot stop it any more than we can calm the ocean. So what should we do? We *must* use it wisely. High technology will require even more thought by the physicians who use it than has been required in the past. We may argue over the type of data that should be collected, but I believe all will agree that simple, painless, and relatively inexpensive techniques will be used initially to screen patients in an effort to find abnormalities. Such screening should either solve the patient's problems or place the physician in a position to determine if additional data are needed for clarification. If more data are needed, physicians must formulate the questions they have about their patients with great precision. The answers to the questions must really matter. The next step will be to select the high technology that is likely to answer the questions. When this approach is used, it will prevent the misuse of high technology that yields results that are interesting but not useful to the care of the patient. Such an approach will prevent the use of many types of procedures when only one or two methods are needed. This method of keeping high technology from running rampant is emphasized in this book. The concept must become part of the fabric of our profession, or the waves of the high-technology future will drown us all.

Prediction: High technology will continue to invade our profession, but we will be able to control its use. Such control will permit our patients to profit from the remarkable progress that is certain to come.

Judgment

In the past, when little could be done, the physician needed less judgment about what to do. As it becomes possible to do more diagnostically and therapeutically, a physician's judgment must be sharpened to a fine edge. Since the future will bring us more diagnostic tests and more therapeutic measures, it follows that a physician will need to determine not only if something *can* be done but if it *should* be done. Such judgment cannot be made without mental skills that were not needed in the past. These include decision analysis, understanding of experimental design, statistics, computers, and many other skills.

Prediction: The cardiologists of the future will be required to possess much judgment. I believe they will rise to the challenge.

The Maintenance of Humanism

When any inanimate object becomes part of the scene which historically has involved two sensitive persons, the physician and the patient, the object is likely to be viewed as an intruder. Laennec's stethoscope was such an intruder. Some physicians viewed it as a gadget that interfered with the doctor-patient relationship. Some observers of the modern scene would see much of modern technology as responsible for a breakdown in the warm and humane relationship that should exist between the physician and a patient. If this is true, consider how the relationship will be affected when the waves of high technology sweep over us in the future.

I have never believed that the breakdown in the doctor-patient relationship has been caused by machines. After all, the machines just sit there. They do not contribute to anything until a person enters the picture. Machines are not inherently inhumane—only people can be inhumane. The taking of the medical history, which does not involve instruments and machines, can be very inhumane. On the other hand, the proper use of high technology that is explained by a sensitive physician and applied by humane and sensitive technicians can be viewed as an opportunity for people to display that they *are* humane even when the high-technology intruder is part of the action.

Prediction: Physicians, nurses, and technicians will be able to perceive that they can use the high technology of the future as a vehicle to show their humaneness. It will be understood that machines cannot hold a patient's hand—only another person (physician, nurse, and technician) can do that.

Summary

High technology will increase in the future. Physicians (and others) will learn to control its use by becoming exquisitely skilled in screening patients for abnormalities and, when other data are needed, in selecting the high technology that will answer the carefully formuated questions.

The physician of the future will be required to make more *judgments* about which of the available diagnostic and therapeutic measures should be used. The physician will meet this challenge.

Humaneness will be viewed as being of high priority, and physicians, nurses, and technicians will have a warm relationship with patients despite the increasing use of high technology.

Should the above fail to occur, the role of the doctor will be transformed to that of a technician who worries about the maintenance of the machines he or she operates rather than remaining an advocate for the patient's care.

Index

Index

A band, 32–33
a wave:
  atrial, 52
  precordial, 153, 155
  venous pulse, 53, 148–50
    abnormalities, 149, 150
    cannon, 149, 150
    pulmonic stenosis and, 656
    tricuspid stenosis and, 795
Abdomen:
  aneurysm in, 1327–28
    coronary bypass surgery and, 990
  angina of, 1334–35, 1368–70
  bruits in, 205
    arteriosclerosis obliterans and, 1341
    mesenteric ischemia and, 1368
    renovascular hypertension and, 1058
  examination of, 204–5
    heart failure and, 352
  pain in. *See* Pain, abdominal.
Abdominothoracic pump, 55
Aberrant conduction, 412, 457–61. *See also* Intraventricular conduction, aberrant.
Abortifacients, 1394
Abscess:
  cerebral, congenital heart disease and, 1362
  endocarditis and, 1139
  myocardial, 1159, 1161
Acanthocytosis, amyotrophic chorea with, 1231
ACC-9089, 1607, 1610
Accelerated idioventricular rhythm, 456
  myocardial infarction and, 976
Accelerated junctional rhythm, 420, 462, 468, 470
  esophageal ECG and, 1698
  myocardial infarction and, 974
Accessory pathways, 415–16
  ablation, 477
  atrial fibrillation and, 448
  AV junctional tachycardia and, 418
  calcium channel blockers and, 1631
  digitalis and, 1644, 1646
  electrophysiological studies, 294
  procainamide and, 477
  programmed stimulation and, 1737–38
  reciprocating tachycardia and, 447–48
  reentry, 416, 418–20
  right bundle branch block and, 216
Accessory pathways:
  supraventricular tachycardia and, 441
  surgical division of, 2014
  Wolff-Parkinson-White syndrome and, 219–20
Accrochage, 467
Acebutolol, 1607. *See also* Beta-blocking agents.
  pharmacodynamics, 1608, 1613, 1617
  pharmacokinetics, 1610, 1611
  structure, 1608
Acetaminophen, 1237
Acetazolamide, 1658
  dose and duration of action, 1659
  site of action, 1660
  toxin excretion and, 1665
Acetylcarnitine, 92, 93
Acetyl CoA, 92, 93
  pyruvate metabolism and, 90
Acetyldigitoxin. *See* Digitalis.
Acetylstrophanthidin, premature ventricular beats and, 1646
Achalasia, 912
Acidosis:
  diuretic-induced, 1665
  hyperchloremic, heart failure and, 362
  renal failure and, 1460
  shock and, 372, 389
Aconitine, atrial fibrillation and, 415
Acrocyanosis, 1352
  treatment, 1353
Acromegaly, 130, 1422–23
  cardiovascular manifestations, 1422–23
  treatment, 1423
Actin, 32–34
  action potential and, 38
  Starling's law and, 44–45
Actinomycosis, myocarditis and, 1173
Action potential, 37–38, 75–78, 1466
  automaticity and, 78–79, 407–8
  calcium and, 1466, 1473–75
  electrocardiography and, 82–84
  fast-response, 75–76
  impulse conduction and, 410
  potassium and, 1466
  Purkinje fiber, 75–78
  reentry and, 414
  slow-response, 78
  sodium and, 38, 76–77, 1466
  triggered activity and, 408
Activity. *See also* Exercise.
  coronary heart disease and, 825, 829–30
  myocardial infarction and, 969, 972, 1028–29
  progressive, 1028–29
  seven-step program, 1030
Acylanid. *See* Digitalis.
Acylcarnitine, 91–92, 94
Acyl CoA, 91–92, 94
Adams-Stokes syndrome, 523, 1360
Addison's disease, 1423
Adenoids, 131
Adenoma, adrenal, 1063–64, 1081–82
Adenosine:
  coronary blood flow and, 61, 62, 858
  formation and fate of, 62
Adenosine monophosphate (AMP):
  cardiomyopathy and, 1193
  drugs inhibiting, 1675
  glycogen and, 89
  myocardial, 62
    ischemia and, 98
  phosphorylation and, 87, 88
  receptor activity and, 1606
  shock and, 380
Adenosine triphosphatase (ATPase):
  aging and, 1404
  myosin, 86, 98–99
    heart failure and, 330
  sarcolemma, heart failure and, 330
Adenosine triphosphate (ATP):
  concentration of, myocardial, 86
  contractility and, 38
  glucose and, 90
  glycogen and, 89
  hypoxia and, 90
  metabolic disorders and, 97–99
  myocardial ischemia and, 98
  shock and, 378–80
Adipose tissue circulation, 1452
Adrenal glands, 1423–24
  adenoma, aldosteronism and, 1063–64, 1081–82
  emotional stress and, 1520–21
  hyperplasia, aldosteronism and, 1046, 1063–64, 1081–83
  insufficiency, 1423
Adrenergic nervous system. *See* Epinephrine; Norepinephrine; Sympathetic nervous system.
Adrenergic receptors:
  alpha, 376–77

Adrenergic receptors: alpha:
blocking agents, 393, 1010, 1083, 1589, 1609–10
coronary vasoconstriction and, 862
norepinephrine and, 1654
stimulating agents, 391, 1588, 1590
beta, 376–77, 1606–7
aging and, 1404, 1406–7, 1606–7
blocking agents. *See* Beta-blocking agents.
isoproterenol and, 392
norepinephrine and, 1654
shock and, 376–77
Adriamycin, toxicity of, 1233–34
Adson's maneuver, 917
Adventitia, fibrous plaque and, 803
Aerobic metabolism, 1398, 1400
Afterdepolarization, 408–9
Afterload (pressure overload), 40, 41
aging and, 1405
aortic impedance and, 47–48
aortic stenosis and, 274, 331, 332, 730, 732
cardiac output and, 267, 363–65
increased, 395
contractility and, 47–48, 266, 331–32
indexes of, 270–71
echocardiography and, 1953
end-diastolic volume and, 47–48
heart failure and, 266–67, 327, 331–32, 348
management, 363–65
hypertrophy and, 331
preload mismatch with, 266–67
reduction of, 363–65
shock and, 372
stroke volume and, 267, 326
vasodilators and, 268, 364, 392, 866
velocity of shortening and, 41, 43
Afterpotential, calcium and, 1473, 1474
Aging, 1403–11. *See also* Elderly.
aortic valve calcification and, 249, 1410
beta receptors and, 1404, 1406–7, 1606–7
cardiomyopathy and, 1238
congestive heart failure and, 1409–10
contractility and, 1405–6
coronary heart disease and, 1409
difficulties in study of, 1403–4
electrophysiology and, 1410
exercise and, 1407–9
hypertension and, 1409
left ventricular function and, 1405
medial degeneration of aorta and, 1322
myocardial function and, 1404–5
normal, 1404–7
peripheral vasculature and, 1406–7
selectivity of, 1404
valvular heart disease and, 249, 1410–11
Aglycone, 1639, 1640
Agonal rhythm, 471
AH interval, 1729–30
incremental atrial pacing and, 1736
programmed atrial stimulation and, 1736–37
Air embolism, 1115–16
coronary bypass surgery and, 2039
hyperbaric pressure and, 1552
Airway clearance, 549–50
Akinesis, 1804
coronary bypass surgery and, 2038, 2039
Albright's syndrome, 403
Albumin:
fatty acids and, 91
pericardial effusion and, 1250
volume expansion and, 388–89
Albuterol, 1483
Alcohol, 937
abuse of, 1446–48
arrhythmias and, 1447–48
beriberi and, 398
cardiomyopathy and, 1182–83, 1446–48
coronary heart disease and, 826
fetal syndrome and, 135
heart failure and, 1446–47
pathophysiological mechanisms and, 1448
sudden death and, 1447–48
uterine depression and, 1394
Aldomet. *See* Methyldopa.
Aldosterone, 1041
diuretics and, 1062, 1657, 1660
excessive. *See* Aldosteronism.
heart failure and, 324, 325
hypertension and, 1041, 1043–46, 1060–64, 1081–83
renin and, 1062
suppressibility of, 1062
Aldosteronism, 1041, 1046
diagnosis, 1060–64
differential diagnosis, 1063–64
edema and, 1664
glucocorticoid-suppressible, 1063, 1064
hypokalemia and, 1061–62
pathophysiology, 1046
treatment, 1081–83
Aldosteronoma, 1063–64, 1081–82
Alkalosis, diuretic-induced, 1665
Alkaptonuria, 1226
Allantoic veins, 10
Allen's test, 1340
Allergy, drug, 1236–37
streptokinase and, 1919
All-or-nothing law, 42
Alpha-blocking agents, 393, 1589
beta blockers with activity as, 1609–10
coronary artery spasm and, 1010
pheochromocytoma and, 1083
Alpha receptors. *See* Adrenergic receptors, alpha.
Alpha-stimulating agents, 391, 1588, 1590
Altitude (high), 1543–47
cardiac output and, 1544–45
coronary artery disease and, 1546
coronary blood flow and, 1545–46
exercise and, 1544
oxygen transport and, 1543–45
polycythemia and, 1544
pulmonary edema and, 338, 1096, 1547
pulmonary hypertension and, 338, 1093, 1095–96, 1121, 1546–47
stroke volume and, 1545
syncope and, 518
Alveolar hypoxia, 1093, 1095–96
vasoconstriction and, 1121–22
Alveoli, shock and, 378
Ambulation, 1028–29
Amebiasis, 1176
Ameboid cells, myocardial, 31, 32
American Heart Association classification, 932–33
American Society of Anesthesiologists seal, 1499
Amiloride, 1658–61
biochemistry, 1658
dosage, 1072, 1659
duration of action, 1659
pharmacokinetics, 1661
site of action, 1660
Amino acids, 95–96
transport systems, 95
Aminophylline, pulmonary edema and, 367
Aminorex, pulmonary hypertension and, 1101
Amiodarone, 1601–3
cardiomyopathy and, 1206, 1207
clinical application, 1602
digitalis and, 1647
electrophysiologic testing of, 478
pharmacokinetics, 1601–2
pharmacologic properties, 1602
toxicity, 1602–3
Amitriptyline, 1479–80
Amniotic fluid embolism, 1116
Amoxapine, 1480
Amoxicillin, endocarditis and, 1153
Ampicillin, endocarditis and, 1149, 1153
Amplifier, phonocardiography, 1991
Amplitude, sound wave, 157
Amputation:
arteriosclerosis obliterans and, 1346
thromboangiitis obliterans and, 1348
Amrinone, 1655–56
contractility and, 360
heart failure and, 1656
pharmacokinetics, 1655–56
pharmacologic actions, 1655
structure, 1653
Amsacrine, 1482
Amylase, pancreatitis and, 915
Amyl nitrate, angina pectoris and, 887
Amyl nitrite:
auscultation and, 195
chemical structure, 940
dosage, 940
Amyloidosis, 1023, 1213–15
cardiomyopathy and, 569–70
classification, 1213
clinical manifestations, 1214–15
echocardiography and, 1957, 1958
gastrointestinal, 1371
pathology, 1213
pathophysiology, 1213–14
treatment, 1215
Amyotrophic chorea, 1231
Anacrotic limb, 141
Anacrotic notch, 53
aortic stenosis and, 733
Anaphylaxis, 1236
Anatomy, 16–35
aortic, 25–26
aortic valve, 22
arterial, 26
atrial, 16
left, 19–20
right, 18–19
AV node, 19, 30–31
capillary, 26
chordae tendineae, 21, 23
conduction system, 30–31
coronary artery, 27–29, 839–40
coronary vein, 29–30
external features, 16–17

Anatomy:
  fibrous skeleton, 17–18
  gross, 16–31
  His bundle, 30–31
  internodal tract, 30
  lymphatic, 25, 26–27
  mitral valve, 21, 22
  nerve, 24–25
  papillary muscle, 21, 23
  pericardial, 23–24, 1249
  pulmonary valve, 22
  pulmonary vasculature, 27
  sinus node, 18, 30
  tricuspid valve, 22–23
  ultrastructural, 31–34
  venous, 26
  ventricular, 16
    left, 20–22
    right, 19
Anectine. *See* Succinylcholine.
Anemia, 399–400
  cardiac output increase and, 399–400
  clinical manifestations, 400
  endocarditis and, 1144
  management, 400
  pathophysiology, 399–400
  renal failure and, 1460, 1462
  sickle-cell, 399–400, 1226–27
Anesthesia, 1494–1509
  agents, 1495–97
    antagonists to, 1504–5
    intravenous administration of, 1504
  arrhythmias and, 1515
  contractility and, 50
  coronary artery disease and, 1500–1501
  coronary bypass surgery and, 952
  depth of, 1499
  electroconvulsive therapy and, 1488
  fluid balance and, 1505
  general, 1495
  glucose intolerance and, 1431
  hemodynamic problems and, 1505–7
  hypertension and, 1502
  informed consent and, 1503
  intensivist and, 1508–9
  local, 1500
  modern precepts of, 1494–95
  monitoring, 1497–99
  objectives of, 1495
  obstetric, 1394
  plan for, 1503–9
  postponement of elective surgery and, 1503
  preoperative preparation, 1500–1501
    assessment, 1500–1501
    medications, 1501
  recovery from, 1504–5
  regional, 1500
  risk assessment, 1502–3
  valvular heart disease and, 1501
  ventilatory support after, 1507–8
Aneurysms:
  abdominal, coronary bypass surgery and, 990
  aortic. *See* Aortic aneurysm.
  aortic arch, 1325
    repair of, 1326, 2045–46
  celiac artery, 1351
  cerebrovascular, 1143, 1151
    hypertension and, 1357
    myxomatous emboli and, 1286–87
  Charcot-Bouchard, 1357
  coronary artery, 711–12, 1020
  femoral artery, 1326, 1351
Aneurysms:
  iliac artery, 1326, 1351
  mycotic, endocarditis and, 1143–44, 1151
  peripheral, 1350–52
  popliteal artery, 1326, 1351
  renal artery, 1351
  retinal, 200
  sinus of Valsalva. *See* Sinus of Valsalva aneurysm (fistula).
  splenic artery, 1351
  ventricular:
    anticoagulants and, 1673–74
    computed tomography and, 1868
    echocardiography and, 1962
    endocardial fibroelastosis and, 847, 849
    false, 987
    heart failure and, 278
    myocardial infarction and, 847–50, 986–87
    radionuclide studies and, 1820, 1821
    roentgenography and, 232
    surgical treatment, 2041–42
    traumatic, 1279
  visceral, 1351
Anger scintillation camera, 1811
Angina, abdominal, 1334–35, 1368–70
Angina pectoris, 113, 889–93
  anxiety and, 891, 907–8
  aortic stenosis and, 732, 910, 990
  arrhythmias and, 988
  arteriography and, indications, 903–4
  AV block and, 964
  Burns' comments on, 884–85
  cardiomyopathy and, 909–10
  classification, 108, 932–33
    surgical intervention and, 949–50
  clinical recognition, 890–91
  cold exposure and, 891
  coronary artery spasm and. *See* variant *below.*
  diabetes mellitus and, 1430
  digitalis and, 942
  duration of, 890
  dyspnea and, 890
  ECG and, 894–95, 1011
    exercise and, 896, 1707, 1708, 1714
    Q waves, 209
    variant angina and, 963
  effort-induced, 891, 1011–12
  equivalents, 890, 961
    recognition, 961
    treatment, 957–58, 961
  errors in diagnosis of, 1536
  Heberden's description of, 883–84
  historical notes on, 883–86
  history, 889–93
    limitations of, 892–93
  Hunter and, 884
  hypercyanotic, 1098
  hypertension and, right ventricular, 910
  hyperthyroidism and, 1414
  hypothyroidism and, 1420, 1421
  insurance and, 1558–59
  likelihood of coronary artery disease and, 303, 307
  location, 890
  management, 891
    angioplasty, 945–46. *See also* Angioplasty, percutaneous transluminal.
    beta-blocking agents, 1613–15
Angina pectoris: management:
    bypass surgery, 949–50. *See also* Coronary bypass surgery.
    calcium channel blockers, 1628–30
    costs of care, 956
    historical notes on, 887–88
    postinfarction, 962–63
    preoperative, 951
    principles, 957–58
    stable angina and, 959
    unstable angina and, 962
    variant angina and, 963–64
  mitral stenosis and, 991
  morning, 891
  muscle bridges and, 1020
  noncardiac surgery and, 1502–3, 1513
  pathology, 842
  patient's description of, 890
  postinfarction, 962–63, 985
    definition and recognition, 962
    treatment, 962–63
  postprandial, 1449–50
  prognosis, 920–24
  prolonged, 964
  pulmonary hypertension and, 1098
  rehabilitation and, 1026. *See also* Rehabilitation.
  risk reduction and, 827–32
  second wind, 891
  smoking and, 891
  stable, 959
    arteriography and, 903
    assessment, 300, 302
    definition, 959
    ECG and, 894
    prognosis, 920–23
    recognition, 959
    surgical intervention and, 949
    treatment, 959
  syphilitic coronary ostial disease and, 1317–18
  unstable, 962
    arteriography and, 903–4
    assessment, 304
    coronary artery spasm and, 1011
    definition, 962
    pathology, 842
    platelet-controlling drugs and, 1677
    prognosis, 923–24
    recognition, 962
    surgical intervention and, 949
    thallium imaging and, 1834
    treatment, 962
  Valsalva maneuver and, 891
  valvular heart disease and, 732, 910, 990, 991
  variant (Prinzmetal's), 963–64
    arrhythmias and, 988
    coronary artery spasm and, 963–64, 1011
    definition, 963
    ECG and, 209, 895, 1011
    historical notes on, 885–86
    natural history, 1013
    prognosis, 924
    recognition, 113, 963
    treatment, 963–64
Angiodysplasia, colonic, 1371
Angiogenesis, 3
Angiography, 1785–90. *See also* Aortography; Cardiac catheterization; Coronary arteriography.
  aortic atresia and, 1790
  aortic regurgitation and, 747, 1788–89
  arteriosclerosis obliterans and, 1342

Angiography:
AV canal and, 608, 610
balloon catheter for, 1785, 1786
cardiomyopathy and, 1190, 1203–4
cerebral, 1356, 1874–76, 1879
complications, 1790–91
contrast media, 1785
digital, 1858–63
aorta and, 1859
cerebral, 1356, 1875–76, 1879
coarctation of aorta and, 256
coronary artery disease and, 1860–61
filming method, 1786–87
pediatric, 1861–62
physical basis for, 1858–59
pulmonary, 1862–63, 1883
renal artery, 1059
ventricular assessment, 1859–60
endomyocardial fibrosis and, 1211–12
exercise and, 901–2
filming methods, 1786–87
glycogenosis and, 1221
laser therapy and, 1923
mesenteric, 1365, 1366, 1368
mitral regurgitation and, 773–74, 1789–90
myocardial failure and, 272
myocardial infarction and, 848
myxoma and, 1289–90, 1291
positioning for, 1787
prognosis and, 311–12, 921, 922
pulmonary. *See* Pulmonary angiography.
pulmonary artery hypoplasia and, 660
pulmonary valve absence and, 667
pulmonic stenosis and, 656, 657, 1788
radionuclide:
coronary heart disease and, 900–902
equilibrium gated, 1818–23
first-pass, 1813–18, 1823
limitation of, 902
renal:
angioplasty and, 1911
digital subtraction, 1059
nephritis and, 1060, 1061
nephrosclerosis and, 1055, 1056–57
tetralogy of Fallot and, 664–65
thromboangiitis obliterans and, 1347–48
transposition of great arteries and, 693
corrected, 701–2
uses of, 1787–89
ventricular dysplasia and, 424
ventricular septal defect and, 594, 1789
Angiokeratoma corporis diffusum, 572, 1222–23
Angioma, gastrointestinal, 1370
Angioplasty:
coarctation of aorta and, 632, 633, 1897–98
percutaneous transluminal, 945–46, 1897–1912
arteriosclerosis obliterans and, 1346
coarctation of aorta and, 1897–98
complications, 946, 1540, 1907–8, 1910, 1912
coronary artery, 1902–8
equipment for, 1904–5, 1909
femoral artery, 1909
historical note on, 888
iliac artery, 1336, 1346, 1909, 1910
Angioplasty: percutaneous transluminal:
indications, 945, 949–50
limitations, 946
mesenteric artery, 1912
pathology, 854
patient selection, 1902, 1909
peripheral vascular, 1908–10
popliteal artery, 1909, 1910
postoperative care, 946
pulmonic stenosis and, 1898–99
recurrent stenosis after, 1908
renal artery, 1079, 1910–12
results and goals, 945
technique, 1905–7, 1909, 1911
thrombolytic therapy and, 1903
vertebral artery, 1912
subclavian arterial flap, 632, 633
Angiosarcoma, 1294
Angiotensin:
analogs of, 1590–91
coronary blood flow and, 62–63
heart failure and, 324, 325, 335, 347
hypertension and, 1041, 1043–46
shock and, 377
Angiotensin-converting enzyme inhibitors, 365, 1589–90
hypertension and, 1077, 1078
dosage, 1072
renovascular, 1079
pharmacology, 1589–90
Angle of Louis, 147
Anitschkow myocytes, 1307
Ankle-arm index, 1974, 1975
Ankylosing spondylitis, 126, 1440–41
aortic regurgitation and, 740, 1440–41
aortitis and, 1323–24
therapy, 1441
Annuloaortic ectasia, 1322
Annuloplasty:
aortic, 2032
DeVega, 2033–34
mitral, 776–77
tricuspid, 797–99, 2033–34
Annulus fibrosus, 22
Anorexia, 121, 1449, 1450
Anrep effect, 48
anesthesia and, 50
Antabuse, 1447
Antiarrhythmic agents, 476–81, 1593–1603. *See also* specific agent.
beta-blocking, 1598–99, 1615
calcium channel blocker, 1630–31
cardiomyopathy and, 1206, 1207
classification, 1593
complications, 1539
digitalis, 1645–46
electrophysiologic studies and, 294, 1738–39
heart failure and, 358
myocardial infarction and, 830–31, 975
newer, 1600–1603
palpitations and, 284
pregnancy and, 1393
prophylactic, 975
sudden death prevention and, 543–44
surgical procedures and, 1515
Antibodies:
digoxin-specific, 1648
endocarditis and, 1139–40
magnetic resonance imaging and, 1894
myosin-specific, radiolabeled, 1849
shock and, 381
Antibodies:
streptococcal, 1310
streptokinase, 1916, 1919
treponemal, 1319
Anticoagulants, 1667–75. *See also* Heparin; Warfarin.
adverse reactions, 1668–69, 1674
aneurysm and, ventricular, 1673–74
aortic valve disease and, 1671
atrial fibrillation and, 1671–72
cardiomyopathy and, 1193, 1669–70
cardiopulmonary bypass and, 2026
cardioversion and, 1672, 1741–42
cerebral embolism and, 1360
coronary bypass surgery and, 1674
coronary heart disease and, 943
deep venous thrombosis and, 1375
endocarditis and, 1150
heart failure and, 1672
indications, 1669–74
mechanism of action, 1667, 1669
mitral valve disease and, 1670–71
myocardial infarction and, 831, 971–72, 983, 1672–73
new developments in, 1669, 1674–75
peripheral arterial occlusion and, 1350
pregnancy and, 1114, 1386, 1393–94
prosthetic valves and, 1671, 1676
mitral, 779
noncardiac surgery and, 1517
pulmonary embolism and, 1110–11
pulmonary hypertension and, 1103
therapeutic regimens, 1667–68, 1669
vs. thrombolytic agents, 1113
transient ischemic attacks and, 1357
Antidepressants, 1479–80
rehabilitation and, 1532–33
Antidiuretic hormone:
heart failure and, 325
shock and, 375, 377
syncope and, 509
Antigen-antibody complexes, shock and, 381
Antigens, HLA, diabetes and, 575
Antihypertensive agents, 1071–78, 1080–85. *See also* specific agent.
adverse effects, 1073, 1540
depression induced by, 1534
dosage range, 1072
interactions of, 1076
protein-binding and dialysance of, 1082
Antimicrobials:
endocarditis and, 1137, 1148–53
prophylactic, 1151–53
noncardiac surgery and, 1517
pacemaker implantation and, 1747
Antimony, toxicity of, 1234
Antineoplastic agents, 1481–82
Antiplatelet agents. *See* Platelets, drugs affecting.
Antipsychotic agents, 1480–81
Antistreptolysin O titer, 1310
Antistreptozyme test, 1310
Antithrombin III:
heparin and, 1667, 1668
warfarin and, 1669
Antithyroid agents, 1416–17
Anturane. *See* Sulfinpyrazone.
Anus, imperforate, 135
Anxiety. *See also* Emotional stress.
angina pectoris and, 891, 907–8
arrhythmias and, 1527

Anxiety:
chest pain and, 114, 907–8, 1527, 1531
coronary bypass surgery and, 1531
coronary heart disease and, 934–35
dyspnea due to, 116
ECG and, 908
hyperventilation and, 518–19, 907–8
iatrogenic disorders and, 1541
mitral valve prolapse and, 1533
myocardial infarction and, 934–35, 985
neurosis and, 1526–27, 1533
rehabilitation and, 1035
Aorta, 1321–26
anatomy, 25–26
aneurysm. *See* Aortic aneurysm.
arch. *See* Aortic arch.
atherosclerosis, 1321–22, 1334
of terminal portion, 1335–36
balloon pump for. *See* Intraaortic balloon counterpulsation.
biventricular origin of, 669. *See also* Tetralogy of Fallot.
clinical manifestations of disease of, 1324–33
coarctation. *See* Coarctation of aorta.
congenital anomalies, 1324
cystic medial necrosis, 1322, 1330
dissection, 1328–33
beta blockers for, 1617
cardiopulmonary bypass and, 2029, 2039
classification, 1329
clinical manifestations, 1330–32
CT scans and, 1871–72
digital subtraction angiography and, 1859
management, 1333, 1617, 2047–48
Marfan's syndrome and, 1322
myocardial infarction vs., 1322
natural history and prognosis, 1332
pain from, 114, 910, 1331
pathogenesis, 1330
pathology, 1328–30
regurgitant valve and, 743, 749, 1331, 1333, 2047
surgical repair, 2047–48
echocardiography, 1938, 1945
embryology, 13–14
endarterectomy of abdominal, 2058, 2061
etiology and pathogenesis of disease of, 1321–24
femoral shunt with, external, 2047
Florence flask, 1325
fluoroscopy and, 1765
grafts:
aneurysm repair, 1326, 1328, 2043–48
femoral artery, 2059–60
iliac artery, 1335–36, 1345
regurgitation repair, 750
impedance of, 47–48, 1039
inflammation. *See* Aortitis.
kinking (pseudocoarctation), 1324
laceration of, 741–42
Marfan's syndrome and, 1322
medial degeneration, 1322, 1325, 1330
occlusive disease, 1334–36
abdominal angina and, 1334–35
acute, 1336
aortoiliac, 1335–36
arch, 1334

Aorta: occlusive disease:
chronic, 1334–35
renovascular hypertension and, 1335
patent ductus arteriosus and, 614–18
pulmonary artery supply from, anomalous, 621–22
pulse of, 142
radiography of. *See* Aortography.
right ventricular origin of. *See* Double-outlet right ventricle; Transposition of great arteries.
roentgenography and, 232–34, 241, 242
sinus of. *See* Sinus of Valsalva.
surgery for diseases of, 2043–51
systolic flow velocity curve, 1979–80
Takayasu's disease, 1323
transposition of. *See* Transposition of great arteries.
trauma of, 1277, 1278, 1280–81
surgical repair of, 2048–49
truncus arteriosus and, 669
tunnel with left ventricle, 644–45
valve of. *See* Aortic valve.
windkessel effect, 26
Aortic aneurysm, 1324–28
abdominal, 1327–28
caval fistula with, 1380
clinical manifestations, 1327
diagnosis, 1327
etiology, 1327
management, 1328
natural history, 1327–28
pathology, 1327
angiography, 1318
arch, 1325, 1326, 2045–46
calcification, 1317
CT scan and, 1871–72
congenital defects and, 1324
dissecting. *See* Aorta, dissection.
false, trauma and, 1281
fusiform, 1324, 1326
hemoptysis and, 119
mycotic, 1322
pain from, 1325
abdominal, 1327
radionuclide studies and, 1822
roentgenography, 1317
ruptured:
abdominal, 1327
syphilis and, 1317
thoracic, 1326
saccular, 1324
sinus of Valsalva. *See* Sinus of Valsalva aneurysm.
surgical treatment, 2043–48
syphilis and, 1316–17, 1319, 1325
thoracic, 1324–27
clinical manifestations, 1325
diagnosis, 1325
etiology, 1324–25
management, 1326–27, 2043–45
natural history and prognosis, 1325
pathology, 1325
surgical repair, 2043–45, 2047
thrombosis, 1324, 1327
Aortic annulus, small, 2032
Aortic arch:
aneurysm, 1325
repair of, 1326, 2045–46
anomalies, 14–15, 622–27
cervical, 626–27
circumflex, 622

Aortic arch:
double, 14, 624
clinical manifestations, 624
CT scan of, 1872
management, 624, 2051
pathology, 624
embryology, 3, 9, 13–15
interrupted, 15, 634–35
classification, 634
clinical manifestations, 634
cyanosis and, 132
management, 634–35
pathology, 634
occlusive disease, 1334
receptors:
blood pressure control and, 1040
shock and, 374
right, 14, 623
avian and common types, 238
clinical manifestations, 623
defects associated with, 238
pathology, 623
roentgenography and, 233, 238
surgical management, 623
tetralogy of Fallot and, 662
syndrome of, 1323
truncus arteriosus and, 9, 669
Aortic–left ventricular tunnel, 644–45
Aorticopulmonary septal defect (window), 9, 618–19
clinical manifestations, 618–19
management, 619
natural history and prognosis, 619
pathology, 618
Aortic pressure:
coronary blood flow and, 857, 861
CPR and, 547
dissection and, 1333
incisura, 52, 53
protein metabolism and, 97
pulse and, 53, 141–42
tamponade and, 1258–59
Aortic sac, 3, 9, 13
Aortic stenosis, 635–42, 729–39
acquired, 729–39
clinical manifestations, 732–35
cost analysis of treatment, 739
etiology, 729
medical treatment, 736
natural history and prognosis, 735–36
pathology, 729–30
pathophysiology, 730–32
physical examination, 733–34
postoperative management, 737–38
rheumatic, 729, 786
surgical treatment, 736–37
afterload and, 274, 331, 332, 730, 732
aging and, 1410
angina pectoris and, 732, 910, 990
assessment, 248–49
acquired disease and, 732–35
congenital disease and, 635–37
calcific, 730, 734, 787
cardiomyopathy vs., 1205
catheterization studies, 273, 734
congenital disease and, 637, 639–41
cerebral hypoperfusion and, 1361
congenital, 635–39
clinical manifestations, 635–37
medical management, 638
natural history and prognosis, 637–38
pathology, 635

Aortic stenosis: congenital:
pathophysiology, 635
surgical management, 638–39
contractility and, 274, 732
coronary heart disease and, 990–91
definition, 635
Doppler studies, 1981–83
ECG, 248, 734
congenital disease and, 636
echocardiography, 248–49, 734, 1959
congenital disease and, 636–37, 639, 641
ejection fraction and, 268
exercise and, 638, 735
fibrous, 729–30
gallop and, atrial, 179
genetics, 568
heart failure and, 273–74, 733
hypertrophy and, 636, 730–32, 734
mitral regurgitation and, 785–86, 788–90
mitral stenosis and, 785, 786, 788, 789
murmur, 190–91, 635–36, 733–34
noncardiac surgery and, 1516
phonocardiography, 1996
pregnancy and, 1387, 1389
preload and, 274
pulse and, 145
radionuclide studies, 735
roentgenography, 734
congenital disease and, 636
vs. sclerosis, 249
sounds, 173, 636, 733–34
ejection, 183, 184
subvalvular, 639–41. *See also* Cardiomyopathy, hypertrophic.
clinical manifestations, 639–40
management, 640–41
mitral stenosis and, 648
natural history and prognosis, 640
pathology, 639
sudden death and, 531
supravalvular, 641–42
clinical manifestations, 641
facial features and, 128, 129
management, 641–42
natural history and prognosis, 641
pathology, 641
pulse pressure inequality and, 141
syncope and, 522, 524, 732–33
systolic pressure and, 635, 636, 638
thromboembolism and, 1671
ventricular function and, 268
Aortic valve, 729–51
absent, 13
anatomy, 22
area determination, 1785
Doppler studies and, 1982–83
assessment, 247–50
atresia and, 646
bicuspid valve and, 247–48, 642–43
regurgitation and, 249–50, 644, 744–48
stenosis and, 248–49, 635–37, 732–35
atresia, 645–47
angiography and, 1790
associated conditions, 645
clinical manifestations, 646
medical management, 646
prognosis, 645
surgical management, 647
atrioventricular canal and, 9
bicuspid, 13, 642–43
acquired, 729, 730
Aortic valve: bicuspid:
associated conditions, 642
calcification, 643, 730
cerebral embolism and, 1358–59
clinical manifestations, 247–48, 642–43
congenital, 642–43, 741
echocardiography, 247, 643, 1955, 1959–60
endocarditis and, 1163
insurance and, 1560
management, 643
natural history and prognosis, 643
pathology, 642
regurgitation and, 741
sounds, 183–84, 636
stenosis and, 635
calcification, 242, 248–49, 730, 734
bicuspid valve and, 643, 730
mitral stenosis and, 787
surgical management, 2031
cusps, 22
double-outlet right ventricle and, 699
echocardiography, 1934, 1935, 1938, 1940–41, 1959
bicuspid valve and, 247, 643, 1955, 1959–60
regurgitation and, 747, 1959
ventricular performance and, 1963–64
embolism from, 1358–59
embryology, 12–13
endocarditis, 1145
bicuspid valve and, 1163
drug-related, 1132
prosthesis and, 1133
regurgitation and, 740, 749, 1138
fibrous skeleton and, 17, 18
mitral valve disease and, 785–91
clinical manifestations, 786–90
etiology, 785
natural history and prognosis, 790
pathology, 785
pathophysiology, 785–86
treatment, 790–91
murmurs, 163
regurgitation and, 193, 745–46, 1315, 1316
necropsy and, 2078, 2079
preoperative evaluation, 2030
regurgitation, 643–44, 739–51
acute severe, 250
aneurysm repair and, 2043, 2047
angiography, 747, 1789
ankylosing spondylitis and, 740, 1440–41
asymptomatic, 249–50
bicuspid valve and, 741
cardiomegaly and, 274
catheterization studies, 274, 275, 747–48
chronic severe, 249
clinical manifestations, 249–50, 644, 744–48
congenital, 643–44, 741
contractility and, 274–75
coronary heart disease and, 991
cost analysis, 751
dilatation of aorta and, 741
dissection and, 743, 749, 1331, 1333, 2047
Doppler studies, 1983–85
ECG, 747
echocardiography, 747, 1959
endocarditis and, 740, 749, 1138
Aortic valve: regurgitation:
etiology, 739
exercise testing, 748
fluoroscopy, 1765
heart failure and, 274–75, 748, 749
history, 744–45
intrinsic disease and, 740
laceration of aorta and, 741–42
Marfan's syndrome and, 741, 745
medical treatment, 749
mitral regurgitation and, 785–91
mitral stenosis and, 785, 788, 789
murmur, 193, 745–46, 1315, 1316
myxoma and, 741
natural history and prognosis, 748–49
noncardiac surgery and, 1516
pathology, 643, 739–42
pathophysiology, 742–44
phonocardiography, 1996
physical examination, 745–47
postoperative care, 751
pregnancy and, 1387, 1389
pulse and, 144
radionuclide studies, 249, 748, 1822
rheumatic, 740, 1308
roentgenography, 747
sounds, 745–46, 1315, 1316
stroke volume and, 742, 747, 748, 1783–84
surgical management, 644, 749–51, 790–91, 2030–32, 2047
syphilis and, 1315–16, 1319
traumatic, 740, 1280
ventricular performance and, 1826
ventricular septal defect and, 591, 595, 741
replacement, 737–39
aneurysm repair and, 2043, 2044
combined mitral-aortic valve disease and, 790–91
endocarditis and, 1133
regurgitation and, 644, 750–51
results, 738–39, 750–51, 2034
small annulus and, 2032
syphilis and, 1316, 1319
technique, 2030–32
sclerosis, 249
sounds, 160
bicuspid valve and, 183–84, 643
closure, 162, 163, 166–76
ejection, 163, 183–84
regurgitation and, 745–46, 1315, 1316
stenosis and, 173, 183, 184, 636, 733–34
stenosis. *See* Aortic stenosis.
transverse section, 18
Aortitis, 1322–24
ankylosing spondylitis and, 1323–24
bacterial, 1322
giant cell, 1323
nonspecific, 1322–23
regurgitation and, 741
Reiter's syndrome and, 1323–24
sudden death and, 530
syphilitic, 1314–17
Takayasu's, 1323
Aortocaval fistula, 1380
Aortocoronary bypass surgery. *See* Coronary bypass surgery.
Aortofemoral bypass graft, 2059–60
Aortography:
aneurysm and, 1318
sinus of Valsalva, 2044

Aortography:
aortocaval fistula and, 1380
coarctation and, 2050
digital subtraction, 1859
dissection and, 1331, 1332
femoral artery occlusion and, 2058
mesenteric occlusion and, 1365, 1368, 1369
pulmonary atresia and, 1788
rupture and, 1281
Aortoiliac endarterectomy, 2058, 2061
Aortoiliac occlusive disease, 1335–36, 1345
acute, 1336
chronic, 1335–36
surgical treatment, 2058–60
Aortoplasty, coarctation and, 632, 633
Aortotomy:
abdominal, 2058
supravalvular stenosis and, 642
valve surgery and, 2031
Apex beat, 153–55
cardiomyopathy and, 1201
mitral regurgitation and, 770
recording of. *See* Apexcardiography.
Apexcardiography, 1993–95
cardiac cycle and, 52, 53
cardiomyopathy and, 1201, 1203, 1995
mitral stenosis and, 1996
myxoma and, 1288
physiological correlations, 1994–95
technique, 1995
Apnea, sleep, obesity and, 1455
Apoproteins, 574
Appraisal, cardiac, 106–8
Approach to patient, 103–8
Apresoline. *See* Hydralazine.
Arachidonic acid, 814
Arachnodactyly, 132
Aramine, 1653
Aretaeus, 1354
Argon laser, 1922, 1923
Arm exercise, 1027, 1032
ergometry, 1705
Arrest, cardiac, 471. *See also* Sudden death.
approach to patient with, 295
cardiopulmonary bypass and, 2028
contributing factors, 471
coronary bypass surgery and, 2037–38
CPR and, 549, 551
identification of, 549
myocardial infarction and, 982, 986
out-of-hospital survivors of, 478
Arrest, respiratory, 549
Arrhythmias, 406–84. *See also* specific disturbance.
aberrant conduction, 412, 457–61. *See also* Intraventricular conduction, aberrant.
accelerated idioventricular, 456
accelerated junctional rhythm, 420, 468, 470
afterdepolarization and, 408–9
aging and, 1410
alcoholism and, 1447–48
anesthesia and, 1515
angina pectoris and, 988
anxiety neurosis and, 1527
assessment, 281–95, 433–71
athletes and, 1401, 1402
atrial, 413–15, 443–47
extrasystoles, 437–38. *See also* Premature atrial beats.

Arrhythmias:
atrial fibrillation, 415, 446–47. *See also* Atrial fibrillation.
atrial flutter, 414–15, 443–45. *See also* Atrial flutter.
atrial tachycardia, 413–14. *See also* Atrial tachycardia.
automaticity and, 407–8
AV block, 427–28, 462–66. *See also* Atrioventricular block.
AV dissociation, 420, 466–68
AV junctional, 417–20. *See also* Atrioventricular junction.
extrasystoles, 438–39
tachycardia, 417–20, 470
variants, 468–69
bradycardia, 426–28. *See also* Bradycardia.
bundle branch block. *See* Bundle branch block.
caffeine and, 1483
calcium and, 1473, 1475
cardiomyopathy and, 1188, 1204
cardioversion and, 483–84. *See also* Cardioversion.
catheter-induced, 2001–2
cerebrovascular disease and, 1359, 1360–61
circus movement, 413–14
concealed conduction and, 412
coronary artery disease and, 304, 988–89
coronary bypass surgery and, 950, 953
cor pulmonale and, 1126
digitalis-induced, 479, 1647–48
Ebstein's anomaly and, 678, 680
ECG and, 433–34. *See also* Electrocardiography.
electricity-induced, 1487
emotional stress and, 1522–23
escape rhythms, 469–70
exercise and, 1711
Friedreich's ataxia and, 1229
genetics and, 576–77
glossary, 433
graphic methods and, 433–35
group beating, 466
heart failure and, 358
history, 281–82
hyperthyroidism and, 1414, 1415
idioventricular, 456, 470–71
impulse conduction and, 409–12
impulse formation and, 407–9, 412
induction studies of, 1737–38
insurance and, 1561
interference dissociation, 466
intraventricular conduction, 412, 457–61. *See also* Intraventricular conduction.
laboratory tests, 282–83
magnesium and, 1476
management, 475–84, 1593–1603
bradyarrhythmias and conduction defects, 479–82
cardioversion, 483–84. *See also* Cardioversion.
delayed repolarization, 479
pacing modalities, 482–83. *See also* Pacing.
pharmacologic, 476–81, 1593–1603. *See also* Antiarrhythmic agents *and* specific agent.
preexcitation syndromes, 477
surgical, 2013–15
tachyarrhythmias, 476–79

Arrhythmias:
mapping of, 1738
mechanisms, 406–28
basis of determination of, 412–13
metastases and, 1296
monitoring of, 2004
morbidity, 563
muscular dystrophy and, 1227, 1228
myocardial infarction and, 925, 968–69
drug therapy, 830–31
as early complication of, 972–77
as late complication of, 985–86
myocardial ischemia and, 957, 961, 988–89
myocarditis and, 1165, 1168, 1170, 1178
nervous system and, 424
in normal populations, 435
palpitation and, 117, 283–87
parasystole, 412, 456–57
physical examination, 282
postoperative, 1518
psychological factors and, 1532
potassium and, 1467–70
preexcitation syndromes, 415–17, 447–49. *See also* Preexcitation syndromes; Wolff-Parkinson-White syndrome.
pregnancy and, 1392
programmed stimulation and, 1737. *See also* Pacing; Stimulation techniques.
pulse and, 146, 150
reciprocal, 468
reentry and, 410–11. *See also* Reentry.
reflection and, 412
repolarization and, 411–12
sarcoidosis and, 1217–18
shock and, 371, 389–90
sick-sinus syndrome, 449–50
sinoatrial block, 461–62
sinus node, 436–37. *See also* Sinus arrhythmias.
dysfunction and, 426–27, 449–50
supraventricular tachycardia, 439–43. *See* Tachycardia, supraventricular.
surgical procedures and, noncardiac, 1514–15, 1518
syncope and, 287, 523–24, 988, 1360, 1361. *See also* Syncope.
diagnosis, 525–27
treatment, 527–28
tachycardia, 413–26. *See also* Tachycardia.
torsades de pointes, 424, 455–56
triggered activity and, 408–9, 413
unidirectional block, 410–11
venous pulse and, 150
ventricular extrasystoles, 450–52. *See also* Premature ventricular beats.
ventricular fibrillation, 425–26, 446–47. *See also* Ventricular fibrillation.
ventricular tachycardia, 420–24, 452–56. *See also* Tachycardia, ventricular.
wandering pacemaker, 468–69
Wolff-Parkinson-White syndrome, 416–17. *See also* Wolff-Parkinson-White syndrome.
Arsenic poisoning, 1234
Arsine poisoning, 1234
Arterial pressure. *See also* Blood pressure; Hypertension; Hypotension.

Arterial pressure:
CPR and, 549
mean, 1038
shock and, 370, 372
Arterial valves. *See* Aortic valve; Pulmonary valve.
Arteries, 26. *See also* specific artery *and* Vasculature.
catheterization, pressure monitoring and, 386
cutdown of, cardiac catheterization and, 1772
Doppler studies and, 1974–76
hyperdynamic state and, 395–96
pulse of. *See* Pulse, arterial.
shock and, 372–73
Arteriography. *See* Angiography; Coronary arteriography; Pulmonary angiography.
Arterioles, 26
shock and, 373
Arteriosclerosis, retinal, 199, 203
Arteriosclerosis obliterans, 1339–46
amputation and, 1346
angioplasty for, 1346
claudication and, 1340
clinical manifestations, 1339–41
diagnosis, 1341–42
differential diagnosis, 1342–43
etiology, 1339
medical treatment, 1343–45
pathology and pathophysiology, 1339
physical examination, 1340–41
prognosis, 1343
rest pain and, 1340
surgical treatment, 1345–46
sympathectomy for, 1346
thrombolytic therapy, 1346
Arteriospasm. *See* Coronary arteries, spasm; Spasm.
Arteriotomy:
aortoiliac, 2058
carotid, 2053
Arteriovenous fistula, 400–402
aortocaval, 1380
cardiac output increase and, 400–402
coronary, 707–8, 1019
clinical manifestations, 257, 708
management, 708
murmur, 194, 257
pathology, 707–8
dialysis, 401, 1462
endocarditis and, 1460
physical examination and, 204
pulmonary, 680–81, 1896–97
systemic, 125, 400–402
clinical manifestations, 401
diagnosis and treatment, 402
Arteritis. *See also* Polyarteritis; Vasculitis.
arteriosclerosis obliterans vs., 1342
coronary, sudden death and, 530
mesenteric, postoperative, 1371
pulmonary, 588
temporal (giant cell), 201, 1323
Arthritis:
gouty, 134
inspection for, 133–34
Jaccoud's, 133, 134
rheumatic fever and, 1308
rheumatoid, 1439–40
inspection for, 133
myocardial nodules and, 1439
pericarditis and, 1269, 1439
therapy, 1440
valvular nodules and, 1439, 1440
Arthropod venom, 1489
Artificial heart, 2069–76
candidate selection, 2075
complications, 2074–75
drive system, 2069, 2071, 2072
historical background, 2069
implantation technique, 2069–70
model, 2069
suspected results, 2070–73
Aschoff body, 1307
Ascites, 118
diuretics and, 1662
endomyocardial fibrosis and, 1211, 1212
physical examination and, 204
Ashman's phenomenon, 447
aberrant conduction and, 458
Aspergillosis:
endocarditis and, 1136
myocarditis and, 1175
Aspirin:
adverse reactions to, 1678
angina pectoris and, 1677
coronary bypass surgery and, 954–55, 1677
coronary heart disease prognosis and, 923
myocardial infarction and, 831, 944, 1677–78
pericarditis and, 1254
prosthetic valves and, 1676
rheumatic fever and, 1311
thromboxane and, 1675
transient ischemic attacks and, 1357
Asplenia, 135, 689–90
Asthenia:
neurocirculatory, 1526, 1533
vasoregulatory, 910–11
Asthma:
beta-blocking agents and, 1618
cardiac, 349
wheezing and, 115–16
Asymmetric septal hypertrophy. *See* Cardiomyopathy, hypertrophic; Hypertrophy, asymmetric septal.
Asynergy, ventricular, 1803–4
Asystole, 471. *See also* Sudden death.
AV block and, 462, 463
cardiopulmonary bypass and, 2028
CPR and, 551
syncope and, 523
Ataxia, Friedreich's, 126, 1229
genetics, 569
Atenolol, 1607. *See also* Beta-blocking agents.
dosage, 941, 1072
hypertension and, 1081
gestational, 1085
pharmacodynamics, 1608, 1613, 1617
pharmacokinetics, 1610, 1611
protein-binding and dialysance, 1082
structure, 1608
Atherosclerosis, 801–992. *See also* Coronary heart disease; Occlusive disease.
acromegaly and, 1422–23
advanced (complicated) lesions, 802–3, 841
aortic, 1321–22, 1334
arch, 1334
terminal portion, 1335–36
arteriography and. *See* Coronary arteriography.
asymptomatic, 958, 959–61
Atherosclerosis:
bypass surgery for. *See* Coronary bypass surgery.
calcification and, 802
cardiomyopathy and, 1187, 1190–91, 1206
carotid artery, 1334, 1355, 1356, 1875
Doppler studies and, 1975
endarterectomy for, 2052–56
catecholamines and, 1524
cellular modulations in, 809–15
cerebrovascular, 1355–57
diagnosis, 1355–56
management, 1356–57
manifestations, 1355
cholesterol and, 807–8, 812–13
preventive measures, 820–22, 828–29
regression and, 819
corticosteroids and, 1524
diabetes mellitus and, 808–9, 825, 829, 1428–29
diet and, 820–22, 828
Doppler studies and, 1975, 1976
emotional stress and, 1523–24
endothelium and, 803, 804, 809–11
barrier role, 809–10
response-to-injury hypothesis, 804–6
exercise and, management and, 933
experimentally induced, 803–4
regression and, 819
fatty streak, 801, 814. *See also* Fatty streak.
fibrous plaque, 801–2, 841
rupture of, 870–71
genetics, 573
glucose (intolerance) and, 825, 829
historical view of, 804
hyperlipidemia and, 807–8, 812–13
preventive measures, 820–23, 828–29
regression and, 819
hypertension and, 808, 823–24, 828
hypotheses of, 804–9, 841–42
hypothyroidism and, 1420
iliac, 1335–36
laser therapy of, 1922–25
lesions of, 801–15
lipogenic theory of, 807, 841
lipoproteins and, 807, 813. *See also* Lipoprotein.
macrophages and, 805, 813
male sex and, 808
mesenteric, 1364, 1368
micrograph, 802
monoclonal theory of, 806–7, 842
myocardial ischemia and, 842, 856. *See also* Myocardial ischemia.
natural history, 817–18
obesity and, 824–25, 829, 936, 1453
obliterative. *See* Arteriosclerosis obliterans.
pathology, 841–55
pediatric beginnings of, 818
peripheral arterial, 2057. *See also* Occlusive disease.
platelets and, 804, 805, 813–14
growth factor from, 806, 812, 813–14
prevention, 817–32, 958
basis for, 817–20
community approach, 817, 819–20, 827
high-risk individual and, 817

Atherosclerosis: prevention:
multifactorial approach, 826–27, 831–32
physician's role in, 826–27
primary, 818, 820–27
secondary, 818, 827–32
validation problems, 818–19
prostaglandins and, 814
radiation and, 1023
regression of, 819
renal failure and, 1463–64
renovascular, 1058–59, 1079–80
research needs and, 814
response-to-injury theory of, 804–6
retinal, 199
risk factors, 807–9, 889
alterable vs. unalterable, 819, 820
evidence for, 819
intervention principle, 817
legal issues and, 1571–72
physician's role and, 826–27
populations and, 817, 819
preventive measures, 820–32
saphenous vein graft, 853, 854
smoking and, 808, 823, 827–28
smooth-muscle cells and, 805, 806, 811–13
spasm of coronary arteries and, 1010
stages in development, 803
sudden death and, 530, 535, 540, 850
thrombosis and, 802, 804–5, 809, 842
transplanted heart and, 2066–67
von Willebrand's disease and, 812
Athletes, 1398–1402
arrhythmias and, 1401, 1402
congenital heart disease and, 1402
ECG and, 1052, 1401
echocardiography and, 1052, 1401
examination of, 1401–2
exercise and, 1398–1400
hypertension and, 1052–53
murmurs in, 1400–1401
stress tests and, 1402
sudden death in, 1401
training effect and, 1400
Ativan, 1496
Atracurium, 1497
Atria (atrium):
action potential, 75, 76
activation sequence, 81, 82
alignment of, 686, 687
anatomy, 16, 18–20
appendages, 18, 20
tricuspid atresia and, 673
balloon septostomy, transposition of great arteries and, 694
bigeminy, 438, 439, 445
compliance, heart failure and, 333
conduction pathways, 30, 73
contractility, 48
depolarization, 206
digitalis effects on, 1643
echocardiographic dimensions, 1936, 1946, 1947
electrocardiography and, 80–81, 1690–1703
embryology, 5, 11–12
failure, 322, 333
fibrillation. *See* Atrial fibrillation.
flutter. *See* Atrial flutter.
gallop. *See* Gallop, atrial.
inexcitable, 490
left:
anatomy, 19–20
Atria: left:
appendage, 20
catheterization of, 1772
enlarged, 758, 764, 772
hypertension and, 1053–54
membrane dividing. *See* Cor triatriatum.
myxoma, 1287–90. *See also* Myxoma.
vena cava union with, 684–85
mechanical function, 48–49
myxoma, 1287–92. *See also* Myxoma.
natriuretic factor, 325, 326
pacing. *See* Pacing, atrial.
premature beats. *See* Premature atrial beats.
programmed stimulation of, 1736–37
refractory period, 1736–37
repolarization, 206
right:
anatomy, 18–19
appendage, 18
Ebstein's anomaly and, 678
electrogram, 1729
frontal view, 18
left ventricular communication with, 613–14
metastases to, 1297
myxoma, 1290–91
pulmonary artery anastomosis to, 676, 706
pulmonary venous connection anomaly and, 682
roentgenography and, 241–43
septum. *See* Atrial septal defect; Interatrial septum.
single, 612
diagnosis and management, 612
transverse sections of, 17, 18
Atrial fibrillation, 415, 446–47
aberrant conduction and, 447, 458, 461
aortic-mitral combined valvular disease and, 789, 790
cardiomyopathy and, 1188, 1204
coronary bypass surgery and, 953
digoxin and, 943
ECG, 446–47
embolism and, 1671–72
heart failure and, 333, 358
hyperthyroidism and, 396–97, 1414
lone, 446, 449
management, 477
calcium channel blockers in, 1630
cardioversion, 483, 1742–44
digitalis in, 1645
mechanism, 415
mitral regurgitation and, 772, 775
mitral stenosis and, 758, 760–61
myocardial infarction and, 974
nuclear probe technique and, 1830
potassium and, 1469
slow, 490
tricuspid regurgitation and, 795
WPW syndrome and, 416, 448
Atrial flutter, 414–15, 441–45
AV block and, 445, 446
calcium channel blockers and, 1631
cardioversion for, 1744
digitalis and, 943, 1645
ECG and, 443–45
entrainment and, 414–15
ladder diagrams and, 434
management, 476
Atrial flutter:
mechanism, 414–15
myocardial infarction and, 974
slow, 490
Wenckebach periods and, 445
Atrial kick, 20, 48
Atrial premature beats. *See* Premature atrial beats.
Atrial pressure, 1091–92
cardiac cycle and, 52
mitral stenosis and, 755
normal, 55
pericarditis and, constrictive, 1257, 1263
tamponade and, 1257
tricuspid regurgitation and, 150
tricuspid stenosis and, 794
venous pulse and, 147, 148
Atrial septal defect, 597–603
anatomic types, 598–99
AV canal and, 605–12
catheterization studies, 601
chambers and, 599
clinical manifestations, 599–600
definition, 597
Doppler studies, 1986–87
Ebstein's anomaly and, 678
ECG, 224, 600–601
echocardiography, 601, 1944
embryology, 9, 12
fossa ovalis and, 598
genetics, 568, 599–600, 602
history, 600
indicator-dilution technique and, 1782
medical management, 602
mitral stenosis and, 599
murmur, 600
natural history and prognosis, 601–2
ostium primum type, 9, 605–6, 611
pathology, 597–99
pathophysiology, 599
physical examination, 600
pulmonary hypertension and, 599
pulmonary venous connection anomaly and, 598, 601, 603–5
pulmonic stenosis and, 655
roentgenography, 234, 235, 600
secundum type, 12, 598, 599
assessment, 255–56, 600, 601
management, 602, 603
sinus venosus type, 598, 603
sounds, 600
ejection, 182
opening snap, 185
second, 167–68, 174
surgical management, 602–3
venous pulse and, 602–3
Atrial tachycardia. *See* Tachycardia, atrial; Tachycardia, supraventricular.
Atrio-Hisian fibers, 415, 416
Atriopeptin, 49
heart failure and, 326
Atriopulmonary anastomosis, 676
univentricular heart and, 706
Atriotomy, myxoma and, 1293
Atrioventricular accessory pathway. *See* Accessory pathways.
Atrioventricular block (AV block), 427–28, 462–66
approach to patient with, 289–91
asystole and, 462, 463
atrial flutter and, 445, 446
atrial tachycardia and, 440
AV dissociation and, 466, 467

Atrioventricular block:
block/acceleration dissociation, 462
causes, 463–64
classification, 462
congenital, 488–89, 576
decremental conduction and, 410
digitalis-induced, 479
ECG and, 290, 464–66
esophageal, 1696, 1697
myocardial infarction and, 977
electrophysiological studies and, 290
His bundle recordings and, 1730–32
HV interval and, 291
management, 480–81
mechanism, 427–28
myocardial infarction and, 427–28, 977
pacing and, 489
in normal populations, 435
pacing and, 480–81, 488–89
potassium and, 1467–69
shock and, 389
surgical procedures and, 1515
syncope and, 287, 288, 516, 523, 524, 526
transposition of great arteries and, 701, 702
Atrioventricular canal, 8–9, 605–12
anatomic types, 605–6
aortic valve and, 9
associated conditions, 606
catheterization studies, 608
clinical manifestations, 607–8
common, 605–12
complete, 606
definition, 605, 686
ECG, 607–8
echocardiography, 608
embryology, 8–9
genetics, 610
history, 607
hypertrophy and, 607–8
medical management, 609–10
murmur, 607
natural history and prognosis, 608–9
partial, 605–6
pathology, 605–6
pathophysiology, 606–7
physical examination, 607
roentgenography, 607
sounds, 607
surgical management, 610–12
Atrioventricular concordance and discordance, 686
corrected transposition of great arteries and, 700
crisscross heart and, 706
Atrioventricular dissociation, 466–68
AV junctional tachycardia and, 420
block/acceleration, 462
definition, 466
ECG, 466–68
escape beats and, 469
isorhythmic, 467, 468
management, 481
potassium and, 1468
retrograde, 1696, 1697
Atrioventricular junction:
accelerated rhythm, 420, 462, 468, 470
esophageal ECG and, 1698
myocardial infarction and, 974
escape rhythm, 435, 469–70
extrasystoles, 438–39
reciprocal rhythm, 468, 469
Atrioventricular junction:
rhythm, 470
tachycardia, 417–20, 470
with AV dissociation, 420
ECG, 419, 441–43
ectopic, 440
myocardial infarction and, 974
nonparoxysmal, 420
with 1:1 AV association, 418–20
paroxysmal, 418–20
reentry and, 418–20
wandering pacemaker and, 469
Atrioventricular node (AV node):
anatomy, 19, 30–31
artery, 29, 427
polyarteritis nodosa and, 1439
calcium channel blockers and, 1627, 1631
conduction time, 1729–30, 1736–37
digitalis and, 1644, 1645
electrophysiology, 73, 80, 1736–37
enhanced conduction (EAVNC), 449
His bundle recording and, 1727, 1730–32
impulse conduction, 410, 1730–32
innervation, 25, 49
internodal pathways and, 30
junction with His bundle. *See* Atrioventricular junction.
mesothelioma of, 1294
pacing and. *See also* Pacing.
incremental, 1736
programmed stimulation and, 1736–37
reentry, 418–20, 440, 441
refractory period, 1736–37
surgical division of, 2015
Atrioventricular sulcus, 16
Atrioventricular valves:
embryology, 12–13
left. *See* Mitral valve.
right. *See* Tricuspid valve.
Atrium. *See* Atria.
Atropine:
bradycardia and, 389, 973
coronary arteriography and, 1792
morphine therapy and, 939
Aureomycin, hypersensitivity to, 1237
Auscultation, 157–95
aids to, 195
blood pressure measurement and, 139–40
drugs and, 195
evolution of, 157
handgrip maneuver and, 195
heart sounds and, 158–61, 164–88. *See also* Sounds, heart.
hyperdynamic state and, 396
murmurs and, 158, 188–95. *See also* Murmurs.
perception of sound and, 158
phonocardiography and, 1992–93
physical properties of, 161–62
physics of, 157
squatting and, 195
stethoscope qualities and, 162
technique, 162–64
transmission of sounds and, 160–61
Valsalva maneuver and, 195
Austin Flint murmur, 193
aortic regurgitation and, 746, 1316
Austrian's syndrome, 1136
Automaticity, 78–79, 407–8
abnormal, 408
atrial pacing and, 1735
Automaticity:
atrial tachycardia and, 413
calcium and, 1473
enhanced, 407
normal, 407–8
reentry vs., 412–13
Automobile safety regulations, 1578
Autonomic nervous system, 24–25. *See also* Parasympathetic nervous system; Sympathetic nervous system.
arrhythmias and, 424
asthenia and, vasoregulatory, 910–11
diabetes mellitus and, 1427–28
heart failure and, 323–24
shock and, 374–76
sinus node dysfunction and, 288–89
syncope and, 511–13
thyroid hormone and, 1415
Autoregulation:
coronary blood flow, 61, 857–58
neurogenic vasoconstriction and, 862
steal and, 864
redistribution of blood flow and, 51
shock and, 377–78
Azotemia, 1460
intact nephron, 1060
Azygos vein:
cardiac catheterization and, 1770
dilatation, heart failure and, 355
roentgenography and, 231, 241
vena caval continuity with, 686
CT scan and, 1872

Bachman's bundle, 30
Back, straight, syndrome of, 134
Bacteremia:
drug abuse and, 1132
endocarditis and, 1144
postoperative, 1151–53
prophylaxis, 1151–53
Bacteria:
aortitis, 1322
endocarditis, 1135–36. *See also* Endocarditis.
myocarditis, 1173
pericarditis, 1270
staphylococcal. *See* Staphylococcal infections.
streptococcal. *See* Streptococcal infections.
Bactericidal titer, endocarditis and, 1148
Baffle, interatrial, 695
Bainbridge reflex, 50
exercise and, 55
Balke test, 1705
Balloon catheter, 1772
angiographic, 1785, 1786
angioplasty. *See* Angioplasty, percutaneous transluminal.
Datascope, 2021–22
embolization therapy and, 1896
flotation, 1999–2002. *See also* Swan-Ganz catheterization.
complications, 2001–2
data collection, 2000
indications, 2000–2001
insertion technique, 1999–2000
Kontron, 2022
monitoring and, 1999–2002
S.M.E.C., 2021
Balloon pump. *See* Intraaortic balloon counterpulsation.
Balloon septostomy, transposition of great arteries and, 694

Barbiturates, anesthetic use of, 1496
Barometric pressure, increased. *See* Hyperbaric pressure.
Baroreceptors:
  digitalis and, 1642
  shock and, 374–75
Batteries, pacemaker, 490–91
Bayer-2052, 1179
Bayes' theorem, 103, 304–6
Beading, retinal vascular, 198–99
Beck's triad, 1260
Bee venom, 1489
Behavioral factors. *See* Emotional stress; Psychological factors.
Behçet's disease, 124, 1238
Bendroflumethiazide, 1659, 1660
  dosage, 1072
Bennett's formula, 248
Benzodiazepines:
  anesthetic use of, 1496
  rehabilitation and, 1532
Benzothiadiazines, 1658–60
Benzthiazide, 1072, 1659
Bergmeister's papilla, 199
Beriberi, 397–99, 1218, 1448–49
  clinical manifestations, 398
  diagnosis and treatment, 399
  laboratory studies, 398–99
Berman balloon catheter, 1786
Beta-blocking agents, 1602–21. *See also* Propranolol and other specific agents.
  adverse effects, 940–41, 1073, 1539, 1617–21
  alpha-blocking activity of, 1609–10
  angina pectoris and, 1613–15
  aortic dissection and, 1617
  arrhythmias and, 1598–99, 1615
  asthma and, 1618
  calcium channel blockers and, 1614, 1629, 1630, 1635
  cardiomyopathy and, 1192–93, 1206–7, 1616
  cardiovascular effects, 1612–17
  central nervous system and, 1612–13, 1620
  choice of, 1620, 1621
  combined therapy with, 1614
  contraindications, 940
  coronary artery spasm and, 1015, 1614–15
  coronary heart disease and, 939–41
  diabetes mellitus and, 1075, 1430
  dosage, 941, 1611
  heart failure and, 358
    induction of, 1618
  hypertension and, 1071–75, 1612–13
    clinical settings and, 1071, 1074
    dosage, 1072
    gestational, 1085
    hyperlipemia and, 1074
    premature ventricular beats and, 1074
    renoparenchymal, 1080–81
  hyperthyroidism and, 1417–18
  hypoglycemia induced by, 1620
  indications, 940, 1612–17
  interactions, 1619, 1621
  membrane-stabilizing activity, 1607
  mitral valve prolapse and, 1616–17
  myocardial infarction and, 830, 967, 1615–16
    historical note on, 887
    long-term use in, 971
  myocardial ischemia and, 866
Beta-blocking agents:
  nitrates and, 1614
  noncardiovascular applications, 1617
  oculomucocutaneous syndrome induced by, 1621
  pharmacokinetics, 940, 1610–11
  pharmacology, 1607–11
  pheochromocytoma and, 1083
  plasma level-dose-efficacy relations, 1611
  postoperative, 953
  potency, 1607, 1608
  pregnancy and, 1393
  protein-binding and dialysance, 1082
  renin and, 1612
  selectivity, 1609
  sinus node dysfunction induced by, 1618
  structure-activity relations, 1607, 1608
  sudden death prevention and, 543
  surgical procedures and, 1514
  sympathomimetic activity, 1609
  syncope and, 528
  tetralogy of Fallot and, 1617
  therapeutic applications, 940, 1612–17
  withdrawal, 1618
Beta receptors. *See* Adrenergic receptors, beta; Beta-blocking agents.
Bethanidine, 1588
Bevantolol, 1607
Bezold-Jarisch reflex, 62
  myocardial infarction and, 981
  shock and, 375
Bicarbonate:
  acidosis correction and, 389
  CPR and, 552
  diuretics and, 1658, 1660
Bicycle ergometry, 1704–5
  catheterization studies and, 1776
  guidelines for, 1032
  radionuclide studies and, 1825
Bierce, Ambrose, 1556
Bigeminy:
  atrial, 438, 439, 445
  ventricular:
    aberrant conduction and, 460
    parasystolic, 456
Bile, lithogenic, 913, 914
Biopsy:
  endomyocardial, 1772–73
    cardiomyopathy and, 1190, 1204
    fibrosis and, 1209–10
    myocarditis and, 1168
    transplanted heart and, 2065
  myocardial, 272
  pericardial, 2009
Bipolar leads, 207
  esophageal, 1691, 1692
  pacemaker, 491
Bipyridine, contractility and, 360
Bisferiens pulse, 144–45
Bjork modification of Fontan shunt, 676
Bjork-Shiley valve, 778, 2034
  broken strut of, 2074
  thromboembolism and, 779, 1671
Blalock-Taussig shunt, 666
Bland-White-Garland syndrome, 708
Blastomycosis, 1175
Blocarden. *See* Timolol.
Block. *See* Atrioventricular block; Bundle branch block; Sinoatrial block; Wenckebach phenomenon.
Blood flow, 57–63
  autoregulation and, 51, 377–78
Blood flow:
  capillary, 26
  cardiac output. *See* Cardiac output.
  cardiopulmonary bypass and, 2027
  cerebral, 1360–61
    CPR and, 547, 548, 552
  coronary. *See* Coronary blood flow.
  CPR and, 547–49, 552
  distribution, 56
  Doppler studies and, 1974–88
  exercise and, 56, 1398
  Fick method for calculating, 1779–80
  heart failure and, 335–36, 347
  heat stress and, 1547–50
  hydrodynamics of, 1038
  indicator-dilution technique and, 1780–82
  intestinal, 1367
  intracardiac, 18, 21, 22
  magnetic resonance imaging and, 1892
  mapping, regurgitant valve and, 1984
  obesity and, 1452, 1454
  organ, 370
  physiology, 57–63
  pulmonary. *See* Pulmonary vasculature, blood flow.
  redistribution of, 51
  regulation of regional, 57–60
  renal, 325
  resistance, 1784
  shock and, 371–74
  shunt, 1779–80, 1781
  ulnar artery, 386
  uterine, pregnancy and, 1384–85
Blood gases. *See* Carbon dioxide tension; Hypercapnia; Hypoxia; Oxygen tension.
Blood pool imaging, 1818–23
Blood pressure, 138–41. *See also* Diastolic pressure; Hypertension; Hypotension; Systolic pressure.
  abnormal, 140–41
  aging and, 1406, 1409
  auscultatory gap and, 1048
  autoregulation and, 377
  cardiac output and, 1038, 1039
  cardiopulmonary bypass and, 2027
  circadian rhythm and, 1049
  coarctation of aorta and, 629, 630
  control systems, 1039–41
  diastolic arterial volume and, 1039
  exercise and, 55, 1399, 1708
  flow-resistance relations and, 58
  heart failure and, 347
  hemodynamics, 1039–40
  hydrodynamics and, 1038
  measurement, 138–40, 1048–49
    direct methods, 138–39
    errors in, 139–40
    indirect methods, 139–40
    obesity and, 1452–53
  monitoring, 1999
    computer-assisted, 2006
    shock and, 384, 386
  neural mechanism, 1040
  normal, 55, 140, 1042
  perioperative, 1498, 1502
    noncardiac surgery and, 1515–16
  physical determinants of, 138
  shock and, 370, 372
    monitoring, 384, 386
  standing position and, 1049
  variability in, 1049
Blood-retina barrier, 200

Blood volume:
aldosteronism and, 1046
exercise and, 55
heat stress and, 1548
hypertension and, 1040–41, 1043–44, 1046
hypotension and, 510, 511
obesity and, 1452, 1453–54
pulmonary, 27
radionuclide studies and, 1822–23
reduced. *See* Hypovolemia.
surgical procedures and, 1505
syncope and, 508, 510, 511
vasodilators and, 1584
venous, 26
Blue bloaters, 1123–24
Blumgart, H. L., 1809
Blunt injuries, 1021, 1276, 1278–81
Body configuration, 122
Body girth enlargement, 118
heart failure and, 350
Bone:
Paget's disease of, 402–3
pyrophosphate uptake by, 1846
roentgenography and, 236
Boot-shaped heart, 234, 663, 664
Bowditch phenomenon, 39, 46, 48
anesthesia and, 50
Brachial artery:
catheterization, 1771, 1772
coronary arteriography and, 1791
pressure, 55
pulse, 143
aortic stenosis and, 733
Brachiocephalic artery:
aortic aneurysm and, 1325, 1326
aortic arch aneurysm repair and, 2045–46
echocardiography, 1945
embryology, 1313, 1314
occlusive disease, 1334
Takayasu's disease and, 1323
tracheal compression by, 627
Brachiocephalic vein:
lymphatics and, 26, 27
pulmonary venous anomaly and, 681–82, 684
Bradycardia, 426–28
approach to patient with, 288–89
artifactual, 1725
atrial pacing techniques and, 1740
AV block. *See* Atrioventricular block.
beta-blocker-induced, 1618
bundle branch block and, 458
carotid sinus reflex and, 515
digitalis-induced, 479
hypotension and, 981
hypothyroidism and, 1420
management, 479–82
mechanisms, 426–28
pregnancy and, 1392
pulse and, 146
shock and, 371, 375, 389
sinus, 426–27, 436–37
approach to patient with, 288–89
athletes and, 1401
management, 479
myocardial infarction and, 436–37, 973
pacing and, 489
shock and, 389
syncope and, 508, 509, 516, 523, 524, 528
-tachycardia syndrome, 449, 450
esophageal ECG and, 1698, 1699
Bradycardia: -tachycardia syndrome:
management, 480
pacing and, 489–90
syncope and, 523, 528
Bradykinin, 59
converting enzyme inhibitors and, 1589
shock and, 376
Brain. *See also* Cerebrovascular disease; Cerebrum; Nervous system.
shock and, 379
Branham's sign, 401
Breathing. *See* Respiration.
difficult. *See* Dyspnea.
Brecher, G. A., 2025
Bridge, muscle, of coronary artery, 1019–20
arteriography and, 1800
Bronchi:
carcinoid of, 1298
heterotaxia and, 689
situs determination and, 687
suis, 625, 626
Bronchial arteries:
collateral flow, hemorrhage and, 1106
pulmonary artery origin from, 670
pulmonary atresia and, 670
Bronchitis:
cor pulmonale and, 1123–24
history, 120
Bruce test, 1705, 1710
Bruits:
abdominal, 205
arteriosclerosis obliterans and, 1341
mesenteric ischemia and, 1368
renovascular hypertension and, 1058
carotid, 1334
asymptomatic, 990, 1355
diagnositc studies and, 1879–80
Budd-Chiari syndrome, 1379–80
Buerger's disease, 1346–48
Bulboventricular fold, 3, 7, 8
Bulboventricular foramen, 703, 705
Bulboventricular sulcus, 3
Bulboventricular tube, 3
Bulbus cordis, 3, 5
septation and, 9
Bullet wounds, 1277, 1278
Bumetanide, 1658. *See also* Diuretics.
dosage, 1072, 1659
duration of action, 1659
hypertension and, 1080
pharmacokinetics, 1661
protein-binding and dialysance, 1082
site of action, 1660
Bundle branch(es). *See also* His bundle.
anatomy, 31
block. *See* Bundle branch block.
blood supply, 427
fibrosis, 427
left, 31, 206
anterior hemiblock and, 213, 214
right, 31, 206
recording from, 1727, 1729
Bundle branch block, 215–19
aberrant conduction and, 457–60
bilateral, 427
bradycardia-dependent, 458
diphtheritic myocarditis and, 1168
electrograms (His bundle) and, 1731–32
HV interval and, 291
left, 217–19
complete, 217–19
Bundle branch block: left:
incomplete, 219
left axis deviation and, 218–19
myocardial infarction and, 218
pacemakers and, 494, 495
masquerading, 215
mechanism, 427–28
myocardial infarction and, 218, 427–28, 977
pacing and, 481–82, 488
right, 215–16
complete, 215
concealed, 216
first heart sound and, 165
incomplete, 215
premature atrial beats and, 215, 218
second heart sound and, 169
Bundle of His. *See* His bundle.
Buproprion, 1480, 1533
Burns:
electrical, 1486–87
endocarditis and, 1134
Burst pacing, 1737
Burwell, C. Sidney, 1383
Buschke's scleredema, 1239
Buthus tamulus, 1235
Bypass grafts:
aortic arch occlusion and, 1334
aortofemoral, 2059–60
aortoiliac occlusive disease and, 1345
coronary artery. *See* Coronary bypass surgery.
femoropopliteal, 1345–46, 2060–61
ileal, 957
renovascular hypertension and, 1335
Bypass tracts. *See* Accessory pathways.

c wave:
atrial, 52
venous pulse, 54, 148
Cachexia, 121, 1449, 1450
heart failure and, 351
Café au lait spots, 124
Café coronary, 915
Caffeine, 1483
Cage, John, 247
Calcification:
aortic aneurysm, 1317
CT scan and, 1871–72
aortic valve, 248–49, 730, 734
bicuspid valve and, 643, 730
combined mitral valve disease and, 787
roentgenography and, 242
surgical management, 2031
atherosclerosis and, 802
coronary artery:
CT scans and, 1867
fluoroscopy and, 894, 1765–67
mitral annulus, echocardiography and, 1959
mitral valve, 764, 767–68, 772
surgical treatment, 777–78
myocardial, infarction and, 873
myxomatous, 1288, 1291
pericardial, 262, 1264
renal failure and, 1459
roentgenography and, 231
Calcium, 1473–76
alcoholism and, 1448
antagonists. *See* Calcium channel blockers.
arrhythmias and, 1473, 1475
conductance, 78

Calcium:
  contractility and, 34, 37–39, 49, 1476, 1653
  digitalis and, 1642
  diuretics and, 1664, 1665
  ECG and, 224–25, 1475–76
  hypervitaminosis D and, 1219
  hypotension and, 1459–60
  norepinephrine and, 1654
  parathyroid hormone and, 1422
  pyrophosphate uptake and, 1844
  relaxation of myocardium and, 38–39
  renal failure and, 1459–60, 1463
  sarcoplasmic reticulum, 330–31
  shock and, 380
  smooth-muscle contraction and, 1009–10
  transmembrane potential and, 1466, 1473–75
Calcium channel blockers, 941, 1624–35
  adverse effects, 941, 1539, 1634–35
  angina pectoris and, 1628–30
  arrhythmias and, 1630–31
  beta blockers and, 1614, 1629, 1630, 1635
  cardiomyopathy and, 1206, 1207, 1632
  cardiovascular effects, 1625–27
  cerebral arterial spasm and, 1633–34
  clinical applications, 941, 1628–34
  combined therapy with, 1630
  contractility and, myocardial, 1626
  coronary artery spasm and, 1014–15, 1629, 1634
  coronary heart disease and, 941
  CPR and, 552–53
  differential effects on slow channels, 1625
  digitalis and, 941, 1631, 1635, 1647
  dosage and therapeutic levels, 1627–28
  electrophysiologic effects, 1626–27
  heart failure and, 1632–33
  historical note on, 887
  hypertension 1072, 1588, 1631–32
  interactions, 1588, 1635
  intracellular effects, 1625
  muscle contraction and, 1625–26
  myocardial infarction and, 830
  myocardial preservation and, 1633
  nitrates and, 1630
  noncardiovascular effects, 1627, 1634
  pharmacodynamics, 1625–27
  pharmacokinetics, 1627–28
  pharmacology, 1587–88, 1624–28
  physiologic principles, 1624
  pregnancy and, 1393
  pulmonary hypertension and, 1633
  structure, 1624–25
  surgical procedures and, 1514
  vasoactivity, 1587–88
  withdrawal of, 1635
Calcium oxalate deposition, 1226
Calmodulin, smooth muscle and, 1009
Cameras, scintillation, 1811–12
Canadian Cardiovascular Society classification, 108, 932–33
Cancer, pulmonary embolism and, 1109, 1117
Candida:
  endocarditis and, 1136
    drug-related, 1132
  myocarditis and, 1161, 1175
Candy cane deformity, 686
Cannon's law, 912
Cannon waves, venous pulse, 149, 150
Cantrell's pentalogy, 707
Capacitance, membrane, 80
Capacitance vessels, 26
Capillaries:
  anatomy, 26
  leak syndrome, 338
  lymphatic, 25, 26
  myocardial:
    infarction and, 867–69
    oxygen supply and, 861–62
  permeability of, shock and, 373–74
  pulmonary. *See* Pulmonary vasculature.
  sphincters and, precapillary, 373
Capillary pressure, 26
  pulmonary. *See* Pulmonary capillary pressure.
  shock and, 373
  vasodilators and, 1584
Captopril, 1589–90
  dosage, 1072, 1587
  heart failure and, 365
  hypertension and, 1077, 1078
    renovascular, 1079
  pharmacology, 1589–90
  protein-binding and dialysance, 1082
  renal vein renin and, 1059
  side effects, 1073
Capture beats:
  AV dissociation and, 466, 467
  definition, 433
  esophageal ECG and, 1696, 1697
Carbohydrates, 89–91
  integrated control of, 90–91
Carbon dioxide:
  laser, 1922
  tension:
    elevated. *See* Hypercapnia.
    vasodilatation and, 59
Carbon disulfide, 1577–78
Carbonic anhydrase inhibitors, 1658–60
Carbon monoxide poisoning, 1235, 1489
  hyperbaric oxygen therapy and, 1554
  occupational, 1577
Carcinoid, 124, 1298–99
  cardiac output increase and, 403
  clinical manifestations, 1298–99
  myocardial, 1215
  pulmonary valve, 793, 795
  treatment, 1299
Carcinoma:
  endometrial, estrogen therapy and, 1425
  metastases from, 1296. *See also* Metastases.
Cardiac catheterization, 1768–1805
  angiography and, 1785–90. *See also* Angiography; Coronary arteriography.
  aortic atresia and, 646
  aortic-mitral combined valvular disease and, 789–90
  aortic regurgitation and, 274, 275, 747–48
  aortic stenosis and, 273, 734
    congenital, 637, 639–41
  arrhythmias induced by, 2001–2
  arteriovenous fistula and, systemic, 401
  atrial septal defect and, 601
  AV canal and, 608
  beriberi and 398–99
  biopsy and, 1772–73
Cardiac catheterization:
  cardiac output and, 1779–81
    dye method for, 1780–81
    Fick method for, 1779
    thermodilution technique for, 1781
  cardiomyopathy and, 276–77, 1203–4
  coarctation of aorta and, 630
  complications, 311–12, 1540, 1790–91
  coronary artery disease and, 299
  cor pulmonale and, 1126
  cor triatriatum and, 651
  crisscross heart and, 706–7
  cutdown for, 1770–72
    arterial, 1772
    venous, 1770–71
  double-outlet right ventricle and, 698
  Ebstein's anomaly and, 678–79
  endocarditis and, 1146
  equipment for, 1772–74
  Fick method and, 1779–80
  first documented, 1768, 1769
  flow calculations, 1779–82
  heart failure and, 270, 272, 276–77, 355–56
  hyperthyroidism and, 397
  indicator-dilution technique and, 1780–82
  interventions during, 1776
  left side, 1771–72
  mitral-aortic combined valvular disease and, 789–90
  mitral regurgitation and, 772–74
    congenital, 650
  mitral stenosis and, 759–60
    congenital, 649
  myocardial failure and, 272, 276–77
  myocarditis and, 1168
  myxoma and, 1288–89, 1291
  neurological complications, 1361
  oxygen analysis and, 1774, 1776–77
  pacing and, atrial, 1776
  patent ductus arteriosus and, 616, 1777–78
  percutaneous venous, 1769–72
  pericarditis and, constrictive, 1263
  position (of catheter) in, 1777–79
  pregnancy and, 1394
  preparations for, 1768–69
  pressure measurements, 1774–76
    recording system for, 1773–74
  prognosis and, 311
  pulmonary atresia and, 661
  pulmonary hypertension and, 1098
  pulmonary venocclusive disease and, 652
  pulmonary venous connection anomaly and, 604–5, 683
  pulmonic stenosis and, 656–57
  radiation exposure and, 1773
  resistance and, 1784
  right side, 1769–71
    monitoring and, 1999–2002
  risks, 311–12, 1540, 1790–91
  shunts and, 1779–82
    calculations, 1779–80
    detection, 1776–77, 1781–82
    quantification, 1781
  single atrium and, 612
  single ventricle and, 704
  techniques, 1769–72
  tetralogy of Fallot and, 664–65
  transposition of great arteries and, 693–94
    corrected, 701–2

Cardiac catheterization:
transseptal, 1772
trauma during, 1022
tricuspid atresia and, 675
tricuspid regurgitation and, 796
tricuspid stenosis and, 796
truncus arteriosus and, 671
valve area calculations and, 1784–85
ventricular septal defect and, 594, 1777
ventricular volume measurements, 1782–84
Cardiac cycle, 52–53
apexcardiography and, 1994
phases, 52
radionuclide studies and, 1815–16, 1820
Cardiac index, 54–55
myocardial infarction and, 979, 980
pulmonary artery occlusion pressure and, 1507
renal failure and, 1462
Cardiac nerves, 24–25
Cardiac output:
afterload and, 267
decrease in, 363–65
hyperdynamic state and, 395
altitude and, 1544–45
aortic stenosis and, 734
blood pressure and, 1038, 1039
digitalis and, 359
dye method for, 1780–81
exercise and, 55, 335, 1398–99
aging and, 1407–8
Fick method for, 1779
heart failure and, 335
enhancement measures, 358–60
heart rate and, 51, 395
heat stress and, 1547–49
hypertension and, 404, 1042–46
hypothyroidism and, 1420
increased (hyperdynamic states, high-output states), 395–404
anemia and, 399–400
arteriovenous fistula and, 400–402
beriberi and, 397–99
carcinoid syndrome and, 403
cor pulmonale and, 403
cutaneous diseases and, 404
drug-induced, 404
environmental factors, 403
hemangiomatosis and, hepatic, 401
hemodialysis and, 401
hepatic disease and, 402
hyperdynamic heart syndrome and, 403
hypertension and, 404, 1042–46
hyperthyroidism and, 396–97
obesity and, 404, 1454
Paget's disease of bone and, 402–3
physical findings, 395–96
physiologic mechanisms, 395
polycythemia vera and, 404
polyostotic fibrous dysplasia and, 403
pregnancy and, 404, 1384, 1385
renal disease and, 404
indicator-dilution technique and, 1780–81
mechanical heart and, 2070, 2072
monitoring, 385–86, 2000
obesity and, 404, 1454
pacing and, 498
pericarditis and, 1256
perioperative, 1506, 1507
Cardiac output:
postoperative, 1518
pregnancy and, 404, 1384, 1385
pulmonary hypertension and, 1093–94
redistribution of, 51
shock and, 371–72, 384
management, 385–86
Swan-Ganz catheterization and, 385, 2000
sympathetic stimulation and, 44
tamponade and, 1256
thermodilution technique for, 385, 1781, 2000
Cardiac plexuses, 25
Cardiac status and prognosis, 101, 106–8
Cardiac veins, 29–30
Cardinal veins, 10, 11
Cardiofacial syndrome, 130
Cardiomegaly. *See also* Dilatation of heart; Hypertrophy.
acromegaly and, 1422, 1423
amyloidosis and, 1213, 1214
aortic regurgitation and, 274
atrial septal defect and, 599
cardiomyopathy and, 1184–86. *See also* Cardiomyopathy, dilated.
Ebstein's anomaly and, 678, 679
glycogenosis and, 1221
Hurler's syndrome and, 1224
hypertension and, 1053–54
insurance and, 1561
mitral regurgitation and, 275
muscular dystrophy and, 1228
roentgenography and, 230–31, 243
Cardiomyopathy, 1181–1215
aging and, 1238
alcoholic, 1182–83, 1446–48
amyloidosis and, 569–70, 1213–15
anticoagulants and, 1669–70
assessment, 259–62
dilated disease and, 259–60, 1187–90
hypertrophic disease and, 259, 1200–1204
restrictive/obliterative disease and, 262, 1210–11
carnitine deficiency and, 568–69
catheterization studies, 276–77, 1203–4
characteristics of, 1182
cobalt, 1183, 1235, 1446
contractility and, 1184, 1187
coronary arteries and, 1187, 1190–91, 1197–98
daunorubicin and, 1183, 1481
diabetes mellitus and, 1428
in fetus, 1429
dilated (congestive), 1181–93
alcohol abuse and, 1182–83
angiocardiography, 1190
atherosclerosis and, 1187, 1190–91
biopsy and, endomyocardial, 1190
catecholamines and, 1184
clinical manifestations, 259–60, 1187–90
differential diagnosis, 1190–91
ECG, 1188, 1189
echocardiography, 260, 261, 1189, 1956
epidemiology, 1184
etiology, 1181–84
genetics, 1183
history, 1187–88
Cardiomyopathy: dilated:
hypertension and, 1183, 1191
hypertrophic cardiomyopathy vs., 1191
idiopathic, 261
immunologic aspects, 1183
infection and, 1183
laboratory studies, 1188–90
natural history and prognosis, 1190
pathology, 1184–87
pathophysiology, 1187
physical examination, 1188
pregnancy and, 1183, 1391–92
radionuclide studies, 261–62, 1189
roentgenography, 1188
thyroid hormone and, 1184
treatment, 1191–93
doxorubicin, 1481, 1826–28
drug-induced, 1236–37, 1481, 1826–28
embolism and, 1670
energy supply defect and, 568–69
Friedreich's ataxia and, 569, 1229
gallop and, atrial, 178
genetics, 568–72, 1181, 1183, 1193
glycogenosis and, 570, 1219, 1220
heart failure and, 1191
dilated disease and, 1187, 1190
hypertrophic disease and, 1204–5, 1207–8
senile, 331
hemochromatosis and, 570, 1221–22
hyperthyroidism and, 1415–16
hypertrophic, 1193–1208
arrhythmias and, 1204
beta blockers and, 1616
biopsy and, endomyocardial, 1204
calcium channel blockers for, 1632
catheterization studies, 1203–4
clinical manifestations, 259, 1200–1204
differential diagnosis, 1205–6
dilated cardiomyopathy vs., 1191
ECG, 1201–2
echocardiography, 259, 1202–3, 1956–58
etiology, 1193–94
fibrous plaque and, 1198
genetics, 569
heart failure and, 1204–5, 1207–8
history, 1200
laboratory studies, 1202–4
natural history and prognosis, 1204
nomenclature, 1193
noncardiac surgery and, 1517
nonobstructive, 1195
pathology, 1194–99
pathophysiology, 1199–1200
physical examination, 1200–1201
pregnancy and, 1205, 1388, 1391
pulse and, 145
radionuclide studies, 260, 1203
roentgenography, 1201
syncope and, 522, 524
treatment, 1206–8
infectious. *See* Myocarditis.
infiltrative, 569–70
insurance and, 1561
ischemic, 989, 1181
assessment, 277–78
pathology, 850–51
prognosis, 930–31
treatment, 989
lentiginosis and, 1239
metabolic disorders and, 99

Cardiomyopathy:
mitochondrial myopathy and, 569
mitral regurgitation and, 766–67, 1184, 1201, 1205
murmurs and, 1191, 1201, 1204
muscular dystrophy and, 571–72, 1228
myocarditis and, 1183
necropsy and, 2079
nonobstructive vs. obstructive, 1200
Noonan's syndrome and, 1238
obesity and, 1453–55
pain from, 909–10
phytanic acid storage disease and, 570
rejection, 1237–38
restrictive/obliterative, 277, 1208–13. *See also* Endomyocardial fibrosis.
assessment, 262, 1210–11
echocardiography and, 1958
pericarditis vs., 262, 1264
selenium deficiency and, 1183–84, 1449
senile, 331
sickle cell trait, 1227
sudden death and, 531, 544, 1204, 1206
thrombosis and, 1184, 1190
toxic, 1233–35
tricuspid regurgitation and, 1184
uremic, 1226, 1462–63
Cardioplegia, 2028
aortic valve surgery and, 2031
ATP and, 98
coronary bypass surgery and, 2037–38
Cardiopulmonary bypass, 2025–29
aortic dissection and, 2029, 2039
aortic valve surgery and, 2031
blood pressure and, 2027
cardioplegia and. *See* Cardioplegia.
complications, 2029
coronary bypass surgery and, 2036
future of, 2029
goals of, 2026
historical notes on, 2025–26
hypothermia and, 2027, 2028
ischemic arrest and, 2028
mechanics of, 2026–27
myocardial protection and, 2027–29
perfusion technique, 2027
reperfusion and, 2028–29
ventricular septal defect and, 596
Cardiopulmonary resuscitation (CPR), 546–53
airway clearance and, 549–50
asystole and, 551
blood flow during, 547–49
bystander-initiated, 541
chest compression during, 550
drugs used in, 552–53
electrical injuries and, 1487
electromechanical dissociation and, 551
exercise testing and, 1711–12
identification of arrest and, 549
intravenous line and, 551
outcome of, 553
postarrest care and, 553
respiratory arrest and, 549
termination of, 553
ventilation during, 550
ventricular fibrillation and, 550–51
Cardiothoracic ratio, 1053
Cardiotonic agents. *See* Digitalis; Inotropic agents.
Cardiotoxins, 1488–89, 1540
radionuclide monitoring of, 1826–28
Cardioversion, 483–84, 1741–46
anticoagulants and, 1672, 1741–42
atrial fibrillation and, 1742–44
atrial flutter and, 1744
complications, 483–84, 1540–41, 1745–46
CPR and, 550
digitalis toxicity and, 1745
energy doses, 1742
implantable device for, 478, 582, 1761–63
mortality and, 1763
patient selection, 1761–62
results and complications, 1762–63
surgical technique, 1762
indications and contraindications, 483
supraventricular tachycardia and, 1744
technique, 1741–42
ventricular fibrillation and, 1744–45
ventricular tachycardia and, 1744
Carditis, 1308–9. *See also* Rheumatic heart disease.
acute, 1308
chronic, 1309
course, 1310–11
management, 1311–12
pathology, 1307
Carey Coombs murmur, 1308
Carnitine:
deficiency, 568–69, 1220
fatty acids and, 91–93
fibroelastosis and, 654
Carotid arteries, 1874–80
angiography, 1874–76
aortic aneurysm and, 1326
aortic arch aneurysm and, 2045–46
atherosclerosis, 1334, 1875
Doppler studies and, 1975
endarterectomy for, 2052–56
transient ischemic attacks and, 1355, 1356
baroreceptors, shock and, 374
bruits, 1334
asymptomatic, 990, 1355
diagnostic studies and, 1879–80
collateral, 1875
computed tomography and, 1876
coronary artery disease and, 990
diagnostic studies, 1874–80
applications, 1879–80
complications, 1879
Doppler studies, 1878–79, 1975–76
duplex scan, 1878–79
embryology, 13, 14
endarterectomy, 1356–57, 2052–56
complications, 2055–56
indications, 2056
results, 2055
technique, 2052–55
fibromuscular dysplasia, 1358
laboratory tests, 1877–79
mechanical obstruction of, 1358
pulse, 143, 144
aortic regurgitation and, 745
aortic stenosis and, 733
cardiomyopathy and, 1201
mitral stenosis and, 757
normal tracing of, 1992
recording of, 1992, 1993
tracheal compression by, 627
Carotid ducts, 13, 14
Carotid sinus, 49
angina relief by massage of, 891
blood pressure control and, 1040
gallop and, 181
hypersensitivity, 490
syncope and, 514–16
pacemaker assessment and, 1759
shock and, 374, 375
sinus tachycardia and, 292
Carotid sinus nerve, 515
Carotid-vertebrobasilar system, syncope and, 513–14
Carpentier ring, 777, 778
tricuspid valve and, 797, 798
Carvallo's sign, 795
Catapres. *See* Clonidine.
Cataracts, 130
Catecholamines. *See also* Dopamine; Epinephrine; Norepinephrine.
aging and, 1405–6
beta-blocking agents and, 1609
beta receptors and, 1606–7
biochemistry and pharmacokinetics, 1654
cardiomyopathy and, 1184
hypertrophic, 1193–94
contractility and, 1653–55
coronary blood flow and, 62
CPR and, 552
emotional stress and, 1522, 1523–24
pheochromocytoma and, 1046, 1065
shock and, 376–77
sudden death and, 1522
syncope and, 511, 512
Catechol-*O*-methyltransferase, 1040, 1654
Cathepsin D, 96
Catheter(s), 1772–73
angioplasty, 1904–5, 1909
balloon. *See* Balloon catheter; Intraaortic balloon counterpulsation; Swan-Ganz catheterization.
flotation. *See* Swan-Ganz catheterization.
Catheterization:
arterial, pressure monitoring and, 386
blood pressure measurement, 138–39
cardiac. *See* Cardiac catheterization.
coronary artery, 1791–93
electrophysiologic study, 1734
His bundle, 1727–29
infection from, 1518
pulmonary artery. *See* Pulmonary artery catheterization.
Swan-Ganz. *See* Swan-Ganz catheterization.
thrombosis induced by, 1373, 1790
urinary, shock monitoring and, 385
Cauda equina syndrome, 1342
Causality assessment, medicolegal, 1569–72
Cedilanid. *See* Digitalis.
Cefazolin, endocarditis and, 1149, 1153
Celiac artery:
aneurysm, 1351
compression syndrome, 1369
stenosis, 1369, 1370
Celiprolol, 1607
Cells:
atherosclerosis and, 809–15
death of, 380
myocardial. *See* Myocardial infarction.
shock and, 380–81, 384

Cephalic vein, pacemaker implantation and, 1748
Cerebral angiography, 1356, 1874–76
complications, 1879
Cerebritis, endocarditis and, 1143
Cerebrovascular disease, 1354–62
aneurysmal:
endocarditis and, 1143, 1151
hypertension and, 1357
myxomatous emboli and, 1286–87
angiography, 1874–76, 1879
arrhythmias and, 1359, 1360–61
atherosclerotic, 1355–57
diagnosis, 1355–56
management, 1356–57
manifestations, 1355
catheterization studies and, 1361
computed tomography and, 1876
congenital heart disease and, 1362
contraceptive agents and, 1482
disability and, 562
dissection, 1358
Doppler studies and, 1976
embolism, 1358–60
atherosclerosis and, 1355
causes, 1358–59
clinical manifestations, 1358
coronary bypass surgery and, 2039
diagnosis, 1359–60
management, 1360
myxoma and, 1286–87, 1359
postoperative, 1361–62
syncope and, 514
endarterectomy and, 2055–56
fibromuscular dysplasia, 1358
hemorrhagic, 1054, 1357
hyperbaric oxygen therapy and, 1533
hypertensive, 1054, 1357–58
hypoperfusion, 1360–61
incidence, 562
infarction, 1355
congenital heart defects and, 1362
embolic. *See* embolism *above.*
endocarditis and, 1143
hypertension and, 1054
lacunar, 1357
myocardial infarction and, 1359
treatment, 1357
watershed, 1361
mechanical obstruction, 1358
mortality, 562
noninvasive vascular laboratory tests and, 1877–79
postoperative, 1361–62
prevalence, 562
spasm, 1633–34
syncope and, 513–14
thrombotic, 1355
venous, 1358
transient ischemia and. *See* Ischemia, transient attacks of.
vasculitis, 1358
venous occlusion, 1358
Cerebrum:
abscess, congenital heart disease and, 1362
blood flow, 1360–61
CPR and, 547, 548, 552
history taking and, 120
shock and, 379
sound perception and, 158
Cervical ganglia, 24–25
Cervical rib syndrome, 916–18
Chagas' disease, 1158
acute, 1169
Chagas' disease:
chronic, 1169–70
clinical manifestations, 1169
laboratory studies, 1169–70
pathology, 1159–60, 1162
pathophysiology, 1165
prognosis, 1177
treatment, 1179
Charcoal, activated, digitalis toxicity and, 1648–49
Charcot-Bouchard microaneurysms, 1357
CHARGE syndrome, 135
Chemical agents:
myocardial effects of, 1231–37
occupational exposure to, 1577–78
Chemoreceptors, 25
shock and, 375
Chemotherapy, 1481–82
Chenodeoxycholic acid, 914
Chest. *See also* Precordium.
compression of, CPR and, 550
blood flow and, 547
inspection of, 134–35
pain in. *See* Pain, chest.
physical examination, 204
roentgenography. *See* Roentgenography.
trauma, 1276–81
blunt, 1278–81
penetrating, 1277–78
Chest wall:
pain, 918
stimulation of, pacemaker assessment and, 1758–59
transmission of sound, 161
Cheyne-Stokes respiration, 116, 350
Chief complaint, 110
Chills, 121
Chlamydial endocarditis, 1136
Chloride, diuretics and, 1658, 1660
Chloroquine, toxicity of, 1231–32
Chlorothiazide, 1658
dosage, 1072, 1659
duration of action, 1659
heart failure in infant and, 585
Chlorpromazine, 1480–81
anesthesia and, 1496
cardiac catheterization and, 1769
toxicity, 1232
Chlortetracycline, hypersensitivity to, 1237
Chlorthalidone, 1658, 1659
cholesterol and, 1074–75
dosage, 1072
hypertension and, 1071
pharmacokinetics, 1660
site of action, 1660
Choking on food, 915
Cholecystitis and cholelithiasis, 913–14
Cholera vaccine, 1237
Cholesterol:
atherosclerosis and, 807–8, 812–13
preventive measures, 820–22, 828–29
regression of, 819
dietary, 807–8, 820–22, 828
diuretics and, 1074–75
drugs lowering, 821, 822–23, 829
emotional stress and, 1523
experimental studies, 803, 804
gallstones and, 913, 914
genetics and, 574
ileal bypass and, 957
pericarditis and, 1271
Cholesterol:
plasma, 820–21
smooth-muscle cells and, 812–13
Cholestyramine:
cholesterol and, 821, 822
digitalis and, 1647, 1649
Chordae tendineae:
anatomy, 21, 23
AV canal and, 606
embryology, 12
mitral commissurotomy and, 762–63
rheumatic endocarditis and, 754
ruptured:
assessment, 252
mitral regurgitation and, 766, 767
myxoma and, 766, 767
trauma and, 1280
tricuspid regurgitation and, 794
undue restraint on, 767
Chorea:
amyotrophic, 1231
rheumatic fever and, 1309
Chorioepithelioma, embolism from, 1117
Chromaffin cell tumors. *See* Pheochromocytoma.
Chromosomes, 566–67
inspection and disorders of, 135
Lyon (inactive X), 806
nondisjunction, 567
Chylopericardium, 1271
Cimetidine, 1484
Cineangiography, 1786
endocarditis and, 1146
Circadian rhythm, blood pressure and, 1049
Circulatory drift, exercise and, 1399–1400
Circulatory failure, 370–71, 384. *See also* Shock.
definition and classification, 319
Circulatory overload, 319
Circus movement, 413–14
atrial flutter and, 414
tachycardia and, 447–48
Cirrhosis:
cardiac output increase and, 402
diuretics and, 1662
Claims. *See* Legal issues.
Clark, Barney B., 2070, 2075
Claudication:
arteriosclerosis obliterans and, 1340
coronary bypass surgery and, 990
pain from, 114–15
surgical management, 2057
thromboangiitis obliterans and, 1347
Clicks, systolic, 184–85
aortic stenosis and, 636, 733
bicuspid aortic valve and, 636
mitral regurgitation and, 769, 770
prosthetic valves and, 187
pulmonary hypertension and, 1098
Clofibrate, hyperlipidemia and, 821, 823, 829
Clonidine, 1588
beta blockers and, 1619, 1620–21
dosage, 1072, 1587
hypertension and, 1081
protein-binding and dialysance, 1082
side effects, 1073
suppression test, 1065
Clostridium perfringens, myocarditis and, 1163, 1164
Closure pressure, 58

Clubbing, 131–32
  cyanosis and, 132
  endocarditis and, 1142
Coagulation:
  drugs inhibiting. *See* Anticoagulants; Heparin; Warfarin.
  polycythemia and, 587
Coagulation necrosis, myocardial, 531, 532, 844–46, 875
  sudden death and, 1522
Coarctation, pulmonary arterial, 659
Coarctation of aorta, 627–34
  abdominal, 1324
  angioplasty for, 1897–98
  associated conditions, 628–29
  catheterization studies, 630
  clinical manifestations, 256, 629–30
  collateral vessels and, 628, 633
  cyanosis and, 132
  digital vascular imaging and, 256
  ECG, 630
  echocardiography, 630
  ejection sounds and, 184
  heart failure and, 630, 631
  history, 629
  hypertension and, 629–31, 1046–47
  medical management, 631
  mitral stenosis and, 648
  murmur, 629
  natural history and prognosis, 630–31
  pathology, 627–28
  pathophysiology, 629
  physical examination, 629–30
  pregnancy and, 1388, 1390
  roentgenography, 234, 242, 630
  surgical management, 632–34, 2049–51
Cobalt cardiomyopathy, 1183, 1235, 1446
Coccidiodomycosis, 1175
Cochlea, 158
Cochlear nerve, 158
Codeine, rheumatic fever and, 1311
Coenzyme A, fatty acids and, 91–93
Coeur en sabot, 663, 664
Coffee (caffeine), 937
Cogan's syndrome, 1238
Cold exposure:
  angina pectoris and, 891
  arteriospastic diseases and, 1352, 1353
  cardiac output increase and, 403
  hypothyroidism and, 1419
  livedo reticularis and, 1352
Coldness:
  arteriospasm and, 1352
  thromboangiitis obliterans and, 1349
Colestipol, cholesterol and, 822
Colitis:
  ischemic, 1367–68
  ulcerative, 1239
Collagen:
  endocardial fibroelastosis and, 654
  myocardial infarction and, 875, 876
  pericardial, 1249
Collagen vascular diseases. *See also* Ankylosing spondylitis; Arthritis, rheumatoid; Lupus erythematosus, systemic; Polyarteritis nodosa; Sclerosis, progressive systemic.
  cor pulmonale and, 1124
  pericarditis and, 1269
Collateral vessels:
  arteriosclerosis obliterans and, 1339–40
  bronchial, hemorrhage and, 1106
Collateral vessels:
  carotid artery, 1875
  coarctation of aorta and, 628, 633
  coronary, 62
    anomalies and, 709, 1018
    ischemia and, 862–63
    myocardial infarction and, 843, 844
    radiography, 906, 1801
    steal mechanism and, 864
  mesenteric, 1364
  pulmonary atresia and, 670
  sudden death and, 535
Collimators, scintillation camera, 1811
Collin, V., 1251
Colloidal osmotic pressure, shock and, 373
Colloids, shock and, 374, 388
Colon:
  angiodysplasia of, 1371
  distension of splenic flexure of, 915
  ischemic, 1367–68
Coma, 120
  diabetic, 1426
  electricity-induced, 1487
  myxedema, 1419
Commissurotomy:
  aortic, 638–39
  mitral, 649, 762–63, 2032
  tricuspid, 797
Compactin, 823
Complement:
  endocarditis and, 1140
  lupus erythematosus and, 1436
  shock and, 381
Compliance. *See also* Distensibility.
  atrial, heart failure and, 333
  patient, 1534
  pulmonary, heart failure and, 337
  vascular:
    arterial pulse and, 141, 142
    vasodilators and, 1584
  ventricular, 43
    cardiomyopathy and, 1199
    hypertrophy and, 328
    mitral regurgitation and, 768
Compression test of Allen, 1340
Computed tomography (CT), 1864–72
  advantages of, 1864
  aortic arch anomalies and, 1872
  aortic dissection and, 1871–72
  blood flow and, myocardial, 1849, 1865, 1866
  calcification of coronary arteries and, 1867
  cerebrovascular disease and, 1356, 1876
  congenital heart disease and, 1867, 1872
  coronary artery bypass and, 1868
  gating of, 1864, 1866
  lungs and, 1867
  metabolic studies, 1850
  myocardial infarction and, 1867–68
  pericardial, 1869–71
    congenital lesions and, 1871
    effusion and, 1869, 1870
    inflammation and, 1870–71
    metastases and, 1297
  pheochromocytoma and, 1066
  photon emission, 1812–13
  positron emission, 1849–50
  quantitation, 1866–67
  technique, 1866
Computed tomography:
  thrombosis and, 1869
  tumors and, 1868–69
  ventricular aneurysm and, 1868
Computers:
  decision making and, 2004
  ECG and, 227
    prolonged, 1720–21, 1722
  monitoring aided by, 2004–7
    clinical functions afforded by, 2006
    interventions and, 2006
    measurements, 2005–6
    systems and design, 2004–5
    trends in, 2006
  pacemaker assessment by, 1757
  radionuclide studies and, 1812–13
    first-pass, 1814
    gated equilibrium, 1819
  requirements analysis and, 2005
  transfusions and, 2006
Conal septum, 9–10
Concealed pathway, 412
  atrial flutter and, 445
  tachycardia and, 418, 448
  WPW syndrome and, 448
Concordance:
  atrioventricular, 686
    crisscross heart and, 706
  ventriculoarterial, 687
    single ventricle and, 703
Conductance, 76–78
  pulmonary artery, 1092–93
  vascular, 58
Conduction system. *See also* Atrioventricular node; Bundle branches; His bundle; Sinus node.
  aberration, 412, 457–61. *See also* Intraventricular conduction, aberrant.
  accessory pathway. *See* Accessory pathways.
  anatomy, 30–31
  arrhythmias and, 409–12. *See also* Arrhythmias.
  atrial, 30, 73
  concealed pathway. *See* Concealed pathway.
  decremental phenomenon, 410, 427
  electrophysiology, 73, 79–80. *See also* Electrocardiography; Electrophysiology.
  esophageal leads and, 1690–1703
  internodal pathways, 30
  intraventricular. *See* Intraventricular conduction.
  lateral view, 31
  Lev's disease, 464
  potassium and, 1467–69
  radiation damage to, 1485, 1486
  reentry, 410–11. *See also* Reentry.
  reflection, 412
  repolarization abnormalities, 411–12
  sudden death and, 531–33
  surgical interruption of, 2014–15
  timing. *See* Conduction times.
  unidirectional block, 410–11
  velocity, 410
Conduction times:
  AV nodal, 1729–30, 1736–37
  esophageal leads and, 1701–2
  His bundle recording and, 1729–30
  His-Purkinje (HV interval), 291, 488, 1729, 1730, 1736–37
  sinus node, 1735–36

Congenital heart disease, 580–713. *See also* specific condition.
  aortic arch anomalies, 622–27
    interruption, 634–35
  aortic–left ventricular tunnel, 644–45
  aorticopulmonary septal defect, 618–19
  aortic stenosis, 635–42
    subvalvular, 639–41
    supravalvular, 641–42
    valvular, 635–39
  aortic valve, 635–39, 642–44
    atresia, 645–47
    bicuspid, 642–43
    regurgitation, 643–44
    stenosis, 635–39
  asplenia and polysplenia syndromes, 689–90
  athletes and, 1402
  atrial septal defect, 597–603
  atrioventricular canal defects, 605–12
  coarctation of aorta, 627–34
  complications, 584–90
  computed tomography and, 1867, 1872
  coronary artery anomalies, 707–12, 1017–19
  coronary sinus malformations, 712
  cor triatriatum, 651–52
  crisscross heart, 706–7
  critical, 581
  cyanosis and, 586–87
  double-outlet left ventricle, 699–700
  double-outlet right ventricle, 696–99
  Ebstein's anomaly, 677–80
  ectopia cordis, 707
  endocardial fibroelastosis, 653–54
  endocarditis and, 1134
  etiology, 581–82
  exertional intolerance and, 589–90
  fetal circulation and, 582–84
    persistent, 584
  genetics, 566–68
  growth retardation and, 589
  heart failure and, 584–86
  incidence, 564, 581–82
  infantile syndrome, 1018
  insurance and, 1560
  left ventricular–right atrial communication, 613–14
  levocardia, dextrocardia, and mesocardia, 688–89
  magnetic resonance imaging and, 1892
  malpositions of cardiac structures, 686–707
  mitral valve, 647–51
    atresia, 647–48
    regurgitation, 649–51
    stenosis, 648–49
  mortality, 564
  myocardial ischemia and, 1016–20
  necropsy and, 2079
  neurological complications of, 1362
  noncardiac surgery and, 1516
  patent ductus arteriosus, 614–18
  pericardial abnormalities, 712–13, 1266
  pregnancy and, 1390–91, 1392
  prevalence, 563–64
  pulmonary arteriovenous fistula, 680–81
  pulmonary artery anomalies, 668–73
    absence, 681
Congenital heart disease: pulmonary artery anomalies:
    hemitruncus, 619–20
    sling, 625–26
  pulmonary hypertension and, 587–89, 1094–95
  pulmonary valve, 654–62
    absence, 667–68
    atresia, 660–62, 670–71
    stenosis, 654–58
  pulmonary vascular obstruction and, 587–89
  pulmonary venous:
    partial connection anomaly, 603–5
    stenosis, 652–53
    total connection anomaly, 681–84
  pulmonic stenosis, 654–59
    subvalvular, 658–59
    supravalvular, 659
    valvular, 654–58
  single atrium, 612
  single ventricle, 703–6
  sinus of Valsalva fistula, 620–21
  subclavian artery anomalies, 622–25
  systemic-pulmonary connections, 590–622
    extracardiac, 614–22
    intracardiac, 590–614
  tetralogy of Fallot, 662–67
  transposition of great arteries:
    complete (dextro), 691–94
    corrected (levo), 700–703
  tricuspid valve, 673–77
    atresia, 673–76
    regurgitation, 677
  truncus arteriosus, 671–73
  Uhl's malformation, 680
  vena caval anomalies, 684–86
  ventricular performance and, 1828
  ventricular septal defect, 590–97
Congestion, noncardiac circulatory, 396
Congestive heart failure. *See* Heart failure, congestive.
Conjunctiva, endocarditis and, 1142
Connective tissue:
  atherosclerosis and, 805, 806
  fibrous plaque and, 801–2
  genetic disorders of, 573
  Marfan's disorder of. *See* Marfan's syndrome.
Conn's syndrome. *See* Aldosteronism.
Conoventricular groove (sulcus), 3
Consent, informed, 1574
  anesthesia and, 1503
  artificial heart and, 2074–75
Contraceptive agents, 1424, 1482–83
  cerebrovascular accidents and, 1482
  complications, 1424–25, 1540
  coronary heart disease and, 825–26, 829
  hypertension and, 1084, 1482
  myocardial infarction and, 1482
  principles for use of, 1482–83
  thromboembolism and, 1374, 1482
Contractility, 37–50
  afterload and, 47–48, 266, 270–71, 331–32
  aging and, 1405–6
  anesthesia and, 50
  aortic regurgitation and, 274–75
  aortic stenosis and, 274, 732
  atrial, 48
  calcium and, 34, 37–39, 49, 1476, 1653
Contractility:
  calcium channel blockers and, 1626
  cardiomyopathy and, 1184, 1187
  catecholamines and, 1653–55
  contractile element (CE) and, 40, 41
  digitalis and, 358–59, 1642
  dobutamine and, 1654–55
  drugs affecting, 49, 358–60
  ejection phase indexes and, 270–71
  elastic components and, 40
  excitation-contraction coupling, 37–39, 1476
  fiber length and, 43, 45–46
  force-velocity-length relations and, 46, 47
  force-velocity relations and, 40–42, 45–46
  force-velocity-volume relations and, 47
  heart failure and, 266, 328, 330–31, 334
    enhancement measures, 358–60
    indexes, 270–72
  heart rate and, 46
  Hill's model of, 40
  hyperthyroidism and, 98–99, 1415
  hypertrophy and, 328
  hypoxia and, 371–72
  increased, effects of, 46, 47
  indexes, 270–72
  Laplace law and, 329
  mechanics of, 40–50
  mitral regurgitation and, 275
  myocardial infarction and, 942
  myosin ATPase and, 98–99
  oxygen consumption and, 56, 865, 866
  potassium and, 1473
  preload and, 42–46
  sequence of contraction and, 48
  shock and, 371–72, 379
  sliding filament hypothesis and, 33–34
  smooth-muscle, vascular, 1009–11
  sodium and, 39
  sympathetic nervous system and, 44, 49
  ultrastructure, 32–34
Contraction band necrosis, 846, 873–74
Contrast media, 1785–86
  echocardiography and, 1948–50
  magnetic resonance imaging and, 1893–94
  phlebography and, 1886–87
Contusion, myocardial, 1278–80
Conus artery, 22, 29
Conus cordis, 5, 9–10
  atrioventricular canal and, 8
  septation and, 9–10
Conus ligament, 17
Convalescence. *See* Rehabilitation.
Converting-enzyme inhibitors. *See* Angiotensin-converting enzyme inhibitors.
Convulsions, syncope vs., 519
Cordis leads, 493
Corgard. *See* Nadolol.
Cori disease, 123
Cornelia de Lange syndrome, 126–27, 133
Coronary arteries. *See also* Coronary heart disease.
  aging and, 1407
  anatomy, 27–29, 839–40
  aneurysm, 711–12, 1020
  angioplasty, 1902–8
    complications, 1907–8

Coronary arteries: angioplasty:
technique, 1904–7
anomalies, 707–12, 1017–19
atresia of ostium, 1018
contralateral sinus of Valsalva as origin, 1017–18
pulmonary artery origin, 708–11, 1018–19
single ostium, 1018
sudden death and, 530
truncus arteriosus and, 669
aortic valve surgery and, 2030
arteriovenous fistula. *See* Arteriovenous fistula, coronary.
atherosclerosis, 842–55. *See also* Atherosclerosis.
blood flow. *See* Coronary blood flow.
bridge of, muscle, 1019–20, 1800
bypass surgery. *See* Coronary bypass surgery.
calcification:
CT scans and, 1867
fluoroscopy and, 894, 1765–67
calcium channel blockers and, 1626
cardiomyopathy and, 1187, 1190–91, 1197–98
catheterization of, 1791–93
collateral, 62
anomalies and, 709, 1018
ischemia and, 862–63
myocardial infarction and, 843, 844
radiography, 906, 1801
steal mechanism and, 864
sudden death and, 535
compression of, 1019–20, 1024
conus, 22, 29
critical closing of, 860*n*.
diagonal (intermediate), 28, 839
radiography, 1794, 1796, 1797
dissection, 1021
echocardiography and, 1941, 1942, 1962
embolism, 1021
myxomatous, 1287
radiography and, 1803
sudden death and, 530, 534
endarterectomy, 956–57
fatty streaks, 801. *See also* Fatty streaks.
fistula. *See* Arteriovenous fistula, coronary.
infection, 530, 1023
innervation, 25
intimal fibrosis (proliferation), 1023
laceration, 1022
left anterior descending:
anatomy, 16, 28, 839–40
asymptomatic disease, 960
occlusion, 841, 846, 848
radiography, 905–6, 1794, 1797–1801
surgery for disease of, 949, 950
left circumflex:
anatomy, 28–29, 839, 840
anomalous origin, 711
dominant, 1798
occlusion, 846
radiography, 1798
surgery for disease of, 949, 950
left main:
anatomy, 28, 839
angioplasty, 1902
anomalies, 708–11, 1017–18
aortic sinus origin of, 711
asymptomatic disease, 960

Coronary arteries: left main:
atresia of origin of, 711
cannulation of, 1792
preoperative care and, 952
prognosis for disease of, 921
pulmonary artery origin of, 708–10
radiography, 1794–98
surgery for disease of, 949, 950
lymphatics and, 25
marginal, 29, 839
metastases and, 1296–97
"milking" of, 1019–20
mucocutaneous lymph node syndrome and, 1023
necropsy and, 2078
obstruction (narrowing, occlusion), 840–50. *See also* Atherosclerosis.
grading stenosis of, 1800
infarction and, 842–43, 868–70
laser therapy of, 1922–25
pathology, 842–50
risk region and, 843, 868
thrombotic. *See* thrombosis *below.*
polyarteritis nodosa, 1022, 1438–39
posterior descending, 28–29, 839
radiography, 1797–99
radiation damage to, 1485, 1486
radiography. *See* Coronary arteriography.
radionuclide studies, 1835–36
reflexes, 61–62
right:
anatomy, 29, 839, 840
anomalies, 710–11, 1017, 1018
cannulation of, 1792–93
dominant, 1799
fistula, 707, 708
occlusion, 846
pulmonary artery origin of, 710–11
radiography, 906, 1797–1800
septal perforating, 28
AV block and, 427
bypass surgery and, 2039
cardiomyopathy and, 1197
radiography, 1796
single, 1018
sinus of Valsalva aneurysm and, 2043, 2044
spasm, 1009–15
adrenergic (sympathetic) influence, 1010
angina pectoris and, 963–64, 1011–12
atherosclerosis and, 1010
beta-blocking agents and, 1015, 1614–15
calcium channel blockers and, 1014–15, 1629, 1634
clinical presentations, 1011–13
definition, 1009
diagnosis, 1013
ECG, 1011, 1013
ergonovine-provoked, 1013–14
etiology, 1010–11
hyperthyroidism and, 1414
infarction and, 871–72, 1012–13
ischemia and, 862
natural history, 1011
physiologic mechanisms, 1009–11
radiography, 906, 1012, 1800–1801
spontaneous, 1013
sudden death and, 535, 536, 1013
thallium imaging and, 1834
treatment, 1014–15
steal mechanism and, 863–64

Coronary arteries:
surgery. *See also* Coronary bypass surgery.
for anomalies, 710
syphilis and, 1023, 1317–18
Takayasu's (pulseless) disease, 1023
third. *See* Conus artery.
thrombosis, 802, 843, 1022
anticoagulants and, 1672–73
early evolving infarction and, 967–68
echocardiography and, 1962
historical notes on, 885
pathogenesis of infarction and, 870
plaque rupture and, 870–71
sudden death and, 530, 534–35, 540, 850
thrombolytic agents and, 1681–82
trauma of, 1021–22, 1278, 1279
vasculitis, 530, 1022–23
vasoconstriction, 61–63, 862
vasodilatation, 61–63, 858, 861
steal and, 864
vasospasm. *See* spasm *above.*
Wegener's granulomatosis and, 1023
Coronary arteriography, 308–9, 902–7, 1791–1803
aneurysm and, 711
angina pectoris and, 903–4
angioplasty and, 1905
aortic root anatomy and, 1792
aortic stenosis and, 734
benefits, 903
bypass surgery and, 2038–39
collaterals and, 906, 1801
contraindications, 905
diagonal arteries and, 1794, 1796, 1797
digital subtraction, 1860–61
embolism and, 1803
ergonovine and, 309, 906
exercise testing vs., 1709
grading stenoses and, 1800
historical notes on, 886
indications, 300, 301, 903–5
information provided by, 1791
interpretation, 308, 905–6, 1793, 1802
left, 1794–98
anterior descending, 905–6, 1794, 1797–1801
cannulation and, 1792
circumflex, 1798
left anterior oblique, 1794–98
limitations, 906–7, 1802
myocardial infarction and, 904
uncomplicated, 970
myxoma and, 1290
pitfalls in, 1800–1801
posterior descending, 1797–99
prognosis and, 921, 922
radionuclide studies vs., 1836–37
right, 906, 1797–1800
cannulation and, 1792–93
right anterior oblique, 1794, 1797–99
risks, 311–12, 902–3, 1803
sagittal angulation, 1796
segmental approach in, 1793
septal perforating arteries and, 1796
spasm and, 906, 1012, 1800–1801
techniques, 1791–93
thrombosis and, 1803
ventricular function and, 906
wall motion and, 906

Coronary arteriovenous fistula. *See* Arteriovenous fistula.
Coronary blood flow, 60–63, 857–64
adenosine and, 858
altitude and, 1545–46
angioplasty and, 1901, 1907
autoregulation, 61, 857–58
neurogenic vasoconstriction and, 862
steal and, 864
beta-blocking agents and, 1614
bypass surgery and, 947
collateral, 862–63. *See also* Coronary arteries, collateral.
compressive forces and, 60
computed tomography and, 1849, 1865, 1866
CPR and, 548
diastole and, 60
distribution, 63
DPTI and, 859–61
humoral factors and, 62–63
intramyocardial pressure and, 859
ischemia and, 309
subendocardial, 859–61
metabolic factors, 60–61
neural factors, 61–62
oxygen and, 60–61, 861–62
perfusion pressure and, 857–61
physical determinants, 60
positron-emission tomography and, 1849
pyrophosphate uptake and, 1845
shock and, 372
steal phenomenon and, 863–64
systole and, 60, 858–59, 860
tamponade and, 1259
thallium imaging and, 1831–44
exercise and, 1834–38
vasoconstriction and, 862
Coronary bypass surgery, 946–56, 2036–40
anesthesia, 952
aneurysm and, 711–12
abdominal, 990
angioplasty and, 1903
anticoagulants and, 1674
aortic regurgitation and, 991
aortic stenosis and, 991
arrhythmias and, 950, 953
arteriography and, 2038–39
cardiopulmonary bypass and, 2036
carotid artery disease and, 990
choice of graft for, 2036–37
claudication and, 990
complications, 952–54, 2039–40
computed tomography and, 1868
economic costs, 956
exercise and, 949–50, 1028–29
family support and, 951
heart failure and, 950, 951
historical note on, 888
hypothyroidism and, 1421–22
indications, 310, 949–50
infarction and, 950
early evolving, 968
insurance and, 1558
ischemic relief and, 947
mammary artery grafts, 853–54, 2037
medical management during, 952
mitral regurgitation and, 991
mitral stenosis and, 991
monitoring and, 2002
mortality, 952
myocardial preservation and, 2037–38
Coronary bypass surgery:
necropsy and, 2078
noncardiac surgery and, 991
pain after, 989–90
patency of graft, 954–55
pathology, 851–54
acute phase, 852–53
chronic phase, 853–54
patient education and, 950–51
pilot certification and, 1578–79
platelet-controlling drugs and, 1676–77
postoperative management, 952
preoperative management, 951–52
psychological factors, 1531–32
rehabilitation from. *See* Rehabilitation.
reoperations, 854
sequential grafting, 2037
spasm and, 1015
subset identification and, 946–47
sudden death and, 544, 950
survival, 299, 310, 947–49
technique, 2038
variables considered before, 947
work status after, 955–56, 1532, 1578–79
Coronary cusps, 27–28
Coronary heart disease, 801–1036. *See also* Atherosclerosis; Myocardial infarction; Myocardial ischemia.
aging and, 1409
alcohol and, 826
altitude and, 1546
anesthesia and, 1500–1501
angina and. *See* Angina pectoris.
angioplasty indications and, 1902–3
anxiety and, 934–35
aortic regurgitation and, 991
aortic stenosis and, 990–91
arrhythmias and, 304, 988–89
arteriography. *See* Coronary arteriography.
aspirin and, 831, 944, 1677–78
prognosis and, 923
assessment, 299–312, 889–907
decision trees for, 301–3
general approach, 299–300
likelihood of disease and, 300–308
prognosis and, 310–12
severity of disease and, 309–10
asymptomatic, 958, 959–60
arteriography and, 904–5
prognosis, 920
surgical intervention and, 950
treatment, 958, 960–61
cardiomyopathy and, 1187, 1190–91, 1206
prognosis, 930–31
carotid artery disease and, 990
causality assessment, medicolegal, 1571–72
classification, 888–89, 931–33
clinical setting, 889
computed tomography and, 1867–68
contraceptive agents and, 825–26, 829
denial of, 985, 1530
depression and, 934–35, 985, 987, 1531
double-vessel:
angioplasty for, 1903
asymptomatic, 960
prognosis, 921, 922
surgical intervention and, 949, 950
Coronary heart disease:
ECG, 302, 304, 894–96
historical notes on, 885
treatment and, 959–60
echocardiography and, 1960–62
exercise for, 1713
management and, 933
preventive measures and, 825, 829–30
rehabilitative, 1026–28, 1031–34
exercise testing, 896, 1026, 1704, 1709–14, 1825
prognosis and, 310–11, 921, 926, 710, 1712
radionuclide, 899–902, 1832, 1834–38, 1842–43
treatment and, 959–60
uncomplicated infarction and, 969–70
fluoroscopy, 894
genetic factors, 824
heart failure and, 930–31
heart rate and, exercise, 921
historical benchmarks, 883–88
history, 889–93
limitations of, 892–93
incidence, 559–60
infarction and. *See* Myocardial infarction.
initial evaluation, 300–308
insurance and, 1557–59
intermediate ("in-between") syndrome, 885
ischemia and. *See* Myocardial ischemia.
legal issues, 1568–69, 1571–72
lupus erythematosus and, 1022, 1437
menopause and, 826
metabolic disorders and, 1023
mitral regurgitation and, 769, 770, 774, 991
mitral stenosis and, 991
mortality, 560
natural history, 817–18, 919. *See also* *prognosis* below.
necropsy and, 2078
nonatherosclerotic, 1016–24
tabulation of, 1017
noncardiac surgery and, 1513–14, 1518
obesity and, 824–25, 829, 936, 1453
pain from. *See* Angina pectoris; Pain, chest.
pathology, 842–55
physical examination, 893–94
pregnancy and, 1392
premature ventricular beats and, 921
prevalence, 559
prevention, 817–32
basis for, 817–20
community approach, 817, 819–20, 827
high-risk individual and, 817
multifactorial approach, 826–27, 831–32
physician's role in, 826–27
primary, 818, 820–27
secondary, 818, 827–32
validation problems, 818–19
probability analysis, 304–6
prognosis, 560, 918–31
asymptomatic patient and, 920
background and principles, 918–20
cardiomyopathy and, 930–31

Coronary heart disease: prognosis:
catheterization and angiography and, 311–12
ECG and, 896
exercise testing and, 310–11, 1710, 1712
historical notes on, 887
index for, 927–28
irreversible ischemia and, 924–29
myocardial infarction and, 924–29
reversible ischemia and, 920–24
stable angina and, 919, 920–23
sudden death and, 929–30
unstable angina and, 923–24
psychological factors, 826, 934–35, 1521–25, 1530–33
radionuclide studies, 899–902, 1825, 1833–48
prognosis and, 922
rehabilitation. *See* Rehabilitation.
retirement and, 936
risk factors, 807–9, 889
alterable vs. unalterable, 819, 820
evidence for, 819
intervention principle, 817
populations and, 817, 819
preventive measures, 820–32
roentgenography, 894
simulating conditions, 907–18
single-vessel:
angioplasty for, 1902–3
asymptomatic, 960–61
prognosis and, 921, 922
surgical intervention and, 949
skiing and, 1546
smoking and, 937
spasm and. *See* Coronary arteries, spasm.
spousal factors, 826
subset identification, 889–907
prognosis and, 919
surgical treatment and, 946–47
sudden death and, 850, 929–30, 987–88
thrombosis and, 530, 534–35, 540
syncope and, 988
thallium imaging, 899–900
transition zone, 919
treatment, 933–92
asymptomatic disease and, 958, 960–61
dietary, 936
different strategies in, rationale for, 991–92
drug, 937–45
endarterectomy, 956–57
exercise, 933, 1713
exercise testing and, 959–60
historical notes on, 887–88
irreversible disease and, 965–87
medical, 933–45
oxygen, 937–38
psychiatric, 933–35
rehabilitative. *See* Rehabilitation.
rest, 933–34, 969
reversible disease and, 959–65
specific subsets and, 957–91
stable subsets and, 959–61
surgical, 945–57. *See also* Angioplasty, percutaneous transluminal; Coronary bypass surgery.
unstable subsets and, 961–65
triple-vessel:
asymptomatic, 960
Coronary heart disease: triple-vessel:
prognosis, 921, 922
surgical intervention and, 949, 950
type A behavior and, 1524–25
vasculitis and, 1022–23
Coronary plexus, 25
Coronary sinus:
anatomy, 29–30
aneurysm, 620–21
atrial septal defect and, 598
catheterization, 309
inadvertent, 1770–71
embryology, 11
fistula, 707, 708
malformations, 712
ostium, 19
pacing leads and, 493, 1753
pulmonary venous anomaly and, 682, 684
Coronary sulcus, 16
Coronary vascular reserve, 60
Coronary veins:
anatomy, 29–30
anomalies, 712
Cor pulmonale, 1120–27
acute, 1096, 1107
cardiac output increase and, 403
catheterization studies, 1126
chest deformity and, 134
chronic, 1120–27
clinical manifestations, 1124–26
definition, 1120
diffuse interstitial lung disease and, 1123–24, 1126
digitalis for, 1127, 1644
ECG, 1125–26
edema and, 1123
embolism and, pulmonary, 1096, 1107
etiology, 1120
heart failure and, 1122–23, 1125, 1127
history, 1124–25
hypertension and, pulmonary, 1095–97, 1121–23, 1126–27
hypoventilation and, 1124, 1127
hypoxemia and, 1095–96
incidence, 1120
left ventricular function in, 1123
management, 1126–27
mechanical obstruction and, 1096–97
natural history and prognosis, 1127
obstructive pulmonary disease and, 1123–24, 1126
pathophysiology, 1120–23
physical examination, 1125
radionuclide studies, 1126
Corrigan, D. J., 739
Corrigan's pulse, 745, 746
Corticosteroids:
aldosteronism and, 1063, 1064
atherosclerosis and, 1524
cardiomyopathy and, 1192
fat embolism and, 1115
myocarditis and, 1177
pericarditis and, 1254
in myocardial infarction, 982
rheumatic fever and, 1311
salt-active. *See* Aldosterone.
septic shock and, 390
transplantation and, 2065
Cortisol, emotional stress and, 1523, 1524
Cor triatriatum, 651–52
clinical manifestations, 651
Cor triatriatum:
dexter, 11
management, 651–52
pathology, 651
sinister, 12
Cor triloculare biventriculare, 612
Corvisart, Jean Nicolas, 1158
Costochondral joint pain, 918
Costoclavicular syndrome, 916
Costoclavicular test, 917
Costs, economic, of heart disease, 557
coronary bypass surgery and, 956
Cotton-wool spots, 199–200
Cough, 117
bloody. *See* Hemoptysis.
heart failure and, 350
syncope and, 517
Coumadin. *See also* Warfarin.
coronary heart disease and, 943
prosthetic valves and, 1517
aortic, 738
mitral, 779
Coumarin, 1669–75. *See also* Warfarin.
adverse reactions, 1674
indications, 1669–74
mechanisms of action, 1669
new developments, 1674–75
therapeutic regimens, 1669
Counterpulsation, intraaortic. *See* Intraaortic balloon counterpulsation.
Coupling:
definition, 433
excitation-contraction, 37–39, 1476
fixed, premature ventricular beats and, 450, 452
parasystole and, 456
ventricular tachycardia and, 452
Courtroom procedures, 1565–67
Covisart, J. N., 138
Coxsackie virus, myocarditis and, 259–60, 1158, 1177
clinical manifestations, 1169
laboratory studies, 1169
Creatine kinase:
cardioversion and, 483, 1745
isoenzymes, 898
muscular dystrophy and, 571
myocardial infarction and, 897, 898
Creatine phosphate, myocardial, 86
CREST syndrome, 1442
Cretinism, athyreotic, 1418
Crisscross heart, 706–7
clinical manifestations, 706–7
management, 707
pathology, 706
Crista supraventricularis, 19
Crista terminalis, 18
Criteria Committee of N.Y. Heart Association, 106
Crotalidae, 1489
Crux of heart, 17
Cryptococcosis, 1175
Cuff, compression, 139
Curran, William J., 1563
Cushing's syndrome, hypertension and, 1063
Cutis laxa, 124
Cutdown:
arterial, cardiac catheterization and, 1772
venous, cardiac catheterization and, 1770–71
Cyanide poisoning, hyperbaric oxygen therapy and, 1554

Cyanosis:
acrocyanosis and, 1352
clubbing and, 132
congenital heart disease and, 586–87
differential, 132
Ebstein's anomaly and, 678
embolism and, paradoxical, 587
growth retardation and, 589
heart failure and, 351
history, 120
jaundice and, 121
livedo reticularis and, 1352
patent ductus arteriosus and, 615
polycythemia and, 586–87
pulmonary arterial sling and, 626
pulmonary atresia and, 670
pulmonary valve absence and, 667
pulmonic stenosis and, 655
Raynaud's phenomenon and, 1352
tetralogy of Fallot and, 663
transposition of great arteries and, 692
tricuspid atresia and, 673, 675
truncus arteriosus and, 671
Cybertach-60 pacing system, 499
Cycle, sound, 157
Cycle ergometry. *See* Bicycle ergometry.
Cyclophosphamide, 1482
toxicity of, 1232–33
Cyclosporine, transplantation and, 2065, 2066
Cyclothiazide, 1659
dosage, 1072
Cycloxygenase, 814
Cyst:
hydatid, 1161. *See also* Echinococcosis.
pericardial, 712–13, 1266, 1295
CT scan of, 1871
Cysticercosis, 1176
Cystic medial necrosis, aortic, 1322, 1330
regurgitant valve and, 644, 741–43
Cytomegalovirus, 1162

d loop, 686
crisscross heart and, 706
double-outlet right ventricle and, 696
transposition of great arteries and, 691
Dacron graft:
aortic aneurysm repair, 1326, 1328, 2043–47
aortic arch occlusive disease and, 1334
aortofemoral, 2059
aortoiliac, 1335–36
IABP and, 2022
Dacron patch:
aorticopulmonary septal defect and, 619
atrial septal defect and, 602, 603
AV canal and, 610
coarctation of aorta and, 633
pulmonary venous connection anomaly and, 685
univentricular heart and, 705
ventricular septal defect and, 666
ventriculotomy and, right, 659
Dardilate. *See* Erythrityl tetranitrate.
Data:
defined base, 105, 106
misinterpretation of, 1538–39
probability analysis and, 304–6
Datascope balloon, 2021–22
Daunorubicin, cardiomyopathy and, 1183, 1481
da Vinci, Leonardo, 785
Deafness, 130
Death, sudden. *See* Sudden death.
Decision making:
Bayes' theorem and, 304–6
coronary artery disease evaluation and, 301–3
Decompression sickness, 1550–52
Decremental conduction, 410, 427
Defecation syncope, 518
Defibrillation, 483–84, 1741, 1744–45. *See also* Cardioversion.
CPR and, 550
implantable device for, 478, 542, 1761–63
Degos' disease, 125
Dehydroemetine, 1232
de Lange syndrome, 126–27, 133
Delirium, postcardiotomy, 1531–32
Demerol. *See* Meperidine.
Denial, coronary heart disease and, 985, 1520
Dental procedures, endocarditis and, 1152
Deoxyribonucleic acid (DNA), 566
Dephosphorylation, 87
glycogen, 89
Depolarization:
action potential and, 76
atrial, 206
automaticity and, 78–79, 407–8
calcium and, 1473
diastolic, 407–8
impulse conduction and, 410
injury and, 209
pacemakers and, 494
potassium and, 1471
triggered activity and, 408–9
ventricular, 207
Depression (mental):
chest pain and, 908
coronary heart disease and, 934–35, 985, 987, 1531
drugs alleviating, 1479–80
hypertension and, 1534
rehabilitation and, 1035
Dermatomyositis, 124
de Senac, Jean-Baptiste, 1181, 1284
Desipramine, 1479
Deslanoside. *See* Digitalis.
DeVega annuloplasty, 2033–34
Dexamethasone:
aldosteronism and, 1063, 1064
pericarditis and, 982
Dextran, shock and, 374, 388
Dextroamphetamine, 1234
Dextrocardia, dextroversion, dextroposition, 231, 688–89
roentgenography and, 231–32
Dextroisomerism, 687, 689
Diabetes insipidus, diuretics and, 1664
Diabetes mellitus, 1426–31
acromegaly and, 1423
angina pectoris and, 1430
arteriosclerosis obliterans and, 1339, 1342
atherosclerosis and, 808–9, 825, 829, 1428–29
beta-blocking agents and, 1075
cardiomyopathy and, 1428
fetal, 1429–30
classification, 1426
coma and, 1426
Diabetes mellitus:
diuretics and, 1075
fatty acids and, 94
genetics, 575
glucose transport and, 89
heart failure and, 1430–31
hypertension and, 1075, 1430
myocardial function and, 85–86
myocardial infarction and, 829, 1430
silent, 1427–28
neuropathy and, 1427–28
orthostatic hypotension (syncope) and, 512–13, 1427
pregnancy and, 1429–30
protein metabolism and, 97
pyruvate metabolism and, 90
retinopathy and, 202
surgery and, 1431
treatment of heart disease in, 1430–31
vibratory perception and, 1427
wound healing in, 1431
Diagnosis:
approach to, 105–8
athlete's heart and, 1401–2
categories of, 107
complications of procedures, 1540
legal issues and, 1567–68, 1574–75
pregnancy and, 1394
misinterpretation of data and, 1538–39
Diagonal coronary arteries, 28, 839
radiography, 1794, 1796, 1797
Dialysis:
arteriovenous fistula and, 1460, 1462
cardiac output increase and, 401
edema and, 1664
ejection fraction and, 1462–63
endocarditis and, 1135, 1460
etiologic factors in development of cardiovascular disease and, 1464
pericarditis and, 1266–67, 1461
potassium and, 1459
tamponade and, 1267
Diastole, 52
arterial volume and, 1039
cardiomyopathy and, 1199
collapse, 148, 150
coronary blood flow and, 60, 859
failure, 320
gallop of. *See* Gallop.
murmurs of, 192–93
auscultatory principles, 163
precordial movement and, 154, 155
radionuclide studies of, 1830–31
sounds of, 163, 176–82
blow, aortic regurgitation and, 745, 746
early, 186
rumble. *See* Rumble, diastolic.
vs. systolic, 176–77
suction of, 48
Diastolic pressure. *See also* Blood pressure; End-diastolic pressure.
coronary blood flow and, 60, 859–61
hypertension and, 1042
hypertrophy and, 328
measurement of, 139
mitral stenosis and, 759
normal, 55, 140
pericarditis and, constrictive, 1256, 1258, 1263
-time index (DPTI), 859–61
variability in, 1049
Diazepam:
anesthetic use of, 1496

Diazepam:
cardiac catheterization and, 1769
cardioversion and, 1742
coronary heart disease and, 938
Diazoxide, 1587
dosage and effects, 1586
pharmacology, 1587
preeclampsia and, 1085
protein-binding and dialysance, 1082
Dibenzyline, 1589. *See also* Phenoxybenzamine.
Dichloisoproterenol, structure of, 1608
Dichloroisoprenaline, 1609
Dicoumarol, 1669
Dicrotic notch, 53, 142
carotid, 143
IABP and, 2023
Dicrotic pulse, 145
Dicrotic wave, 53, 54, 142
Diet:
arteriosclerosis obliterans and, 1344
atherosclerosis and, 820–22, 828
cholesterol in, 807–8, 820–22, 828
coronary heart disease and, 936
hyperalimentation, 1449–50
hypertension and, 1078
liquid protein, 1484
mesenteric ischemia and, 1368
myocardial disease and, 1218–19
obesity and, 1456
potassium in, 1079
sodium-restricted, 360–61, 1078
Diffusion force, 74
Digitalis, 1639–49
aging and, 1406, 1410, 1641
angina pectoris and, 942
arrhythmias induced by, 479, 1647–48
supraventricular tachycardia, 440
arrhythmias treated by, 1645–46
atrial fibrillation and, 943, 1645
bioavailability, 1640–41
calcium channel blockers and, 941, 1631, 1635, 1647
cardioversion and, 1745
chemistry, 1639–40
children and, 1641, 1644–45
choice of preparation, 1646
clinical uses, 1644–46
contractility and, 358–59, 1642
cor pulmonale and, 1127, 1644
electrophysiologic effects, 1642–44
Frank-Starling compensation and, 359
heart failure and, 358–59, 980, 1644–45
in infants, 585
prevention of, 356–57
hepatic failure and, 1641
interactions of, 1646, 1647
loading dose, 359, 1646
maintenance dose, 1645, 1646
mitral stenosis and, 761
myocardial infarction and, 942, 980, 1644, 1645
uncomplicated, 971
myocarditis and, 1178
obesity and, 1641
pharmacokinetics, 1640–42
pharmacological actions, 1642
potassium and, 479, 1470–71, 1647
pregnancy and, 1393, 1641–42
renal failure and, 1641
sinus node and, 480, 1643
structure-activity relations, 1639–40
surgical procedures and, noncardiac, 1514, 1517
Digitalis:
thyroid function and, 1642
toxicity, 1539, 1647–49
vasoconstrictor effect of, 1642
Digital subtraction angiography. *See* Angiography, digital.
Digitoxin. *See also* Digitalis.
dosage, 1646
pharmacokinetics, 1640
Digoxin. *See also* Digitalis.
arrhythmias and, 943
bioavailability, 1640–41
calcium antagonists and, 941
dosage, 359, 943, 1646
heart failure and, 1645
in infants, 585
interactions of, 1646, 1647
pharmacokinetics, 1640
Dihydroergotamine, venous thrombosis and, 1105
Dilatation of heart. *See also* Cardiomyopathy, dilated.
aortic regurgitation and, 742–45, 747
Chagas' disease and, 1159, 1162
heart failure and, 328–29
ischemia and, 850–51
mitral regurgitation and, 768–72
myocardial infarction and, 847
preload and, 332
pulmonary hypertension and, 1097
Dilevalol, 1609
Diltiazem, 941. *See also* Calcium channel blockers.
adverse effects, 1634
angina pectoris and, 1628, 1629
coronary artery spasm and, 1015
dosage, 1072, 1628
pharmacodynamics, 1625–27
pharmacology, 1587–88
structure, 1624, 1625
surgical procedures and, 1514
therapeutic levels, 1628
Diphenylhydantoin, 1597–98
clinical application and toxicity, 1598
digitalis toxicity and, 1648
pharmacokinetics, 1594, 1597–98
pharmacology, 1598
2,3-Diphosphoglyceric acid, oxygen-hemoglobin affinity and, 379
Diphtheritic myocarditis, 1159
clinical manifestations, 1168
laboratory studies, 1168
pathophysiology, 1163–65
prognosis, 1176
treatment, 1178
Dipole theory, 81–82
Dipyridamole:
adverse reactions to, 1678
AMP levels and, 1675
coronary bypass surgery and, 954–55, 1677
myocardial infarction and, 831, 943, 1677
platelets and, 812
prosthetic valves and, 1676
aortic, 738
stress imaging and, 1838–39
Disability:
causality determination and, 1572
cerebrovascular disease and, 562
evaluation of, 1562, 1572–73
psychological factors, 1537, 1542
retirement and, 1564
Disability:
Social Security criteria for, 1578
workers' compensation and, 1563–64, 1571
Discordance:
atrioventricular, 686
corrected transposition of great arteries and, 700
crisscross heart and, 706
ventriculoarterial, 687
corrected transposition of great arteries and, 700
single ventricle and, 703
Disease vs. disorder, 317
Disopyramide, 1595–96
clinical applications, 1596
pharmacokinetics, 1594, 1596
pharmacology, 1596
toxicity, 1596
Dissection:
aortic. *See* Aorta, dissection.
cerebrovascular disease and, 1358
coronary artery, 1021
Distensibility. *See also* Compliance.
vascular (arterial), 58, 1039
aging and, 1406
factors affecting, 138
pulse and, 141, 142
Diuresis, excessive, management of, 362
Diuretics, 1657–66. *See also* specific agent.
aldosterone and, 1062, 1657, 1660
ascites and, 1662
biochemistry, 1658
carbonic anhydrase inhibitors, 1658–60
clinical uses, 1661–65
complications, 1073, 1539, 1665–66
cor pulmonale and, 1127
diabetes mellitus and, 1075
dose and duration of action, 1659
edema and, 1657, 1661–64
pulmonary, 1661–62
Frank-Starling mechanism and, 361, 362
heart failure and, 361–62, 1661–62
in infant, 585
hyperlipidemia and, 1074–75
hypertension and, 1071, 1072, 1664
dosage, 1072
gestational, 1084
renoparenchymal, 1080
resistant, 1077
loop (high-ceiling), 1658–61
miscellaneous uses of, 1664–65
nephrotic syndrome and, 1662
oliguria and, 1665
pharmacokinetics, 1660–61
potassium and, 361–62, 1658–61, 1665
supplementation of, 1071
pregnancy and, 1393
renal failure and, 1662
site of action of, 1658–60
sodium and, 362, 1657, 1665
thiazide (benzothiadiazine), 1658–60
ventricular performance curves and, 1506
Diverticula, pericardial, 712–13
Diving:
syncope and, 518
underwater, 1550–53
Dizziness, 117, 507
aortic regurgitation and, 745
DNA, 566

Dobutamine, 1654–55
cardiomyopathy and, 1192
contractility and, 360, 1654–55
CPR and, 552
heart failure and, 1655
in infant, 586
shock and, 392
structure, 1653
Dopamine. *See also* Catecholamines.
contractility and, 360, 1653
CPR and, 552
heart failure in infant and, 586
shock and, 377
management of, 391–92
structure, 1653
Dopamine-β-hydroxylase, hyperthyroidism and, 1415
Doppler studies, 1974–88
arterial, 1974–76
arteriosclerosis obliterans and, 1342
atrial septal defect and, 1986–87
B-mode combined with, 1974
carotid artery, 1878–79
cerebrovascular disease and, 1355
clinical applications, 1979–87
color flow imaging, 1988
continuous wave, 1974, 1979
errors in interpreting, 1538–39
general recommendations, 1987–88
instrumentation, 1974
limitations, 1987
patent ductus arteriosus and, 1987
plethysmography and, 1977
pulsed, 1974, 1978–79
sample volume, 1979
shift measurement, 1978
shunt, 1986–87
technique, 1978–79
thrombosis and, 1106, 1374, 1976–77
valvular, 1981–86
mitral, 252
prosthetic, 1985–86
regurgitant lesions and, 1983–85
stenosis and, 255, 256, 1981–83
venous, 1976–77
ventricular performance, 1979–81
ventricular septal defect and, 1986
Double-inlet left ventricle, 8
Double-inlet right ventricle, 8
Double-outlet left ventricle, 699–700
clinical manifestations, 700
pathology, 699–700
surgical management, 700
Double-outlet right ventricle, 8, 696–99
associated conditions, 696
clinical manifestations, 697–98
medical management, 699
natural history and prognosis, 698–99
pathology, 696–97
surgical management, 699
Doughnut sign, radionuclide, 1845
Down's syndrome, 567
facial features in, 128
hand in, 133
Doxepin, 1479–80
Doxorubicin, 1481
cardiomyopathy and, 1481, 1826–28
radionuclide monitoring of, 1826–28
toxicity of, 1233–34
Doyle, Arthur Conan, 230
dP/dt, 48
catheterization studies and, 1775
DPTI (diastolic pressure-time index), 859–61
Dressler beats:
aberrant conduction and, 460
ventricular tachycardia and, 454
Dressler's syndrome, 987, 1267
Drift, circulatory, exercise and, 1399–1400
Drive systems, mechanical heart, 2069, 2071, 2072
Driving eligibility, 1578
Droperidol, 1496
Dropped beats, 464
Drugs, 1583–1682. *See also* specific agent.
abuse of, endocarditis and, 1132
anesthetic, 1495–97, 1504–5
antiarrhythmic, 1593–1603
anticoagulant, 1667–75
antidepressant, 1479–80
antihypertensive, 1071–78, 1080–85
antineoplastic, 1481–82
antithyroid, 1416–17
beta-blocking. *See* Beta-blocking agents; Propranolol.
calcium antagonist. *See* Calcium channel blockers.
cardiac output increased by, 404
cholesterol-lowering, 821, 822–23, 829
contraceptive. *See* Contraceptive agents.
contractility and, 49, 358–60
coronary heart disease treatment, 937–45
diuretic, 1657–66
exercise and, 1027–28
hypersensitivity to, 1236–37
iatrogenic disorders and, 1539–40
inotropic, 1639–56. *See also* Digitalis.
noncardiac, 1479–84
pericarditis induced by, 1269
platelet-controlling, 1675–78
pregnancy and, 1392–94
cardiovascular agents, 1392–94
obstetric agents, 1394
psychotropic, 1479–81
stress induced by, 1838–39
thrombolytic. *See* Thrombolytic agents.
toxic effects of, on myocardium, 1231–36
vasoactive, 1583–91. *See also* Vasoconstrictors; Vasodilators; *and* specific agents.
Drummond's artery, 1369
Duchenne dystrophy, 126, 571, 1227–28
Ductus arteriosus:
aortic atresia and, 646
closure of, 583
embryology, 13, 14
fetal circulation and, 582, 583
interrupted aortic arch and, 634
patent. *See* Patent ductus arteriosus.
pulmonary artery origin from, 15, 670
pulmonary atresia and, 661, 670
right aortic arch and, 623
Ductus venosus, 582
pulmonary venous anomaly and, 682
Duke-Elder, Stewart, 198
Duotrate. *See* Pentaerythrityl tetranitrate.
Duplex scanning, 1975
carotid artery, 1878–79
Duroziez's murmur, 747
Dye-dilution curve, shunt detection and, 1781–82
Dye method, cardiac output and, 1780–81
Dysbetalipoproteinemia, 574
Dysphagia, 121, 911, 912
Dyspnea, 115–17
angina pectoris and, 890
anxiety and, 116, 1526–27
cardiomyopathy and, 1187–88, 1200
cor pulmonale and, 1123–24
decompression sickness and, 1551
edema and, 118
on effort, 115, 349
endomyocardial fibrosis and, 1210
errors in interpreting, 1538
exercise testing and, 1708
heart failure and, 349
hypoxia and, 116
mitral regurgitation and, 769
myocardial ischemia and, 961
myocarditis and, 1165
neonatal, 584
paroxysmal nocturnal, 116, 349
postural. *See* Orthopnea.
pregnancy and, 116
pulmonary arterial sling and, 626
pulmonary edema and, 116
pulmonary embolism and, 116, 1107
pulmonary hypertension and, 1097
tetralogy of Fallot and, 663
Dysrhythmias. *See* Arrhythmias; *also* specific disturbance.

E sign, 630
Ear:
hearing apparatus of, 158
inspection of, 130
Ebstein's anomaly, 677–80
catheterization studies, 678
clinical manifestations, 678–79
ECG, 1778
echocardiography, 251, 253
embryology, 12
medical management, 679
natural history and prognosis, 679
pathology, 677–78
pathophysiology, 678
roentgenography, 237
surgical management, 679–80
ECG. *See* Electrocardiography.
Echinococcosis, 1158, 1177
clinical manifestations, 1172
laboratory studies, 1172
pathology, 1160–61
pathophysiology, 1165
treatment, 1179
Echo beat, 468
Echocardiography, 1926–67
advantages of, 1926
A-mode, 1928
amyloidosis and, 1215, 1957, 1958
aorta and, 1938, 1945
aortic atresia and, 646
aortic-mitral combined valvular disease and, 789
aortic regurgitation and, 747, 1959
aortic stenosis and, 248–49, 734, 1959
congenital disease and, 636–37, 639, 641
aortic valve, 1934, 1935, 1938, 1940–41, 1959
bicuspid, 247, 643, 1955, 1959–60
ventricular performance and, 1963–64
apical views, 1938, 1941–43
artifacts, 1965–66

Echocardiography:
athletes and, 1052, 1401
atrial septal defect and, 601, 1944
AV canal and, 608
basic principles, 1927–28
B-mode, 1928, 1930
Doppler method combined with, 1974
cardiomyopathy and:
dilated, 260, 261, 1189, 1956
hypertrophic, 259, 1202–3, 1956–58
restrictive, 1958
clinical applications, 1952–64
coarctation of aorta and, 630
contrast, 1948–50
controls, 1929–30
coronary arteries and, 1941, 1942, 1962
coronary heart disease and, 1960–62
digital processing, 1966
digital scan converter, 1931
Doppler. *See* Doppler studies.
double-outlet right ventricle and, 698
dropout of target and, 1966
Ebstein's anomaly and, 251, 253
ejection fraction and, 1963
electronic scanner, 1930
endocarditis and, 1145–46, 1960
endomyocardial fibrosis and, 1211, 1212
errors in interpreting, 1538–39
exercise, 1950–51
first heart sound and, 159, 164
four-chamber plane, 1936, 1937, 1941, 1944
future of, 1966–67
gray scale and, 1929
heart failure and, 355
historical perspective, 1927
hyperthyroidism and, 397
hypertrophy and, 1054, 1953
hypothyroidism and, 1420
instrumentation, 1928
intracardiac, 1951
intraoperative, 1952
invasive, 1951–52
limitations, 1964–66
long-axis views, 1936, 1937
apical, 1943
parasternal, 1938–40
suprasternal, 1945
measurements:
M-mode, 1935–36
two-dimensional, 1945–48
mechanical scanner, 1930
mitral annulus calcification and, 1959
mitral valve, 1933–34, 1939, 1940, 1954
aortic valve disease combined with, 789
measurement, 1935
prolapse and, 1958–59
regurgitation and, 251, 252, 650, 772, 1954, 1958
stenosis and, 649, 758, 759, 1958
ventricular performance and, 1963
M-mode, 1932–36
equipment, 1928–30
limitations, 1964–65
myocardial failure and, 272, 276
myocardial infarction and, 970–71, 1953, 1960–62
myocarditis and, 1166
myxoma and, 1288, 1291
normal, 1933–35

Echocardiography:
papillary muscle and, 1940
parasternal views, 1938–41
patent ductus arteriosus and, 616
pericardial effusion and, 262–63, 1254–55, 1953, 1954–55
pericardiocentesis and, 1955, 1956
pharmacologic and physiologic interventions, 1951
phased-array scanner, 1930–31
phonocardiography and, 1948, 1996
pivoting, 1938
positioning for, 1931
postprocessing, 1931
pulmonary artery, 1941
pulmonary hypertension and, 1098
pulmonary valve, 1935, 1941
atresia and, 661
regurgitation and, 255
stenosis and, 656
ventricular performance and, 1964
pulmonary venous connection anomaly and, 604, 683
real-time systems, 1930
recording methods, 1929, 1966
right ventricular inflow tract view, 1939–40
right ventricular outflow tract view, 1944
short-axis views, 1936, 1937
parasternal, 1940–41
suprasternal, 1945
shunts and, 1949
single ventricle and, 704
sliding maneuver, 1937–38
subcostal position, 1938, 1943–44
suprasternal position, 1938, 1944–45
syncope and, 524
systolic time intervals and, 1948
tamponade and, 1261, 1953, 1955
techniques, 1931–52
tetralogy of Fallot and, 258, 664, 1949
three-dimensional, 1966–67
tilting, 1938
time gain compensation, 1930
tissue characterization, 1966
tomographic views, 1938–45
transducer, 1927, 1929
index mark for, 1936–37
transesophageal, 1951–52
transposition of great arteries and, 692–93
corrected, 251, 701
tricuspid valve, 1935, 1940, 1941
atresia and, 675
regurgitation and, 253–54, 795–96, 1949–50
two-dimensional, 1936–48
equipment, 1930–31
limitations, 1965
valve motion and sound phenomena and, 159
ventricular aneurysm and, 1962
ventricular performance and, 1962–64
ventricular septal defect and, 594
Echovirus myocarditis, 1169
Economic costs of heart disease, 557
coronary bypass surgery and, 956
Ectopia cordis, 707
Ectopic beats. *See* Extrasystoles; Parasystoles; Premature atrial beats; Premature ventricular beats.
Edema:
albumin administration and, 1663

Edema:
cor pulmonale and, 1123
diuretics and, 1657, 1661–64
dyspnea and, 118
heart failure and, 118, 350, 352
mechanisms of, 324–25
history, 118
idiopathic, of females, 1662
leg, 205
optic disk, 201, 203
periorbital, 118
potassium and, 1662, 1663
pulmonary, 118, 337–339
acute, 349–50, 366–67
alveolar, 354
cardioversion and, 1745
diuretics and, 1661–62
dyspnea and, 116
heart failure and, 337–38, 349–50, 353
high-altitude, 338, 1096, 1547
interstitial, 353
management, 360–63, 366–67
mitral stenosis and, 756, 758
morphine and, 338, 366
noncardiac, 338–39
renal failure and, 1463
roentgenography and, 239
symptoms and signs, 349–50
refractory, 1662–64
renal failure and, 1463, 1662
sodium and, 1657, 1662
tricuspid regurgitation and, 794
vena caval obstruction and, 1378, 1379
venous hypertension and, 1377
Education, patient. *See* Patient education.
Effort syndrome, 1526
Effusion, pericardial. *See* Pericardial effusion; Tamponade.
Ehlers-Danlos syndrome, 123–24, 573
Eicosapentaenoic acid, 814
Einthoven triangle, 207
Eisenmenger syndrome, 10, 589
clinical picture, 593
hemoptysis and, 119
management, 596
roentgenography and, 235, 239
sounds, 174
single second, 168, 169
transplantation for, cardiopulmonary, 2067
Ejection fraction, 51
aging and, 1409
aortic regurgitation and, 747, 749
aortic stenosis and, 268
contractility and, 270, 271
coronary heart disease prognosis and, 922
cycle length and, 195
dialysis and, 1462–63
digital subtraction angiography and, 1861
doxorubicin cardiotoxicity and, 1827
echocardiography and, 1963
exercise and, 901, 902, 1825
heart failure and, 347, 348
mitral regurgitation and, 269, 275
murmurs and, 189, 190
myocardial infarction and, 302–3, 926, 978, 1824
nuclear probe technique and, 1829, 1830
radionuclide studies and, 272, 901, 902, 1815–17, 1819–22

Ejection murmurs, 188–91, 195
Ejection phases, 52
 indexes of, 270–71
Ejection sounds, 163, 182–84
 aortic, 163, 183–84
 pulmonary, 163, 182–83
Elastic element, contraction and, 40
Elastic lamina, fibrous plaque and, 803
Elderly. *See also* Aging.
 arrhythmias in, 1410
 blood pressure measurement in, 1048
 cardiomyopathy in, 331
 digitalis and, 1641
 orthostatic hypotension and, 511
 rehabilitation and, 1034
 symptoms and, 112
Electrical axis, 208
 left deviation, 213, 214
  bundle branch block and, 218–19
 right deviation, 215, 217
Electrical injuries, 1486–88
Electrocardiography (ECG), 206–27, 433–34
 aberrant conduction and, 458–59, 1694–95
 accelerated idioventricular rhythm and, 456
 accessory pathways and, 219–20
 activation sequence and, 80–82, 206
 ambulatory. *See* prolonged *below*.
 amyloidosis and, 1214, 1215
 angina pectoris and, 894–95
  exercise and, 896, 1707, 1708, 1714
  variant, 209, 963, 1011
 anxiety and, 908
 aortic-mitral combined valvular disease and, 789
 aortic regurgitation and, 747
 aortic stenosis and, 248, 636, 734
 artifacts, 225–27
 athletes and, 1052, 1401
 atrial fibrillation and, 446–47
 atrial flutter and, 443–45
 atrial septal defect and, 224, 600–601
 atrial tachycardia and, 441–44, 1694, 1699
 AV block and, 290, 464–66
  myocardial infarction and, 977
 AV canal and, 607–8
 AV dissociation and, 466–68
 AV junctional extrasystoles and, 439
 AV junctional tachycardia and, 419, 441–43
 bigeminy and, atrial, 439, 445
 bipolar leads, 207
 cable connection errors and, 226
 calcium and, 224–25, 1475–76
 cardiomyopathy and:
  dilated, 1188, 1189
  hypertrophic, 1201–2
 coarctation of aorta and, 630
 computers and, 227
 conduction disturbances and, 212–19
 coronary artery anomalies and, 709
 coronary artery spasm and, 1011, 1013
 coronary heart disease and, 302, 304, 894–96
  historical notes on, 885
  treatment and, 959–60
 cor pulmonale and, 1125–26
 depolarization and, 207
 dipole theory and, 81–82
 double-outlet right ventricle and, 698
 Ebstein's anomaly and, 678, 1778

Electrocardiograhy:
 Einthoven triangle and, 207
 electrical axis, 208
 electrical injury and, 1487
 electrolyte imbalances and, 222–25
 emetine toxicity and, 1232
 emphysema and, 223
 endocardial fibroelastosis and, 653
 endocarditis and, 1145
 errors in interpreting, 225–27, 1538, 1723–26
 escape beats and, 470
 esophageal, 1690–1703
  aberrant conduction and, 1694–95
  accelerated junctional rhythm and, 1698
  atrial pacing and, 1698
  atrial tachycardia and, 1694, 1699
  leads, 1690–94
  pacemaker-mediated tachycardia and, 1698–1701
  "pace out" failure and, 1699, 1700
  premature atrial beats and, 1698, 1699
  recording systems, 1691–92
  supraventricular tachycardia and, 293, 1695, 1696
  timing (RA-LA, LA-LV) and, 1701–2
  ventricular pacing and, 1698
  ventricular tachycardia and, 1694–97
 excitation and, 80–81
 exercise, 1706–10. *See also* Exercise testing.
  likelihood of disease and, 307–8
  myocardial infarction and, 896
  myocardial ischemia and, 306
  palpitations and, 285–86
  vs. prolonged ECG, 286, 1723
 extremity leads, 207, 226
 f waves, 446–47
 F waves, 443–45
 filtering, 1717
 focal block and, 216–17
 Friedreich's ataxia and, 1229
 genesis of recording, 80–84
 glycogenosis and, 1220
 heart failure and, 355
 hemiblock and, 213–15, 218
  left anterior, 213–14
  left posterior, 214–15
 hypertrophy and, 221–22, 1053
  hemiblock and, 214, 216
 infarction and, myocardial, 210–12
  acute, 312
  AV block and, 977
  bundle branch block and, 218
  decision-making and, 302
  exercise and, 312, 896
  hemiblock and, 214, 215, 217
  limitations of, 895
  pacemakers and, 495
  prolonged recording and, 971
  Q waves and, 209–10
  right ventricular, 212, 895
  subendocardial, 211–12
  transmural, 210–11
  vectorcardiography and, 1689–90
  ventricular fibrillation and, 541
 injury and, 208–9
 insurance and, 1561
 intraventricular conduction disturbances and, 213–19
 ischemia and, myocardial, 210, 306

Electrocardiograhy:
 isopotential lines, 82, 83
 ladder diagrams (Lewis lines), 433–34
 late potentials and, 1717–19
 left bundle branch block, 217–19
  complete, 217–19
  incomplete, 219
 magnesium and, 224, 1476
 mitral-aortic combined valvular disease and, 789
 mitral regurgitation and, 772
 mitral stenosis and, 223, 758
 muscular dystrophy and, 1228
 myocarditis and, 1166, 1168
  diphtheritic, 1168, 1170
  echovirus, 1171
 myotonia atrophica and, 1230
 myxoma and, 1287–88, 1291
 nodoventricular (Mahaim) fibers and, 220
 noise and, 1716
 nuclear probe technique and, 1829
 P wave, 73, 206. *See also* P wave.
  esophageal recording and, 1694–1702
  genesis, 82
 pacemakers and, 494–95, 1756
  malfunction of, 502–3
 pacing and, ventricular, 220–21
 palpitations and, 284–86
 parasystole and, 456–57
 patent ductus arteriosus and, 616
 pericarditis and, 909, 1252–53
 perioperative, 1498
  noncardiac surgery and, 1512
 potassium and, 222–24, 1471–73
 PR interval, 73. *See also* PR interval.
 precordial leads, 208, 226–27
 pregnancy and, 1394
 premature atrial beats and, 438
 premature ventricular beats and, 451–52
 prolonged (long-term), 282–83, 1720–26
  artifacts and errors, 1723–26
  cardiomyopathy and, 1189
  comparison of techniques, 1722–23
  continuous recorders, 1720, 1722
  coronary artery spasm and, 1013
  duration of, 1723
  event recorders, 1720, 1722
  vs. exercise testing, 286, 1723
  microcomputers and, 1720–21, 1722
  myocardial infarction and, 971
  pacemakers and, 1759
  palpitations and, 284, 286
  scanning and analysis, 1721–22
  ST-T recording, 1723
  syncope and, 525
 pulmonary atresia and, 660
 pulmonary embolism and, 916, 1108
 pulmonary hypertension and, 1098
 pulmonic stenosis and, 224, 656
 Q waves, 209–11, 302
 QRS complex, 206. *See also* QRS complex.
  genesis, 73, 81–84
  signal averaging, 1716–19
 QT interval, 210. *See also* QT interval.
  calcium and, 224–25, 1475–76
  prolonged, 225, 523–24
 quinidine and, 223, 224
 repolarization and, 207, 225
 resting, 206–27

Electrocardiograhy:
right bundle branch block, 215–16
complete, 215
concealed, 216
incomplete, 215
sarcoidosis and, 1218
signal averaging, 1716–19
single atrium and, 612
single ventricle and, 704
sinoatrial block and, 461–62
sinus arrhythmias and, 436
sinus node dysfunction and, 289
special leads, 434
ST segment, 84. *See also* ST segment.
reciprocal changes, 211
sudden death and, 540
syncope and, 287
T wave, 210. *See also* T wave.
genesis, 84
T_a wave, 206
tachycardia and, 292
atrial, 441–44, 1694, 1699
AV junctional, 419, 441–43
esophageal leads and, 293, 1694–97, 1699
QRS widening, 293
sinus, 436
supraventricular, 293, 417, 421, 441–44
ventricular, 293–94, 422, 453–56, 1717–18
tachycardia-bradycardia syndrome and, 450
tamponade and, 1261
telephone transmission and, 283
tetralogy of Fallot and, 664
thallium imaging and, 900
toxoplasmosis and, 1161
transposition of great arteries and, 692
corrected, 701
tricuspid atresia and, 675
tricuspid stenosis and, 795
U wave, hypokalemia and, 223–224, 1471, 1474
unipolar leads, 207, 208
vasoregulatory asthenia and, 910–11
vectorial, 208, 1687–90
ventricular fibrillation and, 470, 471
ventricular septal defect and, 593–94
ventricular tachycardia and, 293–94, 422, 453–56, 1717–18
wandering pacemaker and, 469
Wenckebach phenomenon and, 464, 465
Wilson central terminal, 207
Wolff-Parkinson-White syndrome and, 219–20, 416–18, 447, 448
Electroconvulsive therapy, 1487–88
Electrodes:
cardioverter, 1741, 1742
implantable, 1761
esophageal, 1690–91
hydrogen, shunt detection by, 1782
pacing, 492
stab-in (fish-hook), 2016, 2017
sutureless (screw-in), 2016
Electroencephalogram, syncope and, 509
Electrograms, 434–35
endocardial, pacemaker assessment and, 1759–60
filtered QRS complex vs., 1717
His bundle. *See* His recordings.
intraoperative, 2013–14
Electrograms:
telemetered, pacemakers and, 1758
ventricular fibrillation, 426
ventricular tachycardia, 424, 425
WPW syndrome, 418
Electrolytes, 1466–77. *See also* Calcium; Magnesium; Phosphorus; Potassium; Sodium.
ECG and, 222–25
Electromanometer, 138
Electromechanical dissociation:
CPR and, 551
myocardial infarction and, 982
Electrophysiology, 73–84. *See also* Electrocardiography.
action potential. *See* Action potential.
aging and, 1410
antiarrhythmic agents and, 1593–1602
assessment, 281–95
automaticity, 78–79
calcium channel blockers and, 1626–27
conduction, 79–80. *See also* Conduction system.
digitalis and, 1642–44
drug testing and, 1738–39
electrical injuries and, 1486–87
excitability, 75–78
genesis of electrocardiogram, 80–84
impulse formation, 407–9
invasive studies, 283, 1734–40
anticipated results, 1739
AV block and, 290
AV node, 1736–37
clinical uses, 526
complications, 1739
His bundle recording, 1727–32
intraoperative, 2013–14
intraventricular conduction defect and, 291
vs. long-term ECG, 286
sinus node, 289, 1734–36
tachycardia and, 294–95, 478
mapping and, 1738
syncope and, 287–88, 526
transmembrane potential, 73–75
triggered activity, 408–9, 413
Elema leads, 492, 493
Eliot, T. S., 1764
Elliot, J. W., 1364
Ellis-van Creveld syndrome:
genetics, 568
inspection and, 122, 131, 132
Embolectomy:
aortoiliac, 1336
pulmonary, 1112–13
Embolism:
air, 1115–16
coronary bypass surgery and, 2039
hyperbaric pressure and, 1552
amniotic fluid, 1116
aortic stenosis and, 1671
aortoiliac, 1336
arteriosclerosis obliterans vs., 1342
atrial fibrillation and, 1671–72
cardiomyopathy and, 1190, 1205, 1670
cardioversion and, 1745–46
cerebral, 1358–60
atherosclerosis and, 1355
causes, 1358–59
clinical manifestations, 1358
coronary bypass surgery and, 2039
Embolism: cerebral:
diagnosis, 1359–60
management, 1360
myxomatous, 1286–87, 1359
postoperative, 1361–62
syncope and, 514
contraceptive agents and, 1482
coronary artery, 1021
myxomatous, 1287
radiography and, 1803
sudden death and, 530, 534
endocarditis and, 1142, 1143, 1151
cerebrovascular disease and, 1359
fat, 1114–15
retinal, 201
mesenteric, 1364–66
mitral valve disease and, 1358, 1670–71
stenotic, 755, 761
myocardial infarction and, 983, 1673
paradoxical, 1109–10
cerebral, 1359
cyanosis and, 587
peripheral, 1349
peripheral arterial, 1348–50
myocardial infarction and, 983
prosthetic valves and, 779, 1359, 1671, 1676
pulmonary. *See* Pulmonary embolism.
retinal, 201
myxomatous, 1287
saddle, 1336
therapeutic production of, 1896–97
thrombolytic agents and, 1681
tumor, 1117, 1286–87, 1291, 1359
Embolization technique, pulmonary circulation and, 1896–97
Embryology, 3–15
aortic arch system, 3, 9, 13–15
arterial valves, 12–13
atria, 5, 11–12
atrioventricular canal, 8–9
atrioventricular valves, 12
conus cordis, 5, 9–10
heart loop formation, 3–5
pulmonary veins, 12
septation, 6–12
sinus venosus, 10–11
truncus arteriosus, 5, 9
vasculogenesis, 3
ventricles, 5–8
Emetine, toxicity of, 1231–32
Emotional stress, 1520–34. *See also* Anxiety; Psychological factors.
animal experiments, 1520–21
arrhythmias and, 1522–23
atherosclerosis and, 1523–24
coronary heart disease and, 826, 933–35, 1521–25, 1530–33
definition, 1520
epidemiology, 1521–22
hypertension and, 1525–26, 1533–34
job-related, 1571, 1572
myocardial infarction and, 985, 987
physiological concomitants of, 1520–21
psychophysiological response pattern, 1525
social hierarchies and, 1520–21
sudden death and, 1522–23
syncope and, 508, 509
type A behavior, 1524–25
bypass surgery and, 1531, 1532
Emphysema:
cor pulmonale and, 1123–24

Emphysema:
ECG and, 223
heart failure and, 237
mediastinal, 916
Employment. *See* Occupation; Work status.
Enalapril, 1072, 1587
heart failure and, 365
hypertension and, renovascular, 1079
pharmacology, 1590
side effects, 1073
Encephalopathy:
anoxic, 553
hypertensive, 1054–55, 1357–58
hypoxic, 1361
Reye's, 1239
Encrustation theory of atherosclerosis, 842
Endarterectomy:
aortoiliac, 2058, 2061
carotid, 1356–57, 2052–56
complications, 2055–56
indications, 2056
results, 2055
technique, 2052–55
coronary, 956–57
Endarteritis, 1135
End-diastolic dimension, echocardiography and, 1935–36, 1953
End-diastolic pressure:
afterload mismatch and, 267
aortic-mitral combined valvular disease and, 789–90
aortic regurgitation and, 742–43, 747, 748
aortic stenosis and, 731, 732, 735
catheterization studies and, 1775, 1776
end-diastolic volume vs., 44, 45
heart failure and, 321, 326, 335, 347
mitral regurgitation and, 773
pulmonary artery, myocardial infarction and, 979–80
stroke volume, and, 44, 45
vasodilators and, 363
End-diastolic volume:
afterload and, 47–48
aortic regurgitation, 742, 744, 748
aortic stenosis and, 734, 735
calculation of, 1783, 1784
contraction and, 42, 43
end-diastolic pressure vs., 44, 45
exercise in heart failure and, 335
force-velocity relations and, 47
heart failure and, 335, 347
mitral regurgitation and, 773–75
normal, 55
stroke volume and, 44, 45
Endocardial tube, 3–5
Endocarditis, 1130–53
abscess and, 1139
acute, 1130
antibiotics and, 1137, 1148–50
prophylactic, 1151–53
anticoagulants and, 1150
aortic valve, 1145
bicuspid valve and, 1163
drug-related, 1132
mitral valve disease and, 785, 786
prosthesis and, 1133
regurgitation and, 740, 749, 1138
burns and, 1134
catheterization and cineangiography, 1146
Endocarditis:
in children, 1134
chlamydial, 1136
clinical manifestations, 1140–43
summary of, 1141
clubbing of fingers and, 1142
complications, 1143–44, 1151
cultures and, blood, 1144–45
negative, 1136
definitions and terminology, 1130
dialysis and, 1135, 1460
differential diagnosis, 1144
drug abuse and, 1132
echocardiography and, 1145–46, 1960
electrocardiography and, 1145
embolism and, 1142, 1143, 1151
cerebrovascular disease and, 1359
endarteritis and, 1135
epidemiology, 1131–35
evolution of, 1131
experimental, 1140
eye lesions and, 1142
fungal, 1136
cure rate, 1147
drug-related, 1132
frequency, 1133
glomerulonephritis and, 1140, 1144, 1151
gram-negative, 1136
cure rate, 1147
frequency, 1133
postoperative, 1133
healed, 1140
heart failure and, 1143, 1151
historical note, 1130–31
history, 1140–41
immunity and, 1139–40
infecting organisms, 1135–37
frequency of, 1133
inspection and, 132
Janeway lesions and, 1142
laboratory tests, 1144
location of, 1138
Loeffler's, 1209
lupus erythematosus and, 1436–37
mitral valve, 1146
drug-related, 1132
prolapse and, 1131–32
prosthesis and, 1133–34
regurgitation and, 764–65, 1138
stenosis and, 754
murmurs and, 1142–43
mycotic aneurysm and, 1143–44, 1151
myocarditis and, 1161
natural history and prognosis, 1146–47
neurological manifestations, 1143, 1359
nosocomial, 1134–35
Osler's nodes and, 1142
pathogenesis and pathology, 1137–40
infective, 1137–40
noninfective, 1137
petechiae, and, 1141–42
physical examination, 1141–43
postsurgical, 1132–34, 1151–53
preexisting heart disease and, 1131–32
pregnancy and, 1134, 1386
prophylaxis, 1151–53
noncardiac surgery and, 1517
regimens for, 1153
prosthetic valve, 1133–34, 1136, 1150
abscess and, 1139
Endocarditis: prosthetic valve:
cure rate, 1147
Q fever, 1136
radionuclide studies, 1146
recurrent, 1147
rheumatic, 1131
mitral regurgitation and, 764
mitral stenosis and, 754
pathology, 1307
roentgenography and, 1146
splenomegaly and, 1142
splinter hemorrhages and, 1142
staphylococcal, 1135, 1136, 1163
cure rate, 1147
dialysis and, 1460
drug-related, 1132
frequency, 1133
postoperative, 1133, 1152
treatment, 1148–50
streptococcal, 1135–36
cure rate, 1147
frequency, 1133
postoperative, 1152
treatment, 1148–50
subacute, 1130
susceptible host, 1131–35
thrombotic, 1130, 1137
cerebral infarction and, 1359
treatment, 1147–53
antimicrobial, 1148–53
complications and, 1151
general principles, 1147–48
prophylactic, 1151–53
surgical, 1150–51
tricuspid valve, 253–54, 793–94, 797–99
drug-related, 1132
ventricular septal defect and, 595
verrucous, 1436–37
Endocardium:
amyloid deposits in, 1213, 1214
cushion defect, 8–9. *See also* Atrioventricular canal.
electrogram, pacemaker assessment and, 1759–60
embryology, 6, 8
fibroelastosis, 653–54, 1215–16
classification, 1215
clinical manifestations, 653–54, 1215–16
genetics, 571
medical management, 654
myocardial infarction and, 847, 849
natural history and prognosis, 654
pathology, 653, 1216
fibrous plaque, cardiomyopathy and, 1198
pacing leads and, 493
rheumatoid nodules of, 1439
Endocrine system, 1412–31. *See also* specific glands and disorders.
adrenal glands, 1423–24
estrogens, 1424–26
pancreas, 1426–31
parathyroid glands, 1422
pituitary gland, 1422–23
thyroid gland, 1412–22
Endolymph, 158
Endometrial carcinoma, estrogen therapy and, 1425
Endomyocardial biopsy, 1772–73
cardiomyopathy and, 1190, 1204
fibrosis and, 1209–10
myocarditis and, 1168
transplanted heart and, 2065

Endomyocardial fibrosis, 1208–13
  clinical manifestations, 1210–11
  differential diagnosis, 1212
  eosinophil and, 1208–9
  etiology, 1208
  laboratory studies, 1211–12
  left ventricular, 1211
  pathology, 1209–10
  pathophysiology, 1210
  right ventricular, 1211
  treatment, 1212–13
Endoperoxides, 814
Endophthalmitis, endocarditis and, 1142
Endorphins:
  corticosteroids and, 390
  shock and, 376
Endothelium:
  atherosclerosis and, 803, 804, 809–11
    response-to-injury hypothesis and, 804–6
  barrier role, 809–10
  cell cultures, 810–11
  double-indicator dilution technique and, 387
  endocarditis and, 1137
  growth factor derived from, 811
  platelets and, 809, 812
  prostaglandins and, 814
  thromboresistance of, 804–5, 809
Endotoxemia, 390
End-systolic dimension:
  aortic regurgitation and, 250, 747, 749
  echocardiography and, 1935–36, 1953
End-systolic pressure-volume relations:
  afterload mismatch and, 267
  aortic regurgitation and, 742–44, 748
  aortic stenosis and, 735
Endurance training, 1400
Energy:
  cardiomyopathy and, 568–69
  heart failure and, 329–30
Enflurane, 1496
Entrainment, atrial flutter and, 414–15
Environment, 1543–54
  cardiac output increase and, 403
  cold. *See* Cold exposure.
  electrical injuries, 1486–87
  genetics and, 566
  heat stress, 1547–50
  high-altitude. *See* Altitude (high).
  hyperbaric pressure, 1550–54
  pacemaker testing and, 1759
  poisons, 1488–89
  social, 1520–21
Enzymes, 86–87
  allosteric modification of, 87
  atherosclerosis and, 806–7
  covalent modification of, 87
  genetics and, 568–70, 572–73
  lysosomal, 95–96
    shock and, 380–81
  myocardial infarction and, 897–99
    histochemical techniques and, 877
    historical notes on, 886
    limitations of assays in, 898–99
    size of, 898
  Na-K pump and, 75
  pericarditis and, 909
  thrombectomy and, 1680, 1681
  trauma and, 1279
Eosinophilia, endomyocardial fibrosis and, 1208–13
Eosinophilic leukemia, 1209, 1212
Eosinophils, myocardial infarction and, 875
Ephedrine:
  diabetic neuropathy and, 1428
  vasoconstriction and, 1590
Epicardium, 24
  electrocardiography and, 82
  mapping of, Wolff-Parkinson-White syndrome and, 2013, 2014
  pacemaker attachment to, 493, 2016–20
  pericarditis and, 1253
Epilepsy, syncope vs., 519
Epinephrine. *See also* Catecholamines.
  asystole and, 551
  beta-blocking agents and, 1609
  beta receptors and, 1606
  cardiomyopathy and, 1184
  CPR and, 548, 552
  heart failure in infant and, 586
  pheochromocytoma and, 1046, 1065
  shock and, 376–77
    management of, 391
  structure of, 1653
  toxicity of, 1234
  ventricular fibrillation and, 550
Epistaxis, 121
  hemoptysis vs., 119
Epstein-Barr virus, 1174
Equalization shunt, 239
Equilibrium potential, 74
Equilibrium radionuclide studies. *See* Radionuclide studies, gated equilibrium.
Erb's dystrophy, 1228
Ergometry:
  arm, 1032, 1705
  bicycle. *See* Bicycle ergometry.
  guidelines for, 1032–33
Ergonovine, 1483
  coronary arteriography and, 309, 906
  coronary artery spasm and, 1013–14
    protocol for testing, 1014
  esophageal spasm and, 912
Ergotamine, 1483
Errors. *See also* Iatrogenic disorders.
  blood pressure measurement, 139–40
  in data interpretation, 1538–39
  ECG, 225–27, 1538
    prolonged recording and, 1723–26
  echocardiographic, 1965–66
  in history taking, 110–11
    chest pain and, 892–93
Erythema, tuft, 132
Erythema marginatum, 125
  rheumatic fever and, 1309
Erythrityl tetranitrate:
  chemical structure, 940
  dosage, 940
Erythrocytes, renal failure and, 1460
Erythrocytosis, cor pulmonale and, 1122
Erythromycin:
  digitalis and, 1647
  endocarditis and, 1153
  streptococcal pharyngitis and, 1312
Escape beats, 469–70
  definition, 433
  esophageal ECG and, 1698, 1700
  junctional, 435
Escherichia coli, endocarditis and, 1136
Esmolol, 1607
  pharmacodynamics, 1608, 1613
  pharmacokinetics, 1610, 1611
  structure, 1608
Esophagitis, reflux, 911–12
Esophagus:
  aortic arch compression of, 623, 624
  ECG. *See* Electrocardiography, esophageal.
  echocardiography from, 1951–52
  nutcracker, 912–13
  roentgenography and, 242, 243
  rupture of, 913
  spasm of, 912–13
  sphincter of, 911–12
Estrogens, 1424–26
  myocardial infarction and, 826, 829
  osteoporosis and, 1426
  therapy with, 1424–26
    complications, 1424–25
    recommendations regarding, 1425–26
Ethacrynic acid:
  biochemistry, 1658
  dosage, 1072, 1659
  duration of action, 1659
  heart failure and, 361, 362
    in infant, 585
  pharmacokinetics, 1661
  protein-binding and dialysance, 1082
  site of action, 1660
Ethambutol, tuberculous pericarditis and, 1270
Ethinyl estradiol, 1424
Ethyl alcohol. *See* Alcohol.
Etomidate, 1496
Eustachian valve, 19
Examination, physical. *See* Physical examination.
Excitability, 75–78
  electrocardiogram and, 80–81
Excitation-contraction coupling, 37–39, 1476
  calcium channel blockers and, 1626
Exercise. *See also* Exercise testing.
  aging and, 1407–9
  altitude and, 1544
  anaerobic metabolism and, 51
  aortic stenosis and, 638, 735
  arm vs. leg, 1027
  arrhythmias and, 1711
  arteriosclerosis obliterans and, 1344
  atherosclerosis management and, 933
  blood flow and, 56, 1398
  blood pressure and, 55, 1399
  cardiac output and, 55, 335, 1398–99
    aging and, 1407–8
  cardiomyopathy and, 1192
  complications, 1711–12
  congenital heart disease and, 589–90
  coronary artery spasm and, 1011–12
  coronary bypass surgery and, 949–50, 1028–29
  coronary heart disease and, 1713
    guidelines for, 1032–33
    management and, 933
    prevention and, 825, 829–30
    rehabilitation and, 1026–28, 1031–34
  drug effects on, 1027–28
  dynamic (isotonic), 1027
  echocardiography and, 1950–51
  ejection fraction and, 901, 902, 1825
  expectations of, 1028
  heart failure and, 270, 335, 1034–35
  heart rate and, 55, 1027, 1398–99
    aging and, 1408
  heat and, 1399, 1549–50
  hypotension and, 1711

Exercise:
individualized (prescriptive), 1027
isometric and isotonic, 1027
maintenance, 1034
myocardial infarction and, 829–30, 1028–29, 1713
seven-step program, 1030
oxygen uptake and, 1398, 1400
pregnancy and, 1384–85
premature ventricular beats and, 285, 286, 1708, 1711
pulmonary obstructive disease and, 1828–29
pulmonary vascular pressure and, 1092
responses to:
disproportionate, 1029
physiologic, 55–56, 1398–1400
stroke volume and, 55, 335, 1398, 1399
sympathetic nervous system and, 55, 1399
temperature (body) and, 1399
testing. *See* Exercise testing.
tetralogy of Fallot and, 663
training, 1026–28, 1031–34, 1713
vasoconstriction and, 1399
ventricular performance and, 1824–26, 1828, 1842–43
wall motion and, 1825
Exercise testing, 306–8, 1704–14. *See also* Exercise.
angina pectoris and, 896, 1707, 1708, 1714
angiography, 901–2
anticipated results of, 1708–11
aortic-mitral combined valvular disease and, 789
aortic regurgitation and, 748
asymptomatic individuals and, 1713–14
athletes and, 1402
blood pressure and, 1708
catheterization studies and, 1776
coronary arteriography vs., 1709
coronary bypass surgery and, 949–50
coronary heart disease and, 896, 1026, 1704, 1709–14, 1825
prognosis and, 310–11, 921, 926, 1710, 1712
radionuclide studies, 899–902, 1832, 1834–38, 1842–43
treatment and, 959–60
uncomplicated infarction and, 969–70
dyspnea and, 1708
ECG and, 1706–10. *See also* Electrocardiography, exercise.
falsely negative, 1709
fatigue and, 1708
heart failure and, 270, 335, 1034–35
likelihood of disease and, 307–8
vs. long-term recording, 1723
lower extremity, 1704–5
mitral stenosis and, 760
modes of, 1704–5
monitoring, 1706–8
myocardial ischemia and, 306–8, 921, 1709–14
myocardial perfusion, 1832, 1834–38, 1842–43
myocarditis and, 1168
noncardiac surgery and, 1512, 1513
oxygen requirements and, 1706
predictive value, 305, 306
predischarge, 1026
Exercise testing:
premature ventricular beats and, 1708, 1711
preparation for, 1706
prognosis and, 310–11, 921, 926, 1710, 1712
protocols for, 1705–6
radionuclide, 306–7, 1824–26, 1828. *See also* Radionuclide studies, exercise.
coronary heart disease and, 899–902, 1832, 1834–38, 1842–43
thallium, 306, 899–900, 970, 1832, 1834–38, 1842–43
rationale for, 306
resuscitation and, 1711–12
routine, 300
serial surveillance, 1026
severity of disease and, 310
ST segment changes and, 306, 1708–10
submaximal, 1708
symptom-limited, 1705, 1706–8
syncope and, 525
treadmill, 1704–6
upper extremity, 1705
ventriculographic, 306
ventricular dysfunction and, 1710–11
Exhaustion, myocardial ischemia and, 961
Exons, 566
Exophthalmos, 1413
Expert testimony, 1565–67
Extracorporeal circulation. *See* Cardiopulmonary bypass
Extrasystoles:
atrial, 437–38. *See also* Premature atrial beats.
AV junctional, 438–39
definition, 433
parasystole. *See* Parasystole.
supraventricular tachycardia and, 440, 441
ventricular, 450–52. *See also* Premature ventricular beats.
Extremities:
arteriospasm and, 1352–53
diabetic neuropathy and, 1428
ECG leads and, 207, 226
exercise for, 1027, 1032
exercise testing and, 1704–5
inspection of, 131–34
ischemia of:
acute occlusion and, 1349
arteriosclerosis obliterans and, 1339–46
thromboangiitis obliterans and, 1347
phlebography of, 1885–86
physical examination of, 205
thrombosis in, 1105–6
Eye:
edema of, 118
endocarditis and, 1142
heart failure and, 352
inspection of, 130
retinal examination. *See* Retina.

f waves, 446–47
F waves, 443–45
cardiac cycle and, 52
Fab fragments, digitalis toxicity and, 1648
Fabry's disease, 125–26, 572, 1222
Face, inspection of, 126–30
Fainting. *See* Syncope.
Fallot:
pentalogy (pentad) of, 662, 663
tetralogy of. *See* Tetralogy of Fallot.
trilogy of, 655
Family, 111
coronary bypass surgery and, 951
rehabilitation and, 1029–31
Fascicular beats, 452
Fasciculoventricular fibers, 415, 416
Fascioscapulohumeral dystrophy, 1228
Fast-response fibers, 75, 407–8
Fat(s). *See also* Cholesterol; Hyperlipidemia; Lipoprotein; Triglycerides.
embolism, 1114–15
retinal, 201
saturated vs. unsaturated, 820
epicardial, fluoroscopy and, 1767
Fatigue, 119
diabetes mellitus and, 1429
exercise testing, and, 1708
heart failure and, 119
myocardial ischemia and, 961
Fatty acids, 91–94
free, 91
glucose and, 93–94
transport, 89
utilization, 90
integrated control of, 92–94
metabolism, 91–94
oxidative pathway, 93, 94
prostaglandins and, 814
radionuclide studies and, 1850
uptake and activation, 91
Fatty streak, 801, 841
aortic, 1321
experimentally induced, 804
fibrous plaque and, 802
Federal Aviation Administration, 1578–79
Federal Motor Carrier Safety Regulations, 1578
Feedback mechanism, coronary blood flow and, 858
Femoral arteriovenous fistula, 401
Femoral artery:
aneurysm, 1326, 1351
angiography, 2058
angioplasty, 1346, 1909
aortic shunt with, external, 2047
cardiac catheterization and, 1771
coronary arteriography and, 1791
embolism, 1349
grafts:
aortofemoral bypass, 2059–60
extraanatomic, 2061
femoropopliteal bypass, 2060–61
IABP insertion and, 2022
occlusive disease, 1345–46
Femoral vein:
cardiac catheterization and, 1769–70
Doppler studies and, 1976
His bundle catheterization and, 1727
ligation of, 1111
Femoropopliteal bypass graft, 2060–61
Femoropopliteal occlusive disease, surgical treatment of, 2060–61
Fenofibrate, 823
Fenoximone, 1655
Fentanyl, 1496
Ferritin, hemochromatosis and, 1222
Fetal circulation, 582–84
anticoagulants and, 1114
persistent, 584

Fetal circulation:
pulmonary, 1093
Fetus, 1383. *See also* Pregnancy.
alcohol syndrome in, 135
cardiomyopathy in, diabetic, 1429–30
Fever, 121
endocarditis and, 1140, 1144
myocarditis and, 1165
Fibers:
contractile, 32
fast-response, 75, 407–8
length of, 43–46
echocardiography and, 1935–36, 1963
end-diastolic. *See* Preload.
force-velocity relations and, 45–46
fractional shortening, 270, 271
overload and, 332
presystolic, 43
stroke volume and, 44
tension and, 44–45, 332
wall force and, 327, 329
Mahaim. *See* Mahaim fibers.
sliding filament hypothesis and, 33–34
slow-response, 75, 407, 408
Fibrillation:
atrial. *See* Atrial fibrillation.
ventricular. *See* Ventricular fibrillation.
Fibrin:
amniotic fluid embolism and, 1116
endocarditis and, 1137, 1138
heparin and, 1667
pericarditis and, 1251
streptokinase and, 1679, 1682
warfarin and, 1669
Fibrinogen:
amniotic fluid embolism and, 1116
radioactive, venous thrombosis and, 1374–75
thrombolytic therapy and, 1679, 1917
uptake test, 1887
Fibrinolytic agents. *See also* Thrombolytic agents.
myocardial infarction and, 943
pulmonary embolism and, 1113–14, 1681, 1916–17
Fibroblasts, atherosclerosis and, 803
Fibroelastoma, papillary, 1294
Fibroelastosis, endocardial. *See* Endocardium, fibroelastosis.
Fibroma, 1293–94
papillary, 1294
Fibromuscular dysplasia:
carotid artery, 1358
renal artery, 1058, 1079
sudden death and, 532–33
Fibromusculoelastic lesion, 802, 810
Fibrosis:
aortic valve, 729–30, 740
bundle branch, 427
cardiomyopathy and, 1199
coronary artery, 1023
endomyocardial. *See* Endomyocardial fibrosis.
mitral valve, 764, 766
cardiomyopathy and, 1199
myocardial, scleroderma and, 1442
radiation-induced, 1485, 1486
tricuspid valve, 792, 793
vein wall, 1377
Fibrous body, central, 17
echocardiography and, 1941
Fibrous plaque, 841
aortic, 1321
Fibrous plaque:
endocardial, cardiomyopathy and, 1198
rupture of, 870–71
stages in development of, 803
Fibrous skeleton of heart, 17–18
Fick method, 1779–80
cardiac output and, 1779
shunt calculations and, 1779–80
Filariasis, 1176
Filling pressure. *See* Ventricular pressure, filling.
Filling wave, precordial, 153
Fingers:
clubbed, 131–32
endocarditis and, 1142
contractures of, 123
cyanotic, 132
gangrenous, arteritis and, 123
inspection of, 132–33
polydactyly, 131, 132
red (tuft erythema), 132
tactile perception of, 152–53
ulcers of, thromboangiitis obliterans and, 1347
ulnar deviation of, 133, 134
First-pass radionuclide angiocardiography. *See* Radionuclide studies, first-pass technique.
Fistula:
aortocaval, 1380
arteriovenous. *See* Arteriovenous fistula.
coronary artery, 1019
sinus of Valsalva, 620–21
Flotation catheters. *See* Swan-Ganz catheterization.
Flow. *See also* Blood flow; Coronary blood flow; Pulmonary vasculature, blood flow.
pressure-resistance relations and, 58
Fluids:
extracellular, 1040–41
hydrodynamics and, 1038
hypertension and, 1040–41, 1045
pericardial, 1250. *See also* Pericardial effusion; Tamponade.
replacement therapy, 388
resistance to flow of, 57
retention of. *See* Edema.
surgery and, 1505
third space, 1505
Fluoride excess, 1235
Fluorocarbons, 1235
Fluorodeoxyglucose, 1850
9α-Fluoroprednisolone, hypertension and, 1062, 1063
Fluoroscopy, 1764–68
anticipated results, 1764–65
aortic valve, 248, 249
calcifications and, 1765–67
cardiac vs. noncardiac disease and, 1767
cineangiography and, 1786
complications, 1765
coronary heart disease and, 894
dynamics and, 1765
fat stripes and, subepicardial, 1767
pacemakers and, 1768
prosthetic valves and, 1767
technique, 1764
5-Fluorouracil, 1482
Flurazepam, coronary heart disease and, 938
Flushing, 120, 124
Flutter:
atrial. *See* Atrial flutter.
ventricular, 455
Flying status, 1578–79
Foam cells, atherosclerosis and, 813
Focal block, 216–17
Fontan operation, 676
univentricular heart and, 706
Foot:
hygienic care of, 1344
ulcers, arteriosclerosis obliterans and, 1341, 1344–45
Foramen ovale, 12
aortic atresia and, 645
closure of, 583
Ebstein's anomaly and, 678
fetal circulation and, 582–83
paradoxical embolism and, 1109
pulmonic stenosis and, 655
Force-frequency relation, 46
Force-velocity relations, 40–42
fiber length and, 45–46
Force-velocity-length relations, 46, 47
Force-velocity-volume relations, 47
Formazan, myocardial infarction and, 877–78
49 XXXXY syndrome, 135
Fossa ovalis, 12
anatomy, 19
atrial septal defect and, 598
myxoma and, 1292
Fractional shortening, 270, 271
echocardiography and, 1935–36, 1963
Frank-Starling law, 42–46
aging and, 1405, 1408
digitalis and, 359
diuretics and, 361, 362
heart failure and, 326–27, 346–47, 360
preload and, 1584
Frank-Straub-Wiggers-Starling principle, 42–46
Frequency, sound wave, 157, 158, 161
Friction rubs:
Dressler's syndrome and, 1267
myocardial infarction and, 1267
pericarditis and, 1251–52
Friedreich's ataxia, 126, 1229
genetics, 569
Fructose-1,6-diphosphate, 89
FTA-ABS, 1319
Fucosidosis, 1225
Functional classification, 106
angina pectoris, 108
Fungal infections:
endocarditis, 1136
cure rate, 1147
drug-related, 1132
frequency, 1133
myocarditis, 1161, 1175
Furosemide. *See also* Diuretics.
biochemistry, 1658
dosage, 1072, 1659
duration of action, 1659
edema and, 1663–64
heart failure and, 361, 362, 1644
in infant, 585
hypertension and, 1077, 1664
gestational, 1084
renoparenchymal, 1080
oliguria and, 1665
pharmacokinetics, 1661
protein-binding and dialysance, 1082
pulmonary edema and, 1662

Furosemide:
renal failure and, 1662
site of action, 1660
toxin excretion and, 1665
Fusion beats:
aberrant conduction and, 460
accelerated idioventricular rhythm and, 456
AV dissociation and, 467
esophageal ECG and, 1696, 1697
pacemakers and, 494
parasystole and, 456, 457
ventricular tachycardia and, 454
Future of cardiology, 2081–82

Gadolinium, MRI and, 1893–94
Gait, 126
Galactosidase deficiency, 1223–24
Gallamine, 1497
Gallbladder disease, 913–14
Galleti, P. M., 2025
Gallop, 176–82
aortic stenosis and, 179
atrial, 177–79
heart failure and, 351
myocardial infarction and, 178
timing, 181
block and, 179
cardiomyopathy and, 1188
classification, 182
combination, 181
detection technique, 176
hypertension and, 178–79
mitral regurgitation and, 770
postextrasystolic accentuation of, 180
protodiastolic, mesodiastolic, and presystolic, 182
summation, 182
systolic, 176
ventricular, 52, 179–81
heart failure and, 180, 351
myocardial infarction and, 180
prognosis, 180
pulsus alternans and, 180
timing, 181
Ganglionectomy, occlusive arterial disease and, 2061
Ganglionic blocking agents, 1588
Gangliosidoses, 1223–24
Gangrene:
acute arterial occlusion and, 1350
arteriosclerosis obliterans and, 1341, 1344–45
gas, myocarditis and, 1163, 1164
intestinal, postoperative, 1371
polyarteritis and, 123
thromboangiitis obliterans and, 1348
Gargoylism, 1224
Gastroesophageal junction, 911
Gastrointestinal tract. *See also* Intestine.
amyloidosis, 1371
angioma, congenital, 1370
carcinoid disease, 1298
chest pain and, 911–15
heart failure and, 350
periarteritis nodosa and, 1370
shock and, 378
vascular disease, 1364–71
Gated equilibrium radionuclide studies. *See* Radionuclide studies, gated equilibrium technique.
Gaucher's disease, 573, 1224
Gay, John, 1372
Gemfibrozil, 823
Genetics, 566–77
aortic stenosis and, 638, 641
arrhythmias and, 576–77
arterial wall and, 573–74
atherosclerosis and, 573–74
atrial septal defect and, 568, 599–600, 602
AV canal and, 610
cardiomyopathies and, 568–72, 1181, 1183, 1193
chromosomal aberrations, 566–67. *See also* Chromosomes.
congenital heart disease and, 566–68, 582
connective tissue disorders and, 573
coronary heart disease and, 824
diabetes mellitus and, 575
dominant inheritance, 568
environment and, 566
hyperlipidemia and, 574–75
hypertension and, 575–76
pulmonary, 576
mucolipidoses and, 572
mucopolysaccharidoses and, 572
muscular dystrophy and, 571–72
myocardial function and, 86
recessive inheritance, 567–68
systemic diseases and, 572–73
ventricular septal defect and, 592, 596
Genin, 1639, 1640
Gentamicin:
endocarditis and, 1149
rheumatic fever prophylaxis and, 761
Giant cell arteritis, 201, 1323
Gifford, R. W., Jr., 1071
Gilbert, W. S., 1885
Gitalin. *See* Digitalis.
Globus hystericus, 907
Glomerular filtration rate, heart failure and, 325
Glomerulonephritis:
cardiac output increase and, 404
endocarditis and, 1140, 1144, 1151
hypertension and, 1045, 1059–60
Glossopharyngeal neuralgia, 516–17
Glucocorticoids. *See also* Corticosteroids.
aldosteronism and, 1063, 1064
atherosclerosis and, 1524
Glucose, 87–91
atherosclerosis and, 825, 829
fatty acids and, 89, 90, 93–94
hypertension and, 1075
integrated control of, 90–91
intolerance to, 85–86, 1426. *See also* Diabetes mellitus.
anesthesia and, 1431
perioperative, 1505
myocardial infarction and, 1430
phosphorylation, 89–90
positron-emission tomography and, 1850
shock and, 378, 379
transport, 87–89
Glucose-6-phosphate, 89
shock and, 379
Glucose-6-phosphate dehydrogenase:
genetics and, 573–74
monoclonal theory and, 806
Glutamic acid, shock and, 379
Glutamic oxaloacetic transaminase:
myocardial infarction and, 897
pericarditis and, 909
Glutathione, shock and, 378
Glyceraldehyde-3-phosphate dehydrogenase, 89
Glycerol trinitrate:
chemical structure, 940
dosage, 940
Glycogen:
integrated control of, 90–91
metabolism, 89
myocardial, 89
nodular infiltration of, 1220
storage disease (glycogenosis), 570, 1219–20
Glycogen phosphorylase, 87, 88
Glycogen synthase, 88, 89
Glycolysis, 87–91
integrated control of, 90–91
Glycoproteinoses, 572–73
Glycosides, 1639–49. *See also* Digitalis.
plants simulating effects of, 1488
Glycosphingolipid disorder, 1223
Glycyrrhizinic acid, hypertension and, 1062
Goiter, 1418–19
Gold-195m first pass studies, 1814
Goldman's constant field equation, 74
Gonadal dysgenesis, 567
Gorlin formula, 1784
Gout, 134, 1225–26
Grafts:
abdominal angina and, 1334–35
aortic, regurgitation repair and, 750
aortic aneurysm repair, 1326, 1328, 2043–48
aortic arch occlusive disease and, 1334
aortofemoral, 2059–60
aortoiliac, 1335–36, 1345
coarctation of aorta repair, 2051
coronary bypass. *See* Coronary bypass surgery.
femoropopliteal, 1345–46
IABP and, 2022, 2024
internal mammary artery, 853–54, 954, 2037
pulmonary artery, stenosis and, 1899, 1900
radial artery, 2037
renal artery, 1335
saphenous vein. *See* Saphenous vein grafts.
Graham Steell murmur, 193
Gram-negative endocarditis, 1136
cure rate, 1147
frequency, 1133
postoperative, 1133
Granuloma, sarcoid, 1216–18
Granulomatosis, Wegener's, 1239
coronary arteries and, 1023
Graves' disease, 1413, 1416
Groenblad-Strandberg syndrome, 1238
Group beating, 466
Growth factor:
endothelial-derived, 811
platelet-derived, 806, 812, 813–14
Growth hormone, acromegaly and, 1422–23
Growth retardation, congenital heart disease and, 589
Guanabenz:
dosage, 1072, 1587
side effects, 1073
Guanadrel:
dosage, 1072
pharmacology, 1588–89
side effects, 1073
Guanethidine:
dosage, 1072, 1587
hypersensitivity to, 1237

Guanethidine:
  pharmacology, 1588–89
  protein-binding and dialysance, 1082
  side effects, 1073
Guanosine triphosphate (GTP), protein synthesis and, 95
Gumma, myocardial, 1318
Gunshot wounds, 1022, 1277, 1278
Guy, W. A., 1577

h wave:
  cardiac cycle and, 52
  venous pulse, 148
H zone, 32, 33
Hall Medtronic prosthesis, 2034, 2069
Halo sheathing, retinal vascular, 199
Halothane, 1495, 1496
  contractility and, 50
Hamman's disease, 916
Hamman's sign, 913
Hand:
  inspection of, 131–33
  occupational trauma to, 1578
  venous pressure estimation and, 147
Handgrip, isometric:
  auscultation and, 195
  ventricular function and, 1826
Hand-Schüller-Christian disease, 1225
Harvey, William, 152, 856, 1120, 1249
Headache, 115
  hypertensive encephalopathy and, 1357–58
  migraine, syncopal, 519
Health insurance, 1561–62
Hearing, physiology of, 158
Heart attack, 924. *See also* Myocardial infarction; Myocardial ischemia.
  patient complaint of, 122
Heart block, 461–66. *See also* Atrioventricular block; Bundle branch block; Sinoatrial block; Wenckebach phenomenon.
  focal, 216–17
  gallop and, 179
Heartburn, 121, 911
Heart failure, 265–78, 319–67
  activity and, 1034–35
  afterload and, 266–67, 327, 331–32, 348
    reduction measures, 363–65
  aging and, 1409–10
  alcoholism and, 1446–47
  aldosterone and, 324, 325
  anemia and, 399
  angiotensin and, 324, 325, 335, 347
  anticoagulants and, 1672
  antidiuretic hormone and, 325
  aortic regurgitation and, 274–75, 748, 749
  aortic stenosis and, 273–74, 733
  arrhythmias and, 358
  arteriovenous fistula and, systemic, 401
  assessment, 265–78, 349–51
    selection of procedures, 268–72
    specific problems and, 172–78
  atrial compliance and, 333
  atrial failure and, 322, 333
  atrial fibrillation and, 333, 358
  backward, 321–22
  basic mechanisms of, 329–31
  beriberi and, 398–99
  beta-blocker-induced, 1618
  biopsy and, myocardial, 272
  cachexia and, 351

Heart failure:
  calcium sequestration rate and, 330–31
  cardiac output and, 335
    enhancement measures, 358–60
  cardiomyopathy and, 1191
    dilated, 1187, 1190
    hypertrophic, 1204–5, 1207–8
    ischemic, 277–78, 930–31
    senile, 331
  catheterization studies, 270, 272, 276–77, 355–56
  coarctation of aorta and, 630, 631
  compensatory mechanisms, 323–28, 346–48
    afterload and, 331–32
    definition, 322, 346
    preload and, 332
    symptoms and, 347–48
    tabulation of, 323
  congenital heart disease and, 584–86
  congestive, 319–20, 346
    compensated, 322, 346
    definition, 319–20
    high-output state and, 396
    pulmonary function and, 337–38
  contractility and, 266, 328, 330–31, 334
    indexes of, 270–72
    measures to increase, 358–60
  contralateral ventricle changes and, 334
  coronary bypass surgery and, 950, 951
  coronary heart disease and, 930–31
  cyanosis and, 351
  definition, 319–22, 345–46
  diabetes mellitus and, 1430–31
  diastolic, 320
  doxorubicin-induced, 1826–28
  echocardiography and, 355
  edema and, 118, 350, 352
    mechanisms of, 324–25
    pulmonary, 337–38, 349–50, 353
  emphysema and, 237
  end-diastolic pressure and, 321, 326, 335, 347
  endocardial fibroelastosis and, 653
  endocarditis and, 1143, 1151
  exercise, 270, 335, 1034–35
  eyes and, 352
  fatigue and, 119
  filling impairment, 267–68
  filling pressure and, 265
  forward, 321, 322
  Frank-Starling law and, 326–27, 346–47, 360
  gallop and, 180, 351
  gastrointestinal symptoms and, 350
  hemodynamics, 333–36
  history, 349–51
  hyperthyroidism and, 1415–16
  hypertrophy and, 327–28
  incidence, 562
  intractable, 346, 367
  kidney and, 324–26, 1460, 1462–63
  laboratory studies, 355–56
  Laplace law and, 328–29
  latent, 322
  left-sided, 322
    roentgenography and, 236, 240
  management, 356–67
    afterload decrease and, 363–65
    amrinone in, 1656
    angiotensin-converting enzyme inhibition and, 365

Heart failure: management:
    calcium channel blockers in, 1632–33
    cardiac output increase and, 358–60, 363–65
    components of, 357, 366–67
    contractility increase and, 358–60
    digitalis in, 358–59, 1644–45
    diuretics in, 361–62, 1661–62
    etiological, 357
    heart rate control, 358
    intractable failure and, 367
    mild failure and, 366
    moderately severe failure and, 366
    physiological basis of, 336–37
    preload decrease and, 360–63
    prophylactic, 356–57
    pulmonary edema and, acute, 366–67
    severe chronic failure and, 366
    sodium restriction in, 360–61
    surgical, 365–66
    tabulation of agents used in, 336
    vasodilators in, 337, 362–65
    venous pooling and, 362–63, 364
    workload decrease, 357–58
  mechanical factors, 266–68, 272–73, 320
  mitochondria and, 330
  mitral regurgitation and, 275, 334, 770, 776
  mitral stenosis and, 760
  myocardial failure and. *See* Myocardium, failure.
  myocardial infarction and, 930, 931
    as early complication, 978–80
    as late complication, 986
  myocarditis and, 1165, 1168, 1178
  neck veins and, 351
  nervous system and, 323–24
  obesity and, 1453–55
  overall, 265, 269–70
  oxygen consumption and, 329–30
  oxygen delivery and, 328
  patent ductus arteriosus and, 615, 617
  pathophysiology, 319–39, 346–48
  peripheral circulation and, 335–36
  physical examination, 204, 351–52
  postoperative, 275–76
  preload and, 44, 273, 326, 327, 332
    reduction measures, 360–63
  prognosis, 356
  prostaglandins and, 326
  protein and, 330
  pulmonary edema and, 337–38, 349–50, 353
  pulmonary embolism and, 1107, 1112
  pulmonary hypertension and, 240, 1097
  pulmonary valve absence and, 667
  pulmonary vasculature and, 239–40, 334
  pulsus alternans and, 334, 351
  radionuclide studies, 355, 1823
  refractory, absolute, 367
  renin and, 324, 325, 347
  respiration and, 337, 349–50
  right-sided, 322
    cor pulmonale and, 1122–23, 1125, 1127
    roentgenography and, 237, 240
    secondary, 334–35
  roentgenography and, 236, 237, 239–40, 352–55
  sarcolemma ATPase and, 330

Heart failure:
sarcomere overstretch and, 330
sarcoplasmic reticulum and, 330–31
senility (presbycardia) and, 331
sodium and, retention of, 324–25
management, 360–61
sounds and, 167
stroke volume and, 326, 335
substrate utilization and, 330
surgical procedures and, noncardiac, 1517
systolic, 320–21
tricuspid regurgitation and, 334, 335, 793
vasoconstriction and, 324, 335–36, 347
ventricular aneurysm and, 278
ventricular septal defect and, 594
weakness and, 350
Heart loop, 3–5
Heart rate:
anesthesia and, 50
cardiac output and, 51
increased, 395
carotid sinus reflex and, 515
contractility and, 46
exercise and, 55, 1027, 1398–99
aging and, 1408
coronary heart disease and, 921
heart failure and, 358
hypertension and, 1042
Karvonen method of calculating, 1027
muscle mechanics and, 48
normal, 435, 437
oxygen consumption and, 864
shock and, 371
training effect and, 1400
Heart tube, 3–5
Heat, 1237
cardiac output increase and, 403
circulatory adjustments to, 1547–50
exercise and, 1399, 1549–50
rest and, 1547–49
Heat exchanger, cardiopulmonary bypass, 2027
Heatstroke, 1237
Heberden, William, 882, 883–84
Heimes drive system, 2072
Heimlich maneuver, 915
Helminthic myocarditis, 1176
Hemangioma, 1294
skin, 125
Hemangiomatosis, hepatic, 401
Hemangiosarcoma, 1294
Hematocrit:
artificial heart and, 2073, 2074
dialysis and, 1462
Hematologic diseases, 1226–27. *See also* Anemia; Leukemia.
Hematoma, dissecting, of aorta, 1328–29
Hematuria, endocarditis and, 1144
Hemiazygos vein:
inferior vena cava continuity with, 686
persistent left superior vena cava and, 685
Hemiblock, 213–15, 218
left anterior, 213–14
left posterior, 214–15
Hemingway, Ernest, 1593
Hemitruncus, 619–20
Hemochromatosis, 124, 1221–22
clinical manifestations, 1222
genetics, 570
pathology, 1221–22
Hemochromatosis:
pathophysiology, 1222
treatment, 1222
Hemodialysis. *See also* Dialysis.
cardiac output increase and, 401
endocarditis and, 1135
pericarditis and, 1266–67
Hemodilution, cardiopulmonary bypass and, 2027
Hemodynamics, 54–55
anesthesia and, 1505–7
artificial heart, 2070–73
cardiomyopathy, dilated, 1187
CPR and, 547–49
Doppler methods and. *See* Doppler studies.
exercise, 1398–1400
heart failure, 333–36
hypertension, 1038–40, 1042–46
monitoring of, 1998–2003. *See also* Monitoring.
indications, 2001
myocardial infarction and, 978–80
normal values, 55
pregnancy and, 1383–86
prognosis and, 311
shock, 370–78
Hemodynamic vise, 682
Hemoglobin:
anemia and, 399, 400
carbon monoxide poisoning and, 1554
cyanosis and, 120
dissociation curve, altitude and, 1543, 1545
oxygen affinity of, 379
Hemoperfusion, digitalis toxicity and, 1649
Hemopericardium, 1280
Hemoptysis, 118–19
aortic aneurysm and, 119
Eisenmenger syndrome and, 119
mitral stenosis and, 119, 756
pulmonary infarction and, 119
Hemorrhage:
cerebral, 1054, 1357
heparin-induced, 1668
myocardial infarction and, 873
peptic ulcer, 914
pulmonary, embolism and, 1106
retinal, 200
splinter, endocarditis and, 1142
thrombolytic therapy inducing, 1919–20
traumatic, 1277
warfarin-induced, 1674
Hemorrhagic fever, 1175
Hemorrhagic telangiectasia, hereditary, 1227
gastrointestinal tract and, 1370
Henle's loop, diuretics and, 1660
Henoch-Schönlein purpura, 1227
Heparin, 1667–69. *See also* Anticoagulants.
adverse reactions, 1668–69
cardiopulmonary bypass and, 2026
cerebral embolism and, 1360
coronary heart disease and, 943
deep venous thrombosis and, 1105, 1110, 1375
dosage, 1110, 1111, 1667–68
endocarditis and, 1150
fat embolism and, 1115
indications, 1669
mechanism of action, 1667
Heparin:
myocardial infarction and, 983
myocarditis and, 1178
peripheral arterial occlusion and, 1350
pregnancy and, 1114, 1394
pulmonary embolism and, 1110–11
thrombocytopenia induced by, 1111
thrombolytic agents and, 1113, 1917, 1919
Hepatic vein occlusion, 1366–67, 1379–80
Hepatitis:
cardiac output increase and, 402
coronary bypass surgery and, 954
Hepatojugular reflux, 147–48
heart failure and, 351
Hepatomegaly, misinterpreting, 1538
Heredity. *See* Genetics.
Heredopathia atactica polyneuritiformis, 1225
Hernia, hiatal, 911
Herpes zoster, 918
Herrick, James, 882
on coronary thrombosis, 885
Heterotoxia, 689
Hexokinase, 89
Hiatal hernia, 911
Hiccups, 121
High-output states. *See* Cardiac output, increased.
Hill's model of muscle, 40
Hill's sign, 747
Hippocrates, 1398, 1452, 2008
His bundle:
ablation of, catheter, 1732
anatomy, 30–31
AV node junction with. *See* Atrioventricular junction.
blood supply, 427
branches. *See* Bundle branches.
calcium channel blockers and, 1627
fibrous skeleton and, 18
recordings, 1727–32
filtered QRS complex vs., 1717
impulse conduction and, 1730–32
impulse formation and, 1730
indications, 1730–32
myotonia atrophica and, 1230
nomenclature, 1729–30
noninvasive, 1732
techniques, 1727–29
therapeutic utility, 1732
validation, 1729
surgical division of, 2015
His-Purkinje system. *See also* Purkinje fibers.
aberrant conduction and, 412
block, 427, 480
approach to patient, with, 290
conduction time, 291, 488, 1729, 1730, 1736–37
Histamine, coronary artery spasm and, 1010
Histocompatibility leukocyte antigen, diabetes and, 575
Histoplasmosis, pericardial, 1270
History, 109–22
bronchitis and pulmonary infection, 120
cerebral symptoms, 120
chief complaint, 110
cough, 117
cyanosis, 120
dysphagia, 121
dyspnea, 115–17

History:
edema, 118
elicitation of, 109–10
epistaxis, 121
errors in, 110–11
fatigue and weakness, 119
fever and chills, 121
heart attack statement by patient, 122
hemoptysis, 118–19
hiccups, 121
hoarseness, 120–21
indigestion, 121
insomnia, 120
interpretation, 111, 112
jaundice, 121
legal issues, and, 1574–75
movement, abnormalities, 122
nausea and vomiting, 121
noises heard by patient, 121
pain, 112–15
palpitation, 117
past, 112
present illness, 110
purpose, 109
questionnaires and, 110–11
skin color, 120
squatting, 120
symptom value, 111–12
syncope, 117–18
urinary symptoms, 121
weight loss, 121
worrisome events, 118
HMG-CoA reductase, 574
Hoarseness, 120–21
mitral stenosis and, 756
Hodkin-Huxley theory, 77
Hodkin-Katz equation, 74
Holiday heart syndrome, 1447
Holism, 105
Hollenhorst plaques, 201, 202
Holmes heart, 703
Holosystolic murmurs, 191–92
Holter monitoring. *See* Electrocardiography, prolonged.
Holt-Oram syndrome, 132
genetics, 568
roentgenography and, 236
Homan's sign, 1374
Homocystinuria:
arteriosclerosis obliterans vs., 1343
inspection and, 122, 126, 132
platelets and, 812
Homogentisic oxidase deficiency, 1226
Honk, precordial, 185
Hope, James, 764
Hormones, 1412–31. *See also* specific hormone; gland, or disorder.
adrenal, 1423–24
coronary blood flow and, 62–63
estrogen, 1424–26
pancreatic, 1426–31
parathyroid, 1422
pituitary, 1422–23
receptors for, 1606
thyroid, 1412–22
Hufnagel valve, sounds of, 187
Humanism, 2081–82
Humeroperoneal neuromuscular disease, 1228
Hunter, John, 1520
angina pectoris and, 884
Hurler's syndrome, 572, 1224–25
face in, 126
HV interval, 488, 1729, 1730
heart block and, 1731–32
HV interval:
incremental atrial pacing and, 1736
programmed atrial stimulation and, 1736–37
prolonged, 291
Hydatid cysts. *See also* Echinococcosis.
myocardial, 1161
Hydralazine, 1586–87
cardiomyopathy and, 1192
dosage, 1072, 1586
heart failure and, 364
in infant, 586
hypertension and, 1077, 1081
gestational, 1084–85
pharmacology, 1586–87
protein-binding and dialysance, 1082
side effects, 1073
Hydrocarbons, 1235, 1489
Hydrochlorothiazide:
dosage, 1072, 1659
duration of action, 1659
hypertension and, 1071, 1077
Hydrocortisone:
fat embolism and, 1115
streptokinase and, 1916–1919
Hydrodynamics, 1038
Hydroflumethiazide, 1072, 1659
Hydrogen electrode, shunt detection by, 1782
Hydrogen ion, coronary artery spasm and, 1011
11-β-Hydroxylase deficiency, 1063, 1083
17-α-Hydroxylase deficiency, 1063, 1083
5-Hydroxytryptamine, carcinoid and, 1298
Hyperabduction syndrome, 916
Hyperabduction test, 917
Hyperaldosteronism. *See* Aldosteronism.
Hyperalimentation, 1449–50
Hyperbaric pressure, 1550–54
air embolism and, 1552
decompression sickness and, 1550–52
hypoxia and, 1552–53
oxygen therapy, 1553–54
carbon monoxide poisoning and, 1554
cerebrovascular disease and, 1553
cyanide poisoning and, 1554
ischemic heart disease and, 1553–54
peripheral vascular insufficiency and, 1553
underwater diving and, 1550–53
Hypercalcemia. *See also* Calcium.
diuretics and, 1664, 1665
ECG and, 224–25
parathyroid hormone and, 1422
Hypercapnia (hypercarbia):
cor pulmonale and, 1123
obesity and, 1455
ventilatory support and, 1507–8
Hyperchloremic acidosis, heart failure and, 362
Hypercholesterolemia. *See also* Hyperlipidemia.
control measures, 820–23, 828–29
emotional stress and, 1523
endothelial changes and, 810
experimental studies, 804
familial, 574
ileal bypass and, 957
Hyperdynamic state, 403, 1526, 1533
apexcardiography and, 1995
hypertension and, 1074
Hypereosinophilic syndrome, 1208–9, 1213
Hyperglycemia, diuretic-induced, 1665–66
Hyperinsulinism, 1426
Hyperkalemia. *See also* Potassium.
AV block and, 1467–69
conduction and, 1467–69
ECG and, 222–23, 1471
treatment of, 551
Hyperkinetic heart. *See* Hyperdynamic state.
Hyperlipidemia:
atherosclerosis and, 807–8
preventive measures, 820–23, 828–29
regression of, 819
combined, 575
diuretics and, 1074–75, 1666
drugs reducing, 822–23, 829
familial, 574–75
hypertension and, 1074–75
sympatholytic agents and, 1074
Hyperlipoproteinemia, 574–75
type II, 574
Hyperparathyroidism, 1422
Hyperphosphatemia, renal failure and, 1459
Hyperpolarization, automaticity and, 79
Hypersensitivity:
drug, 1236–37
pericarditis and, 1269
Hyperstat. *See* Diazoxide.
Hypertension, 1038–1103
acromegaly and, 1422
aging and, 1409
aldosterone and, 1041, 1043–46
aldosteronism and, 1041, 1046
diagnosis, 1060–64
treatment, 1081–83
anesthesia and, 1502, 1515
aortic dissection and, 1330, 1331
atherosclerosis and, 808, 823–24, 828
athlete and, 1052–53
blood volume and, 1040–41, 1043–44, 1046
cardiac output and, 404, 1042–46
cardiomyopathy and, 1183, 1191
cardiovascular disease and, 1053–54
causes, 561
cerebrovascular, 1054, 1357–58
encephalopathy and, 1357–58
hemorrhage and, 1357
lacunar infarction and, 1357
classification, 1042
coarctation of aorta and, 629–31, 1046–47
compliance of patient and, 1534
contraceptive agents and, 1084, 1482
Cushing's syndrome and, 1063
definitions, 1041–42
depression (mental) and, 1534
diabetes mellitus and, 1075, 1430
diagnosis, 1048–66
basic evaluation, 1049–53
of secondary hypertension, 1056–66
of target organ damage, 1053–56
diastolic, 1042
encephalopathy and, 1054–55
essential, 1042–44, 1071–79
vs. renovascular, 1058
fluids and, extracellular, 1040–41
gallop and, 178–79
genetics of, 575–76
glomerulonephritis and, 1045, 1059–60

Hypertension:
heart rate and, 1042
hemodynamic principles and, 1038–40, 1042–46
history, 1050
hygienic measures and, 828
hyperlipemia and, 1074–75
hypertrophy and, left ventricular, 1053–54
incidence, 561
insurance and, 1559–60
labile and borderline, 1042–43, 1052
licorice and, 1062, 1063
mechanisms, 1042–47
mild or moderate, 1042–44, 1049–50
treatment, 1071–75, 1078–79
mortality, 561
myocardial infarction and, 828
nephrosclerosis and, 1055–56
neural mechanisms and, 1040, 1042–46, 1071–74
neuropathy and, 1045
obesity and, 1078–79, 1452–53
orthostatic, 1074
pathophysiology, 1042–47
pheochromocytoma and, 1046
diagnosis, 1064–66
treatment, 1083–84
physical examination, 1050, 1051
portal, Budd-Chiari syndrome and, 1379
pregnancy and, 1084–85
premature ventricular beats and, 1074
pressure levels and, 1041–42
measurement of, 1048–49
variability in, 1049
prevalence, 560–61
psychological factors, 1525–26, 1533–34
pulmonary, 1091–1103. *See also* Pulmonary hypertension.
pyelonephritis and, 1045, 1060
renal parenchymal disease and, 1045–46
diagnosis, 1059–60
pathophysiology, 1045–46
treatment, 1080–81
renin-angiotensin-aldosterone system and, 1041, 1043–46
renoprival, 1045
renovascular, 1044–45
angioplasty for, 1910–12
diagnosis, 1058–59
vs. essential, 1058
pathophysiology, 1044–45
treatment, 1079–80, 1335
resistant, 1076–78
retinal, 203
retinopathy and, 1053
salt-and-water dependent, 1045–46, 1078
secondary, 1056–66
severe, accelerated, or malignant, 1043–44, 1051–52, 1075–78
sodium and, 824, 1040–41, 1078
stroke and, 1054
sudden death and, 538
surgical procedures and, 1502, 1515–16
symptoms, 1050
systemic arterial, 1038–85
systolic, 1042, 1052
surgical procedures and, 1516
treatment, 1071–85
aldosteronism and, 1081–83

Hypertension: treatment:
beta-blocking agents in, 1612–13
calcium channel blockers in, 1631–32
compliance and, 1076
contraceptive-induced disease and, 1084
diuretics in, 1071, 1072, 1080, 1084, 1664
drug, 1071–78, 1080–85
mild or moderate disease and, 1071–75, 1078–79
pheochromocytoma and, 1083–84
potassium supplementation, 1071, 1079
pregnancy and, 1084–85
primary (essential) disease and, 1071–79
renoparenchymal disease and, 1080–81
renovascular disease and, 1079–80, 1335
severe or resistant disease and, 1075–78
sodium restriction, 1078
sympatholytic agents in, 1071–75, 1080–81, 1085, 1612–13
vasodilators in, 1075, 1081, 1084–85
weight reduction, 1080–81
uremia and, 1045–46, 1060
venous, 1376–78
volume-dependent, 1077
Hyperthermia. *See also* Heat.
cardiac output increase and, 403
Hyperthyroidism, 396–97, 1412–18
arrhythmias and, 1414, 1415
cardiac output increase and, 396–97
cardiovascular features, 1414–15
catheterization studies, 397
causes, 1413
clinical manifestations, 396–97, 1413
contractility and, 98–99, 1415
diagnostic criteria, 1412
digitalis and, 1642
echocardiography, 397
inspection and, 130
nervous system and, 1415
physical signs, 1413
practical considerations, 1415–16
symptoms, 1413
treatment, 397, 1416–18
antithyroid drugs, 1416–17
cardiovascular aspects, 1417–18
radioactive iodine, 1417
surgical, 1417
Hypertriglyceridemia:
control measures, 821–23
familial, 575
Hypertrophy. *See also* Cardiomyopathy, hypertrophic.
afterload and, 331
aging and, 1404
aortic atresia and, 645
aortic stenosis and, 636, 730–32, 734
asymmetric septal, 1194–95. *See also* Cardiomyopathy, hypertrophic.
echocardiography and, 1202–3, 1957
AV canal and, 607–8
capillaries and, myocardial, 862
compliance and, 328
concentric, 327, 331
contractility and, 328

Hypertrophy:
contralateral ventricular changes and, 334
cor pulmonale and, 1123, 1125–26
diagnosis, 1053–54
eccentric, 327, 332
ECG and, 221–22, 1053
hemiblock and, 214, 216
echocardiography and, 1054, 1953
exercise and, 1400
glycogenosis and, 1219, 1220
heart failure and, 327–28
hypertension and, 1053–54
mitral regurgitation and, 768, 773
mitral stenosis and, 758
obesity and, 1453, 1454
oxygen consumption and, 865
palpitations and, 285
patent ductus arteriosus and, 616
precordial palpation and, 154, 155
preload and, 269, 332
protein metabolism and, 97
pulmonary hypertension and, 1097, 1098
pulmonic stenosis and, 655
RNA and, 97
sudden death and, 535
tetralogy of Fallot and, 664
ventricular septal defect and, 594
wall tension and, 327
Hyperuricemia, diuretics and, 1664, 1666
Hyperventilation, anxiety and, 518–19, 907–8
Hypervitaminosis D, 1219
Hypervolemia, hypertension and, 1039
Hypesthesia, 114
acute arterial occlusion and, 1349
Hypocalcemia. *See also* Calcium.
ECG and, 225, 1475–76
hypotension and, 1459–60
renal failure and, 1459–60
Hypoglycemia, 1426
beta-blocker-induced, 1620
syncope and, 518
Hypokalemia. *See also* Potassium.
aldosteronism and, 1061–62
conduction and, 1469
digitalis and, 479, 1647
diuretic-induced, 1665
potassium supplementation and, 1071
ECG and, 223–24
edema and, 1662
Hypokinesis, 1804
Hypomagnesemia, 1476
diuretic-induced, 1665
ECG and, 224–25
Hyponatremia, diuretics and, 362, 1665
Hypoparathyroidism, 1422
Hypoperfusion:
cerebral, 1360–61
intestinal, 1367
Hypophosphatemia, 1477
hyperalimentation and, 1450
Hypoplastic left heart syndrome, 645–47
endocardial fibroelastosis and, 653
Hypotension:
aortic dissection and, 1331, 1332
bradycardia and, 981
carotid sinus and, 49, 515
compensated, 370, 383
decompensated, 370, 383
exercise-induced, 1711

Hypotension:
hemodynamic abnormalities, 370–78
hypocalcemic, 1459–60
myocardial infarction and, 375, 980–82
orthostatic (postural), 510–13
diabetes mellitus and, 1427
perioperative, 1506
postoperative, 953
pulmonary embolism and, 1107, 1112
reflexes and, 375
stages of, 370–71, 383
surgical procedures and, 1515, 1516
syncope and, 510–13
vasodepressor, 508–9
Hypothermia, 1237
cardiopulmonary bypass and, 2027, 2028
Hypothyroidism, 1418–22
cardiovascular features, 1419–20
causes, 1418–19
clinical features, 1419–20
contractility and, 98–99
diagnostic criteria, 1418
digitalis and, 1642
face in, 130
treatment, 1420–22
cardiovascular aspects, 1421–22
Hypoventilation:
alveolar, 1096
cor pulmonale and, 1124, 1127
obesity and, 1455–56
Hypovolemia:
capillaries and, 373–74
causes, 383–84
diuretic-induced, 1665
reflexes and, 375
surgery and, 1505
treatment of, 388–89
vasodilatation and, 384
Hypoxanthine, 62
Hypoxemia:
cor pulmonale and, 1095–96, 1123
fat embolism and, 1115
myocarditis and, 1177
obesity and, 1455
pulmonary hypertension and, 1095–96
renal failure and, 1462
Hypoxia:
altitude and, 1543–47
alveolar, 1093, 1095–96
vasoconstriction and, 1121–22
ATP and, 90
cellular damage and, 380
contractility and, 371–72
cor pulmonale and, 1121–22, 1126
dyspnea and, 116
encephalopathy and, 1361
fetal circulation persistence and, 584
glucose transport and, 89
hyperbarism and, 1552–53
opiates and, 939
oxygen therapy and, 938
reflexes and, 375
shock and, 371–72, 380, 389
syncope and, 518
tetralogy of Fallot and, 663, 665
treatment, 389
vasodilatation and, 59
Hysteresis, pacing, 501
Hysterical syncope, 519

I band, 32, 33
Iatrogenic disorders, 1536–42
diagnostic procedures and, 1540–41
endocarditis, 1134
esophageal perforation, 913
misinterpretation of data and, 1538–39
prevention and treatment of, 1541–42
psychological factors, 1536, 1537, 1541
statements or actions of physician or personnel and, 1537
surgical complications and, 1541
traumatic, 1276
treatment-related, 1539–41
Idionodal rhythm, 433
accelerated, 468
Idiopathic hypertrophic subaortic stenosis. *See* Cardiomyopathy, hypertrophic.
Idioventricular kick, 48
Idioventricular rhythm, 470–71
accelerated, 456
myocardial infarction and, 976
AV block and, 466
AV dissociation and, 467
Ileal bypass, 957
Ileum, carcinoids of, 1298, 1299
Iliac artery:
aneurysm, 1326, 1351
angioplasty, 1336, 1346, 1909, 1910
aortic dissection and, 1330
embolism, 1336
endarterectomy, 2058, 2061
occlusive disease, 1335–36, 1345
thrombosis, 1335, 1336
Iliac vein:
Doppler studies, 1976
thrombosis, 1374
Imipramine, 1479–80
Immune complexes, endocarditis and, 1140
Immune response:
cardiomyopathy and, 1183
endocarditis and, 1139–40
myocarditis and, 1159, 1177
Immunosuppression, transplantation and, 2065, 2066
Impedance, 57, 1039
aging and, 1407
aortic, 47–48, 1039
deep venous thrombosis and, 1106
mismatch of, 410
pacemaker, 1751
vasodilators and, 1584
Impulse conduction, 409–12. *See also* Conduction system.
aberrant, 412
abnormal formation of impulse and, 412
concealed, 412
His bundle recording and, 1730–32
reentry and, 410–11
reflection, 412
repolarization abnormalities, 411–12
unidirectional block and, 410–11
Impulse formation, 407–9
abnormal conduction of impulse and, 412
automaticity and, 407–8
His bundle recording and, 1730
triggered activity and, 408–9
Inching, stethoscopic, 176–77

Incidence, 557–64
cardiovascular disease in general, 557–58
cerebrovascular disease, 562
congenital heart disease, 564, 581–82
coronary heart disease, 559–60
heart failure, 562
hypertension, 561
pulmonary embolism, 564
rheumatic heart disease, 563
Incisura, pulse, 52, 53
aortic, 142
Indanedione, 1669
Indapamide, 1072
Inderal. *See* Propranolol.
Indicator-dilution technique, 1780–82
cardiac output and, 1780–81
shunts and, 1781–82
Indifferent clamp, 1754
Indigestion, 121, 911
Indium-111 imaging, 1848–49
platelet, 1848–49
polymorphonuclear leukocyte, 1849
Indocyanine:
endothelial assessment and, 387
lung water measurement and, 386
Indomethacin:
patent ductus arteriosus and, 617
pericarditis and, 1254
Indoramin, 1589
Inertia, arterial pulse and, 141
Infantile syndrome, 1018
Infarct-avid agents, 1844–48
Infarction:
cerebral. *See* Cerebrovascular disease, infarction.
intestinal, 1364
nonocclusive, 1367
venous occlusion and, 1366
myocardial. *See* Myocardial infarction.
pulmonary, 119, 1106–7
Infection:
aortic. *See* Aortitis.
coronary artery, 1023
ductus arteriosus, 616, 617
endocarditis. *See* Endocarditis.
myocardial. *See* Myocarditis.
myxoma, 1286
pericardial, 1269–71
postoperative, 1518–19
pulmonary, history and, 120
rheumatic fever, 1306–12
staphylococcal. *See* Staphylococcal infections.
streptococcal. *See* Streptococcal infections. syphilitic. *See* Syphilis.
transplanted heart and, 2066
Influenza, 1174
Informed consent, 1574
anesthesia and, 1503
artificial heart and, 2074–75
Infundibulum:
anatomy, 19
definition, 686
embryology, 10
tetralogy of Fallot and, 662, 666
Innominate artery. *See* Brachiocephalic artery.
Inocor. *See* Amrinone.
Inosine, 62
Inotropic agents, 1639–56. *See also* Digitalis.
amrinone, 1655–56
cardiomyopathy and, 1192
catecholamine, 1653–55

Inotropic agents:
heart failure and, 358–60
nondigitalis, 1652–56
actions of, 1653
classification of, 1653
pregnancy and, 1393
ventricular performance curves and, 1506
Inotropic state, 46–47. *See also* Contractility.
Insect venom, 1489
Insomnia, 120
heart failure and, 350
Inspection, 122–35
body configuration, 122
ear, 130
extremity, 131–34
face, 126–30
gait, 126
mouth, 131
precordial, 152
skin, 122–26
thorax and neck, 134–35
Inspiration. *See also* Respiration.
Kussmaul's sign and, 148–49
pulsus paradoxus and, 146
Insudation theory of atherosclerosis, 842
Insulating materials, 492
Insulin:
excessive, 1426
glucose transport and, 88–89
insufficient, 88–89. *See also* Diabetes mellitus.
protein metabolism and, 96–97
therapeutic, 1429
myocardial infarction and, 1430
postoperative, 1431
Insurance, 1556–62
angina pectoris and, 1558–59
bypass surgery and, 1558
cardiomegaly and, 1561
cardiomyopathy and, 1561
coronary heart disease and, 1557–59
disability evaluation and, 1562, 1572–73
ECG and, 1561
health, 1561–62
hypertension and, 1559–60
intercompany variations in, 1557
litigation and, 1563–76
mortality, life expectancy, ratings, and premiums, 1556–57
myocardial infarction and, 1558
valvular heart disease and, 1560–61
Intensivist, 1508–9
Interatrial pathways, 30
Interatrial septum. *See also* Atrial septal defect.
absent, 612
anatomy, 19
catheterization studies and, 1772
echocardiography and, 1943, 1944
embryology, 11–12
excision of, myxoma and, 1292, 1293
lipomatous hypertrophy of, 1294
Intercalated disks, 32, 35
Interference dissociation, 466
Intermediary vesicle, 32
Internodal pathways, 30
Intersegmental arteries, 13, 15
Interventricular foramen, 3, 6–8
closure, 10
Interventricular lymphatics, 25
Interventricular septum. *See also* Ventricular septal defect.
Interventricular septum:
activation of, 206
anatomy, 19, 20–21
aortic-left ventricular tunnel and, 644
AV canal and, 608
blood supply, 28, 29
disorganized, 1196–97
echocardiography, 594, 1935–36, 1938, 1943
embryology, 6–7, 10
hypertrophy, 1194–98. *See also* Cardiomyopathy, hypertrophic.
asymmetric, 1194–95, 1202–3
membranous, 17–18
resection, 1208
rupture (perforation):
infarction and, 393–94, 983–84
surgical treatment of, 2041
traumatic, 1279
Interventricular sulci, 16
Interventricular veins, 29–30
Interview, history-taking, 109–10
Intestine. *See also* Gastrointestinal tract.
blood flow, 1367
bypass procedure (ileal), 957
gangrene, postoperative, 1371
infarction, 1364
nonocclusive, 1367
venous occlusion and, 1366
ischemia, 1364–70
recurrent, 1368–70
transient, 1367–68
lipodystrophy of, 1239–40
vasculitis, 1370
Intima:
aortic dissection and, 1328, 1330
atherosclerosis and, 805
coronary artery dissection and, 1021
coronary artery fibrosis and, 1023
endothelial injury and, 810
fibrous plaque and, 801, 803
polyarteritis nodosa and, 1438, 1439
proliferation of, 812
pulmonary vascular, hypertension and, 588
Intraaortic balloon counterpulsation, 2021–24
complications, 1541, 2023–24
equipment, 2021–22
indications, 2021
insertion technique, 2022–23
removal procedure, 2024
septal perforation and, 393, 2040
shock management and, 394
timing, 2023
weaning from, 2024
Intramyocardial pressure, 859
Intrapericardial pressure, filling impairment and, 268
Intrathoracic pressure, CPR and, 547–49
Intravenous line:
anesthetic agents and, 1504
CPR and, 551
fluid replacement and, perioperative, 1505
Intraventricular conduction, 212–19
aberrant, 412, 457–61
atrial fibrillation and, 447, 458, 461
esophageal ECG and, 1694–95
forms of, 457–58
premature atrial beats and, 438
vs. premature ventricular beats, 447, 458–60
tachycardia and, 460–61
Intraventricular conduction:
approach to defects of, 291
ECG and, 212–19
esophageal, 1694–95
myocardial infarction and, 977
Introns, 566
Iodine (iodide):
contrast media and, 1785
hyperthyroidism and, 1416–17
radioactive, 1413, 1417
Ions, transmembrane potential and, 74–75
Iopamidol, 1786
Iritis, relapsing, 1238
Iron, excessive, 1221–22
Iron storage disease, genetics of, 570
Irritable heart syndrome, 1526, 1533
Ischemia:
colonic, 1367–68
extremity:
acute occlusion and, 1349
arteriosclerosis obliterans and, 1339–46
thromboangiitis obliterans and, 1347
fatty acids and, 92, 93
glycolysis and, 91
IABP and, 2023
intestinal, 1364–70
recurrent, 1368–70
transient, 1367–68
mesenteric, 1364–70
nonocclusive, 1367
recurrent, 1368–70
systemic vascular disease and, 1370–71
shock and, 371
subendocardial, 859–61, 865
transient attacks of (TIAs), 1355
coronary heart disease and, 990
endarterectomy and, 2055–56
intestinal, 1367–68
management, 1356–57
syncope and, 513–14
ulcers and, 1341, 1344–45, 1347, 1348
Ischemic heart disease. *See also* Coronary heart disease; Myocardial ischemia.
definition, 299
Ismelin. *See* Guanethidine.
Isoenzymes, myocardial infarction and, 897–98
Isoflurane, 1496
Isometric contraction, 40, 41
Isometric exercise, 1027
Isometric handgrip:
auscultation and, 195
ventricular function and, 1825
Isoniazid, tuberculous pericarditis and, 1270
Isopotential lines, 82, 83
Isoproterenol:
AV block and, 481
contractility and, 360
CPR and, 552
heart failure in infant and, 586
shock and, 392
structure, 1608, 1653
toxicity, 1234
Isorhythmic dissociation, 467, 468
Isosorbide dinitrate:
chemical structure, 940
dosage and effects, 940, 1585, 1586
heart failure and, 363

Isosorbide-5-mononitrate, 1585
Isotonic contraction, 41
Isotonic exercise, 1027
Isovolumic contraction and relaxation, 52
  apexcardiography and, 1994
  cardiomyopathy and, 1199

J lead, atrial, 1751–52
Jaccoud's arthritis, 133, 134
James' internodal pathways, 30
Janeway lesions, 132
  endocarditis and, 1142
Jaundice, 121
Jelly, cardiac, 3
Jenner, Edward, 884
Jessamine, 1489
Jet lesions:
  endocarditis and, 1138
  ventricular septal defect and, 591
Job-related injury. *See* Workers' compensation.
Johnson, Samuel, 1704
Joints:
  pain in, 115
  rheumatoid. *See* Arthritis, rheumatoid.
  roentgenography and, 236
Jones criteria, 1311
Judgment, physician's, 2081
Judkins technique of arteriography, 1791
Jugular lymphatics, 26–27
Jugular vein(s):
  heart failure and, 351
  pacemaker implantation and, 1749
  pressure measurement, 147
  pulse, 54, 147–48
    abnormalities, 148–50
    aortic stenosis and, 1996
    c wave, 54, 148
    endomyocardial fibrosis and, 1210, 1211
    examination, 147–48
    mitral stenosis and, 1996
    normal, 148
    recording of, 1993
    tricuspid endocarditis and, 254
    volume changes, 1993
Junctional rhythms. *See* Atrioventricular junction.

Kabikinase. *See* Streptokinase.
Kaliuresis, edema and, 1663
Kallikrein, 59
Kartagener's syndrome, dextrocardia and, 689
Karvonen method for heart rate, 1027
Kawasaki's disease, 129–30, 1023
Kearns' syndrome, 1231
Kearns-Sayre syndrome, 130
  pacing and, 481
Kent bundles, 415–16
  AV junctional tachycardia and, 418
  reentry, 417, 419
    vs. AV node reentry, 418, 420
  right bundle branch block and, 216
  Wolff-Parkinson-White syndrome and, 219–20
Keratitis, interstitial, 1238
Keratosis blennorrhagica, 126
Kerley lines:
  A, 354
  B, 354
    heart failure and, 236
Keshan disease, 1184
Ketamine, 1496
Kidney:
  diuretics and, 1657–60, 1662
  endocarditis and, 1144, 1151, 1460
  failure, 1458–64. *See also* Uremia.
    acidosis and, 1460
    anemia and, 1460, 1462
    atherosclerosis and, 1463–64
    azotemia and, 1460
    calcium and, 1459–60, 1463
    cardiac output increase and, 404
    chronic, 1460–64
    complications, 1460–64
    dialysis for. *See* Dialysis.
    digitalis and, 1641
    diuretics and, 1662
    edema and, 1662
    endocarditis and, 1460
    hypertension and, 1055, 1056, 1060, 1080–81
    myocardial dysfunction and, 1462–63
    pericarditis and, 1460–62
    physiological consequences, 1458–60
    potassium and, 1459
    pulmonary edema and, 1463
    sodium and, 1458–59
  heart failure and, 324–26, 1460, 1462–63
  hypertension and, 1044–46, 1055, 1056
    diagnosis, 1058–60
    treatment, 1079–81, 1910–12, 1335
  pressor system, 1041
  progressive systemic sclerosis and, 1442
  shock and, 375, 378
  vasoconstriction and, 325
Kim-Ray Greenfield filter, 1111–12
Kinetocardiography, 1994
King, Thomas Wilkinson, 1412
Kinins, shock and, 376
Klebsiella endocarditis, 1136
Klinefelter's syndrome, 122
Klippel-Feil syndrome, inspection and, 128, 130
Knife wounds, 1022, 1276, 1277
Knock, pericardial, 186
Kontron balloon, 2022
Korotkov sounds, 139
Kugelberg-Welander syndrome, 572, 1231
Kugel's artery, 29
Kussmaul's sign, 148–49
Kwashiorkor, 1219

l loop, 686
  corrected transposition of great arteries and, 700
  crisscross heart and, 706
Labetalol, 1607. *See also* Beta-blocking agents.
  alpha-blocking activity of, 1609
  dosage, 941, 1072
  pharmacodynamics, 1608, 1613, 1617
  pharmacokinetics, 1610, 1611
  side effects, 1073
  structure, 1608
Labor, drugs used for, 1394
Laboratory tests and data:
  Bayes' theorem and, 304–5
  predictive value, 103, 304–5
  qualities of, 103
  sensitivity and specificity, 103, 304, 305
Lactate:
  fatty acids and, 92, 93
  myocardial ischemia and, 309
  shock and, 378, 379
Lactic dehydrogenase:
  artificial heart and, 2073, 2074
  isoenzymes, 897
  myocardial infarction and, 897–98
Ladder diagrams, 433–34
Laennec, Rene T. H., 157
Lampit, 1179
Lanatoside-C. *See* Digitalis.
Lancisi, G. M., 529
Laniet, Jacques, 1314
Lanoxin. *See* Digoxin.
Laplace law, 47, 56
  blood pressure and, 138
  heart failure and, 328–29
  wall tension and, 58
Larva migrans, 1176
Laryngeal nerves, recurrent, ductus arteriosus and, 618
Laryngeal vertigo, 517
Laser therapy of coronary obstruction, 1922–25
Lasitrophy, 43
Lateral sacs, myocardial, 34, 38
Lawsuits. *See* Legal issues.
LDL. *See* Lipoprotein, low-density.
Leading circle concept, 413–14
Lead poisoning, 1235
Leeuwenhoek, Anton von, 1339
Left anterior descending artery. *See* Coronary arteries, left anterior descending.
Left circumflex artery. *See* Coronary arteries, left circumflex.
Left main coronary artery. *See* Coronary arteries, left main.
Left-to-right shunt. *See* Shunts; *also* specific disorder, *e.g.,* Atrial septal defect.
Leg. *See also* Extremities.
  edema, 205
  exercise for, 1027
  phlebography, 1885–86
  thrombosis in, 1105–6
Legal issues, 1563–76
  causality assessment, 1569–72
  diagnosis specification, 1567–68
  disability evaluation, 1572–73, 1578–79
  examination for, 1574–75
  expert testimony, 1565–67
  malpractice, 1565, 1573–74
  preexisting conditions and, 1564, 1565, 1570
  reports and, 1575–76
  time-of-onset determinations, 1568–69
  tort claims, 1564–65
  types of actions involving cardiology in, 1563–65
  workers' compensation, 1563–64, 1571, 1575, 1579
Legionnaires' disease, myocarditis and, 1173
Leismaniasis, 1175
Lenègre's disease, 427, 463–64
Length-tension relation, 44–45, 332
Lentiginosis, 125, 1239
Lepidic cells, 1285
Leptospirosis, 1173
Leriche syndrome, 1335–36
Leucine, 95, 96

Leukemia:
cardiac infiltration by, 1297–98
eosinophilic, 1209, 1212
myocarditis and, 1159, 1161
Leukocytes:
endocarditis and, 1144
indium imaging and, 1849
myocardial infarction and, 875
myocarditis and, 1159, 1166
Levocardia, 688, 689
Levodopa, 1483–84
Levoisomerism, 687, 690
Levophed, 391. *See also* Norepinephrine.
Levoversion, 232
Lev's disease, 427, 464
Lewis, Thomas, 1099
Lewis lines, 433–34
Liability, 1564–65. *See also* Legal issues.
Libman-Sacks lesions, 1436
Licorice, hypertension and, 1062, 1063
Lidocaine, 1596–97
cardiac catheterization and, 1769
clinical application, 1597
myocardial infarction and, 975
pharmacokinetic properties, 1594, 1596
pharmacologic properties, 1596–97
pregnancy and, 1393
thrombolytic therapy and, 1920
toxicity, 1597
Lidwill, M. C., 486
Life insurance. *See* Insurance.
Ligamentum arteriosum, 14, 614
aortic arch anomalies and, 623, 624
Lightning injuries, 1486–87
Lignocaine. *See* Lidocaine.
Liljestrand, G., 1768
Limb-girdle dystrophy, 1228
Lip, 131
Lipidosis, isolated cardiac, 1224
Lipids. *See also* Cholesterol.
drugs lowering, 822–23, 829
fatty streaks. *See* Fatty streak.
Refsum's disease and, 1225
smooth-muscle cells and, 812–13
Lipoamide dehydrogenase, Friedreich's ataxia and, 569
Lipodystrophy, intestinal, 1239–40
Lipogenic theory of atherosclerosis, 807, 841
Lipoma, cardiac, 1294
Lipoprotein:
deficiency, familial, 574
diet and, 808
genetics and, 574–75
high-density (HDL):
atherosclerosis and, 813
genetics and, 574
risk status and, 822
low-density (LDL):
atherosclerosis and, 807, 813
genetics and, 574
hypercholesterolemia and, 574
platelet-derived growth factor and, 814
reduction of, 821–23, 828
smooth-muscle cells and, 813
very-low-density (VLDL):
dysbetalipoproteinemia and, 574
reduction of, 822, 823
Lithium, 1477, 1480
Lithium anode battery, 491
Litigation. *See* Legal issues.
Livedo reticularis, 1352
treatment, 1353
Liver:
Budd-Chiari syndrome and, 1379–80
cardiac output increase and decrease of, 402
digitalis and, 1641
hemangiomatosis, 401
malposition, 689
painful, heart failure and, 351
paroxysmal engorgement of, 911
physical examination and, 204
shock and, 379
situs determination and, 687
Loeffler's disease, 1208–13. *See also* Endomyocardial fibrosis.
Longfellow, H. W., 1403
Loniten. *See* Minoxidil.
Lopressor. *See* Metoprolol.
Lorazepam, 1496
Lorelco, 822–23
Louis' angle, 147
Lowenberg's cuff sign, 1374
Lown-Ganong-Levine syndrome, 449
atrio-Hisian fibers and, 417
management, 477
Lucretius, 817
Lues. *See* Syphilis.
Lumbar sympathectomy, occlusive arterial disease and, 2061
Lungs. *See also various* Pulmonary *entries.*
anomalous systemic arterial supply to, 621–22
clouding of, edema and, 353
compliance, heart failure and, 337
computed tomography and, 1867
diffuse interstitial disease, 1124
edema. *See* Edema, pulmonary.
embolism. *See* Pulmonary embolism.
examination, 204
heart failure and, 352
heterotaxia and, 689, 690
infarction:
embolism and, 1106–7
hemoptysis and, 119
infection, history and, 120
interlobar fissure thickening, 354
obstructive disease, chronic:
cor pulmonale and, 1123–24, 1126
exercise and, 1828–29
noncardiac surgery and, 1517
ventricular performance and, 1828–29
parenchyma, roentgenography and, 230, 235–36
radionuclide studies, 1881–82
embolism and, 1108
sequestered, 621, 622
shock and, 378–79
transplantation, 2067–68
water in, extravascular, measurement of, 386
Lupus erythematosus, systemic, 1435–37
coronary heart disease and, 1022, 1437
endocarditis and, 1436–37
genetics, 571
intestinal vasculitis and, 1370
myocarditis and, 1437
pericarditis and, 1269, 1436
skin and, 123, 124
therapy, 1437
Lusitrophy, 328
Lutembacher's syndrome, 599
Lyme disease, 570–71, 1174
Lymphangioepithelioma, AV node, 1294
Lymphatics:
cardiac, 25
metastases and, 1296
systemic, 26–27
Lymphedema, 1377–78
Lymph nodes:
cardiac, 25
mucocutaneous syndrome, 129–30, 1023
Lyon chromosome, 806
Lyon hypothesis, 574
Lysosomes, 95–96
releasing factor (LRF), 381
shock and, 380–81
storage diseases, 572

M line, 32, 33
Mackenzie, James, 109, 345
Macrophages:
atherosclerosis and, 805, 813
fatty streaks and, 801, 804
shock and, 378
MacWilliam, J. A., 538
Magnesium, 1476
alcoholism and, 1447
arrhythmias and, 1476
diuretics and, 1665
ECG and, 224–25, 1476
Magnetic resonance imaging, 1888–94
acquired lesions and, 1890–92
basic physical considerations, 1888–89
cerebrovascular disease and, 1356
clinical experience with, 1890–93
congenital heart disease and, 1892
contrast agents for, 1893–94
flow patterns and, 1892
hazards in, 1894
metabolic studies, 85
myocardial ischemia and, 1892–93
pericardial disease and, 1893
shielding for, 1889
Mahaim fibers, 415, 416
AV junctional tachycardia and, 420
ECG and, 220
escape beats and, 470
reentry and, 417, 419
ventricular tachycardia and, 425
Mahomed, 1048
Malabsorption, mesenteric ischemia and, 1368
Malaria, 1175
Malnutrition, 121, 1449, 1450
Malonyl CoA, 92
Malpositions, 686–707
asplenia and polysplenia syndromes, 689–90
assessment, 257–58
crisscross heart, 706–7
definition and terminology, 686–87, 688
double-outlet left ventricle, 699–700
double-outlet right ventricle, 696–99
ectopic cordis, 707
of great arteries (MGA), 687. *See also* Transposition of great arteries.
anatomically corrected (ACM), 687
tricuspid atresia and, 673, 674
levocardia, dextrocardia, and mesocardia, 688–89
roentgenography and, 231–32
segmental approach to diagnosis, 687–88
single ventricle, 703–6
Malpractice, 1565, 1573–74
Maltase deficiency, 1219

Mammary artery grafts, 853–54, 2037
  patency, 954
Mandible, hypoplastic, 131
Mannitol, hypovolemia and, 388
Manometers, blood pressure, 138–39
Mapping:
  electrophysiologic, 1738
  epicardial, WPW syndrome and, 2013, 2014
  flow, regurgitant valve and, 1984
Maprotiline, 1480, 1533
Marfan's syndrome, 573
  aortic-mitral combined valvular disease and, 785
  aortic regurgitation and, 741, 745
  cystic medial degeneration and, 741, 742, 1322
  inspection and, 122, 126, 127, 132
  myxoma and, 767
  pregnancy and, 1388, 1391
Marginal artery, 29
Marginal lymphatic, 25
Marshall's ligament, 11
Marshall's oblique vein, 30
Master, Arthur M., 883, 885
Maxillary artery, embryology of, 13
McArdle's syndrome, 1220
McDermott, Walsh, 918
Means-Lerman scratch, 1414
Mechanical heart. *See* Artificial heart.
Mechanoreceptors, blood pressure and, 1040
Media:
  atherosclerosis and, 802
  coronary aneurysm and, 711
  cystic necrosis of aortic, 1322, 1330
    regurgitation and, 644, 741–43
  degeneration of aortic, 1322, 1325, 1330
  dissection of aortic, 1328–33
  fibromuscular dysplasia, sudden death and, 532–33
  hypertrophy of pulmonary vascular, 1101
  pulmonary hypertension and, 588
  syphilitic lesions of, 1314
Mediastinum:
  emphysema of, 916
  lymphatics of, 26–27
  phlebography of, 1885
  roentgenography and, 234–35
Medicolegal issues. *See* Legal issues.
Medtronic Hall valve, 2034, 2069
Medtronic leads, 492, 493
Medulla oblongata, 60
Meiosis, 567
Melioidosis, myocarditis and, 1173
Membrane:
  capacitance, 80
  potential across. *See* Transmembrane potential.
  shock and, 380, 384
Mendel, G., 566
Meningitis, endocarditis and, 1143
Meningococcal pericarditis, 1270
Meningococcemia, myocarditis and, 1173
Menopause:
  coronary heart disease and, 826
  estrogen therapy and, 1425
Mental retardation, aortic stenosis and, 641
Mental status:
  fat embolism and, 1115
  heart failure and, 350
Mental status:
  hypertensive encephalopathy and, 1357–58
Meperidine:
  cardiac catheterization and, 1769
  myocardial infarction and, 939
Mercury poisoning, 1235
Meromyosin, 34
Mesenchyme, septation and, 6
Mesenteric angiography, 1365, 1368
Mesenteric arteritis, postoperative, 1371
Mesenteric ischemia, 1364–70
  nonocclusive, 1367
  recurrent, 1368–70
  systemic vascular disease and, 1370–71
Mesenteric vascular occlusion, 1364–70
  atherosclerosis and, 1364, 1368
  inferior, 1367–68
  recurrent, 1368–70
  superior, 1364–66, 1368
    angioplasty and, 1912
  venous, 1366
Mesocardia, 688, 707
Mesothelioma, pericardial, 1295
Mestranol, 1424
Metabolic equivalents (METs), 1706
Metabolism, 85–99
  aerobic, 1398, 1400
  anaerobic, 51
  coronary blood flow and, 60–61
  disorders of, 97–99, 1219–26
    coronary heart disease and, 1023
  fatty acid, 91–94
  general features, 85–86
  glucose phosphorylation, 89–90
  glucose transport, 87–89
  glycogen, 89
  glycolytic pathway, 87–91
  mechanisms, 86–87
  myocardial ischemia and, 97–98
  myosin ATPase activity and, 98–99
  oxidative substrates and, 85–86, 87
  protein, 94–97
  pyruvate, 90
  radionuclide studies and, 1850
  shock and, 378–79
Metanephrine, pheochromocytoma and, 1065
Metaraminol, vasoconstriction and, 1590
Metastases, 1295–98
  atrial, 1297
  carcinoid, 1298–99
  coronary involvement in, 1296–97
  diagnostic studies, 1297
  frequency and origin, 1295–96
  intracavitary, 1297
  leukemic, 1297–98
  lymphatic spread of, 1296
  manifestations, 1296
  myocardial, 1296
  pericardial, 1268, 1296, 1297
  treatment, 1297
Methimazole, 944
  hyperthyroidism and, 1416
Methohexital, 1496
Methoxamine:
  auscultation and, 195
  vasoconstriction and, 1590
Methyclothiazide, 1659
  dosage, 1072
Methyldigoxin, 1643
Methyldopa, 1588
  dosage, 1072, 1587
  hypersensitivity to, 1237
Methyldopa:
  hypertension and, 1078, 1081
    gestational, 1085
  protein-binding and dialysance, 1082
  side effects, 1073
Methylparatyrosine, pheochromocytoma and, 1083–84
Methylprednisolone:
  fat embolism and, 1115
  pericarditis and, 982
  septic shock and, 390
  transplantation and, 2065
Methysergide, 1232, 1484
Metoclopramide, digitalis and, 1647
Metocurine, 1497
Metolazone, 1658
  dosage, 1072, 1659
  duration of action, 1659
  edema and, 1664
  hypertension and, 1077
  pharmacokinetics, 1660–61
  protein-binding and dialysance, 1082
  renal failure and, 1458, 1662
  site of action, 1660
Metoprolol, 1607. *See also* Beta-blocking agents.
  dosage, 941, 1072
  hypertension and, 1081
    gestational, 1085
  myocardial infarction and, 967
    long-term use in, 971
  pharmacodynamics, 1608, 1613, 1617
  pharmacokinetics, 1610, 1611
  protein-binding and dialysance, 1082
  structure, 1608
Metrizamide, 1786
Metyrosine, 1589
Mevinolin, 823
Mexiletine, 1601
  clinical application and toxicity, 1601
  pharmacology, 1601
Microaneurysms, retinal, 200
Microangiopathy, diabetic, 1428
Microphones, phonocardiography, 1991
Micturition syncope, 517–18
Midazolam, 1496
Migraine, syncopal, 519
Milrinone, 1655
  contractility and, 360
  structure, 1653
Mineralocorticoids. *See also* Aldosterone.
  hypertension and, 1062, 1063
Mines, G. R., 406
Minipress. *See* Prazosin.
Minoxidil, 1587
  dosage, 1072, 1586
  heart failure and, 364
  hypertension and, 1078, 1081
  pharmacology, 1587
  protein-binding and dialysance, 1082
  side effects, 1073
Mirowski, M., 1761
Mitochondria:
  contractility and, 38, 39
  exercise and, 1400
  fatty acids and, 91–93
  heart failure and, 330
  myocardial, 34
  myopathy and, 569
  oxygen tension and, 861
  shock and, 380
Mitoxantrone, 1482
Mitral annulus, 17, 21
  calcification, 767–68
    echocardiography, 1959

Mitral annulus:
dilatation, 769
remodeling, 776–77
Mitral valve, 754–80
anatomy, 21, 22
annuloplasty, 776–77
anteromedial leaflet, 21, 22
aortic valve disease, and, 747, 785–91
clinical manifestations, 786–90
etiology, 785
natural history and prognosis, 790
pathology, 785
pathophysiology, 785–86
treatment, 790–91
area determination, 1785, 1935
Doppler studies and, 1983
assessment, 250–53
atresia, 647–48
aortic atresia and, 645
clinical manifestations, 647
embryology, 12
management, 647–48
pathology, 647
atrial myxoma and, 253
billowing (floppy), 184, 765
calcification, 764, 767–68, 772
aortic stenosis and, 787
surgical treatment, 777–78
carcinoid and, 1298
cleft, AV canal and, 605–11
coarctation of aorta and, 628–29
commissurotomy, 762–63, 2032
Doppler studies, 1980
regurgitation and, 1983–85
stenosis and, 1983
velocity profile, 252
double-outlet right ventricle and, 699
dysplastic, 648
E point-septal separation (EPSS), 1935, 1963
echocardiography, 1933–34, 1939, 1940, 1954
measurement and, 1935
prolapse and, 771, 772, 1958–59
regurgitation and, 251, 252, 650, 772, 1954, 1958
stenosis and, 649, 758–59, 1958
ventricular performance and, 1963
embolism and, 755, 761, 1358, 1670–71
embryology, 12
endocarditis, 1146
drug-related, 1132
prolapse and, 1131–32
prosthesis and, 1133–34
regurgitation and, 764–65, 1138
fibrosis, 764, 766
cardiomyopathy and, 1199
fibrous skeleton and, 17, 18
floppy, 184, 765
hypoplastic, aortic atresia and, 645, 646
murmurs, 160, 163
diastolic, 192
regurgitation and, 191, 192, 650, 770
stenosis and, 192, 648, 757–58
myxoma and, 1287, 1288
necropsy and, 2078–79
parachute, 648
posterolateral leaflet, 22
postoperative care, 2033
pressure half-time, 252, 1983
prolapse, 184–85
aortic valve prolapse and, 785
Mitral valve: prolapse:
atrial septal defect and, 602
beta blockers for, 1616–17
catheterization studies, 774
cerebral embolism and, 1358
diagnostic criteria, 250–51
ECG, 772
echocardiography, 771, 772, 1958–59
endocarditis and, 1131–32
genetics, 568
hyperthyroidism and, 1414
insurance and, 1560
management, 776
noncardiac surgery and, 1517
palpitations and, 285
pathophysiology, 768–69
phonocardiogram, 771
physical findings, 770
pregnancy and, 1389
prevalence, 563
prognosis, 775
psychological factors, 1533
roentgenography, 772
symptoms, 769
regurgitation, 649–51, 764–80
acquired, 764–80
acute severe, 252
aging and, 1410–11
angiography and, 1789–90
anticoagulants and, 1670–71
aortic regurgitation and, 785–91
aortic stenosis and, 785–86, 788–90
assessment, 251–52, 650, 769–74
atrial fibrillation and, 772, 775
AV canal and, 607–11
cardiomegaly and, 275
cardiomyopathy and, 766–67, 1184, 1199, 1201, 1205
catheterization studies, 650, 772–74
chronic severe, 251–52
congenital, 649–51
contractility and, 275
coronary heart disease and, 769, 770, 774, 991
cost analysis, 779–80
Doppler studies, 1983–85
ECG, 772
echocardiography, 251, 252, 650, 772, 1954, 1958
ejection fraction and, 275
endocarditis and, 764–65, 1138
endomyocardial fibrosis and, 1211
etiology, 764
heart failure and, 275, 334, 770, 776
history, 769–70
insurance and, 1560
medical management, 650, 775–76
murmurs, 191, 192, 650, 770
myocardial failure and, 268, 269, 275
myocardial infarction and, 767, 984, 2041
myxoma and, 765–66
natural history and prognosis, 650, 774–75
pathology, 649–50, 764–68
pathophysiology, 768–69
phonocardiogram, 773, 1996
physical examination, 770–72
postoperative care, 779
precordial palpation and, 155
pregnancy and, 1387, 1389
preload and, 269, 332, 768, 770, 774
Mitral valve: regurgitation:
radionuclide studies, 774, 1822
rheumatic, 764, 1308
roentgenography, 772
sounds, 171–72, 650, 770
stroke volume and, 773, 775, 1783–84
surgical management, 650–51, 776–79, 790–91, 2032
transposition of great arteries and, 251, 650, 701, 702
traumatic, 767
replacement, 777–79, 2032–33
combined aortic-mitral valve disease and, 790–91
endocarditis, 1133–34
regurgitation and, 650–51
results, 778–79, 2034
stenosis and, 649, 762, 763
rheumatoid nodules, 1440
ring (supravalvular), 648, 649
sounds, 160, 163
click, 184
closure, 163, 164–66
opening snap, 185, 756
regurgitation and, 171–72, 650, 770
stenosis and, 185, 756
spongiosa, 766
stenosis, 648–49, 754–64
acquired, 754–64
angina pectoris and, 991
anticoagulants and, 1670–71
aortic regurgitation and, 785, 788, 789
aortic stenosis and, 648, 785, 786, 788, 789
assessment, 252, 648–49, 755–60
atrial fibrillation and, 758, 760–61
atrial septal defect and, 599
cardiomyopathy vs., 1205
catheterization studies, 649, 759–60
coarctation of aorta and, 648
congenital, 648–49
cost analysis, 763–64
Doppler studies, 1983
ECG, 223, 758
echocardiography, 649, 758–59, 1958
embolism and, 755, 761, 1670–71
etiology, 754
exercise testing, 760
heart failure and, 760
hemoptysis and, 119
history, 755–56
medical management, 649, 761–62
murmurs, 192, 648, 757–58
natural history and prognosis, 649, 760–61
noncardiac surgery and, 1516
pathology, 648, 754–55
pathophysiology, 755
phonocardiography and, 1996
physical examination, 756–58
postoperative care, 763
pregnancy and, 763–64, 1387, 1388–89
radionuclide studies, 760
rheumatic, 754–55, 760, 786, 1311
roentgenography, 235, 237, 758
rumble, 757–58
sounds, 185, 756
surgical management, 649, 762–63
thromboembolism, 755, 761, 1670–71
Mixed venous blood, oxygen and, 1777

Mobin-Uddin filter, 1111
Möbitz block, 480, 488
His bundle recording and, 1731
syncope and, 523
Moderator band, 19
Mondor's syndrome, 910
Monge's disease, 1096
Monitoring, 1998–2007
anesthetic, 1497–99
arrhythmias and, 2004
balloon flotation catheterization (Swan-Ganz) and, 1999–2002
complications, 2001–2
data collection, 2000
indications, 2000–2001
insertion technique, 1999–2000
blood pressure, 1999
computer assisted, 2006
computer-based, 2004–7
clinical functions afforded by, 2006
interventions and, 2006
measurements, 2005–6
systems and design, 2004–5
trends in, 2006
coronary bypass surgery and, 2002
Holter. *See* Electrocardiography, prolonged.
myocardial infarction and, 979–80, 2002–3
respiratory, 2004–5
seriously ill patient and, 1998–2003
shock, 384–87
Monoamine oxidase inhibitors, 1480
Monoclonal theory of atherogenesis, 806–7, 842
Monocytes, atherosclerosis and, 804, 805
Mononucleosis, 1174
Morbidity of cardiovascular disease, 557
Morgagni, John Baptist, 839
Morphine:
anesthetic use of, 1496, 1497
coronary heart disease and, 938–39
heart failure and, 366
pulmonary edema and, 338, 366
Mors subita, 529
Mortality, 557–64
cardiovascular disease in general, 557–59
cerebrovascular disease, 562
congenital heart disease, 564
coronary bypass surgery, 952
coronary heart disease, 560
hypertension, 561
insurance and, 1556–57
pulmonary embolism, 564
rheumatic heart disease, 563
secular trends, 558–59
Motor carrier safety regulations, 1578
Mountain sickness, 1096, 1121
Mouth, inspection of, 131
Movement disorders, 122
gait and, 126
Mucocutaneous lymph node syndrome, 129–30, 1023
Mucolipidoses, 572
Mucopolysaccharidoses, 572, 1224–25
chest deformity and, 134
face in, 126
Mucormycosis, 1175
Mueller's sign, 746–47
Mulibrey nanism, 128, 573, 1239
pericarditis and, 1271
Multiple regression, 305
Multiple system atrophy, 512
Mumps, myocarditis and, 1160
Murmurs, 188–95
anemia and, 400
aortic-left ventricular tunnel, 645
aortic-mitral combined valvular disease, 788–89
aortic regurgitation, 193, 745–46
syphilis and, 1315, 1316
aortic stenosis, 190–91, 635–36, 733–34
athletes and, 1400–1401
atrial septal defect, 600
auscultatory technique and, 163–64
aids to, 195
Austin Flint, 193
aortic regurgitation and, 746, 1316
AV canal, 607
carcinoid and, 1298–99
cardiomyopathy, 1191, 1201, 1204
carditis and, 1308
Carey Coombs, 1308
chest deformities and, 134
clicks and, 184
coarctation of aorta, 629
continuous, 194–95
coronary arteriovenous fistula, 194, 257
coronary artery anomalies, 709
coronary heart disease, 893
cor triatriatum, 651
diastolic, 192–93
auscultatory principles and, 163
Duroziez's, 747
ejection, 188–91, 195
endocarditis and, 1142–43
grading, 195
Graham Steell, 193
heard by patient, 121
high-cardiac-output state and, 396
holosystolic (pansystolic), 191–92
honk and, 185
innocent, 189
insurance and, 1560, 1561
left ventricular-right atrial communication and, 613
mitral valve, 160, 163
diastolic, 192–93
regurgitation, 191, 192, 650, 770
stenosis, 192, 648, 757–58
origin theory of, 160
patent ductus arteriosus, 194, 615
prosthetic valve, 188
pulmonary atresia, 660
pulmonary hypertension, 1098
pulmonary regurgitation, 193
pulmonic stenosis, 189–90, 656, 659
regurgitant, 191
sinus of Valsalva fistula, 621
Still's, 189
systolic, 188–92
auscultatory principles, 163
tetralogy of Fallot, 663
transmission of, 160–61
transposition of great arteries, corrected, 701
tricuspid valve, 160, 163
diastolic, 192–93
regurgitation, 191, 677, 795
stenosis, 192, 193, 795
truncus arteriosus, 671
ventricular filling, 163
ventricular septal defect, 192, 194, 592–93
ventricular septal rupture, 983
Muscle:
bridges of, coronary arteries and, 1019–20, 1800
calcium channel blockers and, 1625–26
cardiac. *See* Myocardium.
exercise and, 1398, 1400
Hill's model of, 40
ischemia, arteriosclerosis obliterans and, 1340
mechanics, 40–50
afterload: aortic impedance, 47–48
anesthesia and, 50
atrial function, 48–49
contractility, 46–47. *See also* Contractility.
drugs and, 49
fundamentals, 40–42
heart rate and, 48
neural control, 49
postextrasystolic potentiation, 50
preload (Starling principle), 41–46
sequence of contraction, 48
suction, ventricular, 48
neurological disorders and, 1227–31
potentials, pacemaker malfunctions and, 504
relaxants, 1497
respiratory, assessment of, 387
shock and, 378
smooth. *See* Smooth-muscle cells.
Muscular dystrophy, 126, 571–72, 1227–28
clinical manifestations, 1227–28
pathology, 1227–28
treatment, 1228
X-linked, 571
Mustard operation, 695
Myasthenia gravis, 1230–31
Mycoplasma pneumoniae, 1174
Mycotic aneurysm, endocarditis and, 1143–44, 1151
Mydriatics, 198
Myeloma, 1226
Myocardial infarction, 842–50
accelerated AV junctional rhythm and, 974
accelerated idioventricular rhythm and, 976
activity level and, 969, 972
acute, 842–50
consequences of, 847–50
data gathering and, 312
aneurysms and, ventricular, 986–87
angina pectoris after, 962–63
definition and recognition, 962
treatment, 962–63
anticoagulants and, 831, 943, 1672–73
anxiety and, 934–35, 985
aortic dissection vs., 910
arrest and, 982, 986
arrhythmias and, 925, 968–69
drug therapy, 830–31
as early complication, 972–77
as late complication, 985–86
arteriography and, 904
uncomplicated disease and, 970
aspirin and, 831, 944, 1677–78
atrial fibrillation and, 974
atrial flutter and, 974
atrial tachycardia and, 973–74
AV block and, 427–28, 977
pacing and, 489
AV junctional tachycardia and, 974
beta blockers and, 1615–16

Myocardial infarction:
bundle branch block and, 977
calcification and, 873
capillaries and, 867–69
cardiomyopathy and, ischemic, 930, 931
cerebrovascular disease and, 1359
chronic phase, 301–4
coagulation necrosis, 531, 532, 844–46, 875, 1522
collateral flow and, 843, 844
completed, 968–87
definition, 968
complications, 927–29, 972–87
definition and recognition, 972
early, 972–85
late, 985–87
computed tomography and, 1867–68
contraceptive agents and, 1482
contractility and, 942
contraction band necrosis, 846, 873–74
coronary bypass surgery and, 950
early evolving lesions and, 968
perioperative infarction and, 2040
creatine kinase and, 897, 898
depression (mental) and, 934–35, 985, 987, 1531
diabetes mellitus and, 829, 1427–28, 1430
digitalis and, 942, 1644, 1645
heart failure and, 980
uncomplicated disease and, 971
Dressler's (postinfarction) syndrome and, 987
drug therapy, 830–31
early evolving disease and, 967–68
lipid-lowering, 829
long-term, 971–72
early phase, 300–301
ECG and, 210–12
acute, 312
AV block and, 977
bundle branch block and, 218
decision-making and, 302
exercise, 312, 896
hemiblock and, 214, 215, 217
limitations of, 895
pacemakers and, 495
prolonged, 971
Q waves, 209–10
right ventricular, 212, 895
subendocardial, 211–12
transmural, 210–11
vectorial, 1689–90
ventricular fibrillation and, 541
echocardiography, 970–71, 1953, 1960–62
ejection fraction and, 302–3, 926, 978, 1824
electromechanical dissociation and, 982
embolism and, 1673
systemic arterial, 983
emotional stress and, 985, 987
enzymes and, 897–99
histochemical techniques and, 877
historical notes on, 886
limitations of assays of, 898–99
size of infarct and, 898
estrogen and, 826, 829
evolving, 924–26, 966–68
definition and recognition, 966
treatment, 966–68

Myocardial infarction:
exercise and, 829–30, 1028–29, 1713
seven-step program, 1030
exercise testing, 312, 1711, 1712
prognosis and, 926
uncomplicated disease and, 969–70
expansion of, 847, 848, 876–77
extension of, 877
prognosis and, 929
fibrinolytic agents and, 943
focal block and, 217
friction rub and, 1267
gallop and, 180
atrial, 178
glucose and, 1430
heart failure and, 930, 931
as early complication, 978–80
as late complication, 986
hemodynamics, 978–80
hemorrhagic, 873
histochemical markers and, 877
hypertension and, 828
hypotension and, 375, 980–82
insurance and, 1558
islands (peninsulas) of normal tissue and, 867–68
lactic dehydrogenase and, 897–98
lateral border zone, 867
legal issues and, 1568–69
magnetic resonance imaging and, 1892–93
mitral regurgitation and, 767, 984, 2041
monitoring, 979–80, 2002–3
morphology, 872–78
methods of studying, 877–78
myocarditis and, 1158
myocytolytic, 846, 875
pain from:
persistent, 978, 985
relief of, 966–67, 978
papillary muscle dysfunction and, 984
papillary muscle rupture and, 393, 394, 984, 2041
prognosis and, 929
pathology, 842–50, 866–78
patterns of, 872–78
pericarditis and, 982–83, 1264, 1267
perioperative, 1513–14, 1518
coronary bypass surgery and, 2040
polyarteritis nodosa and, 1439
premature atrial beats and, 973
premature ventricular beats and, 451, 830–31, 974–75, 986
prognosis, 924–30
index for, 927–28
psychological factors and, 1523, 1530–31
pulmonary embolism and, 983, 1673
radionuclide studies, 312, 899–902, 970, 1824
prognosis and, 927
pyrophosphate imaging, 1844–48
thallium imaging, 899–900, 1833–34
recurrent, preventive measures and, 827–32
rehabilitation after. *See* Rehabilitation.
reperfusion and, 844, 872–74
right ventricular, 846, 981–82
ECG and, 212, 875
hemodynamic assessment, 978–79

Myocardial infarction:
risk region and, 843, 868
risk stratification and, 926–27
rupture of heart and, 393–94, 847, 850, 984–85, 2040–41
sexual activity and, 936
SGOT and, 897
shock and, 371–72, 393, 982
shoulder-hand syndrome and, 987
silent, diabetes mellitus and, 1427–28
sinus bradycardia and, 436–37, 973
sinus node dysfunction and, 973
sinus tachycardia and, 972–73
site of, 846–47
size of:
enzymes and, 898
prognosis and, 925
pyrophosphate imaging and, 1848
skeletal framework and, 876
smoking and, 823, 827–28
spasm of coronary arteries and, 871–72, 1012–13
subendocardial, 846, 872
ECG and, 211–12
sudden death and, 541, 850
pathology, 531, 532, 536
uncomplicated disease and, 969
thrombosis and, 843, 870, 1022
anticoagulants and, 1672–73
early evolving infarction and, 967–68
echocardiography and, 1962
plaque rupture and, 870–71
venous, 983, 1673
transmural, 846–47, 872
ECG and, 210–11
treatment, 965–87. *See also* Coronary heart disease, treatment.
calcium channel blockers in, 1633
digitalis in. *See* digitalis and *above.*
drug, 829–31, 967–68, 971–72
evolving disease and, 966–68
length of hospitalization, 969
lipid-lowering agents in, 829
platelet-controlling agents in, 831, 943–44, 1677–78
thrombolytic agents in, 843–44, 967–68, 1917–19
uncomplicated disease and, 968–72
tricuspid regurgitation and, 794
triphenyl tetrazolium chloride (TTC) stain and, 877–78
uncomplicated, 926–27, 968–72
definition and recognition, 968
treatment, 968–72
vasculitis and, 1022–23
vectorcardiography and, 896–97, 1689–90
ventricular fibrillation and, 541, 542, 975, 976
ventricular functional assessment and, 926, 928–29
ventricular septal rupture and, 393–94, 983–84
ventricular tachycardia and, 975–76, 985–86
wavefront progression of, 872
work status and, 830, 1035
Myocardial ischemia, 856–78. *See also* Atherosclerosis; Coronary heart disease.
arrhythmias and, 957, 961, 988–89
assessment, 299–312
general approach, 299–300

Myocardial ischemia: assessment:
likelihood of disease and, 300–308
prognosis and, 310–12
severity of disease and, 309–10
asymptomatic:
definition and recognition, 958, 959–60
exercise testing and, 1713–14
management, 958, 960–61
prognosis, 920
ATP and, 98
blood flow and, 857–64. *See also* Coronary blood flow.
cardiomyopathy and, 989. *See also* Cardiomyopathy, ischemic.
causes, 856–65
collateral flow and, 862–63
congenital anomalies and, 1016–20
coronary sinus studies and, 309
early profound, 924, 965–66
definition and recognition, 965–66
treatment, 966
ECG and, 210, 894–96
echocardiography and, 1960–62
embolism and, 1021
exercise testing and, 306–8, 921, 1709–14
fatty acids and, 92, 93
hyperbaric oxygen therapy and, 1553–54
irreversible. *See also* Mycardial infarction.
prognosis and, 924–30
magnetic resonance imaging and, 1892–93
metabolic disorders and, 97–98
oxygen consumption and, 864–66
oxygen supply and, 861–62, 865–66
pain from, 113–14, 890–93. *See also* Angina pectoris.
prolonged, 113, 890
recurrent, postinfarction, 978, 985
pathology, 842, 866–78
pathophysiology, 856–66
precordial bulge and, 155
premature ventricular beats and, 284, 285
prolonged, 964–65
definition and recognition, 964–65
prognosis and, 924
treatment, 949, 965
protein metabolism and, 97
pulmonary embolism and, 915–16
pulmonary hypertension and, 915
radionuclide studies, 1835–36
reversible, 958–65
prognosis, 920–24
stable subsets, 958–61
treatment, 959–65
unstable subsets, 961–65
risk region and, 843, 868
severe, 866
silent. *See* asymptomatic *above.*
steal mechanism and, 863–64
subendocardium and, 859–61, 865
sudden death and, 850, 929–30
symptoms, 889–93
treatment, 959–66. *See also* Coronary heart disease, treatment.
angioplasty, 945–46. *See also* Angioplasty, percutaneous transluminal.
asymptomatic disease and, 958, 960–61
bypass surgery, 946–56. *See also* Coronary bypass surgery.

Myocardial ischemia: treatment:
drug, 866, 937–45
early profound disease and, 966
oxygen supply-demand considerations, 865–66, 937–38
prolonged episodes and, 949, 965
reversible disease and, 959–65
vasospasm and, coronary artery, 862
wall motion in, echocardiography and, 1961
Myocarditis, 1158–79
arrhythmias and, 1165, 1168, 1170, 1178
assessment, 259–61, 1165–72
bacterial, 1173
biopsy and, 1168
cardiomyopathy and, 1183
catheterization studies, 1168
Chagas' disease and, 1169–70. *See also* Chagas' disease.
coxsackie virus, 259–60, 1158, 1177
clinical manifestations, 1169
laboratory studies, 1169
diphtheritic, 1159
clinical manifestations, 1168
laboratory studies, 1168
pathophysiology, 1163–65
prognosis, 1176
treatment, 1178
echinococcosis and, 1158, 1177, 1179
clinical manifestations, 1172
laboratory studies, 1172
pathology, 1160–61
pathophysiology, 1165
echocardiography, 1166
echovirus, 1169
electrocardiography, 1166, 1168
diphtheria and, 1168, 1170
echovirus and, 1171
endocarditis and, 1161
etiology, 1158–59
exercise testing and, 1168
fungal, 1161, 1175
gas gangrene and, 1163, 1164
genetics, 570–71
heart failure and, 1165, 1168, 1178
helminthic, 1176
history, 1165
idiopathic, 1158
immunosuppression and, 1159, 1177
infarction and, 1158
laboratory tests, 1166–68
leukemia and, 1159, 1161
lupus erythematosus and, 1437
Lyme disease and, 570–71
mumps, 1160
natural history and prognosis, 1172–77
pain from, 1165
pathology (morphology), 1159–63
pathophysiology, 1163–65
physical examination, 1165–66
pregnancy and, 1386, 1387
protozoal, 1175–76
radionuclide studies, 1166–67
rarer forms of, 1173–76
rheumatic, 1309
rickettsial, 1174
roentgenography, 1166
spirochetal, 1173–74
sudden death and, 531, 1163
syphilitic, 1173, 1318
tachycardia and, 1165, 1170, 1178
toxic, 1233, 1234
treatment, 1177–79

Myocarditis:
trichinosis and, 1158, 1179
clinical manifestations, 1170–72
laboratory studies, 1172
pathology, 1160
pathophysiology, 1165
viral, 1158, 1159, 1163, 1174–75
clinical manifestations, 1165, 1166, 1169
Myocardium. *See also* Cardiomyopathy; Myocardial infarction; Myocardial ischemia; Myocarditis.
abscess, 1159, 1161
action potential. *See* Action potential.
aging and, 1404–5
amyloidosis and, 1213–15
biopsy, 272. *See also* Biopsy, endomyocardial.
blood flow, 857–64. *See also* Coronary blood flow.
bridges of coronary arteries, 1019–20, 1800
capillaries, 861–62
infarction and, 867–69
carcinoid, 1215
cell types in, 31–32
contusion, 1278–80
depressant factor, shock and, 381
diabetes mellitus and, 85–86
drug and chemical toxicity and, 1231–36
drug hypersensitivity and, 1236–37
enzymes, 897–99. *See also* Enzymes.
excitation-contraction coupling, 37–39, 1476
failure (depression, dysfunction), 265–66
assessment, 270–72
catheterization studies, 276–77
cerebral hypoperfusion and, 1361
definition, 320
dysdynamic, 321
echocardiography, 272, 276
hemodynamics, 334
mechanisms of, 329–31
mitral regurgitation and, 268, 269, 275
primary and secondary, 321
renal failure and, 1462–63
sudden death and, 540
tricuspid regurgitation and, 677
valvular disease and, 273–75. *See also* specific valve.
without heart failure, 268
fatty acids and, 91–94
fibers. *See* Fibers; Myofibrils.
glycogen and, 89
disorders of, 1219–20
glycolysis and, 87–91
hematologic diseases and, 1226–27
hydatid cysts, 1161
inflammation. *See* Myocarditis.
iron deposits in, 1221–22
mechanical activity, 40–50
afterload, 40, 41, 47–48
aging and, 1404–5
anesthesia and, 50
aortic impedance and, 47–48
atrial function, 48–49
contractility. *See* Contractility.
drugs and, 49
fundamentals, 40–42
heart rate and, 48
neural control, 49
postextrasystolic potentiation, 50

Myocardium: mechanical activity:
preload, 41–46
sequence of contraction, 48
suction, ventricular, 48
metabolism, 85–99. *See also* Metabolism.
metastases to, 1296
mucopolysaccharidoses and, 1224–25
muscular dystrophy and, 1227–28
myasthenia gravis and, 1230–31
myotonia atrophica and, 1230
necrosis, 844–47. *See also* Myocardia infarction.
coagulation, 531, 532, 844–46, 875, 1522
contraction band, 846, 873–74
histologic pattern, 532
myocytolytic. *See* Myocytolysis.
progressive systemic sclerosis and, 1442–43
site of, 846–47
sudden death and, 531, 536, 1522
Zenker, 531, 532, 536
neuromuscular disease and, 1227–31
norepinephrine and, 323
nutritional disorders and, 1218–19
oxygen consumption, 56–57, 864–66
altitude and, 1545
aortic stenosis and, 732
bypass surgery and, 947
contractility and, 865, 866
determinants of, 57, 864–65
heart failure and, 329–30
heart rate and, 864
systolic wall tension and, 865
therapeutic considerations, 865–66
oxygen supply, 861–62
bypass surgery and, 947
therapeutic considerations, 865–66
perfusion. *See also* Coronary blood flow.
thallium imaging and, 1831–44
pheochromocytoma and, 1219
physical agents damaging, 1237
preservation of:
calcium channel blockers and, 1633
cardiopulmonary bypass and, 2027–29
coronary bypass surgery and, 852–53, 2037–38
primary disease, 276–77. *See also* Cardiomyopathy.
protein turnover, 85, 86, 94–97
pyruvate, 90
radiation damage to, 1485, 1486
Raynaud's phenomenon, 1442
Refsum's disease and, 1225
relaxation, 38–39
aging and, 1404–5
reperfusion, 844, 872–74
cardiopulmonary bypass and, 2028–29
pathology of, 844
thallium imaging and, 1834
thrombolytic therapy and, 1918
rheumatoid nodules of, 1439
ruptured, 1278–79
sarcoidosis and, 1216–18
sliding filament hypothesis and, 33–34
systemic disease and, 1216–40
thyroid hormone and, 1415
ultrastructure, 31–34
Starling's law and, 44–45
Myocytolysis, 846, 875
cardiomyopathy and, 1183
Myocytolysis:
coagulative, sudden death and, 1522
emetine toxicity and, 1231
sudden death and, 531, 532
Myofibrils, 32–35
excitation-contraction coupling and, 38
hypertrophic cardiomyopathy and, 1193, 1196
Myoglobin, 51
Myopathy:
cardiac. *See* Cardiomyopathy.
familial centronuclear, 1231
genetics, 568–72
mitochondrial, 569
Myopotentials, pacemakers and, 504
Myosin, 32–34
action potential and, 38
antibodies to, radiolabeling and, 1849
ATPase, 98–99
heart failure and, 330
isozymes of, 86, 98
light chain kinase, 1009
smooth-muscle contractility and, 1009–10
Starling's law and, 44
Myotonia atrophica, 1230
Myotonia dystrophica, 128, 571
Myxedema, 1418–22
adult idiopathic, 1419
coma, 1419
hoarseness and, 121
juvenile, 1418
pericardial effusion and, 1270, 1420
Myxoma, 1284–92
age, sex, and familial factors, 1285
angiography, 1289–90, 1291
aortic-mitral valve prolapse and, 785
aortic regurgitation and, 741
apexcardiogram, 1288
bilateral atrial, 1292
catheterization studies, 1288–89, 1291
differential diagnosis, 1290, 1292
ECG and x-ray, 1287–88, 1291
echocardiography, 1288, 1291, 1954, 1960
embolism from, 1286–87, 1291, 1359
infected, 1286
left atrial, 1287–90
left ventricular, 1292
manifestations, 1285–86, 1290–91
mitral obstruction and, 253, 759
mitral regurgitation and, 765–66
pathology, 1284–85
physical examination, 1287, 1291
radionuclide studies, 1288
right atrial, 1290–92
right ventricular, 1292
surgical resection, 1292, 1293
syncope and, 522
tricuspid obstruction and, 254–55

NAD, NADH. *See* Nicotine adenine dinucleotide.
Nadolol, 1607. *See also* Beta-blocking agents.
dosage, 941, 1072
hypertension and, 1081
pharmacodynamics, 1608, 1613, 1617
pharmacokinetics, 1610, 1611
protein-binding and dialysance, 1082
structure, 1608
Nafcillin, endocarditis and, 1149
Nails, inspection of, 132
Naloxone, 939, 1504
Nanism, mulibrey, 128, 573, 1239
pericarditis and, 1271
Narcan, 939
Narcotics:
anesthetic, 1496
antagonists to, 1504
National Transportation Safety Board, 1579
Natriuresis, 1658
edema and, 1663
Natriuretic factor, atrial, 325, 326
Natriuretic hormone, 1657
Naughton test, 1705
Nausea, 121
Neck vein distension, 135, 147
heart failure and, 351
Necropsy, 2077–80
cardiomyopathy and, 2079
congenital malformations and, 2079
coronary heart disease and, 2078
hypertension and, 2079
pericardial and pulmonary disease and, 2079
principles of, 2077–78, 2080
Necrosis:
cystic medial, of aorta, 1322, 1330
regurgitation and, 644, 741–43
myocardial, 844–47. *See also* Myocardial infarction; Myocardium, necrosis.
Negligence, 1565, 1573–74
Neodymium-yttrium-aluminum garnet laser, 1922, 1924
Neomycin:
cholesterol and, 823
digitalis and, 1647
Neonate. *See also* Congenital heart disease.
circulation in, 583–84
diabetic mother and, 1429–30
heart failure in, 584–86
pulmonary circulation in, 1093
pulmonary hypertension in, 584, 587
respiratory distress syndrome in, 586
Neoplasia. *See* Tumors.
Neovascularization, retinal, 200
Nephritis, hypertension and, 1060
Nephrosclerosis, 1055–56
benign, 1055
hypertension and, 1055–56
malignant, 1055–56
Nephrotic syndrome:
diuretics and, 1662
hypertension and, 1060
Nernst equation, 74
Nervous system. *See also* Cerebrovascular disease.
arrhythmias and, 424
autonomic. *See* Autonomic nervous system; Parasympathetic nervous system; Sympathetic nervous system.
beta-blocking agents and, 1612–13, 1620
catheterization studies and, 1361
coronary blood flow and, 61–62
decompression sickness and, 1551
diabetes mellitus and, 1427–28
electrical stimulation of, 1487–88
embolization, myxomatous, 1286
endocarditis and, 1143
heart failure and, 323–24
heart innervation, 24–25

Nervous system:
hypertension and, 1040, 1042–46, 1071–74
hyperthyroidism and, 1415
multiple system atrophy and, 512
muscle mechanics and, 49
myocardial disease and, 1227–31
shock and, 374–76
syncope and, 511–13
cerebrovascular, 513–14
thoracic outlet syndrome and, 916–18
vascular control by, 59–60
Neuralgia, glossopharyngeal, 516–17
Neuritis, optic, 201
Neurocirculatory asthenia, 1526, 1533
Neoromuscular disease, 1227–31
chest pain and, 916–18
gait and, 126
X-linked humeroperoneal, 1228
Neuropathy:
diabetic, 1427–28
hypertension and, 1045
Neuropeptide tyrosine Y, 63
Neurosis:
anxiety, 1526–27, 1533
cardiac, 1541
Neuroxanthoendothelioma, 1239
Newton, Isaac, 475
New York Heart Association criteria committee, 106, 931–32
Niacin, pellagra and, 1218
Nicotine adenine dinucleotide:
fatty acids and, 92, 93
myocardial, 86
ischemia and, 98
pyruvate metabolism and, 90
shock and, 378
Nicotinic acid, cholesterol and, 822, 829
Niemann-Pick disease, 1224
Nifedipine, 941. *See also* Calcium channel blockers.
adverse effects, 1073, 1634
angina pectoris and, 1629
arteriospasm and, 1353
coronary artery, 1014–15
cardiomyopathy and, 1207
dosage, 1072
and effects, 1586
and therapeutic levels, 1628
heart failure and, 1632–33
interactions of, 1634
pharmacodynamics, 1625–27
pharmacology, 1587–88
structure, 1624–25
surgical procedures and, 1514
Nifurtimox, 1179
Nimodipine, cerebral arterial spasm and, 1633–34
Nitrates, 1585
adverse reactions, 939, 1539
beta blockers and, 1614
calcium channel blockers and, 1630
cardiomyopathy and, 1192
contraindications, 939
coronary heart disease and, 939
indications, 939
occupational exposure to, 1577
pharmacology, 1585
tabulation of, 940
Nitroglycerin:
angina pectoris and, 887, 891
coronary arteriography and, 1793
coronary artery spasm and, 1014
dosage and effects, 1585
esophageal spasm and, 913
Nitroglycerin:
heart failure and, 363, 366
intravenous, myocardial infarction and, 966–67, 980
pharmacology, 1585
shock and, 393
surgical procedures and, 1514, 1515
Nitroglycol, 1577
Nitroprusside, 1586
aortic dissection and, 1333
cannulation procedures and, 1496
dosage and effects, 1586
heart failure and, 364, 1644
in infant, 586
myocardial infarction and, 980
pharmacology, 1586
preeclampsia and, 1085
protein-binding and dialysance, 1082
shock and, 393
surgical procedures and, 1515, 1516
Nitrous oxide, 1496
Nodoventricular fibers, 415, 416
ECG and, 220
reentry and, 417, 419, 426
ventricular tachycardia and, 425
Nodules:
hemorrhagic, 125
Osler's, 132, 1142
rheumatoid, of myocardium, 1439
subcutaneous, rheumatic fever and, 1309
Nodulus Arantii, 22
Noises heard by patient, 121
Nomenclature and Criteria for Diagnosis of Diseases of the Heart and Great Vessels, 106–8
Nomifensine, 1533
Nondisjunction, chromosomal, 567
Noonan's syndrome, 128, 129
cardiomyopathy and, 1238
Norepinephrine. *See also* Catecholamines.
alpha receptors and, 1654
beta receptors and, 1606, 1654
biochemistry and pharmacokinetics, 1654
calcium and, 1654
cardiomyopathy and, 1184
hypertrophic, 1193
contractility and, 1653, 1654
CPR and, 552
heart failure and, 323, 335, 347
hypertension and, 1040
inhibitors of, 1588–89
muscle physiology and, 49
orthostatic hypotension and, 512
pharmacologic actions, 1654
pheochromocytoma and, 1046, 1065
shock and, 376
management of, 391
structure, 1653
syncope and, 509
thyroid hormone and, 1415
toxicity of, 1234
vasoconstriction and, 59, 1590
Norethisterone, hypertension and, 1084
Normal heart, 1–99
anatomy, 16–35
electrical activity, 73–84
embryology, 3–15
metabolic regulation and myocardial function, 85–99
physiology, 37–63
Normodyne. *See* Labetalol.
Norpace. *See* Disopyramide.
Nortriptyline, 1479–80
Nose, cartilage destruction in, 129
Nosocomial endocarditis, 1134–35
Nuclear magnetic resonance. *See* Magnetic resonance imaging.
Nuclear power cells, 491
Nuclear probe, 1812, 1829–30
ventricular function and, 387
Nuclear studies. *See* Radionuclide studies.
Nucleotides. *See* Adenosine monophosphate; Adenosine triphosphate.
Nutrition, 1448–50. *See also* Diet.
hyperalimentation, 1449–50
myocardial disease and, 1218–19

Obesity, 1452–56
atherosclerosis and, 824–25, 829, 936, 1453
blood flow and, 1452, 1454
blood pressure mesurement and, 1452–53
cardiac output and, 404, 1454
cardiomyopathy and, 1453–55
digitalis and, 1641
hypertension and, 1078–79, 1452–53
hypertrophy and, ventricular, 1453, 1454
hypoventilation and, 1455–56
sleep apnea and, 1455
sudden death and, 1455
therapeutic considerations, 1456
weight reduction and, 1456
Oblique vein of Marshall, 30
Obtuse marginal lymphatic, 25
Occlusive disease, 1339–50. *See also* Atherosclerosis.
acute, 1348–50
angioplasty for. *See* Angioplasty.
aortic arch, 1334
aortoiliac, 1335–36, 1345
surgical treatment of, 2058–60
arteriosclerosis obliterans, 1339–46
carotid-vertebrobasilar, 513–14
cerebral. *See* Cerebrovascular disease.
chronic, 1339–48
Doppler studies and, 1975, 1976
femoropopliteal, 1345–46
surgical treatment of, 2060–61
hepatic vein, 1366–67
hyperbaric oxygen therapy and, 1553
incidence, 558
laser therapy for, 1922–25
lumbar sympathectomy and, 2061
mesenteric, 1364–70. *See also* Mesenteric vascular occlusion.
popliteal-tibial, 1346
portal vein, 1366
pulmonary vein, 1100, 1124
subclavian, 514
surgical procedures for, 2057–62
thromboangiitis obliterans, 1346–48
Occupation, 1577–79. *See also* Work status.
emotional stress and, 1571, 1572
job-related injury and, 1563–64, 1579
causality assessment of, 1571
history and, 1575
rehabilitation and, 1035–36
toxic exposures and, 1577–78
Ochronosis, 1226
Oculomucocutaneous syndrome, beta-blocker-induced, 1621
Oculopneumoplethysmography, 1877–78

Odynophagia, 912
Ohm's law, 1784
Oliguria, 121
  diuretics and, 1665
Omphalocele, 707
Omphalomesenteric veins, 10
Oncotic pressure, shock and, 373–74, 388
Opening snaps, 185–86
  mitral valve, 185
    stenosis and, 756
  tricuspid valve, 186
Ophthalmic artery, 1875
  systolic pressure, 1877–78
Ophthalmitis, endocarditis and, 1142
Ophthalmoplegia, chronic progressive external, 1231
Opiates, coronary heart disease and, 938–39
Optic atrophy, 201
Optic disk edema, 201, 203
Oral contraceptive agents. *See* Contraceptive agents.
Orthopnea, 116
  heart failure and, 349
Orthostatic hypertension, 1074
Orthostatic hypotension, 510–13
  diabetes mellitus and, 1427
Osler, W., 265, 1025
Osler's nodes, 132
  endocarditis and, 1142
Osmotic pressure:
  pulmonary capillary pressure and, 1092
  shock and, 373
Osteogenesis imperfecta, 573
Osteoporosis:
  estrogen therapy and, 1426
  heparin-associated, 1668–69
Ostium primum, 9
  atrial septal defect and, 605–6, 611
  embryology, 11
Ostium secundum:
  atrial septal defect and, 12, 598, 599
    assessment, 255–56, 600, 601
    management, 602, 603
  embryology, 11, 12
Ouabain, 1646
  heart failure and, 1644
Ovaries, estrogen secretion by, 1424
Overload:
  pressure. *See* Afterload.
  volume. *See* Preload.
Overweight. *See* Obesity.
Oxalosis, 1226
Oxidative substrates, 85–86, 87
  fatty acids and, 93
  protein metabolism and, 96
Oxprenolol, 1607. *See also* Beta-blocking agents.
  dosage, 1072
  hypertension and, gestational, 1085
  pharmacodynamics, 1608, 1613, 1618
  pharmacokinetics, 1610, 1611
  structure, 1608
Oxygen:
  altitude (high) and, 1543–45
  arteriovenous difference, 55, 56
  cardiac catheterization and, 1774, 1776–77
  cardiac output calculation and, 1779
  cardiopulmonary bypass and, 2026–27, 2028
  consumption rates, systemic, 56
  coronary blood flow and, 60–61
Oxygen:
  dissociation curve, 379
    altitude and, 1543, 1545
  exercise and, 1398
    capacity, 270
    testing, 1706
  heart failure and, 329–30
    peripheral delivery in, 328
  hemoglobin affinity for, 379
  increased extraction of, 51
  maximal uptake of, 270, 1400
  mixed venous blood and, 385–86, 1777
  myocardial consumption, 56–57 864–66
    altitude and, 1545
    aortic stenosis and, 732
    bypass surgery and, 947
    contractility and, 865, 866
    determinants of, 57, 864–65
    heart failure and, 329–30
    heart rate and, 864
    systolic wall tension and, 865
    therapeutic considerations, 865–66
  myocardial supply, 861–62
    bypass surgery and, 947
    therapeutic considerations, 865–66
  tension:
    altitude and, 1543–45
    decreased. *See* Hypoxia.
    ductus arteriosus closure and, 583
    ischemia and, 861
    mitochondria and, 861
    mixed venous, 385–86
    pulmonary embolism and, 1108
  therapy, 389
    carbon monoxide poisoning and, 1554
    cerebrovascular insufficiency and, 1553
    coronary heart disease and, 937–38
    cor pulmonale and, 1126–27
    fat embolism and, 1115
    hyperbaric, 1553–54
    myocardial ischemia and, 1553–54
Oxygenators, 2026–27

P cells, 31–32
P wave. *See also* Electrocardiography.
  aberranta conduction and, 458
  absent, 461–62
  AV block and, 464, 465
  AV junctional extrasystoles and, 439
  determination of, 73
  esophageal ECG and, 1694–1702
  genesis, 82
  His bundle recording and, 1729
  normal, 206
  potassium and, 1471
  premature atrial beats and, 437
  sinus tachycardia and, 437
  supraventricular tachycardia and, 420, 421, 441–43
  wandering pacemaker and, 469
PA interval, 1729
Pacemakers, 482–83, 486–505. *See also* Pacing.
  artifacts, 1757
  cardiomyopathy and, 1207–8
  carotid sinus pressure and, 1759
  chest wall stimulation and, 1758–59
  classification code, 495
  computer assessment, 1757
  demand, 482, 497
    malfunction, 503
Pacemakers:
  ECG, 494–95, 1756
    malfunction and, 502–3
    prolonged, 1759
  electrodes, 492
  environmental interference with, 504
  epicardial, 2016–20
    complications, 2020
    implantation technique, 2016–20
  fluoroscopy and, 1768
  historical aspects, 487
  impedance, 1751
  implantation, 1747–54
    atrial lead, 1751–53
    coronary sinus lead, 1753
    dual-chamber system, 1753
    epicardial, 2016–20
    personnel and equipment, 1747–48
    postoperative care, 1754
    preoperative preparation, 1747
    pulse generator, 1753
    transvenous, 1747–54
    vein isolation, 1748–49
    ventricular lead, 1747–51
  leads, 491–94
    bipolar and unipolar, 491–92
    conductor, 492
    connector, 493
    epimyocardial, 493–94
    fixation, 493
    insulator, 492
    transvenous atrial, 493
  malfunctions and complications, 501–5, 1540, 1757–60
    epicardial implantation, 2020
    flow diagram for investigating, 502
    tabulation of common, 1760
  noncardiac surgery and, 1515
  oscilloscopic analysis, 1757, 1758
  pace out of tachycardia and, 1699, 1700
  positioning of leads, 1749–50
  programmable, 499–501
  pulse generators, 490–91. *See also* Pulse generators.
  radio-frequency, 482
  radiography and, 1750, 1752, 1758
  reprogramming, 1757, 1758
  R-wave size and, 1750–51
  sensors for, 498–99, 501
    malfunction of, 503–4
  sequential, 482
  slew rate, 1751
  sounds produced by, 188
  syncope and, 288, 524, 528
    carotid sinus syndrome and, 516
    orthostatic hypotension and, 513
  tachycardia and, esophageal leads and, 1698–1701
  telemetry and, 500, 1758
  telephonic monitoring of, 1755–56
  testing, 1755–60
    clinic for, 1755–56
    electronic, 1756–57, 1758
    environmental, 1759
    at implantation, 1750–51
    invasive, 1759–60
    investigative procedures, 1757–60
    noninvasive, 1758–59
    provocative movements and, 1759
    routine follow-up, 1755–57
  thresholds, 1757, 1759
    pacing, 1751
    stimulation, 1751
  twiddler's syndrome, 505

Pacemakers:
vector analysis, 1757
wandering, 468–69
Pacing, 482–83. *See also* Pacemakers.
artifacts, 501–3, 1757
asystole and, 551
atrial, 496
arrhythmias induced by, 1737–38
asynchronous, 496
bradycardia and, 1740
catheterization studies and, 1776
constant, 1736
esophageal lead for, 1698
flutter and, 476
implantation of leads for, 1751–53
incremental, 1736
inexcitability and, 490
inhibited, 496
J lead, 1751–52
leads, 493, 1751–53
premature stimulation, 1735–37
rapid, 1735, 1737
screw-in lead, 1752–53
synchronous, 497–98
tachycardia and, 1740
therapeutaic applications, 1740
triggered, 596
automaticity and, 78–79
AV block and, 480–81, 488–89
bundle branch block and, 481–82, 488, 494, 495
burst, 1737
cardiac output and, 498
contraindications, 487
coronary sinus, 1753
Cybertach-60 system, 499
dual-chamber (atroventricular), 496–98, 501
epicardial, 2019–20
lead implantation, 1753
fully automatic, 498
fusion beats and, 494
hysteresis, 501
indications, 481–82, 487–90
modes of, 482–83, 495–99
overdrive, 482–83
paired stimulation, 483
PASAR system, 499
permanent, 481, 487
physiologic, 498
Purkinje fibers and, 80
rate, 498, 500
reentry and, 482
sick sinus syndrome and, 480, 489–90
simultaneous stimulation, 483
tachycardia and, 482, 490, 499–500, 1740
characteristics of ideal system for, 499
temporary, 481
torsades de pointes and, 479
underdrive, 482
ventricular, 495–96
asynchronous, 495
ECG and, 220–21
esophageal lead for, 1698
inhibited, 496, 497
lead implantation, 1747–51
triggered, 496
ventricular fibrillation and, 543
Paget's disease of bone, 402–3
Pain, 112–15
abdominal, 115
aortic aneurysm and, 1327
heart failure and, 351
Pain: abdominal:
ischemic colitis and, 1367
occlusive vascular disease and, 1334–35, 1364–66, 1368
postprandial, 1368
chest, 113–14. *See also* Angina pectoris.
anxiety and, 114, 907–8, 1527, 1531
aortic aneurysm and, 1325
aortic dissection and, 114, 910, 1331
aortic regurgitation and, 744
cardiomyopathy and, 909–10, 1200
colonic distension and, 915
diabetes mellitus and, 1427
duration of, 890
esophageal spasm and, 912
esophagitis and, 911
exercise testing and, 1714
gastrointestinal origin of, 911–15
history, 889–93
location, 890
mediastinal emphysema and, 916
myocardial infarction and, 966–67, 978, 985
myocardial ischemia and, 113–114, 890–93, 978. *See also* Angina pectoris.
myocarditis and, 1165
neuromuscular-skeletal causes of, 916–18
noncardiovascular, 114
pericarditis and, 114, 909, 982, 1251
pneumothorax and, 916
postsurgical, 989–90
premature beats and, 908–9
prolonged, 113, 890
pulmonary embolism and, 114, 1106
pulmonary hypertension and, 114, 915, 1098
Tietze's syndrome and, 918
trauma and, 1279
chest wall, 918
digital, Raynaud's disease and, 115
epigastric:
cholecystitis and, 913
peptaic ulcer and, 914
extremity, 114–15
acute occlusion and, 1349
aortoiliac occlusion and, 1336
arteriosclerosis obliterans and, 1340, 1344
hyperbarism and, 1551
thoracic outlet syndrome and, 917
thromboangiitis obliterans and, 1347
head, 115
joint, 115
Palate, 131
Pallor:
arteriosclerosis obliterans and, 1341
nail bed, 132
Paynaud's phenomenon and, 1352, 1353
syncope and, 508, 510
Palpation:
heart sounds and, 155–156
precordial, 152–56
pulse, 142–43
Palpitations, 117, 283–87
approach to patient with, 283–87
ECG and, 284–86
history, 283
mitral prolapse and, 285
mitral stenosis and, 756
Pancarditis, rheumatic, 1307
Pancreas, 1426
Pancreatitis, 914–15
Pancuronium, 1497
Panniculitis, relapsing febrile nodular non-suppurative, 1238–39
Panophthalmitis, endocarditis and, 1142
Pansystolic murmurs, 191–92
Papillary muscles:
anatomy, 21, 23
cardiomyopathy and, 1199
contraction, 41
dysfunction, infarction and, 984
echocardiography and, 1940
force-velocity relations, 42, 43, 45–46
frontal view, 20
length-tension relation, 44–45
mitral commissurotomy and, 763
mitral stenosis and, 754–55
ruptured:
assessment, 252
infarction and, 393, 394, 929, 984, 2041
mitral regurgitation and, 767
prognosis and, 929
surgical treatment of, 2041
trauma and, 1280
tricuspid regurgitation and, 794
sarcoidosis and, 1217
Papilledema, 201
Papillitis, 201
Papilloma, 1294
Papulosis, atrophic, 125
Para-aminosalicylic acid, hypersensitivity to, 1237
Paracetamol, 1237
Paradoxical critical rate, 458
Paragangliomas, 1046
Paramedics, 540
Parasympathetic nervous system, 24, 25
cardiomyopathy and, 1184
coronary blood flow and, 61
digitalis and, 1642, 1648
orthostatic hypotension and, 512
vasodilatation and, 59
Parasystole, 412, 456–57
artifactual, 1726
definition, 433
ECG, 456–57
ventricular tachycardia and, 452
Parathyroid glands, 1422
renal failure and, 1459, 1463
Parchment heart, 680
Parry, Caleb Hillier, 884
PASAR, 499
Pasteur, Louis, 557
Patent ductus arteriosus, 614–18
aorta and, 614–18
aortic arch interruption and, 634, 635
assessment, 257, 615–16
associated conditions, 614
catheterization studies, 616, 1777–78
cyanosis and, 615
definition, 614
Doppler studies, 1987
ECG, 616
echocardiography, 616
history, 615
medical management, 617
murmur, 194, 615
natural history and prognosis, 616–17
pathology, 614
pathophysiology, 614–15
physical examination, 615
pregnancy and, 615

Patent ductus arteriosus:
pulmonary artery and, 614–18
roentgenography, 615
surgical management, 617–18
Patient:
angina description by, 890
compliance by, 1534
concerns of, 104–5
feelings of, 111
heart attack description by, 122
living through day with, 111
Patient education:
cardiac catheterization and, 1769
coronary bypass surgery and, 950–51
hypertension and, 1534
iatrogenic heart disease and, 1541
rehabilitation and, 1029–31
Pavulon, 1497
Pectinate muscles, 18
Pectus excavatum, 134
Pellagra, 1218
Penbutolol, 1607
Penetrating injuries, 1022, 1276–78
tabulation of, 1277
Penicillin:
endocarditis and, 1131, 1149, 1153
hypersensitivity to, 1236
rheumatic fever and, 761, 1311, 1312
streptococcal pharyngitis and, 1311, 1312
Pentaerythrityl tetranitrate (Pentritol):
chemical structure, 940
dosage, 940
Pentalogy:
of Cantrell, 707
of Fallot, 662, 663
Pentobarbital, contractility and, 50
Peptic ulcer, 914
Percussion wave, pulse, 143–44
Percutaneous transluminal angioplasty. *See* Angioplasty, percutaneous transluminal.
Performance, cardiac, 266, 267. *See also* Heart failure; Myocardium, failure; Ventricles, functional assessment.
Perfusion. *See also* Blood flow; Coronary blood flow.
cardiopulmonary bypass and, 2027
cerebral, 1360–61
pulmonary. *See also* Pulmonary vasculature, blood flow.
radionuclide studies of, 1881–82
thallium imaging and, 1831–44
-ventilation scans, embolism and, 1108
Perfusion pressure, coronary, 857–61
critical level, 860*n*.
Periarteritis nodosa. *See also* Polyarteritis nodosa.
gastrointestinal, 1370
Pericardial effusion, 1254–56. *See also* Tamponade.
assessment, 262–63, 1254–55
chylous, 1271
CT scans and, 1869, 1870
echocardiography and, 262–63, 1254–55, 1953, 1954–55
etiology, 1254
fat stripe and, 1766, 1767
metastases and, 1268, 1297
myxedema (hypothyroidism) and, 1270, 1420
nature of fluid in, 1256
radiation-induced, 1268–69, 1484
Pericardial effusion:
renal failure and, 1267
silent, 1255
surgical management, 2008–13
Pericardiectomy, 1254, 2009–13
complications, 2012
constrictive disease and, 1265–66
indications, 2010, 2012
parietal, 2010–11
postoperative syndrome, 1267–68
radiation-induced disease and, 1485
results, 2012–13
technique, 2009–12
visceral, 2011–12
Pericardiocentesis, 1541, 2008–9
echocardiography and, 1955, 1956
metastatic disease and, 1268
vs. open drainage, 1262–63
radiation-induced disease and, 1485
technique, 2008–9
traumatic injuries and, 1277
Pericardiostomy, uremic pericarditis and, 1461–62
Pericardiotomy, 2009
technique, 2009
Pericarditis, 1251–66
acute, 1251–54
differential diagnosis, 1253
ECG, 1252–53
etiology, 1252
history, 1251
pathology, 1251
physical examination, 1251–52
treatment, 1253–54
assessment, 262–63, 1251–52, 1263
calcific, 252, 1264
cardiomyopathy vs., 262
cholesterol, 1271
constrictive, 1263–66
catheterization studies, 1263
chronic calcific, 1264
differential diagnosis, 1264
effusive, 1261, 1265
etiology, 1263
historical note on, 1256
localized, 1265
occult, 1265
pathophysiology, 1256–58
physical examination, 1263
postoperative, 1264–65
subacute, 1264
symptoms, 1263
treatment, 1265–66
CT scans and, 1870–71
dialysis and, 1266–67, 1461
drug-induced, 1269
ECG and, 212, 909, 1252–53
enzymes and, 909
histoplasmic, 1270
infectious (nonviral), 1269–71
lupus erythematosus and, 1269, 1436
magnetic resonance imaging and, 1893
meningococcal, 1270
myocardial infarction and, 982–83, 1264, 1267
pain from, 114, 909, 982, 1251
physical examination, 204, 1251–52, 1263
posttraumatic, 1268, 1278, 1280
progressive systemic sclerosis and, 1443–44
radiation-induced, 1268–69, 1484–85, 1486
recurrent, 1254
Pericarditis:
Reiter's disease and, 1238
renal failure and, 1460–62
rheumatic, 1307
rheumatoid arthritis and, 1269, 1439
roentgenography, 240
sounds and, knock, 186
staphylococcal, 1270
treatment, 1253–54, 1265–66, 2008–13
tuberculous, 1269–70
uremic, 1226, 1266–67, 1461
venous pulse and, 149, 150
viral, 1251–54
Pericardium, 1249–71
absence, 1266
anatomy, 23–24, 1249
biopsy, 2009
calcification, 262, 1264
compressive syndromes, 1256–66
computed tomography and, 1869–71
congenital defects, 712–13, 1266
cysts, 712–13, 1266, 1295
CT scan and, 1871
diverticula, 712–13
fluid, 1250. *See also* Pericardial effusion.
friction rubs. *See* Friction rubs.
functions, 1251
inflammation. *See* Pericarditis.
lipoma, 1294
mechanical (viscoelastic) properties, 1250–51
mesothelioma, 1295
operative treatment, 2008–13. *See also* Pericardiectomy; Pericardiocentesis; Pericardiotomy.
parietal, 24, 1249
patch from, AV canal and, 611
pressure, 1250, 1251, 1257
tamponande and. *See* Tamponade.
teratoma, 1295
trauma, 1268, 1278, 1280
tumors, 1268, 1295
metastatic, 1268, 1296, 1297
visceral. *See* Epicardium.
Periinfarction block, 216–17
Perilymph, 158
Periorbital edema, 118
Peripheral circulation, 1339–62
aging and, 1406–7
aneurysms, 1350–52
angioplasty of, 1908–10
Doppler studies, 1974–75
embolism, 1348–50
heart failure and, 335–36
occlusive disease, 1339–50. *See also* Atherosclerosis.
acute, 1348–50
aortoiliac, 1335–36, 1345, 2058–60
arteriosclerosis obliterans, 1339–46
chronic, 1339–48
femoropopliteal, 1345–46, 2060–61
hyperbaric oxygen therapy and, 1553
incidence, 558
popliteal-tibial, 1346
surgical procedures for, 2057–62
sympathectomy and, 2061
thromboangiitis obliterans, 1346–48
radionuclide studies and, 1822–23
spastic diseases, 1352–53
surgical procedures for, 2057–62
complications, 2061
indications, 2061–62

Peripheral circulation: surgical procedures for:
results, 2061
techniques, 2058–61
thrombosis, 1348–50
lytic agents and, 1917
veins, 1372–78
Peritrate, 940
Peroneal muscular atrophy, 572
Persantine. *See* Dipyridamole.
Personality:
coronary heart disease and, 826
type A, 1524–25, 1572
bypass surgery and, 1521, 1532
Petechiae:
endocarditis and, 1141–42
fat embolism and, 1115
Phagocytes, endocarditis and, 1148
Pharyngitis, streptococcal, rheumatic fever and, 1306–7, 1310, 1312
Phenformin, 1540
Phenindione, 1237
Phenothiazines, 1480–81
toxicity, 1232
Phenoxybenzamine, pheochromocytoma and, 1083
Phenprocoumon, myocardial infarction and, 1677
Phentolamine, 1589
dosage and effects, 1587
pheochromocytoma and, 1083
shock and, 393
Phenylbutazone, hypersensitivity to, 1238
Phenylephrine:
auscultation and, 195
cardiomyopathy and, 1184
vasoconstriction and, 1590
Phenylpropanolamine, 1235
Phenytoin. *See* Diphenylhydantoin.
Pheochromocytoma, 1064–66
clonidine suppression test and, 1065
diagnosis, 1064–66
hypertension and, 1046, 1064–66, 1083–84
localization, 1065–66
myocardial disease and, 1219
pericardial, 1295
treatment, 1083–84
Phlebitis, 1372–73
Phlebography, 1375, 1885–87
complications, 1886–87
indications, 1885
lower extremity, 1885–86
mediastinal, 1885
pulmonary embolism and, 1109
relation to other tests, 1887
technique, 1885–86
thrombosis and, 1105, 1106, 1885–87
upper extremity, 1885
Phlebotomy, cor pulmonale and, 1127
Phonocardiography, 1990–97
amplifiers, 1991
aortic regurgitation and, 745, 746, 1996
syphilitic, 1315, 1316
aortic stenosis and, 733, 1996
apexcardiogram, 1993–95
cardiomyopathy and, 1201, 1203
carotid pulse, 1993
echocardiography and, 1948, 1996
electronic filtering, 161
facilities, 1991
gallop and, atrial, 177, 178
Phonocardiography:
instrumentation, 1991–92
jugular venous pulse, 1993
microphones, 1991
mitral regurgitation and, 773, 1996
mitral stenosis and, 757, 1996
mitral valve prolapse and, 771
recorder, 1991
respiration and, 1992
second heart sound and, 166
technique, 1992–95
transducers, 1991–92
tricuspid endocarditis and, 254
tricuspid stenosis and, 795
Phosphofructokinase, 88, 89
allosteric activation of, 87
glucose utilization and, 90
Phosphorus (phosphate), 1476–77
diuretics and, 1658, 1660
hyperalimintation and, 1450
inorganic, 86
glucose and, 90
renal failure and, 1459
toxicity of, 1235
Phosphorylase, 89
allosteric activation of, 87
glucose utilization and, 90
glycogen metabolism and, 89
Phosphorylase kinase, 87, 88
Phosphorylation, 87, 88
glucose, 89–90
glycogen, 89
Photon emission computed tomography, 1812–13
Phrenic nerve, pericardium and, 1249, 2010, 2012
Physical activity. *See* Activity; Exercise.
Physical examination:
abdominal, 204–5
auscultation. *See* Auscultation; Sounds, heart.
blood pressure measurement, 138–41
chest, 204
extremity, 205
inspection. *See* Inspection.
palpation. *See* Palpation.
pulse:
arterial, 142–43
venous, 147–48
Physician:
desirable attributes of, 103–4
as expert witness, 1565–67
iatrogenic disorders and. *See* Iatrogenic disorders.
judgment possessed by, 2081
phobia caused by, 1541
preventive role of, 826–27
statements and actions of, 1537
Physiology, 37–63
afterload, 41, 47–68
anesthesia and, 50
atrial, 48–49
blood flow, 57–63
coronary, 60–63
redistribution, 51
cardiac cycle, 52–53
contractility, 46–47
coronary circulation, 60–63
drugs and, 49
exercise response, 55–56
excitation-contraction coupling, 37–39
heart failure, 319–39, 346–48
heart rate, 45–46, 48, 51
hormones and, 49–50, 62–63
hypertrophy and dilatation, 327–29
Physiology:
metabolic factors, 60–61
anaerobic, 51
muscle mechanics, 40–50
neural control, 49
coronary circulation, 61–62
vascular, 59–60
oxygen consumption, 56–57
oxygen extraction, 51
postextrasystolic potentiation, 50
preload, 41–46
pressures, 54–55
pulse, 53–54
arterial, 53
venous, 53–54
reserve, cardiac, 50–52
sequence of contraction, 48
Starling's law, 42–46
stroke volume, 51
suction, ventricular, 48
Phytanic acid, 1225
storage disease, 570
Pierre Robin syndrome, 131
Pigmentation:
blue-black, 134
urochrome, 126
venous hypertension and, 1377
Pilot certification, 1578–79
Pindolol, 1607. *See also* Beta-blocking agents.
dosage, 941, 1072
hypertension and, 1077
pharmacodynamics, 1608, 1613, 1617
pharmacokinetics, 1610, 1611
protein-binding and dialysance, 1082
structure, 1608
Pink puffers, 1123–24
Pirbuterol, 1653
Piroximone, 1655
Pitfalls in cardiology. *See* Errors; Iatrogenic disorders.
Pituitary gland, 1422–23
Planning, 105
Plants, poisoning from, 1488–89
Plasma volume. *See also* Blood volume.
hypertension and, 1040–41, 1043–44
Plasminogen:
thrombolytic therapy and, 1679, 1680, 1682, 1917
tissue-type activator (TPA), 1682, 1921
Platelets:
artificial heart and, 2073, 2074
atherosclerosis and, 804–6, 812–14
drugs affecting, 1675–78. *See also* Aspirin; Dipyridamole; Sulfinpyrazone.
adverse reactions, 1678
AMP-inhibiting, 1675
angina pectoris and, 1677
clinical uses, 1675–78
coronary bypass occlusion and, 1676–77
myocardial infarction and, 831, 943–44, 1677–78
prosthetic valves and, 1676
thromboxane-inhibiting, 1675
endocarditis and, 1137
endothelial injury and, 809, 812
growth factor and, 806, 812, 813–14
homocystinuria and, 812
indium imaging and, 1848–49
prostaglandins and, 814, 1675
research needs and, 814

Platinum electrode, shunt detection by, 1782, 1783
Plethysmography:
cerebrovascular disease and, 1877–78
Doppler studies and, 1977
impedance, deep venous thrombosis and, 1106
Pleural fluid:
heart failure and, 354
physical examination and, 204
roentgenography and, 236
Pneumocytes, shock and, 378
Pneumothorax, spontaneous, 916
Poiseuille's equation, 57, 1038
pulmonary artery pressure and, 1101
Poisoning, 1488–89
arsenic, 1234
arsine, 1234
carbon monoxide, 1235, 1489
hyperbaric oxygen therapy and, 1554
occupational, 1577
cyanide, 1554
hydrocarbon, 1235, 1489
lead, 1235
mercury, 1235
occupational, 1577–78
phosphorus, 1235
plant, 1488–89
scorpion venom, 1489
snake venom, 1489
Poliomyelitis, 1174
Polyarteritis, skin and, 123
Polyarteritis nodosa, 1437–39
clinical manifestations, 1439
conduction system and, 1439
coronary arteries and, 1022, 1438–39
Polychondritis, facial features and, 129
Polycythemia:
altitude and, 1544
cyanosis and, 586–87
tetralogy of Fallot and, 664, 665
vera, cardiac output and, 404
Polydactyly, 131, 132
Polymyalgia rheumatica, aorta and, 1323
Polyneuropathy, Roussy-Levy, 1229–30
Polyostotic fibrous dysplasia, 403
Polysaccharide storage disease, 1220–21
Polysomes, 95
Polysplenia, 689, 690
Polythiazide, 1659, 1660
dosage, 1072
Polyuria, 121
Pompe's disease, 570, 1219
Pope, Alexander, 1687
Popliteal artery:
aneurysm, 1326, 1351
angioplasty, 1909, 1910
embolism, 1349, 1350
entrapment syndrome, 1343, 1349
femoral bypass graft with, 2060–61
occlusive disease, 1345–46
thrombosis, 1349
Popliteal vein:
Doppler studies, 1976
thrombosis, 1375
Porphyria, 1224
Portal vein:
occlusion, 1366
pulmonary venous connection anomaly and, 682, 684
Posicor, 1655
Positron-emission tomography, 1849–50
coronary blood flow, 1849
metabolism and, myocardial, 1850
Postcoarctation syndrome, 633
Postextrasystolic potentiation, 50
Postinfarction syndrome, 987, 1267
Postoperative care:
arrhythmias and, 1518
psychological factors and, 1532
computer-based monitoring and, 2004–7
coronary bypass surgery, 952
infection and, 1518–19
intensivist and, 1508–9
noncardiac surgery, 1518
pacemaker implantation and, 1754
ventilatory support, 1507–8
Postperfusion syndrome, coronary bypass surgery and, 954
Postpericardiotomy syndrome, 1267–68
Postphlebography syndrome, 1887
Posture:
color changes and, in arteriosclerosis obliterans, 1341
dyspnea and. *See* Orthopnea.
hypertension and, 1074
hypotension and, 510–13
diabetes mellitus and, 1427
thoracic outlet syndrome and, 917
Potassium, 1466–73
action potential and, 77
aldosterone and, 1041, 1061–62
arrhythmias and, 1467–70
atrial fibrillation and, 1469
automaticity and, 79
AV block and, 1467–69
cardioplegic solutions and, 2037
conductance and, 77
conduction system and, 1467–69
contractility and, 1473
CPR and, 551
dialysis and, 1459
dietary, 1079
differential sensitivity of cardiac tissue to, 1470
digitalis and, 479, 1470–71, 1647
diuretics and, 361–62, 1071, 1658–61, 1665
ECG and, 222–24, 1471–73
edema and, 1662, 1663
heart failure in infant and, 585
renal failure and, 1459
supplementation, 361–62, 1071
hypertension and, 1071, 1079
transmembrane potential and, 74–75, 1466
Potassium iodide, hyperthyroidism and, 1416–17
Potentials:
ECG and, 80–84
equilibrium, 74
late, 1717–19
muscle, pacemaker malfunction and, 504
threshold, 75, 76, 1466
impulse conduction and, 410
triggered activity and, 408
transmembrane. *See* Transmembrane potential.
Potentiation, postextrasystolic, 50
PR interval, 73. *See also* Electrocardiography.
floating, 464
gallop and, 179
His bundle recording and, 1727, 1729
potassium and, 1471
PR interval:
short, Lown-Ganong-Levine syndrome and, 449
Practolol, 1621
Prazosin:
dosage, 1072, 1587
heart failure and, 364–65
in infant, 586
hypertension and, 1078, 1081
lipids and, 1074
pharmacology, 1589
pheochromocytoma and, 1083
protein-binding and dialysance, 1082
side effects, 1073
Precordium:
aching in, 907
apex beat, 153–55. *See also* Apex beat; Apexcardiography.
bulging, 152, 155
diastole and, 154, 155
ECG leads and, 208, 226–27
ectopic impulses, 155
heart failure and, 351
honk, 185
inspection of, 152
palpation of, 152–56
pulsations, 152–56. *See* Apex beat; Apexcardiography.
right ventricular impulse and, 155
systole and, 153, 155
thrills, 156
thrombophlebitis of, 910
transmission of sound to, 161
Predictive value of tests, coronary artery disease and, 304–5
Prednisone:
pericarditis and, 1254
rheumatic fever and, 1311
transplantation and, 2065
Preeclampsia, 1084-85
Preejection period, 1190, 1994
Preexcitation syndromes, 415–17, 447–49. *See also* Wolff-Parkinson-White syndrome.
His bundle recordings and, 1730
Lown-Ganong-Levine, 449
management, 477
calcium channel blockers and, 1631
mechanism, 415–17
Preexisting conditions, legal issues and, 1564, 1565, 1570
Pregnancy, 1383–94
adjustment of cardiovascular system to, 1383–85
anticoagulants and, 1386, 1393–94
aortic dissection and, 1330
aortic regurgitation and, 1387, 1389
aortic stenosis and, 1387, 1389
arrhythmias and, 1392
cardiac output and, 404, 1384, 1385
cardiomyopathy and, 1183, 1205, 1391–92
dilated, 1391–92
hypertrophic, 1388, 1391
clinical evaluation, 1385–86
coarctation of aorta and, 1388, 1390
congenital heart disease and, 1390–91, 1392
coronary artery disease and, 1392
diabetes mellitus and, 1429–30
diagnostic procedures for heart disease during, 1394
digitalis and, 1641–42
drugs and, 1392–94
cardiovascular, 1392–94

Pregnancy: drugs and:
obstetric, 1394
dyspnea and, 116
endocarditis and, 1134, 1386
exercise and, 1384–85
health priorities in, 1386
hypertension and, 1084
left-to-right shunts and, 1387, 1390
management, 1386
Marfan's syndrome and, 1388, 1391
mitral prolapse and, 1389
mitral regurgitation and, 1387, 1389
mitral stenosis and, 763–64, 1387, 1388–89
myocarditis and, 1386, 1387
patent ductus arteriosus and, 615
prosthetic valves and, 1392
pulmonary embolism and, 1114
pulmonary hypertension and, 1388, 1390
pulmonary valve disease and, 1387, 1389–90
rheumatic fever and, 1386–88
stroke volume and, 1384
surgery and, cardiac, 1392
tetralogy of Fallot and, 1391
transposition of great arteries and, 1391
tricuspid valve disease and, 1390
uterine blood flow and, 1384–85
Preinfarction syndrome, 842
Preload (volume overload), 41–46
afterload mismatch with, 266–67
aortic regurgitation and, 742–43, 747
aortic stenosis and, 274
AV canal and, 608
contractility and, 42–46
diuretics and, 361–62
echocardiography and, 1953
force-velocity relations and, 40–42, 45–46
force-velocity-volume relation and, 47
heart failure and, 44, 273, 326, 327, 332
management, 360–63
hypertrophy and, 269, 332
mitral regurgitation and, 269, 332, 768, 770, 774
reduction of, 360–63
sarcomere length and, 330
shock and, 371
sodium restriction and, 360–61
vasodilators and, 362–63, 392, 866, 1584
Premature atrial beats, 437–38
atrial flutter and, 414
bundle branch block and, 215, 218
escape beats and, 470
esophageal ECG and, 1698, 1699
myocardial infarction and, 973
in normal populations, 435
stimulation technique, 1735–37
tachycardia and, 441
Premature atrioventricular beats, 438–39
Premature ventricular beats, 450–52
vs. aberrant ventricular conduction, 447, 458–60
compensatory pause, 460
coronary heart disease and, 284, 285
prognosis, 921
digitalis for, 1646
ECG and, 451–52
exercise and, 285, 286
testing, 1708, 1711
Premature ventricular beats:
hypertension and, 1074
management, 478
mechanism, 421
myocardial infarction and, 451, 830–31, 974–75, 986
in normal populations, 435
pain from, 908–9
palpitations and, 283–86
potassium and, 1469
pulse and, 146
sudden death and, 539, 540, 543
tachycardia and, 452, 453
Prenalterol, 1653
Prenylamine, 1624
Presbycardia, 331
Pressures. *See also* Atrial pressure; Blood pressure; End-diastolic pressure, *etc.*
cardiac catheterization and, 1774–76
recording system for, 1773–74
closure, 58
CPR and, 547–49
flow relation to, 1038
intramyocardial, 859
overload. *See* Afterload.
perfusion, coronary, 857–61
pericardial, 1250, 1251, 1257
presystolic, 42, 43
tabulation of normal, 55
transmural, 58
Presyncope, 287, 507
causes, 522
diagnostic evaluation, 520
Presystolic pressure, contraction and, 42, 43
Prevalence, 557–64
cardiovascular disease in general, 557
cerebrovascular disease, 562
congenital heart disease, 563–64
coronary heart disease, 559
hypertension, 560–61
rheumatic heart disease, 563
Preventive approach to cardiovascular disease, 564–65
atherosclerosis and, 817–32
Prinzmetal's angina. *See* Angina pectoris, variant.
Probability analysis, coronary artery disease and, 304–6
Probes, nonimaging nuclear, 387, 1812, 1829–30
Problem list, 105
Probucol, cholesterol and, 822–23
Procainamide, 1594–95
accessory pathway and, 477
clinical application, 1595
myocardial infarction and, 975
pharmacokinetic properties, 1594–95
pharmacologic properties, 1595
pregnancy and, 1393
sudden death prevention and, 543
toxicity, 1595
Procardia. *See* Nifedipine.
Progeria, 130
Progestogen, 1424, 1425
Programmed stimulation, 499–501. *See also* Pulse generators.
atrial, 1736–37
reentry and, 421–23
ventricular, 1738
Progress notes, 105
Promethazine, cardiac catheterization and, 1769
Pronestyl. *See* Procainamide.
Propantheline, digitalis and, 1647
Propranolol, 1598–99, 1607. *See also* Beta-blocking agents.
angina pectoris and, 1613–15
aortic dissection and, 1333
arrhythmias and, 1599, 1615
calcium channel blockers and, 1635
cardiomyopathy and, 1206, 1207, 1616
clinical application, 1599
coronary blood flow and, 1614
dosage, 941, 1072, 1587
hypertension and, 1077, 1612–13
gestational, 1085
renoparenchymal, 1081
hyperthyroidism and, 397, 1416–18
lipids and, 1074
long-acting, 1610
myocardial infarction and, 967
long-term use of, 971
pharmacodynamics, 1608, 1613, 1617
pharmacokinetics, 1594, 1598, 1610, 1611
pharmacologic properties, 1598–99
postoperative, 953
protein-binding and dialysance, 1082
structure, 1608
tetralogy of Fallot and, 665
toxicity, 1599
tracheal intubation and, 1496
withdrawal reaction and, 1618, 1629
Propylthiouracil, hyperthyroidism and, 1416, 1417
Prostacycline, 814
shock and, 376
Prostaglandins, 814
atherosclerosis and, 814
coronary artery spasm and, 1010–11
heart failure and, 326
lysosomal enzymes and, 381
platelets and, 814, 1675
Prosthetic valves:
anticoagulants and, 1671, 1676
aortic, 737–39, 2030–32
aneurysm repair and, 2043, 2044
regurgitation and, 644, 750–51
results, 738–39, 750–51, 2034
small annulus and, 2032
syphilis and, 1316, 1319
ball variance, 187, 2034
Bjork-Shiley, 778, 779, 2034
broken strut of, 2074
thromboembolism and, 1671
carcinoid and, 1299
choice of, 2034–35
Doppler studies and, 1985–86
embolism from, 779, 1359, 1671, 1676
endocarditis, 1133–34, 1136, 1150
abscess and, 1150
cure rate, 1147
fluroroscopy and, 1767
Medtronic Hall, 2034, 2069
mitral, 777–79, 2032–33
combined aortic-mitral disease and, 790–91
regurgitation and, 650–51
results, 778–79, 2034
stenosis and, 649, 762, 763
multiple, 2034
murmurs and, 188
necropsy and, 2079
noncardiac surgery and, 1517
platelet-controlling drugs and, 1676
pregnancy and, 1392
pulmonary, 799

Prosthetic valves:
St. Jude, 644, 2034
sounds of, 186–88
Starr-Edwards, 2034
survival curves, 780
thromboembolism and, 1671
thromboembolism, 779, 1671, 1676
tilting-disk, 778, 2034
tricuspid, 797, 799, 2034
carcinoid and, 1299
Ebstein's anomaly and, 679, 680
Protamine, cardiopulmonary bypass and, 2026
Proteases, 96
Protein:
alcoholism and, 1448
C, warfarin and, 1669
contractile, heart failure and, 330
degradation of, 95–96
half-lives, 85, 86
insulin and, 96–97
liquid dietary, 1484
metabolism, 94–97
integrated control of, 96–97
purified plasma, 388–89
synthetic pathway, 95
thyroid binding by, 1412
Protein-calorie undernutrition, 1449
Protein kinase, phosphorylation and, 87, 88
Proteolysis, 95–96
Prothrombin time, warfarin and, 1669, 1675
Protodiastole, 52
Protozoa, myocarditis and, 1175–76
Protriptyline, 1479
Pseudotruncus arteriosus, 668–70
Pseudoxanthoma elasticum, 124–25, 1238, 1370
Psychiatry, coronary heart disease and, 933–35
Psychological factors, 1520–34. *See also* Anxiety; Depression; Emotional stress.
cardiac phobia and, 1541
coronary bypass surgery and, 1531–32
coronary heart disease and, 826, 934–35, 1521–25, 1530–33
disability and, 1537, 1542
hypertension and, 1525–26, 1533–34
iatrogenic disorders and, 1536, 1537, 1541
mitral valve prolapse and, 1533
myocardial infarction and, 1523, 1530–31
rehabilitation and, 1035, 1532–33
transplantation and, cardiac, 1533
Psychosis, cardiac, 908
Psychotherapy, rehabilitation program and, 1532–33
Psychotropic agents, 1479–81
Pulmonary angiography, 1787–89, 1882–84
clinical use, 1884
complications, 1884
contraindications, 1108–9
digital subtraction, 1862–63, 1883
embolism and, 1108–9, 1882–84
indications, 1109, 1882
interpretation, 1884
technique, 1882–83
venous connection anomaly and, 1788
Pulmonary arteriovenous fistula, 680–81
clinical manifestations, 680–81
Pulmonary arteriovenous fistula:
management, 681
pathology, 680
Pulmonary artery (arteries). *See also* Pulmonary vasculature.
absence of anatomic origin of, from heart, 15, 668–73
unilateral, 681
anatomy, 25–26
atresia, 668, 669
atrial anastomosis to, 676
univentricular heart and, 706
banding:
AV canal and, 610
coarctation repair and, 632
double-outlet right ventricle and, 699
transposition of great arteries and, 695
ventricular septal defect and, 596
bronchial artery origin of, 670
catheterization, 1999–2002
cardiac output and, 2000
complications, 2001–2
heart failure and, 270
indications, 2000–2001
insertion technique, 1999–2000
perioperative, 1506
pressure measurement by, 1775–76, 2000
shock and, 385
coarctations, 659
conductance, 1092–93
confluence of, 669–70
coronary artery origin from, 708–11, 1018–19
dilatation of, heart failure and, 353
ductal origin of, 670
echocardiography and, 1941
embryology, 13, 14
fistula, 680–81
with coronary artery, 707–8, 1019
hemitruncus (one pulmonary artery from ascending aorta), 619–20
left ventricular origin of. *See* Double-outlet left ventricle; Transposition of great arteries.
nonconfluence of, 670
patent ductus arteriosus and, 614–18
precordial pulse, 155
pressure, 1121. *See also* Pulmonary hypertension.
catheterization studies, 1775–76, 2000
cor pulmonale and, 1121, 1126
determinants of, 1091–92, 1101
end-diastolic, 979–80
exercise and, 1092
heart failure and, 334
mitral stenosis and, 759
myocardial infarction and, 979–80
normal, 55
occlusion, cardiac index and, 1507
pericarditis and, 1265
tamponade and, 1259
wedge, 55, 385, 388, 1091, 1775–76. *See also* Pulmonary capillary pressure, wedge.
pseudotruncus arteriosus and, 668–70
radiography. *See* Pulmonary angiography.
roentgenograms and, 232–34, 238, 241
Pulmonary artery (arteries):
sling, 625–26
stenosis:
angioplasty for, 1898–99
graft, 1899, 1900
systolic pressure and, 1775
subclavian artery anastomosis to, 666
transposition of. *See* Transposition of great arteries.
truncus arteriosus and, 668–73
Pulmonary capillaries. *See* Pulmonary vasculature.
Pulmonary capillary pressure, 27, 1091–92
edema and, 337–38
elevated, 1094. *See also* Pulmonary hypertension.
mitral stenosis and, 759, 760
osmotic pressure and, 1092
wedge:
mitral regurgitation and, 772, 774
mitral stenosis and, 759
myocardial infarction and, 979
postcapillary obstruction and, 1094
shock and, 373
Pulmonary edema. *See* Edema, pulmonary.
Pulmonary embolism, 1105–17
air, 1115–16
amniotic fluid, 1116–17
angiography and, 1108–9, 1182–84
digital subtraction, 1862
blood gases and, 1108
cancer and, 1109, 1117
cardiomyopathy and, 1190
cor pulmonale and, 1096, 1107
deep venous thrombosis and, 1105–6, 1374
diagnosis, 1105–6
prevention, 1105, 1110
diagnosis, 1106–9
dyspnea and, 116, 1107
ECG and, 916, 1108
fat, 1114–15
heart failure and, 1107, 1112
hemorrhage and, 1106
hypertension and, pulmonary, 1096, 1100, 1102
hypotension and, 1102, 1107
incidence, 564
infarction (pulmonary) and, 1106–7
mortality, 564
myocardial infarction and, 983, 1673
myocardial ischemia and, 915–16
pain from, 114, 1106
paradoxical, 1109–10
pregnancy and, 1114
prognosis, 1112
radionuclide studies, 1108, 1881–82
rare forms of, 1117
roentgenography, 916, 1108
sounds, 916
treatment, 1110–14
anticoagulant, 1110–11
definitive, 1112–13
embolectomy, 1112–13
fibrinolytic, 1113–14, 1681, 1916–17
prophylactic, 1110–12
venous interruption, 1111–12
tumor, 1117, 1291
venography and, 1109
ventilation/perfusion scans and, 1108

Pulmonary hypertension, 1091–1103
altitude and, 338, 1093, 1095–96, 1121, 1546–47
angiography and, 1884
atrial septal defect and, 599
cardiac output and, 1093–94
clinical recognition, 1097–98, 1102, 1125
conductance and, 1092–93
congenital heart disease and, 587–89, 1094–95
cor pulmonale and, 1095–97, 1121–23
management, 1126–27
definition, 1091, 1093–94
embolism and, 1096, 1100, 1102
genetics, 576
heart failure and, 1097
roentgenography and, 240
hypertrophy and, 1097, 1098
hypoxemia-induced, 1095–96
laboratory studies, 1098
mechanical obstruction and, 1096–97
mechanisms, 1094–97, 1121
mitral stenosis and, 758, 760
myocardial ischemia and, 915
neonatal, 584, 587
normal pressures and, 1091–92
pain from, 114, 915, 1098
physical examination, 1098
postcapillary obstruction and, 1094
precapillary obstruction and, 1095
pregnancy and, 1388, 1390
primary, 1099–1103
clinical diagnosis, 1102
etiology and pathogenesis, 1100–1101
nomenclature and classification, 1100
pathology, 1101–2
pathophysiology, 1101
treatment, 1102–3
progressive systemic sclerosis and, 1444
pulmonary regurgitation and, 255
right ventricle and, 1094, 1097, 1122–23
secondary, 1097
sounds, 173–75, 1098
ejection, 182–83
single second, 168, 169
symptoms, 1097–98
syncope and, 522
transplantation for, cardiopulmonary, 2067
treatment, 1102–3, 1126–27
calcium channel blockers in, 1633
tricuspid regurgitation and, 253
venous, 1094
ventricular septal defect and, 592, 593, 595
Pulmonary valve, 792–96
absent, 13, 667–68
clinical manifestations, 667
management, 667–68
acquired lesions, 793
anatomy, 22
area calculation, 1785
assessment, 255
atresia, 660–62
angiography, 1789
clinical manifestations, 660–61
management, 661–62, 671, 673
pathology, 660
tetralogy of Fallot and, 668, 669
tricuspid valve and, 660, 673, 674
Pulmonary valve: atresia:
ventricular septal defect and, 670–73
bicuspid, 13
carcinoid and, 1298, 1299
cusps, 22
dysplastic, 654, 655
facial features and, 128–29
echocardiography, 1935, 1941
atresia and, 661
regurgitation and, 255
stenosis and, 656
ventricular performance and, 1964
embryology, 12–13
fibrous skeleton and, 18
necropsy and, 2078
pregnancy and, 1387, 1389–90
regurgitation, 792–96
assessment, 794–96
carcinoid and, 793
echocardiography, 255
etiology, 792
hypertension and, 255
low-pressure, 255
medical management, 796
murmur, 193
natural history, 796
pathophysiology, 794
physical examination, 795
surgical management, 799
replacement, 799
sounds, 160
closure, 163, 166–76
ejection, 163, 182–83
stenosis and, 169–71, 656
valvotomy and, 171
stenosis. *See* Pulmonic stenosis.
transverse section and, 18
truncus arteriosus and, 669–70
Pulmonary vasculature. *See also* Pulmonary artery; Pulmonary veins.
anatomy, 27
arteriovenous malformation, 1896–97
arteritis, 588
blood flow:
cephalization or centralization, 239
conductance and, 1092–93
Doppler studies and, 1980
hypertension and, 587–89
lateralization or localization, 239
left-to-right shunt and, 1093, 1095
pulmonary atresia and, 670
roentgenography and, 234, 235, 238–39
shunts and, 1093, 1095, 1779–80, 1781
tetralogy of Fallot and, 663, 665
truncus arteriosus and, 671
blood volume, 27
capillary pressure. *See* Pulmonary capillary pressure.
capillary reserve, 27
embolism. *See* Pulmonary embolism.
embolization technique, 1896–97
fetal, 1093
heart failure and, 239–40, 334
hypertension. *See* Pulmonary hypertension.
normal, 1121
obstructive disease, 1094–97. *See also* Cor pulmonale.
congenital heart disease and, 587–89
mechanical, 1096–97
Pulmonary vasculature: obstructive disease:
postcapillary, 1094
precapillary, 1095
secondary, 1094
ventricular septal defect and, 592–95
plexogenic lesions, 1101
radionuclide studies, 1836, 1838
resistance, 1091–92, 1784. *See also* Pulmonary hypertension.
conductance and, 1092
neonatal, 583, 587
normal, 55, 1121
roentgenography, 230, 238–40
shock and, 378–79
systemic communication with, 590–622
anomalous, from descending aorta, 621–22
Blalock-Taussig shunt, 666
extracardiac, 614–22
Fontan shunt, 676
hypertension and, 587–89
intracardiac, 590–614
pulmonary atresia and, 671
vasoconstriction, 27
hypertension and, 1096, 1097, 1100, 1102, 1121–22
hypoxic, 1121–22
mediators, 1122
Pulmonary veins:
anatomy, 20
atresia, 682
connection anomaly. *See* Pulmonary venous connection anomaly.
cor triatriatum and, 12
dilatation, heart failure and, 352, 353
embryology, 12
occlusive disease, 1100
cor pulmonale and, 1124
pressure, 1091–92
stenosis, 652–53
Pulmonary venous connection anomaly, 12
atrial septal defect, 598, 601, 603–5
hemodynamic vise and, 682
partial, 603–5
angiography and, 1788
clinical manifestations, 604–5
medical management, 605
natural history and prognosis, 605
pathology, 603–4
surgical management, 605
total, 681–84
clinical manifestations, 682–83
medical management, 683
natural history and prognosis, 683
pathology, 681–82
pathophysiology, 682
surgical management, 683–84
Pulmonic stenosis, 654–59
angiography, 1788
assessment, 255, 655–56
associated conditions, 655
carcinoid tumor and, 793
catheterization studies, 656–57
dome-shaped, 654–56
Doppler studies, 255, 256
double-outlet right ventricle and, 697, 699
ECG, 224, 656
echocardiography, 656
history, 655

Pulmonic stenosis:
medical management, 657
mitral atresia and, 647
murmurs, 189–90, 656, 659
natural history and prognosis, 657
pathology, 654–55
pathophysiology, 655
physical examination, 655–56
pregnancy and, 1387
roentgenography, 656
single ventricle and, 703, 704
sounds, 169–71, 656
ejection, 182–83
subvalvular, 658–59
clinical manifestations, 658
pathology and pathophysiology, 658
sounds, 170
surgical management, 658–59, 666
supravalvular, 659
surgical management, 657–59, 666
angioplasty, 1898–99
tetralogy of Fallot and, 662, 663
transposition of great arteries and, 691, 694
corrected, 700–701, 703
tricuspid valve and, 655, 673, 674
trilogy of Fallot and, 655
vectorcardiography, 656
Pulse, 53, 141–50. *See also* Heart rate.
alternans. *See* Pulsus alternans.
anacrotic notch (shoulder), 53
aortic, 142
aortic arch interruption and, 623
aortic regurgitation and, 144, 745, 746
aortic stenosis and, 145, 733
apical, 153–55
recording of. *See* Apexcardiography.
arrhythmias and, 146
arterial, 53, 141–46
abnormal, 144–46
contour, 142, 143
examination, 142–43
normal, 143–44
origin of, 141–42
transmission of, 142
arteriosclerosis obliterans and, 1340–41
bisferiens, 144–45
brachial, 143
bradycardia and, 146
cardiomyopathy and, 145, 1201
carotid, 143, 144. *See also* Carotid arteries, pulse.
coarctation of aorta and, 629–30
collapsing, 144
contours of, 53, 54
Corrigan's, aortic regurgitation and, 745, 746
dicrotic, 145
dicrotic notch (halt), 53, 142, 143
IABP and, 2023
endocarditis and, 1142
hyperkinetic, 144
hypokinetic, 145
incisura, 52, 53, 142
paradoxical. *See* Pulsus paradoxus.
parvus et tardus, 145
patent ductus arteriosus and, 615
percussion wave, 143–44
precordial, 152–56
premature ventricular depolarization and, 146
Pulse:
pulmonary artery, 155
Quincke, 144
radial, contours of, 54
tachycardia and, 146
tidal wave, 143, 144
trisection, 143
venous, 53–54, 146–50
a wave, 53, 148–50
abnormal, 148–50
arrhythmias and, 150
c wave, 54, 148
cannon waves, 149, 150
h wave, 148
jugular. *See* Jugular vein pulse.
normal, 148
v wave, 148, 149–50
waveform analysis, 148
x wave, 54, 148, 149
y wave, 52, 54, 148, 150
water-hammer, 144
wave recording. *See also* Phonocardiography.
carotid artery, 1992, 1993
instrumentation, 1991–92
jugular venous, 1993
Pulse generators, 490–91
cardioverter implant and, 1761, 1762
circuitry, 491
historical aspects, 487
implantation, 1753
malfunctions, 501–4
output, 500–501
power source, 490–91
programmable, 499–501
rate, 500
refractory period, 491
replacement, 1753–54
reprogramming, 1757, 1758
sensors, 498–99, 501
slow or irregular, 503–4
testing, 1758–60
explant, 1760
Pulseless disease, 1323
coronary arteries and, 1023
Pulse pressure, 140–41. *See also* Blood pressure.
aortic, 142
aortic stenosis and, 733
arteriovenous fistula and, 402
catheterization studies and, 1774–75
increased, 140
reduced, 140–41
unequal (right-left), 141
Pulsus alternans, 141, 145–46
gallop and, 180
heart failure and, 334, 351
Pulsus paradoxus, 141, 146
tamponade and, 1258–60
Pump:
abdominothoracic, 55
cardiopulmonary bypass, 2026
intraaortic. *See* Intraaortic balloon counterpulsation.
Pump function, 266
compensatory, 331–32
failure, 320–21. *See also* Heart failure.
causes, 320, 321
definition, 321
hemodynamics, 333–34
Pupils, retinal examination and, 198
Purkinje cells, 31, 32
Purkinje fibers, 73. *See also* His-Purkinje system.
action potential, 75–78
Purkinje fibers:
activation sequence and, 206
afterdepolarizations, 408
automaticity, 78–79, 407
fast-response, 407–8
lidocaine and, 1597
pacemaker activity, 80
procainamide and, 1595
slow-response, 407, 408
Purpura:
anaphylactoid, 1227
pinch, 125
thrombotic thrombocytopenic, 1227
sudden death and, 535
Pyelonephritis, hypertension and, 1045, 1060
Pyrophosphate imaging, 1844–48
clinical results, 1846–47
CCU and, 1847–48
indications, 1847
mechanisms of uptake, 1844–45
sizing of infarct and, 1848
technique and interpretation, 1845–46
Pyruvate, 90
Pyruvate dehydrogenase, 88, 90

Q fever endocarditis, 1136
Q waves, 209–11, 302. *See also* Electrocardiography.
necrosis or infarction and, 895
vectorcardiography and, 1688–90
QRS complex, 206. *See also* Electrocardiography.
aberrant conduction and, 459
bundle branch block and, 215, 217–19
bypass tracts and, 219–20
electrical axis and, 208
epicardial potential distributions, 82
genesis, 73, 81–84
myocardial infarction and, 895
pacemakers and, 494
malfunctions of, 502–3
premature ventricular beats and, 451–52
quinidine and, 223, 224
signal averaging and, 1716–19
tachycardia and, 293
esophageal ECG and, 1694, 1695
supraventricular, 441–42
vectorcardiography and, 1688–90
QT interval, 210. *See also* Electrocardiography.
calcium and, 224–25, 1475–76
long (prolonged), 225, 523–24
beta blockers and, 1617
hereditary, 490, 576
sudden death and, 544
Questionnaires, 110–11
Quincke pulse, 144
Quincke's sign, 747
Quinethazone, 1659
dosage, 1072
Quinidine, 1593–94
cardioversion and, 1742
clinical applications, 1594
digitalis and, 1647
ECG and, 223, 224
mitral stenosis and, 761
pharmacokinetic properties, 1593
pharmacologic properties, 1593–94
pregnancy and, 1393
sudden death prevention and, 543
toxicity, 1594

Rabinov-Paulin phlebography technique, 1885
Radial artery:
  catheterization, pressure monitoring and, 386
  compression test of Allen and, 1340
  grafts from, 2037
  pulse, contours of, 54
Radiation, 1023, 1237, 1484–86
  cardiac catheterization and, 1773
  conduction system effects of, 1485, 1486
  coronary artery effects of, 1485, 1486
  fluoroscopy and, 1765
  laser, 1922–25
  myocardial effects of, 1485, 1486
  pathogenesis of, 1486
  pericardial effects of, 1484–85, 1486
  risk factors of, 1485–86
  valvular effects of, 1485, 1486
Radioactive iodine, 1413, 1417
Radiography. *See* Angiography; Roentgenography.
Radioligands, 1606
Radionuclide studies, 1809–50
  amyloidosis and, 1215
  aneurysms and:
    aortic, 1822
    ventricular, 1820, 1821
  Anger camera and, 1811
  angiography:
    coronary heart disease and, 900–902
    equilibrium gated, 1818–23
    first-pass, 1813–18, 1823
    limitation of, 902
  aortic-mitral combined valvular disease and, 789
  aortic regurgitation and, 249, 748, 1822
  aortic stenosis and, 735
  background corrections, 1814–15
  blood pool imaging, 1818–23
  blood volume and, 1822–23
  cardiac cycle and, 1815–16, 1820
  cardiomyopathy and, 1189, 1203
    dilated, 261–62
    hypertrophic, 260
  clinical applications, 1823–29
  computer systems, 1812–13
    first-pass studies and, 1814
    gated equilibrium study and, 1819
  congenital heart disease and, 1828
  coronary arteriography vs., 1836–37
  coronary heart disease and, 899–902, 1825, 1833–48
    prognosis, 922
  cor pulmonale and, 1126
  deep venous thrombosis and, 1105–6
  diastolic function and, 1830–31
  doughnut sign, 1845
  drug-induced cardiotoxicity and, 1826–28
  ejection fraction and, 272, 901, 902, 1815–17, 1819–22
  endocarditis and, 1146
  exercise, 306–7, 1824–26
    coronary heart disease and, 899–902, 1832, 1834–38, 1842–43
    likelihood of disease and, 307, 308
    myocardial infarction and, 312, 970
    myocardial perfusion and, 1832, 1834–38, 1842–43
Radionuclide studies: exercise:
    prognosis and, 310–11
    thallium, 306, 899–900, 1832, 1834–38, 1842–43
    ventricular performance and, 1824–26, 1828, 1842–43
  first-pass technique, 1813–18
    advantages and limitations, 1818, 1823
    left ventricular performance and, 1815–16
    right ventricular performance and, 1816
    shunt detection and, 1816–17
    technical considerations, 1813–15
  gated equilibrium technique, 1818–23
    advantages and limitations, 1823
    myocardial infarction and, 970
  heart failure and, 355, 1823
  historical background, 1810–11
  indium-111 imaging, 1848–49
  infarct-avid agents, 1844–48
  instrumentation, 1811–13
  leukocyte, 1849
  lung, 1881–82
    embolism and, 1108, 1881–82
  metabolic, 1849–50
  mitral regurgitation and, 774, 1822
  mitral stenosis and, 760
  multicrystal camera and, 1811–12
  myocardial infarction and, 312, 899–902, 970, 1824
    prognosis, 927
    pyrophosphate imaging, 1844–48
    thallium imaging, 899–900, 1833–34
  myocardial ischemia and, 1835–36
  myocardial perfusion studies, 1831–44
    anatomic definition and, 1843–44
    exercise, 1832, 1834–38, 1842–43
    function studies vs., 1842–43
    normal image, 1832–33
    pharmacologic stress, 1838–39
    physiology of uptake, 1831
    quantification, 1839–40
    resting, 1833–34, 1843–44
    technique, 1832
    tomographic, 1840–42
  myocarditis and, 1166–67
  myosin-specific antibody and, 1849
  myxoma and, 1288
  new techniques of, 1848–50
  performance assessment, cardiac, 1813–31
  peripheral circulation and, 1822–23
  platelet, 1848–49
  positron, 1849–50
  probe system, 1812, 1829–30
    ventricular function and, 387
  pulmonary embolism and, 1108, 1881–82
  pulmonary hypertension and, 1098
  pulmonary obstructive disease and, 1828–29
  pyrophosphate (Tc-99m), 1844–48
    clinical results, 1846–47
    CCU and, 1847–48
    indications, 1847
    mechanism of uptake, 1844–45
    sizing of infarct and, 1848
    technique and interpretation, 1845–46
  resting ventricular performance and, 1823–24
Radionuclide studies: pyrophosphate:
    technetium-99m. *See* Technetium-99m.
  time-activity curves, 1815–17, 1819, 1820
  thallium. *See* Thallium imaging.
  tomographic imaging system, 1812–13
    thallium-201 and, 1840–42
  valvular heart disease and, 1826
  ventilation-perfusion, 1108, 1881–82
  ventriculography, myocardial infarction and, 970
  volumes and, ventricular, 1815, 1820–22
  wall motion and, 1816, 1819–20
  washout curves and, 1839–40, 1850
Ranitidine, 1484
Rappaport, Maurice B., 1990
Rash:
  dermatomyositis, 124
  lupus erythematosus and, 123, 124
  Reiter's syndrome, 126
  rheumatic fever, 1309
Raynaud's phenomenon (disease), 1352–53, 1618–19
  beta-blocker-induced, 1618–19
  clinical manifestations, 1352–53
  myocardial, 1442
  pain from, 115
  sclerosis and, progressive systemic, 1442
  treatment, 1353
Receptors, cardiac, 375
  inhibitory and excitatory, 374
Reciprocal rhythm, 468, 469
Reciprocating tachycardia, 447–48, 468
  management, 477
  WPW syndrome and, 416, 418
Recompression therapy, 1552
Recording system:
  ECG, long-term, 1720–21
  echocardiography, 1929, 1966
  His bundle, 1727–29
  phonocardiography, 1991
Records, legal issues and, 1575–76
Reentry, 410–11
  accessory pathway, 416, 418–20
  atrial, 413–14
    fibrillation and, 415
    flutter and, 414
  vs. automaticity, 412–13
  AV junctional tachycardia and, 418
  AV nodal, 418–20, 440, 441
  cardioversion and, 483
  mechanism of, 411
  nodoventricular fibers and, 417, 419, 426
  pacemakers and, 482
  preexcitation and, 416
  programmed stimulation and, 421–23
  sinus node, 413
  supraventricular tachycardia and, 413–20, 440–41
    management, 476
  ventricular tachycardia and, 420–23
Reflection, arrhythmias and, 412, 468
Reflex(es):
  Bainbridge, 50
  Bezold-Jarisch, 62
    myocardial infarction and, 981
    shock and, 375
  blood pressure and, 1040
  carotid sinus, 514–15. *See also* Carotid sinus.

Reflex(es):
coronary, 61–62
heat stress and, 1547
orthostatic hypotension and, 511, 512
shock and, 374–76
syncope and, 516–17
Reflux esophagitis, 911–12
Refractory period, AV node, 1736–37
Refsum's disease, 126, 1225
Regitine. *See* Phentolamine.
Rehabilitation, 1025–36
ambulation and, early, 1028–29
categories of patients eligible for, 1025–26
elderly and, 1034
exercise and, 1026–28, 1031–34
arm vs. leg, 1027
drugs and, 1027–28
expectations and, 1028
guidelines for, 1032–33
maintenance, 1034
prescription, 1027
testing, 1026
training, 1026–28, 1031–34
goals of, 1025
iatrogenic heart disease and, 1542
implementation, 1028
inpatient, 1028–31
outpatient, 1031–34
patient education and, 1029–31
principles of, 935–36
psychological factors in, 1035, 1532–33, 1542
severe ventricular dysfunction and, 1034–35
vocational aspects, 1035–36
Reiter's syndrome, 1238
aortitis and, 1323–24
rash of, 126
Relapsing fever, 1174
Renal angiography:
angioplasty and, 1911
digital subtraction, 1059
nephritis and, 1060, 1061
nephrosclerosis and, 1055, 1056–57
Renal artery:
aneurysm, 1351
angioplasty, 1079, 1910–12
aortic dissection and, 1330
atherosclerosis, 1058–59, 1079–80
fibrous dysplasia, 1058, 1079
stenosis, 1058–59
Renal blood flow, 325
Renal disease. *See* Kidney.
Renal failure. *See* Kidney failure.
Renal vein renin activity, 1059
Renin:
aldosteronism and, 1062
beta-blocking agents and, 1071, 1074, 1612
heart failure and, 324, 325, 347
hypertension and, 1041, 1043–46
renal vein, 1059
shock and, 377
sodium and, 1041
syncope and, 508–9
synthesis of, 1041
Renografin, 1786
Renoprival hypertension, 1045
Renovascular hypertension, 1044–45
angioplasty for, 1910–12
diagnosis, 1059–60
vs. essential hypertension, 1058
treatment, 1079, 1335
Reperfusion, myocardial. *See* Myocardium, reperfusion.
Repolarization:
abnormalities, 411–12
action potential and, 77
atrial, 206
automaticity and, 79, 408
delayed, 225
management of, 479
ECG and, 80
ischemia and, 210
potassium and, 1471
quinidine and, 224, 225
T wave and, 84
triggered activity and, 408
ventricular, 207
Report, medicolegal, 1575–76
Reserpine, 1588
dosage, 1072, 1587
hypersensitivity to, 1237
preeclampsia and, 1085
protein-binding and dialysance, 1082
side effects, 1073
Reserve, cardiac, 50–52
coronary vascular, 60
Resistance, 57–58. *See also* Blood pressure; Hypertension; Hypotension.
afterload and, 372
arterial pulse and, 141
catheterization studies and, 1784
flow-pressure relations and, 58
impulse conduction and, 410
mitral regurgitation and, 776
normal values, 55
pressure-flow relationship to, 1038
pulmonary vascular. *See* Pulmonary hypertension; Pulmonary vasculature, resistance.
shock and, 370, 373
syncope and, 508–9
total peripheral, 1038
units of, 57
Resonance, 157
Respiration:
anxiety neurosis and, 1526–27
arrest of, 549
Cheyne-Stokes, 116, 350
cor pulmonale and, 1096, 1123–24
CPR and, 550
decompression sickness and, 1551
difficult. *See* Dyspnea.
ejection sounds and, 182
heart failure and, 337, 349–50
inspection of, 135
Kussmaul's sign and, 148–49
monitoring of, 2004–5
muscles of, assessment of, 387
postoperative, 1507–8
pulsus paradoxus and, 146
second heart sound and, 162–63, 166–67, 173, 175
tamponade and, 1257
work of, 387
Respiratory distress syndrome:
fat embolism and, 1115
neonatal, 586
patent ductus arteriosus and, 615
Response-to-injury theory of atherogenesis, 806–7
Rest:
coronary heart disease and, 933–34, 969
deep venous thrombosis and, 1375
heart failure and, 358
heat stress and, 1547–49
Rest:
myocarditis and, 1177
pulmonary embolism and, 1111
Resuscitation. *See* Cardiopulmonary resuscitation.
Retina, 198–203
cotton-wool spots, 199–200
diabetes and, 202
endocarditis and, 1142
examination, 198–203
exudates, hard, 200
hypertension and, 203, 1053
optic atrophy, 201
optic disk edema, 201, 203
topography, 198
Retinal vessels, 198–203
arteriosclerosis, 199, 203
atherosclerosis, 199
beading, 198–99
caliber changes, 198–99
compression, 199
embolism, 201
myxomatous, 1287
halo sheathing, 199
hemorrhage, 200
leakage, 200
microaneurysms, 200
neovascularization, 200
occlusion, 201
spasm, 199
wall thickening, 199
Retirement:
coronary heart disease and, 936
bypass surgery and, 955
job-related disability and, 1564
Reye's syndrome, 1239
Rhabdomyoma, 1220, 1292–93
Rhabdomyosarcoma, 1294–95
Rheumatic fever, 1306–12
arthritis and, 1308
carditis and, 1308–9
acute, 1308
chronic, 1309
course of, 1310–11
management, 1311–12
pathology, 1307
chorea and, 1309
clinical features, 1307–9
course and prognosis, 1310–11
definition, 1306
endocarditis and, 1307
erythema marginatum, 1309
etiology, 1306
incidence and epidemiology, 563, 1307
Jones criteria, 1311
laboratory findings, 1309–10
nodules and, subcutaneous, 1309
pathogenesis, 1306
pathology, 1307
pericarditis and, 1307
pregnancy and, 1386–88
prevention, 761, 1312
treatment, 1311–12
Rheumatic heart disease, 1309
aortic-mitral combined valvular disease, 785
aortic regurgitation, 740, 1308
aortic stenosis, 729
course of, 1310–11
endocarditis and, 1131
incidence and prevalence, 563
mitral regurgitation, 764, 1308
mitral stenosis, 754–55, 760, 1311
mortality, 563

Rheumatic heart disease:
pathology, 1307
thromboembolism and, 1670
cerebral, 1358
tricuspid valve, 792–93
Rheumatoid factor, endocarditis and, 1139
Rhythm disturbances. *See* Arrhythmias; *also* specific disturbance.
Rib:
cervical, 916–18
notching of, 236, 242
Ribonucleic acid:
hypertrophy and, cardiac, 97
protein synthesis and, 95
Ribosomes, 95
Ricin, 1489
Rickettsial myocarditis, 1174
Rifampin, tuberculous pericarditis and, 1270
Ring:
Carpentier, 777, 778
tricuspid valve, 797, 798
mitral supravalvular, 648, 649
vascular, 622–24
Ringer, Sydney, 1466
Ringer's lactate, hypovolemia and, 388
Risk factors:
atherosclerotic coronary heart disease, 807–9, 889
alterable vs. unalterable, 819, 820
evidence for, 819
intervention principle, 817
legal issues and, 1571–72
physician's role and, 826–27
populations and, 817
preventive measures, 820–32
deep venous thrombosis, 1105
insurance and, 1556–57
sudden death, 538–40
Risk index, noncardiac surgery, 1511–12
Ritodrine, 1394
Rodbard sounds, 139
Rocky Mountain spotted fever, 1174
Roentgenography, 230–43
abnormal densities, 231
abnormal lucencies, 231
anatomical relations and, 17
aortic aneurysm and, 1317
aortic arch and, right, 233
aortic dissection and, 1330, 1331
aortic-mitral combined valvular disease and, 789
aortic regurgitation and, 747
aortic stenosis and, 734
congenital, 636
artificial heart and, 2073
atrial septal defect and, 234, 235, 600
AV canal and, 607
bones and joints and, 236
cardiomyopathy and, 1188, 1201, 1455
chamber enlargement and, 243
coarctation of aorta and, 234, 242, 630
comparison of films in, 236–37
contour of heart and, 231
coronary heart disease and, 894
cor pulmonale and, 1125
double-outlet right ventricle and, 698
Ebstein's anomaly and, 237, 678, 679
endocarditis and, 1146
errors in interpreting, 1538
Roentgenography:
four-chamber cardiac series, 241–43
great vessels and, 232–34, 241
heart failure and, 236, 237, 239–40, 352–55
interlobar fissure thickening and, 354
malpositions of heart and, 231–32
mediastinal structures and, 234–35
mesenteric venous occlusion and, 1366
mitral regurgitation and, 772
mitral stenosis and, 235, 237, 758
myocarditis and, 1166
myxoma and, 1288, 1291
necropsy and, 2078
obesity cardiomyopathy and, 1455
pacing leads and, 1750, 1752, 1758
parenchyma and, pulmonary, 230, 235–36
patent ductus arteriosus and, 615
pericarditis and, 240
pleura and, 236
pregnancy and, 1394
pulmonary edema and, 353, 354
pulmonary embolism and, 916, 1108
pulmonary vasculature and, 230, 238–40
pulmonary veins and, 352, 353
connection anomaly and, 604, 684
pulmonic stenosis and, 656
silhouette of heart and, 16, 17
single ventricle and, 704
situs solitus and, 231–32
size of heart and, 230–31
statistical guidance in, 237–38
steps in examination, 230–38
tetralogy of Fallot and, 233, 234, 663, 664
transposition of great arteries and, 692
corrected, 701
tricuspid valve disease and, 795
atresia, 673–75
ventricular septal defect and, 593
Roth spots, 201
endocarditis and, 1142
Roussy-Levy polyneuropathy, 1229–30
Routine examination, 101
Rubella, 130
myocarditis and, 1174
patent ductus arteriosus and, 615
Rubinstein-Taybi syndrome, inspection and, 127, 133
Rumble, diastolic, 180, 181, 185, 186
mitral stenosis and, 757–58
tricuspid stenosis and, 795
Rupture:
aortic, 1326, 1327
repair of, 2049
syphilis and, 1317
traumatic, 1280–81
atherosclerotic plaque, 870–71
chordae tendineae. *See* Chordae tendineae, ruptured.
esophageal, 913
external cardiac, myocardial infarction and, 984–85
interventricular septum. *See* Interventricular septum, rupture (perforation).
myocardial infarction and, 393–94, 847, 850, 984–85, 2040–41
papillary muscle. *See* Papillary muscles, ruptured.
traumatic, 1278–81
Sack syndrome, 573
St. Jude prosthesis, 2034
aortic regurgitation and, 644
Salbutamol, 1483
Saline:
echocardiography and, 1948–49
hypovolemia and, 388
Salbutamol, cardiomyopathy and, 1192
Sandhoff's disease, 1223
Sansert, 1232
Saphenous vein grafts:
atherosclerosis of, 853, 854
femoropopliteal, 2060
patency, 954–55
reversed, 2036, 2037
thrombosis, 853, 854
Saphenous vein varicosities, 1376–77
Sarcoidosis, 1216–18
clinical manifestations, 1217–18
natural history and prognosis, 1218
pathology, 1216–17
skin and, 125
treatment, 1218
Sarcolemma, 32
action potential and, 38
ATPase, heart failure and, 330
sodium and, 39
Sarcoma, cardiac, 1294–95
Sarcomere, 32, 33
infarction and, 875
length-tension relation, 44–45
overstretch, heart failure and, 330
preload and, 332
Sarcoplasmic reticulum, 32–35
action potential and, 38
calcium sequestration rate, 330–31
eosinophilia, 875
excitation-contraction coupling and, 38
Sarcosporidiosis, 1176
Sarcotubular system, 32
Sartre, Jean-Paul, 1667
Scalenus anticus syndrome, 916
Scarlet fever, myocarditis and, 1173
Scarring:
cardiomyopathy and, 1184
endocarditis and, 1140
myocardial infarction and, 875
Schafer method, 546
Schechter, David, 1747, 1755
Scheie's syndrome, 572
Schistosomiasis, 1176
Schmitt, Otto H., 1716
Schoonmaker technique of arteriography, 1792
Scimitar syndrome, 604, 605
Scintigraphy. *See* Radionuclide studies.
Scintillation cameras, 1811–12
Anger, 1811
multicrystal, 1811–12
Sclerae, blue, 130
Scleredema of Buschke, 1239
Sclerodactylia, 1353
Sclerosis:
aortic, 249
progressive systemic (scleroderma), 1441–44
myocardial lesions, 1442–43
pericarditis and, 1269, 1443–44
pulmonary hypertension and, 1444
skin and, 123
treatment, 1444
tuberous, 124, 1231
genetics, 571
pulmonary hypertension and, 576

Schlicter test, endocarditis and, 1148
Scorpion venom, 1235, 1489
Scurvy, 1219, 1449
Secundum defect. *See* Atrial septal defect, secundum type.
Sedatives, coronary heart disease and, 935, 938
Sedentary living, coronary heart disease and, 825, 829–30
Seizures:
 cerebral hypoperfusion and, 1361
 electrically induced, 1487–88
 hypertensive encephalopathy and, 1054–55, 1357–58
 syncope vs., 519
Seldinger catheterization technique, 1771
 arteriography and, 1791
 IABP insertion and, 2022
Selenium deficiency, cardiomyopathy and, 1183–84, 1449
Self-gain, coronary heart disease and, 908
Semilunar valves. *See* Aortic valve; Pulmonary valve.
Senescence. *See* Aging; Elderly.
Senile heart disease, 331
Senning, Ake, 1747
Senning operation, 695, 696
Sensitivity of tests, 103
 Bayes' theorem and, 304, 305
Sensors, pacemaker, 498–99, 501
 malfunction of, 503–4
Sensory nerve, cardiac, 375
Septal hypertrophy, asymmetric, 1194–95. *See* Cardiomyopathy, hypertrophic.
Septal perforating arteries, 28
 AV block and, 427
 bypass surgery and, 2039
 cardiomyopathy and, 1197
 radiography, 1796
Septation of heart, embryologic, 6–12
 atria and pulmonary veins, 11–12
 atrioventricular canal, 8–9
 conus cordis, 9–10
 mechanisms, 6
 sinus venosus, 10–11
 truncus arteriosus, 9
 ventricular, 6–8
Septation procedure, univentricular heart and, 705
Septic shock, 390
Septostomy, balloon atrial, transposition of great arteries and, 694
Septum primum:
 atrial septal defect and, 9, 605–6, 611
 atrioventricular canal and, 8
 closure of foramen ovale and, 583
 embryology, 11–12
Septum secundum, 12. *See also* Atrial septal defect, secundum type.
Septum spurium, 11
Serotonin, coronary artery spasm and, 1010
Serpasil. *See* Reserpine.
Serum sickness, 1236
Sex differences in heart disease, 558, 559
Sexual activity, myocardial infarction and, 936
Sheep Fab fragments, digitalis toxicity and, 1648
Shock, 370–94
 acidosis and, 372, 389

Shock:
 afterload and, 372
 arrhythmias and, 371, 389–90
 autoregulation and, 377–78
 blood flow and, 371–74
  coronary, 372
 brain function and, 379
 capillaries and, 373–74
 cardiac output and, 371–72, 384, 385–86
 causes, 383–84
 cellular damage and, 380–81, 384
 clinical picture, 383
 compensated, 370, 383
 complement activation and, 381
 contractility and, 371–72, 379
 coronary bypass surgery and, 951–52
 decompensated, 370, 383
 heart function and, 379
 heart rate and, 371
 hemodynamic abnormalities, 370–78
 hypovolemia and, 373–74, 383–84, 388–89
 hypoxia and, 371–72, 380, 389
 irreversible, 370–71, 383
 ischemia and, 371
 kidney and, 375, 378
 liver and, 379
 lung and, 378–79
 lysosomal enzymes and, 380–81
 management, 384–94
  balloon counterpulsation, 394
  general measures, 387–88
  monitoring, 384–87
  sepsis and, 390
  surgical, 393–94
  sympathomimetic amines in, 390–92
  vasodilators in, 392–93
 metabolism and, 378–79
 mitochondria and, 380
 muscle and, 378
 myocardial depressant factor and, 381
 myocardial infarction and, 371–72, 393, 982
 nervous system and, 374–76
 oxygen-hemoglobin affinity and, 379
 pathophysiology, 370–81
 perfusion of tissue and, 371–74
 preload and, 371
 reflexes and, 375–76
 septic, 390
 stages of, 370–71, 383
 stroke volume and, 371–72
 vascular factors, 372–73
 vasoconstriction and, 376–77, 392–93
 vasodilatation and, 376, 390–92
 venous pressure and, 385
 warm, 383
Shoulder-hand syndrome, 132, 987
Shunts:
 aortic atresia and, 646, 647
 aortic-femoral external, 2047
 aortic stenosis and, 637
 arteriovenous. *See* Arteriovenous fistula.
 bidirectional, flow calculations for, 1780
 Blalock-Taussig, 666
 carotid endarterectomy and, 2053–55
 catheterization studies and, 1776–77, 1779–82
 coronary arteriovenous fistula, 708
 Doppler studies and, 1986–87
 echocardiography and, 1949

Shunts:
 equalization, 239
 extracardiac, 614–22
 Fick principle and, 1779–80
 Fontan, 676
  univentricular heart and, 706
 hydrogen electrode for detection of, 1782
 indicator-dilution technique for, 1781–82
 intracardiac, 590–614
 left-to-right. *See also* specific disorder.
  atrial septal defect and, 599
  AV canal and, 608
  catheterization studies and, 1776–77
  coronary artery anomaly and, 1018–19
  digitalis and, 1644–45
  dye-dilution curve and, 1781–82
  flow calculations for, 1779, 1781
  pregnancy and, 1387, 1390
  pulmonary blood flow and, 1093, 1095
  ventricular septal defect and, 592, 594
 patent ductus arteriosus, 614–18
 platinum electrode for detection of, 1782, 1783
 pulmonary atresia and, 661, 671
 radionuclide studies and, 1816–17
 right-to-left, 584. *See also* specific disorder.
  dye-dilution curve and, 1781
  Ebstein's anomaly and, 678
  flow calculations for, 1779, 1781
  paradoxical embolism and, 1108–9
  pregnancy and, 1387
  pulmonic stenosis and, 655
 systemic-pulmonary. *See* Pulmonary vasculature, systemic communication with.
 truncus arteriosus and, 671, 672
 vascularity, 239
Sickle cell anemia, 399–400, 1226–27
 cor pulmonale and, 1124
Sickle cell trait, 1227
Sick sinus syndrome, 449–50. *See also* Sinus node dysfunction.
 management, 479–80
 pacing and, 489–90
 syncope and, 523, 526
Signal averaging, QRS, 1716–19
Silhouette, cardiac, 16, 17
Simpson's rule, echocardiography and, 1946–48
Single atrium, 612
Single ventricle, 7–8, 703–6
Sinoatrial block, 461–62
 ECG, 461–62
 pacing and, 489
Sinoatrial (sinoauricular) node. *See* Sinus node.
Sinus arrhythmias, 436–37
 AV dissociation and, 467
 bradycardia, 426–27, 436–37
  approach to patient with, 288–89
  athletes and, 1401
  management, 479
  myocardial infarction and, 973
  pacing and, 489
  shock and, 389
 myocardial infarction and, 436–37, 972–73
 tachycardia, 413, 437
  carotid sinus massage and, 292

Sinus arrhythmias: tachycardia:
diagnosis, 437
hyperthyroidism and, 1415
myocardial infarction and, 972–73
shock and, 389
Sinus node:
action potential, 75, 76, 78
anatomy, 18, 30
automaticity, 78–79, 407–8
block. *See* Sinoatrial block.
calcium channel blockers and, 1627, 1631
conduction time, 1735–36
digitalis and, 1643
dysfunction, 426–27, 449–50
approach to patient with, 288–89
beta-blocker-induced, 1618
diagnosis, 450
ECG, 289, 450
management, 479–80
myocardial infarction and, 973
pacemakers and, 489–90
syncope and, 523, 526
ECG and, 206
electrophysiologic study, 1734–36
innervation, 25, 49
internodal pathways and, 30
potassium and, 1468
recovery time, 450, 1735
reentry, 413
rhythm, 436–37. *See also* Sinus arrhythmias.
range of rates, 435, 437
somnolent, 1743
wandering pacemaker and, 468–69
Sinus node artery, 29, 30
muscular dystrophy and, 1227
polyarteritis nodosa and, 1439
Sinus of Valsalva:
anatomy, 22
aneurysm (fistula), 620–21
assessment, 258–59, 621
management, 621, 2043, 2044
murmur, 621
pathology, 620–21
regurgitant valve and, 2043
coronary arteriography and, 1792
coronary artery origin from, 711, 1017–18
embryology, 13
Sinus venosus:
atrial septal defect and, 598, 603
embryology, 10–11
Situs ambiguus, 689
definition, 686
roentgenography and, 232
Situs inversus:
assessment, 257
definition, 686
dextrocardia and, 688–89
Situs solitus:
assessment, 257–58
definition, 686
roentgenography and, 231–32
Size of heart. *See also* Cardiomegaly: Hypertrophy.
echocardiography and, 1935–36
roentgenography and, 230–31
Skiing, coronary artery disease and, 1546
Skin:
cardiac output and disease of, 404
color change, 120. *See also* Cyanosis; Pallor.
arteriosclerosis obliterans and, 1341
Skin: color change:
arteriospasm and, 1352–53
hyperextensible, 124
inspection, 122–26
lupus erythematosus and, 123, 124
polyarteritis and, 123
rash. *See* Rash.
scleroderma, 123, 1442
venous hypertension and, 1377
Sleep apnea, obesity and, 1455
Sleeping sickness, 1175
Slew rate, pacemaker, 1751
Sliding filament hypothesis, 33–34
Slow-response fibers, 75, 407, 408
Smallpox vaccine, 1236–37
S.M.E.C. balloon, 2021
Smith-Lemli-Opitz syndrome, 129
Smoking:
angina pectoris and, 891
arteriosclerosis obliterans and, 1339, 1343
atherosclerosis and, 808, 823, 827–28
coronary heart disease and, 937
cor pulmonale and, 1120
myocardial infarction and, 823, 827–28
sudden death and, 538
thromboangiitis obliterans and, 1346–48
Smooth-muscle cells:
atherosclerosis and, 805, 806, 811–13
calcium and, 1009–10
channel blockers and, 1626
contractility, 1009–11
endothelial injury and, 810
experimental studies, 803–4
fatty streaks and, 801, 804
fibrous plaque and, 801, 803
lipid metabolism and, 812–13
monoclonal theory and, 806
physiology, 1009–10
proliferation of, 811–12
prostaglandins and, 814
vasodilators and, 1584–87
Snake venom, 1489
Social hierarchies, 1520–21
Social Security, 1565, 1572
disability criteria, 1578
Socioeconomic factors, 1521–22
Sodium:
action potential and, 38, 76–77, 1466
channel, 76
conductance, 38, 76
contractility and, 39
diuretics and, 362, 1657, 1665
edema and, 1657, 1662
extracellular, 1040, 1041
heart failure and, retention mechanisms in, 324–25
hypertension and, 824, 1040–41, 1078
pregnancy and, 1384
pump, 75
renal failure and, 1458–59
renin and, 1041
restriction of dietary, 360–61, 1078
sarcolemma and, 39
transmembrane potential and, 74–75, 1466
Sodium nitroprusside. *See* Nitroprusside.
Solanine, 1488
Soldier's heart, 1526
Sones technique of arteriography, 1791
Sorbitrate. *See* Isosorbide dinitrate.
Sotalol:
arrhythmias and, 1615
pharmacodynamics, 1608, 1613, 1617
pharmacokinetics, 1610, 1611
structure, 1608
Sounds, heart, 164–88. *See also* Auscultation.
aortic valve, 160
bicuspid, 183–84, 636
closure, 162, 163, 166–76
ejection, 163, 183–84
regurgitation and, 745–46, 1315, 1316
stenosis and, 173, 183, 184, 636, 733–34
apexcardiography and, 1994–95
athletes and, 1400
atrial septal defect, 600
ejection, 182
opening snap, 185
second, 167–68, 174
AV canal defect, 607
cardiac cycle and, 53
cardiomyopathy and, 1188, 1201
coarctation of aorta and, 184
diastolic, 163, 176–82
early, 186
rumble, 180, 181, 185, 186, 757–58, 795
vs. systolic, 176–77
Eisenmenger's syndrome and, 168, 169, 174
ejection, 163, 182–84
aortic, 163, 183–84
murmurs and, 189, 190
pulmonary, 163, 182–83
first, 164–66
abnormally wide splitting of, 165
auscultatory principles, 163
differential diagnosis of splitting of, 165
echocardiography, 159, 164
intensity of, 165–66
origin of, 158–59
physiological splitting of, 164–65
fourth, 160, 182
origin of, 160
frequency (Hz), 157, 158, 161
gallop, 176–82. *See also* Gallop.
atrial, 177–79, 181
classification, 182
combinations, 181
summation, 182
ventricular diastolic, 179–81
heart failure and, 167
hyperthyroidism and, 1414
Korotkov, 139
mitral valve, 160, 163
clicks, 184
closure, 163, 164–66
opening, 185, 756
regurgitation and, 171–72, 650, 770
stenosis and, 185, 756
murmurs. *See* Murmurs.
myxoma and, 1287, 1291
opening snaps, 185–86
mitral valve, 185
tricuspid valve, 186
origin of, 158–60
pacemaker, 188
palpable, 155–56
pericardial knock, 186
physics of, 157
prosthetic valve, 186–88

Sounds, heart:
pulmonary hypertension and, 173–75, 1098
ejection, 182–83
single second, 168, 169
pulmonary valve, 160
closure, 163, 166–76
ejection, 163, 182–83
stenosis and, 169–71, 656
valvotomy and, 171
recording of. *See* Phonocardiography.
rumble, diastolic, 180, 181, 185, 186, 757–58
tricuspid stenosis and, 795
second, 166–76
auscultatory principles, 162–63
fixed splitting of, 167–68, 175–76
misdiagnosis in splitting of, 175–76
mitral stenosis and, 185
origin of, 158–59
phonocardiography, 166
physiological splitting of, 166–67
relative intensity of components of, 173–75
respiration and, 162–63, 166–67, 173, 175
reversed splitting of, 172–73
single, 175
stroke volume and, 167
wide splitting of, 168–72
systolic, 162–63, 182–85
clicks, 184–85. *See also* Clicks, systolic.
vs. diastolic, 176–77
ejection, 182–84
prolongation and, 173
root, 160
whoops, 185
tetralogy of Fallot and, 169–70
third, 160, 180–81
origin of, 160
pericarditis and, 186
transmission of, 160–61
tricuspid valve, 160, 163
closure, 163, 164–65
opening, 186
regurgitation and, 795
stenosis and, 186, 795
valvular theory of, 158–59
ventricular filling, 160, 163, 176
ventricular septal defect, 171, 172, 593
wavelength, 157
tumor "plop," 1287
Spasm, 1352–53
cardiomyopathy and, 1183
clinical manifestations, 1352–53
coronary artery. *See* Coronary arteries, spasm.
esophageal, 912–13
retinal vascular, 199
treatment, 1353
Specificity of tests, 103
Bayes' theorem and, 304, 305
Sphincters:
precapillary, 373
vascular, 26
Sphygmomanometry, 139–40
Spider vemon, 1236
Spinal muscular atrophy, 1231
Spinocerebellar degeneration, 1229
Spirochetal infections. *See also* Syphilis.
myocarditis, 1173–74
Spironolactone. *See also* Diuretics.
aldosteronism and, 1082
Spironolactone:
biochemistry, 1658
cirrhosis with ascites and, 1662
dosage, 1072, 1659
duration of action, 1659
edema and, 1664
heart failure in infant and, 585
pharmacokinetics, 1661
site of action, 1660
Splanchnic vessels:
heat stress and, 1548–50
occlusive disease, 1364–70
venous, 1366
periarteritis nodosa and, 1370
postoperative arteritis, 1371
reflex, shock and, 374
Spleen:
absent, 690
heart failure and, 352
malpositions of heart and, 257
multiple masses of tissue of (polysplenia), 690
physical examination and, 204
Splenic artery aneurysm, 1351
Splenomegaly, endocarditis and, 1142
Splinter hemorrhages, endocarditis and, 1142
Spondylitis, ankylosing. *See* Ankylosing spondylitis.
Sporotrichosis, 1175
Spousal factors, coronary heart disease and, 826
Sprague, Howard B., 1990
Sputum, bloody, 118–19
Squatting:
auscultation and, 195
tetralogy of Fallot and, 120, 663
ST segment, 84. *See also* Electrocardiography.
calcium and, 225
coronary artery spasm and, 1011
coronary heart disease and, 894–96
exercise testing and, 306, 1708–10
injury and, 209
myocardial infarction and, 210–12
pericarditis and, 212, 213
prolonged recording of, 1723
reciprocal changes, 211
Stab wounds, 1022, 1276, 1277
Staircase phenomenon, 39, 48
Standstill, ventricular, 471, 490
Stapedial artery, 13
Staphylococcal infections:
endocarditis, 1135, 1136, 1163
cure rate, 1147
dialysis and, 1460
drug-related, 1132
frequency, 1133
postoperative, 1133, 1152
treatment, 1148–50
pericarditis, 1270
shock and, 390
Starling law. *See also* Frank-Starling law.
heart failure and, 326–27
ultrastructural basis of, 44–45
Starr-Edwards prosthesis, 2034
sounds of, 187, 188
survival curves, 780
thromboembolism and, 1671
Steal mechanism, 1334
coronary, 863–64
subclavian. *See* Subclavian steal syndrome.
Steell, Graham, 792
Steinert's disease, 1230
Stellate ganglion, 25
Sternotomy, pericardiectomy and, 2010, 2011
Sternum, cleft of, 707
Stethoscope, 161–62
ideal, 162
inching technique, 176–77
Stewart-Hamilton formula, 1781
Stiffness:
length-tension relation and, 45
vascular, 58
aging and, 1406
ventricular, 43
Still's murmur, 189
Stimulation techniques, 283. *See also* Electrophysiology, invasive studies; Pacemakers; Pacing; Pulse generators.
palpitations and, 286
reentry and, 421–23
ventricular tachycardia and, 421–23
Stokes, William, 729
Stokes-Adams syndrome, 523, 1360
Stomach, heterotaxia and, 689, 690
Straight-back syndrome, 134
Streptococcal infections:
antibody test, 1310
culture studies, 1310
endocarditis, 1135–36
cure rate, 1147
frequency, 1133
postoperative, 1152
treatment, 1148–50
rheumatic fever, 1306–7, 1310, 1312
Streptokinase, 1679. *See also* Thrombolytic agents.
actions of, 1679
adverse reactions to, 1539, 1919–20
angioplasty and, 1903
antibodies to, 1916, 1919
arteriosclerosis obliterans and, 1346
coronary thrombosis and, 1681–82
historical note on, 887
loading dose, 1916
myocardial infarction and, 943, 967–68, 1917–19
new developments in, 1682
peripheral infusion of, 1917
pulmonary embolism and, 1113–14
systemic infusion of, 1916–19
Streptomycin:
endocarditis and, 1149
hypersensitivity to, 1237
rheumatic fever prophylaxis and, 761
Stress:
anesthesia and, 1494–95
definition, 1520
emotional. *See* Emotional stress; Psychological factors.
heat, 1547–50
pharmacologic, myocardial perfusion and, 1838–39
testing. *See* Exercise testing.
Stroke. *See* Cerebrovascular disease.
Stroke volume, 51
afterload and, 267, 326
altitude and, 1545
aortic, 1979–80
regurgitation and, 742, 747, 748, 1783–84
artificial heart and, 2069, 2071, 2072
digital subtraction angiography and, 1861
Doppler studies and, 1979–81, 1985
end-diastolic pressure and, 44, 45

Stroke volume:
end-diastolic volume and, 44, 45
exercise and, 55, 335, 1398, 1399
Frank-Starling law and, 43–44
heart failure and, 326, 335
hypertension and, 1042, 1043
mitral regurgitation and, 773, 775, 1783–84
pregnancy and, 1384
regurgitant, 1783–84, 1822
Doppler studies and, 1985
second heart sound and, 167
shock and, 371–72
Subaortic stenosis, idiopathic hypertrophic. *See* Cardiomyopathy, hypertrophic.
Subclavian artery:
aberrant, 622–23
clinical manifestations, 622
management, 623
anomalous, 14–15
coarctation of aorta repair and, 633, 2049–51
compression of, 917
embryology, 13, 14
flap angioplasty, 633
interrupted aortic arch and, 623
isolation of, 624–25
occlusive disease, 1334
pressure pulse and, 54
pulmonary artery anastomosis to, 666
Subclavian lymphatics, 26–27
Subclavian steal syndrome, 514, 1334
pulse pressure inequality and, 141
Subclavian vein, pacemaker implantation and, 1748–49
Subcostal approach, epicardial pacemaker implantation and, 2019
Subcutaneous tissue, heart failure and, 352
Subendocardium:
coronary flow to, 63
infarction, 846, 872
ECG and, 211–12
ischemia, 859–61, 865
Subepicardial fat stripe, fluoroscopy and, 1767
Sublimaze, 1497
Subpleural fluid, 354
Substrates:
heart failure and, 330
oxidative, 85–86, 87
fatty acids and, 93
protein metabolism and, 96
Subxiphoid approach:
pacemaker implantation and, epicardial, 2017–18
pericardiocentesis and, 2008–9
Succinylcholine, 1497
electroconvulsive therapy and, 1487, 1488
Sudden death, 529–45
alcoholism and, 1447–48
antiarrhythmic agents and, 543–44
aortic stenosis and, 531
arrhythmias and, 538
athletes and, 1401
beta-blocking agents and, 543
cardiomyopathies and, 531, 544, 1204, 1206
community impact of, 538
conduction system and, 531–33
coronary arteritis and, 530
coronary artery anomalies and, 530, 709, 711
Sudden death:
coronary artery spasm and, 1013
coronary bypass surgery and, 950
coronary embolism and, 530, 534
coronary heart disease and, 530, 540, 850, 987–88
prognostic considerations, 929–30
definition, 529, 538, 987
ECG and, 540
electrical instability and, 539, 544
emotional stress and, 1522–23
familial, 577
hypertension and, 538–39
manifestations prior to, 539
myocardial infarction and, 531, 536, 541
uncomplicated, 969
myocarditis and, 531, 1163
obesity and, 1455
pathogenetic mechanisms, 533–36
pathological findings, 529–36
premature ventricular beats and, 539, 540, 543
prevention, 542–44
recurrence of syndrome, 541–42
resuscitative techniques and, 541, 988. *See also* Cardiopulmonary resuscitation.
risk factors, 538–40
syncope and, 527
tumors of heart and, 531, 534
ventricular fibrillation and, 533, 538, 540–44
prevention and treatment, 542–44
recurrent syndrome and, 541–42
ventricular tachycardia and, 295
Sufentanil, 1496
Sulcus terminalis, 18
Sulfinpyrazone:
adverse reactions to, 1678
endothelium and, 812
myocardial infarction and, 831, 944, 972, 1677, 1678
prosthetic valves and, 1676
thromboxane and, 1675
Sulfonamides:
diuretic, 1658
hypersensitivity to, 1236
Sulmazole, 1655
Superoinferior heart, 706
Surfactant, shock and, 378
Surgery, 2008–76
anesthesia and. *See* Anesthesia.
angioplasty. *See* Angioplasty.
anomalous systemic arteries to lung, 622
aortic aneurysm, 1326–27, 2043–48
abdominal, 1328
aortic arch aneurysm, 1326, 2045–46
aortic arch anomalies, 623, 624
interruption, 634–35
double, 2051
aortic atresia, 647
aortic dissection, 1333, 2047–48
aortic-left ventricular tunnel, 645
aorticopulmonary septal defect, 619
aortic valve, 2030–32
mitral disease combined with, 790–91
regurgitation, 644, 749–51, 2030–32, 2047
stenosis, 638–42, 736–37
arteriosclerosis obliterans, 1345–46
atrial septal defect, 602–3
AV canal, 610–12
Surgery:
bacteremia after, 1151–53
cardiomyopathy, 1208
cardioverter-defibrillator implantation, 1761–62
carotid artery, 2052–56
cerebrovascular disease after, 1361–62
coarctation of aorta, 632–34, 2049–51
complications, 1541
conduction system, 2014–15
coronary arteriovenous fistula, 708
coronary artery anomalies, 710
coronary artery spasm, 1015
coronary bypass. *See* Coronary bypass surgery.
cor triatriatum, 652
diabetics and, 1431
double-outlet left ventricle, 700
double-outlet right ventricle, 699
Ebstein's anomaly, 679–80
echocardiography during, 1952
electrograms during, 2013–14
for endocarditis, 1150–51
endocarditis after, 1132–34, 1151–53
gallbladder, 914
for heart failure, 365–66
hemitruncus, 620
left ventricular–right atrial communication, 614
mitral valve, 2032–33
aortic valve disease combined with, 790–91
regurgitation, 650–51, 776–79
stenosis, 649, 762–63
myocardial failure after, 275–76
myxoma, 1292, 1293
noncardiac, 1511–19
angina pectoris and, 1502–3, 1513
arrhythmias and, 1514–15, 1518
cardiac output and, 1518
congenital heart disease and, 1516
congestive heart failure and, 1517
coronary heart disease and, 991, 1513–14, 1518
digitalis and, 1514, 1517
hypertension and, 1515–16
postoperative problems, 1518–19
preoperative evaluation, 1512
prosthetic valves and, 1517
pulmonary obstructive disease and, 1517
risk assessment, 1511–14
valvular heart disease and, 1516
pacemaker implantation, 1747–54
patent ductus arteriosus, 617–18
pericardiectomy, 1254, 2009–13
pericardiocentesis, 1541, 2008–9
pericardiotomy, 2009
peripheral vascular, 2057–62
pheochromocytoma, 1083
postoperative care. *See* Postoperative care.
postponement of elective, 1503
pregnancy and, 1392
pulmonary arteriovenous fistula, 681
pulmonary artery banding. *See* Pulmonary artery banding.
pulmonary atresia, 661–62, 671, 673
pulmonary embolectomy, 1112–13
pulmonary regurgitation, 799
pulmonary venous connection anomaly, 605, 683–84
pulmonic stenosis, 657–59
renovascular hypertension, 1079–80, 1335

Surgery:
risk index, 1511–12
rupture repair, 2040–41
papillary muscle, 2041
septal, 2041
ventricular free wall, 2040
for shock, cardiogenic, 393–94
single atrium, 612
single ventricle (univentricular heart), 705–6
sinus of Valsalva aneurysm, 621
subclavian artery aberrancy, 623
tachycardia, 2013–15
tetralogy of Fallot, 665–67
thoracic outlet syndrome, 917
thyroid, 397, 1417
tracheal compression relief, 627
transplant, 2063–65
transposition of great arteries, 695–96
corrected, 703
tricuspid atresia, 676
tricuspid regurgitation, 677, 796–99, 2033–34
tricuspid stenosis, 796–97
truncus arteriosus, 672–73
Uhl's malformation, 680
ventricular septal defect, 596–97
pulmonary atresia and, 671, 673
tetralogy of Fallot and, 666
Swallowing:
pain on, 912
syncope and, 516
Swan-Ganz catheterization, 1999–2002
cardiac output and, 385, 2000
complications, 1540, 2001–2
endothelial assessment and, 387
heart failure and, 270, 355
indications, 2000–2001
insertion technique, 1999–2000
lung water measurement and, 386
pressure mesurements, 2000
Sweat glands, 59
Sweating:
heart failure and, 351
syncope and, 508, 510
Sympathectomy:
acute arterial occlusion and, 1350
arteriosclerosis obliterans and, 1346
arteriospastic disease and, 1353
coronary artery, 1015
lumbar, peripheral occlusive disease and, 2061
Sympathetic nervous system, 24–25. *See also* Adrenergic receptors.
aging and, 1404, 1406–7
agonists. *See* Sympathomimetics.
beta-blocking drugs and. *See* Beta-blocking agents.
blood pressure and, 1040
cardiac outut and, 44
contractility and, 44, 49
coronary artery spasm and, 1010
coronary blood flow and, 61
diabetic neuropathy and, 1428
digitalis and, 1642
emotional stress and, 1520–21, 1523
exercise and, 55, 1399
heat stress and, 1547, 1548
hypertension and, 1040, 1042–46, 1071–74
hyperthyroidism and, 1415
orthostatic hypotension and, 511–12
shock and, 374–77
syncope and, 509
Sympathetic nervous system:
vasoconstriction and, 59, 376–77
inhibition of, 1588–89
stimulation of, 1590
vasodilatation and, 59
Sympatholytic agents. *See also* Beta-blocking agents.
hypertension and, 1071–75
dosage, 1072
Sympathomimetics:
beta-blocking drugs and, 1609
complications, 391
receptor activity, 1654
shock and, 390–92
vasoconstriction and, 1590
Symptoms:
cardiac status and prognosis and, 106–8
determinants and value of, 112
history taking and, 109–22. *See also* History.
interpretation of, 112
errors in, 1538
predictive value of, 111
presence and magnitude of, 111–12
worrisome, to patient, 118
Synchronization, AV dissociation and, 467
Syncope, 117–18, 507–28, 988
aortic dissection and, 1331
aortic stenosis and, 522, 524, 732–33
arrhythmias and, 287, 523–24, 988, 1360, 1361
AV block, 287, 288, 516, 523, 524, 526
bradycardia, 508, 509, 523, 524, 528
diagnosis, 525–27
tachycardia, 523–24, 526
treatment, 527–28, 988
cardiac, 521–28
classification, 522
diagnosis, 524–27
pathophysiology, 522–24
treatment, 527–28
cardiomyopathy and, 522, 524, 1200
carotid sinus, 514–16
cerebrovascular, 513–14
hypoperfusion and, 1360–61
classification, 507, 522
convulsive disorders vs., 519
coronary heart disease and, 988
cough (tussive), 517
defecation, 518
definition, 507, 988
diagnostic procedures, 287–88, 520, 524–27
diver's, 518
ECG and, 287
electrophysiologic studies, 287–88, 1739
glossopharyngeal neuralgia and, 516–17
heat, 1549
history, 287
hyperventilation and, 518–19
hypoglycemia and, 518
hypoxia and, 518
hysterical, 519
micturition, 517–18
migraine, 519
near, 117, 507
noncardiovascular, 518–19
obstructive disease and, 522, 524, 527
Syncope:
orthostatic, 510–13
pacemakers and, 288
premonitory symptoms, 508
pulmonary hypertension and, 522, 1097–98
reflex types of, 516–17
subclavian steal syndrome and, 514
sudden death and, 527
swallow (deglutition), 516
vascular, 510–18
vasodepressor, 508–10, 515
vasovagal, 510, 516, 517
Syphilis, 1314–19
aortic aneurysm and, 1316–17, 1319, 1325
aortic regurgitation and, 1315–16, 1319
aortitis and, 1314–17
clinical manifestations, 1315–18
coronary arteries and, 1023, 1317–18
diagnosis, 1318–19
infectious process and natural history, 1314–15
latent period, 1315
myocarditis and, 1173, 1318
treatment, 1319
Systole, 52–53
apexcardiography and, 1994–95
coronary blood flow and, 60, 858–59, 860
DPTI and, 860
failure (dysfunction), 320–21
murmurs of, 188–92
auscultatory principles, 163
precordial movement and, 153, 155
pressure of. *See* Systolic pressure.
sounds of, 162–63, 182–85
clicks, 184–85. *See also* Clicks, systolic.
vs. diastolic, 176–77
ejection, 182–84
gallop, as misnomer, 176
prolongation and, 173
root, 160
whoops, 185
time intervals:
cardiomyopathy and, 1190, 1203
echocardiography and, 1948
Systolic pressure. *See also* Blood pressure.
afterload mismatch and, 266–67
ankle, arteriosclerosis obliterans and, 1342
ankle-arm index, 1974, 1975
aortic stenosis and, 635, 636, 638, 730–32
cardiomyopathy and, 1199–200
Doppler studies and, 1974–75
heart failure and, 266
hypertension and, 1042, 1052
measurement of, 139
normal, 55, 140
ophthalmic artery, 1877–78
physical determinants of, 138
pulmonary artery stenosis and, 1775
pulmonary valve stenosis and, 655
variability in, 1049

T system, 32, 38, 39
T wave, 210
genesis, 84
hypocalcemia and, 225
long-term recording of, 1723

T wave:
  pacemakers and, 494
    malfunction of, 502–3
  potassium and, 222–23, 1471
T_a wave, 206
Tachycardia, 413–26
  antidromic, 448, 454
  approach to patient with, 291–95
  atrial, 413–14. *See also* supraventricular *below.*
    AV block and, 440
    digitalis and, 1643, 1646
    ectopic, 440, 441
    ECG, 441–44, 1694, 1699
    ectopic, 440, 441
    management, 476
    myocardial infarction and, 973–74
  atrial pacing techniques and, 1740
  AV junctional, 417–20, 470
    with AV dissociation, 420
    ECG, 419, 441–43
    ectopic, 440
    myocardial infarction and, 974
    nonparoxysmal, 420
    with 1:1 AV association, 418–20
    paroxysmal, 418–20
    reentry and, 418–20
  -bradycardia syndrome, 449, 450
    esophageal ECG and, 1698, 1699
    management, 480
    pacing and, 489–90
    syncope and, 523, 528
  cardiomyopathy and, 1188, 1204
  definition, 437
  digitalis and, 440, 479, 1643–46
  ECG, 292
    atrial, 441–44, 1694, 1699
    AV junctional, 419, 441–43
    esophageal leads and, 293, 1694–97, 1699
    QRS widening, 293
    sinus, 436
    supraventricular, 293, 417, 421, 441–44
    ventricular, 293–94, 422, 453–56, 1717–18
  electrophysiological studies, 294–95, 478
  familial, 576
  His bundle recording and, 1730
  hyperthyroidism and, 396
  idioventricular, 456
  induction of, 1737–38
  management, 476–79
    surgical, 2013–15
  mapping of, 1738
  mechanisms, 413–26
  multifocal (chaotic), 440, 443
  myocarditis and, 1165, 1170, 1178
  orthodromic, 448, 477
  pacing and, 482, 490, 499–500
    atrial, 1740
    characteristics of ideal system for, 499
    esophageal leads and, 1698–1701
  palpitation and, 117
  pheochromocytoma and, 1083
  physical examination, 292
  pregnancy and, 1392
  pulse and, 146
  reciprocating, 447–48, 468
    management, 477
    WPW syndrome and, 416, 418
  reentry and. *See* Reentry.
  shock and, 371, 389–90
Tachycardia:
  sinus, 413, 437
    carotid sinus massage and, 292
    diagnosis, 437
    hyperthyroidism and, 1415
    myocardial infarction and, 972–73
    shock and, 389
  supraventricular, 439–43
    aberrant conduction and, 460–61
    accessory pathways and, 417, 418
    artifactual, 1725
    calcium channel blockers and, 1630–31
    cardioversion for, 1744
    digitalis and, 1644, 1645
    ECG, 293, 417, 421, 441–44
    ectopic, 440, 441, 476
    esophageal leads and, 1695, 1696
    management, 476–77
    mechanism, 413–14, 416–20
    reentry, 413–20, 440–41, 476
    WPW syndrome and, 447–48, 461
  syncope and, 523–24, 526
  torsades de pointes, 424, 455–56
  ventricular, 420–24, 452–56
    aberrant conduction and, 460–61
    alternating, 455
    approach to patient with, 291–95
    arrest and, 295
    artifactual, 1724
    beta blockers and, 1615, 1616
    bidirectional, 455
    cardioversion for. *See* Cardioversion.
    dysplasia and, 424
    ECG, 293–94, 422, 453–56, 1717–18
    esophageal leads and, 1694–97
    late potentials and, 1717–19
    management, 478–79, 2014–15
    mechanism, 420–24, 452
    myocardial infarction and, 975–76, 985–86
    nodoventricular fibers and, 425
    pleomorphic and polymorphous, 455
    premature beats and, 452, 453
    programmed stimulation and, 421–23, 1737
    reentry, 420–23
    repetitive, 455
    shock and, 389–90
    slow, 456
    sudden death and, 295
  WPW syndrome and, 416
Tachypnea, 135
  pulmonary embolism and, 1106, 1107
Tactile perception, 152–53
Takayasu's disease, 1323
  arteriosclerosis obliterans vs., 1342
  coronary arteries and, 1023
Tamponade, 1256–63
  acute, 1260
  assessment, 262–63, 1260–62
  atypical, 1262
  dialysis and, 1267
  differential diagnosis, 1262
  echocardiography and, 1261, 1953, 1955
  effusive constrictive pericarditis and, 1261, 1265
  etiology, 1259
  historical note on, 1256
  low-pressure, 1261
  metastases and, 1268
Tamponade:
  pathophysiology, 1256–59
  preexisting heart disease and, 1261–62
  pulsus paradoxus and, 1258–60
  radiation-induced, 1484
  subacute, 1260–61
  traumatic, 1277
  treatment, 1262–63. *See also* Pericardiocentesis.
Tangier disease, 131, 574
Taussig-Bing heart, 696–99
Tay-Sachs disease, 1223
Technetium-99m:
  cardiomyopathy and, 260, 261–62
  coronary heart disease and, 900–902
  fist-pass studies, 1813–14
  gate equilibrium studies, 1818
  lung imaging and, 1881
  pyrophosphate imaging, 1844–48
Technology:
  growth of, 2081
  proper use of, 106
Telangiectasia, 125
  hereditary hemorrhagic, 1227
    gastrointestinal tract and, 1370
Telemetry, pacemakers and, 500, 1758
Telephone:
  electrocardiography and, 283
  pacemaker monitoring by, 1755–56
Teletronics lead, 492
Temperature (body):
  cardiopulmonary bypass and, 2027
  exercise and, 1399
  heat stress and, 1547–50
Temporal arteritis, 201
  aorta and, 1323
Tenormin. *See* Atenolol.
Tension-length relation, 44–45, 332
Tension-time index, 860
Teratoma, pericardial, 1295
Terbutaline, 1394, 1483
Terminal cisternae, myocardial, 34, 38, 39
Testimony, expert, 1565–67
Tetralogy of Fallot, 662–67
  assessment, 257, 663–65
  associated conditions, 662
  catheterization studies, 664–65
  definition, 662
  ECG, 664
  echocardiography, 258, 664, 1949
  hematologic studies, 664
  history, 663
  medical management, 665
    beta blockers in, 1617
  murmur, 663
  natural history and prognosis, 665
  pathology, 662
  pathophysiology, 662–63
  physical examination, 663
  precordial palpation and, 155
  pregnancy and, 1391
  pulmonary atresia and, 668, 669
  pulmonary valve absence and, 667
  pulmonic stenosis and, 662, 663
  roentgenography and, 233, 234, 663, 664
  sounds of, 169–70
  squatting and, 120, 663
  surgical management, 665–67
  syncope and, 522
  ventricular septal defect and, 10, 662, 663, 666
Tetrazolium dyes, myocardium infarction and, 877–78

Tetrodotoxin, action potential and, 78
Thallium imaging, 1831–44
  anatomic definition and, 1843–44
  coronary heart disease and, 899–900, 970
  ECG and, 900
  exercise, 306, 899–900, 970, 1832, 1834–38, 1842–43
  function studies vs., 1842–43
  limitations of, 900
  myocardial perfusion studies, 1831–44
  normal image, 1832–33
  pharmacologic stress, 1838–39
  physiology of uptake, 1831
  quantification, 1839–40
  resting, 1833–34, 1843–44
  technique, 1832
  tomographic, 1840–42
Thebesian valve, 19, 30
Thebesian veins, 30
Theophylline, 1483
Thermodilution technique, 385, 1781, 2000
Thiamine deficiency, 399, 1448–49
Thiazides, 1658–60. *See also* specific agent.
  cholesterol and, 1074–75
  dosage, 1072, 1659
  duration of action, 1659
  heart failure and, 1661
  hypertension and, 1664
    gestational, 1084
  side effects, 1073
Thiopental, 1496
Thioridazine, 1480–81
  toxicity, 1232
Thoracic duct, 26, 27
Thoracic ganglia, 24, 25
Thoracic outlet syndrome, 916–18
Thoracotomy:
  pacemaker implantation and, epicardial, 2016, 2018
  pericardiectomy and, 2010
Thorax. *See* Chest; Precordium.
Thorazine. *See* Chlorpromazine.
Threshold potential, 75, 76, 1466
  impulse conduction and, 410
  triggered activity and, 408
Thrills, 156
  aortic stenosis and, 636, 641
  mitral regurgitation and, 770
  pulmonic stenosis and, 656
Thrombectomy, enzymatic, 1680, 1681
Thrombin:
  heparin and, 1667
  warfarin and, 1669
Thromboangiitis obliterans, 1346–48
  clinical manifestations, 1347
  diagnosis, 1347–48
  differential diagnosis, 1348
  digestive system and, 1370
  etiology, 1346–47
  pathology and pathophysiology, 1347
  treatment, 1348
Thrombocytes. *See* Platelets.
Thrombocytopenia:
  heparin-associated, 1111, 1668
  thrombotic purpura, 1227
    sudden death and, 535
Thromboembolism. *See also* Embolism; Pulmonary embolism; Thrombosis.
  mitral stenosis and, 755, 761
  prophylaxis, 1110–11
  prosthetic valves and, 779
Thrombolytic agents, 1678–82, 1916–21. *See also* Streptokinase; Urokinase.
  adverse effects, 1539, 1919–20
  angioplasty and, 1903
  arterial thrombosis and, 1681
  arteriosclerosis obliterans and, 1346
  contraindications, 1920
  coronary thrombosis and, 1681–82
  deep-vein thrombosis and, 1680–81, 1916–17
  dialysis and, 1682
  general considerations, 1916
  indications, 1680–82
  loading dose, 1916
  monitoring of, 1917
  myocardial infarction and, 843–44, 967–68, 1917–19
  new developments in, 1682, 1921
  peripheral thrombosis and, 1917
  pulmonary embolism and, 1113–14, 1681, 1916–17
  stabilization following, 1919
  systemic infusion of, 1916–19
  therapeutic regimens, 1916–19
Thrombophlebitis, 1372–73
  migrans, 1109
  precordial, 910
Thromboplastin time, activated partial:
  heparin and, 1667, 1668
  thrombolytic agents and, 1916, 1917
Thrombosis:
  aortic aneurysm, 1324, 1327
  aortic dissection and, 1331
  aortic stenosis and, 1671
  aortoiliac, 1335, 1336
  atherosclerosis and, 802, 804–5, 809, 842
  cardiomyopathy and, 1184, 1190
  catheter-induced, 1373, 1790
  cerebral, 1355
    venous, 1358
  computed tomography and, 1869
  contraceptive agents and, 1425, 1482
  coronary artery, 802, 843, 1022
    anticoagulants and, 1672–73
    early evolving infarction and, 967–68
    echocardiography and, 1962
    historical notes on, 885
    pathogenesis of infarction and, 870
    plaque rupture and, 870–71
    sudden death and, 530, 534–35, 540, 850
    thrombolytic agents and, 1681–82
  deep venous, 1105–6, 1373–76
    diagnosis, 1105–6, 1374–75
    etiology, 1373–74
    myocardial infarction and, 983, 1673
    phlebography and, 1885–87
    prevention, 1105, 1110
    thrombolytic agents and, 1680–81, 1916–17
    treatment, 1375–76
  Doppler studies and, 1106, 1374, 1976–77
  drugs affecting. *See also* Anticoagulants; Thrombolytic agents; *and* specific agents.
    platelet-controlling, 1675–78
  endocarditis and, 1130, 1137
    cerebral infarction and, 1359
  endomyocardial fibrosis and, 1209–10
Thrombosis:
  endothelial resistance to, 804–5, 809
  estrogen therapy and, 1425
  iliac vein, 1374
  indium imaging and, 1848–49
  lytic agents for. *See* Thrombolytic agents.
  mesenteric, 1364, 1366
  mitral valve disease and, 1670–71
    stenosis and, 755, 761
  peripheral arterial, 1348–50
  platelets and. *See* Platelets.
  popliteal vein, 1375
  portal vein, 1366
  prostaglandins and, 814
  prosthetic valves and, 1671, 1676
  pulmonary embolism and, 1105–6, 1110, 1374
  saphenous vein graft, 853, 854
  vena caval, 1379
Thrombotic thrombocytopenic purpura, 1227
  sudden death and, 535
Thromboxane, 814
  coronary artery spasm and, 1011
  drugs inhibiting, 1675
  shock and, 376
Thumb:
  broad, 133
  hypoplastic, 132, 133
Thyroidectomy, 397, 1417
Thyroid gland, 1412–18. *See also* Hyperthyroidism; Hypothyroidism.
  cardiomyopathy and, 1184
  enlarged, 1418–19
Thyroiditis, 1413, 1416
Thyroid-stimulating hormone (thyrotropin), 1412
  abnormal levels of, 1413, 1418
  thyroxine replacement therapy and, 1421
Thyrotoxicosis. *See* Hyperthyroidism.
Thyrotropin-releasing hormone, 1412, 1413
Thyroxine:
  contractility and, 99
  deficiency, 1418–22
  elevated levels, 1412–18
  free, 397
  replacement therapy, 1421
  tests, 1412
  total plasma, 397
Tibial artery occlusion, 1346
Tibial veins, Doppler studies and, 1976, 1977
Tick paralysis, 1236
Tidal wave, pulse, 143, 144
Tietze's syndrome, 918
Tilting-disk valve, 778, 2034
Time-activity curves, imaging and, 1815–17, 1819, 1820
Time-of-onset determinations, medicolegal, 1568–69
Timolol, 1607. *See also* Beta-blocking agents.
  dosage, 941, 1072
  long-term use of, 971
  pharmacodynamics, 1608, 1613, 1617
  pharmacokinetics, 1610, 1611
  structure, 1608
Tityus trinitatis, 1235
Tocainide, 1600–1601
  clinical application and toxicity, 1601
  pharmacokinetics, 1600–1601
  pharmacologic properties, 1601

Toe:
broad, 133
clubbed, 132
Tolbutamide, 1429, 1540
Tomography:
computerized axial. *See* Computed tomography.
nuclear magnetic resonance. *See* Magnetic resonance imaging.
positron-emission, 1849–50
thallium imaging, 1840–42
Tone, vascular, 58–59
Tongue, enlarged, 131
Tonsils, 131
Torricelli's orifice equation, 1784
Torsades de points, 455–56
management, 479
mechanism, 424
syncope and, 423, 524
Tort actions, 1564–65
Torus aorticus, 19
Touch, physiology of, 152–53
Toxemia of pregnancy, 1084–85
Toxic agents. *See* Cardiotoxins; Poisoning.
Toxic shock syndrome, 390
Toxoplasmosis, myocarditis and, 1161, 1175
Trabeculae carneae, 19, 21
papillary muscle origin from, 23
Trabecula septomarginalis, 7
Trachea:
aortic arch compression of, 623, 624
innominate or carotid artery compression of, 627
pulmonary artery sling and, 626
Training effect, 1400
Tranquilizers:
anesthetic use of, 1496
coronary heart disease and, 935, 938
Transducers:
echocardiography, 1927, 1929
phonocardiography, 1991–92
Transfusion:
anemia and, 400
computer-monitored, 2006
Transitional cells, 31, 32
Transmembrane potential, 73–75
afterdepolarization and, 408
automaticity and, 78, 79
calcium and, 1466, 1473–75
pacemaker cell, 80
potassium and, 1466
reentry and, 414
resting, 1466
sodium and, 1466
Transmural pressure, 58
Transplantation, cardiac, 2062–68
atherosclerosis and, 2066–67
fibrosis of coronary arteries and, 1023
historical background, 2062–63
infection and, 2066
lung transplant combined with, 2067–68
psychological factors, 1533
rejection, 2065, 2066
cardiomyopathy and, 1237–38
selection criteria, 2063
survival, 2065
technique, 2063–65
Transposition of great arteries, 691–96, 700–703
complete (dextro), 691–96
catheterization studies, 693–94
clinical manifestations, 692–94
Transposition of great arteries: complete:
ECG, 692
echocardiography, 692–93
history, 692
medical management, 694–95
natural history and prognosis, 694
pathology, 691
pathophysiology, 691–92
physical examination, 692
roentgenography, 692
surgical management, 695–96
corrected (levo), 5, 700–703
assessment, 258, 701
associated conditions, 700–701
echocardiography, 251, 701
medical management, 702–3
mitral regurgitation and, 251
natural history and prognosis, 702
pathology, 700
surgical management, 703
definition, 687
embryology, 3–5
pregnancy and, 1391
Transverse sections of heart, 17, 18
Transverse tubules, 32, 33, 38
Trauma, 1276–81
aortic, 1277, 1278, 1280–81
surgical repair of, 2048–49
aortic regurgitation and, 740, 1280
blunt, 1021, 1276, 1278–81
catheterization, cardiac, 1022
coronary artery, 1021–22, 1278, 1279
electrical, 1486–88
fat embolism and, 1114, 1115
iatrogenic, 1276
legal issues and, 1563–65, 1575
mitral regurgitation and, 767
myocardial damage and, 1237, 1278–80
penetrating, 1022, 1276–78
tabulation of, 1277
pericarditis and, 1268, 1278, 1280
rupture of heart and, 1278–81
tamponade and, 1277
tricuspid regurgitation and, 794, 1280
vibration, 1578
Trazodone, 1480, 1533
Treadmill testing, 1704–6. *See also* Exercise testing.
guidelines for, 1032
predischarge, 1026
Tremor, electrocardiography and, 226
Trendelenburg's operation, 1112–13
Treponema pallidum, 1314. *See also* Syphilis.
tests for, 1319
Treppe, 39, 46, 48
Triadic junction, 32, 38
Triamterene. *See also* Diuretics.
biochemistry, 1658
dosage, 1072, 1659
duration of action, 1659
pharmacokinetics, 1661
site of action, 1660
Triazolobenzodiazepines, 1532
Trichinosis, myocarditis and, 1158, 1179
clinical manifestations, 1170–72
laboratory studies, 1172
pathology, 1160
pathophysiology, 1165
Trichlormethiazide, 1659
dosage, 1072
Tricuspid annulus, 17, 797–99
Tricuspid valve, 673–80, 792–99
anatomy, 22–23
Tricuspid valve:
annuloplasty, 797–99
area calculation, 1785
assessment, 253–55
atresia and, 673–75
regurgitation and, 253–54, 677, 794–96
stenosis and, 254, 794–96
atresia, 673–76
atrial appendages and, 673
clinical manifestations, 673–75
embryology, 12
medical management, 675–76
murmur, 673
natural history and prognosis, 675
pathology, 673
pulmonary atresia and, 673, 674
pulmonic stenosis and, 673, 674
surgical management, 676
ventricular septal defect and, 673
atrial myxoma and, 254–55
AV canal and, 606–11
carcinoid and, 1298, 1299
cleft, left ventricular–right atrial communication and, 613–14
commissurotomy, 797
congenital disease, 673–80
double-outlet right ventricle and, 699
dysplastic, 677
Ebstein's anomaly and, 12, 677–80
echocardiography, 1935, 1940, 1941
atresia and, 675
regurgitation and, 253–54, 795–96, 1949–50
embryology, 12
endocarditis, 253–54, 793–94, 797–99
drug-related, 1132
fibrous skeleton and, 17, 18
frontal view, 20
murmurs, 160, 163
atresia and, 673
diastolic, 192–93
regurgitation and, 191, 795
stenosis and, 192, 193, 795
necropsy and, 2078–79
pregnancy and, 1390
prolapse, 794
pulmonary atresia and, 660, 673, 674
pulmonic stenosis and, 655, 673, 674
regurgitation, 677, 792–99
assessment, 253–54, 677, 794–96
atrial fibrillation and, 795
carcinoid tumor and, 793
cardiomyopathy and, 1184
catheterization studies, 796
congenital, 677
echocardiography, 253–54, 795–96, 1949–50
endocarditis and, 793–94
etiology, 792
heart failure and, 334, 335, 793
history, 794
low-pressure, 253–54
medical management, 677, 796
murmur, 191, 795
myocardial infarction and, 794
myxoma and, 1291
natural history and prognosis, 796
pathology, 677, 792–94
physical examination, 795
pulmonary hypertension and, 253
rheumatic, 792
surgical management, 677, 796–99, 2033–34
traumatic, 794, 1280

Tricuspid valve: regurgitation:
venous pulse and, 149, 150
replacement, 797, 799, 2034
carcinoid and, 1299
Ebstein's anomaly and, 679, 680
rheumatoid nodules, 1440
sounds, 160, 163
closure, 163, 164–65
opening snap, 186
regurgitation and, 795
stenosis and, 186, 795
stenosis, 792–97
assessment, 254, 794–96
catheterization studies, 796
ECG, 795
etiology, 792
history, 794
medical management, 796
murmur, 192, 193, 795
natural history and prognosis, 796
pathophysiology, 794
phonocardiogram, 795
physical examination, 795
rheumatic, 792
roentgenography, 795
sounds, 186, 795
surgical management, 796–97
transposition of great arteries and, 650
venous pulse and, 148–50
ventricular septal defect and, 596
Tricyclics, 1479–80
rehabilitation and, 1532–33
Triggered activity, 408–9, 413
Triglycerides:
fatty acids and, 91
as risk factors for atherosclerosis, 821–23
sympatholytic agents and, 1074
Triiodothyronine:
decreased levels, 1418
elevated levels, 1412, 1413
uptake test, 397, 1412
Trilogy of Fallot, 655
Trimazosin, 1589
Trimethaphan:
aortic dissection and, 1333
hypertension and, 1044
Trimipramine, 1479
Triphenyl tetrazolium chloride stain, 877–78
Trisomy syndromes, 567
facial features in, 127–28
hand in, 133
Trophoblastic tumors, embolism from, 1117
Tropomyosin, 38
Troponin C, 38
Truncoaortic sac, 5, 9, 13
Truncoconal area, 5, 8, 9
septation, 9
Truncus arteriosus, 668–73
classification, 668
clinical manifestations, 671
embryology, 5, 9
medical management, 672
natural history and prognosis, 671
pathology, 669–70
persistent, 669–70
septation, 9
surgical management, 672–73
types I, II, and III, 668–73
type IV, 670, 673
Trypanosoma cruzi. *See* Chagas' disease.
Trypanosoma gambiense and *rhodesiense*, 1175
TTC stain, 877–78
TTI (tension-time index), 860
Tuberculosis:
myocardial, 1173
pericardial, 1269–70
Tuberous sclerosis, 124, 1231
genetics, 571
pulmonary hypertension and, 576
Tubocurarine, 1497
Tumors, 1284–99. *See also* specific type.
angiosarcoma, 1294
bilateral, 1292
carcinoid, 1298–99
CT scans, 1868–69
embolism from, 1117, 1286–87, 1291, 1359
fibroelastoma, papillary, 1294
fibroma, 1293–94
hemangioma, 1294
hemangiosarcoma, 1294
infected, 1286
left atrial, 1287–90
left ventricular, 1292
leukemic, 1297–98
lipoma, 1294
malignant primary, 1294–95
manifestations, general, 1285–86, 1296
mesothelioma, 1295
of AV node, 1294
metastatic. *See* Metastases.
myxoma, 1284–92
pericardial, 1268, 1295
pheochromocytoma, 1295
"plop" sound and, 1287
primary, 1284–95
rhabdomyoma, 1292–93
rhabdomyosarcoma, 1294–95
right atrial, 1290–92
right ventricular, 1292
secondary, 1295–98. *See also* Metastases.
sudden death and, 531, 534
surgery for, 1292, 1293
tabulation of, 1285
teratoma, 1295
Turner's syndrome, 567
inspection and, 128, 130, 135
Tuttle, Elbert P., Sr., 103
Type A behavior, 1524–25
bypass surgery and, 1531, 1532
medicolegal issues and, 1572
Typhoid fever, myocarditis and, 1173
Tyrosine:
heart failure and, 326
inhibition of, 1589

U wave, hypokalemia and, 223–24, 1471, 1474
Uhl's malformation, 680
Ulcerative colitis, 1239
Ulcers:
finger, thromboangiitis obliterans and, 1347
foot, arteriosclerosis obliterans and, 1341, 1344–45
ischemic, 1341, 1344–45, 1347, 1348
peptic, 914
venous, 1377, 1378
Ulnar artery:
compression test of Allen and, 1340
flow test, 386
Ultrasonography. *See also* Echocardiography.
basic principles, 1927–28
Ultrasonography:
carotid artery, 1878–79
cerebrovascular disease and, 1355
definition, 1926
Doppler. *See* Doppler studies.
pulse-reflected, 1926
Ultrastructure, myocardial, 31–34
Starling's law and, 44–45
Umbilical vessels, 10, 11, 583
Unconsciousness, transient. *See* Syncope.
Underwater diving, 1550–53
Unidirectional block, 410–11
ventricular tachycardia and, 420–21
Unipolar leads, 207
esophageal, 1692, 1693
extremity, 207
pacemaker, 491–92
precordial, 208
Univentricular heart, 703–6
Upstairs-downstairs heart, 706
Urate (uric acid):
diuretics and, 1664, 1666
excess, 1225–26
Uremia, 1226, 1460
cardiomyopathy and, 1226, 1462–63
etiologic factors in development of cardiovascular disease in, 1464
hypertension and, 1045–46, 1060
pericarditis and, 1226, 1266–67, 1461
pulmonary edema and, 1463
Uric acid. *See* Urate.
Urinary symptoms, 121
Urine:
endocarditis and, 1144
shock and, 385
Urochrome pigmentation, 126
Urokinase, 1679–80. *See also* Thrombolytic agents.
arteriosclerosis obliterans and, 1346
coronary thrombosis and, 1681
loading dose, 1916
myocardial infarction and, 943, 1917, 1918
pulmonary embolism and, 1113–14
systemic infusion of, 1916–17
Ursodeoxycholic acid, 914
Uterus:
blood flow of, in pregnancy, 1384–85
drugs affecting, 1394

v wave, 52, 54
mitral regurgitation and, 772, 774
tricuspid regurgitation and, 795
venous pulse, 148
abnormalities, 149–50
Vaccine:
cholera, 1237
smallpox, 1236–37
Vagus nerves, 24
atrial fibrillation and, 415
automaticity and, 79
coronary blood flow and, 61
digitalis and, 1642, 1648
ductus arteriosus and, 618
muscle mechanics and, 49
pressure test, 515
sensory endings, 375
syncope and, 508, 516–17
Valium. *See* Diazepam.
Valsalva maneuver:
angina pectoris and, 891
auscultation and, 195
blood pressure and, 1040
syncope and, 517
Valsalva's sinus. *See* Sinus of Valsalva.

Valve:
area, calculation of, 1784–85
replacement. *See* Prosthetic valves.
Valvectomy, pulmonary, 658, 661
Valvotomy:
aortic, 639
pulmonary, 657, 658
Valvular heart disease, 729–99. *See also* specific valve.
aging and, 1410–11
anesthesia and, 1501
angina pectoris and, 910
assessment, 247–55
cerebral embolism and, 1358–59
Doppler studies and, 1981–86
endocarditis, 1130, 1135. *See also* Endocarditis.
cure rate, 1147
drug-related, 1132
thrombotic, 1137
insurance and, 1560–61
necropsy and, 2078–79
noncardiac surgery and, 1516
pregnancy and, 1388–90
radiation-induced, 1485, 1486
radionuclide studies, 1826
rheumatoid nodules, 1439, 1441
surgical procedures, 2030–35
historical perspective, 2030
results, 2034–35
techniques, 2030–34
traumatic, 1280
Valvulitis, 1307
Valvuloplasty:
mitral, 649, 2032
pulmonary, 1898
Vancomycin, endocarditis and, 1149, 1153
Vanillylmandelic acid, pheochromocytoma and, 1065
Vaporale. *See* Amyl nitrate.
Vaquez, H., 1446
Varicella, 1174
Varicose veins, 1376–77
Vasculature, 1321–80. *See also* specific vessel *and* disease.
aging and, 1406–7
autoregulation, shock and, 377–78
gastrointestinal, 1364–71
genetics and, 573–76
neural control of, 59–60
peripheral. *See* Peripheral circulation.
pulmonary. *See* Pulmonary vasculature.
rings, 622–24
shock and, 372–73
syncope and, 510–18
waterfall phenomenon, 859
Vasculitis. *See also* Arteritis; Polyarteritis.
coronary artery, 1022–23
intestinal, 1370
neurological deficits and, 1358
Vasculogenesis, 3
Vasoconstriction:
blood pressure and, 1040
coronary, 61–63, 862
exercise and, 56, 1399
heart failure and, 324, 335–36, 347
heat stress and, 1548, 1549
inhibitors of, 1588–89
norepinephrine and, 59, 1590
pulmonary, 27
hypertension and, 1096, 1097, 1100, 1102, 1121–22
hypoxic, 1121–22
Vasoconstriction: pulmonary:
mediators, 1122
renal, 325
retinal, 198, 203
shock and, 376–77, 392–93
sympathetic fibers and, 59
sympathomimetic amines and, 391
Vasoconstrictors, 1590–91. *See also* specific agent.
afterload mismatch and, 267
coronary artery spasm and, 1010
digitalis, 1642
pharmacology, 1590–91
smooth-muscle cells and, 1010
Vasodepressor syncope, 508–10, 515
Vasodilatation:
aging and, 1406–7
carbon dioxide tension and, 59
coronary, 61–63
blood flow and, 858, 861
steal and, 864
exercise and, 55, 56, 1399
heat stress and, 1547
hypovolemia and, 384
hypoxia and, 59
myocardial perfusion studies and, 1838–39
parasympathetic fibers and, 59
retinal, 198
shock and, 376, 390–92
sympathetic fibers and, 59
Vasodilators, 1584–90. *See also* specific agent.
afterload and, 268, 364, 392
arteriosclerosis obliterans and, 1344
auscultation and, 195
cardiomyopathy and, 277, 1192
coronary artery spasm and, 1014–15
cor pulmonale and, 1127
heart failure and, 337, 362–65
in infant, 586
prevention of, 357
hypertension and, 1075
dosage, 1072
pulmonary, 1102–3
renoparenchymal, 1081
impedance and, 1584
intravascular volume and, 1584
myocardial ischemia and, 866
occupational exposure to, 1577
pregnancy and, 1393
preload and, 362–63, 392, 866, 1584
shock and, 392–93
smooth-muscle cells and, 1010
venous pooling and, 362–63, 364
ventricular performance curves and, 1506
Vasomotion, 58–59
Vasopressin. *See also* Antidiuretic hormone.
analogs of, 1591
Vasoregulatory asthenia, 910–11
Vasospasm. *See* Spasm.
coronary. *See* Coronary arteries, spasm.
Vater association, 135
Vectorcardiography, 1687–90
current position of, 1688
definition and features of, 1687–88
myocardial infarction and, 896–97, 1689–90
normal, 1688–89
pulmonic stenosis and, 656
vs. vector electrocardiography, 208
Vecuronium, 1497
Vegetation, endocarditis, 1130. *See also* Endocarditis.
location of, 1138
thrombotic, 1137
Veins, 26. *See also* specific vessels.
cutdown of, cardiac catheterization and, 1770–71
Doppler studies, 1976–77
grafts. *See* Saphenous vein grafts.
hypertension of, 1376–78
inflammation of, 1372–73
interruption of, surgical, 1111–12
peripheral, 1372–78
anatomy, 1372
physiology, 1372
pooling in:
heart failure and, 362–63, 364
syncope and, 510, 511
pulse of. *See* Pulse, venous.
radiography of. *See* Phlebography.
shock and, 374
thrombosis, 1105–6, 1373–76
cerebral, 1358
diagnosis, 1375–76
Doppler studies and, 1976–77
etiology, 1373–74
mesenteric, 1364, 1366
myocardial infarction and, 983, 1673
phlebography and, 1885–87
popliteal, 1375
portal, 1366
prevention, 1105, 1110
pulmonary embolism and, 1105–6, 1110, 1374
thrombolytic agents and, 1680–81, 1916–17
treatment, 1375–76
vena caval, 1379
varicose, 1376–77
Velocardiofacial syndrome, 128
Velocity of shortening, 40–42, 46, 47
Vena cava:
inferior:
aortic fistula with, 1380
azygos vein continuity of, 686, 1872
Budd-Chiari syndrome and, 1379
echocardiography and, 1943, 1944
embryology, 11
filter placement in, 1111–12
interruption of, 231, 1111, 1367
left atrial termination of, 684
obstruction, 1379
orifice, 19
pulmonary venous connection anomaly and, 604, 605
situs determination and, 687
pressure, normal, 55
atrial septal defect and, 598, 603
dilatation, heart failure and, 355
left atrial termination of, 684–85
obstruction, 1378–79
orifice, 19
persistent left, 11, 685–86
pulmonary venous connection anomaly and, 598, 603
Venesection, hemochromatosis and, 1222
Venoconstriction. *See* Vasoconstriction.
Venography. *See* Phlebography.
Venom:
arthropod, 1489
black widow spider, 1236
scorpion, 1235, 1489
snake, 1489

Venous hum, 194
hyperdynamic state and, 395
Venous pressure:
elevated, 148
heart failure and, 347
hepatojugular reflux test and, 147–48
Kussmaul's sign and, 148–49
measurement, 147–48
pericarditis and, 1256, 1257, 1263
peripheral, 1372
shock and, 385
tamponade and, 1256, 1257
Venous pulse. *See* Pulse, venous.
Ventilation. *See also* Respiration.
CPR and, 550
postoperative, 1507–8
radionuclide studies, 1108, 1881–82
Ventilation-perfusion scans, 1108, 1881–82
Ventilators, 389
Ventricle(s):
aberrant conduction. *See* Intraventricular conduction.
action potential, 75
activation sequence, 81, 82
alignment, 686, 688
anatomy, 16, 19–22
aneurysm. *See* Aneurysm, ventricular.
arrhythmias, 420–26, 450–61. *See also* Intraventricular conduction: Premature ventricular beats; Tachycardia, ventricular; Ventricular fibrillation.
asymmetric, 1194–95
asynergic, 1803–4
bigeminy, 446
aberrant conduction and, 460
biopsy, 1773. *See also* Biopsy, endomyocardial.
compliance, 43
cardiomyopathy and, 1199
cross section, 19
depolarization, 207
echocardiographic dimensions of, 1935–36, 1945–48
ejection fraction. *See* Ejection fraction.
ejection phases, 52, 270–71
embryology, 5–8
end-systolic dimensions. *See* End-systolic dimension.
failure. *See* Heart failure.
filling, 48. *See also* Preload.
cardiomyopathy and, 1199
endomyocardial fibrosis and, 1210
impaired, 267–68
murmurs, 163
phases of, 52
pressure. *See* Ventricular pressure, filling.
radionuclide studies, 1830–31
shock and, 371
sounds, 160, 163, 176
functional assessment, 267–68. *See also* Contractility; Heart failure; Myocardium, failure.
aging and, 1405
anesthesia and, 1498, 1501
aortic stenosis and, 268
arteriography and, 906
congenital heart disease and, 1828
curves, 44, 46, 267, 1506
digital subtraction angiography and, 1859–60
Doppler studies and, 1979–81
Ventricle(s): functional assessment:
doxorubicin cardiotoxicity and, 1826–28
drug therapy and, 1502
echocardiography and, 1962–64
ejection phase indexes and, 270–71
exercise and, 1710–11, 1824–26, 1828, 1842–43
mitral regurgitation and, 269
myocardial infarction and, 926, 928–29, 978–79
probe technique, nonimaging nuclear, 387, 1829–30
pulmonary obstructive disease and, 1828–29
radionuclide studies, 1813–31
sudden death and, 540
valvular heart disease and, 268, 269, 1826
gallop. *See* Gallop, ventricular.
left:
anatomy, 20–22
aortic tunnel with, 644–45
apex beat, 153–55
double-inlet, 8
double-outlet, 699–700
endomyocardial fibrosis, 1211
hypoplastic, 645–47, 653
inflow tract, 21
mass index, 1054
myxoma, 1292
outflow tract, 21
obstruction. *See* Aortic stenosis.
primitive, 5
right atrial communication with, 613–14
neonatal, 583–84
oxygen consumption and, 56
pacing. *See* Pacing, ventricular.
programmed stimulation of, 1738
repolarization, 207
right:
anatomy, 19
double-inlet, 8
double-outlet, 8, 696–99
dysplastic, 424, 453, 2015
Ebstein's anomaly and, 678
endomyocardial fibrosis, 1211
frontal view, 18
in heart failure, 322, 334–35
hypoplastic, 660, 675
infarction, 212, 846, 978–79, 981–82
inflow tract, 1292
myxoma, 1292
outflow tract, 19, 20
obstruction. *See* Pulmonic stenosis.
precordial impulse, 155
primitive, 5
pulmonary hypertension and, 1094, 1097, 1022–23
Uhl's malformation, 680
roentgenography and, 241–43
rupture. *See* Rupture.
septum. *See* Interventricular septum; Ventricular septal defect.
sequence of contraction of, 48
single, 7–8, 703–6
clinical manifestations, 704
medical management, 705
natural history and prognosis, 704–5
pathology, 703–4
surgical management, 705–6
small, cardiomyopathy and, 1198
Ventricle(s):
stiffness, 43
standstill, 471, 490
suction of, 48
time-activity curves, 1815–17, 1819, 1820
volumes. *See also* End-diastolic volume; End-systolic pressure-volume relations.
catheterization studies and, 1782–84
echocardiography and, 1946–48, 1962–63
exercise and, 1400
radionuclide studies and, 1815, 1820–22
tamponade and, 1258
ventriculography and, 1783–84, 1805
wall force, fiber length and, 327, 329
wall motion. *See* Wall motion.
wall tension (stress). *See* Afterload; Wall tension (stress).
Ventricular aneurysm. *See* Aneurysm, ventricular.
Ventricular arteries, 28, 29
Ventricular fibrillation, 425–26, 471
arrest and, 295
contributing factors, 471
CPR and, 550–51
ECG, 470, 471
management, 542, 976–77
beta blockers in, 1616
cardioversion, 1744–45. *See also* Cardioversion.
implantable device for, 1761–63
paramedics and, 540
preventive, 542–44
mechanism, 425–26
myocardial infarction and, 541, 542, 975, 976
pacing and, 543
reperfusion and, 425, 426
sudden death and, 533, 538, 540–44
prevention and treatment, 542–44
recurrent syndrome and, 541–42
WPW syndrome and, 416, 419
Ventricular flutter, 455
Ventricular premature beats. *See* Premature ventricular beats.
Ventricular pressure:
aortic regurgitation and, 744, 748
aortic stenosis and, 731–32, 735
catheterization studies and, 1775
coronary blood flow and, 859–60
filling, 1091. *See also* Atrial pressure; End-diastolic pressure; Preload.
drug therapy and, 1506
heart failure and, 267, 327
myocardial infarction and, 979, 980
mitral regurgitation and, 773
normal, 55
tricuspid regurgitation and, 150, 253
Ventricular septal defect, 590–97
anatomic types, 590
angiography, 594, 1789
aortic arch interruption and, 634, 635
aortic regurgitation and, 591, 595, 741
associated conditions, 591
AV canal and, 606, 608, 609
catheterization studies, 594, 1777
chambers and, 591
clinical manifestations, 592–94
congestive failure and, 594
definition, 590

Ventricular septal defect:
Doppler studies, 1986
double-outlet left ventricle and, 700
double-outlet right ventricle and, 696–99
ECG, 593–94
echocardiography, 594
Eisenmenger's syndrome and, 10, 593
embryology, 9, 10
endocarditis and, 595
genetics, 592, 596
history, 592
hypertrophy and, 594
left ventricular–right atrial communication and, 613–14
medical management, 595–96
murmur, 192, 194, 592–93
natural history and prognosis, 594–95
pathology, 590–91
pathophysiology, 591–92
physical examination, 592–93
pulmonary artery anomalies and, 668, 669
pulmonary atresia and, 670–73
roentgenography, 593
sinus of Valsalva aneurysm and, 621
sounds, 171, 172, 593
supracristal, 10
surgical management, 596–97
pulmonary atresia and, 671, 673
tetralogy of Fallot and, 666
tetralogy of Fallot and, 10, 662, 663, 666
transposition of great arteries, 691–94
corrected, 700–703
tricuspid atresia and, 673
truncus arteriosus and, 671, 672
Ventricular septum. *See* Interventricular septum; Ventricular septal defect.
Ventriculoarterial concordance and discordance, 687
corrected transposition of great arteries and, 700
single ventricle and, 703
Ventriculography, 1803–5
benefits, 903
digital, 1859–60
exercise, 306
infarction and, 312
information provided by, 1791
intervention, 311
left, 1803–5
limitations, 906–7
myocarditis and, 1166–67
myxoma and, 1290
prognosis and, 311
radionuclide, infarction and, 970
volume measurements and, 1783–84, 1805
Ventriculoradial dysplasia, 132, 133
Ventriculotomy:
double-outlet right ventricle and, 699
right, pulmonic stenosis and, 658–59
Venturi waves, pulmonic stenosis and, 655
Venules:
pulmonary occlusive disease and, 652–53
shock and, 373
Verapamil, 941, 1600. *See also* Calcium channel blockers.
action potential and, 78
angina pectoris and, 1628, 1629
Verapamil:
arrhythmias and, 1600, 1630–31
atrial fibrillation and, 1630
atrial flutter and, 1631
atrial tachycardia and, 476
cardiomyopathy and, 1206, 1207, 1632
clinical application, 1600
coronary artery spasm and, 1015
CPR and, 553
dosage, 1072, 1628
electrophysiologic effects, 1626–27
hypertension and, 1631–32
interactions of, 1634
pharmacodynamics, 1625–27
pharmacokinetics, 1594, 1600
pharmacologic properties, 1587–88, 1600
physiologic principles, 1624
preexcitation syndromes and, 1631
protein-binding and dialysance, 1082
structure, 1625
supraventricular tachycardia and, 1630–31
toxicity, 1600, 1634
Veratridine, Bezold-Jarisch reflex and, 62
Verrucous endocarditis, 1436–37
Vertebral artery:
angiography, 1875, 1876
angioplasty, 1912
Vertebrobasilar arteries, syncope and, 513–14
Vertigo, 519
laryngeal, 517
Vibration disease, 1578
Vibratory perception, diabetes and, 1427
Vieussens, Raymond, 754
Vincristine, 1482
Vindesine, 1482
Virchow, Rudolf, 1105
Viruses:
cardiomyopathy and, 1183
myocarditis, 1158, 1159, 1163, 1174–75
clinical manifestations, 1165, 1166, 1169
pericarditis, 1251–54
Viscosity, blood flow and, 57, 58
Visken. *See* Pindolol.
Vitamin D excess, 1219
Vitamin deficiencies, 1448–49
Vitamin K, warfarin and, 1669
Vitatron electrode, 492
Vitelline veins, 10, 11
Vocation. *See* Occupation; Work status.
Volume overload. *See* Preload.
Vomiting, 121
von Jurgensen, Theodor, 1978
von Willebrand's disease, atherosclerosis and, 812

Walking:
claudication and, 1340, 1347
guidelines for, 1032
rehabilitation and, 1028–29
Wall force, fiber length and, 327, 329
Wall motion:
arteriography and, 906
digital subtraction angiography and, 1860, 1862
echocardiography and, 1961, 1963
exercise and, 1825
Wall motion:
mitral regurgitation and, 772, 774
myocarditis and, 1166
radionuclide studies and, 1816, 1819–20
ventriculography and, 1803–4
Wall tension (stress):
afterload and, 331. *See also* Afterload.
aortic regurgitation and, 743, 744
aortic stenosis and, 268, 636, 731–32
calculation of, 271
heart failure and, 329
hypertrophy and, 327
mitral regurgitation and, 269, 773–74
obesity and, 1454
oxygen consumption and, 56, 865
preload and, 332
pulmonary hypertension and, 1097
vascular, 58
Wandering pacemaker, 468–69
Warfarin, 1669–75
adverse reactions, 1674
aneurysm and, ventricular, 1673–74
aortic valve disease and, 1671
atrial fibrillation and, 1671–72
cardiomyopathy and, 1669–70
cardioversion and, 1672
cerebral embolism and, 1360
coronary heart disease and, 943, 1672–73
bypass surgery and, 1674
endocarditis and, 1150
heart failure and, 1672
heparin vs., 1668
indications, 1669–74
mechanism of action, 1669
mitral valve disease and, 1670–71
myocardial infarction and, 1672–73
new developments and, 1674–75
pregnancy and, 1114, 1393–94
prosthetic valves and, 1671, 1676
pulmonary embolism and, 1110
therapeutic regimens, 1669
Washout curves, radionuclide, 1839–40, 1850
Waterfall phenomenon, vascular, 859
Water-hammer pulse, 144
Wavelength, sound, 157
Weakness, 119
heart failure and, 350
myocardial ischemia and, 961
Weber-Christian disease, 1238–39
Wedge pressure. *See* Pulmonary artery pressure, wedge; Pulmonary capillary pressure, wedge.
Wegener's granulomatosis, 1239
coronary arteries and, 1023
Weight:
excessive. *See* Obesity.
gain:
heart failure and, 350
history and, 118
perioperative, 1505
loss (reduction), 121, 936, 1449
diuretics and, 361
hypertension and, 1078
obesity and, 1456
Weiss, S., 1809
Wenckebach phenomenon:
atrial flutter and, 445
ECG, 464, 465
group beating and, 466
management, 480
Werner's syndrome, 573
inspection and, 123, 126

Westermark sign, 239
Wheezing, 115–16
  heart failure and, 349
Whipple's disease, 134, 1239–40
Whoops, systolic, 185
Williams' syndrome, 641
  pulmonic stenosis and, 659
Wilson, Frank, 206, 1536
Wilson central terminal, 207
Windkessel effect, 26
Wolff-Parkinson-White syndrome, 447–49
  atrial fibrillation and, 416, 448
  concealed, 448
  ECG and, 219–20, 416–18, 447, 448
  epicardial mapping and, intraoperative, 2013, 2014
  management, 477
    calcium channel blockers in, 1631
    digitalis in, 1646
Wolff-Parkinson-White syndrome:
  mechanism, 416–17
  supraventricular tachycardia and, 416, 447–48, 461
  ventricular fibrillation and, 416, 419
Woodworth phenomenon, 48
Workers' compensation, 1563–64, 1579
  causality assessment and, 1571
  history and, 1575
Work status, 1578–79
  coronary bypass surgery and, 955–56, 1532, 1578–79
  disability evaluation and, 1562, 1572–73
  guidelines for, 1578
  motor vehicle operators and, 1578
  myocardial infarction and, 830, 1035
  pilot certification and, 1578–79

x wave (descent), 54, 148
  abnormalities, 149
Xanthogranuloma, juvenile, 1239
Xanthomatosis, 122–23, 1225
Xenon imaging of lung, 1881
X-ray. *See* Roentgenography.
Xylocaine. *See* Lidocaine.

y descent (wave), 52, 54, 148
  abnormalities, 150

Z band, 32, 33, 38
z point, cardiac cycle and, 52
Zenker necrosis, sudden death and, 536, 591, 592

Tomographic ^{201}Tl images in a patient with critical disease of the left anterior descending coronary artery. The format is the same as the illustrations shown in the front endpaper. A large perfusion defect is demonstrated in the anterior wall, septum, and apex. There is complete redistribution demonstrated. The bull's-eye displays show abnormal ^{201}Tl uptake at stress with virtually complete normalization at delayed imaging (Plates D-2 and E-2). In the bull's-eye shown in Plate F-2, there is abnormal ^{201}Tl washout depicted as dark blue and black, defining the precise zone of myocardial ischemia. (See Chapter 109, "Techniques of Nuclear Cardiology," by Zaret and Berger).